SHARE THE VITAL INFORMATION IN PDR'S 1987 EDITION WITH A FRIEND OR COLLEAGUE

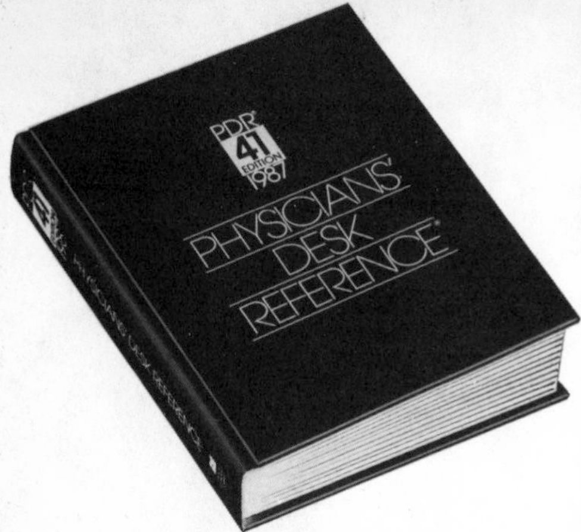

See other side for other PDR reference volumes

1. Payment Enclosed

Send _____ copies of Physicians' Desk Reference .... ([illegible] each)
Send _____ copies of PDR for Nonprescription Drugs .... ($19.95 each)
Send _____ copies of PDR for Ophthalmology .... ($25.95 each)

2. Bill Me

Send _____ copies of Physicians' Desk Reference .... ($34.95 each)
Send _____ copies of PDR for Nonprescription Drugs .... ($21.95 each)
Send _____ copies of PDR for Ophthalmology .... ($27.95 each)

10% discount granted on orders of 26 copies or more (per title)
NJ, IL, and CA residents add applicable sales tax

Signature ____________________
Name ____________________
Institution ____________________
Address ____________________
City ____________________ State ________ Zip ________
Occupation ____________________

Detach along dotted line and mail in envelope to: PDR®, P.O. Box 2017, Mahopac, New York 10541 7R-AN-0
These prices apply to 1987 Editions only. You may use this card to order PDR Editions after 1987, but we will send bill (only) at the prices then in effect.

USE THIS CARD TO ORDER EXTRA COPIES OF PHYSICIANS' DESK REFERENCE

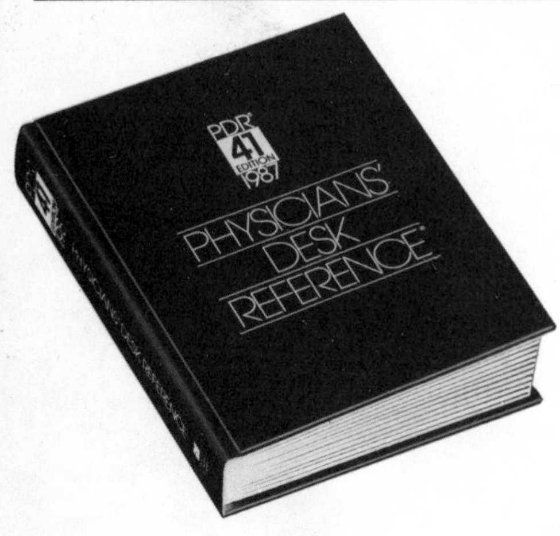

See other side for other PDR reference volumes

1. Payment Enclosed

Send _____ copies of Physicians' Desk Reference .... ($32.95 each)
Send _____ copies of PDR for Nonprescription Drugs .... ($19.95 each)
Send _____ copies of PDR for Ophthalmology .... ($25.95 each)

2. Bill Me

Send _____ copies of Physicians' Desk Reference .... ($34.95 each)
Send _____ copies of PDR for Nonprescription Drugs .... ($21.95 each)
Send _____ copies of PDR for Ophthalmology .... ($27.95 each)

10% discount granted on orders of 26 copies or more (per title)
NJ, IL, and CA residents add applicable sales tax

Signature ____________________
Name ____________________
Institution ____________________
Address ____________________
City ____________________ State ________ Zip ________
Occupation ____________________

Detach along dotted line and mail in envelope to: PDR®, P.O. Box 2017, Mahopac, New York 10541 7R-AN-0
These prices apply to 1987 Editions only. You may use this card to order PDR Editions after 1987, but we will send bill (only) at the prices then in effect.

STAY UP-TO-THE-MINUTE! RESERVE YOUR 1987 PDR SUPPLEMENTS TODAY!

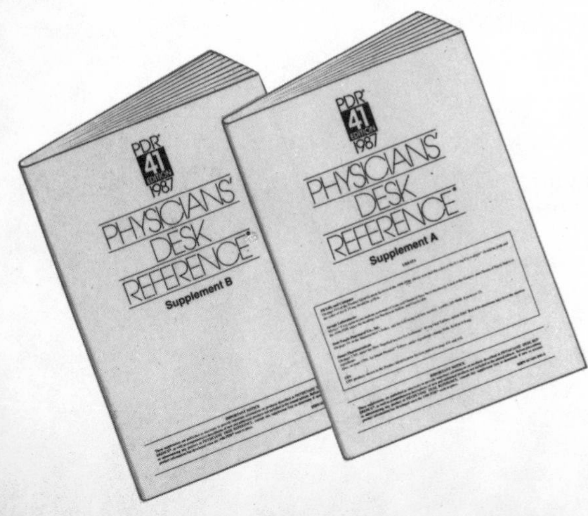

These two supplements keep your 1987 Physicians' Desk Reference up-to-the-minute throughout the year. Every important update between annual editions of the PDR is included in these supplements.

Send me 1 copy of Supplements A & B at $3.99 for both. I understand I may not receive the Spring supplement if I order late in the year. We do not bill for Supplement orders. Please include check or money order for $3.99.

Signature ____________________
Name ____________________
Institution ____________________
Address ____________________
City ____________________ State ________ Zip ________
Occupation ____________________

7R-AN-0

FILL OUT AND MAIL IN AN ENVELOPE WITH CHECK FOR $3.99 TO:
PDR, BOX 2017, MAHOPAC, NEW YORK 10541

COMPLETE YOUR DRUG REFERENCE LIBRARY TODAY!

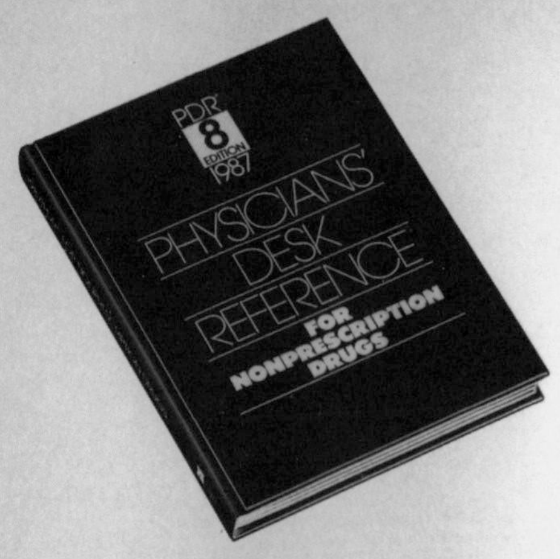

1987 PDR FOR NONPRESCRIPTION DRUGS

The perfect companion volume for your 1987 PDR, the PDR for Nonprescription Drugs provides detailed, accurate information–including ingredients, indications, drug interactions, dosages, and more–on hundreds of over-the-counter drug products and preparations.

1987 PDR FOR OPHTHALMOLOGY

This is the volume the eye-care professionals reach for. PDR for Ophthalmology offers complete information on products and drugs relating to ophthalmology and optometry, plus a manufacturer's section on specialized instrumentation, equipment, and lenses. Charts, tables, bibliography, educational materials.

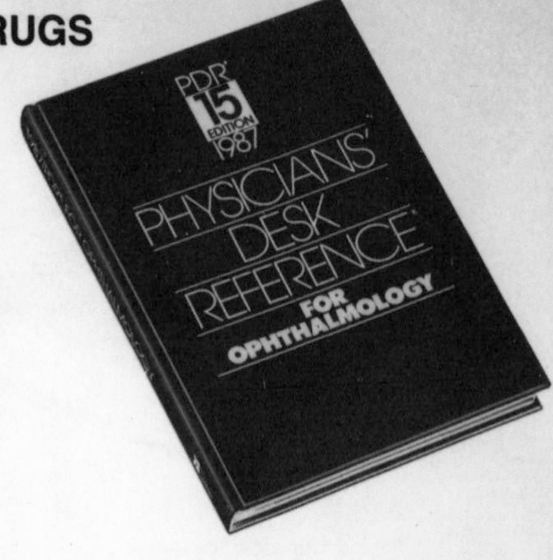

FILL OUT THE OTHER SIDE AND MAIL IN AN ENVELOPE TO:
PHYSICIANS' DESK REFERENCE, BOX 2017, MAHOPAC, NEW YORK 10541

NO DRUG REFERENCE LIBRARY IS COMPLETE WITHOUT THESE VOLUMES

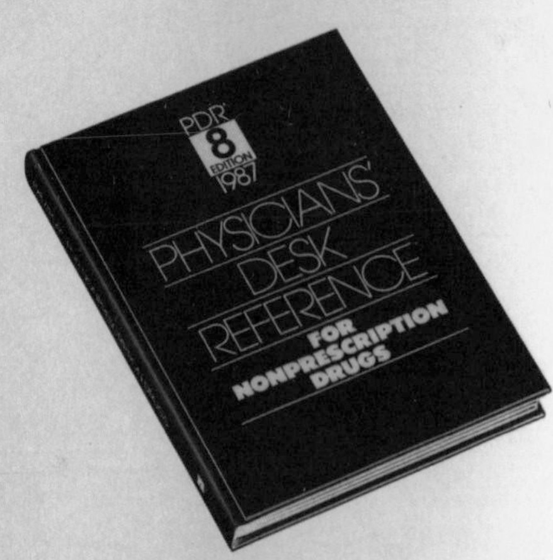

1987 PDR FOR NONPRESCRIPTION DRUGS

The perfect companion volume for your 1987 PDR, the PDR for Nonprescription Drugs provides detailed, accurate information–including ingredients, indications, drug interactions, dosages, and more–on hundreds of over-the-counter drug products and preparations.

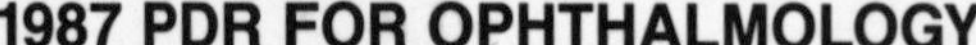

1987 PDR FOR OPHTHALMOLOGY

This is the volume the eye-care professionals reach for. PDR for Ophthalmology offers complete information on products and drugs relating to ophthalmology and optometry, plus a manufacturer's section on specialized instrumentation, equipment, and lenses. Charts, tables, bibliography, educational materials.

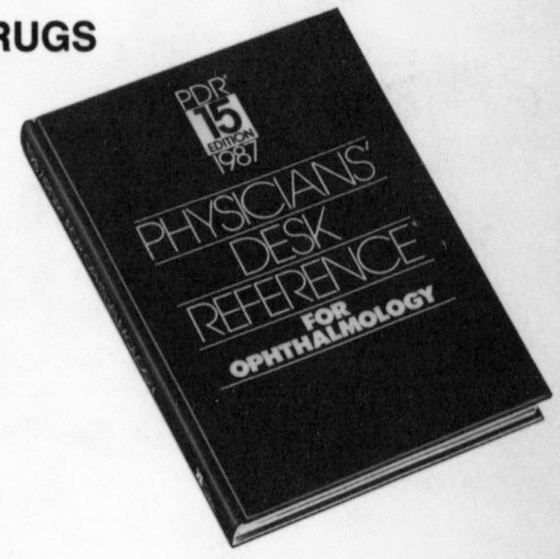

FILL OUT THE OTHER SIDE AND MAIL IN AN ENVELOPE TO:
PHYSICIANS' DESK REFERENCE, BOX 2017, MAHOPAC, NEW YORK 10541

PDR Supplements Order Card
Use the other side to stay up-to-date with Physicians' Desk Reference 1987 Supplements. Only $3.99.

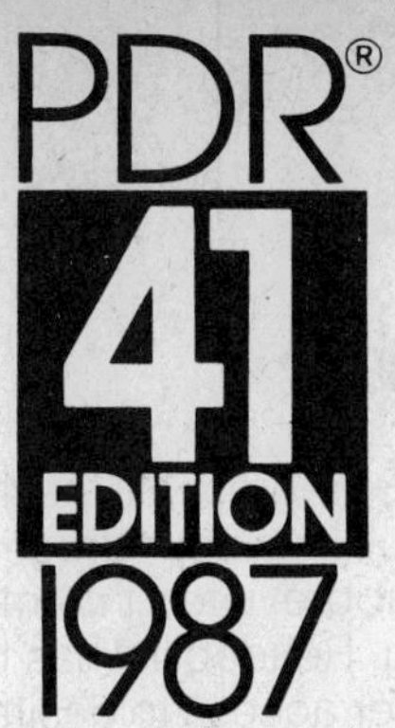

PHYSICIANS' DESK REFERENCE®

Publisher • EDWARD R. BARNHART

Director of Production
MARY TRELEWICZ

Managing Editor
BARBARA B. HUFF

Medical Consultant
NATHAN W. NEMIROFF, M.D.

Manager of Production Services
ELIZABETH H. CARUSO

Index Editor
ADELE L. DOWD

Editorial Assistants
JOAN AKERLIND
BEVERLY PFOHL

Administrative Assistants
ROSEMARIE MCGREGOR
MARGARET SIEKMANN

Art Associate
JOYCE L. WOOD

Director of Manufacturing
RALPH G.PELUSO

Marketing and Circulation Director
THOMAS C. MILLER

Assistant Circulation Director
ANNETTE G. VERNON

Research Director
CHARLOTTE E. SIBLEY

National Sales Manager
SHAWN MEEHAN

Account Managers
JEFF BONISTALLI
PAUL L. SCALITI
DANIEL W. STEEL

Design Director
JOHN NEWCOMB

Assistant Design Director
WILLIAM KUHN

Editorial Consultant
DAVID W. SIFTON

Officers of Medical Economics Company Inc.: President and Chief Executive Officer, Thomas J. McGill; Senior Vice Presidents: Jack E. Angel, Howard C. Clutterbuck, Robert B. Doll; Senior Vice President/Secretary, Stephen J. Sorkenn; Vice Presidents: Jeffrey M. Fass, James H. Jenkins, Willliam J. Reynolds, Lewis A. Scaliti.

ISBN-0-87489-835-8

Foreword to the Forty-first Edition

The 1987 PHYSICIANS' DESK REFERENCE® represents the 41st edition of the publication. This edition has been improved to make it more useful in fulfilling your drug information needs. Product overviews for selected drugs have been included to give abbreviated information about the product's use. These appear immediately before the full product labeling. Readability has been improved by rearranging labeling paragraph headings, in all caps, allowing quicker access to desired drug information. An explanation for pregnancy categories as used in drug labeling has also been included, along with definitions for the various classes of controlled drug substances. Information on inactive ingredients, educational materials (for you and your patients), bibliographies and phonetic spellings all join to make the book even more valuable. Special features also include. . .Guide to the Management of Drug Overdose and a listing of Regional Poison Control Centers.

PHYSICIANS' DESK REFERENCE® is published annually by Medical Economics Company Inc. with the cooperation of the manufacturer whose products appear in the Product Identification (Gray Section), the Product Information (White Section), and the Diagnostic Product Information (Green Section). Intended primarily for physicians, PDR's purpose is to make available essential information on major pharmaceutical and diagnostic products. In addition to this volume, two other editions of PHYSICIANS' DESK REFERENCE will be published in 1987: PDR® FOR NONPRESCRIPTION DRUGS and PDR® FOR OPHTHALMOLOGY.

This edition of PHYSICIANS' DESK REFERENCE® includes the latest available information on over 2,500 products. During the year ahead as important new or revised information about these products becomes available to us, it will be published periodically in a PDR® Supplement. Retain the Supplement with PDR and before prescribing or administering any product described in PHYSICIANS' DESK REFERENCE, consult the latest PDR Supplement to determine if new information about the product has been published.

The function of the Publisher is the compilation, organization and distribution of this information. Product descriptions have been prepared by manufacturers, edited and approved by their medical department and/or medical consultant. Manufacturers suggest headings under which products should appear in the Product Category Index (Blue Section) and the Generic and Chemical Name Index (Yellow Section).

Under the federal Food, Drug & Cosmetic (FD&C) Act, a drug approved for marketing may be labeled, promoted, and advertised by the manufacturer only for those uses for which the drug's safety and effectiveness have been established and which FDA has approved. The Code of Federal Regulations 201.100 (d) (1) pertaining to labeling for prescription products requires that for PDR content, "indications, effects, dosages, routes, methods, and frequency and duration of administration and any relevant warnings, hazards, contraindications, side effects, and precautions" must be the *"same in language and emphasis"* as the approved labeling for the product. FDA regards the words *"same in language and emphasis"* as requiring VERBATIM use of the approved labeling providing such information. Furthermore, information in the approved labeling that is emphasized by the use of type set in a box or in capitals, bold face, or italics must also be given the same emphasis in PDR.

The FDA has also announced that the FD&C Act "does not, however, limit the manner in which a physician may use an approved drug. Once a product has been approved for marketing, a physician may prescribe it for uses or in treatment regimens or patient populations that are not included in approved labeling." Thus, the FDA states also that "accepted medical practice" often includes drug use that is not reflected in approved drug labeling.

For products which do not have official package circulars, the Publisher has emphasized to manufacturers the necessity of describing such products comprehensively so that physicians would have access to all information essential for intelligent and informed prescribing. In organizing and presenting the material in PHYSICIANS' DESK REFERENCE®, the Publisher is providing all the information made available to PDR® by manufacturers. Additional information on any product may be obtained from the manufacturer. In making this material available, the Publisher does not advocate the use of any described product.

EDWARD R. BARNHART
Publisher

Contents

Discontinued Products

Listed below are products discontinued by manufacturers this past year. Please check the Product Name Index to determine if marketing has been assumed by another manufacturer.

Ar-Ex Ltd.
Brush-On-Complexion Coloring—Unscented
Cream for Oily Skin—Unscented
Protein Hair Dressing & Conditioner—Unscented

B.F. Ascher & Company, Inc.
Furose Tablets
Metronid Tablets

Ayerst Laboratories
Anacin-3 With Codeine Tablets
Thiosulfil Tablets

Barry Laboratories, Inc.
Stinging Insect Antigen #108

Burroughs Wellcome Company
A.P.C. with Codeine Tablets Tabloid Brand
Antepar Syrup & Tablets
Cardilate Chewable Tablets

Dermik Laboratories, Inc.
Klaron Acne Lotion

Du Pont Pharmaceuticals
Endecon Tablets
Remsed Tablets

Elkins-Sinn, Inc.
Chloramphenicol Sodium Succinate Injection (Sterile) USP

Forest Laboratories
ACTH 40
ACTH 80
Enzymet Tablets
Heparin Sodium Injectable
Panol Injectable
Panvitex Prenatal Tablets
Sulfaloid Suspension
Sulfaloid 500 Tablets
Tralmag Suspension

Geriatric Pharmaceutical Corp.
Gaysal S

Glaxo Inc.
Corticaine Suppositories
Tri-Cone Capsules

Hyland Therapeutics Division
Hemofil, Antihemophilic Factor (Human), Method Four, Dried
Hu-Tet, Tetanus Immune Globulin (Human), USP
Immune Serum Globulin (Human), USP Gamma Globulin
Proplex, Factor IV Complex (Human) (Factors II, VII, IX & X) Dried
Proplex SX, Factor IX Complex (Human) (Factors II, VII, IX & X) Dried

Hynson, Westcott & Dunning
Phenosulfonphthalein (PSP) Sodium Injection

Kramer Pharmacal Inc.
Sulfadrin Nasal Drops
Vagisulf Cream

Lakeside Pharmaceuticals
Novahistine Cough Formula

Marion Laboratories, Inc.
Ambenyl Cough Syrup
Ambenyl-D Decongestant Cough Formula
Nico-400
Os-Cal-Gesic Tablets

Merck Sharp & Dohme
Cyclaine Topical Solution

Merrell Dow Pharmaceuticals Inc.
Neo-Polycin
Novafed Liquid
Novafed A Liquid

Ortho Diagnostic Systems Inc.
Fetaldex Quantitative Test for Fetal Red Blood Cells in the Maternal Blood Circulation

Ortho Pharmaceutical Corp., Dermatological Division
Cloderm (clocortolone pivalate) Cream

Parke-Davis
Nitrostat SR Capsules
Papase
Povan Filmseals

Pedinol Pharmacal Inc.
Hydrisea Lotion

Reid-Rowell, Inc.
Acetospan Injection
Alermine Tablets
Analone Injection
Appi-Plex Tablets
Baltron Injection
Bendylate Capsules
Bendylate Injection
C-BE Zinc Tablets
C-Ron FA
C-Ron Freckles
Cabadon-M Injection
Colrex Capsules
Colrex Decongestant
Dentavite Chewable Tablets
Drozine Injection
E-Ionate P.A. Injection
Enoxa Tablets
Escot Capsules
Ganphen Injection
I.D. 50 Injection
Irolong II Capsules
Mity-Micin Ointment
Mity-Quin Cream
Nandrolin Injection
Nautrol Injection
Neotep Granucaps
Nospaz Injection
P.S.P. IV (four) Injection
Prednisolone Acetate Injections
Prednisone Tablets
Quinite Tablets
RP-Mycin Tablets
Repen-VK Tablets
SPRX-1 Tablets
Sumox Capsules
Sumox Oral Suspensions
Supen Capsules
Supen Oral Suspensions
T.D. Alermine Granucaps
T.D. Therals Granucaps
T-E Ionate P.A. Injection
T-Ionate P.A. Injection
Tagatap Tablets
Testosterone Aqueous Injection
Testostroval P.A. Injection
Thyroid Injection
Tora Tablets
Tora-30 Capsules
Trates Granucaps
Tuzyme Tablets
Vernate Injection
X-Otag Injection
Zide Tablets

Roche Laboratories
Gantrisin Injectable
Lipo Gantrisin
Nisentil

Rystan Company, Inc.
Derifil Powder

Schering Corporation
Coricidin Medilets Tablets
Corilin Infant Liquid
Metreton Ophthalmic/Otic Solution
My Own Feminine Spray Mist
Sunril Capsules

SmithKline Consumer Products
Contact Cough Capsules
Contact Severe Cold Formula Non Drowsy Capsules
Dietac
Hemoccult Home Test
Sine-Off Extra Strength Non-Aspirin Tablets
Teldrin Multi-Symptom Allergy Reliever

Smith Kline &French Laboratories
Combid Spansule Capsules
Compazine Injection 2 ml. Ampuls
SK-Amitriptyline HC1 Tablets 50 mg. & 150 mg.
SK-Chlorothiazide Tablets 250 mg.
SK-Dexamethasone Tablets 0.5 mg., 0.75 mg. & 1.5 mg.
SK-Doxycycline Hyclate Capsules 50 mg. & 100 mg.
SK-Hydrochlorothiazide Tablets 25 mg. & 50 mg.
SK-Metronidazole Tablets 250 mg.
SK-Penicillin G Tablets, 800,000 units
SK-Propantheline Bromide Tablets 15 mg.
Sk-Reserpine Tablets, 0.25 mg.
Sk-Tetracycline Syrup 125 mg./5 ml.
SK-Thioridazine HC1 Tablets 10 mg., 25 mg., 50 mg. & 100 mg.
Temaril Spansule Capsules 5 mg.
Temaril Tablets 2.5 mg.

UAD Laboratories, Inc.
UAD Lotion Forte

Wallace Laboratories
Dainite Tablets
Dainite-KI Tablets
Milpath Tablets
Miltrate Tablets

Wyeth Laboratories
Aspirin Rectal Suppositories
Atropine Sulfate Injection
Cerose Compound Capsules
Cetro Cirose
Chlorpromazine HC1 Injection, USP
Dexamethasone Sodium Phosphate Injection, USP
Petrogalar, Phenolphthalein
Polymagma Plain Tablets
Potassium Penicillin G Tablets, Buffered
Purodigin Tablets
Sparine Concentrate

SECTION 1

Manufacturers' Index

The manufacturers appearing in this index (white pages) have provided information concerning their pharmaceutical products in either the Product Information or Diagnostic Product Information Section. It is through their patronage that PHYSICIANS' DESK REFERENCE® is made available to you.

Included in this index are the names and addresses of manufacturers, individuals or departments to whom you may address inquiries, a partial list of products as well as emergency telephone numbers wherever available. The symbol ◆ indicates the product is shown in the Product Identification Section. The symbol ▣ indicates the product is described in PDR® FOR NONPRESCRIPTION DRUGS.

Part 1

PAGE

ABBOTT LABORATORIES 403, 502
North Chicago, IL 60064
Address Medical Information inquiries to:
Pharmaceutical Products Division
(312) 937-7069
Hospital Products Division
(312) 937-3806
Consumer Products Division
(312) 937-3806
Distribution Centers
ATLANTA
Stone Mountain, GA 30083
P.O. Box 5049 (404) 493-8330
CHICAGO
Abbott Laboratories
North Chicago, IL 60064
P.O. Box 68 (312) 937-5153
DALLAS
Farmers Branch, TX 75234
4653 Nall Rd. (214) 387-1350
LOS ANGELES
Los Angeles, CA 90060
P.O. Box 60162, Terminal Station
(213) 921-0321
PHILADELPHIA
King of Prussia, PA 19406
920 Eighth Ave., East
(215) 265-9100
Products Available
Abbokinase
Abbokinase Open-Cath
Abbo-Pac
Abbott Unit Dose Packages
Depakene Capsules
Depakote Tablets
E.E.S. Chewable Tablets, 400 Filmtab & Granules
Enduron Tablets
Enduronyl Tablets
EryPed Granules
Ery-Tab Tablets
Erythrocin Stearate Filmtab
Erythromycin Base Filmtab
Fero-Grad-500 Filmtab
Iberet-500 Filmtab
K-Lor
K-Tab Filmtab
Nembutal Sodium Capsules
Oretic Tablets
Panwarfin Tablets
Placidyl Capsules
Surbex-T Filmtab
Tranxene Capsules
Acetic Acid Irrigation
A-hydroCort
Alcohol, Absolute, Ampoules
5% Alcohol & 5% Dextrose Injection
A-methaPred
Amidate (Etomidate Injection) Ampul, Abboject
Aminophyllin 250 mg., 10 ml., Ampul & Vial
Aminophyllin 500 mg., 20 ml., Ampul & Vial
Aminosyn 3.5% M
Aminosyn 5%
Aminosyn 7%
Aminosyn 7% Kit
Aminosyn 7% with Electrolytes
Aminosyn 7% with Electrolytes TPN Kit
Aminosyn 8.5%
Aminosyn 8.5% TPN Kit
Aminosyn 8.5% with Electrolytes
Aminosyn 10%
Aminosyn 10% TPN Kit
Aminosyn with Dextrose, Nutrimix Dual Chamber
Ammonium Chloride
Atropine 0.1 mg./ml., 5 ml., Abboject Syringe
Atropine 0.1 mg./ml., 10 ml., Abboject Syringe
Bupivacaine Hydrochloride Injection, USP, 0.25%, 0.5%, 0.75%, Ampul, Abboject Syringe
Butesin Picrate Ointment
Butyn Dental Ointment
Calcidrine Syrup
Calcium Chloride 10%, Abboject
Calcium Gluceptate Injection Ampul & Abboject
Cecon Solution
◆ Cefol Filmtab
Cenolate Ampules
◆ Chlorthalidone Tablets
Chromium 10 ml. (4 mg./ml.)
Colchicine Tablets
Copper 10 ml. (4 mg./ml.)
Covicone Cream
◆ Cylert Chewable Tablets
◆ Cylert Tablets
Cysteine Hydrochloride Injection
▣ Dayalets Filmtab
▣ Dayalets plus Iron Filmtab
◆ Depakene Capsules & Syrup
◆ Depakote Tablets
Desoxyn
◆ Desoxyn Gradumet Tablets
6% Dextran w/v & 5% Dextrose Injection
6% Dextran w/v & 0.9% Sodium Chloride Injection
2.5% Dextrose & ½ Str Lact Ringer's Injection
5% Dextrose & Lact Ringer's Injection
5% Dextrose & Ringer's Injection
2.5% Dextrose & 0.45% Sodium Chloride Injection
5% Dextrose & 0.225% Sodium Chloride Injection
5% Dextrose & 0.3% Sodium Chloride Injection
5% Dextrose & 0.45% Sodium Chloride Injection
5% Dextrose & 0.9% Sodium Chloride Injection
10% Dextrose & 0.9% Sodium Chloride Injection
2.5% Dextrose Injection
5% Dextrose Injection
5% Dextrose Injection (Partial fill)
10% Dextrose Injection
20% Dextrose Injection
50% Dextrose Injection
5% Dextrose & 0.075% Pot Chl Injection (10 mEq)
5% Dextrose & 0.15% Pot Chl Injection (20 mEq)
5% Dextrose & 0.224% Pot Chl Injection (30 mEq)
5% Dextrose & 0.3% Pot Chl Injection (40 mEq)
5% Dextrose & 0.225% Sodium Chloride with 0.075% Potassium Chloride Injection (10 mEq)
5% Dextrose & 0.225% Sodium Chloride with 0.15% Potassium Chloride Injection (20 mEq)
5% Dextrose & 0.225% Sodium Chloride with 0.224% Potassium Chloride Injection (30 mEq)
5% Dextrose & 0.225% Sodium Chloride with 0.3% Potassium Chloride Injection (40 mEq)
5% Dextrose & 0.45% Sodium Chloride with 0.075% Potassium Chloride Injection (10 mEq)
5% Dextrose & 0.45% Sodium Chloride with 0.15% Potassium Chloride Injection (20 mEq)
5% Dextrose & 0.45% Sodium Chloride with 0.224% Potassium Chloride Injection (30 mEq)
5% Dextrose & 0.45% Sodium Chloride with 0.3% Potassium Chloride Injection (40 mEq)
10% Dextrose Injection
20% Dextrose Injection
30% Dextrose Injection
40% Dextrose Injection
50% Dextrose Injection
60% Dextrose Injection
70% Dextrose Injection
Dical-D Capsules & Wafers
Dical-D with Vitamin C Capsules
◆ Dicumarol Tablets
◆ E.E.S. Chewable Tablets
E.E.S. Drops
E.E.S. Granules
E.E.S. 200 Liquid
◆ E.E.S. 400 Filmtab
E.E.S. 400 Liquid
Empty Evacuated Container
Endrate Solution, Ampoules
◆ Enduron Tablets
◆ Enduronyl Forte Tablets
◆ Enduronyl Tablets
Ephedrine Sulfate, Injection
Epinephrine 1:10,000, 10 ml., Abboject
EryDerm
◆ EryPed Granules
◆ Ery-Tab Tablets
Erythrocin Lactobionate-I.V.
Erythrocin Piggyback
◆ Erythrocin Stearate Filmtab
◆ Erythromycin Base Filmtab
◆ Eutonyl Filmtab
◆ Eutron Filmtab Tablets
Fentonyl Injection, Ampul, Vial
◆ Fero-Folic-500 Filmtab
◆ Fero-Grad-500 Filmtab
Fero-Gradumet Filmtab
10% Fructose Injection
Gemonil Tablets
Gerilets Filmtab
Gerix Elixir
1.5% Glycine Irrigation/Aqualite
H-BIG
Halazone Tablets
Halothane
Harmonyl Tablets
Hydroxyzine HCl Injection, Abbojects, Ampuls, Vials, Syringes
Iberet Filmtab
◆ Iberet-500 Filmtab
Iberet-500 Liquid
◆ Iberet-Folic-500 Filmtab
Iberet Liquid
Iberol Filmtab
Iberol-F Filmtab
Inpersol & 1.5% Dextrose
Inpersol & 2.5% Dextrose
Inpersol & 4.25% Dextrose
Inpersol-LM with 1.5% Dextrose
Inpersol-LM with 2.5% Dextrose
Inpersol-LM with 4.5% Dextrose
10% Invert Sugar Injection
Ionosol B & 5% Dextrose Injection

(◆ Shown in Product Identification Section)

(▣ Described in PDR For Nonprescription Drugs)

Ionosol B & 10% Invert Sugar Injection
Ionosol D & 10% Invert Sugar Injection
Ionosol D-CM & 5% Dextrose Injection
Ionosol G & 10% Dextrose Injection
Ionosol G & 10% Invert Sugar Injection
Ionosol MB & 5% Dextrose Injection
Ionosol T & 5% Dextrose Injection
Isoproterenol HCl 1:5,000 5 ml., Universal Add Syringe
Isoproterenol HCl 1:5,000 10 ml., Universal Add Syringe
Isoproterenol HCl 1:50,000, 10 ml., Abboject
◆ Janimine Filmtab
◆ K-Lor Powder
◆ K-Tab Filmtab
10% LMD w/v in 5% Dextrose Injection
10% LMD w/v with 0.9% Sodium Chloride Injection
LTA Kit, Preattached
LTA II Kit
LTA Pediatric Kit
Lactated Ringer's Injection
Lidocaine HCl Injection, USP, 0.2% in 5% Dextrose
Lidocaine HCl Injection, USP, 0.4% in 5% Dextrose
Lidocaine HCl Injection, USP, 1%, 5 ml., Abboject
Lidocaine HCl Injection, USP, 1%, 5 ml., Sterile Pack Abboject
Lidocaine HCl Injection, USP, 2%, 5 ml., Abboject
Lidocaine HCl Injection, USP, 2%, 5 ml., Sterile Pack Abboject
Lidocaine HCl Injection, USP, 20%, 5 ml., 1 gram-Pintop, U.A.S.
Lidocaine HCl Injection, USP, 20%, 10 ml., 2 gram-Pintop, U.A.S.
Lidocaine HCl Injection, USP, 5% with 7.5% Dextrose
Lidocaine Hydrochloride Injection, U.S.P.
Liposyn II 10% and 20%
Lubritine
Magnesium Sulfate 12.5%, 8 ml., Pintop
Magnesium Sulfate 50% w/v Ampoules & Abboject
Mammol Ointment
Manganese 10 ml. (1 mg./ml.)
5% Mannitol Injection
10% Mannitol Injection
15% Mannitol Injection
20% Mannitol Injection
25% Mannitol Injection
◆ Nembutal Sodium Capsules
Nembutal Sodium Solution
Nembutal Sodium Suppositories
Neut Abbo-Vial & Pintop
Nitropress
Norisodrine Aerotrol
Norisodrine w/Calcium Iodide Syrup
Normosol-M 900 CAL
Normosol-M & 5% Dextrose Injection
Normosol-M & Surbex-T & 5% Dextrose Injection
Normosol-R & 5% Dextrose Injection
Normosol-R/K+ & 5% Dextrose Injection
◆ Ogen Tablets
◆ Ogen Vaginal Cream
◆ Optilets-500 Filmtab
◆ Optilets-M-500 Filmtab
◆ Oretic Tablets
Oreticyl Tablets
Oreticyl Forte Tablets
Panhematin
◆ Panwarfin Tablets
◆ Paradione Capsules & Oral Solution
◆ Peganone Tablets
Penthrane
Pentothal Kit
Pentothal RTM Syringe
Pentothal Rectal Suspension in Syringe
Pentothal (Sodium Thiopental for Injection)
Pentothal (Sterile Powder)
Phenobarbital Sodium Ampoules
Phenurone Tablets
Physiosol Irrigation/Aqualite
◆ Placidyl Capsules
Potassium Acetate 40 mEq Vial, Pintop & Fliptop
Potassium Chloride Injection Ampoules & Vials, Pintop & Universal Additive Syringe
Potassium Chloride 20 mEq. in D-5 W in Abbo-Vac
Potassium Phosphate 15 mM Vial, Pintop & Fliptop
Potassium Phosphate 45 mM Vial
Procaine Hydrochloride Injection 1% & 2% Vial
Quelicin (Succinylcholine Chloride Injection) Ampul & Vial, Pintop
Quelidrine Syrup
Ringer's Injection
Selsun Lotion
Selsun Suspension
Sodium Acetate 40 mEq Vial
5% Sodium Bicarbonate Injection
0.45% Sodium Chloride
5% Sodium Chloride
20% Sodium Chloride
0.9% Sodium Chloride Injection
Sorbitol-Mannitol Irrigation Solution/Aqualite
Sterile Urea
▣ Surbex Filmtab
▣ Surbex w/C Filmtab
◆ Surbex-750 with Iron Filmtab
◆ Surbex-750 with Zinc Filmtab
◆ Surbex-T Filmtab
Surbex-T & 5% Dextrose Injection
TPN Electrolytes
Tham E
Tham Solution
Tral Filmtab
Tral Gradumet Tablets
◆ Tranxene Capsules & Tablets
◆ Tranxene-SD Half Strength Tablets
◆ Tranxene-SD Tablets
◆ Tridione Capsules
◆ Tridione Dulcet Tablets
Tridione Solution
Tronothane Hydrochloride Cream
Tubocurarine Chloride Injection, USP
Ureaphil
Urological Solution G
Vercyte Tablets
Vita-Kaps Filmtab
Vita-Kaps M Filmtab
Vitamin C Filmtab
Water for Injection, Ampoules, Vial
Water for Injection Bacteriostatic 30 ml. Fliptop
Water for Injection, Sterile, Sterile Water
Water, for Irrigation, Sterile/Aqualite
Zinc 10 ml. (1 mg./1 ml.)

ABBOTT LABORATORIES DIAGNOSTICS DIVISION 2220
Abbott Park
Abbott Park, IL 60064
Outside Illinois call toll free
(800) 323-9100
Address inquiries to:
Marketing Services Dept. 49B
Products Available
Thypinone

ADAMS LABORATORIES, INC. 558
P.O. Box 487
10800 S. Pipeline Road
Hurst, TX 76053
Address inquiries to:
John Q. Adams (817) 267-3907
For Medical Emergencies Contact:
John Q. Adams (817) 267-3907
Products Available
Atrohist L.A. Tablets
Atrohist Sprinkle Capsules
Deconsal Capsules
Deconsal L.A. Tablets
Deconsal Sprinkle Capsules
Humibid L.A. Tablets

ADRIA LABORATORIES 403, 561
Division of Erbamont Inc.
Administrative Offices:
5000 Post Road
Dublin, OH 43017
Mailing Address:
P. O. Box 16529
Columbus, OH 43216
Address inquiries to:
Medical Department
(614) 764-8100
Products Available
Adriamycin
Adrucil
◆ Axotal
Chymex
Evac-Q-Kit
Evac-Q-Kwik
Folex for Injection
Folex PFS Injection, USP
Ilopan Injection (Ampuls & Vials)
Ilopan Stat-Pak (Disposable Syringes)
Ilopan-Choline Tablets
Ilozyme Tablets
Kaochlor 10% Liquid
Kaochlor-Eff Tablets
Kaochlor S-F 10% Liquid
◆ Kaon Cl-10
Kaon Elixir, Grape Flavor
Kaon Elixir, Lemon-Lime Flavor
Kaon Tablets
◆ Kaon-Cl
Kaon-Cl 20%
Magan Tablets
Modane Bulk
Modane Liquid
Modane Mild Tablets
Modane Plus
Modane Soft
Modane Tablets
Myoflex Creme
Neosar for Injection
◆ Octamide
Taloin Ointment
Tympagesic Otic Solution
Vincasar
Xylo-Pfan

ADVANCED MEDICAL NUTRITION, INC. 580
2247 National Avenue
Hayward, CA 94545
Address inquiries to:
P.O. Box 5012
Hayward, CA 94540-5012
(415) 783-6969
Products Available
Aler-gest Chewable Digestive Enzymes
Amnidophilus Acidophilus Powder
Balance - Gamma Linolenic Acid
Basic Preventive Junior Children's Multiple Supplement
Basic Preventive Multiple Vitamin-Mineral-Trace Element Supplement
Betaine HCl Capsules
Bioflavonoid Complex (1000 mg.)
C-Plex Powder (Buffered Vitamin C, Bioflavonoids and Trace Elements)
Calcigard 250 Acidified Calcium Citrate Tablets (Vitamin D_3 Optional)
Calcigard One-to-One Calcium-Magnesium Supplement (Vitamin D_3 Optional)
Calcigard Two-to-One Calcium-Magnesium Supplement (Vitamin D_3 Optional)
Candistat 300
Copper Amino Acid Chelate
Fiber-Plex Capsules
Folamint Natural Mouthwash
L-Glutathione Capsules
Hypoaller-C Buffered Vitamin C, Tablets or Powder
Immune-aid Natural Fatty Acids
Iron Amino Acid Chelate
Lipanase High Lipase Pancreatin
Lipex Natural Lipotropic Supplement
Mg-K Aspartate
MaxEPA Capsules
Peptonic Natural Digestive Aid
Professional Garlic Formulas
Protect! Antioxidant Formula
Zinc Picolinate

ALCON LABORATORIES, INC. 581
Alcon Laboratories, Inc.
And its affiliates Inc.
Corporate Headquarters
P.O. Box 6600
6201 South Freeway
Fort Worth, TX 76134
Address inquiries to:
Sales Services (817) 293-0450
Products Available
A.I.D.S. (Alcon Instrument Delivery System)
Alcon Closure System, A.C.S.
Alcon Indirect Ophthalmoscope/Camera
Alcon Surgical System (Irrigation/Aspiration Kits; Phacoemulsification Kits)
BSS (15ml, 250ml, 500ml)
BSS Plus
BSS and BSS Plus Irrigation Solution Administration Set
Betopic Solution
Cetamide Ointment
Cetapred Ointment
Cryophake
Cyclogyl
Cyclomydril
Digilab Model 30D Pneuma-Tonometer
Digilab Model 30R Pneuma-Tonometer
Digilab Model 30R/T Pneuma-Tonometer-Tonographer
Duratears
Enuclene
Epinal
Eye Pak
Eye Stream
Fluorescite
Gonioscopic Prism Solution
I-Knife
Ismotic
Maxidex Ointment
Maxitrol Ointment
Microphake
Microsponge
Miostat
Naphcon-A
Natacyn
Optemp
Osmoglyn
PTG
Pilopine HS Gel
Steri-Units
Tears Naturale
Terry Keratometer
Tobrex Ointment & Solution
Zolyse

ALCON (PUERTO RICO) INC. 584
P.O. Box 3000
Humacao, Puerto Rico 00661
Address inquiries to:
Medical Department
P.O. Box 6380
Fort Worth, TX 76115
(817) 293-0450
Products Available
Adsorbocarpine
Adsorbonac
Adsorbotear
Alcaine
Avitene
Econopred
Econopred Plus
Glaucon
Isopto Atropine
Isopto Carbachol
Isopto Carpine
Isopto Cetamide
Isopto Cetapred
Isopto Homatropine
Isopto Hyoscine
Maxidex Suspension
Maxitrol Suspension
Mydfrin 2.5%
Mydrapred
Mydriacyl
Naphcon
Naphcon Forte
Zincfrin

ALLERGAN PHARMACEUTICALS, INC. 584
2525 Dupont Drive
Irvine, CA 92715
Address inquiries to:
(714) 752-4500
(See also Herbert Laboratories)
Products Available
Albalon Liquifilm ophthalmic solution
Albalon-A Liquifilm ophthalmic solution
Allergan Hydrocare Cleaning & Disinfecting Solution
Allergan Hydrocare Preserved Saline Solution
Allergan Soft Lens Enzymatic Contact Lens Cleaner
Allergan Sorbi-Care Saline Solution
Atropine Sulfate ½% S.O.P. ophthalmic ointment
Atropine Sulfate 1.0% S.O.P. ophthalmic ointment
Atropine Sulfate 1% ophthalmic solution
Betagan Liquifilm ophthalmic solution
Bleph-10 Liquifilm ophthalmic solution
Bleph-10 S.O.P. ophthalmic ointment
Blephamide Liquifilm ophthalmic suspension
Blephamide S.O.P. ophthalmic ointment
Blink-N-Clean hard contact lens solution
Chloroptic ophthalmic solution
Chloroptic S.O.P. ophthalmic ointment
Clean-N-Soak hard contact lens cleaning & soaking solution
Clean-N-Soakit hard contact lens storage case
Clean-N-Stow hard contact lens storage case
Epifrin ophthalmic solution
Extenzyme Protein Cleaner
FML Forte Liquifilm ophthalmic suspension
FML Liquifilm ophthalmic suspension
FML S.O.P. ophthalmic ointment
Genoptic Liquifilm ophthalmic solution
Genoptic S.O.P. ophthalmic ointment
HMS Liquifilm ophthalmic suspension
Herplex Liquifilm ophthalmic solution
LC-65 Daily Contact Lens Cleaner for Polycon & Paraperm rigid gas permeable lenses & all hard & soft lenses
Lacril artificial tears
▣ Lacri-Lube S.O.P. ophthalmic ointment
Lens Clear Soft Lens Cleaner
Lens Fresh Lubricating & Rewetting Drops
LensKeeper contact lens storage case
Lens Plus Saline Solution (preservative-free)
Lensrins preserved saline solution
Lens-Wet lubricating & rewetting solution
▣ Liquifilm Forte enhanced artificial tears
▣ Liquifilm Tears Artificial Tears
Liquifilm Wetting Solution hard contact lens solution
Ophthetic ophthalmic solution
P.V. Carpine Liquifilm ophthalmic solution
Poly-Pred Liquifilm ophthalmic suspension
Pred Forte ophthalmic suspension
Pred Mild ophthalmic suspension
▣ Prefrin Liquifilm Eye Drops
Prefrin-A ophthalmic solution
Propine ophthalmic solution
Refresh artificial tears preservative-free
Relief eye drops for red eyes (preservative-free)
Soakare hard contact lens soaking solution
StyleKeeper contact lens storage case
Surgisol Balanced Salt Solution
▣ Tears Plus Artificial Tears
Total all-in-one hard contact lens solution
Wet-N-Soak wetting and soaking solution for hard contact lenses & Polycon & Paraperm rigid gas permeable lenses

ALPHA THERAPEUTIC CORPORATION 584
5555 Valley Boulevard
Los Angeles, CA 90032
Address inquiries to:
2410 Lillyvale Avenue
Los Angeles, CA 90032
(213) 227-7526
For Medical Emergencies Contact:
Dr. Clyde McAuley (213) 227-7419
Products Available
Albutein 5%
Albutein 25%
HT Profilate
Plasmatein 5%
Profilate Heat-Treated
Profilnine Heat-Treated

ALTO PHARMACEUTICALS, INC. 404, 585
15509 Casey Rd. Ext.
Tampa, FL 33624
Address inquiries to:
Professional Services
P.O. Box 271369
Tampa, FL 33688 (813) 961-1010
Products Available
Akne Drying Lotion
Akne Kaps
Amino G Tablets
Anabolin IM Injection
Anabolin LA-100 Injection
Cefinal II Tablets
◆ Efed II Capsules (Black)
◆ Efed II Capsules (Yellow)
Microcort Lotion
Tri Enz Tablets
Zinc-220 Capsules (Zinc Sulfate Capsules)

ALZA CORPORATION 404, 585
950 Page Mill Road
P.O. Box 10950
Palo Alto, California 94303-0802
Address inquiries to:
Marie E. Barry, Product Manager
(415) 494-5575
For Medical Emergencies Contact:
Virgil A. Place, Medical Director
(415) 494-5310
Products Available
Ocusert Ocular Therapeutic Systems
Pilo-20
Pilo-40
◆ Progestasert Intrauterine Contraceptive System

AMERICAN CRITICAL CARE 590
American Hospital Supply Corp.
McGaw Park, IL 60085
Address inquiries to:
Medical Director or in Emergency
Call: (312) 473-3000
Products Available
Bretylol Injection
Calciparine Injection
Hespan Injection
Intropin Injection
Inulin and Sodium Chloride Injection, USP
Tridil

AMERICAN DERMAL CORPORATION 596
12 Worlds Fair Drive
Somerset New Jersey 08873
Address inquiries to:
Professional Services Department
(800) 526-0199
In New Jersey call: (201) 356-5544
Products Available
Drithocreme
Dritho-Scalp
Viranol

ARCO PHARMACEUTICALS, INC. 597
105 Orville Drive
Bohemia, NY 11716
Address inquiries to:
Professional Service Dept.
(516) 567-9500
Products Available
Arco-Cee Tablets
Arco-Lase Tablets
Arco-Lase Plus Tablets
Arcoret Tablets
Arcoret w/Iron Tablets
Arcotinic Liquid
Arcotinic Tablets
C-B Time Capsules
C-B Time 500 Tablets
C-B Time Liquid
Co-Gel Tablets
Mega-B
Mega-B with C
Megadose
Spantuss Liquid
Spantuss Tablets

AR-EX LTD. 598
233 East Erie Street
Chicago, IL 60611
Address inquiries to:
Andrea Seidner (312) 943-6066
Products Available
Ar-Ex Hypo-Allergenic Cosmetics
Bath Oil - unscented
Body Lotion - unscented
Brush-On Complexion Coloring - unscented
Chap Cream - unscented
Cleansing Cream - unscented
Cold Cream - unscented
Compact Powder - unscented
Cream for Dry Skin - unscented
Cream for Oily Skin - unscented
Deodorant (Cream, Spray, Roll-On) - unscented
Disappear (Blemish Stick) - unscented
Face Powder - unscented
Foundation Lotion - unscented
Lip Gloss - unscented
Moisture Cream - unscented
Moisture Lotion - unscented
Night Cream - unscented
Protein Hair Dressing & Conditioner - unscented
Roll-On Mascara - unscented
Shampoo - unscented
Special Formula Lipstick - unscented
Superfatted Soap - unscented
Safe Suds - unscented

ARMOUR PHARMACEUTICAL COMPANY 404, 598
Executive Office
Suite 4000
One Sentry Parkway
Blue Bell, PA 19422
(215) 834-3850
Eastern Distribution Center
P.O. Box 397
Langhorne, PA 19047
(215) 752-8555
Midwest Distribution Center
4325 Frontage Road
Oak Forest, IL 60452
(312) 687-7440
Western Distribution Center
4902 Ampere Drive
Reno, NV 89502 (702) 348-7666
Southeastern Distribution Center
4660 Hammermill Road
Tucker, GA 30084
(810) 766-3961
Products Available
Acthar
◆ Aquasol A Capsules
Aquasol A Drops
Aquasol A Parenteral
◆ Aquasol E Capsules
Aquasol E Drops
Arm-a-Flow - I.V. Flow Regulator
Arm-a-Med
Isoetharine Hydrochloride
Isoproterenol Hydrochloride
Arm-a-Vial
Sodium Chloride 0.45%
Sodium Chloride 0.9%
Sterile Water
Arm-a-Vial LV
Heater
Humidifier
Nebulizer
Sodium Chloride 0.45%
Sodium Chloride 0.9%
Sterile Water for Inhalation
Barotrast
Biozyme-C
C-B Vone Capsules
C.V.P. Capsules
Chrometrace
Clysodrast
Coppertrace
◆ Dialume
duo-C.V.P. Capsules
Esophotrast
HP Acthar Gel
Lufa Capsules
M.V.I. Pediatric
M.V.I.-12 (Multi-Vitamin Infusion)
M.V.I.-12 Lyophilized (Multi-Vitamin Infusion)
M.V.I.-12 Multi-Dose
M.V.I.-12 UNIT VIAL
Mangatrace
Methischol Capsules
Multitrace 5
Multitrace Pediatric
Multitrace Solution & Concentrate
Oratrast
Plasma Derivative Products
Albuminar-5, Albumin (Human) U.S.P. 5%
Albuminar-25, Albumin (Human) U.S.P. 25%
Gammar, Immune Globulin (Human) U.S.P.
Gamulin Rh
H.T. Factorate, Antihemophilic Factor (Human) Dried, Heat Treated
H.T. Factorate Generation II
Humate-P, Antihemophilic Factor (Human), Pasteurized
Mini-Gamulin Rh
Plasma Plex
Thrombinar
Selenitrace
◆ Stimate Injection
Thrombinar
Thytropar
Trace Elements
Chrometrace
Coppertrace
Mangatrace
Multitrace 5
Multitrace Pediatric
Multitrace Solution & Concentrate
Selenitrace
Zinctrace
Vi-Aqua Capsules
Vi-Aqua Forte Capsules
Vi-Aquamin Forte Capsules
Zinctrace

ARTHER, INC. 606
Box 335
Mountain Lakes, NJ 07046
Address inquiries to:
A. Arthur Lowenthal, President
(800) 327-7914
(201) 226-5288
Products Available
Tryptacin

B. F. ASCHER & COMPANY, INC. 606
15501 W 109th St.
Lenexa, KS 66219
Address inquiries to:
Product Information Dept.
(913) 888-1880
Products Available
Adipost Capsules
Anaspaz PB Tablets
Anaspaz Tablets
▣ Ayr Saline Nasal Drops
▣ Ayr Saline Nasal Mist
Converspaz Improved Capsules
Converzyme Improved Capsules
Drize Capsules
Drotic Ear Drops
Ethaquin Tablets
Hy-Phen Tablets (formerly Hycodaphen)
Kwelcof Liquid
Mobidin Tablets
▣ Mobigesic Tablets
▣ Mobisyl Creme
Niloric Tablets
▣ Pen•Creme
Soft 'N Soothe Creme
Tolfrinic Tablets
▣ Unilax Tablets

ASTRA PHARMACEUTICAL PRODUCTS INC. 608
50 Otis Street
Westboro, MA 01581-4428
Address inquiries to:
Professional Information Department
(617) 366-1100
Products Available
Atropine Sulfate Injection
Calcium Chloride 10% Injection
Calcium Gluconate 10% Injection
Citanest Solutions
Dextrose 50% Injection
Dopamine Solutions
Duranest Hydrochloride & Duranest Hydrochloride with Epinephrine 1:200,000
Dyclone 0.5% and 1% Topical Solutions
Epinephrine Injection
Furosemide Injection, U.S.P.
Nesacaine Solutions
Nesacaine-CE Solutions
Sensorcaine Hydrochloride & Sensorcaine Hydrochloride with Epinephrine 1:200,000
Sodium Bicarbonate Injection
Xylocaine 2% Jelly
▣ Xylocaine 2.5% Ointment
Xylocaine 5% Ointment
Xylocaine 10% Oral Spray
Xylocaine Hydrochloride, Xylocaine Hydrochloride with Epinephrine 1:100,000, & Xylocaine Hydrochloride with Epinephrine 1:200,000
Xylocaine Solution for Ventricular Arrhythmias-Intravenous Injection or Continuous Infusion; or Intramuscular Injection
Xylocaine 1.5% Solution with Dextrose 7.5%
Xylocaine 4% Sterile Solution
Xylocaine 5% Solution with Glucose 7.5%
Xylocaine 4% Topical Solution
Xylocaine 2% Viscous Solution
Yutopar Intravenous Injection
Yutopar Tablets

AYERST LABORATORIES 404, 632, 2221
Division of American Home Products Corp.
685 Third Ave.
New York, NY 10017-4071
For Medical Information
Business hours only (9:00 a.m. to 5:00 p.m. EST), call
(212) 878-5900
For Medical Emergency Information After Hours or On Weekends, call
(212) 986-1000
(212) 878-5000
(212) 878-5900
Regional Sales Offices
South Plainfield, NJ 07080
4000 Hadley Rd. (201) 754-6220 (NJ)
(212) 964-3903 (NY)
Rockville, MD 20852
6252 Montrose Rd.
(301) 984-9140
Chamblee, GA (Atlanta) 30341
3600 American Drive
(404) 451-9578
Mobile, AL 36617
1110 Montlimar Dr.
Suite 720 (205) 344-1282
Mesquite, TX (Dallas) 75149
3601 Executive Blvd.
(214) 285-8741
Ontario, CA 91764
2151 East "D" St.
Suite 121C (714) 984-2426
Foster City, CA 94404
1147 Chess Dr. (415) 574-6065
Overland Park, KS 66214
10300 W. 103rd St.
Bldg. F, Suite 302 (913) 492-0802
Chicago, IL 60648
7545 N. Natchez Ave.
(312) 647-8948
Lakewood, OH 44107
14701 Detroit Ave.
Suite 440 (216) 226-4128
Blue Ash, OH 45242
West Lake Center
4555 Lake Forest Dr.
Suite 460 (513) 563-0040
Springfield, MA 01115
Bay Bank Tower, Suite 1906
P.O. Box 15707
1500 Main St. (413) 737-4594
Distribution Centers
South Plainfield, NJ 07080
4000 Hadley Rd. (201) 754-6220 (NJ)
(212) 964-3903 (NY)
Chamblee, GA 30341
3600 American Dr.
(404) 457-2518
Mesquite, TX 75149
3601 Executive Blvd.
(214) 285-8741
Foster City, CA 94404
1147 Chess Dr. (415) 574-6061
Lenexa, KS 66210
10700 Pflumm Rd.
(913) 888-4310
Chicago, IL 60648
7545 N. Natchez Ave.
(312) 763-0888 (Chicago)
(312) 647-8840 or 8841 (Niles)
Cleveland, OH 44135
15620 Industrial Parkway
(216) 267-9090
Products Available
A.P.L.
Almocarpine
◆ Antabuse
◆ Atromid-S
Auralgan Otic Solution
◆ Aygestin
◆ Beminal-500
Beminal Forte w/Vitamin C
◆ Beminal Stress Plus with Iron
◆ Beminal Stress Plus with Zinc
Clusivol Capsules
Clusivol Syrup
Clusivol 130 Tablets
Dermoplast Aerosol
◆ Diucardin
Enzactin Cream
Ayerst Epitrate
Estradurin
Estrogenic Substance (estrone) In Aqueous Suspension
◆ Factrel Injectable
Fluor-I-Strip Applicators
Fluor-I-Strip-A.T. Applicators
Fluothane
◆ Grisactin
◆ Grisactin Ultra
◆ Inderal Injectable
◆ Inderal Tablets
◆ Inderal LA Long Acting Capsules
◆ Inderide
◆ Inderide LA Long Acting Capsules
Kerodex Cream 51 (water-miscible)
Kerodex Cream 71 (water-repellent)
Larylgan Throat Spray
◆ Mediatric Capsules
Mediatric Liquid
◆ Mediatric Tablets
Mysoline Suspension
◆ Mysoline Tablets
Ophthalgan
◆ PMB 200 & PMB 400
Peptavlon
Phospholine Iodide
◆ Plegine
◆ Posture 300 mg
◆ Posture 600 mg
◆ Posture-D 300 mg Tablets
◆ Posture-D 600 mg Tablets
Premarin Intravenous
◆ Premarin Tablets
◆ Premarin Vaginal Cream
◆ Premarin w/Methyltestosterone
Protopam Chloride for Injection
Protopam Chloride Tablets
◆ Riopan Antacid Chew Tablets
Riopan Antacid Chew Tablets in Rollpack
Riopan Antacid Suspension
◆ Riopan Antacid Swallow Tablets
◆ Riopan Plus Chew Tablets
Riopan Plus Chew Tablets in Rollpack
Riopan Plus Suspension
◆ Extra Strength Riopan Plus Chew Tablets
Extra Strength Riopan Plus Suspension
Sonacide
Testuria
Thiosulfil Duo-Pak Package
◆ Thiosulfil Forte Tablets
◆ Thiosulfil-A Forte Tablets
◆ Thiosulfil-A Tablets
Turgasept Aerosol

BAKER/CUMMINS 676
Dermatological Division of Key Pharmaceuticals, Inc.
4400 Biscayne Blvd.
Miami, FL 33137 (305) 578-5800
(800) 327-0592
Products Available
Acno Lotion & Cleanser

Acticort Lotion 100
▣Complex 15 Lotion, Cream & Face Cream
▣P&S Liquid
▣P&S Plus Tar Gel
▣P&S Shampoo
Panscol Lotion & Ointment
Phacid Shampoo
Ultra Derm Moisturizer
▣Ultra Mide 25 Moisturizer
▣X•seb Shampoo
▣X•seb-T Shampoo

BARNES-HIND, INC. 676
A Revlon Vision Care Company
895 Kifer Road
Sunnyvale, CA 94086
Address inquiries to:
Customer Services Dept.
(800) 854-5615
In CA (800) 542-0195
Products Available
OPHTHALMIC
Alpha Chymar (enzymatic zonulysis)
Blinx (irrigating solution)
Cleaning & Soaking Solution (hard contact lenses)
Comfort Drops (for hard contact lenses)
Comfort Eye Drops (decongestant)
Comfort Tears (lubricant)
Degest 2 (decongestant)
Eppy/N (epinephryl borate)
Fluress (fluorescein-benoxinate combination)
Ful-Glo (fluorescein strips)
Gas Permeable Daily Cleaner (for gas permeable lenses)
Gas Permeable Wetting & Soaking Solution
Gel Clean (for hard contact lenses)
Lyteers (lubricant)
Neo-Tears (lubricant)
One Solution (for hard contact lenses)
Rose Bengal Strips
SOFT MATE Comfort Drops (for soft lenses)
SOFT MATE Daily Cleaning Solution (soft lenses)
SOFT MATE Daily Cleaning Solution II (soft lenses)
SOFT MATE Disinfecting Solution (for soft lenses)
SOFT MATE Disinfection & Storage Solution
SOFT MATE Lens Drops (for soft lenses)
SOFT MATE Preservative-Free Saline Solution
SOFT MATE Rinsing Solution (for soft lenses)
SOFT MATE Saline Solution (for soft lenses)
SOFT MATE Salt Tablets (for soft lenses)
SOFT MATE Weekly Cleaning Solution (soft lenses)
SOFT MATE ps Comfort Drops (for soft lenses)
SOFT MATE ps Daily Cleaning Solution
SOFT MATE ps Saline Solution (for soft lenses)
Soquette Storage Solution (for hard lenses)
Titan Cleaning Solution (for hard lenses)
Titan II Weekly Cleaning Solution (hard lenses)
Wetting Solution (for hard lenses)
Wetting & Soaking Solution (for hard lenses)
DERMATOLOGICAL
Barseb HC Scalp Lotion
Barseb Thera-Spray
HEB Cream Base
Komed Acne Lotion
Komed HC Lotion
Komex
Tinver Lotion

BARR LABORATORIES, INC. 677
265 Livingston Street
Northvale, NJ 07647
Address inquiries to:
(201) 767-1900
Products Available
Acetaminophen Tablets
Acetaminophen w/Codeine Tablets
Allopurinol Tablets
Aminophylline Tablets
Amitriptyline HCl Tablets
Aspirin w/Codeine Tablets
Bisacodyl Tablets
Chlordiazepoxide HCl Capsules
Chlordiazepoxide HCl w/Clidinium Bromide Capsules
Chlorpropamide Tablets
Chlorthalidone Tablets
Chlorzoxazone w/Acetaminophen Tablets
Colchicine Tablets
Dexamethasone Tablets
Diazepam Tablets
Dicyclomine HCl Capsules
Dimenhydrinate Tablets
Diphenhydramine Capsules
Diphenoxylate HCl w/Atropine Sulfate Tablets
Dipyridamole Tablets
Disopyramide Phosphate Capsules
Doxycycline Capsules (DOXY-CAPS)
Doxycycline Tablets (DOXY-TABS)
Ergoloid Mesylates Tablets
Erythromycin Estolate Capsules
Erythromycin Ethylsuccinate Granules
Erythromycin Stearate Tablets
Folic Acid Tablets
Furosemide Tablets
Hydralazine HCl Tablets
Hydrochlorothiazide HCl Tablets
Hydrocodone Bitartrate w/Acetaminophen Tablets
Hydroxyzine HCl Tablets
Hydroxyzine Pamoate Capsules
Ibuprofen Tablets
Isoniazid Tablets
Isosorbide Dinitrate Tablets Oral & S/L
Lorazepam Tablets
Meperidine HCl Tablets
Meprobamate Tablets
Methocarbamol Tablets
Metronidazole Tablets
Oxycodone w/Acetaminophen Tablets
Oxycodone w/Aspirin Tablets
Phenobarbital Tablets
Phenylbutazone Tablets
Prednisone Tablets
Propoxyphene Napsylate and Acetaminophen Tablets
Propranolol HCl Tablets
Propylthiouracil Tablets
Quinidine Sulfate Tablets
Reserpine/Hydralazine HCl/Hydrochlorothiazide Tablets
Reserpine/Hydrochlorothiazide Tablets
Spironolactone Tablets
Spironolactone w/Hydrochlorothiazide Tablets
Sulfamethoxazole Tablets
Sulfamethoxazole w/Trimethoprim Tablets
Sulfinpyrazone Capsules
Sulfisoxazole Tablets
Temazepam Capsules
Tetracycline Capsules
Thioridazine HCl Tablets
Tolazamide Tablets
Tolbutamide Tablets
Trimethoprim Tablets

BARRY LABORATORIES, INC. 678
461 N.E. 27th Street
P.O. Box 1967
Pompano Beach, FL 33061
In Florida call (1-305) 943-7722
Outside of Florida
Toll Free WATS Line (1-800) 327-1141
Address inquiries to:
Special Services Department
Products Available
Allergenic Extracts, Diagnosis and/or Immunotherapy
Dusts
Epidermals
Foods
Fungi (molds & smuts)
Inhalents
Insects
Poison Ivy, Oak, Sumac combined, (Rhus All Antigen)
Pollens
Allergenic Extracts for Immunotherapy
Immunorex-Prescription allergy treatment sets
Rhus All Antigen (Poison Ivy, Oak. Sumac combined)
Diagnostic Allegenic Extracts
Cutaneous
Intracutaneous
Diagnostic Allergenic Test Sets
"50 Plus" Includes a selection of perennial and seasonal allergens for each of 5 botanical zones
Sensi-Test Kit (Disposable Allergy Scarifier)
Merphene Germicidal Concentrate
Rhus All Antigen - Poison Ivy, Oak, Sumac Combined

A. J. BART, INC. 678
Gurabo Industrial Park
P.O. Box 813
Gurabo, Puerto Rico 00658
(809) 737-8445
(809) 737-8446
(809) 737-8447
Address inquiries to:
(809) 737-8445
Products Available
Alba-3 Ointment
Alba-3 Ophthalmic Ointment
Alba-3 Ophthalmic Solution
Alba-Ce Liquid, Drops, Tablets
Albacort Cream
Alba-Dex Injectable, Liquid & Tablets
Albaform-HC Cream
Albafort Injectable
Alba-Gyn Vaginal Cream
Alba-Lybe
Alba-Temp Suppositories, Liquid & Tablets
Albatussin (Sugar Free)
Albatussin Pediatric
Benzotic Ear Drops
Dextrotussin Syrup
Dramatrol Injectable
Iron Cacodylate
Migralam Capsules
Myoforte Tablets
Myophen Injectable
Nervidox
Nervidox-6
Neuro B-12 Forte Injectable
Neuro B-12 Injectable
Pasmin Injectable, Liquid, Capsules
Reocyl Injection
Sedaril
Tia-Doce Injectable Solution
Vita-Numonyl Injectable

BEACH PHARMACEUTICALS 405, 679
Division of Beach Products, Inc.
Executive Office
5220 S. Manhattan Ave.
Tampa, FL 33611 (813) 839-6565
Manufacturing and Distribution
Main St. at Perimeter Rd.
Conestee, SC 29605
Toll Free 1-(800) 845-8210
Address inquiries to:
Richard Stephen Jenkins
(813) 839-6565
Products Available
◆ Beelith Tablets
Citrolith Tablets
◆ K-Phos M.F. Tablets
◆ K-Phos Neutral
◆ K-Phos No. 2 Tablets
◆ K-Phos Original Formula 'Sodium Free' Tablets
◆ Thiacide Tablets
◆ Uroqid-Acid
◆ Uroqid-Acid No. 2

BEECHAM PRODUCTS 681
Division of Beecham Inc.
P.O. Box 1467
Pittsburgh, PA 15230
Address inquiries to:
Professional Services Dept.
800-BEECHAM
PA Residents: 800-242-1718
Products Available
Massengill Disposable Douche
Massengill Liquid Concentrate
Massengill Medicated Disposable Douche
Massengill Powder

BEECHAM LABORATORIES 405, 682
Division of Beecham, Inc.
Bristol, TN 37620
Address inquiries to:
Director, Professional Relations
Beecham Laboratories
501 Fifth Street
Bristol, TN 37620 (615) 764-5141
Products Available
◆ Amoxil Capsules, Oral Suspension & Chewable Tablets
Amoxil Pediatric Drops for Oral Suspension
Anexsia w/Codeine Tablets
Anexsia-D Tablets
◆ Augmentin Tablets, Powder for Oral Suspension, and Chewable Tablets
◆ Bactocill Capsules
Bactocill for Injection
Beepen-VK Oral Solution & Tablets
◆ Cloxapen Capsules
Conar Expectorant Syrup
Conar Suspension
Conar-A Tablets
Corrective Mixture w/Paregoric
Daricon
Daricon PB
Dasin Capsules
◆ Dycill Capsules
Enarax Tablets
◆ Fastin Capsules
Hybephen Tablets
Hycal Liquid
Klebcil for Injection
Livitamin Capsules
Livitamin Capsules w/Intrinsic Factor
Livitamin Chewable Tablets
Livitamin Liquid
Menest Tablets
Morphine & Atropine Injectable
Nallpen for Injection
◆ Nucofed Capsules
Nucofed Expectorant
Nucofed Pediatric Expectorant
Nucofed Syrup
Pyopen Injectable
Semets Troches
Theralax Suppositories
Ticar for Injection
◆ Tigan Capsules
Tigan Injectable
Tigan Suppositories
◆ Timentin for Injection
Totacillin Capsules
Totacillin For Oral Suspension
Totacillin-N Injectable

BEIERSDORF, INC. 694
BDF Plaza
P. O. Box 5529
Norwalk, CT 06856-5529
Address inquiries to:
Medical Division (203) 853-8008
Products Available
Aquaphor
Coverlet
Coverlet Eye Occlusor
Elastoplast
Eucerin Cleansing Bar
Eucerin Creme
Eucerin Lotion
Gelocast
Mediplast

BERLEX LABORATORIES, INC. 405, 694
Wayne, NJ 07470
Address inquiries to:
Educational Services
300 Fairfield Road
Wayne, NJ 07470 (201) 694-4100
For Medical Information
Professional Services Department
110 East Hanover Avenue
Cedar Knolls, NJ 07927
(201) 292-3008
Products Available
◆ Deconamine SR Capsules
Deconamine Syrup
◆ Deconamine Tablets
◆ Levlen 21 Tablets
◆ Levlen 28 Tablets
◆ Quinaglute Dura-Tabs Tablets
Tri-Levlen 21 Tablets
◆ Tri-Levlen 28 Tablets

BEUTLICH, INC. 709
7149 North Austin
Niles, IL 60648 (312) 647-8110
(800) 238-8542
Telex: 5101002772 Topical CGO
Products Available
Ceo-Two Rectal Suppositories
Hurricaine Topical Anesthetic Aerosol Spray
Hurricaine Topical Anesthetic Gel
Hurricaine Topical Anesthetic Liquid
Hurricaine Topical Anesthetic Spray Extension Tubes
Hurricaine Topical Anesthetic Spray Kit
Mevanin-C Capsules
Peridin-C Tablets

BIOCRAFT LABORATORIES, INC. 709
92 Route 46
Elmwood Park, NJ 07407
Address inquiries to:
(201) 796-3434
Products Available
Amitriptyline HCl Tablets
Amoxicillin Capsules
Amoxicillin Suspension
Ampicillin Capsules
Ampicillin Suspension
Ampicillin-Probenecid Suspension
Chloroquine Phosphate Tablets
Clonidine Hydrochloride Tablets
Cloxacillin Capsules
Cloxacillin Solution
Dicloxacillin Capsules
Disopyramide Phosphate Capsules
Hydrocortisone Topical Cream
Imipramine HCl Tablets
Metoclopramide Hydrochloride Tablets
Neomycin Sulfate Tablets
Oxacillin Capsules
Oxacillin Solution
Penicillin G Potassium Tablets
Penicillin V Potassium Solution
Penicillin V Potassium Tablets
Sulfamethoxazole & Trimethoprim Pediatric Suspension
Sulfamethoxazole and Trimethoprim Tablets
Trimethoprim Tablets

BOCK PHARMACAL COMPANY 710
P.O. Box 8519
St. Louis, MO 63126-0519
Address inquiries to:
Professional Services Dept.
(314) 343-0994
Products Available
Broncholate Capsules
Broncholate Syrup
Dolprn #3 Tablets
Hemaspan Tablets
Onset-5 Tablets
Pavadyl Capsules
Poly-Histine CS
Poly-Histine Capsules
Poly-Histine Elixir
Poly-Histine Expectorant Plain
Poly-Histine-D Capsules
Poly-Histine-D Elixir
Poly-Histine-D Ped Caps
Poly-Histine DM Syrup
Poly-Histine-DX Capsules
Prenate 90 Tablets
Theon Syrup
Zephrex Tablets
Zephrex-LA Tablets

BOEHRINGER INGELHEIM PHARMACEUTICALS, INC. 405, 710
A subsidiary of Boehringer Ingelheim Corporation
90 East Ridge
P.O. Box 368
Ridgefield, CT 06877
Address inquiries to:
Medical Services Dept.
(203) 438-0311
Products Available
Alupent Inhalant Solution 5% & Solution Unit Dose 0.6%
Alupent Metered Dose Inhaler
Alupent Syrup

◆ Alupent Tablets
◆ Catapres Tablets
◆ Catapres-TTS
◆ Combipres Tablets
◆ Dulcolax Suppositories
◆ Dulcolax Tablets
◆ Mexitil Capsules
◆ Persantine Tablets
◆ Prelu-2 Capsules
◆ Preludin Endurets
◆ Respbid
Serentil Ampuls
Serentil Concentrate
◆ Serentil Tablets
◆ Thalitone Tablets
Torecan Ampuls
Torecan Suppositories
◆ Torecan Tablets

BOEHRINGER MANNHEIM DIAGNOSTICS 2223
9115 Hague Road
Indianapolis, IN 46250
(317) 845-2000
Products Available
Chemstrip bG Blood Glucose Test
Chemstrip Urine Testing System

BOOTS PHARMACEUTICALS, INC. 406, 724
8800 Ellerbe Road
Shreveport, LA 71106
Address inquiries to:
Medical Director (318) 861-8200
Products Available
F-E-P Creme
◆ Lopurin Tablets
◆ Rufen Tablets
Ru-Tuss Expectorant
Ru-Tuss Liquid
◆ Ru-Tuss Tablets
◆ Ru-Tuss II Capsules
Ru-Tuss with Hydrocodone
Twin-K Liquid
Twin-K-Cl Liquid
◆ Zorprin Tablets

BOYLE & COMPANY 732
1030 South Arroyo Parkway
Pasadena, CA 91105
Address inquiries to:
Susan M. Boyle (818) 441-0284
Products Available
Citra Forte Syrup
Triva Douche Powder

BRAINTREE LABORATORIES, INC. 406, 732
285 Washington Street
Braintree, MA 02184
Address inquiries to:
Mr. Harry P. Keegan, President
(617) 843-2202
For Medical Emergencies Contact:
Geoffrey E. Clark, M.D.
(603) 749-2417
Products Available
◆ GoLYTELY

BRISTOL LABORATORIES 406, 733
(Div. of Bristol-Myers Co.)
2404 W. Pennsylvania St.
Evansville, IN 47721
Address medical inquiries to:
Dept. of Medical Services
(812) 429-5000
Orders may be placed by calling the following toll free numbers:
Within New York State
1-(800) 962-7200
Continental U.S. 1-(800) 448-7700
Alaska - Hawaii 1-(800) 448-1100
Mail orders and all inquiries should be sent to:
Bristol Laboratories Pharmaceutical Division
Order Entry Department
2404 W. Pennsylvania St.
Evansville, IN 47721
Products Available
Amikin
◆ Betapen-VK Tablets and Oral Solution
Cefadyl for Intramuscular or Intravenous Injection
◆ Dynapen Capsules and Powder for Oral Suspension
◆ Kantrex Capsules
Kantrex Injection and Pediatric Injection
Nafcil
◆ Naldecon Syrup, Tablets, Pediatric Drops and Pediatric Syrup
■ Naldecon-CX Adult Liquid
■ Naldecon-DX Adult Liquid
■ Naldecon-DX Children's Syrup
■ Naldecon-DX Pediatric Drops
■ Naldecon-EX Children's Syrup
■ Naldecon-EX Pediatric Drops
◆ Naldegesic Tablets
◆ Polycillin Capsules, for Oral Suspension, and Pediatric Drops
Polycillin-N for Intramuscular or Injection
Polycillin-PRB (ampicillin-probenecid) for Oral Suspension
◆ Polymox Capsules, for Oral Suspension, and Pediatric Drops
Precef
◆ Prostaphlin Capsules, Oral Solution
Prostaphlin for Injection
◆ Saluron
◆ Salutensin/Salutensin-Demi
Stadol
Staphcillin Injection—Buffered
◆ Tegopen Capsules and For Oral Solution
◆ Ultracef Capsules, Tablets & Oral Suspension

BRISTOL-MYERS ONCOLOGY DIVISION 406, 759
(Bristol-Myers Company)
2404 W. Pennsylvania St.
Evansville, IN 47721
Address medical inquiries to:
Dept. of Medical Services
(812) 429-5000
Orders may be placed by calling the following toll free numbers:
Continental US 1-(800) 448-7700
Alaska-Hawaii 1-(800) 448-1100
Mail orders and all inquiries should be sent to:
Bristol Laboratories
Order Entry Department
2404 W. Pennsylvania St.
Evansville, IN 47721
Products Available
BiCNU
Blenoxane
◆ CeeNU
◆ Cytoxan
◆ Lysodren
◆ Megace Tablets
◆ Mexate and Mexate-AQ
Mutamycin
Platinol
VePesid Injection

BRISTOL-MYERS PRODUCTS 770
(Div. of Bristol-Myers Co.)
345 Park Avenue
New York, NY 10154
Address inquiries to:
Alphonse Flora, M.D.
1350 Liberty Avenue
Hillside, NJ 07207
In Emergencies Call:
(212) 546-4616 (9AM-5PM)
(212) 546-4700 (Other times)
Products Available
Ammens Medicated Powder
B.Q. Cold Tablets
Ban Antiperspirant Cream Deodorant
Ban Basic Non-aerosol Antiperspirant Spray
Ban Roll-on Antiperspirant
Ban Solid Antiperspirant Deodorant
Ban Wide Ball Antiperspirant
Bufferin Arthritis Strength Tablets
Bufferin Extra-Strength Analgesic Tablets
Bufferin Tablets
Comtrex Multi-Symptom Cold Reliever Tablets/Caplets/Liquid
Congespirin For Children Aspirin Free Chewable Cold Tablets
Congespirin For Children Aspirin Free Liquid Cold Medicine
Congespirin For Children Cough Syrup
Datril Extra-Strength Tablets & Caplets
Excedrin Extra-Strength Tablets & Caplets
Excedrin P.M. Analgesic/Sleeping Aid Tablets
4-Way Cold Tablets
4-Way Fast Acting Nasal Spray (regular & mentholated)
4-Way Long Acting Nasal Spray
Minit-Rub Greaseless Analgesic Ointment
Mum Antiperspirant Cream Deodorant
No Doz Fast Acting Keep Alert Tablets
Nuprin Ibuprofen/Analgesic Tablets
Pazo Hemorrhoid Ointment & Suppositories
Tickle Antiperspirant
Ultra Ban Aerosol Antiperspirant
Ultra Ban Roll-on Antiperspirant
Ultra Ban Solid Antiperspirant/ Deodorant

THE BROWN PHARMACEUTICAL COMPANY, INC. 406, 773
P.O. Box 1529
Costa Mesa, CA 92628-1529
(800) 556-1937
In CA (800) 331-2331
Address inquiries to:
Professional Service Department
Products Available
◆ Android-5 Buccal
◆ Android-10 Tablets
◆ Android-25 Tablets
◆ Android-F Tablets
Calphosan I.M.
Lipo-Nicin/100 mg.
Lipo-Nicin/250 mg. Tablets

BURROUGHS WELLCOME CO. 406, 775
3030 Cornwallis Road
Research Triangle Park, NC 27709
(919) 248-3000
Address inquiries to:
G. Ed Collins, Pharm. M.S.
(919) 248-3085
Branch Office
Burlingame, CA 94010
1760 Rollins Rd. (415) 697-5630
Products Available
◆ Actidil Tablets & Syrup
◆ Actifed Capsules
◆ Actifed 12-Hour Capsules
◆ Actifed Tablets & Syrup
Actifed with Codeine Cough Syrup
Aerosporin Powder
◆ Alkeran Tablets
Ammonia Aromatic, Vaporole
Amyl Nitrite, Vaporole
Anectine Flo-Pack
Anectine Injection
Atropine Sulfate Injection, Wellcome
Borofax Ointment
◆ Cardilate Oral/Sublingual Tablets
Cortisporin Cream
Cortisporin Ointment
Cortisporin Ophthalmic Ointment Sterile
Cortisporin Ophthalmic Suspension Sterile
Cortisporin Otic Solution Sterile
Cortisporin Otic Suspension Sterile
◆ Daraprim Tablets
Digoxin (See Lanoxin)
◆ Empirin Aspirin Tablets
◆ Empirin w/Codeine Phosphate Nos. 2, 3 & 4
◆ Empracet with Codeine Phosphate Nos. 3 & 4
Erythrityl Tetranitrate (See Cardilate)
◆ Fedrazil Tablets
Imuran Injection
◆ Imuran Tablets
◆ Kemadrin Tablets
Lanoline, Wellcome
◆ Lanoxicaps
◆ Lanoxin—Tablets, Injection & Elixir Pediatric
◆ Leukeran Tablets
Lubafax Surgical Lubricant, Sterile
Mantadil Cream
◆ Marezine Tablets & Injection
◆ Myleran Tablets
■ Neosporin Cream
Neosporin G.U. Irrigant
■ Neosporin Ointment
Neosporin Ophthalmic Ointment Sterile
Neosporin Ophthalmic Solution Sterile
Nix 1% Creme Rinse
Polymyxin B Sulfate (see Aerosporin)
■ Polysporin Ointment, Powder & Spray
Polysporin Ophthalmic Ointment Sterile
◆ Proloprim Tablets
◆ Purinethol Tablets
Scopolamine Hydrobromide Injection, Wellcome
◆ Septra DS Tablets
Septra I.V. Infusion
Septra Suspension
◆ Septra Tablets
◆ Sudafed (Pseudoephedrine HCl) Children's Liquid & Tablets
■ Sudafed Cough Syrup
◆ Sudafed Plus Liquid & Tablets
◆ Sudafed 12 Hour Capsules
◆ Tabloid Brand Thioguanine
Tracrium Injection
Vasoxyl Injection
Viroptic Ophthalmic Solution
Wellcovorin Injection
◆ Wellcovorin Tablets
◆ Zovirax Capsules
Zovirax Ointment 5%
Zovirax Sterile Powder
◆ Zyloprim Tablets

C & M PHARMACAL, INC. 821
1519 E. Eight Mile Rd.
Hazel Park, MI 48030-2696
Address inquiries to:
C & M Pharmacal, Inc.
(800) 423-5173
In MI call collect: (313) 548-7846
For Medical Emergencies Contact:
C & M Pharmacal, Inc.
(800) 423-5173
In MI call collect: (313) 548-7864
Or any Poison Control Center (All products have full ingredient disclosure)
Products Available
Pod-Ben-25
Verr-Canth
Verrex
Verrusol

CAMPBELL LABORATORIES INC. 821
300 East 51st Street
New York, NY 10022
(212) 688-7684
Address inquiries to:
Richard C. Zahn, President
P.O. Box 812, FDR Station
New York, NY 10150
Products Available
Herpecin-L Cold Sore Lip Balm

THE CARLTON CORPORATION 821
See GLENWOOD, INC.

CARNRICK LABORATORIES, INC. 407, 821
65 Horse Hill Road
Cedar Knolls, NJ 07927
(201) 267-2670
Address inquiries to:
Medical Director (201) 267-2670
Products Available
◆ Amen
◆ Bontril PDM
◆ Bontril Slow-Release
◆ Capital and Codeine Suspension
◆ Capital and Codeine Tablets
◆ Hydrocet
◆ Midrin
◆ Nolahist
◆ Nolamine
◆ Phrenilin Forte
◆ Phrenilin
◆ Phrenilin with Codeine No. 3
◆ Propagest
◆ Sinulin (*New Formulation*)
◆ Skelaxin

CENTER LABORATORIES 827
Division of EM Industries, Inc.
35 Channel Drive
Port Washington, NY 11050
Address inquiries to:
Customer Services
Call Toll Free (800) 645-6335
In N.Y. (516) 767-1800
For Medical Emergencies Contact:
Technical Services (516) 767-1800
Products Available
Center-Al—Allergenic Extracts Alum Precipitated
EpiPen—Epinephrine Auto-Injector
EpiPen Jr.

CENTRAL PHARMACEUTICALS, INC. 407, 828
120 East Third St.
Seymour, IN 47274
Address inquiries to:
Daniel J. Desmond (812) 522-3915
Products Available
Analbalm, Liquid
Andronaq-50 Sterile Suspension
Andronaq-LA Injectable
Cenocort A-40 Sterile Suspension
Cenocort Forte Sterile Suspension
Codiclear DH Syrup
Codimal DH Syrup
Codimal DM Syrup
Codimal Expectorant
Codimal PH Syrup
Codimal Tablets & Capsules
Codimal-A Injectable
◆ Codimal-L.A. Capsules
◆ Co-Gesic Tablets
Co-Xan Syrup
Cyclocen Injectable
Dexacen LA-8 Sterile Suspension
Dexacen-4 Injectable
◆ Dia-Gesic
Diphenacen-10 and -50 Injectables
Dramocen Injectable
Estronol Aqueous Sterile Suspension
Estronol-LA Injectable
GG-Cen Syrup/Capsules
Hexalol Tablets
Hydroxacen Injectable
Lifolbex Injectable
◆ Mono-Gesic Tablets
Neocyten Injection
Neolax Tablets
Niferex Elixir
Niferex Forte Elixir
Niferex Tablets
Niferex w/Vitamin C Tablets
◆ Niferex-150 Capsules
◆ Niferex-150 Forte Capsules
◆ Niferex-PN Tablets
◆ Niferex-PN Forte Tablets
Pavacen Capsules
Phencen-50 Injectable
Prednicen-M Tablets
Prednicen-M 21-Pak
Prednisolone Acetate Sterile Suspension
Progestronaq-LA Injectable
Rep-Pred 40 Sterile Suspension
Rep-Pred 80 Sterile Suspension
Rubesol-1000 Injectable
Synophylate Elixir
Synophylate-GG Syrup
Synophylate-GG Tablets
◆ Theoclear L.A.-130 & -260 Capsules
Theoclear-80 Syrup

CETYLITE INDUSTRIES, INC. 831
P.O. Box CN6
9051 River Road
Pennsauken, NJ 08110
Address inquiries to:
Mr. Stanley L. Wachman, President
(609) 665-6111
(800) 257-7740
Products Available
Cetacaine Topical Anesthetic
Cetylcide Germicidal Concentrate
Protexin Oral Breath Spray
Protexin Oral Rinse Concentrate
Skin Screen Protective Skin Lotion

CIBA CONSUMER PHARMACEUTICALS 407, 831
Division of CIBA-GEIGY Corporation
Raritan Plaza III
Edison, NJ 08837
Address inquiries to:
(201) 225-6000
Products Available
Acutrim 16 Hour Appetite Suppressant
Nupercainal Cream & Ointment
Nupercainal Suppositories
Otrivin Nasal Spray & Nasal Drops
Otrivin Pediatric Nasal Drops
PBZ Cream

(◆ Shown in Product Identification Section) **(■ Described in PDR For Nonprescription Drugs)**

PBZ Hydrochloride Cream
Privine Nasal Solution
Privine Nasal Spray
◆ Slow Fe Tablets

CIBA PHARMACEUTICAL COMPANY 407, 832
Division of CIBA-GEIGY Corporation
Address inquiries to:
556 Morris Avenue
Summit, NJ 07901
New Jersey (201) 277-5000
New York (212) 267-6615
Division Offices
Warehouse Offices and Shipping Branches
Eastern
14 Henderson Drive
West Caldwell, NJ 07006
(201) 575-6510
Central
7530 No. Natchez Ave.
Niles, IL 60648 Niles (312) 647-9332
Chicago (312) 763-8700
Western
12850 Moore St.
P.O. Box 6300
Cerritos, CA 90701
Cerritos (213) 404-2651
Products Available
◆ Antrenyl Tablets
◆ Anturane Capsules
◆ Anturane Tablets
◆ Apresazide Capsules
Apresoline Ampuls
◆ Apresoline Tablets
◆ Apresoline-Esidrix Tablets
Cibalith-S Syrup
Coramine Oral Solution
◆ Cytadren Tablets
Desferal Vials
◆ Esidrix Tablets
◆ Esimil Tablets
INH Tablets
◆ Ismelin Tablets
◆ Lithobid Tablets
◆ Ludiomil Tablets
◆ Metandren Linguets & Tablets
◆ Metopirone Tablets
Nupercainal Cream
Nupercainal Ointment
Nupercainal Suppositories
Percorten Pellets
Percorten Pivalate Multiple-dose Vials
Priscoline Hydrochloride Ampuls
Privine Nasal Solution
Privine Nasal Spray
Regitine
Regitine Hydrochloride Tablets
◆ Rimactane Capsules
Rimactane/INH Dual Pack
◆ Ritalin Tablets
◆ Ritalin-SR Tablets
◆ Ser-Ap-Es Tablets
Serpasil Parenteral Solution
◆ Serpasil Tablets
◆ Serpasil-Apresoline Tablets
◆ Serpasil-Esidrix Tablets
◆ Slow-K Tablets
◆ Transderm-Nitro Transdermal Therapeutic System
◆ Transderm Scōp Transdermal Therapeutic System
Vioform Cream
Vioform Ointment
Vioform-Hydrocortisone Cream
Vioform-Hydrocortisone Lotion
Vioform-Hydrocortisone Mild Cream
Vioform-Hydrocortisone Mild Ointment
Vioform-Hydrocortisone Ointment

COLGATE-HOYT LABORATORIES 408, 867
Division of Colgate-Palmolive Company
1 Colgate Way
Canton MA 02021 USA
Address inquiries to:
Professional Services Dept.
(800) 225-3756
Products Available
Luride Drops
◆ Luride Lozi-Tabs Tablets
◆ Full-strength 1.0 mg F
◆ Luride-SF (no artificial flavor or color) 1.0 mg F
◆ Half-strength 0.5 mg F
◆ Quarter-strength 0.25 mg F
Orabase HCA Oral Paste
Phos-Flur Oral Rinse/Supplement
Point-Two Dental Rinse
PreviDent Brush-On Gel
Thera-Flur Topical Gel-Drops
Thera-Flur-N Topical Gel-Drops

CONNAUGHT LABORATORIES, INC. 870
Swiftwater, PA 18370
Address inquiries to:
Biologicals Product Mgr.
(717) 839-7187
For Medical Emergencies Contact:
Medical Director (717) 839-7187
Direct orders to:
Connaught Laboratories, Inc.
Customer Services (800) 538-7678
or (717) 839-7187
Products Available
Diphtheria Antitoxin (Purified, Concentrated Globulin-Equine)
Diphtheria & Tetanus Toxoids Adsorbed USP (For Pediatric Use) (DT)
Diphtheria and Tetanus Toxoids and Pertussis Vaccine Adsorbed USP (For Pediatric Use)
HibVAX (Haemophilus b Polysaccharide Vaccine)
MSTA(TM) (Mumps Skin Test Antigen. USP)
Menomune (Meningococcal Polysaccharide Vaccine, Groups A,C,Y,W-135 Combined)
Poliomyelitis Vaccine (Purified) (For the Prevention of Poliomyelitis) Inactivated, Salk-type
Tetanus Toxoid
Tetanus Toxoid Adsorbed
Tetanus & Diphtheria Toxoids Adsorbed For Adult Use Td
Tubersol (Tuberculin Purified Protein Derivative [Mantoux])
YF-VAX (Yellow Fever Vaccine)(Live, 17D Virus, Avian Leukosis-Free, Stabilized)

COOK-WAITE LABORATORIES, INC. 870
90 Park Avenue
New York, NY 10016
(212) 907-2712
Products Available
Carbocaine Hydrochloride 3% Injection
Carbocaine Hydrochloride 2% with Neo-Cobefrin 1:20,000 Injection
Marcaine Hydrochloride 0.5% with Epinephrine

COOPERVISION PHARMACEUTICALS INC 872
San German, Puerto Rico 00753
Address inquiries to:
Professional Services
San German, Puerto Rico or call
(800) 468-8586
For Medical or Contact Lens Solution Information
Write: Medical Department
2610 Orchard Parkway
San Jose, CA 95134
Call: *(Business Hours Only)*
Joseph Krezanoski, Ph.D.
(800) 538-7834
For Medical Emergency Information After Hours or on Weekends, call
Jerome F. Grattan (201) 821-8846
Products Available
Argyrol Stabilized Solution 10%
Atropisol Ophthalmic Solution 1%
Catarase 1:5,000 & 1:10,000
CooperVision Balanced Salt Solution
Cystex Tablets
Dacriose Ophthalmic Irrigating Solution
Dexacidin Ophthalmic Ointment
Dexacidin Ophthalmic Suspension
Dropperettes:
Argyrol S.S. 20%
Atropisol 0.5%, 1%, 2%
Epinephrine 1:1000
Fluorescein Sodium 2%
Homatropine HBr 2%, 5%
Phenylephrine HCl 10%
Pilocar 1%, 2%, 4%
Sulf-10 (Sodium Sulfacetamide 10%)
Tetracaine HCl 0.5%
E-Pilo Ophthalmic Solutions 1, 2, 3, 4, 6
Eserine Sulfate Ophthalmic Ointment ¼%
Funduscein-10 or -25 (Fluorescein sodium I.V.)
Gentacidin Ophthalmic Ointment
Gentacidin Ophthalmic Solution
Glucose-40 Ophthalmic Ointment 40%
Glyrol Solution
Goniosol Solution
Homatropine Hydrobromide Ophthalmic Solution 2%, 5%
Hypotears Lubricating Eye Drops
Hypotears Ointment (ocular lubricant)
Inflamase Forte 1% Ophthalmic Solution
Inflamase Mild ⅛% Ophthalmic Solution
Lens Care Products:
Clerz
Clerz 2
d-Film
duo-Flow
HGP Cleaner
HGP Conditioning Solution
hy-Flow
Lensine-5
MiraFlow
MiraSept Disinfecting Solution
MiraSept Rinsing & Neutralizing Solution
Pliagel
Unisol
Unisol 4
Lipoflavonoid Vitamin Supplement (Capsule)
Lipotriad Vitamin Supplement (Capsule, Liquid)
Lydia Pinkham (Tablets, Liquid)
Miochol Intraocular
Phenylzin Ophthalmic Solution
Pilocar Ophthalmic Solutions 0.5%, 1%, 2%, 3%, 4%, 6%
Pilocar Ophthalmic Solutions Twin Pack 0.5%, 1%, 2%, 3%, 4%, 6%
Schirmer Tear Test
Sulf-10 Ophthalmic Solution 10%
Tearisol Ophthalmic Solution
Vasocidin Ophthalmic Ointment
Vasocidin Ophthalmic Solution
VasoClear Decongestant Eye Drops
VasoClear A Decongestant Astrigent Lubricating Eye Drops
Vasocon Regular Ophthalmic Solution
Vasocon-A Ophthalmic Solution
Vasosulf Ophthalmic Solution

CUTTER BIOLOGICAL 872
Division of Miles Laboratories, Inc.
2200 Powell Street
Emeryville, CA 94662
Written inquiries to:
Professional Services Manager
Technical & Medical Inquiries:
(800) 227-1762 (outside CA)
(800) 227-3219 (within CA)
Branch Offices
To Order Call:
CHICAGO OFFICE
1852 Brummel Drive
Elk Grove Village IL 60007
(800) 323-2549 (outside IL)
(312) 228-6466 (in IL)
DALLAS TX 75240
P.O. Box 400358
(214) 661-5850 (Within AC 214)
(800) 527-0382 (Outside TX)
(800) 442-5701 (In TX, except AC 214)
LOS ANGELES OFFICE
15320 East Salt Lake Avenue
City of Industry, CA 91744
(818) 968-8561 (within AC 818)
(800) 423-9429 (outside CA)
(800) 352-5495 (in CA, except AC 818)
NEW YORK OFFICE
11 Harts Lane Ste D
East Brunswick, NJ 08816
(800) 221-0831 (outside NJ)
(201) 238-0140 (in NJ)
Products Available
Antihemophilic Factor Koāte-HT
Factor IX Complex (Human) Konȳne-HT
Gamastan (Immune Globulin-Human)
Gamimune N (Immune Globulin Intravenous, 5% in 10% Maltose) pH 4.25
Hepatitis B Immune Globulin (Human) HyperHep
Hyperab (Rabies Immune Globulin-Human)
HyperHep (Hepatitis B Immune Globulin-Human)
Hyper-Tet (Tetanus Immune Globulin-Human)
HypRho-D (Rh_o-D Immune Globulin-Human)
HypRho-D Mini-Dose (Rh_o-D Immune Globulin-Human)
Immune Globulin Intravenous, 5% (In 10% Maltose) pH 4.25, Gamimune N
Immune Globulin (Human) Gamastan
Koate-HT (Antihemophic Factor)
Konȳne-HT (Factor IX Complex-Human)
Plague Vaccine (Human)
Rh_o-D Immune Globulin (Human) HypRho-D
Rh_o-D Immune Globulin (Human) HypRho-D Mini-Dose
Rabies Immune Globulin (Human) Hyperab
Tetanus Immune Globulin (Human) Hyper-Tet

DANBURY PHARMACAL, INC. 876
131 West Street
P.O. Box 296
Danbury, CT 06810
Address Inquiries to:
Nessim Maleh
Ira Sacks
Milton Blitz (203) 744-7200
Products Available
Acetazolamide
Allopurinol Tablets
Bethanechol Chloride Tablets
Butalbital and Acetaminophen Tablets
Carisoprodol Tablets
Chloroquine Phosphate Tablets
Chlorothiazide Tablets
Chlorpropamide Tablets
Chlorthalidone Tablets
Chlorzoxazone Tablets
Chlorzoxazone with APAP Tablets
Clonidine HCl Tablets
Colchicine Tablets
Col-Probenecid Tablets
Cyproheptadine HCl Tablets
Diazepam Tablets
Dicyclomine HCl Capsules
Dicyclomine HCl Tablets
Diphenhydramine HCl Capsules
Dipyridamole Tablets
Disopyramide Phosphate Capsules
Disulfiram Tablets
Doxycycline Hyclate Capsules
Doxycycline Hyclate Tablets
Ergoloid Mesylates Oral Tablets
Ergoloid Mesylates Sublingual Tablets
Erythromycin Estolate Capsules
Flurazepam HCl Tablets
Folic Acid Tablets
Furosemide Tablets
Glutethimide Tablets
Glycopyrrolate Tablets
Hydralazine HCl Tablets
Hydrochlorothiazide, Hydralazine HCl, Reserpine Tablets
Hydrochlorothiazide/Reserpine Tablets
Hydrochlorothiazide Tablets
Hydrocortisone Tablets
Hydroxyzine Hydrochloride Tablets
Hydroxyzine Pamoate Capsules
Ibuprofen Tablets
Isoniazid Tablets
Isosorbide Dinitrate Oral Tablets
Isosorbide Dinitrate Sublingual Tablets
Isoxsuprine HCl Tablets
Lorazepam Tablets
Meprobamate Tablets
Methocarbamol Tablets
Methyldopa Tablets
Metoclopramide HCl Tablets
Metronidazole Tablets
Nylidrin HCl Tablets
Papaverine HCl T.D. Capsules
Papaverine HCl Tablets
Phenobarbital Tablets
Phenylbutazone Tablets
Prednisolone Tablets
Prednisone Tablets
Primidone Tablets
Probenecid Tablets
Procainamide HCl Capsules
Procainamide Hydrochloride S.R. Tablets
Propantheline Bromide Tablets
Propranolol HCl Tablets
Pseudoephedrine HCl Tablets
Quindan Tablets
Quinidine Gluconate Sustained Action Tablets
Quinidine Sulfate Tablets
Spironolactone/Hydrochlorothiazide Tablets
Sulfamethoxazole with Trimethoprim Tablets
Sulfamethoxazole with Trimethoprim Tablets (Double Strength)
Sulfasalazine Tablets
Sulfinpyrazone Tablets
Tetracycline HCl Capsules
Theofedral Tablets
Thioridazine HCl Tablets
Tolazamide Tablets
Tolbutamide Tablets
Triamcinolone Tablets
Trihexyphenidyl HCl Tablets
Trimethoprim Tablets
Tripelennamine HCl Tablets
Tripodrine Tablets
Verapamil HCl Tablets

DELMONT LABORATORIES, INC. 877
P.O. Box AA
Swarthmore, PA 19081
Address inquiries to:
(215) 543-3365
(215) 543-2747
Products Available
Staphage Lysate (SPL)

DERMIK LABORATORIES, INC. 877
790 Penllyn Pike
Blue Bell, PA 19422
Distribution Centers
Langhorne, PA 19047
P.O. Box 247 (215) 752-1211
Oak Forest, IL 60452
P.O. Box 280 (800) 323-4474
Reno, NV 89502
4902 Ampere Drive
(702) 348-7666
Tucker, GA 30084
4660 Hammermill Road
(800) 241-9120
Products Available
Anthra-Derm Ointment 1%, ½%, ¼%, 1/10%
5 Benzagel (5% benzoyl peroxide) & 10 Benzagel (10% benzoyl peroxide), Acne Gels, Microgel Formula
Benzamycin Topical Gel
Drest Gel
Durrax Tablets 10mg, 25mg
Florone Cream 0.05%
Florone Ointment 0.05%
Hytone Cream 1%, 2 ½%
Hytone Lotion 1%, 2 ½%
Hytone Ointment 1%, 2 ½%
Jeri-Bath
Jeri-Lotion
Loroxide Acne Lotion
Psorcon Ointment 0.05%
Psorcon E Emollient Cream 0.05%
Rezamid Acne Lotion
Shepard's Cream Lotion
Shepard's Moisturizing Soap
Shepard's Skin Cream
Sulfacet-R Acne Lotion
Vanoxide Acne Lotion
Vanoxide-HC Acne Lotion
Vlemasque
Vytone Cream ½%, 1%
Zetar Emulsion
Zetar Shampoo

DISTA PRODUCTS COMPANY 408, 882
Division of Eli Lilly and Company
General Offices
Lilly Corporate Center
Indianapolis, IN 46285
For Medical Information, Write:
Medical Department
Lilly Corporate Center
Indianapolis, IN 46285
(317) 261-4000
Sales Offices
Aurora, CO 80014
Suite 111, Cherry Creek Place I
3131 South Vaughn Way
(303) 695-7733
Braintree, MA 02184
Suite 104, Braintree Office Park
35 Braintree Hill Park
(617) 849-0693
*Chicago, IL 60631
Suite 270, O'Hare Plaza
5735 East River Road
(312) 693-8360
Cincinnati, 4 45241
Suite 413, 4055 Executive Park Drive
(513) 563-7010
Cleveland, OH 44130
Suite 395, Interstate Plaza
16600 W. Sprague Road
(216) 243-0047
Dallas, TX 75244-3290
4404 Beltwood Parkway, South
(214) 661-5669
Houston, TX 77042
Suite 360, Richmond Plaza I
9800 Richmond Ave.
(713) 975-6822
Indianapolis, IN 46268
Suite 235, Northwest Plaza
3901 West 86th St.
(317) 261-5770
Jacksonville, FL 32216
Suite 319-A, The Center Building
7825 Baymeadows Way
(904) 731-8530
Kansas City, MO 64114
Suite 610, 9200 Ward Parkway
(816) 361-1020
Melville, NY 11747
Suite 3S02
One Huntington Quadrangle
(516) 752-9839
Memphis, TN 38117
Suite 224, 755 Crossover Lane
(901) 767-3988
Metairie, LA 70006
Suite 508, Security Homestead Bldg.
4900 Veterans Memorial Boulevard
(504) 455-0339
Morristown, NJ 07960
Morristown Centre
10 Madison Avenue
(201) 898-9507
Nashville, TN 37210
Suite 310, 555 Marriott Drive
(615) 885-2700
*Norcross, GA 30091
5944 Peachtree Corners, East
(404) 441-5404
*Pasadena, CA 91101
Suite 916, Mutual Savings Bldg.
301 East Colorado Blvd.
(818) 792-3197
Pittsburgh, PA 15220
Suite 602, Manor Oak Two
1910 Cochran Road
(412) 561-5044
Raleigh, NC 27625
Suite 103, 3109 Poplarwood Court
(919) 872-5210
Redmond, WA 98052
11811 Willows Road
(206) 881-6163
San Francisco, CA 94111
Suite 1170, 100 California St.
(415) 391-2767
Silver Spring, MD 20903
Suite 111, Executive Court
1734 Elton Road (301) 439-1109
Southfield, MI 48075
Suite 940, 3000 Town Center
(313) 358-2278
St. Louis, MO 63131
Suite 325, Corporate Hill II
1633 Des Peres Rd.
(314) 821-0996
St. Paul, MN 55164
4100 North Hamline Ave.
(612) 638-4074
*Stamford, CT 06905
Suite 301, 1600 Summer St.
(203) 357-8872
Tampa, FL 33609
Suite 1060, Lincoln Center
5401 West Kennedy Boulevard
(813) 870-3086
Wynnewood, PA 19096
Suite 202, Seven Wynnewood Road
(215) 642-0438
*Regional Office
Products Available
Becotin Pulvules
Becotin with Vitamin C Pulvules
Becotin-T Tablets
◆ Cinobac Pulvules
Co-Pyronil 2, Pulvules, Pediatric Pulvules, and Liquid
Cordran Ointment & Lotion
Cordran SP Cream
Cordran Tape
Cordran-N Cream and Ointment
Ilosone Chewable Tablets
Ilosone, for Oral Suspension
Ilosone Liquids, Oral Suspensions
◆ Ilosone Pulvules & Tablets
Ilosone Ready-Mixed Drops
Ilotycin Gluceptate, IV, Vials
Ilotycin Ophthalmic Ointment
Ilotycin Tablets
Keflex, for Oral Suspension
Keflex, for Pediatric Drops
◆ Keflex, Pulvules & Tablets
Mi-Cebrin Tablets
Mi-Cebrin T Tablets
◆ Nalfon Pulvules & Tablets
◆ Nalfon 200 Pulvules
◆ Valmid Pulvules

DORSEY LABORATORIES 892
Division of Sandoz, Inc.
P.O. Box 83288
Lincoln, NE 68501
Address Medical inquiries to:
Medical Department
Sandoz Pharmaceuticals
East Hanover, NJ 07936
(201) 386-7500
Other Inquiries to:
Dorsey Laboratories
(402) 464-6311
Products Available
Acid Mantle Creme
▣ Cama Arthritis Pain Reliever
Chexit Tablets
Dorcol Children's Cough Syrup
Dorcol Children's Decongestant Liquid
Dorcol Children's Fever & Pain Reducer
Dorcol Children's Liquid Cold Formula
Eclipse After Sun Moisturizer
Eclipse Lip and Face Protectant, SPF 15
Eclipse Partial Suntan Lotion, SPF 5
Eclipse Original Sunscreen Moisturizing Lotion, SPF 10
Eclipse Total Sunscreen Cooling Alcohol Lotion, SPF 15
Eclipse Total Sunscreen Moisturizing Lotion, SPF 15
Kanulase Tablets
▣ Triaminic Allergy Tablets
▣ Triaminic Chewables
Triaminic Cold Syrup
Triaminic Cold Tablets
Triaminic Expectorant
Triaminic Expectorant DH
Triaminic Expectorant w/Codeine
Triaminic Oral Infant Drops
Triaminic TR Tablets (Timed Release)
Triaminic-12 Tablets
Triaminic-DM Cough Formula
▣ Triaminicin Tablets
Triaminicol Multi-Symptom Cold Syrup
Triaminicol Multi-Symptom Cold Tablets
▣ Tussagesic Tablets
▣ Ursinus Inlay-Tabs

DORSEY PHARMACEUTICALS 897
See SANDOZ PHARMACEUTICALS CORPORATION

DU PONT PHARMACEUTICALS 408, 897
E.I. du Pont de Nemours & Co. (Inc.)
Wilmington, Delaware 19898
Address inquiries to:
Director, Professional Services
1 (800) 441-9861
In Delaware (302) 992-3273
Distribution Centers
Garden City, NY 11530
1000 Stewart Ave.
1 (800) 645-3546
1 (800) 645-3547
In New York State call:
(516) 832-2029
(516) 832-2030
(516) 832-2031
Claremont, CA 91711
1480 N. Claremont Blvd.
(714) 621-7986
(714) 621-7987

DU PONT PHARMACEUTICALS CARIBE, INC.
Subsidiary of E.I. du Pont de Nemours & Company (Inc.)
Post Office Box 12
Manati, Puerto Rico 00701
Address inquiries to:
Du Pont Pharmaceuticals
E.I. du Pont de Nemours & Co. (Inc.)
Wilmington, Delaware 19898
Director, Professional Services
1 (800) 441-9861
In Delaware (302) 992-3273

DU PONT PHARMACEUTICALS, INC.
Subsidiary of E.I. du Pont de Nemours & Company (Inc.)
Post Office Box 363
Manati, Puerto Rico 00701
Address Inquiries to:
Du Pont Pharmaceuticals
E.I. du Pont de Nemours & Co. (Inc.)
Wilmington, Delaware 19898
Director, Professional Services
1 (800) 441-9861
In Delaware (302) 992-3273

Products Available
◆ Coumadin Injection & Tablets
◆ Hycodan Syrup, Tablets
Hycomine Compound Tablets
Hycomine Pediatric Syrup
Hycomine Syrup
Hycotuss Expectorant Syrup
◆ Moban Tablets & Concentrate
◆ Narcan Injection
◆ Nubain Injection
Numorphan Hydrochloride Injection
◆ Numorphan Suppositories
◆ Percocet Tablets
◆ Percodan Tablets
◆ Percodan-Demi Tablets
◆ Symmetrel Capsules & Syrup
◆ Tessalon Perles
◆ Trexan Tablets
Valpin 50 Tablets
◆ Zydone Capsules

DURA PHARMACEUTICALS, INC 912
P.O. Box 28331
San Diego, CA 92128
Address inquiries to:
Same as above (619) 789-6840
For Medical Emergencies Contact:
Craig Wheeler (619) 789-6840
Tom Evangelisti
Products Available
Dura-Gest
Dura Tap-PD
Dura-Vent
Dura-Vent/A
Dura-Vent/DA

EDWARDS PHARMACAL, INC. 913
100 East Hale
Osceola, AR 72370-9990
Address inquiries to:
Professional Services Dept.
P.O. Drawer 129
Osceola, AR 72370-9990
(501) 563-1144
For Medical Emergencies Contact:
Mr. John Newcomb
(501) 563-1144
Or your nearest Poison Control Center
Products Available
Blanex Capsules
C-Span Capsules
Doxy-Caps
ECEE Plus Tablets
E.P. Mycin Capsules
E-Tapp Elixir
Hydrogesic Capsules
Nico-Vert Capsules
Rymed Capsules
Rymed Liquid
Rymed-Jr. Capsules
Rymed-TR Tablets
SRC Expectorant
Senilezol Elixir
Slyn-LL Capsules
Urogesic Tablets
Uromide Tablets

ELDER PHARMACEUTICALS, INC. 409, 913
A subsidiary of the ICN Pharmaceuticals, Inc. Group
ICN Plaza
3300 Hyland Avenue
Costa Mesa, CA 92626
Address inquiries to:
3300 Hyland Avenue
Costa Mesa, CA 92626
(800) 556-1937
In CA (800) 331-2331
(714) 545-0100
Products Available
Benoquin Cream 20%
Elder Psoralite
Eldopaque 2% Cream
Eldopaque Forte 4% Cream
Eldoquin 2% Cream
Eldoquin 2% Lotion
Eldoquin Forte 4% Cream
Fototar Cream
Fototar Stik 6.25%
◆ Oxsoralen Capsule
Oxsoralen Lotion 1%
Pabanol Lotion
RVP Ointment
RVPaba Lip Stick
RVPaque Ointment
Solaquin 2% Cream
Solaquin Forte 4% Cream
Solaquin Forte 4% Gel
◆ Trisoralen Tablets
Vitadye Lotion

ELKINS-SINN, INC. 921
A subsidiary of A.H. Robins Company
2 Esterbrook Lane
Cherry Hill, NJ 08003-4099
(800) 257-8349
Address price and packaging inquiries to:
Marketing Department
Address scientific information inquiries to:
Professional Services Department
Products Available
Aminocaproic Acid Injection
Aminophylline Injection
Atropine Sulfate Injection
Bretylium Tosylate Injection (Preservative-Free)
Calcium Chloride Injection
Calcium Gluconate Injection
Chlorpromazine HCl Injection
Codeine Phosphate Injection
Cyanocobalamin (Vit. B_{12}) Injection
Dexamethasone Sodium Phosphate Injection
Dexpanthenol Injection (d-Pantothenyl Alcohol)
Dextrose Injection
Diazepam Injection
Digoxin Injection
Diphenhydramine HCl Injection
Dopamine HCl Injection
Doxycycline Hyclate for Injection
Duramorph (Preservative-free morphine sulfate injection)
Epinephrine Injection
Erythromycin Lactobionate for Injection
Fentanyl Citrate Injection
Furosemide Injection
Gentamicin Sulfate Injection
Heparin Sodium Injection
Hep-Lock (Heparin Lock Flush Solution)
Hep-Lock U/P (Preservative-Free Heparin Lock Flush Solution)
Hydrocortisone Sodium Succinate for Injection
Hydromorphone HCl Injection
Hydroxyzine HCl Intramuscular Injection
Isoproterenol HCl Injection
Lidocaine HCl Injection
Lidocaine HCl Injection (Preservative-free)
Lidocaine Hydrochloride Injection for Cardiac Arrhythmias
Liodocaine Hydrochloride & Epinephrine Injection
Magnesium Sulfate Injection
Meperidine HCl Injection
Methylene Blue Injection
Methylprednisolone Sodium Succinate for Injection
Metronidazole Redi-Infusion
Mineral Oil, Sterile Light
Morphine Sulfate Injection
Naloxone Hydrochloride Injection, USP
Neostigmine Methylsulfate Injection
Paraldehyde (Sterile)
Pentobarbital Sodium Injection
Phenobarbital Sodium Injection
Phenytoin Sodium Injection
Potassium Chloride Injection
Potassium Chloride Injection (Preservative-Free)
Procainamide Hydrochloride Injection
Procaine HCl Injection
Prochlorperazine Edisylate Injection
Promethazine HCl Injection
Scopolamine Hydrobromide Injection
Sodium Chloride Injection (Preservative-free)
Sodium Chloride Injection, Bacteriostatic
Sodium Nitroprusside Injection
Sotradecol (Sodium Tetradecyl Sulfate Injection)
Thiamine HCl Injection
Vials, Sterile Empty
Water For Injection, Bacteriostatic
Water for Injection, Sterile (Preservative-Free)

ETHITEK PHARMACEUTICALS COMPANY 924
8104 North Lawndale Ave.
Skokie, IL 60076
Address inquiries to:
(312) 675-6616
For Medical Emergencies Contact:
Anne L. Barlow, M.D., Medical Director
(312) 675-6616
Products Available
Moctanin

EVERETT LABORATORIES, INC. 925
76 Franklin Street
East Orange, NJ 07017
Address inquiries to:
Professional Service Dept.
(201) 674-8455

FERNDALE LABORATORIES, INC. 925
780 W. Eight Mile Road
Ferndale, MI 48220
Address inquiries to:
Professional Service Dept.
(313) 548-0900
(800) 621-6003
Products Available
Adphen Tablets
Analpram-HC Rectal Cream
Aquaphyllin Syrup
Benase Tablets
Betuline Liniment
Dapa Tablets
Dapacin Capsules
Dapex 37.5 mg Capsules
Delaxin Tablets
Detachol Adhesive Remover
Doss 300 Capsule
Fastamine Tablets
Ferndex Tablets
Kronofed-A-Jr. Kronocaps
Kronofed-A Kronocaps
Kronohist Kronocaps
Liqui-Doss
Maigret-50 Tablets
Mastisol Liquid Adhesive

(◆ Shown in Product Identification Section)

(▣ Described in PDR For Nonprescription Drugs)

Obestin-30 Capsules
Oxychinol Tablets
Phenobella Tablets
Pramosone Cream, Lotion & Ointment
Prax Cream & Lotion
Procute Cream & Lotion
Rhinocaps Capsules
Salatin Capsules
Strifon Forte Tablets
Synabrom Capsules
T/Prep Skin Degreaser
Tin-Ben Dispenser
Tin-Co-Ben Dispenser
Tri-Pain Tablets
Vio-Pramosone Cream
Vio-Pramosone Lotion

THE FIELDING COMPANY 926
2384 Centerline Industrial Drive
St. Louis, MO 63146
Address inquiries to:
Professional Services Dept.
(314) 567-5462
For Medical Emergencies Contact:
(314) 567-5462
Products Available
Duracid
Gerimed Tablets
Irospan Capsules
Irospan Tablets
Metric 21 Tablets
Nestabs Tablets
Nestabs FA Tablets
Nestrex Tablets

FISONS CORPORATION 926
Pharmaceutical Division
Two Preston Court
Bedford, MA 01730
Address inquiries to:
Professional Services Dept.
(617) 275-1000
Distribution Centers
ATLANTA
James M. Hogan Co., Inc.
5356 Ponce de Leon Ave.
Stone Mountain, GA 30083
(404) 938-7901
BEDFORD
Fisons Corporation
2 Preston Court
Bedford, MA 01730
(617) 275-1000
LOS ANGELES
Obergfel Brothers
2660 East 37th Street
Vernon, CA 90058
(213) 583-8981
Products Available
Bacid Capsules
Ergomar Sublingual Tablets
Intal Capsules
Intal Inhaler
Intal Nebulizer Solution
Isoclor Expectorant
Isoclor Liquid
Isoclor Tablets
Isoclor Timesule Capsules
Kondremul
Kondremul with Cascara
Kondremul with Phenolphthalein
Nasalcrom Nasal Solution
Neo-Cultol
Opticrom 4%
Pediapred Oral Liquid
Persistin
Proferdex
Somophyllin Oral Liquid
Somophyllin Rectal Solution
Somophyllin-CRT Capsules
Somophyllin-DF Oral Liquid
Somophyllin-T Capsules
Vapo-Iso Solution
Vaponefrin Solution
Vitron-C
Vitron-C-Plus

C. B. FLEET CO., INC. 931, 2223
4615 Murray Pl.
Lynchburg, VA 24502-2235
Address inquiries to:
Fred T. Wickis, Jr. (804) 528-4000
Products Available
Fleet Babylax
Fleet Bisacodyl Enema
Fleet Detecatest
Fleet Enema
Fleet Enema Pediatric
Fleet Flavored Castor Oil Emulsion
Fleet Mineral Oil Enema
Fleet Phospho-Soda
Fleet Prep Kits
Fleet Relief
Summer's Eve Medicated Douche

FLEMING & COMPANY 933
1600 Fenpark Dr.
Fenton, MO 63026
Address inquiries to:
John J. Roth, M.D. (314) 343-8200
Products Available
Aerolate Liquid
Aerolate III T.D. Capsules
Aerolate Jr. T.D. Capsules
Aerolate Sr. T.D. Capsules
Alumadrine Tablets
Congess Jr. T.D. Capsules
Congess Sr. T.D. Capsules
▣ Deter T.D. Tablets
Ectasule Minus III T.D. Capsules
Ectasule Minus Jr. T.D. Capsules
Ectasule Minus Sr. T.D. Capsules
Ectasule III T.D. Capsules
Ectasule Jr. T.D. Capsules
Ectasule Sr. T.D. Capsules
Extendryl Chewable Tablets
Extendryl Sr. & Jr. T.D. Capsules
Extendryl Syrup
Impregon Concentrate
Magonate Tablets
▣ Marblen Suspension Peach/Apricot
▣ Marblen Suspension Unflavored
▣ Marblen Tablets
Nephrocaps
▣ Nephrox Suspension
▣ Nicotinex Elixir
▣ Ocean Mist
Ocean A/S Mist
Ocean-A/S Nasal Spray
Ocean-Plus Mist
Pima Syrup
▣ Purge Liquid
Rum-K Syrup
S-P-T "Liquid" Capsules

FLINT 409, 934
Division of Travenol Laboratories, Inc.
One Baxter Parkway
Deerfield, IL 60015
(312) 940-5209
Address inquiries to:
Product Management
Products Available
◆ Choloxin
◆ Flint SSD Cream
◆ Synthroid Injection
◆ Synthroid Tablets
◆ Travase Ointment

FLUORITAB CORPORATION 937
P.O. Box 381
Flint, MI 48501-0381
Address inquiries to:
J. A. Vogt, Manager
(1-313) 239-9770
Products Available
Fluoritab Liquid
Fluoritab Tablets

FOREST PHARMACEUTICALS, INC. 409, 937
Subsidiary of FOREST LABORATORIES, INC.
2510 Metro Blvd.
St. Louis, MO 63043
Address inquiries to:
Professional Services Department
(314) 569-3610
Products Available
◆ AeroBid Inhaler System
Almora Tablets
Ambenyl Cough Syrup
Ambenyl-D Decongestant Cough Formula
Amonidrin Tablets
Anaids Tablets
Andro L.A. "200" Injectable
Andro "100" Injectable
Androgyn L.A. Injectable
Anergan "25" & "50" Injectable
Anodynos-DHC Tablets 100's
Antilirium Injectable
Arbon Plus Tablets
Arbon Tablets
B-12 Plus Injectable
▣ Banalg Hospital Strength Arthritic Pain Reliever
▣ Banalg Liniment
Bancap Capsules
◆ Bancap HC Capsules
Banesin Tablets
Banflex Injectable
Beesix Injectable
Belfer Tablets
Betaprone Liquid
Biamine Injectable
Calscorbate Tablets
Caquin Cream
Cebocap Capsules
Cetane Injection (w/o preservative)
Cetane Timed Capsules
Choron "10" Injectable Pak
Codroxomin Injectable
Conex DA Tablet
Conex Liquid
Conex Lozenges
Conex Plus Tablets
Conex c Codeine Liquid
Cyomin Injectable
Dalalone Injectable
Dalalone D.P. Injectable
Dalalone L.A. Injectable
Dalcaine Injection
Dehist Capsules
Dehist Injectable
depAndro "100" & "200" Injectable
depAndrogyn Injectable
depGynogen Injectable
depMedalone "40" Injectable
depMedalone "80" Injectable
Diabismul Suspension
Diabismul Tablets
Disotate Injectable
Dommanate Injectable
Duradyne DHC Tablets
Duradyne Tablets
Duraphyl Controlled Release Tablets
Eferol Ointment
Eferol Succinate Capsules
Elixophyllin Dye-Free Capsules
Elixophyllin Elixir
Elixophyllin SR Capsules
Elixophyllin-GG Oral Solution
Elixophyllin-KI Elixir
◆ Esgic Tablets & Capsules
Feostat Drops
Feostat Injectable
Feostat Suspension
Feostat Tablets
G.B.S. Tablets
Gesterol "50" Injectable
Gesterol L.A. "250" Injectable
Glycate Tablets
Gynogen Injectable
Gynogen L.A. "10", "20" & "40" Injectable
Hista-Derfule Capsules
Iodo-Niacin Tablets
KBP/O Capsules
Kay Ciel Oral Solution 10%
Kay Ciel Powder
Lidocaine 1% & 2% Injectable
Livroben Injectable
Magnesium Sulfate Injectable
Metra Tablets
N.B.P. Ointment
Nandrobolic Injectable
Nandrobolic L.A. Injectable
Neoquess Injectable
Neoquess Tablets
Niac Capsules
Obermine Capsules
Oxymycin Injectable
Paral Liquid
Pedameth Capsules
Pedameth Liquid
Predalone 50 Injectable
Predalone T.B.A. Injectable
Proklar Tablets
Pyocidin-Otic Solution
Queltuss Tablets
Quiess Injectable
Rauverid Tablets
Rogenic Injectable
Rogenic Tablets
Solu-Eze Solvent
Soniphen Tablets
◆ Sus-Phrine Injection
Tetracycline HCl Capsules
Triamolone "40" Injectable
Triamonide "40" Injectable
Urithol Tablets
Verazinc Capsules
Wolfina "100" Tablets

E. FOUGERA & COMPANY 949
a Division of Altana Inc.
60 Baylis Road
Melville, NY 11747
Address inquiries to:
Customer Service (800) 645-9833
For Medical Emergencies Contact:
E. Fougera (800) 645-9833
Products Available
Analgesic Balm
Analgesic Balm (Greaseless)
Atropine Sulfate Ophthalmic Ointment 1%
Bacitracin-Neomycin-Polymyxin Ointment
Bacitracin-Neomycin-Polymyxin Ophthalmic Ointment
Bacitracin Ointment U.S.P.
Bacitracin Ophthalmic Ointment U.S.P.
Bacitracin Zinc-Polymyxin B Sulfate Ointment
Betamethasone Dipropionate Cream, Ointment & Lotion, U.S.P., 0.05%
Betamethasone Valerate Cream, Lotion & Ointment 0.1%
Boric Acid Ophthalmic Ointment 5%
Cold Cream U.S.P.
Dibucaine Ointment, U.S.P. 1%
Efodine Ointment
Erythromycin Ophthalmic Ointment U.S.P.
Fluocinolone Acetonide Cream & Topical Solution, U.S.P. 0.01%
Fluocinolone Acetonide Cream & Ointment, U.S.P. 0.025%
Geliperm Wound Management System
Geliperm Granulate
Geliperm Wet
Gentamicin Sulfate Cream & Ointment, U.S.P. 0.1%
Hydrocortisone Cream & Ointment, U.S.P. 0.5% & 1%
Hydrocortisone Cream, U.S.P. 2.5%
Hydrophylic Ointment
Ichthammol Ointment 10% & 20%
Iodochlorhydroxyquin 3% with Hydrocortisone Creams
Lanolin U.S.P.
Lidocaine Ointment, U.S.P. 5%
Nitroglycerin Ointment 2%
Nystatin Cream, Ointment, Vaginal Tablets & Oral Suspension U.S.P.
Nystatin-Trimacinolone Acetonide Cream & Ointment
Petrolatum (White) & Petrolatum (White) Ophthalmic Ointment
Polysorb Hydrate Cream
Sulfacetamide Sodium Ophthalmic Ointment
Surgilube Surgical Lubricant
Swim Ear
Tolnaftate Cream & Solution 1% (Antifungal)
Triamcinolone Acetonide Cream, U.S.P. 0.5%
Triamcinolone Acetonide Cream & Ointment, U.S.P. 0.025% & 0.1%
Triple Sulfa Vaginal Cream
Vitamin A + Vitamin D Ointment
Whitfield's Ointment
Yellow Mercuric Oxide Ophthalmic Ointment 1% & 2%
Zinc Oxide Ointment U.S.P.

GEIGY PHARMACEUTICALS 409, 950
Division of CIBA-GEIGY Corporation
Ardsley, NY 10502
Address inquiries to:
Medical Services Dept.
(201) 277-5000
Products Available
Brethaire Inhaler
Brethancer Inhaler
Brethine Ampuls
◆ Brethine Tablets
◆ Butazolidin Capsules & Tablets
◆ Constant-T Tablets
◆ Lioresal Tablets
Lopressor Ampuls
Lopressor Prefilled Syringes
◆ Lopressor Tablets
◆ Lopressor HCT Tablets
Otrivin Nasal Solution
Otrivin Nasal Spray
Otrivin Pediatric Solution
PBZ Elixir
◆ PBZ Tablets
◆ PBZ-SR Tablets
◆ Tegretol Chewable Tablets
◆ Tegretol Tablets
Tofranil Ampuls
◆ Tofranil Tablets
◆ Tofranil-PM Capsules

GENDERM CORPORATION 968
425 Huehl Road
Northbrook, IL 60062
Address inquiries to:
Professional Services Department
(312) 564-5435
Products Available
A-Fil
Maxafil
Meted Shampoo
Meted 2 Shampoo
Occlusal
Packer's Pine Tar Shampoo
Packer's Pine Tar Soap
Pentrax Tar Shampoo with Fractar
PrameGel
SalAc
Texacort
Zostrix

GENENTECH, INC. 970
460 Point San Bruno Blvd.
South San Francisco, CA 94080
Address inquiries to:
Mr. Richard B. Brewer
(415) 952-1000
Products Available
Protropin

GERIATRIC PHARMACEUTICAL CORP. 971
1249 North Franklin Place
Milwaukee, WI 53202
(414) 272-2552
Products Available.
B-C-Bid Capsules (sustained release)
Bilezyme Tablets
Cal-Bid
Cal-Plus
Cevi-Bid Capsules (sustained release)
Cevi-Fer Capsules (sustained release)
Gaysal-S Tablets
Geritonic Liquid
Gen-O-Foam Aerosol
Gustalac Tablets
Gustase Tablets
Gustase Plus Tablets
Iso-Bid Capsules (sustained release)

GILBERT LABORATORIES 972
(Affiliate of FOREST PHARMACEUTICALS, INC.)
2510 Metro Blvd.
St. Louis, MO 63043
Address inquiries to:
Professional Service Dept.
(314) 569-3610
Products Available
Esgic-See listing under Forest Pharmaceuticals, Inc.

GLAXO INC. 410, 972
Five Moore Drive
Research Triangle Park
North Carolina 27709
(919) 248-2100
Address inquiries to:
Medical Services Department
For Medical Emergencies Contact:
(800) 334-0089
In NC (800) 334-0089
Products Available
Amesec Capsules
Atrocholin Tablets
BCG Vaccine
◆ Beclovent Oral Inhaler

◆ Beclovent Oral Inhaler Refill
◆ Beconase Nasal Inhaler
◆ Corticaine Cream
Ethatab Tablets
◆ Fortaz
Seffin, Neutral
◆ Temovate Cream & Ointment
◆ Theobid Duracap Capsules
◆ Theobid Jr. Duracap Capsules
◆ Trandate Injection
◆ Trandate Tablets
◆ Trinsicon/Trinsicon M Capsules
◆ Ventolin Inhaler
◆ Ventolin Inhaler Refill
◆ Ventolin Syrup
◆ Ventolin Tablets
◆ Vicon Forte Capsules
◆ Vicon-C Capsules
◆ Vicon Plus Capsules
◆ Vi-Zac Capsules
◆ Zantac Injection
◆ Zantac 150 & 300 Tablets
◆ Zinacef

GLENBROOK LABORATORIES 410, 996
Division of Sterling Drug Inc.
90 Park Avenue
New York, NY 10016
Address inquiries to:
Medical Director (212) 907-2764
Products Available
◆ Genuine Bayer Aspirin
◆ Bayer Children's Chewable Aspirin
◆ Children's Panadol Chewable Tablets, Liquid, Infants Drops
Diaparene Line
◆ 8 Hour Bayer Timed-Release Aspirin
◆ Maximum Bayer Aspirin
◆ Maximum Strength Midol for Cramps
◆ Maximum Strength Midol PMS
◆ Maximum Strength Panadol Capsules, Tablets & Caplets
◆ Midol-Original Formula
◆ Panadol Jr.
◆ Phillips' Laxcaps
◆ Phillips' Milk of Magnesia Liquid
◆ Phillips' Milk of Magnesia Tablets
Vanquish

GLENWOOD, INC. 410, 998
83 North Summit Street
Tenafly, NJ 07670
Address inquiries to:
Professional Services Dept. 1A
(201) 569-0050
Products Available
Calphosan
Myotonachol
◆ Potaba
Primer Unna Boot
Renoquid
◆ Yodoxin

GRAY PHARMACEUTICAL CO. 999
Affiliate, The Purdue Frederick Company
100 Connecticut Avenue
Norwalk, CT 06856
Address inquiries to:
Medical Department
(203) 853-0123
Products Available
X-Prep Bowel Evacuant Kit #1
X-Prep Bowel Evacuant Kit #2
X-Prep Liquid

GUARDIAN CHEMICAL 1000
A Division of United-Guardian, Inc.
230 Marcus Boulevard
P.O. Box 2500
Smithtown, NY 11787
(516) 273-0900
(800) 645-5566
Address inquiries to:
Director of Medical Research
Products Available
Clorpactin WCS-90
Clorpactin XCB
Lubrajel
Lubraseptic Jelly
pHos-pHaid Tablets
Renacidin
Warexin

W. E. HAUCK, INC. 1000
P.O. Box 1065
Roswell, GA 30075
Address inquiries to:
Warren E. Hauck (404) 475-4758
Products Available
Anuject Injection
Beta-C-Plex Injection
Besta Capsules
Butatran Tablets 30mg.
Cantri Vaginal Cream
Chlorafed H.S. Timecelles
Chlorafed Liquid
Chlorafed Timecelles
Diaqua Tablets
Dolacet Capsules
Entuss Expectorant
Entuss Tablets
Entuss-D Liquid & Tablets
G-1 Capsules
G-2 Capsules
G-3 Capsules
Geravite Elixir
Histor-D Syrup
Histor-D Timecelles
Isotrate Timecelles
Otic-HC Ear Drops
Otic-Plain Ear Drops
Palmiron Tablets
Palmiron-C Tablets
Sinufed Timecelles
Vitormains
Wehless Capsules 35mg.
Wehless-105 Timecelles

HELENA LABORATORIES 2223
1530 Lindbergh Drive
P.O. Box 752
Beaumont, TX 77704
Address inquiries to:
(800) 231-5663
In TX (800) 392-3126
Products Available
ColoScreen Fecal Occult Blood Test
ColoScreen Self-Test (CS-T) Fecal Occult Blood Test
ColoScreen/VPI Fecal Occult Blood Test

HERBERT LABORATORIES 1001
Dermatology Division of Allergan Pharmaceuticals, Inc.
2525 Dupont Drive
Irvine, CA 92715 (714) 752-4500
Products Available
Aeroseb-Dex Topical Aerosol Spray
Aeroseb-HC Topical Aerosol Spray
▣ Aquacare Dry Skin Cream, 2% Urea
▣ Aquacare Dry Skin Lotion
▣ Aquacare/HP Dry Skin Cream & Lotion, 10% Urea
▣ Aquatar Therapeutic Tar Gel
▣ Bluboro Powder Astringent Soaking Solution
▣ Clear By Design Acne Skin Medication
▣ Danex Protein Enriched Dandruff Shampoo
Erymax Topical Solution
Exsel Lotion
Fluonid Cream, Ointment & Topical Solution
Fluoroplex Topical Solution & Cream
Gris-PEG Tablets, 125 mg & 250 mg
Maxiflor Cream
Maxiflor Ointment
Penecort Cream (1% and 2.50%) & Ointment (2.5%)
Penecort Topical Solution 1%
Temaril Tablets, Syrup and Spansule Sustained Release Capsules
▣ Vanseb Cream Dandruff Shampoo
▣ Vanseb Lotion Dandruff Shampoo
▣ Vanseb-T Cream Tar Shampoo
▣ Vanseb-T Lotion Tar Shampoo

DOW B. HICKAM, INC. 1008
P.O. Box 2006
Sugar Land, TX 77487-2006
Address inquiries to:
Professional Service Dept.
(713) 240-1000
Products Available
Granulex
Proderm Topical Dressing

HIGH CHEMICAL COMPANY 1008
Div. Day & Frick, Inc.
1760 N. Howard St.
Philadelphia, PA 19122
Address inquiries to:
Professional Service Dept.
(215) 634-2224
Products Available
Amo-Derm
Klorlyptus
Mus-L-Tone
Sarapin

HOECHST-ROUSSEL PHARMACEUTICALS INC. 411, 1008, 2224
Route 202-206 North
Somerville, NJ 08876
Address medical inquiries to:
Scientific Services Dept.
(8:30AM-5:00PM EST)
(201) 231-2611
For medical emergency information only, after hours and on weekends, call:
(201) 231-2000
Products Available
◆ A/T/S
Claforan
◆ DiaBeta
◆ Doxidan
Doxinate
Doxinate Solution
Duadacin
◆ Festal II
◆ Festalan
◆ Lasix Oral Solution
◆ Lasix Tablets and Injection
◆ Loprox
Relefact TRH
Streptase
◆ Surfak
◆ Topicort Cream
◆ Topicort Gel
◆ Topicort LP
◆ Topicort Ointment
◆ Trental

HOFFMANN-LA ROCHE INC.
See ROCHE LABORATORIES & ROCHE PRODUCTS INC.

HOLLISTER-STIER 1018
Division of Miles Laboratories, Inc.
400 Morgan Lane
West Haven, CT 06516
Products Available
Ana-Kit Insect Sting Treatment Kit

HOYT LABORATORIES 1020
See COLGATE-HOYT LABORATORIES

HUFFMAN LABORATORIES 1020
7360 N.W. 35th Terrace
Miami, FL 33122
Address inquiries to:
Jorge de Cespedes (305) 591-8037
Products Available
Gerobion Geriatric Elixir

HYLAND THERAPEUTICS DIVISION 1020
Travenol Laboratories, Inc.
444 W. Glenoaks Blvd.
Glendale, CA 91202
Address inquiries to:
Product Management
(toll free) (800) 423-2862
For Medical Emergencies Contact:
Medical Director,
Hyland Therapeutics Div.
(818) 956-3200
Branch Offices
Los Angeles, CA
4501 Colorado (800) 423-2862
(818) 240-5600
Coagulation Products Distributed By:
Hyland Therapeutics Division
Travenol Laboratories, Inc.
Glendale, CA 91202
(800) 423-2862
Plasma Extenders & Gamma Globulin Products Distributed By:
Hyland Therapeutic Division
Travenol Laboratories, Inc.
Glendale, CA 91202
(818) 507-5472
Products Available
Autoplex, Anti-Inhibitor Coagulant Complex, Dried
Buminate 5%, Albumin (Human), USP, 5% Solution
Buminate 25%, Albumin (Human), USP, 25% Solution
Hemofil T, Antihemophilic Factor (Human), Method Four, Dried, Heat Treated
Immune Globulin, Intravenous (Human) Gammagard
Proplex SX-T, Factor IX Complex, Heat Treated
Proplex T, Factor IX Complex, Heat Treated
Protenate 5%, Plasma Protein Fraction (Human), USP, 5% Solution

HYNSON, WESTCOTT & DUNNING PRODUCTS 1022
BBL Microbiology Systems
Division of Becton Dickinson and Company
P.O. Box 243
Cockeysville, MD 21030
(800) 638-8663
Products Available
BAL in Oil Ampules
Cardio-Green Vials
Indigo Carmine Ampules
▣ Lactinex Tablets & Granules

ICN PHARMACEUTICALS, INC. 411, 1022
ICN Plaza
3300 Hyland Avenue
Costa Mesa, CA 92626
Address inquiries to:
Professional Service Dept.
(800) 556-1937
In CA (800) 331-2331
(714) 545-0100
Products Available
KATO Potassium Supplement
◆ Testred Capsules
◆ Testred Cypionate 200 Injection
Virazole

IVES LABORATORIES INC. 1026
See WYETH LABORATORIES

JACOBUS PHARMACEUTICAL CO., INC. 1026
37 Cleveland Lane
P.O. Box 5290
Princeton, NJ 08540
Address inquiries to:
Professional Services
(609) 921-7447
For Medical Emergencies Contact:
Medical Department
(609) 921-7447
Products Available
Dapsone USP

JAMOL LABORATORIES INC. 1027
13 Ackerman Avenue
Emerson, NJ 07630
Address inquiries to:
(201) 262-6363
Products Available
Bahim Foot-Aide
Bahim Oil
Otide
Ponaris Nasal Mucosal Emollient
Prep-Aide
Roma-Nol Antiseptic

JANSSEN PHARMACEUTICA INC. 411, 1028
40 Kingsbridge Road
Piscataway, NJ 08854
(201) 524-9881
Products Available
◆ Imodium Capsules/Liquid
Inapsine Injection
Innovar Injection
Monistat I.V.
Nizoral 2% Cream
◆ Nizoral Tablets
Sublimaze Injection
Sufenta Injection
◆ Vermox Chewable Tablets

JOHNSON & JOHNSON PRODUCTS INC. 1037
A Johnson & Johnson Company
Patient Care Division
501 George Street
New Brunswick, NJ 08903
(201) 524-0400
Products Available
Debrisan Wound Cleaning Beads
Debrisan Wound Cleaning Paste
Instat Collagen Absorbable Hemostat
Surgicel Absorbable Hemostat
Surgicel Nu-Knit Absorbable Hemostat

KABIVITRUM, INC. 1040
1131 Harbor Bay Parkway
Alameda, CA 94501
Address inquires to:
Ronald G. Leonardi, Ph.D.
1 (800) 227-1518
For Medical Emergencies Contact
John E. Canham, M.D.
1 (800) 227-1512
Products Available
Kabikinase
Rhesonativ

KENWOOD LABORATORIES 1040
A division of BRADLEY PHARMACEUTICALS, INC.
383 Route 46 West
Fairfield, NJ 07006-2402
Address inquiries to:
(201) 882-1505
Products Available
Apatate Liquid
Bonacal Plus Tablets
Glutofac Tablets
I.L.X. B_{12} Elixir
I.L.X. B_{12} Tablets Crystalline
I.L.X. Elixir
Kenwood Therapeutic Liquid
Posterisan Ointment
Posterisan Suppositories

KEY PHARMACEUTICALS 411, 1040
Galloping Hill Road
Kenilworth, NJ 07033
(201) 558-4000
Address inquiries to:
Professional Services Department
9:00 AM to 5:00 PM EST:
(800) 526-4099
After regular hours and on weekends:
(201) 558-4000
Products Available
Genapax Tampons
Guanidine HCl Tablets
Inhal-Aid
InspirEase
Ipsatol Expectorant Syrup
Ircon Tablets
Ircon-FA Tablets
◆ K-Dur Microburst Release System (potassium chloride) S.R. Tablets
◆ Nitro-Dur (nitroglycerin) Transdermal Infusion System
◆ Nitro-Dur II (nitroglycerin) Transdermal Infusion System
Nitroglyn Capsules
Quinora (quinidine sulfate tablets, USP)
◆ Theo-Dur Sprinkle
◆ Theo-Dur Tablets
Tyzine Nasal Solution
Tyzine Pediatric Nasal Drops

KNOLL PHARMACEUTICALS 411, 1051
A Unit of BASF K&F Corporation
30 North Jefferson Road
Whippany, NJ 07981
Main Switchboard (201) 887-8300
Customer Service (800) 526-0710
Medical Information
(800) 526-0221
NJ (201) 428-8250
Products Available
Akineton Injection
◆ Akineton Tablets
Codeine Sulfate Tablets
Dilaudid Cough Syrup
Dilaudid Injection
◆ Dilaudid-HP Injection
Dilaudid Multiple Dose Vials (Sterile Solution)
Dilaudid Powder
Dilaudid Rectal Suppositories
◆ Dilaudid Tablets
◆ Isoptin Ampules

(◆ Shown in Product Identification Section)

(▣ Described in PDR For Nonprescription Drugs)

◆ Isoptin for Intravenous Injection
◆ Isoptin Oral Tablets
◆ Quadrinal Tablets
Santyl Ointment
◆ Vicodin Tablets

KRAMER PHARMACAL, INC. 1062
8778 S.W. 8th Street
Miami, FL 33174
Address inquiries to:
8778 S.W. 8th Street
Miami, FL 33174 1 (800) 824-4894
For Medical Emergencies Contact:
Professional Director
1 (800) 824-4894
Products Available
Banquin Cream
Cortixin Otic Suspension
Epatrol Capsules
Fungi-Nail Tincture
Lysiplex Syrup
Nasylin Drops
Otipyrin Ear Drops
Simetyl Elixir
Uroseptic D-S Tablets
Vasoflex Tablets
Versisol Lotion
Yohimex Tablets
Yohimex P-Z (Dual Pack) Tablets
Zinckel-220 Tablets

KREMERS URBAN COMPANY 412, 1062
P.O. Box 2038
5600 W. County Line Rd.
Milwaukee, WI 53201
Address inquiries to:
Professional Services Department
(414) 354-4300
(800) 558-5114
For Medical Emergencies Contact:
Professional Services Department
(414) 354-4300
(800) 558-5114
Products Available
◆ Calciferol Drops (Ergocalciferol Oral Solution USP)
◆ Calciferol in Oil Injection (Ergocalciferol USP)
◆ Calciferol Tablets (Ergocalciferol USP)
Chardonna-2 Tablets
Fedahist Expectorant
◆ Fedahist Gyrocaps
Fedahist Syrup
◆ Fedahist Tablets
▣ Gemnisyn Tablets
▣ Kudrox Suspension (Double Strength)
Kutapressin Injection
◆ Kutrase Capsules
◆ Ku-Zyme Capsules
◆ Ku-Zyme HP Capsules
◆ Lactrase Capsules
◆ Levsin Drops
◆ Levsin Elixir
◆ Levsin Injection
◆ Levsin Tablets
Levsin PB Drops
Levsin Phenobarbital Elixir
Levsin Phenobarbital Tablets
◆ Levsinex Timecaps
Levsinex Phenobarbital Timecaps
▣ Milkinol
Pre-Pen
Salimeph Forte

LACTAID INC. 412, 1067
P.O. Box 111
Pleasantville, NJ 08232-0111
Address inquiries to:
Alan E. Kligerman (609) 645-7500
Products Available
◆ Lactaid brand lactase enzyme tablets
◆ Lactaid brand lactase liquid enzyme

LAFAYETTE PHARMACAL, INC. 1067
4200 South Hulen Street
Fort Worth, TX 76109
Address inquiries to:
Lafayette Pharmacal, Inc.
4200 South Hulen Street
Fort Worth, TX 76109
(817) 763-8011
Products Available
▣ Konsyl
▣ Konsyl-D (formerly L. A. Formula)

LAKESIDE PHARMACEUTICALS 412, 1067
Division of Merrell Dow Pharmaceuticals Inc.
2110 E. Galbraith Road
Cincinnati, OH 45215
Address inquiries to:
Professional Information Department
Business hours only (8:15 AM to 5:00 PM EST)
(513) 948-6040
For Medical Emergency Information
After hours or on weekends only,
(513) 948-9111
Products Available
◆ Bentyl 10 mg Capsules
Bentyl Injection
Bentyl Syrup
◆ Bentyl 20 mg Tablets
◆ Bricanyl Injection
◆ Bricanyl Tablets
▣ Cēpacol Anesthetic Lozenges (Troches)
▣ Cēpacol Mouthwash/Gargle
▣ Cēpacol Throat Lozenges
▣ CĒPASTAT Sore Throat Lozenges
▣ CĒPASTAT Sore Throat Lozenges, Cherry Flavor
▣ Delcid
▣ Kolantyl Gel
▣ Kolantyl Wafers
◆ Nicorette
▣ Novahistine Cough & Cold Formula
◆ Novahistine DH
▣ Novahistine DMX
▣ Novahistine Elixir
◆ Novahistine Expectorant
▣ Singlet
◆ Tenuate Dospan Tablets
◆ Tenuate Tablets

LAMBDA PHARMACAL CORPORATION
See A. J. BART, INC.

THE LANNETT COMPANY, INC. 1074
9000 State Road
Philadelphia, PA 19136
Address inquiries to:
Medical Service Dept.
(215) 333-9000
Products Available
Acetazolamide Tablets
▣ Acnederm Lotion & Soap
Adalan Lanatabs
Alphamul Suspension
Amtren Tablets
Arithmin Tablets
Baroflave Powder
Bellafedrol AH Tablets
Bethanechol Chloride Tablets
Bisacodyl Suppositories & Tablets
Brompheniramine Maleate Tablets
Castaderm
Chlorpromazine Tablets
Chlorulan Tablets
Codalan Tablets
Dicalsonate Capsules
Diphenoxylate & Atropine Tablets
Disanthrol Capsules
Disolan Capsules
Disonate Capsules, Liquid & Syrup
Efricon Expectorant
Glutethimide Tablets
Hydrochlorulan Tablets
Isoniazid Tablets & Syrup
Kaylixir
Lanacillin "400"
Lanahex Liquid
Lanamin Capsules
Lanatuss Expectorant
Laniazid Tablets & Syrup
Lanorinal Capsules & Tablets
Lanvisone Cream
Lofene Tablets
Lycolan Elixir
▣ Magnatril Suspension & Tablets
Neocastaderm
Nitrofurantoin Tablets
Obalan Tablets
Orcophen Capsules
Paverolan Lanacaps
Potasalan Elixir
Primidone Tablets
Probenecid Tablets
Promethazine Syrup
Promethazine Tablets
Pyrralan Expectorant DM
Quinalan Sustained Release Tablets
Rufolex Capsules
S-A-C Tablets
Salatar Cream
Sedragesic Tablets
Trichlorex Tablets
Trichlormethiazide Tablets
Veltane Tablets & Expectorant

LASALLE LABORATORIES, INC. 1074
Subsidiary of Mallard, Inc.
3021 Wabash Avenue
Detroit, MI 48216
Address inquiries to:
Mallard, Inc. (313) 964-3910
Products Available
Fetrin
Pacaps
Protid Tablets, Improved Formula

LASER, INC. 1075
2000 N. Main Street,
P.O. Box 905
Crown Point, IN 46307
Address inquiries to:
Donald A. Laser (219) 663-1165
Products Available
Dallergy Capsules, Tablets, Syrup
Dallergy-D Capsules
Dallergy-D Syrup
Dallergy-JR Capsules
Donatussin DC Syrup
Donatussin Drops
Fumatinic Capsules
Fumerin Tablets
Lactocal-F Tablets
Respaire-SR Capsules 60, 120
Theospan-SR Capsules 130 mg., 260 mg.
Theostat 80 Syrup
Trimstat Tablets

LEDERLE LABORATORIES 412, 1075, 2225
Division of American Cyanamid Co.
One Cyanamid Plaza
Wayne, NJ 07470
LEDERLE PARENTERALS, INC.
Carolina, Puerto Rico 00630
LEDERLE PIPERACILLIN, INC.
Carolina, Puerto Rico 00630
Address medical/pharmacy inquiries on marketed products only to:
Professional Services Department
Lederle Laboratories
Pearl River, NY 10965
During business hours (8 AM to 4:30 PM E.S.T.)
(914) 735-2815
After hours emergencies
(914) 735-5000
Distribution Centers
ATLANTA
Bulk Address
Chamblee (Atlanta), GA 30341
5180 Peachtree Industrial Blvd.
Mail Address
Atlanta, GA 30302
P.O. Box 4272
GA Only (800) 282-0399
(All Other) (800) 533-3753
(404) 455-0320
CHICAGO
Bulk Address
Mt. Prospect, IL 60056
1100 E. Business Center Drive
Mail Address
Mt. Prospect, IL 60056-7614
P.O. Box 7614 (312) 827-8871
IL Only (800) 942-1493
(All Other) (800) 533-3753
DALLAS
Bulk Address
Dallas, TX 75247
7611 Carpenter Freeway
Mail Address
Dallas, TX 75265
P.O. Box 225731 (214) 631-2130
(All Other) (800) 533-3753
LOS ANGELES
Bulk Address
Los Angeles, CA 90040
2300 S. Eastern Ave.
Mail Address
Los Angeles, CA 90051
T.A. Box 2202 (213) 726-1016
CA Only (800) 372-6325
(All Other) (800) 533-3753
PHILADELPHIA
Fort Washington, PA 19034
185 Commerce Drive
(Phila. Only) (215) 646-7000
(All Other) (800) 533-3753
(NY-NJ-MD-DE) (800) 533-3753
(CT-VA-WV-DC) (800) 533-3753
Products Available
◆ Acetaminophen Capsules, Tablets, Liquid
Acetaminophen w/Codeine Tablets
Achromycin Intramuscular
Achromycin Intravenous
Achromycin Ophthalmic Ointment 1%
◆ Achromycin Ophthalmic Suspension 1%
Achromycin 3% Ointment
◆ Achromycin V Capsules
Achromycin V Oral Suspension
◆ Allopurinol Tablets
◆ Amicar Intravenous, Syrup & Tablets
◆ Amitriptyline HCl Tablets
◆ Amoxicillin Capsules, Suspension
◆ Ampicillin Trihydrate Capsules, Oral Suspension
◆ Aristocort A Topical Cream
◆ Aristocort A Topical Ointment
Aristocort Forte Parenteral
Aristocort Intralesional
Aristocort Syrup
◆ Aristocort Tablets
◆ Aristocort Topical Cream
◆ Aristocort Topical Ointment
Aristospan Suspension (Intraarticular)
Aristospan Suspension (Intralesional)
◆ Artane Elixir
◆ Artane Sequels
◆ Artane Tablets
Ascorbic Acid Tablets
◆ Asendin
Aureomycin Ointment 3%
Aureomycin Ointment (Ophthalmic) 1%
Benztropine Mesylate Tablets
Brompheniramine Maleate with Codeine, Phenylephrine & Phenylpropanolamine Sequels, Elixir
▣ Caltrate 600
▣ Caltrate 600 + Iron and Vitamin D
▣ Caltrate 600+Vitamin D
▣ Centrum
▣ Centrum, Jr. (Childrens' Chewable) + Iron
▣ Centrum, Jr. (Children's Chewable) Vitamin/Mineral Formula + Extra C
Chlordiazepoxide HCl Capsules
Chlorothiazide Tablets
Chlorpheniramine Maleate Tablets & T.D. Capsules
◆ Chlorpromazine HCl Tablets, Liquid Concentrate
◆ Chlorpropamide Tablets
◆ Chlorthalidone Tablets
Chlorzoxazone with Acetaminophen Tablets
Cholera Vaccine (India Strains)
Cloxacillin Sodium Capsules
◆ Cyclocort Cream
◆ Cyclocort Ointment
◆ Declomycin Capsules and Tablets
Diamox Parenteral
◆ Diamox Sequels
◆ Diamox Tablets
◆ Diazepam Tablets
Dicloxacillin Sodium Capsules
Dicyclomine HCl Capsules, Tablets
Diphenhydramine HCl Cough Syrup
Diphenoxylate HCl 2.5 mg & Atropine Sulfate 0.025 mg
Diphtheria & Tetanus Toxoids, Adsorbed Purogenated
Diphtheria & Tetanus Toxoids & Pertussis Vaccine, Adsorbed
◆ Dipyridamole Tablets
Disopyramide Phosphate Capsules
Docusate Sodium, USP (DSS) Capsules, Syrup
Docusate Sodium, USP w/Casanthranol Capsules, Syrup
Dolene AP-65 Tablets
Dolene Capsules
Dolene Compound-65 Capsules
◆ Doxycycline Hyclate Capsules, Tablets
◆ Ergoloid Mesylates Tablets, Sublingual
Erythromycin Estolate Oral Suspension
◆ Erythromycin Ethylsuccinate Oral Suspension & Tablets
◆ Erythromycin Stearate Tablets
◆ Ferro-Sequels
Ferrous Gluconate Iron Supplement Tablets
Ferrous Sulfate Tablets, Elixir
◆ Filibon F.A. Prenatal Vitamin Tablets
◆ Filibon Forte
◆ Filibon Prenatal Vitamin Tablets
Flurazepam Capsules
Folvite Parenteral & Tablets
▣ Footwork Athlete's Foot Remedy
◆ Furosemide Tablets
▣ Gevrabon Liquid
Gevral Protein Powder
▣ Gevral T Tablets
▣ Gevral Tablets
Guaifenesin Syrup
Guaifenesin w/D-Methorphan Hydrobromide Syrup
Hib-Imune Haemophilus b Polysaccharide Vaccine
◆ Hydralazine HCl Tablets
◆ Hydrochlorothiazide Tablets
◆ Hydromox R Tablets
◆ Hydromox Tablets
◆ Hydroxyzine HCl Tablets
◆ Ibuprofen Tablets
Imipramine HCl Tablets
▣ Incremin w/Iron Syrup
◆ Indomethacin Capsules
Isosorbide Dinitrate Tablets
Isosorbide Dinitrate S.A. Tablets
Isosorbide Dinitrate, Sublingual, Oral
Isoxsuprine HCl Tablets
◆ Ledercillin VK Oral Solution & Tablets
▣ Lederplex Capsules, Liquid
◆ Leucovorin Calcium Injection
◆ Leucovorin Calcium Tablets
Levoprome
Levothyroxine Sodium Tablets
◆ Lorazepam Tablets
◆ Loxitane C Oral Concentrate
◆ Loxitane Capsules
◆ Loxitane IM
◆ Materna 1•60 Tablets
◆ Maxzide Tablets
◆ Meclizine HCl Tablets
Medroxyprogesterone Acetate Tablets
Methenamine Mandelate Suspension Forte
◆ Methocarbamol Tablets
◆ Methotrexate Tablets & Parenteral
Methyclothiazide Tablets
◆ Methyldopa Tablets
◆ Metoclopramide Tablets
◆ Metronidazole Tablets
◆ Minocin Capsules
Minocin Intravenous
Minocin Oral Suspension
◆ Minocin Tablets
◆ Myambutol Tablets
Neoloid Emulsified Castor Oil
Neomycin Sulfate Tablets
◆ Neptazane Tablets
Nilstat for Preparation of Oral Suspension
Nilstat Oral Suspension
◆ Nilstat Oral Tablets
◆ Nilstat Topical Cream
◆ Nilstat Topical Ointment
◆ Nilstat Vaginal Tablets
◆ Nitroglycerin S.R. Capsules
Nylidrin HCl Tablets
Orimune Poliovirus Vaccine, Live, Oral, Trivalent
◆ Papaverine HCl T.R. Capsules
Papaverine HCL Tablets
◆ Pathibamate Tablets
◆ Pathilon Tablets
Penicillin G Potassium Tablets
Penicillin V Potassium
Perihemin Capsules
Peritinic Tablets
Phenobarbital Tablets
◆ Pipracil
Pnu-Imune 23 Pneumococcal Vaccine Polyvalent
Potassium Chloride Liquid
Potassium Gluconate Elixir
Prednisone Tablets
Probenecid Tablets

(◆ **Shown in Product Identification Section**)

(▣ **Described in PDR For Nonprescription Drugs**)

Probenecid with Colchicine Tablets
Procainamide HCl Capsules
◆ Procainamide Hydrochloride S.R. Tablets
Promethazine HCl Syrup Plain
Promethazine HCl Syrup V.C. Plain
Promethazine HCl Syrup V.C. w/Codeine
Promethazine HCl Syrup w/Codeine
Pronemia Capsules
Propoxyphene HCl
◆ Propoxyphene Napsylate with Acetaminophen Tablets
◆ Propranolol Hydrochloride Tablets
Propylthiouracil Tablets
Pseudoephedrine HCl Tablets & Syrup
◆ Pyrazinamide Tablets
Pyridoxine HCl Tablets (Vitamin B_6)
◆ Quinidine Gluconate Sustained Release Tablets
◆ Quinidine Sulfate Tablets
Quinine Sulfate Capsules
Reserpine, Hydrochlorothiazide & Hydralazine Tablets
▣ Spartus High Potency Vitamins & Minerals plus Electrolytes Tablets
▣ Spartus + Iron High Potency Vitamins & Minerals plus Electrolytes Tablets
◆ Spironolactone Tablets
◆ Spironolactone with Hydrochlorothiazide Tablets
▣ Stresscaps Capsules
▣ Stresstabs 600 Tablets, Advanced Formula
▣ Stresstabs 600 with Iron, Advanced Formula
▣ Stresstabs 600 with Zinc, Advanced Formula
◆ Sulfamethoxazole & Trimethoprim Tablets and Pediatric Suspension
◆ Sulfasalazine Tablets
Tetanus Toxoid, Adsorbed
Tetanus Toxoid Purogenated
Tetanus & Diphtheria Toxoids, Combined Purogenated
Thiamine HCl (Vitamin B-1) Tablets
◆ Thioridazine HCl Tablets
◆ Thiotepa Parenteral
Thyroid Tablets
◆ Tolazamide Tablets
◆ Tolbutamide Tablets
◆ TriHemic 600 Tablets
Tri-Immunol Diphtheria & Tetanus Toxoids & Pertussis Vaccine, Adsorbed
Triprolidine HCl with Pseudoephedrine HCl Tablets, Syrup
Tuberculin, Old, Tine Test
Tuberculin Purified Protein Derivative Tine Test (PPD)
Vitamin A, Natural Capsules
Vitamin C Chewable Tablets
Vitamin E, Natural USP Capsules
Vitamin E USP Capsules
▣ Zincon Dandruff Shampoo

LEEMING DIVISION 1121
Pfizer Inc.
100 Jefferson Rd.
Parsippany, NJ 07054
Address inquiries to:
Research and Development Dept.
(201) 887-2100
Products Available
▣ Ben Gay External Analgesic Products
Bonine Tablets
▣ Coryban-D Capsules
▣ Coryban-D Cough Syrup
▣ Desitin Ointment
Li-Ban Lice Control Spray
RID Lice Treatment Kit
▣ Rheaban Tablets
▣ Terramycin Topical Ointment
Unisom Nighttime Sleep-Aid
▣ Visine A.C. Eye Drops
▣ Visine Eye Drops
Wart-Off Wart Remover

LEGERE PHARMACEUTICALS 1122
7326 E. Evans Road
Scottsdale, AZ 85260
(602) 991-4033
Address Inquiries to:
Customer Service & Product Information
Toll Free 1(800) 528-3144
Products Available
ACE + Z Tablets
Acetaco Tablets
Allerdryl 50
B-S-P LA
Cee-500 (Ascorbic Acid)
Cee-1000 T.D. Tablets
Cinalone 40
Cinonide 40
Cobolin-M
Depo-Predate 40
Depo-Predate 80
Dexasone 4
Dexasone 10
Dexasone LA
Dexol T.D. Tablets
Dexol 300
Dextraron
Di-Atro Tablets
Dieutrim Capsules
Di-Hydrotic
E-Cypionate
Estrone
Kabolin
Lidocaine 1% and 2%
Lipo B-C
Livolex
Menaval 20 & Menaval 40
Mersalyl-Theophylline
Myotrol
Natural Estrogenic Substance
Neucalm 50
O. B. Thera Tablets
PT 105 Capsules
Phenazine Tablets & Capsules
Predate 50
Predate S
Predate TBA
Prevenzyme Tablets
Probahist Capsules
Probahist Injectable
Prodrox 250
Progesterone 50
Promet 50
Rodex
Rodex T.D. Capsules
Spasgesic
Stemetic
T-Cypionate
T-E-Cypionate
T-Quil
Teramine Capsules
Testaval 90/4
Testosterone Suspension
Thera-Ron Tablets
Triazide
Vagimide Cream
Vitabese Capsules

LEMMON COMPANY ETHICAL DIVISION 415, 1123
Post Office Box 630
Sellersville, PA 18960
Address inquiries to:
Toll Free (800) 523-6542
(215) 723-5544
Products Available
Acetaminophen Tablets and Capsules
Acetaminophen and Codeine Tablets
◆ Adipex-P Tablets and Capsules
Beta-Val Cream, Lotion & Ointment 0.1%
Chlordiazepoxide Hydrochloride Capsules
Cotrim Tablets & Pediatric Suspension
◆ Cotrim D.S. Tablets
◆ Cotrim S.S. Tablets
Dexampex Tablets and Capsules
Donphen Tablets
Doxy-Lemmon Capsules & Tablets
◆ Epitol
Glucamide Tablets
Indo-Lemmon Capsules
Methampex Tablets
Metryl and Metryl 500 Tablets
Myco-Triacet II Cream and Ointment
Neothylline Tablets and Injection
Neothylline-GG Tablets
Nu'Leven Tablets
Nystatin Cream, Oral Tablets, and Vaginal Tablets
Otocort Sterile Ear Drops, Solution and Suspension
Phentermine HCl Capsules
Potage
◆ Propacet 100
Racet Cream
Racet LCD Cream
Racet-1% Cream
Rhinex D Lay Tablets
Rhus Tox Antigen Injection
S.B.P. Tablets
◆ Sofarin
Statobex G Tablets
Triacet Cream
Triphed Tablets
Urinary #2 Tablets
Vagitrol Vaginal Cream

ELI LILLY AND COMPANY 415, 1124, 2226
For Medical Information, Write
Medical Department
(317) 261-2000
Lilly Corporate Center
Indianapolis, IN 46285
Lilly Regional & District Offices
*Aurora, CO 80014
Suite 111, Cherry Creek Place I
3131 South Vaughn Way
(303) 695-7730
Birmingham, AL 35223
Suite 309, Shades Brook Bldg.
3300 Cahaba Road
(205) 879-2441
Braintree, MA 02184
Suite 104, 35 Braintree Hill Park
(617) 848-6967
(617) 848-9896
Charlotte, NC 28209
Suite 207, Park Seneca Bldg.
1515 Mockingbird Lane
(704) 525-8905
*Chicago, IL 60631
Suite 270, O'Hare Plaza
5735 East River Road
(312) 693-8740
Cincinnati, OH 45241
Suite 413, 4055 Executive Park Dr.
(513) 563-0720
Cleveland, OH 44130
Suite 395, Interstate Plaza
16600 West Sprague Rd.
(216) 243-3600
*Dallas, TX 75244-3290
4404 Beltwood Parkway, South
(214) 661-5620
Enfield, CT 06082
150 Freshwater Boulevard
(203) 741-0761
Honolulu, HI 96825
6838 Niumalu Loop
(808) 396-8444
Houston, TX 77042
Suite 360, Richmond Plaza I
9800 Richmond Ave.
(713) 975-6766
Indianapolis, IN 46268
Suite 235, Northwest Plaza
3901 West 86th Street
(317) 261-2512
Jacksonville, FL 32216
Suite 319-A, The Center Building
7825 Baymeadows Way
(904) 731-7124
Kansas City, MO 64114
Suite 610, 9200 Ward Parkway
(816) 361-6116
Louisville, KY 40223
Suite 133, Wing C
Plainview Triad North
10401 Linn Station Road
(502) 425-2372
Melville, NY 11747
Suite 3S02, One Huntington Quadrangle
(516) 752-9797
Metarie, LA 70006
Suite 508, Security Homestead Bldg.
4900 Veterans Memorial Blvd.
(504) 885-9645
Miami, FL 33156
Suite 412, Dadeland Square
7700 North Kendall Drive
(305) 596-9015
Morristown, NJ 07960
Morristown Centre
10 Madison Avenue
(201) 898-9505
Nashville, TN 37210
Suite 310, 555 Marriott Drive
(615) 889-6010
*Norcross, GA 30091
5944 Peachtree Corners, East
(404) 441-5400
Oklahoma City, OK 73112
Suite 325, Grand Centre
5400 N.W. Grand Blvd.
(405) 947-2482
*Pasadena, CA 91101
Suite 916, Mutual Savings Bldg.
301 E. Colorado Blvd.
(818) 792-5121
Pittsburgh, PA 15220
Suite 602, Manor Oak Two
1910 Cochran Rd.
(412) 922-9770
Raleigh, NC 27625
Suite 103, 3109 Poplarwood Ct.
(919) 872-4836
Redmond, WA 98052
11811 Willows Road
(206) 881-5796
Richmond, VA 23229
Suite 105, Henrico Corporate Center
7798 Carousel Lane
(804) 747-7160
St. Louis, MO 63131
Suite 325, Corporate Hill II
1633 Des Peres Road
(314) 821-0190
St. Paul, MN 55164
4100 North Hamline Ave.
(612) 638-4073
Sacramento, CA 95814
Suite 715, 555 Capitol Mall
(916) 444-2173
San Antonio, TX 78216
Suite 636 North Tower
GPM Life Bldg.
800 N.W. Loop 410
(512) 341-2211
San Diego, CA 92121-1579
(619) 458-7833
San Francisco, CA 94111
Suite 1170, 100 California St.
(415) 362-0559
Silver Spring, MD 20903
Suite 111, Executive Court
1734 Elton Road (301) 439-7991
*Southfield, MI 48075
Suite 940, 3000 Town Center
(313) 358-2208
*Stamford, CT 06905
Suite 301, 1600 Summer St.
(203) 357-1422
Tampa, FL 33609
Suite 1060, Lincoln Center
5401 W. Kennedy Blvd.
(813) 870-2036
Williamsville, NY 14221
Suite 204, 5820 Main St.
(716) 634-0178
Worthington, OH 43085
Suite 250, 300 E. Wilson Bridge Rd.
(614) 846-5090
Wynnewood, PA 19096
Suite 202, Seven Wynnewood Rd
(215) 477-8739
*Regional office also
Products Available
A.S.A. & Codeine Compound Pulvules & Tablets
A.S.A. Enseals, Pulvules, Suppositories & Tablets
Acidulin Pulvules
Aerolone Solution
Alphalin Gelseals
Amertan Jelly
Ammoniated Mercury Ointment
Ammonium Chloride Enseals
Ampicillin Sodium Faspak, USP (sterile)
Amyl Nitrite, Aspirols
Amytal Tablets
Amytal Sodium Ampoules & Vials
Amytal Sodium Pulvules
Analgesic Balm Ointment
Anhydron Tablets
Apomorphine Hydrochloride Soluble Tablets
Arnica Tincture
Aromatic Ammonia Aspirols & Spirit
Aromatic Elixir
Atropine Sulfate Vials, Sterile Ophthalmic Ointment, Tablets & Soluble Tablets
Aventyl HCl Liquid & Pulvules
Bacitracin Ointment & Sterile Ophthalmic Ointment
Belladonna Extract Tablets
Belladonna Tincture
Benzoin Tincture
Betalin Complex Elixir
Betalin Compound Pulvules
Betalin S Ampoules, Vials, Elixir & Tablets
Betalin 12 Crystalline Vials
Bilron Pulvules
Boric Acid Ointment & Sterile Ophthalmic Ointments
Brevital Sodium Vials
Calcium Carbonate Tablets, Aromatic
Calcium Gluceptate, Ampoules
Calcium Gluconate Tablets
Calcium Gluconate w/Vitamin D Pulvules & Tablets
Calcium Hydroxide Powder
Calcium Lactate Tablets
Capastat Sulfate Vials
Capsules, Empty Gelatin
Carbarsone Capsules
Cascara, Aromatic, Fluid Extract
Cascara Sagrada Fluid Extract
Cascara Tablets
Castor Oil Elastic Filled Capsules
◆ Ceclor Pulvules & Suspension
Cevalin Ampoules & Tablets
Citrated Caffeine Tablets
Cocaine Hydrochloride Solvets
Codeine Phosphate Vials & Soluble Tablets
Codeine Sulfate Tablets & Soluble Tablets
Colchicine Ampoules & Tablets
Cologel Liquid
Compound Benzoin Tincture
Copavin, Pulvules
◆ Crystodigin Tablets
Cyanide Antidote Package
◆ Darvocet-N 50 Tablets
◆ Darvocet-N 100 Tablets
◆ Darvon Pulvules
◆ Darvon Compound Pulvules
◆ Darvon Compound-65 Pulvules
◆ Darvon with A.S.A. Pulvules
◆ Darvon-N Suspension & Tablets
◆ Darvon-N with A.S.A. Tablets
Deltalin Gelseals
Dibasic Calcium Phosphate Tablets
Dibasic Calcium Phosphate w/Vitamin D Pulvules
Diethylstilbestrol Enseals, Suppositories & Tablets
Dobutrex Vials
Dolophine Hydrochloride Ampoules, Vials & Tablets
Drolban Vials
Duracillin A.S. Vials
◆ Dymelor Tablets
Emetine Hydrochloride Ampoules
En-Cebrin Pulvules
En-Cebrin F Pulvules
Ephedrine & Amytal Pulvules
Ephedrine Sulfate Ampoules, Pulvules, & Syrups
Eprolin Gelseals
Ergotrate Maleate Ampoules & Tablets
Extralin Pulvules
Ferrous Gluconate Pulvules
Ferrous Sulfate Enseals & Tablets
Folic Acid Tablets
Glucagon for Injection Vials
Green Soap Tincture
Haldrone Tablets
Heparin Sodium Vials
Hepicebrin Tablets
Hexa-Betalin Vials & Tablets
Histadyl E.C. Syrup
Histamine Phosphate (For Gastric Histamine Test) Vials & Ampoules
Histamine Phosphate (Histamine Test for Pheochromocytoma) Ampoules
Homicebrin
Humulin L, 100 Units
Humulin N, 100 Units

Humulin R, 100 Units
Hydriodic Acid Syrup
Ichthammol Ointments
Lente Iletin I, 40 & 100 units
Regular Iletin I, 40 & 100 units
Regular Iletin II (Concentrated), 500 units
Semilente Iletin I, 40 & 100 units
Ultralente Iletin I, 40 & 100 units
NPH Iletin I, 40 & 100 units
Protamine, Zinc & Iletin I, 40 & 100 units
Beef Regular Iletin II, 100 units
Beef Lente Iletin II, 100 units
Beef NPH Iletin II, 100 units
Beef Protamine Zinc & Iletin II, 100 units
Pork Regular Iletin II, 100 units
Pork Lente Iletin II, 100 units
Pork NPH Iletin II, 100 units
Pork Protamine, Zinc & Iletin II, 100 units
Ipecac Syrup
Isoniazid Tablets
Isopropyl Alcohol, 91%
Keflin, Neutral, Vials & Faspak
Kefurox ADD-Vantage
Kefzol Vials, Faspak & ADD-Vantage
Lextron Ferrous Pulvules
Lextron Pulvules
Liver Injection Vials
Magnesium Sulfate Ampoules
Mandol Vials, Faspak & ADD-Vantage
Mercuric Oxide, Yellow, Sterile Ophthalmic Ointments
Merthiolate, Aeropump, Solution & Tincture
◆ Methadone Hydrochloride Diskets
Methyltestosterone Tablets
Metubine Iodide Vials
Milk of Bismuth
Morphine Sulfate Vials & Soluble Tablets
Moxam Vials
Multicebrin Tablets
Myrrh Tincture
Nebcin Vials & Hyporets
Neomycin Sulfate Ointment
Neomycin Sulfate Tablets
Neotrizine Suspension & Tablets
Niacin Tablets
Niacinamide Tablets
Nitroglycerin Sublingual Tablets
Oncovin Solution Vials & Hyporets
Opium (Deodorized) Tincture
Ox Bile Extract Enseals
Pancreatin Enseals & Tablets
Papaverine Hydrochloride, Ampoules, Powder, Tablets & Vials
Paregoric Tincture
Penicillin G Potassium Vials (Buffered)
Penicillin G Procaine Suspension, Sterile, Vials
Phenobarbital Elixir & Tablets
Phenobarbital Sodium Vials
Potassium Chloride Ampoules & Enseals
Potassium Iodide Enseals
Powder Papers
Progesterone Vials
Propylthiouracil Tablets
Protamine Sulfate Ampoules & Vials
Prunicodeine
Pyridoxine Hydrochloride Tablets
Quinidine Gluconate Vials
Quinidine Sulfate Pulvules & Tablets
Quinine Sulfate Pulvules & Tablets
Reserpine Tablets
Reticulex Pulvules
Reticulogen Vials
Reticulogen Fortified Vials
Riboflavin Tablets
Rose, Soluble, for Making Artificial Rose Water
Scarlet Red Ointment
◆ Seconal Sodium Pulvules & Vials
Seconal Sodium Suppositories
Seromycin Pulvules
Silver Nitrate Wax Ampoules
Soda Mint Tablets
Sodium Bicarbonate Tablets
Sodium Chloride Vials, Enseals & Tablets
Sodium Iodide Ampoules
Sodium Salicylate Enseals
Streptomycin Sulfate Vials
Sulfadiazine Tablets
Sulfapyridine Tablets
Sulfur Ointment
Surfadil Cream & Lotion
Tapazole Tablets
Tazidime Vials & ADD-Vantage
Terpin Hydrate & Codeine Elixir
Terpin Hydrate Elixir
Tes-Tape
Testosterone Propionate Vials
Theracebrin Pulvules
Thiamine Hydrochloride Ampoules, Elixer, Tablets, & Vials
Thyroid Enseals & Tablets
Trikates Oral Solution
Tubocurarine Chloride Vials
◆ Tuinal Pulvules
Tycopan Pulvules
Tylosterone, Tablets
V-Cillin K for Oral Solution & Tablets
Vancocin HCl, for Oral Solution
Vancocin HCl, Vials
Velban Vials
Vitamin A, Gelseals
Vitamin B Complex, Elixir & Pulvules
Vitamin C, Tablets
Vitamin D, Gelseals
Vitamin E, Gelseals
Whitfield's Ointment (Double Strength)
Wild Cherry Syrup
Zentinic Pulvules
Zentron Chewable Tablets
Zentron Liquid
Zinc Oxide Ointments
Zinc Oxide Paste Ointment
Zinc Sulfate Compound Powder

LYPHOMED, INC. 1172
10401 W. Touhy Ave.
Rosemont, IL 60018
(312) 390-6500
(except IL) (800) 621-3334
PENTAM Hotline (312) 345-9746
Address medical or scientific inquiries to:
Director, Professional Relations
Marketing Department
Distribution Centers
CHICAGO
Melrose Park, IL 60160
2020 Ruby Street
NEW YORK
Dayton, NJ 08810
P.O. Box 422
LOS ANGELES
Los Angeles, CA 90051
P.O. Box 4029
Products Available
Aminocaproic Acid 250mg/mL
Aminophylline Injection, USP, 25mg/mL
Ascorbic Acid Injection, USP, 250mg/mL
Atropine Sulfate Injection, USP, 0.3/0.4/0.5/1.0mg per ampoule
B Complex Injection with Ascorbic Acid $+B_{12}$- 10,000 units
Bretylium Tosylate 50mg/mL
Bristoject Emergency Syringe System
Aminophylline 25mg/mL
Atropine 0.5mg, 1mg
Calcium Chloride 10%
Dexamethasone Sodium Phosphate 4mg/mL
Dextrose 50%
Diphenhydramine 50mg
Dopamine 40mg/mL
Ephedrine 1mg
Epinephrine 1mg
Lidocaine 1, 2, 4%
Magnesium Sulfate 50%
Metaraminol Bitartrate 1%
Sodium Bicarbonate 4.2, 7.5, 8.4%
Calcium Chloride Injection, USP, 10%
Calcium Gluconate Injection, USP, 10%
Cefazolin Sodium for Injection, USP, 500mg, 1gm, 10gm
Cephalothin Sodium for Injection, USP, 1gm, 2gm
Chloramphenicol Sodium Succinate for Injection, USP, 1 gm
Chorionic Gonadotropin for Injection, USP, 5,000/10,000/20,000 USP units
Chromic Chloride Injection, USP, 4mcg, 20mcg/mL
Cupric Sulfate Injection, USP, 0.4mg, 2mg/mL
Cyanocobalamin Injection, USP, 100mcg/1,000mcg
Dacarbazine 100mg/200mg per vial
Dexamethasone Sodium Phosphate Injection, USP, 4mg/mL, 10mg/mL
Dextrose Injection, USP, 10%, 50%
Dopamine HCl Injection, USP, 200, 400 & 800mg
Doxy-100 & Doxy-200 (Doxycycline Hyclate for Injection, USP)
Ephedrine Injection, USP, 50mg/mL
Erythromycin Lactobionate Injection, USP, 500mg/1,000mg per vial
Fluorouracil Injection, USP, 50mg/mL
Folic Acid Injection, USP, 5mg/mL
Furosemide Injection, USP, 10mg/mL
Gentamicin Sulfate Injection, USP, 10mg/mL, 40mg/mL
Glycopyrrolate Injection, USP, 0.2mg/mL
Heparin Lock Flush Solution, USP, 100u/mL
Heparin Sodium Injection, USP, 1,000u/mL Preservative Free
Heparin Sodium Injection, USP, 1,000/5,000/10,000 units per mL
Heparin Sodium Injection, USP (Beef Lung Origin) 1,000, 10,000, 20,000 units per mL
HepFlush Kit (Heparin Lock Flush Solution, USP, 10u/mL)
HepFlush-10 (Heparin Lock Flush Solution, USP, 10u/mL)
Hydrocortisone Sodium Succinate for Injection, USP, 100, 250, 500 & 1,000mg
Hydroxycobalamin Injection, USP, 1,000 mcg/mL
Hydroxyzine Hydrochloride Injection, USP 25mg/mL, 50mg/mL
I.V. Transfer Spikes
Iodopen (Sodium Iodide Injection) 100mcg/mL
Kanamycin Sulfate Injection, USP, 75mg/2mL, 500mg/2mL, 1gm/3mL
Leukovorin Calcium Injection, USP
Lidocaine Hydrochloride Injection, USP, 1%, 2%, 4%, 20%
Lyphocin P (Vancomycin Hydrochloride Injection, USP) 500mg
LyphoLyte & LyphoLyte-II (Multielectrolyte Concentrate)
MTE-2 (Multiple Trace Elements)
MTE-3 (Multiple Trace Elements)
MTE-4 & MTE-4 Concentrated (Multiple Trace Elements)
MTE-5 & MTE-5 Concentrated (Multiple Trace Elements)
MTE-6 & MTE-6 Concentrated (Multiple Trace Elements)
MTE 7 (Multiple Trace Elements)
MVC (Multivitamin Concentrate)
MVC 9+3 and MVC 9+3 VitaGard
MVC 10+3 Pediatric
Magnesium Sulfate Injection, USP, 10% & 50%
Manganese Sulfate Injection, USP, 0.1, 0.5mg/mL
Mannitol Injection, USP, 25%
Maxifill Transfer Set
Methotrexate Sodium Injection, USP, 20, 50 & 100mg
Methyldopate Hydrochloride Injection 50mg/mL
Methylprednisolone Sodium Succinate for Injection, USP, 40, 125, 500, 1000mg
Metoclopramide Injection 50mg/mL
Metronidazole Injection 500mg
Molypen (Ammonium Molybdate Injection, USP) 25mcg/mL
Multilyte-20 (Multi-Electrolyte Concentrate)
Muri-Lube (mineral oil, sterile, light)
Nalbuphine Injection 10mg/mL, 20mg/mL
Nandrolone Decanoate Injection, USP, 100 mg/mL
NeoTrace-4 (neonatal multiple trace elements)
Nitroglycerin Injection 5mg/mL
Oxytocin Injection, USP, Synthetic, 10 USP Units/mL
PTE-4 (pediatric multiple trace elements)
PTE-5 (pediatric multiple trace elements)
PedTrace-4 (pediatric multiple trace elements)
Pentam 300
Phenytoin Sodium Injection, USP, 50mg/mL
Potassium Acetate Injection, USP, 2, 4mEq/mL
Potassium Chloride Injection, USP, 2, 3mEq/mL
Potassium Phosphates Injection, USP, 3mM phosphate/mL
Procainamide Hydrochloride Injection, 100mg/mL, 500mg/mL
Procaine Hydrochloride Injection, USP, 1%
Pyridoxine Hydrochloride Injection, USP, 100mg/mL
Scopolamine Hydrobromide Injection, USP, 0.3mg/mL, 0.4mg/mL, 1.0mg/mL
Selepen (Selenious Acid Injection) 40mcg/mL
Sodium Acetate Injection, USP, 2, 4mEq/mL
Sodium Bicarbonate Injection, USP, 4%, 7.5%, 8.4%
Sodium Chloride Injeoction, USP, 0.9%, 14.6%, 23.4%
Sodium Nitroprusside Injection, USP, 50mg
Sodium Phosphates Injection, USP, 3mM/phosphate/mL
Soyacal 10%, 20% (intravenous lipids)
Sterile Empty Vials 5, 10, 30mL
Sterile Water for Injection, USP
Thiamine Hydrochloride Injection, USP, 100mg/mL
TraceLyte & TraceLyte-II (Trace elements & electrolytes additive)
TraceLyte with Double Electrolytes & TraceLyte-II with Double Electrolytes
Transfer Needles, thin wall, 19 gauge
Verapamil Hydrochloride Injection 2.5 mg/mL
Vinblastine Sulfate Injection, USP, 10mg
Vincristine Sulfate Injection, USP, 1mg/2mg/5mg per vial
Water (Bacteriostatic) for Injection, USP
Zinc Sulfate Injection, USP, 1, 5mg/mL

MACSIL, INC. 1172
1326 Frankford Avenue
Philadelphia, PA 19125
(215) 739-7300
Products Available
▣ Balmex Baby Powder
▣ Balmex Emollient Lotion
▣ Balmex Ointment

MALLARD INCORPORATED 1172
3021 Wabash Ave.
Detroit, MI 48216-9986
Address inquiries to:
Sales Department (313) 964-3910
Products Available
Allersone
Anoquan
Phenate

MARION LABORATORIES, INC. 415, 1173
Pharmaceutical Division
Marion Industrial Park
Marion Park Drive
Kansas City, MO 64137
Address inquiries to:
Product Surveillance Dept.
P.O. Box 9627
Kansas City, MO 64134
(816) 966-5000
Products Available
◆ Carafate Tablets
◆ Cardizem 30-mg Tablets
◆ Cardizem 60-mg Tablets
Debrox Drops
Ditropan Syrup
◆ Ditropan Tablets
Gaviscon Liquid
◆ Gaviscon Tablets
◆ Gaviscon-2 Tablets
Gly-Oxide Liquid
Nitro-Bid IV
Nitro-Bid Ointment
◆ Nitro-Bid 2.5 Plateau Caps
◆ Nitro-Bid 6.5 Plateau Caps
◆ Nitro-Bid 9 Plateau Caps
◆ Os-Cal 250 Tablets
◆ Os-Cal 500 Chewable Tablets
◆ Os-Cal 500 Tablets
◆ Os-Cal Forte Tablets
◆ Os-Cal Plus Tablets
◆ Pavabid Capsules
◆ Pavabid HP Capsulets
◆ Silvadene Cream
Throat Discs Throat Lozenges

MARION SCIENTIFIC 2227
A Division of Marion Laboratories, Inc.
P. O. Box 8480
Kansas City, MO 64114
Address product inquiries to:
Scientific Technical Services
(800) 821-7772
Products Available
Anaerobic Culturette
Culturette
Culturette II
Culturette Brand 10-Minute Group A Strep ID
Mini-Tip Culturette
Viral Culturette

MARLYN COMPANY, INC. 1180
350 Pauma Place
Escondido, CA 92025
(619) 489-6115
Products Available
Albumin 500 Tablets
C Speridin Tablets, Sustained Release
Daily Nutritional Paks
..... Boosters
..... Care-4
▣ ..... MARLYN PMS
..... Pro-Formance
..... Soft Stress
Hep-Forte Capsules
Marbec Tablets
MARLYN Formula 50 Capsules
MARLYN Prolonged Release Vitamins
Balanced B 125
Clock E, 400 I.U.
Iron-L-99
Niacin, 400 mg.
Super One Daily
Super Citro Cee
Ultimate One
Vitamin B 12, 1000 mcg.
Vitamin C, 1000 mg.

MASON PHARMACEUTICALS, INC. 415, 1180
1201 Dove Street, Suite 520
Newport Beach, CA 92660
(714) 851-6860
Products Available
◆ Damacet-P
◆ Damason-P

MAYRAND, INC. 1181
P.O. Box 8869
4 Dundas Circle
Greensboro, NC 27419
(919) 292-5347
Products Available
Anamine Syrup
Anamine T. D. Caps
Anatuss Tablets & Syrup
Anatuss with Codeine Tablets & Syrup
B.A.C.Tablets
B.A.C. No. 3 Tablets (with Codeine)
Becomject
Benoject-10
Benoject-50
Corgonject-5
Cyanoject
Decaject
Decaject-L.A.
Depoject-40 & Depoject-80
Dramoject
Eldercaps
Eldertonic
Estroject-2
Estroject-LA
Flexoject
Glytuss Tabs
Histaject
Hydrotensin-50 Tablets

(◆ Shown in Product Identification Section)

(▣ Described in PDR For Nonprescription Drugs)

Hydro-Z-50 Tablets
Kenaject-40
Lidoject-1 & Lidoject-2
Lifoject
May-Vita Elixir
Menoject-LA
Nu-Iron Elixir
Nu-Iron 150 Caps
Nu-Iron Plus Elixir
Nu-Iron-V Tablets
Phenoject-50
Predaject-50
Progestaject-50
Sedapap #3 Capsules
Sedapap-10 Tablets
Selestoject
Sorbide T.D. Caps
Spasmoject
Stera-Form Cream
Sterapred Uni-Pak
Sterapred DS Uni-Pak
Sulfa-Gyn
Testoject-50
Testoject-100 L.A. & Testoject-200 L.A.
Tiject-20
Trimcaps
Trimtabs
Tristoject
Vistaject-25 & Vistaject-50

McGREGOR PHARMACEUTICALS INC. 1183
32580 Grand River Avenue
Farmington, MI 48024
Address inquiries to:
Mr. Edward McGregor
(313) 474-8727
Products Available
Rhindecon Capsules
Rhinolar Capsules
Rhinolar-EX Capsules
Rhinolar-EX 12 Capsules

McNEIL CONSUMER PRODUCTS CO. 416, 1183
McNEILAB, INC.
Fort Washington, PA 19034
Address inquiries to:
Professional Relations Department
Fort Washington, PA 19034
Manufacturing Divisions
Fort Washington, PA 19034
Southwest Manufacturing Plant
4001 N. I-35
Round Rock, TX 78664
Distribution Centers
Order Services
Fort Washington, PA 19034
Camp Hill Road
Local Area (215) 233-7000
Round Rock, TX 78664
2820 Oakmont Drive
(512) 244-0850
Glendale, CA 91201
512 Paula Avenue (213) 245-0217
Montgomeryville, PA 18936
1390 Welsh Road (215) 641-1420
Products Available
◆ Children's CoTylenol Liquid Cold Formula and Chewable Cold Tablet
◆ Children's Tylenol acetaminophen Chewable Tablets & Elixir
◆ CoTylenol Cold Medication Tablets & Caplets
◆ CoTylenol Liquid Cold Medication
◆ Delsym Cough Suppressant Syrup
◆ Extra-Strength Sine-Aid Sinus Headache Caplets
◆ Extra-Strength Tylenol acetaminophen Caplets, Tablets & Liquid
◆ Infants' Tylenol Drops
◆ Junior Strength Tylenol Coated Caplets
◆ Maximum-Strength Tylenol Sinus Medication Tablets & Caplets
◆ Medipren Caplets and Tablets
◆ PediaCare 1 Children's Cough Relief Liquid
◆ PediaCare 2 Children's Cold Relief Liquid
◆ PediaCare 3 Children's Cold Relief Liquid & Chewable Tablets
◆ PediaCare Oral Drops
◆ Regular Strength Tylenol acetaminophen Tablets & Caplets
◆ Sine-Aid Sinus Headache Tablets

McNEIL PHARMACEUTICAL 416, 1189
McNEILAB, INC.
Spring House, PA 19477
Address inquiries to:
Professional Services Department
Spring House, PA 19477
(215) 628-5000
Manufacturing Affiliate
Dorado, Puerto Rico 00646
P.O. Box P
Fort Washington, PA 19034
Distribution Divisions
Burr Ridge, IL 60521
261 Shore Drive (312) 655-0366
Glendale, CA 91201
512 Paula Avenue (213) 245-0217
Montgomeryville PA 18936
Park Drive (215) 641-0250
Products Available
Butibel-Zyme Tablets
Carbinoxamine Maleate, see Clistin
Chlorzoxazone, see Parafiex
Clistin Tablets
◆ Haldol Decanoate Injection
◆ Haldol Injection, Tablets & Concentrate
◆ Haloperidol, see Haldol Orap Tablets
◆ Pancrease
Paraflex Tablets
◆ Parafon Forte Tablets
◆ Suprol Capsules
Theophyl-SR
◆ Tolectin 200 Tablets & DS Capsules
◆ Tolmetin Sodium, see Tolectin Tablets
◆ Tylenol w/Codeine Capsules, Tablets & Elixir
◆ Tylox Capsules

MEAD JOHNSON LABORATORIES 416, 1200
Mead Johnson & Company
2404 West Pennsylvania St.
Evansville, IN 47721
(812) 426-6000
Address inquiries to:
Scientific Information Section
Medical Department
Products Available
◆ Estrace
◆ Estrace Vaginal Cream
◆ K-Lyte & K-Lyte DS
◆ K-Lyte/Cl & K-Lyte/Cl 50
◆ Natalins
◆ Natalins Rx
◆ Ovcon-35
◆ Ovcon-50
Questran
◆ Quibron
Quibron Liquid
◆ Quibron-T
◆ Quibron-T/SR

MEAD JOHNSON NUTRITIONAL DIVISION 1219
Mead Johnson & Company
2404 W. Pennsylvania St.
Evansville, IN 47721
(812) 429-5000
Address inquiries to:
Scientific Information Section
Medical Department
Products Available
b-Capsa I Vaccine
▣ Casec
▣ Ce-Vi-Sol
▣ Criticare HN
▣ Enfamil
▣ Enfamil Nursette
▣ Enfamil Ready-To-Use
▣ Enfamil w/Iron
▣ Enfamil w/Iron Ready-To-Use
▣ Fer-In-Sol
▣ Isocal
Isocal HCN
▣ Lofenalac
▣ Lonalac
▣ Lytren
▣ MCT Oil
▣ Moducal
Naturacil
▣ Nutramigen
Poly-Vi-Flor 0.25 mg Vitamins w/Fluoride Chewable Tablets
Poly-Vi-Flor 0.5 mg Vitamins w/Fluoride Chewable Tablets
Poly-Vi-Flor 1.0 mg Vitamins w/Fluoride Chewable Tablets
Poly-Vi-Flor 0.25 mg Vitamins w/Fluoride Drops
Poly-Vi-Flor 0.5 mg Vitamins w/Fluoride Drops
Poly-Vi-Flor 0.25 mg Vitamins w/Iron & Fluoride Chewable Tablets
Poly-Vi-Flor 0.5 mg Vitamins w/Iron & Fluoride Chewable Tablets & Drops
Poly-Vi-Flor 1.0 Vitamins w/Iron & Fluoride Chewable Tablets
Poly-Vi-Flor 0.25 mg Vitamins w/Iron & Fluoride Drops
▣ Poly-Vi-Sol Vitamins Chewable Tablets & Drops
▣ Poly-Vi-Sol Vitamins with Iron & Zinc
▣ Poly-Vi-Sol Vitamins w/Iron Multivitamin & Iron Supplement Drops
▣ Portagen
▣ Pregestimil
▣ ProSobee
▣ Smurf Chewable Vitamins
Smurf Chewable Vitamins w/Iron & Zinc
▣ Sustacal
▣ Sustacal HC
▣ Sustagen
▣ Tempra
▣ Traumacal
▣ Trind
▣ Trind-DM
Tri-Vi-Flor 1.0 mg Vitamins w/Fluoride Chewable Tablets
Tri-Vi-Flor 0.25 mg Vitamins w/Fluoride Drops
Tri-Vi-Flor 0.5 mg Vitamins w/Fluoride Drops
Tri-Vi-Flor 0.25 mg Vitamins w/Iron & Fluoride Drops
▣ Tri-Vi-Sol Vitamins, Chewable Tablets & Drops
▣ Tri-Vi-Sol Vitamins w/Iron Drops & Chewable Tablets

MEAD JOHNSON PHARMACEUTICAL DIVISION 417, 1225
Mead Johnson & Company
2404 W. Pennsylvania St.
Evansville, IN 47721
(812) 429-5000
Address inquiries to:
Scientific Information Section
Medical Department
Products Available
◆ Colace
◆ Desyrel and Desyrel Dividose
◆ Duricef
◆ Klotrix
Mucomyst
◆ Peri-Colace

MEDICAL MARKET SPECIALTIES INC. 1233
P.O. Box 307
Cedar Grove. NJ 07009
Address inquiries to:
Executive Offices
P.O. Box 150
Boonton, NJ 07005
(201) 263-4243
Products Available
Proglycem Capsules
Proglycem Suspension

MEDICAL PRODUCTS PANAMERICANA, INC. 1233
Post Office Box 771
Coral Gables, FL 33134
Address inquiries to:
Professional Services Dept.
(305) 545-6524
Branch and Distribution Division
San Juan, PR (809) 783-6736
Products Available
Aminobrain Capsules
Aminobrain Plus Capsules
Atoximetin-B Capsules
Broncopectol Syrup
Digesplen Elixir
Digesplen-Plus Tablets
Ferlivit Injection
Medispray
Neurodep-Plus Injection
Novaflor Capsules
Rubroben-1000 Injection Lyophilized
Rutiplen-C
Tempotest 225
Trilycal-12
VG Capsules
Varidin Capsules

MEDICONE COMPANY 417, 1233
225 Varick St.
New York, NY 10014
Address inquiries to:
Professional Service Dept.
(212) 924-5166
Products Available
▣ Medicone Derma Ointment
◆ Medicone Derma-HC Ointment
▣ Medicone Dressing Cream
▣ Medicone Rectal Ointment
◆ Medicone Rectal Suppositories
▣ Mediconet

MERCK SHARP & DOHME 417, 1234
Division of Merck & Co., Inc.
West Point, PA 19486
(215) 661-5000
For Medical or Drug Information
Write: Professional Information
Business hours only (8:30 a.m. to 4:45 p.m. EST), call (215) 661-7300
For Medical Emergency Information after hours or on weekends, call
(215) 661-5000
Address other inquiries to:
Professional Service Department
West Point, PA 19486
Branch Offices
Arlington, TX 76011
Great Southwest Industrial District
925-111th Street (817) 640-5657
Atlanta Area:
See Norcross, GA
Baltimore Area:
see Columbia, MD
Boston Area:
see Needham Heights, MA
Chicago Area:
see Oak Brook, IL
Columbia, MD 21045
9199 Red Branch Rd.
(301) 730-8240
Columbus, OH 43228
4242 Janitrol Road
(614) 276-5308
Dallas/Ft. Worth Area:
see Arlington, TX
Denver, CO 80216
4900 Jackson Street
(303) 355-1601
Kansas City Area:
see Overland Park, KS
Kenner, LA 70062
1431 E. Airline Highway
(504) 464-0111
King of Prussia, PA 19406
1045 First Avenue (215) 962-6900
Los Angeles, CA 90040
6409 E. Gayhart Street
(213) 723-9661
Memphis, TN 38106
1980 Latham Street
(901) 948-8501
Minneapolis, MN 55441
12955 State Highway 55
(612) 559-4445
Needham Heights, MA 02194
40 A Street (617) 444-5510
New Orleans Area:
see Kenner, LA
New York Area:
see Teterboro, NJ
Norcross, GA 30071
2825 Northwoods Parkway
(404) 662-7200
Oak Brook, IL 60521
2010 Swift Drive (312) 920-2160
Overland Park, KS 66215
9001 Quivira Rd. (913) 888-1110
Philadelphia Area:
see King of Prussia, PA
Portland, OR 97211
717 N.E. Lombard St.
(503) 285-2582
Teterboro, NJ 07608
111 Central Avenue
(201) 288-7710
Products Available
◆ Aldoclor Tablets
Aldomet Ester HCl Injection
Aldomet Oral Suspension
◆ Aldomet Tablets
◆ Aldoril Tablets
alphaRedisol Injection
Aminohippurate Sodium Injection
Antivenin (Black Widow Spider)
AquaMEPHYTON Injection
Aramine Injection
Attenuvax
◆ Benemid Tablets
Biavax II
◆ Blocadren Tablets
◆ Clinoril Tablets
◆ Cogentin Tablets & Injection
◆ ColBENEMID Tablets
Cortone Acetate Saline Suspension
Cortone Acetate Tablets
Cosmegen Injection
◆ Cuprid Capsules
◆ Cuprimine Capsules
◆ Daranide Tablets
Decaderm 0.1% Topical
Decadron Elixir
Decadron Phosphate Injection
Decadron Phosphate Respihaler
Decadron Phosphate Sterile Ophthalmic Ointment
Decadron Phosphate Sterile Ophthalmic Solution
Decadron Phosphate Topical Cream
Decadron Phosphate Turbinaire
Decadron Phosphate with Xylocaine Injection
◆ Decadron Tablets
Decadron-LA Suspension
Decaspray Topical Aerosol
◆ Demser Capsules
◆ Diupres Tablets
Diuril Intravenous Sodium
Diuril Oral Suspension
◆ Diuril Tablets
◆ Dolobid Tablets
Edecrin Sodium Intravenous
◆ Edecrin Tablets
Elavil Injection
◆ Elavil Tablets
Elspar
◆ Flexeril Tablets
Floropryl Sterile Ophthalmic Ointment
Hep-B-Gammagee
Heptavax-B
Humorsol Sterile Ophthalmic Solution
Hydeltrasol Injection
Hydeltra-T.B.A. Suspension
Hydrocortone Acetate Saline Suspension
Hydrocortone Phosphate Injection
Hydrocortone Tablets
◆ HydroDIURIL Tablets
◆ Hydropres Tablets
◆ Indocin Capsules
Indocin I.V.
Indocin Oral Suspension
◆ Indocin SR Capsules
◆ Indocin Suppositories
Inversine Tablets
Lacrisert Sterile Ophthalmic Insert
M-M-R II
M-R-VAX II
Mefoxin
Mephyton Tablets
Meruvax II
◆ Midamor Tablets
◆ Mintezol Chewable Tablets
Mintezol Suspension
◆ Moduretic Tablets
Mumpsvax
Mustargen
Myochrysine Injection
Neodecadron Sterile Ophthalmic Ointment
Neodecadron Sterile Ophthalmic Solution
Neodecadron Topical Cream
Noroxin
◆ Pepcid
Periactin Syrup
◆ Periactin Tablets
Pneumovax 23

Primaxin
Redisol Injectable
Redisol Tablets
Respihaler (see Decadron Phosphate Respihaler)
◆ Sinemet Tablets
◆ Timolide Tablets
Timoptic Sterile Ophthalmic Solution
◆ Tonocard
◆ Triavil Tablets
Turbinaire (see Decadron Phosphate Turbinaire)
Urecholine Injection
◆ Urecholine Tablets
◆ Vasotec Tablets
◆ Vivactil Tablets

MERICON INDUSTRIES, INC. 1350
8819 N. Pioneer Road
Peoria, IL 61615
Address inquiries to:
Thomas P. Morrissey
(309) 693-2150
Products Available
■ Orazinc Capsules
■ Orazinc Lozenges

MERIEUX INSTITUTE, INC. 1350, 2227
P.O. Box 52-3980
Miami, FL 33152
Address inquiries to:
P.O. Box 52-3980
Miami, FL 33152-3980
(305) 593-9577
For Medical Emergencies Contact:
Merieux Institute, Inc.
(800) 327-2842
Alaska, FL, & HI, call Collect
(305) 593-9577
Products Available
Imogam Rabies Immune Globulin (Human)
Imovax Rabies I.D.
Imovax Rabies Vaccine
Mono-Vacc Test (O.T.)
Multitest CMI Skin Test Antigens for Cellular Hypersensitivity
Rabies Immune Globulin (Human), Imogam Rabies Vaccine
Rabies Vaccine Human Diploid Cell, Imovax Rabies I.D.
Rabies Vaccine Human Diploid Cell, Imovax Rabies
Skin Test Antigens for Cellular Hypersensitivity, Multitest CMI
Tuberculin, Mono-Vacc Test (O.T.)

MERRELL DOW PHARMACEUTICALS INC. 418, 1350
Subsidiary of The Dow Chemical Company
2110 E. Galbraith Road
Cincinnati, OH 45215
Address inquiries to:
Professional Information Department
Business hours only (8:15 AM to 5:00 PM EST)
(513) 948-6040
For Medical Emergency Information
After hours or on weekends only,
(513) 948-9111
Products Available
AVC Suppositories
AVC Vaginal Cream
Accurbron
◆ Cantil Tablets
◆ Cephulac Syrup
Chloramphenicol Injection
◆ Chronulac Syrup
◆ Clomid Tablets
DV Cream
Dow-Isoniazid
Hesper Bitabs
Hesper Capsules
◆ Hiprex Tablets
Imferon
◆ Lorelco
◆ Metahydrin
◆ Metatensin
◆ Norpramin
◆ Novafed A Capsules
Novafed A Liquid
◆ Novafed Capsules
Novafed Liquid
◆ Quinamm Tablets
◆ Rifadin
◆ Rifamate
◆ Seldane
■ Simron Capsules
■ Simron Plus Capsules
2/G
2/G-DM
◆ TACE 12 mg Capsules
◆ TACE 25 mg Capsules
◆ TACE 72 mg Capsules
Terpin Hydrate & Codeine Elixir
◆ Tussend Expectorant
◆ Tussend Liquid & Tablets

METRO MED, INC. 1375
2201 Denton Drive
Austin, TX 78758
Address inquires to:
Loy Walker (512) 836-1636
For Medical Emergencies Contact:
Medical Services (512) 836-1636
Products Available
Alpha-Phed Capsules
Beta-Phed Capsules
Dibatrol
Digestamic
Digestamic #2
Digestamic Liquid
Esprogyn Pack
Furonatal FA Tablets
Histamic Capsules
Histamic Pedi Syrup
Histamic Syrup
Histamic Tablets
Metrogesic
■ Metrovite H.P.
Otogesic HC
Span-FF Capsules
Span R/D Capsules
Trim Sulf DS
Utex SR
Zantine

MILES LABORATORIES, INC. 1375
P.O. Box 340
Elkhart, IN 46515
Address inquiries to:
Medical Dept. (219) 262-7886
Consumer Health Care Division only
Products Available
Alka-Mints Chewable Antacid
Alka-Seltzer Effervescent Antacid
Alka-Seltzer Effervescent Pain Reliever and Antacid
Flavored Alka Seltzer Effervescent Pain Reliever & Antacid
Alka-Seltzer Plus Cold Medicine
■ Bactine Antiseptic-Anesthetic First Aid Spray
■ Bactine Hydrocortisone Skin Care Cream
Biocal Calcium Supplement Chewable Tablets
Biocal Calcium Supplement Tablets
■ Bugs Bunny Multivitamin Supplement (Sugar Free)
■ Bugs Bunny Plus Iron Multivitamin Supplement (Sugar Free)
■ Bugs Bunny Vitamins Plus Minerals (Sugar Free)
■ Bugs Bunny With Extra C (Sugar Free)
■ Flintstones Complete Multivitamin/Mineral Supplement
■ Flintstones Multivitamin Supplement
■ Flintstones Plus Iron Multivitamin Supplement
■ Flintstones With Extra C
■ Miles Nervine Nighttime Sleep-Aid
One-A-Day Essential Multivitamin Supplement
■ One-A-Day Maximum Formula (Multivitamin/Multimineral)
■ One-A-Day Plus Extra C
■ One-A-Day Stressgard Vitamins
■ Within (Multivitamins with Calcium & Extra Iron)

MILES PHARMACEUTICALS 418, 1377
Division of Miles Laboratories, Inc.
400 Morgan Lane
West Haven, CT 06516
Address inquiries to:
Director, Medical Services
(203) 934-9221
Products Available
◆ Adalat Capsules (10 mg)
Azlin
◆ Biltricide
Cort-Dome ¼%, ½%, and 1% Creme
Cort-Dome ¼%, ½%, and 1% Lotion
Cort-Dome High Potency Suppositories
DTIC-Dome
◆ Decholin Tablets
◆ Domeboro Powder Packets, Effervescent Tablets
Dome-Paste Bandage (Unna's Boot)
Domol Bath & Shower Oil
◆ Lithane Tablets
Mezlin
Mithracin
Mycelex 1% Cream
Mycelex 1% Solution
◆ Mycelex Troches
Mycelex-G 1% Vaginal Cream
◆ Mycelex-G 100mg Vaginal Tablets
◆ Mycelex-G 500mg Vaginal Tablets
Mycelex Twin Pack
Neo Cort-Dome Creme
◆ Niclocide Chewable Tablets
Otic Domeboro Solution
Otic Tridesilon Solution 0.05%
◆ Stilphostrol Tablets and Ampuls
Tridesilon Creme 0.05%
Tridesilon Ointment 0.05%

MILEX PRODUCTS, INC. 1400
5915 Northwest Highway
Chicago, IL 60631 (312) 631-6484
Shipping Offices
Milex Western
Post Office Box 46030
Los Angeles, CA 90046
(213) 651-4301
Milex Michigan
Post Office Box 20264
Ferndale, MI 48220
(313) 399-9223
Milex Puerto Rico
GPO Box 554
San Juan, PR 00936
(809) 791-3309
Milex Hawaii
Box 6337
Honolulu, HI 96818
(808) 422-9581
Milex Southeastern
Post Office Drawer 4647
Clearwater, FL 33518
(813) 461-1949
Milex Southern
Post Office Drawer "M"
Weatherford, TX 76086
(817) 594-6865
Milex Carolinas
Post Office Box 23060
Charlotte, NC 28212
(704) 545-4567
Milex Delaware Valley
350 White Horse Pike
Atco, NJ 08004 (609) 767-4818
Milex Delta
Post Office Drawer 5684
Shreveport, LA 71105
(318) 797-1554
Products Available
Amino-Cerv
Basal Thermometers
Breast Self-Examination Kit
Cannula Curette with Swivel Handle
Dilateria
Endometrial Suction Curettes
Fertility Cannula
Fertilo-Pak
Laminaria Japonica
Oligospermia Cups
Pessaries
Pro-Ception
Seminal Pouches
Shur-Seal Gel
Spatula
Tis-U-Trap
Trimo-San
Wide-Seal Diaphragm

MISSION PHARMACAL COMPANY 1400
1325 E. Durango
San Antonio, TX 78210
Address inquiries to:
Professional Service Dept.
(512) 533-7118
Post Office Box 1676
San Antonio, TX 78296
Products Available
Calcet
Calcet Plus
Calcibind
Citracal
Compete
Ferralet
Fosfree
Iromin-G
Lithostat
Mission Prenatal
Mission Prenatal F.A.
Mission Prenatal H.P.
Mission Prenatal RX
Mission Surgical Supplement
Prulet
Supac
Therabid
Thera-Gesic
Urocit-K

MURO PHARMACEUTICAL, INC. 1403
890 East Street
Tewksbury, MA 01876-9987
Address inquiries to:
Professional Service Dept.
1-(800) 225-0974
(617) 851-5981
Products Available
Bromfed Capsules (Timed Release)
Bromfed-PD Capsules (Timed Release)
Bromfed Tablets
Guaifed Capsules (Timed Release)
Guaifed-PD Capsules (Timed Release)
Liquid Pred Syrup
Prelone Syrup
■ Salinex Nasal Mist and Drops

NATURE'S BOUNTY, INC. 1404
90 Orville Drive
Bohemia, NY 11716
Address inquiries to:
Professional Services Dept.
(516) 567-9500
(800) 645-5412
Products Available
B-12 and B-12 Sublingual Tablets
B-50 Tablets
B-100 Tablets-Ultra B Complex
B-Complex + C (Long Acting) Tablets
Beta Carotene Capsules
Calciday 500 Complete Tablets
Calciday-667
Calmtabs Tablets
Ener-B Intranasal Vitamin B_{12} Gel
KLB6 Capsules
KLB6 Grapefruit Diet
l-Lysine 500 mg Tablets
M-KYA
Nature's Bounty 1 Tablets
Oyster Calcium Tablets
Oystercal-D 250
Oystercal-500
Perk-up Intranasal Vitamin B_{12}
Slim with Fiber Tablets
Stress "1000" Tablets
l-Tryptophan (200, 500 & 667 mg)
Ultra Vita-Times Tablets
Vitamin C with Rose Hips
Vitamin E (d-alpha tocopheryl)
Water Pill (Natural Diuretic)
Zacne Tablets

NEUTROGENA DERMATOLOGICS 1404
Division of Neutrogena Corp.
Mitchell S. Wortzman, Ph.D.
5755 West 96th Street
P.O. Box 45036
Los Angeles, CA 90045
(800) 421-6857
In CA (213) 642-1150
Products Available
Liquid Neutrogena
Melanex (3% Hydroquinone) Topical Solution (Neutrogena)
Neutrogena Acne Cleansing Formula
Neutrogena Acne-Drying Gel
Neutrogena Acne Mask
Neutrogena Baby Cleansing Formula
Neutrogena Body Lotion
Neutrogena Conditioner
Neutrogena Dry Skin Formula
Neutrogena Moisture
Neutrogena Norwegian Formula Hand Cream
Neutrogena Oily Skin Formula
Neutrogena Original Formula
Neutrogena Rainbath Shower and Bath Gel
Neutrogena Sesame Seed Body Oil
Neutrogena Shampoo
Neutrogena Solid Soap Shampoo
T/Derm Tar Emollient
T/Gel Scalp Solution (Neutrogena)
T/Gel Therapeutic Conditioner (Neutrogena)
T/Gel Therapeutic Shampoo (Neutrogena)
Vehicle/N (Neutrogena)
Vehicle/N MILD (Neutrogena)

NORCLIFF THAYER INC. 419, 1405
303 South Broadway
Tarrytown, NY 10591
(914) 631-0033
Products Available
◆ A-200 Pyrinate Pediculicide Shampoo, Liquid & Gel
■ Avail Calcium Intensive Multivitamin & Minerals for Women
■ Esotérica Medicated Fade Cream
■ Liquiprin Acetaminophen
■ Nature's Remedy Laxative
■ NoSalt Salt Alternative, Regular and Seasoned
■ Oxy Clean Lathering Facial Scrub
■ Oxy Clean Medicated Cleanser, Pads & Soap
■ Oxy-5 Lotion with Sorboxyl
■ Oxy-10 Lotion and Cover with Sorboxyl
■ Oxy-10 Wash Antibacterial Skin Wash
■ Tums Antacid Tablets, Regular & Extra Strength

NORDISK-USA 1405
6500 Rock Spring Drive
Suite 304
Bethesda, MD 20817
Address inquiries to:
Medical Director (301) 897-9220
Products Available
Insulatard NPH
Insulatard NPH Human
Mixtard
Velosulin
Velosulin Human

NORWICH EATON PHARMACEUTICALS, INC. 419, 1408
A Procter & Gamble Company
(formerly Eaton Laboratories, Professional Products Group, Norwich Products, or Consumer Products Group)
13-27 Eaton Avenue
Norwich, NY 13815
Also see Procter & Gamble
Address medical inquiries to:
Medical Department
Norwich Eaton Pharmaceuticals, Inc.
P.O. Box 191
Norwich, NY 13815-0191
(607) 335-2565
Refer orders & other inquiries to:
Norwich Eaton Pharmaceuticals, Inc.
17 Eaton Avenue
Norwich, NY 13815-0231
(800) 448-4878
New York State customers only,
(607) 335-2121
Products Available
Buprenex Injectable
Comhist LA Capsules
Comhist Tablets
Dantrium Capsules
Dantrium Intravenous
◆ Didronel
Dopar Capsules
Duvoid Tablets
Entex Capsules
◆ Entex LA Tablets
Entex Liquid
Furacin Preparations
Furacin Soluble Dressing
Furacin Topical Cream
Furadantin Oral Suspension
Furadantin Tablets
Furoxone Liquid Suspension

(◆ Shown in Product Identification Section)

(■ Described in PDR For Nonprescription Drugs)

◆ Furoxone Tablets
◆ Macrodantin Capsules
Topicycline
Vivonex
Standard Vivonex Diet
Vivonex T.E.N.
Flavor Packets
Devices
Vivonex Acutrol Enteral Feeding System
Vivonex Delivery System
Vivonex Jejunostomy Kit
Vivonex Tungsten Tip Tube

NTRON INTERNATIONAL SALES CO. **1422**
3833 Redwood Highway
P.O. Box 7000
San Rafael, CA 94912
Address inquiries to:
Customer Services (415) 472-4600
For Medical Emergencies Contact:
Ken Levin, Biomedical Engineer
(415) 472-4600
Products Available
NTRON Transcutaneous Electrical Nerve Stimulator (TENS)

ORGANON INC. **419, 1422**
375 Mount Pleasant Ave.
West Orange, NJ 07052
(201) 325-4500
Products Available
◆ Calderol Capsules
Cortrophin-Zinc
Cortrosyn
◆ Cotazym
◆ Cotazym-S
Deca-Durabolin
Durabolin
Heparin Sodium (from Beef Lung Sources)
Hexadrol Elixir
◆ Hexadrol Tablets
Hexadrol Phosphate Injection
Hexadrol Strip Packs
◆ Hexadrol Therapeutic Pack
Hydrocortisone USP
Liquaemin Sodium
Maxibolin
Norcuron
Pavulon
Pregnyl
Regonol
Succinylcholine Chloride Injection
◆ Wigraine Tablets & Suppositories

ORTHO DIAGNOSTIC SYSTEMS INC. **1429**
Route 202
Raritan, NJ 08869
Address inquiries to:
Customer Service Div.
In NJ: (201) 524-1732
(201) 524-2374
Outside NJ (toll free)
(800) 631-5807
Products Available
Fetalscreen Qualitative Screening Test for D(Rh_o) Positive Fetal Red Blood Cells in the Maternal Circulation
MICRhoGAM Rh_o(D) Immune Globulin (Human)
RhoGAM Rh_o(D) Immune Globulin (Human)

ORTHO PHARMACEUTICAL CORPORATION **419, 1430**
Raritan, NJ 08869
For Medical Information Call:
(201) 524-8895
(201) 524-0504
For Product Information Call:
(201) 524-2343
Products Available
Aci-Jel Therapeutic Vaginal Jelly
▣ Conceptrol Birth Control Cream
Conceptrol Contraceptive Gel
▣ Conceptrol Contraceptive Gel Disposable
▣ Delfen Contraceptive Foam
▣ Gynol II Contraceptive Jelly
▣ Intercept Contraceptive Inserts
Lippes Loop Intrauterine Double-S
▣ Massé Breast Cream
◆ Micronor Tablets
◆ Modicon 21 Tablets
Modicon 28 Tablets
◆ Monistat 3 Vaginal Suppositories
◆ Monistat 7 Vaginal Cream
◆ Monistat 7 Vaginal Suppositories
◆ Monistat Dual-Pak
Ortho Diaphragm Kit-All Flex
Ortho Diaphragm Kit-Coil Spring
Ortho Dienestrol Cream
▣ Ortho Disposable Applicator
▣ Ortho Personal Lubricant
Orthoclone OKT3 Sterile Solution
▣ Ortho-Creme Contraceptive Cream
▣ Ortho-Gynol Contraceptive Jelly
◆ Ortho-Novum 1/35□21
Ortho-Novum 1/35□28
◆ Ortho-Novum 1/50□21
Ortho-Novum 1/50□28
◆ Ortho-Novum 1/80□21
Ortho-Novum 1/80□28
◆ Ortho-Novum 7/7/7 □21 Tablets
Ortho-Novum 7/7/7 □28 Tablets
◆ Ortho-Novum 10/11□21 Tablets
Ortho-Novum 10/11□28 Tablets
◆ Ortho-Novum Tablets 2 mg□21
Ortho-White Diaphragm Kit-Flat Spring
◆ Protostat Tablets
Sultrin Triple Sulfa Cream
Sultrin Triple Sulfa Vaginal Tablets

ORTHO PHARMACEUTICAL CORPORATION **1448**
Dermatological Division
Route 202, P.O. Box 300
Raritan, NJ 08869-0602
(201) 524-0400
Products Available
Erycette
Grifulvin V (griseofulvin microsize) Tablets/Suspension
Meclan (meclocycline sulfosalicylate) Cream
Monistat-Derm (miconazole nitrate) Cream & Lotion
Persa-Gel (benzoyl peroxide)
Persa-Gel W (benzoyl peroxide)
▣ Purpose Dry Skin Cream
▣ Purpose Shampoo
▣ Purpose Soap
Retin-A (tretinoin) Cream/Gel/Liquid
Spectazole (econazole nitrate) Cream

OWEN LABORATORIES **1451**
Division of Dermatological Products of Texas, Inc.
San Antonio, TX 78296
An Affiliate of Alcon Laboratories, Inc.
Fort Worth, TX 76134
Products Available
Cetaphil Lotion
DesOwen Cream
Ionil Shampoo
Ionil Plus Shampoo
Ionil T Shampoo
Ionil T Plus Shampoo
Locoid Cream & Ointment
Nutracort Cream & Lotion
Nutraderm Cream & Lotion

PADDOCK LABORATORIES, INC. **1453**
3101 Louisiana Avenue North
Minneapolis, MN 55427
(800) 328-5113
In MN call collect (612) 546-4676
Address inquiries to:
Medical Department
Products Available
Acetaminophen Tablets
Acetaminophen with Codeine Tablets
Actidose, Activated Charcoal
Actidose-Aqua, Activated Charcoal
Actihist Tablets
Aluminium Paste
Ascorbic Acid Tablets
Aspirin Tablets
Aspirin Tablets, Enteric-Coated
Bacitracin Powder, USP
Benzoin Compound Tincture, USP
Betamethasone Valerate Powder, USP
Bisacodyl Tablets
Burrows Solution
Castor Oil, USP
Charcoal Tablets
Cyanocob Injectable
Decadrol Injectable
Dexamethasone Acetate Powder USP
Diapa-Kare
Docusate Calcium Tablets
Docusate Sodium Capsules
Docusate Sodium with Casanthranol Capsules
ETS-2%
▣ Emulsoil
Erythromycin Powder, USP
Fattibase
Ferrous Gluconate Tablets
Ferrous Sulfate Tablets
Folic Acid Tablets
Formalin 40% in Aquaphor
Glutol
▣ Glutose
Green Soap Tincture, USP
Hydrocortisone Acetate Powder, USP
Hydrocortisone Powder, USP
▣ Ipecac Syrup, USP
Liqua-Gel
Methylone Injectable
Methyltestosterone Powder, USP
Milk of Magnesia, USP
Neomycin Sulfate Powder, USP
Nystatin, USP, for Extemporaneous Preparation of Oral Suspension
Nystatin Powder, USP
Polybase
Polymyxin B Sulfate Powder, USP
Prednisolone Acetate Powder, USP
Prednisolone Powder, USP, Anhydrous
Prednisone Powder, USP
Progesterone Injectable
Progesterone Powder, USP, Micronized
Progesterone Powder, USP, Wettable, Microcrystalline
Schamberg Lotion
Sebacide
Sorbitol Solution, 70%
Testosterone Crystalline Injectable
Testosterone Powder, USP
Testosterone Propionate Injectable
Testosterone Propionate Powder, USP
Triamcinolone Acetonide Powder, USP
Triamcinolone Diacetate Injectable
Vehicle-S
Water for Injection
Zinc Sulfide Compound Lotion
Zincate Capsules

PALISADES PHARMACEUTICALS, INC. **1454**
219 County Road
Tenafly, NJ 07670
Address inquiries to:
Vice President (201) 569-8502
For Medical Emergencies Contact:
Vice President (201) 569-8502
Products Available
Scleromate
Yocon

PARKE-DAVIS **419, 1455, 2227**
Division of Warner-Lambert Company
201 Tabor Rd
Morris Plains, NJ 07950
(201) 540-2000
During working hours:
Product Information
(800) 223-0432
NJ, AK & HI (201) 540-2000
Medical Information
(201) 540-3950
Regional Sales Offices
Atlanta, GA 30328
1140 Hammond Drive
(404) 396-4080
Baltimore (Hunt Valley), MD 21031
11350 McCormick Road
(301) 666-7810
Chicago (Schaumburg), IL 60195
1111 Plaza Drive (312) 884-6990
Dallas, TX 75234
12200 Ford Road (214) 484-5566
Detroit (Troy), MI 48083-1160
500 Stephenson Highway
(313) 589-3292
Los Angeles (Tustin), CA 92680-2179
17822 East 17th Street
(714) 731-3441
Memphis, TN 38119-5884
1355 Lynnfield Road
(901) 767-1921
New York (Paramus, NJ) 07652
12 Route 17 North
(201) 368-0733
Pittsburgh, PA 15220-1285
Manor Oak Two
1910 Cochran Road
(412) 343-9855
Seattle (Bellevue), WA 98004
301-116th Ave, Southeast
(206) 451-1119
Products Available
ACTH Steri-Vial
Abdec Baby Vitamin Drops
Abdec with Fluoride Baby Vitamin Drops
Acetaminophen (Tapar)
Acetaminophen with Codeine Phosphate Tablets, No. 2
Acetaminophen with Codeine Phosphate Tablets, No. 3
Acetaminophen with Codeine Phosphate Tablets, No. 4
Adrenalin Chloride Solution 1:100 & 1:1,000
Alcohol, Rubbing (Lavacol)
◆ Amcill Capsules
Amcill for Oral Suspension
Amcill Pediatric Drops
◆ Amitriptyline Hydrochloride Tablets (Amitril)
Amoxicillin for Oral Suspension
◆ Amoxicillin (Utimox) Capsules
Antibiotics
◆ Amcill Products
◆ Amoxicillin Products
◆ Chloromycetin Products
Coly-Mycin Products
◆ Erythromycin Stearate Tablets (Erypar)
Humatin
Penicillin Products
◆ Penicillin V Potassium Products (Penapar VK)
◆ Tetracycline Hydrochloride Capsules, (Cyclopar) (Cyclopar 500)
◆ Anusol-HC Cream
◆ Anusol-HC Suppositories
Aplisol (tuberculin PPD, diluted)
Aplitest (tuberculin PPD, multiple-puncture device)
Aspirin Tablets
Aspirin with Codeine Phosphate Tablets, No. 2, No. 3 & No. 4
◆ Benadryl Capsules
Benadryl Elixir
◆ Benadryl Kapseals
Benadryl Parenteral
Benadryl Steri-Vials, Ampoules, and Steri-Dose Syringe
Brondecon Elixir
◆ Brondecon Tablets
Calcium Gluconate Injection
Calcium Lactate Tablets
◆ Celontin (Half Strength) Kapseals
◆ Celontin Kapseals
◆ Centrax Capsules, Tablets
Cherry Syrup
Chloramphenicol (Chloromycetin)
Chlordiazepoxide Hydrochloride Capsules
Chloromycetin Cream, 1%
Chloromycetin Hydrocortisone Ophthalmic
◆ Chloromycetin Kapseals
Chloromycetin Ophthalmic
Chloromycetin Ophthalmic Ointment, 1%
◆ Chloromycetin Ophthalmic Solution (Ophthochlor)
Chloromycetin Otic
Chloromycetin Palmitate, Oral Suspension
Chloromycetin Sodium Succinate
Chloromycetin-Polymyxin-Hydrocortisone Acetate Ophthalmic Ointment (Ophthocort)
Chlorpromazine Hydrochloride Tablets (Promapar)
Chlorthalidone Tablets, USP
Choledyl Elixir
Choledyl Pediatric Syrup
◆ Choledyl Tablets
◆ Choledyl SA Tablets
Coly-Mycin M Parenteral
Coly-Mycin S For Oral Suspension
Coly-Mycin S Otic w/Neomycin & Hydrocortisone
Corticotropin Injection (ACTH)
Cyanocobalamin Injection (Sytobex)
◆ Cyclopar & Cyclopar 500 Capsules (tetracycline hydrochloride, USP)
◆ Diazepam Tablets, USP
◆ Dilantin Infatabs
◆ Dilantin Kapseals
Dilantin, Parenteral
◆ Dilantin with Phenobarbital Kapseals
Dilantin-30 Pediatric/Dilantin-125 Suspension
◆ Diphenhydramine Hydrochloride (Benadryl)
Diphenoxylate Hydrochloride & Atropine Sulfate Tablets, USP
Dispos-A-Med Flow Path Kit
Dispos-A-Med, isoetharine hydrochloride; isoproterenol hydrochloride
Dispos-A-Med Vials, Empty
Dispos-A-Vial: Sterile Water, Normal Saline, Half Normal Saline
Docusate Sodium Capsules (D-S-S Capsules)
Docusate Sodium with Casanthranol Capsules (D-D-S Plus Capsules)
Dopamine Hydrochloride Ampoules & Vials (Dopastat)
◆ Doryx Capsules
Doxycycline Hyclate Capsules & Tablets
◆ Duraquin
◆ Easprin
◆ Elase
◆ Elase Ointment
V-Applicator (for Elase Ointment)
◆ Elase-Chloromycetin Ointment
◆ Eldec Kapseals
Epinephrine (Adrenalin)
◆ Ergostat
◆ ERYC
◆ ERYC 125 Pediatric Pellets
◆ Erythromycin Stearate Tablets (Erypar)
◆ Estrovis
◆ Ethosuximide (see Zarontin)
◆ Euthroid
Ferrous Sulfate Filmseals
Fluogen (influenza virus vaccine)
Furosemide Injection, USP
Furosemide Tablets, USP
◆ Geriplex-FS Kapseals
Geriplex-FS Liquid
Histoplasmin, Diluted
◆ Humatin Capsules
Hydrochlorothiazide Tablets, USP (Thiuretic)
◆ Indomethacin Capsules, USP
◆ Infatabs (Dilantin)
Influenza Virus Vaccine (Fluogen)
Ketalar
Ketamine Hydrochloride Injection (Ketalar)
◆ Loestrin [21] 1/20
◆ Loestrin [Fe] 1/20
◆ Loestrin [21] 1.5/30
◆ Loestrin [Fe] 1.5/30
◆ Lopid Capsules
Mandelamine Granules
Mandelamine Suspension
Mandelamine Suspension Forte
◆ Mandelamine Tablets
◆ Meclomen
◆ Methsuximide (Celontin)
◆ Methyldopa Tablets, USP
◆ Milontin Kapseals
◆ Nardil
◆ Natabec Kapseals
◆ Natabec Rx Kapseals
◆ Natabec with Fluoride Kapseals
Natabec-FA Kapseals
◆ Natafort Filmseal
◆ Nitroglycerin Tablets (Nitrostat)
◆ Nitrostat Ointment 2%
◆ Nitrostat Tablets
◆ Nitrostat IV Ampoules
Nitrostat IV Infusion Kit
◆ Norethindrone Acetate and Ethinyl Estradiol Tablets (Loestrin, Norlestrin)
◆ Norlestrin [21] 1/50
◆ Norlestrin [21] 2.5/50
Norlestrin [28] 1/50
◆ Norlestrin [Fe] 1/50
◆ Norlestrin [Fe] 2.5/50
◆ Norlutate

(◆ Shown in Product Identification Section) (▣ Described in PDR For Nonprescription Drugs)

- ◆ Norlutin
- ◆ Ophthochlor Ophthalmic Solution, 0.5%
- Ophthocort Ophthalmic Ointment
- Oxytocin Injection (Pitocin)
- ◆ Paromomycin (Humatin)
- ◆ Parsidol
- Penicillin G Potassium for Injection
- Penicillin V Potassium for Oral Solution
- ◆ Penicillin V Potassium Tablets (Penapar VK)
- ◆ Peritrate Sustained Action
- ◆ Peritrate Tablets
- Phenobarbital Tablets
- ◆ Phensuximide (Milontin)
- ◆ Phenytoin Sodium (Dilantin)
- Pitocin Injection, Ampoules, Steri-Dose Syringes
- Pitressin Synthetic, Ampoules
- Pitressin Tannate in Oil Ampoules
- Pituitrin-S Ampoules
- Poison Ivy Extract
- ◆ Ponstel
- Prazepam Capsules
- ◆ Procan SR Tablets
- ◆ Proloid Tablets
- Propoxyphene Hydrochloride Capsules
- ◆ Pyridium
- ◆ Pyridium Plus
- Quinidine Sulfate Tablets
- Quinine Sulfate Capsules
- ◆ Sinubid
- Spironolactone Tablets, USP
- Spironolactone w/Hydrochlorothiazide Tablets
- Surital Ampoules, Steri-Vials
- Sytobex (Cyanocobalamin Injection)
- ◆ Tabron Filmseal
- ◆ Tedral
- Tedral Elixir
- ◆ Tedral SA
- Tedral Suspension
- ◆ Tedral Tablets
- ◆ Tedral-25 Tablets
- Terpin Hydrate & Codeine Elixir
- ◆ Tetracycline HCl Capsules (Cyclopar)
- ◆ Tetracycline HCl Capsules (Cyclopar 500)
- Theelin Aqueous Suspension
- Thiamylal Sodium (Surital)
- Thiuretic (Hydrochlorothiazide Tablets)
- Thrombostat
- Tuberculin, Aplisol and Aplitest
- Unibase
- ◆ Uticort Cream, Gel, Lotion & Ointment
- V-Applicators for Elase Ointment
- Vasopressin Injection (Pitressin)
- Vira-A for Infusion
- ◆ Vira-A Ophthalmic Ointment, 3%
- ◆ Zarontin Capsules
- Zarontin Syrup

PEDINOL PHARMACAL INC. 1548
30 Banfi Plaza North
Farmingdale, NY 11735
Address inquiries to:
Director of Professional Services
(516) 293-9500
Products Available
- Alginate Styptic Gauze
- Breezee Mist Foot Powder
- Castellani Paint
- Fungoid Creme & Solution
- Fungoid Tincture
- G-myticin Creme and Ointment 0.1%
- Hydrisalic Gel
- Hydrisea Lotion
- Hydrisinol Creme & Lotion
- Lazer Creme
- LazerFormalyde Solution
- LazerSporin-C Solution
- Osti-Derm Lotion
- PNS Unna Boot
- Pedi-Bath Salts
- Pedi-Boro Soak Paks
- Pedi-Cort V Creme
- Pedi-Dri Foot Powder
- Pedi-Pro Foot Powder
- Pedi-Vit A Creme
- Salactic Film
- Steri Unna Boot
- Ureacin Lotion & Creme

PENNWALT PRESCRIPTION DIVISION 422, 1550
Pennwalt Corporation
755 Jefferson Road
Rochester, NY 14623
Address inquiries to:
Director of Professional Relations
P.O. Box 1766
Rochester, NY 14603
(716) 475-9000
Products Available
- ◆ Adapin Capsules
- ◆ Biphetamine Capsules
- Cholan HMB Tablets
- Cholan-DH Tablets
- Emul-O-Balm Liquid
- ◆ Hylorel Tablets
- Infalyte Powder
- ◆ Ionamin Capsules
- Kolyum Liquid and Powder
- Penntuss Suspension
- Tussionex Capsules
- Tussionex Suspension
- Tussionex Tablets
- ◆ Zaroxolyn Tablets

PERSŌN & COVEY, INC. 1554
616 Allen Avenue
Glendale, CA 91201
Address inquiries to:
Lorne V. Persōn, President
(818) 240-1030
(800) 423-2341
Products Available
- ▣ DHS Conditioning Rinse
- ▣ DHS Shampoo
- ▣ DHS Tar Gel Shampoo
- ▣ DHS Tar Shampoo
- ▣ DHS Zinc Dandruff Shampoo
- ▣ DML Mositurizing Lotion
- Drysol
- ▣ Solbar PF 15 Cream (Paba Free)
- ▣ Solbar PF 15 Liquid (Paba Free)
- ▣ Solbar Plus 15 Cream
- ▣ Xerac
- Xerac AC
- ▣ Xerac BP5 & BP10

PFIPHARMECS DIVISION 1555
Pfizer Inc.
235 E. 42nd St.
New York, NY 10017
Address inquiries to:
Professional Services Dept.
(212) 573-2323
See LEEMING DIVISION, ROERIG & PFIZER

PFIZER LABORATORIES DIVISION 422, 1555
Pfizer Inc.
235 E. 42nd St.
New York, NY 10017
Address inquiries to:
Professional Services Dept.
(212) 573-2422
Medical Emergency Calls (Day or Night) (212) 573-2422
Address Export inquiries to:
Pfizer International Inc.
(212) 573-2323
Distribution Centers
Doraville, GA 30340
4360 Northeast Expressway
(404) 448-6666
Hoffman Estates, IL 60196
2400 W. Central Road
(312) 381-9500
Clifton, NJ 07012
230 Brighton Rd. (201) 546-7700
Grand Prairie, TX 75050
502 Fountain Parkway
(214) 647-0222
Irvine, CA 92714
16700 Red Hill Ave.
(714) 540-9180
Products Available
- ◆ Antiminth Oral Suspension
- Cortril Hydrocortisone Topical Ointment 1%
- ◆ Diabinese Tablets
- ◆ Feldene Capsules
- ◆ Minipress Capsules
- ◆ Minizide Capsules
- ◆ Moderil Tablets
- ◆ Procardia Capsules
- ◆ Renese Tablets
- ◆ Renese-R Tablets
- ◆ Sustaire Sustained Release Tablets
- ◆ Terramycin Capsules
- ◆ Vansil Capsules
- Vibramycin Calcium Syrup
- ◆ Vibramycin Hyclate Capsules
- Vibramycin Monohydrate for Oral Suspension
- ◆ Vibra-Tabs Film Coated Tablets
- ◆ Vistaril Capsules
- Vistaril Oral Suspension

PHARMACIA LABORATORIES 422, 1570
Pharmacia Inc.
800 Centennial Ave.
Piscataway, NJ 08854
Address inquiries to:
Medical Director (201) 457-8000
Products Available
- ◆ Azulfidine Tablets, EN-tabs, Oral Suspension
- Hyskon Hysteroscopy Fluid
- Macrodex
- Rheomacrodex

PHARMACRAFT DIVISION 1572
Pennwalt Corporation
755 Jefferson Road
Rochester, NY 14623
Address inquiries to:
Professional Service Department
P.O. Box 1212
Rochester, NY 14603
(716) 475-9000
Products Available
- ▣ Allerest Tablets, Childrens Chewable Tablets, Headache Strength Tablets, Sinus Pain Formula Tablets, Eye Drops, 12 Hour Capsules, & 12 Hour Nasal Spray
- ▣ CaldeCORT Hydrocortisone Multi-Purpose Anti-Itch Cream and Spray
- ▣ CaldeCORT Light Creme
- ▣ Caldesene Medicated Baby Powder & Ointment
- ▣ Cruex Antifungal Powder, Spray Powder & Cream
- ▣ Desenex Antifungal Powder, Spray Powder, Cream, Ointment, Liquid & Penetrating Foam
- ▣ Sinarest Tablets, Extra Strength Tablets & 12 Hour Nasal Spray

PHARMADERM 1572
a division of Altana Inc.
60 Baylis Road
Melville, NY 11747
Address inquiries to:
Customer Service Dept.
(800) 645-9432
(516) 454-8884
- Betamethasone Dipropionate Cream, Ointment & Lotion
- Betamethasone Valerate Cream, Ointment & Lotion
- Fluocinolone Acetonide Cream, Ointment & Topical Solution
- Gentamicin Sulfate Cream & Ointment USP
- Hydrocortisone Cream & Ointment
- Nystatin Cream, Ointment, Vaginal Tablets & Oral Suspension
- Nystatin-Triamcinolone Acetonide Cream & Ointment
- Triamcinolone Acetonide Cream & Ointment
- Triple Sulfa Vaginal Cream

PHARMAFAIR, INC. 1573
110 Kennedy Drive
Hauppauge, NY 11788
Address inquiries to:
Stuart Shansinger 1-(800) 227-1427
or 1-(516) 231-0707
Products Available
- Aurafair Otic Solution
- Balanced Salt Solution
- Benzoyl Peroxide Gel
- Borofair Otic
- Cortifair Cream 1%
- Ear Drops
- Erythromycin Ethylsuccinate Oral Suspension 200 mg/5 ml & 400 mg/5 ml
- Erythromycin 2% Topical Solution
- Gentafair Cream, Ointment & Injectables
- Nystatin Oral Suspension, USP
- Octicair Otic Solution & Suspension
- Procainamide HCl Pronestyl Injectables
- Tolnaftate 1% Topical Cream & Solution
- Topisporin

POYTHRESS LABORATORIES, INC. 1573
16 N. 22nd St.
Post Office Box 26946
Richmond, VA 23261
(804) 644-8591
Address inquiries to:
Special Services Department
Products Available
- Antrocol Tablets, Capsules & Elixir
- Bensulfoid Lotion
- Bensulfoid Powder
- Bensulfoid Tablets
- Lodrane Capsules (Sustained Release)-130 & 260
- Lodrane CR Tablets (Continuous Release)—100, 200 & 300 mg
- Mudrane GG Elixir
- Mudrane GG Tablets
- Mudrane GG-2 Tablets
- Mudrane Tablets
- Mudrane-2 Tablets
- ▣ Panalgesic Liniment & Cream
- Solfoton Tablets & Capsules
- Uro-Phosphate Tablets

PRINCETON PHARMACEUTICAL PRODUCTS 422, 1574
(A Squibb Company)
P.O. Box 4000
Princeton, NJ 08543-4000
(201) 359-9700
Address inquiries to:
Squibb Professional Services Dept.
P.O. Box 4000
Princeton, NJ 08543-4000
(609) 921-4006
Direct orders to:
E. R. Squibb and Sons, Inc.
(Local Distribution Center)
Products Available
- ◆ Corgard
- ◆ Corzide
- Halog Cream, Ointment, Solution & Emollient
- Halog-E Cream
- ◆ Naturetin Tablets
- Naturetin with K Tablets
- Prolixin Decanoate
- Prolixin Elixir
- Prolixin Enanthate
- Prolixin Injection
- Prolixin Oral Concentrate
- ◆ Prolixin Tablets
- ◆ Pronestyl Capsules and Tablets
- Pronestyl Injection
- ◆ Pronestyl-SR Tablets
- ◆ Raudixin Tablets
- Rautrax Tablets
- Rautrax-N Tablets
- ◆ Rauzide Tablets
- Vesprin Injection

PROCTER & GAMBLE 422, 1588
P.O. Box 171
Cincinnati, OH 45201
Also see Norwich Eaton Pharmaceuticals, Inc. & Vicks Health Care Products
Address inquiries to:
Larry W. Farrell (513) 530-2154
For Medical Emergencies Contact:
J. B. Lucas, M.D. (513) 530-3350
After Hours, call COLLECT
(513) 751-5525
Products Available
- ◆ Head & Shoulders
- ▣ Icy Hot Balm
- ▣ Icy Hot Rub
- ▣ Icy Hot Stick
- Metamucil, Instant Mix, Sugar Free, Lemon-Lime Flavor
- Metamucil, Instant Mix, Sugar Free, Orange Flavor
- Metamucil, Powder, Orange Flavor
- Metamucil, Powder, Regular Flavor
- Metamucil, Powder, Strawberry Flavor
- Metamucil, Powder, Sugar Free, Orange Flavor
- Metamucil, Powder, Sugar Free, Regular Flavor
- Pepto-Bismol Liquid & Tablets
- Peridex
- ▣ Tempo Antacid Tablets

THE PURDUE FREDERICK COMPANY 423, 1591
100 Connecticut Avenue
Norwalk, CT 06856
(203) 853-0123
Address inquiries to:
Medical Department
Products Available
- Arthropan Liquid
- Betadine Aerosol Spray
- Betadine Antiseptic Gauze Pad
- Betadine Antiseptic Gel
- Betadine Antiseptic Lubricating Gel
- Betadine Disposable Medicated Douche
- Betadine Hëlafoam Solution
- Betadine Medicated Douche
- Betadine Medicated Douche Kit
- Betadine Mouthwash/Gargle
- Betadine Ointment
- Betadine Perineal Wash Concentrate Kit
- Betadine Shampoo
- Betadine Skin Cleanser
- Betadine Skin Cleanser Foam
- Betadine Solution
- Betadine Solution Swab Aid
- Betadine Solution Swabsticks
- Betadine Surgical Scrub
- Betadine Surgi-Prep Sponge-Brush
- Betadine Vaginal Suppositories
- Betadine Viscous Formula Antiseptic Gauze Pad
- Betadine Whirlpool Concentrate
- ◆ Cardioquin Tablets
- Cerumenex Drops
- Fibermed High-Fiber Supplements
- Fibermed Snacks
- ◆ MS Contin Tablets
- MSIR Oral Solution
- MSIR Oral Solution Concentrate
- ◆ MSIR Tablets
- Phyllocontin
- Senokap DSS Capsules
- Senokot Granules
- Senokot Suppositories
- Senokot Syrup
- Senokot Tablets
- Senokot Tablets Unit Strip Pack
- Senokot-S Tablets
- Trilisate Liquid
- ◆ Trilisate Tablets
- ◆ Uniphyl 200 mg Tablets
- ◆ Uniphyl 400 mg Tablets

BLAIR LABORATORIES, INC.
- Calamatum Lotion
- Calamatum Ointment
- Calamatum Spray
- Fungacetin Ointment
- Gentlax B Granules
- Gentlax S Tablets
- Kerid Ear Drops
- Saratoga Ointment

RAM LABORATORIES CORPORATION 1601
P. O. Box 559071
Miami, FL 33255
Address inquiries to:
In the United States
(305) 264-6620
In Puerto Rico (809) 792-2002
Products Available
- Algisin Capsules
- Apetil Liquid
- Digepepsin Tablets
- Geroton Forte
- Neurochol Capsules
- Otisan Drops
- Pasmol Tablets
- Tusibron
- Tusibron-DM
- Zincvit Capsules

REED & CARNRICK 423, 1601
1 New England Avenue
Piscataway, NJ 08854
Address inquiries to:
Professional Service Dept.
(201) 981-0070
Products Available
Alphosyl Lotion, Cream
Colyte
◆ Cortifoam
◆ Dilatrate-SR
◆ Epifoam
Kwell Cream
◆ Kwell Lotion
◆ Kwell Shampoo
◆ Phazyme Tablets
◆ Phazyme-95 Tablets
◆ Phazyme-125 Capsules
◆ Phazyme-PB Tablets
Proctofoam-HC
proctoFoam/non-steroid
Proxigel
◆ R&C Shampoo
R&C Spray
Trichotine Liquid, Vaginal Douche
Trichotine Powder, Vaginal Douche

REID-PROVIDENT LABORATORIES, INC.
See REID-ROWELL

REID-ROWELL 423, 1608
Corporate Offices & Manufacturing
901 Sawyer Road
Marietta, GA 30062
(404) 578-9000
Address inquiries to:
Robert E. Matthews
(404) 578-2015
Orders may be placed by calling this toll-free number: (800) 241-1643
Mail orders should be sent to:
Reid-Rowell
Order Entry Department
901 Sawyer Road
Marietta, GA 30062
Manufacturing
210 Main Street, W.
Baudette, MN 56623
Toll Free (800) 346-5040
In MN (800) 542-5012
Products Available
Aquatag Tablets
Bacarate Tablets
▣ Balneol
C-Ron
C-Ron Forte
Calinate-FA Tablets
◆ Chenix
Cino-40 Injection
Cin-Quin
Codap Tablets
Colrex Compound Capsules
Colrex Compound Elixir
Colrex Expectorant
Colrex Syrup
Colrex Troches
◆ Compal Capsules
◆ Cortenema
Crystimin-1000 Injection
◆ Curretab Tablets
Dermacort Cream
Dermacort Lotion-0.5%, 1%
Dexone 0.5, 0.75, 1.5, 4
Dezone Injectable
Duoval P.A. Injection
Estraguard Vaginal Cream
◆ Estratab Tablets
◆ Estratest H.S. Tablets
◆ Estratest Tablets
Estraval 2X Injection
Estraval 4X Injection
Estraval-P.A. Injection
Femguard Vaginal Cream
Fluoxymesterone Tablets
Fumatrin Forte Tablets
Histalet DM Syrup
◆ Histalet Forte Tablets
Histalet Syrup
Histalet X Syrup
◆ Histalet X Tablets
▣ Hydrocil Instant
Hyproval P.A. Injection
L.A. Dezone Injection
Lithonate
Lithotabs
Melfiat Tablets
◆ Melfiat 105 Unicelles
Multivitamins Rowell
Neotep Granucaps
Norlac
Norlac RX
Orasone 1, 5, 10, 20, 50
Otoreid-HC Ear Drops
◆ P-V-Tussin Syrup
◆ P-V-Tussin Tablets
Pavacap Unicelles
Perifoam
Pre-Dep 40 Injection
Pre-Dep 80 Injection
Pre-Enthus FA Capsules
Proaqua Tablets
◆ Proctocort
Proval #3 Capsules
Provigan Injection
Quine Capsules
Quinidine Sulfate Capsules & Tablets
Reidamine Injection
Retet-250 Capsules
Retet-500 Capsules
Ro-Bile
Ru-Vert-M Tablets
SPRX-3 Capsules
SPRX-105 Capsules
Tranmep Tablets
Tuzon Tablets
Unifast Unicelles
Unipres Tablets
Unproco Capsules
Vio-Bec
Vio-Bec Forte
◆ Zenate Tablets

RESEARCH INDUSTRIES CORPORATION 1614
Pharmaceutical Division
1847 West 2300 South
Salt Lake City, UT 84119
Address inquiries to:
Medical Department
(800) 453-8432
(801) 972-5500
For Medical Emergencies Contact:
Medical Department
(800) 453-8432
(801) 972-5500
Products Available
Rimso-50

RICHARDSON-VICKS INC. HEALTH CARE PRODUCTS DIVISION 423, 1614
10 Westport Road
Wilton, CT 06897
Address inquiries to:
Vicks Research Center
(203) 929-2500
For Medical Emergencies Contact
Medical Director
Vicks Research Center
(203) 929-2500
Products Available
Chloraseptic Preparations
Children's Chloraseptic Lozenges
Chloraseptic Liquid
Chloraseptic Lozenges, Cherry or Menthol
▣ Cremacoat 1
▣ Cremacoat 2
▣ Cremacoat 3
▣ Cremacoat 4
Dramamine Liquid
Dramamine Tablets
Head & Chest
◆ Percogesic Analgesic Tablets
▣ Vicks Childrens Cough Syrup
▣ Vicks Cough Silencers Cough Drops
▣ Vicks Daycare Daytime Colds Medicine-liquid
▣ Vicks Daycare Multi-Symptom Colds Medicine-capsules
▣ Vicks Formula 44 Cough Control Disc
▣ Vicks Formula 44 Cough Mixture
▣ Vicks Formula 44D Decongestant Cough Mixture
▣ Vicks Formula 44M Multi-Symptom Cough Mixture
▣ Vicks Inhaler
▣ Vicks Nyquil Nighttime Colds Medicine
Vicks Oracin Cherry Flavor Cooling Throat Lozenges
Vicks Oracin Cooling Throat Lozenges
▣ Vicks Sinex Decongestant Nasal Spray
▣ Vicks Sinex Long-Acting Decongestant Nasal Spray
▣ Vicks Throat Lozenges
▣ Vicks Vaporub
▣ Vicks Vaposteam
▣ Vicks Vatronol Nose Drops

RICHARDSON-VICKS, INC. PERSONAL CARE PRODUCTS DIVISION 1616
10 Westport Road
Wilton, CT 06897
Address inquiries to:
Vicks Research Center
(203) 929-2500
For Medical Emergencies Contact
Medical Information
(301) 528-2425
Products Available
▣ Clearasil Adult Care (Sulfur/Resorcinol)
▣ Clearasil 10% Benzoyl Peroxide Medicated Anti-Acne Lotion
▣ Clearasil Maximum Strength Medicated Anti-Acne Cream (10% Benzoyl Peroxide)
▣ Clearasil Medicated Astrigent (Salicylic Acid 0.5%)
▣ Denquel Sensitive Teeth Toothpaste

RIKER LABORATORIES, INC. 423, 1617
Subsidiary of 3M
225-1S-07 3M Center
St. Paul, MN 55144
For Medical Information
Write: Medical Services Department
Riker Laboratories, Inc.
225-1N-07 3M Center
St. Paul, MN 55144
Call: (612) 736-4930
For Medical Emergencies
Call: (612) 736-4930 (all hours)
Customer Service and other services:
Call: (800) 423-5197
or 423-5146 (Outside of CA only)
(818) 341-1300 (CA Residents)
Products Available
Alu-Cap Capsules
Alu-Tab Tablets
Calcium Disodium Versenate Injection
◆ Disalcid Capsules
◆ Disalcid Tablets
Disipal Tablets
Duo-Medihaler Aerosol
Estomul-M Liquid & Tablets
◆ Medihaler Ergotamine Aerosol
Medihaler-Epi Aerosol
Medihaler-Iso Aerosol
◆ Norflex Injectable
◆ Norflex Sustained-Release Tablets
◆ Norgesic Tablets
◆ Norgesic Forte Tablets
Rauwiloid Tablets
◆ Tambocor Tablets
◆ Tepanil Tablets
◆ Tepanil Ten-tab Tablets
Theolair Liquid
◆ Theolair Tablets
Theolair-Plus Tablets & Liquid
◆ Theolair-SR Tablets
◆ Urex Tablets

A. H. ROBINS COMPANY 424, 1623
Pharmaceutical Division
1407 Cummings Drive
Richmond, VA 23220
Address inquiries to:
The Medical Dept. (804) 257-2000
Medical Emergency calls
(day or night) (804) 257-2000
If no answer, call answering service
(804) 257-7788
Products Available
▣ Allbee C-800 Plus Iron Tablets
▣ Allbee C-800 Tablets
▣ Allbee w/C Capsules
Allbee-T Tablets
Arthralgen Tablets
Cough Calmers
▣ Dimacol Capsules
Dimacol Liquid
Dimetane-DC Cough Syrup
Dimetane-DX Cough Syrup
▣ Dimetane Decongestant Elixir
▣ Dimetane Decongestant Tablets
▣ Dimetane Elixir
▣ Dimetane Extentabs
▣ Dimetane Tablets
Dimetane-Ten Injectable
▣ Dimetapp Elixir
▣ Dimetapp Extentabs
▣ Donnagel
Donnagel-PG
◆ Donnatal Capsules
Donnatal Elixir
◆ Donnatal Extentabs
Donnatal No. 2 Tablets
◆ Donnatal Tablets
◆ Donnazyme Tablets
◆ Dopram Injectable
◆ Entozyme Tablets
◆ Exna Tablets
◆ Micro-K Extencaps
◆ Micro-K 10 Extencaps
◆ Mitrolan Chewable Tablets
◆ Pabalate Tablets
◆ Pabalate-SF Tablets
◆ Phenaphen Capsules
◆ Phenaphen w/Codeine Capsules
◆ Phenaphen-650 with Codeine Tablets
◆ Pondimin Tablets
◆ Quinidex Extentabs
◆ Reglan Injectable
Reglan Syrup
◆ Reglan Tablets
◆ Robaxin Injectable
◆ Robaxin Tablets
◆ Robaxin-750 Tablets
◆ Robaxisal Tablets
Robicillin VK Robitabs
Robimycin Robitabs
◆ Robinul Forte Tablets
◆ Robinul Injectable
◆ Robinul Tablets
Robitet '250' Hydrochloride Robicaps
Robitet '500' Hydrochloride Robicaps
▣ Robitussin
Robitussin A-C
▣ Robitussin-CF
Robitussin-DAC
▣ Robitussin-DM
▣ Robitussin Night Relief
▣ Robitussin-PE
Silain Tablets
Silain-Gel Liquid
Viokase Powder
◆ Viokase Tablets
▣ Z-Bec Tablets

ROCHE LABORATORIES 424, 1641, 2229
Division of Hoffmann-La Roche Inc.
Nutley, NJ 07110 (201) 235-5000
For Medical Information
Write: Professional Services Department
Business hours only (8:30 a.m. to 5:00 p.m. EST), call
(201) 235-2355
For Medical Emergency Information only after hours or on weekends, call
(201) 235-2355
Branch Warehouse
Belvidere, NJ 07823-0200
200 Roche Drive (201) 475-5337
Products Available
◆ Accutane Capsules
Alurate Elixir
◆ Ancobon Capsules
Arfonad Ampuls
◆ Azo Gantanol Tablets
◆ Azo Gantrisin Tablets
◆ Bactrim DS Tablets
Bactrim I.V. Infusion
Bactrim Pediatric Suspension
Bactrim Suspension
◆ Bactrim Tablets
Berocca Parenteral Nutrition
◆ Berocca Plus Tablets
◆ Berocca Tablets
Bumex Injection
◆ Bumex Tablets
◆ Clonopin—see Klonopin
Coactin Injectable
Efudex Cream
Efudex Solution
◆ Emcyt Capsules
FUDR Injectable
◆ Fansidar Tablets
Fluorouracil Injection
◆ Gantanol DS Tablets
Gantanol Suspension
◆ Gantanol Tablets
Gantrisin Ophthalmic Ointment/Solution
Gantrisin Pediatric Suspension
Gantrisin Syrup
◆ Gantrisin Tablets
◆ Klonopin Tablets
Konakion Injectable
◆ Larobec Tablets
◆ Larodopa Capsules
◆ Larodopa Tablets
Levo-Dromoran Injectable
◆ Levo-Dromoran Tablets
◆ Marplan Tablets
◆ Matulane Capsules
Mestinon Injectable
Mestinon Syrup
◆ Mestinon Tablets
◆ Mestinon Timespan
Nipride Injectable
◆ Noludar Tablets
◆ Noludar 300 Capsules
Pantopon Injectable
Prostigmin Injectable
◆ Prostigmin Tablets
◆ Rocaltrol Capsules
Rocephin Injectable
Roferon-A
◆ Solatene Capsules
Synkayvite Injectable
◆ Synkayvite Tablets
Taractan Concentrate
Taractan Injectable
◆ Taractan Tablets
◆ Tel-E-Dose (unit dose) Products:
Bactrim Tablets
Bactrim DS Tablets
Bumex Tablets
Gantanol Tablets
Gantrisin Tablets
Trimpex Tablets
Tensilon Injectable
◆ Trimpex Tablets
◆ Valrelease Capsules
VERSED Injection
◆ Vi-Penta F Chewables
Vi-Penta F Infant Drops
Vi-Penta F Multivitamin Drops
Vi-Penta Infant Drops
Vi-Penta Multivitamin Drops
Vitamin K—see Synkayvite
Vitamin K_1—see Konakion

ROCHE PRODUCTS INC. 424, 1688
Manati, Puerto Rico 00701
Address inquiries to:
Roche Laboratories
(see above)
Products Available
◆ Dalmane Capsules
◆ Endep Tablets
◆ Librax Capsules
◆ Libritabs Tablets
◆ Librium Capsules
Librium Injectable
◆ Limbitrol Tablets
◆ Limbitrol DS Tablets
◆ Menrium Tablets
◆ Quarzan Capsules
◆ Tel-E-Dose (unit dose) Products:
Dalmane Capsules
Endep Tablets
Librax Capsules
Librium Capsules
Limbitrol Tablets
Limbitrol DS Tablets
Valium Tablets
◆ Valium Injectable
◆ Valium Tablets
◆ Valium Tel-E-Ject

ROERIG 425, 1699
A division of Pfizer Pharmaceuticals
235 E. 42nd St.
New York, NY 10017

Address inquiries to:
Medical Department
(212) 573-2187
Branch Offices
Doraville, GA 30340
4360 N.E. Expressway
(Southern Region) (404) 448-6666
Hoffman Estates, IL 60196
2400 W. Central Road
(312) 381-9500
(Midwestern & Great Lakes Regions)
Clifton, NJ 07012
230 Brighton Road
(Metro Region) (201) 546-7700
Dallas, TX 75222
P.O. Box 22249
(Southwestern Region)
(214) 647-0222
Irvine, CA 92705
16700 Red Hill Ave.
(Western Region) (714) 540-9180
Products Available
◆ Antivert, Antivert/25 Tablets, Antivert/25 Chewable Tablets & Antivert/50 Tablets
◆ Atarax Tablets & Syrup
Cefobid Intravenous/Intramuscular
Emete-con Intramuscular/Intravenous
◆ Geocillin Tablets
Geopen Intramuscular/Intravenous
◆ Glucotrol
◆ Heptuna Plus Capsules
◆ Marax Tablets & DF Syrup
◆ Navane Capsules and Concentrate
Navane Intramuscular
Pfizerpen for Injection
Pfizerpen-AS Aqueous Suspension
◆ Sinequan Capsules
Sinequan Oral Concentrate
◆ Spectrobid Tablets & Oral Suspension
Streptomycin Sulfate
◆ Tao Capsules
Terra-Cortril Ophthalmic Suspension
Terramycin Intramuscular Solution
Terramycin with Polymyxin B Sulfate Ophthalmic Ointment
◆ Urobiotic-250 Capsules
Vibramycin Hyclate Intravenous
Vistaril Intramuscular Solution

WILLIAM H. RORER, INC. 426, 1723
500 Virginia Drive
Fort Washington, PA 19034
For Medical Emergencies Contact:
Product Surveillance
(215) 628-6761
For Quality Matters Contact:
Quality Assurance/Regulatory Affairs
(215) 628-6000
For Product Information Contact:
Arnold Yeadon, M.D.
Vice President, Medical Affairs
(215) 628-6159
Products Available
◆ Algicon Tablets
◆ Ascriptin Tablets
◆ Ascriptin A/D Tablets
Ascriptin w/codeine Tablets
◆ Azmacort Inhaler
▣ Camalox Suspension
▣ Camalox Tablets
◆ Double Strength Maalox Tablets
▣ Emetrol Solution
◆ Extra Strength Ascriptin
▣ Fermalox Tablets
▣ Maalox Suspension
◆ Maalox Tablets
▣ Maalox Plus Suspension
◆ Maalox Plus Tablets
▣ Maalox TC Suspension
◆ Maalox TC Tablets
◆ Nitrol IV Concentrate
◆ Nitrol Ointment
◆ Nitrolingual Spray
Parepectolin Suspension
◆ Perdiem Granules
◆ Perdiem Plain Granules
◆ Slo-bid Gyrocaps
◆ Slo-Phyllin Gyrocaps
◆ Slo-Phyllin Tablets
Slo-Phyllin 80 Syrup
◆ Slo-Phyllin GG Capsules
Slo-Phyllin GG Syrup
For the following products, please see Kremers-Urban Company
Calciferol Drops (Ergocalciferol Oral Solution USP)
Calciferol in Oil Injection (Ergocalciferol USP)
Calciferol Tablets (Ergocalciferol USP)
Chardonna-2 Tablets
Fedahist Expectorant
Fedahist Gyrocaps
Fedahist Syrup
Fedahist Tablets
Gemnisyn
Kudrox Suspension (Double Strength)
Kutapressin Injection
Kutrase Capsules
Ku-Zyme Capsules
Ku-Zyme HP Capsules
Lactrase Capsules
Levsin Drops
Levsin Elixir
Levsin Injection
Levsin Tablets
Levsin-PB Drops
Levsin Phenobarbital Elixir
Levsin Phenobarbital Tablets
Levsinex Timecaps
Levsinex Phenobarbital Timecaps
Milkinol
Pre-Pen
Salimeph Forte

ROSS LABORATORIES 426, 1735
Div. Abbott Laboratories
Columbus, OH 43216
Address inquiries to:
Henry S. Sauls, M.D., Vice President, Medical Affairs (614) 227-3333
Products Available
Advance
Clear Eyes
Component Nipple System
Ear Drops by Murine—See Murine Ear Wax Removal System
Enrich
Ensure
Ensure HN
Ensure Plus
Ensure Plus HN
Ensure Pudding
Flexiflo Enteral Delivery System
Flexiflo Enteral Feeding Tube, 8 French
Flexiflo Enteral Feeding Tube, 8 French w/Stylet
Flexiflo Enteral Feeding Tube, 12 French
Flexiflo Enteral Nutrition Pump
Flexiflo Enteral Pump Set
Flexiflo Pump Set with Piercing Pin
Flexiflo-II Enteral Pump Set
Flexiflo-II Portable Enteral Nutrition Pump
Flexiflo-II Pump Set with Piercing Pin
Flexiflo-III Enteral Nutrition Pump
Flexiflo-III Enteral Pump Set
Flexiflo-III Pump Set with Piercing Pin
Flexiflo Gravity Gavage Set
Flexiflo Gravity Feeding Set with Piercing Pin
Flexiflo Top-Fill Enteral Nutrition System
Flexiflo Top-Fill Enteral Nutrition System with Preattached Flexiflo Pump Set
Flexiflo Top-Fill Enteral Nutrition System with Preattached Flexiflo-II Pump Set
Flexiflo Top-Fill Enteral Nutrition System with Preattached Flexiflo-III Pump Set
Flexiflo Top-Fill Enteral Nutrition System with Preattached Gravity Gavage Set
Flexitainer Enteral Nutrition Container
Flexitainer 500 Enteral Nutrition Container
Glucose Water 5% & 10%
Isomil
Isomil 20
Isomil SF
Isomil SF 20
Murine Ear Drops
Murine Ear Wax Removal System
Murine Eye Lubricant (Regular Formula)
Murine Plus Tetrahydrozoline HCl Eye Redness Reliever
Osmolite
Osmolite HN
Pediaflor
Pedialyte
Pedialyte RS
Pediamycin
Pediazole
Polycose
◆ Pramet FA
◆ Pramilet FA
ProMod
Pulmocare
RCF
Rondec Oral Drops
Rondec Syrup
◆ Rondec Tablet
Rondec-DM Oral Drops
Rondec-DM Syrup
◆ Rondec-TR Tablet
Ross Hospital Formula System
Ross SLD
Selsun Blue Dandruff Shampoo
Similac
Similac Natural Care
Similac PM 60/40
Similac 13
Similac 20
Similac 24
Similac 24 LBW
Similac 27
Similac Special Care 20
Similac Special Care 24
Similac With Iron
Similac With Iron 13
Similac With Iron 20
Similac With Iron 24
Similac With Whey + Iron 20
Sterilized Water
Tronolane Anesthetic Hemorrhoidal Cream
Tronolane Anesthetic Hemorrhoidal Suppositories
TwoCal HN
Vari-Flavors Flavor Pacs
Vi-Daylin ADC Vitamins Drops
Vi-Daylin ADC Vitamins + Iron Drops
◆ Vi-Daylin Multivitamin Chewable Tablets
Vi-Daylin Multivitamin Drops
Vi-Daylin Multivitamin Liquid
◆ Vi-Daylin Multivitamin + Iron Chewable Tablets
Vi-Daylin Multivitamin + Iron Drops
Vi-Daylin Multivitamin + Iron Liquid
Vi-Daylin/F ADC Vitamins Drops With Fluoride
Vi-Daylin/F ADC Vitamins + Iron Drops With Fluoride
◆ Vi-Daylin/F Tablets With Fluoride
Vi-Daylin/F Multivitamin Drops With Fluoride
◆ Vi-Daylin/F Multivitamin + Iron Chewable Tablets With Fluoride
Vi-Daylin/F Multivitamin + Iron Drops With Fluoride
Vital High Nitrogen
Volu-Feed

ROWELL LABORATORIES, INC.
See REID-ROWELL

ROXANE LABORATORIES, INC. 426, 1758
1809 Wilson Road
Columbus, OH 43228
Address inquiries to:
Professional Services Department
P.O. 16532
Columbus, OH 43216
(Toll Free) (800) 848-0120
(In Ohio call) (614) 228-5403
Products Available
Acetaminophen Elixir (Cherry)
Acetaminophen Elixir (Lime)
Acetaminophen Suppositories
Acetaminophen Tablets
Acetaminophen and Codeine Phosphate Elixir
Acetaminophen and Codeine Phosphate Tablets
Aluminum Hydroxide Gel
Aluminum Hydroxide Gel Concentrated
Aluminum Hydroxide Tablets
Aluminum & Magnesium Hydroxides with Simethicone I
Aluminum & Magnesium Hydroxides with Simethicone II
Aminophylline Tablets & Oral Solution
Amitriptyline Hydrochloride Tablets
Aromatic Cascara Fluidextract
Aromatic Castor Oil
Ascorbic Acid Tablets
Aspirin Suppositories
Bisacodyl Patient Pack
Bisacodyl Suppositories
Bisacodyl Tablets
Calcium Carbonate Tablets, Chewable Tablets & Oral Suspension
Calcium Gluconate Tablets
Castor Oil
Chloral Hydrate Capsules
Chloral Hydrate Syrup
Chlorpheniramine Maleate Tablets
Chlorpromazine Hydrochloride Intensol
Cocaine Hydrochloride Topical Solution
Codeine Phosphate Oral Solution
Codeine Sulfate Tablets
DHT (Dihydrotachysterol) Tablets, Oral Solution & Intensol
Dexamethasone Tablets, Oral Solution & Intensol
Diazepam Tablets
Diluent (Flavored) for Oral Use
Diphenhydramine Hydrochloride Capsules
Diphenhydramine Hydrochloride Elixir
Diphenoxylate Hydrochloride & Atropine Sulfate Tablets & Oral Solution
Docusate Sodium Capsules
Docusate Sodium Syrup
Docusate Sodium with Casanthranol Capsules
Ferrous Sulfate Oral Solution
Ferrous Sulfate Tablets
Furosemide Tablets
Gentz Wipes
Guaifenesin Syrup
Hydrochlorothiazide Tablets, Oral Solution & Intensol
Hydromorphone Hydrochloride Tablets
Imipramine Hydrochloride Tablets
Indomethacin Capsules
Intensol Concentrated Oral Solutions (Package includes bottle & calibrated dropper)
Chlorpromazine Hydrochloride Intensol
DHT (Dihydrotachysterol) Intensol
Dexamethasone Intensol
Hydrochlorothiazine Intensol
Prednisone Intensol
Roxanol (Morphine Sulfate Concentrated Oral Solution) Intensol
Thioridazine HCl Intensol
Ipecac Syrup
Isoetharine Hydrochloride Inhalation
Isoxsuprine Hydrochloride Tablets
Kaolin-Pectin Suspension
Lidocaine Hydrochloride Topical Solution 4%
Lidocaine Viscous 2%
Lithium Carbonate Capsules & Tablets
Lithium Citrate Syrup
Magaldrate Oral Suspension
Magnesia & Alumina Oral Suspension
◆ Marinol Capsules
Meperidine Hydrochloride Syrup
Methadone Hydrochloride Oral Solution & Tablets
Methyldopa Tablets
Milk of Magnesia
Milk of Magnesia-Concentrated
Milk of Magnesia-Cascara Suspension Concentrated
Milk of Magnesia-Mineral Oil Emulsion & Emulsion (Flavored)
Mineral Oil
Mineral Oil-Light Sterile
Morphine Sulfate Oral Solution
Morphine Sulfate Tablets
Neomycin Sulfate Tablets
Paregoric
Phenobarbital Elixir
Phenobarbital Tablets
Potassium Chloride Oral Solution
Potassium Chloride Powder Unflavored
Potassium Gluconate Elixir
Potassium Iodide Oral Solution
Potassium Phosphates Oral Solution
Prednisolone Tablets
Prednisone Tablets, Oral Solution & Intensol
Propantheline Bromide Tablets
Propoxyphene Hydrochloride Capsules
Pseudoephedrine Hydrochloride Syrup
Pseudoephedrine Hydrochloride Tablets
Quinidine Gluconate Sustained Release Tablets
Quinidine Sulfate Tablets
Roxanol (Morphine Sulfate Concentrated Oral Solution)
◆ Roxanol SR (Morphine Sulfate Sustained Release Tablets)
Roxicodone Tablets & Oral Solution
Saliva Substitute
Sodium Chloride Inhalation
Sodium Phosphates Oral Solution
Sodium Polystyrene Sulfonate Suspension
Terpin Hydrate & Codeine Elixir
Theophylline Oral Solution
Thioridazine Hydrochloride Tablets & Intensol
Triprolidine & Pseudoephedrine Hydrochlorides Syrup
Triprolodine & Pseudoephedrine Hydrochlorides Tablets

RUSS PHARMACEUTICALS, INC. 427, 1765
P.O. Box 20507
Birmingham, AL 35216
Address inquiries to:
(205) 822-2730
Products Available
Lortab Liquid
◆ Lortab Tablets
◆ Lortab ASA Tablets
Lortab 5 Tablets
Lortab 7 Tablets
Precare FA
Promist HD Liquid
Promist LA

RYDELLE LABORATORIES, INC. 1766
Subsidiary of S.C. Johnson & Son, Inc.
1525 Howe Street
Racine, Wisconsin 53403
Address inquiries to:
Carol Hansen, Consumer Affairs Director
(414) 631-4000
For Medical Emergencies Contact:
Richard D. Stewart, M.D.
(414) 631-3675
Products Available
Fiberall Fiber Wafers, Fruit & Nut or Oatmeal Raisin
Fiberall Natural Flavor
Fiberall Orange Flavor

RYSTAN COMPANY, INC. 1766
47 Center Avenue
P.O. Box 214
Little Falls, NJ 07424-0214
Address inquiries to:
Professional Service Dept.
(201) 256-3737
Products Available
Chloresium Ointment
Chloresium Solution
Chloresium Tablets
Chloresium Toothpaste
Derifil Tablets
Panafil Ointment
Panafil-White Ointment
Prophyllin Wet Dressing Powder and Ointment

SANDOZ PHARMACEUTICALS CORPORATION 427, 1767
Route 10, East Hanover, NJ 07936
Address inquiries to:
William F. Westlin, M.D.
(201) 386-7500
New York City (212) 349-1212
Products Available
Asbron G Elixir
◆ Asbron G Inlay-Tabs
◆ Belladenal Tablets
◆ Belladenal-S Tablets
Bellafoline Injection & Tablets
◆ Bellergal-S Tablets
Cafergot Suppositories

◆ Cafergot Tablets
Cafergot P-B Suppositories
◆ Cafergot P-B Tablets
Cedilanid-D Injection
D.H.E. 45 Injection
Diapid Nasal Spray
Embolex Injection
◆ Fiogesic Tablets
◆ Fioricet Tablets
◆ Fiorinal Capsules
◆ Fiorinal Tablets
◆ Fiorinal w/Codeine Capsules
◆ Hydergine Oral Tablets, Sublingual Tablets, & Liquid
◆ Hydergine LC Liquid Capsules
Klorvess Effervescent Granules
◆ Klorvess Effervescent Tablets
Klorvess 10% Liquid
Mellaril Concentrate
Mellaril-S Suspension
◆ Mellaril Tablets
◆ Mesantoin Tablets
◆ Metaprel Tablets
Methergine Injection
◆ Methergine Tablets
Neo-Calglucon Syrup
◆ Pamelor Capsules
Pamelor Solution
◆ Parlodel Capsules
◆ Parlodel Tablets
◆ Restoril Capsules
Sandimmune Ampuls
Sandimmune Oral Solution
Sandoglobulin I.V.
◆ Sanorex Tablets
◆ Sansert Tablets
Syntocinon Injection
Syntocinon Nasal Spray
Tavist Syrup
◆ Tavist Tablets
◆ Tavist-1 Tablets
◆ Tavist-D Tablets
◆ Visken Tablets

SAVAGE LABORATORIES 427, 1796
a division of Altana Inc.
60 Baylis Road
Post Office Box 2006
Melville, NY 11747
(516) 454-7677
Products Available
Alphatrex Cream, Ointment & Lotion
Betatrex Cream, Ointment & Lotion
Brexin E.X. Tablets and Liquid
◆ Brexin L.A. Capsules
◆ Chromagen Capsules
◆ Chromagen OB Capsules
Dilor Elixir
◆ Dilor Injectable
◆ Dilor Tablets
◆ Dilor-400 Tablets
◆ Dilor-G Tablets & Liquid
Ditate-DS
Ethiodol
◆ Mytrex F Cream & Ointment
Nystex Cream & Ointment
Nystex Oral Suspension
◆ Sātric
◆ Sātric-500
Trymex Cream & Ointment
Trysul Vaginal Cream

SCHERING CORPORATION 427, 1801
Galloping Hill Road
Kenilworth, NJ 07033
(201) 558-4000
Address inquiries to:
Professional Services Department
9:00 AM to 5:00 PM EST:
(800) 526-4099
After regular hours and on weekends:
(201) 558-4000
Branch Offices
Southeast Branch
5884 Peachtree Rd., N.E.
Chamblee, GA 30341
(404) 457-6315
Midwest Branch
7500 N. Natchez Ave.
Niles, IL 60648 (312) 647-9363
Southwest Branch
1921 Gateway Dr.
Irving, TX 75062 (214) 258-3545
West Coast Branch
14775 Wicks Blvd.
San Leandro, CA 94577
(415) 357-3125
Products Available
⊞ A and D Hand Cream*
⊞ A and D Ointment*
⊞ Afrin Menthol Nasal Spray, 0.05%
⊞ Afrin Nasal Spray 0.05%
⊞ Afrin Nose Drops 0.05%
⊞ Afrin Pediatric Nose Drops 0.025%
◆ Afrinol Repetabs Tablets Long-Acting Nasal Decongestant
Celestone Phosphate Injection
Celestone Soluspan Suspension
Celestone Syrup
◆ Celestone Tablets
⊞ Chlor-Trimeton Allergy Syrup
◆ Chlor-Trimeton Allergy Tablets 4 mg
◆ Chlor-Trimeton Decongestant Tablets
Chlor-Trimeton Injection
◆ Chlor-Trimeton Long-Acting Allergy Repetabs Tablets 8 mg
◆ Chlor-Trimeton Long-Acting Decongestant Repetabs Tablets
◆ Chlor-Trimeton Maximum Strength Allergy Repetabs Tablets 12 mg
◆ Cod Liver Oil Concentrate Capsules*
◆ Cod Liver Oil Concentrate Tablets*
◆ Cod Liver Oil Concentrate Tablets w/Vitamin C*
⊞ Coricidin Cough Syrup
◆ Coricidin "D" Decongestant Tablets
⊞ Coricidin Decongestant Nasal Mist
◆ Coricidin Demilets Tablets For Children
◆ Coricidin Extra Strength Sinus Headache Tablets
◆ Coricidin Tablets
◆ Demazin Repetabs Tablets
⊞ Demazin Syrup
⊞ Dermolate Anal-Itch Ointment
⊞ Dermolate Anti-Itch Cream
⊞ Dermolate Anti-Itch Spray
⊞ Dermolate Scalp-Itch Lotion
Diprolene Cream 0.05%
Diprolene Ointment 0.05%
Diprosone Cream 0.05%
Diprosone Lotion 0.05% w/w
Diprosone Ointment 0.05%
Diprosone Topical Aerosol 0.1% w/w
◆ Disophrol Chronotab Sustained-Action Tablets*
◆ Disophrol Tablets*
◆ Drixoral Sustained-Action Tablets
Drixoral Syrup
⊞ Emko Because Contraceptor Vaginal Contraceptive Foam
⊞ Emko Pre-Fil Vaginal Contraceptive Foam
⊞ Emko Vaginal Contraceptive Foam
◆ Estinyl Tablets
◆ Etrafon A Tablets (4-10)
◆ Etrafon 2-10 Tablets (2-10)
◆ Etrafon Tablets (2-25)
◆ Etrafon Forte Tablets (4-25)
◆ Fulvicin P/G Tablets
◆ Fulvicin P/G 165 & 330 Tablets
◆ Fulvicin-U/F Tablets
Garamycin Cream 0.1%
Garamycin Injectable
Garamycin Injectable Disposable Syringes
Garamycin Intrathecal Injection
Garamycin I.V. Piggyback Injection
Garamycin Ointment 0.1%
Garamycin Ophthalmic Ointment
Garamycin Ophthalmic Solution
Garamycin Pediatric Injectable
Gyne-Lotrimin Vaginal Cream 1%
◆ Gyne-Lotrimin Vaginal Tablets 100 mg
◆ Gyne-Lotrimin Vaginal Tablets 500 mg
Hyperstat I.V. Injection
Intron A
Lotrimin Cream 1%
Lotrimin Lotion 1%
Lotrimin Solution 1%
Lotrisone Cream
◆ Meticorten Tablets
Metimyd Ophthalmic Ointment
Metimyd Ophthalmic Suspension
◆ Miradon Tablets
◆ Mol-Iron Tablets*
◆ Mol-Iron w/Vitamin C Tablets
◆ Naqua Tablets
◆ Naquival Tablets
Netromycin Injection
Normodyne Injection
◆ Normodyne Tablets
◆ Optimine Tablets
Optimyd Ophthalmic Solution
◆ Oreton Methyl Buccal Tablets
◆ Oreton Methyl Tablets
Otobiotic Otic Solution
◆ Paxipam Tablets
Permitil Oral Concentrate*
◆ Permitil Tablets*
Polaramine Expectorant
◆ Polaramine Repetabs Tablets
Polaramine Syrup
◆ Polaramine Tablets
◆ Proventil Inhaler
Proventil Syrup
◆ Proventil Tablets
◆ Rela Tablets
Sebizon Lotion
Sodium Sulamyd Ophthalmic Ointment 10%
Sodium Sulamyd Ophthalmic Solution 10%
Sodium Sulamyd Ophthalmic Solution 30%
Solganal Suspension
◆ Theovent Long-Acting Capsules
⊞ Tinactin Cream 1%
⊞ Tinactin Jock Itch Cream 1%
⊞ Tinactin Jock Itch Spray Powder 1%
⊞ Tinactin Liquid 1% Aerosol
⊞ Tinactin Powder 1%
⊞ Tinactin Powder 1% Aerosol
⊞ Tinactin Solution 1%
◆ Tindal Tablets
Trilafon Concentrate
Trilafon Injection
◆ Trilafon Repetabs Tablets
◆ Trilafon Tablets
◆ Trinalin Repetabs Tablets
Valisone Cream 0.1%
Valisone Lotion 0.1%
Valisone Ointment 0.1%
Valisone Reduced Strength Cream 0.01%
◆ Vancenase Nasal Inhaler
◆ Vanceril Inhaler
*Schering/White Product Line

SCHMID LABORATORIES, INC. 1860
Route 46 West
Little Falls, NJ 07424-0415
Address inquiries to:
Professional Service Dept.
(201) 256-5500
Products Available
Koro-Flex Arcing Spring Diaphragm
Koromex Coil Spring Diaphragm
Ramses Bendex Flexible Cushioned Diaphragm
Ramses Contraceptive Vaginal Jelly
Ramses Flexible Cushioned Diaphragm
Vagisec Medicated Liquid Douche Concentrate
Vagisec Plus Suppositories

SCLAVO INC. 1861, 2230
5 Mansard Court
Wayne, NJ 07470
Address inquiries to:
Francis J. O'Grady (800) 526-5260
Products Available
Antirabies Serum (equine), Purified
Cholera Vaccine
Diphtheria Antitoxin (equine), Refined
Diphtheria & Tetanus Toxoids, Adsorbed (For Pediatric Use)
Diphtheria Toxoid, Adsorbed
SclavoTest-PPD, Tuberculin PPD Multiple Puncture Device
Tetanus Antitoxin (equine), Refined
Tetanus Toxoid, Adsorbed
Tetanus & Diphtheria Toxoids, Adsorbed For Adult Use

SCOT-TUSSIN PHARMACAL CO., INC. 1861
50 Clemence Street
Cranston, RI 02920-0217
Address inquiries to:
Professional Service Dept.
(401) 942-8555
(800) 245-9898, ext. 15
Products Available
Ferro-Bob Tablets
S-T Cort Lotion
S-T Febrol Tablets & Elixir Sugar-Free & Dye-Free
S-T Forte Sugar-Free
S-T Forte Syrup
Scot-Tussin DM Syrup (with sugar) Cough & Cold Medicine
Scot-Tussin DM 2 Syrup (with sugar)
Scot-Tussin Sugar-Free DM Cough & Cold Medicine
Scot-Tussin Sugar-Free Expectorant, Dye-Free & Sodium-Free Cough Formula
Scot-Tussin Sugar-Free 5-Action Cold Formula
Scot-Tussin Syrup 5-Action Cold Formula
Tussirex Sugar-Free, Alcohol-Free
Tussirex Syrup, Alcohol-Free & Dye-Free
Vita-Bob Capsules
Vita-Natal Capsules
Vita-Plus B 12, 10 ml. Vials, 1000 mcgm./ml.
Vita-Plus E Capsules Natural 400 I.U.
Vita-Plus G (geriatric) Capsules
Vita-Plus H (hematinic) Capsules
Vita-Plus H (hematinic) Sugar-Free Liquid

SEARLE PHARMACEUTICALS INC. 429, 1861
Box 5110
Chicago, IL 60680
Address medical inquiries to:
Medical Communications Department
G.D. Searle & Co.
4901 Searle Pkwy.
Skokie, IL 60077
Outside IL
(800) 323-4204 (business hours)
Within IL
(312) 982-7000 (at other times)
Products Available
Aminophyllin Injection
◆ Calan for IV Injection
Cu-7
◆ Diulo
Dramamine Injection
Dramamine Liquid
◆ Dramamine Tablets
◆ Flagyl I.V.
◆ Flagyl I.V. RTU
◆ Nitrodisc
Tatum-T

SEARLE & CO. 429, 1872
San Juan, Puerto Rico 00936
Address medical inquiries to:
Medical Communications Department
4901 Searle Pkwy.
Skokie, IL 60077
Products Available
◆ Aldactazide
◆ Aldactone
◆ Aminophyllin Tablets
◆ Anavar
◆ Banthīne Tablets
◆ Calan Tablets
◆ Demulen 1/35-21
◆ Demulen 1/35-28
◆ Demulen 1/50-21
◆ Demulen 1/50-28
◆ Enovid 5 mg
◆ Enovid 10 mg
◆ Enovid-E 21
◆ Flagyl Tablets
Lomotil Liquid
◆ Lomotil Tablets
◆ Norpace Capsules
◆ Norpace CR Capsules
◆ Ovulen-21
◆ Ovulen-28
◆ Pro-Banthīne Tablets
◆ Theo-24

SERES LABORATORIES, INC. 1895
3331 Industrial Drive
Box 470
Santa Rosa, CA 95402
Address inquiries to:
Kathryn M. MacLeod, Ph.D.
(707) 526-4526
Products Available
Cantharone
Cantharone Plus
Night Cast Formula R (Medicated Acne Mask)
Night Cast Formula S (Medicated Acne Mask)

SERONO LABORATORIES, INC. 1895
280 Pond Street
Randolph, MA 02368
Address inquiries to:
Medical Information Services
(outside MA) (800) 225-5185
(within MA) (617) 963-8154
For Medical Emergencies Contact 24 Hours:
Vice President, Research and Scientific Affairs
(outside MA) (800) 225-5185
(within MA) (617) 963-8154
Products Available
Pergonal (Menotropins for Injection USP)
Profasil HP (human chorionic gonadotropin, USP)
Serophene (clomiphene citrate tablets, USP)

SIGMA-TAU, INC. 1899
723 North Beers St.
Holmdel, NJ 07733
Address inquiries to:
(201) 264-1200
Products Available
Carnitor

SMITHKLINE CONSUMER PRODUCTS 1899
A SmithKline Beckman Company
P. O. Box 8082
Philadelphia, PA 19101
Address inquiries to:
Medical Department
During business hours:
(215) 768-3600
During nonbusiness hours:
(215) 751-5000
Products Available
A.R.M. Tablets
Acnomel Cream
Benzedrex Inhaler
Congestac Tablets
Contac Continuous Action Decongestant Capsules
Contac Jr.
Contac Severe Cold Formula Night Strength Liquid
Ecotrin Enteric Coated Aspirin Maximum Strength Tablets
Ecotrin Enteric Coated Aspirin Regular Strength Tablets
Ecotrin Maximum Strength Safety-Coated Aspirin Capsules
Ecotrin Regular Strength Safety-Coated Aspirin Capsules
Feosol Capsules
Feosol Elixir
Feosol Plus
Feosol Tablets
Ornacol Capsules
Ornex Capsules
Pragmatar w/Sulfur & Salicylic Acid Ointment
Sine-Off Extra Strength No Drowsiness Capsules
Sine-Off Extra Strength Non-Aspirin Capsules
Sine-Off Extra Strength Non-Aspirin Tablets
Teldrin Timed-Release Allergy Capsules
Troph-Iron Liquid
Trophite Liquids & Tablets

SMITH KLINE &FRENCH LABORATORIES 430, 1901
Division of SmithKline Beckman Corporation
1500 Spring Garden St.
P.O. Box 7929
Philadelphia, PA 19101
Address inquiries to:
Medical Dept. (215) 751-4000
Products Available
◆ Ancef Injection
◆ Anspor Capsules

Anspor for Oral Suspension
◆ Cefizox Injection
◆ Compazine Ampuls
◆ Compazine Injection
◆ Compazine Multiple-dose Vials
◆ Compazine Prefilled Disposable Syringes
◆ Compazine Spansule Capsules
◆ Compazine Suppositories
Compazine Syrup
◆ Compazine Tablets
◆ Cytomel Tablets
◆ Darbid Tablets
Dexedrine Elixir
◆ Dexedrine Spansule Capsules
◆ Dexadrine Tablets
◆ Dibenzyline Capsules
◆ Eskalith Capsules
◆ Eskalith Tablets
◆ Eskalith CR Controlled Release Tablets
◆ Hispril Spansule Capsules
◆ Monocid Injection
◆ Ornade Spansule Capsules
Paredrine 1% w/Boric Acid, Ophthalmic Solution
◆ Parnate Tablets
◆ Ridaura
SK-Amitriptyline HCl Tablets
SK-Ampicillin Capsules
SK-Ampicillin For Oral Suspension
SK-Ampicillin-N for Injection
SK-APAP with Codeine Tablets
SK-Bamate Tablets
SK-Chlorothiazide Tablets
SK-Diphenoxylate Tablets
SK-Dipyridamole Tablets
SK-Erythromycin Tablets
SK-Furosemide Tablets
SK-Lygen Capsules
SK-Oxycodone with Acetaminophen Tablets
SK-Oxycodone with Aspirin Tablets
SK-Penicillin G Tablets
SK-Penicillin VK for Oral Solution
SK-Penicillin VK Tablets
SK-Potassium Chloride Oral Solution
SK-Pramine Tablets
SK-Prednisone Tablets
SK-Quinidine Sulfate Tablets
SK-65 Capsules
SK-65 APAP Tablets
SK-65 Compound Capsules
SK-Terpin Hydrate and Codeine Elixir
SK-Tetracycline HCl Capsules
SK-Tolbutamide Tablets
Spansule, sustained release capsules:
◆ 'Compazine' Spansule Capsules
◆ 'Dexedrine' Spansule Capsules
◆ 'Hispril' Spansule Capsules
◆ 'Ornade' Spansule Capsules
◆ 'Thorazine' Spansule Capsules
◆ 'Tuss-Ornade' Spansule Capsules
◆ Tazicef For Injection
Thorazine Concentrate
Thorazine Injection
◆ Thorazine Spansule Capsules
◆ Thorazine Suppositories
Thorazine Syrup
◆ Thorazine Tablets
Tuss-Ornade Liquid
◆ Tuss-Ornade Spansule Capsules
◆ Urispas Tablets
◆ Vontrol Tablets

SK&F CO. 430, 1901
Carolina, Puerto Rico 00630
Subsidiary of SmithKline Beckman Corporation
Address inquiries to:
Smith Kline &French Laboratories (see above)
Products Available
◆ Dyazide Capsules
◆ Dyrenium Capsules
Stelazine Concentrate
Stelazine Injection
◆ Stelazine Multiple-dose Vials
◆ Stelazine Tablets

SK&F LAB CO. 430, 1901
Carolina, Puerto Rico 00630
Subsidiary of SmithKline Beckman Corporation
Address inquiries to:
Smith Kline &French Laboratories (see above)
Products Available
◆ Tagamet HCl Injection
◆ Tagamet HCl Liquid
◆ Tagamet Tablets

SMITHKLINE DIAGNOSTICS, INC. 2230
A SmithKline Beckman Company
P.O. Box 61947
Sunnyvale, CA 94086
Ordering/Pricing/Technical Information:
Toll-free (800) 538-1581
Call Collect in California, Alaska and Hawaii
(408) 732-6000
Products Available
Gastroccult
Hemoccult
Isocult
RapidTest-Strep

SMITH LABORATORIES, INC. 1937
2215 Sanders Road
Northbrook, IL 60062
Customer Service & Other Inquiries:
(800) 356-2225
(312) 564-5700
For Medical Emergencies Contact:
Medical Department
Products Available
Chymodiactin

SOLGAR VITAMIN COMPANY, INC. 431, 1939
410 Ocean Avenue
Lynbrook, NY 11563
Address inquiries to:
P.O. Box 330
Lynbrook, NY 11563
(516) 599-2442
Branch Offices
Guttenberg, New Jersey
Culver City, California
Berlin, Maryland
Products Available
Acidophilus Capsules
Alfalfa Tablets
Amino 75 Capsules
Antioxidant Factors Tabs
Arginine-Ornithine Capsules
Beta Carotene Capsules
Biotin Tablets
Bran Tablets
Brewers Yeast
Calcium 600
Calcium Citrate
Calcium Magnesium Tablets
l-Carnitine Capsules
Chews-Eze Tablets
Choline/Inositol Tablets
Citrus Bioflavinoids Tablets
◆ Daily Gold Pack
Evening Primrose Oil
Formula B-50 Capsules
Formula VM-75 Tablets
Garlic Oil Capsules
Gelatin Capsules
Hy-C Tablets
Lecithin Capsules
Lecithin Granules
Liver Tablets
Lysine Capsules
Max EPA Capsules
Niacin Tablets
Pantothenic Acid Tablets
Phosphatidyl Choline Capsules
Selenium Tablets
Stress Formula B-Complex with C
l-Tryptophan
Vitamin B-1 Tablets
Vitamin B-2 Tablets
Vitamin B-6 Tablets
Vitamin B-12 Tablets
Vitamin C Tablets & Capsules
Vitamin E Capsules
Vitamin K Tablets
Zinc Citrate
Zinc "50" Tablets

E. R. SQUIBB & SONS INC. 431, 1940
General Offices
Post Office Box 4000
Princeton, NJ 08540
(609) 921-4000
Address inquiries to:
Squibb Professional Services Dept.
P.O. Box 4000
Princeton, NJ 08540
(609) 921-4006
Squibb Diagnostics
P.O. Box 191
New Brunswick, NJ 08903
(201) 545-1300
Distribution Centers
ATLANTA, GEORGIA
Post Office Box 16503
Atlanta, GA 30321
State of Ga. Customers Call
(800) 282-9103
Customers in States of Ala., Fla., Miss., N.C., S.C., and Tenn. Call
(800) 241-1744
All others call (800) 241-5364
CHICAGO, ILLINOIS
Post Office Box 788
Arlington Heights, IL 60006
State of IL Customers Call
(800) 942-0674
All others call (800) 323-0665
DALLAS, TEXAS
Mail or telephone orders and customer service inquiries should be directed to Atlanta, GA (see above)
State of MS Customers Call
(800) 241-1744
All others call (800) 241-5364
LOS ANGELES, CALIFORNIA
Post Office Box 428
La Mirada, CA 90638
State of CA Customers Call
(800) 422-4254
State of HI Customers Call
(714) 521-7050
All others call (800) 854-3050
SEATTLE, WASHINGTON
Mail or telephone orders and customer service inquiries should be directed to Los Angeles, CA (see above)
State of AK and MT Customers Call
(714) 521-7050
State of CA Customers Call
(800) 422-4254
All others call (800) 854-3050
NEW YORK AREA
E. R. Squibb & Sons, Inc.
Post Office Box 2013
New Brunswick, NJ 08903
State of ME Customers Call
(201) 469-5400
State of NJ Customers Call
(800) 352-4865
All others call (800) 631-5244
For listing of standard and purified insulins, see SQUIBB-NOVO, INC.
Products Available
Aspirin Tablets USP
B Complex Vitamin Tablets
Broxodent Automatic-Action Toothbrush
Calcium, Phosphate and Vitamin D Tablets
◆ Capoten
◆ Capozide
Castor Oil USP
Cholografin Meglumine
Cholografin Meglumine for Infusion
Cod Liver Oil Capsules
Cod Liver Oil Plain & Mint Flavored
◆ Comoxol
Crysticillin 300 A.S. & 600 A.S.
Cystografin
Cystografin Dilute
Deladumone
Deladumone OB
Delatestryl
Delestrogen
Diatrizoate Meglumine Injection USP 76%
Engran-HP Tablets
Ethril '250' and Ethril '500' Tablets
Florinef Acetate Tablets
Follutein
Fungizone Cream, Lotion and Ointment
Fungizone for Tissue Culture
Fungizone Intravenous
Gastrografin
◆ Hydrea Capsules
Iron and Vitamin C Tablets
Isovue 300
Isovue 370
Isovue-M 200
Isovue-M 300
Kenacort Diacetate Syrup
Kenacort Tablets
Kenalog Cream, Lotion, Ointment, Spray
Kenalog in Orabase
Kenalog-H Cream
Kenalog-10 Injection
Kenalog-40 Injection
Kinevac
Milk of Magnesia Liquid
Mineral Oil
Mycolog II Cream and Ointment
Mycostatin Cream, Ointment
Mycostatin Oral Suspension
◆ Mycostatin Oral Tablets
Mycostatin Powder (for laboratory use)
Mycostatin Topical Powder
◆ Mycostatin Vaginal Tablets
Mysteclin-F Capsules
Mysteclin-F Syrup
Niacin Tablets USP
Nitrazine Paper
Noctec Capsules & Syrup
Nuclear Medicine Products (Radiopharmaceuticals)
A-C-D Solution Modified
Albumotope I 131 Diagnostic Injection
Chromalbin
Chromitope Sodium Diagnostic Injection
Cobatope-57 Reference Standard Solution
Hipputope I 131 Diagnostic Injection
Intrinsic Factor Concentrate Capsules
Iodotope I 131 Diagnostic Capsules
Iodotope I 131 Therapeutic Capsules
Iodotope I 131 Therapeutic Oral Solution
MDP-Squibb
Macrotec
Minitec
Phosphotec
Rubratope-57 Diagnostic Capsules
Rubratope-57 Diagnostic Kit
Techneplex
Tesuloid
Nydrazid Tablets
O-V Statin
Ophthaine Solution
Oragrafin Calcium Granules
Oragrafin Sodium Capsules
Ora-Testryl Tablets
Penicillin G Potassium for Injection USP
Penicillin G Sodium for Injection USP
Pentids for Syrup
Pentids '400' for Syrup
Pentids '400' & '800' Tablets
Pentids Tablets
◆ Principen Capsules '250' & '500'
Principen for Oral Suspension '125' & '250'
Principen with Probenecid Capsules
Proto-Chol Capsules
Renografin-60
Renografin-76
Reno-M-DIP
Reno-M-30
Reno-M-60
Renovist
Renovist II
Renovue-65
Renovue-DIP
Saccharin Tablets
Sinografin
Spec-T Sore Throat Anesthetic Lozenges
Spec-T Sore Throat/Cough Suppressant Lozenges
Spec-T Sore Throat/Decongestant Lozenges
Spectrocin Ointment
◆ Sumycin '250' & '500' Capsules
◆ Sumycin '250' and '500' Tablets
Sumycin Syrup
Suppositories, Glycerin, USP
Sweeta Liquid
Terfonyl Tablets, Oral Suspension
Teslac Tablets
◆ Theragran Hematinic Tablets
▣ Theragran Liquid
▣ Theragran Stress Formula
▣ Theragran Tablets
▣ Theragran-M Tablets
Trigesic Tablets
◆ Trimox '250' & '500' Capsules
Trimox '125' & '250' For Oral Suspension
Valadol Tablets, Liquid
Veetids '125' & '250' for Oral Solution
◆ Veetids '250' & '500' Tablets
◆ Velosef '250' & '500' Capsules
Velosef for Injection
Velosef '125' & '250' for Oral Suspension
Vigran plus Iron Tablets
Vigran Tablets
Vitamin B_1 Tablets USP
Vitamin C Tablets
Vitamin E Capsules
◆ Vivox
Yeast Tablets & Flavored Powder
Zinc Oxide Ointment USP

SQUIBB-MARSAM, INC.
P.O. Box 3648
Cherry Hill, NJ 08034
Address inquiries to:
(609) 424-8282
For Medical Emergencies Contact:
Squibb Professional Services Dept.
(609) 921-4006
Direct orders to:
E. R. Squibb & Sons, Inc.
(Local Distribution Center)
Products Available
Crysticillin 300 A.S. (Sterile Penicillin G Procaine Suspension USP)
Crysticillin 600 A.S.
Heparin Sodium Injection, USP, Preservative-Free
Nydrazid Injection (Isoniazid Injection USP)
Penicillin G Potassium for Injection USP
Rubramin PC (Cyanocobalamin Injection USP)
Sucostrin High Potency Injection
Sucostrin Injection (Succinylcholine Chloride Injection USP)
Tubocurarine Chloride Injection USP

SQUIBB-NOVO, INC. 431, 1971
120 Alexander Street
Princeton, NJ 08540
Address inquiries to:
Medical Communications
(609) 921-8989
For Medical Emergencies Contact:
Medical Communications
(609) 921-8989
Products Available
Lente Insulin
Lente Purified Pork Insulin
NPH Insulin
NPH Purified Pork Insulin
◆ Novolin L
◆ Novolin N
◆ Novolin R
Novolin 70/30
Regular Insulin
Regular Purified Pork Insulin
Semilente Insulin
Semilente Purified Pork Insulin
Ultralente Insulin
Ultralente Purified Beef Insulin

STANDARD PROCESS LABORATORIES, INC. 1972
Home Office
2023 West Wisconsin Avenue
Milwaukee, WI 53233
(414) 933-2100
Branch Offices
Campbell, CA 95008
501-C Vandell Way
(408) 866-0707
(Los Angeles)
City of Commerce, CA 90040
2401 S. Atlantic Blvd.
(213) 263-6133
Orlando, FL 32809
7653 Currency Dr.
(305) 851-6610
Watertown, MA 02172
76 Coolidge Hill Road
(617) 923-2330

(◆ Shown in Product Identification Section)

(▣ Described in PDR For Nonprescription Drugs)

Distributors
Cedar Hill, TX 75104
1330 E. Wintergreen Road
(214) 291-4258
Fort Collins, CO 80526
500 Apple Blossom Lane
(303) 223-6262
Harrisburg, PA 17112
5145 Jonestown Road
(717) 545-9264
Kansas City, MO 64131
8433 Paseo (816) 523-7600
Kirkland, WA 98034
12521 131st Court, N.E.
(206) 820-1158
Oklahoma City, OK 73112
3419 N. Roff Ave. (405) 943-1056
St. Joseph, MI 49085
413 State Street (616) 983-3014
Products Available
Allorganic Trace Minerals-B12
Antronex
Betaine Hydrochloride
Biost Powder
Cal-Amo
Calcium Lactate (Fortified)
Cardio-Plus
Cardiotrophin (Heart)
Catalyn
Cataplex A-F & Betaris
Cataplex E-2
Cataplex F
Chlorophyll Complex Ointment (Fat Soluble)
Chlorophyll Complex Perles (Fat Soluble)
Choline
Comfrey, Pepsin—Formula E-3
Ferroplus
Inositol
Multizyme
Niacinamide B6
Ovex
Pneumotrophin (Lung)
Prost-X
Ribo-Nucleic Acid (RNA)
Thymex
Vasculin
Vitamin B-6 w/Niacinamide
Zypan Tablets

STAR PHARMACEUTICALS, INC. 431, 1972
1990 N.W. 44th Street
Pompano Beach, FL 33064-1278
Address inquiries to:
Scott L. Davidson, President
(305) 971-9704
Stellar Pharmacal Corp.
A Star Pharmacal Co.,
1990 N.W. 44th St.,
Pompano Beach, FL 33064-1278
For Medical Emergencies Contact:
Scott L. Davidson (305) 972-6060
Branch Office
Panamerican Pharmaceutical Inc.
Marina St., #300
P.O. Box 817
Aguada, PR 00602
Address inquiries to:
Luis Cardona, President
(809) 868-2415
Products Available
Prosed
Uro-KP-Neutral
Urolene Blue
◆ Virilon

STELLAR PHARMACAL CORPORATION 1972
1990 N.W. 44th Street
Pompano Beach, FL 33064-1278
Address inquiries to:
Scott L. Davidson, President
(305) 972-6060
Branch Offices
Panamerican Pharmaceutical Inc.
Marina St., #300
P.O. Box 817
Aguada, PR 00602
(809) 868-2415
Products Available
▣ Star-Otic

STIEFEL LABORATORIES, INC. 1972
2801 Ponce de Leon Blvd.
Coral Gables, FL 33134
Address inquiries to:
Werner K. Stiefel (305) 443-3807
Branch Offices
GEORGIA
Post Office Box 47789
Doraville, GA 30362
(404) 455-1896
NEW YORK
Route 145
Oak Hill, NY 12460
(518) 239-6901
PUERTO RICO
P.O. Box 387
Mayaguez, PR 00708
(809) 832-1376
Products Available
Acne-Aid Cleansing Bar
Acne-Aid Cream
Benoxyl-5 Lotion
Benoxyl-10 Lotion
Brasivol Base
Brasivol Fine
Brasivol Medium
Brasivol Rough
Duofilm
LactiCare Lotion
LactiCare-HC Lotions, 1% and 2 1/2%
Lasan Creams, 0.1, 0.2, 0.4%
Lasan HP-1 Cream
Lasan Ointment
Oilatum Soap (Scented)
Oilatum Soap (Unscented)
PanOxyl 5 Acne Gel
PanOxyl 10 Acne Gel
PanOxyl AQ 2½, 5 & 10 Acne Gels
PanOxyl Bar 5
PanOxyl Bar 10
Polytar Bath
Polytar Shampoo
Polytar Soap
Salicylic Acid Soap
Salicylic Acid & Sulfur Soap
Saligel
Sarna Lotion
SAStid (AL)
SAStid (Plain)
SAStid Soap
Scabene Lotion
Scabene Shampoo
Sulfoxyl Lotion Regular
Sulfoxyl Lotion Strong
Sulfur Soap
Surfol Bath Oil
ZNP Bar
ZeaSORB Powder
ZeaSORB-AF Powder

STUART PHARMACEUTICALS 431, 1976
Div. of ICI Americas Inc.
Wilmington, DE 19897
Address inquiries to:
Yvonne Graham, Manager
Professional Services
(302) 575-2231
For Medical Emergencies Contact:
After Hours or On Weekends, call
(302) 575-3000
Products Available
◆ ALternaGEL Liquid
◆ Bucladin-S Softab
◆ Cefotan
◆ Dialose Capsules
◆ Dialose Plus Capsules
◆ Effer-Syllium Instant Mix
◆ Ferancee Tablets
◆ Ferancee-HP Tablets
◆ Hibiclens
◆ Hibiclens Sponge/Brush with Nail Cleaner
◆ Hibistat
◆ Kasof Capsules
◆ Kinesed Tablets
◆ Mulvidren-F Softab
◆ Mylanta Liquid
◆ Mylanta Tablets
◆ Mylanta-II Liquid
◆ Mylanta-II Tablets
Mylicon Drops
◆ Mylicon Tablets
◆ Mylicon-80 Tablets
◆ Nolvadex Tablets
Orexin Softab
◆ Probec-T Tablets
◆ Sorbitrate Chewable Tablets
◆ Sorbitrate Oral Tablets
◆ Sorbitrate Sublingual Tablets
◆ Sorbitrate Sustained Action Tablets
◆ The Stuart Formula (Tablets)
◆ Stuart Prenatal Tablets
◆ Stuartinic Tablets
◆ Stuartnatal 1+1 Tablets
◆ Tenoretic Tablets
◆ Tenormin Tablets

SWEEN CORPORATION 1989
Sween Building
P.O. Box 980
Lake Crystal, MN 56055
(507) 726-6200
Products Available
Bedside-Care
Fordustin'
Gentle Rain Shampoo
Methylbenzethonium Chloride
Micro-Guard
Peri-Care
Peri-Wash
Peri-Wash II
Puri-Clens
Surgi-Kleen
Sween-A-Peel
Sween Cream
Sween Kind Touch
Sween Prep
Sween Soft Touch
Whirl-Sol
Xtracare II

SYNTEX (F.P.) INC. 432, 1992
Humacao, Puerto Rico 00661
Address inquiries to:
Syntex Laboratories, Inc. (see below)
Products Available
◆ Brevicon 21-Day Tablets
◆ Brevicon 28-Day Tablets
◆ Norinyl 1+35 21-Day Tablets
◆ Norinyl 1+35 28-Day Tablets
◆ Norinyl 1+50 21-Day Tablets
◆ Norinyl 1+50 28-Day Tablets
◆ Norinyl 1+80 21-Day Tablets
◆ Norinyl 1+80 28-Day Tablets
◆ Norinyl 2 mg. Tablets
◆ Nor-Q.D. Tablets
◆ Tri-Norinyl 21-Day Tablets
◆ Tri-Norinyl 28-Day Tablets
◆ Wallette Pill Dispenser

SYNTEX LABORATORIES, INC. 432, 1992
3401 Hillview Ave.
P.O. Box 10850
Palo Alto, CA 94303
Direct General/Sales/Order inquiries for U.S. marketed products to:
Marketing Information
(Specify product) (415) 855-5050
Direct Medical Inquiries on U.S. marketed products to:
Medical Information
General Medical Inquiries
(415) 855-5545
Adverse Reaction Inquiries
(415) 852-1386
Products Available
◆ Anadrol-50 Tablets
Carmol HC Cream
▣ Carmol 10 Lotion
▣ Carmol 20 Cream
Femstat Vaginal Cream
Lidex Cream, Gel, Ointment & Topical Solution
Lidex-E Cream
Nasalide Nasal Solution
Neo-Synalar Cream
Synacort Creams
Synalar Creams, Ointment and Topical Solution
Synalar-HP Cream
Synemol Cream
Topic Gel

SYNTEX PUERTO RICO, INC. 432, 1992
Humacao, Puerto Rico 00661
Address Medical inquires to:
Syntex Laboratories, Inc. (see above)
Products Available
◆ Anaprox Tablets
◆ Naprosyn Tablets

TAP PHARMACEUTICALS 2007
1400 Sheridan Road
North Chicago, IL 60064
Address inquiries to:
Medical Dept. 1(800) 622-2011
For Medical Emergencies Contact:
Medical Dept. 1(800) 622-2011
Products Available
Lupron Injection

THOMPSON MEDICAL COMPANY, INC. 2008
919 Third Avenue
New York, NY 10022
Address inquiries to:
Medical Services (212) 688-4420
For Medical Emergencies Contact
Business Hours Only
(212) 688-4420
After Hours or on Weekends
(212) 594-8855
Products Available
Appedrine Tablets, Maximum Strength
Aspercreme Creme and Lotion Rub
Control Capsules, Maximum Strength
Dexatrim Capsules
Dexatrim Capsules, Extra Strength
Dexatrim Capsules, Extra Strength, Caffeine-Free
Dexatrim Capsules, Extra Strength, Plus Vitamins
Dexatrim Maximum Strength Pre-Meal Caplets
Prolamine Capsules, Maximum Strength

TRIMEN LABORATORIES, INC. 2010
80 - 26th Street
Pittsburgh, PA 15222
Address inquiries to:
Professional Service Dept.
(412) 261-0339
Products Available
Amacodone Tablets
Amaphen Capsules
Amaphen with Codeine #3
Deltavac Cream
Dyrexan-OD Capsules
Korigesic Tablets
Natacomp-FA Tablets
Trimedine Expectorant
Viopan-T Tablets

TYSON and ASSOCIATES, INC. 2010
1661 Lincoln Blvd.
Suite 300
Santa Monica, CA 90404
Address Inquiries to:
Professional Services Dept.
Call Collect within CA (213) 452-7844
(800) 367-7744
Products Available
Alpha Plus Capsules
Aminolete Capsules & Powder
Aminomine Capsules & Powder
Aminoplex Capsules & Powder
Amino-Si Tablets
Aminosine Capsules & Powder
Aminostasis Capsules & Powder
Aminotate Capsules & Powder
Aminoxin Tablets (Coenzymatic B_6)
Capristatin Tablets
EFA Plus Drops
Endorphan Capsules
Endorphenyl Capsules (d-Phenylalanine)
Iso-B Capsules
Kaprycidin-A Capsules
Lyte-C Powder
MVM Capsules
Max EPA Capsules
Maxovite Tablets
Niaplus Capsules
Nutrox Capsules
Optivite Tablets
Pantothenic Acid Capsules
Tryptoplex Capsules
Tyson ATP Tablets
Tyson L-Alanine Capsules & Powder
Tyson Alpha Ketoglutaric Acid Capsules
Tyson L-Arginine Capsules & Powder
Tyson L-Aspartic Acid Capsules & Powder
Tyson L-Carnitine U.S.P. Capsules
Tyson L-Citrulline Capsules & Powder
Tyson L-Cysteine HCl Capsules & Powder
Tyson L-Cystine Capsules & Powder
Tyson GABA Capsules & Powder
Tyson L-Glutamic Acid Capsules & Powder
Tyson L-Glutamine Caps & Powder
Tyson L-Glutathione Powder
Tyson Glycine Capsules & Powder
Tyson L-Histidine Capsules & Powder
Tyson L-Isoleucine Capsules & Powder
Tyson L-Leucine Capsules & Powder
Tyson L-Lysine Powder & Caps
Tyson L-Methionine Powder & Caps
Tyson D-Phenylalanine Capsules (Endorphenyl)
Tyson L-Phenylalanine Capsules & Powder
Tyson Proline Capsules & Powder
Tyson L-Serine Capsules & Powder
Tyson Taurine Capsules & Powder
Tyson L-Threonine Powder & Caps
Tyson L-Tryptophan U.S.P. Capsules & Powder
Tyson L-Tyrosine Capsules & Powder
Tyson L-Valine Capsules & Powder
Ultra Choline (Phosphatide Complex)

UAD LABORATORIES, INC. 2011
6635 Highway 18 West
Jackson, MS 39209
Address inquiries to:
Professional Services Department
(601) 372-7773
For Medical Emergencies Contact:
(601) 372-7773
Products Available
AR-600
Adbeon
Adlone 40 and 80
Bucet
Cezin & Cezin-S
Desone & Desone-LA
Dital
Endafed
Endal
Endal Expectorant
Endal Plain
Eudal-SR
Lorcet
Lorcet-HD
Lorpac
Triad
UAD Cream & Cream Lotion
UAD Pred
Vertab Capsules
Zone-A Cream 1%
Zone-A Lotion 1%

U. S. ETHICALS INC.
37-02 48th Avenue
Long Island City, NY 11101
Address inquiries to:
Medical Director (718) 786-8607
Products Available
Azlytal Tablets
Azmadrine Elixir & Tablets
Bellastal Capsules, Elixir & Tablets
Capa Tablets
Declofen SR Capsules
Eclabron Capsules & Elixir
Etnapa Elixir
Ferbetrin Tablets & Syrup
Gastrical Tablets
Hepaferron Syrup
Histabs Tablets
Klavikordal Tablets
Natalac Capsules
Neodex Tablets & Syrup
Niong Tablets
Nitromed
Nitronet Tablets
Nitrong Ointment (See Wharton Laboratories)
Nitrong Tablets (See Wharton Laboratories)
Supervim Drops, Tablets & Syrup
Vitacoms Capsules

U.S. PHARMACEUTICAL CORPORATION 2012
2500 Park Central Blvd.
Decatur, GA 30035
(404) 987-4745

(◆ Shown in Product Identification Section)

(▣ Described in PDR For Nonprescription Drugs)

Mailing Address:
2500 Park Central Blvd.
Decatur, GA 30035
Address inquiries to:
Marketing Director (404) 987-4745
Products Available
Hemocyte Plus Tabules
Hemocyte Tablets
Hemocyte-F Tablets
Isovex Capsules
Magsal Tablets
Medigesic Plus Capsules

USV LABORATORIES, DIVISION USV PHARMACEUTICAL CORP. 433, 2013
500 Virginia Drive
Fort Washington, PA 19034
Address inquiries to:
Medical Department
(215) 628-6761

USV LABORATORIES Inc. 433, 2013
Manati, Puerto Rico 00701
Address inquiries to:
USV Pharmaceutical Corp.
(see above)

USV (P.R.) DEVELOPMENT CORP. 433, 2013
Manati, Puerto Rico 00701
Address inquiries to:
USV Pharmaceutical Corp.
(see above)
Products Available
◆ Arlidin Tablets
◆ Armour Thyroid Tablets
Azolid Capsules & Tablets
Bi-K
Biopar Forté
◆ Calcimar Injection, Synthetic
◆ Calel-D
Cerespan Capsules
Chymoral
Chymoral-100
◆ DDAVP
◆ DDAVP Injection
◆ Demi-Regroton Tablets
Doriden Tablets
◆ Gastrolyte
Histaspan-D Capsules
Histaspan-Plus Capsules
◆ Hygroton Tablets
◆ Levothroid for Injection
◆ Levothroid Tablets
◆ Lozol Tablets
◆ Nicobid
◆ Nicolar Tablets
Nitrospan Capsules
Oxalid Tablets
Panthoderm Cream
Pentritol
Pertofrane Capsules
◆ Regroton Tablets
Thyrar
◆ Thyrolar Tablets
Tussar DM
Tussar SF
Tussar-2

UNITED 2028
Division of Pfizer Hospital Products Group
11775 Starkey Road
Largo, FL 33543
Address inquiries to:
(813) 392-1261
Products Available
Skin-Prep
UniCare Lotion
Uni Derm Moisturizer
Uni Salve Protective Ointment
Uni Wash Skin Cleanser

THE UPJOHN COMPANY 433, 2029
7000 Portage Road
Kalamazoo, MI 49001
(616) 323-4000
Emergency Medical Information
(616) 323-6615
Address inquiries to:
Medical Information
The Upjohn Company
Kalamazoo, MI 49001
Pharmaceutical Sales Areas and Distribution Centers
Atlanta (Chamblee), GA 30341 (404) 451-4822
Boston (Wellesley), MA 02181
(617) 431-7970
Buffalo (Cheektowaga), NY 14225 (716) 681-7160
Chicago (Oak Brook Terrace), IL 60181 (312) 574-3300
Cincinnati, OH 45237
(513) 242-4574
Dallas, TX 75205 (214) 841-3110
Denver, CO 80216 (303) 399-3113
Hartford (Enfield), CT 06082
(203) 741-3421
Honolulu, HI 96813
(808) 538-1181
Kalamazoo, MI 49001
(616) 323-4000
Kansas City, MO 64131
(816) 361-2286
Los Angeles, CA 90038
(213) 463-8101
Memphis, TN 38138
(901) 756-1476
Minneapolis, MN 55422
(612) 588-2786
New York (Garden City), NY 11530 (516) 294-3530
Orlando, FL 32809
(305) 859-4591
Philadelphia (Wayne), PA 19087 (215) 265-2100
Pittsburgh, (Bridgeville), PA 15017 (412) 257-0200
Portland, OR 97232
(503) 232-2133
St. Louis, MO 63146
(314) 872-8626
San Francisco (Palo Alto), CA 94306 (415) 493-8080
Shreveport, LA 71129
(318) 688-3700
Washington, DC 20011
(202) 882-6163
Products Available
◆ Adeflor Chewable Tablets
Adeflor Drops
Adeflor M Tablets
Albamycin Capsules
Alkets Tablets
Atgam Sterile Solution
▣ Baciguent Antibiotic Ointment
Bacitracin, USP, Sterile Powder
Berubigen Sterile Solution
Calcium Chloride Injection, USP, Sterile Solution
Calcium Gluconate Injection, USP, Sterile Solution
Calcium Gluconate Tablets, USP
Calcium Lactate Tablets, USP
Cebenase Tablets
Cheracol Cough Syrup
▣ Cheracol D Cough Formula
▣ Cheracol Plus Head Cold/Cough Formula
▣ Citrocarbonate Antacid
◆ Cleocin HCl Capsules
Cleocin Pediatric Flavored Granules
◆ Cleocin Phosphate Sterile Solution
◆ Cleocin T Topical Solution
Clocream Skin Cream
Colestid Granules
▣ Cortaid Cream
Cortaid Cream with Aloe
▣ Cortaid Lotion
▣ Cortaid Ointment
▣ Cortaid Spray
Cortef Acetate Ointment
▣ Cortef Feminine Itch Cream
Cortef Oral Suspension
Cortef Tablets
Cortisone Acetate Tablets, USP
Cytosar-U Sterile Powder
Delta-Cortef Tablets
◆ Deltasone Tablets
Depo-Estradiol Sterile Solution
◆ Depo-Medrol Sterile Aqueous Suspension
Depo-Provera Sterile Aqueous Suspension
Depo-Testadiol Sterile Solution
Depo-Testosterone Sterile Solution
◆ Didrex Tablets
Diostate D Tablets
E-Mycin E Liquid
E-Mycin Tablets
Erythromycin Tablets (E-Mycin)
Feminone Tablets
Gelfilm Sterile Film
Gelfilm Sterile Ophthalmic Film
Gelfoam Dental Packs
Gelfoam Packs
Gelfoam Prostatectomy Cones
Gelfoam Sterile Compressed Sponge
Gelfoam Sterile Powder
Gelfoam Sterile Sponge
◆ Halcion Tablets
Halodrin Tablets
◆ Halotestin Tablets
Heparin Sodium Injection, USP, Sterile Solution
Hydrocortisone Acetate, U.S.P.; Micronized, Nonsterile Powder (For Prescription Compounding)
Hydrocortisone, U.S.P. Micronized, Nonsterile Powder (For Prescription Compounding)
▣ Kaopectate Anti-Diarrhea Medicine
Kaopectate Anti-Diarrhea Medicine (Bilingual) (English & Spanish labeling)
▣ Kaopectate Concentrate Anti-Diarrhea Medicine
▣ Kaopectate Tablet Formula
Lincocin Capsules
Lincocin Pediatric Capsules
Lincocin Sterile Solution
Lipomul Oral Liquid
◆ Loniten Tablets
◆ Maolate Tablets
Medrol Acetate Topical
◆ Medrol Dosepak Unit of Use
Medrol Enpak Kit
Medrol Enpak Kit (Refill)
◆ Medrol Tablets
◆ Micronase Tablets
◆ Motrin Tablets
Mycifradin Oral Solution
Mycifradin Sterile Powder
Mycifradin Tablets
▣ Myciguent Antibiotic Cream & Ointment
Mycitracin Ophthalmic Ointment
▣ Mycitracin Triple Antibiotic Ointment
Neo-Cortef Cream
Neo-Cortef Ointment
Neo-Cortef Ophthalmic Suspension
Neo-Delta-Cortef Ointment
Neo-Delta-Cortef Ophthalmic Suspension
Neo-Medrol Acetate Topical
Orinase Diagnostic Sterile Powder
◆ Orinase Tablets
Orthoxicol Cough Syrup
P-A-C Revised Formula Analgesic Tablets
Pamine Tablets
Panmycin Capsules
Phenolax Wafers
Prostin VR Pediatric Sterile Solution
Protamine Sulfate for Injection, USP, Sterile Powder
◆ Provera Tablets
▣ Pyrroxate Capsules
▣ Sigtab Tablets
Sodium Chloride Injection, (Bacteriostatic) USP, Sterile Solution
Solu-Cortef Sterile Powder
◆ Solu-Medrol Act-O-Vial & Vials
◆ Solu-Medrol Sterile Powder
Super D Perles
◆ Tolinase Tablets
Trobicin Sterile Powder
▣ Unicap Capsules & Tablets
▣ Unicap Jr Chewable Tablets
▣ Unicap M Tablets
▣ Unicap Plus Iron Tablets
▣ Unicap Senior Tablets
▣ Unicap T Tablets
Uracil Mustard Capsules
Uticillin VK Tablets
Water for Injection (Bacteriostatic), USP, Sterile Solution
◆ Xanax Tablets
Zanosar Sterile Powder
Zymacap Capsules

UPSHER-SMITH LABORATORIES, INC. 2071
14905 23rd Avenue North
Minneapolis, MN 55441
Address inquiries to:
Professional Service Department
(612) 473-4412
For Medical Emergencies Contact:
Scientific Affairs Department
(612) 473-4412
Products Available
Acetaminophen Uniserts Suppositories
Aspirin Delayed-release Tablets
Aspirin Uniserts Suppositories
Bisacodyl Tablets
Bisacodyl Uniserts Suppositories
Docusate Sodium Capsules
Docusate Sodium with Casanthranol Capsules
Ferrous Gluconate Tablets
Ferrous Sulfate Tablets
Hemorrhoidal Uniserts Suppositories
Hexavitamin Tablets
Histatapp Elixir
Kerasol Therapeutic Bath Oil
Klor-10% Solution
Klor-Con Powder
Klor-Con/25 Powder
Klor-Con 20% Solution
Klor-Con/EF Effervescent Tablets
Klor-Con 8/Klor-Con 10 Extended-release Tablets
▣ Lubrin Vaginal Lubricating Inserts
RMS Suppositories
SSKI Solution
Sorbitol Solution
Stress-600 Tablets
Stress-600 with Zinc
Therapeutic B Complex with C Capsules
Therapeutic Multivitamin Tablets
Therapeutic Multivitamin with Mineral Tablets
Trofan Tablets (L-Tryptophan)
Trofan DS Tablets (L-Tryptophan)
Zinc Sulfate Capsules

VITALINE FORMULAS 2073
P.O. Box 6757
Incline Village, NV 89450
Address inquiries to:
Jed D. Meese, Technical Director (702) 831-5656
Products Available
Alka Aid (antacid)
B Complex 50 & 100
B Complex 50 & 100 (controlled time release)
Biotin Forte & Extra Strength 5mg Biotin Forte
Bromelain 500 mg (2400 mcu/gm)
Calcium (oyster shell)
Calcium (Chewable, Vita Calcium)
Calcium Citrate
Cal-Mag Aspartate (calcium/magnesium)
Chromium 1mg
Digestive Enzymes (chewable)
Digestive Supplement (glutamic acid HCl & pepsin)
E-Pherol (dry, d-alpha tocopheral succinate)
Enviro-Stress with zinc & selenium
Free Form Amino Acids
Fructose Wafers (orange & strawberry flavors)
L-Glutamine & Choline
Iron (Chelated Iron Plus)
K-MAG Aspartate (potassium & magnesium aspartates)
LMP Special Formula (natural lipotropic & fiber supplement)
Magna Zinc (30mg elemental zinc)
Magnesium (Cal-Mag Aspartate)
Magnesium (Vita-Mag)
Manganese
Maximum Formula
Maximum Formula (no iron/no copper)
Multimineral Plus
Pancreatin 900mg 8X USP (High Lipase)
Pancreatin Tablets 2400mg USP (High Lipase)
Pantothenic Acid
Potassium Gluconate
Selenium Tablets 200mcg (yeast free)
StimuLean (appetite suppressant)
Total Formula (multivitamin/multimineral)
Vitamin A (with Beta-carotene)
Vitamin B-6 200mg
Vitamin B-6 200mg (controlled time release)
Viatmin C Powder, Buffered
Vitamin C 1000mg (controlled time release)
Vitamin C 1000mg with Bioflavonoids
Vitamin E 400 I.U. Capsules
Vitamin E 400 I.U. Tablets
Zinc 220mg (50mg elemental zinc)

VIVAN PHARMACOL, INC. 2074
1000 Bennett Boulevard
Lakewood, NJ 08701
Address inquiries to:
Professional Services Dept.
(201) 364-9700
For Medical Emergencies Contact:
(201) 364-9701
Products Available
Alphaderm Cream

WALLACE LABORATORIES 434, 2075
P.O. Box 1
Cranbury, NJ 08512
Address inquiries to:
Professional Services
(609) 655-6000
Night and Weekend Emergencies
(609) 799-1167
Send all orders to:
Wallace Laboratories
Div. of Carter-Wallace, Inc.
Post Office Drawer 5
Cranbury, NJ 08512
Products Available
◆ Aquatensen Tablets
Avazyme/Avazyme-100 Tablets
Barbidonna Elixir & Tablets
Barbidonna No. 2 Tablets
Butibel Elixir & Tablets
Buticaps
◆ Butisol Sodium Elixir & Tablets
Covanamine Liquid
Covangesic Tablets
Depen Titratable Tablets
Deprol Tablets
Diutensen Tablets
◆ Diutensen-R Tablets
Lufyllin Elixir
◆ Lufyllin Injection
◆ Lufyllin & Lufyllin-400 Tablets
Lufyllin-EPG Elixir & Tablets
◆ Lufyllin-GG Elixir & Tablets
▣ Maltsupex Liquid, Powder & Tablets
Meprospan Capsules
Micrainin
Milprem Tablets
◆ Miltown Tablets
◆ Miltown 600 Tablets
◆ Organidin Elixir, Solution & Tablets
◆ Rondomycin Capsules
▣ Ryna Liquid
▣ Ryna-C Liquid
▣ Ryna-CX Liquid
◆ Rynatan Pediatric Suspension
◆ Rynatan Tablets
◆ Rynatuss Pediatric Suspension
◆ Rynatuss Tablets
◆ Soma Tablets
◆ Soma Compound Tablets
◆ Soma Compound w/Codeine Tablets
▣ Syllact Powder
Syllamalt Powder
◆ Theo-Organidin Elixir
◆ Tussi-Organidin DM Liquid
◆ Tussi-Organidin Liquid
◆ VōSol HC Otic Solution
◆ VōSol Otic Solution

WEBCON PHARMACEUTICALS 2093
Division of Alcon (Puerto Rico) Inc.
Post Office Box 3000
Humacao, Puerto Rico 00661
Address inquiries to:
Medical Department
Post Office Box 6380
Fort Worth, TX 76115
(817) 293-0450
Products Available
Alconefrin 12 Drops
Alconefrin 25 Drops

Alconefrin 50 Drops
Alconefrin 25 Spray
Anestacon Sterile Solution
Aquachloral Suppositories
Azo-Standard Tablets
B & O No. 15A & No. 16A Supprettes
Cystospaz Tablets
Cystospaz-M Capsules
Neopap Suppositories
Urised Tablets
Urisedamine Tablets

WESTWOOD PHARMACEUTICALS INC. 434, 2095
100 Forest Avenue
Buffalo, NY 14213
(716) 887-3400
Address inquiries to:
Consumer Affairs Department
(716) 887-3773
Products Available
Alpha Keri Moisturizing Bar
Alpha Keri Shower and Bath Oil
Balnetar
Capitrol Cream Shampoo
Desquam-X 10 Bar
Desquam-X 2.5 Gel
Desquam-X 5 Gel
Desquam-X 10 Gel
Desquam-X 5 Wash
Desquam-X 10 Wash
Estar Gel
Eurax Cream & Lotion
Halotex Cream & Solution
Keralyt Gel
Lac-Hydrin 12% Lactate Lotion
Lowila Cake
Maxivate Cream, Lotion & Ointment
Moisturel
PreSun 4 Creamy Sunscreen
PreSun 8 Lotion and Creamy Sunscreens
PreSun 15 Lotion and Creamy Sunscreens
PreSun 15 Facial Stick/Lip Protector Sunscreen
PreSun Facial Sunscreen 15
Sebulex & Sebulex Cream Shampoo
Sebulex Shampoo with Conditioners
Sebutone & Sebutone Cream Shampoo
T-Stat (erythromycin) 2.0% Topical Solution
◆ Tacaryl Chewable Tablets
◆ Tacaryl Syrup & Tablets
Westcort Cream
Westcort Ointment 0.2%

WHARTON LABORATORIES, INC. 2104
37-02 48th Ave.
Long Island City, NY 11101
Address inquiries to:
Medical Director (718) 786-8607
Products Available
Nitrong Ointment
Nitrong Ointment, Unit Dose
Nitrong 2.6 mg. Tablets
Nitrong 6.5 mg. Tablets
Nitrong 9 mg. Tablets

WHITEHALL LABORATORIES INC. 434, 2104
Division of American Home Products Corporation
685 Third Avenue
New York, NY 10017
Address inquiries to:
Medical Department
(212) 878-5508
Products Available
◆ Advil Ibuprofen Caplets and Tablets
◆ Anacin Analgesic Caplets
◆ Anacin Analgesic Tablets
◆ Anacin Maximum Strength Analgesic Coated Tablets
◆ Anacin-3, Children's Acetaminophen Chewable Tablets, Liquid, Infants' Drops
◆ Anacin-3, Maximum Strength Acetaminophen Film-Coated Caplets
◆ Anacin-3, Maximum Strength Acetaminophen Film Coated Tablets
◆ Anacin-3, Regular Strength Acetaminophen Film Coated Tablets
◆ Anbesol Baby Teething Gel Anesthetic
◆ Anbesol Gel Antiseptic Anesthetic
◆ Anbesol Liquid Antiseptic Anesthetic
◆ Arthritis Pain Formula By the Makers of Anacin Analgesic Tablets
◆ Arthritis Pain Formula Aspirin-Free By the Makers of Anacin Analgesic Tablets
Bisodol Antacid Powder
Bisodol Antacid Tablets
Bronitin Asthma Tablets
Bronitin Mist
Compound W Solution & Gel
Denalan Denture Cleanser
◆ Denorex Medicated Shampoo and Conditioner
◆ Denorex Medicated Shampoo, Regular & Mountain Fresh Herbal Scent
◆ Dristan, Advanced Formula Decongestant/Antihistamine/Analgesic Caplets
◆ Dristan Advanced Formula Decongestant/Antihistamine/Analgesic Tablets
Dristan Inhaler
◆ Dristan Long Lasting Nasal Spray, Regular & Menthol
◆ Dristan Nasal Spray, Regular & Menthol
Dristan Room Vaporizer
Dristan-AF Decongestant/Antihistamine/Analgesic Tablets
Dry and Clear Acne Medication Lotion
Dry and Clear Double Strength Cream
Freezone Solution
Heather Feminine Deodorant Spray
Heet Analgesic Liniment
Heet Spray Analgesic
InfraRub Analgesic Cream
◆ Medicated Cleansing Pads By the Makers of Preparation H Hemorrhoidal Remedies
Momentum Muscular Backache Formula
Neet Bikini Line Hair Remover Kit
Neet Depilatory Cream
Neet Depilatory Lotion
Outgro Solution
Oxipor VHC Lotion for Psoriasis
◆ Preparation H Hemorrhoidal Ointment
◆ Preparation H Hemorrhoidal Suppositories
Prepcort Hydrocortisone Cream 0.5%
◆ Primatene Mist
Primatene Mist Suspension
◆ Primatene Tablets-M Formula
◆ Primatene Tablets-P Formula
Quiet World Analgesic/Sleeping Aid
◆ Semicid Vaginal Contraceptive Inserts
Sleep-eze 3 Tablets
Sudden Action Breath Freshener
Sudden Beauty Country Air Mask
Sudden Beauty Hair Spray
◆ Trendar Ibuprofen Tablets
Viro-Med Liquid
Viro-Med Tablets

WILLEN DRUG COMPANY 2108
18 North High St.
Baltimore, MD 21202
Address inquiries to:
Professional Services Dept.
(800) 336-7000
In MD (301) 752-1865
Products Available
Bicitra—Sugar-Free
Neutra-Phos Powder & Capsules
Neutra-Phos-K Powder & Capsules
Polycitra Syrup
Polycitra-K—Sugar-Free
Polycitra-LC—Sugar-Free

WINTHROP-BREON LABORATORIES 435, 2110, 2232
90 Park Avenue
New York, NY 10016
(212) 907-2000
For Medical Information only:
Call toll-free (800) 446-6267
Products Available
Amipaque
Anti-Rust Tablets
Aralen Hydrochloride Injection
◆ Aralen Phosphate Tablets
Aralen Phosphate w/Primaquine Phosphate Tablets
Atabrine Hydrochloride Tablets
Atropine & Demerol Carpuject
◆ Bilopaque Sodium Capsules
⊞ Breonesin Capsules
Bronkephrine Injection
Bronkodyl Capsules
⊞ Bronkolixir
Bronkometer Aerosol
Bronkosol
⊞ Bronkotabs Tablets
Carbocaine Hydrochloride Injection
Codeine Phosphate Carpuject
◆ Danocrine
◆ Demerol APAP Tablets
Demerol Carpuject
Demerol Hydrochloride Injection
Demerol Hydrochloride Syrup
◆ Demerol Hydrochloride Tablets
Demerol Uni-Amp
Dextrose Injection, 10%
Drisdol 50,000 Unit Capsules
Drisdol in Propylene Glycol
Empty Sterile Carpuject
Heparin Lock Flush Solution Carpuject
Heparin Sodium Carpuject
HEP-PAK Convenience Package
Hydromorphone Carpuject
Hydroxyzine Carpuject
Hypaque Meglumine 30%
Hypaque Meglumine 60%
Hypaque Sodium Oral Powder
Hypaque Sodium Oral Solution
Hypaque Sodium 20%
Hypaque Sodium 25%
Hypaque Sodium 50% Injection
Hypaque-Cysto
Hypaque-M, 75% Injection
Hypaque-M, 90% Injection
Hypaque-76 Injection
Hytakerol Capsules & Liquid
Inocor Lactate Injection
Isuprel Hydrochloride Glossets
Isuprel Hydrochloride Injection 1:5000
Isuprel Hydrochloride Mistometer
Isuprel Hydrochloride Solution 1:200 & 1:100
Kayexalate
Levophed Bitartrate Injection
Lotusate Caplets
Luminal Sodium Injection
Marcaine Hydrochloride Injection
Marcaine Hydrochloride with Epinephrine 1:200,000
Marcaine Spinal
Measurin Tablets
Mebaral Tablets
◆ Modrastane Capsules
Morphine Sulfate Carpuject
Mytelase Chloride Caplets
Naloxone Hydrochloride Injection, USP
Naloxone Hydrochloride Injection, USP (Neonatal)
◆ NegGram Caplets
NegGram Suspension
Neo-Synephrine Hydrochloride 1% Carpuject
Neo-Synephrine Hydrochloride 1% Injection
Neo-Synephrine Hydrochloride (Ophthalmic)
Novocain Hydrochloride for Spinal Anesthesia
Novocain Hydrochloride Injection
Omnipaque
Pediacof Cough Syrup
pHisoDerm
pHisoHex
◆ Plaquenil Sulfate Tablets
Pontocaine Hydrochloride Eye Ointment
Pontocaine Hydrochloride for Spinal Anesthesia
Pontocaine Hydrochloride Topical Solution
Primaquine Phosphate Tablets
Sodium Chloride Carpuject
Sulfamylon Acetate Cream
◆ Talacen
Talwin Ampuls
Talwin Carpuject
Talwin Compound
Talwin Injection
◆ Talwin Nx
◆ Telepaque Tablets
◆ Tornalate
◆ Trancopal Caplets
Vitamins
Vitamin D, USP
Drisdol 50,000 Unit Capsules
Drisdol in Propylene Glycol
◆ Winstrol Tablets
⊞ Zephiran Chloride Aqueous Solution
⊞ Zephiran Chloride Concentrate Solution
⊞ Zephiran Chloride Spray
⊞ Zephiran Chloride Tinted Tincture
⊞ Zephiran Towelettes

WINTHROP CONSUMER PRODUCTS 2145
Division of Sterling Drug Inc.
90 Park Avenue
New York, NY 10016
Address inquiries to:
Winthrop Consumer Products
For Medical Emergencies Contact:
Medical Department
(212) 907-3027
(212) 907-3029
Products Available
⊞ Bronkaid Mist
⊞ Bronkaid Mist Suspension
⊞ Bronkaid Tablets
⊞ Campho-Phenique Liquid & Gel
Fergon Capsules
Fergon Elixir
Fergon Tablets
⊞ Haley's M-O, Regular & Flavored
⊞ NTZ Long Acting Spray & Drops
⊞ NāSal Saline Nasal Spray
⊞ NāSal Saline Nose Drops
Neo-Synephrine Jelly
Neo-Synephrine Nasal Spray (Mentholated)
Neo-Synephrine Nasal Sprays
Neo-Synephrine Nose Drops
Neo-Synephrine 12 Hour Nasal Spray
Neo-Synephrine 12 Hour Nose Drops (Adult & Children's Strengths)
Neo-Synephrine 12 Hour Vapor Nasal Spray
⊞ Neo-Synephrine II Long Acting Nasal Spray
⊞ Neo-Synephrine II Long Acting Nose Drops (Adult & Children's Strengths)
⊞ Neo-Synephrine II Long Acting Vapor Nasal Spray
⊞ pHisoAc BP
pHisoDan
⊞ pHisoDerm Regular & Fresh Scent
⊞ pHisoPUFF
Soapure
⊞ WinGel Liquid & Tablets

WYETH LABORATORIES 435, 2146
Division of American Home Products Corporation
P.O. Box 8299
Philadelphia, PA 19101
Address inquiries to:
Professional Service
For General Information call:
(215) 688-4400
For Medical Emergency Information
Day or night call (215) 688-4400
Wyeth Distribution Centers:
Andover, MA 01810
P.O. Box 1776 (617) 475-9075
Atlanta, GA 30302
P.O. Box 4365 (404) 873-1681
Baltimore, MD 21224
101 Kane St. (301) 633-4000
Boston Distribution Center, see under Andover, MA
Buena Park, CA 90622-5000
P.O. Box 5000 (714) 523-5500
(Los Angeles) (213) 627-5374
Chicago Distribution Center, see under Wheaton, IL
Cleveland, OH 44101
P.O. Box 91549 (216) 238-9450
Dallas, TX 75238
P.O. Box 38200 (214) 341-2299
Kansas City Distribution Center, see under North Kansas City, MO
Kent, WA 98064-5609
P.O. Box 5609 (206) 872-8790
Los Angeles Distribution Center, see under Buena Park, CA
Memphis, TN 38101
P.O. Box 1698 (901) 353-4680
North Kansas City, MO 64116
P.O. Box 7588 (816) 842-0680
Pearl City, HI 96782
96-1185 Waihona St., Unit C1
(808) 456-4567
Philadelphia Distribution Center
Paoli, PA 19301
P.O. Box 61 (215) 644-8000
Philadelphia (215) 878-9500
Seattle Distribution Center, see under Kent, WA
Wheaton, IL 60189-0140
P.O. Box 140 (312) 462-7200
Products Available
Alcohol Sponges
⊞ Aludrox Suspension
⊞ Aludrox Tablets
Aminophylline Rectal Suppositories
⊞ Amphojel Suspension
⊞ Amphojel Suspension w/o Flavor
⊞ Amphojel Tablets
Antisnakebite Serum (see Antivenin)
Antivenin (Crotalidae) Polyvalent
Antivenin (Micrurus Fulvius)
Aspirin Tablets, Redipak
Ativan Injection
◆ Ativan Tablets
⊞ Basaljel Capsules
⊞ Basaljel Suspension
⊞ Basaljel Suspension, Extra Strength
⊞ Basaljel Swallow Tablets
Benzathine Penicillin G (see Bicillin)
Bicillin C-R Injection
Bicillin C-R 900/300 Injection
Bicillin Long-Acting Injection
Bicillin Tablets
Biologicals
Bisacodyl Suppositories
CVC Heparin Flush Kits
Cerose-DM
Cerubidine
Cholera Vaccine
Clinipak Unit Dose Medications
Isordil Chewable Tablets 10 mg
Isordil Sublingual Tablets 2.5 mg
Isordil Sublingual Tablets 5 mg
Isordil Sublingual Tablets 10 mg
Isordil 5 Titradose Tablets 5 mg
Isordil 10 Titradose Tablets 10 mg
Isordil 20 Titradose Tablets 20 mg
Isordil 30 Titradose Tablets 30 mg
Isordil 40 Titradose Tablets 40 mg
Sectral Capsules 200 mg
Sectral Capsules 400 mg
Surmontil Capsules 25 mg
Surmontil Capsules 50 mg
Synalgos-DC Capsules
Codeine Phosphate Injection
Codeine Sulfate Tablets, Redipak
⊞ Collyrium Eye Lotion
⊞ Collyrium Eye Drops with Tetrahydrozoline
◆ Cordarone Tablets
Cyanocobalamin Injection
Cyclapen-W for Oral Suspension
◆ Cyclapen-W Tablets
◆ Cyclospasmol Capsules & Tablets
Deponit NTG Film Transdermal Delivery System
◆ Dicloxacillin Sodium Monohydrate (see Pathocil)
Digoxin Injection
Dimenhydrinate Injection
Diphenhydramine HCl Injection
Diphtheria and Tetanus Toxoids Adsorbed (Adult Use) (see Tetanus and Diphtheria Toxoids Adsorbed)
Diphtheria & Tetanus Toxoids Adsorbed
Epinephrine Injection (1:1000)
◆ Equagesic Tablets
◆ Equanil Tablets
◆ Equanil Wyseals
Erythromycin Ethylsuccinate Oral Suspension (See Wyamycin E Liquid)
Erythromycin Stearate Tablets (see Wyamycin S Tablets)
Heparin Flush Kits
Heparin Lock Flush Solution
Heparin Sodium Injection
Hydromorphone HCl Injection
Hydroxyzine HCl Injection
Influenza Virus Vaccine, Trivalent, Subvirion Type
◆ Isordil Chewable Tablets
◆ Isordil Oral Titradose Tablets
◆ Isordil Sublingual Tablets

(◆ Shown in Product Identification Section)

(⊞ Described in PDR For Nonprescription Drugs)

◆ Isordil Tembids Capsules
◆ Isordil Tembids Tablets
Largon Injection
◆ Lo/Ovral Tablets
◆ Lo/Ovral-28 Tablets
◆ Mazanor Tablets
◆ Mepergan Fortis Capsules
Mepergan Injection
Meperidine HCl Injection
Meperidine HCl Tablets, Redipak
Morphine Sulfate Injection
◆ Nordette-21 Tablets
◆ Nordette-28 Tablets
▣ Nursoy, Soy Protein Formula for Infants, Concentrated Liquid, Ready-to-Feed, and Powder
◆ Omnipen Capsules
Omnipen for Oral Suspension
Omnipen Pediatric Drops
Omnipen-N Injection
Opium & Belladonna Rectal Suppositories
◆ Orudis Capsules
◆ Ovral Tablets
◆ Ovral-28 Tablets
Ovrette Tablets
Oxytocin Injection, Synthetic
◆ Pathocil Capsules
Pathocil for Oral Suspension
Penicillin Preparations:
Bicillin Products
Penicillin G Potassium Tablets
◆ Pen • Vee K Products
Wycillin Products
Pentobarbital Sodium Injection
Pen • Vee K for Oral Solution
◆ Pen • Vee K Tablets
Petrogalar, Plain
Phenergan Injection
◆ Phenergan Suppositories
Phenergan Syrup Fortis
Phenergan Syrup Plain
◆ Phenergan Tablets
Phenergan VC
Phenergan VC with Codeine
Phenergan with Codeine
Phenergan with Dextromethorphan
◆ Phenergan-D Tablets
Phenobarbital Sodium Injection
Phenobarbital Tablets, Redipak
Phosphaljel
Prochlorperazine Edisylate Injection
Redipak Unit Dose Medications (Strip Pack and/or Individually Wrapped)
Products:
Aspirin Tablets
Ativan Tablets
Codeine Sulfate Tablets
Equagesic Tablets
Equanil Tablets
Meperidine HCl Tablets
Pen • Vee K Tablets
Phenergan Tablets
Phenobarbital Tablets
Serax Capsules
Unipen Capsules
Wygesic Tablets
Wytensin Tablets
Redipak (Unit of Use Suppository Pack)
Products:
◆ Phenergan Rectal Suppositories
Redipak (Respiratory Therapy Unit)
Products:
Sodium Chloride 0.9% and 0.45%
Sterile Distilled Water
RediTemp-C, Disposable Cold Pack
Resol Oral Electrolyte & Maintenance Solution
▣ SMA Infant Formula, Liquid Concentrated
▣ SMA Infant Formula, Powder
▣ SMA Infant Formula, Ready-to-Feed
Saline Solution (see Sodium Chloride Injection)
Secobarbital Sodium Injection
◆ Sectral Capsules
◆ Serax Capsules
◆ Serax Tablets
▣ Simeco Suspension
Snakebite Serum (see Antivenin)
Sodium Chloride Injection, Bacteriostatic
Sodium Chloride Solution, 0.9% & 0.45%
Sopronol Ointment, Powder & Solution
Sparine Injection
Sparine Syrup
◆ Sparine Tablets
◆ Surmontil Capsules
Synalgos Capsules
◆ Synalgos-DC Capsules
Tetanus & Diphtheria Toxoids Adsorbed for Adult Use
Tetanus & Diphtheria Toxoids Adsorbed (Ultrafined Pediatric) (see Diphtheria & Tetanus Toxoids Adsorbed)
Tetanus Toxoid Adsorbed, Aluminum Phosphate
Tetanus Toxoid Fluid, Purified
◆ Tetracycline HCl Capsules
Thiamine HCl Injection
Trecator-SC Tablets
◆ Triphasil-21
◆ Triphasil-28
◆ Tubex Closed Injection System
Products:
Ativan
Bicillin C-R
Bicillin C-R 900/300
Bicillin L-A
Codeine Phosphate
◆ Cyanocobalamin (Vitamin B_{12})
Digoxin
Dimenhydrinate
Diphenhydramine HCl
Diphtheria & Tetanus Toxoids Adsorbed, Ultrafined Pediatric
Epinephrine
Heparin Flush Kits
Heparin Lock Flush Solution
Heparin Sodium
Hydromorphone HCl
Hydroxyzine HCl
Influenza Virus Vaccine, Trivalent, Purified, Subvirion
Mepergan
Meperidine HCl
Morphine Sulfate
Oxytocin, Synthetic
Pentobarbital Sodium
Phenergan
Phenobarbital Sodium
Prochlorperazine Edisylate
Secobarbital Sodium
Sodium Chloride, Bacteriostatic
Sparine HCl
Tetanus & Diphtheria Toxoids Adsorbed (Adult)
Tetanus Toxoid, Aluminum Phosphate Adsorbed
Tetanus Toxoid Fluid, Purified
Thiamine HCl
Vitamin B_{12} (Cyanocobalamin)
Wycillin
◆ Tubex Fast Trak Syringe
◆ Tubex Hypodermic Syringe
Tubex Sterile Cartridge-Needle Unit Empty
Typhoid Vaccine
◆ Unipen Capsules
Unipen Injection
Unipen for Oral Solution
◆ Unipen Tablets
◆ Vitamin B_{12} Injection (see Cyanocobalamin)
Wyamine Sulfate Injection
Wyamycin E Liquid
◆ Wyamycin S Tablets
◆ Wyanoids Hemorrhoidal Suppositories
Wycillin Injection
Wycillin Injection & Probenecid Tablets
Wydase, Lyophilized
Wydase, Stabilized Solution
◆ Wygesic Tablets
◆ Wymox Capsules
Wymox for Oral Suspension
Wyseals (see Equanil)
◆ Wytensin Tablets

ZENITH LABORATORIES, INC. **2217**
50 Williams Drive
Ramsey, NJ 07446

Address inquiries to:
(201) 327-3100

Products Available
ABC Compound & Codeine Phosphate Capsules No. 3
Acetaminophen and Codeine Phosphate Tablets
Aspirin and Codeine Phosphate Tablets
Azpan Tablets
Butalbital Compound Tablets
Chloramphenicol Capsules
Chlordiazepoxide Hydrochloride Capsules
Chlordiazepoxide HCl & Clidinium Capsules
Chlorpropamide Tablets
Chlorthalidone Tablets
Chlorzoxazone & Acetaminophen Tablets
Clonidine Hydrochloride Tablets
Colchicine Tablets
Conjugated Estrogen Tablets
Cyclandelate Capsules
Cyproheptadine Tablets
Decontabs Tablets
Detuss Capsules (Formula Modified)
Diazepam Tablets
Digoxin Tablets
Diphenhydramine HCl Capsules
Diphenoxylate HCl and Atropine Sulfate Tablets
Dipyridamole Tablets
Disopyramide Phosphate Capsules
Doxycycline Hyclate Capsules
Ergoloid Mesylates Sublingual Tablets
Erythromycin Stearate Tablets
Furosemide Tablets
Hydralazine HCl Tablets
Hydralazine and Hydrochlorothiazide Capsules
Hydrochlorothiazide Tablets
Hydroserpine Tablets, No. 1 & No. 2
Hydroserpine Plus Tablets (R.H.H.)
Hydroxy Compound Tablets
Hydroxyzine HCl Tablets
Hydroxyzine Pamoate Capsules
Indomethacin Capsules
Indomethacin (Zendole) Capsules
Isosorbide Dinitrate Tablets, Oral & Sublingual
Isoxsuprine HCl Tablets
Lorazepam Tablets
Meclizine HCl Tablets
Meprobamate Tablets
Methocarbamol Tablets
Methocarbamol and Aspirin Tablets
Methyclothiazide Tablets
Methyldopa Tablets
Methyldopa & Hydrochlorothiazide Tablets
Metronidazole Tablets
Nitroglycerin Capsules
Nylidrin HCl Tablets
Oxazepam Capsules
Papaverine HCl Capsules
Perphenazine & Amitriptyline HCl Tablets
Phentermine HCl Capsules
Phenylbutazone Capsules
Phenytoin Sodium Capsules, Prompt
Probenecid Tablets
Probenecid and Colchicine Tablets
Procainamide HCl Capsules
Propoxyphene Compound Capsules
Propoxyphene HCl Capsules
Propoxyphene Napsylate and Acetaminophen Tablets
Propranolol Hydrochloride Tablets
Propylthiouracil Tablets
Quinidine Sulfate Tablets
Quinine Sulfate Capsules & Tablets
Reserpine and Hydroflumethiazide Tablets
Spironolactone Tablets
Spironolactone and Hydrochlorothiazide Tablets
Sulfinpyrazone Capsules & Tablets
Sulfisoxazole Tablets
Tetracycline HCl Capsules
Thioridazine HCl Tablets
Tolazamide Tablets
Tolbutamide Tablets
Trifluoperazine HCl Tablets
Triprolidine HCl & Pseudoephedrine HCl Tablets
Verapamil HCl Tablets

SECTION 2

Product Name Index

Part1—In this section products are listed in alphabetical sequence by brand name or (if described) generic name. Only described products have page numbers to assist you in locating additional information. For additional information on other products, you may wish to contact the manufacturer directly.

The symbol ◆ indicates the product is shown in the Product Identification Section. The symbol ▣ indicates the product is described in PDR® FOR NONPRESCRIPTION DRUGS.

Part 2—A list of products that have been discontinued by manufacturers during the past year.

A

(◆ Shown in Product Identification Section)

(▣ Described in PDR For Nonprescription Drugs)

B

(◆ Shown in Product Identification Section)

(▣ Described in PDR For Nonprescription Drugs)

C

D

(◆ Shown in Product Identification Section)

(📖 Described in PDR For Nonprescription Drugs)

E

(◆ Shown in Product Identification Section)

(▣ Described in PDR For Nonprescription Drugs)

F

G

(◆ Shown in Product Identification Section)

(▣ Described in PDR For Nonprescription Drugs)

N

(◆ Shown in Product Identification Section)

(▣ Described in PDR For Nonprescription Drugs)

O

(◆ Shown in Product Identification Section)

(▣ Described in PDR For Nonprescription Drugs)

Q

R

S

(◆ Shown in Product Identification Section)

(▣ Described in PDR For Nonprescription Drugs)

T

(◆ Shown in Product Identification Section)

(▣ Described in PDR For Nonprescription Drugs)

SECTION 3

Product Category Index

Products described in the Product Information (White) or Diagnostic Product Information (Green) Sections are listed according to their classifications. The headings and sub-headings have been determined by the Publisher with the cooperation of the individual manufacturers. In cases where there were differences of opinion or where the manufacturer had no opinion, the Publisher made the final decision. A QUICK-REFERENCE INDEX of headings and sub-headings can be found below.

Product Category Quick-Reference

Product Category Index

U

X

SECTION 4

Generic and Chemical Name Index

In this section the products described in the Product Information (White) and Diagnostic Product Information (Green) Sections are listed under generic and chemical name headings according to the principal ingredient(s). The headings under which products are listed have been determined by the Publisher with the cooperation of the individual manufacturers.

A

E

T

W

X

Product Identification Section

Designed to help you identify products, this section contains actual size, full-color reproductions selected for inclusion by participating manufacturers.

Because tablets and capsules, for the most part, are shown here, you should not infer that these are the only dosage forms. Where other dosage forms are available, the product name is preceded by the † symbol. Refer to the product's description in the PRODUCT INFORMATION (White Section) or check directly with manufacturer.

Letters and/or numbers followed by an asterisk (*) accompanying a product photograph designate the manufacturers' identification code.

While every effort has been made to reproduce products faithfully, this section should be considered only as a quick reference identification aid.

If overdosage is suspected, the user may wish to consult Guide to Management of Drug Overdose printed inside the back cover.

INDEX BY MANUFACTURER

This section is made possible through the courtesy of the manufacturers whose products appear on the following pages. Page numbers of individual products included can be found in the Product Name, Generic and Product Category Indices.

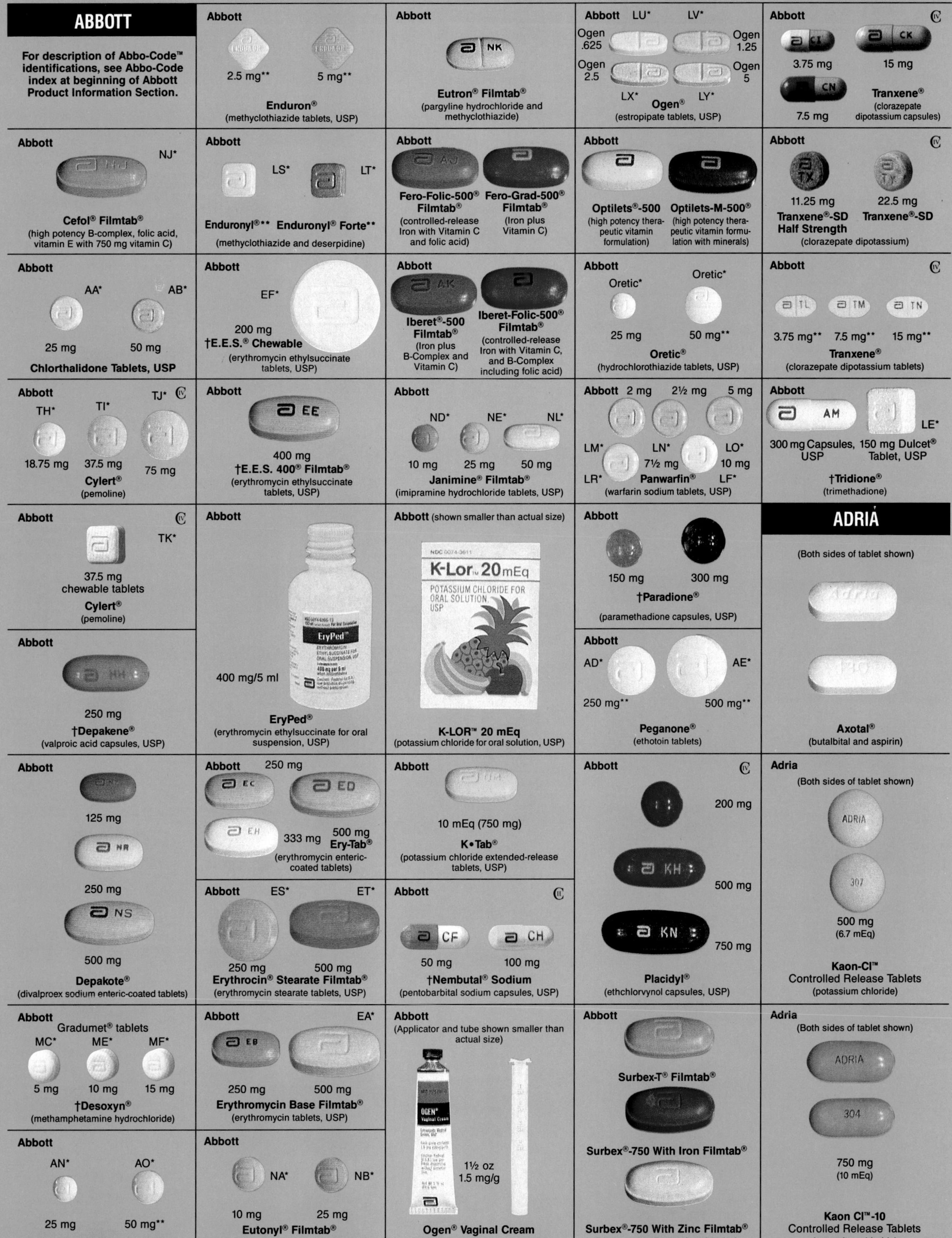

*Abbott Abbo-Code identification letters. Filmtab®—Film-sealed tablets, Abbott. **Grooved tablets.

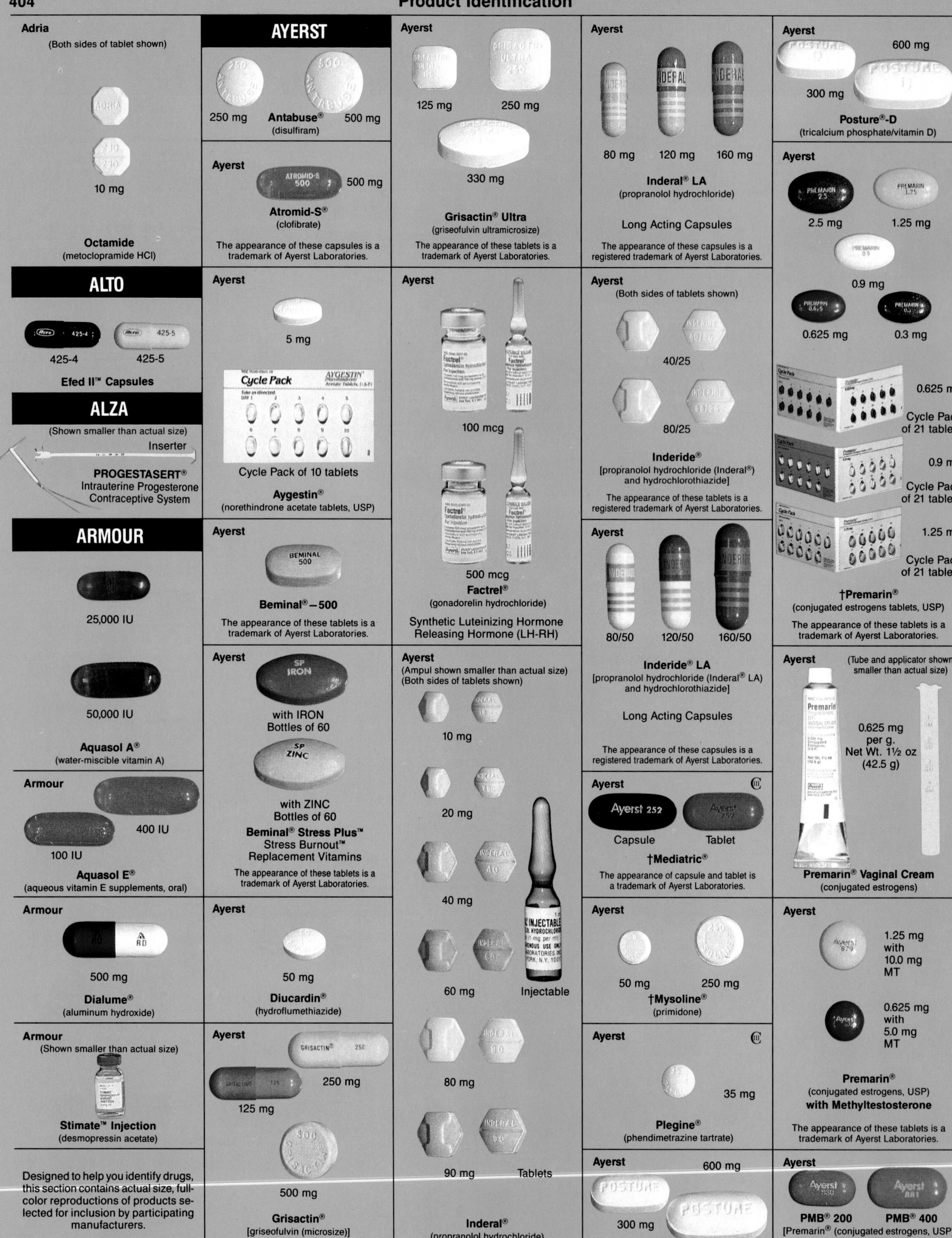

Adria
(Both sides of tablet shown)
10 mg
Octamide
(metoclopramide HCl)
ALTO
425-4
425-5
Efed II™ Capsules
ALZA
(Shown smaller than actual size)
Inserter
PROGESTASERT®
Intrauterine Progesterone
Contraceptive System
ARMOUR
25,000 IU
50,000 IU
Aquasol A®
(water-miscible vitamin A)
Armour
400 IU
100 IU
Aquasol E®
(aqueous vitamin E supplements, oral)
Armour
500 mg
Dialume®
(aluminum hydroxide)
Armour
(Shown smaller than actual size)
Stimate™ Injection
(desmopressin acetate)
Designed to help you identify drugs, this section contains actual size, full-color reproductions of products selected for inclusion by participating manufacturers.
AYERST
250 mg
Antabuse®
500 mg
(disulfiram)
Ayerst
ATROMID-S 500
500 mg
Atromid-S®
(clofibrate)
The appearance of these capsules is a trademark of Ayerst Laboratories.
Ayerst
5 mg
Cycle Pack
AYGESTIN
Cycle Pack of 10 tablets
Aygestin®
(norethindrone acetate tablets, USP)
Ayerst
BEMINAL 500
Beminal® – 500
The appearance of these tablets is a trademark of Ayerst Laboratories.
Ayerst
SP IRON
with IRON
Bottles of 60
SP ZINC
with ZINC
Bottles of 60
Beminal® Stress Plus™
Stress Burnout™
Replacement Vitamins
The appearance of these tablets is a trademark of Ayerst Laboratories.
Ayerst
50 mg
Diucardin®
(hydroflumethiazide)
Ayerst
GRISACTIN® 250
250 mg
125 mg
500 mg
Grisactin®
[griseofulvin (microsize)]
The appearance of capsules and tablet is a trademark of Ayerst Laboratories.
Ayerst
125 mg
250 mg
330 mg
Grisactin® Ultra
(griseofulvin ultramicrosize)
The appearance of these tablets is a trademark of Ayerst Laboratories.
Ayerst
Factrel®
100 mcg
500 mcg
Factrel®
(gonadorelin hydrochloride)
Synthetic Luteinizing Hormone
Releasing Hormone (LH-RH)
Ayerst
(Ampul shown smaller than actual size)
(Both sides of tablets shown)
10 mg
20 mg
40 mg
60 mg
Injectable
80 mg
90 mg
Tablets
Inderal®
(propranolol hydrochloride)
The appearance of these tablets is a registered trademark of Ayerst Laboratories.
Ayerst
80 mg
120 mg
160 mg
Inderal® LA
(propranolol hydrochloride)
Long Acting Capsules
The appearance of these capsules is a registered trademark of Ayerst Laboratories.
Ayerst
(Both sides of tablets shown)
40/25
80/25
Inderide®
[propranolol hydrochloride (Inderal®) and hydrochlorothiazide]
The appearance of these tablets is a registered trademark of Ayerst Laboratories.
Ayerst
80/50
120/50
160/50
Inderide® LA
[propranolol hydrochloride (Inderal® LA) and hydrochlorothiazide]
Long Acting Capsules
The appearance of these capsules is a registered trademark of Ayerst Laboratories.
Ayerst
Ayerst 252
Capsule
Tablet
†Mediatric®
The appearance of capsule and tablet is a trademark of Ayerst Laboratories.
Ayerst
50 mg
250 mg
†Mysoline®
(primidone)
Ayerst
35 mg
Plegine®
(phendimetrazine tartrate)
Ayerst
600 mg
300 mg
Posture®
(tricalcium phosphate)
Ayerst
600 mg
300 mg
Posture®-D
(tricalcium phosphate/vitamin D)
Ayerst
2.5 mg
1.25 mg
0.9 mg
0.625 mg
0.3 mg
0.625 mg
Cycle Pack of 21 tablets
0.9 mg
Cycle Pack of 21 tablets
1.25 mg
Cycle Pack of 21 tablets
†Premarin®
(conjugated estrogens tablets, USP)
The appearance of these tablets is a trademark of Ayerst Laboratories.
Ayerst
(Tube and applicator shown smaller than actual size)
Premarin
0.625 mg
per g.
Net Wt. 1½ oz
(42.5 g)
Premarin® Vaginal Cream
(conjugated estrogens)
Ayerst
1.25 mg with 10.0 mg MT
0.625 mg with 5.0 mg MT
Premarin®
(conjugated estrogens, USP)
with Methyltestosterone
The appearance of these tablets is a trademark of Ayerst Laboratories.
Ayerst
PMB® 200
PMB® 400
[Premarin® (conjugated estrogens, USP) with meprobamate]
The appearance of these tablets is a trademark of Ayerst Laboratories.

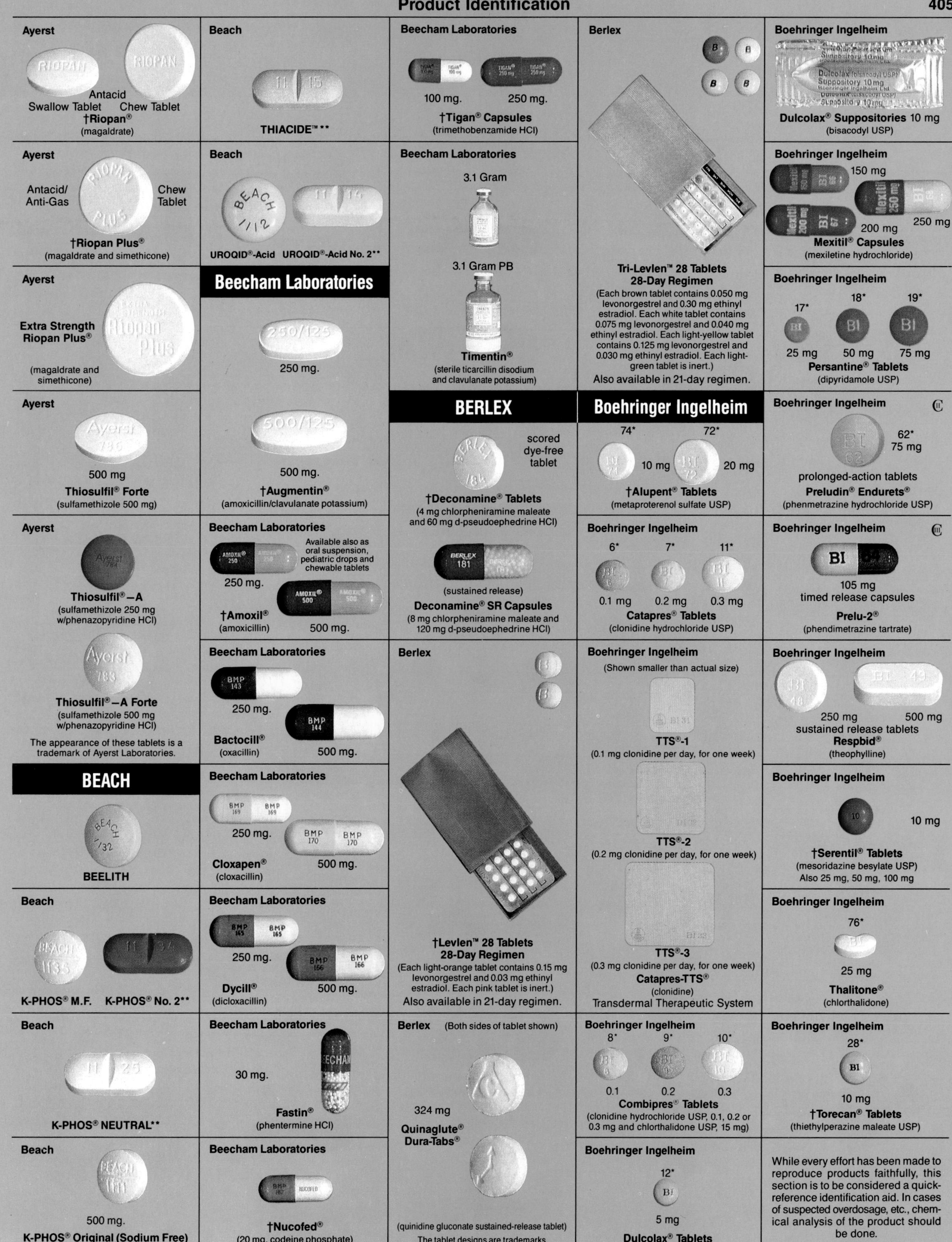

Ayerst

Antacid
Swallow Tablet Chew Tablet
†Riopan®
(magaldrate)

Ayerst

Antacid/ Anti-Gas Chew Tablet
†Riopan Plus®
(magaldrate and simethicone)

Ayerst

Extra Strength Riopan Plus®
(magaldrate and simethicone)

Ayerst

500 mg
Thiosulfil® Forte
(sulfamethizole 500 mg)

Ayerst

Thiosulfil®–A
(sulfamethizole 250 mg w/phenazopyridine HCl)

Thiosulfil®–A Forte
(sulfamethizole 500 mg w/phenazopyridine HCl)

The appearance of these tablets is a trademark of Ayerst Laboratories.

BEACH

BEELITH

Beach

K-PHOS® M.F. K-PHOS® No. 2**

Beach

K-PHOS® NEUTRAL**

Beach

500 mg.
K-PHOS® Original (Sodium Free)
(Potassium Acid Phosphate)

Beach

THIACIDE™**

Beach

UROQID®-Acid UROQID®-Acid No. 2**

Beecham Laboratories

250 mg.

500 mg.
†Augmentin®
(amoxicillin/clavulanate potassium)

Beecham Laboratories

Available also as oral suspension, pediatric drops and chewable tablets
250 mg. 500 mg.
†Amoxil®
(amoxicillin)

Beecham Laboratories

250 mg. 500 mg.
Bactocill®
(oxacillin)

Beecham Laboratories

250 mg. 500 mg.
Cloxapen®
(cloxacillin)

Beecham Laboratories

250 mg. 500 mg.
Dycill®
(dicloxacillin)

Beecham Laboratories

30 mg.
Fastin®
(phentermine HCl)

Beecham Laboratories

†Nucofed®
(20 mg. codeine phosphate)
(60 mg. pseudoephedrine HCl)

Beecham Laboratories

100 mg. 250 mg.
†Tigan® Capsules
(trimethobenzamide HCl)

Beecham Laboratories

3.1 Gram
3.1 Gram PB
Timentin®
(sterile ticarcillin disodium and clavulanate potassium)

BERLEX

scored dye-free tablet
†Deconamine® Tablets
(4 mg chlorpheniramine maleate and 60 mg d-pseudoephedrine HCl)

(sustained release)
Deconamine® SR Capsules
(8 mg chlorpheniramine maleate and 120 mg d-pseudoephedrine HCl)

Berlex

†Levlen™ 28 Tablets
28-Day Regimen
(Each light-orange tablet contains 0.15 mg levonorgestrel and 0.03 mg ethinyl estradiol. Each pink tablet is inert.)
Also available in 21-day regimen.

Berlex (Both sides of tablet shown)

324 mg
Quinaglute® Dura-Tabs®
(quinidine gluconate sustained-release tablet)
The tablet designs are trademarks of Berlex Laboratories, Inc.

Berlex

Tri-Levlen™ 28 Tablets
28-Day Regimen
(Each brown tablet contains 0.050 mg levonorgestrel and 0.30 mg ethinyl estradiol. Each white tablet contains 0.075 mg levonorgestrel and 0.040 mg ethinyl estradiol. Each light-yellow tablet contains 0.125 mg levonorgestrel and 0.030 mg ethinyl estradiol. Each light-green tablet is inert.)
Also available in 21-day regimen.

Boehringer Ingelheim

74* 72*
10 mg 20 mg
†Alupent® Tablets
(metaproterenol sulfate USP)

Boehringer Ingelheim

6* 7* 11*
0.1 mg 0.2 mg 0.3 mg
Catapres® Tablets
(clonidine hydrochloride USP)

Boehringer Ingelheim

(Shown smaller than actual size)
TTS®-1
(0.1 mg clonidine per day, for one week)
TTS®-2
(0.2 mg clonidine per day, for one week)
TTS®-3
(0.3 mg clonidine per day, for one week)
Catapres-TTS®
(clonidine)
Transdermal Therapeutic System

Boehringer Ingelheim

8* 9* 10*
0.1 0.2 0.3
Combipres® Tablets
(clonidine hydrochloride USP, 0.1, 0.2 or 0.3 mg and chlorthalidone USP, 15 mg)

Boehringer Ingelheim

12*
5 mg
Dulcolax® Tablets
(bisacodyl USP)

Boehringer Ingelheim

Dulcolax® Suppositories 10 mg
(bisacodyl USP)

Boehringer Ingelheim

150 mg 200 mg 250 mg
Mexitil® Capsules
(mexiletine hydrochloride)

Boehringer Ingelheim

17* 18* 19*
25 mg 50 mg 75 mg
Persantine® Tablets
(dipyridamole USP)

Boehringer Ingelheim ©

62*
75 mg
prolonged-action tablets
Preludin® Endurets®
(phenmetrazine hydrochloride USP)

Boehringer Ingelheim ©

105 mg
timed release capsules
Prelu-2®
(phendimetrazine tartrate)

Boehringer Ingelheim

250 mg 500 mg
sustained release tablets
Respbid®
(theophylline)

Boehringer Ingelheim

10 mg
†Serentil® Tablets
(mesoridazine besylate USP)
Also 25 mg, 50 mg, 100 mg

Boehringer Ingelheim

76*
25 mg
Thalitone®
(chlorthalidone)

Boehringer Ingelheim

28*
10 mg
†Torecan® Tablets
(thiethylperazine maleate USP)

While every effort has been made to reproduce products faithfully, this section is to be considered a quick-reference identification aid. In cases of suspected overdosage, etc., chemical analysis of the product should be done.

**The name BEACH appears on the reverse side of these tablets.

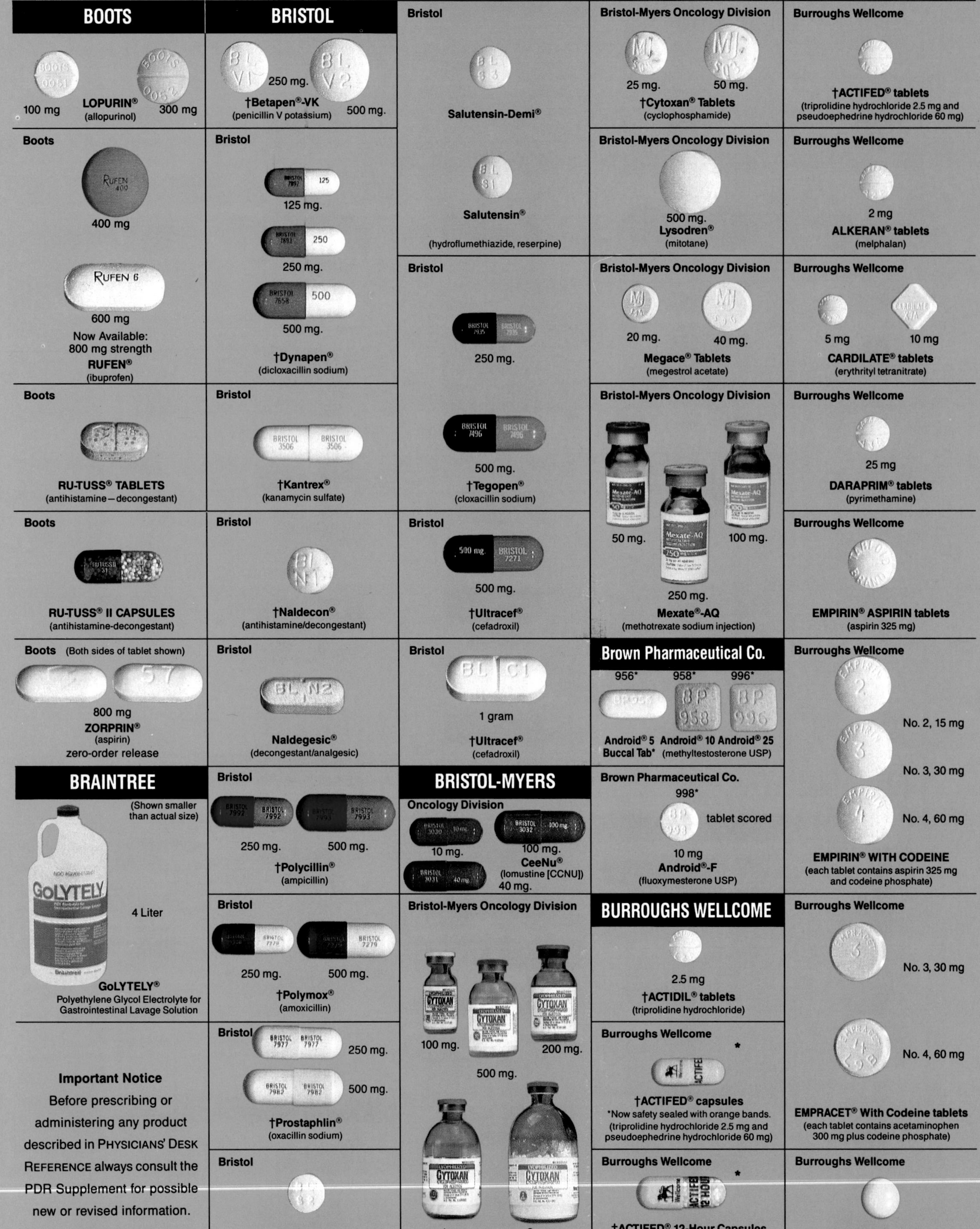
BOOTS
100 mg
LOPURIN®
(allopurinol)
300 mg
BRISTOL
250 mg.
†Betapen®-VK
(penicillin V potassium)
500 mg.
Bristol
Salutensin-Demi®
Bristol-Myers Oncology Division
25 mg.
50 mg.
†Cytoxan® Tablets
(cyclophosphamide)
Burroughs Wellcome
†ACTIFED® tablets
(triprolidine hydrochloride 2.5 mg and pseudoephedrine hydrochloride 60 mg)
Boots
400 mg
600 mg
Now Available:
800 mg strength
RUFEN®
(ibuprofen)
Bristol
125 mg.
250 mg.
500 mg.
†Dynapen®
(dicloxacillin sodium)
Salutensin®
(hydroflumethiazide, reserpine)
Bristol-Myers Oncology Division
500 mg.
Lysodren®
(mitotane)
Burroughs Wellcome
2 mg
ALKERAN® tablets
(melphalan)
Bristol
250 mg.
500 mg.
†Tegopen®
(cloxacillin sodium)
Bristol-Myers Oncology Division
20 mg.
40 mg.
Megace® Tablets
(megestrol acetate)
Burroughs Wellcome
5 mg
10 mg
CARDILATE® tablets
(erythrityl tetranitrate)
Boots
RU-TUSS® TABLETS
(antihistamine—decongestant)
Bristol
†Kantrex®
(kanamycin sulfate)
Bristol-Myers Oncology Division
50 mg.
100 mg.
250 mg.
Mexate®-AQ
(methotrexate sodium injection)
Burroughs Wellcome
25 mg
DARAPRIM® tablets
(pyrimethamine)
Boots
RU-TUSS® II CAPSULES
(antihistamine-decongestant)
Bristol
†Naldecon®
(antihistamine/decongestant)
Bristol
500 mg.
†Ultracef®
(cefadroxil)
Burroughs Wellcome
EMPIRIN® ASPIRIN tablets
(aspirin 325 mg)
Boots (Both sides of tablet shown)
800 mg
ZORPRIN®
(aspirin)
zero-order release
Bristol
Naldegesic®
(decongestant/analgesic)
Bristol
1 gram
†Ultracef®
(cefadroxil)
Brown Pharmaceutical Co.
956* 958* 996*
Android® 5 Buccal Tab*
Android® 10
Android® 25
(methyltestosterone USP)
Burroughs Wellcome
No. 2, 15 mg
No. 3, 30 mg
No. 4, 60 mg
EMPIRIN® WITH CODEINE
(each tablet contains aspirin 325 mg and codeine phosphate)
BRAINTREE
(Shown smaller than actual size)
4 Liter
GoLYTELY®
Polyethylene Glycol Electrolyte for Gastrointestinal Lavage Solution
Bristol
250 mg.
500 mg.
†Polycillin®
(ampicillin)
BRISTOL-MYERS
Oncology Division
10 mg.
100 mg.
40 mg.
CeeNu®
(lomustine [CCNU])
Brown Pharmaceutical Co.
998*
tablet scored
10 mg
Android®-F
(fluoxymesterone USP)
Bristol
250 mg.
500 mg.
†Polymox®
(amoxicillin)
Bristol-Myers Oncology Division
100 mg.
500 mg.
200 mg.
1 gm.
2 gm.
Cytoxan® Injection
(cyclophosphamide)
BURROUGHS WELLCOME
2.5 mg
†ACTIDIL® tablets
(triprolidine hydrochloride)
Burroughs Wellcome
No. 3, 30 mg
No. 4, 60 mg
EMPRACET® With Codeine tablets
(each tablet contains acetaminophen 300 mg plus codeine phosphate)
Important Notice
Before prescribing or administering any product described in PHYSICIANS' DESK REFERENCE always consult the PDR Supplement for possible new or revised information.
Bristol
250 mg.
500 mg.
†Prostaphlin®
(oxacillin sodium)
Burroughs Wellcome
*
†ACTIFED® capsules
*Now safety sealed with orange bands.
(triprolidine hydrochloride 2.5 mg and pseudoephedrine hydrochloride 60 mg)
Bristol
50 mg.
Saluron®
(hydroflumethiazide)
Burroughs Wellcome
*
†ACTIFED® 12-Hour Capsules
*Now safety sealed with orange bands.
(triprolidine hydrochloride 5 mg and pseudoephedrine hydrochloride 120 mg)
Burroughs Wellcome
FEDRAZIL® tablets
(pseudoephedrine hydrochloride 30 mg and chlorcyclizine hydrochloride 25 mg)

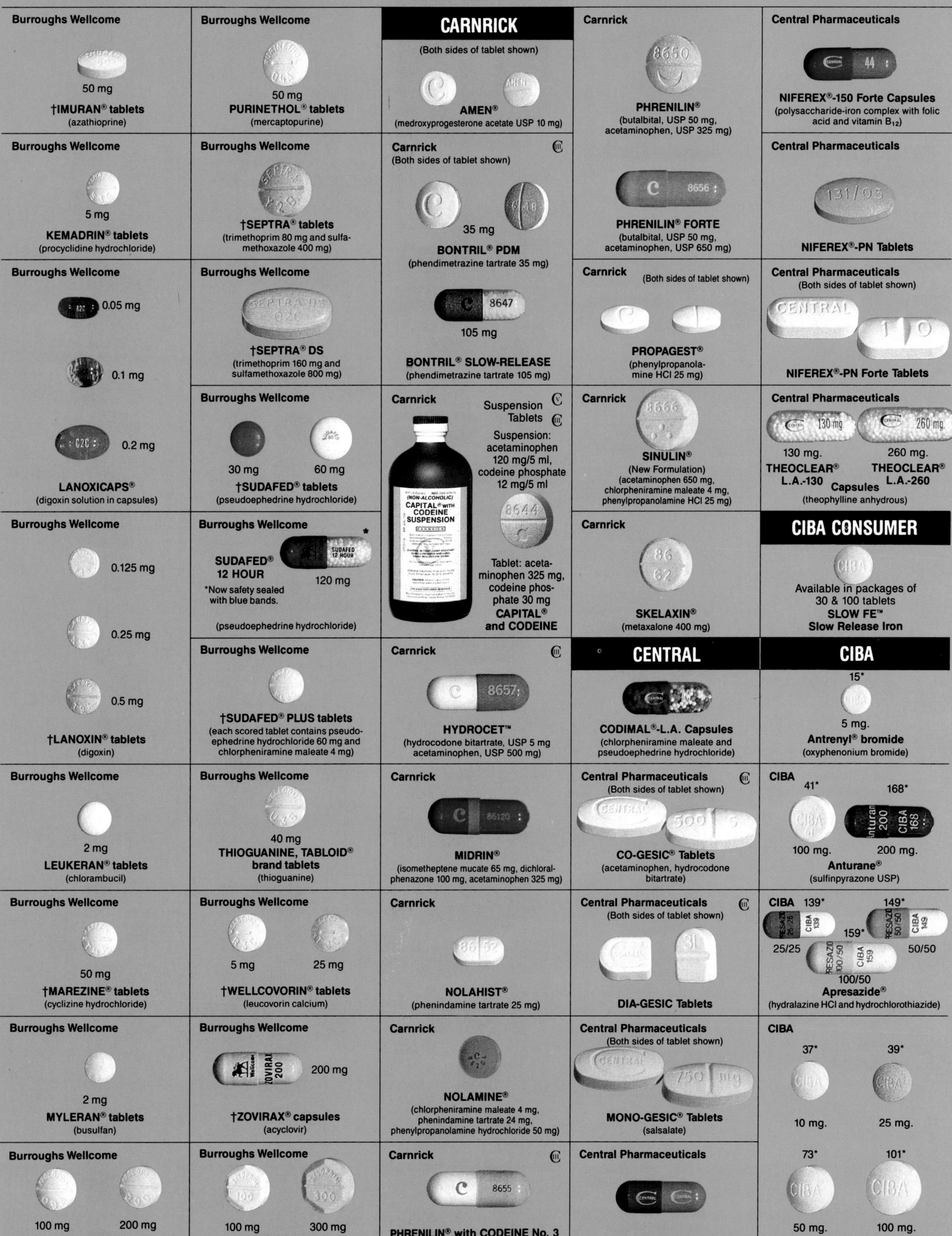
Burroughs Wellcome
50 mg
†IMURAN® tablets
(azathioprine)
Burroughs Wellcome
5 mg
KEMADRIN® tablets
(procyclidine hydrochloride)
Burroughs Wellcome
0.05 mg
0.1 mg
0.2 mg
LANOXICAPS®
(digoxin solution in capsules)
Burroughs Wellcome
0.125 mg
0.25 mg
0.5 mg
†LANOXIN® tablets
(digoxin)
Burroughs Wellcome
2 mg
LEUKERAN® tablets
(chlorambucil)
Burroughs Wellcome
50 mg
†MAREZINE® tablets
(cyclizine hydrochloride)
Burroughs Wellcome
2 mg
MYLERAN® tablets
(busulfan)
Burroughs Wellcome
100 mg
200 mg
PROLOPRIM®
(trimethoprim)
Burroughs Wellcome
50 mg
PURINETHOL® tablets
(mercaptopurine)
Burroughs Wellcome
†SEPTRA® tablets
(trimethoprim 80 mg and sulfa-methoxazole 400 mg)
Burroughs Wellcome
†SEPTRA® DS
(trimethoprim 160 mg and sulfamethoxazole 800 mg)
Burroughs Wellcome
30 mg
60 mg
†SUDAFED® tablets
(pseudoephedrine hydrochloride)
Burroughs Wellcome
*
SUDAFED®
12 HOUR
120 mg
*Now safety sealed with blue bands.
(pseudoephedrine hydrochloride)
Burroughs Wellcome
†SUDAFED® PLUS tablets
(each scored tablet contains pseudo-ephedrine hydrochloride 60 mg and chlorpheniramine maleate 4 mg)
Burroughs Wellcome
40 mg
THIOGUANINE, TABLOID® brand tablets
(thioguanine)
Burroughs Wellcome
5 mg
25 mg
†WELLCOVORIN® tablets
(leucovorin calcium)
Burroughs Wellcome
200 mg
†ZOVIRAX® capsules
(acyclovir)
Burroughs Wellcome
100 mg
300 mg
ZYLOPRIM® tablets
(allopurinol)
CARNRICK
(Both sides of tablet shown)
AMEN®
(medroxyprogesterone acetate USP 10 mg)
Carnrick
(Both sides of tablet shown)
35 mg
BONTRIL® PDM
(phendimetrazine tartrate 35 mg)
105 mg
BONTRIL® SLOW-RELEASE
(phendimetrazine tartrate 105 mg)
Carnrick
Suspension
Tablets
Suspension: acetaminophen 120 mg/5 ml, codeine phosphate 12 mg/5 ml
Tablet: acetaminophen 325 mg, codeine phosphate 30 mg
CAPITAL® and CODEINE
Carnrick
HYDROCET™
(hydrocodone bitartrate, USP 5 mg acetaminophen, USP 500 mg)
Carnrick
MIDRIN®
(isometheptene mucate 65 mg, dichloral-phenazone 100 mg, acetaminophen 325 mg)
Carnrick
NOLAHIST®
(phenindamine tartrate 25 mg)
Carnrick
NOLAMINE®
(chlorpheniramine maleate 4 mg, phenindamine tartrate 24 mg, phenylpropanolamine hydrochloride 50 mg)
Carnrick
PHRENILIN® with CODEINE No. 3
(acetaminophen, USP 325 mg, butalbital, USP 50 mg, codeine phosphate, USP 30 mg)
Carnrick
PHRENILIN®
(butalbital, USP 50 mg, acetaminophen, USP 325 mg)
PHRENILIN® FORTE
(butalbital, USP 50 mg, acetaminophen, USP 650 mg)
Carnrick
(Both sides of tablet shown)
PROPAGEST®
(phenylpropanolamine HCl 25 mg)
Carnrick
SINULIN®
(New Formulation)
(acetaminophen 650 mg, chlorpheniramine maleate 4 mg, phenylpropanolamine HCl 25 mg)
Carnrick
SKELAXIN®
(metaxalone 400 mg)
CENTRAL
CODIMAL®-L.A. Capsules
(chlorpheniramine maleate and pseudoephedrine hydrochloride)
Central Pharmaceuticals
(Both sides of tablet shown)
CO-GESIC® Tablets
(acetaminophen, hydrocodone bitartrate)
Central Pharmaceuticals
(Both sides of tablet shown)
DIA-GESIC Tablets
Central Pharmaceuticals
(Both sides of tablet shown)
MONO-GESIC® Tablets
(salsalate)
Central Pharmaceuticals
NIFEREX®-150 Capsules
(polysaccharide-iron complex)
Central Pharmaceuticals
NIFEREX®-150 Forte Capsules
(polysaccharide-iron complex with folic acid and vitamin B_{12})
Central Pharmaceuticals
NIFEREX®-PN Tablets
Central Pharmaceuticals
(Both sides of tablet shown)
NIFEREX®-PN Forte Tablets
Central Pharmaceuticals
130 mg.
260 mg.
THEOCLEAR® L.A.-130
THEOCLEAR® L.A.-260
Capsules
(theophylline anhydrous)
CIBA CONSUMER
Available in packages of 30 & 100 tablets
SLOW FE™
Slow Release Iron
CIBA
15*
5 mg.
Antrenyl® bromide
(oxyphenonium bromide)
CIBA
41*
168*
100 mg.
200 mg.
Anturane®
(sulfinpyrazone USP)
CIBA
139*
149*
159*
25/25
50/50
100/50
Apresazide®
(hydralazine HCl and hydrochlorothiazide)
CIBA
37*
39*
10 mg.
25 mg.
73*
101*
50 mg.
100 mg.
Apresoline® hydrochloride
(hydralazine hydrochloride)

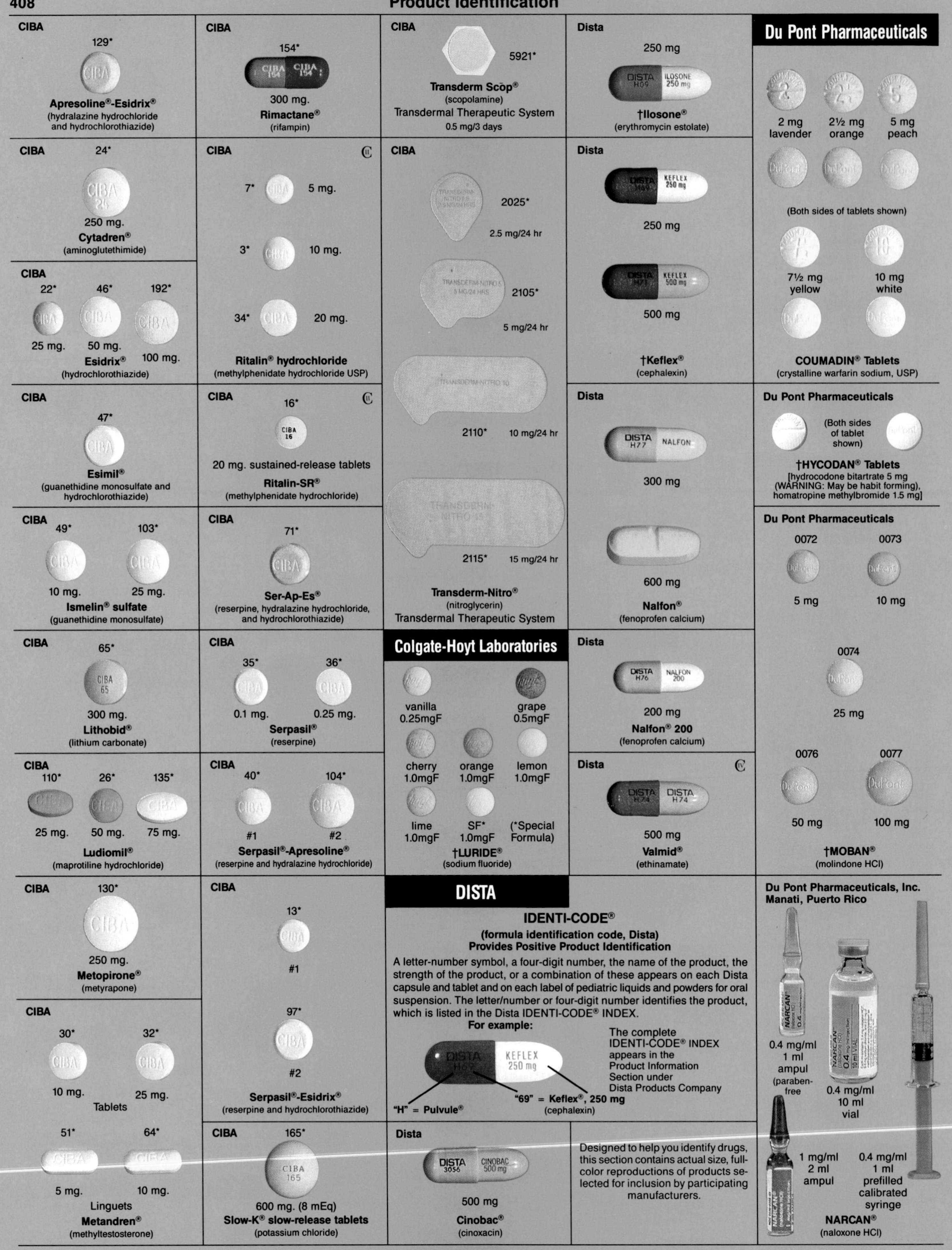
CIBA
129*
Apresoline®-Esidrix®
(hydralazine hydrochloride and hydrochlorothiazide)
CIBA
24*
250 mg.
Cytadren®
(aminoglutethimide)
CIBA
22* 46* 192*
25 mg. 50 mg. 100 mg.
Esidrix®
(hydrochlorothiazide)
CIBA
47*
Esimil®
(guanethidine monosulfate and hydrochlorothiazide)
CIBA
49* 103*
10 mg. 25 mg.
Ismelin® sulfate
(guanethidine monosulfate)
CIBA
65*
300 mg.
Lithobid®
(lithium carbonate)
CIBA
110* 26* 135*
25 mg. 50 mg. 75 mg.
Ludiomil®
(maprotiline hydrochloride)
CIBA
130*
250 mg.
Metopirone®
(metyrapone)
CIBA
30* 32*
10 mg. 25 mg.
Tablets
51* 64*
5 mg. 10 mg.
Linguets
Metandren®
(methyltestosterone)
CIBA
154*
300 mg.
Rimactane®
(rifampin)
CIBA
7* 5 mg.
3* 10 mg.
34* 20 mg.
Ritalin® hydrochloride
(methylphenidate hydrochloride USP)
CIBA
16*
20 mg. sustained-release tablets
Ritalin-SR®
(methylphenidate hydrochloride)
CIBA
71*
Ser-Ap-Es®
(reserpine, hydralazine hydrochloride, and hydrochlorothiazide)
CIBA
35* 36*
0.1 mg. 0.25 mg.
Serpasil®
(reserpine)
CIBA
40* 104*
#1 #2
Serpasil®-Apresoline®
(reserpine and hydralazine hydrochloride)
CIBA
13*
#1
97*
#2
Serpasil®-Esidrix®
(reserpine and hydrochlorothiazide)
CIBA
165*
600 mg. (8 mEq)
Slow-K® slow-release tablets
(potassium chloride)
CIBA
5921*
Transderm Scōp®
(scopolamine)
Transdermal Therapeutic System
0.5 mg/3 days
CIBA
2025*
2.5 mg/24 hr
2105*
5 mg/24 hr
2110* 10 mg/24 hr
2115* 15 mg/24 hr
Transderm-Nitro®
(nitroglycerin)
Transdermal Therapeutic System
Colgate-Hoyt Laboratories
vanilla 0.25mgF
grape 0.5mgF
cherry 1.0mgF
orange 1.0mgF
lemon 1.0mgF
lime 1.0mgF
SF* 1.0mgF
(*Special Formula)
†LURIDE®
(sodium fluoride)
DISTA
IDENTI-CODE®
(formula identification code, Dista)
Provides Positive Product Identification
A letter-number symbol, a four-digit number, the name of the product, the strength of the product, or a combination of these appears on each Dista capsule and tablet and on each label of pediatric liquids and powders for oral suspension. The letter/number or four-digit number identifies the product, which is listed in the Dista IDENTI-CODE® INDEX.
For example:
The complete IDENTI-CODE® INDEX appears in the Product Information Section under Dista Products Company
"H" = Pulvule®
"69" = Keflex®, 250 mg
(cephalexin)
Dista
500 mg
Cinobac®
(cinoxacin)
Designed to help you identify drugs, this section contains actual size, full-color reproductions of products selected for inclusion by participating manufacturers.
Dista
250 mg
†Ilosone®
(erythromycin estolate)
Dista
250 mg
500 mg
†Keflex®
(cephalexin)
Dista
300 mg
600 mg
Nalfon®
(fenoprofen calcium)
Dista
200 mg
Nalfon® 200
(fenoprofen calcium)
Dista
500 mg
Valmid®
(ethinamate)
Du Pont Pharmaceuticals
2 mg lavender
2½ mg orange
5 mg peach
(Both sides of tablets shown)
7½ mg yellow
10 mg white
COUMADIN® Tablets
(crystalline warfarin sodium, USP)
Du Pont Pharmaceuticals
(Both sides of tablet shown)
†HYCODAN® Tablets
[hydrocodone bitartrate 5 mg (WARNING: May be habit forming), homatropine methylbromide 1.5 mg]
Du Pont Pharmaceuticals
0072 0073
5 mg 10 mg
0074
25 mg
0076 0077
50 mg 100 mg
†MOBAN®
(molindone HCl)
Du Pont Pharmaceuticals, Inc.
Manati, Puerto Rico
0.4 mg/ml 1 ml ampul (paraben-free
0.4 mg/ml 10 ml vial
1 mg/ml 2 ml ampul
0.4 mg/ml 1 ml prefilled calibrated syringe
NARCAN®
(naloxone HCl)

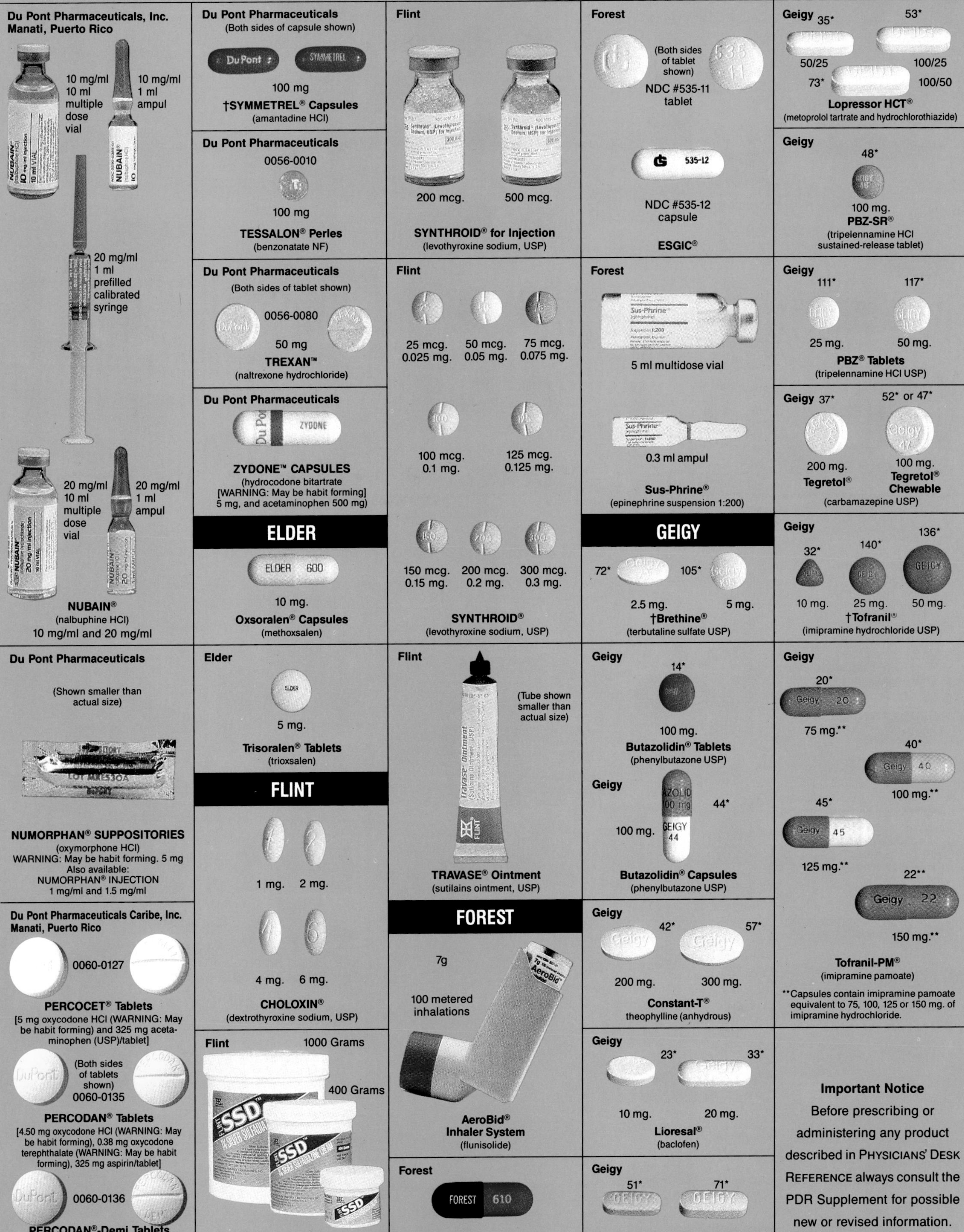

Du Pont Pharmaceuticals, Inc.
Manati, Puerto Rico

10 mg/ml 10 ml multiple dose vial
10 mg/ml 1 ml ampul
20 mg/ml 1 ml prefilled calibrated syringe
20 mg/ml 10 ml multiple dose vial
20 mg/ml 1 ml ampul

NUBAIN®
(nalbuphine HCl)
10 mg/ml and 20 mg/ml

Du Pont Pharmaceuticals
(Both sides of capsule shown)
100 mg
†SYMMETREL® Capsules
(amantadine HCl)

Du Pont Pharmaceuticals
0056-0010
100 mg
TESSALON® Perles
(benzonatate NF)

Du Pont Pharmaceuticals
(Both sides of tablet shown)
0056-0080
50 mg
TREXAN™
(naltrexone hydrochloride)

Du Pont Pharmaceuticals
ZYDONE™ CAPSULES
(hydrocodone bitartrate [WARNING: May be habit forming] 5 mg, and acetaminophen 500 mg)

ELDER

10 mg.
Oxsoralen® Capsules
(methoxsalen)

Flint
200 mcg. 500 mcg.
SYNTHROID® for Injection
(levothyroxine sodium, USP)

Flint
25 mcg. 0.025 mg. 50 mcg. 0.05 mg. 75 mcg. 0.075 mg.
100 mcg. 0.1 mg. 125 mcg. 0.125 mg.
150 mcg. 0.15 mg. 200 mcg. 0.2 mg. 300 mcg. 0.3 mg.
SYNTHROID®
(levothyroxine sodium, USP)

Forest
(Both sides of tablet shown)
NDC #535-11 tablet
NDC #535-12 capsule
ESGIC®

Forest
5 ml multidose vial
0.3 ml ampul
Sus-Phrine®
(epinephrine suspension 1:200)

GEIGY

72* 105*
2.5 mg. 5 mg.
†Brethine®
(terbutaline sulfate USP)

Geigy
35* 53*
50/25 100/25
73* 100/50
Lopressor HCT®
(metoprolol tartrate and hydrochlorothiazide)

Geigy
48*
100 mg.
PBZ-SR®
(tripelennamine HCl sustained-release tablet)

Geigy
111* 117*
25 mg. 50 mg.
PBZ® Tablets
(tripelennamine HCl USP)

Geigy
37* 52* or 47*
200 mg. **Tegretol®**
100 mg. **Tegretol® Chewable**
(carbamazepine USP)

Geigy
32* 140* 136*
10 mg. 25 mg. 50 mg.
†Tofranil®
(imipramine hydrochloride USP)

Du Pont Pharmaceuticals
(Shown smaller than actual size)
NUMORPHAN® SUPPOSITORIES
(oxymorphone HCl)
WARNING: May be habit forming. 5 mg
Also available:
NUMORPHAN® INJECTION
1 mg/ml and 1.5 mg/ml

Du Pont Pharmaceuticals Caribe, Inc.
Manati, Puerto Rico

0060-0127
PERCOCET® Tablets
[5 mg oxycodone HCl (WARNING: May be habit forming) and 325 mg acetaminophen (USP)/tablet]

(Both sides of tablets shown)
0060-0135
PERCODAN® Tablets
[4.50 mg oxycodone HCl (WARNING: May be habit forming), 0.38 mg oxycodone terephthalate (WARNING: May be habit forming), 325 mg aspirin/tablet]

0060-0136
PERCODAN®-Demi Tablets
[2.25 mg oxycodone HCl (WARNING: May be habit forming), 0.19 mg oxycodone terephthalate (WARNING: May be habit forming), 325 mg aspirin/tablet]

Elder
5 mg.
Trisoralen® Tablets
(trioxsalen)

FLINT

1 mg. 2 mg.
4 mg. 6 mg.
CHOLOXIN®
(dextrothyroxine sodium, USP)

Flint
1000 Grams
400 Grams
50 Grams
Flint SSD™
1% Silver Sulfadiazine Cream
For Topical Use Only

Flint
(Tube shown smaller than actual size)
TRAVASE® Ointment
(sutilains ointment, USP)

FOREST

7g
100 metered inhalations
AeroBid®
Inhaler System
(flunisolide)

Forest
Bancap HC®
(hydrocodone bitartrate, 5 mg and acetaminophen, 500 mg)

Geigy
14*
100 mg.
Butazolidin® Tablets
(phenylbutazone USP)

Geigy
100 mg. 44*
Butazolidin® Capsules
(phenylbutazone USP)

Geigy
42* 57*
200 mg. 300 mg.
Constant-T®
theophylline (anhydrous)

Geigy
23* 33*
10 mg. 20 mg.
Lioresal®
(baclofen)

Geigy
51* 71*
50 mg. 100 mg.
Lopressor®
(metoprolol tartrate)

Geigy
20*
75 mg.**
40*
100 mg.**
45*
125 mg.**
22**
150 mg.**
Tofranil-PM®
(imipramine pamoate)
**Capsules contain imipramine pamoate equivalent to 75, 100, 125 or 150 mg. of imipramine hydrochloride.

Important Notice
Before prescribing or administering any product described in PHYSICIANS' DESK REFERENCE always consult the PDR Supplement for possible new or revised information.

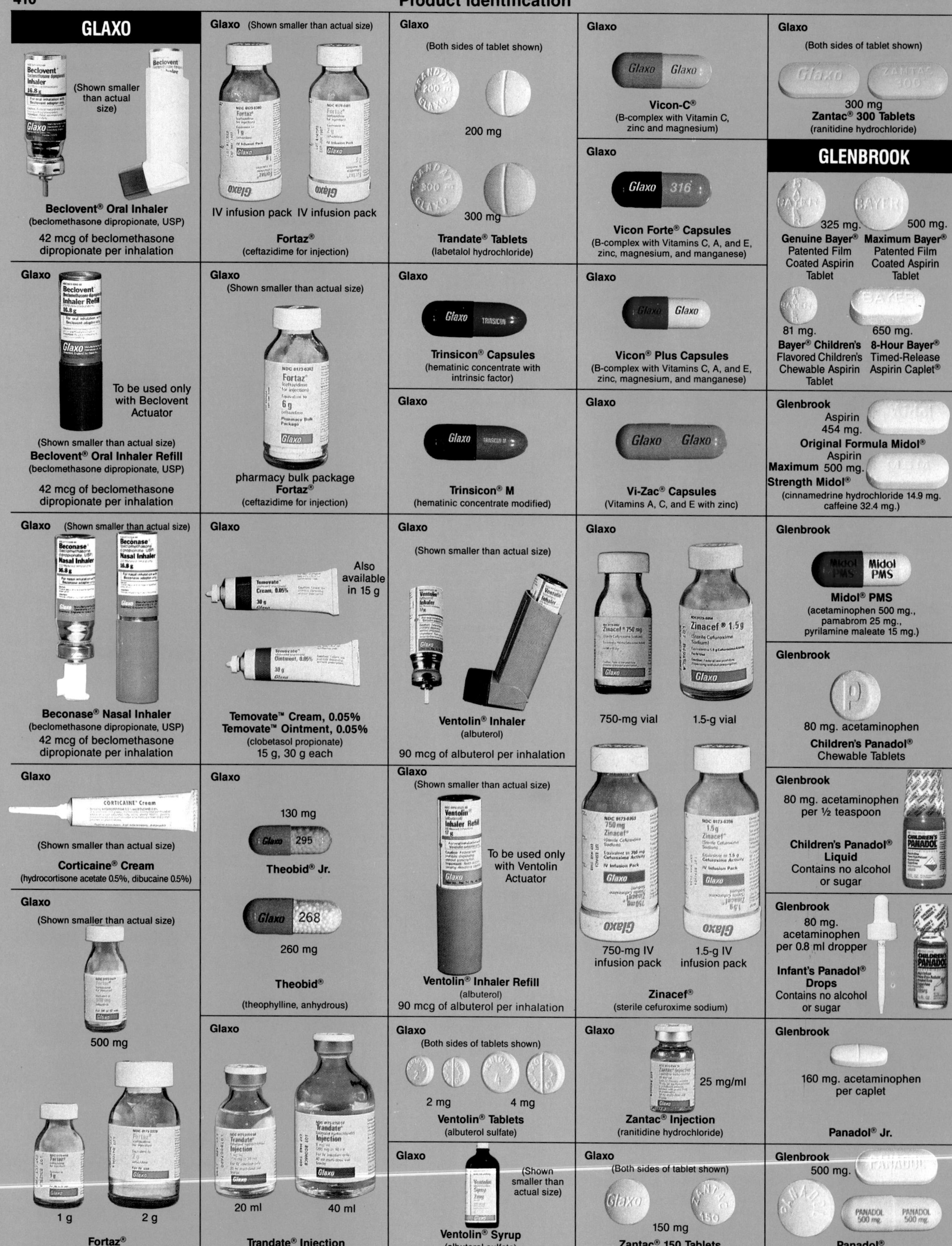

GLAXO

(Shown smaller than actual size)

Beclovent® Oral Inhaler
(beclomethasone dipropionate, USP)
42 mcg of beclomethasone dipropionate per inhalation

Glaxo

To be used only with Beclovent Actuator

(Shown smaller than actual size)
Beclovent® Oral Inhaler Refill
(beclomethasone dipropionate, USP)
42 mcg of beclomethasone dipropionate per inhalation

Glaxo (Shown smaller than actual size)

Beconase® Nasal Inhaler
(beclomethasone dipropionate, USP)
42 mcg of beclomethasone dipropionate per inhalation

Glaxo

(Shown smaller than actual size)
Corticaine® Cream
(hydrocortisone acetate 0.5%, dibucaine 0.5%)

Glaxo
(Shown smaller than actual size)

500 mg

1 g 2 g

Fortaz®
(ceftazidime for injection)

Glaxo (Shown smaller than actual size)

IV infusion pack IV infusion pack
Fortaz®
(ceftazidime for injection)

Glaxo
(Shown smaller than actual size)

pharmacy bulk package
Fortaz®
(ceftazidime for injection)

Glaxo

Also available in 15 g

Temovate™ Cream, 0.05%
Temovate™ Ointment, 0.05%
(clobetasol propionate)
15 g, 30 g each

Glaxo

130 mg
Theobid® Jr.

260 mg
Theobid®
(theophylline, anhydrous)

Glaxo

20 ml 40 ml
Trandate® Injection
(labetalol hydrochloride)

Glaxo
(Both sides of tablet shown)

200 mg

300 mg
Trandate® Tablets
(labetalol hydrochloride)

Glaxo

Trinsicon® Capsules
(hematinic concentrate with intrinsic factor)

Glaxo

Trinsicon® M
(hematinic concentrate modified)

Glaxo
(Shown smaller than actual size)

Ventolin® Inhaler
(albuterol)
90 mcg of albuterol per inhalation

Glaxo
(Shown smaller than actual size)

To be used only with Ventolin Actuator

Ventolin® Inhaler Refill
(albuterol)
90 mcg of albuterol per inhalation

Glaxo
(Both sides of tablets shown)

2 mg 4 mg
Ventolin® Tablets
(albuterol sulfate)

Glaxo

(Shown smaller than actual size)
Ventolin® Syrup
(albuterol sulfate)
2 mg/5 ml

Glaxo

Vicon-C®
(B-complex with Vitamin C, zinc and magnesium)

Glaxo

Vicon Forte® Capsules
(B-complex with Vitamins C, A, and E, zinc, magnesium, and manganese)

Glaxo

Vicon® Plus Capsules
(B-complex with Vitamins C, A, and E, zinc, magnesium, and manganese)

Glaxo

Vi-Zac® Capsules
(Vitamins A, C, and E with zinc)

Glaxo

750-mg vial 1.5-g vial

750-mg IV infusion pack 1.5-g IV infusion pack
Zinacef®
(sterile cefuroxime sodium)

Glaxo

25 mg/ml
Zantac® Injection
(ranitidine hydrochloride)

Glaxo
(Both sides of tablet shown)

150 mg
Zantac® 150 Tablets
(ranitidine hydrochloride)

Glaxo
(Both sides of tablet shown)

300 mg
Zantac® 300 Tablets
(ranitidine hydrochloride)

GLENBROOK

325 mg. **Genuine Bayer®** Patented Film Coated Aspirin Tablet

500 mg. **Maximum Bayer®** Patented Film Coated Aspirin Tablet

81 mg. **Bayer® Children's** Flavored Children's Chewable Aspirin Tablet

650 mg. **8-Hour Bayer®** Timed-Release Aspirin Caplet®

Glenbrook

Aspirin 454 mg.
Original Formula Midol®

Aspirin 500 mg.
Maximum Strength Midol®
(cinnamedrine hydrochloride 14.9 mg. caffeine 32.4 mg.)

Glenbrook

Midol® PMS
(acetaminophen 500 mg., pamabrom 25 mg., pyrilamine maleate 15 mg.)

Glenbrook

80 mg. acetaminophen
Children's Panadol®
Chewable Tablets

Glenbrook

80 mg. acetaminophen per ½ teaspoon
Children's Panadol® Liquid
Contains no alcohol or sugar

Glenbrook

80 mg. acetaminophen per 0.8 ml dropper
Infant's Panadol® Drops
Contains no alcohol or sugar

Glenbrook

160 mg. acetaminophen per caplet
Panadol® Jr.

Glenbrook

500 mg.
Panadol®
Acetaminophen Tablet, Capsule & Caplet

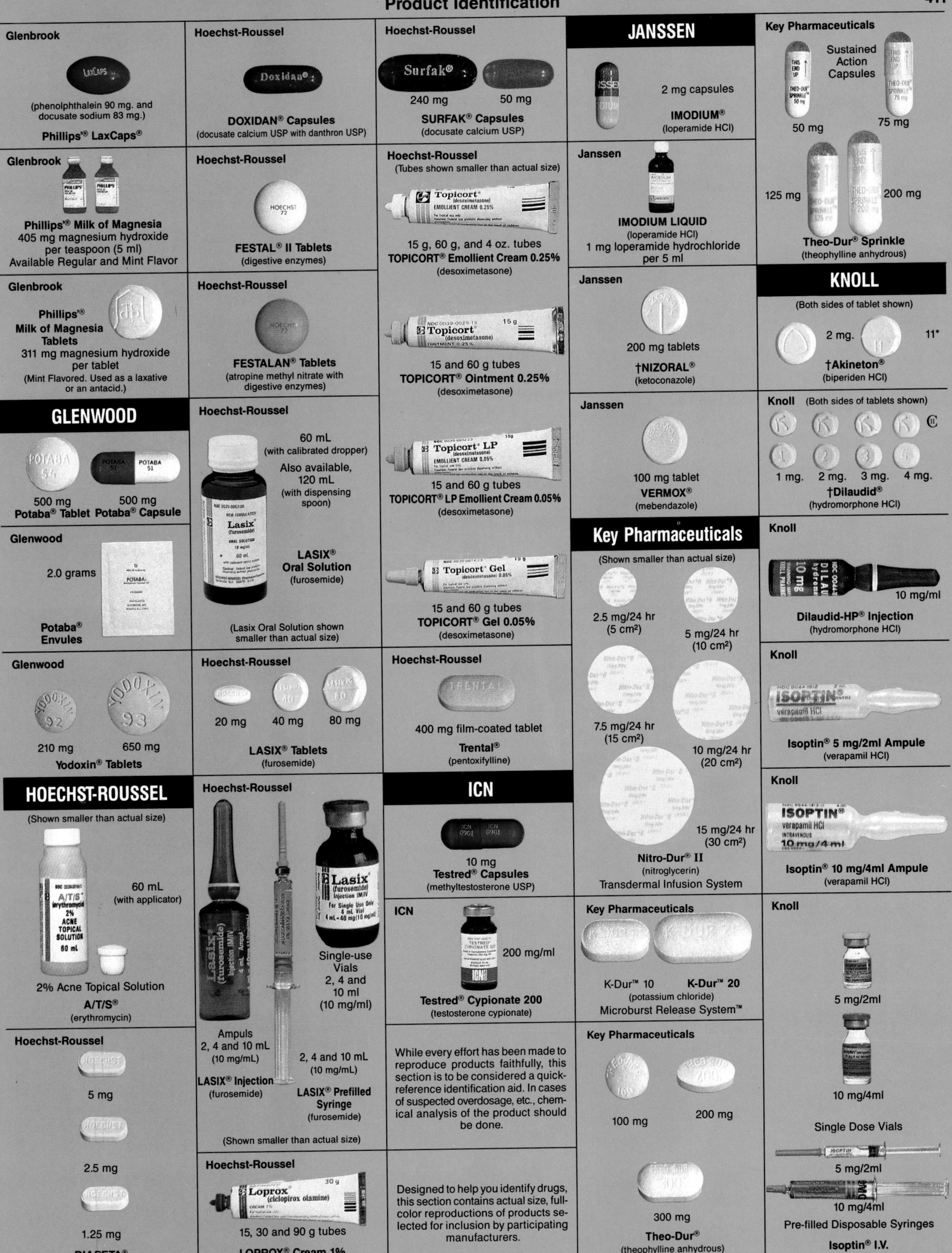

Glenbrook

(phenolphthalein 90 mg. and docusate sodium 83 mg.)

Phillips'® LaxCaps®

Glenbrook

Phillips'® Milk of Magnesia
405 mg magnesium hydroxide per teaspoon (5 ml)
Available Regular and Mint Flavor

Glenbrook

Phillips'® Milk of Magnesia Tablets
311 mg magnesium hydroxide per tablet
(Mint Flavored. Used as a laxative or an antacid.)

GLENWOOD

500 mg Potaba® Tablet
500 mg Potaba® Capsule

Glenwood

2.0 grams
Potaba® Envules

Glenwood

210 mg
650 mg
Yodoxin® Tablets

HOECHST-ROUSSEL

(Shown smaller than actual size)

60 mL (with applicator)
2% Acne Topical Solution
A/T/S®
(erythromycin)

Hoechst-Roussel

5 mg
2.5 mg
1.25 mg
DIABETA®
(glyburide)

Hoechst-Roussel

DOXIDAN® Capsules
(docusate calcium USP with danthron USP)

Hoechst-Roussel

FESTAL® II Tablets
(digestive enzymes)

Hoechst-Roussel

FESTALAN® Tablets
(atropine methyl nitrate with digestive enzymes)

Hoechst-Roussel

60 mL (with calibrated dropper)
Also available, 120 mL (with dispensing spoon)
LASIX® Oral Solution
(furosemide)
(Lasix Oral Solution shown smaller than actual size)

Hoechst-Roussel

20 mg
40 mg
80 mg
LASIX® Tablets
(furosemide)

Hoechst-Roussel

Ampuls 2, 4 and 10 mL (10 mg/mL)
LASIX® Injection
(furosemide)

2, 4 and 10 mL (10 mg/mL)
LASIX® Prefilled Syringe
(furosemide)

Single-use Vials 2, 4 and 10 ml (10 mg/ml)

(Shown smaller than actual size)

Hoechst-Roussel

15, 30 and 90 g tubes
LOPROX® Cream 1%
(ciclopirox olamine)

Hoechst-Roussel

240 mg
50 mg
SURFAK® Capsules
(docusate calcium USP)

Hoechst-Roussel
(Tubes shown smaller than actual size)

15 g, 60 g, and 4 oz. tubes
TOPICORT® Emollient Cream 0.25%
(desoximetasone)

15 and 60 g tubes
TOPICORT® Ointment 0.25%
(desoximetasone)

15 and 60 g tubes
TOPICORT® LP Emollient Cream 0.05%
(desoximetasone)

15 and 60 g tubes
TOPICORT® Gel 0.05%
(desoximetasone)

Hoechst-Roussel

400 mg film-coated tablet
Trental®
(pentoxifylline)

ICN

10 mg
Testred® Capsules
(methyltestosterone USP)

ICN

200 mg/ml
Testred® Cypionate 200
(testosterone cypionate)

While every effort has been made to reproduce products faithfully, this section is to be considered a quick-reference identification aid. In cases of suspected overdosage, etc., chemical analysis of the product should be done.

Designed to help you identify drugs, this section contains actual size, full-color reproductions of products selected for inclusion by participating manufacturers.

JANSSEN

2 mg capsules
IMODIUM®
(loperamide HCl)

Janssen

IMODIUM LIQUID
(loperamide HCl)
1 mg loperamide hydrochloride per 5 ml

Janssen

200 mg tablets
†NIZORAL®
(ketoconazole)

Janssen

100 mg tablet
VERMOX®
(mebendazole)

Key Pharmaceuticals

(Shown smaller than actual size)

2.5 mg/24 hr (5 cm²)
5 mg/24 hr (10 cm²)
7.5 mg/24 hr (15 cm²)
10 mg/24 hr (20 cm²)
15 mg/24 hr (30 cm²)
Nitro-Dur® II
(nitroglycerin)
Transdermal Infusion System

Key Pharmaceuticals

K-Dur™ 10
K-Dur™ 20
(potassium chloride)
Microburst Release System™

Key Pharmaceuticals

100 mg
200 mg
300 mg
Theo-Dur®
(theophylline anhydrous)
Sustained Action Tablets

Key Pharmaceuticals

Sustained Action Capsules
50 mg
75 mg
125 mg
200 mg
Theo-Dur® Sprinkle
(theophylline anhydrous)

KNOLL

(Both sides of tablet shown)

2 mg.
11*
†Akineton®
(biperiden HCl)

Knoll (Both sides of tablets shown)

1 mg.
2 mg.
3 mg.
4 mg.
†Dilaudid®
(hydromorphone HCl)

Knoll

10 mg/ml
Dilaudid-HP® Injection
(hydromorphone HCl)

Knoll

Isoptin® 5 mg/2ml Ampule
(verapamil HCl)

Knoll

Isoptin® 10 mg/4ml Ampule
(verapamil HCl)

Knoll

5 mg/2ml
10 mg/4ml
Single Dose Vials

5 mg/2ml
10 mg/4ml
Pre-filled Disposable Syringes

Isoptin® I.V.
(verapamil HCl)

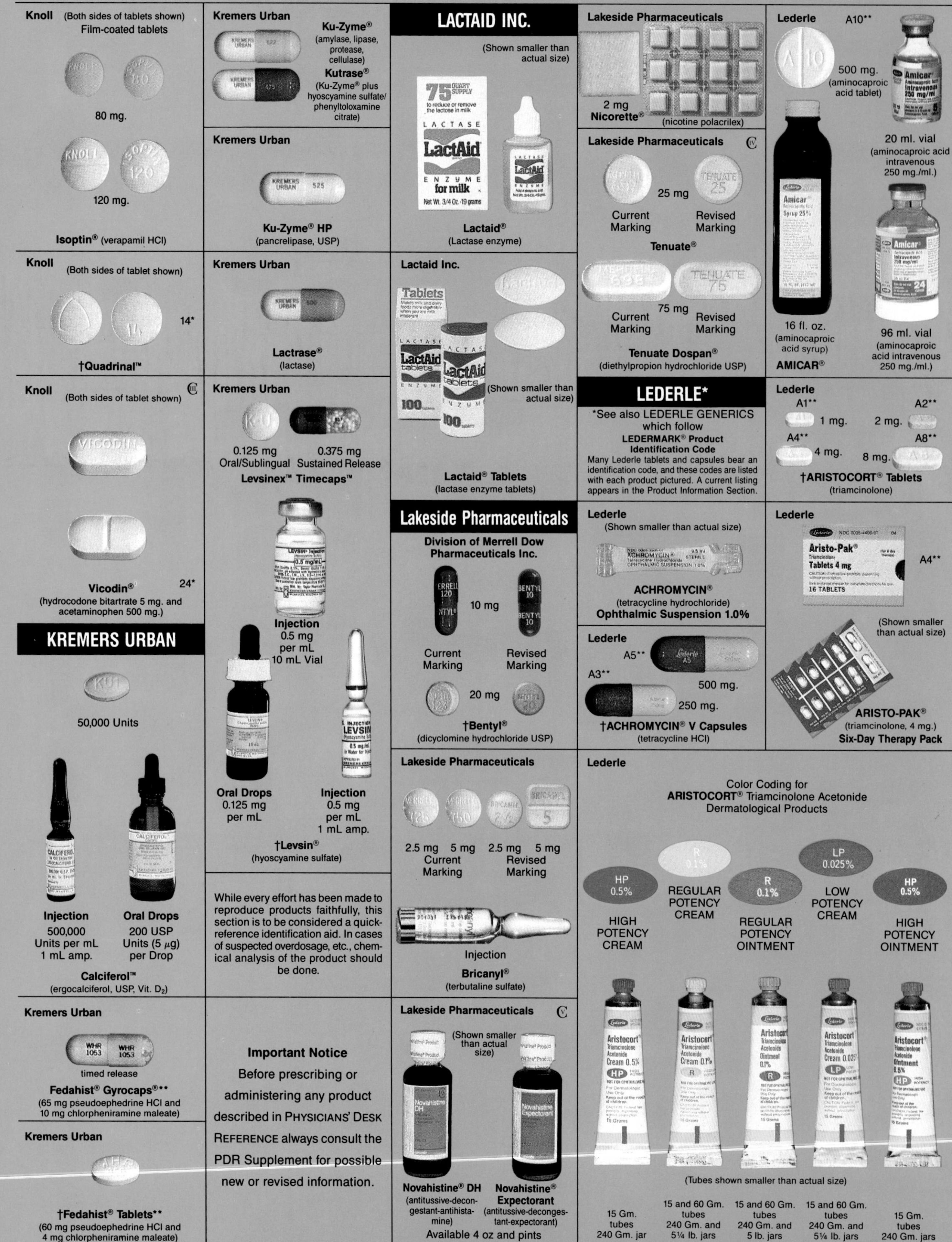

**During the next year, Kremers Urban identification may appear on these products. **Ledermark Product Identification Codes.

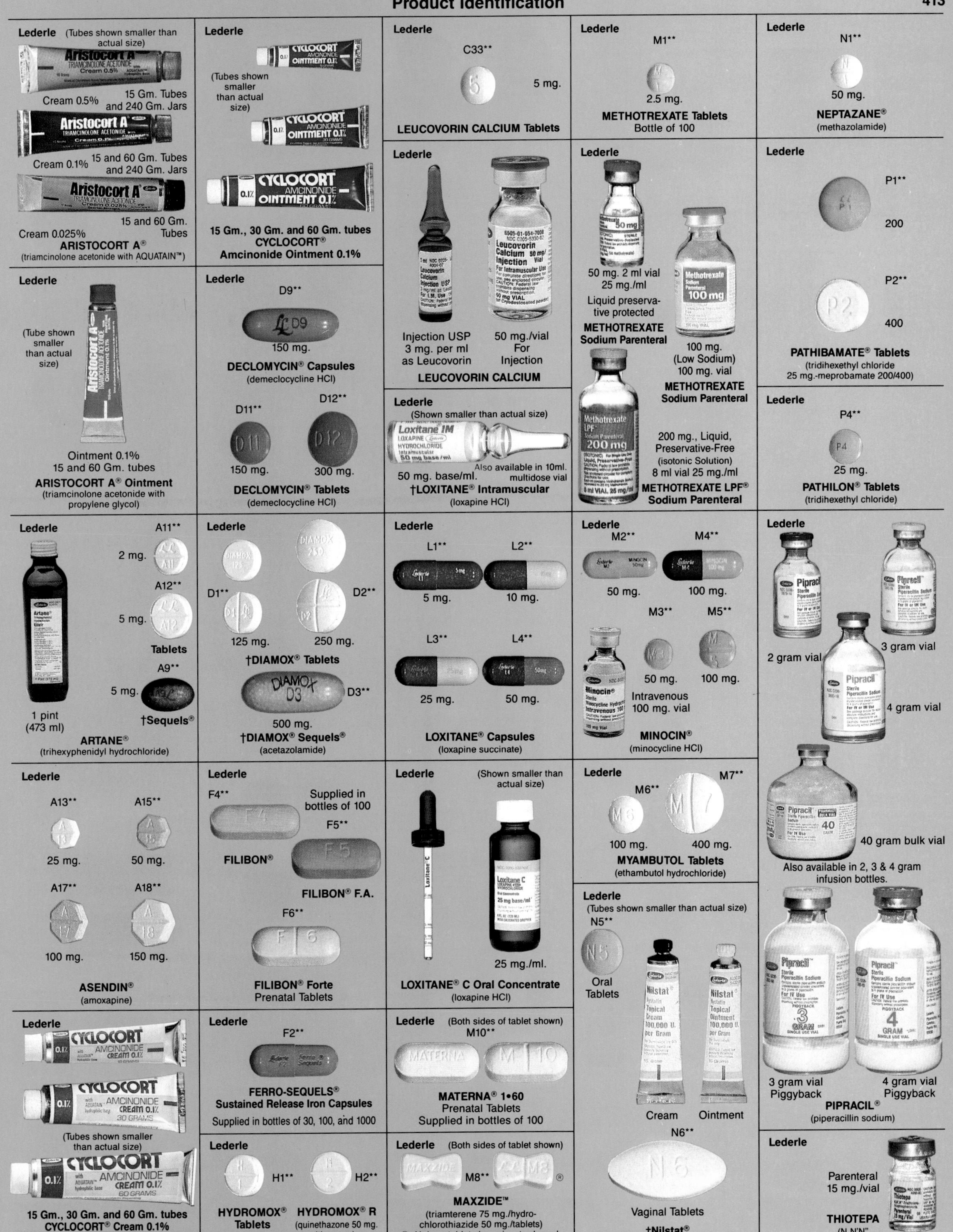

**Ledermark Product Identification Codes.

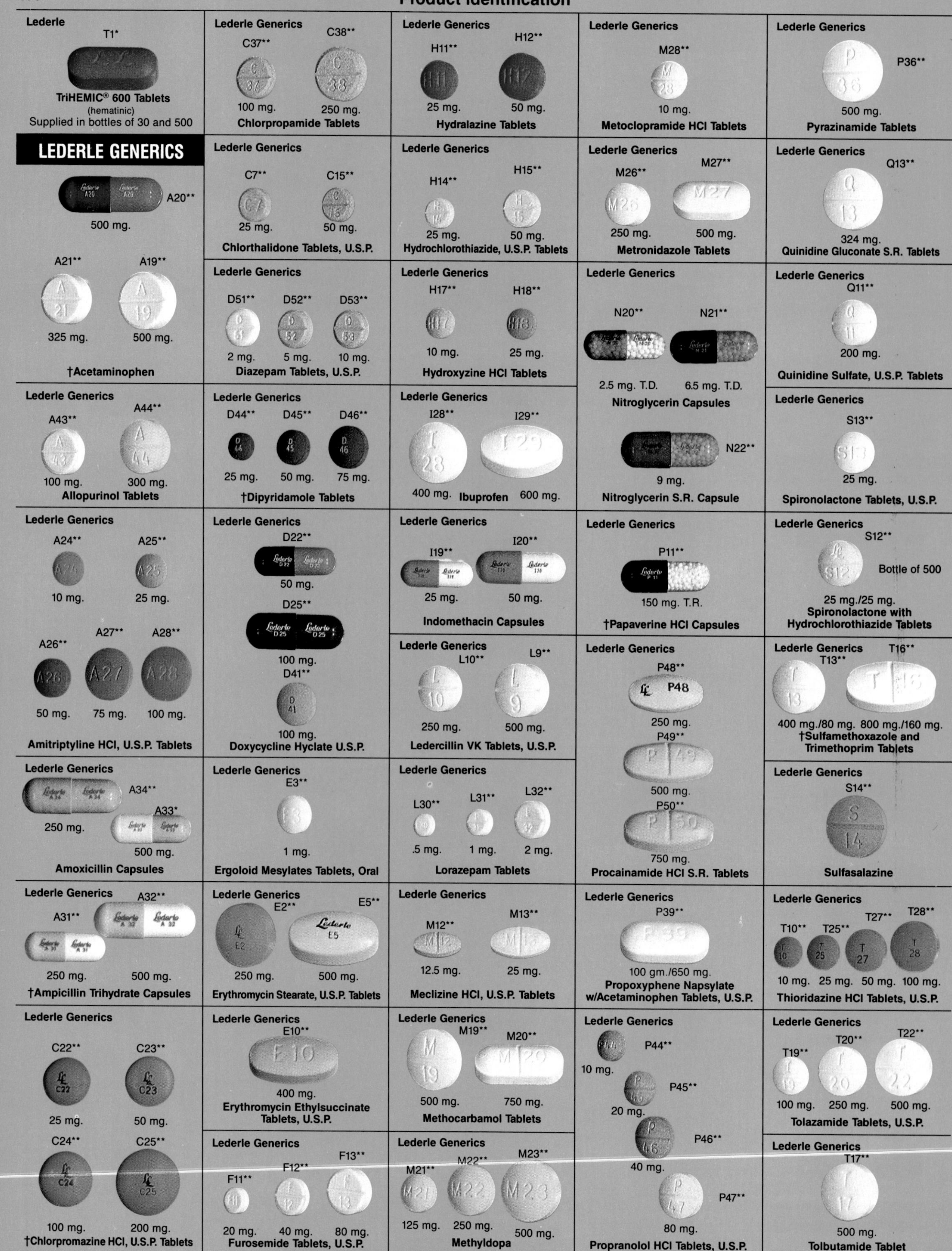

**Ledermark Product Identification Codes.

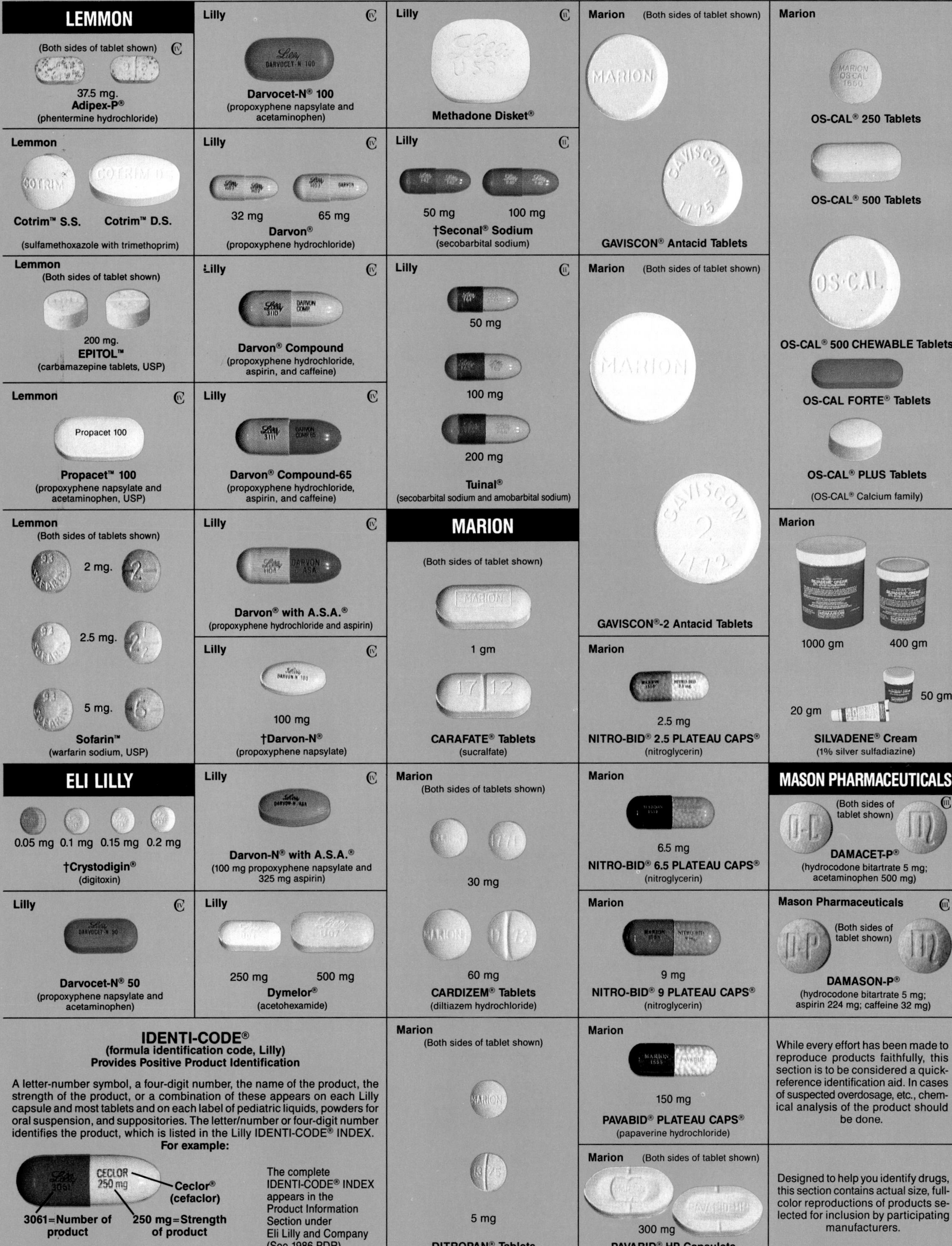

LEMMON

(Both sides of tablet shown) CIV
37.5 mg.
Adipex-P®
(phentermine hydrochloride)

Lemmon
Cotrim™ S.S. **Cotrim™ D.S.**
(sulfamethoxazole with trimethoprim)

Lemmon
(Both sides of tablet shown)
200 mg.
EPITOL™
(carbamazepine tablets, USP)

Lemmon CIV
Propacet 100
Propacet™ 100
(propoxyphene napsylate and acetaminophen, USP)

Lemmon
(Both sides of tablets shown)
2 mg.
2.5 mg.
5 mg.
Sofarin™
(warfarin sodium, USP)

ELI LILLY

0.05 mg 0.1 mg 0.15 mg 0.2 mg
†Crystodigin®
(digitoxin)

Lilly CIV
Darvocet-N® 50
(propoxyphene napsylate and acetaminophen)

Lilly CIV
Darvocet-N® 100
(propoxyphene napsylate and acetaminophen)

Lilly CIV
32 mg 65 mg
Darvon®
(propoxyphene hydrochloride)

Lilly CIV
Darvon® Compound
(propoxyphene hydrochloride, aspirin, and caffeine)

Lilly CIV
Darvon® Compound-65
(propoxyphene hydrochloride, aspirin, and caffeine)

Lilly CIV
Darvon® with A.S.A.®
(propoxyphene hydrochloride and aspirin)

Lilly CIV
100 mg
†Darvon-N®
(propoxyphene napsylate)

Lilly CIV
Darvon-N® with A.S.A.®
(100 mg propoxyphene napsylate and 325 mg aspirin)

Lilly
250 mg 500 mg
Dymelor®
(acetohexamide)

Lilly CII
Methadone Disket®

Lilly CII
50 mg 100 mg
†Seconal® Sodium
(secobarbital sodium)

Lilly CII
50 mg
100 mg
200 mg
Tuinal®
(secobarbital sodium and amobarbital sodium)

IDENTI-CODE®
(formula identification code, Lilly)
Provides Positive Product Identification

A letter-number symbol, a four-digit number, the name of the product, the strength of the product, or a combination of these appears on each Lilly capsule and most tablets and on each label of pediatric liquids, powders for oral suspension, and suppositories. The letter/number or four-digit number identifies the product, which is listed in the Lilly IDENTI-CODE® INDEX.
For example:

CECLOR 250 mg 3061
Ceclor®
(cefaclor)
3061=Number of product
250 mg=Strength of product

The complete IDENTI-CODE® INDEX appears in the Product Information Section under Eli Lilly and Company (See 1986 PDR)

MARION

(Both sides of tablet shown)
1 gm
CARAFATE® Tablets
(sucralfate)

Marion
(Both sides of tablets shown)
30 mg
60 mg
CARDIZEM® Tablets
(diltiazem hydrochloride)

Marion
(Both sides of tablet shown)
5 mg
DITROPAN® Tablets
(oxybutynin chloride)

Marion (Both sides of tablet shown)
GAVISCON® Antacid Tablets

Marion (Both sides of tablet shown)
GAVISCON®-2 Antacid Tablets

Marion
2.5 mg
NITRO-BID® 2.5 PLATEAU CAPS®
(nitroglycerin)

Marion
6.5 mg
NITRO-BID® 6.5 PLATEAU CAPS®
(nitroglycerin)

Marion
9 mg
NITRO-BID® 9 PLATEAU CAPS®
(nitroglycerin)

Marion
150 mg
PAVABID® PLATEAU CAPS®
(papaverine hydrochloride)

Marion (Both sides of tablet shown)
300 mg
PAVABID® HP Capsulets
(papaverine hydrochloride)

Marion
OS-CAL® 250 Tablets
OS-CAL® 500 Tablets
OS-CAL® 500 CHEWABLE Tablets
OS-CAL FORTE® Tablets
OS-CAL® PLUS Tablets
(OS-CAL® Calcium family)

Marion
1000 gm 400 gm
20 gm 50 gm
SILVADENE® Cream
(1% silver sulfadiazine)

MASON PHARMACEUTICALS

(Both sides of tablet shown) CIII
DAMACET-P®
(hydrocodone bitartrate 5 mg; acetaminophen 500 mg)

Mason Pharmaceuticals CIII
(Both sides of tablet shown)
DAMASON-P®
(hydrocodone bitartrate 5 mg; aspirin 224 mg; caffeine 32 mg)

While every effort has been made to reproduce products faithfully, this section is to be considered a quick-reference identification aid. In cases of suspected overdosage, etc., chemical analysis of the product should be done.

Designed to help you identify drugs, this section contains actual size, full-color reproductions of products selected for inclusion by participating manufacturers.

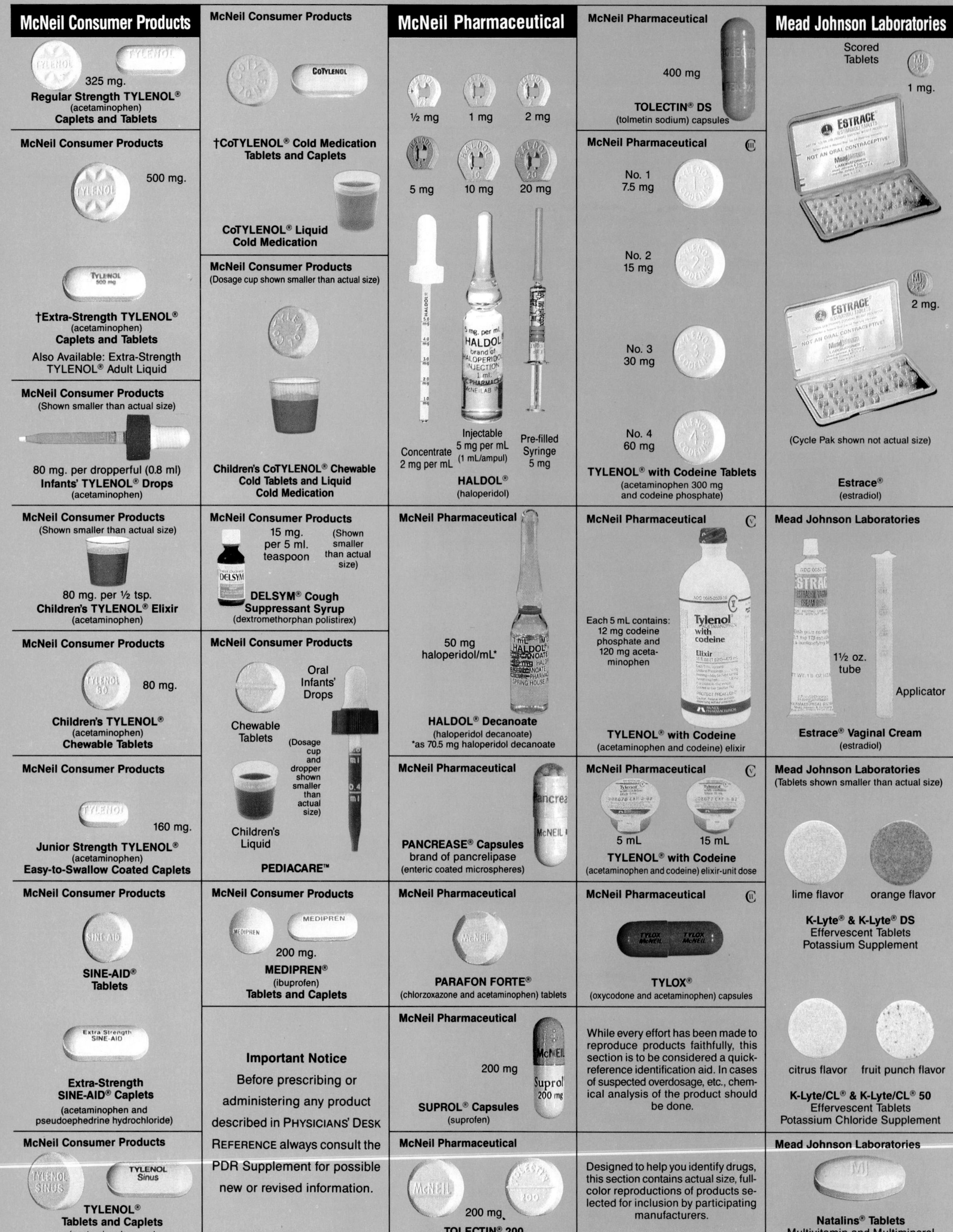

McNeil Consumer Products

325 mg.
Regular Strength TYLENOL®
(acetaminophen)
Caplets and Tablets

McNeil Consumer Products

500 mg.
†Extra-Strength TYLENOL®
(acetaminophen)
Caplets and Tablets
Also Available: Extra-Strength TYLENOL® Adult Liquid

McNeil Consumer Products
(Shown smaller than actual size)

80 mg. per dropperful (0.8 ml)
Infants' TYLENOL® Drops
(acetaminophen)

McNeil Consumer Products
(Shown smaller than actual size)

80 mg. per ½ tsp.
Children's TYLENOL® Elixir
(acetaminophen)

McNeil Consumer Products

80 mg.
Children's TYLENOL®
(acetaminophen)
Chewable Tablets

McNeil Consumer Products

160 mg.
Junior Strength TYLENOL®
(acetaminophen)
Easy-to-Swallow Coated Caplets

McNeil Consumer Products

SINE-AID®
Tablets

Extra-Strength
SINE-AID® Caplets
(acetaminophen and pseudoephedrine hydrochloride)

McNeil Consumer Products

TYLENOL®
Tablets and Caplets
(acetaminophen and pseudoephedrine hydrochloride)

McNeil Consumer Products

†CoTYLENOL® Cold Medication Tablets and Caplets

CoTYLENOL® Liquid Cold Medication

McNeil Consumer Products
(Dosage cup shown smaller than actual size)

Children's CoTYLENOL® Chewable Cold Tablets and Liquid Cold Medication

McNeil Consumer Products

15 mg. per 5 ml. teaspoon
(Shown smaller than actual size)
DELSYM® Cough Suppressant Syrup
(dextromethorphan polistirex)

McNeil Consumer Products

Chewable Tablets
Oral Infants' Drops
Children's Liquid
(Dosage cup and dropper shown smaller than actual size)
PEDIACARE™

McNeil Consumer Products

200 mg.
MEDIPREN®
(ibuprofen)
Tablets and Caplets

Important Notice
Before prescribing or administering any product described in PHYSICIANS' DESK REFERENCE always consult the PDR Supplement for possible new or revised information.

McNeil Pharmaceutical

½ mg 1 mg 2 mg
5 mg 10 mg 20 mg
Concentrate 2 mg per mL
Injectable 5 mg per mL (1 mL/ampul)
Pre-filled Syringe 5 mg
HALDOL®
(haloperidol)

McNeil Pharmaceutical

50 mg haloperidol/mL*
HALDOL® Decanoate
(haloperidol decanoate)
*as 70.5 mg haloperidol decanoate

McNeil Pharmaceutical

PANCREASE® Capsules
brand of pancrelipase
(enteric coated microspheres)

McNeil Pharmaceutical

PARAFON FORTE®
(chlorzoxazone and acetaminophen) tablets

McNeil Pharmaceutical

200 mg
SUPROL® Capsules
(suprofen)

McNeil Pharmaceutical

200 mg
TOLECTIN® 200
(tolmetin sodium) tablets

McNeil Pharmaceutical

400 mg
TOLECTIN® DS
(tolmetin sodium) capsules

McNeil Pharmaceutical Ⓒ III

No. 1 7.5 mg
No. 2 15 mg
No. 3 30 mg
No. 4 60 mg
TYLENOL® with Codeine Tablets
(acetaminophen 300 mg and codeine phosphate)

McNeil Pharmaceutical Ⓒ V

Each 5 mL contains: 12 mg codeine phosphate and 120 mg acetaminophen
TYLENOL® with Codeine
(acetaminophen and codeine) elixir

McNeil Pharmaceutical Ⓒ V

5 mL 15 mL
TYLENOL® with Codeine
(acetaminophen and codeine) elixir-unit dose

McNeil Pharmaceutical Ⓒ II

TYLOX®
(oxycodone and acetaminophen) capsules

While every effort has been made to reproduce products faithfully, this section is to be considered a quick-reference identification aid. In cases of suspected overdosage, etc., chemical analysis of the product should be done.

Designed to help you identify drugs, this section contains actual size, full-color reproductions of products selected for inclusion by participating manufacturers.

Mead Johnson Laboratories

Scored Tablets
1 mg.
2 mg.
(Cycle Pak shown not actual size)
Estrace®
(estradiol)

Mead Johnson Laboratories

1½ oz. tube
Applicator
Estrace® Vaginal Cream
(estradiol)

Mead Johnson Laboratories
(Tablets shown smaller than actual size)

lime flavor orange flavor
K-Lyte® & K-Lyte® DS
Effervescent Tablets
Potassium Supplement

citrus flavor fruit punch flavor
K-Lyte/CL® & K-Lyte/CL® 50
Effervescent Tablets
Potassium Chloride Supplement

Mead Johnson Laboratories

Natalins® Tablets
Multivitamin and Multimineral Supplement

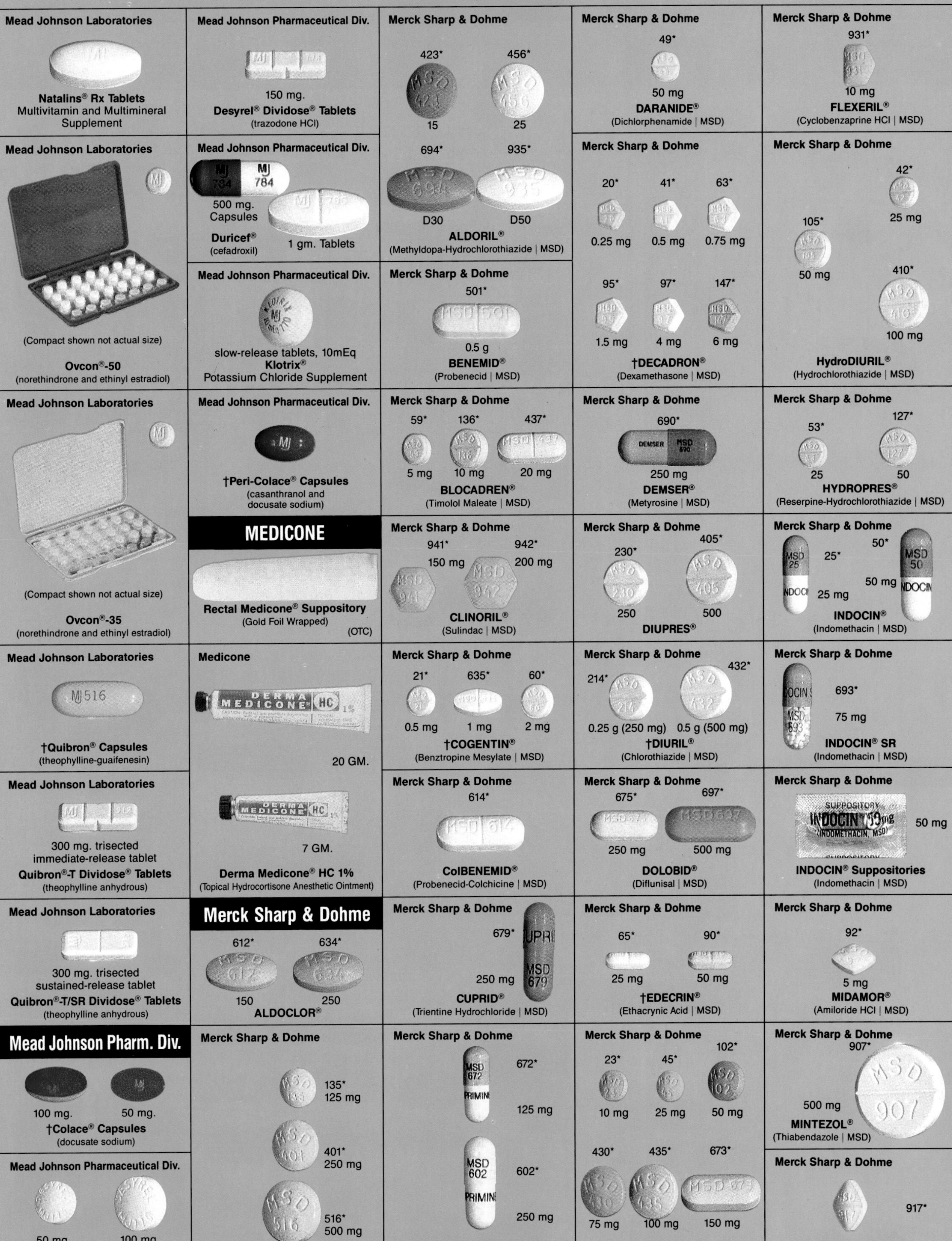

Mead Johnson Laboratories
Natalins® Rx Tablets
Multivitamin and Multimineral Supplement

Mead Johnson Laboratories
(Compact shown not actual size)
Ovcon®-50
(norethindrone and ethinyl estradiol)

Mead Johnson Laboratories
(Compact shown not actual size)
Ovcon®-35
(norethindrone and ethinyl estradiol)

Mead Johnson Laboratories
†Quibron® Capsules
(theophylline-guaifenesin)

Mead Johnson Laboratories
300 mg. trisected immediate-release tablet
Quibron®-T Dividose® Tablets
(theophylline anhydrous)

Mead Johnson Laboratories
300 mg. trisected sustained-release tablet
Quibron®-T/SR Dividose® Tablets
(theophylline anhydrous)

Mead Johnson Pharm. Div.

100 mg. 50 mg.
†Colace® Capsules
(docusate sodium)

Mead Johnson Pharmaceutical Div.
50 mg. 100 mg.
Desyrel® Tablets
(trazodone HCl)

Mead Johnson Pharmaceutical Div.
150 mg.
Desyrel® Dividose® Tablets
(trazodone HCl)

Mead Johnson Pharmaceutical Div.
500 mg. Capsules
1 gm. Tablets
Duricef®
(cefadroxil)

Mead Johnson Pharmaceutical Div.
slow-release tablets, 10mEq
Klotrix®
Potassium Chloride Supplement

Mead Johnson Pharmaceutical Div.
†Peri-Colace® Capsules
(casanthranol and docusate sodium)

MEDICONE

Rectal Medicone® Suppository
(Gold Foil Wrapped)
(OTC)

Medicone
20 GM.
7 GM.
Derma Medicone® HC 1%
(Topical Hydrocortisone Anesthetic Ointment)

Merck Sharp & Dohme

612* 634*
150 250
ALDOCLOR®

Merck Sharp & Dohme
135* 125 mg
401* 250 mg
516* 500 mg
†ALDOMET®
(Methyldopa | MSD)

Merck Sharp & Dohme
423* 456* 15 25
694* 935* D30 D50
ALDORIL®
(Methyldopa-Hydrochlorothiazide | MSD)

Merck Sharp & Dohme
501*
0.5 g
BENEMID®
(Probenecid | MSD)

Merck Sharp & Dohme
59* 136* 437*
5 mg 10 mg 20 mg
BLOCADREN®
(Timolol Maleate | MSD)

Merck Sharp & Dohme
941* 150 mg
942* 200 mg
CLINORIL®
(Sulindac | MSD)

Merck Sharp & Dohme
21* 635* 60*
0.5 mg 1 mg 2 mg
†COGENTIN®
(Benztropine Mesylate | MSD)

Merck Sharp & Dohme
614*
ColBENEMID®
(Probenecid-Colchicine | MSD)

Merck Sharp & Dohme
679*
250 mg
CUPRID®
(Trientine Hydrochloride | MSD)

Merck Sharp & Dohme
672* 125 mg
602* 250 mg
CUPRIMINE®
(Penicillamine | MSD)

Merck Sharp & Dohme
49*
50 mg
DARANIDE®
(Dichlorphenamide | MSD)

Merck Sharp & Dohme
20* 41* 63*
0.25 mg 0.5 mg 0.75 mg
95* 97* 147*
1.5 mg 4 mg 6 mg
†DECADRON®
(Dexamethasone | MSD)

Merck Sharp & Dohme
690*
250 mg
DEMSER®
(Metyrosine | MSD)

Merck Sharp & Dohme
230* 405*
250 500
DIUPRES®

Merck Sharp & Dohme
214* 432*
0.25 g (250 mg) 0.5 g (500 mg)
†DIURIL®
(Chlorothiazide | MSD)

Merck Sharp & Dohme
675* 697*
250 mg 500 mg
DOLOBID®
(Diflunisal | MSD)

Merck Sharp & Dohme
65* 90*
25 mg 50 mg
†EDECRIN®
(Ethacrynic Acid | MSD)

Merck Sharp & Dohme
23* 45* 102*
10 mg 25 mg 50 mg
430* 435* 673*
75 mg 100 mg 150 mg
†ELAVIL®
(Amitriptyline HCl | MSD)

Merck Sharp & Dohme
931*
10 mg
FLEXERIL®
(Cyclobenzaprine HCl | MSD)

Merck Sharp & Dohme
42* 25 mg
105* 50 mg
410* 100 mg
HydroDIURIL®
(Hydrochlorothiazide | MSD)

Merck Sharp & Dohme
53* 127*
25 50
HYDROPRES®
(Reserpine-Hydrochlorothiazide | MSD)

Merck Sharp & Dohme
25* 25 mg
50* 50 mg
INDOCIN®
(Indomethacin | MSD)

Merck Sharp & Dohme
693*
75 mg
INDOCIN® SR
(Indomethacin | MSD)

Merck Sharp & Dohme
50 mg
INDOCIN® Suppositories
(Indomethacin | MSD)

Merck Sharp & Dohme
92*
5 mg
MIDAMOR®
(Amiloride HCl | MSD)

Merck Sharp & Dohme
907*
500 mg
MINTEZOL®
(Thiabendazole | MSD)

Merck Sharp & Dohme
917*
MODURETIC®
(Amiloride HCl-Hydrochlorothiazide | MSD)

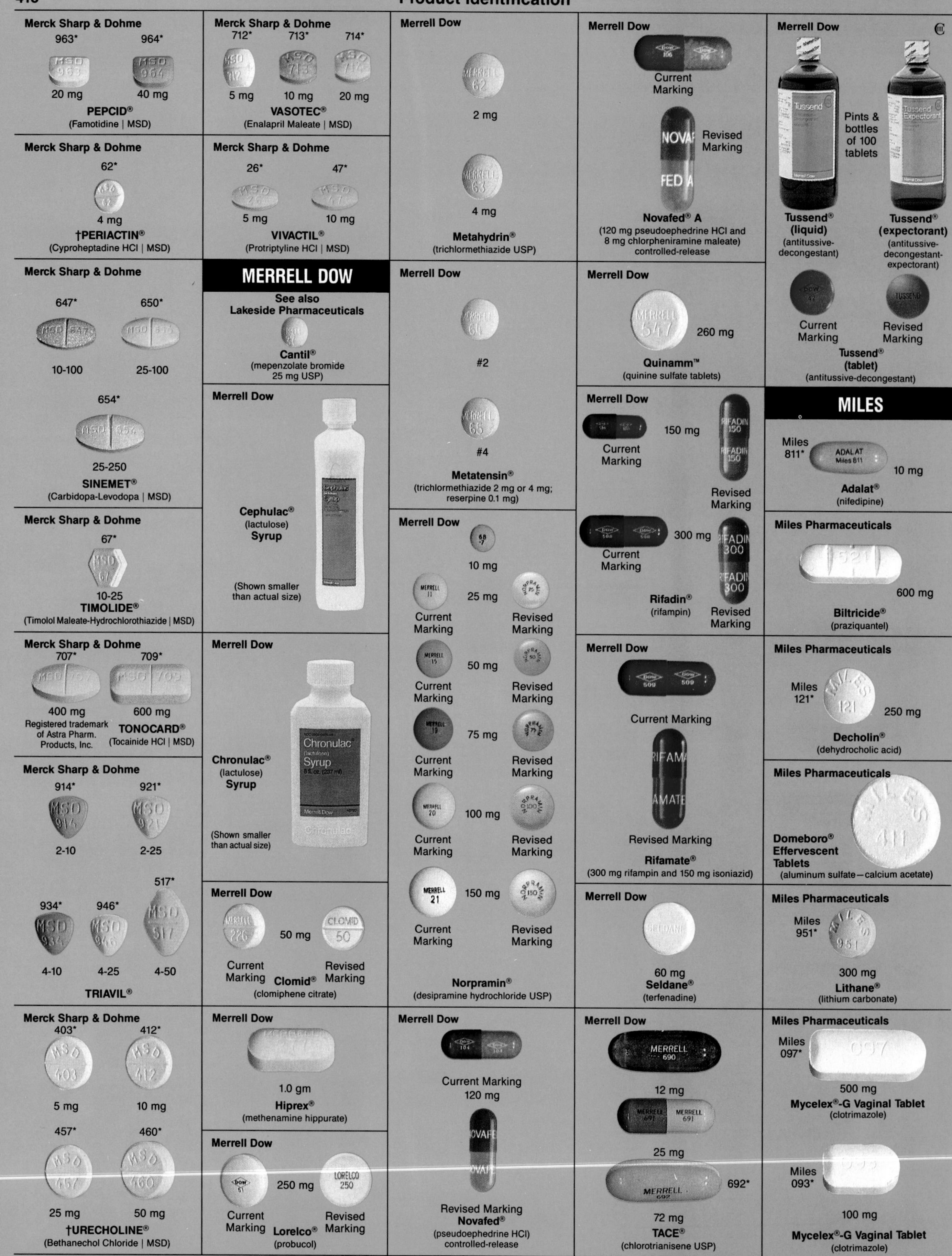
Merck Sharp & Dohme
963* 964*
20 mg 40 mg
PEPCID®
(Famotidine | MSD)
Merck Sharp & Dohme
62*
4 mg
†PERIACTIN®
(Cyproheptadine HCl | MSD)
Merck Sharp & Dohme
647* 650*
10-100 25-100
654*
25-250
SINEMET®
(Carbidopa-Levodopa | MSD)
Merck Sharp & Dohme
67*
10-25
TIMOLIDE®
(Timolol Maleate-Hydrochlorothiazide | MSD)
Merck Sharp & Dohme
707* 709*
400 mg 600 mg
Registered trademark of Astra Pharm. Products, Inc.
TONOCARD®
(Tocainide HCl | MSD)
Merck Sharp & Dohme
914* 921*
2-10 2-25
517*
934* 946*
4-10 4-25 4-50
TRIAVIL®
Merck Sharp & Dohme
403* 412*
5 mg 10 mg
457* 460*
25 mg 50 mg
†URECHOLINE®
(Bethanechol Chloride | MSD)
Merck Sharp & Dohme
712* 713* 714*
5 mg 10 mg 20 mg
VASOTEC®
(Enalapril Maleate | MSD)
Merck Sharp & Dohme
26* 47*
5 mg 10 mg
VIVACTIL®
(Protriptyline HCl | MSD)
MERRELL DOW
See also
Lakeside Pharmaceuticals
Cantil®
(mepenzolate bromide 25 mg USP)
Merrell Dow
Cephulac®
(lactulose)
Syrup
(Shown smaller than actual size)
Merrell Dow
Chronulac®
(lactulose)
Syrup
(Shown smaller than actual size)
Merrell Dow
50 mg
Current Marking
Revised Marking
Clomid®
(clomiphene citrate)
Merrell Dow
1.0 gm
Hiprex®
(methenamine hippurate)
Merrell Dow
250 mg
Current Marking
Revised Marking
Lorelco®
(probucol)
Merrell Dow
2 mg
4 mg
Metahydrin®
(trichlormethiazide USP)
Merrell Dow
#2
#4
Metatensin®
(trichlormethiazide 2 mg or 4 mg; reserpine 0.1 mg)
Merrell Dow
10 mg
25 mg
50 mg
75 mg
100 mg
150 mg
Current Marking
Revised Marking
Norpramin®
(desipramine hydrochloride USP)
Merrell Dow
Current Marking
120 mg
Revised Marking
Novafed®
(pseudoephedrine HCl)
controlled-release
Merrell Dow
Current Marking
Revised Marking
Novafed® A
(120 mg pseudoephedrine HCl and 8 mg chlorpheniramine maleate)
controlled-release
Merrell Dow
260 mg
Quinamm™
(quinine sulfate tablets)
Merrell Dow
150 mg
Current Marking
Revised Marking
300 mg
Current Marking
Revised Marking
Rifadin®
(rifampin)
Merrell Dow
Current Marking
Revised Marking
Rifamate®
(300 mg rifampin and 150 mg isoniazid)
Merrell Dow
60 mg
Seldane®
(terfenadine)
Merrell Dow
12 mg
25 mg
692*
72 mg
TACE®
(chlorotrianisene USP)
Merrell Dow
Pints & bottles of 100 tablets
Tussend®
(liquid)
(antitussive-decongestant)
Tussend®
(expectorant)
(antitussive-decongestant-expectorant)
Current Marking
Revised Marking
Tussend®
(tablet)
(antitussive-decongestant)
MILES
Miles 811*
10 mg
Adalat®
(nifedipine)
Miles Pharmaceuticals
600 mg
Biltricide®
(praziquantel)
Miles Pharmaceuticals
Miles 121*
250 mg
Decholin®
(dehydrocholic acid)
Miles Pharmaceuticals
Domeboro®
Effervescent
Tablets
(aluminum sulfate—calcium acetate)
Miles Pharmaceuticals
Miles 951*
300 mg
Lithane®
(lithium carbonate)
Miles Pharmaceuticals
Miles 097*
500 mg
Mycelex®-G Vaginal Tablet
(clotrimazole)
Miles 093*
100 mg
Mycelex®-G Vaginal Tablet
(clotrimazole)

Miles Pharmaceuticals

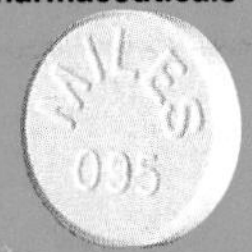

Miles 095* 10 mg

Mycelex® Troche
(clotrimazole)

Miles Pharmaceuticals

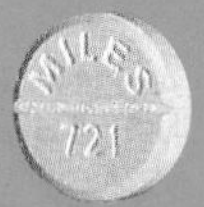

Miles 721* 500 mg

Niclocide® Chewable Tablets
(niclosamide)

Miles Pharmaceuticals

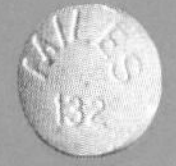

Miles 132*

50 mg
Stiphostrol®
(diethyl stilbestrol diphosphate)

NORCLIFF THAYER

Special Comb Included

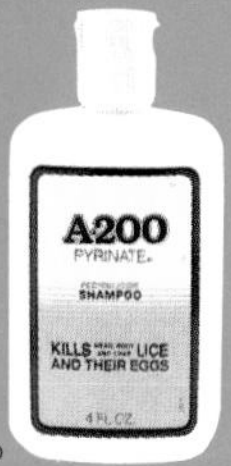

4 fl. oz.

A-200 Pyrinate® Pediculicide Shampoo
Also available:
A-200 Pyrinate Shampoo, 2 fl. oz.
A-200 Pyrinate Shampoo Gel, 1 oz.

NORWICH EATON

scored tablet — sustained release

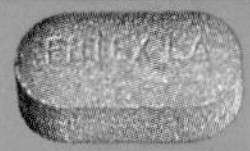

Entex® LA Tablets
(guaifenesin 400 mg.
phenylpropanolamine HCl 75 mg.)

Norwich Eaton

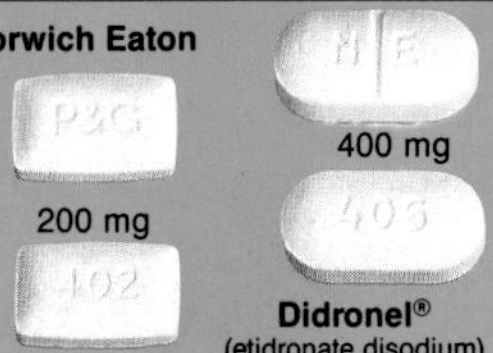

400 mg
200 mg

Didronel®
(etidronate disodium)

Norwich Eaton

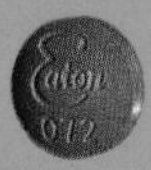

100 mg
Furoxone® Tablets
(furazolidone)

Eaton Laboratories Inc.
Manati, Puerto Rico

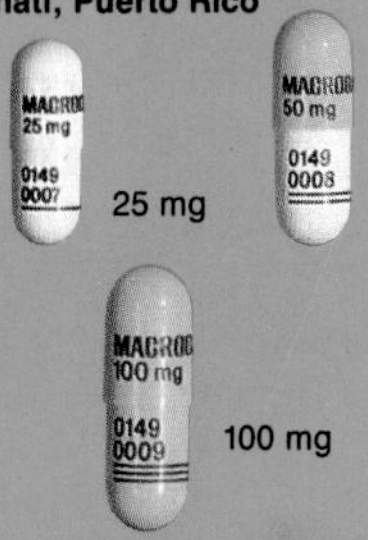

25 mg — 50 mg

100 mg

Macrodantin® Capsules
(nitrofurantoin macrocrystals)

ORGANON

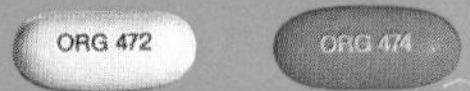

20 mcg — 50 mcg
Calderol®
(calcifediol capsules, USP)

Organon

388*

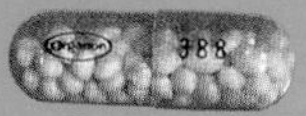

Cotazym-S™
enteric coated spheres
(pancrelipase, USP)

Organon

381*

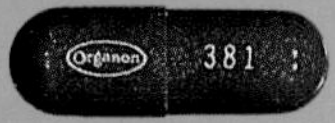

†Cotazym®
(pancrelipase capsules, USP)

Organon

795*

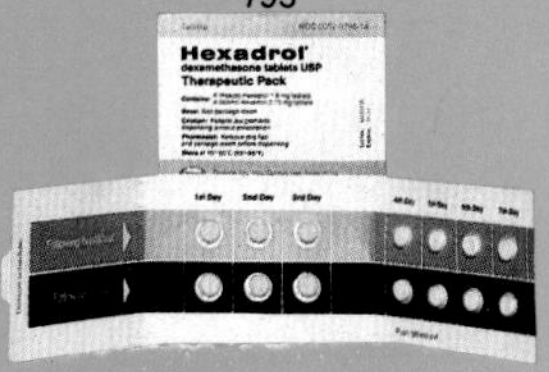

(pack shown smaller than actual size)

6 Hexadrol 1.5 mg. tablets and
8 Hexadrol 0.75 mg. tablets

Hexadrol® Therapeutic Pack
(dexamethasone tablets, USP)

Organon

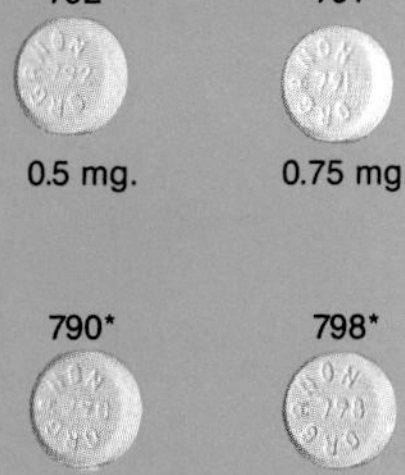

792* — 791*

0.5 mg. — 0.75 mg.

790* — 798*

1.5 mg. — 4.0 mg.

†Hexadrol®
(dexamethasone tablets, USP)

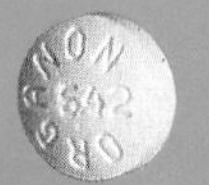

Organon 542*

Wigraine®
(ergotamine tartrate and caffeine tablets, USP)

Organon

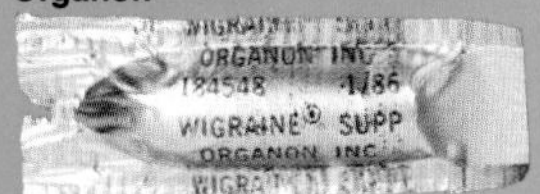

Wigraine®
(ergotamine tartrate and caffeine suppositories, USP)

Designed to help you identify drugs, this section contains actual size, full-color reproductions of products selected for inclusion by participating manufacturers.

ORTHO

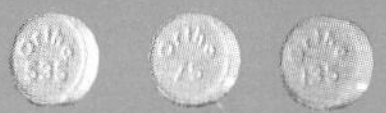

Ortho compacts shown smaller than actual size

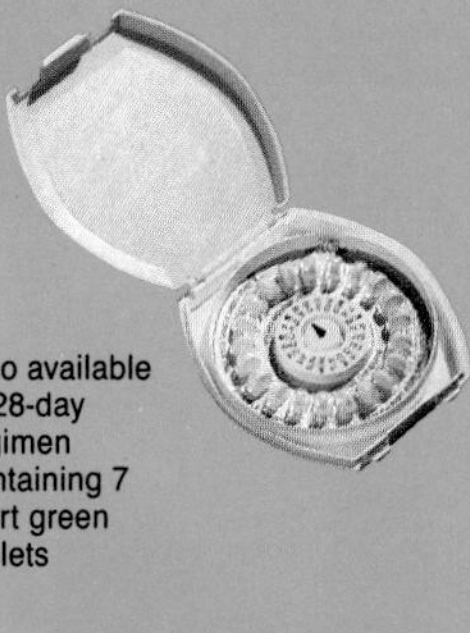

Also available in 28-day regimen containing 7 inert green tablets

ORTHO-NOVUM™ 7/7/7□21 Day Regimen
(Each white tablet contains 0.5 mg of norethindrone and 0.035 mg of ethinyl estradiol)
(Each light peach tablet contains 0.75 mg of norethindrone and 0.035 of ethinyl estradiol)
(Each peach tablet contains 1 mg of norethindrone and 0.035 mg of ethinyl estradiol)

Ortho

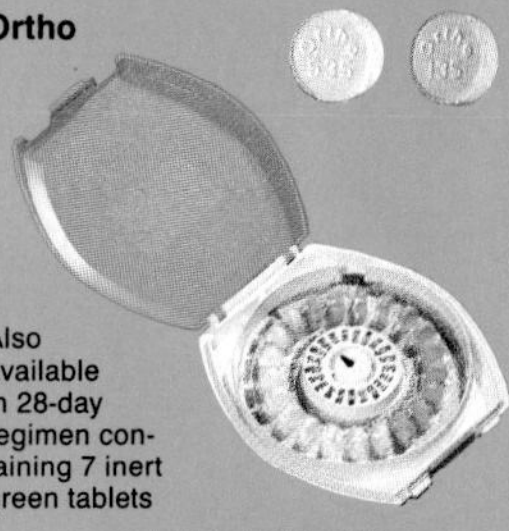

Also available in 28-day regimen containing 7 inert green tablets

ORTHO-NOVUM™ 10/11□21 Day Regimen
(Each white tablet contains 0.5 mg of norethindrone with 0.035 mg of ethinyl estradiol)
(Each peach tablet contains 1 mg of norethindrone with 0.035 mg of ethinyl estradiol)

Ortho

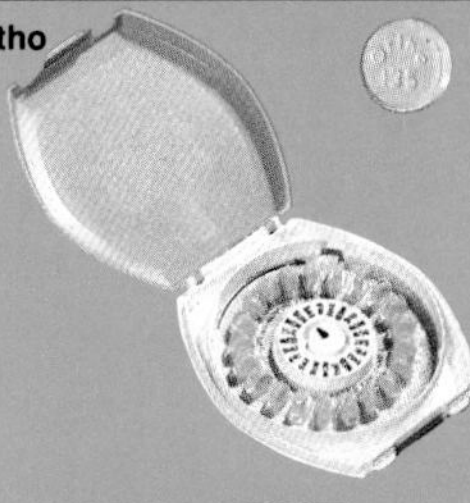

ORTHO-NOVUM™ 1/35□21 Day Regimen
(1 mg of norethindrone with 0.035 mg of ethinyl estradiol)

Also available in 28-day regimen containing 7 inert green tablets

Ortho

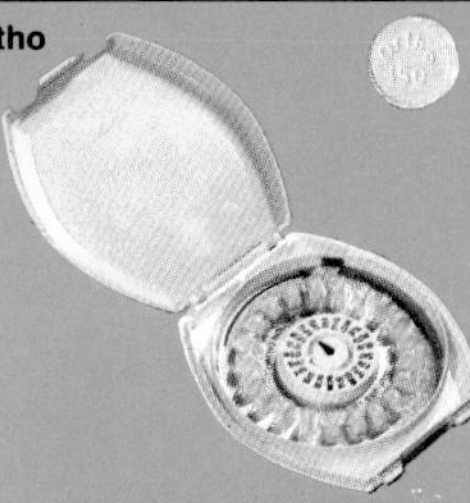

ORTHO-NOVUM™ 1/50□21 Day Regimen
(1 mg of norethindrone with 0.05 mg of mestranol)

Also available in 28-day regimen containing 7 inert green tablets

Ortho

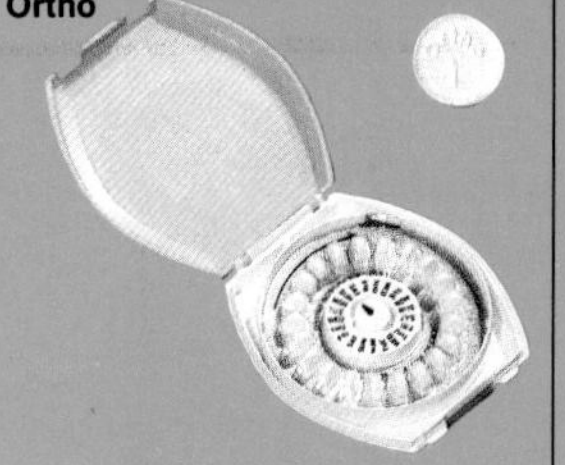

ORTHO-NOVUM™ 1/80□21 Day Regimen
(1 mg of norethindrone with 0.08 mg of mestranol)

Also available in 28-day regimen containing 7 inert green tablets

Ortho

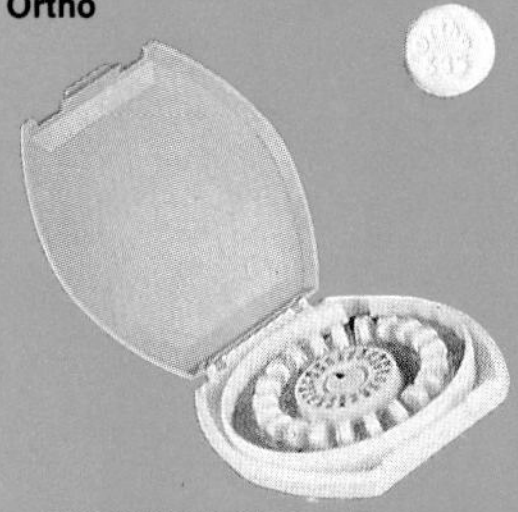

MODICON™ 21 Day Regimen
(0.5 mg of norethindrone with 0.035 mg of ethinyl estradiol)

Also available in 28-day regimen containing 7 inert green tablets

Ortho

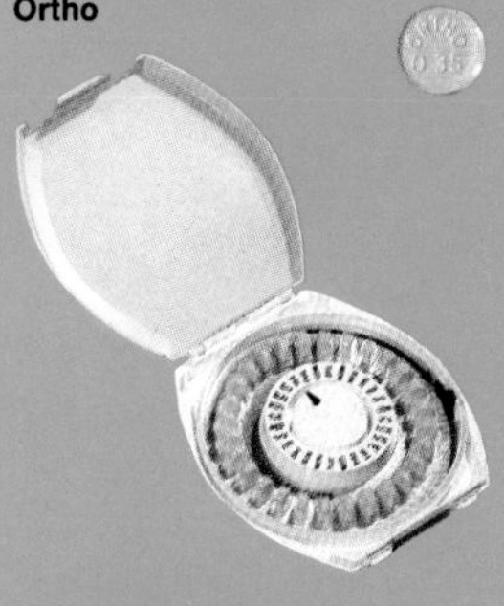

MICRONOR™ 28 Day Regimen
(0.35 mg of norethindrone)

Ortho

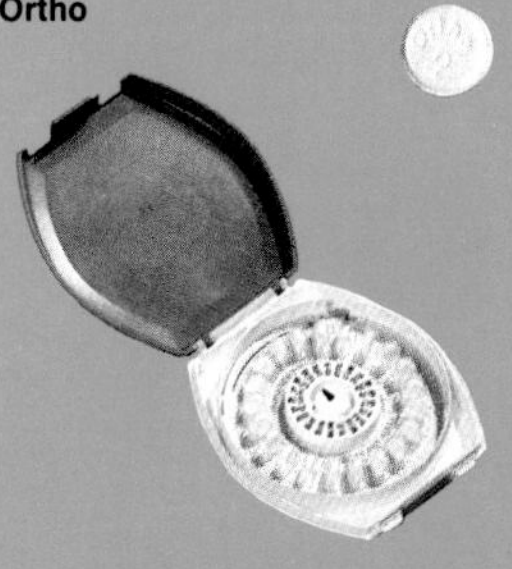

ORTHO-NOVUM™ 2 mg□21 Day Regimen
(2 mg of norethindrone with 0.10 mg of mestranol)

Ortho

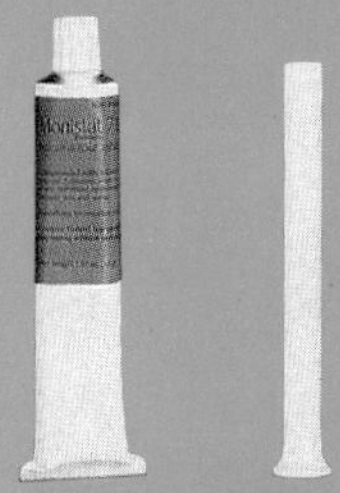

MONISTAT™ 7 VAGINAL Cream
(miconazole nitrate 2%)

Ortho

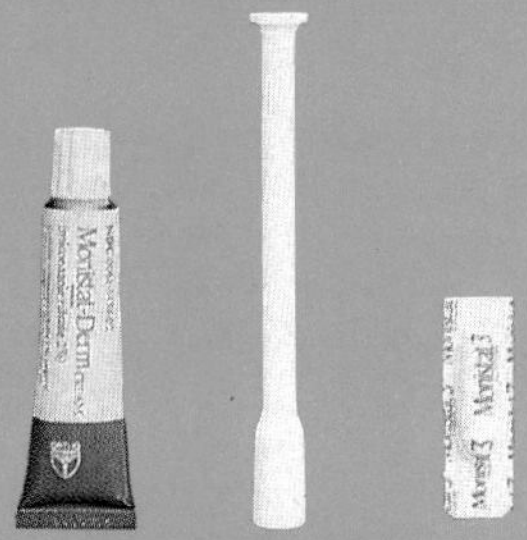

MONISTAT™ Dual-Pak™
(miconazole nitrate)

Ortho

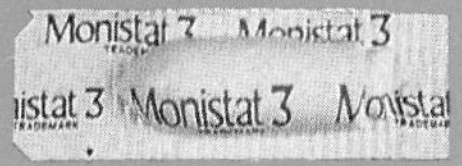

Vaginal Suppositories
MONISTAT™ 3
(200 mg miconazole nitrate)

Ortho

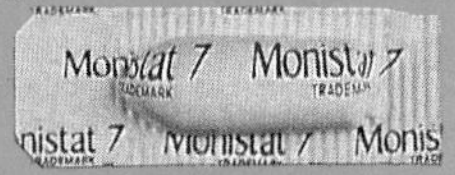

Vaginal Suppositories
MONISTAT™ 7
(100 mg miconazole nitrate)

Ortho

250 mg

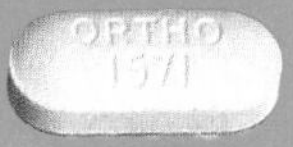

500 mg

PROTOSTAT™
(metronidazole) tablets

PARKE-DAVIS

PARCODE®
(Parke-Davis Accurate Recognition Code) For Prompt, Accurate Product Identification

The imprinted P-D identifies the product as manufactured by Parke-Davis.
The imprinted number designates the particular Parke-Davis Product.

A complete listing of PARCODE numbers appears at the beginning of Parke-Davis Product monographs in the white section.

Parke-Davis

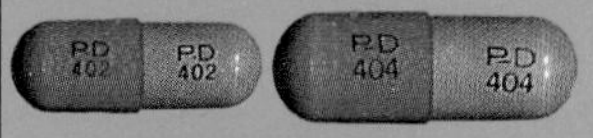

250 mg. — 500 mg.
†Amcill® Capsules
(ampicillin capsules, USP) as the trihydrate

Parke-Davis

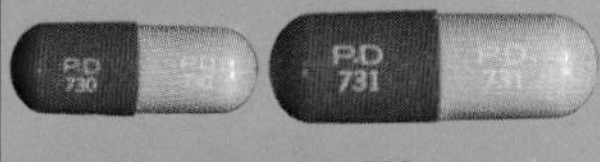

250 mg. — 500 mg.
†Amoxicillin
(Utimox®)

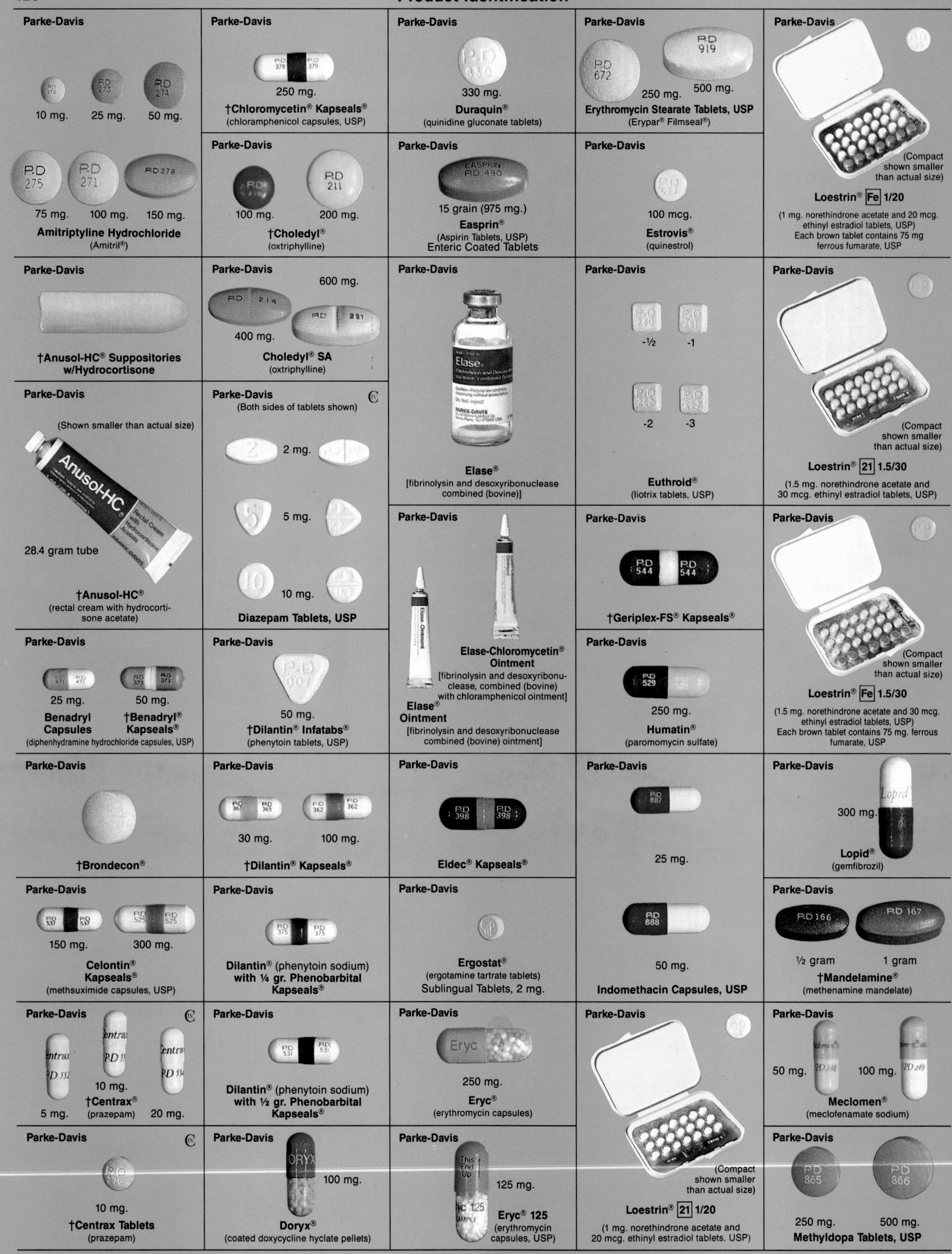

Parke-Davis
10 mg.
25 mg.
50 mg.
75 mg.
100 mg.
150 mg.
Amitriptyline Hydrochloride
(Amitril®)
Parke-Davis
250 mg.
†Chloromycetin® Kapseals®
(chloramphenicol capsules, USP)
Parke-Davis
330 mg.
Duraquin®
(quinidine gluconate tablets)
Parke-Davis
250 mg.
500 mg.
Erythromycin Stearate Tablets, USP
(Erypar® Filmseal®)
Parke-Davis
(Compact shown smaller than actual size)
Loestrin® Fe 1/20
(1 mg. norethindrone acetate and 20 mcg. ethinyl estradiol tablets, USP)
Each brown tablet contains 75 mg ferrous fumarate, USP
Parke-Davis
100 mg.
200 mg.
†Choledyl®
(oxtriphylline)
Parke-Davis
EASPRIN
15 grain (975 mg.)
Easprin®
(Aspirin Tablets, USP)
Enteric Coated Tablets
Parke-Davis
100 mcg.
Estrovis®
(quinestrol)
Parke-Davis
†Anusol-HC® Suppositories w/Hydrocortisone
Parke-Davis
600 mg.
400 mg.
Choledyl® SA
(oxtriphylline)
Parke-Davis
Elase
Elase®
[fibrinolysin and desoxyribonuclease combined (bovine)]
Parke-Davis
-½
-1
-2
-3
Euthroid®
(liotrix tablets, USP)
Parke-Davis
(Compact shown smaller than actual size)
Loestrin® 21 1.5/30
(1.5 mg. norethindrone acetate and 30 mcg. ethinyl estradiol tablets, USP)
Parke-Davis
(Shown smaller than actual size)
Anusol-HC
28.4 gram tube
†Anusol-HC®
(rectal cream with hydrocortisone acetate)
Parke-Davis
(Both sides of tablets shown)
2 mg.
5 mg.
10 mg.
Diazepam Tablets, USP
Parke-Davis
Elase Ointment
Elase-Chloromycetin® Ointment
[fibrinolysin and desoxyribonuclease, combined (bovine) with chloramphenicol ointment]
Elase® Ointment
[fibrinolysin and desoxyribonuclease combined (bovine) ointment]
Parke-Davis
†Geriplex-FS® Kapseals®
Parke-Davis
(Compact shown smaller than actual size)
Loestrin® Fe 1.5/30
(1.5 mg. norethindrone acetate and 30 mcg. ethinyl estradiol tablets, USP)
Each brown tablet contains 75 mg. ferrous fumarate, USP
Parke-Davis
25 mg.
50 mg.
Benadryl Capsules
†Benadryl® Kapseals®
(diphenhydramine hydrochloride capsules, USP)
Parke-Davis
50 mg.
†Dilantin® Infatabs®
(phenytoin tablets, USP)
Parke-Davis
250 mg.
Humatin®
(paromomycin sulfate)
Parke-Davis
†Brondecon®
Parke-Davis
30 mg.
100 mg.
†Dilantin® Kapseals®
Parke-Davis
Eldec® Kapseals®
Parke-Davis
25 mg.
50 mg.
Indomethacin Capsules, USP
Parke-Davis
Lopid
300 mg.
Lopid®
(gemfibrozil)
Parke-Davis
150 mg.
300 mg.
Celontin® Kapseals®
(methsuximide capsules, USP)
Parke-Davis
Dilantin® (phenytoin sodium) with ¼ gr. Phenobarbital Kapseals®
Parke-Davis
Ergostat®
(ergotamine tartrate tablets)
Sublingual Tablets, 2 mg.
Parke-Davis
½ gram
1 gram
†Mandelamine®
(methenamine mandelate)
Parke-Davis
Centrax
5 mg.
10 mg.
20 mg.
†Centrax®
(prazepam)
Parke-Davis
Dilantin® (phenytoin sodium) with ½ gr. Phenobarbital Kapseals®
Parke-Davis
Eryc
250 mg.
Eryc®
(erythromycin capsules)
Parke-Davis
(Compact shown smaller than actual size)
Loestrin® 21 1/20
(1 mg. norethindrone acetate and 20 mcg. ethinyl estradiol tablets, USP)
Parke-Davis
50 mg.
100 mg.
Meclomen®
(meclofenamate sodium)
Parke-Davis
10 mg.
†Centrax Tablets
(prazepam)
Parke-Davis
ORYX
100 mg.
Doryx®
(coated doxycycline hyclate pellets)
Parke-Davis
This End Up
125 mg.
Eryc® 125
(erythromycin capsules, USP)
Parke-Davis
250 mg.
500 mg.
Methyldopa Tablets, USP

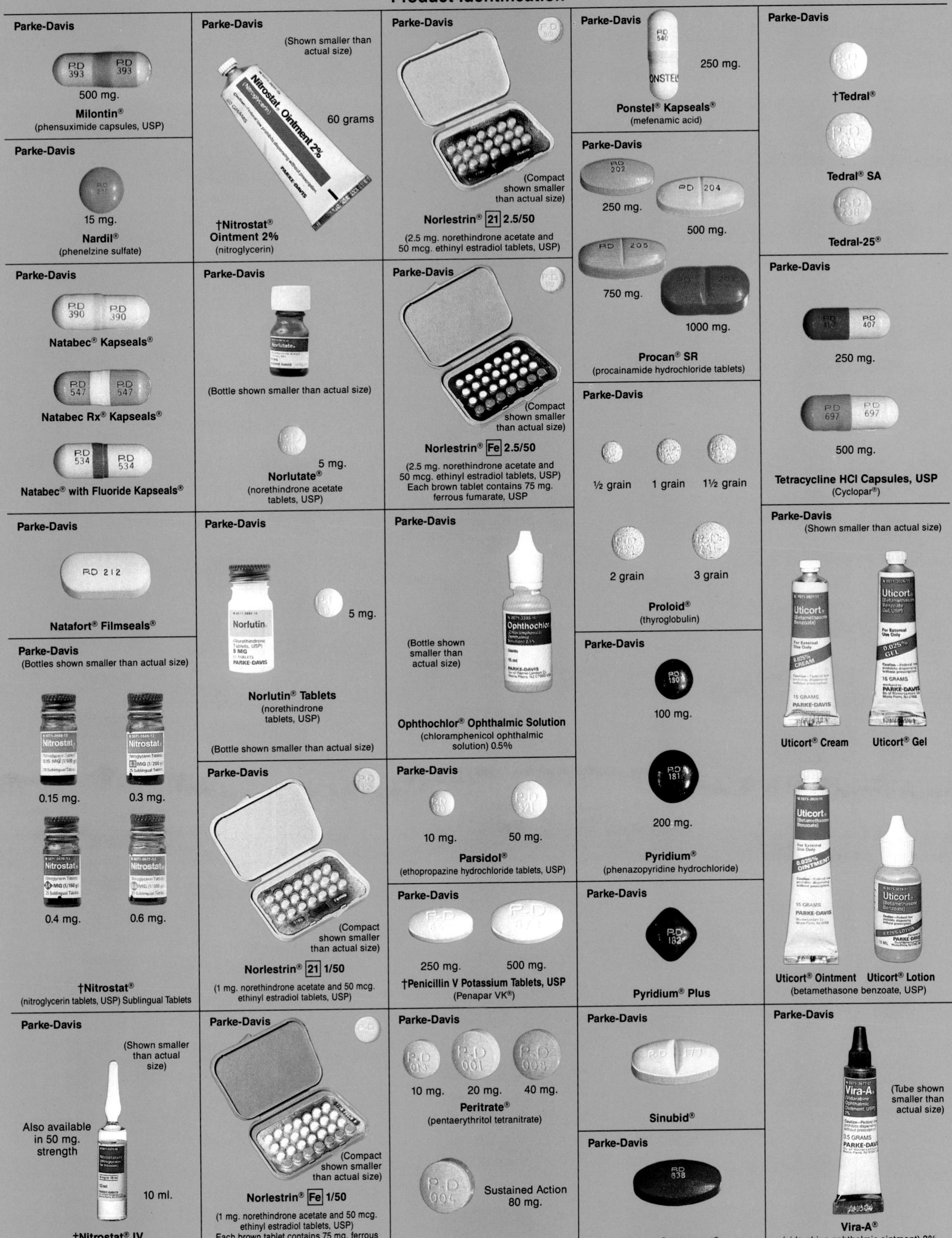

Parke-Davis
500 mg.
Milontin®
(phensuximide capsules, USP)
Parke-Davis
15 mg.
Nardil®
(phenelzine sulfate)
Parke-Davis
Natabec® Kapseals®
Natabec Rx® Kapseals®
Natabec® with Fluoride Kapseals®
Parke-Davis
Natafort® Filmseals®
Parke-Davis
(Bottles shown smaller than actual size)
0.15 mg.
0.3 mg.
0.4 mg.
0.6 mg.
†Nitrostat®
(nitroglycerin tablets, USP) Sublingual Tablets
Parke-Davis
(Shown smaller than actual size)
Also available in 50 mg. strength
10 ml.
†Nitrostat® IV
(nitroglycerin for infusion)
Parke-Davis
(Shown smaller than actual size)
60 grams
†Nitrostat® Ointment 2%
(nitroglycerin)
Parke-Davis
(Bottle shown smaller than actual size)
5 mg.
Norlutate®
(norethindrone acetate tablets, USP)
Parke-Davis
5 mg.
Norlutin® Tablets
(norethindrone tablets, USP)
(Bottle shown smaller than actual size)
Parke-Davis
(Compact shown smaller than actual size)
Norlestrin® 21 1/50
(1 mg. norethindrone acetate and 50 mcg. ethinyl estradiol tablets, USP)
Parke-Davis
(Compact shown smaller than actual size)
Norlestrin® Fe 1/50
(1 mg. norethindrone acetate and 50 mcg. ethinyl estradiol tablets, USP) Each brown tablet contains 75 mg. ferrous fumarate, USP
Parke-Davis
(Compact shown smaller than actual size)
Norlestrin® 21 2.5/50
(2.5 mg. norethindrone acetate and 50 mcg. ethinyl estradiol tablets, USP)
Parke-Davis
(Compact shown smaller than actual size)
Norlestrin® Fe 2.5/50
(2.5 mg. norethindrone acetate and 50 mcg. ethinyl estradiol tablets, USP) Each brown tablet contains 75 mg. ferrous fumarate, USP
Parke-Davis
(Bottle shown smaller than actual size)
Ophthochlor® Ophthalmic Solution
(chloramphenicol ophthalmic solution) 0.5%
Parke-Davis
10 mg.
50 mg.
Parsidol®
(ethopropazine hydrochloride tablets, USP)
Parke-Davis
250 mg.
500 mg.
†Penicillin V Potassium Tablets, USP
(Penapar VK®)
Parke-Davis
10 mg.
20 mg.
40 mg.
Peritrate®
(pentaerythritol tetranitrate)
Sustained Action 80 mg.
Peritrate® SA
Parke-Davis
250 mg.
Ponstel® Kapseals®
(mefenamic acid)
Parke-Davis
250 mg.
500 mg.
750 mg.
1000 mg.
Procan® SR
(procainamide hydrochloride tablets)
Parke-Davis
½ grain
1 grain
1½ grain
2 grain
3 grain
Proloid®
(thyroglobulin)
Parke-Davis
100 mg.
200 mg.
Pyridium®
(phenazopyridine hydrochloride)
Parke-Davis
Pyridium® Plus
Parke-Davis
Sinubid®
Parke-Davis
Tabron® Filmseal®
Parke-Davis
†Tedral®
Tedral® SA
Tedral-25®
Parke-Davis
250 mg.
500 mg.
Tetracycline HCl Capsules, USP
(Cyclopar®)
Parke-Davis
(Shown smaller than actual size)
Uticort® Cream
Uticort® Gel
Uticort® Ointment
Uticort® Lotion
(betamethasone benzoate, USP)
Parke-Davis
(Tube shown smaller than actual size)
Vira-A®
(vidarabine ophthalmic ointment) 3%

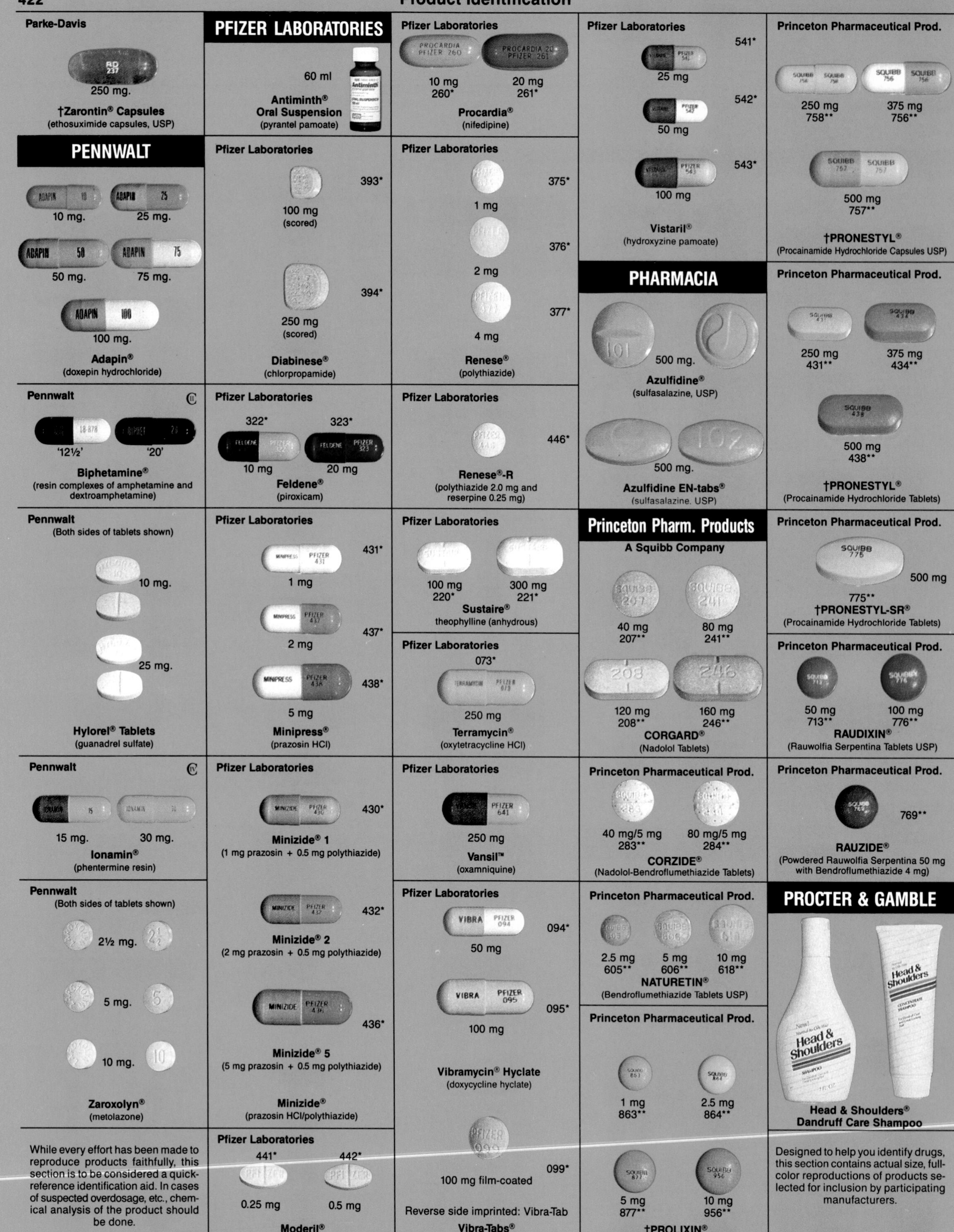

Parke-Davis
250 mg.
†Zarontin® Capsules
(ethosuximide capsules, USP)

PENNWALT

250 mg.

10 mg. 25 mg.
50 mg. 75 mg.
100 mg.
Adapin®
(doxepin hydrochloride)

Pennwalt Ⓒ
'12½' '20'
Biphetamine®
(resin complexes of amphetamine and dextroamphetamine)

Pennwalt
(Both sides of tablets shown)
10 mg.
25 mg.
Hylorel® Tablets
(guanadrel sulfate)

Pennwalt Ⓒ
15 mg. 30 mg.
Ionamin®
(phentermine resin)

Pennwalt
(Both sides of tablets shown)
2½ mg.
5 mg.
10 mg.
Zaroxolyn®
(metolazone)

While every effort has been made to reproduce products faithfully, this section is to be considered a quick-reference identification aid. In cases of suspected overdosage, etc., chemical analysis of the product should be done.

PFIZER LABORATORIES

60 ml
Antiminth®
Oral Suspension
(pyrantel pamoate)

Pfizer Laboratories
100 mg (scored) 393*
250 mg (scored) 394*
Diabinese®
(chlorpropamide)

Pfizer Laboratories
322* 323*
10 mg 20 mg
Feldene®
(piroxicam)

Pfizer Laboratories
1 mg 431*
2 mg 437*
5 mg 438*
Minipress®
(prazosin HCl)

Pfizer Laboratories
430*
Minizide® 1
(1 mg prazosin + 0.5 mg polythiazide)
432*
Minizide® 2
(2 mg prazosin + 0.5 mg polythiazide)
436*
Minizide® 5
(5 mg prazosin + 0.5 mg polythiazide)
Minizide®
(prazosin HCl/polythiazide)

Pfizer Laboratories
441* 442*
0.25 mg 0.5 mg
Moderil®
(rescinnamine)

Pfizer Laboratories
10 mg 260* 20 mg 261*
Procardia®
(nifedipine)

Pfizer Laboratories
1 mg 375*
2 mg 376*
4 mg 377*
Renese®
(polythiazide)

Pfizer Laboratories
446*
Renese®-R
(polythiazide 2.0 mg and reserpine 0.25 mg)

Pfizer Laboratories
100 mg 220* 300 mg 221*
Sustaire®
theophylline (anhydrous)

Pfizer Laboratories
073*
250 mg
Terramycin®
(oxytetracycline HCl)

Pfizer Laboratories
250 mg
Vansil™
(oxamniquine)

Pfizer Laboratories
50 mg 094*
100 mg 095*
Vibramycin® Hyclate
(doxycycline hyclate)
099*
100 mg film-coated
Reverse side imprinted: Vibra-Tab
Vibra-Tabs®
(doxycycline hyclate)

Pfizer Laboratories
25 mg 541*
50 mg 542*
100 mg 543*
Vistaril®
(hydroxyzine pamoate)

PHARMACIA

500 mg.
Azulfidine®
(sulfasalazine, USP)
500 mg.
Azulfidine EN-tabs®
(sulfasalazine, USP)

Princeton Pharm. Products

A Squibb Company
40 mg 207** 80 mg 241**
120 mg 208** 160 mg 246**
CORGARD®
(Nadolol Tablets)

Princeton Pharmaceutical Prod.
40 mg/5 mg 283** 80 mg/5 mg 284**
CORZIDE®
(Nadolol-Bendroflumethiazide Tablets)

Princeton Pharmaceutical Prod.
2.5 mg 605** 5 mg 606** 10 mg 618**
NATURETIN®
(Bendroflumethiazide Tablets USP)

Princeton Pharmaceutical Prod.
1 mg 863** 2.5 mg 864**
5 mg 877** 10 mg 956**
†PROLIXIN®
(Fluphenazine Hydrochloride Tablets USP)

Princeton Pharmaceutical Prod.
250 mg 758** 375 mg 756**
500 mg 757**
†PRONESTYL®
(Procainamide Hydrochloride Capsules USP)

Princeton Pharmaceutical Prod.
250 mg 431** 375 mg 434**
500 mg 438**
†PRONESTYL®
(Procainamide Hydrochloride Tablets)

Princeton Pharmaceutical Prod.
500 mg
775**
†PRONESTYL-SR®
(Procainamide Hydrochloride Tablets)

Princeton Pharmaceutical Prod.
50 mg 713** 100 mg 776**
RAUDIXIN®
(Rauwolfia Serpentina Tablets USP)

Princeton Pharmaceutical Prod.
769**
RAUZIDE®
(Powdered Rauwolfia Serpentina 50 mg with Bendroflumethiazide 4 mg)

PROCTER & GAMBLE

Head & Shoulders®
Dandruff Care Shampoo

Designed to help you identify drugs, this section contains actual size, full-color reproductions of products selected for inclusion by participating manufacturers.

**Princeton, A Squibb Company, product identification number.

PURDUE FREDERICK

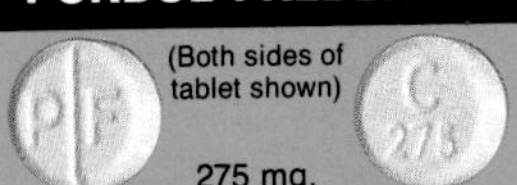

(Both sides of tablet shown)
275 mg.
Bottles of 100 and 500 tablets
CARDIOQUIN® Tablets
(quinidine polygalacturonate)

Purdue Frederick (Both sides of tablet shown)
Bottles of 50, 100, and 250 tablets and also in unit dose packaging.
30 mg.
MS CONTIN® Tablets
(morphine sulfate pentahydrate)

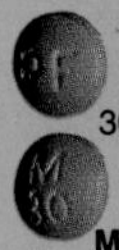

Purdue Frederick (Both sides of tablets shown)
15 mg. 30 mg.
MSIR® Tablets (morphine sulfate, immediate release) bottle of 50 tablets; Also available MSIR® Oral Solution Concentrate and MSIR® Oral Solution Unit Dose.

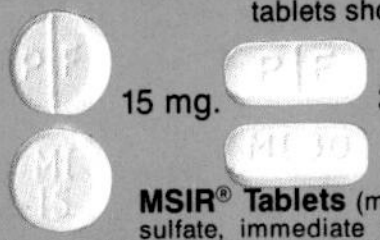

Purdue Frederick
(Both sides of tablets shown)
Trilisate Tablets 500 mg. and 750 mg. available in bottles of 100 tablets and in unit dose packaging. Trilisate 1000 mg. available in bottles of 60 tablets. Trilisate Liquid 500 mg. available in bottles of 8 fluid ounces.
500 mg. 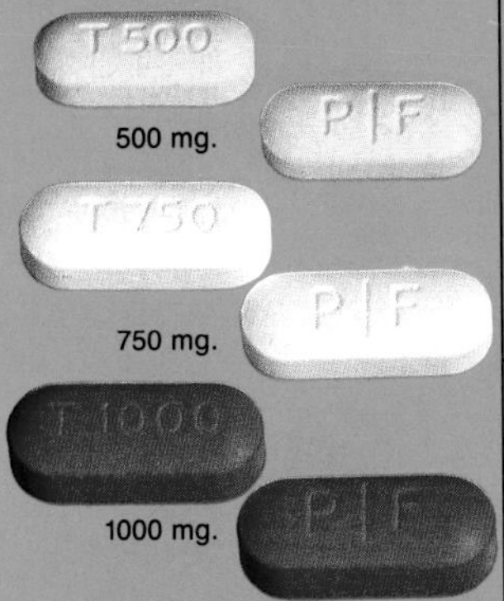
750 mg.
1000 mg.
TRILISATE® Tablets
(choline magnesium trisalicylate)

Purdue Frederick (Both sides of tablets shown)
Uniphyl 200 mg. and 400 mg. available in bottles of 100 tablets. Also available, Uniphyl 400 mg. tablets in bottles of 500 and in unit dose packaging.
200 mg. 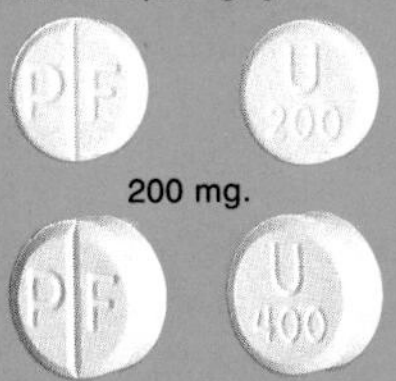
400 mg.
UNIPHYL® Tablets
(theophylline, anhydrous)

Important Notice
Before prescribing or administering any product described in PHYSICIANS' DESK REFERENCE always consult the PDR Supplement for possible new or revised information.

REED & CARNRICK

(Shown smaller than actual size)
Cortifoam® 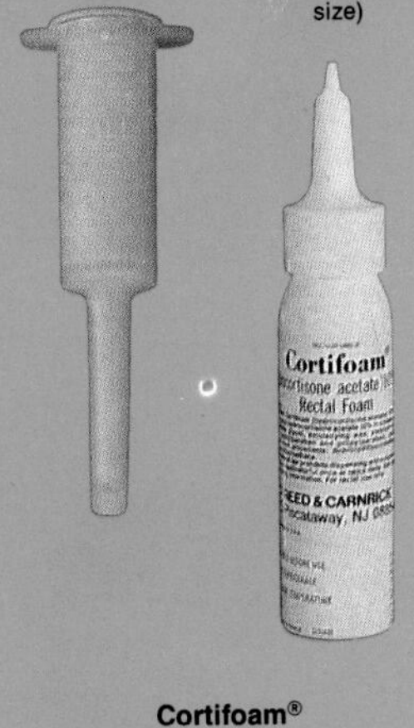
(hydrocortisone acetate) 10%

Reed & Carnrick
40 mg. 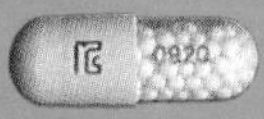
Sustained Release Capsules
Dilatrate®-SR
(isosorbide dinitrate)

Reed & Carnrick
(Shown smaller than actual size)
Epifoam® 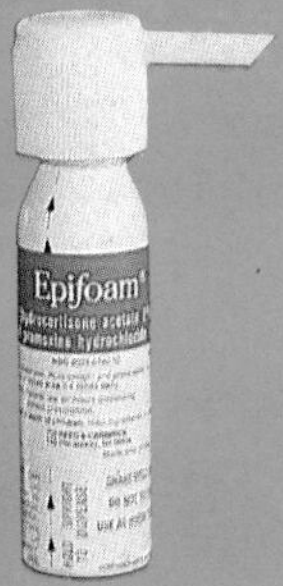
(hydrocortisone acetate) 1%

Reed & Carnrick
Kwell® Lotion **Kwell® Shampoo** 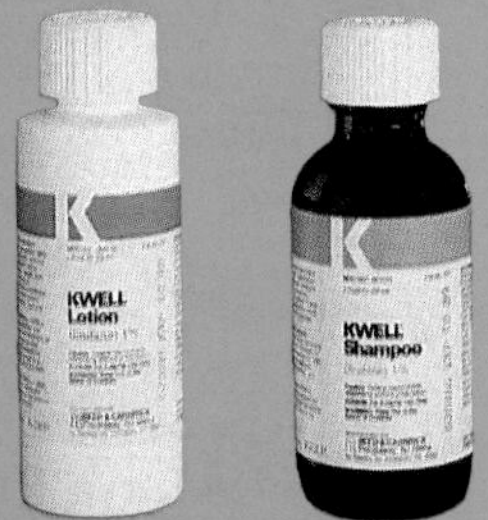
(lindane) 1%

Reed & Carnrick
Phazyme® 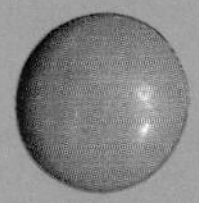

Reed & Carnrick
Phazyme®-95 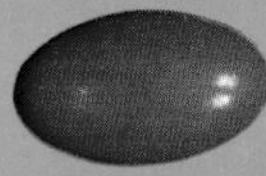

Reed & Carnrick
Phazyme®-125 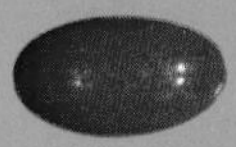

Reed & Carnrick
Phazyme®-PB 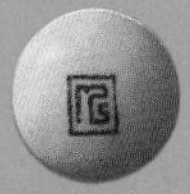

Reed & Carnrick
(Shown smaller than actual size)
Proctofoam®-HC 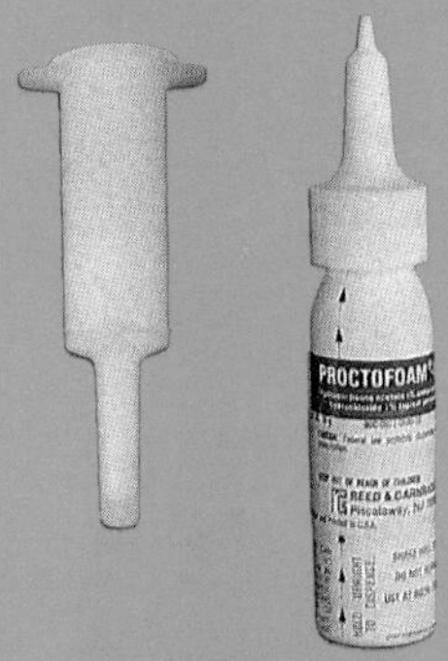
(hydrocortisone acetate) 1%

Reed & Carnrick
Available in 2 and 4 fl. oz. sizes
R&C SHAMPOO® 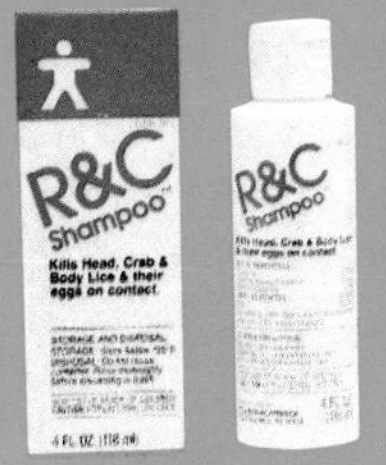
Kills head, crab and body lice and their eggs on contact. Effective nit comb included.

REID-ROWELL

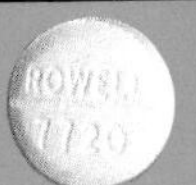

*7720 250 mg.
Chenix®
(chenodiol)

Reid-Rowell
*1290
Compal

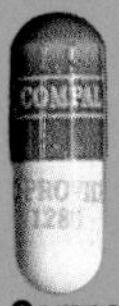

Reid-Rowell
(Shown smaller than actual size)
*1904 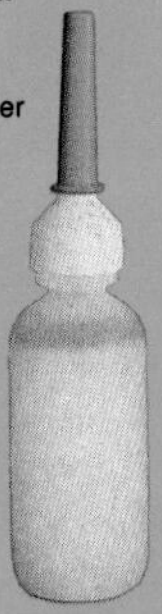
Cortenema®
(hydrocortisone retention enema)

Reid-Rowell
*1007 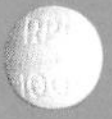
10 mg.
Curretab®
(medroxyprogesterone acetate 10 mg.)

Reid-Rowell
*1014 *1022 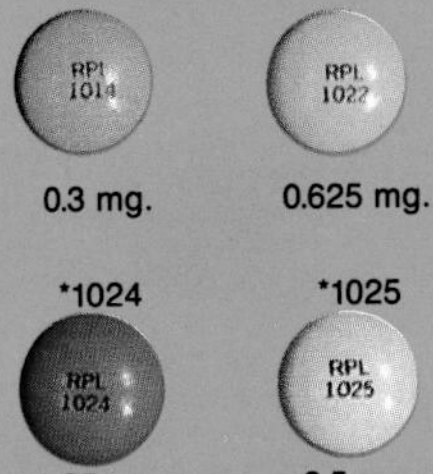
0.3 mg. 0.625 mg.
*1024 *1025
1.25 mg. 2.5 mg.
Estratab®
(esterified estrogens)

Reid-Rowell
*1026 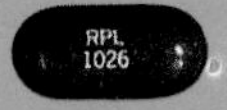
Estratest®
(esterified estrogens 1.25 mg. with methyltestosterone 2.5 mg.)

Reid-Rowell
*1023 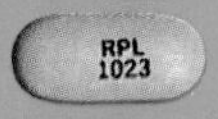
Estratest® H.S.
(esterified estrogens 0.625 mg. with methyltestosterone 1.25 mg.)

Reid-Rowell
*1039 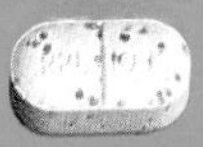
Histalet® Forte

Reid-Rowell *1050 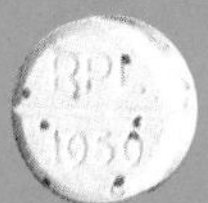
Histalet® X

Reid-Rowell
*1082 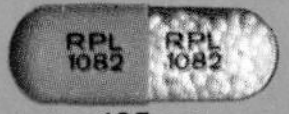
105 mg.
Melfiat®-105 Unicelles®
(phendimetrazine tartrate 105 mg.)

Reid-Rowell
(Shown smaller than actual size)
*1920 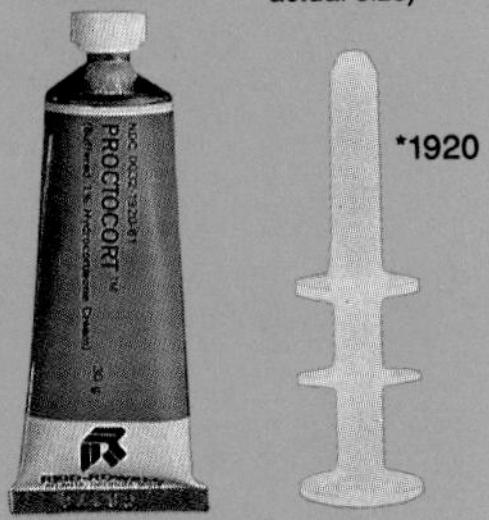
Proctocort™
(buffered 1% hydrocortisone cream)

Reid-Rowell
(Bottle shown smaller than actual size)
*1087 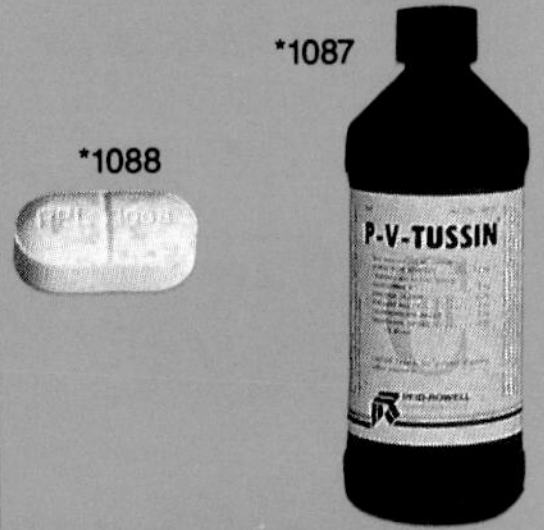
*1088
P-V-Tussin®
Syrup and Tablets

Reid-Rowell
*1146 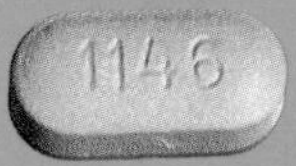
Zenate®

RICHARDSON-VICKS

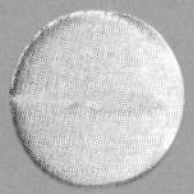

Available in bottles of 24, 50 and 90 tablets
Percogesic®
acetaminophen, phenyltoloxamine citrate

RIKER

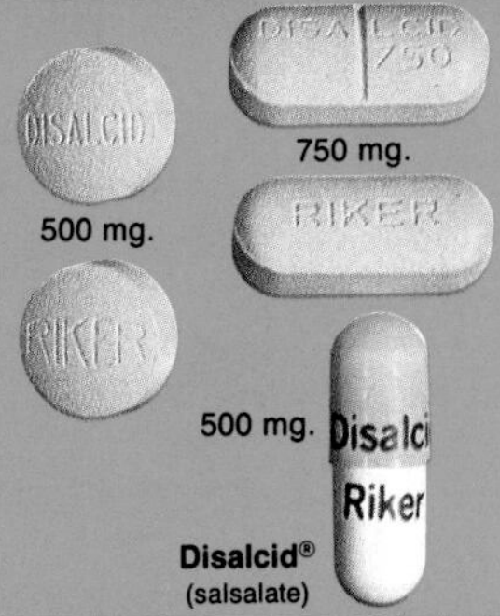

750 mg.
500 mg.
500 mg.
Disalcid®
(salsalate)

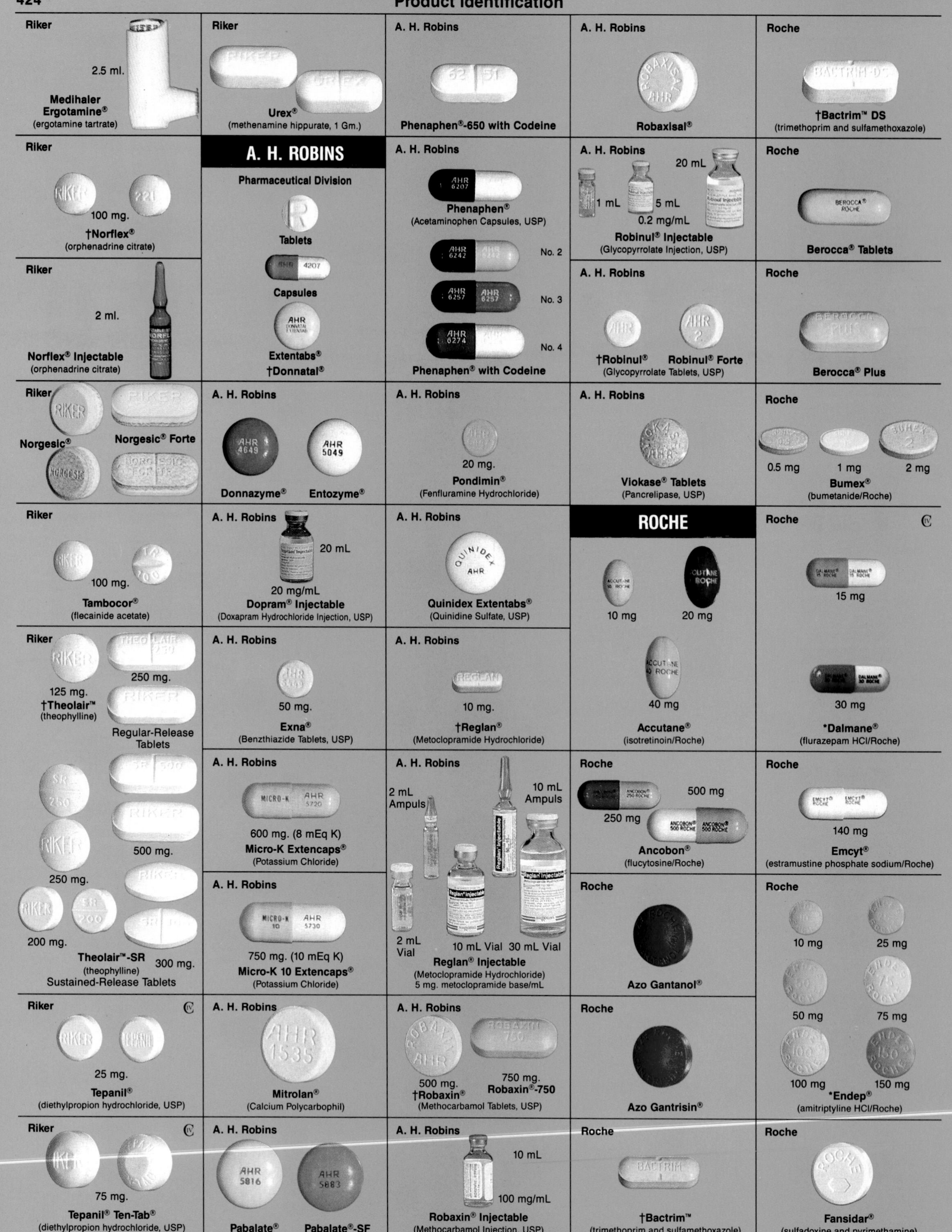

*Dalmane, Endep, Librax, Libritabs, Librium, Limbitrol, Menrium, Quarzan and Valium are products of Roche Products Inc., Manati, PR 00701.

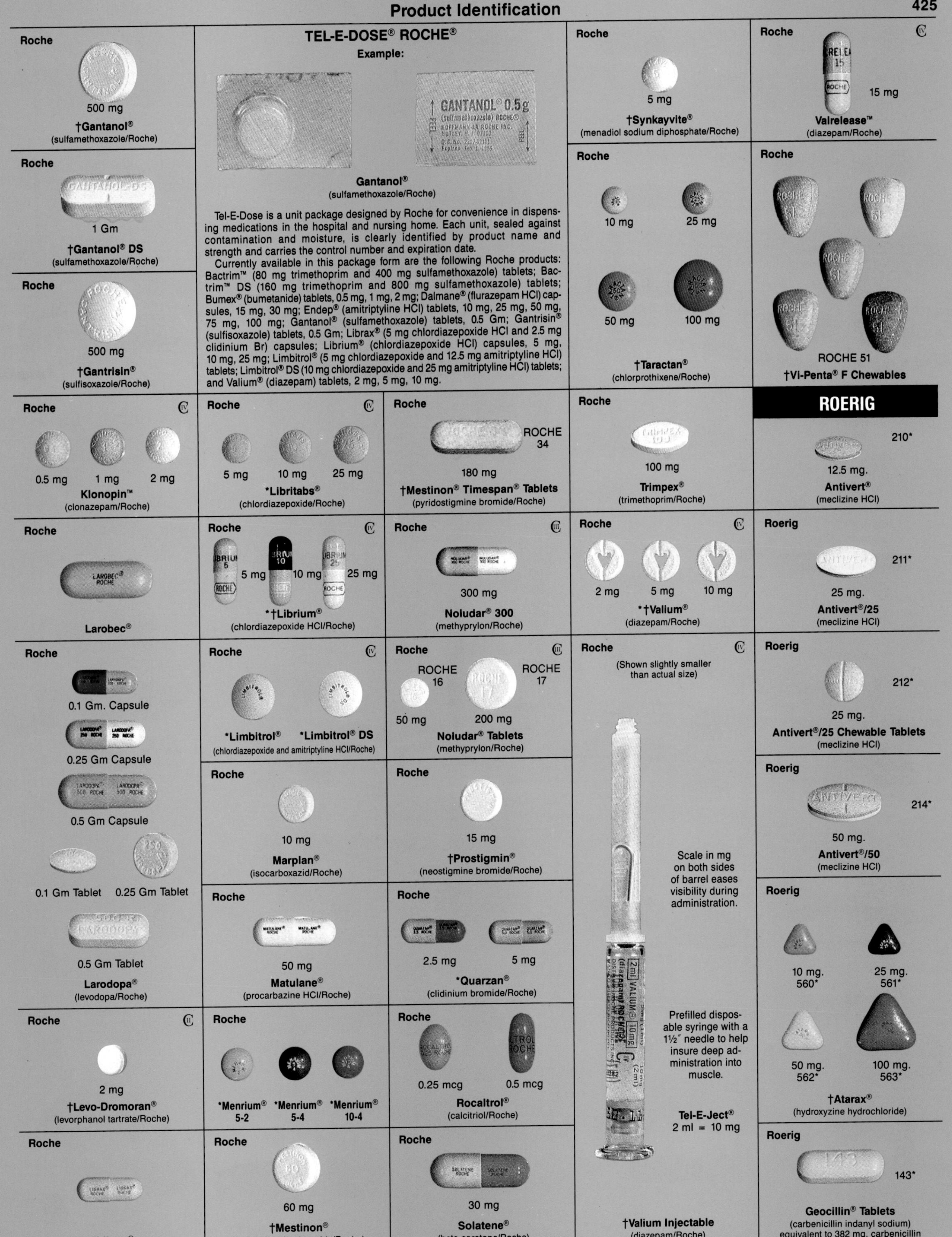

Roche

500 mg

†Gantanol®
(sulfamethoxazole/Roche)

Roche

1 Gm

†Gantanol® DS
(sulfamethoxazole/Roche)

Roche

500 mg

†Gantrisin®
(sulfisoxazole/Roche)

TEL-E-DOSE® ROCHE®

Example:

Gantanol®
(sulfamethoxazole/Roche)

Tel-E-Dose is a unit package designed by Roche for convenience in dispensing medications in the hospital and nursing home. Each unit, sealed against contamination and moisture, is clearly identified by product name and strength and carries the control number and expiration date.

Currently available in this package form are the following Roche products: Bactrim™ (80 mg trimethoprim and 400 mg sulfamethoxazole) tablets; Bactrim™ DS (160 mg trimethoprim and 800 mg sulfamethoxazole) tablets; Bumex® (bumetanide) tablets, 0.5 mg, 1 mg, 2 mg; Dalmane® (flurazepam HCl) capsules, 15 mg, 30 mg; Endep® (amitriptyline HCl) tablets, 10 mg, 25 mg, 50 mg, 75 mg, 100 mg; Gantanol® (sulfamethoxazole) tablets, 0.5 Gm; Gantrisin® (sulfisoxazole) tablets, 0.5 Gm; Librax® (5 mg chlordiazepoxide HCl and 2.5 mg clidinium Br) capsules; Librium® (chlordiazepoxide HCl) capsules, 5 mg, 10 mg, 25 mg; Limbitrol® (5 mg chlordiazepoxide and 12.5 mg amitriptyline HCl) tablets; Limbitrol® DS (10 mg chlordiazepoxide and 25 mg amitriptyline HCl) tablets; and Valium® (diazepam) tablets, 2 mg, 5 mg, 10 mg.

Roche

5 mg

†Synkayvite®
(menadiol sodium diphosphate/Roche)

Roche

10 mg 25 mg 50 mg 100 mg

†Taractan®
(chlorprothixene/Roche)

Roche C-IV

15 mg

Valrelease™
(diazepam/Roche)

Roche

ROCHE 51

†Vi-Penta® F Chewables

Roche C-IV

0.5 mg 1 mg 2 mg

Klonopin™
(clonazepam/Roche)

Roche C-IV

5 mg 10 mg 25 mg

***Libritabs®**
(chlordiazepoxide/Roche)

Roche

ROCHE 34

180 mg

†Mestinon® Timespan® Tablets
(pyridostigmine bromide/Roche)

Roche

100 mg

Trimpex®
(trimethoprim/Roche)

ROERIG

210*

12.5 mg.

Antivert®
(meclizine HCl)

Roche

Larobec®

Roche C-IV

5 mg 10 mg 25 mg

***†Librium®**
(chlordiazepoxide HCl/Roche)

Roche C-III

300 mg

Noludar® 300
(methyprylon/Roche)

Roche C-IV

2 mg 5 mg 10 mg

***†Valium®**
(diazepam/Roche)

Roerig

211*

25 mg.

Antivert®/25
(meclizine HCl)

Roche

0.1 Gm. Capsule

0.25 Gm Capsule

0.5 Gm Capsule

0.1 Gm Tablet 0.25 Gm Tablet

0.5 Gm Tablet

Larodopa®
(levodopa/Roche)

Roche C-IV

***Limbitrol®** ***Limbitrol® DS**
(chlordiazepoxide and amitriptyline HCl/Roche)

Roche C-III

ROCHE 16 ROCHE 17

50 mg 200 mg

Noludar® Tablets
(methyprylon/Roche)

Roche

10 mg

Marplan®
(isocarboxazid/Roche)

Roche

15 mg

†Prostigmin®
(neostigmine bromide/Roche)

Roche

50 mg

Matulane®
(procarbazine HCl/Roche)

Roche

2.5 mg 5 mg

***Quarzan®**
(clidinium bromide/Roche)

Roche C-IV

(Shown slightly smaller than actual size)

Scale in mg on both sides of barrel eases visibility during administration.

Prefilled disposable syringe with a 1½″ needle to help insure deep administration into muscle.

Tel-E-Ject®
2 ml = 10 mg

†Valium Injectable
(diazepam/Roche)

Roerig

212*

25 mg.

Antivert®/25 Chewable Tablets
(meclizine HCl)

Roerig

214*

50 mg.

Antivert®/50
(meclizine HCl)

Roerig

10 mg. 560* 25 mg. 561* 50 mg. 562* 100 mg. 563*

†Atarax®
(hydroxyzine hydrochloride)

Roche C-II

2 mg

†Levo-Dromoran®
(levorphanol tartrate/Roche)

Roche

***Menrium® 5-2** ***Menrium® 5-4** ***Menrium® 10-4**

Roche

0.25 mcg 0.5 mcg

Rocaltrol®
(calcitriol/Roche)

Roche

***Librax®**

Roche

60 mg

†Mestinon®
(pyridostigmine bromide/Roche)

Roche

30 mg

Solatene®
(beta-carotene/Roche)

Roerig

143*

Geocillin® Tablets
(carbenicillin indanyl sodium) equivalent to 382 mg. carbenicillin

*Dalmane, Endep, Librax, Libritabs, Librium, Limbitrol, Menrium, Quarzan and Valium are products of Roche Products Inc., Manati, PR 00701.

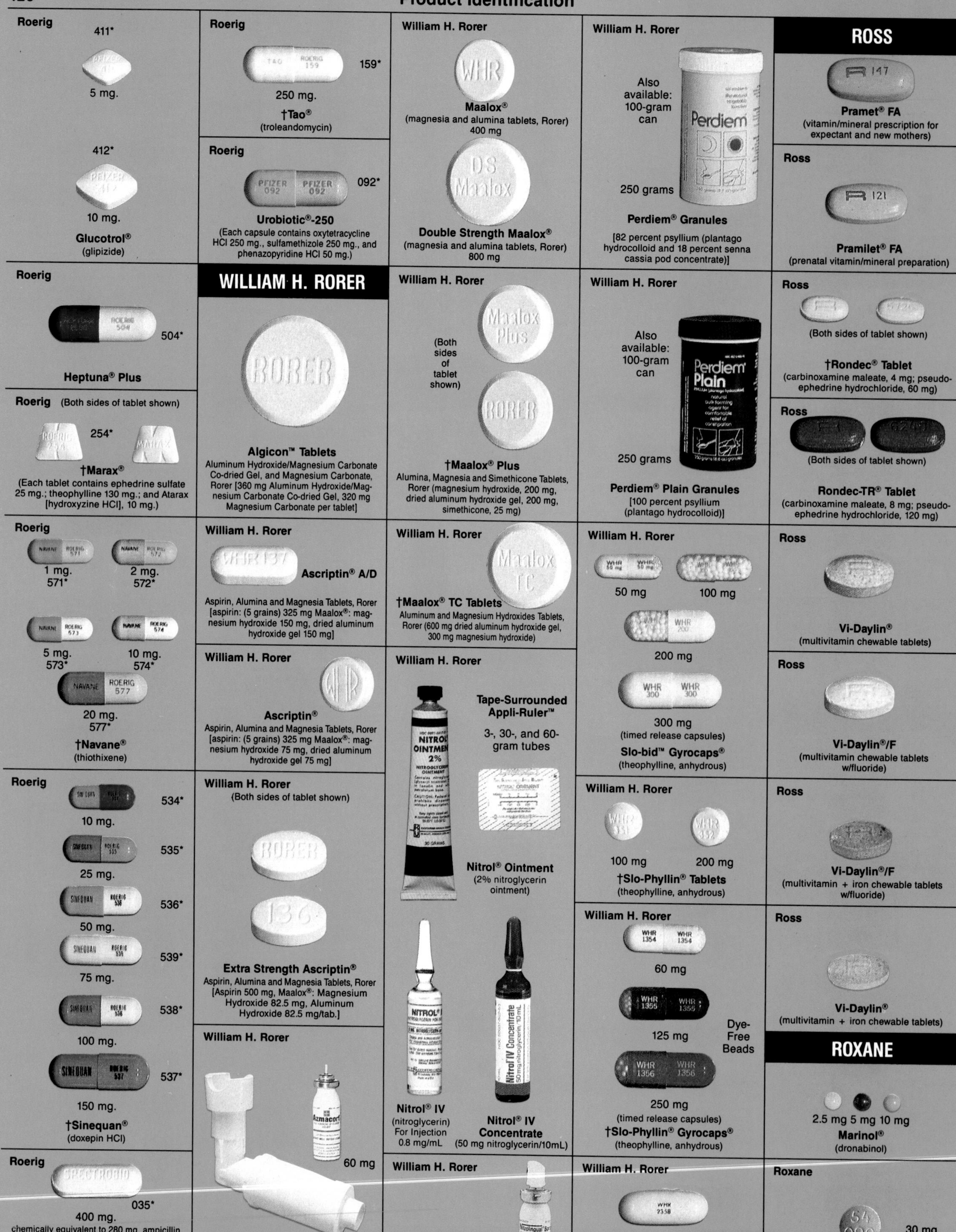

Roerig
411*
5 mg.
412*
10 mg.
Glucotrol®
(glipizide)
Roerig
504*
Heptuna® Plus
Roerig (Both sides of tablet shown)
254*
†Marax®
(Each tablet contains ephedrine sulfate 25 mg.; theophylline 130 mg.; and Atarax [hydroxyzine HCl], 10 mg.)
Roerig
1 mg. 571*
2 mg. 572*
5 mg. 573*
10 mg. 574*
20 mg. 577*
†Navane®
(thiothixene)
Roerig
534*
10 mg.
535*
25 mg.
536*
50 mg.
539*
75 mg.
538*
100 mg.
537*
150 mg.
†Sinequan®
(doxepin HCl)
Roerig
035*
400 mg.
chemically equivalent to 280 mg. ampicillin
†Spectrobid®
(bacampicillin HCl)
Roerig
159*
250 mg.
†Tao®
(troleandomycin)
Roerig
092*
Urobiotic®-250
(Each capsule contains oxytetracycline HCl 250 mg., sulfamethizole 250 mg., and phenazopyridine HCl 50 mg.)
WILLIAM H. RORER
Algicon™ Tablets
Aluminum Hydroxide/Magnesium Carbonate Co-dried Gel, and Magnesium Carbonate, Rorer [360 mg Aluminum Hydroxide/Magnesium Carbonate Co-dried Gel, 320 mg Magnesium Carbonate per tablet]
William H. Rorer
Ascriptin® A/D
Aspirin, Alumina and Magnesia Tablets, Rorer [aspirin: (5 grains) 325 mg Maalox®: magnesium hydroxide 150 mg, dried aluminum hydroxide gel 150 mg]
William H. Rorer
Ascriptin®
Aspirin, Alumina and Magnesia Tablets, Rorer [aspirin: (5 grains) 325 mg Maalox®: magnesium hydroxide 75 mg, dried aluminum hydroxide gel 75 mg]
William H. Rorer
(Both sides of tablet shown)
Extra Strength Ascriptin®
Aspirin, Alumina and Magnesia Tablets, Rorer [Aspirin 500 mg, Maalox®: Magnesium Hydroxide 82.5 mg, Aluminum Hydroxide 82.5 mg/tab.]
William H. Rorer
60 mg
Azmacort™ Inhaler
(triamcinolone acetonide)
William H. Rorer
Maalox®
(magnesia and alumina tablets, Rorer)
400 mg
Double Strength Maalox®
(magnesia and alumina tablets, Rorer)
800 mg
William H. Rorer
(Both sides of tablet shown)
†Maalox® Plus
Alumina, Magnesia and Simethicone Tablets, Rorer (magnesium hydroxide, 200 mg, dried aluminum hydroxide gel, 200 mg, simethicone, 25 mg)
William H. Rorer
†Maalox® TC Tablets
Aluminum and Magnesium Hydroxides Tablets, Rorer (600 mg dried aluminum hydroxide gel, 300 mg magnesium hydroxide)
William H. Rorer
Tape-Surrounded Appli-Ruler™
3-, 30-, and 60-gram tubes
Nitrol® Ointment
(2% nitroglycerin ointment)
Nitrol® IV
(nitroglycerin)
For Injection
0.8 mg/mL
Nitrol® IV Concentrate
(50 mg nitroglycerin/10mL)
William H. Rorer
Nitrolingual® Spray
(nitroglycerin lingual aerosol)
William H. Rorer
Also available: 100-gram can
250 grams
Perdiem® Granules
[82 percent psyllium (plantago hydrocolloid and 18 percent senna cassia pod concentrate)]
William H. Rorer
Also available: 100-gram can
250 grams
Perdiem® Plain Granules
[100 percent psyllium (plantago hydrocolloid)]
William H. Rorer
50 mg
100 mg
200 mg
300 mg
(timed release capsules)
Slo-bid™ Gyrocaps®
(theophylline, anhydrous)
William H. Rorer
100 mg
200 mg
†Slo-Phyllin® Tablets
(theophylline, anhydrous)
William H. Rorer
60 mg
125 mg
Dye-Free Beads
250 mg
(timed release capsules)
†Slo-Phyllin® Gyrocaps®
(theophylline, anhydrous)
William H. Rorer
†Slo-Phyllin® GG Capsules
(theophylline, anhydrous w/guaifenesin)
ROSS
Pramet® FA
(vitamin/mineral prescription for expectant and new mothers)
Ross
Pramilet® FA
(prenatal vitamin/mineral preparation)
Ross
(Both sides of tablet shown)
†Rondec® Tablet
(carbinoxamine maleate, 4 mg; pseudoephedrine hydrochloride, 60 mg)
Ross
(Both sides of tablet shown)
Rondec-TR® Tablet
(carbinoxamine maleate, 8 mg; pseudoephedrine hydrochloride, 120 mg)
Ross
Vi-Daylin®
(multivitamin chewable tablets)
Ross
Vi-Daylin®/F
(multivitamin chewable tablets w/fluoride)
Ross
Vi-Daylin®/F
(multivitamin + iron chewable tablets w/fluoride)
Ross
Vi-Daylin®
(multivitamin + iron chewable tablets)
ROXANE
2.5 mg 5 mg 10 mg
Marinol®
(dronabinol)
Roxane
30 mg
Roxanol SR™
(morphine sulfate sustained release)

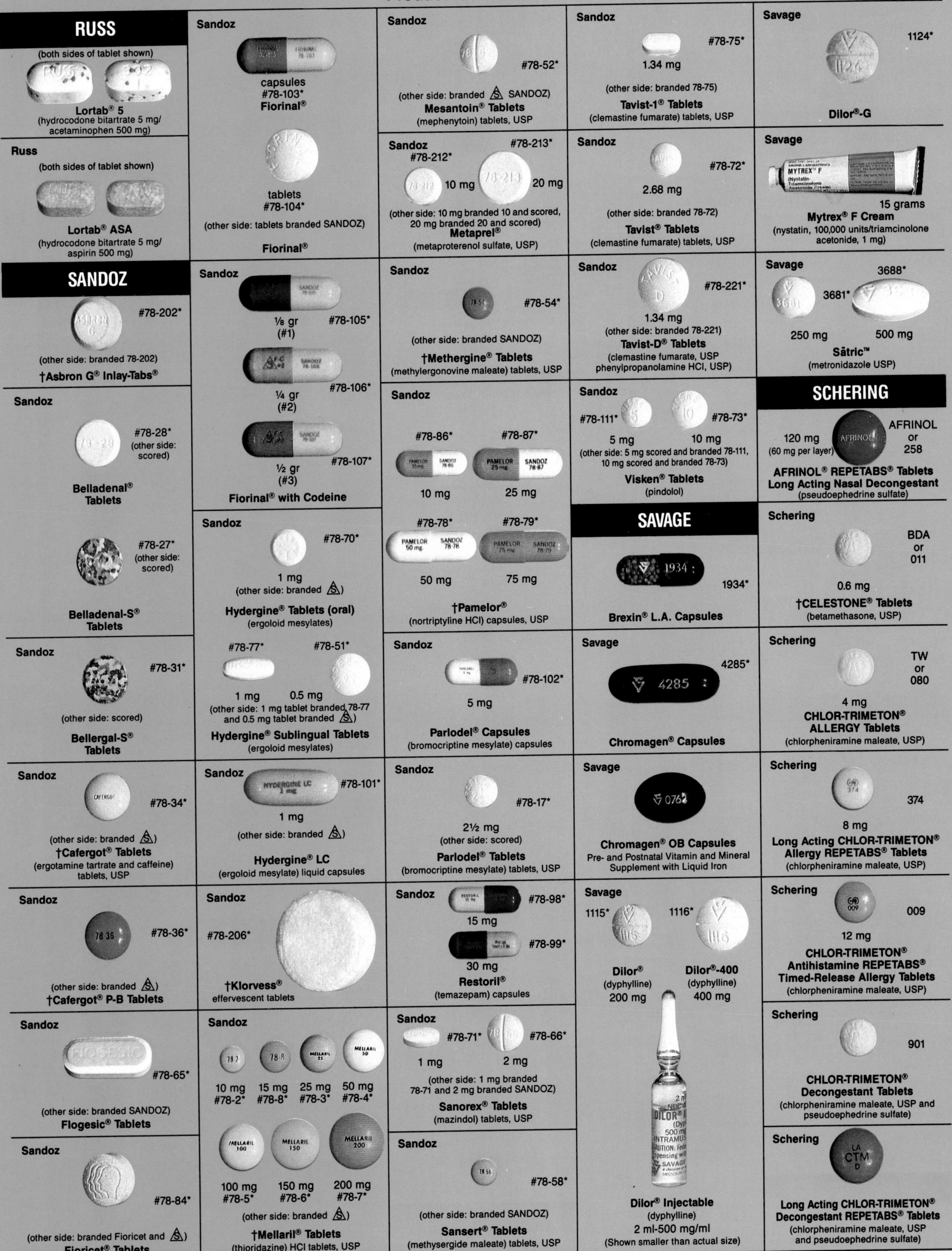
RUSS
(both sides of tablet shown)
Lortab® 5
(hydrocodone bitartrate 5 mg/ acetaminophen 500 mg)
Russ
(both sides of tablet shown)
Lortab® ASA
(hydrocodone bitartrate 5 mg/ aspirin 500 mg)
SANDOZ
#78-202*
(other side: branded 78-202)
†Asbron G® Inlay-Tabs®
Sandoz
#78-28* (other side: scored)
Belladenal® Tablets
#78-27* (other side: scored)
Belladenal-S® Tablets
Sandoz
#78-31*
(other side: scored)
Bellergal-S® Tablets
Sandoz
#78-34*
(other side: branded)
†Cafergot® Tablets
(ergotamine tartrate and caffeine) tablets, USP
Sandoz
#78-36*
(other side: branded)
†Cafergot® P-B Tablets
Sandoz
#78-65*
(other side: branded SANDOZ)
Flogesic® Tablets
Sandoz
#78-84*
(other side: branded Fioricet and)
Fioricet® Tablets
Sandoz
capsules #78-103*
Fiorinal®
tablets #78-104*
(other side: tablets branded SANDOZ)
Fiorinal®
Sandoz
⅛ gr (#1) #78-105*
¼ gr (#2) #78-106*
½ gr (#3) #78-107*
Fiorinal® with Codeine
Sandoz
#78-70*
1 mg
(other side: branded)
Hydergine® Tablets (oral)
(ergoloid mesylates)
#78-77* #78-51*
1 mg 0.5 mg
(other side: 1 mg tablet branded 78-77 and 0.5 mg tablet branded)
Hydergine® Sublingual Tablets
(ergoloid mesylates)
Sandoz
#78-101*
1 mg
(other side: branded)
Hydergine® LC
(ergoloid mesylate) liquid capsules
Sandoz
#78-206*
†Klorvess®
effervescent tablets
Sandoz
10 mg #78-2* 15 mg #78-8* 25 mg #78-3* 50 mg #78-4*
100 mg #78-5* 150 mg #78-6* 200 mg #78-7*
(other side: branded)
†Mellaril® Tablets
(thioridazine) HCl tablets, USP
Sandoz
#78-52*
(other side: branded SANDOZ)
Mesantoin® Tablets
(mephenytoin) tablets, USP
Sandoz
#78-212* #78-213*
10 mg 20 mg
(other side: 10 mg branded 10 and scored, 20 mg branded 20 and scored)
Metaprel®
(metaproterenol sulfate, USP)
Sandoz
#78-54*
(other side: branded SANDOZ)
†Methergine® Tablets
(methylergonovine maleate) tablets, USP
Sandoz
#78-86* #78-87*
10 mg 25 mg
#78-78* #78-79*
50 mg 75 mg
†Pamelor®
(nortriptyline HCl) capsules, USP
Sandoz
#78-102*
5 mg
Parlodel® Capsules
(bromocriptine mesylate) capsules
Sandoz
#78-17*
2½ mg
(other side: scored)
Parlodel® Tablets
(bromocriptine mesylate) tablets, USP
Sandoz
#78-98*
15 mg
#78-99*
30 mg
Restoril®
(temazepam) capsules
Sandoz
#78-71* #78-66*
1 mg 2 mg
(other side: 1 mg branded 78-71 and 2 mg branded SANDOZ)
Sanorex® Tablets
(mazindol) tablets, USP
Sandoz
#78-58*
(other side: branded SANDOZ)
Sansert® Tablets
(methysergide maleate) tablets, USP
Sandoz
#78-75*
1.34 mg
(other side: branded 78-75)
Tavist-1® Tablets
(clemastine fumarate) tablets, USP
Sandoz
#78-72*
2.68 mg
(other side: branded 78-72)
Tavist® Tablets
(clemastine fumarate) tablets, USP
Sandoz
#78-221*
1.34 mg
(other side: branded 78-221)
Tavist-D® Tablets
(clemastine fumarate, USP phenylpropanolamine HCl, USP)
Sandoz
#78-111* #78-73*
5 mg 10 mg
(other side: 5 mg scored and branded 78-111, 10 mg scored and branded 78-73)
Visken® Tablets
(pindolol)
SAVAGE
1934*
Brexin® L.A. Capsules
Savage
4285*
Chromagen® Capsules
Savage
Chromagen® OB Capsules
Pre- and Postnatal Vitamin and Mineral Supplement with Liquid Iron
Savage
1115* 1116*
Dilor® (dyphylline) 200 mg
Dilor®-400 (dyphylline) 400 mg
Dilor® Injectable
(dyphylline)
2 ml-500 mg/ml
(Shown smaller than actual size)
Savage
1124*
Dilor®-G
Savage
15 grams
Mytrex® F Cream
(nystatin, 100,000 units/triamcinolone acetonide, 1 mg)
Savage
3688*
3681*
250 mg 500 mg
Sâtric™
(metronidazole USP)
SCHERING
120 mg (60 mg per layer)
AFRINOL or 258
AFRINOL® REPETABS® Tablets
Long Acting Nasal Decongestant
(pseudoephedrine sulfate)
Schering
BDA or 011
0.6 mg
†CELESTONE® Tablets
(betamethasone, USP)
Schering
TW or 080
4 mg
CHLOR-TRIMETON® ALLERGY Tablets
(chlorpheniramine maleate, USP)
Schering
374
8 mg
Long Acting CHLOR-TRIMETON® Allergy REPETABS® Tablets
(chlorpheniramine maleate, USP)
Schering
009
12 mg
CHLOR-TRIMETON® Antihistamine REPETABS® Timed-Release Allergy Tablets
(chlorpheniramine maleate, USP)
Schering
901
CHLOR-TRIMETON® Decongestant Tablets
(chlorpheniramine maleate, USP and pseudoephedrine sulfate)
Schering
Long Acting CHLOR-TRIMETON® Decongestant REPETABS® Tablets
(chlorpheniramine maleate, USP and pseudoephedrine sulfate)

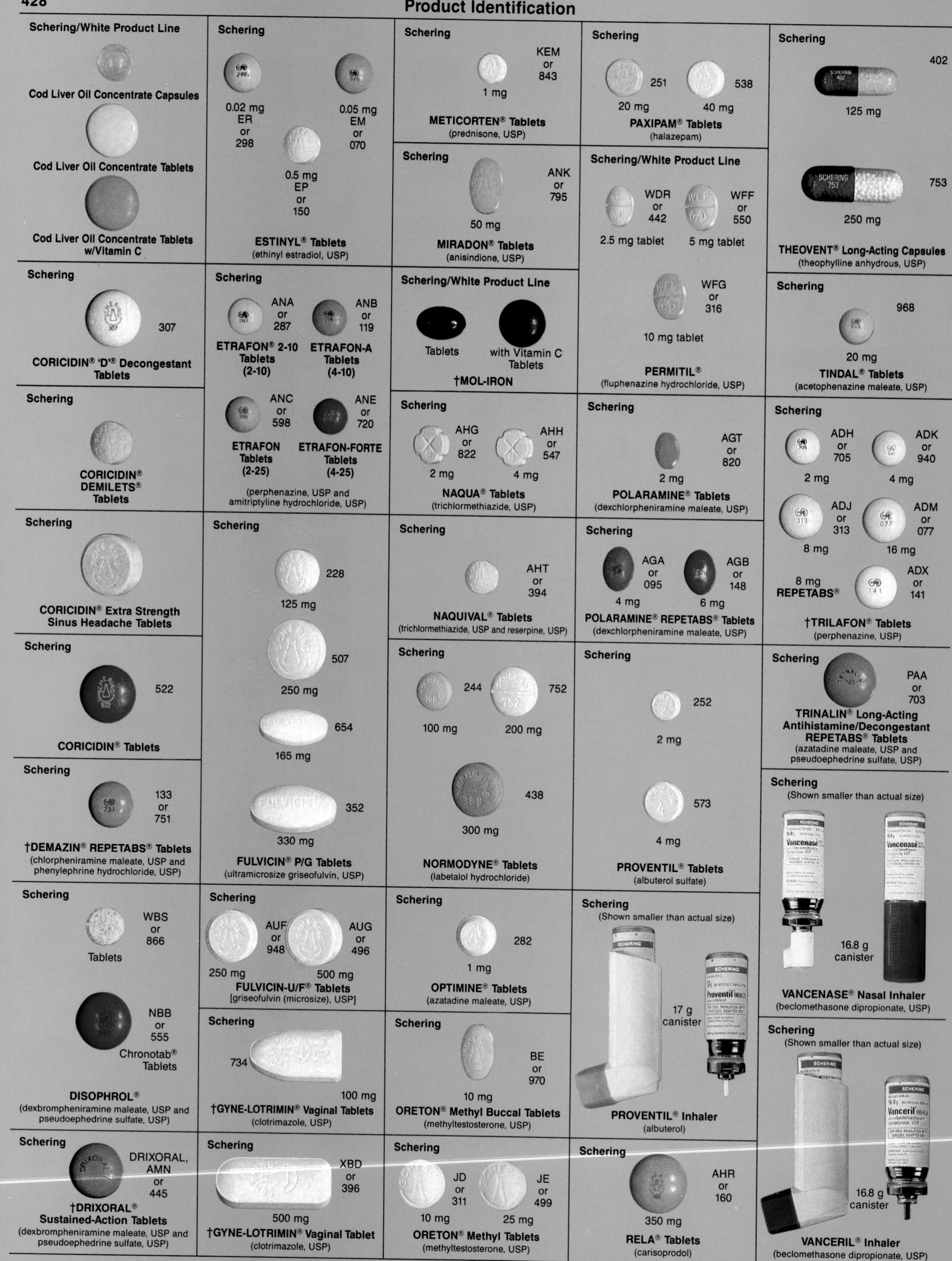
Schering/White Product Line
Cod Liver Oil Concentrate Capsules
Cod Liver Oil Concentrate Tablets
Cod Liver Oil Concentrate Tablets w/Vitamin C
Schering
0.02 mg ER or 298
0.05 mg EM or 070
0.5 mg EP or 150
ESTINYL® Tablets
(ethinyl estradiol, USP)
Schering
KEM or 843
1 mg
METICORTEN® Tablets
(prednisone, USP)
Schering
251 538
20 mg 40 mg
PAXIPAM® Tablets
(halazepam)
Schering
402
125 mg
753
250 mg
THEOVENT® Long-Acting Capsules
(theophylline anhydrous, USP)
Schering
ANK or 795
50 mg
MIRADON® Tablets
(anisindione, USP)
Schering/White Product Line
WDR or 442
WFF or 550
2.5 mg tablet
5 mg tablet
WFG or 316
10 mg tablet
PERMITIL®
(fluphenazine hydrochloride, USP)
Schering
307
CORICIDIN® 'D'® Decongestant Tablets
Schering
ANA or 287
ANB or 119
ETRAFON® 2-10 Tablets (2-10)
ETRAFON-A Tablets (4-10)
ANC or 598
ANE or 720
ETRAFON Tablets (2-25)
ETRAFON-FORTE Tablets (4-25)
(perphenazine, USP and amitriptyline hydrochloride, USP)
Schering/White Product Line
Tablets
with Vitamin C Tablets
†MOL-IRON
Schering
968
20 mg
TINDAL® Tablets
(acetophenazine maleate, USP)
Schering
CORICIDIN® DEMILETS® Tablets
Schering
AHG or 822
AHH or 547
2 mg 4 mg
NAQUA® Tablets
(trichlormethiazide, USP)
Schering
AGT or 820
2 mg
POLARAMINE® Tablets
(dexchlorpheniramine maleate, USP)
Schering
ADH or 705
ADK or 940
2 mg 4 mg
ADJ or 313
ADM or 077
8 mg 16 mg
8 mg REPETABS®
ADX or 141
†TRILAFON® Tablets
(perphenazine, USP)
Schering
CORICIDIN® Extra Strength Sinus Headache Tablets
Schering
228
125 mg
507
250 mg
654
165 mg
352
330 mg
FULVICIN® P/G Tablets
(ultramicrosize griseofulvin, USP)
Schering
AHT or 394
NAQUIVAL® Tablets
(trichlormethiazide, USP and reserpine, USP)
Schering
AGA or 095
AGB or 148
4 mg 6 mg
POLARAMINE® REPETABS® Tablets
(dexchlorpheniramine maleate, USP)
Schering
522
CORICIDIN® Tablets
Schering
244 752
100 mg 200 mg
438
300 mg
NORMODYNE® Tablets
(labetalol hydrochloride)
Schering
252
2 mg
573
4 mg
PROVENTIL® Tablets
(albuterol sulfate)
Schering
PAA or 703
TRINALIN® Long-Acting Antihistamine/Decongestant REPETABS® Tablets
(azatadine maleate, USP and pseudoephedrine sulfate, USP)
Schering
133 or 751
†DEMAZIN® REPETABS® Tablets
(chlorpheniramine maleate, USP and phenylephrine hydrochloride, USP)
Schering
(Shown smaller than actual size)
16.8 g canister
VANCENASE® Nasal Inhaler
(beclomethasone dipropionate, USP)
Schering
WBS or 866
Tablets
NBB or 555
Chronotab® Tablets
DISOPHROL®
(dexbrompheniramine maleate, USP and pseudoephedrine sulfate, USP)
Schering
AUF or 948
AUG or 496
250 mg 500 mg
FULVICIN-U/F® Tablets
[griseofulvin (microsize), USP]
Schering
282
1 mg
OPTIMINE® Tablets
(azatadine maleate, USP)
Schering
(Shown smaller than actual size)
17 g canister
PROVENTIL® Inhaler
(albuterol)
Schering
734
100 mg
†GYNE-LOTRIMIN® Vaginal Tablets
(clotrimazole, USP)
Schering
BE or 970
10 mg
ORETON® Methyl Buccal Tablets
(methyltestosterone, USP)
Schering
(Shown smaller than actual size)
16.8 g canister
VANCERIL® Inhaler
(beclomethasone dipropionate, USP)
Schering
DRIXORAL, AMN or 445
†DRIXORAL® Sustained-Action Tablets
(dexbrompheniramine maleate, USP and pseudoephedrine sulfate, USP)
Schering
XBD or 396
500 mg
†GYNE-LOTRIMIN® Vaginal Tablet
(clotrimazole, USP)
Schering
JD or 311
JE or 499
10 mg 25 mg
ORETON® Methyl Tablets
(methyltestosterone, USP)
Schering
AHR or 160
350 mg
RELA® Tablets
(carisoprodol)

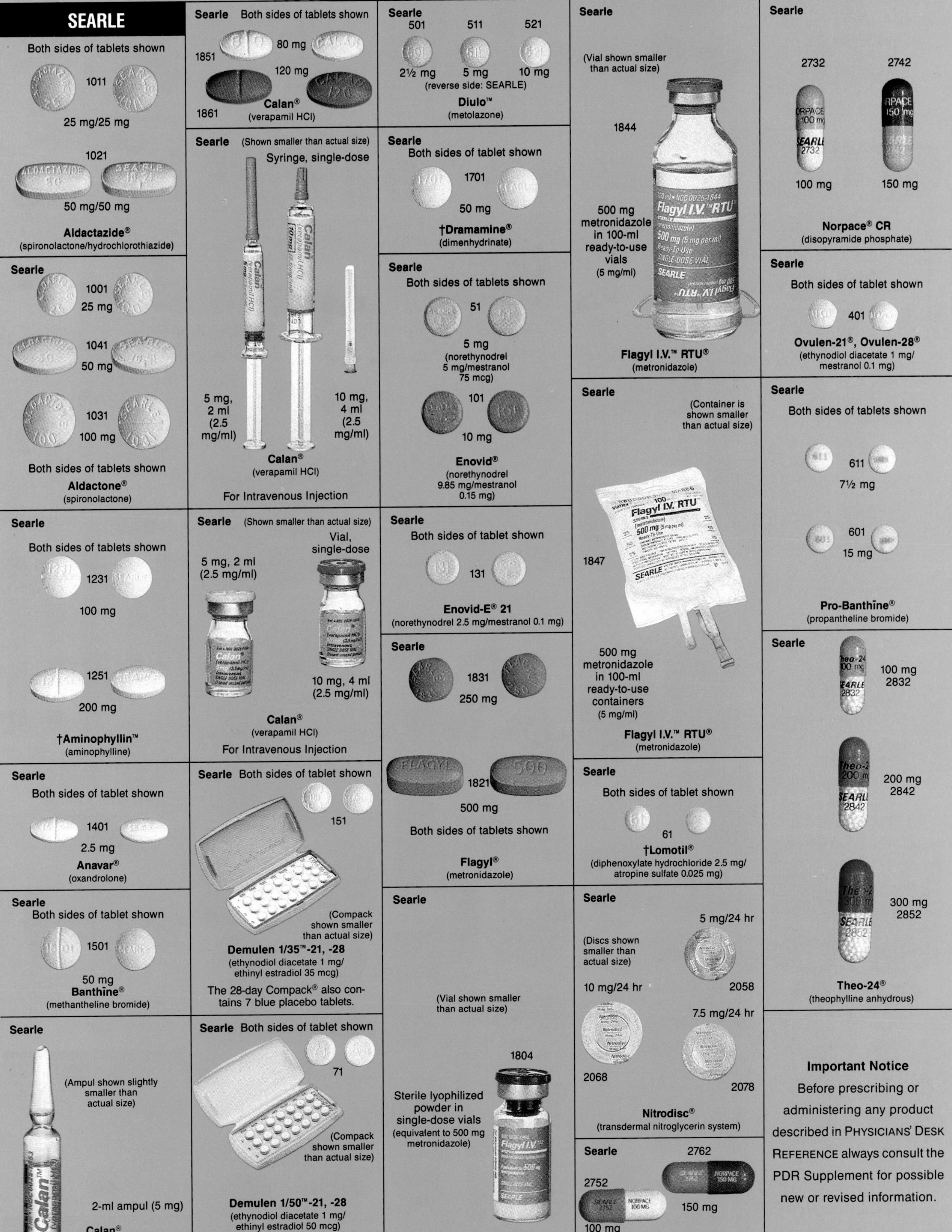
SEARLE
Both sides of tablets shown
1011
25 mg/25 mg
1021
50 mg/50 mg
Aldactazide®
(spironolactone/hydrochlorothiazide)
Searle
1001
25 mg
1041
50 mg
1031
100 mg
Both sides of tablets shown
Aldactone®
(spironolactone)
Searle
Both sides of tablets shown
1231
100 mg
1251
200 mg
†Aminophyllin™
(aminophylline)
Searle
Both sides of tablet shown
1401
2.5 mg
Anavar®
(oxandrolone)
Searle
Both sides of tablet shown
1501
50 mg
Banthine®
(methantheline bromide)
Searle
(Ampul shown slightly smaller than actual size)
2-ml ampul (5 mg)
Calan®
(verapamil HCl)
For Intravenous Injection
Searle Both sides of tablets shown
1851
80 mg
120 mg
1861
Calan®
(verapamil HCl)
Searle (Shown smaller than actual size)
Syringe, single-dose
5 mg, 2 ml (2.5 mg/ml)
10 mg, 4 ml (2.5 mg/ml)
Calan®
(verapamil HCl)
For Intravenous Injection
Searle (Shown smaller than actual size)
Vial, single-dose
5 mg, 2 ml (2.5 mg/ml)
10 mg, 4 ml (2.5 mg/ml)
Calan®
(verapamil HCl)
For Intravenous Injection
Searle Both sides of tablet shown
151
(Compack shown smaller than actual size)
Demulen 1/35™-21, -28
(ethynodiol diacetate 1 mg/ ethinyl estradiol 35 mcg)
The 28-day Compack® also contains 7 blue placebo tablets.
Searle Both sides of tablet shown
71
(Compack shown smaller than actual size)
Demulen 1/50™-21, -28
(ethynodiol diacetate 1 mg/ ethinyl estradiol 50 mcg)
The 28-day Compack® also contains 7 pink placebo tablets.
Searle
501 511 521
2½ mg 5 mg 10 mg
(reverse side: SEARLE)
Diulo™
(metolazone)
Searle
Both sides of tablet shown
1701
50 mg
†Dramamine®
(dimenhydrinate)
Searle
Both sides of tablets shown
51
5 mg
(norethynodrel 5 mg/mestranol 75 mcg)
101
10 mg
Enovid®
(norethynodrel 9.85 mg/mestranol 0.15 mg)
Searle
Both sides of tablet shown
131
Enovid-E® 21
(norethynodrel 2.5 mg/mestranol 0.1 mg)
Searle
1831
250 mg
1821
500 mg
Both sides of tablets shown
Flagyl®
(metronidazole)
Searle
(Vial shown smaller than actual size)
Sterile lyophilized powder in single-dose vials (equivalent to 500 mg metronidazole)
1804
Flagyl I.V.™
(metronidazole HCl)
Searle
(Vial shown smaller than actual size)
1844
500 mg metronidazole in 100-ml ready-to-use vials (5 mg/ml)
Flagyl I.V.™ RTU®
(metronidazole)
Searle
(Container is shown smaller than actual size)
1847
500 mg metronidazole in 100-ml ready-to-use containers (5 mg/ml)
Flagyl I.V.™ RTU®
(metronidazole)
Searle
Both sides of tablet shown
61
†Lomotil®
(diphenoxylate hydrochloride 2.5 mg/ atropine sulfate 0.025 mg)
Searle
5 mg/24 hr
(Discs shown smaller than actual size)
10 mg/24 hr
2058
7.5 mg/24 hr
2068
2078
Nitrodisc®
(transdermal nitroglycerin system)
Searle
2762
2752
150 mg
100 mg
Norpace®
(disopyramide phosphate)
Searle
2732 2742
100 mg 150 mg
Norpace® CR
(disopyramide phosphate)
Searle
Both sides of tablet shown
401
Ovulen-21®, Ovulen-28®
(ethynodiol diacetate 1 mg/ mestranol 0.1 mg)
Searle
Both sides of tablets shown
611
7½ mg
601
15 mg
Pro-Banthine®
(propantheline bromide)
Searle
100 mg 2832
200 mg 2842
300 mg 2852
Theo-24®
(theophylline anhydrous)
Important Notice
Before prescribing or administering any product described in PHYSICIANS' DESK REFERENCE always consult the PDR Supplement for possible new or revised information.

SMITH KLINE & FRENCH

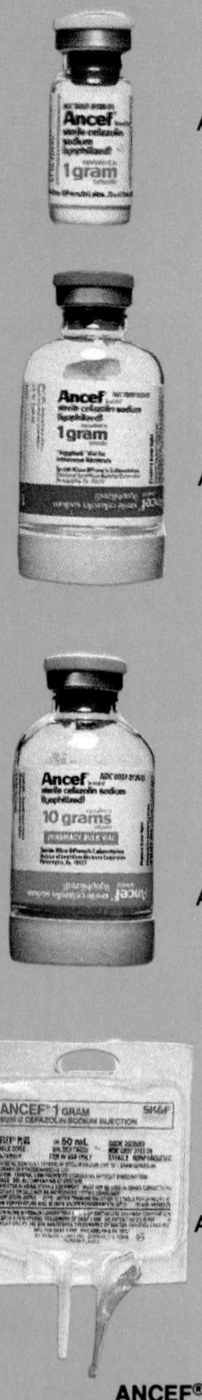

1 gram
Also 250 mg., 500 mg.

1 gram
Also 500 mg.

10 grams
Also 5 grams

1 gram
Also 500 mg.

ANCEF®
(sterile cefazolin sodium, SK&F and cefazolin sodium injection, SK&F)

Smith Kline & French

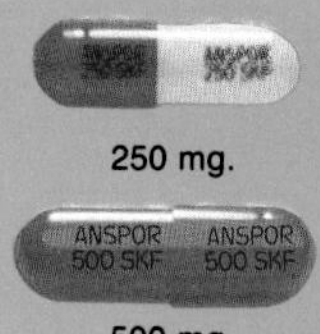

ANSPOR
250 mg.

ANSPOR
500 mg.

Also oral suspension 125 mg. or 250 mg. per 5 ml. teaspoonful (in 100 ml. bottles).

ANSPOR® Capsules
(cephradine, SK&F)

Smith Kline & French

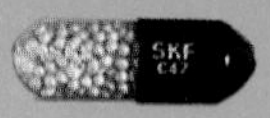

C47
30 mg.

Also 10 mg. C44, 15 mg. C46
†COMPAZINE® SPANSULE® Capsules
(prochlorperazine, SK&F)

Smith Kline & French

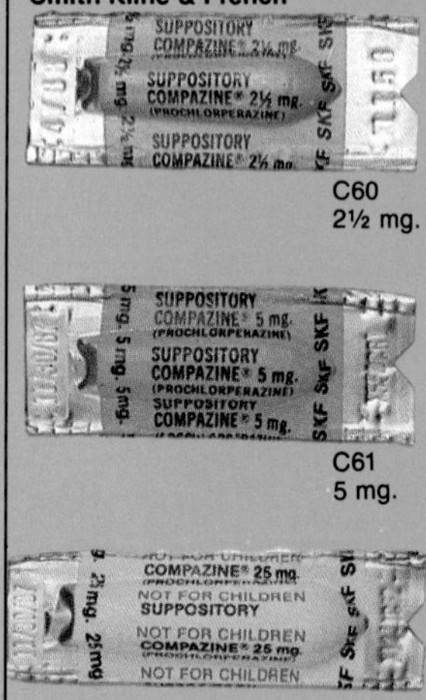

C60
2½ mg.

C61
5 mg.

C62
25 mg.

†COMPAZINE® Suppositories
(prochlorperazine, SK&F)

Smith Kline & French

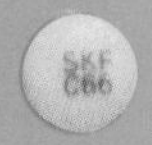

C66
5 mg.

Also 10 mg. C67, 25 mg. C69
†COMPAZINE® Tablets
(prochlorperazine, SK&F)

Smith Kline & French

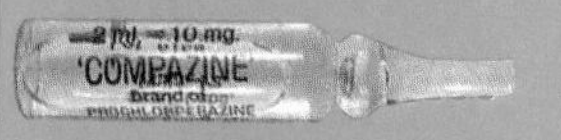

†COMPAZINE®
(prochlorperazine, SK&F)
2 ml. (5 mg./ml.) Ampuls

Smith Kline & French

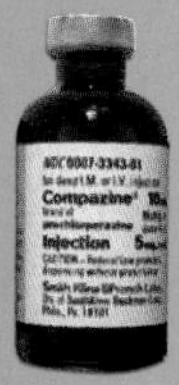

†COMPAZINE®
(prochlorperazine, SK&F)
10 ml. (5 mg./ml.)
Multiple-dose Vials

Smith Kline & French

†COMPAZINE®
(prochlorperazine, SK&F)
2 ml. (5 mg./ml.)
Prefilled Disposable Syringes

FSK

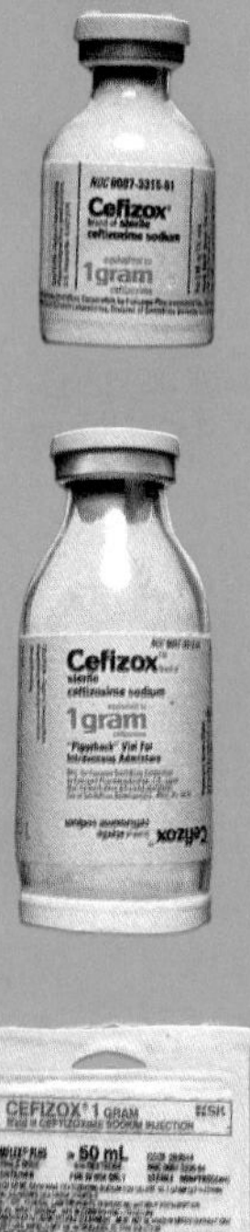

1 gram
Also 2 grams

1 gram
Also 2 grams

1 gram
Also 2 grams

CEFIZOX®
(sterile ceftizoxime sodium, FSK and ceftizoxime sodium injection, FSK)

Smith Kline & French

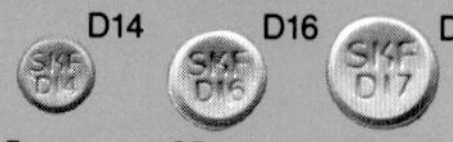

D14 D16 D17
5 mcg. 25 mcg. 50 mcg.
liothyronine as the sodium salt
CYTOMEL® Tablets
(liothyronine sodium, SK&F)

Smith Kline & French

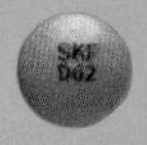

D62
5 mg.
DARBID® Tablets
(isopropamide iodide, SK&F)

Smith Kline & French Ⓒ

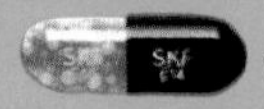

E14
15 mg.

Also 5 mg. E12, 10 mg. E13
†DEXEDRINE® SPANSULE® Capsules
(dextroamphetamine sulfate, SK&F)

Smith Kline & French Ⓒ

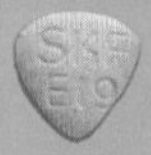

E19
5 mg.
†DEXEDRINE® Tablets
(dextroamphetamine sulfate, SK&F)

Smith Kline & French

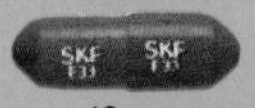

E33
10 mg.
DIBENZYLINE® Capsules
(phenoxybenzamine hydrochloride, SK&F)

SK&F Co.

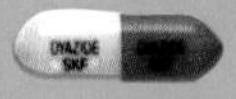

DYAZIDE

DYAZIDE® Capsules

SK&F Co.

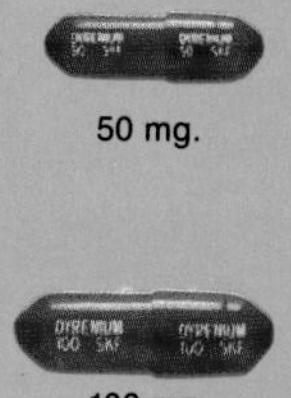

DYRENIUM
50 mg.

DYRENIUM
100 mg.

DYRENIUM® Capsules
(triamterene, SK&F)

Smith Kline & French

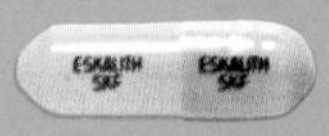

ESKALITH
300 mg.
ESKALITH® Capsules
(lithium carbonate, SK&F)

Smith Kline & French

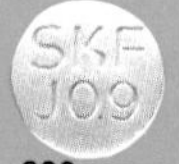

J09
300 mg.
ESKALITH® Tablets
(lithium carbonate, SK&F)

Smith Kline & French

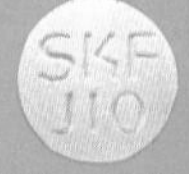

J10
450 mg.
ESKALITH CR®
(lithium carbonate, SK&F)
Controlled Release Tablets

Smith Kline & French

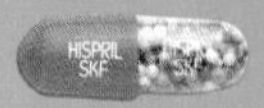

HISPRIL
5 mg.
HISPRIL® SPANSULE® Capsules
(diphenylpyraline hydrochloride, SK&F)

Smith Kline & French

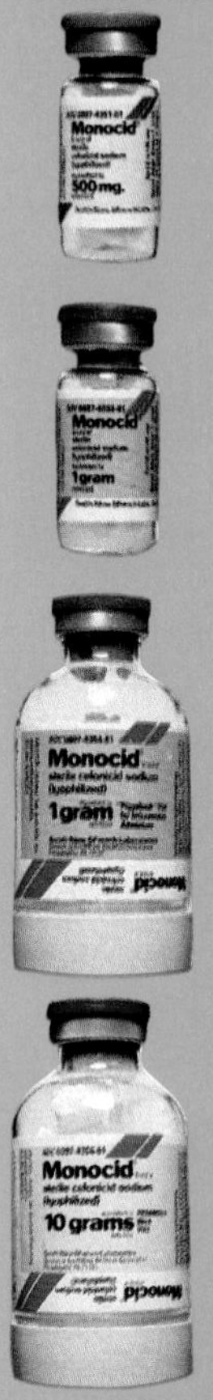

500 mg.

1 gram

1 gram

10 grams

MONOCID®
(sterile cefonicid sodium, SK&F)
(lyophilized)

Smith Kline & French

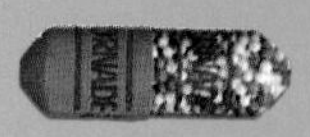

ORNADE
ORNADE® SPANSULE® Capsules

Smith Kline & French

PARNATE
10 mg.
PARNATE® Tablets
(tranylcypromine sulfate, SK&F)

Smith Kline & French

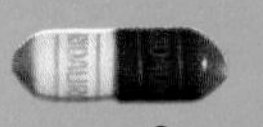

RIDAURA
3 mg.
RIDAURA® Capsules
(auranofin, SK&F)

SMITH KLINE & FRENCH LABORATORIES
Division of SmithKline Beckman Corporation
TABLET & CAPSULE IDENTIFICATION

The unique "taper-end" shape of SK&F capsules is a trademark that quickly identifies them as products of Smith Kline & French Laboratories.

Product Identification Code: Each SK&F capsule and tablet bears a monogram consisting of a three-character code or the name of the specific product. A product-by-product listing of identification codes, including SK-Line® products, appears in SK&F's complete list of products in the Product Information section.

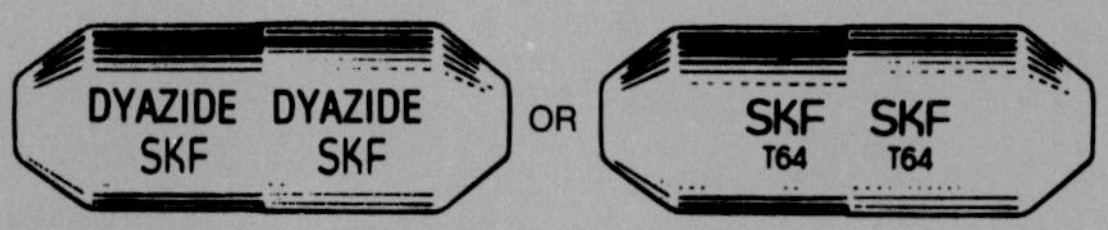

DYAZIDE DYAZIDE SKF SKF OR SKF SKF T64 T64

Capsule Shape: Trademark

The three-unit product identification codes or names that appear beside products in the photo blocks are the same as those imprinted on the pictured products because the codes may be difficult to read in the photo reproductions.

NOTE: Dyazide®, Dyrenium® and Stelazine® are products of SK&F Co., Carolina, P.R. 00630, a subsidiary of SmithKline Beckman Corporation. Tagamet® is a product of SK&F Lab Co., Carolina, P.R. 00630, a subsidiary of SmithKline Beckman Corporation. Cefizox® is manufactured for Fujisawa SmithKline, distributed by SK&F Laboratories, Division of SmithKline Beckman Corporation.

*Smith, Kline & French logo only may appear on tablets. **Logo only may appear on capsules.

SK&F Co.

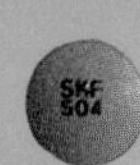

2 mg. S04
Also 1 mg. S03,
5 mg. S06,
10 mg. S07

†STELAZINE® Tablets
(trifluoperazine HCl, SK&F)

SK&F Co.

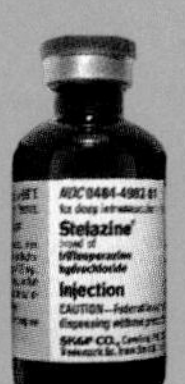

10 ml.
(2 mg./ml.)
Multiple-dose Vials

†STELAZINE®
(trifluoperazine HCl, SK&F)

SK&F Lab Co.

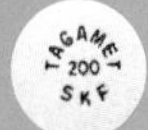

TAGAMET 200 mg.

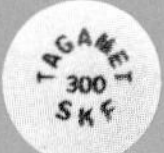

TAGAMET 300 mg.

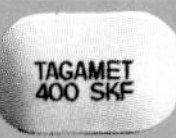

TAGAMET 400 mg.

TAGAMET® Tablets
(cimetidine, SK&F)

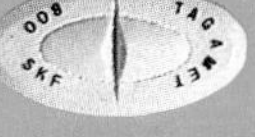

TAGAMET 800 mg.

TAGAMET® TILTAB™ Tablets
(cimetidine, SK&F)

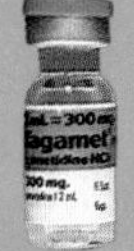

2 ml.
Single-dose

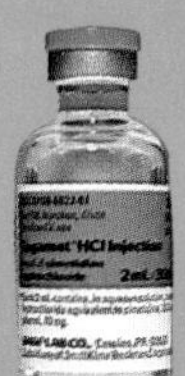

8 ml.
Multiple-dose

Prefilled Disposable Syringe

TAGAMET® HCl INJECTION
(cimetidine hydrochloride, SK&F)
300 mg./2 ml.

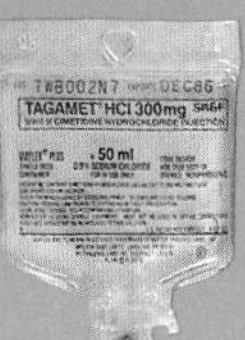

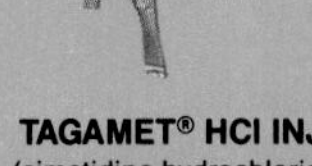

300 mg./50 ml.

TAGAMET® HCl INJECTION
(cimetidine hydrochloride, SK&F)

SK&F Lab Co.

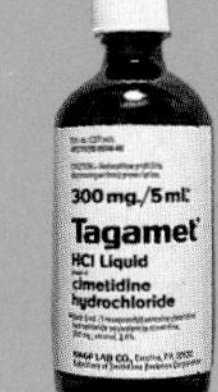

8 fl. oz.

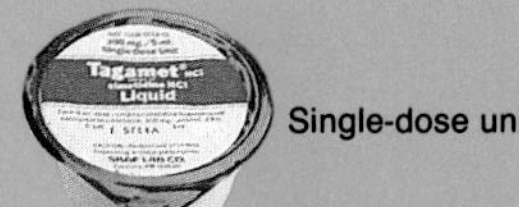

Single-dose unit

Each 5 ml. contains cimetidine hydrochloride equivalent to cimetidine, 300 mg.
TAGAMET® LIQUID
(cimetidine hydrochloride, SK&F)

Smith Kline & French

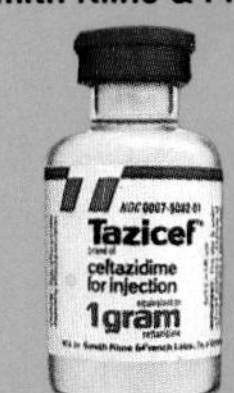

1 gram
Also 2 grams

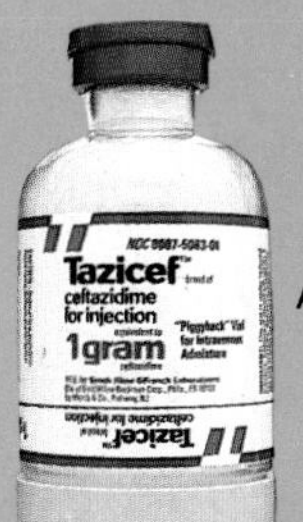

1 gram
Also 2 grams

TAZICEF™
(ceftazidime for injection, SK&F)

Smith Kline & French

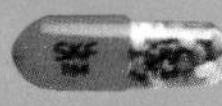

T64
75 mg.

Also 30 mg. T63, 150 mg. T66,
200 mg. T67, 300 mg. T69
†THORAZINE® SPANSULE®
(chlorpromazine hydrochloride, SK&F)
Capsules

Smith Kline & French

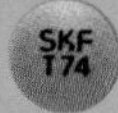

T74
25 mg.

Also 10 mg. T73, 50 mg. T76,
.100 mg. T77, 200 mg. T79
†THORAZINE® Tablets
(chlorpromazine hydrochloride, SK&F)

Smith Kline & French

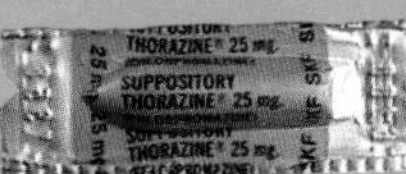

T70
25 mg

Also available 100 mg. T71
†THORAZINE® Suppositories
(chlorpromazine, SK&F)

Smith Kline & French

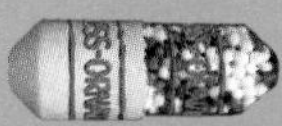

TUSS-ORNADE

†TUSS-ORNADE®
SPANSULE® Capsules

Smith Kline & French

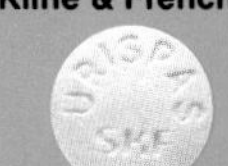

URISPAS

100 mg.
URISPAS® Tablets
(flavoxate HCl, SK&F)

Smith Kline & French

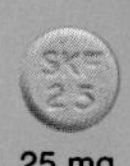

25 mg.
VONTROL® Tablets
(diphenidol as the hydrochloride, SK&F)

SOLGAR

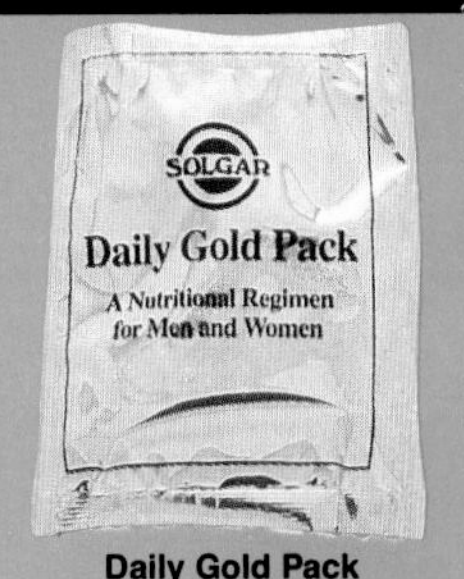

Daily Gold Pack
Complete Multivitamin and Mineral Regimen

E. R. SQUIBB & SONS

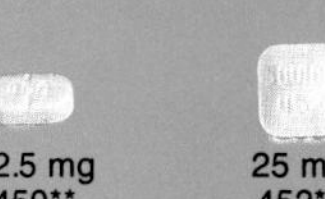

12.5 mg
450**

25 mg
452**

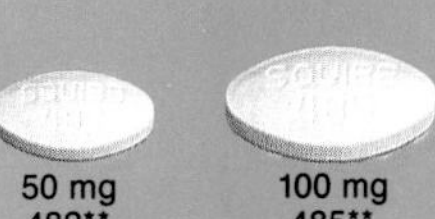

50 mg
482**

100 mg
485**

CAPOTEN®
(Captopril Tablets)

E. R. Squibb & Sons

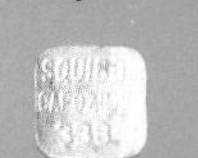

25 mg/15 mg
338**

25 mg/25 mg
349**

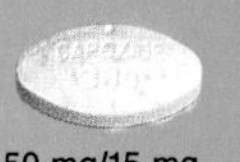

50 mg/15 mg
384**

50 mg/25 mg
390**

CAPOZIDE®
(Captopril-Hydrochlorothiazide Tablets)

E. R. Squibb & Sons

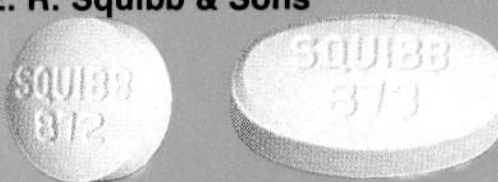

400 mg/80 mg
872**

800 mg/160 mg
873**

COMOXOL™
(Sulfamethoxazole-Trimethoprim Tablets USP)

E. R. Squibb & Sons

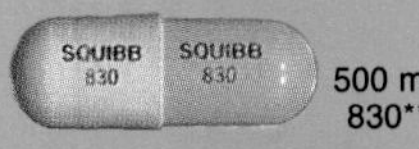

500 mg
830**

HYDREA®
(Hydroxyurea Capsules USP)

E. R. Squibb & Sons

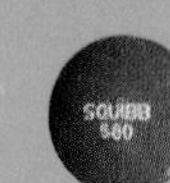

500,000 u
580**

†MYCOSTATIN®
(Nystatin Tablets USP)

E. R. Squibb & Sons

100,000 u
457**

MYCOSTATIN® Vaginal Tablets
(Nystatin Vaginal Tablets USP)

E. R. Squibb & Sons

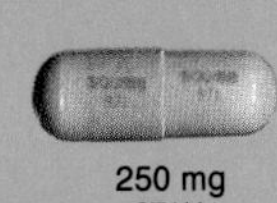

250 mg
971**

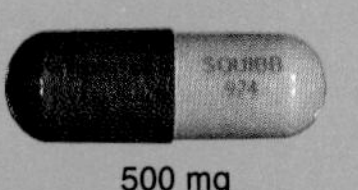

500 mg
974**

†PRINCIPEN®
(Ampicillin Capsules USP)

E. R. Squibb & Sons

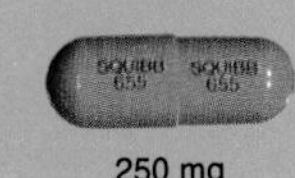

250 mg
655**

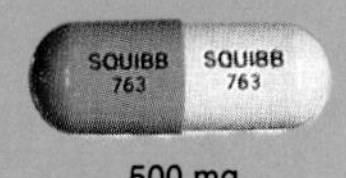

500 mg
763**

†SUMYCIN®
(Tetracycline Hydrochloride Capsules USP)

E. R. Squibb & Sons

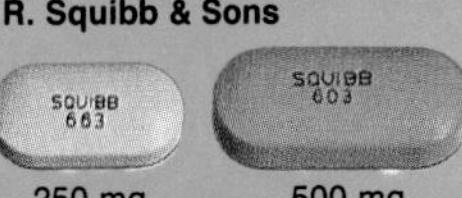

250 mg
663**

500 mg
603**

†SUMYCIN®
(Tetracycline Hydrochloride Tablets USP)

E. R. Squibb & Sons

535**

THERAGRAN HEMATINIC®
(Therapeutic Formula Vitamin Tablets with Hematinics)

E. R. Squibb & Sons

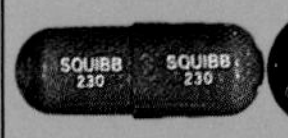

250 mg
230**

500 mg
231**

†TRIMOX®
(Amoxicillin Capsules USP)

E. R. Squibb & Sons

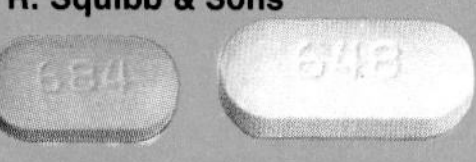

250 mg
684**

500 mg
648**

†VEETIDS®
(Penicillin V Potassium Tablets USP)

E. R. Squibb & Sons

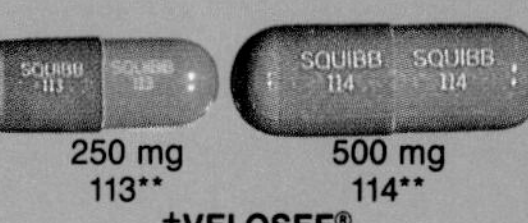

250 mg
113**

500 mg
114**

†VELOSEF®
(Cephradine Capsules USP)

E. R. Squibb & Sons

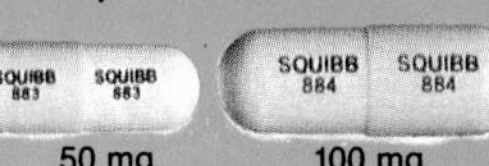

50 mg
883**

100 mg
884**

†VIVOX™
(Doxycycline Hyclate Capsules USP)

E. R. Squibb & Sons

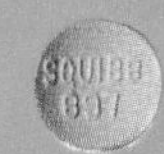

100 mg
897**

†VIVOX™
(Doxycycline Hyclate Tablets USP)

SQUIBB-NOVO

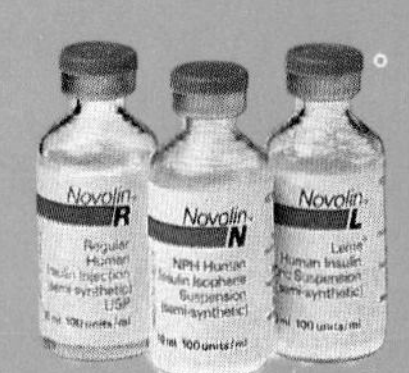

NOVOLIN®
10 ml/100 units/ml
Human insulin (semi-synthetic)
Also available: NOVOLIN® 70/30

STAR

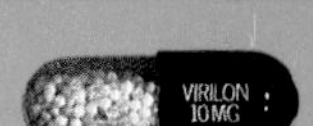

10 mg.

Virilon® Capsules
(macro bead methyltestosterone USP)

STUART

12 oz.

NDC 38-860

5 oz.

30 ml.
unit dose

ALternaGEL® Liquid
(Each 5 ml. contains aluminum hydroxide, 600 mg.)

Stuart

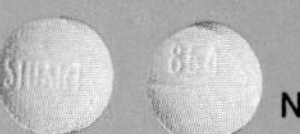

NDC 38-864

(Both sides of tablet shown)
BUCLADIN®-S Softab®
(buclizine hydrochloride, 50 mg.)

**Squibb product identification number.

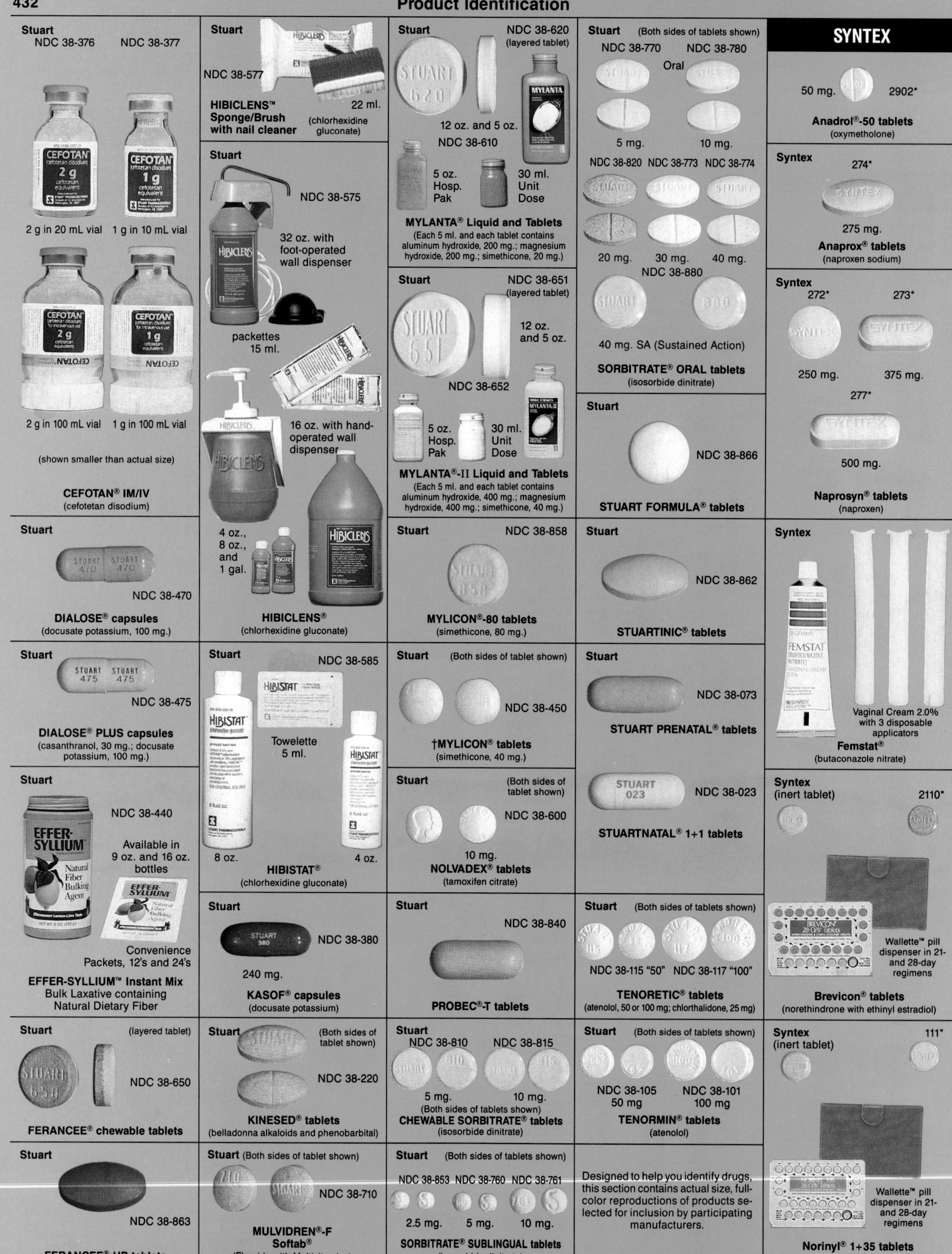
Stuart
NDC 38-376 NDC 38-377
2 g in 20 mL vial 1 g in 10 mL vial
2 g in 100 mL vial 1 g in 100 mL vial
(shown smaller than actual size)
CEFOTAN® IM/IV
(cefotetan disodium)
Stuart
NDC 38-577
22 ml.
HIBICLENS™ Sponge/Brush with nail cleaner
(chlorhexidine gluconate)
Stuart
NDC 38-575
32 oz. with foot-operated wall dispenser
packettes 15 ml.
16 oz. with hand-operated wall dispenser
4 oz., 8 oz., and 1 gal.
HIBICLENS®
(chlorhexidine gluconate)
Stuart
NDC 38-620
(layered tablet)
12 oz. and 5 oz.
NDC 38-610
5 oz. Hosp. Pak
30 ml. Unit Dose
MYLANTA® Liquid and Tablets
(Each 5 ml. and each tablet contains aluminum hydroxide, 200 mg.; magnesium hydroxide, 200 mg.; simethicone, 20 mg.)
Stuart
NDC 38-651
(layered tablet)
12 oz. and 5 oz.
NDC 38-652
5 oz. Hosp. Pak
30 ml. Unit Dose
MYLANTA®-II Liquid and Tablets
(Each 5 ml. and each tablet contains aluminum hydroxide, 400 mg.; magnesium hydroxide, 400 mg.; simethicone, 40 mg.)
Stuart (Both sides of tablets shown)
NDC 38-770 NDC 38-780
Oral
5 mg. 10 mg.
NDC 38-820 NDC 38-773 NDC 38-774
20 mg. 30 mg. 40 mg.
NDC 38-880
40 mg. SA (Sustained Action)
SORBITRATE® ORAL tablets
(isosorbide dinitrate)
Stuart
NDC 38-866
STUART FORMULA® tablets
SYNTEX
50 mg. 2902*
Anadrol®-50 tablets
(oxymetholone)
Syntex
274*
275 mg.
Anaprox® tablets
(naproxen sodium)
Syntex
272* 273*
250 mg. 375 mg.
277*
500 mg.
Naprosyn® tablets
(naproxen)
Stuart
NDC 38-470
DIALOSE® capsules
(docusate potassium, 100 mg.)
Stuart
NDC 38-858
MYLICON®-80 tablets
(simethicone, 80 mg.)
Stuart
NDC 38-862
STUARTINIC® tablets
Syntex
Vaginal Cream 2.0% with 3 disposable applicators
Femstat®
(butaconazole nitrate)
Stuart
NDC 38-475
DIALOSE® PLUS capsules
(casanthranol, 30 mg.; docusate potassium, 100 mg.)
Stuart
NDC 38-585
Towelette 5 ml.
8 oz. 4 oz.
HIBISTAT®
(chlorhexidine gluconate)
Stuart (Both sides of tablet shown)
NDC 38-450
†MYLICON® tablets
(simethicone, 40 mg.)
Stuart
NDC 38-073
STUART PRENATAL® tablets
Stuart
NDC 38-440
Available in 9 oz. and 16 oz. bottles
Convenience Packets, 12's and 24's
EFFER-SYLLIUM™ Instant Mix
Bulk Laxative containing Natural Dietary Fiber
Stuart
(Both sides of tablet shown)
NDC 38-600
10 mg.
NOLVADEX® tablets
(tamoxifen citrate)
Stuart
NDC 38-023
STUARTNATAL® 1+1 tablets
Syntex
(inert tablet) 2110*
Stuart
NDC 38-380
240 mg.
KASOF® capsules
(docusate potassium)
Stuart
NDC 38-840
PROBEC®-T tablets
Stuart (Both sides of tablets shown)
NDC 38-115 "50" NDC 38-117 "100"
TENORETIC® tablets
(atenolol, 50 or 100 mg; chlorthalidone, 25 mg)
Wallette™ pill dispenser in 21- and 28-day regimens
Brevicon® tablets
(norethindrone with ethinyl estradiol)
Stuart (layered tablet)
NDC 38-650
FERANCEE® chewable tablets
Stuart (Both sides of tablet shown)
NDC 38-220
KINESED® tablets
(belladonna alkaloids and phenobarbital)
Stuart
NDC 38-810 NDC 38-815
5 mg. 10 mg.
(Both sides of tablets shown)
CHEWABLE SORBITRATE® tablets
(isosorbide dinitrate)
Stuart (Both sides of tablets shown)
NDC 38-105 50 mg
NDC 38-101 100 mg
TENORMIN® tablets
(atenolol)
Syntex
(inert tablet) 111*
Stuart
NDC 38-863
FERANCEE®-HP tablets
Stuart (Both sides of tablet shown)
NDC 38-710
MULVIDREN®-F Softab®
(Fluoride with Multivitamins)
Stuart (Both sides of tablets shown)
NDC 38-853 NDC 38-760 NDC 38-761
2.5 mg. 5 mg. 10 mg.
SORBITRATE® SUBLINGUAL tablets
(isosorbide dinitrate)
Designed to help you identify drugs, this section contains actual size, full-color reproductions of products selected for inclusion by participating manufacturers.
Wallette™ pill dispenser in 21- and 28-day regimens
Norinyl® 1+35 tablets
(norethindrone with ethinyl estradiol)

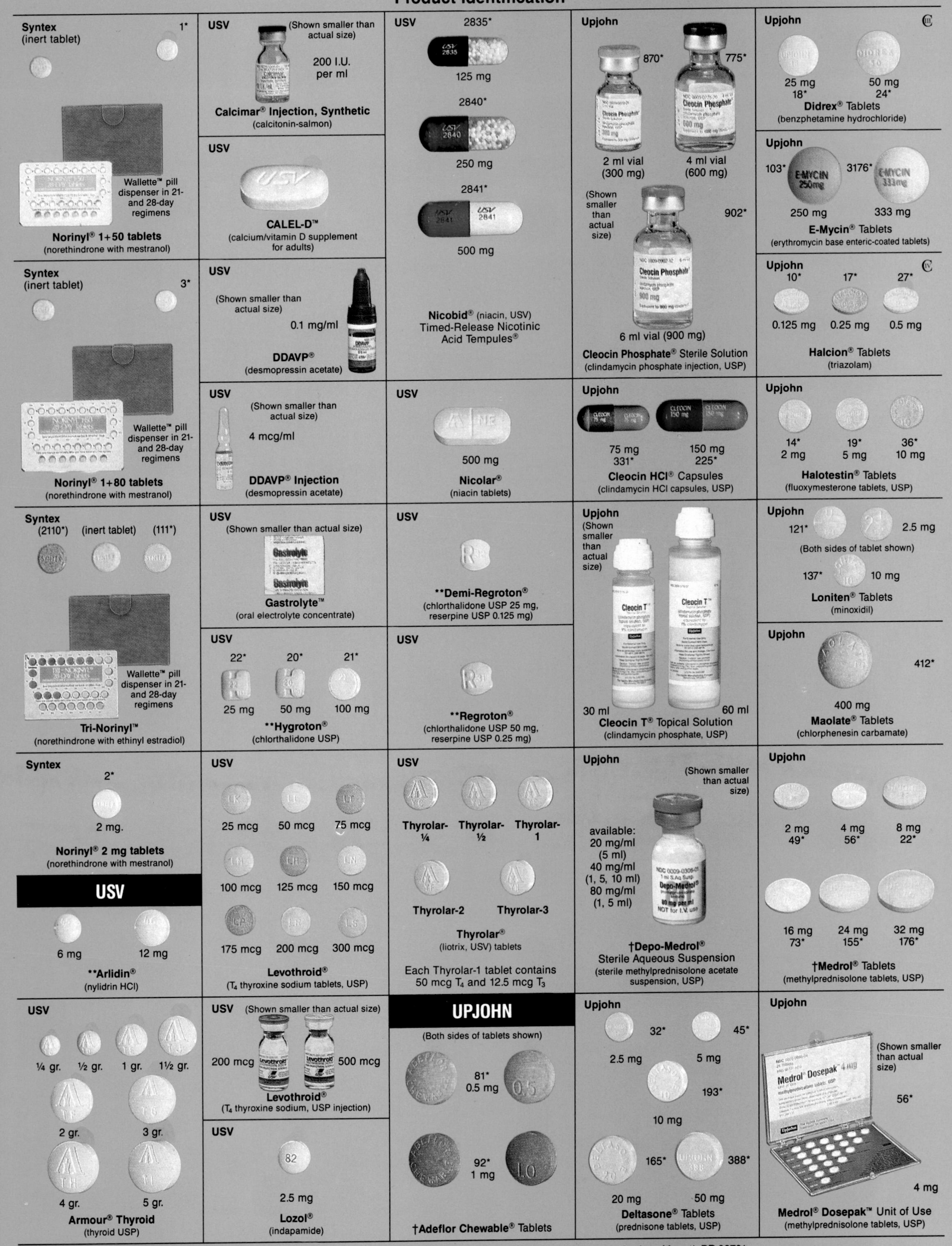

**Arlidin®, Hygroton®, Demi-Regroton® and Regroton® are products of USV Laboratories Inc., Manati, PR 00701.

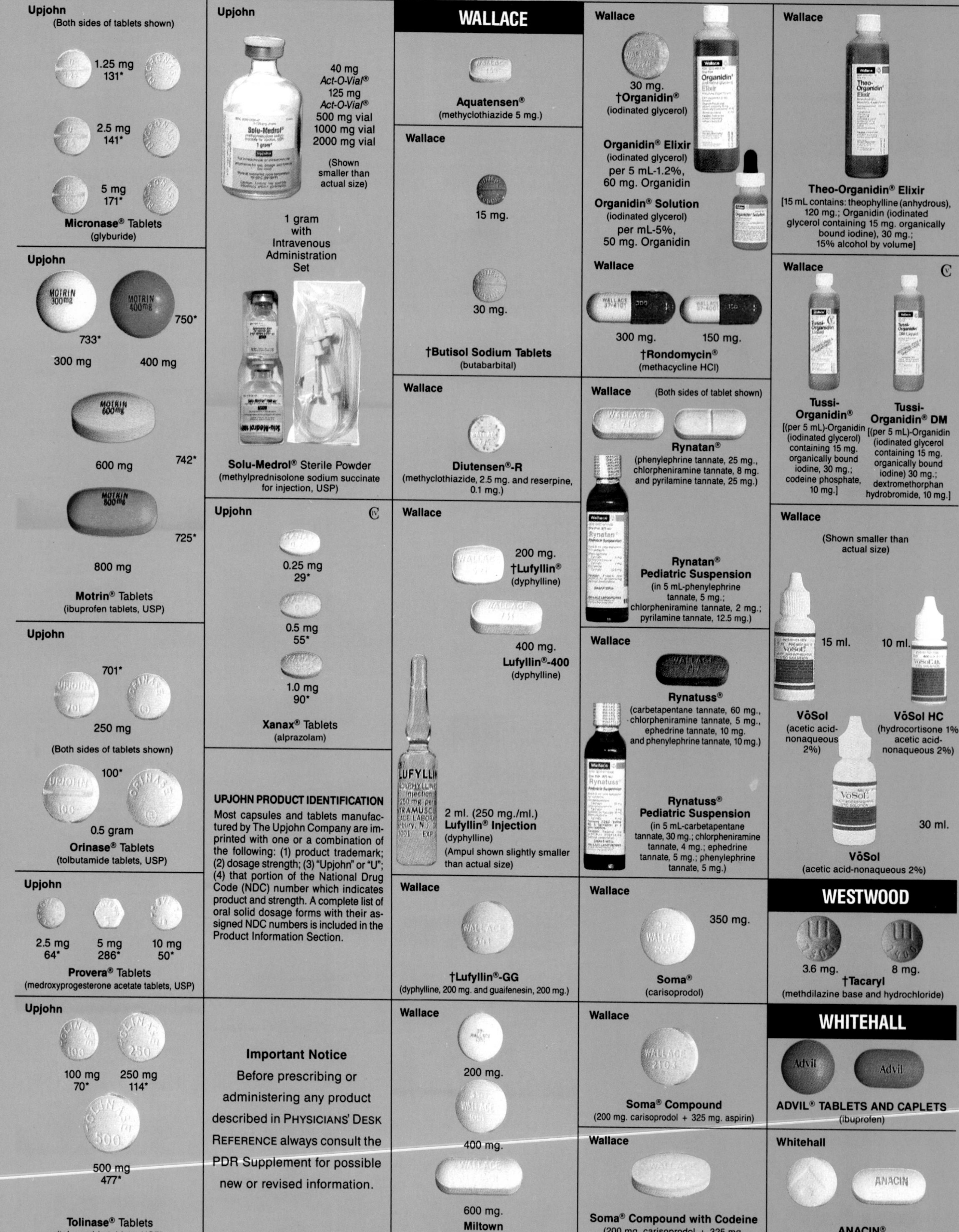

Upjohn
(Both sides of tablets shown)

1.25 mg 131*
2.5 mg 141*
5 mg 171*

Micronase® Tablets
(glyburide)

Upjohn

733* 300 mg
750* 400 mg
600 mg 742*
800 mg 725*

Motrin® Tablets
(ibuprofen tablets, USP)

Upjohn

701*
250 mg
(Both sides of tablets shown)
100*
0.5 gram

Orinase® Tablets
(tolbutamide tablets, USP)

Upjohn

2.5 mg 64*
5 mg 286*
10 mg 50*

Provera® Tablets
(medroxyprogesterone acetate tablets, USP)

Upjohn

100 mg 70*
250 mg 114*
500 mg 477*

Tolinase® Tablets
(tolazamide tablets, USP)

Upjohn

40 mg *Act-O-Vial®*
125 mg *Act-O-Vial®*
500 mg vial
1000 mg vial
2000 mg vial
(Shown smaller than actual size)

1 gram with Intravenous Administration Set

Solu-Medrol® Sterile Powder
(methylprednisolone sodium succinate for injection, USP)

Upjohn ©IV

0.25 mg 29*
0.5 mg 55*
1.0 mg 90*

Xanax® Tablets
(alprazolam)

UPJOHN PRODUCT IDENTIFICATION
Most capsules and tablets manufactured by The Upjohn Company are imprinted with one or a combination of the following: (1) product trademark; (2) dosage strength; (3) "Upjohn" or "U"; (4) that portion of the National Drug Code (NDC) number which indicates product and strength. A complete list of oral solid dosage forms with their assigned NDC numbers is included in the Product Information Section.

Important Notice
Before prescribing or administering any product described in PHYSICIANS' DESK REFERENCE always consult the PDR Supplement for possible new or revised information.

WALLACE

Aquatensen®
(methyclothiazide 5 mg.)

Wallace

15 mg.
30 mg.

†Butisol Sodium Tablets
(butabarbital)

Wallace

Diutensen®-R
(methyclothiazide, 2.5 mg. and reserpine, 0.1 mg.)

Wallace

200 mg.
†Lufyllin®
(dyphylline)

400 mg.
Lufyllin®-400
(dyphylline)

2 ml. (250 mg./ml.)
Lufyllin® Injection
(dyphylline)
(Ampul shown slightly smaller than actual size)

Wallace

†Lufyllin®-GG
(dyphylline, 200 mg. and guaifenesin, 200 mg.)

Wallace

200 mg.
400 mg.
600 mg.
Miltown
(meprobamate)

Wallace

30 mg.
†Organidin®
(iodinated glycerol)

Organidin® Elixir
(iodinated glycerol)
per 5 mL-1.2%,
60 mg. Organidin

Organidin® Solution
(iodinated glycerol)
per mL-5%,
50 mg. Organidin

Wallace

300 mg.
150 mg.
†Rondomycin®
(methacycline HCl)

Wallace (Both sides of tablet shown)

Rynatan®
(phenylephrine tannate, 25 mg., chlorpheniramine tannate, 8 mg. and pyrilamine tannate, 25 mg.)

Rynatan® Pediatric Suspension
(in 5 mL-phenylephrine tannate, 5 mg.; chlorpheniramine tannate, 2 mg.; pyrilamine tannate, 12.5 mg.)

Wallace

Rynatuss®
(carbetapentane tannate, 60 mg., chlorpheniramine tannate, 5 mg., ephedrine tannate, 10 mg. and phenylephrine tannate, 10 mg.)

Rynatuss® Pediatric Suspension
(in 5 mL-carbetapentane tannate, 30 mg.; chlorpheniramine tannate, 4 mg.; ephedrine tannate, 5 mg.; phenylephrine tannate, 5 mg.)

Wallace

350 mg.
Soma®
(carisoprodol)

Wallace

Soma® Compound
(200 mg. carisoprodol + 325 mg. aspirin)

Wallace

Soma® Compound with Codeine
(200 mg. carisoprodol + 325 mg. aspirin + 16 mg. codeine phosphate)

Wallace

Theo-Organidin® Elixir
[15 mL contains: theophylline (anhydrous), 120 mg.; Organidin (iodinated glycerol containing 15 mg. organically bound iodine), 30 mg.; 15% alcohol by volume]

Wallace ©

Tussi-Organidin®
[(per 5 mL)-Organidin (iodinated glycerol) containing 15 mg. organically bound iodine, 30 mg.; codeine phosphate, 10 mg.]

Tussi-Organidin® DM
[(per 5 mL)-Organidin (iodinated glycerol containing 15 mg. organically bound iodine) 30 mg.; dextromethorphan hydrobromide, 10 mg.]

Wallace

(Shown smaller than actual size)

15 ml.
VōSol
(acetic acid-nonaqueous 2%)

10 ml.
VōSol HC
(hydrocortisone 1% acetic acid-nonaqueous 2%)

30 ml.
VōSol
(acetic acid-nonaqueous 2%)

WESTWOOD

3.6 mg.
8 mg.
†Tacaryl
(methdilazine base and hydrochloride)

WHITEHALL

ADVIL® TABLETS AND CAPLETS
(ibuprofen)

Whitehall

ANACIN®
Coated Tablets and Caplets

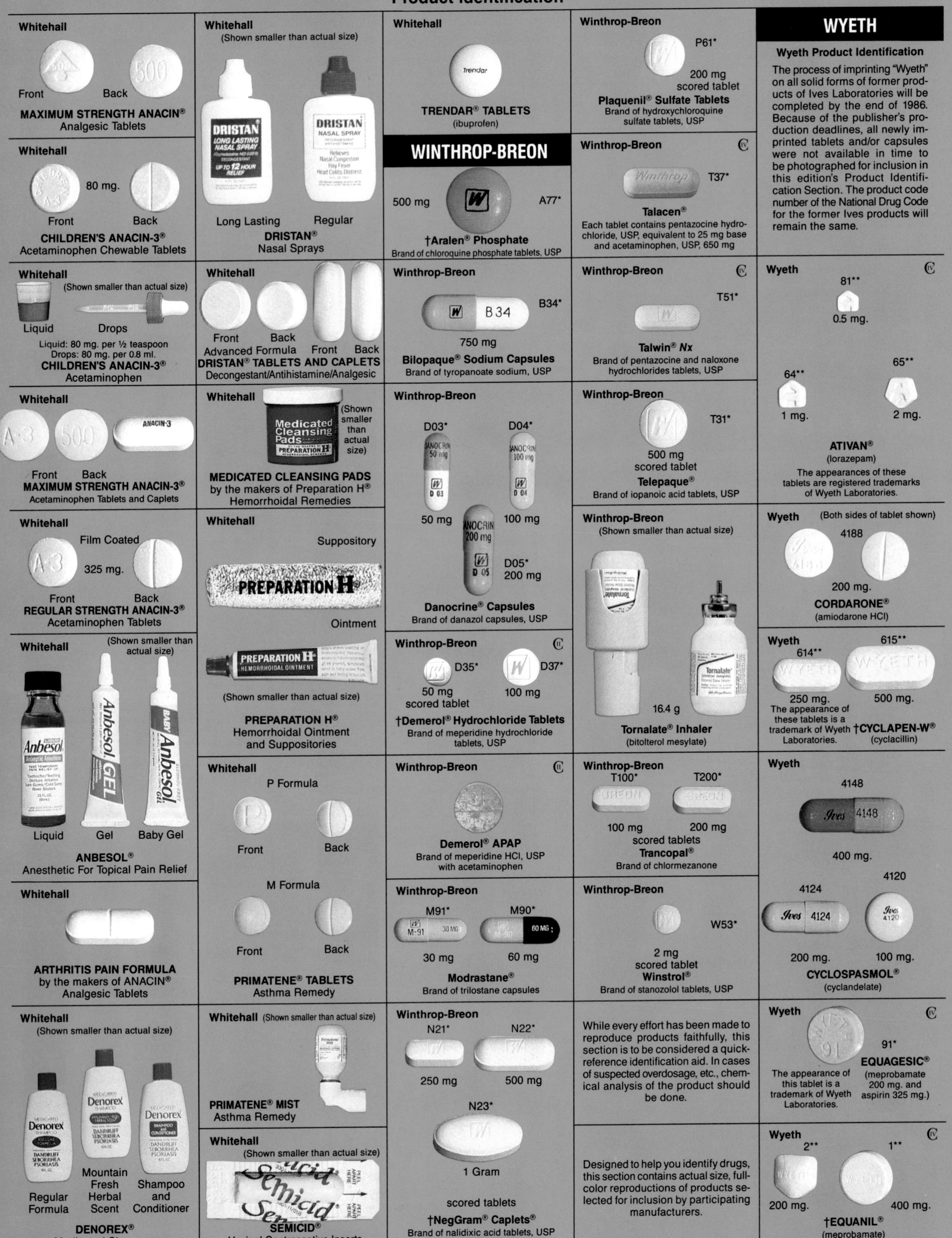

**Product identification number on reverse side of tablet.

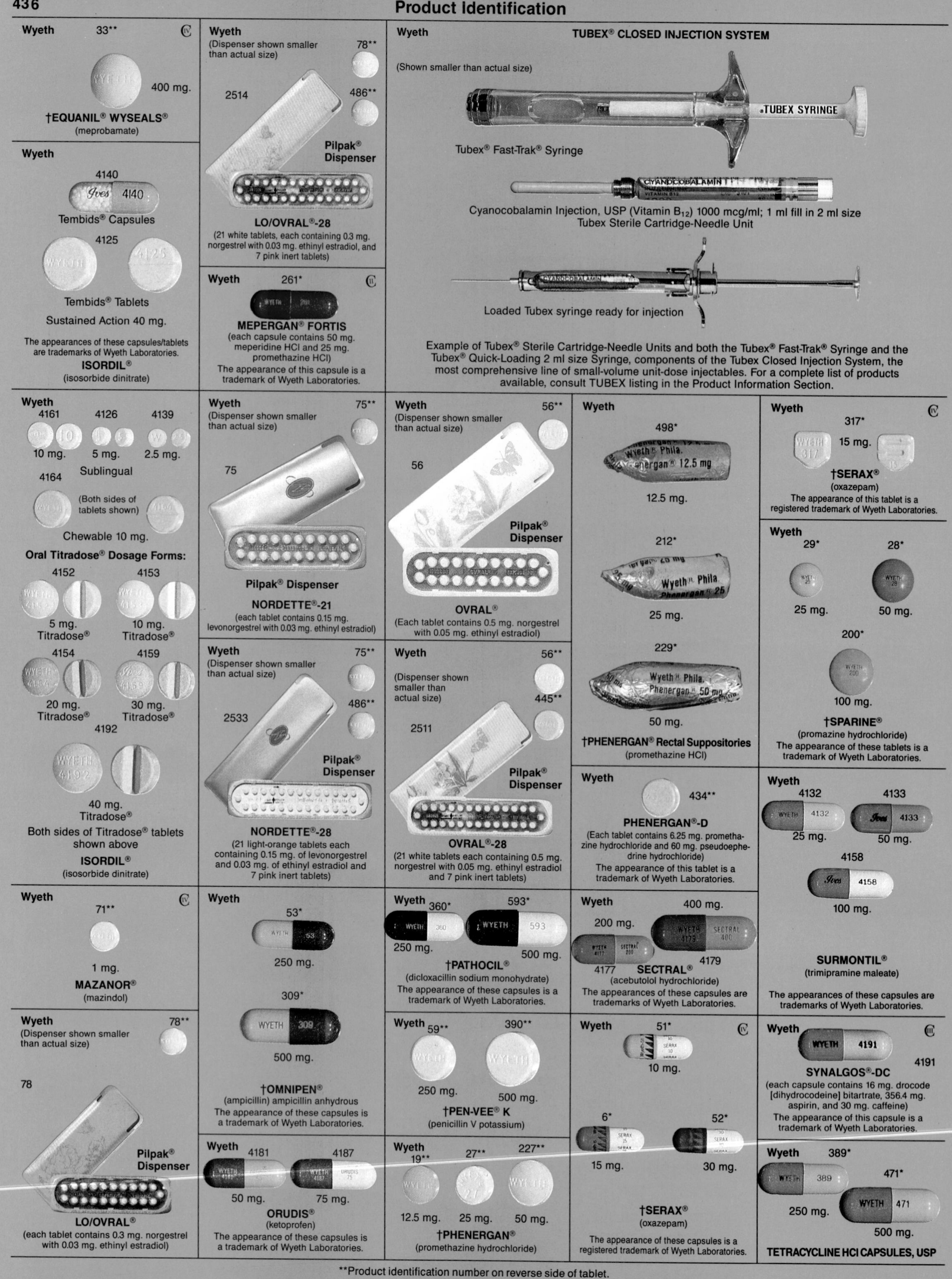

**Product identification number on reverse side of tablet.

Wyeth

** ** **

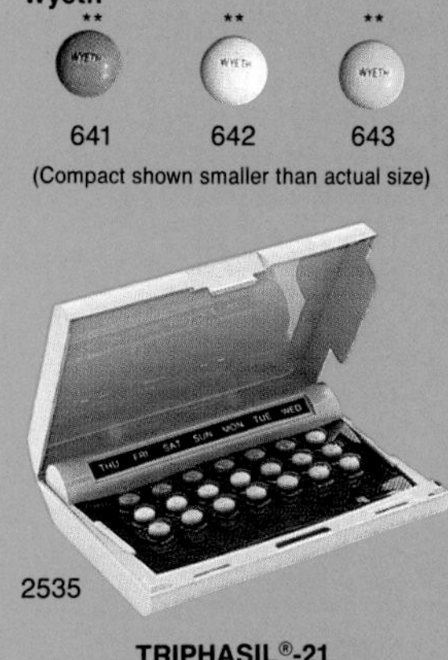

641 642 643

(Compact shown smaller than actual size)

2535

TRIPHASIL®-21

(21 tablets containing the following: 6 brown tablets—0.050 mg. levonorgestrel + 0.030 mg. ethinyl estradiol; 5 white tablets—0.075 mg. levonorgestrel + 0.040 mg. ethinyl estradiol; 10 light-yellow tablets—0.125 mg. levonorgestrel + 0.030 mg. ethinyl estradiol)

Wyeth

** ** ** **

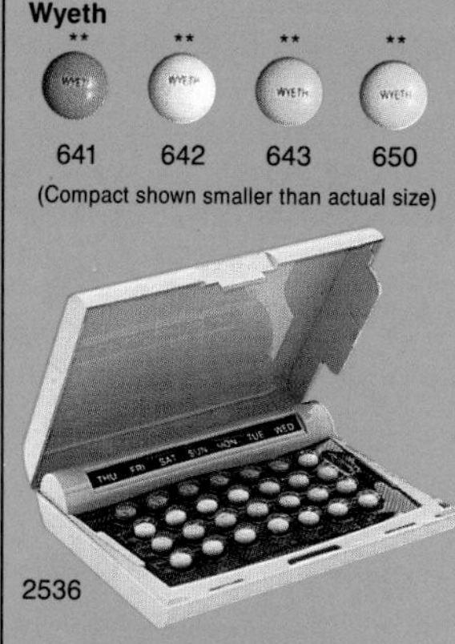

641 642 643 650

(Compact shown smaller than actual size)

2536

TRIPHASIL®-28

(28 tablets containing the following: 6 brown tablets—0.050 mg. levonorgestrel + 0.030 mg. ethinyl estradiol; 5 white tablets—0.075 mg. levonorgestrel + 0.040 mg. ethinyl estradiol; 10 light-yellow tablets—0.125 mg. levonorgestrel + 0.030 mg. ethinyl estradiol; 7 light-green tablets—inert)

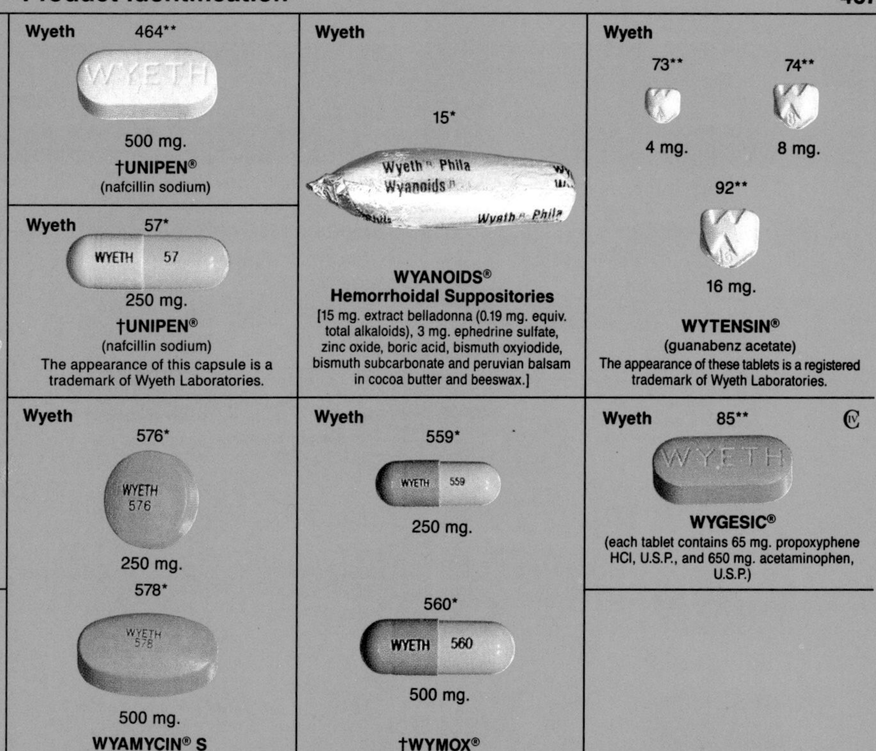

Wyeth 464**

500 mg.

†UNIPEN®

(nafcillin sodium)

Wyeth 57*

250 mg.

†UNIPEN®

(nafcillin sodium)

The appearance of this capsule is a trademark of Wyeth Laboratories.

Wyeth

15*

WYANOIDS®
Hemorrhoidal Suppositories

[15 mg. extract belladonna (0.19 mg. equiv. total alkaloids), 3 mg. ephedrine sulfate, zinc oxide, boric acid, bismuth oxyiodide, bismuth subcarbonate and peruvian balsam in cocoa butter and beeswax.]

Wyeth

73** 74**

4 mg. 8 mg.

92**

16 mg.

WYTENSIN®

(guanabenz acetate)

The appearance of these tablets is a registered trademark of Wyeth Laboratories.

Wyeth

576*

250 mg.

578*

500 mg.

WYAMYCIN® S

(erythromycin stearate)

Wyeth

559*

250 mg.

560*

500 mg.

†WYMOX®

(amoxicillin)

Wyeth 85** C-IV

WYGESIC®

(each tablet contains 65 mg. propoxyphene HCl, U.S.P., and 650 mg. acetaminophen, U.S.P.)

**Product identification number on reverse side of tablet.

Directory of Regional Poison Control Centers

The following list of Regional Poison Control Centers has been compiled from information furnished by the American Association of Poison Control Centers, 20 N. Pine, Baltimore, MD 21202. Telephone number: (301) 528-7604.

It includes those facilities which provide for the medical profession, on a 24-hour basis, information concerning the prevention and treatment of accidents involving ingestion of poisonous and potentially poisonous substances. Unless otherwise noted, inquiries should be addressed to:

Poison Control Center

Alabama Poison Center
809 University Blvd., East
Tuscaloosa, AL 35401
(205) 345-0600
(800) 462-0800

Arizona Poison & Drug Information Center
AZ Health Sciences Center, Room 3204K
University of Arizona
Tucson, AZ 85724
(602) 626-6016
(800) 362-0101

Blodgett Regional Poison Center
1840 Wealthy Street, SE
Grand Rapids, MI 49506
(616) 774-7854
(800) 632-2727

Cardinal Glennon Children's Hospital
Regional Poison Center
1465 S. Grand Avenue
St. Louis, MO 63104
(314) 772-5200
(800) 392-9111

Central & Southern Illinois Poison Resource Center
800 E. Carpenter St.
Springfield, IL 62769
(217) 753-3330
(800) 252-2022

Central Ohio Poison Control Center
700 Children's Drive
Columbus, OH 43205
(614) 228-1323
(800) 682-7625

Duke Poison Control Center
Box 3007
Duke University Medical Center
Durham, NC 27710
(919) 684-8111
(800) 672-1697

Georgia Poison Control Center
Grady Memorial Hospital
Box 26066
80 Butler Street, SE
Atlanta, GA 30335
(404) 589-4400
(800) 282-5846

Hennepin Poison Center
701 Park
Minneapolis, MN 55415
(612) 347-3141

Indiana Poison Center
1001 W. Tenth Street
Indianapolis, IN 46202
(317) 630-7351
(800) 382-9097

Intermountain Regional Poison Control Center
50 N. Medical Drive, Bldg. 428
Salt Lake City, UT 84132
(801) 581-2151
(800) 662-0062

Kentucky Regional Poison Center of Kosair Children's Hospital
P.O. Box 35070
Louisville, KY 40232
(502) 589-8222
(800) 722-5725

Los Angeles County Medical Association Regional Poison Information Center
1925 Wilshire Blvd.
Los Angeles, CA 90057
(213) 484-5151

Louisiana Regional Poison Control Center
1501 Kings Highway
P.O. Box 33932
Shreveport, LA 71130
(318) 425-1524
(800) 535-0525

Maryland Poison Center
120 N. Pine Street Center
Baltimore, MD 21201
(301) 528-7701
(800) 492-2414

Mid Plains Poison Control Center
Children's Memorial Hospital
8301 Dodge Street
Omaha, NE 68114
(402) 390-5400
(800) 642-9999

Minnesota Poison Control System
640 Jackson St.
St. Paul, MN 55101
(612) 221-2113
(800) 222-1222

Nassau County Medical Center Long Island Regional Poison Control Center
2201 Hempstead Turnpike
East Meadow, NY 11554
(516) 542-2323

National Capital Poison Center
3800 Reservoir Road, NW
Washington, DC 20007
(202) 625-3333

New Jersey Poison Information and Education System
201 Lyons Avenue
Newark, NJ 07112
(201) 926-8005
(800) 962-1253

New Mexico Poison and Drug Information Center
University of New Mexico
Albuquerque, NM 87131
(505) 843-2551
(800) 432-6866

New York City Poison Center
455 First Avenue, Room 123
New York, NY 10016
(212) 340-4494
(212) 764-7667

Pittsburgh Poison Center
125 DeSoto Street
Pittsburgh, PA 15213
(412) 647-5600

Poison Control Center Children's Hospital of Michigan
3901 Beaubien Blvd.
Detroit, MI 48201
(313) 494-5711
(800) 572-1655

Rocky Mountain Poison Center
645 Bannock St.
Denver, CO 80204
(303) 893-7774
(800) 332-3073
In Wyoming (800) 442-2701
In Montana (800) 525-5042

San Diego Regional Poison Center
University of California Medical Center
225 Dickinson St., H925
San Diego, CA 92103
(619) 294-6000

San Francisco Bay Area Regional Poison Center
1E86, San Francisco General Hospital
1001 Potrero Avenue
San Francisco, CA 94110
(415) 476-6600
(800) 233-3360

Seattle Poison Center
Children's Orthopedic Hospital and Medical Center, Box 5371
4800 Sand Point Way, NE
Seattle, WA 98105
(206) 526-2121
(800) 732-6985

Southwest Ohio Regional Poison Control System, Drug & Poison Information Center
University of Cincinnati, College of Medicine
231 Bethesda Avenue ML 144
Cincinnati, OH 45267
(513) 872-5111
(800) 872-5111

Tampa Bay Regional Poison Control Center
P.O. Box 18582
Tampa, FL 33679
(813) 253-4444
(800) 282-3171

University of California Davis Medical Center
Regional Poison Control Center
2315 Stockton Blvd.
Sacramento, CA 95817
(916) 453-3692

University of Iowa Hospitals and Clinics Poison Control Center
Pharmacy Department
Iowa City, IA 52242
(319) 356-2922
(800) 272-6477

SECTION 6

Product Information Section

This section is made possible through the courtesy of the manufacturers whose products appear on the following pages. The information concerning each product has been prepared, edited and approved by the medical department, medical director, and/or medical counsel of each manufacturer.

Products described in PHYSICIANS' DESK REFERENCE® which have official package circulars must be in full compliance with Food & Drug Administration regulations pertaining to labeling for prescription drugs. These regulations require that for PDR copy, "indications, effects, dosages, routes, methods, and frequency and duration of administration, and any relevant warnings, hazards, contraindications, side effects, and precautions" must be the *"same in language and emphasis"* as the approved labeling for the product. FDA regards the words *"same language and emphasis"* as requiring VERBATIM use of the approved labeling providing such information. Furthermore, information in the approved labeling that is emphasized by the use of type set in a box or in capitals, bold face, or italics must also be given the same emphasis in PDR. For products which do not have official package circulars, the Publisher has emphasized to manufacturers the necessity of describing such products comprehensively so that physicians would have access to all information essential for intelligent and informed prescribing. In organizing and presenting the material in PHYSICIANS' DESK REFERENCE, the Publisher is providing all the information made available to PDR by manufacturers.

This edition of PHYSICIANS' DESK REFERENCE contains the latest product information available at press-time. During the year, however, new and revised information about the products described herein may be furnished us. This information will be published in the PDR Supplement. Therefore, before prescribing or administering any product described in the following pages, you should first consult the PDR Supplement.

In presenting the following material to the medical profession, the Publisher is not necessarily advocating the use of any product listed.

Abbott Laboratories
Pharmaceutical Products Division
NORTH CHICAGO, IL 60064

ABBO-CODE™ INDEX

The Abbo-Code identification system provides positive identification of a drug and dosage strength. The following Abbott products are imprinted or debossed with an Abbo-Code designation:

PRODUCT	*ABBO-CODE*
Cefol® Filmtab® Tablets	
B-complex vitamins with folic acid, vitamin E, and vitamin C	NJ
Chlorthalidone Tablets, USP	
25 mg	AA
50 mg	AB
Colchicine Tablets, USP	
0.6 mg	AF
Cylert® Tablets Ⓒ **(pemoline)**	
18.75 mg	TH
37.5 mg	TI
75 mg	TJ
37.5 mg Chewable	TK
Depakene® Capsules (valproic acid capsules, USP)	
250 mg	HH
Depakote® Tablets (divalproex sodium enteric-coated tablets)	
125 mg	NT
250 mg	NR
500 mg	NS
Desoxyn® Ⓒ **(methamphetamine hydrochloride)**	
5 mg Tablet	TE
5 mg Gradumet®	MC
10 mg Gradumet	ME
15 mg Gradumet	MF
Dicumarol Tablets, USP	
25 mg	AN
50 mg	AO
E.E.S.® Chewable Tablets (erythromycin ethylsuccinate tablets, USP)	
200 mg erythromycin activity	EF
E.E.S. 400® Filmtab® Tablets (erythromycin ethylsuccinate tablets, USP)	
400 mg erythromycin activity	EE
Enduron® Tablets (methyclothiazide tablets, USP)	
2.5 mg	ENDURON
5 mg	ENDURON
Enduronyl® Tablets	
5 mg methyclothiazide and 0.25 mg deserpidine	LS
Enduronyl® Forte Tablets	
5 mg methyclothiazide and 0.5 mg deserpidine	LT
Ery-Tab® Tablets (erythromycin enteric-coated tablets)	
250 mg	EC
333 mg	EH
500 mg	ED
Erythrocin® Stearate Filmtab® Tablets (erythromycin stearate tablets, USP)	
250 mg erythromycin activity	ES
500 mg erythromycin activity	ET
Erythromycin Base Filmtab® Tablets (erythromycin tablets, USP)	
250 mg	EB
500 mg	EA
Eutonyl® Filmtab® Tablets (pargyline hydrochloride tablets, USP)	
10 mg	NA
25 mg	NB
Eutron® Filmtab® Tablets	
25 mg pargyline hydrochloride and 5 mg methyclothiazide	NK
Fero-Folic-500® Filmtab® Tablets controlled-release iron, folic acid, and vitamin C	AJ
Gemonil® Tablets Ⓒ **(metharbital tablets, USP)**	
100 mg	TF
Harmonyl® Tablets (deserpidine tablets)	
0.25 mg	LK
Iberet-Folic-500® Filmtab® Tablets controlled-release iron, B-complex vitamins with folic acid, and vitamin C	AK
Janimine® Filmtab® Tablets (imipramine hydrochloride tablets, USP)	
10 mg	ND
25 mg	NE
50 mg	NL
K·Tab® Filmtab® Tablets (potassium chloride extended-release tablets, USP)	
10 mEq (750 mg)	NM
Nembutal® Sodium Capsules Ⓒ **(pentobarbital sodium capsules, USP)**	
50 mg	CF
100 mg	CH
Ogen® Tablets (estropipate tablets, USP)	
0.625 tablet (0.75 mg estropipate)	LU
1.25 tablet (1.5 mg estropipate)	LV
2.5 tablet (3 mg estropipate)	LX
5 tablet (6 mg estropipate)	LY
Oretic® Tablets (hydrochlorothiazide tablets, USP)	
25 mg	ORETIC
50 mg	ORETIC
Oreticyl® 25 Tablets	
25 mg hydrochlorothiazide and 0.125 mg deserpidine	AH
Oreticyl® 50 Tablets	
50 mg hydrochlorothiazide and 0.125 mg deserpidine	AI
Oreticyl® Forte Tablets	
25 mg hydrochlorothiazide and 0.25 mg deserpidine	LL
Panwarfin® Tablets (warfarin sodium tablets, USP)	
2 mg	LM
2.5 mg	LN
5 mg	LO
7.5 mg	LR
10 mg	LF
Peganone® Tablets (ethotoin tablets)	
250 mg	AD
500 mg	AE
Phenurone® Tablets (phenacemide tablets, USP)	
500 mg	II
Placidyl® Capsules Ⓒ **(ethchlorvynol capsules, USP)**	
500 mg	KH
750 mg	KN
Tral® Filmtab® Tablets (hexocyclium methylsulfate tablets)	
25 mg	NF
Tranxene® Ⓒ **(clorazepate dipotassium)**	
3.75 mg Capsule	CI
7.5 mg Capsule	CN
15 mg Capsule	CK
3.75 mg Tablet	TL
7.5 mg Tablet	TM
15 mg Tablet	TN
Tranxene®-SD Ⓒ **Single Dose Tablets (clorazepate dipotassium)**	
22.5 mg	TY
11.25 mg Half Strength	TX
Tridione® Dulcet® Tablets (trimethadione tablets, USP)	
150 mg	LE
Tridione® Capsules (trimethadione capsules, USP)	
300 mg	AM
Vercyte® Tablets (pipobroman tablets, USP)	
25 mg	AT

ABBO-PAC®
Unit Dose Packages

The Abbo-Pac unit dose system from Abbott Laboratories offers a wide range of drugs.
Each individual dose is clearly identified by generic name, Abbott name, strength, NDC identification number, expiration date and lot number. Abbo-Pac unit dose containers are designed to accommodate virtually all hospital pharmacy storage racks and to provide maximum accessibility and ease of handling.
The following is a list of products which are now available:

PRODUCT	*DOSAGE STRENGTH*
Depakene® Capsules (valproic acid capsules, USP)	250 mg
Depakote® Tablets (divalproex sodium enteric-coated tablets)	250 mg
Depakote Tablets	500 mg
Enduron® Tablets (methyclothiazide tablets, USP)	5 mg
Enduronyl® Tablets (methyclothiazide 5 mg and deserpidine 0.25 mg)	
E.E.S.® Chewable Tablets (erythromycin ethylsuccinate tablets, USP)	200 mg
E.E.S. 400® Filmtab (erythromycin ethylsuccinate tablets, USP)	400 mg
E.E.S.® Granules (erythromycin ethylsuccinate for oral suspension, USP)	200 mg/5 ml
EryPed® Granules (erythromycin ethylsuccinate for oral suspension, USP)	400 mg/5 ml
Ery-Tab® (erythromycin enteric-coated tablets)	250 mg
Ery-Tab	333 mg
Ery-Tab	500 mg
Erythrocin® Stearate Filmtab (erythromycin stearate tablets, USP)	250 mg
Erythromycin Base Filmtab® (erythromycin tablets, USP)	250 mg
Fero-Grad-500® Filmtab Controlled-Release Iron plus Vitamin C	
Iberet®-500 Filmtab Controlled-Release Iron plus B-Complex and Vitamin C	
K-Lor™ 20 mEq (potassium chloride for oral solution, USP)	20 mEq Potassium 20 mEq Chloride/Packet
K-Lor™ 15 mEq	15 mEq Potassium 15 mEq Chloride/Packet
K·Tab® Filmtab® (potassium chloride extended-release tablets, USP)	10 mEq (750 mg)
Nembutal® Sodium Capsules Ⓒ (pentobarbital sodium capsules, USP)	100 mg
Oretic® Tablets (hydrochlorothiazide tablets, USP)	25 mg
Oretic® Tablets	50 mg
Panwarfin® Tablets (warfarin sodium tablets, USP)	2 mg
Panwarfin® Tablets	2.5 mg
Panwarfin® Tablets	5 mg
Panwarfin® Tablets	7.5 mg
Panwarfin® Tablets	10 mg
Placidyl® Capsules Ⓒ (ethchlorvynol capsules, USP)	500 mg
Surbex-T® Filmtab High-Potency B-Complex Vitamins with Vitamin C	
Tranxene® Capsules Ⓒ (clorazepate dipotassium)	3.75 mg
Tranxene® Capsules Ⓒ	7.5 mg
Tranxene® Capsules Ⓒ	15 mg

ABBOKINASE® ℞
[ab-bo-kī ′nāze]
Urokinase For Injection

ABBOKINASE (urokinase for injection) should be used in hospitals where the recommended diagnostic and monitoring techniques are available. Thrombolytic therapy should be considered in all situations where the benefits to be achieved outweigh the risk of potentially serious hemorrhage. When internal bleeding does occur, it may be more difficult to manage than that which occurs with conventional anticoagulant therapy.
Urokinase treatment should be instituted as soon as possible after onset of pulmonary embolism, preferably no later than seven days after onset. Any delay in instituting lytic therapy to evaluate the effect of heparin decreases the potential for optimal efficacy.[1]
When urokinase is used for treatment of coronary artery thrombosis associated with evolving transmural myocardial infarction, therapy should be instituted within six hours of symptom onset.

DESCRIPTION
Urokinase is an enzyme (protein) produced by the kidney, and found in the urine. There are two forms of urokinase differing in molecular weight but having similar clinical effects. ABBOKINASE (urokinase for injection) is a thrombolytic agent obtained from human kidney cells by tissue culture techniques and is primarily the low molecular weight form. It is supplied as a sterile lyophilized white powder containing mannitol (25 mg/vial) and sodium chloride (45 mg/vial).
Thin translucent filaments may occasionally occur in reconstituted ABBOKINASE vials, but do not indicate any decrease in potency of this product. No clinical problems have been associated with these filaments. See "Dosage and Administration" section.
Following reconstitution with 5.2 ml of Sterile Water for Injection, USP, it is a clear, practically colorless solution; each ml contains 50,000 IU of urokinase activity, 0.5% mannitol, and 0.9% sodium chloride. The pH is adjusted with

sodium hydroxide and/or hydrochloric acid prior to lyophilization.
ABBOKINASE is for intravenous and intracoronary infusion only.

CLINICAL PHARMACOLOGY

Urokinase acts on the endogenous fibrinolytic system. It converts plasminogen to the enzyme plasmin. Plasmin degrades fibrin clots as well as fibrinogen and other plasma proteins.
Intravenous infusion of urokinase in doses recommended for lysis of pulmonary embolism is followed by increased fibrinolytic activity. This effect disappears within a few hours after discontinuation, but a decrease in plasma levels of fibrinogen and plasminogen and an increase in the amount of circulating fibrin (ogen) degradation products may persist for 12–24 hours.[3,4] There is a lack of correlation between embolus resolution and changes in coagulation and fibrinolytic assay results.
Information is incomplete about the pharmacokinetic properties in man. Urokinase administered by intravenous infusion is cleared rapidly by the liver. The serum half-life in man is 20 minutes or less. Patients with impaired liver function (e.g., cirrhosis) would be expected to show a prolongation in half-life. Small fractions of an administered dose are excreted in bile and urine.

INDICATIONS AND USAGE

Pulmonary Embolism: ABBOKINASE (urokinase for injection) is indicated in adults:
—For the lysis of acute massive pulmonary emboli, defined as obstruction of blood flow to a lobe or multiple segments.
—For the lysis of pulmonary emboli accompanied by unstable hemodynamics, i.e., failure to maintain blood pressure without supportive measures.
The diagnosis should be confirmed by objective means, such as pulmonary angiography via an upper extremity vein, or non-invasive procedures such as lung scanning.
Angiographic and hemodynamic measurements demonstrate a more rapid improvement with lytic therapy than with heparin therapy.[5,6,7,8,9]
Coronary Artery Thrombosis: ABBOKINASE has been reported to lyse acute thrombi obstructing coronary arteries, associated with evolving transmural myocardial infarction.[2] The majority of patients who received ABBOKINASE by intracoronary infusion within six hours following onset of symptoms showed recanalization of the involved vessel.
IT HAS NOT BEEN ESTABLISHED THAT INTRACORONARY ADMINISTRATION OF ABBOKINASE DURING EVOLVING TRANSMURAL MYOCARDIAL INFARCTION RESULTS IN SALVAGE OF MYOCARDIAL TISSUE, NOR THAT IT REDUCES MORTALITY. THE PATIENTS WHO MIGHT BENEFIT FROM THIS THERAPY CANNOT BE DEFINED.
I.V. Catheter Clearance: ABBOKINASE is indicated for the restoration of patency to intravenous catheters, including central venous catheters, obstructed by clotted blood or fibrin.[10,11] (See separate section at end of insert concerning I.V. catheter clearance for information regarding warnings, precautions, adverse reactions, and dosage and administration.)

CONTRAINDICATIONS

Because thrombolytic therapy increases the risk of bleeding, urokinase is contraindicated in the following situations: (See WARNINGS.)
—Active internal bleeding
—Recent (within two months) cerebrovascular accident, intracranial or intraspinal surgery
—Intracranial neoplasm

WARNINGS

Bleeding: The aim of urokinase is the production of sufficient amounts of plasmin for lysis of intravascular deposits of fibrin; however, fibrin deposits which provide hemostasis, for example, at sites of needle puncture, will also lyse, and bleeding from such sites may occur.
Intramuscular injections and nonessential handling of the patient must be avoided during treatment with urokinase. Venipunctures should be performed carefully and as infrequently as possible.
Should an arterial puncture be necessary (except for intracoronary administration), upper extremity vessels are preferable. Pressure should be applied for at least 30 minutes, a pressure dressing applied, and the puncture site checked frequently for evidence of bleeding.
In the following conditions, the risks of therapy may be increased and should be weighed against the anticipated benefits:
—Recent (within 10 days) major surgery, obstetrical delivery, organ biopsy, previous puncture of non-compressible vessels
—Recent (within 10 days) serious gastrointestinal bleeding
—Recent trauma including cardiopulmonary resuscitation
—Severe uncontrolled arterial hypertension
—High likelihood of a left heart thrombus, e.g., mitral stenosis with atrial fibrillation
—Subacute bacterial endocarditis
—Hemostatic defects including those secondary to severe hepatic or renal disease
—Pregnancy
—Cerebrovascular disease
—Diabetic hemorrhagic retinopathy
—Any other condition in which bleeding might constitute a significant hazard or be particularly difficult to manage because of its location
Should serious spontaneous bleeding (not controllable by local pressure) occur, the infusion of urokinase should be terminated immediately, and treatment instituted as described under ADVERSE REACTIONS.
Use of Anticoagulants: Concurrent use of anticoagulants with intravenous administration of ABBOKINASE is not recommended. However, concurrent use of heparin may be required during intracoronary administraion of ABBOKINASE. A clinical study[2] with concurrent use of heparin and ABBOKINASE during intracoronary administration has demonstrated no tendency toward increased bleeding that would not be attributable to the procedure or ABBOKINASE alone. Nevertheless, careful monitoring for excessive bleeding is advised.
Arrhythmias: Rapid lysis of coronary thrombi has been reported occasionally to cause atrial or ventricular dysrhythmias as a result of reperfusion requiring immediate treatment. Careful monitoring for arrhythmias should be maintained during and immediately following intracoronary administration of ABBOKINASE.

PRECAUTIONS

Laboratory Tests: Before commencing thrombolytic therapy, obtain a hematocrit, platelet count, and a thrombin time (TT), activated partial thromboplastin time (APTT), or prothrombin time (PT). If heparin has been given, it should be discontinued unless it is to be used in conjunction with ABBOKINASE for intracoronary administration. TT or APTT should be less than twice the normal control value before thrombolytic therapy is started.
During the infusion, coagulation tests and/or measures of fibrinolytic activity may be performed if desired. Results do not, however, reliably predict either efficacy or a risk of bleeding. The clinical response should be observed frequently, and vital signs, i.e., pulse, temperature, respiratory rate and blood pressure, should be checked at least every four hours. The blood pressure should not be taken in the lower extremities to avoid dislodgment of possible deep vein thrombi.
Following the intravenous infusion, *before (re)instituting heparin*, the TT or APTT should be less than twice the upper limits of normal. Following intracoronary infusion of ABBOKINASE, blood coagulation parameters should be determined and heparin therapy continued as appropriate.
Drug Interactions: The interaction of urokinase with other drugs has not been studied. Drugs that alter platelet function should not be used. Common examples are: aspirin, indomethacin and phenylbutazone.
Although a bolus dose of heparin is recommended prior to intracoronary use of urokinase, oral anticoagulants or heparin should not be given concurrently with large doses of urokinase such as those used for pulmonary embolism. Concomitant use of intravenous urokinase and oral anticoagulants or heparin may increase the risk of hemorrhage. (See "WARNINGS" section.)
Carcinogenicity: Adequate data is not available on the long-term potential for carcinogenicity in animals or humans.
Pregnancy: Pregnancy category B. Reproduction studies have been performed in mice and rats at doses up to 1,000 times the human dose and have revealed no evidence of impaired fertility or harm to the fetus due to urokinase. There are, however, no adequate and well-controlled studies in pregnant women. Because animal reproduction studies are not always predictive of human response, this drug should be used during pregnancy only if clearly needed.
Nursing Mothers: It is not known whether this drug is excreted in human milk. Because many drugs are excreted in human milk, caution should be exercised when urokinase is administered to a nursing woman.
Pediatric Use: Safety and effectiveness in children have not been established.

ADVERSE REACTIONS

The following adverse reactions have been associated with intravenous therapy but may also occur with intracoronary artery infusion.
Bleeding: The type of bleeding associated with thrombolytic therapy can be placed into two broad categories:
—Superficial or surface bleeding, observed mainly at invaded or disturbed sites (e.g., venous cutdowns, arterial punctures, sites of recent surgical intervention, etc.).
—Internal bleeding, involving, e.g., the gastrointestinal tract, genitourinary tract, vagina, or intramuscular, retroperitoneal, or intracerebral sites.
Several fatalities due to cerebral or retroperitoneal hemorrhage have occurred during thrombolytic therapy.
Should serious bleeding occur, urokinase infusion should be discontinued and, if necessary, blood loss and reversal of the bleeding tendency can be effectively managed with whole blood (fresh blood preferable), packed red blood cells and cryoprecipitate or fresh frozen plasma. Dextran should not be used. Although the use of aminocaproic acid (ACA, AMICAR®) in humans as an antidote for urokinase has not been documented, it may be considered in an emergency situation.
Allergic Reactions: *In vitro* tests with urokinase, as well as intradermal tests in humans, gave no evidence of induced antibody formation. Relatively mild allergic type reactions, e.g., bronchospasm and skin rash, have been reported rarely. When such reactions occur, they usually respond to conventional therapy.
Fever: Febrile episodes have occurred in approximately 2–3% of treated patients. A cause and effect relationship has not been established. Symptomatic treatment with acetaminophen is usually sufficient to alleviate discomfort. Aspirin is not recommended.

DOSAGE AND ADMINISTRATION

ABBOKINASE IS INTENDED FOR INTRAVENOUS AND INTRACORONARY INFUSION ONLY.

A. Pulmonary Embolism:
Preparation: Reconstitute ABBOKINASE (urokinase for injection) by aseptically adding 5.2 ml of Sterile Water for Injection, USP, to the vial. (It is important that ABBOKINASE be reconstituted *only* with Sterile Water for Injection, USP, *without* preservatives. Bacteriostatic Water for Injection should not be used.) Each vial should be visually inspected for discoloration (practically colorless solution) and for the presence of particulate material. Highly colored solutions should not be used. Because ABBOKINASE contains no preservatives, it should not be reconstituted until immediately before using. Any unused portion of the reconstituted material should be discarded.
To minimize formation of filaments, avoid shaking the vial during reconstitution. Roll and tilt the vial to enhance reconstitution. The solution may be terminally filtered, e.g., through a 0.45 micron or smaller cellulose membrane filter. No other medication should be added to this solution.
Reconstituted ABBOKINASE is diluted with 0.9% Sodium Chloride Injection, USP or 5% Dextrose Injection, USP, prior to intravenous infusion. (See Table I, **Dose Preparation.**)
Administration: Administer ABBOKINASE (urokinase for injection) by means of a constant infusion pump that is capable of delivering a total volume of 195 ml. The following table may be used as an aid in the preparation of ABBOKINASE (urokinase for injection) for administration.
A priming dose of 2,000 IU/lb (4,400 IU/kg) of ABBOKINASE is given as the ABBOKINASE -0.9% Sodium Chloride Injection or 5% Dextrose Injection admixture at a rate of 90 ml/hour over a period of 10 minutes. This is followed by a continuous infusion of 2,000 IU/lb/hr (4,400 IU/kg/hr) of ABBOKINASE at a rate of 15 ml/hour for 12 hours. Since some ABBOKINASE admixture will remain in the tubing at the end of an infusion pump delivery cycle, the following flush procedure should be performed to insure that the total dose of ABBOKINASE is administered. A solution of 0.9% Sodium Chloride Injection or 5% Dextrose Injection approximately equal in amount to the volume of the tubing in the infusion set should be administered via the pump to flush the ABBOKINASE admixture from the entire length of the infusion set. The pump should be set to administer the flush solution at the continuous infusion rate of 15 ml/hour.
Anticoagulation After Terminating Urokinase Treatment: At the end of urokinase therapy, treatment with heparin by continuous intravenous infusion is recommended to prevent recurrent thrombosis. Heparin treatment, without a loading dose, should not begin until the thrombin time has decreased to *less than twice* the normal control value (approximately 3 to 4 hours after completion of the infusion). See manufacturer's prescribing information for proper use of heparin. This should then be followed by oral anticoagulants in the conventional manner.

B. Lysis of Coronary Artery Thrombi:[2]
Preparation: Reconstitute three (3) 250,000 I.U. vials of ABBOKINASE by aseptically adding 5.2 ml of Sterile Water for Injection, USP, to the vial. (It is important that ABBOKINASE be reconstituted *only* with Sterile Water for Injection, USP, *without* preservatives. Bacteriostatic Water for Injection should *not* be used.) Each vial should be visually inspected for discoloration (practically colorless solution) and for the presence of particulate material. Highly colored solutions should not be used. Because ABBOKINASE contains no preservatives, it should not be reconstituted until immediately before using. Any unused portion of the reconstituted material should be discarded.

Continued on next page

If desired, additional literature on any Abbott Product will be provided upon request to Abbott Laboratories.

Abbott—Cont.

To minimize formation of filaments, avoid shaking the vial during reconstitution. Roll and tilt the vial to enhance reconstitution. The solution may be terminally filtered, e.g., through a 0.45 micron or smaller cellulose membrane filter. Add the contents of the three (3) reconstituted ABBOKINASE vials to 500 ml of 5% Dextrose Injection, USP. The resulting solution admixture will have a concentration of approximately 1500 I.U. per ml. No other medication should be added to the solution.
The admixture should be administered immediately as described under Administration. Any solution remaining after administration should be discarded.
NOTE: Adsorption of drug from dilute protein solutions to various materials has been reported in the literature. Therefore, the directions for Preparation and Administration must be followed to assure that significant drug loss does not occur.
Administration: Prior to the infusion of ABBOKINASE, a bolus dose of heparin ranging from 2500 to 10,000 units should be administered intravenously. Prior heparin administration should be considered when calculating the heparin dose for this procedure. Following the bolus dose of heparin, the prepared ABBOKINASE solution should be infused into the occluded artery at a rate of 4 ml per minute (6000 I.U. per minute) for periods up to 2 hours. In a clinical study, the average total dose of ABBOKINASE utilized for lysis of coronary artery thrombi was 500,000 I.U.[2]
To determine response to ABBOKINASE therapy, periodic angiography during the infusion is recommended. It is suggested that the angiography be repeated at approximately 15 minute intervals. ABBOKINASE therapy should be continued until the artery is maximally opened, usually 15 to 30 minutes after the initial opening. Following the infusion, coagulation parameters should be determined. It is advisable to continue heparin therapy after the artery is opened by ABBOKINASE.
When ABBOKINASE was administered selectively into thrombosed coronary arteries via coronary catheter within 6 hours following onset of symptoms of acute transmural myocardial infarction, 60% of the occlusions were opened.[2]
I.V. Catheter Clearance:
Warnings: Excessive pressure should be avoided when ABBOKINASE is injected into the catheter. Such force could cause rupture of the catheter or expulsion of the clot into the circulation.
Precautions: Catheters may be occluded by substances other than blood products, such as drug precipitate. ABBOKINASE is not effective in such a case, and there is a possibility that the precipitate may be forced into the vascular system.
Adverse Reactions: Although there have been no adverse reactions reported as a result of using ABBOKINASE for the removal of clot obstruction from I.V. catheters, the possibility of reactions should nevertheless be considered.
Dosage and Administration:
Preparation: Reconstitute ABBOKINASE (urokinase for injection) by aseptically adding 5.2 ml of Sterile Water for Injection, USP, to the vial. (It is important that ABBOKINASE be reconstituted *only* with Sterile Water for Injection, USP, *without* preservatives. Bacteriostatic Water for Injection should *not* be used.) Add 1 ml of the reconstituted drug to 9.0 ml Sterile Water for Injection, USP, to make a final dilution equivalent to 5,000 IU/ml. One ml of this preparation is to be utilized for each catheter clearing procedure. BECAUSE ABBOKINASE CONTAINS NO PRESERVATIVES, IT SHOULD NOT BE RECONSTITUTED UNTIL IMMEDIATELY BEFORE USING.
Administration: NOTE: When the following procedure is used to clear a central venous catheter, the patient should be instructed to exhale and hold his breath any time the catheter is not connected to I.V. tubing or a syringe. This is to prevent air from entering the open catheter.
Aseptically disconnect the I.V. tubing connection at the catheter hub and attach a 10 ml syringe. Determine occlusion of the catheter by *gently* attempting to aspirate blood from the catheter with the 10 ml syringe. If aspiration is not possible, remove the 10 ml syringe and attach a 1 ml tuberculin syringe filled with prepared ABBOKINASE to the catheter. Slowly and gently inject an amount of ABBOKINASE equal to the volume of the catheter. Aseptically remove the tuberculin syringe and connect a 5 ml syringe to the catheter. Wait at least 5 minutes before attempting to aspirate the drug and residual clot with the 5 ml syringe. Repeat aspiration attempts every 5 minutes. If the catheter is not open within 30 minutes, the catheter may be capped allowing ABBOKINASE to remain in the catheter for 30 to 60 minutes before again attempting to aspirate. A second injection of ABBOKINASE may be necessary in resistant cases.
When patency is restored, aspirate 4 to 5 ml of blood to assure removal of all drug and clot residual. Remove the blood-filled syringe and replace it with a 10 ml syringe filled with 0.9% Sodium Chloride Injection, USP. The catheter should then be gently irrigated with this solution to assure patency of the catheter. After the catheter has been irrigated, remove the 10 ml syringe and aseptically reconnect sterile I.V. tubing to the catheter hub.
[See table below].

HOW SUPPLIED

ABBOKINASE (urokinase for injection) is supplied as a sterile lyophilized preparation (**NDC** 0074-6109-05). Each vial contains 250,000 IU urokinase activity, 25 mg mannitol, and 45 mg sodium chloride. Store ABBOKINASE powder at 2° to 8°C.

REFERENCES

1. Sherry, S., *et al:* Thrombolytic Therapy in Thrombosis: A National Institutes of Health Consensus Development Conference. Ann. Intern. Med. *93*:141–144 (1980).
2. Tennant, S. N., Campbell, W.B., *et al:* Intracoronary Thrombolysis In Acute Myocardial Infarction: Comparison of the Efficacy of Urokinase to Streptokinase. Accepted for Publication, Circulation.
3. Bang, N. U.: Physiology and Biochemistry of Fibrinolysis in *Thrombosis and Bleeding Disorders* (Bang, N. U., Beller, F. K., Deutsch, E., Mammen, E. F., eds.). Academic Press (1971). pp. 292–327.
4. McNicol, G. P.: The Fibrinolytic Enzyme System. Postgrad. Med. J. (August Suppl. 5). *49*:10–12 (1973).
5. Sasahara, A. A., Hyers, T. M., Cole, C. M., *et al.:* The Urokinase Pulmonary Embolism Trial Circulation, (Suppl. II) *47*:1–108 (1973).
6. Urokinase pulmonary embolism trial study group: Urokinase-Streptokinase Embolism Trial. JAMA *229*:1606-1613 (1974).
7. Sasahara, A. A., Bell, W. R., Simon, T. L., Stengle, J. M. and Sherry, S.: The Phase II Urokinase-Streptokinase Pulmonary Embolism Trial. Thrombos. Diathes. Haemorrh. (Stuttg.) *33*:464–476 (1975).
8. Bell, W. R.: Thrombolytic Therapy: A Comparison Between Urokinase and Streptokinase. Sem. Thromb. Hemost. *2*:1–13 (1975).
9. Fratantoni, J. C., Ness, P., Simon, T. L.: Thrombolytic Therapy: Current Status. N. Eng. J. Med., *293*:1073–1078 (1975).
10. Lawson, M., *et al:* The Use of Urokinase to Restore the Patency of Occluded Central Venous Catheters. Am J. Intravenous Therapy and Clinical Nutrition, 9:29–32 (Oct. 1982).
11. Glynn, M.F.X., *et al:* Therapy for Thrombotic Occlusion of Long-term Intravenous Alimentation Catheters, Journal of Parenteral and Enteral Nutrition, *4* (4):387–390 (July/Aug. 1980).

Abbott Laboratories
North Chicago, IL 60064
Ref. 01-2307-R6

TABLE 1
Dose Preparation–Pulmonary Embolism

Weight (pounds)	Total Dose* Urokinase (IU)	Number Vials ABBOKINASE (urokinase for injection)	Volume of ABBOKINASE After Reconstitution (ml)**	+	Volume of Diluent (ml)	=	Final Volume (ml)
81–90	2,250,000	9	45		150		195
91–100	2,500,000	10	50		145		195
101–110	2,750,000	11	55		140		195
111–120	3,000,000	12	60		135		195
121–130	3,250,000	13	65		130		195
131–140	3,500,000	14	70		125		195
141–150	3,750,000	15	75		120		195
151–160	4,000,000	16	80		115		195
161–170	4,250,000	17	85		110		195
171–180	4,500,000	18	90		105		195
181–190	4,750,000	19	95		100		195
191–200	5,000,000	20	100		95		195
201–210	5,250,000	21	105		90		195
211–220	5,500,000	22	110		85		195
221–230	5,750,000	23	115		80		195
231–240	6,000,000	24	120		75		195
241–250	6,250,000	25	125		70		195

Infusion Rate:	Priming Dose	Dose for 12-Hour Period
	15 ml/10 min***	15 ml/hr for 12 hrs

*Priming dose + dose administered during 12-hour period.
**After addition of 5.2 ml of Sterile Water for Injection, USP, per vial (See Preparation.)
***Pump rate = 90 ml/hr

ABBOKINASE® OPEN-CATH® ℞

[*ab-bō-kī'nāze open-cath*]
Urokinase for Catheter Clearance

DESCRIPTION

Urokinase is an enzyme (protein) produced by the kidney and found in the urine. There are two forms of urokinase differing in molecular weight but having similar clinical effects. Urokinase is a thrombolytic agent obtained from human kidney cells by tissue culture techniques and is primarily the low molecular weight form. It is supplied as a sterile lyophilized white powder. Following reconstitution ABBOKINASE OPEN-CATH is a clear, practically colorless solution.
Each ml of reconstituted ABBOKINASE OPEN-CATH contains 5000 IU of urokinase activity, 5 mg gelatin, 15 mg mannitol, 1.7 mg sodium chloride and 4.6 mg monobasic sodium phosphate anhydrous. The pH of ABBOKINASE is adjusted with sodium hydroxide and/or hydrochloric acid prior to lyophilization.

CLINICAL PHARMACOLOGY

Urokinase acts on the endogenous fibrinolytic system. It converts plasminogen to the enzyme plasmin. Plasmin degrades fibrin clots as well as fibrinogen and other plasma proteins.
When used as directed for I.V. catheter clearance, only small amounts of urokinase may reach the circulation; therefore, therapeutic serum levels are not expected to be achieved. Nevertheless, one should be aware of the clinical pharmacology of urokinase.
Intravenous infusion of urokinase in doses recommended for lysis of pulmonary embolism is followed by increased fibrinolytic activity. This effect disappears within a few hours after discontinuation, but a decrease in plasma levels of fibrinogen and plasminogen and an increase in the amount of circulating fibrin (ogen) degradation products may persist for 12–24 hours.[1,2] There is a lack of correlation between embolus resolution and changes in coagulation and fibrinolytic assay results.
Information is incomplete about the pharmacokinetic properties in man. Urokinase administered by intravenous infusion is cleared rapidly by the liver. The serum half-life in man is 20 minutes or less. Patients with impaired liver function (e.g., cirrhosis) would be expected to show a prolongation in half-life. Small fractions of an administered dose are excreted in bile and urine.

INDICATIONS AND USAGE

ABBOKINASE OPEN-CATH (urokinase for catheter clearance) is indicated for the restoration of patency to intravenous catheters, including central venous catheters, obstructed by clotted blood or fibrin.[3,4,5]

CONTRAINDICATIONS

Because thrombolytic therapy increases the risk of bleeding, urokinase is contraindicated in the following situations:
—Active internal bleeding
—Recent (within two months) cerebrovascular accident, intracranial or intraspinal surgery
—Intracranial neoplasm
There have been no reports, however, which would suggest a contraindication for the use of urokinase for I.V. catheter clearance.

WARNINGS

Excessive pressure should be avoided when ABBOKINASE is injected into the catheter. Such force could cause rupture of

the catheter or expulsion of the clot into the circulation. During attempts to determine catheter occlusion, vigorous suction should not be applied due to possible damage to the vascular wall or collapse of soft-wall catheters.
Catheters may be occluded by substances other than fibrin clots, such as drug precipitates. ABBOKINASE is not effective in such cases and there is the possibility that the substances may be forced into the vascular system.

PRECAUTIONS

Carcinogenicity: Adequate data is not available on the long-term potential for carcinogenicity in animals or humans.
Pregnancy: Pregnancy category B. Reproduction studies have been performed in mice and rats at doses up to 1,000 times the human therapeutic dose and have revealed no evidence of impaired fertility or harm to the fetus due to urokinase. There are, however, no adequate and well-controlled studies in pregnant women. Because animal reproduction studies are not always predictive of human response, this drug should be used during pregnancy only if clearly needed.
Nursing Mothers: It is not known whether this drug is excreted in human milk. Because many drugs are excreted in human milk, caution should be exercised when urokinase is administered to a nursing woman.
Pediatric Use: Safety and effectiveness in children have not been established.

ADVERSE REACTIONS

Although there have been no adverse reactions reported as a result of using ABBOKINASE for the removal of clot obstruction from I.V. catheters, the possibility of reactions should nevertheless be considered. The following reactions have been associated with ABBOKINASE in doses recommended for lysis of pulmonary embolism.
Bleeding: The type of bleeding associated with thrombolytic therapy can be placed into two broad categories:
—Superficial or surface bleeding, observed mainly at invaded or disturbed sites (e.g., venous cutdowns, arterial punctures, sites of recent surgical intervention, etc.).
—Internal bleeding, involving, e.g., the gastrointestinal tract, genitourinary tract, vagina, or intramuscular, retroperitoneal, or intracerebral sites.
Several fatalities due to cerebral or retroperitoneal hemorrhage have occurred during thrombolytic therapy.
Should serious bleeding occur, urokinase infusion should be discontinued and, if necessary, blood loss and reversal of the bleeding tendency can be effectively managed with whole blood (fresh blood preferable), packed red blood cells and cryoprecipitate or fresh frozen plasma. Dextran should not be used. Although the use of aminocaproic acid (ACA, AMICAR®) in humans as an antidote for urokinase has not been documented, it may be considered in an emergency situation.
Allergic Reactions: *In vitro* tests with urokinase, as well as intradermal tests in humans, gave no evidence of induced antibody formation. Relatively mild allergic type reactions, e.g., bronchospasm and skin rash, have been reported rarely. When such reactions occur, they usually respond to conventional therapy.
Fever: Febrile episodes have occurred in approximately 2–3% of treated patients. A cause and effect relationship has not been established. Symptomatic treatment with acetaminophen is usually sufficient to alleviate discomfort. Aspirin is not recommended.

DOSAGE AND ADMINISTRATION

CONTAINS NO PRESERVATIVE.
USE IMMEDIATELY AFTER RECONSTITUTION. DISCARD ANY UNUSED PORTION.
Preparation of Solution: *Univial:*
1. Remove protective cap. Turn plunger-stopper a quarter turn and press to force diluent into lower chamber.
2. Roll and tilt to effect solution. Use only a clear, colorless solution.
3. Sterilize top of stopper with a suitable germicide.
4. Insert needle through the center of stopper until tip is barely visible. Withdraw dose.

It is recommended that vigorous shaking be avoided during reconstitution; roll and tilt to enhance reconstitution.
Parenteral drug products should be inspected visually for particulate matter and discoloration prior to administration, whenever solution and container permit.

ADMINISTRATION

When the following procedure is used to clear a central venous catheter, the patient should be instructed to exhale and hold his breath any time the catheter is not connected to I.V. tubing or a syringe. This is to prevent air from entering the open catheter.
Aseptically disconnect the I.V. tubing connection at the catheter hub and attach an empty 10 ml syringe. Determine occlusion of the catheter by *gently* attempting to aspirate blood from the catheter with the 10 ml syringe. If aspiration is not possible, remove the 10 ml syringe and attach a 1 ml tuberculin syringe filled with prepared ABBOKINASE OPEN-CATH to the catheter. Slowly and gently inject an amount of ABBOKINASE equal to the volume of the catheter. Aseptically remove the tuberculin syringe and connect an empty syringe (e.g., 5 ml) to the catheter. Wait at least 5 minutes before attempting to aspirate the drug and residual clot with the empty syringe. Repeat aspiration attempts every 5 minutes. If the catheter is not open within 30 minutes, the catheter may be capped allowing ABBOKINASE to remain in the catheter for 30 to 60 minutes before again attempting to aspirate. A second injection of ABBOKINASE may be necessary in resistant cases. When patency is restored, aspirate 4 to 5 ml of blood to assure removal of all drug and clot residual. Remove the blood-filled syringe and replace it with a 10 ml syringe filled with 0.9% Sodium Chloride Injection, USP. The catheter should then be gently irrigated with this solution to assure patency of the catheter. After the catheter has been irrigated, remove the 10 ml syringe and aseptically reconnect sterile I.V. tubing to the catheter hub.

HOW SUPPLIED

ABBOKINASE OPEN-CATH (urokinase for catheter clearance) is supplied as a sterile lyophilized preparation in a 1-ml single dose Univial® package (**NDC** 0074-6111-01). Store powder below 77°F (25°C). Avoid freezing.

REFERENCES

1. Bang, N. U.: Physiology and Biochemistry of Fibrinolysis In *Thrombosis and Bleeding Disorders* (Bang, N. U., Beller, F. K., Deutsch, E., Mammen, E. F., eds.). Academic Press (1971). pp. 292–327.
2. McNicol, G. P.: The Fibrinolytic Enzyme System. Postgrad. Med. J. (August Suppl. 5). *49* :10–12 (1973).
3. Hurtubise, Michel R., M.D., Bottino, Joseph C., M.D., Lawson, Millie, R.N., McCredie, Kenneth B., M.D.: Restoring Patency of Occluded Central Venous Catheters. Arch. Surg. *115* :212–213 (1980).
4. Glynn, M. F. X., *et al:* Therapy for Thrombotic Occlusion of Long-term Intravenous Alimentation Catheters. Journal of Parenteral and Enteral Nutrition. *4* (4):387–390 (July/Aug. 1980).
5. Lawson, M., Bottino, J. C., Hurtubise, M. R., McCredie, K. B.: The Use of Urokinase to Restore the Patency of Occluded Central Venous Catheters. Am. J. I.V. Ther. and Clin. Nutr., 9(9):29–30,32 (October, 1982).

Abbott Laboratories
North Chicago, IL 60064
Ref. 01-2384-R3

A-HYDROCORT™ ℞

[*ā-hī'dro-cort"*]
(hydrocortisone sodium succinate for injection, USP)
For Intravenous or Intramuscular Use

DESCRIPTION

Hydrocortisone sodium succinate, USP, an adrenocortical-like steroid, is the sodium succinate ester of hydrocortisone. It occurs as a white, or nearly white, odorless hygroscopic amorphous solid. Hydrocortisone sodium succinate is very soluble in water and in alcohol; it is insoluble in chloroform and is very slightly soluble in acetone.
Hydrocortisone sodium succinate is soluble in water and is especially well suited for intravenous use in situations in which high blood levels of hydrocortisone are required rapidly.
A-HYDROCORT (hydrocortisone sodium succinate for injection, USP) is available as:
100 mg Univial®—Each 2 ml (when mixed) contains hydrocortisone sodium succinate equivalent to 100 mg hydrocortisone; also 0.8 mg monobasic sodium phosphate anhydrous; 8.73 mg dibasic sodium phosphate anhydrous; and 18 mg of benzyl alcohol.
250 mg Univial—Each 2 ml (when mixed) contains hydrocortisone sodium succinate equivalent to 250 mg hydrocortisone; also 2 mg monobasic sodium phosphate anhydrous; 21.8 mg dibasic sodium phosphate anhydrous; and 18 mg of benzyl alcohol.
500 mg Univial—Each 4 ml (when mixed) contains hydrocortisone sodium succinate equivalent to 500 mg hydrocortisone; also 4 mg monobasic sodium phosphate anhydrous; 44 mg dibasic sodium phosphate anhydrous; and 36 mg benzyl alcohol.
1000 mg Univial—Each 8 ml (when mixed) contains hydrocortisone sodium succinate equivalent to 1000 mg hydrocortisone; also 8 mg monobasic sodium phosphate anhydrous; 88 mg dibasic sodium phosphate anhydrous; and 72 mg benzyl alcohol.
The pH of each formula was adjusted with sodium hydroxide and/or hydrochloric acid.

IMPORTANT

The solid contents of A-HYDROCORT should not be used with any diluent other than that provided. **Use within 3 days after mixing.**
When reconstituted as directed, the pH of the solutions ranges from 7–8 and the tonicities are, for the 100 mg per 2 ml solution, 0.36 osmolar; for the 250 mg per 2 ml, 500 mg per 4 ml, and 1000 mg per 8 ml solutions, 0.57 osmolar. [Isotonic saline (0.9% Sodium Chloride Injection, USP) = 0.28 osmolar.]

CLINICAL PHARMACOLOGY

Hydrocortisone sodium succinate has potent anti-inflammatory effects. Because it is an adrenocortical-like steroid, hydrocortisone sodium succinate may cause profound and varied metabolic effects in addition to modifying the body's immune response to diverse stimuli.
When given parenterally and in equimolar quantitites, hydrocortisone sodium succinate and hydrocortisone are equivalent in biologic activity.
Following intravenous injection of hydrocortisone sodium succinate, demonstrable effects are evident within one hour and persist for a variable period. Excretion of the administered dose is nearly complete within 12 hours. Thus, if constantly high blood levels are required, injections should be made every four to six hours.
This preparation is also rapidly absorbed when administered intramuscularly and is excreted in a pattern similar to that observed after intravenous injection.

INDICATIONS

Sterile A-HYDROCORT (hydrocortisone sodium succinate) is indicated in situations requiring a rapid and intense hormonal effect.
Intravenous administration of A-HYDROCORT is most appropriate for the following indications:

1. **Endocrine disorders:**
   a. Acute adrenocortical insufficiency (hydrocortisone or cortisone is the drug of choice; mineralocorticoid supplementation may be necessary, particularly when synthetic analogs are used).
   b. Preoperatively and in the event of serious trauma or illness, in patients with known adrenal insufficiency or when adrenocortical reserve is doubtful.
   c. Shock unresponsive to conventional therapy if adrenocortical insufficiency exists or is suspected.
2. **Collagen diseases**—During an exacerbation or as maintenance therapy in selected cases of:
   a. Acute rheumatic carditis.
3. **Allergic states**—Control of severe or incapacitating allergic conditions intractable to adequate trials of conventional treatment in:
   a. Bronchial asthma.
   b. Serum sickness.
   c. Drug hypersensitivity reactions.
   d. Urticarial transfusion reactions.
   e. Acute noninfectious laryngeal edema (epinephrine is the drug of first choice).
4. **Hematologic disorders:**
   a. Idiopathic thrombocytopenic purpura in adults (I.M. administration is contraindicated).

Intramuscular administration of A-HYDROCORT is appropriate for the following indications:

1. **Endocrine disorders:**
   a. Primary or secondary adrenocortical insufficiency (hydrocortisone or cortisone is the drug of choice; synthetic analogs may be used in conjunction with mineralocorticoids where applicable; in infancy, mineralocorticoid supplementation is of particular importance).
   b. Acute adrenocortical insufficiency (hydrocortisone or cortisone is the drug of choice; mineralocorticoid supplementation may be necessary, particularly when synthetic analogs are used).
   c. Preoperatively and in the event of serious trauma or illness, in patients with known adrenal insufficiency or when adrenocortical reserve is doubtful.
   d. Shock unresponsive to conventional therapy if adrenocortical insufficiency exists or is suspected.
   e. Congenital adrenal hyperplasia.
   f. Nonsuppurative thyroiditis.
   g. Hypercalcemia associated with cancer.
2. **Rheumatic disorders**—As adjunctive therapy for short-term administration (to tide the patient over an acute episode or exacerbation) in:
   a. Post-traumatic osteoarthritis.
   b. Synovitis of osteoarthritis.
   c. Rheumatoid arthritis, including juvenile rheumatoid arthritis (selected cases may require low-dose maintenance therapy).
   d. Acute and subacute bursitis.
   e. Epicondylitis.
   f. Acute nonspecific tenosynovitis.
   g. Acute gouty arthritis.

Continued on next page

Abbott—Cont.

h. Psoriatic arthritis.
i. Ankylosing spondylitis.

3. **Collagen diseases**—During an exacerbation or as maintenance therapy in selected cases of:
a. Systemic lupus erythematosus.
b. Acute rheumatic carditis.

4. **Dermatologic diseases:**
a. Severe erythema multiforme (Stevens-Johnson syndrome).
b. Exfoliative dermatitis.
c. Bullous dermatitis herpetiformis.
d. Severe seborrheic dermatitis.
e. Severe psoriasis.
f. Pemphigus.
g. Mycosis fungoides.
h. Systemic dermatomyositis (polymyositis).

5. **Allergic states**—Control of severe or incapacitating allergic conditions intractable to adequate trials of conventional treatment in:
a. Bronchial asthma.
b. Contact dermatitis.
c. Atopic dermatitis.
d. Serum sickness.
e. Seasonal or perennial allergic rhinitis.
f. Drug hypersensitivity reactions.
g. Urticarial transfusion reactions.
h. Acute noninfectious laryngeal edema (epinephrine is the drug of first choice).

6. **Ophthalmic diseases**—Severe acute and chronic allergic and inflammatory processes involving the eye, such as:
a. Herpes zoster ophthalmicus.
b. Iritis, iridocyclitis.
c. Chorioretinitis.
d. Diffuse posterior uveitis and choroiditis.
e. Optic neuritis.
f. Sympathetic ophthalmia.
g. Anterior segment inflammation.
h. Allergic conjunctivitis.
i. Allergic corneal marginal ulcers.

7. **Gastrointestinal diseases**—To tide the patient over a critical period of disease in:
a. Ulcerative colitis—(Systemic therapy).
b. Regional enteritis—(Systemic therapy).

8. **Respiratory diseases:**
a. Symptomatic sarcoidosis.
b. Berylliosis.
c. Fulminating or disseminated pulmonary tuberculosis when concurrently accompanied by appropriate antituberculous chemotherapy.
d. Aspiration pneumonitis.
e. Loeffler's syndrome not manageable by other means.

9. **Hematologic disorders:**
a. Acquired (autoimmune) hemolytic anemia.
b. Secondary thrombocytopenia in adults.
c. Erythroblastopenia (RBC anemia).
d. Congenital (erythroid) hypoplastic anemia.

10. **Neoplastic diseases**—For palliative management of:
a. Leukemias and lymphomas in adults.
b. Acute leukemia of childhood.

11. **Edematous state**—To induce diuresis or remission of proteinuria in the nephrotic syndrome, without uremia, of the idiopathic type or that due to lupus erythematosus.

12. **Nervous system**—Acute exacerbations of multiple sclerosis.

13. **Miscellaneous:**
a. Tuberculous meningitis with subarachnoid block or impending block when used concurrently with appropriate antituberculous chemotherapy.
b. Trichinosis with neurologic or myocardial involvement.

CONTRAINDICATIONS

Systemic fungal infections.

Not for use in newborns. Benzyl alcohol, a preservative in the Bacteriostatic Water for Injection provided with these products, has been associated with toxicity in newborns. Data are unavailable on the toxicity of other preservatives in this age group.

WARNINGS

In patients on corticosteroid therapy subjected to any unusual stress, increased dosage of rapidly acting corticosteroids before, during, and after the stressful situation is indicated.

Corticosteroids may mask some signs of infection, and new infections may appear during their use. There may be decreased resistance and inability to localize infection when corticosteroids are used.

Prolonged use of corticosteroids may produce posterior subcapsular cataracts, glaucoma with possible damage to the optic nerves, and may enhance the establishment of secondary ocular infections due to fungi or viruses.

Average and large doses of cortisone or hydrocortisone can cause elevation of blood pressure, salt and water retention, and increased excretion of potassium. These effects are less likely to occur with the synthetic derivatives except when used in large doses. Dietary salt restriction and potassium supplementation may be necessary. All corticosteroids increase calcium excretion.

While on corticosteroid therapy patients should not be vaccinated against smallpox. Other immunization procedures should not be undertaken in patients who are on corticosteroids, especially on high dose, because of possible hazards of neurological complications and a lack of antibody response.

The use of A-HYDROCORT (hydrocortisone sodium succinate) in active tuberculosis should be restricted to those cases of fulminating or disseminated tuberculosis in which the corticosteroid is used for the management of the disease in conjunction with appropriate antituberculous regimen.

If corticosteroids are indicated in patients with latent tuberculosis or tuberculin reactivity, close observation is necessary as reactivation of the disease may occur. During prolonged corticosteroid therapy, these patients should receive chemoprophylaxis.

Because rare instances of anaphylactoid reactions have occurred in patients receiving parenteral corticosteroid therapy, appropriate precautionary measures should be taken prior to administration, especially when the patient has a history of allergy to any drug.

USAGE IN PREGNANCY

Since adequate human reproduction studies have not been done with corticosteroids, the use of these drugs in pregnancy, nursing mothers, or women of childbearing potential requires that the possible benefits of the drug be weighed against the potential hazards to the mother and embryo or fetus. Infants born of mothers who have received substantial doses of corticosteroids during pregnancy should be carefully observed for signs of hypoadrenalism.

PRECAUTIONS

Drug-induced secondary adrenocortical insufficiency may be minimized by gradual reduction of dosage. This type of relative insufficiency may persist for months after discontinuation of therapy; therefore, in any situation of stress occurring during that period, hormone therapy should be reinstituted. Since mineralocorticoid secretion may be impaired, salt and / or a mineralocorticoid should be administered concurrently.

There is an enhanced effect of corticosteroids in patients with hypothyroidism and in those with cirrhosis.

Corticosteroids should be used cautiously in patients with ocular herpes simplex because of possible corneal perforation.

The lowest possible dose of corticosteroid should be used to control the condition under treatment, and when reduction in dosage is possible, the reduction should be gradual.

Psychic derangements may appear when corticosteroids are used, ranging from euphoria, insomnia, mood swings, personality changes and severe depression, to frank psychotic manifestations. Also, existing emotional instability or psychotic tendencies may be aggravated by corticosteroids.

Aspirin should be used cautiously in conjunction with corticosteroids in hypoprothrombinemia.

Steroids should be used with caution in nonspecific ulcerative colitis, if there is a probability of impending perforation, abscess or other pyogenic infection; diverticulitis; fresh intestinal anastomoses; active or latent peptic ulcer; renal insufficiency; hypertension; osteoporosis; and myasthenia gravis.

Growth and development of infants and children on prolonged corticosteroid therapy should be carefully observed.

Although controlled clinical trials have shown corticosteroids to be effective in speeding the resolution of acute exacerbations of multiple sclerosis they do not show that they affect the ultimate outcome or natural history of the disease. The studies do show that relatively high doses of corticosteroids are necessary to demonstrate a significant effect. (See "Dosage and Administration" section).

Since complications of treatment with glucocorticoids are dependent on the size of the dose and the duration of treatment a risk/benefit decision must be made in each individual case as to dose and duration of treatment and as to whether daily or intermittent therapy should be used.

ADVERSE REACTIONS

Fluid and Electrolyte Disturbances

Sodium retention
Fluid retention
Congestive heart failure in susceptible patients
Potassium loss
Hypokalemic alkalosis
Hypertension

Musculoskeletal

Muscle weakness
Steroid myopathy
Loss of muscle mass
Osteoporosis
Vertebral compression fractures
Aseptic necrosis of femoral and humeral heads
Pathologic fracture of long bones

Gastrointestinal

Peptic ulcer with possible perforation and hemorrhage
Pancreatitis
Abdominal distention
Ulcerative esophagitis

Dermatologic

Impaired wound healing
Thin fragile skin
Petechiae and ecchymoses
Facial erythema
Increased sweating
May suppress reactions to skin tests

Neurological

Increased intracranial pressure with papilledema (pseudo-tumor cerebri) usually after treatment
Convulsions
Vertigo
Headache

Endocrine

Development of Cushingoid state
Suppression of growth in children
Secondary adrenocortical and pituitary unresponsiveness, particularly in times of stress, as in trauma, surgery or illness
Menstrual irregularities
Decreased carbohydrate tolerance
Manifestations of latent diabetes mellitus
Increased requirements for insulin or oral hypoglycemic agents in diabetics

Ophthalmic

Posterior subcapsular cataracts
Increased intraocular pressure
Glaucoma
Exophthalmos

Metabolic

Negative nitrogen balance due to protein catabolism

The following additional adverse reactions are related to parenteral corticosteroid therapy:

Hyperpigmentation or hypopigmentation
Subcutaneous and cutaneous atrophy
Sterile abscess

DOSAGE AND ADMINISTRATION

This preparation may be administered by intravenous injection, by intravenous infusion, or by intramuscular injection; the preferred method for initial emergency use being intravenous injection. Following the initial emergency period, consideration should be given to employing a longer acting injectable preparation or an oral preparation.

Therapy is initiated by administering hydrocortisone sodium succinate intravenously over a period of 30 seconds (e.g., 100 mg) to 10 minutes (e.g., 500 mg or more). In general, high dose corticosteroid therapy should be continued only until the patient's condition has stabilized—usually not beyond 48 to 72 hours. Although adverse effects associated with high dose, short-term corticoid therapy are uncommon, peptic ulceration may occur. Prophylactic antacid therapy may be indicated.

When high dose hydrocortisone therapy must be continued beyond 48 to 72 hours, hypernatremia may occur. Under such circumstances it may be desirable to replace hydrocortisone sodium succinate with a corticoid which causes little or no sodium retention.

The initial dose of hydrocortisone sodium succinate is 100 mg to 500 mg depending upon the severity of the condition. This dose may be repeated at intervals of 2, 4 or 6 hours as indicated by the patient's response and clinical condition. While the dose may be reduced for infants and children, it is governed more by the severity of the condition and response of the patient than by age or body weight but should not be less than 25 mg daily. Patients subjected to severe stress following corticosteroid therapy should be observed closely for signs and symptoms of adrenocortical insufficiency.

Corticoid therapy is an adjunct to, and not a replacement for, conventional therapy.

Multiple Sclerosis:

In the treatment of acute exacerbations of multiple sclerosis, daily doses of 200 mg of prednisolone for a week followed by 80 mg every other day for one month have been shown to be effective (20 mg of hydrocortisone is equivalent to 5 mg of prednisolone).

PREPARATION OF SOLUTIONS

Univial:

1. Remove protective cap, give the plunger-stopper a quarter turn and press to force diluent into lower compartment.
2. Gently agitate to effect solution. Use solution within 72 hours.

3. Sterilize top of plunger-stopper with a suitable germicide.
4. Insert needle squarely through center of plunger-stopper until tip is just visible. Invert vial and withdraw dose.

Further dilution is not necessary for intravenous or intramuscular injection.

For Intravenous Infusion:

Prepare solution as described above. The 100 mg solution may then be added to 100 to 1000 ml (but not less than 100 ml) of 5% Dextrose Injection (or 0.9% Sodium Chloride Injection or 5% Dextrose and 0.9% Sodium Chloride Injection if patient is not on sodium restriction). The 250 mg solution may be added to 250 to 1000 ml (but not less than 250 ml), the 500 mg solution may be added to 500 to 1000 ml (but not less than 500 ml) and the 1000 mg solution to not less than 1000 ml of the same diluents.

HOW SUPPLIED

Sterile A-HYDROCORT (hydrocortisone sodium succinate for injection, USP) is available in the following packages:

100 mg/2 ml Univial **NDC** 0074-5671-02;
250 mg/2 ml Univial **NDC** 0074-5672-02;
500 mg/4 ml Univial **NDC** 0074-5673-04;
1000 mg/8 ml Univial **NDC** 0074-5674-08.

Exposure of pharmaceutical products to heat should be minimized. Avoid excessive heat. Protect from freezing. It is recommended that unreconstituted product be stored below 86°F (30°C); however, brief exposure up to 104°F (40°C) does not adversely affect the product. Protect from light.

Abbott Laboratories
North Chicago, IL 60064
Ref. 01-2332-RI

A–METHAPRED® ℞

[ă-meth 'a-pred "]
(methylprednisolone sodium succinate for injection, USP)
For Intravenous or Intramuscular Use

DESCRIPTION

Methylprednisolone sodium succinate, USP, an adrenocortical-like steroid, is the sodium succinate ester of methylprednisolone.

It occurs as a white, or nearly white, odorless hygroscopic, amorphous solid.

Methylprednisolone sodium succinate is extremely soluble in water and is especially well suited for intravenous use in situations in which high blood levels of methylprednisolone are required rapidly.

A-METHAPRED (methylprednisolone sodium succinate for injection, USP) is available as:

40 mg Univial®—Each 1 ml (when mixed) contains methylprednisolone sodium succinate equivalent to 40 mg methylprednisolone; also 1.6 mg monobasic sodium phosphate anhydrous; 17.46 mg dibasic sodium phosphate anhydrous; 25 mg lactose anhydrous; and 9 mg of benzyl alcohol.

125 mg Univial—Each 2 ml (when mixed) contains methylprednisolone sodium succinate equivalent to 125 mg methylprednisolone; also 1.6 mg monobasic sodium phosphate anhydrous; 17.4 mg dibasic sodium phosphate anhydrous; and 18 mg of benzyl alcohol.

500 mg Univial—Each 4 ml (when mixed) contains methylprednisolone sodium succinate equivalent to 500 mg methylprednisolone; also 6.4 mg monobasic sodium phosphate anhydrous; 69.6 mg dibasic sodium phosphate anhydrous; and 36 mg of benzyl alcohol.

1000 mg Univial—Each 8 ml (when mixed) contains methylprednisolone sodium succinate equivalent to 1000 mg methylprednisolone; also 12.8 mg monobasic sodium phosphate anhydrous; 139.2 mg dibasic sodium phosphate anhydrous; and 72 mg of benzyl alcohol.

The pH of each formula was adjusted with sodium hydroxide and/or hydrochloric acid.

NOTE: The 40 mg and 125 mg Univial should be used within 48 hours after mixing. The 500 mg and 1000 mg Univial should be used within 72 hours after mixing.

CLINICAL PHARMACOLOGY

Methylprednisolone sodium succinate is a potent anti-inflammatory steroid. It has a greater anti-inflammatory potency than prednisolone and even less tendency than prednisolone to induce sodium and water retention. Like the adrenocortical steroids, methylprednisolone sodium succinate may cause profound and varied metabolic effects in addition to modifying the body's immune response to diverse stimuli.

When given parenterally and in equimolar quantities, methylprednisolone sodium succinate and methylprednisolone are equivalent in biologic activity.

The relative potency of methylprednisolone sodium succinate and hydrocortisone sodium succinate, as indicated by depression of eosinophil count, following intravenous administration, is at least four to one. This is in good agreement with the relative oral potency of methylprednisolone and hydrocortisone.

INDICATIONS

When oral therapy is not feasible, and the strength, dosage form and route of administration of the drug reasonably lend the preparation to the treatment of the condition, A-METHAPRED (methylprednisolone sodium succinate) is indicated for intravenous or intramuscular use in the following conditions:

1. **Endocrine disorders:**
   a. Primary or secondary adrenocortical insufficiency (hydrocortisone or cortisone is the drug of choice, synthetic analogs may be used in conjunction with mineralocorticoids where applicable; in infancy, mineralocorticoid supplementation is of particular importance).
   b. Acute adrenocortical insufficiency (hydrocortisone or cortisone is the drug of choice; mineralocorticoid supplementation may be necessary, particularly when synthetic analogs are used).
   c. Preoperatively and in the event of serious trauma or illness, in patients with known adrenal insufficiency or when adrenocortical reserve is doubtful.
   d. Shock unresponsive to conventional therapy if adrenocortical insufficiency exists or is suspected.
   e. Congenital adrenal hyperplasia.
   f. Hypercalcemia associated with cancer.
   g. Nonsuppurative thyroiditis.
2. **Rheumatic disorders**—As adjunctive therapy for short-term administration (to tide the patient over an acute episode or exacerbation) in:
   a. Post-traumatic osteoarthritis.
   b. Synovitis of osteoarthritis.
   c. Rheumatoid arthritis, including juvenile rheumatoid arthritis (selected cases may require low-dose maintenance therapy).
   d. Acute and subacute bursitis.
   e. Epicondylitis.
   f. Acute nonspecific tenosynovitis.
   g. Acute gouty arthritis.
   h. Psoriatic arthritis.
   i. Ankylosing spondylitis.
3. **Collagen diseases** — During an exacerbation or as maintenance therapy in selected cases of:
   a. Systemic lupus erythematosus.
   b. Acute rheumatic carditis.
   c. Systemic dermatomyositis (polymyositis).
4. **Dermatologic diseases:**
   a. Severe erythema multiforme (Stevens-Johnson syndrome).
   b. Exfoliative dermatitis.
   c. Bullous dermatitis herpetiformis.
   d. Severe seborrheic dermatitis.
   e. Severe psoriasis.
   f. Pemphigus.
   g. Mycosis fungoides.
5. **Allergic states** — Control of severe or incapacitating allergic conditions intractable to adequate trials of conventional treatment in:
   a. Bronchial asthma.
   b. Contact dermatitis.
   c. Atopic dermatitis.
   d. Serum sickness.
   e. Seasonal or perennial allergic rhinitis.
   f. Drug hypersensitivity reactions.
   g. Urticarial transfusion reactions.
   h. Acute noninfectious laryngeal edema (epinephrine is the drug of first choice).
6. **Ophthalmic diseases** — Severe acute and chronic allergic and inflammatory processes involving the eye, such as:
   a. Herpes zoster ophthalmicus.
   b. Iritis, iridocyclitis.
   c. Chorioretinitis.
   d. Diffuse posterior uveitis and choroiditis.
   e. Optic neuritis.
   f. Sympathetic ophthalmia.
   g. Anterior segment inflammation.
   h. Allergic conjunctivitis.
   i. Allergic corneal marginal ulcers.
   j. Keratitis.
7. **Gastrointestinal diseases** — To tide the patient over a critical period of disease in:
   a. Ulcerative colitis — (Systemic therapy).
   b. Regional enteritis — (Systemic therapy).
8. **Respiratory diseases:**
   a. Symptomatic sarcoidosis.
   b. Berylliosis.
   c. Fulminating or disseminated pulmonary tuberculosis when concurrently accompanied by appropriate antituberculous chemotherapy.
   d. Aspiration pneumonitis.
   e. Loeffler's syndrome not manageable by other means.
9. **Hematologic disorders:**
   a. Acquired (autoimmune) hemolytic anemia.
   b. Idiopathic thrombocytopenic purpura in adults (IV only; IM administration is contraindicated).
   c. Secondary thrombocytopenia in adults.
   d. Erythroblastopenia (RBC anemia).
   e. Congenital (erythroid) hypoplastic anemia.
10. **Neoplastic diseases** — For palliative management of:
   a. Leukemias and lymphomas in adults.
   b. Acute leukemia of childhood.
11. **Edematous state** — To induce diuresis or remission of proteinuria in the nephrotic syndrome, without uremia, of the idiopathic type or that due to lupus erythematosus.
12. **Nervous System:**
   a. Acute exacerbations of multiple sclerosis.
13. **Miscellaneous:**
   a. Tuberculous meningitis with subarachnoid block or impending block when used concurrently with appropriate antituberculous chemotherapy.
   b. Trichinosis with neurologic or myocardial involvement.

CONTRAINDICATIONS

Systemic fungal infections.

Not for use in newborns. Benzyl alcohol, a preservative in the Bacteriostatic Water for Injection provided with these products, has been associated with toxicity in newborns. Data are unavailable on the toxicity of other preservatives in this age group.

WARNINGS

In patients on corticosteroid therapy subjected to any unusual stress, increased dosage of rapidly acting corticosteroids before, during, and after the stressful situation is indicated.

Corticosteroids may mask some signs of infection, and new infections may appear during their use. There may be decreased resistance and inability to localize infection when corticosteroids are used.

Prolonged use of corticosteroids may produce posterior subcapsular cataracts, glaucoma with possible damage to the optic nerves, and may enhance the establishment of secondary ocular infections due to fungi or viruses.

Average and large doses of cortisone or hydrocortisone can cause elevation of blood pressure, salt and water retention, and increased excretion of potassium. These effects are less likely to occur with the synthetic derivatives except when used in large doses. Dietary salt restriction and potassium supplementation may be necessary. All corticosteroids increase calcium excretion.

While on corticosteroid therapy patients should not be vaccinated against smallpox. Other immunization procedures should not be undertaken in patients who are on corticosteroids, especially on high dose, because of possible hazards of neurological complications and a lack of antibody response.

The use of A-METHAPRED (methylprednisolone sodium succinate) in active tuberculosis should be restricted to those cases of fulminating or disseminated tuberculosis in which the corticosteroid is used for the management of the disease in conjunction with appropriate antituberculous regimen.

If corticosteroids are indicated in patients with latent tuberculosis or tuberculin reactivity, close observation is necessary as reactivation of the disease may occur. During prolonged corticosteroid therapy, these patients should receive chemoprophylaxis.

Because rare instances of anaphylactoid reactions have occurred in patients receiving parenteral corticosteroid therapy, appropriate precautionary measures should be taken prior to administration, especially when the patient has a history of allergy to any drug.

There are reports of cardiac arrhythmias and/or circulatory collapse and/or cardiac arrest following the rapid administration of large IV doses of methylprednisolone sodium succinate (greater than 0.5 gram administered over a period of less than 10 minutes).

USAGE IN PREGNANCY

Since adequate human reproduction studies have not been done with corticosteroids, the use of these drugs in pregnancy, nursing mothers, or women of childbearing potential requires that the possible benefits of the drug be weighed against the potential hazards to the mother and embryo or fetus. Infants born of mothers who have received substantial doses of corticosteroids during pregnancy should be carefully observed for signs of hypoadrenalism.

PRECAUTIONS

Drug-induced secondary adrenocortical insufficiency may be minimized by gradual reduction of dosage. This type of relative insufficiency may persist for months after discontinua-

Continued on next page

Abbott—Cont.

tion of therapy; therefore, in any situation of stress occurring during that period, hormone therapy should be reinstituted. Since mineralocorticoid secretion may be impaired, salt and/or a mineralocorticoid should be administered concurrently.
There is an enhanced effect of corticosteroids on patients with hypothyroidism and in those with cirrhosis.
Corticosteroids should be used cautiously in patients with ocular herpes simplex because of possible corneal perforation.
The lowest possible dose of corticosteroid should be used to control the condition under treatment, and when reduction in dosage is possible, the reduction should be gradual.
Psychic derangements may appear when corticosteroids are used, ranging from euphoria, insomnia, mood swings, personality changes and severe depression, to frank psychotic manifestations. Also, existing emotional instability or psychotic tendencies may be aggravated by corticosteroids.
Aspirin should be used cautiously in conjunction with corticosteroids in hypoprothrombinemia.
Steroids should be used with caution in nonspecific ulcerative colitis, if there is a probability of impending perforation, abscess or other pyogenic infection; diverticulitis; fresh intestinal anastomoses; active or latent peptic ulcer; renal insufficiency; hypertension; osteoporosis, and myasthenia gravis.
Growth and development of infants and children on prolonged corticosteroid therapy should be carefully observed.
Although controlled clinical trials have shown corticosteroids to be effective in speeding the resolution of acute exacerbations of multiple sclerosis, they do not show that corticosteroids affect the ultimate outcome or natural history of the disease. The studies do show that relatively high doses of corticosteroids are necessary to demonstrate a significant effect. (See "Dosage and Administration" section).
Since complications of treatment with glucocorticoids are dependent on the size of the dose and the duration of treatment, a risk/benefit decision must be made in each individual case as to dose and duration of treatment and as to whether daily or intermittent therapy should be used.

ADVERSE REACTIONS

Fluid and Electrolyte Disturbances
- Sodium retention
- Fluid retention
- Congestive heart failure in susceptible patients
- Potassium loss
- Hypokalemic alkalosis
- Hypertension

Musculoskeletal
- Muscle weakness
- Steroid myopathy
- Loss of muscle mass
- Severe arthralgia
- Osteoporosis
- Vertebral compression fractures
- Aseptic necrosis of femoral and humeral heads
- Pathologic fracture of long bones

Gastrointestinal
- Peptic ulcer with possible perforation and hemorrhage
- Pancreatitis
- Abdominal distention
- Ulcerative esophagitis

Dermatologic
- Impaired wound healing
- Thin fragile skin
- Petechiae and ecchymoses
- Facial erythema
- Increased sweating
- May suppress reactions to skin tests

Neurological
- Increased intracranial pressure with papilledema (pseudo-tumor cerebri) usually after treatment
- Convulsions
- Vertigo
- Headache

Endocrine
- Development of Cushingoid state
- Suppression of growth in children
- Secondary adrenocortical and pituitary unresponsiveness particularly in times of stress, as in trauma, surgery or illness
- Menstrual irregularities
- Decreased carbohydrate tolerance
- Manifestations of latent diabetes mellitus
- Increased requirements for insulin or oral hypoglycemic agents in diabetics

Ophthalmic
- Posterior subcapsular cataracts
- Increased intraocular pressure
- Glaucoma
- Exophthalmos

Metabolic
- Negative nitrogen balance due to protein catabolism

The following additional adverse reactions are related to parenteral corticosteroid therapy:
- Hyperpigmentation or hypopigmentation
- Subcutaneous and cutaneous atrophy
- Sterile abscess
- Anaphylactic reaction with or without circulatory collapse, cardiac arrest, bronchospasm
- Urticaria
- Nausea and vomiting
- Cardiac arrhythmias, hypotension or hypertension

DOSAGE AND ADMINISTRATION

When high dose therapy is desired, the recommended dose of methylprednisolone as the sodium succinate is 30 mg/kg administered intravenously over a 10 to 20-minute period. This dose may be repeated every 4 to 6 hours. In general, high dose corticosteroid therapy should be continued only until the patient's condition has stabilized, usually not beyond 48 to 72 hours.
Although adverse effects associated with high dose short-term corticoid therapy are uncommon, peptic ulceration may occur. Prophylactic antacid therapy may be indicated.
In other indications initial dosage will vary from 10 to 40 mg of methylprednisolone depending on the clinical problem being treated. The larger doses may be required for short-term management of severe, acute conditions. The initial dose usually should be given intravenously over a period of one to several minutes. Subsequent doses may be given intravenously or intramuscularly at intervals dictated by the patient's response and clinical condition. Corticoid therapy is an adjunct to, and not replacement for conventional therapy.
Dosage may be reduced for infants and children but should be governed more by the severity of the condition and response of the patient than by age or size. It should not be less than 0.5 mg/kg every 24 hours.
Dosage must be decreased or discontinued gradually when the drug has been administered for more than a few days. If a period of spontaneous remission occurs in a chronic condition, treatment should be discontinued. Routine laboratory studies, such as urinalysis, two-hour postprandial blood sugar, determination of blood pressure and body weight, and a chest X-ray should be made at regular intervals during prolonged therapy. Upper GI X-rays are desirable in patients with an ulcer history or significant dyspepsia.
Methylprednisolone may be administered intravenously by direct push, or by intermittent or continuous infusion; or by intramuscular injection. The preferred method for initial emergency use is either direct I.V. push or intermittent infusion. To administer by intravenous (or intramuscular) injection, prepare solution as directed. The desired dose may be administered intravenously over a period of one to several minutes (for doses of 40 mg or less).
Multiple Sclerosis: In treatment of acute exacerbations of multiple sclerosis, daily doses of 200 mg of prednisolone for a week followed by 80 mg every other day for 1 month have been shown to be effective (4 mg of methylprednisolone is equivalent to 5 mg of prednisolone).

PREPARATION OF UNIVIAL SOLUTIONS

1. Remove protective cap, give the plunger-stopper a quarter turn and press to force diluent into the lower compartment.
2. Agitate immediately to effect solution. With the 1000 mg Univial, for best results, shake continuously for a minimum of 45 seconds before inspecting solution. If necessary, continue shaking to effect complete solution. The Univial should be agitated in a manner which insures mixing throughout both compartments.
3. Use solutions in 40 mg and 125 mg Univials within 48 hours. Use solutions in 500 mg and 1000 mg Univials within 72 hours.
4. Sterilize top of plunger-stopper with a suitable germicide.
5. Insert needle squarely through center of plunger-stopper until tip is just visible. Withdraw dose.

Storage: After mixing, store solution below 86°F; avoid freezing. Refrigeration not required.
For Intravenous Infusion:
To prepare solutions for intravenous infusion, first prepare the solution for injection as directed. This solution may then be added to indicated amounts of 5% Dextrose Injection, 0.9% Sodium Chloride Injection, USP or 5% Dextrose and 0.9% Sodium Chloride Injection, USP.

HOW SUPPLIED

Sterile A-METHAPRED (methylprednisolone sodium succinate for injection, USP) is available in the following packages:
40 mg/ml Univial **NDC** 0074-5684-01;
125 mg/2 ml Univial **NDC** 0074-5685-02;
500 mg/4 ml Univial **NDC** 0074-5630-04;
1000 mg/8 ml Univial **NDC** 0074-5631-08.
Exposure of pharmaceutical products to heat should be minimized. Avoid excessive heat. Protect from freezing. It is recommended that unreconstituted product be stored below 86°F (30°C); however, brief exposure up to 104°F (40°C) does not adversely affect the product. Protect from light.
Abbott Laboratories
North Chicago, IL 60064
Ref. 01-2331-R1

BUTESIN® PICRATE Ointment

[*bū 'ti-sin pick 'rate*]
(butamben picrate)

DESCRIPTION

Butesin Picrate is an anesthetic ointment containing Butesin Picrate (Butamben Picrate), 1%.
Inactive Ingredients: Anhydrous lanolin, ceresin wax, methylparaben, mineral oil, mixed triglycerides, potassium chloride, propylparaben, sodium borate, water, white wax and other ingredients.

INDICATION

For temporary relief of pain due to minor burns.

WARNING

Certain persons, due to idiosyncrasy, are sensitive to this ointment and may develop a rash following its application. In such cases its use should be discontinued, and the ointment remaining on the skin removed with soap and water.

PRECAUTIONS

Should not be applied repeatedly or to large areas except under a physician's instructions. As Butesin Picrate stains cannot be removed from animal fibers, contact with silk or wool fabrics and hair should be avoided.

DOSAGE AND ADMINISTRATION

Spread thinly on painful or denuded lesions of the skin, if these are small. Apply a loose bandage to protect the clothing.

HOW SUPPLIED

1 oz tube (**NDC** 0074-4392-01).
Abbott Laboratories
North Chicago, IL 60064
Ref. 09-5975-3/R5

CALCIDRINE® SYRUP ℞ Ⓒ

[*cal 'si-drīne*]

DESCRIPTION

Calcidrine is an oral antitussive, expectorant syrup. Each 5 ml (teaspoonful) contains Codeine, USP, 8.4 mg, (Warning—May be habit forming); Calcium Iodide, anhydrous 152 mg. The chemical formula for calcium iodide is CaI_2. Codeine is methylmorphine, a natural alkaloid of opium. The chemical formula for codeine is $C_{18}H_{21}NO_3 \cdot H_2O$.

INACTIVE INGREDIENTS

Alcohol 6%, FD&C Yellow No. 6, glycerin, liquid glucose, sucrose, water, natural and artificial flavors and other ingredients to form a palatable syrup.

CLINICAL PHARMACOLOGY

The major effects of codeine in man are on the central nervous system. The antitussive effect is produced by depression of the cough reflex. Codeine is rapidly absorbed from the gastrointestinal tract and is metabolized in the liver.
Iodides are readily absorbed from the gastrointestinal tract and are distributed to extracellular fluid as well as gastric and salivary secretions. Iodides are accumulated by the thyroid gland. Excretion occurs mainly through the kidneys.

INDICATIONS AND USAGE

In adults and children as an expectorant, and for symptomatic relief of coughs.

CONTRAINDICATIONS

Calcidrine should not be used in patients with a history of iodism, or with known hypersensitivity to iodides or codeine. Long-term use of iodide-containing preparations is contraindicated during pregnancy.

WARNINGS

Physiological dependence may develop with the use of codeine.
Usage During Pregnancy: Calcidrine Syrup can cause fetal harm when administered to a pregnant woman. Maternal ingestion of large amounts of iodides during pregnancy has been associated with development of fetal goiter and resultant acute respiratory distress of the neonate. If this drug is used during pregnancy, or if the patient becomes pregnant while taking this drug, the patient should be apprised of the potential hazard to the fetus.

Severe and occasionally fatal skin eruptions have been reported rarely in patients receiving prolonged administration of iodides.

PRECAUTIONS

Laboratory Tests: Patients who must receive prolonged iodide therapy should be evaluated periodically for possible depression of thyroid function.

Drug Interactions: The concurrent administration of calcium iodide and lithium carbonate may enhance the hypothyroid and goitrogenic effects of either drug.

Laboratory Test Interactions: Elevated values may be obtained on thyroid function tests or protein-bound iodine tests when iodide-containing compounds have been ingested. False positive results may be obtained if iodides have been ingested prior to guaiac or benzidine testing.

Carcinogenesis: No data is available on long-term carcinogenicity in animals or humans.

Pregnancy: Pregnancy Category D. See "WARNINGS" section.

Nursing Mothers: Iodine is excreted in breast milk. Caution should be exercised when Calcidrine is administered to a nursing woman.

ADVERSE REACTIONS

In decreasing order of severity: severe and sometimes fatal skin eruptions (ioderma) occur rarely after the prolonged use of iodides. Iodism can occur. Symptoms of iodism include metallic taste, acneform skin lesions, mucous membrane irritation, salivary gland swelling, and gastric distress. These side effects subside quickly upon discontinuance of the iodide-containing drug.

Codeine may produce vomiting, nausea, and constipation.

OVERDOSAGE

Symptoms of acute codeine poisoning include respiratory and central nervous system depression, pinpoint pupils and coma. Blood pressure and body temperature may fall.

Acute iodide poisoning is associated with gastrointestinal irritation. Angioedema with laryngeal swelling may develop. Shock may also occur.

Treatment for overdose of Calcidrine is:

a. Establish a patent airway and ventilate if needed. b. Gastric evacuation. c. Treatment for shock. d. General supportive measures including replacement of fluids and electrolytes may be indicated. e. The use of naloxone to antagonize the narcotic depression of the central nervous system should be considered.

DOSAGE AND ADMINISTRATION

Adults and children over ten years of age, usual dose, 1 to 2 teaspoonfuls every 4 hours. Children 6 to 10 years of age, ½ to 1 teaspoonful every 4 hours. Children 2 to 6 years of age, ½ teaspoonful every 4 hours.

HOW SUPPLIED

Orange-colored syrup in 4 fl oz (**NDC** 0074-5763-04) and pint (**NDC** 0074-5763-16) bottles.

Calcidrine must be dispensed in USP tight, light-resistant glass containers.

Abbott Laboratories
North Chicago, IL 60064
Ref. 02-6645-2/R7

CEFOL® Filmtab® Tablets ℞

[*c'full*]

(B-Complex, folic acid, vitamin E with 750 mg vitamin C)

DESCRIPTION

Each oral Cefol Filmtab vitamin tablet provides:

Ascorbic Acid (C)	750 mg
Niacinamide	100 mg
Calcium Pantothenate	20 mg
Thiamine Mononitrate (B_1)	15 mg
Riboflavin (B_2)	10 mg
Pyridoxine Hydrochloride (B_6)	5 mg
Folic Acid	500 mcg
Cyanocobalamin (B_{12})	6 mcg
Vitamin E (as dl-alpha tocopheryl acetate)	30 IU

INACTIVE INGREDIENTS

Cellulosic polymers, colloidal silicon dioxide, corn starch, D&C Yellow No. 10, FD&C Blue No. 1, magnesium stearate, microcrystalline cellulose, polyethylene glycol, povidone, propylene glycol, titanium dioxide, vanillin and other ingredients.

CLINICAL PHARMACOLOGY

The vitamin components of Cefol are absorbed by the active transport process. All but Vitamin E are rapidly eliminated and not stored in the body. Vitamin E is stored in body tissues.

INDICATIONS AND USAGE

Cefol is indicated in non-pregnant* adults for the treatment of Vitamin C deficiency states with an associated deficient intake or increased need for Vitamin B-Complex, Folic Acid, and Vitamin E.

*Pregnancy may require greater Folic Acid intake.

CONTRAINDICATIONS

Rare hypersensitivity to Folic Acid.

WARNINGS

Folic Acid alone is improper treatment of pernicious anemia and other megaloblastic anemias where Vitamin B_{12} is deficient.

PRECAUTIONS

Folic Acid above 0.1 mg daily may obscure pernicious anemia (hematologic remission may occur while neurological manifestations remain progressive).

ADVERSE REACTIONS

Allergic sensitization has been reported following oral and parenteral administration of Folic Acid.

DOSAGE

Usual adult dose is one tablet daily.

HOW SUPPLIED

Cefol is supplied as green Filmtab tablets in bottles of 100 (NDC 0074-6089-13).

Filmtab—Film-sealed tablets, Abbott.

Shown in Product Identification Section, page 403

Abbott Pharmaceuticals, Inc.
North Chicago, IL 60064
Ref. 03-1305-2/R15

CHLORTHALIDONE Tablets, USP ℞

[*clor-thal'i-dōne*]

HOW SUPPLIED

Abbott Chlorthalidone Tablets, USP are available as scored tablets in two dosage strengths:

25 mg, peach-colored:
Bottles of 100 (**NDC** 0074-4325-13).
50 mg, lavender-colored:
Bottles of 100 (**NDC** 0074-4338-13).
Bottles of 500 (**NDC** 0074-4338-53).

Shown in Product Identification Section, page 403

CYLERT® Tablets ℞ Ⓒ

[*cī'lert*]

(Pemoline)

DESCRIPTION

CYLERT (pemoline) is a central nervous system stimulant. Pemoline is structurally dissimilar to the amphetamines and methylphenidate.

It is an oxazolidine compound and is chemically identified as 2-amino-5-phenyl-2-oxazolin-4-one.

Pemoline is a white, tasteless, odorless powder, relatively insoluble (less than 1 mg/ml) in water, chloroform, ether, acetone, and benzene; its solubility in 95% ethyl alcohol is 2.2 mg/ml.

CYLERT (pemoline) is supplied as tablets containing 18.75 mg, 37.5 mg or 75 mg of pemoline for oral administration. CYLERT is also available as chewable tablets containing 37.5 mg of pemoline.

INACTIVE INGREDIENTS

18.75 mg tablet: corn starch, gelatin, lactose, magnesium hydroxide, polyethylene glycol, talc and other ingredients.

37.5 mg tablet: corn starch, FD&C Yellow No. 6, gelatin, lactose, magnesium hydroxide, polyethylene glycol, talc and other ingredients.

37.5 mg chewable tablet: corn starch, FD&C Yellow No. 6, magnesium hydroxide, magnesium stearate, mannitol, polyethylene glycol, povidone, talc, artificial flavor and other ingredients.

75 mg tablet: corn starch, gelatin, iron oxide, lactose, magnesium hydroxide, polyethylene glycol, talc and other ingredients.

CLINICAL PHARMACOLOGY

CYLERT (pemoline) has a pharmacological activity similar to that of other known central nervous system stimulants; however, it has minimal sympathomimetic effects. Although studies indicate that pemoline may act in animals through dopaminergic mechanisms, the exact mechanism and site of action of the drug in man is not known.

There is neither specific evidence which clearly establishes the mechanism whereby CYLERT produces its mental and behavioral effects in children, nor conclusive evidence regarding how these effects relate to the condition of the central nervous system.

Pemoline is rapidly absorbed from the gastrointestinal tract. Approximately 50% is bound to plasma proteins. The serum half-life of pemoline is approximately 12 hours. Peak serum levels of the drug occur within 2 to 4 hours after ingestion of a single dose. Multiple dose studies in adults at several dose levels indicate that steady state is reached in approximately 2 to 3 days. In animals given radiolabeled pemoline, the drug was widely and uniformly distributed throughout the tissues, including the brain.

Pemoline is metabolized by the liver. Metabolites of pemoline include pemoline conjugate, pemoline dione, mandelic acid, and unidentified polar compounds. CYLERT is excreted primarily by the kidneys with approximately 50% excreted unchanged and only minor fractions present as metabolites.

CYLERT (pemoline) has a gradual onset of action. Using the recommended schedule of dosage titration, significant clinical benefit may not be evident until the third or fourth week of drug administration.

INDICATIONS AND USAGE

CYLERT (pemoline) is indicated in Attention Deficit Disorder (ADD) with hyperactivity as an integral part of a total treatment program which typically includes other remedial measures (psychological, educational, social) for a stabilizing effect in children with a behavioral syndrome characterized by the following group of developmentally inappropriate symptoms: moderate to severe distractibility, short attention span, hyperactivity, emotional lability, and impulsivity. The diagnosis of this syndrome should not be made with finality when these symptoms are only of comparatively recent origin. Nonlocalizing (soft) neurological signs, learning disability, and abnormal EEG may or may not be present, and a diagnosis of central nervous system dysfunction may or may not be warranted.

CONTRAINDICATIONS

CYLERT (pemoline) is contraindicated in patients with known hypersensitivity or idiosyncrasy to the drug. CYLERT should not be administered to patients with impaired hepatic function. (See "ADVERSE REACTIONS" section.)

WARNINGS

Decrements in the predicted growth (i.e., weight gain and/or height) rate have been reported with the long-term use of stimulants in children. Therefore, patients requiring long-term therapy should be carefully monitored.

PRECAUTIONS

General: Clinical experience suggests that in psychotic children, administration of CYLERT may exacerbate symptoms of behavior disturbance and thought disorder.

CYLERT should be administered with caution to patients with significantly impaired renal function.

Laboratory Tests: Liver function tests should be performed prior to and periodically during therapy with CYLERT. The drug should be discontinued if abnormalities are revealed and confirmed by follow-up tests. (See "ADVERSE REACTIONS" section regarding reports of abnormal liver function tests, hepatitis and jaundice.)

Drug Interactions: The interaction of CYLERT (pemoline) with other drugs has not been studied in humans. Patients who are receiving CYLERT concurrently with other drugs, especially drugs with CNS activity, should be monitored carefully.

Decreased seizure threshold has been reported in patients receiving CYLERT concomitantly with *antiepileptic medications.*

Carcinogenesis: Long-term studies have been conducted in rats with doses as high as 150 mg/kg/day for eighteen months. There was no significant difference in the incidence of any neoplasm between treated and control animals.

Mutagenesis: Data are not available concerning long-term effects on mutagenicity in animals or humans.

Impairment of Fertility: The results of studies in which rats were given 18.75 and 37.5 mg/kg/day indicated that pemoline did not affect fertility in males or females at those doses.

Pregnancy: Teratogenic effects: Pregnancy Category B. Reproduction studies have been performed in rats and rabbits at doses of 18.75 and 37.5 mg/kg/day and have revealed no evidence of impaired fertility or harm to the fetus. There are, however, no adequate and well-controlled studies in pregnant women. Because animal reproduction studies are not always predictive of human response, this drug should be used during pregnancy only if clearly needed.

Nonteratogenic effects: Studies in rats have shown an increased incidence of stillbirths and cannibalization when pemoline was administered at a dose of 37.5 mg/kg/day. Postnatal survival of offspring was reduced at doses of 18.75 and 37.5 mg/kg/day.

Nursing Mothers: It is not known whether this drug is excreted in human milk. Because many drugs are excreted in human milk, caution should be exercised when CYLERT is administered to a nursing woman.

Pediatric Use: Safety and effectiveness in children below the age of 6 years have not been established.

Long-term effects of CYLERT in children have not been established (See "WARNINGS" section).

Continued on next page

Abbott—Cont.

CNS stimulants, including pemoline, have been reported to precipitate motor and phonic tics and Tourette's syndrome. Therefore, clinical evaluation for tics and Tourette's syndrome in children and their families should precede use of stimulant medications.
Drug treatment is not indicated in all cases of ADD with hyperactivity and should be considered only in light of complete history and evaluation of the child. The decision to prescribe CYLERT (pemoline) should depend on the physician's assessment of the chronicity and severity of the child's symptoms and their appropriateness for his/her age. Prescription should not depend solely on the presence of one or more of the behavioral characteristics.

ADVERSE REACTIONS

The following are adverse reactions in decreasing order of severity within each category associated with CYLERT:
Hepatic: There have been reports of hepatic dysfunction including elevated liver enzymes, hepatitis and jaundice in patients taking CYLERT. The occurrence of elevated liver enzymes is not rare and these reactions appear to be reversible upon drug discontinuance. Most patients with elevated liver enzymes were asymptomatic. Although no causal relationship has been established, two hepatic-related fatalities have been reported involving patients taking CYLERT.
Hematopoietic: There have been isolated reports of aplastic anemia.
Central Nervous System: The following CNS effects have been reported with the use of CYLERT: convulsive seizures; literature reports indicate that CYLERT may precipitate attacks of Gilles de la Tourette syndrome; hallucinations; dyskinetic movements of the tongue, lips, face and extremities; abnormal oculomotor function including nystagmus and oculogyric crisis; mild depression; dizziness; increased irritability; headache; and drowsiness.
Insomnia is the most frequently reported side effect of CYLERT; it usually occurs early in therapy prior to an optimum therapeutic response. In the majority of cases it is transient in nature or responds to a reduction in dosage.
Gastrointestinal: Anorexia and weight loss may occur during the first weeks of therapy. In the majority of cases it is transient in nature; weight gain usually resumes within three to six months.
Nausea and stomach ache have also been reported.
Miscellaneous: Suppression of growth has been reported with the long-term use of stimulants in children. (See "WARNINGS" section.) Skin rash has been reported with CYLERT.
Mild adverse reactions appearing early during the course of treatment with CYLERT often remit with continuing therapy. If adverse reactions are of a significant or protracted nature, dosage should be reduced or the drug discontinued.

DRUG ABUSE AND DEPENDENCE

Controlled Substance: CYLERT is subject to control under DEA schedule IV.
Abuse: CYLERT failed to demonstrate a potential for self-administration in primates. However, the pharmacologic similarity of pemoline to other psychostimulants with known dependence liability suggests that psychological and/or physical dependence might also occur with CYLERT. There have been isolated reports of transient psychotic symptoms occurring in adults following the long-term misuse of excessive oral doses of pemoline. CYLERT should be given with caution to emotionally unstable patients who may increase the dosage on their own initiative.

OVERDOSAGE

Signs and symptoms of acute overdosage, resulting principally from overstimulation of the central nervous system and from excessive sympathomimetic effects, may include the following: vomiting, agitation, tremors, hyperreflexia, muscle twitching, convulsions (may be followed by coma), euphoria, confusion, hallucinations, delirium, sweating, flushing, headache, hyperpyrexia, tachycardia, hypertension and mydriasis. Treatment consists of appropriate supportive measures. The patient must be protected against self-injury and against external stimuli that would aggravate overstimulation already present. If signs and symptoms are not too severe and the patient is conscious, gastric contents may be evacuated. Chlorpromazine has been reported in the literature to be useful in decreasing CNS stimulation and sympathomimetic effects.
Efficacy of peritoneal dialysis or extracorporeal hemodialysis for CYLERT overdosage has not been established.

DOSAGE AND ADMINISTRATION

CYLERT (pemoline) is administered as a single oral dose each morning. The recommended starting dose is 37.5 mg/day. This daily dose should be gradually increased by 18.75 mg at one week intervals until the desired clinical response is obtained. The effective daily dose for most patients will range from 56.25 to 75 mg. The maximum recommended daily dose of pemoline is 112.5 mg.
Clinical improvement with CYLERT is gradual. Using the recommended schedule of dosage titration, significant benefit may not be evident until the third or fourth week of drug administration.
Where possible, drug administration should be interrupted occasionally to determine if there is a recurrence of behavioral symptoms sufficient to require continued therapy.

HOW SUPPLIED

CYLERT (pemoline) is supplied as monogrammed, grooved tablets in three dosage strengths:
18.75 mg tablets (white) in bottles of 100 (**NDC** 0074-6025-13)
37.5 mg tablets (orange-colored) in bottles of 100 (**NDC** 0074-6057-13)
75 mg tablets (tan-colored) in bottles of 100 (**NDC** 0074-6073-13)
CYLERT (pemoline) Chewable is supplied as 37.5 mg monogrammed, grooved tablets (orange-colored) in bottles of 100 (**NDC** 0074-6088-13)

Shown in Product Identification Section, page 403

Abbott Pharmaceuticals, Inc.
North Chicago, IL 60064

DAYALETS® Filmtab®

[*dāy 'a-lets*]
Multivitamin Supplement for adults and children 4 or more years of age

DAYALETS® PLUS IRON Filmtab®

Multivitamin Supplement with Iron for adults and children 4 or more years of age

(See PDR For Nonprescription Drugs)

DEPAKENE® Capsules and Syrup ℞

[*dep 'a-kāne*]
(Valproic Acid)

> **WARNING**
> HEPATIC FAILURE RESULTING IN FATALITIES HAS OCCURRED IN PATIENTS RECEIVING DEPAKENE. EXPERIENCE HAS INDICATED THAT CHILDREN UNDER THE AGE OF TWO YEARS ARE AT A CONSIDERABLY INCREASED RISK OF DEVELOPING FATAL HEPATOTOXICITY. ESPECIALLY THOSE ON MULTIPLE ANTICONVULSANTS, THOSE WITH CONGENITAL METABOLIC DISORDERS, THOSE WITH SEVERE SEIZURE DISORDERS ACCOMPANIED BY MENTAL RETARDATION, AND THOSE WITH ORGANIC BRAIN DISEASE. WHEN DEPAKENE IS USED IN THIS PATIENT GROUP, IT SHOULD BE USED WITH EXTREME CAUTION AND AS A SOLE AGENT. THE BENEFITS OF SEIZURE CONTROL SHOULD BE WEIGHED AGAINST THE RISKS ABOVE THIS AGE GROUP. EXPERIENCE HAS INDICATED THAT THE INCIDENCE OF FATAL HEPATOTOXICITY DECREASES CONSIDERABLY IN PROGRESSIVELY OLDER PATIENT GROUPS. THESE INCIDENTS USUALLY HAVE OCCURRED DURING THE FIRST SIX MONTHS OF TREATMENT WITH DEPAKENE. SERIOUS OR FATAL HEPATOTOXICITY MAY BE PRECEDED BY NON-SPECIFIC SYMPTOMS SUCH AS LOSS OF SEIZURE CONTROL, MALAISE, WEAKNESS, LETHARGY, FACIAL EDEMA, ANOREXIA AND VOMITING. PATIENTS SHOULD BE MONITORED CLOSELY FOR APPEARANCE OF THESE SYMPTOMS. LIVER FUNCTION TESTS SHOULD BE PERFORMED PRIOR TO THERAPY AND AT FREQUENT INTERVALS THEREAFTER. ESPECIALLY DURING THE FIRST SIX MONTHS.

DESCRIPTION

DEPAKENE (valproic acid) is a carboxylic acid designated as 2-propylpentanoic acid. It is also known as dipropylacetic acid.
Valproic acid (pKa 4.8) has a molecular weight of 144 and occurs as a colorless liquid with a characteristic odor. It is slightly soluble in water (1.3 mg/ml) and very soluble in organic solvents.
DEPAKENE is supplied as soft elastic capsules and syrup for oral administration. Each capsule contains 250 mg valproic acid. The syrup contains the equivalent of 250 mg valproic acid per 5 ml as the sodium salt.

INACTIVE INGREDIENTS

250 mg capsules: corn oil, FD&C Yellow No. 6, gelatin, glycerin, iron oxide, methylparaben, propylparaben, titanium dioxide, and other ingredients.
Syrup: FD&C Red No. 40, glycerin, methylparaben, propylparaben, sorbitol, sucrose, water, natural and artificial flavors, and other ingredients.

CLINICAL PHARMACOLOGY

DEPAKENE is an antiepileptic agent which is chemically unrelated to other drugs used to treat seizure disorders. It has no nitrogen or aromatic moiety characteristic of other antiepileptic drugs. The mechanism by which DEPAKENE exerts its antiepileptic effects has not been established. It has been suggested that its activity is related to increased brain levels of gamma-aminobutyric acid (GABA). The effect on the neuronal membrane is unknown.
DEPAKENE is rapidly absorbed after oral administration. Peak serum levels of valproic acid occur approximately one to four hours after a single oral dose of DEPAKENE. The serum half-life of the parent compound is typically in the range of six to sixteen hours. Half-lives in the lower part of the above range are usually found in patients taking other antiepileptic drugs. A slight delay in absorption occurs when the drug is administered with meals but this does not affect the total absorption.
Valproic acid is rapidly distributed and at therapeutic drug concentrations, drug is highly bound (90%) to human plasma proteins. Increases in dose may result in decreases in the extent of protein binding and variable changes in valproate clearance and elimination.
Elimination of DEPAKENE and its metabolites occurs principally in the urine, with minor amounts in the feces and expired air. Very little unmetabolized parent drug is excreted in the urine. The drug is primarily metabolized in the liver and is excreted as the glucuronide conjugate. Other metabolites in the urine are products of beta, omega-1, and omega oxidation (C-3, C-4, and C-5 positions). The major oxidative metabolite in the urine is 2-propyl-3-keto-pentanoic acid; minor metabolites are 2-propyl-glutaric acid, 2-propyl-5-hydroxypentanoic acid, 2-propyl-3-hydroxypentanoic acid and 2-propyl-4-hydroxypentanoic acid.

INDICATIONS

DEPAKENE (valproic acid) is indicated for use as sole and adjunctive therapy in the treatment of simple (petit mal) and complex absence seizures. DEPAKENE may also be used adjunctively in patients with multiple seizure types which include absence seizures.
In accordance with the International Classification of Seizures, simple absence is defined as very brief clouding of the sensorium or loss of consciousness (lasting usually 2–15 seconds), accompanied by certain generalized epileptic discharges without other detectable clinical signs. Complex absence is the term used when other signs are also present.
SEE "WARNINGS" SECTION FOR STATEMENT REGARDING FATAL HEPATIC DYSFUNCTION.

CONTRAINDICATIONS

DEPAKENE (VALPROIC ACID) SHOULD NOT BE ADMINISTERED TO PATIENTS WITH HEPATIC DISEASE OR SIGNIFICANT DYSFUNCTION.
DEPAKENE is contraindicated in patients with known hypersensitivity to the drug.

WARNINGS

Hepatic failure resulting in fatalities has occurred in patients receiving DEPAKENE. These incidents usually have occurred during the first six months of treatment with DEPAKENE. Serious or fatal hepatotoxicity may be preceded by non-specific symptoms such as loss of seizure control, malaise, weakness, lethargy, facial edema, anorexia and vomiting. Patients should be monitored closely for appearance of these symptoms. Liver function tests should be performed prior to therapy and at frequent intervals thereafter, especially during the first six months. However, physicians should not rely totally on serum biochemistry since these tests may not be abnormal in all instances, but should also consider the results of careful interim medical history and physical examination. Caution should be observed when administering DEPAKENE to patients with a prior history of hepatic disease. Patients on multiple anticonvulsants, children, those with congenital metabolic disorders, those with severe seizure disorders accompanied by mental retardation, and those with organic brain disease may be at particular risk. Experience has indicated that children under the age of two years are at considerably increased risk of developing fatal hepatotoxicity, especially those with the aforementioned conditions. When DEPAKENE is used in this patient group, it should be used with extreme caution and as a sole agent. The benefits of seizure control should be weighed against the risks. Above this age group, experience has indicated that the incidence of fatal hepatotoxicity decreases considerably in progressively older patient groups.
The drug should be discontinued immediately in the presence of significant hepatic dysfunction, suspected or apparent. In some cases, hepatic dysfunction has progressed in spite of discontinuation of drug.
The frequency of adverse effects (particularly elevated liver enzymes) may be dose-related. The benefit of improved seizure control which may accompany the higher doses should therefore be weighed against the possibility of a greater incidence of adverse effects.

Recommended Initial Dosages for Depakene

Weight (kg)	Weight (lb)	Total Daily Dose (mg)	Number of Capsules or Teaspoonfuls of Syrup: Dose 1	Dose 2	Dose 3
10—24.9	22— 54.9	250	0	0	1
25—39.9	55— 87.9	500	1	0	1
40—59.9	88—131.9	750	1	1	1
60—74.9	132—164.9	1,000	1	1	2
75—89.9	165—197.9	1,250	2	1	2

Usage in Pregnancy: ACCORDING TO PUBLISHED AND UNPUBLISHED REPORTS DEPAKENE MAY PRODUCE TERATOGENIC EFFECTS IN THE OFFSPRING OF HUMAN FEMALES RECEIVING THE DRUG DURING PREGNANCY.

THERE ARE MULTIPLE REPORTS IN THE CLINICAL LITERATURE WHICH INDICATE THAT THE USE OF ANTIEPILEPTIC DRUGS DURING PREGNANCY RESULTS IN AN INCREASED INCIDENCE OF BIRTH DEFECTS IN THE OFFSPRING. ALTHOUGH DATA ARE MORE EXTENSIVE WITH RESPECT TO TRIMETHADIONE, PARAMETHADIONE, PHENYTOIN, AND PHENOBARBITAL, REPORTS INDICATE A POSSIBLE SIMILAR ASSOCIATION WITH THE USE OF OTHER ANTIEPILEPTIC DRUGS. THEREFORE, ANTIEPILEPTIC DRUGS SHOULD BE ADMINISTERED TO WOMEN OF CHILDBEARING POTENTIAL ONLY IF THEY ARE CLEARLY SHOWN TO BE ESSENTIAL IN THE MANAGEMENT OT THEIR SEIZURES.

THE INCIDENCE OF NEURAL TUBE DEFECTS IN THE FETUS MAY BE INCREASED IN MOTHERS RECEIVING VALPROATE DURING THE FIRST TRIMESTER OF PREGNANCY. THE CENTERS FOR DISEASE CONTROL (CDC) HAS ESTIMATED THE RISK OF VALPROIC ACID EXPOSED WOMEN HAVING CHILDREN WITH SPINA BIFIDA TO BE APPROXIMATELY 1 to 2%.[1] THIS RISK IS SIMILAR TO THAT FOR NONEPILEPTIC WOMEN WHO HAVE HAD CHILDREN WITH NEURAL TUBE DEFECTS (ANENCEPHALY AND SPINA BIFIDA).

ANIMAL STUDIES HAVE ALSO DEMONSTRATED DEPAKENE INDUCED TERATOGENICITY. Studies in rats and human females demonstrated placental transfer of the drug. Doses greater than 65 mg/kg/day given to pregnant rats and mice produced skeletal abnormalities in the offspring, primarily involving ribs and vertebrae; doses greater than 150 mg/kg/day given to pregnant rabbits produced fetal resorptions and (primarily) soft-tissue abnormalities in the offspring. In rats a dose-related delay in the onset of parturition was noted. Postnatal growth and survival of the progeny were adversely affected, particularly when drug administration spanned the entire gestation and early lactation period.

Antiepileptic drugs should not be discontinued in patients in whom the drug is administered to prevent major seizures because of the strong possibility of precipitating status epilepticus with attendant hypoxia and threat to life. In individual cases where the severity and frequency of the seizure disorder are such that the removal of medication does not pose a serious threat to the patient, discontinuation of the drug may be considered prior to and during pregnancy, although it cannot be said with any confidence that even minor seizures do not pose some hazard to the developing embryo or fetus.

The prescribing physician will wish to weigh these considerations in treating or counseling epileptic women of childbearing potential.

PRECAUTIONS

Hepatic dysfunction: See "Boxed Warning," "Contraindications" and "Warnings" sections.

General: Because of reports of thrombocytopenia, inhibition of the secondary phase of platelet aggregation, and abnormal coagulation parameters, platelet counts and coagulation tests are recommended before initiating therapy and at periodic intervals. It is recommended that patients receiving Depakene be monitored for platelet count and coagulation parameters prior to planned surgery. Evidence of hemorrhage, bruising or a disorder of hemostasis/coagulation is an indication for reduction of Depakene dosage or withdrawal of therapy.

Hyperammonemia with or without lethargy or coma has been reported and may be present in the absence of abnormal liver function tests. If clinically significant elevation occurs, Depakene should be discontinued.

Since Depakene (valproic acid) may interact with concurrently administered antiepileptic drugs, periodic serum level determinations of concomitant antiepileptic drugs are recommended during the early course of therapy. (See "Drug Interactions" section.)

Depakene is partially eliminated in the urine as a keto-metabolite which may lead to a false interpretation of the urine ketone test.

There have been reports of altered thyroid function tests associated with Depakene. The clinical significance of these is unknown.

Information for Patients: Since Depakene may produce CNS depression, especially when combined with another CNS depressant (e.g., alcohol), patients should be advised not to engage in hazardous occupations, such as driving an automobile or operating dangerous machinery, until it is known that they do not become drowsy from the drug.

Drug Interactions: Depakene may potentiate the CNS depressant activity of alcohol.

The concomitant administration of valproic acid with drugs that exhibit extensive protein binding (e.g., aspirin, carbamazepine, and dicumarol) may result in alteration of serum drug levels.

THERE IS EVIDENCE THAT DEPAKENE CAN CAUSE AN INCREASE IN SERUM PHENOBARBITAL LEVELS BY IMPAIRMENT OF NONRENAL CLEARANCE. THIS PHENOMENON CAN RESULT IN SEVERE CNS DEPRESSION. THE COMBINATION OF DEPAKENE AND PHENOBARBITAL HAS ALSO BEEN REPORTED TO PRODUCE CNS DEPRESSION WITHOUT SIGNIFICANT ELEVATIONS OF BARBITURATE OR VALPROATE SERUM LEVELS. ALL PATIENTS RECEIVING CONCOMITANT BARBITURATE THERAPY SHOULD BE CLOSELY MONITORED FOR NEUROLOGICAL TOXICITY. SERUM BARBITURATE LEVELS SHOULD BE OBTAINED, IF POSSIBLE, AND THE BARBITURATE DOSAGE DECREASED, IF APPROPRIATE.

Primidone is metabolized into a barbiturate and, therefore, may also be involved in a similar or identical interaction.

THERE HAVE BEEN REPORTS OF BREAKTHROUGH SEIZURES OCCURRING WITH THE COMBINATION OF DEPAKENE AND PHENYTOIN. MOST REPORTS HAVE NOTED A DECREASE IN TOTAL PLASMA PHENYTOIN CONCENTRATION. HOWEVER, INCREASES IN TOTAL PHENYTOIN SERUM CONCENTRATION HAVE BEEN REPORTED. AN INITIAL FALL IN TOTAL PHENYTOIN LEVELS WITH SUBSEQUENT INCREASE IN PHENYTOIN LEVELS HAS ALSO BEEN REPORTED. IN ADDITION, A DECREASE IN TOTAL SERUM PHENYTOIN WITH AN INCREASE IN THE FREE VS. PROTEIN BOUND PHENYTOIN LEVELS HAS BEEN REPORTED. THE DOSAGE OF PHENYTOIN SHOULD BE ADJUSTED AS REQUIRED BY THE CLINICAL SITUATION.

THE CONCOMITANT USE OF VALPROIC ACID AND CLONAZEPAM MAY PRODUCE ABSENCE STATUS.

There is inconclusive evidence regarding the effects of valproate on serum ethosuximide levels. Patients receiving valproate and ethosuximide, especially along with other anticonvulsants, should be monitored for alterations in serum concentrations of both drugs.

Caution is recommended when Depakene (valproic acid) is administered with drugs affecting coagulation, e.g., aspirin and warfarin. (See "Adverse Reactions" section.)

Carcinogenesis: Depakene was administered to Sprague Dawley rats and ICR (HA/ICR) mice at doses of 0, 80 and 170 mg/kg/day for two years. Although a variety of neoplasms were observed in both species, the chief findings were a statistically significant increase in the incidence of subcutaneous fibrosarcomas in high dose male rats receiving Depakene and a statistically significant dose-related trend for benign pulmonary adenomas in male mice receiving Depakene. The significance of these findings for man is unknown at present.

Mutagenesis: Studies on Depakene have been performed using bacterial and mammalian systems. These studies have provided no evidence of a mutagenic potential for Depakene.

Fertility: Chronic toxicity studies in juvenile and adult rats and dogs demonstrated reduced spermatogenesis and testicular atrophy at doses greater than 200 mg/kg/day in rats and greater than 90 mg/kg/day in dogs. Segment I fertility studies in rats have shown doses up to 350 mg/kg/day for 60 days to have no effect on fertility. THE EFFECT OF DEPAKENE (VALPROIC ACID) ON THE DEVELOPMENT OF THE TESTES AND ON SPERM PRODUCTION AND FERTILITY IN HUMANS IS UNKNOWN.

Pregnancy: See "WARNINGS" section.

Nursing Mothers: Depakene is excreted in breast milk. Concentrations in breast milk have been reported to be 1–10% of serum concentrations. It is not known what effect this would have on a nursing infant. Caution should be exercised when Depakene is administered to a nursing woman.

ADVERSE REACTIONS

Since Depakene (valproic acid) has usually been used with other antiepileptic drugs, it is not possible, in most cases, to determine whether the following adverse reactions can be ascribed to Depakene alone, or the combination of drugs.

Gastrointestinal: The most commonly reported side effects at the initiation of therapy are nausea, vomiting and indigestion. These effects are usually transient and rarely require discontinuation of therapy. Diarrhea, abdominal cramps and constipation have been reported. Both anorexia with some weight loss and increased appetite with weight gain have also been reported. Some patients experiencing gastrointestinal side effects may benefit by converting therapy from Depakene to Depakote (divalproex sodium enteric-coated tablets).[2]

CNS Effects: Sedative effects have been noted in patients receiving valproic acid alone but are found most often in patients receiving combination therapy. Sedation usually disappears upon reduction of other antiepileptic medication. Tremor has been reported in patients receiving valproate and may be dose related. Ataxia, headache, nystagmus, diplopia, asterixis, "spots before eyes", dysarthria, dizziness, and incoordination have rarely been noted. Rare cases of coma have been noted in patients receiving valproic acid alone or in conjunction with phenobarbital.

Dermatologic: Transient increases in hair loss have been observed. Skin rash and erythema multiforme have rarely been noted.

Psychiatric: Emotional upset, depression, psychosis, aggression, hyperactivity and behavioral deterioration have been reported.

Musculoskeletal: Weakness has been reported.

Hematologic: Thrombocytopenia has been reported. Valproic acid inhibits the secondary phase of platelet aggregation. (See "Drug Interactions" section.) This may be reflected in altered bleeding time. Petechiae, bruising, hematoma formation and frank hemorrhage have been reported. (see "Precautions" section.) Relative lymphocytosis and hypofibrinogenemia have been noted. Leukopenia and eosinophilia have also been reported. Anemia and bone marrow suppression have been reported.

Hepatic: Minor elevations of transaminases (e.g., SGOT and SGPT) and LDH are frequent and appear to be dose related. Occasionally, laboratory test results include, as well, increases in serum bilirubin and abnormal changes in other liver function tests. These results may reflect potentially serious hepatoxicity. (See "Warnings" section.)

Endocrine: There have been reports of irregular menses and secondary amenorrhea, and rare reports of breast enlargement and galactorrhea occurring in patients receiving Depakene.

Abnormal thyroid function tests have been reported. (see "Precautions" section.)

Pancreatic: There have been reports of acute pancreatitis, including rare fatal cases, occurring in patients receiving Depakene.

Metabolic: Hyperammonemia. (See "Precautions" section.) Hyperglycinemia has been reported and has been associated with a fatal outcome in a patient with preexistent nonketotic hyperglycinemia.

Other: Edema of the extremities has been reported.

OVERDOSAGE

Overdosage with valproic acid may result in deep coma.

Since Depakene is absorbed very rapidly, the value of gastric evacuation will vary with the time since ingestion. General supportive measures should be applied with particular attention being given to the maintenance of adequate urinary output.

Naloxone has been reported to reverse the CNS depressant effects of Depakene overdosage. Because naloxone could theoretically also reverse the antiepileptic effects of Depakene it should be used with caution.

DOSAGE AND ADMINISTRATION

Depakene (valproic acid) is administered orally. The recommended initial dose is 15 mg/kg/day, increasing at one week intervals by 5 to 10 mg/kg/day, until seizures are controlled or side effects preclude further increases. The maximum recommended dosage is 60 mg/kg/day. If the total daily dose exceeds 250 mg, it should be given in a divided regimen.

The following table is a guide for the initial daily dose of Depakene (valproic acid) (15 mg/kg/day):

[See table above].

The frequency of adverse effects (particularly elevated liver enzymes) may be dose-related. The benefit of improved seizure control which may accompany the higher doses should therefore be weighed against the possibility of a greater incidence of adverse reactions.

Continued on next page

Abbott—Cont.

A good correlation has not been established between daily dose, serum level and therapeutic effect. However, therapeutic serum levels for most patients will range from 50 to 100 mcg/ml. Occasional patients may be controlled with serum levels lower or higher than this range.

As the DEPAKENE dosage is titrated upward, blood levels of phenobarbital and/or phenytoin may be affected. (See "Precautions" section.)

Patients who experience G.I. irritation may benefit from administration of the drug with food or by slowly building up the dose from an initial low level.

THE CAPSULES SHOULD BE SWALLOWED WITHOUT CHEWING TO AVOID LOCAL IRRITATION OF THE MOUTH AND THROAT.

HOW SUPPLIED

DEPAKENE (valproic acid) is available as orange-colored soft gelatin capsules of 250 mg valproic acid in bottles of 100 capsules (**NDC** 0074-5681-13), in ABBO-PAC® unit dose packages of 100 capsules (**NDC** 0074-5681-11), and as a red syrup containing the equivalent of 250 mg valproic acid per 5 ml as the sodium salt in bottles of 16 ounces (**NDC** 0074-5682-16).

REFERENCES

1. Centers for Disease Control, Valproate: A New Cause of Birth Defects—Report from Italy and Follow-Up from France, *Morbidity and Mortality Weekly Report,* 32(33): 438–439, August 26, 1983.
2. Wilder, B.J., et al, Gastrointestinal Tolerance of Divalproex Sodium, *Neurology* 33:808–811, June, 1983

Shown in Product Identification Section, page 403

Abbott Laboratories
North Chicago, IL 60064
Ref. 01-2381-R15

DEPAKOTE® ℞

[dep 'ā-cōat]

(Divalproex Sodium Enteric-Coated Tablets)

WARNING

HEPATIC FAILURE RESULTING IN FATALITIES HAS OCCURRED IN PATIENTS RECEIVING VALPROIC ACID AND ITS DERIVATIVES. EXPERIENCE HAS INDICATED THAT CHILDREN UNDER THE AGE OF TWO YEARS ARE AT A CONSIDERABLY INCREASED RISK OF DEVELOPING FATAL HEPATOTOXICITY, ESPECIALLY THOSE ON MULTIPLE ANTICONVULSANTS, THOSE WITH CONGENITAL METABOLIC DISORDERS, THOSE WITH SEVERE SEIZURE DISORDERS ACCOMPANIED BY MENTAL RETARDATION, AND THOSE WITH ORGANIC BRAIN DISEASE. WHEN DEPAKOTE IS USED IN THIS PATIENT GROUP, IT SHOULD BE USED WITH EXTREME CAUTION AND AS A SOLE AGENT. THE BENEFITS OF SEIZURE CONTROL SHOULD BE WEIGHED AGAINST THE RISKS. ABOVE THIS AGE GROUP, EXPERIENCE HAS INDICATED THAT THE INCIDENCE OF FATAL HEPATOTOXICITY DECREASES CONSIDERABLY IN PROGRESSIVELY OLDER PATIENT GROUPS.

THESE INCIDENTS USUALLY HAVE OCCURRED DURING THE FIRST SIX MONTHS OF TREATMENT. SERIOUS OR FATAL HEPATOTOXICITY MAY BE PRECEDED BY NON-SPECIFIC SYMPTOMS SUCH AS LOSS OF SEIZURE CONTROL, MALAISE, WEAKNESS, LETHARGY, FACIAL EDEMA, ANOREXIA AND VOMITING. PATIENTS SHOULD BE MONITORED CLOSELY FOR APPEARANCE OF THESE SYMPTOMS. LIVER FUNCTION TESTS SHOULD BE PERFORMED PRIOR TO THERAPY AND AT FREQUENT INTERVALS THEREAFTER, ESPECIALLY DURING THE FIRST SIX MONTHS.

DESCRIPTION

Divalproex sodium is a stable co-ordination compound comprised of sodium valproate and valproic acid in a 1:1 molar relationship and formed during the partial neutralization of valproic acid with 0.5 equivalent of sodium hydroxide. Chemically it is designated as sodium hydrogen bis (2-propylpentanoate).

Divalproex sodium has a molecular weight of 310.41 and occurs as a white powder with a characteristic odor.

DEPAKOTE is an oral antiepileptic supplied as enteric-coated tablets in three dosage strengths containing divalproex sodium equivalent to 125 mg, 250 mg or 500 mg of valproic acid.

INACTIVE INGREDIENTS

125 mg tablets: cellulosic polymers, diacetylated monoglycerides, FD&C Blue No. 1, FD&C Red No. 40, povidone, pregelatinized starch (contains corn starch), silica gel, talc, titanium dioxide, vanillin and other ingredients.

250 mg tablets: cellulosic polymers, diacetylated monoglycerides, FD&C Yellow No. 6, iron oxide, povidone, pregelatinized starch (contains corn starch), silica gel, talc, titanium dioxide, vanillin and other ingredients.

500 mg tablets: cellulosic polymers, diacetylated monoglycerides, D&C Red No. 30, FD&C Blue No. 2, iron oxide, povidone, pregelatinized starch (contains corn starch), silica gel, talc, titanium dioxide, vanillin and other ingredients.

CLINICAL PHARMACOLOGY

DEPAKOTE is an antiepileptic agent which is chemically related to valproic acid. It has no nitrogen or aromatic moiety characteristic of other antiepileptic drugs. The mechanism by which DEPAKOTE exerts its antiepileptic effects has not been established. It has been suggested that its activity is related to increased brain levels of gamma-aminobutyric acid (GABA). The effect on the neuronal membrane is unknown. DEPAKOTE dissociates into valproate in the gastrointestinal tract.

Because of the enteric coating of DEPAKOTE, absorption is delayed one hour following oral administration. Thereafter, DEPAKOTE is uniformly and reliably absorbed, as shown by studies in normal volunteers. Peak serum levels of valproate occur in 3 to 4 hours. Bioavailability of divalproex sodium tablets was found to be equivalent to that of DEPAKENE ® (valproic acid) capsules. Concomitant administration with food would be expected to slow absorption but not affect the extent of absorption. The serum half-life of valproate is typically in the range of six to sixteen hours. Half-lives in the lower part of the above range are usually found in patients taking other antiepileptic drugs capable of enzyme induction.

Enteric-coated divalproex sodium may reduce the incidence of the irritative gastrointestinal effects of valproate as compared to valproic acid capsules.

Valproate is rapidly distributed and at therapeutic drug concentrations, drug is highly bound (90%) to human plasma proteins. Increases in dose may result in decreases in the extent of protein binding and increased valproate clearance and elimination.

Elimination of DEPAKOTE and its metabolites occurs principally in the urine, with minor amounts in the feces and expired air. Very little unmetabolized parent drug is excreted in the urine. The drug is primarily metabolized in the liver and is excreted as the glucuronide conjugate. Other metabolites in the urine are products of beta, omega-1, and omega oxidation (C-3, C-4 and C-5 positions). The major oxidative metabolite in the urine is 2-propyl-3-keto-pentanoic acid; minor metabolites are 2-propyl-glutaric acid, 2-propyl-5-hydroxypentanoic acid, 2-propyl-3-hydroxypentanoic acid and 2-propyl-4-hydroxypentanoic acid.

INDICATIONS AND USAGE

DEPAKOTE (divalproex sodium) is indicated for use as sole and adjunctive therapy in the treatment of simple (petit mal) and complex absence seizures. DEPAKOTE may also be used adjunctively in patients with multiple seizure types which include absence seizures.

In accordance with the International Classification of Seizures, simple absence is defined as very brief clouding of the sensorium or loss of consciousness (lasting usually 2–15 seconds), accompanied by certain generalized epileptic discharges without other detectable clinical signs. Complex absence is the term used when other signs are also present.

SEE "WARNINGS" SECTION FOR STATEMENT REGARDING FATAL HEPATIC DYSFUNCTION.

CONTRAINDICATIONS

DEPAKOTE (DIVALPROEX SODIUM) SHOULD NOT BE ADMINISTERED TO PATIENTS WITH HEPATIC DISEASE OR SIGNIFICANT DYSFUNCTION.

DEPAKOTE is contraindicated in patients with known hypersensitivity to the drug.

WARNINGS

Hepatic failure resulting in fatalities has occurred in patients receiving valproic acid. These incidents usually have occurred during the first six months of treatment. Serious or fatal hepatotoxicity may be preceded by nonspecific symptoms such as loss of seizure control, malaise, weakness, lethargy, facial edema, anorexia and vomiting. Patients should be monitored closely for appearance of these symptoms. Liver function tests should be performed prior to therapy and at frequent intervals thereafter, especially during the first six months. However, physicians should not rely totally on serum biochemistry since these tests may not be abnormal in all instances, but should also consider the results of careful interim medical history and physical examination. Caution should be observed when administering DEPAKOTE to patients with a prior history of hepatic disease. Patients on multiple anticonvulsants, children, those with congenital metabolic disorders, those with severe seizure disorders accompanied by mental retardation, and those with organic brain disease may be at particular risk. Experience has indicated that children under the age of two years are at considerably increased risk of developing fatal hepatotoxicity, especially those with the aforementioned conditions. When DEPAKOTE is used in this patient group, it should be used with extreme caution and as a sole agent. The benefits of seizure control should be weighed against the risks. Above this age group, experience has indicated that the incidence of fatal hepatotoxicity decreases considerably in progressively older patient groups.

The drug should be discontinued immediately in the presence of significant hepatic dysfunction, suspected or apparent. In some cases, hepatic dysfunction has progressed in spite of discontinuation of drug.

The frequency of adverse effects (particularly elevated liver enzymes) may be dose-related. The benefit of improved seizure control which may accompany the higher doses should therefore be weighed against the possibility of a greater incidence of adverse effects.

Usage in Pregnancy: ACCORDING TO PUBLISHED AND UNPUBLISHED REPORTS, VALPROIC ACID MAY PRODUCE TERATOGENIC EFFECTS IN THE OFFSPRING OF HUMAN FEMALES RECEIVING THE DRUG DURING PREGNANCY.

THERE ARE MULTIPLE REPORTS IN THE CLINICAL LITERATURE WHICH INDICATE THAT THE USE OF ANTIEPILEPTIC DRUGS DURING PREGNANCY RESULTS IN AN INCREASED INCIDENCE OF BIRTH DEFECTS IN THE OFFSPRING. ALTHOUGH DATA ARE MORE EXTENSIVE WITH RESPECT TO TRIMETHADIONE, PARAMETHADIONE, PHENYTOIN, AND PHENOBARBITAL, REPORTS INDICATE A POSSIBLE SIMILAR ASSOCIATION WITH THE USE OF OTHER ANTIEPILEPTIC DRUGS. THEREFORE, ANTIEPILEPTIC DRUGS SHOULD BE ADMINISTERED TO WOMEN OF CHILDBEARING POTENTIAL ONLY IF THEY ARE CLEARLY SHOWN TO BE ESSENTIAL IN THE MANAGEMENT OF THEIR SEIZURES.

THE INCIDENCE OF NEURAL TUBE DEFECTS IN THE FETUS MAY BE INCREASED IN MOTHERS RECEIVING VALPROATE DURING THE FIRST TRIMESTER OF PREGNANCY. THE CENTERS FOR DISEASE CONTROL (CDC) HAS ESTIMATED THE RISK OF VALPROIC ACID EXPOSED WOMEN HAVING CHILDREN WITH SPINA BIFIDA TO BE APPROXIMATELY 1 to 2%.[1] THIS RISK IS SIMILAR TO THAT FOR NONEPILEPTIC WOMEN WHO HAVE HAD CHILDREN WITH NEURAL TUBE DEFECTS (ANENCEPHALY AND SPINA BIFIDA).

ANIMAL STUDIES HAVE ALSO DEMONSTRATED VALPROIC ACID INDUCED TERATOGENICITY. Studies in rats and human females demonstrated placental transfer of the drug. Doses greater than 65 mg/kg/day given to pregnant rats and mice produced skeletal abnormalities in the offspring, primarily involving ribs and vertebrae; doses greater than 150 mg/kg/day given to pregnant rabbits produced fetal resorptions and (primarily) soft-tissue abnormalities in the offspring. In rats a dose-related delay in the onset of parturition was noted. Postnatal growth and survival of the progeny were adversely affected, particularly when drug administration spanned the entire gestation and early lactation period.

Antiepileptic drugs should not be discontinued in patients in whom the drug is administered to prevent major seizures because of the strong possibility of precipitating status epilepticus with attendant hypoxia and threat to life. In individual cases where the severity and frequency of the seizure disorder are such that the removal of medication does not pose a serious threat to the patient, discontinuation of the drug may be considered prior to and during pregnancy, although it cannot be said with any confidence that even minor seizures do not pose some hazard to the developing embryo or fetus.

The prescribing physician will wish to weigh these considerations in treating or counseling epileptic women of childbearing potential.

PRECAUTIONS

Hepatic Dysfunction: See "Boxed Warning," "Contraindications" and "Warnings" sections.

General: Because of reports of thrombocytopenia, inhibition of the secondary phase of platelet aggregation, and abnormal coagulation parameters, platelet counts and coagulation tests are recommended before initiating therapy and at periodic intervals. It is recommended that patients receiving DEPAKOTE (divalproex sodium) be monitored for platelet count and coagulation parameters prior to planned surgery. Evidence of hemorrhage, bruising or a disorder of hemostasis/coagulation is an indication for reduction of DEPAKOTE dosage or withdrawal of therapy.

Hyperammonemia with or without lethargy or coma has been reported and may be present in the absence of abnormal liver function tests. If clinically significant elevation occurs, DEKAPOTE should be discontinued.

Since DEPAKOTE (divalproex sodium) may interact with concurrently administered antiepileptic drugs, periodic serum level determinations of concomitant antiepileptic drugs are recommended during the early course of therapy. (See "Drug Interactions" section).

Valproate is partially eliminated in the urine as a keto-metabolite which may lead to a false interpretation of the urine ketone test.

There have been reports of altered thyroid function tests associated with valproate. The clinical significance of these is unknown.

Information for Patients: Since DEPAKOTE may produce CNS depression, especially when combined with another CNS depressant (e.g., alcohol), patients should be advised not to engage in hazardous occupations, such as driving an automobile or operating dangerous machinery, until it is known that they do not become drowsy from the drug.

Drug Interactions: Valproic acid may potentiate the CNS depressant activity of alcohol.

The concomitant administration of valproic acid with drugs that exhibit extensive protein binding (e.g., aspirin, carbamazepine, and dicumarol) may result in alteration of serum drug levels.

THERE IS EVIDENCE THAT VALPROIC ACID CAN CAUSE AN INCREASE IN SERUM PHENOBARBITAL LEVELS BY IMPAIRMENT OF NONRENAL CLEARANCE. THIS PHENOMENON CAN RESULT IN SEVERE CNS DEPRESSION. THE COMBINATION OF VALPROIC ACID AND PHENOBARBITAL HAS ALSO BEEN REPORTED TO PRODUCE CNS DEPRESSION WITHOUT SIGNIFICANT ELEVATIONS OF BARBITURATE OR VALPROATE SERUM LEVELS. ALL PATIENTS RECEIVING CONCOMITANT BARBITURATE THERAPY SHOULD BE CLOSELY MONITORED FOR NEUROLOGICAL TOXICITY. SERUM BARBITURATE LEVELS SHOULD BE OBTAINED, IF POSSIBLE, AND THE BARBITURATE DOSAGE DECREASED, IF APPROPRIATE.

Primidone is metabolized into a barbiturate and, therefore, may also be involved in a similar or identical interaction.

THERE HAVE BEEN REPORTS OF BREAK-THROUGH SEIZURES OCCURRING WITH THE COMBINATION OF VALPROIC ACID AND PHENYTOIN. MOST REPORTS HAVE NOTED A DECREASE IN TOTAL PLASMA PHENYTOIN CONCENTRATION. HOWEVER, INCREASES IN TOTAL PHENYTOIN SERUM CONCENTRATION HAVE BEEN REPORTED. AN INITIAL FALL IN TOTAL PHENYTOIN LEVELS WITH SUBSEQUENT INCREASE IN PHENYTOIN LEVELS HAS ALSO BEEN REPORTED. IN ADDITION, A DECREASE IN TOTAL SERUM PHENYTOIN WITH AN INCREASE IN THE FREE VS. PROTEIN BOUND PHENYTOIN LEVELS HAS BEEN REPORTED. THE DOSAGE OF PHENYTOIN SHOULD BE ADJUSTED AS REQUIRED BY THE CLINICAL SITUATION.

THE CONCOMITANT USE OF VALPROIC ACID AND CLONAZEPAM MAY PRODUCE ABSENCE STATUS.

There is inconclusive evidence regarding the effect of valproate on serum ethosuximide levels. Patients receiving valproate and ethosuximide, especially along with other anticonvulsants, should be monitored for alterations in serum concentrations of both drugs.

Caution is recommended when DEPAKOTE (divalproex sodium) is administered with drugs affecting coagulation, e.g., aspirin and warfarin. (See "Adverse Reactions" section).

Carcinogenesis: Valproic acid was administered to Sprague Dawley rats and ICR (HA /ICR) mice at doses of 0, 80 and 170 mg/kg/day for two years. Although a variety of neoplasms were observed in both species, the chief findings were a statistically significant increase in the incidence of subcutaneous fibrosarcomas in high dose male rats receiving valproic acid and a statistically significant dose-related trend for benign pulmonary adenomas in male mice receiving valproic acid. The significance of these findings for man is unknown at present.

Mutagenesis: Studies on valproic acid have been performed using bacterial and mammalian systems. These studies have provided no evidence of a mutagenic potential for DEPAKOTE.

Fertility: Chronic toxicity studies in juvenile and adult rats and dogs demonstrated reduced spermatogenesis and testicular atrophy at doses greater than 200 mg/kg/day in rats and greater than 90 mg/kg/day in dogs. Segment I fertility studies in rats have shown doses up to 350 mg/kg/day for 60 days to have no effect on fertility. THE EFFECT OF DEPAKOTE (DIVALPROEX SODIUM) ON THE DEVELOPMENT OF THE TESTES AND ON SPERM PRODUCTION AND FERTILITY IN HUMANS IS UNKNOWN.

Pregnancy: Pregnancy Category D: See "Warnings" section.

Nursing Mothers: Valproate is excreted in breast milk. Concentrations in breast milk have been reported to be 1–10% of serum concentrations. It is not known what effect this would have on a nursing infant. Caution should be exercised when DEPAKOTE is administered to a nursing woman.

ADVERSE REACTIONS

Since valproic acid and its derivatives have usually been used with other antiepileptic drugs, it is not possible, in most cases, to determine whether the following adverse reactions can be ascribed to valproic acid alone, or the combination of drugs.

Gastrointestinal: The most commonly reported side effects at the initiation of therapy are nausea, vomiting and indigestion. These effects are usually transient and rarely require discontinuation of therapy. Diarrhea, abdominal cramps and constipation have been reported. Both anorexia with some weight loss and increased appetite with weight gain have also been reported. The administration of enteric-coated divalproex sodium may result in reduction of gastrointestinal side effects in some patients.[2]

CNS Effects: Sedative effects have been noted in patients receiving valproic acid alone but are found most often in patients receiving combination therapy. Sedation usually disappears upon reduction of other antiepileptic medication. Tremor has been reported in patients receiving valproate and may be dose-related. Ataxia, headache, nystagmus, diplopia, asterixis, "spots before eyes," dysarthria, dizziness, and incoordination have rarely been noted. Rare cases of coma have been noted in patients receiving valproic acid alone or in conjunction with phenobarbital.

Dermatologic: Transient increases in hair loss have been observed. Skin rash and erythema multiforme rarely have been noted.

Psychiatric: Emotional upset, depression, psychosis, aggression, hyperactivity and behavioral deterioration have been reported.

Musculoskeletal: Weakness has been reported.

Hematologic: Thrombocytopenia has been reported. Valproic acid inhibits the secondary phase of platelet aggregation. (See "Drug Interactions" section). This may be reflected in altered bleeding time. Petechiae, bruising, hematoma formation, and frank hemorrhage have been reported. (See "Precautions" section). Relative lymphocytosis and hypofibrinogenemia have been noted. Leukopenia and eosinophilia have also been reported. Anemia and bone marrow suppression have been reported.

Hepatic: Minor elevations of transaminases (e.g., SGOT and SGPT) and LDH are frequent and appear to be dose related. Occasionally, laboratory test results include, as well, increases in serum bilirubin and abnormal changes in other liver function tests. These results may reflect potentially serious hepatotoxicity. (See "Warnings" section).

Endocrine: There have been reports of irregular menses and secondary amenorrhea, and rare reports of breast enlargement and galactorrhea occurring in patients receiving valproic acid and its derivatives.

Abnormal thyroid function tests have been reported. (See "Precautions" section).

Pancreatic: There have been reports of acute pancreatitis, including rare fatal cases, occurring in patients receiving valproic acid and its derivatives.

Metabolic: Hyperammonemia. (See "Precautions" section). Hyperglycinemia has been reported and has been associated with a fatal outcome in a patient with preexistent nonketotic hyperglycinemia.

Other: Edema of the extremities has been reported.

OVERDOSAGE

Overdosage with valproic acid may result in deep coma. Since DEPAKOTE tablets are enteric-coated, the benefit of gastric lavage or emesis will vary with the time since ingestion. General supportive measures should be applied with particular attention being given to the maintenance of adequate urinary output.

Naloxone has been reported to reverse the CNS depressant effects of valproate overdosage. Because naloxone could theoretically also reverse the antiepileptic effects of DEPAKOTE it should be used with caution.

DOSAGE AND ADMINISTRATION

DEPAKOTE is administered orally. The recommended initial dose is 15 mg/kg/day, increasing at one week intervals by 5 to 10 mg/kg/day until seizures are controlled or side effects preclude further increases. The maximum recommended dosage is 60 mg/kg/day. If the total daily dose exceeds 250 mg, it should be given in a divided regimen.

Conversion from DEPAKENE to DEPAKOTE: In patients previously receiving DEPAKENE (valproic acid) therapy, DEPAKOTE should be initiated at the same total daily dose and dosing schedule.[3] After the patient is stabilized on DEPAKOTE, a twice-a-day or three-times-a-day schedule may be instituted in selected patients.

The frequency of adverse effects (particularly elevated liver enzymes) may be dose-related. The benefit of improved seizure control which may accompany higher doses should therefore be weighed against the possibility of a greater incidence of adverse reactions.

A good correlation has not been established between daily dose, serum level and therapeutic effect. However, therapeutic valproate serum levels for most patients will range from 50 to 100 mcg/ml. Occasional patients may be controlled with serum levels lower or higher than this range.

As the DEPAKOTE dosage is titrated upward, blood levels of phenobarbital and/or phenytoin may be affected. (See "Precautions" section).

Patients who experience G. I. irritation may benefit from administration of the drug with food or by slowly building up the dose from an initial low level.

HOW SUPPLIED

DEPAKOTE (divalproex sodium enteric-coated tablets) are supplied as:

125 mg salmon pink-colored tablets in bottles of 100 (**NDC** 0074-6212-13).

250 mg peach-colored tablets in bottles of 100 (**NDC** 0074-6214-13) and Abbo-Pac® unit dose packages of 100 (**NDC** 0074-6214-11).

500 mg lavender-colored tablets in bottles of 100 (**NDC** 0074-6215-13) and Abbo-Pac® unit dose packages of 100 (**NDC** 0074-6215-11).

REFERENCES

1. Centers for Disease Control, Valproate: A New Cause of Birth Defects—Report from Italy and Follow-up from France, *Morbidity and Mortality Weekly Report* 32(33):438–439, August 26, 1983.
2. Wilder, B.J., et al, Gastrointestinal Tolerance of Divalproex Sodium, *Neurology* 33:808–811, June, 1983.
3. Wilder, B.J., et al, Twice-Daily Dosing of Valproate with Divalproex, *Clin Pharmacol Ther* 34(4): 501–504, 1983.

Abbott Laboratories
North Chicago, IL 60064
Ref. 03-4295-R8

Shown in Product Identification Section, page 403

DESOXYN® ℞ Ⓒ

(methamphetamine hydrochloride)
Tablets—Gradumet® Tablets

METHAMPHETAMINE HAS A HIGH POTENTIAL FOR ABUSE. IT SHOULD THUS BE TRIED ONLY IN WEIGHT REDUCTION PROGRAMS FOR PATIENTS IN WHOM ALTERNATIVE THERAPY HAS BEEN INEFFECTIVE. ADMINISTRATION OF METHAMPHETAMINE FOR PROLONGED PERIODS OF TIME IN OBESITY MAY LEAD TO DRUG DEPENDENCE AND MUST BE AVOIDED. PARTICULAR ATTENTION SHOULD BE PAID TO THE POSSIBILITY OF SUBJECTS OBTAINING METHAMPHETAMINE FOR NON-THERAPEUTIC USE OR DISTRIBUTION TO OTHERS, AND THE DRUG SHOULD BE PRESCRIBED OR DISPENSED SPARINGLY.

DESCRIPTION

DESOXYN (methamphetamine hydrochloride), chemically known as (S)-N, α-dimethylbenzeneethanamine hydrochloride, is a member of the amphetamine group of sympathomimetic amines.

DESOXYN is available as Gradumet sustained-release tablets containing 5 mg, 10 mg or 15 mg of methamphetamine hydrochloride and as conventional tablets containing 5 mg methamphetamine hydrochloride, for oral administration. The Gradumet is an inert, porous, plastic matrix, which is impregnated with DESOXYN. The drug is leached slowly from the Gradumet as it passes through the gastrointestinal tract. The expended matrix is not absorbed and is excreted in the stool.

INACTIVE INGREDIENTS

5 mg Gradumet tablet: magnesium stearate, methyl acrylate-methyl methacrylate copolymer, povidone, talc and other ingredients.

10 mg Gradumet tablet: FD&C Yellow No. 6, magnesium stearate, methyl acrylate-methyl methacrylate copolymer, povidone, talc and other ingredients.

15 mg Gradumet tablet: FD&C Yellow No. 5 (tartrazine), magnesium stearate, methyl acrylate-methyl methacrylate copolymer, povidone, talc and other ingredients.

5 mg tablet: corn starch, lactose, sodium paraminobenzoate, stearic acid, talc and other ingredients.

CLINICAL PHARMACOLOGY

DESOXYN (methamphetamine hydrochloride) is a sympathomimetic amine with CNS stimulant activity. Peripheral actions include elevation of systolic and diastolic blood pressures and weak bronchodilator and respiratory stimulant action. Drugs of this class used in obesity are commonly known as "anorectics" or "anorexigenics." It has not been established, however, that the action of such drugs in treating obesity is primarily one of appetite suppression. Other central nervous system actions, or metabolic effects, may be involved, for example.

Continued on next page

If desired, additional literature on any Abbott Product will be provided upon request to Abbott Laboratories.

Abbott—Cont.

Adult obese subjects instructed in dietary management and treated with "anorectic" drugs, lose more weight on the average than those treated with placebo and diet, as determined in relatively short-term clinical trials.

The magnitude of increased weight loss of drug-treated patients over placebo-treated patients is only a fraction of a pound a week. The rate of weight loss is greatest in the first weeks of therapy for both drug and placebo subjects and tends to decrease in succeeding weeks. The origins of the increased weight loss due to the various possible drug effects are not established. The amount of weight loss associated with the use of an "anorectic" drug varies from trial to trial, and the increased weight loss appears to be related in part to variables other than the drug prescribed, such as the physician-investigator, the population treated, and the diet prescribed. Studies do not permit conclusions as to the relative importance of the drug and non-drug factors on weight loss.

The natural history of obesity is measured in years, whereas the studies cited are restricted to a few weeks duration; thus, the total impact of drug-induced weight loss over that of diet alone must be considered clinically limited.

The mechanism of action involved in producing the beneficial behavioral changes seen in hyperkinetic children receiving DESOXYN is unknown.

In humans, methamphetamine is rapidly absorbed from the gastrointestinal tract. The primary site of metabolism is in the liver by aromatic hydroxylation, N-dealkylation and deamination. At least seven metabolites have been identified in the urine. The biological half-life has been reported in the range of 4 to 5 hours. Excretion occurs primarily in the urine and is dependent on urine pH. Alkaline urine will significantly increase the drug half-life. Approximately 62% of an oral dose is eliminated in the urine within the first 24 hours with about one-third as intact drug and the remainder as metabolites.

INDICATIONS AND USAGE

Attention Deficit Disorder with Hyperactivity—DESOXYN is indicated as an integral part of a total treatment program which typically includes other remedial measures (psychological, educational, social) for a stabilizing effect in children over 6 years of age with a behavioral syndrome characterized by the following group of developmentally inappropriate symptoms: moderate to severe distractibility, short attention span, hyperactivity, emotional lability, and impulsivity. The diagnosis of this syndrome should not be made with finality when these symptoms are only of comparatively recent origin. Nonlocalizing (soft) neurological signs, learning disability, and abnormal EEG may or may not be present, and a diagnosis of central nervous system dysfunction may or may not be warranted.

Exogenous Obesity—as a short-term (i.e., a few weeks) adjunct in a regimen of weight reduction based on caloric restriction, for patients in whom obesity is refractory to alternative therapy, e.g., repeated diets, group programs, and other drugs. The limited usefulness of DESOXYN (see "Clinical Pharmacology" section) should be weighed against possible risks inherent in use of the drug, such as those described below.

CONTRAINDICATIONS

DESOXYN is contraindicated during or within 14 days following the administration of monoamine oxidase inhibitors; hypertensive crises may result. It is also contraindicated in patients with glaucoma, advanced arteriosclerosis, symptomatic cardiovascular disease, moderate to severe hypertension, hyperthyroidism or known hypersensitivity or idiosyncrasy to sympathomimetic amines. Methamphetamine should not be given to patients who are in an agitated state or who have a history of drug abuse.

WARNINGS

Tolerance to the anorectic effect usually develops within a few weeks. When this occurs, the recommended dose should not be exceeded in an attempt to increase the effect; rather, the drug should be discontinued (see "Drug Abuse and Dependence" section).

Decrements in the predicted growth (i.e., weight gain and/or height) rate have been reported with the long-term use of stimulants in children. Therefore, patients requiring long-term therapy should be carefully monitored.

PRECAUTIONS

General: DESOXYN (methamphetamine hydrochloride) should be used with caution in patients with even mild hypertension.

Methamphetamine should not be used to combat fatigue or to replace rest in normal persons.

Prescribing and dispensing of methamphetamine should be limited to the smallest amount that is feasible at one time in order to minimize the possibility of overdosage.

The 15 mg dosage strength of DESOXYN Gradumet tablets contains FD&C Yellow No. 5 (tartrazine) which may cause allergic-type reactions (including bronchial asthma) in certain susceptible individuals. Although the overall incidence of FD&C Yellow No. 5 (tartrazine) sensitivity in the general population is low, it is frequently seen in patients who also have aspirin hypersensitivity.

Information for Patients: The patient should be informed that methamphetamine may impair the ability to engage in potentially hazardous activities, such as, operating machinery or driving a motor vehicle.

The patient should be cautioned not to increase dosage, except on advice of the physician.

Drug Interactions: Insulin requirements in diabetes mellitus may be altered in association with the use of methamphetamine and concomitant dietary regimen.

Methamphetamine may decrease the hypotensive effect of *guanethidine.*

DESOXYN should not be used concurrently with *monoamine oxidase inhibitors* (see "Contraindications" section).

Concurrent administration of *tricyclic antidepressants* and indirect-acting sympathomimetic amines such as amphetamines, should be closely supervised and dosage carefully adjusted.

Phenothiazines are reported in the literature to antagonize the CNS stimulant action of the amphetamines.

Drug/Laboratory Test Interactions: Literature reports suggest that amphetamines may be associated with significant elevation of plasma corticosteroids. This should be considered if determination of plasma corticosteroid levels is desired in a person receiving amphetamines.

Carcinogensis, Mutagenesis, Impairment of Fertility: Data are not available on long-term potential for carcinogenicity, mutagenicity, or impairment of fertility.

Pregnancy: Teratogenic effects: Pregnancy Category C. Methamphetamine has been shown to have teratogenic and embryocidal effects in mammals given high multiples of the human dose. There are no adequate and well-controlled studies in pregnant women. DESOXYN should not be used during pregnancy unless the potential benefit justifies the potential risk to the fetus.

Nonteratogenic effects: Infants born to mothers dependent on amphetamines have an increased risk of premature delivery and low birth weight. Also, these infants may experience symptoms of withdrawal as demonstrated by dysphoria, including agitation and significant lassitude.

Nursing Mothers: It is not known whether this drug is excreted in human milk. Because many drugs are excreted in human milk, caution should be exercised when DESOXYN is administered to a nursing woman.

Pediatric Use: Safety and effectiveness for use as an anorectic agent in children below the age of 12 years have not been established.

Long-term effects of DESOXYN in children have not been established (see "Warnings" section).

Drug treatment is not indicated in all cases of the behavioral syndrome characterized by moderate to severe distractibility, short attention span, hyperactivity, emotional lability and impulsivity. It should be considered only in light of the complete history and evaluation of the child. The decision to prescribe DESOXYN should depend on the physician's assessment of the chronicity and severity of the child's symptoms and their appropriateness for his/her age. Prescription should not depend solely on the presence of one or more of the behavioral characteristics.

When these symptoms are associated with acute stress reaction, treatment with DESOXYN is usually not indicated.

Clinical experience suggests that in psychotic children, administration of DESOXYN may exacerbate symptoms of behavior disturbance and thought disorder.

Amphetamines have been reported to exacerbate motor and phonic tics and Tourette's syndrome. Therefore, clinical evaluation for tics and Tourette's syndrome in children and their families should precede use of stimulant medications.

ADVERSE REACTIONS

The following are adverse reactions in decreasing order of severity within each category that have been reported with DESOXYN:

Cardiovascular: Elevation of blood pressure, tachycardia and palpitation.

Central Nervous System: Psychotic episodes have been rarely reported at recommended doses. Dizziness, dysphoria, overstimulation, euphoria, insomnia, tremor, restlessness and headache. Exacerbation of motor and phonic tics and Tourette's syndrome.

Gastrointestinal: Diarrhea, constipation, dryness of mouth, unpleasant taste and other gastrointestinal disturbances.

Hypersensitivity: Urticaria.

Endocrine: Impotence and changes in libido.

Miscellaneous: Suppression of growth has been reported with the long-term use of stimulants in children (see "Warnings" section).

DRUG ABUSE AND DEPENDENCE

Controlled Substance: DESOXYN (methamphetamine hydrochloride) is subject to control under DEA schedule II.

Abuse: DESOXYN has been extensively abused. Tolerance, extreme psychological dependence, and severe social disability have occurred. There are reports of patients who have increased the dosage to many times that recommended. Abrupt cessation following prolonged high dosage administration results in extreme fatigue and mental depression; changes are also noted on the sleep EEG. Manifestations of chronic intoxication with DESOXYN include severe dermatoses, marked insomnia, irritability, hyperactivity, and personality changes. The most severe manifestation of chronic intoxication is psychosis, often clinically indistinguishable from schizophrenia.

OVERDOSAGE

Manifestations of acute overdosage with methamphetamine include restlessness, tremor, hyperreflexia, rapid respiration, confusion, assaultiveness, hallucinations, and panic states. Fatigue and depression usually follow the central stimulation. Cardiovascular effects include arrhythmias, hypertension or hypotension, and circulatory collapse. Gastrointestinal symptoms include nausea, vomiting, diarrhea, and abdominal cramps. Fatal poisoning usually terminates in convulsions and coma.

Management of acute methamphetamine intoxication is largely symptomatic and includes gastric evacuation and sedation with a barbiturate. Experience with hemodialysis or peritoneal dialysis is inadequate to permit recommendations in this regard.

Acidification of urine increases methamphetamine excretion. Intravenous phentolamine (Regitine®) has been suggested for possible acute, severe hypertension, if this complicates methamphetamine overdosage. Usually a gradual drop in blood pressure will result when sufficient sedation has been achieved. Chlorpromazine has been reported to be useful in decreasing CNS stimulation and sympathomimetic effects.

Since the Gradumet tablet releases methamphetamine gradually, therapy should be directed at reversing the effects of the ingested drug and at supporting the patient until symptoms subside. Saline cathartics are useful for hastening the evacuation of the tablets that have not already released medication.

DOSAGE AND ADMINISTRATION

DESOXYN (methamphetamine hydrochloride) is given orally. Methamphetamine should be administered at the lowest effective dosage, and dosage should be individually adjusted. Late evening medication should be avoided because of the resulting insomnia.

Attention Deficit Disorder with Hyperactivity:

For treatment of children 6 years or older with a behavioral syndrome characterized by moderate to severe distractibility, short attention span, hyperactivity, emotional lability and impulsivity: an initial dose of 5 mg DESOXYN (methamphetamine hydrochloride) once or twice a day is recommended. Daily dosage may be raised in increments of 5 mg at weekly intervals until optimum clinical response is achieved. The usual effective dose is 20 to 25 mg daily. The total daily dose may be given as conventional tablets in two divided doses daily or once daily using the Gradumet tablet. The Gradumet form should not be utilized for initiation of dosage nor until the conventional titrated daily dosage is equal to or greater than the dosage provided in a Gradumet tablet.

Where possible, drug administration should be interrupted occasionally to determine if there is a recurrence of behavioral symptoms sufficient to require continued therapy.

For obesity: one Gradumet tablet, 10 or 15 mg, once a day in the morning. When the conventional tablet form is prescribed, 5 mg should be taken one-half hour before each meal. Treatment should not exceed a few weeks in duration. Methamphetamine is not recommended for use as an anorectic agent in children under 12 years of age.

HOW SUPPLIED

DESOXYN (methamphetamine hydrochloride) is supplied as follows:

Gradumet Tablets, 5 mg, white, in bottles of 100 (**NDC** 0074-6941-04); 10 mg, orange, in bottles of 100 (**NDC** 0074-6948-08) and 500 (**NDC** 0074-6948-09); and 15 mg, yellow, in bottles of 100 (**NDC** 0074-6959-07) and 500 (**NDC** 0074-6959-08).

Tablets, 5 mg, white, in bottles of 100 (**NDC** 0074-3377-04).

Shown in Product Identification Section, page 403

Abbott Pharmaceuticals Inc.
North Chicago, IL 60064
Ref. 03-4265-R8

DICAL-D® CAPSULES—WAFERS

[dī'cal-d]

(Dibasic Calcium Phosphate with Vitamin D)

DESCRIPTION

Capsules

Daily dosage (three capsules) provides:

Vitamin D	399 IU (10 mcg)	99% USRDA*
Calcium	0.35 g	35% USRDA
Phosphorous	0.27 g	27% USRDA

Each gelatin capsule contains:
Dibasic Calcium Phosphate, hydrous (as anhydrous form) .... 500 mg
Cholecalciferol .... 3.33 mcg (133 IU)
Corn starch, talc and magnesium stearate added.
Calcium to phosphorous ratio 1.3 to 1.

Wafers

Daily dosage (two wafers) provides:

Vitamin D	400 IU (10 mcg)	100% USRDA
Calcium	0.464 g	46% USRDA
Phosphorous	0.36 g	36% USRDA

Each wafer contains:
Cholecalciferol .... 5 mcg (200 IU)
Dibasic Calcium Phosphate, hydrous .... 1 g
Added dextrose, sucrose, talc, stearic acid, mineral oil, salt, and natural and artificial flavorings.
Calcium to phosphorous ratio 1.29 to 1.
*% U.S. Recommended Daily Allowance for adults and children 4 or more years of age.

INDICATIONS

For those individuals who must restrict their intake of dairy products.

DOSAGE AND ADMINISTRATION

Usual dose for adults and children 4 years and older:
Wafers—Chew 1 wafer twice daily with meals, or as directed by the physician or dentist.
Capsules—1 capsule 3 times daily with meals, or as directed by the physician or dentist.

HOW SUPPLIED

Dical-D Capsules in bottles of 100 (NDC 0074-3594-04) and 500 (NDC 0074-3594-02).
Dical-D Wafers in box of 51 (NDC 0074-3589-01).
Abbott Laboratories/
Abbott Pharmaceuticals, Inc.
North Chicago, IL 60064
Ref. 03-1294-6/R16 & 09-5876-5/R9

DICUMAROL Tablets, USP ℞

[dĭ-coo 'mu-rawl]

HOW SUPPLIED

Dicumarol tablets are supplied as:
25 mg tablets:
bottles of 100 (NDC 0074-3794-01);
bottles of 1000 (**NDC** 0074-3794-06).
50 mg tablets:
bottles of 100 (**NDC** 0074-3773-01);
bottles of 1000 (**NDC** 0074-3773-02).

INACTIVE INGREDIENTS

25 mg tablets: corn starch, lactose, magnesium stearate, talc and other ingredients.
50 mg tablets: corn starch, D&C Red No. 30, lactose, stearic acid, talc and other ingredients.

Shown in Product Identification Section, page 403

Abbott Pharmaceuticals, Inc.
North Chicago, IL 60064

ENDURON® ℞

[en 'de-ron]
(methyclothiazide tablets, USP)

DESCRIPTION

ENDURON (methyclothiazide) is a member of the benzothiadiazine (thiazide) family of drugs. It is an analogue of hydrochlorothiazide.
Clinically, ENDURON is an oral diuretic-antihypertensive agent.

INACTIVE INGREDIENTS

2.5 mg tablets: corn starch, FD&C Yellow No. 6, lactose, magnesium stearate, talc and other ingredients.
5 mg tablets: corn starch, D&C Red No. 36, FD&C Red No. 3, lactose, magnesium stearate, talc and other ingredients.

ACTIONS

The diuretic and saluretic effects of ENDURON result from a drug-induced inhibition of the renal tubular reabsorption of electrolytes. The excretion of sodium and chloride is greatly enhanced. Potassium excretion is also enhanced to a variable degree, as it is with the other thiazides. Although urinary excretion of bicarbonate is increased slightly, there is usually no significant change in urinary pH. Methyclothiazide has a per mg natriuretic activity approximately 100 times that of the prototype thiazide, chlorothiazide. At maximal therapeutic dosages, all thiazides are approximately equal in their diuretic/natriuretic effects.
There is significant natriuresis and diuresis within two hours after administration of a single dose of methyclothiazide. These effects reach a peak in about six hours and persist for 24 hours following oral administration of a single dose.
Like other benzothiadiazines, ENDURON also has antihypertensive properties, and may be used for this purpose either alone or to enhance the antihypertensive action of other drugs. The mechanism by which the benzothiadiazines, including methyclothiazide, produce a reduction of elevated blood pressure is not known. However, sodium depletion appears to be involved.
ENDURON is rapidly absorbed and slowly eliminated by the kidneys as both intact drug and as a metabolite showing no diuretic activity in a rat model.

INDICATIONS

ENDURON is indicated in the management of hypertension either as the sole therapeutic agent or to enhance the effect of other antihypertensive drugs in the more severe forms of hypertension.
ENDURON (methyclothiazide) is indicated as adjunctive therapy in edema associated with congestive heart failure, hepatic cirrhosis, and corticosteroid and estrogen therapy.
ENDURON has also been found useful in edema due to various forms of renal dysfunction such as the nephrotic syndrome, acute glomerulonephritis, and chronic renal failure.
Usage in Pregnancy: The routine use of diuretics in an otherwise healthy pregnant woman is inappropriate and exposes mother and fetus to unnecessary hazard. Diuretics do not prevent development of toxemia of pregnancy, and there is no satisfactory evidence that they are useful in the treatment of developed toxemia.
Edema during pregnancy may arise from pathological causes or from the physiological and mechanical consequences of pregnancy. Thiazides are indicated in pregnancy when edema is due to pathological causes, just as they are in the absence of pregnancy (however, see Warnings, below). Dependent edema in pregnancy, resulting from restriction of venous return by the expanded uterus, is properly treated through elevation of the lower extremities and use of support hose; use of diuretics to lower intravascular volume in this case is illogical and unnecessary. There is hypervolemia during normal pregnancy which is harmful to neither the fetus nor the mother (in the absence of cardiovascular disease), but which is associated with edema, including generalized edema, in the majority of pregnant women. If this edema produces discomfort, increased recumbency will often provide relief. In rare instances, this edema may cause extreme discomfort which is not relieved by rest. In these cases, a short course of diuretics may provide relief and may be appropriate.

CONTRAINDICATIONS

Renal decompensation.
Hypersensitivity to this or other sulfonamide-derived drugs.

WARNINGS

Methyclothiazide shares with other thiazides the propensity to deplete potassium reserves to an unpredictable degree.
Thiazides should be used with caution in patients with renal disease or significant impairment of renal function, since azotemia may be precipitated and cumulative drug effects may occur.
Thiazides should be used with caution in patients with impaired hepatic function or progressive liver disease, since minor alterations of fluid and electrolyte balance may precipitate hepatic coma.
Thiazides may be additive or potentiative of the action of other antihypertensive drugs. Potentiation occurs with ganglionic or peripheral adrenergic blocking drugs.
Sensitivity reactions may occur in patients with a history of allergy or bronchial asthma.
The possibility of exacerbation or activation of systemic lupus erythematosus has been reported.
Usage in Pregnancy: Thiazides cross the placental barrier and appear in cord blood. The use of thiazides in pregnant women requires that the anticipated benefit be weighed against possible hazards to the fetus. These hazards include fetal or neonatal jaundice, thrombocytopenia, and possible other adverse reactions that have occurred in the adult.
Nursing Mothers: Thiazides appear in breast milk. If use of the drug is deemed essential, the patient should stop nursing.

PRECAUTIONS

Periodic determinations of serum electrolytes should be performed at appropriate intervals for the purpose of detecting possible electrolyte imbalances such as hyponatremia, hypochloremic alkalosis, and hypokalemia. Serum and urine electrolyte determinations are particularly important when a patient is vomiting excessively or receiving parenteral fluids. All patients should be observed for other clinical signs of electrolyte imbalances such as dryness of mouth, thirst, weakness, lethargy, drowsiness, restlessness, muscle pains or cramps, muscular fatigue, hypotension, oliguria, tachycardia, and gastrointestinal disturbances such as nausea and vomiting.
Hypokalemia may develop with thiazides as with any other potent diuretic, especially when brisk diuresis occurs, severe cirrhosis is present, or when corticosteroids or ACTH are given concomitantly. Interference with the adequate oral intake of electrolytes will also contribute to the possible development of hypokalemia. Potassium depletion, even of a mild degree, resulting from thiazide use, may sensitize a patient to the effects of cardiac glycosides such as digitalis.
Any chloride deficit is generally mild and usually does not require specific treatment except under extraordinary circumstances (as in liver disease or renal disease). Dilutional hyponatremia may occur in edematous patients in hot weather; appropriate therapy is water restriction rather than administration of salt, except in rare instances when the hyponatremia is life threatening.
In actual salt depletion, appropriate replacement is the therapy of choice.
Hyperuricemia may occur or frank gout may be precipitated in certain patients receiving thiazide therapy.
Insulin requirements in diabetic patients may be increased, decreased, or unchanged. Latent diabetes mellitus may become manifest during thiazide administration.
Thiazide drugs may increase the responsiveness to tubocurarine.
The antihypertensive effects of the drug may be enhanced in the postsympathectomy patient.
Thiazides may decrease arterial responsiveness to norepinephrine. This diminution is not sufficient to preclude effectiveness of the pressor agent for therapeutic use.
If progressive renal impairment becomes evident as indicated by a rising nonprotein nitrogen or blood urea nitrogen, a careful reappraisal of therapy is necessary with consideration given to withholding or discontinuing diuretic therapy.
Thiazides may decrease serum PBI levels without signs of thyroid disturbance.
Thiazides have been reported, on rare occasions, to have elevated serum calcium to hypercalcemic levels. The serum calcium levels have returned to normal when the medication has been stopped. This phenomenon may be related to the ability of the thiazide diuretics to lower the amount of calcium excreted in the urine.

ADVERSE REACTIONS

Gastrointestinal system reactions: Anorexia, gastric irritation, nausea, vomiting, cramping, diarrhea, constipation, jaundice (intrahepatic cholestatic jaundice), pancreatitis.
Central nervous system reactions: Dizziness, vertigo, paresthesias, headache, xanthopsia.
Hematologic reactions: Leukopenia, agranulocytosis, thrombocytopenia, aplastic anemia.
Dermatologic—hypersensitivity reactions:
Purpura, photosensitivity, rash, urticaria, necrotizing angiitis (vasculitis) (cutaneous vasculitis).
Cardiovascular reaction: Orthostatic hypotension may occur and may be aggravated by alcohol, barbiturates, or narcotics.
Other: Hyperglycemia, glycosuria, hypercalcemia, hyperuricemia, muscle spasm, weakness, restlessness.
There have been isolated reports that certain nonedematous individuals developed severe fluid and electrolyte derangements after only brief exposure to normal doses of thiazide and non-thiazide diuretics. The condition is usually manifested as severe dilutional hyponatremia, hypokalemia, and hypochloremia. It has been reported to be due to inappropriately increased ADH secretion and appears to be idiosyncratic. Potassium replacement is apparently the most important therapy in the treatment of this syndrome along with removal of the offending drug.
Whenever adverse reactions are severe, treatment should be discontinued.

DOSAGE AND ADMINISTRATION

ENDURON (methyclothiazide) is administered orally. Therapy should be individualized according to patient response. This therapy should be titrated to gain maximal therapeutic response as well as the minimal dose possible to maintain that therapeutic response.
For edematous conditions: The usual adult dose ranges from 2.5 to 10 mg once daily. Maximum effective single dose is 10 mg; larger single doses do not accomplish greater diuresis, and are not recommended.
For the treatment of hypertension: The usual adult dose ranges from 2.5 to 5 mg once daily.
If control of blood pressure is not satisfactory after 8 to 12 weeks of therapy with 5 mg once daily, another antihypertensive drug should be added. Increase of the dosage of ENDURON will usually not result in further lowering of blood pressure.
Methyclothiazide may be either employed alone for mild to moderate hypertension or concurrently with other antihypertensive drugs in the management of more severe forms of hypertension. Combined therapy may provide adequate control of hypertension with lower dosage of the component drugs and fewer or less severe side effects. An enhanced response frequently follows its concurrent administration with

Continued on next page

If desired, additional literature on any Abbott Product will be provided upon request to Abbott Laboratories.

Abbott—Cont.

Harmonyl® (deserpidine) so that dosage of both drugs may be reduced.
When other antihypertensive agents are to be added to the regimen, this should be accomplished gradually. Ganglionic blocking agents should be given at only half the usual dose since their effect is potentiated by pretreatment with ENDURON.

OVERDOSAGE

Symptoms of overdosage include electrolyte imbalance and signs of potassium deficiency such as confusion, dizziness, muscular weakness, and gastrointestinal disturbances. General supportive measures including replacement of fluids and electrolytes may be indicated in treatment of overdosage.

HOW SUPPLIED

ENDURON (methyclothiazide tablets, USP) is provided in two dosage sizes as monogrammed, grooved, square-shaped tablets:

2.5 mg, orange-colored:
bottles of 100 (NDC 0074-6827-01),
bottles of 1000 (NDC 0074-6827-02).
5 mg, salmon-colored:
bottles of 100 (NDC 0074-6812-01),
bottles of 1000 (NDC 0074-6812-02),
bottles of 5000 (NDC 0074-6812-03),
Abbo-Pac® unit dose packages of 100 (NDC 0074-6812-10).

Shown in Product Identification Section, page 403

Abbott Pharmaceuticals, Inc.
North Chicago, IL 60064
Ref. 03-4282-R6

ENDURONYL® Tablets ℞

[en-du 're-nil]
(methyclothiazide and deserpidine)

Oral thiazide-rauwolfia therapy for hypertension.

> **WARNING**
> This fixed combination drug is not indicated for initial therapy of hypertension. Hypertension requires therapy titrated to the individual patient. If the fixed combination represents the dosage so determined, its use may be more convenient in patient management. The treatment of hypertension is not static, but must be reevaluated as conditions in each patient warrant.

DESCRIPTION

ENDURONYL is an orally-administered combination of Enduron® (methyclothiazide) and Harmonyl® (deserpidine). Methyclothiazide is an oral diuretic-antihypertensive of the benzothiadiazine (thiazide) class. Deserpidine is a purified rauwolfia alkaloid, chemically identified as 11-desmethoxyreserpine, which produces antihypertensive effects.

INACTIVE INGREDIENTS

Enduronyl tablets: corn starch, D&C Yellow No. 10, FD&C Yellow No. 6, lactose, magnesium stearate, talc and other ingredients.
Enduronyl Forte tablets: corn starch, iron oxide, lactose, magnesium stearate, talc and other ingredients.

ACTIONS

The combined antihypertensive actions of methyclothiazide and deserpidine result in a total clinical antihypertensive effect which is greater than can ordinarily be achieved by either drug given individually.
The diuretic and saluretic effects of methyclothiazide result from a drug-induced inhibition of the renal tubular reabsorption of electrolytes. The excretion of sodium and chloride is greatly enhanced. Potassium excretion is also enhanced to a variable degree, as it is with the other thiazides. Although urinary excretion of bicarbonate is increased slightly, there is usually no significant change in urinary pH. Methyclothiazide has a per mg natriuretic activity approximately 100 times that of the prototype thiazide, chlorothiazide. At maximal therapeutic dosages, all thiazides are approximately equal in their diuretic/natriuretic effects.
There is significant natriuresis and diuresis within two hours after administration of a single dose of methyclothiazide. These effects reach a peak in about six hours and persist for 24 hours following oral administration of a single dose.
Like other benzothiadiazines, methyclothiazide also has antihypertensive properties, and may be used for this purpose either alone or to enhance the antihypertensive action of other drugs. The mechanism by which the benzothiadiazines, including methyclothiazide, produce a reduction of elevated blood pressure is not known. However, sodium depletion appears to be involved.
Methyclothiazide is rapidly absorbed and slowly eliminated by the kidney as both intact drug and as a metabolite showing no diuretic activity in a rat model.
The pharmacologic actions of Harmonyl (deserpidine) are essentially the same as those of other active rauwolfia alkaloids. Deserpidine probably produces its antihypertensive effects through depletion of tissue stores of catecholamines (epinephrine and norepinephrine) from peripheral sites. The antihypertensive effect is often accompanied by bradycardia. There is no significant alteration in cardiac output or renal blood flow. The carotid sinus reflex is inhibited, but postural hypotension is rarely seen with the use of conventional doses of Harmonyl alone.
Deserpidine, like other rauwolfia alkaloids, is characterized by slow onset of action and sustained effect which may persist following withdrawal of the drug.

INDICATIONS

ENDURONYL (methyclothiazide and deserpidine) is indicated in the treatment of mild to moderately severe hypertension (see boxed warning). In many cases ENDURONYL alone produces an adequate reduction of blood pressure. In resistant or unusually severe cases ENDURONYL also may be supplemented by more potent antihypertensive agents. When administered with ENDURONYL, more potent agents can be given at reduced dosage to minimize undesirable side effects.

CONTRAINDICATIONS

Methyclothiazide is contraindicated in patients with renal decompensation and in those who are hypersensitive to this or other sulfonamide-derived drugs.
Deserpidine is contraindicated in patients with known hypersensitivity, mental depression especially with suicidal tendencies, active peptic ulcer, and ulcerative colitis. It is also contraindicated in patients receiving electroconvulsive therapy.

WARNINGS

Methyclothiazide
Methyclothiazide shares with other thiazides the propensity to deplete potassium reserves to an unpredictable degree.
Thiazides should be used with caution in patients with renal disease or significant impairment of renal function, since azotemia may be precipitated and cumulative drug effects may occur.
Thiazides should be used with caution in patients with impaired hepatic function or progressive liver disease, since minor alterations of fluid and electrolyte balance may precipitate hepatic coma.
Thiazides may be additive or potentiative of the action of other antihypertensive drugs. Potentiation occurs with ganglionic or peripheral adrenergic blocking drugs.
Sensitivity reactions may occur in patients with a history of allergy or bronchial asthma.
The possibility of exacerbation or activation of systemic lupus erythematosus has been reported.
Deserpidine
Extreme caution should be exercised in treating patients with a history of mental depression. Discontinue the drug at the first sign of despondency, early morning insomnia, loss of appetite, impotence, or self-deprecation. Drug-induced depression may persist for several months after drug withdrawal and may be severe enough to result in suicide.

Usage in Pregnancy and Lactation:
Methyclothiazide
Thiazides cross the placental barrier and appear in cord blood. The use of thiazides in pregnant women requires that the anticipated benefit be weighed against possible hazards to the fetus. These hazards include fetal or neonatal jaundice, thrombocytopenia, and possible other adverse reactions that have occurred in the adult.
Thiazides appear in breast milk. If use of the drug is deemed essential, the patient should stop nursing.
Deserpidine
The safety of deserpidine for use during pregnancy or lactation has not been established; therefore, it should be used in pregnant women or in women of childbearing potential only when in the judgment of the physician its use is deemed essential to the welfare of the patient. Increased respiratory secretions, nasal congestion, cyanosis, and anorexia may occur in infants born to rauwolfia alkaloid-treated mothers, since these preparations are known to cross the placental barrier to enter the fetal circulation and appear in cord blood. They also are secreted by nursing mothers into breast milk.
Reproductive and teratology studies in rats reduced the mating index and neonatal survival indices; the no-effect dosage has not been established.

PRECAUTIONS

Periodic determinations of serum electrolytes should be performed at appropriate intervals for the purpose of detecting possible electrolyte imbalances such as hyponatremia, hypochloremic alkalosis, and hypokalemia. Serum and urine electrolyte determinations are particularly important when a patient is vomiting excessively or receiving parenteral fluids. All patients should be observed for other clinical signs of electrolyte imbalances such as dryness of mouth, thirst, weakness, lethargy, drowsiness, restlessness, muscle pains or cramps, muscular fatigue, hypotension, oliguria, tachycardia, and gastrointestinal disturbances such as nausea and vomiting.
Hypokalemia may develop with thiazides as with any other potent diuretic, especially when brisk diuresis occurs, severe cirrhosis is present, or when corticosteroids or ACTH are given concomitantly. Interference with the adequate oral intake of electrolytes will also contribute to the possible development of hypokalemia. Potassium depletion, even of a mild degree, resulting from thiazide use, may sensitize a patient to the effects of cardiac glycosides such as digitalis.
Any chloride deficit is generally mild and usually does not require specific treatment except under extraordinary circumstances (as in liver disease or renal disease). Dilutional hyponatremia may occur in edematous patients in hot weather; appropriate therapy is water restriction rather than administration of salt, except in rare instances when the hyponatremia is life threatening.
In actual salt depletion, appropriate replacement is the therapy of choice.
Hyperuricemia may occur or frank gout may be precipitated in certain patients receiving thiazide therapy.
Insulin requirements in diabetic patients may be increased, decreased, or unchanged. Latent diabetes mellitus may become manifest during thiazide administration.
Thiazide drugs may increase the responsiveness to tubocurarine.
The antihypertensive effects of the drug may be enhanced in the postsympathectomy patient.
Thiazides may decrease arterial responsiveness to norepinephrine. This diminution is not sufficient to preclude effectiveness of the pressor agent for therapeutic use.
If progressive renal impairment becomes evident as indicated by a rising nonprotein nitrogen or blood urea nitrogen, a careful reappraisal of therapy is necessary with consideration given to withholding or discontinuing diuretic therapy.
Thiazides may decrease serum PBI levels without signs of thyroid disturbance.
Thiazides have been reported, on rare occasions, to have elevated serum calcium to hypercalcemic levels. The serum calcium levels have returned to normal when the medication has been stopped. This phenomenon may be related to the ability of the thiazide diuretics to lower the amount of calcium excreted in the urine.
Because rauwolfia preparations increase gastrointestinal motility and secretion, this drug should be used cautiously in patients with a history of peptic ulcer, ulcerative colitis, or gallstones, where biliary colic may be precipitated.
Caution should be exercised when treating hypertensive patients with renal insufficiency since they adjust poorly to lowered blood pressure levels.
Use deserpidine cautiously with digitalis and quinidine since cardiac arrhythmias have occurred with rauwolfia preparations.
Preoperative withdrawal of deserpidine does not assure that circulatory instability will not occur. It is important that the anesthesiologist be aware of the patient's drug intake and consider this in the overall management, since hypotension has occurred in patients receiving rauwolfia preparations.
Anticholinergic and/or adrenergic drugs (metaraminol, norepinephrine) have been employed to treat adverse vagocirculatory effects.
Animal tumorigenicity: There are no studies demonstrating that deserpidine is an animal tumorigen, although it is a prolactin stimulator and structurally related to reserpine. Rodent studies with reserpine, however, have shown that reserpine is an animal tumorigen, causing an increased incidence of mammary fibroadenomas in female mice, malignant tumors of the seminal vesicles in male mice, and malignant adrenal medullary tumors in male rats. These findings arose in 2 year studies in which the drug was administered in the feed at concentrations of 5 to 10 ppm—about 100 to 300 times the usual human dose. The breast neoplasms are thought to be related to reserpine's prolactin-elevating effect. Several other prolactin-elevating drugs have also been associated with an increased incidence of mammary neoplasia in rodents.
The extent to which these findings indicate a risk to humans is uncertain. Tissue culture experiments show that about one-third of human breast tumors are prolactin-dependent *in vitro,* a factor of considerable importance if the use of the drug is contemplated in a patient with previously detected breast cancer. The possibility of an increased risk of breast cancer in reserpine users has been studied extensively; however, no firm conclusion has emerged. Although a few epidemiologic studies have suggested a slightly increased risk (less than twofold in all studies except one) in women who have used reserpine, other studies of generally similar design have not confirmed this. Epidemiologic studies conducted using other drugs (neuroleptic agents) that, like reserpine, increase prolactin levels and, therefore, would be considered rodent mammary carcinogens, have not shown an association between chronic administration of the drug and human mammary tumorigenesis. While long-term clinical observa-

tion has not suggested such an association, the available evidence is considered too limited to be conclusive at this time. An association of reserpine intake with pheochromocytoma or tumors of the seminal vesicles has not been explored.

ADVERSE REACTIONS

Methyclothiazide

Gastrointestinal System Reactions: Anorexia, gastric irritation, nausea, vomiting, cramping, diarrhea, constipation, jaundice (intrahepatic cholestatic jaundice), pancreatitis.
Central Nervous System Reactions: Dizziness, vertigo, paresthesias, headache, xanthopsia.
Hematologic Reactions: Leukopenia, agranulocytosis, thrombocytopenia, aplastic anemia.
Dermatologic — Hypersensitivity Reactions: Purpura, photosensitivity, rash, urticaria, necrotizing angiitis (vasculitis) (cutaneous vasculitis).
Cardiovascular Reaction: Orthostatic hypotension may occur and may be aggravated by alcohol, barbiturates, or narcotics.
Other: Hyperglycemia, glycosuria, hypercalcemia, hyperuricemia, muscle spasm, weakness, restlessness.
There have been isolated reports that certain nonedematous individuals developed severe fluid and electrolyte derangements after only brief exposure to normal doses of thiazide and non-thiazide diuretics. The condition is usually manifested as severe dilutional hyponatremia, hypokalemia, and hypochloremia. It has been reported to be due to inappropriately increased ADH secretion and appears to be idiosyncratic. Potassium replacement is apparently the most important therapy in the treatment of this syndrome along with removal of the offending drug.
Whenever adverse reactions are severe, treatment should be discontinued.

Deserpidine

The following adverse reactions have been reported with rauwolfia preparations. These reactions are usually reversible and disappear when the drug is discontinued.
Gastrointestinal: Including hypersecretion, anorexia, diarrhea, nausea, and vomiting.
Cardiovascular: Including angina-like symptoms, arrhythmias (particularly when used concurrently with digitalis or quinidine), and bradycardia.
Central Nervous System: Including drowsiness, depression, nervousness, paradoxical anxiety, nightmares, extrapyramidal tract symptoms, CNS sensitization manifested by dull sensorium, and deafness.
Dermatologic—Hypersensitivity: Including pruritus, rash, and asthma in asthmatic patients.
Ophthalmologic: Including glaucoma, uveitis, optic atrophy, and conjunctival injection.
Hematologic: Thrombocytopenic purpura.
Miscellaneous: Nasal congestion, weight gain, impotence or decreased libido, dysuria, dyspnea, muscular aches, dryness of mouth, dizziness, and headache.

DOSAGE AND ADMINISTRATION

Dosage should be determined by individual titration of ingredients (see boxed warning). Dosage of both components should be carefully adjusted to the needs of the individual patient. Since at least ten days to two weeks may elapse before the full effects of the drugs become manifest, the dosage of the drugs should not be adjusted more frequently.
Two tablet strengths, ENDURONYL (methyclothiazide 5 mg, deserpidine 0.25 mg) and ENDURONYL FORTE (methyclothiazide 5 mg, deserpidine 0.5 mg), each grooved, are provided to permit considerable latitude in meeting the dosage requirements of individual patients.*
The following table will help in determining which dose of ENDURONYL or ENDURONYL FORTE best represents the equivalent of the titrated dose.

Daily Dosage of ENDURONYL	methyclothiazide	deserpidine
½ tablet	2.5 mg	0.125 mg
1 tablet	5.0 mg	0.250 mg
1½ tablet	7.5 mg	0.375 mg
2 tablets	10.0 mg	0.500 mg

Daily Dosage of ENDURONYL FORTE	methyclothiazide	deserpidine
½ tablet	2.5 mg	0.250 mg
1 tablet	5.0 mg	0.500 mg
1½ tablet	7.5 mg	0.750 mg
2 tablets	10.0 mg	1.000 mg

The appropriate dose of ENDURONYL is administered orally, once daily. The usual adult dosage is one lower-strength ENDURONYL tablet daily.
There is no contraindication to combining the administration of ENDURONYL with other antihypertensive agents. When other antihypertensive agents are to be added to the regimen, this should be accomplished gradually. Ganglionic blocking agents should be given at only half the usual dose since their effect is potentiated by pretreatment with ENDURONYL.

OVERDOSAGE

Symptoms of thiazide overdosage include electrolyte imbalance and signs of potassium deficiency such as confusion, dizziness, muscular weakness, and gastrointestinal disturbances. General supportive measures including replacement of fluids and electrolytes may be indicated in treatment of overdosage.
An overdosage of deserpidine is characterized by flushing of the skin, conjunctival injection, and pupillary constriction. Sedation ranging from drowsiness to coma may occur. Hypotension, hypothermia, central respiratory depression and bradycardia may develop in cases of severe overdosage. Treatment consists of the careful evacuation of stomach contents followed by the usual procedures for the symptomatic management of CNS depressant overdosage. If severe hypotension occurs it should be treated with a direct acting vasopressor such as norepinephrine bitartrate injection.

HOW SUPPLIED

ENDURONYL (methyclothiazide and deserpidine) is supplied as monogrammed, grooved, square-shaped tablets in the following dosage sizes and quantities:
ENDURONYL (5 mg of methyclothiazide and 0.25 mg of deserpidine) yellow tablets in bottles of 100 (**NDC** 0074-6838-01) and 1000 (**NDC** 0074-6838-02). Also available in ABBO-PAC® unit dose packages, 100 tablets (**NDC** 0074-6838-06), in strips of 10 tablets.
ENDURONYL FORTE (5 mg of methyclothiazide and 0.5 mg of deserpidine) gray-colored tablets in bottles of 100 (**NDC** 0074-6854-01) and 1000 (**NDC** 0074-6854-02).

*Each component is separately available as ENDURON (methyclothiazide) and HARMONYL (deserpidine).

Shown in Product Identification Section, page 403

Abbott Pharmaceuticals, Inc.
North Chicago, IL 60064
Ref. 03-4284-R6

ERYDERM® 2% ℞
[*e'ry-derm*]
erythromycin topical solution, USP

DESCRIPTION

Erythromycin is an antibiotic produced from a strain of *Streptomyces erythraeus*. It is basic and readily forms salts with acids. Each ml of ERYDERM 2% (erythromycin topical solution) contains 20 mg of erythromycin base in a vehicle consisting of polyethylene glycol, acetone, and alcohol 77%.

ACTIONS

Although the mechanism by which ERYDERM acts in reducing inflammatory lesions of acne vulgaris is unknown, it is presumably due to its antibiotic action.

INDICATIONS

ERYDERM is indicated for the topical control of acne vulgaris.

CONTRAINDICATIONS

ERYDERM is contraindicated in persons who have shown hypersensitivity to any of its ingredients.

WARNINGS

The safe use of ERYDERM during pregnancy or lactation has not been established.

PRECAUTIONS

ERYDERM is for external use only and should be kept away from the eyes and mucous membranes including those of the nose and mouth. Do not allow solution to contact clothing and furniture. Concomitant topical acne therapy should be used with caution because a cumulative irritant effect may occur, especially with the use of peeling, desquamating, or abrasive agents.
The use of antimicrobial agents may be associated with the overgrowth of antibiotic resistant organisms. If this occurs, administration of this drug should be discontinued and appropriate measures taken.

ADVERSE REACTIONS

Adverse conditions experienced included dryness, pruritus, erythema, desquamation, and burning sensation.

DOSAGE AND ADMINISTRATION

ERYDERM should be applied with applicator or pad to the affected area twice a day after the skin is thoroughly washed with warm water and soap. The solution should be applied with a dabbing action when the applicator is used. Use enough solution to cover the affected area lightly.

HOW SUPPLIED

ERYDERM 2% (erythromycin topical solution, USP) is supplied in 60 ml bottles with applicator (**NDC** 0074-2698-02). Store at temperatures below 86°F (30°C).
Abbott Laboratories
North Chicago, IL 60064
Ref. 09-5849-3/R1

ERYPED® ℞
[*erē'ped*]
(erythromycin ethylsuccinate for oral suspension, USP)

DESCRIPTION

Erythromycin is produced by a strain of *Streptomyces erythraeus* and belongs to the macrolide group of antibiotics. It is basic and readily forms salts with acids. The base, the stearate salt, and the esters are poorly soluble in water. Erythromycin ethylsuccinate is an ester of erythromycin suitable for oral administration.
EryPed (erythromycin ethylsuccinate for oral suspension) is for reconstitution with water to form a suspension containing erythromycin ethylsuccinate equivalent to 400 mg of erythromycin per 5 ml (teaspoonful) with an appealing banana flavor. After mixing, EryPed must be stored below 77°F (25°C) and used within 35 days; refrigeration is not required. This product is intended primarily for pediatric use but can also be used in adults.

INACTIVE INGREDIENTS

Caramel, polysorbate, sodium citrate, sucrose, xanthan gum, artificial flavors and other ingredients.

ACTIONS

Microbiology: Biochemical tests demonstrate that erythromycin inhibits protein synthesis of the pathogen without directly affecting nucleic acid synthesis. Antagonism has been demonstrated between clindamycin and erythromycin.
NOTE: Many strains of *Hemophilus influenzae* are resistant to erythromycin alone, but are susceptible to erythromycin and sulfonamides together. Staphylococci resistant to erythromycin may emerge during a course of erythromycin therapy. Culture and susceptibility testing should be performed.
Disc Susceptibility Tests: Quantitative methods that require measurement of zone diameters give the most precise estimates of antibiotic susceptibility. One recommended procedure (21 CFR section 460.1) uses erythromycin class discs for testing susceptibility; interpretations correlate zone diameters of this disc test with MIC values for erythromycin. With this procedure, a report from the laboratory of "susceptible" indicates that the infecting organism is likely to respond to therapy. A report of "resistant" indicates, that the infective organism is not likely to respond to therapy. A report of "intermediate susceptibility" suggests that the organism would be susceptible if higher doses were used.

CLINICAL PHARMACOLOGY

Erythromycin binds to the 50 S ribosomal subunits of susceptible bacteria and suppresses protein synthesis.
Orally administered erythromycin ethylsuccinate suspension is readily and reliably absorbed under both fasting and nonfasting conditions.
Erythromycin diffuses readily into most body fluids. Only low concentrations are normally achieved in the spinal fluid, but passage of the drug across the blood-brain barrier increases in meningitis. In the presence of normal hepatic function, erythromycin is concentrated in the liver and excreted in the bile; the effect of hepatic dysfunction on excretion of erythromycin by the liver into the bile is not known. Less than 5 percent of the orally administered dose of erythromycin is excreted in active form in the urine.
Erythromycin crosses the placental barrier and is excreted in breast milk.

INDICATIONS

Streptococcus pyogenes (Group A beta-hemolytic streptococcus): Upper and lower respiratory tract, skin, and soft tissue infections of mild to moderate severity.
Injectable benzathine penicillin G is considered by the American Heart Association to be the drug of choice in the treatment and prevention of streptococcal pharyngitis and in long-term prophylaxis of rheumatic fever.
When oral medication is preferred for treatment of the above conditions, penicillin G, V, or erythromycin are alternate drugs of choice.
When oral medication is given, the importance of strict adherence by the patient to the prescribed dosage regimen must be stressed. A therapeutic dose should be administered for at least 10 days.
Alpha-hemolytic streptococci (viridans group): Although no controlled clinical efficacy trials have been conducted, oral erythromycin has been suggested by the American Heart Association and American Dental Association for use in a regimen for prophylaxis against bacterial endocarditis in patients hypersensitive to penicillin who have congenital heart disease, or rheumatic or other acquired valvular heart disease when they undergo dental procedures and surgical procedures of the upper respiratory tract.[1] Erythromycin is

Continued on next page

Abbott—Cont.

not suitable prior to genitourinary or gastrointestinal tract surgery. NOTE: When selecting antibiotics for the prevention of bacterial endocarditis the physician or dentist should read the full joint statement of the American Heart Association and the American Dental Association.[1]

Staphylococcus aureus: Acute infections of skin and soft tissue of mild to moderate severity. Resistant organisms may emerge during treatment.

Streptococcus pneumoniae (Diplococcus pneumoniae): Upper respiratory tract infections (e.g., otitis media, pharyngitis) and lower respiratory tract infections (e.g., pneumonia) of mild to moderate degree.

Mycoplasma pneumoniae (Eaton agent, PPLO): For respiratory infections due to this organism.

Hemophilus influenzae: For upper respiratory tract infections of mild to moderate severity when used concomitantly with adequate doses of sulfonamides. (See sulfonamide labeling for appropriate prescribing information). The concomitant use of the sulfonamides is necessary since not all strains of *Hemophilus influenzae* are susceptible to erythromycin at the concentrations of the antibiotic achieved with usual therapeutic doses.

Chlamydia trachomatis: For the treatment of urethritis in adult males due to *Chlamydia trachomatis.*

Ureaplasma urealyticum: For the treatment of urethritis in adult males due to *Ureaplasma urealyticum.*

Treponema pallidum: Erythromycin is an alternate choice of treatment for primary syphilis in patients allergic to the penicillins. In treatment of primary syphilis, spinal fluid examinations should be done before treatment and as part of follow-up after therapy.

Corynebacterium diphtheriae: As an adjunct to antitoxin, to prevent establishment of carriers, and to eradicate the organism in carriers.

Corynebacterium minutissimum: For the treatment of erythrasma.

Entamoeba histolytica: In the treatment of intestinal amebiasis only. Extraenteric amebiasis requires treatment with other agents.

Listeria monocytogenes: Infections due to this organism.

Bordetella pertussis: Erythromycin is effective in eliminating the organism from the nasopharynx of infected individuals, rendering them non-infectious. Some clinical studies suggest that erythromycin may be helpful in the prophylaxis of pertussis in exposed susceptible individuals.

Legionnaires' Disease: Although no controlled clinical efficacy studies have been conducted, *in vitro* and limited preliminary clinical data suggest that erythromycin may be effective in treating Legionnaires' Disease.

CONTRAINDICATIONS

Erythromycin is contraindicated in patients with known hypersensitivity to this antibiotic.

PRECAUTIONS

Erythromycin is principally excreted by the liver. Caution should be exercised in administering the antibiotic to patients with impaired hepatic function. There have been reports of hepatic dysfunction, with or without jaundice occurring in patients receiving oral erythromycin products.

Areas of localized infection may require surgical drainage in addition to antibiotic therapy.

Recent data from studies of erythromycin reveal that its use in patients who are receiving high doses of theophylline may be associated with an increase of serum theophylline levels and potential theophylline toxicity. In case of theophylline toxicity and/or elevated serum theophylline levels, the dose of theophylline should be reduced while the patient is receiving concomitant erythromycin therapy.

Usage during pregnancy and lactation: The safety of erythromycin for use during pregnancy has not been established. Erythromycin crosses the placental barrier. Erythromycin also appears in breast milk.

ADVERSE REACTIONS

The most frequent side effects of erythromycin preparations are gastrointestinal, such as abdominal cramping and discomfort, and are dose related. Nausea, vomiting, and diarrhea occur infrequently with usual oral doses.

During prolonged or repeated therapy, there is a possibility of overgrowth of nonsusceptible bacteria or fungi. If such infections occur, the drug should be discontinued and appropriate therapy instituted.

Allergic reactions ranging from urticaria and mild skin eruptions to anaphylaxis have occurred.

There have been isolated reports of reversible hearing loss occurring chiefly in patients with renal insufficiency and in patients receiving high doses of erythromycin.

DOSAGE AND ADMINISTRATION

EryPed (erythromycin ethylsuccinate for oral suspension) may be administered without regard to meals.

Children: Age, weight, and severity of the infection are important factors in determining the proper dosage. In mild to moderate infections the usual dosage of erythromycin ethylsuccinate for children is 30 to 50 mg/kg/day in equally divided doses. For more severe infections this dosage may be doubled.

The following dosage schedule is suggested for mild to moderate infections:

Body Weight	Total Daily Dose
Under 10 lbs	30-50 mg/kg/day 15-25 mg/lb/day
10 to 15 lbs	200 mg
16 to 25 lbs	400 mg
26 to 50 lbs	800 mg
51 to 100 lbs	1200 mg
over 100 lbs	1600 mg

Adults: 400 mg erythromycin ethylsuccinate every 6 hours is the usual dose. Dosage may be increased up to 4 g per day according to the severity of the infection.

If twice-a-day dosage is desired in either adults or children, one-half of the total daily dose may be given every 12 hours. Doses may also be given three times daily if desired by administering one-third of the total daily dose every 8 hours.

In the treatment of streptococcal infections, a therapeutic dosage of erythromycin ethylsuccinate should be administered for at least 10 days. In continuous prophylaxis against recurrences of streptococcal infections in persons with a history of rheumatic heart disease, the usual dosage is 400 mg twice a day.

For prophylaxis against bacterial endocarditis[1] in patients with congenital heart disease, or rheumatic or other acquired valvular heart disease when undergoing dental procedures or surgical procedures of the upper respiratory tract, give 1.6 g (20 mg/kg for children) orally 1 ½ to 2 hours before the procedure, and then, 800 mg (10 mg/kg for children) orally every 6 hours for 8 doses.

For treatment of urethritis due to *C. trachomatis* or *U. urealyticum:* 800 mg three times a day for 7 days.

For treatment of primary syphilis: Adults: 48 to 64 g given in divided doses over a period of 10 to 15 days.

For intestinal amebiasis: Adults: 400 mg four times daily for 10 to 14 days. Children: 30 to 50 mg/kg/day in divided doses for 10 to 14 days.

For use in pertussis: Although optimal dosage and duration have not been established, doses of erythromycin utilized in reported clinical studies were 40 to 50 mg/kg/day, given in divided doses for 5 to 14 days.

For treatment of Legionnaires' Disease: Although optimal doses have not been established, doses utilized in reported clinical data were 1.6 to 4 g daily in divided doses.

HOW SUPPLIED

EryPed (erythromycin ethylsuccinate for oral suspension, USP), 400 mg per 5 ml, is supplied in 60-ml (**NDC** 0074-6305-60), 100-ml (**NDC** 0074-6305-13) and 200-ml (**NDC** 0074-6305-53) bottles, and 5-ml unit dose in ABBO-PAC® packages of 100 bottles (**NDC** 0074-6305-05). After reconstitution, EryPed must be stored below 77°F (25°C) and used within 35 days; refrigeration not required.

Reference: 1. American Heart Association. 1977. Prevention of bacterial endocarditis. Circulation 56:139A-143A.

Shown in Product Identification Section, page 403

Abbott Laboratories
North Chicago, IL 60064
Ref. 01-2366-R4

ERY-TAB® ℞

[ĕrē'tab]

(erythromycin enteric-coated tablets)

DESCRIPTION

Erythromycin is produced by a strain of *Streptomyces erythraeus* and belongs to the macrolide group of antibiotics. It is basic and readily forms salts with acids. The base is white to off-white crystals or powder slightly soluble in water, soluble in alcohol, in chloroform, and in ether. ERY-TAB (erythromycin enteric-coated tablets) is specially coated to protect the contents from the inactivating effects of gastric acidity and to permit efficient absorption of the antibiotic in the small intestine.

ERY-TAB is available in three dosage strengths containing either 250 mg, 333 mg, or 500 mg of erythromycin as the free base.

INACTIVE INGREDIENTS

250 mg tablet: cellulosic polymers, diacetylated monoglycerides, D&C red no. 30, iron oxide, magnesium stearate, microcrystalline cellulose, povidone, sodium citrate, soybean derivatives, talc, titanium dioxide, vanillin and other ingredients.

333 mg tablet: cellulosic polymers, diacetylated monoglycerides, FD&C blue no. 1, magnesium stearate, microcrystalline cellulose, povidone, sodium citrate, soybean derivatives, talc, titanium dioxide, vanillin and other ingredients.

500 mg tablet: cellulosic polymers, diacetylated monoglycerides, FD&C red no. 40, iron oxide, magnesium stearate, microcrystalline cellulose, povidone, sodium citrate, soybean derivatives, talc, titanium dioxide, vanillin and other ingredients.

ACTIONS

The mode of action of erythromycin is inhibition of protein synthesis without affecting nucleic acid synthesis. Resistance to erythromycin of some strains of *Hemophilus influenzae* and staphylococci has been demonstrated. Culture and susceptibility testing should be done. If the Kirby-Bauer method of disc susceptibility is used, a 15 mcg erythromycin disc should give a zone diameter of at least 18 mm when tested against an erythromycin susceptible organism.

Bioavailability data are available from Abbott Laboratories, Dept. 498.

ERY-TAB is well absorbed and may be given without regard to meals.

After absorption, erythromycin diffuses readily into most body fluids. In the absence of meningeal inflammation, low concentrations are normally achieved in the spinal fluid but passage of the drug across the blood-brain barrier increases in meningitis. In the presence of normal hepatic function, erythromycin is concentrated in the liver and excreted in the bile; the effect of hepatic dysfunction on excretion of erythromycin by the liver into the bile is not known. After oral administration, less than 5 percent of the activity of the administered dose can be recovered in the urine.

Erythromycin crosses the placental barrier but fetal plasma levels are low.

INDICATIONS

Streptococcus pyogenes (Group A beta-hemolytic streptococcus): For upper and lower respiratory tract, skin, and soft tissue infections of mild to moderate severity.

Injectable benzathine penicillin G is considered by the American Heart Association to be the drug of choice in the treatment and prevention of streptococcal pharyngitis and in long-term prophylaxis of rheumatic fever.

When oral medication is preferred for treatment of the above conditions, penicillin G, V, or erythromycin are alternate drugs of choice.

When oral medication is given, the importance of strict adherence by the patient to the prescribed dosage regimen must be stressed. A therapeutic dose should be administered for at least 10 days.

Alpha-hemolytic streptococci (viridans group): Although no controlled clinical efficacy trials have been conducted, oral erythromycin has been suggested by the American Heart Association and American Dental Association for use in a regimen for prophylaxis against bacterial endocarditis in patients hypersensitive to penicillin who have congenital heart disease, or rheumatic or other acquired valvular heart disease when they undergo dental procedures and surgical procedures of the upper respiratory tract.[1] Erythromycin is not suitable prior to genitourinary or gastrointestinal tract surgery. NOTE: When selecting antibiotics for the prevention of bacterial endocarditis the physician or dentist should read the full joint statement of the American Heart Association and the American Dental Association.[1]

Staphylococcus aureus: For acute infections of skin and soft tissue of mild to moderate severity. Resistant organisms may emerge during treatment.

Streptococcus pneumoniae (Diplococcus pneumoniae): For upper respiratory tract infections (e.g., otitis media, pharyngitis) and lower respiratory tract infections (e.g., pneumonia) of mild to moderate degree.

Mycoplasma pneumoniae (Eaton agent, PPLO): For respiratory infections due to this organism.

Hemophilus influenzae: For upper respiratory tract infections of mild to moderate severity when used concomitantly with adequate doses of sulfonamides. Not all strains of this organism are susceptible at the erythromycin concentrations ordinarily achieved (see appropriate sulfonamide labeling for prescribing information).

Chlamydia trachomatis: Erythromycin is indicated for treatment of the following infections caused by *Chlamydia trachomatis:* conjunctivitis of the newborn, pneumonia of infancy and urogenital infections during pregnancy. When tetracyclines are contraindicated or not tolerated, erythromycin is indicated for the treatment of uncomplicated urethral, endocervical, or rectal infections in adults due to *Chlamydia trachomatis.*[2]

Treponema pallidum: Erythromycin is an alternate choice of treatment for primary syphilis in patients allergic to the penicillins. In treatment of primary syphilis, spinal fluid examinations should be done before treatment and as part of follow-up after therapy.

Corynebacterium diphtheriae and C. minutissimum: As an adjunct to antitoxin, to prevent establishment of carriers, and to eradicate the organism in carriers.

In the treatment of erythrasma.
Entamoeba histolytica: In the treatment of intestinal amebiasis only. Extra-enteric amebiasis requires treatment with other agents.
Listeria monocytogenes: Infections due to this organism.
Neisseria gonorrhoeae: Erythrocin® Lactobionate-I.V. (erythromycin lactobionate for injection, USP) in conjunction with erythromycin base orally, as an alternative drug in treatment of acute pelvic inflammatory disease caused by *N. gonorrhoeae* in female patients with a history of sensitivity to penicillin. Before treatment of gonorrhea, patients who are suspected of also having syphilis should have a microscopic examination for *T. pallidum* (by immunofluorescence or darkfield) before receiving erythromycin, and monthly serologic tests for a minimum of 4 months.
Bordetella pertussis: Erythromycin is effective in eliminating the organism from the nasopharynx of infected individuals, rendering them non-infectious. Some clinical studies suggest that erythromycin may be helpful in the prophylaxis of pertussis in exposed susceptible individuals.
Legionnaires' Disease: Although no controlled clinical efficacy studies have been conducted, *in vitro* and limited preliminary clinical data suggest that erythromycin can be effective in treating Legionnaires' Disease.

CONTRAINDICATIONS

Erythromycin is contraindicated in patients with known hypersensitivity to this antibiotic.

WARNING

Usage in pregnancy: Safety for use in pregnancy has not been established.

PRECAUTIONS

Erythromycin is principally excreted by the liver. Caution should be exercised in administering the antibiotic to patients with impaired hepatic function.
There have been reports of hepatic dysfunction, with or without jaundice, occurring in patients receiving oral erythromycin products.
Recent data from studies of erythromycin reveal that its use in patients who are receiving high doses of theophylline may be associated with an increase of serum theophylline levels and potential theophylline toxicity. In cases of theophylline toxicity and/or elevated serum theophylline levels, the dose of theophylline should be reduced while the patient is receiving concomitant erythromycin therapy.
Surgical procedures should be performed when indicated.

ADVERSE REACTIONS

The most frequent side effects of erythromycin preparations are gastrointestinal, such as abdominal cramping and discomfort, and are dose-related. Nausea, vomiting, and diarrhea occur infrequently with usual oral doses.
During prolonged or repeated therapy, there is a possibility of overgrowth of nonsusceptible bacteria or fungi. If such infections occur, the drug should be discontinued and appropriate therapy instituted.
Mild allergic reactions such as urticaria and other skin rashes have occurred. Serious allergic reactions, including anaphylaxis, have been reported. Allergic reactions should be handled in the usual manner.
There have been isolated reports of reversible hearing loss occurring chiefly in patients with renal insufficiency and in patients receiving high doses of erythromycin.

DOSAGE AND ADMINISTRATION

ERY-TAB (erythromycin enteric-coated tablets) is well absorbed and may be given without regard to meals.
Adults: The usual dose is 250 mg four times daily in equally spaced doses. The 333 mg tablet is recommended if dosage is desired every 8 hours. If twice-a-day dosage is desired, the recommended dose is 500 mg every 12 hours.
Dosage may be increased up to 4 or more grams per day according to the severity of the infection. Twice-a-day dosing is not recommended when doses larger than 1 gram daily are administered.
Children: Age, weight, and severity of the infection are important factors in determining the proper dosage. 30 to 50 mg/kg/day, in divided doses, is the usual dose. For more severe infections, this dose may be doubled.
In the treatment of streptococcal infections, a therapeutic dosage of erythromycin should be administered for at least 10 days. In continuous prophylaxis of streptococcal infections in persons with a history of rheumatic heart disease, the dose is 250 mg twice a day.
For prophylaxis against bacterial endocarditis[1] in patients with congenital heart disease, or rheumatic or other acquired valvular heart disease when undergoing dental procedures or surgical procedures of the upper respiratory tract, give 1 g (20 mg/kg for children) orally 1½ to 2 hours before the procedure, and then, 500 mg (10 mg/kg in children) orally every 6 hours for 8 doses.
For conjunctivitis of the newborn caused by *Chlamydia trachomatis:* Oral erythromycin suspension 50 mg/kg/day in 4 divided doses for at least 2 weeks.[2]
For pneumonia of infancy caused by *Chlamydia trachomatis:* Although the optimal duration of therapy has not been established, the recommended therapy is oral erythromycin suspension 50 mg/kg/day in 4 divided doses for at least 3 weeks.[2]
For urogenital infections during pregnancy due to *Chlamydia trachomatis:* Although the optimal dose and duration of therapy have not been established, the suggested treatment is erythromycin 500 mg, by mouth, 4 times a day for at least 7 days. For women who cannot tolerate this regimen, a decreased dose of 250 mg, by mouth, 4 times a day should be used for at least 14 days.[2]
For adults with uncomplicated urethral, endocervical, or rectal infections caused by *Chlamydia trachomatis* in whom tetracyclines are contraindicated or not tolerated: 500 mg, by mouth, 4 times a day for at least 7 days.[2]
For treatment of primary syphilis: 30 to 40 grams given in divided doses over a period of 10 to 15 days.
For treatment of acute pelvic inflammatory disease caused by *N. gonorrhoeae:* After initial treatment with Erythrocin® Lactobionate-I.V. (erythromycin lactobionate for injection, USP) 500 mg every 6 hours for 3 days, the oral dosage recommendation is 250 mg every 6 hours for 7 days.
For dysenteric amebiasis: 250 mg four times daily for 10 to 14 days, for adults; 30 to 50 mg/kg/day in divided doses for 10 to 14 days, for children.
For use in pertussis: Although optimal dosage and duration have not been established, doses of erythromycin utilized in reported clinical studies were 40 to 50 mg/kg/day, given in divided doses for 5 to 14 days.
For treatment of Legionnaires' Disease: Although optimal doses have not been established, doses utilized in reported clinical data were 1 to 4 grams erythromycin base daily in divided doses.

OVERDOSAGE

Gastrointestinal side effects of erythromycin are dose related. Some individuals may exhibit gastric intolerance to even therapeutic amounts.
Erythromycin serum levels are not appreciably affected by hemodialysis or peritoneal dialysis.

HOW SUPPLIED

ERY-TAB (erythromycin enteric-coated tablets), 250 mg, is supplied as pink tablets in bottles of 100 (**NDC** 0074-6304-13), bottles of 500 (**NDC** 0074-6304-53), and Abbo-Pac® unit dose packages of 100 (**NDC** 0074-6304-11).
ERY-TAB, 333 mg, is supplied as white tablets in bottles of 100 (**NDC** 0074-6320-13), bottles of 500 (**NDC** 0074-6320-53), and Abbo-Pac® unit dose packages of 100 (**NDC** 0074-6320-11).
ERY-TAB, 500 mg, is supplied as pink tablets in bottles of 100 (**NDC** 0074-6321-13) and Abbo-Pac® unit dose packages of 100 (**NDC** 0074-6321-11).

REFERENCES

1. American Heart Association. 1977. Prevention of bacterial endocarditis. Circulation 56:139A-143A.
2. CDC Sexually Transmitted Diseases Treatment Guidelines 1982.

U.S. Pat. No. 4,340,582.
Shown in Product Identification Section, page 403
Abbott Laboratories
North Chicago, IL 60064
Ref. 01-2374-R9

E.E.S.® ℞
[ē-ē-s]
(erythromycin ethylsuccinate)

DESCRIPTION

Erythromycin is produced by a strain of *Streptomyces erythraeus* and belongs to the macrolide group of antibiotics. It is basic and readily forms salts with acids. The base, the stearate salt, and the esters are poorly soluble in water. Erythromycin ethylsuccinate is an ester of erythromycin suitable for oral administration.
The cherry-flavored, chewable tablets are easily ingested and are particularly acceptable for the administration of antibiotic medication to young children who are unable to swallow regular tablets or in whom persuasion of a pleasant taste insures cooperation. Each chewable tablet, providing the equivalent of 200 mg of erythromycin, is conveniently scored for division into half-dose (100 mg) portions.
The granules and drops are intended for reconstitution with water. When reconstituted, they are palatable cherry-flavored suspensions.
The pleasant tasting, fruit-flavored liquids are supplied ready for oral administration.
Granules, drops and ready-made suspensions are intended primarily for pediatric use but can also be used in adults.
The Filmtab® tablets are intended primarily for adults or older children.

INACTIVE INGREDIENTS

E.E.S. 200 Liquid: FD&C Red No. 40, methylparaben, polysorbate 60, propylparaben, sodium citrate, sucrose, water, xanthan gum, natural and artificial flavors and other ingredients.
E.E.S. 400 Liquid: D&C Yellow No. 10, FD&C Yellow No. 6, methylparaben, polysorbate 60, propylparaben, sodium citrate, sucrose, water, xanthan gum, natural and artificial flavors and other ingredients.
E.E.S. Granules and Drops: Citric acid, FD&C Red No. 3, magnesium aluminum silicate, sodium carboxymethyl cellulose, sodium citrate, sucrose, artificial flavor, and other ingredients.
E.E.S. Chewable Tablets: Citric acid, confectioner's sugar (contains corn starch), magnesium aluminum silicate, magnesium stearate, sodium carboxymethyl cellulose, sodium citrate, artificial flavor and other ingredients.
E.E.S. 400 Filmtab Tablets: Cellulosic polymers, confectioner's sugar (contains corn starch), corn starch, D&C Red No. 30, D&C Yellow No. 10, FD&C Red No. 40, iron oxide, magnesium stearate, polacrilin potassium, polyethylene glycol, propylene glycol, sodium citrate, sorbic acid, sorbitan monooleate, titanium dioxide, vitamin E and other ingredients.

ACTIONS

Microbiology: Biochemical tests demonstrate that erythromycin inhibits protein synthesis of the pathogen without directly affecting nucleic acid synthesis. Antagonism has been demonstrated between clindamycin and erythromycin.
NOTE: Many strains of *Hemophilus influenzae* are resistant to erythromycin alone, but are susceptible to erythromycin and sulfonamides together. Staphylococci resistant to erythromycin may emerge during a course of erythromycin therapy. Culture and susceptibility testing should be performed.
Disc Susceptibility Tests: Quantitative methods that require measurement of zone diameters give the most precise estimates of antibiotic susceptibility. One recommended procedure (21 CFR section 460.1) uses erythromycin class discs for testing susceptibility; interpretations correlate zone diameters of this disc test with MIC values for erythromycin. With this procedure, a report from the laboratory of "susceptible" indicates that the infecting organism is likely to respond to therapy. A report of "resistant" indicates that the infective organism is not likely to respond to therapy. A report of "intermediate susceptibility" suggests that the organism would be susceptible if higher doses were used.
Clinical Pharmacology: Erythromycin binds to the 50 S ribosomal subunits of susceptible bacteria and suppresses protein synthesis.
Orally administered erythromycin ethylsuccinate suspensions and Filmtab tablets are readily and reliably absorbed. Erythromycin ethylsuccinate chewable tablets are readily and reliably absorbed when chewed. Comparable serum levels of erythromycin are achieved in the fasting and nonfasting states.
Erythromycin diffuses readily into most body fluids. Only low concentrations are normally achieved in the spinal fluid, but passage of the drug across the blood-brain barrier increases in meningitis. In the presence of normal hepatic function, erythromycin is concentrated in the liver and excreted in the bile; the effect of hepatic dysfunction on excretion of erythromycin by the liver into the bile is not known. Less than 5 percent of the orally administered dose of erythromycin is excreted in active form in the urine.
Erythromycin crosses the placental barrier and is excreted in breast milk.

INDICATIONS

Streptococcus pyogenes (Group A beta-hemolytic streptococcus): Upper and lower respiratory tract, skin, and soft tissue infections of mild to moderate severity.
Injectable benzathine penicillin G is considered by the American Heart Association to be the drug of choice in the treatment and prevention of streptococcal pharyngitis and in long-term prophylaxis of rheumatic fever.
When oral medication is preferred for treatment of the above conditions, penicillin G, V, or erythromycin are alternate drugs of choice.
When oral medication is given, the importance of strict adherence by the patient to the prescribed dosage regimen must be stressed. A therapeutic dose should be administered for at least 10 days.
Alpha-hemolytic streptococci (viridans group): Although no controlled clinical efficacy trials have been conducted, oral erythromycin has been suggested by the American Heart Association and American Dental Association for use in a regimen for prophylaxis against bacterial endocarditis in patients hypersensitive to penicillin who have congenital heart disease, or rheumatic or other acquired valvular heart disease when they undergo dental procedures and surgical procedures of the upper respiratory tract.[1] Erythromycin is not suitable prior to genitourinary or gastrointestinal tract

Continued on next page

Abbott—Cont.

surgery. NOTE: When selecting antibiotics for the prevention of bacterial endocarditis the physician or dentist should read the full joint statement of the American Heart Association and the American Dental Association.[1]
Staphylococcus aureus: Acute infections of skin and soft tissue of mild to moderate severity. Resistant organisms may emerge during treatment.
Streptococcus pneumoniae (Diplococcus pneumoniae): Upper respiratory tract infections (e.g., otitis media, pharyngitis) and lower respiratory tract infections (e.g., pneumonia) of mild to moderate degree.
Mycoplasma pneumoniae (Eaton agent, PPLO): For respiratory infections due to this organism.
Hemophilus influenzae: For upper respiratory tract infections of mild to moderate severity when used concomitantly with adequate doses of sulfonamides. (See sulfonamide labeling for appropriate prescribing information). The concomitant use of the sulfonamides is necessary since not all strains of *Hemophilus influenzae* are susceptible to erythromycin at the concentrations of the antibiotic achieved with usual therapeutic doses.
Chlamydia trachomatis: For the treatment of urethritis in adult males due to *Chlamydia trachomatis.*
Ureaplasma urealyticum: For the treatment of urethritis in adult males due to *Ureaplasma urealyticum.*
Treponema pallidum: Erythromycin is an alternate choice of treatment for primary syphilis in patients allergic to the penicillins. In treatment of primary syphilis, spinal fluid examinations should be done before treatment and as part of follow-up after therapy.
Corynebacterium diphtheriae: As an adjunct to antitoxin, to prevent establishment of carriers, and to eradicate the organism in carriers.
Corynebacterium minutissimum: For the treatment of erythrasma.
Entamoeba histolytica: In the treatment of intestinal amebiasis only. Extraenteric amebiasis requires treatment with other agents.
Listeria monocytogenes: Infections due to this organism.
Bordetella pertussis: Erythromycin is effective in eliminating the organism from the nasopharynx of infected individuals, rendering them non-infectious. Some clinical studies suggest that erythromycin may be helpful in the prophylaxis of pertussis in exposed susceptible individuals.
Legionnaires' Disease: Although no controlled clinical efficacy studies have been conducted, *in vitro* and limited preliminary clinical data suggest that erythromycin may be effective in treating Legionnaires' Disease.

CONTRAINDICATIONS

Erythromycin is contraindicated in patients with known hypersensitivity to this antibiotic.

PRECAUTIONS

Erythromycin is principally excreted by the liver. Caution should be exercised in administering the antibiotic to patients with impaired hepatic function. There have been reports of hepatic dysfunction, with or without jaundice occurring in patients receiving oral erythromycin products.
Areas of localized infection may require surgical drainage in addition to antibiotic therapy.
Recent data from studies of erythromycin reveal that its use in patients who are receiving high doses of theophylline may be associated with an increase of serum theophylline levels and potential theophylline toxicity. In case of theophylline toxicity and/or elevated serum theophylline levels, the dose of theophylline should be reduced while the patient is receiving concomitant erythromycin therapy.
Usage during pregnancy and lactation: The safety of erythromycin for use during pregnancy has not been established. Erythromycin crosses the placental barrier. Erythromycin also appears in breast milk.

ADVERSE REACTIONS

The most frequent side effects of erythromycin preparations are gastrointestinal, such as abdominal cramping and discomfort, and are dose related. Nausea, vomiting, and diarrhea occur infrequently with usual oral doses.
During prolonged or repeated therapy, there is a possibility of overgrowth of nonsusceptible bacteria or fungi. If such infections occur, the drug should be discontinued and appropriate therapy instituted.
Allergic reactions ranging from urticaria and mild skin eruptions to anaphylaxis have occurred.
There have been isolated reports of reversible hearing loss occurring chiefly in patients with renal insufficiency and in patients receiving high doses of erythromycin.

DOSAGE AND ADMINISTRATION

Erythromycin ethylsuccinate suspensions, Filmtab tablets and chewable tablets may be administered without regard to meals. For full therapeutic effect, the chewable tablets must be chewed.
Children: Age, weight, and severity of the infection are important factors in determining the proper dosage. In mild to moderate infections the usual dosage of erythromycin ethylsuccinate for children is 30 to 50 mg/kg/day in equally divided doses. For more severe infections this dosage may be doubled.
The following dosage schedule is suggested for mild to moderate infections:

Body Weight	Total Daily Dose
Under 10 lbs	30–50 mg/kg/day 15–25 mg/lb/day
10 to 15 lbs	200 mg
16 to 25 lbs	400 mg
26 to 50 lbs	800 mg
51 to 100 lbs	1200 mg
over 100 lbs	1600 mg

Adults: 400 mg erythromycin ethylsuccinate every 6 hours is the usual dose. Dosage may be increased up to 4 g per day according to the severity of the infection.
If twice-a-day dosage is desired in either adults or children, one-half of the total daily dose may be given every 12 hours. Doses may also be given three times daily if desired by administering one-third of the total daily dose every 8 hours.
In the treatment of streptococcal infections, a therapeutic dosage of erythromycin ethylsuccinate should be administered for at least 10 days. In continuous prophylaxis against recurrences of streptococcal infections in persons with a history of rheumatic heart disease, the usual dosage is 400 mg twice a day.
For prophylaxis against bacterial endocarditis[1] in patients with congenital heart disease, or rheumatic or other acquired valvular heart disease when undergoing dental procedures or surgical procedures of the upper respiratory tract, give 1.6 g (20 mg/kg for children) orally 1½ to 2 hours before the procedure, and then, 800 mg (10 mg/kg for children) orally every 6 hours for 8 doses.
For treatment of urethritis due to *C. trachomatis* or *U. urealyticum:* 800 mg three times a day for 7 days.
For treatment of primary syphilis: Adults: 48 to 64 g given in divided doses over a period of 10 to 15 days.
For intestinal amebiasis: Adults: 400 mg four times daily for 10 to 14 days. Children: 30 to 50 mg/kg/day in divided doses for 10 to 14 days.
For use in pertussis: Although optimal dosage and duration have not been established, doses of erythromycin utilized in reported clinical studies were 40 to 50 mg/kg/day, given in divided doses for 5 to 14 days.
For treatment of Legionnaires' Disease: Although optimal doses have not been established, doses utilized in reported clinical data were those recommended above (1.6 to 4 g daily in divided doses).

HOW SUPPLIED

E.E.S. 200 LIQUID (erythromycin ethylsuccinate oral suspension, USP) is supplied in 1 pint bottles (**NDC** 0074-6306-16) and in packages of six 100-ml bottles (**NDC** 0074-6306-13). Each 5-ml teaspoonful of fruit-flavored suspension contains activity equivalent to 200 mg of erythromycin.
E.E.S. 400® LIQUID (erythromycin ethylsuccinate oral suspension, USP) is supplied in 1 pint bottles (**NDC** 0074-6373-16) and in packages of six 100-ml bottles (**NDC** 0074-6373-13). Each 5-ml teaspoonful of orange, fruit-flavored suspension contains activity equivalent to 400 mg of erythromycin.
Both liquid products require refrigeration to preserve taste until dispensed. Refrigeration by patient is not required if used within 14 days.
E.E.S. GRANULES (erythromycin ethylsuccinate for oral suspension, USP) is supplied in 60-ml (**NDC** 0074-6369-01), 100-ml (**NDC** 0074-6369-02) and 200-ml (**NDC** 0074-6369-10) size bottles. Each 5-ml teaspoonful of reconstituted cherry-flavored suspension contains activity equivalent to 200 mg of erythromycin. E.E.S. GRANULES is also available in 5-ml bottles (when reconstituted) in the ABBO-PAC® unit dose packages of 100 bottles (**NDC** 0074-6369-05).
E.E.S. DROPS (erythromycin ethylsuccinate for oral suspension, USP) is supplied in 50-ml size bottles (**NDC** 0074-6360-50). Each 2.5-ml dropperful (½ teaspoonful) of reconstituted cherry-flavored suspension contains activity equivalent to 100 mg of erythromycin.
E.E.S. CHEWABLE (erythromycin ethylsuccinate tablets, USP) cherry-flavored wafers containing the equivalent of 200 mg of erythromycin are available in packages of 50 (**NDC** 0074-6371-50). Each wafer is individually sealed in a blister package.
E.E.S. 400 Filmtab tablets (erythromycin ethylsuccinate tablets, USP) 400 mg, are available in bottles of 100 (**NDC** 0074-5729-13) and 500 (**NDC** 0074-5729-53), and in ABBO-PAC® unit dose strip packages of 100 (**NDC** 0074-5729-11). Tablets are pink in color.

REFERENCE

1. American Heart Association. 1977. Prevention of bacterial endocarditis. Circulation 56: 139A-143A.

Filmtab—Film-sealed tablets, Abbott.
Shown in Product Identification Section, page 403
Abbott Laboratories
North Chicago, IL 60064
Ref. 01-2371-R10

ERYTHROCIN® LACTOBIONATE-I.V. ℞

[e-rith 'ro-sin lac-tō-bī 'ō-nāte ī. v.]
(erythromycin lactobionate for injection, USP)
Vials For I.V. use only

DESCRIPTION

Erythromycin is produced by a strain of *Streptomyces erythraeus* and belongs to the macrolide group of antibiotics. It is basic and readily forms salts with acids.
ERYTHROCIN LACTOBIONATE (erythromycin lactobionale for injection) is a soluble salt of erythromycin suitable for intravenous administration.

ACTIONS

Microbiology: Biochemical tests demonstrate that erythromycin inhibits protein synthesis of the pathogen without directly affecting nucleic acid synthesis. Antagonism has been demonstrated between clindamycin and erythromycin.
NOTE: Many strains of *Hemophilus influenzae* are resistant to erythromycin alone, but are susceptible to erythromycin and sulfonamides together. Staphylococci resistant to erythromycin may emerge during a course of erythromycin therapy. Culture and susceptibility testing should be performed.
Disc Susceptibility Tests: Quantitative methods that require measurement of zone diameters give the most precise estimates of antibiotic susceptibility. One recommended procedure (21 CFR section 460.1) uses erythromycin class discs for testing susceptibility; interpretations correlate zone diameters of this disc test with MIC values for erythromycin. With this procedure, a report from the laboratory of "susceptible" indicates that the infecting organism is likely to respond to therapy. A report of "resistant" indicates that the infective organism is not likely to respond to therapy. A report of "intermediate susceptibility" suggests that the organism would be susceptible if higher doses were used.
Clinical Pharmacology: Erythromycin binds to the 50 S ribosomal subunits of susceptible bacteria and suppresses protein synthesis.
Intravenous infusion of 500 mg erythromycin lactobionate at a constant rate over 1 hour in fasting adults produced a mean serum erythromycin level of approximately 7 mcg/ml at 20 minutes, 10 mcg/ml at 1 hour, 2.6 mcg/ml at 2.5 hours, and 1 mcg/ml at 6 hours.
Erythromycin diffuses readily into most body fluids. Only low concentrations are normally achieved in the spinal fluid, but passage of the drug across the blood-brain barrier increases in meningitis. In the presence of normal hepatic function, erythromycin is concentrated in the liver and excreted in the bile; the effect of hepatic dysfunction on excretion of erythromycin by the liver into the bile is not known. From 12 to 15 percent of intravenously administered erythromycin is excreted in active form in the urine.
Erythromycin crosses the placental barrier and is excreted in breast milk.

INDICATIONS

ERYTHROCIN LACTOBIONATE is indicated in the treatment of patients where oral administration is not possible or where the severity of the infection requires immediate high serum levels of erythromycin. Intravenous therapy should be replaced by oral administration at the appropriate time.
Streptococcus pyogenes (Group A beta hemolytic streptococcus): Upper and lower respiratory tract, skin, and soft tissue infections of mild to moderate severity.
Injectable benzathine penicillin G is considered by the American Heart Association to be the drug of choice in the treatment and prevention of streptococcal pharyngitis and in long-term prophylaxis of rheumatic fever.
When oral medication is preferred for treatment of the above conditions, penicillin G, V, or erythromycin are alternate drugs of choice.
Staphylococcus aureus: Acute infections of skin and soft tissue of mild to moderate severity. Resistant organisms may emerge during treatment.
Streptococcus pneumoniae (Diplococcus pneumoniae): For upper respiratory tract infections (e.g., otitis media, pharyngitis) and lower respiratory tract infections (e.g., pneumonia) of mild to moderate severity.
Mycoplasma pneumoniae (Eaton agent, PPLO): For respiratory infections due to this organism.
Hemophilus influenzae: For upper respiratory tract infections of mild to moderate severity when used concomitantly

with adequate doses of sulfonamides. (See sulfonamide labeling for appropriate prescribing information). The concomitant use of the sulfonamides is necessary since not all strains of *Hemophilus influenzae* are susceptible to erythromycin at the concentrations of the antibiotic achieved with usual therapeutic doses.

Corynebacterium diphtheriae: As an adjunct to antitoxin, to prevent the establishment of carriers, and to eradicate the organism in carriers.

Corynebacterium minutissimum: In the treatment of erythrasma.

Listeria monocytogenes: Infections due to this organism.

Neisseria gonorrhoeae: ERYTHROCIN PIGGYBACK (erythromycin lactobionate for injection) in conjunction with erythromycin stearate or base orally, as an alternative drug in treatment of acute pelvic inflammatory disease caused by *N. gonorrhoeae* in female patients with a history of sensitivity to penicillin. Before treatment of gonorrhea, patients who are suspected of also having syphilis should have a microscopic examination for *T. pallidum* (by immunofluorescence or darkfield) before receiving erythromycin, and monthly serologic tests for a minimum of 4 months.

Legionnaires' Disease: Although no controlled clinical efficacy studies have been conducted, *in vitro* and limited preliminary clinical data suggest that erythromycin may be effective in treating Legionnaires' Disease.

CONTRAINDICATIONS

Erythromycin is contraindicated in patients with known hypersensitivity to this antibiotic.

PRECAUTIONS

Since erythromycin is principally excreted by the liver, caution should be exercised when erythromycin is administered to patients with impaired hepatic function.

Prolonged or repeated use of erythromycin may result in an overgrowth of non-susceptible bacteria or fungi. If superinfection occurs, erythromycin should be discontinued and appropriate therapy instituted.

Areas of localized infection may require surgical drainage in addition to antibiotic therapy.

Recent data from studies of erythromycin reveal that its use in patients who are receiving high doses of theophylline may be associated with an increase of serum theophylline levels and potential theophylline toxicity. In case of theophylline toxicity and/or elevated serum theophylline levels, the dose of theophylline should be reduced while the patient is receiving concomitant erythromycin therapy.

Usage during pregnancy and lactation: The safety of erythromycin for use during pregnancy has not been established. Erythromycin crosses the placental barrier. Erythromycin also appears in breast milk.

ADVERSE REACTIONS

Side effects following the use of intravenous erythromycin are rare. Occasional venous irritation has been encountered, but if the infusion is given slowly, in dilute solution, preferably by continuous intravenous infusion or intermittent infusion in no less than 20 to 60 minutes, pain and vessel trauma are minimized.

Allergic reactions, ranging from urticaria and mild skin eruptions to anaphylaxis, have occurred with intravenously administered erythromycin.

Reversible hearing loss associated with the intravenous infusion of 4 g or more per day of erythromycin lactobionate has been reported rarely.

DOSAGE AND ADMINISTRATION

For the treatment of severe infections in adults and children, the recommended intravenous dose of erythromycin lactobionate is 15 to 20 mg/kg/day. Higher doses, up to 4 g/day, may be given for very severe infections. ERYTHROCIN LACTOBIONATE-I.V. must be administered by continuous or intermittent intravenous infusion only. Due to the irritative properties of erythromycin, I.V. push is an unacceptable route of administration.

Continuous infusion of erythromycin lactobionate is preferable due to the slower infusion rate and lower concentration of erythromycin; however, intermittent infusion at intervals not greater than every six hours is also effective. Intravenous erythromycin should be replaced by oral erythromycin as soon as possible.

For slow continuous infusion: The final diluted solution of erythromycin lactobionate is prepared to give a concentration of 1 g per liter (1 mg/ml).

For intermittent infusion: Administer one-fourth the total daily dose of erythromycin lactobionate by intravenous infusion in 20 to 60 minutes at intervals not greater than every six hours. The final diluted solution of erythromycin lactobionate is prepared to give a concentration of 1 to 5 mg/ml. No less than 100 ml of I.V. diluent should be used. Infusion should be sufficiently slow to minimize pain along the vein.

For treatment of acute pelvic inflammatory disease caused by *N. gonorrhoeae*, in female patients hypersensitive to penicillins, administer 500 mg erythromycin lactobionate every six hours for three days, followed by oral administration of 250 mg erythromycin stearate or base every six hours for seven days.

For treatment of Legionnaires' Disease: Although optimal doses have not been established, doses utilized in reported clinical data were 1 to 4 grams daily in divided doses.

Preparation of Solution:

1. PREPARE THE INITIAL SOLUTION OF ERYTHROCIN® LACTOBIONATE-I.V. BY ADDING 10 ML OF STERILE WATER FOR INJECTION, USP, TO THE 500 MG VIAL OR 20 ML OF STERILE WATER FOR INJECTION, USP, TO THE 1 G VIAL. Use only Sterile Water for Injection, USP, as other diluents may cause precipitation during reconstitution. Do not use diluents containing preservatives or inorganic salts. Note: When the product is reconstituted as directed above, the resulting solution contains an effective microbial preservative.

After reconstitution, each ml contains 50 mg of erythromycin activity. The initial solution is stable at refrigerator temperature for two weeks, or for 24 hours at room temperature.

2. ADD THE INITIAL DILUTION TO ONE OF THE FOLLOWING DILUENTS BEFORE ADMINISTRATION to give a concentration of 1 g of erythromycin activity per liter (1 mg/ml) for continuous infusion or 1 to 5 mg/ml for intermittent infusion:

0.9% SODIUM CHLORIDE INJECTION, USP
LACTATED RINGER'S INJECTION, USP
NORMOSOL®-R

3. THE FOLLOWING SOLUTIONS MAY ALSO BE USED PROVIDING THEY ARE FIRST BUFFERED WITH NEUT® (4% SODIUM BICARBONATE, ABBOTT) by adding 1 ml of Neut per 100 ml of solution:

5% DEXTROSE INJECTION, USP
5% DEXTROSE AND LACTATED RINGER'S INJECTION
5% DEXTROSE AND 0.9% SODIUM CHLORIDE INJECTION, USP

Neut® (4% sodium bicarbonate, Abbott) must be added to these solutions so that their pH is in the optimum range for erythromycin lactobionate stability. Acidic solutions of erythromycin lactobionate are unstable and lose their potency rapidly. A pH of at least 5.5 is desirable for the final diluted solution of erythromycin lactobionate.

No drug or chemical agent should be added to an erythromycin lactobionate-I.V. fluid admixture unless its effect on the chemical and physical stability of the solution has first been determined.

Stability: The final diluted solution of erythromycin lactobionate should be completely administered within 8 hours, since it is not suitable for storage.*

HOW SUPPLIED

ERYTHROCIN LACTOBIONATE-I.V. (erythromycin lactobionate for injection, USP) is supplied as a sterile, lyophilized powder in packages of 5 vials (**NDC** 0074-6342-05), each vial containing the equivalent of 1 g of erythromycin with 180 mg benzyl alcohol added as preservative; and in packages of 5 vials (**NDC** 0074-6365-02), each vial containing the equivalent of 500 mg of erythromycin with 90 mg benzyl alcohol added as preservative.

Exposure of pharmaceutical products to heat should be minimized. Prior to reconstitution avoid excessive heat. Brief exposure up to 104°F (40°C) does not adversely affect the product.

*Contact Abbott Laboratories, Dept. 498 for additional stability data.

Abbott Laboratories
North Chicago, IL 60064
Ref. 01-2163-R14

ERYTHROCIN® PIGGYBACK ℞

[e-rith 'ro-sin pig 'gy back]
(erythromycin lactobionate for injection, USP)
Single Dose Dispensing Vial
For I.V. use only

DESCRIPTION

Erythromycin is produced by a strain of *Streptomyces erythraeus* and belongs to the macrolide group of antibiotics. It is basic and readily forms salts with acids.

Erythromycin lactobionate is a soluble salt of erythromycin. ERYTHROCIN PIGGYBACK is a dosage form suitable for intermittent intravenous administration.

ACTIONS

Microbiology: Biochemical tests demonstrate that erythromycin inhibits protein synthesis of the pathogen without directly affecting nucleic acid synthesis. Antagonism has been demonstrated between clindamycin and erythromycin.

NOTE: Many strains of *Hemophilus influenzae* are resistant to erythromycin alone, but are susceptible to erythromycin and sulfonamides together. Staphylococci resistant to erythromycin may emerge during a course of erythromycin therapy. Culture and susceptibility testing should be performed.

Disc Susceptibility Tests: Quantitative methods that require measurement of zone diameters give the most precise estimates of antibiotic susceptibility. One recommended procedure (21 CFR section 460.1) uses erythromycin class discs for testing susceptibility; interpretations correlate zone diameters of this disc test with MIC values for erythromycin. With this procedure, a report from the laboratory of "susceptible" indicates that the infecting organism is likely to respond to therapy. A report of "resistant" indicates that the infective organism is not likely to respond to therapy. A report of "intermediate susceptibility" suggests that the organism would be susceptible if higher doses were used.

CLINICAL PHARMACOLOGY

Erythromycin binds to the 50 S ribosomal subunits of susceptible bacteria and suppresses protein synthesis.

Intravenous infusion of 500 mg erythromycin lactobionate at a constant rate over 1 hour in fasting adults produced a mean serum erythromycin level of approximately 7 mcg/ml at 20 minutes, 10 mcg/ml at 1 hour, 2.6 mcg/ml at 2.5 hours, and 1 mcg/ml at 6 hours.

Erythromycin diffuses readily into most body fluids. Only low concentrations are normally achieved in the spinal fluid, but passage of the drug across the blood-brain barrier increases in meningitis. In the presence of normal hepatic function, erythromycin is concentrated in the liver and excreted in the bile; the effect of hepatic dysfunction on excretion of erythromycin by the liver into the bile is not known. From 12 to 15 percent of intravenously administered erythromycin is excreted in active form in the urine.

Erythromycin crosses the placental barrier and is excreted in breast milk.

INDICATIONS

ERYTHROCIN PIGGYBACK (erythromycin lactobionate for injection) is indicated in the treatment of patients where oral administration is not possible or where the severity of the infection requires immediate high serum levels of erythromycin. Intravenous therapy should be replaced by oral administration at the appropriate time.

Steptococcus pyogenes (Group A betahemolytic streptococcus): Upper and lower respiratory tract, skin, and soft tissue infections of mild to moderate severity.

Injectable benzathine penicillin G is considered by the American Heart Association to be the drug of choice in the treatment and prevention of streptococcal pharyngitis and in long-term prophylaxis of rheumatic fever.

When oral medication is preferred for treatment of the above conditions, penicillin G, V, or erythromycin are alternate drugs of choice.

Staphylococcus aureus: Acute infections of skin and soft tissue of mild to moderate severity. Resistant organisms may emerge during treatment.

Streptococcus pneumoniae (Diplococcus pneumoniae): For upper respiratory tract infections (e.g., otitis media, pharyngitis) and lower respiratory tract infections (e.g., pneumonia) of mild to moderate severity.

Mycoplasma pneumoniae (Eaton agent, PPLO): For respiratory infections due to this organism.

Hemophilus influenzae: For upper respiratory tract infections of mild to moderate severity when used concomitantly with adequate doses of sulfonamides. (See sulfonamide labeling for appropriate prescribing information). The concomitant use of the sulfonamides is necessary since not all strains of *Hemophilus influenzae* are susceptible to erythromycin at the concentrations of the antibiotic achieved with usual therapeutic doses.

Corynebacterium diphtheriae: As an adjunct to antitoxin, to prevent the establishment of carriers, and to eradicate the organism in carriers.

Corynebacterium minutissimum: In the treatment of erythrasma.

Listeria monocytogenes: Infections due to this organism.

Neisseria gonorrhoeae: ERYTHROCIN PIGGYBACK (erythromycin lactobionate for injection) in conjunction with erythromycin stearate or base orally, as an alternative drug in treatment of acute pelvic inflammatory disease caused by *N. gonorrhoeae* in female patients with a history of sensitivity to penicillin. Before treatment of gonorrhea, patients who are suspected of also having syphilis should have a microscopic examination for *T. pallidum* (by immunofluorescence or darkfield) before receiving erythromycin, and monthly serologic tests for a minimum of 4 months.

Legionnaires' Disease: Although no controlled clinical efficacy studies have been conducted, *in vitro* and limited preliminary clinical data suggest that erythromycin may be effective in treating Legionnaires' Disease.

CONTRAINDICATIONS

Erythromycin is contraindicated in patients with known hypersensitivity to this antibiotic.

Continued on next page

Abbott—Cont.

PRECAUTIONS

Since erythromycin is principally excreted by the liver, caution should be exercised when erythromycin is administered to patients with impaired hepatic function.

Prolonged or repeated use of erythromycin may result in an overgrowth of nonsusceptible bacteria or fungi. If superinfection occurs, erythromycin should be discontinued and appropriate therapy instituted.

Areas of localized infection may require surgical drainage in addition to antibiotic therapy.

Recent data from studies of erythromycin reveal that its use in patients who are receiving high doses of theophylline may be associated with an increase of serum theophylline levels and potential theophylline toxicity. In case of theophylline toxicity and/or elevated serum theophylline levels, the dose of theophylline should be reduced while the patient is receiving concomitant erythromycin therapy.

Usage during pregnancy and lactation: The safety of erythromycin for use during pregnancy has not been established. Erythromycin crosses the placental barrier. Erythromycin also appears in breast milk.

ADVERSE REACTIONS

Side effects following the use of intravenous erythromycin are rare. Occasional venous irritation has been encountered. Allergic reactions, ranging from urticaria and mild skin eruptions to anaphylaxis, have occurred with intravenously administered erythromycin.

Reversible hearing loss associated with the intravenous infusion of 4 Gm or more per day of erythromycin lactobionate has been reported rarely.

DOSAGE AND ADMINISTRATION

For the treatment of severe infections in adults and children, the recommended intravenous dose of erythromycin lactobionate is 15 to 20 mg/kg/day. Higher doses, up to 4 Gm/day, may be given for very severe infections. ERYTHROCIN PIGGYBACK should be administered by intravenous infusion. Due to the high concentration of erythromycin, I.V. push is not an acceptable route of administration. Intravenous erythromycin should be replaced by oral erythromycin as soon as possible.

After reconstitution each ml of ERYTHROCIN PIGGYBACK solution contains 5 mg of erythromycin activity (500 mg in 100 ml). The drug may be administered directly from the vial. When this preparation is administered by intermittent infusion one-fourth the total daily dose of erythromycin lactobionate should be administered over a 20 to 60 minute period at intervals not greater than every 6 hours. The infusion should be sufficiently slow to minimize pain along the vein.

For treatment of acute pelvic inflammatory disease caused by *N. gonorrhoeae,* in female patients hypersensitive to penicillins, administer 500 mg erythromycin lactobionate every 6 hours for 3 days, followed by oral administration of 250 mg erythromycin stearate or base every 6 hours for 7 days.

For treatment of Legionnaires' Disease: Although optimal doses have not been established, doses utilized in reported clinical data were 1 to 4 grams daily in divided doses.

Preparation of Solution: Prepare the ERYTHROCIN PIGGYBACK (erythromycin lactobionate for injection) solution by adding 100 ml of 0.9% Sodium Chloride Injection, USP, or Lactated Ringer's Injection, USP, or Normosol®-R Solution to the dispensing vial. Immediately after adding diluent, the product should be shaken well to aid dissolution. Lack of immediate agitation will greatly increase time required for complete dissolution. Reconstitution may also be made using 100 ml of the following solutions to which 1 ml of Neut® (4% sodium bicarbonate, Abbott) has first been added:

5% Dextrose Injection, USP
5% Dextrose and Lactated Ringer's Injection
5% Dextrose and 0.9% Sodium Chloride Injection, USP
Normosol®-M and 5% Dextrose Injection
Normosol®-R and 5% Dextrose Injection

Neut® (4% sodium bicarbonate, Abbott) must be added to these solutions so that their pH is in the optimum range for erythromycin lactobionate stability. Acidic solutions of erythromycin lactobionate are unstable and lose their potency rapidly. A pH of at least 5.5 is desirable.

No drug or chemical agent should be added to an erythromycin lactobionate-I.V. fluid admixture unless its effect on the chemical and physical stability of the solution has first been determined.

Stability: The solution should be used within 8 hours if stored at room temperature and 24 hours if stored in the refrigerator. If the solution is to be frozen, it should be frozen (−10°C to −20°C) within 4 hours of preparation. Frozen solution may be stored for 30 days. Frozen solution should be thawed in the refrigerator and used within 8 hours after thawing is completed. THAWED SOLUTION MUST NOT BE REFROZEN.

HOW SUPPLIED

ERYTHROCIN PIGGYBACK (erythromycin lactobionate for injection, USP) is supplied as a sterile, lyophilized powder in packages of 5 single dose dispensing vials (**NDC** 0074-6368-13). Each vial contains the equivalent of 500 mg of erythromycin with 90 mg of benzyl alcohol.

Exposure of pharmaceutical products to heat should be minimized. Prior to reconstitution avoid excessive heat. Brief exposure up to 104°F (40°C) does not adversely affect the product.

Abbott Laboratories
North Chicago, IL 60064
Ref. 01-2161-R5

ERYTHROCIN® STEARATE ℞

[e-ry'thrō-sin]
(erythromycin stearate tablets, USP)
Filmtab® Tablets

DESCRIPTION

Erythromycin is produced by a strain of *Streptomyces erythraeus* and belongs to the macrolide group of antibiotics. It is basic and readily forms salts with acids. The base, the stearate salt, and the esters are poorly soluble in water, and are suitable for oral administration.

ERYTHROCIN STEARATE Filmtab tablets contain the stearate salt of the antibiotic in a unique film coating.

INACTIVE INGREDIENTS

250 mg tablet: Cellulosic polymers, corn starch, D&C Red No. 7, polacrilin potassium, polyethylene glycol, povidone, propylene glycol, sodium carboxymethylcellulose, sodium citrate, sorbic acid, sorbitan monooleate, titanium dioxide and other ingredients.

500 mg tablet: Cellulosic polymers, corn starch, FD&C Red No. 3, magnesium hydroxide, polacrilin potassium, povidone, propylene glycol, sorbitan monooleate, titanium dioxide, vanillin and other ingredients.

ACTIONS

Microbiology: Biochemical tests demonstrate that erythromycin inhibits protein synthesis of the pathogen without directly affecting nucleic acid synthesis. Antagonism has been demonstrated between clindamycin and erythromycin.

NOTE: Many strains of *Hemophilus influenzae* are resistant to erythromycin alone, but are susceptible to erythromycin and sulfonamides together. Staphylococci resistant to erythromycin may emerge during a course of erythromycin therapy. Culture and susceptibility testing should be performed.

Disc Susceptibility Tests: Quantitative methods that require measurement of zone diameters give the most precise estimates of antibiotic susceptibility. One recommended procedure (21 CFR section 460.1) uses erythromycin class discs for testing susceptibility; interpretations correlate zone diameters of this disc test with MIC values for erythromycin. With this procedure, a report from the laboratory of "susceptible" indicates that the infecting organism is likely to respond to therapy. A report of "resistant" indicates that the infective organism is not likely to respond to therapy. A report of "intermediate susceptibility" suggests that the organism would be susceptible if higher doses were used.

Clinical Pharmacology: Erythromycin binds to the 50 S ribosomal subunits of susceptible bacteria and suppresses protein synthesis.

Orally administered ERYTHROCIN STEARATE tablets are readily and reliably absorbed. Optimal serum levels of erythromycin are reached when the drug is taken in the fasting state or immediately before meals.

Erythromycin diffuses readily into most body fluids. Only low concentrations are normally achieved in the spinal fluid, but passage of the drug across the blood-brain barrier increases in meningitis. In the presence of normal hepatic function, erythromycin is concentrated in the liver and excreted in the bile; the effect of hepatic dysfunction on excretion of erythromycin by the liver into the bile is not known. Less than 5 percent of the orally administered dose of erythromycin is excreted in active form in the urine.

Erythromycin crosses the placental barrier and is excreted in breast milk.

INDICATIONS

Streptococcus pyogenes (Group A beta-hemolytic streptococcus): Upper and lower respiratory tract, skin, and soft tissue infections of mild to moderate severity.

Injectable benzathine penicillin G is considered by the American Heart Association to be the drug of choice in the treatment and prevention of streptococcal pharyngitis and in long-term prophylaxis of rheumatic fever.

When oral medication is preferred for treatment of the above conditions, penicillin G, V, or erythromycin are alternate drugs of choice.

When oral medication is given, the importance of strict adherence by the patient to the prescribed dosage regimen must be stressed. A therapeutic dose should be administered for at least 10 days.

Alpha-hemolytic streptococci (viridans group): Although no controlled clinical efficacy trials have been conducted, oral erythromycin has been suggested by the American Heart Association and American Dental Association for use in a regimen for prophylaxis against bacterial endocarditis in patients hypersensitive to penicillin who have congenital heart disease, or rheumatic or other acquired valvular heart disease when they undergo dental procedures and surgical procedures of the upper respiratory tract.[1] Erythromycin is not suitable prior to genitourinary or gastrointestinal tract surgery. NOTE: When selecting antibiotics for the prevention of bacterial endocarditis the physician or dentist should read the full joint statement of the American Heart Association and the American Dental Association.[1]

Staphylococcus aureus: Acute infections of skin and soft tissue of mild to moderate severity. Resistant organisms may emerge during treatment.

Streptococcus pneumoniae (Diplococcus pneumoniae): Upper respiratory tract infections (e.g., otitis media, pharyngitis) and lower respiratory tract infections (e.g., pneumonia) of mild to moderate degree.

Mycoplasma pneumoniae (Eaton agent, PPLO): For respiratory infections due to this organism.

Hemophilus influenzae: For upper respiratory tract infections of mild to moderate severity when used concomitantly with adequate doses of sulfonamides. (See sulfonamide labeling for appropriate prescribing information). The concomitant use of the sulfonamides is necessary since not all strains of *Hemophilus influenzae* are susceptible to erythromycin at the concentrations of the antibiotic achieved with usual therapeutic doses.

Chlamydia trachomatis: Erythromycin is indicated for treatment of the following infections caused by *Chlamydia trachomatis:* conjunctivitis of the newborn, pneumonia of infancy and urogenital infections during pregnancy. When tetracyclines are contraindicated or not tolerated, erythromycin is indicated for the treatment of uncomplicated urethral, endocervical, or rectal infections in adults due to *Chlamydia trachomatis.*[2]

Treponema pallidum: Erythromycin is an alternate choice of treatment for primary syphilis in patients allergic to the penicillins. In treatment of primary syphilis, spinal fluid examinations should be done before treatment and as part of follow-up after therapy.

Corynebacterium diphtheriae: As an adjunct to antitoxin, to prevent establishment of carriers, and to eradicate the organism in carriers.

Corynebacterium minutissimum: For the treatment of erythrasma.

Entamoeba histolytica: In the treatment of intestinal amebiasis only. Extra-enteric amebiasis requires treatment with other agents.

Listeria monocytogenes: Infections due to this organism.

Neisseria gonorrhoeae: Erythrocin Lactobionate-I.V. (erythromycin lactobionate for injection) in conjunction with erythromycin stearate orally, as an alternative drug in treatment of acute pelvic inflammatory disease caused by *N. gonorrhoeae* in female patients with a history of sensitivity to penicillin. Before treatment of gonorrhea, patients who are suspected of also having syphilis should have a microscopic examination for *T. pallidum* (by immunofluorescence or darkfield) before receiving erythromycin, and monthly serologic tests for a minimum of 4 months.

Bordetella pertussis: Erythromycin is effective in eliminating the organism from the nasopharynx of infected individuals, rendering them non-infectious. Some clinical studies suggest that erythromycin may be helpful in the prophylaxis of pertussis in exposed susceptible individuals.

Legionnaires' Disease: Although no controlled clinical efficacy studies have been conducted, *in vitro* and limited preliminary clinical data suggest that erythromycin may be effective in treating Legionnaires' Disease.

CONTRAINDICATIONS

Erythromycin is contraindicated in patients with known hypersensitivity to this antibiotic.

PRECAUTIONS

Erythromycin is principally excreted by the liver. Caution should be exercised in administering the antibiotic to patients with impaired hepatic function. There have been reports of hepatic dysfunction, with or without jaundice occurring in patients receiving oral erythromycin products.

Areas of localized infection may require surgical drainage in addition to antibiotic therapy.

Recent data from studies of erythromycin reveal that its use in patients who are receiving high doses of theophylline may be associated with an increase of serum theophylline levels and potential theophylline toxicity. In case of theophylline toxicity and/or elevated serum theophylline levels, the dose of theophylline should be reduced while the patient is receiving concomitant erythromycin therapy.

Usage during pregnancy and lactation: The safety of erythromycin for use during pregnancy has not been established.

Erythromycin crosses the placental barrier. Erythromycin also appears in breast milk.

ADVERSE REACTIONS

The most frequent side effects of oral erythromycin preparations are gastrointestinal, such as abdominal cramping and discomfort, and are dose-related. Nausea, vomiting, and diarrhea occur infrequently with usual oral doses.

During prolonged or repeated therapy, there is a possibility of overgrowth of nonsusceptible bacteria or fungi. If such infections occur, the drug should be discontinued and appropriate therapy instituted.

Allergic reactions ranging from urticaria and mild skin eruptions to anaphylaxis have occurred.

There have been isolated reports of reversible hearing loss occurring chiefly in patients with renal insufficiency and in patients receiving high doses of erythromycin.

DOSAGE AND ADMINISTRATION

Optimal serum levels of erythromycin are reached when ERYTHROCIN STEARATE (erythromycin stearate) is taken in the fasting state or immediately before meals.

Adults: The usual dosage is 250 mg every 6 hours; or 500 mg every 12 hours, taken in the fasting state or immediately before meals. Up to 4 g per day may be administered, depending upon the severity of the infection.

Children: Age, weight, and severity of the infection are important factors in determining the proper dosage. For the treatment of mild to moderate infections, the usual dosage is 30 to 50 mg/kg/day in 3 or 4 divided doses. When dosage is desired on a twice-a-day schedule, one-half of the total daily dose may be taken every 12 hours in the fasting state or immediately before meals. For the treatment of more severe infections the total daily dose may be doubled.

In the treatment of streptococcal infections, a therapeutic dosage of erythromycin should be administered for at least 10 days. In continuous prophylaxis of streptococcal infections in persons with a history of rheumatic heart disease, the dose is 250 mg twice a day.

For prophylaxis against bacterial endocarditis[1] in patients with congenital heart disease, or rheumatic or other acquired valvular heart disease when undergoing dental procedures or surgical procedures of the upper respiratory tract, give 1 g (20 mg/kg for children) orally 1½ to 2 hours before the procedure, and then, 500 mg (10 mg/kg for children) orally every 6 hours for 8 doses.

For conjunctivitis of the newborn caused by *Chlamydia trachomatis:* Oral erythromycin suspension 50 mg/kg/day in 4 divided doses for at least 2 weeks.[2]

For pneumonia of infancy caused by *Chlamydia trachomatis:* Although the optimal duration of therapy has not been established, the recommended therapy is oral erythromycin suspension 50 mg/kg/day in 4 divided doses for at least 3 weeks.[2]

For urogenital infections during pregnancy due to *Chlamydia trachomatis:* Although the optimal dose and duration of therapy have not been established, the suggested treatment is erythromycin 500 mg, by mouth, 4 times a day on an empty stomach for at least 7 days. For women who cannot tolerate this regimen, a decreased dose of 250 mg, by mouth, 4 times a day should be used for at least 14 days.[2]

For adults with uncomplicated urethral, endocervical, or rectal infections caused by *Chlamydia trachomatis* in whom tetracyclines are contraindicated or not tolerated: 500 mg, by mouth, 4 times a day for at least 7 days.[2]

For treatment of primary syphilis: 30 to 40 g given in divided doses over a period of 10 to 15 days.

For treatment of acute pelvic inflammatory disease caused by *N. gonorrhoeae:* 500 mg Erythrocin Lactobionate-I.V. (erythromycin lactobionate for injection) every 6 hours for 3 days, followed by 250 mg ERYTHROCIN STEARATE every 6 hours for 7 days.

For intestinal amebiasis: Adults: 250 mg four times daily for 10 to 14 days. Children: 30 to 50 mg/kg/day in divided doses for 10 to 14 days.

For use in pertussis: Although optimal dosage and duration have not been established, doses of erythromycin utilized in reported clinical studies were 40 to 50 mg/kg/day, given in divided doses for 5 to 14 days.

For treatment of Legionnaires' Disease: Although optimal doses have not been established, doses utilized in reported clinical data were 1 to 4 g daily in divided doses.

HOW SUPPLIED

ERYTHROCIN STEARATE Filmtab Tablets (erythromycin stearate tablets, USP) are supplied as:

Erythrocin Stearate Filmtab, 250 mg

Bottles of 100 ....(**NDC 0074-6346-20**)

Bottles of 500 ....(**NDC 0074-6346-53**)

ABBO-PAC® unit dose strip packages of
100 tablets ....(**NDC 0074-6346-38**)

Erythrocin Stearate Filmtab, 500 mg

Bottles of 100 ....(**NDC 0074-6316-13**)

REFERENCES

1. American Heart Association. 1977. Prevention of bacterial endocarditis. Circulation 56: 139A-143A.

2. CDC Sexually Transmitted Diseases Treatment Guidelines 1982.

FILMTAB—Film-sealed tablets, Abbott

Shown in Product Identification Section, page 403

Abbott Laboratories
North Chicago, IL 60064
Ref. 07-5360-R9

ERYTHROMYCIN BASE FILMTAB® ℞

[e-ri-thrō-mī′sin]
(erythromycin tablets, USP)

DESCRIPTION

Erythromycin is produced by a strain of *Streptomyces erythraeus* and belongs to the macrolide group of antibiotics. It is basic and readily forms salts with acids. The base, the stearate salt, and the esters are poorly soluble in water, and are suitable for oral administration.

ERYTHROMYCIN BASE FILMTAB tablets contain erythromycin, USP, in a unique, nonenteric film coating.

INACTIVE INGREDIENTS

250 mg tablet: Cellulosic polymers, corn starch, D&C Red No. 30, iron oxide, magnesium hydroxide, magnesium stearate, polyethylene glycol, propylene glycol, sodium starch glycolate, sorbic acid, sorbitan monooleate, titanium dioxide and other ingredients.

500 mg tablet: Castor oil, cellulosic polymers, D&C Red No. 30, magnesium stearate, microcrystalline cellulose, monobasic potassium phosphate, polacrilin potassium, povidone, sodium citrate, titanium dioxide, vanillin and other ingredients.

ACTIONS

Microbiology: Biochemical tests demonstrate that erythromycin inhibits protein synthesis of the pathogen without directly affecting nucleic acid synthesis. Antagonism has been demonstrated between clindamycin and erythromycin. NOTE: Many strains of *Hemophilus influenzae* are resistant to erythromycin alone, but are susceptible to erythromycin and sulfonamides together. Staphylococci resistant to erythromycin may emerge during a course of erythromycin therapy. Culture and susceptibility testing should be performed.

Disc Susceptibility Tests: Quantitative methods that require measurement of zone diameters give the most precise estimates of antibiotic susceptibility. One recommended procedure (21 CFR section 460.1) uses erythromycin class discs for testing susceptibility; interpretations correlate zone diameters of this disc test with MIC values for erythromycin. With this procedure, a report from the laboratory of "susceptible" indicates that the infecting organism is likely to respond to therapy. A report of "resistant" indicates that the infective organism is not likely to respond to therapy. A report of "intermediate susceptibility" suggests that the organism would be susceptible if higher doses were used.

Clinical Pharmacology: Erythromycin binds to the 50 S ribosomal subunits of susceptible bacteria and suppresses protein synthesis.

Orally administered erythromycin is readily absorbed by most patients, especially on an empty stomach, but patient variation is observed. Due to its formulation and nonenteric coating, this erythromycin tablet gives reliable blood levels in the average subject; however, the levels may vary with the individual.

Erythromycin diffuses readily into most body fluids. Only low concentrations are normally achieved in the spinal fluid, but passage of the drug across the blood-brain barrier increases in meningitis. In the presence of normal hepatic function, erythromycin is concentrated in the liver and excreted in the bile; the effect of hepatic dysfunction on excretion of erythromycin by the liver into the bile is not known. Less than 5 percent of the orally administered dose of erythromycin is excreted in active form in the urine.

Erythromycin crosses the placental barrier and is excreted in breast milk.

INDICATIONS

Streptococcus pyogenes (Group A beta-hemolytic streptococcus): Upper and lower respiratory tract, skin, and soft tissue infections of mild to moderate severity.

Injectable benzathine penicillin G is considered by the American Heart Association to be the drug of choice in the treatment and prevention of streptococcal pharyngitis and in long-term prophylaxis of rheumatic fever.

When oral medication is preferred for treatment of the above conditions, penicillin G, V, or erythromycin are alternate drugs of choice.

When oral medication is given, the importance of strict adherence by the patient to the prescribed dosage regimen must be stressed. A therapeutic dose should be administered for at least 10 days.

Alpha-hemolytic streptococci (viridans group): Although no controlled clinical efficacy trials have been conducted, oral erythromycin has been suggested by the American Heart Association and American Dental Association for use in a regimen for prophylaxis against bacterial endocarditis in patients hypersensitive to penicillin who have congenital heart disease, or rheumatic or other acquired valvular heart disease when they undergo dental procedures and surgical procedures of the upper respiratory tract.[1] Erythromycin is not suitable prior to genitourinary or gastrointestinal tract surgery. NOTE: When selecting antibiotics for the prevention of bacterial endocarditis the physician or dentist should read the full joint statement of the American Heart Association and the American Dental Association.[1]

Staphylococcus aureus: Acute infections of skin and soft tissue of mild to moderate severity. Resistant organisms may emerge during treatment.

Streptococcus pneumoniae (Diplococcus pneumoniae): Upper respiratory tract infections (e.g., otitis media, pharyngitis) and lower respiratory tract infections (e.g., pneumonia) of mild to moderate degree.

Mycoplasma pneumoniae (Eaton agent, PPLO): For respiratory infections due to this organism.

Hemophilus influenzae: For upper respiratory tract infections of mild to moderate severity when used concomitantly with adequate doses of sulfonamides. (See sulfonamide labeling for appropriate prescribing information). The concomitant use of the sulfonamides is necessary since not all strains of *Hemophilus influenzae* are susceptible to erythromycin at the concentrations of the antibiotic achieved with usual therapeutic doses.

Chlamydia trachomatis: Erythromycin is indicated for treatment of the following infections caused by *Chlamydia trachomatis:* conjunctivitis of the newborn, pneumonia of infancy and urogenital infections during pregnancy. When tetracyclines are contraindicated or not tolerated, erythromycin is indicated for the treatment of uncomplicated urethral, endocervical, or rectal infections in adults due to *Chlamydia trachomatis.*[2]

Treponema pallidum: Erythromycin is an alternate choice of treatment for primary syphilis in patients allergic to the penicillins. In treatment of primary syphilis, spinal fluid examinations should be done before treatment and as part of follow-up after therapy.

Corynebacterium diphtheriae: As an adjunct to antitoxin, to prevent establishment of carriers, and to eradicate the organism in carriers.

Corynebacterium minutissimum: For the treatment of erythrasma.

Entamoeba histolytica: In the treatment of intestinal amebiasis only. Extra-enteric amebiasis requires treatment with other agents.

Listeria monocytogenes: Infections due to this organism.

Neisseria gonorrhoeae: Erythrocin® Lactobionate-I.V. (erythromycin lactobionate for injection) in conjunction with erythromycin base orally, as an alternative drug in treatment of acute pelvic inflammatory disease caused by *N. gonorrhoeae* in female patients with a history of sensitivity to penicillin. Before treatment of gonorrhea, patients who are suspected of also having syphilis should have a microscopic examination for *T. pallidum* (by immunofluorescence or darkfield) before receiving erythromycin, and monthly serologic tests for a minimum of 4 months.

Bordetella pertussis: Erythromycin is effective in eliminating the organism from the nasopharynx of infected individuals, rendering them non-infectious. Some clinical studies suggest that erythromycin may be helpful in the prophylaxis of pertussis in exposed susceptible individuals.

Legionnaires' Disease: Although no controlled clinical efficacy studies have been conducted, *in vitro* and limited preliminary clinical data suggest that erythromycin may be effective in treating Legionnaires' Disease.

CONTRAINDICATIONS

Erythromycin is contraindicated in patients with known hypersensitivity to this antibiotic.

PRECAUTIONS

Erythromycin is principally excreted by the liver. Caution should be exercised in administering the antibiotic to patients with impaired hepatic function. There have been reports of hepatic dysfunction, with or without jaundice occurring in patients receiving oral erythromycin products.

Areas of localized infection may require surgical drainage in addition to antibiotic therapy.

Recent data from studies of erythromycin reveal that its use in patients who are receiving high doses of theophylline may be associated with an increase of serum theophylline levels and potential theophylline toxicity. In case of theophylline toxicity and/or elevated serum theophylline levels, the dose of theophylline should be reduced while the patient is receiving concomitant erythromycin therapy.

Usage during pregnancy and lactation: The safety of erythromycin for use during pregnancy has not been established.

Continued on next page

Abbott—Cont.

Erythromycin crosses the placental barrier. Erythromycin also appears in breast milk.

ADVERSE REACTIONS

The most frequent side effects of oral erythromycin preparations are gastrointestinal, such as abdominal cramping and discomfort, and are dose-related. Nausea, vomiting, and diarrhea occur infrequently with usual oral doses.

During prolonged or repeated therapy, there is a possibility of overgrowth of nonsusceptible bacteria or fungi. If such infections occur, the drug should be discontinued and appropriate therapy instituted.

Allergic reactions ranging from urticaria and mild skin eruptions to anaphylaxis have occurred.

There have been isolated reports of reversible hearing loss occurring chiefly in patients with renal insufficiency and in patients receiving high doses of erythromycin.

DOSAGE AND ADMINISTRATION

Optimum blood levels are obtained when doses are given on an empty stomach.

Adults: 250 mg every 6 hours is the usual dose; or 500 mg every 12 hours one hour before meals. Dosage may be increased up to 4 g per day according to the severity of the infection.

Children: Age, weight, and severity of the infection are important factors in determining the proper dosage. 30 to 50 mg/kg/day, in divided doses, is the usual dose. For more severe infections this dose may be doubled. If dosage is desired on a twice-a-day schedule, one-half of the total daily dose may be given every 12 hours, one hour before meals.

For the treatment of streptococcal infections: a therapeutic dosage should be administered for at least 10 days. In continuous prophylaxis of streptococcal infections in persons with rheumatic heart disease history, the dose is 250 mg twice a day.

For prophylaxis against bacterial endocarditis[1] in patients with congenital heart disease, or rheumatic or other acquired valvular heart disease when undergoing dental procedures or surgical procedures of the upper respiratory tract, give 1 g (20 mg/kg for children) orally 1½ to 2 hours before the procedure, and then, 500 mg (10 mg/kg for children) orally every 6 hours for 8 doses.

For conjunctivitis of the newborn caused by *Chlamydia trachomatis:* Oral erythromycin suspension 50 mg/kg/day in 4 divided doses for at least 2 weeks.[2]

For pneumonia of infancy caused by *Chlamydia trachomatis:* Although the optimal duration of therapy has not been established, the recommended therapy is oral erythromycin suspension 50 mg/kg/day in 4 divided doses for at least 3 weeks.[2]

For urogenital infections during pregnancy due to *Chlamydia trachomatis:* Although the optimal dose and duration of therapy have not been established, the suggested treatment is erythromycin 500 mg, by mouth, 4 times a day on an empty stomach for at least 7 days. For women who cannot tolerate this regimen, a decreased dose of 250 mg, by mouth 4 times a day should be used for at least 14 days.[2]

For adults with uncomplicated urethral, endocervical, or rectal infections caused by *Chlamydia trachomatis* in whom tetracyclines are contraindicated or not tolerated: 500 mg, by mouth, 4 times a day for at least 7 days.[2]

For treatment of primary syphilis: 30 to 40 g given in divided doses over a period of 10 to 15 days.

For treatment of acute pelvic inflammatory disease caused by *N. gonorrhoeae:* 500 mg Erythrocin Lactobionate-I.V. (erythromycin lactobionate for injection) every 6 hours for 3 days, followed by 250 mg erythromycin base every 6 hours for 7 days.

For intestinal amebiasis: Adults: 250 mg four times daily for 10 to 14 days. Children: 30 to 50 mg/kg/day in divided doses for 10 to 14 days.

For use in pertussis: Although optimal dosage and duration have not been established, doses of erythromycin utilized in reported clinical studies were 40 to 50 mg/kg/day, given in divided doses for 5 to 14 days.

For treatment of Legionnaires' Disease: Although optimal doses have not been established, doses utilized in reported clinical data were 1 to 4 g daily in divided doses.

HOW SUPPLIED

ERYTHROMYCIN BASE FILMTAB tablets (erythromycin tablets, USP) are supplied as pink capsule-shaped tablets in two dosage strengths:

250 mg tablets:

Bottles of 100 ....(**NDC** 0074-6326-13)

Bottles of 500 ....(**NDC** 0074-6326-53)

ABBO-PAC® unit dose strip packages of

100 tablets ....(**NDC** 0074-6326-11)

500 mg tablets:

Bottles of 100 ....(**NDC** 0074-6227-13).

REFERENCES

1. American Heart Association. 1977. Prevention of bacterial endocarditis. Circulation. 56: 139A-143A.
2. CDC Sexually Transmitted Diseases Treatment Guidelines 1982.

FILMTAB—Film-sealed tablets, Abbott.

Shown in Product Identification Section, page 403

Abbott Laboratories
North Chicago, IL 60064
Ref: 01-2382-R11

EUTONYL® Filmtab® Tablets ℞
(pargyline hydrochloride tablets, USP)

DESCRIPTION

EUTONYL (pargyline hydrochloride) is a non-hydrazine monoamine oxidase (MAO) inhibitor with hypotensive activity and is chemically identified as N-methyl-N-2-propynylbenzylamine hydrochloride. Clinically, EUTONYL is an effective oral antihypertensive agent which is primarily useful in the treatment of moderate to severe hypertension. EUTONYL is available as Filmtab tablets in two strengths containing 10 mg or 25 mg of pargyline hydrochloride.

INACTIVE INGREDIENTS

10 mg tablet: Castor oil, cellulosic polymers, corn starch, D&C Red No. 30, lactose, polyethylene glycol, povidone, propylene glycol, sorbitan monooleate, stearic acid, talc, titanium dioxide and other ingredients.

25 mg tablet: Castor oil, cellulosic polymers, corn starch, D&C Red No. 30, FD&C Yellow No. 5 (tartrazine), FD&C Yellow No. 6, lactose, polyethylene glycol, povidone, propylene glycol, sorbitan monooleate, stearic acid, talc, titanium dioxide and other ingredients.

CLINICAL PHARMACOLOGY

EUTONYL is a MAO inhibitor which has a potent antihypertensive action. Its exact mode of action is uncertain. The antihypertensive effect of pargyline is greatest when the patient is in the standing position. In about half of the patients treated, reduction of blood pressure in the sitting and supine positions was nearly as great as in the standing position. An interval of four days to three weeks or more may elapse following initiation of therapy before the full therapeutic effects of a given dosage schedule become manifest. A similar interval may be required for effects to subside after withdrawal of the drug, because the termination of drug effect is dependent on the regeneration of inhibited enzymes.

Information is limited on human pharmacokinetics for pargyline hydrochloride. It is extensively metabolized in the liver. The metabolites N-methyl benzylamine and propioladehyde have been identified. Pargyline passes the blood-brain barrier in rats and has been found in most tissues. In humans less than one percent of a given dose is excreted unchanged in the urine. Studies in the dog indicate that metabolic products are extensively eliminated in the urine.

INDICATIONS AND USAGE

EUTONYL is indicated in the treatment of moderate to severe hypertension. *It is not recommended for use in patients with mild or labile hypertension.* EUTONYL does not interfere with or obviate the use of diuretic therapy in hypertensive patients who may have an associated edema.

EUTONYL may be used alone or concurrently with most other antihypertensive agents. It is often effective at reduced dosage when administered with one of the thiazides and/or rauwolfia alkaloids.

CONTRAINDICATIONS

EUTONYL (pargyline hydrochloride) is contraindicated in patients with pheochromocytoma, paranoid schizophrenia, hyperthyroidism, and advanced renal failure.

EUTONYL should not be administered to those with malignant hypertension or to children under twelve years of age because significant clinical information concerning the use of the drug in these conditions is not available.

In general, the following drugs or agents are contraindicated in patients receiving EUTONYL due to the possibility of precipitating a sudden rise in blood pressure, including hypertensive crisis (see "Warnings" section):

Centrally acting sympathomimetic amines such as amphetamine and related compounds (includes most anorectic agents).

Peripherally acting sympathomimetic drugs such as ephedrine and its derivatives (also found in nasal decongestants, cold remedies, and hay fever preparations).

In some patients receiving pargyline, tyramine may precipitate an abrupt rise in blood pressure, including hypertensive crisis. Therefore, aged cheese (e.g., Cheddar, Camembert, and Stilton), processed cheese, beer and wine (especially, Chianti wine), and other foods which require the action of bacteria or molds for their preparation or preservation because of the presence of pressor substances such as tyramine should be avoided. Other foods which should be avoided during pargyline therapy because of their high pressor amine content include chocolate, yeast extract, avocado, pickled herring, pods of broad beans, ripened bananas, papaya products (including certain meat tenderizers), and chicken livers. Cream cheese, ricotta, and cottage cheese can be allowed in the diet during pargyline therapy since tyramine content is inconsequential.

Parenteral reserpine or guanethidine. Parenteral use of these drugs in patients receiving monoamine oxidase inhibitors results in a sudden release of accumulated catecholamines which may cause a hypertensive reaction. Reserpine and guanethidine should not be given parenterally during, and for at least one week following, treatment with pargyline.

Imipramine, amitriptyline, desipramine, nortriptyline, protriptyline, doxepin, or their analogues. The use of these drugs with a monoamine oxidase inhibitor has been reported to cause vascular collapse and hyperthermia which may be fatal. A drug-free interval (about two weeks) should separate therapy with EUTONYL (pargyline hydrochloride) and use of these agents.

Other monoamine oxidase inhibitors. These may augment the effects of pargyline.

Methyldopa or dopamine. These drugs may cause hyperexcitability in patients receiving pargyline.

L-dopa. There have been several reports of potentiation of the pressor effects of this drug by various monoamine oxidase inhibitors. At least one month should elapse after the discontinuation of pargyline before L-dopa is given.

WARNINGS

The most serious reactions to EUTONYL involve changes in blood pressure.

Hypertensive Crises: The most important reaction associated with EUTONYL administration is the occurrence of hypertensive crises precipitated by its interaction with numerous drug and food substances (see "Contraindications" and "Precautions" sections). These reactions have sometimes been fatal.

These crises are characterized by some or all of the following symptoms: occipital headache which may radiate frontally, palpitation, neck stiffness or soreness, nausea, vomiting, sweating (sometimes with fever and sometimes with cold, clammy skin), dilated pupils, photophobia, visual disturbances, stertorous breathing and coma. Either tachycardia or bradycardia may be present and can be associated with constricting chest pain.

NOTE: Intracranial bleeding has been reported in association with the increase in blood pressure.

Blood pressure should be observed frequently to detect evidence of any pressor response in all patients receiving EUTONYL. Therapy should be discontinued immediately upon the occurrence of palpitation or frequent headaches during therapy.

Recommended Treatment in Hypertensive Crisis: If a hypertensive crisis occurs, EUTONYL should be discontinued and therapy to lower blood pressure should be instituted immediately. Headache tends to abate as blood pressure is lowered. On the basis of present evidence, phentolamine is recommended. (The dosage reported for phentolamine is 5 mg. I.V.). Care should be taken to administer this drug slowly in order to avoid producing an excessive hypotensive effect. Fever should be managed by means of external cooling. Other symptomatic and supportive measures may be desirable in particular cases. Do not use parenteral reserpine.

PRECAUTIONS

General: All patients with impaired circulation to vital organs from any cause including those with angina pectoris, coronary artery disease, and cerebral arteriosclerosis should be closely observed for symptoms of orthostatic hypotension. If hypotension develops in these patients, EUTONYL (pargyline hydrochloride) dosage should be reduced or therapy discontinued since severe and/or prolonged hypotension may precipitate cerebral or coronary vessel thrombosis.

The hypotensive effect of EUTONYL may be augmented by febrile illnesses. It may be advisable to withdraw the drug during such diseases.

Care should be exercised in using EUTONYL in patients with impaired renal function. Since pargyline is excreted primarily in the urine, patients with impaired renal function may experience cumulative drug effects. Such patients should also be watched for elevations of blood urea nitrogen and other evidence of progressive renal failure. If such alterations should persist and progress, the drug should be discontinued.

EUTONYL should not be used in individuals with hyperactive or hyperexcitable personalities, as some of these patients show an undesirable increase in motor activity with restlessness, confusion, agitation, and disorientation. Clinical studies have shown that pargyline may unmask severe psychotic symptoms such as hallucinations or paranoid delusions in some patients with pre-existing serious emotional problems. This can usually be controlled by judicious administration of chlorpromazine intramuscularly, or other phenothiazines, the patient remaining supine for one hour after administration.

Pargyline should be used with caution in patients with Parkinsonism, as it may increase symptoms. In addition, great

care is required if pargyline is administered in conjunction with anti-parkinsonian agents.
Documented cases of eye changes or optic atrophy have not been reported with the use of pargyline as they have with the use of certain other monoamine oxidase inhibitors. However, since non-specific visual disturbances and aggravation of glaucoma have occurred occasionally, it is advisable that patients receiving EUTONYL be examined for changes in color perception, visual fields, fundi, and visual acuity.
The 25 mg dosage strength of EUTONYL tablets contains FD&C Yellow No. 5 (tartrazine) which may cause allergic-type reactions (including bronchial asthma) in certain susceptible individuals. Although the overall incidence of FD&C Yellow No. 5 (tartrazine) sensitivity in the general population is low, it is frequently seen in patients who also have aspirin hypersensitivity.
Information for Patients:
1. PATIENTS SHOULD BE WARNED AGAINST THE USE OF ANY OVER-THE-COUNTER PREPARATIONS, PARTICULARLY "COLD PREPARATIONS" AND ANTIHISTAMINES, OR PRESCRIPTION DRUGS WITHOUT THE KNOWLEDGE AND CONSENT OF THE PHYSICIAN.
2. PATIENTS SHOULD BE CAUTIONED ON THE USE OF CHEESE AND OTHER FOODS WITH HIGH TYRAMINE CONTENT (See "Contraindications" section) AND ALCOHOLIC BEVERAGES IN ANY FORM.
3. PATIENTS SHOULD BE WARNED ABOUT THE LIKELIHOOD OF THE OCCURRENCE OF ORTHOSTATIC HYPOTENSION.
4. PATIENTS SHOULD BE INSTRUCTED TO REPORT PROMPTLY THE OCCURRENCE OF SEVERE HEADACHE OR OTHER UNUSUAL SYMPTOMS.
5. PATIENTS WITH ANGINA PECTORIS OR CORONARY ARTERY DISEASE SHOULD BE ESPECIALLY WARNED NOT TO INCREASE THEIR PHYSICAL ACTIVITIES IN RESPONSE TO A DIMINUTION IN ANGINAL SYMPTOMS OR AN INCREASE IN WELL-BEING OCCURRING DURING TREATMENT WITH EUTONYL.

Laboratory Tests: There have been no substantiated reports of hepatotoxicity associated with pargyline therapy. However, since liver damage has resulted from use of certain other monoamine oxidase inhibitors, and since transient alterations in liver enzyme levels have occasionally occurred with pargyline, it is advisable that patients receiving EUTONYL (pargyline hydrochloride) have periodic liver function tests.
Drug Interactions: The therapeutic response to a variety of drugs may be changed or exaggerated in patients receiving a monoamine oxidase inhibitor such as pargyline hydrochloride. *Caffeine, alcohol, antihistamines, barbiturates, chloral hydrate* and other *hypnotics, sedatives, tranquilizers,* and *narcotics* (*meperidine* should not be used) should be used cautiously and at reduced dosage in patients who are taking pargyline. (See "Contraindications" section).
An increased response to *central depressants* may be manifested by acute hypotension and increased sedative effect. EUTONYL also may augment the hypotensive effects of anesthetic agents, and surgery. For this reason, the drug should be discontinued at least two weeks prior to surgery.
In the event of emergency surgery, ¼ to ⅕ of the usual dose of narcotics, sedatives, analgesics and other premedications should be used. If severe hypotension should occur, this can be controlled by small doses of a vasopressor agent such as norepinephrine.
EUTONYL may induce hypoglycemia. Therefore, EUTONYL should be given with caution to diabetics receiving *hypoglycemic agents* because severe hypoglycemia may occur. If it is necessary to administer EUTONYL to patients receiving insulin or other hypoglycemic agents, the dose of these agents should be reduced accordingly and the patient carefully monitored.
Clinical reports state that certain individuals receiving pargyline for a prolonged period of time are refractory to the nerve-blocking effects of *local anesthetics,* e.g., lidocaine.
Foods containing pressor substances, such as tyramine, should be avoided during pargyline therapy. (See "Contraindications" section).
Carcinogenesis, Mutagenesis, Impairment of Fertility: Adequate data are not available on long-term potential for carcinogenicity in animals or humans for pargyline hydrochloride.
The results of one study in which rats were injected with pargyline 15 mg/kg for ten days revealed seminiferous tubular degeneration with depletion of spermatogenic elements.
Pregnancy: Pregnancy Category C. Inadequate animal data is available to determine teratogenic potential for pargyline hydrochloride. However, limited studies reported in the literature indicate an embryocidal potential.
In one study, two groups of pregnant mice were given pargyline hydrochloride 2 mg/day subcutaneously during either early or late pregnancy. The results indicated that only three out of nineteen in the group treated during early pregnancy had normal litters. The remainder exhibited no signs of implantation. Four out of five litters in the group treated during late pregnancy were normal.
In another study pregnant rats were injected intraamniotically with a single 2.8–4.6 mg/kg dose of pargyline hydrochloride during various stages of pregnancy. Fetal death was noted following pargyline injection during every stage of pregnancy.
One study has been reported in which the intraamniotic administration of 50 to 100 mg of EUTONYL produced abortion in 19 out of 20 pregnant human females during the tenth to twenty-fourth week of gestation.
There are no adequate and well-controlled studies of systemically administered EUTONYL in pregnant women. EUTONYL should be used during pregnancy only if the potential benefit justifies the potential risk to the fetus.
Nursing Mothers: It is not known whether this drug is excreted in human milk. Because many drugs are excreted in human milk and because of the potential for serious adverse reactions in nursing infants from EUTONYL, a decision should be made whether to discontinue nursing or to discontinue the drug, taking into account the importance of the drug to the mother.
Pediatric Use: Safety and effectiveness in children below the age of 12 years have not been established.

ADVERSE REACTIONS

Generally side effects are not severe or serious when the recommended dosages are used and necessary precautions are observed. If side effects are severe or persist the drug should be discontinued. See also "Warnings" and "Precautions" sections. The following adverse reactions are listed by order of decreasing severity within each category.
Cardiovascular: Hypertensive crisis has been precipitated by concurrent use of sympathomimetic drugs or foods containing tyramine. (See "Contraindications" and "Warnings" sections).
Congestive heart failure has been reported in patients with reduced cardiac reserve.
The most frequently occurring side effects are those associated with orthostatic hypotension (dizziness, weakness, palpitation, or fainting). These usually respond to a reduction of dosage. Patients should be warned against rising to a standing position too quickly, especially when getting out of bed. Severe and persistent orthostatic hypotension should be avoided by reduction in dosage or discontinuation of therapy.
Central Nervous System: Increased neuromuscular activity (muscle twitching) and other extrapyramidal symptoms have been reported. Hyperexcitability, insomnia and headache have also occurred.
Gastrointestinal: Vomiting, nausea, mild constipation, increased appetite and dry mouth.
Genitourinary: Difficulty in micturition, impotence and delayed ejaculation.
Dermatologic: Purpura, rash and sweating.
Miscellaneous: In some patients reduction of blood sugar has been noted. Although the significance of this has not been elucidated, the possibility of hypoglycemic effects should be borne in mind. Aggravation of glaucoma, blurred vision, fluid retention, arthralgia, drug fever (rare) and nightmares have been reported. Gain in weight may be due to either edema or increased appetite.

OVERDOSAGE

The characteristic symptoms that may be caused by overdosage are usually those described on the preceding pages. However, an intensification of these symptoms and sometimes severe additional manifestations may be seen, depending on the degree of overdosage and on individual susceptibility. Some patients exhibit insomnia, restlessness and anxiety, progressing in severe cases to agitation, mental confusion and incoherence. Hypotension, dizziness, weakness and drowsiness may occur, progressing in severe cases to extreme dizziness and shock. A few patients have displayed hypertension with severe headache and other symptoms. Rare instances have been reported in which hypertension was accompanied by twitching or myoclonic fibrillation of skeletal muscles with hyperpyrexia, sometimes progressing to generalized rigidity and coma.
Gastric evacuation is helpful if performed early. Treatment should normally consist of general supportive measures, close observation of vital signs and steps to counteract specific symptoms as they occur, since MAO inhibition may persist. The management of hypertensive crises is described under Hypertensive Crises. (See "Warnings" section).
External cooling is recommended if hyperpyrexia occurs. Barbiturates have been reported to help relieve myoclonic reaction, but frequency of administration should be controlled carefully because EUTONYL (pargyline hydrochloride) may prolong barbiturate activity. When hypotension requires treatment, the standard measures for managing circulatory shock should be initiated. If pressor agents are used, the rate of infusion should be regulated by careful observation of the patient because an exaggerated pressor response sometimes occurs in the presence of MAO inhibition. Remember that the toxic effect of EUTONYL may be delayed or prolonged following the last dose of the drug. Therefore, the patient should be closely observed for at least a week.

DOSAGE AND ADMINISTRATION

EUTONYL is orally administered as a single daily dose; there is no known advantage in prescribing the drug more frequently than once daily. Clinical response to the drug is not immediate. Four days to three weeks or more may be required to produce the full effects of a given daily dosage. *For this reason it is generally unwise to increase dosage more frequently than once a week.* Likewise the effects of the drug may persist following reduction of dosage or withdrawal. If therapy must be interrupted because of undesirable side effects, the drug should be withheld until all such effects have disappeared. Therapy is then reinstituted at a lower dosage. Because the drug exerts an orthostatic effect on blood pressure, dosage adjustments should be based upon the blood pressure response *in the standing position.*
The usual adult dosage for initiating therapy in hypertensive patients not receiving other antihypertensive agents is 25 mg once daily. This dosage may be increased once a week by 10 mg increments until the desired response is obtained. The total daily dose of pargyline should not exceed 200 mg if excessive side effects are to be avoided.
Patients over age 65, or those who have undergone sympathectomy may be unusually sensitive to the antihypertensive properties of the drug. In such patients the initial daily dosage should be 10 to 25 mg. When EUTONYL is added to an established antihypertensive regimen, the initial dose should not exceed 25 mg daily (less in sympathectomized or elderly patients).
EUTONYL should not be administered to children under 12 years of age because of limited experience with the drug in this group.
Reduction of blood pressure is often maintained in hypertensive patients with a daily dose of 25 to 50 mg of EUTONYL alone. Larger doses may be tried in resistant cases. In general, dosage should be kept at the minimum level required to maintain a desirable reduction in blood pressure without encountering undue side effects. A few patients may develop a relative tolerance to the antihypertensive effects of the drug. The administration of additional antihypertensive agents may be considered in cases not controlled by EUTONYL alone.

HOW SUPPLIED

EUTONYL (pargyline hydrochloride tablets, USP) is available in Filmtab tablet strengths of 10 mg and 25 mg. The tablets are available in the following packages: 10 mg pink tablets in bottles of 100 (**NDC** 0074-6876-02) and 25 mg apricot-colored tablets in bottles of 100 (**NDC** 0074-6878-01).

Shown in Product Identification Section, page 403

Abbott Pharmaceuticals, Inc.
North Chicago, IL 60064
Ref. 03-4267-R7

FERO-FOLIC-500® Filmtab® Tablets ℞
[*fe'ro fo-lic*]
Controlled-Release Iron with Folic Acid and Vitamin C

IBERET-FOLIC-500® Filmtab® Tablets ℞
Controlled-Release Iron with Vitamin C, and B-Complex, including Folic Acid

DESCRIPTION

FERO-FOLIC-500 Filmtab is a hematinic for oral administration containing 525 mg of ferrous sulfate (equivalent to 105 mg of elemental iron) in a unique controlled-release vehicle, the Gradumet®. In addition, this product contains 800 mcg of folic acid and 500 mg of ascorbic acid present as sodium ascorbate.

INACTIVE INGREDIENTS

Cellulosic polymers, D&C Red No. 30, FD&C Blue No. 1, magnesium stearate, methyl acrylate-methyl methacrylate copolymer, pregelatinized starch (contains corn starch), polyethylene glycol, povidone, propylene glycol, talc, titanium dioxide, vanillin and other ingredients.
IBERET-FOLIC-500 is an Abbott hematinic containing iron in the Gradumet® controlled-release vehicle; vitamin C for enhancement of iron absorption; and the B-Complex vitamins including folic acid. The IBERET-FOLIC-500 Filmtab is for oral use.
Each Filmtab tablet provides:
*Ferrous Sulfate .... 525 mg
(equivalent to 105 mg of elemental iron)
Ascorbic Acid (present as sodium ascorbate) (C) .... 500 mg

Continued on next page

Abbott—Cont.

Niacinamide	30 mg
Calcium Pantothenate	10 mg
Thiamine Mononitrate (B_1)	6 mg
Riboflavin (B_2)	6 mg
Pyridoxine Hydrochloride (B_6)	5 mg
Folic Acid	800 mcg
Cyanocobalamin (B_{12})	25 mcg

*In controlled-release form (Gradumet)

INACTIVE INGREDIENTS

Cellulosic polymers, corn starch, D&C Red No. 7, FD&C Blue No. 1, FD&C Blue No. 2, FD&C Red No. 3, magnesium stearate, methyl acrylate-methyl methacrylate copolymer, polyethylene glycol, povidone, propylene glycol, stearic acid, talc, titanium dioxide, vanillin and other ingredients.

Controlled-release of iron from the Gradumet protects against gastric side effects. The Gradumet is an inert, porous, plastic matrix which is impregnated with ferrous sulfate. Iron is leached from the Gradumet as it passes through the gastrointestinal tract, and the expended matrix is excreted harmlessly in the stool. Controlled-release iron is particularly helpful in patients who have demonstrated intolerance to oral iron preparations.

CLINICAL PHARMACOLOGY

Oral iron is absorbed most efficiently when it is administered between meals. Conventional iron preparations, however, frequently cause gastric irritation when taken on an empty stomach. Studies with iron in the Gradumet have indicated that relatively little of the iron is released in the stomach, gastric intolerance is seldom encountered, and hematologic response ranks with that obtained from plain ferrous sulfate.

Iron is found in the body principally as hemoglobin. Storage in the form of ferritin occurs in the liver, spleen, and bone marrow. Concentrations of plasma iron and the total iron-binding capacity of plasma vary greatly in different physiological conditions and disease states.

Large amounts of ascorbic acid administered orally with ferrous sulfate have been shown to enhance iron absorption. Apparently this is due to the ability of ascorbic acid to prevent the oxidation of ferrous iron to the less effectively absorbed ferric form.

Folic acid and iron are absorbed in the proximal small intestine, particularly the duodenum. Folic acid is absorbed maximally and rapidly at this site, and iron is absorbed in a descending gradient from the duodenum distally.

After absorption folic acid is rapidly converted into its metabolically active forms. Approximately two-thirds is bound to plasma protein. Half of the folic acid stored in the body is found in the liver. Folic acid is also concentrated in spinal fluid.

Except for the folates ingested in liver, yeast, and egg yolk, the percentage of absorption of food folates averages about 10%.

The B-complex vitamins in IBERET-FOLIC-500 are absorbed by the active transport process. B-complex vitamins are rapidly eliminated and therefore are not stored in the body.

Calcium pantothenate is absorbed readily from the gastrointestinal tract and distributed to all body tissues.

INDICATIONS AND USAGE

FERO-FOLIC-500 is indicated for the treatment of iron deficiency and prevention of concomitant folic acid deficiency in nonpregnant adults. FERO-FOLIC-500 is also indicated in pregnancy for the prevention and treatment of iron deficiency and to supply a maintenance dosage of folic acid.

IBERET-FOLIC-500 is indicated in non-pregnant adults for the treatment of iron deficiency and prevention of concomitant folic acid deficiency where there is an associated deficient intake or increased need for the B-complex vitamins. IBERET-FOLIC-500 is also indicated in pregnancy for the prevention and treatment of iron deficiency where there is a concomitant deficient intake or increased need for the B-complex vitamins (including folic acid).

CONTRAINDICATIONS

FERO-FOLIC-500 and IBERET-FOLIC-500 are contraindicated in patients with pernicious anemia.

FERO-FOLIC-500 and IBERET-FOLIC-500 are also contraindicated in the rare instance of hypersensitivity to folic acid.

WARNINGS

Folic acid alone is improper therapy in the treatment of pernicious anemia and other megaloblastic anemias where vitamin B_{12} is deficient.

PRECAUTIONS

Where anemia exists, its nature should be established and underlying causes determined.

FERO-FOLIC-500 and IBERET-FOLIC-500 contain 800 mcg of folic acid per tablet. Folic acid especially in doses above 0.1 mg daily may obscure pernicious anemia, in that hematologic remission may occur while neurological manifestations remain progresssive. Concomitant parenteral therapy with vitamin B_{12} may be necessary in patients with deficiency of vitamin B_{12}. Pernicious anemia is rare in women of childbearing age, and the likelihood of its occurrence along with pregnancy is reduced by the impairment of fertility associated with vitamin B_{12} deficiency.

Like other oral iron preparations, FERO-FOLIC-500 and IBERET-FOLIC-500 should be stored out of the reach of children to guard against accidental iron poisoning (see Overdosage).

Laboratory Tests: In older patients and those with conditions tending to lead to vitamin B_{12} depletion, serum B_{12} levels should be regularly assessed during treatment with FERO-FOLIC-500 or IBERET-FOLIC-500.

Drug Interactions: Absorption of iron is inhibited by *magnesium trisilicate* and *antacids containing carbonates.*

Ferrous sulfate may interfere with the absorption of *tetracyclines.*

The antiparkinsonism effects of *levodopa* may be reversed by pyridoxine.

Iron absorption is inhibited by the ingestion of eggs or milk.

Carcinogenesis: Adequate data are not available on long-term potential for carcinogenesis in animals or humans.

Pregnancy: Pregnancy Category A. Studies in pregnant women have not shown that FERO-FOLIC-500 or IBERET-FOLIC-500 increase the risk of fetal abnormalities if administered during pregnancy. If either of these drugs is used during pregnancy, the possibility of fetal harm appears remote. Because studies cannot rule out the possibility of harm, however, FERO-FOLIC-500 or IBERET-FOLIC-500 should be used during pregnancy only if clearly needed.

Nursing Mothers: Folic acid, ascorbic acid, and B-complex vitamins are excreted in breast milk.

ADVERSE REACTIONS

The likelihood of gastric intolerance to iron in the controlled-release Gradumet vehicle is remote. If such should occur, the tablet may be taken after a meal. Allergic sensitization has been reported following both oral and parenteral administration of folic acid.

OVERDOSAGE

Signs of serious toxicity may be delayed because the iron is in a controlled-release dose form. Increased capillary permeability, reduced plasma volume, increased cardiac output, and sudden cardiovascular collapse may occur in acute iron intoxication. In overdosage, efforts should be made to hasten the elimination of the Gradumet tablets ingested. An emetic should be administered as soon as possible, followed by gastric lavage if indicated. Immediately following emesis, a large dose of a saline cathartic should be used to speed passage through the intestinal tract. X-ray examination may then be considered to determine the position and number of Gradumet tablets remaining in the gastrointestinal tract.

DOSAGE AND ADMINISTRATION

FERO-FOLIC-500 is administered orally and may be taken on an empty stomach.

Adults: For treatment of iron deficiency and prevention of folic acid deficiency, the recommended dose is one tablet daily.

Pregnant Adults: For prevention and treatment of iron deficiency and to supply a maintenance dosage of folic acid, the recommended dose is one tablet daily.

IBERET-FOLIC-500 is administered orally and may be taken on an empty stomach.

Adults: For the treatment of iron deficiency and prevention of concomitant folic acid deficiency where there is an associated deficient intake or increased need for the B-complex vitamins, the recommended dose is one tablet daily.

Pregnant Adults: For the prevention and treatment of iron deficiency where there is a concomitant deficient intake or increased need for the B-complex vitamins including folic acid, the recommended dose is one tablet daily.

HOW SUPPLIED

FERO-FOLIC-500 is supplied as red Filmtab tablets in bottles of 100 (**NDC** 0074-7079-13) and 500 (**NDC** 0074-7079-53).

IBERET-FOLIC-500 is supplied as red Filmtab tablets in bottles of 60 (**NDC** 0074-7125-60).

Abbott Pharmaceuticals, Inc.
North Chicago, IL 60064

Shown in Product Identification Section, page 403

FERO-GRAD-500® Filmtab® tablets

[fe'ro-grad]

IRON plus Vitamin C

Well-tolerated once-daily hematinic with controlled-release iron.

FERO-GRADUMET® Filmtab® tablets

Hematinic supplying controlled-release iron

DESCRIPTION

Each Fero-Gradumet and Fero-Grad-500 tablet contains the equivalent of 105 mg of elemental iron (525 mg of ferrous sulfate) in a unique controlled-release vehicle, the Gradumet®. In addition, each Fero-Grad-500 tablet contains 500 mg of vitamin C (as sodium ascorbate) to improve iron absorption.

The Gradumet, an inert, porous, plastic matrix, is impregnated with ferrous sulfate. Iron is leached from the Gradumet as it passes through the gastrointestinal tract, and the expended matrix is excreted harmlessly in the stool. Controlled-release iron is particularly helpful in patients who have demonstrated intolerance to other oral iron preparations.

INACTIVE INGREDIENTS

Fero-Grad-500: Castor oil, cellulosic polymers, D&C Red No. 7, FD&C Blue No. 1, magnesium stearate, methyl acrylate-methyl methacrylate copolymer, polyethylene glycol, povidone, pregelatinized starch (contains corn starch), propylene glycol, talc, titanium dioxide, vanillin and other ingredients.

Fero-Gradumet: Castor oil, cellulosic polymers, FD&C Red No. 40, FD&C Yellow No. 6, magnesium stearate, methyl acrylate-methyl methacrylate copolymer, polyethylene glycol, povidone, sorbitan monooleate, titanium dioxide, vanillin and other ingredients.

INDICATIONS

Fero-Grad-500: For the treatment of iron deficiency or iron deficiency anemia. Fero-Gradumet: For the prevention and treatment of iron deficiency.

PRECAUTIONS

Where anemia exists, its nature should be established and underlying cause determined.

Like other oral iron preparations Fero-Gradumet and Fero-Grad-500 should be stored out of the reach of children to protect against accidental iron poisoning (see Overdosage).

ADVERSE REACTIONS

The likelihood of gastric intolerance to iron in the controlled-release Gradumet vehicle is slight. If it should occur, the tablet may be taken after a meal.

DOSAGE AND ADMINISTRATION

Fero-Gradumet and Fero-Grad-500 are administered orally and may be taken on an empty stomach. The Gradumet controlled-release vehicle reduces the incidence of gastric side effects by delaying the release of almost all the iron until the tablet has passed the stomach.

Fero-Grad-500: Usual adult dose, including pregnant females: One tablet daily, or as directed by the physician.

Fero-Gradumet: Usual adult dose: Prevention: One tablet daily; Treatment: One tablet twice daily, or as directed by the physician. Pregnant females: Prevention: One tablet daily, or as directed by physician.

OVERDOSAGE

Signs of serious toxicity may be delayed because the iron is in a controlled-release dose form. Increased capillary permeability, reduced plasma volume, increased cardiac output, and sudden cardiovascular collapse may occur in acute iron intoxication. In overdosage, efforts should be made to hasten the elimination of the Gradumet tablets ingested. An emetic should be administered as soon as possible, followed by gastric lavage if indicated. Immediately following emesis, a large dose of a saline cathartic should be used to speed passage through the intestinal tract. X-ray examination may then be considered to determine the position and number of Gradumet tablets remaining in the gastrointestinal tract.

HOW SUPPLIED

Fero-Gradumet is supplied as red tablets in bottles of 100 (**NDC** 0074-6852-02); Fero-Grad-500 is supplied as red tablets in bottles of 30 (**NDC** 0074-7238-30), 100 (**NDC** 0074-7238-01) and 500 (**NDC** 0074-7238-02). The ingredients of these products are listed in one or more of the Medicare designated compendia.

Abbott Pharmaceuticals, Inc.
North Chicago, IL 60064

Shown in Product Identification Section, page 403

GEMONIL® ℞ Ⓒ III

[ge'mō-nil]

(metharbital tablets, USP)

DESCRIPTION

GEMONIL (metharbital) is a synthetic, N-methylated derivative of barbital which is identified chemically as 5,5-diethyl-1-methyl-barbituric acid.

INACTIVE INGREDIENTS

Corn starch, gelatin, lactose, stearic acid, talc and other ingredients.

ACTIONS

GEMONIL produces anticonvulsant effects which are similar to those produced by phenobarbital and mephobarbital. In experimental animals the drug has been shown to be unusually effective against pentylenetetrazol-induced convulsions. GEMONIL is less effective against convulsions induced by electroshock. Toxicity studies in mice, rats, cats and dogs indicate that the drug is less toxic and has less sedative effect than phenobarbital.

GEMONIL is adequately absorbed from the gastrointestinal tract following oral administration. It is demethylated in the liver to barbital, and is excreted largely in this form by the kidneys.

INDICATIONS

GEMONIL is indicated for the control of grand mal, petit mal, myoclonic and mixed types of seizures.

CONTRAINDICATIONS

GEMONIL is contraindicated in patients with known hypersensitivity to barbiturates, and in those with a history of manifest or latent porphyria.

WARNINGS

Metharbital may be habit forming.

USAGE DURING PREGNANCY AND LACTATION: THERE ARE MULTIPLE REPORTS IN THE CLINICAL LITERATURE WHICH INDICATE THAT THE USE OF ANTICONVULSANT DRUGS DURING PREGNANCY RESULTS IN AN INCREASED INCIDENCE OF BIRTH DEFECTS IN THE OFFSPRING. ALTHOUGH DATA ARE MORE EXTENSIVE WITH RESPECT TO TRIMETHADIONE, PARAMETHADIONE, PHENYTOIN, AND PHENOBARBITAL, REPORTS INDICATE A POSSIBLE SIMILAR ASSOCIATION WITH THE USE OF OTHER ANTICONVULSANT DRUGS. THEREFORE, ANTICONVULSANT DRUGS SHOULD BE ADMINISTERED TO WOMEN OF CHILDBEARING POTENTIAL ONLY IF THEY ARE CLEARLY SHOWN TO BE ESSENTIAL IN THE MANAGEMENT OF THEIR SEIZURES.

ANTICONVULSANT DRUGS SHOULD NOT BE DISCONTINUED IN PATIENTS IN WHOM THE DRUG IS ADMINISTERED TO PREVENT MAJOR SEIZURES BECAUSE OF THE STRONG POSSIBILITY OF PRECIPITATING STATUS EPILEPTICUS WITH ATTENDANT HYPOXIA AND RISK TO BOTH MOTHER AND THE UNBORN CHILD. CONSIDERATION SHOULD, HOWEVER, BE GIVEN TO DISCONTINUATION OF ANTICONVULSANTS PRIOR TO AND DURING PREGNANCY WHEN THE NATURE, FREQUENCY AND SEVERITY OF THE SEIZURES DO NOT POSE A SERIOUS THREAT TO THE PATIENT. IT IS NOT, HOWEVER, KNOWN WHETHER EVEN MINOR SEIZURES CONSTITUTE SOME RISK TO THE DEVELOPING EMBRYO OR FETUS.

REPORTS HAVE SUGGESTED THAT THE MATERNAL INGESTION OF ANTICONVULSANT DRUGS, PARTICULARLY BARBITURATES, IS ASSOCIATED WITH A NEONATAL COAGULATION DEFECT THAT MAY CAUSE BLEEDING DURING THE EARLY (USUALLY WITHIN 24 HOURS OF BIRTH) NEONATAL PERIOD. THE POSSIBILITY OF THE OCCURRENCE OF THIS DEFECT WITH THE USE OF GEMONIL SHOULD BE KEPT IN MIND. THE DEFECT IS CHARACTERIZED BY DECREASED LEVELS OF VITAMIN K-DEPENDENT CLOTTING FACTORS, AND PROLONGATION OF EITHER THE PROTHROMBIN TIME OR THE PARTIAL THROMBOPLASTIN TIME, OR BOTH. IT HAS BEEN SUGGESTED THAT VITAMIN K BE GIVEN PROPHYLACTICALLY TO THE MOTHER ONE MONTH PRIOR TO AND DURING DELIVERY, AND TO THE INFANT, INTRAVENOUSLY, IMMEDIATELY AFTER BIRTH.

THE SAFETY OF GEMONIL FOR USE DURING LACTATION HAS NOT BEEN ESTABLISHED.

THE PHYSICIAN SHOULD WEIGH THESE CONSIDERATIONS IN TREATMENT AND COUNSELING OF EPILEPTIC WOMEN OF CHILDBEARING POTENTIAL.

PRECAUTIONS

There is evidence that some barbiturates stimulate hepatic microsomal enzymes and therefore may increase the rate of metabolism of some drugs including the coumarin anticoagulants. Although metharbital has not been directly associated with such effect, caution is advised in patients receiving such anticoagulants.

Since metharbital is detoxified primarily in the liver, GEMONIL should be used with caution in patients with hepatic impairment.

In patients with convulsive disorders who have been taking regular daily doses, withdrawal of GEMONIL should be gradual since abrupt discontinuation of barbiturates given for the treatment of epilepsy may result in status epilepticus.

ADVERSE REACTIONS

GEMONIL (metharbital) has a low toxicity, and side effects are usually infrequent and mild. Gastric distress, dizziness, increased irritability, skin rash and drowsiness (large doses) may occur. If side effects become severe or cannot be controlled by dosage adjustment, the drug should be gradually withdrawn.

DOSAGE AND ADMINISTRATION

GEMONIL is administered orally. As with all antiepileptic therapy, it is particularly important to adjust the dosage for each patient to obtain optimal effect. For adults, the usual starting dose is 100 mg, one to three times daily. The usual initial pediatric dose should be one-half of a 100 mg tablet, one to three times daily, depending on the age and weight of the patient. A dose of 5 to 15 mg/kg per day has been recommended for children. According to the patient's tolerance these dosages may be gradually increased to the level required to control seizures. In some cases very small doses may be effective, whereas in other instances as much as 600 to 800 mg daily are required for adequate control.

GEMONIL may be used alone or in conjunction with other antiepileptic drugs such as Tridione® (trimethadione), Paradione® (paramethadione), Phenurone® (phenacemide), Peganone® (ethotoin), phenytoin sodium, or mephenytoin. Frequently, more effective control of seizures can be achieved by a combination of drugs. When added to an established regimen to replace or supplement other anticonvulsant therapy, the dosage of other medication should be gradually reduced while increasing that of GEMONIL so as to avoid or minimize recurrence of seizures.

OVERDOSAGE

Symptoms of overdosage include drowsiness, irritability, dizziness, and gastric distress. Loss of consciousness and coma may occur following very high doses. Treatment is the same as that for barbiturate intoxication.

HOW SUPPLIED

GEMONIL (metharbital tablets, USP) is supplied as grooved, 100 mg tablets in bottles of 100 (**NDC 0074-6401-01**).

This product is listed in USP, a Medicare designated compendium.

Abbott Laboratories
North Chicago, IL 60064
Ref. 01-2356-R4

H-BIG®
(Hepatitis B Immune Globulin [Human])

DESCRIPTION

Hepatitis B Immune Globulin (Human)—H-BIG®—is a sterile solution of immunoglobulin (10–18% protein) which is prepared by cold alcohol fractionation from pooled venous plasma of individuals with high titers of antibody to the hepatitis B suface antigen (anti-HBs). The product is stabilized with 0.3 M glycine and contains 1:10,000 Thimerosal (a mercury derivative) as a preservative. The solution has a pH of 6.8 ± 0.4. Each vial contains anti-HBs antibody equivalent to or exceeding the potency of anti-HBs in a U.S. reference hepatitis B immune globulin (Office of Biologics Research and Review, FDA).

This product has been prepared from large pools of human venous plasma. Each individual unit of plasma has been found nonreactive for hepatitis B surface antigen (HBsAg) using a U.S. Federally approved test with third-generation sensitivity.

CLINICAL PHARMACOLOGY

Hepatitis B Immune Globulin (Human) provides passive immunization for individuals exposed to the hepatitis B virus (HBV) as evidenced by a reduction in the attack rate of hepatitis B following its use. Clinical studies indicate the advantage of simultaneous administration of Hepatitis B Vaccine and Hepatitis B Immune Globulin (Human). Neonatal studies demonstrated the combined use of Hepatitis B Vaccine and Hepatitis B Immune Globulin (Human) to be more effective in the maintenance of protective antibody levels than prophylactic administration of Hepatitis B Vaccine or Hepatitis B Immune Globulin (Human) alone.

No prospective studies have been performed on the efficacy of concurrent Hepatitis B Vaccine and Hepatitis B Immune Globulin (Human) administration following parenteral exposure, mucous membrane contact or oral ingestion in adults; however, the Recommendation of the Immunization Practices Advisory Committee (ACIP) advises that the combination prophylaxis be provided based upon the increased efficiency found with that regimen in neonates.

In passive immunization with the administration of the recommended dose of Hepatitis B Immune Globulin (Human), a detectable level of circulating anti-HBs persists for approximately two months or longer. Cases of type B hepatitis are rarely seen following exposure to HBV in persons with pre-existing anti-HBs. No confirmed instance of transmission of hepatitis B has been associated with this product.

INDICATIONS AND USAGE

H-BIG® in conjunction with Hepatitis B Vaccine is indicated for post-exposure prophylaxis following either parenteral exposure, e.g., by accidental "needle-stick," or direct mucous membrane contact (accidental splash), or oral ingestion (pipetting accident) involving HBsAg positive materials such as blood, plasma or serum.

H-BIG® is also indicated for prophylaxis of infants born to HBsAg positive mothers. Such infants are at risk of being infected with hepatitis B virus and becoming chronic carriers. The risk is especially great if the mother is HBeAg positive. The carrier state can be prevented in about 75% of such exposures if newborns are given H-BIG® immediately after birth and in the early months of life. Concurrent H-BIG® and Hepatitis B Vaccine administration does not appear to interfere with antibody responses to Hepatitis B Vaccine and increases efficacy to about 94%.

CONTRAINDICATIONS

There are no specific contraindications for H-BIG®. No adverse reactions have been seen in individuals with preexisting hepatitis B surface antigen (HBsAg) although data regarding this occurrence are limited.

WARNINGS

H-BIG® should be given with caution to patients with a history of prior systemic allergic reactions following the administration of human immune globulin preparations.

In patients who have severe thrombocytopenia or any coagulation disorder that would contraindicate intramuscular injections, Hepatitis B Immune Globulin (Human) should be given only if the expected benefits outweigh the risks.

PRECAUTIONS

General

Hepatitis B Immune Globulin (Human) should *not* be administered intravenously because of the potential for serious reactions. Injections should be made intramuscularly, and care should be taken to draw back on the plunger of the syringe before injection in order to be certain that the needle is not in a blood vessel. Although systemic reactions to immune globulin preparations are rare, epinephrine should be available.

CLINICALLY SIGNIFICANT PRODUCT INTERACTIONS

Although administration of Hepatitis B Immune Globulin (Human) did not interfere with measles vaccination it is not known whether H-BIG® may interfere with the immune response to vaccination with other live virus vaccines. Hepatitis B Vaccine may be administered at the same time, but at a different injection site, without interference.

No interactions with other products are known.

Pregnancy Category C

Animal reproduction studies have not been conducted with H-BIG®. It is also not known whether Hepatitis B Immune Globulin (Human) can cause fetal harm when administered to a pregnant woman or can affect reproduction capacity. H-BIG® should be given to a pregnant woman only if clearly needed.

ADVERSE REACTIONS

Local pain and tenderness at the injection site, and urticaria and angioedema may occur; anaphylactic reactions, although rare, have been reported following the injection of human immune globulin preparations.

OVERDOSAGE

Although no data are available, clinical experience with other immunoglobulin preparations suggests that the only manifestations would be pain and tenderness at the injection site.

DOSAGE AND ADMINISTRATION

ADULTS

The Immunization Practices Advisory Committee (ACIP) recommends that Hepatitis B Immune Globulin (Human) and Hepatitis B Vaccine be given concurrently. The recommended dose of H-BIG® is 0.06 mL/kg (usually 3–5mL), administered as soon as possible after exposure (within 24 hours if possible). Immunization with Hepatitis B Vaccine should begin as soon as possible, but within 7 days of exposure. For use of vaccine, see manufacturer's literature. For persons who do not receive the vaccine, a second dose of H-BIG® (0.06 mL/kg) should be given 1 month after the first dose.

NEWBORNS

It is recommended that H-BIG® and Hepatitis B Vaccine be given concurrently to infants born to HBsAg positive mothers (especially those mothers who are HBeAg positive). The recommended dose of H-BIG® for at-risk newborns is 0.5 ml, as soon after birth as possible, preferably no later than 12 hours. Immunization with Hepatitis B Vaccine should begin promptly (within 7 days of birth). For information on Hepatitis B Vaccine refer to appropriate manufacturer's literature. A 0.5 ml dose of H-BIG® should be repeated at 3 and 6 months if Hepatitis B Vaccine is not given.

Parenteral drug products should be inspected visually for particulate matter and discoloration prior to administration, whenever solution and container permit.

HOW SUPPLIED

No. 8399—H-BIG®—is supplied in 0.5 ml syringe, 1 mL, 4 mL and 5 mL vials.

STORAGE

Store at 2 to 8°C (35 to 46°F). Do not freeze. Do not use after expiration date.

Continued on next page

If desired, additional literature on any Abbott Product will be provided upon request to Abbott Laboratories.

Abbott—Cont.

HARMONYL® Tablets ℞
[har'mō-nĭl]
(deserpidine)

DESCRIPTION
Harmonyl (deserpidine) is a purified rauwolfia alkaloid chemically identified as 11-desmethoxyreserpine.

INACTIVE INGREDIENTS
Corn starch, D&C Red No. 36, lactose, magnesium stearate, stearic acid, talc and other ingredients.

ACTIONS
The pharmacologic actions of HARMONYL (deserpidine) are essentially the same as those of other active rauwolfia alkaloids. Deserpidine probably produces its antihypertensive effects through depletion of tissue stores of catecholamines (epinephrine and norepinephrine) from peripheral sites. By contrast, its sedative and tranquilizing properties are thought to be related to depletion of 5-hydroxytryptamine from the brain.
The antihypertensive effect is often accompanied by bradycardia. There is no significant alteration in cardiac output or renal blood flow. The carotid sinus reflex is inhibited, but postural hypotension is rarely seen with the use of conventional doses of HARMONYL alone.
Deserpidine, like other rauwolfia alkaloids, is characterized by slow onset of action and sustained effect which may persist following withdrawal of the drug.

INDICATIONS
HARMONYL (deserpidine) is indicated for the treatment of mild essential hypertension. It is also useful as adjunctive therapy with other antihypertensive agents in the more severe forms of hypertension.
The drug is also indicated for the relief of symptoms in agitated psychotic states, e.g., schizophrenia—primarily in those individuals unable to tolerate phenothiazine derivatives or those who also require antihypertensive medication.

CONTRAINDICATIONS
HARMONYL (deserpidine) is contraindicated in patients with known hypersensitivity, mental depression especially with suicidal tendencies, active peptic ulcer, and ulcerative colitis. It is also contraindicated in patients receiving electroconvulsive therapy.

WARNINGS
Extreme caution should be exercised in treating patients with a history of mental depression. Discontinue the drug at the first sign of despondency, early morning insomnia, loss of appetite, impotence, or self-deprecation. Drug-induced depression may persist for several months after drug withdrawal and may be severe enough to result in suicide.

Usage in Pregnancy and Lactation
The safety of deserpidine for use during pregnancy or lactation has not been established; therefore, it should be used in pregnant women or in women of childbearing potential only when, in the judgment of the physician, its use is deemed essential to the welfare of the patient. Increased respiratory secretions, nasal congestion, cyanosis, and anorexia may occur in infants born to rauwolfia alkaloid-treated mothers since these preparations are known to cross the placental barrier to enter the fetal circulation and appear in cord blood. They also are secreted by nursing mothers into breast milk.
Reproductive and teratology studies in rats reduced the mating index and neonatal survival indices; the no-effect dosage has not been established.

PRECAUTIONS
Because rauwolfia preparations increase gastrointestinal motility and secretion, this drug should be used cautiously in patients with a history of peptic ulcer, ulcerative colitis, or gallstones, where biliary colic may be precipitated.
Caution should be exercised when treating hypertensive patients with renal insufficiency since they adjust poorly to lowered blood pressure levels.
Use HARMONYL (deserpidine) cautiously with digitalis and quinidine since cardiac arrhythmias have occurred with rauwolfia preparations.
Preoperative withdrawal of deserpidine does not assure that circulatory instability will not occur. It is important that the anesthesiologist be aware of the patient's drug intake and consider this in the overall management, since hypotension has occurred in patients receiving rauwolfia preparations.
Anticholinergic and/or adrenergic drugs (metaraminol, norepinephrine) have been employed to treat adverse vagocirculatory effects.
Animal tumorigenicity: There are no studies demonstrating that deserpidine is an animal tumorigen, although it is a prolactin stimulator and structurally related to reserpine. Rodent studies with reserpine, however, have shown that reserpine is an animal tumorigen, causing an increased incidence of mammary fibroadenomas in female mice, malignant tumors of the seminal vesicles in male mice, and malignant adrenal medullary tumors in male rats. These findings arose in 2 year studies in which the drug was administered in the feed at concentrations of 5 and 10 ppm—about 100 to 300 times the usual human dose. The breast neoplasms are thought to be related to reserpine's prolactin-elevating effect. Several other prolactin-elevating drugs have also been associated with an increased incidence of mammary neoplasia in rodents.
The extent to which these findings indicate a risk to humans is uncertain. Tissue culture experiments show that about one-third of human breast tumors are prolactin-dependent *in vitro*, a factor of considerable importance if the use of the drug is contemplated in a patient with previously detected breast cancer. The possibility of an increased risk of breast cancer in reserpine users has been studied extensively; however, no firm conclusion has emerged. Although a few epidemiologic studies have suggested a slightly increased risk (less than twofold in all studies except one) in women who have used reserpine, other studies of generally similar design have not confirmed this. Epidemiologic studies conducted using other drugs (neuroleptic agents) that, like reserpine, increase prolactin levels and, therefore, would be considered rodent mammary carcinogens, have not shown an association between chronic administration of the drug and human mammary tumorigenesis. While long-term clinical observation has not suggested such an association, the available evidence is considered too limited to be conclusive at this time. An association of reserpine intake with pheochromocytoma or tumors of the seminal vesicles has not been explored.

ADVERSE REACTIONS
The following adverse reactions have been reported with rauwolfia preparations. These reactions are usually reversible and disappear when the drug is discontinued.
Gastrointestinal: Including hypersecretion, anorexia, diarrhea, nausea, and vomiting.
Cardiovascular: Including angina-like symptoms, arrhythmias (particularly when used concurrently with digitalis or quinidine), and bradycardia.
Central Nervous System: Including drowsiness, depression, nervousness, paradoxical anxiety, nightmares, extrapyramidal tract symptoms, CNS sensitization manifested by dull sensorium, and deafness.
Dermatologic-Hypersensitivity: Including pruritus, rash, and asthma in asthmatic patients.
Ophthalmologic: Including glaucoma, uveitis, optic atrophy, and conjunctival injection.
Hematologic: Thrombocytopenic purpura.
Miscellaneous: Nasal congestion, weight gain, impotence or decreased libido, dysuria, dyspnea, muscular aches, dryness of mouth, dizziness, and headache.
Water retention with edema in patients with hypertensive vascular disease may occur rarely, but the condition generally clears with cessation of therapy or with the administration of a diuretic agent.

DOSAGE AND ADMINISTRATION
HARMONYL (deserpidine) is administered orally. For the management of mild essential hypertension in the average patient not receiving other antihypertensive agents, the usual initial adult dose is 0.75 to 1 mg daily. Because 10 to 14 days are required to produce the full effects of the drug, adjustments in dosage should not be made more frequently. If the therapeutic response is not adequate, it is generally advisable to add another antihypertensive agent to the regimen. For maintenance, dosage should be reduced. A single daily dose of 0.25 mg of deserpidine may suffice for some patients.
Concomitant use of deserpidine with ganglionic blocking agents, guanethidine, veratrum, hydralazine, methyldopa, chlorthalidone, or thiazides necessitates careful titration of dosage with each agent.
For psychiatric disorders: The average initial oral dose is 0.5 mg daily with a range of 0.125 to 1 mg. Adjust dosage upward or downward according to the patient's response.

OVERDOSAGE
An overdosage of deserpidine is characterized by flushing of the skin, conjunctival injection, and pupillary constriction. Sedation ranging from drowsiness to coma may occur. Hypotension, hypothermia, central respiratory depression and bradycardia may develop in cases of severe overdosage.
Treatment consists of the careful evacuation of stomach contents followed by the usual procedures for the symptomatic management of CNS depressant overdosage. If severe hypotension occurs, it should be treated with a direct acting vasopressor such as Levophed® (norepinephrine bitartrate injection, USP).

HOW SUPPLIED
HARMONYL (deserpidine) Tablets (grooved), 0.25 mg, are salmon-pink and supplied in bottles of 100 (**NDC** 0074-6906-07).
Abbott Laboratories
North Chicago, IL 60064
Ref. 01-2358-R2

IBERET®-500 Filmtab® tablets
[ī'be-ret]
IRON plus B-complex and Vitamin C
Well-tolerated once-daily hematinic with controlled-release iron.
IBERET® Filmtab® tablets
Hematinic Supplying Controlled-Release Iron, Vitamin C and Vitamin B-Complex

DESCRIPTION
Each Iberet-500 and Iberet Filmtab tablet contains 525 mg of ferrous sulfate (equivalent to 105 mg elemental iron) in the Gradumet® controlled-release vehicle. To enhance iron absorption, 500 mg of vitamin C has been added to each Iberet-500 Filmtab.
The Gradumet is an inert, porous, plastic matrix which is impregnated with ferrous sulfate. Iron is leached from the Gradumet as it passes through the gastrointestinal tract, and the expended matrix is excreted harmlessly in the stool.
Controlled-release iron is particularly helpful in patients who have demonstrated intolerance to other oral iron preparations.
Each Iberet-500 Filmtab tablet contains:

Ferrous Sulfate	525 mg
(equivalent to 105 mg of elemental iron)	
Vitamin C (as Sodium Ascorbate)	500 mg
Niacinamide	30 mg
Calcium Pantothenate	10 mg
Vitamin B_1 (Thiamine Mononitrate)	6 mg
Vitamin B_2 (Riboflavin)	6 mg
Vitamin B_6 (Pyridoxine Hydrochloride)	5 mg
Vitamin B_{12} (Cyanocobalamin)	25 mcg

The formulation of Iberet differs from Iberet-500 only in that it contains a lesser amount of vitamin C, 150 mg per Filmtab tablet.

INACTIVE INGREDIENTS
(Iberet and Iberet-500 Filmtabs): Albumen, castor oil, cellulosic polymers, corn starch, FD&C Red No. 40, FD&C Yellow No. 6, iron oxide, magnesium stearate, methyl acrylate-methyl methacrylate copolymer, polyethylene glycol, povidone, stearic acid, talc, titanium dioxide, vanillin and other ingredients.

INDICATIONS
Iberet-500: For the treatment of iron deficiency or iron deficiency anemia when there is a deficient intake or increased need for B-complex vitamins. Iberet: For conditions in which iron deficiency and vitamin C deficiency occur concomitantly with deficient intake or increased need for the B-complex vitamins.

PRECAUTIONS
Where anemia exists, its nature should be established and underlying cause determined.
Like other oral iron preparations, Iberet-500 and Iberet should be stored out of the reach of children to protect against accidental iron poisoning (see Overdosage).

ADVERSE REACTIONS
The likelihood of gastric intolerance to iron in the controlled-release Gradumet vehicle is slight. If it should occur, the tablet may be taken after a meal.

DOSAGE AND ADMINISTRATION
Iberet-500 and Iberet are administered orally and may be taken on an empty stomach. Usual Adult Dose, including pregnant females: One tablet daily, or as directed by the physician.

OVERDOSAGE
Signs of serious iron toxicity may be delayed because the iron is in a controlled-release dose form. Increased capillary permeability, reduced plasma volume, increased cardiac output, and sudden cardiovascular collapse may occur in acute iron intoxication. In overdosage, efforts should be made to hasten the elimination of the Gradumet tablets ingested. An emetic should be administered as soon as possible, followed by gastric lavage if indicated. Immediately following emesis, a saline cathartic should be administered to hasten passage through the intestinal tract. X-ray examination may then be considered to determine the position and number of Gradumet tablets remaining in the gastrointestinal tract.

HOW SUPPLIED
Iberet-500 is supplied as red, oval shaped tablets in bottles of 30 (**NDC** 0074-7235-30), 60 (**NDC** 0074-7235-01) and 500 (**NDC** 0074-7235-03), and in Abbo-Pac® unit dose packages of 100 (**NDC** 0074-7235-11); Iberet is supplied as red, round tablets in bottles of 60 (**NDC** 0074-6863-01).
Shown in Product Identification Section, page 403
Abbott Pharmaceuticals, Inc.
North Chicago, IL 60064

IBERET–FOLIC–500® ℞
Controlled-Release Iron with Vitamin C, and B-Complex, including Folic Acid)
Filmtab® Tablets

See combined listing under FERO-FOLIC-500.
Shown in Product Identification Section, page 403

IBERET®–500 LIQUID
[ī'bĕ-rĕt]
Hematinic Supplying Iron, Vitamin C and Vitamin B-Complex
IBERET®–LIQUID
Hematinic Supplying Iron, Vitamin C and Vitamin B-Complex

DESCRIPTION
Iberet-500 Liquid and Iberet-Liquid are hematinic preparations of ferrous sulfate, B-complex vitamins and ascorbic acid. Each teaspoonful (5 ml) of Iberet-500 Liquid provides:

Elemental Iron (as ferrous sulfate)	26.25 mg
Vitamin C (Ascorbic Acid)	125 mg
Niacinamide	7.5 mg
Dexpanthenol	2.5 mg
Vitamin B_1 (Thiamine Hydrochloride)	1.5 mg
Vitamin B_2 (Riboflavin)	1.5 mg
Vitamin B_6 (Pyridoxine Hydrochloride)	1.25 mg
Vitamin B_{12} (Cyanocobalamin)	6.25 mcg

In a citrus-flavored vehicle.
Iberet-Liquid has a raspberry-mint flavored vehicle; Iberet-500 Liquid has a smaller amount of ascorbic acid: 37.5 mg per teaspoonful.

INACTIVE INGREDIENTS
Iberet-Liquid: Alcohol 1%, methylparaben, propylparaben, sorbitol, water, natural and artificial flavors and other ingredients.
Iberet-500 Liquid: Glycerin, methylparaben, propylene glycol, propylparaben, sodium bicarbonate, sorbitol, sucrose, water, artificial flavor and other ingredients.

INDICATIONS
Iberet-500 Liquid: For conditions in which iron deficiency occurs concomitantly with deficient intake or increased need for the B-complex vitamins. Iberet-Liquid: For conditions in which iron deficiency and vitamin C deficiency occur concomitantly with deficient intake or increased need for the B-complex vitamins.

PRECAUTIONS
Where anemia exists, its nature should be established and underlying cause determined. Iberet-500 Liquid and Iberet-Liquid should be stored out of the reach of children because of the possibility of iron intoxication from accidental overdosage.

ADVERSE REACTIONS
If gastrointestinal symptoms appear as a sign of iron intolerance, smaller individual doses may be given at more frequent intervals to provide the desired daily amount. Administering Iberet-500 Liquid or Iberet-Liquid after meals may also reduce such effects.
Like other liquid iron preparations, Iberet-500 Liquid or Iberet-Liquid may stain the teeth on continued use. Stains may be prevented to a large extent by taking the dose through a straw, first mixing it with water or fruit juice, and by following the dose with a drink of plain water or juice. Brushing the teeth with sodium bicarbonate or hydrogen peroxide will usually remove existing stains.

DOSAGE AND ADMINISTRATION
Iberet-500 Liquid and Iberet-Liquid are administered orally, preferably after meals. Each has a fruit-flavored vehicle, and is suitable for pediatric patients who are unable to take tablets or capsules, and for patients who prefer or can better tolerate liquid medication. Iberet-500 Liquid and Iberet-Liquid may be administered by spoon or incorporated into infant formulas, water, or fruit juices. Iberet-500 Liquid: Usual dosage; Adults, including pregnant females and children 4 years of age and older—2 teaspoonfuls (10 ml) twice daily, after meals; Children 1–3 years of age—1 teaspoonful (5 ml) twice daily, after meals. Otherwise as directed by the physician. Iberet-Liquid: Usual dosage: Adults including pregnant females and children 4 years of age and older—2 teaspoonfuls (10 ml) three times daily, after meals; Children 1–3 years of age—1 teaspoonful (5 ml) three times daily, after meals. Otherwise as directed by the physician.

HOW SUPPLIED
Iberet-500 Liquid (**NDC** 0074-8422-02) and Iberet-Liquid (**NDC** 0074-7173-01) are supplied in 8 fl oz bottles.
Abbott Laboratories
North Chicago, IL 60064
Ref. 02-6647-3/R17 & 02-6648-4/R14

JANIMINE® Filmtab® Tablets ℞
[*ja-ni-mīne*]
(imipramine hydrochloride tablets, USP)

HOW SUPPLIED
JANIMINE is provided in three dosage sizes as monogrammed tablets:
10 mg, round-shaped, orange-colored, in bottles of 100 (**NDC** 0074-1897-13) and bottles of 1000 (**NDC** 0074-1897-19).
25 mg, round-shaped, yellow, in bottles of 100 (**NDC** 0074-1898-13) and bottles of 1000 (**NDC** 0074-1898-19).
50 mg, ovaloid-shaped, peach-colored, in bottles of 100 (**NDC** 0074-1899-13) and bottles of 1000 (**NDC** 0074-1899-19).
Inactive Ingredients: 10 mg tablet: Castor oil, cellulosic polymers, corn starch, FD&C Yellow No. 5 (tartrazine), FD&C Yellow No. 6, microcrystalline celulose, propylene glycol, stearic acid, talc, titanium dioxide, vanillin and other ingredients.
25 mg tablet: Castol oil, cellulosic polymers, corn starch, FD&C Yellow No. 5 (tartrazine), microcrystalline cellulose, propylene glycol, stearic acid, talc, titanium dioxide, vanillin and other ingredients.
50 mg tablet: Castor oil, cellulosic polymers, corn starch, FD&C Yellow No. 6, microcrystalline cellulose, stearic acid, talc, titanium dioxide, vanillin and other ingredients.
Shown in Product Identification Section, page 403
Abbott Laboratories
North Chicago, IL 60064

K-LOR™ Powder ℞
[*k'lor*]
(potassium chloride for oral solution, USP)

DESCRIPTION
Natural fruit-flavored K-LOR (potassium chloride for oral solution, USP) is an oral potassium supplement offered in individual packets as a powder for reconstitution. Each packet of K-LOR 20 mEq contains potassium 20 mEq and chloride 20 mEq provided by potassium chloride 1.5 g. Each packet of K-LOR 15 mEq contains potassium 15 mEq and chloride 15 mEq provided by potassium chloride 1.125 g.

INACTIVE INGREDIENTS
FD&C Yellow No. 6, maltodextrin (contains corn derivative), malic acid, saccharin, silica gel, natural flavoring and other ingredients.

CLINICAL PHARMACOLOGY
Potassium ion is the principal intracellular cation of most body tissues. Potassium ions participate in a number of essential physiological processes, including the maintenance of intracellular tonicity, the transmission of nerve impulses, the contraction of cardiac, skeletal, and smooth muscle and the maintenance of normal renal function.
Potassium depletion may occur whenever the rate of potassium loss through renal excretion and/or loss from the gastrointestinal tract exceeds the rate of potassium intake. Such depletion usually develops slowly as a consequence of prolonged therapy with oral diuretics, primary or secondary hyperaldosteronism, diabetic ketoacidosis, severe diarrhea, or inadequate replacement of potassium in patients on prolonged parenteral nutrition. Potassium depletion due to these causes is usually accompanied by a concomitant deficiency of chloride and is manifested by hypokalemia and metabolic alkalosis. Potassium depletion may produce weakness, fatigue, disturbances of cardiac rhythm (primarily ectopic beats), prominent U-waves in the electrocardiogram, and in advanced cases, flaccid paralysis and/or impaired ability to concentrate urine.
Potassium depletion associated with metabolic alkalosis is managed by correcting the fundamental causes of the deficiency whenever possible and administering supplemental potassium chloride, in the form of high-potassium food or potassium chloride solution or tablets. In rare circumstances, (e.g., patients with renal tubular acidosis) potassium depletion may be associated with metabolic acidosis and hyperchloremia. In such patients potassium replacement should be accomplished with potassium salts other than the chloride, such as potassium bicarbonate, potassium citrate, potassium gluconate, or potassium acetate.

INDICATIONS AND USAGE
1. For therapeutic use in patients with hypokalemia with or without metabolic alkalosis, in digitalis intoxication, and in patients with hypokalemic familial periodic paralysis.
2. For prevention of potassium depletion when the dietary intake of potassium is inadequate in the following conditions: patients receiving digitalis and diuretics for congestive heart failure; hepatic cirrhosis with ascites; states of aldosterone excess with normal renal function; potassium-losing nephropathy, and certain diarrheal states.
3. The use of potassium salts in patients receiving diuretics for uncomplicated essential hypertension is often unnecessary when such patients have a normal dietary pattern. Serum potassium should be checked periodically, however, and, if hypokalemia occurs, dietary supplementation with potassium-containing foods may be adequate to control milder cases. In more severe cases supplementation with potassium salts may be indicated.

CONTRAINDICATIONS
Potassium supplements are contraindicated in patients with hyperkalemia since a further increase in serum potassium concentration in such patients can produce cardiac arrest. Hyperkalemia may complicate any of the following conditions: chronic renal failure, systemic acidosis such as diabetic acidosis, acute dehydration, extensive tissue breakdown as in severe burns or adrenal insufficiency. Potassium supplements are contraindicated in patients receiving potassium-sparing diuretics (e.g., spironolactone, triamterene), since such use may produce severe hyperkalemia.
K-LOR (potassium chloride for oral solution) is contraindicated in patients with known hypersensitivity to any ingredient in this product.
Potassium chloride supplements are contraindicated in hypokalemic patients with metabolic acidosis. These patients should be treated with an alkalinizing potassium salt such as potassium bicarbonate, potassium citrate, potassium gluconate, or potassium acetate.

WARNINGS
Hyperkalemia: In patients with impaired mechanisms for excreting potassium, the administration of potassium salts can produce hyperkalemia and cardiac arrest. This occurs most commonly in patients given potassium intravenously, but may also occur in patients given potassium orally. Potentially fatal hyperkalemia can develop rapidly and can be asymptomatic.
Interaction with Potassium-Sparing Diuretics: Hypokalemia should not be treated by the concomitant administration of potassium salts and a potassium-sparing diuretic (e.g., spironolactone or triamterene), since the simultaneous administration of these agents can produce severe hyperkalemia.

PRECAUTIONS
The diagnosis of potassium depletion is ordinarily made by demonstrating hypokalemia in a patient with a clinical history suggesting some cause for potassium depletion. In interpreting the serum potassium level, the physician should bear in mind that acute alkalosis *per se* can produce hypokalemia in the absence of a deficit in total body potassium, while acute acidosis *per se* can increase the serum potassium concentration to within the normal range even in the presence of a reduced total body potassium. The treatment of potassium depletion, particularly in the presence of cardiac disease, renal disease, or acidosis, requires careful attention to acid-base balance and appropriate monitoring of serum electrolytes, the electrocardiogram, and the clinical status of the patient.
The use of potassium salts in patients with chronic renal disease, or any other condition which impairs potassium excretion, requires particularly careful monitoring of the serum potassium concentration and appropriate dosage adjustment.
Carcinogenesis: No data are available on long-term potential for carcinogenicity in animals or humans.
Pregnancy: K-LOR (potassium chloride for oral solution) is not expected to cause fetal harm when administered in dosages which will not result in hyperkalemia.
Nursing Mothers: Although no studies have been done, it is presumed that potassium chloride is excreted in human milk. Caution should be exercised when K-LOR is administered to a nursing woman.
Pediatric Use: Safety and effectiveness in children have not been established.

ADVERSE REACTIONS
One of the most severe adverse effects is hyperkalemia (see CONTRAINDICATIONS, WARNINGS and OVERDOSAGE).
The most common adverse reactions to oral potassium salts are nausea, vomiting, abdominal discomfort, and diarrhea. These symptoms are due to irritation of the gastrointestinal tract and are best managed by diluting the preparation further, taking the dose with meals, or reducing the dose.
Skin rash has been reported rarely.

OVERDOSAGE
The administration of oral potassium salts to persons with normal excretory mechanisms for potassium rarely causes serious hyperkalemia. However, if excretory mechanisms

Continued on next page

Abbott—Cont.

are impaired or if intravenous administration is too rapid, potentially fatal hyperkalemia can result (see Contraindications and Warnings). It is important to recognize that hyperkalemia is usually asymptomatic and may be manifested only by an increased serum potassium concentration and characteristic electrocardiographic changes (peaking of T-waves, loss of P-waves, depression of S-T segments, and prolongation of QT intervals). Late manifestations include muscle paralysis and cardiovascular collapse from cardiac arrest.

Treatment measures for hyperkalemia include the following: (1) elimination of foods and medications containing potassium and of potassium-sparing diuretics; (2) intravenous administration of 300 to 500 ml/hr of dextrose injection (10%–25%), containing 10 units of insulin/20 g dextrose; (3) correction of acidosis, if present, with intravenous sodium bicarbonate; (4) use of exchange resins, hemodialysis, or peritoneal dialysis. In treating hyperkalemia, it should be recalled that in patients who have been stabilized on digitalis, lowering the serum potassium concentration too rapidly can produce digitalis toxicity.

DOSAGE AND ADMINISTRATION

The dosage depends on the severity of the condition. The usual adult dose is 20 to 80 mEq of potassium per day (1 K-Lor 20 mEq packet 1 to 4 times daily after meals, or 1 K-Lor 15 mEq packet 2 to 5 times daily after meals).

Each 20 mEq (one K-Lor 20 mEq packet) of potassium should be dissolved in at least 4 oz (approximately ½ glassful) cold water or juice. Each 15 mEq (one K-Lor 15 mEq packet) of potassium should be dissolved in at least 3 oz (approximately ½ glassful) cold water or juice. These preparations, like other potassium supplements, must be properly diluted to avoid the possibility of gastrointestinal irritation.

HOW SUPPLIED

K-Lor 20 mEq (potassium chloride for oral solution, USP) is supplied in cartons of 30 packets (**NDC** 0074-3611-01), and cartons of 100 packets (**NDC** 0074-3611-02). Each packet contains potassium, 20 mEq, and chloride, 20 mEq, provided by potassium chloride, 1.5 g.

K-Lor 15 mEq (potassium chloride for oral solution, USP) is supplied in cartons of 100 packets (**NDC** 0074-3633-11). Each packet contains potassium, 15 mEq, and chloride, 15 mEq, provided by potassium chloride, 1.125 g.

Shown in Product Identification Section, page 403

Abbott Laboratories
North Chicago, IL 60064
Ref. 01-2367-R10
TM—Trademark

K•Tab® ℞

[k'tâb]

(Potassium Chloride Extended-Release Tablets, USP)

DESCRIPTION

K-Tab (potassium chloride extended-release tablets) is a film-coated (not enteric-coated) tablet containing 750 mg of potassium chloride (equivalent to 10 mEq) in an inert, porous, wax/polymer matrix. This oral potassium supplement formulation is intended to provide a controlled release of potassium from the matrix to minimize the likelihood of producing high localized concentrations of potassium within the gastrointestinal tract. The expended inert, porous, wax/polymer matrix is not absorbed and may be excreted intact in the stool.

INACTIVE INGREDIENTS

Castor oil, cellulosic polymers, colloidal silicon dioxide, D&C Yellow No. 10, magnesium stearate, paraffin, polyvinyl acetate, titanium dioxide, vanillin and other ingredients.

CLINICAL PHARMACOLOGY

Potassium ion is the principal intracellular cation of most body tissues. Potassium ions participate in a number of essential physiological processes, including the maintenance of intracellular tonicity, the transmission of nerve impulses, the contraction of cardiac, skeletal, and smooth muscle and the maintenance of normal renal function.

Potassium depletion may occur whenever the rate of potassium loss through renal excretion and/or loss from the gastrointestinal tract exceeds the rate of potassium intake. Such depletion usually develops slowly as a consequence of prolonged therapy with oral diuretics, primary or secondary hyperaldosteronism, diabetic ketoacidosis, severe diarrhea, or inadequate replacement of potassium in patients on prolonged parenteral nutrition. Potassium depletion due to these causes is usually accompanied by a concomitant deficiency of chloride and is manifested by hypokalemia and metabolic alkalosis. Potassium depletion may produce weakness, fatigue, disturbances of cardiac rhythm (primarily ectopic beats), prominent U-waves in the electrocardiogram, and in advanced cases, flaccid paralysis and/or impaired ability to concentrate urine.

Potassium depletion associated with metabolic alkalosis is managed by correcting the fundamental causes of the deficiency whenever possible and administering supplemental potassium chloride, in the form of high-potassium food or potassium chloride solution or tablets. In rare circumstances, (e.g., patients with renal tubular acidosis) potassium depletion may be associated with metabolic acidosis and hyperchloremia. In such patients potassium replacement should be accomplished with potassium salts other than the chloride, such as potassium bicarbonate, potassium citrate, potassium gluconate, or potassium acetate.

Bioavailability: Studies of urinary potassium excretion in subjects with potassium balance controlled by dietary measures were used to determine bioavailability of K-Tab (potassium chloride extended-release tablets). There were no significant differences in the cumulative amount of potassium excreted over 48 hours between K-Tab and 10% potassium chloride liquid demonstrating the bioequivalence of K-Tab to the 10% liquid.

INDICATIONS AND USAGE

BECAUSE OF REPORTS OF INTESTINAL AND GASTRIC ULCERATION AND BLEEDING WITH EXTENDED-RELEASE POTASSIUM CHLORIDE PREPARATIONS, THESE DRUGS SHOULD BE RESERVED FOR THOSE PATIENTS WHO CANNOT TOLERATE OR REFUSE TO TAKE LIQUID OR EFFERVESCENT POTASSIUM PREPARATIONS, OR FOR PATIENTS WITH WHOM THERE IS A PROBLEM OF COMPLIANCE WITH THESE PREPARATIONS.

1. For therapeutic use in patients with hypokalemia with or without metabolic alkalosis, in digitalis intoxication, and in patients with hypokalemic familial periodic paralysis.
2. For prevention of potassium depletion when the dietary intake of potassium is inadequate in the following conditions: patients receiving digitalis and diuretics for congestive heart failure; hepatic cirrhosis with ascites; states of aldosterone excess with normal renal function; potassium-losing nephropathy, and certain diarrheal states.
3. The use of potassium salts in patients receiving diuretics for uncomplicated essential hypertension is often unnecessary when such patients have a normal dietary pattern. Serum potassium should be checked periodically, however, and, if hypokalemia occurs, dietary supplementation with potassium-containing foods may be adequate to control milder cases. In more severe cases supplementation with potassium salts may be indicated.

CONTRAINDICATIONS

Potassium supplements are contraindicated in patients with hyperkalemia since a further increase in serum potassium concentration in such patients can produce cardiac arrest. Hyperkalemia may complicate any of the following conditions: chronic renal failure, systemic acidosis such as diabetic acidosis, acute dehydration, extensive tissue breakdown as in severe burns, or adrenal insufficiency. Potassium supplements are contraindicated in patients receiving potassium-sparing diuretics (e.g., spironolactone, triamterene), since such use may produce severe hyperkalemia.

K-Tab is contraindicated in patients with known hypersensitivity to any ingredient in this product.

Wax matrix potassium chloride preparations have produced esophageal ulceration in certain cardiac patients with esophageal compression due to an enlarged left atrium. Their use in such patients is contraindicated.

All solid dosage forms of potassium supplements are contraindicated in any patient in whom there is cause for arrest or delay in tablet passage through the gastrointestinal tract. These patients should take a liquid potassium preparation.

Potassium chloride supplements are contraindicated in hypokalemic patients with metabolic acidosis. These patients should be treated with an alkalinizing potassium salt such as potassium bicarbonate, potassium citrate, potassium gluconate, or potassium acetate.

WARNINGS

Hyperkalemia: In patients with impaired mechanisms for excreting potassium, the administration of potassium salts can produce hyperkalemia and cardiac arrest. This occurs most commonly in patients given potassium intravenously, but may also occur in patients given potassium orally. Potentially fatal hyperkalemia can develop rapidly and can be asymptomatic.

Interaction with Potassium-Sparing Diuretics: Hypokalemia should not be treated by the concomitant administration of potassium salts and a potassium-sparing diuretic (e.g., spironolactone or triamterene), since the simultaneous administration of these agents can produce severe hyperkalemia.

Gastrointestinal lesions:

Potassium chloride tablets have produced stenotic and/or ulcerative lesions of the small bowel and death. These lesions are caused by a high localized concentration of potassium ion in the region of a rapidly dissolving tablet, which in turn injures the bowel wall and thereby produces obstruction, hemorrhage, or perforation. K-Tab (potassium chloride extended-release tablets) is an inert, porous, wax/ polymer matrix tablet formulated to provide a controlled rate of release of potassium chloride and thus to minimize the possibility of a high local concentration of potassium ion near the bowel wall. While the reported frequency of small-bowel lesions is much less with wax matrix tablets (less than one per 100,000 patient-years) than with enteric-coated potassium chloride tablets (40–50 per 100,000 patient-years), cases associated with wax matrix tablets have been reported both in foreign countries and in the United States. In addition, perhaps because the wax matrix tablet preparations are not enteric-coated and therefore release potassium in the stomach, there have been reports of upper gastrointestinal bleeding associated with these products. The total number of gastrointestinal lesions remains less than one per 100,000 patient-years. If severe vomiting, abdominal pain, distention, or gastrointestinal bleeding occurs, potassium chloride extended-release tablets should be discontinued immediately, and the possibility of bowel obstruction or perforation should be considered.

PRECAUTIONS

The diagnosis of potassium depletion is ordinarily made by demonstrating hypokalemia in a patient with a clinical history suggesting some cause for potassium depletion. In interpreting the serum potassium level, the physician should bear in mind that acute alkalosis *per se* can produce hypokalemia in the absence of a deficit in total body potassium, while acute acidosis *per se* can increase the serum potassium concentration to within the normal range even in the presence of a reduced total body potassium. The treatment of potassium depletion, particularly in the presence of cardiac disease, renal disease, or acidosis, requires careful attention to acid-base balance and appropriate monitoring of serum electrolytes, the electrocardiogram, and the clinical status of the patient.

The use of potassium salts in patients with chronic renal disease, or any other condition which impairs potassium excretion, requires particularly careful monitoring of the serum potassium concentration and appropriate dosage adjustment.

Carcinogenesis: No data are available on long-term potential for carcinogenicity in animals or humans.

Pregnancy: K-Tab tablets are not expected to cause fetal harm when administered in dosages which will not result in hyperkalemia.

Nursing Mothers: Although no studies have been done, it is presumed that potassium chloride is excreted in human milk. Caution should be exercised when K-Tab is administered to a nursing woman.

Pediatric use: Safety and effectiveness in children have not been established.

ADVERSE REACTIONS

One of the most severe adverse effects is hyperkalemia (see Contraindications, Warnings, and Overdosage). There also have been reports of upper and lower gastrointestinal conditions including obstruction, bleeding, ulceration, and perforation (see Contraindications and Warnings); other factors known to be associated with such conditions were present in many of these patients.

The most common adverse reactions to oral potassium salts are nausea, vomiting, abdominal discomfort, and diarrhea. These symptoms are due to irritation of the gastrointestinal tract and are best managed by taking the dose with meals, or reducing the dose.

Skin rash has been reported rarely.

OVERDOSAGE

The administration of oral potassium salts to persons with normal excretory mechanisms for potassium rarely causes serious hyperkalemia. However, if excretory mechanisms are impaired or if intravenous administration is too rapid, potentially fatal hyperkalemia can result (see Contraindications and Warnings). It is important to recognize that hyperkalemia is usually asymptomatic and may be manifested only by an increased serum potassium concentration and characteristic electrocardiographic changes (peaking of T-waves, loss of P-waves, depression of S-T segments, and prolongation of QT intervals). Late manifestations include muscle paralysis and cardiovascular collapse from cardiac arrest.

Treatment measures for hyperkalemia include the following: (1) elimination of foods and medications containing potassium and of potassium-sparing diuretics; (2) intravenous administration of 300 to 500 ml/hr of dextrose injection (10%–25%) containing 10 units of insulin/20 g dextrose; (3) correction of acidosis, if present, with intravenous sodium bicarbonate; (4) use of exchange resins, hemodialysis, or peritoneal dialysis. In treating hyperkalemia, it should be recalled that in patients who have been stabilized on digitalis, lowering the serum potassium concentration too rapidly can produce digitalis toxicity.

DOSAGE AND ADMINISTRATION

The usual dietary intake of potassium by the average adult is 40 to 80 mEq per day. Potassium depletion sufficient to cause hypokalemia usually requires the loss of 200 or more mEq of potassium from the total body store. Dosage must be adjusted to the individual needs of each patient, but the usual adult dose is 20–80 mEq of potassium per day.

NOTE: K-TAB IS TO BE SWALLOWED WHOLE AND NOT CRUSHED OR CHEWED.

HOW SUPPLIED

K-TAB (potassium chloride extended-release tablets, USP) contains 750 mg of potassium chloride (equivalent to 10 mEq). K-TAB is provided as yellow, ovaloid, extended-release Filmtab® tablets in bottles of 100 (**NDC** 0074-7804-13) and 1000 (**NDC** 0074-7804-19) and in ABBO-PAC® unit dose packages of 100 (**NDC** 0074-7804-11).

Shown in Product Identification Section, page 403

Filmtab—Film-sealed tablets, Abbott
Abbott Pharmaceuticals, Inc.
North Chicago, IL 60064
Ref. 03-4299-R10

LIDOCAINE HYDROCHLORIDE INJECTION, USP ℞

[*līe 'dō-cāne*]

AQUEOUS SOLUTIONS FOR ACUTE MANAGEMENT OF CARDIAC ARRHYTHMIAS OR FOR LOCAL ANESTHESIA.

Abboject® Unit of Use Syringe
Ampul
Fliptop Vial
Multiple-dose Fliptop Vial
Pintop Vial
Pressurized Pintop Vial
Universal Additive Syringe

DESCRIPTION

Lidocaine Hydrochloride Injection, USP is a sterile, nonpyrogenic solution of lidocaine hydrochloride in water for injection for parenteral administration in various concentrations with characteristics as follows:

	Lidocaine HCl (anhydrous)						
Conc.	**0.5%**	**1%**	**1.5%**	**2%**	**4%**	**10%***	**20%***
mg/mL (anhyd.)	5	10	15	20	40	100	200
pH (approx.)	6.5	6.5	6.5	6.5	6.5	5.7	5.7

*10% and 20% concentrations FOR DILUTION ONLY. **Must not be administered without proper dilution prior to injection.**

Multiple-dose vials contain 0.1% of methylparaben added as preservative. Single-dose vials contain no preservative and unused portions must be discarded after use. May contain sodium hydroxide and hydrochloric acid for pH adjustment. May contain sodium chloride to adjust tonicity.

Lidocaine has cardiac antiarrhythmic properties and is a local anesthetic of the amide type.

Lidocaine Hydrochloride, USP is chemically designated 2-(diethylamino)-2',6'-acetoxylidide monohydrochloride monohydrate, a white powder freely soluble in water. It has the following structural formula:

CH_3

$-NHCOCH_2N(C_2H_5)_2 \cdot HCl \cdot H_2O$

CH_3

FOR CARDIAC ARRHYTHMIAS

CLINICAL PHARMACOLOGY

Mechanism of Action and Electrophysiology:

Studies of the effects of therapeutic concentrations of lidocaine on the electrophysiological properties of mammalian Purkinje fibers have shown that lidocaine attenuates phase 4 diastolic depolarization, decreases automaticity and causes a decrease or no change in excitability and membrane responsiveness. Action potential duration and effective refractory period of Purkinje fibers are decreased while the ratio of effective refractory period to action potential duration is increased. Action potential duration and effective refractory period of ventricular muscle are also decreased. Effective refractory period of the AV node may increase, decrease or remain unchanged and atrial effective refractory period is unchanged. Lidocaine raises the ventricular fibrillation threshold. No significant interactions between lidocaine and the autonomic nervous system have been described and consequently lidocaine has little or no effect on autonomic tone. Clinical electrophysiological studies with lidocaine have demonstrated no change in sinus node recovery time or sinoatrial conduction time, AV nodal conduction time is unchanged or shortened and His-Purkinje conduction time is unchanged.

Hemodynamics:

At therapeutic doses, lidocaine has minimal hemodynamic effects in normal subjects and in patients with heart disease. Lidocaine has been shown to cause no, or minimal decrease in ventricular contractility, cardiac output, arterial pressure or heart rate.

Pharmacokinetics and Metabolism:

Lidocaine is rapidly metabolized by the liver and less than 10% of a dose is excreted unchanged in the urine. Oxidative N-dealkylation, a major pathway of metabolism, results in the metabolites monoethylglycinexylidide and glycinexylidide. The pharmacological/toxicological activities of these metabolites are similar to but less potent than lidocaine. The primary metabolite in urine is a conjugate of 4-hydroxy-2,6-dimethylaniline.

The elimination half-life of lidocaine following an intravenous bolus injection is typically 1.5 to 2.0 hours. There are data that indicate that the half-life may be 3 hours or longer following infusions of greater than 24 hours.

Because of the rapid rate at which lidocaine is metabolized, any condition that alters liver function, including changes in liver blood flow which could result from severe congestive heart failure or shock may alter lidocaine kinetics. The half-life may be two-fold or more greater in patients with liver dysfunction. Renal dysfunction does not affect lidocaine kinetics, but may increase the accumulation of metabolites.

Therapeutic effects of lidocaine are generally associated with plasma levels of 6 to 25 μmole/L (1.5 to 6 μg free base per mL). The blood to plasma distribution ratio is approximately 0.84. Objective adverse manifestations become increasingly apparent with increasing plasma levels above 6.0 μg free base per mL.

The plasma protein binding of lidocaine is dependent on drug concentration and the fraction bound decreases with increasing concentration. At concentrations of 1 to 4 μg free base per mL, 60 to 80 percent of lidocaine is protein bound. In addition to lidocaine concentration, the binding is dependent on the plasma concentration of the α-1-acid glycoprotein.

Lidocaine readily crosses the placental and blood-brain barriers. Dialysis has negligible effects on the kinetics of lidocaine.

INDICATIONS AND USAGE

Lidocaine hydrochloride administered intravenously, is specifically indicated in the acute management of ventricular arrhythmias such as those occurring in relation to acute myocardial infarction, or during cardiac manipulation, such as cardiac surgery.

CONTRAINDICATIONS

Lidocaine hydrochloride is contraindicated in patients with a known history of hypersensitivity to local anesthetics of the amide type. Lidocaine hydrochloride should not be used in patients with Stokes-Adams syndrome, Wolff-Parkinson-White syndrome or with severe degrees of sinoatrial, atrioventricular or intraventricular block in the absence of an artificial pacemaker.

WARNINGS

IN ORDER TO MANAGE POSSIBLE ADVERSE REACTIONS, RESUSCITATIVE EQUIPMENT, OXYGEN AND OTHER RESUSCITATIVE DRUGS SHOULD BE IMMEDIATELY AVAILABLE WHEN LIDOCAINE HYDROCHLORIDE INJECTION IS USED.

THE 10% AND 20% CONCENTRATED SOLUTIONS MUST NOT BE INJECTED UNDILUTED. See DOSAGE AND ADMINISTRATION.

Systemic toxicity may result in manifestations of central nervous system depression (sedation) or irritability (twitching), which may progress to frank convulsions accompanied by respiratory depression and/or arrest. Early recognition of premonitory signs, assurance of adequate oxygenation and, where necessary, establishment of artificial airway with ventilatory support are essential to management of this problem. Should convulsions persist despite ventilatory therapy with oxygen, *small* increments of anticonvulsant drugs may be used intravenously. Examples of such agents include benzodiazepines (e.g., diazepam), ultrashort-acting barbiturates (e.g., thiopental or thiamylal) or a short-acting barbiturate (e.g., pentobarbital or secobarbital). If the patient is under anesthesia, a short-acting muscle relaxant (e.g., succinylcholine) may be used. Longer acting drugs should be used only when recurrent convulsions are evidenced.

Should circulatory depression occur, vasopressors may be used.

Constant electrocardiographic monitoring is essential to the proper administration of lidocaine hydrochloride. Signs of excessive depression of cardiac electrical activity such as sinus node dysfunction, prolongation of the P-R interval and QRS complex or the appearance or aggravation of arrhythmias, should be followed by flow adjustment and, if necessary, prompt cessation of the intravenous infusion of this agent. Occasionally, acceleration of ventricular rate may occur when lidocaine hydrochloride is administered to patients with atrial flutter or fibrillation.

PRECAUTIONS

1. **General:** Caution should be employed in the use of lidocaine hydrochloride in patients with severe liver or kidney disease because accumulation of the drug or metabolites may occur. Lidocaine Hydrochloride Injection, USP should be used with caution in the treatment of patients with hypovolemia, severe congestive heart failure, shock and all forms of heart block. In patients with sinus bradycardia or incomplete heart block, the administration of lidocaine hydrochloride intravenously for the elimination of ventricular ectopic beats without prior acceleration in heart rate (e.g., by atropine, isoproterenol or electric pacing) may promote more frequent and serious ventricular arrhythmias or complete heart block. (See CONTRAINDICATIONS).

Dosage should be reduced for children and for debilitated and/or elderly patients, commensurate with their age and physical status.

The safety of amide local anesthetic agents in patients with genetic predisposition of malignant hyperthermia has not been fully assessed; therefore, lidocaine should be used with caution in such patients.

In hospital environments where drugs known to be triggering agents for malignant hyperthermia (fulminant hypermetabolism) are administered, it is suggested that a standard protocol for management should be available.

It is not known whether lidocaine may trigger this reaction, however, large doses resulting in significant plasma concentrations, as may be achieved by intravenous infusion, pose potential risk to these individuals. Recognition of early unexplained signs of tachycardia, tachypnea, labile blood pressure and metabolic acidosis may precede temperature elevation. Successful outcome is dependent on early diagnosis, prompt discontinuance of the triggering agent and institution of treatment including oxygen therapy, supportive measures and dantrolene (for details see dantrolene package insert).

2. **Patient Information:** The patient should be advised of the possible occurrence of the experiences listed under ADVERSE REACTIONS.
3. **Laboratory Tests:** None known.
4. **Drug Interactions:** Lidocaine Hydrochloride Injection, USP should be used with caution in patients with digitalis toxicity accompanied by atrioventricular block. Concomitant use of beta-blocking agents may reduce hepatic blood flow and thereby reduce lidocaine clearance.
5. **Carcinogenesis, Mutagenesis, Impairment of Fertility:** Long term studies in animals to evaluate the carcinogenic and mutagenic potential or the effect on fertility of lidocaine HCl have not been conducted.
6. **Pregnancy:**
   Teratogenic Effects: *Pregnancy Category B.* Reproduction studies have been performed in rats at doses up to 6.6 times the maximum human doses and have revealed no significant findings. There are, however, no adequate and well-controlled studies in pregnant women. Because animal reproduction studies are not always predictive of human response, this drug should be used during pregnancy only if clearly needed.
7. **Labor and Delivery:** The effects of lidocaine HCl on the mother and the fetus, when used in the management of cardiac arrhythmias during labor and delivery are not known. Lidocaine readily crosses the placental barrier.
8. **Nursing Mothers:** It is not known whether this drug is excreted in human milk. Because many drugs are excreted in human milk, caution should be exercised when lidocaine is administered to a nursing woman.
9. **Pediatric Use:** Safety and effectiveness in children have not been established by controlled clinical studies. (See DOSAGE AND ADMINISTRATION).

ADVERSE REACTIONS

Adverse experiences following the administration of lidocaine are similar in nature to those observed with other amide local anesthetic agents. Adverse experiences may result from high plasma levels caused by excessive dosage or may result from a hypersensitivity, idiosyncrasy or diminished tolerance on the part of the patient. Serious adverse experiences are generally systemic in nature. The following types are those most commonly reported. The adverse experiences under Central Nervous System and Cardiovascular System are listed in general in a progression from mild to severe.

Continued on next page

Abbott—Cont.

1. **Central Nervous System**
CNS reactions are excitatory and/or depressant and may be characterized by light-headedness, nervousness, apprehension, euphoria, confusion, dizziness, drowsiness, tinnitus, blurred or double vision, vomiting, sensations of heat, cold or numbness, twitching, tremors, convulsions, unconsciousness, respiratory depression and arrest. The excitatory reactions may be very brief or may not occur at all, in which case, the first manifestation of toxicity may be drowsiness, merging into unconsciousness and respiratory arrest.
2. **Cardiovascular System**
Cardiovascular reactions are usually depressant in nature and are characterized by bradycardia, hypotension and cardiovascular collapse, which may lead to cardiac arrest.
3. Allergic reactions as a result of sensitivity to lidocaine are extremely rare and, if they occur, should be managed by conventional means.

DRUG ABUSE AND DEPENDENCE

Although specific studies have not been conducted, lidocaine HCl has been used clinically without evidence of abuse of this drug or of psychological or physical dependence as a result of its use.

OVERDOSAGE

Overdosage of lidocaine HCl usually results in signs of central nervous system or cardiovascular toxicity. See ADVERSE REACTIONS.

Should convulsions or signs of respiratory depression and arrest develop, the patency of the airway and adequacy of ventilation must be assured immediately. Should convulsions persist despite ventilatory therapy with oxygen, small increments of anticonvulsive agents may be given intravenously. Examples of such agents include a benzodiazepine (e.g., diazepam), an ultrashort-acting barbiturate (e.g., thiopental or thiamylal) or a short-acting barbiturate (e.g., pentobarbital or secobarbital). If the patient is under general anesthesia, a short-acting muscle relaxant (e.g., succinylcholine) may be administered.

Should circulatory depression occur, vasopressors may be used.

Dialysis is of negligible value in the treatment of acute overdosage from lidocaine HCl.

DOSAGE AND ADMINISTRATION

Adults

Single Direct Intravenous Injection (bolus): The usual dose is 50 to 100 mg of lidocaine hydrochloride (0.70 to 1.4 mg/kg; 0.32 to 0.63 mg/lb) administered intravenously under ECG monitoring. This dose may be administered at the rate of approximately 25 to 50 mg/min (0.35 to 0.70 mg/kg/min; 0.16 to 0.32 mg/lb/min). Sufficient time should be allowed to enable a slow circulation to carry the drug to the site of action. If the initial injection of 50 to 100 mg does not produce a desired response, a second dose may be injected after five minutes. NO MORE THAN 200 to 300 MG OF LIDOCAINE HYDROCHLORIDE SHOULD BE ADMINISTERED DURING A ONE HOUR PERIOD.

Continuous Intravenous Infusion: Following bolus administration, intravenous infusions of lidocaine hydrochloride may be initiated at the rate of 1 to 4 mg/min of lidocaine hydrochloride (0.014 to 0.057 mg/kg/min; 0.006 to 0.026 mg/lb/min). The rate of intravenous infusions should be reassessed as soon as the patient's basic cardiac rhythm appears to be stable or at the earliest signs of toxicity. It should rarely be necessary to continue intravenous infusions of lidocaine for prolonged periods.

Solutions for intravenous infusion may be prepared by the addition of one gram (or two grams) of lidocaine hydrochloride to one liter of 5% dextrose in water using aseptic technique. Approximately a 0.1% (or 0.2%) solution will result from this procedure; that is, each milliliter will contain approximately 1 (or 2 mg) of lidocaine hydrochloride. In those cases in which fluid restriction is medically appropriate, a more concentrated solution may be prepared.

The 20% concentration of lidocaine hydrochloride should be diluted with a suitable large volume parenteral as follows to achieve the above final concentrations for continuous infusion:

20% (200 mg/mL)	LVP Size	Final Conc.
1 g in 5 mL	1000 mL	0.1%
1 g in 5 mL	500 mL	0.2%
1 g in 5 mL	250 mL	0.4%
2 g in 10 mL	1000 mL	0.2%
2 g in 10 mL	500 mL	0.4%

The 10% concentration of lidocaine hydrochloride should be diluted with a suitable large volume parenteral as follows to achieve the above final concentrations for continuous infusion:

10% (100 mg/mL)	LVP Size	Final Conc.
1 g in 10 mL	1000 mL	0.1%
1 g in 10 mL	500 mL	0.2%
1 g in 10 mL	250 mL	0.4%

Lidocaine Hydrochloride Injection, USP has been found to be chemically stable for 24 hours after dilution in 5% dextrose in water. However, as with all intravenous admixtures, dilution of the solution should be made just prior to its administration.

When administering lidocaine hydrochloride (or any potent medication) by continuous intravenous infusion, it is advisable to use a precision volume control I.V. set.

Pediatric

Although controlled clinical studies to establish pediatric dosing schedules have not been conducted, the American Heart Association's *Standards and Guidelines* recommends a bolus dose of 1 mg/kg followed by an infusion rate of 3 μg/kg/min.

NOTE

Regarding Prolonged Infusions. There are data that indicate the half-life may be 3 hours or longer following infusions of greater than 24 hours in duration.

Parenteral drug products should be inspected visually for particulate matter and discoloration prior to administration, whenever solution and container permit.

FOR LOCAL ANESTHESIA

CLINICAL PHARMACOLOGY

Lidocaine stabilizes the neuronal membrane and prevents the initiation and conduction of nerve impulses, thereby effecting local anesthetic action.

Lidocaine is metabolized mainly in the liver and excreted via the kidneys. Approximately 90% of lidocaine administered is excreted in the form of various metabolites, while less than 10% is excreted unchanged.

INDICATIONS

Lidocaine Hydrochloride Injection, USP is indicated for production of local or regional anesthesia, by infiltration techniques, including percutaneous injection and intravenous regional anesthesia by peripheral nerve block techniques such as brachial plexus and intercostal blocks and by central neural techniques, including epidural and caudal blocks, when the accepted procedures for these techniques as described in standard textbooks are followed.

CONTRAINDICATIONS

Lidocaine hydrochloride is contraindicated in patients with a known history of hypersensitivity either to local anesthetic agents of the amide type or to other components of the injectable formulations.

WARNINGS

1. RESUSCITATIVE EQUIPMENT AND DRUGS, INCLUDING OXYGEN, SHOULD BE IMMEDIATELY AVAILABLE WHEN ANY LOCAL ANESTHETIC AGENT IS USED.
2. **Use in Pregnancy:** Reproductive studies have been performed in rats and rabbits without evidence of harm to the animal fetus. However, the safe use of lidocaine in humans has not been established with respect to possible adverse effects upon fetal development. Careful consideration should be given to this fact before administering this drug to women of childbearing potential, particularly during early pregnancy. This does not exclude the use of the drug at term for obstetrical analgesia. Lidocaine HCl has been used effectively for obstetrical analgesia. Adverse effect on the fetus, course of labor or delivery have rarely been observed when proper dosage and proper technique have been employed.
3. Local anesthetic procedures should be used with caution when there is inflammation and/or sepsis in the region of the proposed injection.
4. Vasopressor agents (administered for the treatment of hypotension related to caudal or other epidural blocks) should be used with caution in the presence of oxytocic drugs, as a severe persistent hypertension and even rupture of a cerebral blood vessel may occur.
5. The solutions which contain a vasoconstrictor should be used with extreme caution for patients whose medical history and physical evaluation suggest the existence of hypertension, arteriosclerotic heart disease, cerebral vascular insufficiency, heart block, thyrotoxicosis or diabetes, etc. The solutions which contain a vasoconstrictor should also be used with extreme caution in patients receiving drugs known to produce blood pressure alterations (e.g., MAO inhibitors, tricyclic antidepressants, phenothiazines, etc.) as either sustained hypotension or hypertension may occur.

PRECAUTIONS

The safety and effectiveness of Lidocaine Hydrochloride Injection, USP depends on proper dosage, correct technique, adequate precautions and readiness for emergencies. Standard textbooks should be consulted for specific techniques and precautions for various regional anesthetic procedures. The lowest dosage that results in effective anesthesia should be used. Injection of repeated doses of lidocaine HCl may cause significant increases in blood levels with each repeated dose due to slow accumulation of lidocaine or its metabolites. Tolerance varies with the status of the patient. Debilitated, elderly patients, acutely ill patients and children should be given reduced doses commensurate with their age and physical status. Lidocaine HCl should also be used with caution in patients with severe shock or heart block.

In using lidocaine HCl for infiltration or regional nerve block anesthesia, injection should always be made slowly and with frequent aspirations. Proper tourniquet technique is essential in the performance of intravenous regional anesthesia. Solutions containing epinephrine or other vasoconstrictors should not be used for this technique.

Epidural anesthesia and caudal anesthesia should be used with extreme caution in persons with the following conditions: Existing neurological disease, spinal deformities, septicemia, severe hypertension and extreme youth.

Fetal bradycardia frequently follows paracervical block and may be associated with fetal acidosis. Fetal heart rate should always be monitored during paracervical anesthesia. Added risk appears to be present in prematurity, postmaturity, toxemia of pregnancy, uteroplacental insufficiency and fetal distress. The physician should weigh the possible advantages against dangers when considering paracervical block in these conditions. When the recommended dose is exceeded, the incidence of fetal bradycardia increases. Short-term neonatal neurobehavioral alterations have been observed in association with some local anesthetics administered during labor and delivery. The short-term and long-term significance of these alterations is not known.

Solutions containing a vasoconstrictor should be used cautiously and in carefully circumscribed quantities in areas of the body supplied by end arteries or having otherwise compromised blood supply (e.g., digits, nose, external ear, penis, etc.). Serious cardiac arrhythmias may occur if preparations containing a vasoconstrictor are employed in patients during or following the administration of chloroform, halothane, cyclopropane, trichloroethylene or other related agents.

Lidocaine Hydrochloride Injection, USP should be used with caution in persons with known drug sensitivities. Patients allergic to para-aminobenzoic acid derivatives (procaine, tetracaine, benzocaine, etc.) have not shown cross sensitivity to lidocaine.

The safety of amide local anesthetics in patients with malignant hyperthermia has not been assessed, and therefore, these agents should be used with caution in such patients.

Drowsiness following an injection of lidocaine HCl is usually an early indication of a high blood level of the drug and may occur following inadvertent intravascular administration or rapid absorption of lidocaine. Local anesthetics react with certain metals and cause the release of their respective ions which, if injected, may cause severe local irritation. Adequate precautions should be taken to avoid this type of interaction. (See STERILIZATION, STORAGE AND TECHNICAL PROCEDURES).

ADVERSE REACTIONS

Reactions to lidocaine HCl are similar in character to those observed with other local anesthetic agents. Adverse reactions may be due to high plasma levels as a result of excessive dosage, rapid absorption or inadvertent intravascular injection. Such reactions are systemic in nature and involve the central nervous system and/or the cardiovascular system.

Rarely, reactions may result from hypersensitivity, idiosyncrasy or diminished tolerance on the part of the patient.

CNS reactions are excitatory and/or depressant, and may be characterized by nervousness, dizziness, blurred vision and tremors, followed by drowsiness, convulsions, unconsciousness and, possibly, respiratory arrest. The excitatory reactions may be very brief or may not occur at all, in which case the first manifestations of toxicity may be drowsiness, merging into unconsciousness and respiratory arrest.

Hypotension and bradycardia may occur as normal physiological phenomena following sympathetic block with central neural blocks. Toxic cardiovascular reactions to local anesthetics are usually depressant in nature and are characterized by peripheral vasodilation, hypotension, myocardial depression, bradycardia and, possibly cardiac arrest.

Treatment of a patient with toxic manifestations consists of assuring and maintaining a patent airway, supporting ventilation with oxygen, and assisted or controlled ventilation (respiration) as required. This usually will be sufficient in the management of most reactions.

Should a convulsion persist despite ventilatory therapy with oxygen, small increments of anticonvulsive agents may be given intravenously. Examples of such agents include a benzodiazepine (e.g., diazepam), ultrashort-acting barbiturates (e.g., thiopental or thiamylal) or a short-acting barbiturate (e.g., pentobarbital or secobarbital). Cardiovascular depression may require circulatory assistance with intravenous fluids and/or vasopressors (e.g., ephedrine) as dictated by the clinical situation.

Allergic reactions may occur as a result of sensitivity either to local anesthetics or to the methylparaben used as a preservative in multiple-dose vials. Anaphylactoid type symptomatology and reactions, characterized by cutaneous lesions, urticaria, and edema should be managed by conventional means. The detection of potential sensitivity by skin testing is of limited value.

DOSAGE AND ADMINISTRATION

Table I (Recommended Dosages) summarizes the recommended volumes and concentrations of Lidocaine Hydrochloride Injection, USP for various types of anesthetic procedures. The dosages suggested in this table are for normal healthy adults and refer to the use of epinephrine-free solutions. When larger dosages are required, only solutions containing epinephrine should be used except in those cases where vasopressor drugs may be contraindicated.

These recommended doses serve only as a guide to the amount of anesthetic required for most routine procedures. The actual volume and concentrations to be used depend on a number of factors, such as type and extent of surgical procedure, degree of muscular relaxation required, duration of anesthesia required, the physical state of the patient, etc. In all cases the lowest concentration and smallest dose that will produce the desired result should be given. Dosages should be reduced for children and for elderly and debilitated patients. The onset of anesthesia, the duration of anesthesia and the degree of muscular relaxation are proportional to the volume and concentration of local anesthetic solution used. Thus, an increase in concentration and volume of lidocaine HCl administered will decrease the onset of anesthesia, prolong the duration of anesthesia, provide a greater degree of muscular relaxation and increase the segmental spread of anesthesia. However, increasing the concentration and volume of lidocaine HCl administered may result in a more profound fall in blood pressure when used in epidural anesthesia. Although the incidence of side effects with lidocaine HCl is quite low, caution should be exercised particularly when employing large volumes and concentrations of lidocaine HCl, since the incidence of side effects is directly related to the total dose of local anesthetic agent injected.

It is important that a single-dose container be employed for epidural anesthesia and major peripheral nerve block.

FOR EPIDURAL OR SPINAL ANESTHESIA, USE ONLY SOLUTIONS WITHOUT PRESERVATIVES.

IMPORTANT: *A test dose of 2 to 5 mL should be administered at least 5 minutes prior to injecting the total required volume for central neural blocks (e.g., epidural or caudal anesthesia).*

Maximum Recommended Dosages

For normal healthy adults, the individual dose of lidocaine hydrochloride with epinephrine should be such that the dose of lidocaine hydrochloride is kept below 500 mg and, in any case, should not exceed 7 mg/kg (3.2 mg/lb) of body weight. When used without epinephrine, the amount of Lidocaine Hydrochloride Injection, USP administered should be such that the dose of lidocaine hydrochloride is kept below 300 mg, and in any case, should not exceed 4.5 mg/kg (2.0 mg/lb) of body weight. For continuous epidural or caudal anesthesia, the maximum recommended dosage should not be administered at intervals of less than 90 minutes. For paracervical block for obstetrical analgesia, (including abortion) the maximum recommended dosage (200 mg) should not be administered at intervals of less than 90 minutes. When paracervical block is used for non-obstetrical procedures, more drug may be administered if required to obtain adequate anesthesia. For intravenous regional anesthesia in adults (using lidocaine hydrochloride 0.5% solution without epinephrine), the dose administered should not exceed 4 mg/kg (1.8 mg/lb) of body weight.

Children:

It is difficult to recommend a maximum dose of any drug for children since this varies as a function of age and weight. For children of less than ten years who have a normal lean body mass and normal body development, the maximum dose may be determined by the application of one of the standard pediatric drug formulas (e.g., Clark's rule). For example, in a child of five years weighing 50 lbs, the dose of lidocaine hydrochloride should not exceed 75 to 100 mg when calculated according to Clark's rule. In any case, the maximum dose of lidocaine HCl with epinephrine should not exceed 7 mg/kg (3.2 mg/lb) of body weight. When used without epinephrine, the amount of lidocaine HCl administered should not exceed 4.5 mg/kg (2.0 mg/lb) of body weight. In order to minimize the possibility of toxic reactions, the use of lidocaine HCl 0.5% or 1.0% is recommended for most anesthetic procedures involving pediatric patients. The use of even more dilute solutions (e.g., 0.25% to 0.5%) and total dosages not to exceed 3 mg/kg (1.4 mg/lb) are recommended for induction of intravenous regional anesthesia in children.

Table I
Recommended Dosages of Lidocaine Hydrochloride Injection, USP for Various Anesthetic Procedures in Normal Healthy Adults

Procedure	Conc. (%)	Lidocaine Hydrochloride Injection, USP (without Epinephrine)	
		Vol. (mL)	Total Dose (mg)
Infiltration			
Percutaneous	0.5 or 1.0	1–60	5–300
Intravenous Regional	0.5	10–60	50–300
Peripheral Nerve Blocks, e.g.			
Brachial	1.5	15–20	225–300
Dental	2.0	1–5	20–100
Intercostal	1.0	3	30
Paravertebral	1.0	3–5	30–50
Pudendal (each side)	1.0	10	100
Paracervical			
Obstetrical Analgesia (each side)	1.0	10	100
Sympathetic Nerve Blocks, e.g.			
Cervical (stellate ganglion)	1.0	5	50
Lumbar	1.0	5–10	50–100
Central Neural Blocks			
Epidural*			
Thoracic	1.0	20–30	200–300
Lumbar			
Analgesia	1.0	25–30	250–300
Anesthesia	1.5	15–20	225–300
	2.0	10–15	200–300
Caudal			
Obstetrical Analgesia	1.0	20–30	200–300
Surgical Anesthesia	1.5	15–20	225–300

* Dose determined by number of dermatomes to be anesthetized (2 to 3 mL/dermatome).

THE ABOVE SUGGESTED CONCENTRATIONS AND VOLUMES SERVE ONLY AS A GUIDE. OTHER VOLUMES AND CONCENTRATIONS MAY BE USED PROVIDED THE TOTAL MAXIMUM RECOMMENDED DOSE IS NOT EXCEEDED.

Parenteral drug products should be inspected visually for particulate matter and discoloration prior to administration, whenever solution and container permit.

[See table above].

Sterilization, Storage and Technical Procedures:

Disinfecting agents containing heavy metals, which cause release of respective ions (mercury, zinc, copper, etc.) should not be used for skin or mucous membrane disinfection as they have been related to incidence of swelling and edema. When chemical disinfection of multi-dose vials is desired, either isopropyl alcohol (91%) or 70% ethyl alcohol is recommended. Many commercially available brands of rubbing alcohol, as well as solutions of ethyl alcohol not of USP grade, contain denaturants which are injurious to rubber and, therefore, are not to be used. It is recommended that chemical disinfection be accomplished by wiping the vial or ampul thoroughly with cotton or gauze that has been moistened with the recommended alcohol just prior to use.

HOW SUPPLIED

Lidocaine Hydrochloride Injection, USP is available in a variety of dosage strengths, containers and sizes. Consult Abbott Laboratories, Hospital Products Division for a current listing.

Exposure of pharmaceutical products to heat should be minimized. Avoid excessive heat. Protect from freezing. It is recommended that the product be stored at room temperature (25° C); however, brief exposure up to 40° C does not adversely affect the product.

CAUTION

Federal (USA) law prohibits dispensing without prescription.

06-3508 R16 Rev. Apr., 1984

NEMBUTAL® SODIUM CAPSULES ℞ Ⓒ

[*nêm-bū-tal sō-dī-um*]

(pentobarbital sodium capsules, USP)

WARNING: MAY BE HABIT FORMING

DESCRIPTION

The barbiturates are nonselective central nervous system depressants which are primarily used as sedative hypnotics. The barbiturates and their sodium salts are subject to control under the Federal Controlled Substances Act (See "Drug Abuse and Dependence" section).

Barbiturates are substituted pyrimidine derivatives in which the basic structure common to these drugs is barbituric acid, a substance which has no central nervous system (CNS) activity. CNS activity is obtained by substituting alkyl, alkenyl, or aryl groups on the pyrimidine ring. Nembutal (pentobarbital sodium) is chemically represented by sodium 5-ethyl-5-(1-methylbutyl) barbiturate.

The sodium salt of pentobarbital occurs as a white, slightly bitter powder which is freely soluble in water and alcohol but practically insoluble in benzene and ether. Nembutal Sodium capsules for oral administration contain either 50 mg or 100 mg of pentobarbital sodium.

INACTIVE INGREDIENTS

50 mg Capsule: FD&C Blue No. 1, FD&C Red No. 3, FD&C Yellow No. 6, gelatin, lactose, magnesium stearate, polacrilin potassium, potassium chloride and other ingredients.

100 mg Capsule: colloidal silicon dioxide, corn starch, FD&C Blue No. 1, FD&C Red No. 3, FD&C Yellow No. 5 (tartrazine), FD&C Yellow No. 6, gelatin, magnesium stearate, potassium chloride, and other ingredients.

CLINICAL PHARMACOLOGY

Barbiturates are capable of producing all levels of CNS mood alteration from excitation to mild sedation, to hypnosis, and deep coma. Overdosage can produce death. In high enough therapeutic doses, barbiturates induce anesthesia.

Barbiturates depress the sensory cortex, decrease motor activity, alter cerebellar function, and produce drowsiness, sedation, and hypnosis.

Barbiturate-induced sleep differs from physiological sleep. Sleep laboratory studies have demonstrated that barbiturates reduce the amount of time spent in the rapid eye movement (REM) phase of sleep or dreaming stage. Also, Stages III and IV sleep are decreased. Following abrupt cessation of barbiturates used regularly, patients may experience markedly increased dreaming, nightmares, and/or insomnia. Therefore, withdrawal of a single therapeutic dose over 5 or 6 days has been recommended to lessen the REM rebound and disturbed sleep which contribute to drug withdrawal syndrome (for example, decrease the dose from 3 to 2 doses a day for 1 week).

In studies, secobarbital sodium and pentobarbital sodium have been found to lose most of their effectiveness for both inducing and maintaining sleep by the end of 2 weeks of continued drug administration at fixed doses. The short-, intermediate-, and, to a lesser degree, long-acting barbiturates have been widely prescribed for treating insomnia. Although the clinical literature abounds with claims that the short-acting barbiturates are superior for producing sleep while the intermediate-acting compounds are more effective in maintaining sleep, controlled studies have failed to demonstrate these differential effects. Therefore, as sleep medications, the barbiturates are of limited value beyond short-term use.

Barbiturates have little analgesic action at subanesthetic doses. Rather, in subanesthetic doses these drugs may increase the reaction to painful stimuli. All barbiturates exhibit anticonvulsant activity in anesthetic doses. However,

Continued on next page

If desired, additional literature on any Abbott Product will be provided upon request to Abbott Laboratories.

Abbott—Cont.

of the drugs in this class, only phenobarbital, mephobarbital, and metharbital have been clinically demonstrated to be effective as oral anticonvulsants in subhypnotic doses.

Barbiturates are respiratory depressants. The degree of respiratory depression is dependent upon dose. With hypnotic doses, respiratory depression produced by barbiturates is similar to that which occurs during physiologic sleep with slight decrease in blood pressure and heart rate.

Studies in laboratory animals have shown that barbiturates cause reduction in the tone and contractility of the uterus, ureters, and urinary bladder. However, concentrations of the drugs required to produce this effect in humans are not reached with sedative-hypnotic doses.

Barbiturates do not impair normal hepatic function, but have been shown to induce liver microsomal enzymes, thus increasing and/or altering the metabolism of barbiturates and other drugs. (See "Precautions—*Drug Interactions*" section).

Pharmacokinetics: Barbiturates are absorbed in varying degrees following oral, rectal, or parenteral administration. The salts are more rapidly absorbed than are the acids. The rate of absorption is increased if the sodium salt is ingested as a dilute solution or taken on an empty stomach.

The onset of action for oral or rectal administration varies from 20 to 60 minutes.

Duration of action, which is related to the rate at which the barbiturates are redistributed throughout the body, varies among persons and in the same person from time to time. In Table 1, the barbiturates are classified according to their duration of action. This classification should not be used to predict the exact duration of effect, but the grouping of drugs should be used as a guide in the selection of barbiturates.

No studies have demonstrated that the different routes of administration are equivalent with respect to bioavailability.

[See Table 1 below].

Barbiturates are weak acids that are absorbed and rapidly distributed to all tissues and fluids with high concentrations in the brain, liver, and kidneys. Lipid solubility of the barbiturates is the dominant factor in their distribution within the body. The more lipid soluble the barbiturate, the more rapidly it penetrates all tissues of the body. Barbiturates are bound to plasma and tissue proteins to a varying degree with the degree of binding increasing directly as a function of lipid solubility. The plasma half-life for pentobarbital in adults is 15 to 50 hours and appears to be dose dependent.

Barbiturates are metabolized primarily by the hepatic microsomal enzyme system, and the metabolic products are excreted in the urine, and less commonly, in the feces. Approximately 25 to 50 percent of a dose of aprobarbital or phenobarbital is eliminated unchanged in the urine, whereas the amount of other barbiturates excreted unchanged in the urine is negligible. The excretion of unmetabolized barbiturate is one feature that distinguishes the long-acting category from those belonging to other categories which are almost entirely metabolized. The inactive metabolites of the barbiturates are excreted as conjugates of glucuronic acid.

INDICATIONS AND USAGE

Oral:

a. Sedatives.
b. Hypnotics, for the short-term treatment of insomnia, since they appear to lose their effectiveness for sleep induction and sleep maintenance after 2 weeks (See "Clinical Pharmacology" section).
c. Preanesthetics.

CONTRAINDICATIONS

Barbiturates are contraindicated in patients with known barbiturate sensitivity. Barbiturates are also contraindicated in patients with a history of manifest or latent porphyria.

WARNINGS

1. *Habit forming:* Barbiturates may be habit forming. Tolerance, psychological and physical dependence may occur with continued use. (See "Drug Abuse and Dependence" and "Pharmacokinetics" sections). Patients who have psychological dependence on barbiturates may increase the dosage or decrease the dosage interval without consulting a physician and may subsequently develop a physical dependence on barbiturates. To minimize the possibility of overdosage or the development of dependence, the prescribing and dispensing of sedative-hypnotic barbiturates should be limited to the amount required for the interval until the next appointment. Abrupt cessation after prolonged use in the dependent person may result in withdrawal symptoms, including delirium, convulsions, and possibly death. Barbiturates should be withdrawn gradually from any patient known to be taking excessive dosage over long periods of time. (See "Drug Abuse and Dependence" section).
2. *Acute or chronic pain:* Caution should be exercised when barbiturates are administered to patients with acute or chronic pain, because paradoxical excitement could be induced or important symptoms could be masked. However, the use of barbiturates as sedatives in the postoperative surgical period and as adjuncts to cancer chemotherapy is well established.
3. *Use in pregnancy:* Barbiturates can cause fetal damage when administered to a pregnant woman. Retrospective, case-controlled studies have suggested a connection between the maternal consumption of barbiturates and a higher than expected incidence of fetal abnormalities. Following oral or parenteral administration, barbiturates readily cross the placental barrier and are distributed throughout fetal tissues with highest concentrations found in the placenta, fetal liver, and brain.
Withdrawal symptoms occur in infants born to mothers who receive barbiturates throughout the last trimester of pregnancy. (See "Drug Abuse and Dependence" section). If this drug is used during pregnancy, or if the patient becomes pregnant while taking this drug, the patient should be apprised of the potential hazard to the fetus.
4. *Synergistic effects:* The concomitant use of alcohol or other CNS depressants may produce additive CNS depressant effects.

PRECAUTIONS

General: Barbiturates may be habit forming. Tolerance and psychological and physical dependence may occur with continuing use. (See "Drug Abuse and Dependence" section). Barbiturates should be administered with caution, if at all, to patients who are mentally depressed, have suicidal tendencies, or a history of drug abuse.

Elderly or debilitated patients may react to barbiturates with marked excitement, depression, and confusion. In some persons, barbiturates repeatedly produce excitement rather than depression.

In patients with hepatic damage, barbiturates should be administered with caution and initially in reduced doses. Barbiturates should not be administered to patients showing the premonitory signs of hepatic coma.

The 100 mg dosage strength of Nembutal Sodium capsules contains FD&C Yellow No. 5 (tartrazine) which may cause allergic-type reactions (including bronchial asthma) in certain susceptible individuals. Although the overall incidence of FD&C Yellow No. 5 (tartrazine) sensitivity in the general population is low, it is frequently seen in patients who also have aspirin hypersensitivity.

Information for the patient: Practitioners should give the following information and instructions to patients receiving barbiturates.

1. The use of barbiturates carries with it an associated risk of psychological and/or physical dependence. The patient should be warned against increasing the dose of the drug without consulting a physician.
2. Barbiturates may impair mental and/or physical abilities required for the performance of potentially hazardous tasks (e.g., driving, operating machinery, etc.).
3. Alcohol should not be consumed while taking barbiturates. Concurrent use of the barbiturates with other CNS depressants (e.g., alcohol, narcotics, tranquilizers, and antihistamines) may result in additional CNS depressant effects.

Laboratory tests: Prolonged therapy with barbiturates should be accompanied by periodic laboratory evaluation of organ systems, including hematopoietic, renal, and hepatic systems. (See "Precautions—*General*" and "Adverse Reactions" sections).

Table 1.—*Classification, Onset, and Duration of Action of Commonly used Barbiturates Taken Orally*

Classification	Onset of action	Duration of action
Long-acting Phenobarbital.	1 hour or longer	10 to 12 hours
Intermediate Amobarbital Butabarbital.	¾ to 1 hour	6 to 8 hours
Short-acting Pentobarbital Secobarbital.	10 to 15 minutes	3 to 4 hours

Drug interactions: Most reports of clinically significant drug interactions occurring with the barbiturates have involved phenobarbital. However, the application of these data to other barbiturates appears valid and warrants serial blood level determinations of the relevant drugs when there are multiple therapies.

1. *Anticoagulants:* Phenobarbital lowers the plasma levels of dicumarol (name previously used: bishydroxycoumarin) and causes a decrease in anticoagulant activity as measured by the prothrombin time. Barbiturates can induce hepatic microsomal enzymes resulting in increased metabolism and decreased anticoagulant response of oral anticoagulants (e.g., warfarin, acenocoumarol, dicumarol, and phenprocoumon). Patients stabilized on anticoagulant therapy may require dosage adjustments if barbiturates are added to or withdrawn from their dosage regimen.
2. *Corticosteroids:* Barbiturates appear to enhance the metabolism of exogenous corticosteroids probably through the induction of hepatic microsomal enzymes. Patients stabilized on corticosteroid therapy may require dosage adjustments if barbiturates are added to or withdrawn from their dosage regimen.
3. *Griseofulvin:* Phenobarbital appears to interfere with the absorption of orally administered griseofulvin, thus decreasing its blood level. The effect of the resultant decreased blood levels of griseofulvin on therapeutic response has not been established. However, it would be preferable to avoid concomitant administration of these drugs.
4. *Doxycycline:* Phenobarbital has been shown to shorten the half-life of doxycycline for as long as 2 weeks after barbiturate therapy is discontinued.
This mechanism is probably through the induction of hepatic microsomal enzymes that metabolize the antibiotic. If phenobarbital and doxycycline are administered concurrently, the clinical response to doxycycline should be monitored closely.
5. *Phenytoin, sodium valproate, valproic acid:* The effect of barbiturates on the metabolism of phenytoin appears to be variable. Some investigators report an accelerating effect, while others report no effect. Because the effect of barbiturates on the metabolism of phenytoin is not predictable, phenytoin and barbiturate blood levels should be monitored more frequently if these drugs are given concurrently. Sodium valproate and valproic acid appear to decrease barbiturate metabolism; therefore, barbiturate blood levels should be monitored and appropriate dosage adjustments made as indicated.
6. *Central nervous system depressants:* The concomitant use of other central nervous system depressants including other sedatives or hypnotics, antihistamines, tranquilizers, or alcohol, may produce additive depressant effects.
7. *Monoamine oxidase inhibitors (MAOI):* MAOI prolong the effects of barbiturates probably because metabolism of the barbiturate is inhibited.
8. *Estradiol, estrone, progesterone and other steroidal hormones:* Pretreatment with or concurrent administration of phenobarbital may decrease the effect of estradiol by increasing its metabolism. There have been reports of patients treated with antiepileptic drugs (e.g., phenobarbital) who became pregnant while taking oral contraceptives. An alternate contraceptive method might be suggested to women taking phenobarbital.

Carcinogenesis: Adequate data are not available on long-term potential for carcinogenicity in humans or animals for pentobarbital.

Data from one retrospective study of 235 children in which the types of barbiturates are not identified suggested an association between exposure to barbiturates prenatally and an increased incidence of brain tumor. (Gold, E., et al., "Increased Risk of Brain Tumors in Children Exposed to Barbiturates," Journal of National Cancer Institute, 61:1031–1034, 1978).

Pregnancy: 1. *Teratogenic effects.* Pregnancy Category D—See "Warnings—Use in Pregnancy" section.
2. *Nonteratogenic effects.* Reports of infants suffering from long-term barbiturate exposure in utero included the acute withdrawal syndrome of seizures and hyperirritability from birth to a delayed onset of up to 14 days. (See "Drug Abuse and Dependence" section).

Labor and delivery: Hypnotic doses of these barbiturates do not appear to significantly impair uterine activity during labor. Full anesthetic doses of barbiturates decrease the force and frequency of uterine contractions. Administration of sedative-hypnotic barbiturates to the mother during labor may result in respiratory depression in the newborn. Premature infants are particularly susceptible to the depressant effects of barbiturates. If barbiturates are used during labor and delivery, resuscitation equipment should be available.

Data are currently not available to evaluate the effect of these barbiturates when forceps delivery or other intervention is necessary. Also, data are not available to determine the effect of these barbiturates on the later growth, development, and functional maturation of the child.

Nursing mothers: Caution should be exercised when a barbiturate is administered to a nursing woman since small amounts of barbiturates are excreted in the milk.

ADVERSE REACTIONS

The following adverse reactions and their incidence were compiled from surveillance of thousands of hospitalized patients. Because such patients may be less aware of certain of the milder adverse effects of barbiturates, the incidence of these reactions may be somewhat higher in fully ambulatory patients.

More than 1 in 100 patients. The most common adverse reaction estimated to occur at a rate of 1 to 3 patients per 100 is:
Nervous System: Somnolence.

Less than 1 in 100 patients. Adverse reactions estimated to occur at a rate of less than 1 in 100 patients listed below, grouped by organ system, and by decreasing order of occurrence are:
Nervous system: Agitation, confusion, hyperkinesia, ataxia, CNS depression, nightmares, nervousness, psychiatric disturbance, hallucinations, insomnia, anxiety, dizziness, thinking abnormality.
Respiratory system: Hypoventilation, apnea.
Cardiovascular system: Bradycardia, hypotension, syncope.
Digestive system: Nausea, vomiting, constipation.
Other reported reactions: Headache, injection site reactions, hypersensitivity reactions (angioedema, skin rashes, exfoliative dermatitis), fever, liver damage, megaloblastic anemia following chronic phenobarbital use.

DRUG ABUSE AND DEPENDENCE

Pentobarbital sodium capsules are subject to control by the Federal Controlled Substances Act under DEA schedule II.
Barbiturates may be habit forming. Tolerance, psychological dependence, and physical dependence may occur especially following prolonged use of high doses of barbiturates. Daily administration in excess of 400 mg of pentobarbital or secobarbital for approximately 90 days is likely to produce some degree of physical dependence. A dosage of from 600 to 800 mg taken for at least 35 days is sufficient to produce withdrawal seizures. The average daily dose for the barbiturate addict is usually about 1.5 grams. As tolerance to barbiturates develops, the amount needed to maintain the same level of intoxication increases; tolerance to a fatal dosage, however, does not increase more than two-fold. As this occurs, the margin between an intoxicating dosage and fatal dosage becomes smaller.
Symptoms of acute intoxication with barbiturates include unsteady gait, slurred speech, and sustained nystagmus. Mental signs of chronic intoxication include confusion, poor judgment, irritability, insomnia, and somatic complaints.
Symptoms of barbiturate dependence are similar to those of chronic alcoholism. If an individual appears to be intoxicated with alcohol to a degree that is radically disproportionate to the amount of alcohol in his or her blood the use of barbiturates should be suspected. The lethal dose of a barbiturate is far less if alcohol is also ingested.
The symptoms of barbiturate withdrawal can be severe and may cause death. Minor withdrawal symptoms may appear 8 to 12 hours after the last dose of a barbiturate. These symptoms usually appear in the following order: anxiety, muscle twitching, tremor of hands and fingers, progressive weakness, dizziness, distortion in visual perception, nausea, vomiting, insomnia, and orthostatic hypotension. Major withdrawal symptoms (convulsions and delirium) may occur within 16 hours and last up to 5 days after abrupt cessation of these drugs. Intensity of withdrawal symptoms gradually declines over a period of approximately 15 days. Individuals susceptible to barbiturate abuse and dependence include alcoholics and opiate abusers, as well as other sedative-hypnotic and amphetamine abusers.
Drug dependence to barbiturates arises from repeated administration of a barbiturate or agent with barbiturate-like effect on a continuous basis, generally in amounts exceeding therapeutic dose levels. The characteristics of drug dependence to barbiturates include: (a) a strong desire or need to continue taking the drug; (b) a tendency to increase the dose; (c) a psychic dependence on the effects of the drug related to subjective and individual appreciation of those effects; and (d) a physical dependence on the effects of the drug requiring its presence for maintenance of homeostasis and resulting in a definite, characteristic, and self-limited abstinence syndrome when the drug is withdrawn.
Treatment of barbiturate dependence consists of cautious and gradual withdrawal of the drug. Barbiturate-dependent patients can be withdrawn by using a number of different withdrawal regimens. In all cases withdrawal takes an extended period of time. One method involves substituting a 30 mg dose of phenobarbital for each 100 to 200 mg dose of barbiturate that the patient has been taking. The total daily amount of phenobarbital is then administered in 3 to 4 divided doses, not to exceed 600 mg daily. Should signs of withdrawal occur on the first day of treatment, a loading dose of 100 to 200 mg of phenobarbital may be administered IM in addition to the oral dose. After stabilization on phenobarbital, the total daily dose is decreased by 30 mg a day as long as withdrawal is proceeding smoothly. A modification of this regimen involves initiating treatment at the patient's regular dosage level and decreasing the daily dosage by 10 percent if tolerated by the patient.
Infants physically dependent on barbiturates may be given phenobarbital 3 to 10 mg/kg/day. After withdrawal symptoms (hyperactivity, disturbed sleep, tremors, hyperreflexia) are relieved, the dosage of phenobarbital should be gradually decreased and completely withdrawn over a 2 week period.

Table 2.—*Concentration of Barbiturate in the Blood Versus Degree of CNS Depression*

Barbiturate	Onset/ duration	Blood barbiturate level in ppm (μg/ml) — Degree of depression in nontolerant persons* 1	2	3	4	5
Pentobarbital	Fast/short	≤2	0.5 to 3	10 to 15	12 to 25	15 to 40
Secobarbital	Fast/short	≤2	0.5 to 5	10 to 15	15 to 25	15 to 40
Amobarbital	Intermediate/ intermediate	≤3	2 to 10	30 to 40	30 to 60	40 to 80
Butabarbital	Intermediate/ intermediate	≤5	3 to 25	40 to 60	50 to 80	60 to 100
Phenobarbital	Slow/long	≤10	5 to 40	50 to 80	70 to 120	100 to 200

* Categories of degree of depression in nontolerant persons.
1. Under the influence and appreciably impaired for purposes of driving a motor vehicle or performing tasks requiring alertness and unimpaired judgment and reaction time.
2. Sedated, therapeutic range, calm, relaxed, and easily aroused.
3. Comatose, difficult to arose, significant depression of respiration.
4. Compatible with death in aged or ill persons or in presence of obstructed airway, other toxic agents, or exposure to cold.
5. Usual lethal level, the upper end of the range includes those who received some supportive treatment.

OVERDOSAGE

The toxic dose of barbiturates varies considerably. In general, an oral dose of 1 g of most barbiturates produces serious poisoning in an adult. Death commonly occurs after 2 to 10 g of ingested barbiturate. Barbiturate intoxication may be confused with alcoholism, bromide intoxication, and with various neurological disorders.
Acute overdosage with barbiturates is manifested by CNS and respiratory depression which may progress to Cheyne-Stokes respiration, areflexia, constriction of the pupils to a slight degree (though in severe poisoning they may show paralytic dilation), oliguria, tachycardia, hypotension, lowered body temperature, and coma. Typical shock syndrome (apnea, circulatory collapse, respiratory arrest, and death) may occur.
In extreme overdose, all electrical activity in the brain may cease, in which case a "flat" EEG normally equated with clinical death cannot be accepted. This effect is fully reversible unless hypoxic damage occurs. Consideration should be given to the possibility of barbiturate intoxication even in situations that appear to involve trauma.
Complications such as pneumonia, pulmonary edema, cardiac arrhythmias, congestive heart failure, and renal failure may occur. Uremia may increase CNS sensitivity to barbiturates. Differential diagnosis should include hypoglycemia, head trauma, cerebrovascular accidents, convulsive states, and diabetic coma. Blood levels from acute overdosage for some barbiturates are listed in Table 2.
[See table above].
Treatment of overdosage is mainly supportive and consists of the following:

1. Maintenance of an adequate airway, with assisted respiration and oxygen administration as necessary.
2. Monitoring of vital signs and fluid balance.
3. If the patient is conscious and has not lost the gag reflex, emesis may be induced with ipecac. Care should be taken to prevent pulmonary aspiration of vomitus. After completion of vomiting, 30 g activated charcoal in a glass of water may be administered.
4. If emesis is contraindicated, gastric lavage may be performed with a cuffed endotracheal tube in place with the patient in the face down position. Activated charcoal may be left in the emptied stomach and a saline cathartic administered.
5. Fluid therapy and other standard treatment for shock, if needed.
6. If renal function is normal, forced diuresis may aid in the elimination of the barbiturate. Alkalinization of the urine increases renal excretion of some barbiturates, especially phenobarbital, also aprobarbital, and mephobarbital (which is metabolized to phenobarbital).
7. Although not recommended as a routine procedure, hemodialysis may be used in severe barbiturate intoxications or if the patient is anuric or in shock.
8. Patient should be rolled from side to side every 30 minutes.
9. Antibiotics should be given if pneumonia is suspected.
10. Appropriate nursing care to prevent hypostatic pneumonia, decubiti, aspiration, and other complications of patients with altered states of consciousness.

DOSAGE AND ADMINISTRATION

Adults: The usual hypnotic dose consists of 100 mg at bedtime.
Children: The preoperative dose is 2 to 6 mg/kg/24 hours (maximum 100 mg), depending on age, weight, and the desired degree of sedation.
The proper hypnotic dose for children must be judged on the basis of individual age and weight.
Dosages of barbiturates must be individualized with full knowledge of their particular characteristics and recommended rate of administration. Factors of consideration are the patient's age, weight, and condition.
Special patient population: Dosage should be reduced in the elderly or debilitated because these patients may be more sensitive to barbiturates. Dosage should be reduced for patients with impaired renal function or hepatic disease.

HOW SUPPLIED

NEMBUTAL Sodium Capsules (pentobarbital sodium capsules, USP) are supplied as follows:
50 mg transparent and orange-colored capsules in bottles of 100 (**NDC** 0074-3150-11);
100 mg yellow capsules in bottles of 100 (**NDC** 0074-3114-01), 500 (**NDC** 0074-3114-02) and in the Abbo-Pac® unit dose packages of 100 (**NDC** 0074-3114-21).
Abbott Pharmaceuticals, Inc.
North Chicago, IL 60064
Shown in Product Identification Section, page 403

NEMBUTAL® SODIUM SOLUTION ℞ Ⓒ
[nem'-bū-tal]
(pentobarbital sodium injection, USP)
Ampuls—Vials

WARNING: MAY BE HABIT FORMING. DO NOT USE IF MATERIAL HAS PRECIPITATED.

DESCRIPTION

The barbiturates are nonselective central nervous system depressants which are primarily used as sedative hypnotics and also anticonvulsants in subhypnotic doses. The barbiturates and their sodium salts are subject to control under the Federal Controlled Substances Act (See "Drug Abuse and Dependence" section).
The sodium salts of amobarbital, pentobarbital, phenobarbital, and secobarbital are available as sterile parenteral solutions.
Barbiturates are substituted pyrimidine derivatives in which the basic structure common to these drugs is barbituric acid, a substance which has no central nervous system (CNS) activity. CNS activity is obtained by substituting alkyl, alkenyl, or aryl groups on the pyrimidine ring.
NEMBUTAL Sodium Solution (pentobarbital sodium injection) is a sterile solution for intravenous or intramuscular injection. Each ml contains pentobarbital sodium 50 mg, in a vehicle of propylene glycol, 40%, alcohol, 10% and water for injection, to volume. The pH is adjusted to approximately 9.5 with hydrochloric acid and/or sodium hydroxide.
NEMBUTAL Sodium is a short-acting barbiturate, chemically designated as sodium 5-ethyl-5-(1-methylbutyl) barbiturate. The sodium salt occurs as a white, slightly bitter powder which is freely soluble in water and alcohol but practically insoluble in benzene and ether.

Continued on next page

If desired, additional literature on any Abbott Product will be provided upon request to Abbott Laboratories.

Abbott—Cont.

CLINICAL PHARMACOLOGY

Barbiturates are capable of producing all levels of CNS mood alteration from excitation to mild sedation, to hypnosis, and deep coma. Overdosage can produce death. In high enough therapeutic doses, barbiturates induce anesthesia.

Barbiturates depress the sensory cortex, decrease motor activity, alter cerebellar function, and produce drowsiness, sedation, and hypnosis.

Barbiturate-induced sleep differs from physiological sleep. Sleep laboratory studies have demonstrated that barbiturates reduce the amount of time spent in the rapid eye movement (REM) phase of sleep or dreaming stage. Also, Stages III and IV sleep are decreased. Following abrupt cessation of barbiturates used regularly, patients may experience markedly increased dreaming, nightmares, and/or insomnia. Therefore, withdrawal of a single therapeutic dose over 5 or 6 days has been recommended to lessen the REM rebound and disturbed sleep which contribute to drug withdrawal syndrome (for example, decrease the dose from 3 to 2 doses a day for 1 week).

In studies, secobarbital sodium and pentobarbital sodium have been found to lose most of their effectiveness for both inducing and maintaining sleep by the end of 2 weeks of continued drug administration at fixed doses. The short-, intermediate-, and, to a lesser degree, long-acting barbiturates have been widely prescribed for treating insomnia. Although the clinical literature abounds with claims that the short-acting barbiturates are superior for producing sleep while the intermediate-acting compounds are more effective in maintaining sleep, controlled studies have failed to demonstrate these differential effects. Therefore, as sleep medications, the barbiturates are of limited value beyond short-term use.

Barbiturates have little analgesic action at subanesthetic doses. Rather, in subanesthetic doses these drugs may increase the reaction to painful stimuli. All barbiturates exhibit anticonvulsant activity in anesthetic doses. However, of the drugs in this class, only phenobarbital, mephobarbital, and metharbital have been clinically demonstrated to be effective as oral anticonvulsants in subhypnotic doses.

Barbiturates are respiratory depressants. The degree of respiratory depression is dependent upon dose. With hypnotic doses, respiratory depression produced by barbiturates is similar to that which occurs during physiologic sleep with slight decrease in blood pressure and heart rate.

Studies in laboratory animals have shown that barbiturates cause reduction in the tone and contractility of the uterus, ureters, and urinary bladder. However, concentration of the drugs required to produce this effect in humans are not reached with sedative-hypnotic doses.

Barbiturates do not impair normal hepatic function, but have been shown to induce liver microsomal enzymes, thus increasing and/or altering the metabolism of barbiturates and other drugs. (See "Precautions—*Drug Interactions*" section).

Pharmacokinetics: Barbiturates are absorbed in varying degrees following oral, rectal, or parenteral administration. The salts are more rapidly absorbed than are the acids.

The onset of action for oral or rectal administration varies from 20 to 60 minutes. For IM administration, the onset of action is slightly faster. Following IV administration, the onset of action ranges from almost immediately for pentobarbital sodium to 5 minutes for phenobarbital sodium. Maximal CNS depression may not occur until 15 minutes or more after IV administration for phenobarbital sodium.

Duration of action, which is related to the rate at which the barbiturates are redistributed throughout the body, varies among persons and in the same person from time to time.

No studies have demonstrated that the different routes of administration are equivalent with respect to bioavailability.

Barbiturates are weak acids that are absorbed and rapidly distributed to all tissues and fluids with high concentration in the brain, liver, and kidneys. Lipid solubility of the barbiturates is the dominant factor in their distribution within the body. The more lipid soluble the barbiturate, the more rapidly it penetrates all tissues of the body. Barbiturates are bound to plasma and tissue proteins to a varying degree with the degree of binding increasing directly as a function of lipid solubility. The plasma half-life for pentobarbital in adults is 15 to 50 hours and appears to be dose-dependent.

Barbiturates are metabolized primarily by the hepatic microsomal enzyme system, and the metabolic products are excreted in the urine, and less commonly, in the feces. Approximately 25 to 50 percent of a dose of aprobarbital or phenobarbital is eliminated unchanged in the urine, whereas the amount of other barbiturates excreted unchanged in the urine is negligible. The excretion of unmetabolized barbiturate is one feature that distinguishes the long-acting category from those belonging to other categories which are almost entirely metabolized. The inactive metabolites of the barbiturates are excreted as conjugates of glucuronic acid.

INDICATIONS AND USAGE

Parenteral:

a. Sedatives.
b. Hypnotics, for the short-term treatment of insomnia, since they appear to lose their effectiveness for sleep induction and sleep maintenance after 2 weeks (See "Clinical Pharmacology" section).
c. Preanesthetics.
d. Anticonvulsant, in anesthetic doses, in the emergency control of certain acute convulsive episodes, e.g., those associated with status epilepticus, cholera, eclampsia, meningitis, tetanus, and toxic reactions to strychnine or local anesthetics.

CONTRAINDICATIONS

Barbiturates are contraindicated in patients with known barbiturate sensitivity. Barbiturates are also contraindicated in patients with a history of manifest or latent porphyria.

WARNINGS

1. *Habit forming:* Barbiturates may be habit forming. Tolerance, psychological and physical dependence may occur with continued use. (See "Drug Abuse and Dependence" and "Pharmacokinetics" sections). Patients who have psychological dependence on barbiturates may increase the dosage or decrease the dosage interval without consulting a physician and may subsequently develop a physical dependence on barbiturates. To minimize the possibility of overdosage or the development of dependence, the prescribing and dispensing of sedative-hypnotic barbiturates should be limited to the amount required for the interval until the next appointment. Abrupt cessation after prolonged use in the dependent person may result in withdrawal symptoms, including delirium, convulsions, and possibly death. Barbiturates should be withdrawn gradually from any patient known to be taking excessive dosage over long periods of time. (See "Drug Abuse and Dependence" section).
2. *IV administration:* Too rapid administration may cause respiratory depression, apnea, laryngospasm, or vasodilation with fall in blood pressure.
3. *Acute or chronic pain:* Caution should be exercised when barbiturates are administered to patients with acute or chronic pain, because paradoxical excitement could be induced or important symptoms could be masked. However, the use of barbiturates as sedatives in the postoperative surgical period and as adjuncts to cancer chemotherapy is well established.
4. *Use in pregnancy:* Barbiturates can cause fetal damage when administered to a pregnant woman. Retrospective, case-controlled studies have suggested a connection between the maternal consumption of barbiturates and a higher than expected incidence of fetal abnormalities. Following oral or parenteral administration, barbiturates readily cross the placental barrier and are distributed throughout fetal tissues with highest concentrations found in the placenta, fetal liver, and brain. Fetal blood levels approach maternal blood levels following parenteral administration.

   Withdrawal symptoms occur in infants born to mothers who receive barbiturates throughout the last trimester of pregnancy. (See "Drug Abuse and Dependence" section). If this drug is used during pregnancy, or if the patient becomes pregnant while taking this drug, the patient should be apprised of the potential hazard to the fetus.
5. *Synergistic effects:* The concomitant use of alcohol or other CNS depressants may produce additive CNS depressant effects.

PRECAUTIONS

General: Barbiturates may be habit forming. Tolerance and psychological and physical dependence may occur with continuing use. (See "Drug Abuse and Dependence" section). Barbiturates should be administered with caution, if at all, to patients who are mentally depressed, have suicidal tendencies, or a history of drug abuse.

Elderly or debilitated patients may react to barbiturates with marked excitement, depression, and confusion. In some persons, barbiturates repeatedly produce excitement rather than depression.

In patients with hepatic damage, barbiturates should be administered with caution and initially in reduced doses. Barbiturates should not be administered to patients showing the premonitory signs of hepatic coma.

Parenteral solutions of barbiturates are highly alkaline. Therefore, extreme care should be taken to avoid perivascular extravasation or intra-arterial injection. Extravascular injection may cause local tissue damage with subsequent necrosis; consequences of intra-arterial injection may vary from transient pain to gangrene of the limb. Any complaint of pain in the limb warrants stopping the injection.

Information for the patient: Practitioners should give the following information and instructions to patients receiving barbiturates.

1. The use of barbiturates carries with it an associated risk of psychological and/or physical dependence. The patient should be warned against increasing the dose of the drug without consulting a physician.
2. Barbiturates may impair mental and/or physical abilities required for the performance of potentially hazardous tasks (e.g., driving, operating machinery, etc.).
3. Alcohol should not be consumed while taking barbiturates. Concurrent use of the barbiturates with other CNS depressants (e.g., alcohol, narcotics, tranquilizers, and antihistamines) may result in additional CNS depressant effects.

Laboratory tests: Prolonged therapy with barbiturates should be accompanied by periodic laboratory evaluation of organ systems, including hematopoietic, renal, and hepatic systems. (See "Precautions-*General*" and "Adverse Reactions" sections).

Drug interactions: Most reports of clinically significant drug interactions occurring with the barbiturates have involved phenobarbital. However, the application of these data to other barbiturates appears valid and warrants serial blood level determinations of the relevant drugs when there are multiple therapies.

1. *Anticoagulants:* Phenobarbital lowers the plasma levels of dicumarol (name previously used: bishydroxycoumarin) and causes a decrease in anticoagulant activity as measured by the prothrombin time. Barbiturates can induce hepatic microsomal enzymes resulting in increased metabolism and decreased anticoagulant response of oral anticoagulants (e.g., warfarin, acenocoumarol, dicumarol, and phenprocoumon). Patients stabilized on anticoagulant therapy may require dosage adjustments if barbiturates are added to or withdrawn from their dosage regimen.
2. *Corticosteroids:* Barbiturates appear to enhance the metabolism of exogenous corticosteroids probably through the induction of hepatic microsomol enzymes. Patients stabilized on corticosteroid therapy may require dosage adjustments if barbiturates are added to or withdrawn from their dosage regimen.
3. *Griseofulvin:* Phenobarbital appears to interfere with the absorption of orally administered griseofulvin, thus decreasing its blood level. The effect of the resultant decreased blood levels of griseofulvin on therapeutic response has not been established. However, it would be preferable to avoid concomitant administration of these drugs.
4. *Doxycycline:* Phenobarbital has been shown to shorten the half-life of doxycycline for as long as 2 weeks after barbiturate therapy is discontinued.

This mechanism is probably through the induction of hepatic microsomal enzymes that metabolize the antibiotic. If phenobarbital and doxycycline are administered concurrently, the clinical response to doxycycline should be monitored closely.

5. *Phenytoin, sodium valproate, valproic acid:* The effect of barbiturates on the metabolism of phenytoin appears to be variable. Some investigators report an accelerating effect, while others report no effect. Because the effect of barbiturates on the metabolism of phenytoin is not predictable, phenytoin and barbiturate blood levels should be monitored more frequently if these drugs are given concurrently. Sodium valproate and valproic acid appear to decrease barbiturate metabolism; therefore, barbiturate blood levels should be monitored and appropriate dosage adjustments made as indicated.
6. *Central nervous system depressants:* The concomitant use of other central nervous system depressants, including other sedatives or hypnotics, antihistamines, tranquilizers, or alcohol, may produce additive depressant effects.
7. *Monoamine oxidase inhibitors (MAOI):* MAOI prolong the effects of barbiturates probably because metabolism of the barbiturate is inhibited.
8. *Estradiol, estrone, progesterone and other steroidal hormones:* Pretreatment with or concurrent administration of phenobarbital may decrease the effect of estradiol by increasing its metabolism. There have been reports of patients treated with antiepileptic drugs (e.g., phenobarbital) who became pregnant while taking oral contraceptives. An alternate contraceptive method might be suggested to women taking phenobarbital.

Carcinogenesis: Adequate data are not available on long-term potential for carcinogenicity in humans or animals for pentobarbital.

Data from one retrospective study of 235 children in which the types of barbiturates are not identified suggested an association between exposure to barbiturates prenatally and an increased incidence of brain tumor. (Gold, E., et al., "Increased Risk of Brain Tumors in Children Exposed to Barbiturates," Journal of National Cancer Institute, 61:1031–1034, 1978).

Pregnancy: 1. *Teratogenic effects.* Pregnancy Category D—See "Warnings—Use in Pregnancy" section.

2. *Nonteratogenic effects.* Reports of infants suffering from long-term barbiturate exposure in utero included the acute withdrawal syndrome of seizures and hyperirritability from birth to a delayed onset of up to 14 days. (See "Drug Abuse and Dependence" section).

Labor and delivery: Hypnotic doses of these barbiturates do not appear to significantly impair uterine activity during labor. Full anesthetic doses of barbiturates decrease the force and frequency of uterine contractions. Administration of sedative-hypnotic barbiturates to the mother during labor may result in respiratory depression in the newborn. Premature infants are particularly susceptible to the depressant effects of barbiturates. If barbiturates are used during labor and delivery, resuscitation equipment should be available. Data are currently not available to evaluate the effect of these barbiturates when forceps delivery or other intervention is necessary. Also, data are not available to determine the effect of these barbiturates on the later growth, development, and functional maturation of the child.
Nursing mothers: Caution should be exercised when a barbiturate is administered to a nursing woman since small amounts of barbiturates are excreted in the milk.

ADVERSE REACTIONS

The following adverse reactions and their incidence were compiled from surveillance of thousands of hospitalized patients. Because such patients may be less aware of certain of the milder adverse effects of barbiturates, the incidence of these reactions may be somewhat higher in fully ambulatory patients.
More than 1 in 100 patients. The most common adverse reaction estimated to occur at a rate of 1 to 3 patients per 100 is: *Nervous System:* Somnolence.
Less than 1 in 100 patients. Adverse reactions estimated to occur at a rate of less than 1 in 100 patients listed below, grouped by organ system, and by decreasing order of occurrence are:
Nervous system: Agitation, confusion, hyperkinesia, ataxia, CNS depression, nightmares, nervousness, psychiatric disturbance, hallucinations, insomnia, anxiety, dizziness, thinking abnormality.
Respiratory system: Hypoventilation, apnea.
Cardiovascular system: Bradycardia, hypotension, syncope.
Digestive system: Nausea, vomiting, constipation.
Other reported reactions: Headache, injection site reactions, hypersensitivity reactions (angioedema, skin rashes, exfoliative dermatitis), fever, liver damage, megaloblastic anemia following chronic phenobarbital use.

DRUG ABUSE AND DEPENDENCE

Pentobarbital sodium injection is subject to control by the Federal Controlled Substances Act under DEA schedule II.
Barbiturates may be habit forming. Tolerance, psychological dependence, and physical dependence may occur especially following prolonged use of high doses of barbiturates. Daily administration in excess of 400 mg of pentobarbital or secobarbital for approximately 90 days is likely to produce some degree of physical dependence. A dosage of from 600 to 800 mg taken for at least 35 days is sufficient to produce withdrawal seizures. The average daily dose for the barbiturate addict is usually about 1.5 g. As tolerance to barbiturates develops, the amount needed to maintain the same level of intoxication increases; tolerance to a fatal dosage, however, does not increase more than two-fold. As this occurs, the margin between an intoxicating dosage and fatal dosage becomes smaller.
Symptoms of acute intoxication with barbiturates include unsteady gait, slurred speech, and sustained nystagmus. Mental signs of chronic intoxication include confusion, poor judgment, irritability, insomnia, and somatic complaints.
Symptoms of barbiturate dependence are similar to those of chronic alcoholism. If an individual appears to be intoxicated with alcohol to a degree that is radically disproportionate to the amount of alcohol in his or her blood the use of barbiturates should be suspected. The lethal dose of a barbiturate is far less if alcohol is also ingested.
The symptoms of barbiturate withdrawal can be severe and may cause death. Minor withdrawal symptoms may appear 8 to 12 hours after the last dose of a barbiturate. These symptoms usually appear in the following order: anxiety, muscle twitching, tremor of hands and fingers, progressive weakness, dizziness, distortion in visual perception, nausea, vomiting, insomnia, and orthostatic hypotension. Major withdrawal symptoms (convulsions and delirium) may occur within 16 hours and last up to 5 days after abrupt cessation of these drugs. Intensity of withdrawal symptoms gradually declines over a period of approximately 15 days. Individuals susceptible to barbiturate abuse and dependence include alcoholics and opiate abusers, as well as other sedative-hypnotic and amphetamine abusers.
Drug dependence to barbiturates arises from repeated administration of a barbiturate or agent with barbiturate-like effect on a continuous basis, generally in amounts exceeding therapeutic dose levels. The characteristics of drug dependence to barbiturates include: (a) a strong desire or need to continue taking the drug; (b) a tendency to increase the dose; (c) a psychic dependence on the effects of the drug related to subjective and individual appreciation of those effects; and (d) a physical dependence on the effects of the drug requiring its presence for maintenance of homeostasis and resulting in a definite, characteristic, and self-limited abstinence syndrome when the drug is withdrawn.
Treatment of barbiturate dependence consists of cautious and gradual withdrawal of the drug. Barbiturate-dependent patients can be withdrawn by using a number of different withdrawal regimens. In all cases withdrawal takes an extended period of time. One method involves substituting a 30 mg dose of phenobarbital for each 100 to 200 mg dose of barbiturate that the patient has been taking. The total daily amount of phenobarbital is then administered in 3 to 4 divided doses, not to exceed 600 mg daily. Should signs of withdrawal occur on the first day of treatment, a loading dose of 100 to 200 mg of phenobarbital may be administered IM in addition to the oral dose. After stabilization on phenobarbital, the total daily dose is decreased by 30 mg a day as long as withdrawal is proceeding smoothly. A modification of this regimen involves initiating treatment at the patient's regular dosage level and decreasing the daily dosage by 10 percent if tolerated by the patient.
Infants physically dependent on barbiturates may be given phenobarbital 3 to 10 mg/kg/day. After withdrawal symptoms (hyperactivity, disturbed sleep, tremors, hyperreflexia) are relieved, the dosage of phenobarbital should be gradually decreased and completely withdrawn over a 2-week period.

OVERDOSAGE

The toxic dose of barbiturates varies considerably. In general, an oral dose of 1 g of most barbiturates produces serious poisoning in an adult. Death commonly occurs after 2 to 10 g of ingested barbiturate. Barbiturate intoxication may be confused with alcoholism, bromide intoxication, and with various neurological disorders.
Acute overdosage with barbiturates is manifested by CNS and respiratory depression which may progress to Cheyne-Stokes respiration, areflexia, constriction of the pupils to a slight degree (though in severe poisoning they may show paralytic dilation), oliguria, tachycardia, hypotension, lowered body temperature, and coma. Typical shock syndrome (apnea, circulatory collapse, respiratory arrest, and death) may occur.
In extreme overdose, all electrical activity in the brain may cease, in which case a "flat" EEG normally equated with clinical death cannot be accepted. This effect is fully reversible unless hypoxic damage occurs. Consideration should be given to the possibility of barbiturate intoxication even in situations that appear to involve trauma.
Complications such as pneumonia, pulmonary edema, cardiac arrhythmias, congestive heart failure, and renal failure may occur. Uremia may increase CNS sensitivity to barbiturates. Differential diagnosis should include hypoglycemia, head trauma, cerebrovascular accidents, convulsive states, and diabetic coma. Blood levels from acute overdosage for some barbiturates are listed in Table 2. [See Table 2 in Nembutal Capsules prescribing information.]
Treatment of overdosage is mainly supportive and consists of the following:

1. Maintenance of an adequate airway, with assisted respiration and oxygen administration as necessary.
2. Monitoring of vital signs and fluid balance.
3. Fluid therapy and other standard treatment for shock, if needed.
4. If renal function is normal, forced diuresis may aid in the elimination of the barbiturate. Alkalinization of the urine increases renal excretion of some barbiturates, especially phenobarbital, also aprobarbital, and mephobarbital (which is metabolized to phenobarbital).
5. Although not recommended as a routine procedure, hemodialysis may be used in severe barbiturate intoxications or if the patient is anuric or in shock.
6. Patient should be rolled from side to side every 30 minutes.
7. Antibiotics should be given if pneumonia is suspected.
8. Appropriate nursing care to prevent hypostatic pneumonia, decubiti, aspiration, and other complications of patients with altered states of consciousness.

DOSAGE AND ADMINISTRATION

Dosages of barbiturates must be individualized with full knowledge of their particular characteristics and recommended rate of administration. Factors of consideration are the patient's age, weight, and condition. Parenteral routes should be used only when oral administration is impossible or impractical.
Intramuscular Administration: IM injection of the sodium salts of barbiturates should be made deeply into a large muscle, and a volume of 5 ml should not be exceeded at any one site because of possible tissue irritation. After IM injection of a hypnotic dose, the patient's vital signs should be monitored. The usual adult dosage of NEMBUTAL Sodium Solution is 150 to 200 mg as a single IM injection; the recommended pediatric dosage ranges from 2 to 6 mg/kg as a single IM injection not to exceed 100 mg.
Intravenous Administration: IV injection is restricted to conditions in which other routes are not feasible, either because the patient is unconscious (as in cerebral hemorrhage, eclampsia, or status epilepticus, or because the patient resists (as in delirium), or because prompt action is imperative. Slow IV injection is essential and patients should be carefully observed during administration. This requires that blood pressure, respiration, and cardiac function be maintained, vital signs be recorded, and equipment for resuscitation and artificial ventilation be available. The rate of IV injection should not exceed 50 mg/min for pentobarbital sodium.
There is no average intravenous dose of NEMBUTAL Sodium Solution (pentobarbital sodium injection) that can be relied on to produce similar effects in different patients. The possibility of overdose and respiratory depression is remote when the drug is injected slowly in fractional doses.
A commonly used initial dose for the 70 kg adult is 100 mg. Proportional reduction in dosage should be made for pediatric or debilitated patients. At least one minute is necessary to determine the full effect of intravenous pentobarbital. If necessary, additional small increments of the drug may be given up to a total of from 200 to 500 mg for normal adults.
Anticonvulsant use: In convulsive states, dosage of NEMBUTAL Sodium Solution should be kept to a minimum to avoid compounding the depression which may follow convulsions. The injection must be made slowly with due regard to the time required for the drug to penetrate the blood-brain barrier.
Special patient population: Dosage should be reduced in the elderly or debilitated because these patients may be more sensitive to barbiturates. Dosage should be reduced for patients with impaired renal function or hepatic disease.
Inspection: Parenteral drug products should be inspected visually for particulate matter and discoloration prior to administration, whenever solution containers permit. Solutions for injection showing evidence of precipitation should not be used.

HOW SUPPLIED

NEMBUTAL Sodium Solution (pentobarbital sodium injection, USP) is available in the following sizes:
2-ml ampul, 100 mg ($1\frac{1}{2}$ gr), in boxes of 25 (**NDC** 0074-6899-04); 20-ml multiple-dose vial, 1 g, in boxes of 5 (**NDC** 0074-3778-04); and 50-ml multiple-dose vial, 2.5 g, in boxes of 5 (**NDC** 0074-3778-05).
Each ml contains:
Pentobarbital Sodium,
derivative of barbituric acid ....50 mg ($\frac{3}{4}$ gr)
Warning—May be habit forming.
Propylene glycol ....40% v/v
Alcohol 10%
Water for Injection ....qs
(pH adjusted to approximately 9.5 with hydrochloric acid and/or sodium hydroxide.)
Exposure of pharmaceutical products to heat should be minimized. Avoid excessive heat. Protect from freezing. It is recommended that the product be stored at room temperature 86°F (30°C), however, brief exposure up to 104°F (40°C) does not adversely affect the product.
Abbott Laboratories
North Chicago, IL 60064

NEMBUTAL® SODIUM SUPPOSITORIES ℞ Ⓒ

[*nĕm-bū 'tal*]
(pentobarbital sodium suppositories)

WARNING: MAY BE HABIT FORMING

DESCRIPTION

The barbiturates are nonselective central nervous system depressants which are primarily used as sedative hypnotics. The barbiturates and their sodium salts are subject to control under the Federal Controlled Substances Act (See "Drug Abuse and Dependence" section).
Barbiturates are substituted pyrimidine derivatives in which the basic structure common to these drugs is barbituric acid, a substance which has no central nervous system (CNS) activity. CNS activity is obtained by substituting alkyl, alkenyl, or aryl groups on the pyrimidine ring. Nembutal (pentobarbital sodium) is chemically represented by sodium 5-ethyl-5-(1-methylbutyl) barbiturate.
The sodium salt of pentobarbital occurs as a white, slightly bitter powder which is freely soluble in water and alcohol but practically insoluble in benzene and ether. Each rectal suppository contains either 30 mg, 60 mg, 120 mg, or 200 mg of pentobarbital sodium.

Continued on next page

Abbott—Cont.

INACTIVE INGREDIENTS
Semi-synthetic glycerides and other ingredients.

CLINICAL PHARMACOLOGY
Barbiturates are capable of producing all levels of CNS mood alteration from excitation to mild sedation, to hypnosis, and deep coma. Overdosage can produce death. In high enough therapeutic doses, barbiturates induce anesthesia.
Barbiturates depress the sensory cortex, decrease motor activity, alter cerebellar function, and produce drowsiness, sedation, and hypnosis.
Barbiturate-induced sleep differs from physiological sleep. Sleep laboratory studies have demonstrated that barbiturates reduce the amount of time spent in the rapid eye movement (REM) phase of sleep or dreaming stage. Also, Stages III and IV sleep are decreased. Following abrupt cessation of barbiturates used regularly, patients may experience markedly increased dreaming, nightmares, and/or insomnia. Therefore, withdrawal of a single therapeutic dose over 5 or 6 days has been recommended to lessen the REM rebound and disturbed sleep which contribute to drug withdrawal syndrome (for example, decrease the dose from 3 to 2 doses a day for 1 week).
In studies, secobarbital sodium and pentobarbital sodium have been found to lose most of their effectiveness for both inducing and maintaining sleep by the end of 2 weeks of continued drug administration at fixed doses. The short-, intermediate-, and, to a lesser degree, long-acting barbiturates have been widely prescribed for treating insomnia. Although the clinical literature abounds with claims that the short-acting barbiturates are superior for producing sleep while the intermediate-acting compounds are more effective in maintaining sleep, controlled studies have failed to demonstrate these differential effects. Therefore, as sleep medications, the barbiturates are of limited value beyond short-term use.
Barbiturates have little analgesic action at subanesthetic doses. Rather, in subanesthetic doses these drugs may increase the reaction to painful stimuli. All barbiturates exhibit anticonvulsant activity in anesthetic doses. However, of the drugs in this class, only phenobarbital, mephobarbital, and metharbital have been clinically demonstrated to be effective as oral anticonvulsants in subhypnotic doses.
Barbiturates are respiratory depressants. The degree of respiratory depression is dependent upon dose. With hypnotic doses, respiratory depression produced by barbiturates is similar to that which occurs during physiologic sleep with slight decrease in blood pressure and heart rate.
Studies in laboratory animals have shown that barbiturates cause reduction in the tone and contractility of the uterus, ureters, and urinary bladder. However, concentrations of the drugs required to produce this effect in humans are not reached with sedative-hypnotic doses.
Barbiturates do not impair normal hepatic function, but have been shown to induce liver microsomal enzymes, thus increasing and/or altering the metabolism of barbiturates and other drugs. (See "Precautions—*Drug Interactions*" section).
Pharmacokinetics: Barbiturates are absorbed in varying degrees following oral, rectal, or parenteral administration. The onset of action for oral or rectal administration varies from 20 to 60 minutes.
Duration of action, which is related to the rate at which the barbiturates are redistributed throughout the body, varies among persons and in the same person from time to time.
No studies have demonstrated that the different routes of administration are equivalent with respect to bioavailability.
Barbiturates are weak acids that are absorbed and rapidly distributed to all tissues and fluids with high concentrations in the brain, liver, and kidneys. Lipid solubility of the barbiturates is the dominant factor in their distribution within the body. The more lipid soluble the barbiturate, the more rapidly it penetrates all tissues of the body. Barbiturates are bound to plasma and tissue proteins to a varying degree with the degree of binding increasing directly as a function of lipid solubility. The plasma half-life for pentobarbital in adults is 15 to 50 hours and appears to be dose dependent.
Barbiturates are metabolized primarily by the hepatic microsomal enzyme system, and the metabolic products are excreted in the urine, and less commonly, in the feces. Approximately 25 to 50 percent of a dose of aprobarbital or phenobarbital is eliminated unchanged in the urine, whereas the amount of other barbiturates excreted unchanged in the urine is negligible. The excretion of unmetabolized barbiturate is one feature that distinguishes the long-acting category from those belonging to other categories which are almost entirely metabolized. The inactive metabolites of the barbiturates are excreted as conjugates of glucuronic acid.

INDICATIONS AND USAGE
Rectal: Barbiturates administered rectally are absorbed from the colon and are used when oral or parenteral administration may be undesirable.
1. Sedative.
2. Hypnotic, for the short-term treatment of insomnia, since they appear to lose their effectiveness for sleep induction and sleep maintenance after 2 weeks (See "Clinical Pharmacology" section).

CONTRAINDICATIONS
Barbiturates are contraindicated in patients with known barbiturate sensitivity. Barbiturates are also contraindicated in patients with a history of manifest or latent porphyria.

WARNINGS
1. *Habit forming:* Barbiturates may be habit forming. Tolerance, psychological and physical dependence may occur with continued use. (See "Drug Abuse and Dependence" and "Pharmacokinetics" sections). Patients who have psychological dependence on barbiturates may increase the dosage or decrease the dosage interval without consulting a physician and may subsequently develop a physical dependence on barbiturates. To minimize the possibility of overdosage or the development of dependence, the prescribing and dispensing of sedative-hypnotic barbiturates should be limited to the amount required for the interval until the next appointment. Abrupt cessation after prolonged use in the dependent person may result in withdrawal symptoms, including delirium, convulsions, and possibly death. Barbiturates should be withdrawn gradually from any patient known to be taking excessive dosage over long periods of time. (See "Drug Abuse and Dependence" section).
2. *Acute or chronic pain:* Caution should be exercised when barbiturates are administered to patients with acute or chronic pain, because paradoxical excitement could be induced or important symptoms could be masked. However, the use of barbiturates as sedatives in the postoperative surgical period and as adjuncts to cancer chemotherapy is well established.
3. *Use in pregnancy:* Barbiturates can cause fetal damage when administered to a pregnant woman. Retrospective, case-controlled studies have suggested a connection between the maternal consumption of barbiturates and a higher than expected incidence of fetal abnormalities. Following oral or parenteral administration, barbiturates readily cross the placental barrier and are distributed throughout fetal tissues with highest concentrations found in the placenta, fetal liver, and brain. It is presumed that this effect will also be seen following rectal administration.
Withdrawal symptoms occur in infants born to mothers who receive barbiturates throughout the last trimester of pregnancy. (See "Drug Abuse and Dependence" section). If this drug is used during pregnancy, or if the patient becomes pregnant while taking this drug, the patient should be apprised of the potential hazard to the fetus.
4. *Synergistic effects:* The concomitant use of alcohol or other CNS depressants may produce additive CNS depressant effects.

PRECAUTIONS
General: Barbiturates may be habit forming. Tolerance and psychological and physical dependence may occur with continuing use. (See "Drug Abuse and Dependence" section). Barbiturates should be administered with caution, if at all, to patients who are mentally depressed, have suicidal tendencies, or a history of drug abuse.
Elderly or debilitated patients may react to barbiturates with marked excitement, depression, and confusion. In some persons, barbiturates repeatedly produce excitement rather than depression.
In patients with hepatic damage, barbiturates should be administered with caution and initially in reduced doses. Barbiturates should not be administered to patients showing the premonitory signs of hepatic coma.
Information for the patient: Practitioners should give the following information and instructions to patients receiving barbiturates.
1. The use of barbiturates carries with it an associated risk of psychological and/or physical dependence. The patient should be warned against increasing the dose of the drug without consulting a physician.
2. Barbiturates may impair mental and/or physical abilities required for the performance of potentially hazardous tasks (e.g., driving, operating machinery, etc.)
3. Alcohol should not be consumed while taking barbiturates. Concurrent use of the barbiturates with other CNS depressants (e.g., alcohol, narcotics, tranquilizers, and antihistamines) may result in additional CNS depressant effects.

Laboratory tests: Prolonged therapy with barbiturates should be accompanied by periodic laboratory evaluation of organ systems, including hematopoietic, renal, and hepatic systems. (See "Precautions — *General*" and "Adverse Reactions" sections).
Drug interactions: Most reports of clinically significant drug interactions occurring with the barbiturates have involved phenobarbital. However, the application of these data to other barbiturates appears valid and warrants serial blood level determinations of the relevant drugs when there are multiple therapies.
1. *Anticoagulants:* Phenobarbital lowers the plasma levels of dicumarol (name previously used: bishydroxycoumarin) and causes a decrease in anticoagulant activity as measured by the prothrombin time. Barbiturates can induce hepatic microsomal enzymes resulting in increased metabolism and decreased anticoagulant response of oral anticoagulants (e.g., warfarin, acenocoumarol, dicumarol, and phenprocoumon). Patients stabilized on anticoagulant therapy may require dosage adjustments if barbiturates are added to or withdrawn from their dosage regimen.
2. *Corticosteroids:* Barbiturates appear to enhance the metabolism of exogenous corticosteroids probably through the induction of hepatic microsomal enzymes. Patients stabilized on corticosteroid therapy may require dosage adjustments if barbiturates are added to or withdrawn from their dosage regimen.
3. *Griseofulvin:* Phenobarbital appears to interfere with the absorption of orally administered griseofulvin, thus decreasing its blood level. The effect of the resultant decreased blood levels of griseofulvin on therapeutic response has not been established. However, it would be preferable to avoid concomitant administration of these drugs.
4. *Doxycycline:* Phenobarbital has been shown to shorten the half-life of doxycycline for as long as 2 weeks after barbiturate therapy is discontinued.
This mechanism is probably through the induction of hepatic microsomal enzymes that metabolize the antibiotic. If phenobarbital and doxycycline are administered concurrently, the clinical response to doxycycline should be monitored closely.
5. *Phenytoin, sodium valproate, valproic acid:* The effect of barbiturates on the metabolism of phenytoin appears to be variable. Some investigators report an accelerating effect, while others report no effect. Because the effect of barbiturates on the metabolism of phenytoin is not predictable, phenytoin and barbiturate blood levels should be monitored more frequently if these drugs are given concurrently. Sodium valproate and valproic acid appear to decrease barbiturate metabolism; therefore, barbiturate blood levels should be monitored and appropriate dosage adjustments made as indicated.
6. *Central nervous system depressants:* The concomitant use of other central nervous system depressants, including other sedatives or hypnotics, antihistamines, tranquilizers, or alcohol, may produce additive depressant effects.
7. *Monoamine oxidase inhibitors (MAOI):* MAOI prolong the effects of barbiturates probably because metabolism of the barbiturate is inhibited.
8. *Estradiol, estrone, progesterone and other steroidal hormones:* Pretreatment with or concurrent administration of phenobarbital may decrease the effect of estradiol by increasing its metabolism. There have been reports of patients treated with antiepileptic drugs (e.g., phenobarbital) who became pregnant while taking oral contraceptives. An alternate contraceptive method might be suggested to women taking phenobarbital.

Carcinogenesis: Adequate data are not available on long-term potential for carcinogenicity in humans or animals for pentobarbital.
Data from one retrospective study of 235 children in which the types of barbiturates are not identified suggested an association between exposure to barbiturates prenatally and an increased incidence of brain tumor. (Gold, E., et al, "Increased Risk of Brain Tumors in Children Exposed to Barbiturates," Journal of National Cancer Institute, 61:1031–1034, 1978).
Pregnancy: 1. Teratogenic effects. Pregnancy Category D — See "Warnings — Use in Pregnancy" section.
2. *Nonteratogenic effects.* Reports of infants suffering from long-term barbiturate exposure in utero included the acute withdrawal syndrome of seizures and hyperirritability from birth to a delayed onset of up to 14 days. (See "Drug Abuse and Dependence" section).
Labor and delivery: Hypnotic doses of these barbiturates do not appear to significantly impair uterine activity during labor. Full anesthetic doses of barbiturates decrease the force and frequency of uterine contractions. Administration of sedative-hypnotic barbiturates to the mother during labor may result in respiratory depression in the newborn. Premature infants are particularly susceptible to the depressant effects of barbiturates. If barbiturates are used during labor and delivery, resuscitation equipment should be available. Data are currently not available to evaluate the effect of these barbiturates when forceps delivery or other intervention is necessary. Also, data are not available to determine

the effect of these barbiturates on the later growth, development, and functional maturation of the child.

Nursing mothers: Caution should be exercised when a barbiturate is administered to a nursing woman since small amounts of barbiturates are excreted in the milk.

ADVERSE REACTIONS

The following adverse reactions and their incidence were compiled from surveillance of thousands of hospitalized patients. Because such patients may be less aware of certain of the milder adverse effects of barbiturates, the incidence of these reactions may be somewhat higher in fully ambulatory patients.

More than 1 in 100 patients. The most common adverse reaction estimated to occur at a rate of 1 to 3 patients per 100 is:

Nervous System: Somnolence.

Less than 1 in 100 patients. Adverse reactions estimated to occur at a rate of less than 1 in 100 patients listed below, grouped by organ system, and by decreasing order of occurrence are:

Nervous system: Agitation, confusion, hyperkinesia, ataxia, CNS depression, nightmares, nervousness, psychiatric disturbance, hallucinations, insomnia, anxiety, dizziness, thinking abnormality.

Respiratory system: Hypoventilation, apnea.

Cardiovascular system: Bradycardia, hypotension, syncope.

Digestive system: Nausea, vomiting, constipation.

Other reported reactions: Headache, injection site reactions, hypersensitivity reactions (angioedema, skin rashes, exfoliative dermatitis), fever, liver damage, megaloblastic anemia following chronic phenobarbital use.

DRUG ABUSE AND DEPENDENCE

Pentobarbital sodium suppositories are subject to control by the Federal Controlled Substances Act under DEA schedule III.

Barbiturates may be habit forming. Tolerance, psychological dependence, and physical dependence may occur especially following prolonged use of high doses of barbiturates. Daily administration in excess of 400 mg of pentobarbital or secobarbital for approximately 90 days is likely to produce some degree of physical dependence. A dosage of from 600 to 800 mg taken for at least 35 days is sufficient to produce withdrawal seizures. The average daily dose for the barbiturate addict is usually about 1.5 grams. As tolerance to barbiturates develops, the amount needed to maintain the same level of intoxication increases; tolerance to a fatal dosage, however, does not increase more than two-fold. As this occurs, the margin between an intoxicating dosage and fatal dosage becomes smaller.

Symptoms of acute intoxication with barbiturates include unsteady gait, slurred speech, and sustained nystagmus. Mental signs of chronic intoxication include confusion, poor judgment, irritability, insomnia, and somatic complaints.

Symptoms of barbiturate dependence are similar to those of chronic alcoholism. If an individual appears to be intoxicated with alcohol to a degree that is radically disproportionate to the amount of alcohol in his or her blood the use of barbiturates should be suspected. The lethal dose of a barbiturate is far less if alcohol is also ingested.

The symptoms of barbiturate withdrawal can be severe and may cause death. Minor withdrawal symptoms may appear 8 to 12 hours after the last dose of a barbiturate. These symptoms usually appear in the following order: anxiety, muscle twitching, tremor of hands and fingers, progressive weakness, dizziness, distortion in visual perception, nausea, vomiting, insomnia, and orthostatic hypotension. Major withdrawal symptoms (convulsions and delirium) may occur within 16 hours and last up to 5 days after abrupt cessation of these drugs. Intensity of withdrawal symptoms gradually declines over a period of approximately 15 days. Individuals susceptible to barbiturate abuse and dependence include alcoholics and opiate abusers, as well as other sedative-hypnotic and amphetamine abusers.

Drug dependence to barbiturates arises from repeated administration of a barbiturate or agent with barbiturate-like effect on a continuous basis, generally in amounts exceeding therapeutic dose levels. The characteristics of drug dependence to barbiturates include: (a) a strong desire or need to continue taking the drug; (b) a tendency to increase the dose; (c) a psychic dependence on the effects of the drug related to subjective and individual appreciation of those effects; and (d) a physical dependence on the effects of the drug requiring its presence for maintenance of homeostasis and resulting in a definite, characteristic, and self-limited abstinence syndrome when the drug is withdrawn.

Treatment of barbiturate dependence consists of cautious and gradual withdrawal of the drug. Barbiturate-dependent patients can be withdrawn by using a number of different withdrawal regimens. In all cases withdrawal takes an extended period of time. One method involves substituting a 30 mg dose of phenobarbital for each 100 to 200 mg dose of barbiturate that the patient has been taking. The total daily amount of phenobarbital is then administered in 3 to 4 divided doses, not to exceed 600 mg daily. Should signs of withdrawal occur on the first day of treatment, a loading dose of 100 to 200 mg of phenobarbital may be administered IM in addition to the oral dose. After stabilization on phenobarbital, the total daily dose is decreased by 30 mg a day as long as withdrawal is proceeding smoothly. A modification of this regimen involves initiating treatment at the patient's regular dosage level and decreasing the daily dosage by 10 percent if tolerated by the patient.

Infants physically dependent on barbiturates may be given phenobarbital 3 to 10 mg/kg/day. After withdrawal symptoms (hyperactivity, disturbed sleep, tremors, hyperreflexia) are relieved, the dosage of phenobarbital should be gradually decreased and completely withdrawn over a 2 week period.

OVERDOSAGE

The toxic dose of barbiturates varies considerably. In general, an oral dose of 1 g of most barbiturates produces serious poisoning in an adult. Death commonly occurs after 2 to 10 g of ingested barbiturate. Barbiturate intoxication may be confused with alcoholism, bromide intoxication, and with various neurological disorders.

Acute overdosage with barbiturates is manifested by CNS and respiratory depression which may progress to Cheyne-Stokes respiration, areflexia, constriction of the pupils to a slight degree (though in severe poisoning they may show paralytic dilation), oliguria, tachycardia, hypotension, lowered body temperature, and coma. Typical shock syndrome (apnea, circulatory collapse, respiratory arrest, and death) may occur.

In extreme overdose, all electrical activity in the brain may cease, in which case a "flat" EEG normally equated with clinical death cannot be accepted. This effect is fully reversible unless hypoxic damage occurs. Consideration should be given to the possibility of barbiturate intoxication even in situations that appear to involve trauma.

Complications such as pneumonia, pulmonary edema, cardiac arrhythmias, congestive heart failure, and renal failure may occur. Uremia may increase CNS sensitivity to barbiturates. Differential diagnosis should include hypoglycemia, head trauma, cerebrovascular accidents, convulsive states, and diabetic coma. Blood levels from acute overdosage for some barbiturates are listed in Table 2. [See Table 2 shown in Nembutal Capsules prescribing information.]

Treatment of overdosage is mainly supportive and consists of the following:

1. Maintenance of an adequate airway, with assisted respiration and oxygen administration as necessary.
2. Monitoring of vital signs and fluid balance.
3. Fluid therapy and other standard treatment for shock, if needed.
4. If renal function is normal, forced diuresis may aid in the elimination of the barbiturate. Alkalinization of the urine increases renal excretion of some barbiturates, especially phenobarbital, also aprobarbital, and mephobarbital (which is metabolized to phenobarbital).
5. Although not recommended as a routine procedure, hemodialysis may be used in severe barbiturate intoxications or if the patient is anuric or in shock.
6. Patient should be rolled from side to side every 30 minutes.
7. Antibiotics should be given if pneumonia is suspected.
8. Appropriate nursing care to prevent hypostatic pneumonia, decubiti, aspiration, and other complications of patients with altered states of consciousness.

DOSAGE AND ADMINISTRATION

Typical hypnotic doses for adults and children are given below. These are intended only as a guide, and administration should be adjusted to the individual needs of each patient. For sedation, in children 5–14 years and in adults, reduce dose appropriately.

Adults (average to above average weight)— one 120 mg or one 200 mg suppository.

Children —

12–14 years (80–110 lbs)	one 60 mg or one 120 mg suppository
5–12 years (40–80 lbs)	one 60 mg suppository
1–4 years (20–40 lbs)	one 30 mg or one 60 mg suppository
2 months–1 year (10–20 lbs)	one 30 mg suppository

Suppositories should not be divided.

Dosages of barbiturates must be individualized with full knowledge of their particular characteristics and recommended rate of administration. Factors of consideration are the patient's age, weight, and condition.

Special patient population: Dosage should be reduced in the elderly or debilitated because these patients may be more sensitive to barbiturates. Dosage should be reduced for patients with impaired renal function or hepatic disease.

HOW SUPPLIED

NEMBUTAL Sodium Suppositories (pentobarbital sodium suppositories) are available as suppositories containing pentobarbital sodium in the amount of 30 mg (½ gr) (NDC 0074-3272-01); 60 mg (1 gr) (NDC 0074-3148-01); 120 mg (2 gr) (NDC 0074-3145-01) and 200 mg (3 gr) (NDC 0074-3164-01). Supplied in boxes of 12 suppositories.

Store in a refrigerator (36°–46°F).

Abbott Laboratories
North Chicago, IL 60064
Ref. 07-5369-R10

NITROPRESS® ℞

[nī'tro-press]

(sterile sodium nitroprusside, USP)

> NITROPRESS is only to be used as an infusion with sterile 5% dextrose injection. Not for direct injection.
> NITROPRESS should be used only when the necessary facilities and equipment for continuous monitoring of blood pressure are available.
> If at infusion rates of up to 10 mcg/kg/min- ute, an adequate reduction of blood pressure is not obtained within ten minutes, administration of NITROPRESS should be stopped.
> The instructions included herein should be reviewed thoroughly before administration of NITROPRESS.

DESCRIPTION

This antihypertensive agent is for intravenous infusion only. When mixed, each 2 ml of NITROPRESS (sterile sodium nitroprusside, USP) in injectable form contains the equivalent of 50 mg of sodium nitroprusside dihydrate (sodium nitrosylpentacyanoferrate [III]) in sterile water for injection in an amber-colored, single dose Univial.®

Chemically, sodium nitroprusside is Na_2 [Fe(CN)$_5$NO]·$2H_2O$. It is a reddish-brown powder which is soluble in water. In aqueous solution, it is photosensitive and should be protected from light.

CLINICAL PHARMACOLOGY

NITROPRESS is a potent, immediate acting, intravenous hypotensive agent. This action is probably due to the nitroso (NO) group. Its effect is almost immediate and ends when the IV infusion is stopped. Generally, NITROPRESS is rapidly metabolized to cyanide and subsequently converted to thiocyanate through the mediation of a hepatic enzyme, rhodanase. The rate of conversion from cyanide to thiocyanate is dependent on the availability of sulfur, usually thiosulfate. The hypotensive effect is augmented by ganglionic blocking agents, volatile liquid anesthetics (such as halothane and enflurane), and by most other circulatory depressants.

The hypotensive effects of NITROPRESS are caused by peripheral vasodilation as a result of a direct action on the blood vessels, independent of autonomic innervation. No relaxation is seen in the smooth muscle of the uterus or duodenum *in situ* in animals.

Sodium nitroprusside administered intravenously to hypertensive and normotensive patients produced a marked lowering of the arterial blood pressure, slight increase in heart rate, a mild decrease in cardiac output and a moderate diminution in calculated total peripheral vascular resistance.

The decrease in calculated total peripheral vascular resistance suggests arteriolar vasodilatation. The decreases in cardiac and stroke index noted may be due to the peripheral vascular pooling of blood.

In hypertensive patients, moderate depressor doses induce renal vasodilatation roughly equivalent to the decrease in pressure without an appreciable increase in renal blood flow or a decrease in glomerular filtration.

In normotensive subjects, acute reduction of mean arterial pressure to 60 to 75 mmHg by infusion of sodium nitroprusside caused a significant increase in renin activity of renal venous plasma in correlation with the degree of reduction in pressure. Renal response to reduction in pressure was more striking in renovascular hypertensive patients, with significant increase in renin release occurring from the involved kidney at mean arterial pressures ranging from 90 to 137 mmHg. Furthermore, the magnitude of renin release from the involved kidney was significantly greater when compared with that in normotensive subjects, while in the contralateral, uninvolved kidney, no significant release of renin was detected during the reduction of pressure.

INDICATIONS AND USAGE

NITROPRESS (sterile sodium nitroprusside) is indicated for the immediate reduction of blood pressure of patients in hypertensive crises. Concomitant oral antihypertensive medication should be started while the hypertensive emergency is being brought under control with NITROPRESS.

NITROPRESS is also indicated for producing controlled hypotension during anesthesia in order to reduce bleeding in sur-

Continued on next page

Abbott—Cont.

gical procedures where surgeon and anesthesiologist deem it appropriate.

CONTRAINDICATIONS

NITROPRESS should not be used in the treatment of compensatory hypertension, *e.g.,* arteriovenous shunt or coarctation of the aorta.
The use of NITROPRESS to produce controlled hypotension during surgery is contraindicated in patients with known inadequate cerebral circulation. NITROPRESS is not intended for use during emergency surgery in moribund patients (A.S.A. Class 5E).

WARNINGS

> If excessive amounts of NITROPRESS are used and/or sulfur—usually thiosulfate—supplies are depleted, cyanide toxicity can occur. (See Overdosage.)
> If sodium nitroprusside infusion is to be extended, particularly if renal impairment is present, close attention should be given to not exceeding the recommended maximum infusion rate of 10 mcg/kg/min. If in the course of therapy increased tolerance to the drug (as shown by the need for higher infusion rate) develops, it is essential to monitor blood acid-base balance, as metabolic acidosis is the earliest and most reliable evidence of cyanide toxicity. If signs of metabolic acidosis appear, NITROPRESS should be discontinued and an alternate drug administered.
> Serum thiocyanate levels do not reflect cyanide toxicity. However, serum thiocyanate levels should be monitored daily if treatment is to be extended, especially in patients with renal dysfunction. Thiocyanate accumulation and toxicity may manifest itself as tinnitus, blurred vision, delirium.

The following warnings apply to use of NITROPRESS for controlled hypotension during anesthesia:
1. Tolerance to blood loss, anemia and hypovolemia may be diminished. If possible, pre-existing anemia and hypovolemia should be corrected prior to employing controlled hypotension.
2. Hypotensive anesthetic techniques may alter pulmonary ventilation perfusion ratio. Patients intolerant of additional dead air space at ordinary oxygen partial pressure may benefit from higher oxygen partial pressure.
3. Extreme caution should be exercised in patients who are especially poor surgical risks (A.S.A. Class 4 and 4E).

NITROPRESS IS ONLY TO BE USED AS AN INFUSION WITH 5% DEXTROSE INJECTION. NOT FOR DIRECT INJECTION.
Infusion rates greater than 10 mcg/kg/minute are rarely required. If, at this rate, an adequate reduction in blood pressure is not obtained within 10 minutes, administration of NITROPRESS (sterile sodium nitroprusside) should be stopped.

PRECAUTIONS

General: Adequate facilities, equipment and personnel should be available for frequent and vigilant monitoring of blood pressure, since the hypotensive effect of NITROPRESS occurs rapidly.
When the infusion is slowed or stopped, blood pressure usually begins to rise immediately and returns to pretreatment levels within one to ten minutes. It should be used with caution and initially in low doses in elderly patients, since they may be more sensitive to the hypotensive effects of the drug. Young, vigorous males may require somewhat larger than ordinary doses of sodium nitroprusside for hypotensive anesthesia; however, the infusion rate of 10 mcg/kg/minute should not be exceeded. Deepening of anesthesia, if indicated, might permit satisfactory conditions to exist within the recommended dosage range.
Because of the rapid onset of action and potency of NITROPRESS, it should preferably be administered with the use of an infusion pump, micro-drip regulator, or any similar device that would allow precise measurement of the flow rate.
Since cyanide is converted into thiocyanate through the mediation of a hepatic enzyme, rhodanase, NITROPRESS should be used with caution in patients with hepatic insufficiency.
Since thiocyanate inhibits both the uptake and binding of iodine, caution should be exercised in using NITROPRESS in patients with hypothyroidism or severe renal impairment.
Hypertensive patients are more sensitive to the intravenous effect of sodium nitroprusside than are normotensive subjects. Patients who are receiving concomitant antihypertensive medications are more sensitive to the hypotensive effect of sodium nitroprusside and the dosage should be adjusted accordingly.
Once dissolved in solution, NITROPRESS tends to deteriorate in the presence of light. Therefore, it must be protected from light by covering the container of the prepared solution with the light-protective sleeve supplied with the product, or aluminum foil, or other opaque materials. If properly protected from light, the freshly reconstituted and diluted solution is stable for 24 hours.
NITROPRESS in aqueous solution yields the nitroprusside ion which reacts with even minute quantities of a wide variety of inorganic and organic substances to form usually highly colored reaction products (blue, green or dark red). If this occurs, the infusion should be replaced.
Drug Interactions: The hypotensive effect of sodium nitroprusside is augmented by *ganglionic blocking agents. Volatile liquid anesthetics* (such as halothane and enflurane) also augment the hypotensive effect. Most other *circulatory depressants* will augment the hypotensive effect of sodium nitroprusside.
Carcinogenesis: No data are available on long-term potential for carcinogenicity in animals or humans for sodium nitroprusside.
Usage During Pregnancy: Pregnancy Category C. Animal reproduction studies have not been conducted with NITROPRESS. It is also not known whether NITROPRESS (sterile sodium nitroprusside) can cause fetal harm when administered to a pregnant woman or can affect reproduction capacity. NITROPRESS should be given to a pregnant woman only if clearly needed.
Nursing Mothers: It is not known whether this drug is excreted in human milk. Because many drugs are excreted in human milk, caution should be exercised when NITROPRESS is administered to a nursing woman.

ADVERSE REACTIONS

Nausea, retching, diaphoresis, apprehension, headache, restlessness, muscle twitching, retrosternal discomfort, palpitations, dizziness and abdominal pain have been noted with too rapid reduction in blood pressure, but these symptoms rapidly disappeared with slowing of the rate of the infusion or temporary discontinuation of infusion and did not reappear with continued slower rate of administration. Irritation at the infusion site may occur.
One case of hypothyroidism following prolonged therapy with intravenous sodium nitroprusside has been reported. A patient with severe hypertension with uremia received 3900 mg of sodium nitroprusside intravenously over a period of 21 days. This is one of the longest reported intravenous uses of this agent. There was no tachyphylaxis, but the patient developed evidence of hypothyroidism, together with retention of thiocyanate (9.5 mg/100 ml). With peritoneal dialysis the thiocyanate level diminished and the signs of hypothyroidism subsided.

OVERDOSAGE

The first signs of sodium nitroprusside overdosage are those of profound hypotension. As with instances of depletion of thiosulfate supplies, overdosage may lead to cyanide toxicity. Metabolic acidosis and increasing tolerance to the drug are early indications of overdosage. These may be associated with or followed by dyspnea, headache, vomiting, dizziness, ataxia and loss of consciousness. Sodium nitroprusside should then be immediately discontinued. Other signs of cyanide poisoning are coma, imperceptible pulse, absent reflexes, widely dilated pupils, pink color, distant heart sounds, and shallow breathing. Oxygen alone will not provide relief. Nitrites should be administered to induce methemoglobin formation. Methemoglobin, in turn, combines with cyanide bound to cytochrome oxidase to liberate cytochrome oxidase and form a non-toxic complex, cyanmethemoglobin. Cyanide then gradually dissociates from the latter and is converted by administration of thiosulfate to sodium thiocyanate in the presence of rhodanase.
Treatment: In cases of massive overdosage when signs of cyanide toxicity are present use the following regimen:
1. Discontinue administration of NITROPRESS.
2. Administer amyl nitrite inhalations for 15 to 30 seconds each minute until 3% sodium nitrite solution can be prepared for I.V. administration.
3. Sodium nitrite 3% solution should be injected intravenously at a rate not exceeding 2.5 to 5 ml/minute up to a total dose of 10 to 15 ml with careful monitoring of the blood pressure.
4. Following the above steps, inject sodium thiosulfate intravenously, 12.5 g in 50 ml of 5% dextrose injection over a ten-minute period.
5. Since signs of overdosage may reappear, the patient must be observed for several hours.
6. If signs of overdosage reappear, sodium nitrite and sodium thiosulfate injections are repeated in one-half of the above doses.
7. During the administration of nitrites and later when thiocyanate formation is taking place, blood pressure may drop but can be corrected with vasopressor agents.

DOSAGE AND ADMINISTRATION

Reconstitution Directions for Univial:
1. Remove protective cap.
   Turn plunger-stopper a quarter turn and press to force sterile water for injection into lower chamber.
2. Shake gently to effect solution.
   Use only a clear solution.
3. Sterilize top of stopper with a suitable germicide.
4. Insert needle through the center of stopper until tip is barely visible. Withdraw dose.

Depending on the desired concentration, all of the reconstituted Univial solution should be diluted in 250 to 1000 ml of 5% dextrose injection and promptly covered with light-protective sleeve supplied with the product, or aluminum foil, or other opaque materials to protect from light. *If properly protected from light, the freshly reconstituted and diluted solution is stable for 24 hours.* The freshly prepared solution for infusion has a very faint brownish tint. If it is highly colored, it should be discarded (see Precautions). *The infusion fluid used for the administration of NITROPRESS should not be employed as a vehicle for simultaneous administration of any other drug.*
In patients who are not receiving antihypertensive drugs, the average dose of NITROPRESS (sterile sodium nitroprusside) for both adults and children is 3 mcg/kg/minute (range of 0.5 to 10 mcg/kg/minute). Usually, at 3 mcg/kg/minute, blood pressure can be lowered by about 30 to 40% below the pretreatment diastolic levels and maintained. In hypertensive patients receiving concomitant antihypertensive medications, smaller doses are required. In order to avoid excessive levels of thiocyanate and lessen the possibility of a precipitous drop in blood pressure, infusion rates greater than 10 mcg/kg/minute should rarely be used. If, at this rate, an adequate reduction of blood pressure is not obtained within 10 minutes, administration of NITROPRESS should be stopped.
One Univial (50 mg) NITROPRESS in 1000 ml 5% dextrose injection provides a concentration of 50 mcg/ml.
One Univial (50 mg) NITROPRESS in 500 ml 5% dextrose injection provides a concentration of 100 mcg/ml.
One Univial (50 mg) NITROPRESS in 250 ml 5% dextrose injection provides a concentration of 200 mcg/ml.

Dose	mcg/kg/min.
Average	3
Range	0.5 to 10

The intravenous infusion of NITROPRESS should be administered by an infusion pump, micro-drip regulator or any similar device that will allow precise measurement of the flow rate. Care should be taken to avoid extravasation. The rate of administration should be adjusted to maintain the desired antihypertensive or hypotensive effect, as determined by frequent blood pressure determinations. It is recommended that the blood pressure should not be allowed to drop at a too rapid rate and the systolic pressure not be lowered below 60 mmHg. In hypertensive emergencies NITROPRESS infusion may be continued until the patient can safely be treated with oral antihypertensive medications.

HOW SUPPLIED

NITROPRESS (sterile sodium nitroprusside, USP) is supplied in an amber-colored, single dose Univial (**NDC** 0074-3019-02), each 2 ml (when mixed) containing the equivalent of 50 mg sodium nitroprusside dihydrate in sterile water for injection. Exposure of pharmaceutical products to heat should be minimized. Avoid excessive heat. Protect from freezing. It is recommended that reconstituted product be stored below 86°F (30°C); however, brief exposure up to 104°F (40°C) does not adversely affect the product. Protect from light—store in carton until use.

Univial®—Sterile two-compartment vial, Abbott.
Abbott Laboratories
North Chicago, IL 60064
Ref. 01-2313-R6

NORISODRINE® AEROTROL® ℞

[no-ris'o-drene air'ō-trol]
(isoproterenol hydrochloride inhalation aerosol, USP)
In a Controlled-Dose Nebulizer

DESCRIPTION

Isoproterenol HCl 0.25% w/w (=2.8 mg/ml) in inert chlorofluorohydrocarbon propellants; alcohol 33%; ascorbic acid 0.1% as preservative; and artificial and natural flavors.
Each depression of the valve delivers approximately 0.12 mg to the patient.

ACTIONS

Isoproterenol is a short-acting sympathomimetic drug. It produces pharmacologic response in the cardiovascular system and on the smooth muscles of the bronchial tree. The drug will prevent or overcome histamine-induced asthma in both experimental animals and man, and is effective when used prophylactically. It is one of the most potent bronchodilators known and can be used in patients who do not respond to the bronchodilating action of epinephrine. Isoproterenol has a cardio-accelerating effect, but its vasoconstricting action is less pronounced than that of epinephrine. Therapeutic doses may produce a slight increase in systolic blood pressure, but a slight decrease in diastolic. Larger doses may cause peripheral vasodilatation in the renal, mesenteric and femoral beds and some patients respond with a decrease in diastolic, but no change in systolic pressure. Such effects are usually of very short duration.

INDICATIONS

For the treatment of bronchospasm associated with acute and chronic bronchial asthma, pulmonary emphysema, bronchitis, and bronchiectasis.

CONTRAINDICATIONS

Use of isoproterenol in patients with pre-existing cardiac arrhythmias associated with tachycardia is contraindicated because the cardiac stimulant effects of the drug may aggravate such disorders.

WARNINGS

Excessive use of an adrenergic aerosol should be discouraged, as it may lose its effectiveness. Occasional patients have been reported to develop severe paradoxical airway resistance with repeated excessive use of isoproterenol inhalation preparations. The cause of this refractory state is unknown. It is advisable that in such instances the use of this preparation be discontinued immediately and alternative therapy instituted, since in the reported cases the patients did not respond to other forms of therapy until the drug was withdrawn.

Deaths have been reported following excessive use of isoproterenol inhalation preparations and the exact cause is unknown. Cardiac arrest was noted in several instances.

PRECAUTIONS

Isoproterenol and epinephrine may be used interchangeably if the patient becomes unresponsive to one or the other but should not be used concurrently. If desired, these drugs may be alternated, provided an interval of at least four hours has elapsed.

As with all sympathomimetic drugs, isoproterenol should be used with great caution in the presence of cardiovascular disorders, including coronary insufficiency, hypertension, hyperthyroidism and diabetes, or when there is a sensitivity to sympathomimetic amines.

Although there has been no evidence of teratogenic effects with this drug, use of any drug in pregnancy, lactation, or in women of childbearing age requires that the potential benefit of the drug be weighed against its possible hazard to the mother and child.

ADVERSE REACTIONS

Only a small percentage of patients experience any side effects following oral inhalation of aerosolized isoproterenol. Overdosage may produce tachycardia with resultant coronary insufficiency, palpitations, vertigo, nausea, tremors, headache, insomnia, central excitation, and blood pressure changes. These reactions are similar to those produced by other sympathomimetic agents.

DOSAGE AND ADMINISTRATION

The usual dose for the relief of dyspnea in the acute episode is 1 to 2 inhalations. Start with one inhalation. If no relief is evident after 2 to 5 minutes, a second inhalation may be taken. For daily maintenance, use 1 to 2 inhalations 4 to 6 times daily, or as directed by the physician. The physician should be careful to instruct the patient in the proper technique of administration so that the number of inhalations per treatment and the frequency of treatment may be titrated to the patient's response.

No more than two inhalations should be taken at any one time, or more than 6 inhalations in any hour during a 24-hour period, unless advised by physician.

DIRECTIONS FOR USE

Before each use, remove cap and assemble.

1. Breathe out fully. Place mouthpiece well into the mouth, aimed at the back of the throat.
2. As you begin to breathe in deeply, press the vial firmly down into the adapter. This releases one dose. Continue to breathe in until your lungs are completely filled.
3. Remove from mouth. Hold your breath for several seconds, then breathe out slowly.

WARNING

Do not exceed the dose prescribed by your physician. If difficulty in breathing persists, contact your physician immediately.

HOW SUPPLIED

NORISODRINE AEROTROL (isoproterenol hydrochloride inhalation aerosol, USP), 0.25% w/w, is supplied in a 15 ml controlled-dose nebulizer (NDC 0074-6869-03).

Manufactured for
Abbott Laboratories
North Chicago, IL 60064
Ref. 01-2149-R3

NORISODRINE® WITH CALCIUM IODIDE SYRUP ℞

[*nō-rī 'sō-drēn*]
(isoproterenol sulfate and calcium iodide)

HOW SUPPLIED

Each teaspoonful of NORISODRINE WITH CALCIUM IODIDE SYRUP contains 3 mg of isoproterenol sulfate, 150 mg of anhydrous calcium iodide. Norisodrine with Calcium Iodide Syrup is supplied in pint (NDC 0074-6953-01) bottles.

INACTIVE INGREDIENTS

Alcohol 6%, ascorbic acid, caramel coloring, glycerin, liquid glucose, sucrose, water, artificial flavors and other ingredients forming a palatable, aromatic syrup.

Abbott Laboratories
North Chicago, IL 60064

OGEN® ℞

[*ō 'gên*]
(estropipate tablets, USP)
(estropipate vaginal cream, USP)

WARNING:

1. ESTROGENS HAVE BEEN REPORTED TO INCREASE THE RISK OF ENDOMETRIAL CARCINOMA.

Three independent case control studies have shown an increased risk of endometrial cancer in postmenopausal women exposed to exogenous estrogens for prolonged periods.[1–3] This risk was independent of the other known risk factors for endometrial cancer. These studies are further supported by the finding that incidence rates of endometrial cancer have increased sharply since 1969 in eight different areas of the United States with population-based cancer reporting systems, an increase which may be related to the rapidly expanding use of estrogens during the last decade.[4]

The three case control studies reported that the risk of endometrial cancer in estrogen users was about 4.5 to 13.9 times greater than in nonusers. The risk appears to depend on both duration of treatment[1] and on estrogen dose.[3] In view of these findings, when estrogens are used for the treatment of menopausal symptoms, the lowest dose that will control symptoms should be utilized and medication should be discontinued as soon as possible. When prolonged treatment is medically indicated, the patient should be reassessed on at least a semiannual basis to determine the need for continued therapy. Although the evidence must be considered preliminary, one study suggests that cyclic administration of low doses of estrogen may carry less risk than continuous administration;[3] it therefore appears prudent to utilize such a regimen.

Close clinical surveillance of all women taking estrogens is important. In all cases of undiagnosed persistent or recurring abnormal vaginal bleeding, adequate diagnostic measures should be undertaken to rule out malignancy.

There is no evidence at present that "natural" estrogens are more or less hazardous than "synthetic" estrogens at equiestrogenic doses.

2. OGEN SHOULD NOT BE USED DURING PREGNANCY.

According to some investigators, the use of female sex hormones, both estrogens and progestogens, during early pregnancy may seriously damage the offspring. Studies have reported that females exposed in utero to diethylstilbestrol, a non-steroidal estrogen, have an increased risk of developing in later life a form of vaginal or cervical cancer that is ordinarily extremely rare.[5,6] In one of these studies, this risk was estimated as not greater than 4 per 1000 exposures.[7] Furthermore, there are reports that a high percentage of such exposed women (from 30 to 90 percent) have been found to have vaginal adenosis,[8–12] epithelial changes of the vagina and cervix. Although these reported changes are histologically benign, the investigators have not determined whether they are precursors of adenocarcinoma.

Several reports suggest an association between intrauterine exposure to female sex hormones and congenital anomalies in the offspring, including heart defects and limb reduction defects.[13–16] One case control study[16] estimated a 4.7 fold increased risk of limb reduction defects in infants exposed in utero to sex hormones (oral contraceptives, hormone withdrawal tests for pregnancy, or attempted treatment for threatened abortion). Some of these exposures were very short and involved only a few days of treatment. The data suggest that the risk of limb reduction defects in exposed fetuses is somewhat less than 1 per 1000.

In the past, female sex hormones have been used during pregnancy in an attempt to treat threatened or habitual abortion. OGEN is not intended for these uses nor has it been studied for these uses, and therefore should not be used during pregnancy. There is no evidence from well controlled studies that progestogens are effective for these uses.

If OGEN (estropipate) is used during pregnancy, or if the patient becomes pregnant while taking the tablets or using the vaginal cream, she should be apprised of the potential risks to the fetus, and the question of continuation of the pregnancy should be addressed.

DESCRIPTION

OGEN (estropipate), (formerly piperazine estrone sulfate), is a natural estrogenic substance prepared from purified crystalline estrone, solubilized as the sulfate and stabilized with piperazine. It is appreciably soluble in water and has almost no odor or taste. The amount of piperazine in OGEN is not sufficient to exert a pharmacological action. Its addition ensures solubility, stability, and uniform potency of the estrone sulfate. Chemically estropipate is represented by estra 1,3,5(10) -trien-17-one, 3-(sulfooxy)-, compound with piperazine (1:1).

OGEN is available as tablets for oral administration containing either 0.75 mg (OGEN .625), 1.5 mg (OGEN 1.25), 3 mg (OGEN 2.5) or 6 mg (OGEN 5) estropipate.

Each gram of Ogen Vaginal Cream contains 1.5 mg estropipate.

INACTIVE INGREDIENTS

OGEN .625 tablet: Acacia, corn starch, D&C Yellow No. 10, FD&C Yellow No. 6, lactose, methylparaben, piperazine, propylparaben, stearic acid, talc and other ingredients.

OGEN 1.25 tablet: Acacia, corn starch, FD&C Yellow No. 6, lactose, methylparaben, piperazine, propylparaben, stearic acid, talc and other ingredients.

OGEN 2.5 tablet: Acacia, corn starch, FD&C Blue No. 2, lactose, methylparaben, piperazine, propylparaben, stearic acid, talc and other ingredients.

OGEN 5 tablet: Acacia, corn starch, D&C Yellow No. 10, FD&C Blue No. 2, lactose, methylparaben, piperazine, propylparaben, stearic acid, talc and other ingredients.

The base of OGEN Vaginal Cream is composed of the following ingredients: glycerin, mineral oil, glyceryl monostearate, polyethylene glycol ether complex of higher fatty alcohols, cetyl alcohol, anhydrous lanolin, sodium biphosphate, cis-N-(3-chloroallyl) hexaminium chloride, propylparaben, methylparaben, piperazine hexahydrate, citric acid and water.

CLINICAL PHARMACOLOGY

Estrogens are important in the development and maintenance of the female reproductive system and secondary sex characteristics. They promote growth and development of the vagina, uterus, and fallopian tubes, and enlargement of the breasts. Indirectly, they contribute to the shaping of the skeleton, maintenance of tone and elasticity of urogenital structures, changes in the epiphyses of the long bones that allow for the pubertal growth spurt and its termination, growth of axillary and pubic hair, and pigmentation of the nipples and genitals. Along with other hormones such as progesterone, estrogens are intricately involved in the process of menstruation. Estrogens also affect the release of pituitary gonadotropins.

OGEN (estropipate) owes its therapeutic action to estrone, one of the three principal estrogenic steroid hormones of man: estradiol, estrone, and estriol. Estradiol is rapidly hydrolyzed in the body to estrone, which in turn may be hydrated to the less active estriol. These transformations occur readily, mainly in the liver, where there is also free interconversion between estrone and estradiol.

A depletion of endogenous estrogens occurs postmenopausally as a result of a decline in ovarian function, and may cause symptomatic vulvovaginal atrophy. The signs and symptoms of these atrophic changes in the vaginal and vulval epithelia may be alleviated by the topical application of an estrogenic hormone such as OGEN.

Gastrointestinal absorption of orally administered estrogens is usually prompt and complete. OGEN Vaginal Cream may be absorbed transmucosally and may produce systemic estrogenic effects. Inactivation of estrogens in the body occurs mainly in the liver. During cyclic passage through the liver, estrogens are degraded to less active estrogenic compounds and conjugated with sulfuric and glucuronic acids. Estrone is 50–80% bound to protein as it circulates in the blood, primarily as a conjugate with sulfate.

INDICATIONS AND USAGE

The cyclic administration (See "DOSAGE AND ADMINISTRATION" section) of OGEN Tablets is indicated for the treatment of estrogen deficiency associated with:

Continued on next page

Abbott—Cont.

1. Moderate to severe *vasomotor* symptoms of menopause. (There is no evidence that estrogens are effective for nervous symptoms or depression which might occur during menopause, and they should not be used to treat these conditions.)
2. Atrophic vaginitis.
3. Kraurosis vulvae.
4. Female hypogonadism.
5. Female castration.
6. Primary ovarian failure.

The cyclic administration of OGEN Vaginal Cream is indicated for the treatment of atrophic vaginitis or kraurosis vulvae. (See "DOSAGE AND ADMINISTRATION" section.)

OGEN (ESTROPIPATE) HAS NOT BEEN TESTED FOR EFFICACY FOR ANY PURPOSE DURING PREGNANCY. SINCE ITS EFFECT UPON THE FETUS IS UNKNOWN, IT CANNOT BE RECOMMENDED FOR ANY CONDITION DURING PREGNANCY (SEE BOXED WARNING).

CONTRAINDICATIONS

OGEN should not be used in women with any of the following conditions:

1. Known or suspected cancer of the breast.
2. Known or suspected estrogen-dependent neoplasia.
3. OGEN may cause fetal harm when administered to a pregnant woman. OGEN is contraindicated in women who are or may become pregnant (See Boxed Warning).
4. Undiagnosed abnormal genital bleeding.
5. Active thrombophlebitis or thromboembolic disorders.
6. A past history of thrombophlebitis, thrombosis, or thromboembolic disorders associated with previous estrogen use.

OGEN Vaginal Cream is contraindicated in patient's hypersensitive to its ingredients.

WARNINGS

1. *Induction of malignant neoplasms.* Long-term continuous administration of natural and synthetic estrogens in certain animal species has been reported by some investigators to increase the frequency of carcinomas of the breast, cervix, vagina, and liver. There is now evidence that estrogens increase the risk of carcinoma of the endometrium in humans. (See Boxed Warning).

At the present time there is no conclusive evidence that estrogens given to postmenopausal women increase the risk of cancer of the breast.[17,40,41] There are, however, a few retrospective studies which suggest a small but statistically significant increase in the risk factor for breast cancer among these women.[18,42–44] Therefore, caution should be exercised when administering estrogens to women with a strong family history of breast cancer or who have breast nodules, fibrocystic disease, or abnormal mammograms. Careful breast examinations should be performed periodically.

2. *Gallbladder disease.* A recent study has reported a 2 to 3-fold increase in the risk of surgically confirmed gallbladder disease in women receiving postmenopausal estrogens,[17] similar to the 2-fold increase previously noted in users of oral contraceptives.[19,22] In the case of oral contraceptives, the increased risk appeared after two years of use.[22]

3. *Effects similar to those caused by estrogen-progestogen oral contraceptives.* There are several serious adverse effects of oral contraceptives, most of which have not, up to now, been documented as consequences of postmenopausal estrogen therapy. This may reflect the comparatively low doses of estrogen used in postmenopausal women. It would be expected that the larger doses of estrogen used to treat postpartum breast engorgement would be more likely to result in these adverse effects, and, in fact, it has been shown that there is an increased risk of thrombosis in women receiving estrogens for postpartum breast engorgement.[20,21]

a. *Thromboembolic disease.* It is now well established that users of oral contraceptives have an increased risk of various thromboembolic and thrombotic vascular diseases, such as thrombophlebitis, pulmonary embolism, stroke, and myocardial infarction.[22–29] Cases of retinal thrombosis, mesenteric thrombosis, and optic neuritis have been reported in oral contraceptive users. There is evidence that the risk of several of these adverse reactions is related to the dose of the drug.[30,31] An increased risk of post-surgery thromboembolic complications has also been reported in users of oral contraceptives.[32,33] If feasible, estrogen should be discontinued at least 4 weeks before surgery of the type associated with an increased risk of thromboembolism; it should also be discontinued during periods of prolonged immobilization.

While an increased rate of thromboembolic and thrombotic disease in postmenopausal users of estrogens has not been found[17,34] this does not rule out the possibility that such an increase may be present or that subgroups of women who have underlying risk factors or who are receiving relatively large doses of estrogens may have increased risk. Therefore estrogens should not be used in persons with active thrombophlebitis or thromboembolic disorders, and they should not be used in persons with a history of such disorders in association with estrogen use. They should be used with caution in patients with cerebral vascular or coronary artery disease and only for those in whom estrogens are clearly needed.

Large doses of estrogen (5 mg conjugated estrogens per day), comparable to those used to treat cancer of the prostate and breast, have been shown in a large prospective clinical trial in men[35] to increase the risk of nonfatal myocardial infarction, pulmonary embolism and thrombophlebitis. When estrogen doses of this size are used, any of the thromboembolic and thrombotic adverse effects associated with oral contraceptive use should be considered a clear risk.

b. *Hepatic adenoma.* Benign hepatic adenomas appear to be associated with the use of oral contraceptives.[36–38] Although benign, and rare, these may rupture and cause death through intraabdominal hemorrhage. Such lesions have not yet been reported in association with other estrogen or progestogen preparations but should be considered in estrogen users having abdominal pain and tenderness, abdominal mass, or hypovolemic shock. Hepatocellular carcinoma has also been reported in women taking estrogen-containing oral contraceptives.[37] The relationship of this malignancy to these drugs is not known at this time.

c. *Elevated blood pressure.* Increased blood pressure is not uncommon in women using oral contraceptives. There is now a report that this may occur with use of estrogens in the menopause[39] and blood pressure should be monitored with estrogen use, especially if high doses are used.

d. *Glucose tolerance.* A worsening of glucose tolerance has been observed in a significant percentage of patients on estrogen-containing oral contraceptives. For this reason, diabetic patients should be carefully observed while receiving estrogen.

4. *Hypercalcemia.* Administration of estrogens may lead to severe hypercalcemia in patients with breast cancer and bone metastases. If this occurs, the drug should be stopped and appropriate measures taken to reduce the serum calcium level.

PRECAUTIONS

A. General Precautions.

1. A complete medical and family history should be taken prior to the initiation of any estrogen therapy. The pretreatment and periodic physical examinations should include special reference to blood pressure, breasts, abdomen, and pelvic organs, and should include a Papanicolau smear. As a general rule, estrogen should not be prescribed for longer than one year without another physical examination being performed.
2. Diagnostic measures should be taken to rule out gonorrhea or neoplasia before prescribing OGEN Vaginal Cream. Trichomonal, monilial, or bacterial infection should be treated by appropriate anti-microbial therapy.
3. Fluid retention—Estrogens may cause some degree of fluid retention. Therefore, patients with conditions such as epilepsy, migraine, and cardiac or renal dysfunction, which might be influenced by this factor, require careful observation.
4. Certain patients may develop undesirable manifestations of excessive estrogenic stimulation, such as abnormal or excessive uterine bleeding, mastodynia, etc.
5. Oral contraceptives appear to be associated with an increased incidence of mental depression.[22] Although it is not clear whether this is due to the estrogenic or progestogenic component of the contraceptive, patients with a history of depression should be carefully observed.
6. Preexisting uterine leiomyomata may increase in size during estrogen use.
7. The pathologist should be advised of the patient's use of estrogen therapy when relevant specimens are submitted.
8. Patients with a past history of jaundice during pregnancy have an increased risk of recurrence of jaundice while receiving estrogen-containing oral contraceptive therapy. If jaundice develops in any patient receiving estrogen, the medication should be discontinued while the cause is investigated.
9. Estrogens may be poorly metabolized in patients with impaired liver function and they should be administered with caution in such patients.
10. Because estrogens influence the metabolism of calcium and phosphorus, they should be used with caution in patients with metabolic bone diseases that are associated with hypercalcemia or in patients with renal insufficiency.

B. Information for the Patient. See text of Patient Package Insert which appears after PHYSICIAN REFERENCES.

C. Drug Interactions. The concomitant use of any drugs which can induce hepatic microsomal enzymes with estrogens may produce estrogen levels which are lower than would be expected from the dose of estrogen administered.

The use of *broad spectrum antibiotics* which profoundly effect intestinal flora may influence the oral absorption of steroidal compounds including the estrogens.

Diabetics receiving *insulin* may have increased insulin requirements when receiving estrogens.

Laboratory Test Interference. Certain endocrine and liver function tests may be affected by estrogen-containing oral contraceptives. The following similar changes may be expected with larger doses of estrogen:

a. Increased sulfobromophthalein retention.
b. Increased prothrombin and factors VII, VIII, IX, and X; decreased antithrombin 3; increased norepinephrine-induced platelet aggregability.
c. Increased thyroid binding globulin (TBG) leading to increased circulating total thyroid hormone, as measured by PBI, T4 by column, or T4 by radioimmunoassay. Free T3 resin uptake is decreased, reflecting the elevated TBG; free T4 concentration is unaltered.
d. Abnormal glucose tolerance test results.
e. Decreased pregnanediol excretion.
f. Reduced response to metyrapone test.
g. Reduced serum folate concentration.
h. Increased serum triglyceride and phospholipid concentration.

D. Carcinogenesis. Studies have shown an increased risk of endometrial cancer in postmenopausal women exposed to exogenous estrogens for prolonged periods (see Boxed Warning). At the present time there is no conclusive evidence that estrogens given to postmenopausal women increase the risk of cancer of the breast.[17,40,41] There are, however, a few retrospective studies which suggest a small but statistically significant increase in the risk factor for breast cancer among these women.[18,42–44] (See "WARNINGS" section.)

E. Pregnancy. Pregnancy Category X. See "CONTRAINDICATIONS" section and Boxed Warning.

F. Nursing Mothers. Estrogens have been reported to be excreted in human breast milk. Caution should be excercised when OGEN (estropipate) is administered to a nursing woman.

G. Pediatric Use. Because of the effects of estrogens on epiphyseal closure, they should be used judiciously in young patients in whom bone growth is not complete.

ADVERSE REACTIONS

Hypersensitivity reactions, systemic effects such as breast tenderness, and rarely, withdrawal bleeding, have occurred with the use of topical estrogens. Local irritation (especially when prior inflammation is present) has occurred at initiation of therapy.

(See Warnings regarding reports of possible induction of neoplasia, unknown effects upon the fetus, increased incidence of gallbladder disease, and adverse effects similar to those of oral contraceptives, including thromboembolism.)

The following additional adverse reactions in decreasing order of severity within each category have been reported with estrogenic therapy, including oral contraceptives:

1. *Genitourinary system.*
Increase in size of uterine fibromyomata.
Vaginal candidiasis.
Cystitis-like syndrome.
Dysmenorrhea.
Amenorrhea during and after treatment.
Change in cervical eversion and in degree of cervical secretion.
Breakthrough bleeding, spotting, change in menstrual flow.
Premenstrual-like syndrome.

2. *Breast.*
Tenderness, enlargement, secretion.

3. *Gastrointestinal.*
Cholestatic jaundice.
Vomiting, nausea.
Abdominal cramps, bloating.

4. *Skin.*
Hemorrhagic eruption.
Erythema nodosum.
Erythema multiforme.
Hirsutism.
Chloasma or melasma which may persist when drug is discontinued.
Loss of scalp hair.

5. *Eyes.*
Steepening of corneal curvature.
Intolerance to contact lenses.

6. *CNS.*
Chorea.
Mental depression.
Migraine, dizziness, headache.

7. *Miscellaneous.*
Aggravation of porphyria.
Edema.
Reduced carbohydrate tolerance.
Increase or decrease in weight.
Changes in libido.

OVERDOSAGE

Numerous reports of ingestion of large doses of estrogen-containing oral contraceptives by young children indicate that serious ill effects do not occur. Overdosage of estrogen may cause nausea and withdrawal bleeding may occur in females.

DOSAGE AND ADMINISTRATION

OGEN (estropipate) Tablets:

1. *Given cyclically for short-term use:*

For treatment of moderate to severe *vasomotor* symptoms, atrophic vaginitis, or kraurosis vulvae associated with the menopause.

The lowest dose that will control symptoms should be chosen and medication should be discontinued as promptly as possible.

Administration should be cyclic (e.g., 3 weeks on and 1 week off).

Attempts to discontinue or taper medication should be made at 3 to 6 month intervals.

Usual dosage ranges:

Vasomotor symptoms—One OGEN .625 (estropipate) Tablet to one OGEN 5 Tablet per day. The lowest dose that will control symptoms should be chosen. If the patient has not menstruated within the last two months or more, cyclic administration is started arbitrarily. If the patient is menstruating, cyclic administration is started on day 5 of bleeding.

Atrophic vaginitis and kraurosis vulvae—One OGEN .625 Tablet to one OGEN 5 Tablet daily, depending upon the tissue response of the individual patient. The lowest dose that will control symptoms should be chosen. Administer cyclically.

2. *Given cyclically:*

Female hypogonadism; female castration; primary ovarian failure.

Usual dosage ranges:

Female hypogonadism—A daily dose of one OGEN 1.25 Tablet to three OGEN 2.5 Tablets may be given for the first three weeks of a theoretical cycle, followed by a rest period of eight to ten days. The lowest dose that will control symptoms should be chosen. If bleeding does not occur by the end of this period, the same dosage schedule is repeated. The number of courses of estrogen therapy necessary to produce bleeding may vary depending on the responsiveness of the endometrium. If satisfactory withdrawal bleeding does not occur, an oral progestogen may be given in addition to estrogen during the third week of the cycle.

Female castration and primary ovarian failure—A daily dose of one OGEN 1.25 Tablet to three OGEN 2.5 Tablets may be given for the first three weeks of a theoretical cycle, followed by a rest period of eight to ten days. Adjust dosage upward or downward according to severity of symptoms and response of the patient. For maintenance, adjust dosage to lowest level that will provide effective control.

Treated patients with an intact uterus should be monitored closely for signs of endometrial cancer and appropriate diagnostic measures should be taken to rule out malignancy in the event of persistent or recurring abnormal vaginal bleeding.

OGEN (estropipate) Vaginal Cream:

To be administered cyclically for short-term use only:

For treatment of atrophic vaginitis or kraurosis vulvae.

The lowest dose that will control symptoms should be chosen and medication should be discontinued as promptly as possible.

Administration should be cyclic (e.g., three weeks on and one week off).

Attempts to discontinue or taper medication should be made at three to six-month intervals.

Treated patients with an intact uterus should be monitored closely for signs of endometrial cancer and appropriate diagnostic measures should be taken to rule out malignancy in the event of persistent or recurring abnormal vaginal bleeding.

Usual dosage: Intravaginally, 2 to 4 grams of OGEN Vaginal Cream daily, depending upon the severity of the condition.

The following instructions for use are intended for the patient and are printed on the carton label for OGEN Vaginal Cream (estropipate).

1. Remove cap from tube.
2. Make sure plunger of applicator is all the way into the barrel.
3. Screw nozzle end of applicator onto the tube.
4. Squeeze tube to force sufficient cream into applicator so that number on plunger indicating prescribed dose is level with top of barrel.
5. Unscrew applicator from tube and replace cap on tube.
6. To deliver medication, insert end of applicator into vagina and push plunger all the way down.

Between uses, pull plunger out of barrel and wash applicator in warm, soapy water. DO NOT PUT APPLICATOR IN HOT OR BOILING WATER.

HOW SUPPLIED

OGEN (estropipate tablets, USP) is supplied as OGEN .625 (0.75 mg estropipate), yellow tablets, **NDC** 0074-3943-04; OGEN 1.25 (1.5 mg estropipate), peach-colored tablets, **NDC** 0074-3946-04; OGEN 2.5 (3 mg estropipate), blue tablets, **NDC** 0074-3951-04; and OGEN 5 (6 mg estropipate), light green tablets, **NDC** 0074-3958-13. Tablets of all four dosage levels are standardized to provide uniform estrone activity and are grooved (Divide-Tab®) to provide dosage flexibility. All tablet sizes of OGEN are available in bottles of 100.

OGEN (estropipate vaginal cream, USP), 1.5 mg estropipate per gram, is available in packages containing a 1½ oz (42.5 Gm) tube with one plastic applicator calibrated at 1, 2, 3, and 4 Gm levels. (**NDC** 0074-2467-42).

PHYSICIAN REFERENCES

[1]Ziel, H. K., Finkel, W. D., "Increased Risk of Endometrial Carcinoma Among Users of Conjugated Estrogens", *New England-Journal of Medicine*, 293:1167–1170, 1975.

[2]Smith, D. C., Prentic, R., Thompson, D. J., et al., "Association of Exogenous Estrogen and Endometrial Carcinoma," *New England Journal of Medicine*, 293:1164–1167, 1975.

[3]Mack, T. M., Pike, M. C., Henderson, B. E., et al., "Estrogens and Endometrial Cancer in a Retirement Community," *New England Journal of Medicine*, 294:1262–1267, 1976.

[4]Weiss, N. S., Szekely, D. R., Austin, D. F., "Increasing Incidence of Endometrial Cancer in the United States," *New England Journal of Medicine*, 294:1259–1262, 1976.

[5]Herbst, A. L., Ulfelder, H., Poskanzer, D. C., "Adenocarcinoma of Vagina," *New England Journal of Medicine*, 284:878–881, 1971.

[6]Greenwald, P., Barlow, J., Nasca, P., et al., "Vaginal Cancer after Maternal Treatment with Synthetic Estrogens," *New England Journal of Medicine*, 285:390–392, 1971.

[7]Lanier, A., Noller, K., Decker, D., et al., "Cancer and Stilbestrol. A Follow-up of 1719 Persons Exposed to Estrogens In Utero and Born 1943–1959," *Mayo Clinic Proceedings*, 48:793–799, 1973.

[8]Herbst, A., Kurman, R., Scully, R., "Vaginal and Cervical Abnormalities After Exposure to Stilbestrol In Utero" *Obstetrics and Gynecology*, 40:287–298, 1972.

[9]Herbst, A., Robboy, S., Madonald, G., et al., "The Effects of Local Progesterone on Stilbestrol-Associated Vaginal Adenosis," *American Journal of Obstetrics and Gynecology*, 118:607–615, 1974.

[10]Herbst, A., Poskanzer, D., Robboy, S., et al., "Prenatal Exposure to Stilbestrol, A Prospective Comparison of Exposed Female Offspring with Unexposed Controls," *New England Journal of Medicine*, 292:334–339, 1975.

[11]Stafl, A., Mattingly, R., Foley, D., et al., "Clinical Diagnosis of Vaginal Adenosis," *Obstetrics and Gynecology*, 43:118–128, 1974.

[12]Sherman, A. I., Goldrath, M., Berlin, A., et al., "Cervical-Vaginal Adenosis After *In Utero* Exposure to Synthetic Estrogens," *Obstetrics and Gynecology*, 44:531–545, 1974.

[13]Gal, I., Kirman, B., Stern, J., "Hormone Pregnancy Tests and Congenital Malformation," *Nature*, 216:83, 1967.

[14]Levy, E. P., Cohen, A., Fraser, F. C., "Hormone Treatment During Pregnancy and Congenital Heart Defects," *Lancet* 1:611, 1973.

[15]Nora, J., Nora, A., "Birth Defects and Oral Contraceptives," *Lancet*, 1:941–942, 1973.

[16]Janerich, D. T., Piper, J. M., Clebatis, D. M., "Oral Contraceptives and Congenital Limb-Reduction Defects," *New England Journal of Medicine*, 291:697–700, 1974.

[17]Boston Collaborative Drug Surveillance Program "Surgically Confirmed Gall Bladder Disease, Venous Thromboembolism and Breast Tumors in Relation to Post-Menopausal Estrogen Therapy," *New England Journal of Medicine*, 290:15–19, 1974.

[18]Brinton, L. A., Hoover, R. N., Szklo, M., et al., "Menopausal Estrogen Use and Risk of Breast Cancer," *Cancer*, 47(10): 2517–2522, 1981.

[19]Boston Collaborative Drug Surveillance Program, "Oral Contraceptives and Venous Thromboembolic Disease, Surgically Confirmed Gall Bladder Disease and Breast Tumors," *Lancet* 1:1399–1404, 1973.

[20]Daniel, D. G., Campbell, H., Turnbull, A. C., "Puerperal Thromboembolism and Suppression of Lactation," *Lancet*, 2:287–289, 1967.

[21]Bailar, J. C., "Thromboembolism and Oestrogen Therapy," *Lancet*, 2:560, 1967.

[22]Royal College of General Practitioners, "Oral Contraception and Thromboembolic Disease," *Journal of the Royal College of General Practitioners*, 13:267–279, 1967.

[23]Inman, W. H. W., Vessey, M. P., "Investigation of Deaths from Pulmonary, Coronary, and Cerebral Thrombosis and Embolism in Women of Child-Bearing Age," *British Medical Journal*, 2:193–199, 1968.

[24]Vessey, M. P., Doll, R., "Investigation of Relation Between Use of Oral Contraceptives and Thromboembolic Disease. A Further Report," *British Medical Journal*, 2:651–657, 1969.

[25]Sartwell, P. E., Masi, A. T., Arthes, F. G., et al., "Thromboembolism and Oral Contraceptives: An Epidemiological Case Control Study," *American Journal of Epidemiology*, 90:365–380, 1969.

[26]Collaborative Group for the Study of Stroke in Young Women, "Oral Contraception and Increased Risk of Cerebral Ischemia or Thrombosis," *New England Journal of Medicine*, 288:871–878, 1973.

[27]Collaborative Group for the Study of Stroke in Young Women, "Oral Contraceptives and Stroke in Young Women: Associated Risk Factors," *Journal of the American Medical Association*, 231:718–722, 1975.

[28]Mann, J. I., Inman, W. H. W., "Oral Contraceptives and Death from Myocardial Infarction," *British Medical Journal*, 2:245–248, 1975.

[29]Mann, J. I., Vessey, M. P., Thorogood, M., et al., "Myocardial Infarction in Young Women with Special Reference to Oral Contraceptive Practice," *British Medical Journal*, 2:241–245, 1975.

[30]Inman, W. H. W., Vessey, M. P., Westerholm, B., et al., "Thromboembolic Disease and the Steroidal Content of Oral Contraceptives," *British Medical Journal*, 2:203–209, 1970.

[31]Stolley, P. D., Tonascia, J. A., Tockman, M. S., et al., "Thrombosis with Low-Estrogen Oral Contraceptives," *American Journal of Epidemiology*, 102:197–208, 1975.

[32]Vessey, M. P., Doll, R., Fairbairn, A. S., et al., "Post-Operative Thromboembolism and the Use of the Oral Contraceptives," *British Medical Journal*, 3:123–126, 1970.

[33]Greene, G. R., Sartwell, P. E., "Oral Contraceptive Use in Patients with Thromboembolism Following Surgery, Trauma or Infection," *American Journal of Public Health*, 62:680–685, 1972.

[34]Rosenberg, L., Armstrong, M. B., Jick, H., "Myocardial Infarction and Estrogen Therapy in Postmenopausal Women," *New England Journal of Medicine*, 294:1256–1259, 1976.

[35]Coronary Drug Project Research Group, "The Coronary Drug Project: Initial Findings Leading to Modifications of Its Research Protocol," *Journal of the American Medical Association*, 214:1303–1313, 1970.

[36]Baum, J., Holtz, F., Bookstein, J. J., et al., "Possible Association Between Benign Hepatomas and Oral Contraceptives," *Lancet*, 2:926–928, 1973.

[37]Mays, E. T., Christopherson, W. M., Mahr, M. M., et al., "Hepatic Changes in Young Women Ingesting Contraceptive Steroids, Hepatic Hemorrhage and Primary Hepatic Tumors," *Journal of the American Medical Association*, 235:730–782, 1976.

[38]Edmondson, H. A., Henderson, B., Benton, B., "Liver Cell Adenomas Associated with the Use of Oral Contraceptives," *New England Journal of Medicine*, 294:470–472, 1976.

[39]Pfeffer, R. I., Van Den Noort, S., "Estrogen Use and Stroke Risk in Postmenopausal Women," *American Journal of Epidemiology*, 103:445–456, 1976.

[40]Gambrell, R. D., Massey, F. M., Castaneda, T. A., et al., "Estrogen Therapy and Breast Cancer in Postmenopausal Women," *Journal of the American Geriatrics Society*, 28(6): 251–257, 1980.

[41]Kelsey, J. L., Fischer, D. B., Holford, T. R., et al., "Exogenous Estrogens and Other Factors in the Epidemiology of Breast Cancer," *Journal of the National Cancer Institute*, 57(2):327–333, 1981.

[42]Ross, R. K., Paganini-Hill, A., Gerkins, V., et al., "A Case-Control Study of Menopausal Estrogen Therapy and Breast Cancer," *Journal of the American Medical Association*, 243(16):1635–1639, 1980.

[43]Hoover, R., Glass, A., Finkle, W. D., et al., "Conjugated Estrogens and Breast Cancer Risk in Women," *Journal of the National Cancer Institute*, 67(4):815–820, 1981.

[44]Lawson, D. H., Jick, H., Hunter, J. R., et al., "Exogenous Estrogens and Breast Cancer," *American Journal of Epidemiology*, 114(5):710, 1981.

INFORMATION FOR PATIENTS
OGEN®

(estropipate tablets and vaginal cream, USP)

Estrogen cream is used for the local treatment of certain symptoms of estrogen deficiency: the soreness and itching of the vagina and vulva caused by drying and thinning (atrophy) of these tissues.

The discussion that follows is about estrogens that are taken internally for the treatment of symptoms of estrogen deficiency. Some or all of the information below on the systemic use of estrogens may also apply to the estrogen cream.

WHAT YOU SHOULD KNOW ABOUT ESTROGENS: Estrogens are female hormones produced by the ovaries. The ovaries make several different kinds of estrogens. In addition, scientists have been able to make a variety of synthetic estrogens. As far as we know, all these estrogens have similar properties and therefore much the same usefulness, side effects, and risks. This leaflet is intended to help you understand what estrogens are used for, the risks involved in their use, and how to use them as safely as possible.

This leaflet includes the most important information about estrogens, but not all the information. If you want to know more, you can ask your doctor or pharmacist to let you read the package insert prepared for the doctor.

Uses of Estrogen: Estrogens are prescribed by doctors for a number of purposes, including:

1. To provide estrogen during a period of adjustment when a women's ovaries no longer produce it, in order to prevent certain uncomfortable symptoms of estrogen deficiency. (All

Continued on next page

Abbott—Cont.

women normally stop producing estrogens, generally between the ages of 45 and 55; this is called the menopause.)
2. To prevent symptoms of estrogen deficiency when a woman's ovaries have been removed surgically before the natural menopause.
3. To prevent pregnancy. (Estrogens are given along with a progestogen, another female hormone; these combinations are called oral contraceptives or birth control pills. Patient labeling is available to women taking oral contraceptives and they will not be discussed in this leaflet.)

THERE IS NO PROPER USE OF OGEN (ESTROPIPATE) IN A PREGNANT WOMAN.

Estrogens in the Menopause: In the natural course of their lives, all women eventually experience a decrease in estrogen production. This usually occurs between ages 45 and 55 but may occur earlier or later. Sometimes the ovaries may need to be removed before natural menopause by an operation, producing a "surgical menopause."

When the amount of estrogen in the blood begins to decrease, many women may develop typical symptoms: Feelings of warmth in the face, neck, and chest or sudden intense episodes of heat and sweating throughout the body (called "hot flashes" or "hot flushes"). These symptoms are sometimes very uncomfortable. A few women eventually develop changes in the vagina (called "atrophic vaginitis") which cause discomfort, especially during and after intercourse.

Estrogens can be prescribed to treat these symptoms of the menopause. It is estimated that considerably more than half of all women undergoing the menopause have only mild symptoms or no symptoms at all and therefore do not need estrogens. Other women may need estrogens for a few months, while their bodies adjust to lower estrogen levels. Sometimes the need will be for periods longer than six months. In an attempt to avoid over-stimulation of the uterus (womb), estrogens are usually given cyclically during each month of use, that is three weeks of pills followed by one week without pills.

Sometimes women experience nervous symptoms or depression during menopause. There is no evidence that estrogens are effective for such symptoms and they should not be used to treat them, although other treatment may be needed.

You may have heard that taking estrogens for long periods (years) after the menopause will keep your skin soft and supple and keep you feeling young. There is no evidence that this is so, however, and such long-term treatment carries important risks.

The Dangers of Estrogens: 1. *Cancer of the uterus.* If estrogens are used in the postmenopausal period for more than a year, there is an increased risk of *endometrial cancer* (cancer of the uterus). Women taking estrogens have roughly 5 to 10 times as great a chance of getting this cancer as women who take no estrogens. To put this another way, while a postmenopausal woman not taking estrogens has 1 chance in 1,000 each year of getting cancer of the uterus, a woman taking estrogens has 5 to 10 chances in 1,000 each year. For this reason *it is important to take estrogens only when you really need them.*

The risk of this cancer is greater the longer estrogens are used and also seems to be greater when larger doses are taken. For this reason *it is important to take the lowest dose of estrogen that will control symptoms and to take it only as long as it is needed.* If estrogens are needed for longer periods of time, your doctor will want to reevaluate your need for estrogens at least every six months.

Women using estrogens should report any irregular vaginal bleeding to their doctors; such bleeding may be of no importance, but it can be an early warning of cancer of the uterus. If you have undiagnosed vaginal bleeding, you should not use estrogens until a diagnosis is made and you are certain there is no cancer of the uterus.

If you have had your uterus completely removed (total hysterectomy), there is no danger of developing cancer of the uterus.

2. *Other possible cancers.* Estrogens can cause development of other tumors in animals, such as tumors of the breast, cervix, vagina, or liver, when given for a long time. At present there is no good evidence that women using estrogen in the menopause have an increased risk of such tumors, but there is no way yet to be sure they do not; and one study raises the possibility that use of estrogens in the menopause may increase the risk of breast cancer many years later. This is a further reason to use estrogens only when clearly needed. While you are taking estrogens, it is important that you go to your doctor at least once a year for a physical examination. Also, if members of your family have had breast cancer or if you have breast nodules or abnormal mammograms (breast x-rays), your doctor may wish to carry out more frequent examinations of your breasts.

3. *Gallbladder disease.* Women who use estrogens after menopause are more likely to develop gallbladder disease needing surgery than women who do not use estrogens. Birth control pills have a similar effect.

4. *Abnormal blood clotting.* Oral contraceptives increase the risk of blood clotting in various parts of the body. This can result in a stroke (if the clot is in the brain), a heart attack (clot in a blood vessel of the heart), or a pulmonary embolus (a clot which forms in the legs or pelvis, then breaks off and travels to the lungs). Any of these can be fatal.

At this time use of estrogens in the menopause is not known to cause such blood clotting, but this has not been fully studied and there could still prove to be such a risk. It is recommended that if you have had clotting in the legs or lungs or a heart attack or stroke while you were using estrogens or birth control pills, you should not use estrogens. If you have had a stroke or heart attack or if you have angina pectoris, estrogens should be used with great caution and only if clearly needed (for example, if you have severe symptoms of the menopause).

Special Warning About Pregnancy: You should not receive OGEN (estropipate) if you are pregnant. Some scientists have reported that if estrogens are used during pregnancy, there may be a greater than usual chance that the developing baby will be born with a birth defect, although the risk remains small. In addition, other scientists have reported that there is an association between another estrogen-type product (diethylstilbestrol) and appearance of a particular cancer of the vagina or cervix (adenocarcinoma) in young women whose mothers took that drug in pregnancy. Every effort should be made to avoid exposure to OGEN in pregnancy. If exposure occurs, see your doctor.

Other Effects of Estrogens: In addition to the serious known risks of estrogens described above estrogens have the following side effects and potential risks:

1. *Nausea and vomiting.* The most common side effect of estrogen therapy is nausea. Vomiting is less common.
2. *Effects on breasts.* Estrogens may cause breast tenderness or enlargement and may cause the breasts to secrete a liquid. These effects are not dangerous.
3. *Effects on the uterus.* Estrogens may cause benign fibroid tumors of the uterus to get larger.

Some women will have menstrual bleeding when estrogens are stopped. But if the bleeding occurs on days you are still taking estrogens you should report this to your doctor.

4. *Effects on liver.* Women taking oral contraceptives develop on rare occasions a tumor of the liver which can rupture and bleed into the abdomen. So far, these tumors have not been reported in women using estrogens in the menopause, but you should report any swelling or unusual pain or tenderness in the abdomen to your doctor immediately.

Women with a past history of jaundice (yellowing of the skin and white parts of the eyes) may get jaundice again during estrogen use. If this occurs, stop taking estrogens and see your doctor.

5. *Other effects.* Estrogens may cause excess fluid to be retained in the body. This may make some conditions worse, such as epilepsy, migraine, heart disease, or kidney disease.

SUMMARY

Estrogens have important uses, but they have serious risks as well. You must decide, with your doctor, whether the risks are acceptable to you in view of the benefits of treatment. You should not use OGEN (estropipate) if you have cancer of the breast or uterus, are pregnant, have undiagnosed abnormal vaginal bleeding, clotting in the legs or lungs, or have had a stroke, heart attack or angina, or clotting in the legs or lungs in the past while you were taking estrogens.

You can use estrogens as safely as possible by understanding that your doctor will require regular physical examinations while you are taking them and will try to discontinue the drug as soon as possible and use the smallest dose possible. Be alert for signs of trouble including:

1 Abnormal bleeding from the vagina.
2. Pains in the calves or chest or sudden shortness of breath, or coughing blood (indicating possible clots in the legs, heart or lungs).
3. Severe headache, dizziness, faintness, or changes in vision (indicating possible developing clots in the brain or eye).
4. Breast lumps (you should ask your doctor how to examine your own breasts).
5. Jaundice (yellowing of the skin).
6. Mental depression.

Based on his or her assessment of your medical needs, your doctor has prescribed this drug for you. Do not give the drug to anyone else.

Shown in Product Identifictaion Section, page 403

Abbott Laboratories/
Abbott Pharmaceuticals, Inc.
North Chicago, IL 60064

OPTILETS®-500
[*ōp 'ti-lets*]
High potency multivitamin for use in treatment of multivitamin deficiency.

OPTILETS-M-500®
High potency multivitamin for use in treatment of multivitamin deficiency. Mineral supplementation added.

(See PDR For Nonprescription Drugs)
Shown in Product Identification Section, page 403

ORETIC® ℞
[*ō-re 'tic*]
(hydrochlorothiazide tablets, USP)

DESCRIPTION

ORETIC (hydrochlorothiazide) is a member of the benzothiadiazine (thiazide) family of drugs. It is closely related to chlorothiazide. Clinically, ORETIC is an orally active diuretic-antihypertensive agent.

INACTIVE INGREDIENTS

25 and 50 mg tablets: corn starch, lactose, magnesium stearate, talc and other ingredients.

ACTIONS

The diuretic and saluretic effects of ORETIC result from a drug-induced inhibition of the renal tubular reabsorption of electrolytes. The excretion of sodium and chloride is greatly enhanced. Potassium excretion is also enhanced to a variable degree, as it is with the other thiazides. Although urinary excretion of bicarbonate is increased slightly, there is usually no significant change in urinary pH. Hydrochlorothiazide has a per mg natriuretic activity approximately 10 times that of the prototype thiazide, chlorothiazide. At maximal therapeutic dosages, all thiazides are approximately equal in their diuretic/natriuretic effects.

There is significant natriuresis and diuresis within two hours after administration of a single oral dose of hydrochlorothiazide. These effects reach a peak in about six hours and persist for about 12 hours following oral administration of a single dose.

Like other benzothiadiazines, ORETIC also has antihypertensive properties, and may be used for this purpose either alone or to enhance the antihypertensive action of other drugs. The mechanism by which the benzothiadiazines, including hydrochlorothiazide, produce a reduction of elevated blood pressure is not known. However, sodium depletion appears to be involved.

ORETIC (hydrochlorothiazide) is readily absorbed from the gastrointestinal tract and is excreted unchanged by the kidneys.

INDICATIONS

ORETIC is indicated in the management of hypertension either as the sole therapeutic agent or to enhance the effect of other antihypertensive drugs in the more severe forms of hypertension.

ORETIC is indicated as adjunctive therapy in edema associated with congestive heart failure, hepatic cirrhosis, and corticosteroid and estrogen therapy.

ORETIC has also been found useful in edema due to various forms of renal dysfunction such as the nephrotic syndrome, acute glomerulonephritis and chronic renal failure.

Usage in Pregnancy: The routine use of diuretics in an otherwise healthy pregnant woman is inappropriate and exposes mother and fetus to unnecessary hazard. Diuretics do not prevent development of toxemia of pregnancy, and there is no satisfactory evidence that they are useful in the treatment of developed toxemia.

Edema during pregnancy may arise from pathological causes or from the physiological and mechanical consequences of pregnancy. Thiazides are indicated in pregnancy when edema is due to pathological causes, just as they are in the absence of pregnancy (however, see Warnings, below). Dependent edema in pregnancy, resulting from restriction of venous return by the expanded uterus, is properly treated through elevation of the lower extremities and use of support hose; use of diuretics to lower intravascular volume in this case is illogical and unnecessary. There is hypervolemia during normal pregnancy which is harmful to neither the fetus nor the mother (in the absence of cardiovascular disease), but which is associated with edema, including generalized edema, in the majority of pregnant women. If this edema produces discomfort, increased recumbency will often provide relief. In rare instances, this edema may cause extreme discomfort which is not relieved by rest. In these cases, a short course of diuretics may provide relief and may be appropriate.

CONTRAINDICATIONS

Renal decompensation.
Hypersensitivity to this or other sulfonamide-derived drugs.

WARNINGS

Hydrochlorothiazide shares with other thiazides the propensity to deplete potassium reserves to an unpredictable degree.
Thiazides should be used with caution in patients with renal disease or significant impairment of renal function, since azotemia may be precipitated and cumulative drug effects may occur.
Thiazides should be used with caution in patients with impaired hepatic function or progressive liver disease, since minor alterations of fluid and electrolyte balance may precipitate hepatic coma.
Thiazides may be additive or potentiative of the action of other antihypertensive drugs. Potentiation occurs with ganglionic or peripheral adrenergic blocking drugs.
Sensitivity reactions may occur in patients with a history of allergy or bronchial asthma.
The possibility of exacerbation or activation of systemic lupus erythematosus has been reported.
Usage in Pregnancy: Thiazides cross the placental barrier and appear in cord blood. The use of thiazides in pregnant women requires that the anticipated benefit be weighed against possible hazards to the fetus. These hazards include fetal or neonatal jaundice, thrombocytopenia, and possible other adverse reactions that have occurred in the adult.
Nursing Mothers: Thiazides appear in breast milk. If use of the drug is deemed essential, the patient should stop nursing.

PRECAUTIONS

Periodic determinations of serum electrolytes should be performed at appropriate intervals for the purpose of detecting possible electrolyte imbalances such as hyponatremia, hypochloremic alkalosis, and hypokalemia. Serum and urine electrolyte determinations are particularly important when a patient is vomiting excessively or receiving parenteral fluids. All patients should be observed for other clinical signs of electrolyte imbalances such as dryness of mouth, thirst, weakness, lethargy, drowsiness, restlessness, muscle pains or cramps, muscular fatigue, hypotension, oliguria, tachycardia, and gastrointestinal disturbances such as nausea and vomiting.
Hypokalemia may develop with thiazides as with any other potent diuretic, especially when brisk diuresis occurs, severe cirrhosis is present, or when corticosteroids or ACTH are given concomitantly. Interference with the adequate oral intake of electrolytes will also contribute to the possible development of hypokalemia. Potassium depletion, even of a mild degree, resulting from thiazide use, may sensitize a patient to the effects of cardiac glycosides such as digitalis.
Any chloride deficit is generally mild and usually does not require specific treatment except under extraordinary circumstances (as in liver disease or renal disease). Dilutional hyponatremia may occur in edematous patients in hot weather; appropriate therapy is water restriction rather than administration of salt, except in rare instances when the hyponatremia is life threatening.
In actual salt depletion, appropriate replacement is the therapy of choice.
Hyperuricemia may occur or frank gout may be precipitated in certain patients receiving thiazide therapy.
Insulin requirements in diabetic patients may be increased, decreased, or unchanged. Latent diabetes mellitus may become manifest during thiazide administration.
Thiazide drugs may increase the responsiveness to tubocurarine.
The antihypertensive effects of the drug may be enhanced in the postsympathectomy patient.
Thiazides may decrease arterial responsiveness to norepinephrine. This diminution is not sufficient to preclude effectiveness of the pressor agent for therapeutic use.
If progressive renal impairment becomes evident as indicated by a rising-nonprotein nitrogen or blood urea nitrogen, a careful reappraisal of therapy is necessary with consideration given to withholding or discontinuing diuretic therapy.
Thiazides may decrease serum PBI levels without signs of thyroid disturbance.
Thiazides have been reported, on rare occasions, to have elevated serum calcium to hypercalcemic levels. The serum calcium levels have returned to normal when the medication has been stopped. This phenomenon may be related to the ability of the thiazide diuretics to lower the amount of calcium excreted in the urine.

ADVERSE REACTIONS

Gastrointestinal system reactions: Anorexia, gastric irritation, nausea, vomiting, cramping, diarrhea, constipation, jaundice (intrahepatic cholestatic jaundice), pancreatitis.
Central nervous system reactions: Dizziness, vertigo, paresthesias, headache, xanthopsia.
Hematologic reactions: Leukopenia, agranulocytosis, thrombocytopenia, aplastic anemia.
Dermatologic — hypersensitivity reactions: Purpura, photosensitivity, rash, urticaria, necrotizing angiitis (vasculitis) (cutaneous vasculitis).
Cardiovascular reaction: Orthostatic hypotension may occur and may be aggravated by alcohol, barbiturates, or narcotics.
Other: Hyperglycemia, glycosuria, hypercalcemia, hyperuricemia, muscle spasm, weakness, restlessness.
There have been isolated reports that certain nonedematous individuals developed severe fluid and electrolyte derangements after only brief exposure to normal doses of thiazide and non-thiazide diuretics. The condition is usually manifested as severe dilutional hyponatremia, hypokalemia, and hypochloremia. It has been reported to be due to inappropriately increased ADH secretion and appears to be idiosyncratic. Potassium replacement is apparently the most important therapy in the treatment of this syndrome along with removal of the offending drug.
Whenever adverse reactions are severe, treatment should be discontinued.

DOSAGE AND ADMINISTRATION

ORETIC (hydrochlorothiazide) is administered orally. Therapy should be individualized according to patient response. This therapy should be titrated to gain maximal therapeutic response as well as the minimal dose possible to maintain that therapeutic response.
For the management of edema the adult dosage ranges from 25 to 200 mg daily and may be given in single or divided doses. Usually 75 to 100 mg will produce the desired diuretic effect.
For the management of hypertension the usual initial adult dosage is 25 to 50 mg two times daily. The dosage may be increased if necessary to a maximum of 100 mg twice daily.
When therapy is prolonged or large doses are used, particular attention should be given to the patient's electrolyte status. Supplemental potassium may be required.
In the treatment of hypertension hydrochlorothiazide may be either employed alone or concurrently with other antihypertensive drugs. Combined therapy may provide adequate control of hypertension with lower dosage of the component drugs and fewer or less severe side effects. An enhanced response frequently follows its concurrent administration with Harmonyl® (deserpidine) so that dosage of both drugs may be reduced.
For treatment of moderately severe or severe hypertension, supplemental use of other more potent antihypertensive agents such as Eutonyl® (pargyline hydrochloride) may be indicated.
When other antihypertensive agents are to be added to the regimen, this should be accomplished gradually. Additional potent antihypertensive agents should be given at only half the usual dose since their effect is potentiated by pretreatment with ORETIC.

OVERDOSAGE

Symptoms of overdosage include electrolyte imbalance and signs of potassium deficiency such as confusion, dizziness, muscular weakness, and gastrointestinal disturbances. General supportive measures including replacement of fluids and electrolytes may be indicated in treatment of overdosage.

HOW SUPPLIED

ORETIC (hydrochlorothiazide tablets, USP) is provided in two dosage sizes as white tablets:
25 mg tablets:
bottles of 100 (**NDC** 0074-6978-01),
bottles of 1000 (**NDC** 0074-6978-02),
Abbo-Pac® unit dose packages, 100 tablets (**NDC** 0074-6978-05).
50 mg tablets:
bottles of 100 (**NDC** 0074-6985-01),
bottles of 1000 (**NDC** 0074-6985-02),
Abbo-Pac unit dose packages, 100 tablets (**NDC** 0074-6985-06).
Shown in Product Identification Section, page 403
Abbott Laboratories
North Chicago, IL 60064
Ref. 01-2362-R4

ORETICYL® ℞
[ō-re'ti-sill]
(hydrochlorothiazide and deserpidine tablets)

Oral thiazide-rauwolfia therapy for hypertension.

WARNING

This fixed combination drug is not indicated for initial therapy of hypertension. Hypertension requires therapy titrated to the individual patient. If the fixed combination represents the dosage so determined, its use may be more convenient in patient management. The treatment of hypertension is not static, but must be reevaluated as conditions in each patient warrant.

DESCRIPTION

ORETICYL is an orally administered combination of Oretic® (hydrochlorothiazide) and Harmonyl® (deserpidine). Hydrochlorothiazide is a diuretic-antihypertensive agent of the benzothiadiazine (thiazide) class. Deserpidine is a purified rauwolfia alkaloid, chemically identified as 11-desmethoxyreserpine, which produces antihypertensive effects.

INACTIVE INGREDIENTS

Oreticyl 25 and Oreticyl 50 tablets: corn starch, lactose, magnesium stearate, red ferric oxide, talc and other ingredients.
Oreticyl Forte tablets: corn starch, iron oxide, lactose, magnesium stearate, talc and other ingredients.

ACTIONS

The combined antihypertensive actions of hydrochlorothiazide and deserpidine result in a total clinical antihypertensive effect which is greater than can ordinarily be achieved by either drug given individually.
The diuretic and saluretic effects of hydrochlorothiazide result from a drug-induced inhibition of the renal tubular reabsorption of electrolytes. The excretion of sodium and chloride is greatly enhanced. Potassium excretion is also enhanced to a variable degree, as it is with the other thiazides. Although urinary excretion of bicarbonate is increased slightly, there is usually no significant change in urinary pH. Hydrochlorothiazide has a per mg natriuretic activity approximately 10 times that of the prototype thiazide, chlorothiazide. At maximal therapeutic dosages, all thiazides are approximately equal in their diuretic/natriuretic effects.
There is significant natriuresis and diuresis within two hours after administration of a single oral dose of hydrochlorothiazide. These effects reach a peak in about six hours and persist for about 12 hours following oral administration of a single dose.
Like other benzothiadiazines, hydrochlorothiazide also has antihypertensive properties, and may be used for this purpose either alone or to enhance the antihypertensive action of other drugs. The mechanism by which the benzothiadiazines, including hydrochlorothiazide, produce a reduction of elevated blood pressure is not known. However, sodium depletion appears to be involved.
Hydrochlorothiazide is readily absorbed from the gastrointestinal tract and is excreted unchanged by the kidneys.
The pharmacologic actions of Harmonyl (deserpidine) are essentially the same as those of other active rauwolfia alkaloids. Deserpidine probably produces its antihypertensive effects through depletion of tissue stores of catecholamines (epinephrine and norepinephrine) from peripheral sites. The antihypertensive effect is often accompanied by bradycardia. There is no significant alteration in cardiac output or renal blood flow. The carotid sinus reflex is inhibited, but postural hypotension is rarely seen with the use of conventional doses of Harmonyl alone.
Deserpidine, like other rauwolfia alkaloids, is characterized by slow onset of action and sustained effect which may persist following withdrawal of the drug.

INDICATIONS

ORETICYL (hydrochlorothiazide and deserpidine) is indicated in the treatment of patients with mild to moderately severe hypertension (see boxed warning). It may be used alone for this purpose or added to other antihypertensive agents for the management of more severe hypertension. When administered with ORETICYL, more potent agents can be given at reduced dosage to minimize undesirable side effects.

CONTRAINDICATIONS

Hydrochlorothiazide is contraindicated in patients with renal decompensation and in those who are hypersensitive to this or other sulfonamide-derived drugs.
Deserpidine is contraindicated in patients with known hypersensitivity, mental depression especially with suicidal tendencies, active peptic ulcer, and ulcerative colitis. It is also contraindicated in patients receiving electroconvulsive therapy.

WARNINGS

Hydrochlorothiazide
Hydrochlorothiazide shares with other thiazides the propensity to deplete potassium reserves to an unpredictable degree.
Thiazides should be used with caution in patients with renal disease or significant impairment of renal function, since azotemia may be precipitated and cumulative drug effects may occur.
Thiazides should be used with caution in patients with impaired hepatic function or progressive liver disease, since

Continued on next page

Abbott—Cont.

minor alterations of fluid and electrolyte balance may precipitate hepatic coma.
Thiazides may be additive or potentiative of the action of other antihypertensive drugs. Potentiation occurs with ganglionic or peripheral adrenergic blocking drugs.
Sensitivity reactions may occur in patients with a history of allergy or bronchial asthma.
The possibility of exacerbation or activation of systemic lupus erythematosus has been reported.
Deserpidine
Extreme caution should be exercised in treating patients with a history of mental depression. Discontinue the drug at the first sign, of despondency, early morning insomnia, loss of appetite, impotence, or self-deprecation. Drug-induced depression may persist for several months after drug withdrawal and may be severe enough to result in suicide.
Usage in Pregnancy and Lactation:
Hydrochlorothiazide
Thiazides cross the placental barrier and appear in cord blood. The use of thiazides in pregnant women requires that the anticipated benefit be weighed against possible hazards to the fetus. These hazards include fetal or neonatal jaundice, thrombocytopenia, and possible other adverse reactions that have occurred in the adult.
Thiazides appear in breast milk. If use of the drug is deemed essential, the patient should stop nursing.
Deserpidine
The safety of deserpidine for use during pregnancy or lactation has not been established; therefore, it should be used in pregnant women or in women of childbearing potential only when in the judgment of the physician its use is deemed essential to the welfare of the patient. Increased respiratory secretions, nasal congestion, cyanosis, and anorexia may occur in infants born to rauwolfia alkaloid-treated mothers, since these preparations are known to cross the placental barrier to enter the fetal circulation and appear in cord blood. They also are secreted by nursing mothers into breast milk.
Reproductive and teratology studies in rats reduced the mating index and neonatal survival indices. The no-effect dosage has not been established.

PRECAUTIONS

Periodic determinations of serum electrolytes should be performed at appropriate intervals for the purpose of detecting possible electrolyte imbalances such as hyponatremia, hypochloremic alkalosis, and hypokalemia. Serum and urine electrolyte determinations are particularly important when a patient is vomiting excessively or receiving parenteral fluids. All patients should be observed for other clinical signs of electrolyte imbalances such as dryness of mouth, thirst, weakness, lethargy, drowsiness, restlessness, muscle pains or cramps, muscular fatigue, hypotension, oliguria, tachycardia, and gastrointestinal disturbances such as nausea and vomiting.
Hypokalemia may develop with thiazides as with any other potent diuretic, especially when brisk diuresis occurs, severe cirrhosis is present, or when corticosteroids or ACTH are given concomitantly. Interference with the adequate oral intake of electrolytes will also contribute to the possible development of hypokalemia. Potassium depletion, even of a mild degree, resulting from thiazide use, may sensitize a patient to the effects of cardiac glycosides such as digitalis.
Any chloride deficit is generally mild and usually does not require specific treatment except under extraordinary circumstances (as in liver disease or renal disease). Dilutional hyponatremia may occur in edematous patients in hot weather; appropriate therapy is water restriction rather than administration of salt, except in rare instances when the hyponatremia is life threatening.
In actual salt depletion, appropriate replacement is the therapy of choice.
Hyperuricemia may occur or frank gout may be precipitated in certain patients receiving thiazide therapy.
Insulin requirements in diabetic patients may be increased, decreased, or unchanged. Latent diabetes mellitus may become manifest during thiazide administration.
Thiazide drugs may increase the responsiveness to tubocurarine.
The antihypertensive effects of the drug may be enhanced in the postsympathectomy patient.
Thiazides may decrease arterial responsiveness to norepinephrine. This diminution is not sufficient to preclude effectiveness of the pressor agent for therapeutic use.
If progressive renal impairment becomes evident as indicated by a rising-nonprotein nitrogen or blood urea nitrogen, a careful reappraisal of therapy is necessary with consideration given to withholding or discontinuing diuretic therapy.
Thiazides may decrease serum PBI levels without signs of thyroid disturbance.
Thiazides have been reported, on rare occasions, to have elevated serum calcium to hypercalcemic levels. The serum calcium levels have returned to normal when the medication has been stopped. This phenomenon may be related to the ability of the thiazide diuretics to lower the amount of calcium excreted in the urine.
Because rauwolfia preparations increase gastrointestinal motility and secretion, this drug should be used cautiously in patients with a history of peptic ulcer, ulcerative colitis, or gallstones, where biliary colic may be precipitated.
Caution should be exercised when treating hypertensive patients with renal insufficiency since they adjust poorly to lowered blood pressure levels.
Use deserpidine cautiously with digitalis and quinidine since cardiac arrhythmias have occurred with rauwolfia preparations.
Preoperative withdrawal of deserpidine does not assure that circulatory instability will not occur. It is important that the anesthesiologist be aware of the patient's drug intake and consider this in the overall management, since hypotension has occurred in patients receiving rauwolfia preparations. Anticholinergic and/ or adrenergic drugs (metaraminol, norepinephrine) have been employed to treat adverse vagocirculatory effects.
Animal tumorigenicity: There are no studies demonstrating that deserpidine is an animal tumorigen, although it is a prolactin stimulator and structurally related to reserpine. Rodent studies with reserpine, however, have shown that reserpine is an animal tumorigen, causing an increased incidence of mammary fibroadenomas in female mice, malignant tumors of the seminal vesicles in male mice, and malignant adrenal medullary tumors in male rats. These findings arose in 2 year studies in which the drug was administered in the feed at concentrations of 5 and 10 ppm—about 100 to 300 times the usual human dose. The breast neoplasms are thought to be related to reserpine's prolactin-elevating effect. Several other prolactin-elevating drugs have also been associated with an increased incidence of mammary neoplasia in rodents.
The extent to which these findings indicate a risk to humans is uncertain. Tissue culture experiments show that about one-third of human breast tumors are prolactin-dependent *in vitro*, a factor of considerable importance if the use of the drug is contemplated in a patient with previously detected breast cancer. The possibility of an increased risk of breast cancer in reserpine users has been studied extensively; however, no firm conclusion has emerged. Although a few epidemiologic studies have suggested a slightly increased risk (less than twofold in all studies except one) in women who have used reserpine, other studies of generally similar design have not confirmed this. Epidemiologic studies conducted using other drugs (neuroleptic agents) that, like reserpine, increase prolactin levels and, therefore, would be considered rodent mammary carcinogens, have not shown an association between chronic administration of the drug and human mammary tumorigenesis. While long-term clinical observation has not suggested such an association, the available evidence is considered too limited to be conclusive at this time. An association of reserpine intake with pheochromocytoma or tumors of the seminal vesicles has not been explored.

ADVERSE REACTIONS

Hydrochlorothiazide
Gastrointestinal System Reactions: Anorexia, gastric irritation, nausea, vomiting, cramping, diarrhea, constipation, jaundice (intrahepatic cholestatic jaundice), pancreatitis.
Central Nervous System Reactions: Dizziness, vertigo, paresthesias, headache, xanthopsia.
Hematologic Reactions: Leukopenia, agranulocytosis, thrombocytopenia, aplastic anemia.
Dermatologic — Hypersensitivity Reactions: Purpura, photosensitivity, rash, urticaria, necrotizing angitis (vasculitis) (cutaneous vasculitis).
Cardiovascular Reaction: Orthostatic hypotension may occur and may be aggravated by alcohol, barbiturates, or narcotics.
Other: Hyperglycemia, glycosuria, hypercalcemia, hyperuricemia, muscle spasm, weakness, restlessness.
There have been isolated reports that certain nonedematous individuals developed severe fluid and electrolyte derangements after only brief exposure to normal doses of thiazide and non-thiazide diuretics. The condition is usually manifested as severe dilutional hyponatremia, hypokalemia, and hypochloremia. It has been reported to be due to inappropriately increased ADH secretion and appears to be idiosyncratic. Potassium replacement is apparently the most important therapy in the treatment of this syndrome along with the removal of the offending drug.
Whenever adverse reactions are severe, treatment should be discontinued.
Deserpidine
The following adverse reactions have been reported with rauwolfia preparations. These reactions are usually reversible and disappear when the drug is discontinued.
Gastrointestinal: Including hypersecretion, anorexia, diarrhea, nausea, and vomiting.
Cardiovascular: Including angina-like symptoms, arrhythmias (particularly when used concurrently with digitalis or quinidine), and bradycardia.
Central Nervous System: Including drowsiness, depression, nervousness, paradoxical anxiety, nightmares, extrapyramidal tract symptoms, CNS sensitization manifested by dull sensorium, and deafness.
Dermatologic—Hypersensitivity: Including pruritus, rash, and asthma in asthmatic patients.
Ophthalmologic: Including glaucoma, uveitis, optic atrophy, and conjunctival injection.
Hematologic: Thrombocytopenic purpura.
Miscellaneous: Nasal congestion, weight gain, impotence or decreased libido, dysuria, dyspnea, muscular aches, dryness of mouth, dizziness and headache.

DOSAGE AND ADMINISTRATION

Dosage should be determined by individual titration of ingredients (see boxed warning). Dosage of both components should be carefully adjusted to the needs of the individual patient. Since at least ten days to two weeks may elapse before the full effects of the drugs become manifest, the dosage should not be adjusted more frequently.
Three tablet strengths, ORETICYL 25 (hydrochlorothiazide 25 mg, deserpidine 0.125 mg); ORETICYL 50 (hydrochlorothiazide 50 mg, deserpidine 0.125 mg); and ORETICYL FORTE (hydrochlorothiazide 25 mg, deserpidine 0.25 mg), all grooved, are provided to permit considerable latitude in meeting the dosage requirements of individual patients.
The table below will help in determining which dose of ORETICYL 25, ORETICYL 50, or ORETICYL FORTE best represents the equivalent of the titrated dose.

ORETICYL 25	hydro-chlorothiazide	deserpidine
1 tablet bid	25.0 mg bid	0.125 mg bid
1½ tablet bid	37.5 mg bid	0.188 mg bid
2 tablets bid	50.0 mg bid	0.250 mg bid

ORETICYL 50	hydro-chlorothiazide	deserpidine
1 tablet bid	50 mg bid	0.125 mg bid
1½ tablet bid	75 mg bid	0.188 mg bid
2 tablets bid	100 mg bid	0.250 mg bid

ORETICYL FORTE	hydro-chlorothiazide	deserpidine
1 tablet bid	25.0 mg bid	0.250 mg bid
1½ tablet bid	37.5 mg bid	0.375 mg bid
2 tablets bid	50.0 mg bid	0.500 mg bid

The usual adult dosage is one ORETICYL 50 two times daily.
When other antihypertensive agents are to be added to the regimen, this should be accomplished gradually. Ganglionic blocking agents should be given at only half the usual dose since their effect is potentiated by pretreatment with ORETICYL (hydrochlorothiazide and deserpidine).

OVERDOSAGE

Symptoms of thiazide overdosage include electrolyte imbalance and signs of potassium deficiency such as confusion, dizziness, muscular weakness, and gastrointestinal disturbances. General supportive measures including replacement of fluids and electrolytes may be indicated in treatment of overdosage.
An overdosage of deserpidine is characterized by flushing of the skin, conjunctival injection, and pupillary constriction. Sedation ranging from drowsiness to coma may occur. Hypotension, hypothermia, central respiratory depression and bradycardia may develop in cases of severe overdosage. Treatment consists of the careful evacuation of stomach contents followed by the usual procedures for the symptomatic management of CNS depressant overdosage. If severe hypotension occurs it should be treated with a direct acting vasopressor such as norepinephrine bitartrate injection.

HOW SUPPLIED

ORETICYL is supplied as grooved tablets in the following dosage sizes:
Rose-colored ORETICYL 25, contains hydrochlorothiazide 25 mg, deserpidine 0.125 mg, in bottles of 100 (**NDC** 0074-6922-01).
Rose-colored ORETICYL 50, contains hydrochlorothiazide 50 mg, deserpidine 0.125 mg, in bottles of 100 (**NDC** 0074-6931-01).
Gray-colored ORETICYL FORTE, contains hydrochlorothiazide 25 mg, deserpidine 0.25 mg, in bottles of 100 (**NDC** 0074-6927-01).
Abbott Laboratories
North Chicago, IL 60064
Ref. 01-2361-R6

PANHEMATIN® ℞

[pan-hē'ma-tin]
(hemin for injection)
For I.V. Use Only

> PANHEMATIN (hemin for injection) should only be used by physicians experienced in the management of porphyrias in hospitals where the recommended clinical and laboratory diagnostic and monitoring techniques are available.
> PANHEMATIN therapy should be considered after an appropriate period of alternate therapy (i.e., 400 g glucose/day for 1 to 2 days). (See "WARNINGS", "PRECAUTIONS" and "DOSAGE AND ADMINISTRATION" sections.)

DESCRIPTION

PANHEMATIN (hemin for injection) is an enzyme inhibitor derived from processed red blood cells. Hemin for injection was known previously as hematin. The term hematin has been used to describe the chemical reaction product of hemin and sodium carbonate solution. Hemin is an iron containing metalloporphyrin. Chemically hemin is represented as chloro[7,12-diethenyl-3,8,13,17-tetramethyl-21H,23H-porphine-2,18-dipropanoato (2-)-N^{21},N^{22}, N^{23}, N^{24}] iron.

PANHEMATIN is a sterile, lyophilized powder suitable for intravenous administration after reconstitution. Each dispensing vial of PANHEMATIN contains the equivalent of 313 mg hemin, 215 mg sodium carbonate and 300 mg of sorbitol. The pH may have been adjusted with hydrochloric acid; the product contains no preservatives. When mixed as directed with 43 ml Sterile Water for Injection, USP, hemin 313 mg/43 ml is approximately equivalent to hematin 7 mg/ml.

CLINICAL PHARMACOLOGY

Heme acts to limit the hepatic and/or marrow synthesis of porphyrin. This action is likely due to the inhibition of delta-aminolevulinic acid synthetase, the enzyme which limits the rate of the porphyrin/heme biosynthetic pathway. The exact mechanism by which hematin produces symptomatic improvement in patients with acute episodes of the hepatic porphyrias has not been elucidated.[1,9]

Following intravenous administration of hematin in non-jaundiced human patients, an increase in fecal urobilinogen can be observed which is roughly proportional to the amount of hematin administered. This suggests an enterohepatic pathway as at least one route of elimination. Bilirubin metabolites are also excreted in the urine following hematin injections.[2]

PANHEMATIN (hemin for injection) therapy for the acute porphyrias is not curative. After discontinuation of PANHEMATIN treatment, symptoms generally return although in some cases remission is prolonged. Some neurological symptoms have improved weeks to months after therapy although little or no response was noted at the time of treatment.

Other aspects of human pharmacokinetics have not been defined.

INDICATIONS AND USAGE

PANHEMATIN (hemin for injection) is indicated for the amelioration of recurrent attacks of acute intermittent porphyria temporarily related to the menstrual cycle in susceptible women.

Manifestations such as pain, hypertension, tachycardia, abnormal mental status and mild to progressive neurologic signs may be controlled in selected patients with this disorder.

Similar findings have been reported in other patients with acute intermittent porphyria, porphyria variegata and hereditary coproporphyria. PANHEMATIN is not indicated in porphyria cutanea tarda.

CONTRAINDICATIONS

Hemin for injection is contraindicated in patients with known hypersensitivity to this drug.

WARNINGS

PANHEMATIN (hemin for injection) therapy is intended to limit the rate of porphyria/heme biosynthesis possibly by inhibiting the enzyme delta-aminolevulinic acid synthetase. For this reason, drugs such as estrogens, barbituric acid derivatives and steroid metabolites which increase the activity of delta-aminolevulinic acid synthetase should be avoided.

Also, because PANHEMATIN has exhibited transient, mild anticoagulant effects during clinical studies, concurrent anticoagulant therapy should be avoided.[9] The extent and duration of the hypocoagulable state induced by PANHEMATIN has not been established.

PRECAUTIONS

General:

Clinical benefit from PANHEMATIN depends on prompt administration. Attacks of porphyria may progress to a point where irreversible neuronal damage has occurred. PANHEMATIN therapy is intended to prevent an attack from reaching the critical stage of neuronal degeneration. PANHEMATIN is not effective in repairing neuronal damage.[9]

Recommended dosage guidelines should be strictly followed. Reversible renal shutdown has been observed in a case where an excessive hematin dose (12.2 mg/kg) was administered in a single infusion. Oliguria and increased nitrogen retention occurred although the patient remained asymptomatic.[4] No worsening of renal function has been seen with administration of recommended dosages of hematin.[9]

A large arm vein or a central venous catheter should be utilized for the administration of hemin for injection to avoid the possibility of phlebitis.

Since reconstituted PANHEMATIN is not transparent, any undissolved particulate matter is difficult to see when inspected visually. Therefore, terminal filtration through a sterile 0.45 micron or smaller filter is recommended.

Tests for Diagnosis and Monitoring of Therapy: Before PANHEMATIN therapy is begun, the presence of acute porphyria must be diagnosed using the following criteria:[9]

a. Presence of clinical symptoms.

b. Positive Watson-Schwartz or Hoesch test. (A negative Watson-Schwartz or Hoesch test indicates a porphyric attack is highly unlikely. When in doubt quantitative measures of delta-aminolevulinic acid and porphobilinogen in serum or urine may aid in diagnosis.)

Urinary concentrations of the following compounds may be *monitored* during PANHEMATIN therapy. Drug effect will be demonstrated by a decrease in one or more of the following compounds:[3–6] ALA—delta-aminolevulinic acid, UPG —uroporphyrinogen, PBG—porphobilinogen or coproporphyrin.

Carcinogenesis, Mutagenesis, Impairment of Fertility: No data are available on potential for carcinogenicity, mutagenicity or impairment of fertility in animals or humans.

Pregnancy: Teratogenic effects: Pregnancy Category C. Animal reproduction studies have not been conducted with hematin. It is also not known whether hematin can cause fetal harm when administered to a pregnant woman or can affect reproduction capacity. For this reason hemin for injection should not be given to a pregnant woman unless the expected benefits are sufficiently important to the health and welfare of the patient to outweigh the unknown hazard to the fetus.

Nursing Mothers: It is not known whether this drug is excreted in human milk. Because many drugs are excreted in human milk, caution should be exercised when hemin for injection is administered to a nursing woman.

Pediatric Use: Safety and effectiveness in children have not been established.

ADVERSE REACTIONS

Reversible renal shutdown has occurred with administration of excessive doses (See "PRECAUTIONS" section).

Phlebitis with or without leucocytosis and with or without mild pyrexia has occurred after administration of hematin through small arm veins.

There has been one report in the literature[8] of coagulopathy occurring in a patient receiving hematin therapy. This patient exhibited prolonged prothrombin time and partial thromboplastin time, thrombocytopenia, mild hypofibrinogenemia, mild elevation of fibrin split products and a 10% fall in hematocrit.

OVERDOSAGE

Reversible renal shutdown has been observed in a case where an excessive hematin dose (12.2 mg/kg) was administered in a single infusion. Treatment of this case consisted of ethacrynic acid and mannitol.[7]

DOSAGE AND ADMINISTRATION

Before administering hemin for injection, an appropriate period of alternate therapy (i.e., 400 g glucose/day for 1 to 2 days) must be considered. If improvement is unsatisfactory for the treatment of acute attacks of porphyria, an intravenous infusion of PANHEMATIN containing a dose of 1 to 4 mg/kg/day of hematin should be given over a period of 10 to 15 minutes for 3 to 14 days based on the clinical signs. In more severe cases this dose may be repeated no earlier than every 12 hours. No more than 6 mg/kg of hematin should be given in any 24-hour period.

After reconstitution each ml of PANHEMATIN contains the equivalent of approximately 7 mg of hematin (313 mg hemin/43 ml), 5 mg sodium carbonate (215 mg/43 ml) and 7 mg sorbitol. The drug may be administered directly from the vial.

Dosage Calculation Table

1 mg hematin equivalent	=	0.14 ml PANHEMATIN
2 mg hematin equivalent	=	0.28 ml PANHEMATIN
3 mg hematin equivalent	=	0.42 ml PANHEMATIN
4 mg hematin equivalent	=	0.56 ml PANHEMATIN

Since reconstituted PANHEMATIN is not transparent, any undissolved particulate matter is difficult to see when inspected visually. Therefore, terminal filtration through a sterile 0.45 micron or smaller filter is recommended.

Preparation of Solution: Reconstitute PANHEMATIN by aseptically adding 43 ml of Sterile Water for Injection, USP, to the dispensing vial. Immediately after adding diluent, the product should be shaken well for a period of 2 to 3 minutes to aid dissolution. **NOTE:** Because PANHEMATIN contains no preservative and because PANHEMATIN undergoes rapid chemical decomposition in solution, it should not be reconstituted until immediately before use. After the first withdrawal from the vial, any solution remaining must be discarded.

No drug or chemical agent should be added to a PANHEMATIN fluid admixture unless its effect on the chemical and physical stability has first been determined.

HOW SUPPLIED

PANHEMATIN (hemin for injection) is supplied as a sterile, lyophilized black powder in single dose dispensing vials (**NDC** 0074-2000-43). Each dispensing vial contains the equivalent of 313 mg hemin, 215 mg sodium carbonate and 300 mg sorbitol (43 ml when mixed as directed). The pH may have been adjusted with hydrochloric acid; the product contains no preservatives. Hemin 313 mg/43 ml is approximately equivalent to 7 mg hematin/ml. Store lyophilized powder frozen until time of use.

REFERENCES

1. Bickers, D., Treatment of the Porphyrias: Mechanisms of Action, *J Invest Dermatol* 77(1):107–113, 1981.
2. Watson, C. J., Hematin and Porphyria, editorial, *N Engl J Med* 293(12):605–607, September 18, 1975.
3. Lamon, J. M., Hematin Therapy for Acute Porphyria, *Medicine* 58(3):252–269, 1979.
4. Dhar, G. J., et al., Effects of Hematin in Hepatic Porphyria, *Ann Intern Med* 83:20–30, 1975.
5. Watson, C. J., et al., Use of Hematin in the Acute Attack of the "Inducible" Hepatic Porphyrias, *Adv Intern Med* 23:265–286, 1978.
6. McColl, K. E., et al., Treatment with Haematin in Acute Hepatic Porphyria, *Q J Med*, New Series L (198):161–174, Spring, 1981.
7. Dhar, G. J., et al., Transitory Renal Failure Following Rapid Administration of a Relatively Large Amount of Hematin in a Patient with Acute Intermittent Porphyria in Clinical Remission, *Acta Med Scand* 203:437–443, 1978.
8. Morris, D. L., et al., Coagulopathy Associated with Hematin Treatment for Acute Intermittent Porphyria, *Ann Intern Med* 95:700–701, 1981.
9. Pierach, C. A., Hematin Therapy for the Porphyric Attack, *Semin Liver Dis* 2(2):125–131, May, 1982.

Abbott Laboratories
North Chicago, IL 60064

PANWARFIN® ℞

[păn-wăr'fin]
(warfarin sodium tablets, USP)

HOW SUPPLIED

PANWARFIN (warfarin sodium tablets, USP) for oral administration, grooved and bearing dosage strength numerals are available as follows:

2 mg, lavender-colored: bottles of 100 (**NDC** 0074-6626-03), and ABBO-PAC® unit dose packages of 100 tablets (**NDC** 0074-6626-07).

2½ mg, orange-colored: bottles of 100 (**NDC** 0074-7202-01), and ABBO-PAC unit dose packages of 100 tablets (**NDC** 0074-7202-05).

5 mg, peach-colored: bottles of 100 (**NDC** 0074-7210-01), 500 (**NDC** 0074-7210-09), and ABBO-PAC unit dose packages of 100 tablets (**NDC** 0074-7210-05).

7½ mg, yellow: bottles of 100 (**NDC** 0074-6638-03), and ABBO-PAC unit dose packages of 100 tablets (**NDC** 0074-6638-07).

10 mg, white: bottles of 100 (**NDC** 0074-7218-01), and ABBO-PAC unit dose packages of 100 tablets (**NDC** 0074-7218-05).

INACTIVE INGREDIENTS

2 mg tablets: corn starch, D&C Red No. 30, FD&C Blue No. 1, lactose, magnesium stearate, microcrystalline cellulose, polacrilin potassium and other ingredients.

2.5 mg tablets: corn starch, FD&C Yellow No. 6, lactose, magnesium stearate, microcrystalline cellulose, polacrilin potassium and other ingredients.

5 mg tablets: corn starch, D&C Red No. 30, FD&C Yellow No. 6, lactose, magnesium stearate, microcrystalline cellulose, polacrilin potassium and other ingredients.

7.5 mg tablets: corn starch, FD&C Yellow No. 5 (tartrazine), lactose, magnesium stearate, microcrystalline cellulose, polacrilin potassium and other ingredients.

10 mg tablets: corn starch, lactose, magnesium stearate, microcrystalline cellulose, polacrilin potassium and other ingredients.

Shown in Product Identification Section, page 403

Abbott Pharmaceuticals, Inc.
North Chicago, IL 60064

If desired, additional literature on any Abbott Product will be provided upon request to Abbott Laboratories.

Continued on next page

Abbott—Cont.

PARADIONE® ℞
[*pă-ră-dī 'own*]
(paramethadione)
Capsules and Oral Solution

> BECAUSE OF ITS POTENTIAL TO PRODUCE FETAL MALFORMATIONS AND SERIOUS SIDE EFFECTS, PARADIONE (paramethadione) SHOULD ONLY BE UTILIZED WHEN OTHER LESS TOXIC DRUGS HAVE BEEN FOUND INEFFECTIVE IN CONTROLLING ABSENCE (PETIT MAL) SEIZURES.

DESCRIPTION

PARADIONE (paramethadione) is an antiepileptic agent. An oxazolidinedione compound, it is chemically identified as 5-Ethyl-3,5-dimethyl-2,4-oxazolidinedione. PARADIONE is a synthetic, oily, slightly water-soluble liquid. It is supplied in capsular and liquid forms for oral use only. The capsules are available in two dosage strengths. One strength contains 150 mg the other 300 mg of paramethadione per capsule. Each ml of the liquid contains 300 mg of paramethadione.

INACTIVE INGREDIENTS

150 mg capsule: FD&C Yellow No. 6, gelatin, glycerin, methylparaben, olive oil ethyl ester, propylparaben and other ingredients.
300 mg capsule: FD&C Blue No. 1, FD&C Yellow No. 5 (tartrazine), FD&C Yellow No. 6, gelatin, glycerin, methylparaben, olive oil ethyl ester, propylparaben and other ingredients.
Paradione Solution: Alcohol 65%, water and other ingredients.

CLINICAL PHARMACOLOGY

PARADIONE has been shown to prevent pentylenetetrazol-induced and thujone-induced seizures in experimental animals; the drug has a less marked effect on seizures induced by picrotoxin, procaine, cocaine, or strychnine. Unlike the hydantoins and antiepileptic barbiturates, PARADIONE does not modify the maximal seizure pattern in patients undergoing electroconvulsive therapy. PARADIONE has a sedative effect that may increase to the point of ataxia when excessive doses are used. A toxic dose of the drug in animals (approximately 1 g/kg) produced sleep, unconsciousness, and respiratory depression.
Paramethadione is rapidly absorbed from the gastrointestinal tract. It is demethylated by liver microsomes to an active N-demethylated metabolite, and is excreted slowly in this form by the kidney; almost no unmetabolized PARADIONE is excreted.

INDICATIONS AND USAGE

PARADIONE (paramethadione) is indicated for the control of absence (petit mal) seizures that are refractory to treatment with other drugs.

CONTRAINDICATIONS

PARADIONE is contraindicated in patients with a known hypersensitivity to the drug.

WARNINGS

PARADIONE may cause serious side effects. Strict medical supervision of the patient is mandatory, especially during the initial year of therapy.
USAGE DURING PREGNANCY: THERE ARE MULTIPLE REPORTS IN THE CLINICAL LITERATURE WHICH INDICATE THAT THE USE OF ANTIEPILEPTIC DRUGS DURING PREGNANCY RESULTS IN AN INCREASED INCIDENCE OF BIRTH DEFECTS IN THE OFFSPRING. DATA ARE MORE EXTENSIVE WITH RESPECT TO TRIMETHADIONE, PARAMETHADIONE, PHENYTOIN AND PHENOBARBITAL THAN WITH OTHER ANTIEPILEPTIC DRUGS.
THEREFORE, ANTIEPILEPTIC DRUGS SUCH AS PARADIONE (PARAMETHADIONE) SHOULD BE ADMINISTERED TO WOMEN OF CHILDBEARING POTENTIAL ONLY IF THEY ARE CLEARLY SHOWN TO BE ESSENTIAL IN THE MANAGEMENT OF THEIR SEIZURES. EFFECTIVE MEANS OF CONTRACEPTION SHOULD ACCOMPANY THE USE OF PARADIONE IN SUCH PATIENTS. IF A PATIENT BECOMES PREGNANT WHILE TAKING PARADIONE, TERMINATION OF THE PREGNANCY SHOULD BE CONSIDERED. A PATIENT WHO REQUIRES THERAPY WITH PARADIONE AND WHO WISHES TO BECOME PREGNANT SHOULD BE ADVISED OF THE RISKS.
REPORTS HAVE SUGGESTED THAT THE MATERNAL INGESTION OF ANTIEPILEPTIC DRUGS, PARTICULARLY BARBITURATES, IS ASSOCIATED WITH A NEONATAL COAGULATION DEFECT THAT MAY CAUSE BLEEDING DURING THE EARLY (USUALLY WITHIN 24 HOURS OF BIRTH) NEONATAL PERIOD. THE POSSIBILITY OF THE OCCURRENCE OF THIS DEFECT WITH THE USE OF PARADIONE SHOULD BE KEPT IN MIND. THE DEFECT IS CHARACTERIZED BY DECREASED LEVELS OF VITAMIN K-DEPENDENT CLOTTING FACTORS, AND PROLONGATION OF EITHER THE PROTHROMBIN TIME OR THE PARTIAL THROMBOPLASTIN TIME, OR BOTH. IT HAS BEEN SUGGESTED THAT PROPHYLACTIC VITAMIN K BE GIVEN TO THE MOTHER ONE MONTH PRIOR TO, AND DURING DELIVERY, AND TO THE INFANT, INTRAVENOUSLY, IMMEDIATELY AFTER BIRTH.

PRECAUTIONS

General: Abrupt discontinuation of PARADIONE may precipitate absence (petit mal) status. PARADIONE (paramethadione) should always be withdrawn gradually unless serious adverse effects dictate otherwise. In the latter case, another antiepileptic may be substituted to protect the patient.
PARADIONE (paramethadione) should be withdrawn promptly if skin rash appears, because of the grave possibility of the occurrence of exfoliative dermatitis or severe forms of erythema multiforme. Even a minor acneiform or morbilliform rash should be allowed to clear completely before treatment with PARADIONE is resumed; reinstitute therapy cautiously.
PARADIONE should ordinarily not be used in patients with severe blood dyscrasias.
Hepatitis has been associated rarely with the use of oxazolidinediones. Jaundice or other signs of liver dysfunction are an indication for withdrawal of PARADIONE. PARADIONE should ordinarily not be used in patients with severe hepatic impairment.
Fatal nephrosis has been reported with the use of oxazolidinediones. Persistent or increasing albuminuria, or the development of any other significant renal abnormality, is an indication for withdrawal of the drug. PARADIONE should ordinarily not be used in patients with severe renal dysfunction.
Hemeralopia has occurred with the use of oxazolidinedione compounds; this appears to be an effect of the drugs on the neural layers of the retina, and usually can be reversed by a reduction in dosage. Scotomata are an indication for withdrawal of the drug. Caution should be observed when treating patients who have diseases of the retina or optic nerve.
Manifestations of systemic lupus erythematosus have been associated with the use of the oxazolidinediones, as they have with the use of certain other antiepileptics. Lymphadenopathies simulating malignant lymphoma have also occurred. Lupus-like manifestations or lymph node enlargement are indications for withdrawal of PARADIONE. Signs and symptoms may disappear after discontinuation of therapy, and specific treatment may be unnecessary.
A myasthenia gravis-like syndrome has been associated with the chronic use of the oxazolidinediones. Symptoms suggestive of this condition are indications for withdrawal of PARADIONE.
The 300 mg capsule of PARADIONE contains FD&C Yellow No. 5 (tartrazine) which may cause allergic-type reactions (including bronchial asthma) in certain susceptible individuals. Although the overall incidence of FD&C Yellow No. 5 (tartrazine) sensitivity in the general population is low, it is frequently seen in patients who also have aspirin hypersensitivity.
Information for Patients: Patients should be advised to report immediately such signs and symptoms as sore throat, fever, malaise, easy-bruising, petechiae, or epistaxis, or others that may be indicative of an infection or bleeding tendency.
Laboratory Tests: A complete blood count should be done prior to initiating therapy with PARADIONE, and at monthly intervals thereafter. A marked depression of the blood count is an indication for withdrawal of the drug. If no abnormality appears within 12 months, the interval between blood counts may be extended. A moderate degree of neutropenia with or without a corresponding drop in the leukocyte count is not uncommon. Therapy need not be withdrawn unless the neutrophil count is 2500 or less; more frequent blood examinations should be done when the count is less than 3,000. Other blood dyscrasias, including leukopenia, eosinophilia, thrombocytopenia, pancytopenia, agranulocytosis, hypoplastic anemia, and fatal aplastic anemia, have occurred with the use of oxazolidinediones.
Liver function tests should be done prior to initiating therapy with PARADIONE, and at monthly intervals thereafter.
A urinalysis should be done prior to initiating therapy with PARADIONE and at monthly intervals thereafter.
Drug Interactions: Drugs known to cause toxic effects similar to those of the oxazolidinediones should be avoided or used only with extreme caution during therapy with PARADIONE.
Carcinogenesis: No data are available on long-term potential for carcinogenicity in animals or humans.
Pregnancy: Pregnancy Category D. See "Warnings" section.
Nursing Mothers: It is not known whether this drug is excreted in human milk. Because many drugs are excreted in human milk and because of the potential for serious adverse reactions in nursing infants from PARADIONE, a decision should be made whether to discontinue nursing or to discontinue the drug, taking into account the importance of the drug to the mother.

ADVERSE REACTIONS

The following side effects, in decreasing order of severity, have been associated with the use of oxazolidinedione compounds. Although not all of them have been reported with the use of PARADIONE, the possibility of their occurrence should be kept in mind when the drug is prescribed.
Renal: Fatal nephrosis has occurred. Albuminuria.
Hematologic: Fatal aplastic anemia, hypoplastic anemia, pancytopenia, agranulocytosis, leukopenia, neutropenia, thrombocytopenia, eosinophilia, retinal and petechial hemorrhages, vaginal bleeding, epistaxis, and bleeding gums.
Hepatic: Hepatitis has been reported rarely.
Dermatologic: Acneiform or morbilliform skin rash that may progress to severe forms of erythema multiforme or to exfoliative dermatitis. Hair loss.
CNS/Neurologic: A myasthenia gravis-like syndrome has been reported. Precipitation of tonic-clonic (grand mal) seizures, vertigo, personality changes, increased irritability, drowsiness, headache, parasthesias, fatigue, malaise, and insomnia.
Drowsiness usually subsides with continued therapy. If it persists, a reduction in dosage is indicated.
Ophthalmologic: Diplopia, hemeralopia, and photophobia.
Cardiovascular: Changes in blood pressure.
Gastrointestinal: Vomiting, abdominal pain, gastric distress, nausea, anorexia, weight loss, and hiccups.
Other: Lupus erythematosus, and lymphadenopathies simulating malignant lymphoma, have been reported. Pruritus associated with lymphadenopathy and hepatosplenomegaly has occurred in hypersensitive individuals.

OVERDOSAGE

Symptoms of acute PARADIONE overdosage include drowsiness, nausea, dizziness, ataxia, visual disturbances. Coma may follow massive overdosage.
Gastric evacuation, either by induced emesis, or by lavage, or both, should be done immediately. General supportive care, including frequent monitoring of the vital signs and close observation of the patient, are required.
It has been reported that alkalinization of the urine may be expected to increase the excretion of the N-demethylated metabolite of PARADIONE.
A blood count and a careful evaluation of hepatic and renal function should be done following recovery.

DOSAGE AND ADMINISTRATION

PARADIONE is administered orally.
Because PARADIONE Oral Solution contains alcohol 65%, it may be desirable to dilute the preparation with water before administering it to small children.
Usual Adult Dosage: 0.9–2.4 g daily in 3 or 4 equally divided doses (i.e., 300–600 mg 3 or 4 times daily).
Initially, give 0.9 g daily; increase this dose by 300 mg at weekly intervals until therapeutic results are seen or until toxic symptoms appear.
Maintenance dosage should be the least amount of drug required to maintain control.
Children's Dosage: Usually 0.3–0.9 g daily in 3 or 4 equally divided doses.

HOW SUPPLIED

PARADIONE Capsules (paramethadione capsules, USP) are round capsules supplied as 150 mg (orange color) (**NDC** 0074-3976-01), and 300 mg (green color) (**NDC** 0074-3838-01) in bottles of 100.

Shown in Product Identification Section, page 403

PARADIONE Solution (paramethadione oral solution, USP), 300 mg per ml, is supplied in 50-ml bottles (**NDC** 0074-3860-01). A dropper is provided with each bottle, which is marked to permit easy measurement of 0.5 ml and 1 ml doses. The solution is clear and colorless.
Abbott Laboratories
North Chicago, IL 60064

PEGANONE® ℞
[*pĕg 'ă-noon*]
(ethotoin tablets)

DESCRIPTION

PEGANONE (ethotoin) is an oral antiepileptic of the hydantoin series and is chemically identified as 3-ethyl-5-phenyl-2, 4-imidazolidinedione. PEGANONE tablets are available in two dosage strengths of 250 mg and 500 mg respectively.

INACTIVE INGREDIENTS

250 mg and 500 mg tablets: Acacia, lactose, sodium carboxymethylcellulose, stearic acid, talc and other ingredients.

CLINICAL PHARMACOLOGY

PEGANONE (ethotoin) exerts an antiepileptic effect without causing general central nervous system depression. The mechanism of action is probably very similar to that of phenytoin. The latter drug appears to stabilize rather than to raise the normal seizure threshold, and to prevent the spread of seizure activity rather than to abolish the primary focus of seizure discharges.

In laboratory animals, the drug was found effective against electroshock convulsions, and to a lesser extent, against complex partial (psychomotor) and pentylenetetrazol-induced seizures.

In mice, the duration of antiepileptic activity was prolonged by hepatic injury but not by bilateral nephrectomy; the drug is apparently biotransformed by the liver.

Ethotoin is fairly rapidly absorbed; the extent of oral absorption is not known. The drug exhibits saturable metabolism with respect to the formation of N-deethyl and p-hydroxyl-ethotoin, the major metabolites. Where plasma concentrations are below about 8 mg/l, the elimination half-life of ethotoin is in the range of 3 to 9 hours. Above this concentration, the dose-dependent, nonlinear kinetics of the drug preclude definition of any conventional half-life. Experience suggests that therapeutic plasma concentrations fall in the range of 15 to 50 mg/l; however, this range is not as extensively documented as those quoted for other antiepileptics.

INDICATIONS AND USAGE

PEGANONE (ethotoin) is indicated for the control of tonic-clonic (grand mal) and complex partial (psychomotor) seizures.

CONTRAINDICATIONS

PEGANONE (ethotoin) is contraindicated in patients with hepatic abnormalities or hematologic disorders.

WARNINGS

USAGE DURING PREGNANCY— THERE ARE MULTIPLE REPORTS IN THE CLINICAL LITERATURE WHICH INDICATE THAT THE USE OF ANTIEPILEPTIC DRUGS DURING PREGNANCY RESULTS IN AN INCREASED INCIDENCE OF BIRTH DEFECTS IN THE OFFSPRING. ALTHOUGH DATA ARE MORE EXTENSIVE WITH RESPECT TO TRIMETHADIONE, PARAMETHADIONE, PHENYTOIN, AND PHENOBARBITAL, REPORTS INDICATE A POSSIBLE SIMILAR ASSOCIATION WITH THE USE OF OTHER ANTIEPILEPTIC DRUGS. THEREFORE, ANTIEPILEPTIC DRUGS SHOULD BE ADMINISTERED TO WOMEN OF CHILDBEARING POTENTIAL ONLY IF THEY ARE CLEARLY SHOWN TO BE ESSENTIAL IN THE MANAGEMENT OF THEIR SEIZURES.

ANTIEPILEPTIC DRUGS SHOULD NOT BE DISCONTINUED IN PATIENTS IN WHOM THE DRUG IS ADMINISTERED TO PREVENT MAJOR SEIZURES BECAUSE OF THE STRONG POSSIBILITY OF PRECIPITATING STATUS EPILEPTICUS WITH ATTENDANT HYPOXIA AND RISK TO BOTH MOTHER AND THE UNBORN CHILD. CONSIDERATION SHOULD, HOWEVER, BE GIVEN TO DISCONTINUATION OF ANTIEPILEPTICS PRIOR TO AND DURING PREGNANCY WHEN THE NATURE, FREQUENCY AND SEVERITY OF THE SEIZURES DO NOT POSE A SERIOUS THREAT TO THE PATIENT. IT IS NOT, HOWEVER, KNOWN WHETHER EVEN MINOR SEIZURES CONSTITUTE SOME RISK TO THE DEVELOPING EMBRYO OR FETUS.

REPORTS HAVE SUGGESTED THAT THE MATERNAL INGESTION OF ANTIEPILEPTIC DRUGS, PARTICULARLY BARBITURATES, IS ASSOCIATED WITH A NEONATAL COAGULATION DEFECT THAT MAY CAUSE BLEEDING DURING THE EARLY (USUALLY WITHIN 24 HOURS OF BIRTH) NEONATAL PERIOD. THE POSSIBILITY OF THE OCCURRENCE OF THIS DEFECT WITH THE USE OF PEGANONE SHOULD BE KEPT IN MIND. THE DEFECT IS CHARACTERIZED BY DECREASED LEVELS OF VITAMIN K-DEPENDENT CLOTTING FACTORS, AND PROLONGATION OF EITHER THE PROTHROMBIN TIME OR THE PARTIAL THROMBOPLASTIN TIME, OR BOTH. IT HAS BEEN SUGGESTED THAT VITAMIN K BE GIVEN PROPHYLACTICALLY TO THE MOTHER ONE MONTH PRIOR TO, AND DURING DELIVERY, AND TO THE INFANT, INTRAVENOUSLY, IMMEDIATELY AFTER BIRTH.

THE PHYSICIAN SHOULD WEIGH THESE CONSIDERATIONS IN TREATMENT AND COUNSELING OF EPILEPTIC WOMEN OF CHILDBEARING POTENTIAL.

PRECAUTIONS

General: Blood dyscrasias have been reported in patients receiving PEGANONE. Although the etiologic role of PEGANONE has not been definitely established, physicians should be alert for general malaise, sore throat and other symptoms indicative of possible blood dyscrasia.

There is some evidence suggesting that hydantoin-like compounds may interfere with folic acid metabolism, precipitating a megaloblastic anemia. If this should occur during gestation, folic acid therapy should be considered.

Information for Patients: Patients should be advised to report immediately such signs and symptoms as sore throat, fever, malaise, easy bruising, petechiae, epistaxis, or others that may be indicative of an infection or bleeding tendency.

Laboratory Tests: Liver function tests should be performed if clinical evidence suggests the possibility of hepatic dysfunction. Signs of liver damage are indication for withdrawal of the drug.

It is recommended that blood counts and urinalyses be performed when therapy is begun and at monthly intervals for several months thereafter. As in patients receiving other hydantoin compounds and other antiepileptic drugs, blood dyscrasias have been reported in patients receiving PEGANONE (ethotoin). Marked depression of the blood count is indication for withdrawal of the drug.

Drug Interactions: PEGANONE used in combination with other drugs known to adversely affect the hematopoietic system should be avoided if possible.

Considerable caution should be exercised if PEGANONE is administered concurrently with *Phenurone (phenacemide)* since paranoid symptoms have been reported during therapy with this combination.

A two-way interaction between the hydantoin antiepileptic, *phenytoin,* and the *coumarin anticoagulants* has been suggested. Presumably, phenytoin acts as a stimulator of coumarin metabolism and has been reported to cause decreased serum levels of the coumarin anticoagulants and increased prothrombin-proconvertin concentrations. Conversely, the coumarin anticoagulants have been reported to increase the serum levels and prolong the serum half-life of phenytoin by inhibiting its metabolism. Although there is no documentation of such, a similar interaction between ethotoin and the coumarin anticoagulants may occur. Caution is therefore advised when administering PEGANONE to patients receiving coumarin anticoagulants.

Carcinogenesis: No data are available on long-term potential for carcinogenicity in animals or humans.

Pregnancy: Pregnancy Category C. See "Warnings" section.

Nursing Mothers: Ethotoin is excreted in breast milk. Because of the potential for serious adverse reactions in nursing infants from ethotoin, a decision should be made whether to discontinue nursing or to discontinue the drug, taking into account the importance of the drug to the mother.

ADVERSE REACTIONS

Adverse reactions associated with PEGANONE, in decreasing order of severity, are:

Isolated cases of lymphadenopathy and systemic lupus erythematosus have been reported in patients taking hydantoin compounds, and lymphadenopathy has occurred with PEGANONE. Withdrawal of therapy has resulted in remission of the clinical and pathological findings. Therefore, if a lymphoma-like syndrome develops, the drug should be withdrawn and the patient should be closely observed for regression of signs and symptoms before treatment is resumed.

Ataxia and gum hypertrophy have occurred only rarely—usually only in patients receiving an additional hydantoin derivative. It is of interest to note that ataxia and gum hypertrophy have subsided in patients receiving other hydantoins when PEGANONE was given as a substitute antiepileptic.

Occasionally, vomiting or nausea after ingestion of PEGANONE has been reported, but if the drug is administered after meals, the incidence of gastric distress is reduced. Other side effects have included chest pain, nystagmus, diplopia, fever, dizziness, diarrhea, headache, insomnia, fatigue, numbness and skin rash.

OVERDOSAGE

Symptoms of acute overdosage include drowsiness, visual disturbance, nausea and ataxia. Coma is possible at very high dosage.

Treatment should be begun by inducing emesis; gastric lavage may be considered as an alternative. General supportive measures will be necessary. A careful evaluation of blood-forming organs should be made following recovery.

DOSAGE AND ADMINISTRATION

PEGANONE is administered orally in 4 to 6 divided doses daily. The drug should be taken after food, and doses should be spaced as evenly as practicable. Initial dosage should be conservative. For adults, the initial daily dose should be 1 g or less, with subsequent gradual dosage increases over a period of several days. The optimum dosage must be determined on the basis of individual response. The usual adult maintenance dose is 2 to 3 g daily. Less than 2 g daily has been found ineffective in most adults.

Pediatric dosage depends upon the age and weight of the patient. The initial dose should not exceed 750 mg daily. The usual maintenance dose in children ranges from 500 mg to 1 g daily, although occasionally 2 or (rarely) 3 g daily may be necessary.

If a patient is receiving another antiepileptic drug, it should not be discontinued when PEGANONE therapy is begun. The dosage of the other drug should be reduced gradually as that of PEGANONE is increased. PEGANONE may eventually replace the other drug or the optimal dosage of both antiepileptics may be established.

PEGANONE is compatible with all commonly employed antiepileptic medications with the possible exception of Phenurone® (phenacemide). In tonic-clonic (grand mal) seizures, use of the drug with Gemonil® (metharbital) or phenobarbital may be beneficial. PEGANONE may be used in combination with drugs such as Tridione® (trimethadione) or Paradione® (paramethadione), as an adjunct in those patients with absence (petit mal) associated with tonic-clonic (grand mal).

HOW SUPPLIED

PEGANONE (ethotoin) grooved, white tablets are supplied in two dosage strengths: 250 mg, bottles of 100 (**NDC** 0074-6902-01); 500 mg, bottles of 100 (**NDC** 0074-6905-04).

This product is listed in N.D., a Medicare designated compendium.

Abbott Laboratories
North Chicago, IL 60064
Ref. 01-2360-R5

Shown in Product Identification Section, page 403

PENTHRANE® ℞

[pen'thrāne]
(methoxyflurane, USP)

DESCRIPTION

PENTHRANE® (Methoxyflurane, USP), a volatile liquid, is intended only for vaporization at suitable concentrations for administration by inhalation with appropriate anesthesia equipment or devices.

PENTHRANE is an inhalation anesthetic/analgesic which belongs to the fluorinated hydrocarbon group of volatile anesthetics. It is chemically designated 2,2 - dichloro -1, 1 - difluoroethyl methyl ether and has the following structural formula:

$$CH\ CL_2CF_2 - O - CH_3$$

PENTHRANE has a mildly pungent odor.

Some of the physical constants are:

Molecular weight	164.97
Boiling point at 760 mm Hg	104.6° C
Partition coefficients at 37° C	
Water/gas	4.5
Blood/gas (mean range)	10.20 to 14.06
Oil/gas	825
Vapor Pressure 17.7° C	20 mm Hg
Flash points	
in air	62.8° C
in oxygen (closed system)	32.8° C
in nitrous oxide 50% with 50% oxygen	28.2° C
Lower limits of flammability of vapor concentration	
in air	7.0%
in oxygen	5.4%
in N_2O 50%	4.6%

PENTHRANE (Methoxyflurane, USP) is stable and does not decompose in contact with soda lime. An antioxidant, butylated hydroxytoluene 0.01% w/w is added to insure stability on standing. This slowly oxidizes to a yellow pigment that progressively turns to brown, and which may accumulate on the vaporizer wick. The colored matter may be removed by rinsing the wick with diethyl ether. The wick must be dried after cleaning to avoid introducing diethyl ether into the system.

Polyvinyl chloride plastics are extracted by PENTHRANE, therefore, contact should be avoided. PENTHRANE does not extract polyethylene plastics, polypropylene plastics, fluorinated hydrocarbon plastics or nylon. It is very soluble in rubber and soda lime. Disposable conductive plastic circuits should be discarded after a single use to avoid cross contamination and because PENTHRANE may reduce conductivity of such materials below safe limits for subsequent administration of a flammable anesthetic.

The vapor concentration of PENTHRANE is limited by its vapor pressure at room temperature to a maximum of about 3.5% at 23° C. In practice, this concentration is not easily reached due to the cooling effect of vaporization. PENTHRANE is not flammable except at vapor concentrations well above those recommended for its use. Recommended concentrations are nonflammable and nonexplosive in air, oxygen and nitrous oxide mixtures at ordinary room temperature.

Continued on next page

Abbott—Cont.

CLINICAL PHARMACOLOGY

PENTHRANE provides anesthesia and/or analgesia.

After surgical anesthesia with PENTHRANE, analgesia and drowsiness may persist after consciousness has returned. This may obviate or reduce the need for narcotics in the immediate postoperative period.

When used alone in safe concentration, PENTHRANE (Methoxyflurane, USP) will not produce appreciable skeletal muscle relaxation. A muscle relaxing agent, e.g., succinylcholine chloride (Quelicin®) or tubocurarine chloride should be used as an adjunct.

Bronchiolar constriction or laryngeal spasm is not ordinarily provoked by PENTHRANE.

During PENTHRANE anesthesia, the cardiac rhythm is usually regular. The myocardium is only minimally sensitized by PENTHRANE to epinephrine. Some decrease in blood pressure often accompanies light planes of anesthesia. This may be accompanied by bradycardia. The hypotension noted is accompanied by reduced cardiac contractile force and reduced cardiac output.

When used for obstetrical delivery, light planes of PENTHRANE anesthesia have little effect on uterine contractions. There are no known contraindications to the concomitant use of PENTHRANE and oxytocic agents.

Biotransformation of PENTHRANE occurs in man. Approximately 20% of PENTHRANE uptake is recovered in the exhaled air, while urinary excretion of organic fluorine, fluoride and oxalic acid accounts for about 30% of the PENTHRANE uptake.

Studies have shown that higher peak blood fluoride levels are obtained earlier in obese patients than in non-obese.

INDICATIONS AND USAGE

1. PENTHRANE is indicated usually in combination with oxygen and nitrous oxide to provide anesthesia for surgical procedures in which total duration of PENTHRANE administration is anticipated to be 4 hours or less, and in which PENTHRANE is not to be used in concentrations that will provide skeletal muscle relaxation; see WARNINGS regarding time and dose relationships.
2. PENTHRANE (Methoxyflurane, USP) may be used alone with hand held inhalers or in combination with oxygen and nitrous oxide for analgesia in obstetrics and in minor surgical procedures.

CONTRAINDICATIONS

See WARNINGS.

WARNINGS

SEQUENTIAL ANESTHESIA WITH PENTHRANE AND HALOTHANE, OR HALOTHANE AND PENTHRANE, IN EITHER ORDER, HAS BEEN FOLLOWED BY JAUNDICE IN A FEW RARE CASES. WHEN A PREVIOUS EXPOSURE TO PENTHRANE (METHOXYFLURANE, USP) OR HALOTHANE HAS BEEN FOLLOWED BY UNEXPLAINED HEPATIC DYSFUNCTION AND/OR JAUNDICE, CONSIDERATION SHOULD BE GIVEN TO THE USE OF OTHER AGENTS.

THE NEPHROTOXICITY ASSOCIATED WITH PENTHRANE ADMINISTRATION APPEARS TO BE RELATED TO THE TOTAL DOSE (TIME AND CONCENTRATION). SEE PARAGRAPH 5. THE MANIFESTATIONS RANGE IN SEVERITY FROM REVERSIBLE ALTERATIONS IN LABORATORY FINDINGS TO POLYURIC OR OLIGURIC RENAL FAILURE, SOMETIMES FATAL.

POLYURIC RENAL FAILURE IS CHARACTERIZED BY THE DEVELOPMENT, EARLY IN THE POSTOPERATIVE PERIOD, OF THE FOLLOWING:

WEIGHT LOSS

URINE: LOW SPECIFIC GRAVITY, LARGE VOLUME EQUAL TO OR IN EXCESS OF FLUID INTAKE, DECREASED OSMOLALITY.

SERUM/BLOOD: ELEVATION OF SODIUM, CHLORIDE, URIC ACID, BUN, CREATININE.

THIS SYNDROME IS BELIEVED TO BE RELATED TO RELEASE OF THE FLUORIDE ION, A METABOLIC PRODUCT OF PENTHRANE AND TO BE RELATED TO THE TOTAL DOSAGE ADMINISTERED. THEREFORE, THE LOWEST EFFECTIVE DOSAGE SHOULD BE ADMINISTERED, ESPECIALLY IN AGED OR OBESE PATIENTS AND IN SURGICAL, PROCEDURES OF LONG DURATION, BEARING IN MIND THAT THE TOTAL DOSE DELIVERED TO THE PATIENT IS A FACTOR OF DURATION OF ADMINISTRATION AND CONCENTRATION OF VAPOR.

OXALATE CRYSTALS AND/OR ACUTE TUBULAR NECROSIS HAVE BEEN NOTED AT AUTOPSY.

The guiding principles in minimizing the possibility of renal injury are:

1. AVOID USING PENTHRANE (METHOXYFLURANE, USP) AS THE SOLE OR PRINCIPLE AGENT TO ACHIEVE MUSCULAR RELAXATION.
2. PATIENTS WITH PRE-EXISTING RENAL DISEASE, IMPAIRMENT OF RENAL FUNCTION, TOXEMIA OF PREGNANCY, AND PATIENTS UNDERGOING VASCULAR SURGERY AT OR NEAR THE RENAL VESSELS SHOULD NOT RECEIVE PENTHRANE UNLESS IN THE JUDGMENT OF THE PHYSICIAN THE BENEFITS OUTWEIGH THE INCREASED RISK OF NEPHROTOXIC EFFECT.
3. URINARY OUTPUT SHOULD BE MONITORED IN ALL PATIENTS IF EXCESSIVE URINE OUTPUT OCCURS, APPROPRIATE LABORATORY STUDIES SHOULD BE DONE TO ASSESS RENAL FUNCTION. IN HIGH RISK PATIENTS (SEE 2, ABOVE) SERIAL TESTS OF RENAL FUNCTION AND MEASUREMENTS OF FLUID AND ELECTROLYTE BALANCE ARE IMPERATIVE. ALL FLUID AND ELECTROLYTE LOSSES SHOULD BE PROMPTLY REPLACED.
4. THE CONCURRENT USE OF TETRACYCLINE AND PENTHRANE HAS BEEN REPORTED TO RESULT IN FATAL RENAL TOXICITY. THE POSSIBILITY EXISTS THAT PENTHRANE MAY ENHANCE THE ADVERSE RENAL EFFECTS OF OTHER DRUGS INCLUDING CERTAIN ANTIBIOTICS OF KNOWN NEPHROTOXIC POTENTIAL SUCH AS GENTAMICIN, KANAMYCIN, COLISTIN, POLYMYXIN B, CEPHALORIDINE AND AMPHOTERICIN B. THIS SHOULD BE CAREFULLY CONSIDERED WHEN PRESCRIBING SUCH DRUGS DURING THE PREOPERATIVE, OPERATIVE AND POSTOPERATIVE PERIODS.
5. BECAUSE OF THE DOSE-RELATED NEPHROTOXICITY POTENTIAL OF PENTHRANE (METHOXYFLURANE, USP), IT IS SUGGESTED THAT THE TOTAL DURATION OF LIGHT ANESTHETIC DEPTH WITH PENTHRANE NOT EXCEED APPROXIMATELY 4 HOURS AT A SINGLE ADMINISTRATION.

PRECAUTIONS

Diabetic patients may have an increased likelihood of developing nephropathy if they have impaired renal function or polyuria, are obese, or are not optimally controlled.

Caution should be exercised in using PENTHRANE in patients under treatment with enzyme inducing drugs (e.g., barbiturates) as such agents may enhance the metabolism of PENTHRANE, resulting in increased fluoride levels.

Ventilation should be assessed carefully and, if depressed, should be augmented to insure adequate oxygenation and carbon dioxide removal. Parenteral anesthetic adjuncts (e.g., barbiturates, narcotics and neuromuscular blocking agents) may also cause depression of respiration requiring assisted or controlled ventilation. A sufficient reduction in respiratory minute volume occurs during deep anesthesia to produce a significant respiratory acidosis if ventilation is not adequately assisted. PENTHRANE causes a slight metabolic acidosis.

PENTHRANE augments the effect of nondepolarizing muscle relaxants so that their usual dosage should be reduced by approximately one-half.

Epinephrine or levarterenol (norepinephrine) should be employed cautiously during PENTHRANE anesthesia.

When PENTHRANE is used under the conditions of dosage and administration shown below, in surgery or obstetrics, inorganic fluoride levels may infrequently reach those at which changes in renal laboratory values have been seen.

General anesthesia, including general anesthesia with PENTHRANE (Methoxyflurane, USP), has been associated in susceptible individuals with the acute onset of fulminant hypermetabolism of skeletal muscle known as *malignant hyperthermic crisis.* This syndrome is characterized by the acute onset of skeletal muscle overactivity and resulting high oxygen demand which usually exceeds supply. TACHYCARDIA and TACHYPNEA are the most important early signs; these may be associated with increased utilization of anesthesia circuit carbon dioxide absorber, arrhythmias, cyanosis, skin mottling, profuse sweating, unstable blood pressure, rapidly rising body temperature (usually appearing sometime after the first signs, when noted) and other indications of markedly increased oxygen demand. Laboratory tests usually confirm the excessive oxygen demand and resulting metabolic acidosis (blood gases); hyperkalemia and myoglobinemia are also frequently noted. Hypoglobinuria and renal failure may develop later. When these signs suggests a diagnosis of malignant hyperthermic crisis, it is important to terminate the anesthetic, cancel the surgery when possible, confirm the diagnosis and initiate management of the condition.

Dantrolene sodium intravenous is indicated, along with supportive measures, in the management of malignant hyperthermic crisis. These necessary supportive measures must be individualized, but will usually involve discontinuance of the suspect triggering agents, attendance to increased oxygen requirements and carbon dioxide production, management of metabolic acidosis, assurance of adequate urinary output, management of electrolyte imbalance and institution of measures to control rising temperature, when indicated. Consult literature references and the prescribing information for dantrolene sodium intravenous for additional information about the management of malignant hyperthermic crisis.

Information for patients:

When appropriate, as in some cases where discharge is anticipated soon after methoxyflurane anesthesia, patients should be cautioned not to drive an automobile, operate hazardous machinery or engage in hazardous sports for 24 hours or more (depending upon total dosage of methoxyflurane, condition of the patient and consideration given to other drugs administered) after anesthesia.

Carcinogenesis, mutagenesis, impairment of fertility:

A 15 month transplacental inhalation study of methoxyflurane at a subanesthetic concentration of 0.13% in the mouse revealed no evidence of anesthetic-related carcinogenesis. This concentration is equivalent to 36 hours of 0.2% methoxyflurane.

Mutagenesis testing of methoxyflurane was negative. Tests included: Ames bacterial assay, mouse sperm morphology assay and sister chromatied exchange in Chinese hamster ovary cells.

Studies of the effect on fertility have not been reported.

Pregnancy Category C: Methoxyflurane has been shown to cause fetal growth retardation in the rat at levels equivalent to 67 hours exposure of 0.2% methoxyflurane. There are no adequate and well-controlled studies in pregnant women. Methoxyflurane should be used during pregnancy only if the potential benefit justifies the potential risk to the fetus.

Nursing Mothers: Caution should be exercised when PENTHRANE (Methoxyflurane, USP) is administered to a nursing mother.

Labor and Delivery: In obstetrics attention should be given to the directions for Dosage and Administration shown below. Fluoride levels in cord blood are usually less than, but may equal those of the mother at delivery. The effect of inorganic fluoride on the infant is not known. However, clinical experience has demonstrated that cases of high output renal failure in either mother or child must be considered unlikely.

Pediatric Use: Safety and effectiveness of PENTHRANE (Methoxyflurane, USP) in children have not been established.

ADVERSE REACTIONS

Renal dysfunction: See WARNINGS.

Hepatic dysfunction, jaundice, and fatal hepatic necrosis have occurred following PENTHRANE anesthesia. Also as with other anesthetics, transient alterations in liver function tests may follow PENTHRANE administration. Hepatic complications rarely have involved reported cross reactions between PENTHRANE and Halothane.

Some patients exhibit pallor during recovery from PENTHRANE anesthesia.

Other adverse reactions which have been reported include cardiac arrest, malignant hyperpyrexia, prolonged postoperative somnolence, respiratory depression laryngospasm, bronchospasm, nausea, vomiting postoperative headache, hypotension and emergence delirium.

OVERDOSAGE

Patients should be closely observed for signs of excessive dosage during administration of PENTHRANE. PENTHRANE overdosage is characterized by decrease in tidal and minute volume; decrease in blood pressure, pallor, cyanosis and muscle relaxation. If the above signs are observed, turn off vaporizer and increase ventilation. If anesthesia exceeds light levels, vapor concentration should be reduced promptly. Prolonged administration (beyond four hours) and/or excessive vapor concentration beyond the equivalent of four hours of 0.25% delivered methoxyflurane may cause nephrotoxic effects attributable to metabolic release of free fluoride ion. See WARNINGS, PRECAUTIONS and DOSAGE AND ADMINISTRATION.

In the event of postoperative excessive urine output, fluid and electrolyte losses should be promptly replaced.

DOSAGE AND ADMINISTRATION

THE LOWEST EFFECTIVE DOSAGE OF PENTHRANE (METHOXYFLURANE, USP) SHOULD BE USED IN ORDER TO MINIMIZE THE POSSIBILITY OF NEPHROPATHY AND TO ALLOW FOR OPTIMAL RECOVERY TIME. IN CASES OF UNUSUALLY HIGH MAINTENANCE REQUIREMENTS, THE USE OF ANESTHETIC ADJUNCTS OR ANOTHER AGENT MAY BE INDICATED. THE ABSENCE OF HYPOTENSION CANNOT BE RELIED UPON AS EVIDENCE THAT DOSAGE HAS NOT BEEN EXCESSIVE DURING MAINTENANCE.

Analgesia

For analgesia, intermittent inhalation of vapor concentrations in the range of 0.3 to 0.8% are recommended. PENTHRANE may be self administered by hand held inhalers (e.g., Analgizer, Cyprane) if the patient is kept under close observation.

For intermittent administration from the hand-held inhaler, dosage for each patient is limited to not more than a single 15 mL charge of liquid PENTHRANE. Such analgesia in labor should not be instituted before relief becomes necessary. Use of the hand-held inhaler does not preclude transfer of the patient to a conventional anesthesia machine for inhalation anesthesia, but concentrations should be kept at the lowest effective dosage. Total time for anesthesia combined with analgesia should be as short as possible, bearing in mind the recommended duration for continuous anesthesia (four hours).

Anesthesia

A light level of anesthesia should be used. The use of deeper levels to achieve muscle relaxation should be avoided.

Apparatus: PENTHRANE should be vaporized by calibrated, temperature compensated, out of circle vaporizers (e.g., Pentec II, Pentomatic) or other methods which provide accurate delivered vapor concentration. Anesthetic uptake by rubber tubing, bags and soda lime which may prolong induction and recovery time can be reduced by the use of nonabsorptive plastic circuit material (not polyvinyl chloride) and fresh moist Baralyme. The fresh gas inlet should be located downstream of the CO_2 absorber in order to avoid excessive anesthetic absorption, and the rebreathing bag and pop-off valve should be located on the expiratory side.

Premedication: The usual preanesthetic medications may be administered prior to PENTHRANE (Methoxyflurane, USP) anesthesia, see PRECAUTIONS.

Induction: Use of a parenteral induction agent (such as an ultra-short acting barbiturate) is recommended unless contraindicated in an individual patient.

Carrier Gases: For general surgery, PENTHRANE should usually be administered with a carrier gas flow consisting of oxygen and at least 50% nitrous oxide in order to minimize the total PENTHRANE dose unless nitrous oxide is contraindicated.

Muscle Relaxation: PENTHRANE should not be administered at levels required to achieve muscle relaxation. Adequate relaxation should be obtained from adjunctive use of a muscle relaxant, e.g., succinylcholine chloride (Quelicin®) or tubocurarine chloride. The usual dosage of nondepolarizing muscle relaxants should be reduced by approximately one-half.

Vapor Concentrations: Initially PENTHRANE concentrations may be increased as tolerated to a maximum of approximately 2.0%. This concentration should only be continued for about two to five minutes, or until patient signs of light anesthesia are evident. The concentration of PENTHRANE should then be reduced by frequent decrements to the lowest possible levels consistent with the maintenance of adequate anesthesia. For example, in a 70 kg patient, the following sequential reduction in the delivered vapor concentration of PENTHRANE (Methoxyflurane, USP) may be appropriate:

Elapsed Minutes				
0 to 5	5 to 20	20 to 60	60 to 120	120 to 240
Vapor Conc.*				
2.0%	0.6%	0.4%	0.2%	0.1%

* Concentrations are approximate and subject to adjustment according to patient signs of anesthesia. Based on 5 liters per minute gas flow and ventilation rate throughout procedure, 50/50 N_2O and oxygen.

Concentration may be increased or decreased according to the requirements of the individual patient. Four hours of 0.25% delivered methoxyflurane should not be exceeded in normal adult patients unless in the opinion of the clinician, the anticipated benefits outweigh the increased risk of dose related nephrotoxicity. The product of these two factors (four hours of 0.25% delivered methoxyflurane) may be used to estimate other combinations of time and dose: Thus two hours of 0.5%, for example, should not ordinarily be exceeded. In sufficiently long cases, PENTHRANE should be discontinued 30 to 40 minutes before the end of surgery. Rapid flushing will not remove PENTHRANE absorbed by rubber circuit components.

Patient signs and levels: The PENTHRANE level of conscious analgesia is suited for pain relief, as in labor and uncomplicated vaginal deliveries. The level of unconscious analgesia is suitable for many minor surgical procedures. The level of light anesthesia is recommended for general surgical use. Deep anesthesia with PENTHRANE (Methoxyflurane, USP) is not recommended.

Appropriate patient signs of PENTHRANE anesthesia should be observed closely as a guide to proper depth. A blood pressure decrease of about 22 mm Hg may be seen during induction. A greater decrease may occur in hypertensive patients. Blood pressure usually recovers as a level of light anesthesia is reached. The absence of hypotension cannot be relied upon as evidence that dosage has not been excessive during maintenance.

HOW SUPPLIED

PENTHRANE (Methoxyflurane, USP) is supplied in 125 ml and 15 ml bottles, List 6864.

Preserve in tight, light-resistant containers and avoid exposure to excessive heat.

Protect from light. Protect from freezing and extreme heat.

Caution: Federal (USA) law prohibits dispensing without prescription.

06-3179-R26-3/82

Marketed by

Abbott Laboratories

PENTOTHAL® Ⓒ III

[*pen 'tōe-thal*]

(thiopental sodium for injection, USP)

WARNING: MAY BE HABIT FORMING.

DESCRIPTION

Pentothal (Thiopental Sodium for Injection, USP) is a thiobarbiturate, the sulfur analogue of sodium pentobarbital. The drug is prepared as a sterile powder and after reconstitution with an appropriate diluent is administered by the intravenous route.

Pentothal is chemically designated sodium 5-ethyl-5-(1-methylbutyl)-2-thiobarbiturate and has the following structural formula:

H N SNa O C_2H_5 $CH_3(CH_2)_2CH$ N CH O

The drug is a yellowish, hygroscopic powder, stabilized with anhydrous sodium carbonate as a buffer (60 mg/g of thiopental sodium).

CLINICAL PHARMACOLOGY

Pentothal (Thiopental Sodium for Injection, USP) is an ultrashort-acting depressant of the central nervous system which induces hypnosis and anesthesia, but not analgesia. It produces hypnosis within 30 to 40 seconds of intravenous injection. Recovery after a small dose is rapid, with some somnolence and retrograde amnesia. Repeated intravenous doses lead to prolonged anesthesia because fatty tissues act as a reservoir; they accumulate Pentothal in concentrations 6 to 12 times greater than the plasma concentration, and then release the drug slowly to cause prolonged anesthesia.

The half-life of the elimination phase after a single intravenous dose is three to eight hours.

The distribution and fate of Pentothal (as with other barbiturates) is influenced chiefly by its lipid solubility (partition coefficient), protein binding and extent of ionization. Pentothal has a partition coefficient of 580.

Approximately 80% of the drug in the blood is bound to plasma protein. Pentothal is largely degraded in the liver and to a smaller extent in other tissues, especially the kidney and brain. It has a pk_a of 7.4.

Concentration in spinal fluid is slightly less than in the plasma.

Biotransformation products of thiopental are pharmacologically inactive and mostly excreted in the urine.

INDICATIONS AND USAGE

Pentothal (Thiopental Sodium for Injection, USP) is indicated (1) as the sole anesthetic agent for brief (15 minute) procedures, (2) for induction of anesthesia prior to administration of other anesthetic agents, (3) to supplement regional anesthesia, (4) to provide hypnosis during balanced anesthesia with other agents for analgesia or muscle relaxation, (5) for the control of convulsive states during or following inhalation anesthesia, local anesthesia, or other causes, (6) in neurosurgical patients with increased intracranial pressure, if adequate ventilation is provided, and (7) for narcoanalysis and narcosynthesis in psychiatric disorders.

Contraindications:

Absolute Contraindications:

(1) Absence of suitable veins for intravenous administration,

(2) hypersensitivity (allergy) to barbiturates, (3) status asthmaticus, and (4) latent or manifest porphyria.

Relative Contraindications:

(1) Severe cardiovascular disease, (2) hypotension or shock, (3) conditions in which the hypnotic effect may be prolonged or potentiated — excessive premedication, Addison's disease, hepatic or renal dysfunction, myxedema, increased blood urea, severe anemia, asthma and myasthenia gravis.

WARNINGS

KEEP RESUSCITATIVE AND ENDOTRACHEAL INTUBATION EQUIPMENT AND OXYGEN READILY AVAILABLE. MAINTAIN PATENCY OF THE AIRWAY AT ALL TIMES.

This drug should be administered only by persons qualified in the use of intravenous anesthetics.

Avoid extravasation or intra-arterial injection.

WARNING: MAY BE HABIT FORMING.

PRECAUTIONS

Observe aseptic precautions at all times in preparation and handling of Pentothal (Thiopental Sodium for Injection, USP) solutions.

If used in conditions involving relative contraindications, reduce dosage and administer slowly.

Care should be taken in administering the drug to patients with advanced cardiac disease, increased intracranial pressure, asthma, myasthenia gravis and endocrine insufficiency (pituitary, thyroid, adrenal, pancreas).

Nursing Mothers: Thiopental sodium readily crosses the placental barrier and small amounts may appear in the milk of nursing mothers following administration of large doses.

Pregnancy Category C. Animal reproduction studies have not been conducted with Pentothal. It is also not known whether Pentothal can cause fetal harm when administered to a pregnant woman or can affect reproduction capacity. Pentothal should be given to a pregnant woman only if clearly needed.

ADVERSE REACTIONS

Adverse reactions include respiratory depression, myocardial depression, cardiac arrhythmias, prolonged somnolence and recovery, sneezing, coughing, bronchospasm, laryngospasm and shivering. Hypersensitivity reactions to barbiturates, including Pentothal (Thiopental Sodium for Injection, USP), have been reported.

DRUG ABUSE AND DEPENDENCE

WARNING: MAY BE HABIT FORMING.

Thiopental sodium is classified as a Schedule III controlled substance.

OVERDOSAGE

Overdosage may occur from too rapid or repeated injections. Too rapid injection may be followed by an alarming fall in blood pressure even to shock levels. Apnea, occasional laryngospasm, coughing and other respiratory difficulties with excessive or too rapid injections may occur. In the event of suspected or apparent overdosage, the drug should be discontinued, a patent airway established (intubate if necessary) or maintained, and oxygen should be administered, with assisted ventilation if necessary. The lethal dose of barbiturates varies and cannot be stated with certainty. Lethal blood levels may be as low as 1 mg/100 ml for short-acting barbiturates; less if other depressant drugs or alcohol are also present.

DOSAGE AND ADMINISTRATION

Pentothal (Thiopental Sodium for Injection, USP) is administered by the intravenous route only. Individual response to the drug is so varied that there can be no fixed dosage. The drug should be titrated against patient requirements as governed by age, sex and body weight. Younger patients require relatively larger doses than middle-aged and elderly persons; the latter metabolize the drug more slowly. Pre-puberty requirements are the same for both sexes, but adult females require less than adult-males. Dose is usually proportional to body weight and obese patients require a larger dose than relatively lean persons of the same weight.

Premedication

Premedication usually consists of atropine or scopolamine to suppress vagal reflexes and inhibit secretions. In addition, a barbiturate or an opiate is often given. Sodium pentobarbital injection (Nembutal®) is suggested because it provides a preliminary indication of how the patient will react to barbiturate anesthesia. Ideally, the peak effect of these medications should be reached shortly before the time of induction.

Test Dose

It is advisable to inject a small "test" dose of 25 to 75 mg (1 to 3 mL of a 2.5% solution) of Pentothal (Thiopental Sodium for Injection, USP) to assess tolerance or unusual sensitivity to Pentothal, and pausing to observe patient reaction for at least 60 seconds. If unexpectedly deep anesthesia develops or if respiratory depression occurs, consider these possibilities: (1) the patient may be unusually sensitive to Pentothal, (2) the solution may be more concentrated than had been assumed, or (3) the patient may have received too much premedication.

Use in Anesthesia

Moderately slow induction can usually be accomplished in the "average" adult by injection of 50 to 75 mg (2 to 3 mL of a 2.5% solution) at intervals of 20 to 40 seconds, depending on the reaction of the patient. Once anesthesia is established, additional injections of 25 to 50 mg can be given whenever the patient moves.

Slow injection is recommended to minimize respiratory depression and the possibility of overdosage. The smallest dose consistent with attaining the surgical objective is the desired

Continued on next page

Abbott—Cont.

goal. Momentary apnea following each injection is typical, and progressive decrease in the amplitude of respiration appears with increasing dosage. Pulse remains normal or increases slightly and returns to normal. Blood pressure usually falls slightly but returns toward normal. Muscles usually relax about 30 seconds after unconsciousness is attained, but this may be masked if a skeletal muscle relaxant is used. The tone of jaw muscles is a fairly reliable index. The pupils may dilate but later contract; sensitivity to light is not usually lost until a level of anesthesia deep enough to permit surgery is attained. Nystagmus and divergent strabismus are characteristic during early stages, but at the level of surgical anesthesia, the eyes are central and fixed. Corneal and conjunctival reflexes disappear during surgical anesthesia.
When Pentothal (Thiopental Sodium for Injection, USP) is used for induction in balanced anesthesia with a skeletal muscle relaxant and an inhalation agent, the total dose of Pentothal can be estimated and then injected in two to four fractional doses. With this technique, brief periods of apnea may occur which may require assisted or controlled pulmonary ventilation. As an initial dose, 210 to 280 mg (3 to 4 mg/kg) of Pentothal is usually required for rapid induction in the average adult (70 kg).
When Pentothal (Thiopental Sodium for Injection, USP) is used as the sole anesthetic agent, the desired level of anesthesia can be maintained by injection of small repeated doses as needed or by using a continuous intravenous drip in a 0.2% or 0.4% concentration. (Sterile water should not be used as the diluent in these concentrations, since hemolysis will occur). With continuous drip, the depth of anesthesia is controlled by adjusting the rate of infusion.

Use in Convulsive States

For the control of convulsive states following anesthesia (inhalation or local) or other causes, 75 to 125 mg (3 to 5 mL of a 2.5% solution) should be given as soon as possible after the convulsion begins. Convulsions following the use of a local anesthetic may require 125 to 250 mg of Pentothal (Thiopental Sodium for Injection), given over a ten minute period. If the convulsion is caused by a local anesthetic, the required dose of Pentothal will depend upon the amount of local anesthetic given and its convulsant properties.

Use in Neurosurgical Patients with Increased Intracranial Pressure

In neurosurgical patients, intermittent bolus injections of 1.5 to 3.5 mg/kg of body weight may be given to reduce intraoperative elevations of intracranial pressure, if adequate ventilation is provided.

Use in Psychiatric Disorders

For narcoanalysis and narcosynthesis in psychiatric disorders, premedication with an anticholinergic agent may precede administration of Pentothal. After a test dose, Pentothal is injected at a slow rate of 100 mg/min (4 mL/min of a 2.5% solution) with the patient counting backwards from 100. Shortly after counting becomes confused but before actual sleep is produced, the injection is discontinued. Allow the patient to return to a semidrowsy state where conversation is coherent. Alternatively, Pentothal (Thiopental Sodium for Injection, USP) may be administered by rapid I.V. drip using a 0.2% concentration in 5% dextrose and water. At this concentration, the rate of administration should not exceed 50 mL/min.

Management of Some Complications: *Respiratory depression* (hypoventilation, apnea), which may result from either unusual responsiveness to Pentothal (Thiopental Sodium for Injection, USP) or overdosage, is managed as stated above. Pentothal should be considered to have the same potential for producing respiratory depression as an inhalation agent, and patency of the airway must be protected at all times.
Laryngospasm may occur with light Pentothal narcosis at intubation, or in the absence of intubation if foreign matter or secretions in the respiratory tract create irritation. Laryngeal and bronchial vagal reflexes can be suppressed, and secretions minimized by giving atropine or scopolamine premedication and a barbiturate or opiate. Use of a skeletal muscle relaxant or positive pressure oxygen will usually relieve laryngospasm. Tracheostomy may be indicated in difficult cases.
Myocardial depression, proportioned to the amount of drug in direct contact with the heart, can occur and may cause hypotension, particularly in patients with an unhealthy myocardium. Arrhythmias may appear if P_{CO_2} is elevated, but they are uncommon with adequate ventilation. Management of myocardial depression is the same as for overdosage. Pentothal (Thiopental Sodium for Injection, USP) does not sensitize the heart to epinephrine or other sympathomimetic amines.
Extravascular infiltration should be avoided. Care should be taken to insure that the needle is within the lumen of the vein before injection of Pentothal. Extravascular injection may cause chemical irritation of the tissues varying from slight tenderness to venospasm, extensive necrosis and sloughing. This is due primarily to the high alkaline pH (10 to 11) of clinical concentrations of the drug. If extravasation occurs, the local irritant effects can be reduced by injection of 1% procaine locally to relieve pain and enhance vasodilatation. Local application of heat also may help to increase local circulation and removal of the infiltrate.
Intra-arterial injection can occur inadvertently, especially if an aberrant superficial artery is present at the medical aspect of the antecubital fossa. The area selected for intravenous injection of the drug should be palpated for detection of an underlying pulsating vessel. Accidental intra-arterial injection can cause arteriospasm and severe pain along the course of the artery with blanching of the arm and fingers. Appropriate corrective measures should be instituted promptly to avoid possible development of gangrene. Any patient complaint of pain warrants stopping the injection. Methods suggested for dealing with this complication vary with the severity of symptoms. The following have been suggested:

1. Dilute the injected Pentothal (Thiopental Sodium for Injection, USP) by removing the tourniquet and any restrictive garments.
2. Leave the needle in place, if possible.
3. Inject the artery with a dilute solution of papaverine, 40 to 80 mg, or 10 mL of 1% procaine, to inhibit smooth muscle spasm.
4. If necessary, perform sympathetic block of the brachial plexus and/or stellate ganglion to relieve pain and assist in opening collateral circulation. Papaverine can be injected into the subclavian artery, if desired.
5. Unless otherwise contraindicated, institute immediate heparinization to prevent thrombus formation.
6. Consider local infiltration of an alpha-adrenergic blocking agent such as phentolamine into the vasospastic area.
7. Provide additional symptomatic treatment as required.

Shivering after Pentothal anesthesia, manifested by twitching face muscles and occasional progression to tremors of the arms, head, shoulder and body, is a thermal reaction due to increased sensitivity to cold. Shivering appears if the room environment is cold and if a large ventilatory heat loss has been sustained with balanced inhalation anesthesia employing nitrous oxide. Treatment consists of warming the patient with blankets, maintaining room temperature near 22° C (72°F), and administration of chlorpromazine or methylphenidate.

PREPARATION OF SOLUTIONS

Pentothal (Thiopental Sodium for Injection, USP) is supplied as a yellowish, hygroscopic powder in a variety of different containers. Solutions should be prepared aseptically with one of the three following diluents. Sterile Water for Injection, USP, Sodium Chloride Injection, USP or 5% Dextrose Injection, USP. Clinical concentrations used for intermittent intravenous administration vary between 2.0% and 5.0%. A 2.0% or 2.5% solution is most commonly used. A 3.4% concentraton in sterile water for injection is isotonic; concentrations less than 2.0% in this diluent are not used because they cause hemolysis. For continuous intravenous drip administration, concentrations of 0.2% or 0.4% are used. Solutions may be prepared by adding Pentothal to 5% Dextrose Injection, USP, Sodium Chloride Injection, USP or Normosol® R pH 7.4.
Since Pentothal (Thiopental Sodium for Injection, USP) contains no added bacteriostatic agent, extreme care in preparation and handling should be exercised at all times to prevent the introduction of microbial contaminants. Solutions should be freshly prepared and used promptly: when reconstituted for administration to several patients, unused portions should be discarded after 24 hours. Sterilization by heating should not be attempted.

WARNING

The 2.5 g and larger sizes contain adequate medication for several patients.

COMPATIBILITY

Any solution of Pentothal (Thiopental Sodium for Injection, USP) with a visible precipitate should not be administered. The stability of Pentothal solutions depends upon several factors, including the diluent, temperature of storage and the amount of carbon dioxide from room air that gains access to the solution. Any factor or condition which tends to lower pH (increase acidity) of Pentothal solutions will increase the likelihood of precipitation of thiopental acid. Such factors include the use of diluents which are too acid and the absorption of carbon dioxide which can combine with water to form carbonic acid.
Solutions of succinylcholine, tubocurarine or other drugs which have an acid pH should not be mixed with Pentothal solutions. The most stable solutions are those reconstituted in water or isotonic saline, kept under refrigeration and tightly stoppered. The presence or absence of a visible precipitate offers a practical guide to the physical compatibility of prepared solutions of Pentothal (Thiopental Sodium for Injection, USP).

Calculations for Various Concentrations:

Concentration Desired Percent	mg/mL	Amounts to Use Pentothal g	Diluent mL
0.2	2	1	500
0.4	4	1	250
		2	500
2.0	20	5	250
		10	500
2.5	25	1	40
		5	200
5	50	1	20
		5	100

Reconstituted solutions of Pentothal should be inspected visually for particulate matter and discoloration, whenever solution and container permit.

HOW SUPPLIED

Pentothal (Thiopental Sodium for Injection, USP) is available in a variety of sizes and containers in combination packages with diluent as shown at the end of this insert.

Diluents in Pentothal® Kits

READY-TO-MIX SYRINGES AND VIALS

(For preparing solutions of Thiopental Sodium for Injection, USP)

DESCRIPTION

The following diluents in various container, syringe and vial sizes are provded in Pentothal Kits, Pentothal Ready-to-Mix Syringes and Vials for preparing solutions of Pentothal (Thiopental Sodium for Injection, USP) for clinical use:
Sterile Water for Injection, USP is sterile, nonpyrogenic preparation of water for injection which contains no bacteriostat, antimicrobial agents or added buffers. The pH is 5.7 (approximate).
Sterile Water for Injection, USP is a pharmaceutic aid (solvent) for intravenous administration only after addition of a solute.
Water is chemically designated H_2O.
0.9% Sodium Chloride Injection, USP is a sterile, nonpyrogenic, isotonic solution of sodium chloride and water for injection. Each mL contains sodium chloride 9 mg (308 mOsm/liter calc). It contains no bacteriostat, antimicrobial agents or added buffers except for pH adjustment. May contain hydrochloric acid or sodium hydroxide for pH adjustment. Approximate pH 5.7.
0.9% Sodium Chloride Injection, USP is an isotonic vehicle fo intravenous administration of another solute.
Sodium chloride is chemically designated NaCl, a white crystalline compound freely soluble in water.
The semi-rigid vial contained in List Nos. 3329, 6435, 6418, 6419 and 6420 is fabricated from a specially formulated polyolefin. It is a copolymer of ethylene and propylene. The safety of the plastic has been confirmed by tests in animals according to USP biological standards for plastic containers. The container requires no vapor barrier to maintain the proper labeled volume.

CLINICAL PHARMACOLOGY

Sterile Water for Injection, USP serves only as a pharmaceutic aid for diluting or dissolving drugs prior to administration.
Water is an essential constituent of all body tissues and accounts for approximately 70% of total body weight. Average normal adult daily requirement ranges from two to three liters (1.0 to 1.5 liters each for insensible water loss by perspiration and urine excretion).
Water balance is maintained by various regulatory mechanisms. Water distribution depends primarily on the concentration of dissociated electrolytes in the body compartments and sodium (Na+) plays a major role in maintaining a physiologic equilibrium between fluid intake and output.
0.9% Sodium Chloride Injection, USP serves only as an isotonic vehicle for drugs prior to administration.
Sodium chloride in water is an electrolyte solution of sodium (Na+) and chloride (Cl−) ions. These ions are normal constituents of the body fluids (principally extracellular) and are essential for maintaining electrolyte balance.
The distribution and excretion of sodium (Na+) and chloride (Cl−) are largely under the control of the kidney which maintains a balance between intake and output of these ions. The small volumes of fluid and amounts of sodium chloride provided by 0.9% Sodium Chloride Injection in Ready-to-Mix Syringes are unlikely to produce a significant effect on fluid or electrolyte balance.

INDICATIONS AND USAGE

These products are indicated only for preparing Pentothal (Thiopental Sodium for Injection, USP) solutions for clinical use.

CONTRAINDICATIONS

Do not use unless the diluent is clear and the bottle or vial seal or syringe package is undamaged.
Diluents in Pentothal Kits, Ready-to-Mix Syringes or Vials should not be used for fluid or sodium chloride replacement.

WARNINGS

Intravenous administration of Sterile Water for Injection, USP without a solute may result in hemolysis.
Use aseptic technique for preparing Pentothal (Thiopental Sodium for Injection, USP) solutions when using Pentothal Kits, Syringes or Vials and during withdrawal from reconstituted single or multiple use containers.
Administer only clear reconstituted solutions.
Use within 24 hours after reconstitution. Discard unused portions.

PRECAUTIONS

Inspect reconstituted (mixed) solutions of Pentothal (Thiopental Sodium for Injection, USP) for clarity and freedom from precipitation or discoloration prior to administration.
Use Transfer Label in each Pentothal Kit and affix to container of reconstituted solution to show concentration and time of preparation.
Pregnancy Category C. Animal reproduction studies have not been conducted with sodium chloride. It is also not known whether sodium chloride can cause fetal harm when administered to a pregnant woman or can affect reproduction capacity. Sodium chloride should be given a pregnant woman only if clearly needed.

ADVERSE REACTIONS

Reactions which may occur because of the diluents, technique of preparation or mixing, or administration of reconstituted solutions of Pentothal (Thiopental Sodium for Injection, USP) include febrile response or infection at the site of injection, venous thrombosis or phlebitis extending from the site of injection and extravasation.
If an adverse reaction does occur, discontinue the injection, evaluate the patient, institute appropriate therapeutic countermeasures and save the remainder of unused solution (or the used container or syringe) for examination if deemed necessary.

DRUG ABUSE AND DEPENDENCE

None known.

OVERDOSAGE

Used as diluents for preparing solutions of Pentothal (Thiopental Sodium for Injection, USP) the small volumes of administered fluid (from Sterile Water for Injection in bottles and vials) and amounts of sodium chloride (from 0.9% Sodium Chloride Injection in Ready-to-Mix Syringes) are unlikely to pose a threat of fluid or sodium chloride overload.

DOSAGE AND ADMINISTRATION

Pentothal (Thiopental Sodium for Injection, USP) solutions should be administered only by intravenous injection and by individuals experienced in the conduct of intravenous anesthesia.
The volume of choice of diluent for preparing Pentothal (Thiopental Sodium for Injection, USP) solutions for clinical use depends on the concentration and vehicle desired. Pentothal Kits provide only Sterile Water for Injection as the diluent for individual or multi-patient use; Pentothal Ready-to-Mix Syringes provide 0.9% Sodium Chloride Injection, USP or Sterile Water for Injection as the diluent for individual patient use; vials provide only Sterile Water for Injection, USP as the diluent for individual patient use.
Parenteral drug products should be inspected visually for particulate matter and discoloration prior to administration, whenever solution and container permit. See PRECAUTIONS.

HOW SUPPLIED

The diluent in Pentothal Kits is supplied in various size partial-fill glass containers with various dosage sizes of Pentothal (Thiopental Sodium for Injection, USP). Kits include all items needed for aseptic transfer of Pentothal powder from a squeeze bottle into the diluent partial-fill container.
The diluent in Pentothal Ready-to-Mix Syringes is supplied in a separate vial injector or vial to permit intrasyringe mixing with the Pentothal in a powder vial which is then removed to permit immediate intravenous injection of reconstituted solution into a vein or attachment to a standard stopcock assembly.
Vials are supplied in cartons with different dosage sizes of Pentothal (Thiopental Sodium for Injection, USP) for preparing 2.0% or 2.5% concentrations by using a separate syringe (not supplied) for mixing.
See attached table above for list of sizes available.
Exposure of pharmaceutical products to heat should be minimized. Avoid excessive heat. Protect from freezing. It is recommended that the product be stored at room temperature (25° C); however, brief exposure up to 40° C does not adversely affect the product.
Keep reconstituted solution in a cool place.

CAUTION

Federal (USA) law prohibits dispensing without prescription.
06-3806-R4-5/86

Pentothal® and Diluent in Kits, Ready-to-Mix Syringes and Vials

List No.	Pentothal	Pentothal Container	Diluent (mL)*	Diluent Container	Theoretical Reconstituted Conc. (%)
6259	2.5 g	Squeeze Bottle	W (125)	PF Bottle	2.0
6108	5.0 g	Squeeze Bottle	W (250)	PF Bottle	2.0
6244	1.0 g	Squeeze Bottle	W (40)	PF Bottle	2.5
6260	2.5 g	Squeeze Bottle	W (100)	PF Bottle	2.5
6504	5.0 g	Squeeze Bottle	W (200)	PF Bottle	2.5
6435	1.0 g	Vial	W (50)	Plastic Vial	2.0
3329	500 mg	Vial	W (20)	Plastic Vial	2.5
6246	400 mg	Syringe	S (20)	Syringe	2.0
6241	250 mg	Syringe	S (10)	Syringe	2.5
6243	500 mg	Syringe	S (20)	Syringe	2.5

PF — denotes Partial Fill
W — denotes Sterile Water for Injection, USP
S — denotes 0.9% Sodium Chloride Injection, USP

*Diluent containers are slighlty overfilled to assure compliance with USP minimum fill volume requirements.

PHENURONE® ℞

[fĕn ′ū-rōne]
(phenacemide tablets, USP)

DESCRIPTION

PHENURONE (phenacemide) is a valuable antiepileptic drug for use in selected patients with epilepsy. Since therapy with PHENURONE involves certain risks, *physicians should thoroughly familiarize themselves with the undesirable side effects which may occur and the precautions to be observed.* PHENURONE (phenacemide) is a substituted acetylurea derivative. Chemically PHENURONE is identified as N-(aminocarbonyl)-benzeneacetamide. PHENURONE tablets contain 500 mg phenacemide for oral administration.

INACTIVE INGREDIENTS

Corn starch, lactose, talc and other ingredients.

CLINICAL PHARMACOLOGY

In experimental animals, PHENURONE in doses well below those causing neurological signs, elevates the threshold for minimal electroshock convulsions and abolishes the tonic phase of maximal electroshock seizures. The drug prevents or modifies seizures induced by pentylenetetrazol or other convulsants. In comparative tests, PHENURONE was found to be equal or more effective than other commonly used antiepileptics against complex partial (psychomotor) seizures which were induced in mice by low frequency stimulation of the cerebral cortex. Studies in mice have shown that PHENURONE exerts a synergistic antiepileptic effect with mephenytoin, phenobarbital, or trimethadione.
Given orally to laboratory animals, PHENURONE has a low acute toxicity. In mice, slight ataxia appears at 400 mg/kg and light sleep occurs at 800 mg/kg. In high doses the drug causes marked ataxia and coma, the fatal dose being in the range of 3 to 5 g/kg for mice, rats, and cats.
PHENURONE is metabolized by the liver, however, further definition of human pharmacokinetics has not been determined.

INDICATIONS AND USAGE

PHENURONE (phenacemide) is indicated for the control of severe epilepsy, particularly mixed forms of complex partial (psychomotor) seizures, refractory to other drugs.

CONTRAINDICATIONS

PHENURONE should not be administered unless other available antiepileptics have been found to be ineffective in satisfactorily controlling seizures.

WARNINGS

PHENURONE (phenacemide) can produce serious side effects as well as direct organ toxicity. As a consequence its use entails the assumption of certain risks which must be weighed against the benefit to the patient. *Ordinarily* PHENURONE *should not be administered unless other available antiepileptics have been found to be ineffective in controlling seizures.*
Death attributable to liver damage during therapy with PHENURONE has been reported. PHENURONE should be used with caution in patients with a history of previous liver dysfunction. If jaundice or other signs of hepatitis appear, the drug should be discontinued.
Aplastic anemia has occurred in association with PHENURONE therapy and death from this condition has been reported. PHENURONE should ordinarily not be used in patients with severe blood dyscrasias. Marked depression of the blood count is an indication for withdrawal of the drug.
Usage During Pregnancy: PHENURONE can cause fetal harm when administered to a pregnant woman. There are multiple reports in the clinical literature which indicate that the use of antiepileptic drugs during pregnancy results in an increased incidence of birth defects in the offspring. Reports have also suggested that the maternal ingestion of antiepileptic drugs, particularly barbiturates, is associated with a neonatal coagulation defect that may cause bleeding during the early (usually within 24 hours of birth) neonatal period. The possibility of the occurrence of this defect with the use of PHENURONE should be kept in mind. The defect is characterized by decreased levels of vitamin K-dependent clotting factors, and prolongation of either the prothrombin time or the partial thromboplastin time, or both. It has been suggested that vitamin K be given prophylactically to the mother one month prior to and during delivery, and to the infant, intravenously, immediately after birth. If this drug is used during pregnancy, or if the patient becomes pregnant while taking this drug, the patient should be apprised of the potential hazard to the fetus.

PRECAUTIONS

General: Extreme caution must be exercised in treating patients who previously have shown personality disorders. It may be advisable to hospitalize such patients during the first week of treatment. Personality changes, including attempts at suicide and the occurrence of psychoses requiring hospitalization, have been reported during therapy with PHENURONE (phenacemide). Severe or exacerbated personality changes are an indication for withdrawal of the drug.
PHENURONE (phenacemide) should be used with caution in patients with a history of previous liver dysfunction.
PHENURONE should be administered with caution to patients with a history of allergy, particularly in association with the administration of other antiepileptics. The drug should be discontinued at the first sign of a skin rash or other allergic manifestation.
Information for Patients: The patient and his family should be aware of the possibility of personality changes so the family can watch for changes in the behavior of the patient such as decreased interest in surroundings, depression, or aggressiveness.
The patient should be told to report immediately any symptoms indicative of a developing blood dyscrasia such as malaise, sore throat, or fever.
Laboratory Tests: Liver function tests should be performed before and during therapy. Death attributable to liver damage during therapy with PHENURONE has been reported. If jaundice or other signs of hepatitis appear, the drug should be discontinued.
Complete blood counts should be made before instituting PHENURONE, and at monthly intervals thereafter. If no abnormality appears within 12 months, the interval between blood counts may be extended. Blood changes have been reported with leukopenia (leukocyte count of 4,000 or less per cubic millimeter of blood) as the most commonly observed effect. However, aplastic anemia has occurred in association with PHENURONE therapy, and death from this condition has been reported. *The total number of each cellular element per cubic millimeter is a better index of possible blood dyscrasia than the percentage of cells.* Marked depression of the blood count is an indication for withdrawal of the drug.
Similarly, as nephritis has occasionally occurred in patients on PHENURONE, the urine should be examined at regular intervals. Abnormal urinary findings are an indication for discontinuance of therapy.
Drug Interactions: Extreme caution is essential if PHENURONE is administered with any other antiepileptic which is known to cause similar toxic effects.
Considerable caution should be exercised if PHENURONE (phenacemide) is administered concurrently with *Peganone (ethotoin)* since paranoid symptoms have been reported during therapy with this combination.
Carcinogenesis: No data are available on long-term potential for carcinogenicity in animals or humans.
Pregnancy: Pregnancy Category D. See "Warnings" section.
Nursing Mothers: It is not known whether this drug is excreted in human milk. Because many drugs are excreted in human milk and because of the potential for serious adverse

Continued on next page

If desired, additional literature on any Abbott Product will be provided upon request to Abbott Laboratories.

Abbott—Cont.

reactions in nursing infants from PHENURONE, a decision should be made whether to discontinue nursing or to discontinue the drug, taking into account the importance of the drug to the mother.

Pediatric Use: Safety and effectiveness in children below the age of 5 years have not been established.

ADVERSE REACTIONS

The following adverse effects associated with PHENURONE are listed by decreasing order of frequency based on data from one large clinical study.[1]

Psychiatric: Psychic changes (17 in 100 patients).

Gastrointestinal: Gastrointestinal disturbances (8 in 100 patients), including anorexia (5 in 100 patients) and weight loss (less than 1 in 100 patients).

Dermatologic: Skin rash (5 in 100 patients).

CNS: Drowsiness (4 in 100 patients), headache (2 in 100 patients), insomnia (1 in 100 patients), dizziness and paresthesias (less than 1 in 100 patients).

Hematopoietic: Blood dyscrasias (primarily leukopenia), including fatal aplastic anemia (2 in 100 patients).

Hepatic: Hepatitis, including fatalities (2 in 100 patients).

Renal: Abnormal urinary findings, including a rise in serum creatinine[2], and nephritis (1 in 100 patients or less).

Other: Fatigue, fever, muscle pain and palpitation (less than 1 in 100 patients).

OVERDOSAGE

Symptoms of acute overdosage include excitement or mania, followed by drowsiness, ataxia and coma. In one case of acute overdosage, dizziness was followed by coma which lasted nearly 24 hours. Treatment should be started by inducing emesis; gastric lavage may be considered as an alternative or adjunct. General supportive measures will be necessary. A careful evaluation of liver and kidney function, mental state, and the blood-forming organs should be made following recovery.

DOSAGE AND ADMINISTRATION

PHENURONE is administered orally.

Since PHENURONE may produce serious toxic effects, it is strongly recommended that the dosage be held to the minimum amount necessary to achieve an adequate therapeutic effect.

For adults the usual starting dose is 1.5 g daily, administered in three divided doses of 500 mg each. After the first week, if seizures are not controlled and the drug is well tolerated, an additional 500 mg tablet may be taken upon arising. In the third week, if necessary, the dosage may be further increased by another 500 mg at bedtime. Satisfactory results have been noted in some patients on an initial dose of 250 mg three times per day. The effective total daily dose for adults usually ranges from 2 to 3 g, although some patients have required as much as 5 g daily.

For the pediatric patient from 5 to 10 years of age, approximately one-half the adult dose is recommended. It should be given at the same intervals as for adults.

PHENURONE may be administered alone or in conjunction with other antiepileptics. However, extreme caution must be exercised if other antiepileptics cause toxic effects similar to PHENURONE.

When PHENURONE is to replace other antiepileptic medication, the latter should be withdrawn gradually as the dosage of PHENURONE is increased to maintain seizure control.

HOW SUPPLIED

PHENURONE (Phenacemide Tablets, USP), grooved, white, 500 mg are supplied in bottles of 100 (**NDC** 0074-3971-05).

REFERENCES

1. Tyler, M. W., King, E. Q.: Phenacemide in Treatment of Epilepsy. JAMA 147: 17–21 (1951).
2. Richards, R.K., Bjornsson, T. D., Waterbury, L. D.: Rise in Serum and Urine Creatinine After Phenacemide. Clin. Pharmacol. Ther. 23: 430–437 (1978).

Abbott Laboratories
North Chicago, IL 60064
Ref. 01-2350-R8

PLACIDYL® ℞ Ⓒ

[pla'ci-dil]
(ethchlorvynol capsules, USP)
Oral hypnotic

DESCRIPTION

PLACIDYL (ethchlorvynol) is a tertiary carbinol. It is chemically designated as 1-chloro-3-ethyl-1-penten-4-yn-3-ol. Ethchlorvynol occurs as a liquid which is immiscible with water and miscible with most organic solvents. PLACIDYL is an oral hypnotic available in capsule form containing either 200 mg, 500 mg or 750 mg of ethchlorvynol.

INACTIVE INGREDIENTS

200 mg capsule: FD&C Red No. 40, gelatin, glycerin, methylparaben, polyethylene glycol, propylparaben, sorbitol, titanium dioxide and other ingredients.

500 mg capsule: FD&C Red No. 40, gelatin, glycerin, iron oxide, methylparaben, polyethylene glycol, propylparaben, sorbitol, titanium dioxide and other ingredients.

750 mg capsule: FD&C Blue No. 1, FD&C Yellow No. 5 (tartrazine), FD&C Yellow No. 6, gelatin, glycerin, iron oxide, methylparaben, polyethylene glycol, propylparaben, sorbitol, titanium dioxide and other ingredients.

CLINICAL PHARMACOLOGY

The usual hypnotic dose of PLACIDYL induces sleep within 15 minutes to one hour. The duration of the hypnotic effect is about five hours. The mechanism of action is unknown.

PLACIDYL is rapidly absorbed from the gastrointestinal tract with peak plasma concentrations usually occurring within two hours after a single oral fasting dose. Plasma concentrations required for hypnotic effects are unknown. The plasma half-life ($t_{1/2}$, β) of the parent compound is approximately ten to twenty hours. Studies with ^{14}C-PLACIDYL have demonstrated that within 24 hours, 33% of a single 500 mg dose is excreted in the urine mostly as metabolites. The major plasma and urinary metabolite is the secondary alcohol of PLACIDYL. The free and conjugated forms of this metabolite in the urine account for about 40% of the dose. Other minor metabolites have been identified as the primary alcohol and a secondary alcohol with an altered acetylene group. Studies with ^{14}C-PLACIDYL in animals indicate that the parent compound and its metabolites undergo extensive enterohepatic recirculation.

Distribution studies indicate that there is extensive tissue localization of ethchlorvynol, particularly in adipose tissue. Ethchlorvynol and/or its metabolites have also been detected in liver, kidneys, spleen, brain, bile and cerebrospinal fluid.

INDICATIONS AND USAGE

PLACIDYL is indicated as short-term hypnotic therapy for periods up to one week in duration for the management of insomnia. If retreatment becomes necessary, after drug-free intervals of one or more weeks, it should only be undertaken upon further evaluation of the patient.

CONTRAINDICATIONS

PLACIDYL is contraindicated in patients with known hypersensitivity to the drug and in patients with porphyria.

WARNINGS

PLACIDYL SHOULD BE ADMINISTERED WITH CAUTION TO MENTALLY DEPRESSED PATIENTS WITH OR WITHOUT SUICIDAL TENDENCIES. IT SHOULD ALSO BE ADMINISTERED WITH CAUTION TO THOSE WHO HAVE A PSYCHOLOGICAL POTENTIAL FOR DRUG DEPENDENCE. THE LEAST AMOUNT OF DRUG THAT IS FEASIBLE SHOULD BE PRESCRIBED FOR THESE PATIENTS.

Psychological and Physical Dependence: PROLONGED USE OF PLACIDYL MAY RESULT IN TOLERANCE AND PSYCHOLOGICAL AND PHYSICAL DEPENDENCE. PROLONGED ADMINISTRATION OF THE DRUG IS NOT RECOMMENDED. (See "Drug Abuse and Dependence" section.)

PRECAUTIONS

General: Elderly or debilitated patients should receive the smallest effective amount of PLACIDYL (ethchlorvynol).

Caution should be exercised when treating patients with impaired hepatic or renal function.

Patients who exhibit unpredictable behavior, or paradoxical restlessness or excitement in response to barbiturates or alcohol may react in this manner to PLACIDYL.

PLACIDYL should not be used for the management of insomnia in the presence of pain unless insomnia persists after pain is controlled with analgesics.

The 750 mg dosage strength of PLACIDYL contains FD&C Yellow No. 5 (tartrazine) which may cause allergic-type reactions (including bronchial asthma) in certain susceptible individuals. Although the overall incidence of FD&C Yellow No. 5 (tartrazine) sensitivity in the general population is low, it is frequently seen in patients who also have aspirin hypersensitivity.

Information for Patients: The use of ethchlorvynol carries with it an associated risk of psychological and/or physical dependence. The patient should be warned against increasing the dose of the drug without consulting a physician.

Patients should be advised that, for the duration of the effect of PLACIDYL, mental and/or physical abilities required for the performance of potentially hazardous tasks such as the operation of dangerous machinery including motor vehicles, may be impaired.

Patients should be cautioned to avoid the concomitant use of PLACIDYL with alcohol, barbiturates, other CNS depressants, or MAO inhibitors.

Drug Interactions: The concomitant use of PLACIDYL with alcohol, barbiturates, other CNS depressants, or MAO inhibitors may produce exaggerated depressant effects.

Ethchlorvynol may cause a decreased prothrombin time response to coumarin anticoagulants; therefore, the dosage of these drugs may require adjustment when therapy with ethchlorvynol is initiated and after it is discontinued.

Transient delirium has been reported with the concomitant use of PLACIDYL and amitriptyline; therefore, PLACIDYL should be administered with caution to patients receiving tricyclic antidepressants.

Carcinogenesis: A study in mice receiving oral doses of PLACIDYL up to 7 times the maximum human daily dose for 22 to 24 months produced equivocal results. When compared to controls, a statistically significant increase in total lung tumors was found in female mice given the high dose of PLACIDYL. However, the 48% incidence is not substantially higher than the high value (39%) reported for the historical laboratory controls.

No evidence of carcinogenic potential was observed in rats given PLACIDYL at 5 to 15 times the maximum human daily dose for up to 2 years.

Usage During Pregnancy: 1. Teratogenic—Pregnancy Category C. Ethchlorvynol has been associated with a higher percentage of stillbirths and a lower survival rate of progeny among rats given 40 mg/kg/day. There are no adequate and well-controlled studies in pregnant women. Therefore, ethchlorvynol is not recommended for use during the first and second trimesters of pregnancy. Ethchlorvynol should be used during pregnancy only if the potential benefit justifies the potential risk to the fetus.

2. Non-teratogenic—Clinical experience has indicated that ethchlorvynol taken during the third trimester of pregnancy may produce CNS depression and transient withdrawal symptoms in the newborn. These symptoms resemble congenital narcotic withdrawal symptoms (See "Drug Abuse and Dependence" section).

Nursing Mothers: It is not known whether this drug is excreted in breast milk. Because many drugs are excreted in human milk and because of the potential for serious adverse reactions in nursing infants from PLACIDYL, a decision should be made whether to discontinue nursing or to discontinue the drug, taking into account the importance of the drug to the mother.

Pediatric Use: PLACIDYL is not recommended for use in children since its safety and effectiveness in the pediatric age group has not been determined.

ADVERSE REACTIONS

Adverse effects in decreasing order of severity within each of the following categories are:

Hypersensitivity: cholestatic jaundice, urticaria and rash.

Hematologic: thrombocytopenia—one case of fatal immune thrombocytopenia due to ethchlorvynol has been reported.

Gastrointestinal: vomiting, gastric upset, nausea and aftertaste.

Neurologic: dizziness and facial numbness.

Miscellaneous: blurred vision, hypotension and mild "hangover".

The following idiosyncratic responses have been reported occasionally: syncope without marked hypotension, profound muscular weakness, hysteria, marked excitement, prolonged hypnosis and mild stimulation.

Transient ataxia and giddiness have occurred in patients in whom absorption of the drug is especially rapid. These effects can sometimes be controlled by giving PLACIDYL with food.

(See "Drug Abuse and Dependence" section for the signs and symptoms of chronic intoxication).

DRUG ABUSE AND DEPENDENCE

PLACIDYL is subject to control by the Federal Controlled Substances Act under DEA schedule IV.

Abuse: Pulmonary edema of rapid onset has resulted from the I.V. abuse of PLACIDYL (ethchlorvynol).

Dependence: Signs and symptoms of intoxication have been reported with the prolonged use of doses as low as 1 g/day. Signs and symptoms of chronic intoxication may include incoordination, tremors, ataxia, confusion, slurred speech, hyperreflexia, diplopia, and generalized muscle weakness. Toxic amblyopia, scotoma, nystagmus, and peripheral neuropathy have also been reported with prolonged use of ethchlorvynol; these symptoms are usually reversible.

Severe withdrawal symptoms similar to those seen during barbiturate and alcohol withdrawal have been reported following abrupt discontinuance of prolonged use of PLACIDYL. These symptoms may appear as late as nine days after sudden withdrawal of the drug. Signs and symptoms of PLACIDYL withdrawal may include convulsions, delirium, schizoid reaction, perceptual distortions, memory loss, ataxia, insomnia, slurring of speech, unusual anxiety, irritability, agitation, and tremors. Other signs and symptoms may include anorexia, nausea, vomiting, weakness, dizziness, sweating, muscle twitching, and weight loss.

Management of a patient who manifests withdrawal symptoms from PLACIDYL involves readministration of the drug to approximately the same level of chronic intoxication which existed before the abrupt discontinuance. (Phenobarbital may be substituted for PLACIDYL.) A gradual, stepwise reduction of dosage may then be made over a period of days or weeks. A phenothiazine compound may be used in addition to this regimen for those patients who exhibit psychotic symptoms during the withdrawal period. The patient undergoing withdrawal from PLACIDYL must be hospitalized or closely observed, and given general supportive care as indicated.

In one report an infant born to a mother who received 500 mg PLACIDYL at bedtime daily throughout the third trimester, exhibited withdrawal symptoms on the second day of life. The symptoms included episodic jitteriness, hyperactivity, restlessness, irritability, disturbed sleep and hunger. The neonate responded to a single oral dose of phenobarbital (3 mg/kg). The withdrawal symptoms gradually decreased and completely disappeared by the tenth day of life.

OVERDOSAGE

Acute intoxication is characterized by prolonged deep coma, severe respiratory depression, hypothermia, hypotension, and relative bradycardia. Nystagmus and pancytopenia resulting from acute PLACIDYL overdose have been reported.

Although death has occurred following the ingestion of 6 g of PLACIDYL, there have been reports of patients who have survived overdoses of 50 g and more with intensive care. Fatal blood concentrations usually range from 20 to 50 μg/ml.[1] Because large amounts of ethchlorvynol are taken up by adipose tissue, the blood concentration is an unreliable indicator of the magnitude of overdose.

Management of acute PLACIDYL intoxication is similar to that of acute barbiturate intoxication.[2] Gastric evacuation should be performed immediately. (In the unconscious patient, gastric lavage should be preceded by tracheal intubation with a cuffed tube.) Supportive care (assisted ventilation, frequent and careful monitoring of vital signs, control of blood pressure) is essential. Emphasis should be placed on pulmonary care and monitoring of blood gases. Hemoperfusion utilizing the Amberlite column technique has been reported in the literature to be the most effective method in the management of acute PLACIDYL overdose.[3] In addition, hemodialysis and peritoneal dialysis have each been reported to be of some value. (Aqueous and oil dialysates have been used. Forced diuresis with maintenance of a high urinary output has also been reported of some value.) (See "Drug Abuse and Dependence" section for the signs and symptoms of chronic intoxication.)

DOSAGE AND ADMINISTRATION

The usual adult hypnotic dose of PLACIDYL (ethchlorvynol) is 500 mg taken orally at bedtime. A dose of 750 mg may be required for patients whose sleep response to a 500 mg capsule is inadequate, or for patients being changed from barbiturates or other nonbarbiturate hypnotics. Up to 1000 mg may be given as a single bedtime dose when insomnia is unusually severe. A single supplemental dose of 200 mg may be given to reinstitute sleep in patients who may awaken after the original bedtime dose of 500 or 750 mg.

For patients whose insomnia is characterized only by untimely awakening during the early morning hours, a single dose of 200 mg taken upon awakening may be adequate for relief.

The smallest effective dose of PLACIDYL should be given to elderly or debilitated patients.

PLACIDYL should not be prescribed for periods exceeding one week. (See "Drug Abuse and Dependence" section.)

HOW SUPPLIED

PLACIDYL (ethchlorvynol capsules, USP) is supplied as:

200 mg red capsules:
Bottles of 100 .... (**NDC** 0074-6661-08).

500 mg red capsules:
Bottles of 100 .... (**NDC** 0074-6685-15).
Bottles of 500 .... (**NDC** 0074-6685-02).
ABBO-PAC® unit dose strip packages of 100 .... (**NDC** 0074-6685-10).

750 mg green capsules:
Bottles of 100 .... (**NDC** 0074-6630-01).

REFERENCES

1. AMA Dept. of Drugs. *AMA Drug Evaluations,* Massachusetts: Publishing Sciences Group, Inc., 1980.
2. Khantzian, E. J., McKenna, G. J., Acute Toxic and Withdrawal Reactions Associated with Drug Abuse, *Annals of Internal Medicine,* 90:361–372, 1979.
3. Lynn, R.I., et al. Resin Hemoperfusion for Treatment of Ethchlorvynol Overdose, *Annals of Internal Medicine,* 91:549–553, 1979.

Shown in Product Identification Section, page 403

Abbott Laboratories
North Chicago, IL 60064
Ref. 01-2363-R7

QUELIDRINE® SYRUP

[quel 'i-drēn]
(non-narcotic, antihistaminic cough suppressant)

COMPOSITION

Each teaspoonful (5 ml) contains:

Dextromethorphan Hydrobromide	10 mg
Chlorpheniramine Maleate	2 mg
Ephedrine Hydrochloride	5 mg
Phenylephrine Hydrochloride	5 mg
Ammonium Chloride	40 mg
Ipecac Fluidextract	0.005 ml

INACTIVE INGREDIENTS

Alcohol 2%, D&C Red No. 33, glycerin, liquid glucose, magnesium carbonate, methylparaben, propylparaben, sucrose, tolu balsam tincture, water, artificial flavors and other ingredients forming a palatable, aromatic syrup.

ACTION AND INDICATIONS

Quelidrine is designed as an aid in the management of cough associated with acute or subacute simple respiratory infections. Quelidrine provides a wide range of therapeutic action against the cough complex—without the risk of addiction or the production of undue central depression.

WARNINGS

As with any drug, if you are pregnant or nursing a baby, seek the advice of a health professional before using this product. Keep this and all medicines out of the reach of children.

PRECAUTIONS

Quelidrine should be administered with caution to patients with hypertension, serious organic heart disease, angina pectoris, diabetes, thyroid disease, or to persons receiving digitalis. When cough persists or accompanies a high fever, the underlying cause and need for other medication should be reevaluated.

SIDE EFFECTS

Quelidrine is safe for patients of all ages, but professional supervision of dosage for young patients is essential. Side effects are infrequent. Drowsiness, nausea, vomiting, nervousness, palpitation, blurred vision and insomnia may occur in susceptible patients. Constipation is seldom a problem. If side effects are encountered, dosage should be reduced or medication withdrawn.

DOSAGE AND ADMINISTRATION

Adults—1 teaspoonful, one to four times daily. Children 6 years of age or older, ½ teaspoonful, one to four times daily. Children 2 to 6 years old, ¼ teaspoonful one to four times daily. Under 2, as directed by physician. Quelidrine may be diluted with Syrup, NF in order to facilitate pediatric administration.

HOW SUPPLIED

Quelidrine Syrup is supplied in bottles of 4 fluid ounces (**NDC** 0074-6883-04), with or without a prescription.
Store below 77°F (25°C).
Abbott Laboratories
North Chicago, IL 60064
Ref. 07-5368-R20

SELSUN® ℞

[sel 'sun]
(selenium sulfide lotion, USP)

DESCRIPTION

SELSUN (selenium sulfide lotion) is a liquid antiseborrheic, antifungal preparation for topical application, containing selenium sulfide 2 ½% w/v in aqueous suspension; also contains: bentonite, lauric diethanolamide, ethylene glycol monostearate, titanium dioxide, amphoteric-2, sodium lauryl sulfate, sodium phosphate (monobasic), glyceryl monoricinoleate, citric acid, captan, and perfume.

Clinical Pharmacology: Selenium sulfide appears to have a cytostatic effect on cells of the epidermis and follicular epithelium, thus reducing corneocyte production.

INDICATIONS AND USAGE

For the treatment of dandruff and seborrheic dermatitis of the scalp.
For treatment of tinea versicolor.

CONTRAINDICATIONS

SELSUN should not be used by patients allergic to any of its components.

PRECAUTIONS

General: Should not be used when acute inflammation or exudation is present as increased absorption may occur.

Information for Patients: Application to skin or scalp may produce skin irritation or sensitization. If sensitivity reactions occur, use should be discontinued. May be irritating to mucous membranes of the eyes and contact with this area should be avoided. When applied to the body for treatment of tinea versicolor, SELSUN may produce skin irritation especially in the genital area and where skin folds occur. These areas should be thoroughly rinsed after application.

Carcinogenesis: Studies in mice using dermal application of 25% and 50% solutions of 2.5% selenium sulfide lotion over an 88 week period, indicated no carcinogenic effects.

Pregnancy: WHEN USED ON BODY SURFACES FOR THE TREATMENT OF TINEA VERSICOLOR, SELSUN IS CLASSIFIED AS PREGNANCY CATEGORY C. Animal reproduction studies have not been conducted with SELSUN. It is also not known whether SELSUN can cause fetal harm when applied to body surfaces of a pregnant woman or can affect reproduction capacity. Under ordinary circumstances SELSUN should not be used for the treatment of tinea versicolor in pregnant women.

Pediatric Use: Safety and effectiveness in infants have not been established.

ADVERSE REACTIONS

In decreasing order of severity: skin irritation; occasional reports of increase in amount of normal hair loss; discoloration of hair (can be avoided or minimized by thorough rinsing of hair after treatment). As with other shampoos, oiliness or dryness of hair and scalp may occur.

OVERDOSAGE

Accidental Oral Ingestion:
Selsun is intended for external use only. There have been no documented reports of serious toxicity in humans resulting from acute ingestion of SELSUN, however, acute toxicity studies in animals suggest that ingestion of large amounts could result in potential human toxicity. For this reason, evacuation of the stomach contents should be considered in cases of acute oral ingestion.

DOSAGE AND ADMINISTRATION

For treatment of dandruff and seborrheic dermatitis:

1. Massage about 1 or 2 teaspoonfuls of shampoo into wet scalp.
2. Allow to remain on the scalp for 2 to 3 minutes.
3. Rinse scalp thoroughly.
4. Repeat application and rinse thoroughly.
5. After treatment, wash hands well.

For the usual case, two applications each week for two weeks will afford control. After this, the lotion may be used at less frequent intervals—weekly, every two weeks, or even every 3 or 4 weeks in some cases. The preparation should not be applied more frequently than required to maintain control.

For treatment of tinea versicolor: Apply to affected areas and lather with a small amount of water. Allow product to remain on skin for 10 minutes, then rinse the body thoroughly. Repeat this procedure once a day for 7 days. The product may damage jewelry; jewelry should be removed before use.

HOW SUPPLIED

SELSUN (selenium sulfide lotion, USP) is supplied in 4-fluidounce nonbreakable plastic bottles (**NDC** 0074-2660-04). SELSUN is to be dispensed only on the prescription of a physician.
Abbott Laboratories
North Chicago, IL 60064

SURBEX®

[sir 'bex]
Vitamin B-Complex

SURBEX® with C

Vitamin B-Complex with Vitamin C

(See PDR For Nonprescription Drugs)

SURBEX-T®

[sir 'bex-t]
High-Potency Vitamin B-Complex with 500 mg of Vitamin C

(See PDR For Nonprescription Drugs)
Shown in Product Identification Section, page 403

SURBEX®-750 with IRON

[sir 'bex ī-ron]
High-potency B-complex with iron, vitamin E and 750 mg vitamin C

(See PDR For Nonprescription Drugs)
Shown in Product Identification Section, page 403

Continued on next page

If desired, additional literature on any Abbott Product will be provided upon request to Abbott Laboratories.

Abbott—Cont.

SURBEX®-750 with ZINC
[*sir'bex zinc*]
High-potency B-complex with zinc, vitamin E and 750 mg vitamin C

(See PDR For Nonprescription Drugs)
Shown in Product Identification Section, page 403

TRAL® Filmtab® Tablets ℞
[*trăl*]
(hexocyclium methylsulfate)

DESCRIPTION

TRAL (hexocyclium methylsulfate) is a quaternary ammonium salt. Chemically, it is designated as N-(beta-cyclohexyl-beta-hydroxy-beta-phenylethyl)-N′-methylpiperazine methosulfate. Physically, TRAL is a white powder soluble in water or physiological saline yielding a stable solution.

INACTIVE INGREDIENTS

Albumen, castor oil, cellulosic polymers, corn starch, FD&C Blue No. 1, FD&C Blue No. 2, FD&C Yellow No. 5 (tartrazine), lactose, polyethylene glycol, povidone, propylene glycol, sodium citrate, sorbitan monooleate, stearic acid, talc, titanium dioxide and other ingredients.

ACTIONS

Clinically, TRAL is an effective anticholinergic agent which inhibits gastric secretion and gastrointestinal motility.
The drug has an antimuscarinic action similar to that of other quaternary ammonium compounds which produce anticholinergic effects. In experimental animals the drug has been shown to decrease gastric secretion, prevent gastric ulceration, decrease gastrointestinal motility, dilate the pupils, inhibit salivation, increase the heart rate, and counteract the peripheral muscarinic effect of choline esters. With massive overdosage the drug also may produce a peripheral curare-like neuromuscular block and ganglionic blockade. In studies with human subjects, TRAL produced a decrease in gastric acidity, and a decrease in the volume of gastric secretion.
TRAL is absorbed from the gastrointestinal tract but the degree of absorption varies. Following oral administration of a single dose of the drug in conventional tablet form, its effects persist for 3 to 4 hours. The metabolic fate and route of excretion are unknown.

INDICATIONS

TRAL is indicated as adjunctive therapy in the treatment of peptic ulcer. IT SHOULD BE NOTED AT THIS POINT IN TIME THAT THERE IS A LACK OF CONCURRENCE AS TO THE VALUE OF ANTICHOLINERGICS IN THE TREATMENT OF GASTRIC ULCER. IT HAS NOT BEEN SHOWN WHETHER ANTICHOLINERGIC DRUGS AID IN THE HEALING OF A PEPTIC ULCER, DECREASE THE RATE OF RECURRENCES OR PREVENT COMPLICATION. To be effective the dosage must be titrated to the individual patient's needs.

CONTRAINDICATIONS

TRAL is contraindicated in patients with glaucoma; obstructive uropathy (for example, bladder neck obstruction due to prostatic hypertrophy); obstructive disease of the gastrointestinal tract (as in achalasia, paralytic ileus, pyloroduodenal stenosis, etc.); intestinal atony of the elderly or debilitated patient; unstable cardiovascular status; in acute hemorrhage; severe ulcerative colitis; toxic megacolon complicating ulcerative colitis; myasthenia gravis.

WARNINGS

In the presence of a high environmental temperature, heat prostration can occur with drug use (fever and heat stroke due to decreased sweating).
TRAL may produce drowsiness or blurred vision. In this event, the patient should be warned not to engage in activities requiring mental alertness such as operating a motor vehicle or other machinery, or perform hazardous work while taking this drug.
Usage in Pregnancy and Lactation: The safety of TRAL for use during pregnancy or lactation has not been established. When given to pregnant rabbits at daily oral doses of 2.5 and 40 mg/kg/day, which are 1.2 and 20 times the human dose, TRAL increased the rate of abortion and fetal resorption.
As with all anticholinergic drugs, an inhibitory effect on lactation may occur.

PRECAUTIONS

TRAL should be used with caution in patients with:
Autonomic neuropathy.
Hepatic or renal disease.
Ulcerative colitis—large doses may suppress intestinal motility to the point of producing a paralytic ileus and the use of this drug may precipitate or aggravate the serious complication of toxic megacolon.
Hyperthyroidism, coronary heart disease, congestive heart failure, cardiac arrhythmias, hypertension and non-obstructing prostatic hypertrophy.
Hiatal hernia associated with reflux esophagitis since anticholinergic drugs may aggravate this condition.
It should be noted that the use of anticholinergic drugs in the treatment of gastric ulcer may produce a delay in gastric emptying time and may complicate such therapy (antral stasis).
Investigate any tachycardia before giving anticholinergic (atropine-like) drugs since they may increase the heart rate.
With overdosage, a curare-like action may occur.
This product contains FD&C Yellow No. 5 (tartrazine) which may cause allergic-type reactions (including bronchial asthma) in certain susceptible individuals. Although the overall incidence of FD&C Yellow No. 5 (tartrazine) sensitivity in the general population is low, it is frequently seen in patients who also have aspirin hypersensitivity.

ADVERSE REACTIONS

Adverse reactions may include xerostomia, urinary hesitancy and retention, blurred vision, mydriasis, cycloplegia, increased intraocular tension, tachycardia, palpitations, headaches, nervousness, drowsiness, weakness, dizziness, insomnia, nausea, vomiting, impotency, dysphagia, altered taste perception, heartburn, bloated feeling, constipation, paralytic ileus, flushing, decreased sweating, urticaria and other dermal manifestations, severe allergic reaction or drug idiosyncrasies, and some degree of mental confusion and/or excitement especially in elderly persons.
When side effects are severe and cannot be controlled by reduction of dosage, the medication should be withdrawn.

DOSAGE AND ADMINISTRATION

TRAL is administered orally. The usual recommended adult dose of TRAL is one 25 mg Filmtab tablet four times daily, taken before meals and at bedtime.
For optimal therapeutic effect, dosage should be adjusted to the patient's response.
TRAL is not for use in children.

OVERDOSAGE

The first sign of overdosage may be indicated by an atropine-like flush, particularly in the blush areas. Other manifestations of overdosage are revealed by the appearance or an increase in intensity of dryness of the mouth or other side effects.
With unusually large doses the quaternary ammonium type of anticholinergic agent may produce a curare-like action and ganglionic blockade manifested by respiratory paralysis and circulatory collapse. This is unlikely to occur with therapeutic doses. Neostigmine methylsulfate at a dose of 0.5 to 2 mg given by slow intravenous injection and repeated as required may be administered as an antidote. Only in exceptional cases should the total dose of neostigmine methylsulfate exceed 5 mg. Artificial respiration and other supportive measures should be applied if needed.

HOW SUPPLIED

TRAL (hexocyclium methylsulfate) Filmtab tablets, 25 mg, green, (NDC 0074-6698-02) are supplied in bottles of 100.
Abbott Laboratories
North Chicago, IL 60064

TRANXENE® ℞ Ⓒ
[*tran'zēen*]
(clorazepate dipotassium)
Capsules
Tablets
TRANXENE®-SD
& TRANXENE-SD HALF STRENGTH
(clorazepate dipotassium)
Tablets

DESCRIPTION

Chemically, TRANXENE (clorazepate dipotassium) is a benzodiazepine. The empirical formula is $C_{16}H_{11}ClK_2N_2O_4$; the molecular weight is 408.92.
The compound occurs as a fine, light yellow, practically odorless powder. It is insoluble in the common organic solvents, but very soluble in water. Aqueous solutions are unstable, clear, light yellow, and alkaline.

INACTIVE INGREDIENTS

3.75 mg Capsule: FD&C Blue No. 1, FD&C Red No. 3, FD&C Yellow No. 6, gelatin, iron oxide, magnesium stearate, microcrystalline cellulose, potassium carbonate, potassium chloride, talc, titanium dioxide and other ingredients.
7.5 mg Capsule: D&C Yellow No. 10, FD&C Blue No. 1, FD&C Red No. 3, FD&C Red No. 33, FD&C Yellow No. 6, gelatin, iron oxide, magnesium stearate, microcrystalline cellulose, potassium carbonate, potassium chloride, talc, titanium dioxide and other ingredients.
15 mg Capsule: FD&C Blue No. 1, FD&C Red No. 3, FD&C Yellow No. 6, gelatin, iron oxide, magnesium stearate, microcrystalline cellulose, potassium carbonate, potassium chloride, talc, titanium dioxide and other ingredients.
3.75 mg Tablet: Colloidal silicon dioxide, FD&C Blue No. 2, magnesium oxide, magnesium stearate, microcrystalline cellulose, potassium carbonate, potassium chloride, talc and other ingredients.
7.5 mg Tablet: Colloidal silicon dioxide, FD&C Yellow No. 6, magnesium oxide, magnesium stearate, microcrystalline cellulose, potassium carbonate, potassium chloride, talc and other ingredients.
15 mg Tablet: Colloidal silicon dioxide, FD&C Red No. 3, magnesium oxide, magnesium stearate, microcrystalline cellulose, potassium carbonate, potassium chloride, talc and other ingredients.
Tranxene-SD Tablet 22.5 mg: Castor oil wax, iron oxide, lactose, magnesium oxide, magnesium stearate, potassium carbonate, potassium chloride, talc and other ingredients.
Tranxene-SD Half Strength Tablet 11.25 mg: Castor oil wax, FD&C Blue No. 2, lactose, magnesium oxide, magnesium stearate, potassium carbonate, potassium chloride, talc and other ingredients.

ACTIONS

Pharmacologically, clorazepate dipotassium has the characteristics of the benzodiazepines. It has depressant effects on the central nervous system. The primary metabolite, nordiazepam, quickly appears in the blood stream. The serum half-life is about 2 days. The drug is metabolized in the liver and excreted primarily in the urine. (See ANIMAL AND CLINICAL PHARMACOLOGY section).

INDICATIONS

TRANXENE is indicated for the management of anxiety disorders or for the short-term relief of the symptoms of anxiety. Anxiety or tension associated with the stress of everyday life usually does not require treatment with an anxiolytic.
TRANXENE is indicated as adjunctive therapy in the management of partial seizures.
The effectiveness of TRANXENE in long-term management of anxiety, that is, more than 4 months, has not been assessed by systematic clinical studies. Long-term studies in epileptic patients, however, have shown continued therapeutic activity. The physician should reassess periodically the usefulness of the drug for the individual patient.
TRANXENE is indicated for the symptomatic relief of acute alcohol withdrawal.

CONTRAINDICATIONS

TRANXENE is contraindicated in patients with a known hypersensitivity to the drug, and in those with acute narrow angle glaucoma.

WARNINGS

TRANXENE is not recommended for use in depressive neuroses or in psychotic reactions.
Patients on TRANXENE should be cautioned against engaging in hazardous occupations requiring mental alertness, such as operating dangerous machinery including motor vehicles.
Since TRANXENE has a central nervous system depressant effect, patients should be advised against the simultaneous use of other CNS-depressant drugs, and cautioned that the effects of alcohol may be increased.
Because of the lack of sufficient clinical experience, TRANXENE is not recommended for use in patients less than 9 years of age.
Physical and Psychological Dependence: Withdrawal symptoms (similar in character to those noted with barbiturates and alcohol) have occurred following abrupt discontinuance of clorazepate. Symptoms of nervousness, insomnia, irritability, diarrhea, muscle aches and memory impairment have followed abrupt withdrawal after long-term use of high dosage. Withdrawal symptoms have also been reported following abrupt discontinuance of benzodiazepines taken continuously at therapeutic levels for several months.
Caution should be observed in patients who are considered to have a psychological potential for drug dependence.
Evidence of drug dependence has been observed in dogs and rabbits which was characterized by convulsive seizures when the drug was abruptly withdrawn or the dose was reduced; the syndrome in dogs could be abolished by administration of clorazepate.
Usage in Pregnancy: **An increased risk of congenital malformations associated with the use of minor tranquilizers (chlordiazepoxide, diazepam, and meprobamate) during the first trimester of pregnancy has been suggested in several studies. TRANXENE, a benzodiazepine derivative, has not been studied adequately to determine whether it, too, may be associated with an increased risk of fetal abnormality. Because use of these drugs is rarely a matter of urgency, their use during this period should almost always be avoided. The possibility that a woman of childbearing potential may be pregnant at the time of institution of therapy should be considered. Patients should be advised that if they become pregnant during therapy or intend to become pregnant they should communicate with their physician about the desirability of discontinuing the drug.**
Usage during Lactation: TRANXENE should not be given to nursing mothers since it has been reported that nordiazepam is excreted in human breast milk.

PRECAUTIONS

In those patients in which a degree of depression accompanies the anxiety, suicidal tendencies may be present and protective measures may be required. The least amount of drug that is feasible should be available to the patient.

Patients on TRANXENE for prolonged periods should have blood counts and liver function tests periodically. The usual precautions in treating patients with impaired renal or hepatic function should also be observed.

In elderly or debilitated patients, the initial dose should be small, and increments should be made gradually, in accordance with the response of the patient, to preclude ataxia or excessive sedation.

ADVERSE REACTIONS

The side effect most frequently reported was drowsiness. Less commonly reported (in descending order of occurrence) were: dizziness, various gastrointestinal complaints, nervousness, blurred vision, dry mouth, headache, and mental confusion. Other side effects included insomnia, transient skin rashes, fatigue, ataxia, genitourinary complaints, irritability, diplopia, depression and slurred speech.

There have been reports of abnormal liver and kidney function tests and of decrease in hematocrit.

Decrease in systolic blood pressure has been observed.

DOSAGE AND ADMINISTRATION

For the symptomatic relief of anxiety: TRANXENE capsules and tablets are administered orally in divided doses. The usual daily dose is 30 mg. The dose should be adjusted gradually within the range of 15 to 60 mg daily in accordance with the response of the patient. In elderly or debilitated patients it is advisable to initiate treatment at a daily dose of 7.5 to 15 mg.

TRANXENE capsules and tablets may also be administered in a single dose daily at bedtime; the recommended initial dose is 15 mg. After the initial dose, the response of the patient may require adjustment of subsequent dosage. Lower doses may be indicated in the elderly patient. Drowsiness may occur at the initiation of treatment and with dosage increment.

TRANXENE-SD (22.5 mg tablets) may be administered as a single dose every 24 hours. This tablet is intended as an alternate dosage form for the convenience of patients stabilized on a dose of 7.5 mg capsules or tablets three times a day. TRANXENE-SD should not be used to initiate therapy.

TRANXENE-SD HALF STRENGTH (11.25 mg tablets) may be administered as a single dose every 24 hours.

For the symptomatic relief of acute alcohol withdrawal:
The following dosage schedule is recommended:

1st 24 hours (Day 1)	30 mg Tranxene, initially; followed by 30 to 60 mg in divided doses
2nd 24 hours (Day 2)	45 to 90 mg in divided doses
3rd 24 hours (Day 3)	22.5 to 45 mg in divided doses
Day 4	15 to 30 mg in divided doses

Thereafter, gradually reduce the daily dose to 7.5 to 15 mg. Discontinue drug therapy as soon as patient's condition is stable.

The maximum recommended total daily dose is 90 mg. Avoid excessive reductions in the total amount of drug administered on successive days.

As an Adjunct to Antiepileptic Drugs:
In order to minimize drowsiness, the recommended initial dosages and dosage increments should not be exceeded.

Adults: The maximum recommended initial dose in patients over 12 years old is 7.5 mg three times a day. Dosage should be increased by no more than 7.5 mg every week and should not exceed 90 mg/day.

Children (9-12 years): The maximum recommended initial dose is 7.5 mg two times a day. Dosage should be increased by no more than 7.5 mg every week and should not exceed 60 mg/day.

Drug Interactions: If TRANXENE is to be combined with other drugs acting on the central nervous system, careful consideration should be given to the pharmacology of the agents to be employed. Animal experience indicates that TRANXENE prolongs the sleeping time after hexobarbital or after ethyl alcohol, increases the inhibitory effects of chlorpromazine, but does not exhibit monoamine oxidase inhibition. Clinical studies have shown increased sedation with concurrent hypnotic medications. The actions of the benzodiazepines may be potentiated by barbiturates, narcotics, phenothiazines, monoamine oxidase inhibitors or other antidepressants.

If TRANXENE is used to treat anxiety associated with somatic disease states, careful attention must be paid to possible drug interaction with concomitant medication.

In bioavailability studies with normal subjects, the concurrent administration of antacids at therapeutic levels did not significantly influence the bioavailability of TRANXENE.

Management of Overdosage: Overdosage is usually manifested by varying degrees of CNS depression ranging from slight sedation to coma. As in the management of overdosage with any drug, it should be borne in mind that multiple agents may have been taken.

There are no specific antidotes for the benzodiazepines. The treatment of overdosage should consist of the general measures employed in the management of overdosage of any CNS depressant. Gastric evacuation either by the induction of emesis, lavage, or both, should be performed immediately. General supportive care, including frequent monitoring of the vital signs and close observation of the patient, is indicated. Hypotension, though rarely reported, may occur with large overdoses. In such cases the use of agents such as Levophed® Bitartrate (norepinephrine bitartrate injection, USP) or Aramine® Injection (metaraminol bitartrate injection, USP) should be considered.

While reports indicate that individuals have survived overdoses of TRANXENE as high as 450 to 675 mg, these doses are not necessarily an accurate indication of the amount of drug absorbed since the time interval between ingestion and the institution of treatment was not always known. Sedation in varying degrees was the most common physiological manifestation of TRANXENE overdosage. Deep coma when it occurred was usually associated with the ingestion of other drugs in addition to TRANXENE.

Animal and Clinical Pharmacology: Studies in rats and monkeys have shown a substantial difference between doses producing tranquilizing, sedative and toxic effects. In rats, conditioned avoidance response was inhibited at an oral dose of 10 mg/kg; sedation was induced at 32 mg/kg; the LD_{50} was 1320 mg/kg. In monkeys aggressive behavior was reduced at an oral dose of 0.25 mg/kg; sedation (ataxia) was induced at 7.5 mg/kg; the LD_{50} could not be determined because of the emetic effect of large doses, but the LD_{50} exceeds 1600 mg/kg.

Twenty-four dogs were given TRANXENE orally in a 22-month toxicity study; doses up to 75 mg/kg were given. Drug-related changes occurred in the liver; weight was increased and cholestasis with minimal hepatocellular damage was found, but lobular architecture remained well preserved.

Eighteen rhesus monkeys were given oral doses of TRANXENE from 3 to 36 mg/kg daily for 52 weeks. All treated animals remained similar to control animals. Although total leucocyte count remained within normal limits it tended to fall in the female animals on the highest doses.

Examination of all organs revealed no alterations attributable to TRANXENE. There was no damage to liver function or structure.

Reproduction Studies: Standard fertility, reproduction, and teratology studies were conducted in rats and rabbits. Oral doses in rats up to 150 mg/kg and in rabbits up to 15 mg/kg produced no abnormalities in the fetuses. TRANXENE (clorazepate dipotassium) did not alter the fertility indices or reproductive capacity of adult animals. As expected, the sedative effect of high doses interfered with care of the young by their mothers (see Usage in Pregnancy).

Clinical Pharmacology: Studies in healthy men have shown that TRANXENE has depressant effects on the central nervous system. Prolonged administration of single daily doses as high as 120 mg was without toxic effects. Abrupt cessation of high doses was followed in some patients by nervousness, insomnia, irritability, diarrhea, muscle aches, or memory impairment.

Absorption—Excretion: After oral administration of TRANXENE there is essentially no circulating parent drug. Nordiazepam, its primary metabolite, quickly appears in the blood stream. In 2 volunteers given 15 mg (50 μC) of ^{14}C-TRANXENE, about 80% was recovered in the urine and feces within 10 days. Excretion was primarily in the urine with about 1% excreted per day on day 10.

HOW SUPPLIED

TRANXENE (clorazepate dipotassium) is supplied as:
3.75 mg gray and white capsules:
Bottles of 100 .... (**NDC** 0074-3417-13)
Bottles of 500 .... (**NDC** 0074-3417-53)
ABBO-PAC® unit dose packages:
100 .... (**NDC** 0074-3417-11).
7.5 mg gray and maroon capsules:
Bottles of 100 .... (**NDC** 0074-3418-13)
Bottles of 500 .... (**NDC** 0074-3418-53)
ABBO-PAC unit dose packages:
100 .... (**NDC** 0074-3418-11).
15 mg gray capsules:
Bottles of 100 .... (**NDC** 0074-3419-13)
Bottles of 500 .... (**NDC** 0074-3419-53)
ABBO-PAC unit dose packages:
100 .... (**NDC** 0074-3419-11).
3.75 mg blue-colored, scored tablets:
Bottles of 100 .... (**NDC** 0074-4389-13).
7.5 mg peach-colored, scored tablets:
Bottles of 100 .... (**NDC** 0074-4390-13).
15 mg lavender-colored, scored tablets:
Bottles of 100 .... (**NDC** 0074-4391-13).
TRANXENE-SD 22.5 mg tan-colored, single dose tablets:
Bottles of 100 .... (**NDC** 0074-2997-13).
TRANXENE-SD HALF STRENGTH 11.25 mg blue-colored, single dose tablets:
Bottles of 100 .... (**NDC** 0074-2699-13).

Shown in Product Identification Section, page 403

Abbott Pharmaceuticals, Inc.
North Chicago, IL 60064
Ref. 03-4288-R5

TRIDIONE® ℞

[*try'dē-own*]
(trimethadione)
Tablets, Capsules, and Oral Solution

BECAUSE OF ITS POTENTIAL TO PRODUCE FETAL MALFORMATIONS AND SERIOUS SIDE EFFECTS, TRIDIONE (trimethadione) SHOULD ONLY BE UTILIZED WHEN OTHER LESS TOXIC DRUGS HAVE BEEN FOUND INEFFECTIVE IN CONTROLLING PETIT MAL SEIZURES.

DESCRIPTION

TRIDIONE (trimethadione) is an antiepileptic agent. An oxazolidinedione compound, it is chemically identified as 3,5,5-trimethyloxozolidine-2,4-dione.

TRIDIONE is a synthetic, water-soluble, white, crystalline powder. It is supplied in capsular, tablet, and liquid forms for oral use only.

INACTIVE INGREDIENTS

300 mg Capsule: Corn starch, FD&C Blue No. 1, FD&C Red No. 3, FD&C Yellow No. 6, gelatin, titanium dioxide, artificial flavor and other ingredients.

150 mg Dulcet Tablet: Corn starch, lactose, magnesium stearate, magnesium trisilicate, sucrose, natural/synthetic flavor and other ingredients.

Solution: FD&C Yellow No. 6, methylparaben, sucrose, water, natural/synthetic flavors and other ingredients.

CLINICAL PHARMACOLOGY

TRIDIONE has been shown to prevent pentylenetetrazol-induced and thujone-induced seizures in experimental animals; the drug has a less marked effect on seizures induced by picrotoxin, procaine, cocaine, or strychnine. Unlike the hydantoins and antiepileptic barbiturates, TRIDIONE does not modify the maximal seizure pattern in patients undergoing electroconvulsive therapy.

TRIDIONE has a sedative effect that may increase to the point of ataxia when excessive doses are used. A toxic dose of the drug in animals (approximately 2 g/kg) produced sleep, unconsciousness, and respiratory depression.

Trimethadione is rapidly absorbed from the gastrointestinal tract. It is demethylated by liver microsomes to the active metabolite, dimethadione.

Approximately 3% of a daily dose of TRIDIONE is recovered in the urine as unchanged drug. The majority of trimethadione is excreted slowly by the kidney in the form of dimethadione.

INDICATIONS

TRIDIONE (trimethadione) is indicated for the control of petit mal seizures that are refractory to treatment with other drugs.

CONTRAINDICATIONS

TRIDIONE is contraindicated in patients with a known hypersensitivity to the drug.

WARNINGS

TRIDIONE may cause serious side effects. Strict medical supervision of the patient is mandatory, especially during the initial year of therapy.

TRIDIONE (trimethadione) should be withdrawn promptly if skin rash appears, because of the grave possibility of the occurrence of exfoliative dermatitis or severe forms of erythema multiforme. Even a minor acneiform or morbilliform rash should be allowed to clear completely before treatment with TRIDIONE is resumed; reinstitute therapy cautiously.

A complete blood count should be done prior to intiating therapy with TRIDIONE, and at monthly intervals thereafter. A marked depression of the blood count is an indication for withdrawal of the drug. If no abnormality appears within 12 months, the interval between blood counts may be extended. A moderate degree of neutropenia with or without a corresponding drop in the leukocyte count is not uncommon. Therapy need not be withdrawn unless the neutrophil count is 2500 or less; more frequent blood examinations should be

Continued on next page

Abbott—Cont.

done when the count is less than 3,000. Other blood dyscrasias, including leukopenia, eosinophilia, thrombocytopenia, pancytopenia, agranulocytosis, hypoplastic anemia, and fatal aplastic anemia, have occurred. Patients should be advised to report immediately such signs and symptoms as sore throat, fever, malaise, easy bruising, petechiae, or epistaxis, or others that may be indicative of an infection or bleeding tendency. TRIDIONE should ordinarily not be used in patients with severe blood dyscrasias.

Liver function tests should be done prior to initiating therapy with TRIDIONE, and at monthly intervals thereafter. Hepatitis has been reported rarely. Jaundice or other signs of liver dysfunction are an indication for withdrawal of the drug. TRIDIONE should ordinarily not be used in patients with severe hepatic impairment.

A urinalysis should be done prior to initiating therapy with TRIDIONE and at monthly intervals thereafter. Fatal nephrosis has been reported. Persistent or increasing albuminuria, or the development of any other significant renal abnormality, is an indication for withdrawal of the drug. TRIDIONE should ordinarily not be used in patients with severe renal dysfunction.

Hemeralopia has occurred; this appears to be an effect of TRIDIONE on the neural layers of the retina, and usually can be reversed by a reduction in dosage. Scotomata are an indication for withdrawal of the drug. Caution should be observed when treating patients who have diseases of the retina or optic nerve.

Manifestations of systemic lupus erythematosus have been associated with the use of TRIDIONE, as they have with the use of certain other anticonvulsants. Lymphadenopathies simulating malignant lymphoma have occurred. Lupus-like manifestations or lymph node enlargement are indications for withdrawal of the drug. Signs and symptoms may disappear after discontinuation of therapy, and specific treatment may be unnecessary.

A myasthenia gravis-like syndrome has been associated with the chronic use of trimethadione. Symptoms suggestive of this condition are indications for withdrawal of the drug.

Drugs known to cause toxic effects similar to those of TRIDIONE should be avoided or used only with extreme caution during therapy with TRIDIONE.

USAGE DURING PREGNANCY AND LACTATION:

THERE ARE MULTIPLE REPORTS IN THE CLINICAL LITERATURE WHICH INDICATE THAT THE USE OF ANTICONVULSANT DRUGS DURING PREGNANCY RESULTS IN AN INCREASED INCIDENCE OF BIRTH DEFECTS IN THE OFFSPRING. DATA ARE MORE EXTENSIVE WITH RESPECT TO TRIMETHADIONE, PARAMETHADIONE, PHENYTOIN AND PHENOBARBITAL THAN WITH OTHER ANTICONVULSANT DRUGS.

THEREFORE, ANTICONVULSANT DRUGS SUCH AS TRIDIONE (TRIMETHADIONE) SHOULD BE ADMINISTERED TO WOMEN OF CHILDBEARING POTENTIAL ONLY IF THEY ARE CLEARLY SHOWN TO BE ESSENTIAL IN THE MANAGEMENT OF THEIR SEIZURES. EFFECTIVE MEANS OF CONTRACEPTION SHOULD ACCOMPANY THE USE OF TRIDIONE IN SUCH PATIENTS. IF A PATIENT BECOMES PREGNANT WHILE TAKING TRIDIONE, TERMINATION OF THE PREGNANCY SHOULD BE CONSIDERED. A PATIENT WHO REQUIRES THERAPY WITH TRIDIONE AND WHO WISHES TO BECOME PREGNANT SHOULD BE ADVISED OF THE RISKS.

REPORTS HAVE SUGGESTED THAT THE MATERNAL INGESTION OF ANTICONVULSANT DRUGS, PARTICULARLY BARBITURATES, IS ASSOCIATED WITH A NEONATAL COAGULATION DEFECT THAT MAY CAUSE BLEEDING DURING THE EARLY (USUALLY WITHIN 24 HOURS OF BIRTH) NEONATAL PERIOD. THE POSSIBILITY OF THE OCCURRENCE OF THIS DEFECT WITH THE USE OF TRIDIONE SHOULD BE KEPT IN MIND. THE DEFECT IS CHARACTERIZED BY DECREASED LEVELS OF VITAMIN K-DEPENDENT CLOTTING FACTORS, AND PROLONGATION OF EITHER THE PROTHROMBIN TIME OR THE PARTIAL THROMBOPLASTIN TIME, OR BOTH. IT HAS BEEN SUGGESTED THAT PROPHYLACTIC VITAMIN K BE GIVEN TO THE MOTHER ONE MONTH PRIOR TO, AND DURING DELIVERY, AND TO THE INFANT, INTRAVENOUSLY, IMMEDIATELY AFTER BIRTH.

THE SAFETY OF TRIDIONE FOR USE DURING LACTATION HAS NOT BEEN ESTABLISHED.

PRECAUTIONS

Abrupt discontinuation of TRIDIONE may precipitate petit mal status. TRIDIONE should always be withdrawn gradually unless serious adverse effects dictate otherwise. In the latter case, another anticonvulsant may be substituted to protect the patient.

Usage during Pregnancy and Lactation:
See WARNINGS.

ADVERSE REACTIONS

The following side effects, some of them serious, have been associated with the use of TRIDIONE.

Gastrointestinal: nausea, vomiting, abdominal pain, gastric distress.

CNS/Neurologic: drowsiness, fatigue, malaise, insomnia, vertigo, headache, paresthesias, precipitation of grand mal seizures, increased irritability, personality changes.

Drowsiness usually subsides with continued therapy. If it persists, a reduction in dosage is indicated.

Hematologic: bleeding gums, epistaxis, retinal and petechial hemorrhages, vaginal bleeding; neutropenia, leukopenia, eosinophilia, thrombocytopenia, pancytopenia, agranulocytosis, hypoplastic anemia, and fatal aplastic anemia.

Dermatologic: acneiform or morbilliform skin rash that may progress to exfoliative dermatitis or to severe forms of erythema multiforme.

Other: hiccups, anorexia, weight loss, hair loss, changes in blood pressure, albuminuria, hemeralopia, photophobia, diplopia.

Fatal nephrosis has occurred.

Hepatitis has been reported rarely.

Lupus erythematosus, and lymphadenopathies simulating malignant lymphoma, have been reported.

Pruritus associated with lymphadenopathy and hepatosplenomegaly has occurred in hypersensitive individuals.

A myasthenia gravis-like syndrome has been reported.

OVERDOSAGE

Symptoms of acute TRIDIONE overdosage include drowsiness, nausea, dizziness, ataxia, visual disturbances. Coma may follow massive overdosage.

Gastric evacuation, either by induced emesis, or by lavage, or both, should be done immediately. General supportive care, including frequent monitoring of the vital signs and close observation of the patient, are required.

Alkalinization of the urine has been reported to enhance the renal excretion of dimethadione, the active metabolite of TRIDIONE.

A blood count and a careful evaluation of hepatic and renal function should be done following recovery.

DOSAGE AND ADMINISTRATION

TRIDIONE is administered orally.

Usual Adult Dosage: 0.9–2.4 g daily in 3 or 4 equally divided doses (i.e. 300–600 mg 3 or 4 times daily).

Initially, give 0.9 g daily; increase this dose by 300 mg at weekly intervals until therapeutic results are seen or until toxic symptoms appear.

Maintenance dosage should be the least amount of drug required to maintain control.

Children's Dosage: Usually 0.3–0.9 g daily in 3 or 4 equally divided doses.

HOW SUPPLIED

TRIDIONE Capsules (trimethadione capsules, USP), 300 mg (white) are supplied in bottles of 100 (**NDC** 0074-3709-01).

TRIDIONE Dulcet® Tablets (trimethadione tablets, USP), 150 mg (white) chewable tablets are supplied in bottles of 100 (**NDC** 0074-3753-01).

Shown in Product Identification Section, page 403

TRIDIONE Solution (trimethadione oral solution, USP), 1.2 g per fluidounce (40 mg per ml), is supplied in pint bottles (**NDC** 0074-3721-01).

Abbott Laboratories/
Abbott Pharmaceuticals, Inc.
North Chicago, IL 60064
®Dulcet—Sweetened tablets, Abbott.
Ref. 01-2368-R4

TRONOTHANE® HYDROCHLORIDE

[*tro 'nō-thāne hy-drō-clō 'rīde*]
(pramoxine hydrochloride)
Cream

DESCRIPTION

Tronothane Hydrochloride (pramoxine hydrochloride) is a surface anesthetic agent, chemically unrelated to the benzoate esters of the "caine" type. It is chemically designated as 4-n-butoxyphenyl gammamorpholinopropyl ether hydrochloride.

INDICATIONS

Tronothane Hydrochloride is indicated for temporary relief of pain and itching due to minor burns, sunburn, minor cuts, abrasions, insect bites, minor skin irritations, hemorrhoids and other anorectal disorders.

CONTRAINDICATIONS

Tronothane Hydrochloride is not suitable for and should not be injected into the tissues. It should not be used for bronchoscopy or gastroscopy, or in patients who are hypersensitive to the drug.

WARNINGS

Tronothane Hydrochloride is not intended for prolonged use. Do not apply to large areas of the body. Do not use in the eyes or nose.

If condition worsens, or persists for 7 days, consult physician. If bleeding or increased pain occurs when using the product in the rectum, consult physician promptly.

For topical use in children under 2 years or anorectal use in children under 12 years, use only as directed by physician. Keep out of reach of children.

ADVERSE REACTIONS

Local skin reactions, e.g. stinging and burning. Discontinue use if redness, irritation, swelling or pain occur.

DOSAGE AND ADMINISTRATION

Topical—Adults and children 2 years of age or older: Apply to affected area 3 to 4 times daily, or as directed by a physician.

Anorectal—When practical, wash the area with soap and warm water, and rinse off all soap before application. Adults and children 12 years of age or older: Apply up to 5 times daily, especially morning, night and after bowel movements, or as directed by a physician.

External—Apply liberally to affected area.

Intrarectal—Remove cap from tube and attach clean applicator. Squeeze tube to fill and lubricate applicator. Gently insert applicator into rectum and squeeze tube. Thoroughly cleanse applicator with soap and warm water after use.

HOW SUPPLIED

Tronothane Hydrochloride 1% Cream (pramoxine hydrochloride cream, USP), pramoxine hydrochloride 1% in a water miscible base containing cetyl alcohol, cetyl esters wax, glycerin, sodium lauryl sulfate, methylparaben, and propylparaben, is supplied in a 1-oz tube with rectal applicator (**NDC** 0074-6645-01).

These products are listed in USP, a Medicare designated compendium.

Abbott Laboratories
North Chicago, IL 60064

If desired, additional literature on any Abbott Product will be provided upon request to Abbott Laboratories.

Adams Laboratories, Inc.

P.O. BOX 487
10800 S. PIPELINE ROAD
HURST, TX 76053

ATROHIST® L.A. Tablets ℞

HOW SUPPLIED

Bottles of 100 tablets (NDC 53014-0021-1).

ATROHIST® SPRINKLE Capsules ℞

DESCRIPTION

Each ATROHIST® SPRINKLE Capsule provides 2 mg brompheniramine maleate, 25 mg phenyltoloxamine citrate, and 10 mg phenylephrine hydrochloride in a sustained-release formulation intended for oral administration. The microencapsulated contents of a capsule may be sprinkled on a small amount of soft food immediately prior to ingestion, making the product ideal for children and other patients unable to swallow capsules or tablets. Capsules are oversized to facilitate opening but may also be swallowed whole.

ATROHIST® SPRINKLE Capsules have antihistaminic and nasal decongestant effects. The components of ATROHIST® SPRINKLE Capsules have the following chemical names and structural formula:

Brompheniramine Maleate:

2-[p-bromo-α-[2-(dimethylamino) ethyl] benzyl] pyridimaleate

$C_{16}H_{19}BrN_2 \cdot C_4H_4O_4$ MW = 435.32

Phenyltoloxamine Citrate:

N,N-dimethyl-2(alpha phenyl-ortho-toloxy)-ethylamine

$C_{17}H_{21}NO \cdot C_6H_8O_7$ MW = 447.5

Phenylephrine Hydrochloride:
(R)-3-hydroxy-α-[(methylamino) methyl] benzenemethanol hydrochloride

$C_9H_{13}NO_2 \cdot HCl$ MW =203.67

CLINICAL PHARMACOLOGY

Brompheniramine maleate and phenyltoloxamine citrate are antihistamines which act on H_1 receptors as antagonists and interfere with the action of histamine, primarily in capillaries surrounding mucous tissues and sensory nerves of nasal and adjacent areas. Both drugs are rapidly and almost completely absorbed from the gastrointestinal tract and distributed throughout the body, including the central nervous system (CNS). Little, if any, of the drugs is excreted unchanged in the urine; most is apparently metabolized by the liver and excreted as degradation products within 24 hours.
Alkylamine-type antihistamines such as brompheniramine maleate are among the most potent H_1 blockers and are generally effective in relatively low doses. Although brompheniramine is not so prone as other types of antihistamines to cause drowsiness, a significant proportion of patients do experience this effect. CNS stimulation is more common with alkylamines. Ethanolamine-type antihistamines such as phenyltoloxamine citrate are potent and effective H_1 blockers that possess significant antimuscarinic activity and have a pronounced tendency to induce sedation.
Phenylephrine hydrochloride effects its vasoconstrictor activity by releasing noradrenaline from sympathetic nerve endings, and from direct stimulation of α-adrenoreceptors in blood vessels. Following oral administration, constriction of blood vessels in the nasal mucosa helps relieve nasal congestion. In therapeutic doses the drug causes little, if any, central nervous system stimulation.

INDICATIONS AND USAGE

ATROHIST® SPRINKLE Capsules are indicated for symptomatic relief of seasonal and perennial allergic rhinitis, vasomotor rhinitis, and eustachian tube congestion. The product is particularly suitable for use in children and other patients unable to swallow tablets or capsules.

CONTRAINDICATIONS

This product is contraindicated in patients with hypersensitivity to antihistamines or sympathomimetic amines, and in patients receiving monoamine oxidase (MAO) inhibitor therapy (see **Drug Interactions** section).
Patients known to be hypersensitive to other sympathomimetic amines may exhibit cross sensitivity to phenylephrine. Phenylephrine is contraindicated in patients with severe hypertension or severe coronary artery disease. Patient idiosyncrasy to adrenergic agents may be manifested by insomnia, dizziness, weakness, tremors or arrhythmias.

WARNINGS

Antihistamines should be used with considerable caution in patients with: narrow angle glaucoma; stenosing peptic ulcer; pyloroduodenal obstruction; symptomatic prostatic hypertrophy; bladder neck obstruction.
Sympathomimetic amines should be used with caution in patients with hypertension, ischemic heart disease, diabetes mellitus, increased intraocular pressure, hyperthyroidism, or prostatic hypertropy. Sympathomimetics may produce central nervous system stimulation with convulsions or cardiovascular collapse with accompanying hypotension. **Do not exceed recommended dosage.**
Hypertensive crises can occur with concurrent use of phenylephrine and monoamine oxidase (MOA) inhibitors, indomethacin or with beta-blockers and methyldopa. If a hypertensive crisis occurs, these drugs should be discontinued immediately and therapy to lower blood pressure should be instituted. Fever should be managed by means of external cooling.

PRECAUTIONS

General: Antihistamines have an atropine-like action and therefore should be used with caution in patients with a history of bronchial asthma, increased intraocular pressure, hyperthyroidism, cardiovascular disease and hypertension. Phenylephrine should be used with caution in patients with diabetes, hypertension, cardiovascular disease and hyperreactivity to ephedrine.
Information for Patients: Antihistamines may impair mental and physical abilities required for the performance of potentially hazardous tasks, such as driving a vehicle or operating machinery. Patients should be warned accordingly. Capsules may be swallowed whole or the entire contents sprinkled on a small amount of soft food (jam etc.) immediately prior to ingestion. Capsule contents should not be subdivided. Capsule contents should not be crushed or chewed.
Pediatric Use: This product is not recommended for use in children under 2 years of age. In infants and children, antihistamines in **overdosage** may cause hallucinations, convulsions or death. As in adults, antihistamines may diminish mental alertness in children. In the young child particularly, they may produce excitation.
Use in Elderly: The elderly (60 years and older) are more likely to experience adverse reactions to sympathomimetics. Overdosage of sympathomimetics in this age group may cause hallucinations, convulsions, CNS depression, and death.
Drug Interactions: MAO inhibitors and tricyclic antidepressants may prolong and intensify the anticholinergic (drying) effects of antihistamines. Beta-adrenergic blockers and MAO inhibitors may potentiate the pressor effect of phenylephrine (see **WARNINGS**). Concurrent use of digitalis glycosides may increase the possibility of cardiac arrhythmias. Sympathomimetics may reduce the hypotensive effects of guanethidine, mecamylamine, methyldopa, reserpine and veratrum alkaloids. Concurrent use of tricyclic anticdepressants may antagonize the effects of phenylephrine. Concomitant use of antihistamines with alcohol, tricyclic antidepressants, barbiturates and other CNS depressants may have an additive effect.
Carcinogenesis, Mutagenesis, Impairment of Fertility: No data are available on the long-term potential of the components of this product for carcinogenesis, mutagenesis, or impairment of fertility in animals or humans.
Pregnancy: Category C: Animal reproduction studies have not been conducted with the components of this product. It is also not known whether these drugs can cause fetal harm when administered to a pregnant woman or can effect reproduction capacity. Accordingly, this product should be given to a pregnant woman only if clearly needed.
Nursing Mothers: Use of this product by nursing mothers is not recommended because of the higher than usual risk for infants from sympathomimetic amines.

ADVERSE REACTIONS

Hyper-reactive individuals may display ephedrine-like reactions such as tachycardia, palpitations, headache, dizziness, or nausea. Sympathomimetics have been associated with certain untoward reactions including fear, anxiety, nervousness, restlessness, tremor, weakness, pallor, respiratory difficulty, dysuria, insomnia, hallucinations, convulsions, CNS depression, arrhythmias, and cardiovascular collapse with hypotension.
Possible side effects of antihistamines are drowsiness, dry mouth, anorexia, nausea, vomiting, headache and nervousness, blurring of vision, polyuria, heartburn, dysuria and very rarely, dermatitis.

OVERDOSAGE

Since ATROHIST® SPRINKLE Capsules contain pharmacologically different compounds, treatment of overdosage should be based upon the symptomatology of the patient as it relates to the individual ingredients. A detailed description of the symptoms which are likely to appear after ingestion of an excess of the individal components follows:
Manifestations of antihistamine overdosage may vary from CNS depression (sedation, apnea, cardiovascular collapse) to stimulation (insomnia, hallucinations, tremors or convulsions). Other signs and symptoms may be dizziness, tinnitus, ataxia, blurred vision, and hypotension. Stimulation is particularly likely in children, as are atropine-like signs and symptoms (dry-mouth; fixed, dilated pupils; flushing; hyperthermia and gastrointestinal symptoms).
Overdosage with phenylephrine may manifest itself as excessive CNS stimulation resulting in excitment, tremor, restlessness and insomnia. Other effects may include tachycardia, hypertension, pallor, mydriasis, hyperglycemia and urinary retention. Severe overdosage may cause tachypnea or hypernea, hallucination, convulsions or delirium, but in some individuals there may be CNS depression with somnolence, stupor or respiratory depression. Arrhythmias (including ventricular fibrillation) may lead to hypotension and circulatory collapse. Severe hypokalemia can occur, probably due to a compartmental shift rather than a depletion of potassium.
The LD_{50} of phenylephrine (single oral dose) has been reported to be 120 mg/kg in the mouse and 350 mg/kg in the rat. The toxic and lethal concentrations in human biologic fluids are not known. No information is available regarding the LD_{50} of brompheniramine maleate and phenyltoloxamine citrate, and their toxic and lethal concentrations in human biologic fluids are not known. Cases of fatal overdosage with antihistamines have been reported in the literature.
In the event of overdosage, emergency treatment should be started immediately. Since the action of sustained release products may continue for as long as 12 hours, treatment of overdosage should be directed toward reducing further absorption and supporting the patient for at least that length of time. Gastric emptying (Syrup of Ipecac) and/or lavage is recommended as soon as possible after ingestion, even if the patient has vomited spontaneously. Either isotonic or half-isotonic saline may be used for lavage. Administration of an activated charcoal slurry is benefical after lavage and/or emesis if less than 4 hours have passed since ingestion. Saline cathartics, such as Milk of Magnesia, are useful for hastening the evacuation of unreleased medication.
Adrenergic receptor blocking agents are antidotes to phenylephrine. In practice, the most useful is the beta-blocker propanolol which is indicated when there are signs of cardiac toxicity. Theoretically, phenylephrine is dialyzable but procedures have not been clinically established.
In severe cases of overdosage, it is essential to monitor both the heart (by electrocardiograph) and plasma electrolytes, and to give intravenous potassium as indicated. Vasopressors may be used to treat hypotension. Excessive CNS stimulation may be counteracted with parenteral diazepam. Stimulants should not be used. Hyperpyrexia, especially in children, may require treatment with tepid water sponge baths or a hyperthermic blanket. Apnea is treated with ventilatory support.

DOSAGE AND ADMINISTRATION

Adults and children over 12 years of age: Three capsules every 12 hours not to exceed 6 capsules in 24 hours. **Children 6 to 12 years:** One or two capsules every 12 hours not to exceed 4 capsules in 24 hours. **Children 2 to 6 years:** One capsule every 12 hours not to exceed 2 capsules in 24 hours. Capsules may be swallowed whole or the entire contents sprinkled on a small amount of soft food immediately prior to ingestion. **Subdividing the contents of a capsule is not recommended.**

HOW SUPPLIED

Bottles of 100 capsules (NDC 53014-0022-1). White beads in a yellow and clear capsule imprinted with "Adams/0022". Store at controlled room temperature between 15° C and 30° C (59° F and 86° F). Dispense in tight, light-resistant containers.
CAUTION: Federal law prohibits dispensing without prescription.

DECONSAL® Capsules ℞

HOW SUPPLIED

Bottles of 100 capsules (NDC 53014-0014-1).

DECONSAL® L.A. Tablets ℞

HOW SUPPLIED

Bottles of 100 tablets (NDC 53014-0015-1).

DECONSAL® SPRINKLE Capsules ℞

DESCRIPTION

Each DECONSAL® SPRINKLE Capsule provides 10 mg phenylephrine hydrochloride and 200 mg guaifenesin in a sustained-release formulation intended for oral administration. The microencapsulated contents of a capsule may be sprinkled on a small amount of soft food immediately prior to ingestion, making the product ideal for children and other patients unable to swallow capsules or tablets. Capsules are oversized to facilitate opening but may also be swallowed whole.
Phenylephrine hydrochloride is an orally effective nasal decongestant. Chemically, it is (R)-3-hydroxy-α-[(methylamino) methyl] benzenemethanol hydrochloride and has the following structural formula:

$C_9H_{13}NO_2 \cdot HCl$ MW = 203.67
Guaifenesin is an expectorant. Chemically, it is 3-(2-methoxyphenoxy)-1, 2-propanediol and has the following structural formula:

$C_{10}H_{14}O_4$ MW = 198.22

Continued on next page

Adams Laboratories—Cont.

CLINICAL PHARMACOLOGY

Phenylephrine hydrochloride effects its vasoconstrictor activity by releasing noradrenaline from sympathetic nerve endings, and from direct stimulation of α-adrenoreceptors in blood vessels. Following oral administration, constriction of blood vessels in the nasal mucosa helps relieve nasal congestion. In therapeutic doses the drug causes little, if any, central nervous system stimulation.
Guaifenesin is an expectorant which increases respiratory tract fluid secretions and helps to loosen phlegm and bronchial secretions. By reducing the viscosity of secretions, guaifenesin increases the efficiency of the cough reflex and of ciliary action in removing accumulated secretions from the trachea and bronchi. Guaifenesin is readily absorbed from the gastrointestinal tract and is rapidly metabolized and excreted in the urine. Guaifenesin has a plasma half-life of one hour. The major urinary metabolite is β-(2-methoxyphenoxy) lactic acid.

INDICATIONS AND USAGE

DECONSAL ® SPRINKLE Capsules are indicated for the temporary relief of nasal congestion and cough associated with respiratory tract infections such as sinusitis, pharyngitis, bronchitis, and asthma, when these conditions are complicated by tenacious mucous and/or mucous plugs and congestion. The product is effective in productive as well as non-productive cough, but is of particular value in dry, non-productive cough which tends to injure the mucous membrane of the air passages. DECONSAL® SPRINKLE Capsules are particularly suitable for use in children and other patients unable to swallow tablets or capsules.

CONTRAINDICATIONS

This product is contraindicated in patients with hypersensitivity to guaifenesin, or with hypersensitivity or idiosyncrasy to sympathomimetic amines which may be manifested by insomnia, dizziness, weakness, tremor or arrhythmias.
Patients known to be hypersensitive to other sympathomimetic amines may exhibit cross sensitivity with phenylephrine. Phenylephrine is contraindicated in patients with severe hypertension, severe coronary artery disease and patients on monoamine oxidase (MAO) inhibitor therapy. (see **Drug Interactions** section).

WARNINGS

Sympathomimetic amines should be used with caution in patients with hypertension, ischemic heart disease, diabetes mellitus, increased intraocular pressure, hyperthyroidism, or prostatic hypertrophy. Sympathomimetics may produce central nervous system stimulation with convulsions or cardiovascular collapse with accompanying hypotension. **Do not exceed recommended dosage.**
Hypertensive crises can occur with concurrent use of phenylephrine and monoamine oxidase (MAO) inhibitors, indomethacin or with beta-blockers and methyldopa. If a hypertensive crisis occurs, these drugs should be discontinued immediately and therapy to lower blood pressure should be instituted. Fever should be managed by means of external cooling.

PRECAUTIONS

General: Use with caution in patients with diabetes, hypertension, cardiovascular disease and hyperreactivity to ephedrine.
Before prescribing medication to suppress or modify cough, it is important to ascertain that the underlying cause of cough is identified, that modification of cough does not increase the risk of clinical or physiologic complications, and that appropriate therapy for the primary disease is instituted.
Information for Patients: Capsules may be swallowed whole or the entire contents sprinkled on a small amount of soft food (jam etc.) immediately prior to ingestion. Capsule contents should not be subdivided. Capsule contents should not be crushed or chewed. Patients should be instructed to check with physician if symptoms do not improve within 5 days or if fever is present.
Pediatric Use: This product in not recommended for use in children under 2 years of age.
Use in Elderly: The elderly (60 years and older) are more likely to experience adverse reactions to sympathomimetics. Overdosage of sympathomimetics in this age group may cause hallucinations, convulsions, CNS depression, and death.
Drug Interactions: Beta-adrenergic blockers and MAO inhibitors may poteniate the pressor effect of phenylephrine (see **WARNINGS**). Concurrent use of digitalis glycosides may increase the possibility of cardiac arrhythmias. Sympathomimetics may reduce the hypotensive effects of guanethidine, mecamylamine, methyldopa, reserpine and veratrum alkaloids. Concurrent use of tricyclic antidepressants may antagonize the effects of phenylephrine.
Drug/Laboratory Test Interactions: Guaifenesin may increase renal clearance for urate and thereby lower serum uric acid levels. Guaifenesin may produce an increase in urinary 5-hydroxy-indoleacetic acid and may therefore interfere with the interpretation of this test for the diagnosis of carcinoid syndrome. It may also falsely elevate the VMA test for catechols. Administration of this drug should be discontinued 48 hours prior to the collection of urine specimens for such tests.
Carcinogenesis, Mutagenesis, Impairment of Fertility: No data are available on the long-term potential of the components of this product for carcinogenesis, mutagenesis, or impairment of fertility in animals or humans.
Pregnancy: Category C: Animal reproduction studies have not been conducted with the components of this product. It is also not known whether these drugs can cause fetal harm when administered to a pregnant woman or can affect reproduction capacity. Accordingly, this product should be given to a pregnant woman only if clearly needed.
Nursing Mothers: Use of this product by nursing mothers is not recommended because of the higher than usual risk for infants from sympathomimetic amines.

ADVERSE REACTIONS

Hyper-reactive individuals may display ephedrine-like reactions such as tachycardia, palpitations, headache, dizziness, or nausea. Sympathomimetics have been associated with certain untoward reactions including fear, anxiety, nervousness, restlessness, tremor, weakness, pallor, respiratory difficulty, dysuria, insomnia, hallucinations, convulsions, CNS depression arrhythmias, and cardiovascular collapse with hypotension. No serious side effects have been reported with the use of guaifenesin.

OVERDOSAGE

Since DECONSAL® SPRINKLE Capsules contain two pharmacologically different compounds, treatment of overdosage should be based upon the symptamatology of the patient as it relates to the individual ingredients. Treatment of acute overdosage would probably be based upon treating the patient for phenylephrine toxicity which may manifest itself as excessive CNS stimulation resulting in excitement, tremor, restlessness, and insomnia. Other effects may include tachycardia, hypertension, pallor, mydriasis, hyperglycemia and urinary retention. Severe overdosage may cause tachypnea or hypernea, hallucinations, convulsions or delirium, but in some individuals there may be CNS depression with somnolence, stupor or respiratory depression. Arrhythmias (including ventricular fibrillation) may lead to hypotension and circulatory collapse. Severe hypokalemia can occur, probably due to a compartmental shift rather than a depletion of potassium. Overdosage with guaifenesin is unlikely to produce toxic effects since its toxicity is much lower that that of phenylephrine.
The LD_{50} of phenylephrine (single oral dose) had been reported to be 120 mg/kg in the mouse and 350 mg/kg in the rat. The toxic and lethal concentrations in human biologic fluids are not known. Guaifenesin, when administered by stomach tube to test animals in doses up to 5 grams/kg, produced no signs of toxicity.
Since the action of sustained-release products may continue for as long as 12 hours, treatment of overdosage should be directed toward reducing futher absorption and supporting the patient for at least that length of time. Gastric emptying (Syrup of Ipecac) and/or lavage is recommended as soon as possible after ingestion, even if the patient has vomited spontaneously. Either isotonic or half-isotonic saline may be used for lavage. Administration of an activated charcoal slurry is beneficial after lavage and/or emesis if less than 4 hours have passed since ingestion. Saline cathartics, such as Milk of Magnesia, are useful for hastening the evacuation of unreleased medication.
Adrenergic receptor blocking agents are antidotes to phenylephrine. In practice, the most useful is the beta-blocker propanolol which is indicated when there are signs of cardiac toxicity. Theoretically, phenylephrine is dialyzable but procedures have not been clinically established.
In severe cases of overdosage, it is essential to monitor both the heart (by electrocardigraph) and plasma electrolytes, and to give intravenous potassium as indicated. Vasopressors may be used to treat hypotension. Excessive CNS stimulation may be counteracted with parenteral diazepam. Stimulants should not be used.

DOSAGE AND ADMINISTRATION

Adults and children over 12 years of age: Three capsules every 12 hours not to exceed 6 capsules in 24 hours. **Children 6 to 12 years:** One or two capsules every 12 hours not to exceed 4 capsules in 24 hours. **Children 2 to 6 years:** One capsule every 12 hours not to exceed 2 capsules in 24 hours. Capsules may be swallowed whole or the entire contents sprinkled on a small amount of soft food immediately prior to ingestion. **Subdividing the contents of a capsule is not recommended.**

HOW SUPPLIED

Bottles of 100 capsules (NDC 53014-0016-1). White beads in a blue and clear capsule imprinted with "Adams/0016". Store at controlled room temperature between 15° and 30° C (59° F and 86° F). Dispense in tight, light-resistant containers.
CAUTION: Federal law prohibits dispensing without prescription.

HUMIBID® L.A. Tablets ℞
(Guaifenesin)

DESCRIPTION

Each light green scored, sustained-release tablet provides 600 mg guaifenesin.
Chemically, guaifenesin is 3-(2-methoxyphenoxy)-1, 2-propanediol and has the following structural formula:

OH
OCH_2CHCH_2OH
OCH_3

$C_{10}H_{14}O_4$ MW = 198.22

CLINICAL PHARMACOLOGY

Guaifenesin is an expectorant which increases respiratory tract fluid secretions and helps to loosen phlegm and bronchial secretions. By reducing the viscosity of secretions, guaifenesin increases the efficiency of the cough reflex and of ciliary action in removing accumulated secretions from the trachea and bronchi. Guaifenesin is readily absorbed from the gastrointestinal tract and is rapidly metabolized and excreted in the urine. Guaifenesin has a plasma half-life of one hour. The major urinary metabolite is β-(2-methoxyphenoxy) lactic acid.

INDICATIONS AND USAGE

HUMIBID® L.A. Tablets are indicated for the temporary relief of coughs associated with respiratory tract infections and related conditions such as sinusitis, pharyngitis, bronchitis, and asthma, when these conditions are complicated by tenacious mucous and/or mucous plugs and congestion. The drug is effective in productive as well as non-productive cough, but is of particular value in dry, non-productive cough which tends to injure the mucous membrane of the air passages.

CONTRAINDICATIONS

This drug is contraindicated in patients with hypersensitivity to guaifenesin.

PRECAUTIONS

General: Before prescribing medication to suppress or modify cough, it is important to ascertain that the underlying cause of cough is identified, that modification of cough does not increase the risk of clinical or physiological complications, and that appropriate therapy for the primary disease is instituted.
Drug/Laboratory Test Interactions: Guaifenesin may increase renal clearance for urate and thereby lower serum uric acid levels. Guaifenesin may produce an increase in urinary 5-hydroxyindoleacetic acid and may therefore interfere with the interpretation of this test for the diagnosis of carcinoid syndrome. It may also falsely elevate the VMA test for catechols. Administration of this drug should be discontinued 48 hours prior to the collection of urine specimens for such tests.
Carcinogenesis, Mutagenesis, Impairment of Fertility: No data are available on the long-term potential for carcinogenesis, mutagenesis, or impairment of fertility in animals or humans.
Pregnancy: Category C: Animal reproduction studies have not been conducted with guaifenesin. It is also not known whether guaifenesin can cause fetal harm when administered to a pregnant woman or can affect reproduction capacity. Guaifenesin should be given to a pregnant woman only if clearly needed.
Nursing Mothers: It is not known whether guaifenesin is excreted in human milk. Because many drugs are excreted in human milk, caution should be exercised when guaifenesin is administered to a nursing woman and a decision should be made whether to discontinue nursing or to discontinue the drug, taking into account the importance of the drug to the mother.

ADVERSE REACTIONS

No serious side effects from guaifenesin have been reported.

OVERDOSAGE

Overdosage with guaifenesin is unlikely to produce toxic effects since its toxicity is low. Guaifenesin, when administered by stomach tube to test animals in doses up to 5 grams/kg, produced no signs of toxicity. In severe cases of overdosage, treatment should be aimed at reducing further absorption of the drug. Gastric emptying (Syrup of Ipecac) and/or lavage is recommended as soon as possible after ingestion.

DOSAGE AND ADMINISTRATION

Adults and children over 12 years of age: One or two tablets every 12 hours not to exceed 4 tablets (2400 mg) in 24 hours. **Children 6 to 12 years:** One tablet every 12 hours not to exceed 2 tablets (1200 mg) in 24 hours. **Children 2 to 6 years:** ½ tablet every 12 hours not to exceed 1 tablet (600 mg) in 24 hours.

HOW SUPPLIED

Bottles of 100 tablets (NDC 53014-0012-1). Light green, scored tablets are embossed with "Adams/0012". Store at controlled room temperature between 15° C and 30° C (59° F and 86° F). Dispense in tight containers.

CAUTION: Federal law prohibits dispensing without prescription.

Adria Laboratories

Division of Erbamont Inc.
5000 POST ROAD
DUBLIN, OH 43017

PRODUCT IDENTIFICATION CODES

To provide quick and positive identification of Adria Laboratories Inc. products, we have imprinted the product identification number on one side of all tablets and capsules. The other side of the tablet displays the name "ADRIA".

In order that you may quickly identify a product by its code number, we have compiled below a numerical list of code numbers of prescription products with their corresponding product names:

[See table above].

PRODUCT IDENTIFICATION CODE	PRODUCT INDEX
130	Axotal® (butalbital, USP, 50 mg and aspirin, USP, 650 mg. Warning: May be habit forming)
200	Ilozyme® (pancrelipase, USP) Tablets
230	Octamide™ (metoclopramide hydrochloride) Tablets, 10 mg
231	Ilopan-Choline® Tablets (dexpanthenol 50 mg./choline bitartrate 25 mg)
304	Kaon CL-10™ (potassium chloride) Controlled Release Tablets, 750 mg. (10 mEq)
307	Kaon-CL® (potassium chloride) Controlled Release Tablets, 500 mg (6.7 mEq)
312	Kaon® (potassium gluconate) Tablets, 1.7 g (5 mEq)
412	Magan® (magnesium salicylate) Tablets, 545 mg.

ADRIAMYCIN® ℞
[a 'dreeah-mī "sin]
(doxorubicin hydrochloride)
for injection
FOR INTRAVENOUS USE ONLY

PRODUCT OVERVIEW

KEY FACTS

ADRIAMYCIN is a cytotoxic agent active against a variety of hematologic malignancies and solid tumors. The active ingredient, doxorubicin hydrochloride, is an anthracycline antibiotic that selectively kills malignant cells and causes tumor regression.

MAJOR USES

ADRIAMYCIN is clinically effective against disseminated neoplastic conditions including acute lymphoblastic and myeloblastic leukemia, Wilm's tumor, neuroblastoma, soft tissue and bone sarcomas, breast carcinoma, ovarian carcinoma, transitional cell bladder carcinoma, thyroid carcinoma, Hodgkin's and non-Hodgkin's lymphoma, bronchogenic carcinoma and gastric carcinoma.

SAFETY INFORMATION

ADRIAMYCIN is intended for intravenous use only. Care must be taken to avoid extravasation. Patients must be carefully monitored and doses adjusted to avoid too severe myelosuppression or mucositis. Too large cumulative doses may cause cardiomyopathy leading to congestive heart failure.

PRESCRIBING INFORMATION

ADRIAMYCIN® ℞
[a 'dreeah-mī "sin]
(doxorubicin hydrochloride)
for injection
FOR INTRAVENOUS USE ONLY

WARNINGS

1. Severe local tissue necrosis will occur if there is extravasation during administration (See Dosage and Administration). ADRIAMYCIN must not be given by the intramuscular or subcutaneous route.
2. Serious irreversible myocardial toxicity with delayed congestive failure often unresponsive to any cardiac supportive therapy may be encountered as total dosage approaches 550 mg/m^2. This toxicity may occur at lower cumulative doses in patients with prior mediastinal irradiation or on concurrent cyclophosphamide therapy.
3. Dosage should be reduced in patients with impaired hepatic function.
4. Severe myelosuppression may occur.
5. ADRIAMYCIN should be administered only under the supervision of a physician who is experienced in the use of cancer chemotherapeutic agents.

DESCRIPTION

Doxorubicin is a cytotoxic anthracycline antibiotic isolated from cultures of **Streptomyces peucetius** var. **caesius.** Doxorubicin consists of a naphthacenequinone nucleus linked through a glycosidic bond at ring atom 7 to an amino sugar, daunosamine. The structural formula is as follows:

Doxorubicin binds to nucleic acids, presumably by specific intercalation of the planar anthracycline nucleus with the DNA double helix. The anthracycline ring is lipophilic but the saturated end of the ring system contains abundant hydroxyl groups adjacent to the amino sugar, producing a hydrophilic center. The molecule is amphoteric, containing acidic functions in the ring phenolic groups and a basic function in the sugar amino group. It binds to cell membranes as well as plasma proteins. It is supplied in the hydrochloride form as a freeze-dried powder containing lactose.

CLINICAL PHARMACOLOGY

Though not completely elucidated, the mechanism of action of doxorubicin is related to its ability to bind to DNA and inhibit nucleic acid synthesis. Cell culture studies have demonstrated rapid cell penetration and perinucleolar chromatin binding, rapid inhibition of mitotic activity and nucleic acid synthesis, mutagenesis and chromosomal aberrations.

Animal studies have shown activity in a spectrum of experimental tumors, immunosuppression, carcinogenic properties in rodents, induction of a variety of toxic effects, including delayed and progressive cardiac toxicity, myelosuppression in all species and atrophy to testes in rats and dogs.

Pharmacokinetic studies show the intravenous administration of normal or radiolabeled ADRIAMYCIN (doxorubicin hydrochloride) for injection is followed by rapid plasma clearance and significant tissue binding. Urinary excretion, as determined by fluorimetric methods, accounts for approximately 4-5% of the administered dose in five days. Biliary excretion represents the major excretion route, 40-50% of the administered dose being recovered in the bile or the feces in seven days. Impairment of liver function results in slower excretion, and consequently, increased retention and accumulation in plasma and tissues. ADRIAMYCIN does not cross the blood brain barrier.

INDICATIONS AND USAGE

ADRIAMYCIN has been used successfully to produce regression in disseminated neoplastic conditions such as acute lymphoblastic leukemia, acute myeloblastic leukemia, Wilms' tumor, neuroblastoma, soft tissue and bone sarcomas, breast carcinoma, ovarian carcinoma, transitional cell bladder carcinoma, thyroid carcinoma, lymphomas of both Hodgkin and non-Hodgkin types, bronchogenic carcinoma in which the small cell histologic type is the most responsive compared to other cell types and gastric carcinoma.

A number of other solid tumors have also shown some responsiveness but in numbers too limited to justify specific recommendation. Studies to date have shown malignant melanoma, kidney carcinoma, large bowel carcinoma, brain tumors and metastases to the central nervous system not to be significantly responsive to ADRIAMYCIN therapy.

CONTRAINDICATIONS

ADRIAMYCIN therapy should not be started in patients who have marked myelosuppression induced by previous treatment with other antitumor agents or by radiotherapy. Conclusive data are not available on pre-existing heart disease as a co-factor of increased risk of ADRIAMYCIN induced cardiac toxicity. Preliminary data suggest that in such cases cardiac toxicity may occur at doses lower than the recommended cumulative limit. It is therefore not recommended to start ADRIAMYCIN in such cases. ADRIAMYCIN treatment is contraindicated in patients who received previous treatment with complete cumulative doses of ADRIAMYCIN and/or daunorubicin.

WARNINGS

Special attention must be given to the cardiac toxicity exhibited by ADRIAMYCIN. Although uncommon, acute left ventricular failure has occurred, particularly in patients who have received total dosage of the drug exceeding the currently recommended limit of 550 mg/m^2. This limit appears to be lower (400 mg/m^2) in patients who received radiotherapy to the mediastinal area or concomitant therapy with other potentially cardiotoxic agents such as cyclophosphamide. The total dose of ADRIAMYCIN administered to the individual patient should also take into account a previous or concomitant therapy with related compounds such as daunorubicin. Congestive heart failure and/or cardiomyopathy may be encountered several weeks after discontinuation of ADRIAMYCIN therapy.

Cardiac failure is often not favorably affected by presently known medical or physical therapy for cardiac support. Early clinical diagnosis of drug induced heart failure appears to be essential for successful treatment with digitalis, diuretics, low salt diet and bed rest. Severe cardiac toxicity may occur precipitously without antecedent EKG changes. A baseline EKG and EKGs performed prior to each dose or course after 300 mg/m^2 cumulative dose has been given is suggested. Transient EKG changes consisting of T-wave flattening, S-T depression and arrhythmias lasting for up to two weeks after a dose or course of ADRIAMYCIN are presently not considered indications for suspension of ADRIAMYCIN therapy. ADRIAMYCIN cardiomyopathy has been reported to be associated with a persistent reduction in the voltage of the QRS wave, a prolongation of the systolic time interval and a reduction of the ejection fraction as determined by echocardiography or radionuclide angiography. None of these tests have yet been confirmed to consistently identify those individual patients that are approaching their maximally tolerated cumulative dose of ADRIAMYCIN. If test results indicate change in cardiac function associated with ADRIAMYCIN the benefit of continued therapy must be carefully evaluated against the risk of producing irreversible cardiac damage.

Acute life-threatening arrhythmias have been reported to occur during or within a few hours after ADRIAMYCIN administration.

There is a high incidence of bone marrow depression, primarily of leukocytes, requiring careful hematologic monitoring. With the recommended dosage schedule, leukopenia is usually transient, reaching its nadir at 10-14 days after treatment with recovery usually occurring by the 21st day. White blood cell counts as low as 1000 mm^3 are to be expected during treatment with appropriate doses of ADRIAMYCIN. Red blood cell and platelet levels should also be monitored since they may also be depressed. Hematologic toxicity may require dose reduction or suspension or delay of ADRIAMYCIN therapy. Persistent severe myelo-suppression may result in superinfection or hemorrhage.

ADRIAMYCIN may potentiate the toxicity of other anticancer therapies. Exacerbation of cyclophosphamide induced hemorrhagic cystitis and enhancement of the hepatotoxicity of 6-mercaptopurine have been reported. Radiation induced toxicity to the myocardium, mucosae, skin and liver have been reported to be increased by the administration of ADRIAMYCIN.

Toxicity to recommended doses of ADRIAMYCIN is enhanced by hepatic impairment, therefore, prior to the individual dosing, evaluation of hepatic function is recommended using conventional clinical laboratory tests such as SGOT, SGPT, alkaline phosphatase and bilirubin. (See Dosage and Administration).

Necrotizing colitis manifested by typhlitis (cecal inflammation), bloody stools and severe and sometimes fatal infections have been associated with a combination of ADRIAMYCIN given by i.v. push daily for 3 days and cytarabine given by continuous infusion daily for 7 or more days.

On intravenous administration of ADRIAMYCIN extravasation may occur with or without an accompanying stinging or burning sensation and even if blood returns well on aspira-

Continued on next page

Adria—Cont.

tion of the infusion needle (See Dosage and Administration). If any signs or symptoms of extravasation have occurred the injection or infusion should be immediately terminated and restarted in another vein.
ADRIAMYCIN and related compounds have also been shown to have mutagenic and carcinogenic properties when tested in experimental models.
Usage in Pregnancy—Safe use of ADRIAMYCIN in pregnancy has not been established. ADRIAMYCIN is embryotoxic and teratogenic in rats and embryotoxic and abortifacient in rabbits. Therefore, the benefits to the pregnant patient should be carefully weighed against the potential toxicity to fetus and embryo. The possible adverse effects on fertility in males and females in humans or experimental animals have not been adequately evaluated.

PRECAUTIONS

Initial treatment with ADRIAMYCIN requires close observation of the patient and extensive laboratory monitoring. It is recommended, therefore, that patients be hospitalized at least during the first phase of the treatment.
Like other cytotoxic drugs, ADRIAMYCIN may induce hyperuricemia secondary to rapid lysis of neoplastic cells. The clinician should monitor the patient's blood uric acid level and be prepared to use such supportive and pharmacologic measures as might be necessary to control this problem.
ADRIAMYCIN imparts a red coloration to the urine for 1-2 days after administration and patients should be advised to expect this during active therapy.
ADRIAMYCIN is not an anti-microbial agent.

ADVERSE REACTIONS

Dose limiting toxicities of therapy are myelosuppression and cardiotoxicity (See Warnings). Other reactions reported are:
Cutaneous—Reversible complete alopecia occurs in most cases. Hyperpigmentation of nailbeds and dermal creases, primarily in children, and onycholysis have been reported in a few cases. Recall of skin reaction due to prior radiotherapy has occurred with ADRIAMYCIN administration.
Gastrointestinal—Acute nausea and vomiting occurs frequently and may be severe. This may be alleviated by antiemetic therapy. Mucositis (stomatitis and esophagitis) may occur 5–10 days after administration. The effect may be severe leading to ulceration and represents a site of origin for severe infections. The dose regimen consisting of administration of ADRIAMYCIN on three successive days results in the greater incidence and severity of mucositis. Ulceration and necrosis of the colon, especially the cecum, may occur leading to bleeding or severe infections which can be fatal. This reaction has been reported in patients with acute non-lymphocytic leukemia treated with a 3-day course of ADRIAMYCIN combined with cytarabine. Anorexia and diarrhea have been occasionally reported.
Vascular—Phlebosclerosis has been reported especially when small veins are used or a single vein is used for repeated administration. Facial flushing may occur if the injection is given too rapidly.
Local—Severe cellulitis, vesication and tissue necrosis will occur if ADRIAMYCIN is extravasated during administration. Erythematous streaking along the vein proximal to the site of the injection has been reported (See Dosage and Administration).
Hypersensitivity—Fever, chills and urticaria have been reported occasionally. Anaphylaxis may occur. A case of apparent cross sensitivity to lincomycin has been reported.
Other—Conjunctivitis and lacrimation occur rarely.

OVERDOSAGE

Acute overdosage with ADRIAMYCIN enhances the toxic effects of mucositis, leukopenia and thrombopenia. Treatment of acute overdosage consists of treatment of the severely myelosuppressed patient with hospitalization, antibiotics, platelet and granulocyte transfusions and symptomatic treatment of mucositis.
Chronic overdosage with cumulative doses exceeding 550 mg/m^2 increases the risk of cardiomyopathy and resultant congestive heart failure. Treatment consists of vigorous management of congestive heart failure with digitalis preparations and diuretics. The use of peripheral vasodilators has been recommended.

DOSAGE AND ADMINISTRATION

Care in the administration of ADRIAMYCIN will reduce the chance of perivenous infiltration. It may also decrease the chance of local reactions such as urticaria and erythematous streaking. On intravenous administration of ADRIAMYCIN, extravasation may occur with or without an accompanying stinging or burning sensation and even if blood returns well on aspiration of the infusion needle. If any signs or symptoms of extravasation have occurred, the injection or infusion should be immediately terminated and restarted in another vein. If it is known or suspected that subcutaneous extravasation has occurred, local infiltration with an injectable corticosteroid and flooding the site with normal saline has been reported to lessen the local reaction. Because of the progressive nature of extravasation reactions, the area of injection should be frequently examined and plastic surgery consultation obtained. If ulceration begins, early wide excision of the involved area should be considered.[1]
The most commonly used dosage schedule is 60-75 mg/m^2 as a single intravenous injection administered at 21-day intervals. The lower dose should be given to patients with inadequate marrow reserves due to old age, or prior therapy, or neoplastic marrow infiltration. An alternative dose schedule is weekly doses of 20 mg/m^2 which has been reported to produce a lower incidence of congestive heart failure. Thirty mg/m^2 on each of three successive days repeated every 4 weeks has also been used. ADRIAMYCIN dosage must be reduced if the bilirubin is elevated as follows: Serum Bilirubin 1.2-3.0 mg/dl-give $\frac{1}{2}$ normal dose, > 3 mg/dl—give $\frac{1}{4}$ normal dose.
Preparation of Solution: ADRIAMYCIN 10 mg, 20 mg and 50 mg vials should be reconstituted with 5 ml, 10 ml and 25 ml respectively of Sodium Chloride Injection USP (0.9%) or Sterile Water for Injection USP to give a final concentration of 2 mg/ml of doxorubicin hydrochloride. If Sterile Water for Injection USP is used for reconstitution, the resulting solution must be brought towards isotonicity before injection by adding 2 to 3 times the volume of 0.9% Sodium Chloride Injection USP to the aqueous solution. An appropriate volume of air should be withdrawn from the vial during reconstitution to avoid excessive pressure build-up. Bacteriostatic diluents are not recommended.
After adding the diluent, the vial should be shaken and the contents allowed to dissolve. The reconstituted solution is stable for 24 hours at room temperature and 48 hours under refrigeration (4-10°C). It should be protected from exposure to sunlight and any unused solution should be discarded.
It is recommended that ADRIAMYCIN be slowly administered into the tubing of a freely running intravenous infusion of Sodium Chloride Injection USP or 5% Dextrose Injection USP. The tubing should be attached to a Butterfly® needle inserted preferably into a large vein. If possible, avoid veins over joints or in extremities with compromised venous or lymphatic drainage. The rate of administration is dependent on the size of the vein and the dosage. However the dose should be administered in not less than 3 to 5 minutes. Local erythematous streaking along the vein as well as facial flushing may be indicative of too rapid an administration. A burning or stinging sensation may be indicative of perivenous infiltration and the infusion should be immediately terminated and restarted in another vein. Perivenous infiltration may occur painlessly.
ADRIAMYCIN should not be mixed with heparin or 5-fluorouracil since it has been reported that these drugs are incompatible to the extent that a precipitate may form. Until specific compatibility data are available, it is not recommended that ADRIAMYCIN be mixed with other drugs.
ADRIAMYCIN has been used concurrently with other approved chemotherapeutic agents. Evidence is available that in some types of neoplastic disease combination chemotherapy is superior to single agents. The benefits and risks of such therapy continue to be elucidated; listed in CLINICAL STUDIES are combinations that have been reported to be clinically superior to any agent in the combination used alone.
Handling and Disposal: Skin reactions associated with ADRIAMYCIN have been reported. Caution in the handling and preparation of the powder and solution must be exercised and the use of gloves is recommended. If ADRIAMYCIN powder or solution contacts the skin or mucosae, immediately wash thoroughly with soap and water.
Procedures for proper handling and disposal of anti-cancer drugs should be considered. Several guidelines on this subject have been published.[2–7] There is no general agreement that all of the procedures recommended in the guidelines are necessary or appropriate.

HOW SUPPLIED

ADRIAMYCIN® (doxorubicin hydrochloride) for injection is available as follows:
10 mg—Each vial contains 10 mg of doxorubicin HCl and 50 mg of lactose USP as a sterile red-orange lyophilized powder. Packaged and supplied in 10-vial packs NDC 0013-1006-91.
20 mg—Each vial contains 20 mg of doxorubicin HCl and 100 mg of lactose USP as a sterile red-orange lyophilized powder. Packaged and supplied in 5-vial packs NDC 0013-1076-94.
50 mg—Each vial contains 50 mg of doxorubicin HCl and 250 mg of lactose USP as a sterile red-orange lyophilized powder. Packaged and supplied in a single vial pack NDC 0013-1016-79.
Protect from exposure to sunlight and discard any unused solution.

CLINICAL STUDIES

Clinical studies support the efficacy of ADRIAMYCIN used concurrently with other chemotherapeutic agents. Listed below are tumor types and drugs used concurrently with ADRIAMYCIN.
Acute lymphocytic leukemia in adults. ADRIAMYCIN with vincristine and prednisone[8,9] or with cytosine arabinoside, vincristine and prednisone[14].
Acute lymphocytic leukemia in children. ADRIAMYCIN with vincristine and prednisone[10,11]
Acute non-lymphocytic leukemia. ADRIAMYCIN with arabinosyl cytosine[12] or with arabinosyl cytosine, vincristine and prednisone[13,14].
Carcinoma of the breast. ADRIAMYCIN with 5-fluorouracil and/or cyclophosphamide[15,16] or with vincristine with or without cyclophosphamide[17].
Bronchogenic carcinoma, non-small cell: ADRIAMYCIN with cyclophosphamide, methotrexate and procarbazine[18] or with cyclophosphamide and cisplatin[19]. Bronchogenic carcinoma, small cell: ADRIAMYCIN with vincristine and cyclophosphamide[20,21,22].
Hodgkin disease: ADRIAMYCIN with bleomycin, vincristine and dacarbazine[23,24].
Non-Hodgkin lymphoma: ADRIAMYCIN with cyclophosphamide, vincristine and prednisone[25], or bleomycin, cyclophosphamide, vincristine and prednisone[26].
Carcinoma of the ovary. ADRIAMYCIN with cisplatin[27,28].
Soft tissue sarcoma: ADRIAMYCIN with dacarbazine or with dacarbazine, cyclophosphamide and vincristine[29,30].
Carcinoma of the bladder. ADRIAMYCIN with cisplatin and cyclophosphamide[31] or with 5-flourouracil[32].
Carcinoma of the stomach. ADRIAMYCIN with 5-fluorouracil and Mitomycin-C[33,34].

REFERENCES

1. Rudolph R et al: Skin Ulcers Due to ADRIAMYCIN. Cancer 38: 1087-1094, Sept. 1976.
2. Recommendations for the Safe Handling of Parenteral Antineoplastic Drugs. NIH Publication No. 83-2621. For sale by the Superintendent of Documents, U.S. Government Printing Office, Washington, D.C. 20402.
3. AMA Council Report. Guidelines for Handling Parenteral Antineoplastics. JAMA, March 15, 1985.
4. National Study Commission on Cytotoxic Exposure—Recommendations for Handling Cytotoxic Agents. Available from Louis P. Jeffrey, Sc. D., Director of Pharmacy Services, Rhode Island Hospital, 593 Eddy Street, Providence, Rhode Island 02902.
5. Clinical Oncological Society of Australia: Guidelines and recommendations for safe handling of antineoplastic agents. Med J Australia 1:426-428 1983.
6. Jones R. B., et al. Safe handling of chemotherapeutic agents: A report from the Mount Sinai Medical Center. CA—A Cancer Journal for Clinicians Sept/Oct, 258-263 1983.
7. American Society of Hospital Pharmacists technical assistance bulletin on handling cytotoxic drugs in hospitals. Am J Hosp Pharm 42:131-137, 1985.
8. Muriel FS, Pavlovsky S, Penalver JA et al: Evaluation of Induction of Remission, Intensification, and Central Nervous System Prophylactic Treatment in Acute Lymphoblastic Leukemia. Cancer 34:418-426, 1974.
9. Shaw MT, Raab SO: ADRIAMYCIN in Combination Chemotherapy of Adult Acute Lymphoblastic Leukemia: A Southwest Oncology Group Study. Med Pediatr Oncol 3:261-266, 1977.
10. Sallan SE, Camitta BM, Cassady JR et al: Intermittent Combination Chemotherapy with ADRIAMYCIN for Childhood Acute Lymphoblastic Leukemia: Clinical Results. Blood 51:425-433, 1978.
11. Rivera G, Aur RJA, Dahl GV: Second Cessation of Therapy in Childhood Lymphocytic Leukemia. Blood 53:1114-1120, 1979.
12. Preisler HD, Rustum Y, Henderson ES, et al: Treatment of Acute Non-Lymphocytic Leukemia: Use of Anthracycline-Cytosine Arabinoside Induction Therapy and Comparison of Two Maintenance Regimens. Blood 53:455-464, 1979.
13. Weinstein HJ, Mayer RJ, Rosenthal DS: Treatment of Acute Myelogenous Leukemia in Children and Adults. N. Engl J Med 303:473-478, 1980.
14. McCredie KB, Bodey GP, Freireich EJ, et al: Chemoimmunotherapy of Adult Acute Leukemia. Cancer 47:1256-1261, 1981.
15. Bull JM, Tormey DC, Li S-H, et al: A Randomized Comparative Trial of ADRIAMYCIN Versus Methotrexate in Combination Drug Therapy. Cancer 41:1649-1657, 1978.
16. Smalley RV, Bartolucci AA: Variations in Responsiveness and Survival of Clinical Subsets of Patients with Metastatic Breast Cancer to Two Chemotherapy Combinations. Eur J Cancer (Suppl 1) 141-146, 1980.
17. Brambilla C, Valagussa P, Bonadonna G: Sequential combination Chemotherapy in Advanced Breast Cancer. Cancer Chemother Pharmacol 1:35-39, 1978.
18. Bitran JD, Desser RK, DeMeester TR, et al: Cyclophosphamide, ADRIAMYCIN, Methotrexate and Procarbazine (CAMP)-Effective Four-Drug Combination Chemotherapy for Metastatic Non-Oat Cell Bronchogenic Carcinoma. Cancer Treat Rep 60:1225-1230, 1976.

19. Eagan RT, Frytak S, Creagan ET: Phase II Study of Cyclophosphamide, ADRIAMYCIN and Cis-dichlorodiamineplatinum II by Infusion in Patients with Adenocarcinoma and Large Cell Carcinoma of the Lung. Cancer Treat Rep 63:1589-1591, 1979.
20. Livingston RB, Moore TN, Heilbrun L, et al: Small Cell Carcinoma of the Lung: Combined Chemotherapy and Radiation, Ann Intern Med 88:194-199, 1978.
21. Lyman GH, Hartmann RC, Hussain IS, et al: Combination Chemotherapy and Radiation Therapy of Undifferentiated Small Cell Bronchogenic Carcinoma. South Med J 71:519-524, 1978.
22. Greco FA, Richardson RL, Snell JD, et al: Small Cell Lung Cancer. Am J Med 66:625-630, 1979.
23. Bonadonna G, DeLena M, Monfardini S, et al: Combination Usage of ADRIAMYCIN (NSC 123127) in Malignant Lymphomas. Cancer Chemother Rep Part 3. Vol 6:381-388, 1975.
24. Case DC, Young CW, Nisce L, et al: Eight-Drug Combination Chemotherapy (MOPP and ABVD) and Local Radiotherapy for Advanced Hodgkin's Disease. Cancer Treat Rep 60:1217-1223, 1976.
25. McKelvey EM, Gottlieb JA, Wilson HE, et al: Hydroxyldaunomycin (ADRIAMYCIN) Combination Chemotherapy in Malignant Lymphoma. Cancer 38:1484-1493, 1976.
26. Schein PS, DeVita VT, Hubbard S, et al: Bleomycin, ADRIAMYCIN, Cyclophosphamide, Vincristine, and Prednisone (BACOP) Combination Chemotherapy in the Treatment of Advanced Diffuse Histiocytic Lymphoma. Ann Intern Med 85:417-422, 1976.
27. Briscoe KE, Pasmantier MW, Ohnuma T, Kennedy BJ: Cis-Dichlorodiammine platinum (II) and ADRIAMYCIN Treatment of Advanced Ovarian Cancer. Cancer Treat Rep 62:2027-2030, 1978.
28. Bruckner HW, Cohen CJ, Goldberg JD, et al: Improved Chemotherapy for Ovarian Cancer with Cis-diamminedichloroplatinum and ADRIAMYCIN. Cancer 47:2288-2294, May 1, 1981.
29. Gottlieb JA, Baker LH, O'Bryan RM, et al: ADRIAMYCIN (NSC-123127) Used Alone and in Combination for Soft Tissue and Bony Sarcoma. Cancer Chemother Rep Part 3 Vol 6:271-282, 1975.
30. Yap BS, Baker LH, Sinkovics JG, et al: Cyclophosphamide, Vincristine, ADRIAMYCIN and DTIC (CYVADIC) Combination Chemotherapy for the Treatment of Advanced Sarcomas. Cancer Treat Rep 64:93-98, 1980.
31. Kedia KR, Gibbons C, Persky L: The Management of Advanced Bladder Carcinoma. J Urol 125:655-658, 1981.
32. Martino S, Samal B, Al-Sarraf M: Phase II Study of 5-Fluorouracil and ADRIAMYCIN in Transitional Cell Carcinoma of the Urinary Tract. Cancer Treat Rep 64:161-163, 1980.
33. Macdonald JS, Schein PS, Woolley PV, et al: 5-Fluorouracil, Doxorubicin and Mitomycin (FAM) Combination Chemotherapy for Advanced Gastric Cancer. Ann Intern Med 93:533-536, 1980.
34. Panettiere FJ, Heilbran L: Experiences with two treatment Schedules in the Combination Chemotherapy of Advanced Gastric Carcinoma. In: Mitomycin C. Current Status and New Developments. Schein PS ed., New York, Academic Press 1979 pp. 145-157.

Distributed by: ADRIA LABORATORIES, Division of Erbamont Inc., COLUMBUS, OHIO 43215. Manufactured by: FARMITALIA CARLO ERBA S.p.A., MILAN, ITALY

ADRUCIL® ℞
[a 'drew-sill"]
(fluorouracil)
INJECTION, USP
FOR INTRAVENOUS USE ONLY

PRODUCT OVERVIEW

KEY FACTS

ADRUCIL is a cytotoxic agent active against a variety of solid tumors. The active ingredient, fluorouracil, is a fluorinated pyrimidine antimetabolite that kills malignant cells and causes tumor regression.

MAJOR USES

ADRUCIL is clinically effective in the palliative management of carcinoma of the colon, rectum, breast, stomach and pancreas.

SAFETY INFORMATION

ADRUCIL is intended for intravenous use only. Patients must be carefully monitored and the dose adjusted to avoid too severe myelosuppression, diarrhea or gastrointestinal hemorrhage, especially in patients with previous irradiation of the pelvis, use of alkylating agents or who have widespread involvement of bone marrow by metastatic tumors or impaired hepatic or renal function.

PRESCRIBING INFORMATION

ADRUCIL® ℞
[a 'drew-sill"]
(fluorouracil)
INJECTION, USP
FOR INTRAVENOUS USE ONLY

WARNINGS

Adrucil should be administered only by or under the supervision of a qualified physician who is experienced in cancer chemotherapy and the use of potent antimetabolites. Because severe toxic reactions may occur, it is recommended that patients be hospitalized during the initial course of therapy. Before administering Adrucil, the contents of this insert should be thoroughly reviewed.

DESCRIPTION

Fluorouracil is a fluorinated pyrimidine belonging to the category of antimetabolites. Fluorouracil resembles the natural uracil molecule except it has been fluorinated in the 5 position; it has the following structural formula:

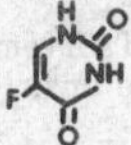

Molecular formula: $C_4H_3FN_2O_2$
Molecular Weight: 130.08

It is sparingly soluble in water (12.2 mg/ml) at pH 7 and has pK's of 8.0 and 13.0.

Adrucil (Fluorouracil) Injection, USP is supplied as a sterile aqueous solution for intravenous injection. It has a pH of 8.6 to 9.0. The ampules are filled with a 5% excess to permit withdrawal and administration of the labeled volume.

A precipitate may form as a result of exposure to low temperatures. Redissolve by heating to 140°F (60°C) with vigorous shaking, and allow to cool to body temperature prior to use.

ACTIONS

The mechanism of action of fluorouracil is mainly related to competitive inhibition of thymidylate synthetase, the enzyme catalyzing the methylation of deoxyuridylic acid to thymidylic acid. The consequent thymidine deficiency results in inhibition of deoxyribonucleic acid (DNA) synthesis, thus inducing cell death. Also, moderate inhibition of ribonucleic acid (RNA) and incorporation of fluorouracil into RNA have been observed, but these effects do not appear to play a significant role in the determination of the antitumor action of fluorouracil.

The effects of DNA and RNA deprivation are most marked on those cells which grow rapidly and which take up fluorouracil at a more rapid pace. Inactive degradation products (e.g., CO_2, urea, α-fluoro-β-alanine) result from the extensive catabolic metabolism of fluorouracil. Following intravenous injection, no intact drug can be detected in the plasma after 3 hours and 60 to 80% of the dose is excreted as respiratory CO_2 in 8 to 12 hours. Within 6 hours approximately 15% of the total drug administered is excreted unchanged in the urine with over 90% of this excretion occurring in the first hour.

INDICATIONS

Adrucil is effective in the palliative management of carcinoma of the colon, rectum, breast, stomach and pancreas in patients who are considered incurable by surgery or other means.

CONTRAINDICATIONS

Adrucil therapy should not be started in patients with a poor nutritional state, depressed bone marrow function, or potentially serious infections.

WARNINGS

THE DAILY DOSE OF ADRUCIL IS NOT TO EXCEED 800 MG AND IT IS RECOMMENDED THAT PATIENTS BE HOSPITALIZED DURING THEIR FIRST COURSE OF TREATMENT.

Adrucil (Fluorouracil) Injection, USP should be used with extreme caution in poor risk patients with a history of high-dose pelvic irradiation, previous use of alkylating agents, or who have a widespread involvement of bone marrow by metastatic tumors, or impaired hepatic or renal function. The drug is not intended as an adjuvant to surgery. Although severe toxicity and fatalities are more likely to occur in poor risk patients, these effects have occasionally been encountered in patients in relatively good condition. Severe hematologic toxicity, gastrointestinal hemorrhage, and even death may result from use of Adrucil (Fluorouracil) Injection, USP despite meticulous selection of patients and careful adjustment of dosage.

Usage in Pregnancy: Safe use of Adrucil (Fluorouracil) Injection, USP has not been established with respect to adverse effects on fetal development. Therefore, this drug should not be used during pregnancy, particularly in the first trimester, unless in the judgement of the physician the potential benefits to the patient outweigh the hazards.

Because the risk of mutagenesis has not been evaluated, such possible effects on males and females must be considered.

Combination Therapy: Any form of therapy which adds to the stress of the patient, interferes with nutrition or depresses bone marrow function will increase the toxicity of Adrucil (Fluorouracil) Injection, USP.

PRECAUTIONS

Adrucil (Fluorouracil) Injection, USP is a highly toxic drug with a narrow margin of safety. Special attention must be given to the toxicity exhibited by fluorouracil. Patients should be carefully supervised since it must be recognized that therapeutic response is unlikely to occur without some evidence of toxicity. Patients should be advised of expected toxic effects, especially oral manifestations. White blood counts with differential are recommended before each dose. Knowledge of WBC nadir is necessary for eventual subsequent dosage adjustments.

Administration of Adrucil (Fluorouracil) Injection, USP is to be discontinued promptly when one of the following signs appear:

1. Stomatitis or esophagopharyngitis (at first visible sign)
2. Leukopenia (WBC < 3500 mm^3) or rapidly falling white blood count
3. Vomiting (intractable)
4. Diarrhea (frequent bowel movements or watery stools)
5. Gastrointestinal ulceration and bleeding
6. Thrombocytopenia (platelets < 100,000 mm^3)
7. Hemorrhage (from any site)

Drug Interactions: Adrucil (Fluorouracil) with leucovorin, the latter usually given 24 hours after sequential administration of methotrexate and 5-FU, may result in increased potency and toxicity.

ADVERSE REACTIONS

Stomatitis and esophagopharyngitis (which may lead to sloughing and ulceration), diarrhea, anorexia, nausea and emesis are common.

Myelosuppression almost uniformly accompanies a course of adequate therapy with fluorouracil. Low WBC counts are usually first observed between the 9th and 14th day after the first course of treatment with nadir occurring during the third week, although at times delayed for as long as 25 days. By the 30th day the count is usually within the normal range. Thrombocytopenia also may occur.

Alopecia and dermatitis are seen in a substantial number of cases and patients should be advised of this consequence of treatment. The alopecia is reported to be reversible. The dermatitis is often a pruritic maculopapular rash generally appearing on the extremities and less frequently on the trunk. It is usually reversible and responsive to symptomatic treatment. Dry skin and fissuring have also been noted.

Photosensitivity, as manifested by erythema or increased pigmentation of the skin, may occasionally occur. Also reported were photophobia, lacrimation, epistaxis, euphoria, acute cerebellar syndrome (which may persist following discontinuation of treatment) and nail changes including loss of nails. Myocardial ischemia has also been reported.

DOSAGE AND ADMINISTRATION

Note:

The recommended route of administration of Adrucil is only by intravenous injection, using care to avoid extravasation. No dilution of Adrucil is required.

It is recommended that all dosages be based on the patient's actual weight. However, if the patient is obese or if there has been a spurious weight gain due to edema, ascites, or other forms of abnormal fluid retention, then the estimated lean body mass (dry weight) should be used.

Prior to treatment, it is recommended that each patient be carefully evaluated to accurately estimate the optimum initial dosage of Adrucil.

Initial Therapy (See Contraindications, Warnings and Precautions before prescribing):

I. A dose of 12 mg/kg is given intravenously once daily for 4 successive days. The daily dose should not be more than 800 mg. If no toxicity is observed at any time during the course of therapy, 6 mg/kg are given on the 6th, 8th, 10th and 12th days. No therapy is given on the 5th, 7th, 9th or 11th days. Therapy is to be discontinued at the end of the 12th day, even if no toxicity has become apparent.

II. In poor risk patients or those who are not in an adequate nutritional state, a dose level of 6 mg/kg/day for 3 days is recommended. If no toxicity is observed at any time during the treatment, 3 mg/kg may be given on the 5th, 7th and 9th days. No therapy is given on the 4th, 6th or 8th days. The daily dose should not exceed 400 mg.

A sequence of injections on either schedule constitutes a "course of therapy."

Therapy should be discontinued promptly when any of the signs of toxicity listed under PRECAUTIONS appears.

Continued on next page

Adria—Cont.

Maintenance Therapy: When toxicity has not been a problem, or after the toxic signs from the initial course of therapy have subsided, therapy should be continued using either of the following schedules:

A. Repeat dosage of the first course, beginning 30 days after the last day of the previous course of treatment.
B. Administer a maintenance dosage of 10 to 15 mg/kg/week. Do not exceed 1 gram per week. Reduced doses should be used for poor risk patients.

The dosage of drug to be used should take into account the patient's reaction to the previous course of therapy and be adjusted accordingly. Some patients have received from 9 to 45 courses of treatment during periods which ranged from 12 to 60 months.

Adrucil (Fluorouracil) Injection, USP should not be mixed with IV additives or chemotherapeutic agents.

Handling and Disposal: Procedures for proper handling and disposal of anti-cancer drugs should be considered. Several guidelines on this subject have been published.[1–6] There is no general agreement that all of the procedures recommended in the guidelines are necessary or appropriate.

HOW SUPPLIED

Adrucil (Fluorouracil) Injection, USP is available in 10 ml ampules, as a colorless to faint yellow aqueous solution containing 500 mg of fluorouracil and pH adjusted with sodium hydroxide to 8.6 to 9.0. Packaged and supplied in individual cartons, there are 10 ampules per shelf container NDC 0013-1026-91.

NOTE: Although Adrucil ampule solution may discolor slightly during storage, the potency and safety are not adversely affected. Store at room temperature 59–86°F (15–30°C) and protect from light. If a precipitate occurs due to exposure to low temperatures, re-solubilize by heating to 140°F (60°C) with vigorous shaking; allow to cool to body temperature before using.

REFERENCES

1. Recommended for the Safe Handling of Parenteral Antineoplastic Drugs. NIH Publication No. 83-2621. For sale by the Superintendent of Documents, U.S. Government Printing Office, Washington, D.C. 20402.
2. AMA Council Report. Guidelines for Handling Parenteral Antineoplastics. JAMA, March 15, 1985.
3. National Study Commission on Cytotoxic Exposure—Recommendations for Handling Cytotoxic Agents. Available from Louis P. Jeffrey, Sc. D., Director of Pharmacy Services, Rhode Island Hospital, 593 Eddy Street, Providence, Rhode Island 02902.
4. Clinical Oncological Society of Australia: Guidelines and recommendations for safe handling of antineoplastic agents. Med J Australia 1:426–428 1983.
5. Jones R. B., et al. Safe handling of chemotherapeutic agents: A report from the Mount Sinai Medical Center, Ca—A Cancer Journal for Clinicians Sept/Oct, 258–263 1983.
6. American Society of Hospital Pharmacists technical assistance bulletin on handling cytotoxic drugs in hospitals. Am J Hosp Pharm 42:131–137, 1985.

Distributed by:
ADRIA LABORATORIES
Division of Erbamont Inc.
COLUMBUS, OHIO 43215
Manufactured by:
Taylor Pharmacal Co.
Decatur, Illinois 62525

AXOTAL® ℞

[ax 'ō-tall"]
(Butalbital and Aspirin), Tablets, USP

PRODUCT OVERVIEW

KEY FACTS

Analgesic and anxiolytic drug for treatment of tension headaches (muscle contraction headaches). Aspirin is the analgesic component. Butalbital provides the anxiolytic action and has a muscle relaxant effect. AXOTAL does not contain caffeine.

MAJOR USES

For the relief of the symptom complex of tension headaches.

SAFETY INFORMATION

Contraindicated for patients hypersensitive to aspirin or barbiturates or patients with porphyria. Caution is necessary for patients with asthma, allergies, nasal polyps, bleeding problems, peptic ulcer, renal impairment or drug abuse problems. May impair mental or physical abilities required for driving or operating machinery.

PRESCRIBING INFORMATION

AXOTAL® ℞

[ax 'ō-tall"]
(Butalbital and Aspirin), Tablets, USP

WARNING

May be habit forming.

DESCRIPTION

Each AXOTAL tablet for oral administration contains: butalbital, USP, 50 mg (Warning: May be habit forming) and aspirin, USP, 650 mg.

Butalbital, 5-allyl-5-isobutyl barbituric acid, a white odorless crystalline powder, is a short to intermediate-acting barbiturate. Its molecular formula is $C_{11}H_{16}N_2O_3$ and molecular weight 224.26. The chemical structure of butalbital is:

$H_2C{=}CHCH_2$, $(CH_3)_2CHCH_2$ [structure: pyrimidinetrione ring with H, O, N, O, NH, O]

ACTIONS

Pharmacologically, AXOTAL combines the analgesic properties of aspirin with the anxiolytic and muscle relaxant properties of butalbital.

INDICATIONS

AXOTAL is indicated for the relief of the symptom complex of tension (or muscle contraction) headaches.

CONTRAINDICATIONS

Hypersensitivity to aspirin or barbiturates. Patients with porphyria.

PRECAUTIONS

General—AXOTAL should be used with caution in patients with certain medical problems, including those with a history of asthma, allergies and nasal polyps. Also, the drug must be prescribed carefully for patients with hemophilia or other bleeding problems, peptic ulcer, renal impairment, or a history of drug abuse or dependence.

Information for patients—AXOTAL may impair the mental and/or physical abilities required for the performance of potentially hazardous tasks, such as driving a car or operating machinery. The patient should be cautioned accordingly.

Drug Interactions—Patients receiving narcotic analgesics, antipsychotics, antianxiety agents, or other CNS depressants (including alcohol) concomitantly with AXOTAL may exhibit additive CNS depressant effects. When combined therapy is contemplated, the dose of one or both agents should be reduced.

Drugs	Effect
Aspirin with anti-inflammatory agents	Increased ulcerogenic effects
Butalbital with coumarin anticoagulants	Decreased effect of anti-coagulant because of increased metabolism resulting from enzyme induction.
Butalbital with tricyclic anti-depressants	Decreased blood levels of anti-depressant

Usage in Pregnancy—Adequate studies have not been performed in animals to determine whether this drug affects fertility in males or females, has teratogenic potential or has other adverse effects on the fetus. Although there is no clearly defined risk, experience cannot exclude the possibility of infrequent or subtle damage to the human fetus. AXOTAL should be used in pregnant women only when clearly needed.

Nursing Mothers—The effects of AXOTAL on infants of nursing mothers are not known. Salicylates and barbiturates are excreted in the breast milk of nursing mothers. The serum levels in infants are believed to be insignificant with therapeutic doses.

Pediatric Use—Safety and effectiveness in children below the age of 12 have not been established.

ADVERSE REACTIONS

The most frequent adverse reactions are drowsiness and dizziness. Less frequent adverse reactions are lightheadness and gastrointestinal disturbances including nausea, vomiting and flatulence. Mental confusion or depression can occur due to intolerance or overdosage of butalbital.

DRUG ABUSE AND DEPENDENCE

Prolonged use of barbiturates can produce drug dependence, characterized by psychic dependence, and less frequently, physical dependence, and tolerance. The abuse liability of AXOTAL is similar to that of other barbiturate-containing drug combinations. Caution should be exercised when prescribing medication for patients with a known propensity for taking excessive quantities of drugs which is not uncommon in patients with chronic tension headaches.

OVERDOSAGE

The toxic effects of acute overdosage of AXOTAL are attributable mainly to its barbiturate component and, to a lesser extent, aspirin. Symptoms attributable to acute *barbiturate poisoning* include drowsiness, confusion and coma, respiratory depression, hypertension and shock. Symptoms of *salicylate overdosage* include central nausea and vomiting, tinnitus and deafness, vertigo and headaches, mental dullness and confusion, diaphoresis, rapid pulse and increased respiration leading to respiratory alkalosis. Treatment consists primarily of management of barbiturate intoxication and the correction of acid-base imbalance due to salicylism. Vomiting should be induced mechanically or with emetics, such as ipecac syrup, in the conscious patient. Gastric lavage may be used if the pharyngeal and laryngeal reflexes are present and if less than 4 hours have elapsed since ingestion. A cuffed endotracheal tube should be inserted before gastric lavage of the unconscious patient and when necessary to provide assisted respiration. Gastric lavage followed by activated charcoal is recommended regardless of time since ingestion. Diuresis, alkalinization of the urine, and correction of electrolyte disturbances should be accomplished through administration of intravenous fluids such as 1% sodium bicarbonate in 5% dextrose in water. Meticulous attention should be given to maintaining adequate pulmonary ventilation. Exchange transfusion is most feasible for a small infant while intermittent peritoneal dialysis is useful for cases of moderate severity in adults. Hemodialysis with the artifical kidney is the most effective means of removing salicylate and is indicated for the very severe cases of salicylate intoxication. Hypoprothrombinemia should be treated with intravenous Vitamin K (phytonadione). Methemoglobinemia over 30% should be treated with methylene blue administered slowly intravenously.

In all cases of suspected overdose, immediately call your regional poison center for assistance.

DOSAGE AND ADMINISTRATION

One tablet every four hours as needed. Do not exceed 6 tablets per day.

Medication should be taken with food or a full glass of water or milk to lessen gastric irritation caused by aspirin.

HOW SUPPLIED

Each AXOTAL tablet contains butalbital USP, 50 mg, and aspirin 650 mg.

AXOTAL is available for oral administration as uncoated, white, capsule-shaped tablets coded ADRIA, 130.

Tablets are supplied as follows:
NDC 0013-1301-17 in bottles of 100
NDC 0013-1301-21 in bottles of 500

Store in a tight container below 30°C (86°F). Protect from moisture.

Shown in Product Identification Section, page 403

EVAC-Q-KIT®

[ē-vak 'cue-kit]

PRODUCT OVERVIEW

KEY FACTS

EVAC-Q-KIT is a bowel evaculant kit containing magnesium citrate, phenolphthalein tablets and a gas-releasing suppository.

MAJOR USES

Preparation of the colon for radiologic examinations.

SAFETY INFORMATION

The EVAC-Q-MAG solution is contraindicated in the presence of severe renal insufficiency. Do not use any of the components when abdominal pain, nausea or vomiting are present.

PRESCRIBING INFORMATION

EVAC-Q-KIT®

[ē-vak 'cue-kit]

DESCRIPTION

Each EVAC-Q-KIT® contains:

1. EVAC-Q-MAG®—10 fl. oz. Sugar-Free. Ingredients: Magnesium citrate, citric acid and potassium citrate in cherry flavored base. Carbonated.
2. EVAC-Q-TABS® — 2 tablets. Ingredients: Each tablet contains 2 grains (130 mg) of phenolphthalein.
3. EVAC-Q-SERT®—2 suppositories. Ingredients: Potassium bitartrate and sodium bicarbonate in polyethylene glycol base.
4. 1 Instruction Sheet (In English and Spanish)

ACTIONS

Bowel Evacuant.

INDICATIONS

Preparations of the colon for single and multiple radiology examinations requiring a clean colon.

CONTRAINDICATIONS

EVAC-Q-MAG is contraindicated in the presence of severe renal insufficiency.

WARNINGS

Do not use any of these preparations when abdominal pain, nausea, or vomiting are present. Frequent and continued use may cause dependence upon laxatives. Rectal bleeding or failure to respond may indicate a serious condition. Consult physician. As with any drug, if you are pregnant or nursing a baby, seek the advice of a health professional before using this product. KEEP OUT OF REACH OF CHILDREN.

PRECAUTIONS

If skin rash appears, do not use this or any other preparation containing phenolphthalein.

DOSAGE AND ADMINISTRATION

Instructions for Patients—early schedule* Your physician is preparing you for an X-ray examination that requires thorough clearing of the intestinal tract. He is using this EVAC-Q-KIT® routine to make this procedure more comfortable for you.

BE SURE TO FOLLOW EACH STEP AND COMPLETE ALL INSTRUCTIONS OR ENTIRE X-RAY EXAMINATION MAY HAVE TO BE REPEATED.

DAY BEFORE EXAMINATION

IMPORTANT: A high fluid intake is essential to the success of this regimen. You MUST take a large glass (8 oz.) of fluid at specified times. (=8 oz. fluid.) Drink only black coffee, plain tea, strained fruit juice, soft drinks or water at the times indicated. NO MILK OR CREAM.

- ☐ **Noon.** Light lunch. Clear soup, two hardboiled eggs, plain Jell-O, fluid.
- ☐ **12:30 P.M.** (or ½ hr. after lunch) Drink entire contents—EVAC-Q-MAG® (#1 in your kit), over ice.
- ☐ **1:00 P.M.** + .
- ☐ **3:00 P.M.** Take two (2) EVAC-Q-TABS® laxative tablets (#2 in your kit) with large glass of water.
- ☐ **4:00 P.M.** + .
- ☐ **5:00 P.M.** Liquid dinner. Clear Soup, plain Jell-O + .
- ☐ **6:00 P.M.** + .
- ☐ **9:00 P.M.** + .
- ☐ **10:00 P.M.** Remove cover from EVAC-Q-SERT® suppository (#3 in your kit). Moisten the suppository in tap water. Insert suppository into rectum. Wait at least 10–15 minutes before evacuating, even if urge is strong.
- ☐ **BEDTIME:** + .

DAY OF TEST. No breakfast.

- ☐ **6:00 A.M.** (must be at least 2 hours before test). Use remaining EVAC-Q-SERT® suppository (#4 in your kit). Follow same directions as 10:00 P.M. night before.

BE SURE TO DRINK ALL THE FLUID SPECIFIED.

NOTE: This product information is for professional use only.

HOW SUPPLIED

Each EVAC-Q-KIT NDC 0013-2199-76 contains:
1. One 10 fl. oz. EVAC-Q-MAG
2. Two tablets—EVAC-Q-TABS
3. Two suppositories—EVAC-Q-SERT
4. 1 Instruction Sheet

Shipping Unit: 12 EVAC-Q-KIT units per carton.

*Late schedule also available. See Instruction Sheet in EVAC-Q-KIT. (Instruction sheet printed in both English and Spanish.)

EVAC-Q-MAG
Manufactured by:
NATIONAL MAGNESIA CO., INC.
GLENDALE, NEW YORK 11385
EVAC-Q-KWIK SUPPOSITORY
Manufactured by:
G & W LABORATORIES, INC.
SOUTH PLAINFIELD, NJ 07050
Distributed by:
ADRIA LABORATORIES
Division of Erbamont Inc.
COLUMBUS, OHIO 43215

EVAC-Q-KWIK®

[ē-vak 'cue-kwik]
Bowel Evacuant System

PRODUCT OVERVIEW

KEY FACTS

EVAC-Q-KWIK is a bowel evacuant kit containing magnesium citrate, phenolphthalein tablets and a bisacodyl suppository.

MAJOR USES

Preparation of the colon for radiologic examinations.

SAFETY INFORMATION

The EVAC-Q-MAG solution is contraindicated in the presence of severe renal insufficiency. Do not use any of the components when abdominal pain, nausea or vomiting are present.

PRESCRIBING INFORMATION

EVAC-Q-KWIK®

[ē-vak 'cue-kwik]
Bowel Evacuant System

DESCRIPTION

EVAC-Q-KWIK is a bowel evacuant system comprised of three separate products that are intended to be administered sequentially at intervals intended to minimize the overlap of pharmacological activity. These three products are augmented by the sequential administration of liquids in a manner to promote the flushing of the G.I. tract. Together, the products and the liquids comprise the bowel evacuant system.

1. EVAC-Q-MAG®—Each bottle contains 10 fl. oz., magnesium citrate oral solution, USP, in a cherry flavored base, sugar-free, carbonated base. It contains sodium 0.84 mEq, potassium 2.1 mEq, magnesium 254 mEq ml/bottle and 66.7 calories.
2. EVAC-Q-TABS®—2 tablets. Each tablet contains phenolphthalein 130 mg.
3. EVAC-Q-KWIK® SUPPOSITORY—bisacodyl 10 mg.
4. Illustrated bilingual instruction sheet.

Magnesium citrate is a saline laxative and has a mild purgative action. It is chemically 2-hydroxy-1,2,3-propanetricarboxylic acid, magnesium salt and has the following structure:

Magnesium citrate occurs as white crystalline powder or granules, slightly soluble in water, soluble in dilute acids. Its molecular weight citrate is 451.12.

Phenolphthalein, a contact laxative, is a diphenylmethane derivative. It is chemically 3,3-bis(4-hydroxyphenyl)-1(3H)-isobenzofuranone and has the following structure:

It occurs as a white, or yellowish-white, crystalline powder and is practically insoluble in water, soluble in alcohol and dilute alkali solutions. Its molecular weight is 318.33.

Bisacodyl, a contact laxative, is also a diphenylmethane derivative. It is chemically 4,4′-(2-pyridylmethylene) diphenol diacetate and has the following structure:

Bisacodyl occurs as a white or off-white crystalline powder, practically insoluble in water, sparingly soluble in alcohol and soluble in chloroform. Its molecular weight is 361.40.

CLINICAL PHARMACOLOGY

Magnesium citrate is a saline laxative. It acts mainly on the small intestine by drawing water into the gut thus increasing intraluminal pressure and intestinal motility, resulting in evacuation of the bowel usually in 3–6 hours or less. Substantial fluid intake is required for this purpose. Approximately 15–30% of the magnesium present in its salts may be absorbed. The magnesium and potassium ions are excreted primarily by the kidney and may accumulate in patients with impaired renal function, in the newborn and in the elderly.

Phenolphthalein, a contact laxative, acts primarily on the large intestine to produce a semifluid stool usually in 4–8 hours. It is dissolved by bile salts and alkaline intestinal secretions and may impart a red color to alkaline feces and urine. Up to 15% of the dose may be absorbed and excreted mainly by the kidney in the conjugated glucuronide form.

Bisacodyl is also a contact laxative which acts on the large intestine to produce brief and strong peristaltic movements resulting in evacuation usually within 15–60 minutes after rectal administration. It is minimally (about 5%) absorbed and excreted mainly in the feces and partly in the urine as the glucuronide.

INDICATIONS AND USAGE

EVAC-Q-KWIK is indicated for use as a bowel evacuant in the preparation of the colon for single or multiple radiological examination requiring a clean colon.

CONTRAINDICATIONS

The EVAC-Q-MAG component is contraindicated in patients with severe renal insufficiency.

WARNINGS

Do not use any laxative preparations when abdominal pain, nausea or vomiting are present. Frequent and continued use may cause dependence upon laxatives. Rectal bleeding or failure to respond may indicate a serious underlying condition and require a physician's consultation. KEEP THIS PRODUCT OUT OF REACH OF CHILDREN.

As with any drug, if the patient is pregnant or nursing a baby, she should consult a health professional before using. (See Precautions: Pregnancy, Nursing Mothers.)

PRECAUTIONS

General—If skin rash appears, do not use EVAC-Q-TABS or any other preparation containing phenolphthalein. The EVAC-Q-KWIK SUPPOSITORY should be used with caution in patients with rectal fissures or ulcerated hemorrhoids.

Phenolphthalein, the active ingredient of EVAC-Q-TABS, may color alkaline feces and urine red.

Laboratory Test Interactions—Phenolphthalein in EVAC-Q-TABS may interfere with the ACETEST® and KETOSTIX® urine tests for ketones to produce a pink color. It may also give false-positive test results for urinary urobilinogen and for estrogens measured by the Kober procedure.

Carcinogenesis, Mutagenesis, Impairment of Fertility—There have been no studies in animals or humans to evaluate the carcinogenesis, mutagenesis or impairment of fertility potential of the EVAC-Q-KWIK.

Pregnancy—Category C. Animal reproduction studies have not been conducted with any of the components of EVAC-Q-KWIK. It is also not known whether the EVAC-Q-KWIK can cause fetal harm when administered to a pregnant woman or can affect reproduction capacity. EVAC-Q-KWIK should be given to a pregnant woman only if clearly needed.

Nursing Mothers—Small amounts of magnesium are excreted in the milk and saliva. Phenolphthalein and bisacodyl are also excreted in human milk. Therefore, caution should be exercised when EVAC-Q-KWIK is administered to a nursing woman.

Pediatric Use—Safety and effectiveness in children below the age of 12 has not been established.

ADVERSE REACTIONS

Excessive bowel activity, usually diarrhea or abdominal discomfort, nausea, vomiting, cramps, weakness, dizziness, palpitations, sweating and fainting may follow the administration of an evacuant. Diarrhea may lead to fluid and electrolyte deficits. Allergic reactions, mainly skin rashes attributed to phenolphthalein, have been reported. Bisacodyl in the EVAC-Q-KWIK SUPPOSITORY may cause irritation or a sensation of burning of the rectal mucosa.

OVERDOSAGE

Accidental or intentional overdosage may lead to severe diarrhea and excessive loss of body fluids and electrolytes, muscle weakness and tremor, gastrointestinal disturbances and fainting. Depressed deep tendon reflexes, sedation, EKG changes or heart block and respiratory paralysis may occur with high plasma magnesium levels.

The excretion of magnesium may be increased by the administration of a diuretic. Only small amounts of phenolphthalein or bisacodyl are absorbed. If ingestion is recent or food is present in the stomach, induction of emesis with ipecac syrup, gastric emptying and lavage and introduction of activated charcoal may be recommended. Fluid and electrolyte administration is also recommended to correct dehydration and electrolyte imbalance.

DOSAGE AND ADMINISTRATION

A high fluid intake and a low residue diet are essential for a successful colon preparation. Recommended liquids are black coffee, plain tea, strained fruit juice, soft drinks or water and NO MILK OR CREAM. The directions provided in the Instruction Sheet and the following schedule should be adhered to closely.

TIME SCHEDULE

NOON	Light lunch: clear soup, plain gelatin, fluid.
4:00 P.M.	Drink entire contents of EVAC-Q-MAG (#1 in the kit), over ice.
5:00 P.M.	8 oz. of fluid.
6:00 P.M.	Liquid dinner. Clear soup, plain gelatin, 8 oz. of fluid.
7:00 P.M.	Take two (2) EVAC-Q-TABS laxative tablets (#2 in the kit) with a large glass of water.

Continued on next page

Adria—Cont.

8:00 P.M.	8 oz. of fluid.
9:00 P.M.	8 oz. of fluid.
10:00 P.M.	Insert one EVAC-Q-KWIK SUPPOSITORY (#3 in the kit) into rectum as far as possible, retain as long as comfort will permit—usually 10–15 minutes—before defecating. Nothing by mouth, after 10:00 P.M. until x-ray examination. Prescription medications can be taken as scheduled with a glass of water.

DRINK ALL THE FLUID SPECIFIED.

ALTERNATE SCHEDULE

(For patients admitted in the afternoon on the day before examination.)

6:00 P.M.	Liquid dinner. Clear soup, plain gelatin, 8 oz. of fluid.
7:00 P.M.	Drink entire contents of EVAC-Q-MAG (#1 in the kit), over ice.
8:00 P.M.	8 oz. of fluid.
9:00 P.M.	8 oz. of fluid.
10:00 P.M.	Take two (2) EVAC-Q-TABS laxative tablets (#2 in the kit) with a large glass of water. Nothing by mouth, after 10:00 p.m. until x-ray examination. Prescription medications can be taken as scheduled with a glass of water.
6:00 A.M.	Insert one EVAC-Q-KWIK SUPPOSITORY (#3 in the kit) into rectum as far as possible, retain as long as comfort will permit—usually 10–15 minutes—before defecating.

DRINK ALL THE FLUID SPECIFIED.

See also: Illustrated Multilingual Instruction Sheet.

NOTE: This product information is for professional use only.

HOW SUPPLIED

Each EVAC-Q-KWIK, NDC 0013-2189-76 contains:

1. One 10 fl. oz. EVAC-Q-MAG
2. Two tablets EVAC-Q-TABS
3. One EVAC-Q-KWIK SUPPOSITORY
4. Instruction Sheet.

Store at controlled room temperature (15–30°C, 59–86°F). Avoid freezing.

EVAC-Q-MAG
Manufactured by:
NATIONAL MAGNESIA CO., INC.
GLENDALE, NEW YORK 11385

EVAC-Q-KWIK SUPPOSITORY
Manufactured by:
G & W LABORATORIES, INC.
SOUTH PLAINFIELD, NJ 07050

Distributed by:
ADRIA LABORATORIES
Division of Erbamont Inc.
COLUMBUS, OHIO 43215

FOLEX® FOR INJECTION ℞

[fō ′lĕx]

(methotrexate sodium)

PRODUCT OVERVIEW

KEY FACTS

FOLEX is a cytotoxic agent active against a variety of hematologic malignancies and solid tumors. The active ingredient, methotrexate sodium, is an anti folic acid antimetabolite that selectively kills malignant cells and causes tumor regression.

MAJOR USES

FOLEX is clinically effective in the treatment of gestational choriocarcinoma, chorioadenoma destruans and hydatidiform mole. It is indicated for the palliation of acute lymphocytic leukemia and is used intrathecally in the treatment of meningeal leukemia. It is effective in the treatment of advanced malignant lymphoma and in the symptomatic control of severe, recalcitrant, disabling psoriasis.

SAFETY INFORMATION

FOLEX is intended for intravenous or intrathecal use only. Patients must be carefully monitored and the dose adjusted to avoid too severe myelosuppression or mucositis especially in patients with impaired renal function. If too large doses are administered, calcium leucovorin may be used to neutralize the immediate toxic effects of FOLEX.

PRESCRIBING INFORMATION

FOLEX® FOR INJECTION ℞

[fōl ′ĕx]

(methotrexate sodium)

WARNINGS

METHOTREXATE MUST BE USED ONLY BY PHYSICIANS EXPERIENCED IN ANTIMETABOLITE CHEMOTHERAPY.

BECAUSE OF THE POSSIBILITY OF FATAL OR SEVERE TOXIC REACTIONS THE PATIENT SHOULD BE FULLY INFORMED BY THE PHYSICIAN OF THE RISKS INVOLVED AND SHOULD BE UNDER HIS CONSTANT SUPERVISION.

DEATHS HAVE BEEN REPORTED WITH THE USE OF METHOTREXATE IN THE TREATMENT OF PSORIASIS.

IN THE TREATMENT OF PSORIASIS METHOTREXATE SHOULD BE RESTRICTED TO SEVERE, RECALCITRANT, DISABLING PSORIASIS WHICH IS NOT ADEQUATELY RESPONSIVE TO OTHER FORMS OF THERAPY, BUT ONLY WHEN THE DIAGNOSIS HAS BEEN ESTABLISHED AS BY BIOPSY AND/OR AFTER DERMATOLOGIC CONSULTATION.

1. Methotrexate may produce marked depression of bone marrow, anemia, leukopenia, thrombocytopenia and bleeding.
2. Methotrexate may be hepatotoxic, particularly at high dosage or with prolonged therapy. Liver atrophy, necrosis, cirrhosis, fatty changes, and periportal fibrosis have been reported. Since changes may occur without previous signs of gastrointestinal or hematologic toxicity, it is imperative that hepatic function be determined prior to initiation of treatment and monitored regularly throughout therapy. Special caution is indicated in the presence of preexisting liver damage or impaired hepatic function. Concomitant use of other drugs with hepatotoxic potential (including alcohol) should be avoided.
3. Methotrexate has caused fetal death and/or congenital anomalies, therefore, it is not recommended in women of childbearing potential unless there is appropriate medical evidence that the benefits can be expected to outweigh the considered risks. Pregnant psoriatic patients should not receive methotrexate. If methotrexate is used during pregnancy or if the patient becomes pregnant while taking the drug, the patient should be apprised of the potential hazard to the fetus.
4. Impaired renal function is usually a contraindication.
5. Diarrhea and ulcerative stomatitis are frequent toxic effects and require interruption of therapy, otherwise hemorrhagic enteritis and death from intestinal perforation may occur.

METHOTREXATE HAS BEEN ADMINISTERED IN VERY HIGH DOSAGE FOLLOWED BY LEUCOVORIN RESCUE IN EXPERIMENTAL TREATMENT OF CERTAIN NEOPLASTIC DISEASES. THIS PROCEDURE IS INVESTIGATIONAL AND HAZARDOUS.

DESCRIPTION

FOLEX (methotrexate sodium) is an antimetabolite used in the treatment of certain neoplastic diseases. Chemically methotrexate is N-[p[[(2,4-diamino-6-pteridinyl) methyl] methylamino] benzoyl] glutamic acid.

Molecular weight: 454.44 $C_{20}H_{22}N_8O_5$

FOLEX FOR INJECTION is available in 25, 50, 100 and 250 mg strengths, each available as sterile lyophilized powder in vials, containing no preservatives, for single use only.

Each 25 mg vial contains methotrexate USP, 25 mg, prepared as the sodium salt, sodium hydroxide to adjust pH to about 8.5.

Each 50 mg vial contains methotrexate USP, 50 mg, prepared as the sodium salt, sodium hydroxide to adjust pH to about 8.5.

Each 100 mg vial contains methotrexate USP, 100 mg, prepared as the sodium salt, sodium hydroxide to adjust pH to about 8.5.

Each 250 mg vial contains methotrexate USP, 250 mg, prepared as the sodium salt, sodium hydroxide to adjust pH to about 8.5.

CLINICAL PHARMACOLOGY

See Folex PFS™ Injection, USP

INDICATIONS AND USAGE

See Folex PFS™ Injection, USP

CONTRAINDICATIONS

See Folex PFS™ Injection, USP

WARNINGS

See box warnings

PRECAUTIONS

See Folex PFS™ Injection, USP

ADVERSE REACTIONS

See Folex PFS™ Injection, USP

OVERDOSAGE

See Folex PFS™ Injection, USP

DOSAGE AND ADMINISTRATION

See Folex PFS™ Injection, USP

CAUTION

Pharmacist—Because of its potential to cause severe toxicity, methotrexate therapy requires close supervision of the patient by the physician. Pharmacists should dispense no more than a seven (7) day supply of the drug at one time. Refill of such prescriptions should be by direct order (written or oral) of the physician only.

DIRECTIONS FOR USE

FOLEX FOR INJECTION (methotrexate sodium)—Reconstitute immediately prior to use with 2 to 25 ml depending on the route of administration, of an appropriate preservative-free medium such as 0.9% Sodium Chloride Injection, USP. FOLEX FOR INJECTION does not contain an antimicrobial agent and care must be taken to ensure the sterility of prepared solutions.

Although the sterile reconstituted solution has been shown to be stable for 24 hours at room temperature; since the product does not contain a preservative, any unused portion should be discarded immediately after use.

HANDLING AND DISPOSAL

See Folex PFS™ Injection

REFERENCES

See Folex PFS™ Injection

HOW SUPPLIED

FOLEX® FOR INJECTION (methotrexate sodium)
Sterile, Preservative Free, Lyophilized Powder
NDC 0013-2226-86 25 mg vial
NDC 0013-2236-86 50 mg vial
NDC 0013-2246-86 100 mg vial
NDC 0013-2256-86 250 mg vial

Store products at room temperature and protect from light.

Manufactured by:
BEN VENUE LABORATORIES
BEDFORD, OHIO 44146
for:
ADRIA LABORATORIES
Division of Erbamont Inc.
COLUMBUS, OHIO 43215

FOLEX PFS™ ℞

[fo ′lex]

(methotrexate sodium)

INJECTION, USP

PRODUCT OVERVIEW

KEY FACTS

FOLEX is a cytotoxic agent active against a variety of hematologic malignancies and solid tumors. The active ingredient, methotrexate sodium, is an anti folic acid antimetabolite that selectively kills malignant cells and causes tumor regression.

MAJOR USES

FOLEX is clinically effective in the treatment of gestational choriocarcinoma, chorioadenoma destruans and hydatidiform mole. It is indicated for the palliation of acute lymphocytic leukemia and is used intrathecally in the treatment of meningeal leukemia. It is effective in the treatment of advanced malignant lymphoma and in the symptomatic control of severe, recalcitrant, disabling psoriasis.

SAFETY INFORMATION

FOLEX is intended for intravenous or intrathecal use only. Patients must be carefully monitored and the dose adjusted to avoid too severe myelosuppression or mucositis especially in patients with impaired renal function. If too large doses are administered, calcium leucovorin may be used to neutralize the immediate toxic effects of FOLEX.

PRESCRIBING INFORMATION

FOLEX PFS™ ℞

[fō ′lĕx]

(methotrexate sodium)

INJECTION, USP

WARNINGS

METHOTREXATE MUST BE USED ONLY BY PHYSICIANS EXPERIENCED IN ANTIMETABOLITE CHEMOTHERAPY.

BECAUSE OF THE POSSIBILITY OF FATAL OR SEVERE TOXIC REACTIONS THE PATIENT SHOULD

BE FULLY INFORMED BY THE PHYSICIAN OF THE RISKS INVOLVED AND SHOULD BE UNDER HIS CONSTANT SUPERVISION.

DEATHS HAVE BEEN REPORTED WITH THE USE OF METHOTREXATE IN THE TREATMENT OF PSORIASIS.

IN THE TREATMENT OF PSORIASIS METHOTREXATE SHOULD BE RESTRICTED TO SEVERE, RECALCITRANT, DISABLING PSORIASIS WHICH IS NOT ADEQUATELY RESPONSIVE TO OTHER FORMS OF THERAPY, BUT ONLY WHEN THE DIAGNOSIS HAS BEEN ESTABLISHED AS BY BIOPSY AND/OR AFTER DERMATOLOGIC CONSULTATION.

1. Methotrexate may produce marked depression of bone marrow, anemia, leukopenia, thrombocytopenia and bleeding.
2. Methotrexate may be hepatotoxic, particularly at high dosage or with prolonged therapy. Liver atrophy, necrosis, cirrhosis, fatty changes, and periportal fibrosis have been reported. Since changes may occur without previous signs of gastrointestinal or hematologic toxicity, it is imperative that hepatic function be determined prior to initiation of treatment and monitored regularly throughout therapy. Special caution is indicated in the presence of preexisting liver damage or impaired hepatic function. Concomitant use of other drugs with hepatotoxic potential (including alcohol) should be avoided.
3. Methotrexate has caused fetal death and/or congenital anomalies, therefore, it is not recommended in women of childbearing potential unless there is appropriate medical evidence that the benefits can be expected to outweigh the considered risks. Pregnant psoriatic patients should not receive methotrexate. If methotrexate is used during pregnancy or if the patient becomes pregnant while taking the drug, the patient should be apprised of the potential hazard to the fetus.
4. Impaired renal function is usually a contraindication.
5. Diarrhea and ulcerative stomatitis are frequent toxic effects and require interruption of therapy, otherwise hemorrhagic enteritis and death from intestinal perforation may occur.

METHOTREXATE HAS BEEN ADMINISTERED IN VERY HIGH DOSAGE FOLLOWED BY LEUCOVORIN RESCUE IN EXPERIMENTAL TREATMENT OF CERTAIN NEOPLASTIC DISEASES. THIS PROCEDURE IS INVESTIGATIONAL AND HAZARDOUS.

DESCRIPTION

FOLEX (methotrexate sodium) is an antimetabolite used in the treatment of certain neoplastic diseases. Chemically methotrexate is N-[p[[(2,4-diamino-6-pteridinyl) methyl] methylamino] benzoyl] glutamic acid.

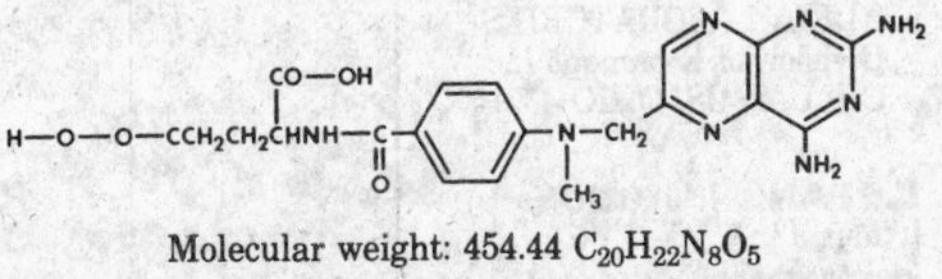

Molecular weight: 454.44 $C_{20}H_{22}N_8O_5$

FOLEX PFS INJECTION, Parenteral, isotonic, preservative-free, single use only, is available in 5 ml (50 and 100 mg), and 10 ml (200 mg) vials.

Each 25 mg/ml, 2 ml (50 mg) vial contains: Methotrexate Sodium equivalent to 50 mg Methotrexate, and the following inactive ingredients: Sodium Chloride 0.490% w/v and Water for Injection qs ad 100% V. Sodium Hydroxide and, if necessary, Hydrochloric Acid to adjust pH to approximately 8.5. Contains approximately 0.43 milliequivalents of sodium per vial and is an isotonic solution.

Each 25 mg/ml, 4 ml (100 mg) vial contains: Methotrexate Sodium equivalent to 100 mg Methotrexate, and the following inactive ingredients: Sodium Chloride 0.490% w/v and Water for Injection qs ad 100% V. Sodium Hydroxide and, if necessary, Hydrochloric Acid to adjust pH to approximately 8.5. Contains approximately 0.86 milliequivalents of sodium per vial and is an isotonic solution.

Each 25 mg/ml, 8 ml (200 mg) vial contains: Methotrexate Sodium equivalent to 200 mg Methotrexate, and the following inactive ingredients: Sodium Chloride 0.490% w/v and Water for Injection qs ad 100% V. Sodium Hydroxide and, if necessary, Hydrochloric Acid to adjust pH to approximately 8.5. Contains approximately 1.72 milliequivalents of sodium per vial and is an isotonic solution.

If desired, the solution may be futhered diluted immediately prior to use with an appropriate sterile, preservative-free medium such as 5% Dextrose Solution, USP or Sodium Chloride Injection, USP.

CLINICAL PHARMACOLOGY

Methotrexate has as its principal mechanism of action the competitive inhibition of the enzyme dihydrofolate reductase. Folic acid must be reduced to tetrahydrofolic acid by this enzyme in the process of DNA synthesis and cellular replication. Methotrexate binds almost irreversibly to dihydrofolate reductase and inhibits the formation of tetrahydrofolates necessary for the metabolic transfer of one-carbon units in a variety of intracellular biochemical processes. The conversion of deoxyuridylate to thymidylate by one-carbon transfer is required for DNA synthesis. One-carbon transfer is also necessary for purine, RNA, amino acid and protein synthesis, thus methotrexate can disrupt several biological processes involved in cell growth.

Actively proliferating tissues such as malignant cells, bone marrow, fetal cells, dermal epithelium, buccal and intestinal mucosa and cells of the urinary bladder are in general more sensitive to this effect of methotrexate than slowly proliferating tissues. Cellular proliferation in malignant tissue is greater than in most normal tissue and thus methotrexate may impair malignant growth without causing irreversible damage to normal tissues.

After parenteral injection, peak serum levels are seen in about 30 to 60 minutes. After injection approximately one half the methotrexate is reversibly bound to serum protein, but exchanges with body fluids easily and diffuses into the body tissue cells. Metabolism of methotrexate in man does not seem to occur to a significant degree.

Excretion of single daily doses occurs through the kidneys in amounts from 55% to 88% or higher within 24 hours. Repeated doses daily result in more sustained serum levels and some retention of methotrexate over each 24-hour period which may result in accumulation of the drug within the tissues. The liver cells appear to retain certain amounts of the drug for prolonged periods even after a single therapeutic dose.

Methotrexate is retained in the presence of impaired renal function and may increase rapidly in the serum and in the tissue cells under such conditions. Methotrexate does not penetrate the blood cerebrospinal fluid barrier in therapeutic amounts when given parenterally. High concentrations of the drug when needed may be attained by direct intrathecal administration.

In psoriasis, the rate of production of epithelial cells in the skin is greatly increased over normal skin. This differential in reproductive rates is the basis for use of methotrexate to control the psoriatic process.

INDICATIONS AND USAGE

Anti-neoplastic Chemotherapy—FOLEX is indicated for the treatment of gestational choriocarcinoma, and in patients with chorioadenoma destruens and hydatidiform mole.

FOLEX is indicated for the palliation of acute lymphocytic leukemia. It is also indicated in the treatment and prophylaxis of meningeal leukemia. In combination with other anticancer drugs or suitable agents, FOLEX may be used for induction of remission, but it is most commonly used, as described in the literature, in the maintenance of induced remissions.

Methotrexate may be used alone or in combination with other anticancer agents in the management of breast cancer, epidermoid cancers of the head and neck, and lung cancer, particularly squamous cell and small cell types.

FOLEX is also effective in the treatment of the advanced stages (III and IV, Ann Arbor Staging System) of malignant lymphoma, particularly in children; and in advanced cases of mycosis fungoides.

Psoriasis Chemotherapy—(See box warnings.) Because of high risk attending its use, FOLEX is only indicated in the symptomatic control of severe, recalcitrant, disabling psoriasis which is not adequately responsive to other forms of therapy, *but only when the diagnosis has been established, as by biopsy and/or after dermatologic consultation.*

CONTRAINDICATIONS

Pregnant psoriatic patients should not receive FOLEX. Psoriatic patients with severe renal or hepatic disorders should not receive FOLEX. Psoriatic patients with preexisting blood dyscrasias, such as bone marrow hypoplasia, leukopenia, thrombocytopenia or anemia, should not receive FOLEX.

WARNINGS

See box warnings.

PRECAUTIONS

Methotrexate has a high potential toxicity, usually dose-related. The physician should be familiar with the various characterisitics of the drug and its established clinical usage. Patients undergoing therapy should be subject to appropriate supervision so the signs or symptoms of possible toxic effects of adverse reactions may be detected and evaluated with minimal delay. Pretreatment and periodic hematologic studies are essential to the use of methotrexate in chemotherapy because of its common effect of hematopoetic suppression. This may occur abruptly and on apparent safe dosage, and any profound drop in blood cell count indicates immediate stopping of the drug and appropriate therapy in patients with malignant disease who have preexisting bone marrow aplasia, leukopenia, thrombocytopenia or anemia, the drug should be used with caution, if at all.

Methotrexate is excreted principally by the kidneys. Its use in the presence of impaired renal function may result in accumulation of toxic amounts or even additional renal damage. The patient's renal status should be determined prior to and during methotrexate therapy and proper caution exercised should significant renal impairment be disclosed. Drug dosage should be reduced or discontinued until renal function is improved or restored.

In general, the following laboratory tests are recommended as part of essential clinical evaluation and appropriate monitoring of patients chosen for or receiving methotrexate therapy; complete hemogram, hematocrit, urinalysis, renal function tests, and liver function tests. A chest x-ray is also recommended. The purpose is to determine any existing organ dysfunction or system impairment. The tests should be performed prior to therapy, at appropriate periods during therapy and after termination of therapy. It may be useful or important to perform liver biopsy or bone marrow aspiration studies where high dose or long-term therapy is being followed.

Methotrexate is bound in part to serum albumin after absorption, and toxicity may be increased because of displacement by certain drugs such as salicylates, sulfonamides, diphenylhydantoin, phenylbutazone, and some antibacterials such as tetracycline, chloramphenicol and para-amino-benzoic acid. These drugs, especially salicylates, phenylbutazone, and sulfonamides, whether antibacterial, hypoglycemic or diuretic, should not be given concurrently until the significance of these findings is established.

Vitamin preparations containing folic acid or its derivatives may alter responses to methotrexate.

Methotrexate should be used with extreme caution in the presence of infection, peptic ulcer, ulcerative colitis, debility and in extreme youth or old age.

If profound leukopenia occurs during therapy, bacterial infection may occur or become a threat. Cessation of the drug and appropriate antibiotic therapy is usually indicated. In severe bone marrow depression, blood or platelet transfusions may be necessary.

Since it is reported that methotrexate may have an immunosuppressive action, this factor must be taken into consideration in evaluating the use of the drug where immune responses in a patient may be important or essential.

In all instances where the use of methotrexate is considered for chemotherapy, the physician must evaluate the need and usefulness of the drug against the risks of toxic effects or adverse reaction. Most such adverse reactions are reversible if detected early. When such effects or reactions do occur, the drug should be reduced in dosage or discontinued and appropriate corrective measures should be taken, according to the clinical judgment of the physician. Reinstitution of methotrexate therapy should be carried out with caution, with adequate consideration of further need for the drug and alertness as to possible recurrence of toxicity.

Tests were negative for carcinogenesis in the Ames test and by sister chromatid exchange in lymphocyte cultures of patients receiving methotrexate. Weak carcinogenesis was reported in one animal study and no carcinogenesis in another.

Usage in Pregnancy—Category D. (See box warnings.) Defective oogenesis or spermatogenesis caused by methotrexate has been reported.

Methotrexate is excreted in breast milk and although no problem in humans have been documented, caution should be exercised when methotrexate is administered to a nursing woman.

ADVERSE REACTIONS

The most common adverse reactions include ulcerative stomatitis, leukopenia, nausea and abdominal distress. Others reported are malaise, undue fatigue, chills and fever, dizziness and decreased resistance to infection. In general, the incidence and severity of side effects are considered to be dose-related. Adverse reactions as reported for the various systems are as follows.

Skin—erythematous rashes, pruritus, urticaria, photosensitivity, depigmentation, alopecia, ecchymosis, telangiectasia, acne, furunculosis. Lesions of psoriasis may be aggravated by concomitant exposure to ultraviolet radiation.

Blood—bone marrow depression, leukopenia, thrombocytopenia, anemia, hypogammaglobulinemia, hemorrhage from various sites, septicemia.

Pulmonary System—interstitial pneumonitis deaths have been reported and chronic interstitial obstructive pulmonary disease has occasionally occurred.

Alimentary System—gingivitis, pharyngitis, stomatitis, anorexia, vomiting, diarrhea, hematemesis, melena, gastrointestinal ulceration and bleeding, enteritis, hepatic toxicity resulting in acute liver atrophy, necrosis, fatty metamorphosis, periportal fibrosis, or hepatic cirrhosis.

Urogenital System—renal failure, azotemia, cystitis, hematuria, defective oogenesis or spermatogenesis, transient oligospermia, menstrual dysfunction, infertility, abortion, fetal defects, severe nephropathy.

Continued on next page

Adria—Cont.

Central Nervous System—headaches, drowsiness, blurred vision. Aphasia, hemiparesis, paresis and convulsions have also occurred following administration of methotrexate.
There have been reports of leucoencephalopathy following intravenous administration of methotrexate to patients who have had craniospinal irradiation.
After the intrathecal use of methotrexate, the central nervous system toxicity which may occur can be classified as follows: (1) chemical arachnoiditis manifested by such symptoms as headache, back pain, nuchal rigidity, and fever; (2) paresis, usually transient, manifested by paraplegia associated with involvement of one or more spinal nerve roots; (3) leucoencephalopathy manifested by confusion, irritability, somnolence, ataxia, dementia, and occasionally major convulsions.
Other reactions related to or attributed to the use of methotrexate such as metabolic changes, precipitating diabetes, osteoporotic effects, abnormal tissue cell changes, and even sudden death have been reported.

OVERDOSAGE

Overdosage may lead to severe toxicity, especially to the hematopoetic and gastrointestinal systems and death may result. Leucovorin (citrovorum factor) is a potent agent for neutralizing the immediate toxic effects of methotrexate. Where large doses or overdoses are given, calcium leucovorin may be administered by intravenous infusion in doses up to 75 mg within 12 hours, followed by 12 mg intramuscularly every 6 hours for 4 doses. Where average doses of methotrexate appear to have an adverse effect, 6 to 12 mg of calcium leucovorin may be given intramuscularly every 6 hours for 4 doses. In general, where overdosage is suspected, the doses of leucovorin should be equal to or higher than the offending dose of methotrexate and should best be administered within the first hour. Use of calcium leucovorin after an hour delay is much less effective.

DOSAGE AND ADMINISTRATION

Anti-neoplastic chemotherapy—FOLEX may be given by intramuscular, intravenous, intraarterial or intrathecal routes. Initial treatment is usually undertaken with the patient under hospital care. Choriocarcinoma and similar trophoblastic diseases—FOLEX is administered intramuscularly in doses of 15 to 30 mg daily for a 5 day course. Such courses are usually repeated for 3 to 5 times as required, with rest periods of one or more weeks interposed between courses, until any manifesting toxic symptoms subside. The effectiveness of therapy is ordinarily evaluated by quantitative analysis of the beta subunit of the serum human chorionic gonadotropin (hCG), which should return to less than 5 mIU/ml usually after the 3rd or 4th course and should usually be followed by a complete resolution of measurable lesions in 4 to 6 weeks. One to two courses of methotrexate after normalization of hCG is usually recommended. Before each course of the drug careful clinical assessment is essential. Cyclic combination therapy of methotrexate with other antitumor drugs has been reported as being useful.
Since hydatidiform mole may precede or be followed by choriocarcinoma, prophylactic chemotherapy with methotrexate has been recommended. Chorioadenoma destruens is considered to be an invasive form of hydatidiform mole. Methotrexate is administered in these disease states in doses similar to those recommended for choriocarcinoma.
Leukemia—Acute lymphatic (lymphoblastic) leukemia in children and young adolescents is the most responsive to present day chemotherapy. In young adults and older patients, clinical remission is more difficult to obtain and early relapse is more common. In chronic lymphatic leukemia, the prognosis for adequate response is less encouraging. Methotrexate alone or in combination with steroids was used initially for induction of remission of lymphoblastic leukemias. More recently corticosteroid therapy in combination with other antileukemic drugs or in cyclic combinations with methotrexate included appears to produce rapid and effective remissions. When used for induction, methotrexate in doses of 3.3 mg/M^2 in combination with prednisone 60 mg/M^2, given daily, produced remission in 50% of patients treated, usually within a period of 4 to 6 weeks. Methotrexate alone or in combination with other agents appears to be the drug of choice for securing maintenance of drug-induced remissions. When remission is achieved and supportive care has produced general clinical improvement, maintenance therapy is initiated as follows: FOLEX is administered two times weekly either by mouth or intramuscularly in doses of 30 mg/M^2. It has also been given in doses of 2.5 mg/kg intravenously every 14 days. If and when relapse does occur, reinduction of remission can again usually be obtained by repeating the initial induction regimen. Various experts have recently introduced a variety of dosage schedules for both induction and maintenance of remission with various combinations of alkylating and antifolic agents. Multiple drug therapy with several agents, including methotrexate, given concomitantly is gaining increasing support in both the acute and chronic forms of leukemia. The physician should familiarize himself with the new advances in antileukemic therapy.
Acute granulocytic leukemia is rare in children but common in adults. This form of leukemia responds poorly to chemotherapy and remissions are short with relapses common, and resistance to therapy develops rapidly.
Meningeal leukemia—Patients with leukemia are subject to leukemic invasion of the central nervous system. This may manifest characteristic signs or symptoms or may remain silent and be diagnosed only by examination of the cerebrospinal fluid which contains leukemic cells in such cases. Therefore, CSF should be examined in all leukemic patients. Since passage of methotrexate from blood serum to the cerebrospinal fluid is minimal, for adequate therapy the drug is administered intrathecally. It is now common practice because of the noted increased frequency of meningeal leukemia to administer methotrexate intrathecally as prophylaxis in all cases of lymphocytic leukemia.
By intrathecal injection, FOLEX is administered in solution in doses of 12 mg per square meter of body surface or in an empirical dose of 15 mg. The solution is made in a strength of 1 mg per ml with an appropriate, sterile, preservative-free medium such as 0.9% Sodium Chloride Injection, USP.
For the treatment of meningeal leukemia, methotrexate is given at intervals of 2 to 5 days. Methotrexate is administered until the cell count of the cerebrospinal fluid returns to normal. At this point one additional dose is advisable.
For prophylaxis against meningeal leukemia, the dosage is the same as for treatment except for the intervals of administration. On this subject, it is advisable for the physician to consult the medical literature.
Large doses may cause convulsions. Untoward side effects may occur with any given intrathecal injection and are commonly neurological in character. Methotrexate given by the intrathecal route appears significantly in the systemic circulation and may cause systemic methotrexate toxicity. Therefore, systemic antileukemic therapy with the drug should be appropriately adjusted, reduced or discontinued. Focal leukemic involvement of the central nervous system may not respond to intrathecal chemotherapy and is best treated with radiotherapy.
Lymphomas—In Burkitt's Tumor, Stages I–II, methotrexate has produced prolonged remissions in some cases. In Stage III, methotrexate is commonly given concomitantly with other antitumor agents. Treatment in all stages usually consists of several courses of the drug interposed with 7 to 10 day rest periods. Malignant lymphomas in Stage III may respond to combined drug therapy with methotrexate given in doses of 0.625 mg to 2.5 mg/kg daily. Hodgkin's Disease responds poorly to methotrexate and to most types of chemotherapy.
Mycosis fungoides—Therapy with methotrexate appears to produce clinical remissions in about one half of the cases treated. Although dosage is usually daily by mouth for weeks or months, methotrexate has also been given intramuscularly in doses of 50 mg once weekly or 25 mg 2 times weekly. Dose levels of drug and adjustment of dose regimen by reduction or cessation of drug are guided by patient response and hematologic monitoring.
Psoriasis Chemotherapy—The patient should be fully informed of the risks involved and should be under constant supervision of the physician.
Assessment of renal function, liver function, and blood elements should be made by history, physical examination, and laboratory tests (such as CBC, urinalysis, serum creatinine, liver function studies, and liver biopsy if indicated) periodically and before reinstituting methotrexate therapy after a rest period. Blood counts should be taken weekly during treatment. Appropriate steps should be taken to avoid conception during and for at least eight weeks following methotrexate therapy.
There are three commonly used general types of dosage schedules:
1. weekly oral or parenteral intermittent large doses
2. divided dose intermittent oral schedule over a 36-hour period
3. daily oral with a rest period

All schedules should be continually tailored to the individual patient. Dose schedules cited below pertain to an average 70 kg adult. An initial test dose one week prior to initiation of therapy is recommended to detect any idiosyncrasy. A suggested dose range is 5 to 10 mg parenterally.
The recommended starting i.v. or i.m. dose schedule is 10 to 25 mg per week until adequate response is achieved. With this dosage schedule, 50 mg per week should ordinarily not be exceeded.
Dosages may be gradually adjusted to achieve optimal clinical response, but not to exceed the maximum stated in the schedule.
Once an optimal clinical response has been achieved, the dosage schedule should be reduced to the lowest possible amount of drug and to the longest rest period. The use of methotrexate may permit the return to conventional topical therapy, which should be encouraged.

CAUTION

Pharmacist—Because of its potential to cause severe toxicity, methotrexate therapy requires close supervision of the patient by the physician. Pharmacists should dispense no more than a seven (7) day supply of the drug at one time. Refill of such prescriptions should be by direct order (written or oral) of the physician only.

DIRECTIONS FOR USE

FOLEX PFS INJECTION (methotrexate sodium)—If dilutions are required, they *should be made immediately* prior to use depending on the route of administration, using an appropriate preservative-free medium such as 0.9% Sodium Chloride Injection, USP. FOLEX PFS INJECTION does not contain an antimicrobial agent and care must be taken to ensure the sterility of prepared solutions. Discard unused portion.
Handling and Disposal: Procedures for proper handling and disposal of anti-cancer drugs should be considered. Several guidelines on this subject have been published.[1–6] There is no general agreement that all of the procedures recommended in the guidelines are necessary or appropriate.

REFERENCES

1. Recommendations for the Safe Handling of Parenteral Antineoplastic Drugs, NIH Publication No. 83-2621. For sale by the Superintendent of Documents, U.S. Government Printing Office, Washington, D.C. 20402.
2. AMA Council Report. Guidelines for Handling Parenteral Antineoplastics. JAMA, March 15, 1985.
3. National Study Commission on Cytotoxic Exposure—Recommendations for Handling Cytotoxic Agents. Available from Louis P. Jeffrey, Sc. D., Director of Pharmacy Services, Rhode Island Hospital, 593 Eddy Street, Providence, Rhode Island 02902.
4. Clinical Oncological Society of Australia: Guidelines and recommendations for safe handling of antineoplastic agents. Med J Australia 1:426–428, 1983.
5. Jones R.B., et al. Safe handling of chemotherapeutic agents: A report from the Mount Sinai Medical Center. Ca—A Cancer Journal for Clinicians Sept/Oct, 258–263, 1983.
6. American Society of Hospital Pharmacists technical assistance bulletin on handling cytotoxic drugs in hospitals. Am J Hosp Pharm 42:131–137, 1985.

HOW SUPPLIED

FOLEX PFS™ (methotrexate sodium) INJECTION, USP
Sterile, Isotonic, Preservative Free Solution
NDC 0013-2266-91 50 mg vial
NDC 0013-2276-91 100 mg vial
NDC 0013-2286-91 200 mg vial
Store products at controlled room temperature 15–30°C (59–86°F) and protect from light.
Manufactured by:
TAYLOR PHARMACAL CO.
DECATUR, ILLINOIS 62525
for:
ADRIA LABORATORIES
Division of Erbamont Inc.
COLUMBUS, OHIO 43215

ILOPAN® INJECTION ℞

[ī'lō-pan]
(dexpanthenol)

DESCRIPTION

ILOPAN® INJECTION (dexpanthenol) is a derivative of pantothenic acid, a member of the B complex of vitamins. ILOPAN INJECTION is a sterile aqueous solution indicated for use as a gastrointestinal stimulant. The chemical name is D-(+)-2, 4-dihydroxy-N-(3-hydroxypropyl)-3,3-dimethylbutyramide. The structural formula is

$$HOCH_2-\overset{CH_3}{\underset{CH_3}{C}}-\overset{OH}{\underset{H}{C}}-CONHCH_2CH_2CH_2OH$$

The empirical formula is $C_9H_{19}NO_4$.
Each ml contains dexpanthenol 250 mg in distilled water for injection.

CLINICAL PHARMACOLOGY

Pantothenic acid is a precursor of coenzyme A, which serves as a cofactor for a variety of enzyme-catalyzed reactions involving transfer of acetyl groups. The final step in the synthesis of acetylcholine consists of the choline acetylase transfer of an acetyl group from acetylcoenzyme A to choline. Acetylcholine is the neurohumoral transmitter in the parasympathetic system and as such maintains the normal functions of the intestine. Decrease in acetylcholine content would result in decreased peristalsis and in extreme cases adynamic ileus. The pharmacological mode of action of the drug is unknown. Pharmacokinetic data in humans are unavailable.

INDICATIONS AND USAGE

Prophylactic use immediately after major abdominal surgery to minimize the possibility of paralytic ileus. Intestinal atony causing abdominal distention; postoperative or postpartum retention of flatus, or postoperative delay in resumption of intestinal motility; paralytic ileus.

CONTRAINDICATIONS

There are no known contraindications to the use of ILOPAN INJECTION.

WARNINGS

There have been rare instances of allergic reactions of unknown cause during the concomitant use of ILOPAN INJECTION with drugs such as antibiotics, narcotics and barbiturates.

Administration of ILOPAN INJECTION directly into the vein is not advised (See Dosage and Administration).

ILOPAN INJECTION should not be administered within one hour of succinylcholine.

PRECAUTIONS

General—If any signs of a hypersensitivity reaction appear, ILOPAN INJECTION should be discontinued. If ileus is a secondary consequence of mechanical obstruction, primary attention should be directed to the obstruction.

The management of adynamic ileus includes the correction of any fluid and electrolyte imbalance (especially hypokalemia), anemia and hypoproteinemia, treatment of infection, avoidance where possible of drugs which are known to decrease gastrointestinal motility and decompression of the gastrointestinal tract when considerably distended by nasogastric suction or use of a long intestinal tube.

Drug Interactions—The effects of succinylcholine appeared to have been prolonged in a woman administered dexpanthenol.

Carcinogenicity, Mutagenicity, and Impairment of Fertility—There have been no studies in animals to evaluate the carcinogenic, mutagenic, or impairment of fertility potential of dexpanthenol.

Pregnancy—Category C. Animal reproduction studies have not been conducted with ILOPAN INJECTION. It is also not known whether ILOPAN INJECTION can cause fetal harm when administered to a pregnant woman or can affect reproduction capacity. ILOPAN INJECTION should be given to a pregnant woman only if clearly needed.

Nursing Mothers—It is not known whether this drug is excreted in human milk. Because many drugs are excreted in human milk, caution should be exercised when ILOPAN INJECTION is administered to a nursing woman.

Pediatric Use—Safety and effectiveness in children have not been established.

ADVERSE REACTIONS

There have been a few reports of allergic reactions and single reports of several other adverse events in association with the administration of dexpanthenol. A causal relationship is uncertain. One patient experienced itching, tingling, difficulty in breathing. Another patient had red patches of skin. Two patients had generalized dermatitis and one patient urticaria.

One patient experienced temporary respiratory difficulty following administration of ILOPAN INJECTION 5 minutes after succinylcholine was discontinued.

One patient experienced a noticeable but slight drop in blood pressure after administration of dexpanthenol while in the recovery room.

One patient experienced intestinal colic one-half hour after the drug was administered.

Two patients vomited following administration and two patients had diarrhea 10 days post-surgery and after ILOPAN INJECTION.

One elderly patient became agitated after administration of the drug.

DOSAGE AND ADMINISTRATION

Prevention of post-operative adynamic ileus: 250 mg (1 ml) or 500 mg (2 ml) intramuscularly. Repeat in 2 hours and then every 6 hours until all danger of adynamic ileus has passed.

Treatment of adynamic ileus: 500 mg (2 ml) intramuscularly. Repeat in 2 hours and then every 6 hours as needed.

Intravenous administration: ILOPAN INJECTION 2 ml (500 mg) may be mixed with bulk I.V. solutions such as glucose or lactate-Ringer's and slowly infused intravenously.

Parenteral drug products should be inspected visually for particulate matter and discoloration prior to administration, whenever solution and container permit.

HOW SUPPLIED

Each milliliter of ILOPAN INJECTION contains dexpanthenol, 250 mg in Water for Injection. ILOPAN INJECTION is available as follows:

ILOPAN INJECTION

NDC 0013-2356-95 2 ml Ampuls, Box of 25

ILOPAN INJECTION STAT-PAK® (unit dose)

NDC 0013-2366-95 Disposable Syringe 2 ml, Box of 25

Mfd. by:
TAYLOR PHARMACAL CO.
DECATUR, ILLINOIS 62525
For:
ADRIA LABORATORIES
Division of Erbamont Inc.
COLUMBUS, OHIO 43215

KAOCHLOR® ℞

[*ka'ō-kloor*]
(Potassium Chloride)
10% Liquid
Contains Sugar

DESCRIPTION

Each 15 ml (tablespoonful) of KAOCHLOR 10% Liquid supplies 20 mEq each of potassium and chloride (as potassium chloride, 1.5 g) with sugar, saccharin, flavoring, and alcohol 5%. Contains FD&C Yellow No. 5 (tartrazine) as a color additive. The chemical name of the drug is potassium chloride.

CLINICAL PHARMACOLOGY

Potassium ion is the principal intracellular cation of most body tissues. Potassium ions participate in a number of essential physiological processes including the maintenance of intracellular tonicity, the transmission of nerve impulses, the contraction of cardiac, skeletal and smooth muscle and the maintenance of normal renal function.

Potassium depletion may occur whenever the rate of potassium loss through renal excretion and/or loss from the gastrointestinal tract exceeds the rate of potassium intake. Such depletion usually develops slowly as a consequence of prolonged therapy with oral diuretics, primary or secondary hyperaldosteronism, diabetic ketoacidosis, or inadequate replacement of potassium in patients on prolonged parenteral nutrition. Such depletion can develop rapidly with severe diarrhea, especially if associated with vomiting. Potassium depletion due to these causes is usually accompanied by a concomitant loss of chloride and is manifested by hypokalemia and metabolic alkalosis. Potassium depletion may produce weakness, fatigue, disturbances of cardiac rhythm (primarily ectopic beats), prominent U-waves in the electrocardiogram, and in advanced cases, flaccid paralysis and/or impaired ability to concentrate urine.

Potassium depletion associated with metabolic alkalosis is managed by correcting the fundamental cause of the deficiency whenever possible and administering supplemental potassium chloride, in the form of high potassium food or potassium chloride solution or tablets.

In rare circumstances (e.g., patients with renal tubular acidosis) potassium depletion may be associated with metabolic acidosis and hyperchloremia. In such patients potassium replacement should be accomplished with potassium salts other than the chloride, such as potassium bicarbonate, potassium citrate, potassium acetate, or potassium gluconate.

INDICATIONS AND USAGE

1. For therapeutic use in patients with hypokalemia with or without metabolic alkalosis, in digitalis intoxication and in patients with hypokalemic familial periodic paralysis.
2. For the prevention of potassium depletion when the dietary intake is inadequate in the following conditions: Patients receiving digitalis and diuretics for congestive heart failure, hepatic cirrhosis with ascites, states of aldosterone excess with normal renal function, potassium-losing nephropathy, and with certain diarrheal states.
3. The use of potassium salts in patients receiving diuretics for uncomplicated essential hypertension is often unnecessary when such patients have a normal dietary pattern. Serum potassium should be checked periodically, however, and if hypokalemia occurs, dietary supplementation with potassium-containing foods may be adequate to control milder cases. In more severe cases supplementation with potassium salts may be indicated.

CONTRAINDICATIONS

Potassium supplements are contraindicated in patients with hyperkalemia since a further increase in serum potassium concentration in such patients can produce cardiac arrest. Hyperkalemia may complicate any of the following conditions: Chronic renal failure, systemic acidosis such as diabetic acidosis, acute dehydration, extensive tissue breakdown as in severe burns, adrenal insufficiency, or the administration of a potassium-sparing diuretic (e.g., spironolactone, triamterene).

WARNINGS

Do not administer full strength. KAOCHLOR 10% Liquid will cause gastrointestinal irritation if administered undiluted. For details regarding adequate dilution, see Dosage and Administration.

Hyperkalemia—In patients with impaired mechanisms for excreting potassium, the administration of potassium salts can produce hyperkalemia and cardiac arrest. This occurs most commonly in patients given potassium by the intravenous route but may also occur in patients given potassium orally. Potentially fatal hyperkalemia can develop rapidly and be asymptomatic. The use of potassium salts in patients with chronic renal disease, or any other condition which impairs potassium excretion, requires particularly careful monitoring of the serum potassium concentration and appropriate dosage adjustment.

Interaction with Potassium Sparing Diuretics—Hypokalemia should not be treated by the concomitant administration of potassium salts and a potassium-sparing diuretic (e.g., spironolactone or triamterene) since the simultaneous administration of these agents can produce severe hyperkalemia.

Metabolic Acidosis—Hypokalemia in patients with metabolic acidosis should be treated with an alkalinizing potassium salt such as potassium bicarbonate, potassium citrate, potassium acetate or potassium gluconate.

PRECAUTIONS

General—The diagnosis of potassium depletion is ordinarily made by demonstrating hypokalemia in a patient with a clinical history suggesting some cause for potassium depletion.

This product contains FD&C Yellow No. 5 (tartrazine) which may cause allergic-type reactions (including bronchial asthma) in certain susceptible individuals. Although the overall incidence of FD&C Yellow No. 5 (tartrazine) sensitivity in the general population is low, it is frequently seen in patients who also have aspirin hypersensitivity.

Laboratory Tests—In interpreting the serum potassium level, the physician should bear in mind that acute alkalosis *per se* can produce hypokalemia in the absence of a deficit in total body potassium while acute acidosis *per se* can increase the serum potassium concentration into the normal range even in the presence of a reduced total body potassium. The treatment of potassium depletion, particularly in the presence of cardiac disease, renal disease, or acidosis, requires careful attention to acid-base balance and appropriate monitoring of serum electrolytes, the electrocardiogram, and the clinical status of the patient.

It is important to recognize that hyperkalemia is usually asymptomatic and may be manifested only by an increased serum potassium concentration and characteristic electrocardiographic changes (peaking of T-waves, loss of P-wave, depression of S-T segment, and prolongation of the QT interval). (See Contraindications, Warnings and Overdosage.)

The use of potassium salts in patients with chronic renal disease, or any other condition which impairs potassium excretion, requires particularly careful monitoring of the serum potassium concentration and appropriate dosage adjustment.

When blood is drawn for analysis of plasma potassium levels, it is important to recognize that artifactual elevations do occur after repeated fist clenching to make veins more prominent during application of a tourniquet.

Carcinogenesis, Mutagenesis, Impairment of Fertility—There have been no studies in animals or humans to evaluate the carcinogenesis, mutagenesis or impairment of fertility for potassium.

Pregnancy—Category C. Animal reproduction studies have not been conducted with KAOCHLOR 10% Liquid. It is also not known whether KAOCHLOR 10% Liquid can cause fetal harm when administered to a pregnant woman or can affect reproduction capacity. KAOCHLOR 10% Liquid should be given to a pregnant woman only if clearly needed.

Nursing Mothers—It is not known whether this drug is excreted in human milk. Because many drugs are excreted in human milk, caution should be exercised when KAOCHLOR 10% Liquid is administered to a nursing woman.

Pediatric Use—Safety and effectiveness in children have not been established.

ADVERSE REACTIONS

The most severe effect is hyperkalemia (see Contraindications, Warnings and Overdosage).

The most common adverse reactions to oral potassium salts are nausea, vomiting, abdominal discomfort, and diarrhea. These symptoms are due to irritation of the gastrointestinal tract and are best managed by diluting the preparation further, taking the dose with meals, or reducing the dose.

OVERDOSAGE

The administration of oral potassium salts to persons with normal excretory mechanisms for potassium rarely causes serious hyperkalemia. However, if excretory mechanisms are impaired or if potassium is administered too rapidly intravenously, potentially fatal hyperkalemia can result (see Contraindications and Warnings). It is important to recognize that hyperkalemia is usually asymptomatic and may be manifested only by an increased serum potassium concentration and characteristic electrocardiographic changes (peaking of T-waves, loss of P-wave, depression of S-T segment, and prolongation of the QT interval). Late manifestations include muscle-paralysis and cardiovascular collapse from cardiac arrest.

Continued on next page

Adria—Cont.

Treatment for hyperkalemia includes the following:

1. Elimination of foods and medications containing potassium and potassium-sparing diuretics.
2. Intravenous administration of 300 to 500 ml/hr of 10% dextrose solution containing 10-20 units of crystalline insulin per 1,000 ml.
3. Correction of acidosis, if present, with intravenous sodium bicarbonate.
4. Use of exchange resins, hemodialysis, or peritoneal dialysis.

In treating hyperkalemia, it should be recalled that in patients who have been stabilized on digitalis, too rapid a lowering of the serum potassium concentration can produce digitalis toxicity.

DOSAGE AND ADMINISTRATION

The usual dietary intake of potassium by the average adult is 40 to 80 mEq per day. Potassium depletion sufficient to cause hypokalemia usually requires the loss of 200 or more mEq of potassium from the total body store.

Dosage must be adjusted to the individual needs of each patient but is typically in the range of 20 mEq per day for the prevention of hypokalemia to 40-100 mEq per day or more for the treatment of potassium depletion.

To minimize gastrointestinal irritation, patients must follow directions regarding dilution. Each tablespoonful (15 ml) should be diluted with three (3) fluid ounces or more of water or other liquid.

One (1) tablespoonful (15 ml) twice daily (after morning and evening meals) supplies 40 mEq of potassium. Deviations from this recommendation may be indicated, since no average total daily dose can be defined but must be governed by close observation for clinical effects. However, potassium intoxication may result from any therapeutic dosage. See "Overdosage" and "Precautions".

HOW SUPPLIED

KAOCHLOR 10% Liquid supplies 20 mEq each of potassium and chloride per tablespoonful (15 ml).

NDC 0013-3103-51 Pint

Storage Conditions—Preserve in tight, light resistant containers. Store at room temperature and protect from cold.

KAOCHLOR® S-F ℞

[*ka'ō-kloor s-f*]

(Potassium Chloride)
10% Liquid
Sugar-Free

DESCRIPTION

Each 15 ml (tablespoonful) of KAOCHLOR S-F 10% Liquid supplies 20 mEq each of potassium and chloride (as potassium chloride, 1.5g) with saccharin, flavoring, and alcohol 5%. The chemical name of the drug is potassium chloride.

CLINICAL PHARMACOLOGY

See KAOCHLOR 10% LIQUID

INDICATIONS AND USAGE

See KAOCHLOR 10% LIQUID

CONTRAINDICATIONS

See KAOCHLOR 10% LIQUID

WARNINGS

See KAOCHLOR 10% LIQUID

PRECAUTIONS

General—The diagnosis of potassium depletion is ordinarily made by demonstrating hypokalemia in patients with a clinical history suggesting some cause for potassium depletion.

Laboratory Tests—See KAOCHLOR 10% LIQUID

Carcinogenesis, Mutagenesis, Impairment of Fertility—See KAOCHLOR 10% LIQUID

Pregnancy—See KAOCHLOR 10% LIQUID

Nursing Mothers—See KAOCHLOR 10% LIQUID

Pediatric Use—See KAOCHLOR 10% LIQUID

ADVERSE REACTIONS

See KAOCHLOR 10% LIQUID

OVERDOSAGE

See KAOCHLOR 10% LIQUID

DOSAGE AND ADMINISTRATION

See KAOCHLOR 10% LIQUID

HOW SUPPLIED

KAOCHLOR S-F 10% Liquid supplies 20 mEq each of potassium and chloride per tablespoonful (15 ml).

NDC 0013-3093-51 Pint

NDC 0013-3093-56 Bottle of 4 Fl. Oz. (36's only).

Storage Conditions—Preserve in tight, light resistant containers. Store at room temperature and protect from cold.

KAON® ELIXIR ℞

[*kā'ŏn*]

(Potassium Gluconate)
Grape Flavor
Sugar-Free

DESCRIPTION

Each 15 ml (tablespoonful) supplies 20 mEq of potassium (as potassium gluconate, 4.68 g) with saccharin and aromatics and alcohol 5%. The chemical name of the drug is gluconic acid potassium salt. The structural formula is:

```
          H    H   OH   H
          |    |    |    |
HOCH2 -  C  -  C  -  C  -  C-COOK
          |    |    |    |
          OH   OH   H    OH
```

CLINICAL PHARMACOLOGY

Potassium ion is the principal intracellular cation of most body tissues. Potassium ions participate in a number of essential physiological processes including the maintenance of intracellular tonicity, the transmission of nerve impulses, the contraction of cardiac, skeletal and smooth muscle and the maintenance of normal renal function.

Potassium depletion may occur whenever the rate of potassium loss through renal excretion and/or loss from the gastrointestinal tract exceeds the rate of potassium intake. Potassium depletion sufficient to cause hypokalemia usually requires the loss of 200 or more mEq of potassium from the total body store. Such depletion usually develops slowly as a consequence of prolonged therapy with oral diuretics, primary or secondary hyperaldosteronism, diabetic ketoacidosis, or inadequate replacement of potassium in patients on prolonged parenteral nutrition. Such depletion can develop rapidly with severe diarrhea, especially if associated with vomiting. Potassium depletion may produce weakness, fatigue, disturbances of cardiac rhythm (primarily ectopic beats), prominent U-waves in the electrocardiogram, and in advanced cases, flaccid paralysis and/or impaired ability to concentrate urine.

INDICATIONS AND USAGE

1. For therapeutic use in patients with hypokalemia with or without metabolic alkalosis, in digitalis intoxication and in patients with hypokalemic familial periodic paralysis.
2. For the prevention of potassium depletion when the dietary intake is inadequate in the following conditions: Patients receiving digitalis and diuretics for congestive heart failure; hepatic cirrhosis with ascites, states of aldosterone excess with normal renal function, potassium-losing nephropathy, and with certain diarrheal states.
3. The use of potassium salts in patients receiving diuretics for uncomplicated essential hypertension is often unnecessary when such patients have a normal dietary pattern. Serum potassium should be checked periodically, however, and if hypokalemia occurs, dietary supplementation with potassium-containing foods may be adequate to control milder cases. In more severe cases supplementation with potassium salts may be indicated.
4. Hypokalemia in patients with metabolic acidosis should be treated with an alkalinizing potassium salt such as potassium gluconate.

CONTRAINDICATIONS

Potassium supplements are contraindicated in patients with hyperkalemia since a further increase in serum potassium concentration in such patients can produce cardiac arrest. Hyperkalemia may complicate any of the following conditions: Chronic renal failure, systemic acidosis such as diabetic acidosis, acute dehydration, extensive tissue breakdown as in severe burns, adrenal insufficiency, or the administration of a potassium-sparing diuretic (e.g., spironolactone, triamterene).

WARNINGS

Do not administer full strength. KAON ELIXIR may cause gastrointestinal irritation if administered undiluted. For details regarding adequate dilution, see Dosage and Administration.

Hyperkalemia—In patients with impaired mechanisms for excreting potassium, the administration of potassium salts can produce hyperkalemia and cardiac arrest. This occurs most commonly in patients given potassium by the intravenous route but may also occur in patients given potassium orally. Potentially fatal hyperkalemia can develop rapidly and be asymptomatic. The use of potassium salts in patients with chronic renal disease, or any other condition which impairs potassium excretion, requires particularly careful monitoring of the serum potassium concentration and appropriate dosage adjustment.

Interaction with Potassium Sparing Diuretics—Hypokalemia should not be treated by the concomitant administration of potassium salts and a potassium-sparing diuretic (e.g., spironolactone or triamterene) since the simultaneous administration of these agents can produce severe hyperkalemia.

PRECAUTIONS

General—The diagnosis of potassium depletion is ordinarily made by demonstrating hypokalemia in a patient with a clinical history suggesting some cause for potassium depletion.

In hypokalemic states, especially in patients on a low-salt diet, hypochloremic alkalosis is a possibility that may require chloride as well as potassium supplementation. In these circumstances, potassium replacement with potassium chloride may be more advantageous than with other potassium salts.

However, KAON ELIXIR can be supplemented with chloride. Ammonium chloride is an excellent source of chloride ion (18.7 mEq per gram) but it should not be used in patients with hepatic cirrhosis where ammonium salts are contraindicated.

Laboratory Tests—In interpreting the serum potassium level, the physician should bear in mind that acute alkalosis *per se* can produce hypokalemia in the absence of a deficit in total body potassium while acute acidosis *per se* can increase the serum potassium concentration into the normal range even in the presence of a reduced total body potassium. The treatment of potassium depletion, particularly in the presence of cardiac disease, renal disease, or acidosis, requires careful attention to acid-base balance and appropriate monitoring of serum electrolytes, the electrocardiogram, and the clinical status of the patient.

It is important to recognize that hyperkalemia is usually asymptomatic and may be manifested only by an increased serum potassium concentration and characteristic electrocardiographic changes (peaking of T-waves, loss of P-wave, depression of S-T segment, and prolongation of the QT interval). (See Contraindications, Warnings, and Overdosage.)

The use of potassium salts in patients with chronic renal disease, or any other condition which impairs potassium excretion, requires particularly careful monitoring of the serum potassium concentration and appropriate dosage adjustment.

When blood is drawn for analysis of plasma potassium levels, it is important to recognize that artifactual elevations do occur after repeated fist clenching to make veins more prominent during application of a tourniquet.

Carcinogenesis, Mutagenesis, Impairment of Fertility—There have been no studies in animals or humans to evaluate the carcinogenesis, mutagenesis or impairment of fertility for potassium.

Pregnancy—Category C. Animal reproduction studies have not been conducted with KAON ELIXIR. It is also not known whether KAON ELIXIR can cause fetal harm when administered to a pregnant woman or can affect reproduction capacity. KAON ELIXIR should be given to a pregnant woman only if clearly needed.

Nursing Mothers—It is not known whether this drug is excreted in human milk. Because many drugs are excreted in human milk, caution should be exercised when KAON ELIXIR is administered to a nursing woman.

Pediatric Use—Safety and effectiveness in children have not been established.

ADVERSE REACTIONS

The most severe adverse effect is hyperkalemia (see Contraindications, Warnings and Overdosage).

The most common adverse reactions to oral potassium salts are nausea, vomiting, abdominal discomfort, and diarrhea. These symptoms are due to irritation of the gastrointestinal tract and are best managed by diluting the preparation further, taking the dose with meals, or reducing the dose.

OVERDOSAGE

The administration of oral potassium salts to persons with normal excretory mechanisms for potassium rarely causes serious hyperkalemia. However, if excretory mechanisms are impaired or if potassium is administered too rapidly intravenously, potentially fatal hyperkalemia can result (see Contraindications and Warnings). It is important to recognize that hyperkalemia is usually asymptomatic and may be manifested only by an increased serum potassium concentration and characteristic electrocardiographic changes (peaking of T-waves, loss of P-wave, depression of S-T segment, and prolongation of the QT interval). Late manifestations include muscle-paralysis and cardiovascular collapse from cardiac arrest.

Treatment for hyperkalemia includes the following:

1. Elimination of foods and medications containing potassium and potassium-sparing diuretics.
2. Intravenous administration of 300 to 500 ml/hr of 10% dextrose solution containing 10–20 units of crystalline insulin per 1,000 ml.
3. Correction of acidosis, if present, with intravenous sodium bicarbonate.
4. Use of exchange resins, hemodialysis, or peritoneal dialysis.

In treating hyperkalemia, it should be recalled that in patients who have been stabilized on digitalis, too rapid a lowering of the serum potassium concentration can produce digitalis toxicity.

DOSAGE AND ADMINISTRATION

The usual dietary intake of potassium by the average adult is 40 to 80 mEq per day. Potassium depletion sufficient to cause hypokalemia usually requires the loss of 200 or more mEq of potassium from the total body store.

Dosage must be adjusted to the individual needs of each patient but is typically in the range of 20 mEq per day for the prevention of hypokalemia to 40–100 mEq per day or more for the treatment of potassium depletion.

To minimize gastrointestinal irritation, patients must follow directions regarding dilution. Each tablespoonful (15 ml) should be diluted with one fluid ounce or more of water or other liquid.

One tablespoonful twice daily (after morning and evening meals) supplies 40 mEq of potassium. Deviations from this recommendation may be indicated, since no average total daily dose can be defined but must be governed by close observation for clinical effects. However, potassium intoxication may result from any therapeutic dosage. See "Overdosage" and "Precautions".

HOW SUPPLIED

KAON ELIXIR (potassium gluconate), Grape, supplies 20 mEq of potassium (as potassium gluconate, 4.68g) per tablespoonful (15 ml).

NDC 0013-3203-51 Pint
NDC 0013-3203-53 Gallon

Storage Conditions—Preserve in tight, light resistant containers. Store at room temperature and protect from cold.

KAON® ℞

[*kā'ŏn*]
(Potassium Gluconate)
Sugar Coated Tablets

DESCRIPTION

Each sugar coated tablet supplies 5 mEq of potassium (as potassium gluconate 1.17g). KAON tablets are sugar coated, not enteric coated, which favors dissolution in the stomach and absorption before reaching the small intestine where the lesions with enteric potassium chloride have occurred. The sugar coating merely adds to palatability and ease of swallowing, not to delay absorption as does the enteric coating. Potassium gluconate is an electrolyte replenisher. The chemical name of the drug is gluconic acid potassium salt. The structural formula is:

```
        H  H  OH H
        |  |  |  |
HOCH2—C—C—C—C—COOK
        |  |  |  |
        OH OH H  OH
```

CLINICAL PHARMACOLOGY

Potassium ion is the principal intracellular cation of most body tissues. Potassium ions participate in a number of essential physiological processes including the maintenance of intracellular tonicity, the transmission of nerve impulses, the contraction of cardiac, skeletal and smooth muscle and the maintenance of normal renal function.

Potassium depletion may occur whenever the rate of potassium loss through renal excretion and/or loss from the gastrointestinal tract exceeds the rate of potassium intake. Potassium depletion sufficient to cause hypokalemia usually requires the loss of 200 or more mEq of potassium from the total body store. Such depletion usually develops slowly as a consequence of prolonged therapy with oral diuretics, primary or secondary hyperaldosteronism, diabetic ketoacidosis, or inadequate replacement of potassium in patients on prolonged parenteral nutrition. Such depletion can develop rapidly with severe diarrhea, especially if associated with vomiting. Potassium depletion may produce weakness, fatigue, disturbances of cardiac rhythm (primarily ectopic beats), prominent U-waves in the electrocardiogram, and in advanced cases, flaccid paralysis and/or impaired ability to concentrate urine.

INDICATIONS AND USAGE

BECAUSE OF REPORTS OF INTESTINAL AND GASTRIC ULCERATION AND BLEEDING WITH SOLID POTASSIUM PREPARATIONS, THESE DRUGS SHOULD BE RESERVED FOR THOSE PATIENTS WHO CANNOT TOLERATE OR REFUSE TO TAKE LIQUIDS OR EFFERVESCENT POTASSIUM PREPARATIONS OR FOR PATIENTS IN WHOM THERE IS A PROBLEM OF COMPLIANCE WITH THESE PREPARATIONS.

1. For therapeutic use in patients with hypokalemia with or without metabolic alkalosis, in digitalis intoxication and in patients with hypokalemic familial periodic paralysis.
2. For the prevention of potassium depletion when the dietary intake is inadequate in the following conditions: Patients receiving digitalis and diuretics for congestive heart failure, hepatic cirrhosis with ascites, states of aldosterone excess with normal renal function, potassium-losing nephropathy, and with certain diarrheal states.
3. The use of potassium salts in patients receiving diuretics for uncomplicated essential hypertension is often unnecessary when such patients have a normal dietary pattern. Serum potassium should be checked periodically, however, and if hypokalemia occurs, dietary supplementation with potassium-containing foods may be adequate to control milder cases. In more severe cases supplementation with potassium salts may be indicated.
4. Hypokalemia in patients with metabolic acidosis should be treated with an alkalinizing potassium salt such as potassium gluconate.

CONTRAINDICATIONS

Potassium supplements are contraindicated in patients with hyperkalemia since a further increase in serum potassium concentration in such patients can produce cardiac arrest. Hyperkalemia may complicate any of the following conditions: Chronic renal failure, systemic acidosis such as diabetic acidosis, acute dehydration, extensive tissue breakdown as in severe burns, adrenal insufficiency, or the administration of a potassium-sparing diuretic (e.g., spironolactone, triamterene).

All solid dosage forms of potassium supplements are contraindicated in any patient in whom there is cause for arrest or delay in tablet passage through the gastrointestinal tract. In these instances, potassium supplementation should be with a liquid preparation.

WARNINGS

Hyperkalemia —In patients with impaired mechanisms for excreting potassium, the administration of potassium salts can produce hyperkalemia and cardiac arrest. This occurs most commonly in patients given potassium by the intravenous route but may also occur in patients given potassium orally. Potentially fatal hyperkalemia can develop rapidly and be asymptomatic. The use of potassium salts in patients with chronic renal disease, or any other condition which impairs potassium excretion, requires particularly careful monitoring of the serum potassium concentration and appropriate dosage adjustment.

Interaction with Potassium Sparing Diuretics —Hypokalemia should not be treated by the concomitant administration of potassium salts and a potassium-sparing diuretic (e.g., spironolactone or triamterene) since the simultaneous administration of these agents can produce severe hyperkalemia.

Gastrointestinal Lesions —Potassium chloride tablets have produced stenotic and/or ulcerative lesions of the small bowel and deaths. These lesions are caused by a high localized concentration of potassium ion in the region of a rapidly dissolving tablet, which injures the bowel wall and thereby produces obstruction, hemorrhage, or perforation. While the reported frequency of small bowel lesions is much less with KAON (potassium gluconate) tablets (less than 2 per 1,000,000 patient years) than with enteric coated tablets (400–500 per 1,000,000 patient years) cases associated with the product have been reported. KAON (potassium gluconate) tablets should be discontinued immediately and the possibility of bowel obstruction or perforation considered if severe vomiting, abdominal pain, distention, or gastrointestinal bleeding occurs.

PRECAUTION

General —The diagnosis of potassium depletion is ordinarily made by demonstrating hypokalemia in a patient with a clinical history suggesting some cause for potassium depletion.

In hypokalemic states, especially in patients on a low-salt diet, hypochloremic alkalosis is a possibility that may require chloride as well as potassium supplementation. In these circumstances, potassium replacement with potassium chloride may be more advantageous than with other potassium salts. However, KAON tablets can be supplemented with chloride. Ammonium chloride is an excellent source of chloride ion (18.7 mEq per gram) but it should not be used in patients with hepatic cirrhosis where ammonium salts are contraindicated.

Information for Patients —KAON (potassium gluconate) tablets should be taken with or immediately after food and with a full glass of water or other liquid.

Laboratory Tests —In interpreting the serum potassium level, the physician should bear in mind that acute alkalosis per se can produce hypokalemia in the absence of a deficit in total body potassium while acute acidosis per se can increase the serum potassium concentration into the normal range even in the presence of a reduced total body potassium. The treatment of potassium depletion, particularly in the presence of cardiac disease, renal disease, or acidosis requires careful attention to acid-base balance and appropriate monitoring of serum electrolytes, the electrocardiogram, and the clinical status of the patient.

It is important to recognize that hyperkalemia is usually asymptomatic and may be manifested only by an increased serum potassium concentration and characteristic electrocardiographic changes (peaking of T-waves, loss of P-wave, depression of S-T segment, and prolongation of the QT interval). (See Contraindications, Warnings and Overdosage.)

The use of potassium salts in patients with chronic renal disease, or any other condition which impairs potassium excretion, requires particularly careful monitoring of the serum potassium concentration and appropriate dosage adjustment.

When blood is drawn for analysis of plasma potassium levels, it is important to recognize that artifactual elevations do occur after repeated fist clenching to make veins more prominent during application of a tourniquet.

Drug Interactions —Concomitant administration of potassium supplements and a potassium-sparing diuretic (e.g., aldosterone antagonists or triamterene) can lead to severe hyperkalemia (see Warnings). Potassium supplements should be used cautiously in patients who are using salt substitutes because most of the latter contain substantial amounts of potassium.

Carcinogenesis, Mutagenesis, Impairment of Fertility —No data are available on long term potential for carcinogenicity in animals or humans.

Pregnancy —Category C. Animal reproduction studies have not been conducted with KAON tablets. It is also not known whether KAON tablets can cause fetal harm when administered to a pregnant woman or can affect reproduction capacity. KAON tablets should be given to a pregnant woman only if clearly needed.

Nursing Mothers —It is not known whether this drug is excreted in human milk. Because many drugs are excreted in human milk, caution should be exercised when KAON tablets are administered to a nursing woman.

Pediatric Use —Safety and effectiveness in children have not been established.

ADVERSE REACTIONS

The most severe adverse effects are hyperkalemia (see Contraindications, Warnings and Overdosage), and gastrointestinal obstruction, bleeding or perforation (see Warnings).

The most common adverse reactions to oral potassium salts are nausea, vomiting, abdominal discomfort, and diarrhea. These symptoms are due to irritation of the gastrointestinal tract and are best managed by diluting the preparation further, taking the dose with meals, or reducing the dose.

OVERDOSAGE

The administration of oral potassium salts to persons with normal excretory mechanisms for potassium rarely causes serious hyperkalemia. However, if excretory mechanisms are impaired or if potassium is administered too rapidly intravenously, potentially fatal hyperkalemia can result (see Contraindications and Warnings). It is important to recognize that hyperkalemia is usually asymptomatic and may be manifested only by an increased serum potassium concentration and characteristic electrocardiographic changes (peaking of T-waves, loss of P-wave, depression of S-T segment, and prolongation of the QT interval). Late manifestations include muscle-paralysis and cardiovascular collapse from cardiac arrest.

Treatment measures for hyperkalemia include the following:

1. Elimination of foods and medications containing potassium and potassium-sparing diuretics.
2. Intravenous administration of 300 to 500 ml/hr of 10% dextrose solution containing 10–20 units of crystalline insulin per 1,000 ml.
3. Correction of acidosis, if present, with intravenous sodium bicarbonate.
4. Use of exchange resins, hemodialysis, or peritoneal dialysis.

In treating hyperkalemia, it should be recalled that in patients who have been stabilized on digitalis, too rapid a lowering of the serum potassium concentration can produce digitalis toxicity.

DOSAGE AND ADMINISTRATION

The usual dietary intake of potassium by the average adult is 40 to 80 mEq per day. Potassium depletion sufficient to cause hypokalemia usually requires the loss of 200 or more mEq of potassium from the total body store.

Dosage must be adjusted to the individual needs of each patient but is typically in the range of 20 mEq per day for the prevention of hypokalemia to 40–100 mEq per day or more for the treatment of potassium depletion.

The usual adult dosage is 2 tablets four times daily (after meals and at bedtime). This supplies 40 mEq of elemental potassium, the approximate minimum adult daily requirement for potassium. Deviations from this recommendation may be indicated, since no average total daily dose can be defined but must be governed by close observation for clinical effects. However, potassium intoxication may result from any therapeutic dosage (see Overdosage and Precautions).

Tablets should be taken with or immediately after food and with a full glass of water or other liquid.

Continued on next page

Adria—Cont.

HOW SUPPLIED

KAON (potassium gluconate) sugar coated tablets supply 5 mEq of potassium (as potassium gluconate 1.17g). KAON tablets are available for oral administration as purple, capsule-shaped sugar coated tablets coded ADRIA, 312.
Tablets are supplied as follows:
NDC 0013-3121-17 in bottles of 100.
NDC 0013-3121-21 in bottles of 500.
Storage Conditions—Store at room temperature.

KAON-CL® ℞
[*kā 'ŏn-sēe-ĕl "*]
(Potassium Chloride)
CONTROLLED RELEASE TABLETS

PRODUCT OVERVIEW

KEY FACTS

KAON-CL is a non-enteric-coated slow release potassium product containing 6.7 mEq or 500 mg of potassium chloride. The potassium is released from a wax matrix. The tablet is sugar coated to increase palatability. Such preparations should be reserved for patients who cannot or will not use liquid or effevescent potassium products.

MAJOR USES

KAON-CL is used in the treatment and prevention of hypokalemia. This may occur in any condition in which renal or gastrointestinal potassium loss exceeds intake.

SAFETY INFORMATION

Contraindicated in hyperkalemia from any cause and in patients in whom tablet passage through the GI tract may be delayed. This product should not be used concomitantly with potassium-sparing diuretics. Small bowel lesions and upper GI bleeding are infrequent with wax matrix preparations.

PRESCRIBING INFORMATION

KAON-CL® ℞
[*kā 'ŏn sēe-ĕl "*]
(Potassium Chloride)
CONTROLLED RELEASE TABLETS

DESCRIPTION

KAON-CL 6.7 mEq is a sugar coated (not enteric-coated) tablet containing 500 mg potassium chloride (equivalent to 6.7 mEq potassium chloride) in a wax matrix. Contains color additives including FD&C Yellow No. 5 (tartrazine). This formulation is intended to provide a controlled release of potassium from the matrix to minimize the likelihood of producing high localized concentrations of potassium within the gastrointestinal tract.

ACTIONS

Potassium ion is the principal intracellular cation of most body tissues. Potassium ions participate in a number of essential physiological processes including the maintenance of intracellular tonicity, the transmission of nerve impulses, the contraction of cardiac, skeletal and smooth muscle and the maintenance of normal renal function.
Potassium depletion may occur whenever the rate of potassium loss through renal excretion and/or loss from the gastrointestinal tract exceeds the rate of potassium intake. Such depletion usually develops slowly as a consequence of prolonged therapy with oral diuretics, primary or secondary hyperaldosteronism, diabetic ketoacidosis, severe diarrhea, or inadequate replacement of potassium in patients on prolonged parenteral nutrition. Potassium depletion due to these causes is usually accompanied by a concomitant deficiency of chloride and is manifested by hypokalemia and metabolic alkalosis. Potassium depletion may produce weakness, fatigue, disturbances of cardiac rhythm (primarily ectopic beats), prominent U-waves in the electrocardiogram, and in advanced cases, flaccid paralysis and/or impaired ability to concentrate urine.
Potassium depletion associated with metabolic alkalosis is managed by correcting the fundamental cause of the deficiency whenever possible and administering supplemental potassium chloride, in the form of high potassium food or potassium chloride solution or tablets. In rare circumstances (e.g., patients with renal tubular acidosis) potassium depletion may be associated with metabolic acidosis and hyperchloremia. In such patients potassium replacement should be accomplished with potassium salts other than the chloride, such as potassium bicarbonate, potassium citrate, potassium acetate, or potassium gluconate.

INDICATIONS

BECAUSE OF REPORTS OF INTESTINAL AND GASTRIC ULCERATION AND BLEEDING WITH SLOW RELEASE POTASSIUM CHLORIDE PREPARATIONS, THESE DRUGS SHOULD BE RESERVED FOR THOSE PATIENTS WHO CANNOT TOLERATE OR REFUSE TO TAKE LIQUIDS OR EFFERVESCENT POTASSIUM PREPARATIONS OR FOR PATIENTS IN WHOM THERE IS A PROBLEM OF COMPLIANCE WITH THESE PREPARATIONS.

1. For therapeutic use in patients with hypokalemia with or without metabolic alkalosis, in digitalis intoxication and in patients with hypokalemic familial periodic paralysis.
2. For the prevention of potassium depletion when the dietary intake is inadequate in the following conditions: Patients receiving digitalis and diuretics for congestive heart failure, hepatic cirrhosis with ascites, states of aldosterone excess with normal renal function, potassium-losing nephropathy, and with certain diarrheal states.
3. The use of potassium salts in patients receiving diuretics for uncomplicated essential hypertension is often unnecessary when such patients have a normal dietary pattern. Serum potassium should be checked periodically, however, and if hypokalemia occurs, dietary supplementation with potassium-containing foods may be adequate to control milder cases. In more severe cases supplementation with potassium salts may be indicated.

CONTRAINDICATIONS

Potassium supplements are contraindicated in patients with hyperkalemia since a further increase in serum potassium concentration in such patients can produce cardiac arrest. Hyperkalemia may complicate any of the following conditions: Chronic renal failure, systemic acidosis such as diabetic acidosis, acute dehydration, extensive tissue breakdown as in severe burns, adrenal insufficiency, or the administration of a potassium-sparing diuretic (e.g., spironolactone, triamterene).
Wax-matrix potassium chloride preparations have produced esophageal ulceration in certain cardiac patients with esophageal compression due to enlarged left atrium. Potassium supplementation, when indicated in such patients, should be with a liquid preparation.
All solid dosage forms of potassium chloride supplements are contraindicated in any patient in whom there is cause for arrest or delay in tablet passage through the gastrointestinal tract. In these instances, potassium supplementation should be with a liquid preparation.

WARNINGS

Hyperkalemia—In patients with impaired mechanisms for excreting potassium, the administration of potassium salts can produce hyperkalemia and cardiac arrest. This occurs most commonly in patients given potassium by the intravenous route but may also occur in patients given potassium orally. Potentially fatal hyperkalemia can develop rapidly and be asymptomatic. The use of potassium salts in patients with chronic renal disease, or any other condition which impairs potassium excretion, requires particularly careful monitoring of the serum potassium concentration and appropriate dosage adjustment.
Interaction with Potassium Sparing Diuretics—Hypokalemia should not be treated by the concomitant administration of potassium salts and a potassium-sparing diuretic (e.g., spironolactone or triamterene) since the simultaneous administration of these agents can produce severe hyperkalemia.
Gastrointestinal Lesions—Potassium chloride tablets have produced stenotic and/or ulcerative lesions of the small bowel and deaths. These lesions are caused by a high localized concentration of potassium ion in the region of a rapidly dissolving tablet, which injures the bowel wall and thereby produces obstruction, hemorrhage or perforation. KAON-CL 6.7 mEq (potassium chloride) is a wax-matrix tablet formulated to provide a controlled rate of release of potassium chloride and thus to minimize the possibility of a high local concentration of potassium ion near the bowel wall. While the reported frequency of small bowel lesions is much less with wax-matrix tablets (less than one per 100,000 patient years) than with enteric-coated potassium chloride tablets (40-50 per 100,000 patient years) cases associated with wax-matrix tablets have been reported both in foreign countries and in the United States. In addition, perhaps because the wax-matrix preparations are not enteric-coated and release potassium in the stomach, there have been reports of upper gastrointestinal bleeding associated with these products. The total number of gastrointestinal lesions remains less than one per 100,000 patient years. KAON-CL 6.7 mEq should be discontinued immediately and the possibility of bowel obstruction or perforation considered if severe vomiting, abdominal pain, distention, or gastrointestinal bleeding occurs.
Metabolic Acidosis—Hypokalemia in patients with metabolic acidosis should be treated with an alkalinizing potassium salt such as potassium bicarbonate, potassium citrate, potassium acetate, or potassium gluconate.

PRECAUTIONS

The diagnosis of potassium depletion is ordinarily made by demonstrating hypokalemia in a patient with a clinical history suggesting some cause for potassium depletion. In interpreting the serum potassium level, the physician should bear in mind that acute alkalosis *per se* can produce hypokalemia in the absence of a deficit in total body potassium while acute acidosis *per se* can increase the serum potassium concentration into the normal range even in the presence of a reduced total body potassium. The treatment of potassium depletion, particularly in the presence of cardiac arrest, renal disease, or acidosis requires careful attention to acid-base balance and appropriate monitoring of serum electrolytes, the electrocardiogram, and the clinical status of the patient.
This product contains FD&C Yellow No. 5 (tartrazine) which may cause allergic-type reactions (including bronchial asthma) in certain susceptible individuals. Although the overall incidence of FD&C Yellow No. 5 (tartrazine) sensitivity in the general population is low, it is frequently seen in patients who also have aspirin hypersensitivity.

ADVERSE REACTIONS

The most common adverse reactions to oral potassium salts are nausea, vomiting, abdominal discomfort and diarrhea. These symptoms are due to irritation of the gastrointestinal tract and are best managed by diluting the preparation further, taking the dose with meals, or reducing the dose. The most severe adverse effects are hyperkalemia (see Contraindications, Warnings and Overdosage) and gastrointestinal obstruction, bleeding or perforation (see Warnings).

OVERDOSAGE

The administration of oral potassium salts to persons with normal excretory mechanisms for potassium rarely causes serious hyperkalemia. However, if excretory mechanisms are impaired or if potassium is administered too rapidly intravenously, potentially fatal hyperkalemia can result (see Contraindications and Warnings). It is important to recognize that hyperkalemia is usually asymptomatic and may be manifested only by an increased serum potassium concentration and characteristic electrocardiographic changes (peaking of T-waves, loss of P-wave, depression of S-T segment, and prolongation of the QT interval). Late manifestations include muscle-paralysis and cardiovascular collapse from cardiac arrest.
Treatment measures for hyperkalemia include the following:

1. Elimination of foods and medications containing potassium and of potassium-sparing diuretics.
2. Intravenous administration of 300 to 500 ml/hr of 10% dextrose solution containing 10–20 units of crystalline insulin per 1,000 ml.
3. Correction of acidosis, if present, with intravenous sodium bicarbonate.
4. Use of exchange resins, hemodialysis, or peritoneal dialysis.

In treating hyperkalemia, it should be recalled that in patients who have been stabilized on digitalis, too rapid a lowering of the serum potassium concentration can produce digitalis toxicity.

DOSAGE AND ADMINISTRATION

The usual dietary intake of potassium by the average adult is 40 to 80 mEq per day. Potassium depletion sufficient to cause hypokalemia usually requires the loss of 200 or more mEq of potassium from the total body store.
Dosage must be adjusted to the individual needs of each patient but is typically in the range of 20 mEq per day for the prevention of hypokalemia to 40–100 mEq per day or more for the treatment of potassium depletion.
One KAON-CL 6.7 mEq three times daily provides 20 mEq of potassium chloride. Two KAON-CL 6.7 mEq three times daily provides 40 mEq of potassium chloride.
Tablets should be taken with a glass of water or other liquid.

HOW SUPPLIED

NDC 0013-3071-17 Bottle of 100 Tablets.
NDC 0013-3071-19 Bottle of 250 Tablets.
NDC 0013-3071-23 Bottle of 1000 Tablets.
Shown in Product Identification Section, page 403

KAON CL-10™ ℞
[*kā 'ŏn see-el "ten*]
(Potassium Chloride)
CONTROLLED RELEASE TABLETS

PRODUCT OVERVIEW

KEY FACTS

KAON CL-10 is a non-enteric-coated slow release potassium product containing 10 mEq or 750 mg of potassium chloride. The potassium is released from a wax matrix. The tablet is sugar coated to increase palatability. Such preparations should be reserved for patients who cannot or will not use liquid or effervescent potassium products.

MAJOR USES

KAON CL-10 is used in the treatment and prevention of hypokalemia. This may occur in any condition in which renal or gastrointestinal potassium loss exceeds intake.

SAFETY INFORMATION

Contraindicated in hyperkalemia from any cause and in patients in whom tablet passage through the GI tract may be delayed. This product should not be used concomitantly with potassium-sparing diuretics. Small bowel lesions and upper GI bleeding are infrequent with wax matrix preparations.

PRESCRIBING INFORMATION

KAON CL-10™ ℞
[kā'ŏn see-el"ten]
(Potassium Chloride)
CONTROLLED RELEASE TABLETS

DESCRIPTION
KAON CL-10 mEq is a sugar coated (not enteric-coated) tablet containing 750 mg potassium chloride (equivalent to 10 mEq potassium chloride) in a wax matrix. This formulation is intended to provide a controlled release of potassium from the matrix to minimize the likelihood of producing high localized concentrations of potassium within the gastrointestinal tract.

ACTIONS
See KAON-CL® TABLETS

INDICATIONS
See KAON-CL TABLETS

CONTRAINDICATIONS
See KAON-CL TABLETS

WARNINGS
See KAON-CL TABLETS

PRECAUTIONS
The diagnosis of potassium depletion is ordinarily made by demonstrating hypokalemia in a patient with a clinical history suggesting some cause for potassium depletion. In interpreting the serum potassium level, the physician should bear in mind that acute alkalosis *per se* can produce hypokalemia in the absence of a deficit in total body potassium while acute acidosis *per se* can increase the serum potassium concentration into the normal range even in the presence of a reduced total body potassium. The treatment of potassium depletion, particularly in the presence of cardiac disease, renal disease, or acidosis requires careful attention to acid-base balance and appropriate monitoring of serum electrolytes, the electrocardiogram, and the clinical status of the patient.

ADVERSE REACTIONS
See KAON-CL TABLETS

OVERDOSAGE
See KAON-CL TABLETS

DOSAGE AND ADMINISTRATION
The usual dietary intake of potassium by the average adult is 40 to 80 mEq per day. Potassium depletion sufficient to cause hypokalemia usually requires the loss of 200 or more mEq of potassium from the total body store.
Dosage must be adjusted to the individual needs of each patient but is typically in the range of 20 mEq per day for the prevention of hypokalemia to 40–100 mEq per day or more for the treatment of potassium depletion.
One KAON CL-10 mEq two times daily provides 20 mEq of potassium chloride. Two KAON CL-10 mEq two times daily provides 40 mEq of potassium chloride.
Tablets should be taken with a glass of water or other liquid.

CAUTION
Federal law prohibits dispensing without prescription.

HOW SUPPLIED
NDC 0013-3041-17 Bottles of 100 Tablets
NDC 0013-3041-21 Bottle of 500 Tablets
NDC 0013-3041-18 Stat-Pak® (Unit Dose) Box of 100 Tablets
Shown in Product Identification Section, page 403

KAON-CL 20%® ℞
[kā'ŏn-see-el"20%]
(Potassium Chloride)
Sugar-Free

DESCRIPTION
Each 15 ml (tablespoonful) of KAON-CL 20% supplies 40 mEq each of potassium and chloride (as potassium chloride, 3g) with saccharin, flavoring, and alcohol 5%. The chemical name of the drug is potassium chloride.

CLINICAL PHARMACOLOGY
See KAOCHLOR 10% LIQUID

INDICATIONS AND USAGE
See KAOCHLOR 10% LIQUID

CONTRAINDICATIONS
See KAOCHLOR 10% LIQUID

WARNINGS
See KAOCHLOR 10% LIQUID

PRECAUTIONS
General: The diagnosis of potassium depletion is ordinarily made by demonstrating hypokalemia in a patient with a clinical history suggesting some cause for potassium depletion.
Laboratory Tests—See KAOCHLOR 10% LIQUID
Carcinogenesis, Mutagenesis, Impairment of Fertility—See KAOCHLOR 10% LIQUID
Pregnancy—See KAOCHLOR 10% LIQUID
Nursing Mothers:—See KAOCHLOR 10% LIQUID
Pediatric Use:—See KAOCHLOR 10% LIQUID

ADVERSE REACTIONS
See KAOCHLOR 10% LIQUID

OVERDOSAGE
See KAOCHLOR 10% LIQUID

DOSAGE AND ADMINISTRATION
The usual dietary intake of potassium by the average adult is 40 to 80 mEq per day. Potassium depletion sufficient to cause hypokalemia usually requires the loss of 200 or more mEq of potassium from the total body store.
Dosage must be adjusted to the individual needs of each patient but is typically in the range of 20 mEq per day for the prevention of hypokalemia to 40-100 mEq per day or more for the treatment of potassium depletion.
To minimize gastrointestinal irritation, patients must follow directions regarding dilution. Each tablespoonful (15 ml) should be diluted with six (6) fluid ounces or more of water or other liquid.
One (1) tablespoonful (15 ml) per day (after the morning meal) supplies 40 mEq of potassium. One tablespoonful twice a day, in six (6) or more fluid ounces of water or other fluid, provides 80 mEq potassium chloride. Deviations from these recommendations may be indicated, since no average total daily dose can be defined but must be governed by close observation for clinical effects. However, potassium intoxication may result from any therapeutic dosage. See "Overdosage" and "Precautions".

HOW SUPPLIED
KAON-CL 20% supplies 40 mEq each of potassium and chloride per tablespoonful (15 ml).
NDC 0013-3113-51 Pint
Storage Conditions—Preserve in tight, light resistant containers. Store at room temperature and protect from cold.

MAGAN® ℞
[mā-găn']
(Magnesium Salicylate)

PRODUCT OVERVIEW

KEY FACTS
MAGAN tablets contain magnesium salicylate, a nonsteroidal anti-inflammatory agent with analgesic and antipyretic properties.

MAJOR USES
MAGAN is used for the relief of the signs and symptoms of rheumatoid arthritis, osteoarthritis, bursitis and other musculoskeletal disorders.

SAFETY INFORMATION
MAGAN is contraindicated in advanced renal insufficiency. It should not be used with uricosuric agents. Avoid or administer with caution to patients with liver damage, hypoprothrombinemia or vitamin K deficiency and before surgery.

PRESCRIBING INFORMATION

MAGAN® ℞
[mā-găn']
(Magnesium Salicylate)

DESCRIPTION
Each MAGAN uncoated, pink, capsule-shaped tablet for oral administration contains 545 mg of magnesium salicylate equivalent to 500 mg of salicylate. Magnesium salicylate is a non-steroidal, antiinflammatory agent with antipyretic and analgesic properties. Its molecular weight is 298.54. It has the following structural formula:

O O
‖ ‖
C—O—Mg—O—C
OH HO

Magnesium salicylate is a white, odorless, crystalline powder with a sweet taste. It is soluble in water and alcohol.

CLINICAL PHARMACOLOGY
Salicylic acid is the active moiety released into the plasma by MAGAN (magnesium salicylate). Salicylic acid is enzymatically biotransformed through two pathways to salicyluric acid and salicylphenolic glucuronide and eliminated in the urine.
Oral salicylates are absorbed rapidly, partly from the stomach but mostly from the upper intestine. Salicylic acid is rapidly distributed throughout all body tissues and most transcellular fluids, mainly by pH-dependent passive processes. It can be detected in synovial, spinal and peritoneal fluid, in saliva and in milk. It readily crosses the placental barrier. From 50% to 90% of salicylic acid is bound to plasma proteins, especially albumin.
Following the ingestion of a single dose of 524 mg of magnesium salicylate, a peak concentration of 3.6 mg/dl salicylic acid is reached in 1.5 hours with a T ½ of 2 hours. The major biotransformation paths for the elimination of salicylic acid from the plasma become saturated by low doses of salicylic acid. As a result, repeated doses of MAGAN increase the plasma concentration and markedly prolong the plasma half-time. The plasma concentration of salicylic acid is increased by conditions that reduce the glomerular filtration rate or tubular secretion such as renal disease or the presence of inhibitors that compete for the transport system such as probenecid.
Therapeutic plasma concentrations of salicylic acid for an adequate antiinflammatory effect needed for the treatment of rheumatoid arthritis range between 20–30 mg/dl. Effective analgesia is achieved at lower concentrations. Salicylates relieve pain by both a peripheral and a CNS effect. Salicylates inhibit the synthesis of prostaglandins; the importance of this mechanism in analgesia and antiinflammation has not been fully elucidated. Salicylates have a antipyretic effect in febrile patients but little in subjects with normal temperatures. This appears to be due to the inhibition of the synthesis of prostaglandins which are powerful pyrogens that affect the hypothalamus. Higher therapeutic concentrations cause reversible tinnitus and high tone hearing loss. Full therapeutic doses of salicylates increase oxygen consumption and CO_2 production. They cause an extracellular and intracellular respiratory alkalosis which is rapidly compensated. Salicylates irritate the gastric mucosa and frequently lead to blood loss in the stool; this effect is more pronounced with aspirin than magnesium salicylate. Salicylates in large doses (over 6 g/day) reduce the plasma prothrombin level. In contrast to aspirin, magnesium salicylate does not affect platelets. Salicylic acid increases the urinary excretion of urates at higher doses but may decrease excretion at lower doses.

INDICATIONS AND USAGE
MAGAN is indicated for the relief of the signs and symptoms of rheumatoid arthritis, osteoarthritis, bursitis and other musculoskeletal disorders.

CONTRAINDICATIONS
MAGAN is contraindicated in patients with advanced chronic renal insufficiency. It may counteract the effect of uricosuric agents and should not be prescribed for patients on such drugs.

WARNINGS
As with all salicylates, MAGAN should be avoided or administered with caution to patients with liver damage, pre-existing hypoprothrombinemia, vitamin K deficiency and before surgery.

PRECAUTIONS
General—Appropriate precautions should be taken in prescribing MAGAN for persons known to be sensitive to salicylates and in patients with erosive gastritis or peptic ulcer. If a reaction develops, the drug should be discontinued. MAGAN should be used with caution, if at all, concomitantly with anticoagulants. Appropriate precautions should be taken in administering MAGAN to patients with any impairment of renal function including discontinuing other drugs containing magnesium and monitoring serum magnesium levels if dosage levels of MAGAN are high.
Drug Interactions—Even small doses of MAGAN should not be given with uricosuric agents such as probenecid that decrease tubular reabsorption because it counteracts their effect. Large doses of MAGAN cause hypoprothrombinemia. Lower doses enhance the effects of anticoagulants such as coumadin and must be used with caution in patients receiving anticoagulants that affect the prothrombin time. Caution should also be exercised in patients concurrently treated with a sulfonylurea hypoglycemic agent or methotrexate because of the drug's capability of displacing them from the plasma protein binding sites, resulting in enhanced action of these agents. A similar displacement of barbiturates and diphenylhydantoin may occur; diphenylhydantoin intoxication has been precipitated by the consumption of aspirin. Salicylates inhibit the diuretic action of spironolactone.
Carcinogenesis, Mutagenesis, Impairment of Fertility—There have been no studies in animals or humans to evaluate the carcinogenesis, mutagenesis or impairment of fertility for magnesium salicylate. Aspirin causes testicular atrophy and inhibition of spermatogenesis in animals.
Pregnancy—Category C.
1. *Teratogenic effects*—Aspirin has been shown to be teratogenic in animals and to increase the incidence of still births and neonatal deaths in women. There are no adequate or well-controlled studies of MAGAN in pregnant women.

Continued on next page

Adria—Cont.

MAGAN should be used during pregnancy only if the potential benefit justifies the potential risk to the fetus.
2. *Non-Teratogenic effects*—Chronic, high dose salicylate therapy of pregnant women increases the length of gestation and the frequency of post maturity and prolongs spontaneous labor. It is recommended MAGAN be taken during the last three months of pregnancy only under the close supervision of a physician.
Nursing Mothers—Since salicylates are excreted in human milk, caution should be exercised when MAGAN is administered to a nursing woman.
Pediatric Use—Safety and effectiveness of MAGAN in children have not been established.

ADVERSE REACTIONS

Magnesium salicylate in large doses has a hypoprothrombinemic effect and should be given with caution in patients receiving anticoagulant drugs, patients with liver damage, pre-existing hypoprothrombinemia, vitamin K deficiency or before surgery.
Salicylates given in overdose produce stimulation (often manifested as tinnitus) followed by depression of the central nervous system. The dosage should be lowered at the onset of tinnitus.
Salicylates may cause gastric mucosal irritation and bleeding. However, fecal blood loss in patients taking MAGAN is significantly less than in those taking aspirin.
MAGAN should not be given to patients with severe renal damage because of the possibility of hypermagnesemia.
In moderate to high doses, salicylates lower the blood glucose in diabetics. Aspirin-induced hypoglycemia has been described in adults undergoing hemodialysis.
Unlike aspirin, magnesium salicylate is not known to affect the platelet adhesiveness involved in the clotting mechanism; and therefore, does not prolong bleeding time. MAGAN has not been associated with reactions causing asthmatic attacks in susceptible people.

OVERDOSAGE

Acute overdosage results in salicylate toxicity. Early signs and symptoms from repeated larger doses as well as a large single dose consist of headache, dizziness, tinnitus (which may be absent in children or the elderly), difficulty in hearing, dimness of vision, mental confusion, lassitude, drowsiness, sweating, thirst, hyperventilation, nausea, vomiting and occasionally diarrhea. More severe salicylate poisoning is manifested by CNS disturbances including EEG abnormalities. Hyperventilation occurs producing initial respiratory alkalosis. This is followed by severe metabolic acidosis with dehydration and loss of potassium. Restlessness, garrulity, incoherent speech, apprehension, vertigo, tremor, diplopia, maniacal delirium, hallucinations, generalized convulsions and coma may occur. Toxic symptoms may occur at serum levels greater than 20 mg/dl in patients over 60 years of age. Hyperventilation may occur at plasma salicylate levels over 35 mg/dl. Death may result from salicylate levels between 45–75 mg/dl. As with other salicylates, 10 to 30 g of the drug may be fatal. Renal or hepatic insufficiency and fever and dehydration in children enhance the acute toxicity of salicylate overdoses. Treatment of acute poisoning is a medical emergency and should be undertaken in a hospital. Serum Na, K, Cl, CO_2 levels, pH, BUN, blood glucose and urine pH and specific gravity should be obtained. Emesis should be induced or gastric lavage performed. Activated charcoal may be administered. Hyperthermia should be controlled with tepid water sponging. Dehydration should be treated and acid-base imbalance corrected. A high concentration of salicylic acid in the brain may be fatal. Correction of acidosis shifts salicylate from the brain to the plasma. A bicarbonate solution should be infused to maintain an alkaline diuresis. Care should be taken to avoid pulmonary edema. The blood pH, plasma pCO_2 and plasma glucose level should be monitored frequently. Ketosis and hypoglycemia may be corrected by glucose infusions and hypokalemia by potassium chloride added to the intravenous infusate. Avoid respiratory depressants. Shock may be combatted by plasma infusions. Hemorrhagic phenomena may necessitate whole blood transfusions or vitamin K_1. In severe intoxication, exchange transfusion, peritoneal dialysis, hemodialysis or hemoperfusion should be performed to remove plasma salicylic acid. Dialysis should be seriously considered if the patient's condition is worsening despite appropriate therapy.

DOSAGE AND ADMINISTRATION

The dosage for MAGAN in the treatment of musculoskeletal disorders such as arthritis should be adjusted according to individual patient's needs. The recommended initial regimen is two tablets three times per day. Dosage may be increased, if necessary, to achieve the desired therapeutic effect. In adjusting the dosage, the physician should monitor the dose limiting parameters such as tinnitus and/or serum salicylate over 30 mg/dl.

HOW SUPPLIED

Each MAGAN tablet contains 545 mg of magnesium salicylate equivalent to 500 mg salicylate. MAGAN is available for oral administration as uncoated, pink, capsule-shaped tablets coded Adria 412. They are supplied as follows:
NDC 0013-4121-17 in bottles of 100
NDC 0013-4121-21 in bottles of 500
Store at room temperature and protect from light.

MODANE® SOFT

[*mō'dāne soft*]
(docusate sodium)
Capsules

PRODUCT OVERVIEW

KEY FACTS

MODANE SOFT is a stool softener which has surface active properties. Each soft-gelatin capsule contains 100 mg. docusate sodium. Effect on stool may not be apparent until 1–3 days after first dose.

MAJOR USES

MODANE SOFT is indicated for the management of functional constipation associated with dry hard stools. It is particularly useful when it is desirable to lessen the strain of defecation. Recommended dosage is 1–3 capsules per day for adults, 1 capsule for children 6–12 years of age.

SAFETY INFORMATION

MODANE SOFT is contraindicated when abdominal pain, nausea, vomiting or other signs of appendicitis are present. It should not be used concomitantly with mineral oil.

PRESCRIBING INFORMATION

MODANE® SOFT

[*mō'dāne soft*]
(docusate sodium)
Capsules

DESCRIPTION

Each MODANE SOFT capsule contains docusate sodium 100 mg in a soft gelatin capsule. Docusate sodium is classified as a stool softener. Chemically, docusate sodium is sulfobutanedioic acid 1,4-bis (2-ethylhexyl) ester sodium salt. The chemical structure is:

```
           C2H5
           |
COOCH2CH(CH2)3CH3
|
CH2
|
CH—SO3Na
|
COOCH2CH(CH2)3CH3
           |
           C2H5
```

docusate sodium

The empirical formula is $C_{20}H_{37}O_7SNa$ and the molecular weight is 444.56. At 25°C the solubility of docusate sodium in water is 15 g/l.

CLINICAL PHARMACOLOGY

Hydration of the stool has been attributed to the drug's surfactant effect on the intestinal contents which was assumed to facilitate penetration of the fecal mass by water and lipids. Although this emollient effect may exist, there is evidence that mucosal permeability is increased and water absorption is inhibited in the jejunum. Similar concentrations inhibit colonic absorption and/or increase intraluminal water and electrolytes. In these respects, it is similar to bile salts and in this manner, may also be considered as a stimulant laxative. Docusate sodium is absorbed to some extent in the duodenum and proximal jejunum. It appears in the bile.

INDICATIONS AND USAGE

MODANE SOFT is indicated for the management of functional constipation associated with dry hard stools. It is especially useful when it is desirable to lessen the strain of defecation (e.g. in persons with painful rectal lesions, hernia or cardiovascular disease). The effect on the stools may not be apparent until 1–3 days after the first dose.

CONTRAINDICATIONS

Mineral oil administration or when abdominal pain, nausea, vomiting, or other signs and/or symptoms of appendicitis are present.

PRECAUTIONS

Drug Interactions—MODANE SOFT may increase the intestinal absorption of mineral oil and may increase the intestinal absorption and/or hepatic uptake of other drugs administered concurrently.
Carcinogenesis, Mutagenesis, Impairment of Fertility—There have been no long term studies of docusate to evaluate carcinogenic potential. There have been no studies to evaluate mutagenic potential or to determine whether docusate has the potential to impair fertility.
Teratogenic Effects—Pregnancy Category C. Animal reproduction studies have not been conducted with docusate. It is also not known whether MODANE SOFT can cause fetal harm when administered to a pregnant woman or can affect reproductive capacity. MODANE SOFT should be given to a pregnant woman only if clearly needed.
Nursing Mothers—It is not known whether this drug is excreted in human milk. Caution should be exercised when MODANE SOFT is administered to a nursing woman.
Pediatric Use—Because of its dosage size, MODANE SOFT is not recommended for use by children less than 6 years of age.

ADVERSE REACTIONS

Adverse reactions are uncommon. Diarrhea, cramping pains and rash have been reported.

OVERDOSAGE

Docusates have a low potential for toxicity. Single doses as large as 50 mg/kg have not produced adverse effects in children. Anorexia, vomiting and diarrhea may result from overdosage.

DOSAGE AND ADMINISTRATION

Adults and children over 12 years of age—1 to 3 capsules daily. Children 6–12 years of age—one capsule daily.

HOW SUPPLIED

Each MODANE SOFT green, soft gelatin capsule contains docusate sodium 100 mg coded 13 503.
NDC 0013-5031-13 Package of 30 Capsules
Store at controlled room temperature (59°- 86°F, 15°-30°C).
Mfd by:
R.P. SCHERER
ST. PETERSBURG, FLORIDA 33702
for:
ADRIA LABORATORIES
Division of Erbamont Inc.
COLUMBUS, OHIO 43215

MODANE®

[*mō'dāne*]
(danthron)
Tablets and Liquid

PRODUCT OVERVIEW

KEY FACTS

MODANE is classified as a stimulant laxative. A soft, semi-fluid stool is passed 6–8 hours after administration. Available in tablets, MODANE contains 75 mg. danthron and MODANE MILD contains 37.5 mg. danthron. Also available in liquid form with each teaspoon containing 37.5 mg. danthron.

MAJOR USES

MODANE is indicated for the management of constipation. MODANE may be useful in geriatric, cardiac, surgical and post partum patients. It may be useful for constipation occurring with or during concomitant use of ganglionic blocking agents, antihistamines, tranquilizers, sympathominetics, anticholinergics. Usual dosage is one MODANE tablet with evening meal, 1–2 MODANE MILD tablets with evening meal, or 1–2 teaspoons of the liquid form.

SAFETY INFORMATION

As with all laxatives, MODANE is contraindicated when abdominal pain, nausea, vomiting or other signs of appendicitis are present. Prolonged use of a laxative may result in dependency.

PRESCRIBING INFORMATION

MODANE®

[*mō'dāne*]
(danthron)
Tablets and Liquid

DESCRIPTION

MODANE® Tablets (yellow)—Each tablet contains danthron 75 mg.
MODANE® MILD Tablets—Each tablet contains danthron 37.5 mg.
MODANE® Liquid—Each 5 ml (teaspoonful) contains danthron 37.5 mg and alcohol 5%.
Danthron is classified as a stimulant laxative and is chemically 1,8-dihydroxyanthraquinone. Its chemical structure is:

HO O OH

O

danthron

The empirical formula is $C_{14}H_8O_4$ and the molecular weight is 240.21. It is practically insoluble in water.

CLINICAL PHARMACOLOGY

Stimulant cathartics act on the intestinal mucosa and have effects both on the net absorption of electrolytes and water and on motility. This group includes danthron, the docusates, castor oil, and bile acids. Despite similarity of their mechanism of action, there are differences among these drugs which are due, for the most part, to dosage and the major site of action, i.e. small intestine or colon.

Anthraquinone cathartics vary in their effects depending upon their anthraquinone content and the ease of liberation of the active constituents from their inactive precursor glycosides. Danthron, although a free anthraquinone, is similar to the pro-drug glycosides in its pharmacological properties. A soft or semifluid stool is passed 6 to 8 hours after administration of an anthraquinone glycoside cathartic such as danthron.

Danthron is absorbed from the small intestine to a limited extent, circulated through the portal system and into the general circulation and excreted in the bile, urine, saliva, colonic mucosa and milk.

INDICATIONS AND USAGE

MODANE is indicated for the management of constipation. It may be useful in the management of constipation in geriatric, cardiac, surgical and postpartum patients. MODANE may be useful in the management of constipation which may occur with or during the concomitant use of antihypertensive agents, ganglionic blocking agents, antihistamines, tranquilizers, sympathomimetics and anticholinergics. A soft or semifluid stool is passed 6 to 8 hours after administration.

Adequate bulk should be provided in the diet and, if the diet does not provide sufficient bulk, by hydrophilic bulking agents. Poor bowel habits should be corrected.

CONTRAINDICATIONS

Should not be used when abdominal pain, nausea, vomiting or other signs and/or symptoms of appendicitis are present.

PRECAUTIONS

General —MODANE may cause harmless pink discoloration of urine (the urine may be pink-red, red-violet or red-brown if alkaline).

As with all laxatives, frequent or prolonged use may result in dependence.

Drug Interactions —The absorption of danthron from the gastrointestinal tract and/or its uptake by hepatic cells may be increased by the co-administration of docusate.

Carcinogenesis, Mutagenesis, Impairment of Fertility —There have been no long term studies of MODANE to evaluate carcinogenic potential. There have been no studies to evaluate mutagenic potential or whether MODANE has the potential to impair fertility.

Teratogenic Effects —Pregnancy Category C. Animal reproduction studies have not been conducted with danthron. It is also not known whether danthron can cause fetal harm when administered to a pregnant woman or can affect reproductive capacity. MODANE should be given to a pregnant woman only if clearly needed.

Nursing Mothers —Danthron is excreted in human milk and has been reported to increase bowel activity in infants nursed by women taking it. Caution should be exercised when MODANE is administered to a nursing woman.

Pediatric Use —In general stimulant cathartics should seldom be used in children.

ADVERSE REACTIONS

Adverse reactions are uncommon. These are in order of frequency: excessive bowel activity (griping, diarrhea, nausea, vomiting), peri-anal irritation, weakness, dizziness, palpitations and sweating. Temporary brownish mucosal staining has occurred with prolonged use. There has also been reported a suspected allergic reaction with facial swelling, redness and discomfort.

OVERDOSAGE

The lowest reported lethal dose in mice and rats is 500 mg/kg. Overdosage may be expected to result in excessive bowel activity. Treatment is symptomatic when the duration of effects is prolonged.

DOSAGE AND ADMINISTRATION

MODANE Tablet (yellow)-Adults—1 tablet with evening meal.

MODANE MILD Tablets (half-strength, pink)-Adults—1 or 2 tablets with the evening meal. For adults who have previously responded with excessive bowel activity to a mild laxative or who are diet-restricted or who are bedfast and for children 6–12 years of age—1 tablet with the evening meal.

MODANE Liquid-Adults—1 to 2 teaspoonfuls with the evening meal. For adults who have previously responded with excessive bowel activity to a mild laxative or who are diet-restricted or who are bedfast and children who are 6–12 years of age—1 teaspoonful with the evening meal.

HOW SUPPLIED

Each MODANE Tablet contains danthron 75 mg in a yellow, round, sugar coated tablet, coded 13 501.
NDC 0013-5011-17 Bottle of 100 Tablets
NDC 0013-5011-23 Bottle of 1000 Tablets
NDC 0013-5011-18 STAT-PAK® (unit dose) 100 Tablets
NDC 0013-5011-07 Package of 10 Tablets
NDC 0013-5011-13 Package of 30 Tablets
Store at room temperature.
Each MODANE MILD Tablet contains danthron 37.5 mg in a pink, round, sugar coated tablet, coded 13 502.
NDC 0013-5021-17 Bottle of 100 Tablets
Store at room temperature.
Each 5 ml (teaspoonful) of MODANE Liquid contains danthron 37.5 mg in a red liquid.
NDC 0013-5033-51 Pint Bottles
Protect from cold.

MODANE® PLUS

[*mō 'dāne plŭs*]
(danthron and docusate sodium)
Tablets

PRODUCT OVERVIEW

KEY FACTS

MODANE PLUS is a combination laxative containing a stimulant cathartic and a stool softener. Danthron is the stimulant component. Docusate sodium is a stool softener. Each tablet contains 50 mg. danthron and 100 mg. docusate sodium.

MAJOR USES

MODANE PLUS is indicated for the management of constipation where a combination of a stimulant plus a stool softener is needed. It may be useful in geriatric, inactive and post surgical patients as well as in patients refractory to other laxatives. Recommended dosage is one tablet with the evening meal for adults and children over 12 years of age.

SAFETY INFORMATION

As with all laxatives, MODANE PLUS is contraindicated when abdominal pain, nausea, vomting or other signs of appendicitis are present. Also, contraindicated with mineral oil administration. Prolonged use of a laxative may result in dependency.

PRESCRIBING INFORMATION

MODANE® PLUS

[*mō 'dāne plŭs*]
(danthron and docusate sodium)
Tablets

DESCRIPTION

Each MODANE PLUS tablet contains danthron 50 mg and docusate sodium 100 mg. Danthron is classified as a stimulant cathartic and docusate sodium is a stool softener. Chemically docusate sodium is sulfobutanedioic acid 1,4-bis (2-ethylhexyl) ester sodium salt and danthron is 1,8-dihydroxyanthraquinone. The empirical formula of docusate sodium is $C_{20}H_{37}O_7SNa$ and its molecular weight is 444.56. The empirical formula of danthron is $C_{14}H_8O_4$ and its molecular weight is 240.21.

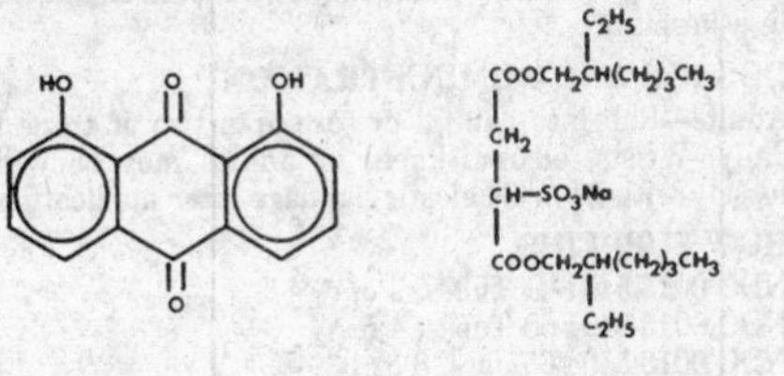

danthron docusate sodium

Danthron is practically insoluble in water. At 25°C the solubility of docusate sodium in water is 15 g/1.

CLINICAL PHARMACOLOGY

Contact cathartics act on the intestinal mucosa and have effects both on the net absorption of electrolytes and water and on motility. This group includes danthron, the docusates, castor oil, and bile acids. Despite similarity of their mechanism of action, there are differences among these drugs which are due, for the most part, to dosage and the major site of action, i.e. small intestine or colon.

Anthraquinone cathartics vary in their effects depending upon their anthraquinone content and the ease of liberation of the active constituents from their precursor glycosides. Danthron, although a free anthraquinone, is similar to the pro-drug glycosides in its pharmacological properties. A soft or semifluid stool is passed 6 to 8 hours after administration of an anthraquinone glycoside cathartic or danthron.

Hydration of the stool has been attributed to docusate sodium's surfactant effect on the intestinal contents which was assumed to facilitate penetration of the fecal mass by water and lipids. Although this emollient effect may exist, there is evidence that mucosal permeability is increased and water absorption is inhibited in the jejunum. Similar concentrations inhibit colonic absorption and/or increase intraluminal water and electrolytes. In these respects docusate sodium is similar to bile salts and in this manner may also be considered as a stimulant laxative.

Danthron is absorbed from the small intestine to a limited extent, circulated through the portal system and into the general circulation and excreted in the bile, urine, saliva, colonic mucosa and milk.

Docusate sodium is absorbed to some extent in the duodenum and proximal jejunum. It appears in the bile.

INDICATIONS AND USAGE

MODANE PLUS is indicated for the management of constipation where a combination of a stimulant plus a stool softener is needed. It may be useful in geriatric or inactive patients, following surgery, and in patients refractory to other laxatives (see MODANE, MODANE SOFT and MODANE BULK). Adequate bulk should be provided in the diet and, if the diet does not provide sufficient bulk, by hydrophilic bulking agents (MODANE BULK). Poor bowel habits should be corrected.

CONTRAINDICATIONS

Mineral oil administration, or when abdominal pain, nausea, vomiting or other signs and/or symptoms of appendicitis are present.

PRECAUTIONS

General —It may cause harmless discoloration of urine (the urine may be pink-red, red-violet or red-brown if alkaline).

As with all laxatives, frequent or prolonged use may result in dependence.

Drug Interactions —Docusate sodium may increase the intestinal absorption and/or hepatic uptake of other drugs administered concurrently.

Carcinogenesis, Mutagenesis, Impairment of Fertility —There have been no long term studies of MODANE PLUS to evaluate carcinogenic potential. There have been no studies to evaluate mutagenic potential or to determine whether MODANE PLUS has the potential to impair fertility.

Teratogenic Effects —Pregnancy Category C. Animal reproduction studies have not been conducted with danthron and docusate sodium. It is also not known whether MODANE PLUS can cause fetal harm when administered to a pregnant woman or can affect reproductive capacity. MODANE PLUS should be given to a pregnant woman only if clearly needed.

Nursing Mothers —Danthron is excreted in human milk and has been reported to increase bowel activity in infants nursed by women taking it. Caution should be exercised when MODANE PLUS is administered to a nursing woman.

Pediatric Use —Because of its dosage size, MODANE PLUS is not recommended for use by children less than 12 years.

ADVERSE REACTIONS

Adverse reactions are uncommon. These are in order of frequency: Excessive bowel activity (griping, diarrhea, nausea, vomiting), peri-anal irritation, weakness, dizziness, palpitations and sweating. Temporary brownish mucosal staining has occurred with prolonged use. There have also been reports of rash and a report of facial swelling, redness and discomfort.

OVERDOSAGE

Docusates and danthron have low potential for toxicity. The oral LD_{50} values of danthron, docusate sodium and danthron— docusate sodium combination in mice were greater than 7 g/kg, 2.64 g/kg and 3.44 g/kg, respectively. The lowest reported lethal dose of danthron in mice and rats is 500 mg/kg. Single doses of docusate sodium, as large as 50 mg/kg, have not produced adverse effects in children. Overdosage may be expected to result in anorexia, vomiting and diarrhea. Treatment is symptomatic when the duration of effects is prolonged.

DOSAGE AND ADMINISTRATION

Adults and children over 12 years of age—1 tablet daily with evening meal.

HOW SUPPLIED

Each MODANE PLUS tablet contains a combination of danthron 50 mg and docusate sodium 100 mg in a brown, round, sugar coated tablet coded 13 504.
NDC 0013-5041-13 30 Tablet Package
NDC 0013-5041-17 Bottle of 100 Tablets
Store at room temperature
AHFS 56:12

Continued on next page

Adria—Cont.

MYOFLEX® CREME
[*mī 'ō-flex*]
(Trolamine Salicylate)

PRODUCT OVERVIEW

KEY FACTS

MYOFLEX is classified as a topical analgesic. With trolamine salicylate (10%) the active ingredient, MYOFLEX is a non-irritating, non-burning, odorless, stainless cream which is readily absorbed. MYOFLEX is not a counterirritant and will not block neuronal membranes. Its formula allows loose wrapping after application. Available in tubes, jars and pump.

MAJOR USES

MYOFLEX is indicated as a topical analgesic for the temporary relief of minor aches and pains of muscles and joints due to muscle strain, sprains and bruises or overexertion. It is a useful topical adjunct in arthritis and rheumatism as a cream for patients with minor stiffness or sore hands and feet.

SAFETY INFORMATION

MYOFLEX is contraindicated in patients sensitive to its ingredients and those with advanced chronic renal insufficiency. As with any drug its use by pregnant or nursing mothers should be on the advice of a physician. Avoid or use with caution in patients with liver damage, hypoprothrombinemia, vitamin K deficiency and before surgery.

PRESCRIBING INFORMATION

MYOFLEX® CREME
[*mī 'ō-flex*]
(Trolamine Salicylate)

DESCRIPTION

Trolamine (formerly Triethanolamine) salicylate 10% in a nongreasy base is a nonirritating, nonburning, odorless, stainless, readily absorbed cream. Trolamine salicylate is a topical analgesic. The empirical formula of trolamine salicylate is $C_6H_{15}NO_3 \cdot C_7H_6O_3$, molecular weight 287.31. Its chemical structure is:

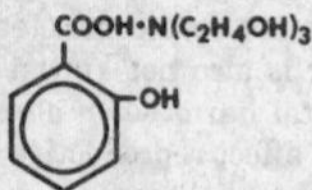

Trolamine salicylate is a light reddish viscous liquid with a faint odor. It is miscible in all proportions with water, glycerin, propylene glycol, and ethyl alcohol.

CLINICAL PHARMACOLOGY

Salicylic acid is the active moiety of MYOFLEX. Salicylic acid is enzymatically biotransformed to salicyluric acid and salicylphenolic glucuronide and eliminated in the urine. Salicylic acid is rapidly distributed throughout all body tissues, mainly by pH-dependent passive processes. It can be detected in synovial, spinal and peritoneal fluids, in saliva and in milk. It readily crosses the placental barrier. About 50% to 90% of salicylic acid is bound to plasma proteins, mainly to albumin.

The urinary excretion of salicylic acid equivalents was studied in 12 normal, healthy male subjects after MYOFLEX application. Salicylic acid was absorbed from MYOFLEX in 11 of 12 normal subjects over the 24-hour period post-application with a mean salicylic acid excretion of 13.5%.

Trolamine salicylate does not block neuronal membranes as do topical anesthetics. Some degree of percutaneous absorption occurs through the skin and blood levels have been demonstrated following topical application in animals and humans. Trolamine salicylate is not a counterirritant analgesic.

INDICATIONS

MYOFLEX is indicated as a topical analgesic for the temporary relief of minor aches and pains of muscles and joints due to muscle strains, sprains and bruises or overexertion. It is a useful topical adjunct in arthritis and rheumatism as a cream for patients with minor rheumatic stiffness or sore hands and feet.

CONTRAINDICATIONS

MYOFLEX is contraindicated in patients sensitive to its ingredients and patients with advanced chronic renal insufficiency.

WARNINGS

For external use only. Avoid contact with eyes or mucous membranes. Keep out of the reach of children.

If condition worsens, or if symptoms persist for more than 7 days, or clear up and occur again within a few days, discontinue use and consult a doctor.

As with any drug, if you are pregnant or nursing a baby, seek the advice of a health professional before using this product.

As with all salicylates, MYOFLEX should be avoided or used with caution in patients with liver damage, pre-existing hypoprothrombinemia, vitamin K deficiency and before surgery.

PRECAUTIONS

General—Apply to affected parts only. Do not apply to broken or irritated skin.

Appropriate precautions should be taken by persons known to be sensitive to salicylates or with impairment of renal function. If a reaction develops, the drug should be discontinued.

Drug Interactions—There are no known drug interactions with MYOFLEX. However, salicylates may counteract the effects of uricosuric agents such as probenecid and enhance the effects of oral anticoagulants such as coumadin. Therefore, they must be used with caution in patients on anticoagulants that affect the prothrombin time. Caution should also be exercised in patients concurrently treated with a sulfonylurea hypoglycemic agent, methotrexate, barbiturates and diphenylhydantoin, because these drugs may be displaced from plasma protein binding sites by salicylate resulting in an enhanced effect. Diphenylhydantoin intoxication has been precipitated by concomitant use of aspirin. The diuretic action of spironolactone is inhibited by salicylates.

Usage in Pregnancy (Category C)—Studies have not been performed in animals or humans to determine whether this drug affects fertility in males or females, has mutagenic, carcinogenic or teratogenic potential or other adverse effects on the fetus. Aspirin causes testicular atrophy and inhibition of spermatogenesis in animals and has been shown to be teratogenic in animals and to increase the incidence of still births and neonatal deaths in pregnant women. As with other salicylates, MYOFLEX should be used during pregnancy only if the potential benefit justifies the potential risk to the fetus.

Chronic, high dose salicylate therapy of pregnant women increases the length of gestation and the frequency of postmaturity and prolongs spontaneous labor. It is, therefore, recommended that MYOFLEX be used during the last three months of pregnancy only under the close supervision of a physician.

Nursing Mothers—Salicylates are excreted in the breast milk of nursing mothers. Caution should be therefore exercised when MYOFLEX is administered to a nursing woman.

Pediatric Use—Safety and effectiveness of MYOFLEX in children have not been established.

ADVERSE REACTIONS

If applied to large skin areas, the absorbed salicylate may cause typical salicylate side effects such as tinnitus, nausea, or vomiting.

OVERDOSAGE

Acute overdosage with MYOFLEX is unlikely. A 2 oz. MYOFLEX tube contains the salicylate equivalent of about 56 grains of aspirin. Early signs and symptoms from repeated large doses consist of headache, dizziness, tinnitus (which may be absent in children or the elderly), difficulty in hearing, dimness of vision, mental confusion, lassitude, drowsiness, sweating, thirst, hyperventilation, nausea, vomiting and occasionally diarrhea. Treatment of acute salicylate poisoning is a medical emergency and should be undertaken in a hospital.

DOSAGE AND ADMINISTRATION

Adults—Rub into painful or sore area two or three times daily. Wrists, elbows, knees or ankles may be wrapped loosely with 2″ or 3″ elastic bandage after application.

HOW SUPPLIED

NDC 0013-5404-61 Tubes, 2 oz.
NDC 0013-5404-60 Tubes, 4 oz.
NDC 0013-5404-65 Jars, 8 oz.
NDC 0013-5404-74 Jars, 1 lb.
NDC 0013-5404-62 Pump Bottle, 3 oz.

Store at controlled room temperature (15–30°C, 59–86°F) (jars).

Protect from freezing or excessive heat (tubes).

NEOSAR® FOR INJECTION ℞
[*nē 'ō-săr*]
(cyclophosphamide USP)

PRODUCT OVERVIEW

KEY FACTS

NEOSAR is a cytotoxic agent active against a variety of hematologic malignancies and solid tumors. The active ingredient, cyclophosphamide, is an alkylating agent of the nitrogen mustard class of drugs. It selectively kills malignant cells and causes tumor regression.

MAJOR USES

NEOSAR alone or with other neoplastic agents is effective against the malignant lymphomas, multiple myeloma, chronic and acute leukemias, mycosis fungoides, neuroblastoma, adenocarcinoma of the ovary, retinoblastoma and carcinoma of the breast.

SAFETY INFORMATION

NEOSAR is intended for intravenous use only. Patients must be carefully monitored and doses adjusted to avoid too severe myelosuppression. Patients should be instructed to increase fluid intake for 24 hours before, during and for 24 hours after receiving cyclophosphamide to help prevent hemorrhagic cystitis that is associated especially with high doses or prolonged use.

PRESCRIBING INFORMATION

NEOSAR® FOR INJECTION ℞
[*nē 'ō-săr*]
(cyclophosphamide USP)

DESCRIPTION

NEOSAR® FOR INJECTION (cyclophosphamide USP) is supplied as a sterile powder, containing sufficient sodium chloride to produce an isotonic solution for parenteral use when reconstituted as directed with Sterile Water for Injection USP. NEOSAR is cyclophosphamide, a member of the nitrogen mustard class of antineoplastic drugs. It is a white crystalline powder which is soluble in water, physiological saline, or alcohol. Cyclophosphamide is 2-[Bis(2-chloroethyl)-amino] tetrahydro-2H-1,3,2-oxazaphospho- rine 2-oxide monohydrate. The structural formula is:

$N(CH_2CH_2Cl)_2 \cdot H_2O$

CLINICAL PHARMACOLOGY

Cyclophosphamide is first hydroxylated by hepatic mixed function oxidases to the intermediate metabolites 4-hydroxycyclophosphamide and aldophosphamide. These are enzymatically oxidized to several inactive metabolites and to the active antineoplastic alkylating compounds nor-nitrogen mustard and phosphoramide mustard. Acrolein is also formed. The mechanism of action of the active metabolites is alkylation, principally of DNA, which interferes with growth of susceptible neoplasms and to some extent, normal tissues. Acrolein has no antineoplastic activity but is considered responsible for irritation of the bladder mucosa. The t ½ of cyclophosphamide ranges from 6 to 12 hours with a volume (Vc) of the central compartment of 0.2 to 0.6 L/kg. The t ½ is shortened by barbiturate and previous cyclophosphamide administration. It is not known whether the rate of activation and metabolism of cyclophosphamide has any clinical significance. Cyclophosphamide or its metabolites do not readily cross the blood brain barrier. Cyclophosphamide is excreted in breast milk. It, or its active metabolites cross the placenta. Cyclophosphamide and its metabolites are excreted by the kidneys.

INDICATIONS

Cyclophosphamide, though effective alone in susceptible malignancies, is more frequently used concurrently or sequentially with other antineoplastic drugs. The following malignancies are often susceptible to cyclophosphamide treatment:

1. Malignant lymphomas (Stages III and IV, Ann Arbor Staging System).
   a. Hodgkin's disease
   b. Lymphoma (nodular or diffuse)
   c. Mixed-cell type lymphoma
   d. Histiocytic lymphoma
   e. Burkitt's lymphoma.
2. Multiple myeloma.
3. Leukemias:
   a. Chronic lymphocytic leukemia.
   b. Chronic granulocytic leukemia (it is ineffective in acute blastic crises).
   c. Acute myelogenous and monocytic leukemia.
   d. Acute lymphoblastic (stem-cell) leukemia in children (cyclophosphamide given during remission is effective in prolonging its duration).
4. Mycosis fungoides (advanced disease).
5. Neuroblastoma.
6. Adenocarcinoma of the ovary.
7. Retinoblastoma.
8. Carcinoma of the breast.

CONTRAINDICATIONS

None known.

WARNINGS

Since cyclophosphamide has been reported to be more toxic in adrenalectomized dogs, adjustment of the doses of both replacement steroids and cyclophosphamide may be necessary for the adrenalectomized patient.

The rate of metabolism and the leukopenic activity of cyclophosphamide reportedly are increased by chronic administration of high doses of phenobarbital. The physician should be alert for possible combined drug actions, desirable or undesirable, involving cyclophosphamide even though cyclophosphamide has been used successfully concurrently with other drugs, including other cytotoxic drugs.

Cyclophosphamide may interfere with normal wound healing.

PRECAUTIONS

Cyclophosphamide should be given cautiously to patients with any of the following conditions:

1. Leukopenia
2. Thrombocytopenia
3. Tumor cell infiltration of bone marrow
4. Previous X-ray therapy
5. Previous therapy with other cytotoxic agents
6. Impaired hepatic function
7. Impaired renal function

Because cyclophosphamide may exert a suppressive action on immune mechanisms, interruption or modification of dosage should be considered for patients who develop bacterial, fungal or viral infections. This is especially true for patients receiving concomitant steroid therapy and perhaps those with a recent history of steroid therapy, since infections in some of these patients have been fatal. Varicella zoster infections appear to be particularly dangerous under these circumstances.

Patients should be instructed to increase their fluid intake for 24 hours before, during, and for at least 24 hours after receiving cyclophosphamide. They should also be instructed to void frequently for 24 hours after receiving cyclophosphamide.

Patients should be informed of the possibility of hair loss.

A white blood count should be obtained regularly while treating patients with cyclophosphamide.

Secondary Neoplasia: Secondary malignancies have developed in some patients treated with cyclophosphamide alone or in association with other antineoplastic drugs and/or modalities. These malignancies most frequently have been urinary bladder, myeloproliferative, and lymphoproliferative malignancies. Secondary malignancies most frequently have developed in the cyclophosphamide-treated patients with primary myeloproliferative and lymphoproliferative malignancies and primary non-malignant diseases in which immune processes are believed to be involved pathologically. In some cases, the secondary malignancy was detected up to several years after cyclophosphamide treatment was discontinued. The secondary urinary bladder malignancies generally have occurred in patients who previously developed hemorrhagic cystitis (see Genitourinary under Adverse Reactions). Although no cause-effect relationship has been established between cyclophosphamide and the development of malignancy in humans, the possibility of secondary malignancy, based on available data, should be considered in any benefit-to-risk assessment for the use of the drug.

Pregnancy Category C. Cyclophosphamide has been shown to be teratogenic and embryotoxic in mice, rats, rabbits, and monkeys when given respectively, in doses 0.02, 0.08, 0.5 and 0.07 times the human dose.

There are no adequate and well-controlled studies in pregnant women. Cyclophosphamide should not be used in pregnancy, particularly in early pregnancy, unless in the judgment of the physician the potential benefits outweigh the possible risks. Cyclophosphamide is excreted in breast milk and breast feeding should be terminated prior to institution of cyclophosphamide therapy.

Patients, male or female, capable of conception ordinarily should be advised of the mutagenic potential of cyclophosphamide. Adequate methods of contraception appear desirable for such patients receiving cyclophosphamide.

ADVERSE REACTIONS

Hematopoietic: Leukopenia is an expected effect and ordinarily is used as a guide to therapy. Thrombocytopenia or anemia may occur in a few patients. These effects are almost always reversible when therapy is interrupted.

Gastrointestinal: Anorexia, nausea, or vomiting are common and related to dose as well as individual susceptibility. There are isolated reports of hemorrhagic colitis, oral mucosal ulceration and jaundice occurring during therapy.

Genitourinary: Sterile hemorrhagic cystitis can result from the administration of cyclophosphamide. THIS CAN BE SEVERE, EVEN FATAL, and is probably due to metabolites in the urine. Nonhemorrhagic cystitis and/or fibrosis of the bladder also have been reported to result from cyclophosphamide administration. Atypical epithelial cells may be found in the urinary sediment. **Ample fluid intake and frequent voiding help to prevent the development of cystitis,** but when it occurs it is ordinarily necessary to interrupt cyclophosphamide therapy. Hematuria usually resolves spontaneously within a few days after cyclophosphamide therapy is discontinued, but may persist for several months. In severe cases replacement of blood loss may be required. The application of electrocautery to telangiectatic areas of the bladder and diversion of urine flow have been successful methods used in treatment of protracted cases. Cryosurgery has also been used. (See also Secondary Neoplasia under Precautions.) Nephrotoxicity, including hemorrhage and clot formation in the renal pelvis, have been reported.

Gonadal suppression, resulting in amenorrhea or azoospermia, has been reported in a number of patients treated with cyclophosphamide and appears to be related to dosage and duration of therapy. This side effect, possibly irreversible, should be anticipated in patients treated with cyclophosphamide. It is not known to what extent cyclophosphamide may affect prepuberal gonads. Fibrosis of the ovary following cyclophosphamide therapy has been reported also.

Integument: It is ordinarily advisable to inform patients in advance of possible alopecia, a frequent complication of cyclophosphamide therapy. Regrowth of hair can be expected although occasionally the new hair may be of a different color or texture. The skin and fingernails may become darker during therapy. Non-specific dermatitis has been reported to occur with cyclophosphamide.

Pulmonary: Interstitial pulmonary fibrosis has been reported in patients receiving high doses of cyclophosphamide over a prolonged period.

OVERDOSAGE

No reports of cyclophosphamide overdosage have been published and no reports of overdosage from NEOSAR have been received. It is expected that acute overdosage of cyclophosphamide will cause severe leukopenia and thrombocytopenia. Cardiac damage, manifested by heart failure has been reported to occur within 15 days of the initial dose of 4 to 10 day courses of cyclophosphamide at total doses per course greater than 140 mg/kg (5.2 g/m^2). Impairment of water excretion with hyponatremia, weight gain and inappropriately concentrated urine has been reported after cyclophosphamide doses greater than 50 mg/kg (2 g/m^2). Patients in whom overdosage is known or suspected should be hospitalized for supportive therapy. No specific antidote is known. Cyclophosphamide is theoretically dialyzable but no studies have been performed to confirm the efficacy of dialysis in a clinical situation.

DOSAGE AND ADMINISTRATION

Chemotherapy with NEOSAR, as with other drugs used in cancer chemotherapy, is potentially hazardous and fatal complications can occur. It is recommended that it be administered only by physicians aware of the associated risks. Therapy may be aimed at either induction or maintenance of remission.

Induction Therapy: The usual initial intravenous loading dose for patients with no hematologic deficiency is 40–50 mg/kg (1500–1800 mg/m^2). This total initial intravenous loading dose usually is given in divided doses over a period of two to five days.

Patients with any previous treatment that may have compromised the functional capacity of the bone marrow, such as X-ray or cytotoxic drugs, and patients with tumor infiltration of the bone marrow may require reduction of the initial loading dose by $\frac{1}{3}$ to $\frac{1}{2}$.

A marked leukopenia is usually associated with the above doses, but recovery usually begins after 7–10 days. The white blood cell count should be monitored closely during induction therapy.

Maintenance Therapy: It is frequently necessary to maintain chemotherapy in order to suppress or retard neoplastic growth. A variety of schedules has been used:

1. 10–15 mg/kg (350–550 mg/m^2) i.v. every 7–10 days
2. 3–5 mg/kg (110–185 mg/m^2) i.v. twice weekly

Unless the disease is unusually sensitive to NEOSAR, it is advisable to give the largest maintenance dose that can be reasonably tolerated by the patient. The total leukocyte count is a good objective guide for regulating the maintenance dose. Ordinarily a leukopenia of 3000–4000 cells/mm^3 can be maintained without undue risk of serious infection or other complications.

Preparation of Solutions: Parenteral drug products should be inspected visually for particulate matter and discoloration prior to administration, whenever solution and container permit. NEOSAR should be prepared for parenteral use by adding. Sterile Water for Injection USP or Bacteriostatic Water for Injection USP (paraben preserved only) to the vial and shaking to dissolve. Use 5 ml for the 100 mg vial, 10 ml for the 200 mg vial, 25 ml for the 500 mg vial, or 50 ml for the 1 g vial. Solutions of NEOSAR may be injected intravenously, intramuscularly, intraperitoneally or intrapleurally or they may be infused intravenously in Dextrose 5% Injection USP or Dextrose 5% and Sodium Chloride 0.9% Injection USP. The reconstituted solution should be used within 24 hours if stored at room temperature or within 6 days if stored under refrigeration (2–8°C; 36–46°F). NEOSAR does not contain an anti-microbial agent and *care must be taken to insure the sterility of prepared solutions.* Solutions reconstituted with Sterile Water for Injection, USP should be used promptly.

HANDLING AND DISPOSAL

Procedures for proper handling and disposal of anti-cancer drugs should be considered. Several guidelines on this subject have been published.[1–6] There is no general agreement that all the procedures recommended in the guidelines are necessary or appropriate.

HOW SUPPLIED

NEOSAR FOR INJECTION (cyclophosphamide USP) contains 45 mg sodium chloride per 100 mg cyclophosphamide (anhydrous) and is available as follows:

NDC 0013-5606-93 100 mg vials (yellow cap), cartons of 12
NDC 0013-5616-93 200 mg vials (blue cap), cartons of 12
NDC 0013-5626-93 500 mg vials (red cap), cartons of 12
NDC 0013-5636-73 1 g vials (gray cap), cartons of 6

Store at a temperature not exceeding 25°C (77°F) is recommended. It will withstand brief exposure to temperatures up to 30°C (86°F), but is to be protected from temperatures above 30°C (86°F).

Use reconstituted solution within 24 hours if stored at room temperature or within 6 days at 2–8°C (36–46°F).

References on selected topics and a physician's brochure are available by writing to: Medical Oncology Section, Adria Laboratories, P.O. Box 16529, Columbus, OH 43216.

1. Recommendations for the Safe Handling of Parenteral Antineoplastic Drugs. NIH Publication No. 83-2621. For sale by the Superintendent of Documents, U.S. Government Printing Office, Washington, D.C. 20402.
2. AMA Council Report. Guidelines for Handling Parenteral Antineoplastics, JAMA, March 15, 1985.
3. National Study Commission on Cytotoxic Exposure—Recommendations for Handling Cytotoxic Agents. Available from Louis P. Jeffrey, Sc. D., Director of Pharmacy Services, Rhode Island Hospital, 593 Eddy Street, Providence, Rhode Island 02902.
4. Clinical Oncological Society of Australia: Guidelines and recommendations for safe handling of antineoplastic agents. Med J Australia 1:426–428 1983.
5. Jones R. B., et al. Safe handling of chemotherapeutic agents: A report from the Mount Sinai Medical Center. CA—A Cancer Journal for Clinicians Sept./Oct. 258–263, 1983.
6. American Society of Hospital Pharmacists technical assistance bulletin on handling cytotoxic drugs in hospitals. Am J Hosp Pharm 42:131–137, 1985.

Manufactured by:
ASTA-WERKE A.G.
BIELEFELD, GERMANY
for:
ADRIA LABORATORIES
Division of Erbamont Inc.
COLUMBUS, OHIO 43215

OCTAMIDE™ ℞
[ŏk 'tuh-mīde]
(metoclopramide hydrochloride)
Tablets

PRODUCT OVERVIEW

KEY FACTS:

Metoclopramide, the active ingredient of OCTAMIDE, stimulates motility of the upper gastrointestinal tract. It seems to sensitize tissues to the action of acetylcholine.

MAJOR USES:

Diabetic gastroparesis.

SAFETY INFORMATION:

Contraindicated whenever stimulation of gastrointestinal motility might be dangerous, as in the presence of hemorrhage, mechanical obstruction or perforation, in patients with pheochromocytoma or with known hypersensitivity to metoclopramide. Extrapyramidal symptoms and depression have been reported.

PRESCRIBING INFORMATION

OCTAMIDE™ ℞
[ŏk 'tuh-mīde]
(metochlopramide hydrochloride)
Tablets

DESCRIPTION

Each tablet contains:
Metoclopramide base ....10 mg.
(as the monohydrochloride monohydrate)

Metoclopramide hydrochloride is a white crystalline, odorless substance, freely soluble in water. Chemically, it is 4-amino-5-chloro-N-[2-(diethylamino)ethyl]-2-methoxy benzamide monohydrochloride monohydrate. Molecular weight 354.3 and the structural formula is:

$CONHCH_2CH_2N(C_2H_5)_2$; OCH_3 ; Cl ; NH_2 ; $\cdot HCl \cdot H_2O$

Continued on next page

Adria—Cont.

CLINICAL PHARMACOLOGY

Metoclopramide stimulates motility of the upper gastrointestinal tract without stimulating gastric, biliary, or pancreatic secretions. Its mode of action is unclear. It seems to sensitize tissues to the action of acetylcholine. The effect of metoclopramide on motility is not dependent on intact vagal innervation, but it can be abolished by anticholinergic drugs. Metoclopramide increases the tone and amplitude of gastric (especially antral) contractions, relaxes the pyloric sphincter and the duodenal bulb, and increases peristalsis of the duodenum and jejunum resulting in accelerated gastric emptying and intestinal transit. It increases the resting tone of the lower esophageal sphincter. It has little, if any, effect on the motility of the colon or gallbladder.
Like the phenothiazines and related drugs, which are also dopamine antagonists, metoclopramide produces sedation and may produce extrapyramidal reactions, although these are comparatively rare (See Warnings). Metoclopramide inhibits the central and peripheral effects of apomorphine, induces release of prolactin and causes a transient increase in circulating aldosterone levels, which may be associated with transient fluid retention.
The onset of pharmacological action of metoclopramide is 30 to 60 minutes following an oral dose; pharmacological effects persist for 1 to 2 hours.
Approximately 85% of the radioactivity of an orally administered radioactive dose appears in the urine within 72 hours. Of the 85% eliminated in the urine, about half was present as free or conjugated metoclopramide.

INDICATIONS AND USAGE

Diabetic, gastroparesis (diabetic gastric stasis)—Metoclopramide hydrochloride is indicated for the relief of symptoms associated with acute and recurrent diabetic gastric stasis. The usual manifestations of delayed gastric emptying (e.g., nausea, vomiting, heartburn, persistent fullness after meals and anorexia) appear to respond to metoclopramide within different time intervals. Significant relief of nausea occurs early and continues to improve over a three-week period. Relief of vomiting and anorexia may precede the relief of abdominal fullness by one week or more.

CONTRAINDICATIONS

Metoclopramide should not be used whenever stimulation of gastrointestinal motility might be dangerous, e.g., in the presence of gastrointestinal hemorrhage, mechanical obstruction, or perforation.
Metoclopramide is contraindicated in patients with pheochromocytoma because the drug may cause a hypertensive crisis, probably due to release of catecholamines from the tumor. Such hypertensive crises may be controlled by phentolamine.
Metoclopramide is contraindicated in patients with known sensitivity or intolerance to the drug.
Metoclopramide should not be used in epileptics or patients receiving other drugs which are likely to cause extrapyramidal reactions, since the frequency and severity of seizures or extrapyramidal reactions may be increased.

WARNINGS

Extrapyramidal symptoms, manifested primarily as acute dystonic reactions, occur in approximately 1 in 500 patients treated with metoclopramide. These occur more frequently in children and young adults. These symptoms may include involuntary movements of limbs and facial grimacing, torticollis, oculogyric crisis, rhythmic protrusion of tongue, bulbar type of speech, trismus, or dystonic reactions resembling tetanus. Rarely, dystonic reactions may be present as stridor and dyspnea. If these symptoms should occur, inject 50 mg Diphenhydramine Hydrochloride intramuscularly, and they usually will subside. Parkinsonism as well as rare persistent dyskinesias have been reported.
Depression bearing a temporal relationship to metoclopramide hydrochloride administration has been reported. The significance of this association is not known.
Tardive Dyskinesia—Tardive Dyskinesia, a syndrome consisting of potentially irreversible, involuntary dyskinetic movements may develop in patients treated with metoclopramide. Although the prevalence of the syndrome appears to be highest among the elderly, especially elderly women, it is impossible to rely upon prevalence estimates to predict, at the inception of neuroleptic treatment, which patients are likely to develop the syndrome.
Both the risk of developing the syndrome and the likelihood that it will become irreversible are believed to increase as the duration of treatment and the total cumulative dose administered to the patient increase. However, the syndrome can develop, although much less commonly, after relatively brief treatment periods at low doses.
There is no known treatment for established cases of tardive dyskinesia although the syndrome may remit, partially or completely, if treatment is withdrawn. Metoclopramide, itself, however, may suppress (or partially suppress) the signs and symptoms of the syndrome and thereby may possibly mask the underlying disease process. The effect that symptomatic suppression has upon the long-term course of the syndrome is unknown.

PRECAUTIONS

General—Patients should be cautioned about engaging in activities requiring mental alertness for a few hours after the drug has been administered.
Drug Interactions—The effects of metoclopramide on gastrointestinal motility are antagonized by anti-cholinergic drugs and narcotic analgesics. Additive sedative effects can occur when metoclopramide is given with alcohol, sedatives, hypnotics, narcotics or tranquilizers. Absorption of drugs from the stomach may be diminished (e.g., digoxin) by metoclopramide, whereas absorption of drugs from the small bowel may be accelerated (e.g., acetaminophen, tetracycline, levodopa, ethanol).
Gastroparesis (gastric stasis) may be responsible for poor diabetic control in some patients. Exogenously administered insulin may begin to act before food has left the stomach and lead to hypoglycemia. Because the action of metoclopramide will influence the delivery of food to the intestines and thus the rate of absorption, insulin dosage or timing of dosage may require adjustment.
Carcinogenesis, Mutagenesis, Impairment of Fertility—Metoclopramide elevates prolactin levels and the elevation persists during chronic administration. Tissue culture experiments indicate that approximately one-third of human breast cancers are prolactin-dependent *in vitro*, a factor of potential importance if the prescription of metoclopramide is contemplated in a patient with previously detected breast cancer. Although disturbances such as galactorrhea, amenorrhea, gynecomastia, and impotence have been reported with prolactin-elevating drugs, the clinical significance of elevated serum prolactin levels is unknown for most patients. An increase in mammary neoplasms has been found in rodents after chronic administration of prolactin-stimulating neuroleptic drugs. Neither clinical studies nor epideminologic studies conducted to date, however, have shown an association between chronic administration of these drugs and mammary tumorigenesis; the available evidence is too limited to be conclusive at this time.
An Ames mutagenicity test performed on metoclopramide was negative.
Pregnancy—Category B—Reproduction studies performed in rats, mice, and rabbits by the i.v., i.m., s.c. and oral routes at maximum levels ranging from 12 to 250 times the human dose have demonstrated no impairment of fertility or significant harm to the fetus due to metoclopramide. There are, however, no adequate and well-controlled studies in pregnant women. Because animal reproduction studies are not always predictive of human response, this drug should be used during pregnancy only if clearly needed.
Nursing Mothers—It is not known whether this drug is excreted in human milk. Because many drugs are excreted in human milk, caution should be exercised when metoclopramide is administered to a nursing mother.

ADVERSE REACTIONS

The most frequent adverse reactions to metoclopramide are restlessness, drowsiness, fatigue and lassitude, which occur in approximately ten percent of patients. Less frequently, insomnia, headache, dizziness, nausea, transient fluid retention, bowel disturbances, rash or extrapyramidal symptoms may occur. Rarely, depression, persistent dyskinesia, stridor and dyspnea have been reported. (See Warnings and Precautions sections).

OVERDOSAGE

Symptoms of overdosage may include drowsiness, disorientation and extra-pyramidal reactions. Anticholinergic or antiparkinson drugs or antihistamines with anti-cholinergic properties may be helpful in controlling the extrapyramidal reactions. Symptoms are self-limiting and usually disappear within 24 hours.

DOSAGE AND ADMINISTRATION

For the relief of symptoms associated with diabetic gastroparesis (diabetic gastric stasis)—In patients who can tolerate oral metoclopramide, administer 10 mg (1 tablet) 30 minutes before each meal and at bedtime (4 doses daily) for 2–8 weeks, depending on response for early manifestations or for mild symptoms and the likelihood of continued well-being upon drug discontinuation. Since diabetic gastric stasis is frequently recurrent, metoclopramide therapy should be reinstituted at the earliest manifestation.

HOW SUPPLIED

Each Octamide™ tablet contains 10 mg metoclopramide base (as the monohydrochloride monohydrate). Octamide™ is available for oral administration as a yellow, scored, octagonal compressed tablet, debossed with ADRIA on one side and 230 on the other side. Octamide™ is available in bottles of 100 (NDC 0013-2301-17) and 500 (NDC 0013-2301-21).

STORAGE CONDITIONS

Store in a tight, light resistant container at controlled room temperature 15°–30°C (59°–86°F).
Manufactured by:
QUANTUM PHARMICS, LTD.
AMITYVILLE, NEW YORK 11701
For:
ADRIA LABORATORIES
Division of Erbamont Inc.
COLUMBUS, OHIO 43215
Shown in Product Identification Section, page 404

TYMPAGESIC® ℞

[*tim "pah-jē 'sik*]
Otic Solution

Analgesic-Decongestant Ear Drops

DESCRIPTION

TYMPAGESIC Otic Solution, analgesic-decongestant ear drops, contains phenylephrine hydrochloride USP 0.25%, antipyrine USP 5% and benzocaine USP 5% v/v in propylene glycol USP.
Phenylephrine hydrochloride is a sympathomimetic amine with local vasoconstriction or decongestant action. It is chemically (R)-3-hydroxy-α-[(methylamino)methyl] benzenemethanol hydrochloride and has the following structure:

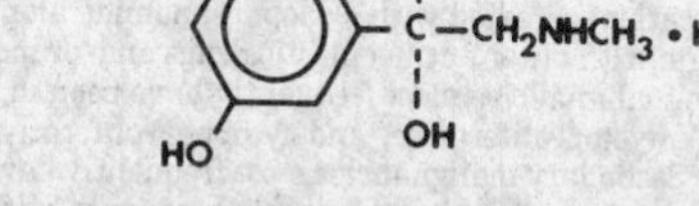

(HO-C₆H₄)–C(H)(OH)–CH_2NHCH_3 • HCl

It occurs as white crystals, has bitter taste and is freely soluble in water and alcohol. Its molecular weight is 203.67.
Antipyrine is an analgesic with local anesthetic action. It is chemically 2:3-dimethyl-1-phenyl-3-pyrazolin-5-one and has the following structure:

[structure: CH_3, CH_3, N, N, O — pyrazolone ring with N-phenyl]

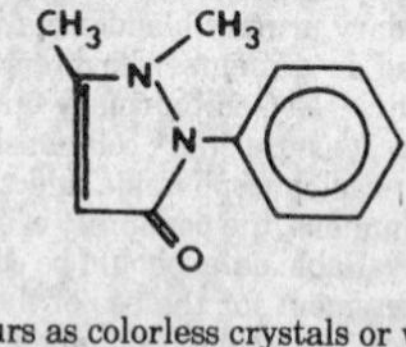

Antipyrine occurs as colorless crystals or white powder, has a slightly bitter taste and is soluble in water and alcohol. Its molecular weight is 188.23.
Benzocaine is a local anesthetic. It is chemically ethyl p-aminobenzoate and has the following structure:

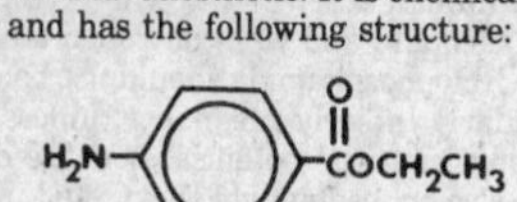

H_2N–C₆H₄–$COCH_2CH_3$ (C=O)

It occurs as white crystals or white crystalline powder and is slightly soluble in water and soluble in organic solvents. Its molecular weight is 165.19.

CLINICAL PHARMACOLOGY

Topical application of phenylephrine produces vasoconstriction mainly by a direct effect on α-adrenergic receptors. The effects of phenylephrine are similar to those of epinephrine. However, phenylephrine is considered less CNS and cardiostimulatory than epinephrine. Phenylephrine, after its absorption, is metabolized in the liver and the intestine by the enzyme monoamine oxidase (MAO). The type, route and rate of excretion of metabolites have not been defined.
Like other local anesthetics, benzocaine acts by blocking nerve conduction first in autonomic, then in sensory and finally in motor nerve fibers. Its effect appears to be due to decreased nerve cell membrane permeability to sodium ions or competition with calcium ions for membrane binding sites. A vasoconstrictor, such as phenylephrine, is added to decrease the rate of absorption and prolong the duration of action of the anesthetic. Ester-type anesthetics, which include benzocaine, after absorption are comparatively rapidly degraded by esterases mainly in the liver and excreted in the urine as metabolites and in small amounts as the unchanged drug.
Antipyrine is believed to have analgesic and local anesthetic effects on the nerve endings. After absorption, it is slowly metabolized in the liver by oxidation and conjugation with glucuronic acid and is excreted in the urine mainly in the conjugated form.

INDICATIONS AND USAGE

TYMPAGESIC Otic Solution may be used as a topical anesthetic in the external auditory canal to relieve ear pain.

It may be used concomitantly with systemic antibiotics as in the treatment of acute otitis media.

CONTRAINDICATIONS

TYMPAGESIC is contraindicated in the presence of a perforated tympanic membrane or ear discharge and in individuals with a history of hypersensitivity to any of its ingredients.

WARNINGS

As with all drugs containing a sympathomimetic or an anesthetic, systemic reactions may occur after local application. Phenylephrine may cause blanching and a feeling of coolness in the skin. Allergic and idiosyncratic reactions to local anesthetics have been observed infrequently. Such reactions are unlikely because absorption from the skin of the ear drum or the external ear canal is minimal.
Cross-sensitivity reactions between members of the *caine* group of local anesthetics have been reported.

PRECAUTIONS

General—Drugs containing a sympathomimetic should be used with caution in the elderly and in patients with hypertension, increased intraocular pressure, diabetes mellitus, ischemic heart disease, hyperthyroidism and prostatic hypertrophy.
High plasma levels of benzocaine and antipyrine may cause CNS stimulation with nausea and vomiting. Such levels, however, are unlikely to be attained following local application in the external ear.
Drug Interactions—MAO inhibitors and β-adrenergic blockers enhance the effects of sympathomimetics. Benzocaine is hydrolyzed in the body to p-aminobenzoic acid which competes with the antibacterial action of sulfonamides. However, these are unlikely to occur because of limited absorption from the external ear canal.
Carcinogenesis, Mutagenesis, Impairment of Fertility—There have been no studies in animals or humans to evaluate the carcinogenesis, mutagenesis or impairment of fertility for TYMPAGESIC.
Pregnancy—Category C. Animal reproduction studies have not been conducted with TYMPAGESIC. It is also not known whether TYMPAGESIC can cause fetal harm when administered to a pregnant woman or can effect reproduction capacity. TYMPAGESIC should be given to a pregnant woman only if clearly needed.
Nursing Mothers—It is not known whether this drug is excreted in human milk. Because many drugs are excreted in human milk, caution should be exercised when TYMPAGESIC is administered to a nursing woman.
Pediatric Use—Safety and effectiveness in children below the age of 12 has not been established.

ADVERSE REACTIONS

Following its absorption, phenylephrine may produce a pressor response or cause restlessness, anxiety, nervousness, weakness, pallor, headache and dizziness. Absorption of benzocaine and antipyrine in the plasma may cause chills, nausea, vomiting, tinnitus and agranulocytosis. Such reactions are unlikely following application of TYMPAGESIC on the external ear canal.
Benzocaine can cause a hypersensitivity reaction consisting of rash, urticaria and edema. Individuals frequently exposed to ester-type local anesthetics can develop contact dermatitis characterized by erythema and pruritus which may progress to vesiculation and oozing.

OVERDOSAGE

It is more likely to be associated with accidental or deliberate ingestion rather than cutaneous absorption. Phenylephrine present in a bottle (13 ml) of TYMPAGESIC, if absorbed, may cause hypertension, headache, vomiting and palpitations. Effects of benzocaine overdosage may include yawning, restlessness, excitement, nausea and vomiting. Antipyrine overdosage may cause giddiness, tremor, sweating and skin eruptions.
Treatment is symptomatic. If ingestion of the contents of a bottle or more of TYMPAGESIC is recent or food is present in the stomach, induction of emesis with ipecac syrup, gastric emptying and lavage and introduction of activated charcoal may be recommended.

DOSAGE AND ADMINISTRATION

Using the dropper, instill TYMPAGESIC Otic Solution in the external ear canal allowing the solution to run into the canal until filled. Insert a cotton pledget into the meatus after moistening with the otic solution. Repeat every 2 to 4 hours, if necessary, until pain is relieved.
Replace dropper in bottle without rinsing.

HOW SUPPLIED

TYMPAGESIC Otic Solution is supplied in 13 ml amber glass dropper bottles (NDC 0013-7363-39).
Store at 15–30°C (59–86°F).

VINCASAR™ ℞

[vin 'kuh-sar"]
(vincristine sulfate)
Injection, USP

PRODUCT OVERVIEW

KEY FACTS

VINCASAR is a cytotoxic agent active against a variety of hematologic malignancies and solid tumors. The active ingredient, vincristine, is a plant alkaloid whose primary mechanism of action in malignant cells is likely the arrest of cellular division during metaphase.

MAJOR USES

VINCASAR is effective against acute leukemia or, together with other antineoplastic agents, against Hodgkin's disease, lymphosarcoma, reticulum-cell sarcoma, rhabdomyosarcoma, neuroblastoma and Wilm's tumor.

SAFETY INFORMATION

VINCASAR is intended for intravenous use only. Care must be taken to avoid extravasation. Neurotoxicity is dose dependent and dose limiting.

PRESCRIBING INFORMATION

VINCASAR™ ℞

[vin 'kuh-sar"]
(vincristine sulfate)
Injection, USP

DESCRIPTION

VINCASAR™ (Vincristine Sulfate) Injection, USP is the salt of an alkaloid obtained from a common flowering herb, the periwinkle plant (*Vinca rosea* Linn.). Originally known as leurocristine, it has also been referred to as LCR and VCR. The molecular weight for Vincristine Sulfate is 923.04. The structural formula is as follows:

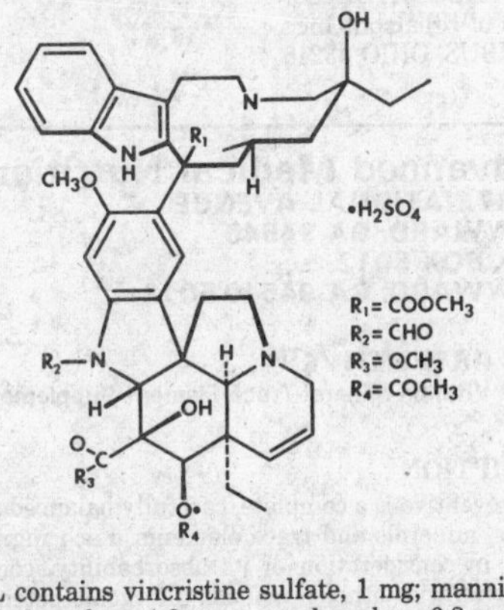

$\cdot H_2SO_4$

$R_1 = COOCH_3$
$R_2 = CHO$
$R_3 = OCH_3$
$R_4 = COCH_3$

Each mL contains vincristine sulfate, 1 mg; mannitol, 100 mg; methylparaben, 1.3 mg; propylparaben, 0.2 mg; water for injection, q.s. Acetic acid and sodium acetate have been added for pH control. The pH of VINCASAR ranges from 3.5 to 5.5.

CLINICAL PHARMACOLOGY

The mode of action of VINCASAR is unknown but is under investigation. Treatment of neoplastic cells *in vitro* with vincristine sulfate demonstrated that it may cause an arrest of mitotic division at the stage of metaphase.
Central-nervous-system leukemia has been reported in patients undergoing otherwise successful therapy with vincristine sulfate. This suggests that VINCASAR does not penetrate well into the cerebrospinal fluid.

INDICATIONS AND USAGE

VINCASAR is indicated in acute leukemia.
It has also been shown to be useful in combination with other oncolytic agents in Hodgkin's disease, lymphosarcoma, reticulum-cell sarcoma, rhabdomyosarcoma, neuroblastoma, and Wilms' tumor.

CONTRAINDICATIONS

There are no contraindications to the use of VINCASAR but careful attention should be given to those conditions listed under Warnings and Precautions.

WARNINGS

This preparation is for intravenous use only. The intrathecal administration of VINCASAR is uniformly fatal. Syringes containing this product should be labeled "VINCASAR FOR INTRAVENOUS USE ONLY."
Since reproduction studies have not been performed in animals, there is insufficient information as to whether this drug may affect fertility in men and women or have teratogenic or other adverse effects on the fetus. The physician should weigh the benefits in relation to the risks when using this and other chemotherapeutic agents in populations in which reproduction may be a factor.

PRECAUTIONS

Acute uric acid nephropathy, which may occur after the administration of oncolytic agents, has also been reported with vincristine sulfate. In the presence of leukopenia or a complicating infection, administration of the next dose of VINCASAR warrants careful consideration.
If central-nervous-system leukemia is diagnosed, additional agents may be required, since VINCASAR does not appear to cross the blood-brain barrier in adequate amounts.
Particular attention should be given to dosage and neurologic side effects if VINCASAR is administered to patients with preexisting neuromuscular disease and also when other drugs with neurotoxic potential are being used.
Acute shortness of breath and severe bronchospasm have been reported following the administration of vinca alkaloids. These reactions have been encountered most frequently when the vinca alkaloid was used in combination with mitomycin-C. The onset may be within minutes or several hours after the vinca is injected.

ADVERSE REACTIONS

In general, adverse reactions are reversible and are related to dosage. The most common adverse reaction is hair loss; the most troublesome are neuromuscular in origin.
When single weekly doses of the drug are employed, the adverse reactions of leukopenia, neuritic pain, constipation, and difficulty in walking are usually of short duration (i.e., less than 7 days). When the dosage is reduced, these reactions may lessen or disappear. They seem to be increased when the calculated amount of drug is given in divided doses. Other adverse reactions, such as hair loss, sensory loss, paresthesia, slapping gait, loss of deep-tendon reflexes, and muscle wasting, may persist for at least as long as therapy is continued. In most instances, they have disappeared by about the sixth week after discontinuance of treatment, but in some patients the neuromuscular difficulties may persist for prolonged periods.
In addition to constipation (mentioned below), paralytic ileus may occur, particularly in young children. The ileus will reverse itself upon temporary discontinuance of VINCASAR and with symptomatic care. It mimics the "surgical abdomen".
Frequently, there is a sequence in the development of neuromuscular side effects. Initially, only sensory impairment and paresthesias may be encountered. With continued treatment, neuritic pain may appear and, later, motor difficulties. No reports have yet been made of any agent that can reverse the neuromuscular manifestations accompanying therapy with VINCASAR.
Convulsions, frequently with hypertension, have been reported in a few patients receiving vincristine sulfate.
Rare occurrences of the syndrome attributed to inappropriate antidiuretic hormone secretion have been observed in patients treated with vincristine sulfate. The syndrome has been described in association with several disease states. There is high urinary sodium excretion in the presence of hyponatremia; renal or adrenal disease, hypotension, dehydration, azotemia, and clinical edema are absent. With fluid deprivation, improvement occurs in the hyponatremia and in the renal loss of sodium.
Constipation may take the form of upper-colon impaction, and, on physical examination, the rectum may be found to be empty. Colicky abdominal pain coupled with an empty rectum may mislead the physician. A flat film of the abdomen is useful in demonstrating this condition. All cases have responded to high enemas and laxatives. A routine prophylactic regimen against constipation is recommended for all patients receiving VINCASAR.
Other adverse reactions that have been reported are abdominal cramps, ataxia, foot drop, weight loss, hypertension, hypotension, rash, optic atrophy with blindness, transient cortical blindness, fever, paresthesia and numbness of the digits, oral ulceration, headache, vomiting, diarrhea, and intestinal necrosis and/or perforation. Polyuria, dysuria, and urinary retention due to bladder atony have occurred. Other drugs known to cause urinary retention particularly in the elderly should, if possible, be discontinued for the first few days following administration of VINCASAR.
Cranial nerve manifestations including isolated paresis and /or paralysis of muscles controlled by cranial motor nerves may occur in absence of motor impairment elsewhere; extraocular muscles and laryngeal muscles are most commonly involved.
Jaw pain, pharyngeal pain, parotid gland pain, bone pain, back pain, limb pain, and myalgias have been reported; pain in these areas may be severe.
VINCASAR does not appear to have any constant or significant effect on the platelets or the red blood cells.
Serious bone-marrow depression is usually not a major dose-limiting event. However, anemia, leukopenia, and thrombocytopenia have been reported. Thrombocytopenia, if present when therapy with VINCASAR is begun, may actually improve before the appearance of marrow remission.

Continued on next page

Adria—Cont.

OVERDOSAGE

Side effects following the use of VINCASAR are dose related. Therefore, following administration of an overdose, patients can be expected to experience side effects in an exaggerated fashion. Supportive care should include the following: (1) prevention of side effects resulting from the syndrome of inappropriate secretion of antidiuretic hormone (this would include restriction of fluid intake and perhaps the administration of a diuretic affecting the function of the loop of Henle and the distal tubule); (2) administration of anticonvulsant doses of phenobarbital; (3) use of enemas to prevent ileus (in some instances, decompression of the gastrointestinal tract may be necessary); (4) monitoring the cardiovascular system; and (5) determining daily blood counts for guidance in transfusion requirements.

Folinic acid has been observed to have a protective effect in normal mice which were administered lethal doses of vincristine sulfate (Cancer Res. 23:1390, 1963). Isolated case reports suggest that folinic acid may be helpful in treating humans who have received an overdose of VINCASAR. A suggested schedule is to administer 15 mg of folinic acid intravenously every 3 hours for 24 hours and then every 6 hours for at least 48 hours. Theoretical tissue levels of vincristine sulfate derived from pharmacokinetic data are predicted to remain significantly elevated for at least 72 hours. Treatment with folinic acid does not eliminate the need for the above-mentioned supportive measures.

DOSAGE AND ADMINISTRATION

This preparation is for intravenous use only (see "Warnings").

Neurotoxicity appears to be dose related. Extreme care must be used in calculating and administering the dose of VINCASAR, since overdosage may have a very serious or fatal outcome.

The concentration of vincristine sulfate is 1 mg/mL. Do not add extra fluid to the vial prior to removal of the dose, withdraw the solution of VINCASAR into an accurate dry syringe, measuring the dose of VINCASAR carefully. Do not add extra fluid to the vial in an attempt to empty it completely.

The drug is administered intravenously *at weekly intervals.* The usual dose of VINCASAR for children is 2 mg/m^2; for adults 1.4 mg/m^2. Various dosage schedules have been used (see references 1–7).

The solution may be injected either directly into a vein or into the tubing of a running intravenous infusion. Injection of VINCASAR may be completed in about 1 minute.

Caution: It is extremely important that the needle be properly positioned in the vein before any vincristine is injected. If leakage into surrounding tissue should occur during intravenous administration of VINCASAR, it may cause considerable irritation. The injection should be discontinued immediately, and any remaining portion of the dose should then be introduced into another vein. Local injection of hyaluronidase and the application of moderate heat to the area of leakage help disperse the drug and are thought to minimize discomfort and the possibility of cellulitis.

Parenteral drug products should be inspected visually for particulate matter and discoloration prior to administration whenever solution and container permits.

Handling and Disposal: Procedures for proper handling and disposal of anti-cancer drugs should be considered. Several guidelines on this subject have been published (8-13). There is no general agreement that all of the procedures recommended in the guidelines are necessary or appropriate.

HOW SUPPLIED

NDC 0013-7426-86 1 mg/1 mL, 1 mL (multiple dose), flip-top vial (mist gray cap)

NDC 0013-7436-86 2 mg/2 mL, 2 mL (multiple dose), flip-top vial (blue cap)

NDC 0013-7446-86 5 mg/5 mL, 5 mL (multiple dose), flip-top vial (red cap)

This product should be **refrigerated** between 2°–8°C (36°–46°F).

REFERENCES

1. Bagley CM Jr, DeVita VT Jr, Berard CW, Canellos GP. Advanced lymphosarcoma: Intensive cyclical combination chemotherapy with cyclophosphamide, vincristine and prednisone. Ann Intern Med 1972; 76:227.
2. DeVita VT Jr, Serpick AA, Carbone PP. Combination chemotherapy in the treatment of advanced Hodgkin's disease. Ann Intern Med 1970;73:881.
3. Lownbraun S, DeVita VT, Serpick AA. Combination chemotherapy with nitrogen mustard, vincristine, procarbazine, and prednisone in lymphosarcoma and reticulum cell sarcoma. Cancer 1970;25:1018.
4. Luce JK, Gamble JF, Wilson HE, Monto RW, Isaacs BL, Palmer FL, Coltman CA Jr, Hewlett JS, Gehan EA, Frei E III. Combined cyclophosphamide, vincristine, and prednisone therapy of malignant lymphoma. Cancer 1971;28:306.
5. Sullivan MP, Nora AH, Kulapongs P, Lane DM, Windmiller J, Thurman WG. Evaluation of vincristine sulfate and cyclophosphamide chemotherapy for metastatic neuroblastoma pediatrics. 1969;44:685.
6. Vietti TJ, Sullivan MP, Haggard ME, Holcumb TM, Berry DH. Vincristine Sulfate and radiation therapy in metastatic Wilms' tumor. Cancer 1970;25:12.
7. Wilbur JR, Sutow WW, Sullivan MP, Castro JR, Taylor HG. Successful treatment of rhabdomyosarcoma with combination chemotherapy and radiotherapy. Am Soc Clin Oncology, April 7, 1971.
8. Recommendations for the Safe Handling of Parenteral Antineoplastic Drugs. NIH Publication No. 893-2621. For sale by the Superintendent of Documents, U.S. Government Printing Office, Washington, D.C. 20402.
9. AMA Council Report. Guideline for Handling Parenteral Antineoplastics. JAMA, March 15, 1985.
10. National Study Commission on Cytotoxic Exposure—Recommendations for Handling Cytotoxic Agents. Available from Louis P. Jeffrey, Sc. D., Director of Pharmacy Services, Rhode Island Hospital, 593 Eddy Street, Providence, Rhode Island 02902.
11. Clinical Oncological Society of Australia: Guidelines and recommendations for safe handling of antineoplastic agents. Med J Australia 1983;1:426-428.
12. Jones RB, et al. Safe handling of chemotherapeutic agents: A report from the Mount Sinai Medical Center, Ca—A Cancer Journal for Clinicians, Sept/Oct, 1983:258-263.
13. American Society of Hospital Pharmacists technical assistance bulletin on handling cytotoxic drugs in hospitals. Am J Hospi Pharm 1985;42:131-137/

Manufactured by:
QUAD PHARMACEUTICALS
INDIANAPOLIS, INDIANA 46268
For:
ADRIA LABORATORIES
Division of Erbamont Inc.
COLUMBUS, OHIO 43215

Advanced Medical Nutrition, Inc.

2247 NATIONAL AVENUE
HAYWARD, CA 94545
P.O. BOX 5012
HAYWARD, CA 94540-5012

BASIC PREVENTIVE™

Multiple Vitamin-Mineral-Trace Element Supplement

DESCRIPTION

Basic Preventive is a complete, carefully balanced source of vitamins, minerals and trace elements. Each ingredient is selected in consideration of its absorbability, competitive relationship with other nutrients, allergenic potential, and long-term safety. Every batch is assayed by an independent laboratory to guarantee potency and shelf-life.

SIX TABLETS PROVIDE:			% US RDA
Vitamin A (fish liver oil)	10,000	I.U.	200
Beta-carotene	15,000	I.U.	
Vitamin D_3 (fish liver oil)	100	I.U.	25
Vitamin E (d-Alpha tocopheryl succinate)	400	I.U.	1333
Vitamin C (Ascorbic acid, corn-free)	1200	mg.	2000
Vitamin B_1 (Thiamine mononitrate)	100	mg.	6666
Vitamin B_2 (Riboflavin)	50	mg.	2940
Vitamin B_6 (Pyridoxine HCl)	100	mg.	5000
Vitamin B_{12} (on ion exchange resin)	100	mcg.	1666
Niacin	50	mg.	250
Niacinamide	150	mg.	750
Panthothenic acid (Ca-salt)	500	mg.	5000
Folic acid	800	mcg.	100
Biotin	300	mcg.	100
Choline (bitartrate)	100	mg.	
Inositol	100	mg.	
para-Amino benzoic acid	50	mg.	
Calcium (oyster shell)	500	mg.	50
Magnesium (aspartate complex)	500	mg.	125
Potassium (aspartate)	99	mg.	
Iron (fumarate)*	20	mg.	110
Iodine (kelp)	244	mcg.	160
Copper (gluconate)*	2	mg.	100
Manganese (aspartate complex)	20	mg.	
Zinc (gluconate)	20	mg.	133
Molybdenum (kelp, chelate)	100	mcg.	
Chromium (SeaSEL-1000™ kelp)	200	mcg.	
Selenium (SeaSEL-1000™ kelp)	200	mcg.	
Bioflavonoids	100	mg.	

*Optional formulas also available without iron and without copper.

Basic Preventive contains no yeast, lactose, wheat, corn, or other starch, sugar or sweeteners, artificial colors or preservatives.

INDICATIONS

Individuals with vitamin, mineral and trace element deficiencies due to sub-optimal dietary intake, age, life style, and special conditions of increased need including pregnancy, illness and medication.

ADMINISTRATION AND DOSAGE

Two tablets three times daily with meals, or as directed by a physician.

SIDE EFFECTS

None reported.

HOW SUPPLIED

Bottles of 180 capsule-shaped tablets; 12 bottles per case.

LITERATURE AND SAMPLES

On request by physician.

STORAGE

In a cool, dry place, away from direct light.
Keep out of reach of children.
NDC #54343-103-01; NDC #54343-104-01; NDC #54343-105-01

CALCIGARD™ 250

Specially acidified calcium citrate

DESCRIPTION

CALCIGARD 250 provides an exceptionally absorbable source of calcium for long-term calcium supplementation. Each tablet provides 250 mg of elemental calcium as calcium citrate. Calcium citrate is significantly better absorbed than calcium carbonate, the range of superiority being from 20–66% in healthy individuals and up to 1000% greater absorption in achlorhydric individuals. Since calcium absorption requires gastric acidification, CALCIGARD 250 is supplied in a unique acidifying base to enhance absorption and bioavailability. Calcigard formulas are also available with magnesium and with magnesium plus vitamin D.

Two CALCIGARD 250 tablets daily provide:			% US RDA
Elemental calcium	500	mg.	50* 38**
Vitamin D_3 (optional)	100	I.U.	25*
Four CALCIGARD 250 tablets daily provide:			
Elemental calcium	1000	mg.	100* 77**
Vitamin D_3 (optional)	200	I.U.	50*

*For adults and children 12 or more years of age.
**For pregnant and lactating women.

INDICATIONS

CALCIGARD 250 and CALCIGARD 250 plus vitamin D provide a daily supplemental source of calcium for use in the prevention of calcium deficiency or when it is desired or recommended by a physician to increase the dietary intake of this mineral.

ADMINISTRATION AND DOSAGE

One to two tablets twice daily with meals or as directed by a physician. For individuals who have difficulty swallowing tablets, CALCIGARD tablets may also be dissolved in a glass of water or other suitable liquid.

SIDE EFFECTS

None reported.

DRUG INTERACTIONS

Antibiotics, anticonvulsants, diuretics, digitalis, corticosteroids, and calcium channel blockers can interfere with calcium absorption.

HOW SUPPLIED

Bottles of 90 oval-shaped tablets; 12 bottles per case.

LITERATURE AND SAMPLES

On request by physician.

STORAGE

In a cool, dry place, away from direct light.
Keep out of reach of children.
NDC #54343-800-01; NDC #54343-801-01

CANDISTAT 300™
Controlled-release caprylic acid supplement

DESCRIPTION
Candistat 300's controlled-release formula provides for uniform dispersion of caprylic acid throughout the small and large intestine where *Candida albicans* proliferation is most prevalent. The inert cellulose coating on each tablet ensures that it will not break down and release caprylic acid in the stomach so that gastric irritation and after-taste following consumption are eliminated.

Each tablet provides:
Caprylic acid (non-phenolic organic complex)......... 300 mg.

INDICATIONS
As part of a dietary program to assist in the management of infections of the intestinal tract caused by *Candida albicans*.

ADMINISTRATION AND DOSAGE
One to three tablets three times daily, or as directed by a physician.

SIDE EFFECTS
None reported.

HOW SUPPLIED
Bottles of 90 tablets; 12 bottles per case.

LITERATURE AND SAMPLES
On request by physician.

STORAGE
In a cool, dry place, away from direct light.
Keep out of reach of children.

IMMUNE-AID™
100% Natural Fatty Acids

DESCRIPTION
IMMUNE-AID is a pure source of omega-3 and omega-6 polyunsaturated fatty acids. MAX-EPA®* and gamma linolenic acid (GLA) are each highly concentrated in IMMUNE-AID. Each soft gelatin capsule also provides carefully balanced amounts of the nutrients the body needs to properly metabolize these fatty acids. These nutrients include niacin, zinc, and vitamins B_6, C and E.

THREE CAPSULES CONTAIN:		% US RDA
MaxEPA™*	1500 mg.	
(containing 270 mg. EPA and 180 mg. DHA)		
Gamma linolenic acid oil	525 mg.	
(containing 63 mg. GLA)		
Vitamin E	45 I.U.	150
(d-alpha tocopherol)		
Vitamin C (ascorbic acid)	187.5 mg.	313
Niacin	15 mg.	75
Vitamin B_6	37.5 mg.	1875
(pyridoxine HCl)		
Zinc (gluconate)	3 mg.	20

Other ingredients: gelatin; natural glycerin; beeswax; water; lecithin; soybean oil; carob coloring.

Nutritional information per serving:

Serving size	3 capsules
Servings per container	30
Calories	24
Protein	less than 1 gram
Carbohydrates	less than 1 gram
Fat** (81% of calories from fat)	less than 2 grams
Polyunsaturated	less than 1 gram
Saturated	less than 1 gram
Cholesterol**	18 mg.

Contains less than 2% of the U.S. RDA of protein, vitamin A, thiamine, riboflavin, calcium, iron.

*MaxEPA is a registered trademark of Seven Seas Health Care, Ltd., Hull, England.

**Information on fat and cholesterol content is provided for individuals who, on the advice of their physician, are modifying their total dietary intake of fat and cholesterol.

INDICATIONS
A nutritional supplement providing a complete, balanced spectrum of polyunsaturated fatty acids for individuals who wish to increase their regular consumption of or who have an increased need for polyunsaturates as may occur with age or disease.

ADMINISTRATION AND DOSAGE
3 capsules daily, with meals. Individual needs, as determined by a physician, may be higher, up to 16 capsules.

SIDE EFFECTS
Softening of stool without increase in frequency. May cause nausea in some individuals if taken on an empty stomach.

HOW SUPPLIED
Bottles containing 90 soft gelatin capsules; 12 bottles per case.

LITERATURE AND SAMPLES
On request by physician.

STORAGE
In a cool, dry place, away from direct light.
Keep out of reach of children.
NDC #54343-400-01

LIPEX™
Natural Lipotropic Nutritional Supplement

DESCRIPTION
LIPEX is specially formulated to provide a unique balance of water soluble dietary fiber and specific nutrients utilized by the body in its natural function of lipid excretion.

Each table provides:

Lecithin	450 mg.
Supplying (approximately)	
Phosphatidylcholine	116 mg.
Phosphatidylethanolamine	91 mg.
Phosphatidylinositol	58 mg.
Carrageenan	390 mg.
(as a source of polysaccharides)	
Guar gum	100 mg.
Niacin	10 mg.*
Vitamin B_6 (pyridoxine HCl)	10 mg.**
Connective tissue (as a source of elastase)	50 mg.
Papain	50 mg.
Silicon dioxide	20 mg.

*Provides 50% of the U.S. Recommended Daily Allowance.
**Provides 500% of the U.S. Recommended Daily Allowance.

INDICATIONS
As a nutritional supplement for individuals wishing to increase their daily dietary intake of water soluble dietary fibers and other nutrients utilized by the body in its natural function of lipid excretion.

ADMINISTRATION AND DOSAGE
2 to 4 tablets daily. Individual needs, as determined by a physician, may be higher in the range of 5 to 20 tablets per day.

SIDE EFFECTS
Large doses may cause mild gastric upset or niacin flush. Increased lipid and bile salt excretion may be accompanied by reduced absorption of fat-soluble vitamins (A, D, and E) and some mineral elements such as calcium and magnesium.

HOW SUPPLIED
Bottles containing 100 tablets; 12 bottles per case.

LITERATURE AND SAMPLES
On request by physician.

STORAGE
In a cool, dry place, away from direct light.
Keep out of reach of children.
NDC #54343-310-01

MAXEPA®
A Natural Source of Omega-3 Polyunsaturates

DESCRIPTION
MAXEPA is a rich source of omega-3 polyunsaturated fatty acids (not less than 30%)—includes EPA (eicosapentaenoic acid, 18%) and DHA (docosahexaenoic acid, 12%) in a natural triglyceride form. As part of a total dietary plan to reduce fat consumption and increase the ratio of polyunsaturated to saturated fats, an increased intake of fish rich in omega-3 polyunsaturated fats can help lower plasma lipid levels and reduce the risk of atherosclerotic disease. MaxEPA fish oil concentrate is obtained only from the flesh of cold water marine fish and, therefore contains very low levels of vitamins A (< 100 I.U./gm) and D (< 10 I.U./gm). MaxEPA is strictly screened to eliminate toxic metals and chemicals.

Each capsule provides:

EPA (eicosapentaenoic acid)	180 mg.
DHA (docosahexaenoic acid)	120 mg.

Nutritional information per serving:

Serving size	2 capsules
Servings per container	50
Calories	21
Protein	less than 1 gram
Carbohydrates	less than 1 gram
Fat* (86% of calories from fat)	**2 grams**
Polyunsaturated	1 gram
Saturated	less than 1 gram
Cholesterol* (600 mg. per 100 gm. or 100 capsules)	12 mg.

Percentages of U. S. Recommended Daily Allowance:
Vitamin E 6%

Contains less than 2% of the US RDA of protein, vitamin A, vitamin C, thiamine, riboflavin, niacin, calcium and iron.
MaxEPA is a registered trademark of Seven Seas Health Care, Ltd., Hull, England.

*Information on fat and cholesterol content is provided for individuals who, on the advice of their physician, are modifying their total dietary intake of fat and cholesterol.

INDICATIONS
For individuals who wish to supplement their regular consumption of oily fish or who do not consume enough oily fish in their diet to receive sufficient quantities of omega-3 polyunsaturated fatty acids. MaxEPA is best taken as part of a total dietary plan to reduce total fat consumption and increase the ratio of polyunsaturated to saturated fats.

ADMINISTRATION AND DOSAGE
One to two capsules daily, or as directed by a physician.

SIDE EFFECTS
None reported.

HOW SUPPLIED
Bottles of 100 soft gelatin capsules; 12 bottles per case.

LITERATURE AND SAMPLES
On request by physician.

STORAGE
In a cool, dry place, away from direct light.
Keep out of reach of children.
NDC #54343-420-01

Alcon Laboratories, Inc.
and its affiliates
CORPORATE HEADQUARTERS:
PO BOX 6600
6201 SOUTH FREEWAY
FORT WORTH, TX 76134

OPHTHALMIC PRODUCTS

For information on Alcon ophthalmic products, consult the PDR for Ophthalmology. See a complete listing of products in the Manufacturer's Index Section of this book. For information, literature, samples or service items contact Alcon Sales Services.

BETOPTIC® ℞
(betaxolol hydrochloride)
0.5% as base
Sterile Ophthalmic Solution

DESCRIPTION
BETOPTIC® Sterile Ophthalmic Solution contains betaxolol hydrochloride, a cardioselective beta-adrenergic receptor blocking agent, in a sterile isotonic solution. Betaxolol hydrochloride is a white, crystalline powder, soluble in water, with a molecular weight of 343.89. The chemical structure is presented below:

$(CH_3)_2CHNHCH_2CHCH_2O$–[benzene ring]–$CH_2CH_2OCH_2$–[cyclopropyl] •HCl (OH on CH)

Empirical Formula:
$C_{18}H_{29}NO_3 \cdot HCl$
Chemical Name
(±)-1-[p-[2-(Cyclopropylmethoxy)ethyl]-3-(isopropylamino)-2-propanol hydrochloride.

Each ml of BETOPTIC Ophthalmic Solution (0.5%) contains: Active: 5.6 mg betaxolol hydrochloride equivalent to betaxolol base 5 mg. Preservative: Benzalkonium Chloride 0.01%. Inactive: Edetate Disodium, Sodium Chloride, Hydrochloric Acid and/or Sodium Hydroxide (to adjust pH) and Purified Water. DM-00

CLINICAL PHARMACOLOGY
Betaxolol HCl, a cardioselective (beta-1-adrenergic) receptor blocking agent, does not have significant membrane-stabilizing (local anesthetic) activity and is devoid of intrinsic sympathomimetic action. Orally administered beta-adrenergic blocking agents reduce cardiac output in healthy subjects and patients with heart disease. In patients with severe impairment of myocardial function beta-adrenergic receptor antagonists may inhibit the sympathetic stimulatory effect necessary to maintain adequate cardiac function.
When instilled in the eye, BETOPTIC Ophthalmic Solution has the action of reducing elevated as well as normal intraocular pressure, whether or not accompanied by glaucoma. Ophthalmic betaxolol has minimal effect on pulmonary and cardiovascular parameters.
Ophthalmic betaxolol (one drop in each eye) was compared to timolol and placebo in a three-way crossover study challenging nine patients with reactive airway disease who were selected on the basis of having at least a 15% reduction in the forced expiratory volume in one second (FEV_1) after admin-

Continued on next page

Alcon Labs.—Cont.

istration of ophthalmic timolol. Betaxolol HCl had no significant effect on pulmonary function as measured by FEV_1, Forced Vital Capacity (FVC) and FEV_1/VC. Additionally, the action of isoproterenol, a beta stimulant, administered at the end of the study was not inhibited by ophthalmic betaxolol. In contrast, ophthalmic timolol signficantly decreased these pulmonary functions.
[See table below].
No evidence of cardiovascular beta-adrenergic blockade during exercise was observed with betaxolol in a double masked, three-way crossover study in 24 normal subjects comparing ophthalmic betaxolol, timolol and placebo for effect on blood pressure and heart rate. Mean arterial blood pressure was not affected by any treatment; however, ophthalmic timolol produced a significant decrease in the mean heart rate.
[See table right].

Clinical Studies: Optic nerve head damage and visual field loss are the result of a sustained elevated intraocular pressure and poor ocular perfusion. BETOPTIC Ophthalmic Solution has the action of reducing elevated as well as normal intraocular pressure and the mechanism of ocular hypotensive action appears to be a reduction of aqueous production as demonstrated by tonography and aqueous fluorophotometry. The onset of action with BETOPTIC Ophthalmic Solution can generally be noted within 30 minutes and the maximal effect can usually be detected 2 hours after topical administration. A single dose provides a 12-hour reduction in intraocular pressure. Clinical observation of glaucoma patients treated with BETOPTIC Ophthalmic Solution for up to three years shows that the intraocular pressure lowering effect is well maintained.
Clinical studies show that topical BETOPTIC Ophthalmic Solution reduces mean intraocular pressure 25% from baseline. In trials using 22 mmHg as a generally accepted index of intraocular pressure control, BETOPTIC Ophthalmic Solution was effective in more than 94% of the population studied, of which 73% were treated with the beta blocker alone. In controlled, double-masked studies, the magnitude and duration of the ocular hypotensive effect of BETOPTIC Ophthalmic Solution and ophthalmic timolol solution were clinically equivalent.
BETOPTIC Ophthalmic Solution has also been used successfully in glaucoma patients who have undergone a laser trabeculoplasty and have needed additional long-term ocular hypotensive therapy.
BETOPTIC Ophthalmic Solution has been well-tolerated in glaucoma patients wearing hard or soft contact lenses and in aphakic patients.
BETOPTIC Ophthalmic Solution does not produce miosis or accommodative spasm which are frequently seen with miotic agents. The blurred vision and night blindness often associated with standard miotic therapy are not associated with BETOPTIC Ophthalmic Solution. Thus, patients with central lenticular opacities avoid the visual impairment caused by a constricted pupil.

INDICATIONS AND USAGE

BETOPTIC® Ophthalmic Solution has been shown to be effective in lowering intraocular pressure and is indicated in the treatment of ocular hypertension and chronic open-angle glaucoma. It may be used alone or in combination with other anti-glaucoma drugs.
In clinical studies BETOPTIC safely controlled the intraocular pressure of 47 patients with glaucoma and reactive airway disease followed for a mean period of 15 months. However, caution should be used in treating patients with severe reactive airway disease.

CONTRAINDICATIONS

Hypersensitivity to any component of this product.
BETOPTIC Ophthalmic Solution is contraindicated in patients with sinus bradycardia, greater than a first degree atrioventricular block, cardiogenic shock, or patients with overt cardiac failure.

Mean Heart Rates[1]

Bruce Stress Exercise Test Minutes	Betaxolol 1%[a]	Timolol 0.5%	Placebo
	TREATMENT		
0	79.2	79.3	81.2
2	130.2	126.0	130.4
4	133.4	128.0*	134.3
6	136.4	129.2*	137.9
8	139.8	131.8*	139.4
10	140.8	131.8*	141.3

[1] Atkins, J. M. *et. al.* Am. J. Oph. 99:173–175, Feb., 1985.
[a] Twice the clinical concentration
* Mean pulse rate significantly lower for timolol than betaxolol or placebo ($p < 0.05$).

WARNING

Although BETOPTIC Ophthalmic Solution has had little or no effect on heart rate or blood pressure in clinical studies, caution should be observed in treating patients with a history of cardiac failure. Treatment with BETOPTIC Ophthalmic Solution should be discontinued at the first signs of cardiac failure.

PRECAUTIONS

Patients who are receiving a beta-adrenergic blocking agent orally and BETOPTIC Ophthalmic Solution should be observed for a potential additive effect either on the intraocular pressure or on the known systemic effects of beta blockade.
While BETOPTIC Ophthalmic Solution has demonstrated a low potential for systemic effect, it should be used with caution in patients with diabetes (especially labile diabetes) because of possible masking of signs and symptoms of acute hypoglycemia. Beta-adrenergic blocking agents may mask certain signs and symptoms of hyperthyroidism and their abrupt withdrawal might precipitate a thyroid storm.
Consideration should be given to the gradual withdrawal of beta-adrenergic blocking agents prior to general anesthesia because of the reduced ability of the heart to respond to beta-adrenergically mediated sympathetic reflex stimuli.
Pulmonary: BETOPTIC Ophthalmic Solution, a cardioselective beta-blocker, has produced only minimal effects in patients with reactive airway disease; however, caution should be exercised in the treatment of patients with excessive restriction of pulmonary function.
Drug Interactions: Although BETOPTIC Ophthalmic Solution used alone has little or no effect on pupil size, mydriasis resulting from concomitant therapy with BETOPTIC Ophthalmic Solution and epinephrine has been reported occasionally. Close observation of the patient is recommended when a beta-blocker is administered to patients receiving catecholamine-depleting drugs such as reserpine, because of possible additive effects and the production of hypotension and/or bradycardia. Caution should be exercised in patients using concomitant adrenergic psychotropic drugs.
Ocular: In patients with angle-closure glaucoma, the immediate treatment objective is to re-open the angle by constriction of the pupil with a miotic agent. Betaxolol has no effect on the pupil; therefore, BETOPTIC Ophthalmic Solution should be used with a miotic to reduce elevated intraocular pressure in angle-closure glaucoma.
As with the use of other antiglaucoma drugs, diminished responsiveness to BETOPTIC Ophthalmic Solution after prolonged therapy has been reported in some patients. However in one long-term study in which 250 patients have been followed for a mean period of two years, no significant difference in mean intraocular pressure has been observed after initial stabilization.

Animal Studies:
No adverse ocular effects were observed following topical ocular administration of BETOPTIC Ophthalmic Solution to rabbits for one year.

Carcinogenesis, Mutagenesis, Impairment of Fertility:
Lifetime studies with betaxolol HCl have been completed in mice at oral doses of 6, 20 or 60 mg/kg/day and in rats at 3, 12 or 48 mg/kg/day; betaxolol HCl demonstrated no carcinogenic effect. Higher dose levels were not tested. In a variety of *in vitro* and *in vivo* bacterial and mammalian cell assays, betaxolol HCl was nonmutagenic.
Pregnancy Category C: Reproduction, teratology, and peri- and post-natal studies have been conducted with orally administered betaxolol HCl in rats and rabbits. There was evidence of drug related post-implantation loss in rabbits and rats at dose levels above 12 mg/kg and 128 mg/kg, respectively. Betaxolol HCl was not shown to be teratogenic, however, and there were no other adverse effects on reproduction at subtoxic dose levels. There are, however, no adequate and well-controlled studies in pregnant women. Because animal reproductive studies are not always predictive of human response, this drug should be used during pregnancy only if clearly indicated.
Nursing Mothers: It is not known whether BETOPTIC Ophthalmic Solution is excreted in human milk. Because many drugs are excreted in human milk, caution should be exercised when BETOPTIC Ophthalmic Solution is administered in nursing women.
Usage in Children: Clinical studies to establish the safety and efficacy in children have not been performed.

ADVERSE REACTIONS

The following adverse reactions have been reported in clinical trials with BETOPTIC Ophthalmic Solution.
Ocular: BETOPTIC Ophthalmic Solution has been well tolerated. Discomfort of short duration was experienced by one in four patients, but none discontinued therapy; occasional tearing has been reported. Rare instances of decreased corneal sensitivity, erythema, itching sensation, corneal punctate staining, keratitis, anisocoria and photophobia have been reported.
Systemic: Systemic reactions following topical administration of BETOPTIC Ophthalmic Solution have been reported rarely (e.g., insomnia and depressive neurosis).

OVERDOSAGE

No information is available on overdosage of humans. The oral LD_{50} of the drug ranged from 350–920 mg/kg in mice and 860–1050 mg/kg in rats. The symptoms which might be expected with an overdose of a systemically administered beta-1-adrenergic receptor blocker agent are bradycardia, hypotension and acute cardiac failure.
A topical overdose of BETOPTIC Ophthalmic Solution may be flushed from the eye(s) with warm tap water.

DOSAGE AND ADMINISTRATION

The usual dose is one drop of BETOPTIC Ophthalmic Solution in the affected eye(s) twice daily. In some patients, the intraocular pressure lowering response to BETOPTIC Ophthalmic Solution may require a few weeks to stabilize. Clinical follow-up should include a determination of the intraocular pressure during the first month of treatment with BETOPTIC Ophthalmic Solution. Thereafter, intraocular pressures should be determined on an individual basis at the judgment of the physician.
When a patient is transferred from a single anti-glaucoma agent, continue the agent already used and add one drop of

FEV_1 —Percent Change from Baseline[1]

	Betaxolol 1.0%[a]	Timolol 0.5%	Placebo
		Means	
Baseline	1.6	1.4	1.4
60 Minutes	2.3	−25.7*	5.8
120 Minutes	1.6	−27.4*	7.5
240 Minutes	−6.4	−26.9*	6.9
Isoproterenol[b]	36.1	−12.4*	42.8

[1] Schoene, R. B., *et. al.* Am. J. Ophthal. 97:86, 1984.
[a] Twice the clinical concentration.
[b] Inhaled at 240 minutes; measurement at 270 minutes.
* Timolol statistically different from betaxolol and placebo ($p < 0.05$).

BETOPTIC Ophthalmic Solution in the affected eye(s) twice a day. On the following day, discontinue the previous anti-glaucoma agent completely and continue with BETOPTIC Ophthalmic Solution.

Because of diurnal variations of intraocular pressure in individual patients, satisfactory response to twice a day therapy is best determined by measuring intraocular pressure at different times during the day. Intraocular pressures ≤ 22 mmHg may not be optimal for control of glaucoma in each patient; therefore, therapy should be individualized.

If the intraocular pressure of the patient is not adequately controlled on this regimen, concomitant therapy with pilocarpine, other miotics, epinephrine or systemically administered carbonic anhydrase inhibitors can be instituted.

When a patient is transferred from several concomitantly administered anti-glaucoma agents, individualization is required. Adjustment should involve one agent at a time made at intervals of not less than one week. A recommended approach is to continue the agents being used and add one drop of BETOPTIC Ophthalmic Solution in the affected eye(s) twice a day. On the following day, discontinue one of the other anti-glaucoma agents. The remaining anti-glaucoma agents may be decreased or discontinued according to the patient's response to treatment. The physician may be able to discontinue some or all of the other anti-glaucoma agents.

HOW SUPPLIED

BETOPTIC Ophthalmic Solution is a sterile, isotonic, aqueous solution of betaxolol hydrochloride. Supplied as follows: 2.5, 5 and 10 ml in plastic ophthalmic DROP-TAINER® dispensers.

2.5 ml: **NDC** 0065-0245-20
5 ml: **NDC** 0065-0245-05
10 ml: **NDC** 0065-0245-10

U.S. Patent Nos. 4,252,984; 4,311,708; 4,342,783

STORAGE

Store at room temperature.

NAPHCON-A® ℞

(naphazoline hydrochloride and pheniramine maleate)
Sterile Ophthalmic Solution

DESCRIPTION

NAPHCON-A® (naphazoline hydrochloride, pheniramine maleate) is a combination of an antihistamine and a decongestant prepared as a sterile topical ophthalmic solution. The active ingredients are represented by the chemical structures:

• HCl

Established name:
Naphazoline Hydrochloride
Chemical name:
1*H*-Imidazole, 4, 5-dihydro-2(1-naphthalenylmethyl)-monohydrochloride.

C_6H_5 — $CHCH_2CH_2N(CH_3)_2$ • HC-COOH ‖ HC-COOH

Established name:
Pheniramine Maleate
Chemical name:
N,N-Dimethyl-γ-phenyl-2-pyridine-propanamine, (Z)-Butenedioic acid.

Each ml contains: Active: Naphazoline Hydrochloride 0.025%, Pheniramine Maleate 0.3%. Preservative: Benzalkonium Chloride 0.01%. Inactive: Boric Acid, Sodium Borate, Edetate Disodium, Sodium Chloride, Sodium Hydroxide and/or Hydrochloric Acid (to adjust pH), and Purified Water.

CLINICAL PHARMACOLOGY

NAPHCON-A® combines the effects of the antihistamine, pheniramine maleate, and the decongestant, naphazoline.

INDICATIONS AND USAGE: Based on a review of a related combination of drugs by the National Academy of Sciences—National Research Council and/or other information, FDA has classified the indications as follows: "Possibly" effective: For relief of ocular irritation and/or congestion or for the treatment of allergic or inflammatory ocular conditions. Final classification of the less-than-effective indication requires further investigation.

CONTRAINDICATIONS

Hypersensitivity to one or more of the components of this preparation.

WARNINGS

Do not use in the presence of narrow angle glaucoma or in patients predisposed to narrow angle glaucoma. Patients under MAO inhibitors may experience a severe hypertensive crisis if given a sympathomimetic drug such as Naphazoline HCl. Use in infants and children may result in CNS depression leading to coma and marked reduction in body temperature.

PRECAUTIONS

For topical use only—not for injection. This preparation should be used with caution in elderly patients with severe cardiovascular disease including cardiac arrhythmias, patients with poorly controlled hypertension, patients with diabetes, especially those with a tendency toward diabetic ketoacidosis. To prevent contaminating the dropper tip and solution, care should be taken not to touch the eyelids or surrounding area with the dropper tip of the bottle.

ADVERSE REACTIONS

The following adverse reactions may occur: Pupillary dilation, increase in intraocular pressure, systemic effects due to absorption (i.e., hypertension, cardiac irregularities, hyperglycemia).

DOSAGE AND ADMINISTRATION

One or two drops instilled in each eye every 3 to 4 hours or less frequently, as required to relieve symptoms.

HOW SUPPLIED

In 15ml plastic DROP-TAINER® Dispenser.
NDC 0998-0080-15

STORAGE

Store at 36° to 80°F. Keep bottle tightly closed when not in use. Protect from light and excessive heat.

TEARS NATURALE®

Artificial Tears

TEARS NATURALE® is a sterile, soothing solution for use as an artificial tear and lubricant in relief of symptoms due to Dry Eye Syndromes. This unique solution contains DUASORB®, a water soluble polymeric system which combines with the existing tears of the eye to promote corneal wetting.

TEARS NATURALE provides extended retention time in the eye even though it is not a highly viscous solution. TEARS NATURALE also reduces the discomfort normally associated with dry eye conditions. Clinical studies have shown it to be more comfortable than other tear substitutes.

Caution: To avoid contamination, do not touch dropper tip to any surface. Keep container tightly closed. Keep out of reach of children. If irritation persists, discontinue use and consult physician. FOR TOPICAL EYE USE ONLY.

DIRECTIONS FOR USE

Instill one or two drops as frequently as required to relieve eye irritation symptoms or as directed by your doctor.

The following attributes of TEARS NATURALE have been demonstrated:

- Synergistically utilizes existing tear components to provide a hydrophilic surface on the cornea through normal precorneal tearfilm—corneal surface adsorptive processes.
- Enhances precorneal tearfilm stability and promotes corneal wetting through physiological blending with the precorneal tearfilm.
- Extends retention time without increased viscosity.
- Increases corneal wetting as judged by a greatly reduced contact angle on the clean corneal surface (18–21°) (Normal saline = 48–52°).
- Increases precorneal tearfilm stability as evidenced by tearfilm breakup time studies.
- Statistically shown in double masked studies more comfortable than any other tear substitutes reported to possess prolonged retention time as well as mucomimetic activity.*

*Mimics the action of conjunctival mucus.

CONTAINS

Active: DUASORB® (Dextran 70, Hydroxypropyl Methylcellulose), water soluble polymeric system. Preservatives: Benzalkonium Chloride 0.01%, Edetate Disodium 0.05%. U.S. Patent 4,039,662

HOW SUPPLIED

In 15 ml and 30 ml DROP-TAINER® dispensers.
15 ml: NDC 0998-0413-15
30 ml: NDC 0998-0413-30
Store at room temperature.

TOBREX® ℞

(tobramycin 0.3%)
Ophthalmic Solution and Ointment

DESCRIPTION

TOBREX® (tobramycin 0.3%) is a sterile topical ophthalmic antibiotic formulation prepared specifically for topical therapy of external infections. This product is supplied in solution and ointment forms. Each ml of solution contains: Tobramycin 0.3% (3 mg/ml), Boric Acid, Sodium Sulfate, Sodium Chloride, Tyloxapol, Sodium Hydroxide and/or Sulfuric Acid (to adjust pH), Purified Water, and Benzalkonium Chloride (0.01%) as a preservative. DM-00

Each gram of ointment contains: Tobramycin 0.3% (3 mg/g), Mineral Oil, Petrolatum base, and Chlorobutanol (0.5%) as a preservative. DM-00

Tobramycin is a water-soluble aminoglycoside antibiotic active against a wide variety of gram-negative and gram-positive ophthalmic pathogens.

The chemical structure of tobramycin is presented below.

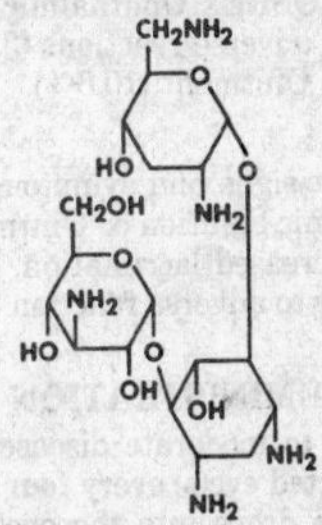

Chemical name:
0-{3-amino-3-deoxy-α-D-gluco-pyranosyl-(1→4)}-O-{2, 6-di-amino-2, 3, 6-trideoxy-α-D-ribohexo-pyranosyl-(1→6)}-2-deoxystreptamine.

CLINICAL PHARMACOLOGY

In Vitro Data: In vitro studies have demonstrated tobramycin is active against susceptible strains of the following microorganisms:

Staphylococci, including *S. aureus* and *S. epidermidis* (coagulase-positive and coagulase-negative), including penicillin-resistant strains.

Streptococci, including some of the Group A— betahemolytic species, some nonhemolytic species, and some *Streptococcus pneumoniae.*

Pseudomonas aeruginosa, Escherichia coli, Klebsiella pneumoniae, Enterobacter aerogenes, Proteus mirabilis (indole-negative) and indole-positive *Proteus* species, *Haemophilis influenzae* and *H. aegyptius, Moraxella lacunata,* and *Acinetobacter calcoaceticus (Herellea vaginacola)* and some *Neisseria* species. Bacterial susceptibility studies demonstrate that in some cases microorganisms resistant to gentamicin retain susceptibility to tobramycin. A significant bacterial population resistant to tobramycin has not yet emerged; however, bacterial resistance may develop upon prolonged use.

INDICATIONS AND USAGE

TOBREX is a topical antibiotic indicated in the treatment of external infections of the eye and its adnexa caused by susceptible bacteria. Appropriate monitoring of bacterial response to topical antibiotic therapy should accompany the use of TOBREX.

Clinical studies have shown tobramycin to be safe and effective for use in children.

CONTRAINDICATIONS

TOBREX Ophthalmic Solution and Ointment are contraindicated in patients with known hypersensitivity to any of their components.

WARNINGS

NOT FOR INJECTION INTO THE EYE. Sensitivity to topically applied aminoglycosides may occur in some patients. If a sensitivity reaction to TOBREX occurs, discontinue use.

PRECAUTIONS

As with other antibiotic preparations, prolonged use may result in overgrowth of nonsusceptible organisms including fungi. If superinfection occurs, appropriate therapy should be initiated. Ophthalmic ointments may retard corneal wound healing.

Pregnancy Category B. Reproduction studies in three types of animals at doses up to thirty-three times the normal human systemic dose have revealed no evidence of impaired fertility or harm to the fetus due to tobramycin. There are, however, no adequate and well-controlled studies in pregnant women. Because animal studies are not always predictive of human response, this drug should be used during pregnancy only if clearly needed.

Continued on next page

Alcon Labs.—Cont.

Nursing Mothers: Because of the potential for adverse reactions in nursing infants from TOBREX, a decision should be made whether to discontinue nursing the infant or discontinue the drug, taking into account the importance of the drug to the mother.

ADVERSE REACTIONS

The most frequent adverse reactions to TOBREX Ophthalmic Solution and Ointment are localized ocular toxicity and hypersensitivity, including lid itching and swelling and conjunctival erythema. These reactions occur in less than three of 100 patients treated with TOBREX. Similar reactions may occur with the topical use of other aminoglycoside antibiotics.

Other adverse reactions have not been reported from TOBREX therapy, however, if topical ocular tobramycin is administered concomitantly with systemic aminoglycoside antibiotics, care should be taken to monitor the total serum concentration.

In clinical trials, TOBREX Ophthalmic Ointment produced significantly fewer adverse reactions (3.7%) than did Garamycin Ophthalmic Ointment (10.6%).

OVERDOSAGE

Clinically apparent signs and symptoms of an overdose of TOBREX Ophthalmic Solution or Ointment (punctate keratitis, erythema, increased lacrimation, edema and lid itching) may be similar to adverse reaction effects seen in some patients.

DOSAGE AND ADMINISTRATION

Solution: In mild to moderate disease, instill one or two drops into the affected eye(s) every four hours. In severe infections, instill two drops into the eye(s) hourly until improvement, following which treatment should be reduced prior to discontinuation.

Ointment: In mild to moderate disease, apply a half-inch ribbon into the affected eye(s) two or three times per day. In severe infections, instill a half-inch ribbon into the affected eye(s) every three to four hours until improvement, following which treatment should be reduced prior to discontinuation.

TOBREX Ointment may be used in conjunction with TOBREX Solution.

HOW SUPPLIED

STERILE solution in 5 ml DROP-TAINER® dispenser (NDC 0998-0643-05), containing tobramycin 0.3% (3 mg/ml) and STERILE ointment in 3.5 g ophthalmic ointment tube (NDC 0065-0644-35) containing tobramycin 0.3% (3 mg/g).

STORAGE

Store at 46°–80°F.

Alcon (Puerto Rico) Inc.

P.O. BOX 3000
HUMACAO, PUERTO RICO 00661

AVITENE® ℞

[ăv 'itēne]
(Microfibrillar Collagen Hemostat)

DESCRIPTION

AVITENE® (Microfibrillar Collagen Hemostat, or MCH), is an absorbable topical hemostatic agent prepared as a dry, sterile, fibrous, water insoluble partial hydrochloric acid salt of purified bovine corium collagen. It is prepared in a loose fibrous form and in a compacted "non-woven" web form. In its manufacture, swelling of the native collagen fibrils is controlled by ethyl alcohol to permit non-covalent attachment of hydrochloric acid to amine groups on the collagen molecule and preservation of the essential morphology of native collagen molecules. Dry heat sterilization causes some cross-linking which is evidenced by reduction of hydrating properties, and a decrease of molecular weight which implies some degradation of collagen molecules. However, the characteristics of collagen which are essential to its effect on the blood coagulation mechanisms are preserved.

ACTIONS

AVITENE (MCH), in contact with a bleeding surface, attracts platelets which adhere to the fibrils and undergo the release phenomenon to trigger aggregation of platelets into thrombi in the interstices of the fibrous mass. The effect on platelet adhesion and aggregation is not inhibited by heparin *in vitro*. It has been found effective in heparinized dogs and in eight of nine fully heparinized human subjects. Platelets of patients with clinical thrombasthenia do not adhere to MCH *in vitro*. However, in clinical trials it was effective in 50 of 68 patients receiving aspirin. MCH cannot control bleeding due to systemic coagulation disorders. Appropriate therapy to correct the underlying coagulopathy should be instituted prior to use of the product. MCH is tenaciously adherent to surfaces wet with blood but excess material not involved in the hemostatic clot may be removed by teasing or irrigation, usually without causing rebleeding. In animal and human studies, it has been shown to stimulate a mild, chronic cellular inflammatory response. When implanted in animal tissues, it is absorbed in less than 84 days. In human studies of hemostasis in osteotomy cuts, it has been shown not to interfere with bone regeneration or healing. In animal studies, it has been demonstrated that MCH does not predispose to stenosis at vascular anastomotic sites. These findings have not been confirmed in human use. Studies have been performed using MCH (fibrous form) in experimental wounds contaminated with hemolytic *Staphylococcus aureus*. The presence of MCH does not enhance or initiate staphylococcus wound infections to a greater or lesser extent than control agents employed for the same purpose. The effects of MCH (fibrous form) on experimental wounds contaminated with a gram-negative aerobic rod and an anaerobic non-spore forming bacteria are currently under investigation.

INDICATIONS

AVITENE (MCH) is used in surgical procedures as an adjunct to hemostasis when control of bleeding by ligature or conventional procedures is ineffective or impractical.

CONTRAINDICATIONS

AVITENE (MCH) should not be used in the closure of skin incisions as it may interfere with the healing of the skin edges. This is due to simple mechanical interposition of dry collagen and not to any intrinsic interference with wound healing. By filling porosities of cancellous bone, MCH may significantly reduce the bond strength of methylmethacrylate adhesives. MCH should not, therefore, be employed on bone surfaces to which prosthetic materials are to be attached with methylmethacrylate adhesives.

WARNINGS

AVITENE (MCH) is inactivated by autoclaving. Ethylene oxide reacts with bound hydrochloric acid to form ethylene chlorohydrin. This product should not be resterilized. MCH is not for injection or intraocular use. Moistening MCH or wetting with saline or thrombin impairs its hemostatic efficacy. It should be used dry. Discard any unused portion. As with any foreign substance use in contaminated wounds may enhance infection.

PRECAUTIONS

Only that amount of AVITENE (MCH) necessary to produce hemostasis should be used. After several minutes, excess material should be removed; this is usually possible without the re-initiation of active bleeding. Failure to remove excess MCH may result in bowel adhesion or mechanical pressure sufficient to compromise the ureter. In otolaryngological surgery, precautions against aspiration should include removal of all excess dry material and thorough irrigation of the pharynx. MCH contains a low, but detectable, level of intercalated bovine serum protein which reacts immunologically as does beef serum albumin. Increases in anti-BSA titer have been observed following treatment with MCH. About two-thirds of individuals exhibit antibody titers because of ingestion of food products of bovine origin. Intradermal skin tests have occasionally shown a weak positive reaction to BSA or MCH but these have not been correlated with IgG titers to BSA. Tests have failed to demonstrate clinically significant elicitation of antibodies of the IgE class against BSA following MCH therapy. Care should be exercised to avoid spillage on nonbleeding surfaces, particularly in abdominal or thoracic viscera. It has been suggested that fragments of MCH may pass through filters of blood scavenging systems. Therefore the reintroduction of blood from operative sites treated with MCH should be avoided. Teratology studies in rats and rabbits have revealed no harm to the animal fetus. There are no well-controlled studies in pregnant women; therefore, MCH should be used in pregnant women only when clearly needed. AVITENE (MCH) should not be used in conjunction with autologous blood salvage circuits.

ADVERSE REACTIONS

The most serious adverse reactions reported which may be related to the use of AVITENE (MCH) are potentiation of infection including abscess formation, hematoma, wound dehiscence and mediastinitis. Other reported adverse reactions possibly related are adhesion formation, allergic reaction, foreign body reaction and subgaleal seroma (report of a single case). The use of MCH in dental extraction sockets has been reported to increase the incidence of alveolalgia. Transient laryngospasm due to aspiration of dry material has been reported following use of MCH in tonsillectomy.

DOSAGE AND ADMINISTRATION

AVITENE (MCH) must be applied directly to the source of bleeding. Because of its adhesiveness, it may seal over the exit site of deeper hemorrhage and conceal an underlying hematoma as in penetrating liver wounds. Surfaces to be treated should be compressed with dry sponges immediately prior to application of the dry MCH. It is then necessary to apply pressure over the MCH with a dry sponge for a period of time which varies with the force and severity of bleeding. A minute may suffice for capillary bleeding (e.g., skin graft donor sites, dermatologic curettage) but three to five or more minutes may be required for brisk bleeding (e.g., splenic tears) or high pressure leaks in major artery suture holes. For control of oozing from cancellous bone, it should be firmly packed into the spongy bone surface. After five to ten minutes, excess MCH should be teased away (see **Precautions**); this can usually be accomplished with blunt forceps and is facilitated by wetting with sterile 0.9% saline solution and irrigation. If breakthrough bleeding occurs in areas of thin application, additional MCH may be applied. The amount required depends, again, on the severity of bleeding. In capillary bleeding, one gram will usually be sufficient for a 50 cm^2 area. Thicker coverage will be required for more brisk bleeding. MCH will adhere to wet gloves, instruments, or tissue surfaces. To facilitate handling, dry smooth forceps should be used. Gloved fingers should not be used to apply pressure. In neurosurgical and other procedures the non-woven web may conveniently be used by applying small squares to bleeding areas and then covering the sites with moist cottonoid "patties". To prevent wetting of the MCH, and to apply needed pressure, a suction tip should be held against the cottonoid for one to several minutes, depending on the briskness of bleeding. After five to ten minutes excess MCH may be removed by teasing and irrigation.

HOW SUPPLIED

Fibrous Form; in 1 g and 5 g sterile jars of sterile microfibrillar collagen hemostat all contained in a sealed can. Sterility of the jar exterior cannot be guaranteed if can seal is broken. Content of jar is sterile until opened. Non-woven Web form; as 70 mm × 70 mm × 1 mm (2.75″ × 2.75″ × .04″) and 70 mm × 35 mm × 1 mm (2.75″ × 1.4″ × .04″) sheets, each contained in a sterile blister pack within a foil pouch. Sterility of the blister pack cannot be guaranteed after the pouch is opened. Content of the blister pack is sterile until adhesive backing is removed.

"AVITENE" is a registered trademark of ALCON (Puerto Rico) INC.

Allergan Pharmaceuticals, Inc.

2525 DUPONT DRIVE
IRVINE, CA 92715

OPHTHALMIC PRODUCTS

For information on Allergan prescription and OTC ophthalmic products, consult the Physicians' Desk Reference For Ophthalmology. For literature, service items or sample material, contact Allergan directly. See a complete listing of products in the Manufacturers' Index section of this book.

Alpha Therapeutic Corporation

5555 VALLEY BOULEVARD
LOS ANGELES, CA 90032

ALBUTEIN® 5% ℞

Albumin (Human), USP, 5% Solution

HOW SUPPLIED

A 5% solution in 250 ml and 500 ml bottles. For use with intravenous administration set.

ALBUTEIN® 25% ℞

Albumin (Human), USP, 25% Solution

HOW SUPPLIED

A 25% solution in 20 ml, 50 ml, and 100 ml vials. For use with intravenous administration set.

HT PROFILATE® dry method Antihemophilic Factor (Human), Factor VIII, AHF, heat-treated

HOW SUPPLIED

In single dose 10 ml and 30 ml size (AHF activity is stated on label of each vial) with sterile diluent and microaggregate filter for withdrawl.

PLASMATEIN® 5% ℞

Plasma Protein Fraction (Human), USP, 5% Solution

HOW SUPPLIED

A 5% solution in 250 ml and 500 ml bottles. For use with intravenous administration set.

PROFILATE HEAT-TREATED® wet method ℞
Antihemophilic Factor (Human), Factor VIII, AHF, heat-treated

HOW SUPPLIED
In single dose 10 ml and 25 ml size (AHF activity is stated on label of each vial) with sterile diluent and microaggregate filter for withdrawal.

PROFILNINE HEAT-TREATED® wet method ℞
Factor IX Complex

HOW SUPPLIED
In single dose 10 ml and 25 ml size (Factor IX activity is stated on label of each vial) with sterile diluent and microaggregate filter for withdrawal.

Alto Pharmaceuticals, Inc.
PO BOX 271369
TAMPA, FL 33688

EFED II™ CAPSULES (Black)
[e'fed]

DESCRIPTION
Each Efed II Black capsule contains: Theionized® caffeine 200 mg.

INDICATIONS
Efed II capsules are safe, effective, and non-habit forming. Efed II fast acting ingredient give immediate relief from fatigue, drowsiness and stuffiness. Use as a stimulant to aid in mental alertness.

WARNINGS
Keep this and all medications out of the reach of small children. Do not exceed recommended dosage. Reduce dosage if nervousness, or restlessness, or sleeplessness occurs. As with any drug, if you are pregnant or nursing a baby, seek the advice of a health professional before using this product.

CAUTION
If under medical care do not take without consulting a pharmacist or physician. Do not take as a substitute for normal sleep. May interfere with sleep if taken within four (4) hours of bedtime.

ADULT DOSAGE
One capsule every four hours, not to exceed four (4) capsules in a 24 hour period. Not recommended for children under 12 years of age.

HOW SUPPLIED
Packages of 24 capsules and bottles of 100.
Capsule imprint #425-4
Shown in Product Identification Section, page 404

EFED II™ CAPSULES (Yellow)
[e'fed]

ACTIVE INGREDIENT
Each Efed II Yellow capsule contains Theionized phenylpropanolamine HCl 37.5 mg.

INDICATIONS
Efed II fast acting ingredient give immediate relief from stuffiness. Use for the symptomatic relief of nasal and sinus congestion, allergic conditions such as hay fever and bronchial asthma. Also effective as a short acting anorexic adjunct in weight control.

CAUTION
If under medical care do not take without consulting a physician or pharmacist. Individuals with high blood pressure, heart disease, diabetes or thyroid disease should use only as directed by a physician.

WARNING
Do not exceed recommended dosage. Reduce dosage if nervousness or restlessness or sleeplessness occurs. This product should not be used by pregnant or lactating women. In case of accidental overdose, seek professional assistance or contact a poison control center immediatey.

ADULT DOSAGE
One capsule twice daily. Not recommended for children under 12 years of age.

HOW SUPPLIED
Package of 24 capsules and bottles of 100.
Capsule imprint #425-5
Shown in Product Identification Section, page 404

ZINC-220® CAPSULES
[zĭnk]
(zinc sulfate 220 mg.)

COMPOSITION
Each opaque blue and pink capsule contains zinc sulfate 220 mg. delivering 55 mg. of elemental zinc. Zinc-220 Capsules do not contain dextrose or glucose.

ACTION AND USES
Zinc-220 Capsules are indicated as a dietary supplement. Normal growth and tissue repair are directly dependent upon an adequate supply of zinc in the diet. Zinc functions as an integral part of a number of enzymes important to protein and carbohydrate metabolism. Zinc-220 Capsules are recommended for deficiencies or the prevention of deficiencies of zinc.

WARNINGS
Zinc-220 if administered in stat dosages of 2 grams (9 capsules) will cause an emetic effect. This product should not be used by pregnant or lactating women.

PRECAUTION
It is recommended that Zinc-220 Capsules be taken with meals or milk to avoid gastric distress.

DOSAGE
One capsule daily with milk or meals. One capsule daily provides approximately 5.3 times the recommended adult requirement for zinc.

HOW SUPPLIED
Bottles of 100 and 1000 capsules and Unit Dose Strips boxes of 100 capsules. (NDC 0731-0401)

Alza Corporation
950 PAGE MILL ROAD
P.O. BOX 10950
PALO ALTO, CA 94303-0802

PROGESTASERT® ℞
[prō-jes-ta-sert]
Intrauterine Progesterone Contraceptive System
Release rate 65 μg/day progesterone for one year

NOTICE
You have received Patient Information Leaflets that Federal Regulations (21 CFR 310.502) require you to furnish to each patient who is considering the use of the PROGESTASERT system.
The Patient Information Leaflet contains information on the safety and efficacy of the system. It also contains the Patient Consent. You must not insert the PROGESTASERT system until:

- You have read this physician prescription labeling and are familiar with all the information it contains.
- You and the patient have read and she has initialed each section of the Patient Information Leaflet.
- You have counseled the patient and answered her questions about contraception, the PROGESTASERT system, and the material in the Leaflet.
- You and the patient have reviewed and signed the Patient Consent.

The completely initialed and signed Leaflet, including the signed Patient Consent, should be retained in the patient's records and a second copy of the initialed and signed Leaflet given to the patient for her records.
The Leaflet is also available in Spanish should you practice require it. Address requests to: Director, Customer Services, ALZA Corporation, 950 Page Mill Road, P.O. Box 10950, Palo Alto, CA 94303-0802. Telephone (800) 227-9953.

DESCRIPTION
The PROGESTASERT system is a white, T-shaped unit constructed of ethylene/vinyl acetate copolymer (EVA) containing titanium dioxide. The 36-mm tubular vertical stem of the T contains a reservoir of 38 mg of progesterone, together with barium sulfate for radiopacity; both are dispersed in medical grade silicone fluid. The 32-mm horizontal crossarms are solid EVA. Two monofilament blue-black nylon indicator/retrieval threads are fastened to the base of the T stem.

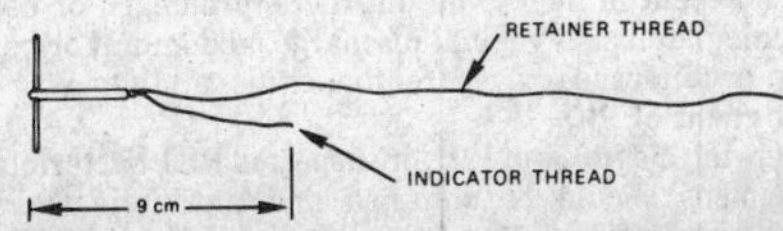

The tip of the shorter indicator thread is 9 cm from the top or leading end of the system and is used to ascertain correct placement at insertion. The long thread extends the length of the inserter, to which it is anchored by a plug that retains the system in the inserter.
The PROGESTASERT system is packaged sterile within its curved, malleable inserter. Progesterone is released from the system *in situ* at an average rate of 65 μg/day for one year by membrane-controlled diffusion from the reservoir. Inert ingredients of the reservoir or membrane—barium sulfate, silicone fluid, titanium dioxide, or EVA—are not released.

CLINICAL PHARMACOLOGY
Compared to an otherwise identical system without progesterone, contraceptive effectiveness of the PROGESTASERT system is enhanced by its continuous release of progesterone into the uterine cavity. The mechanism by which progesterone enhances the contraceptive effectiveness of the T is local, not systemic. The concentrations of luteinizing hormone, estradiol, and progesterone in systemic venous plasma follow regular cyclic patterns indicative of ovulation during use of the PROGESTASERT system. Blood chemistry studies related to liver, kidney, and thyroid function also reveal no clinically meaningful changes.
During use of the PROGESTASERT system, the endometrium shows progestational influence. Progesterone released from the system at an average rate of 65 μg/day suppresses endometrial proliferation (an anti-estrogenic effect). Following system removal, the cyclic endometrial pattern rapidly returns to normal. The local mechanism by which continuously released progesterone enhances the contraceptive effectiveness of the T has not been conclusively demonstrated. Two hypotheses have been offered: progesterone-induced inhibition of sperm capacitation or survival; and alteration of the uterine milieu so as to prevent nidation.

INDICATIONS AND USAGE
The PROGESTASERT system is indicated for intrauterine contraception and must be replaced every 12 months for continued contraceptive effect. The PROGESTASERT system is most appropriately used by multiparious women who have completed their families and are in the latter part of their reproductive years.

CONTRAINDICATIONS
The PROGESTASERT system is contraindicated when the following conditions exist:

1. Pregnancy or suspected pregnancy.
2. History of ectopic pregnancy or a condition that predisposes to ectopic pregnancy (see WARNINGS—Ectopic Pregnancy).
3. Presence of—or a history of—pelvic inflammatory disease (PID) or factors that predispose to PID (See WARNINGS—Pelvic Infection).
4. Patient or her partner has multiple sexual partners.
5. Presence of—or a history of—venereal disease (one or more episodes), including but not limited to gonorrhea or chlamydial infections of the genital tract.
6. Postpartum endometritis or infected abortion.
7. Incomplete involution of the uterus following abortion or childbirth.
8. A previously inserted IUD is still in place.
9. History of pelvic surgery that may be associated with an increased risk of ectopic pregnancy, such as surgery of the fallopian tubes or surgery for pelvic adhesions or endometriosis.
10. Abnormalities of the uterus resulting in distortion of the uterine cavity.
11. Known or suspected uterine or cervical malignancy including an unresolved, abnormal "Pap" smear.
12. Genital bleeding of unknown etiology.
13. Acute cervicitis unless and until infection has been completely controlled and has been shown to be non-gonococcal and non-chlamydial.
14. Genital actinomycosis.
15. Conditions or treatments associated with increased susceptibility to infections with microorganisms that might be introduced into the uterus during IUD insertion; such conditions or treatments include leukemia, certain types of valvular heart disease, acquired immune deficiency syndrome (AIDS), and chronic corticosteroid therapy.

WARNINGS
1. Ectopic Pregnancy
The PROGESTASERT system is contraindicated in patients who, in the physician's judgement, are at special risk of having an ectopic pregnancy. Ectopic pregnancy is potentially fatal and appears to occur more frequently with PROGESTASERT system use than with other IUDs and other contraceptives. Therefore, the possibility of ectopic pregnancy must always be considered in PROGESTASERT system users—including those lacking the specific risk factors described below.
The material that follows is intended to aid the physician in the following:

Continued on next page

Alza—Cont.

- Understanding the risks of ectopic pregnancy in PROGESTASERT system users (Section 1a).
- Proper selection of women for PROGESTASERT system use by identifying and excluding those at special risk to ectopic pregnancy (Section 1b).
- Diagnosing and managing ectopic pregnancy in IUD users (Sections 1c and 1d).
- Informing patients of ectopic pregnancy risks (Section 1e).

a. Risks of ectopic pregnancy with PROGESTASERT system use

Should a woman become pregnant while using the PROGESTASERT system, the pregnancy is more likely to be ectopic than pregnancy in a woman using no contraception, ovulation-suppressing oral contraception, or barrier methods. This is because the PROGESTASERT system acts in the uterus to prevent uterine pregnancy, but it does not prevent either ovulation or ectopic pregnancy. Thus, each month that a PROGESTASERT system is used, there is protection against uterine pregnancy but not against ectopic pregnancy. In clinical trials of the PROGESTASERT system 1 of 3.6 pregnancies in parous women and 1 of 6.2 pregnancies in nulliparous women were ectopic.

The per-year risk of ectopic pregnancy in PROGESTASERT system users is approximately 5 per 1,000 or 1 ectopic pregnancy in 200 users per year. This risk is approximately the same as in noncontracepting, sexually active women. In contrast, barrier contraceptives, which prevent fertilization, or oral contraceptives that prevent ovulation, reduce the risk of ectopic pregnancy to a few percent of the risk in noncontracepting, sexually active women.

Two clinical studies conducted by the World Health Organization compared the risk of ectopic pregnancies among 2,239 women wearing a progesterone-releasing IUD similar to the PROGESTASERT system with the risk in 3,303 women wearing a copper-releasing IUD. For the first year the risk of ectopic pregnancy was approximately 6 times higher among women using progesterone systems than among women using copper systems. Over the two years that the studies ran, the risk of an ectopic pregnancy with the progesterone-releasing IUD was about 10 times higher than that with copper-releasing IUDs.

b. Women at special risk to ectopic pregnancy

Several factors have been identified as placing a woman at special risk to ectopic pregnancy. The presence of any of these factors contraindicates use of the PROGESTASERT system. Factors indicating high risk to ectopic pregnancy include a history of ectopic pregnancy or a history or presence of a condition predisposing to ectopic pregnancy such as PID. A prospective clinical study was conducted over 9.5 years in 415 women who had had verified PID and 100 healthy control subjects. The ratio between ectopic and intrauterine pregnancies after PID was 1/24. In contrast, the ratio in the controls was 1/147. Further analysis of these data suggests that women who have had PID subsequently have an 8- to 10-fold greater risk of ectopic pregnancy than sexually active noncontracepting women who have never had PID.

Factors other than PID may also indicate a high risk to ectopic pregnancy. These factors include multiple sexual partners or a partner with multiple sexual partners, pelvic surgery of certain types, retrograde menstruation, endometritis, and endometriosis.

c. Diagnosis of ectopic pregnancy

The absence of risk factors for ectopic pregnancy described above does not rule out ectopic pregnancy. In every instance of pregnancy occurring in a PROGESTASERT system user it is essential that proper measures be taken to determine if the pregnancy is ectopic.

To determine whether ectopic pregnancy has occurred, special attention should be directed to patients with any of the following symptoms or conditions: unusual, abnormal, or irregular vaginal bleeding; delayed or missed menses; pelvic pain, usually unilateral, which may be associated with fainting or the urge to defecate; unexplained pain in the shoulder; or pain associated with bleeding if not part of the usual menstrual cycle. Ectopic pregnancy should be strongly suspected in patients with a positive pregnancy test or elevated β-HCG values but who lack ultrasonographic or other evidence of intrauterine pregnancy.

d. Management of diagnosed or suspected ectopic pregnancy

When ectopic pregnancy is suspected, diagnostic uncertainty should be resolved as quickly as possible, in view of the life-threatening risk of ruptured ectopic pregnancy. When ectopic pregnancy is diagnosed, immediate surgery is often required because a ruptured ectopic pregnancy may occur at any time.

e. Ectopic pregnancy warning to PROGESTASERT system users

All women who choose the PROGESTASERT system must be informed before insertion that a pregnancy occurring in a PROGESTASERT system user is more likely to be ectopic than one occurring in users of ovulation-preventing oral contraceptives or barrier modes, or other IUDs. They should be taught to recognize and report to their physician promptly any symptoms of ectopic pregnancy. Women should also be informed that ectopic pregnancy has been associated with complications leading to loss of fertility.

2. Intrauterine Pregnancy

Intrauterine pregnancy can occur during use of the PROGESTASERT system (see CLINICAL STUDIES section for pregnancy rates). It has been reported that IUDs may be less effective in insulin-dependent diabetics than in nondiabetic women.

a. Long-term effects and congenital anomalies

When pregnancy occurs or proceeds with the PROGESTASERT system in place, long-term effects on the offspring are unknown. Congenital anomalies have occurred under such conditions. Their relationship to the PROGESTASERT system has not been established. Systemically administered sex steroids, including progestational agents, have been associated with an increased risk of congenital anomalies. It is not known whether an increased risk of such anomalies exists when pregnancy continues with a PROGESTASERT system in place. The decision to continue or terminate pregnancy should take into account this unknown risk.

b. Septic abortion

Reports have indicated an increased incidence of septic abortion—associated in some instances with septicemia, septic shock, and death—in patients becoming pregnant with an IUD in place. Most of these reports have been associated with the mid-trimester of pregnancy. In some cases, the initial symptoms have been insidious and not easily recognized. If pregnancy should occur with a PROGESTASERT system *in situ*, the system should be removed if the thread is visible. Removal of the PROGESTASERT system may precipitate abortion. If removal proves to be or would be difficult, termination of the pregnancy should be considered and offered to the patient as an option, bearing in mind that the risks associated with an elective abortion increase with gestational age.

c. Continuation of pregnancy

If the patient chooses to continue the pregnancy with the system in place, she must be warned that this increases the risk of spontaneous abortion and sepsis, which may cause death. The patient must be closely observed, and she must be advised to report immediately all symptoms such as flu-like syndrome, fever, chills, abdominal cramping and pain, bleeding, or unusual vaginal discharge, because generalized symptoms of septicemia may be insidious.

3. Pelvic Infection (Pelvic Inflammatory Disease, PID)

The PROGESTASERT system is contraindicated in the presence of PID or suspected PID or in women with a history of PID. Use of IUDs has been associated with an increased incidence of PID. Therefore a decision to use the PROGESTASERT system must include consideration of the risks of PID. In clinical trials of the PROGESTASERT system, the risk of confirmed PID was 1.1 per 100 women per year. PID can necessitate hysterectomy; can lead to tubo-ovarian abscesses, tubal occlusion and infertility, and tubal damage that predisposes to ectopic pregnancy; can result in peritonitis; and can cause death in infrequent cases.

The effect of PID on fertility is especially important for women who may wish to have children at a later date. The study of 415 women with confirmed PID (see Ectopic Pregnancy) showed that 12% of women who had PID once developed permanently bilaterally occluded fallopian tubes and infertility. After a second occurrence of PID, 37% of women developed permanently bilaterally occluded tubes. After a third occurrence of PID the percentage of women with bilaterally occluded tubes rose to 75%.

a. Women at special risk to PID

PID is usually a sexually transmitted disease. The risk of PID appears to be greater for women who have multiple sexual partners and for women whose sexual partners have multiple sexual partners. Women who have ever had PID are at high risk for a recurrence or re-infection.

b. PID warning to PROGESTASERT system users

All women who choose the PROGESTASERT system must be informed prior to insertion that IUD use has been associated with an increased incidence of PID and that PID can necessitate hysterectomy, can cause tubal damage leading to ectopic pregnancy or infertility, or in infrequent cases can cause death. Patients must be taught to recognize and report to their physician promptly any symptoms of pelvic inflammatory disease. These symptoms include development of menstrual disorders (prolonged or heavy bleeding), unusual vaginal discharge, abdominal or pelvic pain or tenderness, dyspareunia, chills, and fever.

c. Treatment of PID

Following diagnosis of PID, or suspected PID, bacteriologic specimens should be obtained and antibiotic therapy should be initiated promptly. Removal of the PROGESTASERT system soon after initiation of antibiotic therapy is required. Minimal therapy for PID requires at least 10–14 days of high-dose antibiotic. If specific infection and antibiotic sensitivities are obtained, the therapy can be directed to those results. However, PID frequently involves multiple organisms, both aerobic and anaerobic, and combined drug therapy may be indicated even if only one organism is identified.

Genital actinomycosis has been associated primarily with long-term IUD use. If it occurs, promptly institute appropriate antibiotic therapy and remove the PROGESTASERT system.

Guidelines for PID treatment are available from the Center for Disease Control (CDC), Atlanta, Georgia. A copy of the printed guidelines has been provided to you by ALZA Corporation. The guidelines were established after deliberation by a group of experts and staff of the CDC but they should not be construed as rules suitable for use in all patients. Adequate PID treatment requires the application of current standards of therapy prevailing at the time of occurrence of the infection and reference to the specific antibiotic's prescription labeling.

4. Embedment

Partial penetration or lodging of the PROGESTASERT system in the endometrium may decrease contraceptive effectiveness and can result in difficult removals.

5. Fragmentation

If fragmentation of the PROGESTASERT system occurs, all pieces should be removed if possible. Verification of removal should take into account that the horizontal crossarms are not radiopaque.

6. Perforation

Partial or total perforation of the uterine wall or cervix may occur with the use of the PROGESTASERT system. The possibility of perforation must be kept in mind during insertion and at the time of any subsequent examination. It is recommended that the PROGESTASERT system insertion be postponed postpartum, or postabortion with a conceptus of more than 12 weeks gestation, until involution of the uterus is complete. (Involution may be delayed in nursing mothers.) The incidence of perforation and expulsion is greater if involution is not complete. If perforation occurs, the system should be removed. Adhesions, foreign body reactions, peritonitis, cystic masses in the pelvis, intestinal penetrations, and intestinal obstruction may result if an IUD is left in the peritoneal cavity.

PRECAUTIONS

1. Patient Counseling

a. Patients must be informed of the availability, effectiveness, and risks of the PROGESTASERT system and other forms of contraception. They should also be informed of the health risks associated with pregnancy resulting from failure to use any contraception.

b. Prior to insertion of the PROGESTASERT system, the physician or nurse-practitioner must provide the patient with the Patient Information Leaflet. The patient must read the leaflet in its entirety and discuss fully any questions she has concerning the PROGESTASERT system and other methods of contraception. She must then initial and sign the leaflet, including the Patient Consent, where indicated.

2. Patient Evaluation and Clinical Considerations

a. A complete medical history should be obtained to determine conditions that might influence the selection of the PROGESTASERT system or contraindicate its use (see CONTRAINDICATIONS). Physical examination should include a pelvic examination, Pap smear, N. gonorrhoeae and Chlamydia culture and, if indicated, appropriate tests for other forms of venereal disease. **Special attention must be given to ascertaining whether the woman is at a high risk to ectopic pregnancy or to PID. The PROGESTASERT system is contraindicated in these women.**

b. The PROGESTASERT system is not intended for postabortion or postpartum insertion. It should not be inserted until involution of the uterus is complete. (Involution may be delayed in nursing mothers.) The incidence of perforation and expulsion is greater if involution is not completed.

c. The possibility of insertion in the presence of an existing undetermined pregnancy is reduced if insertion is performed during or shortly following a menstrual period.

d. Patients with valvular or congenital heart disease are more prone to develop subacute bacterial endocarditis than patients who do not have valvular or congenital heart disease. Use of a PROGESTASERT system in these patients may represent a potential source of septic emboli. Other conditions predisposing to infection (see CONTRAINDICATIONS) are also contraindications to PROGESTASERT system insertion.

e. IUDs should be used with caution in those patients who have an anemia or a history of menorrhagia or hypermenorrhea. Patients experiencing menorrhagia and/or metrorrhagia following IUD insertion may be at risk for the development of hypochromic microcytic anemia. Also, IUDs should be used with caution in patients who have a coagulopathy or are receiving anticoagulants.

f. Use of the PROGESTASERT system in patients with acute cervicitis should be postponed until proper treatment has cleared up the infection and until the cervicitis has been shown not to be due to gonorrhea or chlamydia (see CONTRAINDICATIONS).

3. Insertion Precautions

a. Because the presence of organisms capable of establishing PID cannot be determined by appearance, and because IUD insertion may be associated with introduction of vaginal bacteria into the uterus, administration of prophylactic antibiotics should be strongly considered. The preferred regimen is doxycycline 200 mg orally 1 hour before insertion. An alternative is erythromycin 500 mg orally 1 hour before insertion and 500 mg orally 6 hours after insertion. Consult an infectious disease specialist regarding other acceptable alternatives. The use of antibiotics in nursing mothers is not recommended. Before prescribing the above mentioned antibiotics, refer to their prescription drug labeling.

b. The uterus should be carefully sounded prior to insertion to determine the degree of patency of the endocervical canal and the internal os, and the direction and depth of the uterine cavity. In occasional cases, severe cervical stenosis may be encountered. Do not use excessive force to overcome this resistance.

c. The uterus should sound to a depth of 6 to 10 centimeters (cm). Insertion of the PROGESTASERT system into a uterine cavity measuring less than 6.5 cm by sounding may increase the incidence of expulsion, bleeding, and pain.

d. Syncope, bradycardia, or other neurovascular episodes may occur during insertion or removal of the PROGESTASERT system, especially in patients with a previous disposition to these conditions. If decreased pulse, perspiration, or pallor are observed, the patient should remain supine until these signs have disappeared.

e. The patient should be told that some bleeding and cramps may occur during the first few weeks after insertion, but if her symptoms continue or are severe she should report them to her physician. She should also be given instructions on what other symptoms require her to call her physician. She should be instructed on how to check after her menstrual period to make certain that the thread still protrudes from the cervix and cautioned not to pull on the thread and displace the PROGESTASERT system. She should be informed that there is no contraceptive protection if the PROGESTASERT system is displaced or expelled.

f. The patient must be told to return within 3 months for a checkup and at 12 months after insertion for removal of the PROGESTASERT system. Patient reminder cards should be properly completed and given to the patient.

4. Follow-up

a. Any inquiries regarding pain, odorous discharge, bleeding, fever, genital lesions or sores, or a missed period should be promptly responded to and prompt examination recommended.

b. If examination during visits subsequent to insertion reveals that the length of the threads has visibly or palpably changed from their length at time of insertion, the system should be considered displaced and should be removed. A new system may be inserted at that time or during the next menses or when it is certain that conception has not occurred. When the thread cannot be visualized by the physician, further investigation is necessary.

c. Since the PROGESTASERT system may be expelled or displaced, patients should be reexamined and evaluated shortly after the post insertion menses, but definitely within 3 months after insertion. **The PROGESTASERT system must be removed every 12 months because of diminished contraceptive effectiveness thereafter.** At the time of reinsertion, appropriate medical and laboratory examinations should be carried out.

d. In the event a pregnancy is confirmed during PROGESTASERT system use, the following steps should be taken:

- Determine whether pregnancy is ectopic and take appropriate measures if it is.
- Inform patient of the risks of leaving an IUD *in situ* or removing it during pregnancy and of the lack of data on the PROGESTASERT system's long-term effects on the offspring of women who had it *in utero* during conception or gestation (see WARNINGS).
- If possible the PROGESTASERT system should be removed after the patient has been warned of the risks of removal. If removal is difficult, the patient should be counseled about and offered pregnancy termination.
- If the PROGESTASERT system is left in place, the patient's course should be followed closely.

ADVERSE REACTIONS

These adverse reactions are not listed in any order of frequency or severity.

Reported adverse reactions with intrauterine contraceptives include: endometritis; spontaneous abortion; septic abortion; septicemia; perforation of the uterus and cervix, embedment; fragmentation of the IUD; pelvic infection; tubo-ovarian abscess; vaginitis; leukorrhea; cervical erosion; pregnancy; ectopic pregnancy; congenital anomalies; difficult removal; complete or partial expulsion of the IUD; intermenstrual spotting; prolongation of menstrual flow; anemia; amenorrhea or delayed menses; pain and cramping; dysmenorrhea; backaches; dyspareunia; neurovascular episodes, including bradycardia and syncope secondary to insertion. Uterine perforation and IUD displacement into the abdomen have been followed by peritonitis, abdominal adhesions, intestinal penetration, intestinal obstruction, and cystic masses in the pelvis. Certain of these adverse reactions can lead to loss of fertility, partial or total removal of reproductive organs, hormonal imbalance, or death.

DIRECTIONS FOR USE

A single PROGESTASERT system is to be inserted into the uterine cavity (see PRECAUTIONS). The system must be removed one year after insertion and replaced for continued contraceptive effectiveness. See INSERTION AND REMOVAL INSTRUCTIONS.

CLINICAL STUDIES

Different event rates have been reported with the use of different IUDs. Inasmuch as these rates are usually derived from separate studies conducted by different investigators in several population groups, they cannot be compared with precision. Clinical trials of the PROGESTASERT system were conducted by ALZA and the World Health Organization from 1970 to 1981; use-effectiveness was determined from combined data as tabulated by the life table method. (Rates are expressed as events per 100 women through 12 months of use.) This experience is based on 117,166 woman months of use, including 5,996 women who completed 12 months of use.

	12 months	
	Parous*	Nulliparous*
Pregnancy		
Intrauterine	1.3	2.1
Extrauterine (ectopic)	0.5	0.4
Total	1.8	2.5
Expulsion	2.7	7.6
Medical Removals	9.3	12.0
Continuation Rate	81.2	73.4

*Columns do not total 100 because rates are not included for the following: scheduled removals, removals for planned pregnancy, release from studies, and lost-to-follow-up.

HOW SUPPLIED

Available in cartons containing six packages, each with a sterile system and sterile inserter.

INSERTION AND REMOVAL INSTRUCTIONS

NOTE: Physicians are cautioned to become thoroughly familiar with the insertion instructions in their entirety before attempting placement of the PROGESTASERT intrauterine progesterone contraceptive system.

DESCRIPTION OF INSERTER

The inserter is a malleable, curved tube designed to conform to the anatomical configuration of most cervical-uterine cavities. The horizontal arms of the T are positioned outside of the inserter and are folded by an arm-cocker attachment immediately prior to insertion. The inserter does not contain a plunger.

DO NOT REMOVE ANY COMPONENT FROM THE INSERTER BEFORE INSERTION OF THE SYSTEM INTO THE UTERUS.

CURVED PORTION OF TUBE
GRADUATION (in cm)
ARM – COCKER
THREAD
ARMS OF PROGESTASERT® SYSTEM
THREAD – RETAINING PLUG

The PROGESTASERT system inserter permits determination of the depth of uterine placement of the PROGESTASERT system. The curvature of the inserter conforms with the usual orientation of the uterus; however, in cases of extreme flexion, the malleable inserter may need to be gently shaped to the desired curvature prior to insertion.

PRELIMINARY PREPARATION

1. Before insertion, the patient must read and initial each section of the Patient Information Leaflet; the medical history and counseling of the patient must be completed; and the Patient Consent must be signed by the patient and by the doctor.
2. Refer to CONTRAINDICATIONS, WARNINGS, and PRECAUTIONS.
3. Prior to insertion of the PROGESTASERT system, a cervical Pap smear, N. gonorrhoeae and Chlamydia cultures, and pelvic examination are to be performed.
4. If used, commence antibiotic prophylaxis one hour before insertion.
5. Use of aseptic technique during insertion is essential.
6. The endocervix should be cleansed with an antiseptic solution and a tenaculum applied to the cervix with downward traction for correction of the angulation of the cervix and stabilization of the cervix.
7. Prior to insertion, determine by uterine sounding the depth and position of the uterus and the patency of the cervical canal. Insertion is not recommended into a uterus that sounds less than 6 cm or more than 10 cm.
8. THE PROGESTASERT SYSTEM MUST BE USED ONLY WITH ITS SPECIALLY DESIGNED INSERTER. This inserter will facilitate fundal placement and is designed to decrease the possibility of uterine perforation. No component should be removed from the inserter before insertion of the system into the uterus.

NOTE: Any intrauterine procedure can result in severe pain, bradycardia, and syncope.

SYSTEM INSERTION

1. Open the PROGESTASERT intrauterine progesterone contraceptive system pouch by COMPLETELY removing the clear cover.

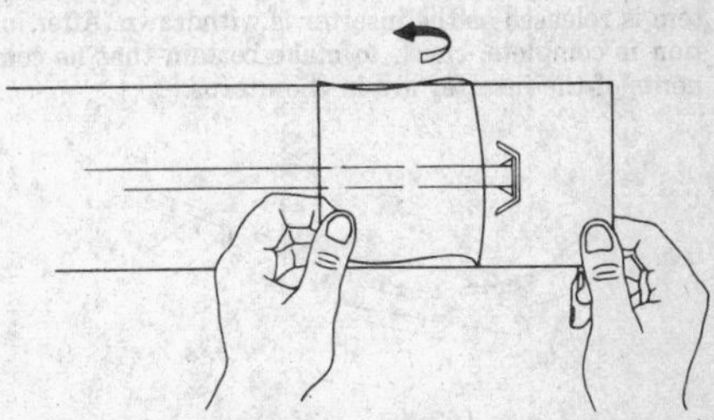

Remove the system and inserter by grasping the handle of the inserter. DO NOT CONTAMINATE THE END CONTAINING THE SYSTEM.

2. IMMEDIATELY PRIOR TO INSERTION, cock the arms of the PROGESTASERT system by pressing straight down on the inserter onto a sterile field as shown. This will cause the arms to fold against the side of the inserter.

NOTE: To avoid alteration of system shape, do not leave the system in the folded position for more than a few minutes.

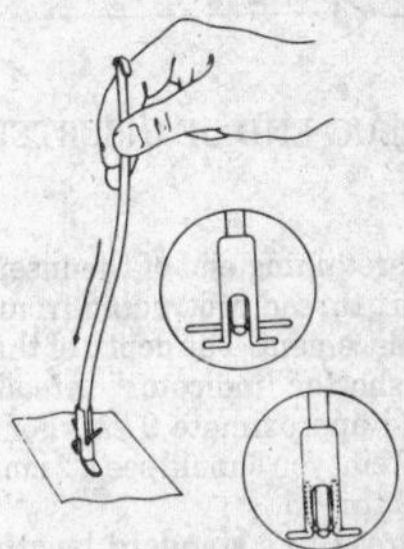

3. Examine the curvature of the inserter. If necessary, it can be easily reshaped to fit the flexion of the uterus. After aligning the curvature of the inserter with the direction of uterine flexion, introduce the inserter into the cervical canal. Be certain that the thread-retaining plug is still secure in the end of the inserter. The arm-cocker will slide along the inserter shaft as the inserter moves through the cervical canal.

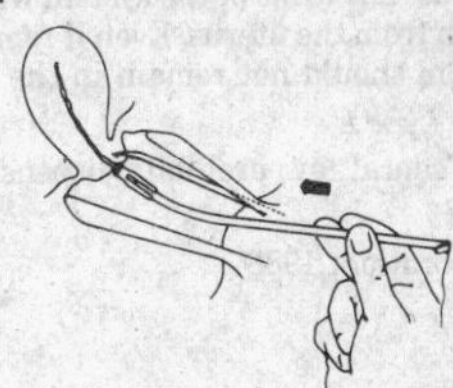

4. Sound steadily but gently with the inserter until the fundus is reached. While the inserter is in this position, note the number seen on the shaft at the base of the arm-cocker. This number approximates the depth in centimeters of the uterus and should equal the previously sounded uterine depth.

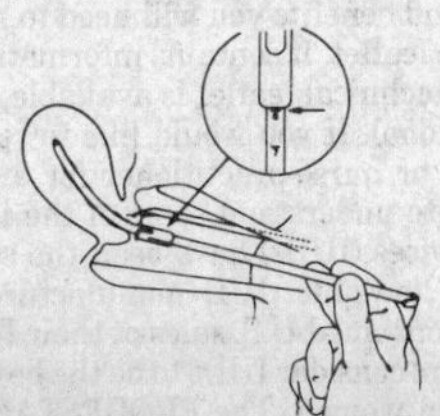

Continued on next page

Alza—Cont.

5. With the inserter still at the fundus, release the retaining thread by squeezing the wings of the thread-retaining plug and removing it.

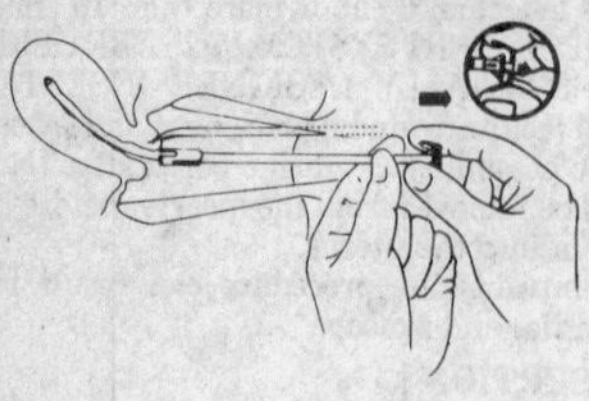

6. Slowly withdraw the inserter. The PROGESTASERT system is released as the inserter is withdrawn. After insertion is complete, check to make certain that no components of the inserter are in the uterus.

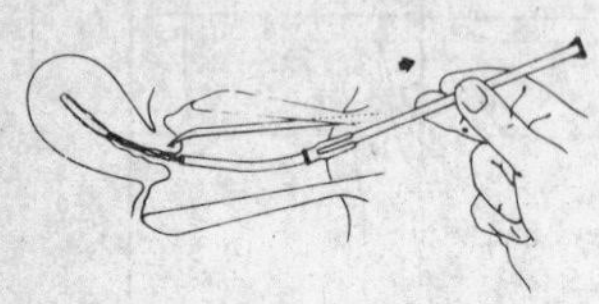

CORRECT FUNDAL PLACEMENT

To be fully effective, the PROGESTASERT system must be placed at the fundus.

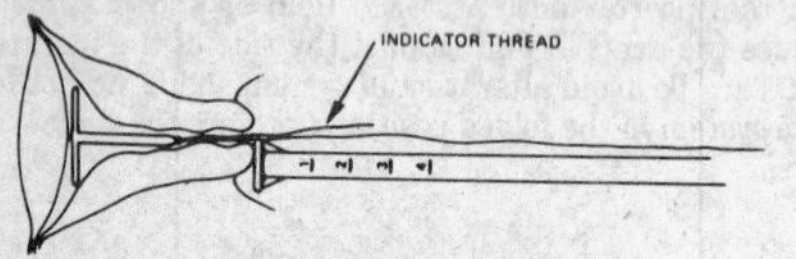

PLUG END OF INSERTER

Using the thread-retaining end of the inserter, estimate the length of the short thread protruding from the cervix to determine correct placement. The depth of the uterus, added to the length of the shorter "indicator" thread protruding from the cervix, should approximate 9 cm. For example, with a uterine depth of 7 cm, you should see a 2 cm protrusion of the short "indicator" thread.
Trim the long thread to a standard length from the cervix (for all your patients) that can be used for future reference in determining continued fundal placement. This length should be at least 3 cm. (If pregnancy or perforation occurs, the thread may be drawn up through the cervix.) Uterine depth and length of trimmed threads should be recorded.

SYSTEM REMOVAL

To remove the PROGESTASERT system, pull gently on the exposed threads. The arms of the system will fold upward as it is withdrawn from the uterus. Even if removal proves difficult, the system should not remain in the uterus after one year.

CAUTION: Federal law prohibits dispensing without prescription.

PROGESTASERT® ℞

Intrauterine Progesterone Contraceptive System
PATIENT INFORMATION

IMPORTANT NOTICE

ALZA's intrauterine device, the PROGESTASERT system, has been available in the United States since 1976. To understand its risks and benefits you will need to read and understand this entire leaflet. It contains information vital to your health. A more technical leaflet is available, written for the medical professional. If you would like to read that leaflet, ask your doctor or nurse-practitioner for a copy. You may need their help to understand some of the information.
Intrauterine devices (IUDs) have been the subject of many personal injury lawsuits. IUD manufacturers other than ALZA have discontinued U.S. sales of their IUDs. Nevertheless, many doctors consider IUDs to be the best contraceptive choice for certain women. The PROGESTASERT system is most appropriately used in women who have had more than one child, who have no desire for future children, and who are in the latter part of their reproductive years.
In addition to reading this leaflet, you should also learn about sterilization and other birth control methods. One of these methods may be more suitable or safer for you than the PROGESTASERT system. To decide, discuss your questions about the PROGESTASERT system and other kinds of birth control with your doctor or nurse-practitioner. Also, have the doctor or nurse-practitioner explain to your satisfaction anything you do not understand in this leaflet.
Under certain conditions you should not have the PROGESTASERT system inserted; the risks to your health or your ability to bear children may be too great. Such conditions are described under SPECIAL RISK FACTORS and WHAT YOU SHOULD DISCUSS WITH YOUR DOCTOR OR NURSE-PRACTITIONER. Even if none of these conditions applies to you, you may still experience serious problems while using the PROGESTASERT system. These problems require immediate medical attention. They can be associated with damage to your reproductive organs and ability to bear children or in infrequent cases can cause death. You may have to undergo major surgery, and you may become temporarily or permanently sterile (see SPECIAL RISK FACTORS). Prompt medical treatment, though absolutely necessary, may not always be effective.
To become familiar with the danger signs of IUD use read ADVERSE REACTIONS, SIDE EFFECTS, and WARNINGS. Then discuss these sections of the leaflet with your doctor or nurse-practitioner.
I have read this notice, and I understand it; I must initial all sections of the leaflet where indicated and will discuss its contents with my doctor or nurse-practitioner. I will not use the PROGESTASERT system without fully understanding this information.

SIGNATURE

DATE

DESCRIPTION

Intrauterine devices (IUDs) are small units inserted into the uterus (womb) to prevent pregnancy. The PROGESTASERT system is one type of IUD. Like other contraceptives, it is not 100% effective. (See USE EFFECTIVENESS for pregnancy rates during its use.)
The PROGESTASERT system is small, flexible, and T-shaped, with a hollow stem containing the hormone progesterone. The T itself is made of a flexible material (ethylene/vinyl acetate copolymer). This material permits the continuous release of progesterone into the uterus for one year. The PROGESTASERT system must be replaced once a year to maintain its contraceptive effect. Two blue-black threads extend from the base of the T. They will extend into your vagina, indicate the presence of the system, and aid in its removal.

THE PROGESTERONE IN THE PROGESTASERT SYSTEM

The PROGESTASERT system is the only intrauterine contraceptive to use progesterone, a hormone chemically identical to a hormone that your ovaries make. In one year the PROGESTASERT system releases only a little more progesterone than your body produces in one day during the latter part of a normal menstrual cycle.
Other contraceptive methods rely on different principles and materials to help prevent pregnancy. For instance, birth control pills rely on substances (progestins and estrogens) that differ from those made by your body.
The PROGESTASERT system is also unique in another way. The hormone it delivers does not travel through the bloodstream. Instead, the progesterone acts locally, directly on the lining of your uterus.

HOW THE PROGESTASERT SYSTEM ACTS AS A CONTRACEPTIVE

How IUDs act as contraceptives is not completely understood. Several theories have been suggested. IUDs seem to interfere in some manner with fertilization, or they may prevent the fertilized egg from remaining in the uterus. IUDs do not prevent ovulation (release of an egg by the ovary).
The PROGESTASERT system acts only within the uterus. Thus, it does not prevent ectopic pregnancy (pregnancy outside the uterus). Ectopic pregnancy can require surgery and can make you unable to bear children; in infrequent cases it can cause death. (See SPECIAL RISK FACTORS—Ectopic Pregnancy.)
I have read this section and understand it or will discuss it with my doctor or nurse-practitioner.

Initials

USE-EFFECTIVENESS

The effectiveness of an IUD is described in several ways: by the number of women who get pregnant while using it; by the number of women who expel the IUD from the uterus; and by the number of removals of the IUD for medical reasons. Different rates of pregnancy, expulsion, and medical removal have been reported for different IUDs. These rates usually come from separate studies conducted by different physicians in several population groups. Therefore the rates cannot be compared with precision.
Clinical studies of the PROGESTASERT system included 5,996 women who used it for one year. The studies included a total of 117,166 woman months of use. (Some women did not use the PROGESTASERT system for a full year.)
In the studies the incidence of unplanned pregnancies was 2 to 3 per 100 woman years, or 2 to 3 women out of 100 became pregnant in a year while using the PROGESTASERT intrauterine progesterone contraceptive system. The number of pregnancies includes both uterine and ectopic (outside the uterus).
In these studies 3 to 8 women out of 100 expelled the system during the first year. Nine to 12 women per year had an adverse reaction requiring system removal. Some of these adverse reactions were pelvic inflammatory disease (PID), an infection of the reproductive organs. The number of women in the studies who used the system for one year was 73 to 81 out of 100.
I have read this section and understand it or will discuss it with my doctor or nurse-practitioner.

Initials

LOSS OF CONTRACEPTIVE EFFECT AFTER PROGESTASERT SYSTEM REMOVAL

Soon after discontinuation of PROGESTASERT system use, its contraceptive effects on the uterus are reversed. In a study of 154 women, 76% of women seeking pregnancy became pregnant within a year following discontinuation.
I have read this section and understand it or will discuss it with my doctor or nurse-practitioner.

Initials

SPECIAL RISK FACTORS

The conditions discussed below can significantly increase your chances of developing serious complications while using an IUD. Some of these conditions can necessitate surgery, can make you unable to have children, or can cause death. Read the information carefully and discuss it with your doctor or nurse-practitioner.

Special Risk Factors for Ectopic Pregnancy

Ectopic pregnancy is a dangerous type of pregnancy that develops outside the uterus. The PROGESTASERT system —unlike most other contraceptives—does not prevent ectopic pregnancy. Studies indicate that PROGESTASERT system users have about the same risk of ectopic pregnancy as sexually active women using no contraception. But among women in the clinical studies who became pregnant while using the PROGESTASERT system, 1 out of 3 to 4 pregnancies among women who had borne one or more children was ectopic; among women who had not had children, 1 out of 6 pregnancies was ectopic.
PROGESTASERT system users are also more apt to have an ectopic pregnancy than users of other IUDs. Two clinical studies conducted by the World Health Organization compared the risk of ectopic pregnancies among women wearing a progesterone-releasing IUD similar to the PROGESTASERT system with the risk in women wearing a copper-releasing IUD. From the combined data of the two studies, the risk of an ectopic pregnancy in the first year was approximately 6 times higher among women using progesterone systems than among women using copper IUDs. Over the two years that the studies ran, the risk of an ectopic pregnancy with the progesterone IUD was about 10 times higher than that with copper-releasing IUDs.
If you have ever had an ectopic pregnancy, you have an increased risk of having another one. You also have an increased risk of an ectopic pregnancy if you have ever had certain infections. These infections include PID or a venereal disease (VD) caused by gonorrhea or chlamydia. **If you have ever had an ectopic pregnancy or these kinds of infections, you must not use the PROGESTASERT system.** Some other contraceptive methods reduce the risk of pregnancy both inside and outside the uterus and may be more suitable for you. Discuss this matter with your doctor or nurse-practitioner.
If you are using the PROGESTASERT system, you should immediately call your doctor if you develop any of the following symptoms, which may indicate ectopic pregnancy:

- A missed period, or a delayed period followed by spotting or scanty or irregular bleeding
- Cramping, tenderness, or sharp pain in your pelvis or lower abdomen
- Fainting associated with pelvic or lower abdominal pain or with an urge to have a bowel movement

- Pelvic or lower abdominal pain radiating down your legs
- Pain in your shoulder
- Pain associated with vaginal bleeding
- Any unusual or abnormal vaginal bleeding

Failure to seek and receive prompt and adequate treatment could greatly increase the chances of sterility or the need for surgery, or could result in death.

Special Risk Factors for Pelvic Infection (Pelvic Inflammatory Disease)

Evidence indicates that IUD users are more likely than other women to suffer a serious infection called pelvic inflammatory disease (PID). PID is the medical term for infection in the upper pelvic area. This area includes the uterus (womb), fallopian tubes, ovaries, and surrounding tissues. (Vaginitis, a local infection of the vagina, is not PID.) PID can lead to permanent blockage of the tubes and sterility, to ectopic pregnancy, or in infrequent cases to death. **If you have or ever have had PID, you must not use the PROGESTASERT system.**

PID is caused by infection with gonorrhea, chlamydia, or other bacteria. PID is usually a sexually transmitted disease, and your chances of getting PID increase greatly if you have more than one sexual partner. Your risk of getting PID also increases if you have a sexual partner who has sexual intercourse with others. **If you have an increased risk of getting PID, you must not use the PROGESTASERT system.**

Treatment of PID may require surgical removal of your uterus (hysterectomy), tubes, and ovaries. Removing the ovaries may result in lifelong need for hormonal treatments to correct the resulting deficiency of the hormones estradiol and progesterone. Such surgery may have to be done on an emergency basis and may result in death.

Symptoms of PID include pelvic or lower abdominal pain, chills, fever, abnormal vaginal discharge, abnormal menstrual bleeding, or painful sexual intercourse. Damage to your tubes can occur even without these symptoms.

If you are using the PROGESTASERT system and develop any of these symptoms, see your doctor as soon as possible. If you have PID, you should promptly receive at least 10–14 days of high-dose antibiotic therapy, and the PROGESTASERT system should be removed. **Failure to seek and receive prompt and adequate treatment will greatly increase the chances that you will become sterile, require surgery, or have life-threatening or fatal PID.**

Other Conditions That Increase Risk of Infection

Some conditions make you susceptible to infection during IUD use or following IUD insertion. These conditions include leukemia, acquired immune deficiency syndrome (AIDS), or long-term corticosteroid therapy. In addition, certain defects or diseases of the heart valves make you more likely than other IUD users to develop heart inflammation or infection. If you have any of these conditions you should not use the PROGESTASERT system.

I have read this section and understand it or will discuss it with my doctor or nurse-practitioner.

____
Initials

SIDE EFFECTS

The following may occur while the PROGESTASERT intrauterine progesterone contraceptive system is being inserted or afterward:

1. Pain, usually uterine cramps or low backache, occurs at the time of insertion and may last for a few days. (Pain and cramping may also occur at removal.) Mild pain medication usually relieves postinsertion and removal pain.
2. Fainting may occur at the time of insertion or removal of an IUD. This normally passes quickly and is not usually serious.
3. Some bleeding occurs following insertion in most women. Because of this, your doctor may choose to insert your system during or at the end of your menstrual period. This timing also reduces the possibility that you could be pregnant at the time of insertion.
4. Partial or total perforation of the uterus may occur at the time of or after PROGESTASERT system insertion. If you think the system may be displaced check with your doctor (see WARNINGS—Tail or thread disappearance). Perforation could result in abdominal adhesions, intestinal obstruction or penetration, inflammation, serious infection, and loss of contraceptive protection. Perforation and its complications may require surgery and in infrequent cases may result in death.
5. Bleeding between menstrual periods—usually just spotting—may occur during the first 2 or 3 months after insertion. The first few menstrual periods after insertion may be heavier and longer than usual. If these conditions continue for longer than 2 or 3 months, consult your doctor.
6. Occasionally you may miss a menstrual period while using the PROGESTASERT intrauterine progesterone contraceptive system. To determine if you are pregnant, report without delay to your doctor.
7. The PROGESTASERT system may come out of your uterus through the cervical opening. Expulsion is most likely to occur during the first 2 or 3 menstrual cycles following insertion. Expulsion leaves you unprotected against the risk of an unplanned pregnancy. Refer to the section called DIRECTIONS FOR USE for information on how to check to see if your system is properly positioned. If you think the IUD has come out or has been displaced, use another birth control method, such as contraceptive vaginal foam, cream, or jelly, or condoms (rubbers), until you can be checked. (These alternative methods are not as effective against uterine pregnancy as the PROGESTASERT system.) Call your doctor for an examination.

I have read this section and understand it or will discuss it with my doctor or nurse-practitioner.

____
Initials

	Yes	No	Don't know—will discuss with my doctor or nurse-practitioner
• **Abnormalities of the uterus (womb)**	☐	☐	☐
• Anemia or blood clotting problems	☐	☐	☐
• Bleeding between periods	☐	☐	☐
• **Cancer of the uterus (womb) or cervix**	☐	☐	☐
• **Corticosteroid therapy**	☐	☐	☐
• **Current suspected or possible pregnancy**	☐	☐	☐
• Diabetes	☐	☐	☐
• **Ectopic pregnancy (pregnancy outside of the uterus)**	☐	☐	☐
• Fainting attacks	☐	☐	☐
• Genital sores or lesions	☐	☐	☐
• **Heart disease**	☐	☐	☐
• **Heart murmur**	☐	☐	☐
• Heavy menstrual flow	☐	☐	☐
• **Infection of the uterus (womb) or cervix**	☐	☐	☐
• IUD in place now	☐	☐	☐
• **Leukemia**	☐	☐	☐
• **Multiple sexual partners**	☐	☐	☐
• **A sexual partner who has multiple sexual partners**	☐	☐	☐
• **Pelvic infection (including pus in fallopian tubes)**	☐	☐	☐
• Prior IUD use	☐	☐	☐
• **Recent abortion or miscarriage**	☐	☐	☐
• **Recent pregnancy**	☐	☐	☐
• Severe menstrual cramps	☐	☐	☐
• **Sexually transmitted disease (venereal disease), such as gonorrhea, chlamydia, or acquired immune deficiency syndrome (AIDS)**	☐	☐	☐
• **Suspicious or abnormal Pap smear**	☐	☐	☐
• **Unexplained genital bleeding**	☐	☐	☐
• **Uterine or pelvic surgery**	☐	☐	☐
• **Vaginal discharge or infection**	☐	☐	☐

WHAT YOU SHOULD DISCUSS WITH YOUR DOCTOR OR NURSE-PRACTITIONER

Before you have the PROGESTASERT system inserted, you should discuss your plans for having children with your doctor or nurse-practitioner. Also indicate below if you have ever had—or suspect you have ever had—any of the conditions listed below. **Some of these conditions, especially those in dark type, might make the PROGESTASERT system an unsuitable contraceptive for you:**

[See table above].

I have read this section and understand it or will discuss it with my doctor or nurse-practitioner.

____
Initials

ADVERSE REACTIONS

The following adverse reactions have been reported and may occur after an IUD is inserted:

- Abdominal infection or adhesions (scar tissue)
- Anemia
- Backache
- Birth defects
- Blood poisoning (septicemia)
- Bowel obstruction
- Cervical infection or erosion
- Cysts on ovaries and tubes
- Death in infrequent cases
- Delayed menstruation
- Difficult removal
- Ectopic pregnancy
- Embedment (IUD surrounded by uterine tissue)
- Expulsion (IUD comes completely or partially out of the uterus)
- Fainting and pain at the time of insertion or removal
- Fragmentation (break-up) of the IUD
- Infertility
- Intermenstrual spotting
- Miscarriage (spontaneous abortion)
- Pain and cramps
- Painful intercourse
- Pelvic infection (PID), which may result in surgical removal of your reproductive organs (hysterectomy)
- Perforation of the uterus (womb) or cervix (IUD passes through uterine tissue)
- Pregnancy
- Prolonged or heavy menstrual flow
- Septic abortion (infected miscarriage) followed in some cases by blood poisoning (septicemia), which can lead to death
- Vaginal discharge and infection

I have read this section and understand it or will discuss it with my doctor or nurse-practitioner.

____
Initials

WARNINGS

If you have a PROGESTASERT system inserted call your doctor immediately for any of the following reasons:

1. **A missed period.** This may mean you are pregnant and the IUD should be removed.
2. **Unexplained or abnormal vaginal bleeding or discharge.** This could indicate a serious complication such as an infection or ectopic pregnancy.
3. **A delayed period followed by scanty or irregular bleeding.** This could indicate an ectopic pregnancy.
4. **Pelvic or lower abdominal pain or cramps or unexplained fever.** Such symptoms could mean an ectopic pregnancy or infection has developed requiring immediate treatment.
5. **Exposure to venereal disease (VD).** The use of the PROGESTASERT intrauterine progesterone contraceptive system does not prevent venereal disease. If exposure to venereal disease is suspected, report for examination and treatment promptly. Failure to do so could result in serious pelvic infection.
6. **Genital sores or lesions, or fever with vaginal discharge.** These may indicate an infection.
7. **Severe or prolonged menstrual bleeding.** If the flow is heavier and lasts much longer than your usual menstrual flow, you may need to have the PROGESTASERT system removed to prevent anemia.
8. **Thread disappearance or pain during sex.** If you cannot feel the tail or thread coming through the cervix, or have pain during sex, the PROGESTASERT system may have been expelled or displaced or may have perforated the uterus. If any of these has occurred, you are no longer protected from pregnancy. Use another birth control method, such as contraceptive vaginal foam, cream, or jelly, or condoms (rubbers) until you can be checked. (These alternative methods are not as effective against uterine pregnancy as the PROGESTASERT system.) If perforation has occurred removal of the PROGESTASERT system is necessary, usually by surgery.

I have read this section and understand it or will discuss it with my doctor or nurse-practitioner.

____
Initials

HOW THE PROGESTASERT SYSTEM IS INSERTED AND REMOVED

Insertion of the PROGESTASERT system takes only a few minutes. Before insertion, your doctor will perform a pelvic examination. Its purpose is to determine the size, shape, and position of the uterus. An instrument called a speculum will hold your vagina open so that the cervix (the entrance to the

Continued on next page

Alza—Cont.

uterus) can be easily seen. (You will probably feel pressure from the speculum throughout the insertion procedure.)
The cervix is then cleaned with an antiseptic solution and an instrument called a tenaculum is attached to it. This instrument holds the uterus steady and in the proper position during insertion. You may feel pain or a pinching sensation as the tenaculum is attached. Then the physician will guide a narrow instrument called a sound through the opening of the cervix into the uterus. The sound measures the depth and position of the uterus. You can expect to feel cramping similar in severity to menstrual cramps as the sound is inserted and withdrawn.
Immediately thereafter, your doctor will guide the PROGESTASERT system (with the cross-arms of the T folded down) through the vagina and the cervix into the uterus.

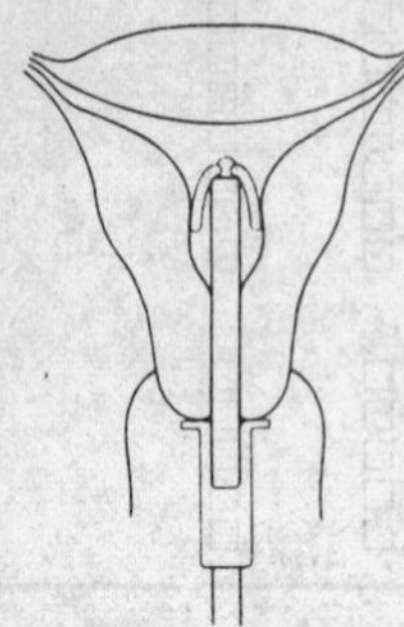

PROGESTASERT® System being inserted

As the system is inserted, the arms of the T will unfold. During insertion you will have some pain or cramping. You may feel nauseous, weak, or faint. After the inserter is removed, the threads attached to the end of the system will be clipped. They will then extend about an inch into the vagina from the cervical opening. During intercourse, neither you nor your partner should be aware of these threads. You should also not be aware of any other part of the system. If you are, promptly follow the instructions under the heading, "Checking Your PROGESTASERT System," in the section DIRECTIONS FOR USE.

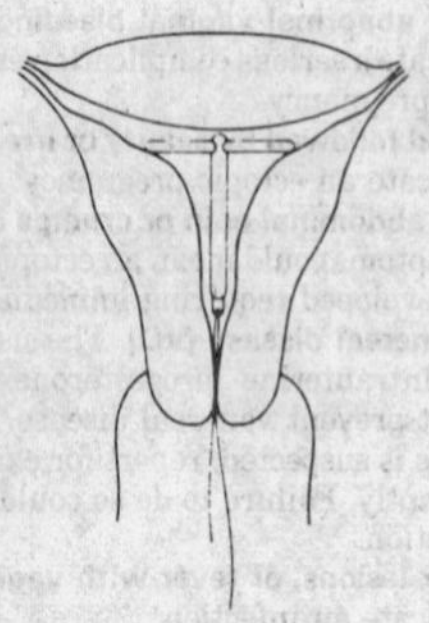

PROGESTASERT® System in place

When it is time to remove the PROGESTASERT system, your doctor must remove it. Its removal usually takes a few minutes and may cause pain or cramping. The system's arms will fold upward as it is withdrawn from your uterus.
I have read this section and understand it or will discuss it with my doctor or nurse-practitioner.

Initials

DIRECTIONS FOR USE

Please read the following information and instructions carefully. Keep a copy of this leaflet so that you may refer to it. If you have any questions, consult your doctor.

Checking Your PROGESTASERT System

The PROGESTASERT system can come out of the uterus (womb) without your knowing it. This occurs most often during or right after a menstrual period. Therefore after each menstrual period, check to make sure the tail or thread is in place in the cervix. You may check more often if you have some concern.
Follow these steps to make sure your PROGESTASERT system is in place:

1. Wash your hands.
2. Squat down or seat yourself on the toilet.
3. Insert the index or middle finger high into your vagina and locate your cervix. The cervix is the mouth of the uterus (womb). If feels firm, like the tip of your nose.

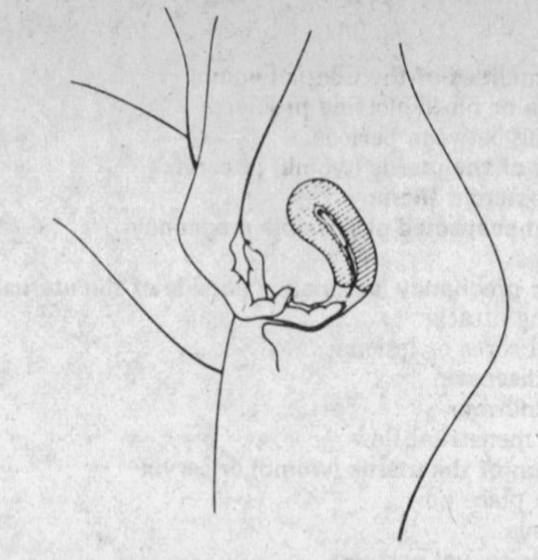

4. Feel for the tails or threads of the system. The threads should be extending from the cervix high in your vagina. The tails or threads may be difficult to feel.
5. If you can feel the tail or threads, the system is probably in place and working. You should **not** pull on the tail or threads. Doing so may displace the system.
6. If you cannot feel the tail or threads, or if you can feel the PROGESTASERT system itself, it may have come out or have been displaced from the uterus. Also, if you or your partner can feel the system during intercourse, it has been displaced. If so, you are not being protected against pregnancy. Until you can be examined, use another birth control method, such as a contraceptive vaginal foam, cream, or jelly, or condoms (rubbers). (These alternatve methods are not as effective against uterine pregnancy as the PROGESTASERT system.) Call your doctor for an examination.

Follow-up Visits to the Doctor

1. You should return to see your doctor as soon as possible after your first menstrual period following insertion of your IUD, but no later than 3 months after insertion. This will allow the doctor to check whether the PROGESTASERT system is in the correct position.
2. **The PROGESTASERT intrauterine progesterone contraceptive system requires replacement once a year because contraceptive effectiveness diminishes thereafter. Check with your doctor or nurse-practitioner concerning an appointment to have the system replaced or removed.**
3. The PROGESTASERT system does not interfere with the proper use of tampons and douches. You may want to discuss this with your doctor or nurse-practitioner.

I have read this section and understand it or will discuss it with my doctor or nurse-practitioner.

Initials

SPECIAL WARNING ABOUT UTERINE PREGNANCY WITH A PROGESTASERT SYSTEM IN PLACE

Some women become pregnant while using the PROGESTASERT intrauterine progesterone contraceptive system. If you miss your menstrual period, or if you suspect you are pregnant, see your doctor or nurse-practitioner right away.
When a pregnancy continues with an IUD in place, serious complications have occurred in some cases: sepsis, (severe blood infection); spontaneous miscarriage (abortion); septic abortion (infected miscarriage); and death. Most of these serious complications have been reported in the middle 3 months of pregnancy.
When the PROGESTASERT system remains in the uterus during conception or pregnancy, the long-term effects on the child (or fetus) are not known. Under such conditions some birth defects have occurred. The relationship to the PROGESTASERT system has not been established. Systemically administered sex steroids, some of which have effects similar to progesterone, have been associated with an increased risk of birth defects. You should discuss all your questions about this with your doctor.
If your doctor confirms that you are pregnant, the PROGESTASERT system should be removed provided the threads are visible. Removal of the system may cause a miscarriage. However, successful IUD removal in pregnancy decreases the likelihood of subsequent complications, including miscarriage.
In some cases removal of the PROGESTASERT system may prove to be difficult. If so, you and your doctor or nurse-practitioner should discuss at that time the question of continuing the pregnancy in view of the serious complications (described above) that may occur. In reaching a decision about abortion, you should be aware that the risks associated with abortion increase with the length of time you have been pregnant.
If you continue your pregnancy with the PROGESTASERT system in place, you will need your physician to follow your course closely throughout your pregnancy. Be sure to report immediately to the doctor if you have any of the following symptoms or signs:

- Bleeding from the vagina
- Pelvic or lower abdominal pain or cramping
- Flu-like symptoms such as chills or fever
- Unusual vaginal discharge

Any of these symptoms could indicate that you are having a miscarriage that may be complicated by an infection. Such an infection can cause infertility or death. Therefore, report any of these symptoms without delay to your doctor, so that you can obtain immediate treatment.
I have read this section and understand it or will discuss it with my doctor or nurse-practitioner.

Initials

PATIENT CONSENT

I have read this leaflet in its entirety and discussed its contents with my doctor or nurse-practitioner. My doctor or nurse-practitioner has answered all my questions and has advised me of the risks and benefits associated with the use of the PROGESTASERT system, with other forms of contraception, and with no form of contraception. I understand that while using the PROGESTASERT system I may experience serious medical problems that may not be caused by any defect in the PROGESTASERT system or inadequacy of medical care. These problems could lead to surgery, sterility, permanent hormonal imbalance, or death.
I have considered all factors and voluntarily choose to have the PROGESTASERT system inserted by

Dr. ....on date ....

Patient Signature

The patient has signed this leaflet in my presence after I counseled her and answered all her questions.

Doctor

Date

This system is scheduled for removal

Date

....

I have chosen not to use the PROGESTASERT system.

Patient Signature

Edition Date: 7/86

Shown in Product Identification Section, page 404

EDUCATIONAL MATERIAL

Booklets - Brochures

A. Progestasert® System Clinical Evidence
(free to physicians)
B. Patient Information Leaflet
(free to patients)

Films - Slides - Videos

A. Progestasert® System Insertion Technique Videocassette
(free for loan of 1 month)

American Critical Care
American Hospital Supply Corporation
McGAW PARK, IL 60085

BRETYLOL® ℞
[*bre'tĭ-lol"*]
(bretylium tosylate)
INJECTION

For Intramuscular or Intravenous Use

DESCRIPTION

BRETYLOL (bretylium tosylate) is o-Bromobenzyl ethyldimethylammonium p-toluene sulfonate.
BRETYLOL is a white, crystalline powder with an extremely bitter taste. It is freely soluble in water and alcohol. Each mL of sterile, non-pyrogenic solution contains 50 mg bretylium tosylate in Water for Injection, USP. The pH is adjusted when necessary, with dilute hydrochloric acid or sodium hydroxide. BRETYLOL contains no preservative.

CLINICAL PHARMACOLOGY

BRETYLOL (bretylium tosylate) is a bromobenzyl quaternary ammonium compound which selectively accumulates in sympathetic ganglia and their postganglionic adrenergic neurons where it inhibits norepinephrine release by depressing adrenergic nerve terminal excitability.

BRETYLOL also suppresses ventricular fibrillation and ventricular arrhythmias. The mechanisms of the antifibrillatory and antiarrhythmic actions of BRETYLOL are not established. In efforts to define these mechanisms, the following electrophysiologic actions of BRETYLOL have been demonstrated in animal experiments:

1. Increase in ventricular fibrillation threshold.
2. Increase in action potential duration and effective refractory period without changes in heart rate.
3. Little effect on the rate of rise or amplitude of the cardiac action potential (Phase 0) or in resting membrane potential (Phase 4) in normal myocardium. However, when cell injury slows the rate of rise, decreases amplitude, and lowers resting membrane potential, BRETYLOL transiently restores these parameters toward normal.
4. In canine hearts with infarcted areas BRETYLOL decreases the disparity in action potential duration between normal and infarcted regions.
5. Increase in impulse formation and spontaneous firing rate of pacemaker tissue as well as increased ventricular conduction velocity.

The restoration of injured myocardial cell electrophysiology toward normal, as well as the increase of the action potential duration and effective refractory period without changing their ratio to each other, may be important factors in suppressing re-entry of aberrant impulses and decreasing induced dispersion of local excitable states.

BRETYLOL induces a chemical sympathectomy-like state which resembles a surgical sympathectomy. Catecholamine stores are not depleted by BRETYLOL, but catecholamine effects on the myocardium and on peripheral vascular resistance are often seen shortly after administration because BRETYLOL causes an early release of norepinephrine from the adrenergic postganglionic nerve terminals. Subsequently, BRETYLOL blocks the release of norepinephrine in response to neuron stimulation. Peripheral adrenergic blockade regularly causes orthostatic hypotension but has less effect on supine blood pressure. The relationship of adrenergic blockade to the antifibrillatory and antiarrhythmic actions of BRETYLOL is not clear. In a study in patients with frequent ventricular premature beats, peak plasma concentration of BRETYLOL and peak hypotensive effects were seen within one hour of intramuscular administration, presumably reflecting adrenergic neuronal blockade. However, suppression of premature ventricular beats was not maximal until 6–9 hours after dosing, when mean plasma concentration had declined to less than one-half of peak level. This suggests a slower mechanism, other than neuronal blockade, was involved in suppression of the arrhythmia. On the other hand, antifibrillatory effect can be seen within minutes of an intravenous injection, suggesting that the effect on the myocardium may occur quite rapidly.

BRETYLOL has a positive inotropic effect on the myocardium, but it is not yet certain whether this effect is direct or is mediated by catecholamine release.

BRETYLOL is eliminated intact by the kidneys. No metabolites have been identified following administration of BRETYLOL in man and laboratory animals. In man, approximately 70 to 80% of a ^{14}C-labelled intramuscular dose is excreted in the urine during the first 24 hours, with an additional 10% excreted over the next three days.

The terminal half-life in four normal volunteers averaged 7.8 ± 0.6 hrs (range 6.9–8.1). In one patient with a creatinine clearance of 21.0 ml/min x 1.73 m^2, the half-life was 16 hours. In one patient with a creatinine clearance of 1.0 ml/min x 1.73 m^2 the half-life was 31.5 hours. During hemodialysis, this patient's arterial and venous BRETYLOL concentrations declined rapidly, resulting in a half-life of 13 hours. During dialysis there was a two-fold increase in total BRETYLOL clearance.

Effect on Heart Rate: There is sometimes an initial small increase in heart rate when BRETYLOL is administered, but this is an inconsistent and transient occurrence.

Hemodynamic Effects: Following intravenous administration of 5 mg/kg of BRETYLOL to patients with acute myocardial infarction, there was a mild increase in arterial pressure, followed by a modest decrease, remaining within normal limits throughout. Pulmonary artery pressures, pulmonary capillary wedge pressure, right atrial pressure, cardiac index, stroke volume index, and stroke work index were not significantly changed. These hemodynamic effects were not correlated with antiarrhythmic activity.

Onset of Action: Suppression of ventricular fibrillation is rapid, usually occurring within minutes following intravenous administration. Suppression of ventricular tachycardia and other ventricular arrhythmias develops more slowly, usually 20 minutes to 2 hours after parenteral administration.

INDICATIONS

BRETYLOL is indicated in the prophylaxis and therapy of ventricular fibrillation.

BRETYLOL is also indicated in the treatment of life-threatening ventricular arrhythmias, such as ventricular tachycardia, that have failed to respond to adequate doses of a first-line antiarrhythmic agent, such as lidocaine.

Use of BRETYLOL should be limited to intensive care units, coronary care units or other facilities where equipment and personnel for constant monitoring of cardiac arrhythmias and blood pressure are available.

Following injection of BRETYLOL there may be a delay of 20 minutes to 2 hours in the onset of antiarrhythmic action, although it appears to act within minutes in ventricular fibrillation. The delay in effect appears to be longer after intramuscular than after intravenous injection.

CONTRAINDICATIONS

There are no contraindications to use in treatment of ventricular fibrillation or life-threatening refractory ventricular arrhythmias.

WARNINGS

1. Hypotension

Administration of BRETYLOL regularly results in postural hypotension, subjectively recognized by dizziness, light-headedness, vertigo or faintness. Some degree of hypotension is present in about 50% of patients while they are supine. Hypotension may occur at doses lower than those needed to suppress arrhythmias.

Patients should be kept in the supine position until tolerance to the hypotensive effect of BRETYLOL develops. Tolerance occurs unpredictably but may be present after several days.

Hypotension with supine systolic pressure greater than 75 mm Hg need not be treated unless there are associated symptoms. If supine systolic pressure falls below 75 mm Hg, an infusion of dopamine or norepinephrine may be used to raise blood pressure. When catecholamines are administered, a dilute solution should be employed and blood pressure monitored closely because the pressor effects of the catecholamines are enhanced by BRETYLOL. Volume expansion with blood or plasma and correction of dehydration should be carried out where appropriate.

2. Transient Hypertension and Increased Frequency of Arrhythmias

Due to the initial release of norepinephrine from adrenergic postganglionic nerve terminals by BRETYLOL, transient hypertension or increased frequency of premature ventricular contractions and other arrhythmias may occur in some patients.

3. Caution During Use with Digitalis Glycosides

The initial release of norepinephrine caused by BRETYLOL may aggravate digitalis toxicity. When a life-threatening cardiac arrhythmia occurs in a digitalized patient, BRETYLOL should be used only if the etiology of the arrhythmia does not appear to be digitalis toxicity and other antiarrhythmic drugs are not effective. Simultaneous initiation of therapy with digitalis glycosides and BRETYLOL (bretylium tosylate) should be avoided.

4. Patients with Fixed Cardiac Output

In patients with fixed cardiac output (i.e., severe aortic stenosis or severe pulmonary hypertension) BRETYLOL should be avoided since severe hypotension may result from a fall in peripheral resistance without a compensatory increase in cardiac output. If survival is threatened by the arrhythmia, BRETYLOL may be used but vasoconstrictive catecholamines should be given promptly if severe hypotension occurs.

Use in Pregnancy: The safety of BRETYLOL in human pregnancy has not been established. However, as the drug is intended for use only in life-threatening situations, it may be used in pregnant women when its benefits outweigh the potential risk to the fetus.

Use in Children: The safety and efficacy of this drug in children has not been established. BRETYLOL has been administered to a limited number of pediatric patients, but such use has been inadequate to define fully proper dosage and limitations for use.

PRECAUTIONS

1. Dilution for Intravenous Use

BRETYLOL should be diluted (one part BRETYLOL with four parts of Dextrose Injection, USP or Sodium Chloride Injection, USP) prior to intravenous use. Rapid intravenous administration may cause severe nausea and vomiting. Therefore, the diluted solution should be infused over a period greater than 8 minutes. In treating existing ventricular fibrillation BRETYLOL should be given as rapidly as possible and may be given without dilution.

2. Use Various Sites for Intramuscular Injection

When injected intramuscularly, not more than 5 mL should be given in a site, and injection sites should be varied since repeated intramuscular injection into the same site may cause atrophy and necrosis of muscle tissue, fibrosis, vascular degeneration and inflammatory changes.

3. Reduce Dosage in Impaired Renal Function

Since BRETYLOL is excreted principally via the kidney, the dosage interval should be increased in patients with impaired renal function. See 'Clinical Pharmacology' section for information on the effect of reduced renal function on half-life.

ADVERSE REACTIONS

Hypotension and postural hypotension have been the most frequently reported adverse reactions (see Warnings section). Nausea and vomiting occurred in about three percent of patients, primarily when BRETYLOL was administered rapidly by the intravenous route (see Precautions section). Vertigo, dizziness, light-headedness and syncope, which sometimes accompanied postural hypotension, were reported in about 7 patients in 1000.

Bradycardia, increased frequency of premature ventricular contractions, transitory hypertension, initial increase in arrhythmias (see Warnings section), precipitation of anginal attacks, and sensation of substernal pressure have also been reported in a small number of patients, i.e., approximately 1–2 patients in 1000.

Renal dysfunction, diarrhea, abdominal pain, hiccups, erythematous macular rash, flushing, hyperthermia, confusion, paranoid psychosis, emotional lability, lethargy, generalized tenderness, anxiety, shortness of breath, diaphoresis, nasal stuffiness and mild conjunctivitis, have been reported in about 1 patient in 1000. The relationship of BRETYLOL administration to these reactions has not been clearly established.

DOSAGE AND ADMINISTRATION

BRETYLOL is to be used clinically only for treatment of life-threatening ventricular arrhythmias under constant electrocardiographic monitoring. The clinical use of BRETYLOL is for short-term use only. Patients should either be kept supine during the course of BRETYLOL therapy or be closely observed for postural hypotension. The optimal dose schedule for parenteral administration of BRETYLOL has not been determined. There is comparatively little experience with dosages greater than 40 mg/kg/day, although such doses have been used without apparent adverse effects. The following schedule is suggested.

A. For immediately Life-threatening Ventricular Arrhythmias such as Ventricular Fibrillation or Hemodynamically Unstable Ventricular Tachycardia:

Administer undiluted BRETYLOL at a dosage of 5 mg/kg of body weight by rapid intravenous injection. Other usual cardiopulmonary resuscitative procedures, including electrical cardioversion, should be employed prior to and following the injection in accordance with good medical practice. If ventricular fibrillation persists, the dosage may be increased to 10 mg/kg and repeated as necessary.

For continuous suppression, dilute 10 mL BRETYLOL containing 500 mg bretylium tosylate to a minimum of 50 mL with Dextrose (5%) Injection, USP, or Sodium Chloride Injection, USP, and administer the diluted solution as a constant infusion of 1 to 2 mg BRETYLOL per minute. An alternative maintenance schedule is to infuse the diluted solution at a dosage of 5 to 10 mg BRETYLOL per kg body weight, over a period greater than 8 minutes, every 6 hours. More rapid infusion may cause nausea and vomiting.

B. Other Ventricular Arrhythmias:

1. Intravenous Use: **BRETYLOL must be diluted as described above before intravenous use.**

   Administer the diluted solution at a dosage of 5 to 10 mg BRETYLOL per kg of body weight by intravenous infusion over a period greater than 8 minutes. More rapid infusion may cause nausea and vomiting. Subsequent doses may be given at 1 to 2 hour intervals if the arrhythmia persists.

   For maintenance therapy, the same dosage may be administered every 6 hours, or a constant infusion of 1 to 2 mg BRETYLOL per minute may be given.

2. For intramuscular Injection: **Do not dilute BRETYLOL prior to intramuscular injection.** Inject 5 to 10 mg BRETYLOL per kg of body weight. Subsequent doses may be given at 1 to 2 hour intervals if the arrhythmia persists. Thereafter maintain the same dosage every 6 to 8 hours.

   Intramuscular injection should not be made directly into or near a major nerve, and the site of injection should be varied on repeated injection.

As soon as possible, and when indicated, patients should be changed to an oral antiarrhythmic agent for maintenance therapy.

HOW SUPPLIED

NDC 0094-0012-10: 10 mL ampul; NDC 0094-0012-37 10 mL prefilled syringe; NDC 0094-0012-71: 10 mL single use vial,

Continued on next page

American Critical—Cont.

each containing 500 mg bretylium tosylate in Water for Injection, USP. pH adjusted, when necessary, with dilute hydrochloric acid or sodium hydroxide. Sterile, non-pyrogenic.

Re. Pat. No. 29,618

CALCIPARINE® ℞
[*cal-cĭ'pŭ-rin*]
(heparin calcium)
INJECTION

For Subcutaneous and IV Use

DESCRIPTION
Heparin is a heterogenous group of straight-chain anionic mucopolysaccharides, called glycosaminoglycans having anticoagulant properties. Although others may be present, the main sugars occurring in heparin are: (1) α-L-iduronic acid 2-sulfate, (2) 2-deoxy-2-sulfamino-α-D-glucose 6-sulfate, (3) β-D-glucuronic acid, (4) 2-acetamido-2-deoxy-α-D-glucose, and (5) α-L-iduronic acid. These sugars are present in decreasing amounts, usually in the order (2) > (1) > (4) > (3) > (5), and are joined by glycosidic linkages, forming polymers of varying sizes. Heparin is strongly acidic because of its content of covalently linked sulfate and carboxylic acid groups. In heparin calcium, the acidic protons of the sulfate units are replaced by calcium ions.
Structure of Heparin Calcium (representative subunits):

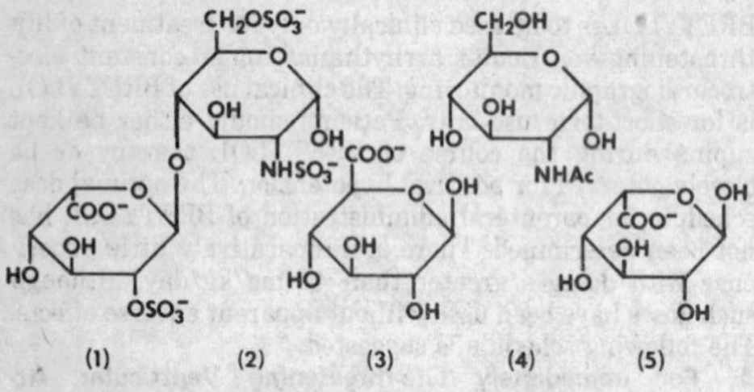

(1) (2) (3) (4) (5)

Calciparine (heparin calcium injection) is a sterile solution of heparin calcium derived from porcine intestinal mucosa, standardized for anticoagulant activity. It is to be administered by intravenous or deep subcutaneous routes. The potency is determined by a biological assay using a USP reference standard based on units of heparin activity per milligram. Each mL of Calciparine contains 25,000 USP heparin units in Water for Injection. Calcium hydroxide and/or hydrochloric acid may have been added during manufacture to adjust pH to approximately 7.

CLINICAL PHARMACOLOGY
Heparin inhibits reactions that lead to the clotting of blood and the formation of fibrin clots both *in vitro* and *in vivo*. Heparin acts at multiple sites in the normal coagulation system. Small amounts of heparin in combination with antithrombin III (heparin cofactor) can inhibit thrombosis by inactivating activated Factor X and inhibiting the conversion of prothrombin to thrombin. Once active thrombosis has developed, larger amounts of heparin can inhibit further coagulation by inactivating thrombin and preventing the conversion of firbrinogen to fibrin. Heparin also prevents the formation of a stable fibrin clot by inhibiting the activation of the fibrin stabilizing factor.
Bleeding time is usually unaffected by heparin. Clotting time is prolonged by full therapeutic doses of heparin; in most cases, it is not measurably affected by low doses of heparin. Peak plasma levels of heparin are achieved 2–4 hours following subcutaneous administration, although there are considerable individual variations. Loglinear plots of heparin plasma concentrations with time for a wide range of dose levels are linear which suggests the absence of zero order processes. Liver and the reticulo-endothelial system are the site of biotransformation. The biphasic elimination curve, a rapidly declining alpha phase ($t_{1/2}$ = 10 minutes) and after the age of 40 a slower beta phase, indicates uptake in organs. The absence of a relationship between anticoagulant half-life and concentration half-life may reflect factors such as protein binding of heparin.
Heparin does not have fibrinolytic activity; therefore, it will not lyse existing clots.

INDICATIONS AND USAGE
Calciparine is indicated for:
Anticoagulant therapy in prophylaxis and treatment of venous thrombosis and its extension;
In a low-dose regimen for prevention of postoperative deep venous thrombosis and pulmonary embolism in patients undergoing major abdomino-thoracic surgery or who for other reasons are at risk of developing thromboembolic disease (see DOSAGE AND ADMINISTRATION);
Prophylaxis and treatment of pulmonary embolism;
Atrial fibrillation with embolization;
Diagnosis and treatment of acute and chronic consumption coagulopathies (disseminated intravascular coagulation);
Prevention of clotting in arterial and heart surgery;
Prophylaxis and treatment of peripheral arterial embolism;
As an anticoagulant in blood transfusions, extracorporeal circulation, and dialysis procedures and in blood samples for laboratory purposes.

CONTRAINDICATIONS
Heparin calcium should not be used in patients:
With severe thrombocytopenia;
In whom suitable blood coagulation tests—e.g., the whole-blood clotting time, partial thromboplastin time, etc.—cannot be performed at appropriate intervals (this contraindication refers to full-dose heparin; there is usually no need to monitor coagulation parameters in patients receiving low-dose heparin);
With an uncontrollable active bleeding state (see WARNINGS), except when this is due to disseminated intravascular coagulation.

WARNINGS
Heparin is not intended for intramuscular use.
Hypersensitivity: Patients with documented hypersensitivity to heparin should be given the drug only in clearly life-threatening situations.
Hemorrhage: Hemorrhage can occur at virtually any site in patients receiving heparin. An unexplained fall in hematocrit, fall in blood pressure, or any other unexplained symptom should lead to serious consideration of a hemorrhagic event.
Heparin calcium should be used with extreme caution in disease states in which there is increased danger of hemorrhage. Some of the conditions in which increased danger of hemorrhage exists are:
Cardiovascular—Subacute bacterial endocarditis. Severe hypertension.
Surgical—During and immediately following (a) spinal tap or spinal anesthesia or (b) major surgery, especially involving the brain, spinal cord, or eye.
Hematologic—Conditions associated with increased bleeding tendencies, such as hemophilia, thrombocytopenia, and some vascular purpuras.
Gastrointestinal—Ulcerative lesions and continuous tube drainage of the stomach or small intestine.
Other—Menstruation, liver disease with impaired hemostasis.
Coagulation Testing: When Calciparine is administered in therapeutic amounts, its dosage should be regulated by frequent blood coagulation tests. If the coagulation test is unduly prolonged or if hemorrhage occurs, Calciparine should be discontinued promptly (see OVERDOSAGE).
Thrombocytopenia: Thrombocytopenia has been reported to occur in patients receiving heparin with a reported incidence of 0 to 30%. Mild thrombocytopenia (count greater than 100,000/mm^3) may remain stable or reverse even if heparin is continued. However, thrombocytopenia of any degree should be monitored closely. If the count falls below 100,000/mm^3 or if recurrent thrombosis develops (see White Clot Syndrome, PRECAUTIONS). Calciparine should be discontinued. If continued heparin therapy is essential, administration of heparin from a different organ source can be reinstituted with caution.

PRECAUTIONS
1. *General:*
a. White Clot Syndrome:
Rare patients on heparin may develop new thrombus formation in association with thrombocytopenia resulting from irreversible aggregation of platelets induced by heparin, the so-called "white clot syndrome." The process may lead to severe thromboembolic complications like skin necrosis, gangrene of the extremities, myocardial infarction, pulmonary embolism, and stroke. Therefore, heparin administration should be promptly discontinued if a patient develops new thrombosis in association with thrombocytopenia.
b. Heparin Resistance:
Increased resistance to heparin is frequently encountered in fever, thrombosis, thrombophlebitis, infections with thrombosing tendencies, myocardial infarction, cancer and in postsurgical patients.
c. Increased Risk in Older Women:
A higher incidence of bleeding has been reported in women over 60 years of age.
2. *Laboratory Tests:*
Periodic platelet counts, hematocrits, and tests for occult blood in stool are recommended during the entire course of heparin therapy, regardless of the route of administration (see DOSAGE AND ADMINISTRATION).
3. *Drug Interactions:*
Oral anticoagulants: Calciparine may prolong the one-stage prothrombin time. Therefore, when Calciparine is given with dicumarol or warfarin sodium, a period of at least 5 hours after the last intravenous dose or 24 hours after the last subcutaneous dose should elapse before blood is drawn if a valid prothrombin time is to be obtained.
Platelet inhibitors: Drugs such as acetylsalicylic acid, dextran, phenylbutazone, ibuprofen, indomethacin, dipyridamole, hydroxychloroquine and others that interfere with platelet-aggregation reactions (the main hemostatic defense of heparinized patients) may induce bleeding and should be used with caution in patients receiving heparin calcium.
Other interactions: Digitalis, tetracyclines, nicotine, or antihistamines may partially counteract the anticoagulant action of heparin calcium.
4. *Drug/Laboratory Tests Interactions:*
Hyperaminotransferasemia:
Significant elevations of aminotransferase (SGOT [S-AST] and SGPT [S-ALT]) levels have occurred in a high percentage of patients (and healthy subjects) who have received heparin. Since aminotransferase determinations are important in the differential diagnosis of myocardial infarction, liver disease, and pulmonary emboli, rises that might be caused by drugs (like heparin) should be interpreted with caution.
5. *Carcinogenesis, Mutagenesis, Impairment of Fertility:*
No long-term studies in animals have been performed to evaluate carcinogenic potential of heparin. Also, no reproduction studies in animals have been performed concerning mutagenesis or impairment of fertility.
6. *Pregnancy:*
Teratogenic Effects: Pregnancy Category C. Animal reproduction studies have not been conducted with heparin calcium. It is also not known whether heparin calcium can cause fetal harm when administered to a pregnant woman or can affect reproduction capacity. Calciparine should be given to a pregnant woman only if clearly needed.
Nonteratogenic Effects: Heparin does not cross the placental barrier.
7. *Nursing Mothers:*
Heparin is not excreted in human milk.
8. *Pediatric Use:*
See DOSAGE AND ADMINISTRATION.

ADVERSE REACTIONS
1. Hemorrhage.
Hemorrhage is the chief complication that may result from heparin therapy (see WARNINGS). An overly prolonged clotting time or minor bleeding during therapy can usually be controlled by withdrawing the drug (see OVERDOSAGE). *It should be appreciated that gastrointestinal or urinary tract bleeding during anticoagulant therapy may indicate the presence of an underlying occult lesion.* Bleeding can occur at any site but certain specific hemorrhagic complications may be difficult to detect:
a. Adrenal hemorrhage, with resultant acute adrenal insufficiency, has occurred during anticoagulant therapy. Therefore, such treatment should be discontinued in patients who develop signs and symptoms of acute adrenal hemorrhage and insufficiency. Intiation of corrective therapy should not depend on laboratory confirmation of the diagnosis, since any delay in an acute situation may result in the patient's death.
b. Ovarian (corpus luteum) hemorrhage developed in a number of women of reproductive age receiving short- or long-term anticoagulant therapy. This complication if unrecognized may be fatal.
c. Retroperitoneal hemorrhage.
2. Local Irritation.
Local irritation, erythema, mild pain, hematoma or ulceration may follow deep subcutaneous (intrafat) injection of heparin calcium. These complications are much more common after intramuscular use, and such use is not recommended.
3. Hypersensitivity.
Generalized hypersensitivity reactions have been reported, with chills, fever, and urticaria as the most usual manifestations, and asthma, rhinitis, lacrimation, headache, nausea and vomiting, and anaphylactoid reactions, including shock, occurring more rarely. Itching and burning, especially on the plantar site of the feet, may occur.
Thrombocytopenia has been reported to occur in patients receiving heparin with a reported incidence of 0–30%. While often mild and of no obvious clinical significance, such thrombocytopenia can be accompanied by severe thromboembolic complications such as skin necrosis, gangrene of the extremities, myocardial infarction, pulmonary embolism, and stroke. (See WARNINGS, PRECAUTIONS).
Certain episodes of painful, ischemic, and cyanosed limbs have in the past been attributed to allergic vasopastic reactions. Whether these are in fact identical to the thrombocytopenia associated complications remains to be determined.
4. Miscellaneous
Osteoporosis following long-term administration of high-doses of heparin, cutaneous necrosis after systemic administration, suppression of aidosterone synthesis, delayed transient alopecia, priapism, and rebound hyperlipemia on discontinuation of heparin calcium have also been reported.
Significant elevations of aminotransferase (SGOT [S-AST] and SGPT [S-ALT]) levels have occurred in a high percentage

of patients (and healthy subjects) who have received heparin.

OVERDOSAGE

Symptoms: Bleeding is the chief sign of heparin overdosage. Nosebleeds, blood in urine or tarry stools may be noted as the first sign of bleeding. Easy bruising or petechial formations may precede frank bleeding.

Treatment: Neutralization of heparin effect:

When clinical circumstances (bleeding) require reversal of heparinization, protamine sulfate (1% solution) by slow infusion will neutralize heparin calcium. *No more than 50 mg* should be administered, *very slowly,* in any 10 minute period. Each mg of protamine sulfate neutralizes approximately 100 USP heparin units. The amount of protamine required decreases over time as heparin is metabolized. Although the metabolism of heparin is complex, it may, for the purpose of choosing a protamine dose, be assumed to have a half-life of about ½ hour after intravenous injection.

Administration of protamine sulfate can cause severe hypotensive and anaphylactoid reactions. Because fatal reactions often resembling anaphylaxis have been reported, the drug should be given only when resuscitation techniques and treatment of anaphylactoid shock are readily available.

For additional information the labeling of Protamine Sulfate Injection, USP products should be consulted.

DOSAGE AND ADMINISTRATION

Parenteral drug products should be inspected visually for particulate matter and discoloration prior to administration, whenever solution and container permit. Slight discoloration does not alter potency.

When heparin is added to an infusion solution for continuous intravenous administration, the container should be inverted at least six times to insure adequate mixing and prevent pooling of the heparin in the solution.

Calciparine (heparin calcium) is not effective by oral administration and should be given by intermittent intravenous injection, intravenous infusion, or deep subcutaneous (intrafat, i.e., above the iliac crest or abdominal fat layer) injection. *The intramuscular route of administration should be avoided because of the frequent occurrence of hematoma at the injection site.*

The dosage of Calciparine should be adjusted according to the patient's coagulation test results. When heparin is given by continuous intravenous infusion, the coagulation time should be determined approximately every 4 hours in the early stages of treatment. When the drug is administered intermittently by intravenous injection, coagulation tests should be performed before each injection during the early stages of treatment and at appropriate intervals thereafter. Dosage is considered adequate when the activated partial thromboplastin time (APTT) is 1.5 to 2 times normal or when the whole blood clotting time is elevated approximately 2.5 to 3 times the control value. After deep subcutaneous (intrafat) injections, tests for adequacy of dosage are best performed on samples drawn 4–6 hours after the injections.

Periodic platelet counts, hematocrits, and tests for occult blood in stool are recommended during the entire course of heparin therapy, regardless of the route of administration.

Converting to Oral Anticoagulant: When an oral anticoagulant of the coumarin or similar type is to be begun in patients already receiving Calciparine, baseline and subsequent tests of prothrombin activity must be determined at a time when heparin activity is too low to affect the prothrombin time. This is about 5 hours after the last I.V. bolus and 24 hours after the last subcutaneous dose. If continuous I.V. heparin infusion is used, prothrombin time can usually be measured at any time.

In converting from Calciparine to an oral anticoagulant, the dose of the oral anticoagulant should be the usual initial amount and thereafter prothrombin time should be determined at the usual intervals. To ensure continuous anticoagulation, it is advisable to continue full Calciparine therapy for several days after the prothrombin time has reached the therapeutic range. Calciparine therapy may then be discontinued without tapering.

Therapeutic Anticoagulant Effect with Full-Dose Calciparine

Although dosage must be adjusted for the individual patient according to the results of suitable laboratory tests, the following dosage schedules may be used as guidelines:

[See table above].

METHOD OF ADMINISTRATION	FREQUENCY	RECOMMENDED DOSE*
Deep Subcuatneous (Intrafat) Injection A different site should be used for each injection to prevent the development of massive hematoma.	Initial Dose	5,000 units by I.V. injection, followed by 10,000–20,000 units of a concentrated solution, subcutaneously
	Every 8 hours	8,000–10,000 units of a concentrated solution
	or Every 12 hours	15,000–20,000 units of a concentrated solution
Intermittent Intravenous Injection	Initial dose	10,000 units, either undiluted or in 50–100 mL of 0.9% Sodium Chloride Injection, USP
	Every 4 to 6 Hours	5,000–10,000 units, either undiluted or in 50–100 mL of 0.9% Sodium Chloride Injection, USP
Continuous Intravenous Infusion	Initial Dose	5,000 units by I.V. Injection
	Continuous	20,000–40,000 units/24 hours in 1,000 mL of 0.9% Sodium Chloride Injection, USP (or in any compatible solution) for infusion

*Based on 150-lb. (68-kg) patient.

Pediatric Use Follow recommendations of appropriate pediatric reference texts. In general, the following dosage schedule may be used as a guideline:

Intial Dose: 50 units/kg (I.V. drip)

Maintenance Dose: 100 units/kg (I.V. drip) every four hours, or 20,000 units/M^2/24 hours continuously

Surgery of the Heart and Blood Vessels Patients undergoing total body perfusion for open-heart surgery should receive an initial dose of not less than 150 units of heparin calcium per kilogram of body weight. Frequently, a dose of 300 units per kilogram is used for procedures estimated to last less than 60 minutes or 400 units per kilogram for those estimated to last longer than 60 minutes.

Low-Dose Prophylaxis of Postoperative Thromboembolism: A number of well-controlled clinical trials have demonstrated that low-dose heparin prophylaxis, given just prior to and after surgery, will reduce the incidence of postoperative deep vein thrombosis in the legs (as measured by the I-125 fibrinogen technique and venography) and of clinical pulmonary embolism. The most widely used dosage has been 5,000 units 2 hours before surgery and 5,000 units every 8 to 12 hours thereafter for 7 days or until the patient is fully ambulatory, whichever is longer. The heparin is given by deep subcutaneous (intrafat, i.e., above the iliac crest or abdominal fat layer, arm or thigh) injection with a fine (25 to 26 gauge) needle to minimize tissue trauma. A concentrated solution of Calciparine (heparin calcium) is recommended. Such prophylaxis should be reserved for patients over the age of 40 who are undergoing major surgery. Patients with bleeding disorders and those having brain or spinal cord surgery, spinal anesthesia, eye surgery, or potentially sanguineous operations should be excluded, as should patients receiving oral anticoagulants or platelet-active drugs (see WARNINGS). The value of such prophylaxis in hip surgery has not been established. The possibility of increased bleeding during surgery or postoperatively should be borne in mind. If such bleeding occurs, discontinuance of Calciparine and neutralization with protamine sulfate are advisable. If clinical evidence of thromboembolism develops despite low-dose prophylaxis, full therapeutic doses of anticoagulants should be given unless contraindicated. Prior to initiating heparinization, the physician should rule out bleeding disorders by appropriate history and laboratory tests, and appropriate coagulation tests should be repeated just prior to surgery. Coagulation tests values should be normal or only slightly elevated at these times.

Extracorporeal Dialysis Follow equipment manufacturers' operating directions carefully.

Blood Transfusion: Addition of 400 to 600 USP units per 100 mL of whole blood is usually employed to prevent coagulation. Usually, 7,500 USP units of heparin calcium are added to 100 mL of 0.9% Sodium Chloride Injection, USP (or 75,000 USP units per 1,000 mL of 0.9% Sodium Chloride Injection, USP) and mixed; from this sterile solution, 6 to 8 mL are added per 100 mL of whole blood.

Laboratory Samples: Addition of 70 to 150 units of heparin calcium per 10 to 20 mL sample of whole blood is usually employed to prevent coagulation of the sample. Leukocyte counts should be performed on heparinized blood within 2 hours after addition of the Calciparine. Heparinized blood should not be used for isoagglutinin, complement, or erythrocyte fragility tests or platelet counts.

Clearing Intermittent Infusion (Heparin Lock) Sets: To prevent clot formation in a heparin lock set following its proper insertion, dilute heparin solution (Heparin Lock Flush Solution, USP) is injected via the injection hub in a quantity sufficient to fill the entire set to the needle tip. This solution should be replaced each time the heparin lock is used. Aspirate before administering any solution via the lock in order to confirm patency and location of needle or catherter tip. If the drug to be administered is incompatible with heparin, the entire heparin lock set should be flushed with sterile water or normal saline before and after the medication is administered; following the second flush, the dilute heparin solution may be reinstilled into the set. The set manufacturer's instructions should be consulted for specifics concerning the heparin lock set in use at a given time.

NOTE: Since repeated injections of small doses of heparin can alter tests for activated partial thromboplastin time (APTT), a baseline value for APTT should be obtained prior to insertion of a heparin lock set.

HOW SUPPLIED

Calciparine (heparin calcium injection) is available as follows:

Calciparine 5,000 USP heparin units, 0.2 mL pre-filled disposable syringe, carton of 10, NDC 0094-0030-02.

Calciparine 12,500 USP heparin units, 0.5 mL ampule with sterile syringe and attached 25-gauge, ⅝ inch needle, carton of 10, NDC 0094-0030-05.

Calciparine 20,000 USP heparin units, 0.8 mL ampule with sterile syringe and attached 25-gauge, ⅝ inch needle, carton of 10, NDC 0094-0030-08.

HESPAN® ℞

[hes'pan]

6% Hetastarch in 0.9% Sodium Chloride Injection

DESCRIPTION

Composition per 100 mL:

Hetastarch .... 6.0 g

Sodium Chloride USP .... 0.90 g

Water for Injection USP .... qs

pH adjusted with Sodium Hydroxide

Concentration of Electrolytes (mEq/liter): Sodium 154, Chloride 154

pH: Approx. 5.5

Calculated Osmolarity: Approximately 310 mOsm/Liter

Hetastarch is an artificial colloid derived from a waxy starch composed almost entirely of amylopectin. Hydroxyethyl ether groups are introduced into the glucose units of the starch and the resultant material is hydrolyzed to yield a product with a molecular weight suitable for use as a plasma expander. Clinical Hetastarch is characterized by its molecular weight and its degree of substitution. The weight average molecular weight is approximately 450,000 with 90% of the polymer units falling within the range of 10,000 to 1,000,000. The degree of substitution is 0.7 which means Hetastarch has 7 hydroxyethyl groups for every 10 glucose units. The polymerized glucose units in Hetastarch are joined primarily by 1–4 linkages with hydroxyethyl groups being attached primarily at the No. 2 position. The polymer closely resembles glycogen.

The Hespan dosage form is a clear, pale yellow to amber solution. Exposure to prolonged adverse storage conditions (temperatures above 40°C or below freezing) may result in a change to a turbid deep brown or the formation of a crystalline precipitate. Do not use the solution if these conditions are evident.

ACTIONS

The colloidal properties of 6% Hetastarch approximate those of human albumin. Intravenous infusion of Hetastarch results in expansion of plasma volume slightly in excess of the volume infused which decreases from this maximum over the succeeding 24 to 36 hours. This expansion of plasma volume may improve the hemodynamic status for 24 hours and longer. Hetastarch molecules below 50,000 molecular weight are rapidly eliminated by renal excretion with approximately 40% of a given total dose appearing in the urine in 24 hours. This is a variable process but generally results in an intravascular Hetastarch concentration of less than 1% of the total dose injected by two weeks. The hydroxyethyl group is not cleaved by the body, but remains intact and attached to glucose units when excreted.

The addition of Hetastarch to whole blood increases the erythrocyte sedimentation rate. Therefore, Hetastarch is used to improve the efficiency of granulocyte collection by centrifugal means.

INDICATIONS

Hetastarch is indicated when plasma volume expansion is desired as an adjunct in the treatment of shock due to hem-

Continued on next page

American Critical—Cont.

orrhage, burns, surgery, sepsis or other trauma. It is not a substitute for blood or plasma.

The adjunctive use of Hetastarch in leukapheresis has also been shown to be safe and efficacious in improving the harvesting and increasing the yield of granulocytes by centrifugal means.

CONTRAINDICATIONS

Hetastarch is contraindicated in patients with severe bleeding disorders or with severe congestive cardiac and renal failure with oliguria or anuria.

WARNINGS

Large volumes may alter the coagulation mechanism. Thus, administration of Hetastarch may result in transient prolongation of prothrombin, partial thromboplastin and clotting times. With administration of large doses, the physician should also be alert to the possibility of transient prolongation of bleeding time.

Hematocrit may be decreased and plasma proteins diluted excessively by administration of large volumes of Hetastarch.

Usage of Leukapheresis: Significant declines in platelet counts and hemoglobin levels have been observed in donors undergoing repeated leukapheresis procedures due to the volume expanding effects of Hetastarch. Hemoglobin levels usually return to normal within 24 hours. Hemodilution by Hetastarch and saline may also result in 24 hour declines of total protein, albumin, calcium and fibrinogen values.

Usage in Pregnancy: Reproduction studies have been done in mice with no evidence of fetal damage. Relevance to humans is not known since Hetastarch has not been given to pregnant women. Therefore, it should not be used in pregnant women, particularly during early pregnancy, unless in the judgment of the physician the potential benefits outweigh the potential hazards.

Usage in Children: No data are available pertaining to use in children.

The safety and compatibility of additives have not been established.

PRECAUTIONS

The possibility of circulatory overload should be kept in mind. Special care should be exercised in patients who have impaired renal clearance since this is the principal way in which Hetastarch is eliminated. Caution should be used when the risk of pulmonary edema and/or congestive heart failure is increased. Indirect bilirubin levels of 0.83 mg % (normal 0.0–0.7 mg %) have been reported in 2 out of 20 normal subjects who received multiple Hetastarch infusions. Total bilirubin was within normal limits at all times; indirect bilirubin returned to normal by 96 hours following the final infusion. The significance, if any, of these elevations is not known; however, caution should be observed before administering Hetastarch to patients with a history of liver disease.

Regular and frequent clinical evaluation and laboratory determinations are necessary for proper monitoring of Hetastarch use during leukapheresis. Studies should include CBC, total leukocyte and platelet counts, leukocyte differential count, hemoglobin, hematocrit, prothrombin time (PT), and partial thromboplastin time (PTT).

Hetastarch is nonantigenic. However, allergic or sensitivity reactions have been reported (see **Adverse Reactions**). If such reactions occur, they are readily controlled by discontinuation of the drug and, if necessary, administration of an antihistaminic agent.

ADVERSE REACTIONS

The following have been reported: vomiting, mild temperature elevation, chills, itching, submaxillary and parotid glandular enlargement, mild influenza-like symptoms, headaches, muscle pains, peripheral edema of the lower extremities, and anaphylactoid reactions consisting of periorbital edema, urticaria, and wheezing.

DOSAGE AND ADMINISTRATION

Dosage in Plasma Volume Expansion: Hetastarch is administered by intravenous infusion only. Total dosage and rate of infusion depend upon the amount of blood lost and the resultant hemoconcentration. In adults, the amount usually administered is 500 to 1000 mL. Total dosage does not usually exceed 1500 mL per day or approximately 20 mL per kg of body weight for the typical 70 kg patient. In acute hemorrhagic shock, an administration rate approaching 20 mL per kg per hour may be used; in burn or septic shock it is usually administered at slower rates.

Dosage in Leukapheresis: In continuous-flow centrifugation (CFC) procedures, 250 to 700 mL Hetastarch is typically infused at a constant fixed ratio, usually 1:8, to venous whole blood.

Multiple CFC procedures using Hetastarch of up to 2 per week and a total of 7 to 10 have been reported to be safe and effective. Adequate data are not available to establish the safety of more frequent or a greater number of procedures.

HOW SUPPLIED

NDC **0094-0037-05-Hespan®** (6% Hetastarch in 0.9% Sodium Chloride Injection) is supplied sterile and nonpyrogenic in 500 mL intravenous infusion bottles.

INTROPIN® ℞

[*in-trō'pin*]

(dopamine HCl injection, USP) 5 mL VIAL and RAP-ADD® Syringe—
200 mg, 400 mg and 800 mg
5 mL AMPUL—200 mg

DESCRIPTION

INTROPIN (dopamine HCl injection, USP) is a clear, practically colorless, aqueous, additive solution for intravenous infusion after dilution. Each mL contains either 40 mg, 80 mg or 160 mg dopamine hydrochloride, USP (equivalent to 32.3 mg, 64.6 mg and 129.2 mg dopamine base, respectively) in Water for Injection, USP containing 1% sodium bisulfite as an antioxidant. Hydrochloric acid or sodium hydroxide added to adjust pH when necessary. The solution is sterile and non-pyrogenic. The pH is 2.5-4.5. INTROPIN, a naturally-occurring catecholamine, is an inotropic vasopressor agent. Its chemical name is 3,4 dihydroxyphenethylamine hydrochloride.

INTROPIN is sensitive to alkalis, iron salts and oxidizing agents. **It must be diluted in an appropriate, sterile parenteral solution** (see Dosage and Administration section) **before intravenous administration.**

ACTIONS

INTROPIN exerts an inotropic effect on the myocardium resulting in an increased cardiac output. INTROPIN produces less increase in myocardial oxygen consumption than isoproterenol and its use is usually not associated with a tachyarrhythmia. Clinical studies indicate that INTROPIN usually increases systolic and pulse pressure with either no effect or a slight increase in diastolic pressure. Total peripheral resistance at low and intermediate therapeutic doses is usually unchanged. Blood flow to peripheral vascular beds may decrease while mesenteric flow increases. INTROPIN has also been reported to dilate the renal vasculature presumptively by activation of a "dopaminergic" receptor. This action is accompanied by increases in glomerular filtration rate, renal blood flow, and sodium excretion. An increase in urinary output produced by dopamine is usually not associated with a decrease in osmolality of the urine.

INDICATIONS

INTROPIN is indicated for the correction of hemodynamic imbalances present in the shock syndrome due to myocardial infarctions, trauma, endotoxic septicemia, open heart surgery, renal failure, and chronic cardiac decompensation as in congestive failure.

Where appropriate, restoration of blood volume with a suitable plasma expander or whole blood should be instituted or completed prior to administration of INTROPIN.

Patients most likely to respond adequately to INTROPIN are those in whom physiological parameters, such as urine flow, myocardial function, and blood pressure, have not undergone profound deterioration. Multiclinic trials indicate that the shorter the time interval between onset of signs and symptoms and initiation of therapy with volume correction and INTROPIN, the better the prognosis.

Poor Perfusion of Vital Organs—Urine flow appears to be one of the better diagnostic signs by which adequacy of vital organ perfusion can be monitored. Nevertheless, the physician should also observe the patient for signs of reversal of confusion or comatose condition. Loss of pallor, increase in toe temperature, and/or adequacy of nail bed capillary filling may also be used as indices of adequate dosage. Clinical studies have shown that when INTROPIN is administered before urine flow has diminished to levels approximately 0.3 mL/minute, prognosis is more favorable. Nevertheless, in a number of oliguric or anuric patients, administration of INTROPIN has resulted in an increase in urine flow which in some cases reached normal levels. INTROPIN may also increase urine flow in patients whose output is within normal limits and thus may be of value in reducing the degree of preexisting fluid accumulation. It should be noted that at doses above those optimal for the individual patient, urine flow may decrease, necessitating reduction of dosage. Concurrent administration of INTROPIN and diuretic agents may produce an additive or potentiating effect.

Low Cardiac Output—Increased cardiac output is related to INTROPIN's direct inotropic effect on the myocardium. Increased cardiac output at low or moderate doses appears to be related to a favorable prognosis. Increase in cardiac output has been associated with either static or decreased systemic vascular resistance (SVR). Static or decreased SVR associated with low or moderate increments in cardiac output is believed to be a reflection of differential effects on specific vascular beds with increased resistance in peripheral beds (e.g. femoral) and concomitant decreases in mesenteric and renal vascular beds. Redistribution of blood flow parallels these changes so that an increase in cardiac output is accompanied by an increase in mesenteric and renal blood flow. In many instances the renal fraction of the total cardiac output has been found to increase. Increase in cardiac output produced by INTROPIN is not associated with substantial decreases in systemic vascular resistance as may occur with isoproterenol.

Hypotension—Hypotension due to inadequate cardiac output can be managed by administration of low to moderate doses of INTROPIN, which have little effect on SVR. At high therapeutic doses, INTROPIN's alpha adrenergic activity becomes more prominent and thus may correct hypotension due to diminished SVR. As in the case of other circulatory decompensation states, prognosis is better in patients whose blood pressure and urine flow have not undergone profound deterioration. Therefore, it is suggested that the physician administer INTROPIN as soon as a definite trend toward decreased systolic and diastolic pressure becomes evident.

CONTRAINDICATIONS

INTROPIN should not be used in patients with pheochromocytoma.

WARNINGS

INTROPIN should not be administered in the presence of uncorrected tachyarrhythmias or ventricular fibrillation.

Do **NOT** add INTROPIN to any alkaline diluent solution, since the drug is inactivated in alkaline solution.

Patients who have been treated with monoamine oxidase (MAO) inhibitors prior to the administration of INTROPIN will require substantially reduced dosage. Dopamine is metabolized by MAO, and inhibition of this enzyme prolongs and potentiates the effect of INTROPIN. The starting dose in such patients should be reduced to at least one-tenth ($\frac{1}{10}$) of the usual dose.

Usage in Pregnancy—Animal studies have revealed no evidence of teratogenic effects from INTROPIN. In one study, administration of INTROPIN to pregnant rats resulted in a decreased survival rate of the newborn and a potential for cataract formation in the survivors. The drug may be used in pregnant women when, in the judgment of the physician, the expected benefits outweigh the potential risk to the fetus.

Usage in Children—The safety and efficacy of this drug in children has not been established. INTROPIN has been used in a limited number of pediatric patients, but such use has been inadequate to fully define proper dosage and limitations for use. Further studies are in progress.

PRECAUTIONS

Avoid Hypovolemia—Prior to treatment with INTROPIN, hypovolemia should be fully corrected, if possible, with either whole blood or plasma as indicated.

Decreased Pulse Pressure—If a disproportionate rise in the diastolic pressure (i.e., a marked decrease in the pulse pressure) is observed in patients receiving INTROPIN, the infusion rate should be decreased and the patient observed carefully for further evidence of predominant vasoconstrictor activity, unless such an effect is desired.

Extravasation—INTROPIN should be infused into a large vein whenever possible to prevent the possibility of extravasation into tissue adjacent to the infusion site. Extravasation may cause necrosis and sloughing of surrounding tissue. Large veins of the antecubital fossa are preferred to veins in the dorsum of the hand or ankle. Less suitable infusion sites should be used only if the patient's condition requires immediate attention. The physician should switch to more suitable sites as rapidly as possible. The infusion site should be continuously monitored for free flow.

Occlusive Vascular Disease—Patients with a history of occlusive vascular disease (for example, atherosclerosis, arterial embolism, Raynaud's disease, cold injury, diabetic endarteritis, and Buerger's disease) should be closely monitored for any changes in color or temperature of the skin in the extremities. If a change in skin color or temperature occurs and is thought to be the result of compromised circulation to the extremities, the benefits of continued INTROPIN infusion should be weighed against the risk of possible necrosis. This condition may be reversed by either decreasing or discontinuing the rate of infusion.

> **IMPORTANT—Antidote for Peripheral Ischemia: To prevent sloughing and necrosis in ischemic areas, the area should be infiltrated as soon as possible with 10 to 15 mL. of saline solution containing from 5 to 10 mg. of Regitine® (brand of phentolamine), an adrenergic blocking agent. A syringe with a fine hypodermic needle should be used, and the solution liberally infiltrated throughout the ischemic area. Sympathetic blockade with phentolamine causes immediate and conspicuous local hyperemic changes if the area is infiltrated within 12 hours. Therefore, phentolamine should be given as soon as possible after the extravasation is noted.**

Avoid Cyclopropane or Halogenated Hydrocarbon Anesthetics—Cyclopropane or halogenated hydrocarbon anesthetics increase cardiac autonomic irritability and therefore may sensitize the myocardium to the action of certain intravenously administered catecholamines. This interaction appears to be related both to pressor activity and to beta adrenergic stimulating properties of these catecholamines. Therefore, as with certain other catecholamines, and because of the theoretical arrhythmogenic potential, INTROPIN should be used with EXTREME CAUTION in patients inhaling cyclopropane or halogenated hydrocarbon anesthetics.

Careful Monitoring Required—Close monitoring of the following indices—urine flow, cardiac output and blood pressure—during INTROPIN infusion is necessary as in the case of any adrenergic agent.

ADVERSE REACTIONS

The most frequent adverse reactions observed in clinical evaluation of INTROPIN included ectopic beats, nausea, vomiting, tachycardia, anginal pain, palpitation, dyspnea, headache, hypotension, and vasoconstriction. Other adverse reactions which have been reported infrequently were aberrant conduction, bradycardia, piloerection, widened QRS complex, azotemia, and elevated blood pressure.

DOSAGE AND ADMINISTRATION

WARNING: This is a potent drug: It must be diluted before administration to patient.

Suggested Dilution—Transfer contents of one or more ampuls, vials or additive syringes by aseptic technique to either a 250 mL or 500 mL bottle of one of the following sterile intravenous solutions:

1) Sodium Chloride Injection, USP
2) Dextrose (5%) Injection, USP
3) Dextrose (5%) and Sodium Chloride (0.9%) Injection, USP
4) Dextrose (5%) in Sodium Chloride (0.45%) Solution
5) Dextrose (5%) in Lactated Ringer's Solution
6) Sodium Lactate (1/6 Molar) Injection, USP
7) Lactated Ringer's Injection, USP

INTROPIN has been found to be stable for a minimum of 24 hours after dilution in the sterile intravenous solutions listed above. However, as with all intravenous admixtures, dilution should be made just prior to administration.

Do **NOT** add INTROPIN to 5% Sodium Bicarbonate or other alkaline intravenous solutions, since the drug is inactivated in alkaline solution.

Rate of Administration—INTROPIN, after dilution, is administered intravenously through a suitable intravenous catheter or needle. An i.v. drip chamber or other suitable metering device is essential for controlling the rate of flow in drops/minute. Each patient must be individually titrated to the desired hemodynamic and/or renal response with INTROPIN. In titrating to the desired increase in systolic blood pressure, the optimum dosage rate for renal response may be exceeded, thus necessitating a reduction in rate after the hemodynamic condition is stablized.

Administration at rates greater than 50 mcg/kg/min has safely been used in advanced circulatory decompensation states. If unnecessary fluid expansion is of concern, adjustment of drug concentration may be preferred over increasing the flow rate of a less concentrated dilution.

Suggested Regimen:

1. When appropriate, increase blood volume with whole blood or plasma until central venous pressure is 10 to 15 cm H_2O or pulmonary wedge pressure is 14–18 mm Hg.
2. Begin administration of diluted solution at doses of 2–5 mcg/kg/minute INTROPIN in patients who are likely to respond to modest increments of heart force and renal perfusion. In more seriously ill patients, begin administration of diluted solution at doses of 5 mcg/kg/minute INTROPIN and increase gradually using 5 to 10 mcg/kg/minute increments up to 20 to 50 mcg/kg/minute as needed. If doses of INTROPIN in excess of 50 mcg/kg/minute are required, it is suggested that urine output be checked frequently. Should urine flow begin to decrease in the absence of hypotension, reduction of INTROPIN dosage should be considered. Multiclinic trials have shown that more than 50% of the patients were satisfactorily maintained on doses of INTROPIN less than 20 mcg/kg/minute. In patients who do not respond to these doses with adequate arterial pressures or urine flow, additional increments of INTROPIN may be employed in an effort to produce an appropriate arterial pressure and central perfusion.
3. Treatment of all patients requires constant evaluation of therapy in terms of the blood volume, augmentation of myocardial contractility, and distribution of peripheral perfusion. Dosage of INTROPIN should be adjusted according to the patient's response, with particular attention to diminution of established urine flow rate, increasing tachycardia or development of new dysrhythmias as indices for decreasing or temporarily suspending the dosage.
4. As with all potent intravenously administered drugs, care should be taken to control the rate of administration so as to avoid inadvertent administration of a bolus of drug.

OVERDOSAGE

In case of accidental overdosage, as evidenced by excessive blood pressure elevation, reduce rate of administration or temporarily discontinue INTROPIN until patient's condition stabilizes. Since INTROPIN's duration of action is quite short, no additional remedial measures are usually necessary. If these measures fail to stabilize the patient's condition, use of the short-acting alpha adrenergic blocking agent, phentolamine, should be considered.

HOW SUPPLIED

—200 mg (5 mL containing 40 mg dopamine HCl, USP per mL)
5 mL Ampul
5 mL Single-dose vial (color coded white)
5 mL RAP-ADD® Additive Syringe (color coded white)
—400 mg (5 mL containing 80 mg dopamine HCl, USP per mL)
5 mL Single-dose vial (color coded green)
5 mL RAP-ADD® Additive Syringe (color coded green)
—800 mg (5 mL containing 160 mg dopamine HCl, USP per mL)
5 mL Single-dose vial (color coded yellow)
5 mL RAP-ADD® Additive Syringe (color coded yellow)

WARNING

NOT FOR DIRECT INTRAVENOUS INJECTION. MUST BE DILUTED BEFORE USE.

TRIDIL® ℞

[tri 'dil]
(nitroglycerin)

FOR INTRAVENOUS USE ONLY. NOT FOR DIRECT INTRAVENOUS INJECTION. TRIDIL® MUST BE DILUTED IN DEXTROSE (5%) INJECTION, USP OR SODIUM CHLORIDE (0.9%) INJECTION, USP PRIOR TO ITS INFUSION (SEE DOSAGE AND ADMINISTRATION SECTION). THE ADMINISTRATION SET USED FOR INFUSION WILL AFFECT THE AMOUNT OF TRIDIL DELIVERED TO THE PATIENT. (SEE WARNINGS, AND DOSAGE AND ADMINISTRATION SECTIONS).

Caution SEVERAL PREPARATIONS OF NITROGLYCERIN FOR INJECTION ARE AVAILABLE. THEY DIFFER IN CONCENTRATION AND/OR VOLUME PER VIAL. WHEN SWITCHING FROM ONE PRODUCT TO ANOTHER ATTENTION MUST BE PAID TO THE DILUTION AND DOSAGE AND ADMINISTRATION INSTRUCTIONS.

DESCRIPTION

TRIDIL (nitroglycerin) is a clear, practically colorless additive solution for intravenous infusion after dilution. Each mL of TRIDIL 5 mg contains 0.5 mg Nitroglycerin with 4.5 mg Lactose, USP; 10% Alcohol, USP; and 13.8 mg Monobasic Sodium Phosphate, USP as a buffer in Water for Injection, USP. Each mL of TRIDIL 25 mg or TRIDIL 50 mg contains 5 mg Nitroglycerin in 30% Alcohol, USP; 30% Propylene Glycol, USP; and Water for Injection, USP.

The solution is sterile, nonpyrogenic, and nonexplosive. TRIDIL, an organic nitrate, is a vasodilator. The chemical name for nitroglycerin is 1,2,3 propanetriol, trinitrate and its chemical structure is:

$$\begin{array}{l} CH_2 - ONO_2 \\ | \\ CH - ONO_2 \\ | \\ CH_2 - ONO_2 \end{array}$$

$C_3H_5N_3O_9$ MOL. WT. 227.09

CLINICAL PHARMACOLOGY

Relaxation of vascular smooth muscle is the principal pharmacologic action of TRIDIL (nitroglycerin). Although venous effects predominate, nitroglycerin produces, in a dose-related manner, dilation of both arterial and venous beds. Dilation of the post-capillary vessels, including large veins, promotes peripheral pooling of blood and decreases venous return to the heart, reducing left ventricular end-diastolic pressure (pre-load). Arteriolar relaxation reduces systemic vascular resistance and arterial pressure (afterload). Myocardial oxygen consumption or demand (as measured by the pressure-rate product, tension-time index and stroke work index) is decreased by both the arterial and venous effects of nitroglycerin, and a more favorable supply-demand ratio can be achieved. Therapeutic doses of intravenous nitroglycerin reduce systolic, diastolic and mean arterial blood pressure. Effective coronary perfusion pressure is usually maintained, but can be compromised if blood pressure falls excessively or increased heart rate decreases diastolic filling time.

Elevated central venous and pulmonary capillary wedge pressures, pulmonary vascular resistance and systemic vascular resistance are also reduced by nitroglycerin therapy. Heart rate is usually slightly increased, presumably a reflex response to the fall in blood pressure. Cardiac index may be increased, decreased, or unchanged. Patients with elevated left ventricular filling pressure and systemic vascular resistance values in conjunction with a depressed cardiac index are likely to experience an improvement in cardiac index. On the other hand, when filling pressures and cardiac index are normal, cardiac index may be slightly reduced by intravenous nitroglycerin.

Nitroglycerin is widely distributed in the body with an apparent volume of distribution of approximately 200 liters in adult male subjects, and is rapidly metabolized to dinitrates and mononitrates, with a short half-life estimated at 1–4 minutes. This results in a low plasma concentration after intravenous infusion. At plasma concentrations of between 50 and 500 ng/ml, the binding of nitroglycerin to plasma proteins is approximately 60%, while that of 1,2 dinitroglycerin and 1,3 dinitroglycerin is 60% and 30% respectively. The activity and half-life of the dinitroglycerin metabolites are not well characterized. The mononitrate is not active.

INDICATIONS AND USAGE

TRIDIL is indicated for:

1. **Control of blood pressure in perioperative hypertension,** i.e., hypertension associated with surgical procedures, especially cardiovascular procedures, such as the hypertension seen during intratracheal intubation, anesthesia, skin incision, sternotomy, cardiac bypass, and in the immediate postsurgical period.
2. **Congestive Heart Failure Associated with Acute Myocardial Infarction.**
3. **Treatment of Angina Pectoris** in patients who have not responded to recommended doses of organic nitrates and/or a beta blocker.
4. **Production of controlled hypotension during surgical procedures.**

CONTRAINDICATIONS

TRIDIL should not be administered to individuals with:

1. A known hypersensitivity to nitroglycerin or a known idiosyncratic reaction to organic nitrates.
2. Hypotension or uncorrected hypovolemia, as the use of TRIDIL in such states could produce severe hypotension or shock.
3. Increased intracranial pressure (e.g., head trauma or cerebral hemorrhage).
4. Constrictive pericarditis and pericardial tamponade.

WARNINGS

1. Nitroglycerin readily migrates into many plastics. To avoid absorption of nitroglycerin into plastic parenteral solution containers, the dilution and storage of TRIDIL for intravenous infusion should be made only in *glass* parenteral solution bottles.
2. Some filters absorb nitroglycerin; they should be avoided.
3. Forty to 80% of the total amount of nitroglycerin in the final diluted solution for infusion is absorbed by the polyvinyl chloride (PVC) tubing of the intravenous administration sets currently in general use. The higher rates of absorption occur when flow rates are low, nitroglycerin concentrations are high, and the administration set is long. Although the rate of loss is highest during the early phase of infusion (when flow rates are lowest) the loss is neither constant nor self-limiting; consequently no simple calculation or correction can be performed to convert the theoretical infusion rate (based on the concentration of the infusion solution) to the actual delivery rate.

Because of this problem, American Critical Care has developed TRIDILSET® i.v. administration set and TRIDILSET V.I.P.® volumetric infusion pump connector set in which loss of TRIDIL is minimal. TRIDILSET or TRIDILSET V.I.P. are recommended for infusions of TRIDIL (see DOSAGE AND ADMINISTRATION).

DOSING INSTRUCTIONS MUST BE FOLLOWED WITH CARE. IT SHOULD BE NOTED THAT WHEN TRIDILSET/TRIDILSET V.I.P. IS USED, THE CALCULATED DOSE WILL BE DELIVERED TO THE PATIENT BECAUSE THE LOSS OF TRIDIL DUE TO ABSORPTION IN STANDARD PVC TUBING WILL BE KEPT TO A MINIMUM. NOTE THAT THE DOSAGES COMMONLY USED IN PUBLISHED STUDIES UTILIZED GENERAL-USE PVC ADMINISTRATION SETS AND RECOMMENDED DOSES BASED ON THIS EXPERIENCE ARE TOO HIGH WHEN TRIDILSET/TRIDILSET V.I.P. IS USED.

PRECAUTIONS

TRIDIL (nitroglycerin) should be used with caution in patients with severe liver or renal disease. Safety of intracoronary injection of this preparation has not been shown.

Excessive hypotension, especially for prolonged periods of time, must be avoided because of possible deleterious effects on the brain, heart, liver, and kidney from poor perfusion and the attendant risk of ischemia, thrombosis, and altered function of these organs. Paradoxical bradycardia and increased angina pectoris may accompany nitroglycerin-induced hypotension. Patients with normal or low pulmonary capillary wedge pressure are especially sensitive to the hypotensive effects of TRIDIL. If pulmonary capillary wedge pressure is being monitored, it will be noted that a fall in wedge pressure precedes the onset of arterial hypotension, and the

Continued on next page

American Critical—Cont.

pulmonary capillary wedge pressure is thus a useful guide to safe titration of the drug.

Carcinogenesis, mutagenesis, impairment of fertility

No long-term studies in animals were performed to evaluate carcinogenic potential of TRIDIL.

Pregnancy

Category C. Animal reproduction studies have not been conducted with TRIDIL. It is also not known whether TRIDIL can cause fetal harm when administered to a pregnant woman or can affect reproduction capacity. TRIDIL should be given to a pregnant woman only if clearly needed.

Nursing Mothers

It is not known whether nitroglycerin is excreted in human milk. Because many drugs are excreted in human milk, caution should be exercised when TRIDIL is administered to a nursing woman.

Pediatric Use

The safety and effectiveness of TRIDIL in children have not been established.

ADVERSE REACTIONS

The most frequent adverse reaction in patients treated with TRIDIL is headache, which occurs in approximately 2% of patients. Other adverse reactions occuring in less than 1% of patients are the following: tachycardia, nausea, vomiting, apprehension, restlessness, muscle twitching, retrosternal discomfort, palpitations, dizziness and abdominal pain.

The following additional adverse reactions have been reported with the oral and/or topical use of nitroglycerin: cutaneous flushing, weakness and occasionally drug rash or exfoliative dermatitis.

OVERDOSAGE

Accidental overdosage of TRIDIL may result in severe hypotension and reflex tachycardia which can be treated by elevating the legs and decreasing or temporarily terminating the infusion until the patient's condition stabilizes. Since the duration of the hemodynamic effects following TRIDIL administration is quite short, additional corrective measures are usually not required. However, if further therapy is indicated, administration of an intravenous alpha adrenergic agonist (e.g. methoxamine or phenylephrine) should be considered.

DOSAGE AND ADMINISTRATION

NOT FOR DIRECT INTRAVENOUS INJECTION

TRIDIL IS A CONCENTRATED, POTENT DRUG WHICH MUST BE DILUTED IN DEXTROSE (5%) INJECTION, USP OR SODIUM CHLORIDE (0.9%) INJECTION, USP PRIOR TO ITS INFUSION. TRIDIL SHOULD NOT BE ADMIXED WITH OTHER DRUGS.

1. Initial Dilution:

Aseptically transfer the contents of one TRIDIL ampul or vial (containing 25 or 50 mg of nitroglycerin) into a 500 mL *glass* bottle of either Dextrose (5%) Injection, USP or Sodium Chloride Injection (0.9%), USP. This yields a final concentration of 50 or 100 mcg/mL. Diluting 5 mg TRIDIL into 100 mL will also yield a final concentration of 50 mcg/mL.

2. Maintenance Dilution:

It is important to consider the fluid requirements of the patient as well as the expected duration of infusion in selecting the appropriate dilution of TRIDIL.

After the initial dosage titration, the concentration of the admixture solution may be increased, if necessary, to limit fluids given to the patient. The TRIDIL concentration should not exceed 400 mcg/mL. See chart.

[See table below].

Note: If the concentration is adjusted, it is imperative to flush TRIDILSET®/TRIDILSET VIP® before a new concentration is utilized. The dead-space of the set is approximately 15 mL, and depending on the flow rate it could take from 10 minutes to 3 hours for the new concentration to reach the patient if the set were not flushed.

Invert the glass parenteral bottle several times following admixture to assure uniform dilution of TRIDIL. When stored in *glass* containers, the diluted solution is physically and chemically stable for up to 48 hours at room temperature, and up to seven days under refrigeration.

Dosage is affected by the type of container and administration set used. See WARNINGS.

Although the usual starting adult dose range reported in clinical studies was 25 mcg/min or more, these studies used PVC ADMINISTRATION SETS. THE USE OF NON-ABSORBING TUBING WILL RESULT IN THE NEED FOR REDUCED DOSES.

If a peristaltic action infusion pump is used, a TRIDILSET i.v. administration set should be selected. As the TRIDILSET drip chamber delivers approximately 60 microdrops/mL, the TRIDIL DILUTION AND ADMINISTRATION TABLE may be used to calculate TRIDIL dilution and admixture flow rate in microdrops/minute to achieve the desired TRIDIL administration rate. If a volumetric infusion pump is used, a TRIDILSET V.I.P. volumetric infusion pump connector set should be selected. The TRIDIL DILUTION AND ADMINISTRATION TABLE may still be used; however, admixture flow rate will be determined directly by the infusion pump and is independent of the drop size of the TRIDILSET V.I.P. drip chamber, which is approximately 15 drops/mL. Thus, the reference to "MICRODROPS/MIN" is not applicable and the corresponding flow rate in ML/HR should be used to determine pump settings. NOTE: the TRIDILSET V.I.P. is not intended for use as an i.v. administration set independent of a volumetric infusion pump.

The dosage for TRIDILSET/TRIDILSET VIP should initially be 5 mcg/min delivered through an infusion pump capable of exact and constant delivery of the drug. Subsequent titration must be adjusted to the clinical situation, with dose increments becoming more cautious as partial response is seen. Initial titration should be in 5 mcg/min increments with increases every 3–5 minutes until some response is noted. If no response is seen at 20 mcg/min, increments of 10 and later 20 mcg/min can be used. Once a partial blood pressure response is observed, the dose increase should be reduced and the interval between increases should be lengthened. Some patients with normal or low left ventricular filling pressures or pulmonary capillary wedge pressure (e.g. angina patients without other complications) may be hypersensitive to the effects of TRIDIL and may respond fully to doses as small as 5 mcg/min. These patients require especially careful titration and monitoring.

There is no fixed optimum dose of TRIDIL. Due to variations in the responsiveness of individual patients to the drug, each patient must be titrated to the desired level of hemodynamic function. Therefore, continuous monitoring of physiologic parameters (e.g. blood pressure and heart rate in all patients, other measurement such as pulmonary capillary wedge pressure, as appropriate MUST BE PERFORMED to achieve the correct dose. Adequate systemic blood pressure and coronary perfusion pressure must be maintained.

HOW SUPPLIED

NDC 0094-0073-10, 5 mg-10 mL ampul.
NDC 0094-0085-05, 25 mg-5 mL ampul.
NDC 0094-0085-86, 25 mg-5 mL single use vial.
NDC 0094-0090-10, 50 mg-10 mL ampul.
NDC 0094-0090-66, 50 mg-10 mL single use vial.

Protect from freezing.

American Dermal Corporation

12 WORLDS FAIR DRIVE
SOMERSET, NJ 08873

DRITHOCREME® ℞

(anthralin) 0.1%, 0.25%, 0.5%, 1.0% (HP)

DESCRIPTION

Drithocreme is a pale yellow topical cream containing 0.1%, 0.25%, 0.5% or 1.0% (HP) anthralin USP in a base of white petrolatum, sodium lauryl sulfate, cetostearyl alcohol, ascorbic acid, salicylic acid, chlorocresol and purified water. The chemical name of anthralin is 1,8,dihydroxy-9-anthrone or 1,8,9-trihydroxyanthracene.

CLINICAL PHARMACOLOGY

Although the precise mechanism of anthralin's anti-psoriatic action is not fully understood, in vitro evidence suggests that its antimitotic effect results from inhibition of DNA synthesis. Additionally, the chemically reducing properties of anthralin may upset oxidative metabolic processes, providing a further slowing down of epidermal mitosis.

Absorption in man has not been finally determined, but in a limited clinical study of Drithocreme, no traces of anthraquinone metabolites were detected in the urine of subjects treated. However, caution is advised in patients with renal disease.

INDICATIONS AND USAGE

An aid in the topical treatment of quiescent or chronic psoriasis. Treatment should be continued until the skin is entirely clear i.e. when there is nothing to feel with the fingers and the texture is normal.

CONTRAINDICATIONS

In patients with acute or actively inflamed psoriatic eruptions, or a history of hypersensitivity to any of the ingredients.

WARNINGS

Avoid contact with the eyes or mucous membranes. Exercise care when applying Drithocreme to the face or intertriginous skin areas, and do not use high strengths in these sites. Discontinue use if a sensitivity reaction occurs or if excessive irritation develops on uninvolved skin areas.

PRECAUTIONS

For external use only. Keep out of the reach of children. To prevent the possibility of staining clothing or bed linen while gaining experience in using Drithocreme, it may be advisable to use protective dressings. To prevent the possibility of discoloration of the bath/shower, particularly where Drithocreme HP (1.0%) has been used, always rinse the bath/-shower with hot water immediately after washing/showering and then use a suitable cleanser to remove any deposit on the surface of the bath or shower. Contact with fabrics, plastics and other materials may cause staining and should be avoided. Always wash hands thoroughly after use. Long-term studies in animals have not been performed to evaluate the carcinogenic potential of the drug. Although anthralin has been found to have tumor-promoting properties on mouse skin, there have been no reports to suggest carcinogenic effects in humans after many years of clinical use.

TRIDIL DILUTION AND ADMINISTRATION TABLE

	DILUTE			
	5 MG TRIDIL IN 100 ML OR 25 MG TRIDIL IN 500 ML	5 MG TRIDIL IN 50 ML OR 25 MG TRIDIL IN 250 ML OR 50 MG TRIDIL IN 500 ML	10 MG TRIDIL IN 50 ML OR 50 MG TRIDIL IN 250 ML OR 100 MG TRIDIL IN 500 ML	100 MG TRIDIL IN 250 ML OR 200 MG TRIDIL IN 500 ML
	TO YIELD			
	50 MCG/ML	100 MCG/ML	200 MCG/ML	400 MCG/ML
TRIDILSET ADMIXTURE FLOW RATE MICRO DROPS/ MIN=ML/HR	TRIDIL ADMINISTRATION RATE MCG I.V. NITROGLYCERIN/MIN			
3	—	5	10	20
6	5	10	20	40
12	10	20	40	80
24	20	40	80	160
48	40	80	160	320
72	60	120	240	480
96	80	160	320	640

PREGNANCY
Pregnancy Category C. Animal reproduction studies have not been conducted with Drithocreme. It is also not known whether Drithocreme can cause fetal harm when administered to a pregnant woman or can affect reproduction capacity. Drithocreme should be given to a pregnant woman only if clearly needed.

NURSING MOTHERS
It is not known whether this drug is excreted in human milk. Because many drugs are excreted in milk and because of the potential for tumorigenicity shown for anthralin in animal studies, a decision should be made whether to discontinue nursing or to discontinue the drug, taking into account the importance of the drug to the mother.

PEDIATRIC USE
Safety and effectiveness in children have not been specifically established.

ADVERSE REACTIONS
Very few instances of contact allergic reactions to anthralin have been reported. However, transient primary irritation of normal skin or uninvolved skin surrounding the treated lesions is more frequently seen. If the initial treatment produces excessive soreness or if the lesions spread, reduce frequency of application and, in extreme cases, discontinue use and consult physician. Some temporary discoloration of hair and fingernails may arise during the period of treatment but should be minimized by careful application. Drithocreme may stain skin, hair or fabrics.

DOSAGE AND ADMINISTRATION
Generally, it is recommended that Drithocreme be applied once a day. The irritant potential of anthralin is directly related to the strength being used and each patient's individual tolerance. Therefore, where the response to anthralin treatment has not previously been established, always commence treatment for at least one week using 0.1% Drithocreme. Increase to the 0.25%, 0.5% or 1.0% (HP) strengths if appropriate. To open the tube, unscrew the cap and invert to pierce membrane.
Drithocreme should normally be applied once daily and removed by washing or showering. The optimal period of contact will vary according to the strength used and the patient's response to treatment.
For The Skin: Apply sparingly only to the psoriatic lesions and rub gently and carefully into the skin until absorbed. It is most important to avoid applying an excessive quantity which may cause unnecessary soiling and staining of the clothing and/or bed linen. At the end of each period of treatment, a bath or shower should be taken to remove any surplus cream which may have become red/brown in color. The margins of the lesions may gradually become stained purple/brown as treatment progresses, but this will disappear after cessation of treatment.
For The Scalp: Comb the hair to remove scalar debris and, after suitably parting, rub the cream well into the lesions. Keep Drithocreme away from the eyes. Care should be taken to avoid application of the cream to uninvolved scalp margins. Remove any unintended residue which may be deposited behind the ears. At the end of each period of contact, wash the hair and scalp to remove any surplus cream (which may have become red/brown in color).
Keep tightly capped when not in use.
Store in a cool place (46°–59°F)

HOW SUPPLIED
50g tubes
Drithocreme 0.1% NDC 51201-0029-1
Drithocreme 0.25% NDC 51201-0028-1
Drithocreme 0.5% NDC 51201-0027-1
Drithocreme HP 1.0% NDC 51201-0026-1

CAUTION
Federal law prohibits dispensing without prescription.
Revised 5/86
AMERICAN DERMAL CORPORATION
Somerset, New Jersey 08873

DRITHO-SCALP® ℞
(anthralin) 0.25%, 0.5%

DESCRIPTION
Dritho-Scalp is a pale yellow topical cream containing 0.25% or 0.5% anthralin USP in a base of white petrolatum, mineral oil, sodium lauryl sulfate, cetostearyl alcohol, ascorbic acid, salicylic acid, chlorocresol and purified water.
The chemical name of anthralin is 1,8,dihydroxy-9-anthrone.

CLINICAL PHARMACOLOGY
Although the precise mechanism of anthralin's anti-psoriatic action is not fully understood, in vitro evidence suggests that its antimitotic effect results from inhibition of DNA synthesis. Additionally, the chemically reducing properties of anthralin may upset oxidative metabolic processes, providing a further slowing down of epidermal mitosis.
Absorption in man has not been finally determined.

INDICATIONS AND USAGE
An aid in the topical treatment of quiescent or chronic psoriasis of the scalp. Treatment should be continued until the skin is entirely clear i.e. when there is nothing to feel with the fingers and the texture is normal.

CONTRAINDICATIONS
In patients with acute or actively inflamed psoriatic eruptions or a history of hypersensitivity to any of the ingredients.

WARNINGS
Avoid contact with the eyes or mucous membranes. Discontinue use if a sensitivity reaction occurs or if excessive irritation develops on uninvolved skin areas.

PRECAUTIONS
For external use only. Keep out of the reach of children. Dritho-Scalp may stain the hair and should be applied sparingly and carefully to psoriasis lesions only. Contact with fabrics, plastics and other materials may cause staining and should be avoided. To prevent the possibility of discoloration, always rinse the bath/shower with hot water immediately after washing/showering and then use a suitable cleanser to remove any deposit on the surface of the bath or shower. Always wash hands thoroughly after use. Long-term studies in animals have not been performed to evaluate the carcinogenic potential of the drug. Although anthralin has been found to have tumor-promoting properties on mouse skin, there have been no reports to suggest carcinogenic effects in humans after many years of clinical use.
Pregnancy: Pregnancy Category C. Animal reproduction studies have not been conducted with Dritho-Scalp. It is also not known whether Dritho-Scalp can cause fetal harm when administered to a pregnant woman or can affect reproduction capacity. Dritho-Scalp should be given to a pregnant woman only if clearly needed.
Nursing Mothers: It is not known whether this drug is excreted in human milk. Because many drugs are excreted in milk and because of the potential for tumorigenicity shown for anthralin in animal studies, a decision should be made whether to discontinue nursing or to discontinue the drug, taking into account the importance of the drug to the mother.
Pediatric Use: Safety and effectiveness in children have not been specifically established.

ADVERSE REACTIONS
Very few instances of contact allergic reactions to anthralin have been reported. However, transient primary irritation of normal skin or uninvolved skin surrounding the treated lesions is more frequently seen. If the initial treatment produces excessive soreness or if the lesions spread, reduce frequency of application and, in extreme cases, discontinue use and consult physician. Some temporary discoloration of hair and fingernails may arise during the period of treatment but should be minimized by careful application. Dritho-Scalp may stain skin, hair or fabrics.

DOSAGE AND ADMINISTRATION
Before initial use, the tube membrane should be pierced by inverting the white cap, which should then be discarded. The black applicator should then be screwed firmly onto the tube. This applicator includes a black cap which should always be replaced between treatments. Generally, it is recommended that Dritho-Scalp be applied once a day. The irritant potential of anthralin is directly related to the strength being used and each patient's individual tolerance. Therefore, where the response to anthralin treatment has not previously been established, always commence treatment for at least one week using 0.25% Dritho-Scalp. Increase to the 0.5% strength only if appropriate.
Dritho-Scalp should normally be applied once daily and removed by washing or showering. The optimal period of contact will vary according to the strength used and the patient's response to treatment.
Comb the hair to remove scalar debris and, after suitably parting, apply Dritho-Scalp only to the lesions and rub in well, taking care to prevent the cream spreading onto the forehead. **Keep Dritho-Scalp well away from the eyes.** Avoid application of the cream to uninvolved scalp margins. Remove any unintended residue which may be deposited behind the ears. At the end of each period of contact, wash the hair and scalp to remove any surplus cream (which may have become red/brown in color). **Always wash hands thoroughly after use.**
Store in a cool place (46°—59°F)

HOW SUPPLIED
50g tube with special applicator
Dritho-Scalp 0.25% NDC 51201-0024-1
Dritho-Scalp 0.5% NDC 51201-0023-1

CAUTION
Federal law prohibits dispensing without prescription.
Printed 5/86

Distributed by:
AMERICAN DERMAL CORPORATION
Somerset, New Jersey 08873

VIRANOL® ℞

DESCRIPTION
Viranol® is a solution for topical application containing 16.7% Salicylic Acid U.S.P., and 16.7% Lactic Acid U.S.P. in a vehicle of Flexible Collodion U.S.P.

ACTION
The active ingredients, Salicylic Acid and Lactic Acid are believed to exert a keratolytic action which effects the removal of wart epidermal cells infected by deoxyribonucleic acid viruses.

INDICATIONS
Viranol® is indicated as an aid in the treatment and removal of plantar warts and other common warts.

CONTRAINDICATIONS
Viranol® should not be used by diabetics or individuals with impaired blood circulation.

WARNINGS
Viranol® should not be applied to moles, birthmarks, unusual warts with protruding hair, genital warts, or warts on the face.

PRECAUTIONS
Viranol® is for external use only. Discontinue use if excessive irritation occurs on normal skin areas. Avoid contact with eyes or on mucous membranes. If contact with eyes or mucous membranes should occur, flush with water to remove Collodion film and continue rinsing for an additional 15 minutes. Viranol® is highly flammable and should not be used or stored near fire or flame. Avoid inhaling vapors.

ADVERSE REACTIONS
Viranol® may cause local irritation on normal skin. Care should be used to avoid contact with normal surrounding skin areas while applying Viranol® directly to wart.

DOSAGE AND ADMINISTRATION
Wash affected area and soak wart in hot water for 5 minutes. Dry thoroughly, then gently remove softened area of the wart by rubbing with a pumice stone, emery board or washcloth. Using the special applicator provided, apply 2 to 4 drops to the wart only. Keep Viranol® away from surrounding skin (preferably by encircling the wart with a ring of petrolatum). Allow to dry before covering with a waterproof bandage. Repeat the above procedure once daily and continue as directed by physician. Discontinue treatment if skin irritation develops or if no improvement occurs after two months' use.

HOW SUPPLIED
10 ml bottle with applicator. NDC #51201-5006-1 Keep bottle tightly capped and store in an upright position at controlled room temperature. Keep out of reach of children.

CAUTION
Federal law prohibits dispensing without prescription.

Arco Pharmaceuticals, Inc.
105 ORVILLE DRIVE
BOHEMIA, NY 11716

ARCO-LASE®
(broad pH spectrum digestant)

COMPOSITION
Each soft, mint flavored tablet contains Trizyme*, 38 mg., and Lipase, 25 mg.
*Contains the following standardized enzymes: amylolytic 30 mg.; proteolytic 6 mg.; cellulolytic 2 mg.

ACTION AND USES
Indicated for most gastrointestinal disorders due to poor digestion. Flatulence, gas and bloating, dyspepsia, distention, fullness, heartburn, or in any condition where normal digestion is impaired by digestive insufficiencies. Arcolase provides the highest standardized enzymatic activity, plus the protective action of the widest pH range. Thus it is effective throughout the entire G.I. tract. Requiring no enteric coating, there is assurance of a positive breakdown of its factors. This is advantageous, because quite often patients with digestive disorders cannot digest their food properly, let alone hard, or enteric coated capsules or tablets.

Continued on next page

Arco—Cont.

SIDE EFFECTS
None.

ADMINISTRATION AND DOSAGE
One tablet with or immediately following meals. Tablet may be swallowed or chewed.

SUPPLIED
Bottles of 50's. NDC 275-4040.

ARCO-LASE® PLUS ℞

COMPOSITION
Same as Arco-Lase, plus the addition of Hyoscyamine sulfate 0.10 mg., atropine sulfate 0.02 mg. and phenobarbital ⅛ gr. (Warning: may be habit forming.)

ACTION AND USES
Gastrointestinal disturbances, such as cramps, bloating, spasms, diarrhea, nausea, vomiting and peptic ulcer. The enzymes correct the digestive insufficiencies.
The antispasmodic and phenobarbital contribute to the symptomatic relief of hypermotility and nervous tension, which usually accompanies functional disturbances of the bowel.

ADMINISTRATION AND DOSAGE
One tablet following meals.

SIDE EFFECTS
May cause rapid pulse, dryness of mouth and blurred vision.

CONTRAINDICATIONS
This product is contraindicated in the presence of glaucoma or prostatic hypertrophy.

SUPPLIED
Bottles of 50's. NDC 275-45-45.

LITERATURE AVAILABLE
Yes.

MEGA-B®
(super potency vitamin B complex, sugar & starch free)

COMPOSITION
Each Mega-B Tablet contains the following Mega Vitamins:

B_1 (Thiamine Mononitrate)	100 mg.
B_2 (Riboflavin)	100 mg.
B_6 (Pyridoxine Hydrochloride)	100 mg.
B_{12} (Cyanocobalamin)	100 mcg.
Choline Bitartrate	100 mg.
Inositol	100 mg.
Niacinamide	100 mg.
Folic Acid	100 mcg.
Pantothenic Acid	100 mg.
d-Biotin	100 mcg.
Para-Aminobenzoic Acid (PABA)	100 mg.

In a base of yeast to provide the identified and unidentified B-Complex Factors.

ADVANTAGES
Each Mega-B capsule-shaped tablet provides the highest vitamin B complex available in a single dose.
Mega-B was designed for those patients who require truly Mega vitamin potencies with the convenience of minimum dosage.

INDICATIONS
Mega-B is indicated in conditions characterized by depletions or increased demand of the water-soluble B-complex vitamins. It may be useful in the nutritional management of patients during prolonged convalescence associated with major surgery. It is also indicated for stress conditions, as an adjunct to antibiotics and diuretic therapy, pre and post operative cases, liver conditions, gastro-intestinal disorders interferring with intake or absorbtion of water-soluble vitamins, prolonged or wasting diseases, diabetes, burns, fractures, severe infections, and some psychological disorders.

WARNING
NOT INTENDED FOR TREATMENT OF PERNICIOUS ANEMIA, OR OTHER PRIMARY OR SECONDARY ANEMIAS.

DOSAGE
Usual dosage is one Mega-B tablet daily, or varied, depending on clinical needs.

SUPPLIED
Yellow capsule shaped tablets in bottles of 30, 100 and 500.

MEGADOSE™
(multiple mega-vitamin formula with minerals, sugar and starch free)

COMPOSITION

Vitamin A	25,000 USP Units
Vitamin D	1,000 USP Units
Vitamin C w/Rose Hips	250 mg.
Vitamin E	100 IU
Folic Acid	400 mcg.
Vitamin B_1	80 mg.
Vitamin B_2	80 mg.
Niacinamide	80 mg.
Vitamin B_6	80 mg.
Vitamin B_{12}	80 mcg.
Biotin	80 mcg.
Pantothenic Acid	80 mg.
Choline Bitartrate	80 mg.
Inositol	80 mg.
Para-Aminobenzoic Acid	80 mg.
Rutin	30 mg.
Citrus Bioflavonoids	30 mg.
Betaine Hydrochloride	30 mg.
Glutamic Acid	30 mg.
Hesperidin Complex	5 mg.
Iodine (from Kelp)	0.15 mg.
Calcium Gluconate*	50 mg.
Zinc Gluconate*	25 mg.
Potassium Gluconate*	10 mg.
Ferrous Gluconate*	10 mg.
Magnesium Gluconate*	7 mg.
Manganese Gluconate*	6 mg.
Copper Gluconate*	0.5 mg.

*Natural mineral chelates in a base containing natural ingredients.

DOSAGE
One tablet daily.

SUPPLIED
Capsule shaped tablets in bottles of 30, 100 and 250.

Ar-Ex Ltd.
233 E. ERIE STREET
CHICAGO, IL 60611

AR-EX HYPO-ALLERGENIC COSMETICS

COMPOSITION
Formulated so you can prescribe cosmetics as you prescribe medications or other therapeutic regimen in dermatological, respiratory, gastrointestinal and other allergies where usual cosmetics are contraindicated.

ACTION AND USES
To provide safe beauty aids and eliminate a whole field of potential irritants and sensitizers that may aggravate or precipitate allergic conditions, as: skin irritations and erythema, contact dermatitis, photosensitivity, dry, chapped skin, lipstick cheilitis, eyelid dermatitis, chronic coryza, chronic vasomotor rhinitis, chronic conjunctivitis, asthma, urticaria, colitis and other G-I symptoms, also other conditions where cosmetics may be prime or contributing offenders.

UNSCENTED COSMETICS
Perfumes, natural or synthetic, and essential oils are known to be capable of irritating the skin, causing Berloque dermatitis (photosensitivity), and causing or aggravating respiratory symptoms simulating asthma and hay fever. For these persons, all AR-EX Cosmetics are available Unscented, and contain absolutely no perfume, natural or synthetic.

A COMPLETE LINE
Following is a list of AR-EX Cosmetics, together with a partial list of potential irritants and allergens which they do NOT contain. When these substances are suspected etiological agents, you can rule them out of your diagnoses when you prescribe AR-EX Cosmetics *by brand name.*

CREAMS AND LOTIONS
Contain no soap, almond oil, oil of orris, coconut oil, bergamot or other citrus oils, lanolin, cocoa butter, karaya gum, gum arabic, tragacanth, rose water or phenol. Unscented.

DEODORANTS
Cream, Spray and Roll-On. Contain no aluminum chloride, aluminum chlorhydroxide, aluminum acetate, aluminum sulfate, alum, salicylic acid, formaldehyde, alcohol or hexachlorophene.

HAIR PREPARATIONS
Contain no soap, lanolin, sulfonated oil, palm or coconut oil, gum karaya, gum arabic, tragacanth, resin, lacquer, shellac. Unscented.

POWDERS
Contain no orris root, oil of orris, bergamot or other citrus oils, corn starch, rice starch, wheat starch, powdered gums or lanolin.

SOAP
Low in excess alkali, superfatted. Contains no lanolin, perfumes, essential oils.

FOUNDATION LOTION
Liquid makeup. Contains no gum acacia, karaya or tragacanth, lanolin, corn oil or other vegetable oils, oil of orris, perfumes or essential oils.

AR-EX SPECIAL FORMULA LIPSTICK
Contains no indelible dyes, eosin, mono-di-tri-or-tetra-brom-fluorescein compounds, but achieves shades through use of lake pigments. Contains no perfumes or essential oils, lanolin, almond oil or cocoa butter.

LITERATURE AVAILABLE
For precise prescription of hypo-allergenic cosmetics in indicated conditions, refer to the AR-EX Ingredient Listing. Sent on request.

SAFE SUDS

COMPOSITION
Hypo-allergenic, all-purpose detergent for patients whose hands or respiratory membranes are irritated by soaps or detergents. For dishes, laundry, floors, rugs, upholstery, etc. Suds in hard or soft water, with pH approximately 6.8. Contains no enzymes, phosphates, lanolin, fillers or bleaches. Biodegradable. NOT scented.

Armour Pharmaceutical Company
SUITE 4000
ONE SENTRY PARKWAY
BLUE BELL, PA 19422

H.P. ACTHAR® GEL* ℞
[āch pē āk 'thär jĕl]
(repository corticotropin injection)
and
ACTHAR® ℞
(corticotropin for injection)

DESCRIPTION
H.P. ACTHAR® GEL (Repository Corticotropin Injection) is a highly purified sterile preparation of the adrenocorticotropic hormone in 16% gelatin to provide a prolonged release after intramuscular or subcutaneous injection.
ACTHAR® (Corticotropin for Injection) is a sterile lyophilized ACTH which in dry form is stable at room temperature. Each vial contains 25 or 40 Units of Corticotropin U.S.P. and approximately 9 and 14 milligrams of hydrolyzed gelatin respectively. After reconstitution, this product is administered in the intravenous, intramuscular, or subcutaneous route.

CLINICAL PHARMACOLOGY
ACTH stimulates the adrenal cortex to secrete cortisol, corticosterone, aldosterone, and a number of weakly androgenic substances. Although ACTH does stimulate secretion of aldosterone, the rate is relatively independent. Prolonged administration of large doses of ACTH induces hyperplasia and hypertrophy of the adrenal cortex and continuous high output of cortisol, corticosterone, and weak androgens. The release of ACTH is under the influence of the nervous system via the corticotropin regulatory hormone released from the hypothalamus and by a negative corticosteroid feedback mechanism. Elevated plasma cortisol suppresses ACTH release.
The trophic effects of ACTH on the adrenal cortex are not understood beyond the fact that they appear to be mediated by cyclic AMP.
ACTH rapidly disappears from the circulation following its intravenous administration; in man the plasma half-life is about 15 minutes.
The maximal effects of a trophic hormone on a target organ are achieved when optimal amounts of hormone are acting continuously. Thus, a fixed dose of ACTH will demonstrate a linear increase in adrenocortical secretion with increasing duration of the infusion.

INDICATIONS AND USAGE
ACTHAR® (Corticotropin for Injection) and H.P. ACTHAR® GEL (Repository Corticotropin Injection) are indicated for diagnostic testing of adrenocortical function.
ACTHAR® (Corticotropin for Injection) and H.P. ACTHAR® GEL (Repository Corticotropin Injection) have limited therapeutic value in those conditions responsive to corticosteroid therapy; in such case, corticosteroid therapy is considered to be the treatment of choice. ACTHAR® (Cortic-

otropin for Injection) and H.P. ACTHAR® GEL (Repository Corticotropin Injection) may be employed in the following disorders:

ENDOCRINE DISORDERS: Nonsuppurative thyroiditis; Hypercalcemia associated with cancer.

NERVOUS SYSTEM DISEASES: Acute exacerbations of multiple sclerosis.

RHEUMATIC DISORDERS: As adjunctive therapy for short-term administration (to tide the patient over an acute episode or exacerbation) in:

Psoriatic arthritis; Rheumatoid arthritis, including juvenile rheumatoid arthritis (selected cases may require low-dose maintenance therapy); Ankylosing spondylitis; Acute and subacute bursitis; Acute nonspecific tenosynovitis; Acute gouty arthritis; Post-traumatic arthritis; Synovitis of osteoarthritis; Epicondylitis.

COLLAGEN DISEASES: During an exacerbation or as maintenance therapy in selected cases of:

Systemic lupus erythematosus; Systemic dermatomyositis (polymyositis); Acute rheumatic carditis.

DERMATOLOGIC DISEASES: Pemphigus; Bullous dermatitis herpetiformis; Severe erythema multiforme (Stevens-Johnson syndrome); Exfoliative dermatitis; Severe psoriasis; Severe seborrheic dermatitis; Mycosis fungoides.

ALLERGIC STATES: Control of severe or incapacitating allergic conditions intractable to adequate trials of conventional treatment—

Seasonal or perennial allergic rhinitis; Bronchial asthma; Contact dermatitis; Atopic dermatitis; Serum sickness.

OPHTHALMIC DISEASES: Severe acute and chronic allergic and inflammatory processes involving the eye and its adnexa such as:

Allergic conjunctivitis; Keratitis; Herpes zoster ophthalmicus; Iritis and iridocyclitis; Diffuse posterior uveitis and choroiditis; Optic neuritis; Sympathetic ophthalmia; Chorioretinitis; Anterior segment inflammation; Allergic corneal marginal ulcers.

RESPIRATORY DISEASES: Symptomatic sarcoidosis; Loeffler's syndrome not manageable by other means; Berylliosis; Fulminating or disseminated pulmonary tuberculosis when used concurrently with antituberculous chemotherapy; Aspiration pneumonitis.

HEMATOLOGIC DISORDERS: Acquired (autoimmune) hemolytic anemia; Secondary thrombocytopenia in adults; Erythroblastopenia (RBC anemia); Congenital (erythroid) hypoplastic anemia.

NEOPLASTIC DISEASES: For palliative management of: Leukemias and lymphomas in adults; Acute leukemia of childhood.

EDEMATOUS STATE: To induce a diuresis or a remission of proteinuria in the nephrotic syndrome without uremia of the idiopathic type or that due to lupus erythematosus.

GASTROINTESTINAL DISEASES: To tide the patient over a critical period of the disease in: Ulcerative colitis; Regional enteritis.

MISCELLANEOUS: Tuberculous meningitis with subarachnoid block or impending block when used concurrently with appropriate anti-tuberculous chemotherapy; Trichinosis with neurologic or myocardial involvement.

CONTRAINDICATIONS

Corticotropin is contraindicated in patients with scleroderma, osteoporosis, systemic fungal infections, ocular herpes simplex, recent surgery, history of or the presence of a peptic ulcer, congestive heart failure, hypertension, or sensitivity to proteins of porcine origin.

Treatment of conditions listed within the INDICATIONS section (see above) is contraindicated when they are accompanied by primary adrenocortical insufficiency or adrenocortical hyperfunction.

Intravenous administration of corticotropin is contraindicated for treatment of conditions listed within the indications section, but Acthar is used intravenously for diagnostic purposes (see DOSAGE AND ADMINISTRATION).

WARNINGS

Chronic administration of corticotropin may lead to adverse effects which are not reversible. Corticotropin may only suppress symptoms and signs of chronic diseases without altering the natural course of the disease. Neither H.P. ACTHAR® GEL (Repository Corticotropin Injection) nor ACTHAR® (Corticotropin for Injection) should be administered for treatment until adrenal responsiveness has been verified with the route of administration which will be utilized during treatment, intramuscularly or subcutaneously. A rise in urinary and plasma corticosteroid values provides direct evidence of a stimulatory effect. Prolonged administration of corticotropin increases the risk of hypersensitivity reactions. Although the action of corticotropin is similar to that of exogenous adrenocortical steroids the quantity of adrenocorticoid may be variable. In patients who receive prolonged corticotropin therapy the additional use of rapidly acting corticosteroids before, during, and after an unusual stressful situation is indicated.

Prolonged use of corticotropin may produce posterior subcapsular cataracts and glaucoma with possible damage to the optic nerves.

Corticotropin may mask some signs of infection, and new infections including those of the eye due to fungi or viruses may appear during its use. There may be decreased resistance and inability to localize infection when corticotropin is used.

Corticotropin can cause elevation of blood pressure, salt and water retention, and increased excretion of potassium. Dietary salt restriction and potassium supplementation may be necessary. Corticotropin increases calcium excretion.

While on corticotropin therapy, patients should not be vaccinated against smallpox. Other immunization procedures should be undertaken with caution in patients who are receiving corticotropin, especially when high doses are administered because of the possible hazards of neurological complications and lack of antibody response.

PRECAUTIONS

1. General

Corticotropin injection should be used in the lowest dose for the shortest period of time to accomplish the therapeutic goal. Corticotropin should be used for treatment only when the disease is intractable to non-steroid treatment. There is an enhanced effect in patients with hypothyroidism and in those with cirrhosis of the liver. Sensitivity to porcine protein should be considered before starting therapy and during the course of treatment should symptoms arise.

When an infection is present, appropriate antibiotic therapy should be given. Patients with latent tuberculosis should be observed closely and if therapy is prolonged, chemoprophylaxis should be instituted.

Psychic symptoms may appear with use of corticotropin or pre-existing symptoms may be enhanced. These may range from mood alteration to a psychotic state.

Patients with a secondary disease may have that disease worsened. Caution should be used when prescribing corticotropin in patients with diabetes, renal insufficiency, diverticulitis, and myasthenia gravis.

Corticotropin often acts by suppressing symptoms without altering the course of the underlying disease. Since complications with corticotropin use are dependent on the dose and duration of treatment, a risk/benefit decision must be made in each case.

Suppression of the pituitary adrenal axis occurs following prolonged therapy which may be slow in returning to normal. Patients should be protected from the stress of trauma or surgery by the use of corticosteroids during the period of stress.

Since maximal corticotropin stimulation of the adrenals may be limited during the first few days of treatment, other drugs should be administered when an immediate therapeutic effect is desirable.

Although controlled clinical trials have shown ACTH to be effective in speeding the resolution of acute exacerbations of multiple sclerosis they do not show that it affects the ultimate outcome or natural history of the disease. The studies do show that relatively high doses of ACTH are necessary to demonstrate a significant effect. (See DOSAGE AND ADMINISTRATION section.)

Treatment of acute gouty arthritis should be limited to a few days. Since rebound attacks may occur when corticotropin is discontinued, conventional concomitant therapy should be administered during corticotropin treatment and for several days after it is stopped.

Aspirin should be used cautiously in conjunction with corticotropin in hypoprothrombinemia.

2. Drug Interactions

Corticotropin may accentuate the electrolyte loss associated with diuretic therapy.

3. Carcinogenesis, Mutagenesis, Impairment of Fertility

Adequate and well controlled studies have not been done in animals. Human use has not been associated with an increase in malignant disease. See Pregnancy warning below.

4. Pregnancy

Pregnancy Class C. Corticotropin has been shown to have an embryocidal effect. There are no adequate and well-controlled studies in pregnant women. Corticotropin should be used during pregnancy only if the potential benefit justifies the potential risk to the fetus.

5. Nursing Mothers

It is not known whether this drug is excreted in human milk. Because many drugs are excreted in human milk and because of the potential for serious adverse reactions in nursing infants from corticotropin, a decision should be made whether to discontinue nursing or to discontinue the drug, taking into account the importance of the drug to the mother.

6. Pediatric Use

Prolonged use of corticotropin in children will inhibit skeletal growth. If use is necessary, it should be given intermittently and the child carefully observed.

ADVERSE REACTIONS

Fluid and electrolyte disturbances:

Sodium retention; fluid retention; potassium loss; hypokalemic alkalosis; calcium loss.

Musculoskeletal:

Muscle weakness; steroid myopathy; loss of muscle mass; osteoporosis; vertebral compression fractures; aseptic necrosis of femoral and humeral heads; pathologic fracture of long bones.

Gastrointestinal:

Peptic ulcer with possible perforation and hemorrhage; pancreatitis; abdominal distention; ulcerative esophagitis.

Dermatologic:

Impaired wound healing; thin fragile skin; petechiae and ecchymoses; facial erythema; increased sweating; suppression of skin test reactions; acne; hyperpigmentation.

Cardiovascular:

Hypertension, necrotizing angiitis; congestive heart failure.

Neurological:

Convulsions; increased intracranial pressure with papilledema, (pseudo-tumor cerebri) usually after treatment; headache, vertigo.

Endocrine:

Menstrual irregularities; development of Cushingoid state; suppression of growth in children; secondary adrenocortical pituitary unresponsiveness, particularly in times of stress, as in trauma, surgery or illness; decreased carbohydrate tolerance; manifestations of latent diabetes mellitus; increased requirements for insulin or oral hypoglycemic agents in diabetics; hirsutism.

Ophthalmic:

Posterior subcapsular cataracts; increased intraocular pressure; glaucoma with possible damage to optic nerve; exophthalmos.

Metabolic:

Negative nitrogen balance due to protein catabolism.

Allergic reactions:

Especially in patients with allergic responses to proteins manifesting as dizziness, nausea and vomiting, shock, skin reactions.

Miscellaneous:

Abscess: prolonged use of ACTH may result in antibodies to it and resulting loss of stimulatory effect.

Drug Abuse and Dependence:

Although drug dependence does not occur, sudden withdrawal of corticotropin after prolonged use may lead to recurrent symptoms which make it difficult to stop. It may be necessary to taper the dose and increase the injection interval to gradually discontinue the medication.

OVERDOSAGE

An acute overdose would present no different adverse reactions.

DOSAGE AND ADMINISTRATION

Standard tests for verification of adrenal responsiveness to corticotropin may utilize as much as 80 units as a single injection or one or more injections of a lesser dosage. Verification tests should be performed prior to treatment with corticotropins. The test should utilize the route(s) of administration proposed for treatment. Following verification, dosage should be individualized according to the disease under treatment and the general medical condition of each patient. Frequency and dose of the drug should be determined by considering severity of the disease, plasma and urine corticosteroid levels and the initial response of the patient. Only gradual change in dosage schedules should be attempted, after full drug effects have become apparent.

The chronic administration of more than 40 units daily may be associated with uncontrollable adverse effects.

When reduction in dosage is indicated this should be done gradually by either reducing the amount of each injection, or administering injections at longer intervals, or by a combination of both of the above. During reduction of dosage careful consideration should be given to the disease being treated, the general medical conditions of the patient and the duration over which corticotropin was administered.

Acthar must be reconstituted at the time of use by dissolving in a convenient volume of Sterile Water for Injection or Sodium Chloride Injection in such a manner that the individual dose will be contained in 1–2 ml of solution. The reconstituted solution should be refrigerated and used within 24 hours.

H.P. ACTHAR® GEL (Repository Corticotropin Injection) and ACTHAR® (Corticotropin for Injection) may be administered intramuscularly or subcutaneously.

H.P. ACTHAR® GEL (Repository Corticotropin Injection) is given intramuscularly or subcutaneously every 24-72 hours in doses of 40-80 units.

The usual intramuscular or subcutaneous dose for ACTHAR® (Corticotropin for Injection) is 20 units four times a day.

Continued on next page

Armour—Cont.

In the treatment of acute exacerbations of multiple sclerosis daily intramuscular doses of 80–120 units for 2–3 weeks may be administered.
For diagnostic purposes, ACTHAR® (Corticotropin for Injection) may be given intravenously in doses of 10-25 units dissolved in 500 ml of 5% glucose infused over an 8-hour period.

HOW SUPPLIED

H.P. ACTHAR® GEL (Repository Corticotropin Injection) is supplied in 5 milliliter multiple dose vials in strengths of 40 and 80 U.S.P. Units per milliliter and 1 milliliter vials containing 40 and 80 U.S.P. Units per milliliter.
ACTHAR® (Corticotropin for Injection) is supplied as a lyophilized powder in vials containing 25 and 40 U.S.P. Units per vial.
H.P. ACTHAR® GEL (Repository Corticotropin Injection) is stable for the period indicated on the label when stored under refrigeration between 2°–8°C (36°–46°F).
ACTHAR® (Corticotropin For Injection) is stable for the period indicated on the label when stored at controlled room temperature between 15°–30°C (59°–86°F).
*U.S. PAT. NO. 2,992,165
Revised: January 1983

AQUASOL A® ℞
[*ăk 'we-sŏl "ā*]
water-miscible vitamin A
50,000 USP Units (15 mg retinol)
vitamin A per capsule
25,000 USP Units (7.5 mg retinol)
vitamin A per capsule

DESCRIPTION

AQUASOL A (water-miscible vitamin A) Capsules provide 50,000 USP Units (15 mg retinol) or 25,000 USP Units (7.5 mg retinol) of vitamin A per capsule as retinol in the form of vitamin A alcohol, a light yellow to amber oil. One USP Unit is equivalent to one international unit (IU) and to 0.3 mcg of retinol or 0.6 mcg of beta-carotene. One molecule of beta-carotene yields two molecules of retinol, which is known as provitamin A.
Vitamin A, one of the fat-soluble vitamins, includes vitamin A itself as well as its precursors, alpha, beta, and gamma-carotene and cryptoxanthin. Of the precursors, beta-carotene predominates in nature and is the most active; on splitting, it forms two molecules of vitamin A, whereas the other precursors form only one molecule of vitamin A.
Ordinarily fat-soluble, the vitamin A in this product has been water solubilized by special processing* to enable better absorption and utilization particularly in conditions in which absorption or utilization of fats and fat-soluble substances is impaired. The capsules also contain ethyl vanillin, FD&C Red #40, gelatin, glycerin, methylparaben, polysorbate 80, and propylparaben.
*Oil-soluble vitamin A water solubilized with polysorbate 80.

CLINICAL PHARMACOLOGY

Retinol combines with opsin, the rod pigment in the retina, to form rhodopsin, which is necessary for visual adaptation to darkness.
Vitamin A prevents retardation of growth and preserves the integrity of the epithelial cells.
Vitamin A deficiency is characterized by nyctalopia, keratomalacia, keratinization and drying of the skin, lowered resistance to infection, retardation of growth, thickening of bone, diminished production of cortical steroids, and fetal malformations. Vitamin A absorption requires bile salts, pancreatic lipase, and dietary fat. The vitamin is stored (primarily as the palmitate) in the Kupffer cells of the liver. The minimum daily requirement is approximately 20 units of vitamin A or 40 units of beta-carotene per kg of body weight. The daily Recommended Dietary Allowances (RDA) established by the National Academy of Sciences for selected categories of population are as follows: children 4-10 years of age, 2,500-3,000 units; adult males, 5,000 units; adult females, 4,000 units; pregnant women, 5,000 units; lactating women, 6,000 units.
The fat-soluble vitamins (A, D, E, and K) are absorbed by complex processes that parallel the absorption of fat. Thus, any condition that causes malabsorption of fat (e.g., celiac disease, tropical sprue, regional enteritis) may result in deficiency of one or all of these vitamins. Fat-soluble vitamins affect permeability or transport in various cell membranes and act as oxidation-reduction agents, coenzymes, or enzyme inhibitors. They are stored principally in the liver and excreted in the feces. Because these vitamins are metabolized very slowly, overdosage may produce toxic effects. Dietary fat is necessary for effective absorption of carotene, and protein is required for absorption of retinols. Protein and, possibly, zinc may be required to mobilize vitamin A reserves in the liver.
Vitamin A is more rapidly absorbed than carotene. Absorption of vitamin A from an aqueous vehicle is appreciably greater than when the drug is given in an oily solution. Carotene is converted to vitamin A in the intestinal wall and in the liver. Vitamin A itself is found only in animal sources; it occurs in high concentrations in the liver of the cod, halibut, tuna, and shark. It is also prepared synthetically. Carotene is found only in plants.

INDICATIONS AND USAGE

AQUASOL A (water-miscible vitamin A) Capsules are effective for the treatment of vitamin A deficiency. Unlike fat-soluble vitamin A products, AQUASOL A Capsules are not contraindicated in the malabsorption syndrome, because of the water-solubilizing process.

CONTRAINDICATIONS

Hypervitaminosis A. Sensitivity to any of the ingredients of this preparation.

WARNINGS

Avoid overdosage. Keep out of the reach of children.
Use in Pregnancy: Safety of amounts exceeding 5,000 units of vitamin A daily during pregnancy has not been established at this time. Therefore, for the protection of the fetus, the use of vitamin A in excess of the recommended dietary allowance should be avoided during normal pregnancy. Animal reproduction studies have shown fetal abnormalities associated with overdosage in several species. Malformations of the central nervous system, eye, palate, and genitourinary tract have been recorded.

PRECAUTIONS

General: Protect from light. Vitamin A ingestion from fortified foods, dietary supplements, self-administered drugs and prescription drug sources should be evaluated. Prolonged daily dose administration of over 25,000 units vitamin A should be under close supervision. Blood level assays are not a direct measure of liver storage. Liver storage should be adequate before discontinuing therapy. Single vitamin A deficiency is rare. Multiple vitamin deficiency is expected in any dietary deficiency.
Drug Interactions: Women receiving oral contraceptives have shown a significant increase in plasma vitamin A levels.
Pregnancy Category C: See Warnings section.
Nursing Mothers: The U.S. Recommended Dietary Allowance of vitamin A (6,000 units) is recommended for nursing mothers. Human milk supplies sufficient vitamin A for infants unless the maternal diet is grossly inadequate.

ADVERSE REACTIONS

See Overdosage section.

OVERDOSAGE

The following amounts have been found to be toxic orally. Toxicity manifestations depend on the age, dosage units, and duration of administration.
Acute toxicity—single dose (25,000 units/kg body weight)
Infant: 350,000 units
Adult: Over 2 million units
Chronic toxicity (4,000 units/kg body weight for 6 to 15 months)
Infants 3 to 6 months old: 18,500 units (water dispersed) per day for one to three months
Adult: 1 million units daily for three days, or 50,000 units daily for longer than 18 months, or 500,000 units daily for two months

Hypervitaminosis A Syndrome:
1. *General manifestations:* Fatigue, malaise, lethargy, abdominal discomfort, anorexia, and vomiting.
2. *Specific manifestations:*
a. Skeletal: slow growth, hard tender cortical thickening over the radius and tibia, migratory arthralgia, and premature closure of the epiphysis:
b. Central Nervous System: irritability, headache, and increased intracranial pressure as manifested by bulging fontanels, papilledema, and exophthalmos.
c. Dermatologic: fissures of the lips, drying and cracking of the skin, alopecia, scaling, massive desquamation, and increased pigmentation.
d. Systemic: hypomenorrhea, hepatosplenomegaly, jaundice, leukopenia, vitamin A plasma level over 1,200 units.

The treatment of hypervitaminosis A consists of immediate withdrawal of the vitamin along with symptomatic and supportive treatment.

DOSAGE AND ADMINISTRATION

For adults and children over eight years of age:
1. Severe deficiency with xerophthalmia: 500,000 units daily for three days, followed by 50,000 units daily for two weeks.
2. Severe deficiency: 100,000 units daily for three days followed by 50,000 units daily for two weeks.
3. Follow-up therapy: 10,000 to 20,000 units daily for two months.
Poor dietary habits should be corrected and an abundant and well-balanced dietary intake should be prescribed.

HOW SUPPLIED

AQUASOL A Capsules (water-miscible vitamin A) 50,000 USP Units vitamin A, bottles of 100 (NDC 0053-0104-00) and 500 (NDC 0053-0104-05); 25,000 USP Units vitamin A, bottles of 100 (NDC 0053-0103-00). These products are dark red, soft gelatin capsules.
These products are manufactured for Armour Pharmaceutical Company, Kankakee, Illinois 60901 by R. P. Scherer Corp., Clearwater, FL 33518.
Shown in Product Identification Section, page 404
Revised: April, 1986

AQUASOL A® DROPS
[*ăk 'we-sŏl "ā*]

COMPOSITION

Oil-soluble vitamin A water solubilized with polysorbate 20 for faster, better absorption and utilization. Drops provide 5,000 IU vitamin A per 0.1 ml.

ACTIONS

There is evidence that aqueous vitamin A produces a more rapid increase in the blood concentration and higher blood levels than the oily form of the vitamin.

ADMINISTRATION AND DOSAGE

As a dietary supplement 0.1 ml (3 drops) daily for adults and children 4 or more years of age provides 100% of the U.S. RDA; 2 drops daily for children under 4, 133%.

HOW SUPPLIED

Drops: 5,000 IU per 0.1 ml, bottles of 30 ml, with dropper.
Issued 12/82

AQUASOL E®
[*ăk 'we-sŏl ē*]
(Aqueous Vitamin E Supplements, Oral)

COMPOSITION

Capsules, 100 IU or 400 IU vitamin E; Drops, 15 IU vitamin E per 0.3 ml. Oil-soluble vitamin E water solubilized with polysorbate 80 for more rapid and more complete absorption.

HOW SUPPLIED

100 IU capsules, bottles of 100; 400 IU capsules, bottles of 30. Drops, 12 ml and 30 ml.
Shown in Product Identification Section, page 404
Issued 12/82

BIOZYME®–C Ointment ℞
[*bī 'ō-zīm-sē "*]
Collagenase

Biozyme®-C Ointment is supplied in 15 gram tubes containing 250 units of collagenase enzyme per gram of white petrolatum USP.

CHROMETRACE™ ℞
[*krōm 'trās*]
Chromic Chloride Injection USP

4 mcg/mL of Chrome

Chrometrace is supplied in 10 mL vials in boxes of 25 (NDC 0053-0830-22).

COPPERTRACE™ ℞
[*kŏp 'er-trās "*]
Cupric Chloride Injection USP

0.4 mg/mL of Copper

Cupric Chloride in Sodium Chloride Solution

Coppertrace is supplied in 10 mL vials in boxes of 25 (NDC 0053-0831-22).

DIALUME® OTC
[*di-a-loom*]
(Aluminum Hydroxide Capsules)

COMPOSITION

Each capsule contains:

Aluminum Hydroxide Powder	500 mg
Sodium Content Not More Than	1.2 mg
Magnesium Content Not More Than	1.0 mg
Calcium Content Not More Than	40 mg
Acid Neutralizing Capacity Per Capsule	10 mEq

INACTIVE INGREDIENT
Calcium Stearate

INDICATIONS
For the relief of heartburn, sour stomach, or acid indigestion.

DRUG INTERACTION PRECAUTION
Do not take this product if you are presently taking a prescription antibiotic drug containing any form of tetracycline.

WARNINGS
Do not take more than six capsules daily for more than 2 weeks, except under the advice and supervision of a physician.
May cause constipation.

DIRECTIONS
One or two capsules three times daily or as directed by a physician.

HOW SUPPLIED
In bottles containing 100 capsules and 500 capsules.
Store and dispense in a tight container as defined in the U.S.P. at controlled room temperature between 15°–30°C (59°–86°F).
Revised 3/85
Shown in Product Identification Section, page 404

For dilution in intravenous infusions only
M.V.I.®-12 ℞
[*ĕm-vē-ī-twĕlv*]
Multi-Vitamin Infusion
M.V.I.®-12 Multi-Dose
Multi-Vitamin Infusion
M.V.I.®-12 UNIT VIAL
Multi-Vitamin Infusion
M.V.I.®-12 Lyophilized
Multi-Vitamins for Infusion

DESCRIPTION
M.V.I.–12 and M.V.I.–12 Multi-Dose are sterile products consisting of two vials labeled Vial 1 and Vial 2 in 5 mL single dose vials and 50 mL multiple dose vials respectively.
Each 5 mL in Vial 1† provides:
ascorbic acid (vitamin C) .... 100 mg
vitamin A* (retinol) .... 1 mg (a)
ergocalciferol* (vitamin D) .... 5 mcg (b)
thiamine (vitamin B_1)
(as the hydrochloride) .... 3 mg
riboflavin (vitamin B_2) (as riboflavin-5-phosphate sodium) .... 3.6 mg
pyridoxine HCl (vitamin B_6) .... 4 mg
niacinamide .... 40 mg
dexpanthenol (d-pantothenyl alcohol) .... 15 mg
vitamin E* (dl-alpha tocopheryl acetate) .... 10 mg (c)
† with propylene glycol 30% and gentisic acid ethanolamide 2% as stabilizers and preservatives, sodium hydroxide for pH adjustment, polysorbate 80 1.6%, polysorbate 20 0.028%, butylated hydroxytoluene 0.002%, butylated hydroxyanisole 0.0005%.
* Oil-soluble vitamins A, D and E water solubilized with polysorbate 80.
(a) 1 mg vitamin A equals 3,300 USP units.
(b) 5 mcg ergocalciferol equals 200 USP units.
(c) 10 mg vitamin E equals 10 USP units.
Each 5 mL in Vial 2 provides:
biotin .... 60 mcg
folic acid .... 400 mcg
cyanocobalamin (vitamin B_{12}) .... 5 mcg
with propylene glycol 30%; and citric acid, sodium citrate, and sodium hydroxide for pH adjustment.
M.V.I.–12 UNIT VIAL is a sterile product in a two-chambered single dose vial which must be mixed just prior to use.
Each 10 mL of the mixed solution provides:
ascorbic acid (vitamin C) .... 100 mg
vitamin A‡ (retinol) .... 1 mg (a)
ergocalciferol‡ (vitamin D) .... 5 mcg (b)
thiamine (vitamin B_1)
(as the hydrochloride) .... 3 mg
riboflavin (vitamin B_2) (as riboflavin-5-phosphate sodium) .... 3.6 mg
pyridoxine HCl (vitamin B_6) .... 4 mg
niacinamide .... 40 mg
dexpanthenol (d-pantothenyl alcohol) .... 15 mg
vitamin E‡ (dl-alpha tocopheryl acetate) .... 10 mg (c)
biotin .... 60 mcg
folic acid .... 400 mcg
cyanocobalamin (vitamin B_{12}) .... 5 mcg
with propylene glycol 30% and gentisic acid ethanolamide 1% as stabilizers and preservatives and citric acid, sodium citrate and sodium hydroxide for pH adjustment, polysorbate 80 0.8%, polysorbate 20 0.014%, butylated hydroxytoluene 0.001%, butylated hydroxyanisole 0.0003%.
‡Oil-soluble vitamins A, D and E water solubilized with polysorbate 80.
(a) 1 mg vitamin A equals 3,300 USP units.
(b) 5 mcg ergocalciferol equals 200 USP units.
(c) 10 mg vitamin E equals 10 USP units.
M.V.I.–12 Lyophilized is a sterile powder intended for reconstitution and dilution in intravenous infusions.
Each vial provides:
ascorbic acid (vitamin C) .... 100 mg
vitamin A† (retinol) .... 1.0 mg (a)
ergocalciferol* (vitamin D) .... 5 mcg (b)
thiamine (vitamin B_1)
(as the base) .... 3.0 mg
riboflavin (vitamin B_2) (as riboflavin-5-phosphate sodium) .... 3.6 mg
pyridoxine (vitamin B_6) .... 4.0 mg
(as the base)
niacinamide .... 40.0 mg
dexpanthenol (d-pantothenyl alcohol) .... 15.0 mg
vitamin E† (dl-alpha tocopheryl acetate) .... 10 mg (c)
biotin .... 60 mcg
folic acid .... 400 mcg
cyanocobalamin (vitamin B_{12}) .... 5 mcg
with mannitol 375 mg, sodium hydroxide for pH adjustment, polysorbate 80 80 mg, polysorbate 20 1.1 mg, butylated hydroxytoluene 82.5 mcg, butylated hydroxyanisole 20.6 mcg.
(a) 1 mg vitamin A equals 3,300 USP units.
(b) 5 mcg ergocalciferol equals 200 USP units.
(c) 10 mg vitamin E equals 10 USP units.
†Oil-soluble vitamins A, D and E water solubilized with polysorbate 80.
"Aqueous" multivitamin formula for intravenous infusion: M.V.I.–12 (Multi-Vitamin Infusion) makes available a combination of important oil-soluble and water-soluble vitamins in an aqueous solution, formulated specially for incorporation into intravenous infusions. Through special processing techniques, the liposoluble vitamins A, D and E have been solubilized in an aqueous medium, permitting intravenous administration of these vitamins.

INDICATIONS AND USAGE
This formulation is indicated as daily multivitamin maintenance dosage for adults and children aged 11 and above receiving parenteral nutrition.
It is also indicated in other situations where administration by the intravenous route is required. Such situations include surgery, extensive burns, fractures and other trauma, severe infectious diseases, and comatose states, which may provoke a "stress" situation with profound alterations in the body's metabolic demands and consequent tissue depletion of nutrients.
The physician should not await the development of clinical signs of vitamin deficiency before initiating vitamin therapy. The use of a multivitamin product obviates the need to speculate on the status of individual vitamin nutriture.
M.V.I.–12 (administered in intravenous fluids under proper dilution) contributes intake of these necessary vitamins, except vitamin K, toward maintaining the body's normal resistance and repair processes.
Patients with multiple vitamin deficiencies or with markedly increased requirements may be given multiples of the daily dosage for two or more days as indicated by the clinical status.
M.V.I.–12 does not contain vitamin K, which may have to be administered separately.
Clinical testing indicates that some patients do not maintain adequate levels of certain vitamins when this formulation in recommended amounts is the sole source of vitamins. No vitamin deficiencies were clinically evident, but blood levels of vitamins A, C, D, and folic acid declined in a number of subjects who received this formulation as the only vitamin source for 4 to 6 months. Therefore, in patients for whom total parenteral nutrition will be continued for long periods of time, these vitamins should be monitored. If deficiencies appear to be developing, multiples of the formulation (1.5 to 3 times) may be needed for a period of time. When multiples of the formulation are used for more than a few weeks, vitamins A and D should be monitored occasionally to be certain that an excess accumulation of these vitamins is not occurring.

CONTRAINDICATIONS
Known hypersensitivity to any of the vitamins in this product or a pre-existing hypervitaminosis.

PRECAUTIONS
Drug Interactions: M.V.I.–12 (Multi-Vitamin Infusion) is not physically compatible with DIAMOX® (acetazolamide) 500 mg, DIURIL® Intravenous Sodium (chlorothiazide sodium) 500 mg, or moderately alkaline solutions. ACHROMYCIN® (tetracycline HCl) 500 mg may not be physically compatible with M.V.I.–12. It has been reported that folic acid is unstable in the presence of calcium salts such as calcium gluconate. Some of the vitamins in M.V.I.–12 may react with vitamin K bisulfite. Direct addition of M.V.I.–12 to intravenous fat emulsions is not recommended.
Carcinogenicity: Carcinogenicity studies have not been performed.
Pregnancy: Pregnant women should follow the U.S. Recommended Daily Allowance for their condition, because their vitamin requirements may exceed those of nonpregnant women.
Nursing Mothers: Lactating women should follow the U.S. Recommended Daily Allowance for their condition, because their vitamin requirements may exceed those of nonlactating women.
Pediatric Use: Safety and effectiveness in children below the age of 11 have not been established.

OVERDOSAGE
The possibility of hypervitaminosis A or D should be borne in mind.

ADVERSE REACTIONS
Allergic reaction has been known to occur following intravenous administration of thiamine. This risk, however, is negligible if the thiamine is administered with other vitamins of the B group.

DOSAGE AND ADMINISTRATION
M.V.I.–12 (Multi-Vitamin Infusion) is ready for immediate use in adults and children aged 11 and above when added to intravenous infusion fluids.
For multiple doses, the Pharmacy Bulk Package is prepared by aseptically transferring the contents of Vial 1 to Vial 2. Mix the solution gently. The mixed solution can be stored in a refrigerator and used within 24 hours. The mixed solution will provide 10–10 mL doses.
Directions for using UNIT VIAL: Remove the protective plastic cap, turn the plunger-stopper 90° and press down firmly to force liquid in the upper chamber and the center seal into the lower compartment. Gently agitate to mix solution. Sterilize the rubber stopper in the usual manner and insert needle squarely though the center of plunger-stopper until tip is just visible. Invert vial and withdraw dose in the usual manner. Vial should be mixed just prior to use. Mixed solution may be stored refrigerated at 2°–8°C for up to 24 hours.
M.V.I.–12 Lyophilized is reconstituted by adding 5 mL of Sterile Water for Injection USP to the 10 mL vial. The vial may be swirled gently after the addition of the water to hasten reconstitution. The reconstituted solution is ready within five minutes for immediate use. The entire contents of the vial should be added to appropriate intravenous infusion fluids.
M.V.I.–12 should not be given as a direct, undiluted intravenous injection as it may give rise to dizziness, faintness, and possible tissue irritation.
For intravenous feeding, one daily dose of M.V.I.–12 (5 mL of Vial 1 plus 5 mL of Vial 2, 10 mL of mixed UNIT VIAL, or 5 mL of reconstituted M.V.I.–12 Lyophilized) is added directly to not less than 500 mL, preferably 1,000 mL, of intravenous dextrose, saline or similar infusion solutions.
Parenteral drug products should be inspected visually for particulate matter and discoloration prior to administration, whenever solution and container permit.
After M.V.I.–12 is diluted in an intravenous infusion, the resulting solution should be refrigerated unless it is to be administered immediately, and in any event should be administered within 48 hours. Some of the vitamins in this product, particularly vitamins A and D, and riboflavin, are light sensitive, and exposure to light should be minimized.
STORE AT 2°–8°C (36°–46°F).

HOW SUPPLIED
M.V.I.–12 —Boxes of 25 and cartons of 100. Each box contains two vials—Vial 1 (5 mL) and Vial 2 (5 mL), both vials to be used for a single dose.
M.V.I.–12 Multi-Dose—Boxes of 20 vials, 50 mL each (10 Vial 1 and Vial 2). Both solutions to be used for a single dose.
M.V.I.–12 UNIT VIAL—Boxes of 25 two-chambered 10 mL vials.
M.V.I.–12 Lyophilized—Boxes of 25 vials.

CAUTION
Federal (USA) law prohibits dispensing without prescription.
Revised: September, 1985

For dilution in intravenous infusions only
M.V.I.® Pediatric ℞
[*ĕm-vē-i pē"dē-ăt'rĭk*]
Multi-Vitamins for Infusion

DESCRIPTION
M.V.I.® Pediatric is a lyophilized, sterile powder intended for reconstitution and dilution in intravenous infusions.

Continued on next page

Armour—Cont.

Each vial provides:
ascorbic acid (vitamin C) .... 80 mg
vitamin A† (retinol) .... 0.7 mg (a)
ergocalciferol† (vitamin D) .... 10 mcg (b)
thiamine (vitamin B_1)
(as the hydrochloride) .... 1.2 mg
riboflavin (vitamin B_2) (as riboflavin-5-phosphate sodium) .... 1.4 mg
pyridoxine (vitamin B_6)
(as the hydrochloride) .... 1.0 mg
niacinamide .... 17.0 mg
dexpanthenol (d-pantothenyl alcohol) .... 5.0 mg
vitamin E† (dl-alpha tocopheryl acetate) .... 7 mg (c)
biotin .... 20 mcg
folic acid .... 140 mcg
cyanocobalamin (vitamin B_{12}) .... 1 mcg
phytonadione (vitamin K_1) .... 200 mcg
with mannitol 375 mg, sodium hydroxide for pH adjustment, polysorbate 80 50 mg, polysorbate 20 0.8 mg, butylated hydroxytoluene 58 mcg, butylated hydroxyanisole 14 mcg.
† Oil-soluble vitamins A, D and E water solubilized with polysorbate 80.
(a) 0.7 mg vitamin A equals 2,300 USP units.
(b) 10 mcg ergocalciferol equals 400 USP units.
(c) 7 mg vitamin E equals 7 USP units.

Multivitamin formula for intravenous infusion:
M.V.I.® Pediatric (Multi-Vitamins for Infusion) provides a combination of important oil-soluble and water-soluble vitamins, formulated especially for incorporation into intravenous infusions after reconstitution. Through special processing techniques, the liposoluble vitamins A, D and E have been water solubilized with polysorbate 80, permitting intravenous administration of these vitamins.

INDICATIONS AND USAGE
This formulation is indicated as daily multivitamin maintenance dosage for infants and children up to 11 years of age receiving parenteral nutrition.
It is also indicated in other situations where administration by the intravenous route is required. Such situations include surgery, extensive burns, fractures and other trauma, severe infectious diseases, and comatose states, which may provoke a "stress" situation with profound alterations in the body's metabolic demands and consequent tissue depletion of nutrients.
The physician should not await the development of clinical signs of vitamin deficiency before initiating vitamin therapy. The use of a multivitamin product obviates the need to speculate on the status of individual vitamin nutriture.
M.V.I.® Pediatric (reconstituted and administered in intravenous fluids under proper dilution) contributes intake of these necessary vitamins toward maintaining the body's normal resistance and repair processes.
Patients with multiple vitamin deficiencies or with markedly increased requirements may be given multiples of the daily dosage for two or more days as indicated by the clinical status.

CONTRAINDICATIONS
Known hypersensitivity to any of the vitamins in this product or a pre-existing hypervitaminosis.

PRECAUTIONS
General: Unlike the adult formulation, M.V.I.®- 12, this product contains phytonadione (vitamin K_1).
Adequate blood levels of vitamin E are achieved when M.V.I.® Pediatric is given to infants at the recommended dosage. Larger doses or supplementation with oral or parenteral vitamin E are not recommended because elevated blood levels of vitamin E may result.
Studies have shown that vitamin A may adhere to plastic resulting in inadequate vitamin A administration in the doses recommended with M.V.I.® Pediatric. Additional vitamin A supplementation may be required.
Drug Interactions: M.V.I.® Pediatric is not physically compatible with DIAMOX® (acetazolamide) 500 mg, DIURIL® Intravenous Sodium (chlorothiazide sodium) 500 mg, aminophylline 125 mg, ampicillin 500 mg, or moderately alkaline solutions. ACHROMYCIN® (tetracycline HCl) 500 mg may not be physically compatible with M.V.I.® Pediatric. It has been reported that folic acid is unstable in the presence of calcium salts such as calcium gluconate. Direct addition of M.V.I.® Pediatric to intravenous fat emulsions is not recommended.
Carcinogenicity: Carcinogenicity studies have not been performed.

ADVERSE REACTIONS
Allergic reaction has been known to occur following intravenous administration of thiamine. This risk, however, is negligible if the thiamine is administered with other vitamins of the B group.

OVERDOSAGE
The possibility of hypervitaminosis A or D should be borne in mind.

DOSAGE AND ADMINISTRATION
M.V.I.® Pediatric is reconstituted by adding 5 ml of Sterile Water for Injection USP, Dextrose Injection USP 5%, or Sodium Chloride Injection to the 10 ml vial. The vial may be swirled gently after the addition of the water to hasten reconstitution. The reconstituted solution is ready within three minutes for immediate use. The amount to be administered should be added to appropriate intravenous infusion fluids (see below).
The reconstituted M.V.I.® Pediatric should not be given as a direct, undiluted intravenous injection as it may give rise to dizziness, faintness and possible tissue irritation.
For intravenous feeding, reconstituted M.V.I.® Pediatric should be added directly to not less than 100 ml of intravenous dextrose, saline or similar infusion solutions.
Infants weighing less than 1 kg: The daily dose is 30% of the contents of the vial. Do not exceed this daily dose.
Infants weighing 1 to 3 kg: The daily dose is 65% of the contents of one vial. Multiples of this recommended dose should not be given to infants weighing less than 3 kg.
Infants and children weighing 3 kg or more up to 11 years of age: The daily dose is the contents of one vial unless there is clinical or laboratory evidence for increasing or decreasing the dosage.
Discard any unused portion.
Parenteral drug products should be inspected visually for particulate matter and discoloration prior to administration, whenever solution and container permit.
After M.V.I.® Pediatric is reconstituted and diluted in an intravenous infusion, the resulting solution should be refrigerated unless it is to be administered immediately, and in any event should be administered within 24 hours. Some of the vitamins in this product, particularly vitamins A and D, and riboflavin, are light sensitive, and exposure to light should be minimized.

HOW SUPPLIED
Boxes of 25 vials (NDC 0053-0815-35).
Revised: 7/85

MANGATRACE™ ℞
[*măng'ga-trās*]
Manganese Chloride Injection USP

0.1 mg/mL of Manganese
Manganese Chloride in Sodium Chloride Solution

Mangatrace is supplied in 10 mL vials in boxes of 25 (NDC 0053-0832-22).

MULTITRACE™ 5 ℞
[*mŭl'tē-trās*]
Trace Element Mixture

DESCRIPTION
Multitrace™ 5, Trace Element Mixture, is a sterile, nonpyrogenic solution containing zinc, copper, manganese, chromium, and selenium for use as an additive to intravenous solutions for total parenteral nutrition (TPN).
Each ml of Multitrace™ 5 contains:
Zinc Chloride* .... 2.08 mg
Copper Chloride dihydrate** .... 1.07 mg
Manganese Chloride tetrahydrate*** .... 0.36 mg
Chromium Chloride hexahydrate**** .... 20.5 mcg
Selenious Acid***** .... 32.7 mcg
Water for Injection .... q.s.
*Equivalent to 1.0 mg Zn
**Equivalent to 0.4 mg Cu
***Equivalent to 0.1 mg Mn
****Equivalent to 4.0 mcg Cr
*****Equivalent to 20 mcg Se
pH adjusted with Hydrochloric Acid and/or Sodium Hydroxide
Zinc Chloride, USP is chemically designated $ZnCl_2$, a white crystalline compound freely soluble in water. Cupric Chloride is chemically designated $CuCl_2$, a crystalline compound freely soluble in water. Manganese Chloride is chemically designated $MnCl_2$, a deliquescent, crystalline compound soluble in water. Chromic Chloride is chemically designated $CrCl_3$, a crystalline compound soluble in water. Selenious Acid is chemically designated H_2Se, white or colorless crystals soluble in water or alcohol.

CLINICAL PHARMACOLOGY
Zinc is an essential nutritional requirement that serves as a cofactor for more than 70 different enzymes including carbonic anhydrase, alkaline phosphatase, lactic dehydrogenase, and both RNA and DNA polymerase. Zinc facilitates wound healing, helps maintain normal growth rates, normal skin hydration, and the senses of taste and smell. Providing zinc during TPN helps prevent development of deficiency symptoms and signs such as: Parakeratosis, hypogeusia, anorexia, dysosmia, geophagia, hypogonadism, growth retardation and hepatosplenomegaly. At plasma levels below 20 mcg zinc/dl, dermatitis followed by alopecia has been reported.
Copper is an essential nutrient that serves as a cofactor for serum ceruloplasmin, an oxidase necessary for proper formation of the iron carrier protein, transferrin. Copper also helps maintain normal rates of red and white blood cell formation. Providing copper during TPN helps prevent development of the following deficiency symptoms and signs: Leukopenia, neutropenia, anemia, depressed ceruloplasmin levels, impaired transferrin formation, and secondary iron deficiency. Normal serum copper values range from 80 to 163 mcg/dl.
Manganese is an essential nutrient that serves as an activator for enzymes such as polysaccharide polymerase, liver arginase, cholinesterase, and pyruvate carboxylase. Providing manganese during TPN helps prevent deficiency symptoms and signs such as nausea and vomiting, weight loss, dermatitis, and changes in growth and color of hair. Assays for manganese in whole blood result in concentrations ranging from 6 to 12 mcg manganese/liter.
Trivalent chromium is part of glucose tolerance factor, an essential activator of insulin-mediated reactions. Chromium helps maintain normal glucose metabolism and peripheral nerve function. Providing chromium during TPN helps prevent deficiency symptoms and signs including impaired glucose tolerance, ataxia, peripheral neuropathy, and a confusional state similar to mild/moderate hepatic encephalopathy. Typical blood levels for chromium range from 1 to 5 mcg/liter, but blood levels are not considered a meaningful index of tissue stores. A normalization of the glucose tolerance curve from the diabetic-like curve typical of chromium deficiency is viewed as a more meaningful indicator of chromium nutriture than serum chromium levels.
Selenium is an essential nutritional requirement that is part of glutathione peroxidase which protects cell components from oxidative damage resulting from peroxidase produced in cellular metabolism. Providing selenium during TPN helps prevent development of deficiency symptoms which include muscle pain and tenderness. Deficiency symptoms in humans have been reported with plasma selenium levels of 0.3 to 0.9 mcg/dl.

INDICATIONS AND USAGE
Multitrace 5 is indicated for use as a supplement to intravenous solutions given for total parenteral nutrition (TPN). Administration helps maintain zinc, copper, manganese, chromium, and selenium blood levels and prevents depletion of endogenous stores and subsequent deficiency states.

CONTRAINDICATIONS
Direct intramuscular or intravenous injection of Multitrace 5, Trace Element Mixture, is contraindicated as the acidic pH of the solution (approximately 2.0) may cause considerable tissue irritation.

WARNINGS
Copper and manganese are eliminated via the bile. In patients with severe liver dysfunction and/or biliary tract obstruction, decreasing or omitting copper and manganese supplements entirely may be necessary.

PRECAUTIONS
Do not use unless the solution is clear and the seal is intact. Multitrace 5, Trace Element Mixture, should be used only in conjunction with a pharmacy-directed admixture program using aseptic technique in a laminar flow environment. Multitrace 5 contains no preservative. Unused portions should be discarded within 24 hours after opening.
Frequent determination of serum levels of the various trace elements is suggested as a guideline for administering Multitrace 5. Zinc is eliminated via the kidneys and the possibility of retention should be considered in patients with renal dysfunction. Copper and manganese are eliminated via the bile and the possibility of retention should be considered in patients with biliary obstruction. In assessing the contribution of chromium supplements to maintenance of glucose homeostasis, consideration should be given to the possibility the patient may be diabetic. The primary route of elimination of selenium is in the urine, but significant losses also occur through feces. Selenium plasma level determinations are suggested as a guideline to adjust, reduce or omit selenium supplements in renal dysfunction and/or gastrointestinal malfunction.
Pregnancy Category C: Animal reproduction studies have not been conducted with Multitrace 5, Trace Element Mixture. It is also not known whether Multitrace 5 can cause fetal harm when administered to a pregnant woman or can affect reproductive capacity. Multitrace 5 should be given to a pregnant woman only if clearly indicated.

ADVERSE REACTIONS
None known.

DRUG ABUSE AND DEPENDENCY
None known.

OVERDOSAGE
Single intravenous doses of 1 to 2 mg zinc/kg body weight have been given to adult leukemic patients without toxic manifestations. However, acute toxicity was reported in an adult when 10 mg zinc was infused over a period of one hour on each of four consecutive days. Symptoms included hypotension, pulmonary edema, diarrhea, vomiting, jaundice, oliguria, blurred vision, tachycardia, decreased level of consciousness, profuse sweating, and hypothermia. Death resulted from an overdose in which 1683 mg zinc was delivered intravenously over the course of 60 hours to a 72-year-old patient. Calcium supplements may confer a protective effect against zinc toxicity.
Copper toxicity can produce prostration, behavior change, diarrhea, progressive marasmus, hypotonia, photophobia, and peripheral edema. Such symptoms have been reported with a serum copper level of 286 mcg/dl. D-penicillamine has been reported effective as an antidote.
Manganese toxicity in TPN patients has not been reported.
Trivalent chromium administered intravenously to TPN patients has been shown to be nontoxic when given at dosage levels of up to 250 mcg/day for two consecutive weeks. Reported toxic reactions to chromium include nausea, vomiting, ulcers of the gastrointestinal tract, renal and hepatic damage, convulsions, and coma.
Exposure to selenium in industrial environments, intake of foods grown in seleniferous soils, application of selenium containing cosmetics, and use of selenium contaminated water have been reported to cause chronic toxicity in humans. Selenium toxicity symptoms include weakened nails, dental defects, hair loss, dermatitis, nervousness, gastrointestinal disorders, mental depression, metallic taste, vomiting and garlic odor of breath and sweat. Death resulted from ingestion of large amounts of selenium compounds. The histopathological changes included fulminating peripheral vascular collapse, internal vascular congestion, diffusely hemorrhagic congested and edematous lungs, and brick-red color gastric mucosa. Coma preceded death. There is no known effective antidote to selenium poisoning in humans.

DOSAGE AND ADMINISTRATION
Each ml of Multitrace 5, Trace Element Mixture contains 1.0 mg Zn, 0.4 mg Cu, 0.1 mg Mn, 4.0 mcg Cr and 20 mcg Se and is administered intravenously only after dilution to a minimum of 1:200.
The following are suggested dosage ranges for the five trace elements:
Zinc: For the metabolically stable adult receiving TPN, the suggested intravenous dosage is 2.5 to 4 mg zinc/day. An additional 2 mg zinc/day is suggested for acute catabolic states. For the stable adult with fluid loss from the small bowel, an additional 12.2 mg zinc/liter of small bowel fluid lost, or an additional 17.1 mg zinc/kg of stool or ileostomy output is recommended. Frequent monitoring of zinc blood levels is suggested for patients receiving more than the usual maintenance dosage level of zinc.
For full term infants and children up to 5 years of age, 100 mcg zinc/kg/day is recommended. For premature infants (birth weight less than 1500 grams) up to 3 kg in body weight, 300 mcg/kg/day is suggested.
Copper: For the adult receiving TPN, the suggested additive dosage is 0.5 to 1.5 mg copper/day.
For pediatric patients, the suggested additive dosage is 20 mcg copper/kg/day.
Manganese: For the adult receiving TPN, the suggested additive dosage for manganese is 0.15 to 0.8 mg/day.
For pediatric patients, a dosage of 2 to 10 mcg manganese/kg/day is recommended.
Chromium: For the adult receiving TPN, the suggested additive dosage is 10 to 15 mcg chromium/ day. The metabolically stable adult with intestinal fluid loss may require 20 mcg chromium/day with frequent monitoring of blood levels as a guideline for subsequent administration.
For pediatric patients, the suggested additive dosage is 0.14 to 0.20 mcg chromium/kg/day.
Selenium: For the metabolically stable adult receiving TPN, the suggested intravenous dosage level is 20 to 40 mcg selenium/day. In adults with selenium deficiency states resulting from long-term TPN support, selenious acid administered intravenously at 100 mcg/day for a period of 24 and 31 days, respectively, has been reported to reverse deficiency symptoms without toxicity.
Frequent monitoring of selenium blood levels is suggested for patients receiving more than the usual maintenance dose. The normal whole blood range for selenium is approximately 10–37 mcg/dl.
Pediatric: For children the suggested dosage level is 3 mcg/kg/day.
Parenteral drug products should be inspected visually for particulate matter and discoloration prior to administration, whenever solution and container permit.

HOW SUPPLIED
Multitrace™ 5, Trace Element Mixture, in 10 ml Unit Dose vials in boxes of 25 (NDC 0053-1457-35).
Store at controlled room temperature between 15°-30°C (59°-86°F); avoid excessive heat.
Revised: March, 1984

MULTITRACE™ PEDIATRIC ℞
[*mŭl 'tē-trās "*]
Trace Element Mixture

DESCRIPTION
Multitrace™ Pediatric, Trace Element Mixture, is a sterile, nonpyrogenic solution containing zinc, copper, manganese and chromium for use as an additive to intravenous solutions for total parenteral nutrition (TPN).
Each ml of Multitrace™ Pediatric contains:

Zinc chloride	2.08 mg
Copper chloride dihydrate	0.27 mg
Manganese chloride tetrahydrate	0.09 mg
Chromium chloride hexahydrate	5.12 mcg
Water for Injection	q.s.
Equivalent to:	
Zn	1.0 mg
Cu	0.1 mg
Mn	25.0 mcg
Cr	1.0 mcg

pH adjusted with sodium hydroxide and/or hydrochloric acid.
Zinc Chloride, USP is chemically designated $ZnCl_2$, a white crystalline compound freely soluble in water. Cupric Chloride is chemically designated $CuCl_2$, a crystalline compound freely soluble in water. Manganese Chloride is chemically designated $MnCl_2$, a deliquescent, crystalline compound soluble in water. Chromic Chloride is chemically designated $CrCl_3$, a crystalline compound soluble in water.

CLINICAL PHARMACOLOGY
Zinc is an essential nutritional requirement that serves as a cofactor for more than 70 different enzymes including carbonic anhydrase, alkaline phosphatase, lactic dehydrogenase, and both RNA and DNA polymerase. Zinc facilitates wound healing, helps maintain normal growth rates, normal skin hydration, and the senses of taste and smell. Providing zinc during TPN helps prevent development of deficiency symptoms and signs such as: Parakeratosis, hypogeusia, anorexia, dysosmia, geophagia, hypogonadism, growth retardation and hepatosplenomegaly. At plasma levels below 20 mcg zinc/dl, dermatitis followed by alopecia has been reported in adults.
Copper is an essential nutrient that serves as a cofactor for serum ceruloplasmin, an oxidase necessary for proper formation of the iron carrier protein, transferrin. Copper also helps maintain normal rates of red and white bood cell formation. Providing copper during TPN helps prevent development of the following deficiency symptoms and signs: Leukopenia, neutropenia, anemia, depressed ceruloplasmin levels, impaired transferrin formation, and secondary iron deficiency. Normal serum copper values range from 80 to 163 mcg/dl in adults.
Manganese is an essential nutrient that serves as an activator for enzymes such as polysaccharide polymerase, liver arginase, cholinesterase, and pyruvate carboxylase. Providing manganese during TPN helps prevent deficiency symptoms and signs such as nausea and vomiting, weight loss, dermatitis, and changes in growth and color of hair. Assays for manganese in whole blood result in concentrations ranging from 6 to 12 mcg manganese/liter in adults.
Trivalent chromium is part of glucose tolerance factor, an essential activator of insulin-mediated reactions. Chromium helps maintain normal glucose metabolism and peripheral nerve function. Providing chromium during TPN helps prevent deficiency symptoms and signs including impaired glucose tolerance, ataxia, peripheral neuropathy, and a confusional state similar to mild/moderate hepatic encephalopathy. Typical blood levels for chromium range from 1 to 5 mcg/liter in adults, but blood levels are not considered a meaningful index of tissue stores. A normalization of the glucose tolerance curve from the diabetic-like curve typical of chromium deficiency is viewed as a more meaningful indicator of chromium nutriture than serum chromium levels.

INDICATIONS AND USAGE
Multitrace™ Pediatric is indicated for use as a supplement to intravenous solutions given for total parenteral nutrition (TPN) for infants and children up to 11 years of age. Administration helps maintain zinc, copper, manganese, and chromium blood levels and prevents depletion of endogenous stores and subsequential deficiency states.

CONTRAINDICATIONS
Direct intramuscular or intravenous injection of Multitrace™ Pediatric, Trace Element Mixture, is contraindicated as the acidic pH of the solution (approximately 2.0) may cause considerable tissue irritation.

WARNINGS
Copper and manganese are eliminated via the bile. In patients with severe liver dysfunction and/or biliary tract obstruction, decreasing or omitting copper and manganese supplements entirely may be necessary.

PRECAUTIONS
Do not use unless the solution is clear and the seal is intact. Multitrace™ Pediatric, Trace Element Mixture, should be used only in conjunction with a pharmacy-directed admixture program using aseptic technique in a laminar flow environment. Single dose vials contain no preservative; unused portions should be discarded within 24 hours after opening.
Frequent determination of serum levels of the various trace elements is suggested as a guideline for administering Multitrace™ Pediatric. Zinc is eliminated via the kidneys and the possibility of retention should be considered in patients with renal dysfunction. Copper and manganese are eliminated via the bile and the possibility of retention should be considered in patients with biliary obstruction. In assessing the contribution of chromium supplements to maintenance of glucose homeostasis, consideration should be given to the possibility the patent may be diabetic.

ADVERSE REACTIONS
None known.

DRUG ABUSE AND DEPENDENCY
None known.

OVERDOSAGE
Zinc toxicity signs and symptoms include hypotension, pulmonary edema, diarrhea, vomiting, jaundice, oliguria, blurred vision, tachycardia, decreased level of consciousness, profuse sweating, and hypothermia.
Copper toxicity can produce prostration, behavior change, diarrhea, progressive marasmus, hypotonia, photophobia, and peripheral edema. Such symptoms have been reported with a serum copper level of 286 mcg/dl. D-penicillamine has been reported effective as an antidote.
Manganese toxicity in TPN patients has not been reported.
Trivalent chromium administered intravenously to TPN patients has been shown to be nontoxic when given at dosage levels of up to 250 mcg/day for two consecutive weeks. Reported toxic reactions to chromium include nausea, vomiting, ulcers of the gastrointestinal tract, renal and hepatic damage, convulsions, and coma.

DOSAGE AND ADMINISTRATION
Each ml of Multitrace™ Pediatric contains 1.0 mg Zn, 0.1 mg Cu, 25.0 mcg Mn, and 1.0 mcg Cr and is administered intravenously only after dilution to a minimum of 1:200. The following are suggested dosage ranges for the four trace elements.
Zinc: For full-term infants and children, 100 mcg zinc/kg/-day is recommended. For premature infants (birth weight less than 1500 grams) up to 3 kg in body weight, 300 mcg/kg/day is suggested.
Copper: For pediatric patients, the suggested additive dosage is 20 mcg copper/kg/day.
Manganese: For pediatric patients, a dosage of 2 to 10 mcg manganese/kg/day is recommended.
Chromium: For pediatric patients, the suggested additive dosage is 0.14 to 0.20 mcg chromium/kg/ day.
Parenteral drug products should be inspected visually for particulate matter and discoloration prior to administration whenever solution and container permit. See Precautions section.

HOW SUPPLIED
Multitrace™ Pediatric, Trace Element Mixture, is supplied in 3 ml single-dose vials in boxes of 25.
Store at controlled room temperature between 15°-30°C (59°-86°F); avoid excessive heat.
Revised: February, 1984

MULTITRACE™ SOLUTION and CONCENTRATE ℞
[*mŭl 'tē-trās "*]
Trace Element Mixture

Multitrace Solution is supplied in 10 mL single dose vials in boxes of 25 and 30 mL multiple dose vials in boxes of 10.
Multitrace Concentrate is supplied in 1 mL single dose vials in boxes of 25 and 5 mL multiple dose vials in boxes of 10.

SELENITRACE™ ℞
[*sĕ-lē 'nē-trās "*]
Selenious Acid Injection

40 mcg/mL of Selenium

Selenitrace is supplied in 10 mL vials in boxes of 25 (NDC 0053-1449-35).

Continued on next page

Armour—Cont.

STIMATE™ ℞
[*stĭm 'āt*]
(desmopressin acetate) INJECTION

DESCRIPTION

Desmopressin acetate is an antidiuretic hormone affecting renal water conservation and is a synthetic analogue of 8-arginine vasopressin. It is chemically defined as follows:
Mol. Wt. 1183.2
Empirical Formula: $C_{48}H_{74}N_{14}O_{17}S_2$
SCH_2CH_2CO-Tyr-Phe-Gln-Asn-Cys-Pro-D-Arg-
Gly-$NH_2 \cdot C_2H_4O_2 \cdot 3H_2O$
1-(3-mercaptopropionic acid)-8-D-arginine vasopressin monoacetate (salt) trihydrate.
Stimate™ (desmopressin acetate) is provided as a sterile, aqueous solution for injection.
Each ml provides: Desmopressin acetate 4.0 mcg Chlorobutanol 5.0 mg Sodium chloride 9.0 mg Hydrochloric acid to adjust pH to 3.5.

CLINICAL PHARMACOLOGY

Stimate™ contains as active substance, 1-(3-mercaptopropionic acid)-8-D-arginine vasopressin, a synthetic analogue of the natural hormone arginine vasopressin. One ml (4 mcg) of Stimate™ has an antidiuretic activity of about 16 IU; 1 mcg of desmopressin acetate is equivalent to 4 IU.
Desmopressin acetate has been shown to be more potent than arginine vasopressin in increasing plasma levels of factor VIII activity in patients with hemophilia A and von Willebrand's disease Type 1.
Dose-response studies were performed in healthy persons, using doses of 0.1 to 0.4 mcg/kg body weight, infused over a 10-minute period. Maximal dose response occurred at 0.3 to 0.4 mcg/kg. The response to desmopressin acetate of factor VIII activity and plasminogen activator is dose-related, with maximal plasma levels of 300 to 400 percent of initial concentrations obtained after infusion of 0.4 mcg/kg body weight. The increase is rapid and evident within 30 minutes reaching a maximum at a point ranging from 90 minutes to two hours. The factor VIII-related antigen and ristocetin cofactor activity were also increased to a smaller degree, but still dose-dependent.
1. The biphasic half-lives of desmopressin acetate were 7.8 and 75.5 minutes for the fast and slow phases, respectively, compared with 2.5 and 14.5 minutes for lysine vasopressin, another form of the hormone. As a result, desmopressin acetate provides a prompt onset of antidiuretic action with a long duration after each administration.
2. The change in structure of arginine vasopressin to desmopressin acetate has resulted in a decreased vasopressor action and decreased actions on visceral smooth muscle relative to the enhanced antidiuretic activity, so that clinically effective antidiuretic doses are usually below threshold levels for effects on vascular or visceral smooth muscle.
3. When administered by injection, desmopressin acetate has an antidiuretic effect about ten times that of an equivalent dose administered intranasally.
4. The percentage increase of factor VIII levels in patients with mild hemophilia A and von Willebrand's disease was not significantly different from that observed in normal healthy individuals when treated with 0.3 mcg/kg of desmopressin acetate infused over 10 minutes. One hemophilia A patient treated with intravenous desmopressin acetate was shown to have a response that reached as much as five times the baseline value, and that occurred at 4½ hours after infusion.
5. Plasminogen activator activity increases rapidly after desmopressin acetate infusion, but there has been no clinically significant fibrinolysis in patients treated with desmopressin acetate.
6. The effect of repeated administration of desmopressin acetate when doses were given every 12 to 24 hours has generally shown a gradual diminution of the factor VIII activity increase noted with a single dose. The initial response is reproducible in any particular patient if there are 2 or 3 days between administration.

INDICATIONS AND USAGE

Hemophilia A
Stimate™ (desmopressin acetate) is indicated for patients with hemophilia A with factor VIII levels greater than 5%.
Stimate™ will often maintain hemostasis in patients with hemophilia A during surgical procedures and postoperatively when administered 30 minutes prior to scheduled procedure.
Stimate™ will also stop bleeding in hemophilia A patients with episodes of spontaneous or trauma-induced injuries such as hemarthroses, intramuscular hematomas or mucosal bleeding.
Stimate™ is not indicated for the treatment of hemophilia A with factor VIII levels equal to or less than 5%, or for the treatment of hemophilia B, or in patients who have factor VIII antibodies.
In certain clinical situations, it may be justified to try Stimate™ in patients with factor VIII levels between 2–5%; however these patients should be carefully monitored.
Von Willebrand's Disease (Type I)
Stimate™ is indicated for patients with mild to moderate classic von Willebrand's disease (Type I) with factor VIII levels greater than 5%. Stimate™ will often maintain hemostasis in patients with mild to moderate von Willebrand's disease during surgical procedures and postoperatively when administered 30 minutes prior to the scheduled procedure.
Stimate™ will usually stop bleeding in mild to moderate von Willebrand's patients with episodes of spontaneous or trauma-induced injuries such as hemarthroses, intramuscular hematomas or mucosal bleeding.
Those von Willebrand's disease patients who are least likely to respond are those with severe homozygous von Willebrand's disease with factor VIII coagulant activity, factor VIII antigen and von Willebrand's factor (ristocetin cofactor) activities less than 1%. Other patients may respond in a variable fashion depending on the type of molecular defect they have. Bleeding time and factor VIII coagulant activity, factor VIII antigen and von Willebrand's factor activities should be checked during administration of Stimate™ to ensure that adequate levels are being achieved.
Stimate™ is not indicated for the treatment of severe classic von Willebrand's disease (Type I) and when there is evidence of an abnormal molecular form of factor VIII antigen. See Warning.
Diabetes Insipidus
Stimate™ is indicated as antidiuretic replacement therapy in the management of central (cranial) diabetes insipidus and for the management of the temporary polyuria and polydipsia following head trauma or surgery in the pituitary region. Stimate™ is ineffective for the treatment of nephrogenic diabetes insipidus.
Desmopressin acetate is also available as an intranasal preparation, DDAVP.® However, this means of delivery can be compromised by a variety of factors that can make nasal insufflation ineffective or inappropriate. These include poor intranasal absorption, nasal congestion and blockage, nasal discharge, atrophy of nasal mucosa, and severe atrophic rhinitis. Intranasal delivery may be inappropriate where there is an impaired level of consciousness. In addition, cranial surgical procedures, such as transphenoidal hypophysectomy, create situations where an alternative route of administration is needed as in cases of nasal packing or recovery from surgery.

CONTRAINDICATIONS

Known hypersensitivity to Stimate™ (desmopressin acetate).

WARNING

Patients who do not have need of antidiuretic hormone for its antidiuretic effect, in particular those who are young or elderly, should be cautioned to ingest only enough fluid to satisfy thirst, in order to decrease the potential occurrence of water intoxication and hyponatremia.
Stimate™ (desmopressin acetate) should not be used to treat patients with Type IIB von Willebrand's disease since platelet aggregation may be induced.

PRECAUTIONS

GENERAL: For injection use only.
Desmopressin acetate has infrequently produced a slight elevation of blood pressure, which disappeared with a reduction in dosage. The drug should be used with caution in patients with coronary artery insufficiency and/or hypertensive cardiovascular disease, because of possible rise in blood pressure.
Severe allergic reactions have not been reported with desmopressin acetate. It is not known whether antibodies to desmopressin acetate are produced after repeated injections.
Hemophilia A
Laboratory tests for assessing patient status include levels of factor VIII coagulant, factor VIII antigen and factor VIII ristocetin cofactor (von Willebrand factor) as well as activated partial thromboplastin time. Factor VIII coagulant activity should be determined before giving desmopressin acetate for hemostasis. If factor VIII coagulant activity is present at less than 5% of normal, desmopressin acetate should not be relied on.
Von Willebrand's Disease
Laboratory tests for assessing patient status include levels of factor VIII coagulant, factor VIII antigen and factor VIII ristocetin cofactor (von Willebrand factor). The skin bleeding time may be helpful in following these patients.
Diabetes Insipidus
Laboratory tests for monitoring the patient include urine volume and osmolality. In some cases, plasma osmolality may be required.
DRUG INTERACTIONS: Although the pressor activity of desmopressin acetate is very low compared with the antidiuretic activity, use of doses as large as 0.3 mcg/kg of desmopressin acetate with other pressor agents should be done only with careful patient monitoring.
Desmopressin acetate has been used with epsilon aminocaproic acid without adverse effects.
CARCINOGENICITY, MUTAGENICITY, IMPAIRMENT OF FERTILITY: Teratology studies in rats have shown no abnormalities. No further data are available.
PREGNANCY CATEGORY B: Reproduction studies performed in rats and rabbits with subcutaneous doses up to 12.5 times the human dose when used for factor VIII stimulation and 125 times the human dose when used in diabetes insipidus have revealed no evidence of harm to the fetus due to desmopressin acetate. There are several publications of management of diabetes insipidus in pregnant women with no harm to the fetus reported; however, there are no adequate and well-controlled studies in pregnant women. Published reports stress that, as opposed to preparations containing the natural hormones, desmopressin acetate in antidiuretic doses has no uterotonic action, but the physician will have to weigh possible therapeutic advantages against possible danger in each case.
NURSING MOTHERS: It is not known whether this drug is excreted in human milk. Because many drugs are excreted in human milk, caution should be exercised when desmopressin acetate is administered to a nursing woman.
PEDIATRIC USE: Use in infants and children will require careful fluid intake restriction to prevent possible hyponatremia and water intoxication. *Stimate™ should not be used in infants younger than three months* in the treatment of hemophilia A or von Willebrand's disease; safety and effectiveness in children under 12 years of age with diabetes insipidus have not been established.

ADVERSE REACTIONS

Infrequently, desmopressin acetate has produced transient headache, nausea, mild abdominal cramps and vulval pain. These symptoms disappeared with reduction in dosage. Occasionally, injection of desmopressin acetate has produced local erythema, swelling or burning pain. Occasional facial flushing has been reported with the administration of desmopressin acetate.
Desmopressin acetate has infrequently produced a slight elevation of blood pressure, which disappeared with a reduction in dosage.
See WARNING for the possibility of water intoxication and hyponatremia.

OVERDOSAGE

See ADVERSE REACTIONS above. In case of overdosage, the dosage should be reduced, frequency of administration decreased, or the drug withdrawn according to the severity of the condition.
There is no known specific antidote for desmopressin acetate.
An oral LD_{50} has not been established. An intravenous dose of 2 mg/kg in mice demonstrated no effect.

DOSAGE AND ADMINISTRATION

Hemophilia A and von Willebrand's Disease (Type I)
Stimate™ is administered as an intravenous infusion at a dose of 0.3 mcg desmopressin acetate/kg body weight diluted in sterile physiological saline and infused slowly over 15 to 30 minutes. In adults and children weighing more than 10 kg, 50 ml of diluent is used; in children weighing 10 kg or less, 10 ml of diluent is used. Blood pressure and pulse should be monitored during infusion. If Stimate™ is used preoperatively, it should be administered 30 minutes prior to the scheduled procedure.
The necessity for repeat administration of Stimate™ or use of any blood products for hemostasis should be determined by laboratory response as well as the clinical condition of the patient. The tendency toward tachyphylaxis (lessening of response) with repeated administration given more frequently than every 48 hours should be considered in treating each patient.
Diabetes Insipidus
This formulation is administered subcutaneously or by direct intravenous injection. Stimate™ (desmopressin acetate) Injection dosage must be determined for each patient and adjusted according to the pattern of response. Response should be estimated by two parameters: adequate duration of sleep and adequate, not excessive, water turnover.
The usual dosage range in adults is 0.5 ml (2.0 mcg) to 1 ml (4.0 mcg) daily, administered intravenously or subcutaneously, usually in two divided doses. The morning and evening doses should be separately adjusted for an adequate diurnal rhythm of water turnover. For patients who have been controlled on intranasal desmopressin acetate and who must be switched to the injection form, either because of poor intranasal absorption or because of the need for surgery, the comparable antidiuretic dose of the injection is about one-tenth the intranasal dose.
Parenteral drug products should be inspected visually for particulate matter and discoloration prior to administration whenever solution and container permit.

HOW SUPPLIED
Stimate™ (desmopressin acetate) Injection is available as a sterile solution in 10 ml multiple-dose vials, (NDC 0053-2451-02) each containing 4.0 mcg desmopressin acetate per ml.
Keep refrigerated at about 4°C.
Manufactured for
Amour Pharmaceutical Company
Kankakee, Illinois 60901, U.S.A.
By Ferring Pharmaceuticals, Malmö, Sweden
Revised: May, 1985
Shown in Product Identification Section, page 404

THYTROPAR® ℞
[thī 'trō-pär "]
(thyrotropin for injection)
U.S. PAT. No. 2,871,159

THYTROPAR® is supplied as a sterile lyophilized powder containing 10 International Units of Thyrotropic activity. Each package contains one vial of THYTROPAR® (Thyrotropin for Injection) and one vial of THYTROPAR® Diluent (Sodium Chloride Injection).

TRACE ELEMENTS See under:

Chrometrace™ (Chromic Chloride Injection USP)
Coppertrace™ (Cupric Chloride Injection USP)
Mangatrace™ (Manganese Chloride Injection USP)
Multitrace™ 5
Multitrace™ Pediatric
Multitrace Solution and Concentrate
Selenitrace™ (Selenious Acid Injection)
Zinctrace™ (Zinc Chloride Injection USP)

ZINCTRACE™ ℞
[zĭngk 'trās]
Zinc Chloride Injection USP

1 mg/mL of Zinc
Zinctrace is supplied in 10 mL vials in boxes of 25 (NDC 00053-0833-22).

PLASMA DERIVATIVE PRODUCTS

ALBUMINAR®-5 ℞
[al-byōō 'mĭn-är]
Albumin
(Human) U.S.P. 5%

ALBUMINAR®-5 Albumin (Human) is supplied as a 5% solution in:
50 mL bottles containing 2.5 grams of albumin
250 mL bottles containing 12.5 grams of albumin
500 mL bottles containing 25.0 grams of albumin
1000 mL bottles containing 50 grams of albumin
For use with intravenous administration set. See directions on set supplied.

ALBUMINAR®-25 ℞
[ăl-byōō 'mĭn-är "]
Albumin
(Human) U.S.P. 25%

ALBUMINAR®-25 Albumin (Human), is supplied as a 25% solution in:
20 mL vials containing 5.0 grams of albumin
50 mL vials containing 12.5 grams of albumin
100 mL vials containing 25.0 grams of albumin
For use with intravenous administration set. See directions on set supplied.

GAMMAR® ℞
[găm 'är]
Immune Globulin
(Human) U.S.P.

GAMMAR® Immune Globulin (Human) U.S.P. is supplied in 2 mL and 10 mL vials.

GAMULIN® Rh ℞
[găm 'yōō-lĭn "]
Rh_o (D) Immune Globulin (Human)

A sterile Immune Globulin Solution containing Rh_o (D) antibodies. Supplied in individual package containing a single dose vial of Gamulin Rh, patient identification card, directions for use, and patient information brochure and cartons containing 25 single dose vials of Gamulin Rh, 25 patient identification cards, 10 sets of directions for use, and 25 patient information brochures and plastic cases containing 6 single dose syringes of Gamulin Rh, 6 patient identification cards, directions for use, 6 patient information brochures, and 6 laboratory control forms.

H.T. FACTORATE™ ℞
[făk 'tôr-āt "]
Antihemophilic Factor (Human) Dried, Heat-Treated

H.T. Factorate™ Antihemophilic Factor (Human), Heat-Treated is supplied in single dose vials (I.U. activity is stated on label of each vial) with sterile diluent and needles for reconstitution and withdrawal.

H.T. FACTORATE™ GENERATION II™ ℞
[făk 'tôr-āt "]
Antihemophilic Factor (Human) Dried, Heat-Treated

H.T. Factorate™ Generation II™ Antihemophilic Factor (Human), Heat-Treated is supplied in single dose vials (I.U. activity, total protein, and specific activity [I.U. per mg protein] are stated on carton label of each vial) with sterile diluent and needles for reconstitution and withdrawal.

HUMATE-P™ ℞
[hyōō 'māt]
Antihemophilic Factor (Human), Pasteurized

Humate-P™, Antihemophilic Factor (Human), Pasteurized, is supplied in single dose vials (I.U. activity is stated on label of each vial) with sterile diluent and needles for reconstitution and withdrawal. Manufactured by Behringwerke AG, Marburg/Lahn West Germany and distributed by Armour Pharmaceutical Company.

MINI-GAMULIN™ Rh ℞
[mĭ-nē "găm 'yoo-lĭn]
Rh_o (D) Immune Globulin (Human)

A sterile Immune Globulin Solution containing Rh_o (D) antibodies. Mini-Gamulin Rh contains one-sixth the quantity of Rh_o (D) antibody contained in a standard dose of Rh_o (D) Immune Globulin (Human). Mini-Gamulin is supplied in individual packages of single dose vials and cartons of 25 single dose vials.

PLASMA-PLEX® ℞
[plăz 'ma-plĕks]
Plasma Protein Fraction (Human) U.S.P.

As a 5% Solution in:
50 mL bottles containing 2.5 g of selected plasma proteins
250 mL bottles containing 12.5 g of selected plasma proteins
500 mL bottles containing 25.0 g of selected plasma proteins.
For use with intravenous administration set. See directions on set supplied.

THROMBINAR® ℞
[thrŏm 'bĭn-är]
THROMBIN, TOPICAL (BOVINE), U.S.P.

Thrombin, Topical (Bovine), U.S.P. Thrombinar® must not be injected! It is for topical use only.

DESCRIPTION
Thrombinar® Thrombin, Topical (Bovine), U.S.P. is a protein product produced through activation of prothrombin of bovine origin by tissue thromboplastin in the presence of calcium chloride. It is supplied as a sterile powder that has been freeze-dried in the final container. Also contained in this preparation are 50% mannitol and 45% sodium chloride. Mannitol is included to make the dried product friable and more readily soluble. The material contains no preservative.
This product is prepared under rigid assay control against U.S. Standard Thrombin.

CLINICAL PHARMACOLOGY
Thrombinar® requires no intermediate physiological agent for its action. It clots the fibrinogen of the blood directly. Failure to clot blood occurs in the rare case where the primary clotting defect is the absence of fibrinogen itself. The speed with which thrombin clots blood is dependent upon its concentration.

INDICATIONS AND USAGE
Thrombinar® Thrombin, Topical (Bovine) U.S.P., is indicated as an aid in hemostasis whenever oozing blood and minor bleeding from capillaries and small venules is accessible.
In various types of surgery solutions of thrombin may be used in conjunction with absorbable gelatin sponge, USP for hemostasis.

CONTRAINDICATIONS
Thrombinar® is contraindicated in persons known to be sensitive to any of its components and/or to material of bovine origin.

WARNING

Because of its action in the clotting mechanism, Thrombinar® must not be injected or otherwise allowed to enter large blood vessels. Extensive intravascular clotting and even death may result.

PRECAUTIONS
General—Consult the absorbable gelatin sponge product labeling for use prior to utilizing a thrombin saturated-sponge procedure.
Pregnancy—Category C—Animal reproduction studies have not been conducted with Thrombin, Topical (Bovine) U.S.P. It is also not known whether Thrombin, Topical (Bovine), U.S.P. can cause fetal harm when administered to a pregnant woman or can affect reproduction capacity. Thrombin, Topical (Bovine), U.S.P. should be given to a pregnant woman only if clearly indicated.
Pediatric Use—Safety and effectiveness in children have not been established.

ADVERSE REACTIONS
Allergic reactions may be encountered in persons known to be sensitive to bovine materials.

DOSAGE AND ADMINISTRATION
Solutions of Thrombinar® Thrombin, Topical (Bovine), U.S.P. may be prepared in Sterile Water for Injection, USP or isotonic saline. Sterile Water for Injection is recommended for reconstitution for 1,000 units per mL or greater, isotonic saline for more dilute solutions. The intended use determines the strength of the solution to prepare. For general use such as plastic surgery, skin grafting, neurosurgery, solutions containing approximately 100 units per mL are frequently used. For this, 10 mL of diluent added to the 1,000 unit vial is suitable. Where bleeding is profuse, concentrations as high as 1,000 to 2,000 units per mL may be required. For this, the 5,000 unit, 10,000 unit, or 20,000 unit vials dissolved in the appropriate amount of diluent supplied in each package is convenient. Other potencies to suit the needs of the case may be prepared by selecting the proper strength package and dissolving the contents in an appropriate volume of diluent. In many situations, it may be advantageous to use Thrombinar® in dry form on oozing surfaces.
Caution: Product contains no preservative. Solution should be used immediately upon reconstitution. However, the solution may be refrigerated at approximately 5°C. Do not use after 3 hours.
The following techniques are suggested for the topical application of thrombin:

1. The recipient surface should be sponged (not wiped) free of blood before thrombin is applied.
2. A spray may be used or the surface may be flooded using a sterile syringe and small gauge needle. The most effective hemostasis results when the thrombin mixes freely with the blood as soon as it reaches the surface.
3. In instances where thrombin in dry form is needed, the vial is opened by removing the metal ring by grasping the edge where it is scored and tearing, using sterile pliers. The rubber-diaphragm cap may be easily removed and the dried thrombin is then broken up into a powder by means of sterile glass rod or other suitable sterile instrument.
4. Sponging of treated surfaces should be avoided in order that the clot remain securely in place.
   Thrombin, Topical (Bovine), U.S.P. may be used in conjunction with absorbable gelatin sponge, USP as follows:
   1. Prepare thrombin solution of the desired strength.
   2. Immerse sponge strips of the desired size in the thrombin solution. Knead the sponge strips vigorously with moistened fingers to remove trapped air, thereby facilitating saturation of the sponge.
   3. Apply saturated sponge to bleeding area. Hold in place for 10 to 15 seconds with a pledget of cotton or a small gauze sponge.

HOW SUPPLIED
Thrombinar® Thrombin, Topical (Bovine), U.S.P. is supplied in 1,000 U.S. Standard unit vials, 5,000 U.S. Standard unit vials, 10,000 U.S. Standard unit vials, 20,000 U.S. Standard unit vials, and 50,000 U.S. Standard unit vials of Thrombin, Topical. The 5,000 U.S. Standard unit vial is supplied with one 5 mL vial of Sterile Water for Injection, U.S.P. The 10,000 U.S. Standard unit vial is supplied with one 10 mL vial of Sterile Water for Injection U.S.P. The 20,000 U.S. Standard unit vial is supplied with one 20 mL vial of Sterile Water for Injection U.S.P.

Continued on next page

Armour—Cont.

STORAGE
Store vials at 2°–8°C (36°–46°F).
Revised: May, 1985

EDUCATIONAL MATERIAL

Albuminar
"The Clinical Uses of normal serum Albumin (human)" (CME—Rutgers) cassette and accompanying brochure.
Available to physicians and pharmacists—contact your local Armour Sales Representative.
Factorate
Hemophilia booklets
—Management of hemophilia
—Boys with hemophilia
—Employment issues in hemophilia
—Employee with hemophilia
—Professional services in hemophilia
—Fluid Management—its a whole new ballgame
Available to physicians, pharmacists and patients—contact your local Armour Sales Representative or Armour Corporate Headquarters.
Gamulin
"Confidence Factor" booklets
—in Rh negative women
—in abortion
—in antepartum prophylaxis
—in prenatal diagnostic testing
The above literature is available to physicians, pharmacists and patients.
Monograph Series—"The Prevention of Rh Isoimmunization"
#1— Amniocentesis and Rh Isoimmunization
#2— Antenatal Rh Immune Globulin Use in an Uneventful Pregnancy
#3— Management of the High-Risk Pregnancy
#4— Massive Transplacental Hemorrhage, the Laboratory and the Blood Bank
Film—"Hemolytic disease of the newborn"
The Monograph Series and film are available to physicians and pharmacists—contact your local Armour Sales Representative or Armour Corporate Headquarters.
M.V.I. Product Line
"Establishing a Nutritional Support Team" —audiovisual presentation and accompanying brochure
Quarterly newsletter—"The Nutritional Support Team"
Available to physicians and pharmacists—contact your local Armour Sales Representative or Armour Corporate Headquarters.
Stimate
Booklets
—Questions and answers
—Mild hemophilia
Available to physicians and pharmacists—contact your local Armour Sales Representative or Armour Corporate Headquarters.
Thrombinar
Surgical casebook series
#1— Banded gastroplasty
#2— Abdominal aortic aneurysm inlay anastomosis
#3— Cholecystectomy
#4— Surgical intervention due to chemical peritonitis
#5— Repair of laceration of inferior vena cava
#6— The Whipple Procedure in chronic pancreatitis
Available to physicians and pharmacists—contact your local Armour Sales Representative or Armour Corporate Headquarters.

IDENTIFICATION PROBLEM?
Consult PDR's
Product Identification Section
where you'll find over 1200
products pictured actual size
and in full color.

Arther, Inc.
BOX 335
MOUNTAIN LAKES, NJ 07046

TRYPTACIN®
[*trip'tă-sin*]
(brand of l-tryptophan)

DESCRIPTION
TRYPTACIN - Chemically, l-tryptophan, aminoindole-3-propionic acid is white to slightly yellowish white crystals or crystalline powder, taste slightly bitter. When dried, contains not less than 98.5% and not more than 100.5% of l-tryptophan($C_{11}H_{12}N_2O_2$).

ACTION AND USES
Dietary supplement, essential amino acid. L-tryptophan is a precursor of the neurotransmitter, serotonin (5-hydroxytryptamine). Some research activities are listed under "References."

ADMINISTRATION AND DOSAGE
2 to 4 500 mg. tablets one half hour before bedtime.

HOW SUPPLIED
Capsule shaped, scored white tablets.
Bottle of 100's—NDC 48558-001-10
Bottle of 250's—NDC 48558-001-25

REFERENCES
Potentiation of the Antidepressant Action of Clomipramine by Tryptophan
Arch. Gen. Psych. 33:1, 384–389. 1976

L-tryptophan in Obsessive-Compulsive Disorders
Am. J. Psych. 134:4 Nov 1977

L-tryptophan: A Rational Hypnotic with Clinical Potential
Am. J. Psych. 134:4, Apr 1977

Tryptophan Antidepressant 'Psychological Sedative': Fact or Fancy?
Psychopharmacology 61: 97–102, 1979

Pain and Tryptophan
J. Neurosurg., 53:44–52, 1980

Tryptophan in the Treatment of Depression
Advances in Experimental Medicine and Biology, 133: 727–737, 1981

Short-term and Repetitive Administration of Oral Tryptophan in Normal Men
Arch. Gen. Psych. 38:619–626, 1981

Effects of L-tryptophan on Sleepiness and on Sleep
J. Psychiatric Research 17(2): 107–113, 1983

Selectivity in Response to L-tryptophan Among Insomniac Subjects: A Preliminary Report
Sleep 6(3): 247–256, 1983

Lithium Carbonate and L-tryptophan in the Treatment of Bipolar and Schizoaffective Disorders
Am. J. Psych. 140:6, 757–760, 1983

The Effects of Tryptophan and Tyrosine on Human Mood and Performance
Psychopharmacology Bulletin 20(3): 595–598, 1984

B.F. Ascher & Company, Inc.
15501 WEST 109TH STREET
LENEXA, KS 66219

ADIPOST™ ℂ℞
[*ad-uh-post*]

Phendimetrazine tartrate slow-release capsules .... 105 mg

HOW SUPPLIED
White/clear capsules with Ascher logo and NDC 225/400 printed in red on each capsule half. Contains blue & white slow-release beads.
Bottles of 100—NDC 0225-0400-15

ANASPAZ® Tablets ℞
[*an'ah-spăz*]

(l-hyoscyamine sulfate) .... 0.125 mg

HOW SUPPLIED
Yellow, compressed, scored tablets with the Ascher logo on one side and the NDC 225/295 on the other.
Bottles of 100—NDC 0225-0295-15
Bottles of 500—NDC 0225-0295-20

AYR® Saline Nasal Mist and Drops

(See PDR For Nonprescription Drugs)

CONVERZYME® ℞
[*con-ver-zyme*]

Each capsule contains the enzymes:
Cellulase .... 5 mg
Protease .... 10 mg
Amylase .... eq. 30 mg
Lipase .... 13 mg

HOW SUPPLIED
Pink, opaque hard gel capsules
Bottles of 100—NDC 0225-0366-15

DRIZE® ℞
[*driz*]
Chlorpheniramine maleate .... 12 mg.
Phenylpropanolamine HCl .... 75 mg.

HOW SUPPLIED
Clear capsules with white slow-release beads with the NDC 225-405 imprinted in iron oxide black to insure the product is dye-free.
Bottles of 100—NDC 0225-0405-15

HY-PHEN® Tablets ℂIII ℞
formerly Hycodaphen
[*hi-fen*]
hydrocodone bitartrate 5 mg
(WARNING: May be habit forming.)
acetaminophen 500 mg

DESCRIPTION
Each HY-PHEN tablet contains:
Hydrocodone Bitartrate* 5 mg.
*WARNING: May be habit forming.
Acetaminophen 500 mg.
Acetaminophen is a nonopiate, non-salicylate analgesic and antipyretic which occurs as a white, odorless crystalline powder possessing a slightly bitter taste. Hydrocodone bitartrate is an opioid analgesic and antitussive and occurs as fine, white crystals or as a crystalline powder. It is affected by light.

INACTIVE INGREDIENTS
Microcrystalline cellulose, NF; magnesium stearate, NF; sodium starch glycolate, NF; pregelatinized starch, NF.

CLINICAL PHARMACOLOGY
Hydrocodone is a semisynthetic narcotic analgesic and antitussive with multiple actions qualitatively similar to those of codeine. Most of these involve the central nervous system and smooth muscle. The precise mechanism of action of hydrocodone and other opiates is not known, although it is believed to relate to the existence of opiate receptors in the central nervous system. In addition to analgesia, narcotics may produce drowsiness, changes in mood and mental clouding.
Radioimmunoassay techniques have recently been developed for the analysis of hydrocodone in human plasma. After a 10 mg oral dose of hydrocodone bitartrate, a mean peak serum drug level of 23.6 ng/ml and an elimination half-life of 3.8 hours were found.
The analgesic action of acetaminophen involves peripheral and central influences, but the specific mechanism is as yet undetermined. Antipyretic activity is mediated through hypothalamic heat regulating centers. Acetaminophen inhibits prostaglandin synthetase. Therapeutic doses of acetaminophen have negligible effects on the cardiovascular or respiratory systems; however, toxic doses may cause circulatory failure and rapid, shallow breathing. Acetaminophen is rapidly and almost completely absorbed from the gastrointestinal tract, producing maximum serum concentrations within 30 minutes to one hour. The plasma half-life in adults and children ranges from 0.90 hours to 3.25 hours with an average of approximately 2 hours. The drug distributes uniformly in most body fluids and is approximately 25% protein bound. Acetaminophen is conjugated in the liver, with less than 3% of the dose excreted unchanged in 24 hours. The primary metabolic pathway is conjugation to sulfate and glucuronide by-products. A minor oxidative pathway forms cysteine and mercapturic acid. These compounds are subsequently excreted by the kidneys into the urine.

INDICATIONS AND USAGE
For the relief of moderate to moderately severe pain.

CONTRAINDICATIONS
Hypersensitivity to acetaminophen or hydrocodone.

WARNINGS

Respiratory Depression: At high doses or in sensitive patients, hydrocodone may produce dose-related respiratory depression by acting directly on brain stem respiratory centers. Hydrocodone also affects centers that control respiratory rhythm, and may produce irregular and periodic breathing.

Head Injury and Increased Intracranial Pressure: The respiratory depressant effects of narcotics and their capacity to elevate cerebrospinal fluid pressure may be markedly exaggerated in the presence of head injury, other intracranial lesions or a pre-existing increase in intracranial pressure. Furthermore, narcotics produce adverse reactions which may obscure the clinical course of patients with head injuries.

Acute Abdominal Conditions: The administration of narcotics may obscure the diagnosis or clinical course of patients with acute abdominal conditions.

PRECAUTIONS

Special Risk Patients: As with any narcotic analgesic agent, HY-PHEN should be used with caution in elderly or debilitated patients and those with severe impairment of hepatic or renal function, hypothyroidism. Addison's disease, prostatic hypertrophy or urethral stricture. The usual precautions should be observed and the possibility of respiratory depression should be kept in mind.

Information for Patients: HY-PHEN, like all narcotics, may impair the mental and/or physical abilities required for the performance of potentially hazardous tasks such as driving a car or operating machinery; patients should be cautioned accordingly.

Cough Reflex: Hydrocodone suppresses the cough reflex; as with all narcotics, caution should be exercised when HY-PHEN is used postoperatively and in patients with pulmonary disease.

Drug Interactions: Patients receiving other narcotic analgesics, antipsychotics, antianxiety agents, or other CNS depressants (including alcohol) concommitantly with HY-PHEN may exhibit an additive CNS depression. When combined therapy is contemplated, the dose of one or both agents should be reduced.

The use of MAO inhibitors or tricyclic antidepressants with hydrocodone preparations may increase the effect of either the antidepressant or hydrocodone.

The concurrent use of anticholinergics with hydrocodone may produce paralytic ileus.

Usage in Pregnancy: Pregnancy Category C. Hydrocodone has been shown to be teratogenic in hamsters when given in doses 700 times the human dose. There are no adequate and well-controlled studies in pregnant women. HY-PHEN should be used during pregnancy only if the potential benefit justifies the potential risk to the fetus.

Nonteratogenic Effects: Babies born to mothers who have been taking opioids regularly prior to delivery will be physically dependent. The withdrawal signs include irritability and excessive crying, tremors, hyperactive reflexes, increased respiratory rate, increased stools, sneezing, yawning, vomiting, and fever. The intensity of the syndrome does not always correlate with the duration of maternal opioid use or dose. There is no consensus on the best method of managing withdrawal. Chlorpromazine 0.7 to 1.0 mg/kg q6h, and paregoric 2 to 4 drops/kg q4h, have been used to treat withdrawal symptoms in infants. The duration of therapy is 4 to 28 days, with the dosage decreased as tolerated.

Labor and Delivery: As with all narcotics, administration of HY-PHEN to the mother shortly before delivery may result in some degree of respiratory depression in the newborn, especially if higher doses are used.

Nursing Mothers: It is not known whether this drug is excreted in human milk. Because many drugs are excreted in human milk and because of the potential for serious adverse reactions in nursing infants from HY-PHEN, a decision should be made whether to discontinue nursing or to discontinue the drug, taking into account the importance of the drug to the mother.

Pediatric Use: Safety and effectiveness in children have not been established.

ADVERSE REACTIONS

Central Nervous System: Sedation, drowsiness, mental clouding, lethargy, impairment of mental and physical performance, anxiety, fear, dysphoria, dizziness, psychic dependence, mood changes.

Gastrointestinal System: Nausea and vomiting may occur; they are more frequent in ambulatory than in recumbent patients. The antiemetic phenothiazines are useful in suppressing these effects; however, some phenothiazine derivatives seem to be antianalgesic and to increase the amount of narcotic required to produce pain relief, while other phenothiazines reduce the amount of narcotic required to produce a given level of analgesia. Prolonged administration of HY-PHEN may produce constipation.

Genitourinary System: Ureteral spasm, spasm of vesical sphincters and urinary retention have been reported.

Respiratory Depression: HY-PHEN may produce dose-related respiratory depression by acting directly on brain stem respiratory centers. Hydrocodone also affects centers that control respiratory rhythm, and may produce irregular and periodic breathing. If significant respiratory depression occurs, it may be antagonized by the use of naloxone hydrochloride. Apply other supportive measures when indicated.

Drug Abuse and Dependence: HY-PHEN is subject to the Federal Controlled Sustance Act (Schedule III). Psychic dependence, physical dependence, and tolerance may develop upon repeated administration of narcotics; therefore, HY-PHEN should be prescribed and administered with caution. However, psychic dependence is unlikely to develop when HY-PHEN is used for a short time for the treatment of pain. Physical dependence, the condition in which continued administration of the drug is required to prevent the appearance of a withdrawal syndrome, assumes clinically significant proportions only after several weeks of continued narcotic use, although some mild degree of physical dependence may develop after a few days of narcotic therapy. Tolerance, in which increasingly large doses are required in order to produce the same degree of analgesia, is manifested initially by a shortened duration of analgesic effect, and subsequently by decreases in the intensity of analgesia. The rate of development of tolerance varies among patients.

OVERDOSAGE

Acetaminophen:

Signs and Symptoms: Acetaminophen in massive overdosage may cause hepatic toxicity in some patients. In cases of suspected overdose, you may wish to call your regional poison center for assistance in diagnosis and for directions in the use of N-acetylcysteine as an antidote.

In adults, hepatic toxicity has rarely been reported with acute overdoses of less than 10 grams and fatalities with less than 15 grams. Importantly, young children seem to be more resistant than adults to the hepatotoxic effect of an acetaminophen overdose. Despite this, the measures outlined below should be initiated in any adult or child suspected of having ingested an acetaminophen overdose.

Early symptoms following a potentially hepatotoxic overdose may include: nausea, vomiting, diaphoresis and general malaise. Clinical and laboratory evidence of hepatic toxicity may not be apparent until 48 to 72 hours postingestion.

Treatment: The stomach should be emptied promptly by lavage or by induction of emesis with syrup of ipecac. Patients' estimates of the quantity of a drug ingested are notoriously unreliable. Therefore, if an acetaminophen overdose is suspected, a serum acetaminophen assay should be obtained as early as possible, but no sooner than four hours following ingestion. Liver function studies should be obtained initially and repeated at 24-hour intervals.

The antidote, N-acetylcysteine, should be administered as early as possible, preferably within 16 hours of the overdose ingestion for optimal results, but in any case, within 24 hours. Following recovery, there are no residual, structural or functional hepatic abnormalities.

Hydrocodone:

Signs and Symptoms: Serious overdose with hydrocodone is characterized by respiratory depression (a decrease in respiratory rate and/or tidal volume, Cheyne-Stokes respiration, cyanosis), extreme somnolence progressing to stupor or coma, skeletal muscle flaccidity, cold and clammy skin, and sometimes bradycardia and hypotension. In severe overdosage, apnea, circulatory collapse, cardiac arrest and death may occur.

Treatment: Primary attention should be given to the reestablishment of adequate respiratory exchange through provision of a patent airway and the institution of assisted or controlled ventilation. The narcotic antagonist naloxone is a specific antidote against respiratory depression which may result from overdosage or unusual sensitivity to narcotics, including hydrocodone. Therefore, an appropriate dose of naloxone (see package insert) should be administered, preferably by the intravenous route, and simultaneously with efforts at respiratory resuscitation. Since the duration of action of hydrocodone may exceed that of the antagonist, the patient should be kept under continued surveillance and repeated doses of the antagonist should be administered as needed to maintain adequate respiration.

An antagonist should not be administered in the absence of clinically significant respiratory or cardiovascular depression. Oxygen, intravenous fluids, vasopressors and other supportive measures should be employed as indicated.

Gastric emptying may be useful in removing unabsorbed drug.

DOSAGE AND ADMINISTRATION

Dosage should be adjusted according to the severity of the pain and the response of the patient. However, it should be kept in mind that tolerance to hydrocodone can develop with continued use and that the incidence of untoward effects is dose related.

The usual dose is one tablet every six hours as needed for pain. If necessary, this dose may be repeated at four hour intervals. In cases of more severe pain, two tablets every six hours (up to 8 tablets in 24 hours) may be required.

HOW SUPPLIED

HY-PHEN is available as a compressed, white, capsule shaped, bisected tablet impressed with two Ascher logos in juxtaposition with the score on one side and 225-450 on the other in bottles of 100 tablets (NDC 0225-0450-15) and 500 tablets (NDC 0225-0450-20) and Hospital Unit Dose Package of 100 Tablets (NDC 0225-0450-21).

Storage: Store HY-PHEN at controlled room temperature 15°–30°C (59°–86°F).

A Schedule Ⓒ III Narcotic.

Mfd. for
B. F. ASCHER & COMPANY, INC.
Lenexa, Kansas 66219

KWELCOF® Ⓒ III ℞
[kwel 'cof]

Each teaspoonful (5 ml) contains:
Hydrocodone bitartrate .... 5 mg
(WARNING: May be habit-forming)
Guaifenesin .... 100 mg

HOW SUPPLIED

Clear, fruit-flavored liquid which is alcohol-free, dye-free, sugar-free and corn products-free.
1 pint bottles—NDC 0225-0420-45
Unit Dose: 10 × 5 ml cups—NDC 0225-0420-75
Unit Dose: 100 × 5 ml cups—NDC 0225-0420-15

MOBIGESIC® Analgesic Tablets

(See PDR For Nonprescription Drugs)

MOBISYL® Analgesic Creme

(See PDR For Nonprescription Drugs)

NILORIC™ ℞
[ni-lor 'ic]

Each sublingual tablet contains ergoloid mesylates 1.0 mg as follows:
dihydroergocornine .... 0.333 mg
dihydroergocristine .... 0.333 mg
dihydroergocryptine .... 0.333 mg
(dihydro-alpha-ergocryptine and dihydro-beta-ergocryptine 2:1)
as methanesulfonates (mesylates)

HOW SUPPLIED

Compressed, white, oval tablet impressed with the Ascher logo on one side and 415 on the other. Bottles of 100—NDC 0225-0415-15

PEN•KERA™ Creme

(See PDR For Nonprescription Drugs)

TOLFRINIC® ℞
[tol-fren-ic]

Each tablet contains:
Ferrous fumarate .... 600 mg
(Provides elemental iron 200 mg)
Vitamin B_{12} (cyanocobalamin) .... 25 mcg
(anyhydrous)
Ascorbic Acid .... 100 mg

HOW SUPPLIED

Brown, sugar-coated tablet with Ascher logo on one side and the NDC 225/105 on the other.
Bottles of 100—NDC 0225-0105-15

UNILAX® Tablets

(See PDR For Nonprescription Drugs)

Products are cross-indexed by
generic and chemical names
in the
YELLOW SECTION

Astra Pharmaceutical Products, Inc.

50 OTIS STREET
WESTBORO, MA 01581-4428

ATROPINE SULFATE ℞

[*ā 'trow-peen*]
Injection, USP
0.1 mg/ml
Adult Strength

(For details of indications, dosage and administration, precautions, and adverse reactions, see circular in package.)

HOW SUPPLIED

Prefilled syringes equipped with 22 g 1¼" needle:
5 ml (0.5 mg) NDC 0186-0648-01
10 ml (1 mg) NDC 0186-0649-01
Solution should be stored at controlled room temperature 15°–30°C (59°–86°F)
021853R00 Iss. 6/85

10% CALCIUM CHLORIDE ℞

[*cal 'cium chlor 'ide*]
Injection, USP
1 gram (100 mg/ml)
27.3 mg (1.4 mEq) Ca++/ml
2.04 mOsm/ml (calc.)
A Hypertonic Solution for Intravenous Injection

Caution: This solution must not be injected intramuscularly or subcutaneously.

(For details of indications, dosage and administration, precautions, and adverse reactions, see circular in package.)

HOW SUPPLIED

10% Calcium Chloride Injection, USP is supplied as follows:
NDC 0186-1165-02 10 ml ampules in packages of 5.
NDC 0186-1166-04 10 ml single dose vials in packages of 25.
NDC 0186-0651-01 10 ml prefilled syringes with 22 g ¼" needle.
The solution should be stored at controlled room temperature 15°–30°C (59°–86°F).
021854R00 Iss. 6/85

10% CALCIUM GLUCONATE ℞

[*cal 'cium glu 'con-ate*]
Injection, USP
0.465 mEq (9.3 mg) Ca++/ml
0.7 mOsm/ml (calculated)
For Intravenous Use Only

(For details of indications, dosage and administration, precautions, and adverse reactions, see circular in package.)

HOW SUPPLIED

Calcium Gluconate USP, 10% is supplied in the following forms:
NDC 0186-1171-02 10 ml Ampule in packages of 5
NDC 0186-1172-04 10 ml Single Dose Vial in packages of 25
Store at controlled room temperature 15°–30°C (59°–86°F).
Note: Supersaturated solutions are prone to precipitation. See PRECAUTIONS for instructions for dissolving crystals.
021858R00 Iss. 8/85

50% DEXTROSE ℞

[*dex 'trose*]
Injection, USP
Concentrated Dextrose
For Intravenous Administration

NOTE: This solution is hypertonic—see Warnings and Precautions

(For details of indications, dosage and administration, precautions, and adverse reactions, see circular in package.)

HOW SUPPLIED

Dextrose Injection USP, 50% is supplied as follows:
50 ml Single Dose Vial, NDC 0186-1170-04
50 ml Prefilled Syringe with 19 g 15/16" needle, NDC 0186-0654-01
The solution should be stored at controlled room temperature 15°–30° (59°–86°F).
021857R00 Iss. 6/85

DOPAMINE HCl Injection, USP ℞

[*dó-pa-mean*]

DESCRIPTION

Dopamine, a sympathomimetic amine vasopressor, is the naturally occurring immediate precursor of norepinephrine. Dopamine hydrochloride is a white to off-white, crystalline powder, which may have a slight odor of hydrochloric acid. It is freely soluble in water and soluble in alcohol. Dopamine HCl is sensitive to alkalies, iron salts, and oxidizing agents. Chemically it is designated as 4-(2-aminoethyl)pyrocatechol hydrochloride, and its molecular formula is $C_8H_{11}NO_2 \bullet HCl$. The chemical structure is:

HO / HO— [benzene ring] —$CH_2CH_2NH_2 \cdot HCl$

Dopamine hydrochloride injection is a clear, practically colorless, sterile, pyrogen-free, aqueous solution of dopamine HCl for intravenous infusion after dilution. Each ml contains either 40 mg, 80 mg or 160 mg dopamine hydrochloride (equivalent to 32.3 mg, 64.6 mg and 129.2 mg dopamine base, respectively) in Water for Injection, USP containing 1% sodium bisulfite as an antioxidant. The pH of the solution may be adjusted with sodium hydroxide and/or hydrochloric acid to pH 2.5–4.5.

Dopamine must be diluted in an appropriate, sterile parenteral solution before intravenous administration. (See DOSAGE AND ADMINISTRATION.)

CLINICAL PHARMACOLOGY

Dopamine is a natural catecholamine formed by the decarboxylation of 3,4-dihydroxyphenylalanine (DOPA). It is a precursor to norepinephrine in noradrenergic nerves and is also a neurotransmitter in certain areas of the central nervous system, especially in the nigrostriatal tract, and in a few peripheral sympathetic nerves.

Dopamine produces positive chronotropic and inotropic effects on the myocardium, resulting in increased heart rate and cardiac contractility. This is accomplished directly by exerting an agonist action on beta-adrenoceptors and indirectly by causing release of norepinephrine from storage sites in sympathetic nerve endings.

Dopamine's onset of action occurs within five minutes of intravenous administration, and with dopamine's plasma half-life of about two minutes, the duration of action is less than ten minutes. However, if monoamine oxidase (MAO) inhibitors are present, the duration may increase to one hour. The drug is widely distributed in the body but does not cross the blood-brain barrier to a significant extent. Dopamine is metabolized in the liver, kidney, and plasma by MAO and catechol-O-methyltransferase to the inactive compounds homovanillic acid (HVA) and 3,4-dihydroxyphenylacetic acid. About 25% of the dose is taken up into specialized neurosecretory vesicles (the adrenergic nerve terminals), where it is hydroxylated to form norepinephrine. It has been reported that about 80% of the drug is excreted in the urine within 24 hours, primarily as HVA and its sulfate and glucuronide conjugates and as 3,4-dihydroxyphenylacetic acid. A very small portion is excreted unchanged.

The predominant effects of dopamine are dose-related, although it should be noted that actual response of an individual patient will largely depend on the clinical status of the patient at the time the drug is administered. At low rates of infusion (0.5–2 mcg/kg/min) dopamine causes vasodilation that is presumed to be due to a specific agonist action on dopamine receptors (distinct from alpha- and beta-adrenoceptors) in the renal, mesenteric, coronary, and intracerebral vascular beds. At these dopamine receptors, haloperidol is an antagonist. The vasodilation in these vascular beds is accompanied by increased glomerular filtration rate, renal blood flow, sodium excretion, and urine flow. Hypotension sometimes occur. An increase in urinary output produced by dopamine is usually not associated with a decrease in osmolality of the urine.

At intermediate rates of infusion (2–10 mcg/kg/min) dopamine acts to stimulate the $beta_1$-adrenoceptors, resulting in improved myocardial contractility, increased SA rate and enhanced impulse conduction in the heart. There is little, if any, stimulation of the $beta_2$-adrenoceptors (peripheral vasodilation). Dopamine causes less increase in myocardial oxygen consumption than isoproterenol, and its use is not usually associated with a tachyarrhythmia. Clinical studies indicate that it usually increases systolic and pulse pressure with either no effect or a slight increase in diastolic pressure. Blood flow to the peripheral vascular beds may decrease while mesenteric flow increases due to increased cardiac output. Total peripheral resistance (alpha effects) at low and intermediate doses is usually unchanged.

At higher rates of infusion (10–20 mcg/kg/min) there is some effect on alpha-adrenoceptors, with consequent vasoconstrictor effects and a rise in blood pressure. The vasoconstrictor effects are first seen in the skeletal muscle vascular beds, but with increasing doses, they are also evident in the renal and mesenteric vessels. At very high rates of infusion (above 20 mcg/kg/min), stimulation of alpha-adrenoceptors predominates and vasoconstriction may compromise the circulation of the limbs and override the dopaminergic effects of dopamine, reversing renal dilation and naturesis.

INDICATIONS AND USAGE

Dopamine HCl is indicated for the correction of hemodynamic imbalances present in the shock syndrome due to myocardial infarction, trauma, endotoxic septicemia, open-heart surgery, renal failure, and chronic cardiac decompensation as in congestive failure.

Patients most likely to respond adequately to dopamine HCl are those in whom physiological parameters, such as urine flow, myocardial function, and blood pressure, have not undergone profound deterioration. Multiclinic trials indicate that the shorter the time interval between onset of signs and symptoms and initiation of therapy with blood volume correction and dopamine HCl, the better the prognosis. Where appropriate, blood volume restoration with a suitable plasma expander or whole blood should be accomplished prior to administration of dopamine HCl.

Poor Perfusion of Vital Organs: Urine flow appears to be one of the better diagnostic signs by which adequacy of vital organ perfusion can be monitored. Nevertheless, the physician should also observe the patient for signs of reversal of confusion or reversal of comatose condition. Loss of pallor, increase in toe temperature, and/or adequacy of nail bed capillary filling may also be used as indices of adequate dosage. Clinical studies have shown that when dopamine HCl is administered before urine flow has diminished to levels of approximately 0.3 mL/minute, prognosis is more favorable. Nevertheless, in a number of oliguric or anuric patients, administration of dopamine HCl has resulted in an increase in urine flow, which in some cases reached normal levels. Dopamine HCl may also increase urine flow in patients whose output is within normal limits and thus may be of value in reducing the degree of preexisting fluid accumulation. It should be noted that at doses above those optimal for the individual patient, urine flow may decrease, necessitating reduction of dosage.

Low Cardiac Output: Increased cardiac output is related to dopamine's direct inotropic effect on the myocardium. Increased cardiac output at low or moderate doses appears to be related to a favorable prognosis. Increase in cardiac output has been associated with either static or decreased systemic vascular resistance (SVR). Static or decreased SVR associated with low or moderate movements in cardiac output is believed to be a reflection of differential effects on specific vascular beds with increased resistance in peripheral beds (e.g., femoral) and concomitant decreases in mesenteric and renal vascular beds.

Redistribution of blood flow parallels these changes so that an increase in cardiac output is accompanied by an increase in mesenteric and renal blood flow. In many instances the renal fraction of the total cardiac output has been found to increase. Increase in cardiac output produced by dopamine is not associated with substantial decreases in systemic vascular resistance as may occur with isoproterenol.

Hypotension: Hypotension due to inadequate cardiac output can be managed by administration of low to moderate doses of dopamine HCl which have little effect on SVR. At high therapeutic doses, dopamine's alpha-adrenergic activity becomes more prominent and thus may correct hypotension due to diminished SVR. As in the case of other circulatory decompensation states, prognosis is better in patients whose blood pressure and urine flow have not undergone profound deterioration. Therefore, it is suggested that the physician administer dopamine HCl as soon as a definite trend toward decreased systolic and diastolic pressure becomes evident.

CONTRAINDICATIONS

Dopamine HCl should not be used in patients with pheochromocytoma.

Dopamine HCl should not be administered to patients with uncorrected tachyarrhythmias or ventricular fibrillation.

WARNINGS

Do NOT add dopamine HCl to any alkaline diluent solution since the drug is inactivated in alkaline solution.

Patients who have been receiving MAO inhibitors prior to the administration of dopamine HCl will require substantially reduced dosage. See *Drug Interactions* below.

Contains sodium bisulfite, a sulfite that may cause serious allergic-type reactions (e.g., hives, itching, wheezing, anaphylaxis) in certain susceptible persons. Although the overall incidence of sulfite sensitivity in the general population is probably low, it is seen more frequently in asthmatics or in atopic nonasthmatic persons.

PRECAUTIONS

General

1. *Monitoring:* Careful monitoring of the following indices is necessary during dopamine HCl infusion, as with any ad-

renergic agent: blood pressure, urine flow, and, when possible, cardiac output and pulmonary wedge pressure.

2. *Hypovolemia:* Prior to treatment with dopamine HCl, hypovolemia should be fully corrected, if possible, with either whole blood or plasma as indicated. Monitoring of central venous pressure or left ventricular filling pressure may be helpful in detecting and treating hypovolemia.
3. *Hypoxia, Hypercapnia, Acidosis:* These conditions which may also reduce the effectiveness and/or increase the incidence of adverse effects of dopamine, must be identified and corrected prior to, concurrently with, administration of dopamine HCl.
4. *Decreased Pulse Pressure:* If a disproportionate increase in diastolic blood pressure and a marked decrease in the pulse pressure are observed in patients receiving dopamine HCl, the rate of infusion should be decreased and the patient observed carefully for further evidence of predominant vasoconstrictor activity, unless such an effect is desired.
5. *Ventricular Arrhythmias:* If an increased number of ectopic beats are observed, the dose should be reduced if possible.
6. *Hypotension:* At lower infusion rates, if hypotension occurs, the infusion rate should be rapidly increased until adequate blood pressure is obtained. If hypotension persists, dopamine HCl should be discontinued and a more potent vasoconstructor agent such as norepinephrine should be administered.
7. *Extravasation:* Dopamine HCl should be infused into a large vein whenever possible to prevent the possibility of extravasation into tissue adjacent to the infusion site. Extravasation may cause necrosis and sloughing of surrounding tissue. Large veins of the antecubital fossa are preferred to veins in the dorsum of the hand or ankle. Less suitable infusion sites should be used only if the patient's condition requires immediate attention. The physician should switch to more suitable sites as rapidly as possible. The infusion site should be continuously monitored for free flow.
8. *Occlusive Vascular Disease:* Patients with a history of occlusive vascular disease (for example, atherosclerosis, arterial embolism, Raynaud's disease, cold injury, diabetic endarteritis, and Buerger's disease) should be closely monitored for any changes in color or temperature of the skin in the extremities. If a change in skin color or temperature occurs and is thought to be the result of compromised circulation in the extremities, the benefits of continued dopamine HCl infusion should be weighed against the risk of possible necrosis. This condition may be reversed by either decreasing the rate or discontinuing the infusion.

IMPORTANT

Antidote for Peripheral Ischemia: To prevent sloughing and necrosis in ischemic areas, the area should be infiltrated as soon as possible with 10 to 15 mL of saline solution containing from 5 to 10 mg of phentolamine mesylate, an adrenergic blocking agent. A syringe with a fine hypodermic needle should be used, and the solution liberally infiltrated throughout the ischemic area. Sympathetic blockade with phentolamine causes immediate and conspicuous local hyperemic changes if the area is infiltrated within 12 hours. Therefore, phentolamine should be given as soon as possible after the extravasation is noted.

9. *Weaning:* When discontinuing the infusion, it may be necessary to gradually decrease the dose of dopamine HCl while expanding blood volume with IV fluids, since sudden cessation may result in marked hypotension.

Drug Interactions

1. Because dopamine is metabolized by monoamine oxidase (MAO), inhibition of this enzyme prolongs and potentiates the effect of dopamine. Patients who have been treated with MAO inhibitors within two to three weeks prior to the administration of dopamine HCl should receive initial doses of dopamine HCl no greater than one tenth (1/10) of the usual dose.
2. Concurrent administration of dopamine HCl and diuretic agents may produce an additive or potentiating effect on urine flow.
3. Tricyclic antidepressants may potentiate the pressor response to adrenergic agents.
4. Cardiac effects of dopamine are antagonized by beta-adrenergic blocking agents, such as propranolol and metoprolol. The peripheral vasoconstriction caused by high doses of dopamine HCl is antagonized by alpha-adrenergic blocking agents. Dopamine-induced renal and mesenteric vasodilation is not antagonized by either alpha- or beta-adrenergic blocking agents.
5. Haloperidol appears to have strong central antidopaminergic properties. Haloperidol and haloperidol-like drugs suppress the dopaminergic renal and mesenteric vasodilation induced at low rates of dopamine infusion.
6. Cyclopropane or halogenated hydrocarbon anesthetics increase cardian autonomic irritability and may sensitize the myocardium to the action of certain intravenously administered catecholamines, such as dopamine. This interaction appears to be related both to pressor activity and to beta-adrenegic stimulating properties of these catecholamines and may produce ventricular arrhythmias and hypertension. Therefore, EXTREME CAUTION should be exercised when administering dopamine HCl to patients receiving cyclopropane or halogenated hydrocarbon anesthetics. It has been reported that results of studies in animals indicate that dopamine-induced ventricular arrhythmias during anesthesia can be reversed by propranolol.
7. The concomitant use of vasopressors and some oxytocic drugs may result in severe persistant hypertension. See Labor and Delivery below.
8. Administration of phenytoin to patients receiving dopamine HCl has been reported to lead to hypotension and bradycardia. It is suggested that in patients receiving dopamine HCl, alternatives to phenytoin should be used if anticonvulsant therapy is needed.

Pregnancy

Pregnancy Category C: Animal studies have revealed no evidence of teratogenic effects due to dopamine. However, in one study, administration of dopamine HCl to pregnant rats resulted in a decreased survival rate of the newborn and a potential for catartact formation in the survivors. There are no adequate and well-controlled studies in pregnant women and it is not known if dopamine crosses the placental barrier. Because animal reproduction studies are not always predictive of human response, this drug should be used during pregnancy only if, in the judgment of the physician, the potential benefit justifies the potential risk to the fetus.

Labor and Delivery

In obstetrics, if vasopressor drugs are used to correct hypotension or are added to a local anesthetic solution, some oxytocic drugs may cause severe persistent hypertension and may even cause rupture of a cerebral blood vessel to occur during the postpartum period.

Nursing Mothers

It is not known whether this drug is excreted in human milk. Because many drugs are excreted in human milk, caution should be exercised when dopamine HCl is administered to a nursing woman.

Pediatric Use

Safety and effectiveness in children have not been established. Dopamine HCl has been used in a limited number of pediatric patients, but such use has been inadequate to fully define proper dosage and limitations for use.

ADVERSE REACTIONS

The following adverse reactions have been observed, but there are not enough data to support an estimate of their frequency.

Cardiovascular System

ventricular arrhythmia (at very high doses)
ectopic beats
tachycardia
anginal pain
palpitation
cardiac conduction abnormalities
widened QRS complex
bradycardia
hypotension
hypertension
vasoconstriction

Respiratory System: dyspnea
Gastrointestinal System: nausea, vomiting
Metabolic/Nutritional System: azotemia
Central Nervous System: headache, anxiety
Dermatological System: piloerection
Other: Gangrene of the extremities has occurred when high doses were administered for prolonged periods or in patients with occlusive vascular disease receiving low doses of dopamine HCl.

OVERDOSAGE

In case of accidental overdosage, as evidenced by excessive elevation of blood pressure, reduce rate of administration or temporarily discontinue dopamine HCl until patient's condition stabilizes. Since dopamine's duration of action is quite short, no additional remedial measures are usually necessary. If these measures fail to stabilize the patient's condition, use of the short-acting alpha-adrenergic blocking agent phentolamine should be considered.

DOSAGE AND ADMINISTRATION

WARNING: This is a potent drug. It must be diluted before administration to patient.

Suggested Dilution

Transfer contents of one or more ampules, vials or additive syringes of dopamine hydrochloride by aseptic technique to either a 250 mL, or 500 mL container of one of the following sterile intravenous solutions:

1. Sodium Chloride Injection, USP
2. Dextrose 5% Injection, USP
3. Dextrose (5%) and Sodium Chloride (0.9%) Injection, USP
4. Dextrose (5%) and Sodium Chloride (0.45%) Injection, USP
5. Dextrose (5%) in Lactated Ringer's Injection
6. Sodium Lactate (1/6 Molar) Injection, USP
7. Lactated Ringer's Injection, USP

Dopamine HCl has been found to be stable for a minimum of 24 hours after dilution in the sterile intravenous solutions listed above. However, as with all intravenous admixtures, dilution should be made just prior to administration.

Do NOT add dopamine HCl to 5% Sodium Bicarbonate or other alkaline intravenous solution, since the drug is inactivated in alkaline solution.

Rate of Administration

Dopamine HCl, after dilution, is administered intravenously through a suitable intravenous catheter or needle. An IV drip chamber or other suitable metering device is essential for controlling the rate of flow in drops/minute. Each patient must be individually titrated to the desired hemodynamic and/or renal response with dopamine HCl. In titrating to the desired increase in systolic blood pressure, the optimum dosage rate for renal response may be exceeded, thus necessitating a reduction in rate after the hemodynamic condition is stabilized.

Administration at rates greater than 50 mcg/kg/minute have safely been used in advanced circulatory decompensation states. If unnecessary fluid expansion is of concern, adjustment of drug concentration may be preferred over increasing the flow rate of a less concentrated dilution.

Suggested Regimen:

1. When appropriate, increase blood volume with whole blood or plasma until central venous pressure is 10 to 15 cm H_2O or pulmonary wedge pressure is 14 to 18 mm Hg.
2. Begin administration of diluted solution at doses of 2–5 mcg/kg/minute dopamine HCl in patients who are likely to respond to modest increments of heart force and renal perfusion.
   In more seriously ill patients, begin administration of diluted solution at doses of 5 mcg/kg/ minute dopamine HCl and increase gradually using 5–10 mcg/kg/minute increments up to 20–50 mcg/kg/minute as needed. If doses of dopamine HCl in excess of 50 mcg/kg/minute are required, it is suggested that urine output be checked frequently. Should urine flow begin to decrease in the absence of hypotension, reduction of dopamine HCl dosage should be considered. Multiclinic trials have shown that more than 50% of the patients were satisfactorily maintained on doses of dopamine HCl of less than 20 mcg/kg/minute. In patients who do not respond to these doses with adequate arterial pressures or urine flow, additional increments of dopamine HCl may be employed in an effort to produce an appropriate arterial pressure and central perfusion.
3. Treatment of all patients requires constant evaluation of therapy in terms of the blood volume, augmentation of myocardial contractility, and distribution of peripheral perfusion. Dosage of dopamine HCl should be adjusted according to the patient's response, with particular attention to diminution of established urine flow rate, increasing tachycardia or development of new dysrhythmias as indices for decreasing or temporarily suspending the dosage.
4. As with all potent intravenously administered drugs, care should be taken to control the rate of administration so as to avoid inadvertent administration of a bolus of drug.

Parenteral drug products should be inspected visually for particulate matter and discoloration prior to administration, whenever solution and container permit.

HOW SUPPLIED

Dopamine HCl 200 mg is supplied in the following forms:
Ampule—5 ml (40 mg/ml) NDC 0186-1050-03
Single Dose Vial—5 ml (40 mg/ml) NDC 0186-1010-13
Additive Syringe—5 ml (40 mg/ml) NDC 0186-0638-01

Dopamine HCl 400 mg is supplied in the following forms:
Ampule —5 ml (80 mg/ml) NDC 0186-1051-03
—10 ml (40 mg/ml) NDC 0186-1055-03
Single Dose Vial—5 ml (80 mg/ml) NDC 0186-1012-13
Additive Syringe —5 ml (80 mg/ml) NDC 0186-0641-01
—10 ml (40 mg/ml) NDC 0186-0639-01

Dopamine HCl 800 mg is supplied in the following forms:
Ampule—5 ml (160 mg/ml) NDC 0186-1052-03
Single Dose Vial—5 ml (160 mg/ml) NDC 0186-1014-13
Additive Syringe—5 ml (160 mg/ml) NDC 0186-0642-01

Packages are color coded according to the total dosage content; 200 mg coded blue/white, 400 mg coded green/white and 800 mg coded yellow/white.

Store at controlled room temperature 15°–30°C (59°–86°F). Protect from light.

Avoid contact with alkalies (including sodium bicarbonate), oxidizing agents, or iron salts.

NOTE: Do not use the Injection if it is darker than slightly yellow or discolored in any other way.

021861R03 Rev. 4/86 (3)

Continued on next page

Astra—Cont.

DURANEST® ℞
[dur'a-nest]
(etidocaine hydrochloride)
Solutions for infiltration and nerve block

DESCRIPTION

Duranest (etidocaine HCl) Solutions are sterile aqueous solutions that contain a local anesthetic agent and are administered parenterally by injection. See INDICATIONS AND USAGE for specific uses. The specific quantitative composition of each available solution is shown in Table 1.
Duranest Solutions contain etidocaine HCl, which is chemically designated as butanamide, N-(2,6-dimethylphenyl)-2-(ethylpropylamine)-, monohydrochloride and has the following structural formula:

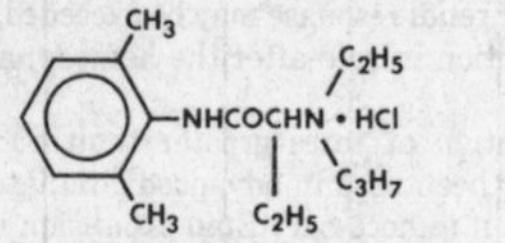

Epinephrine is (-)-3, 4-Dihydroxy-α-[(methylamino) methyl] benzyl alcohol and has the following structural formula:

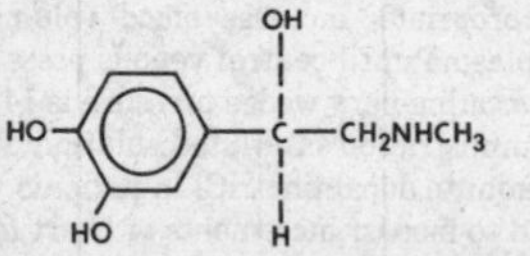

The pKa of etidocaine (7.74) is similar to that of lidocaine (7.86). However, etidocaine possesses a greater degree of lipid solubility and protein binding capacity than does lidocaine.
Duranest Solutions are sterile and, except for the 1.5% concentration, are available with or without epinephrine 1:200,000. Single dose containers of Duranest Solution without epinephrine may be reautoclaved is necessary.
See Table 1 below. Composition of available solutions.

CLINICAL PHARMACOLOGY

Mechanism of action: Etidocaine stabilizes the neuronal membrane by inhibiting the ionic fluxes required for the initiation and conduction of impulses, thereby effecting local anesthetic action.
Onset and duration of action: In vivo animal studies have shown that etidocaine has a rapid onset (3–5 minutes) and a prolonged duration of action (5–10 hours). Based on comparative clinical studies of lidocaine and etidocaine, the anesthetic properties of etidocaine in man may be characterized as follows: Initial onset of sensory analgesia and motor blockade is rapid (usually 3–5 minutes) and similar to that produced by lidocaine. Duration of sensory analgesia is 1.5 to 2 times longer than that of lidocaine by the peridural route. The difference in analgesic duration between etidocaine and lidocaine may be even greater following peripheral nerve blockade than following central neural block. Duration of analgesia in excess of 9 hours is not infrequent when etidocaine is used for peripheral nerve blocks such as brachial plexus blockade. Etidocaine produces a profound degree of motor blockade and abdominal muscle relaxation when used for peridural analgesia.
Hemodynamics: Excessive blood levels may cause changes in cardiac output, total peripheral resistance, and mean arterial pressure. With central neural blockade these changes may be attributable to block of autonomic fibers, a direct depressant effect of the local anesthetic agent on various components of the cardiovascular system, and/or the beta-adrenergic receptor stimulating action of epinephrine when present. The net effect is normally a modest hypotension when the recommended dosages are not exceeded.
Pharmacokinetics and metabolism: Information derived from diverse formulations, concentrations and usages reveals that etidocaine is completely absorbed following parenteral administration, its rate of absorption depending, for example, upon such factors as the site of administration and the presence or absence of a vasconstrictor agent. Except for intravenous administration, the highest blood levels are obtained following intercostal nerve block and the lowest after subcutaneous administration.
The plasma binding of etidocaine is dependent on drug concentration, and the fraction bound decreases with increasing concentration. At 0.5–1.0 μg/ml, 95% is bound to plasma protein.
Etidocaine crosses the blood-brain and placental barriers, presumably by passive diffusion.
Etidocaine is metabolized rapidly by the liver, and metabolites and unchanged drug are excreted by the kidney. Biotransformation includes oxidative N-dealkylation, ring hydroxylation, cleavage of the amide linkage, and conjugation. To date, approximately 20 metabolites of etidocaine have been found in the urine. The percent of dose excreted as unchanged drug is less than 10%.
The mean elimination half-life of etidocaine following a bolus intravenous injection is about 2.5 hours. Because of the rapid rate at which etidocaine is metabolized, any condition that affects liver function may alter etidocaine kinetics. Renal dysfunction may not affect etidocaine kinetics but may increase the accumulation of metabolites.
Factors such as acidosis and the concomitant use of CNS stimulants and depressants affect the CNS levels of etidocaine required to produce overt systemic effects. In the rhesus monkey arterial blood levels of 4.5 μg/ml have been shown to be threshold for convulsive activity.

INDICATIONS AND USAGE

Duranest (etidocaine HCl) Solutions are indicated for infiltration anesthesia, peripheral nerve blocks (e.g., brachial plexus, intercostal, ulnar, inferior alveolar), and central neural block (i.e., lumbar or caudal epidural blocks).

CONTRAINDICATIONS

Etidocaine is contraindicated in patients with a known history of hypersensitivity to local anesthetics of the amide type.

WARNINGS

DURANEST SOLUTIONS FOR INFILTRATION AND NERVE BLOCK SHOULD BE EMPLOYED ONLY BY CLINICIANS WHO ARE WELL VERSED IN DIAGNOSIS AND MANAGEMENT OF DOSE-RELATED TOXICITY AND OTHER ACUTE EMERGENCIES THAT MIGHT ARISE FROM THE BLOCK TO BE EMPLOYED AND THEN ONLY AFTER ENSURING THE *IMMEDIATE* AVAILABILITY OF OXYGEN, OTHER RESUSCITATIVE DRUGS, CARDIOPULMONARY EQUIPMENT, AND THE PERSONNEL NEEDED FOR PROPER MANAGEMENT OF TOXIC REACTIONS AND RELATED EMERGENCIES (See also ADVERSE REACTIONS and PRECAUTIONS). DELAY IN PROPER MANAGEMENT OF DOSE-RELATED TOXICITY, UNDERVENTILATION FROM ANY CAUSE AND/OR ALTERED SENSITIVITY MAY LEAD TO THE DEVELOPMENT OF ACIDOSIS, CARDIAC ARREST AND, POSSIBLY, DEATH.
To avoid intravascular injection, aspiration should be performed before the local anesthetic solution is injected. The needle must be repositioned until no return of blood can be elicited by aspiration. Note, however, that the absence of blood in the syringe does not guarantee that intravascular injection has been avoided.
Local anesthetic solutions containing antimicrobial preservatives (e.g., methylparaben) should not be used for epidural anesthesia because the safety of these agents has not been established with regard to intrathecal injection, either intentional or accidental.
Vasopressor agents administered for the treatment of hypotension related to caudal or other epidural blocks should not be used in the presence of ergot-type oxytocic drugs, since severe persistent hypertension and even rupture of cerebral blood vessels may occur.

PRECAUTIONS

General: The safety and effectiveness of etidocaine depend on proper dosage, correct technique, adequate precautions, and readiness for emergencies. Standard textbooks should be consulted for specific techniques and precautions for various regional anesthetic procedures. Resuscitative equipment, oxygen, and other resuscitative drugs should be available for immediate use (See WARNINGS and ADVERSE REACTIONS.) The lowest dosage that results in effective anesthesia should be used to avoid high plasma levels and serious adverse effects. Syringe aspirations should also be performed before and during each supplemental injection when using indwelling catheter techniques. During the administration of epidural anesthesia, it is recommended that a test dose be administered initially and that the patient be monitored for central nervous system toxicity and cardiovascular toxicity, as well as for signs of unintended intrathecal administration, before proceeding. When clinical conditions permit, consideration should be given to employing local anesthetic solutions that contain epinephrine for the test dose because circulatory changes compatible with epinephrine may also serve as a warning sign of unintended intravascular injection. An intravascular injection is still possible even if aspirations for blood are negative. Repeated doses of etidocaine may cause significant increases in blood levels with each repeated dose because of slow accumulation of the drug or its metabolites. Tolerance to elevated blood levels varies with the status of the patient. Debilitated, elderly patients, acutely ill patients, and children should be given reduced doses commensurate with their age and physical condition. Etidocaine should also be used with caution in patients with severe shock or heart block.
Lumbar and caudal epidural anesthesia should be used with extreme caution in persons with the following conditions: existing neurological disease, spinal deformities, septicemia and severe hypertension.
Local anesthetic solutions containing a vasoconstrictor should be used cautiously and in carefully circumscribed quantities in areas of the body supplied by end arteries or having otherwise compromised blood supply. Patients with peripheral vascular disease and those with hypertensive vascular disease may exhibit exaggerated vasoconstrictor response. Ischemic injury or necrosis may result. Preparations containing a vasoconstrictor should be used with caution in patients during or following the administration of potent general anesthetic agents, since cardiac arrhythmias may occur under such conditions.
Careful and constant monitoring of cardiovascular and respiratory (adequacy of ventilation) vital signs and the patient's state of consciousness should be accomplished after each local anesthetic injection. It should be kept in mind at such times that restlessness, anxiety, tinnitus, dizziness, blurred vision, tremors, depression or drowsiness may be early warning signs of central nervous system toxicity.
Since amide-type local anesthetics are metabolized by the liver, Duranest Solution should be used with caution in patients with hepatic disease.
Patients with severe hepatic disease, because of their inability to metabolize local anesthetics normally, are a greater risk of developing toxic plasma concentrations. Duranest Solution should also be used with caution in patients with impaired cardiovascular function since they may be less able to compensate for functional changes associated with the prolongation of A-V conduction produced by these drugs.
Many drugs used during the conduct of anesthesia are considered potential triggering agents for familial malignant hyperthermia. Since it is not known whether amide-type local anesthetics may trigger this reaction and since the need for supplemental general anesthesia cannot be predicted in advance, it is suggested that a standard protocol for the management of malignant hyperthermia should be available. Early unexplained signs of tachycardia, tachypnea, labile blood pressure and metabolic acidosis may precede temperature elevation. Successful outcome is dependent on early diagnosis, prompt discontinuance of the suspect triggering agent(s) and institution of treatment, including oxygen therapy, indicated supportive measures and dantrolene (consult dantrolene sodium intravenous package insert before using).
Etidocaine should be used with caution in persons with known drug sensitivities. Patients allergic to para-aminobenzoic acid derivatives (procaine, tetracaine, benzocaine, etc.) have not shown cross sensitivity to etidocaine.
Use in the Head and Neck Area: Small doses of local anesthetics injected into the head and neck area, including retrobulbar, dental and stellate ganglion blocks, may produce adverse reactions similar to systemic toxicity seen with unintentional intravascular injections of larger doses. The injection procedures require the utmost care. Confusion, convulsions, respiratory depression and/or respiratory arrest, and cardiovascular stimulation or depression have been reported. These reactions may be due to intra-arterial injection of the local anesthetic with retrograde flow to the cerebral circulation. They may also be due to puncture of the dural sheath of the optic nerve during retrobulbar block with diffusion of any local anesthetic along the subdural space to the midbrain. Patients receiving these blocks should have their circulation and respiration monitored and be constantly observed. Resuscitative equipment and personnel for treating adverse reactions should be immediately available.

Table 1. Composition of Available Solutions

Product Identification		Formula			
Duranest (etidocaine HCl) Concentration %	Epinephrine Dilution (as the bitartrate)	pH	Sodium chloride (mg/ml)	Single Dose Vials/ Dental Cartridge Sodium metabisulfite (mg/ml)	Citric acid (mg/ml)
1.0	None	4.0–5.0	7.1	None	—
1.0	1:200,000	3.0–4.5	7.1	0.5	0.2
1.5	1:200,000	3.0–4.5	6.2	0.5	0.2

NOTE: pH of all solutions adjusted with sodium hydroxide or hydrochloric acid. Duranest dental cartridges are only available as 1.5% solution with epinephrine 1:200,000

Dosage recommendations should not be exceeded. (See DOSAGE AND ADMINISTRATION.)

Use in Dentistry: Because of the long duration of anesthesia, when Duranest 1.5% with epinephrine is used for dental injections, patients should be cautioned about the possibility of inadvertent trauma to tongue, lips and buccal mucosa and advised not to chew solid foods or test the anesthetized area by biting or probing.

Information for Patients: When appropriate, patients should be informed in advance that they may experience temporary loss of sensation and motor activity, usually in the lower half of the body, following proper administration of epidural anesthesia.

Clinically significant drug interactions: The administration of local anesthetic solutions containing epinephrine or norepinephrine to patients receiving monoamine oxidase inhibitors, tricyclic antidepressants or phenothiazines may produce severe, prolonged hypotension or hypertension. Concurrent use of these agents should generally be avoided. In situations when concurrent therapy is necessary, careful patient monitoring is essential.

Concurrent administration of vasopressor drugs (for the treatment of hypotension related to epidural blocks) and ergot-type oxytocic drugs may cause severe, persistent hypertension or cerebrovascular accidents.

Drug Laboratory test interactions: The intramuscular injection of etidocaine may result in an increase in creatine phosphokinase levels. Thus, the use of this enzyme determination, without isoenzyme separation, as a diagnostic test for the presence of acute myocardial infarction may be compromised by the intramuscular injection of etidocaine.

Carcinogenesis, mutagenesis, impairment of fertility: Studies of etidocaine in animals to evaluate the carcinogenic and mutagenic potential have not been conducted. Studies in rats at 1.7 times the maximum recommended human dose have revealed no impairment of fertility.

Use in Pregnancy: Teratogenic Effects. Pregnancy Category B. Reproduction studies have been performed in rats and rabbits at doses up to 1.7 times the human dose and have revealed no evidence of harm to the fetus caused by etidocaine. There are, however, no adequate and well-controlled studies to pregnant women. Animal reproduction studies are not always predictive of human response. General consideration should be given to this fact before administering etidocaine to women of childbearing potential, especially during early pregnancy when maximum organogenesis takes place.

Labor and delivery: Local anesthetics rapidly cross the placenta and when used for epidural, paracervical, pudendal or caudal block anesthesia, can cause varying degrees of maternal, fetal and neonatal toxicity. (See CLINICAL PHARMACOLOGY—Pharmacokinetics). The incidence and degree of toxicity depends upon the procedure performed, the type and amount of drug used, and the technique of drug administration. Adverse reactions in the parturient, fetus and neonate involve alterations of the central nervous system, peripheral vascular tone and cardiac function.

Maternal hypotension has resulted from regional anesthesia. Local anesthetics produce vasodilation by blocking sympathetic nerves. Elevating the patient's legs and positioning her on her left side will help prevent decreases in blood pressure. The fetal heart rate also should be monitored continuously and electronic fetal monitoring is highly advisable.

Epidural anesthesia may alter the forces of parturition through changes in uterine contractility or maternal expulsive efforts. Because Duranest Solution may produce profound motor block, it is not recommended for epidural anesthesia in normal delivery. Duranest Solution is, however, recommended for epidural anesthesia when caesarian section is to be performed.

The use of some local anesthetic drug products during labor and delivery may be followed by diminished muscle strength and tone for the first day or two of life. The long-term significance of these observations is unknown.

Fetal bradycardia may occur in 20 to 30 percent of patients receiving paracervical nerve block anesthesia with the amide-type local anesthetics and may be associated with fetal acidosis. Fetal heart rate should always be monitored during paracervical anesthesia. The physician should weigh the possible advantages against risks when considering paracervical block in prematurity, toxemia of pregnancy, and fetal distress. Careful adherence to recommended dosage is of the utmost importance in obstetrical paracervical block. Failure to achieve adequate analgesia with recommended doses should arouse suspicion of intravascular or fetal intracranial injection. Cases compatible with unintended fetal intracranial injection of local anesthetic solution have been reported following intended paracervical or pudendal block or both. Babies so affected present with unexplained neonatal depression at birth, which correlates with high local anesthetic serum levels, and often manifest seizures within six hours. Prompt use of supportive measures combined with forced urinary excretion of the local anesthetic has been used successfully to manage this complication. Case reports of maternal convulsions and cardiovascular collapse following use of some local anesthetics for paracervical block in early pregnancy (as anesthesia for elective abortion) suggest that systemic absorption under these circumstances may be rapid. There are inadequate data in support of safe and effective use of etidocaine for obstetrical or non-obstetrical paracervical block, therefore, such use is not recommended.

Nursing mothers: It is not known whether this drug is excreted in human milk. Because many drugs are excreted in human milk, caution should be exercised when etidocaine is administered to a nursing woman.

Pediatric use: No information is currently available on appropriate pediatric doses.

ADVERSE REACTIONS

Systemic: Adverse experiences following the administration of etidocaine are similar in nature to those observed with other amide local anesthetic agents. These adverse experiences are, in general, dose-related and may result from high plasma levels caused by excessive dosage, rapid absorption or unintended intravascular injection, or may result from a hypersensitivity, idiosyncrasy or diminished tolerance on the part of the patient. Serious adverse experiences are generally systemic in nature. The following types are those most commonly reported:

Central nervous system: CNS manifestations are excitatory and/or depressant and may be characterized by lightheadedness, nervousness, apprehension, euphoria, confusion, dizziness, drowsiness, tinnitus, blurred or double vision, vomiting, sensations of heat, cold or numbness, twitching, tremors, convulsions, unconsciousness, respiratory depression and arrest. The excitatory manifestations may be very brief or may not occur at all, in which case the first manifestation of toxicity may be drowsiness merging into unconsciousness and respiratory arrest.

Drowsiness following the administration of etidocaine is usually an early sign of a high blood level of the drug and may occur as a consequence of rapid absorption.

Cardiovascular system: Cardiovascular manifestations are usually depressant and are characterized by bradycardia, hypotension, and cardiovascular collapse, which may lead to cardiac arrest.

Allergic: Allergic reactions are characterized by cutaneous lesions, urticaria, edema or anaphylactoid reactions. Allergic reactions may occur as a result of sensitivity either to local anesthetic agents or to the methylparaben used as a preservative in multiple dose vials. The detection of sensitivity by skin testing is of doubtful value.

Neurologic: The incidences of adverse reactions associated with the use of local anesthetics may be related to the total dose of local anesthetic administered and are also dependent upon the particular drug used, the route of administration and the physical status of the patient.

In the practice of caudal or lumbar epidural block, occasional unintentional penetration of the subarachnoid space by the catheter may occur. Subsequent adverse effects may depend partially on the amount of drug administered subdurally. These may include spinal block of varying magnitude (including total spinal block), hypotension secondary to spinal block, loss of bladder and bowel control, and loss of perineal sensation and sexual function. Persistent motor, sensory and/or autonomic (sphincter control) deficit of some lower spinal segments with slow recovery (several months) or incomplete recovery have been reported in rare instances when caudal or lumbar epidural block has been attempted. Backache and headache have also been noted following use of these anesthetic procedures.

OVERDOSAGE

Acute emergencies from local anesthetics are generally related high plasma levels encountered during therapeutic use of local anesthetics or to unintended subarachnoid injection of local anesthetic solution (see ADVERSE REACTIONS, WARNINGS, and PRECAUTIONS).

Management of local anesthetic emergencies: The first consideration is prevention, best accomplished by careful and constant monitoring of cardiovascular and respiratory vital signs and the patient's state of consciousness after each local anesthetic injection. At the first sign of change, oxygen should be administered.

The first step in the management of convulsions, as well as underventilation or apnea due to unintentional subarachnoid injection of drug solution, consists of immediate attention to the maintenance of a patent airway and assisted or controlled ventilation with oxygen and a delivery system capable of permitting immediate positive airway pressure by mask. Immediately after the institution of these ventilatory measures, the adequacy of circulation should be evaluated, keeping in mind that drugs used to treat convulsions sometimes depress the circulation when administered intravenously. Should convulsions persist despite adequate respiratory support, and if the status of the circulation permits, small increments of an ultra-short acting barbiturate (such as thiopental or thiamylal) or a benzodiazepine (such as diazepam) may be administered intravenously. The clinician should be familiar, prior to use of local anesthetics, with these anticonvulsant drugs. Supportive treatment of circulatory depression may require administration of intravenous fluids and, when appropriate, a vasopressor as directed by the clinical situation (e.g., ephedrine).

If not treated immediately, both convulsions and cardiovascular depression can result in hypoxia, acidosis, bradycardia, arrhythmias and cardiac arrest. Underventilation or apnea due to unintentional subarachnoid injection of local anesthetic solution may produce these same signs and also lead to cardiac arrest if ventilatory support is not instituted. If cardiac arrest should occur, standard cardiopulmonary resuscitative measures should be instituted.

Endotracheal intubation, employing drugs and techniques familiar to the clinician, may be indicated, after initial administration of oxygen by mask, if difficulty is encountered in the maintenance of a patent airway or if prolonged ventilatory support (assisted or controlled) is indicated.

Dialysis is of negligible value in the treatment of acute overdosage with etidocaine.

The intravenous LD_{50} of etidocaine HCl in female mice is 7.6 (6.6–8.5) mg/kg and the subcutanous LD_{50} is 112 (96–166) mg/kg.

DOSAGE AND ADMINISTRATION

As with all local anesthetic agents, the dose of Duranest (etidocaine HCl) Solution to be employed will depend upon the area to be anesthetized, the vascularity of the tissues, the number of neuronal segments to be blocked, the type of regional anesthetic technique, and the physical condition and tolerance of the individual patient.

The maximum dose to be employed as a single injection should be determined on the basis of the status of the patient and the type of regional anesthetic technique to be performed. Although single injections of 450 mg have been employed for regional anesthesia without adverse effects, at present it is strongly recommended that the maximal dose as a single injection should not exceed 400 mg (approximately 8.0 mg/kg or 3.6 mg/lb based on a 50 kg person) with epinephrine 1:200,000 and 300 mg (approximately 6 mg/kg and 2.7 mg/lb based on a 50 kg person) without epinephrine. Because etidocaine has been shown to disappear quite rapidly from blood, toxicity is influenced by rapidity of administration, and therefore slow injection in vascular areas is highly recommended. Incremental doses of Duranest Solution may be repeated at 2–3 hour intervals.

Caudal and lumbar epidural block: As a precaution against the adverse experiences sometimes observed following unintentional penetration of the subarachnoid space, a test dose of 2–5 ml should be administered at least 5 minutes prior to injecting the total volume required for a lumbar or caudal epidural block. The test dose should be repeated if the patient is moved in a manner that may have displaced the catheter. Epinephrine, if contained in the test dose (10–15μg have been suggested), may serve as a warning of unintentional intravascular injection. If injected into a blood vessel this amount of epinephrine is likely to produce a transient "epinephrine response" within 45 seconds, consisting of an increase in heart rate and systolic blood pressure, circumoral pallor, palpitations and nervousness in the unsedated patient. The sedated patient may exhibit only a pulse rate increase of 20 or more beats per minute for 15 or more seconds. Patients on beta-blockers may not manifest changes in heart rate, but blood pressure monitoring can detect an evanescent rise in systolic blood pressure. Adequate time should be allowed for onset of anesthesia after administration of each test dose. The rapid injection of a large volume of Duranest Solution through the catheter should be avoided, and when feasible fractional doses should be administered.

In the event of the known injection of a large volume of local anesthetic solution into the subarchnoid space after suitable resuscitation and if the catheter is in place, consider attempting the recovery of drug by draining a moderate amount of cerebrospinal fluid (such as 10 ml) through the epidural catheter.

Use in Dentistry: When used for local anesthesia in dental procedures the dosage of Duranest (etidocaine HCl) Solution depends on the physical status of the patient, the area of the oral cavity to be anesthetized, the vascularity of the oral tissues, and the technique of anesthesia. The least volume of solution that results in effective local anesthesia should be administered. For specific techniques and procedures of local anesthesia in the oral cavity, refer to standard textbooks.

Dosage requirements should be determined on an individual basis. In maxillary infiltration and/or inferior alveolar nerve block, initial dosages of 1.0–5.0 ml ($\frac{1}{2}$–$2\frac{1}{2}$ cartridges) of Duranest Solution 1.5% with epinephrine 1:200,000 are usually effective.

Aspiration is recommended since it reduces the possibility of intravascular injection, thereby keeping the incidence of side effects and anesthetic failures to a minimum.

The following dosage recommendations are intended as guides for the use of Duranest Solution in the average adult patient. As indicated previously, the dosage should be reduced for elderly or debilitated patients or patients with severe renal disease.

Continued on next page

Astra—Cont.

No information is available on appropriate pediatric doses.

NOTE:

Parenteral drug products should be inspected visually for particulate matter and discoloration prior to administration whenever the solution and container permit. Solutions that are discolored and/or contain particulate matter should not be used.

[See table below].

HOW SUPPLIED

[See table above].

Store at controlled room temperature 15°-30°C (59°-86°F).

021842R00 Iss. 7/85

Dosage Form and Volume	Duranest Solution Concentration	Epinephrine Dilution (as the bitartrate)	pH	NDC Number
Single Dose Vials 30 ml	1.0%	None	4.0–5.0	0186-0820-01
	1.0%	1:200,000	3.0–4.5	0186-0825-01
20 ml	1.5%	1:200,000	3.0–4.5	0186-0836-03
Dental Cartridge 1.8 ml	1.5%	1:200,000	3.0–4.5	0186-0840-14

Table 2. Dosage Recommendations

PROCEDURE	Duranest HCl with epinephrine 1:200,000 Conc. (%)	Vol. (ml)	Total Dose (mg)
Peripheral Nerve Block	1.0	5–40	50–400
Central Neural Block			
Lumbar Peridural			
Intraabdominal or Pelvic Surgery	1.0	10–30	100–300
Lower Limb Surgery	or		
Caesarean Section	1.5	10–20	150–300

PROCEDURE	Duranest HCl with epinephrine 1:200,000 Conc. (%)	Vol. (ml)	Total Dose (mg)
Caudal	1.0	10–30	100–300
Maxillary Infiltration and/or Inferior Alveolar Nerve Block	1.5	1–5	15–75

DYCLONE® 0.5% and 1% ℞

[dié-clone]

(dyclonine HCl)

Topical Solutions, U.S.P.

NOT FOR INJECTION OR OPHTHALMOLOGY

Full prescribing information is contained in the package insert.

For additional information, contact Astra's Professional Information Department.

HOW SUPPLIED

Sterile, in one fluid ounce bottles, DYCLONE 0.5% TOPICAL SOLUTION (NDC 0186-3001-01) and DYCLONE 1% TOPICAL SOLUTION (NDC 0186-3002-01). Keep tightly closed. Store at controlled room temperature: 15°-30°C (59°-86°F). Avoid excessive heat (temperatures above 40°C (104°F). Subject to damage by freezing.

EPINEPHRINE ℞

[ep-ĕ-nef′-rin]

Injection, USP

1:10,000 (0.1 mg/ml)

Adult Strength

(For details of indications, dosage and administration, precautions, and adverse reactions, see circular in package.)

HOW SUPPLIED

Epinephrine Injection USP, 1:10,000, is supplied in 10 ml prefilled syringes with a 22 g 1¼″ needle. (NDC 0186-0653-01). The solution should be stored at controlled room temperature 15°-30°C (59°-86°F) and should be protected from light by storage in the original carton until use.

021856R02 Rev. 3/86(2)

FUROSEMIDE INJECTION, U.S.P. ℞

10 mg/ml

PROTECT FROM LIGHT • DO NOT USE IF THE SOLUTION IS DISCOLORED • STORE AT CONTROLLED ROOM TEMPERATURE

> WARNING: Furosemide is a potent diuretic which if given in excessive amounts can lead to a profound diuresis with water and electrolyte depletion. Therefore, careful medical supervision is required, and the individual dose and the dosage schedule have to be adjusted to each patient's needs.
> (See under "DOSAGE AND ADMINISTRATION")

DESCRIPTION

Furosemide is an anthranilic acid derivative, chemically known as 4-chloro-N-furfuryl-5-sulfamoylanthranilic acid, with the following structural formula:

Furosemide injection is a sterile solution of furosemide in Water for injection. Each ml contains 10 mg furosemide, 7.5 mg sodium chloride, and sodium hydroxide and/or hydrochloric acid to adjust pH to 8.5 to 9.3. The single use vials do not contain any antimicrobial preservatives. (See HOW SUPPLIED section).

CLINICAL PHARMACOLOGY

Furosemide has been demonstrated to inhibit primarily the Reabsorption of sodium not only in the proximal and distal tubules but also in the loop of Henle. The high degree of efficacy is largely due to this unique site of action. The action on the distal tubule is independent of any inhibitory effect on carbonic anhydrase and aldosterone.

The diuresis following an intravenous injection commences within five minutes, and somewhat later after intramuscular injection. The diuresis reaches its peak within the first half hour and lasts for two hours.

INDICATIONS

Furosemide is indicated for the treatment of edema associated with congestive heart failure, cirrhosis of the liver, and renal disease, including the nephrotic syndrome. Furosemide is particularly useful when an agent with greater diuretic potential than that of those commonly employed is desired.

Parenteral therapy should be reserved for patients unable to take oral medication or for patients in emergency clinical situations.

Furosemide Injection is also indicted as adjunctive therapy in acute pulmonary edema. The intravenous administration of Furosemide is indicated when a rapid onset of diuresis is desired, eg, in acute pulmonary edema.

If gastrointestinal absorption is impaired or oral medication is not practical for any reason Furosemide is indicated by the intravenous or intramuscular route. Parenteral use should be replaced with oral Furosemide as soon as practical.

CONTRAINDICATIONS

Furosemide is contraindicated in anuria. Furosemide is also contraindicated in patients with a history of hypersensitivity to this compound.

WARNINGS

Excessive diuresis may result in dehydration and reduction in blood volume with circulatory collapse and with the possibility of vascular thrombosis and embolism, particularly in elderly patients. Excessive loss of potassium in patients receiving digitalis glycosides may precipitate digitalis toxicity. Care should also be exercised in patients receiving potassium-depleting steroids.

Frequent serum electrolyte, CO_2, and BUN determinations should be performed during the first few months of therapy and periodically thereafter, and abnormalities corrected or the drug temporarily withdrawn.

In patients with hepatic cirrhosis and ascites, initiation of therapy with Furosemide is best carried out in the hospital. In hepatic coma and in states of electrolyte depletion, therapy should not be instituted until the basic condition is improved. Sudden alterations of fluid and electrolyte balance in patients with cirrhosis may precipitate hepatic coma; therefore, strict observation is necessary during the period of diuresis. Supplemental potassium chloride and, if required, an aldosterone antagonist are helpful in preventing hypokalemia and metabolic alkalosis.

If increasing azotemia and oliguria occur during treatment of severe progressive renal disease, the drug should be discontinued.

As with many other drugs, patients should be observed regularly for the possible occurrence of blood dyscrasias, liver damage, or other idiosyncratic reactions.

Patients with known sulfonamide sensitivity may show allergic reactions to Furosemide.

Furosemide may add to or potentiate the therapeutic effect of other antihypertensive drugs. Potentiation occurs with ganglionic or peripheral adrenergic blocking drugs.

The possibility exists of exacerbation or activation of systemic lupus erythematosus.

Furosemide appears in breast milk. If use of the drug is deemed essential, the patient should stop nursing.

Parenterally administered Furosemide may increase the ototoxic potential of aminoglycoside antibiotics. Especially in the presence of impaired renal function, the use of parenterally administered Furosemide in patients to whom aminoglycoside antibiotics are also being given should be avoided, except in life-threatening situations.

Cases of tinnitus and reversible hearing impairment have been reported with parenteral use of Furosemide. There have also been some reports of cases in which irreversible hearing impairment occurred. Usually, ototoxicity has been reported when Furosemide was injected rapidly in patients with severe impairment of renal function at doses exceeding several times the usual recommended dose and in whom other drugs known to be ototoxic were given. If the physician elects to use high dose parenteral therapy in patients with severely impaired renal function, controlled intravenous infusion is advisable (for adults, an infusion rate not exceeding 4 mg Furosemide per minute has been used).

PRECAUTIONS

As with any effective diuretic, electrolyte depletion may occur during therapy with Furosemide, especially in patients receiving higher doses and a restricted salt intake. Periodic determinations of serum electrolytes to detect possible imbalance should be performed at appropriate intervals.

All patients receiving Furosemide therapy should be observed for signs of fluid or electrolyte imbalance: namely, hyponatremia, hypochloremic alkalosis, and hypokalemia. Serum and urine electrolyte determinations are particularly important when the patient is vomiting excessively or receiving parenteral fluids. Medications such as digitalis may also influence serum electrolytes. Warning signs, irrespective of cause, are: dryness of mouth, thirst, weakness, lethargy, drowsiness, restlessness, muscle pains or cramps, muscular fatigue, hypotension, oliguria, tachycardia, arrhythmia, and gastrointestinal disturbances such as nausea and vomiting.

Hypokalemia may develop with Furosemide as with any other potent diuretic, especially with brisk diuresis, when cirrhosis is present, or during concomitant use of corticosteroids or ACTH.

Interference with adequate oral electrolyte intake will also contribute to hypokalemia. Digitalis therapy may exaggerate metabolic effects of hypokalemia, especially with reference to myocardial activity.

Asymptomatic hyperuricemia can occur and gout may rarely be precipitated.

Periodic checks on urine and blood glucose should be made in diabetics and even those suspected of latent diabetes when receiving Furosemide. Increases in blood glucose and alterations in glucose tolerance tests with abnormalities of the fasting and 2-hour postprandial sugar have been observed, and rare cases of precipitation of diabetes mellitus have been reported.

Furosemide may lower serum calcium levels, and rare cases of tetany have been reported. Accordingly, periodic serum calcium levels should be obtained.

Reversible elevations of BUN may be seen. These have been observed in association with dehydration, which should be avoided, particularly in patients with renal insufficiency.

Patients receiving high doses of salicylates, as in rheumatic disease, in conjunction with Furosemide may experience salicylate toxicity at lower doses because of competitive renal excretory sites.
Furosemide has a tendency to antagonize the skeletal muscle relaxing effect of tubocurarine and may potentiate the action of succinylcholine. Lithium generally should not be given with diuretics because they reduce its renal clearance and add a high risk of lithium toxicity.
It has been reported in the literature that diuretics such as Furosemide may enhance the nephrotoxicity of cephaloridine. Therefore, Furosemide and cephaloridine should not be administered simultaneously.
Furosemide may decrease arterial responsiveness to norepinephrine. This diminution is not sufficient to preclude effectiveness of the pressor agent for therapeutic use.
It has been reported in the literature that coadministration of indomethacin may reduce the natriuretic and antihypertensive effects of Furosemide in some patients. This effect has been attributed to inhibition of prostaglandin synthesis by indomethacin. Indomethacin may also affect plasma renin levels and aldosterone excretion; this should be borne in mind when a renin profile is evaluated in hypertensive patients. Patients receiving both indomethacin and Furosemide should be observed closely to determine if the desired diuretic and/or antihypertensive effect of Furosemide is achieved.
Renal calcifications (from barely visible on x-ray to staghorn) have occurred in some severely premature infants treated with intravenous Furosemide for edema due to patent ductus arteriosus and hyaline membrane disease. The concurrent use of chlorothiazide has been reported to decrease hypercalciuria and to dissolve some calculi.

Pregnancy

Pregnancy Category C
Furosemide has been shown to cause unexplained maternal deaths and abortion in rabbits at 2, 4, and 8 times the human dose. There are no adequate and well-controlled studies in pregnant women. Furosemide should be used during pregnancy only if the potential benefit justifies the potential risk to the fetus.
The effects of furosemide on the embryonic and fetal development and on pregnant dams were studied in mice, rats and rabbits.
Furosemide caused unexplained maternal deaths and abortions in the rabbits when 50 mg/kg (4 times the maximal recommended human dose of 600 mg per day) was administered between days 12 to 17 of gestation. In a previous study the lowest dose of only 25 mg/kg (2 times the maximal recommended human dose of 600 mg per day) caused maternal deaths and abortions. In a third study, none of the pregnant rabbits survived a dose of 100 mg/kg. Data from the above studies indicate fetal lethality which can precede maternal deaths.
The results of the mouse study and one of the three rabbit studies also showed an increased incidence of hydronephrosis (distention of the renal pelvis and, in some cases, of the ureters) in fetuses derived from treated dams as compared to the incidence in fetuses from the control group.

ADVERSE REACTIONS

Gastrointestinal System Reactions
1. anorexia
2. oral and gastric irritation
3. nausea
4. vomiting
5. cramping
6. diarrhea
7. constipation
8. jaundice (intrahepatic cholestatic jaundice)
9. pancreatitis

Central Nervous System Reactions
1. dizziness
2. vertigo
3. paresthesias
4. headache
5. xanthopsia
6. blurred vision
7. tinnitus and hearing loss

Hematologic Reactions
1. anemia
2. leukopenia
3. agranulocytosis (rare)
4. thrombocytopenia
5. aplastic anemia (rare)

Dermatologic—Hypersensitivity Reactions
1. purpura
2. photosensitivity
3. rash
4. urticaria
5. necrotizing angiitis (vasculitis, cutaneous vasculitis)
6. exfoliative dermatitis
7. erythema multiforme
8. pruritus

Cardiovascular Reaction
Orthostatic hypotension may occur and be aggravated by alcohol, barbiturates, or narcotics.

Other
1. hyperglycemia
2. glycosuria
3. hyperuricemia
4. muscle spasm
5. weakness
6. restlessness
7. urinary bladder spasm
8. thrombophlebitis
9. transient pain at the injection site following intramuscular injection

Whenever adverse reactions are moderate or severe furosemide dosage should be reduced or therapy withdrawn.

DOSAGE AND ADMINISTRATION

Adults

Parenteral Administration: Oral medication is not recommended or in emergency situations where prompt diuresis is desired. Parenteral therapy should be replaced with oral therapy, as soon as this is practical, for the continued mobilization of edema.
The usual initial dose of furosemide is 20 to 40 mg given as a single dose, injected intramuscularly or intravenously. The intravenous injection should be given slowly (1 to 2 minutes). Ordinarily, a prompt diuresis ensues. Depending on the patient's response a second dose can be administered two hours after the first dose, or later.
If the diuretic response with a single dose of 20 to 40 mg is not satisfactory, increase the dose by increments of 20 mg, not sooner than two hours after the previous dose, until the desired diuretic effect has been obtained. This individually determined single dose should than be given once or twice daily.
If the physician elects to use high dose parenteral therapy it should be administered as a controlled infusion at a rate not exceeding 4mg/min. Furosemide Injection, USP is a mildly buffered alkaline solution which should not be mixed with acidic solutions of pH below 5.5. To prepare infusion solutions, Sodium Chloride (0.9%) Injection, Lactated Ringers Injection, and Dextrose (5%) Injection have been used after pH has been adjusted when necessary.
Therapy should be individualized according to patient response. This therapy should be titrated to gain maximal therapeutic response as well as the minimal dose possible to maintain that therapeutic response. Close medical supervision is necessary.
Acute Pulmonary Edema: The usual initial dose of furosemide is 40 mg injected intravenously. The injection should be given slowly (1 to 2 minutes). If 40 mg furosemide does not produce a satisfactory response within 1 hour the dose may be increased to 80 mg given intravenously (over 1 to 2 minutes).
If deemed necessary, additional therapy (e.g., digitalis, oxygen) can be administered concomitantly.

Infants and Children

Pediatric Administration: Parenteral administration of furosemide should be reserved for patients in whom oral medication is not recommended. Parenteral therapy should be replaced by oral therapy, as soon as this is practical, for continued mobilization of edema. For maintenance therapy in infants and children the dose should be adjusted to the minimum effective level.
The usual initial dose of Furosemide Injection (intravenously or intramuscularly) in infants and children is 1 mg/kg of body weight and should be given under close medical supervision. If the diuretic response after the initial dose is not satisfactory, dosage may be increased by 1 mg/kg, not sooner than two hours after the previous dose, until the desired effect has been obtained. Doses greater than 6 mg/kg body weight are not recommended.
Parenteral drug products should be inspected visually for particular matter and discoloration prior to administration, whenever solution and container permit.

HOW SUPPLIED

Furosemide injection, U.S.P., 10 mg/ml is supplied in the following forms:
Ampules:
2 ml (20 mg), 10 per package, NDC 0186-1110-03
4 ml (40 mg), 10 per package, NDC 0186-1111-03
10 ml (100 mg), 5 per package, NDC 0186-1113-02
Single Dose Vials:
2 ml (20 mg), 25 per package, NDC 0186-1114-13
4 ml (40 mg), 25 per package, NDC 0186-1115-13
8 ml (80 mg), 25 per package, NDC 0186-1116-12
10 ml (100 mg), 25 per package, NDC 0186-1117-12
Prefilled Syringes:
4 ml (40 mg), NDC 0186-0635-01
10 ml (100 mg), NDC 0186-0636-01
Syringes supplied with 22 gauge × 1 ¼″ needle.
All solutions should be stored at controlled room temperature 15°–30°C (59°–86°F) and should be protected from light. Do not use if the solution is discolored.
021841RO1 Rev. 6/85(1)

NESACAINE® ℞

[nes'a-caine]
(Chloroprocaine HCl) Solution

NESACAINE®–CE ℞

(Chloroprocaine HCl) Solution
for Infiltration and Nerve Block

pH differs from USP, pH 2.7–5.0

DESCRIPTION

Nesacaine and Nesacaine-CE Solutions are local anesthetics. The active ingredient in Nesacaine and Nesacaine-CE Solutions is chloroprocaine HCl (benzoic acid, 4-amino-2-chloro-2-(diethylamino)ethyl ester, monohydrochloride), which is represented by the following structural formula:

$NH_2-C_6H_3(Cl)-COOCH_2CH_2N(C_2H_5)_2 \cdot HCl$

Table 1. Composition of Available Solutions
[See table above].

Product Identification	Formula (mg/ml) Chloroprocaine HCl	Sodium Chloride	Sodium Bisulfite	Calcium Disodium Edetate	Methylparaben
Nesacaine 1%	10	6.7	0.7	0.1	1.0
Nesacaine 2%	20	4.7	0.7	0.1	1.0
Nesacaine-CE 2%	20	4.7	0.7	0.1	—
Nesacaine-CE 3%	30	3.3	0.7	0.1	—

The solutions are adjusted to pH 2.7–5.0 by means of hydrochloric acid. The pH range differs from U.S.P.
Although Nesacaine and Nesacaine-CE Solutions are sterile, the vials may be autoclaved for terminal sterilization, with no significant decrease in potency.

CLINICAL PHARMACOLOGY

Chloroprocaine, like other local anesthetics, blocks the generation and the conduction of nerve impulses, presumably by increasing the threshold for electrical excitation in the nerve, by slowing the propagation of the nerve impulse and by reducing the rate of rise of the action potential. In general, the progression of anesthesia is related to the diameter, myelination and conduction velocity of affected nerve fibers. Clinically, the order of loss of nerve function is as follows: (1) pain, (2) temperature, (3) touch, (4) proprioception, and (5) skeletal muscle tone.
Systemic absorption of local anesthetics produces effects on the cardiovascular and central nervous systems. At blood concentrations achieved with normal therapeutic doses, changes in cardiac conduction, excitability, refractoriness, contractility, and peripheral vascular resistance are minimal. However, toxic blood concentrations depress cardiac conduction and excitability, which may lead to atrioventricular block and ultimately to cardiac arrest. In addition, with toxic blood concentrations myocardial contractility may be depressed and peripheral vasodilation may occur, leading to decreased cardiac output and arterial blood pressure.
Following systemic absorption, toxic blood concentrations of local anesthetics can produce central nervous system stimulation, depression, or both. Apparent central stimulation may be manifested as restlessness, tremors and shivering, which may progress to convulsions. Depression and coma may occur, possibly progressing ultimately to respiratory arrest.
However, the local anesthetics have a primary depressant effect on the medulla and on higher centers. The depressed stage may occur without a prior stage of central nervous system stimulation.

PHARMACOKINETICS

The rate of systemic absorption of local anesthetic drugs is dependent upon the total dose and concentration of drug administered, the route of administration, the vascularity of the administration site, and the presence or absence of epinephrine in the anesthetic solution. Epinephrine usually reduces the rate of absorption and plasma concentration of

Continued on next page

Astra—Cont.

local anesthetics and is sometimes added to local anesthetic solutions in order to prolong the duration of action.
The onset of action with chloroprocaine is rapid (usually within 6 to 12 minutes), and the duration of anesthesia, depending upon the amount used and the route of administration, may be up to 60 minutes.
Local anesthetics appear to cross the placenta by passive diffusion. However, the rate and degree of diffusion varies considerably among the different drugs as governed by: (1) the degree of plasma protein binding, (2) the degree of ionization, and (3) the degree of lipid solubility. Fetal/maternal ratios of local anesthetics appear to be inversely related to the degree of plasma protein binding, since only the free, unbound drug is available for placental transfer. Thus, drugs with the highest protein binding capacity may have the lowest fetal/maternal ratios. The extent of placental transfer is also determined by the degree of ionization and lipid solubility of the drug. Lipid soluble, nonionized drugs readily enter the fetal blood from the maternal circulation.
Depending upon the route of administration, local anesthetics are distributed to some extent to all body tissues, with high concentrations found in highly perfused organs such as the liver, lungs, heart and brain.
Various pharmacokinetic parameters of the local anesthetics can be significantly altered by the presence of hepatic or renal disease, addition of epinephrine, factors affecting urinary pH, renal blood flow, the route of administration, and the age of the patient. The *in vitro* plasma half-life of chloroprocaine in adults is 21 ± 2 seconds for males and 25 ± 1 seconds for females. The *in vitro* plasma half-life in neonates is 43 ± 2 seconds.
Chloroprocaine is rapidly metabolized in plasma by hydrolysis of the ester linkage by pseudocholinesterase. The hydrolysis of chloroprocaine results in the production of β-diethylaminoethanol and 2-chloro-4-aminobenzoic acid, which inhibits the action of the sulfonamides (SEE PRECAUTIONS).
The kidney is the main excretory organ for most local anesthetics and their metabolites. Urinary excretion is affected by urinary perfusion and factors affecting urinary pH.

INDICATIONS AND USAGE

Nesacaine 1% and 2% Solutions, in multidose vials with methylparaben as preservative, are indicated for the production of local anesthesia by infiltration and peripheral nerve block. They are not to be used for lumbar or caudal epidural anesthesia.
Nesacaine-CE 2% and 3% Solutions, in single-dose vials without preservative, are indicated for the production of local anesthesia by infiltration, peripheral and central nerve block, including lumbar and caudal epidural blocks.
Nesacaine and Nesacaine-CE Solutions are not to be used for subarachnoid administration.

CONTRAINDICATIONS

Nesacaine and Nesacaine-CE Solutions are contraindicated in patients hypersensitive (allergic) to drugs of the PABA ester group.
Lumbar and caudal epidural anesthesia should be used with extreme caution in persons with the following conditions; existing neurological disease, spinal deformities, septicemia and severe hypertension.

WARNINGS

LOCAL ANESTHETICS SHOULD ONLY BE EMPLOYED BY CLINICIANS WHO ARE WELL VERSED IN DIAGNOSIS AND MANAGEMENT OF DOSE RELATED TOXICITY AND OTHER ACUTE EMERGENCIES WHICH MIGHT ARISE FROM THE BLOCK TO BE EMPLOYED, AND THEN ONLY AFTER ENSURING THE *IMMEDIATE* AVAILABILITY OF OXYGEN, OTHER RESUSCITATIVE DRUGS, CARDIOPULMONARY RESUSCITATIVE EQUIPMENT, AND THE PERSONNEL RESOURCES NEEDED FOR PROPER MANAGEMENT OF TOXIC REACTIONS AND RELATED EMERGENCIES (See also *ADVERSE REACTIONS and PRECAUTIONS.*) DELAY IN PROPER MANAGEMENT OF DOSE RELATED TOXICITY, UNDERVENTILATION FROM ANY CAUSE AND/OR ALTERED SENSITIVITY MAY LEAD TO THE DEVELOPMENT OF ACIDOSIS, CARDIAC ARREST AND, POSSIBLY, DEATH. NESACAINE (chloroprocaine HCl) SOLUTION contains methylparaben and should not be used for lumbar or caudal epidural anesthesia because safety of this antimicrobial preservative has not been established with regard to intrathecal injection, either intentional or unintended. NESACAINE-CE Solution contains no preservative; discard unused solution remaining in vial after initial use.
Vasopressors should not be used in the presence of ergot-type oxytocic drugs, since a severe persistent hypertension may occur.
To avoid intravascular injection, aspiration should be performed before the anesthetic solution is injected. The needle must be repositioned until no blood return can be elicited. However, the absence of blood in the syringe does not guarantee that intravascular injection has been avoided.
Mixtures of local anesthetics are sometimes employed to compensate for the slower onset of one drug and the shorter duration of action of the second drug. Experiments in primates suggest that toxicity is probably additive when mixtures of local anesthetics are employed, but some experiments in rodents suggest synergism. Caution regarding toxic equivalence should be exercised when mixtures of local anesthetics are employed.
Contains sodium bisulfite, a sulfite that may cause serious allergic-type reactions (e.g., hives, itching, wheezing, anaphylaxis) in certain susceptible persons. Although the overall incidence of sulfite sensitivity in the general population is probably low, it is seen more frequently in asthmatics or in atopic nonasthmatic persons.

PRECAUTIONS

General: The safety and effective use of chloroprocaine depend on proper dosage, correct technique, adequate precautions and readiness for emergencies. Resuscitative equipment, oxygen and other resuscitative drugs should be available for immediate use. (See WARNINGS and ADVERSE REACTIONS). The lowest dosage that results in effective anesthesia should be used to avoid high plasma levels and serious adverse effects. Injections should be made slowly, with frequent aspirations before and during the injection to avoid intravascular injection. Syringe aspirations should also be performed before and during each supplemental injection in continuous (intermittent) catheter techniques. During the administration of epidural anesthesia, it is recommended that a test dose be administered (3 ml of 3% or 5 ml of 2% Nesacaine-CE Solution) initially and that the patient be monitored for central nervous system toxicity and cardiovascular toxicity, as well as for signs of unintended intrathecal administration, before proceeding. When clinical conditions permit, consideration should be given to employing a chloroprocaine solution that contains epinephrine for the test dose because circulatory changes characteristic of epinephrine may also serve as a warning sign of unintended intravascular injection. An intravascular injection is still possible even if aspirations for blood are negative. With the use of continuous catheter techniques, it is recommended that a fraction of each supplemental dose be administered as a test dose in order to verify proper location of the catheter.
Injection of repeated doses of local anesthetics may cause significant increases in plasma levels with each repeated dose due to slow accumulation of the drug or its metabolites. Tolerance to elevated blood levels varies with the physical condition of the patient. Debilitated, elderly patients, acutely ill patients, and children should be given reduced doses commensurate with their age and physical status. Local anesthetics should also be used with caution in patients with hypotension or heart block.
Careful and constant monitoring of cardiovascular and respiratory (adequacy of ventilation) vital signs and the patient's state of consciousness should be accomplished after each local anesthetic injection. It should be kept in mind at such times that restlessness, anxiety, tinnitus, dizziness, blurred vision, tremors, depression or drowsiness may be early warning signs of central nervous system toxicity.
Local anesthetic solutions containing a vasoconstrictor should be used cautiously and in carefully circumscribed quantities in areas of the body supplied by end arteries or having otherwise compromised blood supply. Patients with peripheral vascular disease and those with hypertensive vascular disease may exhibit exaggerated vasoconstrictor response. Ischemic injury or necrosis may result.
Since ester-type local anesthetics are hydrolyzed by plasma cholinesterase produced by the liver, chloroprocaine should be used cautiously in patients with hepatic disease.
Local anesthetics should also be used with caution in patients with impaired cardiovascular function since they may be less able to compensate for functional changes associated with the prolongation of A-V conduction produced by these drugs.
Use in Ophthalmic Surgery: When local anesthetic solutions are employed for retrobulbar block, lack of corneal sensation should not be relied upon to determine whether or not the patient is ready for surgery. This is because complete lack of corneal sensation usually precedes clinically acceptable external ocular muscle akinesia.

INFORMATION FOR PATIENTS

When appropriate, patients should be informed in advance that they may experience temporary loss of sensation and motor activity, usually in the lower half of the body, following proper administration of epidural anesthesia.
Clinically Significant Drug Interactions: The administration of local anesthetic solutions containing epinephrine or norepinephrine to patients receiving monoamine oxidase inhibitors, tricyclic antidepressants or phenothiazines may produce severe, prolonged hypotension or hypertension. Concurrent use of these agents should generally be avoided. In situations when concurrent therapy is necessary, careful patient monitoring is essential.
Concurrent administration of vasopressor drugs (for the treatment of hypotension related to obstetric blocks) and ergot-type oxytocic drugs may cause severe, presistent hypertension or cerebrovascular accidents.
The para-aminobenzoic acid metabolite of chloroprocaine inhibits the action of sulfonamides. Therefore, chloroprocaine should not be used in any condition in which a sulfonamide drug is being employed.
Carcinogenesis, Mutagenesis, and Impairment of Fertility: Long-term studies in animals to evaluate carcinogenic potential and reproduction studies to evaluate mutagenesis or impairment of fertility have not been conducted with chloroprocaine.
Pregnancy Category C: Animal reproduction studies have not been conducted with chloroprocaine. It is also not known whether chloroprocaine can cause fetal harm when administered to a pregnant woman or can affect reproduction capacity. Chloroprocaine should be given to a pregnant woman only if clearly needed. This does not preclude the use of chloroprocaine at term for the production of obstetrical anesthesia.
Labor and Delivery: Local anesthetics rapidly cross the placenta, and when used for epidural, paracervical, pudendal or caudal block anesthesia, can cause varying degrees of maternal, fetal and neonatal toxicity.
(See CLINICAL PHARMACOLOGY—Pharmacokinetics)
The incidence and degree of toxicity depend upon the procedure performed, the type and amount of drug used, and the technique of drug administration. Adverse reactions in the parturient, fetus and neonate involve alterations of the central nervous system, peripheral vascular tone and cardiac function.
Maternal hypotension has resulted from regional anesthesia. Local anesthetics produce vasodilation by blocking sympathetic nerves. Elevating the patient's legs and positioning her on her left side will help prevent decreases in blood pressure. The fetal heart rate also should be monitored continuously, and electronic fetal monitoring is highly advisable.
Epidural, paracervical, or pudendal anesthesia may alter the forces of parturition through changes in uterine contractility or maternal expulsive efforts. In one study, paracervical block anesthesia was associated with a decrease in the mean duration of first stage labor and facilitation of cervical dilation. However, epidural anesthesia has also been reported to prolong the second stage of labor by removing the parturient's reflex urge to bear down or by interfering with motor function. The use of obstetrical anesthesia may increase the need for forceps assistance.
The use of some local anesthetic drug products during labor and delivery may be followed by diminished muscle strength and tone for the first day or two of life. The long-term significance of these observations is unknown.
Careful adherence to recommended dosage is of the utmost importance in obstetrical paracervical block. Failure to achieve adequate analgesia with recommended doses should arouse suspicion of intravascular or fetal intracranial injection. Cases compatible with unintended fetal intracranial injection of local anesthetic solution have been reported following intended paracervical or pudendal block or both. Babies so affected present with unexplained neonatal depression at birth which correlates with high local anesthetic serum levels and usually manifest seizures within six hours. Prompt use of supportive measures combined with forced urinary excretion of the local anesthetic has been used successfully to manage this complication.
Case reports of maternal convulsions and cardiovascular collapse following use of some local anesthetics for paracervical block in early pregnancy (as anesthesia for elective abortion) suggest that systemic absorption under these circumstances may be rapid. The recommended maximum dose of each drug should not be exceeded. Injection should be made slowly and with frequent aspiration. Allow a 5-minute interval between sides.
There are no data concerning use of chloroprocaine for obstetrical paracervical block when toxemia of pregnancy is present or when fetal distress or prematurity is anticipated in advance of the block; such use is, therefore, not recommended.
The following information should be considered by clinicians who select chloroprocaine for obstetrical paracervical block anesthesia: 1) Fetal bradycardia (generally a heart rate of less than 120 per minute for more than 2 minutes) has been noted by electronic monitoring in about 5 to 10 percent of the cases (various studies) where initial total doses of 120 mg to 400 mg of chloroprocaine were employed. The incidence of bradycardia, within this dose range, might not be dose related. 2) Fetal acidosis has not been demonstrated by blood gas monitoring around the time of bradycardia or afterwards. These data are limited and generally restricted to nontoxemic cases where fetal distress or prematurity was not anticipated in advance of the block. 3) No intact chloroprocaine and only trace quantities of a hydrolysis product, 2-chloro-4-aminobenzoic acid, have been demonstrated in umbilical cord arterial or venous plasma following properly administered paracervical block with chloroprocaine. 4) The role of drug factors and non-drug factors associated with fetal bradycardia following paracervical block are unexplained at this time.

Nursing Mothers: It is not known whether this drug is excreted in human milk. Because many drugs are excreted in human milk, caution should be exercised when chloroprocaine is administered to a nursing woman.

Pediatric Use: Guidlines for the administration of Nesacaine and Nesacaine-CE Solutions to children are presented in DOSAGE AND ADMINISTRATION.

ADVERSE REACTIONS

Systemic: The most commonly encountered acute adverse experiences that demand immediate countermeasures are related to the central nervous system and the cardiovascular system. These adverse experiences are generally dose related and may result from rapid absorption from the injection site, diminished tolerance, or from unintentional intravascular injection of the local anesthetic solution. In addition to systemic dose-related toxicity, unintentional subarachnoid injection of drug during the intended performance of caudal or lumbar epidural block or nerve blocks near the vertebral column (especially in the head and neck region) may result in underventilation or apnea ("Total Spinal"). Factors influencing plasma protein binding, such as acidosis, systemic diseases that alter protein production, or competition of other drugs for protein binding sites, may diminish individual tolerance. Plasma cholinesterase deficiency may also account for diminished tolerance to ester type local anesthetics.

Central Nervous System Reactions: These are characterized by excitation and/or depression. Restlessness, anxiety, dizziness, tinnitus, blurred vision or tremors may occur, possibly proceeding to convulsions. However, excitement may be transient or absent, with depression being the first manifestation of an adverse reaction. This may quickly be followed by drowsiness merging into unconsciousness and respiratory arrest.

The incidence of convulsions associated with the use of local anesthetics varies with the procedure used and the total dose administered. In a survey of studies of epidural anesthesia, overt toxicity progressing to convulsions occurred in approximately 0.1 percent of local anesthetic administrations.

Cardiovascular System Reactions: High doses, or unintended intravascular injection, may lead to high plasma levels and related depression of the myocardium, hypotension, bradycardia, ventricular arrhythmias and, possibly, cardiac arrest.

Allergic: Allergic type reactions are rare and may occur as a result of sensitivity to the local anesthetic or to other formulation ingredients, such as the antimicrobial preservative methylparaben, contained in multiple dose vials. These reactions are characterized by signs such as urticaria, pruritis, erythema, angioneurotic edema (including laryngeal edema), tachycardia, sneezing, nausea, vomiting, dizziness, syncope, excessive sweating, elevated temperature, and possibly, anaphylactoid type symptomatology (including severe hypotension). Cross sensitivity among members of the ester-type local anesthetic group has been reported. The usefulness of screening for sensitivity has not been definitely established.

Neurologic: In the practice of caudal or lumbar epidural block, occasional unintentional penetration of the subarachnoid space by the catheter may occur (see PRECAUTIONS). Subsequent adverse observations may depend partially on the amount of drug administered intrathecally. These observations may include spinal block of varying magnitude (including total spinal block), hypotension secondary to spinal block, loss of bladder, and bowel control, and loss of perineal sensation and sexual function. Arachnoiditis, persistent motor, sensory and/or autonomic (sphincter control) deficit of some lower spinal segments with slow recovery (several months) or incomplete recovery have been reported in rare instances. (See DOSAGE AND ADMINISTRATION discussion of Caudal and Lumbar Epidural Block). Backache and headache have also been noted following lumbar epidural or caudal block.

OVERDOSAGE

Acute emergencies from local anesthetics are generally related to high plasma levels encountered during therapeutic use of local anesthetics or to unintended subarachnoid injection of local anesthetic solution (see ADVERSE REACTIONS, WARNINGS, and PRECAUTIONS).

In mice, the intravenous LD_{50} of chloroprocaine HCl is 97 mg/kg and the subcutaneous LD_{50} of chloroprocaine HCl is 950 mg/kg.

Management of Local Anesthetic Emergencies: The first consideration is prevention, best accomplished by careful and constant monitoring of cardiovascular and respiratory vital signs and the patient's state of consciousness after each local anesthetic injection. At the first sign of change, oxygen should be administered.

The first step is the management of convulsions, as well as underventilation or apnea due to unintentional subarachnoid injection of drug solution, consists of immediate attention to the maintenance of a patent airway and assisted or controlled ventilation with oxygen and a delivery system capable of permitting immediate positive airway pressure by mask. Immediately after the institution of these ventilatory measures, the adequacy of the circulation should be evaluated, keeping in mind that drugs used to treat convulsions sometimes depress the circulation when administered intravenously. Should convulsions persist despite adequate respiratory support, and if the status of the circulation permits, small increments of an ultra-short acting barbiturate (such as thiopental or thiamylal) or a benzodiazepine (such as diazepam) may be administered intravenously; the clinician should be familiar, prior to use of local anesthetics, with these anticonvulsant drugs. Supportive treatment of circulatory depression may require administration of intravenous fluids and, when appropriate, a vasopressor dictated by the clinical situation (such as ephedrine to enhance myocardial contractile force).

If not treated immediately, both convulsions and cardiovascular depression can result in hypoxia, acidosis, bradycardia, arrhythmias and cardiac arrest. Underventilation or apnea due to unintentional subarachnoid injection of local anesthetic solution may produce these same signs and also lead to cardiac arrest if ventilatory support is not instituted. If cardiac arrest should occur, standard cardiopulmonary resuscitative measures should be instituted. Recovery has been reported after prolonged resuscitative efforts.

Endotracheal intubation, employing drugs and techniques familiar to the clinician, may be indicated, after initial administration of oxygen by mask, if difficulty is encountered in the maintenance of a patent airway or if prolonged ventilatory support (assisted or controlled) is indicated.

DOSAGE AND ADMINISTRATION

Chloroprocaine may be administered as a single injection or continuously through an indwelling catheter. As with all local anesthetics, the dose administered varies with the anesthetic procedure, the vascularity of the tissues, the depth of anesthesia and degree of muscle relaxation required, the duration of anesthesia desired, and the physical condition of the patient. The smallest dose and concentration required to produce the desired result should be used. Dosage should be reduced for children, elderly and debilitated patients and patients with cardiac and/or liver disease. The maximum single recommended doses of chloroprocaine in adults are: without epinephrine, 11 mg/kg, not to exceed a maximum total dose of 800 mg; with epinephrine (1:200,000), 14 mg/kg, not to exceed a maximum total dose of 1000 mg. For specific techniques and procedures, refer to standard textbooks.

Caudal and Lumbar Epidural Block: In order to guard against adverse experiences sometimes noted following unintended penetration of the subarachnoid space, the following procedure modifications are recommended: 1. Use an adequate test dose (3 ml of Nesacaine-CE 3% Solution or 5 ml of Nesacaine-CE 2% Solution) prior to induction of complete block. This test dose should be repeated if the patient is moved in such a fashion as to have displaced the epidural catheter. Allow adequate time for onset of anesthesia following administration of each test dose. 2. Avoid the rapid injection of a large volume of local anesthetic solution through the catheter. Consider fractional doses, when feasible. 3. In the event of the known injection of a large volume of local anesthetic solution into the subarachnoid space, after suitable resuscitation and if the catheter is in place, consider attempting the recovery of drug by draining a moderate amount of cerebrospinal fluid (such as 10 ml) through the epidural catheter.

As a guide for some routine procedures, suggested doses are given below:

1. Infiltration and Peripheral Nerve Block: NESACAINE or NESACAINE-CE (Chloroprocaine HCl) SOLUTION

[See table above].

Anesthetic Procedure	Solution Concentration %	Volume (ml)	Total Dose (mg)
Mandibular	2	2–3	40–60
Infraorbital	2	0.5–1	10–20
Brachial plexus	2	30–40	600–800
Digital (without epinephrine)	1	3–4	30–40
Pudendal	2	10 each side	400
Paracervical (see also PRECAUTIONS)	1	3 per each of 4 sites	up to 120

2. Caudal and Lumbar Epidural Block: NESACAINE-CE SOLUTION. For caudal anesthesia, the initial dose is 15 to 25 ml of a 2% or 3% solution. Repeated doses may be given at 40 to 60 minutes intervals.

For lumbar epidural anesthesia, 2.0 to 2.5 ml per segment of a 2% or 3% solution can be used. The usual total volume of Nesacaine-CE Solution is from 15 to 25 ml. Repeated doses 2 to 6 ml less than the original dose may be given at 40 to 50 minutes intervals.

The above dosages are recommended as a guide for use in the average adult. Maximum dosages of all local anesthetics must be individualized after evaluating the size and physical condition of the patient and the rate of systemic absorption from a particular injection site.

Pediatric Dosage: It is difficult to recommend a maximum dose of any drug for children, since this varies as a function of age and weight. For children over 3 years of age who have a normal lean body mass and normal body development, the maximum dose is determined by the child's age and weight and should not exceed 11 mg/kg (5 mg/lb). For example, in a child of 5 years weighing 50 lbs (23 kg), the dose of chloroprocaine HCl without epinephrine would be 250 mg. Concentrations of 0.5–1.0% are suggested for infiltration and 1.0–1.5% for nerve block. In order to guard against systemic toxicity, the lowest effective concentration and lowest effective dose should be used at all times. Some of the lower concentrations for use in infants and smaller children are not available in pre-packaged containers; it will be necessary to dilute available concentrations with the amount of 0.9% sodium chloride injection necessary to obtain the required final concentration of chloroprocaine solution.

Preparation of Epinephrine Solutions—To prepare a 1:200,000 epinephrine-chloroprocaine HCl solution, add 0.15 ml of a 1 to 1000 Epinephrine Injection U.S.P. to 30 ml of Nesacaine-CE Solution.

Chloroprocaine is incompatible with caustic alkalis and their carbonates, soaps, silver salts, iodine and iodides.

Parenteral drug products should be inspected visually for particulate matter and discoloration prior to administration, whenever solution and container permit. As with other anesthetics having a free aromatic amino group, Nesacaine and Nesacaine-CE Solutions are slightly photosensitive and may become discolored after prolonged exposure to light. It is recommended that these vials be stored in the original outer containers, protected from direct sunlight. Discolored solution should not be administered. If exposed to low temperature, Nesacaine and Nesacaine-CE Solutions may deposit crystals of chloroprocaine HCl which will redissolve with shaking when returned to room temperature. The product should not be used if it contains undissolved (e.g., particulate) material.

HOW SUPPLIED

NESACAINE (Chloroprocaine HCl) SOLUTION with preservatives is supplied as follows:

1% solution (NDC 0186-0971-66) in 30 ml multiple dose vials, 12 vials per package.

2% solution (NDC 0186-0972-66) in 30 ml multiple dose vials, 12 vials per package.

NESACAINE-CE (Chloroprocaine HCl) SOLUTION without preservatives is supplied as follows:

2% solution (NDC 0186-0993-66) in 30 ml single dose vials, 12 vials per package.

3% solution (NDC 0186-0994-66) in 30 ml single dose vials, 12 vials per package.

Keep from freezing. Protect from light. Store at controlled room temperature: 15°–30°C (59°–86°F).

021849R03 Rev. 1/86(3)

SENSORCAINE® ℞

[*sén-sor-caine*]

(bupivacaine HCl)

Injection for Infiltration and Nerve Block

DESCRIPTION

Sensorcaine® (bupivacaine HCl) injections are sterile isotonic solutions that contain a local anesthetic agent with and without epinephrine (as bitartrate) 1:200,000 and are administered parenterally by injection. See INDICATIONS AND USAGE for specific uses. The quantitative composition of each available solution is shown in Table 1. Solutions of bupivacaine HCl may be autoclaved if they do not contain epinephrine.

Sensorcaine® injections contain bupivacaine HCl which is chemically designated as 2-piperidinecarboxamide, 1-butyl-N-(2,6-dimethylphenyl)-monohydrochloride, monohydrate and has the following structure:

$(CH_2)_3CH_3$ CH_3 N — CONH — · HCl · H_2O CH_3

Continued on next page

Astra—Cont.

Epinephrine is (-)-3,4-Dihydroxy-α-[(methylamino) methyl] benzyl alcohol. It has the following structural formula:

The pKa of bupivacaine (8.1) is similar to that of lidocaine (7.86). However, bupivacaine possesses a greater degree of lipid solubility and is protein bound to a greater extent than lidocaine.

Bupivacaine is related chemically and pharmacologically to the aminoacyl local anesthetics. It is a homologue of mepivacaine and is chemically related to lidocaine. All three of these anesthetics contain an amide linkage between the aromatic nucleus and the amino or piperidine group. They differ in this respect from the procaine-type local anesthetics, which have an ester linkage.

[See table below].

CLINICAL PHARMACOLOGY

Local anesthetics block the generation and the conduction of nerve impulses, presumably by increasing the threshold for electrical excitation in the nerve, by slowing the propagation of the nerve impulse, and by reducing the rate of rise of the action potential. In general, the progression of anesthesia is related to the diameter, myelination and conduction velocity of affected nerve fibers. Clinically, the order of loss of nerve function is as follows: (1) pain, (2) temperature, (3) touch, (4) proprioception, and (5) skeletal muscle tone.

Systemic absorption of local anesthetics produces effects on the cardiovascular and central nervous systems. At blood concentrations achieved with therapeutic doses, changes in cardiac conduction, excitability, refractoriness, contractility, and peripheral vascular resistance are minimal. However, toxic blood concentrations depress cardiac conduction and excitability, which may lead to atrioventricular block, ventricular arrhythmias and to cardiac arrest. In addition, myocardial contractility is depressed and peripheral vasodilation occurs, leading to decreased cardiac output and arterial blood pressure.

Recent clinical reports and animal research suggest that these cardiovascular changes are more likely to occur with bupivacaine.

Following systemic absorption, local anesthetics can produce central nervous system stimulation, depression or both. Apparent central stimulation is usually manifested as restlessness, tremors and shivering, progressing to convulsions, followed by depression and coma, progressing ultimately to respiratory arrest. However, the local anesthetics have a primary depressant effect on the medulla and on higher centers. The depressed stage may occur without a prior excited stage.

Pharmacokinetics: The rate of systemic absorption of local anesthetics is dependent upon the total dose and concentration of drug administered, the route of administration, the vascularity of the administration site, and the presence or absence of epinephrine in the anesthetic solution. A dilute concentration of epinephrine (1:200,000 or 5 μg/ml) usually reduces the rate of absorption and peak plasma concentration of bupivacaine, permitting the use of moderately larger total doses and sometimes prolonging the duration of action.

The onset of action with bupivacaine is rapid and anesthesia is long-lasting. It has also been noted that there is a period of analgesia that persists after the return of sensation, during which time the need for potent analgesics is reduced.

Local anesthetics are bound to plasma proteins in varying degrees. Generally, the lower the plasma concentration of drug, the higher the percentage of drug bound to plasma proteins.

Local anesthetics appear to cross the placenta by passive diffusion. The rate and degree of diffusion is governed by: (1) the degree of plasma protein binding, (2) the degree of ionization, and (3) the degree of lipid solubility. Fetal/maternal ratios of local anesthetics appear to be inversely related to the degree of plasma protein binding, because only the free, unbound drug is available for placental transfer. Bupivacaine, with a high protein binding capacity (95%), has a low fetal/maternal ratio (0.2–0.4). The extent of placental transfer is also determined by the degree of ionization and lipid solubility of the drug. Lipid soluble, nonionized drugs readily enter the fetal blood from the maternal circulation.

Depending upon the route of adminstration, local anesthetics are distributed to some extent to all body tissues, with high concentrations found in highly perfused organs such as the liver, lungs, heart and brain.

Pharmacokinetic studies on the plasma profile of bupivacaine after direct intravenous injection suggest a three-compartment open model. The first compartment is represented by the rapid intravascular distribution of the drug. The second compartment represents the equilibration of the drug throughout the highly perfused organs such as the brain, myocardium, lungs, kidneys and liver. The third compartment represents an equilibration of the drug with poorly perfused tissues, such as muscle and fat. The elimination of drug from tissue depends largely upon the ability of binding sites in the circulation to carry it to the liver where is is metabolized.

After injection of Sensorcaine® (bupivacaine HCl) injection for caudal, epidural or peripheral nerve block in man, peak levels of bupivacaine in the blood are reached in 30 to 45 minutes, followed by a decline to insignificant levels during the next 3 to 6 hours.

Various pharmacokinetic parameters of the local anesthetics can be significantly altered by the presence of hepatic or renal disease, addition of epinephrine, factors affecting urinary pH, renal blood flow, the route of drug administration, and the age of the patient. The half-life of bupivacaine in adults is 3.5 ± 2.0 hours and in neonates 8.1 hours.

Amide-type local anesthetics such as bupivacaine are metabolized primarily in the liver via conjugation with glucuronic acid.

Patients with hepatic disease, especially those with severe hepatic disease, may be more susceptible to the potential toxicities of the amide-type local anesthetics. The major metabolite of bupivacaine is 2,6-pipecoloxylidine.

The kidney is the main excretory organ for most local anesthetics and their metabolites. Urinary excretion is affected by renal perfusion and factors affecting urinary pH. Only 5% of bupivacaine is excreted unchanged in the urine.

When administered in recommended doses and concentrations, Sensorcaine® (bupivacaine HCl) injection does not ordinarily produce irritation or tissue damage and does not cause methemoglobinemia.

INDICATIONS AND USAGE

Sensorcaine® (bupivacaine HCl) injection is indicated for the production of local or regional anesthesia or analgesia for surgery, for oral surgery procedures, for diagnostic and therapeutic procedures and for obstetrical procedures. Only the 0.25% and 0.5% concentrations are indicated for obstetrical anesthesia. (See WARNINGS.)

Experience with non-obstetrical surgical procedures in pregnant patients is not sufficient to recommend use of the 0.75% concentration in these patients. Sensorcaine® (bupivacaine HCl) injection is not recommended for intravenous regional anesthesia (Bier Block). See WARNINGS.

The routes of administration and indicated Sensorcaine® (bupivacaine HCl) concentrations are:

local infiltration	0.25%
peripheral nerve block	0.25%, 0.5%
retrobulbar block	0.75%
sympathetic block	0.25%
lumbar epidural	0.25%, 0.5% and 0.75% (non-obstetrical)
caudal	0.25%, 0.5%

(See DOSAGE AND ADMINISTRATION for additional information.) Standard textbooks should be consulted to detemine the accepted procedures and techniques for the administration of Sensorcaine® (bupivacaine HCl).

CONTRAINDICATIONS

Sensorcaine® (bupivacaine HCl) injection is contraindicated in obstetrical paracervical block anesthesia. Its use by this technique has resulted in fetal bradycardia and death.

Sensorcaine® (bupivacaine HCl) is contraindicated in patients with a known hypersensitivity to it or to any local anesthetic agent of the amide type or to other components of bupivacaine solutions.

WARNINGS

THE 0.75% CONCENTRATION OF SENSORCAINE® (BUPIVACAINE HYDROCHLORIDE) INJECTION IS NOT RECOMMENDED FOR OBSTETRICAL ANESTHESIA. THERE HAVE BEEN REPORTS OF CARDIAC ARREST WITH DIFFICULT RESUSCITATION OR DEATH DURING USE OF BUPIVACAINE FOR EPIDURAL ANESTHESIA IN OBSTETRICAL PATIENTS. IN MOST CASES, THIS HAS FOLLOWED USE OF THE 0.75% CONCENTRATION. RESUSCITATION HAS BEEN DIFFICULT OR IMPOSSIBLE DESPITE APPARENTLY ADEQUATE PREPARATION AND APPROPRIATE MANAGEMENT. CARDIAC ARREST HAS OCCURRED AFTER CONVULSIONS RESULTING FROM SYSTEMIC TOXICITY, PRESUMABLY FOLLOWING UNINTENTIONAL INTRAVASCULAR INJECTION. THE 0.75% CONCENTRATION SHOULD BE RESERVED FOR SURGICAL PROCEDURES WHERE A HIGH DEGREE OF MUSCLE RELAXATION AND PROLONGED EFFECT ARE NECESSARY.

LOCAL ANESTHETICS SHOULD ONLY BE EMPLOYED BY CLINICIANS WHO ARE WELL VERSED IN DIAGNOSIS AND MANAGEMENT OF DOSE-RELATED TOXICITY AND OTHER ACUTE EMERGENCIES WHICH MIGHT ARISE FROM THE BLOCK TO BE EMPLOYED, AND THEN ONLY AFTER ENSURING THE *IMMEDIATE* AVAILABILITY OF OXYGEN, OTHER RESUSCITATIVE DRUGS, CARDIOPULMONARY RESUSCITATIVE EQUIPMENT, AND THE PERSONNEL RESOURCES NEEDED FOR PROPER MANAGEMENT OF TOXIC REACTIONS AND RELATED EMERGENCIES. (See also ADVERSE REACTIONS and PRECAUTIONS.) DELAY IN PROPER MANAGEMENT OF DOSE-RELATED TOXICITY, UNDERVENTILATION FROM ANY CAUSE AND/OR ALTERED SENSITIVITY MAY LEAD TO THE DEVELOPMENT OF ACIDOSIS, CARDIAC ARREST AND, POSSIBLY, DEATH.

Local anesthetic solutions containing antimicrobial preservatives, i.e. those supplied in multiple dose vials, should not be used for epidural or caudal anesthesia because safety has not been established with regard to intrathecal injection, either intentional or unintentional, of such preservatives.

It is essential that aspiration for blood or cerebrospinal fluid (where applicable) be done prior to injecting any local anesthetic, both the original dose and all subsequent doses, to avoid intravascular or subarachnoid injection. However, a negative aspiration does *not* ensure against an intravascular or subarachnoid injection.

Bupivacaine HCl with epinephrine 1:200,000 or other vasopressors should not be used concomitantly with ergot-type oxytocic drugs, because a severe persistent hypertension may occur. Likewise, solutions of bupivacaine containing a vasoconstrictor, such as epinephrine, should be used with extreme caution in patients receiving monoamine oxidase (MAO) inhibitors or antidepressants of the triptyline or imipramine types, because severe prolonged hypertension may result.

Until further experience is gained in children younger than 12 years, administration of bupivacaine in this age group is not recommended.

TABLE 1. COMPOSITION OF AVAILABLE SOLUTIONS*

PRODUCT IDENTIFICATION		FORMULA						
		Multiple Dose Vials				Ampules and Single Dose Vials		
Bupivacaine HCl Concentration %	Epinephrine (as bitratrate) Dilution	Sodium Chloride (mg/ml)	Citric Acid (mg/ml)	Sodium Metabisulfite (mg/ml)	Methylparaben (mg/ml)	Sodium Chloride (mg/ml)	Citric Acid (mg/ml)	Sodium Metabisulfite (mg/ml)
0.25	None	8.0	None	None	1.0	8.0	None	None
0.50	None	8.0	None	None	1.0	8.0	None	None
0.50	1:200,000	Not available				8.0	0.2	0.5
0.75	None	Not available				8.0	None	None
0.75	1:200,000	Not available				8.0	0.2	0.5

*pH of all solutions adjusted to 4.5–6.5 (plain solutions) or to 3.3–5.5 (epinephrine-containing solutions) with sodium hydroxide and/or hydrochloric acid.

Reports of cardiac arrest and death have occurred with the use of bupivacaine for intravenous regional anesthesia (Bier Block). Information on safe dosages or techniques of administration of this product are lacking; therefore bupivacaine is not recommended for use by this technique.

Prior use of chloroprocaine may interfere with subsequent use of bupivacaine. Because of this, and because safety of intercurrent use of bupivacaine and chloroprocaine has not been established, such use is not recommended.

Sensorcaine® Solutions with epinephrine contain sodium metabisulfite, a sulfite that may cause serious allergic-type reactions (e.g., hives, itching, wheezing, anaphylaxis) in certain susceptible persons. Although the overall incidence of sulfite sensitivity in the general population is probably low, it is seen more frequently in asthmatics or in atopic nonasthmatic persons.

PRECAUTIONS

General: The safety and effectiveness of local anesthetics depend on proper dosage, correct technique, adequate precautions and readiness for emergencies. Resuscitative equipment, oxygen and other resuscitative drugs should be available for immediate use. (See WARNINGS and ADVERSE REACTIONS.) During major regional nerve blocks, the patient should have I.V. fluids running via an indwelling catheter to assure a functioning intravenous pathway. The lowest dosage of local anesthetic that results in effective anesthesia should be used to avoid high plasma levels and serious adverse effects. Injections should be made slowly, with frequent aspirations before and during the injection to avoid intravascular injection .

Epidural Anesthesia: During epidural administration of bupivacaine, concentrated solutions (0.5–0.75%) should be administered in incremental doses of 3 to 5 ml with sufficient time between doses to detect toxic manifestations of unintentional intravascular or intrathecal injection . Syringe aspirations should also be performed before and during each supplemental injection in continuous (intermittent) catheter techniques. An intravascular injection is still possible even if aspirations for blood are negative.

During the administration of epidural anesthethesia, it is recommended that a test dose be administered initially and the effects monitored before the full dose is given. When using a "continuous" catheter technique, test doses should be given prior to both the original and all reinforcing doses, because plastic tubing in the epidural space can migrate into a blood vessel or through the dura. When clinical conditions permit, the test dose should contain epinephrine (10 to 15 μg have been suggested) to serve as a warning of unintentional intravascular injection . If injected into a blood vessel, this amount of epinephrine is likely to produce a transient "epinephrine response" within 45 seconds, consisting of an increase in heart rate and systolic blood pressure, circumoral pallor, palpitations and nervousness in the unsedated patient. The sedated patient may exhibit only a pulse rate increase of 20 or more beats per minute for 15 or more seconds. Therefore, following the test dose, the heart rate should be monitored for a heart rate increase. The test dose should also contain 10 to 15 mg of Sensorcaine® (bupivacaine HCl) injection or an equivalent dose of a short-acting amide anesthetic such as 30 to 40 mg of lidocaine, to detect an unintentional intrathecal administration. This will be manifested within a few minutes by signs of spinal block (e.g. decreased sensation of the buttocks, paresis of the legs, or, in the sedated patient, absent knee jerk). Patients on beta-blockers may not manifest changes in heart rate, but blood pressure monitoring can detect an evanescent rise in systolic blood pressure.

Injection of repeated doses of local anesthetics may cause significant increases in plasma levels with each repeated dose due to slow accumulation of the drug or its metabolites or to slow metabolic degradation. Tolerance to elevated blood levels varies with the physical condition of the patient. Debilitated, elderly patients and acutely ill patients should be given reduced doses commensurate with their age and physical condition. Local anesthetics should also be used with caution in patients with hypotension or heart block.

Careful and constant monitoring of cardiovascular and respiratory vital signs (adequacy of ventilation) and the patient's state of consciousness should be performed after each local anesthetic injection . It should be kept in mind at such times that restlessness, anxiety, incoherent speech, light-headedness, numbness and tingling of the mouth and lips, metallic taste, tinnitus, dizziness, blurred vision, tremors, twitching, depression, or drowsiness may be early warning signs of central nervous system toxicity.

Local anesthetic solutions containing a vasoconstrictor should be used cautiously and in carefully restricted quantities in areas of the body supplied by end arteries or having otherwise compromised blood supply such as digits, nose, external ear, penis, etc. Patients with hypertensive vascular disease may exhibit exaggerated vasoconstrictor response. Ischemic injury or necrosis may result.

Because amide-type local anesthetics such as bupivacaine are metabolized by the liver, these drugs, especially repeat doses, should be used cautiously in patients with hepatic disease. Patients with severe hepatic disease, because of their inability to metabolize local anesthetics normally, are at a greater risk of developing toxic plasma concentrations. Local anesthetics should also be used with caution in patients with impaired cardiovascular function because they may be less able to compensate for functional changes associated with the prolongation of A-V conduction produced by these drugs.

Serious dose-related cardiac arrythmias may occur if preparations containing a vasoconstrictor such as epinephrine are employed in patients during or following the administration of potent inhalation anesthetics. In deciding whether to use these products concurrently in the same patients, the combined action of both agents upon the myocardium, the concentration and volume of vasoconstrictor used, and the time since injection , when applicable, should be taken into account.

Many drugs used during the conduct of anesthesia are considered potential triggering agents for familial malignant hyperthermia. Because it is not known whether amide-type local anesthetics may trigger this reaction and because the need for supplemental general anesthesia cannot be predicted in advance, it is suggested that a standard protocol for management should be available. Early unexplained signs of tachycardia, tachypnea, labile blood pressure and metabolic acidosis may precede temperature elevation. Successful outcome is dependent on early diagnosis, prompt discontinuance of the suspect triggering agent(s) and prompt treatment, including oxygen therapy, dantrolene (consult dantrolene sodium intravenous package insert before using) and other supportive measures.

Use in Head and Neck Area: Small doses of local anesthetics injected into the head and neck area, including retrobulbar, dental and stellate ganglion blocks, may produce adverse reactions similar to systemic toxicity seen with unintentional intravascular injection s of larger doses. Confusion, convulsions, respiratory depression and/or respiratory arrest, and cardiovascular stimulation or depression have been reported. These reactions may be due to intraarterial injection of the local anesthetic with retrograde flow to the cerebral circulation. Patients receiving these blocks should have their circulation and respiration monitored and be constantly observed. Resuscitative equipment and personnel for treating adverse reactions should be immediately available. Dosage recommendations should not be exceeded. (See DOSAGE AND ADMINISTRATION.)

Use in Ophthalmic Surgery: When Sensorcaine® (bupivacaine HCl) 0.75% injection is used for retrobulbar block, complete corneal anesthesia usually precedes onset of clinically acceptable external ocular muscle akinesia. Therefore, the presence of akinesia rather than anesthesia alone should determine readiness of the patient for surgery.

Information for Patients: When appropriate, patients should be informed in advance that they may experience temporary loss of sensation and motor activity, usually in the lower half of the body following proper administration of caudal or lumbar epidural anesthesia. Also, when appropriate, the physician should discuss other information including adverse reactions in the Sensorcaine® (bupivacaine HCl) package insert.

Clinically Significant Drug Interactions: The administration of local anesthetic solutions containing epinephrine or norepinephrine to patients receiving monoamine oxidase inhibitors or tricyclic antidepressants may produce severe, prolonged hypertension. Concurrent use of these agents should generally be avoided. In situations in which concurrent therapy is necessary, careful patient monitoring is essential.

Concurrent administration of vasopressor drugs and of ergot-type oxytocic drugs may cause severe, persistent hypertension or cerebrovascular accidents.

Phenothiazines and butyrophenones may reduce or reverse the pressor effect of epinephrine.

Carcinogenesis, Mutagenesis, and Impairment of Fertility: - Long-term studies in animals of most local anesthetics, including bupivacaine, to evaluate the carcinogenic potential have not been conducted. Mutagenic potential or the effect on fertility have not been determined. There is no evidence from human data that bupivacaine may be carcinogenic or mutagenic or that it impairs fertility.

Pregnancy Category C: Decreased pup survival in rats and embryocidal effect in rabbits have been observed when bupivacaine HCl was administered to these species in doses comparable to nine and five times, respectively, the maximum recommended daily human dose (400 mg). There are no adequate and well-controlled studies in pregnant women of the effect of bupivacaine on the developing fetus. Sensorcaine® (bupivacaine HCl) injection should be used during pregnancy only if the potential benefit justifies the potential risk to the fetus. This does not exclude the use of Sensorcaine® (bupivacaine HCl) injection (0.25% and 0.5% concentrations) at term for obstetrical anesthesia or analgesia. (See LABOR AND DELIVERY.)

Labor and Delivery: See Box WARNING regarding obstetrical use of 0.75% concentration.

Sensorcaine® (bupivacaine HCl) injection is contraindicated in obstetrical paracervical block anesthesia.

Local anesthetics rapidly cross the placenta, and when used for epidural, caudal or pudendal block anesthesia, can cause varying degrees of maternal, fetal and neonatal toxicity. (See CLINICAL PHARMACOLOGY.) The incidence and degree of toxicity depend upon the procedure performed, the type and amount of drug used, and the technique of drug administration. Adverse reactions in the parturient, fetus and neonate involve alterations of the central nervous system, peripheral vascular tone and cardiac function.

Maternal hypotension has resulted from regional anesthesia. Local anesthetics produce vasodilation by blocking sympathetic nerves. Elevating the patient's legs and positioning her on her left side will help prevent decreases in blood pressure. The fetal heart rate also should be monitored continuously, and electronic fetal monitoring is highly advisable.

Epidural, caudal, or pudendal anesthesia may alter the forces of parturition through changes in uterine contractility or maternal expulsive efforts. Epidural anesthesia has been reported to prolong the second stage of labor by removing the parturient's reflex urge to bear down or by interfering with motor function. The use of obstetrical anesthesia may increase the need for forceps assistance.

The use of some local anesthetic drug products during labor and delivery may be followed by diminished muscle strength and tone for the first day or two of life. This has not been reported with Sensorcaine® (bupivacaine HCl) injection.

It is extremely important to avoid aortocaval compression by the gravid uterus during administration of regional block to parturients. To do this, the patient must be maintained in the left lateral decubitus position or a blanket roll or sandbag may be placed beneath the right hip and the gravid uterus displaced to the left.

Nursing Mothers: It is not known whether local anesthetic drugs are excreted in human milk. Because many drugs are excreted in human milk, caution should be exercised when local anesthetics are administered to a nursing mother.

Pediatric Use: Until further experience is gained in children younger than 12 years, administration of Sensorcaine® (bupivacaine HCl) injection in this age group is not recommended.

ADVERSE REACTIONS

Reactions to bupivacaine are characteristic of those associated with other amide-type local anesthetics. A major cause of adverse reactions to this group of drugs may be associated with excessive plasma levels,which may be due to overdosage, unintentional intravascular injection or slow metabolic degradation.

Systemic: The most commonly encountered acute adverse experiences that demand immediate countermeasures are related to the central nervous system and the cardiovascular system. These adverse experiences are generally dose related and due to high plasma levels which may result from overdosage, rapid absorption from the injection site, diminished tolerance or from unintentional intravascular injection of the local anesthetic solution. In addition to systemic dose-related toxicity, unintentional subarachnoid injection of drug during the intended performance of caudal or lumbar epidural block or nerve blocks near the vertebral column (especially in the head and neck region) may result in underventilation or apnea ("Total or High Spinal"). Also, hypotension due to loss of sympathetic tone and respiratory paralysis or underventilation due to cephalad extension of the motor level of anesthesia may occur. This may lead to secondary cardiac arrest if untreated. Factors influencing plasma protein binding, such as acidosis, systemic diseases that alter protein production or competition with other drugs for protein binding sites, may diminish individual tolerance.

Central Nervous System Reactions: These are characterized by excitation and/or depression. Restlessness, anxiety, dizziness, tinnitus, blurred vision or tremors may occur, possibly proceeding to convulsions. However, excitement may be transient or absent, with depression being the first manifestation of an adverse reaction. This may quickly be followed by drowsiness merging into unconsciousness and respiratory arrest. Other central nervous system effects may be nausea, vomiting, chills, and constriction of the pupils.

The incidence of convulsions associated with the use of local anesthetics varies with the procedure used and the total dose administered. In a survey of studies of epidural anesthesia, overt toxicity progressing to convulsions occurred in approximately 0.1 percent of local anesthetic administrations.

Cardiovascular System Reactions: High doses or unintentional intravascular injection may lead to high plasma levels and related depression of the myocardium, decreased cardiac

Continued on next page

Astra—Cont.

output, heart block, hypotension, bradycardia, ventricular arrhythmias, including ventricular tachycardia and ventricular fibrillation, and cardiac arrest. (See WARNINGS, PRECAUTIONS, and OVERDOSAGE sections).

Allergic: Allergic type reactions are rare and may occur as a result of sensitivity to the local anesthetic or to other formulation ingredients, such as the antimicrobial preservative methylparaben contained in multiple dose vials or sulfites in epinephrine-containing solutions. These reactions are characterized by signs such as urticaria, pruritis, erythema, angioneurotic edema (including laryngeal edema), tachycardia, sneezing, nausea, vomiting, dizziness, syncope, excessive sweating, elevated temperature, and possibly, anaphylactoid symptomatology (including severe hypotension). Cross sensitivity among members of the amide-type local anesthetic group has been reported. The usefulness of screening for sensitivity has not been definitely established.

Neurologic: The incidence of adverse neurologic reactions associated with the use of local anesthetics may be related to the total dose of local anesthetic administered and are also dependent upon the particular drug used, the route of administraion and the physical status of the patient. Many of these effects may be related to local anesthetic techniques, with or without a contribution from the drug.

In the practice of caudal or lumbar epidural block, occasional unintentional penetration of the subarachnoid space by the catheter or needle may occur. Subsequent adverse effects may depend partially on the amount of drug administered intrathecally and the physiological and physical effects of a dural puncture. A high spinal is characterized by paralysis of the legs, loss of consciousness, respiratory paralysis and bradycardia.

Neurologic effects following unintentional subarachnoid administration during epidural or caudal anesthesia may include spinal block by varying magnitude (including high or total spinal block); hypotension secondary to spinal block; urinary retention; fecal and urinary incontinence; loss of perineal sensation and sexual function; persistent anesthesia, paresthesia, weakness, paralysis of the lower extremities and loss of sphincter control, all of which may have slow, incomplete or no recovery; headache; backache; septic meningitis; meningismus; slowing of labor; increased incidence of forceps delivery; or cranial nerve palsies due to traction on nerves from loss of cerebrospinal fluid.

OVERDOSAGE

Acute emergencies from local anesthetics are generally related to high plasma levels encountered during therapeutic use of local anesthetics or to unintended subarachnoid injection of local anesthetic solution. (See ADVERSE REACTIONS, WARNINGS, and PRECAUTIONS).

Management of Local Anesthetic Emergencies: The first consideration is prevention, best accomplished by careful and constant monitoring of cardiovascular and respiratory vital signs and the patient's state of consciousness after each local anesthetic injection . At the first sign of change, oxygen should be administered.

The first step in the management of systemic toxic reactions, as well as underventilation or apnea due to unintentional subarachnoid injection of drug solution, consists of **immediate** attention to the establishment and maintenance of a patent airway and effective assisted or controlled ventilation with 100% oxygen with a delivery system capable of permitting immediate positive airway pressure by mask. This may prevent convulsions if they have not already occurred.

If necessary, use drugs to control the convulsions. A 50 to 100 mg bolus I.V. injection of succinylcholine will paralyze the patient without depressing the central nervous or cardiovascular systems and facilitate ventilation. A bolus I.V. dose of 5 to 10 mg of diazepam or 50 to 100 mg of thiopental will permit ventilation and counteract central nervous system stimulation, but these drugs also depress the central nervous system, respiratory and cardiac function, add to postictal depression, and may result in apnea. Intravenous barbiturates, anticonsulsant agents, or muscle relaxants should

TABLE 2. DOSAGE RECOMMENDATIONS—SENSORCAINE® (bupivacaine HCl) INJECTIONS WITHOUT EPINEPHRINE

Type of Block	Each Dose conc.(%)	ml.	mg.	Motor Block*
Local infiltration	0.25	up to 70	up to 175	—
Epidural	0.75**	10–20	75–150	Complete
	0.50	10–20	50–100	Moderate to complete
	0.25	10–20	25–50	Partial to moderate
Caudal	0.50	15–30	75–150	Moderate to complete
	0.25	15–30	37.5–75	Moderate
Peripheral	0.50	5–35	25–175	Moderate to complete
	0.25	5–70	12.5–175	Moderate to complete
Retrobulbar†	0.75	2–4	15–30	Complete
Sympathetic†	0.25	20–50	50–125	—

*With continuous techniques, repeat doses increase the degree of motor block. The first repeat dose of 0.5% may produce complete motor block. Intercostal nerve block with 0.25% may also produce complete motor block for intra-abdominal surgery.
**For single dose; not for continuous techniques; not for use in obstetrics.
†See PRECAUTIONS.

only be administered by those familiar with their use. Immediately after the institution of these ventilatory measures, the adequacy of the circulation should be evaluated. Supportive treatment of circulatory depression may require administration of intravenous fluids, and, when appropriate, a vasopressor dictated by the clinical situation (such as ephedrine or epinephrine to enhance myocardial contractile force).

If difficulty is encountered in the maintenance of a patent airway or if prolonged ventilatory support (assisted or controlled) is indicated, endotracheal intubation, employing drugs and techniques familiar to the clinician, may be indicated after initial administration of oxygen by mask.

Recent clinical data from patients experiencing local anesthetic induced convulsions demonstrated rapid development of hypoxia, hypercarbia and acidosis wih bupivacaine within a minute of the onset of convulsions. These observations suggest the oxygen consumption and carbon dioxide production are greatly increased during local anesthetic convulsions and emphasize the importance of immediate and effective ventilation with oxygen which may avoid cardiac arrest.

If not treated immediately, convulsions with simultaneous hypoxia, hypercarbia and acidosis, plus myocardial depression from the direct effects of the local anesthetic may result in cardiac arrhythmias, bradycardia, asystole, ventricular fibrillation, or cardiac arrest. Respiratory abnormalities, includng apnea, may occur. Underventilation or apnea due to unintentional subarachnoid injection of local anesthetic solution may produce these same signs and also lead to cardiac arrest if ventilatory support is not instituted. *If cardiac arrest should occur, a successful outcome may require prolonged resuscitative efforts.*

The supine position is dangerous in pregnant women at term because of aortocaval compression by the gravid uterus. Therefore, during treatment of systemic toxicity, maternal hypotension or fetal bradycardia following regional block, the parturient should be maintained in the left lateral decubitus position if possible, or manual displacement of the uterus off the great vessels be accomplished.

The mean seizure dosage of bupivacaine in rhesus monkeys was found to be 4.4 mg/kg with mean arterial plasma concentration of 4.5 mcg/ml. The intravenous and subcutaneous LD50s in mice are 6 to 8mg/kg and 38 to 54mg/kg respectively.

DOSAGE AND ADMINISTRATION

The dosage varies and depends upon the area to be anesthetized, the vascularity of the tissues, the number of neuronal segments to be blocked, individual tolerance, and the technique of anesthesia. The lowest dosage needed to provide effective anesthesia should be administered. The rapid injection of a large volume of local anesthetic solution should be avoided and fractional doses should be used when feasible. For specific techniques and procedures, refer to standard textbooks.

For most indications, the duration of anesthesia with Sensorcaine® (bupivacaine HCl) injection is such that a single dose is sufficient.

In each case, the maximum dosage limit must be determined by evaluating the size and physical status of the patient and considering the usual rate of systemic absorption from a specific injection site. Most experience to date is with single doses up to 175 mg of bupivacaine HCl without epinephrine or 225 mg with epinephrine 1:200,000. More or less drug may be used depending on the physical condition of each case. The dose may be repeated as often as every 3 hours. In studies to date, total daily doses up to 400 mg have been reported. Until further experience is gained, this dose should not be exceeded in 24 hours. The dosages in the following table are recommended as a guide for use in the average adult. For young, elderly or debilitated patients, these dosages should be reduced. Until further experience is gained, Sensorcaine® injection is not recommended for children younger than 12 years. Sensorcaine® (bupivacaine HCl) is contraindicated in obstetrical paracervial block and is not recommended for use in intravenous regional anesthesia (Bier Block).

Use in Epidural Anesthesia: During epidural administration, Sensorcaine® (bupivacaine HCl) 0.5% and 0.75% injections should be administered in incremental doses of 3 to 5 ml, with sufficient time between doses to detect toxic manifestations of unintentional intravascular or intrathecal injection. In obstetrics, only the 0.5% and 0.25% concentrations should be used; incremental doses of 3 to 5 ml of the 0.5% solution, not exceeding 50–100 mg at any dosing interval, are recommended. Repeat doses should be preceded by a test dose containing epinephrine if the vasoconstrictor is not contraindicated.

UNUSED PORTIONS OF SOLUTIONS IN SINGLE DOSE CONTAINERS SHOULD BE DISCARDED, SINCE THIS PRODUCT FORM CONTAINS NO PRESERVATIVES.

[See table 2 above].

NOTE: Parenteral drug products should be inspected visually for particulate matter and discoloration prior to administration whenever the solution and container permit. Solutions that are discolored and/or contain particulate matter should not be used.

HOW SUPPLIED

SOLUTIONS OF SENSORCAINE® (BUPIVACAINE HYDROCHLORIDE) SHOULD NOT BE USED FOR THE PRODUCTION OF SPINAL ANESTHESIA (SUBARACHNOID BLOCK) BECAUSE OF INSUFFICIENT DATA TO SUPPORT SUCH USE.

[See table to left].

Disinfecting agents containing heavy metals, which cause release of respective ions (mercury, zinc, copper, etc.), should not be used for skin or mucous membrane disinfection since they have been related to incidents of swelling and edema. When chemical disinfection of the container surface is desired, either pure undiluted isopropyl alcohol (91%) or ethyl alcohol (70%) USP is recommended. It is recommended that chemical disinfection be accomplished by wiping the ampule or vial stopper thoroughly with cotton or gauze that has been moistened with the recommended alcohol just prior to use.

Solutions should be stored at controlled room temperature 15° to 30° C (59°–86°F).

Solutions containing epinephrine should be protected from light.

Sensorcaine® (bupivacaine HCl) injections

Dosage Form	Concentrate	Astra Sterile-Pak®
Single Dose Vials, 10 ml	0.25%, 0.5% and 0.75% without epinephrine	
Single Dose Vials, 30 ml	0.25% and 0.5% without epinephrine	x
	0.5% and 0.75% with epinephrine 1:200,000	x
Multiple dose Vials, 50 ml	0.25% and 0.5% without epinephrine	
Single Dose Ampules, 30 ml	0.25%, 0.5%, 0.75% without epinephrine	x
	0.5% and 0.75% with epinephrine 1:200,000	x
Single Dose Ampules, 5 ml	0.5% with epinephrine 1:200,000	

x–Package forms—also available in Astra Sterile-Pak® Pre-sterilized vials or ampules in a Convenient Dispenser Carton.

021851R08 1/86

SODIUM BICARBONATE ℞

[*so'-dēum by-car'-bōw-nāte*]

Injection, USP

FOR CORRECTION OF METABOLIC ACIDOSIS AND OTHER CONDITIONS REQUIRING SYSTEMIC ALKALINIZATION

(For details of indications, dosage and administration, precautions, and adverse reactions, see circular in package.)

HOW SUPPLIED

Sodium Bicarbonate Injection, USP is supplied in the following dosage forms:

[See table to right]

Solutions should be stored at controlled room temperature 15°-30°C (59°-86°F).

021852R00 Iss. 6/85

NDC No. 0186-	Dosage Form	Conc. %	mg/ml ($NaHCO_3$)	mEq/ml; ($Na+$)	mEq/ml (HCO_3)	mEq/Container size (ml)	mOsm
0650-01	Syringe	8.4	84	1.0	1.0	50/50	2/ml
1164-04	Vial	8.4	84	1.0	1.0	50/50	2/ml
0656-01	Syringe (Pediatric)	8.4	84	1.0	1.0	10/10	2/ml
1162-04	Vial	7.5	75	0.9	0.9	44.6/50	1.79/ml
0647-01	Syringe	7.5	75	0.9	0.9	44.6/50	1.79/ml
0646-01	Syringe (Infant)	4.2	42	0.5	0.5	5/10	1/ml
0645-01	Syringe (Infant)	4.2	42	0.5	0.5	2.5/5	1/ml

XYLOCAINE® (lidocaine hydrochloride) ℞

[*zī'lo-caine*]

STERILE AQUEOUS SOLUTIONS

Local anesthetic for infiltration and nerve block

DESCRIPTION

Xylocaine (lidocaine HCl) Solutions are sterile aqueous solutions that contain a local anesthetic agent and are administered parenterally by injection. See INDICATIONS for specific uses. The specific quantitative composition for each available solution is shown in Table 1.

Xylocaine solutions contain lidocaine HCl, which is chemically designated as acetamide 2-(diethylamino)-N-(2,6-dimethylphenyl)-monohydrochloride.

Epinephrine is (−)−3,4-Dihydroxy-α-[(methylamino) methyl] benzyl alcohol.

[See table below].

CLINICAL PHARMACOLOGY

Mechanism of action: Lidocaine stabilizes the neuronal membrane by inhibiting the ionic fluxes required for the initiation and conduction of impulses, thereby effecting local anesthetic action.

Hemodynamics: Excessive blood levels may cause changes in cardiac output, total peripheral resistance, and mean arterial pressure. With central neural blockade these changes may be attributable to block of autonomic fibers, a direct depressant effect of the local anesthetic agent on various components of the cardiovascular system and/or the beta-adrenergic receptor stimulating action of epinephrine when present. The net effect is normally a modest hypotension when the recommended dosages are not exceeded.

Pharmacokinetics and metabolism: Information derived from diverse formulations, concentrations and usages reveals that lidocaine is completely absorbed following parenteral administration, its rate of absorption depending, for example, upon various factors such as the site of administration and the presence or absence of a vasoconstrictor agent. Except for intravascular administration, the highest blood levels are obtained following intercoastal nerve block and the lowest after subcutaneous administration.

The plasma binding of lidocaine is dependent on drug concentration, and the fraction bound decreases with increasing concentration. At concentrations of 1 to 4 μg of free base per ml 60 to 80 percent of lidocaine is protein bound. Binding is also dependent on the plasma concentration of the alpha-1-acid glycoprotein.

Lidocaine crosses the blood-brain and placental barriers, presumably by passive diffusion.

Lidocaine is metabolized rapidly by the liver, and metabolites and unchanged drug are excreted by the kidneys. Biotransformation includes oxidative N-dealkylation, ring hydroxylation, cleavage of the amide linkage, and conjugation. N-dealkylation, a major pathway of biotransformation, yields the metabolites monoethylglycinexylidide and glycinexylidide. The pharmacological/toxicological actions of these metabolites are similar to, but less potent than, those of lidocaine. Approximately 90% of lidocaine administered is excreted in the form of various metabolites, and less than 10% is excreted unchanged. The primary metabolite in urine is a conjugate of 4-hyroxy-2, 6-dimethylaniline.

The elimination half-life of lidocaine following an intravenous bolus injection is typically 1.5 to 2.0 hours. Because of the rapid rate at which lidocaine is metabolized, any condition that affects liver function may alter lidocaine kinetics. The half-life may be prolonged two-fold or more in patients with liver dysfunction. Renal dysfunction does not affect lidocaine kinetics but may increase the accumulation of metabolites.

Factors such as acidosis and the use of CNS stimulants and depressants affect the CNS levels of lidocaine required to produce overt systemic effects. Objective adverse manifestations become increasingly apparent with increasing venous plasma levels above 6.0 μg free base per ml. In the rhesus monkey arterial blood levels of 18–21 μg/ml have been shown to be threshold for convulsive activity.

INDICATIONS AND USAGE

Xylocaine (lidocaine HCl) Solutions are indicated for production of local or regional anesthesia by infiltration techniques such as percutaneous injection and intravenous regional anesthesia by peripheral nerve block techniques such as brachial plexus and intercostal and by central neural techniques such as lumbar and caudal epidural blocks, when the accepted procedures for these techniques as described in standard textbooks are observed.

CONTRAINDICATIONS

Lidocaine is contraindicated in patients with a known history of hypersensitivity to local anesthetics of the amide type.

WARNINGS

XYLOCAINE SOLUTIONS FOR INFILTRATION AND NERVE BLOCK SHOULD BE EMPLOYED ONLY BY CLINICIANS WHO ARE WELL VERSED IN DIAGNOSIS AND MANAGEMENT OF DOSE-RELATED TOXICITY AND OTHER ACUTE EMERGENCIES THAT MIGHT ARISE FROM THE BLOCK TO BE EMPLOYED AND THEN ONLY AFTER ENSURING THE *IMMEDIATE* AVAILABILITY OF OXYGEN. OTHER RESUSCITATIVE DRUGS, CARDIOPULMONARY EQUIPMENT, AND THE PERSONNEL NEEDED FOR PROPER MANAGEMENT OF TOXIC REACTIONS AND RELATED EMERGENCIES (See also ADVERSE REACTIONS and PRECAUTIONS). DELAY IN PROPER MANAGEMENT OF DOSE-RELATED TOXICITY, UNDERVENTILATION FROM ANY CAUSE AND/OR ALTERED SENSITIVITY MAY LEAD TO THE DEVELOPMENT OF ACIDOSIS, CARDIAC ARREST AND, POSSIBLY, DEATH.

To avoid intravascular injection, aspiration should be performed before the local anesthetic solution is injected. The needle must be repositioned until no return of blood can be elicited by aspiration. Note, however, that the absence of blood in the syringe does not guarantee that intravascular injection has been avoided.

Local anesthetic solutions containing antimicrobial preservatives (e.g., methylparaben) should not be used for epidural or spinal anesthesia because the safety of these agents has not been established with regard to intrathecal injection, either intentional or accidental.

Xylocaine Solutions with epinephrine contain sodium metabisulfite, a sulfite that may cause serious allergic-type reactions (e.g., hives, itching, wheezing, anaphylaxis) in certain susceptible persons. Although the overall incidence of sulfite sensitivity in the general population is probably low, it is seen more frequently in asthmatics or in atopic nonasthmatic persons.

PRECAUTIONS

General: The safety and effectivness of lidocaine depend on proper dosage, correct technique, adequate precautions, and readiness for emergencies. Standard textbooks should be consulted for specific techniques and precautions for various regional anesthetic procedures.

Resuscitative equipment, oxygen, and other resuscitative drugs should be available for immediate use. (See WARNINGS and ADVERSE REACTIONS). The lowest dosage that results in effective anesthesia should be used to avoid high plasma levels and serious adverse effects. Syringe aspirations should also be performed before and during each supplemental injection when using indwelling catheter techniques. During the administration of epidural anesthesia, it is recommended that a test dose be administered initially and that the patient be monitored for central nervous system toxicity and cardiovascular toxicity, as well as for signs of unintended intrathecal administration before proceeding. When clinical conditions permit, consideration should be given to employing local anesthetic solutions that contain epinephrine for the test dose because circulatory changes compatible with epinephrine may also serve as a warning sign of unintended intravascular injection. An intravascular injection is still possible even if aspirations for blood are negative. Repeated doses of lidocaine may cause significant increases in blood levels with each repeated dose because of slow accumulation of the drug or its metabolites. Tolerance to elevated blood levels varies with the status of the patient. Debilitated, elderly patients, acutely ill patients and children should be given reduced doses commensurate with their age and physical condition. Lidocaine should also be used with caution in patients with severe shock or heart block.

Lumbar and caudal epidural anesthesia should be used with extreme caution in persons with the following conditions: existing neurological disease, spinal deformities, septicemia and severe hypertension.

Continued on next page

TABLE I COMPOSITION OF AVAILABLE SOLUTIONS

PRODUCT IDENTIFICATION		FORMULA: SINGLE DOSE VIALS AND AMPULES			MULTIPLE DOSE VIALS			
Xylocaine (lidocaine HCl) Solution (Percent)	Epinephrine (dilution)	Sodium Chloride (mg/ml)	Sodium Metabisulfite (mg/ml)	Citric Acid (mg/ml)	Sodium Chloride (mg/ml)	Sodium Metabisulfite (mg/ml)	Citric Acid (mg/ml)	Methyl-Paraben (mg/ml)
0.5	None	8.0	None	None	8.0	None	None	1.0
0.5	1:200,000	N.S.	N.S.	N.S.	8.0	0.5	0.2	1.0
1.0	None	7.0	None	None	7.0	None	None	1.0
1.0	1:200,000	7.0	0.5	0.2	N.S.	N.S.	N.S.	N.S.
1.0	1:100,000	N.S.	N.S.	N.S.	7.0	0.5	0.2	1.0
1.5	None	6.5	None	None	N.S.	N.S.	N.S.	N.S.
1.5	1:200,000	6.5	0.5	0.2	N.S.	N.S.	N.S.	N.S.
2.0	None	6.0	None	None	6.0	None	None	1.0
2.0	1:200,000	6.0	0.5	0.2	N.S.	N.S.	N.S.	N.S.
2.0	1:100,000	N.S.	N.S.	N.S.	6.0	0.5	0.2	1.0

N.S. Not Supplied

NOTE: pH of all solutions adjusted to USP limits with sodium hydroxide and/or hydrochloric acid.

Astra—Cont.

Local anesthetic solutions containing a vasoconstrictor should be used cautiously and in carefully circumscribed quantities in areas of the body supplied by end arteries or having otherwise compromised blood supply. Patients with peripheral vascular disease and those with hypertensive vascular disease may exhibit exaggerated vasoconstrictor response. Ischemic injury or necrosis may result. Preparations containing a vasoconstrictor should be used with caution in patients during or following the administration of potent general anesthetic agents, since cardiac arrhythmias may occur under such conditions.

Careful and constant monitoring of cardiovascular and respiratory (adequacy of ventilation) vital signs and the patient's state of consciousness should be accomplished after each local anesthetic injection. It should be kept in mind at such times that restlessness, anxiety, tinnitus, dizziness, blurred vision, tremors, depression or drowsiness may be early warning signs of central nervous system toxicity.

Since amide-type local anesthetics are metabolized by the liver, Xylocaine Solution should be used with caution in patients with hepatic disease. Patients with severe hepatic disease because of their inability to metabolize local anesthetics normally, are a greater risk of developing toxic plasma concentrations. Xylocaine Solution should also be used with caution in patients with impaired cardiovascular function since they may be less able to compensate for functional changes associated with the prolongation of A-V conduction produced by these drugs.

Many drugs used during the conduct of anesthesia are considered potential triggering agents for familial malignant hyperthermia. Since it is not known whether amide-type local anesthetics may trigger this reaction and since the need for supplemental general anesthesia cannot be predicted in advance, it is suggested that a standard protocol for the management of malignant hyperthermia should be available. Early unexplained signs of tachycardia, tachypnea, labile blood pressure and metabolic acidosis may precede temperature elevation. Successful outcome is dependent on early diagnosis, prompt discontinuance of the suspect triggering agent(s) and institution of treatment, including oxygen therapy, indicated supportive measures and dantrolene (consult dantrolene sodium intravenous package insert before using).

Proper tourniquet technique, as described in publications and standard textbooks, is essential in the performance of intravenous regional anesthesia. Solutions containing epinephrine or other vasoconstrictors should not be used for this technique.

Lidocaine should be used with caution in persons with known drug sensitivities. Patients allergic to para-aminobenzoic acid derivatives (procaine, tetracine, benzocaine, etc.) have not shown cross sensitivity to lidocaine.

Use in the Head and Neck Area: Small doses of local anesthetics injected into the head and neck area, including retrobulbar, dental and stellate ganglion blocks, may produce adverse reactions similar to systemic toxicity seen with unintentional intravascular injections of larger doses. Confusion, convulsions, respiratory depression and/or respiratory arrest, and cardiovascular stimulation or depression have been reported. These reactions may be due to intra-arterial injections of the local anesthetic with retrograde flow to the cerebral circulation. Patients receiving these blocks should have their circulation and respiration monitored and be constantly observed. Resuscitative equipment and personnel for treating adverse reactions should be immediately available. Dosage recommendations should not be exceeded. (See DOSAGE and ADMINISTRATION).

Information for Patients: When appropriate, patients should be informed in advance that they may experience temporary loss of sensation and motor activity, usually in the lower half of the body, following proper administration of epidural anesthesia.

Clinically significant drug interactions: The administration of local anesthetic solutions containing epinephrine or norepinephrine to patients receiving monamine oxidase inhibitors or tricyclic antidepressants may produce severe, prolonged hypertension.

Phenothiazines and butyrophenones may reduce or reverse the pressor effect of epinephrine.

Concurrent use of these agents should generally be avoided. In situations when concurrent therapy is necessary, careful patient monitoring is essential.

Concurrent administration of vasopressor drugs (for the treatment of hypotension related to obstetric blocks) and ergot-type oxytocic drugs may cause severe persistent hypertension or cerebrovascular accidents.

Drug Laboratory test interactions: The intramuscular injection of lidocaine may result in an increase in creatine phosphokinase levels. Thus, the use of this enzyme determination without isoenzyme separation, as a diagnostic test for the presence of acute myocardial infarction may be compromised by the intramuscular injection of lidocaine.

Carcinogenesis, mutagenesis, impairment of fertility: Studies of lidocaine in animals to evaluate the carcinogenic and mutagenic potential or the effect on fertility have not been conducted.

Pregnancy: Teratogenic Effects. Pregnancy Category B. Reproduction studies have been performed in rats at doses up to 6.6 times the human dose and have revealed no evidence of harm to the fetus caused by lidocaine. There are, however, no adequate and well-controlled studies in pregnant women. Animal reproduction studies are not always predictive of human response. General consideration should be given to this fact before administering lidocaine to women of childbearing potential, especially during early pregnancy when maximum organogenesis takes place.

Labor and delivery: Local anesthetics rapidly cross the placenta and when used for epidural, paracervical, pudendal or caudal block anesthesia, can cause varying degrees of maternal, fetal and neonatal toxicity (See CLINICAL PHARMACOLOGY—Pharmacokinetics). The potential for toxicity depends upon the procedure performed, the type and amount of drug used, and the technique of drug administration. Adverse reactions in the parturient, fetus and neonate involve alterations of the central nervous system peripheral vascular tone and cardiac function.

Maternal hypotension has resulted from regional anesthesia. Local anesthetics produce vasodilation by blocking sympathetic nerves. Elevating the patient's legs and positioning her on her left side will help prevent decreases in blood pressure. The fetal heart rate also should be monitored continuously, and electronic fetal monitoring is highly advisable.

Epidural, spinal, paracervical, or pudendal anesthesia may alter the forces of parturition through changes in uterine contractility or maternal expulsive efforts. In one study paracervical block anesthesia was associated with a decrease in the mean duration of first stage labor and facilitation of cervical dilation. However, spinal and epidural anesthesia have also been reported to prolong the second stage of labor by removing the parturient's reflex urge to bear down or by interfering with motor function. The use of obstetrical anesthesia may increase the need for forceps assistance.

The use of some local anesthetic drug products during labor and delivery may be followed by diminished muscle strength and tone for the first day or two of life. The long term significance of these observations is unknown. Fetal bradycardia may occur in 20 to 30 percent of patients receiving paracervical nerve block anesthesia with the amide-type local anesthetics and may be associated with fetal acidosis. Fetal heart rate should always be monitored during paracervical anesthesia. The physician should weigh the possible advantages against risks when considering paracervical block in prematurity, toxemia of pregnancy, and fetal distress. Careful adherence to recommended dosage is of the utmost importance in obstetrical paracervical block. Failure to achieve adequate analgesia with recommended doses should arouse suspicion of intravascular or fetal intracranial injection. Cases compatible with unintended fetal intracranial injection of local anesthetic solution have been reported following intended paracervical or pudendal block or both. Babies so affected present with unexplained neonatal depression at birth, which correlates with high local anesthetic serum levels, and often manifest seizures within six hours. Prompt use of supportive measures combined with forced urinary excretion of the local anesthetic has been used successfully to manage this complication.

Case reports of maternal convulsions and cardiovascular collapse following use of some local anesthetics for paracervical block in early pregnancy (as anesthesia for elective abortion) suggest that systemic absorption under these circumstances may be rapid. The recommended maximum dose of each drug should not be exceeded. Injection should be made slowly and with frequent aspiration. Allow a 5-minute interval between sides.

Nursing mothers: It is not known whether this drug is excreted in human milk. Because many drugs are excreted in human milk, caution should be exercised when lidocaine is administered to a nursing woman.

Pediatric use: Dosages in children should be reduced, commensurate with age, body weight and physical condition. See DOSAGE AND ADMINISTRATION.

ADVERSE REACTIONS

Systemic: Adverse experiences following the administration of lidocaine are similar in nature to those observed with other amide local anesthetic agents. These adverse experiences are, in general, dose-related and may result from high plasma levels caused by excessive dosage, rapid absorption or inadvertent intravascular injection, or may result from a hypersensitivity, idiosyncrasy or diminished tolerance on the part of the patient. Serious adverse experiences are generally systemic in nature. The following types are those most commonly reported:

Central nervous system: CNS manifestations are excitatory and/or depressant and may be characterized by lightheadedness, nervousness, apprehension, euphoria, confusion, dizziness, drowsiness, tinnitus, blurred or double vision, vomiting, sensations of heat, cold or numbness, twitching, tremors, convulsions, unconsciusness, respiratory depression and arrest. The excitatory manifestations may be very brief or may not occur at all, in which case the first manifestation of toxicity may be drowsiness merging into unconsciousness and respiratory arrest.

Drowsiness following the administration of lidocaine is usually an early sign of a high blood level of the drug and may occur as a consequence of rapid absorption.

Cardiovascular system: Cardiovascular manifestations are usually depressant and are characterized by bradycardia, hypotension, and cardiovascular collapse, which may lead to cardiac arrest.

Allergic: Allergic reactions are characterized by cutaneous lesions, urticaria, edema or anaphylactoid reactions. Allergic reactions may occur as a result of sensitivity either to local anesthetic agents or to the methylparaben used as a preservative in multiple dose vials. Allergic reactions as a result of sensitivity to lidocaine are extremely rare and, if they occur, should be managed by conventional means. The detection of sensitivity by skin testing is of doubtful value.

Neurologic: The incidences of adverse reactions associated with the use of local anesthetics may be related to the total dose of local anesthetic administered and are also dependent upon the particular drug used, the route of administration and the physical status of the patient. In a prospective review of 10,440 patients who received lidocaine for spinal anesthesia, the incidences of adverse reactions were reported to be about 3 percent each for positional headaches, hypotension and backache; 2 percent for shivering; and less than 1 percent each for peripheral nerve symptoms, nausea, respiratory inadequacy and double vision. Many of these observations may be related to local anesthetic techniques, with or without a contribution from the local anesthetic.

In the practice of caudal or lumbar epidural block, occasional unintentional penetration of the subarachnoid space by the catheter may occur. Subsequent adverse effects may depend partially on the amount of drug administered subdurally. These may include spinal block of varying magnitude (including total spinal block), hypotension secondary to spinal block, loss of bladder and bowel control, and loss of perineal sensation and sexual function. Persistent motor, sensory and/or autonomic (sphincter control) deficit of some lower spinal segments with slow recovery (several months) or incomplete recovery have been reported in rare instances when caudal or lumbar epidural block has been attempted. Backache and headache have also been noted following use of these anesthetic procedures.

OVERDOSAGE

Acute emergencies from local anesthetics are generally related to high plasma levels encountered during therapeutic use of local anesthetics or to unintended subarachnoid injection of local anesthetic solution (see ADVERSE REACTIONS, WARNINGS and PRECAUTIONS).

Management of local anesthetic emergencies: The first consideration is prevention, best accomplished by careful and constant monitoring of cardiovascular and respiratory vital signs and the patient's state of consciousness after each local anesthetic injection. At the first sign of change, oxygen should be administered.

The first step in the management of convulsions, as well as underventilation or apnea due to unintended subarachnoid injection of drug solution, consists of immediate attention to the maintenance of a patent airway and assisted or controlled ventilation with oxygen and a delivery system capable of permitting immediate positive airway pressure by mask. Immediately after the institution of these ventilatory measures, the adequacy of the circulation should be evaluated, keeping in mind that drugs used to treat convulsions sometimes depress the circulation when administered intravenously. Should convulsions persist despite adequate repiratory support, and if the status of the circulation permits, small increments of an ultra-short acting barbiturate (such as thiopental or thiamylal) or a benzodiazepine (such as diazepam) may be administered intravenously. The clinician should be familiar, prior to use of local anesthetics, with these anticonvulsant drugs. Supportive treatment of circulatory depression may require administration of intravenous fluids and, when appropriate, a vasopressor as directed by the clinical situation (e.g. ephedrine).

If not treated immediately, both convulsions and cardiovascular depression can result in hypoxia, acidosis, bradycardia, arrhythmias and cardiac arrest. Underventilation or apenea due to unintentional subarachnoid injection of local anesthetic solution may produce these same signs and also lead to cardiac arrest if ventilatory support is not instituted. If cardiac arrest should occur standard cardiopulmonary resuscitative measures should be instituted.

Endotracheal intubation, employing drugs and techniques familiar to the clinician, may be indicated, after initial administration of oxygen by mask, if difficulty is encountered in the maintenance of a patent airway or if prolonged ventilatory support (assisted or controlled) is indicated.

Dialysis is of negligible value in the treatment of acute overdosage with lidocaine.

The oral LD_{50} of lidocaine HCl in non-fasted female rats is 459 (346–773) mg/kg (as the salt) and 214 (159–324) mg/kg (as the salt) in fasted female rats.

DOSAGE AND ADMINISTRATION

Table II (Recommended Dosages) summarizes the recommended volumes and concentrations of Xylocaine Solution for various types of anesthetic procedures. The dosages suggested in this table are for normal healthy adults and refer to the use of epinephrine-free solutions. When larger volumes are required only solutions containing epinephrine should be used, except in those cases where vasopressor drugs may be contraindicated.

These recommended doses serve only as a guide to the amount of anesthetic required for most routine procedures. The actual volumes and concentrations to be used depend on a number of factors such as type and extent of surgical procedure, depth of anesthesia and degree of muscular relaxation required, duration of anesthesia required, and the physical condition of the patient. In all cases the lowest concentration and smallest dose that will produce the desired result should be given. Dosages should be reduced for children and for elderly and debilitated patients and patients with cardiac and/or liver disease.

The onset of anesthesia, the duration of anesthesia and the degree of muscular relaxation are proportional to the volume and concentration (i.e. total dose) of local anesthetic used. Thus, an increase in volume and concentration of Xylocaine Solution will decrease the onset of anesthesia, prolong the duration of anesthesia, provide a greater degree of muscular relaxation and increase the segmental spread of anesthesia. However, increasing the volume and concentration of Xylocaine Solution may result in a more profound fall in blood pressure when used in epidural anesthesia. Although the incidence of side effects with lidocaine is quite low, caution should be exercised when employing large volumes and concentrations, since the incidence of side effects is directly proportional to the total dose of local anesthetic agent injected.

For intravenous regional anesthesia, only the 50 ml single dose vial containing Xylocaine (lidocaine HCl) 0.5% Solution should be used.

Epidural Anesthesia

For epidural anesthesia, only the following dosage forms of Xylocaine Solution are recommended:

1% without epinephrine .... 30 ml ampules
30 ml single dose vials
1% with epinephrine 1:200,000 .... 30 ml ampules
30 ml single dose vials
1.5% without epinephrine .... 20 ml ampules
20 ml single dose vials
1.5% with epinephrine 1:200,000 .... 30 ml ampules
30 ml single dose vials
2% without epinephrine .... 10 ml ampules
10 ml single dose vials
2% with epinephrine 1:200,000 .... 20 ml ampules
20 ml single dose vials

Although these solutions are intended specifically for epidural anesthesia, they may also be used for infiltration and peripheral nerve block, provided they are employed as single dose units. These solutions contain no bacteriostatic agent. In epidural anesthesia, the dosage varies with the number of dermatomes to be anesthetized (generally 2-3 ml of the indicated concentration per dermatome).

Caudal and lumbar epidural block: As a precaution against the adverse experiences sometimes observed following unintentional penetration of the subarachnoid space, a test dose of 2–5 ml should be administered at least 5 minutes prior to injecting the total volume required for a lumbar or caudal epidural block. The test dose should be repeated if the patient is moved in a manner that may have displaced the catheter. Epinephine, if contained in the test dose (10–15 µg have been suggested), may serve as a warning of unintentional intravascular injection. If injected into a blood vessel, this amount of epinephrine is likely to produce a transient "epinephrine response" within 45 seconds, consisting of an increase in heart rate and systolic blood pressure, circumoral pallor, palpitations and nervousness in the unsedated patient. The sedated patient may exhibit only a pulse rate increase of 20 or more beats per minutes for 15 or more seconds. Patients on beta-blockers may not manifest changes in heart rate, but blood pressure monitoring can detect an evanescent rise in systolic blood pressure. Adequate time should be allowed for onset of anesthesia after administration of each test dose. The rapid injection of a large volume of Xylocaine Solution through the catheter should be avoided, and, when feasible, fractional doses should be administered.

In the event of the known injection of a large volume of local anesthetic solution into the subarachnoid space, after suitable resuscitation and if the catheter is in place, consider attempting the recovery of drug by draining a moderate amount of cerebrospinal fluid (such as 10 ml) through the epidural catheter.

MAXIMUM RECOMMENDED DOSAGES

Adults: For normal healthy adults, the individual maximum dose of lidocaine HCl with epinephrine should not exceed 7 mg/kg (3.5 mg/lb) of body weight and in general it is recommended that the maximum total dose not exceed 500 mg. When used without epinephrine, the maximum individual dose should not exceed 4.5 mg/kg (2 mg per lb) of body weight, and in general it is recommended that the maximum total dose does not exceed 300 mg. For continuous epidural or caudal anesthesia, the maximum recommended dosage should not be administered at intervals of less than 90 minutes. When continuous lumbar or caudal epidural anesthesia is used for non-obstetrical procedures, more drug may be administered if required to produce adequate anesthesia.

The maximum recommended dose per 90 minute period of lidocaine hydrochloride for paracervical block in obstetrical patients and non-obstetrical patients is 200 mg total. One half of the total dose is usually administered to each side. Inject slowly five minutes between sides. (See also discussion of paracervical block in PRECAUTIONS).

For intravenous regional anesthesia, the dose administered should not exceed 4 mg/kg in adults.

Children: It is difficult to recommend a maximum dose of any drug for children, since this varies as a function of age and weight. For children over 3 years of age who have a normal lean body mass and normal body development, the maximum dose is determined by the child's age and weight. For example, in a child of 5 years weighing 50 lbs., the dose of lidocaine HCl should not exceed 75–100 mg (1.5–2 mg/lb). The use of even more dilute solutions (i.e., 0.25–0.5%) and total dosages not to exceed 3 mg/kg (1.4 mg/lb) are recommended for induction of intravenous regional anesthesia in children.

In order to guard against systemic toxicity, the lowest effective concentration and lowest effective dose should be used at all times. In some cases it will be necessary to dilute available concentrations with 0.9% sodium chloride injection in order to obtain the required final concentration.

NOTE: Parenteral drug products should be inspected visually for particulate matter and discoloration prior to administration whenever the solution and container permit. Solutions that are discolored and/or contain particulate matter should not be used.

TABLE II Recommended Dosages

PROCEDURE	Xylocaine (lidocaine hydrochloride) Solution (without epinephrine) Conc (%)	Vol (ml)	Total Dose (mg)
Infiltration			
Percutaneous	0.5 or 1.0	1–60	5–300
Intravenous regional	0.5	10–60	50–300
Peripheral Nerve Blocks, e.g.			
Brachial	1.5	15–20	225–300
Dental	2.0	1–5	20–100
Intercostal	1.0	3	30
Paravertebral	1.0	3–5	30–50
Pudendal (each side)	1.0	10	100
Paracervical			
Obstetrical analgesia (each side)	1.0	10	100
Sympathetic Nerve Blocks, e.g.			
Cervical (stellate ganglion)	1.0	5	50
Lumbar	1.0	5–10	50–100
Central Neural Blocks			
Epidural*			
Thoracic	1.0	20–30	200–300
Lumbar			
Analgesia	1.0	25–30	250–300
Anesthesia	1.5	15–20	225–300
	2.0	10–15	200–300
Caudal			
Obstetrical analgesia	1.0	20–30	200–300
Surgical anesthesia	1.5	15–20	225–300

* Dose determined by number of dermatomes to be anesthetized (2–3 ml/dermatome).

THE ABOVE SUGGESTED CONCENTRATIONS AND VOLUMES SERVE ONLY AS A GUIDE. OTHER VOLUMES AND CONCENTRATIONS MAY BE USED PROVIDED THE TOTAL MAXIMUM RECOMMENDED DOSE IS NOT EXCEEDED.

Sterilization, Storage and Technical Procedures: Disinfecting agents containing heavy metals, which cause release of respective ions (mercury, zinc, copper, etc.) should not be used for skin or mucous membrane disinfection as they have been related to incidents of swelling and edema. When chemical disinfection of multi-dose vials is desired, either isopropyl alcohol (91%) or ethyl alcohol (70%) is recommended. Many commercially available brands of rubbing alcohol as well as solutions of ethyl alcohol not of U.S.P. grade, contain denaturants which are injurious to rubber and therefore are not to be used.

HOW SUPPLIED

[See table above].

021850R04 Rev. 1/86(4)

HOW SUPPLIED

Xylocaine (lidocaine HCl) Concentration	/Epinephrine Dilution (if present)	Ampules (ml) 2	5	10	20	30	Single Dose Vials (ml) 2*	5	10	20	30	50	Multiple Dose Vials (ml) 10	20	50
0.5%							X	X	X			X	X		X
0.5%	/1:200,000														X
1%		X	X			X	X	X	X		X		X	X	X
1%	/1:100,000													X	X
1%	/1:200,000					X					X				
1.5%					X				X	X					
1.5%	/1:200,000					X					X				
2%		X		X			X	X	X				X	X	X
2%	/1:100,000													X	X
2%	/1:200,000				X					X					

All solutions should be stored at controlled room temperatures 15°–30°C (59°–86°F). * = 3 ml vial with 2 ml fill

XYLOCAINE® SOLUTION ℞

[*zī'lo-caine*]

(lidocaine hydrochloride)

FOR VENTRICULAR ARRHYTHMIAS

DESCRIPTION

Xylocaine (lidocaine hydrochloride) Solution is a sterile solution of an antiarrhythmic agent administered intravenously by either direct injection or continuous infusion, or intramuscularly by injection. The specific quantitative for each available solution appears in Table 1.

[See table 1 next page]

Xylocaine Solutions are composed of aqueous solutions of lidocaine hydrochloride. Lidocaine hydrochloride is chemically designated acetamide, 2-(diethylamino)-N-(2, 6 dimethylphenyl)-, monohydrochloride and is represented by the following structural formula:

CH_3; NH—CO—CH_2—N(C_2H_5)(C_2H_5) • HCl; CH_3

Continued on next page

Astra—Cont.

CLINICAL PHARMACOLOGY

Mechanism of action and electrophysiology:
Studies of the effects of therapeutic concentrations of lidocaine on the electrophysiological properties of mammalian Purkinje fibers have shown that lidocaine attenuates phase 4 diastolic depolarization, decreases automaticity, and causes a decrease or no change in excitability and membrane responsiveness. Action potential duration and effective refractory period of Purkinje fibers are decreased, while the ratio of effective refractory period to action potential duration is increased. Action potential duration and effective refractory period of ventricular muscle are also decreased. Effective refractory period of the AV node may increase, decrease or remain unchanged, and atrial effective refractory period is unchanged. Lidocaine raises the ventricular fibrillation threshold. No significant interactions between lidocaine and the autonomic nervous system have been described and consequently, lidocaine has little or no effect on autonomic tone.
Clinical electrophysiological studies with lidocaine have demonstrated no change in sinus node recovery time or sinoatrial conduction time. AV nodal conduction time is unchanged or shortened, and His-Purkinje conduction time is unchanged.

Hemodynamics:
At therapeutic doses, lidocaine has minimal hemodynamic effects in normal subjects and in patients with heart disease. Lidocaine has been shown to cause no, or minimal, decrease in ventricular contractility, cardiac output, arterial pressure or heart rate.

Pharmacokinetics and metabolism:
Lidocaine is rapidly metabolized by the liver, and less than 10% of a dose is excreted unchanged in the urine. Oxidative N-dealkylation, a major pathway of metabolism, results in the metabolites monoethylglycinexylidide and glycinexylidide. The pharmacological/toxicological activities of these metabolites are similar to, but less potent than, lidocaine. The primary metabolite in urine is a conjugate of 4-hydroxy-2,6-dimethylaniline.
The elimination half-life of lidocaine following an intravenous bolus injection is typically 1.5 to 2.0 hours. There are data that indicate that the half-life may be 3 hours or longer following infusions of greater than 24 hours.
Because of the rapid rate at which lidocaine is metabolized, any condition that alters liver function, including changes in liver blood flow, which could result from severe congestive heart failure or shock, may alter lidocaine kinetics. The half-life may be two-fold or more greater in patients with liver dysfunction. Renal dysfunction does not affect lidocaine kinetics, but may increase the accumulation of metabolites.
Therapeutic effects of lidocaine are generally associated with plasma levels of 6 to 25 μmole/L (1.5 to 6μg free base per ml). The blood to plasma distribution ratio is approximately 0.84. Objective adverse manifestations become increasingly apparent with increasing plasma levels above 6.0 μg free base per ml.
The plasma protein binding of lidocaine is dependent on drug concentration, and the fraction bound decreases with increasing concentration. At concentrations of 1 to 4 μg free base per ml, 60 to 80 percent of lidocaine is protein bound. In addition to lidocaine concentration, the binding is dependent on the plasma concentration of the α-1-acid glycoprotein.
Lidocaine readily crosses the placental and blood-brain barriers. Dialysis has negligible effects on the kinetics of lidocaine.
When an appropriate dose of Xylocaine Solution is administered intramuscularly into the deltoid muscle, effective antiarrhythmic blood levels are usually obtained within 5 to 15 minutes and usually persist for 60 to 90 minutes. Absorption from other intramuscular sites such as the vastus lateralis and gluteus maximus is slower, resulting in significantly lower blood levels during the first hour.

INDICATIONS AND USAGE

Xylocaine Solution, administered intravenously or intramuscularly, is specifically indicated in the acute management of ventricular arrhythmias such as those occurring in relation to acute myocardial infarction, or during cardiac manipulation, such as cardiac surgery.

CONTRAINDICATIONS

Xylocaine Solution is contraindicated in patients with a known history of hypersensitivity to local anesthetics of the amide type. Xylocaine Solution should not be used in patients with Stokes-Adams syndrome, Wolff-Parkinson-White syndrome, or with severe degrees of sinoatrial, atrioventricular, or intraventicular block in the absence of an artificial pacemaker.

WARNINGS

IN ORDER TO MANAGE POSSIBLE ADVERSE REACTIONS, RESUSCITATIVE EQUIPMENT, OXYGEN AND OTHER RESUSCITATIVE DRUGS SHOULD BE IMMEDIATELY AVAILABLE WHEN XYLOCAINE (LIDOCAINE HYDROCHLORIDE) SOLUTION IS USED.
Systemic toxicity may result in manifestations of central nervous sytem depression (sedation) or irritability (twitching), which may progress to frank convulsions accompanied by respiratory depression and/or arrest. Early recognition of premonitory signs, assurance of adequate oxygenation and, where necessary, establishment of artificial airway with ventilatory support are essential to management of this problem. Should convulsions persist despite ventilatory therapy with oxygen, *small* increments of anticonvulsant drugs may be used intravenously. Examples of such agents include benzodiazepines (e.g., diazepam), ultra short-acting barbiturates (e.g., thiopental or thiamylal), or a short-acting barbiturate (e.g., pentobarbital or secobarbital). If the patient is under anesthesia, a short-acting muscle relaxant (e.g., succinylcholine) may be used. Longer acting drugs should be used only when recurrent convulsions are evidenced.
Should circulatory depression occur, vasopressors may be used.
Constant electrocardiographic monitoring is essential to the proper administration of Xylocaine Solutions. Signs of excessive depression of cardiac electrical activity such as sinus node dysfunction, prolongation of the P-R interval and QRS complex or the appearance or aggravation of arrhythmias, should be followed by flow adjustment and, if necessary, prompt cessation of the intravenous infusion of this agent. Occasionally, acceleration of ventricular rate may occur when Xylocaine Solution is administered to patients with atrial flutter or fibrillation.

PRECAUTIONS

1. **General:** Caution should be employed in the use of Xylocaine Solution in patients with severe liver or kidney disease because accumulation of the drug or metabolites may occur.
   Xylocaine Solution should be used with caution in the treatment of patients with hypovolemia, severe congestive heart failure, shock, and all forms of heart block. In patients with sinus bradycardia or incomplete heart block, the administration of Xylocaine Solution intravenously for the elimination of ventricular ectopic beats, without prior acceleration in heart rate (e.g., by atropine, isoproterenol or electric pacing), may promote more frequent and serious ventricular arrhythmias or complete heart block (see CONTRAINDICATIONS).
   Dosage should be reduced for children and for debilitated and/or elderly patients, commensurate with their age and physical status.
   The safety of amide local anesthetic agents in patients with genetic predispositon to malignant hyperthermia has not been fully assessed; therefore, lidocaine should be used with caution in such patients.
   In hospital environments where drugs known to be triggering agents for malignant hyperthermia (fulminant hypermetabolism) are administered, it is suggested that a standard protocol for management should be available.
   It is not known whether lidocaine may trigger this reaction; however, large doses resulting in significant plasma concentrations, as may be achieved by intravenous infusion, pose potential risk to these individuals. Recognition of early unexplained signs of tachycardia, tachypnea, labile blood pressure and metabolic acidosis may precede temperature elevation. Successful outcome is dependent on early diagnosis, prompt discontinuance of the triggering agent and institution of treatment including oxygen therapy, supportive measures and dantrolene (for details see dantrolene package insert).
2. **Patient information:** The patient should be advised of the possible occurrence of the experiences listed under ADVERSE REACTIONS.
3. **Laboratory tests:** None known.
4. a. **Drug interactions:** Xylocaine Solutions should be used with caution in patients with digitalis toxicity accompanied by atrioventricular block. Concomitant use of beta-blocking agents or cimetidine may reduce hepatic blood flow and thereby reduce lidocaine clearance.
   b. **Drug/Laboratory test interactions:** The intramuscular use of Xylocaine Solution may result in an increase in creatine phosphokinase levels. Thus, the use of this enzyme determination, without isoenzyme separation, as a diagnostic test for the presence of acute myocardial infarction may be compromised by the use of intramuscular Xylocaine Solution.
5. **Carcinogenesis, mutagenesis, impairment of fertility:** Long term studies in animals to evaluate the carcinogenic and mutagenic potential or the effect on fertility of Xylocaine Solution have not been conducted.
6. **Pregnancy:**
   a. **Teratogenic effects:** Pregnancy Category B. Reproduction studies have been performed in rats at doses up to 6.6 times the maximum human doses and have revealed no significant findings. There are, however, no adequate and well-controlled studies in pregnant women. Because animal reproduction studies are not always predictive of human response, this drug should be used during pregnancy only if clearly needed.
7. **Labor and delivery:** The effects of Xylocaine Solution on the mother and the fetus, when used in the management of cardiac arrhythmias during labor and delivery, are not known. Lidocaine readily crosses the placental barrier.
8. **Nursing mothers:** It is not known whether this drug is excreted in human milk. Because many drugs are excreted in human milk, caution should be exercised when lidocaine is administered to a nursing woman.
9. **Pediatric use:** Safety and effectiveness in children have not been established by controlled clinical studies. (See DOSAGE AND ADMINISTRATION).

ADVERSE REACTIONS

Adverse experiences following the administration of lidocaine are similar in nature to those observed with other amide local anesthetic agents. Adverse experiences may result from high plasma levels caused by excessive dosage or may result from a hypersensitivity, idiosyncrasy or diminished tolerance on the part of the patient. Serious adverse experiences are generally systemic in nature. The following types are those most commonly reported. The adverse experiences under Central Nervous System and Cardiovascular System are listed, in general, in a progression from mild to severe.

1. **Central Nervous System:**
   CNS reactions are excitatory and/or depressant, and may be characterized by light-headedness, nervousness, apprehension, euphoria, confusion, dizziness, drowsiness, tinnitus, blurred or double vision, vomiting, sensations of heat, cold or numbness, twitching, tremors, convulsions, unconsciousness, respiratory depression and arrest. The excitatory reactions may be very brief or may not occur at all, in which case, the first manifestation of toxicity may be drowsiness, merging into unconsciousness and respiratory arrest.
2. **Cardiovascular System:**
   Cardiovascular reactions are usually depressant in nature and are characterized by bradycardia, hypotension, and cardiovascular collapse, which may lead to cardiac arrest.
3. Allergic reactions as a result of sensitivity to lidocaine are extremely rare and, if they occur, should be managed by conventional means.

DRUG ABUSE AND DEPENDENCE

Although specific studies have not been conducted, Xylocaine Solution has been used clinically without evidence of abuse of this drug or of psychological or physical dependence as a result of its use.

TABLE 1 Composition of available solutions:

Dosage Form		Composition* lidocaine hydrochloride (mg per ml)	sodium chloride (mg per ml)
For Direct Intravenous Injection	5 ml (100 mg) prefilled syringe	20	6
	5 ml (100 mg) ampule	20	6
For Preparation of Intravenous Infusion Solutions	25 ml (One Gram) single use vial	40	None
	50 ml (Two Grams) single use vial	40	None
	5 ml (One Gram) additive syringe	200	None
	10 ml (Two Grams) additive syringe	200	None
For Intramuscular Injection	5 ml (500 mg) ampule	100	None

*pH of all solutions adjusted to 5.0-7.0 with sodium hydroxide and/or hydrochloric acid.
All containers are for single use: solutions do not contain preservatives.

OVERDOSAGE

Overdosage of Xylocaine (lidocaine hydrochloride) Solution usually results in signs of central nervous system or cardiovascular toxicity. See ADVERSE REACTIONS.

Should convulsions or signs of respiratory depression and arrest develop, the patency of the airway and adequacy of ventilation must be assured immediately. Should convulsions persist despite ventilatory therapy with oxygen, small increments of anticonvulsive agents may be given intravenously. Examples of such agents include a benzodiazepine (e.g., diazepam), an ultrashort-acting barbiturate (e.g., thiopental or thiamylal), or a short-acting barbiturate (e.g., pentobarbital or secobarbital). If the patient is under general anesthesia, a short-acting muscle relaxant (e.g., succinylcholine) may be administered.

Should circulatory depression occur, vasopressors may be used. Should cardiac arrest occur, standard CPR procedures should be instituted.

Dialysis is of negligible value in the treatment of acute overdosage from Xylocaine Solution.

DOSAGE AND ADMINISTRATION

Adults

Single Direct Intravenous Injection (bolus):

ONLY THE 5 ML, 100 MG DOSAGE SIZE (20 MG/ML) should be used for direct intravenous injection. The usual dose is 50 to 100 mg of lidocaine hydrochloride (0.70 to 1.4 mg/kg: 0.32 to 0.63 mg/lb) administered intravenously under ECG monitoring. This dose may be administered at the rate of approximately 25 to 50 mg/min (0.35 to 0.70 mg/kg/min; 0.16 to 0.32 mg/lb/min). Sufficient time should be allowed to enable a slow circulation to carry the drug to the site of action. If the initial injection of 50 to 100 mg does not produce a desired response, a second dose may be injected after 5 minutes. The syringe should be activated immediately prior to the injection. (See illustrated instructions for use on produce package.) NO MORE THAN 200 TO 300 MG OF LIDOCAINE HYDROCHLORIDE SHOULD BE ADMINISTERED DURING A ONE HOUR PERIOD.

Continuous Intravenous Infusion:

Following bolus administration, intravenous infusions of Xylocaine Solution may be initiated at the rate of 1 to 4 mg/min of lidocaine hydrochloride (0.014 to 0.057 mg/kg/min; 0.006 to 0.026 mg/lb/min). The rate of intravenous infusions should be reassessed as soon as the patient's basic cardiac rhythm appears to be stable or at the earliest signs of toxicity. It should rarely be necessary to continue intravenous infusions of lidocaine for prolonged periods.

Solutions for intravenous infusion may be prepared by the addition of one gram (or two grams) of lidocaine hydrochloride to one liter of 5% dextrose in water using aseptic technique. Approximately a 0.1% (or 0.2%) solution will result from this procedure; that is, each milliliter will contain approximately 1 (or 2 mg) of lidocaine hydrochloride. In those cases in which fluid restriction is medically appropriate, a more concentrated solution may be prepared.

Xylocaine Solution has been found to be chemically stable for 24 hours after dilution in 5% dextrose in water. However, as with all intravenous admixtures, dilution of the solution should be made just prior to its administration.

Parenteral drug products should be inspected visually for particulate matter and discoloration prior to administration whenever the solution and container permit.

Intramuscular Injection:

The recommended dose of lidocaine hydrochloride by the intramuscular route is 300 mg (approximately 4.3 mg/kg or 2.0 mg/lb). The deltoid muscle is recommended as the preferred site of injection, since therapeutic blood levels of lidocaine occur faster and the peak blood level is significantly higher following deltoid administration as compared to injections into the lateral thigh or gluteus. Injections should be made with frequent aspiration to avoid possible inadvertent intravascular injection.

As soon as possible, and when indicated, patients should be changed to an intravenous infusion of Xylocaine Solution. However, if necessary, an additional intramuscular injection may be made after an interval of 60-90 minutes.

Pediatric

Although controlled clinical studies to establish pediatric dosing schedules have not been conducted, the American Heart Association's *Standards and Guidelines* recommends a bolus dose of 1 mg/kg followed by an infusion rate of 30 µg/kg/min.

Note regarding prolonged infusions: There are data that indicate the half-life may be 3 hours or longer following infusions of greater than 24 hours in duration.

HOW SUPPLIED

For direct intravenous injection, Xylocaine (lidocaine hydrochloride) Solution without preservatives is supplied in 5 ml, 100 mg ampules (20 mg/ml) and in 5 ml, 100 mg prefilled syringes.

For intramuscular injection, Xylocaine Solution without preservatives is supplied in 5 ml, 500 mg ampules (100 mg/ml).

For preparing solutions for intravenous infusions, Xylocaine Solution without sodium chloride or preservatives is supplied in one and two gram additive syringes and in one and two gram single use vials. Vials are available with or without pre-sterilized transfer unit manufactured by the West Company.

Solutions should be stored at controlled room temperature 15°–30°C (59°–86°F).

021834R01 Rev. 6/84

XYLOCAINE® (lidocaine hydrochloride) ℞
[*zī'lo-caine*]
4% STERILE SOLUTION
For transtracheal use, retrobulbar injection, and for topical application

DESCRIPTION

Xylocaine (lidocaine HCl) 4% Sterile Solution contains a local anesthetic agent and is administered topically or by injection. See INDICATIONS for specific uses.

Xylocaine 4% Sterile Solution contains lidocaine HCl, which is chemically designated as acetamide, 2-(diethylamino)-N-(2,6-dimethylphenyl)-monohydrochloride.

Xylocaine 4% Sterile Solution in 5 ml ampules may be autoclaved repeatedly if necessary.

Composition of Xylocaine 4% Sterile Solution

Each ml contains lidocaine HCl, 40.0 mg, and sodium hydroxide and/or hydrochloric acid to adjust pH to 5.0–7.0. A sterile, aqueous solution.

CLINICAL PHARMACOLOGY

Mechanism of action: Lidocaine stabilizes the neuronal membrane by inhibiting the ionic fluxes required for the initiation and conduction of impulses, thereby effecting local anesthetic action.

Onset and duration of anesthesia: The onset of action is rapid. For retrobulbar injection, 4 ml of Xylocaine 4% Sterile Solution provides an average duration of action of 1 to 1 1/2 hours. This duration may be extended for ophthalmic surgery by the addition of epinephrine, the usual recommended dilution being 1:50,000 to 1:100,000.

Hemodynamics: Excessive blood levels may cause changes in cardiac output, total peripheral resistance, and mean arterial pressure. These changes may be attributable to a direct depressant effect of the local anesthetic agent on various components of the cardiovascular system. The net effect is normally a modest hypotension when the recommended dosages are not exceeded.

Pharmacokinetics and metabolism: Information derived from other formulations, concentrations and usages reveals that lidocaine is completely absorbed following parenteral administration, its rate of absorption depending, for example, upon such factors such as the site of administration and the presence or absence of a vasoconstrictor agent. Lidocaine may be absorbed following topical administration to mucous membranes, its rate and extent of absorption depending upon concentration and total dose administered, the specific site of application and duration of exposure. In general, the rate of absorption of local anesthetic agents following topical application occurs most rapidly after intratracheal administration. Lidocaine is also well absorbed from the gastrointestinal tract, but little intact drug appears in the circulation because of biotransformation by the liver.

Lidocaine is metabolized rapidly by the liver, and metabolites and unchanged drug are excreted by the kidneys. Biotransformation includes oxidative N-dealkylation, ring hydroxylation, cleavage of the amide linkage, and conjugation. N-dealkylation, a major pathway of biotransformation, yields the metabolites monoethylglycinexylidide and glycinexylidide. The pharmacological/toxicological actions of these metabolites are similar to, but less potent than, those of lidocaine. Approximately 90% of lidocaine administered is excreted in the form of various metabolites, and less than 10% is excreted unchanged. The primary metabolite in urine is a conjugate of 4-hydroxy-2,6-dimethylaniline.

Studies have shown that peak blood levels of lidocaine may occur as early as 5 and as late as 30 minutes after endotracheal administration of a 4% lidocaine HCl solution.

The plasma binding of lidocaine is dependent on drug concentration, and the fraction bound decreases with increasing concentration. At concentrations of 1 to 4 µg of free base per ml, 60 to 80 percent of lidocaine is protein bound. Binding is also dependent on the plasma concentration of the alpha-1-acid glycoprotein.

Lidocaine crosses the blood-brain and placental barriers, presumably by passive diffusion.

Studies of lidocaine metabolism following intravenous bolus injections have shown that the elimination half-life of this agent is typically 1.5 to 2.0 hours. Because of the rapid rate at which lidocaine is metabolized, any condition that affects liver function may alter lidocaine kinetics. The half-life may be prolonged two-fold or more in patients with liver dysfunction. Renal dysfunction does not affect lidocaine kinetics but may increase the accumulation of metabolites.

Factors such as acidosis and the use of CNS stimulants and depressants affect the CNS levels of lidocaine required to produce overt systemic effects. Objective adverse manifestations become increasingly apparent with increasing venous plasma levels above 6.0 µg free base per ml. In the rhesus monkey arterial blood levels of 18–21 µg/ml have been shown to be threshold for convulsive activity.

INDICATIONS AND USAGE

Xylocaine (lidocaine HCl) 4% Sterile Solution is indicated for the production of topical anesthesia of the mucous membranes of the respiratory tract or the genito-urinary tract. It may be injected trans-tracheally to anesthetize the larynx and trachea, and it may be administered by retrobulbar injection to provide anesthesia for ophthalmic surgery.

CONTRAINDICATIONS

Lidocaine is contraindicated in patients with a known history of hypersensitivity to local anesthetics of the amide type.

WARNINGS

XYLOCAINE 4% STERILE SOLUTION SHOULD BE EMPLOYED ONLY BY CLINICIANS WHO ARE WELL VERSED IN DIAGNOSIS AND MANAGEMENT OF DOSE-RELATED TOXICITY AND OTHER ACUTE EMERGENCIES THAT MIGHT ARISE AND THEN ONLY AFTER ENSURING THE *IMMEDIATE* AVAILABILITY OF OXYGEN, OTHER RESUSCITATIVE DRUGS, CARDIOPULMONARY EQUIPMENT, AND THE PERSONNEL NEEDED FOR PROPER MANAGEMENT OF TOXIC REACTIONS AND RELATED EMERGENCIES (See also ADVERSE REACTIONS and PRECAUTIONS.) DELAY IN PROPER MANAGEMENT OF DOSE-RELATED TOXICITY, UNDERVENTILATION FROM ANY CAUSE AND /OR ALTERED SENSITIVITY MAY LEAD TO THE DEVELOPMENT OF ACIDOSIS, CARDIAC ARREST AND, POSSIBLY, DEATH.

To avoid intravascular injection, aspiration should be performed before the local anesthetic solution is injected. The needle must be repositioned until no return of blood can be elicited by aspiration. Note, however, that the absence of blood in the syringe does not guarantee that intravascular injection has been avoided.

Xylocaine 4% Sterile Solution should be used with extreme caution if there is sepsis or severely traumatized mucosa in the area of application, since under such conditions there is the potential for rapid systemic absorption.

PRECAUTIONS

General: The safety and effectiveness of lidocaine depend on proper dosage, correct technique, adequate precautions, and readiness for emergencies. Resuscitative equipment, oxygen and other resuscitative drugs should be available for immediate use. (See WARNINGS and ADVERSE REACTIONS.) The lowest dosage that results in effective anesthesia should be used to avoid high plasma levels and serious adverse effects. Repeated doses of lidocaine may cause significant increases in blood levels with each repeated dose, because of slow accumulation of the drug or its metabolites. Tolerance to elevated blood levels varies with the status of the patient. Debilitated, elderly patients, acutely ill patients, and children should be given reduced doses commensurate with their age and physical status. Lidocaine should also be used with caution in patients with severe shock or heart block.

Local anesthetic solutions containing a vasoconstrictor should be used cautiously and in carefully circumscribed quantities in areas of the body supplied by end arteries or having otherwise compromised blood supply. Patients with peripheral vascular disease and those with hypertensive vascular disease may exhibit exaggerated vasoconstrictor response. Ischemic injury or necrosis may result. Preparations containing a vasoconstrictor should be used with caution in patients during or following the administration of potent general anesthetic agents, since cardiac arrhythmias may occur under such conditions.

Careful and constant monitoring of cardiovascular and respiratory (adequacy of ventilation) vital signs and the patient's state of consciousness should be accomplished after each local anesthetic injection. It should be kept in mind at such times that restlessness, anxiety, tinnitus, dizziness, blurred vision, tremors, depression or drowsiness may be early warning signs of central nervous system toxicity.

Since amide-type local anesthetics are metabolized by the liver, Xylocaine 4% Sterile Solution should be used with caution in patients with hepatic disease.

Patients with severe hepatic disease, because of their inability to metabolize local anesthetic normally, are a greater risk of developing toxic plasma concentrations. Xylocaine 4% Sterile Solution should also be used with caution in patients with impaired cardiovascular function since they may be less able to compensate for functional changes associated with the prolongation of A-V conduction produced by these drugs.

Use in Ophthalmic Surgery: When local anesthetic solutions are employed for retrobulbar block, lack of corneal

Continued on next page

Astra—Cont.

sensation should not be relied upon to determine whether or not the patient is ready for surgery since corneal sensation usually precedes clinically acceptable external ocular muscle akinesia.
Many drugs used during the conduct of anesthesia are considered potential triggering agents for familial malignant hyperthermia. Since it is not known whether amide-type local anesthetics may trigger this reaction and since the need for supplemental general anesthesia cannot be predicted in advance, it is suggested that a standard protocol for management should be available. Early unexplained signs of tachycardia, tachypnea, labile blood pressure and metabolic acidosis may precede temperature elevation. Successful outcome is dependent on early diagnosis, prompt discontinuance of the suspect triggering agent(s) and institution of treatment, including oxygen theray, indicated supportive measures and dantrolene (consult dantrolene sodium intravenous package insert before using).
Lidocaine should be used with caution in persons with known drug sensitivities. Patients allergic to para-aminobenzoic acid derivatives (procaine, tetracaine, benzocaine, etc.) have not shown cross sensitivity to lidocaine.
Use in the Head and Neck Area: Small doses of local anesthetics injected into the head and neck area, including retrobulbar, dental and stellate ganglion blocks, may produce adverse reactions similar to systemic toxicity seen with unintentional intravascular injections of larger doses. Confusion, convulsions, respiratory depression and/or respiratory arrest, and cardiovascular stimulation or depression have been reported. These reactions may be due to intra-arterial injection of the local anesthetic with retrograde flow to the cerebral circulation. Patients receiving these blocks should have their circulation and respiration monitored and be constantly observed. Resuscitative equipment and personnel for treating adverse reactions should be immediately available. Dosage recommendations should not be exceeded. (See DOSAGE AND ADMINISTRATION.)
Information for Patients: When topical anesthetics are used in the mouth, the patient should be aware that the production of topical anesthesia may impair swallowing and thus enhance the danger of aspiration. For this reason, food should not be ingested for 60 minutes following use of local anesthetic preparations in the mouth or throat area. This is particularly important in children because of their frequency of eating.
Numbness of the tongue or buccal mucosa may enhance the danger of unintentional biting trauma. Food and chewing gum should not be taken while the mouth or throat area is anesthetized.
Clinically significant drug interactions: The administration of local anesthetic solutions containing epinephrine or norepinephrine to patients receiving monoamine oxidase inhibitors, tricyclic antidepressants or phenothiazines may produce severe, prolonged hypotension or hypertension. Concurrent use of these agents should generally be avoided. In situations when concurrent therapy is necessary, careful patient monitoring is essential.
Drug/Laboratory test interactions: The intramuscular injection of lidocaine may result in an increase in creatine phosphokinase levels. Thus, the use of this enzyme determination, without isoenzyme separation, as a diagnostic test for the presence of acute myocardiac infarction may be compromised by the intramuscular injection of lidocaine.
Carcinogenesis, mutagenesis, impairment of fertility: Studies of lidocaine in animals to evaluate the carcinogenic and mutagenic potential or the effect on fertility have not been conducted.
Use in Pregnancy: Teratogenic Effects. Pregnancy Category B. Reproduction studies have been performed in rats at doses up to 6.6 times the human dose and have revealed no evidence of harm to the fetus caused by lidocaine. There are, however, no adequate and well-controlled studied in pregnant women. Animal reproduction studies are not always predictive of human response. General consideration should be given to this fact before administering lidocaine to women of childbearing potential, especially during early pregnancy when maximum organogenesis takes place.
Labor and delivery: Lidocaine is not contraindicated in labor and delivery. Should Xylocaine 4% Sterile Solution be used concomitantly with other products containing lidocaine, the total dose contributed by all formulations must be kept in mind.
Nursing mothers: It is not known whether this drug is excreted in human milk. Because many drugs are excreted in human milk, caution should be exercised when lidocaine is administered to a nursing woman.
Pediatric use: Dosages in children should be reduced, commensurate with age and body weight. See DOSAGE AND ADMINISTRATION.

ADVERSE REACTIONS

Adverse experiences following the administration of lidocaine are similar in nature to those observed with other amide local anesthetic agents. These adverse experiences are, in general, dose-related and may result from high plasma levels caused by excessive dosage, rapid absorption or inadvertent intravascular injection, or may result from a hypersensitivity, idiosyncrasy or diminished tolerance on the part of the patient. Serious adverse experiences are generally systemic in nature. The following types are those most commonly reported:
Central nervous system: CNS manifestations are excitatory and/or depressant and may be characterized by lightheadedness, nervousness, apprehension, euphoria, confusion, dizziness, drowsiness, tinnitus, blurred or double vision, vomiting, sensations of heat, cold or numbness, twitching, tremors, convulsions, unconsciousness, respiratory depression and arrest. The excitatory manifestations may be very brief or may not ocur at all, in which case the first manifestation of toxicity may be drowsiness merging into unconsciousness and respiratory arrest.
Drowsiness following the administration of lidocaine is usually an early sign of a high blood level of the drug and may occur as a consequence of rapid absorption.
Cardiovascular system: Cardiovascular manifestations are usually depressant and are characterized by bradycardia, hypotension, and cardiovascular collapse, which may lead to cardiac arrest.
Allergic: Allergic reactions are characterized by cutaneous lesions, urticaria, edema or anaphylactoid reactions. Allergic reactions as a result of sensitivity to lidocaine are extremely rare and, if they occur, should be managed by conventional means. The detection of sensitivity by skin testing is of doubtful value.
Neurologic: The incidences of adverse reactions associated with the use of local anesthetics may be related to the total dose of local anesthetic administered and are also dependent upon the particular drug used, the route of administration and the physical status of the patient.

OVERDOSAGE

Acute emergencies from local anesthetics are generally related to high plasma levels encountered during therapeutic use of local anesthetics or to unintended subarachnoid injection of local anesthetic solution (see ADVERSE REACTIONS, WARNINGS, and PRECAUTIONS).
Management of local anesthetic emergencies: The first consideration is prevention, best accomplished by careful and constant monitoring of cardiovascular and respiratory vital signs and the patient's state of consciousness after each local anesthetic injection. At the first sign of change, oxygen should be administered.
The first step in the management of convulsions consists of immediate attention to the maintenance of a patent airway and assisted or controlled ventilation with oxygen and a delivery system capable of permitting immediate positive airway pressure by mask. Immediately after the institution of these ventilatory measures, the adequacy of the circulation should be evaluated, keeping in mind that drugs used to treat convulsions sometimes depress the circulation when administered intravenously. Should convulsions persist despite adequate respiratory support, and if the status of the circulation permits, small increments of an ultra-short acting barbiturate (such as thiopental or thiamylal) or a benzodiazepine (such as diazepam) may be administered intravenously. The clinician should be familiar, prior to use of local anesthetics, with these anticonvulsant drugs. Supportive treatment of circulatory depression may require administration of intravenous fluids and, when appropriate, a vasopressor as directed by the clinical situation (e.g., ephedrine).
If not treated immediately, both convulsions and cardiovascular depression can result in hypoxia, acidosis, bradycardia, arrhythmias and cardiac arrest. If cardiac arrest should occur, standard cardiopulmonary resuscitative measures should be instituted.
Endotracheal intubation, employing drugs and techniques familiar to the clinician, may be indicated, after initial administration of oxygen by mask, if difficulty is encountered in the maintenance of a patent airway or if prolonged ventilatory support (assisted or controlled) is indicated.
Dialysis is of negligible value in the treatment of acute overdosage with lidocaine.
The intravenous LD_{50} of lidocaine HCl in female mice is 26 (21–31) mg/kg and the subcutaneous LD_{50} is 264 (203–304) mg/kg.

DOSAGE AND ADMINISTRATION

When Xylocaine 4% Sterile Solution is used concomitantly with other products containing lidocaine, the total dose contributed by all formulations must be kept in mind.
The dosage varies and depends upon the area to be anesthetized, vascularity of the tissues, individual tolerance and the technique of anesthesia. The lowest dosage needed to provide effective anesthesia should be administered. Dosages should be reduced for children and for elderly and debilitated patients.
Although the incidence of adverse effects with Xylocaine 4% Sterile Solution is quite low, caution should be exercised, particularly when employing large volumes and concentrations of Xylocaine 4% Sterile Solution since the incidence of adverse effects is directly proportional to the total dose of local anesthetic agent administered. For specific techniques and procedures refer to standard textbooks.
The dosages below are for normal, healthy adults.
RETROBULBAR INJECTION: The suggested dose for a 70 kg person is 3–5 ml (120–200 mg of lidocaine HCl), i.e., 1.7–3 mg/kg or 0.9–1.5 mg/lb body weight. A portion of this is injected retrobulbarly and the rest may be used to block the facial nerve.
TRANSTRACHEAL INJECTION: For local anesthesia by the transtracheal route 2–3 ml should be injected through a large enough needle so that the injection can be made rapidly. By injecting during inspiration some of the drug will be carried into the bronchi and the resulting cough will distribute the rest of the drug over the vocal cords and the epiglottis.
Occasionally it may be necessary to spray the pharynx by oropharyngeal spray to achieve complete analgesia. For the combination of the injection and spray, it should rarely be necessary to utilize more than 5 ml (200 mg of lidocaine HCl), i.e., 3 mg/kg or 1.5 mg/lb body weight.
TOPICAL APPLICATION: For laryngoscopy, bronchoscopy and endotracheal intubation, the pharynx may be sprayed with 1–5 ml (40–200 mg of lidocaine HCl), i.e., 0.6–3 mg/kg or 0.3–1.5 mg/lb body weight.

MAXIMUM RECOMMENDED DOSAGES

Normal Healthy Adults: The maximum recommended dose of Xylocaine 4% Sterile Solution should be such that the dose of lidocaine HCl is kept below 300 mg and in any case should not exceed 4.5 mg/kg (2 mg/lb) body weight.
Children:
It is difficult to recommend a maximum dose of any drug for children since this varies as a function of age and weight. For children of less than ten years who have a normal lean body mass and normal body development, the maximum dose may be determined by the application of one of the standard pediatric drug formulas (e.g. Clark's rule). For example, in a child of five years weighing 50 lbs., the dose of lidocaine hydrochloride should not exceed 75–100 mg when calculated according to Clark's rule. In any case, the maximum dose of Xylocaine Solution with epinephrine should not exceed 7 mg/kg (3.2 mg/lb.) of body weight. When used without epinephrine, the amount of Xylocaine Solution administered should be such that the dose of lidocaine is kept below 300 mg and in any case should not exceed 4.5 mg/kg (2.0 mg/lb) of body weight.
NOTE: Parenteral drug products should be inspected visually for particulate matter and discoloration prior to administration whenever the solution and container permit. Solutions that are discolored and/or contain particulate matter should not be used.

HOW SUPPLIED

Xylocaine (lidocaine HCl) 4% Sterile Solution, 5 ml ampule (NDC 0186-0235-03) and 5 ml prefilled sterile disposable syringe packaged in a presterilized kit containing a laryngotracheal cannula (NDC 0186-0235-72).
Store at controlled room temperature: 15°C–30°C (59°–86°F).
021562R04 7/84

XYLOCAINE® (lidocaine hydrochloride) ℞

[zī'lo-caine]
4% TOPICAL SOLUTION
For topical application

DESCRIPTION

Xylocaine (lidocaine HCl) 4% Topical Solution contains a local anesthetic agent and is administered topically. See INDICATIONS for specific uses.
Xylocaine 4% Topical Solution contains lidocaine HCL, which is chemically designated as acetamide, 2-(diethylamino)-N-(2,6-dimethylphenyl)-, monohydrochloride.
The 50ml screw-cap bottle should not be autoclaved, because the closure employed cannot withstand autoclaving temperatures and pressures. Composition of Xylocaine (lidocaine HCl) 4% Topical Solution: Each ml contains lidocaine HCl, 40mg, methylparaben, and sodium hydroxide and/or hydrochloric acid to adjust pH to 6.0–7.0.
An aqueous solution. NOT FOR INJECTION

CLINICAL PHARMACOLOGY

Mechanism of action: Lidocaine stabilizes the neuronal membrane by inhibiting the ionic fluxes required for the initiation and conduction of impulses, thereby effecting local anesthetic action.
Hemodynamics: Excessive blood levels may cause changes in cardiac output, total peripheral resistance, and mean arterial pressure. These changes may be attributable to a direct depressant effect of the local anesthetic agent on various components of the cardiovascular system.
Pharmacokinetics and metabolism: Lidocaine may be absorbed following topical administration to mucuous membranes, its rate of absorption and percent of dose absorbed depending upon concentration and total dose administered, the specific site of application and duration of exposure. In

general, the rate of absorption of local anesthetic agents following topical application occurs most rapidly after intratracheal administration. Lidocaine is well-absorbed from the gastrointestinal tract, but little intact drug appears in the circulation because of biotransformation in the liver.
Lidocaine is metabolized rapidly by the liver, and metabolites and unchanged drug are excreted by the kidney. Biotransformation includes oxidative N-dealkylation, ring hydroxylation, cleavage of the amide linkage, and conjugation. N-dealkylation, a major pathway of biotransformation, yields the metabolites monoethylglycinexylidide and glycinexylidide. The pharmacological/toxicological actions of these metabolites are similar to, but less potent than, those of lidocaine. Approximately 90% of lidocaine administered is excreted in the form of various metabolites, and less than 10% is excreted unchanged. The primary metabolite in urine is a conjugate of 4-hydroxy-2, 6-dimethylaniline.
The plasma binding of lidocaine is dependent on drug concentration, and the fraction bound decreases with increasing concentration. At concentrations of 1 to 4 μg of free base per ml, 60 to 80 percent of lidocaine is protein bound. Binding is also dependent on the plasma concentration of the alpha-1-acid glycoprotein.
Lidocaine crosses the blood-brain and placental barriers, presumably by passive diffusion.
Studies of lidocaine metabolism following intravenous bolus injections have shown that the elimination half-life of this agent is typically 1.5 to 2.0 hours. Because of the rapid rate at which lidocaine is metabolized, any condition that affects liver function may alter lidocaine kinetics. The half-life may be prolonged two-fold or more in patients with liver dysfunction. Renal dysfunction does not affect lidocaine kinetics but may increase the accumulation of metabolites.
Factors such as acidosis and the use of CNS stimulants and depressants affect the CNS levels of lidocaine required to produce overt systemic effects. Objective adverse manifestations become increasingly apparent with increasing venous plasma levels above 6.0 μg free base per ml. In the rhesus monkey arterial blood levels of 18-21 μg/ml have been shown to be threshold for convulsive activity.

INDICATIONS AND USAGE

Xylocaine (lidocaine HCl) 4% Topical Solution is indicated for the production of topical anesthesia of accessible mucous membranes of the oral and nasal cavities and proximal portions of the digestive tract.

CONTRAINDICATIONS

Lidocaine is contraindicated in patients with a known history of hypersensitivity to local anesthetics of the amide type or to other components of Xylocaine 4% Topical Solution.

WARNINGS

IN ORDER TO MANAGE POSSIBLE ADVERSE REACTIONS, RESUSCITATIVE EQUIPMENT, OXYGEN AND OTHER RESUSCITATIVE DRUGS MUST BE IMMEDIATELY AVAILABLE WHEN LOCAL ANESTHETIC AGENTS, SUCH AS LIDOCAINE, ARE ADMINISTERED TO MUCUOUS MEMBRANES.
Xylocaine 4% Topical Solution should be used with extreme caution if there is sepsis or severely traumatized mucosa in the area of application, since under such conditions there is the potential for rapid systemic absorption.

PRECAUTIONS

General: The safety and effectiveness of lidocaine depend on proper dosage, correct technique, adequate precautions, and readiness for emergencies. Resuscitative equipment, oxygen, and other resuscitative drugs should be available for immediate use. (See WARNINGS and ADVERSE REACTIONS). The lowest dosage that results in effective anesthesia should be used to avoid high plasma levels and serious adverse effects. Repeated doses of lidocaine may cause significant increases in blood levels with each repeated dose because of slow accumulation of the drug or its metabolites. Tolerance to elevated blood levels varies with the status of the patient. Debilitated, elderly patients, acutely ill patients, and children should be given reduced doses commensurate with their age and physical status. Lidocaine should also be used with caution in patients with severe shock or heart block.
Xylocaine 4% Topical Solution should be used with caution in patients with known drug sensitivities. Patients allergic to para-aminobenzoic acid derivatives (procaine, tetracaine, benzocaine, etc.) have not shown cross sensitivity to lidocaine.
Although it has been shown that the rate of absorption of lidocaine after spraying the laryngo-tracheal mucosa with a solution of the local anesthetic agent is normally relatively slow, there is the attendant risk that occasionally some of the solution may gravitate into the lower respiratory tract where surface area for absorption and tissue blood flow are markedly greater. This can result in unexpectedly rapid and high blood levels, and this possibility must be kept in mind whenever Xylocaine 4% Topical Solution is administered.
Many drugs used during the conduct of anesthesia are considered potential triggering agents for familial malignant hyperthermia. Since it is not known whether amide-type local anesthetics may trigger this reaction and since the need for supplemental general anesthesia cannot be predicted in advance, it is suggested that a standard protocol for management should be available. Early unexplained signs of tachycardia, tachypnea, labile blood pressure and metabolic acidosis may precede temperature elevation. Successful outcome is dependent on early diagnosis, prompt discontinuance of the suspect triggering agent(s) and institution of treatment, including oxygen therapy, indicated supportive measures and dantrolene (consult dantrolene sodium intravenous package insert before using).
Information for Patients: When topical anesthetics are used in the mouth, the patient should be aware that the production of topical anesthesia may impair swallowing and thus enhance the danger of aspiration. For this reason, food should not be ingested for 60 minutes following use of local anesthetic preparations in the mouth or throat area. This is particularly important in children because of their frequency of eating.
Numbness of the tongue or buccal mucosa may enhance the danger of unintentional biting trauma. Food and chewing gum should not be taken while the mouth or throat area is anesthetized.
Carcinogenesis, mutagenesis, impairment of fertility: Studies of lidocaine in animals to evaluate the carcinogenic and mutagenic potential or the effect on fertility have not been conducted.
Use in Pregnancy: Pregnancy Category B. Reproduction studies have been performed in rats at doses up to 6.6 times the human dose and have revealed no evidence of harm to the fetus caused by lidocaine. There are, however, no adequate and well-controlled studies in pregnant women. Animal reproduction studies are not always predictive of human response. General consideration should be given to this fact before administering lidocaine to women of childbearing potential, especially during early pregnancy when maximum organogenesis takes place.
Labor and Delivery: Lidocaine is not contraindicated in labor and delivery. Should Xylocaine 4% Topical Solution be used concomitantly with other products containing lidocaine, the total dose being administered must be kept in mind.
Nursing mothers: It is not known whether this drug is excreted in human milk. Because many drugs are excreted in human milk, caution should be exercised when lidocaine is administered to a nursing woman.
Pediatric use: Dosages in children should be reduced, commensurate with age, body weight and physical condition. See DOSAGE AND ADMINISTRATION.

ADVERSE REACTIONS

Adverse experiences following the administration of lidocaine are similar in nature to those observed with other amide local anesthetic agents. These adverse experiences are, in general, dose-related and may result from high plasma levels caused by excessive dosage or rapid absorption, or may result from a hypersensitivity, idiosyncrasy or diminished tolerance on the part of the patient. Serious adverse experiences are generally systemic in nature. The following types are those most commonly reported:
Central nervous system: CNS manifestations are excitatory and/or depressant and may be characterized by lightheadedness, nervousness, apprehension, euphoria, confusion, dizziness, drowsiness, tinnitus, blurred or double vision, vomiting, sensations of heat, cold or numbness, twitching, tremors, convulsions, unconsciousness, respiratory depression and arrest. The excitatory manifestations may be very brief or may not occur at all, in which case the first manifestation of toxicity may be drowsiness merging into unconsciousness and respiratory arrest.
Drowsiness following the administration of lidocaine is usually an early sign of a high blood level of the drug and may occur as a consequence of rapid absorption.
Cardiovascular system: Cardiovascular manifestations are usually depressant and are characterized by bradycardia, hypotension, and cardiovascular collapse, which may lead to cardiac arrest.
Allergic: Allergic reactions are characterized by cutaneous lesions, urticaria, edema or anaphylactoid reactions. Allergic reactions may occur as a result of sensitivity either to the local anesthetic agent or to other ingredients in the formulation. Allergic reactions as a result of sensitivity to lidocaine are extremely rare and, if they occur, should be managed by conventional means. The detection of sensitivity by skin testing is of doubtful value.

OVERDOSAGE

Acute emergencies from local anesthetics are generally related to high plasma levels encountered during therapeutic use of local anesthetics. (see ADVERSE REACTIONS, WARNINGS, and PRECAUTIONS).
Management of local anesthetic emergencies: The first consideration is prevention, best accomplished by careful and constant monitoring of cardiovascular and respiratory vital signs and the patient's state of consciousness after each local anesthetic administration. At the first sign of change, oxygen should be administered.
The first step in the management of convulsions consists of immediate attention to the maintenance of a patent airway and assisted or controlled ventilation with oxygen and a delivery system capable of permitting immediate positive airway pressure by mask. Immediately after the institution of these ventilatory measures, the adequacy of the circulation should be evaluated, keeping in mind that drugs used to treat convulsions sometimes depress the circulation when administered intravenously. Should convulsions persist despite adequate respiratory support, and if the status of the circulation permits, small increments of an ultra-short acting barbiturate (such as thiopental or thiamylal) or a benzodiazepine (such as diazepam) may be administered intravenously. The clinician should be familiar, prior to use of local anesthetics, with these anticonvulsant drugs. Supportive treatment of circulatory depression may require administration of intravenous fluids and, when appropriate, a vasopressor as directed by the clinical situation (e.g., ephedrine).
If not treated immediately, both convulsions and cardiovascular depression can result in hypoxia, acidosis,, bradycardia, arrhythmias and cardiac arrest. If cardiac arrest should occur, standard cardiopulmonary resuscitative measures should be instituted.
Dialysis is of negligible value in the treatment of acute overdosage with lidocaine.
The intravenous LD_{50} of lidocaine HCl in female mice is 26 (21–31) mg/kg and the subcutaneous LD_{50} is 264 (203–304) mg/kg.

DOSAGE AND ADMINISTRATION

When Xylocaine 4% Topical Solution is used concomitantly with other products containing lidocaine, the total dose contributed by all formulations must be kept in mind.
The dosage varies and depends upon the area to be anesthetized, vascularity of the tissues, individual tolerance, and the technique of anesthesia. The lowest dosage needed to provide effective anesthesia should be administered. Dosages should be reduced for children and for elderly and debilitated patients. The maximum dose should not exceed 4.5 mg/kg (2 mg/lb) of body weight. Although the incidence of adverse effects with Xylocaine 4% Topical Solution is quite low, caution should be exercised, particularly when employing large volumes, since the incidenceof adverse effects is directly proportional to the total dose of local anesthetic agent administered.
The dosages recommended below are for normal, healthy adults:
When used as a spray, or when applied by means of cotton applicators or packs, as when instilled into a cavity, the suggested dosage of Xylocaine 4% Topical Solution is 1–5ml (40–200mg lidocaine HCl), i.e., 0.6–3.0mg/kg or 0.3–1.5mg/lb body weight.
NOTE: The solution may be applied with a sterile swab which is discarded after a single use. When spraying, transfer the solution from the original container to an atomizer.

MAXIMUM RECOMMENDED DOSAGES

Normal healthy adults: The maximum recommended dose of Xylocaine 4% Topical Solution should be such that the dose of lidocaine HCl is kept below 300mg and in any case should not exceed 4.5 mg/kg (2mg/lb) body weight.
Children:
It is difficult to recommend a maximum dose of any drug for children since this varies as a function of age and weight. For children of less than ten years who have a normal lean body mass and normal body development, the maximum dose may be determined by the application of one of the standard pediatric drug formulas (e.g. Clark's rule). For example, in a child of five years weighing 50 lbs., the dose of lidocaine hydrochloride should not exceed 75-100mg when calculated according to Clark's rule. In any case, the maximum dose of Xylocaine Solution with epinephrine should not exceed 7 mg/kg (3.2mg/lb) of body weight. When used without epinephrine, the amount of Xylocaine Solution administered should be such that the dose is kept below 300mg and in any case should not exceed 4.5mg/kg (2.0mg/lb) of body weight.

HOW SUPPLIED

Xylocaine (lidocaine HCl) 4% Topical Solution 50ml screw-cap bottle, cartoned (NDC 0186-0320-01). NOT FOR INJECTION.
Store at controlled room temperature: 15°-30°C (59°-86°F).
021802R01 7/84

Continued on next page

Astra—Cont.

XYLOCAINE® (lidocaine) ℞
[zī'lo-caine]
HYDROCHLORIDE 1.5% WITH DEXTROSE 7.5%
Sterile Aqueous Solution Only for Spinal Anesthesia in Obstetrics

(For details of indications, dosage and administration, precautions, and adverse reactions, see circular in package.)

HOW SUPPLIED

Xylocaine® (lidocaine) Hydrochloride 1.5% Solution with Dextrose 7.5% (NDC 0186-0212-03) is supplied in 2 ml ampules in packages of 10.

XYLOCAINE® (lidocaine hydrochloride) ℞
[zī'lo-cain]
5% SOLUTION WITH GLUCOSE 7.5%
Sterile Aqueous Solution for Spinal Anesthesia

(For details of indications, dosage and administration, precautions, and adverse reactions, see circular in package.)

HOW SUPPLIED

Xylocaine® (lidocaine hydrochloride) 5% solution with Glucose 7.5% (NDC 0186-0225-03) is supplied in 2 ml ampules in packages of 10.

XYLOCAINE® 2% (lidocaine HCl) ℞
[zī'lo-caine]
JELLY
A Topical Anesthetic for Urological Procedures and Lubrication of Endotracheal Tubes

DESCRIPTION

Xylocaine (lidocaine HCl) 2% Jelly is a sterile aqueous product that contans a local anesthetic agent and is administered topically. See INDICATIONS for specific uses.
Xylocaine 2% Jelly contains lidocaine HCl which is chemically designated as acetamide, 2-(diethylamino)-N-(2,6-dimethylphenyl)-, monohydrochloride and has the following structural formula:

CH_3, C_2H_5 — NH-CO-CH_2-N — • HCl — CH_3, C_2H_5

Xylocaine 2% Jelly also contains hydroxypropylmethylcellulose, and the resulting mixture maximizes contact with mucosa and provides lubrication for instrumentation.
The unused portion should be discarded after initial use.
Composition of Xylocaine 2% Jelly:
Each ml contains 20 mg of lidocaine HCl. The formulation also contains methylparaben, propylparaben, hydroxypropylmethylcellulose, and sodium hydroxide and/or hydrochloric acid to adjust pH to 6.0–7.0.

CLINICAL PHARMACOLOGY

Mechanism of action: Lidocaine stabilizes the neuronal membrane by inhibiting the ionic fluxes required for the initiation and conduction of impulses, thereby effecting local anesthetic action.
Onset of action: The onset of action is 3–5 minutes. It is ineffective when applied to intact skin.
Hemodynamics: Excessive blood levels may cause changes in cardiac output, total peripheral resistance, and mean arterial pressure. These changes may be attributable to a direct depressant effect of the local anesthetic agent on various components of the cardiovascular system.
Pharmacokinetics and metabolism: Lidocaine may be absorbed following topical administration to mucous membranes, its rate and extent of absorption depending upon concentration and total dose administered, the specific site of application and duration of exposure. In general, the rate of absorption of local anesthetic agents following topical application occurs most rapidly after intratracheal administration. Lidocaine is also well-absorbed from the gastrointestinal tract, but little intact drug may appear in the circulation because of biotransformation in the liver.
Lidocaine is metabolized rapidly by the liver, and metabolites and unchanged drug are excreted by the kidneys. Biotransformation includes oxidative N-dealkylation, ring hydroxylation, cleavage of the amide linkage, and conjugation. N-dealkylation, a major pathway of biotransformation, yields the metabolites monoethylglycinexylidide and glycinexylidide. The pharmacological/toxicological actions of these metabolites are similar to, but less potent than, those of lidocaine. Approximately 90% of lidocaine administered is excreted in the form of various metabolites, and less than 10% is excreted unchanged. The primary metabolite in urine is a conjugate of 4-hydroxy-2,6-dimethylaniline.
The plasma binding of lidocaine is dependent on drug concentration, and the fraction bound decreases with increasing concentration. At concentrations of 1 to 4 μg of free base per ml, 60 to 80 percent of lidocaine is protein bound. Binding is also dependent on the plasma concentration of the alpha-1-acid glycoprotein.
Lidocaine crosses the blood-brain and placental barriers, presumably by passive diffusion.
Studies of lidocaine metabolism following intravenous bolus injections have shown that the elimination half-life of this agent is typically 1.5 to 2.0 hours. Because of the rapid rate at which lidocaine is metabolized, any condition that affects liver function may alter lidocaine kinetics. The half-life may be prolonged two-fold or more in patients with liver dysfunction. Renal dysfunction does not affect lidocaine kinetics but may increase the accumulation of metabolites.
Factors such as acidosis and the use of CNS stimulants and depressants affect the CNS levels of lidocaine required to produce overt systemic effects. Objective adverse manifestations become increasingly apparent with increasing venous plasma levels above 6.0 μg free base per ml. In the rhesus monkey arterial blood levels of 18–21 μg/ml have been shown to be threshold for convulsive activity.

INDICATIONS AND USAGE

Xylocaine (lidocaine HCl) 2% Jelly is indicated for prevention and control of pain in procedures involving the male and female urethra, for topical treatment of painful urethritis, and as an anesthetic lubricant for endotracheal intubation (oral and nasal).

CONTRAINDICATIONS

Lidocaine is contraindicated in patients with a known history of hypersensitivity to local anesthetics of the amide type or to other components of Xylocaine 2% Jelly.

WARNINGS

EXCESSIVE DOSAGE, OR SHORT INTERVALS BETWEEN DOSES, CAN RESULT IN HIGH PLASMA LEVELS AND SERIOUS ADVERSE EFFECTS. PATIENTS SHOULD BE INSTRUCTED TO STRICTLY ADHERE TO THE RECOMMENDED DOSAGE AND ADMINISTRATION GUIDELINES AS SET FORTH IN THIS PACKAGE INSERT.
THE MANAGEMENT OF SERIOUS ADVERSE REACTIONS MAY REQUIRE THE USE OF RESUSCITATIVE EQUIPMENT, OXYGEN, AND OTHER RESUSCITATIVE DRUGS.
Xylocaine 2% Jelly should be used with extreme caution in the presence of sepsis or severely traumatized mucosa in the area of application, since under such conditions there is the potential for rapid systemic absorption.
When used for endotracheal tube lubrication care should be taken to avoid introducing the product into the lumen of the tube. Do not use the jelly to lubricate the endotracheal stylettes. If allowed into the inner lumen, the jelly may dry on the inner surface leaving a residue which tends to clump with flexion, narrowing the lumen. There have been rare reports in which this residue has caused the lumen to occlude. See also ADVERSE REACTION and DOSAGE & ADMINISTRATION.

PRECAUTIONS

General: The safety and effectiveness of lidocaine depend on proper dosage, correct technique, adequate precautions, and readiness for emergencies. (See WARNINGS and ADVERSE REACTIONS.) The lowest dosage that results in effective anesthesia should be used to avoid high plasma levels and serious adverse effects. Repeated doses of lidocaine may cause significant increases in blood levels with each repeated dose because of slow accumulation of the drug or its metabolites. Tolerance to elevated blood levels varies with the status of the patient. Debilitated, elderly patients, acutely ill patients, and children should be given reduced doses commensurate with their age and physical status. Lidocaine should also be used with caution in patients with severe shock or heart block.
Xylocaine 2% Jelly should be used with caution in patients with known drug sensitivities. Patients allergic to para-aminobenzoic acid derivatives (procaine, tetracaine, benzocaine, etc.) have not shown cross sensitivity to lidocaine.
Many drugs used during the conduct of anesthesia are considered potential triggering agents for familial malignant hyperthermia. Since it is not known whether amide-type local anesthetics may trigger this reaction and since the need for supplemental general anesthesia cannot be predicted in advance, it is suggested that a standard protocol for management should be available. Early unexplained signs of tachycardia, tachypnea, labile blood pressure and metabolic acidosis may precede temperature elevation. Successful outcome is dependent on early diagnosis, prompt discontinuance of the suspect triggering agent(s) and institution of treatment, including oxygen therapy, indicated supportive measures and dantrolene (consult dantrolene sodium intravenous package insert before using).
Information for Patients: When topical anesthetics are used in the mouth, the patient should be aware that the production of topical anesthesia may impair swallowing and thus enhance the danger of aspiration. For this reason, food should not be ingested for 60 minutes following use of local anesthetic preparations in the mouth or throat area. This is particularly important in children because of their frequency of eating.
Numbness of the tongue or buccal mucosa may enhance the danger of unintentional biting trauma. Food and chewing gum should not be taken while the mouth or throat area is anesthetized.
Carcinogenesis, mutagenesis, impairment of fertility: Studies of lidocaine in animals to evauate the carcinogenic and mutagenic potential or the effect on fertility have not been conducted.
Use in Pregnancy: Teratogenic Effects. Pregnancy Category B. Reproduction studies have been performed in rats at doses up to 6.6 times the human dose and have revealed no evidence of harm to the fetus caused by lidocaine. There are, however, no adequate and well-controlled studies in pregnant women. Animal reproduction studies are not always predictive of human response. General consideration should be given to this fact before administering lidocaine to women of childbearing potential, especially during early pregnancy when maximum organogenesis takes place.
Labor and Delivery: Lidocaine is not contraindicated in labor and delivery. Should Xylocaine 2% Jelly be used concomitantly with other products containing lidocaine, the total dose contributed by all formulations must be kept in mind.
Nursing mothers: It is not known whether this drug is excreted in human milk. Because many drugs are excreted in human milk, caution should be exercised when lidocaine is administered to a nursing woman.
Pediatric use: Dosages in children should be reduced, commensurate with age, body weight and physical condition. See DOSAGE AND ADMINISTRATION.

ADVERSE REACTIONS

Adverse experiences following the administration of lidocaine are similar in nature to those observed with other amide local anesthetic agents. These adverse experiences are, in general, dose-related and may result from high plasma levels caused by excessive dosage or rapid absorption, or may result from a hypersensitivity, idiosyncrasy or diminished tolerance on the part of the patient. Serious adverse experiences are generally systemic in nature. The following types are those most commonly reported:
There have been rare reports of endotracheal tube occlusion associated with the presence of dried jelly residue in the inner lumen of the tube. See also WARNINGS and DOSAGE & ADMINISTRATION.
Central nervous system. CNS manifestations are excitatory and/or depressant and may be characterized by lightheadedness, nervousness, apprehension, euphoria, confusion, dizziness, drowsiness, tinnitus, blurred or double vision, vomiting, sensations of heat, cold or numbness, twitching, tremors, convulsions, unconsciousness, respiratory depression and arrest. The excitatory manifestations may be very brief or may not occur at all, in which case the first manifestation of toxicity may be drowsiness merging into unconsciousness and respiratory arrest.
Drowsiness following the administration of lidocaine is usually an early sign of a high blood level of the drug and may occur as a consequence of rapid absorption.
Cardiovascular system: Cardiovascular manifestations are usually depressant and are characterized by bradycardia, hypotension, and cardiovascular collapse, which may lead to cardiac arrest.
Allergic: Allergic reactions are characterized by cutaneous lesions, urticaria, edema or anaphylactoid reactions. Allergic reactions may occur as a result of sensitivity either to the local anesthetic agent or to other components in the formulation. Allergic reactions as a result of sensitivity to lidocaine are extremely rare and, if they occur, should be managed by conventional means. The detection of sensitivity by skin testing is of doubtful value.

OVERDOSAGE

Acute emergencies from local anesthetics are generally related to high plasma levels encountered during therapeutic use of local anesthetics. (See ADVERSE REACTIONS, WARNINGS, and PRECAUTIONS.)
Management of local anesthetic emergencies: The first consideration is prevention, best accomplished by careful and constant monitoring of cardiovascular and respiratory vital signs and the patient's state of consciousness after each local anesthetic administration. At the first sign of change, oxygen should be administered.
The first step in the management of convulsions consists of immediate attention to the maintenance of a patent airway

and assisted or controlled ventilation with oxygen and a delivery system capable of permitting immediate positive airway pressure by mask. Immediately after the institution of these ventilatory measures, the adequacy of the circulation should be evaluated, keeping in mind that drugs used to treat convulsions sometimes depress the circulation when administered intravenously. Should convulsions persist despite adequate respiratory support, and if the status of the circulation permits, small increments of an ultra-short acting barbiturate (such as thiopental or thiamylal) or a benzodiazepine (such as diazepam) may be administered intravenously. The clinician should be familiar, prior to use of local anesthetics, with these anticonvulsant drugs. Supportive treatment or circulatory depression may require administration of intravenous fluids and, when appropriate, a vasopressor as directed by the clinical situation (e.g. ephedrine).

If not treated immediately, both convulsions and cardiovascular depression can result in hypoxia, acidosis, bradycardia, arrhythmias and cardiac arrest. If cardiac arrest should occur, standard cardiopulmonary resuscitative measures should be instituted.

Diallysis is of negligible value in the treatment of acute overdosage with lidocaine.

The oral LD_{50} of lidocaine HCl in non-fasted female rats is 459 (346–773) mg/kg (as the salt) and 214 (159–324) mg/kg as the salt in fasted female rats.

DOSAGE AND ADMINISTRATION

When Xylocaine 2% Jelly is used concomitantly with other products containing lidocaine, the total dose contributed by all formulations must be kept in mind.

The dosage varies and depends upon the area to be anesthetized, vascularity of the tissues, individual tolerance, and the technique of anesthesia. The lowest dosage needed to provide effective anesthesia should be administered. Dosages should be reduced for children and for elderly and debilitated patients. Although the incidence of adverse effects with Xylocaine 2% Jelly is quite low, caution should be exercised, particularly when employing large amounts, since the incidence of adverse effects is directly proportional to the total dose of local anesthetic agent administered.

For surface anesthesia of the male adult urethra: The plastic cone is sterilized for 5 minutes in boiling water, cooled, and attached to the tube. The cone may be gas sterilized or cold sterilized, as preferred. The jelly is instilled slowly into the urethra by gently expressing the contents of the tube until the patient has a feeling of tension or until almost half the tube (15 ml; *i.e.,* 300 mg of lidocaine HCl) is emptied. A penile clamp is then applied for several minutes at the corona and then the remaining contents of the tube are instilled.

Prior to sounding or cystoscopy, a penile clamp should be applied for 5 to 10 minutes to obtain adequate anesthesia. The contents of one tube (30 ml, *i.e.,* 600 mg) are usually required to fill and dilate the male urethra.

Prior to catheterization, smaller volumes (5–10 ml, *i.e.,* 100–200 mg) are usually adequate for lubrication.

For surface anesthesia of the female adult urethra: The plastic cone is sterilized for 5 minutes in boiling water, cooled, and attached to the tube. The cone may be gas sterilized or cold sterilized, as preferred. Three to five ml of the jelly is instilled slowly into the urethra by gently expressing approximately 10–20% of the contents of the tube. If desired, some jelly may be deposited on a cotton swab and introduced into the urethra. In order to obtain adequate anesthesia, several minutes should be allowed prior to performing urological procedures.

Lubrication for endotracheal intubation: Apply a moderate amount of jelly to the external surface of the endotracheal tube shortly before use. Care should be taken to avoid introducing the product into the lumen of the tube. Do not use the jelly to lubricate endotracheal stylettes. See WARNINGS and ADVERSE REACTIONS concerning rare reports of inner lumen occlusion. It is also recommended that use of endotracheal tubes with dried jelly on the external surface be avoided for lack of lubricating effect.

MAXIMUM DOSAGE: No more than one tube (600 mg of lidocaine HCl) should be given in any 12 hour period.

Children: It is difficult to recommend a maximum dose of any drug for children since this varies as a function of age and weight. For children less than ten years who have a normal lean body mass and a normal lean body development, the maximum dose may be determined by the application of one of the standard pediatric drug formulas (e.g., Clark's rule). For example, in a child of five years weighing 50 lbs., the dose of lidocaine hydrochloriide should not exceed 75–100 mg when calculated according to Clark's rule. In any case, the maximum amount of Xylocaine administered should not exceed 4.5 mg/kg (2.0 mg/lb) of body weight.

HOW SUPPLIED

Xylocaine (lidocaine HCl) 2% Jelly (NDC 0186-0330-01) is supplied in collapsible tubes that deliver 30 ml. A detachable applicator cone and a key for expressing the contents are included in each package.

Store at controlled room temperature 15°–30°C (59°–86°F).

021838R09 9/84

5% XYLOCAINE (lidocaine) ℞

[zī′lo-caine]

Ointment

A Water-Soluble Topical Anesthetic Ointment

DESCRIPTION

Xylocaine (lidocaine) 5% Ointment contains a local anesthetic agent and is administered topically. See INDICATIONS for specific uses.

Xylocaine 5% Ointment contains lidocaine, which is chemically designated as acetamide, 2-(diethylamino)-N-(2,6-dimethylphenyl)-, and has the following structural formula:

CH_3, C_2H_5, NH-CO-CH_2-N, CH_3, C_2H_5

Composition of Xylocaine 5% Ointment

Each gram of the plain and flavored ointments contains lidocaine, 50 mg, polyethylene glycol 1500, polyethylene glycol 4000, propylene gylcol and sodium saccharin. The flavored ointment contains peppermint oil and spearmint oil.

CLINICAL PHARMACOLOGY

Mechanism of action:

Lidocaine stabilizes the neuronal membrane by inhibiting the ionic fluxes required for the initiation and conduction of impulses, thereby effecting local anesthetic action.

Onset of anesthesia:

Xylocaine (lidocaine) 5% Ointment effects local, topical anesthesia. The onset of action is 3–5 minutes. It is ineffective when applied to intact skin.

Hemodynamics:

Excessive blood levels may cause changes in cardiac output, total peripheral resistance, and mean arterial pressure. These changes may be attributable to a direct depressant effect of the local anesthetic agent on various components of the cardiovascular system.

Pharmacokinetics and metabolism:

Lidocaine may be absorbed following topical administration to mucous membranes, its rate and extent of absorption depending upon the specific site of application, duration of exposure, concentration, and total dosage. In general, the rate of absorption of local anesthetic agents following topical application occurs most rapidly after intratracheal administration. Lidocaine is also well-absorbed from the gastrointestinal tract, but little intact drug appears in the circulation because of biotransformation in the liver.

Lidocaine is metabolized rapidly by the liver, and metabolites and unchanged drug are excreted by the kidneys. Biotransformation includes oxidative N-dealkylation, ring hydroxylation, cleavage of the amide linkage, and conjugation. N-dealkylation, a major pathway of biotransformation, yields the metabolites monoethylglycinexylidide and glycinexylidide. The pharmacological/toxicological actions of these metabolites are similar to, but less potent than, those of lidocaine. Approximately 90% of lidocaine administered is excreted in the form of various metabolites, and less than 10% is excreted unchanged. The primary metabolite in urine is a conjugate of 4-hydroxy-2, 6-dimethylaniline.

The plasma binding of lidocaine is dependent on drug concentration, and the fraction bound decreases with increasing concentration. At concentrations of 1 to 4 μg of free base per ml, 60 to 80 percent of lidocaine is protein bound. Binding is also dependent on the plasma concentration of the alpha-1-acid glycoprotein.

Lidocaine crosses the blood-brain and placental barriers, presumably by passive diffusion.

Studies of lidocaine metabolism following intravenous bolus injections have shown that the elimination half-life of this agent is typically 1.5 to 2.0 hours. Because of the rapid rate at which lidocaine is metabolized, any condition that affects liver function may alter lidocaine kinetics. The half-life may be prolonged two-fold or more in patients with liver dysfunction. Renal dysfunction does not affect lidocaine kinetics but may increase the accumulation of metabolites.

Factors such as acidosis and the use of CNS stimulants and depressants affect the CNS levels of lidocaine required to produce overt systemic effects. Objective adverse manifestations become increasingly apparent with increasing venous plasma levels above 6.0 μg free base per ml. In the rhesus monkey arterial blood levels of 18–21 μg/ml have been shown to be threshold for convulsive activity.

INDICATIONS AND USAGE

Xylocaine (lidocaine) 5% Ointment is indicated for production of anesthesia of accessible mucous membranes of the oropharynx.

It is also useful as an anesthetic lubricant for intubation and for the temporary relief of pain associated with minor burns, including sunburn, abrasions of the skin, and insect bites.

CONTRAINDICATIONS

Lidocaine is contraindicated in patients with a known history of hyersensitivity to local anesthetics of the amide type or to other components of Xylocaine 5% Ointment.

WARNINGS

EXCESSIVE DOSAGE, OR SHORT INTERVALS BETWEEN DOSES, CAN RESULT IN HIGH PLASMA LEVELS AND SERIOUS ADVERSE EFFECTS, PATIENTS SHOULD BE INSTRUCTED TO STRICTLY ADHERE TO THE RECOMMENDED DOSAGE AND ADMINISTRATION GUIDELINES AS SET FORTH IN THIS PACKAGE INSERT.

THE MANAGEMENT OF SERIOUS ADVERSE REACTIONS MAY REQUIRE THE USE OF RESUSCITATIVE EQUIPMENT, OXYGEN, AND OTHER RESUSCITATIVE DRUGS.

Xylocaine 5% Ointment should be used with extreme caution in the presence of sepsis or severely traumatized mucosa in the area of application, since under such conditions there is the potential for rapid systemic absorption.

PRECAUTIONS

General:

The safety and effectiveness of lidocaine depend on proper dosage, correct technique, adequate precautions, and readiness for emergencies. (See WARNINGS and ADVERSE REACTIONS). The lowest dosage that results in effective anesthesia should be used to avoid high plasma levels and serious adverse effects. Repeated doses of lidocaine may cause significant increases in blood levels with each repeated dose because of slow accumulation of the drug and/or its metabolites. Tolerance to elevated blood levels varies with the status of the patient. Debilitated, elderly patients, acutely ill patients, and children should be given reduced doses commensurate with their age and physical condition. Lidocaine should also be used with caution in patients with severe shock or heart block.

Xylocaine 5% Ointment should be used with caution in patients with known drug sensitivities. Patients allergic to paraaminobenzoic acid derivatives (procaine, tetracaine, benzocaine, etc.) have not shown cross sensitivity to lidocaine. Many drugs used during the conduct of anesthesia are considered potential triggering agents for familial malignant hyperthermia. Since it is not known whether amide-type local anesthetics may trigger this reaction and since the need for supplemental general anesthesia cannot be predicted in advance, it is suggested that a standard protocol for the management of malignant hyperthermia should be available. Early unexplained signs of tachycardia, tachypnea, labile blood pressure and metabolic acidosis may precede temperature elevation. Successful outcome is dependent on early diagnosis, prompt discontinuance of the suspect triggering agent(s) and institution of treatment, including oxygen therapy, indicated supportive measures and dantrolene (consult dantrolene sodium intravenous package insert before using).

Information for Patients:

When topical anesthetics are used in the mouth, the patient should be aware that the production of topical anesthesia may impair swallowing and thus enhance the danger of aspiration. For this reason, food should not be ingested for 60 minutes following the use of local anesthetic preparations in the mouth or throat area. This is particularly important in children because of their frequency of eating.

Numbness of the tongue or buccal mucosa may enhance the danger of unintentional biting trauma. Food and chewing gum should not be taken while the mouth or throat area is anesthetized.

Carcinogenesis, mutagenesis, impairment of fertility:

Studies of lidocaine in animals to evaluate the carcinogenic and mutagenic potential or the effect on fertility have not been conducted.

Use in Pregnancy:

Teratogenic Effects. Pregnancy Category B. Reproduction studies have been performed in rats at doses up to 6.6 times the human dose and have revealed no evidence of harm to the fetus caused by lidocaine. There are, however, no adequate and well-controlled studies in pregnant women. Animal reproduction studies are not always predictive of human response. General consideration should be given to this fact before administering lidocaine to women of childbearing potential, especially during early pregnancy when maximum organogenesis takes place.

Labor and Delivery:

Lidocaine is not contraindicated in labor and delivery. Should Xylocaine 5% Ointment be used concomitantly with other products containing lidocaine, the total dose contributed by all formulations must be kept in mind.

Nursing Mothers:

It is not known whether this drug is excreted in human milk. Because many drugs are excreted in human milk, caution should be exercised when lidocaine is administered to a nursing woman.

Continued on next page

Astra—Cont.

Pediatric use:
Dosage in children should be reduced, commensurate with age, body weight and physical condition. Caution must be taken to avoid overdosage when applying Xylocaine 5% Ointment to large areas of injured or abraded skin, since the systemic absorption of lidocaine may be increased under such conditions. See DOSAGE and ADMINISTRATION.

ADVERSE REACTIONS

Adverse experiences following the administration of lidocaine are similar in nature to those observed with other amide local anesthetic agents. These adverse experiences are, in general, dose-related and may result from high plasma levels caused by excessive dosage or rapid absorption, or may result from a hypersensitivity, idiosyncrasy or diminished tolerance on the part of the patient. Serious adverse experiences are generally systemic in nature. The following types are those most commonly reported:
Central nervous system:
CNS manifestations are excitatory and/or depressant and may be characterized by lightheadedness, nervousness, apprehension, euphoria, confusion, dizziness, drowsiness, tinnitus, blurred or double vision, vomiting, sensations of heat, cold or numbness, twitching, tremors, convulsions, unconsciousness, respiratory depression and arrest. The excitatory manifestations may be very brief or may not occur at all, in which case the first manifestation of toxicity may be drowsiness merging into unconsciousness and respiratory arrest.
Drowsiness following the administration of lidocaine is usually an early sign of a high blood level of the drug and may occur as a consequence of rapid absorption.
Cardiovascular system:
Cardiovascular manifestations are usually depressant and are characterized by bradycardia, hypotension, and cardiovascular collapse, which may lead to cardiac arrest.
Allergic:
Allergic reactions are characterized by cutaneous lesions, urticaria, edema or anaphylactoid reactions. Allergic reactions may occur as a result of sensitivity either to the local anesthetic agent or to other components in the formulation. Allergic reactions as a result of sensitivity to lidocaine are extremely rare and, if they occur, should be managed by conventional means. The detection of sensitivity by skin testing is of doubtful value.

OVERDOSAGE

Acute emergencies from local anesthetics are generally related to high plasma levels encountered during therapeutic use of local anesthetics. (see ADVERSE REACTIONS, WARNINGS, and PRECAUTIONS).
Management of local anesthetic emergencies:
The first consideration is prevention, best accomplished by careful and constant monitoring of cardiovascular and repiratory vital signs and the patient's state of consciousness after each local anethetic administration. At the first sign of change, oxygen should be administered.
The first step in the management of convulsions consists of immediate attention to the maintenance of a patent airway and assisted or controlled ventilation with oxygen and a delivery system capable of permitting immediate positive airway pressure by mask. Immediately after the institution of these ventilatory measures, the adequacy of the circulation should be evaluated, keeping in mind that drugs used to treat convulsions sometimes depress the circulation when administered intravenously. Should convulsions persist despite adequate respiratory support, and if the status of the circulation permits, small increments of an ultra-short acting barbiturate (such as thiopental or thiamylal) or a benzodiazepine (such as diazepam) may be administered intravenously. The clinician should be familiar, prior to use of local anesthetics, with these anticonvulsant drugs. Supportive treatment of circulatory depression may require administration of intravenous fluids and, when appropriate, a vasopressor as directed by the clinical situation (e.g., ephedrine).
If not treated immediately, both convulsions and cardiovascular depression can result in hypoxia, acidosis, bradycardia, arrhythmias and cardiac arrest. If cardiac arrest should occur, standard cardiopulmonary resuscitative measures should be instituted.
Dialysis is of negligible value in the treatment of acute overdosage with lidocaine.
The oral LD_{50} of lidocaine HCI in non-fasted female rats is 459 (346-773) mg/kg (as the salt) and 214 (159-324) mg/kg (as the salt) in fasted female rats.

DOSAGE AND ADMINISTRATION

When Xylocaine 5% Ointment is used concomitantly with other products containing lidocaine, the total dose contributed by all formulations must be kept in mind.
Adult
A single application should not exceed 5 gm of Xylocaine 5% Ointment, containing 250 mg of Xylocaine base (equivalent chemically to approximately 300 mg of Xylocaine hydrochloride). This is roughly equivalent to squeezing a six (6) inch length of ointment from the tube. In a 70 kg adult this dose equals 3.6 mg/kg (1.6 mg/lb) lidocaine base. No more than one-half tube, approximately 17–20 gm of ointment or 850–1000 mg Xylocaine base, should be administered in any one day.
Although the incidence of adverse effects with Xylocaine 5% Ointment is quite low, caution should be exercised, particularly when employing large amounts, since the incidence of adverse effects is directly proportional to the total dose of local anesthetic agent administered.
Dosage for children
It is difficult to recommend a maximum dose of any drug for children since this varies as a function of age and weight. For children less than ten years who have a normal lean body mass and a normal lean body development, the maximum dose may be determined by the application of one of the standard pediatric drug formulas (e.g., Clark's rule). For example, in a child of five years weighing 50 lbs., the dose of lidocaine should not exceed 75–100 mg when calculated according to Clark's rule. In any case, the maximum amount of Xylocaine administered should not exceed 4.5 mg/kg (2.0 mg/lb) of body weight.
Administration
For medical use, apply topically for adequate control of symptoms. The use of a sterile gauze pad is sugested for application to broken skin tissue. Apply to the tube prior to intubation.
In dentistry, apply to previously dried oral mucosa. Subsequent removal of excess saliva with cotton rolls or saliva ejector minimizes dilution of the ointment, permits maximum penetration, and minimizes the possibility of swallowing the topical ointment.
For use in connection with the insertion of new dentures, apply to all denture surfaces contacting mucosa.
IMPORTANT: Patients should consult a dentist at intervals not exceeding 48 hours throughout the fitting period.

HOW SUPPLIED

Xylocaine (lidocaine) 5% Ointment (NDC 0186-0315-21) is available in 35 gm tubes.
Xylocaine (lidocaine) 5% Ointment Flavored for application within the oral cavity, is dispensed in 3.5 gram tubes, 10 tubes per carton (NDC 0186-0350-03), and in 35-gram jars (NDC 0186-0350-01).
KEEP CONTAINER TIGHTLY CLOSED AT ALL TIMES WHEN NOT IN USE.
Store at controlled room temperature 15°C–30°C (59°–86°F).
Manufactured by MK Laboratories, Inc., Fairfield, CT 06430
021709R10 Rev. 8/85 (10)

XYLOCAINE ® (lidocaine)
[*zī'lo-cain*]
2.5% OINTMENT

(See PDR For Nonprescription Drugs)

XYLOCAINE® (lidocaine) ℞
[*zī'lo-caine*]
10% Oral Spray
Flavored Topical Anesthetic Aerosol
For Use In The Oral Cavity

WARNING—CONTENTS UNDER PRESSURE.

DESCRIPTION

Xylocaine (lidocaine) 10% Oral Spray contains a local anesthetic agent and is administered topically in the oral cavity. See INDICATIONS for specific uses.
Xylocaine 10% Oral Spray contains lidocaine, which is chemically designated as acetamide,2-(diethylamino)-N-(2,6-dimethylphenyl)-, and has the following structural formula:

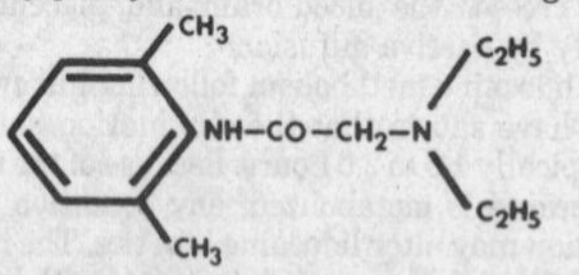

Composition of Xylocaine (lidocaine) 10% Oral Spray
Each actuation of the metered dose valve delivers 0.1ml of solution containing lidocaine, 10mg, cetylpyridinium chloride, absolute alcohol, saccharin, flavor, and polyethylene glycol.
And as propellants: trichlorofluoromethane/dichlorodifluoromethane (65%/35%).

CLINICAL PHARMACOLOGY

Mechanism of action: Lidocaine stabilizes the neuronal membrane by inhibiting the ionic fluxes required for the initiation and conduction of impulses, thereby effecting local anesthetic action.
Onset and duration of action: Xylocaine (lidocaine) 10% Oral Spray acts on intact mucous membranes to produce local anesthesia. Anesthesia occurs usually within 1–2 minutes and persists for approximately 10–15 minutes.
Hemodynamics: Excessive blood levels may cause changes in cardiac output, total peripheral resistance, and mean arterial pressure. These changes may be attributable to a direct depressant effect of the local anesthetic agent on various components of the cardiovascular system.
Pharmacokinetcs and metabolism: Lidocaine may be absorbed following topical administration to mucous membranes, its rate of absorption and percent of dose absorbed depending upon concentration and total dose administered, the specific site of application and duration of exposure. In general, the rate of absorption of local anesthetic agents following topical application occurs most rapidly after intratracheal administration. Lidocaine is well-absorbed from the gastrointestinal tract, but little intact drug appears in the circulation because of biotransformation in the liver.
Lidocaine is metabolized rapidly by the liver, and metabolites and unchanged drug are excreted by the kidney. Biotransformation includes oxidative N-dealkylation, ring hydroxylation, cleavage of the amide linkage, and conjugation. N-dealkylation, a mjaor pathway of biotransformation, yields the metabolites monoethylglycinexylidide and glycinexylidide. The pharmacological/toxicological actions of these metabolites are similar to, but less potent than, those of lidocaine. Approximately 90% of lidocaine administered is excreted in the form of various metabolites, and less than 10% is excreted unchanged. The primary metabolite in urine is a conjugate of 4-hydroxy-2, 6-dimethylaniline.
The plasma binding of lidocaine is dependent on drug concentration, and the fraction bound decreases with increasing concentration. At concentrations of 1 to 4 μg of free base per ml, 60 to 80 percent of lidocaine is protein bound. Binding is also dependent on the plasma concentration of the alpha-1-acid glycoprotein.
Lidocaine crosses the blood-brain and placental barriers, presumably by passive diffusion.
Studies of lidocaine metabolism following intravenous bolus injections have shown that the elimination half-life of this agent is typically 1.5 to 2.0 hours. Because of the rapid rate at which lidocaine is metabolized, any condition that affects liver function may alter lidocaine kinetics. The half-life may be prolonged two-fold or more in patients with liver dysfunction. Renal dysfunction does not affect lidocaine kinetics but may increase the accumulation of metabolites.
Factors such as acidosis and the use of CNS stimulants and depressants affect the CNS levels of lidocaine required to produce overt systemic effects. Objective adverse manifestations become increasingly apparent with increasing venous plasma levels above 6.0 μg free base per ml. In the rhesus monkey arterial blood levels of 18–21 μg/ml have been shown to be threshold for convulsive activity.

INDICATIONS AND USAGE

Xylocaine (lidocaine) 10% Oral Spray is indicated for the production of topical anesthesia of the accessible mucous membranes of the mouth and oropharynx.

CONTRAINDICATIONS

Lidocaine is contraindicated in patients with a known history of hypersensitivity to local anesthetics of the amide type or to other components of Xylocaine 10% Oral Spray.

WARNINGS

IN ORDER TO MANAGE POSSIBLE ADVERSE REACTIONS, RESUSCITATIVE EQUIPMENT, OXYGEN AND OTHER RESUSCITATIVE DRUGS MUST BE IMMEDIATELY AVAILABLE WHEN LOCAL ANESTHETIC AGENTS, SUCH AS LIDOCAINE, ARE ADMINISTERED TO MUCOUS MEMBRANES.
Xylocaine 10% Oral Spray should be used with extreme caution if there is sepsis or extremely traumatized mucosa in the area of application, since under such conditions there is the potential for rapid systemic absorption.

PRECAUTIONS

General: The safety and effectiveness of lidocaine depend on proper dosage, correct technique, adequate precautions, and readiness for emergencies. Resuscitative equipment, oxygen, and other resuscitative drugs should be available for immediate use. (See WARNINGS and ADVERSE REACTIONS). The lowest dosage that result in effective anesthesia should be used to avoid high plasma levels and serious adverse effects. Repeated doses of lidocaine may cause significant increases in blood levels with each repeated dose because of slow accumulation of the drug or its metabolites. Tolerance varies with the status of the patient. Debilitated, elderly patients, acutely ill patients, and children should be given reduced doses commensurate with their age and physical status. Lidocaine should also be used with caution in patients with severe shock or heart block.
Xylocaine 10% Oral Spray should be used with caution in patients with known drug sensitivities. Patients allergic to para-aminobenzoic acid derivatives (procaine, tetracaine, benzocaine, etc.) have not shown cross sensitivity to lidocaine.
Many drugs used during the conduct of anesthesia are considered potential triggering agents for familial malignant hyperthermia. Since it is not known whether amide-type

local anesthetics may trigger this reaction and since the need for supplemental general anesthesia cannot be predicted in advance, it is suggested that a standard protocol for management should be available. Early unexplained signs of tachycardia, tachypnea, labile blood pressure and metabolic acidosis may precede temperature elevation. Successful outcome is dependent on early diagnosis, prompt discontinuance of the suspect triggering agent(s) and institution of treatment, including oxygen therapy, indicated supportive measures and dantrolene (consult dantrolene sodium intravenous package insert before using).

Information for Patients: When topical anesthetics are used in the mouth, the patient should be aware that the production of topical anesthesia may impair swallowing and thus enhance the danger of aspiration. For this reason, food should not be ingested for 60 minutes following use of local anesthetic preprations in the mouth or throat area. This is particularly important in children because of their frequency of eating.

Numbness of the tongue or buccal mucosa may enhance the danger of unintentional biting trauma. Food and chewing gum should not be taken while the mouth or throat area is anesthetized.

Carcinogenesis, mutagenesis, impairment of fertility: Studies of lidocaine in animals to evaluate the carcinogenic and mutagenic potential or the effect on fertility have not been conducted.

Use in Pregnancy: Teratogenic Effects. Pregnancy Category B. Reproduction studies have been performed in rats at doses up to 6.6 times the human dose and have revealed no evidence of harm to the fetus caused by lidocaine. There are, however, no adequate and well-controlled studies in pregnant women. Animal reproduction studies are not always predictive of human response. General consideration should be given to this fact before administering lidocaine to women of childbearing potential, especially during early pregnancy when maximum organogenesis takes place.

Labor and Delivery: Lidocaine is not contraindicated in labor and delivery. Should Xylocaine 10% Oral Spray be used concomitantly with other products containing lidocaine, the total dose contributed by all formulations must be kept in mind.

Nursing mothers: It is not known whether this drug is excreted in human milk. Because many drugs are excreted in human milk, caution should be exercised when lidocaine is administered to a nursing woman.

Pediatric use: Safety and effectiveness in children below the age of 12 years have not been established.

ADVERSE REACTIONS

Adverse experiences following the administration of lidocaine are similar in nature to those observed with other amide local anesthetic agents. These adverse experiences are, in general, dose-related and may result from high plasma levels caused by excessive dosage or rapid absorption, or may result from a hypersensitivity, idiosyncrasy or diminished tolerance on the part of the patient. Serious adverse experiences are generally systemic in nature. The following types are those most commonly reported:

Central nervous system: CNS manifestations are excitatory and/or depressant and may be characterized by lightheadedness, nervousness, apprehension, euphoria, confusion, dizziness, drowsiness, tinnitus, blurred or double vision, vomiting, sensations of heat, cold or numbness, twitching, tremors, convulsions, unconsciousness, respiratory depression and arrest. The excitatory manifestations may be very brief or may not occur at all, in which case the first manifestation of toxicity may be drowsiness merging into unconsciousness and respiratory arrest.

Drowsiness following the administration of lidocaine is usually an early sign of a high blood level of the drug and may occur as a consequence of rapid absorption.

Cardiovascular system: Cardiovascular manifestations are usually depressant and are characterized by bradycardia, hypotension, and cardiovascular collapse, which may lead to cardiac arrest.

Allergic: Allergic reactions are characterized by cutaneous lesions, urticaria, edema or anaphylactoid reactions. Allergic reactions may occur as a result of sensitivity either to the local anesthetic agent or to other ingredients in the formulation. Allergic reactions as a result of sensitivity to lidocaine are extremely rare and, if they occur, should be managed by conventional means. The detection of sensitivity by skin testing is of doubtful value.

OVERDOSAGE

Acute emergencies from local anesthetics are generally related to high plasma levels encountered during therapeutic use of local anesthetics. (see ADVERSE REACTIONS, WARNINGS, and PRECAUTIONS).

Management of local anesthetic emergencies: The first consideration is prevention, best accomplished by careful and constant monitoring of cardiovascular and respiratory vital signs and the patient's state of consciousness after each local anesthetic administration. At the first sign of change, oxygen should be administered.

The first step in the management of convulsions consists of immediate attention to the maintenance of a patent airway and assisted or controlled ventilation with oxygen and a delivery system capable of permitting immediate positive airway pressure by mask. Immediately after the institution of these ventilatory measures, the adequacy of the circulation should be evaluated, keeping in mind that drugs used to treat convulsions sometimes depress the circulation when administered intravenously. Should convulsions persist despite adequate respiratory support, and if the status of the circulation permits, small increments of an ultra-short acting barbiturate (such as thiopental or thiamylal) or a benzodiazepine (such as diazepam) may be administered intravenously. The clinician should be familiar, prior to use of local anesthetics, with these anticonvulsant drugs. Supportive treatment of circulatory depression may require administration of intravenous fluids and, when appropriate, a vasopressor as directed by the clinical situation (e.g., ephedrine).

If not treated immediately, both convulsions and cardiovascular depression can result in hypoxia, acidosis, bradycardia, arrhythmias and cardiac arrest. If cardiac arrest should occur, standard cardiopulmonary resuscitative measures should be instituted.

Dialysis is of negligible value in the treatment of acute overdosage with lidocaine.

The intravenous LD_{50} of lidocaine HCl in female mice is 26(21–31) mg/kg and the subcutaneous LD_{50} is 264(203–304) mg/kg.

DOSAGE AND ADMINISTRATION

When Xylocaine 10% Oral Spray is used concomitantly with other products containing lidocaine, the total dose contributed by all formulations must be kept in mind.

Two metered doses per quadrant are recommended as the upper limit and, *under no circumstances* should one exceed three metered doses per quadrant of oral mucosa over a one-half hour period to produce the desired anesthetic effect. Experience in children is inadequate to recommend a pediatric dose at this time.

HOW SUPPLIED

NDC 0186-0355-01. A 60ml (2 oz.) aerosol container provides a total amount of 8.26gm (w/w) of the active ingredient lidocaine. Each actuation of the metered dose valve delivers 10mg of lidocaine.

Contents under pressure. Do not puncture or incinerate container. Do not expose to heat or store at temperatures above 120°F. Avoid contact with the eyes. Inhalation and swallowing should be avoided.

Keep out of the reach of children.

Use only as directed; intentional misuse by deliberately concentrating and inhaling the contents can be harmful or fatal.

STORE AT CONTROLLED ROOM TEMPERATURE 15°–30°C (59°–86°F).

Manufactured by Armstrong Laboratories, Inc., West Roxbury, MA 02132

021731R04 7/84

XYLOCAINE® 2% (lidocaine ℞
[zī'lo-caine]
hydrochloride) VISCOUS SOLUTION

A Topical Anesthetic for the Mucous Membranes of the Mouth and Pharynx

DESCRIPTION

Xylocaine (lidocaine HCl) 2% Viscous Solution contains a local anesthetic agent and is administered topically. Xylocaine 2% Viscous Solution contains lidocaine HCl, which is chemically designated as acetamide, 2-(diethylamino)-N-(2.6-dimethylphenyl)-, monohydrochloride.

The molecular formula of lidocaine is $C_{14}H_{22}N_2O$. The molecular weight is 234.34.

COMPOSITION OF SOLUTION

Each ml contains 20 mg of lidocaine HCl, flavoring, sodium saccharin, methylparaben, propylparaben and sodium carboxymethylcellulose in purified water. The pH is adjusted to 6.0–7.0 by means of sodium hydroxide and/or hydrochloric acid.

CLINICAL PHARMACOLOGY

Mechanism of action: Lidocaine stabilizes the neuronal membrane by inhibiting the ionic fluxes required for the initiation and conduction of impulses, thereby effecting local anesthetic action.

Hemodynamics: Excessive blood levels may cause changes in cardiac output, total peripheral resistance, and mean arterial pressure. These changes may be attributable to a direct depressant effect of the local anesthetic agent on various components of the cardiovascular system. The net effect is normally a modest hypotension when the recommended dosages are not exceeded.

Pharmacokinetics and metabolism: Lidocaine is absorbed following topical administration to mucous membranes, its rate and extent of absorption being dependent upon concentration and total dose administered, the specific site of application, and duration of exposure. In general, the rate of absorption of local anesthetic agents following topical application occurs most rapidly after intratracheal administration. Lidocaine is also well-absorbed from the gastro-intestinal tract, but little intact drug appears in the circulation because of biotransformation in the liver.

The plasma binding of lidocaine is dependent on drug concentration, and the fraction bound decreases with increasing concentration. At concentrations of 1 to 4 ug of free base per ml, 60 to 80 percent of lidocaine is protein bound. Binding is also dependent on the plasma concentration of the alpha-1-acid glycoprotein.

Lidocaine crosses the blood-brain and placental barriers, presumably by passive diffusion.

Lidocaine is metabolized rapidly by the liver, and metabolites and unchanged drug are excreted by the kidneys. Biotransformation includes oxidative N-dealkylation, ring hydroxylation, cleavage of the amide linkage, and conjugation. N-dealkylation, a major pathway of biotransformation, yields the metabolites monoethylglycinexylidide and glycinexylidide. The pharmacological/ toxicological actions of these metabolites are similar to, but less potent than, those of lidocaine. Approximately 90% of lidocaine administered is excreted in the form of various metabolites, and less than 10% is excreted unchanged. The primary metabolite in urine is a conjugate of 4-hydroxy-2, 6-dimethylaniline.

The elimination half-life of lidocaine following an intravenous bolus injection is typically 1.5 to 2.0 hours. Because of the rapid rate at which lidocaine is metabolized, any condition that affects liver function may alter lidocaine kinetics. The half-life may be prolonged two-fold or more in patients with liver dysfunction. Renal dysfunction does not affect lidocaine kinetics but may increase the accumulation of metabolites.

Factors such as acidosis and the use of CNS stimulants and depressants affect the CNS levels of lidocaine required to produce overt systemic effects. Objective adverse manifestations become increasingly apparent with increasing venous plasma levels above 6.0 ug free base per ml. In the rhesus monkey arterial blood levels of 18–21 ug/ml have been shown to be threshold for convulsive activity.

INDICATIONS AND USAGE

Xylocaine (lidocaine HCl)2% Viscous Solution is indicated for the production of topical anesthesia of irritated or inflamed mucous membranes of the mouth and pharynx. It is also useful for reducing gagging during the taking of X-ray pictures and dental impressions.

CONTRAINDICATIONS

Lidocaine is contraindicated in patients with a known history of hypersensitivity to local anesthetics of the amide type, or to other components of the solution.

WARNINGS

EXCESSIVE DOSAGE, OR SHORT INTERVALS BETWEEN DOSES, CAN RESULT IN HIGH PLASMA LEVELS AND SERIOUS ADVERSE EFFECTS. PATIENTS SHOULD BE INSTRUCTED TO STRICTLY ADHERE TO THE RECOMMENDED DOSAGE AND ADMINISTRATION GUIDELINES AS SET FORTH IN THIS PACKAGE INSERT.

THE MANAGEMENT OF SERIOUS ADVERSE REACTIONS MAY REQUIRE THE USE OF RESUSCITATIVE EQUIPMENT, OXYGEN, AND OTHER RESUSCITATIVE DRUGS.

Xylocaine 2% Viscous Solution should be used with extreme caution if the mucosa in the area of application has been traumatized, since under such conditions there is the potential for rapid systemic absorption.

PRECAUTIONS

General: The safety and effectiveness of lidocaine depend on proper dosage, correct technique, adequate precautions, and readiness for emergencies (See WARNINGS and ADVERSE REACTIONS). The lowest dosage that results in effective anethesia should be used to avoid high plasma levels and serious adverse effects. Repeated doses of lidocaine may cause significant increases in blood levels with each repeated dose because of slow accumulation of the drug and /or its metabolites. Tolerance varies with the status of the patient. Debilitated, elderly patients, acutely ill patients, and children should be given reduced doses commensurate with their age, weight and physical condition. Lidocaine should also be used with caution in patients with severe shock or heart block.

Xylocaine 2% Viscous Solution should be used with caution in persons with known drug sensitivities. Patients allergic to para-aminobenzoic acid derivatives (procaine, tetracaine, benzocaine, etc.) have not shown cross sensitivity to lidocaine.

Information for Patients: When topical anesthetics are used in the mouth or throat, the patient should be aware that the production of topical anesthesia may impair swallowing and

Continued on next page

Astra—Cont.

thus enhance the danger of aspiration. For this reason, food should not be ingested for 60 minutes following use of local anesthetic preparations in the mouth or throat area. This is particularly important in children because of their frequency of eating.
Numbness of the tongue or buccal mucosa may increase the danger of biting trauma. For this reason food and/or chewing gum should not be used while the mouth or throat area is anesthetized.
PATIENTS SHOULD BE INSTRUCTED TO STRICTLY ADHERE TO DOSING INSTRUCTIONS, AND TO KEEP THE SUPPLY OF MEDICATION OUT OF REACH OF CHILDREN.
Carcinogenesis, mutagenesis, impairment of fertility: Studies of lidocaine in animals to evaluate the carcinogenic and mutagenic potential or the effect on fertility have not been conducted.
Pregnancy: Teratogenic Effects. Pregnancy Category B. Reproduction studies have been performed in rats at doses up to 6.6 times the human dose and have revealed no evidence of harm to the fetus caused by lidocaine. There are, however, no adequate and well-controlled studies in pregnant women. Because animal reproduction studies are not always predictive of human response, this drug should be used in pregnancy only if clearly needed.
Nursing mothers: It is not known whether this drug is excreted in human milk. Because many drugs are excreted in human milk, caution should be exercised when lidocaine is administered to nursing women.
Pediatric use: Dosages in children should be reduced, commensurate with age, body weight and physical condition. See DOSAGE AND ADMINISTRATION.

ADVERSE REACTIONS

Adverse experiences following the adminstration of lidocaine are similar in nature to those observed with other amide local anesthetic agents. These adverse experiences are, in general, dose-related and may result from high plasma levels caused by excessive dosage or rapid absorption, or may result from a hypersensitivity, idiosyncrasy or diminished tolerance on the part of the patient. Serious adverse experiences are generally systemic in nature. The following types are those most commonly reported:
Central nervous system: CNS manifestations are excitatory and/or depressant and may be characterized by lightheadedness, nervousness, apprehension, euphoria, confusion, dizziness, drowsiness, tinnitus, blurred or double vision, vomiting, sensations of heat, cold or numbness, twitching, tremors, convulsions, unconsciousness, respiratory depression and arrest. The excitatory manifestations may be very brief or may not occur at all, in which case the first manifestation of toxicity may be drowsiness merging into unconsciousness and respiratory arrest.
Drowsiness following the administration of lidocaine is usually an early sign of a high blood level of the drug and may occur as a consequence of rapid absorption.
Cardiovascular system: Cardiovascular manifestations are usually depressant and are characterized by bradycardia, hypotension, and cardiovascular collapse, which may lead to cardiac arrest.
Allergic: Allergic reactions are characterized by cutaneous lesions, urticaria, edema or anaphylactoid reactions. Allergic reactions may occur as a result of sensitivity either to the local anesthetic agent or to the methylparaben and/or propylparaben used in this formulation. Allergic reactions as a result of sensitivity to lidocaine are extremely rare and, if they occur, should be managed by conventional means. The detection of sensitivity by skin testing is of doubtful value.

OVERDOSAGE

Acute emergencies from local anesthetics are generally related to high plasma levels encountered during therapeutic use of local anesthetics (see ADVERSE REACTIONS, WARNINGS, and PRECAUTIONS).
Management of local anesthetic emergencies: The first consideration is prevention, best accomplished by careful and constant monitoring of cardiovascular and respiratory vital signs and the patient's state of consciousness after each local anesthetic administration.
The first step in the management of convulsions consists of immediate attention to the maintenance of a patent airway and assisted or controlled ventilation with oxygen. In situations where trained personnel are readily available, ventilation should be maintained and oxygen should be delivered by a delivery system capable of permitting immediate positive airway pressure by mask. Immediately after the institution of these ventilatory measures, the adequacy of the circulation should be evaluated, keeping in mind that drugs used to treat convulsions sometimes depress the circulation when administered intravenously. Should convulsions persist despite adequate respiratory support, and if the status of the circulation permits, small increments of an ultra-short acting barbiturate (such as thiopental or thiamylal) or a benzodiazepine (such as diazepam) may be administered intravenously. The clinician should be familiar, prior to use of local anesthetics, with these anticonvulsant drugs. Supportive treatment of circulatory depression may require administration of intravenous fluids and, when appropriate, a vasopressor as indicated by the clinical situation (e.g., ephedrine).
If not treated immediately, both convulsions and cardiovascular depression can result in hypoxia, acidosis, bradycardia, arrhythmias and cardiac arrest. If cardiac arrest should occur, standard cardiopulmonary resuscitative measures should be instituted.
Dialysis is of negligible value in the treatment of acute overdosage with lidocaine.
The oral LD_{50} of lidocaine in non-fasted female rats is 459 (346–773) mg/kg (as the salt) and 214 (159–324) mg/kg (as the salt) in fasted female rats.

DOSAGE AND ADMINISTRATION

Adult
The maximum recommended single dose of Xylocaine (lidocaine HCl) 2% Viscous Solution for healthy adults should be such that the dose of lidocaine HCl does not exceed 4.5 mg/kg or 2 mg/lb body weight and does not in any case exceed a total of 300 mg.
For symptomatic treatment of irritated or inflamed mucous membranes of the mouth and pharynx, the usual adult dose is one 15 ml tablespoonful undiluted. For use in the mouth, the solution should be swished around in the mouth and spit out. For use on the pharynx, the undiluted solution should be gargled and may be swallowed. This dose should not be administered at intervals of less than three hours, and not more than eight doses should be given in a 24-hour period.
The dosage should be adjusted commensurate with the patient's age, weight and physical condition (see PRECAUTIONS).
Pediatric
It is difficult to recommend a maximum dose of any drug for children since this varies as function of age and weight. For children over 3 years of age who have a normal lean body mass and normal body development, the maximum dose is determined by the childs weight or age. For example: in a child of 5 years weighing 50 lbs., the dose of lidocaine hydrochloride should not exceed 75–100 mg (3/4 to 1 teaspoonful).
For infants and in children under 3 years of age, 1/4 teaspoon of the solution should be accurately measured and applied to the immediate area with a cotton-tipped applicator. This dose should not be administered at intervals of less than three hours. Not more than four doses should be given in a 12-hour period.

HOW SUPPLIED

Xylocaine 2% (lidocaine HCl) Viscous Solution is available in 100 ml (NDC 0186-0360-01) and 450 ml (NDC 0186-0360-11) polyethylene squeeze bottles and in unit of use (adult dose) packages of 25 (20 ml) polyethylene bottles (NDC 0186-0361-78).
The solutions should be stored at controlled room temperature 15°–30°C (59°–86°F).
021833-00 1/83

YUTOPAR® ℞

[*yoo̅ 'tow-par*]
(ritodrine hydrochloride)
Sterile Solution and Tablets

CAUTION: Federal law prohibits dispensing without prescription.

DESCRIPTION

Yutopar, which contains the betamimetic (beta sympathomimetic amine) ritodrine hydrochloride, is available in two dosage forms. Yutopar for parenteral (intravenous) use is a clear, colorless, sterile, aqueous solution; each milliliter contains either 10 mg. or 15 mg. of ritodrine hydrochloride, 0.44% (w/v) of acetic acid, 0.24% (w/v) of sodium hydroxide, 0.1% (w/v) of sodium metabisulfite, and 0.29% (w/v) of sodium chloride in water for injection USP. Hydrochloric acid or additional sodium hydroxide is used to adjust pH. **FOR INTRAVENOUS USE ONLY. MUST BE DILUTED BEFORE USE. FOR DOSAGE AND ADMINISTRATION INSTRUCTIONS, SEE PRODUCT INFORMATION BELOW. DO NOT USE IF SOLUTION IS DISCOLORED OR CONTAINS A PRECIPITATE.**
Each Yutopar tablet contains 10 mg. of ritodrine hydrochloride.
Ritodrine hydrochloride is a white, odorless crystalline powder, freely soluble in water, with a melting point between 196° and 205° C. The chemical name of ritodrine hydrochloride is erythro-p-hydroxy-α-[1[(p-hydroxyphenethyl)-amino]ethyl]benzyl alcohol hydrochloride and has the chemical structure:

HO–C₆H₄–CH(OH)–CH(CH₃)–NH–CH₂–CH₂–C₆H₄–OH •HCl

CLINICAL PHARMACOLOGY

Yutopar (ritodrine hydrochloride) is a beta-receptor agonist, which has been shown by *in vitro* and *in vivo* pharmacologic studies in animals to exert a preferential effect on the β_2 adrenergic receptors such as those in the uterine smooth muscle. Stimulation of the β_2 receptors inhibits contractility of the uterine smooth muscle.
In humans, intravenous infusions of 0.05 to 0.30 mg./min. or single oral doses of 10 to 20 mg. decreased the intensity and frequency of uterine contractions. These effects were antagonized by beta-blocking compounds. Intravenous administration induced an immediate dose-related elevation of heart rate with maximum mean increases between 19 and 40 beats per minute. Widening of the pulse pressure was also observed; the average increase in systolic blood pressure was 4.0 mm. Hg, and the average decrease in diastolic pressure was 12.3 mm. Hg. With oral intake, the increase in heart rate was mild and delayed.
During intravenous infusion in humans, transient elevations of blood glucose, insulin, and free fatty acids have been observed. Decreased serum potassium has also been found, but effects on other electrolytes have not been reported.
Serum kinetics in humans (non-pregnant females) of an intravenous infusion of 60 minutes duration were determined by measuring serum ritodrine levels by a radioimmunoassay technique. Three half-lives were calculated: the first of 6 to 9 minutes dominated the ascending phase of the serum drug-level curve; the second phase of 1.7 to 2.6 hours dominated the descending curve; and finally, a third phase, with a half-life of more than 10 hours, was discernible. In a study of serum kinetics after oral ingestion (male subjects), the decline of serum drug levels could be described in terms of a two-phase decay with an initial half-life of 1.3 hours and a final half-life of 12 hours. With either route of administration, 90% of the excretion was completed within 24 hours after the dose.
Comparison of ritodrine serum levels after intravenous administration with those after oral dosage indicates the oral bioavailability is about 30%. Intravenous infusion at a rate of 0.15 mg./min. for 1 hour yielded maximum serum levels ranging between 32 and 52 ng./ml. in a group of 6 non-pregnant female volunteers; maximum serum levels following single and repeated (4 × 10 mg./24 hr.) 10 mg. oral doses ranged between 5 and 15 ng./ml. and were obtained within 30 to 60 minutes after ingestion.
Placental transfer was confirmed by measurement of drug concentrations in cord blood showing that ritodrine and its conjugates reach the fetal circulation.

INDICATIONS AND USAGE

Yutopar is indicated for the management of preterm labor in suitable patients.
Administered intravenously, the drug will decrease uterine activity and thus prolong gestation in the majority of such patients. After intravenous Yutopar has arrested the acute episode, oral administration may help to avert relapse. Additional acute episodes may be treated by repeating the intravenous infusion. The incidence of neonatal mortality and respiratory distress syndrome increases when the normal gestation period is shortened.
Since successful inhibition of labor is more likely with early treatment, therapy with Yutopar should be instituted as soon as the diagnosis of preterm labor is established and contraindications ruled out in pregnancies of 20 or more weeks' gestation. The efficacy and safety of Yutopar in advanced labor, that is, when cervical dilatation is more than 4 cm. or effacement is more than 80%, have not been established.

CONTRAINDICATIONS

Yutopar is contraindicated before the 20th week of pregnancy.
Yutopar is also contraindicated in those conditions of the mother or fetus in which continuation of pregnancy is hazardous; specific contraindications include:

1. Antepartum hemorrhage which demands immediate delivery
2. Eclampsia and severe preeclampsia
3. Intrauterine fetal death
4. Chorioamnionitis
5. Maternal cardiac disease
6. Pulmonary hypertension
7. Maternal hyperthyroidism
8. Uncontrolled maternal diabetes mellitus (See PRECAUTIONS.)
9. Pre-existing maternal medical conditions that would be seriously affected by the known pharmacologic properties of a betamimetic drug; such as: hypovolemia, cardiac arrhythmias associated with tachycardia or digitalis intoxication, uncontrolled hypertension, pheochromocytoma, bronchial asthma already treated by betamimetics and/or steroids
10. Known hypersensitivity to any component of the product

WARNINGS

> Maternal pulmonary edema has been reported in patients treated with Yutopar, sometimes after delivery. It has occurred more often when patients were treated concomitantly with corticosteroids. Maternal death from this condition has been reported with or without corticosteroids given concomitantly with drugs of this class.
>
> Patients so treated must be closely monitored in the hospital. The patient's state of hydration should be carefully monitored; fluid overload must be avoided. (See DOSAGE AND ADMINISTRATION.) Intravenous fluid loading may be aggravated by the use of betamimetics with or without corticosteroids and may turn into manifest circulatory overloading with subsequent pulmonary edema. If pulmonary edema develops during administration, the drug should be discontinued. Edema should be managed by conventional means.

Intravenous administration of Yutopar should be supervised by persons having knowledge of the pharmacology of the drug and who are qualified to identify and manage complications of drug administration and pregnancy. *Because cardiovascular responses are common and more pronounced during intravenous administration of Yutopar, cardiovascular effects, including maternal pulse rate and blood pressure and fetal heart rate, should be closely monitored. Care should be exercised for maternal signs and symptoms of pulmonary edema. A persistent high tachycardia (over 140 beats per minute) may be one of the signs of impending pulmonary edema with drugs of this class. Occult cardiac disease may be unmasked with the use of Yutopar. If the patient complains of chest pain or tightness of chest, the drug should be temporarily discontinued and an ECG should be done as soon as possible.*

The drug should not be administered to patients with mild to moderate preeclampsia, hypertension, or diabetes unless the attending physician considers that the benefits clearly outweigh the risks.

Yutopar Solution contains sodium metabisulfite, a sulfite that may cause serious allergic-type reactions (e.g., hives, itching, wheezing, anaphylaxis) in certain susceptible persons. Although the overall incidence of sulfite sensitivity in the general population is probably low, it is seen more frequently in asthmatics or in atopic nonasthmatic persons.

PRECAUTIONS

When Yutopar is used for the management of preterm labor in a patient with premature rupture of the membranes, the benefits of delaying delivery should be balanced against the potential risks of development of chorioamnionitis.

Among low birth weight infants, approximately 9% may be growth retarded for gestational age. Therefore, Intra-Uterine Growth Retardation (IUGR) should be considered in the differential diagnosis of preterm labor; this is especially important when the gestational age is in doubt. The decision to continue or reinitiate the administration of Yutopar will depend on an assessment of fetal maturity. In addition to clinical parameters, other studies, such as sonography or amniocentesis, may be helpful in establishing the state of fetal maturity if it is in doubt.

Baseline EKG

This should be done to rule out occult maternal heart disease.

Laboratory Tests

Because intravenous administration of Yutopar has been shown to elevate plasma insulin and glucose and to decrease plasma potassium concentrations, monitoring of glucose and electrolyte levels is recommended during protracted infusions. Decrease of plasma potassium concentrations is usually transient, returning to normal within 24 hours. Special attention should be paid to biochemical variables when treating diabetic patients or those receiving potassium-depleting diuretics.

Serial hemograms may be helpful as an index of state of hydration.

Drug Interactions

Corticosteroids used concomitantly may lead to pulmonary edema. (See Warnings.)

Cardiovascular effects of Yutopar solution (especially cardiac arrhythmia or hypotension) may be potentiated by concomitant use of the following drugs.

1. magnesium sulfate
2. diazoxide
3. meperidine
4. potent general anesthetic agents

Systemic hypertension may be exaggerated in the presence of parasympatholytic agents such as atropine.

The effects of other sympathomimetic amines may be potentiated when concurrently administered and these effects may be additive. A sufficient time interval should elapse prior to administration of another sympathomimetic drug.

With either oral or intravenous administration, 90% of the excretion of Yutopar is completed within 24 hours after the dose. (See CLINICAL PHARMACOLOGY.)

Beta-adrenergic blocking drugs inhibit the action of Yutopar; coadministration of these drugs should, therefore, be avoided.

With anesthetics used in surgery, the possibility that hypotensive effects may be potentiated should be considered.

Migraine Headache

Transient cerebral ischemia associated with beta sympathomimetic therapy has been reported in two patients with migraine headache.

Carcinogenesis, Mutagenesis, Impairment of Fertility

In rats given oral doses of 1, 10 and 150 mg./kg./day of ritodrine hydrochloride for 82 weeks, benign and malignant tumors were found in the various dosage groups. Since there were no important differences between untreated controls and treated groups and no dose-related trends, it was concluded that there was no evidence of tumorigenicity. The incidence (2–4%) of tumors of the type found in this study is not unusual in this species.

Reproduction studies in rats and rabbits have revealed no evidence of impaired fertility due to ritodrine hydrochloride.

Pregnancy

Teratogenic Effects

(Pregnancy Category B)

Reproduction studies were performed in rats and rabbits. The doses employed intravenously were 1/9 (1 mg./kg.), 1/3 (3 mg./kg.), and 1 (9 mg./kg.) times the maximum human daily intravenous dose (but given to the animals as a bolus rather than by infusion). The oral doses, 10 and 100 mg./kg. represented 5 and 50 times the maximum human daily oral maintenance dose. The results of these studies have revealed no evidence of impaired fertility or harm to the fetus due to ritodrine hydrochloride.

No adverse fetal effects were encountered when single intravenous doses of 1, 3, and 9 mg./kg./day or oral doses of 10 and 100 mg./kg./day were given to rats and rabbits on Days 6 through 15 and 6 through 18 of gestation, respectively. Intravenous doses of 1 and 8 mg./kg./day or oral doses of 10 and 100 mg./kg./day administered to the mother from Day 15 of pregnancy to Day 21 postpartum did not affect perinatal or postnatal development in rats. A slight increase in fetal weight in the rat was observed. Oral administration to both sexes did not impair fertility or reproductive performance. Lethal doses to pregnant rats did not cause immediate fetal demise. There are no adequate and well-controlled studies of Yutopar effects in pregnant women before 20 weeks' gestation; *therefore, this drug should not be used before the 20th week of pregnancy.* Studies of Yutopar administered to pregnant women from the 20th week of gestation have not shown increased risk of fetal abnormalities. Follow-up of selected variables in a small number of children for up to 2 years has not revealed harmful effects on growth, developmental or functional maturation. Nonetheless, although clinical studies did not demonstrate a risk of permanent adverse fetal effects from Yutopar, the possibility cannot be excluded; therefore, Yutopar should be used only when clearly indicated.

Some studies indicate that infants born before 36 weeks' gestation make up less than 10% of all births but account for as many as 75% of perinatal deaths and one-half of all neurologically handicapped infants. There are data available indicating that infants born at any time prior to full term may manifest a higher incidence of neurologic or other handicaps than occurs in the total population of infants born at or after full term. In delaying or preventing preterm labor, the use of Yutopar should result in an overall increase in neonatal survival. Handicapped infants who might not have otherwise survived may survive.

ADVERSE REACTIONS

The unwanted effects of Yutopar are related to its betamimetic activity and usually are controlled by suitable dosage adjustment.

Effects Associated with Intravenous Administration

Usual effects (80–100% of patients)

Intravenous infusion of Yutopar leads almost invariably to dose-related alterations in maternal and fetal heart rates and in maternal blood pressure. During clinical studies in which the maximum infusion rate was limited to 0.35 mg./min. (one patient received 0.40 mg./min.), the maximum maternal and fetal heart rates averaged, respectively, 130 (range 60 to 180) and 164 (range 130 to 200) beats per minute. The maximum maternal systolic blood pressures averaged 128 mm. Hg (range 96 to 162 mm. Hg), an average increase of 12 mm. Hg from pretreatment levels. The minimum maternal diastolic blood pressures averaged 48 mm. Hg (range 0 to 76 mm. Hg), an average decrease of 23 mm. Hg from pretreatment levels. While the more severe effects were usually managed effectively by dosage adjustments, in less than 1% of patients, persistent maternal tachycardia or decreased diastolic blood pressure required withdrawal of the drug. A persistent high tachycardia (over 140 beats per minute) may be one of the signs of impending pulmonary edema. (See WARNINGS.)

Yutopar infusion is associated with transient elevation of blood glucose and insulin, which decreases toward normal values after 48 to 72 hours despite continued infusion. Elevation of free fatty acids and cAMP has been reported. Reduction of potassium levels should be expected; other biochemical effects have not been reported.

Frequent effects (10–50% of patients)

Intravenous Yutopar, in about one-third of the patients, was associated with palpitation. Tremor, nausea, vomiting, headache, or erythema was observed in 10 to 15% of patients.

Occasional effects (5–10% of patients)

Nervousness, jitteriness, restlessness, emotional upset, or anxiety was reported in 5 to 6% of patients and malaise in similar numbers.

Infrequent effects (1–3% of patients)

Cardiac symptoms including chest pain or tightness (rarely associated with abnormalities of ECG) and arrhythmia were reported in 1 to 2% of patients. (See Warnings.)

Other infrequently reported maternal effects included: anaphylactic shock, rash, heart murmur, epigastric distress, ileus, bloating, constipation, diarrhea, dyspnea, hyperventilation, hemolytic icterus, glycosuria, lactic acidosis, sweating, chills, drowsiness, and weakness.

Neonatal Effects

Infrequently reported neonatal symptoms include hypoglycemia and ileus. In addition, hypocalcemia and hypotension have been reported in neonates whose mothers were treated with other betamimetic agents.

Effects Associated with Oral Administration

Frequent effects (<50% of patients)

Oral ritodrine in clinical studies was often associated with small increases in maternal heart rate, but little or no effect upon either maternal systolic or diastolic blood pressure or upon fetal heart rate was found.

Oral ritodrine in 10 to 15% of patients was associated with palpitation or tremor. Nausea and jitterness were less frequent (5 to 8%), while rash was observed in some patients (3 to 4%), and arrhythmia was infrequent (about 1%).

OVERDOSAGE

The symptoms of overdosage are those of excessive beta-adrenergic stimulation including exaggeration of the known pharmacologic effects, the most prominent being tachycardia (maternal and fetal), palpitation, cardiac arrhythmia, hypotension, dyspnea, nervousness, tremor, nausea, and vomiting. If an excess of ritodrine tablets is ingested, gastric lavage or induction of emesis should be carried out followed by administration of activated charcoal. When symptoms of overdose occur as a result of intravenous administration, ritodrine should be discontinued; an appropriate beta-blocking agent may be used as an antidote. Ritodrine hydrochloride is dialyzable.

Acute intravenous toxicity was studied in rats and rabbits and acute oral toxicity in mice, rats, guinea pigs, and dogs. The LD50 values in the most sensitive of the species used were 64 mg./kg. intravenously in the nonpregnant rabbit and 540 mg./kg. orally in the nonpregnant mouse. The intravenous LD50 value in the pregnant rat was 85 mg./kg. The amount of drug required to produce symptoms of overdose in humans is individually variable. No reports of human mortality due to overdose have been received.

DOSAGE AND ADMINISTRATION

In the management of preterm labor, the initial intravenous treatment should usually be followed by oral administration. The optimum dose of Yutopar is determined by a clinical balance of uterine response and unwanted effects.

Intravenous Therapy

Do not use intravenous Yutopar if the solution is discolored or contains any precipitate or particulate matter. Yutopar solution should be used promptly after preparation, but in no case after 48 hours of preparation.

Method of Administration: To minimize the risks of hypotension, the patient should be maintained in the left lateral position throughout infusion and careful attention given to her state of hydration, but fluid overload must be avoided.

For appropriate control and dose titration, a controlled infusion device is recommended to adjust the rate of flow in drops/minute. An i.v. microdrip chamber (60 drops/ml.) can provide a convenient range of infusion rates within the recommended dose range for Yutopar.

Recommended Dilution: 150 mg. ritodrine hydrochloride in 500 ml. fluid yielding a final concentration of 0.3 mg./ml*. Ritodrine for intravenous infusion should be diluted with 5% w/v dextrose solution. Because of the increased probability of pulmonary edema, saline diluents such as:

—0.9% w/v sodium chloride solution,

—compound sodium chloride solution (Ringer's solution)

—and Hartmann's solution, should be reserved for cases where dextrose solution is medically undesirable e.g. diabetes mellitus.

*In those cases where fluid restriction is medically desirable, a more concentrated solution may be prepared.

Intravenous therapy should be started as soon as possible after diagnosis. The usual initial dose is 0.1 mg./minute (0.33 ml./min., 20 drops/min. using a microdrip chamber at the

Continued on next page

Astra—Cont.

recommended dilution), to be gradually increased according to the results by 0.05 mg./minute (0.17 ml./min., 10 drops/-min. using a microdrip chamber at the recommended dilution) every 10 minutes until the desired result is attained. The effective dosage usually lies between 0.15 and 0.35 mg./minute (0.50 to 1.17 ml./min., 30–70 drops/min. using a microdrip chamber at the recommended dilution). Frequent monitoring of maternal uterine contractions, heart rate, and blood pressure, and of fetal heart rate is required, with dosage individually titrated according to response. If other drugs need to be given intravenously, the use of "piggyback" or other site of intravenous administration permits the continued independent control of the rate of infusion of the Yutopar.
The infusion should generally be continued for at least 12 hours after uterine contractions cease. With the recommended dilution, the maximum volume of fluid that might be administered after 12 hours at the highest dose (0.35 mg./min.) will be approximately 840 ml.
The amount of i.v. fluids administered and the rate of administration should be monitored to avoid circulatory fluid overload (over-hydration). (See PRECAUTIONS, *Laboratory Tests.*)
Oral Maintenance
One tablet (10 mg.) may be given approximately 30 minutes before the termination of intravenous therapy. The usual dosage schedule for the first 24 hours of oral administration is 1 tablet (10 mg.) every two hours. Thereafter, the usual maintenance is 1 or 2 tablets (10 to 20 mg.) every four to six hours, the dose depending on uterine activity and unwanted effects. The total daily dose of oral ritodrine should not exceed 120 mg. The treatment may be continued as long as the physician considers it desirable to prolong pregnancy.
Recurrence of unwanted preterm labor may be treated with repeated infusion of Yutopar.
How Supplied:
NDC 0186-0599-03: 5 ml. ampuls in boxes of 10. Each ampul contains 50 mg. (10 mg./ml.) of ritodrine hydrochloride.
NDC 0186-0597-12: 10 ml vial in boxes of 6. Each vial contains 150 mg (15 mg/ml) of ritodrine hydrochloride.
NDC 0186-0595-60: 10 mg. tablets in bottles of 60. Each round, yellow tablet contains 10 mg. ritodrine hydrochloride and is inscribed YUTOPAR on one side and scored on the other.
NDC 0186-0595-78: 10 mg unit dose tablets in boxes of 100. Each round, yellow tablet contains 10 mg. ritodrine hydrochloride and is inscribed YUTOPAR on one side and scored on the other.
NDC 0186-0644-01: 10 ml syringe in boxes of 10. Each syringe contains 150 mg (15 mg/ml) of ritodrine hydrochloride.
Both the tablet and intravenous dosage forms should be stored at room temperature, preferably below 86°F. (30°C). Protect from excessive heat.
Oral dosage form manufactured by DUPHAR B.V., Amsterdam, Holland for
ASTRA®
Astra Pharmaceuticals Products, Inc.
Westborough MA 01581
Yutopar® licensed by Duphar B. V. Amsterdam, Holland
021843R04 3/86

For information on Astra products, write to:
Professional Information Dept.
Astra Pharmaceutical Products, Inc.
50 Otis Street
Westborough Massachusetts 01581-4428

Important Notice
Before prescribing or administering any product described in PHYSICIANS' DESK REFERENCE always consult the PDR Supplement for possible new or revised information

Ayerst Laboratories
Division of American Home Products Corporation
685 THIRD AVE.
NEW YORK, NY 10017-4071

ANTABUSE® ℞
[*an'tah-būse*]
Brand of disulfiram
In Alcoholism

CAUTION: Federal law prohibits dispensing without prescription.

WARNING
ANTABUSE should never be administered to a patient when he is in a state of alcohol intoxication, or without his full knowledge.
The physician should instruct relatives accordingly.

DESCRIPTION
CHEMICAL NAME: bis(diethylthiocarbamoyl) disulfide
STRUCTURAL FORMULA:

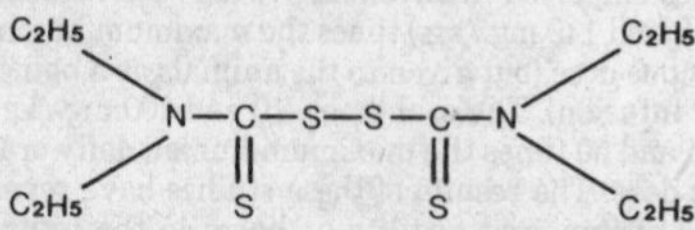

ANTABUSE occurs as a white to off-white, odorless, and almost tasteless powder, soluble in water to the extent of about 20 mg in 100 mL, and in alcohol to the extent of about 3.8 g in 100 mL.
ANTABUSE contains these inactive ingredients:
Magnesium Aluminum Silicate
Magnesium Stearate, NF
Povidone, USP
Starch, NF

ACTION
ANTABUSE produces a sensitivity to alcohol which results in a highly unpleasant reaction when the patient under treatment ingests even small amounts of alcohol.
ANTABUSE blocks the oxidation of alcohol at the acetaldehyde stage. During alcohol metabolism after ANTABUSE intake, the concentration of acetaldehyde occurring in the blood may be 5 to 10 times higher than that found during metabolism of the same amount of alcohol alone.
Accumulation of acetaldehyde in the blood produces the complex of highly unpleasant symptoms referred to hereinafter as the ANTABUSE-alcohol reaction. This reaction, which is proportional to the dosage of both ANTABUSE (disulfiram) and alcohol, will persist as long as alcohol is being metabolized. ANTABUSE does not appear to influence the rate of alcohol elimination from the body.
ANTABUSE is slowly absorbed from the gastrointestinal tract and is slowly eliminated from the body. One (or even two) weeks after a patient has taken his last dose of ANTABUSE, ingestion of alcohol may produce unpleasant symptoms.
Prolonged administration of ANTABUSE does not produce tolerance; the longer a patient remains on therapy, the more exquisitely sensitive he becomes to alcohol.

INDICATION
ANTABUSE (disulfiram) is an aid in the management of selected chronic alcoholic patients who want to remain in a state of enforced sobriety so that supportive and psychotherapeutic treatment may be applied to best advantage. (Used alone, without proper motivation and without supportive therapy, ANTABUSE is not a cure for alcoholism, and it is unlikely that it will have more than a brief effect on the drinking pattern of the chronic alcoholic.)

CONTRAINDICATIONS
Patients who are receiving or have recently received metronidazole, paraldehyde, alcohol, or alcohol-containing preparations, *eg*, cough syrups, tonics and the like, should not be given ANTABUSE.
ANTABUSE is contraindicated in the presence of severe myocardial disease or coronary occlusion, psychoses, and hypersensitivity to disulfiram or to other thiuram derivatives used in pesticides and rubber vulcanization.

WARNINGS

ANTABUSE (disulfiram) should never be administered to a patient when he is in a state of alcohol intoxication, or without his full knowledge.
The physician should instruct relatives accordingly.

The patient must be fully informed of the ANTABUSE-alcohol reaction. He must be strongly cautioned against surreptitious drinking while taking the drug and he must be fully aware of possible consequences. He should be warned to avoid alcohol in disguised form, *ie*, in sauces, vinegars, cough mixtures, and even aftershave lotions and back rubs. He should also be warned that reactions may occur with alcohol up to 14 days after ingesting ANTABUSE.
The ANTABUSE-ALCOHOL REACTION: ANTABUSE plus alcohol, even small amounts, produces flushing, throbbing in head and neck, throbbing headache, respiratory difficulty, nausea, copious vomiting, sweating, thirst, chest pain, palpitation, dyspnea, hyperventilation, tachycardia, hypotension, syncope, marked uneasiness, weakness, vertigo, blurred vision, and confusion. In severe reactions there may be respiratory depression, cardiovascular collapse, arrhythmias, myocardial infarction, acute congestive heart failure, unconsciousness, convulsions, and death.
The intensity of the reaction varies with each individual, but is generally proportional to the amounts of ANTABUSE and alcohol ingested. Mild reactions may occur in the sensitive individual when the blood alcohol concentration is increased to as little as 5 to 10 mg per 100 mL. Symptoms are fully developed at 50 mg per 100 mL and unconsciousness usually results when the blood alcohol level reaches 125 to 150 mg.
The duration of the reaction varies from 30 to 60 minutes, to several hours in the more severe cases, or as long as there is alcohol in the blood.
DRUG INTERACTIONS: Disulfiram appears to decrease the rate at which certain drugs are metabolized and so may increase the blood levels and the possibility of clinical toxicity of drugs given concomitantly.
DISULFIRAM SHOULD BE USED WITH CAUTION IN THOSE PATIENTS RECEIVING PHENYTOIN AND ITS CONGENERS, SINCE THE CONCOMITANT ADMINISTRATION OF THESE TWO DRUGS CAN LEAD TO PHENYTOIN INTOXICATION. PRIOR TO ADMINISTERING DISULFIRAM TO A PATIENT ON PHENYTOIN THERAPY, A BASELINE PHENYTOIN SERUM LEVEL SHOULD BE OBTAINED. SUBSEQUENT TO INITIATION OF DISULFIRAM THERAPY, SERUM LEVELS ON PHENYTOIN SHOULD BE DETERMINED ON DIFFERENT DAYS FOR EVIDENCE OF AN INCREASE OR FOR A CONTINUING RISE IN LEVELS. INCREASED PHENYTOIN LEVELS SHOULD BE TREATED WITH APPROPRIATE DOSAGE ADJUSTMENT.
It may be necessary to adjust the dosage of oral anticoagulants upon beginning or stopping disulfiram, since disulfiram may prolong prothrombin time.
Patients taking isoniazid when disulfiram is given should be observed for the appearance of unsteady gait or marked changes in mental status and the disulfiram discontinued if such signs appear.
In rats, simultaneous ingestion of disulfiram and nitrite in the diet for 78 weeks has been reported to cause tumors, and it has been suggested that disulfiram may react with nitrites in the rat stomach to form a nitrosamine, which is tumorigenic. Disulfiram alone in the diet of rats did not lead to such tumors. The relevance of this finding to humans is not known at this time.
CONCOMITANT CONDITIONS: Because of the possibility of an accidental ANTABUSE-alcohol reaction, ANTABUSE (disulfiram) should be used with extreme caution in patients with any of the following conditions: diabetes mellitus, hypothyroidism, epilepsy, cerebral damage, chronic and acute nephritis, hepatic cirrhosis or insufficiency.
USAGE IN PREGNANCY: The safe use of this drug in pregnancy has not been established. Therefore, ANTABUSE should be used during pregnancy only when, in the judgment of the physician, the probable benefits outweigh the possible risks.

PRECAUTIONS
Patients with a history of rubber contact dermatitis should be evaluated for hypersensitivity to thiuram derivatives before receiving ANTABUSE (see Contraindications).
It is suggested that every patient under treatment carry an Identification Card, stating that he is receiving ANTABUSE and describing the symptoms most likely to occur as a result of the ANTABUSE-alcohol reaction. In addition, this card should indicate the physician or institution to be contacted in emergency. (Cards may be obtained from Ayerst Laboratories upon request.)
Alcoholism may accompany or be followed by dependence on narcotics or sedatives. Barbiturates have been administered concurrently with ANTABUSE without untoward effects, but the possibility of initiating a new abuse should be considered.
Baseline and follow-up transaminase tests (10–14 days) are suggested to detect any hepatic dysfunction that may result with ANTABUSE (disulfiram) therapy. In addition, a complete blood count and a sequential multiple analysis-12 (SMA-12) test should be made every six months.
Patients taking ANTABUSE Tablets should not be exposed to ethylene dibromide or its vapors. This precaution is based on preliminary results of animal research currently in progress which suggests a toxic interaction between inhaled eth-

ylene dibromide and ingested disulfiram resulting in a higher incidence of tumors and mortality in rats. Correlation of this finding to humans, however, has not been demonstrated.

ADVERSE REACTIONS

(See CONTRAINDICATIONS, WARNINGS, and PRECAUTIONS.)

OPTIC NEURITIS, PERIPHERAL NEURITIS, AND POLYNEURITIS MAY OCCUR FOLLOWING ADMINISTRATION OF ANTABUSE.

Multiple cases of both cholestatic and fulminant hepatitis have been reported to be associated with administration of ANTABUSE.

Occasional skin eruptions are, as a rule, readily controlled by concomitant administration of an antihistaminic drug.

In a small number of patients, a transient mild drowsiness, fatigability, impotence, headache, acneform eruptions, allergic dermatitis, or a metallic or garlic-like aftertaste may be experienced during the first two weeks of therapy. These complaints usually disappear spontaneously with the continuation of therapy, or with reduced dosage.

Psychotic reactions have been noted, attributable in most cases to high dosage, combined toxicity (with metronidazole or isoniazid), or to the unmasking of underlying psychoses in patients stressed by the withdrawal of alcohol.

DOSAGE AND ADMINISTRATION

ANTABUSE (disulfiram) should never be administered until the patient has abstained from alcohol for at least 12 hours.

INITIAL DOSAGE SCHEDULE: In the first phase of treatment, a maximum of 500 mg daily is given in a single dose for one to two weeks. Although usually taken in the morning, ANTABUSE may be taken on retiring by patients who experience a sedative effect. Alternatively, to minimize, or eliminate, the sedative effect, dosage may be adjusted downward.

MAINTENANCE REGIMEN: The average maintenance dose is 250 mg daily (range, 125 to 500 mg); it should not exceed 500 mg daily.

NOTE: Occasionally patients, while seemingly on adequate maintenance doses of ANTABUSE, report that they are able to drink alcoholic beverages with impunity and without any symptomatology. All appearances to the contrary, such patients must be presumed to be disposing of their tablets in some manner without actually taking them. Until such patients have been observed reliably taking their daily ANTABUSE tablets (preferably crushed and well mixed with liquid), it cannot be concluded that ANTABUSE is ineffective.

DURATION OF THERAPY: The daily, uninterrupted administration of ANTABUSE (disulfiram) must be continued until the patient is fully recovered socially and a basis for permanent self-control is established. Depending on the individual patient, maintenance therapy may be required for months, or even years.

TRIAL WITH ALCOHOL: During early experience with ANTABUSE, it was thought advisable for each patient to have at least one supervised alcohol-drug reaction. More recently, the test reaction has been largely abandoned. Furthermore, such a test reaction should never be administered to a patient over 50 years of age. A clear, detailed, and convincing description of the reaction is felt to be sufficient in most cases.

However, where a test reaction is deemed necessary, the suggested procedure is as follows:

After the first one to two weeks' therapy with 500 mg daily, a drink of 15 mL (½ oz) of 100 proof whiskey, or equivalent, is taken slowly. This test dose of alcoholic beverage may be repeated once only so that the total dose does not exceed 30 mL (1 oz) of whiskey. Once a reaction develops, no more alcohol should be consumed. Such tests should be carried out only when the patient is hospitalized, or comparable supervision and facilities, including oxygen, are available.

MANAGEMENT OF ANTABUSE-ALCOHOL REACTION: In severe reactions, whether caused by an excessive test dose or by the patient's unsupervised ingestion of alcohol, supportive measures to restore blood pressure and treat shock should be instituted. Other recommendations include: oxygen, carbogen (95% oxygen and 5% carbon dioxide), vitamin C intravenously in massive doses (1 g), and ephedrine sulfate. Antihistamines have also been used intravenously. Potassium levels should be monitored, particularly in patients on digitalis, since hypokalemia has been reported.

HOW SUPPLIED

ANTABUSE—Each tablet (scored) contains 250 mg disulfiram, in bottles of 100 (NDC 0046-0809-81)—Each tablet (scored) contains 500 mg disulfiram, in bottles of 50 (NDC 0046-0810-50) and 1,000 (NDC 0046-0810-91).

Shown in Product Identification Section, page 404

A.P.L.® ℞

Brand of chorionic gonadotropin for injection, USP
For Intramuscular Injection Only

CAUTION: Federal law prohibits dispensing without prescription.

DESCRIPTION

Human chorionic gonadotropin (HCG), a polypeptide hormone produced by the human placenta, is composed of an alpha and a beta subunit. The alpha subunit is essentially identical to the alpha subunits of the human pituitary gonadotropins, luteinizing hormone (LH) and follicle-stimulating hormone (FSH), as well as to the alpha subunit of human thyroid stimulating hormone (TSH). The beta subunits of these hormones differ in amino acid sequence.

A.P.L. (chorionic gonadotropin for injection, USP) is a gonad-stimulating principle obtained from the urine of pregnant women. It is an amorphous powder prepared by cryodesiccation, and is freely soluble in water.

ACTIONS

The action of HCG is virtually identical to that of pituitary LH, although HCG appears to have a small degree of FSH activity as well. It stimulates production of gonadal steroid hormones by stimulating the interstitial cells (Leydig cells) of the testis to produce androgens and the corpus luteum of the ovary to produce progesterone. Androgen stimulation in the male leads to the development of secondary sex characteristics and may stimulate testicular descent when no anatomical impediment to descent is present. This descent is usually reversible when HCG is discontinued. During the normal menstrual cycle, LH participates with FSH in the development and maturation of the normal ovarian follicle, and the midcycle LH surge triggers ovulation. HCG can substitute for LH in this function.

During a normal pregnancy, HCG secreted by the placenta maintains the corpus luteum after LH secretion decreases, supporting continued secretion of estrogen and progesterone, and preventing menstruation. HCG HAS NO KNOWN EFFECT ON FAT MOBILIZATION, APPETITE OR SENSE OF HUNGER, OR BODY FAT DISTRIBUTION.

INDICATIONS

HCG HAS NOT BEEN DEMONSTRATED TO BE EFFECTIVE ADJUNCTIVE THERAPY IN THE TREATMENT OF OBESITY. THERE IS NO SUBSTANTIAL EVIDENCE THAT IT INCREASES WEIGHT LOSS BEYOND THAT RESULTING FROM CALORIC RESTRICTION, THAT IT CAUSES A MORE ATTRACTIVE OR "NORMAL" DISTRIBUTION OF FAT, OR THAT IT DECREASES THE HUNGER AND DISCOMFORT ASSOCIATED WITH CALORIE RESTRICTED DIETS.

1. Cryptorchidism not due to anatomic obstruction. In general, A.P.L. (chorionic gonadotropin for injection, USP) is thought to induce testicular descent in situations when descent would have occurred at puberty. A.P.L. thus may help to predict whether or not orchiopexy will be needed in the future. Although, in some cases, descent following A.P.L. administration is permanent, in most cases the response is temporary. Therapy is usually instituted between the ages of 4 and 9.
2. Selected cases of male hypogonadism secondary to pituitary failure.
3. Induction of ovulation and pregnancy in the anovulatory, infertile woman in whom the cause of anovulation is secondary and not due to ovarian failure, and who has been appropriately pretreated with human menotropins.

CONTRAINDICATIONS

Precocious puberty, prostatic carcinoma or other androgen-dependent neoplasia, prior allergic reaction to chorionic gonadotropin.

WARNINGS

HCG should be used in conjunction with human menopausal gonadotropins only by physicians experienced with infertility problems who are familiar with the criteria for patient selection, contraindications, warnings, precautions, and adverse reactions described in the package insert for menotropins. The principal serious adverse reactions during this use are: (1) ovarian enlargement, ascites with or without pain, and/or pleural effusion, (2) rupture of ovarian cysts with resultant hemoperitoneum, (3) multiple births, and (4) arterial thromboembolism.

PRECAUTIONS

Induction of androgen secretion by chorionic gonadotropin may induce precocious puberty in patients treated for cryptorchidism. If signs of precocious puberty occur, therapy should be discontinued.

Since androgens may cause fluid retention, chorionic gonadotropin should be used with caution in patients with epilepsy, migraine, asthma, cardiac or renal disease.

ADVERSE REACTIONS

Headache
Irritability
Restlessness
Depression
Tiredness
Edema
Precocious puberty
Gynecomastia
Pain at site of injection

DOSAGE AND ADMINISTRATION

There is a marked variance of opinion concerning the dosage regimens to be used. Therefore the regimen employed in any particular case will depend upon the indication for use, the age and weight of the patient, and the physician's preference. The following regimens have been advocated by various authorities.

Cryptorchidism: (Therapy is usually instituted between the ages of 4 and 9.)

(1) 4,000 USP Units three times weekly for three weeks.
(2) 5,000 USP Units every second day for four injections.
(3) 15 injections of 500 to 1,000 USP Units over a period of six weeks.
(4) 500 USP Units three times weekly for four to six weeks. If this course of treatment is not successful, another is begun one month later, giving 1,000 USP Units per injection.

Selected cases of male hypogonadism secondary to pituitary failure:

(1) 500 to 1,000 USP Units three times a week for three weeks, followed by the same dose twice a week for three weeks.
(2) 1,000 to 2,000 USP Units three times weekly.
(3) 4,000 USP Units three times weekly for six to nine months, following which the dosage may be reduced to 2,000 USP Units three times weekly for an additional three months.

Induction of ovulation and pregnancy in the anovulatory, infertile woman in whom the cause of anovulation is secondary:

5,000 to 10,000 USP Units one day following the last dose of menotropins.

HOW SUPPLIED

A.P.L. (chorionic gonadotropin for injection, USP)

NDC 0046-0970-10 — Each package provides:
(1) One vial containing 5,000 USP Units chorionic gonadotropin in dry form, and
(2) One 10 mL ampul sterile diluent.

NDC 0046-0971-10 — Each package provides:
(1) One vial containing 10,000 USP Units chorionic gonadotropin in dry form, and
(2) One 10 mL ampul sterile diluent.

NDC 0046-0972-10 — Each package provides:
(1) One vial containing 20,000 USP Units chorionic gonadotropin in dry form, and
(2) One 10 mL ampul sterile diluent.

When reconstituted with 10 mL of accompanying sterile diluent, the resulting solutions also contain 2.0% benzyl alcohol, not more than 0.2% phenol, and the following concentrations of lactose: No. 970, 0.9%; No. 971, 1.8%; No. 972, 3.6%. The pH is adjusted with sodium hydroxide or hydrochloric acid.

MAY BE STORED FOR 90 DAYS IN A REFRIGERATOR AFTER RECONSTITUTION.

ATROMID-S® ℞

[*ă'trō-mid*]

Brand of clofibrate
Antilipidemic agent for reduction of elevated serum lipids

CAUTION: Federal law prohibits dispensing without prescription.

DESCRIPTION

ATROMID-S is ethyl 2-(p-chlorophenoxy)-2-methyl-propionate.

structural formula

$$Cl-C_6H_4-O-C(CH_3)_2-C(=O)-OC_2H_5$$

Its molecular formula is $C_{12}H_{15}O_3Cl$, molecular weight 242.7, and boiling point 158°–160°C. at 25 mm. It is a stable, colorless to pale yellow liquid with a faint odor and characteristic taste, soluble in common solvents but not in water.

ATROMID-S Capsules contain the following inactive ingredients: D&C Red No. 28, D&C Red No. 30, D&C Yellow No.

Continued on next page

Ayerst—Cont.

10, FD&C Blue No. 1, FD&C Red No. 3, FD&C Yellow No. 6, gelatin.

ACTIONS

ATROMID-S is an antilipidemic agent. It acts to lower elevated serum lipids by reducing the very low density lipoprotein fraction (S_f20–400) rich in triglycerides. Serum cholesterol, especially the low density lipoprotein fraction (S_f0–20), is also decreased, particularly in those whose cholesterol levels are elevated at the outset.

The mechanism of action has not been established definitively. In man, clofibrate reduces cholesterol formation early in the biosynthetic chain. In addition, clofibrate has been shown to cause increased excretion of neutral sterols.

Animal studies suggest that clofibrate interrupts cholesterol biosynthesis prior to mevalonate formation.

INDICATIONS

Drug therapy should not be used for the routine treatment of elevated blood lipids for the prevention of coronary heart disease. Dietary therapy specific for the type of hyperlipidemia is the initial treatment of choice.[1] Excess body weight and alcoholic intake may be important factors in hypertriglyceridemia and should be addressed prior to any drug therapy. Physical exercise can be an important ancillary measure. Contributory diseases such as hypothyroidism or diabetes mellitus should be looked for and adequately treated. The use of drugs should be considered only when reasonable attempts have been made to obtain satisfactory results with nondrug methods. If the decision ultimately is to use drugs, the patient should be instructed that this does not reduce the importance of adhering to diet.

Because ATROMID-S (clofibrate) is associated with certain serious adverse findings reported in two large clinical trials (see WARNINGS), agents other than clofibrate may be more suitable for a particular patient.

ATROMID-S is indicated for Primary Dysbetalipoproteinemia (Type III hyperlipidemia) that does not respond adequately to diet.

ATROMID-S may be considered for the treatment of adult patients with very high serum triglyceride levels (Types IV and V hyperlipidemia) who present a risk of abdominal pain and pancreatitis and who do not respond adequately to a determined dietary effort to control them. Patients with triglyceride levels in excess of 750 mg per deciliter are likely to present such risk.

ATROMID-S has little effect on the elevated cholesterol levels of most subjects with hypercholesterolemia. A minority of subjects show a more pronounced response. However, it must be understood that there is no evidence that use of any lipid-altering agent will be beneficial in preventing death from coronary heart disease (see WARNINGS). Therefore, the physician should be very selective and confine clofibrate treatment to patients with clearly defined risk due to severe hypercholesterolemia (*e.g.* individuals with familial hypercholesterolemia starting in childhood) who inadequately respond to appropriate diet and more effective cholesterol-lowering drugs.

ATROMID-S is not useful for the hypertriglyceridemia of Type I hyperlipidemia.

The biochemical response to ATROMID-S (clofibrate) is variable, and it is not always possible to predict from the lipoprotein type or other factors which patients will obtain favorable results. It is essential that lipid levels be assessed and that the drug be discontinued in any patient in whom lipids do not show significant improvement.

CONTRAINDICATIONS

Clofibrate is contraindicated in pregnant women. While teratogenic studies have not demonstrated any effect attributable to clofibrate, it is known that serum of the rabbit fetus accumulates a higher concentration of clofibrate than that found in maternal serum, and it is possible that the fetus may not have developed the enzyme system required for the excretion of clofibrate.

It is contraindicated in lactating women since it is not known if clofibrate is secreted in the milk.

It is contraindicated in patients with clinically significant hepatic or renal dysfunction.

It is contraindicated in patients with primary biliary cirrhosis since it may raise the already elevated cholesterol in these cases.

WARNINGS

In a large prospective study involving 5,000 patients in a clofibrate-treated group and 5,000 in a placebo-treated group followed for an average of five years on drug or placebo and one year beyond (the WHO study), there was a statistically significant 36% higher mortality due to noncardiovascular causes in the clofibrate-treated group than in a comparable placebo group. Half of this difference was due to malignancy; other causes of death included postcholecystectomy complications and pancreatitis.[2] In another prospective study involving 1,000 clofibrate- and 3,000 placebo-treated patients followed for an average of six years on drug or placebo (the Coronary Drug Project study), the noncardiovascular mortality rate, including that of malignancy, was not significantly different in the clofibrate- and placebo-treated groups.[3] This should not be interpreted to mean that clofibrate is not associated with an increased risk of noncardiovascular death because the patients in the Coronary Drug Project were much older than those in the WHO study and they all had had a previous myocardial infarction so that the deaths in the Coronary Drug Project were overwhelmingly due to cardiovascular causes and it would have been very difficult to discern a clofibrate-associated risk of death due to noncardiovascular causes if it existed. Both studies demonstrated that clofibrate users have twice the risk of developing cholelithiasis and cholecystitis requiring surgery as do nonusers.

A potential benefit of clofibrate was, however, reported in the WHO study which involved patients with hypercholesterolemia and no history of myocardial infarction or angina pectoris. In this study, there was noted a statistically significant 25% decrease in subsequent nonfatal myocardial infarctions in the clofibrate-treated group when compared with the placebo group. There was no difference in incidence of fatal myocardial infarction in the two groups. If the study had been continued longer, had included diet, had been restricted to patients who had both hyperlipidemia and increased risk factors *and* who obtained significant clofibrate-induced reduction in serum lipids, it is possible that it may have shown a decrease in fatal myocardial infarctions. In the Coronary Drug Project study, which involved patients with or without hypercholesterolemia and/or hypertriglyceridemia and with a history of previous myocardial infarction, there was no significant difference in incidence of either nonfatal or fatal myocardial infarction between the clofibrate- and placebo-treated groups.[2]

As a result of these and other studies, the following can be stated:

1. Clofibrate, in general, causes a relatively modest reduction of serum cholesterol and a somewhat greater reduction of serum triglycerides. In Type III hyperlipidemia, however, substantial reductions of both cholesterol and triglycerides can occur with use of clofibrate.
2. No study to date has shown a convincing reduction in incidence of *fatal* myocardial infarction.
3. A significantly increased incidence of cholelithiasis has been demonstrated consistently in clofibrate-treated groups, and an increase in morbidity from this complication and mortality from cholecystectomy must be anticipated during clofibrate treatment.
4. Several types of other undesirable events have been associated in a statistically significant way with clofibrate administration in the WHO or the Coronary Drug Project studies. There was an increase in incidence of noncardiovascular deaths reported in the WHO study. There was an increase in cardiac arrhythmias and intermittent claudication and in definite or suspected thromboembolic events and angina reported in the Coronary Drug Project, which was not, however, reported in the WHO study.
5. Administration of clofibrate to mice and rats in long-term studies at eight times the human dose, and to rats at five times the human dose, resulted in a higher incidence of benign and malignant liver tumors than in controls. Lower doses were not included in these studies.

BECAUSE OF THE HEPATIC TUMORIGENICITY OF CLOFIBRATE IN RODENTS AND THE POSSIBLE INCREASED RISK OF MALIGNANCY ASSOCIATED WITH CLOFIBRATE IN THE HUMAN, AS WELL AS THE INCREASED RISK OF CHOLELITHIASIS, AND BECAUSE THERE IS NOT, TO DATE, SUBSTANTIAL EVIDENCE OF A BENEFICIAL EFFECT ON CARDIOVASCULAR MORTALITY FROM CLOFIBRATE, THIS DRUG SHOULD BE UTILIZED ONLY FOR THOSE PATIENTS DESCRIBED IN THE INDICATIONS SECTION, AND SHOULD BE DISCONTINUED IF SIGNIFICANT LIPID RESPONSE IS NOT OBTAINED.

Concomitant Anticoagulants

CAUTION SHOULD BE EXERCISED WHEN ANTICOAGULANTS ARE GIVEN IN CONJUNCTION WITH ATROMID-S (CLOFIBRATE). THE DOSAGE OF THE ANTICOAGULANT SHOULD BE REDUCED USUALLY BY ONE-HALF (DEPENDING ON THE INDIVIDUAL CASE) TO MAINTAIN THE PROTHROMBIN TIME AT THE DESIRED LEVEL TO PREVENT BLEEDING COMPLICATIONS. FREQUENT PROTHROMBIN DETERMINATIONS ARE ADVISABLE UNTIL IT HAS BEEN DEFINITELY DETERMINED THAT THE PROTHROMBIN LEVEL HAS BEEN STABILIZED.

Avoidance of Pregnancy

Strict birth control procedures must be exercised by women of childbearing potential. In patients who plan to become pregnant, clofibrate should be withdrawn several months before conception. Because of the possibility of pregnancy occurring despite birth control precautions in patients taking clofibrate, the possible benefits of the drug to the patient must be weighed against possible hazards to the fetus.

PRECAUTIONS

Before instituting therapy with clofibrate, attempts should be made to control serum lipids with appropriate dietary regimens, weight loss in obese patients, control of diabetes mellitus, etc.

Because of the long-term administration of a drug of this nature, adequate baseline studies should be performed to determine that the patient has significantly elevated serum lipid levels. Frequent determinations of serum lipids should be obtained during the first few months of ATROMID-S (clofibrate) administration, and periodic determinations thereafter. The drug should be withdrawn after three months if response is inadequate. However, in the case of xanthoma tuberosum, the drug should be employed for longer periods (even up to one year) provided that there is a reduction in the size and/or number of the xanthomata.

Subsequent serum lipid determinations should be done to detect a paradoxical rise in serum cholesterol or triglyceride levels. Clofibrate will not alter the seasonal variations of serum cholesterol peak elevations in midwinter and late summer and decreases in fall and spring. If the drug is discontinued, the patient should be continued on an appropriate hypolipidemic diet, and his serum lipids should be monitored until stabilized, as a rise in these values to or above the original baseline may occur.

During clofibrate therapy, frequent serum transaminase determinations and other liver function tests should be performed since the drug may produce abnormalities in these parameters. These effects are usually reversible when the drug is discontinued. Hepatic biopsies are usually within normal limits. If the hepatic function tests steadily rise or show excessive abnormalities, the drug should be withdrawn. Therefore use with caution in those patients with a past history of jaundice or hepatic disease.

Since cholelithiasis is a possible side effect of clofibrate therapy, appropriate diagnostic procedures should be performed if signs and symptoms related to disease of the biliary system should occur.

Clofibrate may produce "flu-like" symptoms (muscular aching, soreness, cramping). The physician should differentiate this from actual viral and/or bacterial disease.

Use with caution in patients with peptic ulcer since reactivation has been reported. Whether this is drug-related is unknown.

Complete blood counts should be done periodically since anemia, and more frequently, leukopenia have been reported in patients who have been taking clofibrate.

Various cardiac arrhythmias have been reported with the use of clofibrate.

Several investigators have observed in their studies that clofibrate may produce a decrease in cholesterol linoleate but an increase in palmitoleate and oleate, the latter being considered atherogenic in experimental animals. The significance of this finding is unknown at this time.

ADVERSE REACTIONS

Of the pertinent reactions, the most common is nausea. Less frequently encountered gastrointestinal reactions are vomiting, loose stools, dyspepsia, flatulence, and abdominal distress. Reactions reported less often than gastrointestinal ones are headache, dizziness, and fatigue; muscle cramping, aching, and weakness; skin rash, urticaria, and pruritus; dry brittle hair, and alopecia.

The following reported adverse reactions are listed alphabetically by systems:

Cardiovascular
- Increased or decreased angina
- Cardiac arrhythmias
- Both swelling and phlebitis at site of xanthomas

Dermatologic
- Skin rash
- Alopecia
- Allergic reaction including urticaria
- Dry skin and dry brittle hair
- Pruritus

Gastrointestinal
- Nausea
- Diarrhea
- Gastrointestinal upset (bloating, flatulence, abdominal distress)
- Hepatomegaly (not associated with hepatotoxicity)
- Gallstones
- Vomiting
- Stomatitis and gastritis

Genitourinary
- Impotence and decreased libido
- Findings consistent with renal dysfunction as evidenced by dysuria, hematuria, proteinuria, decreased urine output. One patient's renal biopsy suggested "allergic reaction."

Hematologic
- Leukopenia
- Potentiation of anticoagulant effect
- Anemia
- Eosinophilia

Musculoskeletal
- Myalgia (muscle cramping, aching, weakness)
- "Flu-like" symptoms
- Arthralgia

Neurologic
- Fatigue, weakness, drowsiness
- Dizziness
- Headache

Miscellaneous
- Weight gain
- Polyphagia

Laboratory Findings
- Abnormal liver function tests as evidenced by increased transaminase (SGOT and SGPT), BSP retention, and increased thymol turbidity
- Proteinuria
- Increased creatine phosphokinase

Reported adverse reactions whose direct relationship with the drug has not been established: peptic ulcer, gastrointestinal hemorrhage, rheumatoid arthritis, tremors, increased perspiration, systemic lupus erythematosus, blurred vision, gynecomastia, thrombocytopenic purpura.

DOSAGE AND ADMINISTRATION

Initial: The recommended dosage for adults is 2 g daily in divided doses. Some patients may respond to a lower dosage.
Maintenance: Same as for initial dosage.
Note: In children, insufficient studies have been done to show safety and efficacy.

DRUG INTERACTIONS

Caution should be exercised when anticoagulants are given in conjunction with ATROMID-S (clofibrate). The dosage of the anticoagulant should be reduced usually by one-half (depending on the individual case) to maintain the prothrombin time at the desired level to prevent bleeding complications. Frequent prothrombin determinations are advisable until it has been definitely determined that the prothrombin level has been stabilized.

MANAGEMENT OF OVERDOSAGE

While there has been no reported case of overdosage, should it occur, symptomatic supportive measures should be taken.

HOW SUPPLIED

ATROMID-S—Each capsule contains 500 mg clofibrate, in bottles of 100 (NDC 0046-0243-81).

REFERENCES

1. Coronary Risk Handbook (1973), American Heart Association. 2. Report from the Committee of Principal Investigators: A cooperative trial in the primary prevention of ischaemic heart disease using clofibrate, *Br Heart J* 40:1069, 1978. 3. The Coronary Drug Project Research Group: Clofibrate and niacin in coronary heart disease, *JAMA* 231:360, 1975.

Shown in Product Identification Section, page 404

AURALGAN® Otic Solution ℞

[aw-răl'gan]

CAUTION: Federal law prohibits dispensing without prescription.

DESCRIPTION

Each mL contains:

Antipyrine	54.0 mg
Benzocaine	14.0 mg
Glycerin dehydrated q.s. to	1.0 mL

(contains not more than 0.6% moisture)
(also contains oxyquinoline sulfate)

TOPICAL DECONGESTANT AND ANALGESIC

AURALGAN is an otic solution containing antipyrine, benzocaine, and dehydrated glycerin. The solution congeals at 0° C (32° F), but returns to normal consistency, unchanged, at room temperature.

The structures of the components are:

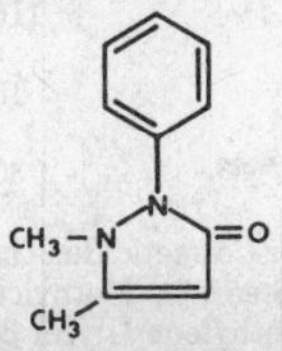

antipyrine 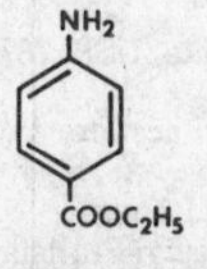 benzocaine 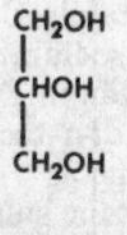 glycerin

CLINICAL PHARMACOLOGY

AURALGAN combines the hygroscopic property of dehydrated glycerin with the analgesic action of antipyrine and benzocaine to relieve pressure, reduce inflammation and congestion, and alleviate pain and discomfort in acute otitis media.
AURALGAN does not blanch the tympanic membrane or mask the landmarks and, therefore, does not distort the otoscopic picture.

INDICATIONS AND USAGE

Acute otitis media of various etiologies
— prompt relief of pain and reduction of inflammation in the congestive and serous stages
— adjuvant therapy during systemic antibiotic administration for resolution of the infection

Because of the close anatomical relationship of the eustachian tube to the nasal cavity, otitis media is a frequent problem, especially in children in whom the tube is shorter, wider, and more horizontal than in adults.

Removal of cerumen
—facilitates the removal of excessive or impacted cerumen.

CONTRAINDICATIONS

Hypersensitivity to any of the components or substances related to them.
In the presence of spontaneous perforation or discharge.

PRECAUTIONS

Carcinogenesis, Mutagenesis, Impairment of Fertility: No long-term studies in animals or humans have been conducted. *Pregnancy Category C:* Animal reproduction studies have not been conducted with AURALGAN. It is also not known whether AURALGAN can cause fetal harm when administered to a pregnant woman, or can affect reproduction capacity. AURALGAN should be given to a pregnant woman only if clearly needed.
Nursing Mothers: It is not known whether this drug is excreted in human milk. Because many drugs are excreted in human milk, caution should be exercised when AURALGAN is administered to a nursing woman.

DOSAGE AND ADMINISTRATION

Acute otitis media: Instill AURALGAN, permitting the solution to run along the wall of the canal until it is filled. Avoid touching the ear with dropper. Then moisten a cotton pledget with AURALGAN and insert into meatus. Repeat every one to two hours until pain and congestion are relieved.

Removal of cerumen
Before: Instill AURALGAN three times daily for two or three days to help detach cerumen from wall of canal and facilitate removal.
After: AURALGAN is useful for drying out the canal or relieving discomfort.

Before and after removal of cerumen, a cotton pledget moistened with AURALGAN should be inserted into the meatus following instillation.
NOTE: Do not rinse dropper after use. Replace in bottle and screw cap tightly.

HOW SUPPLIED

AURALGAN® Otic Solution, in package containing 10 mL bottle with separate dropper-screw cap attachment (NDC 0046-1000-10).

AYGESTIN® ℞

[ā-jĕs'tĭn]

Brand of norethindrone acetate tablets, USP

CAUTION: Federal law prohibits dispensing without prescription.

WARNING:
THE USE OF PROGESTATIONAL AGENTS DURING THE FIRST FOUR MONTHS OF PREGNANCY IS NOT RECOMMENDED.
Progestational agents have been used beginning with the first trimester of pregnancy in an attempt to prevent habitual abortion or treat threatened abortion. There is no adequate evidence that such use is effective and there is evidence of potential harm to the fetus when such drugs are given during the first four months of pregnancy. Furthermore, in the vast majority of women, the cause of abortion is a defective ovum, which progestational agents could not be expected to influence. In addition, the use of progestational agents with their uterine-relaxant properties, in patients with fertilized defective ova may cause a delay in spontaneous abortion. Therefore, the use of such drugs during the first four months of pregnancy is not recommended.
Several reports suggest an association between intrauterine exposure to female sex hormones and congenital anomalies, including congenital heart defects and limb reduction defects.[1-5] One study[4] estimated a 4.7-fold increased risk of limb reduction defects in infants exposed in utero to sex hormones (oral contraceptives, hormone withdrawal tests for pregnancy, or attempted treatment for threatened abortion). Some of these exposures were very short and involved only a few days of treatment. The data suggest that the risk of limb reduction defects in exposed fetuses is somewhat less than 1 in 1,000 if the patient is exposed to AYGESTIN® (norethindrone acetate tablets, USP) during the first four months of pregnancy or if she becomes pregnant while taking this drug, she should be apprised of the potential risks to the fetus.

DESCRIPTION

AYGESTIN®
(norethindrone acetate tablets, USP)—
5 mg oral tablets.

AYGESTIN (17-hydroxy-19-nor-17α-pregn-4-en- 20-yn-3-one acetate), a synthetic, orally active progestin, is the acetic acid ester of norethindrone. On a weight basis it is twice as potent as norethindrone. It is a white, or creamy white, crystalline powder.

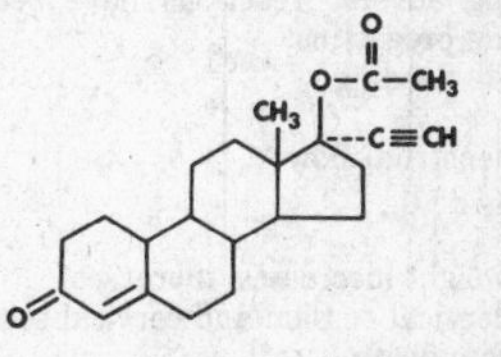

AYGESTIN Tablets contain the following inactive ingredients: lactose, magnesium stearate, and microcrystalline cellulose.

ACTIONS

Norethindrone acetate induces secretory changes in an estrogen-primed endometrium. It acts to inhibit the secretion of pituitary gonadotropins which, in turn, prevent follicular maturation and ovulation.

INDICATIONS

AYGESTIN (norethindrone acetate tablets, USP) is indicated for the treatment of secondary amenorrhea, endometriosis, and abnormal uterine bleeding due to hormonal imbalance in the absence of organic pathology such as submucous fibroids or uterine cancer.

CONTRAINDICATIONS

Thrombophlebitis, thromboembolic disorders, cerebral apoplexy, or a past history of these conditions
Markedly impaired liver function or liver disease
Known or suspected carcinoma of the breast
Undiagnosed vaginal bleeding
Missed abortion
As a diagnostic test for pregnancy

WARNINGS

1. Discontinue medication pending examination if there is a sudden partial or complete loss of vision, or if there is sudden onset of proptosis, diplopia, or migraine. If examination reveals papilledema or retinal vascular lesions, medication should be withdrawn.
2. Detectable amounts of progestogens have been identified in the milk of mothers receiving them. The effect of this on the nursing infant has not been determined.
3. Because of the occasional occurrence of thrombophlebitis and pulmonary embolism in patients taking progestogens, the physician should be alert to the earliest manifestations of the disease.
4. Masculinization of the female fetus has occurred when progestogens have been used in pregnant women.
5. Some beagle dogs treated with medroxy-progesterone acetate developed mammary nodules. Although nodules occasionally appeared in control animals, they were intermittent in nature, whereas nodules in treated animals were larger and more numerous, and persisted. There is no general agreement as to whether the nodules are benign or malignant. Their significance with respect to humans has not been established.

PRECAUTIONS

A. General Precautions.
1. The pretreatment physical examination should include special reference to breasts and pelvic organs, as well as a Papanicolaou smear.
2. Because this drug may cause some degree of fluid retention, conditions which might be influenced by this factor, such as epilepsy, migraine, asthma, cardiac or renal dysfunctions, require careful observation.
3. In cases of breakthrough bleeding, as in all cases of irregular bleeding per vaginam, nonfunctional causes should be borne in mind. In cases of undiagnosed vaginal bleeding, adequate diagnostic measures are indicated.

Continued on next page

Ayerst—Cont.

4. Patients who have a history of psychic depression should be carefully observed and the drug discontinued if the depression recurs to a serious degree.
5. Any possible influence of prolonged progestogen therapy on pituitary, ovarian, adrenal, hepatic, or uterine functions awaits further study.
6. A decrease in glucose tolerance has been observed in a small percentage of patients on estrogen-progestogen combination drugs. The mechanism of this decrease is obscure. For this reason, diabetic patients should be carefully observed while receiving progestogen therapy.
7. The age of the patient constitutes no absolute limiting factor, although treatment with progestogens may mask the onset of the climacteric.
8. The pathologist should be advised of progestogen therapy when relevant specimens are submitted.
B. Information for the Patient. See text which appears after REFERENCES.

ADVERSE REACTIONS
The following adverse reactions have been observed in women taking progestins:
breakthrough bleeding
spotting
change in menstrual flow
amenorrhea
edema
changes in weight (decreases, increases)
changes in cervical erosion and cervical secretions
cholestatic jaundice
rash (allergic) with and without pruritus
melasma or chloasma
mental depression
Progestins may alter the result of pregnanediol determinations. The following laboratory results may be altered by the concomitant use of estrogens with progestins:
hepatic function
coagulation tests—increase in prothrombin, factors VII, VIII, IX, and X
increase in PBI, BEI, and a decrease in T^3 uptake
metyrapone test
A statistically significant association has been demonstrated between use of estrogen-progestogen combination drugs and the following serious adverse reactions: thrombophlebitis, pulmonary embolism, and cerebral thrombosis and embolism. For this reason, patients on progestogen therapy should be carefully observed. Although available evidence is suggestive of an association, such a relationship has been neither confirmed nor refuted for the following serious adverse reactions:
Neuro-ocular lesions, *eg*, retinal thrombosis and optic neuritis.
The following adverse reactions have been observed in patients receiving estrogen-progestogen combination drugs.

1. Rise in blood pressure in susceptible individuals
2. Premenstrual-like syndrome
3. Changes in libido
4. Changes in appetite
5. Cystitis-like syndrome
6. Headache
7. Nervousness
8. Dizziness
9. Fatigue
10. Backache
11. Hirsutism
12. Loss of scalp hair
13. Erythema multiforme
14. Erythema nodosum
15. Hemorrhagic eruption
16. Itching

In view of these observations, patients on progestogen therapy should be carefully observed.

DOSAGE AND ADMINISTRATION
Therapy with AYGESTIN® (norethindrone acetate tablets, USP) must be adapted to the specific indications and therapeutic response of the individual patient. This dosage schedule assumes the interval between menses to be 28 days.
Secondary amenorrhea, abnormal uterine bleeding due to hormonal imbalance in the absence of organic pathology: 2.5 to 10 mg AYGESTIN may be given daily for from 5 to 10 days during the second half of the theoretical menstrual cycle to produce an optimum secretory transformation of an endometrium that has been adequately primed with either endogenous or exogenous estrogen.
Progestin withdrawal bleeding usually occurs within three to seven days after discontinuing AYGESTIN therapy. Patients with a past history of recurrent episodes of abnormal uterine bleeding may benefit from planned menstrual cycling with AYGESTIN.
Endometriosis:
Initial daily dosage of 5 mg AYGESTIN for two weeks. Dosage should be increased by 2.5 mg per day every two weeks until 15 mg per day of AYGESTIN is reached. Therapy may be held at this level for six to nine months or until annoying breakthrough bleeding demands temporary termination.

HOW SUPPLIED
Each scored AYGESTIN tablet contains 5 mg norethindrone acetate, USP, in bottles of 50 (NDC 0046-0894-50). Also available in Cycle Packs of 10 (0046-0894-10).

PHYSICIAN REFERENCES

1. Gal I, Kirman B, Stern J: Hormonal pregnancy tests and congenital malformation. Nature *216*:83, 1967.
2. Levy EP, Cohen A, Fraser FC: Hormone treatment during pregnancy and congenital heart defects. Lancet *1*:611, 1973.
3. Nora JJ, Nora AH: Birth defects and oral contraceptives. Lancet *1*:941-942, 1973.
4. Janerich DT, Piper JM, Glebatis DM: Oral contraceptives and congenital limb-reduction defects. N Engl J Med *291*:697-700, 1974.
5. Hernonen OP, Stone D, Monson RR, et al: Cardiovascular birth defects and antenatal exposure to female sex hormones. N Engl J Med *296*:67-70, 1977.

INFORMATION FOR THE PATIENT
Your doctor has prescribed AYGESTIN® (norethindrone acetate tablets, USP), a progestin, for you. AYGESTIN is similar to the progesterone hormones naturally produced by the body. Progestins are used to treat menstrual disorders and to test if the body is producing certain hormones.

WARNING
There is an increased risk of birth defects in children whose mothers take this drug during the first four months of pregnancy.
Progestins have been used as a test for pregnancy but such use is no longer considered safe because of possible damage to a developing baby. Also, more rapid methods for testing for pregnancy are now available.
These drugs have also been used to prevent miscarriage in the first few months of pregnancy. No adequate evidence is available to show that they are effective for this purpose and there is evidence of an increased risk of birth defects, such as heart or limb defects, if these drugs are taken during the first four months of pregnancy. Furthermore, most cases of early miscarriage are due to causes which could not be helped by these drugs.
The exact risk of taking these drugs early in pregnancy and having a baby with a birth defect is not known. However, one study found that babies born to women who had taken sex hormones (such as progesterone-like drugs) during the first three months of pregnancy were 4 to 5 times more likely to have abnormalities of the arms or legs than if their mothers had not taken such drugs. Some of these women had taken these drugs for only a few days. The chance that an infant whose mother had taken this drug will have this type of defect is about 1 in 1,000. If you take AYGESTIN (norethindrone acetate tablets, USP) and later find you were pregnant when you took it, be sure to discuss this with your doctor as soon as possible.

HOW SUPPLIED
AYGESTIN® (norethindrone acetate tablets, USP)—scored 5 mg tablets, in bottles of 50, for oral administration. Also available in Cycle Packs of 10.
Shown in Product Identification Section, page 404

BEMINAL® 500 — OTC
[*bē 'mĭn-awl*]
High potency vitamin supplement vitamin B complex with 500 mg vitamin C

Each tablet contains:		% U.S. RDA*
Thiamine mononitrate (vit. B_1)	25.0 mg	1717%
Riboflavin (vit. B_2)	12.5 mg	735%
Niacinamide (vit. B_3) as niacinamide ascorbate	100.0 mg	500%
Pyridoxine hydrochloride (vit. B_6)	10.0 mg	500%
Calcium pantothenate	20.0 mg	92%
Ascorbic acid (vit. C) as ascorbic acid and niacinamide ascorbate	500.0 mg	833%
Cyanocobalamin (vit. B_{12})	5.0 mcg	83%

Also contains: Calcium Carboxymethylcellulose, Dioctyl Phthalate, Dye FD&C Yellow No. 6 Aluminum Lake, Ethylcellulose, Flavor, Lactose, Magnesium Stearate, Microcrystalline Cellulose, Polyethylene Glycol 800, Polyethylene Glycol 20000, Titanium Dioxide.
Does not contain saccharin or other sweeteners.
*U.S. Recommended Daily Allowance

DOSAGE
12-year-olds and older, one tablet daily.

HOW SUPPLIED
BEMINAL-500 Tablets, in bottles of 100 (NDC 0046-0830-81).
Shown in Product Identification Section, page 404

BEMINAL® FORTE — OTC
[*bē 'mĭn-awl*]
with VITAMIN C
High potency vitamin supplement vitamin B complex with vitamin C

Each capsule contains:		% U.S. RDA*
Thiamine mononitrate (vit. B_1)	25.0 mg	1717%
Riboflavin (vit. B_2)	12.5 mg	735%
Niacinamide	50.0 mg	250%
Pyridoxine HCl (vit. B_6)	3.0 mg	150%
Calcium pantothenate	10.0 mg	46%
Ascorbic acid (vit. C)	250.0 mg	417%
Cyanocobalamin (vit. B_{12})	2.5 mcg	42%

Also contains: D&C Yellow No. 10, FD&C Blue No. 1, FD&C Red No. 3, FD&C Yellow No. 6, Gelatin Capsule, Lactose, Magnesium Stearate, Mineral Oil Triturate.
*U.S. Recommended Daily Allowance

DOSAGE
12-year-olds and older, 1 capsule daily.

HOW SUPPLIED
BEMINAL FORTE with VITAMIN C Capsules, in bottles of 100 (NDC 0046-0817-81).

BEMINAL STRESS PLUS™ — OTC
[*bē 'mĭn-awl*]
Stress potency replacement vitamins

BEMINAL STRESS PLUS™
with IRON

Each tablet contains:	% U.S. RDA*
vitamin B_1 as thiamine mononitrate, USP, 25.0 mg	1717%
vitamin B_2 as riboflavin, USP, 12.5 mg	735%
vitamin B_3 as niacinamide, 100.0 mg	500%
vitamin B_5 as calcium pantothenate, USP, 20.0 mg	92%
vitamin B_6 as pyridoxine hydrochloride, USP, 10.0 mg	500%
vitamin B_{12} as cyanocobalamin, 25.0 mcg	417%
vitamin Bc as folic acid, USP, 400.0 mcg	100%
vitamin C as sodium ascorbate, USP, 787.0 mg	1167%
vitamin E as *dl-a*-tocopheryl acetate, 45.0 IU	150%
Iron as ferrous fumarate, USP, 82.2 mg	150%

Also contains: Dioctyl Phthalate, Color-Cosmetic Red Oxide, Ethylcellulose, Flavor, Magnesium Stearate, Methylcellulose, Microcrystalline Cellulose, Polyethylene Glycol 8000, Polyethylene Glycol 20000, Titanium Dioxide.
*U.S. Recommended Daily Allowance

BEMINAL STRESS PLUS™
with ZINC

Each tablet contains:	% U.S. RDA*
vitamin B_1 as thiamine mononitrate, USP, 25.0 mg	1717%
vitamin B_2 as riboflavin, USP, 12.5 mg	735%
vitamin B_3 as niacinamide, 100.0 mg	500%
vitamin B_5 as calcium pantothenate, USP, 20.0 mg	92%
vitamin B_6 as pyridoxine hydrochloride, USP, 10.0 mg	500%
vitamin B_{12} as cyanocobalamin, 25.0 mcg	417%
vitamin C as sodium ascorbate, USP, 787.0 mg	1167%
vitamin E as *dl-a*-tocopheryl acetate, 45.0 IU	150%
Zinc as zinc sulfate, 111.1 mg	300%

Also contains: Dioctyl Phthalate, Color-Cosmetic Red Oxide, Ethylcellulose, Flavor, Magnesium Stearate, Methylcellulose, Microcrystalline Cellulose, Polyethylene Glycol 8000, Polyethylene Glycol 20000, Titanium Dioxide.
*U.S. Recommended Daily Allowance

INDICATION
Dietary supplement.

ACTION AND USES
The BEMINAL STRESS PLUS formulas can help replenish the vitamins and minerals depleted by the stress of sickness, infections, and surgery. BEMINAL STRESS PLUS formulas may also be used where the demand on the body's store of vitamins and minerals may be increased by dieting, lack of sleep, the use of alcohol or cigarettes, jogging, and other strenuous physical exercise.

RECOMMENDED INTAKE
12-year-olds and older, one tablet daily.

HOW SUPPLIED
BEMINAL STRESS PLUS with Iron—bottles of 60 tablets.
BEMINAL STRESS PLUS with Zinc—bottles of 60 tablets.
Shown in Product Identification Section, page 404

CLUSIVOL® Capsules OTC

High potency vitamin supplement with minerals
Capsules for 12-year-olds and older

Each capsule contains:		% U.S. RDA*
vitamin A (as palmitate)	10,000 USP Units	200
Ergocalciferol (vit. D_2)	400 USP Units	100
Ascorbic acid (vit. C) (as sodium ascorbate)	150.0 mg	250
Thiamine mononitrate (vit. B_1)	10.0 mg	687
Riboflavin (vit. B_2)	5.0 mg	294
Pyridoxine HCl (vit. B_6)	0.5 mg	25
d-Panthenol	1.0 mg	10.7
Cyanocobalamin (vit. B_{12})	2.5 mcg	42
Niacinamide	50.0 mg	250
vitamin E†	0.5 IU	**
Iron†	15.0 mg	83
Calcium†	120.0 mg	12
Manganese†	0.5 mg	***
Zinc†	0.6 mg	4
Magnesium†	3.0 mg	**

Also contains: D&C Red No. 28, D&C Red No. 33, D&C Yellow No. 10, FD&C Blue No. 1, FD&C Red No. 40, Flavor, Gelatin Capsule, Hydrogenated Soybean Oil, Lecithin, Titanium Dioxide, Yellow Wax.
†Supplied as *d*-α-tocopheryl acetate concentrate, ferrous sulfate, calcium carbonate, manganous sulfate, zinc sulfate, and magnesium sulfate.
*U.S. Recommended Daily Allowance
**Contains less than 2% U.S. RDA
***U.S. RDA not established.

DOSAGE AND ADMINISTRATION
One capsule daily.

HOW SUPPLIED
CLUSIVOL Capsules, bottle of 100 (NDC 0046-0293-81).

CLUSIVOL® 130 Tablets

[*klū'sĭ-vawl*]
High potency vitamin supplement with minerals
Tablets for 12-year-olds and older

Each tablet contains:		% U.S. RDA*
vitamin A (as palmitate)	10,000 USP Units	200
Ergocalciferol (vit. D_2)	400 USP Units	100
Ascorbic acid (vit. C) (as sodium ascorbate)	150.0 mg	250
Thiamine mononitrate (vit. B_1)	10.0 mg	687
Riboflavin (vit. B_2)	5.0 mg	294
Pyridoxine HCl (vit. B_6)	0.5 mg	25
d-Panthenol	1.0 mg	10.7
Cyanocobalamin (vit. B_{12})	2.5 mcg	42
Niacinamide	50.0 mg	250
vitamin E†	0.5 IU	**
Iron†	15.0 mg	83
Calcium†	120.0 mg	12
Manganese†	0.5 mg	***
Zinc†	0.6 mg	4
Magnesium†	3.0 mg	**

Also contains: Calcium Carboxymethylcellulose, Color—Cosmetic Red Oxide, Dioctyl Phthalate, Ethylcellulose, Flavors, Lactose, Magnesium Stearate, Methylcellulose, Polyethylene Glycol, Titanium Dioxide.
†Supplied as *dl*-α-tocopheryl acetate, ferrous fumarate, calcium carbonate, manganese gluconate, zinc oxide, and magnesium oxide.
*U.S. Recommended Daily Allowance
**Contains less than 2% U.S. RDA
***U.S. RDA not established

DOSAGE AND ADMINISTRATION
One tablet daily.

HOW SUPPLIED
CLUSIVOL 130, bottle of 130 tablets (NDC 0046-0270-81).

CLUSIVOL® SYRUP OTC

[*klū'sĭ-vawl*]
Vitamin supplement with minerals
Syrup for children and adults

Each 5 mL (1 teaspoonful) contains:		% U.S. RDA*
vitamin A (as palmitate)	2,500 USP Units	50
Cholecalciferol (vit. D_3)	400 USP Units	100
Ascorbic acid (vit. C)	15.0 mg	25
Cyanocobalamin (vit. B_{12})	2.0 mcg	33
Thiamine HCl (vit. B_1)	1.0 mg	67
Riboflavin (vit. B_2)	1.0 mg	59
Niacinamide (vit. B_3)	5.0 mg	25
d-Panthenol	3.0 mg	32
Pyridoxine HCl (vit. B_6)	0.6 mg	30
Manganese†	0.5 mg	***
Zinc†	0.5 mg	3.3
Magnesium†	3.0 mg	**

Also contains: Acacia, Butylated Hydroxy Anisole, Calcium Hypophosphite, Calcium Lactate, Caramel, Citric Acid, Corn Oil, Cysteine Hydrochloride, Dextrose, Flavors, Lactic Acid, Propylene Glycol, Sodium Lauryl Sulfate, Sucrose, Tragacanth, Viscarin®, Water.
†Supplied as the gluconates of manganese and magnesium, and zinc lactate.
*U.S. Recommended Daily Allowance.
**Contains less than 2% U.S. RDA.
***U.S. RDA not established.

A comprehensive nutritional formula incorporating essential fat- and water-soluble vitamins together with important minerals. Presented in a candy-flavored syrup base; particularly appealing to children, but also enjoyed by older individuals who prefer a liquid preparation.

ACTION AND USES
A vitamin and mineral supplement for better health for the entire family.

DOSAGE
Children and Adults: One teaspoonful (5 mL) daily.

HOW SUPPLIED
CLUSIVOL Syrup, in bottles of 8 fl oz (½ pint) (NDC 0046-0920-08), and 16 fl oz (1 pint) (NDC 0046-0920-16).

DERMOPLAST® Aerosol Spray OTC

[*der'mō-plăst*]
Topical anesthetic and antipruritic

Contains (exclusive of propellants) 20% benzocaine and 0.5% menthol in a water-dispersible base of TWEEN® 85 and polyethylene glycol 400 monolaurate, with methylparaben as a preservative.
A topical anesthetic and antipruritic spray providing soothing, temporary relief of skin pain, itching, and discomfort due to episiotomy, pruritus vulvae, postpartum hemorrhoids, sunburn, abrasions, minor cuts, burns, and insect bites. May be applied without touching sensitive affected areas.

WARNINGS
FOR EXTERNAL USE ONLY. Avoid spraying in eyes. Contents under pressure. Do not puncture or incinerate. Do not expose to heat or temperatures above 120° F. Do not use near open flame. Use only as directed. Intentional misuse by deliberately concentrating and inhaling the contents can be harmful or fatal.
Do not take orally. Not for prolonged use. If the condition for which this preparation is used persists or if a rash or irritation develops, discontinue use and consult physician.

DIRECTIONS FOR USE
Hold can in a comfortable position, 6-12 inches away from affected area. Point spray nozzle and press button. To apply to face, spray in palm of hand. May be administered three or four times daily, or as directed by physician.

HOW SUPPLIED
DERMOPLAST Aerosol Spray, in Net Wt 2-¾ oz (78 g)—NDC 0046-1008-02; Net Wt 3 oz (85 g)—NDC 0046-1008-03; and Net Wt 6 oz (170 g)—NDC 0046-1008-06.

DIUCARDIN® ℞

[*dī"ū-car'din*]
Brand of hydroflumethiazide
A diuretic-antihypertensive agent

CAUTION: Federal law prohibits dispensing without prescription.

DESCRIPTION
DIUCARDIN® (hydroflumethiazide) is an oral thiazide (benzothiadiazide) diuretic-antihypertensive agent.
DIUCARDIN is available in 50 mg tablets.
Chemical name: 3,4-Dihydro-6-(trifluoromethyl)-2H-1,2,4-benzothiadiazine-7-sulfonamide 1,1-dioxide.
Structural formula:

Hydroflumethiazide is an odorless white to cream colored, finely divided, crystalline powder. It has a melting point between 270° and 275° C. Hydroflumethiazide is freely soluble in acetone, soluble in alcohol, and slightly soluble in water.
The inactive ingredients contained in DIUCARDIN Tablets are: lactose, magnesium stearate, microcrystalline cellulose, povidone, and starch.

CLINICAL PHARMACOLOGY
DIUCARDIN is a thiazide diuretic and antihypertensive. DIUCARDIN affects the renal tubular mechanism of electrolyte reabsorption. At maximal therapeutic dosage all thiazides are approximately equal in their diuretic potency.
DIUCARDIN increases excretion of sodium and chloride in approximately equivalent amounts. Natriuresis causes a secondary loss of potassium and bicarbonate.
The mechanism of the antihypertensive effect of DIUCARDIN is unknown. DIUCARDIN does not affect normal blood pressure.
Onset of action of DIUCARDIN occurs in two hours and the peak effect at about four hours. Its action persists for approximately 6 to 12 hours. Thiazides are eliminated rapidly by the kidney.

INDICATIONS AND USAGE
DIUCARDIN is indicated as adjunctive therapy in edema associated with congestive heart failure, hepatic cirrhosis and corticosteroid and estrogen therapy.
DIUCARDIN has also been found useful in edema due to various forms of renal dysfunction as: nephrotic syndrome; acute glomerulonephritis; and chronic renal failure.
DIUCARDIN is indicated in the management of hypertension either as the sole therapeutic agent or to enhance the effect of other antihypertensive drugs in the more severe forms of hypertension.
Usage in Pregnancy: The routine use of diuretics in an otherwise healthy woman is inappropriate and exposes mother and fetus to unnecessary hazard. Diuretics do not prevent development of toxemia of pregnancy, and there is no satisfactory evidence that they are useful in the treatment of developed toxemia.

Edema during pregnancy may arise from pathological causes or from the physiologic and mechanical consequences of pregnancy. Thiazides are indicated in pregnancy when edema is due to pathologic causes just as they are in the absence of pregnancy (however, see WARNINGS, below). Dependent edema in pregnancy, resulting from restriction of venous return by the expanded uterus, is properly treated through elevation of the lower extremities and use of support hose. Use of diuretics to lower intravascular volume in this case is illogical and unnecessary. There is hypervolemia during normal pregnancy which is harmful to neither the fetus nor the mother (in absence of cardiovascular disease), but which is associated with edema, including generalized edema, in the majority of pregnant women. If this edema produces discomfort, increased recumbency will often provide relief. In rare instances, this edema may cause extreme discomfort which is not relieved by rest. In these cases, a short course of diuretics may provide relief and may be appropriate.

Continued on next page

Ayerst—Cont.

CONTRAINDICATIONS

Anuria.
Hypersensitivity to this or other sulfonamide-derived drugs.

WARNINGS

Thiazides should be used with caution in severe renal disease. In patients with renal disease, thiazides may precipitate azotemia. Cumulative effects of the drug may develop in patients with impaired renal function.
Thiazides should be used with caution in patients with impaired hepatic function or progressive liver disease, since minor alterations of fluid and electrolyte balance may precipitate hepatic coma.
Thiazides may add to or potentiate the action of other antihypertensive drugs. Potentiation occurs with ganglionic or peripheral adrenergic blocking drugs.
Sensitivity reactions may occur in patients with or without a history of allergy or bronchial asthma.
The possibility of exacerbation or activation of systemic lupus erythematosus has been reported.
DIUCARDIN (hydroflumethiazide) can cause fetal harm when administered to a pregnant woman. Thiazides cross the placental barrier and appear in cord blood. Hazards to the fetus include fetal or neonatal jaundice, thrombocytopenia, and possibly other adverse reactions which have occurred in the adult. If this drug is used during pregnancy, or if the patient becomes pregnant while taking this drug, the patient should be apprised of the potential hazard to the fetus.
Lithium generally should not be given with diuretics because they reduce its renal clearance and add a high risk of lithium toxicity. Refer to the package insert on lithium before use of such concomitant therapy.

PRECAUTIONS

General:
Periodic determination of serum electrolytes to detect possible electrolyte imbalance should be performed at appropriate intervals.
All patients receiving thiazide therapy should be observed for clinical signs of fluid or electrolyte imbalance: namely, hyponatremia, hypochloremic alkalosis, and hypokalemia. Serum and urine electrolyte determinations are particularly important when the patient is vomiting excessively or receiving parenteral fluids. Medication such as digitalis may also influence serum electrolytes. Warning signs, irrespective of cause, are: dryness of mouth, thirst, weakness, lethargy, drowsiness, restlessness, muscle pains or cramps, muscular fatigue, hypotension, oliguria, tachycardia, and gastrointestinal disturbances such as nausea and vomiting.
Hypokalemia may develop, especially with brisk diuresis, when severe cirrhosis is present, or during concomitant use of corticosteroids or ACTH.
Interference with adequate oral electrolyte intake will also contribute to hypokalemia. Hypokalemia can sensitize or exaggerate the response of the heart to the toxic effects of digitalis (*e.g.,* increased ventricular irritability). Concurrent administration of a potassium sparing diuretic or potassium supplements may be indicated in these patients.
Any chloride deficit is generally mild and usually does not require specific treatment except under extraordinary circumstances (as in liver disease or renal disease). Dilutional hyponatremia may occur in edematous patients in hot weather; appropriate therapy is water restriction, rather than administration of salt, except in rare instances when the hyponatremia is life-threatening. In actual salt depletion, appropriate replacement is the therapy of choice.
Hyperuricemia may occur or frank gout may be precipitated in certain patients receiving thiazide therapy.
Diabetes mellitus which has been latent may become manifest during thiazide administration.
The antihypertensive effects of the drug may be enhanced in the postsympathectomy patient.
If progressive renal impairment becomes evident, consider withholding or discontinuing diuretic therapy.
Drug Interactions: Insulin requirements in diabetic patients may be increased, decreased or unchanged.
Thiazide drugs may increase the responsiveness to tubocurarine.
Thiazides may decrease arterial responsiveness to norepinephrine. This diminution is not sufficient to preclude effectiveness of the pressor agent for therapeutic use.
Drug/laboratory test Interactions: Thiazides may decrease serum PBI levels without signs of thyroid disturbance.
Calcium excretion is decreased by thiazides. Pathological changes in the parathyroid gland with hypercalcemia and hypophosphatemia have been observed in a few patients on prolonged thiazide therapy. The common complications of hyperparathyroidism such as renal lithiasis, bone resorption, and peptic ulceration have not been seen. Thiazides should be discontinued before carrying out tests for parathyroid function.
Carcinogenesis, mutagenesis, impairment of fertility: No long-term reproductive studies have been performed.
Pregnancy: *Teratogenic effects:* Pregnancy category D. See WARNINGS section.
Nonteratogenic effects: See WARNINGS section.
Nursing mothers: Thiazides appear in breast milk. If use of the drug is deemed essential, the patient should stop nursing.
Pediatric use: Safety and effectiveness in children have not been established.

ADVERSE REACTIONS

Gastrointestinal System: anorexia, gastric irritation, nausea, vomiting, cramping, diarrhea, constipation, jaundice (intrahepatic cholestatic jaundice), pancreatitis, sialadenitis
Central Nervous System: dizziness, vertigo, paresthesias, headache, xanthopsia
Hematologic: leukopenia, agranulocytosis, thrombocytopenia, aplastic anemia, hemolytic anemia
Cardiovascular: orthostatic hypotension (may be aggravated by alcohol, barbiturates, or narcotics)
Hypersensitivity: purpura, photosensitivity, rash, urticaria, necrotizing angiitis (vasculitis, cutaneous vasculitis), fever, respiratory distress including pneumonitis, anaphylactic reactions
Other: hyperglycemia, glycosuria, hyperuricemia, muscle spasm, weakness, restlessness, transient blurred vision
Whenever adverse reactions are moderate or severe, thiazide dosage should be reduced or therapy withdrawn.

OVERDOSAGE

The following information is provided to serve as guidelines in treating overdosage.
HYDROFLUMETHIAZIDE
Signs and Symptoms:
Diuresis is to be expected; lethargy of varying degree may appear and may progress to coma within a few hours, with minimal depression of respiration and cardiovascular function, and without significant serum electrolyte changes or dehydration. The mechanism of CNS depression with thiazide overdosage is unknown.
G.I. irritation and hypermotility may occur; temporary elevation of BUN has been reported and serum electrolyte changes could occur, especially in patients with impairment of renal function.
Treatment:
Evacuate gastric contents but take care to prevent aspiration, especially in the stuporous or comatose patient. G.I. effects are usually of short duration, but may require symptomatic treatment.
Monitor serum electrolyte levels and renal function; institute supportive measures as required individually to maintain hydration, electrolyte balance, respiration, and cardiovascular-renal function.
DIUCARDIN (hydroflumethiazide) is slowly dialyzable.

DOSAGE AND ADMINISTRATION

Therapy should be individualized according to patient response. Use the smallest dosage necessary to maintain the required response.
The usual daily dosages for antihypertensive and diuretic effect are:

Diuretic	Antihypertensive
Adult: 25 to 200 mg	50 to 100 mg

Dosage regimens using 25 mg DIUCARDIN may be adequate in some cases.
Dosage should not exceed 200 mg per day.
For Diuresis in the Adult:
Initial recommended dose is 50 mg once or twice a day. Daily maintenance dose may be as little as 25 mg or as much as 200 mg, depending on patient's response. With dosages in excess of 100 mg daily, it is generally preferable to administer DIUCARDIN in divided doses.
Many patients with edema respond to intermittent therapy, i.e., administration on alternate days or on three to five days each week. With an intermittent schedule, excessive response and the resulting undesirable electrolyte imbalance are less likely to occur.
For Control of Hypertension in the Adult:
Usual starting dose is 50 mg twice daily. Dosage is increased or decreased according to the blood pressure response of the patient. Usual maintenance dose is 50 mg to 100 mg per day. Dosage should not exceed 200 mg per day.
Careful observations for changes in blood pressure must be made when this compound is used with other antihypertensive drugs, especially during initial therapy. The dosage of other agents must be reduced by at least 50 percent as soon as it is added to the regimen to prevent excessive drop in blood pressure. As the blood pressure falls under the potentiating effect of this agent, a further reduction in dosage, or even discontinuation, of other antihypertensive drugs may be necessary.

HOW SUPPLIED

DIUCARDIN—Each scored, white oval compressed tablet, inscribed "DIUCARDIN®50," contains 50 mg hydroflumethiazide, in bottles of 100 (NDC 0046-0702-81).
Store at room temperature (approximately 25° C).
Shown in Product Identification Section, page 404

ENZACTIN® Cream OTC

[en-zăc'tin]
Brand of triacetin

Also contains polyethylene glycol 400, polyethylene glycol 4000, and titanium dioxide.

ACTION

For prevention and treatment of athlete's foot and other superficial fungus infections. The "self-regulating" action of ENZACTIN (triacetin) releases a constant effective level of *free* fatty acid at the site of infection, in a concentration that is nonirritating.
"*Self-regulating" action*—At a neutral or higher pH of infected skin and in the presence of the enzyme esterase (found abundantly in skin, serum, and fungi), glycerol and free fatty acid (acetic) are rapidly liberated from triacetin. At this point, the growth of fungi is inhibited by the free acid.
With an accumulation of free acid, the pH drops and esterase activity decreases. Then, as the acid in the skin diffuses or becomes neutralized, the pH rises and esterase is reactivated, to release more free acid for fungistatic control.
Relieves itching and soreness promptly. Helps prevent spread of infection. Nonirritating. Odorless and stainless.

INDICATIONS

Athlete's foot and other superficial fungus infections.

ADMINISTRATION

Thoroughly cleanse affected and adjacent areas with dilute alcohol or a mild soap and warm water. Pat dry. Apply cream liberally twice daily, preferably morning and evening.
Note: Rayon fabrics should not come in contact with ENZACTIN (triacetin) Cream. For protection, cover treated areas with clean cotton cloth or bandage. If infection persists, consult a physician.

HOW SUPPLIED

ENZACTIN Cream—250 mg triacetin per gram (in emollient base), in 1 oz (28.35 g) collapsible tubes (NDC 0046-0201-01).

AYERST EPITRATE® ℞

[ĕp'i-trāt]
Brand of epinephrine bitartrate ophthalmic solution

CAUTION: Federal law prohibits dispensing without prescription.

DESCRIPTION

EPITRATE (epinephrine bitartrate) Ophthalmic Solution is a sterile aqueous solution of levorotatory epinephrine bitartrate, 2% (equivalent to 1.1% base). Inactive ingredients include chlorobutanol (chloral derivative) 0.55%, sodium bisulfite, sodium chloride, polyoxypropylene-polyoxyethylene-diol, and disodium edetate. Epinephrine bitartrate is an adrenergic agent with the chemical name (-)-3,4,-Dihydroxy-α-[(methylamino) methyl] benzyl alcohol (+) tartrate (1:1) salt. It has a low surface tension.

CLINICAL PHARMACOLOGY

EPITRATE lowers intraocular pressure by reducing the rate of aqueous formation. Improvement in outflow facility is also observed in certain cases following prolonged therapy.

INDICATIONS AND USAGE

Useful in management of chronic simple (open-angle) glaucoma, either alone or in combination with miotics. In selected cases, it may also be used with carbonic anhydrase inhibitors.

CONTRAINDICATIONS

Prior to peripheral iridectomy, an epinephrine preparation is contraindicated in eyes that are capable of angle closure since its relatively weak mydriatic action may, nevertheless, precipitate angle block. Gonioscopy should be carried out on all patients before initiating therapy.

WARNINGS

Topical use of epinephrine in any form should be interrupted prior to general anesthesia with certain anesthetics such as cyclopropane or halothane which sensitize the myocardium to sympathomimetics.

PRECAUTIONS

EPITRATE (epinephrine bitartrate) should be used with caution in the presence of hypertension, diabetes, hyperthyroidism, heart disease, and cerebral arteriosclerosis because of the possibility of systemic action.
Do not use the solution if it is brown or contains a precipitate.

Drug Interactions: (See WARNINGS.)
Carcinogenesis, Mutagenesis, Impairment of Fertility: No long-term studies in animals or humans have been conducted.
Pregnancy Category C: Animal reproduction studies have not been conducted with EPITRATE. It is also not known whether EPITRATE can cause fetal harm when administered to a pregnant woman or can affect reproduction capacity. EPITRATE should be given to a pregnant woman only if clearly needed.
Nursing Mothers: It is not known whether this drug is excreted in human milk. Because many drugs are excreted in human milk, caution should be exercised when EPITRATE is administered to a nursing woman.
Pediatric Use: Safety and effectiveness in children have not been established.

ADVERSE REACTIONS

As with other epinephrine solutions, transitory stinging on initial instillation may be expected. Headache or browache frequently occur on beginning EPITRATE therapy, but usually diminish as treatment is continued. Conjunctival allergy occurs occasionally. Pigmentary deposits in the lids, conjunctiva or cornea may occur after prolonged use of epinephrine eyedrops. In rare cases, maculopathy with a central scotoma may result from the use of topical epinephrine in aphakic patients; prompt reversal generally follows discontinuance of the drug. Systemic effects have occasionally been reported, such as: palpitation, tachycardia, extrasystoles, hypertension, trembling, sweating, and pallor.

DOSAGE AND ADMINISTRATION

One drop, with frequency of instillation being individualized, from every two or three days to twice daily. More frequent instillation than one drop four times daily does not usually elicit any further improvement in therapeutic response.

HOW SUPPLIED

AYERST EPITRATE®—ophthalmic solution of epinephrine bitartrate 2% (equivalent to 1.1% base). Package containing 7.5 mL bottle with separate dropper-screw cap attachment (NDC 0046-1015-07).

ESTRADURIN® ℞

[ĕs "tra-dū 'rin]
Brand of polyestradiol phosphate
For Intramuscular Injection Only

CAUTION: Federal law prohibits dispensing without prescription.

DESCRIPTION

ESTRADURIN (polyestradiol phosphate) is a water-soluble, high molecular weight polyester of phosphoric acid and 17β-estradiol. It is provided in a SECULE® containing 40 mg polyestradiol phosphate, 0.022 mg phenylmercuric nitrate, and 5.2 mg sodium phosphate. As solubilizing agents for the active ingredient, 25 mg niacinamide and 4 mg propylene glycol are also present. The pH is adjusted with sodium hydroxide.
One 2 mL ampul of sterile diluent is also provided.

CLINICAL PHARMACOLOGY

Estrogens are important in the development and maintenance of the female reproductive system. In responsive tissues estrogens enter the cell and are transported into the nucleus.
In the male patient with androgenic hormone-dependent conditions, such as metastatic carcinoma of the prostate gland, estrogens counter the androgenic influence by competing for the receptor sites. As a result of treatment with estrogens, metastatic lesions in the bone may also show improvement.
Biologically active estradiol units are gradually split off from the large parent molecule, thus providing a continuous level of active estrogen over a prolonged period. The liberated estradiol is metabolized by the body in the same manner as the endogenous hormone. There is no depot effect at the site of injection—90 percent of injected dose leaves the bloodstream within 24 hours. Passive storage occurs in the reticuloendothelial system. As circulating levels of estradiol drop, more returns to the bloodstream from the site of storage for an even, continuous therapeutic effect. Increasing the dose acts to prolong the duration of pharmacologic action rather than to increase blood levels.
Metabolism and inactivation occur primarily in the liver. Some estrogens are excreted into the bile; however they are reabsorbed from the intestine and returned to the liver through the portal venous system. Water-soluble estrogen conjugates are strongly acidic and are ionized in body fluids, which favor excretion through the kidneys since tubular reabsorption is minimal.

INDICATION

ESTRADURIN (polyestradiol phosphate) is indicated in the treatment of prostatic carcinoma—palliative therapy of advanced disease.

CONTRAINDICATIONS

Estrogens should not be used in men with any of the following conditions:
1. Known or suspected cancer of the breast except in appropriately selected patients being treated for metastatic disease.
2. Known or suspected estrogen-dependent neoplasia.
3. Active thrombophlebitis or thromboembolic disorders.

WARNINGS

1. *Induction of malignant neoplasms.* Long-term, continuous administration of natural and synthetic estrogens in certain animal species increases the frequency of carcinomas of the breast, cervix, vagina, and liver.
2. *Gallbladder disease.* A recent study has reported a 2- to 3-fold increase in the risk of surgically confirmed gallbladder disease in women receiving postmenopausal estrogens,[1] similar to the 2-fold increase previously noted in users of oral contraceptives.[2,7a]
3. *Effects similar to those caused by estrogen-progestogen oral contraceptives.* There are several serious adverse effects of oral contraceptives. It has been shown that there is an increased risk of thrombosis in men receiving estrogens for prostatic cancer and women for postpartum breast engorgement.[3–6]
a. *Thromboembolic disease.* It is now well established that users of oral contraceptives have an increased risk of various thromboembolic and thrombotic vascular diseases, such as thrombophlebitis, pulmonary embolism, stroke, and myocardial infarction.[7–14] Cases of retinal thrombosis, mesenteric thrombosis, and optic neuritis have been reported in oral contraceptive users. There is evidence that the risk of several of these adverse reactions is related to the dose of the drug.[15,16] An increased risk of postsurgery thromboembolic complications has also been reported in users of oral contraceptives.[17,18] If feasible, estrogen should be discontinued at least 4 weeks before surgery of the type associated with an increased risk of thromboembolism, or during periods of prolonged immobilization.
Estrogens should not be used in persons with active thrombophlebitis or thromboembolic disorders. They should be used with caution in patients with cerebral vascular or coronary artery disease and only for those in whom estrogens are clearly indicated.
Large doses of estrogen (5 mg conjugated estrogens per day), comparable to those used to treat cancer of the prostate, have been shown in a large prospective clinical trial in men[19] to increase the risk of nonfatal myocardial infarction, pulmonary embolism and thrombophlebitis. When estrogen doses of this size are used, any of the thromboembolic and thrombotic adverse effects associated with oral contraceptive use should be considered a clear risk.
b. *Hepatic adenoma.* Benign hepatic adenomas appear to be associated with the use of oral contraceptives.[20–22] Although benign, and rare, these may rupture and may cause death through intra-abdominal hemorrhage. Such lesions have not yet been reported in association with other estrogen or progestogen preparations but should be considered in estrogen users having abdominal pain and tenderness, abdominal mass, or hypovolemic shock. Hepatocellular carcinoma has also been reported in women taking estrogen-containing oral contraceptives.[21] The relationship of this malignancy to these drugs is not known at this time.
c. *Elevated blood pressure.* Women using oral contraceptives sometimes experience increased blood pressure which, in most cases, returns to normal on discontinuing the drug. There is now a report that this may occur with use of estrogens in the menopause[23] and blood pressure should be monitored with estrogen use, especially if high doses are used.
d. *Glucose tolerance.* A worsening of glucose tolerance has been observed in a significant percentage of patients on estrogen-containing oral contraceptives. For this reason, diabetic patients should be carefully observed while receiving estrogen.
4. *Hypercalcemia.* Administration of estrogens may lead to severe hypercalcemia in patients with breast cancer and bone metastases. If this occurs, the drug should be stopped and appropriate measures taken to reduce the serum calcium level.

PRECAUTIONS

1. A complete medical and family history should be taken prior to the initiation of any estrogen therapy. The pretreatment and periodic physical examinations should include special reference to blood pressure, breasts, abdomen, and pelvic organs. As a general rule, estrogen should not be prescribed for longer than one year without another physical examination being performed.
2. Fluid retention—Because estrogens may cause some degree of fluid retention, conditions which might be influenced by this factor such as asthma, epilepsy, migraine, and cardiac or renal dysfunction, require careful observation.
3. Certain patients may develop undesirable manifestations of excessive estrogenic stimulation, such as gynecomastia.
4. Oral contraceptives appear to be associated with an increased incidence of mental depression.[7a] Although it is not clear whether this is due to the estrogenic or progestogenic component of the contraceptive, patients with a history of depression should be carefully observed.
5. The pathologist should be advised of estrogen therapy when relevant specimens are submitted.
6. If jaundice develops in any patient receiving estrogen, the medication should be discontinued while the cause is investigated.
7. Estrogens may be poorly metabolized in patients with impaired liver function and they should be administered with caution in such patients.
8. Because estrogens influence the metabolism of calcium and phosphorus, they should be used with caution in patients with metabolic bone diseases that are associated with hypercalcemia or in patients with renal insufficiency.
9. Because of the effects of estrogens on epiphyseal closure, they should be used judiciously in young patients in whom bone growth is not complete.
10. Certain endocrine and liver function tests may be affected by estrogen-containing oral contraceptives. The following similar changes may be expected with larger doses of estrogen:
a. Increased sulfobromophthalein retention.
b. Increased prothrombin and factors VII, VIII, IX, and X; decreased antithrombin 3; increased norepinephrine-induced platelet aggregability.
c. Increased thyroid binding globulin (TBG) leading to increased circulating total thyroid hormone, as measured by PBI, T4 by column, or T4 by radioimmunoassay. Free T3 resin uptake is decreased, reflecting the elevated TBG; free T4 concentration is unaltered.
d. Impaired glucose tolerance.
e. Reduced response to metyrapone test.
f. Reduced serum folate concentration.
g. Increased serum triglyceride and phospholipid concentration.

ADVERSE REACTIONS

(See WARNINGS regarding induction of neoplasia, increased incidence of gallbladder disease, and adverse effects similar to those of oral contraceptives, including thromboembolism.) The following additional adverse reactions have been reported with estrogenic therapy, including oral contraceptives:
1. *Breasts:* Tenderness, enlargement, secretion.
2. *Gastrointestinal:* Nausea, vomiting; abdominal cramps, bloating; cholestatic jaundice.
3. *Skin:* Chloasma or melasma which may persist when drug is discontinued; erythema multiforme; erythema nodosum; hemorrhagic eruption; loss of scalp hair; hirsutism.
4. *Eyes:* Steepening of corneal curvature; intolerance to contact lenses.
5. *CNS:* Headache, migraine, dizziness; mental depression; chorea.
6. *Miscellaneous:* Increase or decrease in weight; reduced carbohydrate tolerance; aggravation of porphyria; edema; changes in libido.

ACUTE OVERDOSAGE

Numerous reports of ingestion of large doses of estrogen-containing oral contraceptives by young children indicate that acute serious ill effects do not occur. Overdosage of estrogen may cause nausea, and withdrawal bleeding may occur in females.

DOSAGE AND ADMINISTRATION

Inoperable progressing prostatic cancer—40 mg intramuscularly every two to four weeks or less frequently, depending on clinical response of the patient. If the response is not satisfactory doses up to 80 mg may be used. Experimental evidence indicates that increasing the dose primarily prolongs the duration of action, but the amount of estrogen available at any one time is not significantly increased. The dosage should be adjusted as indicated by careful observation of the patient.
Deep intramuscular injection only is recommended. (Initially, some patients may experience a burning sensation at site of injection. This is transitory, and it may not recur with subsequent injections, or may be obviated by concomitant administration of a local anesthetic.)
If a response to estrogen therapy is going to occur, it will be apparent within three months of the beginning of therapy. If it does occur, the hormone should be continued until the disease is again progressive. The hormone should then be stopped, and the patient may obtain another period of improvement known as "rebound regression." This occurs in 30% of the patients who show objective improvement on estrogens.

DIRECTIONS FOR USE
Reconstitution for use:
1. Introduce sterile diluent into SECULE, preferably with a 20 gauge needle affixed to a 5 mL syringe.

Continued on next page

Ayerst—Cont.

2. Swirl gently until a solution is effected. (DO NOT AGITATE VIOLENTLY.)

Stability: After reconstitution, if storage is desired, the solution should be kept at room temperature and away from direct light. Under these conditions the solution is stable for about 10 days, so long as cloudiness or evidence of a precipitate has not occurred.

HOW SUPPLIED

NDC 0046-0451-02—Each package provides:

1. One SECULE® containing 40 mg polyestradiol phosphate, 0.022 mg phenylmercuric nitrate, and 5.2 mg sodium phosphate. As solubilizing agents for the active ingredient, 25 mg niacinamide and 4 mg propylene glycol are also present. The pH is adjusted with sodium hydroxide.
2. One 2 mL ampul of sterile diluent.

ESTRADURIN (polyestradiol phosphate) is prepared by cryodesiccation.

PHYSICIAN REFERENCES

1. Boston Collaborative Drug Surveillance Program: N. Engl. J. Med. *290*:15–19, 1974.
2. Boston Collaborative Drug Surveillance Program: Lancet *1*:1399–1404, 1973.
3. Daniel, D. G., *et al.*: Lancet *2*:287–289, 1967.
4. The Veterans Administration Cooperative Urological Research Group: J. Urol. *98*:516–522, 1967.
5. Bailar, J. C.: Lancet *2*:560, 1967.
6. Blackard, C., *et al.*: Cancer *26*:249–256, 1970.
7. Royal College of General Practitioners: J. R. Coll. Gen. Pract. *13*:267–279, 1967.

7a. Royal College of General Practitioners: Oral Contraceptives and Health, New York, Pitman Corp., 1974.

8. Inman, W. H. W., *et al.*: Br. Med. J. *2*:193–199, 1968.
9. Vessey, M. P., *et al.*: Br. Med. J. *2*:651–657, 1969.
10. Sartwell, P. E., *et al.*: Am. J. Epidemiol. *90*:365–380, 1969.
11. Collaborative Group for the Study of Stroke in Young Women: N. Engl. J. Med. *288*:871–878, 1973.
12. Collaborative Group for the Study of Stroke in Young Women: J.A.M.A. *231*:718–722, 1975.
13. Mann, J. I., *et al.*: Br. Med. J. *2*:245–248, 1975.
14. Mann, J. I., *et al.*: Br. Med. J. *2*:241–245, 1975.
15. Inman, W. H. W., *et al.*: Br. Med. J. *2*:203–209, 1970.
16. Stolley, P. D., *et al.*: Am. J. Epidemiol. *102*:197–208, 1975.
17. Vessey, M. P., *et al.*: Br. Med. J. *3*:123–126, 1970.
18. Greene, G. R., *et al.*: Am. J. Public Health *62*:680–685, 1972.
19. Coronary Drug Project Research Group: J.A.M.A. *214*:1303–1313, 1970.
20. Baum, J., *et al.*: Lancet *2*:926–928, 1973.
21. Mays, E. T., *et al.*: J.A.M.A. *235*:730–732, 1976.
22. Edmondson, H. A., *et al.*: N. Engl. J. Med. *294*:470–472, 1976.
23. Pfeffer, R. I., *et al.*: Am. J. Epidemiol. *103*:445–456, 1976.

SECULE®—Trademark to designate a special vial containing an injectable preparation in dry form.

FACTREL® ℞

[făc-trĕl']

(gonadorelin hydrochloride)

Synthetic Luteinizing Hormone Releasing Hormone (LH-RH)

DIAGNOSTIC USE ONLY

CAUTION: Federal law prohibits dispensing without prescription.

DESCRIPTION

An agent for use in evaluating hypothalamic-pituitary gonadotropic function. FACTREL (gonadorelin hydrochloride) injectable is available as a sterile lyophilized powder for reconstitution and administration by subcutaneous or intravenous routes.

Chemical Name: 5-oxo-L-prolyl-L-histidyl -L- tryptophyl -L- seryl -L- tyrosyl-glycyl -L- leucyl-L-argi-nyl-L-prolyl glycinamide hydrochloride

[See structural formula below].

FACTREL is $C_{55}H_{75}N_{17}O_{13}HCl$, as the mono- or dihydrochloride, or their mixture. The gonadorelin base has a molecular weight of 1182.33. It is a white powder, soluble in alcohol and water, hygroscopic and moisture-sensitive, and stable at room temperature. The synthetic decapeptide, FACTREL, has a chemical composition and structure identical to the natural hormone, identified from porcine or ovine hypothalami.

Each vial of FACTREL contains 100 or 500 mcg gonadorelin as the hydrochloride, with 100 mg lactose, USP. Each ampul of sterile diluent contains 2% benzyl alcohol and Water for Injection, USP.

CLINICAL PHARMACOLOGY

FACTREL has been shown to have gonadotropin-releasing effects upon the anterior pituitary. The range for normal baseline LH levels, as determined from the literature, is 5-25 mIU/mL in postpubertal males, and postpubertal and premenopausal females. The standard used is the Second International Reference Preparation—HMC. This range may not correspond in each laboratory performing the assay since the concentration of LH in normal individuals varies with different assay methods. The normal responses to FACTREL analyzed from the results of clinical studies included:

(1) LH peak (mIU/mL)
(highest LH value post-FACTREL administration)
(2) Maximum LH increase (mIU/mL)
(peak LH value—LH baseline value)
(3) LH percent response

$$\frac{\text{peak LH—baseline LH}}{\text{baseline LH}} \times 100\%$$

(4) Time to peak (minutes)
(time required to reach LH peak value)

Normal adult subjects were shown to have these LH responses following FACTREL administration by subcutaneous or intravenous routes.

I. MALE ADULTS:

A) Subcutaneous Administration
The results are based on 18 tests in males between the ages of 18–42 years, inclusive:
(1) LH peak: mean 60.3 ± 26.2 mIU/mL
100% ≥ 24.0 mIU/mL
90% ≥ 32.8 mIU/mL
(2) Maximum LH increase: mean 46.7 ± 20.8 mIU/mL
100% ≥ 12.3 mIU/mL
90% ≥ 20.9 mIU/mL
(3) LH percent response: mean 437 ± 243% range: 66–1853%
90% ≥ 188%

B) Intravenous Administration
The results are based on 26 tests in males between the ages of 19–58 years, inclusive:
(1) LH peak: mean 63.8 ± 40.3 mIU/mL
100% ≥ 12.6 mIU/mL
90% ≥ 26.0 mIU/mL
(2) Maximum LH increase: mean 51.3 ± 35.2 mIU/mL
100% ≥ 7.4 mIU/mL
90% ≥ 14.8 mIU/mL
(3) LH percent response: mean 481 ± 184% range: 67–2139%
90% ≥ 142%
(4) Time to peak: mean 27 ± 14 min.

In males older than 50 years, the LH baseline and peak levels tend to be higher; however, the maximum LH increases do not differ in regard to age.

II. FEMALE ADULTS:

A) Subcutaneous Administration
The results are based on 38 tests in females between the ages of 19–36 years, inclusive:
(1) LH peak: mean 67.9 ± 27.5 mIU/mL
100% ≥ 12.5 mIU/mL
90% ≥ 39.0 mIU/mL
(2) Maximum LH increase: mean 52.8 ± 26.4 mIU/mL
100% ≥ 7.5 mIU/mL
90% ≥ 23.8 mIU/mL
(3) LH percent response: mean 374 ± 221% range: 108–981%
90% ≥ 185%
(4) Time to peak: mean 71.5 ± 49.6 min.

B) Intravenous Administration
The results are based on 31 tests in females between the ages of 20–35 years inclusive:
(1) LH peak: mean 57.6 ± 36.7 mIU/mL
100% ≥ 20.0 mIU/mL
90% ≥ 24.6 mIU/mL
(2) Maximum LH increase: mean 44.5 ± 31.8 mIU/mL
100% ≥ 7.5 mIU/mL
90% ≥ 16.2 mIU/mL
(3) LH percent response: mean 356 ± 282% range: 60–1300%
90% ≥ 142%
(4) Time to peak: mean 36 ± 24 min.

The FACTREL (gonadorelin hydrochloride) tests on which the normal female responses are based were performed in the early follicular phase of the menstrual cycle (Days 1–7).

In menopausal and postmenopausal females, the baseline LH levels are elevated and the maximum LH increases are exaggerated when compared with the premenopausal levels.

Patients with clinically diagnosed or suspected pituitary and/or hypothalamic dysfunction were often shown to have subnormal or no LH responses following FACTREL administration. For example, in clinical tests of 6 patients with known postpubertal panhypopituitarism, and 11 patients with Prader-Willi Syndrome, 100% showed subnormal responses or no rise in LH. Subnormal responses to the FACTREL test also were observed in 21 (95%) of 22 patients with prepubertal panhypopituitarism. In 19 patients with Sheehan's syndrome, 16 (84%) had a subnormal response. In the FACTREL test in 44 patients with Kallmann's syndrome, 33 (77%) had subnormal LH responses.

INDICATIONS AND USAGE

FACTREL as a single injection is indicated for evaluating the functional capacity and response of the gonadotropes of the anterior pituitary. This single injection test does not measure pituitary gonadotropic reserve for which more prolonged or repeated administration may be required. The LH response is useful in testing patients with suspected gonadotropin deficiency, whether due to the hypothalamus alone or in combination with anterior pituitary failure. FACTREL is also indicated for evaluating residual gonadotropic function of the pituitary following removal of a pituitary tumor by surgery and/or irradiation. In clinical studies to date, however, the single injection test has not been useful in differentiating pituitary disorders from hypothalamic disorders. The FACTREL test can be performed concomitantly with other post-treatment evaluations.

The results of the FACTREL test complement the clinical examination and other laboratory tests used to confirm or substantiate hypogonadotropic hypogonadism.

In cases where there is a normal response, it indicates the presence of functional pituitary gonadotropes. The single injection test does not measure pituitary gonadotropic reserve.

CONTRAINDICATIONS

Hypersensitivity to gonadorelin hydrochloride or any of the components.

PRECAUTIONS

Antibody formation has been rarely reported after chronic administration of large doses of FACTREL.

The FACTREL test should be conducted in the absence of other drugs which directly affect the pituitary secretion of the gonadotropins. These would include a variety of preparations which contain androgens, estrogens, progestins, or glucocorticoids. The gonadotropin levels may be transiently elevated by spironolactone, minimally elevated by levodopa, and suppressed by oral contraceptives and digoxin. The response to FACTREL may be blunted by phenothiazines and dopamine antagonists which cause a rise in prolactin.

Pregnancy Category B. Reproduction studies have been performed in mice, rats, and rabbits at doses up to 50 times the human dose, and have revealed no evidence of harm to the fetus due to FACTREL. There are, however, no adequate and well-controlled studies in pregnant women. Because animal reproduction studies are not always predictive of human response, this drug should be used during pregnancy only if clearly needed.

Appropriate precautions should be taken because the effects of LH-RH on the fetus and developing offspring have not been adequately evaluated. Repetitive, high doses of FACTREL may cause luteolysis and inhibition of spermatogenesis.

ADVERSE REACTIONS

Systemic complaints such as headaches, nausea, lightheadedness, abdominal discomfort, and flushing have been re-

Structural Formula:

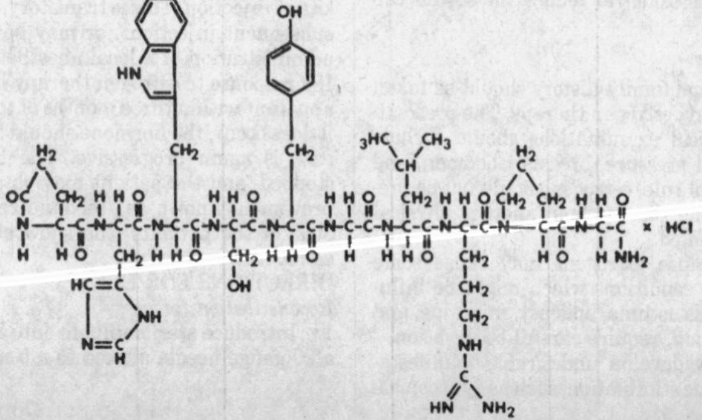

ported rarely following administration of 100 mcg of FACTREL. Local swelling, occasionally with pain and pruritus, at the injection site may occur if FACTREL is administered subcutaneously. Local and generalized skin rash have been noted after chronic subcutaneous administration.
Rare instances of hypersensitivity reaction (bronchospasm, tachycardia, flushing, urticaria, induration at injection site) have been reported following multiple-dose administration.

OVERDOSAGE

FACTREL (gonadorelin hydrochloride) has been administered parenterally in doses up to 3 mg BID for 28 days without any signs or symptoms of overdosage. In case of overdosage or idiosyncrasy, symptomatic treatment should be administered as required.

DOSAGE AND ADMINISTRATION

Adults: 100 mcg dose, subcutaneously or intravenously. In females for whom the phase of the menstrual cycle can be established, the test should be performed in the early follicular phase (Days 1–7).

TEST METHODOLOGY

To determine the status of the gonadotropin secretory capacity of the anterior pituitary, a test procedure requiring seven venous blood samples for LH is recommended.

PROCEDURE:

1. Venous blood samples should be drawn at -15 minutes and immediately prior to FACTREL administration. The LH baseline is obtained by averaging the LH values of the two samples.
2. Administer a bolus of 100 mcg of FACTREL subcutaneously or intravenously.
3. Draw venous blood samples at 15, 30, 45, 60, and 120 minutes after administration.
4. Blood samples should be handled as recommended by the laboratory that will determine the LH content. It must be emphasized that the reliability of the test is directly related to the inter-assay and intra-assay reliability of the laboratory performing the assay.

INTERPRETATION OF TEST RESULTS

Interpretation of the LH response to FACTREL requires an understanding of the hypothalamic-pituitary physiology, knowledge of the clinical status of the individual patient, and familiarity with the normal ranges and the standards used in the laboratory performing the LH assays.
Figures 1 through 4 represent the LH response curves after FACTREL administration in normal subjects. The normal LH response curves were established between the 10th percentile (B line) and 90th percentile (A line) of all LH responses in normal subjects analyzed from the results of clinical studies. LH values are reported in units of mIU/mL and time is displayed in minutes. Individual patient responses should be plotted on the appropriate curve. A subnormal response in patients is defined as three or more LH values which fall below the B line of the normal LH response curve.
In cases where there is a blunted or borderline response, the FACTREL (gonadorelin hydrochloride) test should be repeated.

Fig. 1:
Normal Male LH Response After FACTREL 100 mcg, Subcutaneous Administration 10th and 90th percentiles.

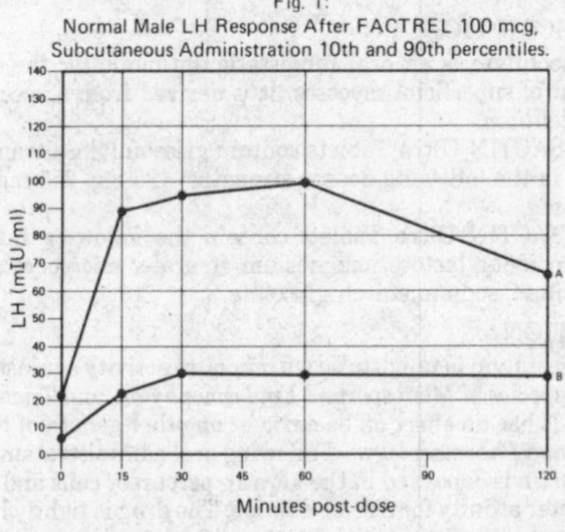

Fig. 2:
Normal Male LH Response After FACTREL 100 mcg, Intravenous Administration 10th and 90th percentiles.

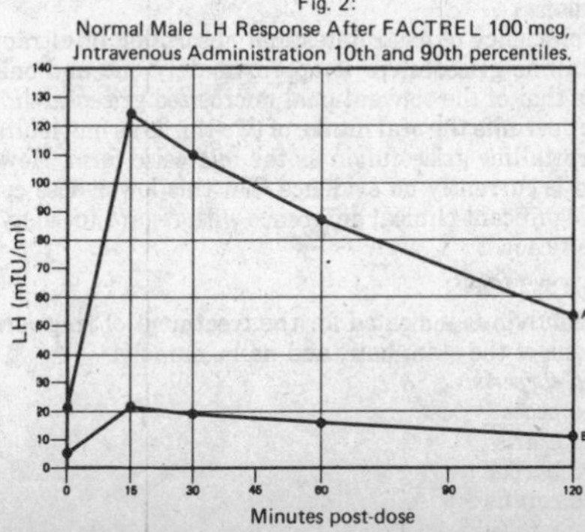

Fig. 3:
Normal Female LH Response After FACTREL 100 mcg, Subcutaneous Administration 10th and 90th percentiles.

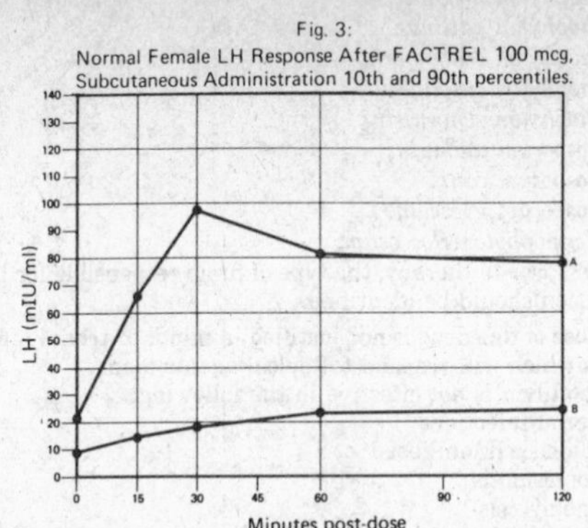

Fig. 4:
Normal Female LH Response After FACTREL 100 mcg, Intravenous Administration 10th and 90th percentiles.

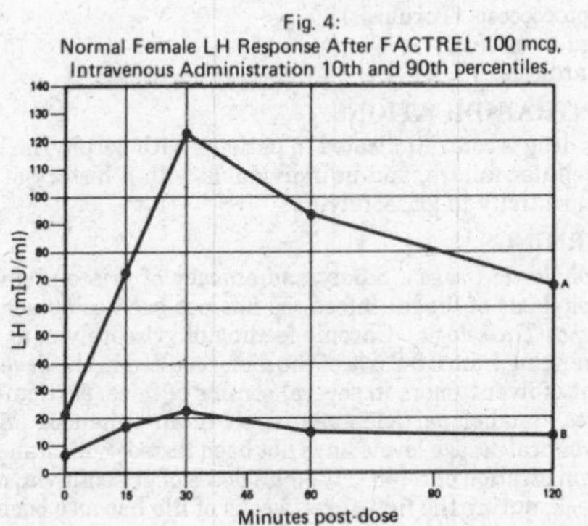

The FACTREL (gonadorelin hydrochloride) test complements the clinical assessment of patients with a variety of endocrine disorders involving the hypothalamic-pituitary axis. In cases where there is a normal response, it indicates the presence of functional pituitary gonadotropes. The single injection test does not determine the pathophysiological cause for the subnormal response and does not measure pituitary gonadotropic reserve.

HOW SUPPLIED

LYOPHILIZED POWDER

in single-dose vials containing 100 mcg (NDC 0046-0507-05) and 500 mcg (NDC 0046-0509-05) gonadorelin as the hydrochloride with 100 mg lactose, USP. Each vial is accompanied by one ampul containing 2 mL sterile diluent of 2% benzyl alcohol in Water for Injection, USP.

DIRECTIONS

Store at room temperature (approximately 25°C).
Reconstitute 100 mcg vial with 1.0 mL of the accompanying sterile diluent.
Reconstitute 500 mcg vial with 2.0 mL of the accompanying sterile diluent.
Prepare solution immediately before use.
After reconstitution, store at room temperature and use within 1 day.
Discard unused reconstituted solution and diluent.
Diagnostic Method of Use Patent 3,947,569

Shown in Product Identification Section, page 404

FLUOTHANE® ℞

[flū'o-thān]
Brand of halothane, USP

CAUTION: Federal law prohibits dispensing without prescription.

DESCRIPTION

FLUOTHANE, brand of halothane, USP, is an inhalation anesthetic. It is 2-bromo-2-chloro-1,1,1-trifluoroethane and has the following structural formula:

```
    F   Br
    |   |
F—C—C—Cl
    |   |
    F   H
```

The specific gravity is 1.872-1.877 at 20° C, and the boiling point (range) is 49° C-51° C at 760 mm Hg. The vapor pressure is 243 mm Hg at 20° C. The blood/gas coefficient is 2.5 at 37° C, and the olive oil/water coefficient is 220 at 37° C. Vapor concentrations within anesthetic range are nonirritating and have a pleasant odor. FLUOTHANE is nonflammable, and its vapors mixed with oxygen in proportions from 0.5 to 50 per cent (v/v) are not explosive.
FLUOTHANE does not decompose in contact with warm soda lime. When moisture is present, the vapor attacks aluminum, brass, and lead, but not copper. Rubber, some plastics, and similar materials are soluble in FLUOTHANE; such materials will deteriorate rapidly in contact with FLUOTHANE vapor or liquid. Stability of FLUOTHANE is maintained by the addition of 0.01 per cent thymol (w/w), up to 0.00025% ammonia (w/w), and storage is in amber-colored bottles.

FLUOTHANE should not be kept indefinitely in vaporizer bottles not specifically designed for its use. Thymol does not volatilize along with FLUOTHANE, and therefore accumulates in the vaporizer, and may, in time, impart a yellow color to the remaining liquid or to wicks in vaporizers. The development of such discoloration may be used as an indicator that the vaporizer should be drained and cleaned, and the discolored FLUOTHANE (halothane, USP) discarded. Accumulation of thymol may be removed by washing with diethyl ether. After cleaning a wick or vaporizer, make certain all the diethyl ether has been removed before reusing the equipment to avoid introducing ether into the system.

ACTIONS

FLUOTHANE is an inhalation anesthetic. Induction and recovery are rapid and depth of anesthesia can be rapidly altered. FLUOTHANE progressively depresses respiration. There may be tachypnea with reduced tidal volume and alveolar ventilation. FLUOTHANE is not an irritant to the respiratory tract, and no increase in salivary or bronchial secretions ordinarily occurs. Pharyngeal and laryngeal reflexes are rapidly obtunded. It causes bronchodilation. Hypoxia, acidosis, or apnea may develop during deep anesthesia.

FLUOTHANE reduces the blood pressure, and frequently decreases the pulse rate. The greater the concentration of the drug, the more evident these changes become. Atropine may reverse the bradycardia. FLUOTHANE does not cause the release of catecholamines from adrenergic stores. FLUOTHANE also causes dilation of the vessels of the skin and skeletal muscles.
Cardiac arrhythmias may occur during FLUOTHANE anesthesia. These include nodal rhythm, AV dissociation, ventricular extrasystoles and asystole. FLUOTHANE sensitizes the myocardial conduction system to the action of epinephrine and norepinephrine, and the combination may cause serious cardiac arrhythmias. FLUOTHANE increases cerebral spinal fluid pressure. FLUOTHANE produces moderate muscular relaxation. Muscle relaxants are used as adjuncts in order to maintain lighter levels of anesthesia. FLUOTHANE augments the action of nondepolarizing relaxants and ganglionic blocking agents. FLUOTHANE is a potent uterine relaxant.

INDICATIONS

FLUOTHANE (halothane, USP) is indicated for the induction and maintenance of general anesthesia.

CONTRAINDICATIONS

FLUOTHANE is not recommended for obstetrical anesthesia except when uterine relaxation is required.

WARNINGS

When previous exposure to FLUOTHANE was followed by unexplained jaundice, consideration should be given to the use of other agents.
FLUOTHANE should be used in vaporizers that permit a reasonable approximation of output, and preferably of the calibrated type. The vaporizer should be placed out of circuit in closed circuit rebreathing systems; otherwise overdosage is difficult to avoid. The patient should be closely observed for signs of overdosage, *i.e.*, depression of blood pressure, pulse rate, and ventilation, particularly during assisted or controlled ventilation.
Usage in Pregnancy. Safe use of FLUOTHANE has not been established with respect to possible adverse effects upon fetal development. Therefore, FLUOTHANE should not be used in women where pregnancy is possible and particularly during early pregnancy, unless, in the judgment of the physician, the potential benefits outweigh the unknown hazards to the fetus.

PRECAUTIONS

The uterine relaxation obtained with FLUOTHANE (halothane, USP), unless carefully controlled, may fail to respond to ergot derivatives and oxytocic posterior pituitary extract.

FLUOTHANE increases cerebrospinal fluid pressure. Therefore, in patients with markedly raised intracranial pressure, if FLUOTHANE is indicated, administration should be preceded by measures ordinarily used to reduce cerebrospinal fluid pressure. Ventilation should be carefully assessed, and it may be necessary to assist or control ventila-

Continued on next page

Ayerst—Cont.

tion to insure adequate oxygenation and carbon dioxide removal.
Epinephrine or norepinephrine should be employed cautiously, if at all, during FLUOTHANE (halothane, USP) anesthesia, since their simultaneous use may induce ventricular tachycardia or fibrillation.
Nondepolarizing relaxants and ganglionic blocking agents should be administered cautiously, since their actions are augmented by FLUOTHANE.
It has been reported that in genetically susceptible individuals, the use of general anesthetics and the muscle relaxant, succinylcholine, may trigger a syndrome known as malignant hyperthermic crisis. Monitoring temperature during surgery will aid in early recognition of this syndrome. Dantrolene sodium and supportive measures are generally indicated in the management of malignant hyperthermia.

ADVERSE REACTIONS

The following adverse reactions have been reported: mild, moderate and severe hepatic dysfunction (including hepatic necrosis), cardiac arrest, hypotension, respiratory arrest, cardiac arrhythmias, hyperpyrexia, shivering, nausea, and emesis.

DOSAGE AND ADMINISTRATION

FLUOTHANE may be administered by the nonrebreathing technic, partial rebreathing, or closed technic. The induction dose varies from patient to patient. The maintenance dose varies from 0.5 per cent to 1.5 per cent.
FLUOTHANE may be administered with either oxygen or a mixture of oxygen and nitrous oxide.

HOW SUPPLIED

Unit packages of 125 mL (NDC 0046-3125-81) and 250 mL (NDC 0046-3125-82) of halothane, USP, stabilized with 0.01% thymol (w/w) and up to 0.00025% ammonia (w/w).

GRISACTIN® ℞

[*grĭz-ăc'tĭn*]
brand of griseofulvin (microsize)

CAUTION: Federal law prohibits dispensing without prescription.

DESCRIPTION

Griseofulvin is an oral fungistatic antibiotic for the treatment of superficial mycoses. It is derived from a species of *Penicillium.*
GRISACTIN is produced by a special process that fractures griseofulvin particles into minute crystals of irregular shape offering a greater and more effective surface area for increased gastrointestinal absorption.
GRISACTIN Capsules and Tablets contain the following inactive ingredients:
—125 mg capsules: black iron oxide, D&C Yellow No. 10, FD&C Blue No. 2, FD&C Red No. 3, FD&C Red No. 40, FD&C Yellow No. 6, gelatin, lactose, talc, water.
—250 mg capsules: black iron oxide, D&C Yellow No. 10, FD&C Blue No. 2, FD&C Red No. 40, FD&C Yellow No. 6, gelatin, lactose, magnesium stearate, titanium dioxide, water.
—500 mg tablets: calcium carboxymethylcellulose, D&C Red No. 36, gelatin, magnesium stearate, starch.

ACTION

Griseofulvin is fungistatic with *in vitro* activity against various species of *Microsporum, Epidermophyton,* and *Trichophyton.* It has no effect on bacteria or on other genera of fungi.
Griseofulvin is deposited in the keratin precursor cells and has a greater affinity for diseased tissue. The drug is tightly bound to the new keratin which becomes highly resistant to fungal invasions.
Griseofulvin absorption from the gastrointestinal tract varies considerably among individuals mainly because of insolubility of the drug in aqueous media of the upper G.I. tract. The peak serum level found in fasting adults given 0.5 g occurs at about four hours and ranges between 0.5 to 2.0 mcg/mL. The serum level may be increased by giving the drug with a meal with a high fat content.

INDICATIONS

Griseofulvin is indicated for the treatment of ringworm infections of the skin, hair, and nails, namely:
Tinea corporis
Tinea pedis
Tinea cruris
Tinea barbae
Tinea capitis
Tinea unguium (onychomycosis) when caused by one or more of the following genera of fungi:
Trichophyton rubrum
Trichophyton tonsurans
Trichophyton mentagrophytes
Trichophyton interdigitalis
Trichophyton verrucosum
Trichophyton megnini
Trichophyton gallinae
Trichophyton crateriform
Trichophyton sulphureum
Trichophyton schoenleini
Microsporum audouini
Microsporum canis
Microsporum gypseum
Epidermophyton floccosum.
NOTE: Prior to therapy, the type of fungi responsible for the infection should be identified.
The use of this drug is not justified in minor or trivial infections which will respond to topical agents alone.
Griseofulvin is *not* effective in the following:
Bacterial infections
Candidiasis (Moniliasis)
Histoplasmosis
Actinomycosis
Sporotrichosis
Chromoblastomycosis
Coccidioidomycosis
North American Blastomycosis
Cryptococcosis (Torulosis)
Tinea versicolor
Nocardiosis

CONTRAINDICATIONS

This drug is contraindicated in patients with porphyria, hepatocellular failure, and in individuals with a history of hypersensitivity to griseofulvin.

WARNINGS

Prophylactic Usage: Safety and efficacy of griseofulvin for prophylaxis of fungal infections has not been established.
Animal Toxicology: Chronic feeding of griseofulvin, at levels ranging from 0.5-2.5% of the diet, resulted in the development of liver tumors in several strains of mice, particularly males. Smaller particle sizes result in an enhanced effect. Lower oral dosage levels have not been tested. Subcutaneous administration of relatively small doses of griseofulvin, once a week, during the first three weeks of life has also been reported to induce hepatomata in mice. Although studies in other animal species have not yielded evidence of tumorigenicity, these studies were not of adequate design to form a basis for conclusions in this regard.
In subacute toxicity studies, orally administered griseofulvin produced hepatocellular necrosis in mice, but this has not been seen in other species. Disturbances in porphyrin metabolism have been reported in griseofulvin-treated laboratory animals. Griseofulvin has been reported to have a colchicine-like effect on mitosis and cocarcinogenicity with methylcholanthrene in cutaneous tumor induction in laboratory animals.
Usage in Pregnancy: The safety of this drug during pregnancy has not been established.
Animal Reproduction Studies: It has been reported in the literature that griseofulvin was found to be embryotoxic and teratogenic on oral administration to pregnant rats. Pups with abnormalities have been reported in the litters of a few bitches treated with griseofulvin. Additional animal reproduction studies are in progress.
Suppression of spermatogenesis has been reported to occur in rats, but investigation in man failed to confirm this.

PRECAUTIONS

Patients on prolonged therapy with any potent medication should be under close observation. Periodic monitoring of organ system function, including renal, hepatic, and hematopoietic, should be done.
Since griseofulvin is derived from species of *Penicillium,* the possibility of cross-sensitivity with penicillin exists; however, known penicillin-sensitive patients have been treated without difficulty.
Since a photosensitivity reaction is occasionally associated with griseofulvin therapy, patients should be warned to avoid exposure to intense natural or artificial sunlight. Lupus erythematosus, lupus-like syndromes, or exacerbation of existing lupus erythematosus have been reported in patients receiving griseofulvin.
Griseofulvin decreases the activity of warfarin-type anticoagulants so that patients receiving these drugs concomitantly may require dosage adjustment of the anticoagulant during and after griseofulvin therapy.
Barbiturates usually depress griseofulvin activity and concomitant administration may require a dosage adjustment of the antifungal agent.
The effect of alcohol may be potentiated by griseofulvin, producing such effects as tachycardia and flush.

ADVERSE REACTIONS

When adverse reactions occur, they are most commonly of the hypersensitivity type such as skin rashes, urticaria, and rarely, angioneurotic edema, and may necessitate withdrawal of therapy and appropriate countermeasures. Paresthesias of the hands and feet have been reported rarely after extended therapy. Other side effects reported occasionally are oral thrush, nausea, vomiting, epigastric distress, diarrhea, headache, fatigue, dizziness, insomnia, mental confusion, and impairment of performance of routine activities.
Proteinuria and leukopenia have been reported rarely. Administration of the drug should be discontinued if granulocytopenia occurs.
When rare, serious reactions occur with griseofulvin, they are usually associated with high dosages, long periods of therapy, or both.

DOSAGE AND ADMINISTRATION

Accurate diagnosis of the infecting organism is essential. Identification should be made either by direct microscopic examination of a mounting of infected tissue in a solution of potassium hydroxide or by culture on an appropriate medium.
Medication must be continued until the infecting organism is completely eradicated as indicated by appropriate clinical or laboratory examination. Representative treatment periods are—*tinea capitis,* 4 to 6 weeks; *tinea corporis,* 2 to 4 weeks; *tinea pedis,* 4 to 8 weeks; *tinea unguium*—depending on rate of growth—fingernails, at least 4 months; toenails, at least 6 months.
General measures in regard to hygiene should be observed to control sources of infection or reinfection. Concomitant use of appropriate topical agents is usually required, particularly in treatment of *tinea pedis.* In some forms of athlete's foot, yeasts and bacteria may be involved as well as fungi. Griseofulvin will not eradicate the bacterial or monilial infection.
Adults: 0.5 g daily (125 mg q.i.d., 250 mg b.i.d., or 500 mg/day). Patients with less severe or extensive infections may require less, whereas those with widespread lesions may require a starting dose of 0.75 g to 1.0 g a day. This may be reduced gradually to 0.5 g or less after a response has been noted. In all cases, the dosage should be individualized.
Children: A dosage of 10 mg/kg daily is usually adequate (children from 30 to 50 lb, 125 mg to 250 mg daily; children over 50 lb, 250 mg to 500 mg daily, in divided doses). Dosage should be individualized, as with adults.
Clinical relapse will occur if the medication is not continued until the infecting organism is eradicated.

HOW SUPPLIED

GRISACTIN [griseofulvin (microsize)]—
GRISACTIN 125, each capsule contains 125 mg, in bottles of 100 (NDC 0046-0442-81).
GRISACTIN 250, each capsule contains 250 mg, in bottles of 100 (NDC 0046-0443-81) and 500 (NDC 0046-0443-85).
GRISACTIN 500, each tablet (scored) contains 500 mg, in bottles of 60 (NDC 0046-0444-60).
Store at room temperature (approximately 25°C).

Shown in Product Identification Section, page 404

GRISACTIN® Ultra ℞

[*grĭz-ăc'tĭn*]
(griseofulvin ultramicrosize)

CAUTION: Federal law prohibits dispensing without prescription.

DESCRIPTION

Griseofulvin is an oral fungistatic antibiotic for the treatment of superficial mycoses. It is derived from a species of *Penicillium.*
GRISACTIN Ultra Tablets contain griseofulvin ultramicrosize in the following dosage strengths: 125 mg, 250 mg, and 330 mg.
GRISACTIN Ultra Tablets contain the following inactive ingredients: lactose, magnesium stearate, microcrystalline cellulose, sodium starch glycolate.

ACTION

Griseofulvin is fungistatic with *in vitro* activity against various species of *Microsporum, Epidermophyton,* and *Trichophyton.* It has no effect on bacteria or on other genera of fungi.
Human Pharmacology: Following oral administration, griseofulvin is deposited in the keratin percursor cells and has a greater affinity for diseased tissue. The drug is tightly bound to the new keratin which becomes highly resistant to fungal invasions.
The efficiency of gastrointestinal absorption of ultramicrocrystalline griseofulvin is approximately one and one-half times that of the conventional microsized griseofulvin. This factor permits the oral intake of two-thirds as much ultramicrocrystalline griseofulvin as the microsize form. However, there is currently no evidence that this lower dose confers any significant clinical difference with regard to safety and/or efficacy.

INDICATIONS

Griseofulvin is indicated for the treatment of ringworm infections of the skin, hair, and nails, namely:
Tinea corporis
Tinea pedis
Tinea cruris
Tinea barbae
Tinea capitis

Tinea unguium (onychomycosis) when caused by one or more of the following genera of fungi:

Trichophyton rubrum
Trichophyton tonsurans
Trichophyton mentagrophytes
Trichophyton interdigitalis
Trichophyton verrucosum
Trichophyton megnini
Trichophyton gallinae
Trichophyton crateriform
Trichophyton sulphureum
Trichophyton schoenleini
Microsporum audouini
Microsporum canis
Microsporum gypseum
Epidermophyton floccosum

NOTE: Prior to therapy, the type of fungi responsible for the infection should be identified.

The use of this drug is not justified in minor or trivial infections which will respond to topical agents alone.

Griseofulvin is *not* effective in the following:

Bacterial infections
Candidiasis (Moniliasis)
Histoplasmosis
Actinomycosis
Sporotrichosis
Chromoblastomycosis
Coccidioidomycosis
North American Blastomycosis
Cryptococcosis (Torulosis)
Tinea versicolor
Nocardiosis

CONTRAINDICATIONS

This drug is contraindicated in patients with porphyria, hepatocellular failure, and in individuals with a history of hypersensitivity to griseofulvin.

WARNINGS

Prophylactic Usage
Safety and efficacy of griseofulvin for prophylaxis of fungal infections has not been established.

Animal Toxicology
Chronic feeding of griseofulvin, at levels ranging from 0.5–2.5% of the diet, resulted in the development of liver tumors in several strains of mice, particularly males. Smaller particle sizes result in an enhanced effect. Lower oral dosage levels have not been tested. Subcutaneous administration of relatively small doses of griseofulvin, once a week, during the first three weeks of life has also been reported to induce hepatomata in mice. Although studies in other animal species have not yielded evidence of tumorigenicity, these studies were not of adequate design to form a basis for conclusions in this regard.

In subacute toxicity studies, orally administered griseofulvin produced hepatocellular necrosis in mice, but this has not been seen in other species. Disturbances in porphyrin metabolism have been reported in griseofulvin-treated laboratory animals. Griseofulvin has been reported to have a colchicine-like effect on mitosis and cocarcinogenicity with methylcholanthrene in cutaneous tumor induction in laboratory animals.

Usage in Pregnancy
The safety of this drug during pregnancy has not been established.

Animal Reproduction Studies
It has been reported in the literature that griseofulvin was found to be embryotoxic and teratogenic on oral administration to pregnant rats. Pups with abnormalities have been reported in the litters of a few bitches treated with griseofulvin. Additional animal reproduction studies are in progress. Suppression of spermatogenesis has been reported to occur in rats, but investigation in man failed to confirm this.

PRECAUTIONS

Patients on prolonged therapy with any potent medication should be under close observation. Periodic monitoring of organ system function, including renal, hepatic, and hematopoietic, should be done.

Since griseofulvin is derived from species of *Penicillium*, the possibility of cross-sensitivity with penicillin exists; however, known penicillin-sensitive patients have been treated without difficulty.

Since a photosensitivity reaction is occasionally associated with griseofulvin therapy, patients should be warned to avoid exposure to intense natural or artificial sunlight.

Lupus erythematosus, lupus-like syndromes, or exacerbation of existing lupus erythematosus have been reported in patients receiving griseofulvin.

Griseofulvin decreases the activity of warfarin-type anticoagulants so that patients receiving these drugs concomitantly may require dosage adjustment of the anticoagulant during and after griseofulvin therapy.

Barbiturates usually depress griseofulvin activity and concomitant administration may require a dosage adjustment of the antifungal agent.

The effect of alcohol may be potentiated by griseofulvin, producing such effects as tachycardia and flush.

ADVERSE REACTIONS

When adverse reactions occur, they are most commonly of the hypersensitivity type such as skin rashes, urticaria, and rarely, angioneurotic edema, and may necessitate withdrawal of therapy and appropriate countermeasures. Paresthesias of the hands and feet have been reported rarely after extended therapy. Other side effects reported occasionally are oral thrush, nausea, vomiting, epigastric distress, diarrhea, headache, fatigue, dizziness, insomnia, mental confusion, and impairment of performance of routine activities. Proteinuria and leukopenia have been reported rarely. Administration of the drug should be discontinued if granulocytopenia occurs.

When rare, serious reactions occur with griseofulvin, they are usually associated with high dosages, long periods of therapy, or both.

DOSAGE AND ADMINISTRATION

Accurate diagnosis of the infecting organism is essential. Identification should be made either by direct microscopic examination of a mounting of infected tissue in a solution of potassium hydroxide or by culture on an appropriate medium.

Medication must be continued until the infecting organism is completely eradicated as indicated by appropriate clinical or laboratory examination. Representative treatment periods are—*tinea capitis*, 4 to 6 weeks; *tinea corporis*, 2 to 4 weeks; *tinea pedis*, 4 to 8 weeks; *tinea unguium* —depending on rate of growth—fingernails, at least 4 months; toenails, at least 6 months.

General measures in regard to hygiene should be observed to control sources of infection or reinfection. Concomitant use of appropriate topical agents is usually required, particularly in treatment of *tinea pedis*. In some forms of athlete's foot, yeasts and bacteria may be involved as well as fungi. Griseofulvin will not eradicate the bacterial or monilial infection.

Adults: Daily administration of 330 mg (as a single dose or in divided doses) will give a satisfactory response in most patients with *tinea corporis, tinea cruris,* and *tinea capitis.* For those fungal infections more difficult to eradicate such as *tinea pedis* and *tinea unguium*, a divided dose of 660 mg is recommended.

Children: Approximately 3.3 mg per pound of body weight per day of ultramicrosize griseofulvin is an effective dose for most children. On this basis the following dosage schedules are suggested:

Children weighing 35 to 50 lbs: 125 mg to 165 mg
Children weighing 50 to 75 lbs: 165 to 250 mg
Children weighing 75 lbs and over: 250 to 330 mg
Children 2 years of age and younger: dosage has not been established.

Clinical experience with griseofulvin in children with *tinea capitis* indicates that a single daily dose is effective. Clinical relapse will occur if the medication is not continued until the infecting organism is eradicated.

HOW SUPPLIED

GRISACTIN® Ultra (griseofulvin ultramicrosize) Tablets, 125 mg: white, square-shaped, compressed tablets impressed with the trade name and dosage strength, in bottles of 100 (NDC 0046-0434-81).

GRISACTIN® Ultra Tablets, 250 mg: white, square-shaped compressed tablets impressed with the trade name and dosage strength, in bottles of 100 (NDC 0046-0435-81).

GRISACTIN® Ultra Tablets, 330 mg: scored, white, wide-oval shaped, compressed tablets impressed with the trade name and dosage strength, in bottles of 100 (NDC 0046-0437-81).

Store at room temperature (approximately 25° C).

Shown in Product Identification Section, page 404

INDERAL® ℞

[*ĭn 'der-al*]
Brand of propranolol hydrochloride

CAUTION: Federal law prohibits dispensing without prescription.

DESCRIPTION

INDERAL (propranolol hydrochloride) is a synthetic beta-adrenergic receptor-blocking agent chemically described as 1-(Isopropylamino)-3-(1-naphthyloxy)-2-propanol hydrochloride. Its structural formula is

$OCH_2CHOHCH_2NHCH(CH_3)_2 \cdot HCl$

INDERAL is a stable, white, crystalline solid which is readily soluble in water and ethanol. Its molecular weight is 295.81.

INDERAL is available as 10 mg, 20 mg, 40 mg, 60 mg, 80 mg, and 90 mg tablets for oral administration and as a sterile injectable solution for intravenous administration.

The inactive ingredients contained in INDERAL Tablets are: lactose, magnesium stearate, microcrystalline cellulose, and stearic acid. In addition, INDERAL 10 mg and 80 mg Tablets contain FD&C Yellow No. 6 and D&C Yellow No. 10; INDERAL 20 mg Tablets contain FD&C Blue No. 1; INDERAL 40 mg Tablets contain FD&C Blue No. 1, FD&C Yellow No. 6, and D&C Yellow No. 10; INDERAL 60 mg Tablets contain D&C Red No. 30; INDERAL 90 mg Tablets contain D&C Red No. 30 and synthetic iron oxide.

CLINICAL PHARMACOLOGY

INDERAL is a nonselective, beta-adrenergic receptor-blocking agent possessing no other autonomic nervous system activity. Its specifically competes with beta-adrenergic receptor-stimulating agents for available receptor sites. When access to beta-receptor sites is blocked by INDERAL, the chronotropic, inotropic, and vasodilator responses to beta-adrenergic stimulation are decreased proportionately.

Propranolol is almost completely absorbed from the gastrointestinal tract, but a portion is immediately bound by the liver. Peak effect occurs in one to one and one-half hours. The biologic half-life is approximately four hours.

There is no simple correlation between dose or plasma level and therapeutic effect, and the dose-sensitivity range as observed in clinical practice is wide. The principal reason for this is that sympathetic tone varies widely between individuals. Since there is no reliable test to estimate sympathetic tone or to determine whether total beta blockade has been achieved, proper dosage requires titration.

The mechanism of the antihypertensive effect of INDERAL has not been established. Among the factors that may be involved in contributing to the antihypertensive action are: (1) decreased cardiac output, (2) inhibition of renin release by the kidneys, and (3) diminution of tonic sympathetic nerve outflow from vasomotor centers in the brain. Although total peripheral resistance may increase initially, it readjusts to or below the pretreatment level with chronic use. Effects on plasma volume appear to be minor and somewhat variable. INDERAL has been shown to cause a small increase in serum potassium concentration when used in the treatment of hypertensive patients.

In angina pectoris, propranolol generally reduces the oxygen requirement of the heart at any given level of effort by blocking the catecholamine-induced increases in the heart rate, systolic blood pressure, and the velocity and extent of myocardial contraction. Propranolol may increase oxygen requirements by increasing left ventricular fiber length, end diastolic pressure, and systolic ejection period. The net physiologic effect of beta-adrenergic blockade is usually advantageous and is manifested during exercise by delayed onset of pain and increased work capacity.

Propranolol exerts its antiarrhythmic effects in concentrations associated with beta-adrenergic blockade and this appears to be its principal antiarrhythmic mechanism of action. In dosages greater than required for beta blockade, INDERAL (propranolol hydrochloride) also exerts a quinidine-like or anesthetic-like membrane action which affects the cardiac action potential. The significance of the membrane action in the treatment of arrhythmias is uncertain.

The mechanism of the antimigraine effect of propranolol has not been established. Beta-adrenergic receptors have been demonstrated in the pial vessels of the brain.

Beta-receptor blockage can be useful in conditions in which, because of pathologic or functional changes, sympathetic activity is detrimental to the patient. But there are also situations in which sympathetic stimulation is vital. For example, in patients with severely damaged hearts, adequate ventricular function is maintained by virtue of sympathetic drive, which should be preserved. In the presence of AV block greater than first degree, beta blockade may prevent the necessary facilitating effect of sympathetic activity on conduction. Beta blockade results in bronchial constriction by interfering with adrenergic bronchodilator activity, which should be preserved in patients subject to bronchospasm.

Propranolol is not significantly dialyzable.

The Beta-Blocker Heart Attack Trial (BHAT) was a National Heart, Lung and Blood Institute-sponsored, multicenter, randomized, double-blind, placebo-controlled trial conducted in 31 U.S. centers (plus one in Canada) in 3,837 persons without history of severe congestive heart failure or presence of recent heart failure; certain conduction defects; angina since infarction, who had survived the acute phase of myocardial infarction. Propranolol was administered at either 60 or 80 mg tid, based on blood levels achieved during an initial trial of 40 mg tid. Therapy with INDERAL, begun 5–21 days following infarction, was shown to reduce overall mortality up to 39 months, the longest period of follow-up. This was pri-

Continued on next page

Ayerst—Cont.

marily attributable to a reduction in cardiovascular mortality. The protective effect of INDERAL was consistent regardless of age, sex, or site of infarction. Compared to placebo, total mortality was reduced 39% at 12 months and 26% over an average follow-up period of 25 months. The Norwegian Multicenter Trial, in which propranolol was administered at 40 mg qid, gave overall results which support the findings in the BHAT.

Although the clinical trials used either tid or qid dosing, clinical, pharmacologic, and pharmacokinetic data provide a reasonable basis for concluding that bid dosing with propranolol should be adequate in the treatment of post-infarction patients.

CLINICAL: In the BHAT, patients on INDERAL were prescribed either 180 mg/day (82% of patients) or 240 mg/day (18% of patients). Patients were instructed to take the medication 3 times a day at mealtimes. This dosing schedule would result in an overnight dosing interval of 12 to 14 hours, which is similar to the dosing interval for a bid regimen. In addition, blood samples were drawn at various times and analyzed for propranolol. When the patients were grouped into tertiles, based on the blood levels observed, and the mortality in the upper and lower tertiles were compared, there was no evidence that blood levels affected mortality.

PHARMACOLOGIC: Studies in normal volunteers have shown that a 90 mg bid regimen maintains beta blockade at, or above, the minimum for 60 mg tid dosing for 24 hours, even though differences occurred at two time intervals. At 10–12 hours after the first dose of the day, tid dosing gave more beta blockade than bid dosing; at 20–24 hours the trend of the relationship was reversed. These relationships were similar in direction to those observed for plasma propranolol levels (see Pharmacokinetic).

PHARMACOKINETIC: A bioavailability study in normal volunteers showed that the blood levels produced by 180 mg/day given bid are below those provided by the same daily dosage given tid at 10–12 hours after the first dose of the day, but above those of a tid regimen at 20–24 hours. However, the blood levels produced by bid dosing were always equivalent to or above the minimum for tid dosing throughout the 24 hours. In addition, the mean AUC on the fourth day for the bid regimen was about 17% greater than for the tid regimen (1,194 *vs.* 1,024 ng/mL·hr).

INDICATIONS AND USAGE

Hypertension

INDERAL is indicated in the management of hypertension. It may be used alone or used in combination with other antihypertensive agents, particularly a thiazide diuretic. INDERAL (propranolol hydrochloride) is not indicated in the management of hypertensive emergencies.

Angina Pectoris Due to Coronary Atherosclerosis

INDERAL is indicated for the long-term management of patients with angina pectoris.

Cardiac Arrhythmias

1.) Supraventricular arrhythmias
  a) Paroxysmal atrial tachycardias, particularly those arrhythmias induced by catecholamines or digitalis or associated with the Wolff-Parkinson-White syndrome. (See W-P-W under WARNINGS.)
  b) Persistent sinus tachycardia, which is noncompensatory and impairs the well-being of the patient.
  c) Tachycardias and arrhythmias due to thyrotoxicosis when causing distress or increased hazard and when immediate effect is necessary as adjunctive, short-term (2–4 weeks) therapy.
  May be used with, but not in place of, specific therapy. (See Thyrotoxicosis under WARNINGS.)
  d) Persistent atrial extrasystoles, which impair the well-being of the patient and do not respond to conventional measures.
  e) Atrial flutter and fibrillation when ventricular rate cannot be controlled by digitalis alone, or when digitalis is contraindicated.

2.) Ventricular tachycardias
  Ventricular arrhythmias do not respond to propranolol as predictably as do the supraventricular arrhythmias.
  a) Ventricular tachycardias
  With the exception of those induced by catecholamines or digitalis, INDERAL is not the drug of first choice. In critical situations when cardioversion techniques or other drugs are not indicated or are not effective, INDERAL may be considered. If, after consideration of the risks involved, INDERAL is used, it should be given intravenously in low dosage and very slowly. (See DOSAGE AND ADMINISTRATION.) *Care in the administration of* INDERAL *with constant electrocardiographic monitoring is essential as the failing heart requires some sympathetic drive for maintenance of myocardial tone.*
  b) Persistent premature ventricular extrasystoles which do not respond to conventional measures and impair the well-being of the patient.

3.) Tachyarrhythmias of digitalis intoxication
  If digitalis-induced tachyarrhythmias persist following discontinuance of digitalis and correction of electrolyte abnormalities, they are usually reversible with *oral* INDERAL. Severe bradycardia may occur (see OVERDOSAGE.)
  Intravenous propranolol hydrochloride is reserved for life-threatening arrhythmias. Temporary maintenance with oral therapy may be indicated. (See DOSAGE AND ADMINISTRATION.)

4.) Resistant tachyarrhythmias due to excessive catecholamine action during anesthesia
  Tachyarrhythmias due to excessive catecholamine action during anesthesia may sometimes arise because of release of endogenous catecholamines or administration of catecholamines. When usual measures fail in such arrhythmias, INDERAL may be given intravenously to abolish them. All general inhalation anesthetics produce some degree of myocardial depression. Therefore, when INDERAL is used to treat arrhythmias during anesthesia, it should be used with extreme caution and constant ECG and central venous pressure monitoring. (See WARNINGS.)

Myocardial Infarction

INDERAL is indicated to reduce cardiovascular mortality in patients who have survived the acute phase of myocardial infarction and are clinically stable.

Migraine

INDERAL is indicated for the prophylaxis of common migraine headache. The efficacy of propranolol in the treatment of a migraine attack that has started has not been established and propranolol is not indicated for such use.

Hypertrophic Subaortic Stenosis

INDERAL is useful in the management of hypertrophic subaortic stenosis, especially for treatment of exertional or other stress-induced angina, palpitations, and syncope. INDERAL also improves exercise performance. The effectiveness of propranolol hydrochloride in this disease appears to be due to a reduction of the elevated outflow pressure gradient which is exacerbated by beta-receptor stimulation. Clinical improvement may be temporary.

Pheochromocytoma

After primary treatment with an alpha-adrenergic blocking agent has been instituted, INDERAL (propranolol hydrochloride) may be useful as *adjunctive* therapy if the control of tachycardia becomes necessary before or during surgery.

It is hazardous to use INDERAL unless alpha-adrenergic blocking drugs are already in use, since this would predispose to serious blood pressure elevation. Blocking only the peripheral dilator (beta) action of epinephrine leaves its constrictor (alpha) action unopposed.

In the event of hemorrhage or shock, there is a disadvantage in having both beta and alpha blockade since the combination prevents the increase in heart rate and peripheral vasoconstriction needed to maintain blood pressure.

With inoperable or metastatic pheochromocytoma, INDERAL may be useful as an adjunct to the management of symptoms due to excessive beta-receptor stimulation.

CONTRAINDICATIONS

INDERAL is contraindicated in 1) cardiogenic shock, 2) sinus bradycardia and greater than first-degree block, 3) bronchial asthma, 4) congestive heart failure (see WARNINGS), unless the failure is secondary to a tachyarrhythmia treatable with INDERAL.

WARNINGS

CARDIAC FAILURE: Sympathetic stimulation may be a vital component supporting circulatory function in patients with congestive heart failure, and its inhibition by beta blockade may precipitate more severe failure. Although beta blockers should be avoided in overt congestive heart failure, if necessary, they can be used with close follow-up in patients with a history of failure who are well compensated and are receiving digitalis and diuretics. Beta-adrenergic blocking agents do not abolish the inotropic action of digitalis on heart muscle.

IN PATIENTS WITHOUT A HISTORY OF HEART FAILURE, continued use of beta blockers can, in some cases, lead to cardiac failure. Therefore, at the first sign or symptom of heart failure, the patient should be digitalized and/or treated with diuretics, and the response observed closely, or INDERAL should be discontinued (gradually, if possible).

IN PATIENTS WITH ANGINA PECTORIS, there have been reports of exacerbation of angina and, in some cases, myocardial infarction, following *abrupt* discontinuance of INDERAL therapy. Therefore, when discontinuance of INDERAL is planned, the dosage should be gradually reduced over at least a few weeks and the patient should be cautioned against interruption or cessation of therapy without the physician's advice. If INDERAL therapy is interrupted and exacerbation of angina occurs, it usually is advisable to reinstitute INDERAL therapy and take other measures appropriate for the management of unstable angina pectoris. Since coronary artery disease may be unrecognized, it may be prudent to follow the above advice in patients considered at risk of having occult atherosclerotic heart disease who are given propranolol for other indications.

Nonallergic Bronchospasm (eg, chronic bronchitis, emphysema)—PATIENTS WITH BRONCHOSPASTIC DISEASES SHOULD, IN GENERAL, NOT RECEIVE BETA BLOCKERS. INDERAL should be administered with caution since it may block bronchodilation produced by endogenous and exogenous catecholamine stimulation of beta receptors.

MAJOR SURGERY: The necessity or desirability of withdrawal of beta-blocking therapy prior to major surgery is controversial. It should be noted, however, that the impaired ability of the heart to respond to reflex adrenergic stimuli may augment the risks of general anesthesia and surgical procedures.

INDERAL (propranolol hydrochloride), like other beta blockers, is a competitive inhibitor of beta-receptor agonists and its effects can be reversed by administration of such agents, eg, dobutamine or isoproterenol. However, such patients may be subject to protracted severe hypotension. Difficulty in starting and maintaining the heartbeat has also been reported with beta blockers.

DIABETES AND HYPOGLYCEMIA: Beta-adrenergic blockade may prevent the appearance of certain premonitory signs and symptoms (pulse rate and pressure changes) of acute hypoglycemia in labile insulin-dependent diabetes. In these patients, it may be more difficult to adjust the dosage of insulin.

THYROTOXICOSIS: Beta blockade may mask certain clinical signs of hyperthyroidism. Therefore, abrupt withdrawal of propranolol may be followed by an exacerbation of symptoms of hyperthyroidism, including thyroid storm. Propranolol does not distort thyroid function tests.

IN PATIENTS WITH WOLFF-PARKINSON-WHITE SYNDROME, several cases have been reported in which, after propranolol, the tachycardia was replaced by a severe bradycardia requiring a demand pacemaker. In one case this resulted after an initial dose of 5 mg propranolol.

PRECAUTIONS

GENERAL: Propranolol should be used with caution in patients with impaired hepatic or renal function. INDERAL is not indicated for the treatment of hypertensive emergencies. Beta-adrenoreceptor blockade can cause reduction of intraocular pressure. Patients should be told that INDERAL may interfere with the glaucoma screening test. Withdrawal may lead to a return of increased intraocular pressure.

CLINICAL LABORATORY TESTS: Elevated blood urea levels in patients with severe heart disease, elevated serum transaminase, alkaline phosphatase, lactate dehydrogenase.

DRUG INTERACTIONS: Patients receiving catecholamine-depleting drugs such as reserpine should be closely observed if INDERAL is administered. The added catecholamine-blocking action may produce an excessive reduction of resting sympathetic nervous activity which may result in hypotension, marked bradycardia, vertigo, syncopal attacks, or orthostatic hypotension.

CARCINOGENESIS, MUTAGENESIS, IMPAIRMENT OF FERTILITY: Long-term studies in animals have been conducted to evaluate toxic effects and carcinogenic potential. In 18-month studies in both rats and mice, employing doses up to 150 mg/kg/day, there was no evidence of significant drug-induced toxicity. There were no drug-related tumorigenic effects at any of the dosage levels. Reproductive studies in animals did not show any impairment of fertility that was attributable to the drug.

PREGNANCY: Pregnancy Category C. INDERAL has been shown to be embryotoxic in animal studies at doses about 10 times greater than the maximum recommended human dose.

There are no adequate and well-controlled studies in pregnant women. INDERAL should be used during pregnancy only if the potential benefit justifies the potential risk to the fetus.

NURSING MOTHERS: INDERAL is excreted in human milk. Caution should be exercised when INDERAL (propranolol hydrochloride) is administered to a nursing woman.

PEDIATRIC USE: Safety and effectiveness in children have not been established.

ADVERSE REACTIONS

Most adverse effects have been mild and transient and have rarely required the withdrawal of therapy.

Cardiovascular: Bradycardia; congestive heart failure; intensification of AV block; hypotension; paresthesia of hands; thrombocytopenic purpura; arterial insufficiency, usually of the Raynaud type.

Central Nervous System: Light-headedness; mental depression manifested by insomnia, lassitude, weakness, fatigue; reversible mental depression progressing to catatonia; visual disturbances; hallucinations; an acute reversible syndrome characterized by disorientation for time and place, short-

term memory loss, emotional lability, slightly clouded sensorium, and decreased performance on neuropsychometrics.
Gastrointestinal: Nausea; vomiting; epigastric distress; abdominal cramping; diarrhea; constipation; mesenteric arterial thrombosis; ischemic colitis.
Allergic: Pharyngitis and agranulocytosis; erythematous rash; fever combined with aching and sore throat; laryngospasm and respiratory distress.
Respiratory: Bronchospasm.
Hematologic: Agranulocytosis; nonthrombocytopenic purpura; thrombocytopenic purpura.
Auto-Immune: In extremely rare instances, systemic lupus erythematosus has been reported.
Miscellaneous: Alopecia; LE-like reactions; psoriasiform rashes; dry eyes; male impotence; and Peyronie's disease have been reported rarely. Oculomucocutaneous reactions involving the skin, serous membranes and conjunctivae reported for a beta blocker (practolol) have not been associated with propranolol.

DOSAGE AND ADMINISTRATION

The dosage range for INDERAL is different for each indication.

ORAL

HYPERTENSION—*Dosage must be individualized.*
The usual initial dosage is 40 mg INDERAL twice daily, whether used alone or added to a diuretic. Dosage may be increased gradually until adequate blood pressure control is achieved. The usual maintenance dosage is 120 to 240 mg per day. In some instances a dosage of 640 mg a day may be required. The time needed for full hypertensive response to a given dosage is variable and may range from a few days to several weeks.
While twice-daily dosing is effective and can maintain a reduction in blood pressure throughout the day, some patients, especially when lower doses are used, may experience a modest rise in blood pressure toward the end of the 12-hour dosing interval. This can be evaluated by measuring blood pressure near the end of the dosing interval to determine whether satisfactory control is being maintained throughout the day. If control is not adequate, a larger dose, or 3-times-daily therapy may achieve better control.

ANGINA PECTORIS—*Dosage must be individualized.*
Starting with 10–20 mg three or four times daily, before meals and at bedtime, dosage should be gradually increased at three- to seven-day intervals until optimal response is obtained. Although individual patients may respond at any dosage level, the average optimal dosage appears to be 160 mg per day. In angina pectoris, the value and safety of dosage exceeding 320 mg per day have not been established.
If treatment is to be discontinued, reduce dosage gradually over a period of several weeks. (See WARNINGS.)

ARRHYTHMIAS—10–30 mg three or four times daily, before meals and at bedtime.

MYOCARDIAL INFARCTION
The recommended daily dosage is 180–240 mg per day, in divided doses. Although a tid regimen was used in the Beta Blocker Heart Attack Trial and a qid regimen in the Norwegian Multicenter Trial, there is a reasonable basis for the use of either a tid or bid regimen (see CLINICAL PHARMACOLOGY). The effectiveness and safety of daily dosages greater than 240 mg for prevention of cardiac mortality have not been established. However, higher dosages may be needed to effectively treat coexisting diseases such as angina or hypertension (see above).

MIGRAINE—*Dosage must be individualized.*
The initial oral dose is 80 mg INDERAL daily, in divided doses. The usual effective dose range is 160–240 mg per day. The dosage may be increased gradually to achieve optimal migraine prophylaxis.
If a satisfactory response is not obtained within four to six weeks after reaching the maximal dose, INDERAL (propranolol hydrochloride) therapy should be discontinued. It may be advisable to withdraw the drug gradually over a period of several weeks.

HYPERTROPHIC SUBAORTIC STENOSIS—20–40 mg three or four times daily, before meals and at bedtime.

PHEOCHROMOCYTOMA—*Preoperatively* — 60 mg daily, in divided doses for three days prior to surgery, concomitantly with an alpha-adrenergic blocking agent.
—*Management of inoperable tumor* —30 mg daily, in divided doses.

PEDIATRIC DOSAGE
At this time the data on the use of the drug in this age group are too limited to permit adequate directions for use.

INTRAVENOUS
Intravenous administration is reserved for life-threatening arrhythmias or those occurring under anesthesia. The usual dose is from 1 to 3 mg administered under careful monitoring, *eg*, electrocardiographic, central venous pressure. The rate of administration should not exceed 1 mg (1 mL) per minute to diminish the possibility of lowering blood pressure and causing cardiac standstill. Sufficient time should be allowed for the drug to reach the site of action even when a slow circulation is present. If necessary, a second dose may be given after two minutes. Thereafter, additional drug should not be given in less than four hours. Additional INDERAL should not be given when the desired alteration in rate and/or rhythm is achieved.
Transference to oral therapy should be made as soon as possible.
The intravenous administration of INDERAL has not been evaluated adequately in the management of hypertensive emergencies.

OVERDOSAGE
INDERAL is not significantly dialyzable. In the event of overdosage or exaggerated response, the following measures should be employed:
GENERAL—If ingestion is or may have been recent, evacuate gastric contents, taking care to prevent pulmonary aspiration.
BRADYCARDIA—ADMINISTER ATROPINE (0.25 to 1.0 mg); IF THERE IS NO RESPONSE TO VAGAL BLOCKADE, ADMINISTER ISOPROTERENOL CAUTIOUSLY.
CARDIAC FAILURE—DIGITALIZATION AND DIURETICS.
HYPOTENSION—VASOPRESSORS, *eg*, LEVARTERENOL OR EPINEPHRINE (THERE IS EVIDENCE THAT EPINEPHRINE IS THE DRUG OF CHOICE).
BRONCHOSPASM—ADMINISTER ISOPROTERENOL AND AMINOPHYLLINE.

HOW SUPPLIED

INDERAL
(propranolol hydrochloride)
Tablets

INDERAL 10—Each hexagonal-shaped, orange, scored tablet, embossed with an "I" and imprinted with "INDERAL 10," contains 10 mg propranolol hydrochloride, in bottles of 100 (NDC 0046-0421-81); 1,000 (NDC 0046-0421-91); and 5,000 (NDC 0046-0421-95). Also in Unit Dose packages of 100 (NDC 0046-0421-99); and in Unit of Use packages of 60 (NDC 0046-0421-60), 90 (NDC 0046-0421-61), 100 (NDC 0046-0421-80), and 120 (NDC 0046-0421-62).

INDERAL 20—Each hexagonal-shaped, blue, scored tablet, embossed with an "I" and imprinted with "INDERAL 20," contains 20 mg propranolol hydrochloride in bottles of 100 (NDC 0046-0422-81), 1,000 (NDC 0046-0422-91), and 5,000 (NDC 0046-0422-95). Also in Unit Dose packages of 100 (NDC 0046-0422-99); and in Unit of Use packages of 60 (NDC 0046-0422-60), 90 (NDC 0046-0422-61), 100 (NDC 0046-0422-80), and 120 (NDC 0046-0422-62).

INDERAL 40—Each hexagonal-shaped, green, scored tablet, embossed with an "I" and imprinted with "INDERAL 40," contains 40 mg propranolol hydrochloride, in bottles of 100 (NDC 0046-0424-81), 1,000 (NDC 0046-0424-91), and 5,000 (NDC 0046-0424-95). Also in Unit Dose packages of 100 (NDC 0046-0424-99); and in Unit of Use packages of 60 (NDC 0046-0424-60), 90 (NDC 0046-0424-61), 100 (NDC 0046-0424-80), and 120 (NDC 0046-0424-62).

INDERAL 60—Each hexagonal-shaped, pink, scored tablet, embossed with an "I" and imprinted with "INDERAL 60," contains 60 mg propranolol hydrochloride in bottles of 100 (NDC 0046-0426-81), and 1,000 (NDC 0046-0426-91). Also in Unit Dose packages of 100 (NDC 0046-0426-99).

INDERAL 80—Each hexagonal-shaped, yellow, scored tablet, embossed with an "I" and imprinted with "INDERAL 80," contains 80 mg propranolol hydrochloride, in bottles of 100 (NDC 0046-0428-81), 1,000 (NDC 0046-0428-91), and 5,000 (NDC 0046-0428-95). Also in Unit Dose packages of 100 (NDC 0046-0428-99); and in Unit of Use packages of 60 (NDC 0046-0428-60), 90 (NDC 0046-0428-61), 100 (NDC 0046-0428-80), and 120 (NDC 0046-0428-62).

INDERAL 90—Each hexagonal-shaped, lavender, scored tablet, embossed with an "I" and imprinted with "INDERAL 90," contains 90 mg propranolol hydrochloride in bottles of 100 (NDC 0046-0439-81), and 1,000 (NDC 0046-0439-91). Also in Unit Dose packages of 100 (NDC 0046-0439-99).

The appearance of these tablets is a registered trademark of Ayerst Laboratories.
Store at room temperature (approximately 25° C).

INJECTABLE
—Each mL contains 1 mg of propranolol hydrochloride in Water for Injection. The pH is adjusted with citric acid. Supplied as: 1 mL ampuls in boxes of 10 (NDC 0046-3265-10).
Store at room temperature (approximately 25° C).

Shown in Product Identification Section, page 404

INDERAL® LA ℞

[*in 'der-al*]
Brand of propranolol hydrochloride
(Long Acting Capsules)

CAUTION: Federal law prohibits dispensing without prescription.

DESCRIPTION

INDERAL (propranolol hydrochloride) is a synthetic beta-adrenergic receptor-blocking agent chemically described as 1-(Isopropylamino)-3-(1-naphthyloxy)-2-propanol hydrochloride. Its structural formula is

$$\text{O}\,CH_2CHOHCH_2NHCH(CH_3)_2 \cdot HCl$$

INDERAL is a stable, white, crystalline solid which is readily soluble in water and ethanol. Its molecular weight is 295.81.
INDERAL LA is formulated to provide a sustained release of propranolol hydrochloride. INDERAL LA is available as 80 mg, 120 mg, and 160 mg capsules.
INDERAL LA contains the following inactive ingredients: ethylcellulose, gelatin capsules, hydroxypropyl methylcellulose, and microcrystalline cellulose. In addition, INDERAL LA 80 mg and 120 mg Capsules contain FD&C Blue No. 1, FD&C Red No. 3, and D&C Red No. 28; INDERAL LA 160 mg Capsules contain FD&C Blue No. 1.

CLINICAL PHARMACOLOGY

INDERAL is a nonselective, beta-adrenergic receptor-blocking agent possessing no other autonomic nervous system activity. It specifically competes with beta-adrenergic receptor-stimulating agents for available receptor sites. When access to beta-receptor sites is blocked by INDERAL, the chronotropic, inotropic, and vasodilator responses to beta-adrenergic stimulation are decreased proportionately.
INDERAL LA Capsules (80, 120, and 160 mg) release propranolol HCl at a controlled and predictable rate. Peak blood levels following dosing with INDERAL LA occur at about 6 hours and the apparent plasma half-life is about 10 hours. When measured at steady state over a 24-hour period, the areas under the propranolol plasma concentration-time curve (AUCs) for the capsules are approximately 60% to 65% of the AUCs for a comparable divided daily dose of INDERAL Tablets. The lower AUCs for the capsules are due to greater hepatic metabolism of propranolol, resulting from the slower rate of absorption of propranolol. Over a twenty-four (24) hour period, blood levels are fairly constant for about twelve (12) hours then decline exponentially.
INDERAL LA should not be considered a simple mg-for-mg substitute for conventional propranolol and the blood levels achieved do not match (are lower than) those of two to four times daily dosing with the same dose. When changing to INDERAL LA from conventional propranolol, a possible need for retitration upwards should be considered, especially to maintain effectiveness at the end of the dosing interval. In most clinical settings, however, such as hypertension or angina where there is little correlation between plasma levels and clinical effect, INDERAL LA has been therapeutically equivalent to the same mg dose of conventional INDERAL as assessed by 24-hour effects on blood pressure and on 24-hour exercise responses of heart rate, systolic pressure, and rate pressure product. INDERAL LA can provide effective beta blockade for a 24-hour period.
The mechanism of the antihypertensive effect of INDERAL has not been established. Among the factors that may be involved in contributing to the antihypertensive action are: (1) decreased cardiac output, (2) inhibition of renin release by the kidneys, and (3) diminution of tonic sympathetic nerve outflow from vasomotor centers in the brain. Although total peripheral resistance may increase initially, it readjusts to or below the pretreatment level with chronic use. Effects on plasma volume appear to be minor and somewhat variable. INDERAL has been shown to cause a small increase in serum potassium concentration when used in the treatment of hypertensive patients.
In angina pectoris, propranolol generally reduces the oxygen requirement of the heart at any given level of effort by blocking the catecholamine-induced increases in the heart rate, systolic blood pressure, and the velocity and extent of myocardial contraction. Propranolol may increase oxygen requirements by increasing left ventricular fiber length, end diastolic pressure, and systolic ejection period. The net physiologic effect of beta-adrenergic blockade is usually advantageous and is manifested during exercise by delayed onset of pain and increased work capacity.
In dosages greater than required for beta blockade, INDERAL (propranolol hydrochloride) also exerts a quinidine-like or anesthetic-like membrane action which affects the cardiac action potential. The significance of the membrane action in the treatment of arrhythmias is uncertain.
The mechanism of the antimigraine effect of propranolol has not been established. Beta-adrenergic receptors have been demonstrated in the pial vessels of the brain.
Beta-receptor blockade can be useful in conditions in which, because of pathologic or functional changes, sympathetic activity is detrimental to the patient. But there are also situations in which sympathetic stimulation is vital. For example, in patients with severely damaged hearts, adequate ven-

Continued on next page

Ayerst—Cont.

tricular function is maintained by virtue of sympathetic drive, which should be preserved. In the presence of AV block, greater than first degree, beta blockade may prevent the necessary facilitating effect of sympathetic activity on conduction. Beta blockade results in bronchial constriction by interfering with adrenergic bronchodilator activity, which should be preserved in patients subject to bronchospasm.

Propranolol is not significantly dialyzable.

INDICATIONS AND USAGE

Hypertension

INDERAL LA is indicated in the management of hypertension; it may be used alone or used in combination with other antihypertensive agents, particularly a thiazide diuretic. INDERAL LA is not indicated in the management of hypertensive emergencies.

Angina Pectoris Due to Coronary Atherosclerosis

INDERAL LA is indicated for the long-term management of patients with angina pectoris.

Migraine

INDERAL LA is indicated for the prophylaxis of common migraine headache. The efficacy of propranolol in the treatment of a migraine attack that has started has not been established and propranolol is not indicated for such use.

Hypertrophic Subaortic Stenosis

INDERAL LA is useful in the management of hypertrophic subaortic stenosis, especially for treatment of exertional or other stress-induced angina, palpitations, and syncope. INDERAL LA also improves exercise performance. The effectiveness of propranolol hydrochloride in this disease appears to be due to a reduction of the elevated outflow pressure gradient which is exacerbated by beta-receptor stimulation. Clinical improvement may be temporary.

CONTRAINDICATIONS

INDERAL is contraindicated in 1) cardiogenic shock; 2) sinus bradycardia and greater than first-degree block; 3) bronchial asthma; 4) congestive heart failure (see WARNINGS), unless the failure is secondary to a tachyarrhythmia treatable with INDERAL (propranolol hydrochloride).

WARNINGS

CARDIAC FAILURE: Sympathetic stimulation may be a vital component supporting circulatory function in patients with congestive heart failure, and its inhibition by beta blockade may precipitate more severe failure. Although beta blockers should be avoided in overt congestive heart failure, if necessary, they can be used with close follow-up in patients with a history of failure who are well compensated and are receiving digitalis and diuretics. Beta-adrenergic blocking agents do not abolish the inotropic action of digitalis on heart muscle.

IN PATIENTS WITHOUT A HISTORY OF HEART FAILURE, continued use of beta blockers can, in some cases, lead to cardiac failure. Therefore, at the first sign or symptom of heart failure, the patient should be digitalized and/or treated with diuretics, and the response observed closely, or INDERAL should be discontinued (gradually, if possible).

IN PATIENTS WITH ANGINA PECTORIS, there have been reports of exacerbation of angina and, in some cases, myocardial infarction, following *abrupt* discontinuance of INDERAL therapy. Therefore, when discontinuance of INDERAL is planned the dosage should be gradually reduced over at least a few weeks, and the patient should be cautioned against interruption or cessation of therapy without the physician's advice. If INDERAL therapy is interrupted and exacerbation of angina occurs, it usually is advisable to reinstitute INDERAL therapy and take other measures appropriate for the management of unstable angina pectoris. Since coronary artery disease may be unrecognized, it may be prudent to follow the above advice in patients considered at risk of having occult atherosclerotic heart disease who are given propranolol for other indications.

Nonallergic Bronchospasm (eg, chronic bronchitis, emphysema)—PATIENTS WITH BRONCHOSPASTIC DISEASES SHOULD IN GENERAL NOT RECEIVE BETA BLOCKERS. INDERAL (propranolol hydrochloride) should be administered with caution since it may block bronchodilation produced by endogenous and exogenous catecholamine stimulation of beta receptors.

MAJOR SURGERY: The necessity or desirability of withdrawal of beta-blocking therapy prior to major surgery is controversial. It should be noted, however, that the impaired ability of the heart to respond to reflex adrenergic stimuli may augment the risks of general anesthesia and surgical procedures.

INDERAL, like other beta blockers, is a competitive inhibitor of beta-receptor agonists and its effects can be reversed by administration of such agents, eg, dobutamine or isoproterenol. However, such patients may be subject to protracted severe hypotension. Difficulty in starting and maintaining the heartbeat has also been reported with beta blockers.

DIABETES AND HYPOGLYCEMIA: Beta-adrenergic blockade may prevent the appearance of certain premonitory signs and symptoms (pulse rate and pressure changes) of acute hypoglycemia in labile insulin-dependent diabetes. In these patients, it may be more difficult to adjust the dosage of insulin.

THYROTOXICOSIS: Beta blockade may mask certain clinical signs of hyperthyroidism. Therefore, abrupt withdrawal of propranolol may be followed by an exacerbation of symptoms of hyperthyroidism, including thyroid storm. Propranolol does not distort thyroid function tests.

IN PATIENTS WITH WOLFF-PARKINSON-WHITE SYNDROME, several cases have been reported in which, after propranolol, the tachycardia was replaced by a severe bradycardia requiring a demand pacemaker. In one case this resulted after an initial dose of 5 mg propranolol.

PRECAUTIONS

GENERAL: Propranolol should be used with caution in patients with impaired hepatic or renal function. INDERAL (propranolol hydrochloride) is not indicated for the treatment of hypertensive emergencies.

Beta-adrenoreceptor blockade can cause reduction of intraocular pressure. Patients should be told that INDERAL may interfere with the glaucoma screening test. Withdrawal may lead to a return of increased intraocular pressure.

CLINICAL LABORATORY TESTS: Elevated blood urea levels in patients with severe heart disease, elevated serum transaminase, alkaline phosphatase, lactate dehydrogenase.

DRUG INTERACTIONS: Patients receiving catecholamine-depleting drugs, such as reserpine, should be closely observed if INDERAL is administered. The added catecholamine-blocking action may produce an excessive reduction of resting sympathetic nervous activity, which may result in hypotension, marked bradycardia, vertigo, syncopal attacks, or orthostatic hypotension.

CARCINOGENESIS, MUTAGENESIS, IMPAIRMENT OF FERTILITY: Long-term studies in animals have been conducted to evaluate toxic effects and carcinogenic potential. In 18-month studies, in both rats and mice, employing doses up to 150 mg/kg/day, there was no evidence of significant drug-induced toxicity. There were no drug-related tumorigenic effects at any of the dosage levels. Reproductive studies in animals did not show any impairment of fertility that was attributable to the drug.

PREGNANCY: Pregnancy Category C. INDERAL (propranolol hydrochloride) has been shown to be embryotoxic in animal studies at doses about 10 times greater than the maximal recommended human dose.

There are no adequate and well-controlled studies in pregnant women. INDERAL should be used during pregnancy only if the potential benefit justifies the potential risk to the fetus.

NURSING MOTHERS: INDERAL is excreted in human milk. Caution should be exercised when INDERAL is administered to a nursing woman.

PEDIATRIC USE: Safety and effectiveness in children have not been established.

ADVERSE REACTIONS

Most adverse effects have been mild and transient and have rarely required the withdrawal of therapy.

Cardiovascular: Bradycardia; congestive heart failure; intensification of AV block; hypotension; paresthesia of hands; thrombocytopenic purpura; arterial insufficiency, usually of the Raynaud type.

Central Nervous System: Light-headedness, mental depression manifested by insomnia, lassitude, weakness, fatigue, reversible mental depression progressing to catatonia; visual disturbances; hallucinations; an acute reversible syndrome characterized by disorientation for time and place, short-term memory loss, emotional lability, slightly clouded sensorium, and decreased performance on neuropsychometrics.

Gastrointestinal: Nausea; vomiting; epigastric distress; abdominal cramping; diarrhea; constipation; mesenteric arterial thrombosis; ischemic colitis.

Allergic: Pharyngitis and agranulocytosis; erythematous rash; fever combined with aching and sore throat; laryngospasm and respiratory distress.

Respiratory: Bronchospasm.

Hematologic: Agranulocytosis, nonthrombocytopenic purpura, thrombocytopenic purpura.

Auto-Immune: In extremely rare instances, systemic lupus erythematosus has been reported.

Miscellaneous: Alopecia; LE-like reactions; psoriasiform rashes; dry eyes; male impotence; and Peyronie's disease have been reported rarely. Oculomucocutaneous reactions involving the skin, serous membranes and conjunctivae reported for a beta blocker (practolol) have not been associated with propranolol.

DOSAGE AND ADMINISTRATION

INDERAL LA provides propranolol hydrochloride in a sustained-release capsule for administration once daily. If patients are switched from INDERAL Tablets to INDERAL LA Capsules, care should be taken to assure that the desired therapeutic effect is maintained. INDERAL LA should not be considered a simple mg-for-mg substitute for INDERAL. INDERAL LA has different kinetics and produces lower blood levels. Retitration may be necessary especially to maintain effectiveness at the end of the 24-hour dosing interval.

HYPERTENSION—*Dosage must be individualized.* The usual initial dosage is 80 mg INDERAL LA (propranolol hydrochloride) once daily, whether used alone or added to a diuretic. The dosage may be increased to 120 mg once daily or higher, until adequate blood pressure control is achieved. The usual maintenance dosage is 120 to 160 mg once daily. In some instances a dosage of 640 mg may be required. The time needed for full hypertensive response to a given dosage is variable and may range from a few days to several weeks.

ANGINA PECTORIS—*Dosage must be individualized.* Starting with 80 mg INDERAL LA once daily, dosage should be gradually increased at three- to seven-day intervals until optimal response is obtained. Although individual patients may respond at any dosage level, the average optimal dosage appears to be 160 mg once daily. In angina pectoris, the value and safety of dosage exceeding 320 mg per day have not been established.

If treatment is to be discontinued, reduce dosage gradually over a period of a few weeks (see WARNINGS).

MIGRAINE—*Dosage must be individualized.* The initial oral dose is 80 mg INDERAL LA once daily. The usual effective dose range is 160-240 mg once daily. The dosage may be increased gradually to achieve optimal migraine prophylaxis. If a satisfactory response is not obtained within four to six weeks after reaching the maximal dose, INDERAL LA therapy should be discontinued. It may be advisable to withdraw the drug gradually over a period of several weeks.

HYPERTROPHIC SUBAORTIC STENOSIS—80-160 mg INDERAL LA once daily.

PEDIATRIC DOSAGE

At this time the data on the use of the drug in this age group are too limited to permit adequate directions for use.

OVERDOSAGE

Inderal is not significantly dialyzable. In the event of overdosage or exaggerated response, the following measures should be employed:

GENERAL—If ingestion is or may have been recent, evacuate gastric contents, taking care to prevent pulmonary aspiration.

BRADYCARDIA—ADMINISTER ATROPINE (0.25 to 1.0 mg); IF THERE IS NO RESPONSE TO VAGAL BLOCKADE, ADMINISTER ISOPROTERENOL CAUTIOUSLY.

CARDIAC FAILURE—DIGITALIZATION AND DIURETICS.

HYPOTENSION—VASOPRESSORS, eg, LEVARTERENOL OR EPINEPHRINE (THERE IS EVIDENCE THAT EPINEPHRINE IS THE DRUG OF CHOICE).

BRONCHOSPASM—ADMINISTER ISOPROTERENOL AND AMINOPHYLLINE.

HOW SUPPLIED

INDERAL LA CAPSULES
(propranolol hydrochloride)

—Each light-blue capsule, identified by 3 narrow bands, 1 wide band, and "INDERAL LA 80," contains 80 mg of propranolol hydrochloride in bottles of 100 (NDC 0046-0471-81) and 1,000 (NDC 0046-0471-91). Also available in a Unit Dose package of 100 (NDC 0046-0471-99).

—Each light-blue/dark-blue capsule, identified by 3 narrow bands, 1 wide band, and "INDERAL LA 120," contains 120 mg of propranolol hydrochloride in bottles of 100 (NDC 0046-0473-81) and 1,000 (NDC 0046-0473-91). Also available in a Unit Dose package of 100 (NDC 0046-0473-99).

—Each dark-blue capsule, identified by 3 narrow bands, 1 wide band, and "INDERAL LA 160," contains 160 mg of propranolol hydrochloride in bottles of 100 (NDC 0046-0479-81) and 1,000 (NDC 0046-0479-91). Also available in a Unit Dose package of 100 (NDC 0046-0479-99).

The appearance of these capsules is a registered trademark of Ayerst Laboratories.

Store at room temperature (approximately 25° C).

Shown in Product Identification Section, page 404

INDERIDE® ℞

[*ĭn 'de-rīde*]

Brand of propranolol hydrochloride (INDERAL®) and hydrochlorothiazide

No. 484—Each INDERIDE® 40/25 tablet contains:
Propranolol hydrochloride
(INDERAL®) .... 40 mg
Hydrochlorothiazide .... 25 mg
No. 488—Each INDERIDE® 80/25 tablet contains:
Propranolol hydrochloride
(INDERAL®) .... 80 mg

Hydrochlorothiazide ....25 mg
CAUTION: Federal law prohibits dispensing without prescription.

Warning

This fixed combination drug is not indicated for initial therapy of hypertension. Hypertension requires therapy titrated to the individual patient. If the fixed combination represents the dosage so determined, its use may be more convenient in patient management. The treatment of hypertension is not static, but must be reevaluated as conditions in each patient warrant.

DESCRIPTION

INDERIDE combines two antihypertensive agents: INDERAL (propranolol hydrochloride), a beta-adrenergic blocking agent, and hydrochlorothiazide, a thiazide diuretic-antihypertensive.
Propranolol hydrochloride is a stable, white to off-white, crystalline powder with a melting point of about 164° C. It is odorless and has a bitter taste. It is readily soluble in water and ethanol, and insoluble in non-polar solvents. Its chemical name is 1-(Isopropylamino)-3-(1-naphthyloxy)-2-propanol hydrochloride.
Hydrochlorothiazide is a white, or practically white, practically odorless, crystalline powder. It is slightly soluble in water, freely soluble in sodium hydroxide solution, sparingly soluble in methanol; insoluble in ether, chloroform, benzene, and dilute mineral acids. Its chemical name is 6-Chloro-3,4-dihydro-2H-1,2,4-benzothiadiazine-7-sulfonamide 1,1-dioxide.
The inactive ingredients contained in INDERIDE Tablets are: lactose, magnesium stearate, microcrystalline cellulose, stearic acid, and yellow ferric oxide.

CLINICAL PHARMACOLOGY

Propranolol hydrochloride (INDERAL®):
Propranolol hydrochloride is a beta-adrenergic receptor-blocking drug, possessing no other autonomic nervous system activity. It specifically competes with beta-adrenergic receptor-stimulating agents for available beta-receptor sites. When access to beta-receptor sites is blocked by propranolol, the chronotropic, inotropic, and vasodilator responses to beta-adrenergic stimulation are decreased proportionately.
Propranolol is almost completely absorbed from the gastrointestinal tract, but a portion is immediately bound by the liver. Peak effect occurs in one to one and one-half hours. The biologic half-life is approximately two to three hours. Propranolol is not significantly dialyzable. There is no simple correlation between dose or plasma level and therapeutic effect, and the dose-sensitivity range, as observed in clinical practice, is wide. The principal reason for this is that sympathetic tone varies widely between individuals. Since there is no reliable test to estimate sympathetic tone or to determine whether total beta blockade has been achieved, proper dosage requires titration.
The mechanism of the antihypertensive effects of propranolol has not been established. Among the factors that may be involved are: (1) decreased cardiac output, (2) inhibition of renin release by the kidneys, and (3) diminution of tonic sympathetic nerve outflow from vasomotor centers in the brain.
Propranolol hydrochloride decreases heart rate, cardiac output, and blood pressure. Although total peripheral vascular resistance may increase initially, it readjusts to or below the pretreatment level with chronic usage. Earlier studies indicate that plasma volume remains unchanged or may decrease. However, there are certain more recent studies suggesting that in the absence of sodium restriction, plasma volume may increase.
Beta-receptor blockade is useful in conditions in which, because of pathologic or functional changes, sympathetic activity is excessive or inappropriate, and detrimental to the patient. But there are also situations in which sympathetic stimulation is vital. For example, in patients with severely damaged hearts, adequate ventricular function is maintained by virtue of sympathetic drive, which should be preserved. In the presence of AV block, beta blockade may prevent the necessary facilitating effect of sympathetic activity on conduction. Beta blockade results in bronchial constriction by interfering with adrenergic bronchodilator activity which should be preserved in patients subject to bronchospasm.
The proper objective of beta-blockade therapy is to decrease adverse sympathetic stimulation, but not to the degree that may impair necessary sympathetic support.
Hydrochlorothiazide:
Hydrochlorothiazide is a benzothiadiazine (thiazide) diuretic closely related to chlorothiazide. The mechanism of the antihypertensive effect of the thiazides is unknown. Thiazides do not affect normal blood pressure.
Thiazides affect the renal tubular mechanism of electrolyte reabsorption. At maximal therapeutic dosage, all thiazides are approximately equal in their diuretic potency.
Thiazides increase excretion of sodium and chloride in approximately equivalent amounts. Natriuresis causes a secondary loss of potassium and bicarbonate.
Onset of diuretic action of thiazides occurs in 2 hours, and the peak effect in about 4 hours. Its action persists for approximately 6 to 12 hours. Thiazides are eliminated rapidly by the kidney.

INDICATION

INDERIDE [propranolol HCl (INDERAL®) and hydrochlorothiazide] is indicated in the management of hypertension. (See Boxed Warning.)

CONTRAINDICATIONS

Propranolol hydrochloride (INDERAL®):
Propranolol hydrochloride is contraindicated in: 1) bronchial asthma; 2) allergic rhinitis during the pollen season; 3) sinus bradycardia and greater than first-degree block; 4) cardiogenic shock; 5) right ventricular failure secondary to pulmonary hypertension; 6) congestive heart failure (see WARNINGS), unless the failure is secondary to a tachyarrhythmia treatable with propranolol; 7) in patients on adrenergic-augmenting psychotropic drugs (including MAO inhibitors), and during the two-week withdrawal period from such drugs.
Hydrochlorothiazide:
Hydrochlorothiazide is contraindicated in patients with anuria or hypersensitivity to this or other sulfonamide-derived drugs.

WARNINGS

Propranolol hydrochloride (INDERAL®):
CARDIAC FAILURE: Sympathetic stimulation is a vital component supporting circulatory function in congestive heart failure, and inhibition with beta blockade always carries the potential hazard of further depressing myocardial contractility and precipitating cardiac failure. Propranolol acts selectively without abolishing the inotropic action of digitalis on the heart muscle (*ie*, that of supporting the strength of myocardial contractions). In patients already receiving digitalis, the positive inotropic action of digitalis may be reduced by propranolol's negative inotropic effect. The effects of propranolol and digitalis are additive in depressing AV conduction.
IN PATIENTS WITHOUT A HISTORY OF CARDIAC FAILURE, continued depression of the myocardium over a period of time can, in some cases, lead to cardiac failure. In rare instances, this has been observed during propranolol therapy. Therefore, at the first sign or symptom of impending cardiac failure, patients should be fully digitalized and/or given a diuretic, and the response observed closely: a) if cardiac failure continues, despite adequate digitalization and diuretic therapy, propranolol therapy should be immediately withdrawn; b) if tachyarrhythmia is being controlled, patients should be maintained on combined therapy and the patient closely followed until threat of cardiac failure is over.

IN PATIENTS WITH ANGINA PECTORIS, there have been reports of exacerbation of angina and, in some cases, myocardial infarction, following *abrupt* discontinuation of propranolol therapy. Therefore, when discontinuance of propranolol is planned the dosage should be gradually reduced and the patient carefully monitored. In addition, when propranolol is prescribed for angina pectoris, the patient should be cautioned against interruption or cessation of therapy without the physician's advice. If propranolol therapy is interrupted and exacerbation of angina occurs, it usually is advisable to reinstitute propranolol therapy and take other measures appropriate for the management of unstable angina pectoris. Since coronary artery disease may be unrecognized, it may be prudent to follow the above advice in patients considered at risk of having occult atherosclerotic heart disease, who are given propranolol for other indications.

IN PATIENTS WITH THYROTOXICOSIS, possible deleterious effects from long-term use have not been adequately appraised. Special consideration should be given to propranolol's potential for aggravating congestive heart failure. Propranolol may mask the clinical signs of developing or continuing hyperthyroidism or complications and give a false impression of improvement. Therefore, abrupt withdrawal of propranolol may be followed by an exacerbation of symptoms of hyperthyroidism, including thyroid storm. This is another reason for withdrawing propranolol slowly. Propranolol does not distort thyroid function tests.
IN PATIENTS WITH WOLFF-PARKINSON-WHITE SYNDROME, several cases have been reported in which, after propranolol, the tachycardia was replaced by a severe bradycardia requiring a demand pacemaker. In one case this resulted after an initial dose of 5 mg propranolol.
IN PATIENTS UNDERGOING MAJOR SURGERY, beta blockade impairs the ability of the heart to respond to reflex stimuli. For this reason, with the exception of pheochromocytoma, propranolol should be withdrawn 48 hours prior to surgery, at which time all chemical and physiologic effects are gone according to available evidence. However, in case of emergency surgery, since propranolol is a competitive inhibitor of beta-receptor agonists, its effects can be reversed by administration of such agents, *eg*, isoproterenol or levarterenol. However, such patients may be subject to protracted severe hypotension. Difficulty in restarting and maintaining the heart beat has also been reported.
IN PATIENTS PRONE TO NONALLERGIC BRONCHOSPASM (*eg*, CHRONIC BRONCHITIS, EMPHYSEMA), propranolol should be administered with caution since it may block bronchodilation produced by endogenous and exogenous catecholamine stimulation of beta receptors.
DIABETICS AND PATIENTS SUBJECT TO HYPOGLYCEMIA: Because of its beta-adrenergic blocking activity, propranolol may prevent the appearance of premonitory signs and symptoms (pulse rate and pressure changes) of acute hypoglycemia. This is especially important to keep in mind in patients with labile diabetes. Hypoglycemic attacks may be accompanied by a precipitous elevation of blood pressure.
Hydrochlorothiazide:
Thiazides should be used with caution in severe renal disease. In patients with renal disease, thiazides may precipitate azotemia. In patients with impaired renal function, cumulative effects of the drug may develop.
Thiazides should also be used with caution in patients with impaired hepatic function or progressive liver disease, since minor alterations of fluid and electrolyte balance may precipitate hepatic coma.
Thiazides may add to or potentiate the action of other antihypertensive drugs. Potentiation occurs with ganglionic or peripheral adrenergic-blocking drugs.
Sensitivity reactions may occur in patients with a history of allergy or bronchial asthma.
The possibility of exacerbation or activation of systemic lupus erythematosus has been reported.
USE IN PREGNANCY:
Propranolol hydrochloride (INDERAL®):
The safe use of propranolol in human pregnancy has not been established. Use of any drug in pregnancy or women of childbearing potential requires that the possible risk to mother and/or fetus be weighed against the expected therapeutic benefit. Embryotoxic effects have been seen in animal studies at doses about 10 times the maximal recommended human dose.
Hydrochlorothiazide:
Thiazides cross the placental barrier and appear in cord blood. The use of thiazides in pregnant women requires that the anticipated benefit be weighed against possible hazards to the fetus. These hazards include fetal or neonatal jaundice, thrombocytopenia, and possibly other adverse reactions which have occurred in the adult.
Nursing Mothers: Thiazides appear in breast milk. If the use of the drug is deemed essential, the patient should stop nursing.

PRECAUTIONS

Propranolol hydrochloride (INDERAL®):
Patients receiving catecholamine-depleting drugs, such as reserpine, should be closely observed if propranolol is administered. The added catecholamine-blocking action of this drug may then produce an excessive reduction of the resting sympathetic nervous activity. Occasionally, the pharmacologic activity of propranolol may produce hypotension and/or marked bradycardia, resulting in vertigo, syncopal attacks, or orthostatic hypotension.
As with any new drug given over prolonged periods, laboratory parameters should be observed at regular intervals. The drug should be used with caution in patients with impaired renal or hepatic function.
Hydrochlorothiazide:
Periodic determination of serum electrolytes to detect possible electrolyte imbalance should be performed at appropriate intervals.
All patients receiving thiazide therapy should be observed for clinical signs of fluid or electrolyte imbalance, namely: Hyponatremia, hypochloremic alkalosis, and hypokalemia. Serum and urine electrolyte determinations are particularly important when the patient is vomiting excessively or receiving parenteral fluids. Medication such as digitalis may also influence serum electrolytes. Warning signs, irrespective of cause are: Dryness of mouth, thirst, weakness, lethargy, drowsiness, restlessness, muscle pains or cramps, muscular fatigue, hypotension, oliguria, tachycardia, and gastrointestinal disturbances such as nausea and vomiting.
Hypokalemia may develop, especially with brisk diuresis, when severe cirrhosis is present, or during concomitant use of corticosteroids or ACTH.
Interference with adequate oral electrolyte intake will also contribute to hypokalemia. Hypokalemia can sensitize or exaggerate the response of the heart to the toxic effects of digitalis (*eg*, increased ventricular irritability). Hypokalemia may be avoided or treated by use of potassium supplements such as foods with a high potassium content.

Continued on next page

Ayerst—Cont.

Any chloride deficit is generally mild and usually does not require specific treatment except under extraordinary circumstances (as in liver or renal disease). Dilutional hyponatremia may occur in edematous patients in hot weather; appropriate therapy is water restriction, rather than administration of salt, except in rare instances when the hyponatremia is life-threatening. In actual salt depletion, appropriate replacement is the therapy of choice.
Hyperuricemia may occur or frank gout may be precipitated in certain patients receiving thiazide therapy.
Insulin requirements in diabetic patients may be increased, decreased, or unchanged. Diabetes mellitus which has been latent may become manifest during thiazide administration.
Thiazide drugs may increase the responsiveness to tubocurarine.
The antihypertensive effects of the drug may be enhanced in the postsympathectomy patient. Thiazides may decrease arterial responsiveness to norepinephrine. This diminution is not sufficient to preclude effectiveness of the pressor agent for therapeutic use.
If progressive renal impairment becomes evident, consider withholding or discontinuing diuretic therapy.
Thiazides may decrease serum PBI levels without signs of thyroid disturbance.
Calcium excretion is decreased by thiazides. Pathologic changes in the parathyroid gland with hypercalcemia and hypophosphatemia have been observed in a few patients on prolonged thiazide therapy. The common complications of hyperparathyroidism, such as renal lithiasis, bone resorption, and peptic ulceration, have not been seen. Thiazides should be discontinued before carrying out tests for parathyroid function.

ADVERSE REACTIONS

Propranolol hydrochloride (INDERAL®):
Cardiovascular: Bradycardia; congestive heart failure; intensification of AV block; hypotension; paresthesia of hands; arterial insufficiency, usually of the Raynaud type; thrombocytopenic purpura.
Central Nervous System: Light-headedness; mental depression manifested by insomnia, lassitude, weakness, fatigue, reversible mental depression progressing to catatonia; visual disturbances; hallucinations; an acute reversible syndrome characterized by disorientation for time and place, short-term memory loss, emotional lability, slightly clouded sensorium, and decreased performance on neuropsychometrics.
Gastrointestinal: Nausea; vomiting; epigastric distress; abdominal cramping; diarrhea; constipation; mesenteric arterial thrombosis; ischemic colitis.
Allergic: Pharyngitis and agranulocytosis; erythematous rash; fever combined with aching and sore throat; laryngospasm and respiratory distress.
Respiratory: Bronchospasm.
Hematologic: Agranulocytosis; nonthrombocytopenic purpura; thrombocytopenic purpura.
Miscellaneous: Reversible alopecia. Oculomucocutaneous reactions involving the skin, serous membranes and conjunctivae reported for a beta blocker (practolol) have not been conclusively associated with propranolol.
Clinical Laboratory Test Findings: Elevated blood urea levels in patients with severe heart disease, elevated serum transaminase, alkaline phosphatase, lactate dehydrogenase.
Hydrochlorothiazide:
Gastrointestinal: Anorexia; gastric irritation; nausea; vomiting; cramping; diarrhea; constipation; jaundice (intrahepatic cholestatic jaundice); pancreatitis; sialadenitis.
Central Nervous System: Dizziness; vertigo; paresthesias; headache; xanthopsia.
Hematologic: Leukopenia; agranulocytosis; thrombocytopenia; aplastic anemia.
Cardiovascular: Orthostatic hypotension (may be aggravated by alcohol, barbiturates, or narcotics).
Hypersensitivity: Purpura; photosensitivity; rash; urticaria; necrotizing angiitis (vasculitis, cutaneous vasculitis); fever; respiratory distress, including pneumonitis; anaphylactic reactions.
Other: Hyperglycemia; glycosuria; hyperuricemia; muscle spasm; weakness; restlessness; transient blurred vision.
Whenever adverse reactions are moderate or severe, thiazide dosage should be reduced, or therapy withdrawn.

DOSAGE AND ADMINISTRATION

The dosage must be determined by individual titration (see Boxed Warning).
Hydrochlorothiazide is usually given at a dose of 50 to 100 mg per day. The initial dose of propranolol is 40 mg twice daily, and it may be increased gradually until optimal blood pressure control is achieved. The usual effective dose is 160 to 480 mg per day.
One to two INDERIDE [propranolol HCl (INDERAL®) and hydrochlorothiazide] Tablets twice daily can be used to administer up to 320 mg of propranolol and 100 mg of hydrochlorothiazide. For doses of propranolol greater than 320 mg, the combination products are not appropriate, because their use would lead to an excessive dose of the thiazide component.
When necessary, another antihypertensive agent may be added gradually, beginning with 50% of the usual recommended starting dose to avoid an excessive fall in blood pressure.

Overdosage or Exaggerated Response:
The propranolol hydrochloride (INDERAL) component may cause bradycardia, cardiac failure, hypotension, or bronchospasm.
The hydrochlorothiazide component can be expected to cause diuresis. Lethargy of varying degree may appear and may progress to coma within a few hours, with minimal depression of respiration and cardiovascular function, and in the absence of significant serum electrolyte changes or dehydration. The mechanism of central nervous system depression with thiazide overdosage is unknown. Gastrointestinal irritation and hypermotility can occur; temporary elevation of BUN has been reported, and serum electrolyte changes could occur, especially in patients with impairment of renal function.
TREATMENT
The following measures should be employed:
GENERAL—If ingestion is, or may have been, recent, evacuate gastric contents taking care to prevent pulmonary aspiration.
BRADYCARDIA—Administer atropine (0.25 to 1.0 mg). If there is no response to vagal blockade, administer isoproterenol cautiously.
CARDIAC FAILURE—Digitalization and diuretics.
HYPOTENSION—Vasopressors, *eg,* levarterenol or epinephrine.
BRONCHOSPASM—Administer isoproterenol and aminophylline.
STUPOR OR COMA—Administer supportive therapy as clinically warranted.
GASTROINTESTINAL EFFECTS—Though usually of short duration, these may require symptomatic treatment.
ABNORMALITIES IN BUN AND/OR SERUM ELECTROLYTES—Monitor serum electrolyte levels and renal function; institute supportive measures, as required individually, to maintain hydration, electrolyte balance, respiration, and cardiovascular-renal function.

HOW SUPPLIED

—Each hexagonal-shaped, off-white, scored INDERIDE 40/25 tablet, embossed with an "I" and imprinted with "INDERIDE 40/25," contains 40 mg propranolol hydrochloride (INDERAL®) and 25 mg hydrochlorothiazide, in bottles of 100 (NDC 0046-0484-81) and 1,000 (NDC 0046-0484-91). Also in Unit Dose packages of 100 (NDC 0046-0484-99).
—Each hexagonal-shaped, off-white, scored INDERIDE 80/25 tablet, embossed with an "I" and imprinted with "INDERIDE 80/25," contains 80 mg propranolol hydrochloride (INDERAL®) and 25 mg hydrochlorothiazide, in bottles of 100 (NDC 0046-0488-81) and 1,000 (NDC 0046-0488-91). Also in Unit Dose packages of 100 (NDC 0046-0488-99).
The appearance of these tablets is a registered trademark of Ayerst Laboratories.
Store at room temperature (approximately 25° C).
Shown in Product Identification Section, page 404

INDERIDE® LA ℞

[*in 'de-rīde*]
Brand of propranolol hydrochloride (INDERAL® LA) and hydrochlorothiazide (Long Acting Capsules)

No. 455—Each INDERIDE® LA 80/50 Capsule contains:
Propranolol hydrochloride (INDERAL® LA) .... 80 mg
Hydrochlorothiazide .... 50 mg
No. 457—Each INDERIDE® LA 120/50 Capsule contains:
Propranolol hydrochloride (INDERAL® LA) .... 120 mg
Hydrochlorothiazide .... 50 mg
No. 459—Each INDERIDE® LA 160/50 Capsule contains:
Propranolol hydrochloride (INDERAL® LA) .... 160 mg
Hydrochlorothiazide .... 50 mg
CAUTION: Federal law prohibits dispensing without prescription.

DESCRIPTION

INDERIDE LA is indicated in the once-daily management of hypertension.
INDERIDE LA combines two antihypertensive agents: INDERAL (propranolol hydrochloride), a beta-adrenergic receptor-blocking agent, and hydrochlorothiazide, a thiazide diuretic-antihypertensive. INDERIDE LA is formulated to provide a sustained release of propranolol hydrochloride. Hydrochlorothiazide in INDERIDE LA exists in a conventional (not sustained-release) formulation.
INDERAL (propranolol hydrochloride) is a synthetic beta-adrenergic receptor-blocking agent chemically described as 1-(isopropylamino)-3-(1-naphthyloxy)-2-propanol hydrochloride. Its structural formula is:

$O\ CH_2CHOHCH_2NHCH(CH_3)_2 \cdot HCl$

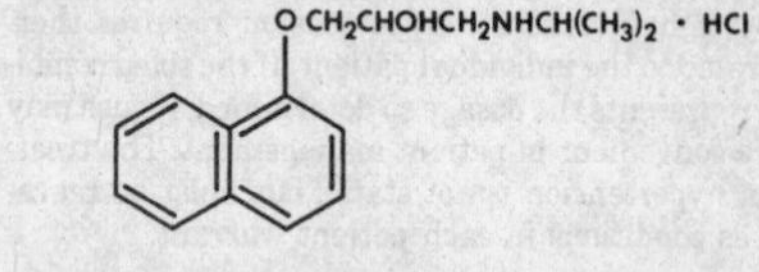

INDERAL is a stable, white, crystalline solid which is readily soluble in water and ethanol. Its molecular weight is 295.81.
Hydrochlorothiazide is a white, or practically white, practically odorless, crystalline powder. It is slightly soluble in water; freely soluble in sodium hydroxide solution; sparingly soluble in methanol; insoluble in ether, chloroform, benzene, and dilute mineral acids. Its chemical name is 6-Chloro-3,4-dihydro-2H-1,2,4-benzothiadiazine-7-sulfonamide 1,1-dioxide. Its structural formula is:

NH_2SO_2, S, O, O, NH, Cl, N, H

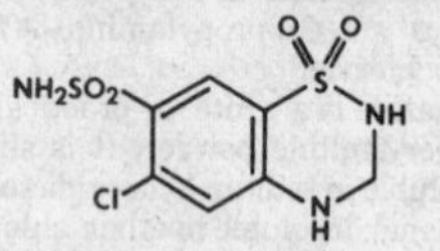

INDERIDE LA contains the following inactive ingredients: calcium carbonate, ethylcellulose, gelatin capsules, hydroxypropyl methylcellulose, lactose, magnesium stearate, microcrystalline cellulose, sodium lauryl sulfate, sodium starch glycolate, titanium dioxide, and D&C Yellow No. 10. In addition, INDERIDE LA 80/50 mg and 120/50 mg Capsules contain D&C Red No. 33; INDERIDE LA 120/50 mg and 160/50 mg Capsules contain FD&C Blue No. 1 and FD&C Red No. 40.

CLINICAL PHARMACOLOGY

Propranolol hydrochloride (INDERAL®):
INDERAL is a nonselective, beta-adrenergic receptor-blocking agent possessing no other autonomic nervous system activity. It specifically competes with beta-adrenergic receptor-stimulating agents for available receptor sites. When access to beta-receptor sites is blocked by INDERAL, the chronotropic, inotropic, and vasodilator responses to beta-adrenergic stimulation are decreased proportionately.
INDERIDE LA Capsules (80/50, 120/50, and 160/50 mg) release propranolol hydrochloride at a controlled and predictable rate. Peak propranolol blood levels following dosing with INDERIDE LA occur at about 6 hours and the apparent plasma half-life is about 10 hours. Over a 24-hour period, propranolol blood levels are fairly constant for about 12 hours, then decline exponentially. When measured at steady state over a 24-hour period, the areas under the propranolol plasma concentration-time curve (AUCs) for the capsules are approximately 60% to 65% of the AUCs for a comparable divided daily dose of INDERAL Tablets. The lower AUCs for the capsules are due to greater hepatic metabolism of propranolol resulting from the slower rate of absorption of propranolol.
INDERIDE LA should not be considered a simple mg-for-mg substitute for conventional INDERIDE Tablets and the propranolol blood levels achieved do not match (are lower than) those of twice-daily dosing of INDERIDE Tablets with the same dose. When changing to INDERIDE LA from conventional INDERIDE Tablets, a possible need for retitration upwards should be considered.
The mechanism of the antihypertensive effect of propranolol has not been established. Among the factors that may be involved in contributing to the antihypertensive action are: (1) decreased cardiac output, (2) inhibition of renin release by the kidneys, and (3) diminution of tonic sympathetic nerve outflow from vasomotor centers in the brain.
Propranolol hydrochloride decreases heart rate, cardiac output, and blood pressure. Although total peripheral vascular resistance may increase initially, it readjusts to or below the pretreatment level with chronic usage. Effects on plasma volume appear to be minor and somewhat variable. INDERAL has been shown to cause a small increase in serum potassium concentration when used in the treatment of hypertensive patients.
Beta-receptor blockade is useful in conditions in which, because of pathologic or functional changes, sympathetic activity is excessive or inappropriate, and detrimental to the patient. But there are also situations in which sympathetic stimulation is vital. For example, in patients with severely damaged hearts, adequate ventricular function is maintained by virtue of sympathetic drive, which should be preserved. In the presence of AV block, beta blockade may prevent the necessary facilitating effect of sympathetic activity on conduction. Beta blockade results in bronchial constriction by interfering with adrenergic bronchodilator activity,

which should be preserved in patients subject to bronchospasm.
The proper objective of beta-blockade therapy is to decrease adverse sympathetic stimulation, but not to the degree that may impair necessary sympathetic support.

Hydrochlorothiazide:
Hydrochlorothiazide is a benzothiadiazine (thiazide) diuretic closely related to chlorothiazide. The mechanism of the antihypertensive effect of the thiazides is unknown. Thiazides usually do not affect normal blood pressure.
Thiazides affect the renal tubular mechanism of electrolyte reabsorption. At maximal therapeutic dosage, all thiazides are approximately equal in their diuretic efficacy.
Thiazides increase excretion of sodium and chloride in approximately equivalent amounts. Natriuresis causes a secondary loss of potassium and bicarbonate.
Onset of diuretic action of thiazides occurs in 2 hours, and the peak effect in about 4 hours. Its action persists for approximately 6 to 12 hours. Thiazides are eliminated rapidly by the kidney. The hydrochlorothiazide in INDERIDE LA is a conventional (not sustained-release) formulation.

INDICATIONS AND USAGE
INDERIDE LA is indicated in the management of hypertension.
This fixed combination drug is not indicated for initial therapy of hypertension. Hypertension requires therapy titrated to the individual patient. If the fixed combination represents the dosage so determined, its use may be more convenient in patient management. The treatment of hypertension is not static, but must be reevaluated as conditions in each patient warrant.

CONTRAINDICATIONS
Propranolol hydrochloride (INDERAL®):
Propranolol is contraindicated in: 1) cardiogenic shock; 2) sinus bradycardia and greater than first-degree block; 3) bronchial asthma; 4) congestive heart failure (see WARNINGS), unless the failure is secondary to a tachyarrhythmia treatable with propranolol.

Hydrochlorothiazide:
Hydrochlorothiazide is contraindicated in patients with anuria or hypersensitivity to this or other sulfonamide-derived drugs.

WARNINGS
Propranolol hydrochloride (INDERAL®):
CARDIAC FAILURE: Sympathetic stimulation may be a vital component supporting circulatory function in patients with congestive heart failure, and its inhibition by beta blockade may precipitate more severe failure. Although beta blockers should be avoided in overt congestive heart failure, if necessary, they can be used with close follow-up in patients with a history of failure who are well compensated, and are receiving digitalis and diuretics. Beta-adrenergic blocking agents do not abolish the inotropic action of digitalis on heart muscle.
IN PATIENTS WITHOUT A HISTORY OF HEART FAILURE, continued use of beta blockers can, in some cases, lead to cardiac failure. Therefore, at the first sign or symptom of heart failure, the patient should be digitalized and/or treated with diuretics, and the response observed closely, or propranolol should be discontinued (gradually, if possible).

IN PATIENTS WITH ANGINA PECTORIS, there have been reports of exacerbation of angina and, in some cases, myocardial infarction, following *abrupt* discontinuance of propranolol therapy. Therefore, when discontinuance of propranolol is planned, the dosage should be gradually reduced and the patient carefully monitored. In addition, when propranolol is prescribed for angina pectoris, the patient should be cautioned against interruption or cessation of therapy without the physician's advice. If propranolol therapy is interrupted and exacerbation of angina occurs, it usually is advisable to reinstitute propranolol therapy and take other measures appropriate for the management of unstable angina pectoris. Since coronary artery disease may be unrecognized, it may be prudent to follow the above advice in patients considered at risk of having occult atherosclerotic heart disease who are given propranolol for other indications.

THYROTOXICOSIS: Beta blockade may mask certain clinical signs of hyperthyroidism. Therefore, abrupt withdrawal of propranolol may be followed by an exacerbation of symptoms of hyperthyroidism, including thyroid storm. Propranolol does not distort thyroid function tests.
IN PATIENTS WITH WOLFF-PARKINSON-WHITE SYNDROME, several cases have been reported in which, after propranolol, the tachycardia was replaced by a severe bradycardia requiring a demand pacemaker. In one case this resulted after an initial dose of 5 mg propranolol.
MAJOR SURGERY: The necessity or desirability of withdrawal of beta-blocking therapy prior to major surgery is controversial. It should be noted, however, that the impaired ability of the heart to respond to reflex adrenergic stimuli may augment the risks of general anesthesia and surgical procedures.
Nonallergic Bronchospasm (eg, chronic bronchitis, emphysema)—PATIENTS WITH BRONCHOSPASTIC DISEASES SHOULD, IN GENERAL, NOT RECEIVE BETA BLOCKERS. INDERAL should be administered with caution since it may block bronchodilation produced by endogenous and exogenous catecholamine stimulation of beta receptors.
DIABETES AND HYPOGLYCEMIA: Beta-adrenergic blockade may prevent the appearance of certain premonitory signs and symptoms (pulse rate and pressure changes) of acute hypoglycemia in labile insulin-dependent diabetes. In these patients, it may be more difficult to adjust the dosage of insulin. Hypoglycemic attacks may be accompanied by a precipitous elevation of blood pressure.

Hydrochlorothiazide:
Thiazides should be used with caution in severe renal disease. In patients with renal disease, thiazides may precipitate azotemia. In patients with impaired renal function, cumulative effects of the drug may develop.
Thiazides should also be used with caution in patients with impaired hepatic function or progressive liver disease, since minor alterations of fluid and electrolyte balance may precipitate hepatic coma.
Thiazides may add to or potentiate the action of other antihypertensive drugs. Potentiation occurs with ganglionic or peripheral adrenergic-blocking drugs.
Sensitivity reactions may occur in patients with a history of allergy or bronchial asthma.
The possibility of exacerbation or activation of systemic lupus erythematosus has been reported.

PRECAUTIONS
Propranolol hydrochloride (INDERAL®):
GENERAL: Propranolol should be used with caution in patients with impaired hepatic or renal function. Propranolol is not indicated for the treatment of hypertensive emergencies.
Beta-adrenoreceptor blockade can cause reduction of intraocular pressure. Patients should be told that propranolol may interfere with the glaucoma screening test. Withdrawal may lead to a return of increased intraocular pressure.
Clinical Laboratory Tests: Elevated blood urea levels in patients with severe heart disease, elevated serum transaminase, alkaline phosphatase, lactate dehydrogenase.
DRUG INTERACTIONS: Patients receiving catecholamine-depleting drugs, such as reserpine, should be closely observed if propranolol is administered. The added catecholamine-blocking action may produce an excessive reduction of resting sympathetic nervous activity, which may result in hypotension, marked bradycardia, vertigo, syncopal attacks, or orthostatic hypotension.
CARCINOGENESIS, MUTAGENESIS, IMPAIRMENT OF FERTILITY: Long-term studies in animals have been conducted to evaluate toxic effects and carcinogenic potential. In 18-month studies, in both rats and mice, employing doses up to 150 mg/kg/day, there was no evidence of significant drug-induced toxicity. There were no drug-related tumorigenic effects at any of the dosage levels. Reproductive studies in animals did not show any impairment of fertility that was attributable to the drug.
PREGNANCY: Pregnancy Category C. Propranolol has been shown to be embryotoxic in animal studies at doses about 10 times greater than the maximal recommended human dose. There are no adequate and well-controlled studies in pregnant women. Propranolol should be used during pregnancy only if the potential benefit justifies the potential risk to the fetus.
NURSING MOTHERS: Propranolol is excreted in human milk. Caution should be exercised when propranolol is administered to a nursing mother.
PEDIATRIC USE: Safety and effectiveness in children have not been established.

Hydrochlorothiazide:
GENERAL: Periodic determination of serum electrolytes to detect possible electrolyte imbalance should be performed at appropriate intervals.
All patients receiving thiazide therapy should be observed for clinical signs of fluid or electrolyte imbalance, namely: Hyponatremia, hypochloremic alkalosis, and hypokalemia. Serum and urine electrolyte determinations are particularly important when the patient is vomiting excessively or receiving parenteral fluids. Medication such as digitalis may also influence serum electrolytes. Warning signs irrespective of cause are: Dryness of mouth, thirst, weakness, lethargy, drowsiness, restlessness, muscle pains or cramps, muscular fatigue, hypotension, oliguria, tachycardia, and gastrointestinal disturbances such as nausea and vomiting.
Hypokalemia may develop, especially with brisk diuresis, when severe cirrhosis is present, or during concomitant use of corticosteroids or ACTH.
Interference with adequate oral electrolyte intake will also contribute to hypokalemia. Hypokalemia can sensitize or exaggerate the response of the heart to the toxic effect of digitalis (eg, increased ventricular irritability). Hypokalemia may be avoided or treated by use of potassium supplements, such as foods with a high potassium content.
Any chloride deficit is generally mild and usually does not require specific treatment, except under extraordinary circumstances (as in liver or renal disease). Dilutional hyponatremia may occur in edematous patients in hot weather; appropriate therapy is water restriction, rather than administration of salt, except in rare instances when the hyponatremia is life-threatening. In actual salt depletion, appropriate replacement is the therapy of choice.
Hyperuricemia may occur or frank gout may be precipitated in certain patients receiving thiazide therapy.
Insulin requirements in diabetic patients may be increased, decreased, or unchanged. Diabetes mellitus which has been latent may become manifest during thiazide administration.
If progressive renal impairment becomes evident, consider withholding or discontinuing diuretic therapy.
Thiazides may decrease serum PBI levels without signs of thyroid disturbance.
Calcium excretion is decreased by thiazides. Pathologic changes in the parathyroid gland with hypercalcemia and hypophosphatemia have been observed in a few patients on prolonged thiazide therapy. The common complications of hyperparathyroidism, such as renal lithiasis, bone resorption, and peptic ulceration have not been seen. Thiazides should be discontinued before carrying out tests for parathyroid function.
DRUG INTERACTIONS: Thiazide drugs may increase the responsiveness to tubocurarine.
The antihypertensive effects of thiazides may be enhanced in the postsympathectomy patient. Thiazides may decrease arterial responsiveness to norepinephrine. This diminution is not sufficient to preclude effectiveness of the pressor agent for therapeutic use.
PREGNANCY: Pregnancy Category C. Thiazides cross the placental barrier and appear in cord blood. The use of thiazides in pregnancy requires that the anticipated benefit be weighed against possible hazards to the fetus. These hazards include fetal or neonatal jaundice, thrombocytopenia, and possibly other adverse reactions which have occurred in the adult.
NURSING MOTHERS: Thiazides appear in human milk. If use of the drug is deemed essential, the patient should stop nursing.
PEDIATRIC USE: Safety and effectivenss in children have not been established.

ADVERSE REACTIONS
Propranolol hydrochloride (INDERAL®):
Most adverse effects have been mild and transient and have rarely required the withdrawal of therapy.
Cardiovascular: Bradycardia; congestive heart failure; intensification of AV block; hypotension; paresthesia of hands; thrombocytopenic purpura; arterial insufficiency, usually of the Raynaud type.
Central Nervous System: Light-headedness; mental depression manifested by insomnia, lassitude, weakness, fatigue, reversible mental depression progressing to catatonia; visual disturbances; hallucinations; an acute reversible syndrome characterized by disorientation for time and place, short-term memory loss, emotional lability, slightly clouded sensorium, and decreased performance on neuropsychometrics.
Gastrointestinal: Nausea, vomiting, epigastric distress, abdominal cramping, diarrhea, constipation, mesenteric arterial thrombosis, ischemic colitis.
Allergic: Pharyngitis and agranulocytosis; erythematous rash; fever combined with aching and sore throat; laryngospasm and respiratory distress.
Respiratory: Bronchospasm.
Hematologic: Agranulocytosis; nonthrombocytopenic purpura, thrombocytopenic purpura.
Auto-Immune: In extremely rare instances, systemic lupus erythematosus has been reported.
Miscellaneous: Alopecia; LE-like reactions; psoriasiform rashes; dry eyes; male impotence; and Peyronie's disease have been reported rarely. Oculomucocutaneous reactions involving the skin, serous membrances, and conjunctivae reported for a beta blocker (practolol) have not been associated with propranolol.

Hydrochlorothiazide:
Gastrointestinal: Anorexia; gastric irritation, nausea, vomiting, cramping; diarrhea; constipation; jaundice (intrahepatic cholestatic jaundice); pancreatitis; sialadenitis.
Central Nervous System: Dizziness, vertigo; paresthesias; headache; xanthopsia.
Hematologic: Leukopenia; agranulocytosis; thrombocytopenia; aplastic anemia.
Cardiovascular: Orthostatic hypotension (may be aggravated by alcohol, barbiturates, or narcotics).
Hypersensitivity: Purpura; photosensitivity; rash; urticaria; necrotizing angiitis (vasculitis, cutaneous vasculitis); fever; respiratory distress, including pneumonitis; anaphylactic reactions.

Continued on next page

Ayerst—Cont.

Other: Hyperglycemia; glycosuria; hyperuricemia; muscle spasm; weakness; restlessness; transient blurred vision.
Whenever adverse reactions are moderate or severe, thiazide dosage should be reduced or therapy withdrawn.

DOSAGE AND ADMINISTRATION

The dosage must be determined by individual titration.
Hydrochlorothiazide can be given at doses of 25–100 mg per day when used alone, but in most patients, 50 mg exerts a maximal effect. The initial dose of propranolol is 80 mg daily, and it may be increased gradually until optimal blood pressure control is achieved. The usual effective dose, when used alone, is 160–480 mg per day.
One INDERIDE LA Capsule once-a-day can be used to administer up to 160 mg of propranolol and 50 mg of hydrochlorothiazide. For doses of propranolol greater than 160 mg, the combination products are not appropriate because their use would lead to an excessive dose of the thiazide component.
INDERIDE LA provides propranolol hydrochloride in a sustained-release form and hydrochlorothiazide in conventional formulation, for once-daily administration. If patients are switched from INDERIDE Tablets (or INDERAL plus hydrochlorothiazide) to INDERIDE LA, care should be taken to ensure that the desired therapeutic effect is maintained. INDERIDE LA should not be considered a mg-for-mg substitute for INDERIDE or INDERAL plus hydrochlorothiazide. INDERIDE LA has different kinetics and produces lower blood levels. Retitration may be necessary, especially to maintain effectiveness at the end of the 24-hour dosing interval.
When necessary, another antihypertensive agent may be added gradually, beginning with 50% of the usual recommended starting dose, to avoid an excessive fall in blood pressure.

OVERDOSAGE OR EXAGGERATED RESPONSE

The propranolol hydrochloride (INDERAL) component may cause bradycardia, cardiac failure, hypotension, or bronchospasm.
The hydrochlorothiazide component can be expected to cause diuresis. Lethargy of varying degree may appear and may progress to coma within a few hours, with minimal depression of respiration and cardiovascular function, and in the absence of significant serum electrolyte changes or dehydration. The mechanism of central nervous system depression with thiazide overdosage is unknown. Gastrointestinal irritation and hypermotility can occur; temporary elevation of BUN has been reported and serum electrolyte changes could occur, especially in patients with impairment of renal function.
TREATMENT
The following measures should be employed:
GENERAL—If ingestion is, or may have been, recent, evacuate gastric contents, taking care to prevent pulmonary aspiration.
BRADYCARDIA—Administer atropine (0.25–1.0 mg). If there is no response to vagal blockade, administer isoproterenol cautiously.
CARDIAC FAILURE—Digitalization and diuretics.
HYPOTENSION—Vasopressors, eg, levarterenol or epinephrine.
BRONCHOSPASM—Administer isoproterenol and aminophylline.
STUPOR OR COMA—Administer supportive therapy as clinically warranted.
GASTROINTESTINAL EFFECTS—Though usually of short duration, these may require symptomatic treatment.
ABNORMALITIES IN BUN AND/OR SERUM ELECTROLYTES—Monitor serum electrolyte levels and renal function; institute supportive measures, as required individually, to maintain hydration, electrolyte balance, respiration, and cardiovascular function.

HOW SUPPLIED

—Each beige capsule, identified by one wide band and 3 narrow bands, all in gold, and "INDERIDE LA 80/50," contains 80 mg of propranolol hydrochloride (INDERAL® LA) and 50 mg of hydrochlorothiazide, in bottles of 100 (NDC 0046-0455-81).
—Each beige/brown capsule, identified by one wide band and 3 narrow bands, all in gold, and "INDERIDE LA 120/50," contains 120 mg of propranolol hydrochloride (INDERAL® LA) and 50 mg of hydrochlorothiazide, in bottles of 100 (NDC 0046-0457-81).
—Each brown capsule, identified by one wide band and 3 narrow bands, all in gold, and "INDERIDE LA 160/50, contains 160 mg of propranolol hydrochloride (INDERAL® LA) and 50 mg of hydrochlorothiazide, in bottles of 100 (NDC 0046-0459-81).
The appearance of these capsules is a registered trademark of Ayerst Laboratories.
Store at room temperature (approximately 25° C).

Shown in Product Identification Section, page 404

KERODEX® OTC

[kĕr′o-dĕx]
Skin Barrier Cream

ACTION AND USES

A specially formulated barrier cream to help protect against potentially irritating chemicals, compounds, and solutions in common use. When applied and used as directed, KERODEX provides a barrier film that helps to block contact with skin irritants. KERODEX No. 71 (water-repellent) is for use in handling or working with *wet* materials; No. 51 is for *dry* or *oily* work. KERODEX is greaseless and stainless.

APPLICATION

1. Wash hands clean and dry *thoroughly*. 2. Squeeze out ½ inch of cream into palm of one hand. Rub hands together with a washing motion until cream is *lightly* and *evenly* distributed, leaving no excess. Make sure cream reaches under nails, around cuticles, between fingers, across wrists and backs of hands (forearms, if necessary). 3. A second application is recommended. **NOTE:** After applying KERODEX 71, "set" by holding hands under cold running water. Pat dry. After applying KERODEX 51, avoid contact with water. If hands become wet during work, reapply.

HOW SUPPLIED

KERODEX 71 (water-repellent cream for wet work), in 4 oz (113 g) tubes (NDC 0046-0071-04), 1 lb. jars (NDC 0046-0071-01), and 8 lb. tins (NDC 0046-0071-08).
KERODEX 51 (water-miscible cream for dry or oily work), in 4 oz (113 g) tubes (NDC 0046-0051-04), 1 lb. jars (NDC 0046-0051-01), and 8 lb. tins (NDC 0046-0051-08).

LARYLGAN® Throat Spray OTC

[lăr′al-gan]

An aqueous solution containing:

Antipyrine	0.30%
Pyrilamine maleate	0.05%
Sodium caprylate	0.50%

Also contains: alcohol, benzyl alcohol, glycerin, methylparaben, PEG-40 castor oil, propylparaben, sodium saccharin, flavors, and other aromatics.

ACTION

The analgesic-like effect of LARYLGAN helps to allay pain of irritated mucosa. The glycerin dehydrated vehicle provides maximum spreading and penetrating properties to help the medication reach the affected areas. It is non-narcotic.

INDICATIONS

A soothing and refreshing spray for dry throat and for minor sore throat due to irritants such as smoking or postnasal drip.

WARNING

Severe and persistent sore throat or sore throat accompanied by high fever, headache, nausea, and vomiting may be serious. Consult physician promptly. Do not use more than two days or administer to children under 3 years of age unless directed by physician.

ADMINISTRATION

Instructions for Use: Adults and children 3 years of age or older. Remove cap. Hold close to mouth. Spray as needed. If throat condition persists, consult a physician.

HOW SUPPLIED

LARYLGAN Throat Spray, in 0.94 fl oz (28 mL) bottles (NDC 0046-1005-01).

MEDIATRIC® Ⓒ℞

[mē″dē-ăt′rik]

Each capsule or tablet contains:

Premarin® (conjugated estrogens, USP)	0.25	mg
Methyltestosterone	2.5	mg
Ascorbic acid (vit. C)*	100.0	mg
Cyanocobalamin	2.5	mcg
Thiamine mononitrate	10.0	mg
Riboflavin	5.0	mg
Niacinamide	50.0	mg
Pyridoxine HCl	3.0	mg
Calc. pantothenate	20.0	mg
Dried ferrous sulfate	30.0	mg
Methamphetamine HCl	1.0	mg

*For Capsules, provided as ascorbic acid, 70 mg, and as sodium ascorbate, 30 mg.

Also available: MEDIATRIC Liquid
Each 15 mL (3 teaspoonfuls) contains:

Premarin® (conjugated estrogens, USP)	0.25	mg
Methyltestosterone	2.5	mg
Thiamine HCl	5.0	mg
Cyanocobalamin	1.5	mcg
Methamphetamine HCl	1.0	mg

Contains 15% alcohol—some loss unavoidable.

CAUTION: Federal law prohibits dispensing without prescription.

1. ESTROGENS HAVE BEEN REPORTED TO INCREASE THE RISK OF ENDOMETRIAL CARCINOMA.
Three independent case control studies have reported an increased risk of endometrial cancer in postmenopausal women exposed to exogenous estrogens for more than one year.[1–3] This risk was independent of the other known risk factors for endometrial cancer. These studies are further supported by the finding that incidence rates of endometrial cancer have increased sharply since 1969 in eight different areas of the United States with population-based cancer reporting systems, an increase which may be related to the rapidly expanding use of estrogens during the last decade.[4]
The three case control studies reported that the risk of endometrial cancer in estrogen users was about 4.5 to 13.9 times greater than in nonusers. The risk appears to depend on both duration of treatment[1] and on estrogen dose.[3] In view of these findings, when estrogens are used for the treatment of menopausal symptoms, the lowest dose that will control symptoms should be utilized and medication should be discontinued as soon as possible. When prolonged treatment is medically indicated, the patient should be reassessed on at least a semiannual basis to determine the need for continued therapy. Although the evidence must be considered preliminary, one study suggests that cyclic administration of low doses of estrogen may carry less risk than continuous administration[3]; it therefore appears prudent to utilize such a regimen.
Close clinical surveillance of all women taking estrogens is important. In all cases of undiagnosed persistent or recurring abnormal vaginal bleeding, adequate diagnostic measures should be undertaken to rule out malignancy.
There is no evidence at present that "natural" estrogens are more or less hazardous than "synthetic" estrogens at equiestrogenic doses.

2. ESTROGENS SHOULD NOT BE USED DURING PREGNANCY.
The use of female sex hormones, both estrogens and progestogens, during early pregnancy may seriously damage the offspring. It has been shown that females exposed in utero to diethylstilbestrol, a non-steroidal estrogen, have an increased risk of developing in later life a form of vaginal or cervical cancer that is ordinarily extremely rare.[5,6] This risk has been estimated as not greater than 4 per 1,000 exposures.[7] Furthermore, a high percentage of such exposed women (from 30% to 90%) have been found to have vaginal adenosis,[8–12] epithelial changes of the vagina and cervix. Although these changes are histologically benign, it is not known whether they are precursors of malignancy. Although similar data are not available with the use of other estrogens, it cannot be presumed they would not induce similar changes.
Several reports suggest an association between intrauterine exposure to female sex hormones and congenital anomalies, including congenital heart defects and limb reduction defects.[13–16] One case control study[16] estimated a 4.7-fold increased risk of limb reduction defects in infants exposed in utero to sex hormones (oral contraceptives, hormone withdrawal tests for pregnancy, or attempted treatment for threatened abortion). Some of these exposures were very short and involved only a few days of treatment. The data suggest that the risk of limb reduction defects in exposed fetuses is somewhat less than 1 per 1,000.
In the past, female sex hormones have been used during pregnancy in an attempt to treat threatened or habitual abortion. There is considerable evidence that estrogens are ineffective for these indications, and there is no evidence from well controlled studies that progestogens are effective for these uses.
If MEDIATRIC is used during pregnancy, or if the patient becomes pregnant while taking this drug, she should be apprised of the potential risks to the fetus, and the advisability of pregnancy continuation.

DESCRIPTION

MEDIATRIC provides estrogen and androgen in small doses, nutritional supplements, together with a mild antidepressant.
MEDIATRIC Tablets contain the following inactive ingredients: alginic acid, calcium phosphate tribasic, calcium sulfate anhydrous, carnauba wax, cosmetic black iron oxide, D&C Red No. 7, D&C Red No. 36, FD&C Blue No. 2, FD&C Red No. 40, FD&C Yellow No. 6, lactose, magnesium stea-

rate, mannitol, methylcellulose, microcrystalline cellulose, pharmaceutical glaze, sorbitan tristearate, sucrose, titanium dioxide.

MEDIATRIC Capsules contain the following inactive ingredients: ethyl vanillin, FD&C Blue No. 1, FD&C Red No. 33, gelatin, lecithin, soybean oil, wax mixture.

ACTION

MEDIATRIC provides (1) *steroids* to help counteract declining gonadal hormone secretion, and as important regulators of metabolic processes; (2) *nutritional supplements* specially selected to meet the needs of the aged and aging patient, and to act as necessary catalysts for the maintenance of efficient enzyme systems; and (3) *a mild antidepressant* to impart a gentle emotional uplift.

INDICATION

For use in aging patients of both sexes.

MEDIATRIC HAS NOT BEEN SHOWN TO BE EFFECTIVE FOR ANY PURPOSE DURING PREGNANCY AND ITS USE MAY CAUSE SEVERE HARM TO THE FETUS (SEE BOXED WARNING).

CONTRAINDICATIONS

Estrogens should not be used in women (or men) with any of the following conditions:

1. Known or suspected cancer of the breast except in appropriately selected patients being treated for metastatic disease.
2. Known or suspected estrogen-dependent neoplasia.
3. Known or suspected pregnancy (See Boxed Warning).
4. Undiagnosed abnormal genital bleeding.
5. Active thrombophlebitis or thromboembolic disorders.
6. A past history of thrombophlebitis, thrombosis, or thromboembolic disorders associated with previous estrogen use (except when used in treatment of breast or prostatic malignancy).

Methyltestosterone should not be used in persons with any of the following conditions:

1. Known or suspected carcinoma of the prostate and in carcinoma of the male breast.
2. Severe liver damage.
3. Pregnancy or in breast-feeding mothers because of the possibility of masculinization of the female fetus or breast-fed infant.

WARNINGS

Associated with Estrogens

1. *Induction of malignant neoplasms.* Long-term continuous administration of natural and synthetic estrogens in certain animal species increases the frequency of carcinomas of the breast, cervix, vagina, and liver. There are now reports that estrogens increase the risk of carcinoma of the endometrium in humans. (See Boxed Warning.)

At the present time there is no satisfactory evidence that estrogens given to postmenopausal women increase the risk of cancer of the breast,[17] although a recent long-term followup of a single physician's practice has raised this possibility.[18] Because of the animal data, there is a need for caution in prescribing estrogens for women with a strong family history of breast cancer or who have breast nodules, fibrocystic disease, or abnormal mammograms.

2. *Gallbladder disease.* A recent study has reported a 2- to 3-fold increase in the risk of surgically confirmed gallbladder disease in women receiving postmenopausal estrogens,[17] similar to the 2-fold increase previously noted in users of oral contraceptives.[19,24a]

3. *Effects similar to those caused by estrogen-progestogen oral contraceptives.* There are several serious adverse effects of oral contraceptives, most of which have not, up to now, been documented as consequences of postmenopausal estrogen therapy. This may reflect the comparatively low doses of estrogen used in postmenopausal women. It would be expected that the larger doses of estrogen used to treat prostatic or breast cancer or postpartum breast engorgement are more likely to result in these adverse effects, and, in fact, it has been shown that there is an increased risk of thrombosis in men receiving estrogens for prostatic cancer and women for postpartum breast engorgement.[20–23]

a. *Thromboembolic disease.* It is now well established that users of oral contraceptives have an increased risk of various thromboembolic and thrombotic vascular diseases, such as thrombophlebitis, pulmonary embolism, stroke, and myocardial infarction.[24–31] Cases of retinal thrombosis, mesenteric thrombosis, and optic neuritis have been reported in oral contraceptive users. There is evidence that the risk of several of these adverse reactions is related to the dose of the drug.[32,33] An increased risk of postsurgery thromboembolic complications has also been reported in users of oral contraceptives.[34,35] If feasible, estrogen should be discontinued at least 4 weeks before surgery of the type associated with an increased risk of thromboembolism, or during periods of prolonged immobilization.

While an increased rate of thromboembolic and thrombotic disease in postmenopausal users of estrogens has not been found,[17–24,25–36] this does not rule out the possibility that such an increase may be present or that subgroups of women who have underlying risk factors or who are receiving relatively large doses of estrogens may have increased risk. Therefore estrogens should not be used in persons with active thrombophlebitis or thromboembolic disorders, and they should not be used (except in treatment of malignancy) in persons with a history of such disorders in association with estrogen use. They should be used with caution in patients with cerebral vascular or coronary artery disease and only for those in whom estrogens are clearly needed.

Large doses of estrogen (5 mg conjugated estrogens per day), comparable to those used to treat cancer of the prostate and breast, have been shown in a large prospective clinical trial in men[37] to increase the risk of nonfatal myocardial infarction, pulmonary embolism and thrombophlebitis. When estrogen doses of this size are used, any of the thromboembolic and thrombotic adverse effects associated with oral contraceptive use should be considered a clear risk.

b. *Hepatic adenoma.* Benign hepatic adenomas appear to be associated with the use of oral contraceptives.[38–40] Although benign, and rare, these may rupture and may cause death through intra-abdominal hemorrhage. Such lesions have not yet been reported in association with other estrogen or progestogen preparations but should be considered in estrogen users having abdominal pain and tenderness, abdominal mass, or hypovolemic shock. Hepatocellular carcinoma has also been reported in women taking estrogen-containing oral contraceptives.[39] The relationship of this malignancy to these drugs is not known at this time.

c. *Elevated blood pressure.* Women using oral contraceptives sometimes experience increased blood pressure which, in most cases, returns to normal on discontinuing the drug. There is now a report that this may occur with use of estrogens in the menopause[41] and blood pressure should be monitored with estrogen use, especially if high doses are used.

d. *Glucose tolerance.* A worsening of glucose tolerance has been observed in a significant percentage of patients on estrogen-containing oral contraceptives. For this reason, diabetic patients should be carefully observed while receiving estrogen.

4. *Hypercalcemia.* Administration of estrogens may lead to severe hypercalcemia in patients with breast cancer and bone metastases. If this occurs, the drug should be stopped and appropriate measures taken to reduce the serum calcium level.

Associated with Methyltestosterone

1. Female patients should be watched carefully for symptoms or signs of virilization such as hoarseness or deepening of the voice, oily skin, acne, hirsutism, enlarged clitoris, stimulation of libido, and menstrual irregularities. At the dosage necessary to achieve a tumor response, androgens will cause masculinization of a female, but occasionally a sensitive female may exhibit one or more of these signs on smaller doses. Some of these changes, such as voice changes, may be irreversible even after drug is stopped.
2. Cholestatic hepatitis with jaundice and altered liver function tests, such as increased BSP retention and rises in SGOT levels, have been reported with methyltestosterone. These changes appear to be related to dosage of the drug. Therefore, in the presence of any changes in liver function tests, the drug should be discontinued.

PRECAUTIONS

Associated with Estrogens

A. General Precautions.

1. A complete medical and family history should be taken prior to the initiation of any estrogen therapy. The pretreatment and periodic physical examinations should include special reference to blood pressure, breasts, abdomen, and pelvic organs, and should include a Papanicolaou smear. As a general rule, estrogen should not be prescribed for longer than one year without another physical examination being performed.
2. Fluid retention—Because estrogens may cause some degree of fluid retention, conditions which might be influenced by this factor such as asthma, epilepsy, migraine, and cardiac or renal dysfunction, require careful observation.
3. Certain patients may develop undesirable manifestations of excessive estrogenic stimulation, such as abnormal or excessive uterine bleeding, mastodynia, etc.
4. Oral contraceptives appear to be associated with an increased incidence of mental depression.[24a] Although it is not clear whether this is due to the estrogenic or progestogenic component of the contraceptive, patients with a history of depression should be carefully observed.
5. Preexisting uterine leiomyomata may increase in size during estrogen use.
6. The pathologist should be advised of estrogen therapy when relevant specimens are submitted.
7. Patients with a past history of jaundice during pregnancy have an increased risk of recurrence of jaundice while receiving estrogen-containing oral contraceptive therapy. If jaundice develops in any patient receiving estrogen, the medication should be discontinued while the cause is investigated.
8. Estrogens may be poorly metabolized in patients with impaired liver function and they should be administered with caution in such patients.
9. Because estrogens influence the metabolism of calcium and phosphorus, they should be used with caution in patients with metabolic bone diseases that are associated with hypercalcemia or in patients with renal insufficiency.
10. Because of the effects of estrogens on epiphyseal closure, they should be used judiciously in young patients in whom bone growth is not complete.
11. Certain endocrine and liver function tests may be affected by estrogen-containing oral contraceptives. The following similar changes may be expected with larger doses of estrogen:

a. Increased sulfobromophthalein retention.
b. Increased prothrombin and factors VII, VIII, IX, and X; decreased antithrombin 3; increased norepinephrine-induced platelet aggregability.
c. Increased thyroid binding globulin (TBG) leading to increased circulating total thyroid hormone, as measured by PBI, T4 by column, or T4 by radioimmunoassay. Free T3 resin uptake is decreased, reflecting the elevated TBG; free T4 concentration is unaltered.
d. Impaired glucose tolerance.
e. Decreased pregnanediol excretion.
f. Reduced response to metyrapone test.
g. Reduced serum folate concentration.
h. Increased serum triglyceride and phospholipid concentration.

B. Information for the Patient. See text which appears after the PHYSICIAN REFERENCES.

C. Pregnancy Category X. See CONTRAINDICATIONS and Boxed Warning.

D. Nursing Mothers. As a general principle, the administration of any drug to nursing mothers should be done only when clearly necessary since many drugs are excreted in human milk.

Associated with Methyltestosterone

A. Prolonged dosage of androgen may result in sodium and fluid retention. This may present a problem, especially in patients with compromised cardiac reserve or renal disease.
B. If priapism or other signs of excessive sexual stimulation develop, discontinue therapy.
C. In the male, prolonged administration or excessive dosage may cause inhibition of testicular function, with resultant oligospermia and decrease in ejaculatory volume. Use cautiously in young boys to avoid possible premature epiphyseal closure or precocious sexual development.
D. Hypersensitivity and gynecomastia may occur rarely.
E. PBI may be decreased in patients taking androgens.
F. Hypercalcemia may occur. If this does occur, the drug should be discontinued.

ADVERSE REACTIONS

Associated with Estrogens

(See Warnings regarding induction of neoplasia, adverse effects on the fetus, increased incidence of gallbladder disease, and adverse effects similar to those of oral contraceptives, including thromboembolism.) The following additional adverse reactions have been reported with estrogenic therapy, including oral contraceptives:

1. *Genitourinary system:* Breakthrough bleeding, spotting, change in menstrual flow; dysmenorrhea; premenstrual-like syndrome; amenorrhea during and after treatment; increase in size of uterine fibromyomata; vaginal candidiasis; change in cervical erosion and in degree of cervical secretion; cystitis-like syndrome.
2. *Breasts:* Tenderness, enlargement, secretion.
3. *Gastrointestinal:* Nausea, vomiting; abdominal cramps, bloating; cholestatic jaundice.
4. *Skin:* Chloasma or melasma which may persist when drug is discontinued; erythema multiforme; erythema nodosum; hemorrhagic eruption; loss of scalp hair; hirsutism.
5. *Eyes:* Steepening of corneal curvature; intolerance to contact lenses.
6. *CNS:* Headache, migraine, dizziness; mental depression; chorea.
7. *Miscellaneous:* Increase or decrease in weight; reduced carbohydrate tolerance; aggravation of porphyria; edema; changes in libido.

Associated with Methyltestosterone

Cholestatic jaundice

Hypercalcemia, particularly in patients with metastatic breast carcinoma. This usually indicates progression of bone metastases.

Sodium and water retention

Priapism

Virilization in female patients

Hypersensitivity and gynecomastia

ACUTE OVERDOSAGE

Numerous reports of ingestion of large doses of estrogen-containing oral contraceptives by young children indicate that acute serious ill effects do not occur. Overdosage of es-

Continued on next page

Ayerst—Cont.

trogen may cause nausea, and withdrawal bleeding may occur in females.

DOSAGE AND ADMINISTRATION

Male and female—1 MEDIATRIC Capsule or Tablet daily. (MEDIATRIC Liquid, 3 teaspoonfuls daily.)

In the female: To avoid continuous stimulation of breast and uterus, cyclic therapy is recommended (3 week regimen with 1 week rest period—Withdrawal bleeding may occur during this 1 week rest period).

Treated patients with an intact uterus should be monitored closely for signs of endometrial cancer and appropriate diagnostic measures should be taken to rule out malignancy in the event of persistent or recurring abnormal vaginal bleeding.

In the male: A careful check should be made on the status of the prostate gland when therapy is given for protracted intervals.

HOW SUPPLIED

MEDIATRIC Capsules, in bottles of 100 (NDC 0046-0252-81).
MEDIATRIC Tablets, in bottles of 100 (NDC 0046-0752-81).
MEDIATRIC Liquid, in bottles of 16 fluid ounces (NDC 0046-0910-16).

PHYSICIAN REFERENCES

1. Ziel, H. K., *et al.*: N. Engl. J. Med. *293*:1167–1170, 1975.
2. Smith, D. C., *et al.*: N. Engl. J. Med. *293*:1164–1167, 1975.
3. Mack, T. M., *et al.*: N. Engl. J. Med. *294*:1262–1267, 1976.
4. Weiss, N. S., *et al.*: N. Engl. J. Med. *294*:1259–1262, 1976.
5. Herbst, A. L., *et al.*: N. Engl. J. Med. *284*:878–881, 1971.
6. Greenwald, P., *et al.*: N. Engl. J. Med. *285*:390–392, 1971.
7. Lanier, A., *et al.*: Mayo Clin. Proc. *48*:793–799, 1973.
8. Herbst, A., *et al.*: Obstet. Gynecol. *40*:287–298, 1972.
9. Herbst, A., *et al.*: Am. J. Obstet. Gynecol. *118*:607–615, 1974.
10. Herbst, A., *et al.*: N. Engl. J. Med. *292*:334–339, 1975.
11. Stafl, A., *et al.*: Obstet. Gynecol. *43*:118–128, 1974.
12. Sherman, A. I., *et al.*: Obstet. Gynecol. *44*:531–545, 1974.
13. Gal, I., *et al.*: Nature *216*:83, 1967.
14. Levy, E. P., *et al.*: Lancet *1*:611, 1973.
15. Nora, J., *et al.*: Lancet *1*:941–942, 1973.
16. Janerich, D. T., *et al.*: N. Engl. J. Med. *291*:697–700, 1974.
17. Boston Collaborative Drug Surveillance Program: N. Engl. J. Med. *290*:15–19, 1974.
18. Hoover, R., *et al.*: N. Engl. J. Med. *295*:401–405, 1976.
19. Boston Collaborative Drug Surveillance Program: Lancet *1*:1399–1404, 1973.
20. Daniel, D. G., *et al.*: Lancet *2*:287–289, 1967.
21. The Veterans Administration Cooperative Urological Research Group: J. Urol. *98*:516–522, 1967.
22. Bailar, J. C.: Lancet *2*:560, 1967.
23. Blackard, C., *et al.*: Cancer *26*:249–256, 1970.
24. Royal College of General Practitioners: J. R. Coll. Gen. Pract. *13*:267–279, 1967.

24a. Royal College of General Practitioners: Oral Contraceptives and Health, New York, Pitman Corp., 1974.

25. Inman, W. H. W., *et al.*: Br. Med. J. *2*:193–199, 1968.
26. Vessey, M. P., *et al.*: Br. Med. J. *2*:651–657, 1969.
27. Sartwell, P. E., *et al.*: Am. J. Epidemiol. *90*:365–380, 1969.
28. Collaborative Group for the Study of Stroke in Young Women: N. Engl. J. Med. *288*:871–878, 1973.
29. Collaborative Group for the Study of Stroke in Young Women: J.A.M.A. *231*:718–722, 1975.
30. Mann, J. I., *et al.*: Br. Med. J. *2*:245–248, 1975.
31. Mann, J. I., *et al.*: Br. Med. J. *2*:241–245, 1975.
32. Inman, W. H. W., *et al.*: Br. Med. J. *2*:203–209, 1970.
33. Stolley, P. D., *et al.*: Am. J. Epidemiol. *102*:197–208, 1975.
34. Vessey, M. P., *et al.*: Br. Med. J. *3*:123–126, 1970.
35. Greene, G. R., *et al.*: Am. J. Public Health *62*:680–685, 1972.
36. Rosenberg, L., *et al.*: N. Engl. J. Med. *294*:1256–1259, 1976.
37. Coronary Drug Project Research Group: J.A.M.A. *214*:1303–1313, 1970.
38. Baum, J., *et al.*: Lancet *2*:926–928, 1973.
39. Mays, E. T., *et al.*: J.A.M.A. *235*:730–732, 1976.
40. Edmondson, H. A., *et al.*: N. Engl. J. Med. *294*:470–472, 1976.
41. Pfeffer, R. I., *et al.*: Am. J. Epidemiol. *103*:445–456, 1976.

INFORMATION FOR THE PATIENT

WHAT YOU SHOULD KNOW ABOUT ESTROGENS

Estrogens are female hormones produced by the ovaries. The ovaries make several different kinds of estrogens. In addition, scientists have been able to make a variety of synthetic estrogens. As far as we know, all these estrogens have similar properties and therefore much the same usefulness, side effects, and risks. This leaflet is intended to help you understand what estrogens are used for, the risks involved in their use, and how to use them as safely as possible.

This leaflet includes the most important information about estrogens, but not all the information. If you want to know more, you should ask your doctor for more information or you can ask your doctor or pharmacist to let you read the package insert prepared for the doctor.

USES OF ESTROGEN

THERE IS NO PROPER USE OF ESTROGENS IN A PREGNANT WOMAN.

Estrogens are prescribed by doctors for a number of purposes, including:

1. To provide estrogen during a period of adjustment when a woman's ovaries stop producing a majority of her estrogens, in order to prevent certain uncomfortable symptoms of estrogen deficiency. (With the menopause, which generally occurs between the ages of 45 and 55, women produce a much smaller amount of estrogens.)
2. To prevent symptoms of estrogen deficiency when a woman's ovaries have been removed surgically before the natural menopause.
3. To prevent pregnancy. (Estrogens are given along with a progestogen, another female hormone; these combinations are called oral contraceptives or birth control pills. Patient labeling is available to women taking oral contraceptives and they will not be discussed in this leaflet.)
4. To treat certain cancers in women and men.
5. To prevent painful swelling of the breasts after pregnancy in women who choose not to nurse their babies.

ESTROGENS IN THE MENOPAUSE

In the natural course of their lives, all women eventually experience a decrease in estrogen production. This usually occurs between ages 45 and 55 but may occur earlier or later. Sometimes the ovaries may need to be removed before natural menopause by an operation, producing a "surgical menopause."

When the amount of estrogen in the blood begins to decrease, many women may develop typical symptoms: feelings of warmth in the face, neck, and chest or sudden intense episodes of heat and sweating throughout the body (called "hot flashes" or "hot flushes"). These symptoms are sometimes very uncomfortable. Some women may also develop changes in the vagina (called "atrophic vaginitis") which cause discomfort, especially during and after intercourse.

Estrogens can be prescribed to treat these symptoms of the menopause. It is estimated that considerably more than half of all women undergoing the menopause have only mild symptoms or no symptoms at all and therefore do not need estrogens. Other women may need estrogens for a few months, while their bodies adjust to lower estrogen levels. Sometimes the need will be for periods longer than six months. In an attempt to avoid overstimulation of the uterus (womb), estrogens are usually given cyclically during each month of use, such as three weeks of pills followed by one week without pills.

Sometimes women experience nervous symptoms or depression during menopause. There is no evidence that estrogens are effective for such symptoms without associated vasomotor symptoms. In the absence of vasomotor symptoms, estrogens should not be used to treat nervous symptoms, although other treatment may be needed.

You may have heard that taking estrogens for long periods (years) after the menopause will keep your skin soft and supple and keep you feeling young. There is no evidence that this is so, however, and such long-term treatment carries important risks.

ESTROGENS TO PREVENT SWELLING OF THE BREASTS AFTER PREGNANCY

If you do not breast-feed your baby after delivery, your breasts may fill up with milk and become painful and engorged. This usually begins about 3 to 4 days after delivery and may last for a few days to up to a week or more. Sometimes the discomfort is severe, but usually it is not and can be controlled by pain-relieving drugs such as aspirin and by binding the breasts up tightly. Estrogens can be used to try to prevent the breasts from filling up. While this treatment is sometimes successful, in many cases the breasts fill up to some degree in spite of treatment. The dose of estrogens needed to prevent pain and swelling of the breasts is much larger than the dose needed to treat symptoms of the menopause and this may increase your chances of developing blood clots in the legs or lungs (see below). Therefore, it is important that you discuss the benefits and the risks of estrogen use with your doctor if you have decided not to breast-feed your baby.

THE DANGERS OF ESTROGENS

1. *Endometrial cancer.* There are reports that if estrogens are used in the postmenopausal period for more than a year, there is an increased risk of *endometrial cancer* (cancer of the lining of the uterus). Women taking estrogens have roughly 5 to 10 times as great a chance of getting this cancer as women who take no estrogens. To put this another way, while a postmenopausal woman not taking estrogens has 1 chance in 1,000 each year of getting endometrial cancer, a woman taking estrogens has 5 to 10 chances in 1,000 each year. For this reason *it is important to take estrogens only when they are really needed.*

The risk of this cancer is greater the longer estrogens are used and when larger doses are taken. Therefore you should not take more estrogen than your doctor prescribes. *It is important to take the lowest dose of estrogen that will control symptoms and to take it only as long as it is needed.* If estrogens are needed for longer periods of time, your doctor will want to reevaluate your need for estrogens at least every six months.

Women using estrogens should report any vaginal bleeding to their doctors; such bleeding may be of no importance, but it can be an early warning of endometrial cancer. If you have undiagnosed vaginal bleeding, you should not use estrogens until a diagnosis is made and you are certain there is no endometrial cancer.

NOTE: If you have had your uterus removed (total hysterectomy), there is no danger of developing endometrial cancer.

2. *Other possible cancers.* Estrogens can cause development of other tumors in animals, such as tumors of the breast, cervix, vagina, or liver, when given for a long time. At present there is no good evidence that women using estrogen in the menopause have an increased risk of such tumors, but there is no way yet to be sure they do not; and one study raises the possibility that use of estrogens in the menopause may increase the risk of breast cancer many years later. This is a further reason to use estrogens only when clearly needed. While you are taking estrogens, it is important that you go to your doctor at least once a year for a physical examination. Also, if members of your family have had breast cancer or if you have breast nodules or abnormal mammograms (breast x-rays), your doctor may wish to carry out more frequent examinations of your breasts.

3. *Gallbladder disease.* Women who use estrogens after menopause are more likely to develop gallbladder disease needing surgery than women who do not use estrogens. Birth control pills have a similar effect.

4. *Abnormal blood clotting.* Oral contraceptives increase the risk of blood clotting in various parts of the body. This can result in a stroke (if the clot is in the brain), a heart attack (clot in a blood vessel of the heart), or a pulmonary embolus (a clot which forms in the legs or pelvis, then breaks off and travels to the lungs). Any of these can be fatal.

At this time use of estrogens in the menopause is not known to cause such blood clotting, but this has not been fully studied and there could still prove to be such a risk. It is recommended that if you have had clotting in the legs or lungs or a heart attack or stroke while you were using estrogens or birth control pills, you should not use estrogens (unless they are being used to treat cancer of the breast or prostate). If you have had a stroke or heart attack or if you have angina pectoris, estrogens should be used with great caution and only if clearly needed (for example, if you have severe symptoms of the menopause).

The larger doses of estrogen used to prevent swelling of the breasts after pregnancy have been reported to cause clotting in the legs and lungs.

SPECIAL WARNING ABOUT PREGNANCY

You should not receive estrogen if you are pregnant. If this should occur, there is a greater than usual chance that the developing child will be born with a birth defect, although the possibility remains fairly small. A female child may have an increased risk of developing cancer of the vagina or cervix later in life (in the teens or twenties). Every possible effort should be made to avoid exposure to estrogens during pregnancy. If exposure occurs, see your doctor.

OTHER EFFECTS OF ESTROGENS

In addition to the serious known risks of estrogens described above, estrogens have the following side effects and potential risks:

1. *Nausea and vomiting.* The most common side effect of estrogen therapy is nausea. Vomiting is less common.
2. *Effects on breasts.* Estrogens may cause breast tenderness or enlargement and may cause the breasts to secrete a liquid. These effects are not dangerous.
3. *Effects on the uterus.* Estrogens may cause benign fibroid tumors of the uterus to get larger.
4. *Effects on liver.* Women taking oral contraceptives develop on rare occasions a tumor of the liver which can rupture and bleed into the abdomen and may cause death. So far, these tumors have not been reported in women using estrogens in the menopause, but you should report any swelling or unusual pain or tenderness in the abdomen to your doctor immediately.

Women with a past history of jaundice (yellowing of the skin and white parts of the eyes) may get jaundice again during estrogen use. If this occurs, stop taking estrogens and see your doctor.

5. *Other effects.* Estrogens may cause excess fluid to be retained in the body. This may make some conditions worse, such as asthma, epilepsy, migraine, heart disease, or kidney disease.

SUMMARY

Estrogens have important uses, but they have serious risks as well. You must decide, with your doctor, whether the risks are acceptable to you in view of the benefits of treatment. Except where your doctor has prescribed estrogens for use in special cases of cancer of the breast or prostate, you should not use estrogens if you have cancer of the breast or uterus, are pregnant, have undiagnosed abnormal vaginal bleeding, clotting in the legs or lungs, or have had a stroke, heart attack or angina, or clotting in the legs or lungs in the past while you were taking estrogens.

You can use estrogens as safely as possible by understanding that your doctor will require regular physical examinations while you are taking them and will try to discontinue the drug as soon as possible and use the smallest dose possible. Be alert for signs of trouble including:

1. Abnormal bleeding from the vagina.
2. Pains in the calves or chest or sudden shortness of breath, or coughing blood.
3. Severe headache, dizziness, faintness, or changes in vision.
4. Breast lumps (you should ask your doctor how to examine your own breasts).
5. Jaundice (yellowing of the skin).
6. Mental depression.

Your doctor has prescribed this drug for you and you alone. Do not give the drug to anyone else.

HOW SUPPLIED

MEDIATRIC®—provides estrogen and androgen in small doses, nutritional supplements, and a mild antidepressant. It is supplied as capsules, tablets, and liquid.

Shown in Product Identification Section, page 404

MYSOLINE® ℞

[mī'sō-lēn]
Brand of primidone
Anticonvulsant

CAUTION: Federal law prohibits dispensing without prescription.

DESCRIPTION

Chemical name: 5-ethyldihydro-5-phenyl-4,6 (1H, 5H) pyrimidine-dione

Structural formula:

MYSOLINE is a white crystalline, highly stable substance, M.P. 279–284°C. It is poorly soluble in water (60 mg per 100 mL at 37°C) and in most organic solvents. It possesses no acidic properties, in contrast to its barbiturate analog.

MYSOLINE 50 mg Tablets contain these inactive ingredients: Gelatin, NF; Lactose, NF; Magnesium Stearate, NF; Polyethylene Glycol 8000, NF; Starch, NF.

MYSOLINE 250 mg Tablets contain these inactive ingredients: Gelatin, NF; Magnesium Stearate, NF; Polyethylene Glycol 8000, NF; Starch, NF.

MYSOLINE Suspension contains these inactive ingredients: Ammonia Solution, Diluted; Citric Acid, USP; D&C Yellow No. 10; FD&C Yellow No. 6; Magnesium Aluminum Silicate; Methylparaben, NF; Propylparaben, NF; Saccharin Sodium, NF; Sodium Alginate; Sodium Citrate; Sodium Hypochlorite Solution, USP; Sorbic Acid, NF; Sorbitan Monolaurate; Water, USP, Purified; Flavors.

ACTIONS

MYSOLINE raises electro- or chemoshock seizure thresholds or alters seizure patterns in experimental animals. The mechanism(s) of primidone's antiepileptic action is not known. Primidone *per se* has anticonvulsant activity as do its two metabolites, phenobarbital and phenylethylmalonamide (PEMA). In addition to its anticonvulsant activity, PEMA potentiates that of phenobarbital in experimental animals.

INDICATIONS

MYSOLINE, either alone or used concomitantly with other anticonvulsants, is indicated in the control of grand mal, psychomotor, and focal epileptic seizures. It may control grand mal seizures refractory to other anticonvulsant therapy.

CONTRAINDICATIONS

Primidone is contraindicated in: 1) patients with porphyria and 2) patients who are hypersensitive to phenobarbital (see ACTIONS).

WARNINGS

The abrupt withdrawal of antiepileptic medication may precipitate status epilepticus.

The therapeutic efficacy of a dosage regimen takes several weeks before it can be assessed.

Usage in pregnancy: The effects of MYSOLINE (primidone) in human pregnancy and nursing infants are unknown.

Recent reports suggest an association between the use of anticonvulsant drugs by women with epilepsy and an elevated incidence of birth defects in children born to these women. Data are more extensive with respect to diphenylhydantoin and phenobarbital, but these are also the most commonly prescribed anticonvulsants; less systematic or anecdotal reports suggest a possible similar association with the use of all known anticonvulsant drugs.

The reports suggesting an elevated incidence of birth defects in children of drug-treated epileptic women cannot be regarded as adequate to prove a definite cause and effect relationship. There are intrinsic methodologic problems in obtaining adequate data on drug teratogenicity in humans; the possibility also exists that other factors, *eg*, genetic factors or the epileptic condition itself, may be more important than drug therapy in leading to birth defects. The great majority of mothers on anticonvulsant medication deliver normal infants. It is important to note that anticonvulsant drugs should not be discontinued in patients in whom the drug is administered to prevent major seizures because of the strong possibility of precipitating status epilepticus with attendant hypoxia and threat to life. In individual cases where the severity and frequency of the seizure disorder are such that the removal of medication does not pose a serious threat to the patient, discontinuation of the drug may be considered prior to and during pregnancy, although it cannot be said with any confidence that even minor seizures do not pose some hazard to the developing embryo or fetus.

The prescribing physician will wish to weigh these considerations in treating or counseling epileptic women of childbearing potential.

Neonatal hemorrhage, with a coagulation defect resembling vitamin K deficiency, has been described in newborns whose mothers were taking primidone and other anticonvulsants. Pregnant women under anticonvulsant therapy should receive prophylactic vitamin K_1 therapy for one month prior to, and during, delivery.

PRECAUTIONS

The total daily dosage should not exceed 2 g. Since MYSOLINE (primidone) therapy generally extends over prolonged periods, a complete blood count and a sequential multiple analysis-12 (SMA-12) test should be made every six months.

In Nursing Mothers: There is evidence that in mothers treated with primidone, the drug appears in the milk in substantial quantities. Since tests for the presence of primidone in biological fluids are too complex to be carried out in the average clinical laboratory, it is suggested that the presence of undue somnolence and drowsiness in nursing newborns of MYSOLINE-treated mothers be taken as an indication that nursing should be discontinued.

ADVERSE REACTIONS

The most frequently occurring early side effects are ataxia and vertigo. These tend to disappear with continued therapy, or with reduction of initial dosage. Occasionally, the following have been reported: nausea, anorexia, vomiting, fatigue, hyperirritability, emotional disturbances, sexual impotency, diplopia, nystagmus, drowsiness, and morbilliform skin eruptions. Occasionally, persistent or severe side effects may necessitate withdrawal of the drug. Megaloblastic anemia may occur as a rare idiosyncrasy to MYSOLINE and to other anticonvulsants. The anemia responds to folic acid without necessity of discontinuing medication.

DOSAGE AND ADMINISTRATION

Adult Dosage: Patients 8 years of age and older who have received no previous treatment may be started on MYSOLINE (primidone) according to the following regimen using either 50 mg or scored 250 mg MYSOLINE Tablets.

Days 1–3: 100 to 125 mg at bedtime
Days 4–6: 100 to 125 mg bid
Days 7–9: 100 to 125 mg tid
Day 10-maintenance: 250 mg tid

For most adults and children 8 years of age and over, the usual maintenance dosage is three to four 250 mg MYSOLINE tablets daily in divided doses (250 mg tid or qid). If required, an increase to five or six 250 mg tablets daily may be made but daily doses should not exceed 500 mg qid.

INITIAL: ADULTS AND CHILDREN OVER 8

KEY: · = 50 mg tablet ● = 250 mg tablet

DAY	1	2	3	4	5	6
AM				··	··	··
NOON						
PM	··	··	··	··	··	··

DAY	7	8	9	10	11	12
AM	··	··	··	●		
NOON	··	··	··	●	Adjust to	
PM	··	··	··	●	Maintenance	

Dosage should be individualized to provide maximum benefit. In some cases, serum blood level determinations of primidone may be necessary for optimal dosage adjustment. The clinically effective serum level for primidone is between 5–12 µg/mL.

In patients already receiving other anticonvulsants: MYSOLINE should be started at 100 to 125 mg at bedtime and gradually increased to maintenance level as the other drug is gradually decreased. This regimen should be continued until satisfactory dosage level is achieved for the combination, or the other medication is completely withdrawn. When therapy with MYSOLINE (primidone) alone is the objective, the transition from concomitant therapy should not be completed in less than two weeks.

Pediatric Dosage: For children under 8 years of age, the following regimen may be used:

Days 1–3: 50 mg at bedtime
Days 4–6: 50 mg bid
Days 7–9: 100 mg bid
Day 10-maintenance: 125 mg tid to 250 mg tid

For children under 8 years of age, the usual maintenance dosage is 125 to 250 mg three times daily, or 10–25 mg/kg/day in divided doses.

HOW SUPPLIED

MYSOLINE (primidone) Tablets

Each tablet contains 250 mg of primidone (scored), in bottles of 100 (NDC 0046-0430-81) and 1,000 (NDC 0046-0430-91).

Also in Unit Dose packages of 100 (NDC 0046-0430-99).

Each tablet contains 50 mg of primidone (scored), in bottles of 100 (NDC 0046-0431-81) and 500 (NDC 0046-0431-85).

MYSOLINE Suspension

Each 5 mL (teaspoonful) contains 250 mg of primidone, in bottles of 8 fluid ounces (NDC 0046-3850-08).

Shown in Product Identification Section, page 404

PEPTAVLON® ℞

[pĕp-tăv'lon]
Brand of
pentagastrin
A diagnostic agent for
evaluation of gastric acid
secretory function.

CAUTION: Federal law prohibits dispensing without prescription.

DESCRIPTION

Chemical name: N-t-butyloxycarbonyl-β-alanyl-L-tryptophyl-L-methionyl-L-aspartyl-L-phenylalanyl amide.

Structural formula:

Pentagastrin is a synthetic pentapeptide containing the carboxyl terminal tetrapeptide, the active portion found in all natural gastrins. Pentagastrin is a colorless crystalline solid. It is soluble in dimethylformamide and dimethylsulfoxide; it is almost insoluble in water, ethanol, ether, benzene, chloroform, and ethyl acetate.

ACTIONS

PEPTAVLON (pentagastrin) contains the C-terminal tetrapeptide responsible for the actions of the natural gastrins and, therefore, acts as a physiologic gastric acid secretagogue. The recommended dose of 6 mcg/kg subcutaneously produces a peak acid output which is reproducible when used in the same individual.

PEPTAVLON stimulates gastric acid secretion approximately ten minutes after subcutaneous injection, with peak responses occurring in most cases twenty to thirty minutes after administration. Duration of activity is usually between sixty and eighty minutes.

Continued on next page

Ayerst—Cont.

INDICATIONS

PEPTAVLON (pentagastrin) is used as a diagnostic agent to evaluate gastric acid secretory function. It is useful in testing for:

Anacidity:—as a diagnostic aid in patients with suspected pernicious anemia, atrophic gastritis, or gastric carcinoma.

Hypersecretion:—as a diagnostic aid in patients with suspected duodenal ulcer or postoperative stomal ulcer, and for the diagnosis of Zollinger-Ellison tumor.

PEPTAVLON (pentagastrin) is also useful in determining the adequacy of acid-reducing operations for peptic ulcer.

CONTRAINDICATIONS

Hypersensitivity or idiosyncrasy to pentagastrin.

WARNINGS

Use in Pregnancy—The use of pentagastrin in pregnancy has NOT been studied, and the benefit of administration of the drug must be weighed against any possible risk to the mother and/or fetus.

Use in Children—There are insufficient data to recommend the use of, or establish a dosage, in children.

****

In amounts in excess of the recommended dose, pentagastrin may cause inhibition of gastric acid secretion.

PRECAUTIONS

Use with caution in patients with pancreatic, hepatic, or biliary disease. Like gastrin, pentagastrin could, in some cases, have the physiologic effect of stimulating pancreatic enzyme and bicarbonate secretion, as well as biliary flow.

ADVERSE REACTIONS

Pentagastrin causes fewer and less severe cardiovascular and other adverse reactions than histamine or betazole. The majority of reactions to pentagastrin are related to the gastrointestinal tract.

The following reactions associated with the use of pentagastrin have been reported.

Gastrointestinal: Abdominal pain, desire to defecate, nausea, vomiting, borborygmi, blood-tinged mucus

Cardiovascular: Flushing, tachycardia

Central Nervous System: Dizziness, faintness or light-headedness, drowsiness, sinking feeling, transient blurring of vision, tiredness, headache

Allergic and Hypersensitivity Reactions: May occur in some patients.

Miscellaneous: Shortness of breath, heavy sensation in arms and legs, tingling in fingers, chills, sweating, generalized burning sensation, warmth, pain at site of injection, bile in collected specimens

DOSAGE AND ADMINISTRATION

Adults: 6 mcg/kg subcutaneously. Effect begins in about ten minutes; peak response usually occurs in twenty to thirty minutes. (For discussion of the test and explicit directions, consult Baron, JH: Gastric function tests, in Wastell, C: *Chronic Duodenal Ulcer,* New York, Appleton-Century-Crofts, 1972, pp 82–114.)

Note: Data are inadequate to recommend the use of, or establish a dosage, in children.

OVERDOSAGE

In case of overdosage or idiosyncrasy, symptomatic treatment should be administered as required.

HOW SUPPLIED

PEPTAVLON—In 2 mL ampuls. Each mL contains 0.25 mg (250 mcg) pentagastrin. Also contains 0.88% sodium chloride, and Water for Injection, USP. The pH is adjusted with ammonium hydroxide and/or hydrochloric acid. Cartons of 10 (NDC 0046-3290-10).

CLINICAL STUDIES

Gastric Acid Secretion: Peak gastric output in mEq/hr caused by subcutaneous injection of 6 mcg/kg pentagastrin does not differ significantly from that caused by the standard subcutaneous injection of the histamine acid phosphate dose used in the augmented histamine test (40 mcg/kg). For example, in 25 normal volunteers, pentagastrin produced an average peak acid output of 28.4 mEq/hr compared with 24.7 mEq/hr by histamine. In 45 patients with duodenal ulcer, or suspected duodenal ulcer, pentagastrin produced an average peak gastric acid output of 39.7 mEq/hr compared with 33.7 mEq/hr by histamine. In 18 patients with gastric ulcer, or suspected gastric ulcer, pentagastrin produced an average peak output of 17.4 mEq/hr compared with 19.4 mEq/hr by histamine. The overall mean for peak acid secretion by pentagastrin was 24.8 mEq/hr compared with 22.6 mEq/hr by histamine. No biochemical abnormality which might indicate specific organ toxicity has been encountered following the administration of pentagastrin.

PHOSPHOLINE IODIDE® ℞

[*fŏs'fo-lĭn ī'o-dīd*]

(echothiophate iodide for ophthalmic solution)

CAUTION: Federal law prohibits dispensing without prescription.

DESCRIPTION

PHOSPHOLINE IODIDE occurs as a white, crystalline, water-soluble, hygroscopic solid having a slight mercaptan-like odor. When freeze-dried in the presence of potassium acetate, the mixture appears as a white amorphous deposit on the walls of the bottle.

Each package contains materials for dispensing 5 mL of eyedrops: (1) bottle containing PHOSPHOLINE IODIDE in one of four potencies [1.5 mg (0.03%), 3.0 mg (0.06%), 6.25 mg (0.125%), or 12.5 mg (0.25%)] as indicated on the label, with 40 mg potassium acetate in each case. Sodium hydroxide or acetic acid may have been incorporated to adjust pH during manufacturing. (2) a 5 mL bottle of diluent containing chlorobutanol (chloral derivative), 0.55%; mannitol, 1.2%; boric acid, 0.06%; and exsiccated sodium phosphate, 0.026% (3) sterilized dropper.

ACTIONS

PHOSPHOLINE IODIDE is a long-acting cholinesterase inhibitor for topical use which enhances the effect of endogenously liberated acetylcholine in iris, ciliary muscle, and other parasympathetically innervated structures of the eye. It thereby causes miosis, increase in facility of outflow of aqueous humor, fall in intraocular pressure, and potentiation of accommodation.

PHOSPHOLINE IODIDE (echothiophate iodide) will depress both plasma and erythrocyte cholinesterase levels in most patients after a few weeks of eyedrop therapy.

INDICATIONS

GLAUCOMA—Chronic open-angle glaucoma. Subacute or chronic angle-closure glaucoma after iridectomy or where surgery is refused or contraindicated. Certain non-uveitic secondary types of glaucoma, especially glaucoma following cataract surgery.

ACCOMMODATIVE ESOTROPIA—Concomitant esotropias with a significant accommodative component.

CONTRAINDICATIONS

1. Active uveal inflammation.
2. Most cases of angle closure glaucoma, due to the possibility of increasing angle block.
3. Hypersensitivity to the active or inactive ingredients.

WARNINGS

1. *Use in Pregnancy:* Safe use of anticholinesterase medications during pregnancy has not been established, nor has the absence of adverse effects on the fetus or on the respiration of the neonate.
2. Succinylcholine should be administered only with great caution, if at all, prior to or during general anesthesia to patients receiving anticholinesterase medication because of possible respiratory or cardiovascular collapse.
3. Caution should be observed in treating glaucoma with PHOSPHOLINE IODIDE (echothiophate iodide) in patients who are at the same time undergoing treatment with systemic anticholinesterase medications for myasthenia gravis, because of possible adverse additive effects.

PRECAUTIONS

1. Gonioscopy is recommended prior to initiation of therapy.
2. Where there is a quiescent uveitis or a history of this condition, anticholinesterase therapy should be avoided or used cautiously because of the intense and persistent miosis and ciliary muscle contraction that may occur.
3. While systemic effects are infrequent, proper use of the drug requires digital compression of the nasolacrimal ducts for a minute or two following instillation to minimize drainage into the nasal chamber with its extensive absorption area. The hands should be washed immediately following instillation.
4. Temporary discontinuance of medication is necessary if salivation, urinary incontinence, diarrhea, profuse sweating, muscle weakness, respiratory difficulties, or cardiac irregularities occur.
5. Patients receiving PHOSPHOLINE IODIDE who are exposed to carbamate or organophosphate type insecticides and pesticides (professional gardeners, farmers, workers in plants manufacturing or formulating such products, etc.) should be warned of the additive systemic effects possible from absorption of the pesticide through the respiratory tract or skin. During periods of exposure to such pesticides, the wearing of respiratory masks, and frequent washing and clothing changes may be advisable.
6. Anticholinesterase drugs should be used with extreme caution, if at all, in patients with marked vagotonia, bronchial asthma, spastic gastrointestinal disturbances, peptic ulcer, pronounced bradycardia and hypotension, recent myocardial infarction, epilepsy, parkinsonism, and other disorders that may respond adversely to vagotonic effects.
7. Anticholinesterase drugs should be employed prior to ophthalmic surgery only as a considered risk because of the possible occurrence of hyphema.
8. PHOSPHOLINE IODIDE (echothiophate iodide) should be used with great caution, if at all, where there is a prior history of retinal detachment.

ADVERSE REACTIONS

1. Although the relationship, if any, of retinal detachment to the administration of PHOSPHOLINE IODIDE has not been established, retinal detachment has been reported in a few cases during the use of PHOSPHOLINE IODIDE in adult patients without a previous history of this disorder.
2. Stinging, burning, lacrimation, lid muscle twitching, conjunctival and ciliary redness, browache, induced myopia with visual blurring may occur.
3. Activation of latent iritis or uveitis may occur.
4. Iris cysts may form, and if treatment is continued, may enlarge and obscure vision. This occurrence is more frequent in children. The cysts usually shrink upon discontinuance of the medication, reduction in strength of the drops or frequency of instillation. Rarely, they may rupture or break free into the aqueous. Regular examinations are advisable when the drug is being prescribed for the treatment of accommodative esotropia.
5. Prolonged use may cause conjunctival thickening, obstruction of nasolacrimal canals.
6. Lens opacities occurring in patients under treatment for glaucoma with PHOSPHOLINE IODIDE have been reported and similar changes have been produced experimentally in normal monkeys. Routine examinations should accompany clinical use of the drug.
7. Paradoxical increase in intraocular pressure may follow anticholinesterase instillation. This may be alleviated by prescribing a sympathomimetic mydriatic such as phenylephrine.

DOSAGE AND ADMINISTRATION

GLAUCOMA—

Selection of Therapy: The *medication prescribed* should be that which will control the intraocular pressure around-the-clock with the least risk of side effects or adverse reactions. "Tonometric glaucoma" (ocular hypertension without other evidence of the disease) is frequently not treated with any medication, and PHOSPHOLINE IODIDE (echothiophate iodide) is certainly not recommended for this condition. In early chronic simple glaucoma with field loss or disc changes, pilocarpine is generally used for initial therapy and can be recommended so long as control is thereby maintained over the 24 hours of the day.

When this is not the case, PHOSPHOLINE IODIDE 0.03% may be effective and probably has no greater potential for side effects. If this dosage is inadequate, epinephrine and a carbonic anhydrase inhibitor may be added to the regimen. When still more effective medication is required, the higher strengths of PHOSPHOLINE IODIDE may be prescribed with the recognition that the control of the intraocular pressure should have priority regardless of potential side effects. In secondary glaucoma following cataract surgery, the higher strengths of the drug are frequently needed and are ordinarily very well tolerated.

The *dosage regimen* prescribed should call for the lowest concentration that will control the intraocular pressure around-the-clock. Where tonometry around-the-clock is not feasible, it is suggested that appointments for tension-taking be made at different times of the day so that inadequate control may be more readily detected. Two doses a day are preferred to one in order to maintain as smooth a diurnal tension curve as possible, although a single dose per day or every other day has been used with satisfactory results. Because of the long duration of action of the drug, it is never necessary or desirable to exceed a schedule of twice a day. The daily dose or one of the two daily doses should always be instilled just before retiring to avoid inconvenience due to the miosis.

Early Chronic Simple Glaucoma: PHOSPHOLINE IODIDE (echothiophate iodide) 0.03% instilled twice a day, just before retiring and in the morning, may be prescribed advantageously for cases of early chronic simple glaucoma that are not controlled around-the-clock with pilocarpine. Because of prolonged action, control during the night and early morning hours may then sometimes be obtained. A change in therapy is indicated if, at any time, the tension fails to remain at an acceptable level on this regimen.

Advanced Chronic Simple Glaucoma and Glaucoma Secondary to Cataract Surgery: These cases may respond satisfactorily to PHOSPHOLINE IODIDE 0.03% twice a day as above. When the patient is being transferred to PHOSPHOLINE IODIDE (echothiophate iodide) because of unsatisfactory control with pilocarpine, carbachol, epinephrine, etc., one of the higher strengths, 0.06%, 0.125%, or 0.25% will usually be needed. In this case, a brief trial with the 0.03% eyedrops will be advantageous in that the higher strengths will then be more easily tolerated.

Concomitant Therapy: PHOSPHOLINE IODIDE may be used concomitantly with epinephrine, a carbonic anhydrase inhibitor, or both.

Technic: Good technic in the administration of PHOSPHOLINE IODIDE requires that finger pressure at the inner canthus should be exerted for a minute or two following instillation of the eyedrops, to minimize drainage into the nose and throat. Excess solution around the eye should be removed with tissue and any medication on the hands should be rinsed off.

ACCOMMODATIVE ESOTROPIA—

In Diagnosis: One drop of 0.125% may be instilled once a day in both eyes on retiring, for a period of two or three weeks. If the esotropia is accommodative, a favorable response will usually be noted which may begin within a few hours.

In Treatment: PHOSPHOLINE IODIDE (echothiophate iodide) is prescribed at the lowest concentration and frequency which gives satisfactory results. After the initial period of treatment for diagnostic purposes, the schedule may be reduced to 0.125% every other day or 0.06% every day. These dosages can often be gradually lowered as treatment progresses. The 0.03% strength has proven to be effective in some cases. The maximum usually recommended dosage is 0.125% once a day, although more intensive therapy has been used for short periods.

Technic: See Dosage and Administration, Section on Glaucoma.

Duration of Treatment

In diagnosis, only a short period is required and little time will be lost in instituting other procedures if the esotropia proves to be unresponsive. In therapy, there is no definite limit so long as the drug is well tolerated. However, if the eyedrops, with or without eyeglasses, are gradually withdrawn after about a year or two and deviation recurs, surgery should be considered. As with other miotics, tolerance may occasionally develop after prolonged use. In such cases, a rest period will restore the original activity of the drug.

OVERDOSAGE

Antidotes are atropine, 2 mg parenterally; PROTOPAM® CHLORIDE (pralidoxime chloride), 25 mg per kg intravenously; artificial respiration should be given if necessary.

Directions for Preparing Eyedrops

1. Use aseptic technic.
2. Tear off aluminum seals, and remove and discard rubber plugs from both drug and diluent containers.
3. Pour diluent into drug container.
4. Remove dropper assembly from its sterile wrapping. Holding dropper assembly by the screw cap and, WITHOUT COMPRESSING RUBBER BULB, insert into drug container and screw down tightly.
5. Shake for several seconds to ensure mixing.
6. Do not cover nor obliterate instructions to patient regarding storage of eyedrops.

Storage and Stability of Eyedrops

Keep eyedrops in refrigerator to obtain maximum useful life of six months. Room temperature is acceptable if drops will be used up within a month.

HOW SUPPLIED

Each package contains PHOSPHOLINE IODIDE (echothiophate iodide), diluent, and dropper for dispensing 5 mL eyedrops of the strength indicated on the label. Four potencies are available:

NDC 0046-1062-05	1.5 mg package for 0.03%
NDC 0046-1064-05	3.0 mg package for 0.06%
NDC 0046-1065-05	6.25 mg package for 0.125%
NDC 0046-1066-05	12.5 mg package for 0.25%

PLEGINE® Tablets Ⓒ℞

[plĕj-ĕn′]

Brand of phendimetrazine tartrate

Anorexiant

CAUTION: Federal law prohibits dispensing without prescription.

DESCRIPTION

Chemical name: (+)-3,4-Dimethyl-2-phenylmorpholine Tartrate

Structural formula:

C_6H_5–CH, CH_2, CH_3–CH, CH_2, N, CH_3, O, $\cdot C_4O_6H_6$

PLEGINE is the dextro isomer of phendimetrazine tartrate. Phendimetrazine tartrate is a white, odorless powder with a bitter taste. It is soluble in water, methanol, and ethanol. PLEGINE contains these inactive ingredients: D&C Yellow #10, FD&C Yellow #6, Lactose, NF, Magnesium Stearate, NF, Polyethylene Glycol 8000, NF.

ACTIONS

PLEGINE is a phenylalkylamine sympathomimetic with pharmacologic activity similar to the prototype drugs of this class used in obesity, the amphetamines. Actions include central nervous system stimulation and elevation of blood pressure. Tachyphylaxis and tolerance have been demonstrated with all drugs of this class in which these phenomena have been looked for.

Drugs of this class used in obesity are commonly known as "anorectics" or "anorexigenics." It has not been established, however, that the action of such drugs in treating obesity is primarily one of appetite suppression. Other central nervous system actions, or metabolic effects, may be involved, for example.

Adult obese subjects instructed in dietary management and treated with "anorectic" drugs, lose more weight on the average than those treated with placebo and diet, as determined in relatively short-term clinical trials.

The magnitude of increased weight loss of drug-treated patients over placebo-treated patients is only a fraction of a pound a week. The rate of weight loss is greatest in the first weeks of therapy for both drug and placebo subjects and tends to decrease in succeeding weeks. The possible origins of the increased weight loss due to the various drug effects are not established. The amount of weight loss associated with the use of an "anorectic" drug varies from trial to trial, and the increased weight loss appears to be related in part to variables other than the drug prescribed, such as the physician-investigator, the population treated, and the diet prescribed. Studies do not permit conclusions as to the relative importance of the drug and non-drug factors on weight loss. The natural history of obesity is measured in years, whereas the studies cited are restricted to a few weeks' duration; thus, the total impact of drug-induced weight loss over that of diet alone must be considered clinically limited.

INDICATIONS

PLEGINE (phendimetrazine tartrate) is indicated in the management of exogenous obesity as a short-term adjunct (a few weeks) in a regimen of weight reduction based on caloric restriction. The limited usefulness of agents of this class should be measured against possible risk factors inherent in their use (see ACTIONS).

CONTRAINDICATIONS

Known hypersensitivity or idiosyncratic reactions to sympathomimetics.

Advanced arteriosclerosis, symptomatic cardiovascular disease, moderate and severe hypertension, hyperthyroidism

Highly nervous or agitated patients

Patients with a history of drug abuse

Patients taking other CNS stimulants, including monamine oxidase inhibitors

WARNINGS

DRUG DEPENDENCE: PLEGINE is related chemically and pharmacologically to the amphetamines. Amphetamines and related stimulant drugs have been extensively abused, and the possibility of abuse of PLEGINE should be kept in mind when evaluating the desirability of including a drug as part of a weight reduction program. Abuse of amphetamines and related drugs may be associated with intense psychological dependence and severe social dysfunction. There are reports of patients who have increased the dosage to many times that recommended. Abrupt cessation following prolonged high dosage administration results in extreme fatigue and mental depression; changes are also noted on the sleep EEG. Manifestations of chronic intoxication with anorectic drugs include severe dermatoses, marked insomnia, irritability, hyperactivity, and personality changes. The most severe manifestation of chronic intoxications is psychosis, often clinically indistinguishable from schizophrenia.

Tolerance to the anorectic effect of PLEGINE (phendimetrazine tartrate) develops within a few weeks. When this occurs, its use should be discontinued; the maximum recommended dose should not be exceeded.

Use of PLEGINE (phendimetrazine tartrate) within 14 days following the administration of monamine oxidase inhibitors may result in a hypertensive crisis.

Abrupt cessation of administration following prolonged high dosage results in extreme fatigue and depression. Because of the effect on the central nervous system, PLEGINE may impair the ability of the patient to engage in potentially hazardous activities such as operating machinery or driving a motor vehicle; the patient should therefore be cautioned accordingly.

Usage in Pregnancy: Safe use in pregnancy has not been established. Until more information is available, phendimetrazine tartrate should not be taken by women who are or may become pregnant unless, in the opinion of the physician, the potential benefits outweigh the possible hazards.

Usage in Children: PLEGINE is not recommended for use in children under 12 years of age.

PRECAUTIONS

Caution is to be exercised in prescribing PLEGINE for patients with even mild hypertension.

Insulin requirements in diabetes mellitus may be altered in association with the use of PLEGINE and the concomitant dietary regimen.

PLEGINE may decrease the hypotensive effect of guanethidine.

The least amount feasible should be prescribed or dispensed at one time in order to minimize the possibility of overdosage.

ADVERSE REACTIONS

Central Nervous System: Overstimulation, restlessness, insomnia, agitation, flushing, tremor, sweating, dizziness, headache, psychotic states, blurring of vision

Cardiovascular: Palpitation, tachycardia, elevated blood pressure

Gastrointestinal: Mouth dryness, nausea, diarrhea, constipation, stomach pain

Genitourinary: Urinary frequency, dysuria, changes in libido

DOSAGE AND ADMINISTRATION

Usual adult dosage: 1 tablet (35 mg) bid or tid, one hour before meals.

Dosage should be individualized to obtain an adequate response with the lowest effective dosage. In some cases, ½ tablet per dose may be adequate; dosage should not exceed 2 tablets tid.

Overdosage: Acute overdosage of phendimetrazine tartrate may manifest itself by the following signs and symptoms: unusual restlessness, confusion, belligerence, hallucinations, and panic states. Fatigue and depression usually follow the central stimulation. Cardiovascular effects include arrhythmias, hypertension, or hypotension and circulatory collapse. Gastrointestinal symptoms include nausea, vomiting, diarrhea, and abdominal cramps. Poisoning may result in convulsions, coma, and death.

The management of overdosage is largely symptomatic. It includes sedation with a barbiturate. If hypertension is marked, the use of a nitrate or rapid-acting alpha receptor-blocking agent should be considered. Experience with hemodialysis or peritoneal dialysis is inadequate to permit recommendations for its use.

HOW SUPPLIED

PLEGINE—Each scored tablet contains 35 mg phendimetrazine tartrate, in bottles of 100 (NDC 0046-0755-81) and 1,000 (NDC 0046-0755-91).

Shown in Product Identification Section, page 404

PMB® 200 ℞

Each tablet contains:

Premarin® (conjugated estrogens, USP) .... 0.45 mg

Meprobamate .... 200.0 mg

PMB® 400

Each tablet contains:

Premarin® (conjugated estrogens, USP) .... 0.45 mg

Meprobamate .... 400.0 mg

CAUTION: Federal law prohibits dispensing without prescription.

1. ESTROGENS HAVE BEEN REPORTED TO INCREASE THE RISK OF ENDOMETRIAL CARCINOMA.

Three independent case control studies have reported an increased risk of endometrial cancer in postmenopausal women exposed to exogenous estrogens for more than one year.[1–3] This risk was independent of the other known risk factors for endometrial cancer. These studies are further supported by the finding that incidence rates of endometrial cancer have increased sharply since 1969 in eight different areas of the United States with population-based cancer reporting systems, an increase which may be related to the rapidly expanding use of estrogens during the last decade.[4]

The three case control studies reported that the risk of endometrial cancer in estrogen users was about 4.5 to 13.9 times greater than in nonusers. The risk appears to depend on both duration of treatment[1] and on estrogen dose.[3] In view of these findings, when estrogens are used for the treatment of menopausal symptoms, the lowest dose that will control symptoms should be utilized and medication should be discontinued as soon as possible. When prolonged treatment is medically indicated, the patient should be reassessed on at least a semiannual basis to determine the need for continued therapy. Although the evidence must be considered preliminary,

Continued on next page

Ayerst—Cont.

one study suggests that cyclic administration of low doses of estrogen may carry less risk than continuous administration;[3] it therefore appears prudent to utilize such a regimen.

Close clinical surveillance of all women taking estrogens is important. In all cases of undiagnosed persistent or recurring abnormal vaginal bleeding, adequate diagnostic measures should be undertaken to rule out malignancy.

There is no evidence at present that "natural" estrogens are more or less hazardous than "synthetic" estrogens at equiestrogenic doses.

2. ESTROGENS SHOULD NOT BE USED DURING PREGNANCY.

The use of female sex hormones, both estrogens and progestogens, during early pregnancy may seriously damage the offspring. It has been shown that females exposed in utero to diethylstilbestrol, a non-steroidal estrogen, have an increased risk of developing in later life a form of vaginal or cervical cancer that is ordinarily extremely rare.[5,6] This risk has been estimated as not greater than 4 per 1,000 exposures.[7] Furthermore, a high percentage of such exposed women (from 30% to 90%) have been found to have vaginal adenosis,[8–12] epithelial changes of the vagina and cervix. Although these changes are histologically benign, it is not known whether they are precursors of malignancy. Although similar data are not available with the use of other estrogens, it cannot be presumed they would not induce similar changes.

Several reports suggest an association between intrauterine exposure to female sex hormones and congenital anomalies, including congenital heart defects and limb reduction defects.[13–16] One case control study[16] estimated a 4.7-fold increased risk of limb reduction defects in infants exposed in utero to sex hormones (oral contraceptives, hormone withdrawal tests for pregnancy, or attempted treatment for threatened abortion). Some of these exposures were very short and involved only a few days of treatment. The data suggest that the risk of limb reduction defects in exposed fetuses is somewhat less than 1 per 1,000.

In the past, female sex hormones have been used during pregnancy in an attempt to treat threatened or habitual abortion. There is considerable evidence that estrogens are ineffective for these indications, and there is no evidence from well-controlled studies that progestogens are effective for these uses.

If PMB is used during pregnancy, or if the patient becomes pregnant while taking this drug, she should be apprised of the potential risks to the fetus, and the advisability of pregnancy continuation.

3. THIS FIXED-COMBINATION DRUG IS NOT INDICATED FOR INITIAL THERAPY.

In cases where estrogen given alone has not alleviated anxiety and tension existing as part of the menopausal symptom complex, therapy may then consist of separate administration of estrogen and meprobamate in order to determine the appropriate dosage of each drug for the patient. If this fixed combination represents the dosage so determined, its use may be more convenient in patient management. The treatment of such patients is not static, but must be reevaluated as conditions in each patient warrant.

DESCRIPTION

PMB is a combination of PREMARIN® (conjugated estrogens, USP) and meprobamate, a tranquilizing agent, in tablet form for oral administration.

PREMARIN (conjugated estrogens, USP) is a mixture of estrogens, obtained exclusively from natural sources, occurring as the sodium salts of water-soluble estrogen sulfates blended to represent the average composition of material derived from pregnant mares' urine. It contains estrone, equilin, and 17α-dihydroequilin, together with smaller amounts of 17α-estradiol, equilenin, and 17 α-dihydroequilenin as salts of their sulfate esters.

Meprobamate is the dicarbamic acid ester of 2-methyl-2-*n*-propyl-1,3-propanediol.

PMB Tablets contain the following inactive ingredients: calcium phosphate tribasic, calcium sulfate anhydrous, carnauba wax, lactose, magnesium stearate, methylcellulose, microcrystalline cellulose, pharmaceutical glaze, sucrose, talc, titanium dioxide.

—PMB 200 Tablets also contain: D&C Yellow No. 10, FD&C Blue No. 1, FD&C Yellow No. 6.

—PMB 400 Tablets also contain: FD&C Blue No. 2, FD&C Red No. 3.

CLINICAL PHARMACOLOGY

Estrogens are important in the development and maintenance of the female reproductive system and secondary sex characteristics. They promote growth and development of the vagina, uterus, and fallopian tubes, and enlargement of the breasts. Indirectly, they contribute to the shaping of the skeleton, maintenance of tone and elasticity of urogenital structures, changes in the epiphyses of the long bones that allow for the pubertal growth spurt and its termination, growth of axillary and pubic hair, and pigmentation of the nipples and genitals. Decline of estrogenic activity at the end of the menstrual cycle can bring on menstruation, although the cessation of progesterone secretion is the most important factor in the mature ovulatory cycle. However, in the preovulatory or nonovulatory cycle, estrogen is the primary determinant in the onset of menstruation. Estrogens also affect the release of pituitary gonadotropins.

The pharmacologic effects of conjugated estrogens are similar to those of endogenous estrogens. They are soluble in water and are well absorbed from the gastrointestinal tract.

In responsive tissues (female genital organs, breasts, hypothalamus, pituitary) estrogens enter the cell and are transported into the nucleus. As a result of estrogen action, specific RNA and protein synthesis occurs.

Metabolism and inactivation occur primarily in the liver. Some estrogens are excreted into the bile; however, they are reabsorbed from the intestine and returned to the liver through the portal venous system. Water-soluble estrogen conjugates are strongly acidic and are ionized in body fluids, which favor excretion through the kidneys since tubular reabsorption is minimal.

Meprobamate is used clinically for the reduction of anxiety and tension. The precise mechanism(s) of its action is not known. It is well absorbed from the gastrointestinal tract and has a physiological half-life of about 10 hours. It is excreted in the urine primarily as hydroxymeprobamate and as a glucuronide.

The combination of PREMARIN with meprobamate as provided in PMB relieves the underlying estrogen deficiency and affords tranquilizing activity to ameliorate the anxiety and tension not due to estrogen deficiency.

INDICATION

For the treatment of moderate-to-severe vasomotor symptoms of the menopause when anxiety and tension are part of the symptom complex and only in those cases in which the use of estrogens alone has not resulted in alleviation of such symptoms.

PMB HAS NOT BEEN SHOWN TO BE EFFECTIVE FOR ANY PURPOSE DURING PREGNANCY AND ITS USE MAY CAUSE SEVERE HARM TO THE FETUS (SEE BOXED WARNING).

Concomitant Propestin Use: The lowest effective dose appropriate for the specific indication should be utilized. Studies of the addition of a progestin for 7 or more days of a cycle of estrogen administration have reported a lowered incidence of endometrial hyperplasia. Morphological and biochemical studies of the endometrium suggest that 10 to 13 days of progestin are needed to provide maximal maturation of the endometrium and to eliminate any hyperplastic changes. Whether this will provide protection from endometrial carcinoma has not been clearly established. There are possible additional risks which may be associated with the inclusion of progestin in estrogen replacement regimens. (See PRECAUTIONS.) The choice of progestin and dosage may be important; produce labeling should be reviewed to minimize possible adverse effects.

CONTRAINDICATIONS

Estrogens should not be used in women with any of the following conditions:

1. Known or suspected cancer of the breast.
2. Known or suspected estrogen-dependent neoplasia.
3. Known or suspected pregnancy (see Boxed Warning).
4. Undiagnosed abnormal genital bleeding.
5. Active thrombophlebitis or thromboembolic disorders.
6. A past history of thrombophlebitis, thrombosis, or thromboembolic disorders associated with previous estrogen use.

Meprobamate should not be used in patients with the following conditions:

1. A history of allergic or idiosyncratic reactions to meprobamate or related compounds such as carisoprodol, mebutamate, tybamate, or carbromal.
2. Acute intermittent porphyria.

WARNINGS

USAGE IN PREGNANCY AND LACTATION.

An increased risk of congenital malformations associated with the use of minor tranquilizers (meprobamate, chlordiazepoxide, and diazepam) during the first trimester of pregnancy has been suggested in several studies. Because use of these drugs is rarely a matter of urgency, their use during this period should almost always be avoided. The possibility that a woman of childbearing potential may be pregnant at the time of institution of therapy should be considered. Patients should be advised that if they become pregnant during therapy or intend to become pregnant they should communicate with their physicians about the desirability of discontinuing the drug.

Meprobamate passes the placental barrier. It is present both in umbilical cord blood at or near maternal plasma levels and in breast milk of lactating mothers at concentrations two to four times that of maternal plasma. When use of meprobamate is contemplated in breast-feeding patients, the drug's higher concentrations in breast milk as compared to maternal plasma levels should be considered.

Usage in Children—PMB is not intended for use in children.

Associated with Estrogen Administration:

1. *Induction of malignant neoplasms.* Long-term continuous administration of natural and synthetic estrogens in certain animal species increases the frequency of carcinomas of the breast, cervix, vagina, and liver. There are now reports that estrogens increase the risk of carcinoma of the endometrium in humans. (see Boxed Warning.)

At the present time there is no satisfactory evidence that estrogens given to postmenopausal women increase the risk of cancer of the breast,[17] although a recent long-term follow-up of a single physician's practice has raised this possibility.[18] Because of the animal data, there is a need for caution in prescribing estrogens for women with a strong family history of breast cancer or who have breast nodules, fibrocystic disease, or abnormal mammograms.

2. *Gallbladder disease.* A recent study has reported a 2- to 3-fold increase in the risk of surgically confirmed gallbladder disease in women receiving postmenopausal estrogens,[17] similar to the 2-fold increase previously noted in users of oral contraceptives.[19,24a]

3. *Effects similar to those caused by estrogen-progestogen oral contraceptives.* There are several serious adverse effects of oral contraceptives, most of which have not, up to now, been documented as consequences of postmenopausal estrogen therapy. This may reflect the comparatively low doses of estrogen used in postmenopausal women. It would be expected that the larger doses of estrogen used to treat prostatic or breast cancer or postpartum breast engorgement are more likely to result in these adverse effects, and, in fact, it has been shown that there is an increased risk of thrombosis in men receiving estrogens for prostatic cancer and women for postpartum breast engorgement.[20–23]

a. *Thromboembolic disease.* It is now well established that users of oral contraceptives have an increased risk of various thromboembolic and thrombotic vascular diseases, such as thrombophlebitis, pulmonary embolism, stroke, and myocardial infarction.[24–31] Cases of retinal thrombosis, mesenteric thrombosis, and optic neuritis have been reported in oral contraceptive users. There is evidence that the risk of several of these adverse reactions is related to the dose of the drug.[32,33] An increased risk of postsurgery thromboembolic complications has also been reported in users of oral contraceptives.[34,35] If feasible, estrogen should be discontinued at least 4 weeks before surgery of the type associated with an increased risk of thromboembolism, or during periods of prolonged immobilization.

While an increased rate of thromboembolic and thrombotic disease in postmenopausal users of estrogens has not been found,[17–24,25–36] this does not rule out the possibility that such an increase may be present or that subgroups of women who have underlying risk factors or who are receiving relatively large doses of estrogens may have increased risk. Therefore estrogens should not be used in persons with active thrombophlebitis or thromboembolic disorders, and they should not be used (except in treatment of malignancy) in persons with a history of such disorders in association with estrogen use. They should be used with caution in patients with cerebral vascular or coronary artery disease and only for those in whom estrogens are clearly needed.

Large doses of estrogen (5 mg conjugated estrogens per day), comparable to those used to treat cancer of the prostate and breast, have been shown in a large prospective clinical trial in men[37] to increase the risk of nonfatal myocardial infarction, pulmonary embolism and thrombophlebitis. When estrogen doses of this size are used, any of the thromboembolic and thrombotic adverse effects associated with oral contraceptive use should be considered a clear risk.

b. *Hepatic adenoma.* Benign hepatic adenomas appear to be associated with the use of oral contraceptives.[38–40] Although benign, and rare, these may rupture and may cause death through intra-abdominal hemorrhage. Such lesions have not yet been reported in association with other estrogen or progestogen preparations but should be considered in estrogen users having abdominal pain and tenderness, abdominal mass, or hypovolemic shock. Hepatocellular carcinoma has also been reported in women taking estrogen-containing oral contraceptives.[39] The relationship of this malignancy to these drugs is not known at this time.

c. *Elevated blood pressure.* Women using oral contraceptives sometimes experience increased blood pressure which, in most cases, returns to normal on discontinuing the drug. There is now a report that this may occur with use of estrogens in the menopause[41] and blood pressure should be monitored with estrogen use, especially if high doses are used.

d. *Glucose tolerance.* A worsening of glucose tolerance has been observed in a significant percentage of patients on estrogen-containing oral contraceptives. For this reason, diabetic patients should be carefully observed while receiving estrogen.

4. *Hypercalcemia.* Administration of estrogens may lead to severe hypercalcemia in patients with breast cancer and bone metastases. If this occurs, the drug should be stopped and appropriate measures taken to reduce the serum calcium level.

Associated with Meprobamate Administration:

1. *Drug Dependence*—Physical dependence, psychological dependence, and abuse have occurred. When chronic intoxication from prolonged use occurs, it usually involves ingestion of greater than recommended doses and is manifested by ataxia, slurred speech, and vertigo. Therefore, careful supervision of dose and amounts prescribed is advised, as well as avoidance of prolonged administration, especially for alcoholics and other patients with a known propensity for taking excessive quantities of drugs.

Sudden withdrawal of the drug after prolonged and excessive use may precipitate recurrence of preexisting symptoms, such as anxiety, anorexia, or insomnia, or withdrawal reactions, such as vomiting, ataxia, tremors, muscle twitching, confusional states, hallucinosis, and, rarely, convulsive seizures. Such seizures are more likely to occur in persons with central nervous system damage or preexistent or latent convulsive disorders. Onset of withdrawal symptoms occurs usually within 12 to 48 hours after discontinuation of meprobamate; symptoms usually cease within the next 12 to 48 hours.

When excessive dosage has continued for weeks or months, dosage should be reduced gradually over a period of one or two weeks rather than abruptly stopped. Alternatively, a short-acting barbiturate may be substituted, then gradually withdrawn.

2. *Potentially Hazardous Tasks*—Patients should be warned that this drug may impair the mental and/or physical abilities required for the performance of potentially hazardous tasks such as driving a motor vehicle or operating machinery.

3. *Additive Effects*—Since the effects of meprobamate and alcohol or meprobamate and other CNS depressants or psychotropic drugs may be additive, appropriate caution should be exercised with patients who take more than one of these agents simultaneously.

PRECAUTIONS

Associated with Estrogen:

A. General Precautions.

1. A complete medical and family history should be taken prior to the initiation of any estrogen therapy. The pretreatment and periodic physical examinations should include special reference to blood pressure, breasts, abdomen, and pelvic organs, and should include a Papanicolaou smear. As a general rule, estrogen should not be prescribed for longer than one year without another physical examination being performed.

2. Fluid retention—Because estrogens may cause some degree of fluid retention, conditions which might be influenced by this factor such as asthma, epilepsy, migraine, and cardiac or renal dysfunction, require careful observation.

3. Certain patients may develop undesirable manifestations of excessive estrogenic stimulation, such as abnormal or excessive uterine bleeding, mastodynia, etc.

4. Oral contraceptives appear to be associated with an increased incidence of mental depression.[24a] Although it is not clear whether this is due to the estrogenic or progestogenic component of the contraceptive, patients with a history of depression should be carefully observed.

5. Preexisting uterine leiomyomata may increase in size during estrogen use.

6. The pathologist should be advised of estrogen therapy when relevant specimens are submitted.

7. Patients with a past history of jaundice during pregnancy have an increased risk of recurrence of jaundice while receiving estrogen-containing oral contraceptive therapy. If jaundice develops in any patient receiving estrogen, the medication should be discontinued while the cause is investigated.

8. Estrogens may be poorly metabolized in patients with impaired liver function and they should be administered with caution in such patients.

9. Because estrogens influence the metabolism of calcium and phosphorus, they should be used with caution in patients with metabolic bone diseases that are associated with hypercalcemia or in patients with renal insufficiency.

10. Because of the effects of estrogens on epiphyseal closure, they should be used judiciously in young patients in whom bone growth is not complete.

11. Certain endocrine and liver function tests may be affected by estrogen-containing oral contraceptives. The following similar changes may be expected with larger doses of estrogen:

a. Increased sulfobromophthalein retention.

b. Increased prothrombin and factors VII, VIII, IX, and X; decreased antithrombin 3; increased norepinephrine-induced platelet aggregability.

c. Increased thyroid binding globulin (TBG) leading to increased circulating total thyroid hormone, as measured by PBI, T4 by column, or T4 by radioimmunoassay. Free T3 resin uptake is decreased, reflecting the elevated TBG; free T4 concentration is unaltered.

d. Impaired glucose tolerance.

e. Decreased pregnanediol excretion.

f. Reduced response to metyrapone test.

g. Reduced serum folate concentration.

h. Increased serum triglyceride and phospholipid concentration.

12. If concomitant progestin therapy is used, potential risks may include adverse effects on carbohydrate and lipid metabolism.

B. Information for the Patient. (See text which appears after the PHYSICIAN REFERENCES.)

C. Pregnancy Category X. (See CONTRAINDICATIONS and Boxed Warning.)

D. Nursing Mothers. As a general principle, the administration of any drug to nursing mothers should be done only when clearly necessary since many drugs are excreted in human milk.

Associated with Meprobamate:

A. The lowest effective dose should be administered, particularly to debilitated patients, in order to preclude oversedation.

B. The possibility of suicide attempts should be considered and the least amount of drug feasible should be dispensed at any one time.

C. Meprobamate is metabolized in the liver and excreted by the kidney; to avoid its excess accumulation, caution should be exercised in administration to patients with compromised liver or kidney function.

D. Meprobamate occasionally may precipitate seizures in epileptic patients.

ADVERSE REACTIONS

Associated with Estrogen Administration:

(See WARNINGS regarding induction of neoplasia, adverse effects on the fetus, increased incidence of gallbladder disease, and adverse effects similar to those of oral contraceptives, including thromboembolism.) The following additional adverse reactions have been reported with estrogenic therapy, including oral contraceptives:

1. *Genitourinary system:* Breakthrough bleeding, spotting, change in menstrual flow; dysmenorrhea; premenstrual-like syndrome; amenorrhea during and after treatment; increase in size of uterine fibromyomata; vaginal candidiasis; change in cervical erosion and in degree of cervical secretion; cystitis-like syndrome.

2. *Breasts:* Tenderness, enlargement, secretion.

3. *Gastrointestinal:* Nausea, vomiting; abdominal cramps, bloating; cholestatic jaundice.

4. *Skin:* Chloasma or melasma which may persist when drug is discontinued; erythema multiforme; erythema nodosum; hemorrhagic eruption; loss of scalp hair; hirsutism.

5. *Eyes:* Steepening of corneal curvature; intolerance to contact lenses.

6. *CNS:* Headache, migraine, dizziness; mental depression; chorea.

7. *Miscellaneous:* Increase or decrease in weight; reduced carbohydrate tolerance; aggravation of porphyria; edema; changes in libido.

The following have been reported with meprobamate therapy:

1. *Central Nervous System*—Drowsiness, ataxia, dizziness, slurred speech, headache, vertigo, weakness, paresthesias, impairment of visual accommodation, euphoria, overstimulation, paradoxical excitement, fast EEG activity.

2. *Gastrointestinal*—Nausea, vomiting, diarrhea.

3. *Cardiovascular*—Palpitations, tachycardia, various forms of arrhythmia, transient ECG changes, syncope; also, hypotensive crises (including one fatal case).

4. *Allergic or Idiosyncratic*—Allergic or idiosyncratic reactions are usually seen within the period of the first to fourth dose in patients having had no previous contact with the drug. Milder reactions are characterized by an itchy, urticarial, or erythematous maculopapular rash which may be generalized or confined to the groin. Other reactions have included leukopenia, acute nonthrombocytopenic purpura, petechiae, ecchymoses, eosinophilia, peripheral edema, adenopathy, fever, fixed drug eruption with cross reaction to carisoprodol, and cross sensitivity between meprobamate/mebutamate and meprobamate/carbromal.

More severe hypersensitivity reactions, rarely reported, include hyperpyrexia, chills, angioneurotic edema, bronchospasm, oliguria, and anuria. Also, anaphylaxis, erythema multiforme, exfoliative dermatitis, stomatitis, proctitis, Stevens-Johnson syndrome, and bullous dermatitis, including one fatal case of the latter, following administration of meprobamate in combination with prednisolone.

In case of allergic or idiosyncratic reactions to meprobamate, discontinue the drug and initiate appropriate symptomatic therapy, which may include epinephrine, antihistamines, and in severe cases corticosteroids. In evaluating possible allergic reactions, also consider allergy to excipients (information on excipients is available to physicians on request).

5. *Hematologic* (See also *Allergic or Idiosyncratic.*)—Agranulocytosis and aplastic anemia have been reported, although no causal relationship has been established. These cases rarely were fatal. Rare cases of thrombocytopenic purpura have been reported.

6. *Other*—Exacerbation of porphyric symptoms.

OVERDOSAGE

Acute overdosage (estrogen alone):

Numerous reports of ingestion of large doses of estrogen-containing oral contraceptives by young children indicate that acute serious ill effects do not occur. Overdosage of estrogen may cause nausea, and withdrawal bleeding may occur in females.

Acute simple overdosage (meprobamate alone): Death has been reported with ingestion of as little as 12 grams meprobamate and survival with as much as 40 grams.

Blood levels: 0.5—2.0 mg% represents the usual blood level range of meprobamate after therapeutic doses. The level may occasionally be as high as 3.0 mg%.

3—10 mg% usually corresponds to findings of mild-to-moderate symptoms of overdosage, such as stupor or light coma.

10—20 mg% usually corresponds to deeper coma, requiring more intensive treatment. Some fatalities occur.

At levels greater than 20 mg%, more fatalities than survivals can be expected.

Acute combined (alcohol or other CNS depressants or psychotropic drugs) **overdosage:** Since effects can be additive, a history of ingestion of a low dose of meprobamate plus any of these compounds (or of a relatively low blood or tissue level) cannot be used as a prognostic indicator.

In cases where excessive doses have been taken, sleep ensues rapidly and blood pressure, pulse, and respiratory rates are reduced to basal levels. Any drug remaining in the stomach should be removed and symptomatic therapy given. Should respiration or blood pressure become compromised, respiratory assistance, central nervous system stimulants, and pressor agents should be administered cautiously as indicated. Meprobamate is metabolized in the liver and excreted by the kidney. Diuresis, osmotic (mannitol) diuresis, peritoneal dialysis, and hemodialysis have been used successfully. Careful monitoring of urinary output is necessary and caution should be taken to avoid overhydration. Relapse and death, after initial recovery, have been attributed to incomplete gastric emptying and delayed absorption. Meprobamate can be measured in biological fluids by two methods: colorimetric[42] and gas chromatographic.[43]

DOSAGE AND ADMINISTRATION

Given cyclically for short-term use only:

For the treatment of moderate-to-severe vasomotor symptoms of the menopause when anxiety and tension are part of the symptom complex and only in those cases in which the use of estrogens alone has not resulted in alleviation of such symptoms.

The lowest dose that will control symptoms should be chosen and medication should be discontinued as promptly as possible. The usual dosage of conjugated estrogen is 1.25 milligrams daily. The usual dosage of meprobamate is 1,200 to 1,600 milligrams daily.

Administration should be cyclic (eg, three weeks on and one week off).

Attempts to discontinue or taper medication should be made at three- to six-month intervals.

PMB® 200 & PMB® 400: The usual dosage is one tablet of either strength three times daily administered cyclically. Use of meprobamate during the rest period should be considered for those patients who may require continuing medication with tranquilizer. After the first few cycles of therapy, the patient's need for continuing the use of the meprobamate component should be reevaluated.

Daily dosage should be adjusted to individual requirements. The daily dosage should not exceed 6 tablets of PMB 200 per day or 4 tablets of PMB 400 per day.

Treated patients with an intact uterus should be monitored closely for signs of endometrial cancer and appropriate diagnostic measures should be taken to rule out malignancy in the event of persistent or recurring abnormal vaginal bleeding.

HOW SUPPLIED

PMB® 200, in bottles of 60 (NDC 0046-0880-60).

PMB® 400, in bottles of 60 (NDC 0046-0881-60).

PHYSICIAN REFERENCES

1. Ziel, H. K., *et al.*: N. Engl. J. Med. *293*:1167–1170, 1975.
2. Smith, D. C., *et al.*: N. Engl. J. Med. *293*:1164–1167, 1975.
3. Mack, T. M., *et al.*: N. Engl. J. Med. *294*:1262–1267, 1976.
4. Weiss, N. S., *et al.*: N. Engl. J. Med. *294*:1259–1262, 1976.

Continued on next page

Ayerst—Cont.

5. Herbst, A. L., *et al.*: N. Engl. J. Med. *284*:878–881, 1971.
6. Greenwald, P., *et al.*: N. Engl. J. Med. *285*:390–392, 1971.
7. Lanier, A., *et al.*: Mayo Clin. Proc. *48*:793–799, 1973.
8. Herbst, A., *et al.*: Obstet. Gynecol. *40*:287–298, 1972.
9. Herbst, A., *et al.*: Am. J. Obstet. Gynecol. *118*:607–615, 1974.
10. Herbst, A., *et al.*: N. Engl. J. Med. *292*:334–339, 1975.
11. Stafl, A., *et al.*: Obstet. Gynecol. *43*:118–128, 1974.
12. Sherman, A. I., *et al.*: Obstet. Gynecol. *44*:531–545, 1974.
13. Gal, I., *et al.*: Nature *216*:83, 1967.
14. Levy, E. P., *et al.*: Lancet *1*:611, 1973.
15. Nora, J., *et al.*: Lancet *1*:941–942, 1973.
16. Janerich, D. T., *et al.*: N. Engl. J. Med. *291*:697–700, 1974.
17. Boston Collaborative Drug Surveillance Program: N. Engl. J. Med. *290*:15–19, 1974.
18. Hoover, R., *et al.*: N. Engl. J. Med. *295*:401–405, 1976.
19. Boston Collaborative Drug Surveillance Program: Lancet *1*:1399–1404, 1973.
20. Daniel, D. G., *et al.*: Lancet *2*:287–289, 1967.
21. The Veterans Administration Cooperative Urological Research Group: J. Urol. *98*:516–522, 1967.
22. Bailar, J. C.: Lancet *2*:560, 1967.
23. Blackard, C., *et al.*: Cancer *26*:249–256, 1970.
24. Royal College of General Practitioners: J. R. Coll. Gen. Pract. *13*:267–279, 1967.

24a. Royal College of General Practitioners: Oral Contraceptives and Health, New York, Pitman Corp., 1974.

25. Inman, W. H. W., *et al.*: Br. Med. J. *2*:193–199, 1968.
26. Vessey, M. P., *et al.*: Br. Med. J. *2*:651–657, 1969.
27. Sartwell, P. E., *et al.*: Am. J. Epidemiol. *90*:365–380, 1969.
28. Collaborative Group for the Study of Stroke in Young Women: N. Engl. J. Med. *288*:871–878, 1973.
29. Collaborative Group for the Study of Stroke in Young Women: J.A.M.A. *231*:718–722, 1975.
30. Mann, J. I., *et al.*: Br. Med. J. *2*:245–248, 1975.
31. Mann, J. I., *et al.*: Br. Med. J. *2*:241–245, 1975.
32. Inman, W. H. W., *et al.*: Br. Med. J. *2*:203–209, 1970.
33. Stolley, P. D., *et al.*: Am. J. Epidemiol. *102*:197–208, 1975.
34. Vessey, M. P., *et al.*: Br. Med. J. *3*:123–126, 1970.
35. Greene, G. R., *et al.*: Am. J. Public Health *62*:680–685, 1972.
36. Rosenberg, L., *et al.*: N. Engl. J. Med. *294*:1256–1259, 1976.
37. Coronary Drug Project Research Group: J.A.M.A. *214*:1303–1313, 1970.
38. Baum, J., *et al.*: Lancet *2*:926–928, 1973.
39. Mays, E. T., *et al.*: J.A.M.A. *235*:730–732, 1976.
40. Edmondson, H. A., *et al.*: N. Engl. J. Med. *294*:470–472, 1976.
41. Pfeffer, R. I., *et al.*: Am. J. Epidemiol. *103*:445–456, 1976.
42. Hoffman, A. J., *et al.*: J. Am. Pharm. Assoc. *48*:740, 1959.
43. Douglas, J. F., *et al.*: Anal. Chem. *39*:956, 1967.

INFORMATION FOR THE PATIENT

WHAT YOU SHOULD KNOW ABOUT ESTROGENS

Estrogens are female hormones produced by the ovaries. The ovaries make several different kinds of estrogens. In addition, scientists have been able to make a variety of synthetic estrogens. As far as we know, all these estrogens have similar properties and therefore much the same usefulness, side effects, and risks. This leaflet is intended to help you understand what estrogens are used for, the risks involved in their use, and how to use them as safely as possible.

This leaflet includes the most important information about estrogens, but not all the information. If you want to know more, you should ask your doctor for more information or you can ask your doctor or pharmacist to let you read the package insert prepared for the doctor.

USES OF ESTROGEN

THERE IS NO PROPER USE OF ESTROGENS IN A PREGNANT WOMAN

Estrogens are prescribed by doctors for a number of purposes, including:

1. To provide estrogen during a period of adjustment when a woman's ovaries stop producing a majority of her estrogens, in order to prevent certain uncomfortable symptoms of estrogen deficiency. (With the menopause, which generally occurs between the ages of 45 and 55, women produce a much smaller amount of estrogens.)
2. To prevent symptoms of estrogen deficiency when a woman's ovaries have been removed surgically before the natural menopause.
3. To prevent pregnancy. (Estrogens are given along with a progestogen, another female hormone; these combinations are called oral contraceptives or birth control pills. Patient labeling is available to women taking oral contraceptives and they will not be discussed in this leaflet.)
4. To treat certain cancers in women and men.
5. To prevent painful swelling of the breasts after pregnancy in women who choose not to nurse their babies.

ESTROGENS IN THE MENOPAUSE

In the natural course of their lives, all women eventually experience a decrease in estrogen production. This usually occurs between ages 45 and 55 but may occur earlier or later. Sometimes the ovaries may need to be removed before natural menopause by an operation, producing a "surgical menopause."

When the amount of estrogen in the blood begins to decrease, many women may develop typical symptoms: feelings of warmth in the face, neck, and chest or sudden intense episodes of heat and sweating throughout the body (called "hot flashes" or "hot flushes"). These symptoms are sometimes very uncomfortable. Some women may also develop changes in the vagina (called "atrophic vaginitis") which cause discomfort, especially during and after intercourse.

Estrogens can be prescribed to treat these symptoms of the menopause. It is estimated that considerably more than half of all women undergoing the menopause have only mild symptoms or no symptoms at all and therefore do not need estrogens. Other women may need estrogens for a few months, while their bodies adjust to lower estrogen levels. Sometimes the need will be for periods longer than six months. In an attempt to avoid overstimulation of the uterus (womb), estrogens are usually given cyclically during each month of use, such as three weeks of pills followed by one week without pills.

Sometimes women experience nervous symptoms or depression during menopause. There is no evidence that estrogens are effective for such symptoms without associated vasomotor symptoms. In the absence of vasomotor symptoms, estrogens should not be used to treat nervous symptoms, although other treatment may be needed.

You may have heard that taking estrogens for long periods (years) after the menopause will keep your skin soft and supple and keep you feeling young. There is no evidence that this is so, however, and such long-term treatment carries important risks.

ESTROGENS TO PREVENT SWELLING OF THE BREASTS AFTER PREGNANCY

If you do not breast-feed your baby after delivery, your breasts may fill up with milk and become painful and engorged. This usually begins about 3 to 4 days after delivery and may last for a few days to up to a week or more. Sometimes the discomfort is severe, but usually it is not and can be controlled by pain-relieving drugs such as aspirin and by binding the breasts up tightly. Estrogens can be used to try to prevent the breasts from filling up. While this treatment is sometimes successful, in many cases the breasts fill up to some degree in spite of treatment. The dose of estrogens needed to prevent pain and swelling of the breasts is much larger than the dose needed to treat symptoms of the menopause and this may increase your chances of developing blood clots in the legs or lungs (see below). Therefore, it is important that you discuss the benefits and the risks of estrogen use with your doctor if you have decided not to breast-feed your baby.

THE DANGERS OF ESTROGENS

1. *Endometrial cancer.* There are reports that if estrogens are used in the postmenopausal period for more than a year there is an increased risk of *endometrial cancer* (cancer of the lining of the uterus). Women taking estrogens have roughly 5 to 10 times as great a chance of getting this cancer as women who take no estrogens. To put this another way, while a postmenopausal woman not taking estrogens has 1 chance in 1,000 each year of getting endometrial cancer, a woman taking estrogens has 5 to 10 chances in 1,000 each year. For this reason *it is important to take estrogens only when they are really needed.*

The risk of this cancer is greater the longer estrogens are used and when larger doses are taken. Therefore you should not take more estrogen than your doctor prescribes. *It is important to take the lowest dose of estrogen that will control symptoms and to take it only as long as it is needed.* If estrogens are needed for longer periods of time, your doctor will want to reevaluate your need for estrogens at least every six months.

Women using estrogens should report any vaginal bleeding to their doctors; such bleeding may be of no importance, but it can be an early warning of endometrial cancer. If you have undiagnosed vaginal bleeding, you should not use estrogens until a diagnosis is made and you are certain there is no endometrial cancer.

NOTE: If you have had your uterus removed (total hysterectomy), there is no danger of developing endometrial cancer.

2. *Other possible cancers.* Estrogens can cause development of other tumors in animals, such as tumors of the breast, cervix, vagina, or liver, when given for a long time. At present there is no good evidence that women using estrogen in the menopause have an increased risk of such tumors, but there is no way yet to be sure they do not; and one study raises the possibility that use of estrogens in the menopause may increase the risk of breast cancer many years later. This is a further reason to use estrogens only when clearly needed. While you are taking estrogens, it is important that you go to your doctor at least once a year for a physical examination. Also, if members of your family have had breast cancer or if you have breast nodules or abnormal mammograms (breast x-rays), your doctor may wish to carry out more frequent examinations of your breasts.

3. *Gallbladder disease.* Women who use estrogens after menopause are more likely to develop gallbladder disease needing surgery then women who do not use estrogens. Birth control pills have a similar effect.

4. *Abnormal blood clotting.* Oral contraceptives increase the risk of blood clotting in various parts of the body. This can result in a stroke (if the clot is in the brain), a heart attack (clot in a blood vessel of the heart), or a pulmonary embolus (a clot which forms in the legs or pelvis, then breaks off and travels to the lungs). Any of these can be fatal.

At this time use of estrogens in the menopause is not known to cause such blood clotting, but this has not been fully studied and there could still prove to be such a risk. It is recommended that if you have had clotting in the legs or lungs or a heart attack or stroke while you were using estrogens or birth control pills, you should not use estrogens (unless they are being used to treat cancer of the breast or prostate). If you have had a stroke or heart attack or if you have angina pectoris, estrogens should be used with great caution and only if clearly needed (for example, if you have severe symptoms of the menopause).

The larger doses of estrogen used to prevent swelling of the breasts after pregnancy have been reported to cause clotting in the legs and lungs.

SPECIAL WARNING ABOUT PREGNANCY

You should not receive estrogen if you are pregnant. If this should occur, there is a greater than usual chance that the developing child will be born with a birth defect, although the possibility remains fairly small. A female child may have an increased risk of developing cancer of the vagina or cervix later in life (in the teens or twenties). Every possible effort should be made to avoid exposure to estrogens during pregnancy. If exposure occurs, see your doctor.

OTHER EFFECTS OF ESTROGENS

In addition to the serious known risks of estrogens described above, estrogens have the following side effects and potential risks:

1. *Nausea and vomiting.* The most common side effect of estrogen therapy is nausea. Vomiting is less common.
2. *Effects on breasts.* Estrogens may cause breast tenderness or enlargement and may cause the breasts to secrete a liquid. These effects are not dangerous.
3. *Effects on the uterus.* Estrogens may cause benign fibroid tumors of the uterus to get larger.
4. *Effects on liver.* Women taking oral contraceptives develop on rare occasions a tumor of the liver which can rupture and bleed into the abdomen and may cause death. So far, these tumors have not been reported in women using estrogens in the menopause, but you should report any swelling or unusual pain or tenderness in the abdomen to your doctor immediately.

Women with a past history of jaundice (yellowing of the skin and white parts of the eyes) may get jaundice again during estrogen use. If this occurs, stop taking estrogens and see your doctor.

5. *Other effects.* Estrogens may cause excess fluids to be retained in the body. This may make some conditions worse, such as asthma, epilepsy, migraine, heart disease, or kidney disease.

SUMMARY

Estrogens have important uses, but they have serious risks as well. You must decide, with your doctor, whether the risks are acceptable to you in view of the benefits of treatment. Except where your doctor has prescribed estrogens for use in special cases of cancer of the breast or prostate, you should not use estrogens if you have cancer of the breast or uterus, are pregnant, have undiagnosed abnormal vaginal bleeding, clotting in the legs or lungs, or have had a stroke, heart attack or angina, or clotting in the legs or lungs in the past while you were taking estrogens.

You can use estrogens as safely as possible by understanding that your doctor will require regular physical examinations while you are taking them and will try to discontinue the drug as soon as possible and use the smallest dose possible. Be alert for signs of trouble including:

1. Abnormal bleeding from the vagina.
2. Pains in the calves or chest or sudden shortness of breath, or coughing blood.
3. Severe headache, dizziness, faintness, or changes in vision.
4. Breast lumps (you should ask your doctor how to examine your own breasts).

5. Jaundice (yellowing of the skin).
6. Mental depression.

Your doctor has prescribed this drug for you and you alone. Do not give the drug to anyone else.

HOW SUPPLIED

PREMARIN® (conjugated estrogens tablets, USP)—tablets for oral administration.

PREMARIN® VAGINAL CREAM—PREMARIN® in a nonliquefying base, designed for vaginal use.

PREMARIN® with METHYLTESTOSTERONE—a combination of PREMARIN and methyltestosterone (an androgen) in tablet form for oral administration.

PMB® 200, 400—a combination of PREMARIN® and meprobamate (a tranquilizing agent) in tablet form for oral administration.

PREMARIN® INTRAVENOUS—PREMARIN® specially prepared for intravenous and intramuscular use.

ESTROGENIC SUBSTANCE (Estrone) in Aqueous Suspension—a sterile aqueous suspension of estrone, a short-acting estrogen, for intramuscular injection only.

Shown in Product Identification Section, page 404

POSTURE® OTC
[*pos 'tūr*]
600 mg
High Potency Calcium Supplement for Healthy Bones
POSTURE® is specially formulated not to produce GAS.

Two tablets contain:		For Adults— % U.S. RDA*
Elemental Calcium (as calcium phosphate)	1200 mg	120%

*Percentage of U.S. Recommended Daily Allowance

INGREDIENTS

Tricalcium phosphate, povidone, microcrystalline cellulose, croscarmellose sodium, talc triturate, sodium lauryl sulfate, magnesium stearate.

RECOMMENDED INTAKE

One or two tablets daily, or as recommended by a physician. Keep Out of Reach of Children.

INDICATION

POSTURE® Tablets provide a daily source of calcium for healthy bones or, when recommended by a physician, to increase dietary intake of calcium.

HOW SUPPLIED

In bottles of 60 tablets (NDC 0046-0275-60).

Shown in Product Identification Section, page 404

POSTURE® OTC
300 mg
Calcium Supplement for Healthy Bones
POSTURE® is specially formulated not to Produce GAS.

Four tablets contain:		For Adults— % U.S. RDA*
Elemental Calcium (as calcium phosphate)	1200 mg	120%

*Percentage of U.S. Recommended Daily Allowance

INGREDIENTS

Tricalcium phosphate, microcrystalline cellulose, croscarmellose sodium, talc triturate, sodium lauryl sulfate, polyethylene glycol 8000, magnesium stearate.

RECOMMENDED INTAKE

2 to 4 tablets daily, or as recommended by a physician. Keep Out of Reach of Children.

HOW SUPPLIED

In bottles of 100 tablets (NDC 0046-0274-81).

Shown in Product Identification Section, page 404

POSTURE®-D OTC
[*pos 'tūr d*]
600 mg
High Potency Calcium Supplement with Vitamin D for Healthy Bones
POSTURE®-D is specially formulated not to produce GAS.

Two tablets contain:		For Adults— % U.S. RDA*
Elemental Calcium (as calcium phosphate)	1200 mg	120%
Vitamin D	250 IU	63%

*Percentage of U.S. Recommended Daily Allowance.

INGREDIENTS

Tricalcium phosphate, vitamin D_3, povidone, microcrystalline cellulose, croscarmellose sodium, talc triturate, sodium lauryl sulfate, magnesium stearate.

RECOMMENDED INTAKE

One or two tablets daily, or as recommended by a physician. Keep Out of Reach of Children.

INDICATION

POSTURE®-D Tablets provide a daily source of calcium for healthy bones or, when recommended by a physician, to increase dietary intake of calcium.

HOW SUPPLIED

In bottles of 60 tablets (NDC 0046-0277-60).

Shown in Product Identification Section, page 404

POSTURE®-D OTC
[*pos 'tūr d*]
300 mg
Calcium Supplement with Vitamin D for Healthy Bones
POSTURE-D is specially formulated not to produce GAS.

Four tablets contain:		For Adults— % U.S. RDA*
Elemental Calcium (as calcium phosphate)	1200 mg	120%
Vitamin D	250 IU	63%

*Percentage of U.S. Recommended Daily Allowance

INGREDIENTS

Tricalcium phosphate, vitamin D_3, microcrystalline cellulose, croscarmellose sodium, talc triturate, sodium lauryl sulfate, polyethylene glycol 8000, magnesium stearate.

RECOMMENDED INTAKE

2 to 4 tablets daily, or as recommended by a physician. Keep Out of Reach of Children.

HOW SUPPLIED

In bottles of 100 tablets (NDC 0046-0276-81).

Shown in Product Identification Section, page 404

PREMARIN® ℞
[*prĕm 'a-rĭn*]
Brand of conjugated estrogens tablets, USP

CAUTION: Federal law prohibits dispensing without prescription.

1. ESTROGENS HAVE BEEN REPORTED TO INCREASE THE RISK OF ENDOMETRIAL CARCINOMA.

Three independent case control studies have reported an increased risk of endometrial cancer in postmenopausal women exposed to exogenous estrogens for more than one year.[1–3] This risk was independent of the other known risk factors for endometrial cancer. These studies are further supported by the finding that incidence rates of endometrial cancer have increased sharply since 1969 in eight different areas of the United States with population-based cancer reporting systems, an increase which may be related to the rapidly expanding use of estrogens during the last decade.[4]

The three case control studies reported that the risk of endometrial cancer in estrogen users was about 4.5 to 13.9 times greater than in nonusers. The risk appears to depend on both duration of treatment[1] and on estrogen dose.[3] In view of these findings, when estrogens are used for the treatment of menopausal symptoms, the lowest dose that will control symptoms should be utilized and medication should be discontinued as soon as possible. When prolonged treatment is medically indicated, the patient should be reassessed on at least a semiannual basis to determine the need for continued therapy. Although the evidence must be considered preliminary, one study suggests that cyclic administration of low doses of estrogen may carry less risk than continuous administration;[3] it therefore appears prudent to utilize such a regimen.

Close clinical surveillance of all women taking estrogens is important. In all cases of undiagnosed persistent or recurring abnormal vaginal bleeding, adequate diagnostic measures should be undertaken to rule out malignancy.

There is no evidence at present that "natural" estrogens are more or less hazardous than "synthetic" estrogens at equiestrogenic doses.

2. ESTROGENS SHOULD NOT BE USED DURING PREGNANCY.

The use of female sex hormones, both estrogens and progestogens, during early pregnancy may seriously damage the offspring. It has been shown that females exposed in utero to diethylstilbestrol, a non-steroidal estrogen, have an increased risk of developing in later life a form of vaginal or cervical cancer that is ordinarily extremely rare.[5,6] This risk has been estimated as not greater than 4 per 1,000 exposures.[7] Furthermore, a high percentage of such exposed women (from 30% to 90%) have been found to have vaginal adenosis,[8–12] epithelial changes of the vagina and cervix. Although these changes are histologically benign, it is not known whether they are precursors of malignancy. Although similar data are not available with the use of other estrogens, it cannot be presumed they would not induce similar changes.

Several reports suggest an association between intrauterine exposure to female sex hormones and congenital anomalies, including congenital heart defects and limb reduction defects.[13–16] One case control study[16] estimated a 4.7-fold increased risk of limb reduction defects in infants exposed in utero to sex hormones (oral contraceptives, hormone withdrawal tests for pregnancy, or attempted treatment for threatened abortion). Some of these exposures were very short and involved only a few days of treatment. The data suggest that the risk of limb reduction defects in exposed fetuses is somewhat less than 1 per 1,000.

In the past, female sex hormones have been used during pregnancy in an attempt to treat threatened or habitual abortion. There is considerable evidence that estrogens are ineffective for these indications, and there is no evidence from well-controlled studies that progestogens are effective for these uses.

If PREMARIN is used during pregnancy, or if the patient becomes pregnant while taking this drug, she should be apprised of the potential risks to the fetus, and the advisability of pregnancy continuation.

DESCRIPTION

PREMARIN (conjugated estrogens tablets, USP) for oral administration contains a mixture of estrogens, obtained exclusively from natural sources, occurring as the sodium salts of water-soluble estrogen sulfates blended to represent the average composition of material derived from pregnant mares' urine. It contains estrone, equilin, and 17 α-dihydroequilin, together with smaller amounts of 17 α-estradiol, equilenin, and 17 α-dihydroequilenin as salts of their sulfate esters. Tablets are available in 0.3 mg, 0.625 mg, 0.9 mg, 1.25 mg, and 2.5 mg strengths of conjugated estrogens.

PREMARIN Tablets contain the following inactive ingredients: calcium phosphate tribasic, calcium sulfate anhydrous, carnauba wax, glyceryl mono-oleate, lactose, magnesium stearate, methylcellulose, microcrystalline cellulose, pharmaceutical glaze, polyethylene glycol, stearic acid, sucrose, talc, titanium dioxide.

—0.3 mg tablets also contain: D&C Yellow No. 10, FD&C Blue No. 1, FD&C Yellow No. 6;

—0.625 mg tablets also contain: FD&C Blue No. 2, FD&C Red No. 3, FD&C Yellow No. 6;

—0.9 mg tablets also contain: D&C Red No. 6, D&C Red No. 7, polysorbate 20;

—1.25 mg tablets also contain: black iron oxide, D&C Yellow No. 10, FD&C Blue No. 1, FD&C Red No. 3, FD&C Yellow No. 6;

—2.5 mg tablets also contain: FD&C Blue No. 2, FD&C Red No. 3.

CLINICAL PHARMACOLOGY

Estrogens are important in the development and maintenance of the female reproductive system and secondary sex characteristics. They promote growth and development of the vagina, uterus, and fallopian tubes, and enlargement of the breasts. Indirectly, they contribute to the shaping of the skeleton, maintenance of tone and elasticity of urogenital structures, changes in the epiphyses of the long bones that allow for the pubertal growth spurt and its termination, growth of axillary and pubic hair, and pigmentation of the nipples and genitals. Decline of estrogenic activity at the end of the menstrual cycle can bring on menstruation, although the cessation of progesterone secretion is the most important factor in the mature ovulatory cycle. However, in the preovulatory or nonovulatory cycle, estrogen is the primary determinant in the onset of menstruation. Estrogens also affect the release of pituitary gonadotropins.

The pharmacologic effects of conjugated estrogens are similar to those of endogenous estrogens. They are soluble in water and are well absorbed from the gastrointestinal tract.

In responsive tissues (female genital organs, breasts, hypothalamus, pituitary) estrogens enter the cell and are transported into the nucleus. As a result of estrogen action, specific RNA and protein synthesis occurs.

Metabolism and inactivation occur primarily in the liver. Some estrogens are excreted into the bile; however, they are reabsorbed from the intestine and returned to the liver

Continued on next page

Ayerst—Cont.

through the portal venous system. Water soluble estrogen conjugates are strongly acidic and are ionized in body fluids, which favor excretion through the kidneys since tubular reabsorption is minimal.

INDICATIONS AND USAGE

1. Moderate-to-severe *vasomotor* symptoms associated with the menopause. (There is no evidence that estrogens are effective for nervous symptoms or depression without associated vasomotor symptoms, and they should not be used to treat such conditions.)
2. **Osteoporosis (Abnormally Low Bone Mass).** PREMARIN (conjugated estrogens tablets, USP) is indicated in postmenopausal women with evidence of loss or deficiency of bone mass, to retard further bone loss and estrogen-deficiency-induced osteoporosis. This product should be used with other important measures such as diet, calcium, and physiotherapy. A more favorable benefit/risk ratio exists in a woman who has had a hysterectomy because she has no risk of endometrial carcinoma (see Boxed Warning).
There is evidence that bone loss is increased in many women following the menopause, but there is no clear way to identify those women who will develop osteoporotic fractures. There is also evidence that the rate of bone loss can be reduced in postmenopausal women by taking estrogens, but substantial evidence is lacking that estrogens decrease the incidence of osteoporotic bone fractures. Women who have had an early surgical menopause (oophorectomy) appear to be at increased risk for the development of osteoporosis.
3. Atrophic vaginitis.
4. Kraurosis vulvae.
5. Female hypogonadism.
6. Female castration.
7. Primary ovarian failure.
8. Breast cancer (for palliation only) in appropriately selected women and men with metastatic disease.
9. Prostatic carcinoma—palliative therapy of advanced disease.
10. Postpartum breast engorgement—Although estrogens have been widely used for the prevention of postpartum breast engorgement, controlled studies have demonstrated that the incidence of significant painful engorgement in patients not receiving such hormonal therapy is low and usually responsive to appropriate analgesic or other supportive therapy. Consequently, the benefit to be derived from estrogen therapy for this indication must be carefully weighed against the potential increased risk of puerperal thromboembolism associated with the use of large doses of estrogens.[20]

PREMARIN (conjugated estrogens tablets, USP) HAS NOT BEEN SHOWN TO BE EFFECTIVE FOR ANY PURPOSE DURING PREGNANCY AND ITS USE MAY CAUSE SEVERE HARM TO THE FETUS (SEE BOXED WARNING).

Concomitant Progestin Use: The lowest effective dose appropriate for the specific indication should be utilized. Studies of the addition of a progestin for 7 or more days of a cycle of estrogen administration have reported a lowered incidence of endometrial hyperplasia. Morphological and biochemical studies of the endometrium suggest that 10 to 13 days of progestin are needed to provide maximal maturation of the endometrium and to eliminate any hyperplastic changes. Whether this will provide protection from endometrial carcinoma has not been clearly established. There are possible additional risks which may be associated with the inclusion of progestin in estrogen replacement regimens. (See PRECAUTIONS.) The choice of progestin and dosage may be important; product labeling should be reviewed to minimize possible adverse effects.

CONTRAINDICATIONS

Estrogens should not be used in women (or men) with any of the following conditions:

1. Known or suspected cancer of the breast except in appropriately selected patients being treated for metastatic disease.
2. Known or suspected estrogen-dependent neoplasia.
3. Known or suspected pregnancy (see Boxed Warning).
4. Undiagnosed abnormal genital bleeding.
5. Active thrombophlebitis or thromboembolic disorders.
6. A past history of thrombophlebitis, thrombosis, or thromboembolic disorders associated with previous estrogen use (except when used in treatment of breast or prostatic malignancy).

WARNINGS

1. *Induction of malignant neoplasms.* Long-term continuous administration of natural and synthetic estrogens in certain animal species increases the frequency of carcinomas of the breast, cervix, vagina, and liver. There are now reports that estrogens increase the risk of carcinoma of the endometrium in humans. (See Boxed Warning.)
At the present time there is no satisfactory evidence that estrogens given to postmenopausal women increase the risk of cancer of the breast,[17] although a recent long-term follow-up of a single physician's practice has raised this possibility.[18] Because of the animal data, there is a need for caution in prescribing estrogens for women with a strong family history of breast cancer or who have breast nodules, fibrocystic disease, or abnormal mammograms.
2. *Gallbladder disease.* A recent study has reported a 2- to 3-fold increase in the risk of surgically confirmed gallbladder disease in women receiving postmenopausal estrogens,[17] similar to the 2-fold increase previously noted in users of oral contraceptives.[19,24a]
3. *Effects similar to those caused by estrogen-progestogen oral contraceptives.* There are several serious adverse effects of oral contraceptives, most of which have not, up to now, been documented as consequences of postmenopausal estrogen therapy. This may reflect the comparatively low doses of estrogen used in postmenopausal women. It would be expected that the larger doses of estrogen used to treat prostatic or breast cancer or postpartum breast engorgement are more likely to result in these adverse effects, and, in fact, it has been shown that there is an increased risk of thrombosis in men receiving estrogens for prostatic cancer and women for postpartum breast engorgement.[20–23]
a. *Thromboembolic disease.* It is now well established that users of oral contraceptives have an increased risk of various thromboembolic and thrombotic vascular diseases, such as thrombophlebitis, pulmonary embolism, stroke, and myocardial infarction.[24–31] Cases of retinal thrombosis, mesenteric thrombosis, and optic neuritis have been reported in oral contraceptive users. There is evidence that the risk of several of these adverse reactions is related to the dose of the drug.[32,33] An increased risk of postsurgery thromboembolic complications has also been reported in users of oral contraceptives.[34,35] If feasible, estrogen should be discontinued at least 4 weeks before surgery of the type associated with an increased risk of thromboembolism, or during periods of prolonged immobilization.
While an increased rate of thromboembolic and thrombotic disease in postmenopausal users of estrogens has not been found,[17–24,25–36] this does not rule out the possibility that such an increase may be present or that subgroups of women who have underlying risk factors or who are receiving relatively large doses of estrogens may have increased risk. Therefore estrogens should not be used in persons with active thrombophlebitis or thromboembolic disorders, and they should not be used (except in treatment of malignancy) in persons with a history of such disorders in association with estrogen use. They should be used with caution in patients with cerebral vascular or coronary artery disease and only for those in whom estrogens are clearly needed.
Large doses of estrogen (5 mg conjugated estrogens per day), comparable to those used to treat cancer of the prostate and breast, have been shown in a large prospective clinical trial in men[37] to increase the risk of nonfatal myocardial infarction, pulmonary embolism and thrombophlebitis. When estrogen doses of this size are used, any of the thromboembolic and thrombotic adverse effects associated with oral contraceptive use should be considered a clear risk.
b. *Hepatic adenoma.* Benign hepatic adenomas appear to be associated with the use of oral contraceptives.[38–40] Although benign, and rare, these may rupture and may cause death through intra-abdominal hemorrhage. Such lesions have not yet been reported in association with other estrogen or progestogen preparations but should be considered in estrogen users having abdominal pain and tenderness, abdominal mass, or hypovolemic shock. Hepatocellular carcinoma has also been reported in women taking estrogen-containing oral contraceptives.[39] The relationship of this malignancy to these drugs is not known at this time.
c. *Elevated blood pressure.* Women using oral contraceptives sometimes experience increased blood pressure which, in most cases, returns to normal on discontinuing the drug. There is now a report that this may occur with use of estrogens in the menopause[41] and blood pressure should be monitored with estrogen use, especially if high doses are used.
d. *Glucose tolerance.* A worsening of glucose tolerance has been observed in a significant percentage of patients on estrogen-containing oral contraceptives. For this reason, diabetic patients should be carefully observed while receiving estrogen.
4. *Hypercalcemia.* Administration of estrogens may lead to severe hypercalcemia in patients with breast cancer and bone metastases. If this occurs, the drug should be stopped and appropriate measures taken to reduce the serum calcium level.

PRECAUTIONS

A. General Precautions.

1. A complete medical and family history should be taken prior to the initiation of any estrogen therapy. The pretreatment and periodic physical examinations should include special reference to blood pressure, breasts, abdomen, and pelvic organs, and should include a Papanicolaou smear. As a general rule, estrogen should not be prescribed for longer than one year without another physical examination being performed.
2. Fluid retention—Because estrogens may cause some degree of fluid retention, conditions which might be influenced by this factor such as asthma, epilepsy, migraine, and cardiac or renal dysfunction, require careful observation.
3. Certain patients may develop undesirable manifestations of excessive estrogenic stimulation, such as abnormal or excessive uterine bleeding, mastodynia, etc.
4. Prolonged administration of unopposed estrogen therapy has been reported to increase the risk of endometrial hyperplasia in some patients.
5. Oral contraceptives appear to be associated with an increased incidence of mental depression.[24a] Although it is not clear whether this is due to the estrogenic or progestogenic component of the contraceptive, patients with a history of depression should be carefully observed.
6. Preexisting uterine leiomyomata may increase in size during estrogen use.
7. The pathologist should be advised of estrogen therapy when relevant specimens are submitted.
8. Patients with a past history of jaundice during pregnancy have an increased risk of recurrence of jaundice while receiving estrogen-containing oral contraceptive therapy. If jaundice develops in any patient receiving estrogen, the medication should be discontinued while the cause is investigated.
9. Estrogens may be poorly metabolized in patients with impaired liver function and they should be administered with caution in such patients.
10. Because estrogens influence the metabolism of calcium and phosphorus, they should be used with caution in patients with metabolic bone diseases that are associated with hypercalcemia or in patients with renal insufficiency.
11. Because of the effects of estrogens on epiphyseal closure, they should be used judiciously in young patients in whom bone growth is not complete.
12. If concomitant progestin therapy is used, potential risks may include adverse effects on carbohydrate and lipid metabolism.

B. Information for the Patient. See text which appears after the PHYSICIAN REFERENCES.

C. Drug/Laboratory Test Interactions: Certain endocrine and liver function tests may be affected by estrogen-containing oral contraceptives. The following similar changes may be expected with larger doses of estrogen:

a. Increased sulfobromophthalein retention.
b. Increased prothrombin and factors VII, VIII, IX, and X; decreased antithrombin 3; increased norepinephrine-induced platelet aggregability.
c. Increased thyroid binding globulin (TBG) leading to increased circulating total thyroid hormone, as measured by PBI, T4 by column, or T4 by radioimmunoassay. Free T3 resin uptake is decreased, reflecting the elevated TBG; free T4 concentration is unaltered.
d. Impaired glucose tolerance.
e. Decreased pregnanediol excretion.
f. Reduced response to metyrapone test.
g. Reduced serum folate concentration.
h. Increased serum triglyceride and phospholipid concentration.

D. Carcinogenesis, Mutagenesis, Impairment of Fertility: See WARNINGS section for information on carcinogenesis.

E. Pregnancy Category X. See CONTRAINDICATIONS and Boxed Warning.

F. Nursing Mothers. It is not known whether this drug is excreted in human milk. Because many drugs are excreted in human milk and because of the potential for serious adverse reactions in nursing infants from estrogens, a decision should be made whether to discontinue nursing or to discontinue the drug, taking into account the importance of the drug to the mother.

G. Pediatric Use: Safety and effectiveness in children have not been established.

ADVERSE REACTIONS

(See Warnings regarding induction of neoplasia, adverse effects on the fetus, increased incidence of gallbladder disease, and adverse effects similar to those of oral contraceptives, including thromboembolism.) The following additional adverse reactions have been reported with estrogenic therapy, including oral contraceptives:

1. *Genitourinary system:* Breakthrough bleeding, spotting, change in menstrual flow; dysmenorrhea; premenstrual-like syndrome; amenorrhea during and after treatment; increase in size of uterine fibromyomata; vaginal candidiasis; change in cervical erosion and in degree of cervical secretion; cystitis-like syndrome.
2. *Breasts:* Tenderness, enlargement, secretion.
3. *Gastrointestinal:* Nausea, vomiting; abdominal cramps, bloating; cholestatic jaundice.
4. *Skin:* Chloasma or melasma which may persist when drug is discontinued; erythema multiforme; erythema nodosum; hemorrhagic eruption; loss of scalp hair; hirsutism.
5. *Eyes:* Steepening of corneal curvature; intolerance to contact lenses.
6. *CNS:* Headache, migraine, dizziness; mental depression; chorea.

7. *Miscellaneous:* Increase or decrease in weight; reduced carbohydrate tolerance; aggravation of porphyria; edema; changes in libido.

ACUTE OVERDOSAGE

Numerous reports of ingestion of large doses of estrogen-containing oral contraceptives by young children indicate that acute serious ill effects do not occur. Overdosage of estrogen may cause nausea, and withdrawal bleeding may occur in females.

DOSAGE AND ADMINISTRATION

1. *Given cyclically for short-term use only:*
For treatment of moderate-to-severe *vasomotor* symptoms, atrophic vaginitis, or kraurosis vulvae associated with the menopause.
The lowest dose that will control symptoms should be chosen and medication should be discontinued as promptly as possible.
Administration should be cyclic (eg, three weeks on and one week off).
Attempts to discontinue or taper medication should be made at three- to six-month intervals.
Usual dosage ranges:
Vasomotor symptoms—1.25 mg daily. If the patient has not menstruated within the last two months or more, cyclic administration is started arbitrarily. If the patient is menstruating, cyclic administration is started on day 5 of bleeding.
Atrophic vaginitis and kraurosis vulvae—0.3 mg to 1.25 mg or more daily, depending upon the tissue response of the individual patient. Administer cyclically.
2. *Given cyclically:* Female hypogonadism; female castration; primary ovarian failure; osteoporosis.
Usual dosage ranges:
Osteoporosis—0.625 mg daily. Administration should be cyclic (eg, three weeks on and one week off).
Female hypogonadism—2.5 to 7.5 mg daily, in divided doses for 20 days, followed by a rest period of 10 days' duration. If bleeding does not occur by the end of this period, the same dosage schedule is repeated. The number of courses of estrogen therapy necessary to produce bleeding may vary depending on the responsiveness of the endometrium.
If bleeding occurs before the end of the 10-day period, begin a 20-day estrogen-progestin cyclic regimen with PREMARIN (conjugated estrogens tablets, USP), 2.5 to 7.5 mg daily in divided doses, for 20 days. During the last five days of estrogen therapy, give an oral progestin. If bleeding occurs before this regimen is concluded, therapy is discontinued and may be resumed on the fifth day of bleeding.
Female castration and primary ovarian failure— 1.25 mg daily, cyclically. Adjust dosage upward or downward according to severity of symptoms and response of the patient. For maintenance, adjust dosage to lowest level that will provide effective control.
3. *Given for a few days:* Prevention of postpartum breast engorgement—3.75 mg every four hours for five doses, or 1.25 mg every four hours for five days.
4. *Given chronically:* Inoperable progressing prostatic cancer—1.25 to 2.5 mg three times daily. The effectiveness of therapy can be judged by phosphatase determinations as well as by symptomatic improvement of the patient.
Inoperable progressing breast cancer in appropriately selected men and postmenopausal women. (See INDICATIONS.)—Suggested dosage is 10 mg three times daily for a period of at least three months.
Treated patients with an intact uterus should be monitored closely for signs of endometrial cancer and appropriate diagnostic measures should be taken to rule out malignancy in the event of persistent or recurring abnormal vaginal bleeding.

HOW SUPPLIED

PREMARIN (conjugated estrogens tablets, USP)
—Each oval *purple* tablet contains 2.5 mg, in bottles of 100 (NDC 0046-0865-81) and 1,000 (NDC 0046-0865-91).
—Each oval *yellow* tablet contains 1.25 mg, in bottles of 100 (NDC 0046-0866-81) and 1,000 (NDC 0046-0866-91); and Unit Dose packages of 100 (NDC 0046-0866-99). Also in Cycle Packs of 21 (NDC 0046-0866-21).
—Each oval *white* tablet contains 0.9 mg, in bottles of 100 (NDC 0046-0864-81). Also in Cycle Packs of 21 (NDC 0046-0864-21).
—Each oval *maroon* tablet contains 0.625 mg, in bottles of 100 (NDC 0046-0867-81), 1,000 (NDC 0046-0867-91); and Unit Dose packages of 100 (NDC 0046-0867-99). Also in Cycle Packs of 21 (NDC 0046-0867-21).
—Each oval *green* tablet contains 0.3 mg, in bottles of 100 (NDC 0046-0868-81) and 1,000 (NDC 0046-0868-91).
The appearance of these tablets is a trademark of Ayerst Laboratories.
Store at room temperature (approximately 25° C).

PHYSICIAN REFERENCES

1. Ziel, H. K., *et al.*: N. Engl. J. Med. *293*:1167–1170, 1975.
2. Smith, D. C., *et al.*: N. Engl. J. Med. *293*:1164–1167, 1975.
3. Mack, T. M., *et al.*: N. Engl. J. Med. *294*:1262–1267, 1976.
4. Weiss, N. S., *et al.*: N. Engl. J. Med. *294*:1259–1262, 1976.
5. Herbst, A. L., *et al.*: N. Engl. J. Med. *284*:878–881, 1971.
6. Greenwald, P., *et al.*: N. Engl. J. Med. *285*:390–392, 1971.
7. Lanier, A., *et al.*: Mayo Clin. Proc. *48*: 793–799, 1973.
8. Herbst, A., *et al.*: Obstet. Gynecol. *40*:287–298, 1972.
9. Herbst, A., *et al.*: Am. J. Obstet. Gynecol. *118*:607–615, 1974.
10. Herbst, A., *et al.*: N. Engl. J. Med. *292*: 334–339, 1975.
11. Stafl, A., *et al.*: Obstet. Gynecol. *43*:118–128, 1974.
12. Sherman, A. I., *et al.*: Obstet. Gynecol. *44*:531–545, 1974.
13. Gal, I., *et al.*: Nature *216*:83, 1967.
14. Levy, E. P., *et al.*: Lancet *1*:611, 1973.
15. Nora, J., *et al.*: Lancet *1*:941–942, 1973.
16. Janerich, D. T., *et al.*: N. Engl. J. Med. *291*:697–700, 1974.
17. Boston Collaborative Drug Surveillance Program: N. Engl. J. Med. *290*:15–19, 1974.
18. Hoover, R., *et al.*: N. Engl. J. Med. *295*:401–405, 1976.
19. Boston Collaborative Drug Surveillance Program: Lancet *1*:1399–1404, 1973.
20. Daniel, D. G., *et al.*: Lancet *2*:287–289, 1967.
21. The Veterans Administration Cooperative Urological Research Group: J. Urol. *98*:516–522, 1967.
22. Bailar, J. C.: Lancet *2*:560, 1967.
23. Blackard, C., *et al.*: Cancer *26*:249–256, 1970.
24. Royal College of General Practitioners: J. R. Coll. Gen. Pract. *13*:267–279, 1967.
24a. Royal College of General Practitioners: Oral Contraceptives and Health, New York, Pitman Corp., 1974.
25. Inman, W. H. W., *et al.*: Br. Med. J. *2*:193–199, 1968.
26. Vessey, M. P., *et al.*: Br. Med. J. *2*:651–657, 1969.
27. Sartwell, P. E., *et al.*: Am. J. Epidemiol. *90*:365–380, 1969.
28. Collaborative Group for the Study of Stroke in Young Women: N. Engl. J. Med. *288*:871–878, 1973.
29. Collaborative Group for the Study of Stroke in Young Women: J.A.M.A. *231*:718–722, 1975.
30. Mann, J. I., *et al.*: Br. Med. J. *2*:245–248, 1975.
31. Mann, J. I., *et al.*: Br. Med. J. *2*:241–245, 1975.
32. Inman, W. H. W., *et al.*: Br. Med. J. *2*:203–209, 1970.
33. Stolley, P. D., *et al.*: Am. J. Epidemiol. *102*:197–208, 1975.
34. Vessey, M. P., *et al.*: Br. Med. J. *3*:123–126, 1970.
35. Greene, G. R., *et al.*: Am. J. Public Health *62*:680–685, 1972.
36. Rosenberg, L., *et al.*: N. Engl. J. Med. *294*:1256–1259, 1976.
37. Coronary Drug Project Research Group: J.A.M.A. *214*:1303–1313, 1970.
38. Baum, J., *et al.*: Lancet *2*:926–928, 1973.
39. Mays, E. T., *et al.*: J.A.M.A. *235*:730–732, 1976.
40. Edmondson, H. A., *et al.*: N. Engl. J. Med. *294*:470–472, 1976.
41. Pfeffer, R. I., *et al.*: Am. J. Epidemiol. *103*:445–456, 1976.

INFORMATION FOR THE PATIENT

WHAT YOU SHOULD KNOW ABOUT ESTROGENS

Estrogens are female hormones produced by the ovaries. The ovaries make several different kinds of estrogens. In addition, scientists have been able to make a variety of synthetic estrogens. As far as we know, all these estrogens have similar properties and therefore much the same usefulness, side effects, and risks. This leaflet is intended to help you understand what estrogens are used for, the risks involved in their use, and how to use them as safely as possible.
This leaflet includes the most important information about estrogens, but not all the information. If you want to know more, you should ask your doctor for more information or you can ask your doctor or pharmacist to let you read the package insert prepared for the doctor.

USES OF ESTROGEN

THERE IS NO PROPER USE OF ESTROGENS IN A PREGNANT WOMAN.
Estrogens are prescribed by doctors for a number of purposes, including:
1. To provide estrogen during a period of adjustment when a woman's ovaries stop producing a majority of her estrogens, in order to prevent certain uncomfortable symptoms of estrogen deficiency. (With the menopause, which generally occurs between the ages of 45 and 55, women produce a much smaller amount of estrogens.)
2. To prevent symptoms of estrogen deficiency when a woman's ovaries have been removed surgically before the natural menopause.
3. To prevent pregnancy. (Estrogens are given along with a progestogen, another female hormone; these combinations are called oral contraceptives or birth control pills. Patient labeling is available to women taking oral contraceptives and they will not be discussed in this leaflet.)
4. To treat certain cancers in women and men.
5. To prevent painful swelling of the breasts after pregnancy in women who choose not to nurse their babies.

ESTROGENS IN THE MENOPAUSE

In the natural course of their lives, all women eventually experience a decrease in estrogen production. This usually occurs between ages 45 and 55 but may occur earlier or later. Sometimes the ovaries may need to be removed before natural menopause by an operation, producing a "surgical menopause."
When the amount of estrogen in the blood begins to decrease, many women may develop typical symptoms: feelings of warmth in the face, neck, and chest or sudden intense episodes of heat and sweating throughout the body (called "hot flashes" or "hot flushes"). These symptoms are sometimes very uncomfortable. Some women may also develop changes in the vagina (called "atrophic vaginitis") which cause discomfort, especially during and after intercourse.
Estrogens can be prescribed to treat these symptoms of the menopause. It is estimated that considerably more than half of all women undergoing the menopause have only mild symptoms or no symptoms at all and therefore do not need estrogens. Other women may need estrogens for a few months, while their bodies adjust to lower estrogen levels. Sometimes the need will be for periods longer than six months. In an attempt to avoid overstimulation of the uterus (womb), estrogens are usually given cyclically during each month of use, such as three weeks of pills followed by one week without pills.
Sometimes women experience nervous symptoms or depression during menopause. There is no evidence that estrogens are effective for such symptoms without associated vasomotor symptoms. In the absence of vasomotor symptoms, estrogens should not be used to treat nervous symptoms, although other treatment may be needed.
You may have heard that taking estrogens for long periods (years) after the menopause will keep your skin soft and supple and keep you feeling young. There is no evidence that this is so, however, and such long-term treatment carries important risks.

ESTROGENS IN POSTMENOPAUSAL OSTEOPOROSIS

Osteoporosis is a thinning of the bones that makes them weaker and more likely to break. The bones that break most commonly in osteoporosis are those of the spine, arms, and upper legs. Both men and women start to lose bone after about age 40, but women seem to lose bone faster after the menopause. Not all women develop osteoporosis after menopause. Adequate calcium in the diet and exercise may help to prevent osteoporosis. Taking estrogens after the menopause seems to slow down the bone loss but there is not enough evidence to show that it prevents the bone from breaking.

ESTROGENS TO PREVENT SWELLING OF THE BREASTS AFTER PREGNANCY

If you do not breast-feed your baby after delivery, your breasts may fill up with milk and become painful and engorged. This usually begins about 3 to 4 days after delivery and may last for a few days to up to a week or more. Sometimes the discomfort is severe, but usually it is not and can be controlled by pain-relieving drugs such as aspirin and by binding the breasts up tightly. Estrogens can be used to try to prevent the breasts from filling up. While this treatment is sometimes successful, in many cases the breasts fill up to some degree in spite of treatment. The dose of estrogens needed to prevent pain and swelling of the breasts is much larger than the dose needed to treat symptoms of the menopause and this may increase your chances of developing blood clots in the legs or lungs (see below). Therefore, it is important that you discuss the benefits and the risks of estrogen use with your doctor if you have decided not to breast-feed your baby.

THE DANGERS OF ESTROGENS

1. *Endometrial cancer.* There are reports that if estrogens are used in the postmenopausal period for more than a year, there is an increased risk of *endometrial cancer* (cancer of the lining of the uterus). Women taking estrogens have roughly 5 to 10 times as great a chance of getting this cancer as women who take no estrogens. To put this another way, while a postmenopausal woman not taking estrogens has 1 chance in 1,000 each year of getting endometrial cancer, a woman taking estrogens has 5 to 10 chances in 1,000 each year. For this reason *it is important to take estrogens only when they are really needed.*
The risk of this cancer is greater the longer estrogens are used and when larger doses are taken. Therefore you should not take more estrogen than your doctor prescribes. *It is important to take the lowest dose of estrogen that will control symptoms and to take it only as long as it is needed.* If estrogens are needed for longer periods of time, your doctor will want to reevaluate your need for estrogens at least every six months.

Continued on next page

Ayerst—Cont.

Women using estrogens should report any vaginal bleeding to their doctors; such bleeding may be of no importance, but it can be an early warning of endometrial cancer. If you have undiagnosed vaginal bleeding, you should not use estrogens until a diagnosis is made and you are certain there is no endometrial cancer.

NOTE: If you have had your uterus removed (total hysterectomy), there is no danger of developing endometrial cancer.

2. *Other possible cancers.* Estrogens can cause development of other tumors in animals, such as tumors of the breast, cervix, vagina, or liver, when given for a long time. At present there is no good evidence that women using estrogen in the menopause have an increased risk of such tumors, but there is no way yet to be sure they do not; and one study raises the possibility that use of estrogens in the menopause may increase the risk of breast cancer many years later. This is a further reason to use estrogens only when clearly needed. While you are taking estrogens, it is important that you go to your doctor at least once a year for a physical examination. Also, if members of your family have had breast cancer or if you have breast nodules or abnormal mammograms (breast x-rays), your doctor may wish to carry out more frequent examinations of your breasts.

3. *Gallbladder disease.* Women who use estrogens after menopause are more likely to develop gallbladder disease needing surgery than women who do not use estrogens. Birth control pills have a similar effect.

4. *Abnormal blood clotting.* Oral contraceptives increase the risk of blood clotting in various parts of the body. This can result in a stroke (if the clot is in the brain), a heart attack (clot in a blood vessel of the heart), or a pulmonary embolus (a clot which forms in the legs or pelvis, then breaks off and travels to the lungs). Any of these can be fatal.

At this time use of estrogens in the menopause is not known to cause such blood clotting, but this has not been fully studied and there could still prove to be such a risk. It is recommended that if you have had clotting in the legs or lungs or a heart attack or stroke while you were using estrogens or birth control pills, you should not use estrogens (unless they are being used to treat cancer of the breast or prostate). If you have had a stroke or heart attack or if you have angina pectoris, estrogens should be used with great caution and only if clearly needed (for example, if you have severe symptoms of the menopause).

The larger doses of estrogen used to prevent swelling of the breasts after pregnancy have been reported to cause clotting in the legs and lungs.

SPECIAL WARNING ABOUT PREGNANCY

You should not receive estrogen if you are pregnant. If this should occur, there is a greater than usual chance that the developing child will be born with a birth defect, although the possibility remains fairly small. A female child may have an increased risk of developing cancer of the vagina or cervix later in life (in the teens or twenties). Every possible effort should be made to avoid exposure to estrogens during pregnancy. If exposure occurs, see your doctor.

OTHER EFFECTS OF ESTROGENS

In addition to the serious known risks of estrogens described above, estrogens have the following side effects and potential risks:

1. *Nausea and vomiting.* The most common side effect of estrogen therapy is nausea. Vomiting is less common.
2. *Effects on breasts.* Estrogens may cause breast tenderness or enlargement and may cause the breasts to secrete a liquid. These effects are not dangerous.
3. *Effects on the uterus.* Estrogens may cause benign fibroid tumors of the uterus to get larger.
4. *Effects on liver.* Women taking oral contraceptives develop on rare occasions a tumor of the liver which can rupture and bleed into the abdomen and may cause death. So far, these tumors have not been reported in women using estrogens in the menopause, but you should report any swelling or unusual pain or tenderness in the abdomen to your doctor immediately.

Women with a past history of jaundice (yellowing of the skin and white parts of the eyes) may get jaundice again during estrogen use. If this occurs, stop taking estrogens and see your doctor.

5. *Other effects.* Estrogens may cause excess fluid to be retained in the body. This may make some conditions worse, such as asthma, epilepsy, migraine, heart disease, or kidney disease.

SUMMARY

Estrogens have important uses, but they have serious risks as well. You must decide, with your doctor, whether the risks are acceptable to you in view of the benefits of treatment. Except where your doctor has prescribed estrogens for use in special cases of cancer of the breast or prostate, you should not use estrogens if you have cancer of the breast or uterus, are pregnant, have undiagnosed abnormal vaginal bleeding, clotting in the legs or lungs, or have had a stroke, heart attack or angina, or clotting in the legs or lungs in the past while you were taking estrogens.

You can use estrogens as safely as possible by understanding that your doctor will require regular physical examinations while you are taking them and will try to discontinue the drug as soon as possible and use the smallest dose possible. Be alert for signs of trouble including:

1. Abnormal bleeding from the vagina.
2. Pains in the calves or chest or sudden shortness of breath, or coughing blood.
3. Severe headache, dizziness, faintness, or changes in vision.
4. Breast lumps (you should ask your doctor how to examine your own breasts).
5. Jaundice (yellowing of the skin).
6. Mental depression.

Your doctor has prescribed this drug for you and you alone. Do not give the drug to anyone else.

Shown in Product Identification Section, page 404

PREMARIN® INTRAVENOUS ℞

[*prĕm ′a-rĭn*]

Brand of conjugated estrogens, USP, for Injection

Specially prepared for Intravenous & Intramuscular use

CAUTION: Federal law prohibits dispensing without prescription.

1. ESTROGENS HAVE BEEN REPORTED TO INCREASE THE RISK OF ENDOMETRIAL CARCINOMA.

Three independent case control studies have reported an increased risk of endometrial cancer in postmenopausal women exposed to exogenous estrogens for more than one year.[1–3] This risk was independent of the other known risk factors for endometrial cancer. These studies are further supported by the finding that incidence rates of endometrial cancer have increased sharply since 1969 in eight different areas of the United States with population-based cancer reporting systems, an increase which may be related to the rapidly expanding use of estrogens during the last decade.[4]

The three case control studies reported that the risk of endometrial cancer in estrogen users was about 4.5 to 13.9 times greater than in nonusers. The risk appears to depend on both duration of treatment[1] and on estrogen dose.[3] In view of these findings, when estrogens are used for the treatment of menopausal symptoms, the lowest dose that will control symptoms should be utilized and medication should be discontinued as soon as possible. When prolonged treatment is medically indicated, the patient should be reassessed on at least a semiannual basis to determine the need for continued therapy. Although the evidence must be considered preliminary, one study suggests that cyclic administration of low doses of estrogen may carry less risk than continuous administration;[3] it therefore appears prudent to utilize such a regimen.

Close clinical surveillance of all women taking estrogens is important. In all cases of undiagnosed, persistent, or recurring abnormal vaginal bleeding, adequate diagnostic measures should be undertaken to rule out malignancy.

There is no evidence at present that "natural" estrogens are more or less hazardous than "synthetic" estrogens at equiestrogenic doses.

2. ESTROGENS SHOULD NOT BE USED DURING PREGNANCY.

The use of female sex hormones, both estrogens and progestogens, during early pregnancy may seriously damage the offspring. It has been shown that females exposed in utero to diethylstilbestrol, a non-steroidal estrogen, have an increased risk of developing, in later life, a form of vaginal or cervical cancer that is ordinarily extremely rare.[5,6] This risk has been estimated as not greater than 4 per 1,000 exposures.[7] Furthermore, a high percentage of such exposed women (from 30% to 90%) have been found to have vaginal adenosis,[8–12] epithelial changes of the vagina and cervix. Although these changes are histologically benign, it is not known whether they are precursors of malignancy. Although similar data are not available with the use of other estrogens, it cannot be presumed they would not induce similar changes.

Several reports suggest an association between intrauterine exposure to female sex hormones and congenital anomalies, including congenital heart defects and limb reduction defects.[13–16] One case control study[16] estimated a 4.7-fold increased risk of limb reduction defects in infants exposed in utero to sex hormones (oral contraceptives, hormone withdrawal tests for pregnancy, or attempted treatment for threatened abortion). Some of these exposures were very short and involved only a few days of treatment. The data suggest that the risk of limb reduction defects in exposed fetuses is somewhat less than 1 per 1,000.

In the past, female sex hormones have been used during pregnancy in an attempt to treat threatened or habitual abortion. There is considerable evidence that estrogens are ineffective for these indications, and there is no evidence from well-controlled studies that progestogens are effective for these uses.

If PREMARIN Intravenous (conjugated estrogens, USP, for injection) is used during pregnancy, or if the patient becomes pregnant while taking this drug, she should be apprised of the potential risks to the fetus, and the advisability of pregnancy continuation.

DESCRIPTION

Each Secule® contains 25 mg of conjugated estrogens, USP, in a sterile lyophilized cake which also contains lactose 200 mg, sodium citrate 12.5 mg and simethicone 0.2 mg. The pH is adjusted with sodium hydroxide or hydrochloric acid. A sterile diluent (5 mL) containing 2% benzyl alcohol and Water for Injection, USP is provided for reconstitution. The reconstituted solution is suitable for intravenous or intramuscular injection.

PREMARIN (conjugated estrogens, USP) is a mixture of estrogens obtained exclusively from natural sources, occurring as the sodium salts of water-soluble estrogen sulfates blended to represent the average composition of material derived from pregnant mares' urine. It contains estrone, equilin, and 17 α-dihydroequilin, together with smaller amounts of 17 α-estradiol, equilenin, and 17 α-dihydroequilenin as salts of their sulfate esters.

CLINICAL PHARMACOLOGY

Estrogens are important in the development and maintenance of the female reproductive system and secondary sex characteristics. They promote growth and development of the vagina, uterus, and fallopian tubes, and enlargement of the breasts. Indirectly, they contribute to the shaping of the skeleton, maintenance of tone and elasticity of urogenital structures, changes in the epiphyses of the long bones that allow for the pubertal growth spurt and its termination, growth of axillary and pubic hair, and pigmentation of the nipples and genitals. Decline of estrogenic activity at the end of the menstrual cycle can bring on menstruation, although the cessation of progesterone secretion is the most important factor in the mature ovulatory cycle. However, in the preovulatory or nonovulatory cycle, estrogen is the primary determinant in the onset of menstruation. Estrogens also affect the release of pituitary gonadotropins.

The pharmacologic effects of conjugated estrogens are similar to those of endogenous estrogens. They are soluble in water and may be administered by intravenous or intramuscular injection.

In responsive tissues (female genital organs, breasts, hypothalamus, pituitary) estrogens enter the cell and are transported into the nucleus. As a result of estrogen action, specific RNA and protein synthesis occurs.

Metabolism and inactivation occur primarily in the liver. Some estrogens are excreted into the bile; however, they are reabsorbed from the intestine and returned to the liver through the portal venous system. Water-soluble estrogen conjugates are strongly acidic and are ionized in body fluids, which favor excretion through the kidneys since tubular reabsorption is minimal.

INDICATION

PREMARIN Intravenous (conjugated estrogens, USP, for injection) is indicated in the treatment of abnormal uterine bleeding due to hormonal imbalance in the absence of organic pathology.

Concomitant Progestin Use: The lowest effective dose appropriate for the specific indication should be utilized. Studies of the addition of a progestin for 7 or more days of a cycle of estrogen administration have reported a lowered incidence of endometrial hyperplasia. Morphological and biochemical studies of the endometrium suggest that 10 to 13 days of progestin are needed to provide maximal maturation of the endometrium and to eliminate any hyperplastic changes. Whether this will provide protection from endometrial carcinoma has not been clearly established. There are possible additional risks which may be associated with the inclusion of progestin in estrogen replacement regimens. (See PRECAUTIONS.) The choice of progestin and dosage may be important; product labeling should be reviewed to minimize possible adverse effects.

CONTRAINDICATIONS

Estrogens should not be used in women with any of the following conditions:

1. Known or suspected cancer of the breast except in appropriately selected patients being treated for metastatic disease.

2. Known or suspected estrogen-dependent neoplasia.
3. Known or suspected pregnancy (see Boxed Warning).
4. Undiagnosed abnormal genital bleeding.
5. Active thrombophlebitis or thromboembolic disorders.
6. A past history of thrombophlebitis, thrombosis, or thromboembolic disorders associated with previous estrogen use (except when used in treatment of breast malignancy).

WARNINGS

1. *Induction of malignant neoplasms.* Long-term continuous administration of natural and synthetic estrogens in certain animal species increases the frequency of carcinomas of the breast, cervix, vagina, and liver. There are now reports that estrogens increase the risk of carcinoma of the endometrium in humans. (See Boxed Warning.)

At the present time there is no satisfactory evidence that estrogens given to postmenopausal women increase the risk of cancer of the breast,[17] although a recent long-term follow-up of a single physician's practice has raised this possibility.[18] Because of the animal data, there is a need for caution in prescribing estrogens for women with a strong family history of breast cancer or who have breast nodules, fibrocystic disease, or abnormal mammograms.

2. *Gallbladder disease.* A recent study has reported a 2- to 3-fold increase in the risk of surgically confirmed gallbladder disease in women receiving postmenopausal estrogens,[17] similar to the 2-fold increase previously noted in users of oral contraceptives.[19,24a]

3. *Effects similar to those caused by estrogen-progestogen oral contraceptives.* There are several serious adverse effects of oral contraceptives, most of which have not, up to now, been documented as consequences of postmenopausal estrogen therapy. This may reflect the comparatively low doses of estrogen used in postmenopausal women. It would be expected that the larger doses of estrogen used to treat prostatic or breast cancer or postpartum breast engorgement are more likely to result in these adverse effects, and, in fact, it has been shown that there is an increased risk of thrombosis in men receiving estrogens for prostatic cancer and women for postpartum breast engorgement.[20–23]

a. *Thromboembolic disease.* It is now well established that users of oral contraceptives have an increased risk of various thromboembolic and thrombotic vascular diseases, such as thrombophlebitis, pulmonary embolism, stroke, and myocardial infarction.[24–31] Cases of retinal thrombosis, mesenteric thrombosis, and optic neuritis have been reported in oral contraceptive users. There is evidence that the risk of several of these adverse reactions is related to the dose of the drug.[32,33] An increased risk of postsurgery thromboembolic complications has also been reported in users of oral contraceptives.[34,35] If feasible, estrogen should be discontinued at least 4 weeks before surgery of the type associated with an increased risk of thromboembolism, or during periods of prolonged immobilization.

While an increased rate of thromboembolic and thrombotic disease in postmenopausal users of estrogens has not been found,[17–24, 25–36] this does not rule out the possibility that such an increase may be present or that subgroups of women who have underlying risk factors or who are receiving relatively large doses of estrogens may have increased risk. Therefore estrogens should not be used in persons with active thrombophlebitis or thromboembolic disorders, and they should not be used (except in treatment of malignancy) in persons with a history of such disorders in association with estrogen use. They should be used with caution in patients with cerebral vascular or coronary artery disease and only for those in whom estrogens are clearly needed.

Large doses of estrogen (5 mg conjugated estrogens per day), comparable to those used to treat cancer of the prostate and breast, have been shown in a large prospective clinical trial in men[37] to increase the risk of nonfatal myocardial infarction, pulmonary embolism and thrombophlebitis. When estrogen doses of this size are used, any of the thromboembolic and thrombotic adverse effects associated with oral contraceptive use should be considered a clear risk.

b. *Hepatic adenoma.* Benign hepatic adenomas appear to be associated with the use of oral contraceptives.[38–40] Although benign, and rare, these may rupture and may cause death through intra-abdominal hemorrhage. Such lesions have not yet been reported in association with other estrogen or progestogen preparations but should be considered in estrogen users having abdominal pain and tenderness, abdominal mass, or hypovolemic shock. Hepatocellular carcinoma has also been reported in women taking estrogen-containing oral contraceptives.[39] The relationship of this malignancy to these drugs is not known at this time.

c. *Elevated blood pressure.* Women using oral contraceptives sometimes experience increased blood pressure which, in most cases, returns to normal on discontinuing the drug. There is now a report that this may occur with use of estrogens in the menopause[41] and blood pressure should be monitored with estrogen use, especially if high doses are used.

d. *Glucose tolerance.* A worsening of glucose tolerance has been observed in a significant percentage of patients on estrogen-containing oral contraceptives. For this reason, diabetic patients should be carefully observed while receiving estrogen.

4. *Hypercalcemia.* Administration of estrogens may lead to severe hypercalcemia in patients with breast cancer and bone metastases. If this occurs, the drug should be stopped and appropriate measures taken to reduce the serum calcium level.

PRECAUTIONS

A. General Precautions.

1. A complete medical and family history should be taken prior to the initiation of any estrogen therapy. The pretreatment and periodic physical examinations should include special reference to blood pressure, breasts, abdomen, and pelvic organs, and should include a Papanicolaou smear. As a general rule, estrogen should not be prescribed for longer than one year without another physical examination being performed.
2. Fluid retention—Because estrogens may cause some degree of fluid retention, conditions which might be influenced by this factor such as asthma, epilepsy, migraine, and cardiac or renal dysfunction, require careful observation.
3. Certain patients may develop undesirable manifestations of excessive estrogenic stimulation, such as abnormal or excessive uterine bleeding, mastodynia, etc.
4. Oral contraceptives appear to be associated with an increased incidence of mental depression.[24a] Although it is not clear whether this is due to the estrogenic or progestogenic component of the contraceptive, patients with a history of depression should be carefully observed.
5. Preexisting uterine leiomyomata may increase in size during estrogen use.
6. The pathologist should be advised of estrogen therapy when relevant specimens are submitted.
7. Patients with a past history of jaundice during pregnancy have an increased risk of recurrence of jaundice while receiving estrogen-containing oral contraceptive therapy. If jaundice develops in any patient receiving estrogen, the medication should be discontinued while the cause is investigated.
8. Estrogens may be poorly metabolized in patients with impaired liver function and they should be administered with caution in such patients.
9. Because estrogens influence the metabolism of calcium and phosphorus, they should be used with caution in patients with metabolic bone diseases that are associated with hypercalcemia or in patients with renal insufficiency.
10. Because of the effects of estrogens on epiphyseal closure, they should be used judiciously in young patients in whom bone growth is not complete.
11. Certain endocrine and liver function tests may be affected by estrogen-containing oral contraceptives. The following similar changes may be expected with larger doses of estrogen:

a. Increased sulfobromophthalein retention.
b. Increased prothrombin and factors VII, VIII, IX, and X; decreased antithrombin 3; increased norepinephrine-induced platelet aggregability.
c. Increased thyroid binding globulin (TBG) leading to increased circulating total thyroid hormone, as measured by PBI, T4 by column, or T4 by radioimmunoassay. Free T3 resin uptake is decreased, reflecting the elevated TBG; free T4 concentration is unaltered.
d. Impaired glucose tolerance.
e. Decreased pregnanediol excretion.
f. Reduced response to metyrapone test.
g. Reduced serum folate concentration.
h. Increased serum triglyceride and phospholipid concentration.

12. If concomitant progestin therapy is used, potential risks may include adverse effects on carbohydrate and lipid metabolism.

B. Information for the Patient. See text which appears after the PHYSICIAN REFERENCES.

C. Pregnancy Category X. See CONTRAINDICATIONS and Boxed Warning.

D. Nursing Mothers. As a general principle, the administration of any drug to nursing mothers should be done only when clearly necessary since many drugs are excreted in human milk.

ADVERSE REACTIONS

(See WARNINGS regarding induction of neoplasia, adverse effects on the fetus, increased incidence of gallbladder disease, and adverse effects similar to those of oral contraceptives, including thromboembolism.) The following additional adverse reactions have been reported with estrogenic therapy, including oral contraceptives:

1. *Genitourinary system:* Breakthrough bleeding, spotting, change in menstrual flow; dysmenorrhea; premenstrual-like syndrome; amenorrhea during and after treatment; increase in size of uterine fibromyomata; vaginal candidiasis; change in cervical erosion and in degree of cervical secretion; cystitis-like syndrome.
2. *Breasts:* Tenderness, enlargement, secretion.
3. *Gastrointestinal:* Nausea, vomiting; abdominal cramps, bloating; cholestatic jaundice.
4. *Skin:* Chloasma or melasma which may persist when drug is discontinued; erythema multiforme; erythema nodosum; hemorrhagic eruption; loss of scalp hair; hirsutism.
5. *Eyes:* Steepening of corneal curvature; intolerance to contact lenses.
6. *CNS:* Headache, migraine, dizziness; mental depression; chorea.
7. *Miscellaneous:* Increase or decrease in weight; reduced carbohydrate tolerance; aggravation of porphyria; edema; changes in libido.

ACUTE OVERDOSAGE

Numerous reports of ingestion of large doses of estrogen-containing oral contraceptives by young children indicate that acute serious ill effects do not occur. Overdosage of estrogen may cause nausea, and withdrawal bleeding may occur in females.

DOSAGE AND ADMINISTRATION

Abnormal uterine bleeding due to hormonal imbalance: One 25 mg injection, intravenously or intramuscularly. Intravenous use is preferred since more rapid response can be expected from this mode of administration. Repeat in 6 to 12 hours if necessary. The use of PREMARIN Intravenous (conjugated estrogens, USP, for injection) does not preclude the advisability of other appropriate measures.

The usual precautionary measures governing intravenous administration should be adhered to. Injection should be made SLOWLY to obviate the occurrence of flushes.

Infusion of PREMARIN Intravenous (conjugated estrogens, USP, for injection) with other agents is not generally recommended. In emergencies, however, when an infusion has already been started, it may be expedient to make the injection into the tubing just distal to the infusion needle. If so used, compatibility of solutions must be considered.

Compatibility of solutions: PREMARIN Intravenous is compatible with normal saline, dextrose, and invert sugar solutions. IT IS NOT COMPATIBLE WITH PROTEIN HYDROLYSATE, ASCORBIC ACID, OR ANY SOLUTION WITH AN ACID pH.

Treated patients with an intact uterus should be monitored closely for signs of endometrial cancer and appropriate diagnostic measures should be taken to rule out malignancy in the event of persistent or recurring abnormal vaginal bleeding.

Directions for Storage and Reconstitution:

Storage before reconstitution: Store package in refrigerator, 2°–8°C (36°–46°F).

To reconstitute: First withdraw air from SECULE so as to facilitate introduction of sterile diluent. Then, flow the sterile diluent slowly against side of SECULE and agitate gently. DO NOT SHAKE VIOLENTLY.

Storage after reconstitution: It is common practice to utilize the reconstituted solution within a few hours. If it is necessary to keep the reconstituted solution for more than a few hours, store the reconstituted solution under refrigeration (2°–8°C). Under these conditions, the solution is stable for 60 days, and is suitable for use unless darkening or precipitation occurs.

HOW SUPPLIED

NDC 0046-0552-05-Each package provides: (1) One SECULE® containing 25 mg of conjugated estrogens, USP, for injection (also lactose 200 mg, sodium citrate 12.5 mg, and simethicone 0.2 mg). The pH is adjusted with sodium hydroxide or hydrochloric acid. (2) One 5 mL ampul sterile diluent with benzyl alcohol 2%, and Water for Injection, USP.

PREMARIN Intravenous (conjugated estrogens, USP, for injection) is prepared by cryodesiccation.

Storage before reconstitution: Store package in refrigerator, 2°–8°C (36°–46°F).

PHYSICIAN REFERENCES

1. Ziel, H. K., *et al.*: N. Engl. J. Med. *293*:1167–1170, 1975.
2. Smith, D. C., *et al.*: N. Engl. J. Med. *293*:1164–1167, 1975.
3. Mack, T. M., *et al.*: N. Engl. J. Med. *294*:1262–1267, 1976.
4. Weiss, N. S., *et al.*: N. Engl. J. Med. *294*:1259–1262, 1976.
5. Herbst, A. L., *et al.*: N. Engl. J. Med. *284*:878–881, 1971.
6. Greenwald, P., *et al.*: N. Engl. J. Med. *285*:390–392, 1971.
7. Lanier, A., *et al.*: Mayo Clin. Proc. *48*:793–799, 1973.
8. Herbst, A., *et al.*: Obstet. Gynecol. *40*:287–298, 1972.
9. Herbst, A., *et al.*: Am. J. Obstet. Gynecol. *118*:607–615, 1974.
10. Herbst, A., *et al.*: N. Engl. J. Med. *292*:334–339, 1975.
11. Stafl, A., *et al.*: Obstet. Gynecol. *43*:118–128, 1974.
12. Sherman, A. I., *et al.*: Obstet. Gynecol. *44*:531–545, 1974.

Continued on next page

Ayerst—Cont.

13. Gal, I., *et al.*: Nature *216*:83, 1967.
14. Levy, E. P., *et al.*: Lancet *1*:611, 1973.
15. Nora, J., *et al.*: Lancet *1*:941–942, 1973.
16. Janerich, D. T., *et al.*: N. Engl. J. Med. *291*:697–700, 1974.
17. Boston Collaborative Drug Surveillance Program: N. Engl. J. Med. *290*:15–19, 1974.
18. Hoover, R., *et al.*: N. Engl. J. Med. *295*:401–405, 1976.
19. Boston Collaborative Drug Surveillance Program: Lancet *1*:1399–1404, 1973.
20. Daniel, D. G., *et al.*: Lancet *2*:287–289, 1967.
21. The Veterans Administration Cooperative Urological Research Group: J. Urol. *98*:516–522, 1967.
22. Bailar, J. C.: Lancet *2*:560, 1967.
23. Blackard, C., *et al.*: Cancer *26*:249–256, 1970.
24. Royal College of General Practitioners: J. R. Coll. Gen. Pract. *13*:267–279, 1967.

24a. Royal College of General Practitioners: Oral Contraceptives and Health, New York, Pitman Corp., 1974.

25. Inman, W. H. W., *et al.*: Br. Med. J. *2*:193–199, 1968.
26. Vessey, M. P., *et al.*: Br. Med. J. *2*:651–657, 1969.
27. Sartwell, P. E., *et al.*: Am. J. Epidemiol. *90*:365–380, 1969.
28. Collaborative Group for the Study of Stroke in Young Women: N. Engl. J. Med. *288*:871–878, 1973.
29. Collaborative Group for the Study of Stroke in Young Women: J.A.M.A. *231*:718–722, 1975.
30. Mann, J. I., *et al.*: Br. Med. J. *2*:245–248, 1975.
31. Mann, J. I., *et al.*: Br. Med. J. *2*:241–245, 1975.
32. Inman, W. H. W., *et al.*: Br. Med. J. *2*:203–209, 1970.
33. Stolley, P. D., *et al.*: Am. J. Epidemiol. *102*:197–208, 1975.
34. Vessey, M. P., *et al.*: Br. Med. J. *3*:123–126, 1970.
35. Greene, G. R., *et al.*: Am. J. Public Health *62*:680–685, 1972.
36. Rosenberg, L., *et al.*: N. Engl. J. Med. *294*:1256–1259, 1976.
37. Coronary Drug Project Research Group: J.A.M.A. *214*:1303–1313, 1970.
38. Baum, J., *et al.*: Lancet *2*:926–928, 1973.
39. Mays, E. T., *et al.*: J.A.M.A. *235*:730–732, 1976.
40. Edmondson, H. A., *et al.*: N. Engl. J. Med. *294*:470–472, 1976.
41. Pfeffer, R. I., *et al.*: Am. J. Epidemiol. *103*:445–456, 1976.

INFORMATION FOR THE PATIENT

WHAT YOU SHOULD KNOW ABOUT ESTROGENS

Estrogens are female hormones produced by the ovaries. The ovaries make several different kinds of estrogens. In addition, scientists have been able to make a variety of synthetic estrogens. As far as we know, all these estrogens have similar properties and therefore much the same usefulness, side effects, and risks. This leaflet is intended to help you understand what estrogens are used for, the risks involved in their use, and how to use them as safely as possible.

This leaflet includes the most important information about estrogens, but not all the information. If you want to know more, you should ask your doctor for more information or you can ask your doctor or pharmacist to let you read the package insert prepared for the doctor.

USES OF ESTROGEN

THERE IS NO PROPER USE OF ESTROGENS IN A PREGNANT WOMAN.

Estrogens are prescribed by doctors for a number of purposes, including:

1. To provide estrogen during a period of adjustment when a woman's ovaries stop producing a majority of her estrogens, in order to prevent certain uncomfortable symptoms of estrogen deficiency. (With the menopause, which generally occurs between the ages of 45 and 55, women produce a much smaller amount of estrogens.)
2. To prevent symptoms of estrogen deficiency when a woman's ovaries have been removed surgically before the natural menopause.
3. To prevent pregnancy. (Estrogens are given along with a progestogen, another female hormone; these combinations are called oral contraceptives or birth control pills. Patient labeling is available to women taking oral contraceptives and they will not be discussed in this leaflet.)
4. To treat certain cancers in women and men.
5. To prevent painful swelling of the breasts after pregnancy in women who choose not to nurse their babies.

ESTROGENS IN THE MENOPAUSE

In the natural course of their lives, all women eventually experience a decrease in estrogen production. This usually occurs between ages 45 and 55 but may occur earlier or later. Sometimes the ovaries may need to be removed before natural menopause by an operation, producing a "surgical menopause."

When the amount of estrogen in the blood begins to decrease, many women may develop typical symptoms: feelings of warmth in the face, neck, and chest or sudden intense episodes of heat and sweating throughout the body (called "hot flashes" or "hot flushes"). These symptoms are sometimes very uncomfortable. Some women may also develop changes in the vagina (called "atrophic vaginitis") which cause discomfort, especially during and after intercourse.

Estrogens can be prescribed to treat these symptoms of the menopause. It is estimated that considerably more than half of all women undergoing the menopause have only mild symptoms or no symptoms at all and therefore do not need estrogens. Other women may need estrogens for a few months, while their bodies adjust to lower estrogen levels. Sometimes the need will be for periods longer than six months. In an attempt to avoid overstimulation of the uterus (womb), estrogens are usually given cyclically during each month of use, such as three weeks of pills followed by one week without pills.

Sometimes women experience nervous symptoms or depression during menopause. There is no evidence that estrogens are effective for such symptoms without associated vasomotor symptoms. In the absence of vasomotor symptoms, estrogens should not be used to treat nervous symptoms, although other treatment may be needed.

You may have heard that taking estrogens for long periods (years) after the menopause will keep your skin soft and supple and keep you feeling young. There is no evidence that this is so, however, and such long-term treatment carries important risks.

ESTROGENS TO PREVENT SWELLING OF THE BREASTS AFTER PREGNANCY

If you do not breast-feed your baby after delivery, your breasts may fill up with milk and become painful and engorged. This usually begins about 3 to 4 days after delivery and may last for a few days to up to a week or more. Sometimes the discomfort is severe, but usually it is not and can be controlled by pain-relieving drugs such as aspirin and by binding the breasts up tightly. Estrogens can be used to try to prevent the breasts from filling up. While this treatment is sometimes successful, in many cases the breasts fill up to some degree in spite of treatment. The dose of estrogens needed to prevent pain and swelling of the breasts is much larger than the dose needed to treat symptoms of the menopause and this may increase your chances of developing blood clots in the legs or lungs (see below). Therefore, it is important that you discuss the benefits and the risks of estrogen use with your doctor if you have decided not to breast-feed your baby.

THE DANGERS OF ESTROGENS

1. *Endometrial cancer.* There are reports that if estrogens are used in the postmenopausal period for more than a year, there is an increased risk of *endometrial cancer* (cancer of the lining of the uterus). Women taking estrogens have roughly 5 to 10 times as great a chance of getting this cancer as women who take no estrogens. To put this another way, while a postmenopausal woman not taking estrogens has 1 chance in 1,000 each year of getting endometrial cancer, a woman taking estrogens has 5 to 10 chances in 1,000 each year. For this reason *it is important to take estrogens only when they are really needed.*

The risk of this cancer is greater the longer estrogens are used and when larger doses are taken. Therefore you should not take more estrogen than your doctor prescribes. *It is important to take the lowest dose of estrogen that will control symptoms and to take it only as long as it is needed.* If estrogens are needed for longer periods of time, your doctor will want to reevaluate your need for estrogens at least every six months.

Women using estrogens should report any vaginal bleeding to their doctors; such bleeding may be of no importance, but it can be an early warning of endometrial cancer. If you have undiagnosed vaginal bleeding, you should not use estrogens until a diagnosis is made and you are certain there is no endometrial cancer.

NOTE: If you have had your uterus removed (total hysterectomy), there is no danger of developing endometrial cancer.

2. *Other possible cancers.* Estrogens can cause development of other tumors in animals, such as tumors of the breast, cervix, vagina, or liver, when given for a long time. At present there is no good evidence that women using estrogen in the menopause have an increased risk of such tumors, but there is no way yet to be sure they do not; and one study raises the possibility that use of estrogens in the menopause may increase the risk of breast cancer many years later. This is a further reason to use estrogens only when clearly needed. While you are taking estrogens, it is important that you go to your doctor at least once a year for a physical examination. Also, if members of your family have had breast cancer or if you have breast nodules or abnormal mammograms (breast x-rays), your doctor may wish to carry out more frequent examinations of your breasts.

3. *Gallbladder disease.* Women who use estrogens after menopause are more likely to develop gallbladder disease needing surgery than women who do not use estrogens. Birth control pills have a similar effect.

4. *Abnormal blood clotting.* Oral contraceptives increase the risk of blood clotting in various parts of the body. This can result in a stroke (if the clot is in the brain), a heart attack (clot in a blood vessel of the heart), or a pulmonary embolus (a clot which forms in the legs or pelvis, then breaks off and travels to the lungs). Any of these can be fatal.

At this time use of estrogens in the menopause is not known to cause such blood clotting, but this has not been fully studied and there could still prove to be such a risk. It is recommended that if you have had clotting in the legs or lungs or a heart attack or stroke while you were using estrogens or birth control pills, you should not use estrogens (unless they are being used to treat cancer of the breast or prostate). If you have had a stroke or heart attack or if you have angina pectoris, estrogens should be used with great caution and only if clearly needed (for example, if you have severe symptoms of the menopause).

The larger doses of estrogen used to prevent swelling of the breasts after pregnancy have been reported to cause clotting in the legs and lungs.

SPECIAL WARNING ABOUT PREGNANCY

You should not receive estrogen if you are pregnant. If this should occur, there is a greater than usual chance that the developing child will be born with a birth defect, although the possibility remains fairly small. A female child may have an increased risk of developing cancer of the vagina or cervix later in life (in the teens or twenties). Every possible effort should be made to avoid exposure to estrogen during pregnancy. If exposure occurs, see your doctor.

OTHER EFFECTS OF ESTROGENS

In addition to the serious known risks of estrogens described above, estrogens have the following side effects and potential risks:

1. *Nausea and vomiting.* The most common side effect of estrogen therapy is nausea. Vomiting is less common.
2. *Effects on breasts.* Estrogens may cause breast tenderness or enlargement and may cause the breasts to secrete a liquid. These effects are not dangerous.
3. *Effects on the uterus.* Estrogens may cause benign fibroid tumors of the uterus to get larger.
4. *Effects on liver.* Women taking oral contraceptives develop on rare occasions a tumor of the liver which can rupture and bleed into the abdomen and may cause death. So far, these tumors have not been reported in women using estrogens in the menopause, but you should report any swelling or unusual pain or tenderness in the abdomen to your doctor immediately.

Women with a past history of jaundice (yellowing of the skin and white parts of the eyes) may get jaundice again during estrogen use. If this occurs, stop taking estrogens and see your doctor.

5. *Other effects.* Estrogens may cause excess fluid to be retained in the body. This may make some conditions worse, such as asthma, epilepsy, migraine, heart disease, or kidney disease.

SUMMARY

Estrogens have important uses, but they have serious risks as well. You must decide, with your doctor, whether the risks are acceptable to you in view of the benefits of treatment. Except where your doctor has prescribed estrogens for use in special cases of cancer of the breast or prostate, you should not use estrogens if you have cancer of the breast or uterus, are pregnant, have undiagnosed abnormal vaginal bleeding, clotting in the legs or lungs, or have had a stroke, heart attack or angina, or clotting in the legs or lungs in the past while you were taking estrogens.

You can use estrogens as safely as possible by understanding that your doctor will require regular physical examinations while you are taking them and will try to discontinue the drug as soon as possible and use the smallest dose possible. Be alert for signs of trouble including:

1. Abnormal bleeding from the vagina.
2. Pains in the calves or chest or sudden shortness of breath, or coughing blood.
3. Severe headache, dizziness, faintness, or changes in vision.
4. Breast lumps (you should ask your doctor how to examine your own breasts).
5. Jaundice (yellowing of the skin).
6. Mental depression.

Your doctor has prescribed this drug for you and you alone. Do not give the drug to anyone else.

PREMARIN® ℞
[*prĕm 'a-rin*]
(CONJUGATED ESTROGENS)
VAGINAL CREAM
in a nonliquefying base

CAUTION: Federal law prohibits dispensing without prescription.

1. ESTROGENS HAVE BEEN REPORTED TO INCREASE THE RISK OF ENDOMETRIAL CARCINOMA.
Three independent case control studies have reported an increased risk of endometrial cancer in postmenopausal women exposed to exogenous estrogens for more than one year.[1–3] This risk was independent of the other known risk factors for endometrial cancer. These studies are further supported by the finding that incidence rates of endometrial cancer have increased sharply since 1969 in eight different areas of the United States with population-based cancer reporting systems, an increase which may be related to the rapidly expanding use of estrogens during the last decade.[4]
The three case control studies reported that the risk of endometrial cancer in estrogen users was about 4.5 to 13.9 times greater than in nonusers. The risk appears to depend on both duration of treatment[1] and on estrogen dose.[3] In view of these findings, when estrogens are used for the treatment of menopausal symptoms, the lowest dose that will control symptoms should be utilized and medication should be discontinued as soon as possible. When prolonged treatment is medically indicated, the patient should be reassessed on at least a semiannual basis to determine the need for continued therapy. Although the evidence must be considered preliminary, one study suggests that cyclic administration of low doses of estrogen may carry less risk than continuous administration;[3] it therefore appears prudent to utilize such a regimen.
Close clinical surveillance of all women taking estrogens is important. In all cases of undiagnosed persistent or recurring abnormal vaginal bleeding, adequate diagnostic measures should be undertaken to rule out malignancy.
There is no evidence at present that "natural" estrogens are more or less hazardous than "synthetic" estrogens at equiestrogenic doses.
2. ESTROGENS SHOULD NOT BE USED DURING PREGNANCY.
The use of female sex hormones, both estrogens and progestogens, during early pregnancy may seriously damage the offspring. It has been shown that females exposed in utero to diethylstilbestrol, a non-steroidal estrogen, have an increased risk of developing in later life a form of vaginal or cervical cancer that is ordinarily extremely rare.[5,6] This risk has been estimated as not greater than 4 per 1,000 exposures.[7] Furthermore, a high percentage of such exposed women (from 30% to 90%) have been found to have vaginal adenosis,[8–12] epithelial changes of the vagina and cervix. Although these changes are histologically benign, it is not known whether they are precursors of malignancy. Although similar data are not available with the use of other estrogens, it cannot be presumed they would not induce similar changes.
Several reports suggest an association between intrauterine exposure to female sex hormones and congenital anomalies, including congenital heart defects and limb reduction defects.[13–16] One case control study[16] estimated a 4.7-fold increased risk of limb reduction defects in infants exposed in utero to sex hormones (oral contraceptives, hormone withdrawal tests for pregnancy, or attempted treatment for threatened abortion). Some of these exposures were very short and involved only a few days of treatment. The data suggest that the risk of limb reduction defects in exposed fetuses is somewhat less than 1 per 1,000.
In the past, female sex hormones have been used during pregnancy in an attempt to treat threatened or habitual abortion. There is considerable evidence that estrogens are ineffective for these indications, and there is no evidence from well-controlled studies that progestogens are effective for these uses.
If PREMARIN (conjugated estrogens) Vaginal Cream is used during pregnancy, or if the patient becomes pregnant while taking this drug, she should be apprised of the potential risks to the fetus, and the advisability of pregnancy continuation.

DESCRIPTION

Each gram of PREMARIN (conjugated estrogens) Vaginal Cream contains 0.625 mg conjugated estrogens. USP, in a nonliquefying base containing cetyl esters wax, cetyl alcohol, white wax, glyceryl monostearate, propylene glycol monostearate, methyl stearate, phenylethyl alcohol, sodium lauryl sulfate, glycerin, and mineral oil. PREMARIN Vaginal Cream is applied intravaginally.
PREMARIN (Conjugated Estrogens) is a mixture of estrogens, obtained exclusively from natural sources, occurring as the sodium salts of water-soluble estrogen sulfates blended to represent the average composition of material derived from pregnant mares' urine. It contains estrone, equilin, and 17 α-dihydroequilin, together with smaller amounts of 17 α-estradiol, equilenin, and 17 α-dihydroequilenin as salts of their sulfate esters.

CLINICAL PHARMACOLOGY

Estrogens are important in the development and maintenance of the female reproductive system and secondary sex characteristics. They promote growth and development of the vagina, uterus, and fallopian tubes, and enlargement of the breasts. Indirectly, they contribute to the shaping of the skeleton, maintenance of tone and elasticity of urogenital structures, changes in the epiphyses of the long bones that allow for the pubertal growth spurt and its termination, growth of axillary and pubic hair, and pigmentation of the nipples and genitals. Decline of estrogenic activity at the end of the menstrual cycle can bring on menstruation, although the cessation of progesterone secretion is the most important factor in the mature ovulatory cycle. However, in the preovulatory or nonovulatory cycle, estrogen is the primary determinant in the onset of menstruation. Estrogens also affect the release of pituitary gonadotropins.
The pharmacologic effects of conjugated estrogens are similar to those of endogenous estrogens. They are soluble in water and may be absorbed from mucosal surfaces after local administration.
In responsive tissues (female genital organs, breasts, hypothalamus, pituitary) estrogens enter the cell and are transported into the nucleus. As a result of estrogen action, specific RNA and protein synthesis occurs.
Metabolism and inactivation occur primarily in the liver. Some estrogens are excreted into the bile; however, they are reabsorbed from the intestine and returned to the liver through the portal venous system. Water-soluble estrogen conjugates are strongly acidic and are ionized in body fluids, which favor excretion through the kidneys since tubular reabsorption is minimal.

INDICATIONS AND USAGE

PREMARIN (Conjugated Estrogen) Vaginal Cream is indicated in the treatment of atrophic vaginitis and kraurosis vulvae.
PREMARIN Vaginal Cream HAS NOT BEEN SHOWN TO BE EFFECTIVE FOR ANY PURPOSE DURING PREGNANCY AND ITS USE MAY CAUSE SEVERE HARM TO THE FETUS (SEE BOXED WARNING).
Concomitant Progestin Use: The lowest effective dose appropriate for the specific indication should be utilized. Studies of the addition of a progestin for 7 or more days of a cycle of estrogen administration have reported a lowered incidence of endometrial hyperplasia. Morphological and biochemical studies of the endometrium suggest that 10 to 13 days of progestin are needed to provide maximal maturation of the endometrium and to eliminate any hyperplastic changes. Whether this will provide protection from endometrial carcinoma has not been clearly established. There are possible additional risks which may be associated with the inclusion of progestin in estrogen replacement regimens. (See PRECAUTIONS.) The choice of progestin and dosage may be important; product labeling should be reviewed to minimize possible adverse effects.

CONTRAINDICATIONS

Estrogens should not be used in women with any of the following conditions:
1. Known or suspected cancer of the breast except in appropriately selected patients being treated for metastatic disease.
2. Known or suspected estrogen-dependent neoplasia.
3. Known or suspected pregnancy (see Boxed Warning).
4. Undiagnosed abnormal genital bleeding.
5. Active thrombophlebitis or thromboembolic disorders.
6. A past history of thrombophlebitis, thrombosis, or thromboembolic disorders associated with previous estrogen use (except when used in treatment of breast malignancy).
PREMARIN Vaginal Cream should not be used in patients hypersensitive to its ingredients.

WARNINGS

1. *Induction of malignant neoplasms.* Long-term continuous administration of natural and synthetic estrogens in certain animal species increases the frequency of carcinomas of the breast, cervix, vagina, and liver. There are now reports that estrogens increase the risk of carcinoma of the endometrium in humans. (see Boxed Warning.)
At the present time there is no satisfactory evidence that estrogens given to postmenopausal women increase the risk of cancer of the breast,[17] although a recent long-term follow-up of a single physician's practice has raised this possibility.[18] Because of the animal data, there is a need for caution in prescribing estrogens for women with a strong family history of breast cancer or who have breast nodules, fibrocystic disease, or abnormal mammograms.
2. *Gallbladder disease.* A recent study has reported a 2- to 3-fold increase in the risk of surgically confirmed gallbladder disease in women receiving postmenopausal estrogens,[17] similar to the 2-fold increase previously noted in users of oral contraceptives.[19,24a]
3. *Effects similar to those caused by estrogen-progestogen oral contraceptives.* There are several serious adverse effects of oral contraceptives, most of which have not, up to now, been documented as consequences of postmenopausal estrogen therapy. This may reflect the comparatively low doses of estrogen used in postmenopausal women. It would be expected that the larger doses of estrogen used to treat prostatic or breast cancer or postpartum breast engorgement are more likely to result in these adverse effects, and, in fact, it has been shown that there is an increased risk of thrombosis in men receiving estrogens for prostatic cancer and women for postpartum breast engorgement.[20–23]
a. *Thromboembolic disease.* It is now well established that users of oral contraceptives have an increased risk of various thromboembolic and thrombotic vascular diseases, such as thrombophlebitis, pulmonary embolism, stroke, and myocardial infarction.[24–31] Cases of retinal thrombosis, mesenteric thrombosis, and optic neuritis have been reported in oral contraceptive users. There is evidence that the risk of several of these adverse reactions is related to the dose of the drug.[32,33] An increased risk of postsurgery thromboembolic complications has also been reported in users of oral contraceptives.[34,35] If feasible, estrogen should be discontinued at least 4 weeks before surgery of the type associated with an increased risk of thromboembolism, or during periods of prolonged immobilization.
While an increased rate of thromboembolic and thrombotic disease in postmenopausal users of estrogens has not been found,[17–24,25–36] this does not rule out the possibility that such an increase may be present or that subgroups of women who have underlying risk factors or who are receiving relatively large doses of estrogens may have increased risk. Therefore estrogens should not be used in persons with active thrombophlebitis or thromboembolic disorders, and they should not be used (except in treatment of malignancy) in persons with a history of such disorders in association with estrogen use. They should be used with caution in patients with cerebral vascular or coronary artery disease and only for those in whom estrogens are clearly needed.
Large doses of estrogen (5 mg conjugated estrogens per day), comparable to those used to treat cancer of the prostate and breast, have been shown in a large prospective clinical trial in men[37] to increase the risk of nonfatal myocardial infarction, pulmonary embolism and thrombophlebitis. When estrogen doses of this size are used, any of the thromboembolic and thrombotic adverse effects associated with oral contraceptive use should be considered a clear risk.
b. *Hepatic adenoma.* Benign hepatic adenomas appear to be associated with the use of oral contraceptives.[38–40] Although benign, and rare, these may rupture and may cause death through intra-abdominal hemorrhage. Such lesions have not yet been reported in association with other estrogen or progestogen preparations but should be considered in estrogen users having abdominal pain and tenderness, abdominal mass, or hypovolemic shock. Hepatocellular carcinoma has also been reported in women taking estrogen-containing oral contraceptives.[39] The relationship of this malignancy to these drugs is not known at this time.
c. *Elevated blood pressure.* Women using oral contraceptives sometimes experience increased blood pressure which, in most cases, returns to normal on discontinuing the drug. There is now a report that this may occur with use of estrogens in the menopause[41] and blood pressure should be monitored with estrogen use, especially if high doses are used.
d. *Glucose tolerance.* A worsening of glucose tolerance has been observed in a significant percentage of patients on estrogen-containing oral contraceptives. For this reason, diabetic patients should be carefully observed while receiving estrogen.
4. *Hypercalcemia.* Administration of estrogens may lead to severe hypercalcemia in patients with breast cancer and bone metastases. If this occurs, the drug should be stopped and appropriate measures taken to reduce the serum calcium level.

PRECAUTIONS

A. General Precautions.
1. A complete medical and family history should be taken prior to the initiation of any estrogen therapy. The pretreatment and periodic physical examinations should include special reference to blood pressure, breasts, abdomen, and pelvic organs, and should include a Papanicolaou smear. As a general rule, estrogen should not be prescribed for longer than one year without another physical examination being performed.
2. Fluid retention—Because estrogens may cause some degree of fluid retention, conditions which might be influ-

Continued on next page

Ayerst—Cont.

enced by this factor such as asthma, epilepsy, migraine, and cardiac or renal dysfunction, require careful observation.
3. Certain patients may develop undesirable manifestations of excessive estrogenic stimulation, such as abnormal or excessive uterine bleeding, mastodynia, etc.
4. Prolonged administration of unopposed estrogen therapy has been reported to increase the risk of endometrial hyperplasia in some patients.
5. Oral contraceptives appear to be associated with an increased incidence of mental depression.[24a] Although it is not clear whether this is due to the estrogenic or progestogenic component of the contraceptive, patients with a history of depression should be carefully observed.
6. Preexisting uterine leiomyomata may increase in size during estrogen use.
7. The pathologist should be advised of estrogen therapy when relevant specimens are submitted.
8. Patients with a past history of jaundice during pregnancy have an increased risk of recurrence of jaundice while receiving estrogen-containing oral contraceptive therapy. If jaundice develops in any patient receiving estrogen, the medication should be discontinued while the cause is investigated.
9. Estrogens may be poorly metabolized in patients with impaired liver function and they should be administered with caution in such patients.
10. Because estrogens influence the metabolism of calcium and phosphorus, they should be used with caution in patients with metabolic bone diseases that are associated with hypercalcemia or in patients with renal insufficiency.
11. Because of the effects of estrogens on epiphyseal closure, they should be used judiciously in young patients in whom bone growth is not complete.
12. If concomitant progestin therapy is used, potential risks may include adverse effects on carbohydrate and lipid metabolism.

B. Information for Patients. See text which appears after the PHYSICIAN REFERENCES.

C. Drug Laboratory Test Interactions. Certain endocrine and liver function tests may be affected by estrogen-containing oral contraceptives. The following similar changes may be expected with larger doses of estrogen:
a. Increased sulfobromophthalein retention.
b. Increased prothrombin and factors VII, VIII, IX, and X; decreased antithrombin 3; increased norepinephrine-induced platelet aggregability.
c. Increased thyroid binding globulin (TBG) leading to increased circulating total thyroid hormone, as measured by PBI, T4 by column, or T4 by radioimmunoassay. Free T3 resin uptake is decreased, reflecting the elevated TBG; free T4 concentration is unaltered.
d. Impaired glucose tolerance.
e. Decreased pregnanediol excretion.
f. Reduced response to metyrapone test.
g. Reduced serum folate concentration.
h. Increased serum triglyceride and phospholipid concentration.

D. Carcinogenesis, Mutagenesis, Impairment of Fertility. See WARNINGS section for information on carcinogenesis.

E. Pregnancy Category X. See CONTRAINDICATIONS and Boxed Warning.

F. Nursing Mothers. It is now known whether this drug is excreted in human milk. Because many drugs are excreted in human milk and because of the potential for serious adverse reactions in nursing infants from estrogens, a decision should be made whether to discontinue nursing or to discontinue the drug, taking into account the importance of the drug to the mother.

G. Pediatric Use. Safety and effectiveness in children have not been established.

ADVERSE REACTIONS

(See WARNINGS regarding induction of neoplasia, adverse effects on the fetus, increased incidence of gallbladder disease, and adverse effects similar to those of oral contraceptives, including thromboembolism.) The following additional adverse reactions have been reported with estrogenic therapy, including oral contraceptives.
1. *Genitourinary system:* Breakthrough bleeding, spotting, change in menstrual flow; dysmenorrhea; premenstrual-like syndrome; amenorrhea during and after treatment; increase in size of uterine fibromyomata; vaginal candidiasis; change in cervical erosion and in degree of cervical secretion; cystitis-like syndrome.
2. *Breasts:* Tenderness, enlargement, secretion.
3. *Gastrointestinal:* Nausea, vomiting; abdominal cramps, bloating; cholestatic jaundice.
4. *Skin:* Chloasma or melasma which may persist when drug is discontinued; erythema multiforme; erythema nodosum; hemorrhagic eruption; loss of scalp hair; hirsutism.
5. *Eyes:* Steepening of corneal curvature; intolerance to contact lenses.
6. *CNS:* Headache, migraine, dizziness; mental depression; chorea.
7. *Miscellaneous:* Increase or decrease in weight; reduced carbohydrate tolerance; aggravation of porphyria; edema; changes in libido.

OVERDOSAGE

Numerous reports of ingestion of large doses of estrogen-containing oral contraceptives by young children indicate that acute serious ill effects do not occur. Overdosage of estrogen may cause nausea, and withdrawal bleeding may occur in females.

DOSAGE AND ADMINISTRATION

Given cyclically for short-term use only:
For treatment of atrophic vaginitis, or kraurosis vulvae.
The lowest dose that will control symptoms should be chosen and medication should be discontinued as promptly as possible.
Administration should be cyclic (e.g., three weeks on and one week off).
Attempts to discontinue or taper medication should be made at three to six month intervals.
Usual dosage range: 2 to 4 g (½ applicatorful to 1 applicatorful) daily, intravaginally or topically, depending on the severity of the condition.
Treated patients with an intact uterus should be monitored closely for signs of endometrial cancer and appropriate diagnostic measures should be taken to rule out malignancy in the event of persistent or recurring abnormal vaginal bleeding.

HOW SUPPLIED

PREMARIN (Conjugated Estrogens) Vaginal Cream—Each gram contains 0.625 mg conjugated estrogens, USP. (Also contains cetyl esters wax, cetyl alcohol, white wax, glyceryl monostearate, propylene glycol monostearate, methyl stearate, phenylethyl alcohol, sodium lauryl sulfate, glycerin, and mineral oil.)
Combination package: Each contains Net Wt. 1½ oz (42.5 g) tube with one plastic applicator calibrated in 1 g increments to a maximum of 4 g (NDC 0046-0872-93).
Also Available—Refill package: Each contains Net Wt. 1½ oz (42.5 g) tube (NDC 0046-0872-01).

PHYSICIAN REFERENCES

1. Ziel, H. K., *et al.*: N. Engl. J. Med. *293*:1167–1170, 1975.
2. Smith, D. C., *et al.*: N. Engl. J. Med. *293*:1164–1167, 1975.
3. Mack, T. M., *et al.*: N. Engl. J. Med *294*:1262–1267, 1976.
4. Weiss, N. S., *et al.*: N. Engl. J. Med. *294*:1259–1262, 1976.
5. Herbst, A. L., *et al.*: N. Engl. J. Med. *284*:878–881, 1971.
6. Greenwald, P., *et al.*: N. Engl. J. Med. *285*:390–392, 1971.
7. Lanier, A., *et al.*: Mayo Clin. Proc. *48*:793–799, 1973.
8. Herbst, A., *et al.*: Obstet. Gynecol. *40*:287–298, 1972.
9. Herbst, A., *et al.*: Am. J. Obstet. Gynecol. *118*:607–615, 1974.
10. Herbst, A., *et al.*: N. Engl. J. Med. *292*:334–339, 1975.
11. Stafl, A., *et al.*: Obstet. Gynecol. *43*:118–128, 1974.
12. Sherman, A. I., *et al.*: Obstet. Gynecol. *44*:531–545, 1974.
13. Gal, I., *et al.*: Nature *216*:83, 1967.
14. Levy, E. P., *et al.*: Lancet *1*:611, 1973.
15. Nora, J., *et al.*: Lancet *1*:941–942, 1973.
16. Janerich, D. T., *et al.*: N. Engl. J. Med. *291*:697–700, 1974.
17. Boston Collaborative Drug Surveillance Program: N. Engl. J. Med. *290*:15–19, 1974.
18. Hoover, R., *et al.*: N. Engl. J. Med. *295*:401–405, 1976.
19. Boston Collaborative Drug Surveillance Program: Lancet *1*:1399–1404, 1973.
20. Daniel, D. G., *et al.*: Lancet *2*:287–289, 1967.
21. The Veterans Administration Cooperative Urological Research Group: J. Urol. *98*:516–522, 1967.
22. Bailar, J. C.: Lancet *2*:560, 1967.
23. Blackard, C., *et al.*: Cancer *26*:249–256, 1970.
24. Royal College of General Practitioners: J. R. Coll. Gen. Pract. *13*:267–279, 1967.

24a. Royal College of General Practitioners: Oral Contraceptives and Health, New York, Pitman Corp., 1974.

25. Inman, W. H. W., *et al.*: Br. Med. J. *2*:193–199, 1968.
26. Vessey, M. P., *et al.*: Br. Med. J. *2*:651–657, 1969.
27. Sartwell, P. E., *et al.*: Am. J. Epidemiol. *90*:365–380, 1969.
28. Collaborative Group for the Study of Stroke in Young Women: N. Engl. J. Med. *288*:871–878, 1973.
29. Collaborative Group for the Study of Stroke in Young Women: J.A.M.A. *231*:718–722, 1975.
30. Mann, J. I., *et al.*: Br. Med. J. *2*:245–248, 1975.
31. Mann, J. I., *et al.*: Br. Med. J. *2*:241–245, 1975.
32. Inman, W. H. W., *et al.*: Br. Med. J. *2*:203–209, 1970.
33. Stolley, P. D., *et al.*: Am. J. Epidemiol. *102*:197–208, 1975.
34. Vessey, M. P., *et al.*: Br. Med. J. *3*:123–126, 1970.
35. Greene, G. R., *et al.*: Am. J. Public Health *62*:680–685, 1972.
36. Rosenberg, L., *et al.*: N. Engl. J. Med. *294*:1256–1259, 1976.
37. Coronary Drug Project Research Group: J.A.M.A. *214*:1303–1313, 1970.
38. Baum, J., *et al.*: Lancet *2*:926–928, 1973.
39. Mays, E. T., *et al.*: J.A.M.A. *235*:730–732, 1976.
40. Edmondson, H. A., *et al.*: N. Engl. J. Med. *294*:470–472, 1976.
41. Pfeffer, R. I., *et al.*: Am. J. Epidemiol. *103*:445–456, 1976.

INFORMATION FOR THE PATIENT

WHAT YOU SHOULD KNOW ABOUT ESTROGENS

Estrogens are female hormones produced by the ovaries. The ovaries make several different kinds of estrogens. In addition, scientists have been able to make a variety of synthetic estrogens. As far as we know, all these estrogens have similar properties and therefore much the same usefulness, side effects, and risks. This leaflet is intended to help you understand what estrogens are used for, the risks involved in their use, and how to use them as safely as possible.
This leaflet includes the most important information about estrogens, but not all the information. If you want to know more, you should ask your doctor for more information or you can ask your doctor or pharmacist to let you read the package insert prepared for the doctor.

USES OF ESTROGEN

THERE IS NO PROPER USE OF ESTROGENS IN A PREGNANT WOMAN

Estrogens are prescribed by doctors for a number of purposes, including:
1. To provide estrogen during a period of adjustment when a woman's ovaries stop producing a majority of her estrogens, in order to prevent certain uncomfortable symptoms of estrogen deficiency. (With the menopause, which generally occurs between the ages of 45 and 55, women produce a much smaller amount of estrogens.)
2. To prevent symptoms of estrogen deficiency when a woman's ovaries have been removed surgically before the natural menopause.
3. To prevent pregnancy. (Estrogens are given along with a progestogen, another female hormone; these combinations are called oral contraceptives or birth control pills. Patient labeling is available to women taking oral contraceptives and they will not be discussed in this leaflet.)
4. To treat certain cancers in women and men.
5. To prevent painful swelling of the breasts after pregnancy in women who choose not to nurse their babies.

ESTROGENS IN THE MENOPAUSE

In the natural course of their lives, all women eventually experience a decrease in estrogen production. This usually occurs between ages 45 and 55 but may occur earlier or later. Sometimes the ovaries may need to be removed before natural menopause by an operation, producing a "surgical menopause".
When the amount of estrogen in the blood begins to decrease, many women may develop typical symptoms: feelings of warmth in the face, neck, and chest or sudden intense episodes of heat and sweating throughout the body (called "hot flashes" or "hot flushes"). These symptoms are sometimes very uncomfortable. Some women may also develop changes in the vagina (called "atrophic vaginitis") which cause discomfort, especially during and after intercourse.
Estrogens can be prescribed to treat these symptoms of the menopause. It is estimated that considerably more than half of all women undergoing the menopause have only mild symptoms or no symptoms at all and therefore do not need estrogens. Other women may need estrogens for a few months, while their bodies adjust to lower estrogen levels. Sometimes the need will be for periods longer than six months. In an attempt to avoid overstimulation of the uterus (womb), estrogens are usually given cyclically during each month of use, such as three weeks of pills followed by one week without pills. Sometimes women experience nervous symptoms or depression during menopause. There is no evidence that estrogens are effective for such symptoms without associated vasomotor symptoms. In the absence of vasomotor symptoms, estrogens should not be used to treat nervous symptoms, although other treatment may be needed.
You may have heard that taking estrogens for long periods (years) after the menopause will keep your skin soft and supple and keep you feeling young. There is no evidence that this is so, however, and such long-term treatment carries important risks.

ESTROGENS TO PREVENT SWELLING OF THE BREASTS AFTER PREGNANCY

If you do not breast feed your baby after delivery, your breasts may fill up with milk and become painful and engorged. This usually begins about 3 to 4 days after delivery and may last for a few days to up to a week or more. Sometimes the discomfort is severe, but usually it is not and can be controlled by pain-relieving drugs such as aspirin and by binding the breasts up tightly. Estrogens can be used to try to prevent the breasts from filling up. While this treatment is sometimes successful, in many cases the breasts fill up to some degree in spite of treatment. The dose of estrogens needed to prevent pain and swelling of the breasts is much larger than the dose needed to treat symptoms of the menopause and this may increase your chances of developing blood clots in the legs or lungs (see below). Therefore, it is important that you discuss the benefits and the risks of estrogen use with your doctor if you have decided not to breast-feed your baby.

THE DANGERS OF ESTROGENS

1. *Endometrial cancer.* There are reports that if estrogens are used in the postmenopausal period for more than a year, there is an increased risk of *endometrial cancer* (cancer of the lining of the uterus). Women taking estrogens have roughly 5 to 10 times as great a chance of getting this cancer as women who take no estrogens. To put this another way, while a postmenopausal woman not taking estrogens has 1 chance in 1,000 each year of getting endometrial cancer, a woman taking estrogens has 5 to 10 chances in 1,000 each year. For this reason, *it is important to take estrogens only when they are really needed.*

The risk of this cancer is greater the longer estrogens are used and when larger doses are taken. Therefore you should not take more estrogen than your doctor prescribes. *It is important to take the lowest dose of estrogen that will control symptoms and to take it only as long as it is needed.* If estrogens are needed for longer periods of time, your doctor will want to reevaluate your need for estrogens at least every six months.

Women using estrogens should report any vaginal bleeding to their doctors; such bleeding may be of no importance, but it can be an early warning of endometrial cancer. If you have undiagnosed vaginal bleeding, you should not use estrogens until a diagnosis is made and you are certain there is no endometrial cancer.

NOTE: If you have had your uterus removed (total hysterectomy), there is no danger of developing endometrial cancer.

2. *Other possible cancers.* Estrogens can cause development of other tumors in animals, such as tumors of the breast, cervix, vagina, or liver, when given for a long time. At present there is no good evidence that women using estrogen in the menopause have an increased risk of such tumors, but there is no way yet to be sure they do not; and one study raises the possibility that use of estrogens in the menopause may increase the risk of breast cancer many years later. This is a further reason to use estrogens only when clearly needed. While you are taking estrogens, it is important that you go to your doctor at least once a year for a physical examination. Also, if members of your family have had breast cancer or if you have breast nodules or abnormal mammograms (breast x-rays), your doctor may wish to carry out more frequent examinations of your breasts.

3. *Gallbladder disease.* Women who use estrogens after menopause are more likely to develop gallbladder disease needing surgery than women who do not use estrogens. Birth control pills have a similar effect.

4. *Abnormal blood clotting.* Oral contraceptives increase the risk of blood clotting in various parts of the body. This can result in a stroke (if the clot is in the brain), a heart attack (clot in a blood vessel of the heart), or a pulmonary embolus (a clot which forms in the legs or pelvis, then breaks off and travels to the lungs). Any of these can be fatal.

At this time use of estrogens in the menopause is not known to cause such blood clotting, but this has not been fully studied and there could still prove to be such a risk. It is recommended that if you have had clotting in the legs or lungs or a heart attack or stroke while you were using estrogens or birth control pills, you should not use estrogens (unless they are being used to treat cancer of the breast or prostate). If you have had a stroke or heart attack or if you have angina pectoris, estrogens should be used with great caution and only if clearly needed (for example, if you have severe symptoms of the menopause).

The larger doses of estrogen used to prevent swelling of the breasts after pregnancy have been reported to cause clotting in the legs and lungs.

SPECIAL WARNING ABOUT PREGNANCY

You should not receive estrogen if you are pregnant. If this should occur, there is a greater than usual chance that the developing child will be born with a birth defect, although the possibility remains fairly small. A female child may have an increased risk of developing cancer of the vagina or cervix later in life (in the teens or twenties). Every possible effort should be made to avoid exposure to estrogens during pregnancy. If exposure occurs, see your doctor.

OTHER EFFECTS OF ESTROGENS

In addition to the serious known risks of estrogens described above, estrogens have the following side effects and potential risks:

1. *Nausea and vomiting.* The most common side effect of estrogen therapy is nausea. Vomiting is less common.
2. *Effects on breasts.* Estrogens may cause breast tenderness or enlargement and may cause the breasts to secrete a liquid. These effects are not dangerous.
3. *Effects on the uterus.* Estrogens may cause benign fibroid tumors of the uterus to get larger.
4. *Effects on liver.* Women taking oral contraceptives develop on rare occasions a tumor of the liver which can rupture and bleed into the abdomen and may cause death. So far, these tumors have not been reported in women using estrogens in the menopause, but you should report any swelling or unusual pain or tenderness in the abdomen to your doctor immediately.

Women with a past history of jaundice (yellowing of the skin and white parts of the eyes) may get jaundice again during estrogen use. If this occurs, stop taking estrogens and see your doctor.

5. *Other effects.* Estrogens may cause excess fluid to be retained in the body. This may make some conditions worse, such as asthma, epilepsy, migraine, heart disease, or kidney disease.

SUMMARY

Estrogens have important uses, but they have serious risks as well. You must decide, with your doctor, whether the risks are acceptable to you in view of the benefits of treatment. Except where your doctor has prescribed estrogens for use in special cases of cancer of the breast or prostate, you should not use estrogens if you have cancer of the breast or uterus, are pregnant, have undiagnosed abnormal vaginal bleeding, clotting in the legs or lungs, or have had a stroke, heart attack or angina, or clotting in the legs or lungs in the past while you were taking estrogens.

You can use estrogens as safely as possible by understanding that your doctor will require regular physical examinations while you are taking them and will try to discontinue the drug as soon as possible and use the smallest dose possible.

Be alert for signs of trouble including:

1. Abnormal bleeding from the vagina.
2. Pains in the calves or chest or sudden shortness of breath, or coughing blood.
3. Severe headache, dizziness, faintness, or changes in vision.
4. Breast lumps (you should ask your doctor how to examine your own breasts).
5. Jaundice (yellowing of the skin).
6. Mental depression.

Your doctor has prescribed this drug for you and you alone. Do not give the drug to anyone else.

HOW SUPPLIED

PREMARIN® (conjugated estrogens tablets, USP)—tablets for oral administration.

Each oval *purple* tablet contains 2.5 mg
Each oval *yellow* tablet contains 1.25 mg
Each oval *white* tablet contains 0.9 mg
Each oval *maroon* tablet contains 0.625 mg
Each oval *green* tablet contains 0.3 mg

PREMARIN® with METHYLTESTOSTERONE—a combination of PREMARIN and methyltestosterone (an androgen), in tablet form for oral administration.

Each round *yellow* tablet contains 1.25 mg PREMARIN and 10 mg methyltestosterone
Each round *maroon* tablet contains 0.625 mg PREMARIN and 5 mg methyltestosterone

PMB® 200, 400—a combination of PREMARIN® and meprobamate (a tranquilizing agent) in tablet form for oral administration.

Each oblong *green* tablet contains 0.45 mg PREMARIN and 200 mg meprobamate
Each oblong *pink* tablet contains 0.45 mg PREMARIN and 400 mg meprobamate

The appearance of these tablets is a trademark of Ayerst Laboratories.

PREMARIN® VAGINAL CREAM—PREMARIN® in a nonliquefying base, designed for vaginal use.

PREMARIN® INTRAVENOUS—PREMARIN® specially prepared for intravenous and intramuscular use.

ESTROGENIC SUBSTANCE (Estrone) in Aqueous Suspension—a sterile aqueous suspension of estrone, a short-acting estrogen, for intramuscular injection only.

Shown in Product Identification Section, page 404

PREMARIN® ℞

[prem 'a-rin with meth "yl-tĕs-tŏs 'ta-rōn]

(conjugated estrogens, USP)
with METHYLTESTOSTERONE

No. 879—Each yellow tablet contains:
Premarin® (conjugated estrogens, USP) .... 1.25 mg
Methyltestosterone .... 10.0 mg
No. 878—Each maroon tablet contains:
Premarin® (conjugated estrogens, USP) .... 0.625 mg
Methyltestosterone .... 5.0 mg

CAUTION: Federal law prohibits dispensing without prescription.

1. ESTROGENS HAVE BEEN REPORTED TO INCREASE THE RISK OF ENDOMETRIAL CARCINOMA.

Three independent case control studies have reported an increased risk of endometrial cancer in postmenopausal women exposed to exogenous estrogens for more than one year.[1-3] This risk was independent of the other known risk factors for endometrial cancer. These studies are further supported by the finding that incidence rates of endometrial cancer have increased sharply since 1969 in eight different areas of the United States with population-based cancer reporting systems, an increase which may be related to the rapidly expanding use of estrogens during the last decade.[4]

The three case control studies reported that the risk of endometrial cancer in estrogen users was about 4.5 to 13.9 times greater than in nonusers. The risk appears to depend on both duration of treatment[1] and on estrogen dose.[3] In view of these findings, when estrogens are used for the treatment of menopausal symptoms, the lowest dose that will control symptoms should be utilized and medication should be discontinued as soon as possible. When prolonged treatment is medically indicated, the patient should be reassessed on at least a semiannual basis to determine the need for continued therapy. Although the evidence must be considered preliminary, one study suggests that cyclic administration of low doses of estrogen may carry less risk than continuous administration;[3] it therefore appears prudent to utilize such a regimen.

Close clinical surveillance of all women taking estrogens is important. In all cases of undiagnosed persistent or recurring abnormal vaginal bleeding, adequate diagnostic measures should be undertaken to rule out malignancy.

There is no evidence at present that "natural" estrogens are more or less hazardous than "synthetic" estrogens at equiestrogenic doses.

2. ESTROGENS SHOULD NOT BE USED DURING PREGNANCY.

The use of female sex hormones, both estrogens and progestogens, during early pregnancy may seriously damage the offspring. It has been shown that females exposed in utero to diethylstilbestrol, a non-steroidal estrogen, have an increased risk of developing in later life a form of vaginal or cervical cancer that is ordinarily extremely rare.[5,6] This risk has been estimated as not greater than 4 per 1,000 exposures.[7] Furthermore, a high percentage of such exposed women (from 30% to 90%) have been found to have vaginal adenosis,[8-12] epithelial changes of the vagina and cervix. Although these changes are histologically benign, it is not known whether they are precursors of malignancy. Although similar data are not available with the use of other estrogens, it cannot be presumed they would not induce similar changes.

Several reports suggest an association between intrauterine exposure to female sex hormones and congenital anomalies, including congenital heart defects and limb reduction defects.[13-16] One case control study[16] estimated a 4.7-fold increased risk of limb reduction defects in infants exposed in utero to sex hormones (oral contraceptives, hormone withdrawal tests for pregnancy, or attempted treatment for threatened abortion). Some of these exposures were very short and involved only a few days of treatment. The data suggest that the risk of limb reduction defects in exposed fetuses is somewhat less than 1 per 1,000.

In the past, female sex hormones have been used during pregnancy in an attempt to treat threatened or habitual abortion. There is considerable evidence that estrogens are ineffective for these indications, and there is no evidence from well-controlled studies that progestogens are effective for these uses.

If PREMARIN with METHYLTESTOSTERONE is used during pregnancy, or if the patient becomes pregnant while taking this drug, she should be apprised of the potential risks to the fetus, and the advisability of pregnancy continuation.

DESCRIPTION

PREMARIN with METHYLTESTOSTERONE is provided in tablets for oral administration.

PREMARIN (conjugated estrogens, USP) is a mixture of estrogens, obtained exclusively from natural sources, occurring as the sodium salts of water-soluble estrogen sulfates blended to represent the average composition of material derived from pregnant mares' urine. It contains estrone,

Continued on next page

Ayerst—Cont.

equilin, and 17 α-dihydroequilin, together with smaller amounts of 17 α-estradiol, equilenin, and 17 α-dihydroequilenin as salts of their sulfate esters.
Methyltestosterone is an androgen.
Androgens are derivatives of cyclopentano-perhydrophenanthrene. Endogenous androgens are C-19 steroids with a side chain at C-17, and with two angular methyl groups. Testosterone is the primary endogenous androgen. Fluoxymesterone and methyltestosterone are synthetic derivatives of testosterone.
Methyltestosterone is a white to light yellow crystalline substance that is virtually insoluble in water but soluble in organic solvents. It is stable in air but decomposes in light.
PREMARIN with METHYLTESTOSTERONE Tablets contain the following inactive ingredients: calcium phosphate tribasic, calcium sulfate anhydrous, carnauba wax, FD&C Blue No. 2, FD&C Yellow No. 6, glyceryl mono-oleate, guar gum, lactose, magnesium stearate, methylcellulose, microcrystalline cellulose, pharmaceutical glaze, polyethylene glycol, stearic acid, sucrose, titanium dioxide.
—0.625 mg PREMARIN with 5.0 mg METHYLTESTOSTERONE. Tablets also contain: FD&C Red No. 3.
—1.25 mg PREMARIN with 10.0 mg METHYLTESTOSTERONE. Tablets also contain: Black iron oxide, D&C Yellow No. 10, FD&C Red No. 40.

CLINICAL PHARMACOLOGY

Estrogens. Estrogens are important in the development and maintenance of the female reproductive system and secondary sex characteristics. They promote growth and development of the vagina, uterus, and fallopian tubes, and enlargement of the breasts. Indirectly, they contribute to the shaping of the skeleton, maintenance of tone and elasticity of urogenital structures, changes in the epiphyses of the long bones that allow for the pubertal growth spurt and its termination, growth of axillary and pubic hair, and pigmentation of the nipples and genitals. Decline of estrogenic activity at the end of the menstrual cycle can bring on menstruation, although the cessation of progesterone secretion is the most important factor in the mature ovulatory cycle. However, in the preovulatory or nonovulatory cycle, estrogen is the primary determinant in the onset of menstruation. Estrogens also affect the release of pituitary gonadotropins.
The pharmacologic effects of conjugated estrogens are similar to those of endogenous estrogens. They are soluble in water and are well absorbed from the gastrointestinal tract.
In responsive tissues (female genital organs, breasts, hypothalamus, pituitary) estrogens enter the cell and are transported into the nucleus. As a result of estrogen action, specific RNA and protein synthesis occurs.

Estrogen Pharmacokinetics

Metabolism and inactivation occur primarily in the liver. Some estrogens are excreted into the bile; however they are reabsorbed from the intestine and returned to the liver through the portal venous system. Water soluble estrogen conjugates are strongly acidic and are ionized in body fluids, which favor excretion through the kidneys since tubular reabsorption is minimal.

Androgens. Endogenous androgens are responsible for the normal growth and development of the male sex organs and for maintenance of secondary sex characteristics. These effects include the growth and maturation of prostate, seminal vesicles, penis, and scrotum; the development of male hair distribution, such as beard, pubic, chest, and axillary hair, laryngeal enlargement, vocal chord thickening, alterations in body musculature, and fat distribution. Drugs in this class also cause retention of nitrogen, sodium, potassium, phosphorus, and decreased urinary excretion of calcium. Androgens have been reported to increase protein anabolism and decrease protein catabolism. Nitrogen balance is improved only when there is sufficient intake of calories and protein.
Androgens are responsible for the growth spurt of adolescence and for the eventual termination of linear growth which is brought about by fusion of the epiphyseal growth centers. In children, exogenous androgens accelerate linear growth rates, but may cause a disproportionate advancement in bone maturation. Use over long periods may result in fusion of the eiphyseal growth centers and termination of growth process. Androgens have been reported to stimulate the production of red blood cells by enhancing the production of erythropoietic stimulating factor.

Androgen Pharmacokinetics

Testosterone given orally is metabolized by the gut and 44 percent is cleared by the liver in the first pass. Oral doses as high as 400 mg per day are needed to achieve clinically effective blood levels for full replacement therapy. The synthetic androgens (methyltestosterone and fluoxymesterone) are less extensively metabolized by the liver and have longer half-lives. They are more suitable than testosterone for oral administration.
Testosterone in plasma is 98% bound to a specific testosterone-estradiol binding globulin, and about 2% is free. Generally, the amount of this sex-hormone binding globulin in the plasma will determine the distribution of testosterone between free and bound forms, and the free testosterone concentration will determine its half-life.
About 90% of a dose of testosterone is excreted in the urine as glucuronic and sulfuric acid conjugates of testosterone and its metabolites; about 6% of a dose is excreted in the feces, mostly in the unconjugated form. Inactivation of testosterone occurs primarily in the liver. Testosterone is metabolized to various 17-keto steroids through two different pathways. There are considerable variations of the half-life of testosterone as reported in the literature, ranging from 10 to 100 minutes.
In many tissues the activity of testosterone appears to depend on reduction to dihydrotestosterone, which binds to cytosol receptor proteins. The steroid-receptor complex is transported to the nucleus where it initiates transcription events and cellular changes related to androgen action.

INDICATIONS

PREMARIN (conjugated estrogens, USP) with METHYLTESTOSTERONE is indicated in the treatment of:
Moderate to severe *vasomotor* symptoms associated with the menopause in those patients not improved by estrogens alone. (There is no evidence that estrogens are effective for nervous symptoms or depression without associated vasomotor symptoms, and they should not be used to treat such conditions.)
PREMARIN with METHYLTESTOSTERONE HAS NOT BEEN SHOWN TO BE EFFECTIVE FOR ANY PURPOSE DURING PREGNANCY AND ITS USE MAY CAUSE SEVERE HARM TO THE FETUS (SEE BOXED WARNING).

CONTRAINDICATIONS

Estrogens should not be used in women with any of the following conditions:
1. Known or suspected cancer of the breast except in appropriately selected patients being treated for metastatic disease.
2. Known or suspected estrogen-dependent neoplasia.
3. Known or suspected pregnancy (see Boxed Warning).
4. Undiagnosed abnormal genital bleeding.
5. Active thrombophlebitis or thromboembolic disorders.
6. A past history of thrombophlebitis, thrombosis, or thromboembolic disorders associated with previous estrogen use (except when used in treatment of breast malignancy).

Methyltestosterone should not be used in:
1. The presence of severe liver damage.
2. Pregnancy and in breast-feeding mothers because of the possibility of masculinization of the female fetus or breast-fed infant.

WARNINGS

Associated with Estrogens

1. *Induction of malignant neoplasms.* Long term continuous administration of natural and synthetic estrogens in certain animal species increases the frequency of carcinomas of the breast, cervix, vagina, and liver. There are now reports that estrogens increase the risk of carcinoma of the endometrium in humans. (See Boxed Warning.)
At the present time there is no satisfactory evidence that estrogens given to postmenopausal women increase the risk of cancer of the breast,[17] although a recent long-term follow-up of a single physician's practice has raised this possibility.[18] Because of the animal data, there is a need for caution in prescribing estrogens for women with a strong family history of breast cancer or who have breast nodules, fibrocystic disease, or abnormal mammograms.
2. *Gallbladder disease.* A recent study has reported a 2- to 3-fold increase in the risk of surgically confirmed gallbladder disease in women receiving postmenopausal estrogens,[17] similar to the 2-fold increase previously noted in users of oral contraceptives.[19,24a]
3. *Effects similar to those caused by estrogen-progestogen oral contraceptives.* There are several serious adverse effects of oral contraceptives, most of which have not, up to now, been documented as consequences of postmenopausal estrogen therapy. This may reflect the comparatively low doses of estrogen used in postmenopausal women. It would be expected that the larger doses of estrogen used to treat prostatic or breast cancer or postpartum breast engorgement are more likely to result in these adverse effects, and, in fact, it has been shown that there is an increased risk of thrombosis in men receiving estrogens for prostatic cancer and women for postpartum breast engorgement.[20–23]
a. *Thromboembolic disease.* It is now well established that users of oral contraceptives have an increased risk of various thromboembolic and thrombotic vascular diseases, such as thrombophlebitis, pulmonary embolism, stroke, and myocardial infarction.[24–31] Cases of retinal thrombosis, mesenteric thrombosis, and optic neuritis have been reported in oral contraceptive users. There is evidence that the risk of several of these adverse reactions is related to the dose of the drug.[32,33] An increased risk of postsurgery thromboembolic complications has also been reported in users of oral contraceptives.[34,35] If feasible, estrogen should be discontinued at least 4 weeks before surgery of the type associated with an increased risk of thromboembolism, or during periods of prolonged immobilization.
While an increased rate of thromboembolic and thrombotic disease in postmenopausal users of estrogens has not been found,[17–24,25–36] this does not rule out the possibility that such an increase may be present or that subgroups of women who have underlying risk factors or who are receiving relatively large doses of estrogens may have increased risk. Therefore estrogens should not be used in persons with active thrombophlebitis or thromboembolic disorders, and they should not be used (except in treatment of malignancy) in persons with a history of such disorders in association with estrogen use. They should be used with caution in patients with cerebral vascular or coronary artery disease and only for those in whom estrogens are clearly needed.
Large doses of estrogen (5 mg conjugated estrogens per day), comparable to those used to treat cancer of the prostate and breast, have been shown in a large prospective clinical trial in men[37] to increase the risk of nonfatal myocardial infarction, pulmonary embolism and thrombophlebitis. When estrogen doses of this size are used, any of the thromboembolic and thrombotic adverse effects associated with oral contraceptive use should be considered a clear risk.
b. *Hepatic adenoma.* Benign hepatic adenomas appear to be associated with the use of oral contraceptives.[38–40] Although benign, and rare, these may rupture and may cause death through intra-abdominal hemorrhage. Such lesions have not yet been reported in association with other estrogen or progestogen preparations but should be considered in estrogen users having abdominal pain and tenderness, abdominal mass, or hypovolemic shock. Hepatocellular carcinoma has also been reported in women taking estrogen-containing oral contraceptives.[39] The relationship of this malignancy to these drugs is not known at this time.
c. *Elevated blood pressure.* Women using oral contraceptives sometimes experience increased blood pressure which, in most cases, returns to normal on discontinuing the drug. There is now a report that this may occur with use of estrogens in the menopause[41] and blood pressure should be monitored with estrogen use, especially if high doses are used.
d. *Glucose tolerance.* A worsening of glucose tolerance has been observed in a significant percentage of patients on estrogen-containing oral contraceptives. For this reason, diabetic patients should be carefully observed while receiving estrogen.
4. *Hypercalcemia.* Administration of estrogens may lead to severe hypercalcemia in patients with breast cancer and bone metastases. If this occurs, the drug should be stopped and appropriate measures taken to reduce the serum calcium level.

Associated with Methyltestosterone

In patients with breast cancer, androgen therapy may cause hypercalcemia by stimulating osteolysis. In this case, the drug should be discontinued.
Prolonged use of high doses of androgens has been associated with the development of peliosis hepatis and hepatic neoplasms including hepatocellular carcinoma. (See PRECAUTIONS—*Carcinogenesis*). Peliosis hepatis can be a life-threatening or fatal complication.
Cholestatic hepatitis and jaundice occur with 17-alpha-alkylandrogens at a relatively low dose. If cholestatic hepatitis with jaundice appears or if liver function tests become abnormal, the androgen should be discontinued and the etiology should be determined. Drug-induced jaundice is reversible when the medication is discontinued.
Edema with or without heart failure may be a serious complication in patients with preexisting cardiac, renal, or hepatic disease. In addition to discontinuation of the drug, diuretic therapy may be required.

PRECAUTIONS

Associated with Estrogens

A. General Precautions.

1. A complete medical and family history should be taken prior to the initiation of any estrogen therapy. The pretreatment and periodic physical examinations should include special reference to blood pressure, breasts, abdomen, and pelvic organs, and should include a Papanicolaou smear. As a general rule, estrogen should not be prescribed for longer than one year without another physical examination being performed.
2. Fluid retention—Because estrogens may cause some degree of fluid retention, conditions which might be influenced by this factor such as asthma, epilepsy, migraine, and cardiac or renal dysfunction, require careful observation.
3. Certain patients may develop undesirable manifestations of excessive estrogenic stimulation, such as abnormal or excessive uterine bleeding, mastodynia, etc.
4. Prolonged administration of unopposed estrogen therapy has been reported to increase the risk of endometrial hyperplasia in some patients.
5. Oral contraceptives appear to be associated with an increased incidence of mental depression.[24a] Although it is not clear whether this is due to the estrogenic or progestogenic component of the contraceptive, patients with a history of depression should be carefully observed.

6. Preexisting uterine leiomyomata may increase in size during estrogen use.
7. The pathologist should be advised of estrogen therapy when relevant specimens are submitted.
8. Patients with a past history of jaundice during pregnancy have an increased risk of recurrence of jaundice while receiving estrogen-containing oral contraceptive therapy. If jaundice develops in any patient receiving estrogen, the medication should be discontinued while the cause is investigated.
9. Estrogens may be poorly metabolized in patients with impaired liver function and they should be administered with caution in such patients.
10. Because estrogens influence the metabolism of calcium and phosphorus, they should be used with caution in patients with metabolic bone diseases that are associated with hypercalcemia or in patients with renal insufficiency.
11. Because of the effects of estrogens on epiphyseal closure, they should be used judiciously in young patients in whom bone growth is not complete.
12. Certain endocrine and liver function tests may be affected by estrogen-containing oral contraceptives. The following similar changes may be expected with larger doses of estrogen.
a. Increased sulfobromophthalein retention.
b. Increased prothrombin and factors VII, VIII, IX, and X; decreased antithrombin 3; increased norepinephrine-induced platelet aggregability.
c. Increased thyroid binding globulin (TBG) leading to increased circulating total thyroid hormone, as measured by PBI, T4 by column, or T4 by radioimmunoassay. Free T3 resin uptake is decreased, reflecting the elevated TBG; free T4 concentration is unaltered.
d. Impaired glucose tolerance.
e. Decreased pregnanediol excretion.
f. Reduced response to metyrapone test.
g. Reduced serum folate concentration.
h. Increased serum triglyceride and phospholipid concentration.

B. Information for the Patient. See text which appears after the PHYSICIAN REFERENCES.

C. Pregnancy Category X. See CONTRAINDICATIONS and Boxed Warning.

D. Nursing Mothers. As a general principle, the administration of any drug to nursing mothers should be done only when clearly necessary since many drugs are excreted in human milk.

Associated with Methyltestosterone

A. General Precautions

1. Women should be observed for signs of virilization (deepening of the voice, hirsutism, acne, clitoromegaly, and menstrual irregularities). Discontinuation of drug therapy at the time of evidence of mild virilism is necessary to prevent irreversible virilization. Such virilization is usual following androgen use at high doses.
2. Prolonged dosage of androgen may result in sodium and fluid retention. This may present a problem, especially in patients with compromised cardiac reserve or renal disease.
3. Hypersensitivity may occur rarely.
4. PBI may be decreased in patients taking androgens.
5. Hypercalcemia may occur. If this does occur, the drug should be discontinued.

B. Information for the Patient

The physician should instruct patients to report any of the following side effects of androgens:

Women: Hoarseness, acne, changes in menstrual periods, or more hair on the face.

All Patients: Any nausea, vomiting, changes in skin color or ankle swelling.

C. Laboratory Tests

1. Women with disseminated breast carcinoma should have frequent determination of urine and serum calcium levels during the course of androgen therapy (See WARNINGS).
2. Because of the hepatotoxicity associated with the use of 17-alpha-alkylated androgens, liver function tests should be obtained periodically.
3. Hemoglobin and hematocrit should be checked periodically for polycythemia in patients who are receiving high doses of androgens.

D. Drug Interactions

1. *Anticoagulants* C-17 substituted derivatives of testosterone, such as methandrostenolone, have been reported to decrease the anticoagulant requirements of patients receiving oral anticoagulants. Patients receiving oral anticoagulant therapy require close monitoring, especially when androgens are started or stopped.
2. *Oxyphenbutazone.* Concurrent administration of oxyphenbutazone and androgens may result in elevated serum levels of oxyphenbutazone.
3. *Insulin.* In diabetic patients the metabolic effects of androgens may decrease blood glucose and insulin requirements.

E. Drug/Laboratory Test Interferences

Androgens may decrease levels of thyroxine-binding globulin, resulting in decreased T_4 serum levels and increased resin uptake of T_3 and T_4. Free thyroid hormone levels remain unchanged, however, and there is no clinical evidence of thyroid dysfunction.

F. Carcinogenesis

Animal Data. Testosterone has been tested by subcutaneous injection and implantation in mice and rats. The implant induced cervical-uterine tumors in mice, which metastasized in some cases. There is suggestive evidence that injection of testosterone into some strains of female mice increases their susceptibility to hepatoma. Testosterone is also known to increase the number of tumors and decrease the degree of differentiation of chemically induced carcinomas of the liver in rats.

Human Data. There are rare reports of hepatocellular carcinoma in patients receiving long-term therapy with androgens in high doses. Withdrawal of the drugs did not lead to regression of the tumors in all cases.

Geriatric patients treated with androgens may be at an increased risk for the development of prostatic hypertrophy and prostatic carcinoma.

G. Pregnancy

Teratogenic Effects. Pregnancy Category X (see CONTRAINDICATIONS).

H. Nursing Mothers

It is not known whether androgens are excreted in human milk. Because many drugs are excreted in human milk and because of the potential for serious adverse reactions in nursing infants from androgens, a decision should be made whether to discontinue nursing or to discontinue the drug, taking into account the importance of the drug to the mother.

ADVERSE REACTIONS

Associated with Estrogens

(See WARNINGS regarding induction of neoplasia, adverse effects on the fetus, increased incidence of gallbladder disease, and adverse effects similar to those of oral contraceptives, including thromboembolism.) The following additional adverse reactions have been reported with estrogenic therapy, including oral contraceptives:

1. *Genitourinary system:* Breakthrough bleeding, spotting, change in menstrual flow; dysmenorrhea; premenstrual-like syndrome; amenorrhea during and after treatment; increase in size of uterine fibromyomata; vaginal candidiasis; change in cervical erosion and in degree of cervical secretion; cystitis-like syndrome.
2. *Breasts:* Tenderness, enlargement, secretion.
3. *Gastrointestinal:* Nausea, vomiting; abdominal cramps, bloating; cholestatic jaundice.
4. *Skin:* Chloasma or melasma which may persist when drug is discontinued; erythema multiforme; erythema nodosum; hemorrhagic eruption; loss of scalp hair; hirsutism.
5. *Eyes:* Steepening of corneal curvature; intolerance to contact lenses.
6. *CNS:* Headache, migraine, dizziness; mental depression; chorea.
7. *Miscellaneous:* Increase or decrease in weight; reduced carbohydrate tolerance; aggravation of porphyria; edema; changes in libido.

Associated with Methyltestosterone

A. Endocrine and Urogenital

1. *Female:* The most common side effects of androgen therapy are amenorrhea and other menstrual irregularities, inhibition of gonadotropin secretion, and virilization, including deepening of the voice and clitoral enlargement. The latter usually is not reversible after androgens are discontinued. When administered to a pregnant woman androgens cause virilization of external genitalia of the female fetus.
2. *Skin and Appendages:* Hirsutism, male pattern of baldness, and acne.
3. *Fluid and Electrolyte Disturbances:* Retention of sodium, chloride, water, potassium, calcium, and inorganic phosphates.
4. *Gastrointestinal:* Nausea, cholestatic jaundice, alterations in liver function test, rarely hepatocellular neoplasms, and peliosis hepatis (see WARNINGS).
5. *Hematologic:* Suppression of clotting factors II, V, VII, and X, bleeding in patients on concomitant anticoagulant therapy, and polycythemia.
6. *Nervous System:* Increased or decreased libido, headache, anxiety, depression, and generalized paresthesia.
7. *Metabolic:* Increased serum cholesterol.
8. *Miscellaneous:* Inflammation and pain at the site of intramuscular injection or subcutaneous implantation of testosterone containing pellets, stomatitis with buccal preparations, and rarely anaphylactoid reactions.

ACUTE OVERDOSAGE

Numerous reports of ingestion of large doses of estrogen-containing oral contraceptives by young children indicate that acute serious ill effects do not occur. Overdosage of estrogen may cause nausea, and withdrawal bleeding may occur in females.

There have been no reports of acute overdosage with the androgens.

DOSAGE AND ADMINISTRATION

Given cyclically for short-term use only:

For treatment of moderate to severe *vasomotor* symptoms associated with the menopause in patients not improved by estrogen alone.

The lowest dose that will control symptoms should be chosen and medication should be discontinued as promptly as possible.

Administration should be cyclic (eg, three weeks on and one week off).

Attempts to discontinue or taper medication should be made at three to six month intervals.

Usual dosage range:

1.25 mg Conjugated Estrogens, USP and 10.0 mg Methyltestosterone (1 yellow tablet, No. 879, or 2 maroon tablets, No. 878), daily and cyclically.

Treated patients with an intact uterus should be monitored closely for signs of endometrial cancer and appropriate diagnostic measures should be taken to rule out malignancy in the event of persistent or recurring abnormal vaginal bleeding.

HOW SUPPLIED

PREMARIN (conjugated estrogens, USP) with METHYLTESTOSTERONE Tablets

—Each round *yellow* tablet contains 1.25 mg PREMARIN and 10.0 mg Methyltestosterone, in bottles of 100 (NDC 0046-0879-81).

—Each round *maroon* tablet contains 0.625 mg PREMARIN and 5.0 mg Methyltestosterone, in bottles of 100 (NDC 0046-0878-81).

The appearance of these tablets is a trademark of Ayerst Laboratories.

Store at room temperature (approximately 25° C).

PHYSICIAN REFERENCES

1. Ziel, H. K., *et al.*: N. Engl. J. Med. *293*:1167–1170, 1975.
2. Smith, D. C., *et al.*: N. Engl. J. Med. *293*:1164–1167, 1975.
3. Mack, T. M., *et al.*: N. Engl. J. Med. *294*:1262–1267, 1976.
4. Weiss, N. S., *et al.*: N. Engl. J. Med. *294*:1259–1262, 1976.
5. Herbst, A. L., *et al.*: N. Engl. J. Med. *284*:878–881, 1971.
6. Greenwald, P., *et al.*: N. Engl. J. Med. *285*:390–392, 1971.
7. Lanier, A., *et al.*: Mayo Clin. Proc. *48*:793–799, 1973.
8. Herbst, A., *et al.*: Obstet. Gynecol. *40*:287–298, 1972.
9. Herbst, A., *et al.*: Am. J. Obstet. Gynecol. *118*:607–615, 1974.
10. Herbst, A., *et al.*: N. Engl. J. Med. *292*:334–339, 1975.
11. Stafl, A., *et al.*: Obstet. Gynecol. *43*:118–128, 1974.
12. Sherman, A. I., *et al.*: Obstet. Gynecol. *44*:531–545, 1974.
13. Gal. I., *et al.*: Nature *216*:83, 1967.
14. Levy, E. P., *et al.*: Lancet *1*:611, 1973.
15. Nora, J., *et al.*: Lancet *1*:941–942, 1973.
16. Janerich, D. T., *et al.*: N. Engl. J. Med. *291*:697–700, 1974.
17. Boston Collaborative Drug Surveillance Program: N. Engl. J. Med. *290*:15–19, 1974.
18. Hoover, R., *et al.*: N. Engl. J. Med. 295: 401–405, 1976.
19. Boston Collaborative Drug Surveillance Program: Lancet *1*:1399–1404, 1973.
20. Daniel, D. G., *et al.*: Lancet *2*:287–289, 1967.
21. The Veterans Administration Cooperative Urological Research Group: J. Urol. *98*:516–522, 1967.
22. Bailar, J. C.: Lancet *2*:560, 1967.
23. Blackard, C., *et al.*: Cancer *26*:249–256, 1970.
24. Royal College of General Practitioners: J. R. Coll. Gen. Pract. *13*:267–279, 1967.

24a. Royal College of General Practitioners: Oral Contraceptives and Health, New York, Pitman Corp., 1974.

25. Inman, W. H. W., *et al.*: Br. Med. J. *2*:193–199, 1968.
26. Vessey, M. P., *et al.*: Br. Med. J. *2*:651–657, 1969.
27. Sartwell, P. E., *et al.*: Am. J. Epidemiol. *90*:365–380, 1969.
28. Collaborative Group for the Study of Stroke in Young Women: N. Engl. J. Med. *288*:871–878, 1973.
29. Collaborative Group for the Study of Stroke in Young Women: J.A.M.A. *231*: 718–722, 1975.
30. Mann, J. I., *et al.*: Br. Med. J. *2*:245–248, 1975.
31. Mann, J. I., *et al.*: Br. Med. J. *2*:241–245, 1975.
32. Inman, W. H. W., *et al.*: Br. Med. J. *2*:203–209, 1970.
33. Stolley, P. D., *et al.*: Am. J. Epidemiol. *102*:197–208, 1975.
34. Vessey, M. P., *et al.*: Br. Med. J. *3*:123–126, 1970.
35. Greene, G. R., *et al.*: Am. J. Public Health *62*:680–685, 1972.
36. Rosenberg, L., *et al.*: N. Engl. J. Med. *294*: 1256–1259, 1976.
37. Coronary Drug Project Research Group: J.A.M.A. *214*:1303–1313, 1970.

Continued on next page

Ayerst—Cont.

38. Baum, J., *et al.*: Lancet *2*:926–928, 1973.
39. Mays, E. T., *et al.*: J.A.M.A. *235*:730–732, 1976.
40. Edmondson, H. A., *et al.*: N. Engl. J. Med. *294*:470–472, 1976.
41. Pfeffer, R. I., *et al.*: Am. J. Epidemiol. *103*:445–456, 1976.

Androgen references available upon request.

INFORMATION FOR THE PATIENT

WHAT YOU SHOULD KNOW ABOUT ESTROGENS

Estrogens are female hormones produced by the ovaries. The ovaries make several different kinds of estrogens. In addition, scientists have been able to make a variety of synthetic estrogens. As far as we know, all these estrogens have similar properties and therefore much the same usefulness, side effects, and risks. This leaflet is intended to help you understand what estrogens are used for, the risks involved in their use, and how to use them as safety as possible.

This leaflet includes the most important information about estrogens, but not all the information. If you want to know more, you should ask your doctor for more information or you can ask your doctor or pharmacist to let you read the package insert prepared for the doctor.

USES OF ESTROGEN

THERE IS NO PROPER USE OF ESTROGENS IN A PREGNANT WOMAN.

Estrogens are prescribed by doctors for a number of purposes, including:

1. To provide estrogen during a period of adjustment when a woman's ovaries stop producing a majority of her estrogens, in order to prevent certain uncomfortable symptoms of estrogen deficiency. (With the menopause, which generally occurs between the ages of 45 and 55, women produce a much smaller amount of estrogens.)
2. To prevent symptoms of estrogen deficiency when a woman's ovaries have been removed surgically before the natural menopause.
3. To prevent pregnancy. (Estrogens are given along with a progestogen, another female hormone; these combinations are called oral contraceptives or birth control pills. Patient labeling is available to women taking oral contraceptives and they will not be discussed in this leaflet.)
4. To treat certain cancers in women and men.
5. To prevent painful swelling of the breasts after pregnancy in women who choose not to nurse their babies.

ESTROGENS IN THE MENOPAUSE

In the natural course of their lives, all women eventually experience a decrease in estrogen production. This usually occurs between ages 45 and 55 but may occur earlier or later. Sometimes the ovaries may need to be removed before natural menopause by an operation, producing a "surgical menopause."

When the amount of estrogen in the blood begins to decrease, many women may develop typical symptoms: feeling of warmth in the face, neck, and chest or sudden intense episodes of heat and sweating throughout the body (called "hot flashes" or "hot flushes"). These symptoms are sometimes very uncomfortable. Some women may also develop changes in the vagina (called "atrophic vaginitis") which cause discomfort, especially during and after intercourse.

Estrogens can be prescribed to treat these symptoms of the menopause. It is estimated that considerably more than half of all women undergoing the menopause have only mild symptoms or no symptoms at all and therefore do not need estrogens. Other women may need estrogens for a few months, while their bodies adjust to lower estrogen levels. Sometimes the need will be for periods longer than six months. In an attempt to avoid overstimulation of the uterus (womb), estrogens are usually given cyclically during each month of use, such as three weeks of pills followed by one week without pills.

Sometimes women experience nervous symptoms or depression during menopause. There is no evidence that estrogens are effective for such symptoms without associated vasomotor symptoms. In the absence of vasomotor symptoms, estrogens should not be used to treat nervous symptoms, although other treatment may be needed.

You may have heard that taking estrogens for long periods (years) after the menopause will keep your skin soft and supple and keep you feeling young. There is no evidence that this is so, however, and such long-term treatment carries important risks.

ESTROGENS TO PREVENT SWELLING OF THE BREASTS AFTER PREGNANCY

If you do not breast-feed your baby after delivery, your breasts may fill up with milk and become painful and engorged. This usually begins about 3 to 4 days after delivery and may last for a few days to up to a week or more. Sometimes the discomfort is severe, but usually it is not and can be controlled by pain-relieving drugs such as aspirin and by binding the breasts up tightly. Estrogens can be used to try to prevent the breasts from filling up. While this treatment is sometimes successful, in many cases the breasts fill up to some degree in spite of treatment. The dose of estrogens needed to prevent pain and swelling of the breasts is much larger than the dose needed to treat symptoms of the menopause and this may increase your chances of developing blood clots in the legs or lungs (see below). Therefore, it is important that you discuss the benefits and the risks of estrogen use with your doctor if you have decided not to breast-feed your baby.

THE DANGERS OF ESTROGENS

1. *Endometrial cancer.* There are reports that if estrogens are used in the postmenopausal period for more than a year, there is an increased risk of *endometrial cancer* (cancer of the lining of the uterus). Women taking estrogens have roughly 5 to 10 times as great a chance of getting this cancer as women who take no estrogens. To put this another way, while a postmenopausal woman not taking estrogens has 1 chance in 1,000 each year of getting endometrial cancer, a woman taking estrogens has 5 to 10 chances in 1,000 each year. For this reason *it is important to take estrogens only when they are really needed.*

The risk of this cancer is greater the longer estrogens are used and when larger doses are taken. Therefore you should not take more estrogen than your doctor prescribes. *It is important to take the lowest dose of estrogen that will control symptoms and to take it only as long as it is needed.* If estrogens are needed for longer periods of time, your doctor will want to reevaluate your need for estrogens at least every six months.

Women using estrogens should report any vaginal bleeding to their doctors; such bleeding may be of no importance, but it can be an early warning of endometrical cancer. If you have undiagnosed vaginal bleeding, you should not use estrogens until a diagnosis is made and you are certain there is no endometrial cancer.

NOTE: If you have had your uterus removed (total hysterectomy), there is no danger of developing endometrial cancer.

2. *Other possible cancers.* Estrogens can cause development of other tumors in animals, such as tumors of the breast, cervix, vagina, or liver, when given for a long time. At present there is no good evidence that women using estrogen in the menopause have an increased risk of such tumors, but there is no way yet to be sure they do not; and one study raises the possibility that use of estrogens in the menopause may increase the risk of breast cancer many years later. This is a further reason to use estrogens only when clearly needed. While you are taking estrogens, it is important that you go to your doctor at least once a year for a physical examination. Also, if members of your family have had breast cancer or if you have breast nodules or abnormal mammograms (breast x-rays), your doctor may wish to carry out more frequent examinations of your breasts.

3. *Gallbladder disease.* Women who use estrogens after menopause are more likely to develop gallbladder disease needing surgery than women who do not use estrogens. Birth control pills have a similar effect.

4. *Abnormal blood clotting.* Oral contraceptives increase the risk of blood clotting in various parts of the body. This can result in a stroke (if the clot is in the brain), a heart attack (clot in a blood vessel of the heart), or a pulmonary embolus (a clot which forms in the legs or pelvis, then breaks off and travels to the lungs). Any of these can be fatal.

At this time use of estrogens in the menopause is not known to cause such blood clotting, but this has not been fully studied and there could still prove to be such a risk. It is recommended that if you have had clotting in the legs or lungs or a heart attack or stroke while you were using estrogens or birth control pills, you should not use estrogens (unless they are being used to treat cancer of the breast or prostate). If you have had a stroke or heart attack or if you have angina pectoris, estrogens should be used with great caution and only if clearly needed (for example, if you have severe symptoms of the menopause).

The larger doses of estrogen used to prevent swelling of the breasts after pregnancy have been reported to cause clotting in the legs and lungs.

SPECIAL WARNING ABOUT PREGNANCY

You should not receive estrogen if you are pregnant. If this should occur, there is a greater than usual chance that the developing child will be born with a birth defect, although the possibility remains fairly small. A female child may have an increased risk of developing cancer of the vagina or cervix later in life (in the teens or twenties). Every possible effort should be made to avoid exposure to estrogens during pregnancy. If exposure occurs, see your doctor.

OTHER EFFECTS OF ESTROGENS

In addition to the serious known risks of estrogens described above, estrogens have the following side effects and potential risks:

1. *Nausea and vomiting.* The most common side effect of estrogen therapy is nausea. Vomiting is less common.
2. *Effects on breasts.* Estrogens may cause breast tenderness or enlargement and may cause the breasts to secrete a liquid. These effects are not dangerous.
3. *Effects on the uterus.* Estrogens may cause benign fibroid tumors of the uterus to get larger.
4. *Effects on liver.* Women taking oral contraceptives develop on rare occasions a tumor of the liver which can rupture and bleed into the abdomen and may cause death. So far, these tumors have not been reported in women using estrogens in the menopause, but you should report any swelling or unusual pain or tenderness in the abdomen to your doctor immediately.

Women with a past history of jaundice (yellowing of the skin and white parts of the eyes) may get jaundice again during estrogen use. If this occurs, stop taking estrogens and see your doctor.

5. *Other effects.* Estrogens may cause excess fluid to be retained in the body. This may make some conditions worse, such as asthma, epilepsy, migraine, heart disease, or kidney disease.

SUMMARY

Estrogens have important uses, but they have serious risks as well. You must decide, with your doctor, whether the risks are acceptable to you in view of the benefits of treatment. Except where your doctor has prescribed estrogens for use in special cases of cancer of the breast or prostrate, you should not use estrogens if you have cancer of the breast or uterus, are pregnant, have undiagnosed abnormal vaginal bleeding, clotting in the legs or lungs, or have had a stroke, heart attack or angina, or clotting in the legs or lungs in the past while you were taking estrogens.

You can use estrogens as safely as possible by understanding that your doctor will require physical examinations while you are taking them and will try to discontinue the drug as soon as possible and use the smallest dose possible. Be alert for signs of trouble including:

1. Abnormal bleeding from the vagina.
2. Pains in the calves or chest or sudden shortness of breath, or coughing blood.
3. Severe headache, dizziness, faintness, or changes in vision.
4. Breast lumps (you should ask your doctor how to examine your own breasts).
5. Jaundice (yellowing of the skin).
6. Mental depression.

Your doctor has prescribed this drug for you and you alone. Do not give the drug to anyone else.

HOW SUPPLIED

PREMARIN® (conjugated estrogens tablets, USP)—tablets for oral administration.

Each oval *purple* tablet contains 2.5 mg
Each oval *yellow* tablet contains 1.25 mg
Each oval *white* tablet contains 0.9 mg
Each oval *maroon* tablet contains 0.625 mg
Each oval *green* tablet contains 0.3 mg

PREMARIN® with METHYLTESTOSTERONE—a combination of PREMARIN and methyltestosterone (an androgen) in tablet form for oral administration.

Each round *yellow* tablet contains 1.25 mg PREMARIN and 10 mg methyltestosterone
Each round *maroon* tablet contains 0.625 mg PREMARIN and 5 mg methyltestosterone

PMB® 200, 400—a combination of PREMARIN® and meprobamate (a tranquilizing agent) in tablet form for oral administration.

Each oblong *green* tablet contains 0.45 mg PREMARIN and 200 mg meprobamate
Each oblong *pink* tablet contains 0.45 mg PREMARIN and 400 mg meprobamate

The appearance of these tablets is a trademark of Ayerst Laboratories.

PREMARIN® VAGINAL CREAM—PREMARIN® in a nonliquefying base, designed for vaginal use.

PREMARIN® INTRAVENOUS—PREMARIN® specially prepared for intravenous and intramuscular use.

ESTROGENIC SUBSTANCE (Estrone) in Aqueous Suspension—a sterile aqueous suspension of estrone, a short-acting estroge, for intramuscular injection only.

Shown in Product Identification Section, page 404

PROTOPAM® CHLORIDE ℞

[*prō"tō-pam klaw'rīde*]

Brand of pralidoxime chloride

CAUTION: Federal law prohibits dispensing without prescription.

DESCRIPTION

PROTOPAM CHLORIDE (pralidoxime chloride) is a cholinesterase reactivator.

Chemically, it is 2-formyl-1-methylpyridinium chloride oxime (pyridine-2-aldoxime methochloride), and has the generic name pralidoxime chloride. It has also been referred to as 2-PAM Chloride.

The chemical structure is:

CH=NOH · Cl (N-CH3 pyridinium structure)

PROTOPAM CHLORIDE occurs as a white, nonhygroscopic, crystalline powder which is soluble in water to the extent of 1 g in less than 1 ml.

The specific activity of the drug resides in the 2-formyl-1-methylpyridinium ion and is independent of the particular salt employed.

PROTOPAM CHLORIDE Tablets contain the following inactive ingredients: critic acid, magnesium stearate, methylcellulose, and microcrystalline cellulose.

ACTIONS

The principal action of PROTOPAM (pralidoxime) is to reactivate cholinesterase (mainly outside of the central nervous system) which has been inactivated by phosphorylation due to an organophosphate pesticide or related compound. The destruction of accumulated acetylcholine can then proceed and neuromuscular junctions will again function normally. PROTOPAM also slows the process of "aging" of phosphorylated cholinesterase to a non-reactivatable form, and detoxifies certain organophosphates by direct chemical reaction. The drug has its most critical effect in relieving paralysis of the muscles of respiration. Because PROTOPAM is less effective in relieving depression of the respiratory center, atropine is always required concomitantly to block the effect of accumulated acetylcholine at this site. PROTOPAM relieves muscarinic signs and symptoms, salivation, bronchospasm, etc., but this action is relatively unimportant since atropine is adequate for this purpose.

PROTOPAM antagonizes the effects on the neuromuscular junction of the carbamate anticholinesterases, neostigmine, pyridostigmine and ambenonium, used in the treatment of myasthenia gravis. However, it is not nearly as effective as an antidote to these drugs as it is to the organophosphates.

PROTOPAM (pralidoxime) is distributed throughout the extracellular water; it is not bound to plasma protein. The drug is rapidly excreted in the urine partly unchanged, and partly as a metabolite produced by the liver. Consequently. PROTOPAM is relatively short acting and repeated doses may be needed, especially where there is any evidence of continuing absorption of the poison.

INDICATIONS

PROTOPAM is indicated as an antidote: (1) in the treatment of poisoning due to those pesticides and chemicals of the organophosphate class which have anticholinesterase activity, and (2) in the control of overdosage by anticholinesterase drugs used in the treatment of myasthenia gravis.

WARNINGS

Use of PROTOPAM should always be under supervision of the subject's personal physician or of the medical department of his employer.

PROTOPAM is not effective in the treatment of poisoning due to phosphorus, inorganic phosphates or organophosphates not having anticholinesterase activity.

Until further information is available, no recommendation is made as to the use of PROTOPAM in intoxication by pesticides of the carbamate class.

PRECAUTIONS

PROTOPAM (pralidoxime) has been very well tolerated in most cases, but it must be remembered that the desperate condition of the organophosphate-poisoned patient will generally mask such minor signs and symptoms as have been noted in normal subjects.

Intravenous administration of PROTOPAM should be carried out slowly and, preferably, by infusion, since certain side effects, such as tachycardia, laryngospasm, and muscle rigidity, have been attributed in a few cases to a too rapid rate of injection. (See DOSAGE AND ADMINISTRATION.)

Because PROTOPAM is excreted in the urine, a decrease in renal function will result in increased blood levels of the drug. Thus, the dosage of PROTOPAM should be reduced in the presence of renal insufficiency.

PROTOPAM should be used with great caution in treating organophosphate overdosage in cases of myasthenia gravis since it may precipitate a myasthenic crisis.

The following precautions should be kept in mind in the treatment of anticholinesterase poisoning, although they do not bear directly on the use of PROTOPAM (pralidoxime): since barbiturates are potentiated by the anticholinesterases, they should be used cautiously in the treatment of convulsions; morphine, theophylline, aminophylline, succinylcholine, reserpine, and phenothiazine-type tranquilizers should be avoided in patients with organophosphate poisoning.

ADVERSE REACTIONS

Dizziness, blurred vision, diplopia and impaired accommodation, headache, drowsiness, nausea, tachycardia, hyperventilation, and muscular weakness have been reported after the use of PROTOPAM , but it is very difficult to differentiate the toxic effects produced by atropine or the organophosphate compounds from those of the drug. When atropine and PROTOPAM are used together, the signs of atropinization may occur earlier than might be expected when atropine is used alone. This is especially true if the total dose of atropine has been large and the administration of PROTOPAM has been delayed. Excitement and manic behavior immediately following recovery of consciousness have been reported in several cases. However, similar behavior has occurred in cases of organophosphate poisoning that were not treated with PROTOPAM.

DOSAGE AND ADMINISTRATION

Organophosphate poisoning

Initial measures should include removal of secretions, maintenance of a patent airway and, if necessary, artificial ventilation.

In the absence of cyanosis, atropine should be given intravenously in doses of 2 to 4 mg; where cyanosis is present, this dose of atropine should be given intramuscularly while simultaneously initiating measures for improving ventilation. Atropine administration should be repeated at 5 to 10 minute intervals until signs of atropine toxicity appear. Some degree of atropinization should be maintained for at least 48 hours.

PROTOPAM (pralidoxime) administration should be started at the same time as atropine.

In adults, inject an initial dose of 1 to 2 g of PROTOPAM (pralidoxime), preferably as an infusion in 100 mL of saline, over a 15 to 30 minute period. If this is not practicable or if pulmonary edema is present, the dose should be given slowly by intravenous injection as a 5% solution in water over not less than five minutes. After about an hour, a second dose of 1 to 2 g will be indicated if muscle weakness has not been relieved. Additional doses may be given cautiously if muscle weakness persists. If intravenous administration is not feasible, intramuscular or subcutaneous injection should be used.

In children, the dose should be 20 to 40 mg per kg.

Treatment will be most effective if given within a few hours after poisoning has occurred. Usually, little will be accomplished if the drug is first administered more than 48 hours after exposure, but in severe poisoning, it is, nevertheless, indicated since occasionally patients have responded after such an interval.

In severe cases, especially after ingestion of the poison, it may be desirable to monitor the effect of therapy electrocardiographically because of the possibility of heart block due to the anticholinesterase. Where the poison has been ingested, it is particularly important to take into account the likelihood of continuing absorption from the lower bowel since this constitutes new exposure. In such cases, additional doses of PROTOPAM (pralidoxime) may be needed every three to eight hours. In effect, the patient should be "titrated" with PROTOPAM as long as signs of poisoning recur.

In the absence of severe gastrointestinal symptoms, resulting from the anticholinesterase intoxication, PROTOPAM (pralidoxime) may be administered orally in doses of 1 to 3 g (2 to 6 tablets) every five hours. As in all cases of organophosphate poisoning, care should be taken to keep the patient under observation for at least 24 hours.

If convulsions interfere with respiration, sodium thiopental (2.5% solution) may be given intravenously with care.

Anticholinesterase overdosage

As an antagonist to such anticholinesterases as neostigmine, pyridostigmine, and ambenonium, which are used in the treatment of myasthenia gravis, PROTOPAM may be given in a dosage of 1 to 2 g intravenously followed by increments of 250 mg every five minutes.

OVERDOSAGE

Artificial respiration and other supportive therapy should be administered as needed.

HOW SUPPLIED

NDC 0046-0375-98—*Emergency Kit:* This contains one 20 mL vial of 1 g of sterile PROTOPAM CHLORIDE (pralidoxime chloride) white to off white porous cake*; one 20 mL ampul of Sterile Water for Injection, USP, without preservative to be used as diluent; sterile, disposable 20 mL syringe; needle; alcohol swab. This is a single dose kit for intravenous administration. Intramuscular or subcutaneous injection may be used when intravenous injection is not feasible.

NDC 0046-0374-06—*Hospital Package:* This contains six 20 mL vials of 1 g each of sterile PROTOPAM CHLORIDE (pralidoxime chloride) white to off white porous cake*, without diluent or syringe. Solution may be prepared by adding 20 mL of Sterile Water for Injection, USP. These are single dose vials for intravenous injection or for intravenous infusion after further dilution with physiologic saline. Intramuscular or subcutaneous injection may be used when intravenous injection is not feasible.

*When necessary, sodium hydroxide is added during processing to adjust the pH.

PROTOPAM CHLORIDE for Injection is prepared by cryodesiccation.

NDC 0046-0376-81—*Tablets:* Each tablet contains 500 mg of pralidoxime chloride, in bottles of 100.

A FULL DISCUSSION OF THE ACTIONS AND USES OF PROTOPAM (PRALIDOXIME) IS GIVEN IN A PROFESSIONAL BROCHURE WHICH IS AVAILABLE FROM AYERST LABORATORIES ON REQUEST.

ANIMAL PHARMACOLOGY AND TOXICOLOGY

The following table lists chemical and trade or generic names of pesticides, chemicals, and drugs against which PROTOPAM (usually administered in conjunction with atropine) has been found to have antidotal activity on the basis of animal experiments. All compounds listed are organophosphates having anticholinesterase activity. A great many additional substances are in industrial use but have been omitted because of lack of specific information. The use of PROTOPAM should, nevertheless, be considered in any life-threatening situation resulting from poisoning by these compounds, since the limited and arbitrary conditions of pharmacologic screening do not always accurately reflect the usefulness of PROTOPAM (pralidoxime) in the clinical situation.

AAT—see PARATHION

AFLIX®—see FORMOTHION

ALKRON®—see PARATHION

AMERICAN CYANAMID 3422—see PARATHION

AMITON—diethyl -S- (2-diethyl-aminoethyl) phosphorothiolate

ANTHIO®—see FORMOTHION

APHAMITE—see PARATHION

ARMIN—ethyl-4-nitrophenyl-ethylphosphonate

AZINPHOS-METHYL—dimethyl-S- (4-oxo-1, 2, 3, -benzotriazin-3 (4 H) -ylmethyl) phosphorodithioate

AZODRIN—dimethyl phosphate of 3-hydroxy-N-methyl-cis-crotonamide

BAYER 16259—see ETHYL GUTHION

BAYER 19639—see DISULFOTON

BAYER 25141— diethyl-4-methyl-sulfinyl-phenylphosphorothionate

BAYER 29493—see FENTHION

BAYER L13/59—see TRICHLOROFON

BAYER E605—see PARATHION

BAYTEX®—see FENTHION

CHIPMAN R6199—see AMITON

COMPOUND 3422—see PARATHION

COMPOUND 4049—see MALATHION

COMPOUND 4072— 2-chloro-1-(2,4-dichlorophenyl) vinyl diethyl-phosphate

CO-RAL®—see COUMAPHOS

COROTHION—see PARATHION

COUMAPHOS—3-chloro-4-methyl coumarin-7-yl-diethyl-phosphorothionate

DBD —see AZINPHOS-METHYL

DDVP—see DICHLORVOS

DELNAV—see DIOXATHION

DEMETON—Mixture of SYSTOX® and ISOSYSTOX®

DEMETON-S—see ISOSYSTOX®

DFP—see ISOFLUROPHATE

Continued on next page

Ayerst—Cont.

DIAZINON— diethyl-(2-isopropyl-4-methyl-6-pyrimidyl) phosphorothionate

DICHLORVOS—dimethyl-2, 2-dichloro vinyl phosphate

DIETHYL-p-NITROPHENYL-PHOSPHORO-THIONATE—see PARATHION

DIETHYL -p- NITROPHENYL - THIONO- PHOSPHATE—see PARATHION

DIOXATHION— 2,3-p-dioxanedithio-S, S-bis (0,0-diethyl phosphorodithioate)

DIPTEREX®—see TRICHLOROFON

DISULFOTON—diethyl -S- (2-ethylthioethyl) phosphorodiothiate

DISYSTON®—see DISULFOTON

DITHIOSYSTOX—see DISULFOTON

DNTP—see PARATHION

DPP—see PARATHION

DSDP—see AMITON

DYFLOS—see DFP

DYLOX®—see TRICHLOROFON

E 600—see PARAOXON

E 601—see METHYL PARATHION

E 605—see PARATHION

E 1059—see SYSTOX

ECHOTHIOPHATE IODIDE —diethoxyphosphinylthiocholine iodide

EKATIN®—see MORPHOTHION

ENDOTHION— 2-(dimethoxyphosphinylthiomethyl)-5-methoxy-4-pyrone

ENT 15108—see PARATHION

ENTEX®—see FENTHION

EPN— ethyl-4-nitrophenyl-phenylphospho-nothionate

ETHION—0,0,0',0'-tetraethyl-S,S'-methylene-bis-phosphoro dithioate

ETHYL GUSATHION—see ETHYL GUTHION

ETHYLGUTHION® —diethyl-S-(4-oxo-1,2,3,-benzotriazinyl-3-methyl) phosphorodithioate

ETILON—see PARATHION

FENTHION—dimethyl-(4-methylthio-3-tolyl) phosphorothionate

FLOROPRYL®—see DFP

FOLIDOL®—see PARATHION

FORMOTHION— dimethyl-S-(N-formyl-N-methylcarbamyl-methyl) phosphorodithioate

G 24480—see DIAZINON

GB—see SARIN

GENITHION—see PARATHION

GUSATHION®—see AZINPHOSMETHYL

GUTHION®—see AZINPHOSMETHYL

HETP—see TEPP

I-ARMIN—isopropyl-4-nitro-phenyl methyl-phosphonate

ISOFLUROPHATE— diisopropyl-phosphorofluoridate

ISOSYSTOX®— diethyl-S-(2-ethylmercapto-ethyl)-phosphorothiolate

LEBACYD®—see FENTHION

MACKOTHION—see PARATHION

MALATHION— dimethyl-S-(1, 2-dicarbeth- oxyethyl) -phosphorodithioate

MALATHON—see MALATHION

M-ARMIN—ethyl-4-nitrophenyl methylphosphonate

MECARBAM— 0,0-dimethyl-S-(N-ethoxycarbonyl-N-methyl carbamoylmethyl) phosphorodithioate

METACIDE—see METHYL PARATHION

METASYSTOX®—see METHYL DEMETON

METASYSTOX I®—dimethyl-2-ethyl-mercaptoethylphosphorothiolate

METASYSTOX R®—see OXYDEMETONMETHYL

METHYL DEMETON—mixture of dimethyl(2-ethylmercap-to-ethyl) phosphorothionate and dimethyl-S-(2-ethylmercap-to-ethyl) phosphorothiolate

METHYL PARATHION— dimethyl-(4-nitrophenyl) phosphorothionate

MEVINPHOS— 1-carbomethoxy-1-propen-2-yl-dimethyl-phosphate

MINTACOL®—see PARAOXON

ML 97—see PHOSPHAMIDON

MORPHOTHION— dimethyl-S-2-keto-2-(N-morpholyl ethyl-phosphorodithioate

NEGUVON®—see TRICHLOROFON

NIRAN®—see PARATHION

NITROSTIGMINE—see PARATHION

0, 0-DIETHYL -O- p-NITRO-PHENYL PHOS-PHOROTHIOATE—see PARATHION

0, 0-DIETHYL -O- p-NITRO-PHENYLTHIO- PHOSPHATE —see PARATHION

OR 1191—see PHOSPHAMIDON

OS 1836—see VINYLPHOS

OXYDEMETONMETHYL—dimethyl-S-2-(ethylsulfinyl) ethyl phosphorothiolate

PARAOXON—diethyl (4 - nitro - phenyl) phosphate.

PARATHION—diethyl (4-nitro-phenyl) phosphorothionate

PENPHOS—see PARATHION

PHENCAPTON—diethyl -S- (2, 5-dichloro- phenylmercaptomethyl) phosphorodithioate

PHOSDRIN®—see MEVINPHOS

PHOS-KIL—see PARATHION

PHOSPHAMIDON—1-chloro -1- diethylcarbamoyl -1- propen -2- yl-dimethylphosphate

PHOSPHOLINE IODIDE®—see echothiophate iodide

PHOSPHOROTHIOIC ACID, 0,0-DIETHYL-0-p-NITRO-PHENYL ESTER—see PARATHION

PLANTHION—see PARATHION

QUELETOX—see FENTHION

RHODIATOX®—see PARATHION

RUELENE®— 4-tert-butyl-2-chlorophenyl-methyl-N-methyl-phosphoroamidate

SARIN— isopropyl - methylphos - phonofluo- ridate

SHELL OS 1836—see VINYLPHOS

SHELL 2046—see MEVINPHOS

SNP—see PARATHION

SOMAN—pinacolyl - methyl - phosphonofluo- ridate

SYSTOX®—diethyl - (2-ethyl-mercaptoethyl) phosphorothionate

TEP—see TEPP

TEPP—tetraethylpyro phosphate

THIOPHOS®—see PARATHION

TIGUVON—see FENTHION

TRICHLOROFON—dimethyl-1-hydroxy-2,2,2-trichloro ethylphosphonate

VAPONA®—see DICHLORVOS

VAPOPHOS—see PARATHION

VINYLPHOS—diethyl -2- chloro-vinylphosphate

PROTOPAM appears to be ineffective, or marginally effective, against poisoning by:
CIODRIN® (alpha-methylbenzyl-3-[dimethoxyphosphinyloxy]-cis-crotonate)
DIMEFOX (tetramethylphosphorodiamidic fluoride)
DIMETHOATE (dimethyl-S-[N-methylcarba- moylmethyl]-phosphorodithioate)
METHYL DIAZINON (dimethyl-[2-isopropyl-4-methylpyrimidyl]-phosphorothionate)
METHYL PHENCAPTON (dimethyl-S- [2, 5-dichloro-phenylmercaptomethyl] phosphorodithioate)
PHORATE (diethyl-S-ethylmercaptomethyl- phosphorodithioate)
SCHRADAN (octamethylpyrophosphoramide)
WEPSYN® (5-amino-1-[bis-(dimethylamino)phosphinyl]-3-phenyl-1,2,4-triazole)

CLINICAL STUDIES

The use of PROTOPAM (pralidoxime) has been reported in the treatment of human cases of poisoning by the following substances:

- Azodrin
- Diazinon
- Dichlorvos (DDVP) with chlordane
- Disulfoton
- EPN
- Isoflurophate
- Malathion
- Metasystox I® and Fenthion
- Methyl demeton
- Methyl parathion
- Mevinphos
- Parathion
- Parathion and Mevinphos
- Phosphamidon
- Sarin
- Systox®
- TEPP

Of these cases, over 100 were due to parathion, about a dozen each to malathion, diazinon, and mevinphos, and a few to each of the other compounds.

RIOPAN® OTC

[rī'o pan]
magaldrate
Antacid

RIOPAN is a chemical entity (not a physical mixture), providing the advantages of a true buffer-antacid (not simply a neutralizing agent): (1) rapid action; (2) uniform buffering action; (3) high acid-consuming capacity; (4) no alkalinization or acid rebound.

Each teaspoonful (5 mL) of Suspension contains:
Magaldrate ....540 mg
Also, acacia, hydroxypropyl methylcellulose, menthol, saccharin, water, and flavors.

Each Chew Tablet contains:
Magaldrate ....480 mg
Also, confectioner's sugar, magnesium stearate, polyethylene glycol, sorbitol, titanium dioxide, and flavors.

Each Swallow Tablet contains:
Magaldrate ....480 mg
Also, magnesium stearate, menthol, microcrystalline cellulose, polyethylene glycol, starch, talc, titanium dioxide, and flavors.

LOW SODIUM CONTENT

Not more than 0.004 mEq (0.1 mg) of sodium—per teaspoonful (5 mL) suspension—per chew tablet—per swallow tablet, which is considered dietetically sodium free.

ACID-NEUTRALIZING CAPACITY
15.0 mEq/5 mL; 13.5 mEq per tablet.

INDICATIONS
For the relief of heartburn, sour stomach, acid indigestion and upset stomach associated with these symptoms. For symptomatic relief of hyperacidity associated with the diagnosis of peptic ulcer, gastritis, peptic esophagitis, gastric hyperacidity, and hiatal hernia.

DIRECTIONS
RIOPAN (magaldrate) Antacid *Suspension* —Take one or two teaspoonfuls, between meals and at bedtime, or as directed by the physician. RIOPAN Antacid *Chew Tablets* —Chew one or two tablets, between meals and at bedtime, or as directed by the physician. RIOPAN Antacid *Swallow Tablets* —Take one or two tablets, between meals and at bedtime, or as directed by the physician. Take with enough water to swallow promptly.

DRUG INTERACTION PRECAUTION
Do not use in patients presently taking a prescription antibiotic drug containing any form of tetracycline.

WARNINGS
Patients should not take more than 18 teaspoonfuls or 20 tablets in a 24-hour period or use this maximum dosage for more than two weeks, except under the advice and supervision of a physician. If you have kidney disease, do not use this product except under the advice and supervision of a physician.

HOW SUPPLIED
RIOPAN Antacid *Suspension* in 12 fl oz (355 mL) plastic bottles (NDC 0046-0765-12). Individual Cups, 1 fl oz (30 mL) ea., tray of 10—10 trays per packer (NDC 0046-0765-99). RIOPAN Antacid *Chew Tablets* —in bottles of 60 (NDC 0046-0928-59) and 100 (NDC 0046-0928-80); in individual film strips (10 × 6 and 10 × 10, respectively). Also, single rollpacks of 12 tablets (NDC 0046-0941-12) and 3-roll rollpacks of 36 tablets (NDC 0046-0941-36). RIOPAN Antacid *Swallow Tablets* —Boxes of 60 (NDC 0046-0927-60) and 100 (NDC 0046-0927-81) in individual film strips (6 × 10 and 10 × 10, respectively).
Shown in Product Identification Section, page 405

RIOPAN PLUS® OTC
[*rī'opan*]
magaldrate and simethicone
Antacid/Anti-Gas

Each teaspoonful (5 mL) of Suspension contains:
Magaldrate .... 540 mg
Simethicone .... 20 mg
Also, acacia, hydroxypropyl methylcellulose, menthol, polyoxyl 8 stearate, saccharin, sorbitan monostearate, water, and flavors.
Each Chew Tablet contains:
Magaldrate .... 480 mg
Simethicone .... 20 mg
Also, confectioner's sugar, magnesium stearate, methylcellulose, polyethylene glycol, silicon dioxide-colloidal, sorbitol, titanium dioxide, and flavors.

LOW SODIUM CONTENT
Not more than 0.004 mEq (0.1 mg) per teaspoonful (5 mL) or chew tablet, which is considered dietetically sodium free.

ACID-NEUTRALIZING CAPACITY
15.0 mEq/5 mL; 13.5 mEq per tablet.

INDICATIONS
For the relief of heartburn, sour stomach, acid indigestion and upset stomach associated with these symptoms, accompanied by the symptoms of gas. For symptomatic relief of hyperacidity associated with the diagnosis of peptic ulcer, gastritis, peptic esophagitis, gastric hyperacidity, hiatal hernia, and postoperative gas pain.

DIRECTIONS
RIOPAN PLUS (magaldrate and simethicone) Antacid/Anti-Gas *Suspension* —Take one or two teaspoonfuls between meals and at bedtime, or as directed by the physician.
RIOPAN PLUS Antacid/Anti-Gas *Chew Tablets* —Chew one or two tablets, between meals and at bedtime, or as directed by the physician.

DRUG INTERACTION PRECAUTION
Do not use in patients presently taking a prescription antibiotic drug containing any form of tetracycline.

WARNINGS
Patients should not take more than 18 teaspoonfuls, or 20 tablets, in a 24-hour period or use this maximum dosage for more than two weeks, except under the advice and supervision of a physician. If you have kidney disease, do not use this product except under the advice and supervision of a physician.

HOW SUPPLIED
RIOPAN PLUS Antacid/Anti-Gas *Suspension* —in 12 fl oz (355 mL) plastic bottles (NDC 0046-0768-12) and 6 fl oz (176 mL) plastic bottles (NDC 0046-0768-06). Individual Cups, 1 fl oz (30 mL) ea., tray of 10—10 trays per packer (NDC 0046-0768-99).
RIOPAN PLUS Antacid/Anti-Gas *Chew Tablets* —in bottles of 60 (NDC 0046-0930-60) and 100 (NDC 0046-0930-81). Also single rollpacks of 12 tablets (NDC 0046-0930-12) and 3-roll rollpacks of 36 tablets (NDC 0046-0930-36).
Shown in Product Identification Section, page 405

EXTRA STRENGTH RIOPAN PLUS® OTC
magaldrate and simethicone
Antacid/Anti-Gas

Each teaspoonful (5 mL) of Suspension contains:
Magaldrate .... 1080 mg
Simethicone .... 30 mg
Also, glycerin, polyoxyethylene 8 stearate, potassium citrate, saccharin, sorbitan monostearate, sorbitol solution, xanthan gum, water, and flavors.
Each Chew Tablet contains:
Magaldrate .... 1080 mg
Simethicone .... 30 mg
Also, confectioner's sugar, magnesium stearate, methylcellulose, polyethylene glycol, saccharin, silicon dioxide-colloidal, sorbitol, titanium dioxide, and flavors.

LOW SODIUM CONTENT
Not more than 0.013 mEq (0.3 mg) per teaspoonful (5 mL), or 0.021 mEq (0.5 mg) per chew tablet, which is considered dietetically sodium free.

ACID-NEUTRALIZING CAPACITY
30 mEq/5 mL suspension; 30 mEq per tablet.

INDICATIONS
For the relief of heartburn, sour stomach, acid indigestion, and upset stomach associated with these symptoms, accompanied by the symptoms of gas. For symptomatic relief of hyperacidity associated with the diagnosis of peptic ulcer, gastritis, peptic esophagitis, gastric hyperacidity, hiatal hernia, and postoperative gas pain.

DIRECTIONS
EXTRA STRENGTH RIOPAN PLUS (magaldrate and simethicone) Antacid/Anti-Gas *Suspension* —Take one or two teaspoonfuls between meals and at bedtime, or as directed by the physician.
EXTRA STRENGTH RIOPAN PLUS Antacid/Anti-Gas *Chew Tablets* —Chew one or two tablets, between meals and at bedtime, or as directed by physician.

DRUG INTERACTION PRECAUTION
Do not use in patients presently taking a prescription antibiotic drug containing any form of tetracycline.

WARNINGS
Patients should not take more than 9 teaspoonfuls in a 24-hour period nor use this maximum dosage for more than two weeks, nor use if they have kidney disease, except under the advice and supervision of a physician.

HOW SUPPLIED
EXTRA STRENGTH RIOPAN PLUS Antacid/Anti-Gas *Suspension* —in 12 fl oz (355 mL) plastic bottles (NDC 0046-0779-12) and 6 fl oz (176 mL) plastic bottles (NDC 0046-0779-06). Individual cups, 1 fl oz (30 mL) ea., tray of 10—10 trays per packer (NDC 0046-0779-99).
EXTRA STRENGTH RIOPAN PLUS Antacid/Anti-Gas *Chew Tablets* —in bottles of 60 (NDC 0046-0787-60).
Shown in Product Identification Section, page 405

THIOSULFIL® FORTE ℞
[*thī"o-sul'fil fawrta*]
(sulfamethizole 500 mg)
Bacteriostatic agent for use in Urinary Tract Infection (due to susceptible organisms)

CAUTION: Federal law prohibits dispensing without prescription.

DESCRIPTION
Chemical name: N'-(5-Methyl-1,3,4-thiadiazol-2-yl) sulfanilamide.
Structural formula:

Sulfamethizole is a 5-membered heterocyclic sulfanilamide, occurring as a white or light buff-colored crystalline powder. Solubility in water is dependent upon the pH (1 g/5 mL at pH 7.5; 1 g/4000 mL at pH 6.5). It is soluble in alcohol, and practically insoluble in benzene.
THIOSULFIL FORTE Tablets contain the following inactive ingredients: gelatin, magnesium stearate, microcrystalline cellulose, starch.

ACTIONS
Mechanism of sulfonamide bacteriostatic action: The primary mechanism of bacteriostatic action by THIOSULFIL FORTE (sulfamethizole, 500 mg) is the same as that of most sulfonamides. By competing with the precursor para-aminobenzoic acid, sulfonamides inhibit bacterial synthesis of folic (pteroylglutamic) acid which is required for bacterial growth. Resistant strains are capable of utilizing folic acid precursors or preformed folic acid.
Antibacterial spectrum: The antibacterial spectrum of all sulfonamides is similar. *In vitro* sensitivity of bacteria to sulfonamides does not always reflect *in vivo* sensitivity. Therefore, efficacy must be carefully evaluated with bacteriologic and clinical responses in the individual patient. (See WARNINGS.)
Factors determining efficacy: Efficacy of antimicrobial therapy is dependent upon a number of factors including the *in vivo* sensitivity of the involved organisms, the concentration of the drug required for bacteriostasis, and the achievable concentration of the sulfonamide at the desired site of action. Because of the very rapid renal clearance of sulfamethizole, the blood levels attained are low, and accumulation of the drug in tissues outside the urinary tract is very limited. Therefore, sulfamethizole is not appropriate for treatment of systemic infections such as nocardiosis or for local lesions outside the urinary tract such as chancroid and trachoma. However, its low degree of acetylation and its rapid renal clearance permit high concentrations of active sulfamethizole to occur in the urinary tract, making it especially applicable for the treatment of infections of this tract. In addition, the possibility of crystalluria is minimized because of the high solubility of the drug in urine.
Approximately 95% of a given dose of sulfamethizole is not metabolized; less than 5% is acetylated. As a consequence, almost all of a given dose of THIOSULFIL FORTE (sulfamethizole, 500 mg) is present in its active form in the body. Approximately 80% of an administered dose is recoverable within eight hours; approximately 98% is cleared within 15 to 24 hours. Sulfamethizole is cleared by the kidney at a rate only 10% to 20% lower than that for creatinine.

INDICATIONS
THIOSULFIL FORTE (sulfamethizole, 500 mg) is indicated in the treatment of urinary tract infections (primarily pyelonephritis, pyelitis, and cystitis) in the absence of obstructive uropathy or foreign bodies, when these infections are caused by susceptible strains of the following organisms: *Escherichia coli, Klebsiella-Enterobacter, Staphylococcus aureus, Proteus mirabilis,* and *Proteus vulgaris.*
Important note, *In vitro* sulfonamide sensitivity tests are not always reliable. The test must be carefully coordinated with bacteriologic and clinical reponse. When the patient is already taking sulfonamides, follow-up cultures should have aminobenzoic acid added to the culture media.
Currently, the increasing frequency of resistant organisms is a limitation of the usefulness of antibacterial agents, including the sulfonamides, especially in the treatment of recurrent and complicated urinary tract infections.

Wide variation in blood levels may result with identical doses. Blood levels should be measured in patients receiving sulfonamides for serious infections. Free sulfonamide blood levels of 5–15 mg per 100 mL may be considered therapeutically effective for most infections, with blood levels of 12–15 mg per 100 mL optimal for serious infections; 20 mg per 100 mL should be the maximum total sulfonamide level, as adverse reactions occur more frequently above this level.

CONTRAINDICATIONS
Sulfonamides should not be used in patients hypersensitive to sulfa drugs. They should not be used in infants less than two months of age, in pregnancy at term, and during the nursing period because sulfonamides pass the placenta and are excreted in the milk and may cause kernicterus.

WARNINGS
Sulfonamides should not be used to treat group A streptococci infections or their sequelae. The occurrence of sore throat, fever, pallor, purpura, or jaundice during sulfonamide administration may be an early indication of serious blood dyscrasias.
Deaths associated with the administration of sulfonamides have been reported from hypersensitivity reactions, agranulocytosis, aplastic anemia, and other blood dyscrasias.
Frequent blood counts and renal function tests should be carried out during sulfonamide treatment, especially during prolonged administration. Microscopic urinalyses should be done once a week when a patient is treated for longer than two weeks. Urine cultures should be made to confirm eradication of bacteriuria.

Continued on next page

Ayerst—Cont.

Usage in Pregnancy: The safe use of sulfonamides in pregnancy has not been established. The teratogenicity potential of most sulfonamides has not been thoroughly investigated in either animals or humans. However, a significant increase in the incidence of cleft palate and other bony abnormalities of offspring has been observed when certain sulfonamides of the short-, intermediate-, and long-acting types were given to pregnant rats and mice at high oral doses (7 to 25 times the human dose).

PRECAUTIONS

The usual precautions used in sulfonamide therapy should be observed, including the maintenance of an adequate fluid intake. Sulfonamides should be used with caution in patients with severe allergy or bronchial asthma, severe impairment of hepatic or renal function, and in patients with glucose-6-phosphate dehydrogenase deficiency since sulfas may cause hemolysis in this latter group.

ADVERSE REACTIONS

Blood dyscrasias: Agranulocytosis, aplastic anemia, thrombocytopenia, leukopenia, hemolytic anemia, purpura, hypoprothrombinemia, and methemoglobinemia.
Allergic reactions: Erythema multiforme (Stevens-Johnson syndrome), generalized skin eruptions, epidermal necrolysis, urticaria, serum sickness, pruritus, exfoliative dermatitis, anaphylactoid reactions, periorbital edema, conjunctival and scleral injection, photosensitization, arthralgia, and allergic myocarditis.
Gastrointestinal reactions: Nausea, emesis, abdominal pains, hepatitis, diarrhea, anorexia, pancreatitis, and stomatitis.
C.N.S. reactions: Headache, peripheral neuritis, mental depression, convulsions, ataxia, hallucinations, tinnitus, vertigo, and insomnia.
Miscellaneous reactions: Drug fever, chills, and toxic nephrosis with oliguria and anuria. Periarteritis nodosum and L.E. phenomenon have occurred.
The sulfonamides bear certain chemical similarities to some goitrogens, diuretics (acetazolamide and the thiazides), and oral hypoglycemic agents. Goiter production, diuresis, and hypoglycemia have occurred rarely in patients receiving sulfonamides. Cross-sensitivity may exist with these agents. Rats appear to be especially susceptible to the goitrogenic effects of sulfonamides, and long term administration has produced thyroid malignancies in the species.

DOSAGE AND ADMINISTRATION

Usual dosage: *Adults:* 500 mg to 1 g, three or four times daily.
Children and infants (over 2 months of age): 30 to 45 mg/kg/24 hours, divided into 4 doses.

HOW SUPPLIED

THIOSULFIL FORTE (sulfamethizole, 500 mg)—Each tablet contains sulfamethizole, 500 mg (scored), in bottles of 100 (NDC 0046-0786-81).

CLINICAL STUDIES

Blood concentrations: Following a single 2 g dose of sulfamethizole, peak total drug levels in whole blood are in the range of 6 mg %; the levels fall to about 50% in four hours, and are negligible at eight hours. Approximately the same concentrations are found in children following a single dose of 100 mg/kg.
Urine concentrations: The following average values of free drug in mg/mL were found after a single 4 g dose of sulfamethizole:

0 to 2	hours	— 7.01
2 to 4	"	— 10.97
4 to 6	"	— 5.93
6 to 10	"	— 1.09
10 to 24	"	— 0.31

Following a single 2 g dose, the following average urine concentrations of total drug in mg/mL were found:

0 to 4	hours	— 5.15
4 to 8	"	— 1.8
8 to 12	"	— 0.4
16 to 24	"	— 0.1

Following a single 1 g dose of sulfamethizole, the average concentration of total drug during the first 3.5 hours was 2.9 mg/mL.
Solubility in urine: Sulfamethizole is highly soluble in urine. The solubilities of free and acetylated drug in buffered urine at 37° C at various pHs, in mg/mL, are given below:

pH	*free*	*acetylated*
4.5	108	33
5.3	220	...
5.6	480	278
6.0	729	310
6.5	5,650	380
7.0	8,250	1,500
7.5	54,000	...

Shown in Product Identification Section, page 405

THIOSULFIL®-A Forte ℞

[*thī"o-sul'fil a fawrta*]
(sulfamethizole 500 mg with phenazopyridine HCl)

Each tablet contains:
Sulfamethizole ....500 mg
Phenazopyridine HCl ....50 mg

&

THIOSULFIL®-A

(sulfamethizole 250 mg with phenazopyridine HCl)

Each tablet contains:
Sulfamethizole ....250 mg
Phenazopyridine HCl ....50 mg

Where pain is part of the problem in Urinary Tract Infection (due to susceptible organisms)

CAUTION: Federal law prohibits dispensing without prescription.

DESCRIPTION

Sulfamethizole [N'-(5-Methyl-1,3,4-thiadiazol-2-yl) sulfanilamide] is a 5-membered heterocyclic sulfanilamide, occurring as a white or light buff-colored crystalline powder. Solubility in water is dependent upon the pH (1 g/5 mL at pH 7.5; 1 g/4000 mL at pH 6.5). It is soluble in alcohol, and practically insoluble in benzene.

Phenazopyridine HCl [2, 6-Diamino-3-phenylazopyridine hydrochloride] occurs as brick-red microcrystals with a slight violet luster. It is soluble in boiling water, ethylene and propylene glycols, slightly soluble in alcohol and cold water, and insoluble in acetone and benzene.

THIOSULFIL-A FORTE and THIOSULFIL-A contain the following inactive ingredients: calcium sulfate anhydrous, FD&C Yellow No. 6, lactose, magnesium stearate, methylcellulose, pharmaceutical glaze.
— THIOSULFIL-A FORTE also contains: amberlite resin, D&C Yellow No. 10, glyceryl mono-oleate, guar gum, polyethylene glycol, starch.
— THIOSULFIL-A also contains: black iron oxide, calcium carboxy-methylcellulose, carnauba wax, D&C Red No. 7, FD&C Blue No. 2, FD&C Red No. 40, microcrystalline cellulose, sucrose, talc, titanium dioxide.

CLINICAL PHARMACOLOGY

The combination of sulfamethizole and phenazopyridine HCl acts to eradicate urinary tract infections caused by susceptible organisms and to relieve associated pain and discomfort.
PHENAZOPYRIDINE HCl: Phenazopyridine HCl is an analgesic that acts on the mucosa of the urinary tract providing relief of pain and discomfort caused by inflammation associated with urinary tract infection.
SULFAMETHIZOLE: MECHANISM OF SULFONAMIDE BACTERIOSTATIC ACTION: The primary mechanism of bacteriostatic action by THIOSULFIL is the same as that of most sulfonamides. By competing with the precursor para-aminobenzoic acid, sulfonamides inhibit bacterial synthesis of folic (pteroylglutamic) acid which is required for bacterial growth. Resistant strains are capable of utilizing folic acid precursors or preformed folic acid.
SULFONAMIDE ANTIBACTERIAL SPECTRUM: The antibacterial spectrum of all sulfonamides is similar. *In vitro* sensitivity of bacteria to sulfonamides does not always reflect *in vivo* sensitivity. Therefore, efficacy must be carefully evaluated with bacteriologic and clinical responses in the individual patient. (See WARNINGS.)
FACTORS DETERMINING ANTIBACTERIAL EFFICACY: Efficacy of antimicrobial therapy is dependent upon a number of factors including the *in vivo* sensitivity of the involved organisms, the concentration of the drug required for bacteriostasis, and the achievable concentration of the sulfonamide at the desired site of action.
Because of the very rapid renal clearance of sulfamethizole, the blood levels attained are low, and accumulation of the drug in tissues outside the urinary tract is very limited. Therefore, sulfamethizole is not appropriate for treatment of systemic infections such as nocardiosis or for local lesions outside the urinary tract such as chancroid and trachoma. However, its low degree of acetylation and its rapid renal clearance permit high concentrations of active sulfamethizole to occur in the urinary tract, making it especially applicable for the treatment of infections of this tract. In addition, the possibility of crystalluria is minimized because of the high solubility of the drug in urine.
Approximately 95% of a given dose of sulfamethizole is not metabolized; less than 5% is acetylated. As a consequence, almost all of a given dose of THIOSULFIL is present in its active form in the body.
Approximately 80% of an administered dose is recoverable within eight hours; approximately 98% is cleared within 15 to 24 hours. Sulfamethizole is cleared by the kidney at a rate only 10 to 20% lower than that for creatinine.

INDICATIONS AND USAGE

For the initial treatment of uncomplicated urinary tract infections caused by susceptible strains of the following microorganisms: *Escherichia coli, Klebsiella* species, *Enterobacter* species, *Proteus mirabilis, Proteus vulgaris,* and *Staphylococcus aureus* when relief of symptoms of pain, burning or urgency is needed during the first 2 days of therapy. Treatment with THIOSULFIL-A FORTE (sulfamethizole 500 mg with phenazopyridine HCl) or THIOSULFIL-A (sulfamethizole 250 mg with phenazopyridine HCl) should not exceed 2 days. There is a lack of evidence that the combination of sulfamethizole and phenazopyridine hydrochloride provide greater benefit than sulfamethizole alone after 2 days. Treatment beyond 2 days should only be continued with sulfamethizole. (See DOSAGE AND ADMINISTRATION.)
Important note. *In vitro* sulfonamide sensitivity tests are not always reliable. The test must be carefully coordinated with bacteriologic and clinical reponse. When the patient is already taking sulfonamides, follow-up cultures should have aminobenzoic acid added to the culture media.
Currently, the increasing frequency of resistant organisms is a limitation of the usefulness of antibacterial agents, including the sulfonamides, especially in the treatment of recurrent and complicated urinary tract infections.
Wide variation in blood levels may result with identical doses. Blood levels should be measured in patients receiving sulfonamides for serious infections. Free sulfonamide blood levels of 5–15 mg per 100 mL may be considered therapeutically effective for most infections, with blood levels of 12–15 mg per 100 mL optimal for serious infections; 20 mg per 100 mL should be the maximum total sulfonamide level, as adverse reactions occur more frequently above this level.

CONTRAINDICATIONS

Sulfonamides should not be used in patients hypersensitive to sulfa drugs. They should not be used in infants less than two months of age, in pregnancy at term, and during the nursing period because sulfonamides pass the placenta and are excreted in the milk and may cause kernicterus.
Phenazopyridine HCl is contraindicated in renal or hepatic failure, glomerulonephritis, and pyelonephritis of pregnancy with gastrointestinal disturbances.

WARNINGS

Sulfonamides should not be used to treat group A streptococci infections or their sequelae. The occurrence of sore throat, fever, pallor, purpura, or jaundice during sulfonamide administration may be an early indication of serious blood dyscrasias.
Deaths associated with the administration of sulfonamides have been reported from hypersensitivity reactions, agranulocytosis, aplastic anemia, and other blood dyscrasias.
Frequent blood counts and renal function tests should be carried out during sulfonamide treatment, especially during prolonged administration. Microscopic urinalyses should be done once a week when a patient is treated for longer than two weeks. Urine cultures should be made to confirm eradication of bacteriuria.

PRECAUTIONS

To allay any possible apprehension, patients should be told that this medication may color the urine orange or red.
The usual precautions used in sulfonamide therapy should be observed, including the maintenance of an adequate fluid intake. Sulfonamides should be used with caution in patients with severe allergy or bronchial asthma, severe impairment of hepatic or renal function, and in patients with glucose-6-phosphate dehydrogenase deficiency since sulfas may cause hemolysis in this latter group.
Carcinogenesis: THIOSULFIL-A FORTE (sulfamethizole 500 mg with phenazopyridine HCl) and THIOSULFIL-A (sulfamethizole 250 mg with phenazopyridine HCl) have not undergone adequate trials relating to carcinogenicity; each component, however, has been evaluated separately. Rats appear to be especially susceptible to the goitrogenic effects of sulfonamides, and long-term administration of sulfonamides has resulted in thyroid malignancies in this species. Long-term administration of phenazopyridine hydrochloride has induced neoplasia in rats (large intestine) and mice (liver). Although no association between phenazopyridine hydrochloride and human neoplasia has been reported, adequate epidemiological studies have not been conducted.
Mutagenesis or Impairment of Fertility: No long-term studies in animals or humans have been conducted.
Pregnancy Category C: Certain sulfonamides of the short-, intermediate-, and long-acting types, when given to rats and mice in doses 7 to 25 times the human dose, have been associated with a significant increase in the incidence of cleft pal-

ate and other bony abnormalities of the offspring. There are no adequate and well-controlled studies in pregnant women. THIOSULFIL®-A and THIOSULFIL®-A FORTE should be used during pregnancy only if the potential benefit justifies the potential risk to the fetus.
Nursing Mothers: (See CONTRAINDICATIONS.)

ADVERSE REACTIONS
Blood dyscrasias: Agranulocytosis, aplastic anemia, thrombocytopenia, leukopenia, hemolytic anemia, purpura, hypoprothrombinemia, and methemoglobinemia.
Allergic reactions: Erythema multiforme (Stevens-Johnson syndrome), generalized skin eruptions, epidermal necrolysis, urticaria, serum sickness, pruritus, exfoliative dermatitis, anaphylactoid reactions, periorbital edema, conjunctival and scleral injection, photosensitization, arthralgia, and allergic myocarditis.
Gastrointestinal reactions: Nausea, emesis, abdominal pains, hepatitis, diarrhea, anorexia, pancreatitis, and stomatitis.
C.N.S. reactions: Headache, peripheral neuritis, mental depression, convulsions, ataxia, hallucinations, tinnitus, vertigo, and insomnia.
Miscellaneous reactions: Drug fever, chills, and toxic nephrosis with oliguria and anuria. Periarteritis nodosum and L.E. phenomenon have occurred.
The sulfonamides bear certain chemical similarities to some goitrogens, diuretics (acetazolamide and the thiazides), and oral hypoglycemic agents. Goiter production, diuresis, and hypoglycemia have occurred rarely in patients receiving sulfonamides. Cross-sensitivity may exist with these agents.

DOSAGE AND ADMINISTRATION
Usual dosage in adults (based on sulfamethizole content):
THIOSULFIL-A FORTE (sulfamethizole 500 mg with phenazopyridine HCl):
2 tablets three or four times daily for 2 days.
THIOSULFIL-A (sulfamethizole 250 mg with phenazopyridine HCl):
2–4 tablets three or four times daily for 2 days. Treatment with THIOSULFIL-A FORTE or THIOSULFIL-A should not exceed 2 days. Treatment beyond 2 days should only be continued with sulfamethizole.
If pain persists, other causes for the discomfort should be investigated.

HOW SUPPLIED
THIOSULFIL-A FORTE (sulfamethizole 500 mg, phenazopyridine HCl 50 mg) Tablets, in bottles of 100 (NDC 0046-0783-81).
THIOSULFIL-A (sulfamethizole 250 mg, phenazopyridine HCl 50 mg) Tablets, in bottles of 100 (NDC 0046-0784-81).
Shown in Product Identification Section, page 405

THIOSULFIL® ℞
[*thīo″sul-fil′fil*]
(sulfamethizole)
DUO-PAK®
Package

CAUTION: Federal law prohibits dispensing without prescription.

DESCRIPTION
This package contains 2 products:

Bottle No. 1—16 Tablets (*yellow*)

THIOSULFIL®-A Forte
(sulfamethizole 500 mg with phenazopyridine HCl)
Each tablet contains:
Sulfamethizole .... 500 mg
Phenazopyridine HCl .... 50 mg

Bottle No. 2—40 Tablets (*white*)

THIOSULFIL® Forte
(sulfamethizole 500 mg)
Each tablet contains:
Sulfamethizole .... 500 mg
Sulfamethizole [N′-(5-Methyl-1,3,4-thiadiazol-2-yl) sulfanilamide] is a 5-membered heterocyclic sulfanilamide occurring as a white or light buff-colored crystalline powder. Solubility in water is dependent upon the pH (1 g 5 mL at pH 7.5; 1 g/4000 mL at pH 6.5). It is soluble in alcohol, and practically insoluble in benzene.

$H_2N-C_6H_4-SO_2-NH-C$ (thiadiazole ring: N—N, S) $C-CH_3$

Phenazopyridine HCl [2,6-Diamino-3-phenylazopyridine hydrochloride] occurs as brick-red microcrystals with a slight violet luster. It is soluble in boiling water, ethylene and propylene glycols, slightly soluble in alcohol and cold water, and insoluble in acetone and benzene.

H_2N, NH_2, HCl, $N{=}N-C_6H_5$

THIOSULFIL-A FORTE Tablets contain the following inactive ingredients: amberlite resin, calcium sulfate anhydrous, D&C Yellow No. 10, FD&C Yellow No. 6, glyceryl mono-oleate, guar gum, lactose, magnesium stearate, methylcellulose, pharmaceutical glaze, polyethylene glycol, starch.
THIOSULFIL FORTE Tablets contain the following inactive ingredients: gelatin, magnesium stearate, microcrystalline cellulose, starch.

CLINICAL PHARMACOLOGY
The combination of sulfamethizole and phenazopyridine in THIOSULFIL-A FORTE acts to eradicate urinary tract infections due to susceptible organisms, and relieve pain and discomfort associated with infection. Following relief of pain, THIOSULFIL FORTE (sulfamethizole), containing only sulfamethizole, provides continuing antibacterial therapy.
PHENAZOPYRIDINE HCl: Phenazopyridine HCl is an analgesic that acts on the mucosa of the urinary tract to provide relief of pain and discomfort caused by inflammation associated with urinary tract infection.
SULFAMETHIZOLE:
Mechanism of sulfonamide bacteriostatic action: The primary mechanism of bacteriostatic action by THIOSULFIL (sulfamethizole) is the same as that of most sulfonamides. By competing with the precursor para-aminobenzoic acid, sulfonamides inhibit bacterial synthesis of folic (pteroylglutamic) acid which is required for bacterial growth. Resistant strains are capable of utilizing folic acid precursors or preformed folic acid.
Sulfonamide antibacterial spectrum: The antibacterial spectrum of all sulfonamides is similar. *In vitro* sensitivity of bacteria to sulfonamides does not always reflect *in vivo* sensitivity. Therefore, efficacy must be carefully evaluated with bacteriologic and clinical responses in the individual patient. (See WARNINGS)
Factors determining antibacterial efficacy: Efficacy of antimicrobial therapy is dependent upon a number of factors including the *in vivo* sensitivity of the involved organisms, the concentration of the drug required for bacteriostasis, and the achievable concentration of the sulfonamide at the desired site of action.
Because of the very rapid renal clearance of sulfamethizole, the blood levels attained are low, and accumulation of the drug in tissues outside the urinary tract is very limited. Therefore, sulfamethizole is not appropriate for treatment of systemic infections such as nocardiosis or for local lesions outside the urinary tract such as chancroid and trachoma. However, its low degree of acetylation and its rapid renal clearance permit high concentrations of active sulfamethizole to occur in the urinary tract, making it especially applicable for the treatment of infections of this tract. In addition, the possibility of crystalluria is minimized because of the high solubility of the drug in urine.
Approximately 95% of a given dose of sulfamethizole is not metabolized; less than 5% is acetylated. As a consequence, almost all of a given dose of THIOSULFIL is present in its active form in the body.
Approximately 80% of an administered dose is recoverable within eight hours; approximately 98% is cleared within 15 to 24 hours. Sulfamethizole is cleared by the kidney at a rate only 10 to 20% lower than that for creatinine.

INDICATIONS AND USAGE
THIOSULFIL-A FORTE (sulfamethizole 500 mg with phenazopyridine HCl)—Bottle No. 1—is indicated for the initial treatment of uncomplicated urinary tract infections caused by susceptible strains of the following microorganisms. *Escherichia coli, Klebsiella* species; *Enterobacter* species, *Proteus mirabilis, Proteus vulgaris,* and *Staphylococcus aureus* when relief of symptoms of pain, burning, or urgency is needed during the first 2 days of therapy. Treatment with THIOSULFIL-A FORTE should not exceed 2 days. There is a lack of evidence that the combination of sulfamethizole and phenazopyridine hydrochloride provides greater benefit than sulfamethizole alone after 2 days. Treatment beyond 2 days should only be continued with sulfamethizole. (See DOSAGE AND ADMINISTRATION.)
THIOSULFIL FORTE (sulfamethizole)—Bottle No. 2—is indicated for continuing antibacterial therapy after pain and discomfort have been relieved.
Important note. *In vitro* sulfonamide sensitivity tests are not always reliable. The test must be carefully coordinated with bacteriologic and clinical response. When the patient is already taking sulfonamides, follow-up cultures should have aminobenzoic acid added to the culture media.
Currently the increasing frequency of resistant organisms is a limitation of the usefulness of antibacterial agents, including the sulfonamides, especially in the treatment of recurrent and complicated urinary tract infections.
Wide variation in blood levels may result with identical doses. Blood levels should be measured in patients receiving sulfonamides for serious infections. Free sulfonamide blood levels of 5–15 mg per 100 mL may be considered therapeutically effective for most infections, with blood levels of 12–15 mg per 100 mL optimal for serious infections; 20 mg per 100 mL should be the maximum total sulfonamide level, as adverse reactions occur more frequently above this level.

CONTRAINDICATIONS
Sulfonamides should not be used in patients hypersensitive to sulfa drugs. They should not be used in infants less than two months of age, in pregnancy at term, and during the nursing period because sulfonamides pass the placenta and are excreted in the milk and may cause kernicterus.
Phenazopyridine HCl is contraindicated in renal or hepatic failure, glomerulonephritis, and pyelonephritis of pregnancy with gastrointestinal disturbances.

WARNINGS
Sulfonamides should not be used to treat group A streptococci infections or their sequelae. The occurrence of sore throat, fever, pallor, purpura, or jaundice during sulfonamide administration may be an early indication of serious blood dyscrasias.
Deaths associated with the administration of sulfonamides have been reported from hypersensitivity reactions, agranulocytosis, aplastic anemia, and other blood dyscrasias.
Frequent blood counts and renal function tests should be carried out during sulfonamide treatment, especially during prolonged administration. Microscopic urinalyses should be done once a week when a patient is treated for longer than two weeks. Urine cultures should be made to confirm eradication of bacteriuria.

PRECAUTIONS
To allay any possible apprehension, patients should be told that this medication may color the urine orange or red.
The usual precautions used in sulfonamide therapy should be observed, including the maintenance of an adequate fluid intake. Sulfonamides should be used with caution in patients with severe allergy or bronchial asthma, severe impairment of hepatic or renal function, and in patients with glucose-6-phosphate dehydrogenase deficiency since sulfas may cause hemolysis in this latter group.
Carcinogenesis: THIOSULFIL-A FORTE and THIOSULFIL FORTE have not undergone adequate trials relating to carcinogenicity; each component, however, has been evaluated separately. Rats appear to be especially susceptible to the goitrogenic effects of sulfonamides, and long-term administration of sulfonamides has resulted in thyroid malignancies in this species. Long-term administration of phenazopyridine hydrochloride has induced neoplasia in rats (large intestine) and mice (liver). Although no association between phenazopyridine hydrochloride and human neoplasia has been reported, adequate epidemiological studies have not been conducted.
Mutagenesis or Impairment of Fertility: No long-term studies in animals or humans have been conducted.
Pregnancy Category C: Certain sulfonamides of the short, intermediate, and long-acting types, when given to rats and mice in doses 7 to 25 times the human dose, have been associated with a significant increase in the incidence of cleft palate and other bony abnormalities of the offspring. There are no adequate and well-controlled studies in pregnant women. THIOSULFIL®-FORTE and THIOSULFIL®-A FORTE should be used during pregnancy only if the potential benefit justifies the potential risk to the fetus.
Nursing Mothers: (See CONTRAINDICATIONS.)

ADVERSE REACTIONS
Blood dyscrasias: Agranulocytosis, aplastic anemia, thrombocytopenia, leukopenia, hemolytic anemia, purpura, hypoprothrombinemia, and methemoglobinemia.
Allergic reactions: Erythema multiforme (Stevens-Johnson syndrome), generalized skin eruptions, epidermal necrolysis, urticaria, serum sickness, pruritus, exfoliative dermatitis, anaphylactoid reactions, periorbital edema, conjunctival and scleral injection, photosensitization, arthralgia, and allergic myocarditis.
Gastrointestinal reactions: Nausea, emesis, abdominal pains, hepatitis, diarrhea, anorexia, pancreatitis, and stomatitis.
C.N.S. reactions: Headache, peripheral neuritis, mental depression, convulsions, ataxia, hallucinations, tinnitus, vertigo, and insomnia.
Miscellaneous reactions: Drug fever, chills, and toxic nephrosis with oliguria and anuria. Periarteritis nodosum and L.E. phenomenon have occurred.
The sulfonamides bear certain chemical similarities to some goitrogens, diuretics (acetazolamide and the thiazides), and oral hypoglycemic agents. Goiter production, diuresis, and hypoglycemia have occurred rarely in patients receiving sulfonamides. Cross-sensitivity may exist with these agents.

DOSAGE AND ADMINISTRATION
Adult dosage regimen:
Start—Bottle No. 1 THIOSULFIL-A FORTE (sulfamethizole 500 mg with phenazopyridine HCl)—2 *yellow* tablets three or four times daily for 2 days.

Continued on next page

Ayerst—Cont.

Continue—Bottle No. 2 THIOSULFIL FORTE (sulfamethizole 500 mg)—2 *white* tablets four times daily for 5 days. Continue medication as recommended by physician.
Treatment with THIOSULFIL-A FORTE or THIOSULFIL-A should not exceed 2 days. Treatment beyond 2 days should only be continued with sulfamethizole.
If pain persists, other causes for the discomfort should be investigated.

HOW SUPPLIED

THIOSULFIL® (sulfamethizole) DUO-PAK® NDC 0046-0780-98.
Bottle No. 1—THIOSULFIL®-A FORTE: 16 tablets (yellow).
Bottle No. 2—THIOSULFIL® FORTE: 40 tablets (white).

EDUCATIONAL MATERIAL

Films-Videos-Slides

As a service to the medical profession, Ayerst Laboratories makes available film, audiovisual, and slide programs on a free-loan basis through the local Ayerst representative, or by writing to: AYERST AUDIOVISUAL PROGRAMS, 22 Riverview Drive, Wayne, NJ 07470-3191. A catalog listing programs on alcoholism, anesthesiology, cardiology, endocrinology, neurology, and pharmacology may be obtained by writing to: Director of Audiovisual Services, Ayerst Laboratories, 685 Third Avenue, New York, NY 10017-4071.
A number of Ayerst Audiovisual Educational Programs, particularly in the fields of cardiovascular disease, osteoporosis, and migraine, qualify viewers for CME credits. Related printed materials on these subjects may be available.

Booklets

Patient and consumer booklets, providing useful information on angina, hypertension, post-MI recovery, the menopause, postmenopausal osteoporosis, osteoporosis and calcium deficiency, postpartum care, and vitamins, are also available. Physicians may write to Manager, Professional Services, Medical Department, Ayerst Laboratories, 685 Third Avenue, New York, NY 10017-4071.

Baker/Cummins

Dermatological Div. of
Key Pharmaceuticals, Inc.
4400 BISCAYNE BLVD.
MIAMI, FLORIDA 33137

COMPLEX 15®
Phospholipid Moisturizer

(See PDR For Nonprescription Drugs)

P&S® LIQUID

(See PDR For Nonprescription Drugs)

P&S® PLUS
Tar Gel

(See PDR For Nonprescription Drugs)

P&S® SHAMPOO

(See PDR For Nonprescription Drugs)

ULTRA MIDE™ 25 MOISTURIZER

(See PDR For Nonprescription Drugs)

XSEB® SHAMPOO

(See PDR For Nonprescription Drugs)

XSEB®-T SHAMPOO

(See PDR For Nonprescription Drugs)

Products are cross-indexed by generic and chemical names in the **YELLOW SECTION**

Barnes-Hind, Inc.

A Revlon Vision Care Company
895 KIFER ROAD
SUNNYVALE, CA 94086

OPHTHALMIC PRODUCTS

For information on BARNES-HIND prescription and OTC ophthalmic products consult the PDR For Ophthalmology. See a complete listing of products in the Manufacturer's Index Section of this book. For information or literature contact BARNES-HIND directly.

DERMATOLOGICAL PRODUCTS

BARSEB® HC ℞
[*bar-sĕb hc*]
SCALP LOTION

DESCRIPTION

Contains hydrocortisone 1%, salicylic acid 0.5%, isopropyl alcohol 45%, propylene glycol, isopropyl myristate, ascorbic acid, and citric acid.

ACTIONS

BARSEB® HC Scalp Lotion is primarily effective because of the anti-inflammatory, antipruritic, and vaso-constrictive actions of hydrocortisone, and salicylic acid aids in loosening and removing adherent sebum, crust, and epithelial debris.

INDICATIONS

For the relief of the inflammatory manifestations of corticosteroid-responsive dermatoses of the scalp.

CONTRAINDICATIONS

Topical steroids are contraindicated in those patients with a history of hypersensitivity to any of the components of the preparations.

PRECAUTIONS

If irritation develops, the product should be discontinued and appropriate therapy instituted.
In the presence of an infection, use of an appropriate antifungal or antibacterial agent should be instituted. If a favorable response does not occur promptly, the corticosteroid should be discontinued until the infection has been adequately controlled.
If extensive areas are treated or if the occlusive technique is used, there will be increased systemic absorption of the corticosteroid and suitable precautions should be taken, particularly in children and infants.
Although topical steroids have not been reported to have an adverse effect on human pregnancy, the safety of their use in pregnant women has not absolutely been established. In laboratory animals, increases in incidence of fetal abnormalities have been associated with exposure of gestating females to topical corticosteroids. Therefore, drugs of this class should not be used extensively on pregnant patients, in large amounts, or for prolonged periods of time.
Not for Ophthalmic Use or Use Around the Eyes.

ADVERSE REACTIONS

The following local adverse reactions have been reported with topical corticosteroids especially under occlusive dressings: burning, itching, irritation, dryness, folliculitis, hypertrichosis, acneform eruptions, hypopigmentation, perioral dermatitis, allergic contact dermatitis, maceration of the skin, secondary infection, skin atrophy, striae, and miliaria. Transient discomfort may occur when first applied to an inflamed scalp.

DOSAGE AND ADMINISTRATION

Part hair, apply once or twice a day with gentle rubbing. Use sparingly. When a favorable response is obtained, reduce dosage as necessary.

CAUTION

Federal (U.S.A.) law prohibits dispensing without prescription.
For dermatologic use only.

HOW SUPPLIED

BARSEB® HC is supplied in 1.75 fl. oz. (52 ml) plastic squeeze bottles.
Store at room temperature; avoid excessive heat (104°F.).

BARSEB® THERA=SPRAY® ℞
[*bar-sĕb thĕr-a sprā*]
Topical Aerosol

DESCRIPTION

Each bottle (84 g) contains 360 mg hydrocortisone, 288 mg salicylic acid, 14 mg benzalkonium chloride, 46 g alcohol with propylene glycol, isopropyl myristate, and butane as propellant.
After evaporation of the propellant, the vehicle contains 0.6% hydrocortisone, 0.48% salicylic acid, and 0.024% benzalkonium chloride.

ACTIONS

BARSEB THERA-SPRAY is primarily effective because of the anti-inflammatory, antipruritic, and vasoconstrictive actions of hydrocortisone, and salicylic acid aids in loosening and removing adherent sebum, crusts, and epithelial debris.

INDICATIONS

BARSEB THERA-SPRAY is indicated for the relief of the inflammatory manifestations of corticosteroid-responsive dermatoses of the scalp.

CONTRAINDICATIONS

Contraindicated in those patients with a history of hypersensitivity to any of the components of the aerosol.

PRECAUTIONS

If irritation develops, discontinue use and institute appropriate therapy.
In the presence of an infection, use of an appropriate antifungal or antibacterial agent should be instituted. If a favorable response does not occur promptly, application of Barseb should be discontinued until the infection has been adequately controlled.
If extensive areas are treated or if the occlusive technique is used, there will be increased systemic absorption of the corticosteroid and suitable precautions should be taken, particularly with children and infants.
Avoid inhalation, ingestion or contact with the eyes or nose. If spray accidentally gets into eyes, flush with copious amounts of water.
Although topical steroids have not been reported to have an adverse effect on human pregnancy, the safety of their use in pregnant women has not absolutely been established. In laboratory animals, increases in incidence of fetal abnormalities have been associated with exposure of gestating females to topical corticosteroids, in some cases at rather low dosage levels. Therefore, drugs of this class should not be used extensively on pregnant patients, in large amounts, or for prolonged periods of time.
This product is not for ophthalmic use.

ADVERSE REACTIONS

The following local adverse reactions have been reported with topical corticosteroids, especially under occlusive dressings: burning, itching, irritation, dryness, folliculitis, hypertrichosis, acneform eruptions, hypopigmentation, perioral dermatitis, allergic contact dermatitis, maceration of the skin, secondary infection, skin atrophy, striae, and miliaria. Transient discomfort may occur when first applied to an inflamed scalp.

DOSAGE AND ADMINISTRATION

BARSEB THERA-SPRAY should be applied once daily during the acute phase or as directed by a physician. A maintenance schedule may be adjusted to the patient's response to therapy.

DIRECTIONS FOR USE

Shake well. Hold the bottle upright (being careful not to spray forehead or eyes); insert applicator tube through hair to scalp at front hairline. Then start spraying and moving applicator tube slowly toward the back of the head. Repeat this procedure until all affected areas of the scalp are treated. Because of the spreading and penetrating properties of BARSEB THERA-SPRAY, it is not necessary to rub or massage medication into the scalp. Assembly directions are provided on the aerosol bottles.

HOW SUPPLIED

BARSEB THERA-SPRAY is supplied in 84 g aerosol bottles with applicator tube.

KOMED® Acne Lotion OTC
[*kō-mĕd*]

Sodium thiosulfate	8%
Salicylic acid	2%
Isopropyl alcohol	25%

The above product also contains menthol, camphor, colloidal alumina, edetate disodium, and purified water.

INDICATIONS

Primarily indicated for the treatment of acne associated with oily skin. KOMED Acne Lotion is indicated in more severe conditions or where stronger keratolytic effect is desired. Komed Lotion features a thixotropic gel of colloidal alumina. It is greaseless and dries to an almost invisible film, forming a medicated base over which non-oily cosmetics may be applied.

PRECAUTIONS

Do not use Komed Lotion on or near the eyes.

DOSAGE AND ADMINISTRATION

Wash affected areas thoroughly. Shake lotion well and apply a thin film twice a day.

HOW SUPPLIED

1¾ fl. oz. (52.5 ml.) plastic squeeze bottles.

KOMED® HC Lotion ℞
[*ko-mĕd hc*]
(hydrocortisone)

DESCRIPTION
Contains hydrocortisone acetate 0.5%, sodium thiosulfate 8%, salicylic acid 2%, isopropyl alcohol 25%, menthol, camphor, colloidal alumina, edetate disodium, and purified water.

INDICATIONS
KOMED HC Acne Lotion is indicated for topical treatment of acne conditions when accompanied by inflammation. KOMED HC features a thixotropic gel of colloidal alumina. The lotion is greaseless and dries to an almost invisible film, forming a medicated base over which non-oily cosmetics may be applied.

CONTRAINDICATIONS
Topical steroids are contraindicated in those patients with a history of hypersensitivity to any of the components of the preparation.

PRECAUTIONS
If irritation develops, the product should be discontinued and appropriate therapy instituted.
In the presence of an infection, the use of an appropriate antifungal or antibacterial agent should be instituted. If a favorable response does not occur promptly, the corticosteroid should be discontinued until the infection has been adequately controlled.
If extensive areas are treated or if the occlusive technique is used, there will be increased systemic absorption of the corticosteroid and suitable precautions should be taken, particularly in children and infants.
Although topical steroids have not been reported to have an adverse effect on human pregnancy, the safety of their use in pregnant women has not been absolutely established. In laboratory animals, increases in incidence of fetal abnormalities have been associated with exposure of gestating females to topical corticosteroids. Therefore, drugs of this class should not be used extensively on pregnant patients, in large amounts, or for prolonged periods of time.
Not for Ophthalmic Use or Use Around the Eyes.

ADVERSE REACTIONS
The following local adverse reactions have been reported with topical corticosteroids especially under occlusive dressings: burning, itching, irritation, dryness, folliculitis, hypertrichosis, acneform eruptions, hypopigmentation, perioral dermatitis, allergic contact dermatitis, maceration of the skin, secondary infection, skin atrophy, striae, and miliaria.

DOSAGE AND ADMINISTRATION
Wash affected areas thoroughly. Shake lotion well and apply a thin film twice a day, or as directed.

HOW SUPPLIED
1¾ fl. oz. (52.5 ml.) plastic squeeze bottles. Store at room temperature, avoid excessive heat.

KOMEX® OTC
[*kō-mĕx*]
(Scrub for Oily Skin and Make-up Removal)

DESCRIPTION
KOMEX® is a dissolving cleanser useful as an aid in reducing oily skin conditions associated with acne.

CONTENTS
SCRUBULES, Barnes-Hind brand of dissolving particles (sodium tetraborate decahydrate), in a preserved base containing a unique combination of surface active soapless cleaning agents, and skin conditioners.

DIRECTIONS
Use Komex in place of your usual soap or cleanser.
Skin Cleansing: Wet the face with warm water. Squeeze Komex onto your fingertips, and gently massage into the face. Continue scrubbing and adding water until Scrubules are completely dissolved (about one minute). Rinse thoroughly and dry. Use once or twice daily.

CAUTION
Avoid contact with eyes. If granules get into the eyes, flush thoroughly with water and avoid rubbing eyes. If skin irritation or excessive dryness develops, or increases, discontinue use. For external use only. Keep out of reach of children. Not to be used on infants. Do not use on inflamed skin.

HOW SUPPLIED
2.65 oz. (75 g.) plastic squeeze tube in unit carton.

TINVER® LOTION ℞
[*tin-ver*]

DESCRIPTION
Sodium thiosulfate 25%, salicylic acid 1%, isopropyl alcohol 10%, propylene glycol, menthol, edetate disodium, colloidal alumina, purified water.

INDICATIONS
For topical use in treatment of tinea versicolor infections.

PRECAUTIONS
Discontinue use if irritation or sensitivity develops. Do not use on or about the eyes.

DOSAGE AND ADMINISTRATION
Thoroughly wash, rinse, and dry affected and susceptible areas before application. Apply thin film of TINVER twice a day. Although diagnostic evidence of the disease may disappear in a few days, it is advisable to continue treatment for a much longer period. Clothing should be boiled to prevent reinfection.

HOW SUPPLIED
4 fl. oz. (180 ml.) plastic squeeze bottles. Store at room temperature, avoid excessive heat.

Barr Laboratories, Inc.
265 LIVINGSTON STREET
NORTHVALE, NJ 07647

Barr Product Listing
Barr manufacturers all of its own products so you can be assured of product identification consistency in color and size batch-to-batch, day-to-day, year-to-year.

NDC # 0555	PRODUCT	
0176	Acetaminophen Tablets 325 mg.	—
0326	Acetaminophen Tablets 500 mg.	—
0217	Acetaminophen w/ Codeine Tablets 300 mg./15 mg.	C-III
0198	Acetaminophen w/ Codeine Tablets 300 mg./30 mg.	C-III
0229	Acetaminophen w/ Codeine Tablets 300 mg./60 mg.	C-III
0241	Allopurinol Tablets 100 mg.	℞
0242	Allopurinol Tablets 300 mg.	℞
0282	Aminophylline Tablets 100 mg.	℞
0281	Aminophylline Tablets 200 mg.	℞
0209	Amitriptyline HCL Tablets 10 mg.	℞
0203	Amitriptyline HCL Tablets 25 mg.	℞
0210	Amitriptyline HCL Tablets 50 mg.	℞
0211	Amitriptyline HCL Tablets 75 mg.	℞
0212	Amitriptyline HCL Tablets 100 mg.	℞
0294	Aspirin w/ Codeine Tablets 325 mg./15 mg.	C-III
0264	Aspirin w/ Codeine Tablets 325 mg./30 mg.	C-III
0280	Aspirin w/ Codeine Tablets 325 mg./60 mg.	C-III
0099	Bisacodyl Tablets 5 mg.	—
0158	Chlordiazepoxide HCL Capsules 5 mg.	C-IV
0033	Chlordiazepoxide HCL Capsules 10 mg.	C-IV
0159	Chlordiazepoxide HCL Capsules 25 mg.	C-IV
0214	Chlordiazepoxide HCL w/ Clindinium Bromide Capsules 5 mg./2.5 mg.	C-IV
0347	Chlorpropamide Tablets 100 mg.	℞
0276	Chlorpropamide Tablets 250 mg.	℞
0267	Chlorthalidone Tablets 25 mg.	℞
0268	Chlorthalidone Tablets 50 mg.	℞
0255	Chlorzoxazone w/ Acetaminophen Tablets 250 mg./300 mg.	℞
0030	Colchicine Tablets 0.65 mg.	℞
0129	Dexamethasone Tablets 0.25 mg.	℞
0130	Dexamethasone Tablets 0.50 mg.	℞
0131	Dexamethasone Tablets 0.75 mg.	℞
0132	Dexamethasone Tablets 1.50 mg.	℞
0163	Diazepam Tablets 2 mg.	C-IV
0363	Diazepam Tablets 5 mg.	C-IV
0164	Diazepam Tablets 10 mg.	C-IV
0128	Dicyclomine HCL Capsules 10 mg.	C-IV
0126	Dicyclomine HCL Tablets 20 mg.	C-IV
0057	Dimenhydrinate Tablets 50 mg.	C-IV
0058	Diphenhydramine Capsules 25 mg.	—
0059	Diphenhydramine Capsules 50 mg.	—
0200	Diphenoxylate HCL w/ Atropine Sulfate Tablets 2.5 mg./0.25 mg.	C-V
0252	Dipyridamole Tablets 25 mg.	℞
0285	Dipyridamole Tablets 50 mg.	℞
0286	Dipyridamole Tablets 75 mg.	℞
0331	Disopyramide Phosphate Capsules 100 mg.	℞
0332	Disopyramide Phosphate Capsules 150 mg.	℞
0296	Doxycycline Capsules 50 mg. (DOXY-CAPS)	℞
0297	Doxycycline Capsules 100 mg. (DOXY-CAPS)	℞
0295	Doxycycline Tablets 100 mg. (DOXY-TABS)	℞
0218	Ergoloid Mesylates Tablets 0.5 mg. S/L	℞
0227	Ergoloid Mesylates Tablets 1.0 mg. S/L	℞
0383	Ergoloid Mesylates Tablets 1.0 mg. ORAL	℞
0230	Erythromycin Estolate Capsules 250 mg.	℞
0215	Erythromycin Ethylsuccinate Granules 200 mg./5 ml.	℞
0259	Erythromycin Ethylsuccinate Tablets 400 mg.	℞
0013	Erythromycin Stearate Tablets 250 mg.	℞
0434	Folic Acid Tablets 1 mg.	℞
0170	Furosemide Tablets 20 mg.	℞
0169	Furosemide Tablets 40 mg.	℞
0388	Hydralazine HCL Tablets 10 mg.	℞
0064	Hydralazine HCL Tablets 25 mg.	℞
0065	Hydralazine HCL Tablets 50 mg.	℞
0389	Hydralazine HCL Tablets 100 mg.	℞
0019	Hydrochlorothiazide HCL Tablets 25 mg.	℞
0020	Hydrochlorothiazide HCL Tablets 50 mg.	℞
0192	Hydrochlorothiazide HCL Tablets 100 mg.	℞
0325	Hydrocodone Bitartrate w/ Acetaminophen Tablets 5 mg./500 mg.	C-III
0301	Hydroxyzine HCL Tablets 10 mg.	℞
0298	Hydroxyzine HCL Tablets 25 mg.	℞
0299	Hydroxyzine HCL Tablets 50 mg.	℞
0300	Hydroxyzine HCL Tablets 100 mg.	℞
0323	Hydroxyzine Pamoate Capsules 25 mg.	℞

Continued on next page

Barr—Cont.

Code	Product	
0302	Hydroxyzine Pamoate Capsules 50 mg.	℞
0324	Hydroxyzine Pamoate Capsules 100 mg.	℞
0419	Ibuprofen Tablets 400 mg.	℞
0420	Ibuprofen Tablets 600 mg.	℞
0066	Isoniazid Tablets 100 mg.	℞
0071	Isoniazid Tablets 300 mg.	℞
0174	Isosorbide Dinitrate Tablets 5 mg. ORAL	℞
0175	Isosorbide Dinitrate Tablets 10 mg. ORAL	℞
0186	Isosorbide Dinitrate Tablets 20 mg. ORAL	℞
0279	Isosorbide Dinitrate Tablets 30 mg. ORAL	℞
0172	Isosorbide Dinitrate Tablets 2.5 mg. S/L	℞
0173	Isosorbide Dinitrate Tablets 5 mg. S/L	℞
0277	Isosorbide Dinitrate Tablets 10 mg. S/L	℞
0370	Lorazepam Tablets 0.5 mg.	C-IV
0371	Lorazepam Tablets 1.0 mg.	C-IV
0372	Lorazepam Tablets 2.0 mg.	C-IV
0381	Meperidine HCL Tablets 50 mg.	C-II
0382	Meperidine HCL Tablets 100 mg.	C-II
0035	Meprobamate Tablets 200 mg.	C-IV
0036	Meprobamate Tablets 400 mg.	C-IV
0106	Methocarbamol Tablets 500 mg.	℞
0107	Methocarbamol Tablets 750 mg.	℞
0291	Metronidazole Tablets 250 mg.	℞
0292	Metronidazole Tablets 500 mg.	℞
0278	Oxycodone w/ Acetaminophen Tablets 5 mg./325 mg.	C-III
0293	Oxycodone w/ Aspirin Tablets 4.5 mg./325 mg.	C-III
0152	Phenobarbital Tablets 15 mg.	C-IV
0153	Phenobarbital Tablets 30 mg.	C-IV
0394	Phenobarbital Tablets 60 mg.	C-IV
0395	Phenylbutazone Tablets 100 mg.	℞
0396	Phenylbutazone Capsules 100 mg.	℞
0026	Prednisone Tablets 5 mg.	℞
0233	Prednisone Tablets 10 mg.	℞
0157	Prednisone Tablets 20 mg.	℞
0317	Propoxyphene Napsylate and Acetaminophen Tablets 50 mg./325 mg.	C-IV
0318	Propoxyphene Napsylate and Acetaminophen Tablets 100 mg./650 mg.	C-IV
0470	Propoxyphene Napsylate and Acetaminophen Tablets 100 mg./650 mg.	C-IV
0365	Propranolol HCL Tablets 10 mg.	℞
0366	Propranolol HCL Tablets 20 mg.	℞
0367	Propranolol HCL Tablets 40 mg.	℞
0089	Propylthiouracil Tablets 50 mg.	℞
0188	Quinidine Sulfate Tablets 200 mg.	℞
0114	Reserpine/Hydrochlorothiazide Tablets 0.125 mg./25 mg.	℞
0116	Reserpine/Hydrochlorothiazide Tablets 0.125 mg./50 mg.	℞
0115	Reserpine/Hydralazine HCL/ Hydrochlorothiazide Tablets 0.1 mg./25 mg./15 mg.	℞
0266	Spironolactone Tablets 25 mg.	℞
0265	Spironolactone w/ Hydrochlorothiazide Tablets 25 mg./25 mg.	℞
0314	Sulfamethoxazole Tablets 500 mg.	℞
0321	Sulfamethoxazole w/ Trimethoprim Tablets 400 mg./80 mg.	℞
0322	Sulfamethoxazole w/ Trimethoprim Tablets 800 mg./160 mg.	℞
0272	Sulfinpyrazone Capsules 200 mg.	℞
0271	Sulfinpyrazone Tablets 100 mg.	℞
0024	Sulfisoxazole Tablets 500 mg.	℞
0487	Temazepam Capsules 15 mg	C-IV
0488	Temazepam Capsules 30 mg	C-IV
0011	Tetracycline Capsules 250 mg.	℞
0010	Tetracycline Capsules 500 mg.	℞
0260	Thioridazine HCL Tablets 10 mg.	℞
0329	Thioridazine HCL Tablets 15 mg.	℞
0261	Thioridazine HCL Tablets 25 mg.	℞
0262	Thioridazine HCL Tablets 50 mg.	℞
0263	Thioridazine HCL Tablets 100 mg.	℞
0327	Thioridazine HCL Tablets 150 mg.	℞
0328	Thioridazine HCL Tablets 200 mg.	℞
0415	Tolazamide Tablets 100 mg.	℞
0416	Tolazamide Tablets 250 mg.	℞
0417	Tolazamide Tablets 500 mg.	℞
0251	Tolbutamide Tablets 500 mg.	℞
0429	Trimethoprim Tablets of 100 mg.	℞

Barry Laboratories, Inc.

461 N. E. 27th STREET
P. O. BOX 1967
POMPANO BEACH, FL 33061

ALLERGENIC EXTRACTS, DIAGNOSIS AND/OR IMMUNOTHERAPY ℞

COMPOSITION

Fluid allergens are available from the following categories: pollens, foods, dusts, epidermals, insects, fungi (molds & smuts), yeasts, and others.

ACTION AND USES

For diagnosis and immunotherapy of specific offenders in allergy.

PRECAUTIONS

Usual precautions used in testing or treating hypersenstive individuals. See product information circulars accompanying each product.

HOW SUPPLIED

Diagnostic materials are availabe in liquid form for cutaneous or intracutaneous testing.

Diagnostic Test Sets: The "50 Plus"—includes a comprehensive selection of perennial and seasonal allergens for each of 5 botanical zones.

Immunorex®—Prescription Allergy Treatment Sets—Individualized, four vial treatment sets are prepared from the physician's instructions, based on the patients's skin test reactions and history. Refills of any dilution are available.

LITERATURE AVAILABLE

Send for free descriptive literature, report and case history forms.

RHUS ALL® ANTIGEN (Barry) ℞

Poison Ivy, Oak and Sumac Combined

COMPOSITION

A triple antigen of the active principles (urushiol) of poison ivy, oak and sumac in an oil vehicle.

INDICATIONS

Prophylactic for hyposensitization of Rhus Dermatitis.

CONTRAINDICATIONS

Not recommended for treatment of active Rhus Dermatitis.

ADMINISTRATION AND DOSAGE

Usual adult dosage: 1 ml. intramuscular injection a week, for two to three weeks prior to patient's exposure.

HOW SUPPLIED

5 ml. multiple dose vial.

LITERATURE AVAILABLE

Write for free Rhus All Antigen pamphlet.

A. J. Bart, Inc.

GURABO INDUSTRIAL PARK
POST OFFICE BOX 813
GURABO, PUERTO RICO 00658

ALBAFORT INJECTABLE ℞

(Iron and B Complex)
FOR INTRAMUSCULAR USE

DESCRIPTION

Albafort is a sterile injectable solution of iron and B Complex vitamins*, each mL contains: Cyanocobalamin (Vit. B_{12}) 100 mcg; Ferrous Gluconate 50 mg; Liver Concentrate (with phenol 60 mcg/mL) supplying 2 mcg/mL Vit. B_{12}; Thiamine HCl (Vit. B_1) 12.5 mg; Riboflavin (Vit. B_2) 0.5 mg; Pyridoxine HCl (Vit. B_6) 2 mg; Dexpanthenol (use equivalent as Calcium Pantothenate) 1 mg; Niacinamide 12.5 mg; Phenol (liquified 98%) 0.5%; Benzyl Alcohol 1.5%; Gentisic Acid Ethanolamide 1.0%; Water for Injection USP q.s.

CLINICAL PHARMACOLOGY

Vitamins and Minerals are essential for normal metabolic functions including hematopoiesis. The B Complex vitamins* play vital roles in the conversion of carbohydrates, proteins and fat into tissue and energy.

Thiamine (B_1) acts as a coenzyme in carbohydrate metabolism. Riboflavin (B_2) functions as a coenzyme in the electron transport system associated with conversion of tissue oxidations into usable energy. Pyridoxine Hydrochloride (B_6) is essential for the metabolism of Amino Acids. Pantothenic Acid functions as a coenzyme in various metabolic acetylation reactions. Cyanocobalamin (B_{12}) is essential to nucleic acid synthesis and normal maturation of red blood cells.

Iron is an essential component in the physiological formation of hemoglobin, adequate amounts of which are necessary to effective erythropoiesis and the resultant oxygen transport capacity of the blood. A similar function is provided by iron in myoglobin production. Iron also serves as a cofactor of several essential enzymes.

INDICATIONS AND USAGE

Albafort injection is indicated for adults and children 11 years of age or older for conditions in which (1) intake or absorption of the B-Complex vitamins* and iron is inadequate and oral intake must be supplemented, or (2) there is a known or suspected serious depletion of iron and B-Complex vitamins* and immediate treatment by the intramuscular route is advisable.

Condition which may require parenteral administration may include disorders which can affect oral intake, gastrointestinal absorption or utilization.

CONTRAINDICATIONS

Albafort is contraindicated in individuals known to be hypersensitive to any of its components.

WARNING

Allergic reactions may occur in patients hypersensitive to any of the components of Albafort. Patients who have early Leber's disease (hereditary optic nerve atrophy) have been found to suffer severe, acute optic atrophy when treated with Vitamin B_{12}. Pyridoxine can decrease the efficacy of Levodopa in the treatment of patients with Parkinsonism. This product should not be used as primary treatment for specific vitamin deficiencies such as: beriberi, pellagra, scurvy, pernicious anemia or other megaloblastic anemia, and riboflavin or pyridoxine deficiency. The possibility of injury to the sciatic nerve should be kept in mind when administering vitamins intramuscularly.

This product should not be used when the following medical problems exist: hemocromatosis or hemosiderosis (indicative of existing iron overload), or anemic conditions which are not accompanied by iron deficiency.

PRECAUTIONS
When anemia exists, its nature should be established and underlying cause determined. Caution is recommended with repeated blood transfusions because the addition of high erythrocytic iron content may produce iron overload. The following procedure may be especially useful in patients monitoring: hemoglobin determination and reticulocyte counts, serum ferritin determination and serum iron determination.
Most antibiotics, methotrexate and pyrimethamine invalidate diagnostic microbiological blood assays for Cyanocobalamin.

ADVERSE REACTIONS
Allergic sensitization has been reported following parenteral administration of Thiamine.

OVERDOSAGE
Early signs of iron poisoning: diarrhea, nausea, stomach pain, vomiting.
Late signs of iron poisoning: bluish-colored lips, fingernails, drowsiness, weakness, weak and unusually fast heart beat.

DOSAGE AND ADMINISTRATION
For intramuscular use only. The recommended dose is: children 11 years of age or older: 0.5 mL to 1 mL once or twice a week; adults: 1 to 2 mLs once or twice a week.
Parenteral drugs should be inspected visually for parculate matter and discoloration prior to administration whenever the solution and container permit.
DO NOT USE IF SEDIMENTATION OR PRECIPITATION OCCURS.
Refrigerate at 2–8°C. Protect from light.

CAUTION
Federal Law prohibits dispensing without prescription.

HOW SUPPLIED
Albafort injection: 10 mL multiple dose vials (NDC 10023-100-10).
*Contains no Folic Acid
ALBA PHARMACAL Literature Revised
Penuelas, Puerto Rico 00724 April 1985

ALBA–LYBE® ℞

COMPOSITION
Each 5 cc contains: Lysine Monohydrochloride 275 mg., Vit. B_{12} Crystalline 10 mcq., Thiamine HCl 5 mg., Riboflavin 4 mg., Pyridoxine HCl 1 mg., Niacinamide 35 mg., D-Panthenol 7 mg., Sorbitol q.s. with a palatable orange flavor.

ACTIONS
Alba-Lybe provides lysine as an appetite stimulant and sorbitol q.s. to provide greater absorption of B_{12} and lysine.

INDICATIONS
As dietetic supplement of all ages, especially in states of anorexia and convalescence.

ADVANTAGES
Alba-Lybe can be administered to patients including the diabetic patient since it contains sorbitol. Sorbitol q.s. base has the advantage over the alcohol base since sorbitol is absorbed much more rapidly than alcohol, as well as the fact that the molecules of lysine and B_{12} adhere to sorbitol. This results in greater appetite and fixing of proteins producing weight increase and better anabolic results.

DOSAGE
Children—½ to 1 teaspoonful three times a day. Adults—1 tablespoonful three times a day.

HOW SUPPLIED
6 oz. bottle (NDC 10023-101-06).

IRON CACODYLATE ℞

DESCRIPTION
Each ampule contains: Iron Cacodylate 65 mg., Sodium Chloride 24 mg, Water for Injection q.s.

HOW SUPPLIED
2 ml Amplues: Boxes of 10 and 25 (NDC 49326-155-02).
5 ml Ampules: Boxes of 10 and 25 (NDC 49326-156-05).

MIGRALAM™ CAPSULES ℞

DESCRIPTION
Each white MIGRALAM capsule contains: Isometheptene Mucate 65 mg., Caffeine 100 mg., Acetaminophen 325 mg.

ACTIONS
Isometheptene Mucate, a sympathomimetic amine, acts by constricting dilated cranial and cerebral arterioles, thus reducing the stimuli that lead to vascular headaches. It is particularly desirable in patients predisposed to nausea and vomiting and where ergotamines are precluded. Its action is similar to ergotamine but possessed of a low order of toxicity. Caffeine, also a cranial vasoconstrictor, is added to further enhance the vasoconstrictor effect. Acetaminophen, an effective non-narcotic analgesic, reduces the perception of pain impulses originating from dilated cerebral vessels. It is unlikely to produce many of the side effects associated with aspirin.

INDICATIONS
For relief of vascular and tension headaches.

> Based on a review for this drug (isometheptene mucate), The National Academy of Sciences-National Research Council and/ or other information, FDA has classified the other indications as "Possibly" effective in the treatment of migraine headache.
> Final classification of the less-than-effective indication requires further investigation.

CONTRAINDICATIONS
MIGRALAM is contraindicated in Glaucoma and/or severe cases of renal disease, hypertension, organic heart disease, hepatic disease and in those patients who are on monoamine-oxidase (MAO) inhibitor therapy.

PRECAUTIONS
Caution should be observed in hypertension, peripheral vascular disease and after recent cardiovascular attacks.

ADVERSE REACTIONS
Transient dizziness and skin rash may appear in hypersensitive patients. This can usually be eliminated by reducing the dose.

DOSAGE AND ADMINISTRATION
FOR RELIEF OF MIGRAINE HEADACHE. The usual adult dosage is two capsules at once, followed by one capsule every hour until relieved, up to 5 capsules within a twelve hour period.
FOR RELIEF OF TENSION HEADACHE. The usual adult dose is one or two capsules every four hours up to 8 capsules a day.

HOW SUPPLIED
Bottles of 100 capsules (NDC 49326-116-90) and 500 capsules (NDC 49326-116-75).

REOCYL Injection ℞
(Sodium Thiosalicylate)

DESCRIPTION
Each mL contains: Sodium Thiosalicylate 50 mg. in water for injection.

HOW SUPPLIED
2 mL ampules in boxes of 25 (NDC 10023-255-25).

Beach Pharmaceuticals
Division of BEACH PRODUCTS, INC.
5220 SOUTH MANHATTAN AVE.
TAMPA, FL 33611

BEELITH Tablets OTC

DESCRIPTION
Each tablet contains magnesium oxide 600 mg and pyridoxine hydrochloride (Vitamin B_6) 25 mg equivalent to B_6 20 mg. (See PDR For Nonprescription Drugs)
Shown in Product Identification Section, page 405

K-PHOS® M.F. ℞
K-PHOS® No.2 ℞
Phosphate Urinary Acidifiers

DESCRIPTION
K-PHOS® M.F.: Each tablet contains potassium acid phosphate 155 mg and sodium acid phosphate, anhydrous 350 mg. Each tablet yields approximately 125.6 mg of phosphorus, 44.5 mg of potassium or 1.1 mEq and 67 mg of sodium or 2.9 mEq. **K-PHOS® No.2:** Each tablet contains potassium acid phosphate 305 mg and sodium acid phosphate, anhydrous 700 mg. Each tablet yields approximately 250 mg of phosphorus, 88 mg of potassium or 2.3 mEq and 134 mg of sodium or 5.8 mEq.

ACTIONS
These products are highly effective urinary acidifiers.

INDICATIONS
For use in patients with elevated urinary pH. These products help keep calcium soluble and reduce odor and rash caused by ammoniacal urine. Also, by acidifying the urine they increase the antibacterial activity of methenamine mandelate and methenamine hippurate.

CONTRAINDICATIONS
These products are contraindicated in patients with infected magnesium ammonium phosphate stones; in patients with severely impaired renal function (less than 30% of normal) and in the presence of hyperphosphatemia.

PRECAUTIONS
Drug Interactions: Use of antacids containing magnesium, aluminum or calcium in conjunction with phosphate preparations may bind the phosphate and prevent its absorption. Concurrent use of antihypertensives, especially diazoxide, guanethidine, hydralazine, methyldopa or rauwolfia alkaloids; or corticosteroids, especially mineralocorticoids or corticotropin, with sodium phosphate may result in hypernatremia. Potassium-containing medications or potassium-sparing diuretics may cause hyperkalemia when used with potassium phosphates, Patients should have serum potassium level determinations at periodic intervals. Plasma levels of salicylates may be increased since salicylate excretion is decreased in acidified urine; addition of monobasic phosphates to patients stabilized on salicylates may lead to toxic salicylate levels.
General: Contains potassium and sodium and should be used with caution if regulation of these elements is desired. Occasionally, some individuals may experience a mild laxative effect during the first few days of phosphate therapy. If laxation persists to an unpleasant degree, reduce the daily dosage until the effect subsides or, if necessary, discontinue the use of this product. Use of this medication should be carefully considered when the following medical problems exist: Cardiac disease (particularly in digitalized patients), Addison's disease, acute dehydration, extensive tissue breakdown, myotonia congenita, cardiac failure, cirrhosis of the liver or severe hepatic disease, peripheral and pulmonary edema, hypernatremia, hypertension, toxemia of pregnancy, hypoparathyroidism, osteomalacia, acute pancreatitis, and rickets.
Laboratory Tests: Careful monitoring of renal function and serum electrolytes (calcium, phosphorous, potassium, sodium) may be required at periodic intervals during phosphate therapy. Other tests may be warranted in some patients, depending on conditions. High serum phosphate levels increase the incidence of extraskeletal calcification.
Carcinogenesis, mutagenesis, impairment of fertility: Long term animal studies to evaluate the carcinogenic, mutagenic, or teratogenic potential of these products have not been performed.
Pregnancy: Pregnancy Category C. Animal reproduction studies have not been conducted with these products. It is also not known whether these products can cause fetal harm when administered to a pregnant woman or can effect reproduction capacity. These products should be given to a pregnant woman only if clearly needed.
Nursing Mothers: It is not known whether these drugs are excreted in human milk. Because many drugs are excreted in human milk, caution should be exercised when these products are administered to a nursing woman.

ADVERSE REACTIONS
The following adverse effects have been reported: headaches; dizziness; mental confusion; seizures; weakness of legs; general fatigue or weakness; muscle cramps; numbness of or tingling of hands, lips, or feet; fast or irregular heartbeat; shortness of breath; swelling of feet or legs; unusual weight gain; low urine output; thirst; nausea; vomiting; stomach pain; diarrhea.

DIRECTIONS
K-PHOS® M.F.: Two tablets four times daily with a full glass of water. **K-PHOS® No.2:** One tablet four times daily with a full glass of water. When the urine is difficult to acidify administer one tablet every two hours not to exceed eight tablets in a 24 hour period.

CAUTION
Federal law prohibits dispensing without prescription.

STORAGE
Keep tightly closed. Store at controlled room temperature, 15°C–30°C (59°F–86°F).

HOW SUPPLIED
K-PHOS® M.F.: White scored tablet with the name BEACH and the number 1135 embossed on each tablet. Bottles of 100 (NDC 0486-1135-01) and bottles of 500 (NDC 0486-1135-05) tablets. **K-PHOS® No.2:** Brown capsule shaped tablet with the name BEACH and the number 1134 embossed on each tablet. Bottles of 100 (NDC 0486-1134-01) and bottles of 500 (NDC 0486-1134-05) tablets.
Shown in Product Identification Section, page 405

Continued on next page

Beach—Cont.

K-PHOS® NEUTRAL ℞

Supplies 250 mg of phosphorus per tablet.

DESCRIPTION

Each tablet contains 852 mg dibasic sodium phosphate anhydrous, 155 mg monobasic potassium phosphate, and 130 mg monobasic sodium phosphate monohydrate. Each tablet yields approximately 250 mg of phosphorus, 298 mg of sodium (13.0 mEq) and 45 mg of potassium (1.1 mEq).

INDICATIONS

K-PHOS® NEUTRAL lowers urinary calcium levels and increases phosphate and pyrophosphate. As a phosphorous supplement, each tablet supplies 25% of the U.S. Recommended Daily Allowance (U.S. RDA) of phosphorus for adults.

CONTRAINDICATIONS

This product is contraindicated in patients with infected urolithiasis or struvite stone formation, in patients with severly impaired renal function (less than 30% of normal), or in the presence of hyperphosphatemia.

PRECAUTIONS

General: This product contains potassium and sodium and should be used with caution if regulation of these elements is desired. Occasionally, some individuals may experience a mild laxative effect during the first few days of phosphate therapy. If laxation persists to an unpleasant degree, reduce the daily dosage until this effect subsides, or, if necessary, discontinue the use of this product.

Caution should be exercised when prescribing this product in the following conditions: Cardiac disease (particularly in digitalized patients); severe adrenal insufficiency (Addison's disease); acute dehydration; severe renal insufficiency; renal function impairment or chronic renal disease; extensive tissue breakdown (such as severe burns); myotonia congenita; cardiac failure; cirrhosis of the liver or severe hepatic disease; peripheral or pulmonary edema; hypernatremia; hypertension; toxemia of pregnancy; hypoparathyroidism; osteomalacia; acute pancreatitis; and rickets.

Information for Patients: Patients with kidney stones may pass old stones when phosphate therapy is started and should be warned of this possibility. Patients should be advised to avoid the use of antacids containing aluminum, magnesium or calcium which may prevent the absorption of phosphate.

Laboratory Tests: Careful monitoring of renal function and serum electrolytes (calcium, phosphorus, potassium, sodium) may be required at periodic intervals during phosphate therapy. Other tests may be warranted in some patients, depending on conditions. High serum phosphate levels increase the incidence of extraskeletal calcification.

Drug Interactions: The use of antacids containing magnesium, aluminum or calcium in conjunction with phosphate preparations may bind the phosphate and prevent its absorption. Concurrent use of antihypertensives, especially diazoxide, guanethidine, hydralazine, methyldopa, or rauwolfia alkaloid; or corticosteroids, especially mineralocorticoids or corticotropin, with sodium phosphate may result in hypernatremia. Calcium-containing preparations and/or vitamin D may antagonize the effects of phosphates in the treatment of hypercalcemia. Potassium-containing medications or potassium-sparing diuretics may cause hyperkalemia when used in potassium phosphates. Patients should have serum potassium level determinations at peroidic intervals.

Carcinogenesis, mutagenesis, impairment of fertility: Long term animal studies to evaluate the carcinogenic, mutagenic or teratogenic potential of inorganic phosphate salts have not been performed.

Pregnancy: Pregnancy Category C. Animal reproduction studies have not been conducted with this product. It is also not known whether this product can cause fetal harm when administered to a pregnant woman or can affect reproduction capacity. This product should be given to a pregnant woman only if clearly needed.

Nursing Mothers: It is not known whether this drug is excreted in human milk. Because many drugs are excreted in human milk, caution should be exercised when this product is administered to a nursing woman.

ADVERSE REACTIONS

Gastrointestinal upsets (diarrhea, nausea, stomach pain, and vomiting) may occur with phosphate therapy. The following side effects have been reported with less frequent incidence: headaches; dizziness; mental confusion; seizures; weakness or heaviness of legs; unusual tiredness or weakness; muscle cramps; numbness, tingling, pain, or weakness of hands or feet; numbness or tingling around lips; fast or irregular heartbeat; shortness of breath or troubled breathing; swelling of feet or lower legs; unusual weight gain; low urine output; unusual thirst.

DIRECTIONS

Adults: One or two tablets four times a day with a full glass of water.

HOW SUPPLIED

White, film coated, capsule-shaped tablet with the name "BEACH" and number "1125" embossed on each tablet. Bottles of 100 (NDC 0486-1125-01) and 500 (NDC 0486-1125-05) tablets.

STORAGE

Keep tightly closed. Store at controlled room temperature, 15°C–30°C (59°–86°F). Dispense in tight containers.

CAUTION

Federal law prohibits dispensing without a prescription.

Shown in Product Identification Section, page 405

K-PHOS® ORIGINAL (Sodium Free) ℞

(Potassium Acid Phosphate)
Urinary Acidifier
Supplies 114 mg of phosphorus per tablet.

DESCRIPTION

Each tablet contains potassium acid phosphate 500 mg. Each tablet yields approximately 114 mg of phosphorus and 144 mg of potassium or 3.7 mEq.

ACTIONS

K-PHOS ORIGINAL (Sodium Free) is a highly effective urinary acidifier.

INDICATIONS

For use in patients with elevated urinary pH. Helps keep calcium soluble and reduces odor and rash caused by ammoniacal urine. Also, by acidifying the urine it increases the antibacterial activity of methenamine mandelate and methenamine hippurate.

CONTRAINDICATIONS

This product is contraindicated in patients with infected magnesium ammonium phosphate stones; in patients with severely impaired renal function (less than 30% of normal); in the presence of hyperphosphatemia and hyperkalemia.

PRECAUTIONS

General: This product contains potassium and should be used with caution if regulation of this element is desired. Occasionally, some individuals may experience a mild laxative effect during the first few days of phosphate therapy. If laxation persists to an unpleasant degree, reduce the daily dosage until this effect subsides or, if necessary, discontinue the use of this product.

Caution should be exercised when prescribing this product in the following conditions: Cardiac disease (particularly in digitalized patients); severe adrenal insufficiency (Addison's disease); acute dehydration; severe renal insufficieny or chronic renal disease; extensive tissue breakdown (such as severe burns); myotonia congenita; hypoparathyroidism; osteomalacia; acute pancreatitis; and rickets.

Information for Patients: Patients with kidney stones may pass old stones when phosphate therapy is started and should be warned of this possibility. Patients should be advised to avoid antacids containing aluminum, calcium, or magnesium which may prevent the absorption of phosphate. To assure against gastrointestinal injury associated with oral ingestion of concentrated potassium salt preparations, patients should be instructed to dissolve tablets completely in an appropriate amount of water before taking.

Laboratory Tests: Careful monitoring of renal function and serum electrolytes (calcium, phosphorous, potassium) may be required at periodic intervals during phosphate therapy. Other tests may be warranted in some patients, depending on conditions. High serum phosphate levels increase the incidence of extraskeletal calcification.

Drug Interactions: The use of antacids containing magnesium, calcium, or aluminum in conjunction with phosphate preparations may bind the phosphate and prevent its absorption. Potassium-containing medications or potassium-sparing diuretics may cause hyperkalemia when used concurrently with potassium phosphates. Patients should have serum potassium level determinations at periodic intervals. Concurrent use of salicylates may lead to increased serum salicylate levels since excretion of salicylates is reduced in acidified urine. Serum salicylate levels should be closely monitored to avoid toxicity.

Carcinogenesis, mutagenesis, impairment of fertility: Long term animal studies to evaluate the carcinogenic, mutagenic, or teratogenic potential of this product have not been performed.

Pregnancy: Pregnancy Category C. Animal reproduction studies have not been conducted with this product. It is also not known whether this product can cause fetal harm when administered to a pregnant woman or can effect reproduction capacity. This product should be given to a pregnant woman only if clearly needed.

Nursing Mothers: It is not known whether this drug is excreted in human milk. Because many drugs are excreted in human milk, caution should be exercised when this product is administered to a nursing woman.

ADVERSE REACTIONS

Gastrointestinal upsets (diarrhea, nausea, stomach pain, and vomiting) may occur with the use of potassium phosphates. The following side effects have been reported with less frequent incidence: irregular heartbeat; dizziness; mental confusion; weakness or heaviness of legs; unusual tiredness; muscle cramps; numbness, tingling, pain, or weakness in hands or feet; numbness or tingling around lips; shortness of breath or troubled breathing; bone and joint pain.

DIRECTIONS

Two tablets dissolved in 6–8 oz. of water 4 times daily with meals and at bedtime. For best results let the tablets soak in water for 2 to 5 minutes, or more if necessary, and stir. If any tablet particles remain undissolved they may be crushed and stirred vigorously to speed dissolution.

CAUTION

Federal law prohibits dispensing without prescription.

STORAGE

Keep tightly closed. Store at controlled room temperature, 15°C–30°C (59°F–86°F).

HOW SUPPLIED

White scored tablet with the name BEACH and the number 1111 embossed on each tablet. Bottles of 100 (NDC 0486-1111-01) and bottles of 500 (NDC 0486-1111-05) tablets.

Shown in Product Identification Section, page 405

THIACIDE TABLETS ℞

[*thī-ă-sīd*]
SODIUM FREE

DESCRIPTION

Each tablet contains methenamine mandelate 500 mg. and potassium acid phosphate 250 mg.

Shown in Product Identification Section, page 405

UROQID-Acid® ℞
UROQID-Acid® No. 2 ℞

Tablets

DESCRIPTION

Each **UROQID-Acid®** tablet contains methenamine mandelate 350 mg and sodium acid phosphate, monohydrate 200 mg. Each **UROQID-Acid® No. 2** tablet contains methenamine mandelate 500 mg and sodium acid phosphate, monohydrate 500 mg.

CLINICAL PHARMACOLOGY

Methenamine mandelate is rapidly absorbed and excreted in the urine. Formaldehyde is released by acid hydrolysis from methenamine with bactericidal levels rapidly reached at pH 5.0–5.5. Proportionally less formaldehyde is released as urinary pH approaches 6.0 and insufficient quantities are released above this level for therapeutic response. In acid urine, mandelic acid exerts its antibacterial action and also contributes to the acidification of the urine. Mandelic acid is excreted by both glomerular filtration and tubular excretion. In acid urine, there is equally effective antibacterial activity against both gram-positive and gram-negative organisms, since the antibacterial action of mandelic acid and formaldehyde is nonspecific. With Proteus vulgaris and urea splitting strains of Pseudomonas and Aerobacter results may be discouraging and particular attention is required in monitoring urinary pH and overall management.

INDICATIONS

Long-term Prophylactic Use: For prevention of reinfection of a sterile urine by converting the urine into an antibacterial medium. Particularly suitable for long-term therapy because of safety and because resistance to the nonspecific bactericidal action of formaldehyde does not develop. There is a growing body of evidence that long-term administration can prevent the recurrence of bacteriuria in patients with chronic pyelonephritis.

General Indications: Particularly useful in those infections which are often incurable because of stone or other obstruction, inlying catheter drainage or residual urine in the bladder in neurological disorders. Specifically recommended for the management of chronic urinary tract infection including pyelitis, pyelonephritis, cystitis and infection accompanying neurogenic bladder. Not recommended for acute infection with parenchymal involvement. A thorough diagnostic investigation as a part of the overall management of the urinary tract infection should accompany the use of this product.

CONTRAINDICATIONS

UROQID-Acid® and **UROQID-Acid® No. 2** are contraindicated in patients with renal insufficiency, severe hepatic disease, severe dehydration, hyperphosphatemia, and in patients who have exhibited hypersensitivity to any components of these products.

PRECAUTIONS

General: These products should not be used as the sole therapeutic agent in acute parenchymal infections causing systemic symptoms such as chills anf fever.

UROQID-Acid® and **UROQID-Acid®No. 2** contain approximately 33 mg and 83 mg of sodium per tablet, respectively, and should be used with caution in patients on a sodium-restricted diet.

Sodium phosphates should be used with caution in the following conditions: cardiac failure; peripheral or pulmonary edema; hypernatremia; hypertension; toxemia of pregnancy; hypoparathyroidism; osteomalacia; acute pancreatitis and rickets.

Large doses of methenamine (8 grams daily for 3 to 4 weeks) have caused bladder irritation, painful and frequent micturation, albuminuria and gross hematuria. Dysuria may occur, although usually at higher than recommended doses, and can be controlled by reducing the dosage. These products contain a urinary acidifier and can cause metabolic acidosis. Care should be taken to maintain an acid urinary pH (below 5.5), especially when treating infections due to urea-splitting organisms such as **Proteus** and strains of **Pseudomonas.** Drugs and/or foods which produce an alkaline urine should be restricted. Frequent urine pH tests are essential. If acidification of the urine is contraindicated or unattainable, use of these products should be discontinued.

Information for Patients: To assure an acidic pH, patients should be instructed to restrict or avoid most fruits, milk and milk products, and antacids containing sodium carbonate or bicarbonate.

Laboratory Tests: As with all urinary tract infections, the efficacy of therapy should be monitored by repeated urine cultures. During long-term therapy, careful monitoring of renal function and serum electrolytes (phosphorus, sodium) may be required at periodic intervals. High serum phosphate levels increase the incidence of extraskeletal ossification.

Drug Interactions: Formaldehyde and sulfonamides form an insoluble precipitate in acid urine and also increase the risk of crystalliuria; therefore, these products should not be used concurrently with sulfonamides. Thiazide diuretics, carbonic anhydrase inhibitors, antacids, or urinary alkalinizing agents should not be used concurrently since they may cause the urine to become alkaline and reduce the effectiveness of methenamine by inhibiting its conversion to formaldehyde. Concurrent use of antihypertensives, especially diazoxide, guanethidine, hydralazine, methyldopa, or rauwolfia alkaloids; or corticosteroids, especially mineralocorticoids or corticotropin, with sodium phosphates may result in hypernatremia. Concurrent use of salicylates may lead to increased serum salicylate levels since excretion of salicylates is reduced in acidified urine. Serum salicylate levels should be closely monitored to avoid toxicity.

Laboratory Test Interactions: Formaldehyde interferes with fluorometric procedures for determination of urinary catecholamines and vanilmandelic acid (VMA) causing erroneously high results. Formaldehyde also causes falsely decreased urine estriol levels by reacting with estriol when acid hydrolysis techniques are used; estriol determinations which use enzymatic hydrolysis are unaffected by folmaldehyde. Formaldehyde causes falsely elevated 17-hydroxycorticosteroid levels when the Porter-Silber method is used and falsely decreased 5-hydroxy-indoleacetic acid (5HIAA) levels by inhibiting color development when nitrosonaphthol methods are used.

Carcinogenesis, mutagenesis, impairment of fertility: Long-term animal studies to evaluate the carcinogenic, mutagenic, or teratogenic potential of these products have not been performed.

Pregnancy: Pregnancy Category C. Animal reproduction studies have not been conducted with these products. It is also not known whether these products can cause fetal harm when administered to a pregnant woman or can affect reproduction capacity. Since methenamine is known to cross the placental barrier, these products should be given to a pregnant woman only if clearly needed.

Nursing Mothers: Methenamine is excreted in breat milk. Caution should be exercised when these products are administered to a nursing woman.

ADVERSE REACTIONS

Gastrointestinal disturbances (nausea, stomach upset), generalized skin rash, dysuria, painful or difficult urination may occur occasionally with the use of methenamine preparations. Microscopic and, rarely, gross hematuria have also been reported.

Gastrointestinal upsets (diarrhea, nausea, stomach pain, and vomiting) may occur with the use of sodium phosphates. The following side effects have been encountered less frequently with administration of sodium phosphates; headaches; dizziness; mental confusion; seizures; weakness or heaviness of legs; unusual tiredness or weakness; muscle cramps; numbness, tingling, pain or weakness in hands or feet; numbness or tingling around lips; fast or irregular heartbeat; shortness of breath or troubled breathing; swelling of feet or lower legs; unusual weight gain; low urine output; unusual thirst.

DIRECTIONS

UROQID-Acid®; Initially, 3 tablets 4 times daily. For maintenance, 1 or 2 tablets, 4 times daily. **UROQID-Acid®No. 2**; Initially, 2 tablets 4 times daily. For maintenance, 2 to 4 tablets daily, in divided doses.

HOW SUPPLIED

UROQID-Acid® is a yellow, sugar coated, tablet with the name BEACH and the number 1112 printed on each tablet. Packaged in bottles of 100 (NDC 0486-1112-01) and 500 (NDC 0486-1112-05) tablets. **UROQID-Acid®No. 2** is a yellow, film coated, capsule shaped tablet with the name BEACH and the number 1114 embossed on each tablet. Packaged in bottles of 100 (NDC 0486-1114-01) and 500 (NDC 0486-1114-05) tablets.

STORAGE

Keep tightly closed. Store at controlled room temperature (15°–30°C) (59°–86°F). Dispense in tight containers.

CAUTION

Federal law prohibits dispensing without prescription.

Shown in Product Identification Section, page 405

Beecham Products

DIVISION OF BEECHAM INC.
POST OFFICE BOX 1467
PITTSBURGH, PA 15230

MASSENGILL® Douches

[mas 'sen-gil]

KEY FACTS

Massengill is the brand name for a line of douches which are recommended for routine cleansing and for temporary relief of vaginal itching and irritation. Massengill Disposable douches are available in two Vinegar & Water formulas (Extra Mild and Extra Cleansing), three Cosmetic solutions (Country Flowers, Belle-Mai, and Mountain Herbs) and a Medicated formula (with povidone-iodine). Massengill also is available in a liquid concentrate and powder form.

MAJOR USES

Massengill's Vinegar & Water and Cosmetic douches are recommended for routine douching, or for cleansing following menstruation or the prescribed use of vaginal medication or contraceptives. Massengill Medicated is recommended in a seven day regimen for the symptomatic relief of minor itching and irritation associated with vaginitis due to Candida albicans, Trichomonas vaginalis and Gardnerella vaginalis.

SAFETY INFORMATION

Do not douch during pregnancy unless directed by a physician.

Massengill Vinegar & Water and Cosmetic Douches—If irritation occurs, discontinue use.

Massengill Medicated — Women with iodine-sensitivity should not use this product. If symptoms persist after seven days, or if redness, swelling or pain develop, consult a physician.

MASSENGILL®

[mas 'sen-gil]

Disposable Douches

MASSENGILL®

Liquid Concentrate

MASSENGILL® Powder

INGREDIENTS

DISPOSABLES: Extra Mild Vinegar and Water—Water and Vinegar.

Extra Cleansing Vinegar and Water—Water, Vinegar, Puraclean™ (Cetylpyridinium Chloride), Diazolidinyl Urea, Disodium EDTA.

Belle-Mai—Water, SD Alcohol 40, Lactic Acid, Sodium Lactate, Octoxynol-9, Cetylpyridinium Chloride, Propylene Glycol (and) Diazolidinyl Urea (and) Methyl Paraben (and) Propyl Paraben, Disodium EDTA, Fragrance, FD&C Blue #1.

Country Flowers—Water, SD Alcohol 40, Lactic Acid, Sodium Lactate, Octoxynol-9, Cetylpyridinium Chloride, Propylene Glycol (and) Diazolidinyl Urea (and), Methyl Paraben (and) Propyl Paraben, Disodium EDTA, Fragrance, D&C Red #28, FD&C Blue #1.

Mountain Herbs—Water, SD Alcohol 40, Lactic Acid, Sodium Lactate, Octoxynol-9, Cetylpyridinium Chloride, Propylene Glycol (and) Diazolidinyl Urea (and) Methyl Paraben (and) Propyl Paraben, Disodium EDTA, Fragrance, D&C Yellow #10, FD&C Blue #1.

LIQUID CONCENTRATE: Water, SD Alcohol 40, Lactic Acid, Sodium Bicarbonate, Octoxynol-9, Fragrance, D&C Yellow #10, FD&C Yellow #6.

POWDER: Sodium Chloride, Ammonium alum, PEG-8, Phenol, Methyl Salicylate, Eucalyptus Oil, Menthol, Thymol, D&C Yellow #10, FD&C Yellow #6.

FLORAL POWDER: Sodium Chloride, Ammonium alum, Octoxynol-9, SD Alcohol 23-A, Fragrance, and FD&C Yellow #6.

INDICATIONS

Recommended for routine cleansing at the end of menstruation, after use of contraceptive creams or jellies (check the contraceptive package instructions first) or to rinse out the residue of prescribed vaginal medication (as directed by physician).

ACTIONS

The buffered acid solutions of Massengill Douches are valuable adjuncts to specific vaginal therapy following the prescribed use of vaginal medication or contraceptives and in feminine hygiene.

DIRECTIONS

DISPOSABLES: Twist off flat, wing-shaped tab from bottle containing premixed solution, attach nozzle supplied and use. The unit is completely disposable.

LIQUID CONCENTRATE: Fill cap ¾ full, to measuring line, and pour contents into douche bag containing 1 quart of warm water. Mix thoroughly.

POWDER: Dissolve two rounded teaspoonfuls in a douche bag containing 1 quart of warm water. Mix thoroughly.

WARNING

Vaginal cleansing douches should not be used more than twice weekly except on the advice of a physician. If irritation occurs, discontinue use. Keep out of reach of children. In case of accidental ingestion, seek professional assistance by contacting your physician, the local poison control center, or the Rocky Mt. Poison Control Center at 303-592-1710 (Collect), 24 hours a day.

HOW SUPPLIED

Disposable—6 oz. disposable plastic bottle.
Liquid Concentrate—4 oz., 8 oz., plastic bottles.
Powder—4 oz., 8 oz., 16 oz., 22 oz., Packettes—10's, 12's.

MASSENGILL® Medicated

[mas 'sen-gil]

Disposable Douche

ACTIVE INGREDIENT

Ceptician™ (0.30% povidone-iodine).

INDICATIONS

For symptomatic relief of minor irritation and itching associated with vaginitis due to Candida albicans, Trichomonas vaginalis and Gardnerella vaginalis.

ACTION

Povidone-iodine is widely recognized as an effective broad spectrum microbicide against both gram negative and gram positive bacteria, fungi, yeasts and protozoa. While remaining active in the presence of blood, serum or bodily secretions, it possesses virtually none of the irritating properties of iodine.

WARNINGS

If symptoms persist after seven days of use, or if redness, swelling or pain develop during treatment, consult a physician. Women with iodine-sensitivity should not use this product. Women may douche during menstruation if they douche gently. Do not douche during pregnancy unless directed by a physician. Douching does not prevent pregnancy. Keep out of reach of children. In case of accidental ingestion, seek professional assistance by contacting your physician, the local poison control center, or the Rocky Mt. Poison Control Center at 303-592-1710 (Collect), 24 hours a day.

DOSAGE AND ADMINISTRATION

Dosage is provided as a single unit concentrate to be added to 6 oz. of sanitized water supplied in a disposable bottle. A specially designed nozzle is provided. After use, the unit is discarded. Use one bottle a day for seven days. Even if symptoms are relieved earlier, treatment should be continued for the full seven days.

HOW SUPPLIED

6 oz. bottle of sanitized water with 0.17 oz. vial of povidone-iodine and nozzle.

EDUCATIONAL MATERIAL

Booklet:

"A Personal Guide to Feminine Freshness"

A 16 page illustrated booklet on vaginal infections, feminine hygiene and douching. Free to physicians, pharmacists and

Continued on next page

Beecham Products—Cont.

patients in limited quantities by writing Beecham or calling 800-BEECHAM. (PA residents 800-242-1718)

Film, Video:

"Feminine Hygiene and You"

This 14 minute color film begins with a simple explanation of how a woman's body works (reproductive system, menstrual cycle, and vaginal secretions) then explains douching. Free loan to physicians, pharmacists and clinics. Available in 16mm, 3/4" video, Beta and VHS by writing Beecham or calling 800-BEECHAM. (PA residents 800-242-1718)

Beecham Laboratories

DIV. OF BEECHAM INC.,
501 FIFTH STREET
BRISTOL, TN 37620

PRODUCT IDENTIFICATION CODES

To provide quick and positive identification of Beecham Laboratories' products, we have imprinted a code number or brand name on tablet and capsule products. In order that you may identify a product by its code and number, we have compiled below a numerical list of code numbers with their corresponding product names. The code number as it appears on tablets and capsules bears the letters BMP plus the numerical code. Amoxil® and Fastin® capsules, and Amoxil® Chewable Tablets bear the brand name only. Augmentin swallow tablets have the name scored on one side and the strength on the other side.

BMP Code No.	Product
105	ANEXSIA® w/Codeine Tablets
106	ANEXSIA®-D Tablets
112	DASIN® Capsules
119	HYBEPHEN® Tablets
121	LIVITAMIN® Capsules
122	LIVITAMIN® w/INTRINSIC FACTOR Capsules
123	LIVITAMIN® CHEWABLE Tablets
125	MENEST™ (Esterified Estrogens, U.S.P.) Tablets 0.3 mg.
126	MENEST™ (Esterified Estrogens, U.S.P.) Tablets 0.625 mg.
127	MENEST™ (Esterified Estrogens, U.S.P.) Tablets 1.25 mg.
128	MENEST™ (Esterified Estrogens, U.S.P.) Tablets 2.5 mg.
135	SEMETS®
140	TOTACILLIN® (Ampicillin) Capsules 250 mg.
141	TOTACILLIN® (Ampicillin) Capsules 500 mg.
143	BACTOCILL® (Oxacillin Sodium) Capsules 250 mg.
144	BACTOCILL® (Oxacillin Sodium) Capsules 500 mg.
145	DARICON® (Oxyphencyclimine HCl) Tablets 10 mg.
146	DARICON®-PB (Oxyphencyclimine HCl, 5 mg. and Phenobarbital, 15 mg.) Tablets
156	TIGAN® (Trimethobenzamide HCl) Capsules 100 mg.
157	TIGAN® (Trimethobenzamide HCl) Capsules 250 mg.
165	DYCILL® (Dicloxacillin Sodium) Capsules 250 mg.
166	DYCILL® (Dicloxacillin Sodium) Capsules 500 mg.
169	CLOXAPEN® (Cloxacillin Sodium) Capsules 250 mg.
170	CLOXAPEN® (Cloxacillin Sodium) Capsules 500 mg.
182	NUCOFED® Capsules
185	BEEPEN-VK® (Penicillin V Potassium) Tablets 250 mg.
186	BEEPEN-VK® (Penicillin V Potassium) Tablets 500 mg
189	AUGMENTIN® (Amoxicillin/Clavulanate Potassium) '125' Chewable Tablets
190	AUGMENTIN® (Amoxicillin/Clavulanate Potassium) '250' Chewable Tablets
194	ENARAX®5 (Oxphencyclimine HCl, 5 mg. and Hydroxyzine HCl, 25 mg.) Tablets
195	ENARAX®10 (Oxphencyclimine HCl, 10 mg, and Hydroxyzine HCl, 25 mg.) Tablets
210	CONAR®-A Tablets

AMOXIL® ℞

[ā-mŏx ′ĭl]
(amoxicillin)
capsules, for oral suspension and chewable tablets

DESCRIPTION

AMOXIL (Amoxicillin) is a semisynthetic antibiotic, an analog of ampicillin, with a broad spectrum of bactericidal activity against many Gram-positive and Gram-negative microorganisms. Chemically it is D-(-)-α-amino-p-hydroxybenzyl penicillin trihydrate. **Inactive Ingredients:** Capsules—Magnesium Stearate, and Magnesium Sulfate. Chewable Tablets—Citric Acid, Corn Starch, F D & C Red 3, Flavorings, Glycine, Mannitol, Magnesium Stearate, Saccharin Sodium, Silica Gel and Sucrose. Oral Suspension—F D & C Red 3, Flavorings, Silica Gel, Sodium Benzoate, Sodium Citrate, Sucrose, Xanthan Gum.

ACTIONS

PHARMACOLOGY

Amoxicillin is stable in the presence of gastric acid and may be given without regard to meals. It is rapidly absorbed after oral administration. It diffuses readily into most body tissues and fluids, with the exception of brain and spinal fluid, except when meninges are inflamed. The half-life of Amoxicillin is 61.3 minutes. Most of the Amoxicillin is excreted unchanged in the urine; its excretion can be delayed by concurrent administration of probenecid. Amoxicillin is not highly protein-bound. In blood serum, Amoxicillin is approximately 20% protein-bound as compared to 60% for penicillin G.

Orally administered doses of 250 mg and 500 mg Amoxicillin capsules result in average peak blood levels one to two hours after administration in the range of 3.5 mcg/ml to 5.0 mcg/ml and 5.5 mcg/ml to 7.5 mcg/ml respectively.

Orally administered doses of Amoxicillin suspension 125 mg/5 ml and 250 mg/5 ml result in average peak blood levels one to two hours after administration in the range of 1.5 mcg/ml to 3.0 mcg/ml and 3.5 mcg/ml to 5.0 mcg/ml respectively. Amoxicillin chewable tablets, 125 mg and 250 mg, produced blood levels similar to those achieved with the corresponding doses of Amoxicillin oral suspensions.

Detectable serum levels are observed up to 8 hours after an orally administered dose of Amoxicillin. Following a 1 Gm dose and utilizing a special skin window technique to determine levels of the antibiotic, it was noted that therapeutic levels were found in the interstitial fluid. Approximately 60 percent of an orally administered dose of Amoxicillin is excreted in the urine within six to eight hours.

MICROBIOLOGY:

AMOXIL (Amoxicillin) is similar to ampicillin in its bactericidal action against susceptible organisms during the stage of active multiplication. It acts through the inhibition of biosynthesis of cell wall mucopeptide. *In vitro* studies have demonstrated the susceptibility of most strains of the following Gram-positive bacteria: alpha- and beta-hemolytic streptococci, *Diplococcus pneumoniae,* nonpenicillinase-producing staphylococci, and *Streptococcus faecalis.* It is active *in vitro* against many strains of *Haemophilus influenzae, Neisseria gonorrhoeae, Escherichia coli* and *Proteus mirabilis.* Because it does not resist destruction by penicillinase, it is not effective against penicillinase-producing bacteria, particularly resistant staphylococci. All strains of Pseudomonas and most strains of Klebsiella and Enterobacter are resistant.

DISC SUSCEPTIBILITY TESTS: Quantitative methods that require measurement of zone diameters give the most precise estimates of antibiotic susceptibility. One such procedure* has been recommended for use with discs for testing susceptibility to ampicillin-class antibiotics. Interpretations correlate diameters of the disc test with MIC values for Amoxicillin. With this procedure, a report from the laboratory of "susceptible" indicates that the infecting organism is likely to respond to therapy. A report of "resistant" indicates that the infecting organism is not likely to respond to therapy. A report of "intermediate susceptibility" suggests that the organism would be susceptible if high dosage is used, or if the infection is confined to tissues and fluids (e.g., urine), in which high antibiotic levels are attained.

* Bauer, A. W., Kirby, W. M. M., Sherris, J. C., and Turck, M.: Antibiotic Testing by a Standardized Single Disc Method, Am. J. Clin. Pathol., 45:493, 1966. Standardized Disc Susceptibility Test, FEDERAL REGISTER 37:20527–29, 1972.

INDICATIONS

AMOXIL (Amoxicillin) is indicated in the treatment of infections due to susceptible strains of the following:

Gram-negative organisms—*H. influenzae, E. coli, P. mirabilis* and *N. gonorrhoeae.*

Gram-positive organisms—Streptococci (including *Streptococcus faecalis), D. pneumoniae* and nonpenicillinase-producing staphylococci.

Therapy may be instituted prior to obtaining results from bacteriological and susceptibility studies to determine the causative organisms and their susceptibility to Amoxicillin. Indicated surgical procedures should be performed.

CONTRAINDICATIONS

A history of allergic reaction to any of the penicillins is a contraindication.

WARNINGS

SERIOUS AND OCCASIONALLY FATAL HYPERSENSITIVITY (ANAPHYLACTOID) REACTIONS HAVE BEEN REPORTED IN PATIENTS ON PENICILLIN THERAPY. ALTHOUGH ANAPHYLAXIS IS MORE FREQUENT FOLLOWING PARENTERAL THERAPY, IT HAS OCCURRED IN PATIENTS ON ORAL PENICILLINS. THESE REACTIONS ARE MORE LIKELY TO OCCUR IN INDIVIDUALS WITH A HISTORY OF SENSITIVITY TO MULTIPLE ALLERGENS. THERE HAVE BEEN REPORTS OF INDIVIDUALS WITH A HISTORY OF PENICILLIN HYPERSENSITIVITY WHO HAVE EXPERIENCED SEVERE REACTIONS WHEN TREATED WITH CEPHALOSPORINS. BEFORE THERAPY WITH ANY PENICILLIN, CAREFUL INQUIRY SHOULD BE MADE CONCERNING PREVIOUS HYPERSENSITIVITY REACTIONS TO PENICILLINS, CEPHALOSPORINS, OR OTHER ALLERGENS. IF AN ALLERGIC REACTION OCCURS, APPROPRIATE THERAPY SHOULD BE INSTITUTED AND DISCONTINUANCE OF AMOXICILLIN THERAPY CONSIDERED. **SERIOUS ANAPHYLACTOID REACTIONS REQUIRE IMMEDIATE EMERGENCY TREATMENT WITH EPINEPHRINE, OXYGEN, INTRAVENOUS STEROIDS, AND AIRWAY MANAGEMENT, INCLUDING INTUBATION, SHOULD ALSO BE ADMINISTERED AS INDICATED.**

USAGE IN PREGNANCY

Safety for use in pregnancy has not been established.

PRECAUTIONS

As with any potent drug, periodic assessment of renal, hepatic and hematopoietic function should be made during prolonged therapy.

The possibility of superinfections with mycotic or bacterial pathogens should be kept in mind during therapy. If superinfections occur (usually involving Enterobacter, Pseudomonas or Candida), the drug should be discontinued and/or appropriate therapy instituted.

ADVERSE REACTIONS

As with other penicillins, it may be expected that untoward reactions will be essentially limited to sensitivity phenomena. They are more likely to occur in individuals who have previously demonstrated hypersensitivity to penicillins and in those with a history of allergy, asthma, hay fever or urticaria. The following adverse reactions have been reported as associated with the use of the penicillins:

Gastrointestinal: Nausea, vomiting and diarrhea.

Hypersensitivity Reactions: Erythematous maculopapular rashes and urticaria have been reported.

NOTE: Urticaria, other skin rashes and serum sickness-like reactions may be controlled with antihistamines and, if necessary, systemic corticosteroids. Whenever such reactions occur, Amoxicillin should be discontinued unless, in the opinion of the physician, the condition being treated is life-threatening and amenable only to Amoxicillin therapy.

Liver: A moderate rise in serum glutamic oxaloacetic transaminase (SGOT) has been noted, but the significance of this finding is unknown.

Hemic and Lymphatic Systems: Anemia, thrombocytopenia, thrombocytopenic purpura, eosinophilia, leukopenia and agranulocytosis have been reported during therapy with the penicillins. These reactions are usually reversible on discontinuation of therapy and are believed to be hypersensitivity phenomena.

DOSAGE AND ADMINISTRATION

Infections of the ear, nose and throat due to streptococci, pneumococci, nonpenicillinase-producing staphylococci and *H. influenzae;*
Infections of the genitourinary tract due to *E. coli, Proteus mirabilis* and *Streptococcus faecalis;*
Infections of the skin and soft-tissues due to streptococci, susceptible staphylococci and *E. coli.*

USUAL DOSAGE:
Adults: 250 mg every 8 hours.
Children: 20 mg/kg/day in divided doses every 8 hours.
Children weighing 20 kg or more should be dosed according to the adult recommendations.

In severe infections or those caused by less susceptible organisms:
500 mg every 8 hours for adults and 40 mg/kg/day in divided doses every 8 hours for children may be needed.

Infections of the lower respiratory tract due to streptococci, pneumococci, nonpenicillinase-producing staphylococci and *H. influenzae:*

USUAL DOSAGE:
Adults: 500 mg every 8 hours.
Children: 40 mg/kg/day in divided doses every 8 hours.
Children weighing 20 kg or more should be dosed according to the adult recommendations.

Gonorrhea, acute uncomplicated ano-genital and urethral infections due to *N. gonorrhoeae* (males and females):

USUAL DOSAGE:
Adults: 3 grams as a single oral dose.
Prepubertal children: 50 mg/kg amoxicillin combined with 25 mg/kg probenecid as a single dose.

NOTE: SINCE PROBENECID IS CONTRAINDICATED IN CHILDREN UNDER 2 YEARS, THIS REGIMEN SHOULD NOT BE USED IN THESE CASES.

Cases of gonorrhea with a suspected lesion of syphilis should have dark-field examinations before receiving Amoxicillin, and monthly serological tests for a minimum of four months.

Larger doses may be required for stubborn or severe infections.

The children's dosage is intended for individuals whose weight will not cause a dosage to be calculated greater than that recommended for adults.

It should be recognized that in the treatment of chronic urinary tract infections, frequent bacteriological and clinical appraisals are necessary. Smaller doses than those recommended above should not be used. Even higher doses may be needed at times. In stubborn infections, therapy may be required for several weeks. It may be necessary to continue clinical and/or bacteriological follow-up for several months after cessation of therapy. Except for gonorrhea, treatment should be continued for a minimum of 48 to 72 hours beyond the time that the patient becomes asymptomatic or evidence of bacterial eradication has been obtained. It is recommended that there be at least 10 days' treatment for any infection caused by hemolytic streptococci to prevent the occurrence of acute rheumatic fever or glomerulonephritis.

DOSAGE AND ADMINISTRATION OF PEDIATRIC DROPS

Usual dosage for all indications except infections of the lower respiratory tract:
Under 6 kg (13 lbs): 0.75 ml every 8 hours.
6–7 kg (13–15 lbs): 1.0 ml every 8 hours.
8 kg (16–18 lbs): 1.25 ml every 8 hours.

Infections of the lower respiratory tract:
Under 6 kg (13 lbs): 1.25 ml every 8 hours.
6–7 kg (13–15 lbs): 1.75 ml every 8 hours.
8 kg (16–18 lbs): 2.25 ml every 8 hours.

Children weighing more than 8 kg (18 lbs) should receive the appropriate dose of the Oral Suspension 125 mg or 250 mg/5 ml.

After reconstitution, the required amount of suspension should be placed directly on the child's tongue for swallowing. Alternate means of administration are to add the required amount of suspension to formula, milk, fruit juice, water, ginger ale or cold drinks. These preparations should then be taken immediately. To be certain the child is receiving full dosage, such preparations should be consumed in entirety.

DIRECTIONS FOR MIXING ORAL SUSPENSION

Prepare suspension at time of dispensing as follows: Tap bottle until all powder flows freely. Add approximately ⅓ of the total amount of water for reconstitution (see table below) and shake vigorously to wet powder. Add remainder of the water and again shake vigorously.

125 mg per 5 ml

Bottle Size	Amount of Water Required for Reconstitution
80 ml	62 ml
100 ml	78 ml
150 ml	116 ml

Each teaspoonful (5 ml) will contain 125 mg Amoxicillin.

125 mg unit dose	5 ml

250 mg per 5 ml

80 ml	59 ml
100 ml	74 ml
150 ml	111 ml

Each teaspoonful (5 ml) will contain 250 mg Amoxicillin.

250 mg unit dose	5 ml
3 Gm single dose	40 ml

DIRECTIONS FOR MIXING PEDIATRIC DROPS

Prepare pediatric drops at time of dispensing as follows: Add the required amount of water (see table below) to the bottle and shake vigorously. Each ml of suspension will then contain Amoxicillin Trihydrate equivalent to 50 mg Amoxicillin.

Bottle Size	Amount of Water Required for Reconstitution
15 ml	12 ml
30 ml	23 ml

NOTE: SHAKE BOTH ORAL SUSPENSION AND PEDIATRIC DROPS WELL BEFORE USING. Keep bottle tightly closed. Any unused portion of the reconstituted suspension must be discarded after 14 days. Refrigeration preferable, but not required.

HOW SUPPLIED

AMOXIL (Amoxicillin) **Capsules.** Each capsule contains 250 mg or 500 mg Amoxicillin as the trihydrate.

250 mg/Capsule
NDC 0029-6006-30 ....bottles of 100
NDC 0029-6006-32 ....bottles of 500
NDC 0029-6006-31 ....unit dose carton of 100

500 mg/Capsule
NDC 0029-6007-30 ....bottles of 100
NDC 0029-6007-32 ....bottles of 500
NDC 0029-6007-31 ....unit dose cartons of 100

Therapy Pack:
NDC 0029-6007-79 ....6 × 500 mg Capsules (3 packs per carton)

AMOXIL (Amoxicillin) **Chewable Tablets.** Each scored tablet contains 125 mg or 250 mg Amoxicillin as the trihydrate.

125 mg/Tablet
NDC 0029-6004-39 ....bottles of 60

250 mg/Tablet
NDC 0029-6005-30 ....bottles of 100

AMOXIL (Amoxicillin) **for Oral Suspension.**

125 mg/5 ml
NDC 0029-6008-21 ....80 ml bottle
NDC 0029-6008-23 ....100 ml bottle
NDC 0029-6008-22 ....150 ml bottle

250 mg/5 ml
NDC 0029-6009-21 ....80 ml bottle
NDC 0029-6009-23 ....100 ml bottle
NDC 0029-6009-22 ....150 ml bottle

Each 5 ml of reconstituted suspension contains 125 mg or 250 mg Amoxicillin as the trihydrate.
NDC 0029-6008-18 ....125 mg unit dose bottle
NDC 0029-6009-18 ....250 mg unit dose bottle

3 Gm for Oral Suspension:
NDC 0029-6037-28 ....single dose bottle

Each single dose bottle contains 3 grams Amoxicillin as the trihydrate.

AMOXIL (Amoxicillin) **Pediatric Drops for Oral Suspension.** Each ml of reconstituted suspension contains 50 mg Amoxicillin as the trihydrate.
NDC 0029-6035-20 ....15 ml bottle
NDC 0029-6038-39 ....30 ml bottle

REV. MARCH, 1985
9416641

Shown in Product Identification Section, page 405

AUGMENTIN® ℞

(amoxicillin/clavulanate potassium)
Tablets and Powder for Oral Suspension and Chewable Tablets

DESCRIPTION

AUGMENTIN is an oral antibacterial combination consisting of the semisynthetic antibiotic amoxicillin and the β-lactamase inhibitor, clavulanate potassium (the potassium salt of clavulanic acid). Amoxicillin is an analog of ampicillin, derived from the basic penicillin nucleus, 6-aminopenicillanic acid. Chemically, amoxicillin is D-(-)-α-amino-p-hydroxybenzyl-penicillin trihydrate and may be represented structurally as:

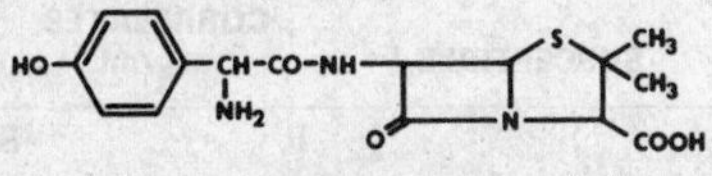

Clavulanic acid is produced by the fermentation of *Streptomyces clavuligerus.* It is a β-lactam structurally related to the penicillins and possesses the ability to inactivate a wide variety of β-lactamases by blocking the active sites of these enzymes. Clavulanic acid is particularly active against the clinically important plasmid mediated β-lactamases frequently responsible for transferred drug resistance to penicillins and cephalosporins. Chemically clavulanate potassium is potassium Z-(3R, 5R)-2-(β-hydroxyethylidene) clavam-3-carboxylate and may be represented structurally as:

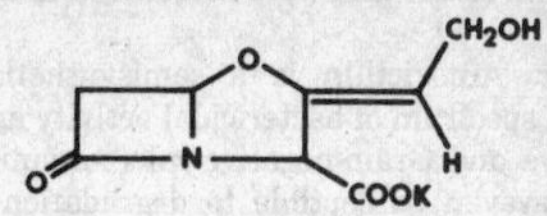

Inactive ingredients: Tablets—Colloidal Silicon Dioxide, Ethyl Cellulose, Hydroxypropyl Cellulose, Hydroxypropyl Methycellulose, Magnesium Stearate, Microcrystalline Cellulose, Sodium Starch Glycolate, and Titanium Dioxide. Powder for Oral Suspension—Colloidal Silicon Dioxide, Flavorings, Mannitol, Silica Gel, Sodium Saccharin, Succinic Acid and Xanthum Gum. Chewable Tablets—Colloidal Silcon Dioxide, D & C Yellow No. 10, Glycine, Magnesium Stearate and Mannitol.

AUGMENTIN is available in '250' and '500' white film-coated tablets and '125' and '250' chewable tablets, and '125' banana flavored and '250' orange flavored oral suspensions. Each AUGMENTIN '250' and '500' tablet contains 250 mg and 500 mg amoxicillin as the trihydrate, respectively, together with 125 mg clavulanic acid as the potassium salt. Each '125' chewable tablet and each teaspoonful (5 mL) of reconstituted AUGMENTIN '125' oral suspension contain 125 mg amoxicillin and 31.25 mg clavulanic acid as the potassium salt while each '250' chewable tablet and each 5 mL of reconstituted AUGMENTIN '250' oral suspension contain 250 mg amoxicillin and 62.5 mg clavulanic acid as the potassium salt.

Each AUGMENTIN tablet contains 0.63 mEq potassium. Each '125' chewable tablet and each 5 mL of reconstituted AUGMENTIN '125' oral suspension contain 0.16 mEq potassium. Each '250' chewable tablet and each 5 mL of reconstituted AUGMENTIN '250' oral suspension contain 0.32 mEq potassium.

CLINICAL PHARMACOLOGY

Amoxicillin and clavulanate, potassium are well absorbed from the gastrointestinal tract after oral administration of AUGMENTIN. AUGMENTIN is stable in the presence of gastric acid and may be given without regard to meals.

Oral administration of one AUGMENTIN '250' or AUGMENTIN '500' tablet provides average peak serum concentrations one to two hours after dosing of 4.4 mcg/mL and 7.6 mcg/mL, respectively, for amoxicillin and 2.3 mcg/mL for clavulanic acid. The areas under the serum concentration curves obtained during the first 6 hours after dosing were 11.4 mcg/mL.hr and 20.2 mcg/mL.hr for amoxicillin, respectively, when one AUGMENTIN '250' or '500' tablet was administered to adult volunteers. The corresponding area under the serum concentration curve for clavulanic acid was 5 mcg/mL.hr. Oral administration of 5 mL of AUGMENTIN '250' suspension or the equivalent dose of 10 mL of AUGMENTIN '125' suspension provides average peak serum concentrations approximately one hour after dosing of 6.9 mcg/mL for amoxicillin and 1.6 mcg/mL for clavulanic acid. The areas under the serum concentration curves obtained during the first 6 hours after dosing were 12.6 mcg/mL.hr for amoxicillin and 2.9 mcg/mL.hr for clavulanic acid when 5 mL of AUGMENTIN '250' suspension or the equivalent dose of 10 mL of AUGMENTIN '125' suspension was administered to adult volunteers. One AUGMENTIN '250' chewable tablet or two AUGMENTIN '125' chewable tablets are equivalent to 5 mL of AUGMENTIN '250' suspension and provide similar serum levels of amoxicillin and clavulanic acid.

Amoxicillin serum concentrations achieved with AUGMENTIN are similar to those produced by the oral administration of equivalent doses of amoxicillin alone. The half life of amoxicillin after the oral administration of AUGMENTIN is 1.3 hours and that of clavulanic acid is 1.0 hour.

Approximately 50–70% of the amoxicillin and approximately 25–40% of the clavulanic acid are excreted unchanged in urine during the first six hours after administration of a single AUGMENTIN '250' or '500' tablet or 10 mL of AUGMENTIN '250' suspension.

Concurrent administration of probenecid delays amoxicillin excretion but does not delay renal excretion of clavulanic acid.

Neither component in AUGMENTIN is highly protein-bound; clavulanic acid has been found to be approximately 30% bound to human serum and amoxicillin approximately 20% bound.

Amoxicillin diffuses readily into most body tissues and fluids with the exception of the brain and spinal fluids. The results of experiments involving the administration of clavulanic acid to animals suggest that this compound, like amoxicillin, is well distributed in body tissues.

Two hours after oral administration of a single 35 mg/kg dose of AUGMENTIN suspension to fasting children, aver-

Continued on next page

Beecham Laboratories—Cont.

age concentrations of 3.0 mcg/mL of amoxicillin and 0.5 mcg/mL of clavulanic acid were detected in middle ear effusions.

Microbiology: Amoxicillin is a semisynthetic antibiotic with a broad spectrum of bactericidal activity against many Gram-positive and Gram-negative microorganisms. Amoxicillin is, however, susceptible to degradation by β-lactamases and therefore the spectrum of activity does not include organisms which produce these enzymes.

Clavulanic acid is a β-lactam, structurally related to the penicillins, which possesses the ability to inactivate a wide range of β-lactamase enzymes commonly found in microorganisms resistant to penicillins and cephalosporins. In particular, it has good activity against the clinically important plasmid mediated β-lactamases frequently responsible for transferred drug resistance.

The formulation of amoxicillin with clavulanic acid in AUGMENTIN protects amoxicillin from degradation by β-lactamase enzymes and effectively extends the antibiotic spectrum of amoxicillin to include many bacteria normally resistant to amoxicillin and other β-lactam antibiotics. Thus AUGMENTIN possesses the distinctive properties of a broad spectrum antibiotic and a β-lactamase inhibitor.

While *in vitro* studies have demonstrated the susceptibility of most strains of the following organisms, clinical efficacy for infections other than those included in the Indications and Usage section has not been documented:

GRAM-POSITIVE BACTERIA: *Staphylococcus aureus* (β-lactamase and non-β-lactamase producing), *Staphylococcus epidermidis* (β-lactamase and non-β-lactamase producing), *Staphylococcus saprophyticus* (β-lactamase and non-β-lactamase producing), *Streptococcus faecalis** (Enterococcus), *Streptococcus pneumoniae** (D. pneumoniae), *Streptococcus pyogenes**, *Streptococcus viridans**

ANAEROBES: *Clostridium* species*, *Peptococcus* species*, *Peptostreptococcus* species*

* These are non-β-lactamase producing strains and therefore are susceptible to amoxicillin alone.

GRAM-NEGATIVE BACTERIA: *Hemophilus influenzae* (β-lactamase and non-B-lactamase producing), *Branhamella catarrhalis (Neisseria catarrhalis)* (β-lactamase and non-β-lactamase producing); *Escherichia coli* (β-lactamase and non-β-lactamase producing), *Klebsiella* species (All known strains are β-lactamase producing), *Enterobacter* species (Although most strains of *Enterobacter* species are resistant *in vitro*, clinical efficacy has been demonstrated with AUGMENTIN in urinary tract infections caused by these organisms.), *Proteus mirabilis* (β-lactamase and non-β-lactamase producing), *Proteus vulgaris* (β-lactamase and non-β-lactamase producing), *Neisseria gonorrhoeae* (β-lactamase and non-β-lactamase producing), *Legionella* species (β-lactamase and non-β-lactamase producing)

ANAEROBES: *Bacteroides* species, including *B. fragilis* (β-lactamase and non-β-lactamase producing).

SUSCEPTIBILITY TESTING

Diffusion Technique: For Kirby-Bauer method of susceptibility testing, a 30 mcg AUGMENTIN (20 mcg amoxicillin + 10 mcg clavulanic acid) diffusion disk should be used. With this procedure, a report from the laboratory of "Susceptible" indicates that the infecting organism is likely to respond to AUGMENTIN therapy and a report of "Resistant" indicates that the infecting organism is not likely to respond to therapy. An "intermediate susceptibility" report suggests that the infecting organism would be susceptible to AUGMENTIN if the higher dosage is used or if the infection is confined to tissues or fluids (e.g. urine) in which high antibiotic levels are attained.

Dilution Techniques: Broth or agar dilution methods may be used to determine the minimal inhibitory concentration (MIC) value for susceptibility of bacterial isolates to AUGMENTIN. Tubes should be inoculated to contain 10^4 to 10^5 organisms/mL or plates "spotted" with 10^3 to 10^4 organisms. The recommended dilution method employs a constant amoxicillin/clavulanic acid ratio of 2 to 1 in all tubes with increasing concentrations of amoxicillin. MIC's are reported in terms of amoxicillin concentration in the presence of clavulanic acid at a constant 2 parts amoxicillin to 1 part clavulanic acid.

[See table below].

[1] The non-β-lactamase-producing organisms which are normally susceptible to ampicillin, such as *Streptococci*, will have similar zone sizes as for ampicillin disks.

[2] The quality control cultures should have the following assigned daily ranges for AUGMENTIN:

		Disks	Mode MIC (mcg/mL)
E. coli	(ATCC 25922)	19–25 mm	4/2–8/4
S. aureus	(ATCC 25923)	28–36 mm	0.25/0.2–0.5/0.25
E. coli	(ATCC 35218)	18–22 mm	4/2–8/4

[3] Expressed as concentration of amoxicillin/clavulanic acid

[4] Organisms which show susceptibility to AUGMENTIN but are resistant to methicillin/oxacillin should be considered resistant.

INDICATIONS AND USAGE

AUGMENTIN is indicated in the treatment of infections caused by susceptible strains of the designated organisms in the conditions listed below:

Lower Respiratory Infections—caused by β-lactamase producing strains of *Hemophilus influenzae.*

Otitis Media—caused by β-lactamse producing strains of *Hemophilus influenzae* and *Branhamella catarrhalis.*

Sinusitis—caused by β-lactamase producing strains of *Hemophilus influenzae* and *Branhamella catarrhalis.*

Skin and Skin Structure Infections—caused by β-lactamase producing strains of *Staphylococcus aureus, Escherichia coli,* and *Klebsiella* spp.

Urinary Tract Infections—caused by β-lactamase producing strains of *Escherichia coli, Klebsiella* spp. and *Enterobacter* spp.

While AUGMENTIN is indicated only for the conditions listed above, infections caused by ampicillin susceptible organisms are also amenable to AUGMENTIN treatment due to its amoxicillin content. Therefore, mixed infections caused by ampicillin susceptible organisms and β-lactamase producing organisms susceptible to AUGMENTIN should not require the addition of another antibiotic.

Bacteriological studies, to determine the causative organisms and their susceptibility to AUGMENTIN, should be performed together with any indicated surgical procedures.

Therapy may be instituted prior to obtaining the results from bacteriological and susceptibility studies to determine the causative organisms and their susceptibility to AUGMENTIN when there is reason to believe the infection may involve any of the β-lactamase producing organisms listed above. Once the results are known, therapy should be adjusted, if appropriate.

CONTRAINDICATIONS

A history of allergic reactions to any penicillin is a contraindication.

WARNINGS

SERIOUS AND OCCASIONALLY FATAL HYPERSENSITIVITY (ANAPHYLACTOID) REACTIONS HAVE BEEN REPORTED IN PATIENTS ON PENICILLIN THERAPY. ALTHOUGH ANAPHYLAXIS IS MORE FREQUENT FOLLOWING PARENTERAL THERAPY, IT HAS OCCURRED IN PATIENTS ON ORAL PENICILLINS. THESE REACTIONS ARE MORE LIKELY TO OCCUR IN INDIVIDUALS WITH A HISTORY OF PENICILLIN HYPERSENSITIVITY AND/OR A HISTORY OF SENSITIVITY TO MULTIPLE ALLERGENS. THERE HAVE BEEN REPORTS OF INDIVIDUALS WITH A HISTORY OF PENICILLIN HYPERSENSITIVITY WHO HAVE EXPERIENCED SEVERE REACTIONS WHEN TREATED WITH CEPHALOSPORINS. BEFORE INITIATING THERAPY WITH ANY PENICILLIN, CAREFUL INQUIRY SHOULD BE MADE CONCERNING PREVIOUS HYPERSENSITIVITY REACTIONS TO PENICILLINS, CEPHALOSPORINS, OR OTHER ALLERGENS. IF AN ALLERGIC REACTION OCCURS, AUGMENTIN SHOULD BE DISCONTINUED AND THE APPROPRIATE THERAPY INSTITUTED. **SERIOUS ANAPHYLACTOID REACTIONS REQUIRE IMMEDIATE EMERGENCY TREATMENT WITH EPINEPHRINE. OXYGEN INTRAVENOUS STEROIDS, AND AIRWAY MANAGEMENT, INCLUDING INTUBATION, SHOULD ALSO BE ADMINISTERED AS INDICATED.**

PRECAUTIONS

General: While AUGMENTIN possesses the characteristic low toxicity of the penicillin group of antibiotics, periodic assessment of organ system functions, including renal, hepatic and hematopoietic function is advisable during prolonged therapy.

A high percentage of patients with mononucleosis who receive ampicillin develop a skin rash. Thus, ampicillin class antibiotics should not be administered to patients with mononucleosis.

The possibility of superinfections with mycotic or bacterial pathogens should be kept in mind during therapy. If superinfections occur (usually involving *Pseudomonas* or *Candida*), the drug should be discontinued and/or appropriate therapy instituted.

Drug Interactions: Probenecid decreases the renal tubular secretion of amoxicillin. Concurrent use with AUGMENTIN may result in increased and prolonged blood levels of amoxicillin.

The concurrent administration of allopurinol and ampicillin increases substantially the incidence of rashes in patients receiving both drugs as compared to patients receiving ampicillin alone. It is not known whether this potentiation of ampicillin rashes is due to allopurinol or the hyperuricemia present in these patients. There are no data with AUGMENTIN and allopurinol administered concurrently.

AUGMENTIN should not be co-administered with ANTABUSE® (disulfiram).

Drug/Laboratory Test Interactions: Oral administraion of AUGMENTIN will result in high urine concentrations of amoxicillin. High urine concentrations of ampicillin may result in false positive reactions when testing for the presence of glucose in urine using Clinitest™, Benedict's Solution or Fehling's Solution. Since this effect may also occur with amoxicillin and therefore AUGMENTIN, it is recommended that glucose tests based on enzymatic glucose oxidase reactions (such as Clinistix™ or Testape™) be used.

Following administration of ampicillin to pregnant women a transient decrease in plasma concentration of total conjugated estriol, estriol-glucuronide, conjugated estrone and estradiol has been noted. This effect may also occur with amoxicillin and therefore AUGMENTIN.

Carcinogenesis, Mutagenesis, Impairment of Fertility: Long-term studies in animals have not been performed to evaluate carcinogenic or mutagenic potential.

Pregnancy (Category B): Reproduction studies have been performed in mice and rats at doses up to ten (10) times the human dose and have revealed no evidence of impaired fertility or harm to the fetus due to AUGMENTIN. There are, however, no adequate and well-controlled studies in pregnant women. Because animal reproduction studies are not always predictive of human response, this drug should be used during pregnancy only if clearly needed.

Labor and Delivery: Oral ampicillin class antibiotics are generally poorly absorbed during labor. Studies in guinea pigs have been shown that intravenous administration of ampicillin decreased the uterine tone, frequency of contractions, height of contractions and duration of contractions. However, it is not known whether the use of AUGMENTIN in humans during labor or delivery has immediate or delayed adverse effects on the fetus, prolongs the duration of labor or increases the likelihood that forceps delivery or other obstretical intervention or resuscitation of the newborn will be necessary.

Nursing Mothers: Ampicillin class antibiotics are excreted in the milk; therefore, caution should be exercised when AUGMENTIN is administered to a nursing woman.

ADVERSE REACTIONS

AUGMENTIN is generally well tolerated. The majority of side effects observed in clinical trials were of a mild and transient nature and less than 3% of patients discontinued therapy because of drug related side effects. The most frequently reported adverse effects were diarrhea/loose stools (9%), nausea (3%), skin rashes and urticaria (3%), vomiting (1%), and vaginitis (1%). The overall incidence of side effects, and in particular diarrhea, increased with the higher recommended dose. Other less frequently reported reactions include: abdominal discomfort, flatulence and headache.

The following adverse reactions have been reported for ampicillin class antibiotics:

Gastrointestinal: Diarrhea, nausea, vomiting, gastritis, stomatitis, glossitis, black "hairy" tongue, enterocolitis and pseudomembraneous colitis.

Hypersensitivity reactions: Skin rashes, urticaria, erythema multiforme and an occasional case of exfoliative dermatitis have been reported. These reactions may be controlled with antihistamines and, if necessary, systemic corticosteroids. Whenever such reactions occur, the drug should be discontinued, unless the opinion of the physician dictates otherwise. Serious and occasional fatal hypersensitivity (anaphylactic) reactions can occur with oral penicillin (See Warnings).

Recommended AUGMENTIN Susceptibility Ranges[1,2]

ORGANISMS	RESISTANT	INTERMEDIATE	SUSCEPTIBLE	MIC[3] CORRELATES mcg/mL	
				R	S
Gram Negative Enteric Bacteria	≤13 mm	14–17 mm	≥18 mm	>32/16	<8/4
Staphylococcus[4] and Hemophilus spp	≤19 mm	—	≥20 mm		≤4/2 ≤4/2

Liver: A moderate rise in SGOT has been noted in patients treated with ampicillin class antibiotics as well as with AUGMENTIN, but the significance of these findings is unknown.
Hemic and Lymphatic Systems: Anemia, thrombocytopenia, thrombocytopenic purpura, eosinophilia, leukopenia and agranulocytosis have been reported during therapy with penicillins. These reactions are usually reversible on discontinuation of therapy and are believed to be hypersensitivity phenomena. A slight thrombocytosis was noted in less than 1% of the patients treated with AUGMENTIN.

OVERDOSAGE

Amoxicillin may be removed from circulation by hemodialysis.
The molecular weight, degree of protein binding and pharmacokinetic profile of clavulanic acid together with information from a single patient with renal insufficiency all suggest that this compound may also be removed by hemodialysis.

DOSAGE AND ADMINISTRATION

Dosage:

Adults: The usual adult dose is one AUGMENTIN '250' tablet every eight hours. For more severe infections and infections of the respiratory tract, the dose should be one AUGMENTIN '500' tablet every eight hours.

Since both the AUGMENTIN '250' and '500' tablets contain the same amount of clavulanic acid (125 mg, as the potassium salt), two AUGMENTIN '250' tablets are not equivalent to one AUGMENTIN '500' tablet. Therefore, two AUGMENTIN '250' tablets should not be substituted for one AUGMENTIN '500' tablet for treatment of more severe infections.

Children: The usual dose is 20 mg/kg/day, based on amoxicillin component, in divided doses every eight hours. For otitis media, sinusitis and lower respiratory infections, the dose should be 40 mg/kg/day, based on the amoxicillin component, in divided doses every eight hours. Severe infections should be treated with the higher recommended dose.

Children weighing 40 kg and more should be dosed according to the adult recommendations.

DIRECTIONS FOR MIXING ORAL SUSPENSION

Prepare a suspension at time of dispensing as follows: Tap bottle until all the powder flows freely. Add approximately ⅔ of the total amount of water for reconstitution (see table below) and shake vigorously to suspend powder. Add remainder of the water and again shake vigorously.

AUGMENTIN '125' Suspension

Bottle Size	Amount of Water Required for Reconstitution
75 mL	67 mL
150 mL	134 mL

Each teaspoonful (5 mL) will contain 125 mg amoxicillin and 31.25 mg of clavulanic acid as the potassium salt.

AUGMENTIN '250' Suspension

Bottle Size	Amount of Water Required for Reconstitution
75 mL	65 mL
150 mL	130 mL

Each teaspoonful (5 mL) will contain 250 mg amoxicillin and 62.5 mg of clavulanic acid as the potassium salt.

Note: SHAKE ORAL SUSPENSION WELL BEFORE USING.

Reconstituted suspension must be stored under refrigeration and discarded after 10 days.

Administration: The absorption of AUGMENTIN is unaffected by food. Therefore, AUGMENTIN may be administered without regard to meals.

HOW SUPPLIED

AUGMENTIN '250' TABLETS: Each white oval filmcoated tablet, debossed with AUGMENTIN on one side and 250/125 on the other side, contains 250 mg amoxicillin as the trihydrate and 125 mg clavulanic acid as the potassium salt.
NDC 0029-6075-27 .... bottles of 30
NDC 0029-6075-30 .... bottles of 100
NDC 0029-6075-31 ....Unit Dose (10×10) 100 tablets
AUGMENTIN '500' TABLETS: Each white oval filmcoated tablet, debossed with AUGMENTIN on one side and 500/125 on the other side, contains 500 mg amoxicillin as the trihydrate and 125 mg clavulanic acid as the potassium salt.
NDC 0029-6080-27 .... bottles of 30
NDC 0029-6080-30 .... bottles of 100
NDC 0029-6080-31 ....Unit Dose (10×10) 100 tablets
AUGMENTIN '125' FOR ORAL SUSPENSION: Each 5 mL of reconstituted banana flavored suspension contains 125 mg amoxicillin and 31.25 mg clavulanic acid as the potassium salt.
NDC 0029-6085-39 .... 75 mL bottle
NDC 0029-6085-22 .... 150 mL bottle
AUGMENTIN '250' FOR ORAL SUSPENSION: Each 5 mL of reconstituted orange flavored suspension contains 250 mg amoxicillin and 62.5 mg clavulanic acid as the potassium salt.
NDC 0029-6090-39 .... 75 mL bottle
NDC 0029-6090-22 .... 150 mL bottle
AUGMENTIN '125' CHEWABLE TABLETS: Each yellow mottled oval tablet, debossed with BMP 189, contains 125 mg amoxicillin as the trihydrate and 31.25 mg clavulanic acid as the potassium salt.
NDC 0029-6073-47 ....carton of 30 (5×6) tablets
AUGMENTIN '250' CHEWABLE TABLETS: Each yellow mottled round tablet, debossed with BMP 190, contains 250 mg amoxicillin as the trihydrate and 62.5 mg clavulanic acid as the potassium salt.
NDC 0029-6074-47 ....carton of 30 (5×6) tablets
REVISED FEB., 1986
9417093

Shown in Product Identification Section, page 405

FASTIN® Capsules Ⓒ
[*făs'tĭn*]
(phentermine hydrochloride)

DESCRIPTION

Each Fastin (phentermine hydrochloride) capsule contains phentermine hydrochloride, 30 mg (equivalent to 24 mg phentermine).
Phentermine Hydrochloride is a white crystalline powder, very soluble in water and alcohol. Chemically, the product is phenyl-tertiary-butyl-amine hydrochloride.
Inactive Ingredients: FD&C Blue 1, Methylcellulose, Polyethylene Glycol and Starch

ACTIONS

FASTIN is a sympathomimetic amine with pharmacologic activity similar to the prototype drugs of this class used in obesity, the amphetamines. Actions include central nervous system stimulation and elevation of blood pressure. Tachyphylaxis and tolerance have been demonstrated with all drugs of this class in which these phenomena have been looked for.
Drugs of this class used in obesity are commonly known as "anorectics" or "anorexigenics." It has not been established that the action of such drugs in treating obesity is primarily one of appetite suppression. Other central nervous system actions, or metabolic effects may be involved, for example.
Adult obese subjects instructed in dietary management and treated with "anorectic" drugs, lose more weight on the average than those treated with placebo and diet, as determined in relatively short-term clinical trials.
The magnitude of increased weight loss of drug-treated patients over placebo-treated patients is only a fraction of a pound a week. The rate of weight loss is greatest in the first weeks of therapy for both drug and placebo subjects and tends to decrease in succeeding weeks. The possible origins of the increased weight loss due to the various drug effects are not established. The amount of weight loss associated with the use of an "anorectic" drug varies from trial to trial, and the increased weight loss appears to be related in part to variables other than the drugs prescribed, such as the physician-investigator, the population treated, and the diet prescribed. Studies do not permit conclusions as to the relative importance of the drug and nondrug factors on weight loss.
The natural history of obesity is measured in years, whereas the studies cited are restricted to a few weeks duration; thus, the total impact of drug-induced weight loss over that of diet alone must be considered clinically limited.

INDICATION

FASTIN is indicated in the management of exogenous obesity as a short term (a few weeks) adjunct in a regimen of weight reduction based on caloric restriction. The limited usefulness of agents of this class (see ACTIONS) should be measured against possible risk factors inherent in their use such as those described below.

CONTRAINDICATIONS

Advanced arteriosclerosis, symptomatic cardiovascular disease, moderate to severe hypertension, hyperthyroidism, known hypersensitivity, or idiosyncrasy to the sympathomimetic amines, glaucoma.
Agitated states.
Patients with a history of drug abuse.
During or within 14 days following the administration of monoamine oxidase inhibitors (hypertensive crises may result).

WARNINGS

Tolerance to the anorectic effect usually develops within a few weeks. When this occurs, the recommended dose should not be exceeded in an attempt to increase the effect; rather, the drug should be discontinued.
FASTIN may impair the ability of the patient to engage in potentially hazardous activities such as operating machinery or driving a motor vehicle; the patient should therefore be cautioned accordingly.
Drug Dependence: FASTIN is related chemically and pharmacologically to the amphetamines. Amphetamines and related stimulant drugs have been extensively abused, and the possibility of abuse of FASTIN should be kept in mind when evaluating the desirability of including a drug as part of a weight reduction program. Abuse of amphetamines and related drugs may be associated with intense psychological dependence and severe social dysfunction. There are reports of patients who have increased the dosage to many times that recommended. Abrupt cessation following prolonged high dosage administration results in extreme fatigue and mental depression; changes are also noted on the sleep EEG. Manifestations of chronic intoxication with anorectic drugs include severe dermatoses, marked insomnia, irritability, hyperactivity, and personality changes. The most severe manifestation of chronic intoxications is psychosis, often clinically indistinguishable from schizophrenia.
Usage in Pregnancy: Safe use in pregnancy has not been established. Use of FASTIN by women who are or who may become pregnant, and those in the first trimester of pregnancy, requires that the potential benefit be weighed against the possible hazard to mother and infant.
Usage in Children: FASTIN is not recommended for use in children under 12 years of age.
Usage with Alcohol: Concomitant use of alcohol with FASTIN may result in an adverse drug interaction.

PRECAUTIONS

Caution is to be exercised in prescribing FASTIN for patients with even mild hypertension.
Insulin requirements in diabetes mellitus may be altered in association with the use of FASTIN and the concomitant dietary regimen.
FASTIN may decrease the hypotensive effect of guanethidine.
The least amount feasible should be prescribed or dispensed at one time in order to minimize the possibility of overdosage.

ADVERSE REACTIONS

Cardiovascular: Palpitation, tachycardia, elevation of blood pressure.
Central Nervous System: Overstimulation, restlessness, dizziness, insomnia, euphoria, dysphoria, tremor, headache, rarely psychotic episodes at recommended doses.
Gastrointestinal: Dryness of the mouth, unpleasant taste, diarrhea, constipation, other gastrointestinal disturbances.
Allergic: Urticaria.
Endocrine: Impotence, changes in libido.

DOSAGE AND ADMINISTRATION

Exogenous Obesity: One capsule at approximately 2 hours after breakfast for appetite control. Late evening medication should be avoided because of the possibility of resulting insomnia.
Administration of one capsule (30 mg.) daily has been found to be adequate in depression of the appetite for twelve to fourteen hours.
FASTIN is not recommended for use in children under 12 years of age.

OVERDOSAGE

Manifestations of acute overdosage with phentermine include restlessness, tremor, hyperreflexia, rapid respiration, confusion, assaultiveness, hallucinations, panic states. Fatigue and depression usually follow the central stimulation. Cardiovascular effects include arrhythmias, hypertension or hypotension, and circulatory collapse. Gastrointestinal symptoms include nausea, vomiting, diarrhea, and abdominal cramps. Fatal poisoning usually terminates in convulsions and coma.
Management of acute phentermine intoxication is largely symptomatic and includes lavage and sedation with a barbiturate. Experience with hemodialysis or peritoneal dialysis is inadequate to permit recommendations in this regard. Acidification of the urine increases phentermine excretion. Intravenous phentolamine (REGITINE) has been suggested for possible acute, severe hypertension, if this complicates phentermine overdosage.

CAUTION

Federal law prohibits dispensing without prescription.

HOW SUPPLIED

Blue and clear capsules with blue and white beads containing 30 mg. phentermine hydrochloride (equivalent to 24 mg. Phentermine).
NDC 0029-2205-30 ....bottles of 100
NDC 0029-2205-39 ....bottles of 450
NDC 0029-2205-31 ....pack 5X30

Shown in Product Identification Section, page 405

Rev. Aug., 1982

Continued on next page

Beecham Laboratories—Cont.

NUCOFED® Ⓒ℞

[nū 'cō-fĕd]

Syrup and Capsules

DESCRIPTION

Nucofed Syrup and Capsules is an antitussive-decongestant containing in each 5 ml (teaspoonful) and each capsule: Codeine Phosphate, 20 mg (Warning: May Be Habit Forming); Pseudoephedrine Hydrochloride, 60 mg. Nucofed Syrup contains no alcohol and contains 2.25 gm of sucrose per 5 ml (teaspoonful). Codeine Phosphate and Pseudoephedrine Hydrochloride may be represented by the following chemical names and structural formulas:

Codeine Phosphate

CH_3 $\overset{+}{N}-H$ $H_2PO_4^- \cdot \frac{1}{2}H_2O$ CH_3O O OH

7,8-didehydro-4,5α-epoxy-3-methoxy-17-methylmorphinan-6α-ol Phosphate (1:1) salt hemihydrate

Pseudoephedrine HCl

H $NHCH_3$ C—C—CH_3 • HCl OH H

[S-(R*,R*)]-α-[1-(methylamino) ethyl]benzene methanol hydrochloride.

Inactive Ingredients, Syrup: Citric Acid, Flavorings, Glycerin, Propylene Glycol, Sodium Benzoate, Sorbitol, Sucrose, D&C Yellow 10, and FD&C Blue 1. **Capsules:** Starch, Lactose and Magnesium Stearate.

CLINICAL PHARMACOLOGY

Nucofed Syrup and Capsules

The clinical pharmacology of this formulated product is thought to be due to the action of its ingredients, Codeine Phosphate and Pseudoephedrine Hydrochloride.

Codeine Phosphate. Codeine causes suppression of the cough reflex by a direct effect on the cough center in the medulla and appears to exert a drying effect on respiratory tract mucosa and to increase viscosity of bronchial secretions.

Codeine is well absorbed from the gastrointestinal tract. Following oral administration, peak antitussive effects usually can be expected to occur within 1–2 hours and may persist for a period of four hours. Codeine is metabolized in the liver. The drug undergoes O-demethylation, N-demethylation, and partial conjugation with glucuronic acid, and is excreted mainly in the urine as norcodeine and morphine in the free and conjugated forms.

Codeine appears in breast milk of nursing mothers and has been reported to cross the placental barrier.

Pseudoephedrine Hydrochloride. Pseudoephedrine is a physiologically active stereoisomer of ephedrine which acts directly on *alpha*, and, to a lesser degree, *beta*-adrenergic receptors. The *alpha*-adrenergic effects are believed to result from the reduced production of cyclic adenosine-3′,5′ monophosphate (cyclic 3′,5′-AMP) by inhibition of the enzyme adenyl cyclase, where *beta*-adrenergic effects appear to be caused by the stimulation of adenyl cyclase activity. Pseudoephedrine acts directly on *alpha*-adrenergic receptors in the respiratory tract mucosa producing vasoconstriction resulting in shrinkage of swollen nasal mucous membranes, reduction of tissue hyperemia, edema, and nasal congestion, and an increase in nasal airway patency. Drainage of sinus secretions is increased and obstructed eustachian ostia may be opened. Relaxation of bronchial smooth muscle by stimulation of $beta_2$ adrenergic receptors may also occur. Following oral administration significant broncho-dilation has not been demonstrated consistently.

Nasal decongestion usually occurs within 30 minutes and persists for 4–6 hours after oral administration of 60 mg of Pseudoephedrine Hydrochloride.

Although specific information is not available, Pseudoephedrine is presumed to cross the placenta and to enter cerebrospinal fluid. It is incompletely metabolized in the liver by N-demethylation to an inactive metabolite. Both are excreted in the urine with 55%–75% of a dose being unchanged.

INDICATIONS AND USAGE

NUCOFED is indicated for symptomatic relief when both coughing and congestion are associated with upper respiratory infections and related conditions such as common cold, bronchitis, influenza, and sinusitis.

CONTRAINDICATIONS

Hypersensitivity to product's active ingredients.

WARNINGS

Persons with persistent cough such as occurs with smoking, asthma, emphysema, or where cough is accompanied by excessive secretions should not take this product except under the advice and supervision of a physician.

May cause or aggravate constipation.

Do not give this product to children taking other drugs except under the advice and supervision of a physician.

Persons with a chronic pulmonary disease or shortness of breath, high blood pressure, heart disease, diabetes or thyroid disease should not take this product except under the advice and supervision of a physician.

Do not exceed recommended dosage because at higher doses nervousness, dizziness, or sleeplessness may occur.

If symptoms do not improve within 7 days or are accompanied by high fever, consult a physician before continuing use.

PRECAUTIONS

General

Inasmuch as the active ingredients of Nucofed Syrup and Capsules consist of Codeine Phosphate and Pseudoephedrine Hydrochloride, this medication should be used with caution in the presence of the following:

- Cardiovascular disease (of any etiology)
- Diabetes mellitus
- Hypertension (of any severity)
- Abnormal thyroid function
- Prostatic hypertrophy
- Addison's disease
- Chronic ulcerative colitis
- History of drug abuse or dependence
- Chronic respiratory disease or impairment
- Functional impairment of the liver or kidney

Patients taking Nucofed Syrup and Capsules should be cautioned when driving or doing jobs requiring alertness and to get up slowly from a lying or sitting position, or to lie down if nausea occurs.

Possible Drug Interactions

Because of the potential for drug interactions, persons currently taking any of the following medications should take Nucofed Syrup and Capsules on the advice and under the supervision of a physician.

- Beta adrenergic blockers—concurrent use may increase the pressor effect of pseudoephedrine.
- Digitalis glycosides—concurrent use with pseudoephedrine may increase the possibility of cardiac arrhythmias.
- Antihypertensive agents including Veratrum alkaloids—hypotensive effects may be decreased by the concurrent use of pseudoephedrine.
- Monoamine oxidase (MAO) inhibitors— these agents may potentiate the pressor effect of Pseudoephedrine and may result in a hypertensive crisis; pseudoephedrine should not be administered during or within 14 days of MAO inhibitors.
- Sympathomimetics, other — sympathomimetics used concurrently may increase the effects either of these agents or of pseudoephedrine, thereby increasing the potential for side effects.
- Tricyclic antidepressants—the concurrent use of tricyclic antidepressants may antagonize the effects of pseudoephedrine and may increase the effects either of the antidepressants themselves or of the codeine component.
- CNS depressants
- Alcohol
- General anesthetics
- Anticholinergics—concurrent use may result in paralytic ileus.

Drug/Laboratory Test Interactions

- Codeine may cause an elevation in serum amylase levels due to the spasm producing potential of narcotic analgesics on the sphincter of Oddi.

Pregnancy: Category C

Animal reproduction studies of the components of Nucofed Syrup and Capsules (Codeine, Pseudoephedrine) have not been conducted. Thus, it is not known whether these agents can cause fetal harm when administered to pregnant women or whether they affect reproductive capacity. Accordingly, Nucofed Syrup and Capsules should be given to pregnant women only where clearly needed.

Nursing Mothers

Codeine and Pseudoephedrine are excreted in breast milk; therefore, caution should be exercised when this medication is prescribed for a nursing mother.

Pediatric Use

Do not give Nucofed Syrup and Capsules to children under two years of age except on the advice and under the supervision of a physician.

ADVERSE REACTIONS

Based on the composition of Nucofed Syrup and Capsules the following side effects may occur: nervousness, restlessness, trouble in sleeping, drowsiness, difficult or painful urination, dizziness or lightheadedness, headache, nausea and vomiting, constipation, trembling, troubled breathing, increase in sweating, unusual paleness, weakness, changes in heart rate.

DRUG ABUSE AND DEPENDENCE

NUCOFED is placed in Schedule III of the Controlled Substances Act.

OVERDOSAGE

Nucofed Syrup and Capsules contain Codeine Phosphate and Pseudoephedrine Hydrochloride. Overdosage as a result of this product should be treated based upon the symptomatology of the patient as it relates to the individual ingredient. Treatment of acute overdosage would probably be based upon treating the patient for codeine toxicity which may be manifested as:

- Gradual drowsiness, dizziness, heaviness of the head, weariness, diminution of sensibility, loss of pain and other modalities of sensation.
- Nausea and vomiting.
- A transient excitement stage, characterized by extreme restlessness, delirium, and rarely epileptiform convulsions, is sometimes seen in children and rarely in adult women.
- Bilateral miosis, progressing to pinpoint pupils, which do not react to light or accommodation. The pupils may dilate during terminal asphyxia.
- Itching of the skin and nose, sometimes with skin rashes and urticaria.
- Coma, with muscular relaxation and depressed or absent superficial and deep reflexes. A Babinski toe sign may appear.
- Marked slowing of the respiratory rate with inadequate pulmonary ventilation and consequent cyanosis. Breathing becomes stertorous and irregular (Cheyne-Stokes or Biot).
- The pulse is slow and the blood pressure gradually falls to shock levels. Urine formation ceases or is reduced to a very low rate.

The lethal dose of codeine for an adult is about 0.5–1.0 gm. Treatment is as recommended for narcotics.

DOSAGE AND ADMINISTRATION

RECOMMENDED DOSAGE: CAPSULE

Adults: 1 capsule every 6 hours, not to exceed 4 capsules in 24 hours.

RECOMMENDED DOSAGE: SYRUP

Adults: 1 teaspoonful every 6 hours, not to exceed 4 teaspoonfuls in 24 hours.

Children:

6 to under 12 years: ½ teaspoonful every 6 hours, not to exceed 2 teaspoonfuls in 24 hours.

2 to under 6 years: ¼ teaspoonful every 6 hours, not to exceed 1 teaspoonful in 24 hours.

Do not give this product to children under 2 years, except under the advice and supervision of a physician.

HOW SUPPLIED

Nucofed Syrup, Green, Mint Flavored

NDC 0029-3135-34 Pints

Nucofed Capsules, Green Top, Clear Bottom

NDC 0029-3138-39 Bottles of 60

CAUTION

Federal law prohibits dispensing without prescription.

DGB—0491/2-85

Revised February, 1985

Shown in Product Identification Section, page 405

NUCOFED® EXPECTORANT Ⓒ℞

[nū 'cō-fĕd]

SYRUP

DESCRIPTION

Nucofed Expectorant is an antitussive-decongestant-expectorant syrup for oral administration containing in each 5 ml (teaspoonful): Codeine Phosphate, 20 mg (Warning: May Be Habit Forming); Pseudoephedrine HCl, 60 mg; Guaifenesin, 200 mg; alcohol, 12.5%.

Codeine Phosphate, Pseudoephedrine Hydrochloride and Guaifenesin may be represented by the following chemical names and structural formulas:

Codeine Phsophate

CH_3 $\overset{+}{N}-H$ $H_2PO_4^- \cdot \frac{1}{2}H_2O$ CH_3O O OH

7,8-didehydro-4,5α-epoxy-3-methoxy-17-methylmorphinan-6α-ol Phosphate (1:1) salt hemihydrate

Pseudoephedrine HCl

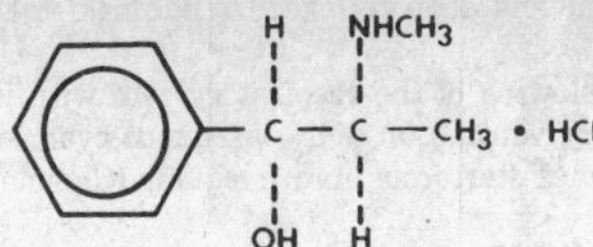

[*S*-(*R**,*R**)]-α-[1-(methylamino) ethyl]benzene methanol hydrochloride

Guaifenesin

$OCH_2CH(OH)CH_2OH$

OCH_3

3-(0-methoxyphenoxy)-1,2-propanediol

Inactive Ingredients: D & C Yellow 10, F D & C Red 40, Flavoring, Glycerin, Saccharin Sodium, Sodium Chloride and Sucrose.

CLINICAL PHARMACOLOGY

Nucofed Expectorant

The clinical pharmacology of this formulated product is thought to be due to the action of its ingredients, Codeine Phosphate, Pseudoephedrine Hydrochloride and Guaifenesin.

Codeine Phosphate. Codeine causes suppression of the cough reflex by a direct effect on the cough center in the medulla and appears to exert a drying effect on respiratory tract mucosa and to increase viscosity of bronchial secretions.

Codeine is well absorbed from the gastrointestinal tract. Following oral administration, peak antitussive effects can be expected to occur within one to two hours and may persist for a period of four hours. Codeine is metabolized in the liver. The drug undergoes O-demethylation, N-demethylation, and partial conjugation with glucuronic acid, and is excreted mainly in the urine as norcodeine and morphine in the free and conjugated forms.

Codeine appears in breast milk of nursing mothers and has been reported to cross the placental barrier.

Pseudoephedrine Hydrochloride. Pseudoephedrine is a physiologically active stereoisomer of ephedrine which acts directly on *alpha*, and to a lesser degree, *beta* -adrenergic receptors. The *alpha* -adrenergic effects are believed to result from the reduced production of cyclic adenosine-3′,5′ monophosphate (cyclic 3′,5′-AMP) by inhibition of the enzyme adenyl cyclase, whereas *beta* -adrenergic effects appear to be caused by the stimulation of adenyl cyclase activity.

Pseudoephedrine acts directly on *alpha* -adrenergic receptors in the respiratory tract mucosa producing vasoconstriction resulting in shrinkage of swollen nasal mucous membranes, reduction of tissue hyperemia, edema, and nasal congestion, and an increase in nasal airway patency. Drainage of sinus secretions is increased and obstructed eustachian ostia may be opened. Relaxation of bronchial smooth muscle by stimulation of *beta* $_2$ adrenergic receptors may also occur. Following oral administration significant broncho-dilation has not been demonstrated consistently.

Nasal decongestion usually occurs within 30 minutes and persists for 4–6 hours after oral administration of 60 mg of pseudoephedrine hydrochloride.

Although specific information is not available, pseudoephedrine is presumed to cross the placenta and to enter cerebrospinal fluid. It is incompletely metabolized in the liver by N-demethylation to an inactive metabolite. Both are excreted in the urine with 55%–75% of a dose being unchanged.

Guaifenesin. Guaifenesin, by increasing respiratory tract fluid, reduces the viscosity of tenacious secretions and acts as an expectorant.

Guaifenesin is excreted in the urine mainly as glucuronates and sulfonates.

INDICATIONS AND USAGE

NUCOFED EXPECTORANT is indicated for symptomatic relief when both coughing and congestion are associated with upper respiratory infections and related conditions such as common colds, bronchitis, influenza, and sinusitis.

CONTRAINDICATIONS

Hypersensitivity to product's active ingredients.

WARNINGS

Persons with persistent cough such as occurs with smoking, asthma, emphysema, or where cough is accompanied by excessive secretions should not take this product except under the advice and supervision of a physician.

Do not give this product to children taking other drugs except under the advice and supervision of a physician.

Persons with a chronic pulmonary disease or shortness of breath, high blood pressure, heart disease, diabetes or thyroid disease should not take this product except under the advice and supervision of a physician.

Do not exceed recommended dosage because at higher doses nervousness, dizziness, or sleeplessness may occur.

If symptoms do not improve within 7 days or are accompanied by high fever, consult a physician before continuing use.

PRECAUTIONS

General. Inasmuch as the active ingredient of Nucofed Expectorant consist of Codeine Phosphate, Pseudoephedrine Hydrochloride and Guaifenesin, this medication should be used with caution in the presence of the following:

- Cardiovascular disease (of any etiology)
- Diabetes mellitus
- Hypertension (of any severity)
- Abnormal thyroid function
- Prostatic hypertrophy
- Addison's disease
- Chronic ulcerative colitis
- History of drug abuse or dependence
- Chronic respiratory disease or impairment
- Functional impairment of the liver or kidney

Patients taking Nucofed Expectorant should be cautioned when driving or doing jobs requiring alertness and to get up slowly from a lying or sitting position, or to lie down if nausea occurs.

Possible Drug Interactions. Because of the potential for drug interactions, persons currently taking any of the following medications should take Nucofed Expectorant only on the advice and under the supervision of a physician.

- Beta adrenergic blockers—concurrent use may increase the pressor effect of pseudoephedrine.
- Digitalis glycosides—concurrent use with pseudoephedrine may increase the possibility of cardiac arrhythmias.
- Antihypertensive agents including Veratrum alkaloids—hypotensive effects may be decreased by the concurrent use of pseudoephedrine.
- Monoamine oxidase (MAO) inhibitors—these agents may potentiate the pressor effect of pseudoephedrine and may result in a hypertensive crisis; pseudoephedrine should not be administered during or within 14 days of MAO inhibitors.
- Sympathomimetics, other—sympathomimetics used concurrently may increase the effects either of these agents or of pseudoephedrine, thereby increasing the potential for side effects.
- Tricyclic antidepressants—the concurrent use of tricyclic antidepressants may antagonize the effects of pseudoephedrine and may increase the effects either of the antidepressants themselves or of the codeine component.
- CNS depressants
- Alcohol
- General anesthetics
- Anticholinergics—concurrent use may result in paralytic ileus.

Drug/Laboratory Test Interactions

- Codeine may cause an elevation in serum amylase levels due to the spasm producing potential of narcotic analgesics on the sphincter of Oddi.
- Guaifenesin is known to interfere with the colorimetric determination of 5-hydroxy-indole-acetic acid (5-HIAA) and vanilmandelic acid (VMA).

Pregnancy: Category C

Animal reproduction studies of the components of Nucofed Expectorants (codeine, pseudoephedrine and guaifenesin) have not been conducted. Thus, it is not known whether these agents can cause fetal harm when administered to pregnant women or whether they affect reproductive capacity. Accordingly, Nucofed Expectorant should be given to pregnant women only where clearly needed.

Nursing Mothers

Codeine and Pseudoephedrine, two of the ingredients in Nucofed Expectorant, are excreted in breast milk; therefore, caution should be exercised when this medication is prescribed for a nursing mother.

Pediatric Use

Do not give Nucofed Expectorant to Children under two years of age except on the advice and under the supervision of a physician.

ADVERSE REACTIONS

Based on the composition of Nucofed Expectorant the following side effects may occur: nervousness, restlessness, trouble in sleeping, drowsiness, difficult or painful urination, dizziness or lightheadedness, headache, nausea or vomiting, constipation, trembling, troubled breathing, increase in sweating, unusual paleness, weakness, changes in heart rate.

DRUG ABUSE AND DEPENDENCE

Nucofed Expectorant has been placed in Schedule III of the Controlled Substances Act.

OVERDOSAGE

Nucofed Expectorant contains Codeine Phosphate, Pseudoephedrine Hydrochloride and Guaifenesin. Overdosage as a result of this product should be treated based upon the symptomatology of the patient as it relates to the individual ingredient. Treatment of acute overdosage would probably be based upon treating the patient for codeine toxicity which may be manifested as:

- Gradual drowsiness, dizziness, heaviness of the head, weariness, diminution of sensibility, loss of pain and other modalities of sensation.
- Nausea and vomiting.
- A transient excitement stage, characterized by extreme restlessness, delirium, and rarely epileptiform convulsions, is sometimes seen in children and rarely in adult women.
- Bilateral miosis, progressing to pinpoint pupils, which do not react to light or accommodation. The pupils may dilate during terminal asphyxia.
- Itching of the skin and nose, sometimes with skin rashes and urticaria.
- Coma, with muscular relaxation and depressed or absent superficial and deep reflexes. A Babinski toe sign may appear.
- Marked slowing of the respiratory rate with inadequate pulmonary ventilation and consequent cyanosis. Breathing becomes stertorous and irregular (Cheyne-Stokes or Biot).
- The pulse is slow and the blood pressure gradually falls to shock levels. Urine formation ceases or is reduced to a very low rate.

The lethal dose of codeine for an adult is about 0.5–1.0 gram. Treatment is as recommended for narcotics.

DOSAGE AND ADMINISTRATION

RECOMMENDED DOSAGE:

Adults: 1 teaspoonful every 6 hours, not to exceed 4 teaspoonfuls in 24 hours.

Children:

6 to under 12 years: $\frac{1}{2}$ teaspoonful every 6 hours, not to exceed 2 teaspoonfuls in 24 hours.

2 to under 6 years: $\frac{1}{4}$ teaspoonful every 6 hours, not to exceed 1 teaspoonful in 24 hours.

Do not give this product to children under 2 years, except under the advice and supervision of a physician.

HOW SUPPLIED

Red, Wintergreen Flavored Syrup

NDC 0029-3142-34 Pints

CAUTION

Federal law prohibits dispensing without prescription.

DGB—1266/3-85

Revised March, 1985

NUCOFED® Ⓒ ℞

[*nū 'cō-fĕd*]

PEDIATRIC EXPECTORANT

SYRUP

DESCRIPTION

Nucofed Pediatric Expectorant is an antitussive-decongestant-expectorant syrup for oral administration containing in each 5 ml (teaspoonful): Codeine Phosphate, 10 mg (Warning: May Be Habit Forming); Pseudoephedrine HCl, 30 mg; Guaifenesin, 100 mg; alcohol, 6%

Codeine Phosphate, Pseudoephedrine Hydrochloride and Guaifenesin may be represented by the following chemical names and structural formulas:

Codeine Phosphate

CH_3 $\overset{+}{N}$—H $H_2PO_4^-$ • $\frac{1}{2}H_2O$ CH_3O OH

7,8-didehydro-4,5α-epoxy-3-methoxy-17-methylmorphinan-6α-ol Phosphate (1:1) salt hemihydrate

Pseudoephedrine HCl

H NHCH3 C—C—CH3 • HCl OH H

[*S*-(*R**,*R**)]-α-[1-(methylamino) ethyl]benzene methanol hydrochloride

Guaifenesin

$OCH_2CH(OH)CH_2OH$

OCH_3

3-(0-methoxyphenoxy)-1,2-propanediol

Continued on next page

Beecham Laboratories—Cont.

Inactive Ingredients: Edetate Disodium, F D & C Red 40, Flavorings, Glycerin, Potassium Sorbate, Saccharin Sodium, Sodium Chloride and Sucrose.

CLINICAL PHARMACOLOGY

Nucofed Pediatric Expectorant
The clinical pharmacology of this formulated product is thought to be due to the action of its ingredients, Codeine Phosphate, Pseudoephedrine Hydrochloride and Guaifenesin.

Codeine Phosphate. Codeine causes suppression of the cough reflex by a direct effect on the cough center in the medulla and appears to exert a drying effect on respiratory tract mucosa and to increase viscosity of bronchial secretions.
Codeine is well absorbed from the gastrointestinal tract. Following oral administration, peak antitussive effect usually can be expected to occur within one to two hours and may persist for a period of four hours. Codeine is metabolized in the liver. The drug undergoes O-demethylation, N-demethylation, and partial conjugation with glucuronic acid, and is excreted mainly in the urine as norcodeine and morphine in the free and conjugated forms.
Codeine appears in breast milk of nursing mothers and has been reported to cross the placental barrier.

Psuedoephedrine Hydrochloride. Pseudoephedrine is a physiologically active stereoisomer of ephedrine which acts directly on *alpha,* and to a lesser degree, *beta* -adrenergic receptors. The *alpha* -adrenergic effects are believed to result from the reduced production of cyclic adenosine-3′,5′ monophosphate (cyclic 3′,5′-AMP) by inhibition of the enzyme adenyl cyclase, whereas *beta* -adrenergic effects appear to be caused by the stimulation of adenyl cyclase activity.
Pseudoephedrine acts directly on *alpha* -adrenergic receptors in the respiratory tract mucosa producing vasoconstriction resulting in shrinkage of swollen nasal mucous membranes, reduction of tissue hyperemia, edema, and nasal congestion, and an increase in nasal airway patency. Drainage of sinus secretions is increased and obstructed eustachian ostia may be opened. Relaxation of bronchial smooth muscle by stimulation of $beta_2$ adrenergic receptors may also occur. Following oral administration significant bronchodilation has not been demonstrated consistently.
Nasal decongestion usually occurs within 30 minutes and persists for 4–6 hours after oral administration of 30 mg of pseudoephedrine hydrochloride.
Although specific information is not available, pseudoephedrine is presumed to cross the placenta and to enter cerebrospinal fluid. It is incompletely metabolized in the liver by N-demethylation to an inactive metabolite. Both are excreted in the urine with 55%–75% of a dose being unchanged.

Guaifenesin. Guaifenesin, by increasing respiratory tract fluid, reduces the viscosity of tenacious secretions and acts as an expectorant.
Guaifenesin is excreted in the urine mainly as glucuronates and sulfonates.

INDICATIONS AND USAGE

NUCOFED PEDIATRIC EXPECTORANT is indicated for symptomatic relief when both coughing and congestion are associated with upper respiratory infections and related conditions such as common cold, bronchitis, influenza, and sinusitis.

CONTRAINDICATIONS

Hypersensitivity to product's active ingredients.

WARNINGS

Persons with persistent cough such as occurs with smoking, asthma, emphysema, or where cough is accompanied by excessive secretions should not take this product except under the advice and supervision of a physician.
Do not give this product to children taking other drugs except under the advice and supervision of a physician.
Persons with a chronic pulmonary disease or shortness of breath, high blood pressure, heart disease, diabetes or thyroid disease should not take this product except under the advice and supervision of a physician.
Do not exceed recommended dosage because at higher doses nervousness, dizziness, or sleeplessness may occur.
If symptoms do not improve within 7 days or are accompanied by high fever, consult a physician before continuing use.

PRECAUTIONS

General. Inasmuch as the active ingredients of Nucofed Pediatric Expectorant consist of Codeine Phosphate, Pseudoephedrine Hydrochloride and Guaifenesin, this medication should be used with caution in the presence of the following:

- Cardiovascular disease (of any etiology)
- Diabetes mellitus
- Hypertension (of any severity)
- Abnormal thyroid function
- Prostatic hypertrophy
- Addison's disease
- Chronic ulcerative colitis
- History of drug abuse or dependence
- Chronic respiratory disease or impairment
- Functional impairment of the liver or kidney

Patients taking Nucofed Pediatric Expectorant should be cautioned when driving or doing jobs requiring alertness and to get up slowly from a lying or sitting position, or to lie down if nausea occurs.

Possible Drug Interactions. Because of the potential for drug interactions, persons currently taking any of the following medications should take Nucofed Pediatric Expectorant only on the advice and under the supervision of a physician.

- Beta adrenergic blockers—concurrent use may increase the pressor effect of pseudoephedrine.
- Digitalis glycosides—concurrent use with pseudoephedrine may increase the possibility of cardiac arrhythmias.
- Antihypertensive agents including Veratrum alkaloids—hypotensive effects may be decreased by the concurrent use of pseudoephedrine.
- Monoamine oxidase (MAO) inhibitors—these agents may potentiate the pressor effect of pseudophedrine and may result in a hypertensive crisis; pseudoephedrine should not be administered during or within 14 days of MAO inhibitors.
- Sympathomimetics, other—sympathomimetics used concurrently may increase the effects either of these agents or of pseudoephedrine, thereby increasing the potential for side effects.
- Tricyclic antidepressants—the concurrent use of tricyclic antidepressants may antagonize the effects of pseudoephedrine and may increase the effects either of the antidepressants themselves or of the codeine component.
- CNS depressants
- Alcohol
- General anesthetics
- Anticholinergics—concurrent use may result in paralytic ileus.

Drug/Laboratory Test Interactions

- Codeine may cause an elevation in serum amylase levels due to the spasm producing potential of narcotic analgesics on the sphincter of Oddi.
- Guaifenesin is known to interfere with the colorimetric determination of 5-hydroxyindole-acetic acid (5-HIAA) and vanilmandelic acid (VMA).

Pregnancy: Category C
Animal reproduction studies of the components of Nucofed Pediatric Expectorant (codeine, pseudoephedrine and guaifensin) have not been conducted. Thus, it is not known whether these agents can cause fetal harm when administered to pregnant women or whether they affect reproductive capacity. Accordingly, Nucofed Pediatric Expectorant should be given to pregnant women only where clearly needed.

Nursing Mothers
Codeine and Pseudoephedrine, two of the ingredients in Nucofed Pediatric Expectorant, are excreted in breast milk; therefore, caution should be exercised when this medication is prescribed for a nursing mother.

Pediatric Use
Do not give Nucofed Pediatric Expectorant to Children under two years of age except on the advice and under the supervision of a physician.

ADVERSE REACTIONS

Based on the composition of Nucofed Pediatric Expectorant the following side effects may occur: nervousness, restlessness, trouble in sleeping, drowsiness, difficult or painful urination, dizziness or lightheadedness, headache, nausea or vomiting, constipation, trembling, troubled breathing, increase in sweating, unusual paleness, weakness, changes in heart rate.

DRUG ABUSE AND DEPENDENCE

Nucofed Pediatric Expectorant has been placed in Schedule V of the Controlled Substances Act.

OVERDOSAGE

Nucofed Pediatric Expectorant contains Codeine Phosphate, Pseudoephedrine Hydrochloride and Guaifenesin. Overdosage as a result of this product should be treated based upon the symptomatology of the patient as it relates to the individual ingredient. Treatment of acute overdosage would probably be based upon treating the patient for codeine toxicity which may be manifested as:

- Gradual drowsiness, dizziness, heaviness of the head, weariness, diminution of sensibility, loss of pain and other modalities of sensation.
- Nausea and vomiting.
- A transient excitement stage, characterized by extreme restlessness, delirium, and rarely epileptiform convulsions, is sometimes seen in children and rarely in adult women.
- Bilateral miosis, progressing to pinpoint pupils, which do not react to light or accommodation. The pupils may dilate during terminal asphyxia.
- Itching of the skin and nose, sometimes with skin rashes and urticaria.
- Coma, with muscular relaxation and depressed or absent superficial and deep reflexes. A Babinski toe sign may appear.
- Marked slowing of the respiratory rate with inadequate pulmonary ventilation and consequent cyanosis. Breathing becomes stertorous and irregular (Cheyne-Stokes or Biot).
- The pulse is slow and the blood pressure gradually falls to shock levels. Urine formation ceases or is reduced to a very low rate.

The lethal dose of codeine for an adult is approximately 0.5–1.0 gm. Reliable information regarding the lethal dose in children is not available. Treatment is as recommended for narcotics.

DOSAGE AND ADMINISTRATION

RECOMMENDED DOSAGE:

Adults and Children 12 years of age and over: 2 teaspoonfuls every 6 hours, not to exceed 8 teaspoonfuls in 24 hours.

Children:

6 to under 12 years: 1 teaspoonful every 6 hours, not to exceed 4 teaspoonfuls in 24 hours.

2 to under 6 years: ½ teaspoonful every 6 hours, not to exceed 2 teaspoonfuls in 24 hours.

Do not give this product to children under 2 years, except under the advice and supervision of a physician.

HOW SUPPLIED

Red, Strawberry Flavored Syrup
NDC 0029-3130-39 Pints

CAUTION

Federal law prohibits dispensing without prescription.
DGB—2010/4-85
Revised April, 1985

TICAR® ℞

[*tī'kar*]
(sterile ticarcillin disodium)
for Intramuscular or Intravenous Administration

DESCRIPTION

TICAR (Ticarcillin Disodium) is a semisynthetic injectable penicillin derived from the penicillin nucleus, 6-aminopenicillanic acid. Chemically, it is 6-[(Carboxy-3-thienylacetyl)amino]3, 3-dimethyl-7-oxo-4-thia-1-azabicyclo [3.2.0]heptane-2-carboxylic acid disodium salt.

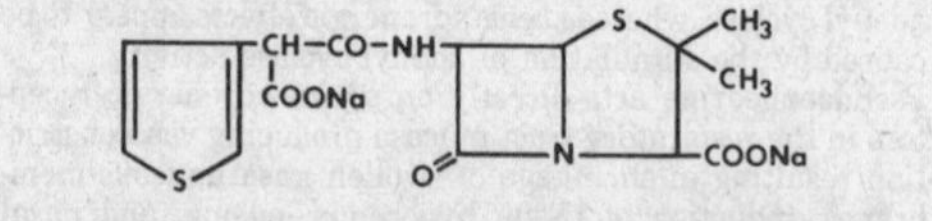

It is supplied as a white to pale yellow powder or lyophilized cake for reconstitution. The reconstituted solution is clear, colorless or pale yellow, having a pH of 6.0–8.0. Ticarcillin is very soluble in water, its solubility is greater than 600 mg/ml.

ACTIONS

PHARMACOLOGY
Ticarcillin is not absorbed orally, therefore, it must be given intravenously or intramuscularly. Following intramuscular administration, peak serum concentrations occur within ½–1 hour. Somewhat higher and more prolonged serum levels can be achieved with the concurrent administration of probenecid.
The minimum inhibitory concentrations (MIC) for many strains of *Pseudomonas* are relatively high by usual standards; serum levels of 60 mcg/ml or greater are required. However, the low degree of toxicity of Ticarcillin permits the use of doses large enough to achieve inhibitory levels for these strains in serum or tissues. Other susceptible organisms usually require serum levels in the 10–25 mcg/ml range.
[See table on top next page].
As with other penicillins, Ticarcillin is eliminated by glomerular filtration and tubular secretion. It is not highly bound to serum protein (approximately 45%) and is excreted unchanged in high concentrations in the urine. After the administration of a 1–2 Gm I.M. dose, a urine concentration of 2000–4000 mcg/ml may be obtained in patients with normal renal function. The serum half-life of Ticarcillin in normal individuals is approximately 70 minutes.
An inverse relationship exists between serum half-life and creatinine clearance, but the dosage of TICAR need only be adjusted in cases of severe renal impairment (see DOSAGE AND ADMINISTRATION). The administered Ticarcillin may be removed from patients undergoing dialysis; the actual amount removed depends on the duration and type of dialysis.
Ticarcillin can be detected in tissues and interstitial fluid following parenteral administration. Penetration into the cerebrospinal fluid, bile and pleural fluid has been demonstrated.

MICROBIOLOGY

Ticarcillin is bactericidal and demonstrates substantial *in vitro* activity against both Gram-positive and Gram-negative organisms. Many strains of the following organisms were found to be susceptible to Ticarcillin *in vitro:*

Pseudomonas aeruginosa (and other species)
Escherichia coli
Proteus mirabilis
Proteus morganii
Proteus rettegri
Proteus vulgaris
Enterobacter species
Haemophilus influenzae
Neisseria species
Salmonella species
Staphylococcus aureus (non-penicillinase producing)
Staphylococcus epidermidis
Beta-hemolytic streptococci (Group A)
Streptococcus faecalis (Enterococcus)
Streptococcus pneumoniae

Anaerobic bacteria, including:
Bacteroides species including *B. fragilis*
Fusobacterium species
Veillonella species
Clostridium species
Eubacterium species
Peptococcus species
Peptostreptococcus species

In vitro synergism between Ticarcillin and gentamicin sulfate, tobramycin sulfate or amikacin sulfate against certain strains of *Pseudomonas aeruginosa* has been demonstrated. Some strains of such microorganisms as *Mima-Herellea (Acinetobacter), Citrobacter* and *Serratia* have shown susceptibility.

Ticarcillin is not stable in the presence of penicillinase. Some strains of *Pseudomonas* have developed resistance fairly rapidly.

DISC SUSCEPTIBILITY TESTS

Susceptibility Tests: Ticarcillin discs or powders should be used for testing susceptibility to ticarcillin. However, organisms, reportedly susceptible to carbenicillin are susceptible to ticarcillin.

Diffusion Techniques: For the disc diffusion method of susceptibility testing a 75 mcg TICAR DISC should be used. The method for this test is the one outlined in NCCLS publication M2-A3* with the following interpretative criteria:
[See table below].

Dilution Techniques: Dilution techniques for determining the MIC (minimum inhibitory concentration) are published by NCCLS for the broth and agar dilution procedures. The MIC data should be interpreted in light of the concentrations present in serum, tissue, and body fluids. Organisms with MIC ≤ 64 are considered susceptible when they are in tissue but organisms with MIC ≤ 128 would be susceptible in urine where the TICAR concentrations are much greater. At present, only dilution methods can be recommended for testing antibiotic susceptibility of obligate anaerobes.

Susceptibility testing methods require the use of control organisms. The 75 mcg ticarcillin disc should give zone diameters between 22 and 28 mm for *P. aeruginosa* ATCC 27853 and 24 and 30 mm for *E. Coli* ATCC 25922. Reference strains are available for dilution testing of ticarcillin. 95% of the MIC's should fall within the following MIC ranges and the majority of MIC's should be at values close to the center of the pertinent range. (Reference NCCLS publication M7-A**)

S. aureus ATCC 29213, 2.0–8.0 mcg/ml; *S. faecalis* ATCC 29212, 16–64 mcg/ml; *E. coli* ATCC 25922, 2.0–8.0 mcg/ml; *P. aeruginosa* ATCC 27853, 8.0–32 mcg/ml.

*Performance standards for Antimicrobiotic Disc Susceptibility Tests, National Committee of Clinical Laboratory Standards, Vol. 4, No. 16, pp. 369–402, 1984.

**Methods for Dilution Antimicrobial Susceptibility Tests for Bacteria That Grow Aerobically, Vol. 5, No. 22, pp. 579–618. 1985.

INDICATIONS

TICAR (Ticarcillin Disodium) is indicated for the treatment of the following infections:

Bacterial septicemia (†)
Skin and soft-tissue infections (†)
Acute and chronic respiratory tract infections (†)(‡)

(†) caused by susceptible strains of *Pseudomonas aeruginosa, Proteus* species (both indole-positive and indole-negative) and *Escherichia coli.*

(‡) (Though clinical improvement has been shown, bacteriological cures cannot be expected in patients with chronic respiratory disease or cystic fibrosis.)

Genitourinary tract infections (complicated and uncomplicated) due to susceptible strains of *Pseudomonas aeruginosa, Proteus* species (both indole-positive and indole-negative), *Escherichia coli, Enterobacter* and *Streptococcus faecalis* (enterococcus).

TICARCILLIN SERUM LEVELS
mcg/ml

Dosage	Route	¼ hr.	½ hr.	1 hr.	2 hr.	3 hr.	4 hr.	6 hr.
Adults:								
500 mg	IM	—	7.7	8.6	6.0	4.0	—	2.9
1 Gm	IM	—	31.0	18.7	15.7	9.7	—	3.4
2 Gm	IM	—	63.6	39.7	32.3	18.9	—	3.4
3 Gm	IV	190.0	140.0	107.0	52.2	31.3	13.8	4.2
5 Gm	IV	327.0	280.0	175.0	106.0	63.0	28.5	9.6
3 Gm + 1 Gm Probenecid	IV Oral	223.0	166.0	123.0	78.0	54.0	35.4	17.1

Neonates:		**½ hr.**	**1 hr.**	**1½ hr.**	**2 hr.**	**4 hr.**	**8 hr.**
50 mg/kg	IM	64.0	70.7	63.7	60.1	33.2	11.6

Ticarcillin is also indicated in the treatment of the following infections due to susceptible anaerobic bacteria:

1. Bacterial septicemia.
2. Lower respiratory tract infections such as empyema, anaerobic pneumonitis and lung abscess.
3. Intra-abdominal infections such as peritonitis and intra-abdominal abscess (typically resulting from anaerobic organisms resident in the normal gastrointestinal tract).
4. Infections of the female pelvis and genital tract, such as endometritis, pelvic inflammatory disease, pelvic abscess and salpingitis.
5. Skin and soft-tissue infections.

Although Ticarcillin is primarily indicated in Gram-negative infections, its *in vitro* activity against Gram-positive organisms should be considered in treating infections caused by both Gram-negative and Gram-positive organisms (see MICROBIOLOGY).

Based on the *in vitro* synergism between Ticarcillin and gentamicin sulfate, tobramycin sulfate or amikacin sulfate against certain strains of *Pseudomonas aeruginosa,* combined therapy has been successful, using full therapeutic dosages. (For additional prescribing information, see the gentamicin sulfate, tobramycin sulfate and amikacin sulfate package inserts.)

NOTE: Culturing and susceptibilty testing should be performed initially and during treatment to monitor the effectiveness of therapy and the susceptibility of the bacteria.

CONTRAINDICATIONS

A history of allergic reaction to any of the penicillins is a contraindication.

WARNINGS

Serious and occasionally fatal hypersensitivity (anaphylactoid) reactions have been reported in patients receiving penicillin. These reactions are more likely to occur in persons with a history of sensitivity to multiple allergens.

There are reports of patients with a history of penicillin hypersensitivity reactions who experience severe hypersensitivity reactions when treated with a cephalosporin. Before therapy with a penicillin, careful inquiry should be made about previous hypersensitivity reactions to penicillins, cephalosporins, and other allergens. If a reaction occurs, the drug should be discontinued unless, in the opinion of the physician, the condition being treated is life-threatening and amenable only to Ticarcillin therapy. **Serious anaphylactoid reactions require immediate emergency treatment with epinephrine. Oxygen, intravenous steroids, airway management, including intubation, should also be administered as indicated.**

Some patients receiving high doses of Ticarcillin may develop hemorrhagic manifestations associated with abnormalities of coagulation tests, such as bleeding time and platelet aggregation. On withdrawal of the drug, the bleeding should cease and coagulation abnormalities revert to normal. Other causes of abnormal bleeding should also be considered. Patients with renal impairment, in whom excretion of Ticarcillin is delayed, should be observed for bleeding manifestations. Such patients should be dosed strictly according to recommendations (see DOSAGE AND ADMINISTRATION). If bleeding manifestations appear, Ticarcillin treatment should be discontinued and appropriate therapy instituted.

PRECAUTIONS

Although TICAR (Ticarcillin Disodium) exhibits the characteristic low toxicity of the penicillins, as with any other potent agent, it is advisable to check periodically for organ system dysfunction (including renal, hepatic and hematopoietic) during prolonged treatment. If overgrowth of resistant organisms occurs, the appropriate therapy should be initiated.

Since the theoretical sodium content is 5.2 milliequivalents (120 mg) per gram of Ticarcillin, and the actual vial content can be as high as 6.5 mEq/Gm, electrolyte and cardiac status should be monitored carefully.

In a few patients receiving intravenous Ticarcillin, hypokalemia has been reported. Serum potassium should be measured periodically, and, if necessary, corrective therapy should be implemented.

As with any penicillin, the possibility of an allergic response, including anaphylaxis, exists, particularly in hypersensitive patients.

USAGE DURING PREGNANCY

Reproduction studies have been performed in mice and rats and have revealed no evidence of impaired fertility or harm to the fetus due to Ticarcillin. There are no well-controlled studies in pregnant women, but investigational experience does not include any positive evidence of adverse effects on the fetus. Although there is no clearly defined risk, such experience cannot exclude the possibility of infrequent or subtle damage to the fetus. Ticarcillin should be used in pregnant women only when clearly needed.

ADVERSE REACTIONS

The following adverse reactions may occur:

Hypersensitivity Reactions: Skin rashes, pruritus, urticaria, drug fever.

Gastrointestinal Disturbances: Nausea and vomiting.

Hemic and Lymphatic Systems: As with other penicillins, anemia, thrombocytopenia, leukopenia, neutropenia and eosinophilia.

Abnormalities of Blood, Hepatic and Renal Laboratory Studies: As with other semisynthetic penicillins, SGOT and SGPT elevations have been reported. To date, clinical manifestations of hepatic or renal disorders have not been observed which could be ascribed solely to Ticarcillin.

CNS: Patients, especially those with impaired renal function, may experience convulsions or neuromuscular excitability when very high doses of the drug are administered.

Other: Local reactions such as pain (rarely accompanied by induration) at the site of the injection have been reported.

Vein irritation and phlebitis can occur, particularly when undiluted solution is directly injected into the vein.
[See table on next page].

DIRECTIONS FOR USE

1 Gm, 3 Gm and 6 Gm Standard Vials

INTRAMUSCULAR USE: (Concentration of approximately 385 mg/ml).

For initial reconstitution use Sterile Water for Injection, U.S.P., Sodium Chloride Injection, U.S.P. or 1% Lidocaine Hydrochloride solution* (without epinephrine).

Each gram of Ticarcillin should be reconstituted with 2 ml of Sterile Water for Injection, U.S.P., Sodium Chloride Injection, U.S.P. or 1% Lidocaine Hydrochloride solution* (without epinephrine) and **used promptly.** Each 2.6 ml of the resulting solution will then contain 1 Gm of Ticarcillin.

*[For full product information, refer to manufacturer's package insert for Lidocaine Hydrochloride.]

As with all intramuscular preparations, TICAR (Ticarcillin Disodium) should be injected well within the body of a relatively large muscle, using usual techniques and precautions.

INTRAVENOUS ADMINISTRATION: (Concentration of approximately 200 mg/ml).

For initial reconstitution use Sodium Chloride Injection, U.S.P., Dextrose Injection 5% or Lactated Ringer's Injection.

Reconstitute each gram of Ticarcillin with 4 ml of the appropriate diluent. After the addition of 4 ml of diluent per gram of Ticarcillin each 1.0 ml of the resulting solution will have an approximate concentration of 200 mg. Once dissolved, further dilute if desired.

Culture	Susceptible	Intermediate	Resistant
P. aeruginosa and *Enterobacteriaceae*	≥ 15 mm	12–14 mm	≤ 11 mm

The MIC Correlates are:

Resistant	> 128 mcg/ml
Susceptible	≤ 64 mcg/ml

Continued on next page

Beecham Laboratories—Cont.

DIRECT INTRAVENOUS INJECTION: In order to avoid vein irritation, administer solution as slowly as possible.

INTRAVENOUS INFUSION: Administer by continuous or intermittent intravenous drip. Intermittent infusion should be administered over a 30 minute to 2 hour period in equally divided doses.

3 Gm Piggyback Bottles:

DIRECT INTRAVENOUS INJECTION: (Concentrations of approximately 29 mg/ml to 100 mg/ml).

The 3 gram bottle should be reconstituted with a minimum of 30 ml of the desired intravenous solution listed below.

Amount of Diluent	Concentration of Solution
100 ml	1 Gm/34 ml (~29 mg/ml)
60 ml	1 Gm/20 ml (50 mg/ml)
30 ml	1 Gm/10 ml (100 mg/ml)

In order to avoid vein irritation, the solution should be administered as slowly as possible. A dilution of approximately 50 mg/ml or more will further reduce the incidence of vein irritation.

INTRAVENOUS INFUSION: Stability studies in the intravenous solutions listed below indicate that Ticarcillin Disodium will provide sufficient activity at room temperature (70°–75°F) within the stated time periods at concentrations between 10 mg/ml and 50 mg/ml—see Stability Period section below.

20 Gm Bulk Pharmacy Package For I.V. Use

RECONSTITUTED STOCK SOLUTION MUST BE TRANSFERRED AND FURTHER DILUTED FOR I.V. INFUSION

Add 85 ml of Sodium Chloride Injection, U.S.P., Dextrose Injection 5% or Lactated Ringer's Injection to the 20 Gm Bulk Pharmacy Package and shake well. For ease of reconstitution, the amount of diluent may be added in two portions. Each 1.0 ml of the resulting concentrated stock solution contains approximately 200 mg of Ticarcillin.

INTRAVENOUS ADMINISTRATION: The desired dosage should be withdrawn from the stock solution and further diluted with Sodium Chloride Injection, U.S.P., Dextrose Injection 5% or Lactated Ringer's Injection to a concentration between 10 mg/ml and 100 mg/ml. If the solution is administered as a direct injection, it should be administered as slowly as possible in order to avoid vein irritation. Using a concentration of 50 mg/ml or less will further reduce the incidence of vein irritation. The solutions can be administered by either a continuous or intermittent intravenous drip. Intermittent infusion should be administered over a 30 minute to 2 hour period in equally divided doses.

30 Gm Bulk Pharmacy Package For I.V. Use

RECONSTITUTED STOCK SOLUTION MUST BE TRANSFERRED AND FURTHER DILUTED FOR I.V. INFUSION

Add 75 ml of Sodium Chloride Injection, U.S.P., Dextrose Injection 5% or Lactated Ringer's Injection to the 30 Gm Bulk Pharmacy Package and shake well. For ease of reconstitution, the amount of diluent may be added in two portions. Each 1.0 ml of the resulting concentrated stock solution contains approximately 300 mg of Ticarcillin.

INTRAVENOUS ADMINISTRATION: The desired dosage should be withdrawn from the stock solution and further diluted with Sodium Chloride Injection, U.S.P., Dextrose Injection 5% or Lactated Ringer's Injection to a concentration between 10 mg/ml and 100 mg/ml. If the solution is administered as a direct injection, it should be administered as slowly as possible in order to avoid vein irritation. Using a concentration of 50 mg/ml or less will further reduce the incidence of vein irritation. The solutions can be administered by either a continuous or intermittent intravenous drip. Intermittent infusion should be administered over a 30 minute to 2 hour period in equally divided doses.

STABILITY/STORAGE CONDITIONS

(For 20 Gm and 30 Gm Bulk Pharmacy Packages)

The concentrated stock solution must be diluted within 24 hours if stored at room temperature (70°–75°F) or within 72 hours if kept under refrigeration (40°F).

Upon further dilution (10 mg/ml to 100 mg/ml), the solutions will provide sufficient activity within an additional 24 hours at room temperature (70°–75°F) or 3 days under refrigeration (40°F).

If the concentrated stock solution is diluted to concentrations between 10 mg/ml and 50 mg/ml within 8 hours with diluents listed below, then the following stability periods apply:

[See table on next page].

Refrigerated solutions stored longer than 72 hours should not be used for multidose purposes.

After reconstitution, the solution can be frozen (approx. 0°F) and stored for up to 30 days. The thawed solution must be

TICAR

DOSAGE AND ADMINISTRATION

Clinical experience indicates that in serious urinary tract and systemic infections, intravenous therapy in the higher doses should be used. Intramuscular injections should not exceed 2 grams per injection.

Adults:

Bacterial Septicemia Respiratory Tract Infections Skin and Soft-Tissue Infections Intra-Abdominal Infections Infections of the Female Pelvis and Genital Tract	200–300 mg/kg/day by I.V. infusion in divided doses every 4 or 6 hours. [The usual dose is 3 gm given every 4 hours (18 gm/day) or 4 gm given every 6 hours (16 gm/day) depending on weight and the severity of the infection.]
Urinary Tract Infections	
Complicated:	150–200 mg/kg/day by I.V. infusion in divided doses every 4 or 6 hours. [Usual recommended dosage for average (70 kg) adults: 3 grams q.i.d.]
Uncomplicated:	1 gram I.M. or direct I.V. every 6 hours.
Infections complicated by renal insuffiency: (1)	Initial loading dose of 3 grams I.V. followed by I.V. doses, based on creatinine clearance and type of dialysis, as indicated below:
Creatinine clearance ml/min.:	
over 60	3 grams every 4 hours
30–60	2 grams every 4 hours
10–30	2 grams every 8 hours
less than 10	2 grams every 12 hours (or 1 gram I.M. every 6 hours)
less than 10 with hepatic dysfunction	2 grams every 24 hours (or 1 gram I.M. every 12 hours)
patients on peritoneal dialysis	3 grams every 12 hours
patients on hemodialysis	2 grams every 12 hours supplemented with 3 grams after each dialysis

To calculate creatinine clearance* from a serum creatinine value use the following formula:

$$C_{cr} = \frac{(140-Age)\ (wt\ in\ kg)}{72 \times S_{cr}(mg/100\ ml)}$$

This is the calculated creatinine clearance for adult males; for females it is 15% less.

* Cockcroft, D.W., et al, "Prediction of Creatinine Clearance from Serum Creatinine" Nephron 16:31–41 (1976).

(1) The half-life of Ticarcillin in patients with renal failure is approximately 13 hours.

Children: Under 40 kg (88 lbs)

The daily dose for children should not exceed the adult dosage.

Bacterial Septicemia Respiratory Tract Infections Skin and Soft-Tissue Infections Intra-Abdominal Infections Infections of the Female Pelvis and Genital Tract	200–300 mg/kg/day by I.V. infusion in divided doses every 4 or 6 hours.
Urinary Tract Infections	
Complicated:	150–200 mg/kg/day by I.V. infusion in divided doses every 4 or 6 hours.
Uncomplicated:	50–100 mg/kg/day I.M. or direct I.V. in divided doses every 6 or 8 hours.
Infections complicated by renal insufficiency:	Clinical data is insufficient to recommend an optimum dose.

Children weighing more than 40 kg (88 lbs) should receive adult dosages.

Neonates: In the neonate, for severe infections (sepsis) due to susceptible strains of *Pseudomonas, Proteus,* and *E. coli*, the following Ticarcillin dosages may be given I.M. or by 10–20 minutes I.V. infusion:

Infants under 2000 grams body weight:		Infants over 2000 grams body weight:	
Aged 0–7 days	75 mg/kg/12 hours (150 mg/kg/day)	Ages 0–7 days	75 mg/kg/8 hours (225 mg/kg/day)
Aged over 7 days	75 mg/kg/8 hours (225 mg/kg/day)	Aged over 7 days	100 mg/kg/8 hours (300 mg/kg/day)

This dosage schedule is intended to produce peak serum concentrations of 125–150 mcg/ml one hour after a dose of Ticarcillin and trough concentrations of 25–50 mcg/ml immediately before the next dose.

NOTE: Gentamicin, tobramycin or amikacin may be used concurrently with Ticarcillin for initial therapy until results of culture and susceptibility studies are known.

Seriously ill patients should receive the higher doses. TICAR has proved to be useful in infections in which protective mechanisms are impaired, such as in acute leukemia and during therapy with immunosuppressive or oncolytic drugs.

used within 24 hours. Unused solutions should be discarded after the time periods mentioned above.

It is recommended that TICAR and gentamicin sulfate, tobramycin sulfate or amikacin sulfate not be mixed together in the same I.V. solution due to the gradual inactivation of gentamicin sulfate, tobramycin sulfate or amikacin sulfate under these circumstances. The therapeutic effect of TICAR and these aminoglycoside drugs remains unimpaired when administered separately.

HOW SUPPLIED

TICAR (Sterile Ticarcillin Disodium). Each vial contains Ticarcillin Disodium equivalent to 1 Gm, 3 Gm, 6 Gm, 20 Gm or 30 Gm Ticarcillin.

NDC 0029-6550-22 ....1 Gm Vial
NDC 0029-6552-26 ....3 Gm Vial
NDC 0029-6555-26 ....6 Gm Vial
NDC 0029-6552-21 ....3 Gm Piggyback Bottle
NDC 0029-6558-21 ....20 Gm Bulk Pharmacy Package
NDC 0029-6559-21 ....30 Gm Bulk Pharmacy Package

January, 1986
7182

TICAR	STABILITY PERIOD	
Intravenous Solution (concentration of 10 mg/ml to 100 mg/ml)	**Room Temperature (70°-75°F).**	**Refrigeration (40°F)**
Sodium Chloride Injection, U.S.P.	72 hours	14 days
Dextrose Injection 5%	72 hours	14 days
Lactated Ringer's Injection	48 hours	14 days

TIGAN® ℞

[tī'găn]

(trimethobenzamide HCl)

DESCRIPTION

Tigan is an antiemetic agent. Chemically, trimethobenzamide HCl is N-[*p*-[2-(di- methylamino)-ethoxy] benzyl]-3,4,5-trimethoxy- benzamide hydrochloride. It has a molecular weight of 424.93.

Capsules; Blue, each containing 250 mg trimethobenzamide hydrochloride; blue and white, each containing 100 mg trimethobenzamide hydrochloride.

INACTIVE INGREDIENTS

Lactose, Magnesium Stearate, and Starch.

Suppositories: (200 mg): Each suppository contains 200 mg trimethobenzamide hydrochloride and 2% benzocaine in a base compounded with polysorbate 80, white beeswax and propylene glycol monostearate.

Suppositories, Pediatric (100 mg): Each suppository contains 100 mg trimethobenzamide hydrochloride and 2% benzocaine in a base compounded with polysorbate 80, white beeswax and propylene glycol monostearate.

Ampuls: Each 2-ml ampul contains 200 mg trimethobenzamide hydrochloride compounded with 0.2% parabens (methyl and propyl) as preservatives, 1 mg sodium citrate and 0.4 mg citric acid as buffers and pH adjusted to approximately 5.0 with sodium hydroxide.

Multiple Dose Vials: Each ml contains 100 mg trimethobenzamide hydrochloride compounded with 0.45% phenol as preservative, 0.5 mg sodium citrate and 0.2 mg citric acid as buffers and pH adjusted to approximately 5.0 with sodium hydroxide.

Thera-Ject ® (Disposable Syringes): Each 2 ml contains 200 mg trimethobenzamide hydrochloride compounded with 0.45% phenol as preservative, 1 mg sodium citrate and 0.4 mg citric acid as buffers, 0.2 mg disodium edetate as stabilizer and pH adjusted to approximately 5.0 with sodium hydroxide.

ACTIONS

The mechanism of action of Tigan as determined in animals is obscure, but may be the chemoreceptor trigger zone (CTZ), an area in the medulla oblongata through which emetic impulses are conveyed to the vomiting center; direct impulses to the vomiting center apparently are not similarly inhibited. In dogs pretreated with trimethobenzamide HCl, the emetic response to apomorphine is inhibited, while little or no protection is afforded against emesis induced by intragastric copper sulfate.

INDICATIONS

Tigan is indicated for the control of nausea and vomiting.

CONTRAINDICATIONS

The injectable form of Tigan in children, the suppositories in premature or newborn infants, and use in patients with known hypersensitivity to trimethobenzamide are contraindicated. Since the suppositories contain benzocaine they should not be used in patients known to be sensitive to this or similar local anesthetics.

WARNINGS

Caution should be exercised when administering Tigan to children for the treatment of vomiting. Antiemetics are not recommended for treatment of uncomplicated vomiting in children and their use should be limited to prolonged vomiting of known etiology. There are three principal reasons for caution:

1. There has been some suspicion that centrally acting antiemetics may contribute, in combination with viral illnesses (a possible cause of vomiting in children), to development of Reye's syndrome, a potentially fatal acute childhood encephalopathy with visceral fatty degeneration, especially involving the liver. Although there is no confirmation of this suspicion, caution is nevertheless recommended.

2. The extrapyramidal symptoms which can occur secondary to Tigan may be confused with the central nervous system signs of an undiagnosed primary disease responsible for the vomiting, e.g., Reye's syndrome or other encephalopathy.

3. It has been suspected that drugs with hepatotoxic potential, such as Tigan, may unfavorably alter the course of Reye's syndrome. Such drugs should therefore be avoided in children whose signs and symptoms (vomiting) could represent Reye's syndrome. It should also be noted that salicylates and acetaminophen are hepatotoxic at large doses. Although it is not known that at usual doses they would represent a hazard in patients with the underlying hepatic disorder of Reye's syndrome, these drugs, too, should be avoided in children whose signs and symptoms could represent Reye's syndrome, unless alternative methods of controlling fever are not successful.

Tigan may produce drowsiness. Patients should not operate motor vehicles or other dangerous machinery until their individual responses have been determined.

Reye's Syndrome has been associated with the use of TIGAN and other drugs, including antiemetics, although their contribution, if any, to the cause and course of the disease hasn't been established. This syndrome is characterized by an abrupt onset shortly following a nonspecific febrile illness, with persistent, severe vomiting, lethargy, irrational behavior, progressive encephalopathy leading to coma, convulsions and death.

Usage in Pregnancy: Trimethobenzamide hydrochloride was studied in reproduction experiments in rats and rabbits and no teratogenicity was suggested. The only effects observed were an increased percentage of embryonic resorptions or stillborn pups in rats administered 20 mg and 100 mg/kg and increased resorptions in rabbits receiving 100 mg/kg. In each study these adverse effects were attributed to one or two dams. The relevance to humans is not known. Since there is no adequate experience in pregnant or lactating women who have received this drug, safety in pregnancy or in nursing mothers has not been established.

Usage with Alcohol: Concomitant use of alcohol with Tigan may result in an adverse drug interaction.

PRECAUTIONS

During the course of acute febrile illness, encephalitides, gastroenteritis, dehydration and electrolyte imbalance, especially in children and the elderly or debilitated, CNS reactions such as opisthotonos, convulsions, coma and extrapyramidal symptoms have been reported with and without use of Tigan or other antiemetic agents. In such disorders caution should be exercised in administering Tigan, particularly to patients who have recently received other CNS-acting agents (phenothiazines, barbiturates, belladonna derivatives). It is recommended that severe emesis should not be treated with an antiemetic drug alone; where possible the cause of vomiting should be established. Primary emphasis should be directed toward the restoration of body fluids and electrolyte balance, the relief of fever and relief of the causative disease process. Overhydration should be avoided since it may result in cerebral edema.

The antiemetic effects of Tigan may render diagnosis more difficult in such conditions as appendicitis and obscure signs of toxicity due to overdosage of other drugs.

ADVERSE REACTIONS

There have been reports of hypersensitivity reactions and Parkinson-like symptoms. There have been instances of hypotension reported following parenteral administration to surgical patients. There have been reports of blood dyscrasias, blurring of vision, coma, convulsions, depression of mood, diarrhea, disorientation, dizziness, drowsiness, headache, jaundice, muscle cramps and opisthotonos. If these occur, the administration of the drug should be discontinued. Allergic-type skin reactions have been observed; therefore, the drug should be discontinued at the first sign of sensitization. While these symptoms will usually disappear spontaneously, symptomatic treatment may be indicated in some cases.

DOSAGE AND ADMINISTRATION

(See WARNINGS and PRECAUTIONS.) Dosage should be adjusted according to the indication for therapy, severity of symptoms and the response of the patient.

Capsules, 250 mg and 100 mg

Usual Adult Dosage

One 250-mg capsule t.i.d. or q.i.d.

Usual Children's Dosage

30 to 90 lbs: One or two 100-mg capsules t.i.d. or q.i.d.

Suppositories, 200 mg (Not to be used in premature or newborn infants.)

Usual Adult Dosage

One suppository (200 mg) t.i.d. or q.i.d.

Usual Children's Dosage

Under 30 lbs: One-half suppository (100 mg) t.i.d. or q.i.d.
30 to 90 lbs: One-half to one suppository (100 to 200 mg) t.i.d. or q.i.d.

SUPPOSITORIES, PEDIATRIC, 100 mg (Not to be used in Premature or newborn infants).

Usual Children's Dosage

Under 30 lbs; One suppository
(100 mg) t.i.d. or q.i.d.
30 to 90 lbs; One to two suppositories
(100 to 200 mg) t.i.d. or q.i.d.

Injectable, 100 mg/ml (Not recommended for use in children.)

Usual Adult Dosage: 2 ml (200 mg) t.i.d. or q.i.d. intramuscularly.

Intramuscular administration may cause pain, stinging, burning, redness and swelling at the site of injection. Such effects may be minimized by deep injection into the upper outer quadrant of the gluteal region, and by avoiding the escape of solution along the route.

Note: The injectable form is intended for intramuscular administration only; it is not recommended for intravenous use.

HOW SUPPLIED

Product	Package Sizes	NDC Numbers
Capsules		
100 mg.	100's	NDC-0029-4082-30
250 mg.	100's	NDC-0029-4083-30
	500's	NDC-0029-4083-32
Suppositories		
200 mg.	10's	NDC-0029-4084-38
	50's	NDC-0029-4084-39
Suppositories Pediatric		
100 mg.	10's	NDC-0029-4088-38
Injectable		
Ampuls		
2 ml, 200 mg.	10's	NDC-0029-4085-22
Vials		
20 ml, 100 mg./ml	Each	NDC-0029-4086-22
Thera-Ject® (Disposable Syringe)		
2 ml, 100 mg./ml	25's	NDC-0029-4087-22

Shown in Product Identification Section, page 405

TIMENTIN® ℞

[tī'mĕn tĭn]

sterile ticarcillin disodium and clavulanate potassium for Intravenous Administration

DESCRIPTION

TIMENTIN is an injectable antibacterial combination consisting of the semisynthetic antibiotic, ticarcillin disodium and the β-lactamase inhibitor, clavulanate potassium (the potassium salt of clavulanic acid) for intravenous administration. Ticarcillin is derived from the basic penicillin nucleus, 6-amino-penicillanic acid. Chemically, it is 6-[(carboxy-3-thienylacetyl)amino]-3,3-dimethyl-7-oxo-4-thia-1-azabicyclo[3.2.0] heptane-2-carboxylic acid disodium salt and may be represented as:

[See Chemical Formula at top of next column].

Clavulanic acid is produced by the fermentation of *Streptomyces clavuligerus.* It is a β-lactam structurally related to the penicillins and possesses the ability to inactivate a wide variety of β-lactamases by blocking the active sites of

Continued on next page

Beecham Laboratories—Cont.

these enzymes. Clavulanic acid is particularly active against the clinically important plasmid mediated β-lactamases frequently responsible for transferred drug resistance to penicillins and cephalosporins.

Chemically, clavulanate potassium is potassium Z-(3R,5R)-2-(β-hydroxyethylidene) clavam-3-carboxylate and may be represented structurally as:

TIMENTIN is supplied as a white to pale yellow powder for reconstitution. TIMENTIN is very soluble in water; its solubility being greater than 600 mg/ml. The reconstituted solution is clear, colorless or pale yellow, having a pH of 5.5 to 7.5. For the TIMENTIN 3.1 Gm and 3.2 Gm vials, the theoretical sodium content is 4.75 mEq (109 mg) per gram of TIMENTIN. The theoretical potassium content is 0.15 mEq (6 mg) and 0.3 mEq (11.9 mg) per gram of TIMENTIN for the 3.1 Gm vial and 3.2 Gm vial, respectively.

CLINICAL PHARMACOLOGY

After an intravenous infusion (30 min.) of 3.1 Gm or 3.2 Gm TIMENTIN, peak serum concentrations of both ticarcillin and clavulanic acid are attained immediately after completion of infusion. Ticarcillin serum levels are similar to those produced by the administration of equivalent amounts of ticarcillin alone with a mean peak serum level of 330 mcg/ml for the 3.1 Gm and 3.2 Gm formulations. The corresponding mean peak serum levels for clavulanic acid were 8 mcg/ml and 16 mcg/ml for the 3.1 Gm and 3.2 Gm formulations, respectively. (See following table.)

[See table below].

The mean area under the serum concentration curves for ticarcillin was 485 mcg/ml.hr for the TIMENTIN 3.1 Gm and 3.2 Gm formulations. The corresponding areas under the serum concentration curves for clavulanic acid were 8.2 mcg/ml.hr and 15.6 mcg/ml.hr for the TIMENTIN 3.1 Gm and 3.2 Gm formulations, respectively.

The mean serum half-lives of ticarcillin and clavulanic acid in healthy volunteers are 68 minutes and 64 minutes, respectively, following administration of 3.1 Gm or 3.2 Gm of TIMENTIN.

Approximately 60-70% of ticarcillin and approximately 35-45% of clavulanic acid are excreted unchanged in urine during the first 6 hours after administration of a single dose of TIMENTIN to normal volunteers with normal renal function. Two hours after an intravenous injection of 3.1 Gm or 3.2 Gm TIMENTIN, concentrations of ticarcillin in urine generally exceed 1500 mcg/ml. The corresponding concentrations of clavulanic acid in urine generally exceed 40 mcg/ml and 70 mcg/ml following administration of the 3.1 Gm and 3.2 Gm doses, respectively. By 4-6 hours after injection, the urine concentrations of ticarcillin and clavulanic acid usually decline to approximately 190 mcg/ml and 2 mcg/ml, respectively, for both doses.

Neither component of TIMENTIN is highly protein bound; ticarcillin has been found to be approximately 45% bound to human serum protein and clavulanic acid approximately 9% bound.

Somewhat higher and more prolonged serum levels of ticarcillin can be achieved with the concurrent administration of probenecid; however, probenecid does not enhance the serum levels of clavulanic acid.

Ticarcillin can be detected in tissues and interstitial fluid following parenteral administration.

Penetration of ticarcillin into the bile, pleural fluid and cerebrospinal fluid with inflamed meninges has been demonstrated. The results of experiments involving the administration of clavulanic acid to animals suggest that this compound, like ticarcillin, is well distributed in body tissues.

An inverse relationship exists between the serum half-life of ticarcillin and creatinine clearance. The dosage of TIMENTIN need only be adjusted in cases of severe renal impairment (see Dosage and Administration).

Ticarcillin may be removed from patients undergoing dialysis; the actual amount removed depends on the duration and type of dialysis.

Microbiology: Ticarcillin is a semisynthetic antibiotic with a broad spectrum of bactericidal activity against many Gram-positive and Gram-negative aerobic and anaerobic bacteria.

Ticarcillin is, however, susceptible to degradation by β-lactamases and therefore the spectrum of activity does not normally include organisms which produce these enzymes

Clavulanic acid is a β-lactam, structurally related to the penicillins, which possesses the ability to inactivate a wide range of β-lactamase enzymes commonly found in microorganisms resistant to penicillins and cephalosporins. In particular, it has good activity against the clinically important plasmid mediated β-lactamases frequently responsible for transferred drug resistance.

The formulation of ticarcillin with clavulanic acid in TIMENTIN protects ticarcillin from degradation by β-lactamase enzymes and effectively extends the antibiotic spectrum of ticarcillin to include many bacteria normally resistant to ticarcillin and other β-lactam antibiotics. Thus TIMENTIN possesses the distinctive properties of a broad spectrum antibiotic and a β-lactamase inhibitor.

While *in vitro* studies have demonstrated the susceptibility of most strains of the following organisms, clinical efficacy for infections other than those included in the Indications section has not been documented.

GRAM-NEGATIVE BACTERIA: *Pseudomonas aeruginosa* (β-lactamase and non-β-lactamase producing), *Pseudomonas* species including *P. maltophilia* (β-lactamase and non-β-lactamase producing), *Escherichia coli* (β-lactamase and non-β-lactamase producing), *Proteus mirabilis* (β-lactamase and non-β-lactamase producing), *Proteus vulgaris* (β-lactamase and non-β-lactamase producing), *Providencia rettgeri* (formerly *Proteus rettgeri*) (β-lactamase and non-β-lactamase producing), *Providencia stuartii* (β-lactamase and non-β-lactamase producing), *Morganella morganii* (formerly *Proteus morganii*) (β-lactamase and non-β-lactamase producing), *Enterobacter* species (Although most strains of *Enterobacter* species are resistant *in vitro*, clinical efficacy has been demonstrated with TIMENTIN in urinary tract infections caused by these organisms). *Acinetobacter* species (β-lactamase and non-β-lactamase producing), *Hemophilus influenzae* (β-lactamase and non-β-lactamase producing), *Branhamella catarrhalis* (β-lactamase and non-β-lactamase producing), *Serratia* species including *S. marcescens* (β-lactamase and non-β-lactamase producing), *Neisseria gonorrhoeae* (β-lactamase and non-β-lactamase producing), *Neisseria meningitidis**, *Salmonella* species (β-lactamase and non-β-lactamase producing), *Klebsiella* species including *K. pneumoniae* (β-lactamase and non-β-lactamase producing), *Citrobacter* species including *C. freundii, C. diversus* and *C. amalonaticus* (β-lactamase and non-β-lactamase producing).

GRAM-POSITIVE BACTERIA: *Staphylococcus aureus* (β-lactamase and non-β-lactamase producing), *Staphylococcus saprophyticus, Staphylococcus epidermidis* (coagulase negative *Staphylococci*) (β-lactamase and non-β-lactamase producing), *Streptococcus pneumoniae** (*D. pneumoniae*), *Streptococcus bovis**, *Streptococcus agalactiae** (Group B), *Streptococcus faecalis** (Enterococcus), *Streptococcus pyogenes** (Group A, β-hemolytic), Viridans group *Streptococci**.

ANAEROBIC BACTERIA: *Bacteroides* species, including *B. fragilis* group (*B. fragilis, B. vulgatus*) (β-lactamase and non-β-lactamase producing), Non-*B. fragilis* (*β-melaninogenicus*) (β-lactamase and non-β-lactamase producing), *B. thetaiotaomicron, B. ovatus, B. distasonis,* (β-lactamase and non-β-lactamase producing), *Clostridium* species including *C. perfringens, C. difficile, C. sporogenes, C. ramosum* and *C. bifermentans**, *Eubacterium* species, *Fusobacterium* species including *F. nucleatum* and *F. necrophorum**, *Peptococcus* species*, *Peptostreptococcus* species*, *Veillonella* species.

*These are non-β-lactamase producing strains and therefore are susceptible to ticarcillin alone. Some of the β-lactamase producing strains are also susceptible to ticarcillin alone.

In vitro synergism between TIMENTIN and gentamicin, tobramycin or amikacin against multi-resistant strains of *Pseudomonas aeruginosa* has been demonstrated.

SUSCEPTIBILITY TESTING:

Diffusion Technique: An 85 mcg TIMENTIN (75 mcg ticarcillin plus 10 mcg clavulanic acid) diffusion disk is available for use with the Kirby-Bauer method. Based on the zone sizes given below, a report of "Susceptible" indicates that the infecting organism is likely to respond to TIMENTIN therapy, while a report of "Resistant" indicates that the organism is not likely to respond to therapy with this antibiotic. A report of "Intermediate" susceptibility indicates that the organism would be susceptible to TIMENTIN at a higher dosage or if the infection is confined to tissues or fluids (e.g., urine) in which high antibiotic levels are attained.

Dilution Technique: Broth or agar dilution methods may be used to determine the minimal inhibitory concentration (MIC) values for bacterial isolates to TIMENTIN. Tubes should be inoculated with the test culture containing 10^4 to 10^5 CFU/ml or plates spotted with a test solution containing 10^3 to 10^4 CFU/ml.

The recommended dilution pattern utilizes a constant level of clavulanic acid, 2 mcg/ml, in all tubes together with varying amounts of ticarcillin. MIC's are expressed in terms of the ticarcillin concentration in the presence of 2 mcg/ml clavulanic acid.

RECOMMENDED RANGES FOR TIMENTIN SUSCEPTIBILITY TESTING[1,2,3]

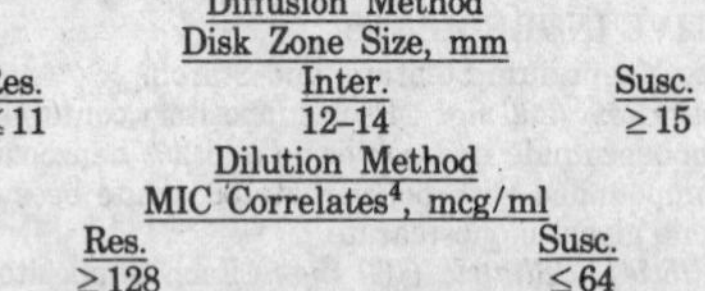

Diffusion Method

Disk Zone Size, mm

Res.	Inter.	Susc.
≤11	12–14	≥15

Dilution Method

MIC Correlates[4], mcg/ml

Res.	Susc.
≥128	≤64

[1] The non-β-lactamase producing organisms which are normally susceptible to ticarcillin will have similar zone sizes as for ticarcillin.

[2] *Staphylococci* which are susceptible to TIMENTIN but resistant to methicillin, oxacillin or nafcillin must be considered as resistant.

[3] The quality control cultures should have the following assigned daily ranges for TIMENTIN:

		Disks	Mode MIC (mcg/ml)
E. coli	(ATCC 25922)	24–30 mm	2/2–8/2
S. aureus	(ATCC 25923)	32–40 mm	—
Ps. aeruginosa	(ATCC 27853)	20–28 mm	8/2–32/2
E. coli	(ATCC 35218)	21–25 mm	4/2–8/2
S. aureus	(ATCC 29213)	—	2/2–8/2

[4] Expressed as concentration of ticarcillin in the presence of a constant 2.0 mcg/ml concentration of clavulanic acid.

INDICATIONS AND USAGE

TIMENTIN is indicated in the treatment of infections caused by susceptible strains of the designated organisms in the conditions listed below:

Bacterial Septicemia: including bacteremia, caused by β-lactamase producing strains of *Klebsiella* spp., *E. coli, Staphylococcus aureus* and *Pseudomonas aeruginosa* (and other *Pseudomonas* species).

Lower Respiratory Infections: caused by β-lactamase producing strains of *Staphylococcus aureus, Hemophilus influenzae* and *Klebsiella* spp.

Bone and Joint Infections: caused by β-lactamase producing strains of *Staphylococcus aureus.*

Skin and Skin Structure Infections: caused by β-lactamase producing strains of *Staphylococcus aureus, Klebsiella* spp. and *E. coli.*

Urinary Tract Infections (complicated and uncomplicated): caused by β-lactamase producing strains of *E. coli, Klebsiella* spp., *Pseudomonas aeruginosa* (and other *Pseudomonas* species), *Citrobacter* spp., *Enterobacter cloacae, Serratia marcescens,* and *Staphylococcus aureus.*

While TIMENTIN is indicated only for the conditions listed above, infections caused by ticarcillin susceptible organisms are also amenable to TIMENTIN treatment due to its ticarcillin content. Therefore, mixed infections caused by ticarcillin susceptible organisms and β-lactamase producing organisms susceptible to TIMENTIN should not require the addition of another antibiotic.

Appropriate culture and susceptibility tests should be performed before treatment in order to isolate and identify organisms causing infection and to determine their susceptibility to TIMENTIN. Because of its broad spectrum of bactericidal activity against Gram-positive and Gram-negative bacteria, TIMENTIN is particularly useful for the treatment of mixed infections and for presumptive therapy prior to the

SERUM LEVELS IN ADULTS
AFTER A 30-MINUTE IV INFUSION OF TIMENTIN

TICARCILLIN SERUM LEVELS (mcg/ml)

Dose	0	15 min.	30 min.	1 hr.	1.5 hr.	3.5 hr.	5.5 hr.
3.1 Gm	324	223	176	131	90	27	6
	(293–388)	(184–293)	(135–235)	(102–195)	(65–119)	(19–37)	(5–7)
3.2 Gm	336	214	186	122	78	29	10
	(301–386)	(180–258)	(160–218)	108–136)	(33–113)	(19–44)	(5–15)

CLAVULANIC ACID SERUM LEVELS (mcg/ml)

Dose	0	15 min.	30 min.	1 hr.	1.5 hr.	3.5 hr.	5.5 hr.
3.1 Gm	8.0	4.6	2.6	1.8	1.2	0.3	0
	(5.3–10.3)	(3.0–7.6)	(1.8–3.4)	(1.6–2.2)	(0.8–1.6)	(0.2–0.3)	
3.2 Gm	15.8	8.3	5.2	3.4	2.5	0.5	0
	(11.7–21.0)	(6.4–10.0)	(3.5–6.3)	(1.9–4.0)	(1.3–3.4)	(0.2–0.8)	

identification of the causative organisms. TIMENTIN has been shown to be effective as single drug therapy in the treatment of some serious infections where normally combination antibiotic therapy might be employed. Therapy with TIMENTIN may be initiated before results of such tests are known when there is reason to believe the infection may involve any of the β-lactamase producing organisms listed above; however, once these results become available, appropriate therapy should be continued.

Based on the *in vitro* synergism between TIMENTIN and aminoglycosides against certain strains of *Pseudomonas aeruginosa*, combined therapy has been successful, especially in patients with impaired host defenses. Both drugs should be used in full therapeutic doses. As soon as results of culture and susceptibility tests become available, antimicrobial therapy should be adjusted as indicated.

CONTRAINDICATIONS

TIMENTIN is contraindicated in patients with a history of hypersensitivity reactions to any of the penicillins.

WARNINGS

SERIOUS AND OCCASIONALLY FATAL HYPERSENSITIVITY (ANAPHYLACTOID) REACTIONS HAVE BEEN REPORTED IN PATIENTS ON PENICILLIN THERAPY. THESE REACTIONS ARE MORE LIKELY TO OCCUR IN INDIVIDUALS WITH A HISTORY OF PENICILLIN HYPERSENSITIVITY AND/OR A HISTORY OF SENSITIVITY TO MULTIPLE ALLERGENS. THERE HAVE BEEN REPORTS OF INDIVIDUALS WITH A HISTORY OF PENICILLIN HYPERSENSITIVITY WHO HAVE EXPERIENCED SEVERE REACTIONS WHEN TREATED WITH CEPHALOSPORINS. BEFORE INITIATING THERAPY WITH TIMENTIN, CAREFUL INQUIRY SHOULD BE MADE CONCERNING PREVIOUS HYPERSENSITIVITY REACTIONS TO PENICILLINS, CEPHALOSPORINS, OR OTHER DRUGS. IF AN ALLERGIC REACTION OCCURS, TIMENTIN SHOULD BE DISCONTINUED AND THE APPROPRIATE THERAPY INSTITUTED. **SERIOUS ANAPHYLACTOID REACTIONS REQUIRE IMMEDIATE EMERGENCY TREATMENT WITH EPINEPHRINE, OXYGEN, INTRAVENOUS STEROIDS, AND AIRWAY MANAGEMENT, INCLUDING INTUBATION, SHOULD ALSO BE PROVIDED AS INDICATED.**

PRECAUTIONS

General: While TIMENTIN possesses the characteristic low toxicity of the penicillin group of antibiotics, periodic assessment of organ system functions, including renal, hepatic and hematopoietic function is advisable during prolonged therapy.

Bleeding manifestations have occurred in some patients receiving beta-lactam antibiotics. These reactions have been associated with abnormalities of coagulation tests such as clotting time, platelet aggregation and prothrombin time and are more likely to occur in patients with renal impairment. If bleeding manifestations appear, TIMENTIN treatment should be discontinued and appropriate therapy instituted.

TIMENTIN has only rarely been reported to cause hypokalemia; however, the possibility of this occurring should be kept in mind particularly when treating patients with fluid and electrolyte imbalance. Periodic monitoring of serum potassium may be advisable in patients receiving prolonged therapy.

The theoretical sodium content is 4.75 mEq (109 mg) per gram of TIMENTIN. This should be considered when treating patients requiring restricted salt intake.

As with any penicillin, an allergic reaction, including anaphylaxis, may occur during TIMENTIN administration, particularly in a hypersensitive individual.

The possibility of superinfections with mycotic or bacterial pathogens should be kept in mind, particularly during prolonged treatment. If superinfections occur, appropriate measures should be taken.

Drug/Laboratory Test Interactions: As with other penicillins, the mixing of TIMENTIN with an aminoglycoside in solutions for parenteral administration can result in substantial inactivation of the aminoglycoside.

Probenecid interferes with the renal tubular secretion of ticarcillin, thereby increasing serum concentrations and prolonging serum half-life of the antibiotic.

High urine concentrations of ticarcillin may produce false positive protein reactions (pseudoproteinuria) with the following methods: sulfosalicylic acid and boiling test, acetic acid test, biuret reaction, and nitric acid test. The bromphenol blue (Multi-stix®) reagent strip test has been reported to be reliable.

The presence of clavulanic acid in TIMENTIN may cause a non-specific binding of IgG and albumin by red cell membranes leading to a false positive Coombs test.

Carcinogenesis, Mutagenesis, Impairment of Fertility: Long-term studies in animals have not been performed to evaluate carcinogenic or mutagenic potential.

Pregnancy (Category B): Reproduction studies have been performed in rats given doses up to 1050 mg/kg/day and have revealed no evidence of impaired fertility or harm to the fetus due to TIMENTIN. There are, however, no adequate and well-controlled studies in pregnant women. Because animal reproduction studies are not always predictive of human response, this drug should be used during pregnancy only if clearly needed.

Nursing Mothers: Caution should be exercised when TIMENTIN is administered to a nursing woman.

Pediatric Use: The efficacy and safety of TIMENTIN have not been established in infants and children under the age of 12.

Drug Abuse and Dependence: Neither TIMENTIN abuse nor TIMENTIN dependence has been reported.

ADVERSE REACTIONS

As with other penicillins, the following adverse reactions may occur:

Hypersensitivity reactions: skin rash, pruritus, urticaria, arthralgia, myalgia, drug fever, chills, chest discomfort, and anaphylactic reactions.

Central nervous system: headache, giddiness, neuromuscular hyperirritability or convulsive seizures.

Gastro-intestinal disturbances: disturbances of taste and smell, stomatitis, flatulence, nausea, vomiting and diarrhea, epigastric pain.

Hemic and Lymphatic systems: thrombocytopenia, leukopenia, neutropenia, eosinophilia and reduction of hemoglobin or hematocrit. Prolongation of prothrombin time and bleeding time.

Abnormalities of hepatic and renal function tests: elevation of serum aspartate aminotransferase (SGOT), serum alanine aminotransferase (SGPT), serum alkaline phosphatase, serum LDH, serum bilirubin. Elevation of serum creatinine and/or BUN, hypernatremia. Reduction in serum potassium and uric acid.

Local reactions: pain, burning, swelling and induration at the injection site and thrombophlebitis with intravenous administration.

Overdosage: As with other penicillins, TIMENTIN in overdosage has the potential to cause neuromuscular hyperirritability or convulsive seizures. Ticarcillin may be removed from circulation by hemodialysis. The molecular weight, degree of protein binding and pharmacokinetic profile of clavulanic acid together with information from a single patient with renal insufficiency all suggest that this compound may also be removed by hemodialysis.

DOSAGE AND ADMINISTRATION

TIMENTIN should be administered by intravenous infusion (30 min.).

Adults: The usual recommended dosage for systemic and urinary tract infections for average (60 kg) adults is 3.1 Gm TIMENTIN (3.1 Gm vial containing 3 Gm ticarcillin and 100 mg clavulanic acid) given every 4 to 6 hours. For patients weighing less than 60 kg, the recommended dosage is 200–300 mg/kg/day, based on ticarcillin content, given in divided doses every 4 to 6 hours.

In urinary tract infections, a dosage of 3.2 Gm TIMENTIN (3.2 Gm vial containing 3 Gm ticarcillin and 200 mg clavulanic acid) given every 8 hours is adequate.

For infections complicated by renal insufficiency[1], an initial loading dose of 3.1 Gm should be followed by doses based on creatinine clearance and type of dialysis as indicated below:

Creatinine clearance ml/min.	Dosage
over 60	3.1 Gm every 4 hrs
30–60	2 Gm every 4 hrs
10–30	2 Gm every 8 hrs
less than 10	2 Gm every 12 hrs
Less than 10 with hepatic dysfunction	2 Gm every 24 hrs
patients on peritoneal dialysis	3.1 Gm every 12 hrs
patients on hemodialysis	2 Gm every 12 hrs supplemented with 3.1 Gm after each dialysis

To calculate creatinine clearance* from a serum creatinine value use the following formula.

$$C_{cr} = \frac{(140\text{-Age})\ (\text{wt in kg})}{72 \times S_{cr}(\text{mg}/100\ \text{ml})}$$

This is the calculated creatinine clearance for adult males, for females it is 15% less.

*Cockcroft, D. W., et al, "Prediction of Creatinine Clearance from Serum Creatinine", *Nephron* 16:31-41 (1976).

[1] The half-life of Ticarcillin in patients with renal failure is approximately 13 hours.

Dosage for any individual patient must take into consideration the site and severity of infection, the susceptibility of the organisms causing infection, and the status of the patient's host defense mechanisms.

The duration of therapy depends upon the severity of infection. Generally, TIMENTIN should be continued for at least 2 days after the signs and symptoms of infection have disappeared. The usual duration is 10 to 14 days; however, in difficult and complicated infections, more prolonged therapy may be required.

Frequent bacteriologic and clinical appraisal is necessary during therapy of chronic urinary tract infection and may be required for several months after therapy has been completed; persistent infections may require treatment for several weeks and doses smaller than those indicated above should not be used.

In certain infections, involving abscess formation, appropriate surgical drainage should be performed in conjunction with antimicrobial therapy.

INTRAVENOUS ADMINISTRATION

Directions: The 3.1 Gm or 3.2 Gm vial should be reconstituted by shaking with approximately 13 ml of Sterile Water for Injection, U.S.P. or Sodium Chloride Injection, U.S.P.; when dissolved, the concentration of ticarcillin will be approximately 200 mg/ml with corresponding concentrations of 6.7 mg/ml and 13.4 mg/ml clavulanic acid for the 3.1 Gm and 3.2 Gm respective doses. Conversely, each 5.0 ml of the 3.1 Gm dose reconstituted with approximately 13 ml of diluent will contain approximately 1 Gm of ticarcillin and 33 mg of clavulanic acid. For the 3.2 Gm dose reconstituted with 13 ml of diluent, each 5.0 ml will contain 1 Gm of ticarcillin and 66 mg of clavulanic acid.

Intravenous Infusion: The dissolved drug should be further diluted to desired volume using a suitable solution listed in the Compatibility and Stability section. The solution of reconstituted drug may then be administered over a period of 30 minutes by direct infusion or through a Y-type intravenous infusion set which may already be in place. If this method or the "piggyback" method of administration is used, it is advisable to discontinue temporarily the administration of any other solutions during the infusion of TIMENTIN.

When TIMENTIN is given in combination with another antimicrobial, such as an aminoglycoside, each drug should be given separately in accordance with the recommended dosage and routes of administration for each drug.

After reconstitution and prior to administration, TIMENTIN, as with other parenteral drugs, should be inspected visually for particulate matter and discoloration.

COMPATIBILITY AND STABILITY

The stock solution at 200 mg/ml is stable for up to 6 hours at room temperature (70°–75°F) or up to 72 hours under refrigeration (40°F). TIMENTIN stability studies in the following intravenous solutions indicate that TIMENTIN will provide sufficient activity at either room temperature or stored under refrigeration within the stated time periods and at concentrations between 10 mg/ml and 100 mg/ml with any of the diluents listed below:

	STABILITY PERIOD	
Intravenous Solution	Room Temp. (70°–75°F)	Refrigeration (40°F)
Sodium Chloride Injection, U.S.P.	24 hours	7 days
Dextrose Injection 5%, U.S.P.	12 hours	3 days
Lactated Ringer's Injection, U.S.P.	24 hours	7 days

Note: TIMENTIN is incompatible with Sodium Bicarbonate.

Unused solutions must be discarded after the time periods stated above.

After reconstitution to a concentration of 100 mg/ml or less, solutions of Sodium Chloride Injection, U.S.P. and Lactated Ringer's Injection, U.S.P. may be frozen and stored for up to 30 days. Solutions prepared from Dextrose Injection 5%, U.S.P. may be stored frozen for 7 days. All thawed solutions should be used within 8 hours.

HOW SUPPLIED

TIMENTIN (Sterile Ticarcillin Disodium and Clavulanate Potassium).

Each 3.1 Gm vial contains sterile ticarcillin disodium equivalent to 3 Gm ticarcillin and sterile clavulanate potassium equivalent to 0.1 Gm clavulanic acid.

NDC 0029-6571-26 .... 3.1 Gm Vial
NDC 0029-6571-21 .... 3.1 Gm Piggyback Bottle

Each 3.2 Gm vial contains sterile ticarcillin disodium equivalent to 3 Gm ticarcillin and sterile clavulanate potassium equivalent to 0.2 Gm clavulanic acid.

NDC 0029-6572-26 .... 3.2 Gm Vial
NDC 0029-6572-21 .... 3.2 Gm Piggyback Bottle

TIMENTIN vials should be stored at room temperature (70°–75°F) or below.

June, 1985
7548/C

Shown in Product Identification Section, page 405

Products are cross-indexed by generic and chemical names in the **YELLOW SECTION**

Beiersdorf, Inc.
BDF PLAZA
P.O. BOX 5529
NORWALK, CT 06856-5529

EUCERIN™ Cleansing Bar
[*ū 'sir-in*]
Unscented Moisturizing Formula

ACTIVE INGREDIENT
Eucerite®

ACTIONS AND USES
Eucerin™ Cleansing Bar has been specially formulated for use on sensitive skin. The formulation contains Eucerite®, a special blend of ingredients that closely resemble the natural oils of the skin, thus providing excellent moisturizing properties. This formulation is unscented and non-comedogenic. Additionally, the ph value of Eucerin Cleansing Bar is maintained at 5.5 in order to match the skin's normal acid mantle.

DIRECTIONS
Use during shower or bath, or as directed by physician

HOW SUPPLIED
3 ounce bar.
List number 3854

EUCERIN® Creme
[*ū 'sir-in*]
Unscented Moisturizing Formula
NDC Numbers–10356-090-01
10356-090-04

COMPOSITION
Water, petrolatum, mineral oil, mineral wax, wool wax alcohol, methylchoroisothiazolinone-methylisothiazolinone.

ACTIONS AND USES
A gentle, non-comedogenic, unscented water-in-oil emulsion, Eucerin helps alleviate excessively dry skin and may be helpful in conditions such as chapped or chafed skin, sunburn, windburn, and itching associated with dryness.

ADMINISTRATION AND DOSAGES
Apply freely to affected areas of the skin as often as necessary or as directed by physician.

PRECAUTIONS
For external use only.

HOW SUPPLIED
16 oz. jar—List Number 0090
4 oz. jar—List Number 3797

EUCERIN® Lotion
[*ū 'sir-in*]
Unscented Moisturizing Formula
NDC Numbers–10356-793-01
10356-793-04
10356-793-06

COMPOSITION
Water, Mineral Oil, Isopropyl Myristate, PEG-40 Sorbitan Peroleate, Lanolin Acid Glycerin Ester, Sorbitol, Propylene Glycol, Cetyl Palmitate, Magnesium Sulfate, Aluminum Stearate, Lanolin Alcohol, BHT, Methylchloroisothiazolinone·Methylisothiazolinone.

ACTIONS AND USES
Eucerin Lotion is a non-comedogenic, unscented, unique water-in-oil formulation that will help to alleviate and soothe the excessively dry skin, and provide long-lasting moisturization.

ADMINISTRATION AND DOSAGE
Apply Eucerin Lotion all over body—hands, arms, legs, and feet—to help moisturize, smooth and soothe rough, dry skin.

PRECAUTIONS
For external use only.

HOW SUPPLIED
4 fluid oz. plastic bottle
List Number 3771
8 fluid oz. plastic bottle.
List Number 3793
16 fluid oz. plastic bottle.
List number 3794

Products are cross-indexed by
generic and chemical names in the
YELLOW SECTION

Berlex Laboratories, Inc.
300 FAIRFIELD ROAD
WAYNE, NJ 07470

DECONAMINE® Tablets ℞
[*dē″con 'uh-mēēn*]
DECONAMINE® SR Capsules ℞
DECONAMINE® Syrup ℞
(chlorpheniramine maleate; d-pseudoephedrine hydrochloride)

DESCRIPTION
Tablets
Each scored, white tablet contains:
chlorpheniramine maleate .... 4 mg
d-pseudoephedrine hydrochloride .... 60 mg
Each DECONAMINE® Tablet also contains the following inactive ingredients: dibasic calcium phosphate, magnesium stearate, microcrystalline cellulose, pregelatinized starch, silica gel, starch (corn), and stearic acid.
SR Capsules
Each sustained-release blue and yellow capsule contains:
chlorpheniramine maleate .... 8 mg
d-pseudoephedrine hydrochloride .... 120 mg
Each DECONAMINE® SR Capsule also contains the following inactive ingredients: coloring agents, gelatin, starch, and sucrose.
Each DECONAMINE® SR Capsule may also contain one or more of the following inactive ingredients: butyl paraben, methyl paraben, propyl paraben, titanium dioxide and other ingredient(s).
The capsules are designed to provide prolonged release of medication.
Syrup—No alcohol, no dye
Each 5 mL (teaspoonful) clear, colorless to slightly yellow liquid contains:
chlorpheniramine maleate .... 2 mg
d-pseudoephedrine hydrochloride .... 30 mg
in a grape-flavored, aromatic vehicle
DECONAMINE® Syrup also contains the following inactive ingredients: citric acid, flavoring agent, glycerin, sodium benzoate, sodium chloride, sorbitol, sucrose, and water.

CLINICAL PHARMACOLOGY
Chlorpheniramine maleate antagonizes the physiological action of histamine by acting as an H_1 receptor blocking agent.
Pseudoephedrine is an orally active sympathomimetic amine and exerts a decongestant action on the nasal mucosa. It does this by vasoconstriction, which results in reduction of tissue hyperemia, edema, nasal congestion and an increase in nasal airway patency. The vasoconstrictive action of pseudoephedrine is similar to that of ephedrine. In the usual dose it has minimal vasopressor effects.

INDICATIONS
For relief of nasal congestion associated with the common cold, hay fever and other allergies, sinusitis, eustachian tube blockage, and vasomotor and allergic rhinitis.

CONTRAINDICATIONS
Patients with severe hypertension, severe coronary artery disease and patients on MAO inhibitor therapy. DECONAMINE® medications are also contraindicated in patients sensitive to antihistamines or sympathomimetic agents.

WARNINGS
Chlorpheniramine maleate should be used with extreme caution in patients with narrow angle glaucoma; stenosing peptic ulcer; pyloroduodenal obstruction; symptomatic prostatic hypertrophy; or bladder neck obstruction. Due to its mild atropine-like action, chlorpheniramine maleate should be used cautiously in patients with bronchial asthma.
Sympathomimetic amines should be used with caution in patients with hypertension, ischemic heart disease, diabetes mellitus, increased intraocular pressure, hyperthyroidism and prostatic hypertrophy. Sympathomimetics may produce central nervous system stimulation with convulsions or cardiovascular collapse with accompanying hypotension.

PRECAUTIONS
Information for patients:
Antihistamines may impair mental and physical abilities required for the performance of potentially hazardous tasks, such as driving a vehicle or operating machinery. Patients should also be warned about possible additive effects with alcohol and other central nervous system depressants (hypnotics, sedatives, tranquilizers).
Drug interactions:
Pseudoephedrine-containing drugs should not be given to patients treated with monoamine oxidase (MAO) inhibitors because of the possibility of precipitating a hypertensive crisis. MAO inhibitors also prolong and intensify the anticholinergic effects of antihistamines. Sympathomimetics may reduce the antihypertensive effect of methyldopa, reserpine, veratrum alkaloids and mecamylamine.
Alcohol and other sedative drugs will potentiate the sedative effects of chlorpheniramine.
Care should be taken in administering DECONAMINE® medications concomitantly with other sympathomimetic amines, since their combined effects on the cardiovascular system may be harmful to the patient.
Pregnancy:
Pregnancy Category C: Animal reproduction studies have not been conducted with DECONAMINE® medications. It is also not known whether DECONAMINE® medications can cause fetal harm when administered to a pregnant woman or can affect reproduction capacity. DECONAMINE® medications should be given to a pregnant woman only if clearly needed.
Nursing Mothers: Due to the possible passage of pseudoephedrine and chlorpheniramine into breast milk, and, because of the higher than usual risk for infants from sympathomimetic amines and antihistamines, the benefit to the mother vs. the potential risk should be considered and a decision should be made whether to discontinue nursing or to discontinue the drug.
Pediatric Use: DECONAMINE® Capsules or Tablets should not be given to children under 12 years of age.

ADVERSE REACTIONS
Chlorpheniramine maleate
Slight to moderate drowsiness may occur and is the most frequent side effect. Other possible side effects of antihistamines in general include:
General: urticaria, drug rash, anaphylactic shock, photosensitivity, excessive perspiration, chills, dryness of mouth, nose and throat;
Cardiovascular: hypotension, headache, palpitation, tachycardia, extrasystoles;
Hematological: hemolytic anemia, thrombocytopenia, agranulocytosis;
CNS: sedation, dizziness, disturbed coordination, fatigue, confusion, restlessness, excitation, nervousness, tremor, irritability, insomnia, euphoria, paresthesia, blurred vision, diplopia, vertigo, tinnitus, hysteria, neuritis, convulsion;
Gastrointestinal: epigastric distress, anorexia, nausea, vomiting, diarrhea, constipation;
Genitourinary: urinary frequency, difficult urination, urinary retention, early menses;
Respiratory: thickening of bronchial secretions, tightness of chest, wheezing and nasal stuffiness.
Pseudoephedrine hydrochloride
Pseudoephedrine may cause mild central nervous system stimulation, especially in those patients who are hypersensitive to sympathomimetic drugs. Nervousness, excitability, restlessness, dizziness, weakness and insomnia may also occur. Headache and drowsiness have also been reported. Large doses may cause lightheadedness, nausea and/or vomiting. Sympathomimetic drugs have also been associated with certain untoward reactions including fear, anxiety, tenseness, restlessness, tremor, weakness, pallor, respiratory difficulty, dysuria, insomnia, hallucination, convulsion, CNS depression, arrhythmias and cardiovascular collapse with hypotension.

OVERDOSAGE
Acute overdosage may produce clinical signs of CNS stimulation and variable cardiovascular effects. Pressor amines should be used with great caution in the presence of pseudoephedrine. Patients with signs of stimulation should be treated conservatively.

DOSAGE AND ADMINISTRATION
Tablets
Adults and children over 12 years, 1 tablet three or four times daily.
Children under 12 years, DECONAMINE® Syrup is recommended.
Syrup
Adults and children over 12 years, 1 to 2 teaspoonfuls (5 to 10 mL) three or four times daily.
Children 6 to 12 years, ½ to 1 teaspoonful (2.5 to 5 mL) three or four times daily, not to exceed 4 teaspoonfuls in 24 hours.
Children 2 to 6 years, ½ teaspoonful (2.5 mL) three or four times daily, not to exceed 2 teaspoonfuls in 24 hours.
Children under two years, as directed by physician.
SR Capsules
Adults and children over 12 years, 1 capsule every 12 hours.
Children under 12 years, DECONAMINE® Syrup is recommended.

HOW SUPPLIED
In bottles of:
Tablets
100 .... NDC 50419-184-10
SR Capsules
100 .... NDC 50419-181-10
500 .... NDC 50419-181-50
Syrup
473 mL .... NDC 50419-185-16
Store at controlled room temperature.
Shown in Product Identification Section, page 405

LEVLEN™ 21 ℞

[*lĕvlĕn*]

Tablets

(levonorgestrel and ethinyl estradiol tablets)

LEVLEN™ 28 ℞

Tablets

(levonorgestrel and ethinyl estradiol tablets)

DESCRIPTION

ORAL CONTRACEPTIVE

LEVLEN™ 21 tablets:

Each LEVLEN™ 21 tablet contains 0.15 mg of levonorgestrel (d(-)-13 beta-ethyl-17-alpha-ethinyl-17-beta-hydroxygon-4-en-3-one), a totally synthetic progestogen, and 0.03 mg of ethinyl estradiol (19-nor-17 α-pregna-1,3,5(10)-trien-20-yne-3, 17-diol). The inactive ingredients present are cellulose, FD&C Yellow 6, lactose, magnesium stearate, and polacrillin potassium.

LEVLEN™ 28 tablets:

21 light-orange LEVLEN™ tablets, each containing 0.15 mg of levonorgestrel (d(-)-13 beta-ethyl-17-alpha-ethinyl-17-beta-hydroxygon-4-en-3-one), a totally synthetic progestogen, and 0.03 mg of ethinyl estradiol (19-nor-17 α-pregna-1,3,5(10)-trien-20-yne-3, 17-diol), and 7 pink inert tablets. The inactive ingredients present are cellulose, FD&C Red 3, FD&C Yellow 6, lactose, magnesium stearate, and polacrillin potassium.

Levonorgestrel　　Ethinyl Estradiol

CLINICAL PHARMACOLOGY

Combination oral contraceptives act primarily through the mechanism of gonadotropin suppression due to the estrogenic and progestational activity of the ingredients. Although the primary mechanism of action is inhibition of ovulation, alterations in the genital tract, including changes in the cervical mucus (which increase the difficulty of sperm penetration) and the endometrium (which reduce the likelihood of implantation), may also contribute to contraceptive effectiveness.

INDICATIONS AND USAGE

LEVLEN™ tablets are indicated for the prevention of pregnancy in women who elect to use oral contraceptives as a method of contraception. Oral contraceptives are highly effective. The pregnancy rate in women using conventional combination oral contraceptives (containing 35 mcg or more of ethinyl estradiol or 50 mcg or more of mestranol) is generally reported as less than one pregnancy per 100 woman-years of use. Slightly higher rates (somewhat more than 1 pregnancy per 100 woman-years of use) are reported for some combination products containing 35 mcg or less of ethinyl estradiol, and rates on the order of 3 pregnancies per 100 woman-years are reported for the progestogen-only oral contraceptives.

These rates are derived from separate studies conducted by different investigators in several population groups and cannot be compared precisely. Furthermore, pregnancy rates tend to be lower as clinical studies are continued, possibly due to selective retention in the longer studies of those patients who accept the treatment regimen and do not discontinue as a result of adverse reactions, pregnancy, or other reasons.

In clinical trials with LEVLEN™ tablets, 1,084 patients completed 8,186 cycles, and a total of three pregnancies were reported. This represents a pregnancy rate of 0.48 per 100 woman-years.

Table 1 gives ranges of pregnancy rates reported in the literature[1] for other means of contraception. The efficacy of these means of contraception (except the IUD) depends upon the degree of adherence to the method.

TABLE 1

PREGNANCIES PER 100 WOMAN-YEARS

IUD, less than 1–6; Diaphragm with spermicidal products (creams or jellies), 2–20; Condom, 3–36; Aerosol foams, 2–29; Jellies and creams, 4–36; Periodic abstinence (rhythm) all types, less than 1–47:

1. Calendar method, 14–47;
2. Temperature method, 1–20;
3. Temperature method—intercourse only in postovulatory phase, less than 1–7;
4. Mucus method, 1–25;

No contraception, 60–80.

Dose-Related Risk of Thromboembolism from Oral Contraceptives: Two studies have shown a positive association between the dose of estrogens in oral contraceptives and the risk of thromboembolism.[2,3] For this reason, it is prudent and in keeping with good principles of therapeutics to minimize exposure to estrogen. The oral-contraceptive product prescribed for any given patient should be that product which contains the least amount of estrogen that is compatible with an acceptable pregnancy rate and patient acceptance. It is recommended that new acceptors of oral contraceptives be started on preparations containing 0.05 mg or less of estrogen.

CONTRAINDICATIONS

Oral contraceptives should not be used in women with any of the following conditions:

1. Thrombophlebitis or thromboembolic disorders.
2. A past history of deep-vein thrombophlebitis or thromboembolic disorders.
3. Cerebral-vascular or coronary-artery disease.
4. Known or suspected carcinoma of the breast.
5. Known or suspected estrogen-dependent neoplasia.
6. Undiagnosed abnormal genital bleeding.
7. Known or suspected pregnancy (see Warning No. 5).
8. Benign or malignant liver tumor which developed during the use of oral contraceptives or other estrogen-containing products.

WARNINGS

Cigarette smoking increases the risk of serious cardiovascular side effects from oral-contraceptive use. This risk increases with age and with heavy smoking (15 or more cigarettes per day) and is quite marked in women over 35 years of age. Women who use oral contraceptives should be strongly advised not to smoke.

The use of oral contraceptives is associated with increased risk of several serious conditions, including thromboembolism, stroke, myocardial infarction, hepatic adenoma, gallbladder disease, hypertension. Practitioners prescribing oral contraceptives should be familiar with the following information relating to these risks.

1. *Thromboembolic Disorders and Other Vascular Problems:* An increased risk of thromboembolic and thrombotic disease associated with the use of oral contraceptives is well-established. Three principal studies in Great Britain[4–6] and three in the United States[7–10] have demonstrated an increased risk of fatal and nonfatal venous thromboembolism and stroke, both hemorrhagic and thrombotic. These studies estimate that users of oral contraceptives are 4 to 11 times more likely than nonusers to develop these diseases without evident cause (Table 2).

CEREBROVASCULAR DISORDERS

In a collaborative American study[9,10] of cerebrovascular disorders in women with and without predisposing causes, it was estimated that the risk of hemorrhagic stroke was 2.0 times greater in users than nonusers and the risk of thrombotic stroke was 4 to 9.5 times greater in users than in nonusers (Table 2).

TABLE 2

SUMMARY OF RELATIVE RISK OF THROMBOEMBOLIC DISORDERS AND OTHER VASCULAR PROBLEMS IN ORAL-CONTRACEPTIVE USERS COMPARED TO NONUSERS

	Relative risk, times greater
Idiopathic thromboembolic disease	4–11
Postsurgery thromboembolic complications	4–6
Thrombotic stroke	4–9.5
Hemorrhagic stroke	2
Myocardial infarction	2–12

MYOCARDIAL INFARCTION

An increased risk of myocardial infarction associated with the use of oral contraceptives has been reported,[11–13] confirming a previously suspected association. These studies, conducted in the United Kingdom, found, as expected, that the greater the number of underlying risk factors for coronary-artery disease (cigarette smoking, hypertension, hypercholesterolemia, obesity, diabetes, history of preeclamptic toxemia) the higher the risk of developing myocardial infarction, regardless of whether the patient was an oral-contraceptive user or not. Oral contraceptives, however, were found to be a clear additional risk factor.

In terms of relative risk, it has been estimated[52] that oral-contraceptive users who do not smoke (smoking is considered a major predisposing condition to myocardial infarction) are about twice as likely to have a fatal myocardial infarction as nonusers who do not smoke. Oral-contraceptive users who are also smokers have about a 5-fold increased risk of fatal infarction compared to users who do not smoke, but about a 10- to 12-fold increased risk compared to nonusers who do not smoke. Furthermore, the amount of smoking is also an important factor. In determining the importance of these relative risks, however, the baseline rates for various age groups, as shown in Table 3, must be given serious consideration. The importance of other predisposing conditions mentioned above in determining relative and absolute risks has not as yet been quantified; it is quite likely that the same synergistic action exists, but perhaps to a lesser extent.

TABLE 3

Estimated annual mortality rate per 100,000 women from myocardial infarction by use of oral contraceptives, smoking habits, and age (in years):

	Myocardial infarction			
	Women aged 30–39		Women aged 40–44	
Smoking habits	Users	Non-users	Users	Non-users
All smokers	10.2	2.6	62.0	15.9
Heavy*	13.0	5.1	78.7	31.3
Light	4.7	0.9	28.6	5.7
Nonsmokers	1.8	1.2	10.7	7.4
Smokers and nonsmokers	5.4	1.9	32.8	11.7

*Heavy smoker: 15 or more cigarettes per day.

From JAIN, A.K., *Studies in Family Planning,* 8:50, 1977.

RISK OF DOSE

In an analysis of data derived from several national adverse-reaction reporting systems,[2] British investigators concluded that the risk of thromboembolism, including coronary thrombosis, is directly related to the dose of estrogen used in oral contraceptives. Preparations containing 100 mcg or more of estrogen were associated with a higher risk of thromboembolism than those containing 50–80 mcg of estrogen. Their analysis did suggest, however, that the quantity of estrogen may not be the sole factor involved. This finding has been confirmed in the United States.[3] Careful epidemiological studies to determine the degree of thromboembolic risk associated with progestogen-only oral contraceptives have not been performed. Cases of thromboembolic disease have been reported in women using these products, and they should not be presumed to be free of excess risk.

ESTIMATE OF EXCESS MORTALITY FROM CIRCULATORY DISEASES

A large prospective study[53] carried out in the U.K. estimated the mortality rate per 100,000 women per year from diseases of the circulatory system for users and nonusers of oral contraceptives according to age, smoking habits, and duration of use. The overall excess death rate annually from circulatory diseases for oral-contraceptive users was estimated to be 20 per 100,000 (ages 15–34—5/100,000; ages 35–44—33/100,000; ages 45–49—140/100,000), the risk being concentrated in older women, in those with a long duration of use, and in cigarette smokers. It was not possible, however, to examine the interrelationships of age, smoking, and duration of use, nor to compare the effects of continuous vs. intermittent use. Although the study showed a 10-fold increase in death due to circulatory diseases in users for 5 or more years, all of these deaths occurred in women 35 or older. Until larger numbers of women under 35 with continuous use for 5 or more years are available, it is not possible to assess the magnitude of the relative risk for this younger age group.

The available data from a variety of sources have been analyzed[14] to estimate the risk of death associated with various methods of contraception. The estimates of risk of death for each method include the combined risk of the contraceptive method (e.g., thromboembolic and thrombotic disease in the case of oral contraceptives) plus the risk attributable to pregnancy or abortion in the event of method failure. This latter risk varies with the effectiveness of the contraceptive method. The findings of this analysis are shown in the bar graph (Figure 1).[14] The study concluded that the mortality associated with all methods of birth control is low and below that associated with childbirth, with the exception of oral contraceptives in women over 40 who smoke. (The rates given for Pill only/smokers for each age group are for smokers as a class. For "heavy" smokers [more than 15 cigarettes a day], the rates given would be about double; for "light" smokers [less than 15 cigarettes a day], about 50 percent.) The lowest mortality is associated with the condom or diaphragm backed up by early abortion. The risk of thromboembolic and thrombotic disease associated with oral contraceptives increases with age after approximately age 30 and, for myocardial infarction, is further increased by hypertension, hypercholesterolemia, obesity, diabetes, or history of preeclamptic toxemia and, especially, by cigarette smoking.

Based on the data currently available, the following chart gives a gross estimate of the risk of death from circulatory disorders associated with the use of oral contraceptives:

Continued on next page

Information on the Berlex products appearing here is based on the labeling in effect on August 1, 1986. Further information for these and other products may be obtained from the Professional Services Department, Berlex Laboratories, Inc., 110 East Hanover Avenue, Cedar Knolls, New Jersey 07927, telephone 201-292-3008.

Berlex—Cont.

SMOKING HABITS AND OTHER PREDISPOSING CONDITIONS—RISK ASSOCIATED WITH USE OF ORAL CONTRACEPTIVES

Age	Below 30	30–39	40+
Heavy smokers	C	B	A
Light smokers	D	C	B
Nonsmokers (no predisposing conditions)	D	C,D	C
Nonsmokers (other predisposing conditions)	C	C,B	B,A

A—Use associated with very high risk.
B—Use associated with high risk.
C—Use associated with moderate risk.
D—Use associated with low risk.

The physician and the patient should be alert to the earliest manifestations of thromboembolic and thrombotic disorders (e.g., thrombophlebitis, pulmonary embolism, cerebrovascular insufficiency, coronary occlusion, retinal thrombosis, and mesenteric thrombosis). Should any of these occur or be suspected, the drug should be discontinued immediately.

A four- to six-fold increased risk of postsurgery thromboembolic complications has been reported in oral-contraceptive users.[15,16] If feasible, oral contraceptives should be discontinued at least 4 weeks before surgery of a type associated with an increased risk of thromboembolism or prolonged immobilization.

Figure 1. Estimated annual number of deaths associated with control of fertility and no control per 100,000 nonsterile women, by regimen of control and age of women.

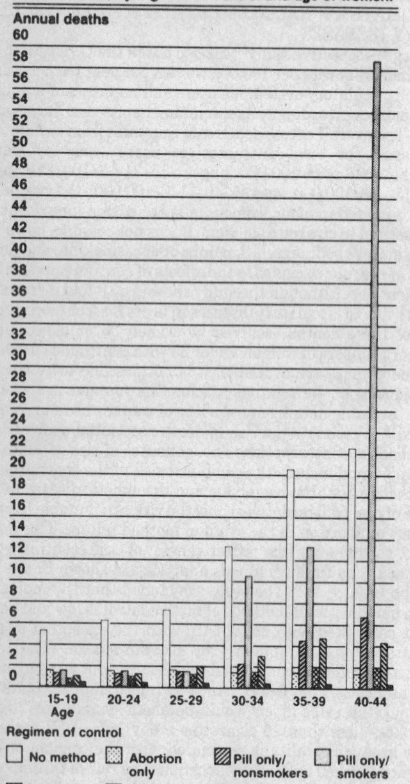

PERSISTENCE OF RISK OF VASCULAR DISORDERS

Findings from one study in Great Britain involving cerebrovascular disease[56] and another study in the United States concerning myocardial infarction[57] suggest that an increased risk of these conditions in users of oral contraceptives persists after discontinuation of the oral contraceptive. In the British study, the risk of cerebrovascular disease remained elevated in former oral-contraceptive users for at least six years after discontinuation. In the U.S. study, an increased risk of myocardial infarction persisted for at least 9 years in women 40- to 49-years-old who had used oral contraceptives for five or more years. The findings in both these studies require confirmation since they are inconsistent with other published information.[9,11,13,58–62]

2. *Ocular Lesions:*

There have been reports of neuro-ocular lesions such as optic neuritis or retinal thrombosis, associated with the use of oral contraceptives. Discontinue oral-contraceptive medication if there is unexplained, sudden or gradual, partial or complete loss of vision; onset of proptosis or diplopia; papilledema; or retinal-vascular lesions, and institute appropriate diagnostic and therapeutic measures.

3. *Carcinoma:*

Long-term continuous administration of either natural or synthetic estrogen in certain animal species increases the frequency of carcinoma of the breast, cervix, vagina, and liver. Certain synthetic progestogens, none currently contained in oral contraceptives, have been noted to increase the incidence of mammary nodules, benign and malignant, in dogs.

In humans, three case-control studies have reported an increased risk of endometrial carcinoma associated with the prolonged use of exogenous estrogen in postmenopausal women.[17–19] One publication[20] reported on the first 21 cases submitted by physicians to a registry of cases of adenocarcinoma of the endometrium in women under 40 on oral contraceptives. Of the cases found in women without predisposing risk factors for adenocarcinoma of the endometrium (e.g., irregular bleeding at the time oral contraceptives were first given, polycystic ovaries), nearly all occurred in women who had used a sequential oral contraceptive. These products are no longer marketed. No evidence has been reported suggesting an increased risk of endometrial cancer in users of conventional combination or progestogen-only oral contraceptives.

Several studies[8,21–24] have found no increase in breast cancer in women taking oral contraceptives or estrogens. One study,[25] however, while also noting no overall increased risk of breast cancer in women treated with oral contraceptives, found an excess risk in the subgroups of oral-contraceptive users with documented benign breast disease. A reduced occurrence of benign breast tumors in users of oral contraceptives has been well-documented.[8,21,25–27]

In summary, there is at present no confirmed evidence from human studies of an increased risk of cancer associated with oral contraceptives. Close clinical surveillance of all women taking oral contraceptives is, nevertheless, essential. In all cases of undiagnosed persistent or recurrent abnormal vaginal bleeding, appropriate diagnostic measures should be taken to rule out malignancy. Women with a strong family history of breast cancer or who have breast nodules, fibrocystic disease, or abnormal mammograms should be monitored with particular care if they elect to use oral contraceptives instead of other methods of contraception.

4. *Hepatic Tumors:*

Benign hepatic adenomas have been found to be associated with the use of oral contraceptives.[28–30,46] One study[46] showed that oral contraceptive formulations with high hormonal potency were associated with a higher risk than lower potency formulations. Although benign, hepatic adenomas may rupture and may cause death through intra-abdominal hemorrhage. This has been reported in short-term as well as long-term users of oral contraceptives. Two studies relate risk with duration of use of the contraceptive, the risk being much greater after 4 or more years of oral-contraceptive use.[30,46] While hepatic adenoma is a rare lesion, it should be considered in women presenting abdominal pain and tenderness, abdominal mass or shock. A few cases of hepatocellular carcinoma have been reported in women taking oral contraceptives. The relationship of these drugs to this type of malignancy is not known at this time.

5. *Use in or Immediately Preceding Pregnancy, Birth Defects in Offspring, and Malignancy in Female Offspring:*

The use of female sex hormones—both estrogenic and progestational agents—during early pregnancy may seriously damage the offspring. It has been shown that females exposed in utero to diethylstilbestrol, a nonsteroidal estrogen, have an increased risk of developing in later life a form of vaginal or cervical cancer that is ordinarily extremely rare.[31,32] This risk has been estimated to be of the order of 1 in 1,000 exposures or less.[33,47] Although there is no evidence at the present time that oral contraceptives further enhance the risk of developing this type of malignancy, such patients should be monitored with particular care if they elect to use oral contraceptives instead of other methods of contraception. Furthermore, a high percentage of such exposed women (from 30 to 90%) have been found to have epithelial changes of the vagina and cervix.[34–38] Although these changes are histologically benign, it is not known whether this condition is a precursor of vaginal malignancy. Male children so exposed may develop abnormalities of the urogenital tract.[48–50] Although similar data are not available with the use of other estrogens, it cannot be presumed that they would not induce similar changes.

An increased risk of congenital anomalies, including heart defects and limb defects, has been reported with the use of sex hormones, including oral contraceptives, in pregnancy.[39–42,51] One case-control study[42] has estimated a 4.7-fold increase in risk of limb-reduction defects in infants exposed in utero to sex hormones (oral contraceptives, hormonal withdrawal tests for pregnancy, or attempted treatment for threatened abortion). Some of these exposures were very short and involved only a few days of treatment. The data suggest that the risk of limb-reduction defects in exposed fetuses is somewhat less than one in 1,000 live births.

In the past, female sex hormones have been used during pregnancy in an attempt to treat threatened or habitual abortion. There is considerable evidence that estrogens are ineffective for these indications, and there is no evidence from well-controlled studies that progestogens are effective for these uses.

There is some evidence that triploidy and possibly other types of polyploidy are increased among abortuses from women who become pregnant soon after ceasing oral contraceptives.[43] Embryos with these anomalies are virtually always aborted spontaneously. Whether there is an overall increase in spontaneous abortion of pregnancies conceived soon after stopping oral contraceptives is unknown. It is recommended that, for any patient who has missed two consecutive periods, pregnancy should be ruled out before continuing the contraceptive regimen. If the patient has not adhered to the prescribed schedule, the possibility of pregnancy should be considered at the time of the first missed period (or after 45 days from the last menstrual period if the progestogen-only oral contraceptives are used), and further use of oral contraceptives should be withheld until pregnancy has been ruled out. If pregnancy is confirmed, the patient should be apprised of the potential risks to the fetus, and the advisability of continuation of the pregnancy should be discussed in the light of these risks.

It is also recommended that women who discontinue oral contraceptives with the intent of becoming pregnant use an alternate form of contraception for a period of time before attempting to conceive. Many clinicians recommend 3 months, although no precise information is available on which to base this recommendation.

The administration of progestogen-only or progestogen-estrogen combinations to induce withdrawal bleeding should not be used as a test of pregnancy.

6. *Gallbladder Disease:*

Studies[8,23,26] report an increased risk of surgically confirmed gallbladder disease in users of oral contraceptives and estrogens. In one study, an increased risk appeared after 2 years of use and doubled after 4 or 5 years of use. In one of the other studies, an increased risk was apparent between 6 and 12 months of use.

7. *Carbohydrate and Lipid Metabolic Effects:*

A decrease in glucose tolerance has been observed in a significant percentage of patients on oral contraceptives. For this reason, prediabetic and diabetic patients should be carefully observed while receiving oral contraceptives.

An increase in triglycerides and total phospholipids has been observed in patients receiving oral contraceptives.[44] The clinical significance of these findings remains to be defined.

8. *Elevated Blood Pressure:*

An increase in blood pressure has been reported in patients receiving oral contraceptives.[26] In some women, hypertension may occur within a few months of beginning oral-contraceptive use. In the first year of use, the prevalence of women with hypertension is low in users and may be no higher than that of a comparable group of nonusers. The prevalence in users increases, however, with longer exposure, and in the fifth year of use is two-and-a-half to three times the reported prevalence in the first year. Age is also strongly correlated with the development of hypertension in oral-contraceptive users. Women who previously have had hypertension during pregnancy may be more likely to develop elevation of blood pressure when given oral contraceptives. Hypertension that develops as a result of taking oral contraceptives usually returns to normal after discontinuing the drug.

9. *Headache:*

The onset or exacerbation of migraine or development of headache of a new pattern which is recurrent, persistent, or severe, requires discontinuation of oral contraceptives and evaluation of the cause.

10. *Bleeding Irregularities:*

Breakthrough bleeding, spotting, and amenorrhea are frequent reasons for patients discontinuing oral contraceptives. In breakthrough bleeding, as in all cases of irregular bleeding from the vagina, nonfunctional causes should be borne in mind. In undiagnosed persistent or recurrent abnormal bleeding from the vagina, adequate diagnostic measures are indicated to rule out pregnancy or malignancy. If pathology has been excluded, time or a change to another formulation may solve the problem. Changing to an oral contraceptive with a higher estrogen content, while potentially useful in minimizing menstrual irregularity, should be done only if necessary, since this may increase the risk of thromboembolic disease.

Women with a past history of oligomenorrhea or secondary amenorrhea or young women without regular cycles may have a tendency to remain anovulatory or to become amenorrheic after discontinuation of oral contraceptives. Women with these preexisting problems should be advised of this possibility and encouraged to use other contraceptive methods. Post-use anovulation, possibly prolonged, may also occur in women without previous irregularities.

11. *Ectopic Pregnancy:*
Ectopic as well as intrauterine pregnancy may occur in contraceptive failures. However, in progestogen-only oral contraceptive failures, the ratio of ectopic to intrauterine pregnancies is higher than in women who are not receiving oral contraceptives, since the drugs are more effective in preventing intrauterine than ectopic pregnancies.

12. *Breast-feeding:*
Oral contraceptives given in the postpartum period may interfere with lactation. There may be a decrease in the quantity and quality of the breast milk. Furthermore, a small fraction of the hormonal agents in oral contraceptives has been identified in the milk of mothers receiving these drugs.[45,54,55] The effects, if any, on the breast-fed child have not been determined. If feasible, the use of oral contraceptives should be deferred until the infant has been weaned.

PRECAUTIONS

GENERAL

1. A complete medical and family history should be taken prior to initiation of oral contraceptives. The pretreatment and periodic physical examinations should include special reference to blood pressure, breasts, abdomen and pelvic organs, including Papanicolaou smear and relevant laboratory tests. As a general rule, oral contraceptives should not be prescribed for longer than 1 year without another physical examination.
2. Under the influence of estrogen-progestogen preparations, preexisting uterine leiomyomata may increase in size.
3. Patients with a history of psychic depression should be carefully observed and the drug discontinued if depression recurs to a serious degree. Patients becoming significantly depressed while taking oral contraceptives should stop the medication and use an alternate method of contraception in an attempt to determine whether the symptom is drug-related.
4. Oral contraceptives may cause some degree of fluid retention. They should be prescribed with caution, and only with careful monitoring, in patients with conditions which might be aggravated by fluid retention, such as convulsive disorders, migraine syndrome, asthma, or cardiac or renal insufficiency.
5. Patients with a past history of jaundice during pregnancy have an increased risk of recurrence of jaundice while receiving oral-contraceptive therapy. If jaundice develops in any patient receiving such drugs, the medication should be discontinued.
6. Steroid hormones may be poorly metabolized in patients with impaired liver function and should be administered with caution in such patients.
7. Oral-contraceptive users may have disturbances in normal tryptophan metabolism which may result in a relative pyridoxine deficiency. The clinical significance of this is yet to be determined.
8. Serum folate levels may be depressed by oral-contraceptive therapy. Since the pregnant woman is predisposed to the development of folate deficiency and the incidence of folate deficiency increases with increasing gestation, it is possible that if a woman becomes pregnant shortly after stopping oral contraceptives, she may have a greater chance of developing folate deficiency and complications attributed to this deficiency.

INFORMATION FOR THE PATIENT
(See patient labeling which follows.)

LABORATORY TESTS

1. The pathologist should be advised of oral-contraceptive therapy when relevant specimens are submitted.
2. Certain endocrine- and liver-function tests and blood components may be affected by estrogen-containing oral contraceptives:

a. Increased sulfobromophthalein retention.
b. Increased prothrombin and factors VII, VIII, IX, and X; decreased antithrombin 3; increased norepinephrine-induced platelet aggregability.
c. Increased thyroid-binding globulin (TBG) leading to increased circulating total-thyroid hormone, as measured by protein-bound iodine (PBI), T4 by column, or T4 by radioimmunoassay. Free T3 resin uptake is decreased, reflecting the elevated TBG; free T4 concentration is unaltered.
d. Decreased pregnanediol excretion.
e. Reduced response to metyrapone test.

DRUG INTERACTIONS
Reduced efficacy and increased incidence of breakthrough bleeding have been associated with concomitant use of rifampin. A similar association has been suggested with barbiturates, phenylbutazone, phenytoin sodium, ampicillin, and tetracycline.

CARCINOGENESIS, MUTAGENESIS, IMPAIRMENT OF FERTILITY
See "Warnings" section #3, 4, and 5 for information on the carcinogenesis, mutagenesis, and impairment of fertility.

PREGNANCY
Pregnancy Category X. See "Contraindications" and "Warnings."

NURSING MOTHERS
See "Warnings." Because of the potential for adverse reactions in nursing infants from oral-contraceptive tablets, a decision should be made whether to discontinue the drug, taking into account the importance of the drug to the mother.

ADVERSE REACTIONS

An increased risk of the following serious adverse reactions has been associated with the use of oral contraceptives (see "Warnings"):

Thrombophlebitis.
Pulmonary embolism.
Coronary thrombosis.
Cerebral thrombosis.
Cerebral hemorrhage.
Hypertension.
Gallbladder disease.
Benign hapatomas.
Congenital anomalies.

There is evidence of an association between the following conditions and the use of oral contraceptives, although additional confirmatory studies are needed:

Mesenteric thrombosis.
Neuro-ocular lesions, e.g., retinal thrombosis and optic neuritis.

The following adverse reactions have been reported in patients receiving oral contraceptives and are believed to be drug-related:

Nausea and/or vomiting, usually the most common adverse reactions, occur in approximately 10% or less of patients during the first cycle. Other reactions, as a general rule, are seen much less frequently or only occasionally.
Gastrointestinal symptoms (such as abdominal cramps and bloating).
Breakthrough bleeding.
Spotting.
Change in menstrual flow.
Dysmenorrhea.
Amenorrhea during and after treatment.
Temporary infertility after discontinuance of treatment.
Edema.
Chloasma or melasma which may persist.
Breast changes: tenderness, enlargement, and secretion.
Change in weight (increase or decrease).
Change in cervical erosion and cervical secretion.
Possible diminution in lactation when given immediately postpartum.
Cholestatic jaundice.
Migraine.
Increase in size of uterine leiomyomata.
Rash (allergic).
Mental depression.
Reduced tolerance to carbohydrates.
Vaginal candidiasis.
Change in corneal curvature (steepening).
Intolerance to contact lenses.

The following adverse reactions have been reported in users of oral contraceptives, and the association has been neither confirmed nor refuted:

Premenstrual-like syndrome.
Cataracts.
Changes in libido.
Chorea.
Changes in appetite.
Cystitis-like syndrome.
Headache.
Nervousness.
Dizziness.
Hirsutism.
Loss of scalp hair.
Erythema multiforme.
Erythema nodosum.
Hemorrhagic eruption.
Vaginitis.
Porphyria.
Hemolytic uremic syndrome.

ACUTE OVERDOSE

Serious ill effects have not been reported following acute ingestion of large doses of oral contraceptives by young children. Overdosage may cause nausea, and withdrawal bleeding may occur in females.

DOSAGE AND ADMINISTRATION

To achieve maximum contraceptive effectiveness, LEVLEN™ 21 tablets and LEVLEN™ 28 tablets must be taken exactly as directed and at intervals not exceeding 24 hours.

The dosage of LEVLEN™ 21 is one tablet daily for 21 consecutive days per menstrual cycle according to prescribed schedule. Tablets are then discontinued for 7 days (three weeks on, one week off).

It is recommended that LEVLEN™ 21 tablets be taken at the same time each day, preferably after the evening meal or at bedtime.

During the first cycle of medication, the patient is instructed to take one LEVLEN™ 21 tablet daily for twenty-one consecutive days beginning on day five of her menstrual cycle. (The first day of menstruation is day one.) The tablets are then discontinued for one week (7 days). Withdrawal bleeding should usually occur within three days following discontinuation of LEVLEN™ 21 tablets.

(If LEVLEN™ 21 tablets are first taken later than the fifth day of the first menstrual cycle of medication or postpartum, contraceptive reliance should not be placed on LEVLEN™ 21 tablets until after the first seven consecutive days of administration. The possibility of ovulation and conception prior to initiation of medication should be considered.)

The patient begins her next and all subsequent 21-day courses of LEVLEN™ 21 tablets on the same day of the week that she began her first course, following the same schedule: 21 days on—7 days off. She begins taking her tablets on the 8th day after discontinuance regardless of whether or not a menstrual period has occurred or is still in progress. Any time a new cycle of LEVLEN™ 21 tablets is started later than the 8th day the patient should be protected by another means of contraception until she has taken a tablet daily for seven consecutive days.

If spotting or breakthrough bleeding occurs, the patient is instructed to continue on the same regimen. This type of bleeding is usually transient and without significance; however, if the bleeding is persistent or prolonged, the patient is advised to consult her physician. Although the occurrence of pregnancy is highly unlikely if LEVLEN™ 21 tablets are taken according to directions, if withdrawal bleeding does not occur, the possibility of pregnancy must be considered. If the patient has not adhered to the prescribed schedule (missed one or more tablets or started taking them on a day later than she should have), the probability of pregnancy should be considered at the time of the first missed period and appropriate diagnostic measures taken before the medication is resumed. If the patient has adhered to the prescribed regimen and misses two consecutive periods, pregnancy should be ruled out before continuing the contraceptive regimen.

The patient should be instructed to take a missed tablet as soon as it is remembered. If two consecutive tablets are missed, they should both be taken as soon as remembered. The next tablet should be taken at the usual time.

Any time the patient misses one or two tablets, she should also use another method of contraception until she has taken a tablet daily for seven consecutive days. If breakthrough bleeding occurs following missed tablets, it will usually be transient and of no consequence. While there is little likelihood of ovulation occurring if only one or two tablets are missed, the possibility of ovulation increases with each successive day that scheduled tablets are missed. If three consecutive tablets are missed, all medication should be discontinued and the remainder of the package discarded. A new tablet cycle should be started on the 8th day after the last tablet was taken, and an alternate means of contraception should be prescribed during the seven days without tablets and until the patient has taken a tablet daily for seven consecutive days. In the nonlactating mother, LEVLEN™ tablets may be prescribed in the postpartum period either immediately or at the first postpartum examination whether or not menstruation has resumed.

LEVLEN™ 28 TABLETS (LEVONORGESTREL AND ETHINYL ESTRADIOL TABLETS)
The dosage of LEVLEN™ 28 tablets is one light-orange tablet daily for 21 consecutive days, followed by one pink inert tablet daily for 7 consecutive days, according to prescribed schedule. It is recommended that tablets be taken at the same time each day, preferably after the evening meal or at bedtime. During the first cycle of medication, the patient is instructed to begin taking LEVLEN™ 28 tablets on the first Sunday after the onset of menstruation. If menstruation begins on a Sunday, the first tablet (light-orange) is taken that day. One light-orange tablet should be taken daily for 21 consecutive days, followed by one pink inert tablet daily for 7 consecutive days. Withdrawal bleeding should usually occur within three days following discontinuation of light-orange tablets.

During the first cycle, contraceptive reliance should not be placed on LEVLEN™ 28 tablets until a light-orange tablet has been taken daily for 7 consecutive days. The possibility of ovulation and conception prior to initiation of medication should be considered.

The patient begins her next and all subsequent 28-day courses of tablets on the same day of the week (Sunday) on

Continued on next page

Information on the Berlex products appearing here is based on the labeling in effect on August 1, 1986. Further information for these and other products may be obtained from the Professional Services Department, Berlex Laboratories, Inc., 110 East Hanover Avenue, Cedar Knolls, New Jersey 07927, telephone 201-292-3008.

Berlex—Cont.

which she began her first course, following the same schedule: 21 days on light-orange tablets—7 days on pink inert tablets. If in any cycle the patient starts tablets later than the proper day, she should protect herself by using another method of birth control until she has taken a light-orange tablet daily for 7 consecutive days.

If spotting or breakthrough bleeding occurs, the patient is instructed to continue on the same regimen. This type of bleeding is usually transient and without significance; however, if the bleeding is persistent or prolonged, the patient is advised to consult her physician. Although the occurrence of pregnancy is highly unlikely if LEVLEN™ 28 tablets are taken according to directions, if withdrawal bleeding does not occur, the possibility of pregnancy must be considered. If the patient has not adhered to the prescribed schedule (missed one or more tablets or started taking them on a day later than she should have), the probability of pregnancy should be considered at the time of the first missed period and appropriate diagnostic measures taken before the medication is resumed. If the patient has adhered to the prescribed regimen and misses two consecutive periods, pregnancy should be ruled out before continuing the contraceptive regimen.

The patient should be instructed to take a missed light-orange tablet as soon as it is remembered. If two consecutive light-orange tablets are missed, they should both be taken as soon as remembered. The next tablet should be taken at the usual time.

Any time the patient misses one or two light-orange tablets, she should also use another method of contraception until she has taken a light-orange tablet daily for seven consecutive days. If the patient misses one or more pink tablets, she is still protected against pregnancy *provided* she begins taking light-orange tablets again on the proper day.

If breakthrough bleeding occurs following missed light-orange tablets, it will usually be transient and of no consequence. While there is little likelihood of ovulation occurring if only one or two light-orange tablets are missed, the possibility of ovulation increases with each successive day that scheduled light-orange tablets are missed. (If three consecutive light-orange LEVLEN™ tablets are missed, all medication should be discontinued and the remainder of the 28-day package discarded. A new tablet cycle should be started on the first Sunday following the last missed tablet, and an alternate means of contraception should be prescribed during the days without tablets and until the patient has taken a light-orange tablet daily for 7 consecutive days.) In the non-lactating mother, LEVLEN™ tablets may be prescribed in the postpartum period either immediately or at the first postpartum examination whether or not menstruation has resumed.

HOW SUPPLIED

LEVLEN™ 21 tablets (0.15 mg levonorgestrel and 0.03 mg ethinyl estradiol), Berlex, are available in packages of 3 SLIDECASE™ dispensers of 21 tablets each as follows:

NDC 50419-021, light orange, round tablet marked "B" on one side and "21" on the other side.

LEVLEN™ 28 tablets (0.15 mg levonorgestrel and 0.03 mg ethinyl estradiol). Berlex, are available in packages of 3 SLIDECASE™ dispensers, each containing 28 tablets as follows:

21 active tablets, NDC 50419-021, light-orange, round tablet marked "B" on one side and "21" on the other side.

7 inert tablet, NDC 50419-028, pink, round tablet marked "B" on one side and "28" on the other side.

REFERENCES

1. "*Population Reports,*" Series H, Number 2, May 1974; Series I, Number 1, June 1974; Series B, Number 2, January 1975; Series H, Number 3, 1975; Series H, Number 4, January 1976 (published by the Population Information Program, The George Washington University Medical Center, 2001 S St. NW., Washington, D.C.).
2. Inman, W. H. W., Vessey, M. P., Westerholm, B., and Engelund, A., "Thromboembolic disease and the steroidal content of oral contraceptives. A report to the Committee on Safety of Drugs," Brit Med J *2*:203–209, 1970.
3. Stolley, P. D., Tonascia, J. A., Tockman, M. S., Sartwell, P. E., Rutledge, A. H., and Jacobs, M. P., "Thrombosis with low-estrogen oral contraceptives," Am J Epidemiol *102*:197–208, 1975.
4. Royal College of General Practitioners, "Oral contraception and thromboembolic disease," J Coll Gen Pract *13*:267–279, 1967.
5. Inman, W. H. W., and Vessey, M. P., "Investigation of deaths from pulmonary, coronary and cerebral thrombosis and embolism in women of childbearing age," Brit Med J *2*:193–199, 1968.
6. Vessey, M. P., and Doll, R., "Investigation of relation between use of oral contraceptives and thromboembolic disease. A further report," Brit Med J *2*:651–657, 1969.
7. Sartwell, P. E., Masi, A. T., Arthes, F. G., Greene, G. R., and Smith, H. E., "Thromboembolism and oral contraceptives: an epidemiological case control study," Am J Epidemiol *90*:365–380, 1969.
8. Boston Collaborative Drug Surveillance Program, "Oral contraceptives and venous thromboembolic disease, surgically confirmed gallbladder disease and breast tumors," Lancet *1*:1399–1404, 1973.
9. Collaborative Group for the Study of Stroke in Young Women, "Oral contraception and increased risk of cerebral ischemia or thrombosis," N Engl J Med *288*:871–878, 1973.
10. Collaborative Group for the Study of Stroke in Young Women, "Oral contraceptives and stroke in young women: associated risk factors," JAMA *231*:718–722, 1975.
11. Mann, J. I., and Inman, W. H. W., "Oral contraceptives and death from myocardial infarction," Brit Med J *2*:245–248, 1975.
12. Mann, J. I., Inman, W. H. W., and Thorogood, M., "Oral contraceptive use in older women and fatal myocardial infarction," Brit Med J *2*:445–447, 1976.
13. Mann, J. I., Vessey, M. P., Thorogood, M., and Doll, R., "Myocardial infarction in young women with special reference to oral contraceptive practice," Brit Med J *2*:241–245, 1975.
14. Tietze, C., "New Estimates of Mortality Associated with Fertility Control," Family Planning Perspectives, *9*:74–76, 1977.
15. Vessey, M. P., Doll, R., Fairbairn, A. S., and Glober, G., "Post-operative thromboembolism and the use of oral contraceptives," Brit Med J *3*:123–126, 1970.
16. Greene, G. R., Sartwell, P. E., "Oral contraceptive use in patients with thromboembolism following surgery, trauma, or infection," Am J Pub Health *62*:680–685, 1972.
17. Smith, D. C., Prentice, R., Thompson, D. J., and Herrmann, W. L., "Association of exogenous estrogen and endometrial carcinoma," N Engl J Med *293*:1164–1167, 1975.
18. Ziel, H. K., and Finkle, W. D., "Increased risk of endometrial carcinoma among users of conjugated estrogens," N Engl J Med *293*:1167–1170, 1975.
19. Mack, T. N., Pike, M. C., Henderson, B. E., Pfeffer, R. I., Gerkins, V. R., Arthur, M., and Brown, S. E., "Estrogens and endometrial cancer in a retirement community," N Engl J Med *294*:1262–1267, 1976.
20. Silverberg, S. G., and Makowski, E. L., "Endometrial carcinoma in young women taking oral contraceptive agents," Obstet Gynecol *46*:503–506, 1975.
21. Vessey, M. P., Doll, R., and Sutton, P. M., "Oral contraceptives and breast neoplasia: a retrospective study," Brit Med J *3*:719–724, 1972.
22. Vessey, M. P., Doll, R., and Jones K., "Oral contraceptives and breast cancer. Progress report of an epidemiological study," Lancet *1*:941–943, 1975.
23. Boston Collaborative Drug Surveillance Program, "Surgically confirmed gallbladder disease, venous thromboembolism and breast tumors in relation to postmenopausal estrogen therapy," N Engl J Med *290*:15–19, 1974.
24. Arthes, F. G., Sartwell, P. E., and Lewison, E. F., "The pill, estrogens, and the breast. Epidemiologic aspects," Cancer *28*:1391–1394, 1971.
25. Fasal, E., and Paffenbarger, R. S., "Oral contraceptives as related to cancer and benign lesions of the breast," J Natl Cancer Inst *55*:767–773, 1975.
26. Royal College of General Practitioners, "Oral Contraceptives and Health," London, Pitman, 1974.
27. Ory, H., Cole P., MacMahon, B., and Hoover, R., "Oral contraceptives and reduced risk of benign breast diseases," N Engl J Med *294*:419–422, 1976.
28. Baum, J., Holtz, F., Bookstein, J. J., and Klein, E. W., "Possible association between benign hepatomas and oral contraceptives," Lancet *2*:926–928, 1973.
29. Mays, E. T., Christopherson, W. M., Mahr, M. M., and Williams, H. C., "Hepatic changes in young women ingesting contraceptive steroids. Hepatic hemorrhage and primary hepatic tumors," JAMA *235*:730–732, 1976.
30. Edmondson, H. A., Henderson, B., and Benton, B., "Liver-cell adenomas associated with use of oral contraceptives," N Engl J Med *294*:470–472, 1976.
31. Herbst, A. L., Ulfedler, H., and Poskanzer, D. C., "Adenocarcinoma of the vagina," N Engl J Med *284*:878–881, 1971.
32. Greenwald, P., Barlow, J. J., Nasca, P. C., and Burnett, W., "Vaginal cancer after maternal treatment with synthetic estrogens," N Engl J Med *285*:390–392, 1971.
33. Lanier, A. P., Noller, K. L., Decker, D. G., Elveback, L., and Kurland, L. T., "Cancer and stilbestrol. A follow-up of 1719 persons exposed to estrogens in utero and born 1943–1959," Mayo Clin Pro *48*:793–799, 1973.
34. Herbst, A. L., Kurman, R. J., and Scully, R. E., "Vaginal and cervical abnormalities after exposure to stilbestrol in utero," Obstet Gynecol *40*:287–298, 1972.
35. Herbst, A. L., Robboy, S. J., Macdonald, G. J., and Scully, R. E., "The effects of local progesterone on stilbestrol-associated vaginal adenosis," Am J Obstet Gynecol *118*:607–615, 1974.
36. Herbst, A. L., Poskanzer, D. C., Robboy, S. J., Friedlander, L., and Scully, R. E., "Prenatal exposure to stilbestrol: a prospective comparison of exposed female offspring with unexposed controls," N Engl J Med *292*:334–339, 1975.
37. Stafl, A., Mattingly, R. F., Foley, D. V., Fetherston, W., "Clinical diagnosis of vaginal adenosis," Obstet Gynecol *43*:118–128, 1974.
38. Sherman, A. I., Goldrath, M., Berlin, A., Vakhariya, V., Banooni, F., Michaels, W., Goodman, P., and Brown, S., "Cervical-vaginal adenosis after in utero exposure to synthetic estrogens," Obstet Gynecol *44*:531–545, 1974.
39. Gal, I., Kirman, B., and Stern, J., "Hormone pregnancy tests and congenital malformation," Nature *216*:83, 1967.
40. Levy, E. P., Cohen, A., and Fraser, F. C., "Hormone treatment during pregnancy and congenital heart defects," Lancet *1*:611, 1973.
41. Nora, J. J., and Nora, A. H., "Birth defects and oral contraceptives," Lancet *1*:941–942, 1973.
42. Janerich, D. T., Piper, J. M., and Glebatis, D. M., "Oral contraceptives and congenital limb-reduction defects," N Engl J Med *291*:697–700, 1974.
43. Carr, D. H., "Chromosome studies in selected spontaneous abortions: I. Conception after oral contraceptives," Canad Med Assoc J *103*:343–348, 1970.
44. Wynn, V., Doar, J. W. H., and Mills, G. L., "Some effects of oral contraceptives on serum-lipid and lipoprotein levels," Lancet *2*:720–723, 1966.
45. Laumas, K. R., Malkani, P. K., Bhatnagar, S., and Laumas, V., "Radioactivity in the breast milk of lactating women after oral administration of 3 H-norethynodrel," Am J Obstet Gynecol *98*:411–413, 1967.
46. Center for Disease Control, "Increased Risk of Hepatocellular Adenoma in Women with Long-term use of Oral Contraceptives," Morbidity and Mortality Weekly Report, *26*:293–294, 1977.
47. Herbst, A. L., Cole, P., Colton, T., Robboy, S. J., Scully, R. E., "Age-incidence and Risk of Diethylstilbestrol-related Clear Cell Adenocarcinoma of the Vagina and Cervix," Am J Obstet Gynecol *128*:43–50, 1977.
48. Bibbo, M., Al-Naqeeb, M., Baccarini, I., Gill, W., Newton, M., Sleeper, K. M., Sonek, M., Wied, G. L., "Follow-up Study of Male and Female Offspring of DES-treated Mothers. A Preliminary Report," J of Repro Med *15*:29–32, 1975.
49. Gill, W. B., Schumacher, G. F. B., Bibbo, M., "Structural and Functional Abnormalities in the Sex Organs of Male Offspring of Mothers Treated with Diethylstilbestrol (DES)," J of Repro Med *16*:147–153, 1976.
50. Henderson, B. E., Senton, B., Cosgrove, M., Baptista, J., Aldrich, J., Townsend, D., Hart, W., and Mack, T., "Urogenital Tract Abnormalities in Sons of Women Treated with Diethylstilbestrol," Pediatrics, *58*:505–507, 1976.
51. Heinonen, O. P., Slone, D., Nonson, R. R., Hook, E. B., and Shapiro, S., "Cardiovascular Birth Defects and Antenatal Exposure to Female Sex Hormones," N Engl J Med *296*:67–70, 1977.
52. Jain, A. K., "Mortality Risk Associated with the Use of Oral Contraceptives," Studies in Family Planning, *8*:50–54, 1977.
53. Beral, V., "Mortality Among Oral Contraceptive Users," Lancet, *2*:727–731, 1977.
54. Nilsson, S., Nygren, K., and Johansson, E., "Ethinyl Estradiol in Human Milk and Plasma after Oral Administration," Contraception *17*:131–139, 1978.
55. Nilsson,S., Nygren, K., and Johansson, E., "d-Norgestrel Concentrations in Maternal Plasma, Milk and Child Plasma During Administration of Oral Contraceptives to Nursing Women," Am J Obstet Gynecol, *129*:178, 1977.
56. Royal College of General Practitioners' Oral contraception study, "Incidence of arterial disease among oral contraceptive users," J Royal Col Gen Pract *33*:75-82, 1983.
57. Slone, D., Shapiro, S., Kaufman, D. W., Rosenberg, L., Miettinen, O., and Stolley, P., "Risk of myocardial infarction in relation to current and discontinued use of oral contraceptives," N Engl J Med *305*:420-424, 1981.
58. Inman, W.H.W., "Oral contraceptives and fatal subarachnoid haemorrhage," Brit Med J *2*:1468-1470, 1979.
59. Petitti, D. B., and Wingerd, J., "Use of oral contraceptives, cigarette smoking and risk of subarachnoid haemorrhage," Lancet *2*:234-236, 1978.
60. Thorogood, M., Adam, S. A., and Mann, J. I., "Fatal subarachnoid haemorrhage in young women: role of oral contraceptives," Brit Med J *283*:762, 1981.
61. Rosenberg, L., Hennekens, C.H., Rosner, B., Belanger, C., Rothman, K. J., and Speizer, F. E., "Oral contraceptive use in relation to nonfatal myocardial infarction," Am J Epidemiol *111*:59-66, 1980.
62. Adam, S. A., Thorogood, M., and Mann, J. I., "Oral contraception and myocardial infarction revisited: the effects of new preparations and prescribing patterns," Brit J Obstet Gynaecol *88*:838-845, 1981.

The patient labeling for oral-contraceptive drug products is set forth below:

Brief Summary Patient Package Insert

Cigarette smoking increases the risk of serious adverse effects on the heart and blood vessels from oral-contraceptive use. This risk increases with age and with heavy

smoking (15 or more cigarettes per day) and is quite marked in women over 35 years of age. Women who use oral contraceptives should not smoke.

Oral contraceptives, taken as directed, are about 99% effective in preventing pregnancy. (The mini-pill, however, is somewhat less effective.) Forgetting to take your pills increases the chance of pregnancy. Women who have or have had clotting disorders, cancer of the breast or sex organs, unexplained vaginal bleeding, a stroke, heart attack, angina pectoris, or who suspect they may be pregnant should not use oral contraceptives. Various drugs, such as some antibiotics, may also decrease the effectiveness of oral contraceptives.

Most side effects of the pill are not serious. The most common side effects are nausea, vomiting, bleeding between menstrual periods, weight gain, and breast tenderness. However, proper use of oral contraceptives requires that they be taken under your doctor's continuous supervision, because they can be associated with serious side effects which may be fatal. Fortunately, these occur very infrequently. The serious side effects are:

1. Blood clots in the legs, lungs, brain, heart, or other organs, and hemorrhage into the brain due to bursting of a blood vessel. Certain of these effects may occur after pill use has been stopped.
2. Liver tumors, which may rupture and cause severe bleeding.
3. Birth defects if the pill is taken while you are pregnant.
4. High blood pressure.
5. Gallbladder disease.

The symptoms associated with these serious side effects are discussed in the detailed leaflet given you with your supply of pills. Notify your doctor if you notice any unusual physical disturbance while taking the pill.

The estrogen in oral contraceptives has been found to cause breast cancer and other cancers in certain animals. These findings suggest that oral contraceptives may also cause cancer in humans. However, studies to date in women taking currently marketed oral contraceptives have not confirmed that oral contraceptives cause cancer in humans.

The detailed leaflet describes more completely the benefits and risks of oral contraceptives. It also provides information on other forms of contraception. Read it carefully. If you have any questions, consult your doctor.

CAUTION

Oral contraceptives are of no value in the prevention or treatment of venereal disease.

DETAILED PATIENT LABELING

WHAT YOU SHOULD KNOW ABOUT ORAL CONTRACEPTIVES

Oral contraceptives ("the pill") are the most effective way (except for sterilization) to prevent pregnancy. They are also convenient and, for most women, free of serious or unpleasant side effects. Oral contraceptives must always be taken under the continuous supervision of a physician.

It is important that any woman who considers using an oral contraceptive understand the risks involved. Although the oral contraceptives have important advantages over other methods of contraception, they have certain risks that no other method has. Only you can decide whether the advantages are worth these risks. This leaflet will tell you about the most important risks. It will explain how you can help your doctor prescribe the pill as safely as possible by telling him about yourself and being alert for the earliest signs of trouble. And it will tell you how to use the pill properly, so that it will be as effective as possible. There is more detailed information available in the leaflet prepared for doctors. Your pharmacist can show you a copy; you may need your doctor's help in understanding parts of it.

WHO SHOULD NOT USE ORAL CONTRACEPTIVES

A. If you have any of the following conditions, you should not use the pill:

1. Clots in the legs or lungs.
2. Angina pectoris.
3. Known or suspected cancer of the breast or sex organs.
4. Unusual vaginal bleeding that has not yet been diagnosed.
5. Known or suspected pregnancy.

B. If you have had any of the following conditions, you should not use the pill:

1. Heart attack or stroke.
2. Clots in the legs or lungs.

C. Cigarette smoking increases the risk of serious adverse effects on the heart and blood vessels from oral-contraceptive use. This risk increases with age and with heavy smoking (15 or more cigarettes per day) and is quite marked in women over 35 years of age. Women who use oral contraceptives should not smoke.

D. If you have scanty or irregular periods or are a young woman without a regular cycle, you should use another method of contraception because, if you use the pill, you may have difficulty becoming pregnant or may fail to have menstrual periods after discontinuing the pill.

DECIDING TO USE ORAL CONTRACEPTIVES

If you do not have any of the conditions listed above and are thinking about using oral contraceptives, to help you decide, you need information about the advantages and risks of oral contraceptives and of other contraceptive methods as well. This leaflet describes the advantages and risks of oral contraceptives. Except for sterilization, the IUD, and abortion, which have their own inherent risks, the only risks of other methods of contraception are those due to pregnancy should the method fail. Your doctor can answer questions you may have with respect to other methods of contraception. He can also answer any questions you may have after reading this leaflet on oral contraceptives.

1. What Oral Contraceptives Are and How They Work. Oral contraceptives are of two types. The most common, often simply called "the pill," is a combination of an estrogen and a progestogen, the two kinds of female hormones. The amount of estrogen and progestogen can vary, but the amount of estrogen is most important because both the effectiveness and some of the dangers of oral contraceptives are related to the amount of estrogen. This kind of oral contraceptive works principally by preventing release of an egg from the ovary. When the amount of estrogen is 50 micrograms or more, and the pill is taken as directed, oral contraceptives are more than 99% effective (i.e., there would be less than 1 pregnancy if 100 women used the pill for 1 year). Pills that contain 20 to 35 micrograms of estrogen vary slightly in effectiveness, ranging from 98% to more than 99% effective.

The second type of oral contraceptive, often called the "mini-pill", contains only a progestogen. It works in part by preventing release of an egg from the ovary, but also by keeping sperm from reaching the egg and by making the uterus (womb) less receptive to any fertilized egg that reaches it. The mini-pill is less effective than the combination oral contraceptive, about 97% effective. In addition, the progestogen-only pill has a tendency to cause irregular bleeding which may be quite inconvenient, or cessation of bleeding entirely. The progestogen-only pill is used despite its lower effectiveness in the hope that it will prove not to have some of the serious side effects of the estrogen-containing pill (see below), but it is not yet certain that the mini-pill does, in fact, have fewer serious side effects. The discussion below, while based mainly on information about the combination pills, should be considered to apply as well to the mini-pill.

2. Other Nonsurgical Ways to Prevent Pregnancy. As this leaflet will explain, oral contraceptives have several serious risks. Other methods of contraception have lesser risks or none at all. They are also less effective than oral contraceptives, but, used properly, may be effective enough for many women.

The following table gives reported pregnancy rates (the number of women out of 100 who would become pregnant in 1 year) for these methods.

PREGNANCIES PER 100 WOMEN PER YEAR

Intrauterine device (IUD), less than 1-6; Diaphragm with spermicidal products (creams or jellies), 2-20; Condom (rubber), 3-36; Aerosol foams, 2-29; Jellies and creams, 4-36; Periodic abstinence (rhythm) all types, less than 1-47:

1. Calendar method, 14-47;
2. Temperature method, 1-20;
3. Temperature method—intercourse only in postovulatory phase, less than 1-7;
4. Mucus method, 1-25;

No contraception, 60-80.

The figures (except for the IUD) vary widely because people differ in how well they use each method. Very faithful users of the various methods obtain very good results, except for users of the calendar method of periodic abstinence (rhythm). Except for the IUD, effective use of these methods requires somewhat more effort than simply taking a single pill every day, but it is an effort that many couples undertake successfully. Your doctor can tell you a great deal more about these methods of contraception.

3. The Dangers of Oral Contraceptives.

a. *Circulatory disorders (abnormal blood clotting and stroke due to hemorrhage).* Blood clots (in various blood vessels of the body) are the most common of the serious side effects of oral contraceptives. A clot can result in a stroke (if the clot is in the brain), a heart attack (if the clot is in a blood vessel of the heart), or a pulmonary embolus (a clot which forms in the legs or pelvis, then breaks off and travels to the lungs). Any of these can be fatal. Clots also occur rarely in the blood vessels of the eye, resulting in blindness or impairment of vision in that eye. There is evidence that the risk of clotting increases with higher estrogen doses. It is, therefore, important to keep the dose of estrogen as low as possible, so long as the oral contraceptive used has an acceptable pregnancy rate and doesn't cause unacceptable changes in the menstrual pattern. Furthermore, cigarette smoking by oral-contraceptive users increases the risk of serious adverse effects on the heart and blood vessels. This risk increases with age and with heavy smoking (15 or more cigarettes per day) and begins to become quite marked in women over 35 years of age. For this reason, women who use oral contraceptives should not smoke.

The risk of abnormal clotting increases with age in both users and nonusers of oral contraceptives, but the increased risk from the contraceptive appears to be present at all ages. For oral-contraceptive users in general, it has been estimated that in women between the ages of 15 and 34 the risk of death due to a circulatory disorder is about 1 in 12,000 per year, whereas for nonusers the risk is about 1 in 50,000 per year. In the age group 35 to 44, the risk is estimated to be about 1 in 2,500 per year for oral-contraceptive users and about 1 in 10,000 per year for nonusers.

Even without the pill the risk of having a heart attack increases with age and is also increased by such heart attack risk factors as high blood pressure, high cholesterol, obesity, diabetes, and cigarette smoking. Without any risk factors present, the use of oral contraceptives alone may double the risk of heart attack. However, the combination of cigarette smoking, especially heavy smoking, and oral contraceptive use greatly increases the risk of heart attack. Oral-contraceptive users who smoke are about 5 times more likely to have a heart attack than users who do not smoke and about 10 times more likely to have a heart attack than nonusers who do not smoke. It has been estimated that users between the ages of 30 and 39 who smoke have about a 1 in 10,000 chance each year of having a fatal heart attack compared to about a 1 in 50,000 chance in users who do not smoke, and about a 1 in 100,000 chance in nonusers who do not smoke. In the age group 40 to 44, the risk is about 1 in 1,700 per year for users who smoke compared to about 1 in 10,000 for users who do not smoke and to about 1 in 14,000 per year for nonusers who do not smoke. Heavy smoking (about 15 cigarettes or more a day) further increases the risk. If you do not smoke and have none of the other heart attack risk factors described above, you will have a smaller risk than listed. If you have several heart attack risk factors, the risk may be considerably greater than listed. In addition to blood-clotting disorders, it has been estimated that women taking oral contraceptives are twice as likely as nonusers to have a stroke due to rupture of a blood vessel in the brain. There is evidence that patients who stop taking oral contraceptives after using them continuously for five or more years may continue to have an increased risk of stroke or heart attack for at least six to nine years after discontinuation.

b. *Formation of tumors.* Studies have found that when certain animals are given the female sex hormone, estrogen, which is an ingredient of oral contraceptives, continuously for long periods, cancers may develop in the breast, cervix, vagina, and liver.

These findings suggest that oral contraceptives may cause cancer in humans. However, studies to date in women taking currently marketed oral contraceptives have not confirmed that oral contraceptives cause cancer in humans. Several studies have found no increase in breast cancer in users, although one study suggested oral contraceptives might cause an increase in breast cancer in women who already have benign breast disease (e.g., cysts).

Women with a strong family history of breast cancer or who have breast nodules, fibrocystic disease, or abnormal mammograms or who were exposed to DES (diethylstilbestrol), an estrogen, during their mother's pregnancy must be followed very closely by their doctors if they choose to use oral contraceptives instead of another method of contraception. Many studies have shown that women taking oral contraceptives have less risk of getting benign breast disease than those who have not used oral contraceptives. Recently, strong evidence has emerged that estrogens (one component of oral contraceptives), when given for periods of more than one year to women after the menopause, increase the risk of cancer of the uterus (womb). There is also some evidence that a kind of oral contraceptive which is no longer marketed, the sequential oral contraceptive, may increase the risk of cancer of the uterus. There remains no evidence, however, that the oral contraceptives now available increase the risk of this cancer. Oral contraceptives do cause, although rarely, a benign (nonmalignant) tumor of the liver. These tumors do not spread, but they may rupture and cause internal bleeding, which may be fatal. A few cases of cancer of the liver have been reported in women using oral contraceptives, but it is not yet known whether the drug caused them.

c. *Dangers to a developing child if oral contraceptives are used in or immediately preceding pregnancy.* Oral contraceptives should not be taken by pregnant women because they may damage the developing child. An increased risk of birth defects, including heart defects and limb defects, has been asso-

Continued on next page

Information on the Berlex products appearing here is based on the labeling in effect on August 1, 1986. Further information for these and other products may be obtained from the Professional Services Department, Berlex Laboratories, Inc., 110 East Hanover Avenue, Cedar Knolls, New Jersey 07927, telephone 201-292-3008.

Berlex—Cont.

ciated with the use of sex hormones, including oral contraceptives, in pregnancy. In addition, the developing female child whose mother has received DES (diethylstilbestrol), an estrogen, during pregnancy has a risk of getting cancer of the vagina or cervix in her teens or young adulthood. This risk is estimated to be about 1 in 1,000 exposures or less. Abnormalities of the urinary and sex organs have been reported in male offspring so exposed. It is possible that other estrogens, such as the estrogens in oral contraceptives, could have the same effect in the child if the mother takes them during pregnancy.

If you stop taking oral contraceptives to become pregnant, your doctor may recommend that you use another method of contraception for a short while. The reason for this is that there is evidence from studies in women who have had "miscarriages" soon after stopping the pill, that the lost fetuses are more likely to be abnormal. Whether there is an overall increase in "miscarriage" in women who become pregnant soon after stopping the pill as compared with women who do not use the pill is not known, but it is possible that there may be. If, however, you do become pregnant soon after stopping oral contraceptives, and do not have a miscarriage, there is no evidence that the baby has an increased risk of being abnormal.

d. *Gallbladder disease.* Women who use oral contraceptives have a greater risk than nonusers of having gallbladder disease requiring surgery. The increased risk may first appear within 1 year of use and may double after 4 or 5 years of use.

e. *Other side effects of oral contraceptives.* Some women using oral contraceptives experience unpleasant side effects that are not dangerous and are not likely to damage their health. Some of these may be temporary. Your breasts may feel tender, nausea and vomiting may occur, you may gain or lose weight, and your ankles may swell. A spotty darkening of the skin, particularly of the face, is possible and may persist. You may notice unexpected vaginal bleeding or changes in your menstrual period. Irregular bleeding is frequently seen when using the mini-pill or combination oral contraceptives containing less than 50 micrograms of estrogen. More serious side effects include worsening of migraine, asthma, epilepsy, and kidney or heart disease because of a tendency for water to be retained in the body when oral contraceptives are used.

Other side effects are growth of preexisting fibroid tumors of the uterus; mental depression, and liver problems with jaundice (yellowing of the skin). Your doctor may find that levels of sugar and fatty substances in your blood are elevated; the long-term effects of these changes are not known. Some women develop high blood pressure while taking oral contraceptives, which ordinarily returns to the original levels when the oral contraceptive is stopped.

Other reactions, although not proved to be caused by oral contraceptives, are occasionally reported. These include more frequent urination and some discomfort when urinating, blood cell breakdown with kidney failure, nervousness, dizziness, some loss of scalp hair, an increase in body hair, an increase or decrease in sex drive, appetite changes, cataracts, and a need for a change in contact lens prescription, or inability to use contact lenses. After you stop using oral contraceptives, there may be a delay before you are able to become pregnant or before you resume having menstrual periods. This is especially true of women who had irregular menstrual cycles prior to the use of oral contraceptives. As discussed previously, your doctor may recommend that you wait a short while after stopping the pill before you try to become pregnant. During this time, use another form of contraception. You should consult your physician before resuming use of oral contraceptives after childbirth, especially if you plan to nurse your baby. Drugs in oral contraceptives are known to appear in the milk, and the long-range effect on infants is not known at this time. Furthermore, oral contraceptives may cause a decrease in your milk supply as well as in the quality of the milk.

4. Comparison of the Risks of Oral Contraceptives and Other Contraceptive Methods. The many studies on the risks and effectiveness of oral contraceptives and other methods of contraception have been analyzed to estimate the risk of death associated with various methods of contraception. This risk has two parts: (a) the risk of the method itself (e.g., the risk that oral contraceptives will cause death due to abnormal clotting), and (b) the risk of death due to pregnancy or abortion in the event the method fails. The results of this analysis are shown in the bar graph (Figure 1). The height of the bars is the number of deaths per 100,000 women each year. There are six sets of bars, each set referring to a specific age group of women. Within each set of bars, there is a single bar for each of the different contraceptive methods. For oral contraceptives, there are two bars—one for smokers and the other for nonsmokers. The analysis is based on present knowledge, and new information could, of course, alter it. The analysis shows that the risk of death from all methods of birth control is low and below that associated with childbirth, except for oral contraceptives in women over 40 who smoke. It shows that the lowest risk of death is associated with the condom or diaphragm (traditional contraception) backed up by early abortion in case of failure of the condom or diaphragm to prevent pregnancy. Also, at any age the risk of death (due to unexpected pregnancy) from the use of traditional contraception, even without a backup of abortion, is generally the same as or less than that from use of oral contraceptives.

Figure 1. Estimated annual number of deaths associated with control of fertility and no control per 100,000 nonsterile women, by regimen of control and age of women.

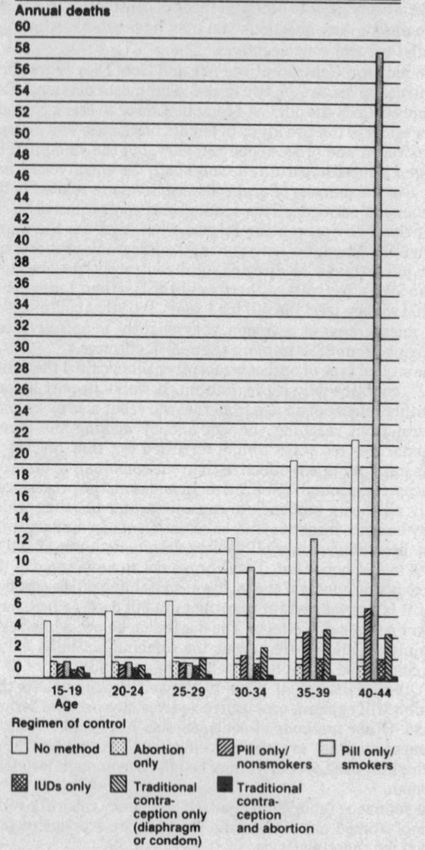

HOW TO USE ORAL CONTRACEPTIVES AS SAFELY AND EFFECTIVELY AS POSSIBLE, ONCE YOU HAVE DECIDED TO USE THEM

1. What to Tell your Doctor.

You can make use of the pill as safely as possible by telling your doctor if you have any of the following:

a. Conditions that mean you should not use oral contraceptives:

Clots in the legs or lungs.
Clots in the legs or lungs in the past.
A stroke, heart attack, or angina pectoris.
Known or suspected cancer of the breast or sex organs.
Unusual vaginal bleeding that has not yet been diagnosed.
Known or suspected pregnancy.

b. Conditions that your doctor will want to watch closely or which might cause him to suggest another method of contraception:

A family history of breast cancer.
Breast nodules, fibrocystic disease of the breast, or an abnormal mammogram.

Diabetes.	Heart or kidney disease.
High blood pressure.	Epilepsy.
High cholesterol.	Mental depression.
Cigarette smoking.	Fibroid tumors of the uterus.
Migraine headaches.	Gallbladder disease.

c. Once you are using oral contraceptives, you should be alert for signs of a serious adverse effect and call your doctor if they occur:

Sharp pain in the chest, coughing blood, or sudden shortness of breath (indicating possible clots in the lungs).
Pain in the calf (possible clot in the leg).
Crushing chest pain or heaviness (indicating possible heart attack).
Sudden severe headache or vomiting, dizziness or fainting, disturbance of vision or speech, or weakness or numbness in an arm or leg (indicating a possible stroke).
Sudden partial or complete loss of vision (indicating a possible clot in the eye).
Breast lumps (you should ask your doctor to show you how to examine your own breasts).
Severe pain in the abdomen (indicating a possible ruptured tumor of the liver).
Severe depression.
Yellowing of the skin (jaundice).

2. How to Take the Pill So That It is Most Effective.

Reduced effectiveness and an increased incidence of breakthrough bleeding have been associated with the use of oral contraceptives with antibiotics such as rifampin, ampicillin, and tetracycline or with certain other drugs such as barbiturates, phenylbutazone or phenytoin sodium. You should use an additional means of contraception during any cycle in which any of these drugs are taken.

To achieve maximum contraceptive effectiveness, oral contraceptives must be taken exactly as directed and at intervals not exceeding 24 hours. It is recommended that tablets be taken at the same time each day, preferably after the evening meal or at bedtime. Taking them on a definite schedule will decrease the chance of forgetting a tablet and also help keep the proper amount of medication in your system. See detailed instructions below for LEVLEN™ 21 and LEVLEN™ 28 tablets.

LEVLEN™ 21 TABLETS (LEVONORGESTREL AND ETHINYL ESTRADIOL TABLETS)

The dosage of LEVLEN™ 21 tablets is one tablet daily for 21 days in a row per mentstrual cycle. Tablets are then discontinued for 7 days. The basic schedule is 21 days on—7 days off.

During the first month, you should begin taking LEVLEN™ 21 tablets on Day 5 of your menstrual cycle whether or not you still have your period. (Day 1 is the first day of menstruation, even if it is almost midnight when you start.) Note: During your first month on LEVLEN™ 21 tablets if you start taking tablets later than Day 5 of your menstrual cycle, you should protect yourself by also using another method of birth control until you have taken a tablet daily for seven consecutive days. Thereafter, if you follow directions carefully you will obtain the full contraceptive benefit. If you begin taking tablets later than the proper day, the possibility of ovulation and pregnancy occurring before beginning medication should be considered. Take one tablet every day until you finish all 21 tablets. No tablets are then taken for one week (7 days). Your period will usually begin about three days after you take the last tablet. Don't be alarmed if the amount of bleeding is not the same as before. On the 8th day, start a new SLIDECASE™ dispenser even if you still have your period. If, for example, you took LEVLEN™ 21 tablets for the first time on a Tuesday, the 8th day will also be a Tuesday. Thus, you will always begin a new cycle on the same day of the week as long as you do not interrupt your original schedule. If you start taking tablets later than the 8th day, you should protect yourself by also using another method of birth control until you have taken a tablet daily for seven days in a row.

LEVLEN™ 28 (LEVONORGESTREL AND ETHINYL ETRADIOL TABLETS)

The dosage of LEVLEN™ 28 tablets is one light-orange active tablet daily for 21 consecutive days followed by one pink inactive tablet daily for 7 consecutive days. The basic schedule is 21 days on light-orange active tablets—7 days on pink inactive tablets. Always take all 21 light-orange tablets in each SLIDECASE™ dispenser before taking the pink tablets.

You should begin taking LEVLEN™ 28 tablets on the first Sunday after your menstrual period begins, whether or not you are still bleeding. If your period begins on a Sunday, take your first tablet that very same day. Your first light-orange tablet is marked with the word "Start". Note: During the first month on LEVLEN™ 28 tablets, you should protect yourself by also using another method of birth control until you have taken a light-orange tablet daily for seven consecutive days. Thereafter, if you follow directions carefully, you will obtain the full contraceptive benefit. If you begin taking tablets later than the proper day, the possibility of ovulation and pregnancy occurring before beginning medication should be considered. Take one tablet every day until you finish all 21 light-orange tablets in a SLIDECASE™ dispenser, followed by all seven pink tablets. Your period will usually begin about three days after you take the last light-orange tablet, which will be during the time you are taking the pink tablets. Don't be alarmed if the amount of bleeding is not the same as before. The day after you have taken your last pink tablet, begin a new SLIDECASE™ dispenser of tablets (taking all 21 light-orange tablets first, just as you did before) so that you will take a tablet every day without interruption. The starting day for each new SLIDECASE™ dispenser will always be Sunday. If in any cycle you start tablets later than the proper day, you should also use another method of birth control until you have taken a light-orange tablet daily for 7 days in a row.

Spotting or Breakthrough Bleeding:

Spotting is slight staining between menstrual periods which may not even require a pad. Breakthrough bleeding is a flow much like a regular period, requiring sanitary protection. Spotting is more common than breakthrough bleeding, and both occur more often in the first few cycles than in later cycles. These types of bleeding are usually temporary and without significance. It is important to continue taking your pills on schedule. If the bleeding persists for more than a few days, consult your doctor.

Forgotten Pills:

LEVLEN™ 21 tablets contain 21 active light-orange tablets per SLIDECASE™ dispenser. LEVLEN™ 28 tablets contain 21 active light-orange tablets plus 7 pink inactive tablets per SLIDECASE™ dispenser.

The chance of becoming pregnant is probably quite small if you miss only one light-orange tablet in a cycle. Of course, with each additional one you skip, the chance increases. If you miss one or more pink tablets (LEVLEN™ 28 tablets), you are still protected against pregnancy as long as you begin taking your next light-orange tablet on the proper day. It is important to take a missed light-orange tablet as soon as it is remembered. If two consecutive light-orange tablets are missed they should both be taken as soon as remembered. The next tablet should then be taken at the usual time. Any time you miss one or two light-orange tablets, or begin a new SLIDECASE™ dispenser after the proper starting day, you should also use another method of birth control until you have taken a light-orange tablet daily for seven consecutive days. If breakthrough bleeding occurs following missed tablets, it will usually be temporary and of no consequence. While there is little likelihood of pregnancy occurring if only one or two light-orange tablets are missed, the possibility of pregnancy increases with each successive day that scheduled light-orange tablets are missed.

If you are taking LEVLEN™ 21 tablets and forget to take three light-orange tablets in a row, do not take them when you remember. Wait four more days—which makes a whole week without tablets. Then begin a new SLIDECASE™ dispenser on the 8th day after the last tablet was taken. During the seven days without tablets, and until you have taken a light-orange tablet daily for seven consecutive days, you should protect yourself from pregnancy by also using another method of birth control.

If you are taking LEVLEN™ 28 tablets and forget to take three light-orange tablets in a row, do not take them when you remember. Stop taking all medication until the first Sunday following the last missed tablet. Then, whether or not you have had your period, and even if you are still bleeding, start a new SLIDECASE™ dispenser. During the days without tablets, and until you have taken a light-orange tablet daily for seven consecutive days, you should protect yourself from pregnancy by also using another method of birth control.

At times there may be no menstrual period after a cycle of pills. Therefore, if you miss one menstrual period but have taken the pills *exactly as you were supposed to,* continue as usual into the next cycle. If you have not taken the pills correctly and miss a menstrual period, you may be pregnant and should stop taking oral contraceptives until your doctor determines whether or not you are pregnant. Until you can get to your doctor, use another form of contraception. If two consecutive menstrual periods are missed, you should stop taking pills until it is determined whether you are pregnant. If you do become pregnant while using oral contraceptives, you should discuss the risks to the developing child with your doctor.

3. Periodic Examination.

Your doctor will take a complete medical and family history before prescribing oral contraceptives. At that time and about once a year thereafter, he will generally examine your blood pressure, breasts, abdomen, and pelvic organs (including a Papanicolaou smear, i.e., test for cancer).

SUMMARY

Oral contraceptives are the most effective method, except sterilization, for preventing pregnancy. Other methods, when used conscientiously, are also very effective and have fewer risks. The serious risks of oral contraceptives are uncommon, and the "pill" is a very convenient method of preventing pregnancy. If you have certain conditions or have had these conditions in the past, you should not use oral contraceptives, because the risk is too great. These conditions are listed in the leaflet. If you do not have these conditions, and decide to use the "pill", please read the leaflet carefully so that you can use the "pill" most safely and effectively. Based on his or her assessment of your medical needs, your doctor has prescribed this drug for you. Do not give the drug to anyone else.

Manufactured for

BERLEX Laboratories, Inc., Wayne, NJ 07470

Issued December 30, 1985 60609-1

Shown in Product Identification Section, page 405

QUINAGLUTE® ℞

[*kwĭn 'uh-glōōt"*]

(quinidine gluconate)

DURA-TABS®

(sustained-release tablets)

DESCRIPTION

Each QUINAGLUTE® (brand of quinidine gluconate) DURA-TABS® (brand of sustained-release tablets) Tablet contains 324 mg quinidine gluconate (equivalent to 202 mg quinidine base) in a tablet matrix specially designed for the sustained-release (8 to 12 hours) of the drug in the gastrointestinal tract. QUINAGLUTE® DURA-TABS® Tablets are to be administered orally.

Quinidine gluconate is the gluconate salt of quinidine [6-methoxy-α-(5-vinyl-2-quinuclidinyl)-4-quinoline-methanol], a dextrorotatory isomer of quinine. Quinidine gluconate is represented by the following structural formula:

Quinidine gluconate contains 62.3% of the anhydrous quinidine alkaloid, whereas quinidine sulfate contains 82.86%. In prescribing QUINAGLUTE® DURA-TABS® Tablets, this factor should be considered.

Therapeutic category: Type I antiarrhythmic.

Each QUINAGLUTE® DURA-TABS® Tablet also contains the following inactive ingredients: confectioner's sugar, magnesium stearate, starch (corn), and other ingredient(s).

CLINICAL PHARMACOLOGY

The antiarrhythmic activity consists of the following basic actions:

1. In arrhythmias due to enhanced automaticity, quinidine decreases the rate of rise of slow diastolic (Phase 4) depolarization, thereby depressing automaticity, particularly in ectopic foci.
2. In addition to the above, quinidine slows depolarization, repolarization and amplitude of the action potential, thus increasing its duration leading to an increase in the refractoriness of atrial and ventricular tissue. Prolongation of the effective refractory period and an increase in conduction time may prevent the reentry phenomenon.
3. Quinidine exerts an indirect anticholinergic effect through blockade of vagal innervation. This anticholinergic effect may facilitate conduction in the atrioventricular junction.

Quinidine absorption from QUINAGLUTE® DURA-TABS® Tablets proceeds at a slower rate than the immediate-release products. In a single-dose pharmacokinetic study conducted in normal volunteers, the time of peak quinidine serum concentration was 1.6 hours for quinidine sulfate tablets and 3.6 hours for QUINAGLUTE® DURA-TABS® Tablets.

The apparent elimination half-life of quinidine ranges from 4 to 10 hours in healthy persons with a usual mean value of 6 to 7 hours. The half-life may be prolonged in elderly persons. From 60% to 80% of the dose is metabolized by the liver. Renal excretion of the intact drug comprises the remainder of the total clearance. Quinidine is approximately 75% bound to serum proteins.

In the past, plasma levels of 1.5 to 5 μg/mL have been reported as therapeutic,[1] based on non-specific assay methodology that quantitates quinidine metabolites as well as intact quinidine. The therapeutic plasma level range using newer, more specific assays has not been definitively established; however, effective reduction of premature ventricular contractions has been reported with blood levels less than 1.0 μg/mL.[2] In general, plasma quinidine levels are lower using specific assays. Clinicians requesting serum quinidine determinations should therefore also ask that the method of analysis be specified.

Due to the wide individual variation in response to quinidine therapy, the usefulness of serum quinidine levels in the planning of optimal quinidine therapy has not been clearly established. A serum quinidine concentration within the reported therapeutic range may not necessarily be the optimal concentration for some patients. In the absence of toxicity, such patients may warrant an increase in dose to achieve the desired therapeutic effect. However, for those patients in whom a high blood level has been achieved without significant therapeutic response, increasing the dose to potentially toxic levels is not warranted and consideration should be given to combination or alternate therapy. In all cases, the physician should carefully consider the patient response and evidence of toxicity along with blood levels in determining optimal quinidine therapy.

[1]Koch-Weser, Arch. Int. Med. 1972, 129:763-772.
[2]Carliner et al, Am. Heart Journ. 1980, 100:483-489.

INDICATIONS AND USAGE

QUINAGLUTE® DURA-TABS® Tablets are indicated in the prevention and/or treatment of:

1. Ventricular arrhythmias
   - Premature ventricular contractions
   - Ventricular tachycardia (when not associated with complete heartblock)
2. Junctional (nodal) arrhythmias
   - AV junctional premature complexes
   - Paroxysmal junctional tachycardia
3. Supraventricular (atrial) arrhythmias
   - Premature atrial contractions
   - Paroxysmal atrial tachycardia
   - Atrial flutter
   - Atrial fibrillation (chronic and paroxysmal)

CONTRAINDICATIONS

1. Idiosyncrasy or hypersensitivity to quinidine.
2. Complete AV block.
3. Complete bundle branch block or other severe intraventricular conduction defects, especially those exhibiting a marked grade of QRS widening.
4. Digitalis intoxication manifested by AV conduction disorders.
5. Myasthenia gravis.
6. Aberrant impulses and abnormal rhythms due to escape mechanisms.

WARNINGS

1. In the treatment of atrial flutter, reversion to sinus rhythm may be preceded by a progressive reduction in the degree of AV block to a 1:1 ratio resulting in an extremely rapid ventricular rate. This possible hazard may be reduced by digitalization prior to administration of quinidine.
2. Recent reports indicate that plasma concentrations of digoxin increase and may even double when quinidine is administered concurrently. Patients on concomitant therapy should be carefully monitored. Reduction of digoxin dosage may have to be considered.
3. Manifestations of quinidine cardiotoxicity such as excessive prolongation of the QT interval, widening of the QRS complex and ventricular tachyarrhythmias mandate immediate discontinuation of the drug and/or close clinical and electrocardiographic monitoring.
4. In susceptible individuals, such as those with marginally compensated cardiovascular disease, quinidine may produce clinically important depression of cardiac function such as hypotension, bradycardia, or heartblock. Quinidine therapy should be carefully monitored in such individuals.
5. Quinidine should be used with extreme caution in patients with incomplete AV block since complete block and asystole may be produced. Quinidine may cause abnormalities of cardiac rhythm in digitalized patients and therefore should be used with caution in the presence of digitalis intoxication.
6. Quinidine should be used with caution in patients exhibiting renal, cardiac or hepatic insufficiency because of potential accumulation of quinidine in plasma leading to toxicity.
7. Patients taking quinidine occasionally have syncopal episodes which usually result from ventricular tachycardia or fibrillation. This syndrome has not been shown to be related to dose or plasma levels. Syncopal episodes frequently terminate spontaneously or in response to treatment, but sometimes are fatal.
8. A few cases of hepatotoxicity, including granulomatous hepatitis, due to quinidine hypersensitivity have been reported in patients taking quinidine. Unexplained fever and/or elevation of hepatic enzymes, particularly in the early stages of therapy, warrant consideration of possible hepatotoxicity. Monitoring liver function during the first 4 to 8 weeks should be considered. Cessation of quinidine in these cases usually results in the disappearance of toxicity.

PRECAUTIONS

General: The precautions to be observed include all those applicable to quinidine. A preliminary test dose of a single tablet of quinidine sulfate may be administered to determine if the patient has an idiosyncrasy to quinidine. Hypersensitivity to quinidine, although rare, should constantly be considered, especially during the first weeks of therapy.

Continued on next page

Information on the Berlex products appearing here is based on the labeling in effect on August 1, 1986. Further information for these and other products may be obtained from the Professional Services Department, Berlex Laboratories, Inc., 110 East Hanover Avenue, Cedar Knolls, New Jersey 07927, telephone 201-292-3008.

Berlex—Cont.

Hospitalization for close clinical observation, electrocardiographic monitoring, and possible determination of plasma quinidine levels is indicated when large doses are used, or with patients who present an increased risk.

Information for Patients: As with all solid oral dosage medications, QUINAGLUTE® DURA-TABS® Tablets should be taken with an adequate amount of fluid, preferably in an upright position, to facilitate swallowing.

Drug Interactions:

Drug	*Effect*
Quinidine with anticholinergic drugs	Additive vagolytic effect
Quinidine with cholinergic drugs	Antagonism of cholinergic effects
Quinidine with carbonic anhydrase inhibitors, sodium bicarbonate, thiazide diuretics	Alkalinization of urine resulting in decreased excretion of quinidine
Quinidine with coumarin anticoagulants	Reduction of clotting factor concentrations
Quinidine with tubocurare, succinylcholine and decamethonium	Potentiation of neuromuscular blockade
Quinidine with phenothiazines and reserpine	Additive cardiac depressive effects
Quinidine with hepatic enzyme-inducing drugs (phenobarbital, phenytoin, rifampin)	Potential for reduction of quinidine plasma levels
Quinidine with cimetidine	Potential for elevation of quinidine plasma levels
Quinidine with digoxin	Increased plasma concentrations of digoxin (See WARNINGS)

Carcinogenesis, Mutagenesis and Impairment of Fertility: Long-term studies in animals have not been performed to evaluate the carcinogenic potential of quinidine. There is currently no evidence of quinidine-induced mutagenesis or impairment of fertility.

Pregnancy: Teratogenic Effects: Pregnancy Category C. Animal reproduction studies have not been conducted with quinidine. There are no adequate and well-controlled studies in pregnant women. QUINAGLUTE® DURA-TABS® Tablets should be administered to a pregnant woman only if clearly indicated.

Nonteratogenic Effects: Like quinine, quinidine has been reported to have oxytocic properties. The significance of this property in the clinical setting has not been established.

Nursing Mothers: Because of passage of the drug into breast milk, caution should be exercised when QUINAGLUTE® DURA-TABS® Tablets are administered to a nursing woman.

Pediatric Use: There are no adequate and well-controlled studies establishing the safety and effectiveness of QUINAGLUTE® DURA-TABS® Tablets in children.

ADVERSE REACTIONS

Symptoms of cinchonism, ringing in ears, headache, nausea, and/or disturbed vision may appear in sensitive patients after a single dose of the drug.

The most frequently encountered side effects to quinidine are gastrointestinal in nature. These gastrointestinal effects include nausea, vomiting, abdominal pain and diarrhea.

Less frequently encountered adverse reactions:

Cardiovascular: Widening of QRS complex, cardiac asystole, ventricular ectopic beats, idioventricular rhythms including ventricular tachycardia and fibrillation, paradoxical tachycardia, arterial embolism and hypotension.

Hematologic: Acute hemolytic anemia, hypoprothrombinemia, thrombocytopenia (purpura), agranulocytosis.

Central Nervous System: Headache, fever, vertigo, apprehension, excitement, confusion, delirium and syncope, disturbed hearing (tinnitus, decreased auditory acuity), disturbed vision (mydriasis, blurred vision, disturbed color perception, reduced vision field, photophobia, diplopia, night blindness, scotomata), optic neuritis.

Dermatologic: Rash, cutaneous flushing with intense pruritus, urticaria. Photosensitivity has also been reported.

Hypersensitivity Reactions: Angioedema, acute asthmatic episode, vascular collapse, respiratory arrest, hepatotoxicity including granulomatous hepatitis (See WARNINGS).

Although rare, there have been reports of lupus erythematosus in patients taking quinidine.

OVERDOSAGE

If ingestion of quinidine is recent, gastric lavage, emesis and / or administration of activated charcoal may reduce absorption. Management of overdosage includes symptomatic treatment, ECG and blood pressure monitoring, cardiac pacing if indicated, and acidification of the urine. Artificial respiration and other supportive measures may be required. IV infusion of 1/6 molar sodium lactate reportedly reduces the cardiotoxic effects of quinidine. Since marked CNS depression may occur even in the presence of convulsions, CNS depressants should not be administered. Hypotension may be treated, if necessary, with metaraminol or norepinephrine after adequate fluid volume replacement. Hemodialysis has been reported to be effective in the treatment of quinidine overdosage in adults and children, but is rarely warranted.

DOSAGE AND ADMINISTRATION

The dosage varies considerably depending upon the general condition and cardiovascular state of the patient. The quantity and frequency of administration of QUINAGLUTE® DURA-TABS® Tablets that will achieve the desired clinical results must be determined for each patient.

The ideal dosage is the minimum amount of total dose and frequency of daily administration that will prevent premature contractions, paroxysmal tachycardias and maintain normal sinus rhythm.

Prevention of premature atrial, nodal or ventricular contractions:

1 to 2 tablets every 8 or 12 hours.

Maintenance of normal sinus rhythm following conversion of paroxysmal tachycardias:

2 tablets every 12 hours or 1 1/2 to 2 tablets every 8 hours are usually required.

Although most patients may be maintained in normal rhythm on a dosage of 1 QUINAGLUTE® DURA-TABS Tablet every 8 or 12 hours; other patients may require larger doses or more frequent administration (ie every 6 hours) than the usually recommended schedule. Such increased dosage should be instituted only after careful clinical and laboratory evaluation of the patient, including monitoring of plasma quinidine levels and, if possible, serial electrocardiograms.

QUINAGLUTE® DURA-TABS® Tablets are generally well tolerated. Gastrointestinal disturbances, if they occur, may be minimized by administering the drug with food.

It is frequently desirable to determine if a patient can tolerate maintenance quinidine therapy prior to electrical conversion. Therefore, maintenance therapy may be initiated 2 to 3 days before electrical conversion is attempted. QUINAGLUTE® DURA-TABS® Tablets are well suited for such a program and can be administered at a maintenance dose felt necessary for a given patient as indicated above.

Note: Dosage may be titrated by breaking the tablet in half. Do not crush or chew since sustained-release properties will be lost.

HOW SUPPLIED

White to off-white round tablet imprinted with:

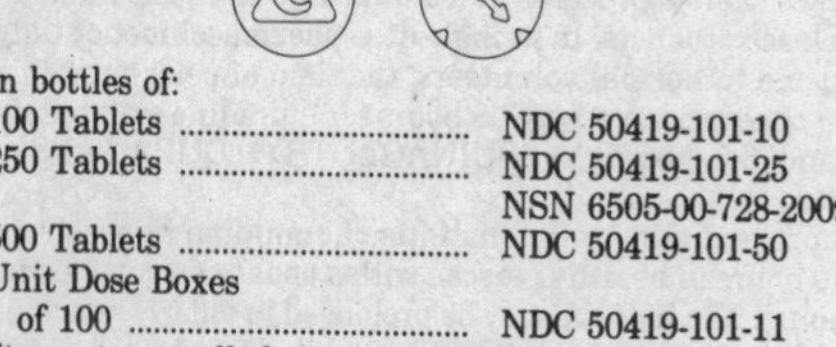

In bottles of:

100 Tablets	NDC 50419-101-10
250 Tablets	NDC 50419-101-25
	NSN 6505-00-728-2009
500 Tablets	NDC 50419-101-50
Unit Dose Boxes of 100	NDC 50419-101-11

Store at controlled room temperature.

Tablet designs are registered trademarks of Berlex Laboratories, Inc.

Shown in Product Identification Section, page 405

TRI-LEVLEN™ 21 ℞

[trī-lĕvlĕn]

Tablets

(levonorgestrel and ethinyl estradiol tablets—triphasic regimen)

TRI-LEVLEN™ 28 ℞

[trī-lĕvlĕn]

Tablets

(levonorgestrel and ethinyl estradiol tablets—triphasic regimen)

DESCRIPTION

TRI-LEVLEN™ 21 tablets

Each cycle of TRI-LEVLEN™ 21 (Levonorgestrel and Ethinyl Estradiol Tablets—Triphasic Regimen) tablets consists of three different drug phases as follows: Phase 1 comprised of 6 brown tablets, each containing 0.050 mg of levonorgestrel (d(-)-13 beta-ethyl-17-alpha-ethinyl-17-beta-hydroxygon-4-en-3-one), a totally synthetic progestogen, and 0.030 mg of ethinyl estradiol (19-nor-17α-pregna-1,3,5(10)-trien-20-yne-3,17-diol); phase 2 comprised of 5 white tablets, each containing 0.075 mg levonorgestrel and 0.040 mg ethinyl estradiol; and, phase 3 comprised of 10 light-yellow tablets, each containing 0.125 mg levonorgestrel and 0.030 mg ethinyl estradiol. The inactive ingredients present are calcium carbonate, glycerin, iron oxides, lactose, magnesium stearate, methylparaben, polyethylene glycol, povidone, propylparaben, sodium benzoate, starch, sucrose, talc, and titanium dioxide.

TRI-LEVLEN™ 28 tablets

Each cycle of TRI-LEVLEN™ 28 (Levonorgestrel and Ethinyl Estradiol Tablets—Triphasic Regimen) tablets consists of three different drug phases as follows: Phase 1 comprised of 6 brown tablets, each containing 0.050 mg of levonorgestrel (d(-)-13 beta-ethyl-17-alpha-ethinyl-17-beta-hydroxygon-4-en-3-one), a totally synthetic progestogen, and 0.030 mg of ethinyl estradiol (19-nor-17 α-pregna-1,3,5(10)-trien-20-yne-3, 17-diol); phase 2 comprised of 5 white tablets, each containing 0.075 mg levonorgestrel and 0.040 mg ethinyl estradiol; and phase 3 comprised of 10 light-yellow tablets, each containing 0.125 mg levonorgestrel and 0.030 mg ethinyl estradiol; then followed by 7 light-green inert tablets. The inactive ingredients present are calcium carbonate, cellulose, FD&C Blue 1, glycerin, iron oxides, lactose, magnesium stearate, methylparaben, polyethylene glycol, povidone, propylparaben, sodium benzoate, starch, sucrose, talc, and titanium dioxide.

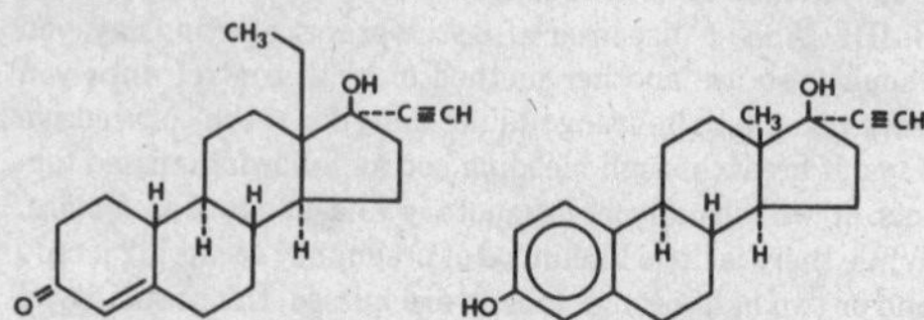

Levonorgestrel Ethinyl Estradiol

CLINICAL PHARMACOLOGY

Combination oral contraceptives act primarily through the mechanism of gonadotropin suppression due to the estrogenic and progestational activity of the ingredients. Although the primary mechanism of action is inhibition of ovulation, alterations in the genital tract, including changes in the cervical mucus (which increase the difficulty of sperm penetration) and the endometrium (which reduce the likelihood of implantation), may also contribute to contraceptive effectiveness.

INDICATIONS AND USAGE

TRI-LEVLEN™ tablets are indicated for the prevention of pregnancy in women who elect to use oral contraceptives as a method of contraception. Oral contraceptives are highly effective. The pregnancy rate in women using conventional combination oral contraceptives (containing 35 mcg or more of ethinyl estradiol or 50 mcg or more of mestranol) is generally reported as less than one pregnancy per 100 woman-years of use. Slightly higher rates (somewhat more than 1 pregnancy per 100 woman-years of use) are reported for some combination products containing 35 mcg or less of ethinyl estradiol, and rates on the order of 3 pregnancies per 100 woman-years are reported for the progestogen-only oral contraceptives.

These rates are derived from separate studies conducted by different investigators in several population groups and cannot be compared precisely. Furthermore, pregnancy rates tend to be lower as clinical studies are continued, possibly due to selective retention in the longer studies of those patients who accept the treatment regimen and do not discontinue as a result of adverse reactions, pregnancy, or other reasons.

In clinical trials with TRI-LEVLEN™ tablets, 3,546 patients completed 35,036 cycles, and a total of nine pregnancies were reported. This represents a pregnancy rate of 0.33 per 100 woman-years. When used as directed, two pregnancies resulted for a corrected pregnancy rate of 0.07 per 100 woman-years.

Table 1 gives ranges of pregnancy rates reported in the literature[1] for other means of contraception. The efficacy of these means of contraception (except the IUD) depends upon the degree of adherence to the method.

TABLE 1

PREGNANCIES PER 100 WOMAN-YEARS

IUD, less than 1–6; Diaphragm with spermicidal products (creams or jellies), 2–20; Condom, 3–36; Aerosol foams, 2–29; Jellies and creams, 4–36; Periodic abstinence (rhythm) all types, less than 1–47:

1. Calendar method, 14–47;
2. Temperature method, 1–20;
3. Temperature method—intercourse only in postovulatory phase, less than 1–7;
4. Mucus method, 1–25;

No contraception, 60–80.

Dose-Related Risk of Thromboembolism from Oral Contraceptives: Two studies have shown a positive association between the dose of estrogens in oral contraceptives and the risk of thromboembolism.[2,3] For this reason, it is prudent and in keeping with good principles of therapeutics to minimize exposure to estrogen. The oral-contraceptive product prescribed for any given patient should be that product which contains the least amount of estrogen that is compatible with an acceptable pregnancy rate and patient acceptance. It is recommended that new acceptors of oral contraceptives be started on preparations containing 0.05 mg or less of estrogen.

CONTRAINDICATIONS

Oral contraceptives should not be used in women with any of the following conditions:

1. Thrombophlebitis or thromboembolic disorders.
2. A past history of deep-vein thrombophlebitis or thromboembolic disorders.
3. Cerebral-vascular or coronary-artery disease.
4. Known or suspected carcinoma of the breast.
5. Known or suspected estrogen-dependent neoplasia.
6. Undiagnosed abnormal genital bleeding.
7. Known or suspected pregnancy (see Warning No. 5).
8. Benign or malignant liver tumor which developed during the use of oral contraceptives or other estrogen-containing products.

WARNINGS

Cigarette smoking increases the risk of serious cardiovascular side effects from oral-contraceptive use. This risk increases with age and with heavy smoking (15 or more cigarettes per day) and is quite marked in women over 35 years of age. Women who use oral contraceptives should be strongly advised not to smoke.

The use of oral contraceptives is associated with increased risk of several serious conditions, including thromboembolism, stroke, myocardial infarction, hepatic adenoma, gallbladder disease, hypertension. Practitioners prescribing oral contraceptives should be familiar with the following information relating to these risks.

1. *Thromboembolic Disorders and Other Vascular Problems:* An increased risk of thromboembolic and thrombotic disease associated with the use of oral contraceptives is well-established. Three principal studies in Great Britain[4–6] and three in the United States[7–10] have demonstrated an increased risk of fatal and nonfatal venous thromboembolism and stroke, both hemorrhagic and thrombotic. These studies estimate that users of oral contraceptives are 4 to 11 times more likely than nonusers to develop these diseases without evident cause (Table 2).

CEREBROVASCULAR DISORDERS

In a collaborative American study[9,10] of cerebrovascular disorders in women with and without predisposing causes, it was estimated that the risk of hemorrhagic stroke was 2.0 times greater in users than nonusers and the risk of thrombotic stroke was 4 to 9.5 times greater in users than in nonusers (Table 2).

TABLE 2
SUMMARY OF RELATIVE RISK OF THROMBOEMBOLIC DISORDERS AND OTHER VASCULAR PROBLEMS IN ORAL-CONTRACEPTIVE USERS COMPARED TO NONUSERS

	Relative risk, times greater
Idiopathic thromboembolic disease	4–11
Postsurgery thromboembolic complications	4–6
Thrombotic stroke	4–9.5
Hemorrhagic stroke	2
Myocardial infarction	2–12

MYOCARDIAL INFARCTION

An increased risk of myocardial infarction associated with the use of oral contraceptives has been reported,[11–13] confirming a previously suspected association. These studies, conducted in the United Kingdom, found, as expected, that the greater the number of underlying risk factors for coronary-artery disease (cigarette smoking, hypertension, hypercholesterolemia, obesity, diabetes, history of preeclamptic toxemia) the higher the risk of developing myocardial infarction, regardless of whether the patient was an oral-contraceptive user or not. Oral contraceptives, however, were found to be a clear additional risk factor.

In terms of relative risk, it has been estimated[52] that oral-contraceptive users who do not smoke (smoking is considered a major predisposing condition to myocardial infarction) are about twice as likely to have a fatal myocardial infarction as nonusers who do not smoke. Oral-contraceptive users who are also smokers have about a 5-fold increased risk of fatal infarction compared to users who do not smoke, but about a 10- to 12-fold increased risk compared to nonusers who do not smoke. Furthermore, the amount of smoking is also an important factor. In determining the importance of these relative risks, however, the baseline rates for various age groups, as shown in Table 3, must be given serious consideration. The importance of other predisposing conditions mentioned above in determining relative and absolute risks has not as yet been quantified; it is quite likely that the same synergistic action exists, but perhaps to a lesser extent.

TABLE 3
Estimated annual mortality rate per 100,000 women from myocardial infarction by use of oral contraceptives, smoking habits, and age (in years):

	Myocardial infarction			
	Women aged 30–39		Women aged 40–44	
Smoking habits	Users	Non-users	Users	Non-users
All smokers	10.2	2.6	62.0	15.9
Heavy*	13.0	5.1	78.7	31.3
Light	4.7	0.9	28.6	5.7
Nonsmokers	1.8	1.2	10.7	7.4
Smokers and nonsmokers	5.4	1.9	32.8	11.7

*Heavy smoker: 15 or more cigarettes per day.
From JAIN, A.K., *Studies in Family Planning, 8*:50, 1977.

RISK OF DOSE

In an analysis of data derived from several national adverse-reaction reporting systems,[2] British investigators concluded that the risk of thromboembolism, including coronary thrombosis, is directly related to the dose of estrogen used in oral contraceptives. Preparations containing 100 mcg or more of estrogen were associated with a higher risk of thromboembolism than those containing 50–80 mcg of estrogen. Their analysis did suggest, however, that the quantity of estrogen may not be the sole factor involved. This finding has been confirmed in the United States.[3] Careful epidemiological studies to determine the degree of thromboembolic risk associated with progestogen-only oral contraceptives have not been performed. Cases of thromboembolic disease have been reported in women using these products, and they should not be presumed to be free of excess risk.

ESTIMATE OF EXCESS MORTALITY FROM CIRCULATORY DISEASES

A large prospective study[53] carried out in the U.K. estimated the mortality rate per 100,000 women per year from diseases of the circulatory system for users and nonusers of oral contraceptives according to age, smoking habits, and duration of use. The overall excess death rate annually from circulatory diseases for oral-contraceptive users was estimated to be 20 per 100,000 (ages 15–34—5/100,000; ages 35–44—33/100,000; ages 45–49—140/100,000), the risk being concentrated in older women, in those with a long duration of use, and in cigarette smokers. It was not possible, however, to examine the interrelationships of age, smoking, and duration of use, nor to compare the effects of continuous vs. intermittent use. Although the study showed a 10-fold increase in death due to circulatory diseases in users for 5 or more years, all of these deaths occurred in women 35 or older. Until larger numbers of women under 35 with continuous use for 5 or more years are available, it is not possible to assess the magnitude of the relative risk for this younger age group.

Figure 1. Estimated annual number of deaths associated with control of fertility and no control per 100,000 non-sterile women, by regimen of control and age of women.

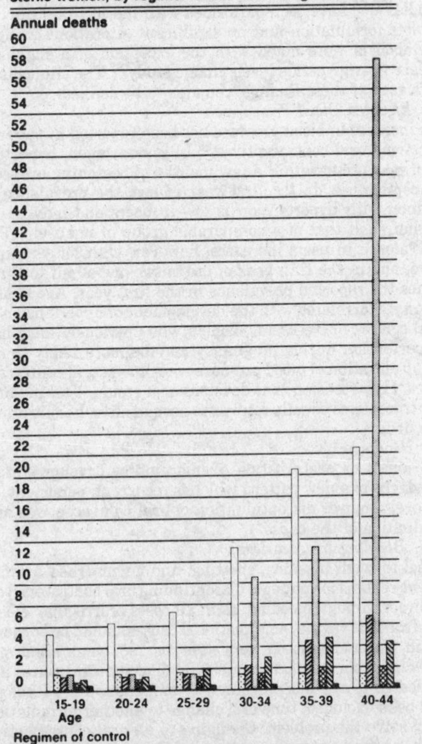

The available data from a variety of sources have been analyzed[14] to estimate the risk of death associated with various methods of contraception. The estimates of risk of death for each method include the combined risk of the contraceptive method (e.g., thromboembolic and thrombotic disease in the case of oral contraceptives) plus the risk attributable to pregnancy or abortion in the event of method failure. This latter risk varies with the effectiveness of the contraceptive method. The findings of this analysis are shown in the bar graph (Figure 1).[14] The study concluded that the mortality associated with all methods of birth control is low and below that associated with childbirth, with the exception of oral contraceptives in women over 40 who smoke. (The rates given for Pill only/smokers for each age group are for smokers as a class. For "heavy" smokers [more than 15 cigarettes a day], the rates given would be about double; for "light" smokers [less than 15 cigarettes a day], about 50 percent.) The lowest mortality is associated with the condom or diaphragm backed up by early abortion. The risk of thromboembolic and thrombotic disease associated with oral contraceptives increases with age after approximately age 30 and, for myocardial infarction, is further increased by hypertension, hypercholesterolemia, obesity, diabetes, or history of preeclamptic toxemia and, especially, by cigarette smoking.

Based on the data currently available, the following chart gives a gross estimate of the risk of death from circulatory disorders associated with the use of oral contraceptives:

SMOKING HABITS AND OTHER PREDISPOSING CONDITIONS—RISK ASSOCIATED WITH USE OF ORAL CONTRACEPTIVES

Age	Below 30	30–39	40+
Heavy smokers	C	B	A
Light smokers	D	C	B
Nonsmokers (no predisposing conditions)	D	C, D	C
Nonsmokers (other predisposing conditions)	C	C, B	B, A

A—Use associated with very high risk.
B—Use associated with high risk.
C—Use associated with moderate risk.
D—Use associated with low risk.

The physician and the patient should be alert to the earliest manifestations of thromboembolic and thrombotic disorders (e.g., thrombophlebitis, pulmonary embolism, cerebrovascular insufficiency, coronary occlusion, retinal thrombosis, and mesenteric thrombosis). Should any of these occur or be suspected, the drug should be discontinued immediately.

A four- to six-fold increased risk of postsurgery thromboembolic complications has been reported in oral-contraceptive users.[15,16] If feasible, oral contraceptives should be discontinued at least 4 weeks before surgery of a type associated with an increased risk of thromboembolism or prolonged immobilization.

PERSISTENCE OF RISK OF VASCULAR DISORDERS

Findings from one study in Great Britain involving cerebrovascular disease[54] and another study in the United States concerning myocardial infarction[55] suggest that an increased risk of these conditions in users of oral contraceptives persists after discontinuation of the oral contraceptive. In the British study, the risk of cerebrovascular disease remained elevated in former oral-contraceptive users for at least six years after discontinuation. In the U.S. study, an increased risk of myocardial infarction persisted for at least 9 years in women 40- to 49-years-old who had used oral contraceptives for five or more years. The findings in both these studies require confirmation since they are inconsistent with other published information.[9,11,13,56–60]

2. *Ocular Lesions:*

There have been reports of neuro-ocular lesions such as optic neuritis or retinal thrombosis associated with the use of oral contraceptives. Discontinue oral-contraceptive medication if

Continued on next page

Information on the Berlex products appearing here is based on the labeling in effect on August 1, 1986. Further information on these and other products may be obtained from the Professional Services Department, Berlex Laboratories, Inc., 110 East Hanover Avenue, Cedar Knolls, New Jersey 07927, telephone 201-292-3008.

Berlex—Cont.

there is unexplained, sudden or gradual, partial or complete loss of vision; onset of proptosis or diplopia; papilledema; or retinal-vascular lesions, and institute appropriate diagnostic and therapeutic measures.

3. *Carcinoma:*

Long-term continuous administration of either natural or synthetic estrogen in certain animal species increases the frequency of carcinoma of the breast, cervix, vagina, and liver. Certain synthetic progestogens, none currently contained in oral contraceptives, have been noted to increase the incidence of mammary nodules, benign and malignant, in dogs.

In humans, three case-control studies have reported an increased risk of endometrial carcinoma associated with the prolonged use of exogenous estrogen in postmenopausal women.[17–19] One publication[20] reported on the first 21 cases submitted by physicians to a registry of cases of adenocarcinoma of the endometrium in women under 40 on oral contraceptives. Of the cases found in women without predisposing risk factors for adenocarcinoma of the endometrium (e.g., irregular bleeding at the time oral contraceptives were first given, polycystic ovaries), nearly all occurred in women who had used a sequential oral contraceptive. These products are no longer marketed. No evidence has been reported suggesting an increased risk of endometrial cancer in users of conventional combination or progestogen-only oral contraceptives.

Several studies[8,21–24] have found no increase in breast cancer in women taking oral contraceptives or estrogens. One study,[25] however, while also noting no overall increased risk of breast cancer in women treated with oral contraceptives, found an excess risk in the subgroups of oral-contraceptive users with documented benign breast disease. A reduced occurrence of benign breast tumors in users of oral contraceptives has been well-documented.[8,21,25–27]

In summary, there is at present no confirmed evidence from human studies of an increased risk of cancer associated with oral contraceptives. Close clinical surveillance of all women taking oral contraceptives is, nevertheless, essential. In all cases of undiagnosed persistent or recurrent abnormal vaginal bleeding, appropriate diagnostic measures should be taken to rule out malignancy. Women with a strong family history of breast cancer or who have breast nodules, fibrocystic disease, or abnormal mammograms should be monitored with particular care if they elect to use oral contraceptives instead of other methods of contraception.

4. *Hepatic Tumors:*

Benign hepatic adenomas have been found to be associated with the use of oral contraceptives.[28–30,46] One study[46] showed that oral contraceptive formulations with high hormonal potency were associated with a higher risk than lower potency formulations. Although benign, hepatic adenomas may rupture and may cause death through intra-abdominal hemorrhage. This has been reported in short-term as well as long-term users of oral contraceptives. Two studies relate risk with duration of use of the contraceptive, the risk being much greater after 4 or more years of oral-contraceptive use.[30,46] While hepatic adenoma is a rare lesion, it should be considered in women presenting abdominal pain and tenderness, abdominal mass or shock. A few cases of hepatocellular carcinoma have been reported in women taking oral contraceptives. The relationship of these drugs to this type of malignancy is not known at this time.

5. *Use in or Immediately Preceding Pregnancy, Birth Defects in Offspring, and Malignancy in Female Offspring:*

The use of female sex hormones—both estrogenic and progestational agents—during early pregnancy may seriously damage the offspring. It has been shown that females exposed in utero to diethylstilbestrol, a non-steroidal estrogen, have an increased risk of developing in later life a form of vaginal or cervical cancer that is ordinarily extremely rare.[31,32] This risk has been estimated to be of the order of 1 in 1,000 exposures or less.[33,47] Although there is no evidence at the present time that oral contraceptives further enhance the risk of developing this type of malignancy, such patients should be monitored with particular care if they elect to use oral contraceptives instead of other methods of contraception. Furthermore, a high percentage of such exposed women (from 30 to 90%) have been found to have epithelial changes of the vagina and cervix.[34–38] Although these changes are histologically benign, it is not known whether this condition is a precursor of vaginal malignancy. Male children so exposed may develop abnormalities of the urogenital tract.[48–50] Although similar data are not available with the use of other estrogens, it cannot be presumed that they would not induce similar changes. An increased risk of congenital anomalies, including heart defects and limb defects, has been reported with the use of sex hormones, including oral contraceptives, in pregnancy.[39–42,51] One case-control study[42] has estimated a 4.7-fold increase in risk of limb-reduction defects in infants exposed in utero to sex hormones (oral contraceptives, hormonal withdrawal tests for pregnancy, or attempted treatment for threatened abortion). Some of these exposures were very short and involved only a few days of treatment. The data suggest that the risk of limb-reduction defects in exposed fetuses is somewhat less than one in 1,000 live births.

In the past, female sex hormones have been used during pregnancy in an attempt to treat threatened or habitual abortion. There is considerable evidence that estrogens are ineffective for these indications, and there is no evidence from well-controlled studies that progestogens are effective for these uses.

There is some evidence that triploidy and possibly other types of polyploidy are increased among abortuses from women who become pregnant soon after ceasing oral contraceptives.[43] Embryos with these anomalies are virtually always aborted spontaneously. Whether there is an overall increase in spontaneous abortion of pregnancies conceived soon after stopping oral contraceptives is unknown. It is recommended that, for any patient who has missed two consecutive periods, pregnancy should be ruled out before continuing the contraceptive regimen. If the patient has not adhered to the prescribed schedule, the possibility of pregnancy should be considered at the time of the first missed period (or after 45 days from the last menstrual period if the progestogen-only oral contraceptives are used), and further use of oral contraceptives should be withheld until pregnancy has been ruled out. If pregnancy is confirmed, the patient should be apprised of the potential risks to the fetus, and the advisability of continuation of the pregnancy should be discussed in the light of these risks.

It is also recommended that women who discontinue oral contraceptives with the intent of becoming pregnant use an alternate form of contraception for a period of time before attempting to conceive. Many clinicians recommend 3 months, although no precise information is available on which to base this recommendation.

The administration of progestogen-only or progestogen-estrogen combinations to induce withdrawal bleeding should not be used as a test of pregnancy.

6. *Gallbladder Disease:*

Studies[8,23,26] report an increased risk of surgically confirmed gallbladder disease in users of oral contraceptives and estrogens. In one study, an increased risk appeared after 2 years of use and doubled after 4 or 5 years of use. In one of the other studies, an increased risk was apparent between 6 and 12 months of use.

7. *Carbohydrate and Lipid Metabolic Effects:*

A decrease in glucose tolerance has been observed in a significant percentage of patients on oral contraceptives. For this reason, prediabetic and diabetic patients should be carefully observed while receiving oral contraceptives.

An increase in triglycerides and total phospholipids has been observed in patients receiving oral contraceptives.[44] Three studies[61–63] have been performed with the TRI-LEVLEN™ tablets formulation and no significant alterations in lipid metabolism were noted with the exception of a slight increase in triglyceride levels in one study.[62] The clinical significance of these findings remains to be defined.

8. *Elevated Blood Pressure:*

An increase in blood pressure has been reported in patients receiving oral contraceptives.[26] In some women, hypertension may occur within a few months of beginning oral-contraceptive use. In the first year of use, the prevalence of women with hypertension is low in users and may be no higher than that of a comparable group of nonusers. The prevalence in users increases, however, with longer exposure, and in the fifth year of use is two-and-a-half to three times the reported prevalence in the first year. Age is also strongly correlated with the development of hypertension in oral-contraceptive users. Women who previously have had hypertension during pregnancy may be more likely to develop elevation of blood pressure when given oral contraceptives. Hypertension that develops as a result of taking oral contraceptives usually returns to normal after discontinuing the drug.

9. *Headache:*

The onset or exacerbation of migraine or development of headache of a new pattern which is recurrent, persistent, or severe, requires discontinuation of oral contraceptives and evaluation of the cause.

10. *Bleeding Irregularities:*

Breakthrough bleeding, spotting, and amenorrhea are frequent reasons for patients discontinuing oral contraceptives. In breakthrough bleeding, as in all cases of irregular bleeding from the vagina, nonfunctional causes should be borne in mind. In undiagnosed persistent or recurrent abnormal bleeding from the vagina, adequate diagnostic measures are indicated to rule out pregnancy or malignancy. If pathology has been excluded, time or a change to another formulation may solve the problem. Changing to an oral contraceptive with a higher estrogen content, while potentially useful in minimizing menstrual irregularity, should be done only if necessary, since this may increase the risk of thromboembolic disease.

Women with a past history of oligomenorrhea or secondary amenorrhea or young women without regular cycles may have a tendency to remain anovulatory or to become amenorrheic after discontinuation of oral contraceptives. Women with these preexisting problems should be advised of this possibility and encouraged to use other contraceptive methods. Post-use anovulation, possibly prolonged, may also occur in women without previous irregularities.

11. *Ectopic Pregnancy:*

Ectopic as well as intrauterine pregnancy may occur in contraceptive failures. However, in progestogen-only oral contraceptive failures, the ratio of ectopic to intrauterine pregnancies is higher than in women who are not receiving oral contraceptives, since the drugs are more effective in preventing intrauterine than ectopic pregnancies.

12. *Breast-feeding:*

Oral contraceptives given in the postpartum period may interfere with lactation. There may be a decrease in the quantity and quality of the breast milk. Furthermore, a small fraction of the hormonal agents in oral contraceptives has been identified in the milk of mothers receiving these drugs.[45,64,65] The effects, if any, on the breast-fed child have not been determined. If feasible, the use of oral contraceptives should be deferred until the infant has been weaned.

PRECAUTIONS

GENERAL

1. A complete medical and family history should be taken prior to initiation of oral contraceptives. The pretreatment and periodic physical examinations should include special reference to blood pressure, breasts, abdomen and pelvic organs, including Papanicolaou smear and relevant laboratory tests. As a general rule, oral contraceptives should not be prescribed for longer than 1 year without another physical examination and PAP smear being performed.
2. Under the influence of estrogen-progestogen preparations, preexisting uterine leiomyomata may increase in size.
3. Patients with a history of psychic depression should be carefully observed and the drug discontinued if depression recurs to a serious degree. Patients becoming significantly depressed while taking oral contraceptives should stop the medication and use an alternate method of contraception in an attempt to determine whether the symptom is drug-related.
4. Oral contraceptives may cause some degree of fluid retention. They should be prescribed with caution, and only with careful monitoring, in patients with conditions which might be aggravated by fluid retention, such as convulsive disorders, migraine syndrome, asthma, or cardiac or renal insufficiency.
5. Patients with a past history of jaundice during pregnancy have an increased risk of recurrence of jaundice while receiving oral-contraceptive therapy. If jaundice develops in any patient receiving such drugs, the medication should be discontinued.
6. Steroid hormones may be poorly metabolized in patients with impaired liver function and should be administered with caution in such patients.
7. Oral-contraceptive users may have disturbances in normal tryptophan metabolism which may result in a relative pyridoxine deficiency. The clinical significance of this is yet to be determined.
8. Serum folate levels may be depressed by oral-contraceptive therapy. Since the pregnant woman is predisposed to the development of folate deficiency and the incidence of folate deficiency increases with increasing gestation, it is possible that if a woman becomes pregnant shortly after stopping oral contraceptives, she may have a greater chance of developing folate deficiency and complications attributed to this deficiency.
9. The pathologist should be advised of oral-contraceptive therapy when relevant specimens are submitted.
10. Certain endocrine- and liver-function tests and blood components may be affected by estrogen-containing oral contraceptives:

a. Increased sulfobromophthalein retention.
b. Increased prothrombin and factors VII, VIII, IX, and X; decreased antithrombin 3; increased norepinephrine-induced platelet aggregability.
c. Increased thyroid-binding globulin (TBG) leading to increased circulating total-thyroid hormone, as measured by protein-bound iodine (PBI), T4 by column, or T4 by radioimmunoassay. Free T3 resin uptake is decreased, reflecting the elevated TBG; free T4 concentration is unaltered.
d. Decreased pregnanediol excretion.
e. Reduced response to metyrapone test.

INFORMATION FOR THE PATIENT

(See patient labeling which follows.)

DRUG INTERACTIONS

Reduced efficacy and increased incidence of breakthrough bleeding have been associated with concomitant use of rifampin. A similar association has been suggested with barbiturates, phenylbutazone, phenytoin sodium, ampicillin, and tetracycline.

CARCINOGENESIS

See "Warnings" section for information on the carcinogenic potential of oral contraceptives.

PREGNANCY

Pregnancy Category X. See "Contraindications" and "Warnings."

NURSING MOTHERS

See "Warnings."

ADVERSE REACTIONS

An increased risk of the following serious adverse reactions has been associated with the use of oral contraceptives (see "Warnings"):

Thrombophlebitis.
Pulmonary embolism.
Coronary thrombosis.
Cerebral thrombosis.
Cerebral hemorrhage.
Hypertension.
Gallbladder disease.
Benign hepatomas.
Congenital anomalies.

There is evidence of an association between the following conditions and the use of oral contraceptives, although additional confirmatory studies are needed:

Mesenteric thrombosis.
Neuro-ocular lesions, e.g., retinal thrombosis and optic neuritis.

The following adverse reactions have been reported in patients receiving oral contraceptives and are believed to be drug-related:

Nausea and/or vomiting, usually the most common adverse reactions, occur in approximately 10 percent or less of patients during the first cycle. Other reactions, as a general rule, are seen much less frequently or only occasionally.
Gastrointestinal symptoms (such as abdominal cramps and bloating).
Breakthrough bleeding.
Spotting.
Change in menstrual flow.
Dysmenorrhea.
Amenorrhea during and after treatment.
Temporary infertility after discontinuance of treatment.
Edema.
Chloasma or melasma which may persist.
Breast changes: tenderness, enlargement, and secretion.
Change in weight (increase or decrease).
Change in cervical erosion and cervical secretion.
Possible diminution in lactation when given immediately postpartum.
Cholestatic jaundice.
Migraine.
Increase in size of uterine leiomyomata.
Rash (allergic).
Mental depression.
Reduced tolerance to carbohydrates.
Vaginal candidiasis.
Change in corneal curvature (steepening).
Intolerance to contact lenses.

The following adverse reactions have been reported in users of oral contraceptives, and the association has been neither confirmed nor refuted:

Premenstrual-like syndrome.
Cataracts.
Changes in libido.
Chorea.
Changes in appetite.
Cystitis-like syndrome.
Headache.
Nervousness.
Dizziness.
Hirsutism.
Loss of scalp hair.
Erythema multiforme.
Erythema nodosum.
Hemorrhagic eruption.
Vaginitis.
Porphyria.
Hemolytic uremic syndrome.

ACUTE OVERDOSE

Serious ill effects have not been reported following acute ingestion of large doses of oral contraceptives by young children. Overdosage may cause nausea, and withdrawal bleeding may occur in females.

DOSAGE AND ADMINISTRATION

To achieve maximum contraceptive effectiveness, TRI-LEVLEN™ tablets (Levonorgestrel and Ethinyl Estradiol Tablets—Triphasic Regimen) must be taken exactly as directed and at intervals not exceeding 24 hours.

TRI-LEVLEN™ 21 TABLETS (LEVONORGESTREL AND ETHINYL ESTRADIOL TABLETS—TRIPHASIC REGIMEN)

TRI-LEVLEN™ 21 tablets are a three-phase preparation. The dosage of TRI-LEVLEN™ 21 tablets is **one tablet daily** for 21 consecutive days per menstrual cycle in the following order: 6 brown tablets (phase 1), followed by 5 white tablets (phase 2), and then followed by the last 10 light-yellow tablets (phase 3), according to the prescribed schedule. Tablets are then discontinued for 7 days (three weeks on, one week off).

It is recommended that TRI-LEVLEN™ 21 tablets be taken at the same time each day, preferably after the evening meal or at bedtime. During the first cycle of medication, the patient should be instructed to take one TRI-LEVLEN™ 21 tablet daily in the order of 6 brown, 5 white and, finally, 10 light-yellow tablets for twenty-one (21) consecutive days, beginning on day one (1) of her menstrual cycle. (The first day of menstruation is day one.) The tablets are then discontinued for one week (7 days). Withdrawal bleeding usually occurs within 3 days following discontinuation of TRI-LEVLEN™ 21 Tablets. (If TRI-LEVLEN™ 21 tablets are first taken later than the first day of the first menstrual cycle of medication or postpartum, contraceptive reliance should not be placed on TRI-LEVLEN™ 21 tablets until after the first 7 consecutive days of administration. The possibility of ovulation and conception prior to initiation of medication should be considered.)

When switching from another oral contraceptive, TRI-LEVLEN™ 21 tablets should be started on the first day of bleeding following the last tablet taken of the previous oral contraceptive.

The patient begins her next and all subsequent 21-day courses of TRI-LEVLEN™ 21 tablets on the same day of the week that she began her first course, following the same schedule: 21 days on—7 days off. She begins taking her brown tablets on the 8th day after discontinuance regardless of whether or not a menstrual period has occurred or is still in progress. Any time the next cycle of TRI-LEVLEN™ 21 tablets are started later than the 8th day, the patient should be protected by another means of contraception until she has taken a tablet daily for seven consecutive days.

If spotting or breakthrough bleeding occurs, the patient is instructed to continue on the same regimen. This type of bleeding is usually transient and without significance; however, if the bleeding is persistent or prolonged, the patient is advised to consult her physician. Although the occurrence of pregnancy is highly unlikely if TRI-LEVLEN™ 21 tablets are taken according to directions, if withdrawal bleeding does not occur, the possibility of pregnancy must be considered. If the patient has not adhered to the prescribed schedule (missed one or more tablets or started taking them on a day later than she should have), the probability of pregnancy should be considered at the time of the first missed period and appropriate diagnostic measures taken before the medication is resumed. If the patient has adhered to the prescribed regimen and misses two consecutive periods, pregnancy should be ruled out before continuing the contraceptive regimen.

The patient should be instructed to take a missed tablet as soon as it is remembered. If two consecutive tablets are missed they should both be taken as soon as remembered. The next tablet should be taken at the usual time.

Any time the patient misses one or two tablets she should also use another method of contraception until she has taken a tablet daily for seven consecutive days. If breakthrough bleeding occurs following missed tablets it will usually be transient and of no consequence. While there is little likelihood of ovulation occurring if only one or two tablets are missed, the possibility of ovulation increases with each successive day that scheduled tablets are missed. If three consecutive tablets are missed, all medication should be discontinued and the remainder of the package discarded. A new package of TRI-LEVLEN™ 21 tablets should be started on the first day of the patient's next bleed after the last tablet was taken. An alternate means of contraception should be prescribed during the days without tablets and continued until the patient has taken a tablet daily for seven consecutive days. In the nonlactating mother, TRI-LEVLEN™ 21 tablets may be prescribed in the postpartum period either immediately or at the first postpartum examination whether or not menstruation has resumed.

TRI-LEVLEN™ 28 TABLETS (LEVONORGESTREL AND ETHINYL ESTRADIOL TABLETS—TRIPHASIC REGIMEN)

TRI-LEVLEN™ 28 tablets are a three-phase preparation plus 7 inert tablets. The dosage of TRI-LEVLEN™ 28 tablets is **one tablet daily** for 28 consecutive days per menstrual cycle in the following order: 6 brown tablets (phase 1), followed by 5 white tablets (phase 2), followed by 10 light-yellow tablets (phase 3), plus 7 light-green inert tablets according to the prescribed schedule.

It is recommended that TRI-LEVLEN™ 28 tablets be taken at the same time each day, preferably after the evening meal or at bedtime. During the first cycle of medication, the patient should be instructed to take one TRI-LEVLEN™ 28 tablet daily in the order of 6 brown, 5 white, 10 light-yellow tablets, and then 7 light-green inert tablets for twenty-eight (28) consecutive days, beginning on day one (1) of her menstrual cycle. (The first day of menstruation is day one). Withdrawal bleeding usually occurs within 3 days following the last light-yellow tablet. (If TRI-LEVLEN™ 28 tablets are first taken later than the first day of the first menstual cycle of medication or postpartum, contraceptive reliance should not be placed on TRI-LEVLEN™ 28 tablets until after the first 7 consecutive days of administration. The possibility of ovulation and conception prior to initiation of medication should be considered.)

When switching from another oral contraceptive, TRI-LEVLEN™ 28 tablets should be started on the first day of bleeding following the last tablet taken on the previous oral contraceptive.

The patient begins her next and all subsequent 28-day courses of TRI-LEVLEN™ 28 tablets on the same day of the week that she began her first course, following the same schedule. She begins taking her brown tablets on the next day after ingestion of the last light-green tablet, regardless of whether or not a menstrual period has occurred or is still in progress. Any time a subsequent cycle of TRI-LEVLEN™ 28 tablets is started later than the next day, the patient should be protected by another means of contraception until she has taken a tablet daily for seven consecutive days.

If spotting or breakthrough bleeding occurs, the patient is instructed to continue on the same regimen. This type of bleeding is usually transient and without significance, however, if the bleeding is persistent or prolonged, the patient is advised to consult her physician. Although the occurrence of pregnancy is highly unlikely if TRI-LEVLEN™ 28 tablets are taken according to directions, if withdrawal bleeding does not occur, the possibility of pregnancy must be considered. If the patient has not adhered to the prescribed schedule (missed one or more tablets or started taking them on a day later than she should have), the probability of pregnancy should be considered at the time of the first missed period and appropriate diagnostic measures taken before the medication is resumed. If the patient has adhered to the prescribed regimen and misses two consecutive periods, pregnancy should be ruled out before continuing the contraceptive regimen.

The patient should be instructed to take a missed brown, white, or light-yellow tablet as soon as it is remembered. If two consecutive brown, white or light-yellow tablets are missed, they should both be taken as soon as remembered. The next tablet should be taken at the usual time.

Any time the patient misses one or two brown, white, or light-yellow tablets, she should also use another method of contraception until she has taken a brown, white, or light-yellow tablet for seven consecutive days. If the patient misses one or more light-green tablets, she is still protected against pregnancy provided she begins taking brown tablets again on the proper day. If breakthrough bleeding occurs following missed brown, white, or light-yellow tablets, it will usually be transient and of no consequence. While there is little likelihood of ovulation occurring if only one or two brown, white or light-yellow tablets are missed, the possibility of ovulation increases with each successive day that scheduled tablets are missed. If three consecutive brown, white, or light-yellow tablets are missed, all medication should be discontinued and the remainder of the package discarded. A new package of TRI-LEVLEN™ 28 tablets should be started on the first day of the patient's next bleed after the last tablet was taken. An alternate means of contraception should be prescribed during the days without tablets and continued until the patient has taken a tablet daily for seven consecutive days. In the nonlactating mother, TRI-LEVLEN™ 28 tablets may be prescribed in the postpartum period either immediately or at the first postpartum examination whether or not menstruation has resumed.

HOW SUPPLIED

TRI-LEVLEN™ 21 tablets (Levonorgestrel and Ethinyl Estradiol Tablets—Triphasic Regimen), Berlex, NDC 50419-430-21, are available in packages of 3 SLIDECASE™ dispensers. Each cycle contains 21 round, coated tablets as follows:

NDC 50419-095, six brown tablets marked "B" on one side and "95" on the other side, each containing 0.050 mg levonorgestrel and 0.030 mg ethinyl estradiol;

NDC 50419-096, five white to off-white tablets marked "B" on one side and "96" on the other side, each containing 0.075 mg levonorgestrel and 0.040 mg ethinyl estradiol; and

NDC 50419-097, ten light-yellow tablets marked "B" on one side and "97" on the other side, each containing 0.125 mg levonorgestrel and 0.030 mg ethinyl estradiol.

TRI-LEVLEN™ 28 tablets (Levonorgestrel and Ethinyl Estradiol Tablets—Triphasic Regimen), Berlex, NDC 50419-431-28, are available in packages of 3 SLIDECASE™ dispensers. Each cycle contains 28 round, coated tablets as follows:

Continued on next page

Information on the Berlex products appearing here is based on the labeling in effect on August 1, 1986. Further information for these and other products may be obtained from the Professional Services Department, Berlex Laboratories, Inc., 110 East Hanover Avenue, Cedar Knolls, New Jersey 07927, telephone 201-292-3008.

Berlex—Cont.

NDC 50419-095, six brown tablets marked "B" on one side and "95" on the other side, each containing 0.050 mg levonorgestrel and 0.030 mg ethinyl estradiol; NDC 50419-096, five white to off-white tablets marked "B" on one side and "96" on the other side, each containing 0.075 mg levonorgestrel and 0.040 mg ethinyl estradiol;
NDC 50419-097, ten light-yellow tablets marked "B" on one side and "97" on the other side, each containing 0.125 mg levonorgestrel and 0.030 mg ethinyl estradiol; and
NDC 50419-011, seven light-green inert tablets marked "B" on one side and "11" on the other side.

REFERENCES

1. "*Population Reports*," Series H, Number 2, May 1974; Series I, Number 1, June 1974; Series B, Number 2, January 1975; Series H, Number 3, 1975; Series H, Number 4, January 1976 (published by the Population Information Program, The George Washington University Medical Center, 2001 S St. NW., Washington, D.C.).
2. Inman, W. H. W., Vessey, M. P., Westerholm, B., and Engelund, A., "Thromboembolic disease and the steroidal content of oral contraceptives. A report to the Committee on Safety of Drugs," Brit Med J *2*:203–209, 1970.
3. Stolley, P. D., Tonascia, J. A., Tockman, M. S., Sartwell, P. E., Rutledge, A. H., and Jacobs, M. P., "Thrombosis with low-estrogen oral contraceptives," Am J Epidemiol *102*:197–208, 1975.
4. Royal College of General Practitioners, "Oral contraception and thromboembolic disease," J Coll Gen Pract *13*:267–279, 1967.
5. Inman, W. H. W., and Vessey, M. P., "Investigation of deaths from pulmonary, coronary and cerebral thrombosis and embolism in women of childbearing age," Brit Med J *2*:193–199, 1968.
6. Vessey, M. P., and Doll, R., "Investigation of relation between use of oral contraceptives and thromboembolic disease. A further report," Brit Med J *2*:651–657, 1969.
7. Sartwell, P. E., Masi, A. T., Arthes, F. G., Greene, G. R., and Smith, H. E., "Thromboembolism and oral contraceptives: an epidemiological case control study," Am J Epidemiol *90*:365–380, 1969.
8. Boston Collaborative Drug Surveillance Program, "Oral contraceptives and venous thromboembolic disease, surgically confirmed gallbladder disease and breast tumors," Lancet *1*:1399–1404, 1973.
9. Collaborative Group for the Study of Stroke in Young Women, "Oral contraception and increased risk of cerebral ischemia or thrombosis," N Engl J Med *288*:871–878, 1973.
10. Collaborative Group for the Study of Stroke in Young Women, "Oral contraceptives and stroke in young women: associated risk factors," JAMA *231*:718–722, 1975.
11. Mann, J. I., and Inman, W. H. W., "Oral contraceptives and death from myocardial infarction," Brit Med J *2*:245–248, 1975.
12. Mann, J. I., Inman, W. H. W., and Thorogood, M., "Oral contraceptive use in older women and fatal myocardial infarction," Brit Med J *2*:445–447, 1976.
13. Mann, J. I., Vessey, M. P., Thorogood, M., and Doll, R., "Myocardial infarction in young women with special reference to oral contraceptive practice," Brit Med J *2*:241–245, 1975.
14. Tietze, C., "New Estimates of Mortality Associated with Fertility Control," Family Planning Perspectives, *9*:74–76, 1977.
15. Vessey, M. P., Doll, R., Fairbairn, A. S., and Glober, G., "Post-operative thromboembolism and the use of oral contraceptives," Brit Med J *3*:123–126, 1970.
16. Greene, G. R., and Sartwell, P. E., "Oral contraceptive use in patients with thromboembolism following surgery, trauma, or infection," Am J Pub Health *62*:680–685, 1972.
17. Smith, D. C., Prentice, R., Thompson, D. J., and Herrmann, W. L., "Association of exogenous estrogen and endometrial carcinoma," N Engl J Med *293*:1164–1167, 1975.
18. Ziel, H. K., and Finkle, W. D., "Increased risk of endometrial carcinoma among users of conjugated estrogens," N Engl J Med *293*:1167–1170, 1975.
19. Mack, T. N., Pike, M. C., Henderson, B. E., Pfeffer, R. I., Gerkins, V. R., Arthur, M., and Brown, S. E., "Estrogens and endometrial cancer in a retirement community," N Engl J Med *294*:1262–1267, 1976.
20. Silverberg, S. G., and Makowski, E. L., "Endometrial carcinoma in young women taking oral contraceptive agents," Obstet Gynecol *46*:503–506, 1975.
21. Vessey, M. P., Doll, R., and Sutton, P. M., "Oral contraceptives and breast neoplasia: a retrospective study," Brit Med J *3*:719–724, 1972.
22. Vessey, M. P., Doll, R., and Jones K., "Oral contraceptives and breast cancer. Progress report of an epidemiological study," Lancet *1*:941–943, 1975.
23. Boston Collaborative Drug Surveillance Program, "Surgically confirmed gallbladder disease, venous thromboembolism and breast tumors in relation to postmenopausal estrogen therapy," N Engl J Med *290*:15–19, 1974.
24. Arthes, F. G., Sartwell, P. E., and Lewison, E. F., "The pill, estrogens, and the breast. Epidemiologic aspects," Cancer *28*:1391–1394, 1971.
25. Fasal, E., and Paffenbarger, R. S., "Oral contraceptives as related to cancer and benign lesions of the breast," J Natl Cancer Inst *55*:767–773, 1975.
26. Royal College of General Practitioners, "Oral Contraceptives and Health," London, Pitman, 1974.
27. Ory, H., Cole P., MacMahon, B., and Hoover, R., "Oral contraceptives and reduced risk of benign breast diseases," N Engl J Med *294*:419–422, 1976.
28. Baum, J., Holtz, F., Bookstein, J. J., and Klein, E. W., "Possible association between benign hepatomas and oral contraceptives," Lancet *2*:926–928, 1973.
29. Mays, E. T., Christopherson, W. M., Mahr, M. M., and Williams, H. C., "Hepatic changes in young women ingesting contraceptive steroids. Hepatic hemorrhage and primary hepatic tumors," JAMA *235*:730–732, 1976.
30. Edmondson, H. A., Henderson, B., and Benton, B., "Liver-cell adenomas associated with use of oral contraceptives," N Engl J Med *294*:470–472, 1976.
31. Herbst, A. L., Ulfedler, H., and Poskanzer, D. C., "Adenocarcinoma of the vagina," N Engl J Med *284*:878–881, 1971.
32. Greenwald, P., Barlow, J. J., Nasca, P. C., and Burnett, W., "Vaginal cancer after maternal treatment with synthetic estrogens," N Engl J Med *285*:390–392, 1971.
33. Lanier, A. P., Noller, K. L., Decker, D. G., Elveback, L., and Kurland, L. T., "Cancer and stilbestrol. A follow-up of 1719 persons exposed to estrogens in utero and born 1943–1959," Mayo Clin Pro *48*:793–799, 1973.
34. Herbst, A. L., Kurman, R. J., and Scully, R. E., "Vaginal and cervical abnormalities after exposure to stilbestrol in utero," Obstet Gynecol *40*:287–298, 1972.
35. Herbst, A. L., Robboy, S. J., Macdonald, G. J., and Scully, R. E., "The effects of local progesterone on stilbestrol-associated vaginal adenosis," Am J Obstet Gynecol *118*:607–615, 1974.
36. Herbst, A. L., Poskanzer, D. C., Robboy, S. J., Friedlander, L., and Scully, R. E., "Prenatal exposure to stilbestrol: a prospective comparison of exposed female offspring with unexposed controls," N Engl J Med *292*:334–339, 1975.
37. Stafl, A., Mattingly, R. F., Foley, D. V., Fetherston, W., "Clinical diagnosis of vaginal adenosis," Obstet Gynecol *43*:118–128, 1974.
38. Sherman, A. I., Goldrath, M., Berlin, A., Vakhariya, V., Banooni, F., Michaels, W., Goodman, P., and Brown, S., "Cervical-vaginal adenosis after in utero exposure to synthetic estrogens," Obstet Gynecol *44*:531–545, 1974.
39. Gal, I., Kirman, B., and Stern, J., "Hormone pregnancy tests and congenital malformation," Nature *216*:83, 1967.
40. Levy, E. P., Cohen, A., and Fraser, F. C., "Hormone treatment during pregnancy and congenital heart defects," Lancet *1*:611, 1973.
41. Nora, J. J., and Nora, A. H., "Birth defects and oral contraceptives," Lancet *1*:941–942, 1973.
42. Janerich, D. T., Piper, J. M., and Glebatis, D. M., "Oral contraceptives and congenital limb-reduction defects," N Engl J Med *291*:697–700, 1974.
43. Carr, D. H., "Chromosome studies in selected spontaneous abortions: I. Conception after oral contraceptives," Canad Med Assoc J *103*:343–348, 1970.
44. Wynn, V., Doar, J. W. H., and Mills, G. L., "Some effects of oral contraceptives on serum-lipid and lipoprotein levels," Lancet *2*:720–723, 1966.
45. Laumas, K. R., Malkani, P. K., Bhatnagar, S., and Laumas, V., "Radioactivity in the breast milk of lactating women after oral administration of 3 H-norethynodrel," Am J Obstet Gynecol *98*:411–413, 1967.
46. Center for Disease Control, "Increased Risk of Hepatocellular Adenoma in Women with Long-term use of Oral Contraceptives," Morbidity and Mortality Weekly Report, *26*:293–294, 1977.
47. Herbst, A. L., Cole, P., Colton, T., Robboy, S. J., and Scully, R. E., "Age-incidence and Risk of Diethylstilbestrol-related Clear Cell Adenocarcinoma of the Vagina and Cervix," Am J Obstet Gynecol *128*:43–50, 1977.
48. Bibbo, M., Al-Naqeeb, M., Baccarini, I., Gill, W., Newton, M., Sleeper, K. M., Sonek, M., and Wied, G. L., "Follow-up Study of Male and Female Offspring of DES-treated Mothers. A Preliminary Report," J of Repro Med *15*:29–32, 1975.
49. Gill, W. B., Schumacher, G. F. B., and Bibbo, M., "Structural and Functional Abnormalities in the Sex Organs of Male Offspring of Mothers Treated with Diethylstilbestrol (DES)," J of Repro Med *16*:147–153, 1976.
50. Henderson, B. E., Senton, B., Cosgrove, M., Baptista, J., Aldrich, J., Townsend, D., Hart, W., and Mack, T., "Urogenital Tract Abnormalities in Sons of Women Treated with Diethylstilbestrol," Pediatrics, *58*:505–507, 1976.
51. Heinonen, O. P., Slone, D., Nonson, R. R., Hook, E. B., and Shapiro, S., "Cardiovascular Birth Defects and Antenatal Exposure to Female Sex Hormones," N Engl J Med *296*:67–70, 1977.
52. Jain, A. K., "Mortality Risk Associated with the Use of Oral Contraceptives," Studies in Family Planning, *8*:50–54, 1977.
53. Beral, V., "Mortality Among Oral Contraceptive Users," Lancet, *2*:727–731, 1977.
54. Royal College of General Practitioners' Oral contraception study, "Incidence of arterial disease among oral contraceptive users," J Royal Col Gen Pract *33*:75–82, 1983.
55. Slone, D., Shapiro, S., Kaufman, D. W., Rosenberg, L., Miettinen, O., and Stolley, P., "Risk of myocardial infarction in relation to current and discontinued use of oral contraceptives," N Engl J Med *305*:420–424, 1981.
56. Inman, W.H.W., "Oral contraceptives and fatal subarachnoid haemorrhage," Brit Med J *2*:1468–1470, 1979.
57. Petitti, D. B., and Wingerd, J., "Use of oral contraceptives, cigarette smoking and risk of subarachnoid haemorrhage," Lancet *2*:234–236, 1978.
58. Thorogood, M., Adam, S. A., and Mann, J. I., "Fatal subarachnoid haemorrhage in young women: role of oral contraceptives," Brit Med J *283*:762, 1981.
59. Rosenberg, L., Hennekens, C.H., Rosner, B., Belanger, C., Rothman, K. J., and Speizer, F. E., "Oral contraceptive use in relation to nonfatal myocardial infarction," Am J Epidemiol *111*:59–66, 1980.
60. Adam, S. A., Thorogood, M., and Mann, J. I., "Oral contraception and myocardial infarction revisited: the effects of new preparations and prescribing patterns," Brit J Obstet Gynaecol *88*:838–845, 1981.
61. Data on file.
62. Briggs, M. H., "Implications and assessment of metabolic effects of oral contraceptives." New considerations in oral contraception. Proceedings of an international symposium, Catholic University-Leuven, Leuven, Belgium. September, 1981 Ed. I. Brosens.
63. Vermeulen, A., and Thiery, M., "Metabolic effects of the triphasic oral contraceptive Trigynon®." Contraception *26*:505–513, 1982.
64. Nilsson, S., Nygren, K., and Johansson, E., "Ethinyl Estradiol in Human Milk and Plasma after Oral Administration." Contraception *17*:131–139, 1978.
65. Nilsson, S., Nygren, K., and Johansson, E., "d-Norgestrel Concentrations in Maternal Plasma, Milk, and Child Plasma During Administration of Oral Contraceptives to Nursing Women." Am J Obstet Gynecol *129*:178, 1977.

The patient labeling for oral-contraceptive drug products is set forth below:

Brief Summary Patient Package Insert

Cigarette smoking increases the risk of serious adverse effects on the heart and blood vessels from oral-contraceptive use. This risk increases with age and with heavy smoking (15 or more cigarettes per day) and is quite marked in women over 35 years of age. Women who use oral contraceptives should not smoke.

Oral contraceptives taken as directed are about 99% effective in preventing pregnancy. (The mini-pill, however, is somewhat less effective.) Forgetting to take your pills increases the chance of pregnancy. Women who have or have had clotting disorders, cancer of the breast or sex organs, unexplained vaginal bleeding, a stroke, heart attack, angina pectoris, or who suspect they may be pregnant should not use oral contraceptives. Various drugs, such as some antibiotics, may also decrease the effectiveness of oral contraceptives.
Most side effects of the pill are not serious. The most common side effects are nausea, vomiting, bleeding between menstrual periods, weight gain, and breast tenderness. However, proper use of oral contraceptives requires that they be taken under your doctor's continuous supervision, because they can be associated with serious side effects which may be fatal. Fortunately, these occur very infrequently. The serious side effects are:

1. Blood clots in the legs, lungs, brain, heart, or other organs, and hemorrhage into the brain due to bursting of a blood vessel. Certain of these effects may occur after pill use has been stopped.
2. Liver tumors, which may rupture and cause severe bleeding.
3. Birth defects if the pill is taken while you are pregnant.
4. High blood pressure.
5. Gallbladder disease.

The symptoms associated with these serious side effects are discussed in the detailed leaflet given you with your supply of pills. Notify your doctor if you notice any unusual physical disturbance while taking the pill.
The estrogen in oral contraceptives has been found to cause breast cancer and other cancers in certain animals. These findings suggest that oral contraceptives may also cause cancer in humans. However, studies to date in women taking currently marketed oral contraceptives have not confirmed that oral contraceptives cause cancer in humans.
The detailed leaflet describes more completely the benefits and risks of oral contraceptives. It also provides information on other forms of contraception. Read it carefully. If you have any questions, consult your doctor.

CAUTION: Oral contraceptives are of no value in the prevention or treatment of venereal disease.

DETAILED PATIENT LABELING

WHAT YOU SHOULD KNOW ABOUT ORAL CONTRACEPTIVES

Oral contraceptives ("the pill") are the most effective way (except for sterilization) to prevent pregnancy. They are also convenient and, for most women, free of serious or unpleasant side effects. Oral contraceptives must always be taken under the continuous supervision of a physician.

It is important that any woman who considers using an oral contraceptive understand the risks involved. Although the oral contraceptives have important advantages over other methods of contraception, they have certain risks that no other method has. Only you can decide whether the advantages are worth these risks. This leaflet will tell you about the most important risks. It will explain how you can help your doctor prescribe the pill as safely as possible by telling him about yourself and being alert for the earliest signs of trouble. And it will tell you how to use the pill properly, so that it will be as effective as possible. There is more detailed information available in the leaflet prepared for doctors. Your pharmacist can show you a copy; you may need your doctor's help in understanding parts of it.

WHO SHOULD NOT USE ORAL CONTRACEPTIVES

A. If you have any of the following conditions, you should not use the pill:

1. Clots in the legs or lungs.
2. Angina pectoris.
3. Known or suspected cancer of the breast or sex organs.
4. Unusual vaginal bleeding that has not yet been diagnosed.
5. Known or suspected pregnancy.

B. If you have had any of the following conditions, you should not use the pill:

1. Heart attack or stroke.
2. Clots in the legs or lungs.

C. Cigarette smoking increases the risk of serious adverse effects on the heart and blood vessels from oral-contraceptive use. This risk increases with age and with heavy smoking (15 or more cigarettes per day) and is quite marked in women over 35 years of age. Women who use oral contraceptives should not smoke.

D. If you have scanty or irregular periods or are a young woman without a regular cycle, you should use another method of contraception because, if you use the pill, you may have difficulty becoming pregnant or may fail to have menstrual periods after discontinuing the pill.

DECIDING TO USE ORAL CONTRACEPTIVES

If you do not have any of the conditions listed above and are thinking about using oral contraceptives, to help you decide, you need information about the advantages and risks of oral contraceptives and of other contraceptive methods as well. This leaflet describes the advantages and risks of oral contraceptives. Except for sterilization, the IUD, and abortion, which have their own inherent risks, the only risks of other methods of contraception are those due to pregnancy should the method fail. Your doctor can answer questions you may have with respect to other methods of contraception. He can also answer any questions you may have after reading this leaflet on oral contraceptives.

1. What Oral Contraceptives Are and How They Work. Oral contraceptives are of two types. The most common, often simply called "the pill," is a combination of an estrogen and a progestogen, the two kinds of female hormones. The amount of estrogen and progestogen can vary, but the amount of estrogen is most important because both the effectiveness and some of the dangers of oral contraceptives are related to the amount of estrogen. This kind of oral contraceptive works principally by preventing release of an egg from the ovary. When the amount of estrogen is 50 micrograms or more, and the pill is taken as directed, oral contraceptives are more than 99% effective (i.e., there would be less than 1 pregnancy if 100 women used the pill for 1 year). Pills that contain 20 to 35 micrograms of estrogen vary slightly in effectiveness, ranging from 98% to more than 99% effective.

The second type of oral contraceptive, often called the "mini-pill", contains only a progestogen. It works in part by preventing release of an egg from the ovary but also by keeping sperm from reaching the egg and by making the uterus (womb) less receptive to any fertilized egg that reaches it. The mini-pill is less effective than the combination oral contraceptive, about 97% effective. In addition, the progestogen-only pill has a tendency to cause irregular bleeding which may be quite inconvenient, or cessation of bleeding entirely. The progestogen-only pill is used despite its lower effectiveness in the hope that it will prove not to have some of the serious side effects of the estrogen-containing pill (see below), but it is not yet certain that the mini-pill does in fact have fewer serious side effects. The discussion below, while based mainly on information about the combination pills, should be considered to apply as well to the mini-pill.

2. Other Nonsurgical Ways to Prevent Pregnancy. As this leaflet will explain, oral contraceptives have several serious risks. Other methods of contraception have lesser risks or none at all. They are also less effective than oral contraceptives, but, used properly, may be effective enough for many women.

The following table gives reported pregnancy rates (the number of women out of 100 who would become pregnant in 1 year) for these methods.

PREGNANCIES PER 100 WOMEN PER YEAR

Intrauterine device (IUD), less than 1–6; Diaphragm with spermicidal products (creams or jellies), 2–20; Condom (rubber), 3–36; Aerosol foams, 2–29; Jellies and creams, 4–36; Periodic abstinence (rhythm) all types, less than 1–47:

1. Calendar method, 14–47;
2. Temperature method, 1–20;
3. Temperature method—intercourse only in postovulatory phase, less than 1–7;
4. Mucus method, 1–25;

No contraception, 60–80.

The figures (except for the IUD) vary widely because people differ in how well they use each method. Very faithful users of the various methods obtain very good results, except for users of the calendar method of periodic abstinence (rhythm). Except for the IUD, effective use of these methods requires somewhat more effort than simply taking a single pill every day, but it is an effort that many couples undertake successfully. Your doctor can tell you a great deal more about these methods of contraception.

3. The Dangers of Oral Contraceptives.

a. *Circulatory disorders (abnormal blood clotting and stroke due to hemorrhage).* Blood clots (in various blood vessels of the body) are the most common of the serious side effects of oral contraceptives. A clot can result in a stroke (if the clot is in the brain), a heart attack (if the clot is in a blood vessel of the heart), or a pulmonary embolus (a clot which forms in the legs or pelvis, then breaks off and travels to the lungs). Any of these can be fatal. Clots also occur rarely in the blood vessels of the eye, resulting in blindness or impairment of vision in that eye. There is evidence that the risk of clotting increases with higher estrogen doses. It is therefore important to keep the dose of estrogen as low as possible, so long as the oral contraceptive used has an acceptable pregnancy rate and doesn't cause unacceptable changes in the menstrual pattern. Furthermore, cigarette smoking by oral-contraceptive users increases the risk of serious adverse effects on the heart and blood vessels. This risk increases with age and with heavy smoking (15 or more cigarettes per day) and begins to become quite marked in women over 35 years of age. For this reason, women who use oral contraceptives should not smoke.

The risk of abnormal clotting increases with age in both users and nonusers of oral contraceptives, but the increased risk from the contraceptive appears to be present at all ages. For oral-contraceptive users in general, it has been estimated that in women between the ages of 15 and 34 the risk of death due to a circulatory disorder is about 1 in 12,000 per year, whereas for nonusers the rate is about 1 in 50,000 per year. In the age group 35 to 44, the risk is estimated to be about 1 in 2,500 per year for oral-contraceptive users and about 1 in 10,000 per year for nonusers.

Even without the pill, the risk of having a heart attack increases with age and is also increased by such heart attack risk factors as high blood pressure, high cholesterol, obesity, diabetes, and cigarette smoking. Without any risk factors present, the use of oral contraceptives alone may double the risk of heart attack. However, the combination of cigarette smoking, especially heavy smoking, and oral contraceptive use greatly increases the risk of heart attack. Oral-contraceptive users who smoke are about 5 times more likely to have a heart attack than users who do not smoke and about 10 times more likely to have a heart attack than nonusers who do not smoke. It has been estimated that users between the ages of 30 and 39 who smoke have about a 1 in 10,000 chance each year of having a fatal heart attack compared to about a 1 in 50,000 chance in users who do not smoke, and about a 1 in 100,000 chance in nonusers who do not smoke. In the age group 40 to 44, the risk is about 1 in 1,700 per year for users who smoke compared to about 1 in 10,000 for users who do not smoke and to about 1 in 14,000 per year for nonusers who do not smoke. Heavy smoking (about 15 cigarettes or more a day) further increases the risk. If you do not smoke and have none of the other heart attack risk factors described above, you will have a smaller risk than listed. If you have several heart attack risk factors, the risk may be considerably greater than listed. In addition to blood-clotting disorders, it has been estimated that women taking oral contraceptives are twice as likely as nonusers to have a stroke due to rupture of a blood vessel in the brain. There is evidence that patients who stop taking oral contraceptives after using them continuously for five or more years may continue to have an increased risk of stroke or heart attack for at least six to nine years after discontinuation.

b. *Formation of tumors.* Studies have found that when certain animals are given the female sex hormone, estrogen, which is an ingredient of oral contraceptives, continuously for long periods, cancers may develop in the breast, cervix, vagina, and liver. These findings suggest that oral contraceptives may cause cancer in humans. However, studies to date in women taking currently marketed oral contraceptives have not confirmed that oral contraceptives cause cancer in humans. Several studies have found no increase in breast cancer in users, although one study suggested oral contraceptives might cause an increase in breast cancer in women who already have benign breast disease (e.g., cysts).

Women with a strong family history of breast cancer or who have breast nodules, fibrocystic disease, or abnormal mammograms or who were exposed to DES (diethylstilbestrol), an estrogen, during their mother's pregnancy must be followed very closely by their doctors if they choose to use oral contraceptives instead of another method of contraception. Many studies have shown that women taking oral contraceptives have less risk of getting benign breast disease than those who have not used oral contraceptives. Recently, strong evidence has emerged that estrogens (one component of oral contraceptives), when given for periods of more than one year to women after the menopause, increase the risk of cancer of the uterus (womb). There is also some evidence that a kind of oral contraceptive which is no longer marketed, the sequential oral contraceptive, may increase the risk of cancer of the uterus. There remains no evidence, however, that the oral contraceptives now available increase the risk of this cancer. Oral contraceptives do cause, although rarely, a benign (nonmalignant) tumor of the liver. These tumors do not spread, but they may rupture and cause internal bleeding, which may be fatal. A few cases of cancer of the liver have been reported in women using oral contraceptives, but it is not yet known whether the drug caused them.

c. *Dangers to a developing child if oral contraceptives are used in or immediately preceding pregnancy.* Oral contraceptives should not be taken by pregnant women because they may damage the developing child. An increased risk of birth defects, including heart defects and limb defects, has been associated with the use of sex hormones, including oral contraceptives, in pregnancy. In addition, the developing female child whose mother has received DES (diethylstilbestrol), an estrogen, during pregnancy has a risk of getting cancer of the vagina or cervix in her teens or young adulthood. This risk is estimated to be about 1 in 1,000 exposures or less. Abnormalities of the urinary and sex organs have been reported in male offspring so exposed. It is possible that other estrogens, such as the estrogens in oral contraceptives, could have the same effect in the child if the mother takes them during pregnancy.

If you stop taking oral contraceptives to become pregnant, your doctor may recommend that you use another method of contraception for a short while. The reason for this is that there is evidence from studies in women who have had "miscarriages" soon after stopping the pill, that the lost fetuses are more likely to be abnormal. Whether there is an overall increase in "miscarriage" in women who become pregnant soon after stopping the pill as compared with women who do not use the pill is not known, but it is possible that there may be. If, however, you do become pregnant soon after stopping oral contraceptives, and do not have a miscarriage, there is no evidence that the baby has an increased risk of being abnormal.

d. *Gallbladder disease.* Women who use oral contraceptives have a greater risk than nonusers of having gallbladder disease requiring surgery. The increased risk may first appear within 1 year of use and may double after 4 or 5 years of use.

e. *Other side effects of oral contraceptives.* Some women using oral contraceptives experience unpleasant side effects that are not dangerous and are not likely to damage their health. Some of these may be temporary. Your breasts may feel tender, nausea and vomiting may occur, you may gain or lose weight, and your ankles may swell. A spotty darkening of the skin, particularly of the face, is possible and may persist. You may notice unexpected vaginal bleeding or changes in your menstrual period. Irregular bleeding is frequently seen when using the mini-pill or combination oral contraceptives containing less than 50 micrograms of estrogen. More serious side effects include worsening of migraine, asthma, epilepsy, and kidney or heart disease because of a tendency for water to be retained in the body when oral contraceptives are used.

Other side effects are growth of preexisting fibroid tumors of the uterus; mental depression, and liver problems with jaundice (yellowing of the skin). Your doctor may find that levels of sugar and fatty substances in your blood are elevated; the long-term effects of these changes are not known. Some women develop high blood pressure while taking oral con-

Continued on next page

Information on the Berlex products appearing here is based on the labeling in effect on August 1, 1986. Further information for these and other products may be obtained from the Professional Services Department, Berlex Laboratories, Inc., 110 East Hanover Avenue, Cedar Knolls, New Jersey 07927, telephone 201-292-3008.

Berlex—Cont.

traceptives, which ordinarily returns to the original levels when the oral contraceptive is stopped.

Other reactions, although not proved to be caused by oral contraceptives, are occasionally reported. These include more frequent urination and some discomfort when urinating, blood-cell breakdown with kidney failure, nervousness, dizziness, some loss of scalp hair, an increase in body hair, an increase or decrease in sex drive, appetite changes, cataracts, and a need for a change in contact lens prescription, or inability to use contact lenses. After you stop using oral contraceptives, there may be a delay before you are able to become pregnant or before you resume having menstrual periods. This is especially true of women who had irregular menstrual cycles prior to the use of oral contraceptives. As discussed previously, your doctor may recommend that you wait a short while after stopping the pill before you try to become pregnant. During this time, use another form of contraception. You should consult your physician before resuming use of oral contraceptives after childbirth, especially if you plan to nurse your baby. Drugs in oral contraceptives are known to appear in the milk, and the long-range effect on infants is not known at this time. Furthermore, oral contraceptives may cause a decrease in your milk supply as well as in the quality of the milk.

4. Comparison of the Risks of Oral Contraceptives and Other Contraceptive Methods. The many studies on the risks and effectiveness of oral contraceptives and other methods of contraception have been analyzed to estimate the risk of death associated with various methods of contraception. This risk has two parts: (a) the risk of the method itself (e.g., the risk that oral contraceptives will cause death due to abnormal clotting), and (b) the risk of death due to pregnancy or abortion in the event the method fails. The results of this analysis are shown in the bar graph (Figure 1). The height of the bars is the number of deaths per 100,000 women each year. There are six sets of bars, each set referring to a specific age group of women. Within each set of bars, there is a single bar for each of the different contraceptive methods. For oral contraceptives, there are two bars—one for smokers and the other for nonsmokers. The analysis is based on present knowledge, and new information could, of course, alter it. The analysis shows that the risk of death from all methods of birth control is low and below that associated with childbirth, except for oral contraceptives in women over 40 who smoke. It shows that the lowest risk of death is associated with the condom or diaphragm (traditional contraception) backed up by early abortion in case of failure of the condom or diaphragm to prevent pregnancy. Also, at any age the risk of death (due to unexpected pregnancy) from the use of traditional contraception, even without a backup of abortion, is generally the same as or less than that from use of oral contraceptives.

Figure 1. Estimated annual number of deaths associated with control of fertility and no control per 100,000 nonsterile women, by regimen of control and age of women.

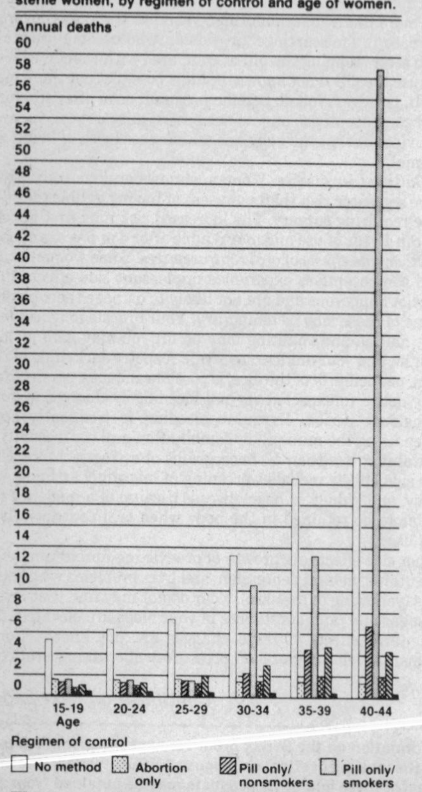

HOW TO USE ORAL CONTRACEPTIVES AS SAFELY AND EFFECTIVELY AS POSSIBLE, ONCE YOU HAVE DECIDED TO USE THEM

1. What to Tell your Doctor.

You can make use of the pill as safely as possible by telling your doctor if you have any of the following:

a. Conditions that mean you should not use oral contraceptives:

Clots in the legs or lungs.
Clots in the legs or lungs in the past.
A stroke, heart attack, or angina pectoris.
Known or suspected cancer of the breast or sex organs.
Unusual vaginal bleeding that has not yet been diagnosed.
Known or suspected pregnancy.

b. Conditions that your doctor will want to watch closely or which might cause him to suggest another method of contraception:

A family history of breast cancer.
Breast nodules, fibrocystic disease of the breast, or an abnormal mammogram.

Diabetes.	Heart or kidney disease.
High blood pressure.	Epilepsy.
High cholesterol.	Mental depression.
Cigarette smoking.	Fibroid tumors of the uterus.
Migraine headaches.	Gallbladder disease.

c. Once you are using oral contraceptives, you should be alert for signs of a serious adverse effect and call your doctor if they occur.

Sharp pain in the chest, coughing blood, or sudden shortness of breath (indicating possible clots in the lungs).
Pain in the calf (possible clot in the leg).
Crushing chest pain or heaviness (indicating possible heart attack).
Sudden severe headache or vomiting, dizziness or fainting, disturbance of vision or speech, or weakness or numbness in an arm or leg (indicating a possible stroke).
Sudden partial or complete loss of vision (indicating a possible clot in the eye).
Breast lumps (you should ask your doctor to show you how to examine your own breasts).
Severe pain in the abdomen (indicating a possible ruptured tumor of the liver).
Severe depression.
Yellowing of the skin (jaundice).

2. How to Take the Pill So That It is Most Effective.

Reduced effectiveness and an increased incidence of breakthrough bleeding have been associated with the use of oral contraceptives with antibiotics such as rifampin, ampicillin, and tetracycline or with certain other drugs such as barbiturates, phenylbutazone or phenytoin sodium. You should use an additional means of contraception during any cycle in which any of these drugs are taken.

To achieve maximum contraceptive effectiveness, oral contraceptives must be taken exactly as directed and at intervals not exceeding 24 hours. It is recommended that tablets be taken at the same time each day, preferably after the evening meal or at bedtime. Taking them on a definite schedule will decrease the chance of forgetting a tablet and also help keep the proper amount of medication in your system. See detailed instructions below for TRI-LEVLEN™ 21 tablets (Levonorgestrel and Ethinyl Estradiol Tablets—Triphasic Regimen) and TRI-LEVLEN™ 28 tablets (Levonorgestrel and Ethinyl Estradiol Tablets—Triphasic Regimen).

For specific instructions on **how to use your particular package**, refer to the Brief Summary Patient Package insert provided with your pill package.

TRI-LEVLEN™ 21 TABLETS (LEVONORGESTREL AND ETHINYL ESTRADIOL TABLETS—TRIPHASIC REGIMEN)

TRI-LEVLEN™ is a three-phased contraceptive, different from the usual same-dose-every-day combination oral contraceptive.

TRI-LEVLEN™ 21 tablets contain 21 active pills divided among 6 brown pills, 5 white pills, and 10 light-yellow pills in each package.

The dosage of TRI-LEVLEN™ 21 tablets is **one pill daily** for 21 days in a row in your menstrual cycle beginning with the first brown pill, continuing through the white pills and finishing the cycle with the light-yellow pills, **in that order.** Pills are then discontinued for 7 days. The basic schedule is 21 days on—7 days off.

In the first month, you should begin taking TRI-LEVLEN™ 21 tablets on day one (1) of your menstrual cycle, which is the first day of your menstruation regardless of the amount of bleeding or spotting. (Day 1 is the first day of menstruation, even if it is almost midnight when you start.) Note: During the first month on TRI-LEVLEN™ 21 tablets, if you start taking pills later than day 1 of your menstrual cycle, you should protect yourself by also using another method of birth control until you have taken a pill daily for seven days in a row (6 brown pills followed by 1 white pill). Thereafter, if you follow directions carefully you will obtain the full contraceptive benefit. If you begin taking pills later than the proper day, the possibility of ovulation and pregnancy occurring before or during the taking of the brown pills should be considered.

Take one pill every day until you finish all 21 pills. No pills are then taken for one week (7 days). Your period will usually begin about three days after you take the last light-yellow pill. Don't be alarmed if the amount of bleeding is not the same as before. On the 8th day, start with a brown pill from a new package, even if you still have your period. If, for example, you took TRI-LEVLEN™ 21 tablets for the first time on a Tuesday, the 8th day will also be a Tuesday. **If you have taken the pills as directed,** you will begin the next cycle on the same day of the week. If you start taking pills later than the 8th day, you should protect yourself by also using another method of birth control until you have taken a pill daily for seven days in a row.

When switching from another oral contraceptive, TRI-LEVLEN™ 21 tablets should be started on the first day of bleeding following the last pill taken of the previous oral contraceptive.

TRI-LEVLEN™ 28 TABLETS (LEVONORGESTREL AND ETHINYL ESTRADIOL TABLETS—TRIPHASIC REGIMEN)

TRI-LEVLEN™ is a three-phased contraceptive, different from the usual same-dose-every-day combination oral contraceptive.

TRI-LEVLEN™ 28 tablets contain active pills divided among 6 brown pills, 5 white pills, and 10 light-yellow pills plus 7 light-green inactive pills per package.

The dosage of TRI-LEVLEN™ 28 tablets is one active pill daily for 21 days in a row beginning with the 6 brown pills, followed by the 5 white pills, followed by the 10 light-yellow pills, and then one of the 7 light-green inactive pills daily for the next 7 days, **in that order,** for a total of 28 days or 4 weeks. The basic schedule is 21 days on active pills (brown, white, and light-yellow)—7 days on light-green inactive pills. Always take all of the 21 active pills (brown, white, and light-yellow) in each package before taking the light-green pills.

When you start your **first** cycle of TRI-LEVLEN™ 28 tablets, you should begin taking your pills on the **first** day of your next menstrual period, regardless of the day of the week or the amount of the bleeding or spotting. Note: During the first month on TRI-LEVLEN™ 28 tablets, if you start taking pills later than day 1 of your menstrual cycle, you should protect yourself by also using another method of birth control until you have taken a pill daily for seven days in a row (6 brown pills followed by 1 white pill). Thereafter, if you follow directions carefully you will obtain the full contraceptive benefit. If you begin taking pills later than the proper day, the possibility of ovulation and pregnancy occurring before or during the taking of the brown pills should be considered. Take one pill every day until you finish all 6 brown, 5 white, and 10 light-yellow pills in a package followed by all 7 light-green pills. Your period will usually begin about three days after you take the last light-yellow pill, which will be during the time you are taking the light-green pills. Don't be alarmed if the amount of bleeding is not the same as before.

The day after you have taken your last light-green pill, begin a new package of pills (first taking the 6 brown, then the 5 white, and then the 10 light-yellow pills one a day just as you did before) so that you will take a pill every day without interruption. **If you have taken the pills as directed,** the starting day for each new package will always be the same day as in the previous cycle. When switching from another oral contraceptive, TRI-LEVLEN™ 28 tablets should be started on the first day of bleeding following the last pill taken of the previous oral contraceptive.

Spotting or Breakthrough Bleeding:

Spotting is slight staining between menstrual periods which may not even require a pad. Breakthrough bleeding is a flow much like a regular period, requiring sanitary protection. Spotting is more common than breakthrough bleeding, and both occur more often in the first few cycles than in later cycles. These types of bleeding are usually temporary and without significance. It is important to continue taking your pills on schedule. If the bleeding persists for more than a few days, consult your doctor.

MISSED PILLS

There is a chance of becoming pregnant if you miss one brown, white, or light-yellow pill, and that chance increases with each additional brown, white, or light-yellow pill missed. If you miss any one of these pills, it is important it be taken as soon as remembered. If you miss any two of these pills consecutively, it is important both be taken as soon as remembered. The next pill should then be taken at the usual time. Any time you miss one or two brown, white, or light-yellow pills, **or begin a new package later than directed,** you should also use another method of birth control until you have taken a brown, white, or light-yellow pill daily for seven consecutive days. If you miss one or more light-green inactive pills (TRI-LEVLEN™ 28 tablets only), you are still protected against pregnancy **provided** you begin taking your next brown pill on the proper day. If breakthrough bleeding occurs following missed pills, it will usually be temporary and of no consequence.

If you forget to take brown, white, or light-yellow pills three days in a row, do not take them when you remember but stop the medication and discard the package. Begin a new package, as directed above, on the first day of bleeding of your next period. During the days without pills, and until you have taken 6 brown and a white pill daily for seven consecutive days, you should protect yourself from pregnancy by also using another method of birth control.

At times there may be no menstrual period after a cycle of pills. Therefore, if you miss one menstrual period but have taken the pills **exactly as you were supposed to,** continue as usual into the next cycle. If you have not taken the pills correctly and miss a menstrual period, you may be pregnant and should stop taking oral contraceptives until your doctor determines whether or not you are pregnant. Until you can get to your doctor, use another form of contraception. If two consecutive menstrual periods are missed, you should stop taking pills until it is determined whether you are pregnant. If you do become pregnant while using oral contraceptives, you should discuss the risks to the developing child with your doctor.

3. Periodic Examination.

Your doctor will take a complete medical and family history before prescribing oral contraceptives. At that time and about once a year thereafter, he will generally examine your blood pressure, breasts, abdomen, and pelvic organs (including a Papanicolaou smear, i.e., test for cancer).

SUMMARY

Oral contraceptives are the most effective method, except sterilization, for preventing pregnancy. Other methods when used conscientiously, are also very effective and have fewer risks. The serious risks of oral contraceptives are uncommon, and the "pill" is a very convenient method of preventing pregnancy. If you have certain conditions or have had these conditions in the past, you should not use oral contraceptives, because the risk is too great. These conditions are listed in the leaflet. If you do not have these conditions, and decide to use the "pill", please read the leaflet carefully so that you can use the "pill" most safely and effectively. Based on his or her assessment of your medical needs, your doctor has prescribed this drug for you. Do not give the drug to anyone else.

Manufactured for
BERLEX Laboratories, Inc., Wayne, NJ 07470
Issued December 30, 1985 60607-1

Shown in Product Identification Section, page 405

Beutlich, Inc.
7149 N. AUSTIN
NILES, IL 60648

CEO-TWO® SUPPOSITORIES

COMPOSITION

Each adult rectal suppository contains sodium bicarbonate and potassium bitartrate in a water soluble polyethylene glycol base.

ACTIONS AND USES

CEO-TWO® is successfully used as a bowel evacuant, and for bowel retraining programs. The gentle pressure of the released CO_2 in the rectum stimulates peristalsis, and defecation usually results in 10 to 20 minutes. CEO-TWO® is especially helpful for spinal cord injury patients. It is gentle as well as safe. Unlike many other rectal suppositories, CEO-TWO® is not an irritant. It is, however, effective and predictable and will not cause an embarrassment at some later inconvenient time and place. Also used pre and post partum, pre and post operatively, or whenever the last 25cm of the lower bowel must be emptied.

ADMINISTRATION AND DOSAGE

One or two suppositories can be used as needed. Moisten CEO-TWO® with warm water before inserting. Patient should retain as long as possible. Dosage can be repeated in 4–6 hours if necessary.

CONTRAINDICATIONS

As with other enemas or laxatives.

HOW SUPPLIED

In packages of 10, white opaque suppositories. Keep in cool, dry place.
DO NOT REFRIGERATE

HURRICAINE® TOPICAL ANESTHETIC LIQUID AND GEL

COMPOSITION

HURRICAINE® (20% Benzocaine)

ACTION AND INDICATION

HURRICAINE® is quick, 15 to 30 seconds, effective and safe topical anesthetic that controls pain on any accessable mucous membrane, as well as to suppress the gag reflex and it tastes good.

ADVANTAGES

Anesthesia is of short duration (12–15 minutes) with virtually no systemic absorption. True allergic reactions are rare. HURRICAINE® is also used in many dental and medical procedures with excellent patient acceptance.
PATIENTS WITH A KNOWN HYPERSENSITIVITY TO BENZOCAINE SHOULD NOT USE HURRICAINE®.
DO NOT USE IN EYES.
NOT FOR INJECTION.
KEEP OUT OF REACH OF CHILDREN.

HOW SUPPLIED

LIQUID or GEL in 1 oz. bottles & ⅛ oz tubes.

HURRICAINE® TOPICAL ANESTHETIC AEROSOL SPRAY

COMPOSITION

20% Benzocaine

ACTION AND INDICATION

HURRICAINE® SPRAY is a good tasting topical anesthetic for oral and mucousal application, will help to control pain as well as to suppress the gag reflex during certain endoscopic procedures.

ADVANTAGES

HURRICAINE® is probably the agent of choice in endoscopy because of its safety, effectiveness, and patients' acceptance. HURRICAINE® provides you with rapid onset of action (15–30 seconds) and short duration (12–15 minutes) with virtually no systemic absorption. True allergic reactions are rare.
PATIENTS WITH A KNOWN HYPERSENSITIVITY TO BENZOCAINE SHOULD NOT USE.
DO NOT USE IN EYES.
NOT FOR INJECTION.
KEEP OUT OF REACH OF CHILDREN.

HOW SUPPLIED

Aerosol SPRAY 2 oz. can

HURRICAINE® TOPICAL ANESTHETIC SPRAY KIT

COMPOSITION

HURRICAINE® SPRAY 2 oz. aerosol can 20% benzocaine with 200 disposable extension tubes.

ADVANTAGES

The use of disposable extention tubes will minimize the risk of infection thru cross contamination. Clean, quick and easy to attach.
PATIENTS WITH A KNOWN HYPERSENSITIVITY TO BENZOCAINE SHOULD NOT USE HURRICAINE®.
DO NOT USE IN EYES.
NOT FOR INJECTION.
KEEP OUT OF REACH OF CHILDREN.

HOW SUPPLIED

2 oz. Aerosol with 200 disposable extension tubes

MEVANIN-C CAPSULES

COMPOSITION

Each capsule contains: Ascorbic Acid 200 mg., Hesperidin Complex 30 mg., Calcium Lactate 300 mg., Cyanocobalamin 1 mcg., Ferrous Sulfate 65 mg., Folic Acid 0.1 mg., Vitamin A 3000 USP units, Vitamin D 300 USP units, Thiamine HCl 2 mg., Riboflavin 2 mg., Pyridoxine HCl 0.5 mg., Niacin 5 mg., plus trace amounts of copper, zinc, manganese, magnesium, potassium and iodine.

ADMINISTRATION AND DOSAGE

One capsule daily.

HOW SUPPLIED

In bottles of 90 and 450 red and white capsules.

PERIDIN-C®

COMPOSITION

Each tablet contains Hesperidin Methyl Chalcone 50 mg., Hesperidin Complex 150 mg., Ascorbic Acid 200 mg.

DOSAGE

1 tablet daily.

HOW SUPPLIED

In bottles of 100 and 500 orange tablets.

Biocraft Laboratories, Inc.
92 ROUTE 46
ELMWOOD PARK, NJ 07407

NDC 0332	PRODUCT	PROD. ID. NO.
	AMITRIPTYLINE HCL TABLETS ℞	
2120	10 mg.	22
2122	25 mg.	23
2124	50 mg.	24
2126	75 mg.	25
2128	100 mg.	26
	AMOXICILLIN CAPSULES ℞	
3107	250 mg.	01
3109	500 mg.	03
	AMOXICILLIN SUSPENSION ℞	
4150	125 mg./5 ml.	
4155	250 mg./5 ml.	
	AMPICILLIN CAPSULES ℞	
3111	250 mg.	05
3113	500 mg.	06
	AMPICILLIN SUSPENSION ℞	
4129	125 mg./5 ml.	
4131	250 mg./5 ml.	
	AMPICILLIN-PROBENECID SUSPENSION ℞	
4140	1 gm. Probenecid; 3.5 gm. Amp	
	CHLOROQUINE PHOSPHATE TABLETS ℞	
2160	250 mg.	38
	CLONIDINE HYDROCHLORIDE TABLETS ℞	
2200	0.1 mg	71
2201	0.2 mg	72
2202	0.3 mg	73
	CLOXACILLIN CAPSULES ℞	
3119	250 mg.	28
3121	500 mg.	30
	CLOXACILLIN SOLUTION ℞	
4159	125 mg./5 ml.	
	DICLOXACILLIN CAPSULES ℞	
3123	250 mg.	02
3125	500 mg.	04
	DISOPYRAMIDE PHOSPHATE CAPSULES ℞	
3127	100 mg	40
3129	150 mg	41
	HYDROCORTISONE TOPICAL CREAM	
5125	1%	
	IMIPRAMINE HCL TABLETS ℞	
2111	10 mg.	19
2113	25 mg.	20
2117	50 mg.	21
	METOCLOPRAMIDE HYDROCHLORIDE TABLETS ℞	
2203	10 mg	93
	NEOMYCIN SULFATE TABLETS ℞	
1177	500 mg.	18
	OXACILLIN CAPSULES ℞	
3115	250 mg.	12
3117	500 mg.	14
	OXACILLIN SOLUTION ℞	
4157	250 mg./5 ml.	
	PENICILLIN G POTASSIUM TABLETS ℞	
1117	200,000 Units	07
1121	250,000 Units	09
1123	400,000 Units	10
	PENICILLIN V POTASSIUM SOLUTION ℞	
4125	125 mg./5 ml.	
4127	250 mg./5 ml.	
	PENICILLIN V POTASSIUM TABLETS ℞	
1171	250 mg. ROUND	15
1172	250 mg. OVAL	16
1173	500 mg. ROUND	17
1174	500 mg. OVAL	49
	SULFAMETHOXAZOLE AND TRIMETHOPRIM TABLETS ℞	
2130	400 mg/80 mg (Single Strength)	32
2132	800 mg/160 mg (Double Strength)	33

Continued on next page

Biocraft—Cont.

SULFAMETHOXAZOLE AND TRIMETHOPRIM PEDIATRIC SUSPENSION ℞

6100 200 mg./40 mg. per 5 ml.

TRIMETHOPRIM TABLETS ℞

2158 100 mg. 34

Bock Pharmacal Company

P.O. BOX 8519
ST. LOUIS, MO 63126-0519

DOLPRN #3 TABLETS ℞ ©III

Analgesic

Each green layered tablet embossed BOCK contains:

Codeine Phosphate	30 mg.
Acetaminophen	400 mg.
Aspirin	250 mg.
Magnesium Hydroxide	60 mg.
Dried Aluminum Hydroxide	60 mg.

HOW SUPPLIED

Bottles of 100.

POLY-HISTINE CS ℞ ©

Each 5 ml. cherry flavored red syrup contains:

Codeine Phosphate	10.0 mg.
(Warning: May be habit forming.)	
Phenylpropanolamine HCl	12.5 mg.
Brompheniramine Maleate	2.0 mg.

HOW SUPPLIED

Bottles of 16 oz.

POLY-HISTINE EXPECTORANT PLAIN

Each 5 ml. cherry flavored red syrup contains:

Phenylpropanolamine HCl	12.5 mg.
Guaifenesin	100.0 mg.

HOW SUPPLIED

Bottles of 16 oz.

POLY-HISTINE-D CAPSULES ℞

Antihistamines + Decongestant

Each red-clear timed release capsule imprinted BOCK contains:

Phenylpropanolamine HCl	50 mg.
Phenyltoloxamine Citrate	16 mg.
Pyrilamine Maleate	16 mg.
Pheniramine Maleate	16 mg.

HOW SUPPLIED

Bottles of 100.

POLY-HISTINE-D ELIXIR ℞

Antihistamines + Decongestant

Each 5 ml. wild cherry flavored red elixir contains:

Phenylpropanolamine HCl	12.5 mg.
Phenyltoloxamine Citrate	4.0 mg.
Pyrilamine Maleate	4.0 mg.
Pheniramine Maleate	4.0 mg.
Alcohol	4%

HOW SUPPLIED

Bottles of 16 oz.

POLY-HISTINE-D PED CAPS ℞

Antihistamine + Decongestant

Each clear timed release capsule imprinted BOCK contains:

Phenylpropanolamine HCl	25 mg.
Phenyltoloxamine Citrate	8 mg.
Pyrilamine Maleate	8 mg.
Pheniramine Maleate	8 mg.

HOW SUPPLIED

Bottles of 100.

POLY-HISTINE DM SYRUP ℞

Each 5 ml. black-raspberry flavored purple syrup contains:

Dextromethorphan HBr	10.0 mg.
Phenylpropanolamine HCl	12.5 mg.
Brompheniramine Maleate	2.0 mg.

HOW SUPPLIED

Bottles of 16 oz.

PRENATE 90® ℞

Vitamin-Mineral Supplement

Each white film coated tablet embossed BOCK contains:

Iron (Ferrous Fumarate)	90 mg.*
Iodine (Potassium Iodine)	0.15 mg.
Calcium (Calcium Carbonate)	250 mg.
Copper (Cupric Oxide)	2 mg.
Zinc (Zinc Oxide)	20 mg.
Folic Acid	1 mg.
Vitamin A (Acetate)	8000 I.U.
Vitamin D (Ergocalciferol)	400 I.U.
Vitamin E (Acetate)	30 I.U.
Vitamin C (Ascorbic Acid)	120 mg.
Vitamin B_1 (Thiamine Mononitrate)	3 mg.
Vitamin B_2 (Riboflavin)	3.4 mg.
Vitamin B_6 (Pyridoxine HCl)	20 mg.
Vitamin B_{12} (Cyanocobalamin)	12 mcg.
Niacinamide	20 mg.
Docusate Sodium	50 mg.

*MICRO IRON (A special base to provide delayed therapeutic action)

HOW SUPPLIED

Bottles of 100.

THEON SYRUP ℞

Each 5 ml. dye-free syrup contains:

Theophylline (Anhydrous)	50 mg.
Alcohol	1%

HOW SUPPLIED

Bottles of 16 oz.

ZEPHREX TABLETS ℞

Each blue film coated tablet embossed BOCK contains:

Pseudoephedrine HCl	60 mg.
Guaifenesin	400 mg.

HOW SUPPLIED

Bottles of 100.

ZEPHREX-LA TABLETS ℞

Each orange timed release tablet embossed BOCK contains:

Pseudoephedrine HCl	120 mg.
Guaifenesin	600 mg.

HOW SUPPLIED

Bottles of 100.

Boehringer Ingelheim Pharmaceuticals, Inc.

A subsidiary of Boehringer Ingelheim Corporation
90 EAST RIDGE
POST OFFICE BOX 368
RIDGEFIELD, CT 06877

ALUPENT® ℞

[al'u-pent]

(metaproterenol sulfate, USP)

Bronchodilator

Tablets 10 mg	**BI-CODE 74**
Tablets 20 mg	**BI-CODE 72**
Metered Dose Inhaler 15 ml	**BI-CODE 70**
Syrup 10 mg/5 ml	**BI-CODE 73**
Inhalant Solution 5%	**BI-CODE 71**
Inhalant Solution Unit Dose Vials 0.6%	**BI-CODE 69**

DESCRIPTION

Alupent® (metaproterenol sulfate USP) Metered Dose Inhaler is administered by oral inhalation. Each Metered Dose Inhaler contains 225 mg of metaproterenol sulfate as a micronized powder. This is sufficient medication for 300 inhalations. Each metered dose expressed from the inhaler delivers at the mouthpiece approximately 0.65 mg of metaproterenol sulfate. The inert ingredients are fluorochlorohydrocarbons as propellants, and sorbitan trioleate.

Alupent Inhalant Solution is administered by oral inhalation with the aid of a hand-bulb nebulizer or an intermittent positive pressure breathing apparatus (IPPB). It contains Alupent 5% in a pH-adjusted aqueous solution containing benzalkonium chloride and edetate disodium as preservatives.

Alupent Inhalant Solution Unit Dose Vial is administered by oral inhalation with the aid of an IPPB. It contains Alupent 0.6% in a sterile pH-adjusted aqueous solution with edetate disodium and sodium chloride.

Alupent Syrup is administered orally. Each teaspoonful (5 ml) of syrup contains metaproterenol sulfate 10 mg. The inactive ingredients are edetate disodium, FD&C Red No. 40, hydroxyethylcellulose, imitation black cherry flavor, methylparaben, propylparaben, saccharin, sorbitol solution.

Alupent Tablets are administered orally. Each tablet contains metaproterenol sulfate 10 mg or 20 mg. The inactive ingredients are colloidal silicon dioxide, corn starch, dibasic calcium phosphate, lactose, magnesium stearate.

Chemically, Alupent is 1-(3,5 dihydroxyphenyl)-2-isopropylaminoethanol sulfate, a white crystalline, racemic mixture of two optically active isomers. It differs from isoproterenol hydrochloride by having two hydroxyl groups attached at the meta positions on the benzene ring rather than one at the meta and one at the para position.

CLINICAL PHARMACOLOGY

Alupent (metaproterenol sulfate USP) is a potent beta-adrenergic stimulator. The Alupent Metered Dose Inhaler and Inhalant Solution have a rapid onset of action. It is postulated that beta-adrenergic stimulants produce many of their pharmacological effects by activation of adenyl cyclase, the enzyme which catalyzes the conversion of adenosine triphosphate to cyclic adenosine monophosphate.

Absorption, biotransformation and excretion studies following administration by inhalation have not been performed. Following oral administration in humans, an average of 40% of the drug is absorbed; it is not metabolized by catechol-O-methyltransferase or sulfatase enzymes in the gut, but is excreted primarily as glucuronic acid conjugates.

When administered orally or by inhalation, Alupent decreases reversible bronchospasm. Pulmonary function tests performed concomitantly usually show improvement following Alupent administration, e.g., an increase in the one-second forced expiratory volume (FEV_1), an increase in maximum expiratory flow rate, an increase in peak expiratory flow rate, an increase in forced vital capacity, and/or a decrease in airway resistance. The resultant decrease in airway obstruction may relieve the dyspnea associated with bronchospasm.

Controlled single- and multiple-dose studies have been performed with pulmonary function monitoring. The duration of effect of a single dose of Alupent Tablets 20 mg or Alupent Syrup (that is, the period of time during which there is a 15% or greater increase in FEV_1.) was up to 4 hours. Four controlled multiple-dose 60-day studies, comparing the effectiveness of Alupent Tablets with ephedrine tablets, have been performed. Because of difficulties in study design, only one study was available which could be analyzed in depth. This study showed a loss of effficacy with time for both Alupent and ephedrine. Therefore, the physician should take this phenomenon into account in evaluating the individual patient's overall management. Further studies are in progress to adequately explain these results.

Controlled single- and multiple-dose studies have been performed with pulmonary function monitoring. The duration of effect of a single dose of two to three inhalations of Alupent Metered Dose Inhaler (MDI) (that is, the period of time during which there is a 20% or greater increase in FEV_1) has varied from 1 to 5 hours.

In repetitive-dosing studies (up to q.i.d.) the duration of effect for a similar dose of Alupent MDI has ranged from about 1 to 2.5 hours. Present studies are inadequate to explain the divergence in duration of the FEV_1 effect between single- and repetitive-dosing studies, respectively.

Following controlled single dose studies with Alupent Inhalant Solution by an intermittent positive pressure breathing apparatus (IPPB) and by hand-bulb nebulizers, significant improvement (15% or greater increase in FEV_1) occurred within 5 to 30 minutes and persisted for periods varying from 2 to 6 hours.

In these studies, the longer duration of effect occurred in the studies in which the drug was administered by IPPB, i.e., 6 hours versus 2 to 3 hours when administered by hand-bulb nebulizer. In these studies the doses used were 0.3 ml by IPPB and 10 inhalations by hand-bulb nebulizer.

In controlled repetitive-dosing studies with Alupent Inhalant Solution by IPPB and by hand-bulb nebulizer the onset of effect occurred within 5 to 30 minutes and duration ranged from 4 to 6 hours. In these studies the doses were 0.3 ml b.i.d. or t.i.d. when given by IPPB, and 10 inhalations q.i.d. (no more often than q4h) when given by hand-bulb nebulizer. As in the single dose studies, effectiveness was measured as a sustained increase in FEV_1, of 15% or greater. In these repetitive-dosing studies there was no apparent difference in duration between the two methods of delivery.

Clinical studies were conducted in which the effectiveness of Alupent Inhalant Solution was evaluated by comparison with that of isoproterenol hydrochloride over periods of two to three months. Both drugs continued to produce significant improvement in pulmonary function throughout this period of treatment.

Recent studies in laboratory animals (minipigs, rodents and dogs) recorded the occurrence of cardiac arrhythmias and sudden deaths (with histologic evidence of myocardial necrosis) when beta agonists and methylxanthines were administered concurrently. The significance of these findings when applied to humans is currently unknown.

INDICATIONS AND USAGE

Alupent® (metaproterenol sulfate USP) is indicated as a bronchodilator for bronchial asthma and for reversible bronchospasm which may occur in association with bronchitis and emphysema.

CONTRAINDICATIONS

Use in patients with cardiac arrhythmias associated with tachycardia is contraindicated.
Although rare, immediate hypersensitivity reactions can occur. Therefore, Alupent® (metaproterenol sulfate USP) is contraindicated in patients with a history of hypersensitivity to any of its components.

WARNINGS

Excessive use of adrenergic aerosols is potentially dangerous. Fatalities have been reported following excessive use of Alupent® (metaproterenol sulfate USP) as with other sympathomimetic inhalation preparations, and the exact cause is unknown. Cardiac arrest was noted in several cases.
Paradoxical bronchoconstriction with repeated excessive administration has been reported with other sympathomimetic agents. Therefore, it is possible that this phenomenon could occur with Alupent.
Patients should be advised to contact their physician in the event that they do not respond to their usual dose of sympathomimetic amine aerosol.

PRECAUTIONS

Because Alupent® (metaproterenol sulfate USP) is a sympathomimetic drug, it should be used with great caution in patients with hypertension, coronary artery disease, congestive heart failure, hyperthyroidism or diabetes, or when there is sensitivity to sympathomimetic amines.
Information for Patients: Extreme care must be exercised with respect to the administration of additional sympathomimetic agents. A sufficient interval of time should elapse prior to administration of another sympathomimetic agent.
Carcinogenesis: Long-term studies in mice and rats to evaluate the oral carcinogenic potential of metaproterenol sulfate have not been completed.
Studies of metaproterenol sulfate have not been conducted to determine mutagenic potential or effect on fertility.
Pregnancy: *Teratogenic Effects: Pregnancy Category C.* Alupent has been shown to be teratogenic and embryocidal in rabbits when given orally in doses 620 times the human inhalation dose and 62 times the human oral dose. There are no adequate and well-controlled studies in pregnant women. Alupent should be used during pregnancy only if the potential benefit justifies the potential risk to the fetus.
Oral reproduction studies in mice, rats and rabbits showed no teratogenic or embryocidal effects at 50 mg/kg corresponding to 310 times the human inhalation dose and 31 times the human oral dose. Teratogenic effects in the rabbit included skeletal abnormalities and hydrocephalus with bone separation.
Nursing Mothers: It is not known whether this drug is excreted in human milk. Because many drugs are excreted in human milk, caution should be exercised when Alupent is administered to a nursing woman.
Pediatric Use: See **DOSAGE AND ADMINISTRATION.**

ADVERSE REACTIONS

Adverse reactions are similar to those noted with other sympathomimetic agents. Adverse reactions such as tachycardia, hypertension, palpitations, nervousness, tremor, nausea and vomiting have been reported.
The most frequent adverse reactions to Alupent Inhalant Solution (metaproterenol sulfate USP) are nervousness and tachycardia which occur in about 1 in 7 patients, tremor which occurs in about 1 in 20 patients and nausea which occurs in about 1 in 50 patients. Less frequent adverse reactions are hypertension, palpitations, vomiting and bad taste which occur in approximately 1 in 300 patients.

OVERDOSAGE

The symptoms of overdosage are those of excessive beta-adrenergic stimulation listed under **ADVERSE REACTIONS.** These reactions usually do not require treatment other than reduction of dosage and/or frequency of administration.

DOSAGE AND ADMINISTRATION

If Alupent® (metaproterenol sulfate USP) is administered before or after other sympathomimetic bronchodilators, caution should be exercised with respect to possible potentiation of adrenergic effects.
Metered Dose Inhaler: The usual single dose is two to three inhalations. With repetitive dosing, inhalation should usually not be repeated more often than about every three to four hours. Total dosage per day should not exceed 12 inhalations. Alupent MDI is not recommended for use in children under 12 years of age.
Inhalant Solution: Usually treatment need not be repeated more often than every four hours to relieve acute attacks of bronchospasm. As part of a total treatment program in chronic bronchospastic pulmonary diseases, Alupent Inhalant Solution may be administered three to four times a day. As with all medications, the physician should begin therapy with the lowest effective dose and then titrate the dosage according to the individual patient's requirements.
Alupent Inhalant Solution is not recommended for use in children under 12 years of age.
Inhalant Solution 5%: Alupent Inhalant Solution is administered by oral inhalation with the aid of a hand bulb nebulizer or an intermittent positive pressure breathing apparatus (IPPB).

Method of Administration	Usual Single Dose	Range	Dilution
Hand-bulb nebulizer	10 inhalations	5–15 inhalations	No dilution
IPPB	0.3 ml	0.2–0.3 ml	Diluted in approx. 2.5 ml of saline solution or other diluent

Inhalation Solution Unit-dose Vial 0.6%: Alupent Inhalant Solution Unit-dose Vial is administered by oral inhalation using an IPPB device. The usual adult dose is one vial per nebulization treatment. Each vial is equivalent to 0.3 ml Alupent Inhalant Solution 5% diluted to 2.5 ml with normal saline.
Syrup: Children aged six to nine years or weight under 60 lbs—one teaspoonful three or four times a day. Children over nine years or weight over 60 lbs—two teaspoonfuls three or four times a day. Experience in children under the age of six is limited to seventy-eight children. Of this number, forty were treated with Alupent syrup for at least one month. In this group daily doses of approximately 1.3 to 2.6 mg/kg were well tolerated. Adults—two teaspoonfuls three or four times a day.
Tablets: *Adults:* The usual dose is 20 mg three or four times a day. *Children:* Aged six to nine years or weight under 60 lbs—10 mg three or four times a day. Over nine years or weight over 60 lbs—20 mg three or four times a day. Alupent tablets are not recommended for use in children under six years at this time.

HOW SUPPLIED

Metered Dose Inhaler: Each Alupent® Metered Dose Inhaler contains 225 mg of metaproterenol sulfate as a micronized powder in inert propellants. Alupent Metered Dose Inhaler with mouthpiece (15 ml). Alupent Metered Dose Inhaler refill (15 ml). Store below 77°F (25°C). Avoid excessive humidity.
Inhalant Solution: Alupent Inhalant Solution is supplied as a 5% solution in bottles of 10 ml or 30 ml with accompanying calibrated dropper. Store below 77°F (25°C). Protect from light. Do not use the solution if it is brown or has a precipitate.
Alupent Inhalant Solution Unit Dose Vial is supplied as a 0.6% clear colorless or nearly colorless solution containing 2.5 ml with 25 vials per box. Store below 77°F (25°C). Protect from light. Do not use the solution if it is brown or has a precipitate.
Syrup: Alupent is available as a cherry-flavored syrup. 10 mg per teaspoonful (5 ml) in 16 fl. oz. bottles. Store below 86°F (30°C). Protect from light.
Tablets: Alupent is supplied in two dosage strengths as scored round white tablets in bottles of 100. Tablets of 10 mg coded BI/74. Tablets of 20 mg coded BI/72. Storage for bottles: Store below 86°F (30°C). Protect from light. Storage for blister samples: Store below 77°F (25°C). Protect from light.
AL-PI 7/86

Shown in Product Identification Section, page 405

CATAPRES® ℞
[kah 'tah-pres]
(clonidine hydrochloride USP)
Oral Antihypertensive
Tablets, 0.1 mg .... BI-CODE 06
Tablets, 0.2 mg .... BI-CODE 07
Tablets, 0.3 mg .... BI-CODE 11

DESCRIPTION

Catapres® (clonidine hydrochloride USP), an antihypertensive agent, is an imidazoline derivative and exists as a mesomeric compound. Its chemical name is 2-(2,6-dichlorophenylamino)-2-imidazoline hydrochloride. It is an odorless, bitter, white crystalline substance soluble in water and alcohol, with a molecular weight of 266.57. The 0.1 mg tablet is equivalent to 0.087 mg of the free base.

ACTIONS

Catapres® (clonidine hydrochloride USP) is an antihypertensive agent whose mechanism of action appears to be central alpha-adrenergic stimulation as demonstrated in animal studies. This results in the inhibition of bulbar sympathetic cardioaccelerator and sympathetic vasoconstrictor centers, thereby causing a decrease in sympathetic outflow from the brain. Initially, Catapres stimulates peripheral alpha-adrenergic receptors producing transient vasoconstriction.
Catapres acts relatively rapidly. The patient's blood pressure declines within 30 to 60 minutes after an oral dose, the maximum decrease occurring within 2 to 4 hours. The antihypertensive effect in humans lasts approximately 6 to 8 hours. The peak plasma level of Catapres occurs in approximately 3 to 5 hours with a plasma half-life of 12 to 16 hours. Catapres, brand of clonidine hydrochloride, and its metabolites are excreted mainly in the urine. When labeled drug was administered, unchanged drug appearing in the urine accounted for about 32 percent of administered radioactivity.
Orthostatic effects are mild and infrequent since supine pressure is reduced to essentially the same extent as standing pressure. Catapres does not alter normal hemodynamic responses to exercise. Acute studies with Catapres in humans have demonstrated a moderate reduction (15 to 20%) of cardiac output in the supine position with no change in the peripheral resistance, while at a 45° tilt there is a smaller reduction in cardiac output and a decrease of peripheral resistance. Renal blood flow and the glomerular filtration rate remain essentially unchanged. During long-term therapy, cardiac output tends to return to control values, while peripheral resistance remains decreased. Slowing of the pulse rate has been observed in most patients given Catapres.
Other studies in humans have provided evidence of a reduction in plasma renin activity and in the excretion of aldosterone and catecholamines in patients treated with Catapres®.
The exact relationship between these pharmacologic actions of Catapres in humans, and its antihypertensive effect in individual patients has not been fully elucidated at this time.
Catapres has been administered together with hydralazine, guanethidine, methyldopa, reserpine, spironolactone, furosemide, chlorthalidone and thiazide diuretics without drug-to-drug interactions. The concomitant administration of a diuretic has been shown to enhance the antihypertensive efficacy of Catapres.

INDICATION

Catapres® (clonidine hydrochloride USP) is indicated in the treatment of hypertension. As an antihypertensive drug, Catapres is mild to moderate in potency. It may be employed in a general treatment program with a diuretic and/or other antihypertensive agents as needed for proper patient response.

WARNINGS

Tolerance may develop in some patients, necessitating a reevaluation of therapy.
Use in Pregnancy: Reproduction studies have been performed with Catapres® (clonidine hydrochloride USP) in three animal species. The findings of these studies reflected no teratogenic effect but some embryotoxicity was evident at doses as low as 0.015 mg/kg (one-third the maximum recommended dose). In view of these findings, and since information on possible adverse effects in pregnant women is limited to uncontrolled clinical data, Catapres is not recommended in women who are or may become pregnant unless the potential benefit outweighs the potential risk to mother and infant.
Use in Children: No clinical experience is available with the use of Catapres in children. Studies are being performed to evaluate its use in the treatment of hypertension in children.

PRECAUTIONS

General: In patients who have developed localized contact sensitization to Catapres-TTS® (clonidine), substitution of oral clonidine hydrochloride therapy may be associated with development of a generalized skin rash.
In patients who develop an allergic reaction to Catapres-TTS that extends beyond the local patch site (such as generalized skin rash, urticaria, or angioedema), oral clonidine hydrochloride substitution may elicit a similar reaction.

WITHDRAWAL

Patients should be instructed not to discontinue therapy without consulting their physician. Sudden cessation of clonidine treatment has resulted in subjective symptoms such as nervousness, agitation and headache, accompanied or followed by a rapid rise in blood pressure and elevated catecholamine concentrations in the plasma, but such occurrences have usually been associated with previous administration of high oral doses (exceeding 1.2 mg/day) and/or with continuation of concomitant beta-blocker therapy. Rare instances of hypertensive encephalopathy and death have been reported. When discontinuing therapy with Catapres, the physician should reduce the dose gradually over 2 to 4 days to avoid withdrawal symptomatology.

Continued on next page

Boehringer Ingelheim—Cont.

An excessive rise in blood pressure following Catapres discontinuation can be reversed by administration of oral clonidine or by intravenous phentolamine. If therapy is to be discontinued in patients receiving beta-blockers and clonidine concurrently, beta-blockers should be discontinued several days before the gradual withdrawal of Catapres.
Patients who engage in potentially hazardous activities, such as operating machinery or driving, should be advised of the sedative effect of Catapres. Like any other antihypertensive agent, Catapres should be used with caution in patients with severe coronary insufficiency, recent myocardial infarction, cerebrovascular disease or chronic renal failure.
As an integral part of their overall long-term care, patients treated with Catapres should receive periodic eye examinations (see Toxicology).

DRUG INTERACTIONS

If a patient receiving clonidine hydrochloride is also taking tricyclic antidepressants, the effect of clonidine may be reduced, thus necessitating an increase in dosage. Clonidine hydrochloride may enhance the CNS-depressive effects of alcohol, barbiturates or other sedatives. Amitriptyline in combination with clonidine enhances the manifestation of corneal lesions in rats (see Toxicology).

ADVERSE REACTIONS

The most common reactions associated with Catapres® (clonidine hydrochloride USP) therapy are dry mouth (about 40%), drowsiness (about 35%), and sedation (about 8%). Constipation, dizziness, headache, and fatigue have been reported. Generally, these effects tend to diminish with continued therapy.
The following reactions have been associated with the drug, some of them rarely. In some instances an exact causal relationship has not been established.
Gastrointestinal: Anorexia, malaise, nausea, vomiting, parotid pain, mild transient abnormalities in liver function tests. There has been one report of possible drug-induced hepatitis without icterus and hyperbilirubinemia in a patient receiving Catapres, chlorthalidone and papaverine hydrochloride.
Metabolic: Weight gain, transient elevation of blood glucose or serum creatine phosphokinase, gynecomastia.
Cardiovascular: Congestive heart failure, Raynaud's phenomenon, and electrocardiographic abnormalities manifested as Wenckebach period or ventricular trigeminy. Rare cases of sinus bradycardia and atrioventricular block have been reported, both with and without the use of concomitant digitalis.
Central Nervous System: Vivid dreams or nightmares, insomnia, other behavioral changes, nervousness, restlessness, anxiety, mental depression.
Dermatologic: Rash, angioneurotic edema, hives, urticaria, thinning of the hair, pruritus not associated with a rash.
Genitourinary: Impotence, urinary retention.
Other: Increased sensitivity to alcohol, dryness, itching or burning of the eyes, dryness of the nasal mucosa, pallor, or weakly positive Coombs' test.

DOSAGE AND ADMINISTRATION

The dose of Catapres® (clonidine hydrochloride USP) must be adjusted according to the patient's individual blood pressure response. The following is a general guide to its administration.
Initial dose: One 0.1 mg tablet twice daily. *Maintenance dose:* Further increments of 0.1 mg or 0.2 mg per day may be made until the desired response is achieved. The therapeutic doses most commonly employed have ranged from 0.2 mg to 0.8 mg per day given in divided doses. Studies have indicated that 2.4 mg is the maximum effective daily dose but doses as high as this have rarely been employed.

OVERDOSAGE

Profound hypotension, weakness, somnolence, diminished or absent reflexes and vomiting followed the accidental ingestion of Catapres® (clonidine hydrochloride USP) by several children from 19 months to 5 years of age. Gastric lavage and administration of an analeptic and vasopressor led to complete recovery within 24 hours. Tolazoline in intravenous doses of 10 mg at 30-minute intervals usually abolishes all effects of Catapres overdosage.

TOXICOLOGY

In several studies Catapres® (clonidine hydrochloride USP) produced a dose-dependent increase in the incidence and severity of spontaneously occurring retinal degeneration in albino rats treated for 6 months or longer. Tissue distribution studies in dogs and monkeys revealed that Catapres was concentrated in the choroid of the eye. In view of the retinal degeneration observed in rats, eye examinations were performed in 908 patients prior to the start of Catapres therapy, who were then examined periodically thereafter. In 353 of these 908 patients, examinations were performed for periods of 24 months or longer. Except for some dryness of the eyes, no drug-related abnormal ophthalmologic findings were recorded and Catapres did not alter retinal function as shown by specialized tests such as the electroretinogram and macular dazzle. In rats, clonidine hydrochloride in combination with amitriptyline produced corneal lesions within 5 days.

HOW SUPPLIED

Catapres® (clonidine hydrochloride USP) is available as 0.1 mg (tan) and 0.2 mg (orange) oval, single-scored tablets in bottles of 100 and 1000 and unit dose packages of 100. Also available as 0.3 mg (peach) oval, single-scored tablets in bottles of 100.
The inactive ingredients are colloidal silicon dioxide, corn starch, dibasic calcium phosphate, FD&C Yellow No. 6, gelatin, glycerin, lactose, magnesium stearate, methyl paraben, propyl paraben. The Catapres 0.1 mg tablet also contains FD&C Blue No. 1 and FD&C Red No. 3.
Store below 86°F (30°C). Avoid excessive humidity.

CAUTION

Federal law prohibits dispensing without prescription.

CA-PI-7/86

Shown in Product Identification Section, page 405

CATAPRES-TTS® ℞

(clonidine) **Catapres-TTS®-1**
Transdermal Therapeutic **Catapres-TTS®-2**
System **Catapres-TTS®-3**
(Programmed delivery *in vivo* of 0.1, 0.2 or 0.3 mg clonidine per day, for one week)

DESCRIPTION

Catapres-TTS® (clonidine) is a transdermal system providing continuous systemic delivery of clonidine for 7 days at an approximately constant rate. Clonidine is a centrally acting alpha agonist and is an antihypertensive agent. It is an imidazoline derivative whose chemical name is 2, 6-dichloro-N-2-imidazolidinylidenebenzenamine.
System Structure and Components: Catapres-TTS® is a multilayered film, 0.2 mm thick, containing clonidine as the active agent. System area is 3.5, 7.0, or 10.5 cm^2 and the amount of drug released is directly proportional to area. (See Release Rate Concept.) The composition per unit area of all three dosages is identical.
Proceeding from the visible surface towards the surface attached to the skin, are four layers: 1) a backing layer of pigmented polyester film; 2) a drug reservoir of clonidine, mineral oil, polyisobutylene, and colloidal silicon dioxide; 3) a microporous polypropylene membrane that controls the rate of delivery of clonidine from the system to the skin surface; 4) an adhesive formulation of clonidine, mineral oil, polyisobutylene, and colloidal silicon dioxide. Prior to use, a protective peel strip of polyester that covers layer 4 is removed.
Release Rate Concept: Catapres-TTS® is programmed to release clonidine at an approximately constant rate for 7 days. The energy source for drug release derives from the concentration gradient existing between a saturated solution of drug in the system and the much lower concentration prevailing in the skin. Clonidine flows in the direction of the lower concentration at a constant rate, limited by the rate-controlling membrane, so long as a saturated solution is maintained in the drug reservoir.
Following system application to intact skin, clonidine in the adhesive layer saturates the skin sites below the system. Clonidine from the drug reservoir then begins to flow through the rate-controlling membrane and the adhesive layer of the system into the systemic circulation via the capillaries beneath the skin. Therapeutic plasma clonidine levels are achieved 2 to 3 days after initial application of Catapres-TTS®.
The 3.5, 7.0 and 10.5 cm^2 systems respectively deliver 0.1, 0.2, and 0.3 mg clonidine per day. To ensure constant release of drug over 7 days, the total drug content of the system is greater than the total amount of drug delivered. Application of a new system to a fresh skin site at weekly intervals continuously maintains therapeutic plasma concentrations of clonidine. If the Catapres-TTS® is removed and not replaced with a new system, therapeutic plasma clonidine levels will persist for about 8 hours and then decline slowly over several days. Over this time period, blood pressure returns gradually to pretreatment levels. If the patient experiences localized skin irritation before completing 7 days of use, the system may be removed and replaced with a new one applied on a fresh skin site.

CLINICAL PHARMACOLOGY

The plasma half-life of clonidine is 12.7 ± 7 hours. Following oral administration, about 40–60% of the absorbed dose is recovered in the urine as unchanged drug in 24 hours. About 50% of the absorbed dose is metabolized in the liver.
Clonidine stimulates alpha-adrenoreceptors in the brain stem, resulting in reduced sympathetic outflow from the central nervous system and a decrease in peripheral resistance, renal vascular resistance, heart rate, and blood pressure. Renal blood flow and glomerular filtration rate remain essentially unchanged. Normal postural reflexes are intact, and therefore orthostatic symptoms are mild and infrequent.
Acute studies with clonidine hydrochloride in humans have demonstrated a moderate reduction (15% to 20%) of cardiac output in the supine position with no change in the peripheral resistance; at a 45° tilt there is a smaller reduction in cardiac output and a decrease of peripheral resistance. During long-term therapy, cardiac output tends to return to control values, while peripheral resistance remains decreased. Slowing of the pulse rate has been observed in most patients given clonidine, but the drug does not alter normal hemodynamic response to exercise.
Other studies in patients have provided evidence of a reduction in plasma renin activity and in the excretion of aldosterone and catecholamines, but the exact relationship of these pharmacologic actions to the antihypertensive effect has not been fully elucidated.
Clonidine acutely stimulates growth hormone release in both children and adults, but does not produce a chronic elevation of growth hormone with long-term use.
Tolerance may develop in some patients, necessitating a reevaluation of therapy.

INDICATIONS FOR USE

Catapres-TTS® (clonidine) is indicated in the treatment of hypertension. It may be employed alone or concomitantly with other antihypertensive agents.

CONTRAINDICATIONS

Catapres-TTS® (clonidine) should not be used in patients with known hypersensitivity to clonidine or to any other component of the adhesive layer of the therapeutic system.

PRECAUTIONS

General: In patients who have developed localized contact sensitization to Catapres-TTS® substitution of oral clonidine hydrochloride therapy may be associated with development of a generalized skin rash.
In patients who develop an allergic reaction to Catapres-TTS® that extends beyond the local patch site (such as generalized skin rash, urticaria, or angioedema) oral clonidine hydrochloride substitution may elicit a similar reaction.
As with all antihypertensive therapy, Catapres-TTS® should be used with caution in patients with severe coronary insufficiency, recent myocardial infarction, cerebrovascular disease, or chronic renal failure.
Transdermal clonidine systems should be removed before attempting defibrillation or cardioversion because of the potential for altered electrical conductivity that may enhance the possibility of arcing, a phenomenon associated with the use of defibrillators.
Withdrawal: Patients should be instructed not to discontinue therapy without consulting their physician. Sudden cessation of clonidine treatment has resulted in subjective symptoms such as nervousness, headache and sweating, accompanied or followed by a rapid rise in blood pressure and elevated catecholamine concentrations in the plasma, but such occurrences have usually been associated with previous administration of high oral doses (exceeding 1.2 mg/day) and/or with continuation of concomitant beta-blocker therapy. Rare instances of hypertensive encephalopathy and death have been reported.
An excessive rise in blood pressure following Catapres-TTS® discontinuance can be reversed by administration of oral clonidine or by intravenous phentolamine. If therapy is to be discontinued in patients receiving beta-blockers and clonidine concurrently, beta-blockers should be discontinued several days before cessation of Catapres-TTS® administration.
Perioperative Use: As with oral clonidine therapy, Catapres-TTS® therapy should not be interrupted during the surgical period. Blood pressure should be carefully monitored during surgery and additional measures to control blood pressure should be available if required. Physicians considering starting Catapres-TTS® therapy during the perioperative period must be aware that therapeutic plasma clonidine levels are not achieved until 2 to 3 days after initial application of Catapres-TTS®. (See Dosage and Administration.)
Information for Patients: Patients who engage in potentially hazardous activities, such as operating machinery or driving, should be advised of a potential sedative effect of clonidine. Patients should be cautioned against interruption of Catapres-TTS® therapy without a physician's advice. Patients should be advised that if the system begins to loosen from the skin after application, the adhesive overlay should be applied directly over the system to ensure good adhesion over its 7-day lifetime. Instructions for using the system are provided. Patients who develop moderate or severe erythema and/or localized vesicle formation at the site of application, or a generalized skin rash, should consult their physician promptly about the possible need to remove the patch.
Drug Interactions: If a patient receiving clonidine is also taking tricyclic antidepressants, the effect of clonidine may be reduced, thus necessitating an increase in dosage. Clonidine may enhance the CNS-depressive effects of alcohol, barbiturates or other sedatives. Amitriptyline in combina-

tion with clonidine enhances the manifestation of corneal lesions in rats. (See Toxicology Section.)

Carcinogenesis, Mutagenesis, Impairment of Fertility: In a 132-week (fixed concentration) dietary administration study in rats, clonidine hydrochloride administered at 111 to 160 times the maximum recommended daily human dose (MRDHD) of Catapres-TTS® was unassociated with evidence of carcinogenic potential. Results from the Ames test with clonidine hydrochloride revealed no evidence of mutagenesis. Fertility of male or female rats was unaffected by doses of clonidine hydrochloride as high as 150 mcg/kg or about 10.5 times the MRDHD of Catapres-TTS®. Fertility of female rats did, however, appear to be affected (in another experiment) by doses of clonidine hydrochloride at 500 to 2000 mcg/kg or 35 to 140 times the MRDHD of Catapres-TTS®.

Pregnancy: Teratogenic Effects Pregnancy Category C. Reproduction studies performed in rabbits at doses up to approximately 10.5 times the maximum recommended daily human dose (MRDHD) of Catapres-TTS® have revealed no evidence of teratogenic or embryotoxic potential in rabbits. In rats, however, doses as low as 1.2 times the MRDHD of clonidine were associated with increased resorptions in a study in which dams were treated continuously from 2 months prior to mating. Increased resorptions were not associated with treatment at the same or at higher dose levels (up to 10.5 times the MRDHD of clonidine) when dams were treated days 6–15 of gestation. Increased resorptions were observed at much higher levels (140 times the MRDHD of clonidine) in rats and mice treated days 1–14 of gestation (lowest dose employed in that study was 500 mcg/kg). There are, however, no adequate and well-controlled studies in pregnant women. Because animal reproduction studies are not always predictive of human response, this drug should be used during pregnancy only if clearly needed.

Nursing Mothers: As clonidine is excreted in human milk, caution should be exercised when Catapres-TTS® is administered to a nursing woman.

Pediatric Use: Safety and effectiveness in children below the age of 12 have not been established.

ADVERSE REACTIONS

Most systemic adverse effects during therapy with Catapres-TTS® (clonidine) have been mild and have tended to diminish with continued therapy. In a 3-month, multiclinic trial of Catapres-TTS® in 101 hypertensive patients, the most frequent systemic reactions were dry mouth (25 patients) and drowsiness (12 patients).

Transient localized skin reactions, primarily localized pruritus, occurred in 51 patients. Twenty-six patients experienced localized erythema. This erythema and pruritus were more common in patients utilizing an adhesive overlay for the entire 7-day treatment period. Allergic contact sensitization to Catapres-TTS® was observed in 5 patients.

In additional clinical experience contact dermatitis was observed in 100 of 631 patients (about 16 in 100) treated for a mean duration of 24 weeks.

The following less frequent adverse experiences were also reported in patients involved in this multiclinic trial with Catapres-TTS®:

Gastrointestinal: Constipation (1 patient); nausea (1); and changes in taste (1).

Central Nervous System: Fatigue (6 patients); headache (5); lethargy (3); sedation (3); insomnia (2); dizziness (2); and nervousness (1).

Genitourinary: Impotence/sexual dysfunction (2 patients).

Dermatological: Localized vesiculation (7 patients); hyperpigmentation (5); edema (3); excoriation (3); burning (3); papules (1); throbbing (1); blanching (1); and generalized macular rash (1).

In additional clinical experience involving 3539 patients, less common dermatological reactions have occurred, where a causal relationship to Catapres-TTS® was not established: maculopapular skin rash (10 cases); urticaria (2 cases); angioedema involving the face (2 cases), one of which also involved the tongue.

Oro-otolaryngeal: Dry throat (2 patients).

In long experience with oral Catapres® (clonidine hydrochloride USP), the most common adverse reactions have been dry mouth (about 40%), drowsiness (about 35%) and sedation (about 8%). In addition, the following adverse reactions have been reported less frequently:

Gastrointestinal: Nausea and vomiting, about 5 in 100 patients; anorexia and malaise, each about 1 in 100; mild transient abnormalities in liver function tests, about 1 in 100; parotitis, rarely.

Metabolic: Weight gain, about 1 in 100 patients; gynecomastia, about 1 in 1000; transient elevation of blood glucose or serum creatine phosphokinase, rarely.

Central Nervous System: Nervousness and agitation, about 3 in 100 patients; mental depression, about 1 in 100 and insomnia, about 5 in 1000. Vivid dreams or nightmares, other behavioral changes, restlessness, anxiety, visual and auditory hallucinations and delirium have been reported.

Cardiovascular: Orthostatic symptoms, about 3 in 100 patients; palpitations and tachycardia, and bradycardia, each about 5 in 1000. Raynaud's phenomenon, congestive heart failure, and electrocardiographic abnormalities (i.e. conduction disturbances and arrythmias) have been reported rarely. Rare cases of sinus bradycardia and atrioventricular block have been reported, both with and without the use of concomitant digitalis.

Dermatological: Rash, about 1 in 100 patients; pruritus, about 7 in 1000; hives, angioneurotic edema and urticaria, about 5 in 1000; alopecia, about 2 in 1000.

Genitourinary: Decreased sexual activity, impotence and loss of libido, about 3 in 100 patients; nocturia, about 1 in 100; difficulty in micturition, about 2 in 1000; urinary retention, about 1 in 1000.

Other: Weakness, about 10 in 100 patients; fatigue, about 4 in 100; headache, and discontinuation syndrome, each about 1 in 100; muscle or joint pain, about 6 in 1000 and cramps of the lower limbs, about 3 in 1000. Dryness, burning of the eyes, dryness of the nasal mucosa, pallor, weakly positive Coombs' test, increased sensitivity to alcohol and fever have been reported.

OVERDOSAGE

If symptoms of overdosage occur, remove all Catapres-TTS® (clonidine) systems. The signs and symptoms of clonidine overdosage include hypotension, bradycardia, lethargy, irritability, weakness, somnolence, diminished or absent reflexes, miosis, vomiting and hypoventilation. With large overdoses, reversible cardiac conduction defects or arrhythmias, apnea, seizures and transient hypertension have been reported. The oral LD_{50} of clonidine in rats was 465 mg/kg, and in mice 206 mg/kg.

The general treatment of Catapres-TTS® overdosage may include intravenous fluids as indicated. Bradycardia can be treated with intravenous atropine sulfate and hypotension with dopamine infusion in addition to intravenous fluids. Hypertension associated with overdosage has been treated with intravenous furosemide or diazoxide or alpha-blocking agents such as phentolamine. Tolazoline, an alpha-blocker, in intravenous doses of 10 mg at 30-minute intervals, may reverse clonidine's effects if other efforts fail. Routine hemodialysis is of limited benefit, since a maximum of 5% of circulating clonidine is removed.

In a patient who ingested 100 mg clonidine hydrochloride, plasma clonidine levels were 60 ng/ml (1 hour), 190 ng/ml (1.5 hours), 370 ng/ml (2 hours) and 120 ng/ml (5.5 and 6.5 hours). This patient developed hypertension followed by hypotension, bradycardia, apnea, hallucinations, semicoma, and premature ventricular contractions. The patient fully recovered after intensive treatment.

DOSAGE AND ADMINISTRATION

Apply Catapres-TTS® (clonidine) to a hairless area of intact skin on the upper arm or torso, once every 7 days. Each new application of Catapres-TTS® should be on a different skin site from the previous location. If the system loosens during 7-day wearing, the adhesive overlay should be applied directly over the system to ensure good adhesion.

To initiate therapy, Catapres-TTS® dosage should be titrated according to individual therapeutic requirements, starting with Catapres-TTS®-1 (clonidine). If after one or two weeks the desired reduction in blood pressure is not achieved, increase the dosage by adding an additional Catapres-TTS®-1 or changing to a larger system. An increase in dosage above two Catapres-TTS®-3 (clonidine) is usually not associated with additional efficacy.

When substituting Catapres-TTS® in patients on prior antihypertensive therapy, physicians should be aware that the antihypertensive effect of Catapres-TTS® may not commence until 2 to 3 days after initial application. Therefore, gradual reduction of prior drug dosage is advised. Some or all previous antihypertensive treatment may have to be continued, particularly in patients with more severe forms of hypertension.

HOW SUPPLIED

Catapres-TTS®-1 (clonidine) and Catapres-TTS®-2 are supplied as 4 pouched systems and 4 adhesive overlays per carton, 3 cartons per shipper. NDC numbers are 0597-0031-12 and 0597-0032-12, respectively. Catapres-TTS®-3 is supplied as 4 pouched systems and 4 adhesive overlays per carton, NDC number 0597-0033-34.

[See table above].

	Programmed Delivery Clonidine *in vivo* Per Day Over 1 Week	Clonidine Content	Size	Code
Catapres-TTS®-1	0.1 mg	2.5 mg	3.5 cm^2	BI-31
Catapres-TTS®-2	0.2 mg	5.0 mg	7.0 cm^2	BI-32
Catapres-TTS®-3	0.3 mg	7.5 mg	10.5 cm^2	BI-33

Storage and Handling: Store below 86°F (30°C).

TOXICOLOGY

In several studies oral clonidine hydrochloride produced a dose-dependent increase in the incidence and severity of spontaneously occurring retinal degeneration in albino rats treated for six months or longer. Tissue distribution studies in dogs and monkeys revealed that clonidine hydrochloride was concentrated in the choroid of the eye. In view of the retinal degeneration observed in rats, eye examinations were performed in 908 patients prior to the start of Catapres® therapy, who were then examined periodically thereafter. In 353 of these 908 patients, examinations were performed for periods of 24 months or longer. Except for some dryness of the eyes, no drug-related abnormal ophthalmologic findings were recorded and Catapres® did not alter retinal function as shown by specialized tests such as the electroretinogram and macular dazzle.

In rats, clonidine hydrochloride in combination with amitriptyline produced corneal lesions within 5 days.

CT-PI -5/86

Shown in Product Identification Section, page 405

COMBIPRES® ℞

[*kom 'be-pres*]

Each tablet contains:
clonidine hydrochloride USP,
0.1 mg or 0.2 mg or 0.3 mg
and chlorthalidone USP, 15 mg
Oral Antihypertensive

Tablets 0.1	**BI-CODE 08**
Tablets 0.2	**BI-CODE 09**
Tablets 0.3	**BI-CODE 10**

WARNING

This fixed combination drug is not indicated for initial therapy of hypertension. Hypertension requires therapy titrated to the individual patient. If the fixed combination represents the dosage so determined, its use may be more convenient in patient management. The treatment of hypertension is not static, but must be reevaluated as conditions in each patient warrant.

DESCRIPTION

Combipres® is a combination of clonidine hydrochloride and chlorthalidone. Clonidine hydrochloride, an antihypertensive agent, is an imidazoline derivative and exists as a mesomeric compound. The chemical name for clonidine hydrochloride is 2-(2,6-dichlorophenylamino)-2-imidazoline hydrochloride. It is an odorless, bitter, white crystalline substance soluble in water and alcohol, with a molecular weight of 266.57. The 0.1 mg tablet is equivalent to 0.087 mg of the free base.

Chlorthalidone is 2-chloro-5-(1-hydroxy-3-oxo-1-isoindolinyl) benzene-sulfonamide. Chlorthalidone is an oral diuretic agent indicated for the treatment of edema and hypertension. The drug has a prolonged action. It differs from other sulfonamide diuretics in that a double ring system is incorporated in its chemical structure.

ACTIONS

Combipres®:

Combipres produces a more pronounced antihypertensive response than occurs after either clonidine hydrochloride or chlorthalidone alone in equivalent doses.

Clonidine hydrochloride:

Clonidine hydrochloride is an antihypertensive agent whose mechanism of action appears to be central alpha-adrenergic stimulation as demonstrated in animal studies. This results in the inhibition of bulbar sympathetic cardioaccelerator and sympathetic vasoconstrictor centers, thereby causing a decrease in sympathetic outflow from the brain. Initially, clonidine hydrochloride stimulates peripheral alpha-adrenergic receptors producing transient vasoconstriction.

Clonidine hydrochloride acts relatively rapidly. The patient's blood pressure declines within 30 to 60 minutes after an oral dose, the maximum decrease occurring within 2 to 4 hours. The antihypertensive effect in humans lasts approximately 6 to 8 hours. The peak plasma level of clonidine hydrochloride occurs in approximately 3 to 5 hours with a plasma half-life of 12 to 16 hours. Clonidine hydrochloride and its metabolites are excreted mainly in the urine. When labeled drug was administered, unchanged drug appearing in the urine accounted for about 32 percent of administered radioactivity.

Orthostatic effects are mild and infrequent since supine pressure is reduced to essentially the same extent as standing pressure. Clonidine hydrochloride does not alter normal

Continued on next page

Boehringer Ingelheim—Cont.

hemodynamic responses to exercise. Acute studies with clonidine hydrochloride in humans have demonstrated a moderate reduction (15 to 20%) of cardiac output in the supine position with no change in the peripheral resistance, while at a 45° tilt there is a smaller reduction in cardiac output and a decrease of peripheral resistance. Renal blood flow and the glomerular filtration rate remain essentially unchanged. During long-term therapy, cardiac output tends to return to control values while peripheral resistance remains decreased. Slowing of the pulse rate has been observed in most patients given clonidine hydrochloride.
Other studies in humans have provided evidence of a reduction in plasma renin activity and in the excretion of aldosterone and catecholamines in patients treated with clonidine hydrochloride.
The exact relationship between these pharmacologic actions of clonidine hydrochloride in humans and its antihypertensive effect in individual patients has not been fully elucidated at this time.
Clonidine hydrochloride has been administered together with hydralazine, guanethidine, methyldopa, reserpine, spironolactone, furosemide, chlorthalidone and thiazide diuretics without drug-to-drug interactions.

Chlorthalidone:
The diuretic action of chlorthalidone is thought to be due to inhibition of sodium and chloride reabsorption in the proximal tubule. It has been suggested that the initial antihypertensive action of the drug is due to a reduction of plasma volume.

INDICATION

Combipres® is indicated in the treatment of hypertension (see box warning).

CONTRAINDICATIONS

Combipres® is contraindicated in patients with known hypersensitivity to chlorthalidone and in patients with severe renal or hepatic diseases.

WARNINGS

Tolerance may develop in some patients treated with Combipres.® When this occurs therapy should be reevaluated.

USE IN PREGNANCY

No teratogenic changes have been observed following concomitant administration of chlorthalidone and clonidine hydrochloride to pregnant rats in doses up to 0.128 mg/kg of clonidine hydrochloride and 32 mg/kg of chlorthalidone. However, when animals were given clonidine hydrochloride alone in doses as low as 0.015 mg/kg (one-third the maximum recommended dose) some embryotoxicity was evident. In view of these findings and since information on possible adverse effects in pregnant women is limited to uncontrolled clinical data, Combipres is not recommended in women who are or may become pregnant, unless the potential benefit outweighs the potential risk to mother and infant.

USE IN CHILDREN

No clinical experience is available with the use of Combipres® in children. Studies are being performed with clonidine hydrochloride to evaluate its use in the treatment of hypertension in children.

PRECAUTIONS

General:
In patients who have developed localized contact sensitization to Catapres-TTS® (clonidine), substitution of oral clonidine hydrochloride therapy may be associated with development of a generalized skin rash.
In patients who develop an allergic reaction to Catapres-TTS that extends beyond the local patch site (such as generalized skin rash, urticaria, or angioedema), oral clonidine hydrochloride substitution may elicit a similar reaction.

WITHDRAWAL

Patients should be instructed not to discontinue therapy without consulting their physician. Sudden cessation of clonidine treatment has resulted in subjective symptoms such as nervousness, agitation and headache, accompanied or followed by a rapid rise in blood pressure and elevated catecholamine concentrations in the plasma, but such occurrences have usually been associated with previous administration of high oral doses (exceeding 1.2 mg/day) and/or with continuation of concomitant beta-blocker therapy. Rare instances of hypertensive encephalopathy and death have been reported. When discontinuing therapy with oral clonidine, the physician should reduce the dose gradually over 2 to 4 days to avoid withdrawal symptomatology.
An excessive rise in blood pressure following oral clonidine discontinuation can be reversed by administration of oral clonidine or by intravenous phentolamine. If therapy is to be discontinued in patients receiving beta-blockers and clonidine concurrently, beta-blockers should be discontinued several days before the gradual withdrawal of oral clonidine.
Patients who engage in potentially hazardous activities, such as operating machinery or driving, should be advised of the sedative effect of the clonidine hydrochloride component.
Like any other antihypertensive agent, Combipres should be used with caution in patients with severe coronary insufficiency, recent myocardial infarction, cerebrovascular disease or chronic renal failure.
As an integral part of their overall long-term care, patients treated with Combipres should receive periodic eye examinations (see Toxicology).

DRUG INTERACTIONS

If a patient receiving clonidine hydrochloride is also taking tricyclic antidepressants, the effect of clonidine may be reduced, thus necessitating an increase in dosage. Clonidine hydrochloride may enhance the CNS-depressive effects of alcohol, barbiturates or other sedatives. Amitriptyline in combination with clonidine enhances the manifestation of corneal lesions in rats (see Toxicology).

Chlorthalidone:
Patients predisposed toward or affected by diabetes should be tested periodically while receiving Combipres, because of the hyperglycemic effect of chlorthalidone.
Because of the possibility of progression of renal failure, periodic determination of the BUN is indicated. If, in the physician's opinion, a rising BUN is significant, the drug should be stopped.
The chlorthalidone component of Combipres may lead to sodium and/or potassium depletion. Muscular weakness, muscle cramps, anorexia, nausea, vomiting, constipation, lethargy or mental confusion may occur. Severe dietary salt restriction is not recommended in patients receiving Combipres.
Periodic determinations of the serum potassium level will aid the physician in the detection of hypokalemia. Extra care should be given to detection of hypokalemia in patients receiving adrenal corticosteroids, ACTH or digitalis. Hypochloremic alkalosis often precedes other evidences of severe potassium deficiency. Frequently, therefore, more sensitive indicators than the potassium serum level are the serum bicarbonate and chloride concentrations. Also indicative of potassium depletion can be electrocardiographic alterations such as changes in conduction time, reduction in amplitude of the T wave, ST segment depression, prominent U wave. These abnormalities may appear with potassium depletion before the serum level of potassium decreases. To lessen the possibility of potassium deficiency, the diet, in addition to meat and vegetables, should include potassium-rich foods such as citrus fruits and bananas. If significant potassium depletion should occur during therapy, oral potassium supplements in the form of potassium chloride (3 to 4.5 g/day), fruit juice and bananas should be given.

ADVERSE REACTIONS

Combipres® is generally well tolerated. The most common reactions associated with Combipres are dry mouth (about 40%), drowsiness (about 35%), and sedation (about 8%). Constipation, dizziness, headache and fatigue have been reported. Generally, these effects tend to diminish with continued therapy.
In addition to the reactions listed above, certain adverse reactions associated with the component drugs of Combipres are shown below.

Clonidine hydrochloride:
Gastrointestinal: Anorexia, malaise, nausea, vomiting, parotid pain, mild transient abnormalities in liver function tests. One case of possible drug-induced hepatitis without icterus or hyperbilirubinemia has been reported in a patient receiving clonidine hydrochloride, chlorthalidone and papaverine hydrochloride.
Metabolic: Weight gain, transient elevation of blood glucose or serum creatine phosphokinase, gynecomastia.
Cardiovascular: Congestive heart failure, Raynaud's phenomenon, and electrocardiographic abnormalities manifested as Wenckebach period or ventricular trigeminy. Rare cases of sinus bradycardia and atrioventricular block have been reported, both with and without the use of concomitant digitalis.
Central Nervous System: Vivid dreams or nightmares, insomnia, other behavioral changes, nervousness, restlessness, anxiety, mental depression.
Dermatologic: Rash, angioneurotic edema, hives, urticaria, thinning of the hair, pruritus not associated with a rash.
Genitourinary: Impotence, urinary retention.
Other: Increased sensitivity to alcohol, dryness, itching or burning of the eyes, dryness of the nasal mucosa, pallor or weakly positive Coombs' test.

Chlorthalidone:
Symptoms such as nausea, gastric irritation, anorexia, constipation and cramping, weakness, dizziness, transient myopia and restlessness are occasionally observed. Headache and impotence or dysuria may occur rarely. Orthostatic hypotension has been reported and may be potentiated when chlorthalidone is combined with alcohol, barbiturates or narcotics. Skin rashes, urticaria and purpura have been reported in a few instances.
A decreased glucose tolerance evidenced by hyperglycemia and glycosuria may develop inconsistently. This condition, usually reversible on discontinuation of therapy, responds to control with antidiabetic treatment. Diabetics and those predisposed should be checked regularly.
As with other diuretic agents, hypokalemia may occur (see Precautions). Hyperuricemia may be observed on occasion and acute attacks of gout have been precipitated. In cases where prolonged and significant elevation of blood uric acid concentration is considered potentially deleterious, concomitant use of a uricosuric agent is effective in reversing hyperuricemia without loss of diuretic and/or antihypertensive activity.
Idiosyncratic drug reactions such as aplastic anemia, thrombocytopenia, leukopenia, agranulocytosis and necrotizing angiitis have occurred, but are rare.
The remote possibility of pancreatitis should be considered when epigastric pain or unexplained gastrointestinal symptoms develop after prolonged administration.
Other adverse reactions which have been reported with this general class of compounds include: jaundice, xanthopsia, paresthesia and photosensitization.

DOSAGE AND ADMINISTRATION

DOSAGE: As determined by individual titration of clonidine hydrochloride and chlorthalidone (see box warning).
The following is a general guide to the administration of the individual components of Combipres®:

Clonidine hydrochloride:
Initial dose: One 0.1 mg tablet twice daily. *Maintenance dose:* Further increments of 0.1 mg or 0.2 mg per day may be made until the desired response is achieved. The therapeutic doses most commonly employed have ranged from 0.2 to 0.8 mg per day, given in divided doses. Studies have indicated that 2.4 mg is the maximum effective daily dose but doses as high as this have rarely been employed.

Chlorthalidone:
The usual initial dose is 50 mg daily, which may be given in divided doses.
If the individual doses of clonidine hydrochloride and chlorthalidone determined by titration represent the dose contained in Combipres, for convenience the patient may then be given Combipres.

OVERDOSAGE

Clonidine hydrochloride:
Profound hypotension, weakness, somnolence, diminished or absent reflexes and vomiting followed the accidental ingestion of clonidine hydrochloride by several children from 19 months to 5 years of age. Gastric lavage and administration of an analeptic and vasopressor led to complete recovery within 24 hours. Tolazoline in intravenous doses of 10 mg at 30-minute intervals usually abolishes all effects of clonidine hydrochloride overdosage.

Chlorthalidone:
Symptoms of overdosage include nausea, weakness, dizziness, and disturbances of electrolyte balance. There is no specific antidote, but gastric lavage is recommended, followed by supportive treatment. Where necessary, this may include intravenous dextrose and saline with potassium, administered with caution.

TOXICOLOGY

In several studies, clonidine hydrochloride produced a dose-dependent increase in the incidence and severity of spontaneously occurring retinal degeneration in albino rats treated for 6 months or longer. Tissue distribution studies in dogs and monkeys revealed that clonidine hydrochloride was concentrated in the choroid of the eye. In view of the retinal degeneration observed in rats, eye examinations were performed in 908 patients prior to the start of clonidine hydrochloride therapy, who were then examined periodically thereafter. In 353 of these 908 patients, examinations were performed for periods of 24 months or longer. Except for some dryness of the eyes, no drug-related abnormal ophthalmologic findings were recorded and clonidine hydrochloride did not alter retinal function as shown by specialized tests such as the electroretinogram and macular dazzle.
In rats, clonidine hydrochloride in combination with amitriptyline produced corneal lesions within 5 days.

HOW SUPPLIED

Combipres® 0.1 (each tablet contains clonidine hydrochloride, 0.1 mg +chlorthalidone, 15 mg). It is available as pink, oval, single-scored compressed tablets in bottles of 100 and 1000.
Combipres® 0.2 (each tablet contains clonidine hydrochloride, 0.2 mg +chlorthalidone, 15 mg). It is available as blue, oval, single-scored compressed tablets in bottles of 100 and 1000.
Combipres® 0.3 (each tablet contains clonidine hydrochloride, 0.3 mg +chlorthalidone, 15 mg). It is available as white, oval, single-scored compressed tablets in bottles of 100.
The inactive ingredients are colloidal silicon dioxide, corn starch, dibasic calcium phosphate, gelatin, glycerin, lactose, magnesium stearate, methyl paraben, propyl paraben. Combipres 0.1 and Combipres 0.2 also contain FD&C Red No. 3 and FD&C Blue No. 1, respectively.

Store below 86°F (30°C). Avoid excessive humidity.

CAUTION

Federal law prohibits dispensing without prescription.

CM-PI-7/86

Shown in Product Identification Section, page 405

DULCOLAX®

[*dul 'co-lax*]
(bisacodyl USP)
Tablets of 5 mg .... BI-CODE 12
Suppositories of 10 mg .... BI-CODE 52
Laxative

DESCRIPTION

Dulcolax is a contact laxative acting directly on the colonic mucosa to produce normal peristalsis throughout the large intestine. Its unique mode of action permits either oral or rectal administration, according to the requirements of the patient. Because of its gentleness and reliability of action, Dulcolax may be used whenever constipation is a problem. In preparation for surgery, proctoscopy, or radiologic examination, Dulcolax provides satisfactory cleansing of the bowel, obviating the need for an enema.

The active ingredient in Dulcolax, bisacodyl, is a colorless, tasteless compound that is practically insoluble in water and alkaline solution. It is designated chemically bis(p-acetoxyphenyl)-2-pyridylmethane.

Active Ingredient: bisacodyl USP 5 mg per tablet.

Also Contains: acacia, acetylated monoglyceride, carnauba wax, cellulose acetate phthalate, corn starch, dibutyl phthalate, docusate sodium, gelatin, glycerin, iron oxides, kaolin, lactose, magnesium stearate, pharmaceutical glaze, polyethylene glycol, povidone, sodium benzoate, sorbitan monooleate, sucrose, talc, titanium dioxide, white wax, Yellow 6. Contains FD&C Yellow No. 5 (tartrazine) as a color additive.

Suppository: Active Ingredient: bisacodyl USP 10 mg per suppository. **Also Contains:** hydrogenated vegetable oil.

ACTIONS

Dulcolax differs markedly from other laxatives in its mode of action: it is virtually nontoxic, and its laxative effect occurs on contact with the colonic mucosa, where it stimulates sensory nerve endings to produce parasympathetic reflexes resulting in increased peristaltic contractions of the colon. Administered orally, Dulcolax is absorbed to a variable degree from the small bowel but such absorption is not related to the mode of action of the compound. Dulcolax administered rectally in the form of suppositories is negligibly absorbed. The contact action of the drug is restricted to the colon, and motility of the small intestine is not appreciably influenced. Local axon reflexes, as well as segmental reflexes, are initiated in the region of contact and contribute to the widespread peristaltic activity producing evacuation. For this reason, Dulcolax may often be employed satisfactorily in patients with ganglionic blockage or spinal cord damage (paraplegia, poliomyelitis, etc.).

INDICATIONS

Acute Constipation: Taken at bedtime, Dulcolax tablets are almost invariably effective the following morning. When taken before breakfast, they usually produce an effect within six hours. For a prompter response and to replace enemas, the suppositories, which are usually effective in 15 minutes to one hour, can be used.

Chronic Constipation and Bowel Retraining: Dulcolax is extremely effective in the management of chronic constipation, particularly in older patients. By gradually lengthening the interval between doses as colonic tone improves, the drug has been found to be effective in redeveloping proper bowel hygiene. There is no tendency to "rebound".

Preparation for Radiography: Dulcolax tablets are excellent in eliminating fecal and gas shadows from x-rays taken of the abdominal area. For barium enemas, no food should be given following the administration of the tablets, to prevent reaccumulation of material in the cecum, and a suppository should be given one to two hours prior to examination.

Preoperative Preparation: Dulcolax tablets have been shown to be an ideal laxative in emptying the G.I. tract prior to abdominal surgery or to other surgery under general anesthesia. They may be supplemented by suppositories to replace the usual enema preparation. Dulcolax will not replace the colonic irrigations usually given patients before intracolonic surgery, but is useful in the preliminary emptying of the colon prior to these procedures.

Postoperative Care: Suppositories can be used to replace enemas, or tablets given as an oral laxative, to restore normal bowel hygiene after surgery.

Antepartum Care: Either tablets or suppositories can be used for constipation in pregnancy without danger of stimulating the uterus.

Preparation for Delivery: Suppositories can be used to replace enemas in the first stage of labor provided that they are given at least two hours before the onset of the second stage.

Postpartum Care: The same indications apply as in postoperative care, with no contraindication in nursing mothers.

Preparation for Sigmoidoscopy or Proctoscopy: For unscheduled office examinations, adequate preparation is usually obtained with a single suppository. For sigmoidoscopy scheduled in advance, however, administration of tablets the night before in addition will result in adequate preparation almost invariably.

Colostomies: Tablets the night before or a suppository inserted into the colostomy opening in the morning will frequently make irrigations unnecessary, and in other cases will expedite the procedure.

CONTRAINDICATION

There is no contraindication to the use of Dulcolax, other than an acute surgical abdomen.

PRECAUTION

Dulcolax tablets contain FD&C Yellow No. 5 (tartrazine) which may cause allergic-type reactions (including bronchial asthma) in certain susceptible individuals. Although the overall incidence of FD&C Yellow No. 5 (tartrazine) sensitivity in the general population is low, it is frequently seen in patients who also have aspirin hypersensitivity.

Caution for Patients: Do not use laxative products when abdominal pain, nausea, or vomiting are present unless directed by a doctor. As with all medicines, keep these tablets/suppositories out of reach of children. Frequent or continued use of this preparation may result in dependence on laxatives.

ADVERSE REACTIONS

As with any laxative, abdominal cramps are occasionally noted, particularly in severely constipated individuals.

DOSAGE

Tablets

Tablets must be swallowed whole, not chewed or crushed, and should not be taken within one hour of antacids or milk.

Adults: Two or three (usually two) tablets suffice when an ordinary laxative effect is desired. This usually results in one or two soft, formed stools.

Up to six tablets may be safely given in preparation for special procedures when greater assurance of complete evacuation of the colon is desired. In producing such thorough emptying, these higher doses may result in several loose, unformed stools.

Children: One or two tablets, depending on age and severity of constipation, administered as above. Tablets should not be given to a child too young to swallow them whole.

Suppositories

Adults: One suppository at the time a bowel movement is required. Usually effective in 15 minutes to one hour.

Children: Half a suppository is generally effective for infants and children under two years of age. Above this age, a whole suppository is usually advisable.

Combined

In preparation for surgery, radiography and sigmoidoscopy, a combination of tablets the night before and a suppository in the morning is recommended (see Indications).

HOW SUPPLIED

Dulcolax (bisacodyl): Yellow, enteric-coated tablets of 5 mg in boxes of 24, bottles of 100, 1000 and unit-strip packages of 100; Suppositories of 10 mg in boxes of 2, 4, 8, 50 and 500.

NOTE

Dulcolax suppositories and tablets should be stored at temperatures below 86°F (30°C) and excessive humidity should be avoided.

CLINICAL APPLICATIONS

Dulcolax can be used in virtually any patient in whom a laxative or enema is indicated. It has no effect on the blood picture, erythrocyte sedimentation rate, urinary findings, or hepatic or renal function. It may be safely given to infants and the aged, pregnant or nursing women, debilitated patients, and may be prescribed in the presence of such conditions as cardiovascular, renal, or hepatic diseases.

ALSO AVAILABLE

Dulcolax® Bowel Prep Kit. Each kit contains:
1 Dulcolax suppository of 10 mg bisacodyl;
4 Dulcolax tablets of 5 mg bisacodyl;
Complete patient instructions.

DU-PI-11/85

Shown in Product Identification Section, page 405

MEXITIL® ℞

(mexiletine hydrochloride)
Oral Antiarrhythmic
Capsules of 150 mg, 200 mg and 250 mg

DESCRIPTION

Mexitil® (mexiletine hydrochloride) is an orally active antiarrhythmic agent available as 150 mg, 200 mg and 250 mg capsules. 100 mg of mexiletine hydrochloride is equivalent to 83.31 mg of mexiletine base. It is a white to off-white crystalline powder with slightly bitter taste, freely soluble in water and in alcohol. Mexitil has a pKa of 8.4.

Chemically, Mexitil is 1-methyl-2-(2,6-xylyloxy)-ethylamine hydrochloride.

Mexitil Capsules contain the following inactive ingredients: colloidal silicon dioxide, corn starch, magnesium stearate.

CLINICAL PHARMACOLOGY

Mechanism of Action: Mexitil® (mexiletine hydrochloride) is a local anesthetic, antiarrhythmic agent, structurally similar to lidocaine, but orally active. In animal studies, Mexitil has been shown to be effective in the suppression of induced ventricular arrhythmias, including those induced by glycoside toxicity and coronary artery ligation. Mexitil, like lidocaine, inhibits the inward sodium current, thus reducing the rate of rise of the action potential, Phase 0. Mexitil decreased the effective refractory period (ERP) in Purkinje fibers. The decrease in ERP was of lesser magnitude than the decrease in action potential duration (APD), with a resulting increase in the ERP/APD ratio.

Electrophysiology in Man: Mexiletine is a Class 1B antiarrhythmic compound with electrophysiologic properties in man similar to those of lidocaine, but dissimilar from quinidine, procainamide, and disopyramide.

In patients with normal conduction systems, Mexitil has a minimal effect on cardiac impulse generation and propagation. In clinical trials, no development of second-degree or third-degree AV block was observed. Mexitil did not prolong ventricular depolarization (QRS duration) or repolarization (QT intervals) as measured by electrocardiography. Theoretically, therefore, Mexitil may be useful in the treatment of ventricular arrhythmias associated with a prolonged QT interval.

In patients with pre-existing conduction defects, depression of the sinus rate, prolongation of sinus node recovery time, decreased conduction velocity and increased effective refractory period of the intraventricular conduction system have occasionally been observed.

The antiarrhythmic effect of Mexitil has been established in controlled comparative trials against placebo, quinidine, procainamide and disopyramide. Mexitil, at doses of 200–400 mg q8h, produced a significant reduction of ventricular premature beats, paired beats, and episodes of non-sustained ventricular tachycardia compared to placebo and was similar in effectiveness to the active agents. Among all patients entered into the studies, about 30% in each treatment group had a 70% or greater reduction in PVC count and about 40% failed to complete the three-month studies because of adverse effects. Follow-up of patients from the controlled trials has demonstrated continued effectiveness of Mexitil in long-term use.

Hemodynamics: Hemodynamic studies in a limited number of patients, with normal or abnormal myocardial function, following oral administration of Mexitil, have shown small, usually not statistically significant, decreases in cardiac output and increases in systemic vascular resistance, but no significant negative inotropic effect. Blood pressure and pulse rate remain essentially unchanged. Mild depression of myocardial function, similar to that produced by lidocaine, has occasionally been observed following intravenous Mexitil therapy in patients with cardiac disease.

Pharmacokinetics: Mexitil is well absorbed (~90%) from the gastrointestinal tract. Unlike lidocaine, its first-pass metabolism is low. Peak blood levels are reached in two to three hours. In normal subjects, the plasma elimination half-life of Mexitil is approximately 10–12 hours. It is 50–60% bound to plasma protein, with a volume of distribution of 5–7 liters/kg. Mexitil is metabolized in the liver. Approximately 10% is excreted unchanged by the kidney. While urinary pH does not normally have much influence on elimination, marked changes in urinary pH influence the rate of excretion: acidification accelerates excretion, while alkalinization retards it.

Several metabolites of mexiletine have shown minimal antiarrhythmic activity in animal models. The most active is the minor metabolite N-methylmexiletine, which is less than 20% as potent as mexiletine. The urinary excretion of N-methylmexiletine in man is less than 0.5%. Thus the therapeutic activity of Mexitil is due to the parent compound.

Hepatic impairment prolongs the elimination half-life of Mexitil. In eight patients with moderate to severe liver disease, the mean half-life was approximately 25 hours.

Consistent with the limited renal elimination of Mexitil, little change in the half-life has been detected in patients with reduced renal function. In eight patients with creatinine clearance less than 10 ml/min, the mean plasma elimination half-life was 15.7 hours; in seven patients with creatinine clearance between 11–40 ml/min, the mean half-life was 13.4 hours.

The absorption rate of Mexitil is reduced in clinical situations such as acute myocardial infarction in which gastric emptying time is increased. Narcotics, atropine and magnesium-aluminum hydroxide have also been reported to slow the absorption of Mexitil. Metoclopramide has been reported to accelerate absorption.

Continued on next page

Boehringer Ingelheim—Cont.

Mexiletine plasma levels of at least 0.5 mcg/ml are generally required for therapeutic response. An increase in the frequency of central nervous system adverse effects has been observed when plasma levels exceed 2.0 mcg/ml. Thus the therapeutic range is approximately 0.5 to 2.0 mcg/ml. Plasma levels within the therapeutic range can be attained with either three times daily or twice daily dosing but peak to trough differences are greater with the latter regimen, creating the possibility of adverse effects at peak and arrhythmic escape at trough. Nevertheless, some patients may be transferred successfully to the twice daily regimen (see DOSAGE AND ADMINISTRATION).

INDICATIONS

Mexitil® (mexiletine hydrochloride) is indicated for the suppression of symptomatic ventricular arrhythmias, including frequent premature ventricular contractions, unifocal or multifocal, couplets and ventricular tachycardia.

Like other antiarrhythmics, mexiletine has not been shown to prevent sudden death in patients with serious ventricular ectopic activity, and also, like other antiarrhythmics, it has potentially serious adverse effects, including the ability to worsen arrhythmias. It is therefore essential that each patient given mexiletine be evaluated electrocardiographically and clinically prior to and during mexiletine therapy to determine whether the response to mexiletine supports continued treatment.

CONTRAINDICATIONS

Mexitil® (mexiletine hydrochloride) is contraindicated in the presence of cardiogenic shock or pre-existing second- or third-degree AV block (if no pacemaker is present).

PRECAUTIONS

General: If a ventricular pacemaker is operative, patients with second or third degree heart block may be treated with Mexitil® (mexiletine hydrochloride) if continuously monitored. A limited number of patients (45 of 475 in controlled clinical trials) with preexisting first degree AV block were treated with Mexitil; none of these patients developed second or third degree AV block. Caution should be exercised when it is used in such patients or in patients with pre-existing sinus node dysfunction or intraventricular conduction abnormalities.

Like other antiarrhythmics Mexitil can cause worsening of arrhythmias. This has been uncommon in patients with less serious arrhythmias (frequent premature beats or nonsustained ventricular tachycardia: see ADVERSE REACTIONS), but is of greater concern in patients with life-threatening arrhythmias such as sustained ventricular tachycardia. In patients with such arrhythmias subjected to programmed electrical stimulation or to exercise provocation, 10–15% of patients had exacerbation of the arrhythmia, a rate not greater than that of other agents.

Mexitil should be used with caution in patients with hypotension and severe congestive heart failure.

Since Mexitil is metabolized in the liver, and hepatic impairment has been reported to prolong the elimination half-life of Mexitil, patients with liver disease should be followed carefully while receiving Mexitil. The same caution should be observed in patients with hepatic dysfunction secondary to congestive heart failure.

Concurrent drug therapy or dietary regimens which may markedly alter urinary pH should be avoided during Mexitil therapy. The minor fluctuations in urinary pH associated with normal diet do not affect the excretion of Mexitil.

SGOT Elevation and Liver Injury: In three-month controlled trials, elevations of SGOT greater than three times the upper limit of normal occurred in about 1% of both mexiletine-treated and control patients. Approximately 2% of patients in the mexiletine compassionate use program had elevations of SGOT greater than or equal to three times the upper limit of normal. These elevations frequently occurred in association with identifiable clinical events and therapeutic measures such as congestive heart failure, acute myocardical infarction, blood transfusions and other medications. These elevations were often asymptomatic and transient, usually not associated with elevated bilirubin levels and usually did not require discontinuation of therapy. Marked elevations of SGOT (>1000 U/L) were seen before death in four patients with end-stage cardiac disease (severe congestive heart failure, cardiogenic shock).

In foreign marketing experience rare instances of severe liver injury, including hepatic necrosis, have been reported in association with Mexitil treatment. It is recommended that patients in whom an abnormal liver test has occurred, or who have signs or symptoms suggesting liver dysfunction, be carefully evaluated. If persistent or worsening elevation of hepatic enzymes is detected, consideration should be given to discontinuing therapy.

Blood dyscrasias: Blood dyscrasias were not seen in the controlled trials. Among 10,867 patients treated with mexiletine in the compassionate use program, marked leukopenia (neutrophils less than 1000/mm^3) or agranulocytosis were seen in 0.06%, and milder depressions of leukocytes were seen in 0.08%, and thrombocytopenia was observed in 0.16%. Many of these patients were seriously ill and received concomitant medications with known hematologic adverse effects. Rechallenge with mexiletine in several cases was negative. Marked leukopenia or agranulocytosis did not occur in any patient receiving Mexitil alone; five of the six cases of agranulocytosis were associated with procainamide (sustained release preparations in four) and one with vinblastine. If significant hematologic changes are observed, the patient should be carefully evaluated, and, if warranted, Mexitil should be discontinued. Blood counts usually return to normal within one month of discontinuation. (See ADVERSE REACTIONS.)

Convulsions (seizures) did not occur in Mexitil controlled clinical trials. In the compassionate use program, convulsions were reported in about 2 of 1000 patients. Twenty-eight percent of these patients discontinued therapy. Convulsions were reported in patients with and without a prior history of seizures. Mexiletine should be used with caution in patients with known seizure disorder.

Drug Interactions: In a large compassionate use program Mexitil has been used concurrently with commonly employed antianginal, antihypertensive, and anticoagulant drugs without observed interactions. A variety of antiarrhythmics such as quinidine or propranolol were also added, sometimes with improved control of ventricular ectopy. When phenytoin or other hepatic enzyme inducers such as rifampin and phenobarbital have been taken concurrently with Mexitil, lowered Mexitil plasma levels have been reported. Monitoring of Mexitil plasma levels is recommended during such concurrent use to avoid ineffective therapy.

In a formal study, benzodiazepines were shown not to affect Mexitil plasma concentrations. ECG intervals (PR, QRS and QT) were not affected by concurrent Mexitil and digoxin, diuretics, or propranolol.

Cimetidine has been shown to raise Mexitil plasma levels. During concurrent therapy, the patient should be monitored carefully for adverse effects.

Mexitil does not alter serum digoxin levels, but magnesium-aluminum hydroxide, when used to treat gastrointestinal symptoms due to Mexitil, has been reported to lower serum digoxin levels.

Carcinogenesis, Mutagenesis and Impairment of Fertility: Studies of carcinogenesis in rats (24 months) and mice (18 months) did not demonstrate any tumorigenic potential. Mexitil was found to be non-mutagenic in the Ames test. Mexitil did not impair fertility in the rat.

Pregnancy/Teratogenic Effects: *Pregnancy Category C:* Reproduction studies performed with Mexitil in rats, mice and rabbits at doses up to four times the maximum human oral dose (20 mg/kg in a 50 kg patient) revealed no evidence of teratogenicity or impaired fertility but did show an increase in fetal resorption. There are no adequate and well-controlled studies in pregnant women; this drug should be used in pregnancy only if the potential benefit justifies the potential risk to the fetus.

Nursing Mothers: Mexitil appears in human milk in concentrations similar to those observed in plasma. Therefore, if the use of Mexitil is deemed essential, an alternative method of infant feeding should be considered.

Pediatric Use: Safety and effectiveness in children have not been established.

ADVERSE REACTIONS

Mexitil® (mexiletine hydrochloride) commonly produces reversible gastrointestinal and nervous system adverse reactions but is otherwise well tolerated. Mexitil has been evaluated in 483 patients in one-month and three-month controlled studies and in over 10,000 patients in a large compassionate use program. Dosages in the controlled studies ranged from 600–1200 mg/day; some patients (8%) in the compassionate use program were treated with higher daily doses (1600–3200 mg/day). In the three-month controlled trials comparing Mexitil to quinidine, procainamide and disopyramide, the most frequent adverse reactions were upper gastrointestinal distress (41%), lightheadedness (10.5%), tremor (12.6%) and coordination difficulties (10.2%). Similar frequency and incidence were observed in the one-month placebo-controlled trial. Although these reactions were generally not serious, and were dose-related and reversible with a reduction in dosage, by taking the drug with food or antacid or by therapy discontinuation, they led to therapy discontinuation in 40% of patients in the controlled trials. A tabulation of the adverse events reported in the one-month placebo-controlled trial follows:

Comparative Incidence (%) of Adverse Events among Patients Treated with Mexiletine and Placebo in the 4-Week, Double-Blind Crossover Trial

	Mexiletine N = 53	*Placebo* N = 49
Cardiovascular		
Palpitations	7.5	10.2
Chest Pain	7.5	4.1
Increased Ventricular Arrhythmias/PVC's	1.9	—
Digestive		
Nausea/Vomiting/Heartburn	39.6	6.1
Central Nervous System		
Dizziness/Lightheadedness	26.4	14.3
Tremor	13.2	—
Nervousness	11.3	6.1
Coordination Difficulties	9.4	—
Changes in Sleep Habits	7.5	16.3
Paresthesias/Numbness	3.8	2.0
Weakness	1.9	4.1
Fatigue	1.9	2.0
Tinnitus	1.9	4.1
Confusion/Clouded Sensorium	1.9	2.0
Other		
Headache	7.5	6.1
Blurred Vison/Visual Disturbances	7.5	2.0
Dyspnea/Respiratory	5.7	10.2
Rash	3.8	2.0
Non-specific Edema	3.8	—

A tabulation of adverse reactions occurring in one percent or more of patients in the three-month controlled studies follows:

[See table on next page].

Less than 1%: Syncope, edema, hot flashes, hypertension, short-term memory loss, loss of conciousness, other psychological changes, diaphoresis, urinary hesitancy/retention, malaise, impotence/decreased libido, pharyngitis.

An additional group of over 10,000 patients has been treated in a program allowing administration of Mexitil under compassionate use circumstances. These patients were seriously ill with the large majority on multiple drug therapy. Twenty-four percent of the patients continued in the program for one year or longer. Adverse reactions leading to therapy discontinuation occurred in 15 percent of patients (usually upper gastrointestinal system or nervous system effects). In general, the more common adverse reactions were similar to those in the controlled trials. Less common adverse events possibly related to Mexitil use include:

Cardiovascular System: Syncope and hypotension, each about 6 in 1000; bradycardia, about 4 in 1000; angina/angina-like pain, about 3 in 1000; edema, atrioventricular block/conduction disturbances and hot flashes, each about 2 in 1000; atrial arrhythmias, hypertension and cardiogenic shock, each about 1 in 1000.

Central Nervous System: Short-term memory loss, about 9 in 1000 patients; hallucinations and other psychological changes, each about 3 in 1000; psychosis and convulsions/seizures, each about 2 in 1000; loss of consciousness, about 6 in 10,000.

Digestive: Dysphagia, about 2 in 1000; peptic ulcer, about 8 in 10,000; upper gastrointestinal bleeding, about 7 in 10,000; esophageal ulceration, about 1 in 10,000.

Laboratory: Abnormal liver function tests, about 5 in 1000 patients; positive ANA and thrombocytopenia, each about 2 in 1000; leukopenia (including neutropenia and agranulocytosis), about 1 in 1000; myelofibrosis, about 2 in 10,000 patients.

Other: Diaphoresis, about 6 in 1000; altered taste, about 5 in 1000; salivary changes, hair loss and impotence/decreased libido, each about 4 in 1000; malaise, about 3 in 1000; urinary hesitancy/retention, each about 2 in 1000; hiccups, dry skin, laryngeal and pharyngeal changes and changes in oral mucous membranes, each about 1 in 1000; SLE syndrome, about 4 in 10,000.

Hematology: Blood dyscrasias were not seen in the controlled trials but did occur among the 10,867 patients treated with mexiletine in the compassionate use program (see PRECAUTIONS).

Myelofibrosis was reported in two patients in the compassionate use prgram; one was receiving long-term thiotepa therapy and the other had pretreatment myeloid abnormalities.

OVERDOSAGE

Marked overdosage in humans has not been reported. On the basis of acute toxicity studies in animals, the major toxicity would be expected to be related to the central nervous system, including ataxia and convulsions.

There is no specific antidote for Mexitil® (mexiletine hydrochloride). Acidification of the urine, which will accelerate the excretion of mexiletine, may be useful. Treatment of overdosage should be suportive, and may include the administration of atropine if hypotension or bradycardia occurs.

DOSAGE AND ADMINISTRATION

The dosage of Mexitil® (mexiletine hydrochloride) must be individualized on the basis of response and tolerance, both of which are dose-related. Administration with food or antacid is recommended. Initiate Mexitil therapy with 200 mg every eight hours when rapid control of arrhythmia is not essential. A minimum of two to three days between dose adjustments is recommended. Dose may be adjusted in 50 or 100 mg increments up or down.

As with any antiarrhythmic drug, clinical and electrocardiographic evaluation (including Holter monitoring if necessary

Comparative Incidence (%) of Adverse Events among Patients Treated with Mexiletine or Control Drugs in the 12-Week, Double-Blind Trials

	Mexiletine N = 430	Quinidine N = 262	Procainamide N = 78	Disopyramide N = 69
Cardiovascular				
Palpitations	4.3	4.6	1.3	5.8
Chest Pain	2.6	3.4	1.3	2.9
Angina/Angina-like Pain	1.7	1.9	2.6	2.9
Increased Ventricular Arrhythmias/PVC's	1.0	2.7	2.6	—
Digestive				
Nausea/Vomiting/ Heartburn	39.3	21.4	33.3	14.5
Diarrhea	5.2	33.2	2.6	8.7
Constipation	4.0	—	6.4	11.6
Changes in Appetite	2.6	1.9	—	—
Abdominal Pain/Cramps/ Discomfort	1.2	1.5	—	1.4
Central Nervous System				
Dizziness/ Lightheadedness	18.9	14.1	14.1	2.9
Tremor	13.2	2.3	3.8	1.4
Coordination Difficulties	9.7	1.1	1.3	—
Changes in Sleep Habits	7.1	2.7	11.5	8.7
Weakness	5.0	5.3	7.7	2.9
Nervousness	5.0	1.9	6.4	5.8
Fatigue	3.8	5.7	5.1	1.4
Speech Difficulties	2.6	0.4	—	—
Confusion/Clouded Sensorium	2.6	—	3.8	—
Paresthesias/Numbness	2.4	2.3	2.6	—
Tinnitus	2.4	1.5	—	—
Depression	2.4	1.1	1.3	1.4
Other				
Blurred Vision/Visual Disturbances	5.7	3.1	5.1	7.2
Headache	5.7	6.9	7.7	4.3
Rash	4.2	3.8	10.3	1.4
Dyspnea/Respiratory	3.3	3.1	5.1	2.9
Dry Mouth	2.8	1.9	5.1	14.5
Arthralgia	1.7	2.3	5.1	1.4
Fever	1.2	3.1	2.6	—

for evaluation) are needed to determine whether the desired antiarrhythmic effect has been obtained and to guide titration and dose adjustment.

Satisfactory control can be achieved in most patients by 200 to 300 mg given every eight hours with food or antacid. If satisfactory response has not been achieved at 300 mg q8h, and the patient tolerates Mexitil well, a dose of 400 mg q8h may be tried. As the severity of CNS side effects increases with total daily dose, the dose should not exceed 1200 mg/day.

In general, patients with renal failure will require the usual doses of Mexitil. Patients with severe liver disease, however, may require lower doses and must be monitored closely. Similarly, marked right-sided congestive heart failure can reduce hepatic metabolism and reduce the needed dose. Plasma level may also be affected by certain concomitant drugs (see PRECAUTIONS: Drug Interactions).

Loading Dose: When rapid control of ventricular arrhythmia is essential, an initial loading dose of 400 mg of Mexitil may be administered, followed by a 200 mg dose in eight hours. Onset of therapeutic effect is usually observed within 30 minutes to two hours.

Q12H Dosage Schedule: Some patients responding to Mexitil may be transferred to a 12-hour dosage schedule to improve convenience and compliance. If adequate suppression is achieved on a Mexitil dose of 300 mg or less every eight hours, the same total daily dose may be given in divided doses every 12 hours while carefully monitoring the degree of suppression of ventricular ectopy. This dose may be adjusted up to a maximum of 450 mg every 12 hours to achieve the desired response.

Transferring to Mexitil: The following dosage schedule, based on theoretical considerations rather than experimental data, is suggested for transferring patients from other Class I oral antiarrhythmic agents to Mexitil: Mexitil treatment may be initiated with a 200 mg dose, and titrated to response as described above 6–12 hours after the last dose of quinidine sulfate, 3–6 hours after the last dose of procainamide, 6–12 hours after the last dose of disopyramide or 8–12 hours after the last dose of tocainide.

In patients in whom withdrawal of the previous antiarrhythmic agent is likely to produce life-threatening arrhythmias, hospitalization of the patient is recommended.

When transferring from lidocaine to Mexitil, the lidocaine infusion should be stopped when the first oral dose of Mexitil is administered. The infusion line should be left open until suppression of the arrhythmia appears to be satisfactorily maintained. Consideration should be given to the similarity of the adverse effects of lidocaine and Mexitil and the possibility that they may be additive.

HOW SUPPLIED

Mexitil® (mexiletine hydrochloride) is supplied in hard gelatin capsules containing 150 mg, 200 mg or 250 mg of mexiletine hydrochloride:

Mexitil® 150 mg capsules are red and caramel with the marking BI 66. Available in bottles of 100 (NDC 0597-0066-01) and individually blister-sealed unit-dose cartons of 100 (NDC 0597-0066-61).

Mexitil® 200 mg capsules are red with the marking BI 67. Available in bottles of 100 (NDC 0597-0067-01) and individually blister-sealed unit-dose cartons of 100 (NDC 0597-0067-61).

Mexitil® 250 mg capsules are red and aqua green with the marking BI 68. Available in bottles of 100 (NDC 0597-0068-01) and individually blister-sealed unit-dose cartons of 100 (NDC 0597-0068-61).

Store below 86°F (30°C).

Caution: Federal law prohibits dispensing without prescription.

ME-PI-1186

Shown in Product Identification Section, page 405

PERSANTINE® ℞

[per-san 'tēn]

(dipyridamole USP)

For Long-Term Therapy of Chronic Angina Pectoris

Tablets of 25 mg .... BI-CODE 17
Tablets of 50 mg .... BI-CODE 18
Tablets of 75 mg .... BI-CODE 19

DESCRIPTION

Persantine® (dipyridamole USP) is classified as a coronary vasodilator. The drug is unrelated chemically to the nitrates or digitalis.

Chemistry: Persantine is a homogeneous yellow crystalline powder, odorless but with a bitter taste. It is soluble in dilute acids, methanol, and chloroform. Its basic structure is a double ring of two condensed pyrimidine rings. It is designated chemically as 2,6-bis-(diethanolamino)-4,8-dipiperidino-pyrimido-(5,4-d) pyrimidine.

ACTIONS

Human: Persantine (dipyridamole USP) in therapeutic doses usually produces no significant alteration of systemic blood pressure or of blood flow in peripheral arteries; it increases coronary blood flow primarily by a selective dilation of the coronary arteries. The drug increases coronary sinus oxygen saturation without significantly altering myocardial oxygen consumption. A mild positive inotropic effect has been demonstrated in animals and man.

Animal: Experimental work in dogs subjected to artificial narrowing of one or both branches of the left coronary artery and chronically fed Persantine has demonstrated an increase in intercoronary collateral circulation greater than that seen in placebo- or nitrate-treated animals exposed to identical conditions. A similar increase in collateral anastomoses over controls has been shown in healthy animals fed the drug.

In studies with heart preparations, the drug has been shown to protect against disturbances in function and fall in high-energy phosphate levels induced by hypoxia.

In animal (rat) studies using combination therapy with digitalis and dipyridamole, potentiation of digitalis toxicity occurred as measured by an augmentation of phosphorus exchange of the phosphorus-containing fractions of the myocardium. Experiments in cats, on the other hand, have shown that dipyridamole decreases the acute toxicity of digitoxin.

Studies with electron microscopy have demonstrated preservation of the anatomic structure of heart mitochondria (sarcosomes) in animals pretreated with the drug and exposed to hypoxia. Untreated animals showed dissolution of mitochondrial structure under similar conditions.

INDICATIONS

Based on a review of this drug by the National Academy of Sciences—National Research Council and/or other information, FDA has classified the indication as follows:

"Possibly" effective: For long-term therapy of chronic angina pectoris. Prolonged therapy may reduce the frequency of, or eliminate, anginal episodes, improve exercise tolerance, and reduce nitroglycerin requirements. The drug is not intended to abort the acute anginal attack.

Final classification of the less-than-effective indications requires further investigation.

CONTRAINDICATIONS

No specific contraindications are known.

PRECAUTIONS

Since excessive doses can produce peripheral vasodilation, the drug should be used cautiously in patients with hypotension.

ADVERSE REACTIONS

Adverse reactions are minimal and transient at recommended dosages.

Instances of headache, dizziness, nausea, flushing, weakness, or syncope, mild gastrointestinal distress and skin rash have been noted during therapy. Rare cases of what appeared to be an aggravation of angina pectoris have been reported, usually at the initiation of therapy.

On those uncommon occasions when adverse reactions have been persistent or intolerable to the patient, withdrawal of the medication has been followed promptly by cessation of the undesirable symptoms.

DOSAGE AND ADMINISTRATION

The recommended dosage is 50 mg three times a day, taken at least one hour before meals. In some cases higher doses may be necessary but should be used with the knowledge that a significantly increased incidence of side effects is associated with increased dosage. Clinical response may not be evident before the second or third month of continuous therapy.

HOW SUPPLIED

Persantine (dipyridamole USP) is available as round, orange, sugar-coated tablets of 25 mg, in bottles of 100 and 1000 and unit-dose packages of 100.

Persantine-50 is available as round, orange, sugar-coated tablets of 50 mg, in bottles of 100 and 1000 and unit dose packages of 100.

Persantine-75 is available as round, orange, sugar-coated tablets of 75 mg, in bottles of 100 and 500 and unit dose packages of 100.

All tablets contain the following as inactive ingredients: acacia, carnauba wax, corn starch, FD&C Blue No. 1 aluminum lake, lactose, magnesium stearate, polyethylene glycol, povidone, shellac, sucrose, talc, titanium dioxide, white wax. In addition, the 25 mg tablets contain: FD&C Red No. 3 aluminum lake, FD&C Yellow No. 6 aluminum lake, and sodium benzoate; the 50 mg tablets contain: FD&C Yellow No. 6; the 75 mg tablets contain: FD&C Yellow No. 6.

PE-PI-10/85

Shown in Product Identification Section, page 405

Continued on next page

Boehringer Ingelheim—Cont.

PRELUDIN® ℂ ℞
[pra-lu'din]
(phenmetrazine hydrochloride USP)
Endurets® (prolonged-action tablets), 75 mg.........BI-CODE 62

DESCRIPTION

Preludin® (phenmetrazine hydrochloride USP) belongs to the oxazine group of compounds and is designated chemically as 2-phenyl-3-methyltetrahydro-1,4-oxazine hydrochloride.
Phenmetrazine hydrochloride is a white, water-soluble, crystalline powder.

ACTIONS

Preludin (phenmetrazine hydrochloride USP) is a sympathomimetic amine with pharmacologic activity similar to the prototype drugs of this class used in obesity, the amphetamines. Actions include central nervous system stimulation and elevation of blood pressure. Tachyphylaxis and tolerance have been demonstrated with all drugs of this class in which these phenomena have been looked for.
Drugs of this class used in obesity are commonly known as "anorectics" or "anorexigenics". It has not been established, however, that the action of such drugs in treating obesity is primarily one of appetite suppression. Other central nervous system actions, or metabolic effects, may be involved, for example.
Adult obese subjects instructed in dietary management and treated with "anorectic" drugs, lose more weight on the average than those treated with placebo and diet, as determined in relatively short-term clinical trials.
The magnitude of increased weight loss of drug-treated patients over placebo-treated patients is only a fraction of a pound a week. The rate of weight loss is greatest in the first weeks of therapy for both drug and placebo subjects and tends to decrease in succeeding weeks. The possible origins of the increased weight loss due to the various drug effects are not established. The amount of weight loss associated with the use of an "anorectic" drug varies from trial to trial, and the increased weight loss appears to be related in part to variables other than the drug prescribed, such as the physician-investigator, the population treated, and the diet prescribed. Studies do not permit conclusions as to the relative importance of the drug and non-drug factors on weight loss.
The natural history of obesity is measured in years, whereas the studies cited are restricted to a few weeks' duration; thus, the total impact of drug-induced weight loss over that of diet alone must be considered clinically limited.
Preludin Endurets are formulated to release the active drug substance *in vivo* in a more gradual fashion than the standard formulation, as demonstrated by blood levels. The formulation has not been shown superior in effectiveness with respect to weight loss over the same dosage of the standard, noncontrolled-release formulations.

INDICATION

Preludin (phenmetrazine hydrochloride USP) is indicated in the management of exogenous obesity as a short-term (a few weeks) adjunct in a regimen of weight reduction based on caloric restriction. The limited usefulness of agents of this class (see Actions) should be measured against possible risk factors inherent in their use such as those described below.

CONTRAINDICATIONS

Advanced arteriosclerosis, symptomatic cardiovascular disease, moderate to severe hypertension, hyperthyroidism, known hypersensitivity or idiosyncrasy to sympathomimetic amines, glaucoma. Agitated states. Patients with a history of drug abuse. Concomitant use of CNS stimulants. During or within 14 days following the administration of monoamine oxidase inhibitors (hypertensive crises may result).

WARNINGS

Tolerance usually develops within a few weeks. When this occurs, the recommended dose should not be exceeded in an attempt to increase anorectic effect; rather, the drug should be discontinued.
Preludin (phenmetrazine hydrochloride USP) may impair the ability of the patient to engage in potentially hazardous activities such as operating machinery or driving a motor vehicle; the patient should therefore be cautioned accordingly.
Drug Dependence: Preludin is related chemically and pharmacologically to the amphetamines. Amphetamines and related stimulant drugs have been extensively abused, and the possibility of abuse of Preludin should be kept in mind when evaluating the desirability of including a drug as part of a weight reduction program. Abuse of amphetamines and related drugs may be associated with intense psychological dependence and severe social dysfunction. There are reports of patients who have increased the dosage to many times that recommended. Abrupt cessation following prolonged high dosage administration results in extreme fatigue and mental depression; changes are also noted on the sleep EEG. Manifestations of chronic intoxication with anorectic drugs include severe dermatoses, marked insomnia, irritability, hyperactivity, and personality changes. The most severe manifestation of chronic intoxication is psychosis, often clinically indistinguishable from schizophrenia.
Usage in Pregnancy: Safe use in pregnancy has not been established. Animal reproductive studies demonstrated no teratogenic effects. However, the conception rate was adversely affected, as well as survival and body weight of pups at weaning. There have been clinical reports of congenital malformation associated with the use of this compound but a causal relationship has not been proved. Until more information is available, Preludin should not be used by women who are or may become pregnant, particularly in the first trimester, unless in the opinion of the prescribing physician the potential benefits outweigh the possible risks.
Usage in Children: Preludin is not recommended for use in children under 12 years of age.

PRECAUTIONS

Caution should be exercised in prescribing Preludin (phenmetrazine hydrochloride USP) for patients with even mild hypertension. Insulin requirements in diabetes mellitus may be altered in association with the use of Preludin, and the concomitant dietary regimen. Preludin may decrease the hypotensive effect of guanethidine. The least amount feasible should be prescribed or dispensed at one time in order to minimize the possibility of overdosage.
Preludin Endurets, 75 mg, contain FD&C Yellow No. 5 (tartrazine) which may cause allergic-type reactions (including bronchial asthma) in certain susceptible individuals. Although the overall incidence of FD&C Yellow No. 5 (tartrazine) sensitivity in the general population is low, it is frequently seen in patients who also have aspirin hypersensitivity.

ADVERSE REACTIONS

Cardiovascular: Palpitation, tachycardia, elevation of blood pressure.
Central Nervous System: Overstimulation, restlessness, dizziness, insomnia, euphoria, dysphoria, tremor, headache; rarely psychotic episodes at recommended doses.
Gastrointestinal: Dryness of the mouth, unpleasant taste, diarrhea, constipation, other gastrointestinal disturbances.
Allergic: Urticaria.
Endocrine: Impotence, changes in libido.

DOSAGE AND ADMINISTRATION

Preludin (phenmetrazine hydrochloride USP) is not recommended for use in children under 12 years of age.
The maximum adult dosage is one 75 mg Endurets prolonged-action tablet taken daily. Since an Endurets tablet provides appetite suppression for approximately 12 hours, the time of administration should be determined by the period of the day over which the anorectic effect is desired.

OVERDOSAGE

Manifestations of acute overdosage with phenmetrazine hydrochloride include restlessness, tremor, hyperreflexia, rapid respiration, confusion, assaultiveness, hallucinations, panic states. Fatigue and depression usually follow the central stimulation. Cardiovascular effects include arrhythmias, hypertension, or hypotension and circulatory collapse. Gastrointestinal symptoms include nausea, vomiting, diarrhea and abdominal cramps. Poisoning may result in convulsions, coma, and death.
Management of acute phenmetrazine hydrochloride intoxication is largely symptomatic and includes lavage and sedation with a barbiturate. Experience with hemodialysis or peritoneal dialysis is inadequate to permit recommendation in this regard. As with the amphetamines, acidification of the urine should increase phenmetrazine hydrochloride excretion. Intravenous phentolamine has been suggested for possible acute, severe hypertension if this complicates phenmetrazine overdosage.

HOW SUPPLIED

Preludin (phenmetrazine hydrochloride USP) is available as pink, round Endurets prolonged-action tablets of 75 mg, for once-a-day administration. Bottles of 100, NDC 0597-0062-01.

ACTIVE INGREDIENT

Each prolonged-action tablet contains phenmetrazine hydrochloride 75 mg.

INACTIVE INGREDIENTS

Aluminum tristearate, confectioner's sugar, corn starch, FD&C Blue No. 2, FD&C Red No. 3, FD&C Yellow No. 5 (tartrazine), FD&C Yellow No. 6, gelatin, magnesium stearate, silica gel, stearic acid, talc and other ingredients.

PR-PI-6/85

Shown in Product Identification Section, page 405

PRELU-2® ℂ ℞
[pra'lu (2)]
(phendimetrazine tartrate USP)
Timed Release Capsules BI-CODE 64
105 mg

DESCRIPTION

Chemical name: phendimetrazine tartrate (+) 3, 4 dimethyl-2-phenylmorpholine tartrate. Phendimetrazine tartrate is a white, odorless powder with a bitter taste. It is soluble in water, methanol and ethanol. It has a molecular weight of 341.
The capsule is manufactured in a special base which is designed for prolonged release.

ACTIVE INGREDIENT

Each timed-release capsule contains phendimetrazine tartrate 105 mg.

INACTIVE INGREDIENTS

D&C Red No. 33, D&C Yellow No. 10, FD&C Blue No. 1, FD&C Yellow No. 6, gelatin, providone, shellac, silica gel, starch, sucrose, talc, titanium dioxide.

CLINICAL PHARMACOLOGY

Phendimetrazine tartrate is a sympathomimetic amine with pharmacologic activity similar to the prototype of drugs of this class used in obesity, the amphetamines. Actions include central nervous system stimulation and elevation of blood pressure. Tachyphylaxis and tolerance have been demonstrated with all drugs of this class in which these phenomena have been looked for.
Drugs of this class used in obesity are commonly known as 'anorectics' or 'anorexigenics.' It has not been established, however, that the action of such drugs in treating obesity is primarily one of appetite suppression. Other central nervous system actions, or metabolic effects, may be involved, for example.
Adult obese subjects instructed in dietary management and treated with 'anorectic' drugs lose more weight on the average than those treated with placebo and diet, as determined in relatively short-term clinical trials.
The magnitude of increased weight loss of drug-treated patients over placebo-treated patients is only a fraction of a pound a week. The rate of weight loss is greatest in the first weeks of therapy for both drug and placebo subjects and tends to decrease in succeeding weeks. The possible origins of the increased weight loss due to the various drug effects are not established. The amount of weight loss associated with the use of an 'anorectic' drug varies from trial to trial, and the increased weight loss appears to be related in part to variables other than the drug prescribed, such as the physician-investigator, the population treated, and the diet prescribed. Studies do not permit conclusions as to the relative importance of the drug and non-drug factors on weight loss.
The natural history of obesity is measured in years, whereas the studies cited are restricted to a few weeks duration; thus, the total impact of drug-induced weight loss over that of diet alone must be considered clinically limited.
The active drug 105 mg of phendimetrazine tartrate in each capsule of this special timed release dosage form approximates the action of three 35 mg non-timed doses taken at four hour intervals.
The major route of elimination is via the kidneys where most of the drug and metabolites are excreted. Some of the drug is metabolized to phenmetrazine and also phendimetrazine-N-oxide.
The average half-life of elimination when studied under controlled conditions is about 3.7 hours for both the timed and non-timed forms. The absorption half-life of the drug from conventional non-timed 35 mg phendimetrazine tablets is appreciably more rapid than the absorption rate of the drug from the timed release formulation.

INDICATIONS AND USAGE

Phendimetrazine tartrate is indicated in the management of exogenous obesity as a short-term adjunct (a few weeks) in a regimen of weight reduction based on caloric restriction. The limited usefulness of agents of this class (see Clinical Pharmacology) should be measured against possible risk factors inherent in their use such as those described below.

CONTRAINDICATIONS

Advanced arteriosclerosis, symptomatic cardiovascular disease, moderate to severe hypertension, hyperthyroidism, known hypersensitivity, or idiosyncrasy to the sympathomimetic amines, glaucoma.
Agitated states.
Patients with a history of drug abuse.
During or within 14 days following the administration of monoamine oxidase inhibitors (hypertensive crises may result).

WARNINGS

Tolerance to the anorectic effect usually develops within a few weeks. When this occurs, the recommended dose should not be exceeded in an attempt to increase the effect; rather, the drug should be discontinued.

Phendimetrazine tartrate may impair the ability of the patient to engage in potentially hazardous activities such as operating machinery or driving a motor vehicle; the patient should therefore be cautioned accordingly.

DRUG DEPENDENCE

Phendimetrazine tartrate is related chemically and pharmacologically to the amphetamines. Amphetamines and related stimulant drugs have been extensively abused, and the possibility of abuse of phendimetrazine tartrate should be kept in mind when evaluating the desirability of including a drug as part of a weight reduction program. Abuse of amphetamines and related drugs may be associated with intense psychological dependence and severe social dysfunction. There are reports of patients who have increased the dosage to many times that recommended. Abrupt cessation following prolonged high dosage administration results in extreme fatigue and mental depression; changes are also noted on the sleep EEG. Manifestations of chronic intoxication with anorectic drugs include severe dermatoses, marked insomnia, irritability, hyperactivity, and personality changes. The most severe manifestation of chronic intoxication is psychosis, often clinically indistinguishable from schizophrenia.

Usage in Pregnancy: The safety of phendimetrazine tartrate in pregnancy and lactation has not been established. Therefore phendimetrazine tartrate should not be taken by women who are or may become pregnant.

Usage in Children: Phendimetrazine tartrate is not recommended for use in children under 12 years of age.

PRECAUTIONS

Caution is to be exercised in prescribing phendimetrazine tartrate for patients with even mild hypertension.

Insulin requirements in diabetes mellitus may be altered in association with the use of phendimetrazine tartrate and the concomitant dietary regimen.

Phendimetrazine tartrate may decrease the hypotensive effect of guanethidine.

The least amount feasible should be prescribed or dispensed at one time in order to minimize the possibility of overdosage.

ADVERSE REACTIONS

Cardiovascular: Palpitation, tachycardia, elevation of blood pressure.

Central Nervous System: Overstimulation, restlessness, dizziness, insomnia, euphoria, dysphoria, tremor, headache; rarely psychotic episodes at recommended doses.

Gastrointestinal: Dryness of the mouth, unpleasant taste, diarrhea, constipation, other gastrointestinal disturbances.

Allergic: Urticaria.

Endocrine: Impotence, changes in libido.

OVERDOSAGE

Manifestations of acute overdosage with phendimetrazine tartrate include restlessness, tremor, hyperreflexia, rapid respiration, confusion, assaultiveness, hallucinations, panic states.

Fatigue and depression usually follow the central stimulation.

Cardiovascular effects include arrhythmias, hypertension or hypotension and circulatory collapse. Gastrointestinal symptoms include nausea, vomiting, diarrhea, and abdominal cramps. Fatal poisoning usually terminates in convulsions and coma. Management of acute phendimetrazine tartrate intoxication is largely symptomatic and includes lavage and sedation with a barbiturate. Experience with hemodialysis or peritoneal dialysis is inadequate to permit recommendation in this regard. Acidification of the urine increases phendimetrazine tartrate excretion. Intravenous phentolamine (Regitine) has been suggested for possible acute, severe hypertension, if this complicates phendimetrazine tartrate overdosage.

DOSAGE AND ADMINISTRATION

Since this product is a timed release dosage form, limit to one timed release capsule (105 mg phendimetrazine tartrate) in the morning.

Phendimetrazine tartrate is not recommended for use in children under 12 years of age.

HOW SUPPLIED

105 mg capsules (celery and green) in bottles of 100.

Federal law prohibits dispensing without a prescription.

PZ-PI-9/85

Shown in Product Identification Section, page 405

RESPBID® ℞

[resp'bid]

(theophylline)

Sustained release

Tablets of 250 mg and 500 mg

Oral Bronchodilator

DESCRIPTION

Respbid® (theophylline) is an oral xanthine bronchodilators. Chemically, theophylline is 3,7-dihydro-1,3-dimethyl-1H-purine-2,6-dione.

Respbid tablets contain 250 or 500 mg anhydrous theophylline, in a sustained-release formulation (see HOW SUPPLIED). Anhydrous theophylline is a white, odorless crystalline powder having a bitter taste.

The inactive ingredients in Respbid tablets are cellulose acetate phthalate, lactose, magnesium stearate.

CLINICAL PHARMACOLOGY

Theophylline directly relaxes the smooth muscle of the bronchial airways and pulmonary blood vessels, thus acting mainly as a bronchodilator and smooth muscle relaxant. The drug also has other actions typical of the xanthine derivatives: coronary vasodilation; diuresis; cardiac, cerebral, and skeletal muscle stimulation. The actions of theophylline may be mediated through inhibition of phosphodiesterase and a resultant increase in intracellular cyclic AMP which could mediate smooth muscle relaxation. At concentrations higher than those attained in vivo, theophylline also inhibits the release of histamine by mast cells.

In vitro, theophylline has been shown to act synergistically with beta agonists that increase intracellular cyclic AMP through the stimulation of adenyl cyclase, but synergism has not been demonstrated in patients. More data are needed to determine if theophylline and beta agonists have a clinically important additive effect in vivo.

Development of tolerance is not known to occur with chronic use of theophylline.

Pharmacokinetics: The half-life of theophylline is influenced by a number of known variables. It is prolonged in patients suffering from chronic alcoholism, impaired hepatic or renal function, congestive heart failure, and in patients receiving some macrolide antibiotics and cimetidine. Older adults (over age 55) and patients with chronic obstructive pulmonary disease, with or without cor pulmonale, may also have much slower clearance rates. For such patients, the theophylline half-life may exceed 24 hours.

Newborns and neonates have extremely slow clearance rates compared with older infants (over 6 months) and children, and may also have a theophylline half-life of over 24 hours. High fever for prolonged periods may also reduce the rate of theophylline elimination. Administration of influenza vaccine and infection with influenza virus have been associated with an impaired rate of theophylline elimination and consequent increases in serum theophylline levels, sometimes with toxic symptoms.

Theophylline Elimination Characteristics

	Theophylline Clearance Rates (mean ± S.D.)	Half-life Average (mean ± S.D.)
Children (over 6 months of age)	1.45 ± 0.58 ml/kg/min	3.7 ± 1.1 hrs.
Adult non-smokers with uncomplicated asthma	0.65 ± 0.19 ml/kg/min	8.7 ± 2.2 hrs.

The half-life of theophylline in smokers (one to two packs/day) averages four to five hours, much shorter than the half-life in nonsmokers which averages seven to nine hours. The increase in theophylline clearance caused by smoking is probably the result of induction of drug-metabolizing enzymes that do not readily normalize after cessation of smoking. It appears that between three months and two years may be necessary for normalization of the effect of smoking on theophylline pharmacokinetics.

In a single-dose study in eight fasted subjects, Respbid (theophylline) tablets, 250 mg given at 7 mg/kg produced peak theophylline plasma levels of 9.1 ± 3.8 (SD) mcg/ml at 5.0 ± 1.5 hours following dose administration. The extent of theophylline absorption from Respbid was complete in these subjects when compared with that from an immediate-release tablet. In a five-day, multiple-dose study involving 18 fasted subjects, Respbid tablets, 250 mg given twice daily (11 mg/kg per day) produced mean minimum and maximum theophylline plasma levels of 7.3 ± 2.3 mcg/ml and 10.8 ± 3.1 mcg/ml, respectively.

INDICATIONS AND USAGE

For relief and/or prevention of symptoms of asthma and reversible bronchospasm associated with chronic bronchitis and emphysema.

CONTRAINDICATIONS

Respbid (theophylline) tablets are contraindicated in individuals who are hypersensitive to any of their components.

WARNINGS

Status asthmaticus should be considered a medical emergency and is defined as that degree of bronchospasm which is not rapidly responsive to usual doses of conventional bronchodilators. Optimal therapy for such patients frequently requires both **additional medication,** parenterally administered, and **close monitoring,** preferably in an intensive care setting.

Although increasing the dose of theophylline may bring about relief, such treatment may be associated with toxicity. The likelihood of such toxicity developing increases significantly when the serum theophylline concentration exceeds 20 mcg/ml. Therefore, determination of serum theophylline levels is recommended to assure maximal benefit without excessive risk.

Serum levels above 20 mcg/ml are rarely found after appropriate administration of the recommended doses. However, in individuals in whom theophylline plasma clearance is reduced **for any reason,** even conventional doses may result in increased serum levels and potential toxicity. Reduced theophylline clearance has been documented in the following readily identifiable groups: 1) patients with impaired renal or liver function; 2) patients over 55 years of age, particularly males and those with chronic lung disease; 3) those with cardiac failure from any cause; 4) neonates; and 5) those patients taking certain drugs (some macrolide antibiotics and cimetidine). Decreased clearance of theophylline may be associated with either influenza immunization or active infection with influenza (see Clinical Pharmacology—Pharmacokinetics).

Reduction of dosage and laboratory monitoring are especially appropriate in the above individuals.

Less serious signs of theophylline toxicity, i.e., nausea and restlessness, may appear in up to 50% of patients. Unfortunately, however, serious side effects such as ventricular arrhythmias, convulsions or even death may appear as the first sign of toxicity without any previous warning. Stated differently, **serious toxicity is not reliably preceded by less severe side effects.**

Many patients who require theophylline may exhibit tachycardia due to their underlying disease process so that the cause/effect relationship to elevated serum theophylline concentrations may not be appreciated.

Theophylline products may cause dysrhythmia and/or worsen pre-existing arrhythmias, and any significant change in rate and/or rhythm warrants monitoring and further investigation.

The occurrence of arrhythmias and sudden death (with histological evidence of necrosis of the myocardium) has been recorded in laboratory animals (minipigs, rodents and dogs) when theophylline and beta agonists were administered concomitantly, although not when either was administered alone. The significance of these findings when applied to human usage is currently unknown.

PRECAUTIONS

General Precautions: The half-life of theophylline is shorter in smokers than in nonsmokers. Therefore smokers may require larger or more frequent doses. Morphine and curare should be used with caution in patients with airway obstruction as they may suppress respiration and stimulate histamine release. Alternative drugs should be used when possible. Theophylline should not be administered concurrently with other xanthine medications. Use with caution in patients with severe cardiac disease, severe hypoxemia, hypertension, hyperthyroidism, acute myocardial injury, cor pulmonale, congestive heart failure, liver disease, in the elderly (especially males) and in neonates. In particular, greater caution should be used in giving theophylline to patients with congestive heart failure. Frequently, such patients have markedly prolonged theophylline serum levels with theophylline persisting in serum for long periods following discontinuation of the drug.

Use theophylline cautiously in patients with a history of peptic ulcer. Theophylline may occasionally act as a local irritant to the G.I. tract, although gastrointestinal symptoms are more commonly centrally mediated and associated with serum concentrations over 20 mcg/ml.

Information for Patients: If nausea, vomiting, restlessness, irregular heartbeat, or convulsions occur, contact a physician immediately.

Take only the amount of drug that has been prescribed. Do not take a larger dose, or take the drug more often, or for a longer time than recommended.

Do not take other medicines, especially those for pulmonary disorders, except on the advice of a physician.

Contact your physician if pulmonary symptoms occur repeatedly, especially at the end of a dosing interval.

Avoid drinking large amounts of caffeine-containing beverages, such as coffee, tea, cocoa, or cola, or eating large quantities of chocolate while taking this medicine, since these foods may increase the side effects of theophylline.

Continued on next page

Boehringer Ingelheim—Cont.

If serum theophylline is:		Directions:
Within normal limits	10 to 20 mcg/ml	Maintain dosage if tolerated. Recheck serum theophylline concentration at 6- to 12-month intervals.*
Too high	20 to 25 mcg/ml	Decrease doses by about 10%. Recheck serum theophylline concentration at 6- to 12-month intervals.*
Too high	25 to 30 mcg/ml	Skip next dose and decrease subsequent doses by about 25%.
Dangerous	Over 30 mcg/ml	Skip next two doses and decrease subsequent doses by 50%. Recheck serum theophylline.
Too low	7.5 to 10 mcg/ml	Increase dose by about 25%.** Recheck serum theophylline concentration at 6- to 12-month intervals.*
Too low	5 to 7.5 mcg/ml	Increase dose by about 25% to the nearest dose increment and recheck serum theophylline for guidance in further dosage adjustment (another increase will probably be needed, but this provides a safety check).

*Finer adjustments in dosage may be needed for some patients.

**If symptoms occur repeatedly at the end of a dosing interval, change the dosing regimen to q 8 hrs, not exceeding the recommended daily dose.

Respbid (theophylline) tablets should not be chewed or crushed.

Laboratory Tests: Serum levels of theophylline should be monitored periodically to maintain optimum levels of 10 to 20 mcg/ml. The incidence of toxicity increases sharply above this range. For such measurements, serum should be obtained four to six hours after administration of Respbid tablets. Patient compliance with the prescribed Respbid regimen should have been good for the 48 hours preceding serum collection (i.e., no missed doses). ANY INCREASE IN DOSAGE BASED ON SERUM THEOPHYLLINE LEVEL WHEN THESE INSTRUCTIONS HAVE NOT BEEN FOLLOWED MAY INCREASE THE RISK OF TOXICITY. Because of the narrow range for therapeutic serum levels and great within-patient and between-patient variation in dosage necessary to produce and maintain such levels, measurement of serum theophylline is advised for individualization of dosage, both initially and during maintenance therapy. Certain patients may have slow elimination rates due to underlying conditions (see CLINICAL PHARMACOLOGY, WARNINGS and PRECAUTIONS, General Precautions); in such patients, conventional doses may produce high serum levels and associated signs of toxicity.

Drug Interactions: ***Drug/Drug:*** Toxic synergism with ephedrine has been documented and may occur with some other sympathomimetic bronchodilators. The administration of theophylline and sympathomimetic drugs concurrently is of particular concern in patients with cardiac arrhythmias. The following table lists drugs known to interact with theophylline and the effects of their concomitant use.

DRUG	EFFECT
Theophylline with lithium carbonate	Increased excretion of lithium carbonate
Theophylline with propranolol	Antagonism of propranolol effect
Theophylline with cimetidine	Increased theophylline blood levels
Theophylline with troleandomycin or erythromycin	Increased theophylline blood levels

Drug/Food: Respbid tablets have not been adequately studied to determine whether their bioavailability is altered when they are given with food.

Available data suggest that drug administration at the time of food ingestion may influence the absorption characteristics of some or all theophylline controlled-release products resulting in serum values different from those found after administration in the fasting state.

A drug-food effect, if any, would likely have its greatest clinical significance when high theophylline serum levels are being maintained and/or when large single doses (greater than 13 mg/kg or 900 mg) of a controlled-release theophylline product are given. The influence of the type and amount of food on performance of controlled-release theophylline products is under study at this time.

Drug/Laboratory Test Interactions: When plasma levels of theophylline are measured by spectrophotometric methods, note that coffee, tea, cola beverages, chocolate, and acetaminophen can produce falsely high values.

Carcinogenesis, Mutagenesis, Impairment of Fertility: Long-term animal studies have not been performed to evaluate the carcinogenic potential, mutagenic potential, or the effect on fertility of xanthine compounds.

Pregnancy: Category C—Animal reproduction studies have not been conducted with theophylline. It is also not known whether theophylline can cause fetal harm when administered to a pregnant woman or can affect reproduction capacity. Xanthines should be given to a pregnant woman only if clearly needed.

Nursing Mothers: It has been reported that theophylline distributes readily into breast milk, and may cause adverse effects in the infant. Caution must be used if prescribing xanthines to a mother who is nursing, taking into account the risk-benefit of this therapy.

Pediatric Use: Respbid tablets are not recommended for administration to children less than six years of age.

ADVERSE REACTIONS

The most consistent adverse reactions are usually due to overdose and are:

1. **Gastrointestinal:** nausea, vomiting, epigastric pain, hematemesis, diarrhea.
2. **Central nervous system:** headaches, irritability, restlessness, insomnia, reflex hyperexcitability, muscle twitching, clonic and tonic generalized convulsions.
3. **Cardiovascular:** palpitation, tachycardia, extrasystoles, flushing, hypotension, circulatory failure, ventricular arrhythmias.
4. **Respiratory:** tachypnea.
5. **Renal:** albuminuria, increased excretion of renal tubular and red blood cells, potentiation of diuresis.
6. **Others:** hyperglycemia and inappropriate ADH syndrome.

DRUG ABUSE AND DEPENDENCE

Drug abuse and dependence have not been reported with theophylline.

OVERDOSAGE

Management: If potential overdose is established and seizure has not occurred:

1. Induce vomiting.
2. Administer a cathartic (this is particularly important if sustained-release preparations have been taken).
3. Administer activated charcoal.

If patient is having a seizure:

1. Establish an airway.
2. Administer oxygen.
3. Treat the seizure with intravenous diazepam, 0.1 to 0.3 mg/kg up to a maximum dose of 10 mg.
4. Monitor vital signs, maintain blood pressure and provide adequate hydration.

Post-seizure coma:

1. Maintain airway and oxygenation.
2. Follow above recommendations to prevent absorption of drug, but intubation and lavage will have to be performed instead of inducing emesis, and the cathartic and charcoal will need to be introduced via a large-bore gastric lavage tube.
3. Continue to provide full supportive care and adequate hydration while waiting for drug to be metabolized. In general, the drug is metabolized sufficiently rapidly so that dialysis is not required.

General: Serum theophylline should be monitored until the level is less than 20 mcg/ml.

Electrolyte balance and hydration should be maintained by intravenous fluids.

If hypotension is not corrected by intravenous fluids, vasopressor drugs may be administered cautiously. (Caution: Sympathomimetic drugs may precipitate cardiac arrhythmia.)

Theophylline is dialyzable. However, in patients with very high serum theophylline levels and severe intoxication, charcoal hemoperfusion may be employed. This procedure is very effective in removing theophylline from the blood, and is to be preferred over peritoneal dialysis or hemodialysis.

DOSAGE AND ADMINISTRATION

For most patients, **effective use** of theophylline, i.e., associated with optimal likelihood of benefit combined with minimal risk of toxicity, is considered to occur when serum levels are maintained between 10 and 20 mcg/ml. Levels above 20 mcg/ml may produce toxicity, and in a small number of patients, toxicity may even be seen with serum levels between 15 and 20 mcg/ml, particularly during initiation of therapy.

There is considerable variation from patient to patient in the dosage required to achieve and maintain therapeutic and safe levels, primarily because of variable rates of elimination. Therefore, it is essential not only that dosage be individualized, but also that titration and monitoring of serum levels be utilized where available. When serum concentration cannot be obtained, restriction of dosage to the amounts and intervals recommended in the guidelines listed below becomes essential.

Dosage should be calculated on the basis of lean (ideal) body weight where mg/kg doses are presented. Theophylline does not distribute into fatty tissue.

Dosage guidelines are approximations only and the wide range of theophylline clearance between individuals (particularly those with concomitant disease) makes indiscriminate usage hazardous.

As a practical consideration, it is not always possible to obtain serum level determinations. Under such conditions, restriction of the daily dose (in otherwise healthy adults) to not greater than 13 mg/kg per day (of anhydrous theophylline) or 900 mg, whichever is less, in divided doses will result in relatively few patients exceeding serum levels of 20 mcg/ml and the resultant risk of toxicity.

Respbid (theophylline) tablets have not been adequately studied for their bioavailability when administered with food (see PRECAUTIONS, Drug/Food Interactions).

Respbid tablets should not be chewed or crushed.

Dosing Guidelines: Acute Symptoms—Respbid tablets are not intended for patients experiencing an acute episode of bronchospasm (associated with asthma, chronic bronchitis, or emphysema). Such patients require **rapid** relief of symptoms and should be treated with an immediate-release theophylline preparation, an intravenous theophylline preparation or other bronchodilators, and not with controlled release products.

Chronic Symptoms—Theophylline administration is a treatment of first choice for the management of chronic asthma (to prevent symptoms and maintain patent airways) and is recommended for chronic bronchitis and emphysema. The appropriate dosage of theophylline can be established using an immediate-release preparation. Slow clinical titration is preferred to help assure acceptance and safety of the medication. When appropriate theophylline serum levels have been attained and clinical improvement has been maintained, the patient can usually be switched to Respbid tablets by dividing the total daily dose of immediate-release theophylline by two and administering the appropriate Respbid tablet every 12 hours (see conversion chart below). However, certain patients, such as the young, smokers, or some nonsmoking adults, are likely to metabolize theophylline rapidly and require the total daily dose administered as three equal doses at eight-hour intervals. Such patients can generally be identified as having trough serum levels lower than desired or repeatedly exhibiting symptoms near the end of a dosing interval.

If the established daily dose is:	The q 12 hr regimen is: No. tablets:	strength:
500 mg	1	Respbid 250 mg
1000 mg	1	Respbid 500 mg

Alternatively, therapy of chronic bronchospasm can be initiated with Respbid if the above dosage strengths permit titration and adjustment of dosage. It is recommended that for children under 25 kg, proper dosage be established with a liquid preparation to permit titration in small increments.

Recommended Doses for Chronic Bronchospasm: Initial Dose—As an initial dose, 16 mg/kg per 24 hours in divided doses at 8- or 12-hour intervals as appropriate.

Increasing Dose—The above daily dosage may be increased in approximately 25% increments at two- to three-day intervals so long as the drug is tolerated, until satisfactory clinical response is observed or the maximum dose indicated in the following section is reached.

Maximum Dose Where the Serum Concentration Is Not Measured:

WARNING: DO NOT ATTEMPT TO MAINTAIN ANY DOSE THAT IS NOT TOLERATED.

Do not exceed the following:

Age <9 years	24 mg/kg/day
Age 9–12 years	20 mg/kg/day
Age 12–16 years	18 mg/kg/day
Age >16 years	13 mg/kg/day or 900 mg, whichever is less

Measurement of Serum Theophylline: For measurement of serum theophylline levels during chronic therapy, see PRECAUTIONS—Laboratory Tests.

Dosage Adjustment after Serum Theophylline Measurement:

[See table above].

IT IS IMPORTANT THAT NO PATIENT BE MAINTAINED ON ANY DOSAGE THAT IS NOT TOLERATED. In instructing patients to increase dosage, they should be instructed not to take a subsequent dose if side effects occur and to resume therapy at a lower dose once adverse effects have disappeared.

Caution should be exercised for younger children who may not complain of minor side effects. Older adults, those with cor pulmonale, congestive heart failure, and/or liver disease may have unusually low dosage requirements and thus may experience toxicity at the maximal dosage recommended above.

HOW SUPPLIED

Respbid® (theophylline) is supplied as 250 mg white, round, scored sustained release tablets imprinted with "BI 48" (NDC 0597-0048-01) and 500 mg white, capsule-shaped, scored sustained release tablets imprinted with "BI 49" (NDC 0597-0049-01) in bottles of 100.

Store below 30°C (86°F).

Caution: Federal law prohibits dispensing without prescription.

RE-PI-5/86

Shown in Product Identification Section, page 405

SERENTIL® ℞

[*seh-ren 'til*]

(mesoridazine USP) besylate

Tablets, 10 mg............BI-CODE 10
Tablets, 25 mg............BI-CODE 25
Tablets, 50 mg............BI-CODE 50
Tablets, 100 mg............BI-CODE 100
Concentrate of 25 mg/ml............BI-CODE 25
Ampuls of 1 ml (25 mg)............BI-CODE 27

DESCRIPTION

Serentil® (mesoridazine USP), the besylate salt of a metabolite of thioridazine, is a phenothiazine tranquilizer which is effective in the treatment of schizophrenia, organic brain disorders, alcoholism and psychoneuroses.

Serentil is 10-[2(1-methyl-2-piperidyl) ethyl]-2-(methyl-sulfinyl)-phenothiazine [as the besylate].

Tablets, 10 mg, for oral administration—Active Ingredient: mesoridazine (as the besylate), 10 mg. Inactive Ingredients: acacia, carnauba wax, colloidal silicon dioxide, FD&C Red No. 40 aluminum lake, lactose, microcrystalline cellulose, povidone, sodium benzoate, starch, stearic acid, sucrose, talc, titanium dioxide.

Tablets, 25 mg, for oral administration—Active Ingredient: mesoridazine (as the besylate), 25 mg. Inactive Ingredients: acacia, carnauba wax, colloidal silicon dioxide, FD&C Red No. 40 aluminum lake, lactose, microcrystalline cellulose, povidone, sodium benzoate, stearic acid, sucrose, talc, titanium dioxide.

Tablets, 50 mg, for oral administration—Active Ingredient: mesoridazine (as the besylate), 50 mg. Inactive Ingredients: acacia, carnauba wax, colloidal silicon dioxide, FD&C Red No. 40 aluminum lake, gelatin, lactose, microcrystalline cellulose, povidone, sodium benzoate, starch, stearic acid, sucrose, talc, titanium dioxide.

Tablets, 100 mg, for oral administration—Active Ingredient: mesoridazine (as the besylate), 100 mg. Inactive Ingredients: acacia, carnauba wax, colloidal silicon dioxide, FD&C Red No. 40 aluminum lake, gelatin, lactose, microcrystalline cellulose, povidone, sodium benzoate, starch, stearic acid, sucrose, talc, titanium dioxide.

Ampuls, 1 ml, for intramuscular administration—Active Ingredient: mesoridazine (as the besylate), 25 mg. Inactive Ingredients: edetate disodium USP, 0.5 mg; sodium chloride USP, 7.2 mg; carbon dioxide gas (bone dry) q.s., water for injection USP, q.s. to 1 ml.

Concentrate, for oral administration—Active Ingredient: mesoridazine (as the besylate), 25 mg per ml. Inactive Ingredients: alcohol, 0.61% by volume; citric acid; FD&C Red No. 40; flavors; methylparaben; propylparaben; purified water; sodium citrate, sorbitol.

ACTIONS

Based upon animal studies Serentil (mesoridazine USP), like other phenothiazines, acts indirectly on reticular formation, whereby neuronal activity into reticular formation is reduced without affecting its intrinsic ability to activate the cerebral cortex. In addition, the phenothiazines exhibit at least part of their activities through depression of hypothalamic centers. Neurochemically, the phenothiazines are thought to exert their effects by a central adrenergic blocking action.

INDICATIONS

In clinical studies Serentil (mesoridazine USP) has been found useful in the following disease states:

Schizophrenia: Serentil is effective in the treatment of schizophrenia. It substantially reduces the severity of emotional withdrawal, conceptual disorganization, anxiety, tension, hallucinatory behavior, suspiciousness and blunted affect in schizophrenic patients. As with other phenothiazines, patients refractory to previous medication may respond to Serentil.

Behavioral Problems in Mental Deficiency and Chronic Brain Syndrome: The effect of Serentil was found to be excellent or good in the management of hyperactivity and uncooperativeness associated with mental deficiency and chronic brain syndrome.

Alcoholism—Acute and Chronic: Serentil ameliorates anxiety, tension, depression, nausea and vomiting in both acute and chronic alcoholics without producing hepatic dysfunction or hindering the functional recovery of the impaired liver.

Psychoneurotic Manifestations: Serentil reduces the symptoms of anxiety and tension, prevalent symptoms often associated with neurotic components of many disorders, and benefits personality disorders in general.

CONTRAINDICATIONS

As with other phenothiazines, Serentil (mesoridazine USP) is contraindicated in severe central nervous system depression or comatose states from any cause. Serentil is contraindicated in individuals who have previously shown hypersensitivity to the drug.

WARNINGS

Tardive Dyskinesia: Tardive dyskinesia, a syndrome consisting of potentially irreversible, involuntary, dyskinetic movements may develop in patients treated with neuroleptic (antipsychotic) drugs. Although the prevalence of the syndrome appears to be highest among the elderly, especially elderly women, it is impossible to rely upon prevalence estimates to predict, at the inception of neuroleptic treatment, which patients are likely to develop the syndrome. Whether neuroleptic drug products differ in their potential to cause tardive dyskinesia is unknown.

Both the risk of developing the syndrome and the likelihood that it will become irreversible are believed to increase as the duration of treatment and the total cumulative dose of neuroleptic drugs administered to the patient increase. However, the syndrome can develop, although much less commonly, after relatively brief treatment periods at low doses.

There is no known treatment for established cases of tardive dyskinesia, although the syndrome may remit, partially or completely, if neuroleptic treatment is withdrawn. Neuroleptic treatment, itself, however, may suppress (or partially suppress) the signs and symptoms of the syndrome and thereby may possibly mask the underlying disease process. The effect that symptomatic suppression has upon the long-term course of the syndrome is unknown.

Given these considerations, neuroleptics should be prescribed in a manner that is most likely to minimize the occurrence of tardive dyskinesia. Chronic neuroleptic treatment should generally be reserved for patients who suffer from a chronic illness 1) that is known to respond to neuroleptic drugs, and 2) for which alternative, equally effective but potentially less harmful treatments are *not* available or appropriate. In patients who do require chronic treatment, the smallest dose and the shortest duration of treatment producing a satisfactory clinical response should be sought. The need for continued treatment should be reassessed periodically.

If signs and symptoms of tardive dyskinesia appear in a patient on neuroleptics, drug discontinuation should be considered. However, some patients may require treatment despite the presence of the syndrome.

(For further information about the description of tardive dyskinesia and its clinical detection, please refer to the sections on Information for Patients and Adverse Reactions.)

Where patients are participating in activities requiring complete mental alertness (e.g., driving), it is advisable to administer the phenothiazines cautiously and to increase the dosage gradually.

Usage in Pregnancy: The safety of this drug in pregnancy has not been established; hence, it should be given only when the anticipated benefits to be derived from treatment exceed the possible risks to mother and fetus.

Usage in Children: The use of Serentil (mesoridazine USP) in children under 12 years of age is not recommended, because safe conditions for its use have not been established.

Attention should be paid to the fact that phenothiazines are capable of potentiating central nervous system depressants (e.g., anesthetics, opiates, alcohol, etc.) as well as atropine and phosphorus insecticides.

PRECAUTIONS

While ocular changes have not to date been related to Serentil (mesoridazine USP), one should be aware that such changes have been seen with other drugs of this class.

Because of possible hypotensive effects, reserve parenteral administration for bedfast patients or for acute ambulatory cases, and keep patient lying down for at least one-half hour after injection.

Leukopenia and/or agranulocytosis have been attributed to phenothiazine therapy. A single case of transient granulocytopenia has been associated with Serentil. Since convulsive seizures have been reported, patients receiving anticonvulsant medication should be maintained on that regimen while receiving Serentil.

Neuroleptic drugs elevate prolactin levels; the elevation persists during chronic administration. Tissue culture experiments indicate that approximately one-third of human breast cancers are prolactin dependent in vitro, a factor of potential importance if the prescription of these drugs is contemplated in a patient with a previously detected breast cancer. Although disturbances such as galactorrhea, amenorrhea, gynecomastia, and impotence have been reported, the clinical significance of elevated serum prolactin levels is unknown for most patients. An increase in mammary neoplasms has been found in rodents after chronic administration of neuroleptic drugs. Neither clinical studies nor epidemiologic studies conducted to date, however, have shown an association between chronic administration of these drugs and mammary tumorigenesis; the available evidence is considered too limited to be conclusive at this time.

Information for Patients: Given the likelihood that some patients exposed chronically to neuroleptics will develop tardive dyskinesia, it is advised that all patients in whom chronic use is contemplated be given, if possible, full information about this risk.

ADVERSE REACTIONS

Drowsiness and hypotension were the most prevalent side effects encountered. Side effects tended to reach their maximum level of severity early with the exception of a few (rigidity and motoric effects) which occurred later in therapy.

With the exceptions of tremor and rigidity, adverse reactions were generally found among those patients who received relatively high doses early in treatment. Clinical data showed no tendency for the investigators to terminate treatment because of side effects.

Serentil (mesoridazine USP) has demonstrated a remarkably low incidence of adverse reactions when compared with other phenothiazine compounds.

Central Nervous System: Drowsiness, Parkinson's syndrome, dizziness, weakness, tremor, restlessness, ataxia, dystonia, rigidity, slurring, akathisia, motoric reactions (opisthotonos) have been reported.

Autonomic Nervous System: Dry mouth, nausea and vomiting, fainting, stuffy nose, photophobia, constipation and blurred vision have occurred in some instances.

Genitourinary System: Inhibition of ejaculation, impotence, enuresis, incontinence have been reported.

Skin: Itching, rash, hypertrophic papillae of the tongue and angioneurotic edema have been reported.

Cardiovascular System: Hypotension and tachycardia have been reported. EKG changes have occurred in some instances (see Phenothiazine Derivatives: Cardiovascular Effects).

Phenothiazine Derivatives: It should be noted that efficacy, indications and untoward effects have varied with the different phenothiazines. The physician should be aware that the following have occurred with one or more phenothiazines and should be considered whenever one of these drugs is used:

Autonomic Reactions: Miosis, obstipation, anorexia, paralytic ileus.

Cutaneous Reactions: Erythema, exfoliative dermatitis, contact dermatitis.

Blood Dyscrasias: Agranulocytosis, leukopenia, eosinophilia, thrombocytopenia, anemia, aplastic anemia, pancytopenia.

Allergic Reactions: Fever, laryngeal edema, angioneurotic edema, asthma.

Hepatotoxicity: Jaundice, biliary stasis.

Cardiovascular Effects: Changes in the terminal portion of the electrocardiogram, including prolongation of the Q-T interval, lowering and inversion of the T wave and appearance of a wave tentatively identified as a bifid T or a U wave have been observed in some patients receiving the phenothiazine tranquilizers, including Serentil (mesoridazine USP). To date, these appear to be due to altered repolarization and not related to myocardial damage. They appear to be reversible. While there is no evidence at present that these changes are in any way precursors of any significant disturbance of cardiac rhythm, it should be noted that sudden and unexpected deaths apparently due to cardiac arrest have occurred in patients previously showing characteristic electrocardiographic changes while taking the drug. The use of periodic electrocardiograms has been proposed but would appear to be of questionable value as a predictive device.

Hypotension, rarely resulting in cardiac arrest, has been noted.

Extrapyramidal Symptoms: Akathisia, agitation, motor restlessness, dystonic reactions, trismus, torticollis, opisthotonos, oculogyric crises, tremor, muscular rigidity, akinesia.

Tardive dyskinesia: Chronic use of neuroleptics may be associated with the development of tardive dyskinesia. The salient features of this syndrome are described in the **Warnings** section and below.

The syndrome is characterized by involuntary choreoathetoid movements which variously involve the tongue, face, mouth, lips, or jaw (e.g., protrusion of the tongue, puffing of cheeks, puckering of the mouth, chewing movements), trunk and extremities. The severity of the syndrome and the degree of impairment produced vary widely.

The syndrome may become clinically recognizable either during treatment, upon dosage reduction, or upon withdrawal of treatment. Movements may decrease in intensity and may disappear altogether if further treatment with neuroleptics is withheld. It is generally believed that reversibility is more likely after short- rather than long-term neuro-

Continued on next page

Boehringer Ingelheim—Cont.

leptic exposure. Consequently, early detection of tardive dyskinesia is important. To increase the likelihood of detecting the syndrome at the earliest possible time, the dosage of neuroleptic drug should be reduced periodically (if clinically possible) and the patient observed for signs of the disorder. This maneuver is critical, for neuroleptic drugs may mask the signs of the syndrome.
Endocrine Disturbances: Menstrual irregularities, altered libido, gynecomastia, lactation, weight gain, edema. False positive pregnancy tests have been reported.
Urinary Disturbances: Retention, incontinence.
Others: Hyperpyrexia. Behavioral effects suggestive of a paradoxical reaction have been reported. These include excitement, bizarre dreams, aggravation of psychoses and toxic confusional states. More recently, a peculiar skin-eye syndrome has been recognized as a side effect following long-term treatment with phenothiazines. This reaction is marked by progressive pigmentation of areas of the skin or conjunctiva and/or accompanied by discoloration of the exposed sclera and cornea. Opacities of the anterior lens and cornea described as irregular or stellate in shape have also been reported. Systemic lupus erythematosus-like syndrome.

DOSAGE AND ADMINISTRATION

The dosage of Serentil (mesoridazine USP), as with most medications, should be adjusted to the needs of the individual. The lowest effective dosage should always be used. When maximum response is achieved, dosage may be reduced gradually to a maintenance level.
Schizophrenia: For most patients, regardless of symptom severity, a starting dose of 50 mg t.i.d. is recommended. The usual optimum total daily dose range is 100-400 mg per day.
Behavioral Problems in Mental Deficiency and Chronic Brain Syndrome: For most patients a starting dose of 25 mg t.i.d. is recommended. The usual optimum total daily dose range is 75-300 mg per day.
Alcoholism: For most patients the usual starting dose is 25 mg b.i.d. The usual optimum total daily dose range is 50-200 mg per day.
Psychoneurotic Manifestations: For most patients the usual starting dose is 10 mg t.i.d. The usual optimum total daily dose range is 30-150 mg per day.

INJECTABLE FORM

In those situations in which an intramuscular form of medication is indicated, Serentil (mesoridazine USP) injectable is available. For most patients a starting dose of 25 mg is recommended. The dose may be repeated in 30 to 60 minutes, if necessary. The usual optimum total daily dose range is 25-200 mg per day.

HOW SUPPLIED

Tablets: 10 mg, 25 mg, 50 mg, and 100 mg mesoridazine (as the besylate). Bottles of 100.
Ampuls: 1 ml [25 mg mesoridazine (as the besylate)]. Boxes of 20 and 100.
Concentrate: Contains 25 mg mesoridazine (as the besylate) per ml; alcohol, USP, 0.61% by volume. Immediate containers: Amber glass bottles of 4 fl oz (118 ml) packaged in cartons of 12 bottles, with an accompanying dropper graduated to deliver 10 mg, 25 mg and 50 mg of mesoridazine (as the besylate).
Storage: Below 77°F. Protect from light. Dispense in amber glass bottles only.
The concentrate may be diluted with distilled water, acidified tap water, orange juice or grape juice.
Each dose should be so diluted just prior to administration. Preparation and storage of bulk dilutions is not recommended.
Additional information available to physicians.

PHARMACOLOGY

Pharmacological studies in laboratory animals have established that Serentil (mesoridazine USP) has a spectrum of pharmacodynamic actions typical of a major tranquilizer. In common with other tranquilizers it inhibits spontaneous motor activity in mice, prolongs thiopental and hexobarbital sleeping time in mice and produces spindles and block of arousal reaction in the EEG of rabbits. It is effective in blocking spinal reflexes in the cat and antagonizes d-amphetamine excitation and toxicity in grouped mice. It shows a moderate adrenergic blocking activity in vitro and in vivo and antagonizes 5-hydroxytryptamine in vivo. Intravenously administered, it lowers the blood pressure of anesthetized dogs. It has a weak antiacetylcholine effect in vitro.
The most outstanding activity of Serentil is seen in tests developed to investigate antiemotive activity of drugs. Such tests are those in which the rat reacts to acute or chronic stress by increased defecation (emotogenic defecation) or tests in which "emotional mydriasis" is elicited in the mouse by an electric shock. In both of these tests Serentil is effective in reducing emotive reactions. Its ED_{50} in inhibiting emotogenic defecation in the rat is 0.053 mg/kg (subcutaneous administration). Serentil has a potent antiemetic action. The intravenous ED_{50} against apomorphine-induced emesis in the dog is 0.64 mg/kg. Serentil, in common with other phenothiazines, demonstrates antiarrhythmic activity in anesthetized dogs.
Metabolic studies in the dog and rabbit with tritium labeled mesoridazine demonstrate that the compound is well absorbed from the gastrointestinal tract. The biological half-life of Serentil in these studies appears to be somewhere between 24 and 48 hours. Although significant urinary excretion was observed following the administration of Serentil, these studies also suggest that biliary excretion is an important excretion route for mesoridazine and/ or its metabolites.

Toxicity Studies
Acute LD_{50} (mg/kg):

Serentil

Route	Mouse	Rat	Rabbit	Dog
Oral	560±62.5	644±48	MLD=800	MLD=800
I.M.	—	509M 584 F	405	—
I.V.	26±0.08	—	—	—

Chronic toxicity studies were conducted in rats and dogs. Rats were administered Serentil (mesoridazine USP), orally seven days per week for a period of seventeen months in doses up to 160 mg/kg per day. Dogs were administered Serentil orally seven days per week for a period of thirteen months. The daily dosage of the drug was increased during the period of this test such that the "top-dose" group received a daily dose of 120 mg/kg of mesoridazine for the last month of the study.
Untoward effects which occurred upon chronic administration of high dose-levels included:
Rats: Reduction of food intake, slowed weight gain, morphological changes in pituitary-supported endocrine organs, and melanin-like pigment deposition in renal tissues.
Dogs: Emesis, muscle tremors, decreased food intake and death associated with aspiration of oral-gastric contents into the respiratory system.
Increased intrauterine resorptions were seen with Serentil in rats at 70 mg/kg and in rabbits at 125 mg/kg but not at 60 and 100 mg/kg, respectively. No drug-related teratology was suggested by these reproductive studies.
Local irritation from the intramuscular injection of Serentil was of the same order of magnitude as with other phenothiazines.

NOTE

Some tablets manufactured in 1985 contain different ingredients, including FD&C Yellow No. 5 (tartrazine) which may cause allergic-type reactions (including bronchial asthma) in certain susceptible individuals. Please check Package Insert for exact formulation.

SE-PI-8/85

Shown in Product Identification Section, page 405

THALITONE® ℞

[*thal'ih-tōn*]
(chlorthalidone USP)
Tablets of 25 mg

DESCRIPTION

Thalitone (chlorthalidone USP) is a monosulfamyl diuretic which differs chemically from thiazide diuretics in that a double-ring system is incorporated in its structure.
Chlorthalidone is 2-chloro-5-(1-hydroxy-3-oxo-1-isoindolinyl) benzenesulfonamide.

ACTIONS

Chlorthalidone is an oral diuretic with prolonged action (48–72 hours) and low toxicity. The diuretic effect of the drug occurs within two hours of an oral dose and continues for up to 72 hours. It produces copious diuresis with greatly increased excretion of sodium and chloride. At maximal therapeutic dosage, chlorthalidone is approximately equal in its diuretic effect to comparable maximal therapeutic doses of benzothiadiazine diuretics. The site of action appears to be the cortical diluting segment of the ascending limb of Henle's loop of the nephron.

INDICATIONS

Diuretics such as Thalitone (chlorthalidone USP) are indicated in the management of hypertension either as the sole therapeutic agent or to enhance the effect of other antihypertensive drugs in the more severe forms of hypertension.
Thalitone is indicated as adjunctive therapy in edema associated with congestive heart failure, hepatic cirrhosis, and corticosteroid and estrogen therapy.
Thalitone has also been found useful in edema due to various forms of renal dysfunction such as nephrotic syndrome, acute glomerulonephritis, and chronic renal failure.
Usage in Pregnancy: The routine use of diuretics in an otherwise healthy woman is inappropriate and exposes mother and fetus to unnecessary hazard. Diuretics do not prevent development of toxemia of pregnancy, and there is no satisfactory evidence that they are useful in the treatment of developed toxemia. Edema during pregnancy may arise from pathological causes or from the physiologic and mechanical consequences of pregnancy. Chlorthalidone is indicated in pregnancy when edema is due to pathologic causes, just as it is in the absence of pregnancy (however, see Warnings below). Dependent edema in pregnancy, resulting from restriction of venous return by the expanded uterus, is properly treated through elevation of the lower extremities and use of support hose; use of diuretics to lower intravascular volume in this case is illogical and unnecessary. There is hypervolemia during normal pregnancy which is harmful to neither the fetus nor the mother (in the absence of cardiovascular disease), but which is associated with edema, including generalized edema, in the majority of pregnant women. If this edema produces discomfort, increased recumbency will often provide relief. In rare instances, this edema may cause extreme discomfort which is not relieved by rest. In these cases, a short course of diuretics may provide relief and may be appropriate.

CONTRAINDICATIONS

Anuria.
Hypersensitivity to chlorthalidone or other sulfonamide-derived drugs.

WARNINGS

Should be used with caution in severe renal disease. In patients with renal disease, chlorthalidone or related drugs may precipitate azotemia. Cumulative effects of the drug may develop in patients with impaired renal function.
Chlorthalidone should be used with caution in patients with impaired hepatic function or progressive liver disease, since minor alterations of fluid and electrolyte balance may precipitate hepatic coma.
Chlorthalidone may add to or potentiate the action of other antihypertensive drugs. Potentiation occurs with ganglionic or peripheral adrenergic blocking drugs.
Sensitivity reactions may occur in patients with a history of allergy or bronchial asthma.
The possibility of exacerbation or activation of systemic lupus erythematosus has been reported with thiazide diuretics, which are structurally related to chlorthalidone. However, systemic lupus erythematosus has not been reported following chlorthalidone administration.
Usage in Pregnancy: Reproduction studies in various animal species at multiples of the human dose showed no significant level of teratogenicity; no fetal or congenital abnormalities were observed. Animal data should not be extrapolated for clinical application.
Thiazides cross the placental barrier and appear in cord blood. The use of chlorthalidone and related drugs in pregnant women requires that the anticipated benefits of the drug be weighed against possible hazards to the fetus. These hazards include fetal or neonatal jaundice, thrombocytopenia, and possibly other adverse reactions which have occurred in the adult.
Nursing Mothers: Thiazides cross the placental barrier and appear in breast milk. If use of the drug is deemed essential, the patient should stop nursing.

PRECAUTIONS

Periodic determination of serum electrolytes to detect possible electrolyte imbalance should be performed at appropriate intervals.
All patients receiving chlorthalidone should be observed for clinical signs of fluid or electrolyte imbalance; namely, hyponatremia, hypochloremic alkalosis, and hypokalemia. Serum and urine electrolyte determinations are particularly important when the patient is vomiting excessively or receiving parenteral fluids. Medication such as digitalis may also influence serum electrolytes. Warning signs, irrespective of cause, are dryness of mouth, thirst, weakness, lethargy, drowsiness, restlessness, muscle pains or cramps, muscular fatigue, hypotension, oliguria, tachycardia, and gastrointestinal disturbances such as nausea and vomiting. Hypokalemia may develop with chlorthalidone as with any other potent diuretic, especially with brisk diuresis, when severe cirrhosis is present, or during concomitant use of corticosteroids or ACTH.
Interference with adequate oral electrolyte intake will also contribute to hypokalemia. Digitalis therapy may exaggerate metabolic effects of hypokalemia, especially with reference to myocardial activity.
Any chloride deficit is generally mild and usually does not require specific treatment except under extraordinary circumstances (as in liver disease or renal disease). Dilutional hyponatremia may occur in edematous patients in hot weather; appropriate therapy is water restriction, rather than administration of salt except in rare instances when

the hyponatremia is life threatening. In actual salt depletion, appropriate replacement is the therapy of choice. Hyperuricemia may occur or frank gout may be precipitated in certain patients receiving chlorthalidone.
Insulin requirements in diabetic patients may be increased, decreased or unchanged. Latent diabetes mellitus may become manifest during chlorthalidone administration.
Chlorthalidone and related drugs may increase the responsiveness to tubocurarine. The antihypertensive effects of the drug may be enhanced in the postsympathectomy patient.
Chlorthalidone and related drugs may decrease arterial responsiveness to norepinephrine. This diminution is not sufficient to preclude effectiveness of the pressor agent for the therapeutic use.
If progressive renal impairment becomes evident, as indicated by a rising non-protein nitrogen or blood urea nitrogen, a careful reappraisal of therapy is necessary with consideration given to withholding or discontinuing diuretic therapy.
Chlorthalidone and related drugs may decrease serum PBI levels without signs of thyroid disturbance.

ADVERSE REACTIONS

Gastrointestinal System Reactions: anorexia, gastric irritation, nausea, vomiting, cramping, diarrhea, constipation, jaundice (intrahepatic cholestatic jaundice), pancreatitis.
Central Nervous System Reactions: dizziness, vertigo, paresthesias, headache, xanthopsia.
Hematologic Reactions: leukopenia, agranulocytosis, thrombocytopenia, aplastic anemia.
Dermatologic-Hypersensitivity Reactions: purpura, photosensitivity, rash, urticaria, necrotizing angiitis (vasculitis) (cutaneous vasculitis), Lyell's syndrome (toxic epidermal necrolysis).
Cardiovascular Reactions: Orthostatic hypotension may occur and may be aggravated by alcohol, barbiturates or narcotics.
Other Adverse Reactions: hyperglycemia, glycosuria, hyperuricemia, muscle spasm, weakness, restlessness, impotence.
Whenever adverse reactions are moderate or severe, chlorthalidone dosage should be reduced or therapy withdrawn.

DOSAGE AND ADMINISTRATION

Therapy should be initiated with the lowest possible dose. This dose should be titrated according to individual patient response to gain maximal therapeutic benefit while maintaining the minimal dosage possible. A single dose given in the morning with food is recommended; divided doses are unnecessary.
Hypertension. Initiation: Therapy, in most patients, should be initiated with a single daily dose of 25 mg. If the response is insufficient after a suitable trial, the dosage may be increased to a single daily dose of 50 mg. If additional control is required, the dosage of Thalitone (chlorthalidone USP) may be increased to 100 mg once daily or a second antihypertensive drug (step-2 therapy) may be added. Dosage above 100 mg daily usually does not increase effectiveness. Increases in serum uric acid and decreases in serum potassium are dose-related over the 25–100 mg/day range.
Maintenance: Maintenance doses may be lower than initial doses and should be adjusted according to individual patient response. Effectiveness is well sustained during continued use.
Edema. Initiation: Adults, initially 50 to 100 mg daily, or 100 mg on alternate days. Some patients may require 150 to 200 mg at these intervals, or up to 200 mg daily. Dosages above this level, however, do not usually produce a greater response.
Maintenance: Maintenance doses may often be lower than initial doses and should be adjusted according to the individual patient. Effectiveness is well sustained during continued use.

OVERDOSAGE

Symptoms of overdosage include nausea, weakness, dizziness and disturbances of electrolyte balance. There is no specific antidote, but gastric lavage is recommended, followed by supportive treatment. Where necessary, this may include intravenous dextrose-saline with potassium, administered with caution.

HOW SUPPLIED

White, kidney-shaped compressed tablets coded BI/76 containing 25 mg of chlorthalidone in bottles of 100, NDC number 0597-0076-01.
The inactive ingredients are colloidal silicon dioxide, lactose, magnesium stearate, microcrystalline cellulose, povidone, sodium starch glycolate.

ANIMAL PHARMACOLOGY

Biochemical studies in animals have suggested reasons for the prolonged effect of chlorthalidone. Absorption from the gastrointestinal tract is slow due to its low solubility. After passage to the liver, some of the drug enters the general circulation, while some is excreted in the bile, to be reabsorbed later. In the general circulation, it is distributed widely to the tissues, but is taken up in highest concentrations by the kidneys, where amounts have been found 72 hours after ingestion, long after it has disappeared from other tissues. The drug is excreted unchanged in the urine.
Store Below 30°C (86°F). TH-PI-8/85
Shown in Product Identification Section, page 405

TORECAN® ℞
[*tor'eh-can*]
thiethylperazine maleate tablets USP **BI-CODE 28**
thiethylperazine malate injection USP **BI-CODE 30**
(for intramuscular use use only)
thiethylperazine maleate suppositories USP **BI-CODE 29**

DESCRIPTION

Torecan (thiethylperazine USP) is a phenothiazine. Thiethylperazine is characterized by a substituted thioethyl group at position 2 in the phenothiazine nucleus, and a piperazine moiety in the side chain. The chemical designation is: 2-ethyl-mercapto-10-[3'-(1"-methyl-piperazinyl-4")-propyl-1'] phenothiazine.
Tablets, 10 mg, for oral administration. Active Ingredient: thiethylperazine maleate USP 10 mg. Inactive Ingredients: acacia, carnauba wax, FD&C Yellow No. 5 aluminum lake (tartrazine), FD&C Yellow No. 6 aluminum lake, gelatin, lactose, magnesium stearate, povidone, sodium benzoate, sorbitol, starch, stearic acid, sucrose, talc, titanium dioxide.
Ampul, 2 ml, for intramuscular administration. Active Ingredient: thiethylperazine malate USP 10 mg per 2 ml. Inactive Ingredients: sodium metabisulfite NF, 0.5 mg; ascorbic acid USP, 2.0 mg, sorbitol NF, 40 mg; carbon dioxide gas q.s.; water for injection USP, q.s.
Suppository, 10 mg, for rectal administration. Active Ingredient: thiethylperazine maleate USP 10 mg. Inactive ingredient: cocoa butter NF.

ACTIONS

The pharmacodynamic action of Torecan (thiethylperazine USP) in humans is unknown. However, a direct action of Torecan (thiethylperazine USP) on both the CTZ and the vomiting center may be concluded from induced vomiting experiments in animals.

INDICATIONS

Torecan (thiethylperazine USP) is indicated for the relief of nausea and vomiting.

CONTRAINDICATIONS

Severe central nervous system (CNS) depression and comatose states. In patients who have demonstrated a hypersensitivity reaction (e.g., blood dyscrasias, jaundice) to phenothiazines.
Because severe hypotension has been reported after the intravenous administration of phenothiazines, this route of administration is contraindicated.
Usage in Pregnancy: Torecan is contraindicated in pregnancy.

WARNINGS

Phenothiazines are capable of potentiating CNS depressants (e.g., anesthetics, opiates, alcohol, etc.) as well as atropine and phosphorous insecticides.
Since Torecan (thiethylperazine USP) may impair mental and/or physical ability required in the performance of potentially hazardous tasks such as driving a car or operating machinery, it is recommended that patients be warned accordingly.
Postoperative Nausea and Vomiting: With the use of this drug to control postoperative nausea and vomiting occurring in patients undergoing elective surgical procedures, restlessness and postoperative CNS depression during anesthesia recovery may occur. Possible postoperative complications of a severe degree of any of the known reactions of this class of drug must be considered.
Postural hypotension may occur after an initial injection, rarely with the tablet or suppository.
The administration of epinephrine should be avoided in the treatment of drug-induced hypotension in view of the fact that phenothiazines may induce a reversed epinephrine effect on occasion.
Should a vasoconstrictive agent be required, the most suitable are levarterenol and phenylephrine.
The use of this drug has not been studied following intracardiac and intracranial surgery.
Usage in Pediatrics: The safety and efficacy of Torecan in children under 12 years of age has not been established.
Nursing Mothers: Information is not available concerning the secretion of Torecan in the milk of nursing mothers. As a general rule, nursing should not be undertaken while a patient is on a drug, since many drugs are secreted in human milk.

PRECAUTIONS

Abnormal movements such as extrapyramidal symptoms (EPS) (e.g., dystonia, torticollis, dysphasia, oculogyric crises, akathisia) have occurred. Convulsions have also been reported. The varied symptom complex is more likely to occur in young adults and children. Extrapyramidal effects must be treated by reduction of dosage or cessation of medication.
Torecan (thiethylperazine maleate USP) tablets contain FD&C Yellow No. 5 (tartrazine) which may cause allergic-type reactions (including bronchial asthma) in certain susceptible individuals. Although the overall incidence of FD&C Yellow No. 5 (tartrazine) sensitivity in the general population is low, it is frequently seen in patients who also have aspirin hypersensitivity.
Postoperative Nausea and Vomiting: When used in the treatment of the nausea and/or vomiting associated with anesthesia and surgery, it is recommended that Torecan should be administered by deep intramuscular injection at or shortly before the termination of anesthesia.

ADVERSE REACTIONS

Central Nervous System: Serious: Convulsions have been reported. Extrapyramidal symptoms (EPS) may occur, such as dystonia, torticollis, oculogyric crises, akathisia, and gait disturbances. Others: Occasional cases of dizziness, headache, fever and restlessness have been reported.
Drowsiness may occur on occasion, following an initial injection. Generally this effect tends to subside with continued therapy or is usually alleviated by a reduction in dosage.
Autonomic Nervous System: Dryness of the mouth and nose, blurred vision, tinnitus. An occasional case of sialorrhea together with altered gustatory sensation has been observed.
Endocrine System: Peripheral edema of the arms, hands and face.
Hepatotoxicity: An occasional case of cholestatic jaundice has been observed.
Others: An occasional case of cerebral vascular spasm and trigeminal neuralgia has been reported.
Phenothiazine Derivatives: The physician should be aware that the following have occurred with one or more phenothiazines and should be considered whenever one of these drugs is used:
Blood Dyscrasias: Serious: Agranulocytosis, leukopenia, thrombocytopenia, aplastic anemia, pancytopenia. Others: Eosinophilia, leukocytosis.
Autonomic Reactions: Miosis, obstipation, anorexia, paralytic ileus.
Cutaneous Reactions: Serious: Erythema, exfoliative dermatitis, contact dermatitis.
Hepatotoxicity: Serious: Jaundice, biliary stasis.
Cardiovascular Effects: Serious: Hypotension, rarely leading to cardiac arrest; electrocardiographic (ECG) changes.
Extrapyramidal Symptoms: Serious: Akathisia, agitation, motor restlessness, dystonic reactions, trismus, torticollis, opisthotonos, oculogyric crises, tremor, muscular rigidity, akinesia—some of which have persisted for several months or years especially in patients of advanced age with brain damage.
Endocrine Disturbances: Menstrual irregularities, altered libido, gynecomastia, weight gain. False positive pregnancy tests have been reported.
Urinary Disturbances: Retention, incontinence.
Allergic Reactions: Serious: Fever, laryngeal edema, angioneurotic edema, asthma.
Others: Hyperpyrexia. Behavioral effects suggestive of a paradoxical reaction have been reported. These include excitement, bizarre dreams, aggravation of psychoses and toxic confusional states. While there is no evidence at present that ECG changes observed in patients receiving phenothiazines are in any way precursors of any significant disturbance of cardiac rhythm, it should be noted that sudden and unexpected deaths apparently due to cardiac arrest have been reported in a few instances in hospitalized psychotic patients previously showing characteristic ECG changes. A peculiar skin-eye syndrome has also been recognized as a side effect following long-term treatment with certain phenothiazines. This reaction is marked by progressive pigmentation of areas of the skin or conjunctiva and/or accompanied by discoloration of the exposed sclera and cornea. Opacities of the anterior lens and cornea described as irregular or stellate in shape have also been reported.
Drug Interactions: Phenothiazines are capable of potentiating CNS depressants (e.g., anesthetics, opiates, alcohol, etc.) as well as atropine and phosphorous insecticides.
Phenothiazines may induce a reversed epinephrine effect on occasion.

DOSAGE AND ADMINISTRATION

Adult: Usual daily dose range is 10 mg to 30 mg.
Oral: One tablet, one to three times daily.
Intramuscular: 2 ml IM, one to three times daily. (See Precautions.)
Suppository: Insert one suppository, one to three times daily.
Children: Appropriate dosage of Torecan (thiethylperazine USP) has not been determined in children.

HOW SUPPLIED

Tablets: Each tablet contains 10 mg thiethylperazine maleate USP, bottles of 100.
Ampuls: Each 2 ml ampul contains in aqueous solution 10 mg thiethylperazine malate, USP. Boxes of 20 and 100.

Continued on next page

Boehringer Ingelheim—Cont.

Storage: Below 86° F; light-resistant container.
Administer only if clear and colorless.
Suppositories: Each containing 10 mg thiethylperazine maleate, USP. Packages of 12.
Storage: Below 77° F; tight container (sealed foil).

TO-PI-5/86

Shown in Product Identification Section, page 405

Boots Pharmaceuticals, Inc.

8800 ELLERBE ROAD
SHREVEPORT, LA 71106 U.S.A.

PRODUCT INFORMATION WAS PREPARED IN APRIL, 1986. FOR FURTHER INFORMATION ON THESE AND OTHER BOOTS PRODUCTS CONTACT YOUR BOOTS REPRESENTATIVE OR WRITE BOOTS PHARMACEUTICALS, INC., P. O. BOX 6750, SHREVEPORT, LA 71136.

F-E-P CREME® ℞

[f-e-p krĕm]

DESCRIPTION

F-E-P Creme is a topical preparation containing Hydrocortisone acetate 1.0% and Pramoxine hydrochloride 1.0% in a hydrophilic cream base containing stearic acid, cetyl alcohol, aquaphor, isopropylpalmitate, polyoxyl-40-stearate, propylene glycol, potassium sorbate 0.1%, sorbic acid 0.1%, triethanolamine lauryl sulfate and water.

Topical corticosteroids are anti-inflammatory and anti-pruritic agents. The chemical structural formulas for active ingredients are presented below.

Hydrocortisone acetate
(Pregn-4-ene-3,20-dione,21-(acetyloxy)
-11,17-dihydroxy-,(11β)-.

Pramoxine Hydrochloride
(4(3-(p-butoxyphenoxyl))-propyl-
morpholine hydrochloride.)

CLINICAL PHARMACOLOGY

Topical corticosteroids share anti-inflammatory, antipruritic and vasoconstrictive actions.

The mechanism of anti-inflammatory activity of the topical corticosteroids is unclear. Various laboratory methods, including vasoconstrictor assays, are used to compare and predict potencies and/or clinical efficacies of the topical corticosteroids. There is some evidence to suggest that a recognizable correlation exists between vasoconstrictor potency and therapeutic efficacy in humans.

Pramoxine hydrochloride is a topical anesthetic agent which provides temporary relief from itching and pain. It acts by stabilizing the neuronal membrane of nerve endings with which it comes into contact.

PHARMACOKINETICS

The extent of percutaneous absorption of topical corticosteroids is determined by many factors including the vehicle, the integrity of the epidermal barrier, and the use of occlusive dressings.

Topical corticosteroids can be absorbed from normal intact skin. Inflammation and/or other disease processes in the skin increase percutaneous absorption. Occlusive dressings substantially increase the percutaneous absorption of topical corticosteroids. Thus, occlusive dressings may be a valuable therapeutic adjunct for treatment of resistant dermatoses. (See **DOSAGE AND ADMINISTRATION**).

Once absorbed through the skin, topical corticosteroids are handled through pharmacokinetic pathways similar to systemically administered corticosteroids. Corticosteroids are bound to plasma proteins in varying degrees. Corticosteroids are metabolized primarily in the liver and are then excreted by the kidneys. Some of the topical corticosteroids and their metabolites are also excreted into the bile.

INDICATIONS AND USAGE

Topical corticosteroids are indicated for the relief of the inflammatory and pruritic manifestations of corticosteroid-responsive dermatoses.

CONTRAINDICATIONS

Topical corticosteroids are contraindicated in those patients with a history of hypersensitivity to any of the components of the preparation.

PRECAUTIONS

General: Systemic absorption of topical corticosteroids has produced reversible hypothalmic-pituitary-adrenal (HPA) axis suppression, manifestations of Cushing's syndrome, hyperglycemia, and glucosuria in some patients.

Conditions which augment systemic absorption include the applications of the more potent steroids, use over large surface areas, prolonged use, and the addition of occlusive dressings.

Therefore patients receiving a large dose of a potent topical steroid applied to a large surface area and under an occlusive dressing should be evaluated periodically for evidence of HPA axis suppression by using the urinary free cortisol and ACTH stimulation tests. If HPA axis suppression is noted, an attempt should be made to withdraw the drug, to reduce the frequency of application, or to substitute a less potent steroid.

Recovery of HPA axis function is generally prompt and complete upon discontinuation of the drug. Infrequently, signs and symptoms of steroid withdrawal may occur, requiring supplemental systemic corticosteroids.

Children may absorb proportionally large amounts of topical corticosteroids and thus be more susceptible to systemic toxicity. (See **PRECAUTIONS—Pediatric Use**).

If irritation develops, topical corticosteroids should be discontinued and appropriate therapy instituted.

In the presence of dermatological infections, the use of an appropriate antifungal or antibacterial agent should be instituted. If a favorable response does not occur promptly, the corticosteroid should be discontinued until the infection has been adequately controlled.

Information for the Patient: Patients using topical corticosteroids should receive the following information and instructions:

1. This medication is to be used as directed by the physician. It is for external use only. Avoid contact with the eyes.
2. Patients should be advised not to use this medication for any disorder other than for which it was prescribed.
3. The treated skin area should not be bandaged or otherwise covered or wrapped as to be occlusive unless directed by the physician.
4. Patients should report any signs of adverse local reactions, especially under occlusive dressing.
5. Parents of pediatric patients should be advised not to use tightfitting diapers or plastic pants on a child being treated in the diaper area, as these garments may constitute occlusive dressings.

Laboratory Tests: The following tests may be helpful in evaluating the HPA axis suppression.
Urinary free cortisol test
ACTH stimulation test

Carcinogenesis, Mutagenesis, and Impairment of Fertility: Long-term animal studies have not been performed to evaluate the carcinogenic potential or the effect on fertility of topical corticosteroids.

Studies to determine mutagencity with prednisolone and hydrocortisone have revealed negative results.

Pregnancy Category C: Corticosteroids are generally teratogenic in laboratory animals when administered systemically at relatively low dosage levels. The more potent corticosteroids have been shown to be teratogenic after dermal application in laboratory animals. There are no adequate and well-controlled studies in pregnant women on teratogenic effects from topically applied corticosteroids. Therefore, topical corticosteroids should be used in pregnancy only if the potential benefit justifies the potential risk to the fetus. Drugs of this class should not be used extensively on pregnant patients, in large amounts, or for prolonged periods of time.

Nursing Mothers: It is not known whether topical administration of corticosteroids could result in sufficient systemic absorption to produce detectable amounts in breast milk. Systemically administered corticosteroids are secreted into breast milk in quantities NOT likely to have a deleterious effect on the infant. Nevertheless, caution should be exercised when topical corticosteroids are administered to a nursing woman.

Pediatric Use: Pediatric patients may demonstrate greater susceptibiliy to topical corticosteroid-induced HPA axis suppression and Cushing's syndrome than mature patients because of a larger skin surface area to body weight ratio.

Hypothalmic-pituitary-adrenal (HPA) axis suppression, Cushing's syndrome, and intracranial hypertension have been reported in children receiving topical corticosteroids. Manifestations of adrenal suppression in children include linear growth retardation delayed weight gain, low plasma cortisol levels, and absence of response to ACTH stimulation. Manifestations of intracranial hypertension include bulging fontanelles, headaches, and bilateral papilledema.

Administration of topical corticosteroids to children should be limited to the least amount compatible with an effective therapeutic regimen. Chronic corticosteroid therapy may intefere with the growth and development of children.

ADVERSE REACTIONS

The following local adverse reactions are reported infrequently with topical corticosteroids, but may occur more frequently with the use of occlusive dressings. These reactions are listed in an approximate decreasing order of occurrence.

Burning
Itching
Irritation
Dryness
Folliculitis
Hypertrichosis
Acneiform eruptions
Hypopigmentation
Perioral dermatitis
Allergic contact dermatitis
Maceration of the skin
Secondary infection
Skin atrophy
Striae
Miliaria

OVERDODAGE

Topically applied corticosteroids can be absorbed in sufficient amounts to produce systemic effects (See **PRECAUTIONS**).

DOSAGE AND ADMINISTRATION

Topical corticosteroids are generally applied to the affected area as a thin film 3–4 times daily depending on the severity of the condition.

Occlusive dressings may be used for the management of psoriasis or recalcitrant conditions.

If an infection develops, the use of occlusive dressings should be discontinued and appropriate antimicrobial therapy instituted.

HOW SUPPLIED

½ oz. (15 gm.) tubes NDC 0524-2026-51

CAUTION

Federal law prohibits dispensng without prescription.

Manufactured by:
Ferndale Laboratories, Inc.
Ferndale, Michigan 48220

Distributed by:
Boots Pharmaceuticals, Inc.
Shreveport, Louisiana 71106 U.S.A.

1/84 2026-01

LOPURIN® ℞

[lō-pyoor-in]
allopurinol Tablets, USP

DESCRIPTION

Lopurin (allopurinol) has the following structural formula:

Lopurin is known chemically as 1,5-dihydro-4*H*-pyrazolo [3,4-*d*]pyrimidin-4-one. It is a xanthine oxidase inhibitor which is administered orally. Its solubility in water at 37°C is 80.0 mg/dl and is greater in an alkaline solution.

CLINICAL PHARMACOLOGY

Loupin (allopurinol) acts on purine catabolism, without disrupting the biosynthesis of purines. It reduces the production of uric acid by inhibiting the biochemical reactions immediately preceding its formation.

Lopurin is a structural analogue of the natural purine base, hypoxanthine. It is an inhibitor of xanthine oxidase, the enzyme responsible for the conversion of hypoxanthine to xanthine and of xanthine to uric acid, the end product of purine metabolism in man. Lopurin is metabolized to the corresponding xanthine analogue, oxipurinol (alloxanthine), which also is an inhibitor of xanthine oxidase.

[See structural formula on next page].

It has been shown that reutilization of both hypoxanthine and xanthine for nucleotide and nucleic acid synthesis is markedly enhanced when their oxidations are inhibited by Lopurin and oxipurinol. This reutilization does not disrupt normal nucleic acid anabolism, however, because feedback inhibition is an integral part of purine biosynthesis. As a result of xanthine oxidase inhibition, the serum concentration of hypoxanthine plus xanthine in patients receiving Lopurin for treatment for hyperuricemia is usually in the range of 0.3 to 0.4 mg/dl compared to a normal level of approximately 0.15 mg/dl. A maximum of 0.9 mg/dl of these oxypurines has been reported when the serum urate was lowered to less than 2 mg/dl by high doses of Lopurin. These values are far below the saturation levels at which point their precipitation would be expected to occur (above 7 mg/dl).

The renal clearance of hypoxanthine and xanthine is at least 10 times greater than that of uric acid. The increased xanthine and hypoxanthine in the urine have not been accompanied by problems of nephrolithiasis. Xanthine crystalluria has been reported in only three patients. Two of the patients had Lesch-Nyhan syndrome, which is characterized by excessive uric acid production combined with a deficiency of the enzyme, hypoxanthine-guanine phosphoribosyltransferase (HGPRTase). This enzyme is required for the conversion of hypoxanthine, xanthine, and guanine to their respective nucleotides. The third patient had lymphosarcoma and produced an extremely large amount of uric acid because of rapid cell lysis during chemotherapy.

Lopurin is approximately 90% absorbed from the gastrointestinal tract. Peak plasma levels generally occur at 1.5 hours and 4.5 hours for Lopurin and oxipurinol respectively, and after a single oral dose of 300 mg Lopurin, maximum plasma levels of about 3 μg/ml of Lopurin and 6.5 μg/ml of oxipurinol are produced.

Approximately 20% of the ingested Lopurin is excreted in the feces. Because of its rapid oxidation to oxipurinol and a renal clearance rate approximately that of glomerular filtration rate, Lopurin has a plasma half-life of about 1–2 hours. Oxypurinol, however, has a longer plasma half-life (approximately 15.0 hours) and therefore effective xanthine oxidase inhibition is maintained over a 24-hour period with single daily doses of Lopurin. Whereas Lopurin is cleared essentially by glomerular filtration, oxipurinol is reabsorbed in the kidney tubules in a manner similar to the reabsorption of uric acid.

The clearance of oxipurinol is increased by uricosuric drugs, and as a consequence, the addition of a uricosuric agent reduces to some degree the inhibition of xanthine oxidase by oxipurinol and increases to some degree the urinary excretion of uric acid. In practice, the net effect of such combined therapy may be useful in some patients in achieving minimum serum uric acid levels provided the total urinary uric acid load does not exceed the competence of the patient's renal function.

Hyperuricemia may be primary, as in gout, or secondary to diseases such as acute and chronic leukemia, polycythemia vera, multiple myeloma, and psoriasis. It may occur with the use of diuretic agents, during renal dialysis, in the presence of renal damage, during starvation or reducing diets and in the treatment of neoplastic disease where rapid resolution of tissue masses may occur. Asymptomatic hyperuricemia is not an indication for Lopurin treatment (see INDICATIONS AND USAGE).

Gout is a metabolic disorder which is characterized by hyperuricemia and resultant deposition of monosodium urate in the tissues, particularly the joints and kidneys. The etiology of this hyperuricemia is the overproduction of uric acid in relation to the patient's ability to excrete it. If progressive deposition of urates is to be arrested or reversed, it is necessary to reduce the serum uric acid level below the saturation point to suppress urate precipitation.

Administration of Lopurin generally results in a fall in both serum and urinary uric acid within two to three days. The degree of this decrease can be manipulated almost at will since it is dose-dependent. A week or more of treatment with Lopurin may be required before its full effects are manifested; likewise, uric acid may return to pretreatment levels slowly (usually after a period of seven to ten days following cessation of therapy). This reflects primarily the accumulation and slow clearance of oxipurinol. In some patients a dramatic fall in urinary uric acid excretion may not occur, particularly in those with severe tophaceous gout. It has been postulated that this may be due to the mobilization of urate from tissue deposits as the serum uric acid level begins to fall.

Lopurin's action differs from that of uricosuric agents, which lower the serum uric acid level by increasing urinary excretion of uric acid. Lopurin reduces both the serum and urinary uric acid levels by inhibiting the formation of uric acid. The use of Lopurin to block the formation of urates avoids the hazard of increased renal excretion of uric acid posed by uricosuric drugs.

Lopurin can substantially reduce serum and urinary uric acid levels in previously refractory patients even in the presence of renal damage serious enough to render uricosuric drugs virtually ineffective. Salicylates may be given conjointly for their antirheumatic effect without compromising the action of Lopurin. This is in contrast to the nullifying effect of salicylates on uricosuric drugs.

Lopurin also inhibits the enzymatic oxidation of mercaptopurine, the sulfur-containing analogue of hypoxanthine, to 6-thiouric acid. This oxidation, which is catalyzed by xanthine oxidase inactivates mercaptopurine. Hence, the inhibition of such oxidation by Lopurin may result in as much as a 75% reduction in the therapeutic dose requirement of mercaptopurine when the two compounds are given together.

Lopurin (allopurinol)
1,5-dihydro-4*H*-pyrazolo-
[3,4-*d*]pyrimidin-4-one

Oxipurinol
1*H* pyrazolo[3,4-*d*]-
pyrimidine, 4,6(5*H*,7*H*)-dione

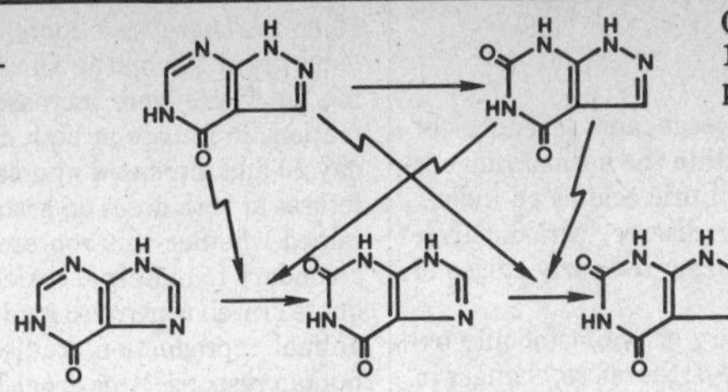

Hypoxanthine
purin-6(1*H*)-one

Xanthine
3,7-dihydro-1*H*-purine-
2,6-dione

Uric Acid
7,9-dihydro-1*H*-purine-
2,6,8(3*H*)-trione

INDICATIONS AND USAGE

THIS IS NOT AN INNOCUOUS DRUG. IT IS NOT RECOMMENDED FOR THE TREATMENT OF ASYMPTOMATIC HYPERURICEMIA.

Lopurin (allopurinol) reduces serum and urinary uric acid concentrations. Its use should be individualized for each patient and requires an understanding of its mode of action and pharmacokinetics (see CLINICAL PHARMACOLOGY, CONTRAINDICATIONS, WARNINGS and PRECAUTIONS).

Lopurin is indicated in:

(1) the management of patients with signs and symptoms of primary or secondary gout (acute attacks, tophi, joint destruction, uric acid lithiasis and/or nephropathy).

(2) the management of patients with leukemia, lymphoma and malignancies who are receiving cancer therapy which causes elevations of serum and urinary acid levels. Lopurin treatment should be discontinued when the potential for overproduction of uric acid is no longer present.

(3) the management of patients with recurrent calcium oxalate calculi whose daily uric acid excretion exceed 800 mg/day in male patients and 750 mg/day in female patients. Therapy in such patients should be carefully assessed initially and reassessed periodically to determine in each case that treatment is beneficial and that the benefits outweigh the risks.

CONTRAINDICATIONS

Patients who have developed a severe reaction to Lopurin (allopurinol) should not be restarted on the drug.

WARNINGS

LOPURIN (ALLOPURINOL) SHOULD BE DISCONTINUED AT THE FIRST APPEARANCE OF SKIN RASH OR OTHER SIGNS WHICH MAY INDICATE AN ALLERGIC REACTION. In some instances a skin rash may be followed by more severe hypersensitivity reactions such as exfoliative, urticarial and purpuric lesions as well as Stevens-Johnson syndrome (erythema multiforme exudativum), and/or generalized vasculitis, irreversible hepatotoxicity and on rare occasions death.

In patients receiving Purinethol® (mercaptopurine) or Imuran® (azathioprine), the concomitant administration of 300–600 mg of Lopurin per day will require a reduction in dose to approximately one-third to one-fourth of the usual dose of mercaptopurine or azathioprine. Subsequent adjustment of doses of mercaptopurine or azathioprine should be made on the basis of therapeutic response and the appearance of toxic effects (see CLINICAL PHARMACOLOGY).

A few cases of reversible clinical hepatotoxicity have been noted in patients taking Lopurin, and in some patients asymptomatic rises in serum alkaline phosphatase or serum transaminase have been observed. If anorexia, weight loss or pruritus develop in patients on Lopurin, evaluation of liver function should be part of their diagnostic workup. In patients with pre-existing liver disease, periodic liver function tests are recommended during the early stages of therapy.

Due to the occasional occurrence of drowsiness, patients should be alerted to the need for due precaution when engaging in activities where alertness is mandatory.

The occurrence of hypersensitivity reactions to Lopurin may be increased in patients with decreased renal function receiving thiazides and Lopurin concurrently. For this reason, in this clinical setting, such combinations should be administered with caution and patients should be observed closely.

PRECAUTIONS

General: An increase in acute attacks of gout has been reported during the early stages of Lopurin (allopurinol) administration, even when normal or subnormal serum uric acid levels have been attained. Accordingly, maintenance doses of colchicine generally should be given prophylactically when Lopurin is begun. In addition, it is recommended that the patient start with a low dose of Lopurin (100 mg daily) and increase at weekly intervals by 100 mg until a serum uric acid level of 6 mg/dl or less is attained but without exceeding the maximum recommended dose (800 mg per day). The use of colchicine or anti-inflammatory agents may be required to suppress gouty attacks in some cases. The attacks usually become shorter and less severe after several months of therapy. The mobilization of urates from tissue deposits which cause fluctuations in the serum uric acid levels may be a possible explanation for these episodes. Even with adequate Lopurin therapy, it may require several months to deplete the uric acid pool sufficiently to achieve control of the acute attacks.

A fluid intake sufficient to yield a daily urinary output of at least two liters and the maintenance of a neutral or, preferably, slightly alkaline urine are desirable to (1) avoid the theoretical possibility of formation of xanthine calculi under the influence of Lopurin therapy and (2) help prevent renal precipitation of urates in patients receiving concomitant uricosuric agents.

Some patients with preexisting renal disease or poor urate clearance have shown a rise in BUN during Lopurin administration. Although the mechanism responsible for this has not been established, patients with impaired renal function should be carefully observed during the early stages of Lopurin administration and dosage decreased or the drug withdrawn if increased abnormalities in renal function appear and persist.

Renal failure in association with Lopurin administration has been observed among patients with hyperuricemia secondary to neoplastic diseases. Concurrent conditions such as multiple myeloma and congestive myocardial disease were present among those patients whose renal dysfunction increased after Lopurin was begun. Renal failure is also frequently associated with gouty nephropathy and rarely with Lopurin-associated hypersensitivity reactions. Albuminuria has been observed among patients who developed clinical gout following chronic glomerulonephritis and chronic pyelonephritis.

Patients with decreased renal function require lower doses of Lopurin than those with normal renal function. Lower than recommended doses should be used to initiate therapy in any patients with decreased renal function and they should be observed closely during the early stages of Lopurin administration. In patients with severely impaired renal function or decreased urate clearance, the half-life of oxipurinol in the plasma is greatly prolonged. Therefore, a dose of 100 mg per day or 300 mg twice a week, or perhaps less, may be sufficient to maintain adequate xanthine oxidase inhibition to reduce serum urate levels.

Bone marrow depression has been reported in patients receiving Lopurin, most of whom received concomitant drugs with the potential for causing this reaction. This has occurred as early as six weeks to as long as six years after the initiation of Lopurin therapy. Rarely a patient may develop varying degrees of bone marrow depression, affecting one or more cell lines, while receiving Lopurin alone.

Information for Patients: Patients should be informed of the following:

(1) They should be cautioned to discontinue Lopurin (allopurinol) and to consult their physician immediately at the first sign of a skin rash, painful urination, blood in the urine, irritation of the eyes, or swelling of the lips or mouth. (2) They should be reminded to continue drug therapy prescribed for gouty attacks since optimal benefit of Lopurin may be delayed for two to six weeks. (3) They should be encouraged to increase fluid intake during therapy to prevent renal stones. (4) If a single dose of Lopurin is occasionally forgotten, there is no need to double the dose at the next scheduled time. (5) There may be certain risks associated with the concomitant use of Lopurin and dicumarol, sulfinpyrazone, mercaptopurine, azathioprine, ampicillin, amoxicillin and thiazide diuretics, and they should follow the instructions of their physician. (6) Due to the occasional occurrence of drowsiness, patients should take precautions when engaging in activities where alertness is mandatory. (7) Patients may wish to take Lopurin after meals to minimize gastric irritation.

Continued on next page

Boots—Cont.

Laboratory Tests: The correct dosage and schedule for maintaining the serum uric acid within the normal range is best determined by using the serum uric acid as an index.
In patients with pre-existing liver disease, periodic liver function tests are recommended during the early stages of therapy (see WARNINGS).
Lopurin (allopurinol) and its primary active metabolite oxipurinol are eliminated by the kidneys; therefore, changes in renal function have a profound effect on dosage. In patients with decreased renal function or who have concurrent illnesses which can affect renal function such as hypertension and diabetes mellitus, periodic laboratory parameters of renal function, particularly BUN and serum creatinine or creatinine clearance, should be performed and the patient's Lopurin dosage reassessed.
The prothrombin time should be reassessed periodically in the patients receiving dicumarol who are given Lopurin.
Drug Interactions: In patients receiving Purinethol® (mercaptopurine) or Imuran® (azathioprine), the concomitant administration of 300–600 mg of Lopurin (allopurinol) per day will require a reduction in dose to approximately one-third to one-fourth of the usual dose of mercaptopurine or azathioprine. Subsequent adjustment of doses of mercaptopurine or azathioprine should be made on the basis of therapeutic response and the appearance of toxic effects (see CLINICAL PHARMACOLOGY.)
It has been reported that Lopurin prolongs the half-life of the anticoagulant, dicumarol. The clinical basis of this drug interaction has not been established but should be noted when Lopurin is given to patients already on dicumarol therapy.
Since the excretion of oxipurinol is similar to that of urate, uricosuric agents, which increase the excretion of urate, are also likely to increase the excretion of oxipurinol and thus lower the degree of inhibition of xanthine oxidase. The concomitant administration of uricosuric agents and Lopurin has been associated with a decrease in the excretion of oxypurines (hypoxanthine and xanthine) and an increase in urinary uric acid excretion compared with that observed with Lopurin alone. Although clinical evidence to date has not demonstrated renal precipitation of oxypurines in patients either on Lopurin alone or in combination with uricosuric agents, the possibility should be kept in mind.
The reports that the concomitant use of Lopurin and thiazide diuretics may contribute to the enhancement of allopurinol toxicity in some patients have been reviewed in an attempt to establish a cause-and-effect relationship and a mechanism of causation. Review of these case reports indicates that the patients were mainly receiving thiazide diuretics for hypertension and that tests to rule out decreased renal function secondary to hypertensive nephropathy were not often performed. In those patients in whom renal insufficiency was documented, however, the recommendation to lower the dose of Lopurin was not followed. Although a causal mechanism and a cause-and-effect relationship have not been established, current evidence suggests that renal function should be monitored in patients on thiazide diuretics and Lopurin even in the absence of renal failure, and dosage levels should be even more conservatively adjusted in those patients on such combined therapy if diminished renal function is detected.
An increase in the frequency of skin rash has been reported among patients receiving ampicillin or amoxicillin concurrently with Lopurin compared to patients who are not receiving both drugs. The cause of the reported association has not been established.
Enhanced bone marrow suppression by cyclophosphamide and other cytotoxic agents has been reported among patients with neoplastic disease, except leukemia, in the presence of Lopurin. However, in a well-controlled study of patients with lymphoma on combination therapy. Lopurin did not increase the marrow toxicity of patients treated with cyclophosphamide, doxorubicin, bleomycin, procarbazine and/or mechlorethamine.
Tolbutamide's conversion to inactive metabolites has been shown to be catalyzed by xanthine oxidase from rat liver. The clinical significance, if any, of these observations is unknown.
Chlorpropamide's plasma half-life may be prolonged by Lopurin, since Lopurin and chlorpropamide may compete for excretion in the renal tubule. The risk of hypoglycemia secondary to this mechanism may be increased if Lopurin and chlorpropamide are given concomitantly in the presence of renal insufficiency.
Drug/Laboratory Test Interactions: Lopurin (allopurinol) is not known to alter the accuracy of laboratory tests.
Pregnancy: *Teratogenic Effects:* Pregnancy Category C. Reproductive studies have been performed in rats and rabbits at doses up to twenty times the usual human dose (5 mg/kg/day), and it was concluded that there was no impaired fertility or harm to the fetus due to allopurinol. There is a published report of a study in pregnant mice given 50 or 100 mg/kg allopurinol intraperitoneally on gestation days 10 or 13. There were increased numbers of dead fetuses in dams given 100 mg/kg allopurinol but not in those given 50 mg/kg. There were increased numbers of external malformations in fetuses at both doses of allopurinol on gestation day 10 and increased numbers of skeletal malformations in fetuses at both doses on gestation day 13. It cannot be determined whether this represented a fetal effect or an effect secondary to maternal toxicity. There are, however, no adequate or well controlled studies in pregnant women. Because animal reproduction studies are not always predictive of human response, this drug should be used during pregnancy only if clearly needed.
Experience with allopurinol during human pregnancy has been limited partly because women of reproductive age rarely require treatment with allopurinol. There are two unpublished reports and one published paper of women giving birth to normal offspring after receiving allopurinol during pregnancy.
Nursing Mothers: Allopurinol and oxipurinol have been found in the milk of a mother who was receiving allopurinol. Since the effect of allopurinol on the nursing infant is unknown, caution should be exercised when allopurinol is administered to a nursing woman.
Pediatric Use: Allopurinol is rarely indicated for use in children with the exception of those with hyperuricemia secondary to malignancy or to certain rare inborn errors of purine metabolism (see INDICATIONS and DOSAGE AND ADMINISTRATION).

ADVERSE REACTIONS

Data upon which the following estimates of incidence of adverse reactions are made are derived from experiences reported in the literature, unpublished clinical trials and voluntary reports since marketing of allopurinol began. Past experience suggested that the most frequent event following the initiation of allopurinol treatment was an increase in acute attacks of gout (average 6% in early studies). An analysis of current usage suggests that the incidence of acute gouty attacks has diminished to less than 1%. The explanation for this decrease has not been determined but may be due in part to initiating therapy more gradually (see PRECAUTIONS and DOSAGE AND ADMINISTRATION).
The most frequent adverse reactions to allopurinol is skin rash. Skin reactions can be severe and sometimes fatal. Therefore, treatment with allopurinol should be discontinued immediately if a rash develops (see WARNINGS). Some patients with the most severe reaction also had fever, chills, arthralgias, cholestatic jaundice, eosinophilia and mild leukocytosis or leukopenia. Among 55 patients with gout treated with allopurinol for 3 to 34 months (average greater than 1 year) and followed prospectively, Rundles observed that 3% of patients developed a type of drug reaction which was predominantly a pruritic maculopapular skin eruption, sometimes scaly or exfoliative. However, with current usage, skin reactions have been observed less frequently than 1%. The explanation for this decrease is not obvious. The incidence of skin rash may be increased in the presence of renal insufficiency. The frequency of skin rash among patients receiving ampicillin or amoxicillin concurrently with allopurinol has been reported to be increased (see PRECAUTIONS).

Most Common Reactions*
Probably Causally Related

Gastrointestinal: diarrhea, nausea, alkaline phosphatase increase, SGOT/SGPT increase
Metabolic and Nutritional: acute attacks of gout
Skin and Appendages: rash, maculopapular rash

*Early clinical studies and incidence rates from early clinical experience with Lopurin suggested that these adverse reactions were found to occur at a rate of greater than 1%. The most frequent event observed was acute attacks of gout following the initiation of therapy. Analyses of current usage suggest that the incidence of these adverse reactions is now less than 1%. The explanation for this decrease has not been determined, but it may be due to following recommended usage (See ADVERSE REACTIONS introduction, INDICATIONS, PRECAUTIONS and DOSAGE AND ADMINISTRATION).

Incidence Less Than 1%
Probably Causally Related

Body as a whole: ecchymosis, fever, headache
Cardiovascular: necrotizing angiitis, vasculitis
Gastrointestinal: hepatic necrosis, granulomatous hepatitis, hepatomegaly, hyperbilirubinemia, cholestatic jaundice, vomiting, intermittent abdominal pain, gastritis, dyspepsia
Hemic and Lymphatic: thrombocytopenia, eosinophilia, leukocytosis, leukopenia
Musculoskeletal: myopathy, arthralgias
Nervous: peripheral neuropathy, neuritis, paresthesia, somnolence
Respiratory: epistaxis
Skin and Appendages: erythema multiforme exudativum (Stevens-Johnson syndrome), toxic epidermal necrolysis (Lyell's syndrome), hypersensitivity vasculitis, purpura, vesicular bullous dermatitis, exfoliative dermatitis, eczematoid dermatitis, pruritus, urticaria, alopecia, onycholysis, lichen planus
Special Senses: taste loss/perversion
Urogenital: renal failure, uremia (see PRECAUTIONS)

Incidence Less Than 1%
Causal Relationship Unknown

Body as a whole: malaise
Cardiovascular: pericarditis, peripheral vascular disease, thrombophlebitis, bradycardia vasodilation
Endocrine: infertility (male), hypercalcemia, gynecomastia (male)
Gastrointestinal: hemorrhagic pancreatitis, gastrointestinal bleeding, stomatitis, salivary gland swelling, hyperlipidemia, tongue edema, anorexia
Hemic and Lymphatic: aplastic anemia, agranulocytosis, eosinophilic fibrohistiocytic lesion of bone marrow, pancytopenia, prothrombin decrease, anemia, hemolytic anemia, reticulocytosis, lymphadenopathy, lymphocytosis
Musculoskeletal: myalgia
Nervous: optic neuritis, confusion, dizziness, vertigo, foot drop, decrease in libido, depression, amnesia, tinnitis, asthenia, insomnia
Respiratory: bronchospasm, asthma, pharyngitis, rhinitis
Skin and Appendages: furunculosis, facial edema, sweating, skin edema
Special Senses: cataracts, macular retinitis, iritis, conjunctivitis, amblyopia
Urogenital: nephritis, impotence, primary hematuria, albuminuria

OVERDOSAGE

Massive overdosing or acute poisoning by Lopurin (allopurinol) has not ben reported. In mice the 50% lethal dose (LD_{50}) is 160 mg/kg given intraperitoneally (i.p.) with deaths delayed up to five days and 700 mg/kg orally (p.o.) (approximately 140 times the usual human dose) with deaths delayed up to three days. In rats the acute LD_{50} is 750 mg/kg i.p. and 6000 mg/kg p.o. (approximately 1200 times the human dose).
In the management of overdosage there is no specific antidote for Lopurin. There has been no clinical experience in the management of a patient who has taken massive amounts of Lopurin.
Both Lopurin and oxipurinol are dialyzable; however, the usefulness of hemodialysis or peritoneal dialysis in the management of a Lopurin overdose is unknown.

DOSAGE AND ADMINISTRATION

The dosage of Lopurin (allopurinol) to accomplish full control of gout and to lower serum uric acid to normal or near-normal levels varies with the severity of the disease. The average is 200 to 300 mg per day for patients with mild gout and 400 to 600 mg per day for those with moderately severe tophaceous gout. The appropriate dosage may be administered in divided doses or as a single equivalent dose with the 300 mg tablet. Dosage requirements in excess of 300 mg should be administered in divided doses. The minimal effective dosage is 100 to 200 mg daily and the maximal recommended dosage is 800 mg daily. To reduce the possibility of flare-up of acute gouty attacks, it is recommended that the patient start with a low dose of Lopurin (100 mg daily) and increase at weekly intervals by 100 mg until a serum uric acid level of 6 mg/dl or less is attained but without exceeding the maximal recommended dosage.
Normal serum urate levels are usually achieved in one to three weeks. The upper limit of normal is about 7 mg/dl for men and postmenopausal women and 6 mg/dl for premenopausal women. Too much reliance should not be placed on a single serum uric acid determination since, for technical reasons, estimation of uric acid may be difficult. By selecting the appropriate dosage and, in certain patients, using uricosuric agents concurrently, it is possible to reduce serum uric acid to normal or, if desired, to as low as 2 to 3 mg/dl and keep it there indefinitely.
While adjusting the dosage of Lopurin in patients who are being treated with colchicine and/or antiinflammatory agents, it is wise to continue the latter therapy until serum uric acid has been normalized and there has been freedom from acute gouty attacks for several months.
In transferring a patient from a uricosuric agent to Lopurin, the dose of the uricosuric agent should be gradually reduced over a period of several weeks and the dose of Lopurin gradually increased to the required dose needed to maintain a normal serum uric acid level.
It should also be noted that Lopurin is generally better tolerated if taken following meals. A fluid intake sufficient to yield a daily urinary output of at least two liters and the maintenance of a neutral, or preferably, slightly alkaline urine are desirable.
Since Lopurin and its metabolites are primarily eliminated only by the kidney, accumulation of the drug can occur in renal failure, and the dose of Lopurin should consequently be reduced. With a creatinine clearance of 10 to 20 ml/min. a daily dosage of 200 mg of Lopurin is suitable. When the creatinine clearance is less than 10 ml/min the daily dosage should not exceed 100 mg. With extreme renal impairment

(creatinine clearance less than 3 ml/min) the interval between doses may also need to be lengthened.
The correct size and frequency of dosage for maintaining the serum uric acid just within the normal range is best determined by using the serum uric acid level as an index.
For the prevention of uric acid nephropathy during the vigorous therapy of neoplastic disease, treatment with 600 to 800 mg daily for two or three days is advisable together with a high fluid intake. Otherwise similar considerations to the above recommendations for treating patients with gout govern the regulation of dosage for maintenance purposes in secondary hyperuricemia.
The dose of Lopurin recommended for management of recurrent calcium oxalate stones in hyperuricosuric patients is 200 to 300 mg/day in divided doses or as the single equivalent. This dose may be adjusted up or down depending upon the resultant control of the hyperuricosia based upon subsequent 24 hour urinary determinations. Clinical experience suggest that patients with recurrent calcium oxalate stones may also benefit from dietary changes such as the reduction of animal protein, sodium, refined sugars, oxalate-rich foods, and excessive calcium intake as well as an increase in oral fluids and dietary fiber.
Children, 6 to 10 years of age, with secondary hyperuricemia associated with malignancies may be given 300 mg Lopurin daily while those under 6 years are generally given 150 mg daily. The response is evaluated after approximately 48 hours of therapy and a dosage adjustment is made if necessary.

HOW SUPPLIED

LOPURIN®
100 mg (white) scored tablets, imprinted BOOTS/0051, unit dose, cartons of 100—NDC 0524-0051-21, bottles of 100—NDC 0524-0051-01, bottles of 1000—NDC 0524-0051-10.
Store at 15° to 30°C (59° to 86°F) in a dry place.
300 mg (peach) scored tablets, imprinted BOOTS/0052, unit dose, cartons of 100—NDC 0524-0052-21, bottles of 30—NDC 0524-0052-30, bottles of 100—NDC 0524-0052-01, bottles of 500—NDC 0524-0052-05.
Store at 15° to 30°C (59° to 86°F) in a dry place and protect from light

CAUTION

Federal Law Prohibits Dispensing Without Prescription.

Distributed by
Boots Pharmaceuticals, Inc.
Shreveport, Louisiana 71106 U.S.A.
Manufactured By:
Boots Laboratories, Incorporated
Palisades Park, N.J. 07650

Boots 0051
0052
Licensed for Use under U.S. Patent 3,624,205
Rev. March 1985
Shown in Product Identification Section, page 406

RUFEN® ℞
[roo-fin]
(ibuprofen)

DESCRIPTION

Rufen (ibuprofen) is (±)-2-(*p*-isobutylphenyl) propionic acid. It is a white powder with a melting point of 74–77°C and is very slightly soluble in water (< 1 mg/ml) and readily soluble in organic solvents such as ethanol and acetone.
Its structural formula is:

$$(CH_3)_2CH-CH_2-C_6H_4-CH(CH_3)-COOH$$

Rufen is a nonsteroidal anti-inflammatory agent. It is available in 400 and 600 mg tablets for oral administration.

CLINICAL PHARMACOLOGY

Rufen (ibuprofen) is a nonsteroidal anti-inflammatory agent that possesses analgesic and antipyretic activities. Its mode of action, like that of other nonsteroidal anti-inflammatory agents, is not completely understood, but may be related to prostaglandin synthetase inhibition. Rufen does not alter the course of the underlying disease.
In patients treated with Rufen for rheumatoid arthritis and osteoarthritis, the anti-inflammatory action of Rufen has been shown by reduction in joint swelling, reduction in pain, reduction in duration of morning stiffness, reduction in disease activity as assessed by both the investigator and patient, and by improved functional capacity as demonstrated by an increase in grip strength, a delay in the time to onset of fatigue, and a decrease in time to walk 50 feet.
In clinical studies in patients with rheumatoid arthritis and osteoarthritis, Rufen has been shown to be comparable to aspirin in controlling the aforementioned signs and symptoms of disease activity and to be associated with a statistically significant reduction in the milder gastrointestinal side effects (see ADVERSE REACTIONS). Rufen may be well tolerated in some patients who have had gastrointestinal side effects with aspirin, but these patients when treated with Rufen should be carefully followed for signs and symptoms of gastrointestinal ulceration and bleeding.
Although it is not definitely known whether ibuprofen causes less peptic ulceration than aspirin, in one study involving 885 patients with rheumatoid arthritis treated for up to one year, there were no reports of gastric ulceration with ibuprofen whereas frank ulceration was reported in 13 patients in the aspirin group (statistically significant $p < .001$).
In clinical studies in patients with rheumatoid arthritis, Rufen has been shown to be comparable to indomethacin in controlling the aforementioned signs and symptoms of disease activity and to be associated with a statistically significant reduction of the milder gastrointestinal (see ADVERSE REACTIONS) and CNS side effects.
Rufen may be used in combination with gold salts and/or corticosteroids. When Rufen and placebo were compared in gold-treated rheumatoid arthritis patients, Rufen was consistently more effective in relieving symptoms than was placebo. However, it cannot be inferred that Rufen potentiates the effect of gold on the underlying disease. Whether or not Rufen can be used in conjunction with partially effective doses of corticosteroid for a "steroid-sparing" effect, and result in greater improvement, has not been adequately studied.
Controlled studies have demonstrated that Rufen is a more effective analgesic than propoxyphene for the relief of episiotomy pain, pain following dental extraction procedures, and for the relief of the symptoms of primary dysmenorrhea.
In patients with primary dysmenorrhea, Rufen has been shown to reduce elevated levels of prostaglandin activity in the menstrual fluid and to reduce resting and active intrauterine pressure, as well as the frequency of uterine contractions. The probable mechanism of action is to inhibit prostaglandin synthesis rather than simply to provide analgesia.
Pharmacokinetics: Rufen is rapidly absorbed when administered orally. Peak serum ibuprofen levels are generally attained one to two hours after administration. With single doses ranging from 200 mg to 800 mg, a dose-response relationship exists between amount of drug administered and the integrated area under the serum drug concentration vs time curve. Above 800 mg, however, the area under the curve increases less than proportional to increases in dose. There is no evidence of drug accumulation or enzyme induction.
The administration of Rufen tablets either under fasting conditions or immediately before meals yields quite similar serum ibuprofen concentration-time profiles. When Rufen is administered immediately after a meal, there is a reduction in the rate of absorption but no appreciable decrease in the extent of absorption. The bioavailability of Rufen is minimally altered by the presence of food.
Rufen is rapidly metabolized and eliminated in the urine. The excretion of Rufen is virtually complete 24 hours after the last dose. The serum half-life of Rufen is 1.8 to 2.0 hours. Studies have shown that following ingestion of the drug 45% to 79% of the dose was recovered in the urine within 24 hours as metabolite A (25%), (+)-2-4'-(2-hydroxy-2-methylpropyl)phenyl propionic acid and metabolite B (37%), (+)-2-4'-(2-carboxypropyl) phenyl propionic acid, the percentages of free and conjugated ibuprofen were approximately 1% and 14%, respectively.

INDICATIONS AND USAGE

Rufen (ibuprofen) is indicated for relief of the signs and symptoms of rheumatoid arthritis and osteoarthritis.
Rufen is indicated for the relief of mild to moderate pain.
Rufen is also indicated for the treatment of primary dysmenorrhea.
Since there have been no controlled trials to demonstrate whether there is any beneficial effect or harmful interaction with the use of Rufen in conjunction with aspirin, the combination cannot be recommended (see **Drug Interactions**).
Controlled clinical trials to establish the safety and effectiveness of Rufen in children have not been conducted.

CONTRAINDICATIONS

Rufen (ibuprofen) should not be used in patients who have previously exhibited hypersensitivity to it, or in individuals with the syndrome of nasal polyps, angioedema and bronchospastic reactivity to aspirin, iodides or other nonsteroidal anti-inflammatory agents. Anaphylactoid reactions have occurred in such patients.

WARNINGS

Peptic ulceration and gastrointestinal bleeding, sometimes severe, have been reported in patients receiving Rufen (ibuprofen). Peptic ulceration, perforation, or severe gastrointestinal bleeding can have a fatal outcome, and although a few such reports have been received with ibuprofen, a cause and effect relationship has not been established. Rufen should be given under close supervision to patients with a history of upper gastrointestinal tract disease, and only after consulting the ADVERSE REACTIONS section.
In patients with active peptic ulcer and active rheumatoid arthritis, attempts should be made to treat the arthritis with nonulcerogenic drugs, such as gold. If Rufen must be given, the patient should be under close supervision for signs of ulcer perforation or gastrointestinal bleeding.
As with other nonsteroidal anti-inflammatory agents, chronic studies in rats and monkeys have shown histologic evidence of mild renal toxicity as demonstrated by papillary edema and papillary necrosis, in some animals. Renal papillary necrosis has been rarely reported in humans in association with Rufen treatment.

PRECAUTIONS

Blurred and/or diminished vision, scotomata, and/or changes in color vision have been reported. If a patient develops such complaints while receiving Rufen (ibuprofen), the drug should be discontinued and the patient should have an ophthalmologic examination which includes central visual fields and color vision testing.
Fluid retention and edema have been reported in association with Rufen; therefore, the drug should be used with caution in patients with a history of cardiac decompensation or hypertension.
As with other nonsteroidal anti-inflammatory drugs, borderline elevations of one or more liver tests may occur in up to 15% of patients. These abnormalities may progress, may remain essentially unchanged, or may be transient with continued therapy. The SGPT (ALT) test is probably the most sensitive indicator of liver dysfunction. Meaningful (3 times the upper limit of normal) elevations of SGPT or SGOT (AST) occurred in controlled clinical trials in less than 1% of patients. A patient with symptoms and/or signs suggesting liver dysfunction, or in whom an abnormal liver test has occurred, should be evaluated for evidence of the development of more severe hepatic reaction while on therapy with Rufen. Severe hepatic reactions, including jaundice and cases of fatal hepatitis, have been reported with ibuprofen as with other nonsteroidal anti-inflammatory drugs. Although such reactions are rare, if abnormal liver tests persist or worsen, if clinical signs and symptoms consistent with liver disease develop, or if systemic manifestations occur (e.g. eosinophilia, rash, etc.), Rufen should be discontinued.
Since Rufen is eliminated primarily by the kidneys, patients with significantly impaired renal function should be closely monitored and a reduction in dosage should be anticipated to avoid drug accumulation. Prospective studies on the safety of Rufen in patients with chronic renal failure have not been conducted.
Rufen, like other nonsteroidal anti-inflammatory agents, can inhibit platelet aggregation but the effect is quantitatively less and of shorter duration than that seen with aspirin. Ibuprofen has been shown to prolong bleeding time (but within the normal range) in normal subjects. Because this prolonged bleeding effect may be exaggerated in patients with underlying hemostatic defects, Rufen should be used with caution in persons with intrinsic coagulation defects and those on anticoagulant therapy.
Patients on Rufen should report to their physicians signs or symptoms of gastrointestinal ulceration or bleeding, blurred vision or other eye symptoms, skin rash, weight gain, or edema.
In order to avoid exacerbation of disease or adrenal insufficiency, patients who have been on prolonged corticosteroid therapy should have their therapy tapered slowly rather than discontinued abruptly when Rufen is added to the treatment program.
The antipyretic and anti-inflammatory activity of ibuprofen may reduce fever and inflammation, thus diminishing their utility as diagnostic signs in detecting complications of presumed noninfectious, noninflammatory painful conditions.
Drug Interactions: *Coumarin-type anticoagulants.* Several short-term controlled studies failed to show that Rufen significantly affected prothrombin times or a variety of other clotting factors when administered to individuals on coumarin-type anticoagulants. However, because bleeding has been reported when Rufen and other nonsteroidal anti-inflammatory agents have been administered to patients on coumarin-type anticoagulants, the physician should be cautious when administering Rufen® (ibuprofen) to patients on anticoagulants.
Aspirin. Animal studies show that aspirin given with nonsteroidal anti-inflammatory agents, including Rufen, yields a net decrease in anti-inflammatory activity with lowered blood levels of the non-aspirin drug. Single dose bioavailability studies in normal volunteers have failed to show an effect of aspirin on ibuprofen blood levels. Correlative clinical studies have not been done.
Pregnancy: Reproductive studies conducted in rats and rabbits at doses somewhat less than the maximal clinical dose did not demonstrate evidence of developmental abnormalities. However, animal reproduction studies, are not always predictive of human response. As there are no adequate and well-controlled studies in pregnant women, this drug should be used during pregnancy only if clearly needed. Because of the known effects of nonsteroidal anti-inflammatory drugs on the fetal cardiovascular system (closure of ductus arteriosus) use during late pregnancy should be avoided. As

Continued on next page

Boots—Cont.

with other drugs known to inhibit prostaglandin synthesis, an increased incidence of dystocia and delayed parturition occurred in rats. Administration of ibuprofen is not recommended during pregnancy.

Nursing Mothers: In limited studies, an assay capable of detecting 1 mcg/ml did not demonstrate ibuprofen in the milk of lactating mothers. However, because of the limited nature of the studies and the possible adverse effects of prostaglandin inhibiting drugs on neonates, Rufen is not recommended for use in nursing mothers.

ADVERSE REACTIONS

The most frequent type of adverse reaction occurring with Rufen (ibuprofen) is gastrointestinal. In controlled clinical trials, the percentage of patients reporting one or more gastrointestinal complaints ranged from 4% to 16%.

In controlled studies when ibuprofen was compared to aspirin and indomethacin in equally effective doses, the overall incidence of gastrointestinal complaints was about half that seen in either the aspirin-, or indomethacin-treated patients.

Reactions observed during controlled clinical trials which occurred in more than 1 in 100 patients were:

Incidence greater than 1%

Gastrointestinal: nausea*, epigastric pain*, heartburn*, diarrhea, abdominal distress, nausea and vomiting, indigestion, constipation, abdominal cramps or pain, fullness of the GI tract (bloating and flatulence).

Central Nervous System: dizziness*, headache, nervousness.

Dermatologic: rash* (including maculopapular type), pruritus.

Special Senses: tinnitus.

Metabolic: decreased appetite.

Cardiovascular: edema, fluid retention (generally responds promptly to drug discontinuation; see PRECAUTIONS).

*Reactions occurring in 3% to 9% of patients treated with Rufen. (Those reactions occurring in less than 3% of the patients are unmarked.)

Incidence less than 1%

The following adverse reactions, occurring less frequently than 1 in 100, have been reported in controlled clinical trials and from marketing experience. The probability of a causal relationship exists between Rufen and these adverse reactions:

Gastrointestinal: gastric or duodenal ulcer with bleeding and/or perforation, gastrointestinal hemorrhage, melena, gastritis, hepatitis, jaundice, abnormal liver function tests.

Dermatologic: vesiculobullous eruptions, urticaria, erythema multiforme, Stevens-Johnson syndrome and alopecia.

Central Nervous System: depression, insomnia, confusion, emotional lability, somnolence, aseptic meningitis with fever and coma.

Special Senses: hearing loss, amblyopia (blurred and/or diminished vision, scotomata and/or changes in color vision). [see PRECAUTIONS].

Hematologic: neutropenia, agranulocytosis, aplastic anemia, hemolytic anemia (sometimes Coombs' positive), thrombocytopenia with or without purpura eosinophilia, decreases in hemoglobin and hematocrit.

Cardiovascular: congestive heart failure in patients with marginal cardiac function, elevated blood pressure and palpitations.

Allergic: syndrome of abdominal pain, fever, chills, nausea and vomiting, anaphylaxis, bronchospasms (see CONTRAINDICATIONS).

Renal: acute renal failure in patients with preexisting significantly impaired renal function, decreased creatinine clearance, polyuria, azotemia, cystitis, hematuria.

Miscellaneous: dry eyes and mouth, gingival ulcers, rhinitis.

Causal relationship unknown

Other reactions have been reported but occurred under circumstances where a causal relationship could not be established. However, in these rarely reported events, the possibility cannot be excluded. Therefore these observations are being listed to serve as alerting information to the physician.

Gastrointestinal: pancreatitis.

Central Nervous System: paresthesias, hallucinations, dream abnormalities, pseudotumor cerebri.

Dermatologic: toxic epidermal necrolysis, photo-allergic skin reactions.

Special Senses: conjunctivitis, diplopia, optic neuritis.

Hematologic: bleeding episodes (e.g., epistaxis, menorrhagia).

Allergic: serum sickness, lupus erythematosus syndrome, Henoch-Schonlein vasculitis.

Endocrine: gynecomastia, hypoglycemic reaction.

Cardiovascular: arrhythmias (sinus tachycardia, sinus bradycardia).

Renal: renal papillary necrosis.

OVERDOSAGE

Approximately 1½ hours after the reported ingestion of from 7 to 10 ibuprofen tablets (400 mg), a 19-month old child weighing 12 kg was seen in the hospital emergency room, apneic and cyanotic, responding only to painful stimuli. This type of stimulus, however, was sufficient to induce respiration. Oxygen and parenteral fluids were given; a greenish-yellow fluid was aspirated from the stomach with no evidence to indicate the presence of ibuprofen. Two hours after ingestion the child's condition seemed stable; she still responded only to painful stimuli and continued to have periods of apnea lasting from 5 to 10 seconds. She was admitted to intensive care and sodium bicarbonate was administered as well as infusions of dextrose and normal saline. By four hours post-ingestion she could be aroused easily, sit by herself and respond to spoken commands. Blood level of ibuprofen was 102.9 mcg/ml approximately 8½ hours after accidental ingestion. At 12 hours she appeared to be completely recovered.

In two other reported cases where children (each weighing approximately 10 kg) had taken six tablets for an estimated acute intake of approximately 120 mg/kg, there were no signs of acute intoxication or late sequelae. Blood level in one child 90 minutes after ingestion was 700 mcg/ml, about 10 times the peak levels seen in absorption-excretion studies.

A 19-year old male who had taken 8,000 mg of ibuprofen over a period of a few hours complained of dizziness, and nystagmus was noted. After hospitalization, parenteral hydration and three days bed rest, he recovered with no reported sequelae.

In cases of acute overdosage, the stomach should be emptied by vomiting or lavage, though little drug will likely be recovered if more than an hour has elapsed since ingestion. Because the drug is acidic and is excreted in the urine, it is theoretically beneficial to administer alkali and induce diuresis.

DOSAGE AND ADMINISTRATION

Rheumatoid arthritis and osteoarthritis, including flareups of chronic disease.

Suggested Dosage: 400 mg or 600 mg t.i.d. or q.i.d. The dose of Rufen (ibuprofen) should be tailored to each patient, and may be lowered or raised from the suggested doses depending on the severity of symptoms either at time of initiating drug therapy or as the patient responds or fails to respond.

In general, patients with rheumatoid arthritis seem to require higher doses of Rufen than do patients with osteoarthritis.

The smallest dose of Rufen that yields acceptable control should be employed.

A therapeutic response to Rufen therapy is sometimes seen in a few days to a week but most often is observed by two weeks. After a satisfactory response has been achieved, the patient's dose should be reviewed and adjusted as required.

Dysmenorrhea: For the treatment of dysmenorrhea, beginning with the earliest onset of such pain, Rufen should be given in a dose of 400 mg every 4 hours as necessary.

Mild to moderate pain: 400 mg every 4 to 6 hours as necessary for the relief of pain.

In controlled analgesic clinical trials, doses of Rufen greater than 400 mg were no more effective than the 400 mg dose.

Do not exceed 2,400 mg total daily dose. If gastrointestinal complaints occur, administer Rufen with meals or milk.

HOW SUPPLIED

Rufen Tablets 400 mg: round magenta sugar-coated tablets printed RUFEN 400.

Bottles of 100	NDC 0524-0039-01
Bottles of 500	NDC 0524-0039-05
Unit Dose Cartons of 100	NDC 0524-0039-21

Rufen Tablets 600 mg: oblong white film-coated tablets printed RUFEN 6.

Bottles of 100	NDC 0524-0062-01
Bottles of 500	NDC 0524-0062-05

Manufactured for:
Boots Pharmaceuticals, Inc.
Shreveport, Louisiana 71106, U.S.A.
by
The Boots Company P.L.C.
Nottingham, England

Rufen Tablets 600 mg: oblong white film-coated tablets printed RUFEN 6.

Bottles of 100	NDC 0524-0062-01
Bottles of 500	NDC 0524-0062-05
Unit Dose Cartons of 100	NDC 0524-0062-21

Manufactured and Distributed by:
Boots Pharmaceuticals, Inc.
Shreveport, Louisiana 71106 U.S.A.

Caution: Federal law prohibits dispensing without prescription.

U.S. Patent No. 3,385,886.

Rev. 2/85 0039-12

Shown in Product Identification Section, page 406

RU-TUSS® EXPECTORANT ℞
[roo-tŭs]

DESCRIPTION

Each 5 ml (teaspoonful) of RU-TUSS® Expectorant contains:

Dextromethorphan Hydrobromide	10 mg
Pseudoephedrine Hydrochloride	30 mg
Guaifenesin	100 mg
Alcohol	10%

RU-TUSS® Expectorant is an oral antitussive nasal decongestant and expectorant combination.

ACTIONS

DEXTROMETHORPHAN HYDROBROMIDE is a centrally acting non-narcotic antitussive. Centrally acting antitussive agents produce cough suppression by acting on the central nervous system to depress the medullary (brain) cough center and thus raise its threshold for afferent (incoming) cough impulses.

PSEUDOEPHEDRINE HYDROCHLORIDE is a nasal decongestant which acts by causing constriction of dilated blood vessels (vasoconstriction) within the nasal mucosa.

GUAIFENESIN is an expectorant which promotes lower respiratory tract drainage by thinning bronchial secretions.

INDICATIONS AND USAGE

For the temporary relief of nonproductive cough, (due to minor throat and bronchial irritation), and nasal congestion as may occur with the common cold; relieves irritated membranes in the respiratory passageways by preventing dryness through increased mucus flow.

WARNINGS

Do not take this product if you have hypersensitivity to any of the components, hypertension, heart disease, diabetes, thyroid disease, glaucoma, difficulty in urination due to enlargement of prostate gland.

May cause marked drowsiness; avoid alcohol, driving a motor vehicle, or operating heavy machinery while taking this medication.

May cause excitability, especially in children.

Do not take this product for persistent or chronic cough such as occurs with smoking, asthma, or emphysema, or if cough is accompanied by excessive secretions except under the advise and supervision of a physician.

A persisent cough may be a sign of a serious condition. If cough persists for more than one week, tends to recur, or is accompanied by high fever, rash, or persistent headaches, consult a physician.

As with any drug, if you are pregnant or nursing a baby, seek the advice of a health professional before using this product.

Do not exceed recommended dosage, because at higher doses nervousness, dizziness, or sleeplessness may occur. Do not give this product to children under two years of age except under the advice and supervision of a physician.

PRECAUTIONS

Drug interactions: Do not take this product if you are presently taking a prescription antihypertensive or antidepressant drug containing a monoamine oxidase inhibitor except under the advice and supervision of a physician. **Drug/laboratory test interactions:** GUAIFENSIN may interfere with certain laboratory tests such as 5-hydroxyindoleacetic acid and vanillyl mandelic acid, which are employed as screening tests for carcinoid tumors and pheochromocytoma. In case of an accidental overdose, seek professional assistance or contact a poison control center immediately.

ADVERSE REACTIONS

Adverse reactions include drowsiness, insomnia, headache, loss of appetite, vomiting, hallucination, urticaria, hysteria, ataxia, edema of the face.

ABUSE

Abuse of dextromethorphan has been reported with doses of 300 to 1500 mg several times daily, resulting in intoxication with bizarre behavior but no physical dependence.

DOSAGE AND ADMINISTRATION

Adults, two teaspoonfuls orally, every 4 to 6 hours, not to exceed 12 teaspoonfuls in any 24 hour period. Children 6 to 12 years, oral dose is one teaspoonful every 4 to 6 hours, not to exceed 6 teaspoonfuls in any 24 hour period. Children 2 to 6 years, oral dosage is one-half teaspoonful every 4 to 6 hours not to exceed 3 teaspoonfuls in any 24 hour period. Do not administer to children under two years of age except under the advice and supervision of a physician.

HOW SUPPLIED

Pint bottles (16 fl. oz)
NDC 0524-3010-16

Manufactured and Distributed by
Boots Pharmaceuticals, Inc.
Shreveport, Louisiana 71106 U.S.A.

Rev. 12/84 3010-01

RU–TUSS®
WITH HYDROCODONE
[roo-tŭs]

DESCRIPTION

Each fluid ounce of RU-TUSS with Hydrocodone contains:

Hydrocodone Bitartrate	10 mg
(WARNING: MAY BE HABIT FORMING)	
Phenylephrine Hydrochloride	30 mg
Phenylpropanolamine Hydrochloride	20 mg
Pheniramine Maleate	20 mg
Pyrilamine Maleate	20 mg
Alcohol	5%

RU-TUSS with Hydrocodone is an oral antitussive, antihistaminic and nasal decongestant preparation.

INDICATIONS AND USAGE

RU-TUSS with Hydrocodone is indicated for the temporary relief of symptoms associated with hay fever, allergies, nasal congestion and cough due to the common cold.

CONTRAINDICATIONS

Hypersensitivity to antihistamines. Concomitant use of an antihypertensive or antidepressant drugs containing a monoamine oxidase inhibitor is contraindicated.
RU-TUSS with Hydrocodone is contraindicated in patients with glaucoma, bronchial asthma and in women who are pregnant.

WARNINGS

Patients should be warned of the potential that RU-TUSS with Hydrocodone may be habit forming.
RU-TUSS with Hydrocodone may cause drowsiness.
Patients should be warned of the possible additive effects caused by taking antihistamines with alcohol, hypnotics, sedatives and tranquilizers.

PRECAUTIONS

Patients taking RU-TUSS with Hydrocodone should avoid driving a motor vehicle or operating dangerous machinery (See Warnings).
Caution should be taken with patients having hypertension and cardiovascular disease.

ADVERSE REACTIONS

RU-TUSS with Hydrocodone may cause drowsiness, lassitude, giddiness, dryness of mucous membranes, tightness of the chest, thickening of bronchial secretions, urinary frequency and dysuria, palpitation, tachycardia, hypotension/hypertension, faintness, dizziness, tinnitus, headache, incoordination, visual disturbances, mydriasis, xerostomia, blurred vision, anorexia, nausea, vomiting, diarrhea, constipation, epigastric distress, hyperirritability, nervousness and insomnia.
Overdoses may cause restlessness, excitation, delirium, tremors, euphoria, stupor, tachycardia and even convulsions.

DOSAGE AND ADMINISTRATION

Adults: 2 teaspoonfuls, orally, every 4 to 6 hours.
Children 6 to 12 years of age: 1 teaspoonful every 4 to 6 hours.
Children 2 to 6 years of age: ½ to 1 teaspoonful every 4 to 6 hours, according to age. Doses for children should not be repeated more than 4 times in any 24-hour period.

HOW SUPPLIED

Pint bottles (16 fl. oz) NDC 0524-1007-16
Federal law prohibits dispensing without prescription.

Manufactured and Distributed by
Boots Pharmaceuticals, Inc.
Shreveport, Louisiana 71106 U.S.A.

Rev. 10/80 1007-03

RU–TUSS® LIQUID
[roo-tŭs]
(Formerly RU-TUSS® Plain)

DESCRIPTION

Each 5 ml (teaspoonful) of RU-TUSS Liquid contains:

Phenylephrine Hydrochloride	5 mg
Chlorpheniramine Maleate	2 mg
Alcohol	5%

RU-TUSS Liquid is an oral antihistaminic and nasal decongestant preparation.

INDICATIONS AND USAGE

RU-TUSS Liquid is indicated for the temporary relief of congestion, runny nose, sneezing, itching of nose or throat and itchy or watery eyes due to hay fever or the common cold.

DRUG INTERACTION PRECAUTIONS

Do not take this product if you are presently taking a prescription antihypertensive or antidepressant drug containing a monoamine oxidase inhibitor, except under the advice and supervision of a doctor.

WARNINGS

Do not exceed recommended dosage because at higher doses, nervousness, dizziness, or sleeplessness may occur.
If symptoms do not improve within 7 days or are accompanied by a high fever, consult a doctor before continuing use.
Do not take this product if you have high blood pressure, heart disease, diabetes, thyroid disease, asthma, glaucoma, or difficulty in urination due to enlargement of the prostate gland, except under the advice and supervision of a doctor.
May cause drowsiness. Avoid alcoholic beverages, driving a motor vehicle or operating heavy machinery while taking this product.
May cause excitability, especially in children.
Do not give to children under 6 years of age, except under the advice and supervision of a doctor.
As with any drug, if you are pregnant or nursing a baby, seek the advice of a doctor before using this product.

PRECAUTIONS

This package is not child resistant. Keep this and all medications out of reach of children.
In case of accidental overdose, seek professional assistance or contact a poison control center immediately.

DOSAGE AND ADMINISTRATION

Adults, 2 teaspoonfuls, orally, every 4 to 6 hours, not to exceed 6 doses every 24 hours.
Children 6 to 12 years of age, 1 teaspoonful every 4 to 6 hours, not to exceed 6 doses every 24 hours.
Children under 6 years of age, consult a doctor before using.

HOW SUPPLIED

Pint bottles (16 fl. oz)
NDC 0524-1009-16

Manufactured and Distributed by:
Boots Pharmaceuticals, Inc.
Shreveport, Louisiana 71106 U.S.A.

Rev. 9-84 1009-03

RU–TUSS® TABLETS ℞
[roo-tŭs]

DESCRIPTION

Each prolonged action tablet contains:

Phenylephrine Hydrochloride	25 mg
Phenylpropanolamine Hydrochloride	50 mg
Chlorpheniramine Maleate	8 mg
Hyoscyamine Sulfate	0.19 mg
Atropine Sulfate	0.04 mg
Scopolamine Hydrobromide	0.01 mg

Ru-Tuss Tablets act continuously for 10 to 12 hours.
Ru-Tuss Tablets are an oral antihistaminic, nasal decongestant and anti-secretory preparation.

INDICATIONS AND USAGE

Ru-Tuss Tablets provide relief of the symptoms resulting from irritation of sinus, nasal and upper respiratory tract tissues. Phenylephrine and phenylpropanolamine combine to exert a vasoconstrictive and decongestive action while chlorpheniramine maleate decreases the symptoms of watering eyes, post nasal drip and sneezing which may be associated with an allergic-like response. The belladonna alkaloids, hyoscyamine, atropine and scopolamine further augment the anti-secretory activity of Ru-Tuss Tablets.

CONTRAINDICATIONS

Hypersensitivity to antihistamines or sympathomimetics. Ru-Tuss Tablets are contraindicated in children under 12 years of age and in patients with glaucoma, bronchial asthma and women who are pregnant. Concomitant use of MAO inhibitors is contraindicated.

WARNINGS

Ru-Tuss Tablets may cause drowsiness. Patients should be warned of the possible additive effects caused by taking antihistamines with alcohol, hypnotics, sedatives or tranquilizers.

PRECAUTIONS

Ru-Tuss Tablets contain belladonna alkaloids, and must be administered with care to those patients with urinary bladder neck obstruction. Caution should be exercised when Ru-Tuss Tablets are given to patients with hypertension, cardiac or peripheral vascular disease or hyperthyroidism. Patients should avoid driving a motor vehicle or operating dangerous machinery (See **WARNINGS:**).

OVERDOSAGE

Since the action of sustained release products may continue for as long as 12 hours, treatment of overdoses directed at reversing the effects of the drug and supporting the patient should be maintained for at least that length of time. Saline cathartics are useful for hastening evacuation of unreleased medication. In children and infants, antihistamine overdosage may produce convulsions and death.

ADVERSE REACTIONS

Hypersensitivity reactions such as rash, urticaria, leukopenia, agranulocytosis, and thrombocytopenia may occur. Other adverse reactions to Ru-Tuss Tablets may be drowsiness, lassitude, giddiness, dryness of the mucous membranes, tightness of the chest, thickening of bronchial secretions, urinary frequency and dysuria, palpitation, tachycardia, hypotension/hypertension, faintness, dizziness, tinnitus, headache, incoordination, visual disturbances, mydriasis, xerostomia, blurred vision, anorexia, nausea, vomiting, diarrhea, constipation, epigastric distress, hyperirritability, nervousness, dizziness and insomnia. Large overdoses may cause tachypnea, delirium, fever, stupor, coma and respiratory failure.

DOSAGE AND ADMINISTRATION

Adults and children over 12 years of age, one tablet morning and evening. Not recommended for children under 12 years of age. Tablets are to be swallowed whole.

HOW SUPPLIED

Bottles of 100 Tablets **NDC** 0524-0058-01
Bottles of 500 Tablets **NDC** 0524-0058-05
Federal law prohibits dispensing without prescription.

Distributed by:
Boots Pharmaceuticals, Inc.
Shreveport, Louisiana 71106
Manufactured by:
Vitarine Company, Inc.
Springfield Gardens, New York, 11413

Rev. 9/81 0058-02
Shown in Product Identification Section, page 406

RU–TUSS® II CAPSULES ℞
[roo-tŭs]

DESCRIPTION

Each sustained release capsule contains 12mg. of Chlorpheniramine Maleate, USP and 75mg. of Phenylpropanolamine Hydrochloride, USP in a base to provide prolonged activity.
CHLORPHENIRAMINE MALEATE
Category: Antihistaminic.
Structural Formula:

Molecular Formula: $C_{16}H_{19}ClN_2 \cdot C_4H_4O_4$
Molecular Weight: 390.87
Chemical Name: 2[p-chloro-α[2-(dimethylamino) ethyl] benzyl] pyridine maleate (1:1).
PHENYLPROPANOLAMINE HYDROCHLORIDE
Category: Adrenergic (vasoconstrictor).
Structural Formula:

Molecular Formula: $C_9H_{13}NO \cdot HCl$
Molecular Weight: 187.67
Chemical name: Benzenemethanol,α-(1-aminoethyl)-,hydrochloride,(R*,S*)-, (±).

CLINICAL PHARMACOLOGY

Chlorpheniramine Maleate is an antihistamine with anticholinergic (drying) and sedative side effects. Antihistamines appear to compete with histamine for H_1 cell receptor sites on effector cells.
Chlorpheniramine Maleate does not prevent the release of histamine in response to injury, drugs, or antigens. Antihistamines effectively block most smooth muscle responses to histamine and act as an antagonism of the constrictor action of histamine on respiratory smooth muscle. Antihistamines counteract edema formation and whealing in response to injury, antigens, or histamine-liberating drugs. Antihistamines are readily absorbed from the gastrointestinal tract. The main site of metabolic transformation is the liver, but the lung and kidney can also metabolize the drug.
Phenylpropanolamine HCl acts similarly to ephedrine. It is effective orally for the symptomatic control of allergic manifestations, such as perennial hay fever and bronchial asthma. Its action is more prolonged than that of ephedrine, and it is not so apt to produce anxiety complex as is ephedrine.

INDICATIONS

For the treatment of the symptoms of seasonal and perennial allergic rhinitis and vasomotor rhinitis, including nasal obstruction (congestion).

Continued on next page

Boots—Cont.

CONTRAINDICATIONS

Hypersensitivity to any of the components, concurrent MAO inhibitor therapy, severe hypertension, bronchial asthma, coronary artery disease, stenosing peptic ulcer, pyloroduodenal or bladder neck obstruction. Do not use in children under 12 years.

Do not use this drug in patients with narrow-angle glaucoma, obstructive or paralytic ileus, intestinal atony of the elderly or debilitated patient, unstable cardiovascular status in acute hemorrhage, severe ulcerative colitis, toxic megacolon complicating ulcerative colitis, myasthenia gravis.

Use In Nursing Mothers: Because of the higher risk of antihistamines for infants generally and for newborns and prematures in particular, antihistamine therapy is contraindicated in nursing mothers.

Use In Lower Respiratory Disease: Antihistamines **should not** be used to treat lower respiratory tract symptoms, including asthma. Antihistamines are also contraindicated in the following conditions: hypersensitivity to Chlorpheniramine Maleate and other antihistamines of similar chemical structure, monoamine oxidase inhibitor therapy. (See Drug Interactions Section.)

Use In The Elderly (Approximately 60 Years Or Older): Antihistamines are more likely to cause dizziness, sedation, and hypotension in elderly patients.

WARNINGS

Caution patients about activities requiring alertness (e.g., operating vehicles or machinery). Patients should also be warned about the possible additive effects of alcohol and other CNS depressants.

Usage In Pregnancy: Safe use in pregnancy has not been established. This drug should be used in pregnancy, nursing mothers or by women who might bear children only when the potential benefits have been weighed against the possible hazards to the mother and child. However, this drug has had extensive clinical use in pregnant patients without known deleterious effect. Rat reproduction studies with low drug doses have shown no teratogenic effect. As with all anticholinergics, an inhibitory effect on lactation may occur.

PRECAUTIONS

Chlorpheniramine Maleate has an atropine-like action and therefore should be used with caution in patients with a history of bronchial asthma, increased intraocular pressure, hyperthyroidism, cardiovascular disease, and/or hypertension.

In patients with functional or organic gastrointestinal hypermotility or malabsorption syndrome, this product is not the preferred therapy.

This drug should be used with caution when the following medical conditions exist: hiatal hernia with reflux esophagitis, intestinal atony of the elderly or debilitated, intestinal obstruction, myasthenia gravis, renal function impairment, and ulcerative colitis (severe).

Drug Interactions: Alcohol or CNS depressants, especially anesthetics, barbiturates, and narcotics.

MAO inhibitors prolong and intensify the anticholinergic (drying) effects of antihistamines.

ADVERSE REACTIONS

Chlorpheniramine Maleate has a cocaine-like effect on sympathetic nervous transmission and thus prolongs the response to nervous stimulation, potentiates the response to norepinephrine, and inhibits the response to tyramine.

Slight to moderate drowsiness occurs relatively infrequently with Chlorpheniramine Maleate. Other possible side effects common to antihistamines in general include:

General: Urticaria, drug rash, anaphylactic shock, photosensitivity, excessive perspiration, chills, dryness of mouth, nose and throat.

Cardiovascular System: Hypotension, hypertension, headache, palpitations, tachycardia, extrasystoles.

Hematologic System: Hemolytic anemia, thrombocytopenia, agranulocytosis, leukopenia.

Nervous System: Sedation, dizziness, disturbed coordination, fatigue, confusion, restlessness, excitation, nervousness, tremor, irritability, insomnia, euphoria, paresthesias, blurred vision, diplopia, vertigo, tinnitus, acute labyrinthitis hysteria, neuritis, convulsions.

Gastrointestinal System: Epigastric distress, anorexia, nausea, vomiting, diarrhea, constipation.

Genitourinary System: Urinary frequency, difficult urination, urinary retention, early menses.

Respiratory System: Thickening of bronchial secretions, tightness of chest and wheezing, nasal stuffiness.

DOSAGE AND ADMINISTRATION

Dosage should be individualized according to the needs and response of the patient. Adults: one capsule every 8 to 12 hours, not to exceed 3 capsules daily. Not for use in children under 12 years of age.

OVERDOSAGE

In the event of overdosage, emergency treatment should be started immediately.

Manifestations: May vary from central nervous system depression (sedation, apnea, cardiovascular collapse) to stimulation (insomnia, hallucination, tremors or convulsions). Other signs and symptoms may be tinnitus, blurred vision, dizziness, ataxia and hypotension. Stimulation is particularly likely in children, as are atropine-like signs and symptoms (dry mouth, fixed dilated pupils, flushing, hyperthermia and gastrointestinal symptoms).

Treatment: The patient should be induced to vomit, even if emesis has occurred spontaneously. Vomiting by the administration of ipecac syrup is a preferred method. However, vomiting should not be induced in patients with impaired consciousness. The action of ipecac is facilitated by physical activity and by administering eight to twelve fluid ounces of water. If emesis does not occur within fifteen minutes, the dose of ipecac should be repeated. Precautions against aspiration must be taken, especially in infants and children. Following emesis, any drug remaining in the stomach may be absorbed by activated charcoal administered as a slurry with water. If vomiting is unsuccessful, or contraindicated, gastric lavage should be performed. Isotonic and one-half isotonic saline are the lavage solutions of choice. Saline cathartics, such as milk of magnesia, draw water into the bowel by osmosis and, therefore, may be valuable for their action in rapid dilution of bowel content. After emergency treatment, the patient should continue to be medically monitored. Treatment of the signs and symptoms of overdosage is symptomatic and supportive.

Special Note on "Sustained Release" Capsules: Since much of the "Sustained Release" capsule medication is coated for gradual release, therapy directed at reversing the effects of the ingested drugs and at supporting the patient should be continued for as long as overdosage symptoms remain. Saline cathartics are useful for hastening evacuation of pellets that have not already released medication.

Stimulants (analeptic agents) should **not** be used. Vasopressors may be used to treat hypotension. Short-acting barbiturates, diazepam or paraldehyde may be administered to control seizures. Hyperpyrexia, especially in children, may require treatment with tepid water sponge baths or a hypothermic blanket. Apnea is treated with ventilatory support. If photophobia occurs, the patient should be kept in a darkened room.

HOW SUPPLIED

Green and clear capsules with green and white beads, in bottles of 100, **NDC** 0524-0031-01.

Store at controlled room temperature 15–30°C (59–86°F). Protect from moisture.

CAUTION

Federal law prohibits dispensing without prescription.

Rev. 84-5B C84/12
PN 10503
9/84 0031-02

Distributed by
Boots Pharmaceuticals, Inc.
Shreveport, LA 71106 U.S.A.
Manufactured by
Cord Laboratories, Inc.
Broomfield, CO 80020

Shown in Product Identification Section, page 406

TWIN-K® ℞

DESCRIPTION

Each 15 ml (one tablespoonful) supplies 20 mEq of potassium ions as a combination of potassium gluconate and potassium citrate in a sorbitol and saccharin solution.

INDICATIONS AND USAGE

For use as oral potassium therapy in the prevention or treatment of hypokalemia which may occur secondary to diuretic or corticosteroid administration. It may be used in the treatment of cardiac arrhythmias due to digitalis intoxication.

CONTRAINDICATIONS

Severe renal impairment with oliguria or azotemia, untreated Addison's disease, adynamia episodica hereditaria, acute dehydration, heat cramps and hyperkalemia from any cause. This product should not be used in patients receiving aldosterone antagonists or triamterene.

WARNINGS

TWIN-K (potassium gluconate and potassium citrate) is a palatable oral potassium replacement. It appears that little if any potassium gluconate-citrate is transported to the jejunum or ileum where enteric coated potassium chloride lesions have been noted. Excessive, undiluted doses of TWIN-K may cause a saline laxative effect.

PRECAUTIONS

Potassium is a major intracellular cation which plays a significant role in body physiology. The serum level of potassium is normally 3.8–5.0 mEq/liter. While the serum or plasma level is a poor indicator of total body stores, a plasma or serum level below 3.5 mEq/liter is considered to be indicative of hypokalemia.

The most common cause of hypokalemia is excessive loss of potassium in the urine. However, hypokalemia can also occur with vomiting, gastric drainage and diarrhea.

Usually a potassium deficiency can be corrected by oral administration of potassium supplements. With normal kidney function, it is difficult to produce potassium intoxication by oral administration. However, potassium supplements must be administered with caution since, usually, the exact amount of the deficiency is not accurately known. Checks on the patient's clinical status and serum potassium levels should be made. High serum potassium levels may cause death by cardiac depression, arrhythmias or arrest.

In patients with hypokalemia who also have alkalosis and a chloride deficiency (hypokalemic-hypochloremic alkalosis), there will be a requirement for chloride ions. TWIN-K is not recommended for use in these patients.

ADVERSE REACTIONS

Symptoms of potassium intoxication include paresthesias of the extremities, flaccid paralysis, listlessness, mental confusion, weakness and heaviness of the legs, fall in blood pressure, cardiac arrhythmias and heart block. Hyperkalemia may exhibit the following electrocardiographic abnormalities: disappearance of the P wave, widening and slurring of the QRS complex, changes of the ST segment and tall peaked T waves.

TWIN-K taken on an empty stomach in undiluted doses larger than 30 ml (two tablespoons) can produce gastric irritation with nausea, vomiting, diarrhea, and abdominal discomfort.

OVERDOSAGE

The administration of oral potassium supplements to persons with normal kidney function rarely causes serious hyperkalemia. However, if the renal excretory function is impaired, potentially fatal hyperkalemia can result. It is important to note that hyperkalemia is usually asymptomatic and may be manifested only by an increased serum potassium concentration and characteristic E.K.G. changes.

Treatment measures include:

1. Elimination of potassium containing drugs or foods.
2. Elimination of potassium-sparing diuretics.
3. Intravenous administration of 300 to 500 ml/hr of a 10% dextrose solution containing 10–20 units of crystalline insulin per 1,000 milliliters.
4. Correction of acidosis, if present, with intravenous sodium bicarbonate.
5. Use of exchange resins, hemodialysis, or peritoneal dialysis.

In treating hyperkalemia, it should be noted that patients stabilized on digitalis can develop digitalis toxicity when the serum potassium concentration is lowered too rapidly.

DOSAGE AND ADMINISTRATION

The usual adult dosage is one tablespoonful (15 ml) in 8 fluid ounces of water or fruit juice, two to four times a day. This will supply 40 to 80 mEq of potassium ions. The usual maintenance dose of potassium is 20 mEq per day while replacement doses range from 30 mEq to 100 mEq per day. Because of the potential for gastrointestinal irritation, undiluted large single doses (more than a tablespoonful or 15 ml) of TWIN-K are to be avoided.

To minimize gastrointestinal irritation, it is recommended that TWIN-K be taken with meals or diluted with water or fruit juice. A tablespoonful (15 ml) in 8 ounces of water is approximately isotonic. More than a single tablespoonful should not be taken without prior dilution.

Deviations from this schedule may be indicated, since no average total daily dose can be defined, but must be governed by close observation for clinical effects.

HOW SUPPLIED

Bottles of 1 pint (16 fl. oz.)
NDC 0524-0021-16
CAUTION: Federal law prohibits dispensing without prescription.

Manufactured and Distributed by
Boots Pharmaceuticals, Inc.
Shreveport, Louisiana 71106 U.S.A.

Rev. 11/83 0021-02

TWIN-K-Cl® ℞

DESCRIPTION

Each 15 ml (one tablespoonful) supplies 15 mEq of potassium ions and 4 mEq of chloride ions as a combination of potassium gluconate, potassium citrate, and ammonium chloride, in a sorbitol and saccharin solution.

INDICATIONS AND USAGE

For use as oral potassium therapy in the prevention or treatment of hypokalemia which may occur secondary to diuretic

or corticosteroid administration. It may be used in the treatment of cardiac arrhythmias due to digitalis intoxication.
Potassium and chloride are usually the salts of choice in the treatment of hypokalemia since chloride and potassium deficiencies are likely to be associated with each other.
In patients with hypokalemia who also have alkalosis and a chloride deficiency (hypokalemic-hypochloremic alkalosis), there will be a requirement for chloride ions. TWIN-K-Cl is recommended for use in these patients.

CONTRAINDICATIONS

Severe renal impairment with oliguria or azotemia, untreated Addison's disease, adynamia episodica hereditaria, acute dehydration, heat cramps and hyperkalemia from any cause. This product should not be used in patients receiving aldosterone antagonists or triamterene.

WARNINGS

TWIN-K-Cl is a palatable oral potassium replacement. Excessive, undiluted doses of TWIN-K-Cl may cause a saline laxative effect.

PRECAUTIONS

Potassium is a major intracellular cation which plays a significant role in body physiology. The serum level of potassium is normally 3.8–5.0 mEq/liter. While the serum or plasma level is a poor indicator of total body stores, a plasma or serum level below 3.5 mEq/liter is considered to be indicative of hypokalemia.
The most common cause of hypokalemia is excessive loss of potassium in the urine. However, hypokalemia can also occur with vomiting, gastric drainage and diarrhea.
Usually a potassium deficiency can be corrected by oral administration of potassium supplements. With normal kidney function, it is difficult to produce potassium intoxication by oral administration. However, potassium supplements must be administered with caution since, usually, the exact amount of the deficiency is not accurately known. Checks on the patient's clinical status and serum potassium levels should be made. High serum potassium levels may cause death by cardiac depression, arrhythmias or arrest.

ADVERSE REACTIONS

Symptoms of potassium intoxication include paresthesias of the extremities, flaccid paralysis, listlessness, mental confusion, weakness and heaviness of the legs, fall in blood pressure, cardiac arrhythmias and heart block. Hyperkalemia may exhibit the following electrocardiographic abnormalities: disappearance of the P wave, widening and slurring of the QRS complex, changes of the ST segment and tall peaked T waves.
TWIN-K-Cl taken on an empty stomach in undiluted doses larger than 30 ml (two tablespoons) can produce gastric irritation with nausea, vomiting, diarrhea, and abdominal discomfort.

OVERDOSAGE

The administration of oral potassium supplements to persons with normal kidney function rarely causes serious hyperkalemia. However, if the renal excretory function is impaired potentially fatal hyperkalemia can result. It is important to note that hyperkalemia is usually asymptomatic and may be manifested only by an increased serum potassium concentration and characteristic E.K.G. changes.
Treatment measures include:

1. Elimination of potassium containing drugs or foods.
2. Elimination of potassium-sparing diuretics.
3. Intravenous administration of 300 to 500 ml/hr of a 10% dextrose solution containing 10–20 units of crystalline insulin per 1,000 milliliters.
4. Correction of acidosis, if present, with intravenous sodium bicarbonate.
5. Use of exchange resins, hemodialysis, or peritoneal dialysis. In treating hyperkalemia, it should be noted that patients stabilized on digitalis can develop digitalis toxicity when the serum potassium concentration is lowered too rapidly.

DOSAGE AND ADMINISTRATION

The usual adult dosage is one tablespoonful (15 ml) in 8 fluid ounces of water or fruit juice, two to four times a day. This will supply 30 to 60 mEq of potassium ions and 8 to 16 mEq of chloride ions. The usual maintenance dose of potassium is 20 mEq per day while replacement doses range from 30 mEq to 100 mEq per day. Because of the potential for gastrointestinal irritation, undiluted large single doses (more than a tablespoonful or 15 ml) of TWIN-K-Cl are to be avoided.
To minimize gastrointestinal irritation, it is recommended that TWIN-K-Cl be taken with meals or diluted with water or fruit juice. A tablespoonful (15 ml) in 8 ounces of water is approximately isotonic. More than a single tablespoonful should not be taken without prior dilution.
Deviations from this schedule may be indicated, since no average total daily dose can be defined, but must be governed by close observation for clinical effects.

HOW SUPPLIED

Bottles of 1 pint (16 fl. oz.)
NDC 0524-0022-16
Caution: Federal law prohibits dispensing without prescription.

Manufactured and Distributed by
Boots Pharmaceuticals, Inc.
Shreveport, Louisiana 71106 U.S.A.

Rev. 11/83 0022-02

ZORprin® ℞
(aspirin)
(Zero-Order Release)

DESCRIPTION

Each capsule-shaped tablet of Zorprin contains 800 mg of aspirin, formulated in a special matrix to control the release of aspirin after ingestion. The in vitro release of aspirin from the tablet matrix is linear and independent of the concentration of the drug.
The structural formula of aspirin is

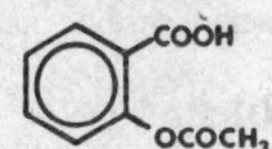

CLINICAL PHARMACOLOGY

Aspirin, as contained in Zorprin, is a salicylate that has demonstrated anti-inflammatory and analgesic activity. Its mode of action as an anti-inflammatory and analgesic agent may be due to the inhibition of synthesis of prostaglandins, although its exact mode of action is not known.
Zorprin dissolution is pH dependent. In vitro studies have shown very little aspirin to be released in acidic solutions; whereas, Zorprin releases the majority of its aspirin (90%) in a zero-order mode at a neutral to alkaline pH. It is this pH dependence of Zorprin that reduces direct contact between aspirin and the gastric mucosa, resulting in a reduction of its gastrointestinal side-effect potential.
Bioavailability data for Zorprin have confirmed that plasma levels of salicylic acid and acetylsalicylic acid can be measured 24 hours after a single oral dose. This substantiates a twice daily dose regimen. Multiple dose bioavailability studies showed similar steady-state salicylate levels for Zorprin as for conventional release aspirin using the same total daily dose. Long-term monitoring of salicylate levels showed no signs of accumulation once steady-state levels were reached (4–6 days).
Studies of in vivo prostaglandin levels (PGE2) have shown Zorprin plasma levels of salicylic acid and acetylsalicylic acid to reduce PGE2 levels 14 hours after a single oral 800 mg dose while an equivalent dose of aspirin produced a reduction of PGE2 levels only through six hours. Zorprin's effect on other prostaglandins than PGE2 has not been determined.
Salicylates are excreted mainly by the kidney, and from studies in humans it appears that salicylate is excreted in the urine as free salicylic acid (10%); salicyluric acid (75%); salicylic phenolic (10%); acyl glucuronides (5%) and gentisic acid (<1%).

INDICATIONS & USAGE

Zorprin is indicated for the treatment of rheumatoid arthritis and osteoarthritis. The safety and efficacy of Zorprin have not been established in those rheumatoid arthritic patients who are designated by the American Rheumatism Association as Functional Class IV (incapacitated, largely or wholly bedridden, or confined to wheelchair, little or no self-care).
In patients treated with Zorprin for rheumatoid arthritis and osteoarthritis, the anti-inflammatory action of Zorprin has been shown by reduction in pain, morning stiffness and disease activity as assessed by both the investigators and patients.
In clinical studies in patients with rheumatoid arthritis and osteoarthritis, Zorprin has been shown to be comparable to conventional release aspirin in controlling the aforementioned signs and symptoms of disease activity and to be associated with a statistically significant reduction in the milder gastrointestinal side effects (see ADVERSE REACTIONS).
Zorprin may be well tolerated in some patients who have had gastrointestinal side effects with conventional release aspirin, but these patients when treated with Zorprin should be carefully followed for signs and symptoms of gastrointestinal bleeding and ulceration.
Since there have been no controlled trials to demonstrate whether or not there is any beneficial effect or harmful interaction with the use of Zorprin in conjunction with other nonsteroidal anti-inflammatory agents (NSAI), the combination cannot be recommended (see **Drug Interactions**).
Because of its relatively long onset of action, Zorprin is not recommended for antipyresis or for short-term analgesia.

CONTRAINDICATIONS

Zorprin should not be used in patients known to be hypersensitive to salicylates or in individuals with the syndrome of nasal polyps, angioedema, bronchospastic reactivity to aspirin, renal or hepatic insufficiency, hypoprothrombinemia or other bleeding disorders. Zorprin is not recommended for children under 12 years of age; it is contraindicated in all children with fever accompanied by dehydration.

WARNINGS

Zorprin should be used with caution when anticoagulants are prescribed concurrently, since aspirin may depress platelet aggregation and increase bleeding time. Large doses of salicylates may have hypoglycemic action and enhance the effect of the oral hypoglycemics; concomitant use therefore is not recommended. However, if such use is necessary, dosage of the hypoglycemic agent must be reduced. The hypoglycemic action of the salicylates may also necessitate adjustment of the insulin requirements of diabetics.
While salicylates in large doses have a uricosuric effect, smaller amounts may reduce urate excretion and increase serum uric acid.
USE IN PREGNANCY: Aspirin can harm the fetus when administered to pregnant women. Aspirin interferes with maternal and infant hemostasis and may lengthen the duration of pregnancy and parturition. Aspirin has produced teratogenic effects and increases the incidence of stillbirths and neonatal deaths in animals.
If this drug is used during pregnancy, or if the patient becomes pregnant while taking this drug, the patient should be apprised of the potential hazard to the fetus.
Aspirin should not be taken during the last 3 months of pregnancy.

PRECAUTIONS

Appropriate precautions should be taken in prescribing Zorprin (aspirin) for patients who are known to be sensitive to aspirin or salicylates. Particular care should be used when prescribing this medication for patients with erosive gastritis, peptic ulcer, mild diabetes or gout. As with all salicylate drugs, caution should be exercised in prescribing Zorprin (aspirin) for those patients with bleeding tendencies or those on anticoagulants.
In order to avoid exacerbation of disease or adrenal insufficiency, patients who have been on prolonged corticosteroid therapy should have their therapy tapered slowly rather than discontinued abruptly when Zorprin is made a part of the treatment program.
Patients receiving large doses of aspirin and/or prolonged therapy may develop mild salicylate intoxication (salicylism) that may be reversed by dosage reduction.
Salicylates can produce changes in thyroid function tests.
Salicylates should be used with caution in patients with severe hepatic damage, preexisting hypoprothrombinemia, Vitamin K deficiency and in those undergoing surgery.
Since aspirin release from Zorprin® (aspirin) is pH dependent, it may change in those conditions where the gastric pH has been increased as a result of antacids, gastric secretion inhibitors or surgical procedures.
Drug Interactions: (See **WARNINGS**) Aspirin may interfere with some anticoagulant and antidiabetic drugs. Drugs which lower serum uric acid by increasing uric acid excretion (uricosurics) may be antagonized by the concomitant use of aspirin, particularly in doses less than 2.0 grams/day. Nonsteroidal anti-inflammatory drugs may be competitively displaced from their albumin binding sites by aspirin. This effect may negate the clinical efficacy of both drugs. Also, the gastrointestinal inflammatory potential of nonsteroidal anti-inflammatory drugs may be potentiated by aspirin. The combination of alcohol and aspirin may increase the risk of gastrointestinal bleeding.
Aspirin may enhance the activity of methotrexate and increase its toxicity.
Sodium excretion produced by spironolactone may be decreased in the presence of salicylates. Concomitant administration of other anti-inflammatory drugs may increase the risk of gastrointestinal ulceration. Urinary alkalinizers decrease aspirin's effectiveness by increasing the rate of salicylate renal excretion. Phenobarbital decreases aspirin's effectiveness by enzyme induction.
Pregnancy Category D. See **WARNINGS** Section.
Nursing Mothers: Salicylates have been detected in the breast milk of nursing mothers. Because of the potential for serious adverse reactions in nursing infants from aspirin, a decision should be made whether to discontinue nursing or discontinue the drug, taking into account the benefit of the drug to the mother.

ADVERSE REACTIONS

Hematologic: Aspirin interferes with hemostasis. Patients with a history of blood coagulation defects or receiving anticoagulant drugs or with severe anemia should avoid Zorprin. Aspirin used chronically may cause a persistent iron deficiency anemia.
Gastrointestinal: Aspirin may potentiate peptic ulcer, and cause stomach distress or heartburn. Aspirin can cause an increase in occult bleeding and in some patients massive gastrointestinal bleeding. However, the greatest release of

Continued on next page

Boots—Cont.

active drug from Zorprin is designed to occur in the small intestine over a period of time. This has resulted in fewer symptomatic gastrointestinal side effects.
Allergic: Allergic and anaphylactic reactions have been noted when hypersensitive individuals have taken aspirin. Fatal anaphylactic shock, while not common, has been reported.
Respiratory: Aspirin intolerance, manifested by exacerbation of bronchospasm and rhinitis, may occur in patients with a history of nasal polyps, asthma, or rhinitis. The mechanism of this intolerance is unknown but may be the result of aspirin-induced shunting of prostaglandin synthesis to the lipoxygenase pathway and the liberation of leukotrienes, e.g., slow-reacting substance of anaphylaxis.
Dermatologic: Hives, rashes, and angioedema may occur, especially in patients suffering from chronic urticaria.
Central Nervous System: Taken in overdoses, aspirin provides stimulation which may be manifested by tinnitus. Following initial stimulation, depression of the central nervous system may be noted.
Renal: Aspirin rarely may aggravate chronic kidney disease.
Hepatic: High doses of aspirin have been reported to produce reversible hepatic dysfunction.

OVERDOSAGE

Overdosage, if it occurs would produce the usual symptoms of salicylism: tinnitus, vertigo, headache, confusion, drowsiness, sweating, hyperventilation, vomiting or diarrhea. Plasma salicylate levels in adults may range from 50 to 80 mg/dl in the mildly intoxicated patient to 110 to 160* mg/dl in the severely intoxicated patient. An arterial blood pH of 7.1 may indicate serious poisoning. The clearance of salicylates in children is much slower than adults and this should receive due consideration when aspirin overdosages occur in infants; salicylate half-lives of 30 hours have been reported in infants 4–8 months old. Treatment for mild intoxication should include emptying the stomach with an emetic, or gastric lavage with 5% sodium bicarbonate. Individuals suffering from severe intoxication should, in addition, have forced diuresis by intravenous infusions of sodium bicarbonate and dextrose or sodium lactate. In extreme cases, hemodialysis or peritoneal dialysis may be required.
(*A plasma salicylate level of 160 mg/dl in an adult is usually considered lethal.)

DOSAGE & ADMINISTRATION

In order to achieve a zero-order release, the tablets of Zorprin should be swallowed intact.
Breaking the tablets or disrupting the structure will alter the release profile of the drug.
It is recommended that Zorprin be taken with sufficient quantities of fluids (8 oz. or more).
Adult Dosage: For mild to moderate pain associated with rheumatoid arthritis and osteoarthritis, the recommended initial dose of Zorprin is 1600 mg (2-800 mg tablets) twice a day. Because of Zorprin's prolonged release of aspirin into the bloodstream, the tablets may be taken as a b.i.d. dose. Further adjustment of the dosage should be determined by the physician, based upon the patient's response and needs. Since it will take 4–6 days to reach steady-state levels of salicylic acid with Zorprin, it is recommended that dosages be given for at least one week before further adjustment. In general, patients with rheumatoid arthritis seem to require higher doses of Zorprin than do patients with osteoarthritis.
Zorprin is not recommended for children below the age of 12.

HOW SUPPLIED

Zorprin Tablets 800 mg; plain, white capsule-shaped tablets. Bottles of 100 Tablets—NDC 0524-0057-01
Caution: Federal law prohibits dispensing without prescription.
U.S. Patent No. 4,308,251

Manufactured by:
Boots Laboratories, Inc.
Palisades Park, New Jersey 07650 USA
Distributed by:
Boots Pharmaceuticals, Inc.
Shreveport, Louisiana 71106 USA

Rev. 3-86 0057-04
Shown in Product Identification Section, page 406

Products are listed alphabetically in the **PINK SECTION.**

Boyle & Company
1030 SO. ARROYO PARKWAY
PASADENA, CA 91105

CITRA® FORTE SYRUP Ⓒ℞
Oral Solution

PRODUCT OVERVIEW

KEY FACTS

Citra Forte Syrup is a unique combination of two antihistamines and a proven antitussive in a sodium free, pleasant tasting vehicle.

MAJOR USES

Citra Forte has been used successfully for many years to provide cough suppressant action where a narcotic antitussive is indicated or where the cough is caused by a histamine response.

SAFETY INFORMATION

Citra Forte is contraindicated in patients with allergies to the formula ingredients and should be used with caution in patients with hypertension, cardiac disease, diabetes or hyperthyroidism.

PRESCRIBING INFORMATION

CITRA® FORTE SYRUP Ⓒ℞
Oral Solution

COMPOSITION

	ea. 5 ml
Hydrocodone Bitartrate (Warning: May be habit forming	5 mg
Pheniramine Maleate	2.5 mg
Pyrilamine Maleate	3.33 mg

Alcohol 2% in a pleasant flavored syrup base with Ascorbic Acid 30 mg and Potassium Citrate 150 mg.

ACTION AND USES

CITRA FORTE SYRUP: Antitussive, Expectorant, Antihistaminic, Provides effective cough suppressant action sodium free. Two antihistamines to help control allergic reactions.

ADMINISTRATION AND DOSAGE

CITRA FORTE SYRUP: Usual Adult Dose.—One or two teaspoonfuls every 3 or 4 hours. *Children* (6-12)—one-half adult dosage. *Children under 6 years*—according to standard method of calculation.

PRECAUTIONS

Patients should be advised to avoid using machinery or driving until response to antihistamines is established. Use with caution in patients with idiosyncrasies to formula ingredients. CITRA FORTE should be used with caution in patients with hypertension, cardiac disease, diabetes or hyperthyroidism.

HOW SUPPLIED

CITRA FORTE SYRUP in pints and gallons.
Caution: Federal (USA) law prohibits dispensing without prescription.

TRIVA® DOUCHE POWDER
FOR VAGINAL USE ONLY

PRODUCT OVERVIEW

KEY FACTS

Triva powder effectively treats Monilial and Trichomonal vaginal infections as well as non-specific Vulvovaginitis. Treatment is antiseptic as well as symptomatic.

MAJOR USES

When used as directed as a douche, chronic, stubborn cases of Monilia and Trichomonas occurring separately or together can be eradicated along with symptoms.

SAFETY INFORMATION

Occasionally irritation occurs at the onset of treatment. Triva is contraindicated in patients with allergies to the formula ingredients.

PRESCRIBING INFORMATION

TRIVA® DOUCHE POWDER
FOR VAGINAL USE ONLY

COMPOSITION

Triva Douche Powder contains (per 3 g packet):

Oxyquinoline Benzoate	60 mg (2%)
Alkyl Aryl Sulfonate	1.05 g (35%)
Disodium Edetate	10 mg (0.33%)
Sodium Sulfate	1.59 g (52.5%)
Lactose (dispersant)	290 mg (9.67%)

ACTION AND USES

TRIVA DOUCHE POWDER effectively treats Monilial and Trichomonal as well as Non-specific Vulvovaginitis. Chronic, stubborn cases as well as Monilia and Trichomonas occurring together can be successfully treated. Organisms are eradicated along with symptoms. Vaginal flora and pH return to normal spontaneously. Trichomonacidal, bactericidal, detergent and chelating agents are provided for a safe, simple, patient-administered treatment without need for restraints on patient's activities. Flushing and detergent action of the douche quickly destroys the infection and stops the symptoms.
Effectiveness of TRIVA DOUCHE POWDER has been demonstrated by clinical tests. Both diagnosis and cure were established by the use of special Papanicolaou smear and Sabouraud culture.

ADMINISTRATION AND DOSAGE

TRIVA DOUCHE POWDER (individual packet dissolved in 1 qt water) is effective in most cases of Monilial, Trichomonal and Non-specific Vulvovaginitis. It provides rapid relief from symptoms. Particularly useful in pre- and post-operative and post-partum care. May be used adjunctively with oral treatment for Trichomonas.
TRIVA DOUCHE POWDER, sig, douche (1 packet in 1 qt water) morning and night for 12 days.
IMPORTANT: During menstruation, continue treatment as instructed.

PRECAUTIONS

Occasionally, irritation occurs at the onset of treatment. In such cases it is recommended that the douche be prescribed in one-half or less than usual strength for a day or two, then treatment resumed as directed.

SIDE EFFECTS

None.

CONTRAINDICATIONS

Allergy or hypersensitivity to any ingredient.

HOW SUPPLIED

TRIVA DOUCHE POWDER—24 individual 3 G packets.

Braintree Laboratories, Inc.
285 WASHINGTON STREET
BRAINTREE, MA 02184

GoLYTELY® ℞
[go-līt ′lē]
Polyethylene Glycol Electrolyte for Gastrointestinal Lavage Solution

DESCRIPTION

A white powder for reconstitution containing 236 g polyethylene glycol 3350, 22.74 g sodium sulfate, 6.74 g sodium bicarbonate, 5.86 g sodium chloride, and 2.97 g potassium chloride. When dissolved in water to a volume of 4 liters, GoLYTELY is an isosmotic solution having a mildly salty taste. For oral administration.

CLINICAL PHARMACOLOGY

Orally administered GoLYTELY induces a diarrhea that rapidly cleanses the bowel, usually within four hours. Polyethylene glycol 3350 acts as an osmotic agent, and the electrolyte concentration results in virtually no net absorption or secretion of ions. Large volumes may be administered without significant changes in water or electrolyte balance.

INDICATION AND USAGE

GoLYTELY is indicated for bowel cleansing prior to colonoscopy and barium enema x-ray examination.

CONTRAINDICATIONS

GoLYTELY is contraindicated in patients with gastrointestinal obstruction, gastric retention, bowel perforation, toxic colitis or megacolon.

WARNINGS

No additional ingredients, flavoring, etc, should be added to the solution before administration.

PRECAUTIONS

Patients with impaired gag reflex or in an unconscious or semiconscious state, or who are otherwise prone to regurgitation or aspiration, should be observed during the administration of GoLYTELY, especially if it is given via nasogastric tube. If gastrointestinal obstruction or perforation is suspected, appropriate studies should be performed to rule out these contraindications before administering GoLYTELY.
Pregnancy Category C. Animal reproduction studies have not been conducted with GoLYTELY. It is also not known whether GoLYTELY can cause fetal harm when administered to a pregnant woman or can affect reproductive capacity. GoLYTELY should be given to a pregnant woman only if clearly needed.
Safety and effectiveness in children have not been established.
Long-term studies have not been done on animals to determine carcinogenic potential or effects on reproduction.

ADVERSE REACTIONS

GoLYTELY administration is associated with a low incidence of side effects—primarily nausea, abdominal fullness and bloating, and occasional cramps and vomiting. These side effects are transient and usually subside rapidly.

DOSAGE AND ADMINISTRATION

The recommended dosage for adults is 4 liters of GoLYTELY solution prior to gastrointestinal examination. GoLYTELY is usually taken orally but may be given via nasogastric tube to patients who are unwilling or unable to drink the preparation. The rate of administration is 8 oz (240 mL) every ten minutes, until the 4 liters is consumed. It is preferred that each portion be ingested rapidly, not taken in small amounts. The first bowel movement should occur approximately one hour after the start of GoLYTELY administration.

Various regimens have been used. Ideally, the patient should fast approximately three to four hours prior to ingesting GoLYTELY, but in no case should solid foods be given for at least two hours before the solution is administered. One method is to schedule patients for examination at midmorning, allowing the patient three hours for drinking and a one-hour waiting period to complete bowel evacuation. Another method is to administer GoLYTELY on the evening before the examination, particularly if the patient is to have a barium enema. No foods except clear liquids are permitted after GoLYTELY administration and prior to examination.

HOW SUPPLIED

In powdered form, for oral administration as a solution following reconstitution. Each disposable jug contains, in powdered form: polyethylene glycol 3350 236 g, sodium sulfate 22.74 g, sodium bicarbonate 6.74 g, sodium chloride 5.86 g, potassium chloride 2.97 g. When made up to 4 L volume with water, the solution contains PEG 3350 17.6 mmol/L, sodium 125 mmol/L, sulfate 40 mmol/L, chloride 35 mmol/L, bicarbonate 20 mmol/L, and potassium 10 mmol/L.

CAUTION

Federal law prohibits dispensing without prescription.

STORAGE

Store in sealed container at 59° to 86°F. When reconstituted, keep solution refrigerated. Use within 48 hours. Discard unused portion. (NDC 52268-0100-01).

Made by Lyne Laboratories,
Stoughton, MA 02072, for
BRAINTREE LABORATORIES, INC.
P.O. Box 361, Braintree, MA 02184
617-843-2202
©1985 Rev. 6-13-85

Shown in Product Identification Section, page 406

EDUCATIONAL MATERIAL

Booklets

Two patient booklets are available: "Bowel Preparation Before Your Barium Enema," and "Bowel Preparation Before Your Colonoscopy." Supplies available to practitioners on request.

Products are
listed alphabetically
in the
PINK SECTION.

Products are cross-indexed
by product classifications
in the
BLUE SECTION

Products are cross-indexed by
generic and chemical names
in the
YELLOW SECTION

Bristol Laboratories

(Division of Bristol-Myers Co.)
EVANSVILLE, IN 47721

AMIKIN® ℞

[*ah-mi 'kin*]
(amikacin sulfate)

This is the full text of the latest Official Package circular dated December 1985 [3015 D1M-09].

WARNINGS

Patients treated with parenteral aminoglycosides should be under close clinical observation because of the potential ototoxicity and nephrotoxicity associated with their use. Safety for treatment periods which are longer than 14 days has not been established.

Neurotoxicity, manifested as vestibular and permanent bilateral auditory ototoxicity, can occur in patients with preexisting renal damage and in patients with normal renal function treated at higher doses and/or for periods longer than those recommended. The risk of aminoglycoside-induced ototoxicity is greater in patients with renal damage. High frequency deafness usually occurs first and can be detected only by audiometric testing. Vertigo may occur and may be evidence of vestibular injury. Other manifestations of neurotoxicity may include numbness, skin tingling, muscle twitching and convulsions. The risk of hearing loss due to aminoglycosides increases with the degree of exposure to either high peak or high trough serum concentrations. Patients developing cochlear damage may not have symptoms during therapy to warn them of developing eighth-nerve toxicity, and total or partial irreversible bilateral deafness may occur after the drug has been discontinued. Aminoglycoside-induced ototoxicity is usually irreversible.

Aminoglycosides are potentially nephrotoxic. The risk of nephrotoxicity is greater in patients with impaired renal function and in those who receive high doses or prolonged therapy.

Neuromuscular blockade and respiratory paralysis have been reported following parenteral injection, topical instillation (as in orthopedic and abdominal irrigation or in local treatment of empyema), and following oral use of aminoglycosides. The possibility of these phenomena should be considered if aminoglycosides are administered by any route, especially in patients receiving anesthetics, neuromuscular blocking agents such as tubocurarine, succinylcholine, decamethonium, or in patients receiving massive transfusions of citrate-anticoagulated blood. If blockage occurs, calcium salts may reverse these phenomena, but mechanical respiratory assistance may be necessary.

Renal and eighth-nerve function should be closely monitored especially in patients with known or suspected renal impairment at the onset of therapy and also in those whose renal function is initially normal but who develop signs of renal dysfunction during therapy. Serum concentrations of amikacin should be monitored when feasible to assure adequate levels and to avoid potentially toxic levels and prolonged peak concentrations above 35 micrograms per ml. Urine should be examined for decreased specific gravity, increased excretion of proteins, and the presence of cells or casts. Blood urea nitrogen, serum creatinine, or creatinine clearance should be measured periodically. Serial audiograms should be obtained where feasible in patients old enough to be tested, particularly high risk patients. Evidence of ototoxicity (dizziness, vertigo, tinnitus, roaring in the ears, and hearing loss) or nephrotoxicity requires discontinuation of the drug or dosage adjustment.

Concurrent and/or sequential systemic, oral or topical use of other neurotoxic or nephrotoxic products, particularly bacitracin, cisplatin, amphotericin B, cephaloridine, paromomycin, viomycin, polymyxin B, colistin, vancomycin, or other aminoglycosides should be avoided. Other factors that may increase risk of toxicity are advanced age and dehydration.

The concurrent use of AMIKIN with potent diuretics (ethacrynic acid, or furosemide) should be avoided since diuretics by themselves may cause ototoxicity. In addition, when administered, intravenously, diuretics may enhance aminoglycoside toxicity by altering antibiotic concentrations in serum and tissue.

DESCRIPTION

Amikacin sulfate is a semi-synthetic aminoglycoside antibiotic derived from kanamycin. It is $C_{22}H_{43}N_5O_{13} \cdot 2H_2SO_4$. D-Streptamine, 0-3-amino-3-deoxy-α-D-glucopyranosyl-(1 → 6)-0-[6-amino-6-deoxy-α-D-glucopyranosyl-(1 → 4)]-N1-(4-amino-2-hydroxyl-1-oxobutyl)-2-deoxy-, (S)-, sulfate (1:2)(salt).

NH₂ NHCOC(OH)(H)CH₂CH₂NH₂ · OH · HO · OH · OH · HOCH₂ · CH₂NH₂ · NH₂ · 2H₂SO₄

The dosage form is supplied as a sterile, colorless to light straw colored solution. The 100 mg per 2 ml vial contains, in addition to amikacin sulfate, 0.13% sodium bisulfite and 0.5% sodium citrate with pH adjusted to 4.5 with sulfuric acid. The 500 mg per 2 ml vial and the 1 gram per 4 ml vial contain 0.66% sodium bisulfite and 2.5% sodium citrate with pH adjusted to 4.5 with sulfuric acid.

CLINICAL PHARMACOLOGY

Intramuscular Administration—AMIKIN is rapidly absorbed after intramuscular administration. In normal adult volunteers, average peak serum concentrations of about 12, 16, and 21 mcg/ml are obtained 1 hour after intramuscular administration of 250-mg (3.7mg/Kg), 375-mg (5 mg/Kg), 500-mg (7.5 mg/Kg), single doses, respectively. At 10 hours, serum levels are about 0.3 mcg/ml, 1.2 mcg/ml, and 2.1 mcg/ml, respectively.

Tolerance studies in normal volunteers reveal that amikacin is well tolerated locally following repeated intramuscular dosing, and when given at maximally recommended doses, no ototoxicity or nephrotoxicity has been reported. There is no evidence of drug accumulation with repeated dosing for 10 days when administered according to recommended doses.

With normal renal function, about 91.9% of an intramuscular dose is excreted unchanged in the urine in the first 8 hours, and 98.2% within 24 hours. Mean urine concentrations for 6 hours are 563 mcg/ml following a 250-mg dose, 697 mcg/ml following a 375-mg dose, and 832 mcg/ml following a 500-mg dose.

Preliminary intramuscular studies in newborns of different weights (less than 1.5 Kg, 1.5 to 2.0 Kg, over 2.0 Kg) at a dose of 7.5 mg/Kg revealed that, like other aminoglycosides, serum half-life values were correlated inversely with postnatal age and renal clearances of amikacin. The volume of distribution indicates that amikacin, like other aminoglycosides, remains primarily in the extracellular fluid space of neonates. Repeated dosing every 12 hours in all the above groups did not demonstrate accumulation after 5 days.

Intravenous Administration—Single doses of 500 mg (7.5 mg/Kg) administered to normal adults as an infusion over a period of 30 minutes produced a mean peak serum concentration of 38 mcg/ml at the end of the infusion, and levels of 24 mcg/ml, 18 mcg/ml, and 0.75 mcg/ml at 30 minutes, 1 hour and 10 hours post-infusion, respectively. Eighty-four percent of the administered dose was excreted in the urine in 9 hours and about 94% within 24 hours.

Repeat infusions of 7.5 mg/Kg every 12 hours in normal adults were well tolerated and caused no drug accumulation.

General—Pharmocokinetic studies in normal adult subjects reveal the mean serum half-life to be slightly over 2 hours with a mean total apparent volume of distribution of 24 liters (28% of the body weight). By the ultrafiltration technique, reports of serum protein binding range from 0 to 11%. The mean serum clearance rate is about 100 ml/min and the renal clearance rate is 94 ml/min in subjects with normal renal function.

Amikacin is excreted primarily by glomerular filtration. Patients with impaired renal function or diminished glomerular filtration pressure excrete the drug much more slowly (effectively prolonging the serum half-life). Therefore, renal function should be monitored carefully and dosage adjusted accordingly (see suggested dosage schedule under "Dosage and Administration").

Following administration at the recommended dose, therapeutic levels are found in bone, heart, gallbladder, and lung tissue in addition to significant concentrations in urine, bile, sputum, bronchial secretions, interstitial, plural and synovial fluids.

Spinal fluid levels in normal infants are approximately 10 to 20% of the serum concentrations and may reach 50% when the meninges are inflamed. AMIKIN has been demonstrated to cross the placental barrier and yield significant concentrations in amniotic fluid. The peak fetal serum concentration is about 16% of the peak maternal serum concentration and maternal and fetal serum half-life values are about 2 and 3.7 hours, respectively.

Microbiology

Gram-negative—Amikacin is active **in vitro** against **Pseudomonas** species, **Escherichia coli, Proteus** species (indole-posi-

Continued on next page

Bristol—Cont.

tive and indole-negative), **Providencia** species, **Klebsiella-Enterobacter-Serratia** species, **Acinetobacter** (formerly **Mima-Herellea**) species, and **Citrobacter freundii.**
When strains of the above organisms are found to be resistant to other aminoglycosides, including gentamicin, tobramycin and kanamycin, many are susceptible to amikacin **in vitro.**
Gram-positive—Amikacin is active **in vitro** against penicillinase and non-penicillinase-producing **Staphylococcus** species including methicillin-resistant strains. However, aminoglycosides in general have a low order of activity against other Gram-positive organisms; viz, **Streptococcus pyogenes,** enterococci, and **Streptococcus pneumoniae** (formerly **Diplococcus pneumoniae**).
Amikacin resists degradation by most aminoglycoside inactivating enzymes known to affect gentamicin, tobramycin, and kanamycin.
In vitro studies have shown that AMIKIN combined with a beta-lactam antibiotic acts synergistically against many clinically significant gram-negative organisms.
Disc Susceptibility Tests—Quantitative methods that require measurement of zone diameters give the most precise estimates of antibiotic susceptibility. One such procedure* has been recommended for use with discs to test susceptibility to amikacin. Interpretation involves correlation of the diameters obtained in the disc test with MIC values for amikacin. When the causative organism is tested by the Kirby-Bauer method of disc susceptibility, a 30-mcg amikacin disc should give a zone of 17 mm or greater to indicate susceptibility. Zone sizes of 14 mm or less indicate resistance. Zone sizes of 15 to 16 mm indicate intermediate susceptibility. With this procedure, a report from the laboratory of "susceptible" indicates that the infecting organism is likely to respond to therapy. A report of "resistant" indicates that the infecting organism is not likely to respond to therapy. A report of "intermediate susceptibility" suggests that the organism would be susceptible if the infection is confined to tissues and fluids (e.g., urine) in which high antibiotic levels are attained.

INDICATIONS AND USAGE

AMIKIN is indicated in the short-term treatment of serious infections due to susceptible strains of Gram-negative bacteria, including **Pseudomonas** species, **Escherichia coli,** species of indole-positive and indole-negative **Proteus, Providencia** species, **Klebsiella-Enterobacter-Serratia** species, and **Acinetobacter (Mima-Herellea)** species.
Clinical studies have shown AMIKIN to be effective in bacterial septicemia (including neonatal sepsis); in serious infections of the respiratory tract, bones and joints, central nervous system (including meningitis) and skin and soft tissue; intra-abdominal infections (including peritonitis); and in burns and post-operative infections (including post-vascular surgery). Clinical studies have shown AMIKIN also to be effective in serious complicated and recurrent urinary tract infections due to these organisms. Aminoglycosides, including AMIKIN injectable, are not indicated in uncomplicated initial episodes of urinary tract infections unless the causative organisms are not susceptible to antibiotics having less potential toxicity.
Bacteriologic studies should be performed to identify causative organisms and their susceptibilities to amikacin. AMIKIN may be considered as initial therapy in suspected Gram-negative infections and therapy may be instituted before obtaining the results of susceptibility testing. Clinical trials demonstrated that AMIKIN was effective in infections caused by gentamicin and/or tobramycin-resistant strains of Gram-negative organisms, particularly **Proteus rettgeri, Providencia stuartii, Serratia marcescens,** and **Pseudomonas aeruginosa.** The decision to continue therapy with the drug should be based on results of the susceptibility tests, the severity of the infection, the response of the patient and the important additional considerations contained in the "Warning" box above.
AMIKIN has also been shown to be effective in staphylococcal infections and may be considered as initial therapy under certain conditions in the treatment of known or suspected staphylococcal disease such as, severe infections where the causative organism may be either a Gram-negative bacterium or a staphylococcus, infections due to susceptible strains of staphylococci in patients allergic to other antibiotics, and in mixed staphylococcal/Gram-negative infections.
In certain severe infections such as neonatal sepsis, concomitant therapy with a penicillin-type drug may be indicated because of the possibility of infections due to Gram-positive organisms such as streptococci or pneumococci.

CONTRAINDICATIONS

A history of hypersensitivity to amikacin is a contraindication for its use. A history of hypersensitivity or serious toxic reactions to aminoglycosides may contraindicate the use of any other aminoglycoside because of the known cross-sensitivities of patients to drugs in this class.

WARNING

See "Warning" box above.
Aminoglycosides can cause fetal harm when administered to a pregnant woman. Aminoglycosides cross the placenta and there have been several reports of total irreversible, bilateral congenital deafness in children whose mothers received streptomycin during pregnancy. Although serious side effects to the fetus or newborns have not been reported in the treatment of pregnant women with other aminoglycosides, the potential for harm exists. Reproduction studies of amikacin have been performed in rats and mice and revealed no evidence of impaired fertility or harm to the fetus due to amikacin. There are no well controlled studies in pregnant women, but investigational experience does not include any positive evidence of adverse effects to the fetus. If this drug is used during pregnancy, or if the patient becomes pregnant while taking this drug, the patient should be apprised of the potential hazard to the fetus.

PRECAUTIONS

Aminoglycosides are quickly and almost totally absorbed when they are applied topically, except to the urinary bladder, in association with surgical procedures. Irreversible deafness, renal failure, and death due to neuromuscular blockade have been reported following irrigation of both small and large surgical fields with an aminoglycoside preparation.
AMIKIN is potentially nephrotoxic, ototoxic and neurotoxic. The concurrent or serial use of other ototoxic or nephrotoxic agents should be avoided either systemically or topically because of the potential for additive effects. Increased nephrotoxicity has been reported following concomitant parenteral administration of aminoglycoside antibiotics and cephalosporins. Concomitant cephalosporins may spuriously elevate creatinine determinations.
Since AMIKIN is present in high concentrations in the renal excretory system, patients should be well-hydrated to minimize chemical irritation of the renal tubules. Kidney function should be assessed by the usual methods prior to starting therapy and daily during the course of treatment.
If signs of renal irritation appear (casts, white or red cells, or albumin), hydration should be increased. A reduction in dosage (see "Dosage and Administration") may be desirable if other evidence of renal dysfunction occurs such as decreased creatinine clearance; decreased urine specific gravity; increased BUN, creatinine, or oliguria. If azotemia increases or if a progressive decrease in urinary output occurs, treatment should be stopped.
Note: When patients are well-hydrated and kidney function is normal the risk of nephrotoxic reactions with amikacin is low if the dosage recomendations (see "Dosage and Administration") are not exceeded.
Elderly patients may have reduced renal function which may not be evident in routine screening tests such as BUN or serum creatinine. A creatinine clearance determination may be more useful. Monitoring of renal function during treatment with aminoglycosides is particularly important.
Aminoglycosides should be used with caution in patients with muscular disorders such as myasthenia gravis or parkinsonism since these drugs may aggravate muscle weakness because of their potential curare-like effect on the neuromuscular junction.
In vitro mixing of aminoglycosides with beta-lactam antibiotics (penicillin or cephalosporins) may result in a significant mutual inactivation. A reduction in serum half-life or serum level may occur when an aminoglycoside or penicillin-type drug is administered by separate routes. Inactivation of the aminoglycoside is clinically significant only in patients with severely impaired renal function. Inactivation may continue in specimens of body fluids collected for assay, resulting in inaccurate aminoglycoside readings. Such specimens should be properly handled (assayed promptly, frozen, or treated with beta-lactamase).
Cross-allergenicity among aminoglycosides has been demonstrated.
As with other antibiotics, the use of amikacin may result in overgrowth of nonsusceptible organisms. If this occurs, appropriate therapy should be instituted.
Aminoglycosides should not be given concurrently with potent diuretics (See box warning).
Carcinogenesis, Mutagenesis, Impairment of Fertility—Studies in humans have not been performed with the aminoglycosides to determine their effect on carcinogenesis, mutagenesis, or impairment of fertility.
Pregnancy—Category D (See Warning section).
Nursing Mothers—It is not known whether this drug is excreted in human milk. As a general rule, nursing should not be undertaken while a patient is on a drug since many drugs are excreted in human milk.
PEDIATRIC USE—Aminoglycosides should be used with caution in premature and neonatal infants because of the renal immaturity of these patients and the resulting prolongation of serum half-life of these drugs

ADVERSE REACTIONS

All aminoglycosides have the potential to induce auditory, vestibular, and renal toxicity and neuromuscular blockade (see Warning Box). They occur more frequently in patients with present or past history of renal impairment, of treatment with other ototoxic or nephrotoxic drugs, and in patients treated for longer periods and /or with higher doses than recommended.
Neurotoxicity-Ototoxicity—Toxic effects on the eighth cranial nerve can result in hearing loss, loss of balance, or both. Amikacin primarily affects auditory function. Cochlear damage includes high frequency deafness and usually occurs before clinical hearing loss can be detected.
Neurotoxicity-Neuromuscular Blockage—Acute muscular paralysis and apnea can occur following treatment with aminoglycoside drugs.
Nephrotoxicity—Elevation of serum creatinine, albuminuria, presence of red and white cells, casts, azotemia, and oliguria have been reported. Renal function changes are usually reversible when the drug is discontinued.
Other—In addition to those described above, other adverse reactions which have been reported on rare occasions are skin rash, drug fever, headache, paresthesia, tremor, nausea and vomiting, eosinophilia, arthralgia, anemia, and hypotension.
Overdosage—In the event of overdosage or toxic reaction, peritoneal dialysis or hemodialysis will aid in the removal of amikacin from the blood. In the newborn infant, exchange transfusion may also be considered.

DOSAGE AND ADMINISTRATION

The patient's pretreatment body weight should be obtained for calculation of correct dosage. AMIKIN may be given intramuscularly or intravenously.
The status of renal function should be estimated by measurement of the serum creatinine concentration or calculation of the endogenous creatinine clearance rate. The blood urea nitrogen (BUN) is much less reliable for this purpose. Reassessment of renal function should be made periodically during therapy.
Whenever possible, amikacin concentrations in serum should be measured to assure adequate but not excessive levels. It is desirable to measure both peak and trough serum concentrations intermittently during therapy. Peak concentrations (30–90 minutes after injection) above 35 micrograms per ml and trough concentrations (just prior to the next dose) above 10 micrograms per ml should be avoided. Dosage should be adjusted as indicated.
Intramuscular Administration for Patients with Normal Renal Function—The recommended dosage for adults, children and older infants (see box "Warning") with normal renal function is 15 mg/Kg/day divided into 2 or 3 equal doses administered at equally-divided intervals, i.e., 7.5 mg/Kg q.12h or 5 mg/Kg q.8h. Treatment of patients in the heavier weight classes should not exceed 1.5 gram/day.
When amikacin is indicated in newborns (see box "Warning"), it is recommended that a loading dose of 10 mg/Kg be administered initially to be followed with 7.5 mg/Kg every 12 hours.
The usual duration of treatment is 7 to 10 days. It is desirable to limit the duration of treatment to short term whenever feasible. The total daily dose by all routes of administration should not exceed 15 mg/Kg/day. In difficult and complicated infections where treatment beyond 10 days is considered, the use of AMIKIN should be reevaluated. If continued, amikacin serum levels, and renal, auditory, and vestibular functions should be monitored. At the recommended dosage level, uncomplicated infections due to amikacin-sensitive organisms should respond in 24 to 48 hours. If definite clinical response does not occur within 3 to 5 days, therapy should be stopped and the antibiotic susceptibility pattern of the invading organism should be rechecked. Failure of the infection to respond may be due to resistance of the organsim or to the presence of septic foci requiring surgical drainage.
When AMIKIN is indicated in uncomplicated urinary tract infections, a dose of 250 mg twice daily may be used.
[See table on next page].
Intramuscular Administration for Patients with Impaired Renal Function—Whenever possible, serum amikacin concentrations should be monitored by appropriate assay procedures. Doses may be adjusted in patients with impaired renal function either by administering normal doses at prolonged intervals or by administering reduced doses at a fixed interval.
Both methods are based on the patient's creatinine clearance or serum creatinine values since these have been found to correlate with aminoglycoside half-lives in patients with diminished renal function. These dosage schedules must be used in conjunction with careful clinical and laboratory observations of the patient and should be modified as necessary. Neither method should be used when dialysis is being performed.
Normal Dosage at Prolonged Intervals—If the creatinine clearance rate is not available and the patient's condition is stable, a dosage interval in hours for the normal dose can be

DOSAGE GUIDELINES

ADULTS AND CHILDREN WITH NORMAL RENAL FUNCTION

Patient Weight		Dosage		
lbs.	kg	7.5 mg/kg q. 12h	OR	5mg/kg q. 8h
99	45	337.5 mg		225 mg
110	50	375 mg		250 mg
121	55	412.5 mg		275 mg
132	60	450 mg		300 mg
143	65	487.5 mg		325 mg
154	70	525 mg		350 mg
165	75	562.6 mg		375 mg
176	80	600 mg		400 mg
187	85	637.5 mg		425 mg
198	90	675 mg		450 mg
209	95	712.5 mg		475 mg
220	100	750 mg		500 mg

Available as: 100 mg/2 ml vial, 500 mg/2 ml vial, 1g/4 ml vial, 500 mg/2 ml Disposable Syringe

calculated by multiplying the patient's serum creatinine by 9, e.g., if the serum creatinine concentration is 2 mg/100 ml, the recommended single dose (7.5 mg/Kg) should be administered every 18 hours.

Reduced Dosage at Fixed Time Intervals—When renal function is impaired and it is desirable to administer AMIKIN at a fixed time interval, dosage must be reduced. In these patients serum AMIKIN concentrations should be measured to assure accurate administration of AMIKIN and to avoid concentrations above 35 mcg/ml. If serum assay determinations are not available and the patient's condition is stable, serum creatinine and creatinine clearance values are the most readily available indicators of the degree of renal impairment to use as a guide for dosage.

First, initiate therapy by administering a normal dose, 7.5 mg/Kg, as a loading dose. This loading dose is the same as the normally recommended dose which would be calculated for a patient with a normal renal function as described above.

To determine the size of maintenance doses administered every 12 hours, the loading dose should be reduced in proportion to the reduction in the patient's creatinine clearance rate:

$$\text{Maintenance Dose Every 12 hours} = \frac{\text{observed CC in ml/min}}{\text{normal CC in ml/min}} \times \text{calculated loading dose in mg}$$

(CC—creatinine clearance rate)

An alternate rough guide for determining reduced dosage at 12 hour intervals (for patients whose steady state serum creatinine values are known) is to divide the normally recommended dose by the patient's serum creatinine.

The above dosage schedules are not intended to be rigid recommendations but are provided as guides to dosage when the measurement of amikacin serum levels is not feasible.

Intravenous Administration—The individual dose, the total daily dose, and the total cumulative dose of AMIKIN are identical to the dose recommended for intramuscular administration. The solution for intravenous use is prepared by adding the contents of a 0.5 gram vial to 100–200 ml of sterile diluent such as Normal Saline or 5% Dextrose in Water or any other compatible solution.

The solution is administered to adults over a 30 to 60 minute period. The total daily dose should not exceed 15 mg/Kg/day and may be divided into either 2 or 3 equally-divided doses at equally-divided intervals.

In pediatric patients the amount of fluid used will depend on the amount ordered for the patient. It should be a sufficient amount to infuse the amikacin over a 30 to 60 minute period. Infants should receive a 1 to 2 hour infusion.

Amikacin should not be physically premixed with other drugs but should be administered separately according to the recommended dose and route.

Stability in IV Fluids—AMIKIN is stable for 24 hours at room temperature at concentrations of 0.25 and 5.0 mg/ml in the following solutions:

5% Dextrose Injection, USP
5% Dextrose and 0.2% Sodium Chloride Injection, USP
5% Dextrose and 0.45% Sodium Chloride Injection, USP
0.9% Sodium Chloride Injection, USP
Lactated Ringer's Injection, USP
Normosol®M in 5% Dextrose Injection, USP (or Plasma-Lyte 56 Injection in 5% Dextrose in Water)
Normosol®R in 5% Dextrose Injection, USP (or Plasma-Lyte 148 Injection in 5% Dextrose in Water)

In the above solutions with AMIKIN concentrations of 0.25 and 5.0 mg/ml, solutions aged for 60 days at 4°C and then stored at 25°C had utility times of 24 hours.

At the same concentrations, solutions frozen and aged for 30 days at −15°C, thawed, and stored at 25°C had utility times of 24 hours.

Parenteral drug products should be inspected visually for particulate matter and discoloration prior to administration whenever the solution and container permit.

Aminoglycosides administered by any of the above routes should not be physically premixed with other drugs but should be administered separately.

Because of the potential toxicity of aminoglycosides, "fixed dosage" recommendations which are not based upon body weight are not advised. Rather, it is essential to calculate the dosage to fit the needs of each patient.

SUPPLY

AMIKIN is supplied as a colorless solution which requires no refrigeration. It is stable at room temperature for at least two years. At times the solution may become a very pale yellow; this does not indicate a decrease in potency.

AMIKIN (amikacin sulfate injection)
NDC 0015-3015-20—100 mg per 2 ml
NDC 0015-3020-20—500 mg per 2 ml
NDC 0015-3020-21—Disposable Syringe (500 mg per 2 ml)
NDC 0015-3023-20—1 gram per 4 ml

*Bauer, A. W., Kirby, W. M. M., Sherris, J. C., and Turck, M.: Antibiotic Testing by a Standardized Single Disc Method, Am. J. Clin. Pathol. 45:493, 1966; Standardized Disc Susceptibility Test, FEDERAL REGISTER, 37:20527–29, 1972.

3015DIM-09 December 1985

BETAPEN®-VK ℞

(penicillin V potassium)
Tablets (Film Coated) and Oral Solution

This is the full text of the latest Official Package Circular dated February 1985 [7506 DIR-08].

DESCRIPTION

Betapen-VK is the potassium salt of penicillin V. The oral solutions contain in each 5 ml. (teaspoonful) 125 mg. or 250 mg. of penicillin V activity, respectively.

Inactive ingredients in Betapen-VK tablets are: Carbowax 8000, carnauba wax, ethyl cellulose, lactose, magnesium stearate, methanol, methyl cellulose, opaspray white, starch and white wax.

Inactive ingredients in Betapen-VK oral solution are: acacia, citric acid, DL-Menthol, FD & C Red No. 40, natural & artificial flavorings, sodium benzoate, sodium citrate, sodium saccharin, sucrose and thymol.

CLINICAL PHARMACOLOGY

Penicillin V exerts a bactericidal action against penicillin-susceptible microorganisms during the stage of active multiplication. It acts through the inhibition of biosynthesis of cell wall mucopeptide. It is not active against the penicillinase-producing bacteria, which include many strains of staphylococci. The drug exerts high **in vitro** activity against staphylococci (except penicillinase-producing strains), streptococci (Groups A, C, G, H, L, and M) and pneumococci. Other organisms susceptible **in vitro** to penicillin V are **Corynebacterium diphtheriae, Bacillus anthracis,** Clostridia, **Actinomyces bovis, Streptobacillus moniliformis, Listeria monocytogenes,** Leptospira and **Neisseria gonorrhoeae. Treponema pallidum** is extremely susceptible.

Penicillin V has the distinct advantage over penicillin G in resistance to inactivation by gastric acid. It may be given with meals; however, blood levels are slightly higher when the drug is given on an empty stomach. Average blood levels are two to five times higher than the levels following the same dose of oral penicillin G and also show much less individual variation.

Once absorbed, penicillin V is about 80% bound to serum protein. Tissue levels are highest in the kidney, with lesser amounts in the liver, skin, and intestines. Small amounts are found in all other body tissues and the cerebrospinal fluid. The drug is excreted as rapidly as it is absorbed in individuals with normal renal function; however, recovery of the drug from the urine indicates that only about 25% of the dose is absorbed. In neonates, young infants, and individuals with impaired renal function, excretion is considerably delayed.

INDICATIONS AND USAGE

Betapen-VK is indicated in the treatment of mild to moderately severe infections due to penicillin G-susceptible microorganisms. Therapy should be guided by bacteriological studies (including susceptibility tests) and by clinical response.

Note: Severe pneumonia, empyema, bacteremia, pericarditis, meningitis, and arthritis should not be treated with oral penicillins during the acute stage.

Indicated surgical procedures should be performed.

The following infections will usually respond to adequate doses of penicillin V: Streptococcal Infections (without bacteremia), mild to moderate infections of the upper respiratory tract, scarlet fever, and mild erysipelas.

Note: Streptococci in Groups A, C, G, H, L, and M are very susceptible to penicillin. Other groups, including Group D (Enterococcus) are resistant.

Pneumococcal Infections—Mild to moderately severe infections of the respiratory tract.

Staphylococcal Infections — penicillin G-susceptible. Mild infections of the skin and soft tissue.

Note: Reports indicate an increasing number of strains of staphylococci resistant to penicillin G, emphasizing the need for culture and susceptibility studies in treating suspected staphylococcal infections.

Fusospirochetosis (Vincent's gingivitis and pharyngitis) —Mild to moderately severe infections of the oropharynx usually respond to therapy with oral penicillin.

Note: Necessary dental care should be accomplished in infections involving gum tissue.

Medical conditions in which oral penicillin therapy is indicated as prophylaxis: For the prevention of recurrence following rheumatic fever and/or chorea. Prophylaxis with oral penicillin on a continuing basis has proven effective in preventing recurrence of these conditions.

Although no controlled clinical efficacy studies have been conducted, penicillin V has been suggested by the American Heart Association and the American Dental Association for use as part of a parenteral-oral regimen and as an alternative oral regimen for prophylaxis against bacterial endocarditis in patients with congenital heart disease or rheumatic or other acquired valvular heart disease when they undergo dental procedures and surgical procedures of the respiratory tract.[1] Since it may happen that **alpha**-hemolytic streptococci, relatively resistant to penicillin, may be found when patients are receiving continuous oral penicillin for secondary prevention of rheumatic fever, prophylactic agents other than penicillin may be chosen for these patients and prescribed in addition to their continuous rheumatic fever prophylactic regimen. Oral penicillin should not be used as adjunctive prophylaxis for genitourinary instrumentation or surgery, lower intestinal tract surgery, sigmoidoscopy, and childbirth.

Note: When selecting antibiotics for the prevention of bacterial endocarditis, the physician or dentist should read the full joint statement of the American Heart Association and the American Dental Association.[1]

CONTRAINDICATIONS

A previous hypersensitivity reaction to any penicillin is a contraindication.

WARNING

Serious and occasionally fatal hypersensitivity (anaphylactoid) reactions have been reported in patients on penicillin therapy. Although anaphylaxis is more frequent following parenteral therapy, it has occurred in patients on oral penicillins. These reactions are more apt to occur in individuals with a history of sensitivity to multiple allergens.

There have been well documented reports of individuals with a history of penicillin hypersensitivity reactions who experienced severe hypersensitivity reactions when treated with cephalosporins. Before therapy with a penicillin, careful inquiry should be made concerning previous hypersensitivity reactions to penicillins, cephalosporins, and other allergens. If an allergic reaction occurs, the drug should be discontinued and the patient treated with the usual agents, e.g., antihistamines, pressor amines, corticosteroids.

PRECAUTIONS

Penicillins should be used with caution in individuals with a history of significant allergies and/or asthma.

The oral route of administration should not be relied upon in patients with severe illness, or with nausea, vomiting, gastric dilatation, cardiospasm or intestinal hypermotility.

Continued on next page

Bristol—Cont.

Occasional patients will not absorb therapeutic amounts of orally administered penicillins.
In streptococcal infections, therapy must be sufficient to eliminate the organism (10 days minimum); otherwise the sequelae of streptococcal disease may occur. Cultures should be taken following completion of treatment to determine whether streptococci have been eradicated.
Prolonged use of antibiotics may promote the overgrowth of nonsusceptible organisms, including fungi. Should superinfection occur, appropriate measures should be taken.

ADVERSE REACTIONS

Although the incidence of reactions to oral penicillins has been reported with much less frequency than following parenteral therapy, it should be remembered that all degrees of hypersensitivity, including fatal anaphylaxis, have been reported with oral penicillin.
The most common reactions to oral penicillin are nausea, vomiting, epigastric distress, diarrhea, and black hairy tongue. The hypersensitivity reactions reported are skin eruptions (maculopapular to exfoliative dermatitis), urticaria and other serum sickness reactions, laryngeal edema and anaphylaxis. Fever and eosinophilia may frequently be the only reaction observed. Hemolytic anemia, leukopenia, thrombocytopenia, neuropathy, and nephropathy are infrequent reactions and usually associated with high doses of parenteral penicillin.

ADMINISTRATION AND DOSAGE

The dosage of Betapen-VK should be determined according to the susceptibility of the causative organism and the severity of infection, and adjusted to the clinical response of the patient.
The usual dosage recommendations for adults and children 12 years and over are as follows:
Streptococcal Infections—mild to moderately severe—of the upper respiratory tract and including scarlet fever and erysipelas: 125 to 250 mg. (200,000 to 400,000 units) every 6 to 8 hours for 10 days.
Pneumococcal Infections—mild to moderately severe—of the respiratory tract, including otitis media: 250 mg. (400,000 units) every 6 hours until the patient has been afebrile for at least 2 days.
Staphylococcal Infections—mild infections of skin and soft tissue (culture and susceptibility tests should be performed): 250 mg. (400,000 units) every 6 to 8 hours.
Fusospirochetosis (Vincent's Infection) of the oropharynx —mild to moderately severe infections: 250 mg. (400,000 units) every 6 to 8 hours.
For the prevention of recurrence following rheumatic fever and/or chorea: 125 mg. (200,000 units) twice daily on a continuing basis.
For prophylaxis against bacterial endocarditis[1] in patients with congenital heart disease or rheumatic or other acquired valvular heart disease when undergoing dental procedures or surgical procedures of the upper respiratory tract, 1 of 2 regimens may be selected:

(1) For the oral regimen, give 2 grams of penicillin V (1 gram for children under 60 lbs) ½ to 1 hour before the procedure, and then, 500 mg (250 mg for children under 60 lbs) every 6 hours for 8 doses; or
(2) For the combined parenteral-oral regimen, give 1 million units of aqueous crystalline penicillin G (30,000 units/kg in children) intramuscularly mixed with 600,000 units procaine penicillin G (600,000 units for children) ½ to 1 hour before the procedure, and then, oral penicillin V, 500 mg for adults or 250 mg for children less than 60 lbs, every 6 hours for 8 doses. Doses for children should not exceed recommendations for adults for a single dose or for a 24-hour period.

DIRECTIONS FOR DISPENSING ORAL SOLUTIONS

Prepare this formulation at the time of dispensing. For ease in preparation, add water to the bottle in two portions and shake well after each addition. Add the total amount of water as directed on the labeling of the package being dispensed. The reconstituted solutions are stable for 14 days under refrigeration.

HOW SUPPLIED

BETAPEN-VK (penicillin V potassium) for Oral Solution. Each 5 ml. of reconstituted solution contains penicillin V potassium equivalent to 125 or 250 mg. penicillin V.
NDC 0015-7506—125 mg
NDC 0015-7507—250 mg
BETAPEN-VK (penicillin V potassium) Tablets (Film Coated). Each tablet contains penicillin V potassium equivalent to 250 or 500 mg. penicillin V.
NDC 0015-7508-250 mg.
NDC 0015-7509-500 mg.
For information on package sizes available, refer to the current price schedule.

Reference:
1. American Heart Association. 1977. Prevention of bacterial endocarditis. Circulation. 56:139A-143A.
Shown in Product Identification Section, page 406

CEFADYL® ℞
[cef-a-dill]
(sterile cephapirin sodium)

This is the full text of the latest Official Package Circular dated October 1983 [7628DIR-25].

DESCRIPTION

Cefadyl (sterile cephapirin sodium) is a cephalosporin antibiotic intended for intramuscular or intravenous administration only. Each 500 mg contains 1.18 milli-equivalents of sodium.
Cefadyl is the sodium salt of 7-α-(4-pyridylthio)-acetamidocephalosporanic acid and has the following structural formula.

[structural formula: pyridyl–S-CH₂-C(=O)-NH– cephem nucleus with CH₂-O-C(=O)-CH₃ and CO₂Na]

CLINICAL PHARMACOLOGY

Human Pharmacology

TABLE I

Duration of Blood Levels of Cephapirin in Normal Volunteers (Figures are mcg/ml)

	Time After Injection in Hours		
	½	4	6
Cefadyl 500 mg. I.M. (single dose)	9.0	0.7	0.2
Cefadyl 1 gram I.M. (single dose)	16.4	1.0	0.3

Cefadyl and its metabolites were excreted primarily by the kidneys. Antibiotic activity in the urine was equivalent to 35% of a 500-mg dose 6 hours after I.M. injection, and to 65% of a 500-mg dose 12 hours after injection. Following an I.M. dose of 500 mg, peak urine levels averaged 900 mcg/ml within the first 6 hours.

TABLE II

Duration of Blood Levels of Cephapirin in Normal Volunteers (Figures are mcg/ml)

	Time After Injection in Minutes		
	5	30	180
Cefadyl 500 mg rapid I.V.	35	6.7	0.27
Cefadyl 1 gram rapid I.V.	67	14.0	0.61
Cefadyl 2 gram rapid I.V.	129	31.7	1.11

Seventy percent of the administered dose was recovered in the urine within 6 hours.
Repetitive intravenous administration of 1-gram doses over 6-hour periods produced serum levels between 4.5 and 5.5 mcg/ml.
At therapeutic drug levels, normal human serum binds Cefadyl to the extent of 44 to 50%. The average serum half-life of Cefadyl in patients with normal renal function is approximately 36 minutes.
The major metabolite of cephapirin is desacetyl cephapirin which has been shown to contribute to antibacterial activity.
Controlled studies in normal adult volunteers revealed that Cefadyl was well tolerated intramuscularly. In controlled studies of volunteers and of patients receiving I.V. Cefadyl, the incidence of venous irritation was low.

Microbiology

In vitro tests demonstrate that the action of cephalosporins results from inhibition of cell-wall synthesis. Cefadyl is active against the following organisms **in vitro:**

Beta-hemolytic streptococci and other streptococci.
(Many strains of enterococci, e.g. **S. faecalis**, are relatively resistant.)
Staphylococcus aureus (penicillinase and nonpenicillinase-producing).
Staphylococcus epidermidis (methicillin-susceptible strains).
Streptococcus pneumoniae
(formerly **Diplococcus pneumoniae)**
Proteus mirabilis
Haemophilus influenzae
Escherichia coli
Klebsiella species

Most strains of Enterobacter and indole-positive Proteus (**P. vulgaris, P. morganii, P. rettgeri**) are resistant to Cefadyl. Methicillin-resistant staphylococci, Serratia, Pseudomonas, Mima, and Herellea species are almost uniformly resistant to Cefadyl.
Disc Susceptibility Tests. — Quantitative methods that require measurement of zone diameters give the most precise estimates of antibiotic susceptibility. One such procedure* has been recommended for use with discs for testing susceptibility to cephalosporin class antibiotics. Interpretations correlate diameters of the disc test with MIC values for Cefadyl. With this procedure, a report from the laboratory of "susceptible" indicates that the infecting organism is likely to respond to therapy. A report of "resistant" indicates that the infecting organism is not likely to respond to therapy. A report of "intermediate susceptibility" suggests that the organism would be susceptible if high dosage is used, or if the infection is confined to tissues and fluid (e.g., urine), in which high antibiotic levels are attained.

INDICATIONS

Cefadyl is indicated in the treatment of infections caused by susceptible strains of the designated microorganisms in the diseases listed below. Culture and susceptibility studies should be performed. Therapy may be instituted before results of susceptibility studies are obtained.
Respiratory tract infections caused by **S. pneumoniae** (formerly **D. pneumoniae**); **Staphylococcus aureus** (penicillinase and nonpenicillinase-producing), Klebsiella species, **H. influenzae** and Group A beta-hemolytic streptococci.
Skin and skin structure infections caused by **Staphylococcus aureus** (penicillinase and nonpenicillinase-producing), **Staphylococcus epidermidis** (methicillin-susceptible strains), **E. coli, P. mirabilis,** Klebsiella species, and Group A beta-hemolytic streptococci.
Urinary tract infections caused by **Staphylococcus aureus** (penicillinase and nonpenicillinase-producing), **E. coli, P. mirabilis,** and Klebsiella species.
Septicemia caused by **Staphylococcus aureus** (penicillinase and nonpenicillinase-producing), **S. viridans, E. coli,** Klebsiella species and Group A beta-hemolytic streptococci.
Endocarditis caused by **Streptococcus viridans** and **Staphylococcus aureus** (penicillinase and nonpenicillinase-producing).
Osteomyelitis caused by **Staphylococcus aureus** (penicillinase and nonpenicillinase-producing), Klebsiella species, **P. mirabilis,** and Group A beta-hemolytic streptococci.
Perioperative Prophylaxis—The prophylactic administration of Cefadyl preoperatively and postoperatively may reduce the incidence of certain postoperative infections in patients undergoing surgical procedures which are classified as contaminated or potentially contaminated, e.g., vaginal hysterectomy.
The perioperative use of Cefadyl may also be effective in surgical patients in whom infection at the operative site would present a serious risk, e.g., during open-heart surgery and prosthetic arthroplasty.
The prophylactic administration of Cefadyl should be discontinued within a 24 hour period after the surgical procedure. In surgery where the occurrence of infection may be particularly devastating, e.g., open-heart surgery and prosthetic arthroplasty, the prophylactic administration of Cefadyl may be continued for 3 to 5 days following completion of surgery. If there are signs of infection, specimens for culture should be obtained for the identification of the causative organism so that appropriate therapy may be instituted (See Dosage and Administration.)
Note: If the susceptibility tests show that the causative organism is resistant to Cefadyl, other appropriate therapy should be instituted.

CONTRAINDICATIONS

Cefadyl is contraindicated in persons who have shown hypersensitivity to cephalosporin antibiotics.

WARNINGS

IN PENICILLIN-ALLERGIC PATIENTS, CEPHALOSPORINS SHOULD BE USED WITH GREAT CAUTION. THERE IS CLINICAL AND LABORATORY EVIDENCE OF PARTIAL CROSS-ALLERGENICITY OF THE PENICILLINS AND THE CEPHALOSPORINS, AND THERE ARE INSTANCES OF PATIENTS WHO HAVE HAD REACTIONS TO BOTH DRUGS (INCLUDING ANAPHYLAXIS AFTER PARENTERAL USE).
Any patient who has demonstrated some form of allergy, particularly to drugs, should receive antibiotics cautiously and then only when absolutely necessary. No exceptions should be made with regard to Cefadyl.

SERIOUS ANAPHYLACTOID REACTIONS REQUIRE IMMEDIATE EMERGENCY TREATMENT WITH EPINEPHRINE. OXYGEN, INTRAVENOUS STEROIDS, AND AIRWAY MANAGEMENT, INCLUDING INTUBATION, SHOULD ALSO BE ADMINISTERED AS INDICATED.

PRECAUTIONS

Usage in Pregnancy—Pregnancy Category B. Reproduction studies have been performed in rats and mice and have revealed no evidence of impaired fertility or harm to the fetus due to Cefadyl. There are however no well controlled studies in pregnant women. Because animal studies are not always predictive of human response, this drug should be used during pregnancy only if clearly indicated.

Nursing Mothers—Cefadyl may be present in human milk in small amounts. Caution should be exercised when Cefadyl is administered to a nursing woman.

The renal status of the patients should be determined prior to and during Cefadyl therapy, since in patients with impaired renal function, a reduced dose may be appropriate (see Dosage, Adults). When Cefadyl was given to patients with marked reduction in renal function and to renal transplant patients, no adverse effects were reported.

Prolonged use of Cefadyl may result in the overgrowth of nonsusceptible organisms. Careful observation of the patient is essential. If superinfection occurs during therapy, appropriate measures should be taken.

With high urine concentrations of cephapirin, false-positive glucose reactions may occur if Clinitest, Benedict's Solution, or Fehling's Solution are used. Therefore, it is recommended that glucose tests based on enzymatic glucose oxidase reactions (such as Clinistix or Tes-Tape) be used.

Increased nephrotoxicity has been reported following concomitant administration of cephalosporins and aminoglycoside antibiotics.

ADVERSE REACTIONS

Hypersensitivity—Cephalosporins were reported to produce the following reactions: maculopapular rash, urticaria, reactions resembling serum sickness, and anaphylaxis. Eosinophilia and drug fever have been observed to be associated with other allergic reactions. These reactions are most likely to occur in patients with a history of allergy, particularly to penicillin.

Blood—During large scale clinical trials, rare instances of neutropenia, leukopenia, and anemia were reported. Some individuals, particularly those with azotemia, have developed positive direct Coombs' test during therapy with other cephalosporins.

Liver—Elevations in SGPT or SGOT, alkaline phosphatase, and bilirubin have been reported.

Kidney—Rises in BUN have been observed; their frequency increases in patients over 50 years old.

DOSAGE AND ADMINISTRATION

Adults—The usual dose is 500 mg to 1 gram every 4 to 6 hours intramuscularly or intravenously. The lower dose of 500 mg is adequate for certain infections, such as skin and skin structure and most urinary tract infections. However, the higher dose is recommended for more serious infections. Very serious or life-threatening infections may require doses up to 12 grams daily. The intravenous route is preferable when high doses are indicated.

Depending upon the causative organism and the severity of infection, patients with reduced renal function (moderately severe oliguria or serum creatinine above 5.0 mg/100 ml) may be treated adequately with a lower dose, 7.5 to 15 mg/Kg of cephapirin every 12 hours. Patients with severely reduced renal function and who are to be dialyzed should receive the same dose just prior to dialysis and every 12 hours thereafter.

Perioperative Prophylactic Use—To prevent postoperative infection in contaminated or potentially contaminated surgery. Recommended doses are:

a. 1 to 2 grams IM or IV administered ½ hour to 1 hour prior to the start of surgery.
b. 1 to 2 grams during surgery (administration modified depending on the duration of the operative procedure).
c. 1 to 2 grams IV or IM every 6 hours for 24 hours postoperatively.

It is important (1) the preoperative dose be given just prior to the start of surgery (½ to 1 hour) so that adequate antibiotic levels are present in the serum and tissues at the time of initial surgical incision, and (2) Cefadyl be administered, if necessary, at appropriate intervals during surgery to provide sufficient levels of the antibiotic at the anticipated moments of greatest exposure to infective organisms.

In surgery where the occurrence of infection may be particularly devastating, e.g., open-heart surgery and prosthetic arthroplasty, the prophylactic administration of Cefadyl may be continued for 3 to 5 days following completion of surgery.

Children—The dosage is in accordance with age, weight, and severity of infection. The recommended total daily dose is 40 to 80 mg/Kg (20 to 40 mg/lb) administered in four equally divided doses.

The drug has not been extensively studied in infants, therefore, in the treatment of children under the age of three months the relative benefit/ risk should be considered.

Therapy in beta-hemolytic streptococcal infections should continue for at least 10 days.

Where indicated surgical procedures should be performed in conjunction with antibiotic therapy. Cefadyl may be administered by the intramuscular or the intravenous routes.

Intramuscular Injection

The 500-mg and 1-gram vials should be reconstituted with 1 or 2 ml of Sterile Water for Injection, U.S.P., or Bacteriostatic Water for Injection, U.S.P., respectively. Each 1.2 ml contains 500 mg of cephapirin. All injections should be deep in the muscle mass.

Intravenous Injection

The intravenous route may be preferable for patients with bacteremia, septicemia, or other severe or life-threatening infections who may be poor risks because of lowered resistance resulting from such debilitating conditions as malnutrition, trauma, surgery, diabetes, heart failure, or malignancy, particularly if shock is present or impending. If patient has impaired renal function, a reduced dose may be indicated (see Dosage, Adults). In conditions such as septicemia, 6 to 8 grams per day may be given intravenously for several days at the beginning of therapy; then, depending on the clinical response and laboratory findings, the dosage may gradually be reduced.

When the infection has been refractory to previous forms of treatment and multiple sites have been involved, daily doses up to 12 grams have been used.

Intermittent Intravenous Injection

The contents of the 500-mg, 1-gram or 2-gram vial should be diluted with 10 ml or more of the specified diluent and administered slowly over a 3- to 5-minute period or may be given with intravenous infusions.

Intermittent Intravenous Infusion with Y-Tube

Intermittent intravenous infusion with a Y-type administration set can also be accomplished while bulk intravenous solutions are being infused. However, during infusion of the solution containing Cefadyl it is desirable to discontinue the other solution. When this technique is employed, careful attention should be paid to the volume of the solution containing Cefadyl so that the calculated dose will be infused. When a Y-tube hookup is used, the contents of the 4-gram vial of cephapirin should be diluted by addition of 40 ml of Bacteriostatic Water for Injection, U.S.P., Dextrose Injection, U.S.P., or Sodium Chloride Injection, U.S.P.

STABILITY

Utility Time For Cefadyl In Various Diluents At Concentrations Ranging From 20 to 400 mg/ml

Diluent	Approximate Concentration (mg/ml)	Utility Time 25°C	4°C
Water for Injection	50 to 400	12 hours	10 days
Bacteriostatic Water for Injection with Benzyl Alcohol or Parabens	250 to 400	48 hours	10 days
Normal Saline	20 to 100	24 hours	10 days
5% Dextrose in Water	20 to 100	24 hours	10 days

All of the above solutions can be frozen immediately after reconstitution and stored at −15°C for 60 days before use. After thawing at room temperature (25°C), all of the solutions are stable for at least 12 hours at room temperature or 10 days under refrigeration (4°C).

The pH of the resultant solution ranges from 6.5 to 8.5. During these storage conditions, no precipitation occurs. A change in solution color during this storage time does not affect the potency.

Compatibility with the Infusion Solution

Cefadyl is stable and compatible for 24 hours at room temperature at concentrations between 2 mg/ml and 30 mg/ml in the following solutions.

Sodium Chloride Injection, U.S.P.
5% W/V Dextrose in Water, U.S.P.
Sodium Lactate Injection, U.S.P.
5% Dextrose in Normal Saline, U.S.P.
10% Invert Sugar in Normal Saline
10% Invert Sugar in Water
5% Dextrose + 0.2% Sodium Chloride Injection, U.S.P.
Lactated Ringer's Injection, U.S.P.
Lactated Ringer's with 5% Dextrose
5% Dextrose + 0.45% Sodium Chloride Injection, U.S.P.
Ringer's Injection, U.S.P.
10% Dextrose Injection, U.S.P.
Sterile Water for Injection, U.S.P.
20% Dextrose Injection, U.S.P.
5% Sodium Chloride in Water
5% Dextrose in Ringer's Injection
Normosol® R
Normosol® R in 5% Dextrose Injection
Ionosol® D-CM
Ionosol® G in 10% Dextrose Injection

In addition, Cefadyl, at a concentration of 4 mg/ml, is stable and compatible for 10 days under refrigeration (4°C) or 14 days in the frozen state (15°C) followed by 24 hours at room temperature (25°C) in all of the intravenous solutions listed above.

"Piggyback" I.V. Package:

This glass vial contains the labeled quantity of Cefadyl and is intended for intravenous administration. The diluent and volume are specified on the label.

Hospital Bulk Package:

This glass vial contains 20 grams Cefadyl and is designed for use in the pharmacy in preparing I.V. additives. Add 67 ml of Sodium Chloride Injection, U.S.P., or Dextrose Injection, U.S.P. The resulting solution will contain 250 mg cephapirin activity per ml. Following reconstitution in this manner, the solutions are stable for 24 hours at room temperature or 10 days under refrigeration.

Caution: Not to be dispensed as a unit.

SUPPLY

Cefadyl (Sterile Cephapirin Sodium) for I.M. or I.V. Injection. Cephapirin sodium equivalent to 500 mg, 1 gram, 2 grams, 4 grams, or 20 grams cephapirin.

NDC 0015-7627-28—500-mg vial
NDC 0015-7628-28—1-gram vial
NDC 0015-7629-30—2-gram vial
NDC 0015-7628-22—1-gram "piggyback" vial
NDC 0015-7629-28—2-gram "piggyback" vial
NDC 0015-7630-20—4-gram "piggyback" vial
NDC 0015-7613-20—20-gram Hospital Bulk Package

For information on package sizes available, refer to the current price schedule.

---

*Bauer, A. W., Kirby, W. M. M., Sherris, J. C. and Turck, M.: Antibiotic Testing by a Standardized Single Disc Method, Am. J. Clin. Pathol., 45:493, 1966; Standardized Disc Susceptibility Test, FEDERAL REGISTER 37:20527–29, 1972.

DYNAPEN® ℞

[dīn'ō-pĕn]
(dicloxacillin sodium)

DICLOXACILLIN SODIUM CAPSULES
125 mg, 250 mg and 500 mg

DICLOXACILLIN SODIUM FOR ORAL SUSPENSION
62.5 mg per 5 ml

This is the full text of the latest official Package Circular dated February 1985 [7856DIR-12].

DESCRIPTION

Dynapen (dicloxacillin sodium) is an antibacterial agent of the isoxazolyl penicillin series. It is a penicillinase-resistant, acid resistant semisynthetic penicillin suitable for oral administration. Dynapen is available as an oral suspension and capsules.

Inactive ingredient in Dynapen capsules is magnesium stearate (may also contain lactose).

Inactive ingredients in Dynapen oral suspension are: avicel, cetyl esters wax, ethyl cellulose, FD & C Red No. 40, kaolin, natural & artificial flavorings, sodium benzoate, sodium chloride, sodium citrate, sodium saccharin and sucrose.

DICLOXACILLIN SODIUM

$C_{19}H_{16}Cl_2N_3NaO_5S \cdot H_2O$ 510.32 [CAS-13412 64-1] 4-Thia-1-azabicyclo [3·2·0]heptane-2-carboxylic acid,6-[[[3-(2,6-dichlorophenyl)-5-methyl-4-isoxazolyl]carbonyl]-amino]-3,3-dimethyl-7-oxo-,monosodium salt, monohydrate, [2S-(2α, 5α, 6β)]

CLINICAL PHARMACOLOGY

Microbiology. Penicillinase-resistant penicillins exert a bactericidal action against penicillin-susceptible microorganisms during the state of active multiplication. All penicillins inhibit the biosynthesis of the bacterial cell wall.

The drugs in this class are highly resistant to inactivation by staphylococcal penicillinase and are active against penicillinase producing and non-penicillinase producing strains of

Continued on next page

Bristol—Cont.

Staphylococcus aureus. The penicillinase-resistant penicillins are active **in vitro** against a variety of other bacteria.

Susceptibility Plate Testing. Quantitative methods of susceptibility testing that require measurement of zone diameters or minimal inhibitory concentrations (M.I.C.'s) give the most precise estimates of antibiotic susceptibility. One such procedure has been recommended for use with discs to test susceptibility to this class of drugs.

Interpretations correlate diameters on the disc test with MIC values. A penicillinase-resistant class disc may be used to determine microbial susceptibility to cloxacillin, dicloxacillin, methicillin, nafcillin, and oxacillin. With this procedure, employing a 5 microgram methicillin sodium disc, a report from the laboratory of "susceptible" (zone of at least 14 mm) indicates that the infecting organism is likely to respond to therapy. A report of "resistant" (zone of less than 10 mm) indicates that the infecting organism is not likely to respond to therapy. A report of "intermediate susceptibility" (zone of 10–13 mm) suggests that the organism might be susceptible if high doses of the antibiotic are used, or if the infection is confined to tissues and fluids (e.g., urine), in which high antibiotic levels are attained.

In general, all staphylococci should be tested against the penicillin G disc and against the methicillin disc. Routine methods of antibiotic susceptibility testing may fail to detect strains of organisms resistant to the penicillinase-resistant penicillins. For this reason, the use of large inocula and 48-hour incubation periods may be necessary to obtain accurate susceptibility studies with these antibiotics. Bacterial strains which are resistant to one of the penicillinase-resistant penicillins should be considered resistant to all of the drugs in the class.

Pharmacokinetics. Dynapen (dicloxacillin sodium) is resistant to destruction by acid. Absorption of Dynapen after oral administration is rapid but incomplete. Studies with an oral dose of 125 mg gave average serum levels at 60 minutes of 4.74 mcg/ml. At four hours, average levels were 0.62 mcg/ml. In one study, single oral doses of Dynapen 500 mg produced peak serum concentrations of 10–17 mcg/ml at 1–1.5 hours.

Once absorbed, Dynapen (dicloxacillin sodium) binds to serum protein, mainly albumin. The degree of protein binding reported varies with the method of study and the investigator, but generally has been found to be $97.9 \pm 0.6\%$. Oral absorption of dicloxacillin is delayed when the drug is administered after meals.

Dynapen, with normal doses, has insignificant concentrations in the cerebrospinal and ascitic fluids. It is found in therapeutic concentrations in the pleural, bile and amniotic fluids. Dynapen is rapidly excreted as unchanged drug in the urine by glomerular filtration and active tubular secretion. The elimination half-life for Dynapen is about 0.7 hours.

INDICATIONS AND USAGE

The penicillinase-resistant penicillins are indicated in the treatment of infections caused by penicillinase-producing staphylococci which have demonstrated susceptibility to the drugs. Cultures and susceptibility tests should be performed initially to determine the causative organism and their sensitivity to the drug (See **CLINICAL PHARMACOLOGY**—Susceptibility Plate Testing).

The penicillinase-resistant penicillins may be used to initiate therapy in suspected cases of resistant staphylococcal infections prior to the availability of laboratory test results. The penicillinase-resistant penicillins should not be used in infections caused by organisms susceptible to penicillin G. If the susceptibility tests indicate that the infection is due to an organism other than a resistant staphylococcus, therapy should not be continued with a penicillinase-resistant penicillin.

CONTRAINDICATIONS

A history of a hypersensitivity (anaphylactic) reaction to any penicillin is a contraindication.

WARNINGS

Serious and occasionally fatal hypersensitivity (anaphylactic shock with collapse) reactions have occurred in patients receiving penicillin. The incidence of anaphylactic shock in all penicillin-treated patients is between 0.015 and 0.04 percent. Anaphylactic shock resulting in death has occurred in approximately 0.002 percent of the patients treated. Although anaphylaxis is more frequent following a parenteral administration, it has occurred in patients receiving oral penicillins.

When penicillin therapy is indicated, it should be initiated only after a comprehensive patient drug and allergy history has been obtained. If an allergic reaction occurs, the drug should be discontinued and the patient should receive supportive treatment, e.g., artificial maintenance of ventilation, pressor amines, antihistamines, and corticosteroids. Individuals with a history of penicillin hypersensitivity may also experience allergic reactions when treated with a cephalosporin.

PRECAUTIONS

General. Penicillinase-resistant penicillins should generally not be administered to patients with a history of sensitivity to any penicillin.

Penicillin should be used with caution in individuals with histories of significant allergies and/or asthma. Whenever allergic reactions occur, penicillin should be withdrawn unless, in the opinion of the physician, the condition being treated is life-threatening and amenable only to penicillin therapy.

The oral route of administration should not be relied upon in patients with severe illness, or with nausea, vomiting, gastric dilation, cardiospasm, or intestinal hypermotility. Occasionally patients will not absorb therapeutic amounts of orally administered penicillin.

The use of antibiotics may result in overgrowth of nonsusceptible organisms. If new infections due to bacteria or fungi occur, the drug should be discontinued and appropriate measures taken.

Information for the Patient. Patients receiving penicillins should be given the following information and instructions by the physician:

1. Patients should be told that penicillin is an antibacterial agent which will work with the body's natural defenses to control certain types of infections. They should be told that the drug should not be taken if they have had an allergic reaction to any form of penicillin previously, and to inform the physician of any allergies or previous allergic reactions to any drugs they may have had (see **WARNINGS**).
2. Patients who have previously experienced an anaphylactic reaction to penicillin should be instructed to wear a medical identification tag or bracelet.
3. Because most antibacterial drugs taken by mouth are best absorbed on an empty stomach, patients should be directed, unless circumstances warrant otherwise, to take penicillin one hour before meals or two hours after eating (See **CLINICAL PHARMACOLOGY**—Pharmacokinetics).
4. Patients should be told to take the entire course of therapy prescribed, even if fever and other symptoms have stopped (See **PRECAUTIONS**—General).
5. If any of the following reactions occur, stop taking your prescription and notify the physician: shortness of breath, wheezing, skin rash, mouth irritation, black tongue, sore throat, nausea, vomiting, diarrhea, fever, swollen joints, or any unusual bleeding or bruising (See **ADVERSE REACTIONS**).
6. Do not take any additional medications without physician approval, including non-prescription drugs such as antacids, laxatives or vitamins.
7. Discard any liquid forms of penicillin after 7 days if stored at room temperature or after 14 days if refrigerated.

Laboratory Tests. Bacteriologic studies to determine the causative organisms and their susceptibility to the penicillinase-resistant penicillins should be performed (See **CLINICAL PHARMACOLOGY**—Microbiology). In the treatment of suspected staphylococcal infections, therapy should be changed to another active agent if culture tests fail to demonstrate the presence of staphylococci.

Periodic assessment of organ system function including renal, hepatic, and hematopoietic should be made during prolonged therapy with the penicillinase-resistant penicillins.

Blood cultures, white blood cell, and differential cell counts should be obtained prior to initiation of therapy and at least weekly during therapy with penicillinase-resistant penicillins.

Periodic urinalysis, blood urea nitrogen, and creatinine determinations should be performed during therapy with the penicillinase-resistant penicillins and dosage alterations should be considered if these values become elevated. If any impairment of renal function is suspected or known to exist, a reduction in the total dosage should be considered and blood levels monitored to avoid possible neurotoxic reactions (See **DOSAGE AND ADMINISTRATION**).

SGOT and SGPT values should be obtained periodically during therapy to monitor for possible liver function abnormalities.

Drug Interactions. Tetracycline, a bacteriostatic antibiotic, may antagonize the bactericidal effect of penicillin and concurrent use of these drugs should be avoided.

Carcinogenesis, Mutagenesis, Impairment of Fertility. No long-term animal studies have been conducted with these drugs.

Studies on reproduction (Nafcillin) in rats and rabbits reveal no fetal or maternal abnormalities before conception and continuously through weaning (one generation).

Pregnancy Category B. Reproduction studies performed in the mouse, rat, and rabbit have revealed no evidence of impaired fertility or harm to the fetus due to the penicillinase-resistant penicillins. Human experience with the penicillins during pregnancy has not shown any positive evidence of adverse effects on the fetus. There are, however, no adequate or well-controlled studies in pregnant women showing conclusively that harmful effects of these drugs on the fetus can be excluded. Because animal reproduction studies are not always predictive of human response, this drug should be used during pregnancy only if clearly needed.

Nursing Mothers. Penicillins are excreted in breast milk. Caution should be exercised when penicillins are administered to a nursing woman.

Pediatric Use. Because of incompletely developed renal function in newborns, penicillinase-resistant penicillins (especially methicillin) may not be completely excreted, with abnormally high blood levels resulting. Frequent blood levels are advisable in this group with dosage adjustments when necessary. All newborns treated with penicillins should be monitored closely for clinical and laboratory evidence of toxic or adverse effects (See **DOSAGE AND ADMINISTRATION**).

ADVERSE REACTIONS

Body as a Whole: The reported incidence of allergic reactions to penicillin ranges from 0.7 to 10 percent (See **WARNINGS**). Sensitization is usually the result of treatment but some individuals have had immediate reactions to penicillin when first treated. In such cases, it is thought that the patients may have had prior exposure to the drug via trace amounts present in milk and vaccines.

Two types of allergic reactions to penicillin are noted clinically, immediate and delayed.

Immediate reactions usually occur within 20 minutes of administration and range in severity from urticaria and pruritus to angioneurotic edema, laryngospasm, bronchospasm, hypotension, vascular collapse, and death. Such immediate anaphylactic reactions are very rare (See **WARNINGS**) and usually occur after parenteral therapy but have occurred in patients receiving oral therapy. Another type of immediate reaction, an accelerated reaction, may occur between 20 minutes and 48 hours after administration and may include urticaria, pruritus, and fever. Although laryngeal edema, laryngospasm, and hypotension occasionally occur, fatality is uncommon.

Delayed allergic reactions to penicillin therapy usually occur after 48 hours and sometimes as late as 2 to 4 weeks after initiation of therapy. Manifestations of this type of reaction include serum sickness-like symptoms (i.e., fever, malaise, urticaria, myalgia, arthralgia, abdominal pain) and various skin rashes. Nausea, vomiting, diarrhea, stomatitis, black or hairy tongue, and other symptoms of gastrointestinal irritation may occur, especially during oral penicillin therapy.

Nervous System Reactions: Neurotoxic reactions similar to those observed with penicillin G may occur with large intravenous doses of the penicillinase-resistant penicillins especially with patients with renal insufficiency.

Urogenital Reactions: Renal tubular damage and interstitial nephritis have been associated with the administration of methicillin sodium and infrequently with the administration of nafcillin and oxacillin. Manifestations of this reaction may include rash, fever, eosinophilia, hematuria, proteinuria, and renal insufficiency. Methicillin-induced nephropathy does not appear to be dose-related and is generally reversible upon prompt discontinuation of therapy.

Metabolic Reactions: Agranulocytosis, neutropenia, and bone marrow depression have been associated with the use of methicillin sodium, nafcillin, oxacillin, and cloxacillin. Hepatotoxicity, characterized by fever, nausea, and vomiting associated with abnormal liver function tests, mainly elevated SGOT levels, has been associated with the use of oxacillin and cloxacillin.

DOSAGE AND ADMINISTRATION

The penicillinase-resistant penicillins are available for oral administration and for intramuscular and intravenous injection. The sodium salts of methicillin, oxacillin, and nafcillin may be administered parenterally and the sodium salts of cloxacillin, dicloxacillin, oxacillin, and nafcillin are available for oral use.

Bacteriologic studies to determine the causative organisms and their sensitivity to the penicillinase-resistant penicillins should always be performed. Duration of therapy varies with the type and severity of infection as well as the overall condition of the patient, therefore it should be determined by the clinical and bacteriological response of the patient. In severe staphylococcal infections, therapy with penicillinase-resistant penicillins should be continued for at least 14 days. Therapy should be continued for at least 48 hours after the patient has become afebrile, asymptomatic, and cultures are negative. The treatment of endocarditis and osteomyelitis may require a longer term of therapy.

Concurrent administration of the penicillinase-resistant penicillins and probenecid increases and prolongs serum penicillin levels. Probenecid decreases the apparent volume of distribution and slows the rate of excretion by competitively inhibiting renal tubular secretion of penicillin. Penicillin-probenecid therapy is generally limited to those infections where very high serum levels of penicillin are necessary.

Oral preparations of the penicillinase-resistant penicillins should not be used as initial therapy in serious, life-threatening infections (see **PRECAUTIONS**—General). Oral ther-

RECOMMENDED DOSAGES FOR DYNAPEN (dicloxacillin sodium) IN MILD TO MODERATE AND SEVERE INFECTIONS

DRUG	ADULTS		CHILDREN	
	Mild to Moderate	Severe	Mild to Moderate	Severe
Dicloxa-cillin	125 mg every 6 hours	250 mg every 6 hours	12.5 mg/kg/day[a] in equally divided doses every 6 hours	25 mg/kg/day[a] in equally divided doses every 6 hours

(a) Patients weighing less than 40 Kg (88 lbs)

apy with the penicillinase-resistant penicillins may be used to follow-up the previous use of a parenteral agent as soon as the clinical condition warrants. For intramuscular gluteal injections, care should be taken to avoid sciatic nerve injury. With intravenous administration, particularly in elderly patients, care should be taken because of the possibility of thrombophlebitis.
[See table above].

DIRECTIONS FOR DISPENSING ORAL SUSPENSION

Prepare these formulations at the time of dispensing. For ease in preparation, add water to the bottle in two portions and shake well after each addition. Add the total amount of water as directed on the labeling of the package being dispensed. The reconstituted formulation is stable for 14 days under refrigeration.

HOW SUPPLIED

Dynapen (dicloxacillin sodium) for Oral Suspension, 62.5 mg per 5 ml.
NDC 0015-7856
Dynapen (dicloxacillin sodium) Capsules. Each capsule contains dicloxacillin sodium equivalent to 125, 250, or 500 mg dicloxacillin.
NDC 0015-7892—125 mg
NDC 0015-7893—250 mg
NDC 0015-7658—500 mg
For information on package sizes available, refer to the current price schedule.
7856DIR-12 **February 1985**
Shown in Product Identification Section, page 406

KANTREX® CAPSULES ℞

[kan 'treks]
(kanamycin sulfate)
Not for Systemic Use

This is the full text of the latest Official Package Circular dated February 1985 [3506 DIR-09].

DESCRIPTION

Kanamycin sulfate is a water soluble aminoglycoside antibiotic derived from **Streptomyces kanamyceticus.** It is supplied in oral formulation for topical effect within the gastrointestinal tract, because it is absorbed only very slightly when administered orally, and is excreted unchanged in the feces.
Inactive ingredients in Kantrex Capsules are: lactose, magnesium stearate and sodium chloride.

ACTIONS

Kanamycin is poorly absorbed from the normal gastrointestinal tract. The small absorbed fraction is rapidly excreted with normal kidney function. The unabsorbed portion of the drug is eliminated unchanged in the feces.
Most intestinal bacteria are eliminated rapidly following oral administration of kanamycin, with bacterial suppression persisting for 48 to 72 hours.

INDICATIONS

Suppression of Intestinal Bacteria—Kanamycin is indicated when supression of the normal bacterial flora of the bowel is desirable for short-term adjunctive therapy.
Hepatic Coma—Prolonged administration has been shown to be effective adjunctive therapy in **Hepatic Coma** by reduction of the ammonia-forming bacteria in the intestinal tract. The subsequent reduction in blood ammonia has resulted in neurologic improvement.

CONTRAINDICATIONS

This drug is contraindicated in the presence of intestinal obstruction and in individuals with a history of hypersensitivity to the drug.

WARNINGS

Although negligible amounts of kanamycin are absorbed through intact intestinal mucosa (approximately 1 percent), the possibility of increased absorption from ulcerated or denuded areas should be considered. If renal insufficiency develops during treatment, the dosage should be reduced or the antibiotic discontinued. Urine and blood examinations and audiometric tests should be given prior to and during extended therapy in individuals with hepatic and/or renal disease.

USAGE IN PREGNANCY

Safety for use in pregnancy has not been established.

PRECAUTIONS

Caution should be taken in concurrent use of other ototoxic and/or nephrotoxic antimicrobial drugs while kanamycin is administered orally. These include streptomycin, neomycin, polymyxin B, colistin, viomycin, gentamicin, and cephaloridine.
The concurrent use of potent diuretics (e.g. ethacrynic acid, furosemide, and mannitol, particularly when the diuretics are given intravenously) should be avoided. They may cause cumulative adverse effects of the kanamycin on the kidney and auditory nerve.
Prolonged use of oral kanamycin may result in overgrowth of nonsusceptible organisms, particularly fungi. If this occurs, appropriate therapy should be instituted.

ADVERSE REACTIONS

The most common adverse reactions to oral kanamycin are nausea, vomiting, and diarrhea. The "Malabsorption Syndrome" characterized by increased fecal fat, decreased serum carotene, and fall in xylose absorption has been reported with prolonged therapy. Nephrotoxicity and ototoxicity have been reported following prolonged and high dosage therapy in hepatic coma.

Dosage and Administration For Oral Use Only:
Suppression of Intestinal Bacteria:

1. As an adjunct in therapy of Hepatic Coma for extended therapy: 8 to 12 Gm. per day in divided doses.
2. As an adjunct to mechanical cleansing of the large bowel in short term therapy: 1.0 Gm. (2 capsules) every hour for 4 hours followed by 1.0 Gm. (2 capsules) every 6 hours for 36 to 72 hours.

Duration of therapy within this range depends on the condition of the patient, the type and amount of concurrent mechanical cleansing (catharsis and enemas), and the customary medical routine.

SUPPLY

KANTREX (kanamycin sulfate) Capsules. Kanamycin sulfate equivalent to 500 mg kanamycin per capsule.
NDC 0015-3506—500mg
For information on package sizes available, refer to the current price schedule.
Shown in Product Identification Section, page 406

KANTREX® INJECTION ℞

[kan 'treks]
(kanamycin sulfate injection)
500 mg. per 2 ml.; 1.0 Gm. per 3 ml.

KANTREX® PEDIATRIC INJECTION ℞

(kanamycin sulfate injection)
75 mg. per 2 ml.

This is the full text of the latest Official Package Circular dated November 1978 [3502DIM-09].

WARNING

Patients treated with aminoglycosides by any route should be under close clinical observation because of the potential toxicity associated with their use. As with other aminoglycosides, the major toxic effects of kanamycin sulfate are its action on the auditory and vestibular branches of the eighth nerve and the renal tubules. Loss of high frequency perception usually occurs before clinical hearing loss and can be detected by audiometric testing. There may not be clinical symptoms to warn of developing cochlear damage. Vertigo may occur and may be evidence of vestibular injury. Renal impairment may be characterized by decreased creatinine clearance, the presence of cells or casts, oliguria, proteinuria, decreased urine specific gravity, or evidence of increasing nitrogen retention (increasing BUN, NPN or serum creatinine).
In patients with impaired kidney function, the risks of severe ototoxic and nephrotoxic reactions are sharply increased. In such cases, either the total daily dosage should be reduced, or the interval between doses lengthened, or both. Assessment of renal function and audiograms should be obtained before treatment if possible and monitored frequently during the course of therapy (see "Precautions"). If there is evidence of progressive renal dysfunction (increasing NPN, BUN, serum creatinine or oliguria) during therapy, audiometric tests are advised and discontinuation of the drug should be considered.
Elderly patients, patients with preexisting tinnitus or vertigo or known subclinical deafness, those having received prior ototoxic drugs, and patients receiving a total dose of more than 15 g of kanamycin sulfate should be carefully observed for signs of eighth nerve damage. Loss of hearing may occur in such patients even with normal renal function.
Neuromuscular blockade with respiratory paralysis may occur when kanamycin sulfate is administered intraperitoneally concomitantly with anesthesia and muscle-relaxing drugs. Although there have been isolated reports of respiratory depression following intraperitoneal instillation of kanamycin, there is no conclusive proof that this side effect can be produced with recommended doses of the drug.
The concurrent and/or sequential systemic or topical use of kanamycin and other potentially ototoxic, nephrotoxic, and/or neurotoxic drugs, particularly streptomycin, polymyxin B, colistin, neomycin, gentamicin, cephaloradine, paromomycin, tobramycin, amikacin, vancomycin and viomycin should be avoided because the toxicity may be additive.
Kanamycin sulfate should not be given concurrently with potent diuretics (ethacrynic acid, furosemide, meralluride sodium, sodium mercaptomerin, or mannitol). Some diuretics themselves cause ototoxicity, and intravenously administered diuretics may enhance aminoglycoside toxicity by altering antibiotic concentrations in serum and tissue.

DESCRIPTION

Kanamycin sulfate is an aminoglycoside antibiotic produced by **Streptomyces kanamyceticus.** It is $C_{18}H_{36}N_4O_{11} \cdot 2H_2SO_4$. D-Streptomine, 0-3-amino-3-deoxy-α-D-glucopyranosyl— (1→6)-0-[6-amino-6-deoxy-α-D-glucopyranosyl-(1→4)]-2-deoxy, sulfate 1:2 (salt). It consists of two amino sugars glycosidically linked to deoxystreptamine.

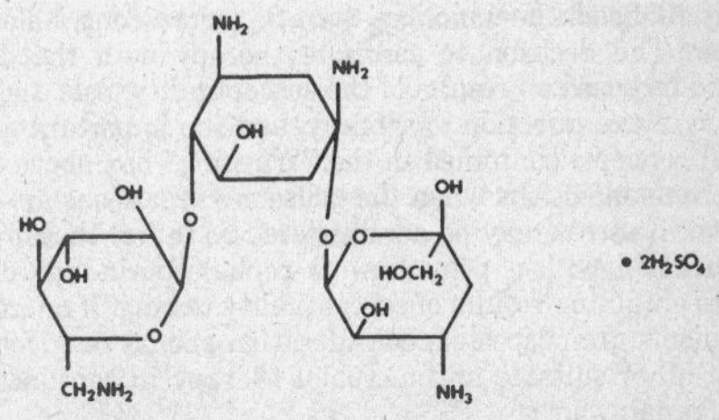

Kanamycin sulfate injection, sterile solution for parenteral administration, contains respectively: kanamycin sulfate 75 mg, 500 mg, and 1 g; sodium bisulfite, an antioxidant, 0.099%, 0.66%, and 0.45%, and sodium citrate, 0.33%, 2.2%, and 2.2% with pH of each dosage form adjusted to 4.5 with sulfuric acid.

ACTION

Clinical Pharmacology

The drug is rapidly absorbed after intramuscular injection and peak serum levels are generally reached within approximately one hour. Doses of 7.5 mg/Kg give mean peak levels of 22 mcg/ml. At 8 hours following a 7.5 mg/Kg dose, mean serum levels are 3.2 mcg/ml. Intravenous administration of kanamycin over a period of one hour resulted in serum concentrations similar to those obtained by intramuscular administration.
Kanamycin diffuses rapidly into most body fluids including synovial and peritoneal fluids and bile. Significant levels of the drug appear in cord blood and amniotic fluid following intramuscular administration to pregnant patients. Spinal fluid concentrations in normal infants are approximately 10 to 20 percent of serum levels and may reach 50 percent when the meninges are inflamed.
Studies in normal adult patients have shown only trace levels of kanamycin in spinal fluid. No data are available on adults with meningitis.
The drug is excreted almost entirely by glomerular filtration and is not reabsorbed by the renal tubules. Hence, high concentrations are attained in the nephron, and the urine may contain levels 10 to 20 times higher than those in serum. Renal excretion is extremely rapid. In patients with normal renal function, approximately one-half of the administered

Continued on next page

Bristol—Cont.

dose is cleared within 4 hours and excretion is complete within 24 to 48 hours. Patients with impaired renal function or with diminished glomerular filtration pressure excrete kanamycin more slowly. Such patients may build up excessively high blood levels which greatly increase the risk of ototoxic reactions.

Microbiology

Kanamycin sulfate is a bactericidal antibiotic which acts by inhibiting the synthesis of protein in susceptible microorganisms. Kanamycin sulfate is active **in vitro** against many strains of **Staphylococcus aureus** (including penicillinase and nonpenicillinase-producing strains). **Staphylococcus epidermidis, N. gonorrhoeae, H. influenzae, E. coli, Enterobacter aerogenes,** Shigella, Salmonella, **K. pneumoniae, Serratia marcescens, Acinetobacter,** and many strains of both indole-positive and indole-negative **Proteus** that are frequently resistant to other antibiotics. Bacterial resistance to kanamycin develops slowly in most susceptible organisms. **In vitro** studies have demonstrated that an aminoglycoside combined with an antibiotic which interferes with cell wall synthesis (i.e., penicillins or cephalosporins) acts synergistically against some strains of Gram-negative organisms and enterococci (**Streptococcus faecalis**).

Susceptibility testing: The infecting organism should be cultured and its susceptibility demonstrated as a guide to therapy. If the Kirby-Bauer method of disc susceptibility is used, a 30-mcg kanamycin disc should give a zone of inhibition of 17 mm or more when tested against a kanamycin-susceptible bacterial strain. A zone of 16 mm or less indicates that the infecting organism is likely to be resistant. In certain conditions, it may be desirable to do additional susceptibility testing by the tube or Agar dilution method. Kanamycin reference standard is available for this purpose.

INDICATIONS AND USAGE

Kanamycin is indicated in the treatment of serious infections caused by susceptible strains of microorganisms. Bacteriological studies to identify the causative organisms and to determine their susceptibility to kanamycin should be performed. Therapy may be instituted prior to obtaining the results of susceptibility testing.

Kanamycin may be considered as initial therapy in the treatment of infections where one or more of the following are the known or suspected pathogens: **E. coli, Proteus** species (both indole-positive and indole-negative), **Enterobacter aerogenes, Klebsiella pneumoniae, Serratia marcescens, Acinetobacter.** The decision to continue therapy with the drug should be based on results of the susceptibility tests, the response of the infection to therapy, and the important additional concepts contained in the "Warning" box above.

In serious infections when the causative organisms are unknown, Kantrex may be administered as initial therapy in conjunction with a penicillin- or cephalosporin-type drug before obtaining results of susceptibility testing. If anaerobic organisms are suspected, consideration should be given to using other suitable antimicrobial therapy in conjunction with kanamycin.

Although kanamycin is not the drug of choice for staphylococcal infections, it may be indicated under certain conditions for the treatment of known or suspected staphylococcal disease. These situations include the initial therapy of severe infections where the organism is thought to be either a Gram-negative bacterium or a staphylococcus, infections due to susceptible strains of staphylococci in patients allergic to other antibiotics, and mixed staphylococcal/Gram-negative infections.

CONTRAINDICATIONS

A history of hypersensitivity or toxic reaction to one aminoglycoside may also contraindicate the use of any other aminoglycoside, because of the known cross-sensitivity and cumulative effects of drugs in this category.

THIS DRUG IS NOT INDICATED IN LONG-TERM THERAPY (e.g. Tuberculosis) BECAUSE OF THE TOXIC HAZARD ASSOCIATED WITH EXTENDED ADMINISTRATION.

WARNING

See "Warning" box above.

PRECAUTIONS

Ototoxicity: In patients with renal dysfunction an audiogram should be obtained before treatment and repeated frequently during therapy. Therapy should be stopped if tinnitus or subjective hearing loss develops, or if follow-up audiograms show loss of high frequency perception.

It should be emphasized that since renal function may alter appreciably during therapy, the serum creatinine should be checked daily or more frequently. Changes in the concentration would, of course, necessitate changes in the dosage frequency.

Nephrotoxicity: Because of the high concentration of kanamycin sulfate in the urinary excretory system, patients should be well-hydrated to prevent chemical irritation of the renal tubules. Kidney function should be assessed by the usual methods, e.g., urinalysis, BUN, serum creatinine, prior to starting therapy and periodically during the course of treatment. If signs of renal irritation appear, such as casts, white or red cells, and albumin, hydration should be increased and a reduction in dosage may be desirable (see "Dosage and Administration"). These signs usually disappear when treatment is completed. However, if azotemia or a progressive decrease in urine output occurs, treatment should be stopped.

The possibility of neuromuscular blockade with respiratory paralysis should be considered if aminoglycosides are administered by any route in patients receiving anesthetics, in patients receiving neuromuscular-blocking agents such as tubocurarine, succinylcholine, decamethonium or in patients receiving massive transfusions of citrate-anticoagulated blood. In all cases, patients should be observed carefully for signs of respiratory depression. If blockade occurs, calcium salts or neostigmine may reverse this phenomenon.

NOTE: The risk of toxic reactions is low in well-hydrated patients with normal kidney function, who receive a total dose of 15 g of kanamycin or less.

Because of the possibility of additive effects of other potentially ototoxic, neurotoxic, and/or nephrotoxic drugs, the concurrent or sequential administration of these drugs with kanamycin sulfate should be avoided (see "Warning" box).

Increased nephrotoxicity has been reported following concomitant parenteral administration of aminoglycoside antibiotics and cephalothin.

Since kanamycin sulfate and methicillin inactivate each other **in vitro**, they should not be physically mixed together in the same solution intended for parenteral administration. However, this inactivation has not been demonstrated in patients who receive both drugs by different routes of administration. (See "Dosage and Administration.")

Elderly patients may have reduced renal function which may not be evident in the results of routine screening tests, such as BUN or serum creatinine. A creatinine clearance determination may be more helpful. Monitoring of renal function during treatment is particularly important in such patients.

Aminoglycosides should be used with caution in patients with myasthenia gravis since these drugs may aggravate muscle weakness because of their curare-like effect on the neuromuscular function.

Kanamycin sulfate should not be given concurrently with potent diuretics (see "Warning" box).

Neurotoxic and nephrotoxic antibiotics may be absorbed from body surfaces after local irrigation or application. The potential toxic effect of aminoglycosides administered in this fashion should be considered (see "Warning" box).

Cross-allergenicity among aminoglycosides has been demonstrated.

As with other antibiotics, kanamycin sulfate administration may result in overgrowth of nonsusceptible organisms, including fungi. If superinfection occurs, appropriate therapy should be instituted.

Pregnancy:

Reproduction studies have been performed in rats and rabbits and have revealed no evidence of impaired fertility or teratogenic effects. Dosages of 200 mg/Kg/day in pregnant rats and pregnant guinea pigs led to hearing impairment in the offspring. There are no well-controlled studies in pregnant women but clinical experience does not include any positive evidence of adverse effects on the fetus. Although there is no clearly defined risk, such experience cannot exclude the possibility of infrequent or subtle damage to the fetus. Kantrex should be used in pregnant women only when clearly needed.

ADVERSE REACTIONS

Nephrotoxicity—Albuminuria, presence of red and white cells, and granular casts; azotemia and oliguria have been reported.

Ototoxicity—Tinnitus, vertigo, and partial reversible to irreversible hearing loss have been reported, usually associated with higher than recommended dosage. Rapid development of hearing loss has been reported in patients with poor kidney function treated concurrently with kanamycin and one of the rapid-acting diuretic agents given intravenously. These have included ethacrynic acid, furosemide, and mannitol.

Other—Some local irritation or pain may follow intramuscular injection. Other adverse reactions of the drug reported on rare occasions are skin rash, drug fever, headache, and paresthesia.

OVERDOSAGE

In the event of overdosage or toxic reaction, hemodialysis or peritoneal dialysis will aid in the removal of kanamycin from the blood. In the newborn infant, exchange transfusions may also be considered.

DOSAGE AND ADMINISTRATION

Intramuscular Route: Inject deeply into the upper outer quadrant of the gluteal muscle. The recommended dose for adults or children is 15 mg/Kg/day in two equally divided dosages administered at equally divided intervals, i.e. 7.5 mg/Kg q12h. If continuously high blood levels are desired, the daily dose of 15 mg/Kg may be given in equally divided doses every 6 or 8 hours. Treatment of patients in the heavier weight classes, i.e. >100 Kg, should not exceed 1.5 g/day.

In patients with impaired renal function, it is desirable to follow therapy by appropriate serum assays. If this is not feasible, a suggested method is to reduce the frequency of administration in patients with renal dysfunction. The interval between doses may be calculated with the following formula:

Serum creatinine (mg/100 ml) $\times$ 9 = Dosage Interval (in hours): e.g., if the serum creatinine is 2 mg, the recommended dose (7.5 mg/Kg) should be administered every 18 hours. Changes in creatinine concentration during therapy would, of course, necessitate changes in the dosage frequency.

The usual duration of treatment is 7 to 10 days. The total daily dose by all routes of administration should not exceed 1.5 g/day.

At the recommended dosage level, uncomplicated infections due to kanamycin-susceptible organisms should respond to therapy in 24 to 48 hours. If definite clinical response does not occur within 3 to 5 days, therapy should be stopped and the antibiotic susceptibility pattern of the invading organism should be rechecked. Failure of the infection to respond may be due to resistance of the organism or to the presence of septic foci requiring surgical drainage.

Intravenous Administration: The dose should not exceed 15 mg/Kg per day and must be administered slowly. The solution for intravenous use is prepared by adding the contents of a 500-mg vial to 100 to 200 ml of sterile diluent such as Normal Saline or 5% Dextrose in Water, or the contents of a 1 g vial to 200 to 400 ml of sterile diluent. The appropriate dose is administered over a 30- to 60-minute period. The total daily dose should be divided into two or three equally divided doses.

In pediatric patients the amount of diluent used should be sufficient to infuse the kanamycin sulfate over a 30- to 60-minute period.

Kanamycin sulfate injection should not be physically mixed with other antibacterial agents but each should be administered separately in accordance with its recommended route of administration and dosage schedule.

Intraperitoneal Use: (following exploration for established peritonitis or after peritoneal contamination due to fecal spill during surgery.)

Adults: 500 mg diluted in 20 ml sterile distilled water may be instilled through a polyethylene catheter sutured into the wound at closure. If possible, instillation should be postponed until the patient has fully recovered from the effects of anesthesia and muscle-relaxing drugs (see "Warning" box).

Aerosol Treatment: 250 mg two to four times a day. Withdraw 250 mg (1 ml) from 500-mg vial and dilute it with 3 ml Physiological Saline and nebulize.

Other Routes of Administration: Kantrex Injection in concentrations of 0.25 percent (2.5 mg/ml) has been used as an irrigating solution in abscess cavities, pleural space, peritoneal and ventricular cavities. Possible absorption of Kantrex by such routes must be taken into account and dosage adjustments should be arranged so that a maximum total dose of 1.5 g/day by all routes of administration is not exceeded.

PEDIATRIC DOSAGE GUIDE FOR
KANTREX PEDIATRIC INJECTION,
75 mg/2 ml—
AMOUNT PER 24 HOURS
TO BE GIVEN IN DIVIDED DOSES

Weight in Pounds	Weight in Kilograms	Daily Dosage in Milligrams	Daily Dosage in Milliliters
2.2	1.00	15.0	0.4
2.8	1.25	18.8	0.5
3.3	1.50	22.5	0.6
3.9	1.75	26.2	0.7
4.4	2.00	30.0	0.8
5.0	2.25	33.8	0.9
5.5	2.50	37.5	1.0
6.0	2.75	41.2	1.1
6.6	3.00	45.0	1.2
7.7	3.50	52.5	1.4
8.8	4.00	60.0	1.6
9.9	4.50	67.5	1.8
11.0	5.00	75.0	2.0

STABILITY

Occasionally, some vials may darken during the shelf-life of the product, but this does not indicate a loss of potency.

HOW SUPPLIED

KANTREX INJECTION (kanamycin sulfate injection)

NDC 0015-3502-20—500 mg per 2 ml

NDC 0015-3502-24—Disposable Syringe (500 mg per 2 ml)

NDC 0015-3503-20—1 g per 3 ml

KANTREX PEDIATRIC INJECTION (kanamycin sulfate injection)
NDC 0015-3512-20—75 mg per 2 ml
(activity assayed as kanamycin base)

NAFCIL™ ℞

[*năf'sĭl*]
(nafcillin sodium for injection)
For Intramuscular or Intravenous Injection

This is the full text of the latest Official Package Circular dated June 1984 [7224DIR-10].

DESCRIPTION

Nafcil (nafcillin sodium) is a semisynthetic antibiotic substance derived from 6-amino-penicillanic acid. It is the sodium salt in a parenteral dosage form.

NAFCILLIN SODIUM

$C_{21}H_{21}N_2NaO_5S \cdot H_2O$ 454.47 [CAS 7177-50-6]
4-Thia-1-azabicyclo [3.2.0] heptane-2-carboxylic acid, 6[[(2-ethoxy-1-naphthalenyl) carbonyl] amino]-3,3-dimethyl-7-oxo-monosodium salt, monohydrate, [2S (2α, 5α, 6β)].

CLINICAL PHARMACOLOGY

Microbiology: Penicillinase-resistant penicillins exert a bactericidal action against penicillin-susceptible microorganisms during the state of active multiplication. All penicillins inhibit the biosynthesis of the bacterial cell wall.
The drugs in this class are highly resistant to inactivation by staphylococcal penicillinase and are active against penicillinase producing and non-penicillinase producing strains of **Staphylococcus aureus.**
The penicillinase-resistant penicillins are active **in vitro** against a variety of other bacteria.
Susceptibility Plate Testing: Quantitative methods of susceptibility testing that require measurement of zone diameters or minimal inhibitory concentrations (M.I.C.s) give the most precise estimates of antibiotic susceptibility. One such procedure has been recommended for use with discs to test susceptibility to this class of drugs. Interpretations correlate diameters on the disc test with MIC values. A penicillinase-resistant class disc may be used to determine microbial susceptibility to cloxacillin, dicloxacillin, methicillin, nafcillin, and oxacillin. With this procedure, employing a 5 microgram methicillin sodium disc, a report from the laboratory of "susceptible" (zone of at least 14 mm) indicates that the infecting organism is likely to respond to therapy. A report of "resistant" (zone of less than 10 mm) indicates that the infecting organism is not likely to respond to therapy. A report of "intermediate susceptibility" (zone of 10 to 13 mm) suggests that the organism might be susceptible if high doses of the antibiotic are used, or if the infection is confined to tissues and fluids (e.g., urine), in which high antibiotic levels are attained.
In general, all staphylococci should be tested against the penicillin G disc and against the methicillin disc. Routine methods of antibiotic susceptibility testing may fail to detect strains of organisms resistant to the penicillinase-resistant penicillins. For this reason, the use of large inocula and 48-hour incubation periods may be necessary to obtain accurate susceptibility studies with these antibiotics. Bacterial strains which are resistant to one of the penicillinase-resistant penicillins should be considered resistant to all of the drugs in the class.

PHARMACOKINETICS

Intramuscular injections of Nafcil (nafcillin sodium) 1 gram produced peak serum levels in 0.5 to 1 hour of 7.61 mcg/ml. The degree of protein binding reported has been 89.9 +/- 1.5%. With normal doses Nafcil is found in therapeutic concentrations in the pleural, bile and amniotic fluids. Insignificant concentrations are found in the cerebrospinal fluid and aqueous humor. Blood concentrations may be tripled by the concurrent use of probenecid. Clinical studies with nafcillin sodium in infants under three days of age and prematures have revealed higher blood levels and slower rates of urinary excretion than in older children and adults. A high concentration of nafcillin sodium is excreted via the bile. About 30% of an intramuscular dose is excreted in the urine.

STABILITY PERIODS FOR NAFCIL (nafcillin sodium)

Concentration Mg/Ml	Sterile H_2O for Injection	Isotonic Sodium Chloride	M/6 Molar Sodium Lactate Solution	5% Dextrose In H_2O	5% Dextrose In 0.45% NaCl	10% Invert Sugar	Lactated Ringers Solution
ROOM TEMPERATURE (25°C)							
10-200	24 Hrs	24 Hrs					
30			24 Hrs				
2-30				24 Hrs	24 Hrs		
10-30						24 Hrs	24 Hrs
REFRIGERATION (4°C)							
10-200	7 Days	7 Days					
10-30			7 Days	7 Days	7 Days	7 Days	7 Days
FROZEN (−15°C)							
250	90 Days	90 Days					
10-250			90 Days	90 Days	90 Days	90 Days	90 Days

INDICATIONS AND USAGE

The penicillinase-resistant penicillins are indicated in the treatment of infections caused by penicillinase-producing staphylococci which have demonstrated susceptibility to the drugs. Cultures and susceptibility tests should be performed initially to determine the causative organisms and their sensitivity to the drug (See **Clinical Pharmacology** — Susceptibility Plate Testing).
The penicillinase-resistant penicillins may be used to initiate therapy in suspected cases of resistant staphylococcal infections prior to the availability of laboratory test results.
The penicillinase-resistant penicillins should not be used in infections caused by organisms susceptible to penicillin G. If the susceptibility tests indicate that the infection is due to an organism other than a resistant staphylococcus, therapy should not be continued with a penicillinase-resistant penicillin.

CONTRAINDICATIONS

A history of a hypersensitivity (anaphylactic) reaction to any penicillin is a contraindication.

WARNINGS

Serious and occasionally fatal hypersensitivity (anaphylactic shock with collapse) reactions have occurred in patients receiving penicillin. The incidence of anaphylactic shock in all penicillin-treated patients is between 0.015 and 0.04 percent. Anaphylactic shock resulting in death has occurred in approximately 0.002 percent of the patients treated. Although anaphylaxis is more frequent following a parenteral administration, it has occurred in patients receiving oral penicillins.
When penicillin therapy is indicated, it should be initiated only after a comprehensive patient drug and allergy history has been obtained. If an allergic reaction occurs, the drug should be discontinued and the patient should receive supportive treatment, e.g., artificial maintenance of ventilations, pressor amines, antihistamines, and corticosteroids. Individuals with a history of penicillin hypersensitivity may also experience allergic reactions when treated with a cephalosporin.

PRECAUTIONS

GENERAL: Penicillinase-resistant penicillins should generally not be administered to patients with a history of sensitivity to any penicillin.
Penicillin should be used with caution in individuals with histories of significant allergies and/or asthma. Whenever allergic reactions occur, penicillin should be withdrawn unless, in the opinion of the physician, the condition being treated is life-threatening and amenable only to penicillin therapy.
The oral route of administration should not be relied upon in patients with severe illness, or with nausea, vomiting, gastric dilation, cardiospasm, or intestinal hypermotility. Occasionally patients will not absorb therapeutic amounts of orally administered penicillin.
The use of antibiotics may result in overgrowth of nonsusceptible organisms. If new infections due to bacteria or fungi occur, the drug should be discontinued and appropriate measures taken.
Laboratory Tests: Bacteriologic studies to determine the causative organisms and their susceptibility to the penicillinase-resistant penicillins should be performed (See **Clinical Pharmacology** —Microbiology). In the treatment of suspected staphylococcal infections, therapy should be changed to another active agent if culture tests fail to demonstrate the presence of staphylococci.
Periodic assessment or organ system function including renal, hepatic, and hematopoietic should be made during prolonged therapy with the penicillinase-resistant penicillins.
Blood cultures, white blood cell, and differential cell counts should be obtained prior to initiation of therapy and at least weekly during therapy with penicillinase-resistant penicillins.
Periodic urinalysis, blood urea nitrogen, and creatinine determinations should be performed during therapy with the penicillinase-resistant penicillins and dosage alterations should be considered if these values become elevated. If any impairment of renal function is suspected or known to exist, a reduction in the total dosage should be considered and blood levels monitored to avoid possible neurotoxic reactions. (See **Dosage and Administration**).
SGOT and SGPT values should be obtained periodically during therapy to monitor for possible liver function abnormalities.
Drug Interactions: Tetracycline, a bacteriostatic antibiotic, may antagonize the bactericidal effect of penicillin and concurrent use of these drugs should be avoided.
Carcinogenesis, Mutagenesis, Impairment of Fertility: No long-term animal studies have been conducted with these drugs.
Studies on reproduction (nafcillin) in rats and rabbits reveal no fetal or maternal abnormalities before conception and continuously through weaning (one generation).
Pregnancy Category B: Reproduction studies performed in the mouse, rat, and rabbit have revealed no evidence of impaired fertility or harm to the fetus due to the penicillinase-resistant penicillins. Human experience with the penicillins during pregnancy has not shown any positive evidence of adverse effects on the fetus. There are, however, no adequate or well-controlled studies in pregnant women showing conclusively that harmful effects of these drugs on the fetus can be excluded. Because animal reproduction studies are not always predictive of human response, this drug should be used during pregnancy only if clearly needed.
Nursing Mothers: Penicillins are excreted in breast milk. Caution should be exercised when penicillins are administered to a nursing woman.
Pediatric Use: Because of incompletely developed renal function in newborns, penicillinase-resistant penicillins (especially methicillin) may not be completely excreted, with abnormally high blood levels resulting. Frequent blood levels are advisable in this group with dosage adjustments when necessary. All newborns treated with penicillins should be monitored closely for clinical and laboratory evidence of toxic or adverse effects (See **Dosage and Administration**).

ADVERSE REACTIONS

Body as a Whole: The reported incidence of allergic reactions to penicillins ranges from 0.7 to 10 percent (See **Warnings**). Sensitization is usually the result of treatment but some individuals have had immediate reactions to penicillin when first treated. In such cases, it is thought that the patients may have had prior exposure to the drug via trace amounts present in milk and vaccines.
Two types of allergic reactions to penicillin are noted clinically, immediate and delayed.
Immediate reactions usually occur within 20 minutes of administration and range in severity from urticaria and pruri-

Continued on next page

Bristol—Cont.

tus to angioneurotic edema, laryngospasm, bronchospasm, hypotension, vascular collapse, and death. Such immediate anaphylactic reactions are very rare (See **Warnings**) and usually occur after parenteral therapy but have occurred in patients receiving oral therapy. Another type of immediate reaction, an accelerated reaction, may occur between 20 minutes and 48 hours after administration and may include urticaria, pruritus, and fever. Although laryngeal edema, larynogospasm, and hypotension occasionally occur, fatality is uncommon.
Delayed allergic reactions to penicillin therapy usually occur after 48 hours and sometimes as late as 2 to 4 weeks after initiation of therapy. Manifestations of this type of reaction include serum sickness-like symptoms (i.e., fever, malaise, urticaria, myalgia, arthralgia, abdominal pain) and various skin rashes. Nausea, vomiting, diarrhea, stomatitis, black or hairy tongue and other symptoms of gastrointestinal irritation may occur, especially during oral penicillin therapy.
Nervous System Reactions: Neurotoxic reactions similar to those observed with penicillin G may occur with large intravenous doses of the penicillinase-resistant penicillins especially with patients with renal insufficiency.
Urogenital Reactions: Renal tubular damage and interstitial nephritis have been associated with the administration of methicillin sodium and infrequently with the administration of nafcillin and oxacillin. Manifestations of this reaction may include rash, fever, eosinophilia, hematuria, proteinuria, and renal insufficiency. Methicillin-induced nephropathy does not appear to be dose-related and is generally reversible upon prompt discontinuation of therapy.
Metabolic Reactions: Agranulocytosis, neutropenia, and bone marrow depression have been associated with the use of methicillin sodium, nafcillin, oxacillin, and cloxacillin. Hepatotoxicity, characterized by fever, nausea, and vomiting associated with abnormal liver function tests, mainly elevated SGOT levels, has been associated with the use of oxacillin and cloxacillin.

DOSAGE AND ADMINISTRATION

The penicillinase-resistant penicillins are available for oral administration and for intramuscular and intravenous injection. The sodium salts of methicillin, oxacillin, and nafcillin may be administered parenterally and the sodium salts of cloxacillin, dicloxacillin, oxacillin, and nafcillin are available for oral use.
Bacteriologic studies to determine the causative organisms and their sensitivity to the penicillinase-resistant penicillins should always be performed. Duration of therapy varies with the type and severity of infection as well as the overall condition of the patient; therefore it should be determined by the clinical and bacteriological response of the patient. In severe staphylococcal infections, therapy with penicillinase-resistant penicillins should be continued for at least 14 days. Therapy should be continued for at least 48 hours after the patient has become afebrile, asymptomatic, and cultures are negative. The treatment of endocarditis and osteomyelitis may require a longer term of therapy.
Concurrent administration of the penicillinase-resistant penicillins and probenecid increases and prolongs serum penicillin levels. Probenecid decreases the apparent volume of distribution and slows the rate of excretion by competitively inhibiting renal tubular secretion of penicillin. Penicillin-probenecid therapy is generally limited to those infections where very high serum levels of penicillin are necessary.
Oral preparations of the penicillinase-resistant penicillins should not be used as initial therapy in serious, life threatening infections (See **Precautions** — General). Oral therapy with the penicillinase-resistant penicillins may be used to follow-up the previous use of a parenteral agent as soon as the clinical condition warrants. For intramuscular gluteal infections, care should be taken to avoid sciatic nerve injury. With intravenous administration, particularly in elderly patients, care should be taken because of the possibility of thrombophlebitis.
[See table below].

DIRECTIONS FOR USE

For Intramuscular Use: Reconstitute with Sterile Water for Injection, USP, 0.9% Sodium Chloride Injection, USP or Bacteriostatic Water for Injection, USP (with benzyl alcohol or parabens); add 1.8 ml to the 500 mg vial for 2 ml resulting solution; 3.4 ml to the 1 g vial for 4 ml resulting solution; 6.6 ml to the 2 g vial for 8 ml resulting solution. All reconstituted vials have a concentration of 250 mg per ml.
The clear solution should be administered by deep intragluteal injection immediately after reconstitution.
Reconstituted Stability: Reconstitute with the required amount of Sterile Water for Injection, USP, 0.9% Sodium Chloride Injection, USP or Bacteriostatic Water for Injection, USP (with benzyl alcohol or parabens). The resulting solutions are stable for 3 days at room temperature or 7 days under refrigeration or 90 days frozen.
For Direct Intravenous Use: The required amount of drug should be diluted in 15 to 30 ml of Sterile Water for Injection, USP or Sodium Chloride Injection, USP and injected over a 5- to 10-minute period. This may be accomplished through the tubing of an intravenous infusion if desirable.
For Administration by Intravenous Drip: Reconstitute as directed above (For Intramuscular Use) prior to diluting with Intravenous Solution.
[See table on preceding page].
Only those solutions listed above should be used for the intravenous infusion of Nafcil (nafcillin sodium). The concentration of the antibiotic should fall within the range specified. The drug concentration and the rate and volume of the infusion should be adjusted so that the total dose of nafcillin is administered before the drug loses its stability in the solution in use.
There is no clinical experience available on the use of this agent in neonates or infants for this route of administration. This route of administration should be used for relatively short-term therapy (24 to 48 hours) because of the occasional occurrence of thrombophlebitis particularly in elderly patients.
If another agent is used in conjunction with nafcillin therapy, **it should not be physically mixed** with nafcillin but should be administered separately.
"Piggyback" I.V. Package: This glass vial contains the labeled quantity of Nafcil and is intended for intravenous administration. The diluent and volume are specified on the label of each package.
When the "piggyback" vial is reconstituted with either Sterile Water for Injection, USP or 0.9% Sodium Chloride Injection, USP and the resulting solutions are in a concentration of 10 to 200 mg/ml, the solutions are stable for 24 hours at room temperature or 7 days under refrigeration and 90 days frozen.
Hospital Bulk Package: This glass vial contains 10 grams Nafcil and is designed for use in the pharmacy in preparing I.V. additives.Add 93 ml Sterile Water for Injection, USP or 0.9% Sodium Chloride Injection, USP. The resulting solution will contain 100 mg nafcillin activity per ml. Solutions in a concentration of 10 mg to 200 mg per ml are stable for 24 hours at room temperature or 7 days under refrigeration. Solutions in a concentration of 250 mg per ml are stable for 3 days at room temperature or 7 days under refrigeration and 90 days frozen.

CAUTION

NOT TO BE DISPENSED AS A UNIT.

SUPPLY

Nafcil (nafcillin sodium) for Injection. Nafcillin sodium equivalent to 500 mg. 1 gram, 2 grams, or 10 grams nafcillin per vial.
NDC 0015-7224-20 — 500 mg vial
NDC 0015-7225-20 — 1 gram vial
NDC 0015-7226-20 — 2 gram vial
NDC 0015-7225-28 — 1 gram "piggyback" vial
NDC 0015-7226-28 — 2 gram "piggyback" vial
NDC 0015-7101-28 — 10 gram Hospital Bulk Package
For information on package sizes available, refer to the current price schedule.

RECOMMENDED DOSAGES FOR NAFCIL (nafcillin sodium)

Drug	Adults	Infants and Children <40 kg (88 lbs)	Other Recommendations
Nafcillin	500 mg IM every 4 to 6 hrs. IV every 4 hrs.	25 mg/kg IM twice daily	Neonates 10 mg/kg IM twice daily
	1 gram IM or IV every 4 hrs. (severe infections)		

NALDECON® ℞

[*nal 'dĕ-cŏn*]
Tablets, Syrup, Pediatric Drops and Pediatric Syrup
For Oral Use Only

This is the full text of the latest Official Package Circular dated October 1985 [5600DIM-17].

DESCRIPTION

Naldecon is a preparation containing:
[See table above].

Naldecon	For immediate action	For delayed action	Total contents
Each sustained-action tablet contains:			
Phenylpropanolamine hydrochloride	20.0 mg	20.0 mg	40.0 mg
Phenylephrine hydrochloride	5.0 mg	5.0 mg	10.0 mg
Phenyltoloxamine citrate	7.5 mg	7.5 mg	15.0 mg
Chlorpheniramine maleate	2.5 mg	2.5 mg	5.0 mg
Each teaspoonful (5 ml) of syrup contains:			
Phenylpropanolamine hydrochloride			20.0 mg
Phenylephrine hydrochloride			5.0 mg
Phenyltoloxamine citrate			7.5 mg
Chlorpheniramine maleate			2.5 mg

	Pediatric Syrup each 5-ml contains:	Pediatric Drops each 1-ml dropper contains:
Each pediatric formulation contains the following ingredients:		
Phenylpropanolamine hydrochloride	5.0 mg	5.0 mg
Phenylephrine hydrochloride	1.25 mg	1.25 mg
Phenyltoloxamine citrate	2.0 mg	2.0 mg
Chlorpheniramine maleate	0.5 mg	0.5 mg

Inactive ingredients in Naldecon tablets are: acacia, Carbowax 8000, gelatin, lactose, magnesium stearate, starch, sucrose and white wax.
Inactive ingredients in Naldecon syrup, pediatric syrup, and pediatric drops are: D & C Red No. 33, D & C Yellow No. 10, natural & artificial flavorings, glycerin, povidone, purified water, sodium benzoate and sorbitol.

CLINICAL PHARMACOLOGY

Phenylpropanolamine Hydrochloride
The drug may directly stimulate adrenergic receptors but probably indirectly stimulates both alpha (α) and beta (β) adrenergic receptors by releasing norepinephrine from its storage sites. Phenylpropanolamine increases heart rate, force of contraction and cardiac output, and excitability. It acts on α receptors in the mucosa of the respiratory tract, producing vasoconstriction which results in shrinkage of swollen mucous membranes, reduction of tissue, hyperemia, edema and nasal congestion, and an increase in nasal airway patency. Phenylpropanolamine causes CNS stimulation and reportedly has an anorexigenic effect.
Phenylephrine Hydrochloride
Phenylephrine acts predominantly by a direct action on alpha (α) adrenergic receptors. In therapeutic doses, the drug has no significant stimulant effect on the beta (β) adrenergic receptors of the heart. Following oral administration, constriction of blood vessels in the nasal mucosa may relieve nasal congestion. In therapeutic doses the drug causes little, if any, central nervous system stimulation.
Phenyltoloxamine Citrate
Phenyltoloxamine is an H_1 blocking agent which interferes with the action of histamine primarily in capillaries surrounding mucous tissues and sensory nerves of nasal and adjacent areas. It has the ability to interfere with certain actions of acetylcholine-inhibiting secretions in the nose, mouth and pharynx. It commonly causes CNS depression.
Chlorpheniramine Maleate
Chlorpheniramine competitively antagonizes most of the smooth muscle stimulating actions of histamine on the H_1 receptors of the GI tract, uterus, large blood vessels and bronchial muscle. It also antagonizes the action of histamine

that results in increased capillary permeability and the formation of edema.

INDICATIONS AND USAGE

For the relief of nasal congestion and eustachian tube congestion associated with the common cold, sinusitis and acute upper respiratory infections. Also indicated symptomatic relief of perennial and seasonal allergic rhinitis, vasomotor rhinitis.

Decongestants in combination with antihistamines have been used to relieve eustachian tube congestion associated with acute eustachian salpingitis, aerotitis and serous otitis media.

CONTRAINDICATIONS

Patients with severe hypertension, severe coronary artery disease, patients on MAO inhibitor therapy; patients with narrow angle glaucoma, urinary retention, peptic ulcer and during an asthmatic attack. Also contraindicated in patients with hypersensitivity or idiosyncrasy to sympathomimetic amines or antihistamines.

WARNINGS

Sympathomimetic amines should be used judiciously and sparingly in patients with hypertension, diabetes mellitus, ischemic heart disease, increased intraocular pressure, hyperthyroidism or prostatic hypertrophy. See, however, CONTRAINDICATIONS. Sympathomimetics may produce central nervous system stimulation with convulsions or cardiovascular collapse with accompanying hypotension.

Antihistamines may impair mental and physical abilities required for the performance of potentially hazardous tasks, such as driving a vehicle or operating machinery, and may impair mental alertness in children. Chlorpheniramine and phenyltoloxamine have an atropine-like action and should be used with caution in patients with increased intraocular pressure, cardiovascular disease, hypertension or in patients with a history of bronchial asthma. See, however, CONTRAINDICATIONS.

Do not exceed recommended dosage.

PRECAUTIONS

Patients with diabetes, hypertension, cardiovascular disease and hyperreactivity to ephedrine. The antihistaminics may cause drowsiness and ambulatory patients who operate machinery or motor vehicles should be cautioned accordingly.

DRUG INTERACTIONS

MAO inhibitors and beta adrenergic blockers increase the effect of sympathomimetics. Sympathomimetics may reduce the antihypertensive effects of methyldopa, mecamylamine, reserpine and veratrum alkaloids. Concomitant use of antihistamines with alcohol, tricyclic antidepressants, barbiturates and other CNS depressants may have an additive effect.

Pregnancy Category C: Animal reproduction studies have not been conducted with Naldecon. It is also not known whether Naldecon can cause fetal harm when administered to a pregnant woman or can effect reproductive capacity. Naldecon should be given to a pregnant woman only if clearly needed.

NURSING MOTHERS

Caution should be exercised when this drug is given to nursing mothers due to the higher than usual risk of the sympathomimetic amines in infants.

ADVERSE REACTIONS

Hyperreactive individuals may display ephedrine-like reactions such as tachycardia, palpitations, headache, dizziness or nausea. Patients sensitive to antihistamines may experience mild sedation. Sympathomimetics have been associated with certain untoward reactions including restlessness, tremor, weakness, pallor, respiratory difficulty, dysuria, insomnia, hallucinations, convulsions, CNS depression, arrhythmias and cardiovascular collapse with hypotension. Possible side effects of antihistamines are drowsiness, restlessness, dizziness, weakness, dry mouth, anorexia, nausea, vomiting, headache, nervousness, blurring of vision, polyuria, heartburn, dysuria and, very rarely, dermatitis.

DOSAGE AND ADMINISTRATION

This chart represents single dosages for the products listed below. Usual dosage schedule for Naldecon Pediatric Drops, Naldecon Pediatric Syrup and Naldecon Syrup is every 3 to 4 hours, not to exceed four doses in a 24-hour period. For sustained-action Naldecon Tablets, doses should be administered on arising, in midafternoon, and at bedtime.

[See table above].

HOW SUPPLIED

NDC 0015-5600—Naldecon Tablets
NDC 0015-5601—Naldecon Syrup
NDC 0015-5615—Naldecon Pediatric Drops
NDC 0015-5616—Naldecon Pediatric Syrup

For information on package sizes available, refer to the current price schedule.

Shown in Product Identification Section, page 406

Single Dosage for ...	Naldecon Pediatric Drops	Naldecon Pediatric Syrup	Naldecon Syrup	Naldecon Tablets
3 to 6 months (12–17 lbs)	¼ ml (0.25 ml)			
6 to 12 months (17–24 lbs)	½ ml (0.5 ml)	½ teaspoonful		
1 to 6 years (24–50 lbs)	1 ml (1.0 ml)	1 teaspoonful		
6 to 12 years (over 50 lbs)		2 teaspoonfuls	½ teaspoonful	½ tablet
over 12 years			1 teaspoonful	1 tablet

NALDECON-CX® ADULT LIQUID Ⓒ

[nal 'dĕ-côn]

DESCRIPTION

Each teaspoonful (5ml) of Naldecon-CX Adult Liquid contains:

Phenylpropanolamine hydrochloride .... 18 mg
Guaifenesin (glyceryl guaiacolate) .... 200 mg
Codeine Phosphate .... 10 mg
(Warning: May be Habit Forming)

INDICATIONS

Provide prompt relief from cough and nasal congestion, due to the common cold, bronchitis, nasopharyngitis, and influenza. Codeine termporarily quiets non-productive coughing by its antitussive action while guaifenesin's expectorant action helps loosen phlegm and bronchial secretions. Phenylpropanolamine reduces swelling of nasal passages and shrinks swollen membranes. This combination production is antihistamine-free and alcohol-free.

CONTRAINDICATIONS

Hypersensitivity of guaifenesin, codeine or sympathomimetic amines.

WARNINGS

Nervousness, dizziness or sleeplessness may occur if recommended dosage is exceeded. Do not give this product to a child with high blood pressure, heart disease, diabetes or thyroid disease except under the advice and supervision of a physician. Do not give this product to a child presently taking a prescription drug containing a monamine oxidase inhibitor except under the advice and supervision of a physician. Do not administer this product for persistent or chronic cough associated with asthma or emphysema or when cough is accompanied by excessive secretions, except under the care and advice of a physician. A persistent cough may be a sign of a serious condition. If cough persists for more than 1 week, tends to recur, or is accompanied by high fever, rash or persistent headaches, consult a physician. Keep this and all drugs out of the reach of children. In case of accidental overdose, seek professional assistance or contact a poison control center immediately.

INACTIVE INGREDIENTS

Avicel, Cough Syrup Flavor, DC Antifoam AF Emulsion, FD&C Blue No. 1, FD&C Red No. 40, Glycerin, Purified Water, Sodium Citrate, Sorbic Acid and Sucrose.

WARNING

As with any drug, if you are pregnant or nursing a baby, seek the advice of a health professional before using this product.

DOSAGE AND ADMINISTRATION

Children 2–6 years of age: ½ teaspoonful every 4 hours. Children 6–12 years of age: 1 teaspoonful every 4 hours. Adults: 2 teaspoonful every 4 hours. Do not exceed 4 doses every 24 hours. This product is a suspension—shake well before using.

HOW SUPPLIED

Naldecon-CX Adult Liquid—4oz. and pint bottles.
Also Described in PDR For Nonprescription Drugs.

NALDECON-DX ADULT LIQUID OTC

[nal 'dĕ-côn Dx]

DESCRIPTION

Each teaspoonful (5ml) of Naldecon-DX Adult Liquid contains:

Phenylpropanolamine hydrochloride 18mg
Guaifenesin (glyceryl guaiacolate) 200mg
Dextromethorphan hydrobromide 15mg

INDICATIONS

Provide prompt relief from cough and nasal congestion due to the common cold, bronchitis, nasopharyngitis, and recurrent bronchial coughing. Dextromethorphan temporarily quiets non-productive coughing by its antitussive action while guaifenesin's expectorant action helps loosen phlegm and bronchial secretions. Phenylpropanolamine reduces swelling of nasal passages: shrinks swollen membranes. This combination product is antihistamine-free, sugar-free and alcohol-free.

CONTRAINDICATIONS

Hypersensitivity to guaifenesin, dextromethorphan, or sympathomimetic amines.

WARNINGS

Nervousness, dizziness or sleeplessness may occur if recommended dosage is exceeded. Do not give this product to a child with high blood pressure, heart disease, diabetes or thyroid disease except under the advice and supervision of a physician. Do not give this product to a child presently taking a prescription drug containing a monamine oxidase inhibitor except under the advice and supervision of a physician. Do not administer this product for persistent or chronic cough such as occurs with asthma or emphysema or when cough is accompanied by excessive secretions except under the care and advice of a physician. A persistent cough may be a sign of a serious condition. If cough persists for more than 1 week, tends to recur, or is accompanied by high fever, rash or persistent headaches, consult a physician. Keep this and all drugs out of the reach of children. In case of accidental overdose, seek professional assistance or contact a Poison Control Center immediately.

INACTIVE INGREDIENTS

Avicel, DC Antifoam AF Emulsion, FD&C Yellow No. 6, Natural and Artificial Flavorings, Povidone, Propylene Glycol, Purified Water, Sodium Citrate, Sorbic Acid and Sorbitol.

WARNING: As with any drug, if you are pregnant or nursing a baby, seek the advice of a health professional before using this product.

DOSAGE AND ADMINISTRATION

12 years and older: 2 teaspoonsful 4 times daily. This product is a suspension—shake well before using.

HOW SUPPLIED

Naldecon-DX Adult Liquid—4oz. and pint bottles.
Also Described in PDR For Nonprescription Drugs

NALDECON-DX® PEDIATRIC DROPS OTC

[nal 'dĕ-côn Dx]

DESCRIPTION

Each 1ml of Naldecon-DX Pediatric Drops contains:

Phenylpropanolamine hydrochloride 9mg
Guaifenesin (glyceryl guaiacolate) 30mg
Dextromethorphan hydrobromide 7.5mg
Alcohol 0.6%

INDICATIONS

Provide prompt relief from cough and nasal congestion due to the common cold, bronchitis, nasopharyngitis and recurrent bronchial coughing. Dextromethorphan temporarily quiets non-productive coughing by its antitussive action while guaifenesin's expectorant action helps loosen phlegm and bronchial secretions. Phenylpropanolamine reduces swelling of nasal passages: shrinks swollen membranes. This combination product is antihistamine-free and sugar-free.

CONTRAINDICATIONS

Hypersensitivity to guaifenesin, dextromethorphan, or sympathomimetic amines.

WARNINGS

Nervousness, dizziness or sleeplessness may occur if recommended dosage is exceeded. Do not give this product to a child with high blood pressure, heart disease, diabetes or thyroid disease except under the advice and supervision of a physician. Do not give this product to a child presently taking a prescription drug containing a monamine oxidase inhibitor except under the advice and supervision of a physician. Do not administer this product for persistent or chronic

Continued on next page

Bristol—Cont.

cough such as occurs with asthma or emphysema or when cough is accompanied by excessive secretions except under the care and advice of a physician. A persistent cough may be a sign of a serious condition. If cough persists for more than 1 week, tends to recur, or is accompanied by high fever, rash or persistent headaches, consult a physician. Keep this and all drugs out of the reach of children. In case of accidental overdose, seek professional assistance or contact a Poison Control Center immediately.

INACTIVE INGREDIENTS

Citric Acid, FD&C Yellow No. 6, Natural and Artificial Flavorings, Propylene Glycol, Purified Water, Sodium Benzoate, Sodium Saccharin and Sorbitol.

DOSAGE AND ADMINISTRATION

Dose should be adjusted to age or weight and be given 4 times a day (see calibrations on dropper). Administer by mouth only.

1–3 Months:	4–6 Months:	7–9 Months:	10 Months or over:
1/4ml	1/2ml	3/4ml	1ml
(8–12 lbs.)	(13–17 lbs.)	(18–20 lbs.)	(21 lbs. or more)

Bottle label dosage reads as follows: Children under 2 years of age: use only as directed by a physician.

HOW SUPPLIED

Naldecon-DX Pediatric Drops—30ml bottle with calibrated dropper.
Also Described in PDR For Nonprescription Drugs

NALDECON-DX® OTC
[nal'dĕ-cŏn Dx]
CHILDREN'S SYRUP

DESCRIPTION

Each teaspoonful (5ml) of Naldecon-DX Children's Syrup contains:

Phenylpropanolamine hydrochloride	9mg
Guaifenesin (glyceryl guaiacolate)	100mg
Dextromethorphan hydrobromide	7.5mg
Alcohol	5%

INDICATIONS

Provide prompt relief from cough and nasal congestion due to the common cold, bronchitis, nasopharyngitis and recurrent bronchial coughing. Dextromethorphan temporarily quiets non-productive coughing by its antitussive action while guaifenesin's expectorant action helps loosen phlegm and bronchial secretions. Phenylpropanolamine reduces swelling of nasal passages: shrinks swollen membranes. This combination product is antihistamine-free.

CONTRAINDICATIONS

Hypersensitivity to guaifenesin, dextromethorphan, or sympathomimetic amines.

WARNINGS

Nervousness, dizziness or sleeplessness may occur if recommended dosage is exceeded. Do not give this product to a child with high blood pressure, heart disease, diabetes or thyroid disease except under the advice and supervision of a physician. Do not give this product to a child presently taking a prescription drug containing a monamine oxidase inhibitor except under the advice and supervision of a physician. Do not administer this product for persistent or chronic cough such as occurs with asthma or emphysema or when cough is accompanied by excessive secretions except under the care and advice of a physician. A persistent cough may be a sign of a serious condition. If cough persists for more than 1 week, tends to recur, or is accompanied by high fever, rash or persistent headaches, consult a physician. Keep this and all drugs out of the reach of children. In case of accidental overdose seek professional assistance or contact a Poison Control Center immediately.

INACTIVE INGREDIENTS

FD&C Yellow No. 6, Fructose, Glycerin, Natural and Artificial Flavorings, Purified Water, Sodium Benzoate, Sucrose and Tartaric Acid.

DOSAGE AND ADMINISTRATION

Children 2–6 years of age (under 50 lbs.): 1 teaspoonful every 4 hours. Children 6–12 years of age (under 100 lbs.): 2 teaspoonful every 4 hours. Do not exceed 4 doses every 24 hours. Under 2 years: use only as directed by a physician.

HOW SUPPLIED

Naldecon-DX Children's Syrup—4oz. and pint bottles.
Also Described in PDR For Nonprescription Drugs

NALDECON-EX® PEDIATRIC DROPS OTC
[nal'dĕ-cŏn Ex]

DESCRIPTION

Each 1ml of Naldecon-EX Pediatric Drops contains:

Phenylpropanolamine hydrochloride	9mg
Guaifenesin (glyceryl guaiacolate)	30mg
Alcohol	0.6%

INDICATIONS

Combined decongestant/expectorant designed specifically to promptly reduce the swelling of nasal membranes and to help loosen phlegm and bronchial secretions through productive coughing. This dual action is of particular value in infants with common cold, acute bronchitis, bronchiolitis, tracheobronchitis, nasopharyngitis and croup. This combination product is antihistamine-free.

CONTRAINDICATIONS

Hypersensitivity to guaifenesin or sympathomimetic amines.

WARNINGS

Nervousness, dizziness or sleeplessness may occur if recommended dosage is exceeded. Do not give this product to a child with high blood pressure, heart disease, diabetes or thyroid disease except under the advice and supervision of a physician. Do not give this product to a child presently taking a prescription drug containing a monamine oxidase inhibitor except under the advice and supervision of a physician. Do not administer this product for persistent or chronic cough such as occurs with asthma or emphysema or when cough is accompanied by excessive secretions except under the care and advice of a physician. A persistent cough may be a sign of a serious condition. If cough persists for more than 1 week, tends to recur, or is accompanied by high fever, rash or persistent headaches, consult a physician.
Keep this and all drugs out of the reach of children. In case of accidental overdose, seek professional assistance or contact a Poison Control Center immediately.

INACTIVE INGREDIENTS

Citric Acid, D&C Yellow No. 10, Natural and Artificial Flavorings, Propylene Glycol, Purified Water, Sodium Benzoate and Sucrose.

DOSAGE AND ADMINISTRATION

Dose should be adjusted to age or weight and be given 4 times a day (see calibrations on dropper). Administer by mouth only.

1–3 Months:	4–6 Months:	7–9 Months:	10 Months or over:
1/4ml	1/2ml	3/4ml	1ml
(8–12 lbs.)	(13–17 lbs.)	(18–20 lbs.)	(21 lbs. or more)

Bottle label dosage reads as follows: Children under 2 years of age: use only as directed by a physician.

HOW SUPPLIED

Naldecon-EX Pediatric Drops—30ml bottle with calibrated dropper.
Also Described in PDR For Nonprescription Drugs

NALDECON-EX® CHILDREN'S SYRUP OTC
[nal'dĕ-cŏn Ex]

DESCRIPTION

Each teaspoonful (5ml) of Naldecon-EX Children's Syrup contains:

Phenylpropanolamine hydrochloride	9mg
Guaifenesin (glyceryl guaiacolate)	100mg
Alcohol	5%

INDICATIONS

Combined decongestant/expectorant designed specifically to promptly reduce the swelling of nasal membranes and to help loosen phlegm and bronchial secretions through productive coughing. This dual action is of particular value in children with common cold, acute bronchitis, bronchiolitis, tracheobronchitis, nasopharyngitis and croup. This combination product is antihistamine-free and sugar-free.

CONTRAINDICATIONS

Hypersensitivity to guaifenesin or sympathomimetic amines.

WARNINGS

Nervousness, dizziness or sleeplessness may occur if recommended dosage is exceeded. Do not give this product to a child with high blood pressure, heart disease, diabetes or thyroid disease except under the advice and supervision of a physician. Do not give this product to a child presently taking a prescription drug containing a monamine oxidase inhibitor except under the advice and supervision of a physician. Do not administer this product for persistent or chronic cough such as occurs with asthma or emphysema or when cough is accompanied by excessive secretions except under the care and advice of a physician. A persistent cough may be a sign of a serious condition. If cough persists for more than 1 week, tends to recur, or is accompanied by high fever, rash or persistent headaches, consult a physician. Keep this and all drugs out of the reach of children. In case of accidental overdose, seek professional assistance or contact a Poison Control Center immediately.

INACTIVE INGREDIENTS

D&C Yellow No. 10, Glycerin, Natural and Artificial Flavorings, Propylene Glycol, Purified Water, Sodium Benzoate, Sodium Saccharin, Sorbitol and Tartaric Acid.

DOSAGE AND ADMINISTRATION

Children 2–6 years of age (under 50 lbs.): 1 teaspoonful every 4 hours. Children 6–12 years of age (under 100 lbs.): 2 teaspoonful every 4 hours. Do not exceed 4 doses every 24 hours. Under 2 years: use only as directed by a physician.

HOW SUPPLIED

Naldecon-EX Children's Syrup—4oz. and pint bottles.
Also Described in PDR For Nonprescription Drugs

POLYCILLIN® ℞
[pol"e-cil'lin]
(ampicillin)
CAPSULES
250 mg. and 500 mg.
For Oral Suspension
125 mg. per 5 ml., 250 mg. per 5 ml., 500 mg. per 5 ml.
Pediatric Drops
100 mg. per ml.

POLYCILLIN-N® ℞
(sterile ampicillin sodium)
For Intramuscular or Intravenous Injection

This is the full text of the latest Combined Official Package Circulars dated February 1985 [7988DIR-17 Polycillin] *and May 1979* [7401DIR-24 Polycillin-N]. (S 9/78)

DESCRIPTION

Polycillin (ampicillin) is a synthetic penicillin with a broad spectrum of bactericidal activity against both penicillin-susceptible Gram-positive organisms and many common Gram-negative pathogens.
Inactive ingredient in Polycillin capsules is: magnesium stearate.
Inactive ingredients in Polycillin for oral suspension and pediatric drops are: Atmos 300, DC antifoam AF emulsion, FD & C Red No. 40, lecithin, natural & artificial flavorings, silicon dioxide colloidal, sodium benzoate, sodium citrate, sucrose and vanillin.
Polycillin-N (sterile ampicillin sodium) contains 2.9 milliequivalents of sodium per 1 gram of drug.

ACTIONS

Pharmacology

Polycillin is stable in the presence of gastric acid and is well-absorbed from the gastrointestinal tract. It diffuses readily into most body tissues and fluids. However, penetration into the cerebrospinal fluid and brain occurs only when the meninges are inflamed. Ampicillin is excreted largely unchanged in the urine and its excretion can be delayed by concurrent administration of probenecid. The active form appears in the bile in higher concentrations than those found in serum. Ampicillin is the least serum-bound of all the penicillins, averaging about 20% compared to approximately 60 to 90% for other penicillins. Polycillin is well-tolerated by most patients and has been given in doses of 2 grams daily for many weeks without adverse reactions.

Microbiology

The following bacteria have been shown in **in vitro** studies to be susceptible to Polycillin:

GRAM-POSITIVE ORGANISMS: Hemolytic and non-hemolytic streptococci, **D. pneumoniae,** non-penicillinase-producing staphylococci, Clostridia spp., **B. anthracis, Listeria monocytogenes,** and most strains of enterococci.

GRAM-NEGATIVE ORGANISMS: H. influenzae, N. gonorrhoeae, N. meningitidis, Proteus mirabilis, and many strains of Salmonella, Shigella, and **E. coli.**

Polycillin does not resist destruction by penicillinase. Polycillin Susceptibility Test Discs, 10 mcg. should be used to estimate the **in vitro** susceptibility of bacteria to Polycillin.

INDICATIONS

Polycillin is indicated for the treatment of infections due to susceptible Gram-positive organisms including streptococci, pneumococci, penicillin G-susceptible staphylococci, and enterococci, and susceptible strains of Gram-negative bacteria including **H. influenzae, E. coli, Proteus mirabilis, N. gonorrhoeae, N. meningitidis,** Shigella, **S. typhosa** and other Salmonella.
Bacteriology studies to determine the causative organisms and their susceptibility to ampicillin should be performed. Therapy may be instituted prior to obtaining results of susceptibility testing.

It is advisable to reserve the parenteral form of this drug for moderately severe and severe infections and for patients who are unable to take the oral forms. A change to oral Polycillin (ampicillin) may be made as soon as appropriate.
Indicated surgical procedures should be performed.

CONTRAINDICATIONS
A history of a previous hypersensitivity reaction to any of the penicillins is a contraindication.

WARNING
Serious and occasionally fatal hypersensitivity (anaphylactoid) reactions have been reported in patients on penicillin therapy. Although anaphylaxis is more frequent following parenteral therapy, it has occurred in patients on oral penicillins. These reactions are more apt to occur in individuals with a history of sensitivity to multiple allergens.
There have been well-documented reports of individuals with a history of penicillin hypersensitivity reactions who have experienced severe hypersensitivity reactions when treated with a cephalosporin. Before therapy with a penicillin, careful inquiry should be made concerning previous hypersensitivity reactions to penicillins, cephalosporins, and other allergens.
Serious anaphylactoid reactions require immediate emergency treatment with epinephrine. Oxygen, intravenous steroids, and airway management, including intubation, should also be administered as indicated.

USAGE IN PREGNANCY
Safety for use in pregnancy has not been established.

PRECAUTIONS
The possibility of superinfections with mycotic organisms or bacterial pathogens should be kept in mind during therapy. In such cases, discontinue the drug and substitute appropriate treatment.
As with any potent drug, periodic assessment of organ system function, including renal, hepatic, and hematopoietic, should be made during prolonged therapy.
With high urine concentrations of ampicillin, false-positive glucose reactions may occur if Clinitest, Benedict's Solution, or Fehling's Solution are used. Therefore, it is recommended that glucose tests based on enzymatic glucose oxidase reactions (such as Clinistix or Tes-Tape) be used.

ADVERSE REACTIONS
As with other penicillins, it may be expected that untoward reactions will be essentially limited to sensitivity phenomena. They are more likely to occur in individuals who have previously demonstrated hypersensitivity to penicillins and in those with a history of allergy, asthma, hay fever, or urticaria.
The following adverse reactions have been reported as associated with the use of ampicillin:
Gastrointestinal—Glossitis, stomatitis, black "hairy" tongue, nausea, vomiting, enterocolitis, pseudomembranous colitis, and diarrhea. (These reactions are usually associated with oral dosage forms.)
Hypersensitivity reactions—Skin rashes and urticaria have been reported frequently. A few cases of exfoliative dermatitis and erythema multiforme have been reported. Anaphylaxis is the most serious reaction experienced and has usually been associated with the parenteral dosage form.

NOTE
Urticaria, other skin rashes, and serum sickness-like reactions may be controlled with antihistamines and, if necessary, systemic corticosteroids. Whenever such reactions occur, ampicillin should be discontinued, unless, in the opinion of the physician, the condition being treated is life threatening and amenable only to ampicillin therapy. Serious anaphylactic reactions require the immediate use of epinephrine, oxygen, and intravenous steroids.
Liver—A moderate rise in serum glutamic oxaloacetic transaminase (SGOT) has been noted, particularly in infants, but the significance of this finding is unknown. Mild transitory SGOT elevations have been observed in individuals receiving larger (two to four times) than usual and oft-repeated intramuscular injections. Evidence indicates that glutamic oxaloacetic transaminase (GOT) is released at the site of intramuscular injection of ampicillin sodium and that the presence of increased amounts of this enzyme in the blood does not necessarily indicate liver involvement.
Hemic and Lymphatic Systems—Anemia, thrombocytopenia, thrombocytopenic purpura, eosinophilia, leukopenia, and agranulocytosis have been reported during therapy with the penicillins. These reactions are usually reversible on discontinuation of therapy and are believed to be hypersensitivity phenomena.
Other—Since infectious mononucleosis is viral in origin, ampicillin should not be used in the treatment. A high percentage of patients with mononucleosis who received ampicillin developed a skin rash.

Polycillin-N—Reconstitution Volumes

NDC 0015	Label Claim	Recommended Amount of Diluent	Withdrawable Volume	Concentration (in mg/ml)
7401-20	125 mg.	1.2 ml.	1.0 ml.	125 mg.
7402-20	250 mg.	1.0 ml.	1.0 ml.	250 mg.
7403-20	500 mg.	1.8 ml.	2.0 ml.	250 mg.
7404-20	1.0 gram	3.5 ml.	4.0 ml.	250 mg.
7405-20	2.0 gram	6.8 ml.	8.0 ml.	250 mg.

DOSAGE
Infections of the respiratory tract and soft tissues:
Oral: Patients weighing 20 Kg. (44 lbs.) or more: 250 mg. every 6 hours.
Patients weighing less than 20 Kg. (44 lbs.): 50 mg./Kg./day in equally divided doses at 6-to 8-hour intervals.
Parenteral: Patients weighing 40 Kg. (88 lbs.) or more: 250 to 500 mg. every 6 hours.
Patients weighing less than 40 Kg. (88 lbs.): 25 to 50 mg./Kg./day in equally divided doses at 6-to 8-hour intervals.
Infections of the gastrointestinal and genitourinary tracts:
Oral: Patients weighing 20 Kg. (44 lbs.) or more: 500 mg. every 6 hours.
Patients weighing less than 20 Kg. (44 lbs.): 100 mg./Kg./day in equally divided doses at 6-to 8-hour intervals.
Infections of the gastrointestinal and genitourinary tracts (including those caused by Neisseria gonorrhoeae in females).
Parenteral: Patients weighing 40 Kg. (88 lbs.) or more: 500 mg. every 6 hours.
Patients weighing less than 40 Kg. (88 lbs.): 50 mg./Kg./day in equally divided doses at 6-to 8-hour intervals.
In the treatment of chronic urinary tract and intestinal infections, frequent bacteriological and clinical appraisal is necessary. Smaller doses than those recommended above should not be used. Higher doses should be used for stubborn or severe infections. In stubborn infections, therapy may be required for several weeks. It may be necessary to continue clinical and/or bacteriological follow-up for several months after cessation of therapy.
Urethritis in males or females due to N. gonorrhoeae:
Oral: 3.5 Grams, with 1.0 Gram probenecid, administered simultaneously.
Urethritis in males due to N. gonorrhoeae:
Parenteral: Adult: Two doses of 500 mg. each at an interval of 8 to 12 hours. Treatment may be repeated if necessary or extended if required.
In the treatment of complications of gonorrheal urethritis, such as prostatitis and epididymitis, prolonged and intensive therapy is recommended. Cases of gonorrhea with a suspected primary lesion of syphilis should have darkfield examinations before receiving treatment. In all other cases where concomitant syphilis is suspected, monthly serological tests should be made for a minimum of four months.
The parenteral doses for the preceding infections may be given by either the intramuscular or intravenous route. A change to oral Polycillin (ampicillin) may be made when appropriate.
Bacterial Meningitis
Parenteral ONLY: Adults and Children: 150 to 200 mg./Kg./day in equally divided doses every 3 to 4 hours. (Treatment may be initiated with intravenous drip therapy and continued with intramuscular injections.) The doses for other infections may be given by either the intravenous or intramuscular route.
Septicemia
Parenteral ONLY: Adults and Children: 150 to 200 mg./Kg./day. Start with intravenous administration for at least three days and continue with the intramuscular route every 3 to 4 hours.
Treatment of all infections should be continued for a minimum of 48 to 72 hours beyond the time that the patient becomes asymptomatic or evidence of bacterial eradication has been obtained. A minimum of 10-days treatment is recommended for any infection caused by Group A beta-hemolytic streptococci to help prevent the occurrence of acute rheumatic fever or acute glomerulonephritis.
The following Dosage chart may be useful as a guide to therapy with the Pediatric Drops.
[See table below].

Pediatric Drops—Dosage Chart

Polycillin Weight Kg.	Lb.	Infection: Respiratory	Infection: GU/GI
Up to 5	Up to 11	62.5 mg. q. 6h. (½ dropperful q. 6h.)	125 mg. q. 6h. (1 dropperful q. 6h.)
5 to 7.5	11 to 16.5	94 mg. q. 6h. (¾ dropperful q. 6h.)	188 mg. q. 6h. (1½ dropperfuls q. 6h.)
7.6 to 10	16.6 to 22	125 mg. q. 6h. (1 dropperful q. 6h.)	250 mg. q. 6h. (2 dropperfuls q. 6h.)

NOTE
For ease in administration, the dropper assembly is calibrated at the 62.5–mg. level (½ dropperful), at the 94–mg. level (¾ dropperful), and at the 125–mg. level (1 dropperful). Children over 10 Kg. (22 pounds) would generally be dosed with Polycillin for Oral Suspension.
Directions for Dispensing Oral Suspension and Pediatric Drops: Prepare these formulations at the time of dispensing. For ease in preparation, add water to the bottle in two portions and shake well after each addition. Add the total amount of water as directed on the labeling of the package being dispensed. The reconstituted formulation is stable for 14 days under refrigeration.
Parenteral—Directions For Use: Use only freshly prepared solutions. Intramuscular and intravenous injections should be administered within one hour after preparation, since the potency may decrease significantly after this period.
For Intramuscular Use: Dissolve contents of a vial with the amount of Sterile Water for Injection, U.S.P. or Bacteriostatic Water for Injection, U.S.P., listed in the table below. [See table above].
While Polycillin-N, 1.0 g. and 2.0 g., are primarily for intravenous use, they may be administered intramuscularly when the 250-mg. or 500-mg. vials are unavailable. In such instances, dissolve in 3.5 or 6.8 ml. Sterile Water for Injection, U.S.P. or Bacteriostatic Water for Injection, U.S.P., respectively. The resulting solution will provide a concentration of 250 mg. per ml.
Polycillin-N, 125 mg., is intended primarily for pediatric use. It also serves as a convenient dosage form when small parenteral doses of the antibiotic are required.
For Direct Intravenous Use: Add 5 ml. Sterile Water for Injection, U.S.P. or Bacteriostatic Water for Injection, U.S.P. to the 125-, 250-, and 500- mg. vials and administer slowly over a 3- to 5- minute period. Polycillin-N, 1.0 Gm. or 2.0 Gm., may also be given by direct intravenous administration. Dissolve in 7.4 or 14.8 ml. Sterile Water for Injection, U.S.P., or Bacteriostatic Water for Injection, U.S.P. respectively, and administer slowly over at least 10 to 15 minutes. CAUTION: More rapid administration may result in convulsive seizures.
For Administration by Intravenous Drip: Reconstitute as directed above (For Direct Intravenous Use) prior to diluting with Intravenous Solution. Stability studies on ampicillin sodium at several concentrations in various intravenous solutions indicate the drug will lose less than 10% activity at the temperatures noted for the time periods stated:
[See table above].
Only those solutions listed above should be used for the intravenous infusion of Polycillin-N. The concentrations should fall within the range specified. The drug concentration and the rate and volume of the infusion should be adjusted so that the total dose of ampicillin is administered before the drug loses its stability in the solution in use.
"Piggyback" I.V. Package: These glass vials contain the labeled quantity of POLYCILLIN-N and are intended for intravenous administration. The diluent and volume are specified on the label of each package.
Hospital Bulk Package: This glass vial contains 10 grams ampicillin and is designed for use in the pharmacy in preparing I.V. additives. Add 94 ml Sterile Water for Injection, U.S.P. The resulting solution will contain 100 milligrams ampicillin activity per ml, and is stable up to one hour at room temperature. Diluting further within one hour to 5 mg to 10 mg per ml, the resulting solution will remain stable for 8 hours at room temperature or 72 hours under refrigeration.
Caution: NOT TO BE DISPENSED AS A UNIT.

Continued on next page

Bristol—Cont.

Polycillin-N IV Stability
Room Temperature (25°C.)

Diluent	Concentrations	Stability Periods
Sterile Water for Injection	up to 30 mg./ml.	8 hours
Isotonic Sodium Chloride	up to 30 mg./ml.	8 hours
M/6 Sodium Lactate Solution	up to 30 mg./ml.	8 hours
5% Dextrose in Water	10 to 20 mg./ml.	2 hours
5% Dextrose in Water	up to 2 mg./ml.	4 hours
5% Dextrose in 0.45% NaCl	up to 2 mg./ml.	4 hours
10% Invert Sugar in Water	up to 2 mg./ml.	4 hours
Lactated Ringer's Solution	up to 30 mg./ml.	8 hours
Refrigerated (4°C.)		
Sterile Water for Injection	30 mg./ml.	48 hours
Sterile Water for Injection	up to 20 mg./ml.	72 hours
Isotonic Sodium Chloride	30 mg./ml.	48 hours
Isotonic Sodium Chloride	up to 20 mg./ml.	72 hours
Lactated Ringer's Solution	up to 30 mg./ml.	24 hours
M/6 Sodium Lactate	up to 30 mg./ml.	8 hours
5% Dextrose in Water	up to 20 mg./ml.	4 hours
5% Dextrose in 0.45% NaCl	up to 10 mg./ml.	4 hours
10% Invert Sugar	up to 20 mg./ml.	3 hours

SUPPLY

Polycillin (ampicillin) for Oral Suspension. Each 5 ml. of reconstituted suspension contains ampicillin trihydrate equivalent to 125, 250, or 500 mg. ampicillin.
NDC 0015-7988—125 mg., 80 ml., 100 ml., 150 ml. and 200 ml. bottles
NDC 0015-7998—250 mg., 80 ml., 100 ml., 150 ml. and 200 ml. bottle
NDC 0015-7884—500 mg., 100 ml. bottle
Polycillin (ampicillin) Capsules. Ampicillin trihydrate equivalent to 250 or 500 mg. ampicillin per capsule.
NDC 0015-7992—250 mg.
NDC 0015-7993—500 mg.
Shown in Product Identification Section, page 406
Polycillin (ampicillin) for oral suspension. Each ml. of reconstituted pediatric drops contains ampicillin trihydrate equivalent to 100 mg. ampicillin.
NDC 0015-7884—100 mg., 20 ml. bottles.
Polycillin-N (sterile ampicillin sodium) for I.M. or I.V. Injection. Ampicillin sodium equivalent to 125, 250, 500 mg., 1.0 Gm., or 2.0 Gm. ampicillin per vial.
NDC 0015-7401-20—125-mg. vial.
NDC 0015-7402-20—250-mg. vial.
NDC 0015-7403-20—500-mg. vial.
NDC 0015-7404-20—1.0-Gm. vial.
NDC 0015-7405-20—2.0 Gm. vial.
NDC 0015-7403-31—500 mg. "piggyback" vial.
NDC 0015-7404-36—1.0 gram "piggyback" vial.
NDC 0015-7405-28—2.0 gram "piggyback" vial.
NDC 0015-7100-28—10 gram Hospital Bulk Package
For information on package sizes available, refer to the current price sheets.

POLYCILLIN-PRB® ℞

[*pol"e-cil'lin*]
(ampicillin-probenecid)
For Oral Suspension
Ampicillin Trihydrate equivalent to 3.5 Grams ampicillin with 1.0 Gram probenecid

This is the full text of the latest Official Package Circular dated February 1985 [7607 DIR-07].

DESCRIPTION

Polycillin-PRB (ampicillin-probenecid) is a semisynthetic penicillin in combination with probenecid.
Inactive ingredients in Polycillin-PRB oral Suspension are: Atmos 300, FD & C Red No. 40, natural & artificial flavorings, sodium saccharin, sucrose and Veegum F.

ACTIONS

Pharmacology
Ampicillin is stable in the presence of gastric acid and is well-absorbed from the gastrointestinal tract. It diffuses readily into most body tissues and fluids. However, penetration into the cerebrospinal fluid and brain occurs only when the meninges are inflamed. Ampicillin is excreted largely unchanged in the urine and its excretion can be delayed by concurrent administration of probenecid. The active form appears in the bile in higher concentrations than those found in serum. Ampicillin is the least serum-bound of all the penicillins, averaging about 20% compared to approximately 60 to 90% for other penicillins. Probenecid inhibits the renal tubular secretion of penicillins causing an increased serum level of the antibiotic.
Microbiology
Neisseria gonorrhoeae has been shown in **in vitro** studies to be susceptible to ampicillin.

INDICATIONS

Ampicillin-probenecid is indicated for the treatment of uncomplicated infections (urethral, endocervical, or rectal) due to **N. gonorrhoeae** in males and females.
Susceptibility studies should be performed with recurrent infections or when resistant strains are encountered. Therapy may be instituted prior to obtaining results of susceptibility testing.

CONTRAINDICATIONS

Ampicillin
A history of previous hypersensitivity reactions to any of the penicillins is a contraindication.
Probenecid
Polycillin-PRB should not be given to individuals with a known hypersensitivity to probenecid. It is not recommended for patients with known blood dyscrasias, uric acid kidney stones or during an acute attack of gout.

WARNINGS

Serious and occasionally fatal hypersensitivity reactions have been reported in patients on penicillin therapy. Although anaphylaxis is more frequent following parenteral therapy, it has occurred in patients on oral penicillins. These reactions are more apt to occur in individuals with a history of sensitivity to multiple allergens.
There have been well-documented reports of individuals with a history of penicillin hypersensitivity reactions who have experienced severe hypersensitivity reactions when treated with a cephalosporin. Before therapy with a penicillin, careful inquiry should be made concerning previous hypersensitivity reactions to penicillins, cephalosporins, and other allergens. If an allergic reaction occurs, the patient should be treated with the usual agents, e.g., pressor amines, antihistamines, and corticosteroids. Serious anaphylactoid reactions require emergency treatment with epinephrine. Oxygen, intravenous steroids, and airway management, including intubation, should also be administered as indicated.
USAGE IN PREGNANCY: Safety for use in pregnancy has not been established.

PRECAUTIONS

Cases of gonococcal infection with a suspected lesion of syphilis should have darkfield examinations ruling out syphilis before receiving ampicillin. Patients who do not have suspected lesions of syphilis and are treated with ampicillin should have a follow-up serologic test for syphilis each month for four months to detect syphilis that may have been masked by treatment for gonorrhea. Patients with gonorrhea who also have syphilis should be given additional appropriate parenteral penicillin treatment.

ADVERSE REACTIONS

As with other penicillins, it may be expected that untoward reactions to ampicillin will be essentially limited to sensitivity phenomena. They are more likely to occur in individuals who have previously demonstrated hypersensitivity to penicillins and in those with a history of allergy, asthma, hay fever, or urticaria.
The following adverse reactions have been reported as associated with the use of ampicillin:
Gastrointestinal—Glossitis, stomatitis, black "hairy" tongue, nausea, vomiting, enterocolitis, pseudomembranous colitis, and diarrhea. (These reactions are usually associated with oral dosage forms.)
Hypersensitivity reactions—Skin rashes and urticaria have been reported frequently. A few cases of exfoliative dermatitis and erythema multiforme have been reported. Anaphylaxis is the most serious reaction experienced and has usually been associated with the parenteral form.
Serious acute hypersensitivity reactions may require the use of epinephrine, oxygen, and airway management, which may include endotracheal intubation, intravenous steroids, and repletion of plasma volume.
Liver—A moderate rise in serum glutamic oxaloacetic transaminase (SGOT) has been noted, but the significance of this finding is unknown.
Hemic and Lymphatic Systems—Anemia, thrombocytopenia, thrombocytopenic purpura, eosinophilia, leukopenia, and agranulocytosis have been reported during therapy with the penicillins. These reactions are usually reversible on discontinuation of therapy and are believed to be hypersensitivity phenomena.

DOSAGE

Acute N. gonorrhoeae infections in adult males and females.
3.5 Grams ampicillin, with 1.0 Gram probenecid, administered simultaneously. One bottle contains enough of each drug for the required single dose.
It is desirable that follow-up cultures be obtained from the original site(s) of infection 7 to 14 days after therapy.
In women, it is also desirable to obtain culture test-of-cure from both the endocervical and anal canal.
Directions For Dispensing Oral Suspension: Prepare this formulation at the time of dispensing. For ease in preparation, add water to the bottle in two portions and shake well after each addition. Add the total amount of water as directed on the labeling of the package being dispensed. The reconstituted formulation is stable for 24 hours at room temperature.

SUPPLY

POLYCILLIN-PRB (Ampicillin-Probenecid) for Oral Suspension. Ampicillin Trihydrate equivalent to 3.5 Grams ampicillin with 1.0 Gram probenecid, single-dose bottle.
NDC 0015-7607

POLYMOX® ℞

[*pol"e-mox*]
(amoxicillin)
CAPSULES
250 mg. and 500 mg.
FOR ORAL SUSPENSION
125 mg. per 5 ml., 250 mg. per 5 ml.
PEDIATRIC DROPS
50 mg. per ml.

This is the full text of the latest Official Package Circular dated February 1985 [7276DIRO-08].

DESCRIPTION

Polymox® (amoxicillin) is a semisynthetic penicillin, an analogue of ampicillin, with a broad spectrum of bactericidal activity against Gram-positive organisms and many Gram-negative pathogens.
Inactive ingredient in Polymox capsules is: magnesium stearate.
Inactive ingredients in Polymox for oral suspension and pediatric drops are: acacia, Atmos 300, DC antifoam AF emulsion, FD & C Red No. 40, lecithin, natural & artificial flavorings, silicon dioxide colloidal, sodium benzoate, sodium citrate and sucrose.

ACTIONS

Pharmacology
Polymox® is stable in the presence of gastric acid and is well absorbed from the gastrointestinal tract and may be given with no regard to food. It diffuses readily into most body tissues and fluids, with the exception of brain and spinal fluid, except when meninges are inflamed. The half-life of amoxicillin is 61.3 minutes. Most of the amoxicillin is excreted unchanged in the urine; its excretion can be delayed by concurrent administration of probenecid. Amoxicillin is not highly protein-bound. In blood serum, amoxicillin is approximately 20% protein-bound as compared to 60% for penicillin-G.
Orally administered doses of 250 mg. and 500 mg. amoxicillin capsules result in average peak blood levels one to two hours after administration in the range of 3.5 mcg./ml. to 5.0 mcg./ml. and 5.5 mcg./ml. to 7.5 mcg./ml. respectively.
Orally administered doses of amoxicillin suspension 125 mg./5 ml., and 250 mg./5 ml., result in average peak blood levels one to two hours after administration in the range of 1.5 mcg./ml. to 3.0 mcg./ml. and 3.5 mcg./ml. to 5.0 mcg./ml. respectively.
Detectable serum levels are observed up to 8 hours after an orally administered dose of amoxicillin. Approximately 60 percent of an orally administered dose of amoxicillin is excreted in the urine within six to eight hours.

Microbiology
Polymox® (amoxicillin) is similar to ampicillin in its bactericidal action against susceptible organisms during the stage of active multiplication. It acts through the inhibition of biosynthesis of cell wall mucopeptides. **In vitro** studies have demonstrated the susceptibility of most strains of the following Gram-positive bacteria: alpha- and beta-hemolytic streptococci, **Diplococcus pneumoniae,** nonpenicillinase-producing **staphylococci,** and **Streptococcus faecalis.** It is

active **in vitro** against many strains of **Haemophilus influenzae, Neisseria gonorrhoeae, Escherichia coli** and **Proteus mirabilis.** Because it does not resist destruction by penicillinase, it is **not** effective against penicillinase-producing bacteria, particularly resistant staphylococci. All strains of Pseudomonas and most strains of Klebsiella and Enterobacter are resistant.

Disc Susceptibility Tests

Quantitative methods that require measurement of zone diameters give the most precise estimates of antibiotic susceptibility. One such procedure* has been recommended for use with discs for testing susceptibility to ampicillin-class antibiotics. Interpretations correlate diameters on the disc test with MIC values for amoxicillin. With this procedure, a report from the laboratory of "susceptible" indicates that the infecting organism is likely to respond to therapy. A report of "resistant" indicates that the infecting organism is not likely to respond to therapy. A report of "intermediate susceptibility" suggests that the organism would be susceptible if high dosage is used, or if the infection is confined to tissues and fluids (e.g., urine), in which high antibiotic levels are attained.

INDICATIONS

Polymox® (amoxicillin) is indicated in the treatment of infections due to susceptible strains of the following:

GRAM-NEGATIVE ORGANISMS—**H. influenzae, E. coli, P. mirabilis** and **N. gonorrhoeae.**

GRAM-POSITIVE ORGANISMS—Streptococci (including **Streptococcus faecalis**), **D. pneumoniae,** and nonpenicillinase-producing staphylococci.

Therapy may be instituted prior to obtaining results from bacteriological and susceptibility studies to determine the causative organisms and their susceptibility to amoxicillin.

Indicated surgical procedures should be performed.

CONTRAINDICATIONS

A history of a previous hypersensitivity reaction to any of the penicillins is a contraindication.

WARNING

Serious and occasionally fatal hypersensitivity (anaphylactoid) reactions have been reported in patients on penicillin therapy. Although anaphylaxis is more frequent following parenteral therapy, it has occurred in patients on oral penicillins. These reactions are more apt to occur in individuals with a history of sensitivity to multiple allergens.

There have been well-documented reports of individuals with a history of penicillin hypersensitivity reactions who have experienced severe hypersensitivity reactions when treated with a cephalosporin. Before therapy with a penicillin, careful inquiry should be made concerning previous hypersensitivity reactions to penicillins, cephalosporins, and other allergens.

SERIOUS ANAPHYLACTOID REACTIONS REQUIRE IMMEDIATE EMERGENCY TREATMENT WITH EPINEPHRINE. OXYGEN, INTRAVENOUS STEROIDS, AND AIRWAY MANAGEMENT, INCLUDING INTUBATION, SHOULD ALSO BE ADMINISTERED AS INDICATED.

USAGE IN PREGNANCY

Safety for use in pregnancy has not been established.

PRECAUTIONS

The possibility of superinfections with mycotic organisms or bacterial pathogens should be kept in mind during therapy. In such cases, discontinue the drug and substitute appropriate treatment.

As with any potent drug, periodic assessment of organ system function, including renal, hepatic, and hematopoietic, should be made during prolonged therapy.

ADVERSE REACTIONS

As with other penicillins, it may be expected that untoward reactions will be essentially limited to sensitivity phenomena. They are more likely to occur in individuals who have previously demonstrated hypersensitivity to penicillins and in those with a history of allergy, asthma, hay fever, or urticaria.

The following adverse reactions have been reported as associated with the use of penicillin:

Gastrointestinal—Glossitis, stomatitis, black "hairy" tongue, nausea, vomiting, and diarrhea. (These reactions are usually associated with oral dosage forms.)

Hypersensitivity Reactions—Skin rashes and urticaria have been reported frequently. A few cases of exfoliative dermatitis and erythema multiforme have been reported. Anaphylaxis is the most serious reaction experienced and has usually been associated with the parenteral dosage form.

NOTE

Urticaria, other skin rashes, and serum sickness-like reactions may be controlled with antihistamines and, if necessary, systemic corticosteroids. Whenever such reactions occur, penicillin should be discontinued unless, in the opinion of the physician, the condition being treated is life threatening and amenable only to penicillin therapy. Serious anaphylactic reactions require the immediate use of epinephrine, oxygen, and intravenous steroids.

Liver—A moderate rise in serum glutamic oxaloacetic transaminase (SGOT) has been noted, particularly in infants, but the significance of this finding is unknown.

Hemic and Lymphatic Systems—Anemia, thrombocytopenia, thrombocytopenic purpura, **eosinophilia,** leukopenia, and agranulocytosis have been reported during therapy with the penicillins. These reactions are usually reversible on discontinuation of therapy and are believed to be hypersensitivity phenomena.

DOSAGE AND ADMINISTRATION

Infections of the ear, nose, and throat due to streptococci, pneumococci, nonpenicillinase-producing staphylococci and **H. influenzae;**

Infections of the genitourinary tract due to **E. coli, Proteus mirabilis,** and **Streptococcus faecalis;**

Infections of the skin and soft-tissues due to streptococci, susceptible staphylococci, and **E. coli:**

Usual Dosage: Adults: 250 mg. every 8 hours.

Children: 20 mg./Kg./day in divided doses every 8 hours. Children weighing 20 Kg. or more should be dosed according to the adult recommendations.

In severe infections or those caused by less susceptible organisms: 500 mg. every 8 hours for adults, and 40 mg./Kg./day in divided doses every 8 hours for children may be needed.

Infections of the lower respiratory tract, due to streptococci, pneumococci, nonpenicillinase-producing staphylococci, and **H. influenzae:**

Usual Dosage: Adults: 500 mg. every 8 hours.

Children: 40 mg./Kg./day in divided doses every 8 hours. Children weighing 20 Kg. or more should be dosed according to the adult recommendations.

Larger doses may be required for stubborn or severe infections.

The children's dosage is intended for individuals whose weight will not cause a dosage to be calculated greater than that recommended for adults.

Gonorrhea, acute uncomplicated ano-genital and urethral infections due to **N. gonorrhoeae:** (males and females) 3 grams as a single oral dose.

Cases of gonorrhea with a suspected lesion of syphilis should have dark-field examinations before receiving amoxicillin, and monthly serological tests for a minimum of four months.

It should be recognized that in the treatment of chronic urinary tract infections, frequent bacteriological and clinical appraisals are necessary. Smaller doses than those recommended above should not be used. Even higher doses may be needed at times. In stubborn infections, therapy may be required for several weeks. It may be necessary to continue clinical and/or bacteriological follow-up for several months after cessation of therapy. Except for gonorrhea, treatment should be continued for a minimum of 48 to 72 hours beyond the time that the patient becomes asymptomatic or evidence of bacterial eradication has been obtained. It is recommended that there be at least 10 days treatment for any infection caused by hemolytic streptococci to prevent the occurrence of acute rheumatic fever or glomerulonephritis.

Dosage and Administration of Pediatric Drops: Usual dosage for all indications except infections of the lower respiratory tract:

Under 6 Kg. (13 lbs.): 0.5 ml. every 8 hours.
6-8 Kg. (13 to 18 lbs.): 1 ml. every 8 hours.

Infections of the lower respiratory tract:

Under 6 Kg. (13 lbs.): 1 ml. every 8 hours.
6-8 Kg. (13 to 18 lbs.): 2 ml. every 8 hours.

Children weighing more than 8 Kg. (18 lbs.) should receive the appropriate dose of the Oral Suspension 125 mg. or 250 mg./5 ml.

After reconstitution, the required amount of suspension should be placed directly on the child's tongue for swallowing. Alternate means of administration are to add the required amount of suspension to formula, milk, fruit juice, water, ginger ale, or cold drinks. These preparations should then be taken immediately. To be certain the child is receiving full dosage, such preparations should be consumed in entirety.

Directions For Dispensing Oral Suspension and Pediatric Drops:

Prepare these formulations at the time of dispensing. For ease in preparation, add water to the bottle in two portions and shake well after each addition. Add the total amount of water as directed on the labeling of the package being dispensed.

The reconstituted formulation is stable for 14 days at either room temperature or refrigeration.

HOW SUPPLIED

Polymox (amoxicillin) Capsules. Each capsule contains amoxicillin trihydrate equivalent to 250 or 500 mg. amoxicillin.

NDC 0015-7278—250 mg., bottles of 100 and 500.

NDC 0015-7279—500 mg., bottles of 50 and 100.

Shown in Product Identification Section, page 406

Polymox (amoxicillin) for Oral Suspension. Each 5 ml. of reconstituted suspension contains amoxicillin trihydrate equivalent to 125 or 250 mg. amoxicillin.

NDC 0015-7276—125 mg., 80 ml., 100 ml. and 150 ml. bottles.

NDC 0015-7277—250 mg., 80 ml., 100 ml. and 150 ml. bottles.

Polymox (amoxicillin) for Oral Suspension. Each ml. of reconstituted pediatric drops contains amoxicillin trihydrate equivalent to 50 mg. amoxicillin.

NDC 0015-7277—50 mg.

For information on package sizes available, refer to the current price sheets.

---

*Bauer, A.W., Kirby, W.M.M., Sherris, J.C., and Turck, M.: Antibiotic Testing by a Standardized Single Disc Method, Am. J. Clin. Pathol., 45:493, 1966; Standardized Disc Susceptibility Test, FEDERAL REGISTER 37:20527–29, 1972.

PRECEF® ℞

[pree-sef]

cefonide for injection

This is the full text of the latest Official Package Circular dated January 1986 [7351DIR-09].

DESCRIPTION

Precef (ceforanide) is a semisynthetic broad spectrum cephalosporin antibiotic for parenteral administration. It is provided as a sterile sodium-free mixture of crystalline 7-[O-(aminomethyl) phenylacetamido]-3[[[1-carboxymethyl)-IH-tetrazol-5-yl]thio]methyl]-3-cephem-4-carboxylic acid and L (+) lysine. When reconstituted a solution of the lysine salt of ceforanide is formed. Solutions of Precef range in color from light yellow to amber depending on the concentration and diluent used. The pH of the solution ranges from 5.5 to 8.5. The structural formula is as shown below:

Clinical Pharmacology: Mean peak plasma concentrations of 40 and 76 mcg/ml occurred at 1 hr. after intramuscular administration of doses of 0.5 and 1.0 gram, respectively, of Precef to normal subjects. These concentrations declined to 3.9 and 6.7 mcg/ml at 12 hours. Following 30-minute intravenous infusions of 1.0 and 2.0 gram doses of Precef, respectively, the mean plasma concentrations were 125 and 240 mcg/ml, declining to 5.9 and 9.0 mcg/ml in 12 hours.

The terminal plasma half-life was 2.9 hours after intravenous and intramuscular administration. Plasma protein binding was 80% at plasma concentrations achieved after 0.5-2.0 gram doses. There was no evidence of drug accumulation and plasma pharmacokinetics did not change after twice daily administration of 0.5-2.0 grams for 9.5 days.

Precef was not metabolized prior to elimination and was primarily excreted by the kidneys. After intramuscular administration of 0.5 and 1.0 gram doses, mean peak urinary concentrations of 1250 and 2900 mcg/ml occurred within 2 hours. Urine levels were 110 and 265 mcg/ml, respectively, at 9–12 hours. Intravenous doses of 1.0 and 2.0 gram of Precef produced mean urinary concentrations of 2550 and 5130 mcg/ml, respectively, within 2 hours after administration. Urine levels were 190 and 440 mcg/ml, respectively, at 9–12 hours. Excretion kinetics and clearance rates did not change following twice daily administration of these doses for 9.5 days. Urinary excretion accounted for 78–95% of the 0.5–2.0 gram intramuscular and/or intravenous dose in 12 hours.

Probenecid has no effect on serum concentrations of Precef. Precef reaches therapeutic levels in the gall bladder, myocardium, bone, skeletal muscle, and vaginal tissue. Therapeutic levels are also achieved in pericardial fluid, synovial fluid and bile.

Microbiology: The bactericidal activity of Precef results from inhibition of cell wall synthesis. Ceforanide has a high degree of stability in the presence of some **beta**-lactamases. Ceforanide is usually active against the following microorganisms **in vitro.**

Aerobes:

Gram-negative:

- **Escherichia coli**
- **Klebsiella** species
- **Proteus mirabilis**
- **Providencia** species (including **Providencia rettgeri,** formerly **Proteus rettgeri**)
- **Citrobacter** species
- **Haemophilus influenzae**
- **Haemophilus parainfluenzae**
- **Enterobacter** species
- **Salmonella typhi**
- **Neisseria gonorrhoeae**

Gram-positive:

- Staphylococci, including penicillinase-producing strains.

Continued on next page

Bristol—Cont.

Note: Methicillin-resistant staphylococci as well as some strains of **Staphylococcus epidermidis** are resistant.

Streptococcus pneumoniae (Formerly **Diplococcus pneumoniae**)

Group A and Group B streptococci

Streptococcus viridans

Note: Most strains of enterococci, e.g. **Streptococcus faecalis, are resistant.**

Anaerobes:

Fusobacterium species

Clostridium species

Note: Most strains of **Clostridium difficile** are resistant.

Peptococcus species

Peptostreptococcus species

While most strains of **B. fragilis** are resistant, ceforanide demonstrates **in vitro** activity against some bacteroides species.

Note: Pseudomonas, Acinetobacter calcoaceticus (formerly **Mima** and **Herellea** species) and most **Serratia** strains are resistant to ceforanide.

Disc susceptibility tests: Quantitative methods that require measurement of zone diameters give the most precise estimate of antibiotic susceptibility. One such procedure† has been recommended for use with discs to test susceptibility to ceforanide.

Reports from laboratory giving results of the standard single-disc susceptibility test with a 30-mcg cefamandole disc should be interpreted according to the following criteria:

Susceptible organisms produce zones of 18 mm or greater, indicating that the test organism is likely to respond to therapy.

Organisms that produce zones of 15 to 17 mm are expected to be susceptible if high dosage is used or if the infection is confined to tissues and fluids (e.g. urine) in which high antibiotic levels are attained.

Resistant organisms produce zones of 14 mm or less, indicating that other therapy should be selected.

For gram-positive isolates, the test may be performed with either the cephalosporin-class disc (30 mcg cephalothin) or the cefamandole disc (30 mcg cefamandole), and a zone of 18 mm is indicative of a ceforanide-susceptible organism. Gram-negative organisms should be tested with the cefamandole disc (using the above criteria) since ceforanide has been shown by **in vitro** tests to have activity against certain strains of **Enterobacteriaceae** found resistant when tested with the cephalosporin-class disc. Gram-negative organisms having zones of less than 18 mm around the cephalothin disc are not necessarily moderately susceptible or resistant to ceforanide.

In other susceptibility testing procedures e.g. ICS agar dilution†† or the equivalent, a bacterial isolate may be considered susceptible if the MIC value for ceforanide is not more than 16 mcg/ml. Organisms are considered resistant to ceforanide if the MIC is greater than 32 mcg/ml. Organisms having an MIC value of 32 mcg/ml or less than 32 mcg/ml, but greater than 16 mcg/ml are expected to be susceptible if high dosage is used or if the infection is confined to tissues and fluids (e.g. urine) in which high antibiotic levels are attained.

INDICATIONS AND USAGE

Precef is indicated for the treatment of serious infections caused by susceptible strains of the designated microorganisms in the diseases listed below:

(1) Bone and Joint Infections—caused by **Staphylococcus aureus** (penicillinase and non-penicillinase producing strains).

(2) Endocarditis—caused by **Staphylococcus aureus** (penicillinase and non-penicillinase producing strains).

(3) Lower Respiratory Tract Infections—caused by **Staphylococcus aureus** (penicillinase and non-penicillinase producing strains), **Streptococcus pneumoniae** (formerly **D. pneumoniae**), **Klebsiella pneumoniae**, and **Haemophilus influenzae.**

(4) Bacterial Septicemia—caused by **Staphylococcus aureus** (penicillinase and non-pencillinase producing strains), **Streptococcus pneumoniae**, and **Escherichia coli.**

(5) Skin and Skin Structure Infections—caused by **Staphylococcus aureus** (penicillinase and non-penicillinase producing strains), **Staphylococcus epidermidis**, Group A and Group B streptococci, **Escherichia coli, Proteus mirabillis**, and **Klebsiella pneumoniae.**

(6) Urinary Tract Infections—caused by **Escherichia coli, Proteus mirabillis**, and **Klebsiella pneumoniae.**

NOTE: Injectable Penicillin G Benzathine is considered to be the drug of choice in the treatment and prevention of streptococcal infections including prophylaxis of rheumatic fever.

Specimens for bacteriologic cultures should be obtained in order to isolate and identify causative organisms and to determine their susceptibilities to ceforanide. Therapy may be instituted before results of susceptibility studies are known; however, once these results become available, the antibiotic treatment should be adjusted accordingly.

Prophylactic Use—PERIOPERATIVE PROPHYLAXIS: The preoperative prophylactic administration of Precef may prevent the growth of susceptible organisms and thereby may reduce the incidence of certain postoperative infections in patients undergoing surgical procedures which are classified as contaminated or potentially contaminated, e.g. vaginal hysterectomy. Effective prophylactic use of an antibiotic in surgery depends upon the time of administration. Precef should usually be administered sixty minutes before the operation to allow sufficient time to achieve an effective antibiotic concentration in the wound tissues during the procedure. Prophylactic administration is usually not required after the surgical procedure ends and should be discontinued within a 24 hour period. In the majority of surgical procedures, continuing prophylactic administration of any antibiotic does not reduce the incidence of subsequent infections but will increase the possibility of adverse reactions and the development of bacterial resistance.

The perioperative use of Precef may also be effective in surgical patients in whom infections at the operative site would present a serious risk, e.g. during prosthetic arthroplasty and open-heart surgery. Although ceforanide has been shown to be as effective as cephalothin in the prevention of infections following coronary artery bypass surgery, no placebo controlled trials have been conducted to evaluate any cephalosporin antibiotic in the prevention of infection following either coronary artery bypass surgery or prosthetic heart valve replacement. In these procedures where the occurrence of infection may be particularly devastating, the prophylactic administration of Precef may be continued for 2 days, administered every 12 hours following completion of surgery. If there are signs of infection, specimens for culture should be obtained for the identification of the causative organism so that the appropriate therapy may be instituted. (See Dosage and Administration.)

CONTRAINDICATION

Precef is contraindicated in patients with known hypersensitivity to ceforanide and the cephalosporin group of antibiotics.

WARNINGS

BEFORE THERAPY WITH PRECEF IS INSTITUTED, CAREFUL INQUIRY SHOULD BE MADE TO DETERMINE WHETHER THE PATIENT HAS HAD PREVIOUS HYPERSENSITIVITY REACTIONS TO CEPHALOSPORINS, PENICILLINS, OR OTHER DRUGS. THIS PRODUCT SHOULD BE GIVEN CAUTIOUSLY TO PENICILLIN-SENSITIVE PATIENTS. ANTIBIOTICS SHOULD BE ADMINISTERED WITH CAUTION TO ANY PATIENT WHO HAS DEMONSTRATED SOME FORM OF ALLERGY, PARTICULARLY TO DRUGS. IF AN ALLERGIC REACTION TO PRECEF OCCURS, DISCONTINUE THE DRUG. SERIOUS ACUTE HYPERSENSITIVITY REACTIONS MAY REQUIRE EPINEPHRINE ADMINISTRATION AND OTHER EMERGENCY MEASURES.

Pseudomembranous colitis has been reported with the use of cephalosporins (and other broad spectrum antibiotics), therefore, it is important to consider its diagnosis in patients in whom diarrhea develops in association with cephalosporin use.

Treatment with broad spectrum antibiotics alters the normal flora of the colon and may permit overgrowth of clostridia. Studies indicate a toxin produced by **Clostridium difficile** is one primary cause of antibiotic-associated colitis. Cholestyramine and colestipol HCl resins have been shown to bind the toxin **in vitro.**

Mild cases of colitis may respond to drug discontinuance alone. Moderate to severe cases should be managed with fluid, electrolyte, and protein supplementation as indicated. When the colitis is not relieved by drug discontinuation or when it is severe, oral vancomycin is effective treatment of the antibiotic-associated pseudomembranous colitis produced by **C. difficile.** Other causes of colitis should also be considered.

PRECAUTIONS

Although Precef rarely produces alterations in kidney function, evaluation of renal status during therapy is recommended, especially in seriously ill patients receiving the maximum dosage. The total daily dose of Precef should be reduced in patients with transient or persistent renal insufficiency (see Dosage) because high and prolonged serum antibiotic concentrations can occur in such individuals from usual dosage.

Cephalosporins should be given with caution to patients receiving concurrent treatment with potent diuretics as these regimens are suspected of adversely affecting renal function. Nephrotoxicity has been reported following concomitant administration of cephalosporins and aminoglycoside antibiotics.

Precef should be prescribed with caution in individuals with a history of gastrointestinal disease, particularly colitis.

As with other antibiotics, prolonged use of Precef may result in overgrowth of non-susceptible organisms. Repeated evaluation of the patient's condition is essential. If superinfection occurs during therapy, appropriate measures should be taken.

Usage in Pregnancy—Pregnancy Category B—In a study in which rats were treated prior to mating and through pregnancy and lactation at dose levels (1600 mg/kg/day) 50 times the usual Precef dose (30 mg/kg/day), there was no evidence of impaired male or female fertility or reproductive performance. Results of teratogenicity tests in mice and rats employing doses as high as 25 times the human dose were also negative. In a peri-postnatal study, female rats treated subcutaneously with Precef at 50 times the usual human dose had a higher number of resorption sites than controls and there was a decrease in viability of the offspring. These phenomena may well have been secondary to the effects on the maternal animals of the high volume of solution injected (8 ml/kg/day), rather than representing a direct effect on the conceptus; neither was evident at lower dosage levels (e.g. 25 times human dose). There are, however, no adequate and well controlled studies in pregnant women. Because animal reproduction studies are not always predictive of human response, Precef should be used during pregnancy only if clearly needed.

Labor and Delivery—There are no data concerning the administration of Precef to women during labor or prior to delivery.

Nursing Mothers—It is not known whether Precef is excreted in human milk. Because many drugs are, caution should be exercised when Precef is administered to a nursing woman.

Pediatric Use—Safety and effectiveness of Precef in children below the age of one year have not been established. Therefore, if Precef is administered to infants, the physician should determine if the potential benefits of the product's use outweigh the possible risk of administration. Precef has been effectively used in children between the ages of 1–17 years.

Certain recent cephalosporins have caused testicular changes in juvenile rats. During animal studies, Precef has not caused testicular changes in juvenile rats at a daily dose of 1,000 mg/Kg/day (25 × the human pediatric dose) for 31 days.

ADVERSE REACTIONS

Allergic Reactions: Rash (one in 45 patients), pruritus (one in 200 patients) and eosinophilia (in about one in 12 patients) have been reported. Reactions are more likely to occur in patients wth a history of hypersensitivity, particularly to penicillins.

Hematopoietic: As occurs during therapy with other cephalosporin antibiotics, therapy with Precef has been associated with transient thrombocytosis (in about one in 5 patients). Some individuals (one in 40 patients) have developed positive direct Coombs Tests during treatment with ceforanide without clinical or laboratory evidence of hemolysis.

Gastrointestinal: Nausea (one in 270 patients), vomiting (one in 2,000 patients) and diarrhea (one in 140 patients) have been reported.

Symptoms of pseudomembranous colitis may appear during or after cephalosporin treatment.

Laboratory Changes: Transient elevation in SGOT (one in 16 patients), SGPT (one in 9 patients), and alkaline phosphatase levels (one in 27 patients) have been reported.

As with other cephaloporins, transient elevations in serum creatinine and BUN levels have been observed (in one in 9 and one in 50 patients, respectively). As may occur with intramuscular injections, the administration of Precef by this route has been associated with an elevation of CPK (in about one in 3 patients).

LOCAL EFFECTS

Local effects were reported in less than one percent of patients and included pain (one in 155 patients) and phlebitis (one in 140 patients).

Other reactions which have been reported in less than one percent of patients are local swelling, lethargy, confusion, headache, and hypotension.

DOSAGE AND ADMINISTRATION

Dosage:

Adults—The usual dose range for Precef is 0.5 to 1.0 gram twice daily depending on the severity of the infection. Precef is administered every 12 hours by either the intramuscular or intravenous route. The route of administration should be dictated by the condition of the patient and anticipated ease of administration.

---

† Bauer, et al., Am J Clin Path 1966; 45:493 and Federal Register 1972 Sep 30; 37:20525-20529.

†† Determine by the ICS agar-dilution method (Ericsson H M, and Sherris J.C. Acta Pathol Microbiol Scand 1971 (B), Supplement No 217 or any other method that has been shown to give equivalent results.

Children—Administration of 20–40 mg/kg/day in equally divided doses every 12 hours has been effective for most infections susceptible to Precef.

Perioperative Prophylactic Use—To prevent postoperative infection in contaminated or potentially contaminated surgery a 0.5 to 1 gram I.M. or I.V. dose administered 1 hour prior to the start of surgery is recommended.

It is important that the preoperative dose be given 1 hour prior to the start of surgery so that adequate antibiotic levels are present in the serum and tissues at the time of initial surgical incision.

In surgery where the occurrence of infection may be particularly devastating e.g. prosthetic arthroplasty and open-heart surgery, the prophylactic administration of Precef may be continued for 2 days following completion of surgery.

Impaired Renal Function—Dosage should be determined by the degree of renal impairment, the severity of infection, the susceptibility of the causative organism, and therapeutic monitoring. If the creatinine clearance rate (Cl_{cr}) is 60 ml/min/1.73m^2 or greater, the normal 12 hour dosing interval is maintained. When Cl_{cr} is 20–59 ml/min/1.73m^2 a 24-hour dosing interval is recommended, and when Cl_{cr} is 5–19 ml/min/1.73m^2 a 48-hour dosing interval is recommended. If Cl_{cr} is less than 5ml/min/1.73m^2, a 48–72 hour dosing interval may be used with monitoring of plasma ceforanide concentrations.

If only serum creatinine is available, creatinine clearance may be calculated from the following formula when renal function and serum creatinine levels are at steady state.

Males: $CL_{cr} = \dfrac{(140 - \text{age}) \times \text{Wt (kg)}}{72 \times \text{serum creatinine (mg/100 ml)}}$

Females: 0.85 of the above value

Note: As with antibiotic therapy in general, administration of Precef should be continued for a minimum of 48 to 72 hours after the patient becomes asymptomatic or after evidence of bacterial eradication has been obtained. A minimum of 10 days of treatment is recommended in infections caused by a group A beta-hemolytic streptococci in order to guard against the risk of rheumatic fever or glomerulonephritis.

Administration: Precef may be administered by either the intramuscular or the intravenous routes. Controlled clinical studies performed in normal adult volunteers and patients demonstrated that ceforanide was very well tolerated intramuscularly. In normal volunteers and patients receiving intravenous therapy, a low incidence of venous irritation was attributed to ceforanide. The intravenous route may be preferable for patients with bacterial septicemia, or other severe or life-threatening infections. These patients may be poor risks because of lowered resistance resulting from such debilitating conditions as malnutrition, trauma, surgery, diabetes, heart failure, or malignancy, particularly if shock is present or impending.

Intramuscular Injection: The 500 mg and 1 gram vials should be reconstituted with 1.7 ml and 3.2 ml, respectively, of Bacteriostatic Water for Injection, 0.9% Sodium Chloride Injection, Sterile Water for Injection, or Bacteriostatic Sodium Chloride Injection. Shake immediately. Each 1.0 ml contains 250 mg of ceforanide. The resulting solutions are stable for 48 hours at room temperature (25°C), 14 days under refrigeration (4°C), and 90 days in the frozen state (−15°C). After thawing, the solution is stable for 48 hours at room temperature. All injections should be administered deep into the muscle mass.

Intravenous Injection: The contents of the 500 mg vial should be diluted in 5 ml or more of the specified diluent; the 1 gram vial should be diluted in 10 ml or more of the specified diluent, and shaken immediately. Both may be administered slowly by direct I.V. administration over a 3 to 5 minute period.

Intravenous Solutions: At concentrations up to 10 mg/ml, Precef is stable and compatible for 48 hours at room temperature (25°C), 14 days under refrigeration (4°C) and 90 days in the frozen state (−15°C) followed by 48 hours at 25°C when thawed, in the following intravenous solutions:

- Sterile Water for Injection, USP
- 0.9% Sodium Chloride Injection, USP
- 5% Dextrose Injection, USP
- Lactated Ringer's Injection, USP
- Lactated Ringer's and 5% Dextrose Injection
- 10% Dextrose Injection, USP
- 5% Dextrose and 0.2% Sodium Chloride Injection, USP
- 5% Dextose and 0.45% Sodium Chloride Injection, USP

StrapKap® Piggyback I.V. Package—Reconstitute up to a concentration of 10 mg/ml with any of the appropriate I.V. solutions listed above.

Shake immediately upon reconstitution. The initial Precef Injection appears somewhat cloudy but will de-aerate upon brief standing to provide a clear solution. Parenteral drug products should be inspected visually for particulate matter and discoloration prior to administration, whenever solution and container permit.

Hospital Bulk Package: The hospital bulk dosage form is available in 10 gram StrapKap piggyback glass containers. This package is designed for use in the pharmacy in preparing I.V. additives. The diluent(s) and appropriate reconstitution volume(s) are specified on the individual container labels. The resulting solution will contain 250 mg of ceforanide activity per ml. Following reconstitution, the solutions are stable for 48 hours at room temperature, 14 days under refrigeration, and 90 days in the frozen state. After thawing, the solutions are stable for 48 hours at room temperature.

Caution: Hospital bulk packages must not be dispensed as a unit.

HOW SUPPLIED

Precef is supplied in 500 mg vials and 500 mg piggybacks equivalent to 500 mg ceforanide and 1 gram vials and 1 gram piggybacks equivalent to 1 gram ceforanide. Also, a Hospital Bulk Package equivalent to 10 grams ceforanide.

NDC 0015-7351-20—500 mg vial
NDC 0015-7351-28—500 mg piggyback vial
NDC 0015-7352-20—1 gram vial
NDC 0015-7352-28—1 gram piggyback vial
NDC 0015-7356-20—10 gram StrapKap Hospital Bulk Package

For information on package sizes available, refer to the current price schedule.

PROSTAPHLIN® ℞

(oxacillin sodium)
Capsules, Oral Solution, I.M. or I.V.

This is the full text of the latest Combined Official Package Circular dated June 1984 [7977DIR-11] *and* [7979DIR-28]

(17) 11/84

DESCRIPTION

Prostaphlin (oxacillin sodium) is an antibacterial agent of the isoxazolyl penicillin series. It is a penicillinase-resistant, acid-resistant, semi-synthetic penicillin. Each 1 gram of Prostaphlin for injection contains approximately 2.5 mEq of sodium and is buffered with 20 mg. of dibasic sodium phosphate.

Inactive ingredient in Prostaphlin capsules is: magnesium stearate.

Inactive ingredients in Prostaphlin oral solution are: FD & C Red No. 40, natural & artificial flavorings, potassium alginate, sodium benzoate, sodium citrate, sodium saccharin and sucrose.

$C_{19}H_{18}N_3NaO_5S \cdot H_2O$ 441.43 [CAS 7240·38 2]
4-Thia-1-azabicyclo[3.2.0]heptane-2-carboxylic acid, 3,3 dimethyl-6-[[(5-methyl-3-phenyl-4-isoxazolyl) carbonyl] amino]-7-oxo-, monosodium salt, monohydrate, [2S (2α,5α, 6β)].

CLINICAL PHARMACOLOGY

Microbiology

Penicillinase-resistant penicillins exert a bactericidal action against penicillin-susceptible microorganisms during the state of active multiplication. All penicillins inhibit the biosynthesis of the bacterial cell wall.

The drugs in this class are highly resistant to inactivation by staphylococcal penicillinase and are active against penicillinase producing and non-penicillinase producing strains of *Staphylococcus aureus*.

The penicillinase-resistant penicillins are active *in vitro* against a variety of other bacteria.

Susceptibility Plate Testing

Quantitative methods of susceptibility testing that require measurement of zone diameters or minimal inhibitory concentrations (M.I.C.s) give the most precise estimates of antibiotic susceptibility. One such procedure has been recommended for use with discs to test susceptibility to this class of drugs. Interpretations correlate diameters on the disc test with MIC values. A penicillinase-resistant class disc may be used to determine microbial susceptibility to cloxacillin, dicloxacillin, methicillin, nafcillin, and oxacillin. With this procedure, employing a 5 microgram methicillin sodium disc, a report from the laboratory of "susceptible" (zone of at least 14 mm) indicates that the infecting organism is likely to respond to therapy. A report of "resistant" (zone of less than 10 mm) indicates that the infecting organism is not likely to respond to therapy. A report of "intermediate susceptibility" (zone of 10–13 mm) suggests that the organism might be susceptible if high doses of the antibiotic are used, or if the infection is confined to tissues and fluids (e.g., urine), in which high antibiotic levels are attained.

In general, all staphylococci should be tested against the penicillin G disc and against the methicillin disc. Routine methods of antibiotic susceptibility testing may fail to detect strains of organisms resistant to the penicillinase-resistant penicillins. For this reason, the use of large inocula and 48-hour incubation periods may be necessary to obtain accurate susceptibility studies with these antibiotics. Bacterial strains which are resistant to one of the penicillinase-resistant penicillins should be considered resistant to all of the drugs in the class.

PHARMACOKINETICS

Prostaphlin, with normal doses, has insignificant concentrations in the cerebrospinal and ascitic fluids. It is found in therapeutic concentrations in the pleural, bile and amniotic fluids. Prostaphlin is rapidly excreted as unchanged drug in the urine by glomerular filtration and active tubular secretion.

Prostaphlin (oxacillin sodium) binds to serum protein, mainly albumin. The degree of protein binding reported varies with the method of study and the investigator, but generally has been found to be 94.2±2.1%.

Prostaphlin (oxacillin sodium) is resistant to destruction by acid. Absorption of Prostaphlin after oral administration is rapid but incomplete. A single 250-mg oral dose gives a 1-hour peak serum level of 1.65 mcg/ml. A 500-mg dose peaks at about 2.6 mcg/ml. Peak serum levels with the oral solution occur somewhat earlier, about one-half hour after dosing. A single dose of 250-mg oral solution gives a peak serum level of 1.9 mcg/ml; of 500-mg, 4.8 mcg/ml. Oral absorption is delayed when the drug is administered after meals.

Intramuscular injections give peak serum levels 30 minutes after injection. A 250 mg dose gives a level of 5.3 mcg/ml while a 500 mg dose peaks at 10.9 mcg/ml. Intravenous injection gives a peak about 5 minutes after the injection is completed. Slow I.V. dosing with 500 mg gives a 5 minute peak of 43 mcg/ml with a half-life of 20 to 30 minutes.

INDICATIONS AND USAGE

The penicillinase-resistant penicillins are indicated in the treatment of infections caused by penicillinase-producing staphylococci which have demonstrated susceptibility to the drugs. Culture and susceptibility tests should be performed initially to determine the causative organisms and their sensitivity to the drug (See CLINICAL PHARMACOLOGY—Susceptibility Plate Testing).

The penicillinase-resistant penicillins may be used to initiate therapy in suspected cases of resistant staphylococcal infections prior to the availability of laboratory test results.

The penicillinase-resistant penicillins should not be used in infections caused by organisms susceptible to penicillin G. If the susceptibility tests indicate that the infection is due to an organism other than a resistant staphylococcus, therapy should not be continued with a penicillinase-resistant penicillin.

CONTRAINDICATIONS

A history of hypersensitivity (anaphylactic) reaction to any penicillin is a contraindication.

WARNINGS

Serious and occasionally fatal hypersensitivity (anaphylactic shock with collapse) reactions have occurred in patients receiving penicillin. The incidence of anaphylactic shock in all penicillin-treated patients is between 0.015 and 0.04 percent. Anaphylactic shock resulting in death has occurred in approximately 0.002 percent of the patients treated. Although anaphylaxis is more frequent following a parenteral administration, it has occurred in patients receiving oral penicillins.

When penicillin therapy is indicated, it should be initiated only after a comprehensive patient drug and allergy history has been obtained. If an allergic reaction occurs, the drug should be discontinued and the patient should receive supportive treatment, e.g., artificial maintenance of ventilation, pressor amines, antihistamines, and corticosteroids. Individuals with a history of penicillin hypersensitivity may also experience allergic reactions when treated with a cephalosporin.

PRECAUTIONS

General

Penicillinase-resistant penicillins should generally not be administered to patients with a history of sensitivity to any penicillin.

Penicillin should be used with caution in individuals with histories of significant allergies and/or asthma. Whenever allergic reactions occur, penicillin should be withdrawn unless, in the opinion of the physician, the condition being treated is life-threatening and amenable only to penicillin therapy.

The oral route of administration should not be relied upon in patients with severe illness, or with nausea, vomiting, gastric dilation, cardiospasm, or intestinal hypermotility. Occasionally patients will not absorb therapeutic amounts of orally administered penicillin.

The use of antibiotics may result in overgrowth of nonsusceptible organisms. If new infections due to bacteria or fungi

Continued on next page

Bristol—Cont.

RECOMMENDED PARENTERAL DOSAGES FOR PROSTAPHLIN (oxacillin sodium)

Drug	Adults	Infants and Children < 40 kg (88 lbs)	Other Recommendations
Oxacillin	250–500 mg IM or IV every 4–6 hours (mild to moderate infections)	50 mg/kg/day IM or IV in equally divided doses every 6 hours (mild to moderate infections)	
	1 gram IM or IV every 4–6 hours (severe infections)	100 mg/kg/day IM or IV in equally divided doses every 4–6 hours (severe infections)	Premature and Neonates 25 mg/kg/day IM or IV

occur, the drug should be discontinued and appropriate measures taken.

Laboratory Tests

Bacteriologic studies to determine the causative organisms and their susceptibility to the penicillinase-resistant penicillins should be performed (See **Clinical Pharmacology—Microbiology**). In the treatment of suspected staphylococcal infections, therapy should be changed to another active agent if culture tests fail to demonstrate the presence of staphylococci.

Periodic assessment of organ system function including renal, hepatic, and hematopoietic should be made during prolonged therapy with the penicillinase-resistant penicillins.

Blood cultures, white blood cell, and differential cell counts should be obtained prior to initiation of therapy and at least weekly during therapy with penicillinase-resistant penicillins.

Periodic urinalysis, blood urea nitrogen; and creatinine determinations should be performed during therapy with the penicillinase-resistant penicillins and dosage alterations should be considered if these values become elevated. If any impairment of renal function is suspected or known to exist, a reduction in the total dosage should be considered and blood levels monitored to avoid possible neurotoxic reactions (See **Dosage and Administration**).

SGOT and SGPT values should be obtained periodically during therapy to monitor for possible liver function abnormalities.

Drug Interactions

Tetracycline, a bacteriostatic antibiotic, may antagonize the bactericidal effect of penicillin and concurrent use of these drugs should be avoided.

Carcinogenesis, Mutagenesis, Impairment of Fertility

No long-term animal studies have been conducted with these drugs. Studies on reproduction (nafcillin) in rats and rabbits reveal no fetal or maternal abnormalities before conception and continuously through weaning (one generation).

Pregnancy Category B

Reproduction studies performed in the mouse, rat, and rabbit have revealed no evidence of impaired fertility or harm to the fetus due to the penicillinase-resistant penicillins. Human experience with the penicillins during pregnancy has not shown any positive evidence of adverse effects on the fetus. There are, however, no adequate or well-controlled studies in pregnant women showing conclusively that harmful effects of these drugs on the fetus can be excluded. Because animal reproduction studies are not always predictive of human response, this drug should be used during pregnancy only if clearly needed.

Nursing Mothers

Penicillins are excreted in breast milk. Caution should be exercised when penicillins are administered to a nursing woman.

Pediatric Use

Because of incompletely developed renal function in newborns, penicillinase-resistant penicillins (especially methicillin) may not be completely excreted, with abnormally high blood levels resulting. Frequent blood levels are advisable in this group with dosage adjustments when necessary. All newborns treated with penicillins should be monitored closely for clinical and laboratory evidence of toxic or adverse effects (See **Dosage and Administration**).

ADVERSE REACTIONS

Body as a Whole:

The reported incidence of allergic reactions to penicillins ranges from 0.7 to 10 percent (See WARNINGS). Sensitization is usually the result of treatment but some individuals have had immediate reactions to penicillin when first treated. In such cases, it is thought that the patients may have had prior exposure to the drug via trace amounts present in milk and vaccines.

Two types of allergic reactions to penicillin are noted clinically, immediate and delayed.

Immediate reactions usually occur within 20 minutes of administration and range in severity from urticaria and pruritus to angioneurotic edema, laryngospasm, bronchospasm, hypotension, vascular collapse, and death. Such immediate anaphylactic reactions are very rare (See WARNINGS) and usually occur after parenteral therapy but have occurred in patients receiving oral therapy. Another type of immediate reaction, an accelerated reaction, may occur between 20 minutes and 48 hours after administration and may include urticaria, pruritus, and fever. Although laryngeal edema, laryngospasm, and hypotension occasionally occur, fatality is uncommon.

Delayed allergic reactions to penicillin therapy usually occur after 48 hours and sometimes as late as 2 to 4 weeks after initiation of therapy. Manifestations of this type of reaction include serum sickness-like symptoms (i.e., fever, malaise, urticaria, myalgia, arthralgia, abdominal pain) and various skin rashes. Nausea, vomiting, diarrhea, stomatitis, black or "hairy" tongue, and other symptoms of gastrointestinal irritation may occur, especially during oral penicillin therapy.

Nervous System Reactions:

Neurotoxic reactions similar to those observed with Penicillin G may occur with large intravenous doses of the penicillinase-resistant penicillins especially in patients with renal insufficiency.

Urogenital Reactions:

Renal tubular damage and interstitial nephritis have been associated with the administration of methicillin sodium and infrequently with the administration of nafcillin and oxacillin. Manifestations of this reaction may include rash, fever, eosinophilia, hematuria, proteinuria, and renal insufficiency. Methicillin-induced nephropathy does not appear to be dose-related and is generally reversible upon prompt discontinuation of therapy.

Gastrointestinal Reactions

Pseudomembranous colitis has been reported with the use of Prostaphlin (and other broad spectrum antibiotics); therefore, it is important to consider its diagnosis in patients who develop diarrhea in association with antibiotic use.

Treatment with broad spectrum antibiotics alters normal flora of the colon and may permit overgrowth of clostridia. Studies indicate a toxin produced by *Clostridium difficile* is one primary cause of antibiotic-associated colitis. Cholestyramine and colestipol resins have been shown to bind the toxin *in vitro*.

Mild cases of colitis may respond to drug discontinuance alone.

Moderate to severe cases should be managed with fluid, electrolyte and protein supplementation as indicated.

When the colitis is not relieved by drug discontinuance or when it is severe, oral vancomycin is the treatment of choice for antibiotic-associated pseudomembranous colitis produced by *C. difficile*. Other causes of colitis should also be considered.

Metabolic Reactions:

Agranulocytosis, neutropenia, and bone marrow depression have been associated with the use of methicillin sodium, nafcillin, oxacillin, and cloxacillin. Hepatotoxicity, characterized by fever, nausea, and vomiting associated with abnormal liver function tests, mainly elevated SGOT levels, has been associated with the use of oxacillin and cloxacillin.

DOSAGE AND ADMINISTRATION

The penicillinase-resistant penicillins are available for oral administration and for intramuscular and intravenous injection. The sodium salts of methicillin, oxacillin, and nafcillin may be administered parenterally and the sodium salts of cloxacillin, dicloxacillin, oxacillin, and nafcillin are available for oral use.

Bacteriologic studies to determine the causative organisms and their sensitivity to the penicillinase-resistant penicillins should always be performed. Duration of therapy varies with the type and severity of infection as well as the overall condition of the patient, therefore it should be determined by the clinical and bacteriological response of the patient. In severe staphylococcal infections, therapy with penicillinase-resistant penicillins should be continued for at least 14 days. Therapy should be continued for at least 48 hours after the patient has become afebrile, asymptomatic, and cultures are negative. The treatment of endocarditis and osteomyelitis may require a longer term of therapy.

Concurrent administration of the penicillinase-resistant penicillins and probenecid increases and prolongs serum penicillin levels. Probenecid decreases the apparent volume of distribution and slows the rate of excretion by competitively inhibiting renal tubular secretion of penicillin. Penicillin-probenecid therapy is generally limited to those infections where very high serum levels of penicillin are necessary.

Oral preparations of the penicillinase-resistant penicillins should not be used as initial therapy in serious, life-threatening infections (See **Precautions—General**). Oral therapy with the penicillinase-resistant penicillins may be used to follow-up the previous use of a parenteral agent as soon as the clinical condition warrants. For intramuscular gluteal injections, care should be taken to avoid sciatic nerve injury. With intravenous administration, particularly in elderly patients, care should be taken because of the possibility of thrombophlebitis.

[See table below].

Directions For Dispensing Oral Solution: Prepare these formulations at the time of dispensing. For ease in preparation, add water to the bottle in two portions and shake well after each addition. Add the total amount of water as directed on the labeling of the package being dispensed. The reconstituted formulation is stable for 3 days at room temperature or 14 days under refrigeration.

[See table above].

DIRECTIONS FOR USE

For Intramuscular Use: Use Sterile Water for Injection, USP. Add 1.4 ml to the 250 mg vial, 2.7 ml to the 500 mg vial, 5.7 ml to the 1 gram vial, 11.5 ml to the 2 gram vial, and 23 ml to the 4 gram vial. Shake well until a clear solution is obtained. After reconstitution, vials will contain 250 mg of active drug per 1.5 ml of solution. The reconstituted solution is stable for 3 days at 70°F or for one week under refrigeration (40°F).

For Direct Intravenous Use: Use Sterile Water for Injection, USP or Sodium Chloride Injection, USP. Add 5 ml to the 250 mg and 500 mg vials; 10 ml to the 1 gram vial; 20 ml to the 2 gram vial; and 40 ml to the 4 gram vial. Withdraw the entire contents and administer slowly over a period of approximately 10 minutes.

For Administration by Intravenous Drip: Reconstitute as directed above (For Direct Intravenous Use) prior to diluting with Intravenous Solution.

[See table top of next page].

Stability studies on Prostaphlin at concentrations of 0.5 mg/ml and 2 mg/ml in various intravenous solutions listed below indicate the drug will lose less than 10% activity at room temperature (70°F) during a 6 hour period.

I.V. Solution:

5% Dextrose in Normal Saline
10% D-Fructose in Water
10% D-Fructose in Normal Saline
Lactated Potassic Saline Injection
10% Invert Sugar in Normal Saline
10% Invert Sugar Plus 0.3% Potassium Chloride in Water
Travert 10% Electrolyte #1
Travert 10% Electrolyte #2
Travert 10% Electrolyte #3

Only those solutions listed above should be used for the intravenous infusion of Prostaphlin. The concentration of the antibiotic should fall within the range specified. The drug concentration and the rate and volume of the infusion should be adjusted so that the total dose of oxacillin is administered before the drug loses its stability in the solution in use.

If another agent is used in conjunction with oxacillin therapy, **it should not be physically mixed** with oxacillin but should be administered separately.

"Piggyback" I.V. Package: This glass vial contains the la-

RECOMMENDED ORAL DOSAGES FOR PROSTAPHLIN (oxacillin sodium) IN MILD TO MODERATE AND SEVERE INFECTIONS

DRUG	ADULTS Mild to Moderate	ADULTS Severe	CHILDREN Mild to Moderate	CHILDREN Severe
Oxacillin	500 mg every 4–6 hours	1 gram every 4–6 hours (follow up of parenteral therapy)	50 mg/kg/day[a] in equally divided doses every 6 hours	100 mg/kg/day[a] in equally divided doses every 4–6 hours (follow up of parenteral therapy)

[a] Patients weighing less than 40 Kg (88 lbs)

beled quantity of Prostaphlin and is intended for intravenous administration. The diluent and volume are specified on the label of each package.
Discard solution after 24 hours at room temperature.
Hospital Bulk Package: This glass vial contains 10 grams Prostaphlin and is designed for use in the pharmacy in preparing I.V. additives. Add 93 ml Sterile Water for Injection, USP or Sodium Chloride Injection, USP. The resulting solution will contain 100 mg oxacillin sodium per ml.
Following reconstitution in this manner, the resulting solutions are stable for 4 days at room temperature or 7 days under refrigeration.
CAUTION: NOT TO BE DISPENSED AS A UNIT.

SUPPLY

Prostaphlin (oxacillin sodium) for Injection. Oxacillin sodium equivalent to 250, 500 mg, 1, 2, 4 or 10 grams oxacillin per vial.
NDC 0015-7978-20—250 mg vial
NDC 0015-7979-20—500 mg vial
NDC 0015-7981-20—1 gram vial
NDC 0015-7970-20—2 gram vial
NDC 0015-7300-20—4 gram vial
NDC 0015-7981-28—1 gram "Piggyback" vial
NDC 0015-7970-28—2 gram "Piggyback" vial
NDC 0015-7300-28—4 gram "Piggyback" vial
NDC 0015-7103-28—10 gram "Hospital Bulk Package"
Also available: PROSTAPHLIN (oxacillin sodium) Capsules. Oxacillin sodium equivalent to 250 or 500 mg oxacillin per capsule.
NDC 0015-7977—250 mg
NDC 0015-7982—500 mg
PROSTAPHLIN (oxacillin sodium) for Oral Solution. Each 5 ml of reconstituted solution contains oxacillin sodium equivalent to 250 mg oxacillin.
NDC 0015-7985—250 mg
For information on package sizes available, refer to the current price schedule.
Shown in Product Identification Section, page 406

STABILITY PERIODS
PROSTAPHLIN

Concentration Mg/Ml	Sterile H_2O for Injection	Isotonic Sodium Chloride	M/6 Molar Sodium Lactate Solution	5% Dextrose in H_2O	5% Dextrose in 0.45% NaCl	10% Invert Sugar	Lactated Ringers Solution
ROOM TEMPERATURE (25°C)							
10–100	4 Days	4 Days					
10–30			24 Hrs		24 Hrs		
0.5–2				6 Hrs		6 Hrs	6 Hrs
REFRIGERATION (4°C)							
10–100	7 Days	7 Days					
10–30			4 Days	4 Days	4 Days	4 Days	4 Days
FROZEN (−15°C)							
50–100	30 Days						
250/1.5 ml	30 Days						
100		30 Days					
10–100			30 Days	30 Days	30 Days	30 Days	30 Days

SALURON® ℞
[*săl-ū-rŏn*]
(hydroflumethiazide)

This is the full text of the latest Official Package Circular dated February 1985 [5410DIR-12].

DESCRIPTION

Saluron (hydroflumethiazide) is a potent oral diuretic-antihypertensive agent of low toxicity. Each tablet contains 50 mg hydroflumethiazide.
Saluron is 3.4-Hydro-7-Sulfamyl-6-Trifluoromethyl-1,2,4-Benzothiadiazine 1,1-Dioxide. Hydroflumethiazide is very slightly soluble in water, soluble in methanol and freely soluble in acetone. Inactive ingredients in Saluron tablets are cellulose microcrystalline, lactose, magnesium stearate, silicon dioxide colloidal and sodium starch glycolate. It has the following structural formulae.

CLINICAL PHARMACOLOGY

Hydroflumethiazide is incompletely but fairly rapidly absorbed from the gastrointestinal tract. It appears to have a biphasic biological half-life with an estimated alpha-phase of about 2 hours and an estimated beta-phase of about 17 hours; it has a metabolite with a longer half-life, which is extensively bound to the red blood cells. Hydroflumethiazide is excreted in the urine; its metabolite has also been detected in the urine.
The mechanism of action results in an interference with the renal tubular mechanism of electrolyte reabsorption. At maximal therapeutic dosage all thiazides are approximately equal in their diuretic potency. The mechanism whereby thiazides function in the control of hypertension is unknown.

INDICATIONS AND USAGE

Saluron is indicated as adjunctive therapy in edema associated with congestive heart failure, hepatic cirrhosis, and corticosteroid and estrogen therapy.
Saluron has also been found useful in edema due to various forms of renal dysfunction such as nephrotic syndrome, acute glomerulonephritis, and chronic renal failure.
Saluron is indicated in the management of hypertension either as the sole therapeutic agent or to enhance the effectiveness of other antihypertensive drugs in the more severe forms of hypertension.
Usage in Pregnancy—The routine use of diurectics in an otherwise healthy woman is inappropriate and exposes mother and fetus to unnecessary hazard. Diuretics do not prevent development of toxemia of pregnancy, and there is no satisfactory evidence that they are useful in the treatment of developed toxemia.
Edema during pregnancy may arise from pathological causes or from the physiologic and mechanical consequences of pregnancy. Thiazides are indicated in pregnancy when edema is due to pathologic causes, just as they are in the absence of pregnancy (however, see **Warnings** below). Dependent edema in pregnancy, resulting from restriction of venous return by the expanded uterus is properly treated through elevation of the lower extremities and use of support hose; use of diuretics to lower intravascular volume in this case is illogical and unnecessary. There is hypervolemia during normal pregnancy which is harmful to neither the fetus nor the mother (in the absence of cardiovascular disease), but which is associated with edema, including generalized edema, in the majority of pregnant women. If this edema produces discomfort, increased recumbency will often provide relief. In rare instances, this edema may cause extreme discomfort which is not relieved by rest. In these cases, a short course of diuretics may provide relief and may be appropriate.

CONTRAINDICATIONS

Saluron is contraindicated in patients with anuria or hypersensitivity to this or other sulfonamide derived drugs.

WARNINGS

Saluron should be used with caution in severe renal disease. In patients with renal disease, thiazide may precipitate azotemia. Cumulative effects of the drug may develop in patients with impaired renal function.
Thiazides should be used with caution in patients with impaired hepatic function or progressive liver disease, since minor alterations of fluid and electrolyte balance may precipitate hepatic coma.
Thiazides may be additive or potentiative of the action of other antihypertensive drugs. Potentiation occurs with ganglionic or peripheral adrenergic blocking drugs.
Sensitivity reactions may occur in patients with a history of allergy or bronchial asthma.
The possibility of exacerbation or activation of systemic lupus erythematosus has been reported.

PRECAUTIONS

General—All patients receiving thiazide therapy should be observed for clinical signs of fluid or electrolyte imbalance; namely, hyponatremia, hypochloremic alkalosis, and hypokalemia. Serum and urine electrolyte determinations are particularly important when the patient is vomiting excessively or receiving parenteral fluids. Medication such as digitalis may also influence serum electrolytes. Warning signs, irrespective of cause, are: dryness of mouth, thirst, weakness, lethargy, drowsiness, restlessness, muscle pains or cramps, muscular fatigue, hypotension, oliguria, tachycardia, and gastrointestinal disurbances such as nausea and vomiting.
Hypokalemia may develop with thiazides as with any other potent diuretic, especially with brisk diuresis, when severe cirrhosis is present, or during concomitant use of corticosteroids or ACTH.
Interference with adequate oral electrolyte intake will also contribute to hypokalemia. Digitalis therapy may exaggerate metabolic effects of hypokalemia especially with reference to myocardial activity.
Any chloride deficit is generally mild and usually does not require specific treatment except under extraordinary circumstances (as in liver disease or renal disease). Dilutional hyponatremia may occur in edematous patients in hot weather; appropriate therapy is water restriction, rather than administration of salt except in rare instances when the hyponatremia is life-threatening. In actual salt depletion, appropriate replacement is the therapy of choice.
Hyperuricemia may occur or frank gout may be precipitated in certain patients receiving thiazide therapy.
Insulin requirements in diabetic patients may be increased, decreased, or unchanged. Latent diabetes mellitus may become manifested during thiazide administration.
Thiazide drugs may increase the responsiveness to tubocurarine.
The antihypertensive effects of the drug may be enhanced in the postsympathectomy patient.
Thiazides may decrease arterial responsiveness to norepinephrine. This diminution is not sufficient to preclude effectiveness of the pressor agent for therapeutic use.
If progressive renal impairment becomes evident, as indicated by a rising nonprotein nitrogen or blood urea nitrogen, a careful reappraisal of therapy is necessary with consideration given to withholding or discontinuing diuretic therapy.
Thiazides may decrease serum PBI levels without signs of thyroid disturbance.
Lithium generally should not be given with diuretics because they reduce its renal clearance and increase the risk of lithium toxicity. Read circulars for lithium preparations before use of such concomitant therapy with "Saluron".
Information for Patients—This medicine may cause a loss of potassium from your body. To help prevent this, your doctor may want you to:

- eat or drink foods that have a high potassium content (for example, orange or other citrus fruit juices), or
- take a potassium supplement, or
- take another medicine to help prevent the loss of the potassium in the first place.

It is very important to follow these directions. Also, it is important not to change your diet on your own. This more important if you are already on a special diet (as for diabetes), or if you are taking a potassium supplement or a medicine to reduce potassium loss. Extra potassium may not be necessary and, in some cases, too much potassium could be harmful.
Check with your doctor if you become sick and have severe or continuing vomiting or diarrhea. These problems may cause you to lose additional water and potassium.
Caution: Diabetics—Thiazide diuretics may raise blood sugar levels. While you are using this medicine, be especially careful in testing for sugar in your urine. If you have any questions about this, check with your doctor.
A few people who take this medicine may become more sensitive to sunlight than they are normally. When you begin to take this medicine, avoid too much sun or use of a sunlamp until you see how you react, especially if you tend to burn easily. If you have a severe reaction, check with your doctor.
For patients taking this medicine for high blood pressure:

- **Do not take other medicines unless they have been discussed with your doctor.**

This especially includes over-the-counter (nonprescription) medicines for appetite control, asthma, colds, cough, hay fever, or sinus.

Continued on next page

Bristol—Cont.

Laboratory Tests—Periodic determination of serum electrolytes to detect possible electrolyte imbalance should be performed at appropriate intervals.

Drug Interactions—Anticoagulants, oral
(effects may be decreased when used concurrently with thiazide diuretics; dosage adjustments may be necessary)
Antigout medications
(thiazide diuretics may raise the level of blood uric acid; dosage adjustment of antigout medications may be necessary to control hyperuricemia and gout)
Antihypertensive medications, other, especially diazoxide, or Preanesthetic and anesthetic agents used in surgery or Skeletal muscle relaxants, nondepolarizing, used in surgery
(effects may be potentiated when used concurrently with thiazide diuretics; dosage adjustments may be necessary)
Amphotericin B or Corticosteroids or Corticotropin (ACTH)
(concurrent use with thiazide diuretics may intensify electrolyte imbalance, particularly hypokalemia)
Cardiac glycosides
(concurrent use with thiazide diuretics may enhance the possibility of digitalis toxicity associated with hypokalemia)
Colestipol
(may inhibit gastrointestinal absorption of the thiazide diuretics; administration 1 hour before or 4 hours after colestipol is recommended)
Hypoglycemics
(thiazide diuretics may raise blood glucose levels; for adult-onset diabetics, dosage adjustment of hypoglycemic medications may be necessary during and after thiazide diuretic therapy; insulin requirements may be increased, decreased, or unchanged)
Lithium salts
(concurrent use with thiazide diuretics is not recommended, as they may provoke lithium toxicity because of reduced renal clearance)
Methenamine
(effectiveness may be decreased when used concurrently with thiazide diuretics because of alkalinization of the urine)

Diagnostic Interference—With expected physiologic effects
Blood and urine glucose levels (usually only in patients with a predisposition to glucose intolerance) and
Serum bilirubin levels (by displacement from albumin binding) and
Serum calcium levels (thiazide diuretics should be discontinued before parathyroid function tests are carried out) and
Serum uric acid levels (may be increased)
Serum magnesium, potassium, and sodium levels (may be decreased; serum magnesium levels may increase in uremic patients)
Serum protein-bound iodine (PBI) levels (may be decreased)

Carcinogenesis, Mutagenesis, Impairment of Fertility—No long-term studies in animals have been performed to evaluate carcinogenic or mutagenic potential or impairment of fertility.

Usage in Pregnancy—Pregnancy Category D:

Teratogenic Effects—Saluron can cause fetal harm when administered to a pregnant woman. These hazards include fetal or neonatal jaundice, thrombocytopenia, and possibly other adverse reactions which have occurred in the adult. If this drug is used in pregnancy, or if the patient becomes pregnant while taking this drug, the patient should be apprised of the potential hazard to the fetus.

Nonteratogenic Effects—Fetal or neonatal jaundice, thrombocytopenia, and possibly other adverse reactions which have occurred in the adult.

Nursing Mothers—Thiazides appear in breast milk. If use of the drug is deemed essential, the patient may consider stopping nursing.

Pediatric Use—Safety and effectiveness in children have not been established.

ADVERSE REACTIONS

The following adverse reactions have been observed, but there is not enough systematic collection of data to support an estimate of their frequency.

A. Gastrointestinal system reactions: Anorexia, gastric irritation, nausea, vomiting, cramping, diarrhea, constipation, jaundice (intrahepatic cholestatic jaundice), pancreatitis.
B. Central nervous system reactions: Dizziness, vertigo, parathesias, headache, xanthopsia.
C. Hematologic reactions: Leukopenia, agranulocytosis, thrombocytopenia, aplastic anemia.
D. Dermatologic-Hypersensitivity reactions: Purpura, photosensitivity, rash, urticaria, necrotizing angiitis (vasculitis) (cutaneous vasculitis).
E. Cardiovascular reaction: Orthostatic hypotension may occur and may be aggravated by alcohol, barbiturates, or narcotics.
F. Other: Hyperglycemia; glycosuria, muscle spasm, weakness, restlessness.

Whenever adverse reactions are moderate or severe, thiazide dosage should be reduced or therapy withdrawn.

OVERDOSAGE

Signs and Symptoms—Diuresis, lethargy progressing to coma, with minimal cardiorespiratory depression and with or without significant serum electrolyte changes or dehydration; GI irritation; hypermotility; transient elevation in BUN level.

Treatment—Empty stomach by gastric lavage, taking care to avoid aspiration. Monitor serum electrolyte levels and renal function, and institute supportive measures, as required to maintain hydration, electrolyte balance, respiration, and cardiovascular and renal function. Treat GI effects symptomatically.

DOSAGE AND ADMINISTRATION

The average adult diuretic dose is 25 to 200 mg per day. The average adult antihypertensive dose is 50 to 100 mg per day. Therapy should be individualized according to patient response. This therapy should be titrated to gain maximal therapeutic response as well as the minimal dose possible to maintain that therapeutic response.

HOW SUPPLIED

NDC 0015-5410—Saluron Tablets, scored, 50 mg
For information on package sizes available, refer to the current price schedule.

Shown in Product Identification Section, page 406

SALUTENSIN®
SALUTENSIN-Demi® ℞

[*săl-ū-tĕn ′sĭn*]

(Hydroflumethiazide, Reserpine Antihypertensive Formulation)

This is the full text of the latest Official Package Circular dated March 1985 [5436 DIR 11]

> **WARNING**
> This fixed combination drug is not indicated for initial therapy of hypertension. Hypertension requires therapy titrated to the individual patient. If the fixed combination represents the dosage so determined, its use may be more convenient in patient management. The treatment of hypertension is not static, but must be reevaluated as conditions in each patient warrant.

DESCRIPTION

Salutensin tablets for oral administration combine two antihypertensive agents: Saluron® (hydroflumethiazide) and reserpine. The chemical name for hydroflumethiazide is 3,4-dihydro-7-sulfamyl-6-trifluoromethyl-2H-1,2,4-benzothiadiazine-1,1-dioxide. Hydroflumethiazide is very slightly soluble in water, soluble in methanol and freely soluble in acetone. It has the following structural formulae:

F_3C H_2NO_2S N H CH_2 N-H S O O

Hydroflumethiazide

Reserpine (3,4,5-trimethoxybenzoyl methyl reserpate) is a crystalline alkaloid derived from Rauwolfia serpentina. It is very slightly soluble in water, slightly soluble in acetone, methanol and ethanol and freely soluble in chloroform and methylene chloride. It has the following structural formulae:

CH_3O N H CH_3O—C O OCH_3 OCH_3 OCH_3 O CH_3

Reserpine

Each Salutensin tablet contains:

Saluron (hydroflumethiazide)	50 mg.
Reserpine	0.125 mg.

Each Salutensin-Demi tablet contains:

Saluron (hydroflumethiazide)	25 mg.
Reserpine	0.125 mg.

Inactive ingredients in Salutensin tablets are: D & C Yellow No. 10 Lake, FD & C Blue 1 Lake 12%, lactose, magnesium stearate, povidone, starch and sucrose.

Inactive ingredients in Salutensin-Demi tablets are: D & C Red No. 30 Lake, D & C Yellow No. 10 Lake, lactose, magnesium stearate, povidone, starch and sucrose.

CLINICAL PHARMACOLOGY

Hydroflumethiazide is incompletely but fairly rapidly absorbed from the gastrointestinal tract. It appears to have a biphasic biological half-life with an estimated alpha-phase of about 2 hours and an estimated beta-phase of about 17 hours; it has a metabolite with a longer half-life, which is extensively bound to the red blood cells. Hydroflumethiazide is excreted in the urine; its metabolite has also been detected in the urine.

Hydroflumethiazide is an oral diuretic-antihypertensive agent. It exerts its effect by inhibiting renal tubular reabsorption, including increased excretion of sodium and chloride and water with variable concomitant loss of potassium and bicarbonate as well. When used alone as an antihypertensive agent, hydroflumethiazide usually induces a gradual but sustained decrease in abnormally elevated blood-pressure—both systolic and diastolic. Hypertensive patients who have been maintained on chlorothiazide or hydrochlorothiazide may also be maintained on hydroflumethiazide.

Reserpine is absorbed from the gastrointestinal tract. About 6% has been reported to be excreted in the urine in the first 24 hours and about 8% in the first 4 days, mainly as the metabolite trimethyoxybenzoic acid. Over 60% is excreted in the faeces in the first 4 days, mainly unchanged. Reserpine crosses the placental barrier and also appears in breast milk. The component, reserpine, probably produces its antihypertensive effects through depletion of tissue stores of catecholamines (epinephrine and norepinephrine) from peripheral sites. By contrast, its sedative and tranquilizing properties are thought to be related to depletion of 5-hydroxytryptamine from the brain.

Reserpine is characterized by slow onset of action and sustained effect. Both its cardiovascular and central nervous system effects may persist following withdrawal of the drug. Careful observation for changes in blood pressure must be made when Salutensin is used with other antihypertensive drugs. The dosage of other agents must be reduced by at least 50 percent as soon as Salutensin is added to the regimen to prevent excessive drop in blood pressure. As the blood pressure falls under the potentiating effect of Salutensin, a further reduction in dosage or even discontinuation of other antihypertensive drugs may be necessary.

Hypertension therapy requires therapy titrated to the individual patient. If a fixed combination represents the dosage so determined its use may be more convenient in patient management.

INDICATIONS AND USAGE

Hypertension (see box warning).

Usage in Pregnancy—The routine use of diuretics in an otherwise healthy woman is inappropriate and exposes mother and fetus to unnecessary hazard. Diuretics do not prevent development of toxemia of pregnancy, and there is no satisfactory evidence that they are useful in the treatment of developed toxemia. Edema during pregnancy may arise from pathological causes or from the physiologic and mechanical consequences of pregnancy. Thiazides are indicated in pregnancy when edema is due to pathologic causes, just as they are in the absence of pregnancy (however, see **Warnings**, below). Dependent edema in pregnancy, resulting from restriction of venous return by the expanded uterus, is properly treated through elevation of the lower extremities and use of support hose; use of diuretics to lower intravascular volume in this case is illogical and unnecessary. There is hypervolemia during normal pregnancy which is harmful to neither the fetus nor the mother (in the absence of cardiovascular disease), but which is associated with edema, including generalized edema, in the majority of pregnant women. If this edema produces discomfort, increased recumbency will often provide relief. In rare instances, this edema may cause extreme discomfort which is not relieved by rest. In these cases, a short course of diuretics may provide relief and may be appropriate.

CONTRAINDICATIONS

Salutensin is contraindicated in patients who have previously demonstrated hypersensitivity to its components. Patients with anuria or oliguria should not be given this medication. The presence of an active peptic ulcer, ulcerative colitis or severe depression contraindicates the use of reserpine. If electroshock therapy is necessary, treatment with Salutensin should be discontinued at least seven (7) days prior to this therapy.

WARNINGS

Azotemia may be precipitated or increased by hydroflumethiazide. Special caution is necessary in patients with impaired renal function to avoid cumulative or toxic effects.

Since in hepatic cirrhosis, minor alterations of fluid and electrolyte balance may precipitate coma, hydroflumethiazide should be given with caution.

The possibility of sensitivity reactions should be considered in patients with a history of allergy or bronchial asthma.

Hydroflumethiazide potentiates the action of other antihypertensive drugs. Therefore, the dosage of these agents, especially the ganglion blockers, must be reduced by at least 50 percent as soon as hydroflumethiazide is added to the regimen.

The possibility of exacerbation or activation of systemic lupus erythematosus has been reported for sulfonamide derivatives (including thiazides) and reserpine.

The occurrence of mental depression due to reserpine in doses of 0.25 mg daily or less is unusual. In any event, Salutensin should be discontinued at the first sign of depression.

PRECAUTIONS

General—Salutensin is a combination product containing hydroflumethiazide and reserpine. Precautions to be observed are associated with the individual components and are listed below.

Hydroflumethiazide—Careful check should be kept for signs of fluid and electrolyte imbalance. Serum and urine electrolyte determinations are particularly important when the patient is vomiting excessively or receiving parenteral fluids. Warning signs, irrespective of cause are: dryness of mouth, thirst, weakness, lethargy, drowsiness, restlessness, muscle pains or cramps, muscular fatigue, hypotension, oliguria, tachycardia, and gastrointestinal disturbances.

Potassium excretion is usually minimal. However, hypokalemia may develop with hydroflumethiazide as with any other potent diuretic, especially with brisk diuresis, when severe cirrhosis is present, or during concomitant use of steroids or ACTH. Interference with adequate electrolyte intake will contribute to hypokalemia. Digitalis therapy may exaggerate metabolic effects of hypokalemia especially with reference to myocardial activity. If dietary salt is unduly restricted, especially during hot weather, in severely edematous patients with congestive failure or renal disease, a low salt syndrome may complicate therapy with thiazides.

Hypokalemia may be avoided or treated by use of potassium chloride or giving foods with a high potassium content. Any chloride deficit may similarly be corrected by use of ammonium chloride (excepting patients with hepatic disease) and largely prevented by a near normal salt intake.

Thiazide drugs may increase the responsiveness to tubocurarine. The antihypertensive effect of the drug may be enhanced in the post-sympathectomy patient. Hydroflumethiazide decreases arterial responsiveness to norepinephrine, as do other thiazides, necessitating due care in surgical patients. It is recommended that thiazides be discontinued 48 hours before elective surgery. Orthostatic hypotension may occur and may be potentiated by alcohol, barbiturates, or narcotics.

Pathological changes in the parathyroid glands with hypercalcemia and hypophosphatemia have been observed in a few patients on prolonged thiazide therapy. The common complications of hyperparathyroidism such as renal lithiasis, bone resorption, and peptic ulceration have not been seen. The effect of discontinuance of thiazide therapy on serum calcium and phosphorus levels may be helpful in assessing the need for parathyroid surgery in such patients. Parathyroidectomy has been followed by subjective clinical improvement in most patients, but is without effect on the hypertension. Following surgery, thiazide therapy may be resumed.

Caution is necessary in patients with hyperuricemia or a history of gout, since gout may be precipitated. Insulin requirements in diabetic patients may be increased, decreased, or unchanged. In latent diabetics, hydroflumethiazide, in common with other benzothiadiazines, may cause hyperglycemia and glycosuria.

Reserpine—Since reserpine may increase gastric secretion and motility, it should be used cautiously in patients with a history of peptic ulcer, ulcerative colitis, or other gastrointestinal disorders. This compound may precipitate biliary colic in patients with gallstones, or bronchial asthma in susceptible persons.

Reserpine may cause hypotension including orthostatic hypotension. In hypertensive patients on reserpine therapy significant hypotension and bradycardia may develop during surgical anesthesia. Therefore, the drug should be discontinued two weeks before giving anesthesia. For emergency surgical procedures, it may be necessary to give vagal blocking agents parenterally to prevent or reverse hypotension and/or bradycardia.

Anxiety or depression, as well as psychosis, may develop during reserpine therapy. If depression is present when therapy is begun, it may be aggravated. Mental depression is unusual with reserpine doses of 0.25 mg daily or less. In any case, Salutensin should be discontinued at the first sign of depression. Extreme caution should be used in treating patients with a history of mental depression, and the possibility of suicide should be kept in mind.

As with most antihypertensive therapy, caution should be exercised when treating hypertensive patients with renal insufficiency, since they adjust poorly to lowered blood pressure levels. Use reserpine cautiously with digitalis and quinidine; cardiac arrhythmias have occurred with reserpine preparations. Thiazides may decrease serum P.B.I. levels without signs of thyroid disturbance.

Information for Patients—If you miss a dose of this medicine, take it as soon as possible. If it is almost time for your next dose, do not take the missed dose at all and do not double the next one. Instead, go back to your regular dosing schedule. If you have any questions about this, check with your doctor.

This medicine may cause a loss of potassium from your body. To help prevent this, your doctor may want you to:

- eat or drink foods that have a high potassium content (for example, orange or other citrus fruit juices,) or
- take a potassium supplement, or
- take another medicine to help prevent the loss of the potassium in the first place.

It is very important to follow these directions. Also, it is important not to change your diet on your own. This is more important if you are already on a special diet (as for diabetes), or if you are taking a potassium supplement or a medicine to reduce potassium loss. Extra potassium may not be necessary and, in some cases, too much potassium could be harmful.

Check with your doctor if you become sick and have severe or continuing vomiting or diarrhea. These problems may cause you to lose additional water and potassium.

Caution: Diabetics—This medicine may raise blood sugar levels. While you are using this medicine, be especially careful in testing for sugar in your urine. If you have any questions about this, check with your doctor.

A few people who take this medicine may become more sensitive to sunlight than they are normally. When you begin to take this medicine, avoid too much sun or use a sunlamp until you see how you react, especially if you tend to burn easily. If you have a severe reaction, check with your doctor.

This medicine may cause some people to become drowsy or less alert than they are normally. This is more likely to happen when you begin to take it or when you increase the amount of medicine you are taking. **Make sure you know how you react to this medicine before you drive, use machines, or do other jobs that require you to be alert.**

Dizziness, lightheadedness, or fainting may occur, especially when you get up from a lying or sitting position. Getting up slowly may help but if the problem continues or gets worse, check with your doctor.

In some patients, this medicine may cause mental depression. **Tell your doctor right away:**

- if you or anyone else notices unusual changes in your moods.
- if you start having early-morning sleeplessness or unusually vivid dreams or nightmares.

This medicine will add to the effects of alcohol and other medicines (CNS depressants) that slow down the nervous system. Some examples of CNS depressants are antihistamines or medicine for hay fever, other allergies, or colds; sedatives, tranquilizers, or sleeping medicine; prescription pain medicine or narcotics; barbiturates; medicine for seizures; tricyclic antidepressants (medicine for depression); or anesthetics, including dental anesthetics. **Check with your doctor before taking any of the above while you are taking this medicine.**

Before having any kind of surgery (including dental surgery), or emergency treatment, **make sure the doctor or dentist in charge knows that you are taking this medicine.**

This medicine may cause stuffiness in the nose. However, do not use nasal decongestant medicines without first checking with your doctor or pharmacist.

Do not take other medicines unless they have been discussed with your doctor. This especially includes over-the-counter (nonprescription) medicines for appetite control, asthma, colds, cough, hay fever, or sinus, since they may tend to increase your blood pressure.

Your mouth, nose, and throat may feel very dry while you are taking this medicine. To help relieve mouth dryness, chew sugarless gum or dissolve bits of ice in your mouth.

Laboratory Tests—Determination of serum electrolytes to detect possible electrolyte imbalance should be performed at appropriate intervals.

DRUG INTERACTIONS

Reserpine

Alcohol or
CNS depressants
(concurrent use may enhance the CNS depressant effects of either these medications or rauwolfia alkaloids)

Antihypertensives, other, or
Diuretics
(antihypertensive effects may be potentiated when used concurrently with rauwolfia alkaloids; although some combinations are frequently used for therapeutic advantage, when used concurrently dosage adjustments may be necessary)

Beta-blockers
(concurrent administration with beta-blockers may result in additive and possible excessive beta-adrenergic blockage. Although this effect is largely theoretical, close observation is recommended)

Digitalis glycosides or
Quinidine
(concurrent use may result in cardiac arrhythmias; although this interaction is controversial and does not appear to be significant with usual doses, caution is recommended, especially when large doses of rauwolfia alkaloids are used in digitalized patients)

Levodopa
(since rauwolfia alkaloids may cause dopamine depletion and parkinsonism effects, concurrent use is not recommended)

Methotrimeprazine
(concurrent use may result in additive hypotension)

Monoamine oxidase (MAO) inhibitors
(concurrent use with rauwolfia alkaloids may result in moderate to sudden and severe hypertension and hyperpyrexia which can reach crisis levels)

Sympathomimetics
Indirect-acting amines such as amphetamines, ephedrine, methylphenidate, phenylpropanolamine, pseudoephedrine, tryamine
(rauwolfia alkaloids inhibit the action of indirect-acting sympathomimetics by depleting catecholamine stores)
Direct-acting amines such as epinephrine isoproterenol and norepinephrine (levarterenol). Included are metaraminol and phenylephrine which are thought to act both directly and indirectly
(Rauwolfia alkaloids may theoretically prolong the action of direct-acting sympathomimetics by preventing uptake into storage granules; a "denervation supersensitivity" response is also possible, although concurrent use with rauwolfia alkaloids is not known to produce severe adverse effects, a significant increase in blood pressure has been documented when phenylephrine ophthalmic drops have been administered to patients taking reserpine, and caution and close observation are recommended)

Tricyclic antidepressants
(concurrent use may decrease the hypotensive effects of rauwolfia alkaloids and interfere with the antidepressant effects of these medications)

Hydroflumethiazide

Antihypertensive medications, other, especially diazoxide, or
Preanesthetic and anesthetic agents used in surgery or
Skeletal muscle relaxants, nondepolarizing, used in surgery
(effects may be potentiated when used concurrently with thiazide diuretics, dosage adjustments may be necessary)

Amphotericin B or
Corticosteroids or
Corticotropin (ACTH)
(concurrent use with thiazide diuretics may intensify electrolyte imbalance, particularly hypokalemia)

Cardiac glycosides
(concurrent use with thiazide diuretics may enhance the possibility of digitalis toxicity associated with hypokalemia)

Colestipol
(may inhibit gastrointestinal absorption of the thiazide diuretics; administration 1 hour before or 4 hours after colestipol is recommended)

Hypoglycemics
(thiazide diuretics may raise blood glucose levels for adult-onset diabetics, dosage adjustment of hypoglycemic medications may be necessary during and after thiazide diuretic therapy; insulin requirements may be increased, decreased, or unchanged)

Lithium salts
(concurrent use with thiazide diuretics is not recommended, as they may provoke lithium toxicity because of reduced renal clearance)

Methenamine
(effectiveness may be decreased when used concurrently with thiazide diuretics because of alkalinization of the urine)

Diagnostic Interference

Reserpine

With diagnostic test results
Urinary steroid colorimetric determinations by modified Glenn-Nelson technique or Holtorff-Koch modification of Zimmerman reaction (falsely low because rauwolfia alkaloids slightly decrease absorbance)

With expected physiologic effects
Serum prolactin levels (may be increased)
Urinary catecholamine excretion (large parenteral doses of reserpine may cause an initial increase, although an overall decrease is usually noted with chronic administration of rauwolfia alkaloids)

Continued on next page

Bristol—Cont.

Urinary vanilmandelic acid (VMA) excretion (intramuscular administration of reserpine causes an initial increase of about 40%, followed by a decrease by the end of the second day, chronic or parenteral administration of rauwolfia alkaloids results in an overall decrease)

Hydroflumethiazide

With expected physiologic effects

Blood and urine glucose levels (usually only in patients with a predisposition to glucose intolerance) and

Serum bilirubin levels (by displacement from albumin binding) and

Serum calcium levels (thiazide diuretics should be discontinued before parathyroid function tests are carried out) and

Serum uric acid levels (may be increased)

Serum magnesium, potassium, and sodium levels (may be decreased; serum magnesium levels may increase in uremic patients)

Serum protein bound iodine (PBI) levels (may be decreased)

Animal Tumorigenicity—Rodent studies have shown that reserpine is an animal tumorigen, causing an increased incidence of mammary fibroadenomas in female mice, malignant tumors of the seminal vesicals in male mice, and malignant adrenal medullary tumors in male rats. These findings arose in 2 year studies in which the drug was administered in the feed at concentrations of 5 and 10 ppm—about 100 to 300 times the usual human dose. The breast neoplasms are thought to be related to reserpine's prolactin-elevating effect. Several other prolactin-elevating drugs have also been associated with an increased incidence of mammary neoplasia in rodents.

The extent to which these findings indicate a risk to humans is uncertain. Tissue culture experiments show that about one-third of human breast tumors are prolactin-dependent **in vitro**, a factor of considerable importance if the use of the drug is contemplated in a patient with previously detected breast cancer. The possibility of an increased risk of breast cancer in reserpine users has been studied extensively; however, no firm conclusion has emerged. Although a few epidemiologic studies have suggested a slightly increased risk (less than two-fold in all studies except one) in women who have used reserpine, other studies of generally similar design have not confirmed this. Epidemiologic studies conducted using other drugs (neuroleptic agents) that, like reserpine, increase prolactin levels and therefore would be considered rodent mammary carcinogens, have not shown an association between chronic administration of the drug and human mammary tumorigenesis. While long-term clinical observation has not suggested such an association, the available evidence is considered too limited to be conclusive at this time. An association of reserpine intake with pheochromocytoma or tumors of the seminal vesicles has not been explored.

Pregnancy: Teratogenic Effects—Pregnancy Category C—Animal reproduction studies have not been conducted with Salutensin. It is also not known whether Salutensin can cause fetal harm when administered to a pregnant woman or can affect reproduction capacity. Salutensin should be given to a pregnant woman only if clearly indicated.

Nonteratogenic Effects—There is some evidence that side effects such as nasal congestion, lethargy, depressed Moro reflex, and bradycardia may appear in infants born of reserpine-treated mothers. Thiazides cross the placental barrier and appear in cord blood. When Salutensin is used in women of childbearing age, the potential benefits of the drug should be weighed against the possible hazards to the fetus. These hazards included fetal or neonatal jaundice, thrombocytopenia, and possibly other adverse reactions which have occurred in the adult.

Nursing Mothers—Thiazides and reserpine appear in breast milk. If use of the drug is deemed essential, the mother may consider stopping nursing.

Pediatric Use—Safety and effectiveness in children have not been established.

ADVERSE REACTIONS

The following adverse reactions have been observed, but there is not enough systematic collection of data to support an estimate of their frequency.

Hydroflumethiazide

A. Gastrointestinal System Reactions: anorexia, gastric irritation, nausea, vomiting, cramping, diarrhea, constipation, jaundice (intrahepatic cholestatic jaundice), pancreatitis, hyperglycemia, and glycosuria.
B. Central Nervous System Reactions: dizziness, vertigo paresthesias, headache and xanthopsia.
C. Hematologic Reactions: leukopenia, thrombocytopenia, agranulocytosis, and aplastic anemia.
D. Dermatologic Hypersensitivity Reactions: purpura, photosensitivity, rash, urticaria, and necrotizing angiitis (vasculitis) (cutaneous vasculitis).
E. Cardiovascular Reaction: orthostatic hypotension may occur and may be aggravated by alcohol, barbiturates or narcotics.
F. Miscellaneous: muscle spasm, weakness, restlessness, fever, respiratory distress including pneumonitis, pulmonary edema and anaphylactic reactions.

Whenever adverse reactions are moderate or severe, thiazide dosage should be reduced or therapy withdrawn.

Reserpine

A. Gastrointestinal System Reactions: anorexia, nausea, increased intestinal motility, diarrhea, dryness of the mouth, increased salivation, vomiting.
B. Central Nervous System Reactions: excessive sedation, nightmares, headaches, dizziness, blurred vision, syncope, impotence or decreased libido, mental depression, nervousness, paradoxical anxiety, dull sensorium, deafness, glaucoma, uveitis, optic atrophy, Parkinsonian-like syndrome.
C. Hematologic Reactions: epistaxis, purpura due to thrombocytopenia.
D. Dermatological Reactions: conjunctival injection, flushing of the skin, pruritus, rash.
E. Cardiovascular Reactions: bradycardia dyspnea, angina pectoris and other direct cardiac effects (e.g., premature ventricular contractions, fluid retention, congestive failure).
F. Miscellaneous: nasal congestion, weight gain, muscular aches, enhanced susceptibility to colds, dysuria, nonpuerperal lactation

OVERDOSAGE

Signs and Symptoms—Hydroflumethiazide-related effects: diuresis, lethargy progressing to coma with minimal cardiorespiratory depression GI irritation, hypermotility, elevated BUN, serum electrolyte changes.

Reserpine-related effects: impairment of consciousness ranging from drowsiness to coma, flushing, conjunctival injection, miosis, hypotension, hypothermia, respiratory depression, bradycardia, diarrhea.

Treatment—Induce emesis or use gastric lavage, followed by activated charcoal, to empty stomach. Treat hypotension by volume expansion, if possible. If a vasopressor is needed, use phenylephrine levarterenol or metarminol. Treat significant bradycardia with vagal blocking agents, along with other appropriate measures. Monitor serum electrolytes and renal function and institute supportive measures, as required. Treat GI effects symptomatically. Observe patient for at least 72 hours.

DOSAGE

As determined by individual titration (see box warning).

The usual adult dose of Salutensin is one tablet once or twice daily. If a smaller amount of thiazide diuretic is desired, Salutensin-Demi, one tablet once or twice daily, can be given. Most patients will respond to this dosage level. In refractory cases, the physician may carefully increase the dose to three or four tablets per day in divided doses providing the proper precautions are observed—careful attention to serum uric acid, fasting blood sugar, BUN or NPN, and serum electrolyte levels. (See sections on **Precautions** and **Warnings** above). When the desired blood pressure reduction has been achieved, the dose should be reduced to the minimum effective dose for the individual patient.

Careful observation for changes in blood pressure must be made when Salutensin is used with other antihypertensive drugs. The dosage of other agents must be reduced by at least 50 percent as soon as Salutensin is added to the regimen to prevent excessive drop in blood pressure. As the blood pressure falls under the potentiating effect of Salutensin, a further reduction in dosage or even a discontinuation of other antihypertensive drugs may be necessary.

SUPPLY

Salutensin Tablets
NDC 0015-5436
Salutensin-Demi Tablets
NDC 0015-5455

For information on package sizes available, refer to the current price schedule.

Shown in Product Identification Section, page 406

STADOL® ℞

[*stā'dōl*]
(butorphanol tartrate)

This is the full text of the latest Official Package Circular dated October 1979 [5644DIM-04].

DESCRIPTION

Stadol (butorphanol tartrate), sterile, parenteral, narcotic agonist-antagonist, analgesic, is a member of the phenanthrene series. The chemical name is levo-N- cyclobutylmethyl-6, 10aβ-dihydroxy-1,2,3,9,10, 10a-hexahydro- (4H) - 10, 4a-iminoethanophenanthrene tartrate. It is a white crystalline substance soluble in aqueous solution. The dose is expressed as the salt. One milligram of tartrate salt is equivalent to 0.68 milligram of base. In addition to Stadol (butorphanol tartrate), each ml contains 3.3 mg citric acid, 6.4 mg sodium citrate and 6.4 mg sodium chloride.

The structural formula is

N-CH₂ · OH · HO · $\cdot C_4H_6O_6$

The molecular weight is 477.56 and the molecular formula is $C_{21}H_{29}NO_2 \cdot C_4H_6O_6$

CLINICAL PHARMACOLOGY

Stadol is a potent analgesic. The duration of analgesia is generally 3 to 4 hours and is approximately equivalent to that of morphine. The onset time for analgesia is within 10 minutes following intramuscular injection and very rapidly following intravenous administration. Peak analgesic activity is obtained at 30 to 60 minutes following intramuscular injection and more rapidly following intravenous administration.

Narcotic Antagonist Activity

Stadol has narcotic antagonist activity which is approximately equivalent to that of nalorphine, 30 times that of pentazocine and 1/40 that of naloxone (Narcan®) as measured by the antagonism of morphine analgesia in the rat tail flick test.

Mechanism of Analgesic Action

The exact mechanism of action of Stadol is unknown. It is felt that the class of narcotic antagonist analgesics exert their analgesic effect via a central nervous system mechanism. Currently, it is believed the site of action of centrally acting analgesics is subcortical, possibly in the limbic system.

Effect on Respiration

At the analgesic dose of 2 mg, Stadol depresses respiration to a degree equal to 10 mg morphine. The magnitude of respiratory depression with Stadol is not appreciably increased at doses of 4 mg. In contrast to the magnitude of respiratory depression, the duration of respiratory depression with Stadol is dose-related. Any respiratory depression produced by Stadol is reversible by naloxone which is a specific antagonist.

Cardiovascular Effects

The hemodynamic changes after the intravenous administration of Stadol are similar to the reported hemodynamic changes after pentazocine. The changes include increased pulmonary artery pressure, pulmonary wedge pressure, left ventricular end-diastolic pressure, systemic arterial pressure, and pulmonary vascular resistance. Although smaller than those following pentazocine, these changes are nevertheless in a direction which increases the work of the heart, especially in the pulmonary circuit.

INDICATIONS AND USAGE

Stadol is recommended for the relief of moderate to severe pain. Stadol can also be used for preoperative or preanesthetic medication, as a supplement to balanced anesthesia, and for the relief of prepartum pain.

CONTRAINDICATIONS

Stadol should not be administered to patients who have been shown to be hypersensitive to it.

WARNINGS

Patients Physically Dependent on Narcotics

Because of its antagonist properties, Stadol is not recommended for patients physically dependent on narcotics. Detoxification in such patients is required prior to use.

Due to the difficulty in assessing addiction in patients who have recently received substantial amounts of narcotic medication, caution should be used in the administration of Stadol. Detoxification of such patients prior to usage should be carefully considered.

Drug Dependence

Special care should be exercised in administering Stadol to emotionally unstable patients and to those with a history of drug misuse. When long-term therapy is contemplated, such patients should be closely supervised. Even though Stadol has a low physical dependence liability, care should be taken that individuals who may be prone to drug abuse are closely supervised. It is important to avoid increases in dose and frequency of injections by the patient and to prevent the use of the drug in anticipation of pain rather than for the relief of pain.

Head Injury and Increased Intracranial Pressure

Although there is no clinical experience in patients with head injury, it can be assumed that Stadol, like other potent analgesics, elevates cerebrospinal fluid pressure. Therefore the use of Stadol in cases of head injury can produce effects (e.g., miosis) which may obscure the clinical course of patients with head injuries. In such patients Stadol must be used with extreme caution and only if its use is deemed essential.

Cardiovascular Effects

Because Stadol increases the work of the heart, especially the pulmonary circuit, (see Clinical Pharmacology), the use of this drug in acute myocardial infarction or in cardiac patients with ventricular dysfunction or coronary insufficiency should be limited to those who are hypersensitive to morphine sulfate or meperidine.

PRECAUTIONS

Certain Respiratory Conditions
Because Stadol causes some respiratory depression, it should be administered only with caution and low dosage to patients with respiratory depression (e.g., from other medication, uremia, or severe infection), severely limited respiratory reserve, bronchial asthma, obstructive respiratory conditions, or cyanosis.

Impaired Renal or Hepatic Function
Although laboratory tests have not indicated that Stadol causes or increases renal or hepatic impairment, the drug should be administered with caution to patients with such impairment. Extensive liver disease may predispose to greater side effects and greater activity from the usual clinical dose, possibly the result of decreased metabolism of the drug by the liver.

Biliary Surgery
Clinical studies have not been done to establish the safety of Stadol administration to patients about to undergo surgery of the biliary tract.

Usage as a Pre-Operative or Pre-Anesthetic Medication
Slight increases in systolic blood pressure may occur, therefore caution should be employed when Stadol is used in the hypertensive patient.

Usage in Balanced Anesthesia
The use of pancuronium in combination with Stadol may cause an increase in conjunctival changes.

Usage in Pregnancy
The safety of Stadol for use in pregnancy prior to the labor period has not been established; therefore, this drug should be used in pregnant patients only when in the judgment of the physician its use is deemed essential to the welfare of the patient.
Reproduction studies have been performed in rats, mice, and rabbits and have revealed no evidence of impaired fertility or harm to the fetus due to Stadol at about 2.5 to 5 times the human dose.

Usage in Labor and Delivery
Safety to the mother and fetus following the administration of Stadol during labor has been established. Patients receiving Stadol during labor have experienced no adverse effects other than those observed with commonly used analgesics. Stadol should be used with caution in women delivering premature infants.

Usage in Nursing Mothers
The use of Stadol in lactating mothers who are nursing their infants is not recommended, since it is not known whether this drug is excreted in milk. Stadol has been used safely for labor pain in mothers who subsequently nursed their infants.

Usage in Children
Safety and efficacy in children below age 18 years have not been established at present.

ADVERSE REACTIONS

The most frequent adverse reactions in 1250 patients treated with Stadol are: sedation (503, 40%), nausea (82, 6%), clammy/sweating (76, 6%).
Less frequent reactions are: headache (35, 3%), vertigo (33, 3%), floating feeling (33, 3%), dizziness (23, 2%), lethargy (19, 2%), confusion (15, 1%), lightheadedness (12, 1%).
Other adverse reactions which may occur (reported incidence of less than 1%) are:
CNS: nervousness, unusual dreams, agitation, euphoria, hallucinations
Autonomic: flushing and warmth, dry mouth, sensitivity to cold
Cardiovascular: palpitation, increase or decrease of blood pressure
Gastrointestinal: vomiting
Respiratory: slowing of respiration, shallow breathing
Dermatological: rash or hives
Eye: diplopia or blurred vision

OVERDOSAGE

Manifestations
Although there have been no experiences of overdosage with Stadol during clinical trials, this may occur due to accidental or intentional misuse as well as therapeutic use. Based on the pharmacology of Stadol, overdosage could produce some degree of respiratory depression and variable cardiovascular and central nervous system effects.

Treatment
The immediate treatment of suspected Stadol overdosage is intravenous naloxone. The respiratory and cardiac status of the patient should be evaluated constantly and appropriate supportive measures instituted, such as oxygen, intravenous fluids, vasopressors, and assisted or controlled respiration.

DOSAGE AND ADMINISTRATION

Adults:
Intramuscular—The usual recommended single dose is 2 mg. This may be repeated every three to four hours, as necessary. The effective dosage range, depending on the severity of pain, is 1 to 4 mg repeated every three to four hours. At this time, there is insufficient clinical data to recommend single doses beyond 4 mg.
Intravenous—The usual recommended single dose for intravenous administration is 1 mg repeated every three to four hours as necessary. The effective dosage range, depending on the severity of pain, is 0.5 to 2 mg repeated every three to four hours.

Concomitant Use with Tranquilizers
According to accepted procedure, the dose of Stadol should be reduced when administered concomitantly with phenothiazines and other tranquilizers which may potentiate the action of Stadol.

Children:
Since there is no clinical experience in children under 18 years, Stadol is not recommended in this age group.

Storage Conditions
Store at room temperature.

SUPPLY

Stadol (butorphanol tartrate) Injection for I.M. or I.V. use is available as follows:
NDC 0015-5644-20—2 mg per ml, 2-ml vial
NDC 0015-5645-20—1 mg per ml, 1-ml vial
NDC 0015-5646-20—2 mg per ml, 1-ml vial
NDC 0015-5646-23—2 mg per ml, 1-ml Disposable Syringe
NDC 0015-5648-20—2 mg per ml, 10-ml multi-dose vial
For information on package sizes available, refer to the current price schedule.

STAPHCILLIN® ℞

[stăf'sĭl-ĭn]
(methicillin sodium for Injection)
Buffered
For I.M. Or I.V. Use

This is the full text of the latest Official Package Circular dated June 1984 [7961DIR-18].

DESCRIPTION

Staphcillin (methicillin sodium) is a semisynthetic antibiotic substance derived from 6-amino penicillanic acid. It is the sodium salt in a parenteral dosage form. Each gram of Staphcillin is equivalent to 900 mg methicillin activity and is buffered with 50 mg sodium citrate.

METHICILLIN SODIUM

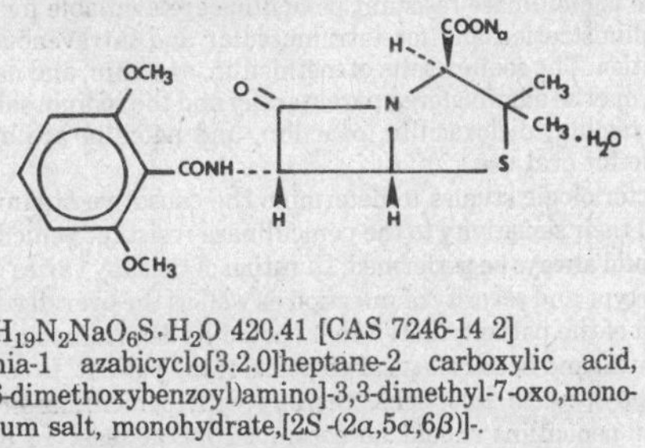

$C_{17}H_{19}N_2NaO_6S \cdot H_2O$ 420.41 [CAS 7246-14 2]
4-Thia-1 azabicyclo[3.2.0]heptane-2 carboxylic acid, 6-[(2,6-dimethoxybenzoyl)amino]-3,3-dimethyl-7-oxo,monosodium salt, monohydrate,[2S-(2α,5α,6β)]-.

CLINICAL PHARMACOLOGY

Microbiology: Penicillinase-resistant penicillins exert a bactericidal action against penicillin-susceptible microorganisms during the state of active multiplication. All penicillins inhibit the biosynthesis of the bacterial cell wall.
The drugs in this class are highly resistant to inactivation by staphylococcal penicillinase and are active against penicillinase producing and non-penicillinase producing strains of **Staphylococcus aureus.**
The penicillinase-resistant penicillins are active *in vitro* against a variety of other bacteria.
Susceptibility Plate Testing: Quantitative methods of susceptibility testing that require measurement of zone diameters or minimal inhibitory concentrations (MIC's) give the most precise estimates of antibiotic susceptibilty. One such procedure has been recommended for use with discs to test susceptibility to this class of drugs. Interpretations correlate diameters on the disc test with MIC values. A penicillinase-resistant class disc may be used to determine microbial susceptibility to cloxacillin, dicloxacillin, methicillin, nafcillin and oxacillin. With this procedure, employing a 5 microgram methicillin sodium disc, a report from the laboratory of "susceptible" (zone of at least 14 mm) indicates that the infecting organism is likely to respond to therapy. A report of "resistant" (zone of less than 10 mm) indicates that the infecting organism is not likely to respond to therapy. A report of "intermediate susceptibility" (zone of 10 to 13 mm) suggests that the organism might be susceptible if high doses of the antibiotic are used, or if the infection is confined to tissues and fluids (e.g., urine), in which high antibiotic levels are attained.
In general, all staphylococci should be tested against the penicillin G disc and against the methicillin disc. Routine methods of antibiotic susceptibility testing may fail to detect strains of organisms resistant to the penicillinase-resistant penicillins. For this reason, the use of large inocula and 48-hour incubation periods may be necessary to obtain accurate susceptibility studies with these antibiotics. Bacterial strains which are resistant to one of the penicillinase-resistant penicillins should be considered resistant to all of the drugs in the class.

PHARMACOKINETICS

Staphcillin (methicillin sodium) is not acid-resistant and must be administered by intramuscular or intravenous injection. A 1-Gram intramuscular dose gives a peak blood level of approximately 12 mcg/ml which drops off to about 1 mcg/ml within a 4-hour period. Methicillin is rapidly excreted unchanged in the urine in individuals with normal kidney function. Impairment in kidney function results in elevated blood levels which may require adjustment of dosage and treatment intervals. Protein binding of methicillin is approximately 40%. The drug penetrates body tissues well, and diffuses readily into pleural, pericardial, and synovial fluids. As with all penicillins, absorption into spinal fluids is poor under normal conditions. However, higher concentrations may be attained in the presence of meningeal inflammation.

INDICATIONS AND USAGE

The penicillinase-resistant penicillins are indicated in the treatment of infections caused by penicillinase-producing staphylococci which have demonstrated susceptibility to the drugs. Culture and susceptibility tests should be performed initially to determine the causative organisms and their sensitivity to the drug (See **Clinical Pharmacology**—Susceptibility Plate Testing).
The penicillinase-resistant penicillins may be used to initiate therapy in suspected cases of resistant staphylococcal infections prior to the availability of laboratory test results.
The penicillinase-resistant penicillins should not be used in infections caused by organisms susceptible to penicillin G. If the susceptibility tests indicate that the infection is due to an organism other than a resistant staphylococcus, therapy should not be continued with a penicillinase-resistant penicillin.

CONTRAINDICATIONS

A history of a hypersensitivity (anaphylactic) reaction to any penicillin is a contraindication.

WARNINGS

Serious and occasionally fatal hypersensitivity (anaphylactic shock with collapse) reactions have occurred in patients receiving penicillin. The incidence of anaphylactic shock in all penicillin-treated patients is between 0.015 and 0.04 percent. Anaphylactic shock resulting in death has occurred in approximately 0.002 percent of the patients treated. Although anaphylaxis is more frequent following a parenteral administration, it has occurred in patients receiving oral penicillins.
When penicillin therapy is indicated, it should be initiated only after a comprehensive patient drug and allergy history has been obtained. If an allergic reaction occurs, the drug should be discontinued and the patient should receive supportive treatment, e.g., artificial maintenance of ventilation, pressor amines, antihistamines, and corticosteroids. Individuals with a history of penicillin hypersensitivity may also experience allergic reactions when treated with a cephalosporin.

PRECAUTIONS

General: Penicillinase-resistant penicillins should generally not be administered to patients with a history of sensitivity to any penicillin.
Penicillin should be used with caution in individuals with histories of significant allergies and/or asthma. Whenever allergic reactions occur, penicillin should be withdrawn unless, in the opinion of the physician, the condition being treated is life-threatening and amenable only to penicillin therapy.
The oral route of administration should not be relied upon in patients with severe illness, or with nausea, vomiting, gastric dilation, cardiospasm, or intestinal hypermotility. Occasionally patients will not absorb therapeutic amounts of orally administered penicillin.
The use of antibiotics may result in overgrowth of nonsusceptible organisms. If new infections due to bacteria or fungi occur, the drug should be discontinued and appropriate measures taken.
Laboratory Tests: Bacteriologic studies to determine the causative organisms and their susceptibility to the penicillinase-resistant penicillins should be performed (See **Clinical Pharmacology**—Microbiology). In the treatment of suspected staphylococcal infections, therapy should be changed

Continued on next page

Bristol—Cont.

to another active agent if culture tests fail to demonstrate the presence of staphylococci.
Periodic assessment of organ system function including renal, hepatic, and hematopoietic should be made during prolonged therapy with the penicillinase-resistant penicillins. Blood cultures, white blood cell, and differential cell counts should be obtained prior to initiation of therapy and at least weekly during therapy with penicillinase-resistant penicillins.
Periodic urinalysis, blood urea nitrogen, and creatinine determinations should be performed during therapy with the penicillinase resistant penicillins and dosage alterations should be considered if these values become elevated. If any impairment of renal function is suspected or known to exist, a reduction in the total dosage should be considered and blood levels monitored to avoid possible neurotoxic reactions (See **DOSAGE AND ADMINISTRATION**).
SGOT and SGPT values should be obtained periodically during therapy to monitor for possible liver function abnormalities.
Drug Interactions: Tetracycline, a bacteriostatic antibiotic, may antagonize the bactericidal effect of penicillin and concurrent use of these drugs should be avoided.
Carcinogenesis, Mutagenesis, Impairment of Fertility: No long-term animal studies have been conducted with these drugs.
Studies on reproduction (nafcillin) in rats and rabbits reveal no fetal or maternal abnormalities before conception and continuously through weaning (one generation).
Pregnancy Category B: Reproduction studies performed in the mouse, rat, and rabbit have revealed no evidence of impaired fertility or harm to the fetus due to the penicillinase-resistant penicillins. Human experience with the penicillins during pregnancy has not shown any positive evidence of adverse effects on the fetus. There are, however, no adequate or well-controlled studies in pregnant women showing conclusively that harmful effects of these drugs on the fetus can be excluded. Because animal reproduction studies are not always predictive of human response, this drug should be used during pregnancy only if clearly needed.
Nursing Mothers: Penicillins are excreted in breast milk. Caution should be exercised when penicillins are administered to a nursing woman.
Pediatric Use: Because of incompletely developed renal function in newborns, penicillinase-resistant penicillins (especially methicillin) may not be completely excreted, with abnormally high blood levels resulting. Frequent blood levels are advisable in this group with dosage adjustments when necessary. All newborns treated with penicillins should be monitored closely for clinical and laboratory evidence of toxic or adverse effects (See **DOSAGE AND ADMINISTRATION**).

ADVERSE REACTIONS

Body as a Whole: The reported incidence of allergic reactions to penicillins ranges from 0.7 to 10 percent (See **WARNINGS**). Sensitization is usually the result of treatment but some individuals have had immediate reactions to penicillin when first treated. In such cases, it is thought that the patients may have had prior exposure to the drug via trace amounts present in milk and vaccines.
Two types of allergic reactions to penicillin are noted clinically, immediate and delayed.
Immediate reactions usually occur within 20 minutes of administration and range in severity from urticaria and pruritus to angioneurotic edema, laryngospasm, bronchospasm, hypotension, vascular collapse, and death. Such immediate anaphylactic reactions are very rare (See **WARNINGS**) and usually occur after parenteral therapy but have occurred in patients receiving oral therapy. Another type of immediate reaction, an accelerated reaction, may occur between 20 minutes and 48 hours after administration and may include urticaria, pruritus, and fever. Although laryngeal edema, laryngospasm, and hypotension occasionally occur, fatality is uncommon.
Delayed allergic reactions to penicillin therapy usually occur after 48 hours and sometimes as late as 2 to 4 weeks after initiation of therapy. Manifestations of this type of reaction include serum sickness-like symptoms (i.e., fever, malaise, urticaria, myalgia, arthralgia, abdominal pain) and various skin rashes. Nausea, vomiting, diarrhea, stomatitis, black or hairy tongue, and other symptoms of gastrointestinal irritation may occur, especially during oral penicillin therapy.
Nervous System Reactions: Neurotoxic reactions similar to those observed with penicillin G may occur with large intravenous doses of the penicillinase-resistant penicillins especially in patients with renal insufficiency.
Urogenital Reactions: Renal tubular damage and interstitial nephritis have been associated with the administration of methicillin sodium and infrequently with the administration of nafcillin and oxacillin. Manifestations of this reaction may include rash, fever, eosinophilia, hematuria, proteinuria, and renal insufficiency. Methicillin-induced nephropathy does not appear to be dose-related and is generally reversible upon prompt discontinuation of therapy.
Metabolic Reactions: Agranulocytosis, neutropenia, and bone marrow depression have been associated with the use of methicillin sodium, nafcillin, oxacillin, and cloxacillin. Hepatotoxicity, characterized by fever, nausea, and vomiting associated with abnormal liver function tests, mainly elevated SGOT levels, has been associated with the use of oxacillin and cloxacillin.

DOSAGE AND ADMINISTRATION

The penicillinase-resistant penicillins are available for oral administration and for intramuscular and intravenous injection. The sodium salts of methicillin, oxacillin, and nafcillin may be administered parenterally and the sodium salts of cloxacillin, dicloxacillin, oxacillin, and nafcillin are available for oral use.
Bacteriologic studies to determine the causative organisms and their sensitivity to the penicillinase-resistant penicillins should always be performed. Duration of therapy varies with the type and severity of infection as well as the overall condition of the patient; therefore it should be determined by the clinical and bacteriological response of the patient. In severe staphylococcal infections, therapy with penicillinase-resistant penicillins should be continued for at least 14 days. Therapy should be continued for at least 48 hours after the patient has become afebrile, asymptomatic, and cultures are negative. The treatment of endocarditis and osteomyelitis may require a longer term of therapy.
Concurrent administration of the penicillinase-resistant penicillins and probenecid increases and prolongs serum penicillin levels. Probenecid decreases the apparent volume of distribution and slows the rate of excretion by competitively inhibiting renal tubular secretion of penicillin. Penicillin-probenecid therapy is generally limited to those infections where very high serum levels of penicillin are necessary.
Oral preparations of the penicillinase-resistant penicillins should not be used as initial therapy in serious, life-threatening infections (See **PRECAUTIONS**—General). Oral therapy with the penicillinase-resistant penicillins may be used to follow up the previous use of a parenteral agent as soon as the clinical condition warrants. For intramuscular gluteal injections, care should be taken to avoid sciatic nerve injury. With intravenous administration, particularly in elderly patients, care should be taken because of the possibility of thrombophlebitis.
[See table below].

RECOMMENDED DOSAGES FOR STAPHCILLIN (methicillin sodium)

Drug	Adults	Infants and Children < 40 kg (88 lbs)
Methicillin Sodium	1 gram IM every 4 or 6 hours IV every 6 hours	25 mg/kg IM every 6 hours IV not recommended

STABILITY PERIODS
STAPHCILLIN

Concentration Mg/Ml	Sterile H_2O for Injection	Isotonic Sodium Chloride	M/6 Molar Sodium Lactate Solution	5% Dextrose in H_2O	5% Dextrose in 0.45% NaCl	10% Invert Sugar	Lactated Ringers Solution
ROOM TEMPERATURE (25°C)							
10–200	24 Hrs	24 Hrs					
2–20			8 Hrs	8 Hrs		8 Hrs	8 Hrs
10–30					24 hrs		
REFRIGERATION (4°C)							
10–200	7 Days	7 Days					
10–30			7 Days	7 Days	7 Days	7 Days	7 Days
FROZEN (−15°C)							
19–500	30 Days						
20–100		30 Days	30 Days	30 Days	30 Days	30 Days	30 Days

DIRECTIONS FOR USE

For Intramuscular Use: Use Sterile Water for Injection, USP or Sodium Chloride Injection, USP. Add 1.5 ml to the 1 gram vial, 5.7 ml to the 4 gram vial, and 8.6 ml to the 6 gram vial and withdraw the entire contents. Each 1 ml will contain approximately 500 mg of Staphcillin. The solutions are stable for 24 hours at room temperature or 4 days under refrigeration.
For Direct Intravenous Use: Further dilute each 1 ml of solution, reconstituted as above, with 25 ml of Sodium Chloride Injection, USP and inject at the rate of 10 ml per minute.
For Administration by Intravenous Drip: Reconstitute as directed above (For Intramuscular Use) prior to diluting with Intravenous Solution.
[See table above].
Stability studies on Staphcillin at concentrations of 2 mg/ml, 10 mg/ml and 20 mg/ml in various intravenous solutions listed below indicate the drug will lose less than 10% activity at room temperature (70°F) during an 8-hour period.
I.V. Solution:
5% Dextrose in Normal Saline
10% D-Fructose in Water
10% D-Fructose in Normal Saline
Lactated Potassic Saline Injection
5% Plasma Hydrolysate in Water
*10% Invert Sugar in Normal Saline
10% Invert Sugar Plus 0.3% Potassium Chloride in Water
Travert 10% Electrolyte #1
Travert 10% Electrolyte #2
Travert 10% Electrolyte #3
Only those solutions listed above should be used for the intravenous infusion of Staphcillin. The concentration of the antibiotic should fall within the range specified. The drug concentration and the rate and volume of the infusion should be adjusted so that the total dose of methicillin is administered before the drug loses its stability in the solution in use. If another agent is used in conjunction with methicillin therapy, **it should not be physically mixed** with methicillin but should be administered separately.
*At a concentration of 2 mg/ml, Staphcillin is stable for only 4 hours in this solution. Concentrations between 10 mg/ml and 30 mg/ml are stable for 8 hours.
"Piggyback" I.V. Package: This glass vial contains the labeled quantity of Staphcillin and is intended for intravenous administration. The diluent and volume are specified on the label of each package.
Discard solution after 24 hours at room temperature.
Hospital Bulk Package: This glass vial contains 10 grams Staphcillin and is designed for use in the pharmacy in preparing I.V. additives. Add 94 ml Sterile Water for Injection, USP or Sodium Chloride Injection, USP. The resulting solution will contain 100 mg methicillin sodium per ml, which is equivalent to 90 mg per ml methicillin activity.
Following reconstitution in this manner, the resulting solutions are stable for 24 hours at room temperature or 7 days under refrigeration.
CAUTION: NOT TO BE DISPENSED AS A UNIT.

SUPPLY

STAPHCILLIN (methicillin sodium for injection) buffered.
NDC 0015-7961-20—1 gram vial
NDC 0015-7964-20—4 gram vial
NDC 0015-7965-20—6 gram vial

NDC 0015-7961-28—1 gram "piggyback" vial
NDC 0015-7964-28—4 gram "piggyback" vial
NDC 0015-7102-28—10 gram Hospital Bulk Package
For information on package sizes available, refer to the current price schedule.

TEGOPEN® ℞

[*tĕg'ō-pĕn*]
Cloxacillin Sodium
CLOXACILLIN SODIUM CAPSULES
250 mg and 500 mg
CLOXACILLIN SODIUM FOR ORAL SOLUTION
125 mg/5 ml

This is the full text of the latest Official Package Circular dated February 1985 [7935 DIR-11].

DESCRIPTION

Tegopen (cloxacillin sodium) is an antibacterial agent of the isoxazolyl penicillin series. It is a penicillinase-resistant, acid resistant semisynthetic penicillin suitable for oral administration. Tegopen is available as an oral solution and capsules.
Inactive ingredient in Tegopen capsules is: magnesium stearate.
Inactive ingredients in Tegopen oral solution are: FD & C Red No. 3, natural & artificial flavorings, sodium benzoate, sodium chloride, sodium citrate, sodium saccharin and sucrose.

CLOXACILLIN SODIUM

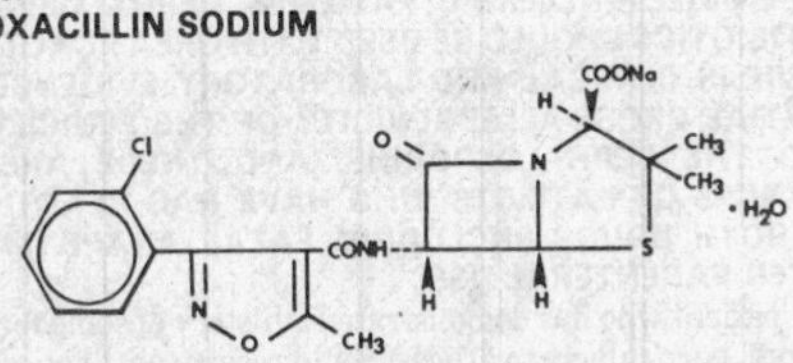

$C_{19}H_{17}ClN_3NaO_5S.H_2O$ 475.88 [CAS 7081 44 9]4-Thia-1-azabicyclo[3.2.0]heptane-2-carboxylic acid, 6 [[[3 (2-chlorophenyl)-5-methyl-4-isoxazolyl] carbonyl] amino] 3,3-dimethyl-7-oxo-, monosodium salt, monohydrate, [2 *S* ($2\alpha 5\alpha$, 6β)]-.

CLINICAL PHARMACOLOGY

Microbiology: Penicillinase-resistant penicillins exert a bactericidal action against penicillin-susceptible microorganisms during the state of active multiplication. All penicillins inhibit the biosynthesis of the bacterial cell wall.
The drugs in this class are highly resistant to inactivation by staphylococcal penicillinase and are active against penicillinase producing and non-penicillinase producing strains of **Staphylococcus aureus.** The penicillinase-resistant penicillins are active **in vitro** against a variety of other bacteria.
Susceptibility Plate Testing: Quantitative methods of susceptibility testing that require measurement of zone diameters or minimal inhibitory concentrations (MIC's) give the most precise estimates of antibiotic susceptibility. One such procedure has been recommended for use with discs to test susceptibility to this class of drugs.
Interpretations correlate diameters on the disc test with MIC values. A penicillinase-resistant class disc may be used to determine microbial susceptibility to cloxacillin, dicloxacillin, methicillin, nafcillin, and oxacillin. With this procedure, employing a 5 microgram methicillin sodium disc, a report from the laboratory of "susceptible" (zone of at least 14 mm) indicates that the infecting organism is likely to respond to therapy. A report of "resistant" (zone of less than 10 mm) indicates that the infecting organism is not likely to respond to therapy. A report of "intermediate susceptibility" (zone of 10 to 13 mm) suggests that the organism might be susceptible if high doses of the antibiotic are used, or if the infection is confined to tissues and fluids (e.g., urine), in which high antibiotic levels are attained.
In general, all staphylococci should be tested against the penicillin G disc and against the methicillin disc. Routine methods of antibiotic susceptibility testing may fail to detect strains of organisms resistant to the penicillinase-resistant penicillins. For this reason, the use of large inocula and 48-hour incubation periods may be necessary to obtain accurate susceptibility studies with these antibiotics. Bacterial strains which are resistant to one of the penicillinase-resistant penicillins should be considered resistant to all of the drugs in the class.
Pharmacokinetics: Tegopen (cloxacillin sodium) is resistant to destruction by acid. Absorption of Tegopen after oral administration is rapid but incomplete. Studies with an oral dose of 1 gram gave average serum levels at 60 minutes of 14.4 mcg/ml. At four hours, average levels were 2 mcg/ml. In one study, single oral doses of Tegopen 500 mg produced peak serum concentrations of 7.5 to 14.4 mcg/ml at 1 to 1.5 hours.
Once absorbed, Tegopen (cloxacillin sodium) binds to serum protein, mainly albumin. The degree of protein binding reported varies with the method of study and the investigator, but generally has been found to be $95.2 \pm 0.5\%$. Oral absorption of cloxacillin is delayed when the drug is administered after meals.
Tegopen, with normal doses, has insignificant concentrations in the cerebrospinal and ascitic fluids. It is found in therapeutic concentrations in the pleural, bile and amniotic fluids. Tegopen is rapidly excreted as unchanged drug in the urine by glomerular filtration and active tubular secretion.

INDICATIONS AND USAGE

The penicillinase-resistant penicillins are indicated in the treatment of infections caused by penicillinase-producing staphylococci which have demonstrated susceptibility to the drugs. Cultures and susceptibility tests should be performed initially to determine the causative organisms and their sensitivity to the drug (See **Clinical Pharmacology—Susceptibility Plate Testing**).
The penicillinase-resistant penicillins may be used to initiate therapy in suspected cases of resistant staphylococcal infections prior to the availability of laboratory test results. The penicillinase-resistant penicillins should not be used in infections caused by organisms susceptible to penicillin G. If the susceptibility tests indicate that the infection is due to an organism other than a resistant staphylococcus, therapy should not be continued with a penicillinase-resistant penicillin.

CONTRAINDICATIONS

A history of a hypersensitivity (anaphylactic) reaction to any penicillin is a contraindication.

WARNINGS

Serious and occasionally fatal hypersensitivity (anaphylactic shock with collapse) reactions have occurred in patients receiving penicillin. The incidence of anaphylactic shock in all penicillin-treated patients is between 0.015 and 0.04 percent. Anaphylactic shock resulting in death has occured in approximately 0.002 percent of the patients treated. Although anaphylaxis is more frequent following a parenteral administration, it has occurred in patients receiving oral penicillins.
When penicillin therapy is indicated, it should be initiated only after a comprehensive patient drug and allergy history has been obtained. If an allergic reaction occurs, the drug should be discontinued and the patient should receive supportive treatment, e.g., artificial maintenance of ventilation, pressor amines, antihistamines, and corticosteroids. Individuals with a history of penicillin hypersensitivity may also experience allergic reactions when treated with a cephalosporin.

PRECAUTIONS

General: Penicillinase-resistant penicillins should generally not be administered to patients with a history of sensitivity to any penicillin.
Penicillin should be used with caution in individuals with histories of significant allergies and/or asthma. Whenever allergic reactions occur, penicillin should be withdrawn unless, in the opinion of the physician, the condition being treated is life-threatening and amenable only to penicillin therapy.
The oral route of administration should not be relied upon in patients with severe illness, or with nausea, vomiting, gastric dilation, cardiospasm, or intestinal hypermotility. Occasionally patients will not absorb therapeutic amounts of orally administered penicillin.
The use of antibiotics may result in overgrowth of nonsusceptible organisms. If new infections due to bacteria or fungi occur, the drug should be discontinued and appropriate measures taken.
Information for the Patient: Patients receiving penicillins should be given the following information and instructions by the physician:
1. Patients should be told that penicillin is an antibacterial agent which will work with the body's natural defenses to control certain types of infections. They should be told that the drug should not be taken if they have had an allergic reaction to any form of penicillin previously, and to inform the physician of any allergies or previous allergic reactions to any drugs they may have had (see **Warnings**).
2. Patients who have previously experienced an anaphylactic reaction to penicillin should be instructed to wear a medical identification tag or bracelet.
3. Because most antibacterial drugs taken by mouth are best absorbed on an empty stomach, patients should be directed, unless circumstances warrant otherwise, to take penicillin one hour before meals or two hours after eating (See **Clinical Pharmacology—Pharmacokinetics**).
4. Patients should be told to take the entire course of therapy prescribed, even if fever and other symptoms have stopped (See **Precautions—General**).
5. If any of the following reactions occur, stop taking your prescription and notify the physician: shortness of breath, wheezing, skin rash, mouth irritation, black tongue, sore throat, nausea, vomiting, diarrhea, fever, swollen joints, or any unusual bleeding or bruising (See **Adverse Reactions**).
6. Do not take any additional medications without physician approval, including non-prescription drugs such as antacids, laxatives or vitamins.
7. Discard any liquid forms of penicillin after 7 days if stored at room temperature or after 14 days if refrigerated.
Laboratory Tests: Bacteriologic studies to determine the causative organisms and their susceptibility to the penicillinase-resistant penicillins should be performed (See **Clinical Pharmacology—Microbiology**). In the treatment of suspected staphylococcal infections, therapy should be changed to another active agent if culture tests fail to demonstrate the presence of staphylococci.
Periodic assessment of organ system function including renal, hepatic, and hematopoietic should be made during prolonged therapy with the penicillinase-resistant penicillins.
Blood cultures, white blood cell, and differential cell counts should be obtained prior to initiation of therapy and at least weekly during therapy with penicillinase-resistant penicillins.
Periodic urinalysis, blood urea nitrogen, and creatinine determinations should be performed during therapy with the penicillinase-resistant penicillins and dosage alterations should be considered if these values become elevated. If any impairment of renal function is suspected or known to exist, a reduction in the total dosage should be considered and blood levels monitored to avoid possible neurotoxic reactions (See **Dosage and Administration**).
SGOT and SGPT values should be obtained periodically during therapy to monitor for possible liver function abnormalities.
Drug Interactions: Tetracycline, a bacteriostatic antibiotic, may antagonize the bactericidal effect of penicillin and concurrent use of these drugs should be avoided.
Carcinogenesis, Mutagenesis, Impairment of Fertility: No long-term animal studies have been conducted with these drugs.
Studies on reproduction (Nafcillin) in rats and rabbits reveal no fetal or maternal abnormalities before conception and continuously through weaning (one generation).
Pregnancy Category B: Reproduction studies performed in the mouse, rat, and rabbit have revealed no evidence of impaired fertility or harm to the fetus due to the penicillinase-resistant penicillins. Human experience with the penicillins during pregnancy has not shown any positive evidence of adverse effects on the fetus. There are, however, no adequate or well-controlled studies in pregnant women showing conclusively that harmful effects of these drugs on the fetus can be excluded. Because animal reproduction studies are not always predictive of human response, this drug should be used during pregnancy only if clearly needed.
Nursing Mothers: Penicillins are excreted in breast milk. Caution should be exercised when penicillins are administered to a nursing woman.
Pediatric Use: Because of incompletely developed renal function in newborns penicillinase-resistant penicillins (especially methicillin) may not be completely excreted, with abnormally high blood levels resulting. Frequent blood levels are advisable in this group with dosage adjustments when necessary. All newborns treated with penicillins should be monitored closely for clinical and laboratory evidence of toxic or adverse effects (See **Dosage and Administration**).

ADVERSE REACTIONS

Body as a Whole: The reported incidence of allergic reactions to penicillin ranges from 0.7 to 10 percent (See **Warnings**). Sensitization is usually the result of treatment but some individuals have had immediate reactions to penicillin when first treated. In such cases, it is thought that the patients may have had prior exposure to the drug via trace amounts present in milk and vaccines.
Two types of allergic reactions to penicillin are noted clinically, immediate and delayed.
Immediate reactions usually occur within 20 minutes of administration and range in severity from urticaria and pruritus to angioneurotic edema, laryngospasm, bronchospasm, hypotension, vascular collapse, and death. Such immediate anaphylactic reactions are very rare (See **Warnings**) and usually occur after parenteral therapy but have occurred in patients receiving oral therapy. Another type of immediate reaction, an accelerated reaction, may occur between 20 minutes and 48 hours after administration and may include urticaria, pruritus, and fever. Although laryngeal edema, laryngospasm, and hypotension occasionally occur, fatality is uncommon.
Delayed allergic reactions to penicillin therapy usually occur after 48 hours and sometimes as late as 2 to 4 weeks after initiation of therapy. Manifestations of this type of reaction include serum sickness-like symptoms (i.e., fever, malaise, urticaria, myalgia, arthralgia, abdominal pain) and various skin rashes. Nausea, vomiting, diarrhea, stomatitis, black or

Continued on next page

Bristol—Cont.

hairy tongue, and other symptoms of gastrointestinal irritation may occur, especially during oral penicillin therapy.

Nervous System Reactions: Neurotoxic reactions similar to those observed with penicillin G may occur with large intravenous doses of the penicillinase-resistant penicillins especially in patients with renal insufficiency.

Urogenital Reactions: Renal tubular damage and interstitial nephritis have been associated with the administration of methicillin sodium and infrequently with the administration of nafcillin and oxacillin. Manifestations of this reaction may include rash, fever, eosinophilia, hematuria, proteinuria, and renal insufficiency. Methicillin-induced nephropathy does not appear to be dose-related and is generally reversible upon prompt discontinuation of therapy.

Metabolic Reactions: Agranulocytosis, neutropenia, and bone marrow depression have been associated with the use of methicillin sodium, nafcillin, oxacillin, and cloxacillin. Hepatotoxicity, characterized by fever, nausea, and vomiting associated with abnormal liver function tests, mainly elevated SGOT levels, has been associated with the use of oxacillin and cloxacillin.

DOSAGE AND ADMINISTRATION

The penicillinase-resistant penicillins are available for oral administration and for intramuscular and intravenous injection. The sodium salts of methicillin, oxacillin, and nafcillin may be administered parenterally and the sodium salts of cloxacillin, dicloxacillin, oxacillin, and nafcillin are available for oral use.

Bacteriologic studies to determine the causative organisms and their sensitivity to the penicillinase resistant penicillins should always be performed. Duration of therapy varies with the type and severity of infection as well as the overall condition of the patient, therefore it should be determined by the clinical and bacteriological response of the patient. In severe staphylococcal infections, therapy with penicillinase-resistant penicillins should be continued for at least 14 days. Therapy should be continued for at least 48 hours after the patient has become afebrile, asymptomatic, and cultures are negative. The treatment of endocarditis and osteomyelitis may require a longer term of therapy.

Concurrent administration of the penicillinase-resistant penicillins and probenecid increases and prolongs serum penicillin levels. Probenecid decreases the apparent volume of distribution and slows the rate of excretion by competitively inhibiting renal tubular secretion of penicillin. Penicillin-probenecid therapy is generally limited to those infections where very high serum levels of penicillin are necessary.

Oral preparations of the penicillinase-resistant penicillins should not be used as initial therapy in serious, life-threatening infections (see **Precautions—General**). Oral therapy with the penicillinase-resistant penicillins may be used to follow up the previous use of a parenteral agent as soon as the clinical condition warrants. For intramuscular gluteal injections, care should be taken to avoid sciatic nerve injury. With intravenous administration, particularly in elderly patients, care should be taken because of the possibility of thrombophlebitis.

[See table below].

Directions For Dispensing Oral Solution: Prepare solution at the time of dispensing. For ease in preparation, add the water in two portions, shaking well after each addition. Add the total amount of water as directed on the labeling of the package being dispensed. Refrigerated, the solution is stable for 14 days.

HOW SUPPLIED

Tegopen (cloxacillin sodium) for Oral Solution, 125 mg per 5 ml.

NDC 0015-7941—125 mg per 5 ml

Tegopen (cloxacillin sodium) Capsules. Each capsule contains cloxacillin sodium equivalent to 250 or 500 mg cloxacillin.

NDC 0015-7935—250 mg
NDC 0015-7496—500 mg

For information on package sizes available, refer to the current price schedule.

Shown in Product Identification Section, page 406

ULTRACEF® ℞

[ul-trah-sef]
cefadroxil
CAPSULES, TABLETS AND ORAL SUSPENSION

This is the full text of the latest Official Package Circular dated February, 1985 [7271DIR-11].

DESCRIPTION

ULTRACEF (cefadroxil) is a semisynthetic cephalosporin antibiotic intended for oral administration. It is a white to yellowish-white crystalline powder. It is soluble in water and it is acid-stable. It is chemically designated as 7- [[D-2-amino-2-(4-hydroxyphenyl) acetyl]amino]-3- methyl-8-oxo-5-thia-1-azabicyclo [4.2.0]oct-2-ene-2- carboxylic acid monohydrate. Inactive ingredient in Ultracef capsules is: magnesium stearate.

Inactive ingredients in Ultracef tablets are: cellulose microcrystalline and magnesium stearate.

Inactive ingredients in Ultracef for oral suspension are: Avicel, FD& C Red No. 40, natural & artificial flavorings, Polysorbate 80, sodium benzoate, sucrose and tragacanth.

It has the following structural formula.

HO — C₆H₄ — CHCNH (C=O, NH₂) … S … N … CH₃ … CO_2H · H_2O

CLINICAL PHARMACOLOGY

ULTRACEF (cefadroxil) is rapidly absorbed after oral administration. Following single doses of 500 and 1000 mg, average peak serum concentrations were approximately 16 and 28 mcg/ml, respectively. Measurable levels were present 12 hours after administration. Over 90 percent of the drug is excreted unchanged in the urine within 24 hours. Peak urine concentrations are approximately 1800 mcg/ml during the period following a single 500-mg oral dose. Increases in dosage generally produce a proportionate increase in ULTRACEF urinary concentration. The urine antibiotic concentration, following a 1-gram dose, was maintained well above the MIC of susceptible urinary pathogens for 20 to 22 hours.

MICROBIOLOGY

In vitro tests demonstrate that the cephalosporins are bactericidal because of their inhibition of cell-wall synthesis. ULTRACEF is active against the following organisms **in vitro:**

- Beta-hemolytic streptococci
- Staphylococci, including coagulase-positive, coagulase-negative, and penicillinase-producing strains
- **Streptococcus (Diplococcus) pneumoniae**
- **Escherichia coli**
- **Proteus mirabilis**
- **Klebsiella** species

Note: Most strains of Enterococci (**Streptococcus faecalis** and **S. faecium**) are resistant to ULTRACEF. It is not active against most strains of **Enterobacter** species. **P. Morganii,** and **P. vulgaris.** It has no activity against **Pseudomonas** species and **Acinetobacter calcoaceticus** (formerly **Mima** and **Herellea** species).

Disc Susceptibility Tests—Quantitative methods that require measurement of zone diameters give the most precise estimates of antibiotic susceptibility. One recommended procedure (CFR Section 460.1) uses a cephalosporin-class disc for testing susceptibility; interpretations correlate zone diameters of this disc test with MIC values for ULTRACEF. With this procedure, a report from the laboratory of "resistant" indicates that the infecting organism is not likely to respond to therapy. A report of "intermediate susceptibility" suggests that the organism would be susceptible if the infection is confined to the urinary tract, as ULTRACEF produces high antibiotic levels in the urine.

INDICATIONS

ULTRACEF (cefadroxil) is indicated for the treatment of the following infections when caused by susceptible strains of the designated microorganisms:

Urinary tract infections caused by **E. coli, P. mirabilis,** and **Klebsiella** species.

Skin and skin structure infections caused by staphylococci and/or streptococci.

Pharyngitis and tonsillitis caused by Group A beta-hemolytic streptococci. (Penicillin is the usual drug of choice in the treatment and prevention of streptococcal infections, including the prophylaxis of rheumatic fever. ULTRACEF is generally effective in the eradication of streptococci from the nasopharynx; however substantial data establishing the efficacy of ULTRACEF in the subsequent prevention of rheumatic fever are not available at present.)

Note: Culture and susceptibility tests should be initiated prior to and during therapy. Renal function studies should be performed when indicated.

CONTRAINDICATIONS

ULTRACEF (cefadroxil) is contraindicated in patients with known allergy to the cephalosporin group of antibiotics.

WARNING

IN PENICILLIN-ALLERGIC PATIENTS, CEPHALOSPORIN ANTIBIOTICS SHOULD BE USED WITH GREAT CAUTION. THERE IS CLINICAL AND LABORATORY EVIDENCE OF PARTIAL CROSS-ALLERGENICITY OF THE PENICILLINS AND THE CEPHALOSPORINS, AND THERE ARE INSTANCES OF PATIENTS WHO HAVE HAD REACTIONS TO BOTH DRUGS (INCLUDING FATAL ANAPHYLAXIS AFTER PARENTERAL USE).

Any patient who has demonstrated a history of some form of allergy, particularly to drugs, should receive antibiotics cautiously and then only when absolutely necessary. No exception should be made with regard to ULTRACEF (cefadroxil).

Pseudomembranous colitis has been reported with the use of cephalosporins (and other broad spectrum antibiotics); therefore, it is important to consider its diagnosis in patients who develop diarrhea in association with antibiotic use.

Treatment with broad spectrum antibiotics alters normal flora of the colon and may permit overgrowth of clostridia. Studies indicate a toxin produced by **Clostridium difficile** is one primary cause of antibiotic-associated colitis. Cholestyramine and colestipol resins have been shown to bind the toxin **in vitro.**

Mild cases of colitis may respond to drug discontinuance alone.

Moderate to severe cases should be managed with fluid, electrolyte and protein supplementation as indicated.

When the colitis is not relieved by drug discontinuance or when it is severe, oral vancomycin is the treatment of choice for antibiotic-associated pseudomembranous colitis produced by **C. difficile.** Other causes of colitis should also be considered.

PRECAUTIONS

Patients should be followed carefully so that any side effects or unusual manifestations of drug idiosyncrasy may be detected. If a hypersensitivity reaction occurs, the drug should be discontinued and the patient treated with the usual agents (e.g., epinephrine or other pressor amines, antihistamines, or corticosteroids).

ULTRACEF (cefadroxil) should be used with caution in the presence of markedly impaired renal function (creatinine clearance rate of less than 50 ml/min/1.73M²). (See DOSAGE AND ADMINISTRATION.) In patients with known or suspected renal impairment, careful clinical observation and appropriate laboratory studies should be made prior to and during therapy.

Prolonged use of ULTRACEF may result in the overgrowth of nonsusceptible organisms. Careful observation of the patient is essential. If superinfection occurs during therapy, appropriate measures should be taken.

Positive direct Coombs' tests have been reported during treatment with the cephalosporin antibiotics. In hematologic studies or in transfusion cross-matching procedures when antiglobulin tests are performed on the minor side or in Coombs' testing of newborns whose mothers have received cephalosporin antibiotics before parturition, it should be recognized that a positive Coombs' test may be due to the drug.

ULTRACEF should be prescribed with caution in individuals with a history of gastrointestinal disease, particularly colitis.

USAGE IN PREGNANCY

Pregnancy Category B: Reproduction studies have been performed in mice and rats at doses up to 11 times the human dose and have revealed no evidence of impaired fertility or harm to the fetus due to cefadroxil. There are, however, no adequate and well controlled studies in pregnant women.

RECOMMENDED DOSAGES FOR TEGOPEN (cloxacillin sodium) IN MILD TO MODERATE AND SEVERE INFECTIONS

DRUG	ADULTS		CHILDREN	
	Mild to Moderate	Severe	Mild to Moderate	Severe
Cloxacillin	250 mg every 6 hours	500 mg or higher every 6 hours	50 mg/kg/day[a] in equally divided doses every 6 hours	100 mg/kg/day[a] or higher in equally divided doses every 6 hours

[a]Patients weighing less than 20 Kg (44 lbs)

Because animal reproduction studies are not always predictive of human response, this drug should be used during pregnancy only if clearly needed.
Nursing Mothers: Caution should be exercised when cefadroxil is administered to a nursing mother.

ADVERSE REACTIONS

Gastrointestinal — Symptoms of pseudomembranous colitis can appear during antibiotic treatment. Nausea and vomiting have been reported rarely. Administration with food decreases nausea and does not decrease absorption. Diarrhea and dysuria have also occurred.
Hypersensitivity — Allergies (in the form of rash, urticaria, and angioedema) have been observed. These reactions usually subsided upon discontinuation of the drug.
Other reactions have included genital pruritus, genital moniliasis, vaginitis, and moderate transient neutropenia.

DOSAGE AND ADMINISTRATION

ULTRACEF (cefadroxil) is acid stable and may be administered orally without regard to meals. Administration with food may be helpful in diminishing potential gastrointestinal complaints occasionally associated with oral cephalosporin therapy.

Adults

Urinary Tract Infections — for uncomplicated lower urinary tract infections (i.e. cystitis) the usual dosage is 1 or 2 grams per day in single (q.d.) or divided doses (b.i.d.).
For all other urinary tract infections the usual dosage is 2 grams per day in divided doses (b.i.d.).
Skin and Skin Structure Infections — For skin and skin structure infections the usual dosage is 1 gram per day in single (q.d.) or divided doses (b.i.d.).
Pharyngitis and Tonsillitis — Treatment of Group A beta-hemolytic streptococcal pharyngitis and tonsillitis — 1 gram per day in divided doses (b.i.d.) for 10 days.
Children — The recommended daily dosage for children is 30 mg/kg/day in divided doses every 12 hours as indicated:

Child's Weight		Ultracef Oral Suspension	
lbs	Kg	125 mg/5 ml	250 mg/5 ml
10	4.5	½ tsp. b.i.d.	
20	9.1	1 tsp. b.i.d.	½ tsp. b.i.d.
30	13.6	1 ½ tsp. b.i.d.	¾ tsp. b.i.d.
40	18.2	2 tsp. b.i.d.	1 tsp. b.i.d.
50	22.7	2 ½ tsp. b.i.d.	1 ¼ tsp. b.i.d.

In the treatment of beta-hemolytic, streptococcal infections, a therapeutic dosage of Ultracef should be administered for at least ten days.
In patients with renal impairment, the dosage of cefadroxil should be adjusted according to creatinine clearance rates to prevent drug accumulation. The following schedule is suggested. In adults, the initial dose is 1000 mg of ULTRACEF (cefadroxil) and the maintenance dose (based on the creatinine clearance rate [ml/min/1.73M^2]) is 500 mg at the time intervals listed below.

Creatinine Clearances	Dosage Interval
0-10 ml/min	36 hours
10-25 ml/min	24 hours
25-50 ml/min	12 hours

Patients with creatinine clearance rates over 50 ml/min may be treated as if they were patients having normal renal function.

HOW SUPPLIED

ULTRACEF (cefadroxil) tablets. Each tablet contains cefadroxil monohydrate equivalent to 1 gram cefadroxil.
NDC 0015-7286—1 gram—Bottles of 24's
ULTRACEF (cefadroxil) capsules. Each capsule contains cefadroxil monohydrate equivalent to 500 mg cefadroxil.
NDC 0015-7271—500 mg—Bottles of 50's and 100's
ULTRACEF (cefadroxil) for oral suspension. Each 5 ml of reconstituted suspension contains cefadroxil monohydrate equivalent to 125 mg or 250 mg cefadroxil.
NDC 0015-7283—125 mg—available in 50 and 100 ml
NDC 0015-7284—250 mg—available in 50 and 100ml
Directions for mixing are included on the label. Shake well before using. Keep container tightly closed.
Store reconstituted suspension in refrigerator, discard unused portion after 14 days.
For information on package sizes available, refer to the current price schedule.

Shown in Product Identification Section, page 406

Bristol-Myers Oncology Division

(Bristol-Myers Company)
2404 W. PENNSYLVANIA STREET
EVANSVILLE, IN 47721

BiCNU® ℞

[*bĭk'nū*]
(carmustine [BCNU])

This is the full text of the latest Official Package Circular dated December 1985 [3012 DIM-09].

WARNING

BiCNU should be administered preferably by individuals experienced in antineoplastic therapy. Since delayed bone marrow toxicity is the major toxicity, complete blood counts should be monitored frequently for at least 6 weeks after a dose. Repeat doses of BiCNU should not be given more frequently than every 6 weeks. The bone marrow toxicity of BiCNU is cumulative, and therefore dosage adjustment must be considered on the basis of nadir blood counts from prior dose (see dosage adjustment table under **Dosage**).
It is recommended that liver function, pulmonary function, and renal function tests also be monitored.

DESCRIPTION

BiCNU (1,3-bis (2-chloroethyl)-1-nitrosourea) is one of the nitrosoureas. It is a white lyophilized powder with a molecular weight of 214.06. It is highly soluble in alcohol and poorly soluble in water. It is also highly soluble in lipids.
The structural formula is:

$$Cl-CH_2-CH_2-\underset{NO}{N}-\overset{O}{\overset{\|}{C}}-NHCH_2-CH_2-Cl$$

ACTION

BiCNU alkylates DNA and RNA and has also been shown to inhibit several enzymes by carbamoylation of amino acids in proteins.
Intravenously administered BiCNU is rapidly degraded, with no intact drug detectable after 15 minutes. However, in studies with C^{14} labeled drug, prolonged levels of the isotope were observed in the plasma and tissue, probably representing radioactive fragments of the parent compound.
It is thought that the antineoplastic and toxic activities of BiCNU may be due to metabolites. Approximately 60 to 70% of a total dose is excreted in the urine in 96 hours and about 10% as respiratory CO_2. The fate of the remainder is undetermined.
Because of the high lipid solubility and the relative lack of ionization at a physiological pH, BiCNU crosses the blood brain barrier quite effectively. Levels of radioactivity in the CSF are 50% or greater than those measured concurrently in plasma.

INDICATIONS

BiCNU is indicated as palliative therapy as a single agent or in established combination therapy with other approved chemotherapeutic agents in the following:

1. **Brain tumors**—glioblastoma, brainstem glioma, medulloblastoma, astrocytoma, ependymoma, and metastatic brain tumors.
2. **Multiple myeloma**—in combination with prednisone.
3. **Hodgkin's Disease**—as secondary therapy in combination with other approved drugs in patients who relapse while being treated with primary therapy, or who fail to respond to primary therapy.
4. **Non-Hodgkin's lymphomas**—as secondary therapy in combination with other approved drugs for patients who relapse while being treated with primary therapy, or who fail to respond to primary therapy.

CONTRAINDICATIONS

BiCNU should not be given to individuals who have demonstrated a previous hypersensitivity to it.
BiCNU should not be given to individuals with decreased circulating platelets, leukocytes, or erythrocytes either from previous chemotherapy or other causes.

WARNINGS

Safe use in pregnancy has not been established. BiCNU is embryotoxic and teratogenic in rats and embryotoxic in rabbits at dose levels equivalent to the human dose. BiCNU also affects fertility in male rats at doses somewhat higher than the human dose.
BiCNU is carcinogenic in rats and mice, producing a marked increase in tumor incidence in doses approximating those employed clinically.
Nitrosourea therapy does have carcinogenic potential. The occurrence of acute leukemia and bone marrow dysplasias have been reported in patients following nitrosourea therapy.

PRECAUTIONS

BiCNU should be administered preferably by individuals experienced in antineoplastic therapy. Since delayed bone marrow toxicity is the major toxicity, complete blood counts should be monitored frequently for at least 6 weeks after a dose. Repeat doses of BiCNU should not be given more frequently than every 6 weeks. The bone marrow toxicity of BiCNU is cumulative, and therefore dosage adjustment must be considered on the basis of nadir blood counts from prior dose (see Dosage Adjustment Table under DOSAGE).
It is recommended that liver function tests also be monitored.
Safe Use in Pregnancy has not been established. Therefore, the benefit to risk of toxicity must be carefully weighed.
See "Warnings" section for information on carcinogenesis.

ADVERSE REACTIONS

Hematopoietic—The most frequent and most serious toxicity of BiCNU is delayed myelosuppression. It usually occurs 4 to 6 weeks after drug administration and is dose-related. Platelet nadirs occur at 4 to 5 weeks; leukocyte nadirs occur at 5 to 6 weeks post therapy. Thrombocytopenia is generally more severe than leukopenia. However both may be dose limiting toxicities. Anemia also occurs, but is generally less severe.
Gastrointestinal—Nausea and vomiting after IV administration of BiCNU are noted frequently. This toxicity appears within 2 hours of dosing, usually lasting 4 to 6 hours, and is dose-related. Prior administration of antiemetics is effective in diminishing and sometimes preventing this side effect.
Hepatic—When high doses of BiCNU have been employed, a reversible type of hepatic toxicity, manifested by increased transaminase, alkaline phosphatase and bilirubin levels, has been reported in a small percentage of patients.
Pulmonary—Pulmonary toxicity characterized by pulmonary infiltrate and/or fibrosis have been reported in some patients receiving prolonged therapy with BiCNU.
Renal—Renal abnormalities consisting of decrease in kidney size, progressive azotemia and renal failure have been reported in patients who received large cumulative doses after prolonged therapy with BiCNU and related nitrosoureas. Kidney damage has also been reported occasionally in patients receiving lower total doses.
Local—Burning at the site of injection is common but true thrombosis is rare.
Other—Rapid IV infusion of BiCNU may produce intensive flushing of the skin and suffusion of the conjunctiva within 2 hours, lasting about 4 hours.
Accidental contact of reconstituted BiCNU with the skin has caused burning and hyperpigmentation of the affected areas.

DOSAGE

The recommended dose of BiCNU as single agent in previously untreated patients is 200 mg/m^2 intravenously every 6 weeks. This may be given as a single dose or divided into daily injections such as 100 mg/m^2 on 2 successive days. When BiCNU is used in combination with other myelosuppressive drugs or in patients in whom bone marrow reserve is depleted, the doses should be adjusted accordingly.
A repeat course of BiCNU should not be given until circulating blood elements have returned to acceptable levels (platelets above 100,000/mm^3; leukocytes above 4,000/mm^3), and this is usually in 6 weeks. Blood counts should be monitored frequently and repeat courses should not be given before 6 weeks because of delayed toxicity.
Doses subsequent to the initial dose should be adjusted according to the hematologic response of the patient to the preceding dose. The following schedule is suggested as a guide to dosage adjustment:

Nadir After Prior Dose		Percentage of Prior Dose to be Given
Leukocytes	Platelets	
>4000 -	>100,000 -	100%
3000-3999	75,000-99,999	100%
2000-2999	25,000-74,999	70%
<2000 -	< 25,000 -	50%

PREPARATION OF INTRAVENOUS SOLUTIONS

Dissolve BiCNU with 3 ml. of the supplied sterile diluent and then aseptically add 27 ml. of Sterile Water for Injection, U.S.P., to the alcohol solution. Each ml of the resulting solution will contain 3.3 mg of BiCNU in 10% ethanol having a pH of 5.6 to 6.0. Accidental contact of reconstituted BiCNU with the skin has caused transient hyperpigmentation of the affected areas.
Reconstitution as recommended results in a clear, colorless solution which may be further diluted with Sodium Chloride for Injection, U.S.P., or 5% Dextrose for Injection, U.S.P.
The reconstituted solution should be used intravenously only and should be administered by IV drip over a 1 to 2 hour period. Injection of BiCNU over shorter periods of time may produce intense pain and burning at the site of injection.

Continued on next page

Bristol-Myers Oncology—Cont.

Important Note: The lyophilized dosage formulation contains no preservatives and is not intended as a multiple dose vial.

STABILITY

Unopened vials of the dry powder must be stored in a refrigerator (2°C to 8°C). The recommended storage of unopened vials prevents significant decomposition for at least 2 years. After reconstitution as recommended, decomposition of BiCNU at room temperature is linear with time. After 3 hours, appoximately 6% of the solution has decomposed and after 6 hours, approximately 8%.

Refrigeration (4°C) of the reconstituted BiCNU significantly increases the stability of the solution. After 24 hours, when protected from light, there is only 4% decomposition. Further dilution of the reconstituted solution with 500 ml. of Sodium Chloride for Injection, U.S.P., or 5% Dextrose for Injection, U.S.P., results in a solution which is stable for 48 hours when protected from light and refrigerated.

Important Note: BiCNU has a low melting point (approximately 30.5°C–32.0°C). Exposure of the drug to this temperature or above will cause the drug to liquify and appear as an oil film in the bottom of the vials. This is a sign of decomposition and vials should be discarded.

Procedures for proper handling and disposal of anti-cancer drugs should be considered. Several guidelines on this subject had been published.[1–6] There is no general agreement that all of the procedures recommended in the guidelines are necessary or appropriate.

REFERENCES

1. Recommendations for the Safe Handling of Parenteral Antineoplastic Drugs. NIH Publication No. 83-2621. For sale by the Superintendent of Documents, U.S. Government Printing Office, Washington, D.C. 20402.
2. AMA Council Report. Guidelines for Handling Parenteral Antineoplastics. JAMA, March 15, 1985.
3. National Study Commission on Cytotoxic Exposure—Recommendations for Handling Cytotoxic Agents. Available from Louis P. Jeffrey, Sc.D., Director of Pharmacy Services, Rhode Island Hospital, 593 Eddy Street, Providence, Rhode Island 02902.
4. Clinical Oncological Society of Australia: Guidelines and Recommendations for Safe Handling of Antineoplastic Agents. Med. J. Australia 1:426–428, 1983.
5. Jones, R. B., et al. Safe Handling of Chemotherapeutic Agents: A Report from the Mount Sinai Medical Center, Ca—A Cancer Journal for Clinicians Sept./Oct., 258–263, 1983.
6. American Society of Hospital Pharmacists Technical Assistance Bulletin on Handling Cytotoxic Drugs in Hospitals. Am. J. Hosp. Pharm. 42:131–137, 1985.

SUPPLY

BiCNU (Carmustine [BCNU]). Each package contains a vial containing 100 mg. carmustine and a vial containing 3 ml. sterile diluent.

NDC 0015-3012

For information on package sizes available, refer to the current price schedule.

BLENOXANE® ℞

[blē-nŏk 'săn]

(sterile bleomycin sulfate)

This is the full text of the latest Official Package Circular dated December 1985 [3010 DIR-16].

> **WARNING**
>
> It is recommended that Blenoxane be administered under the supervision of a qualified physician experienced in the use of cancer chemotherapeutic agents.
> Appropriate management of therapy and complications is possible only when adequate diagnostic and treatment facilities are readily available.
> Pulmonary fibrosis is the most severe toxicity associated with Blenoxane. The most frequent presentation is pneumonitis occasionally progressing to pulmonary fibrosis. Its occurrence is higher in elderly patients and in those receiving greater than 400 units total dose, but pulmonary toxicity has been observed in young patients and those treated with low doses.
> A severe idiosyncratic reaction consisting of hypotension, mental confusion, fever, chills, and wheezing has been reported in approximately 1% of lymphoma patients treated with Blenoxane.

DESCRIPTION

Blenoxane (sterile bleomycin sulfate) is a mixture of cytotoxic glycopeptide antibiotics isolated from a strain of **Streptomyces verticillus.** It is freely soluble in water.

Note: A unit of bleomycin is equal to the formerly used milligram activity. The term milligram activity is a misnomer and was changed to units to be more precise.

ACTION

Although the exact mechanism of action of Blenoxane is unknown, available evidence would seem to indicate that the main mode of action is the inhibition of DNA synthesis with some evidence of lesser inhibition of RNA and protein synthesis.

In mice, high concentrations of Blenoxane are found in the skin, lungs, kidneys, peritoneum, and lymphatics. Tumor cells of the skin and lungs have been found to have high concentrations of Blenoxane in contrast to the low concentrations found in hematopoietic tissue. The low concentrations of Blenoxane found in bone marrow may be related to high levels of Blenoxane degradative enzymes found in that tissue.

In patients with a creatinine clearance of > 35 ml. per minute, the serum or plasma terminal elimination half-life of bleomycin is approximately 115 minutes. In patients with a creatinine clearance of < 35 ml. per minute, the plasma or serum terminal elimination half-life increases exponentially as the creatinine clearance decreases. In humans, 60 to 70% of an administered dose is recovered in the urine as active bleomycin.

INDICATIONS

Blenoxane should be considered a palliative treatment. It has been shown to be useful in the management of the following neoplasms either as a single agent or in proven combinations with other approved chemotherapeutic agents:

Squamous Cell Carcinoma—Head and neck including mouth, tongue, tonsil, nasopharynx, oropharynx, sinus, palate, lip, buccal mucosa, gingiva, epiglottis, skin, larynx, penis, cervix, and vulva. The response to Blenoxane is poorer in patients with head and neck cancer previously irradiated.

Lymphomas—Hodgkin's, reticulum cell sarcoma, lymphosarcoma.

Testicular Carcinoma—Embryonal cell, choriocarcinoma, and teratocarcinoma.

CONTRAINDICATIONS

Blenoxane is contraindicated in patients who have demonstrated a hypersensitive or an idiosyncratic reaction to it.

WARNINGS

Patients receiving Blenoxane must be observed carefully and frequently during and after therapy. It should be used with extreme caution in patients with significant impairment of renal function or compromised pulmonary function.

Pulmonary toxicities occur in 10% of treated patients. In approximately 1%, the nonspecific pneumonitis induced by Blenoxane progresses to pulmonary fibrosis, and death. Although this is age and dose related, the toxicity is unpredictable. Frequent roentgenograms are recommended.

Idiosyncratic reactions similar to anaphylaxis have been reported in 1% of lymphoma patients treated with Blenoxane. Since these usually occur after the first or second dose, careful monitoring is essential after these doses.

Renal or hepatic toxicity, beginning as a deterioration in renal or liver function tests, have been reported, infrequently. These toxicities may occur, however, at any time after initiation of therapy.

Usage in Pregnancy: Safe use of Blenoxane in pregnant women has not been established.

ADVERSE REACTIONS

Pulmonary—This is potentially the most serious side effect, occurring in approximately 10% of treated patients. The most frequent presentation is pneumonitis occasionally progressing to pulmonary fibrosis. Approximately 1% of patients treated have died of pulmonary fibrosis. Pulmonary toxicity is both dose and age-related, being more common in patients over 70 years of age and in those receiving over 400 units total dose. This toxicity, however, is unpredictable and has been seen occasionally in young patients receiving low doses.

Because of lack of specificity of the clinical syndrome, the identification of patients with pulmonary toxicity due to Blenoxane has been extremely difficult. The earliest symptom associated with Blenoxane pulmonary toxicity is dyspnea. The earliest sign is fine rales.

Radiographically, Blenoxane-induced pneumonitis produces nonspecific patchy opacities, usually of the lower lung fields. The most common changes in pulmonary function tests are a decrease in total lung volume and a decrease in vital capacity. However, these changes are not predictive of the development of pulmonary fibrosis.

The microscopic tissue changes due to Blenoxane toxicity include bronchiolar squamous metaplasia, reactive macrophages, atypical alveolar epithelial cells, fibrinous edema, and interstitial fibrosis. The acute stage may involve capillary changes and subsequent fibrinous exudation into alveoli producing a change similar to hyaline membrane formation and progressing to a diffuse interstitial fibrosis resembling the Hamman-Rich syndrome. These microscopic findings are nonspecific, e.g., similar changes are seen in radiation pneumonitis, pneumocystic pneumonitis.

To monitor the onset of pulmonary toxicity, roentgenograms of the chest should be taken every 1 to 2 weeks. If pulmonary changes are noted, treatment should be discontinued until it can be determined if they are drug related. Recent studies have suggested that sequential measurement of the pulmonary diffusion capacity for carbon monoxide (DL_{co}) during treatment with Blenoxane may be an indicator of subclinical pulmonary toxicity. It is recommended that the DL_{co} be monitored monthly if it is to be employed to detect pulmonary toxicities, and thus the drug should be discontinued when the DL_{co} falls below 30 to 35% of the pretreatment value.

Because of bleomycin's sensitization of lung tissue, patients who have received bleomycin are at greater risk of developing pulmonary toxicity when oxygen is administered in surgery. While long exposure to very high oxygen concentrations is a known cause of lung damage, after bleomycin administration, lung damage can occur at lower concentrations that usually would be considered safe. Suggestive preventive measures are:

(1) Maintain $FI\ O_2$ at concentrations approximating that of room air (25%) during surgery and the post operative period.

(2) Monitor carefully fluid replacement, focusing more on colloid administration rather than crystalloid.

Idiosyncratic Reactions—In approximately 1% of the lymphoma patients treated with Blenoxane an idiosyncratic reaction, similar to anaphylaxis clinically, has been reported. The reaction may be immediate or delayed for several hours, and usually occurs after the first or second dose. It consists of hypotension, mental confusion, fever, chills, and wheezing. Treatment is symptomatic including volume expansion, pressor agents, antihistamines, and corticosteroids.

Integument and Mucus Membranes—These are the most frequent side effects, being reported in approximately 50% of treated patients. These consist of erythema, rash, striae, vesiculation, hyperpigmentation, and tenderness of the skin. Hyperkeratosis, nail changes, alopecia, pruritus, and stomatitis have also been reported. It was necessary to discontinue Blenoxane therapy in 2% of treated patients because of these toxicities.

Skin toxicity is a relatively late manifestation usually developing in the 2nd and 3rd week of treatment after 150 to 200 units of Blenoxane has been administered and appears to be related to the cumulative dose.

Other—Fever, chills, and vomiting were frequently reported side effects. Anorexia and weight loss are common and may persist long after termination of this medication. Pain at tumor site, phlebitis, and other local reactions were reported infrequently.

There are isolated reports of Raynaud's phenomenon occurring in patients with testicular carcinomas treated with a combination of Blenoxane and Velban®. It is currently unknown if the cause for the Raynaud's phenomenon in these cases is the disease, Blenoxane, Velban, or a combination of any or all of these.

DOSAGE

Because of the possibility of an anaphylactoid reaction, lymphoma patients should be treated with 2 units or less for the first 2 doses. If no acute reaction occurs, then the regular dosage schedule may be followed.

The following dose schedule is recommended: **Squamous cell carcinoma, lymphosarcoma, reticulum cell sarcoma, testicular carcinoma**—0.25 to 0.50 units/Kg. (10 to 20 units/M.^{2}) given intravenously, intramuscularly, or subcutaneously weekly or twice weekly.

Hodgkin's Disease—0.25 to 0.50 units/Kg. (10 to 20 units/M.^{2}) given intravenously, intramuscularly, or subcutaneously weekly or twice weekly. After a 50% response, a maintenance dose of 1 unit daily or 5 units weekly intravenously or intramuscularly should be given.

Pulmonary toxicity of Blenoxane appears to be dose-related with a striking increase when the total dose is over 400 units. Total doses over 400 units should be given with great caution.

NOTE

When Blenoxane is used in combination with other antineoplastic agents, pulmonary toxicities may occur at lower doses.

Improvement of Hodgkin's Disease and testicular tumors is prompt and noted within two weeks. If no improvement is seen by this time, improvement is unlikely. Squamous cell cancers respond more slowly, sometimes requiring as long as three weeks before any improvement is noted.

ADMINISTRATION

Blenoxane may be given by the intramuscular, intravenous, or subcutaneous routes.

Intramuscular or Subcutaneous—Dissolve the contents of a Blenoxane vial in 1 to 5 ml. of Sterile Water for Injection, U.S.P., Sodium Chloride for Injection, U.S.P., 5% Dextrose Injection, U.S.P., or Bacteriostatic Water for Injection, U.S.P.

Intravenous—Dissolve the contents of the vial in 5 ml. or more of a solution suitable for injection, e.g., physiologic saline or glucose, and administer slowly over a period of ten minutes.

Stability: The sterile powder is stable under refrigeration (2°-8°C) and should not be used after the expiration date is reached.

Blenoxane is stable for 24 hours at room temperature in Sodium Chloride or 5% Dextrose Solution.

Blenoxane is stable for 24 hours in 5% Dextrose containing heparin 100 units per ml. or 1000 units per ml.

Procedures for proper handling and disposal of anti-cancer drugs should be considered. Several guidelines on this subject had been published.[1–6] There is no general agreement that all of the procedures recommended in the guidelines are necessary or appropriate.

REFERENCES

1. Recommendations for the Safe Handling of Parenteral Antineoplastic Drugs. NIH Publication No. 83-2621. For sale by the Superintendent of Documents, U.S. Government Printing Office, Washington, D.C. 20402.
2. AMA Council Report. Guidelines for Handling Parenteral Antineoplastics. JAMA, March 15, 1985.
3. National Study Commission on Cytotoxic Exposure—Recommendations for Handling Cytotoxic Agents. Available from Louis P. Jeffrey, Sc. D., Director of Pharmacy Services, Rhode Island Hospital, 593 Eddy Street, Providence, Rhode Island 02902.
4. Clinical Oncological Society of Australia: Guidelines and Recommendations for Safe Handling of Antineoplastic Agents. Med. J. Australia 1:426–428, 1983.
5. Jones, R. B., et. al. Safe Handling of Chemotherapeutic Agents: A Report from the Mount Sinai Medical Center, Ca—A Cancer Journal for Clinicians Sept./Oct., 258–263, 1983.
6. American Society of Hospital Pharmacists Technical Assistance Bulletin on Handling Cytotoxic Drugs in Hospitals. Am. J. Hosp. Pharm. 42:131–137, 1985.

SUPPLY

Each vial contains 15 units of Blenoxane as sterile bleomycin sulfate.

NDC 0015-3010-20

For information on package sizes available, refer to the current price sheet.

CeeNU® ℞

[*cē'nū*]
(lomustine [CCNU])

This is the full text of the latest Official Package Circular dated February 1983 [3030 CIM-03].

> **WARNING**
>
> CeeNU should be administered by individuals experienced in the use of antineoplastic therapy.
> Since the major toxicity is delayed bone marrow suppression, blood counts should be monitored weekly for at least 6 weeks after a dose. (See "Adverse Reactions.")
> At the recommended dosage, courses of CeeNU should not be given more frequently than 6 weeks.
> Caution should be used in administering CeeNU to patients with decreased circulating platelets, leukocytes, or erythrocytes. (See "Dosage and Administration.")
> Liver function should be monitored periodically. (See "Adverse Reactions.")

DESCRIPTION

CeeNU 1-(2-chloroethyl)-3-cyclohexyl-1-nitrosoureal is one of a group of nitrosoureas. It is a yellow powder with the empirical formula of $C_9H_{16}ClN_3O_2$ and a molecular weight of 233.71. CeeNU is soluble in 10% ethanol (0.05 mg. per ml.) and in absolute alcohol (70 mg. per ml.). CeeNU is relatively insoluble in water (< 0.05 mg. per ml.). It is relatively unionized at a physiological pH.

Inactive ingredients in CeeNU capsules are: magnesium stearate and mannitol.

The structural formula is:

```
      NH—(cyclohexyl)
     /
O=C
     \
      N—CH2—CH2—Cl
      |
      N=O
```

ACTION

It is generally agreed that CeeNU acts as an alkylating agent but, as with other nitrosoureas, it may also inhibit several key enzymatic processes.

CeeNU may be given orally. Following oral administration of radioactive CeeNU at doses ranging from 30 mg/M² to 100 mg/M², about half of the radioactivity given was excreted within 24 hours. The serum half-life of the drug and/or metabolites ranges from 16 hours to 2 days. Tissue levels are comparable to plasma levels at 15 minutes after intravenous administration.

Because of the high lipid solubility and the relative lack of ionization at a physiological pH, CeeNU crosses the blood brain barrier quite effectively. Levels of radioactivity in the CSF are 50% or greater than those measured concurrently in plasma.

INDICATIONS

CeeNU is indicated as palliative therapy to be employed in addition to other modalities, or in established combination therapy with other approved chemotherapeutic agents in the following:

Brain tumors—both primary and metastatic, in patients who have already received appropriate surgical and/or radiotherapeutic procedures;

Hodgkin's Disease—as a secondary therapy.

CONTRAINDICATIONS

CeeNU should not be given to individuals who have demonstrated a previous hypersensitivity to it.

WARNINGS

Safe use in pregnancy has not been established. CeeNU is embryotoxic and teratogenic in rats and embryotoxic in rabbits at dose levels equivalent to the human dose. CeeNU also affects fertility in male rats at doses somewhat higher than the human dose.

CeeNU is carcinogenic in rats and mice, producing a marked increase in tumor incidence in doses approximating those employed clinically.

Nitrosourea therapy does have carcinogenic potential. The occurrence of acute leukemia and bone marrow dysplasias have been reported in patients following nitrosourea therapy.

Pulmonary Toxicity—Three cases of pulmonary infliltrates and/or fibrosis have been reported with CeeNU, to date. Onset of toxicity has occurred after an interval of six months or longer from the start of therapy with cumulative doses ranging from 600 to 1040 mg.

Related nitrosoureas are also associated with pulmonary toxicity.

PRECAUTIONS

CeeNU should be administered by individuals experienced in the use of antineoplastic therapy.

Since the major toxicity is delayed bone marrow suppression blood counts should be monitored weekly for at least 6 weeks after a dose. (See "Adverse Reactions".)

At the recommended dosage, courses of CeeNU should not be given more frequently than every 6 weeks.

Caution should be used in administering CeeNU to patients with decreased circulating platelets, leukocytes, or erythrocytes. (See "Dosage and Administration".)

Liver function should be monitored periodically. (See "Adverse Reactions".)

See "Warnings" section for information on carcinogenesis.

ADVERSE REACTIONS

Nausea and vomiting may occur 3 to 6 hours after an oral dose and usually last less than 24 hours. The frequency and duration may be reduced by the use of antiemetics prior to dosing and by the administration of CeeNU to fasting patients.

Thrombocytopenia occurs at about 4 weeks after a dose of CeeNU and persists for 1 to 2 weeks.

Leukopenia occurs at about 6 weeks after a dose of CeeNU and persists for 1 to 2 weeks. Approximately 65% of patients develop white blood counts below 5000 wbc/mm³ and 36% develop white blood counts below 3000 wbc/mm³.

CeeNU may produce cumulative myelosuppression, manifested by more depressed indices or longer duration of suppression after repeated doses.

Other toxicities: Stomatitis, alopecia, anemia, and hepatic toxicity, manifested by transient reversible elevation of liver function tests, have been reported infrequently.

Neurological reactions such as disorientation, lethargy, ataxia, and dysarthria have been noted in some patients receiving CeeNU. However, the relationship to medication in these patients is unclear.

Renal abnormalities consisting of decrease in kidney size, progressive azotemia and renal failure have been reported in patients who received large cumulative doses after prolonged therapy with CeeNU and related nitrosoureas. Kidney damage has also been reported occasionally in patients receiving lower total doses.

DOSAGE AND ADMINISTRATION

The recommended dose of CeeNU in adults and children is 130 mg/M² as a single dose by mouth every 6 weeks.

In individuals with compromised bone marrow function, the dose should be reduced to 100 mg/M² every 6 weeks.

A repeat course of CeeNU should not be given until circulating blood elements have returned to acceptable levels (platelets above 100,000/mm³; leukocytes above 4,000/mm³). Blood counts should be monitored weekly and repeat courses should not be given before 6 weeks because the hematologic toxicity is delayed and cumulative.

Doses subsequent to the initial dose should be adjusted according to the hematologic response of the patient to the preceding dose. The following schedule is suggested as a guide to dosage adjustment:

Nadir After Prior Dose: Leukocytes	Nadir After Prior Dose: Platelets	Percentage of Prior Dose to be Given
> 4000	> 100,000	100%
3000-3999	75,000-99,999	100%
2000-2999	25,000-74,999	70%
< 2000	< 25,000	50%

When CeeNU is used in combination with myelosuppressive drugs, the doses should be adjusted accordingly.

STABILITY

CeeNU capsules are stable for at least 3 years when stored at room temperature in well closed containers. Avoid excessive heat (over 40°C).

SUPPLY

The dose pack of CeeNU (Lomustine [CCNU]) Capsules contains;

NDC 0015-3032-13—2—100 mg capsules (Green/ Green)
NDC 0015-3031-13—2—40 mg capsules (Purple/ Green)
NDC 0015-3030-13—2—10 mg capsules (Purple/Purple)

Directions to the Pharmacist

The capsules are to provide enough medication for a single dose. The total dose prescribed by the physician can be obtained (to within 10 mg) by determining the appropriate combination of the enclosed capsule strengths.

The appropriate number of capsules of each size should be placed in a single vial to which the patient information label (gummed label provided) explaining the differences in the appearance of the capsules is affixed.

Example: A patient dose of 240 mg can be obtained by combining two 100 mg capsules and one 40 mg capsule. The remaining capsules (if any) should be discarded.

A patient information sticker, to be placed on dispensing container, is enclosed.

Also Available: Individual bottles of 20 capsules each.
NDC 0015-3032-20—20—100 mg. capsules (Green/Green)
NDC 0015-3031-20—20—40 mg. capsules (White/Green)
NDC 0015-3030-20—20—10 mg. capsules (White/White)

Procedures for proper handling and disposal of anti-cancer drugs should be considered. Several guidelines on this subject had been published.[1–6] There is no general agreement that all of the procedures recommended in the guidelines are necessary or appropriate.

REFERENCES

1. Recommendations for the Safe Handling of Parenteral Antineoplastic Drugs. NIH Publication No. 83-2621. For sale by the Superintendent of Documents, U.S. Government Printing Office, Washington, D.C. 20402.
2. AMA Council Report. Guidelines for Handling Parenteral Antineoplastics. JAMA, March 15, 1985.
3. National Study Commission on Cytotoxic Exposure—Recommendations for Handling Cytotoxic Agents. Available from Louis P. Jeffrey, Sc. D., Director of Pharmacy Services, Rhode Island Hospital, 593 Eddy Street, Providence, Rhode Island 02902.
4. Clinical Oncological Society of Australia: Guidelines and Recommendations for Safe Handling of Antineoplastic Agents. Med. J. Australia 1:426–428, 1983.
5. Jones, R. B., et. al. Safe Handling of Chemotherapeutic Agents: A Report from the Mount Sinai Medical Center, Ca—A Cancer Journal for Clinicians Sept./Oct., 258–263, 1983.
6. American Society of Hospital Pharmacists Technical Assistance Bulletin on Handling Cytotoxic Drugs in Hospitals. Am. J. Hosp. Pharm. 42:131–137, 1985.

Shown in Product Identification Section, page 406

CYTOXAN® ℞

[*sī-taks'an*]
(Cyclophosphamide)

This is the full text of the latest official Package Circular dated December 1985 [P 0404-03].

DESCRIPTION

CYTOXAN (cyclophosphamide) is supplied as a sterile powder for parenteral use containing 45 mg sodium chloride per 100 mg cyclophosphamide (anhydrous), a sterile lyophilizate for parenteral use containing 75 mg mannitol per 100 mg cyclophosphamide (anhydrous), a tablet for oral use containing 25 mg cyclophosphamide (anhydrous), and a tablet for oral use containing 50 mg cyclophosphamide (anhydrous). Inactive ingredients in CYTOXAN tablets are: acacia, FD&C Blue No. 1, FD&C Yellow No. 10 Aluminum Lake, lactose, magnesium stearate, starch, stearic acid and talc. Cyclophos-

Continued on next page

Bristol-Myers Oncology—Cont.

phamide is a synthetic antineoplastic drug chemically related to the nitrogen mustards. Cyclophosphamide is a white crystalline powder with the molecular formula of $C_7H_{15}CL_2N_2O_2P \cdot H_2O$ and a molecular weight of 279.1. The chemical name for cyclophosphamide is 2-bis[(2-chloroethyl)-amino] tetrahydro-2H-1, 3, 2-oxazaphosphorine 2-oxide monohydrate. Cyclophosphamide is soluble in water, saline, or ethanol and has the following structural formula:

O, P, O, $N(CH_2CH_2Cl)_2 \cdot H_2O$, NH

ACTIONS

Although it is classified generally as an alkylating agent, cyclophosphamide itself is not an alkylating agent or irritant. It interferes with the growth of susceptible neoplasms and, to some extent, certain normal tissues. Its mechanism of action is not known.

Cyclophosphamide is absorbed from the gastrointestinal tract and parenteral sites. It is metabolized (the details of metabolism are not fully known) and the drug and its metabolites are distributed throughout the body, including the brain. Intravenously administered, cyclophosphamide is reported to have a serum half-life of about four hours; however the drug and/or its metabolites may be detected in plasma up to seventy-two hours.

Cyclophosphamide and its metabolites are excreted by the kidneys, but the extent to which they are excreted by other routes is not known. Of three alkylating metabolites found in urine, only one (nor-nitrogen mustard) has been identified definitely.

INDICATIONS

Cyclophosphamide, though effective alone in susceptible malignancies, is more frequently used concurrently or sequentially with other antineoplastic drugs. The following malignancies are often susceptible to cyclophosphamide treatment:

1. Malignant lymphomas (Stages III and IV of the Ann Arbor staging system); Hodgkin's disease; lymphocytic lymphoma (nodular or diffuse); mixed-cell type lymphoma; histiocytic lymphoma; Burkitt's lymphoma.
2. Multiple myeloma.
3. Leukemias: chronic lymphocytic leukemia; chronic granulocytic leukemia (it is ineffective in acute blastic crisis); acute myelogenous and monocytic leukemia; acute lymphoblastic (stem-cell) leukemia in children (cyclophosphamide given during remission is effective in prolonging its duration).
4. Mycosis fungoides (advanced disease).
5. Neuroblastoma (disseminated disease).
6. Adenocarcinoma of the ovary.
7. Retinoblastoma.
8. Carcinoma of the breast.

WARNINGS

Cardiac Toxicity: Although a few instances of cardiac dysfunction have been reported following use of recommended doses of cyclophosphamide, no causal relationship has been established. Cardiotoxicity has been observed in some patients receiving high doses of cyclophosphamide ranging from 120 to 270 mg/kg administered over a period of a few days, usually as a portion of an intensive antineoplastic multidrug regimen or in conjunction with transplantation procedures. In a few instances with high doses of cyclophosphamide, severe, and sometimes fatal, congestive heart failure has occurred within a few days after the first cyclophosphamide dose. Histopathologic examination has primarily shown hemorrhagic myocarditis.

No residual cardiac abnormalities as evidenced by electrocardiogram or echocardiogram appear to be present in patients surviving episodes of apparent cardiac toxicity associated with high doses of cyclophosphamide.

Cyclophosphamide has been reported to potentiate doxorubicin-induced cardiotoxicity.

Adrenalectomy: Since cyclophosphamide has been reported to be more toxic in adrenalectomized dogs, adjustment of the doses of both replacement steroids and cyclophosphamide may be necessary for the adrenalectomized patient.

OTHER

Barbiturates: The rate of metabolism and the leukopenic activity of cyclophosphamide reportedly are increased by chronic administration of high doses of phenobarbital.

Combined Drug Actions: The physician should be alert for possible combined drug actions, desirable or undesirable, involving cyclophosphamide even though cyclophosphamide has been used successfully concurrently with other drugs, including other cytotoxic drugs.

Wound Healing: Cyclophosphamide may interfere with normal wound healing.

Usage in Pregnancy: Cyclophosphamide can be teratogenic or cause fetal resorption in experimental animals. It should not be used in pregnancy, particularly in early pregnancy, unless in the judgment of the physician the potential benefits outweigh the possible risks. Cyclophosphamide is excreted in breast milk and breast-feeding should be terminated prior to institution of cyclophosphamide therapy.

Patients, male or female, capable of conception ordinarily should be advised of the mutagenic potential of cyclophosphamide. Adequate methods of contraception appear desirable for such patients receiving cyclophosphamide.

PRECAUTIONS

Cyclophosphamide should be given cautiously to patients with any of the following conditions.

1. Leukopenia
2. Thrombocytopenia
3. Tumor cell infiltration of bone marrow
4. Previous X-ray therapy
5. Previous therapy with other cytotoxic agents
6. Impaired hepatic function
7. Impaired renal function

Because cyclophosphamide may exert a suppressive action on immune mechanisms, the interruption or modification of dosage should be considered for patients who develop bacterial, fungal or viral infections. This is especially true for patients receiving concomitant steroid therapy and perhaps those with a recent history of steroid therapy, since infections in some of these patients have been fatal. Varicella zoster infections appear to be particularly dangerous under these circumstances.

ADVERSE REACTIONS

Secondary Neoplasia. Secondary malignancies have developed in some patients treated with cyclophosphamide alone or in association with other antineoplastic drugs and/or modalities. These malignancies most frequently have been urinary bladder, myeloproliferative, and lymphoproliferative malignancies. Secondary malignancies most frequently have developed in the cyclophosphamide-treated patients with primary myeloproliferative and lymphoproliferative malignancies and primary nonmalignant diseases in which immune processes are believed to be involved pathologically. In some cases, the secondary malignancy was detected up to several years after cyclophosphamide treatment was discontinued. The secondary urinary bladder malignancies generally have occurred in patients who previously developed hemorrhagic cystitis (see Genitourinary under Adverse Reactions). Although no cause-effect relationship has been established between cyclophosphamide and the development of malignancy in humans, the possibility of secondary malignancy, based on available data, should be considered in any benefit-to-risk assessment for the use of the drug.

Hematopoietic. Leukopenia is an expected effect and ordinarily is used as a guide to therapy. Thrombocytopenia or anemia may occur in a few patients. These effects are almost always reversible when therapy is interrupted.

Gastrointestinal. Anorexia, nausea, or vomiting are common and related to dose as well as individual susceptibility. There are isolated reports of hemorrhagic colitis, oral mucosal ulceration and jaundice occurring during therapy.

Genitourinary. Sterile hemorrhagic cystitis can result from the administration of cyclophosphamide. **This can be severe, even fatal, and is probably due to metabolites in the urine.** Nonhemorrhagic cystitis and/or fibrosis of the bladder also have been reported to result from cyclophosphamide administration. Atypical epithelial cells may be found in the urinary sediment. **Ample fluid intake and frequent voiding help to prevent the development of cystitis,** but when it occurs it is ordinarily necessary to interrupt cyclophosphamide therapy. Hematuria usually resolves spontaneously within a few days after cyclophosphamide therapy is discontinued, but may persist for several months. In severe cases replacement of blood loss may be required. The application of electrocautery to telangiectatic areas of the bladder and diversion of urine flow have been successful methods used in treatment of protracted cases. Cryosurgery has also been used. (See also Secondary Neoplasia under Adverse Reactions.) Nephrotoxicity, including hemorrhage and clot formation in the renal pelvis, has been reported.

Gonadal suppression, resulting in amenorrhea or azoospermia, has been reported in a number of patients treated with cyclophosphamide and appears to be related to dosage and duration of therapy. This side effect, possibly irreversible, should be anticipated in patients treated with cyclophosphamide. It is not known to what extent cyclophosphamide may affect prepuberal gonads. Fibrosis of the ovary following cyclophosphamide therapy has been reported also.

Integument: It is ordinarily advisable to inform patients in advance of possible alopecia, a frequent complication of cyclophosphamide therapy. Regrowth of hair can be expected although occasionally the new hair may be of a different color or texture. The skin and fingernails may become darker during therapy. Non-specific dermatitis has been reported to occur with cyclophosphamide.

Pulmonary: Interstitial pulmonary fibrosis has been reported in patients receiving high doses of cyclophosphamide over a prolonged period.

DOSAGE AND ADMINISTRATION

Chemotherapy with cyclophosphamide, as with other drugs used in cancer chemotherapy, is potentially hazardous and fatal complications can occur. It is recommended that it be administered only by physicians aware of the associated risks. Therapy may be aimed at either induction or maintenance of remission.

Induction Therapy: The usual initial intravenous loading dose for patients with no hematologic deficiency is 40–50 mg/kg. This total initial intravenous loading dose usually is given in divided doses over a period of two to five days.

Patients with any previous treatment that may have compromised the functional capacity of the bone marrow, such as X ray or cytotoxic drugs, and patients with tumor infiltration of the bone marrow may require reduction of the initial loading dose by $\frac{1}{3}$ to $\frac{1}{2}$.

A marked leukopenia is usually associated with the above doses, but recovery usually begins after 7–10 days. The white blood cell count should be monitored closely during induction therapy.

If initial therapy is given orally, a dose of 1–5 mg/kg/day can be administered depending on tolerance by the patient.

Maintenance Therapy: It is frequently necessary to maintain chemotherapy in order to suppress or retard neoplastic growth. A variety of schedules has been used:

(1) 1–5 mg/kg p.o. daily
(2) 10–15 mg/kg i.v. every 7–10 days
(3) 3–5 mg/kg i.v. twice weekly

Unless the disease is unusually sensitive to cyclophosphamide, it is advisable to give the largest maintenance dose that can be reasonably tolerated by the patient. The total leukocyte count is a good objective guide for regulating the maintenance dose. Ordinarily a leukopenia of 3000–4000 cells/cu. mm. can be maintained without undue risk of serious infection or other complications.

Preparation and Handling of Solutions: Parenteral drug products should be inspected visually for particulate matter and discoloration prior to administration, whenever solution and container permit.

CYTOXAN for Injection and Lyophilized CYTOXAN for Injection should be prepared for parenteral use by adding Bacteriostatic Water for Injection, U.S.P. (paraben preserved only) or Sterile Water for Injection, U.S.P. to the vial and shaking to dissolve. Use the quantity of diluent shown below to reconstitute the product.

Dosage Strength	CYTOXAN for Injection Quantity of Diluent	Lyophilized CYTOXAN for Injection Quantity of Diluent
100 mg	5 ml	—
200 mg	10 ml	—
500 mg	25 ml	20–25 ml
1.0 g	50 ml	50 ml
2.0 g	100 ml	80–100 ml

Solutions of CYTOXAN for Injection and Lyophilized CYTOXAN for Injection may be injected intravenously, intramuscularly, intraperitoneally, or intrapleurally or they may be infused intravenously in the following:

- Dextrose Injection, U.S.P. (5% dextrose)
- Dextrose and Sodium Chloride Injection, U.S.P. (5% dextrose and 0.9% sodium chloride)
- 5% Dextrose and Ringer's Injection
- Lactated Ringer's Injection, U.S.P.
- Sodium Chloride Injection, U.S.P. (0.45% sodium chloride)
- Sodium Lactate Injection, U.S.P. ($\frac{1}{6}$ molar sodium lactate)

Reconstituted CYTOXAN for Injection and Lyophilized CYTOXAN for Injection are chemically and physically stable for 24 hours at room temperature or for six days in the refrigerator; they do not contain any antibacterial agent and thus care must be taken to assure the sterility of prepared solutions.

CYTOXAN for Injection and Lyophilized CYTOXAN for Injection prepared by adding Bacteriostatic Water for Injection U.S.P. (paraben preserved only) should be used within 24 hours if stored at room temperature or within 6 days if stored under refrigeration.

If CYTOXAN for Injection or Lyophilized CYTOXAN for Injection is not prepared by adding Bacteriostatic Water for Injection U.S.P. (paraben preserved only), it is recommended that the solution be used promptly (preferably within six hours). The osmolarities of solutions of CYTOXAN for Injection, Lyophilized CYTOXAN for Injection, and normal saline are compared in the following table:

Lyophilized CYTOXAN for Injection	mOsm/L
4 ml diluent per 100 mg cyclophosphamide	219
5 ml diluent per 100 mg cyclophosphamide	172
CYTOXAN for Injection	352
Normal saline	287

Lyophilized CYTOXAN for Injection is slightly hypotonic with respect to normal saline.
Extemporaneous liquid preparations of CYTOXAN for oral administration may be prepared by dissolving CYTOXAN for Injection or Lyophilized CYTOXAN for Injection in Aromatic Elixir, N.F. Such preparations should be stored under refrigeration and used within 14 days.

OVERDOSAGE

No specific antidote for CYTOXAN products is known. Management of overdosage would include general supportive measures to sustain the patient through any period of toxicity that might occur.

HOW SUPPLIED

CYTOXAN for Injection contains 45 mg of sodium chloride per 100 mg of cyclophosphamide (anhydrous) and is supplied in vials for single dose use.
CYTOXAN® for Injection (cyclophosphamide with sodium chloride).
NDC 0015-0500-41 100 mg vials, carton of 12, case of 1 carton
NDC 0015-0501-41 200 mg vials, carton of 12, case of 1 carton
NDC 0015-0502-41 500 mg vials, carton of 12, case of 1 carton
NDC 0015-0505-41 1.0 g vials, carton of 6
NDC 0015-0506-41 2.0 g vials, carton of 6
Lyophilized CYTOXAN for Injection contains 75 mg of mannitol per 100 mg of cyclophosphamide (anhydrous) and is supplied in vials for single dose use.
Lyophilized CYTOXAN® (cyclophosphamide) for Injection.
NDC 0015-0539-41 100 mg vials, carton of 12, case of 1 carton
NDC 0015-0546-41 200 mg vials, carton of 12, case of 1 carton
NDC 0015-0547-41 500 mg vials, carton of 12, case of 1 carton
NDC 0015-0548-41 1.0 g vials, carton of 6
NDC 0015-0549-41 2.0 g vials, carton of 6
CYTOXAN Tablets, 25 mg, and CYTOXAN Tablets, 50 mg, are white tablets with blue flecks containing 25 mg and 50 mg cyclophosphamide (anhydrous), respectively.
CYTOXAN® (cyclophosphamide) tablets.
NDC 0015-0503-01 50 mg, bottles of 100
NDC 0015-0503-02 50 mg, bottles of 1000
NDC 0015-0503-03 50 mg, Unit Dose cartons of 100
NDC 0015-0503-48 50 mg compliance pack, cartons of 28
NDC 0015-0504-01 25 mg, bottles of 100
Storage at or below 77°F (25°C) is recommended; this product will withstand brief exposure to temperatures up to 86°F (30°C) but should be protected from temperatures above 86°F (30°C).
Procedures for proper handling and disposal of anti-cancer drugs should be considered. Several guidelines on this subject had been published.[1–6] There is no general agreement that all of the procedures recommended in the guidelines are necessary or appropriate.

REFERENCES

1. Recommendations for the Safe Handling of Parenteral Antineoplastic Drugs. NIH Publication No. 83-2621. For sale by the Superintendent of Documents, U.S. Government Printing Office, Washington, D.C. 20402.
2. AMA Council Report. Guidelines for Handling Parenteral Antineoplastics. JAMA, March 15, 1985.
3. National Study Commission on Cytotoxic Exposure—Recommendations for Handling Cytotoxic Agents. Available from Louis P. Jeffrey, Sc. D., Director of Pharmacy Services, Rhode Island Hospital, 593 Eddy Street, Providence, Rhode Island 02902.
4. Clinical Oncological Society of Australia: Guidelines and Recommendations for Safe Handling of Antineoplastic Agents. Med. J. Australia 1:426–428, 1983.
5. Jones, R. B., et. al. Safe Handling of Chemotherapeutic Agents: A Report from the Mount Sinai Medical Center, CA—A Cancer Journal for Clinicians Sept./Oct., 258–263, 1983.
6. American Society of Hospital Pharmacists Technical Assistance Bulletin on Handling Cytotoxic Drugs in Hospitals. Am. J. Hosp. Pharm. 42:131–137, 1985.

References on selected topics and a physician's brochure are available by writing to: Medical Services Department, Bristol Laboratories, Syracuse, NY 13221.
Show in Product Identification Section, page 406

LYSODREN® ℞
[*li 'sō-drĕn ''*]
(mitotane)
Tablets, USP

This is the full text of the latest Official Package Circular dated December 1985 [3080DIM-04].

WARNINGS

Lysodren (mitotane) should be administered under the supervision of a qualified physician experienced in the use of cancer chemotherapeutic agents. Lysodren should be temporarily discontinued immediately following shock or severe trauma since adrenal suppression is its prime action. Exogenous steroids should be administered in such circumstances, since the depressed adrenal may not immediately start to secrete steroids.

DESCRIPTION

Lysodren (mitotane) is an oral chemotherapeutic agent. It is best known by its trivial name, o,p'-DDD, and is chemically, 1,1-dichloro-2-(o-chlorophenyl) -2- (p-chlorophenyl) ethane. The chemical structure is shown below.

$CHCl_2$ — CH — Cl — Cl

Lysodren is a white granular solid composed of clear colorless crystals. It is tasteless and has a slight pleasant aromatic odor. It is soluble in ethanol, isoctane and carbon tetrachloride. It has a molecular weight of 320.05.
Inactive ingredients in Lysodren tablets are: avicel, Polyethylene Glycol 4000, silicon dioxide, and starch.
Lysodren is available as 500 mg scored tablets for oral administration.

CLINICAL PHARMACOLOGY

Lysodren can best be described as an adrenal cytotoxic agent, although it can cause adrenal inhibition, apparently without cellular destruction. Its biochemical mechanism of action is unknown. Data are available to suggest that the drug modifies the peripheral metabolism of steroids as well as directly suppressing the adrenal cortex. The administration of Lysodren alters the extra-adrenal metabolism of cortisol in man, leading to a reduction in measurable 17-hydroxy corticosteroids, even though plasma levels of corticosteroids do not fall. The drug apparently causes increased formation of 6-β-hydroxyl cortisol.
Data in adrenal carcinoma patients indicate that about 40% of oral Lysodren is absorbed and approximately 10% of administered dose is recovered in the urine as a water-soluble metabolite. A variable amount of metabolite (1 to 17%) is excreted in the bile and the balance is apparently stored in the tissues.
Following discontinuation of Lysodren, the plasma terminal half life has ranged from 18 to 159 days. In most patients blood levels become undetectable after six to nine weeks. Autopsy data have provided evidence that Lysodren is found in most tissues of the body; however, fat tissues are the primary site of storage. Lysodren is converted to a water-soluble metabolite.
No unchanged Lysodren has been found in urine or bile.

INDICATIONS AND USAGE

Lysodren is indicated in the treatment of inoperable adrenal cortical carcinoma of both functional and non-functional types.

CONTRAINDICATIONS

Lysodren should not be given to individuals who have demonstrated a previous hypersensitivity to it.

WARNINGS

Lysodren should be temporarily discontinued immediately following shock or severe trauma, since adrenal suppression is its prime action. Exogenous steroids should be administered in such circumstances, since the depressed adrenal may not immediately start to secrete steroids.
Lysodren should be administered with care to patients with liver disease other than metastatic lesions from the adrenal cortex, since the metabolism of Lysodren may be interfered with and the drug may accumulate.
All possible tumor tissues should be surgically removed from large metastatic masses before Lysodren administration is instituted. This is necessary to minimize the possibility of infarction and hemorrhage in the tumor due to a rapid cytotoxic effect of the drug.
Long-term continuous administration of high doses of Lysodren may lead to brain damage and impairment of function. Behavioral and neurological assessments should be made at regular intervals when continuous Lysodren treatment exceeds two years.
A substantial percentage of the patients treated show signs of adrenal insufficiency. It therefore appears necessary to watch for and institute steroid replacement in those patients. However, some investigators have recommended that steroid replacement therapy be administered concomitantly with Lysodren. It has been shown that the metabolism of exogenous steroids is modified and consequently somewhat higher doses than normal replacement therapy may be required.

PRECAUTIONS

General: Adrenal insufficiency may develop in patients treated with Lysodren, and adrenal steroid replacement should be considered for these patients.
Since sedation, lethargy, vertigo, and other CNS side effects can occur, ambulatory patients should be cautioned about driving, operating machinery, and other hazardous pursuits requiring mental and physical alertness.
Carcinogenesis, Mutagenesis, Impairment of Fertility: The carcinogenic and mutagenic potentials of Lysodren are unknown. However, the mechanism of action of this compound suggests that it probably has less carcinogenic potential than other cytotoxic chemotherapeutic drugs.
Pregnancy: Pregnancy "Category C". Animal reproduction studies have not been conducted with Lysodren. It is also not known whether Lysodren can cause fetal harm when administered to a pregnant woman or can affect reproduction capacity. Lysodren should be given to a pregnant woman only if clearly needed.
Nursing Mothers: It is not known whether this drug is excreted in human milk. Because many drugs are excreted in human milk and because of the potential for adverse reactions in nursing infants from mitotane, a decision should be made whether to discontinue nursing or to discontinue the drug, taking into account the importance of the drug to the mother.

ADVERSE REACTIONS

A very high percentage of patients treated with Lysodren have shown at least one type of side effect. The main types of adverse reactions consist of the following:

1. Gastrointestinal disturbances, which consisted of anorexia, nausea or vomiting, and in some cases diarrhea, occur in about 80% of the patients.
2. Central nervous system side effects occur in 40% of the patients. These consist primarily of depression as manifested by lethargy and somnolence (25%), and dizziness or vertigo (15%).
3. Skin toxicity has been observed in about 15% of the cases. These skin changes consist primarily of transient skin rashes which do not seem to be dose-related. In some instances, this side effect subsided while the patients were maintained on the drug without a change of dose.

Infrequently occurring side effects involve the eye (visual blurring, diplopia, lens opacity, toxic retinopathy); the genitourinary system (hematuria, hemorrhagic cystitis, and albuminuria); cardiovascular system (hypertension, orthostatic hypotension, and flushing); and some miscellaneous complaints including generalized aching, hyperpyrexia, and lowered protein bound iodine (PBI).

OVERDOSAGE

No proven antidotes have been established for Lysodren overdosage.

DOSAGE AND ADMINISTRATION

The recommended treatment schedule is to start the patient at 2 to 6 g of Lysodren per day in divided doses, either three or four times a day. Doses are usually increased incrementally to 9 to 10 g per day. If severe side effects appear, the dose should be reduced until the maximum tolerated dose is achieved. If the patient can tolerate higher doses and improved clinical response appears possible, the dose should be increased until adverse reactions interfere. Experience has shown that the maximum tolerated dose (MTD) will vary from 2 to 16 g per day, but has usually been 9 to 10 g per day. The highest doses used in the studies to date were 18 to 19 g per day.
Treatment should be instituted in the hospital until a stable dosage regimen is achieved.
Treatment should be continued as long as clinical benefits are observed. Maintenance of clinical status or slowing of growth of metastatic lesions can be considered clinical benefits if they can clearly be shown to have occurred.
If no clinical benefits are observed after three months at the maximum tolerated dose, the case may be considered a clinical failure. However, 10% of the patients who showed a measurable response required more than three months at the MTD. Early diagnosis and prompt institution of treatment improve the probability of a positive clinical response. Clinical effectiveness can be shown by reduction in tumor mass, reduction in pain, weakness or anorexia and reduction of symptoms and signs due to excessive steroid production.
A number of patients have been treated intermittently with treatment being restarted when severe symptoms have reappeared. Patients often do not respond after the third or fourth such course. Experience accumulated to date suggests that continuous treatment with the maximum possible dosage of Lysodren is the best approach.
Procedures for proper handling and disposal of anti-cancer drugs should be considered. Several guidelines on this subject had been published.[1–6] There is no general agreement that all of the procedures recommended in the guidelines are necessary or appropriate.

Continued on next page

Bristol-Myers Oncology—Cont.

REFERENCES

1. Recommendations for the Safe Handling of Parenteral Antineoplastic Drugs. NIH Publication No. 83-2621. For sale by the Superintendent of Documents, U.S. Government Printing Office, Washington, D.C. 20402.
2. AMA Council Report. Guidelines for Handling Parenteral Antineoplastics. JAMA, March 15, 1985.
3. National Study Commission on Cytotoxic Exposure—Recommendations for Handling Cytotoxic Agents. Available from Louis P. Jeffrey, Sc. D., Director of Pharmacy Services, Rhode Island Hospital, 593 Eddy Street, Providence, Rhode Island 02902.
4. Clinical Oncological Society of Australia: Guidelines and Recommendations for Safe Handling of Antineoplastic Agents. Med. J. Australia 1:426–428, 1983.
5. Jones, R. B., et. al. Safe Handling of Chemotherapeutic Agents: A Report from the Mount Sinai Medical Center, CA—A Cancer Journal for Clinicians Sept./Oct., 258–263, 1983.
6. American Society of Hospital Pharmacists Technical Assistance Bulletin on Handling Cytotoxic Drugs in Hospitals. Am. J. Hosp. Pharm. 42:131–137, 1985.

HOW SUPPLIED

Lysodren (mitotane) Tablets, USP
NDC 0015-3080-60—500 mg Tablets, bottle of 100
Tablets may be stored at room temperature.
Shown in Product Identification Section, page 406

MEGACE® ℞

[mĕg ′ace]
(megestrol acetate)
U.S. Patent No. 3,356,573

This is the full text of the latest Official Package Circular dated February 1985 (P1450-04).

THE USE OF PROGESTATIONAL AGENTS DURING THE FIRST FOUR MONTHS OF PREGNANCY IS NOT RECOMMENDED

Progestational agents have been used beginning with the first trimester of pregnancy in an attempt to prevent habitual abortion or treat threatened abortion. There is no adequate evidence that such use is effective and there is evidence of potential harm to the fetus when such drugs are given during the first four months of pregnancy.

Furthermore, in the vast majority of women, the cause of abortion is a defective ovum, which progestational agents could not be expected to influence. In addition, the use of progestational agents, with their uterine-relaxant properties, in patients with fertilized defective ova may cause a delay in spontaneous abortion. Therefore, the use of such drugs during the first four months of pregnancy is not recommended.

Several reports suggest an association between intrauterine exposure to female sex hormones and congenital anomalies, including congenital heart defects and limb reduction defects.[1-5] One study[4] estimated a 4.7-fold increased risk of limb reduction defects in infants exposed *in utero* to sex hormones (oral contraceptives, hormone withdrawal tests for pregnancy, or attempted treatment for threatened abortion).

Some of these exposures were very short and involved only a few days of treatment. The data suggest that the risk of limb reduction defects in exposed fetuses is somewhat less than 1 to 1,000.

If the patient is exposed to Megace during the first four months of pregnancy or if she becomes pregnant while taking this drug, she should be apprised of the potential risks to the fetus.

DESCRIPTION

Megestrol acetate is a white, crystalline solid chemically described as 17α-acetoxy-6-methylpregna-4, 6-diene-3, 20-dione. Its molecular weight is 384.5. Inactive ingredients in Megace Tablets are: acacia, calcium phosphate, FD&C Blue No. 1, Aluminum Lake, lactose, magnesium stearate, silicon dioxide colloidal and starch. The empirical formula is $C_{24}H_{32}O_4$ and the structural formula is:

CH_3 C=O --OCOCH$_3$ O CH_3

MEGESTROL ACETATE*
***U.S. Patent No. 3,356,573**

ACTIONS

While the precise mechanism by which Megace (megestrol acetate) produces its antineoplastic effects against endometrial carcinoma is unknown at the present time, an antiluteinizing effect mediated via the pituitary has been postulated. There is also evidence to suggest a local effect as a result of the marked changes brought about by the direct instillation of progestational agents into the endometrial cavity. Likewise, the antineoplastic action of Megace (megestrol acetate) on carcinoma of the breast is unclear.

INDICATIONS

Megace (megestrol acetate) is indicated for the palliative treatment of advanced carcinoma of the breast or endometrium (i.e., recurrent, inoperable, or metastatic disease). It should not be used in lieu of currently accepted procedures such as surgery, radiation, or chemotherapy.

CONTRAINDICATIONS

As a diagnostic test for pregnancy.

WARNINGS

Administration for up to 7 years of megestrol acetate to female dogs is associated with an increased incidence of both benign and malignant tumors of the breast. Comparable studies in rats and studies in monkeys are not associated with an increased incidence of tumors. The relationship of the dog tumors to humans is unknown but should be considered in assessing the benefit-to-risk ratio when prescribing Megace and in surveillance of patients on therapy.

The use of Megace (megestrol acetate) in other types of neoplastic disease is not recommended.

PRECAUTIONS

There are no specific precautions identified for the use of Megace (megestrol acetate) when used as recommended. Close, customary surveillance is indicated for any patient being treated for recurrent or metastatic cancer. Use with caution in patients with a history of thrombophlebitis.

ADVERSE REACTIONS

No untoward effects have been ascribed to Megace (megestrol acetate) therapy. Reports have been received of patients developing carpal tunnel syndrome, deep vein thrombophlebitis and alopecia while taking megestrol acetate.

OVERDOSAGE

No serious side effects have resulted from studies involving Megace (megestrol acetate) administered in dosages as high as 800 mg/day.

DOSAGE AND ADMINISTRATION

Breast cancer: 160 mg/day (40 q.i.d.)
Endometrial carcinoma: 40—320 mg/day in divided doses.
At least two months of continuous treatment is considered an adequate period for determining the efficacy of Megace (megestrol acetate).

HOW SUPPLIED

Megace® is available as light blue, scored tablets containing 20 mg or 40 mg megestrol acetate.
NDC 0015-0595-01, Bottles of 100 20 mg tablet
NDC 0015-0596-41, Bottles of 100 40 mg tablet
NDC 0015-0596-45, Bottles of 500 40 mg tablet
NDC 0015-0596-46 Bottles of 250 40 mg tablet

REFERENCES

1. Gal I, Kirman B and Stern J: "Hormonal Pregnancy Tests and Congenital Malformation," Nature 216:83, 1967.
2. Levy EP, Cohen A and Fraser FC: "Hormone Treatment During Pregnancy and Congenital Heart Defects," Lancet 1:611, 1973.
3. Nora J and Nora A: "Birth Defects and Oral Contraceptives," Lancet 1:941, 1973.
4. Janerich DT, Piper JM and Glebatis DM: "Oral Contraceptives and Congenital Limb-Reduction Defects," N Eng J Med, 291:697, 1974.
5. Heinonen OP, Slone D, Monson RR, Hook EB and Shapiro S: "Cardiovascular Birth Defects and Antenatal Exposure to Female Sex Hormones," N Eng J Med, 296:67, 1977.

Shown in Product Identification Section, page 406

MEXATE ℞
MEXATE-AQ ℞

Methotrexate Sodium for Injection

This is the full text of the latest Official Package Circular dated December 1985 (3050DIM-12).

WARNINGS

METHOTREXATE MUST BE USED ONLY BY PHYSICIANS EXPERIENCED IN ANTIMETABOLITE CHEMOTHERAPY.

BECAUSE OF THE POSSIBILITY OF FATAL OR SEVERE TOXIC REACTIONS THE PATIENT SHOULD BE FULLY INFORMED BY THE PHYSICIAN OF THE RISKS INVOLVED AND SHOULD BE UNDER HIS CONSTANT SUPERVISION.

DEATHS HAVE BEEN REPORTED WITH THE USE OF METHOTREXATE IN THE TREATMENT OF PSORIASIS. IN THE TREATMENT OF PSORIASIS METHOTREXATE SHOULD BE RESTRICTED TO SEVERE, RECALCITRANT, DISABLING PSORIASIS WHICH IS NOT ADEQUATELY RESPONSIVE TO OTHER FORMS OF THERAPY, BUT ONLY WHEN THE DIAGNOSIS HAS BEEN ESTABLISHED AS BY BIOPSY AND/OR AFTER DERMATOLOGIC CONSULTATION.

1. Methotrexate may produce marked depression of bone marrow, anemia, leukopenia, thrombocytopenia and bleeding.
2. Methotrexate may be hepatotoxic, particularly at high dosage or with prolonged therapy. Liver atrophy, necrosis, cirrhosis, fatty changes, and periportal fibrosis have been reported. Since changes may occur without previous signs of gastrointestinal or hematologic toxicity, it is imperative that hepatic function be determined prior to initiation of treatment and monitored regularly throughout therapy. Special caution is indicated in the presence of preexisting liver damage or impaired hepatic function. Concomitant use of other drugs with hepatotoxic potential (including alcohol) should be avoided.
3. Methotrexate has caused fetal death and/or congenital anomalies, therefore, it is not recommended in women of childbearing potential unless there is appropriate medical evidence that the benefits can be expected to outweigh the considered risks. Pregnant psoriatic patients should not receive methotrexate.
4. Impaired renal function is usually a contraindication.
5. Diarrhea and ulcerative stomatitis are frequent toxic effects and require interruption of therapy; otherwise hemorrhagic enteritis and death from intestinal perforation may occur.

METHOTREXATE HAS BEEN ADMINISTERED IN VERY HIGH DOSAGE FOLLOWED BY LEUCOVORIN RESCUE IN EXPERIMENTAL TREATMENT OF CERTAIN NEOPLASTIC DISEASES. THIS PROCEDURE IS INVESTIGATIONAL AND HAZARDOUS.

DESCRIPTION

Mexate, Mexate-AQ (Methotrexate Sodium) is an antimetabolite used in the treatment of certain neoplastic diseases. Chemically methotrexate is N-p (2,4-diamino-6-pteridinyl) methyl -methylamino benzoyl glutamic acid.

H_2N N N N N CH_3 CH_2N CONH NH_2 $NaOOCCH_2CH_2$ ---C---COOH H

Molecular weight: 454.46

Mexate for injection is 20, 50, 100 and 250 mg single dose vials of lyophilized sterile powder, containing no preservatives, to be administered parenterally.

Each 20 mg vial contains methotrexate, 20 mg. prepared as the sodium salt, sodium hydroxide to adjust pH to about 8.5.

Each 50 mg vial contains methotrexate, 50 mg, prepared as the sodium salt; sodium hydroxide to adjust pH to about 8.5.

Each 100 mg vial contains methotrexate, 100 mg, prepared as the sodium salt, sodium hydroxide to adjust pH to about 8.5.

Each 250 mg vial contains methotrexate, 250 mg, prepared as the sodium salt; sodium hydroxide to adjust pH to about 8.5.

Mexate-AQ, isotonic, preservative-free, single use only, is available in 2 ml (50 mg), 4 ml (100 mg), and 10 ml (250 mg) vials.

Each 25 mg/ml, 2 ml (50 mg) vial contains: Methotrexate Sodium equivalent to 50 mg Methotrexate, and the following inactive ingredients: Sodium Chloride 0.490% w/v and Water for Injection qs ad 100% V. Sodium Hydroxide and, if necessary, Hydrochloric Acid to adjust pH to approx. 8.5. Contains approximately 0.4 milliequivalents of sodium per vial and is an isotonic solution.

Each 25 mg/ml, 4 ml (100 mg) vial contains: Methotrexate Sodium equivalent to 100 mg Methotrexate, and the following inactive ingredients: Sodium Chloride 0.490% w/v and Water for Injection qs ad 100% V. Sodium Hydroxide, and, if necessary, Hydrochloric Acid to adjust pH to approx. 8.5. Contains approximately 0.87 milliequivalents of sodium per vial and is an isotonic solution.

Each 25 mg/ml, 10 ml (250 mg) vial contains: Methotrexate Sodium equivalent to 250 mg Methotrexate and the following inactive ingredients: Sodium Chloride 0.490% w/v and Water for Injection qs ad 100% V. Sodium Hydroxide and, if necessary, Hydrochloric Acid to adjust pH to approx. 8.5. Contains approximately 2.17 milliequivalents of sodium per vial and is an isotonic solution.

If desired, the solution may be further diluted immediately prior to use with an appropriate sterile preservative-free

medium such as 5% Dextrose Solution, USP or Sodium Chloride Injection, USP.
Mexate for Injection is available in 20, 50, 100 and 250 mg single dose vials of lyophilized sterile powder, containing no preservatives, to be administered parenterally.
Each 20 mg vial contains methotrexate, 20 mg, prepared as the sodium salt; sodium hydroxide to adjust pH to about 8.5.
Each 50 mg vial contains methotrexate, 50 mg, prepared as the sodium salt; sodium hydroxide to adjust pH to about 8.5.
Each 100 mg vial contains methotrexate, 100 mg, prepared as the sodium salt; sodium hydroxide to adjust pH to about 8.5.
Each 250 mg vial contains methotrexate, 250 mg, prepared as the sodium salt; sodium hydroxide to adjust pH to about 8.5.

CLINICAL PHARMACOLOGY

Mexate, Mexate-AQ (Methotrexate Sodium) has as its principle mechanism of action the competitive inhibition of the enzyme folic acid reductase. Folic acid must be reduced to tetrahydrofolic acid by this enzyme in the process of DNA synthesis and cellular replication. Methotrexate inhibits the reduction of folic acid and interferes with tissue-cell reproduction.
Actively proliferating tissues such as malignant cells, bone marrow, fetal cells, dermal epithelium, buccal and intestinal mucosa and cells of the urinary bladder are in general more sensitive to this effect of methotrexate. Cellular proliferation in malignant tissue is greater than in most normal tissue and thus methotrexate may impair malignant growth without irreversible damage to normal tissues.
After intramuscular injection, peak serum levels are seen in about 30 to 60 minutes. Methotrexate is reversibly bound to serum protein, but exchanges with body fluids easily and diffuses into the body tissue cells. Most studies suggest less than 90% protein binding.
Excretion of single daily doses occurs through the kidneys in amounts from 55% to 88% or higher within 24 hours. Repeated doses daily result in more sustained serum levels and some retention of methotrexate over each 24 hour period which may result in accumulation of the drug within the tissues. The liver cells appear to retain certain amounts of the drug for prolonged periods even after a single therapeutic dose. Methotrexate is retained in the presence of impaired renal function and may increase rapidly in the serum and in the tissue cells under such conditions. Methotrexate does not penetrate the blood cerebrospinal fluid barrier in therapeutic amounts when given parenterally. High concentrations of the drug when needed may be attained by direct intrathecal administration.
In psoriasis, the rate of production of epithelial cells in the skin is greatly increased over normal skin. This differential in reproductive rates is the basis for the use of methotrexate to control the psoriatic process.

INDICATIONS

Anti-neoplastic Chemotherapy: Methotrexate is indicated for the treatment of gestational choriocarcinoma, and in patients with chorioadenoma destruens and hydatidiform mole.
Methotrexate is indicated for the palliation of acute lymphocytic leukemia. It is also indicated in the treatment and prophylaxis of meningeal leukemia. Greatest effect has been observed in palliation of acute lymphoblastic (stem-cell) leukemias in children. In combination with other anticancer drugs or suitable agents methotrexate may be used for induction of remission, but it is most commonly used, as described in the literature, in the maintenance of induced remissions.
Methotrexate may be used alone or in combination with other anticancer agents in the management of breast cancer, epidermoid cancers of the head and neck, and lung cancer, particularly squamous cell and small cell types.
Methotrexate is also effective in the treatment of the advanced stages (III and IV, Peters Staging Systems) of lymphosarcoma, particularly in those cases in children; and in advanced cases of mycosis fungoides.
Psoriasis Chemotherapy (See box warnings at top of insert.)
Because of high risk attending its use, methotrexate is only indicated in the symptomatic control of severe, recalcitrant, disabling psoriasis which is not adequately responsive to other forms of therapy, but only when the diagnosis has been established, as by biopsy and/or after dermatologic consultation.

CONTRAINDICATIONS

Patients with known hypersensitivity to methotrexate. Pregnant psoriatic patients should not receive methotrexate. Psoriatic patients with severe renal or hepatic disorders should not receive methotrexate. Psoriatic patients with preexisting blood dyscrasias, such as bone marrow hypoplasia, leukopenia, thrombocytopenia or anemia, should not receive methotrexate.

WARNINGS

See Box Warnings

PRECAUTIONS

Methotrexate has a high potential toxicity, usually dose-related. The physician should be familiar with the various characteristics of the drug and its established clinical usage. Patients undergoing therapy should be subject to appropriate supervision so that signs or symptoms of possible toxic effects or adverse reactions may be detected and evaluated with minimal delay. Pretreatment and periodic hematologic studies are essential to the use of methotrexate in chemotherapy because of its common effect of hematopoietic suppression. This may occur abruptly and with apparent safe dosage, and any profound drop in blood-cell count indicates immediate stopping of the drug and the initiation of appropriate therapy. In patients with malignant disease who have pre-existing bone marrow aplasia, leukopenia, thrombocytopenia or anemia, the drug should be used with caution, if at all.
Methotrexate is excreted principally by the kidneys. Its use in the presence of impaired renal function may result in accumulation of toxic amounts or even additional renal damage. The patient's renal status should be determined prior to and during methotrexate therapy and proper caution excercised should significant renal impairment be disclosed. Drug dosage should be reduced or discontinued until renal function is improved or restored.
In general, the following laboratory tests are recommended as part of essential clinical evaluation and appropriate monitoring of patients chosen for or receiving methotrexate therapy: complete hemogram; hematocrit; urinalysis; renal function test; and liver function tests. A chest x-ray is also recommended. The purpose is to determine any existing organ dysfunction or system impairment. The tests should be performed prior to therapy, at appropriate periods during therapy and after termination of therapy. It may be useful or important to perform liver biopsy or bone marrow aspiration studies where high dose or long-term therapy is being followed.
Methotrexate is predominantly bound to serum albumin and toxicity may be increased because of displacement by certain drugs such as salicylates, sulfonamides, diphenylhydantoin, phenylbutazone, and some antibacterials as tetracycline, chloramphenicol and para-amino-benzoic acid. These drugs, especially salicylates, phenylbutazone and sulfonamides, whether antibacterial, hypoglycemic or diuretic, should not be given concurrently until the significance of these findings is established.
Vitamin preparations containing folic acid or its derivatives may alter responses to methotrexate.
Methotrexate should be used with extreme caution in the presence of infection, peptic ulcer, ulcerative colitis, debility, and in extreme youth and old age.
If profound leukopenia occurs during therapy, bacterial infection may occur or become a threat. Cessation of the drug and appropriate antibiotic therapy is usually indicated. In severe bone marrow depression, blood or platelet transfusions may be necessary.
Since it is reported that methotrexate may have an immunosuppressive action, this factor must be taken into consideration in evaluating the use of the drug where immune responses in a patient may be important or essential.
Carcinogenesis, Mutagenesis, Impairment of Fertility: Like most other anticancer agents, methotrexate might have a carcinogenic potential (See "BOX WARNINGS")
Pregnancy:
Pregnancy "Category D"—Methotrexate has caused fetal death and/or congenital anomalies and is therefore not recommended in women of childbearing potential unless there is appropriate medical evidence that the benefits to the mother can be expected to outweigh the considered risks to the fetus. Pregnant psoriatic patients should not receive methotrexate (see "BOX WARNINGS").
Nursing Mothers:
Because of the potential for serious adverse reactions in nursing infants from methotrexate, a decision should be made whether to discontinue nursing or to discontinue the drug, taking into account the importance of the drug to the mother.
In all instances where the use of methotrexate is considered for chemotherapy, the physician must evaluate the need and usefulness of the drug against the risks of toxic effects or adverse reaction. Most such adverse reactions are reversible if detected early. When such effects or reactions do occur, the drug should be reduced in dosage or discontinued and appropriate corrective measures should be taken, according to the clinical judgment of the physician. Reinstitution of methotrexate therapy should be carried out with caution, with adequate consideration of further need for the drug and alertness as to possible recurrence of toxicity.

ADVERSE REACTIONS

The most common adverse reactions include ulcerative stomatitis, leukopenia, nausea and abdominal distress. Others reported are malaise, undue fatigue, chills and fever, dizziness and decreased resistance to infection. In general, the incidence and severity of side effects are considered to be dose-related. Adverse reactions as reported for the various systems are as follows:
Skin: Erythematous rashes, pruritus, urticaria, photosensitivity, depigmentation, alopecia, ecchymosis, telangiectasia, acne, furunculosis. Lesions of psoriasis may be aggravated by concomitant exposure to ultraviolet radiation.
Blood: bone marrow depression, leukopenia, thrombocytopenia, anemia, hypogammaglobulinemia, hemorrhage from various sites, septicemia.
Alimentary System: gingivitis, pharyngitis, stomatitis, anorexia, vomiting, diarrhea, hematemesis, melena, gastrointestinal ulceration and bleeding, enteritis, hepatic toxicity resulting in acute liver atrophy, necrosis, fatty metamorphosis, periportal fibrosis, or hepatic cirrhosis.
Urogenital System: renal failure, azotemia, cystitis, hematuria; defective oogenesis or spermatogenesis, transient oligospermia, menstrual dysfunction; infertility, abortion, fetal defects, severe nephropathy.
Pulmonary System: Interstitial Pneumonitis. Deaths have been reported and chronic interstitial obstructive pulmonary disease has occasionally occurred.
Central Nervous System: headaches, drowsiness, blurred vision. Aphasia, hemiparesis, paresis and convulsions have also occurred following administration of methotrexate. There have been reports of leucoencephalopathy following intravenous administration of methotrexate to patients who have had craniospinal irradiation.
After the intrathecal use of methotrexate, the central nervous system toxicity which may occur can be classified as follows:
(1) chemical arachnoiditis manifested by such symptoms as headache, back pain, vomiting, nuchal rigidity, fever.
(2) paresis, usually transient, manifested by paraplegia associated with involvement with one or more spinal nerve roots.
(3) leucoencephalopathy manifested by confusion, dysarthria, irritability, somnolence, ataxia, dementia, and occasionally major convulsions and coma.

Other reactions related to or attributed to the use of methotrexate, such as interstitial pneumonitis; metabolic changes precipitating diabetes; osteoporotic effects, abnormal tissue cell changes, and sudden death have been reported.

DOSAGE AND ADMINISTRATION

Anti-neoplastic Chemotherapy
Mexate, Mexate-AQ may be given by intramuscular, intravenous, intra-arterial or intrathecal route. Initial treatment is usually undertaken with the patient under hospital care.
* For conversion of mg/kg b.w. to mg/M2 of body surface or the reverse, a ratio of 1:30 is given as a guideline. The conversion factor varies between 1:20 and 1:40 depending on age and body fluid.

Choriocarcinoma and similar trophoblastic diseases: Methotrexate is administered intramuscularly in doses of 15 to 30 mg daily for a 5-day course. Such courses are usually repeated 3 to 5 times as required, with rest periods of one or more weeks interposed between courses, until any manifesting toxic symptoms subside. The effectiveness of therapy is ordinarily evaluated by 24-hour urine quantitative analysis of urinary chorionic gonadotropin hormone (CGH) which should return to normal or less than 50 IU/24 hours usually after the 3rd or 4th course and usually be followed by a complete resolution of measurable lesions in 4 to 6 weeks. One to 2 courses of methotrexate after normalization of CGH is usually recommended.
Before each course of the drug, careful clinical assessment is essential. Cyclic combination therapy of methotrexate with other antitumor drugs has been reported as being useful.
Since hydatidiform mole may precede choriocarcinoma, prophylactic chemotherapy with methotrexate has been recommended. Chorioadenoma destruens is considered to be an invasive form of hydatidiform mole. Methotrexate is administered in these disease states in doses similar to those recommended for choriocarcinoma.
Leukemia: Acute lymphatic (lymphoblastic) leukemia in children and young adolescents is the most responsive to present-day chemotherapy. In young adults and older patients, clinical remission is more difficult to obtain and early relapse is more common. In chronic lymphatic leukemia, the prognosis for adequate response is less encouraging.
Methotrexate alone or in combination with steroids was used initially for induction of remission of lymphoblastic leukemias. More recently corticosteroid therapy, in combination with other antileukemic drugs or in cyclic combinations with methotrexate included, appears to produce rapid and effective remissions. When used for induction, methotrexate in doses of 3.3 mg/M2 in combination with prednisone 60 mg/M2, given daily, produced remission in 50% of patients treated, usually within a period of 4 to 6 weeks.
Methotrexate alone or in combination with other agents appears to be the drug of choice for securing maintenance of drug induced remissions. When remission is achieved and

Continued on next page

Bristol-Myers Oncology—Cont.

supportive care has produced general clinical improvement, maintenance therapy is initiated, as follows: methotrexate is administered 2 times weekly intramuscularly in doses of 30 mg/M2. It has also been given in doses of 2.5 mg/kg intravenously every 14 days. If and when relapse does occur, reinduction of remission can again usually be obtained by repeating the initial induction regimen. Various experts have recently introduced a variety of dosage schedules for both induction and maintenance of remission with various combinations of alkylating and antifolic agents. Multiple drug therapy with several agents, including methotrexate, given concomitantly is gaining increasing support in both the acute and chronic forms of leukemia.

Acute granulocytic leukemia is rare in children but common in adults. This form of leukemia responds poorly to chemotherapy and remissions are short with relapses common, and resistance to therapy develops rapidly.

Meningeal leukemia: Patients with leukemia are subject to leukemic invasion of the central nervous system. This may manifest characteristic signs or symptoms or may remain silent and be diagnosed only by examination of the cerebrospinal fluid which contains leukemic cells in such cases. Therefore, the CSF should be examined in all leukemic patients. Since passage of methotrexate from blood serum to the cerebrospinal fluid is minimal, for adequate therapy the drug is administered intrathecally. It is now common practice because of the noted increased frequency of meningeal leukemia to administer methotrexate intrathecally as prophylaxis in all cases of lymphocytic leukemia.

By intrathecal injection, the sodium salt of methotrexate is administered in solution in doses of 12 mg per square meter of body surface or in an empirical dose of 15 mg. The solution is made in a strength of 1 mg per ml with an appropriate, sterile, preservative-free medium such as Sodium Chloride Injection, U.S.P.

For the treatment of meningeal leukemia, methotrexate is given at intervals of 2 to 5 days. Methotrexate is administered until the cell count of the cerebrospinal fluid returns to normal. At this point one additional dose is advisable.

For prophylaxis against meningeal leukemia, the dosage is the same as for treatment except for the intervals of administration. On this subject, it is advisable for the physician to consult the medical literature.

Large doses may cause convulsions. Untoward side effects may occur with any given intrathecal injection and are commonly neurological in character. Methotrexate given by the intrathecal route appears significantly in the systemic circulation and may cause systemic methotrexate toxicity. Therefore systemic antileukemic therapy with the drug should be appropriately adjusted, reduced or discontinued. Focal leukemic involvement of the central nervous system may not respond to intrathecal chemotherapy and is best treated with radiotherapy.

Lymphomas: In Burkitt's tumor, stages I—II, methotrexate has produced prolonged remissions in some cases. In stage III methotrexate is often given concomitantly with other antitumor agents. Treatment in all stages usually consists of several courses of the drug interposed with 7 to 10 day rest periods. Lymphosarcomas in stage III may respond to combined drug therapy with methotrexate given in doses of 0.625 mg to 2.5 mg/kg daily.

Mycosis fungoides: Therapy with methotrexate appears to produce clinical remissions in about one half of the cases treated. Dosage is usually 2.5 to 10 mg daily by mouth for weeks or months. Methotrexate has also been given intramuscularly in doses of 50 mg once weekly or 25 mg twice weekly. Drug dose levels and their subsequent adjustment are guided by patient response and hematologic monitoring.

Psoriasis Chemotherapy

The patient should be fully informed of the risks involved and should be under the constant supervision of a physician.

Assessment of renal function, liver function, and blood elements should be made by history, physical examination, and laboratory tests (such as CBC, urinalysis, serum creatinine, liver function studies, and liver biopsy if indicated) before beginning methotrexate, periodically during methotrexate therapy, and before reinstituting methotrexate therapy after a rest period. Appropriate steps should be taken to avoid conception during and for at least 8 weeks following methotrexate therapy.

There are 3 commonly used general types of dosage schedules:

1. weekly oral or parenteral intermittent large doses
2. divided dose intermittent oral schedule over a 36-hour period
3. daily oral dose with a rest period

All schedules should be continually tailored to the individual patient. Dose schedules cited below pertain to an average 70 Kg adult. An initial test dose one week prior to initiation of therapy is recommended to detect any idiosyncrasy. A suggested dose range is 5 to 10 mg parenterally.

Recommended starting dose schedules:

1. Weekly single oral, IM or IV dose schedule: 10–25 mg per week until adequate response is achieved. With this dosage schedule, 50 mg per week should ordinarily not be exceeded.
2. Divided oral dose schedule: 2.5 mg at 12 hour intervals for three doses or at 8 hour intervals for four doses each week. With this dosage schedule, 30 mg per week should not be exceeded.
3. Daily oral dose schedule: 2.5 mg daily for five days followed by at least a two day rest period. With this dosage schedule, 6.25 mg per day should not be exceeded.

Special Note

Available data suggest that schedule 3 (daily oral dose with a rest period) may carry an increased risk of serious liver pathology.

Dosages may be gradually adjusted to achieve optimal clinical response, but not to exceed the maximum stated in the schedule.

Once optimal clinical response has been achieved, the dosage schedule should be reduced to the lowest possible amount of drug and to the longest possible rest period. The use of methotrexate may permit the return to conventional topical therapy, which should be encouraged.

Antidote for Overdosage

Leucovorin (citrovorum factor) is a potent agent for neutralizing the immediate toxic effects of methotrexate on the hematopoietic system. Where large doses or overdoses are given, Calcium Leucovorin may be administered by intravenous infusion in doses up to 75 mg within 12 hours, followed by 12 mg intramuscularly every 6 hours for 4 doses. Where average doses of methotrexate appear to have an adverse effect, 2 to 4 ml (6 to 12 mg) of Calcium Leocovorin may be given intramuscularly every 6 hours for 4 doses. In general, where overdosage is suspected, the dose of Leucovorin should be equal to or higher than the offending dose of methotrexate and should best be administered within the first hour. Use of Calcium Leucovorin after an hour delay is much less effective.

CAUTION

Pharmacist: Because of its potential to cause severe toxicity, methotrexate therapy requires close supervision of the patient by the physician. Pharmacists should dispense no more than a 7-day supply of the drug at one time. Refill of such prescriptions should be by direct order (written or oral) of the physician only.

DIRECTIONS FOR USE

As with other potentially toxic compounds, caution should be exercised in handling the powder or the solution of methotrexate. Skin reactions associated with accidental exposure to Mexate may occur. The use of gloves is recommended. If Mexate powder or solution contact skin or mucosa, immediately wash the skin or mucosa thoroughly with soap and water.

Parenteral drug products should be inspected visually for particulate matter and discoloration prior to administration, whenever solution and container permit.

MEXATE (METHOTREXATE SODIUM) FOR INJECTION

Intramuscular or intravenous administration: reconstitute with 2 to 10 ml of Sterile Water for Injection, USP, 0.9% Sodium Chloride Injection, USP, or Bacteriostatic Water for Injection, USP with Parabens or Benzyl Alcohol.

Intrathecal administration: reconstitute immediately prior to use with an appropriate sterile, preservative-free medium such as 0.9% Sodium Chloride Injection, USP. The concentration for intrathecal injection should be 1 mg to 2.5 mg/ml.

MEXATE-AQ (MEXTHOTREXATE SODIUM) INJECTION

This preservative-free preparation may be given by the intramuscular, intravenous and intrathecal routes.

STABILITY

Mexate (Methotrexate Sodium) for Injection is stable for four weeks at room temperature (25°C) at concentrations of 2 to 125 mg/ml in Bacteriostatic Water for Injection, USP with Parabens or Benzyl Alcohol. These solutions are stable for three months under refrigeration (4°C) or frozen (−15°C).

Mexate-AQ (Methotrexate Sodium) Injection. Vials are stable to expiration date shown on container label.

Procedures for proper handling and disposal of anti-cancer drugs should be considered: Several guidelines on this subject had been published.[1–4] There is no general agreement that all of the procedures recommended in the guidelines are necessary or appropriate.

REFERENCES

1. Recommendations for the Safe Handling of Parenteral Antineoplastic Drugs. NIH Publication No. 83-2621. For sale by the Superintendent of Documents, U.S. Government Printing Office, Washington, D.C. 20402.
2. AMA Council Report. Guidelines for Handling Parenteral Antineoplastics. JAMA, March 15, 1985.
3. National Study Commission on Cytotoxic Exposure—Recommendations for Handling Cytotoxic Agents. Available from Louis P. Jeffrey, Sc. D., Director of Pharmacy Services, Rhode Island Hospital, 593 Eddy Street, Providence, Rhode Island 02902.
4. Clinical Oncological Society of Australia: Guidelines and Recommendations for Safe Handling of Antineoplastic Agents. Med. J. Australia 1:426–428, 1983.
5. Jones, R. B., et. al. Safe Handling of Chemotherapeutic Agents: A Report from the Mount Sinai Medical Center. Ca—A Cancer Journal for Clinicians Sept./Oct., 258–263, 1983.
6. American Society of Hospital Pharmacists Technical Assistance Bulletin on Handling Cytotoxic Drugs in Hospitals. Am. J. Hosp. Pharm. 42:131–137, 1985.

HOW SUPPLIED

Mexate (methotrexate sodium) for Injection.

NDC 0015-3050-20 20 mg vial
NDC 0015-3051-20 50 mg vial
NDC 0015-3052-20 100 mg vial
NDC 0015-3053-20 250 mg vial

Mexate-AQ (methotrexate sodium) for Injection:

NDC-0015-3006-20 Each vial contains 50 mg of methotrexate in 2 ml.
NDC-0015-3007-20 Each vial contains 100 mg of methotrexate in 4 ml.
NDC-0015-3008-20 Each vial contains 250 mg of methotrexate in 10 ml.

Shown in Product Identification Section, page 406

MUTAMYCIN® ℞

[mū″-tē-mī′-sĭn]
(mitomycin for injection)

This is the full text of the latest Official Package Circular dated December 1985 [3001DIM-21].

WARNING

Mutamycin should be administered under the supervision of a qualified physician experienced in the use of cancer chemotherapeutic agents. Appropriate management of therapy and complications is possible only when adequate diagnostic and treatment facilities are readily available.

Bone marrow suppression, notably thrombocytopenia and leukopenia, which may contribute to overwhelming infections in an already compromised patient, is the most common and severe of the toxic effects of Mutamycin (see "Warnings" and "Adverse Reactions" sections).

Hemolytic Uremic Syndrome (HUS)—A serious, and often fatal, syndrome consisting of microangiopathic hemolytic anemia, thrombocytopenia, renal failure and hypertension has been reported in patients receiving Mutamycin. Most of these patients received long-term therapy (6 to 12 months) with Mutamycin in combination with fluorouracil; however, some patients received Mutamycin in combination with other drugs or were treated for less than 6 months.

DESCRIPTION

Mutamycin (also known as mitomycin and/or mitomycin-C) is an antibiotic isolated from the broth of **Streptomyces caespitosus** which has been shown to have antitumor activity. The compound is heat stable, has a high melting point, and is freely soluble in organic solvents.

ACTION

Mutamycin selectively inhibits the synthesis of deoxyribonucleic acid (DNA). The guanine and cytosine content correlates with the degree of Mutamycin-induced cross-linking. At high concentrations of the drug, cellular RNA and protein synthesis are also suppressed.

In humans, Mutamycin is rapidly cleared from the serum after intravenous administration. Time required to reduce the serum concentration by 50% after a 30 mg. bolus injection is 17 minutes. After injection of 30 mg., 20 mg., or 10 mg. I.V., the maximal serum concentrations were 2.4 mcg./ml., 1.7 mcg./ml., and 0.52 mcg./ml., respectively. Clearance is effected primarily by metabolism in the liver, but metabolism occurs in other tissues as well. The rate of clearance is inversely proportional to the maximal serum concentration because, it is thought, of saturation of the degradative pathways.

Approximately 10% of a dose of Mutamycin is excreted unchanged in the urine. Since metabolic pathways are saturated at relatively low doses, the percent of a dose excreted in urine increases with increasing dose. In children, excretion of intravenously administered Mutamycin is similar.

Animal Toxicology—Mutamycin has been found to be carcinogenic in rats and mice. At doses approximating the recommended clinical dose in man, it produces a greater than 100 percent increase in tumor incidence in male Sprague-Dawley rats, and a greater than 50 percent increase in tumor incidence in female Swiss mice.

INDICATIONS
Mutamycin is not recommended as single-agent, primary therapy. It has been shown to be useful in the therapy of disseminated adenocarcinoma of the stomach or pancreas in proven combinations with other approved chemotherapeutic agents and as palliative treatment when other modalities have failed. Mutamycin is not recommended to replace appropriate surgery and /or radiotherapy.

CONTRAINDICATIONS
Mutamycin is contraindicated in patients who have demonstrated a hypersensitive or idiosyncratic reaction to it in the past.
Mutamycin is contraindicated in patients with thrombocytopenia, coagulation disorder, or an increase in bleeding tendency due to other causes.

WARNINGS
Patients being treated with Mutamycin must be observed carefully and frequently during and after therapy.
The use of Mutamycin results in a high incidence of bone marrow suppression, particularly thrombocytopenia and leukopenia. Therefore, the following studies should be obtained repeatedly during therapy and for at least 8 weeks following therapy: platelet count, white blood cell count, differential, and hemoglobin. The occurrence of a platelet count below 150,000/mm^3 or a WBC below 4,000/mm^3 or a progressive decline in either is an indication for interruption of therapy.
Patients should be advised of the potential toxicity of this drug, particularly bone marrow suppression. Deaths have been reported due to septicemia as a result of leukopenia due to the drug.
Patients receiving Mutamycin should be observed for evidence of renal toxicity. Mutamycin should not be given to patients with a serum creatinine greater than 1.7 mg. percent.
Usage in Pregnancy—Safe use of Mutamycin in pregnant women has not been established. Teratological changes have been noted in animal studies. The effect of Mutamycin on fertility is unknown.

ADVERSE REACTIONS
Bone Marrow Toxicity— This was the most common and most serious toxicity, occurring in 605 of 937 patients (64.4%). Thrombocytopenia and/or leukopenia may occur anytime within 8 weeks after onset of therapy with an average time of 4 weeks. Recovery after cessation of therapy was within 10 weeks. About 25% of the leukopenic or thrombocytopenic episodes did not recover. Mutamycin produces cumulative myelosuppression.
Integument and Mucus Membrane Toxicity— This has occurred in approximately 4% of patients treated with Mutamycin. Cellulitis at the injection site has been reported and is occasionally severe. Stomatitis and alopecia also occur frequently. Rashes are rarely reported. The most important dermatological problem with this drug, however, is the necrosis and consequent sloughing of tissue which results if the drug is extravasated during injection. Extravasation may occur with or without an accompanying stinging or burning sensation and even if there is adequate blood return when the injection needle is aspirated. There have been reports of delaying erythema and/or ulceration occurring either at or distant from the injection site, weeks to months after Mutamycin, even when no obvious evidence of extravasation was observed during administration. Skin grafting has been required in some cases.
Renal Toxicity—2% of 1,281 patients demonstrated a statistically significant rise in creatinine. There appeared to be no correlation between total dose administered or duration of therapy and the degree of renal impairment.
Pulmonary Toxicity—This has occurred infrequently but can be severe. Dyspnea with a nonproductive cough and radiographic evidence of pulmonary infiltrates may be indicative of Mutamycin-induced pulmonary toxicity. If other etiologies are eliminated, Mutamycin therapy should be discontinued. Steroids have been employed as treatment of this toxicity, but the therapeutic value has not been determined.
Hemolytic Uremic Syndrome (HUS)—A serious, and often fatal, syndrome consisting of microangiopathic hemolytic anemia, thrombocytopenia, renal failure and hypertension has been reported in patients receiving Mutamycin. Most of these patients received long-term therapy (6 to 12 months) with Mutamycin in combination with fluorouracil; however, some patients received Mutamycin in combination with other drugs or were treated for less than 6 months.
Acute Side Effects Due to Mutamycin were fever, anorexia, nausea, and vomiting. They occurred in about 14% of 1,281 patients.
Other Undesirable Side Effects that have been reported during Mutamycin therapy have been headache, blurring of vision, confusion, drowsiness, syncope, fatigue, edema, thrombophlebitis, hematemesis, diarrhea, and pain. These did not appear to be dose related and were not unequivocally drug related. They may have been due to the primary or metastatic disease processes.

DOSAGE AND ADMINISTRATION
Mutamycin should be given intravenously only, using care to avoid extravasation of the compound. If extravasation occurs, cellulitis, ulceration, and slough may result.
Each vial contains either mitomycin 5 mg. and mannitol 10 mg. or mitomycin 20 mg. and mannitol 40 mg. To administer, add Sterile Water for Injection, 10 ml. or 40 ml. respectively. Shake to dissolve. If product does not dissolve immediately, allow to stand at room temperature until solution is obtained.
After full hematological recovery (see guide to dosage adjustment) from any previous chemotherapy, the following dosage schedule may be used at 6 to 8 week intervals.

20 mg./M.^{2} intravenously as a single dose via a functioning intravenous catheter.

Because of cumulative myelosuppression, patients should be fully reevaluated after each course of Mutamycin, and the dose reduced if the patient has experienced any toxicities. Doses greater than 20 mg./M.^{2} have not been shown to be more effective, and are more toxic than lower doses.
The following schedule is suggested as a guide to dosage adjustment:

Nadir After Prior Dose		Percentage of Prior Dose to be Given
Leukocytes	Platelets	
> 4000	> 100,000	100%
3000–3999	75,000–99,999	100%
2000–2999	25,000–74,999	70%
< 2000	< 25,000	50%

No repeat dosage should be given until leukocyte count has returned to 3000 and platelet count to 75,000.
When Mutamycin is used in combination with other myelosuppressive agents, the doses should be adjusted accordingly. If the disease continues to progress after two courses of Mutamycin, the drug should be stopped since chances of response are minimal.

STABILITY
1. **Unreconstituted** Mutamycin is stable for at least 4 years at room temperature. Avoid excessive heat (over 40°C).
2. **Reconstituted** with Sterile Water for Injection to a concentration of 0.5 mg. per ml., Mutamycin is stable for 14 days refrigerated or 7 days at room temperature.
3. **Diluted** in various IV fluids at room temperature, to a concentration of 20 to 40 micrograms per ml:

IV Fluid	Stability
5% Dextrose Injection	3 hours
0.9% Sodium Chloride Injection	12 hours
Sodium Lactate Injection	24 hours

4. **The combination** of Mutamycin (5 mg. to 15 mg.) and heparin (1,000 units to 10,000 units) in 30 ml. of 0.9% Sodium Chloride Injection is stable for 48 hours at room temperature.

Procedures for proper handling and disposal of anti-cancer drugs should be considered. Several guidelines on this subject had been published.[1–6] There is no general agreement that all of the procedures recommended in the guidelines are necessary or appropriate.

REFERENCES
1. Recommendations for the Safe Handling of Parenteral Antineoplastic Drugs. NIH Publication No. 83-2621. For sale by the Superintendent of Documents, U.S. Government Printing Office, Washington, D.C. 20402.
2. AMA Council Report. Guidelines for Handling Parenteral Antineoplastics, JAMA, March 15, 1985.
3. National Study Commission on Cytotoxic Exposure—Recommendations for Handling Cytotoxic Agents. Available from Louis P. Jeffrey, Sc. D., Director of Pharmacy Services, Rhode Island Hospital, 593 Eddy Street, Providence, Rhode Island 02902.
4. Clinical Oncological Society of Australia: Guidelines and Recommendations for Safe Handling of Antineoplastic Agents. Med. J. Australia 1:426–428, 1983.
5. Jones, R. B., et. al. Safe Handling of Chemotherapeutic Agents: A Report from the Mount Sinai Medical Center, Ca—A Cancer Journal for Clinicians Sept./Oct., 258–263, 1983.
6. American Society of Hospital Pharmacists Technical Assistance Bulletin on Handling Cytotoxic Drugs in Hospitals, Am. J. Hosp. Pharm. 42:131–137, 1985.

SUPPLY
Mutamycin (mitomycin) for Injection.
NDC 0015-3001-20—Each vial contains 5 mg. mitomycin.
NDC 0015-3002-20—Each vial contains 20 mg. mitomycin.

PLATINOL® ℞
[plă 'tĭ-nŏl"]
(cisplatin for injection)

This is the full text of the latest Official Package Circular dated December 1985 (3070 DIM-25).

> **WARNING**
> Platinol (cisplatin) should be administered under the supervision of a qualified physician experienced in the use of cancer chemotherapeutic agents. Appropriate management of therapy and complications is possible only when adequate diagnostic and treatment facilities are readily available.
> Cumulative renal toxicity associated with Platinol is severe. Other major dose-related toxicities are myelosuppression and nausea and vomiting.
> Ototoxicity, which may be more pronounced in children, and is manifested by tinnitus, and/or loss of high frequency hearing and occasionally deafness, is significant.
> *Anaphylactic-like* reactions to Platinol have been reported. Facial edema, bronchoconstriction, tachycardia, and hypotension may occur within minutes of Platinol administration. Epinephrine, corticosteroids, and antihistamines have been effectively employed to alleviate symptoms (see "Warnings" and "Adverse Reactions" sections).

DESCRIPTION
Platinol (cisplatin) (cis-diamminedichloroplatinum) is a heavy metal complex containing a central atom of platinum surrounded by two chloride atoms and two ammonia molecules in the cis position. It is a white lyophylized powder with the molecular formula Pt $Cl_2H_6N_2$, and a molecular weight of 300.1. It is soluble in water or saline at 1 mg/ml and in dimethylformamide at 24 mg/ml. It has a melting point of 207°C.

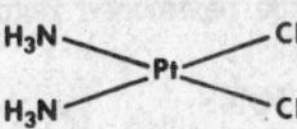

ACTION
Platinol has biochemical properties similar to those of bifunctional alkylating agents producing interstrand and intrastrand crosslinks in DNA. It is apparently cell-cycle nonspecific. Following a single I.V. dose, Platinol concentrates in liver, kidneys, and large and small intestines in animals and humans. Platinol apparently has poor penetration into the CNS.
Plasma levels of radioactivity decay in a biphasic manner after an I.V. bolus dose of radioactive Platinol to patients. The initial plasma half-life is 25 to 49 minutes, and the post-distribution plasma half-life is 58 to 73 hours. During the post-distribution phase, greater than 90% of the radioactivity in the blood is protein bound. Platinol is excreted primarily in the urine. However, urinary excretion is incomplete with only 27 to 43% of the radioactivity being excreted within the first 5 days post-dose in human beings. There are insufficient data to determine whether biliary or intestinal excretion occurs.

INDICATIONS
Platinol is indicated as palliative therapy to be employed as follows:
Metastatic Testicular Tumors—in established combination therapy with other approved chemotherapeutic agents in patients with metastatic testicular tumors who have already received appropriate surgical and/or radiotherapeutic procedures. An established combination therapy consists of Platinol, Blenoxane (Bleomycin Sulfate) and Velban (Vinblastine Sulfate).
Metastatic Ovarian Tumors—in established combination therapy with other approved chemotherapeutic agents in patients with metastatic ovarian tumors who have already received appropriate surgical and/or radiotherapeutic procedures. An established combination consists of Platinol and Adriamycin (Doxorubicin Hydrochloride). Platinol, as a single agent, is indicated as secondary therapy in patients with metastatic ovarian tumors refractory to standard chemotherapy who have not previously received Platinol therapy.
Advanced Bladder Cancer—Platinol is indicated as a single agent for patients with transitional cell bladder cancer which is no longer amenable to local treatments such as surgery and/or radiotherapy.

CONTRAINDICATIONS
Platinol is contraindicated in patients with preexisting renal impairment. Platinal should not be employed in myelosuppressed patients, or patients with hearing impairment.

Continued on next page

Bristol-Myers Oncology—Cont.

Platinol is contraindicated in patients with a history of allergic reactions to Platinol or other platinum-containing compounds.

WARNINGS

Platinol produces cumulative nephrotoxicity which is potentiated by aminoglycoside antibiotics. The serum creatinine, BUN, creatinine clearance and magnesium, potassium and calcium levels should be measured prior to initiating therapy, and prior to each subsequent course. At the recommended dosage, Platinol should not be given more frequently than once every 3 to 4 weeks (see "Adverse Reactions").

There are reports of severe neuropathies in patients in whom regimens are employed using higher doses of Platinol or greater dose frequencies than those recommended herein. These neuropathies may be irreversible and are seen as paresthesias in a stocking-glove distribution, areflexia, and loss of proprioception and vibratory sensation.

Loss of motor function has also been reported.

Anaphylactic-like reactions to Platinol have been reported. These reactions have occurred within minutes of administration to patients with prior exposure to Platinol, and have been alleviated by administration of epinephrine, corticosteroids and antihistamines.

Since ototoxicity of Platinol is cumulative, audiometric testing should be performed prior to initiating therapy and prior to each subsequent dose of drug (see "Adverse Reactions").

Safe use in human pregnancy has not been established.

Platinol is mutagenic in bacteria and produces chromosome aberrations in animal cells in tissue culture. In mice Platinol is teratogenic and embryotoxic.

Platinol has not been studied for its carcinogenic potential but compounds with similar mechanisms of action and mutagenicity have been reported to be carcinogenic.

PRECAUTIONS

Peripheral blood counts should be monitored weekly. Liver function should be monitored periodically. Neurologic examination should also be performed regularly (see "Adverse Reactions").

ADVERSE REACTIONS

Nephrotoxicity

Dose-related and cumulative renal insufficiency is the major dose-limiting toxicity of Platinol. Renal toxicity has been noted in 28 to 36% of patients treated with a single dose of 50 mg/M^2. It is first noted during the second week after a dose and is manifested by elevations in BUN and creatinine, serum uric acid and/or a decrease in creatinine clearance. **Renal toxicity becomes more prolonged and severe with repeated courses of the drug. Renal function must return to normal before another dose of Platinol can be given.**

Impairment of renal function has been associated with renal tubular damage. The administration of Platinol using a 6- to 8-hour infusion with intravenous hydration, and mannitol has been used to reduce nephrotoxicity. However, renal toxicity still can occur after utilization of these procedures.

Ototoxicity

Ototoxicity has been observed in up to 31% of patients treated with a single dose of Platinol 50 mg/M^2, and is manifested by tinnitus and/or hearing loss in the high frequency range (4,000 to 8,000 Hz). Decreased ability to hear normal conversational tones may occur occasionally. Ototoxic effects may be more severe in children receiving Platinol. Hearing loss can be unilateral or bilateral and tends to become more frequent and severe with repeated doses. It is unclear whether Platinol-induced ototoxicity is reversible. Careful monitoring of audiometry should be performed prior to initiation of therapy and prior to subsequent doses of Platinol.

Hematologic

Myelosuppression occurs in 25 to 30% of patients treated with Platinol. The nadirs in circulating platelets and leukocytes occur between days 18 to 23 (range 7.5 to 45) with most patients recovering by day 39 (range 13 to 62). Leukopenia and thrombocytopenia are more pronounced at higher doses (>50 mg/M^2). Anemia (decrease of 2 g hemoglobin/100 ml) occurs at approximately the same frequency and with the same timing as leukopenia and thrombocytopenia.

Gastrointestinal

Marked nausea and vomiting occur in almost all patients treated with Platinol, and are occasionally so severe that the drug must be discontinued. Nausea and vomiting usually begin within one to four hours after treatment and last up to 24 hours. Various degrees of nausea and anorexia may persist for up to one week after treatment.

Other Toxicities:

Serum Electrolyte Disturbances

Hypomagnesemia, hypocalcemia, hypokalemia and hypophosphatemia have been reported to occur in patients treated with Platinol and are probably related to renal tubular damage. Tetany has occasionally been reported in those patients with hypocalcemia and hypomagnesemia. Generally, normal serum electrolyte levels are restored by administering supplemental electrolytes and discontinuing Platinol.

Hyperuricemia

Hyperuricemia has been reported to occur at approximately the same frequency as the increases in BUN and serum creatinine. It is more pronounced after doses greater than 50 mg/M^2, and peak levels of uric acid generally occur between 3 to 5 days after the dose. Allopurinol therapy for hyperuricemia effectively reduces uric acid levels.

Neurotoxicity (see "Warnings" section)—Neurotoxicity, usually characterized by peripheral neuropathies, has occurred in some patients. The neuropathies may occur after prolonged therapy (4 to 7 months): however, neurologic symptoms have been reported to occur after a single dose. Platinol therapy should be discontinued when the symptoms are first observed. Preliminary evidence suggests peripheral neuropathy may be irreversible in some patients.

Loss of taste and seizures have also been reported.

Ocular Toxicity—Optic neuritis, papilledema and cerebral blindness have been reported infrequently in patients receiving standard recommended doses of Platinol. Improvement and/or total recovery usually occurs after discontinuing Platinol. Steroids with or without mannitol have been used: however, efficacy has not been established.

Blurred vision and altered color perception have been reported after the use of regimens with higher doses of Platinol or greater dose frequencies than those recommended in the package insert. The altered color perception manifests as a loss of color discrimination, particularly in the blue-yellow axis. The only finding on fundoscopic exam is irregular retinal pigmentation of the macular area.

Anaphylactic-like Reactions

Anaphylactic-like reactions have been occasionally reported in patients previously exposed to Platinol. The reactions consist of facial edema, wheezing, tachycardia and hypotension within a few minutes of drug administration. Reactions may be controlled by intravenous epinephrine, corticosteroids or antihistamines. Patients receiving Platinol should be observed carefully for possible anaphylactic-like reactions and supportive equipment and medication should be available to treat such a complication.

Other toxicities reported to occur infrequently are cardiac abnormalities, anorexia and elevated SGOT.

DOSAGE AND ADMINISTRATION

Note: Needles or intravenous sets containing aluminum parts that may come in contact with Platinol should not be used for preparation or administration. Aluminum reacts with Platinol, causing precipitate formation and a loss of potency.

Metastatic Testicular Tumors—An effective combination for the treatment of patients with metastatic testicular carcinomas includes Platinol, Blenoxane (Bleomycin Sulfate) and Velban (Vinblastine Sulfate). Remission induction therapy consists of Platinol, Blenoxane (Bleomycin Sulfate) and Velban (Vinblastine Sulfate) in the following doses:

PLATINOL—20 mg/M^2 I.V. daily for 5 days (days 1–5) every three weeks for three courses.

BLENOXANE® (Bleomycin Sulfate)—30 units I.V. weekly (Day 2 of each week) for 12 consecutive doses.

VELBAN® (Vinblastine Sulfate)—0.15 to 0.2 mg/Kg I.V. twice weekly (Days 1 and 2) every three weeks for four courses (a total of eight doses).

Maintenance therapy for patients who respond to the above regimen consists of Velban (Vinblastine Sulfate) 0.3 mg/Kg I.V. every 4 weeks for a total of 2 years.

For directions for the administration of Blenoxane (Bleomycin Sulfate) and Velban (Vinblastine Sulfate), refer to their respective package insert.

Metastatic Ovarian Tumors—An effective combination for the treatment of patients with metastatic ovarian tumors includes Platinol and Adriamycin (Doxorubicin Hydrochloride) in the following doses:

PLATINOL—50 mg/M^2 I.V. once every 3 weeks (Day 1).

ADRIAMYCIN™ (Doxorubicin Hydrochloride)—50 mg/M^2 I.V. once every 3 weeks (Day 1).

For directions for the administration of Adriamycin (Doxorubicin Hydrochloride), refer to the Adriamycin (Doxorubicin Hydrochloride) package insert.

In combination therapy, Platinol and Adriamycin (Doxorubicin Hydrochloride) are administered sequentially.

As a single agent, Platinol should be administered at a dose of 100 mg/M^2 I.V. once every 4 weeks.

Advanced Bladder Cancer—Platinol should be administered as a single agent at a dose of 50–70 mg/M^2 I.V. once every 3 to 4 weeks depending on the extent of prior exposure to radiation therapy and/or prior chemotherapy. For heavily pretreated patients an initial dose of 50 mg/M^2 repeated every 4 weeks is recommended.

Pretreatment hydration with 1 to 2 liters of fluid infused for 8 to 12 hours prior to a Platinol dose is recommended. The drug is then diluted in 2 liters of 5% Dextrose in ½ or ⅓N Saline containing 37.5 g of mannitol, and infused over a 6- to 8-hour period. Adequate hydration and urinary output must be maintained during the following 24 hours.

A repeat course of Platinol should not be given until the serum creatinine is below 1.5 mg/100 ml, and/or the BUN is below 25 mg/100 ml. A repeat course should not be given until circulating blood elements are at an acceptable level (platelets $\geq$100,000/mm^3, WBC $\geq$4,000/mm^3). Subsequent doses of Platinol should not be given until an audiometric analysis indicates that auditory acuity is within normal limits.

As with other potentially toxic compounds, caution should be exercised in handling the powder and preparing the solution of cisplatin. Skin reactions associated with accidental exposure to cisplatin may occur. The use of gloves is recommended. If cisplatin powder or solution contact skin or mucosae, immediately wash the skin or mucosae thoroughly with soap and water.

Preparation of Intravenous Solutions: The 10 mg and 50 mg vials should be reconstituted with 10 ml or 50 ml of Sterile Water for Injection, U.S.P., respectively. Each ml of the resulting solution will contain 1 mg of Platinol.

Reconstitution as recommended results in a clear, colorless solution.

The reconstituted solution should be used intravenously only and should be administered by I.V. infusion over a 6- to 8-hour period. (See "Dosage and Administration".)

STABILITY

Unopened vials of the dry powder are stable for 2 years at room temperature (27°C).

The reconstituted solution is stable for 20 hours at room temperature (27°C).

Important Note: Once reconstituted, the solution should be kept at room temperature (27°C). If the reconstituted solution is refrigerated a precipitate will form.

HOW SUPPLIED

PLATINOL (cisplatin) for Injection

NDC 0015-3070-20—Each amber vial contains 10 mg of cisplatin.

NDC 0015-3072-20—Each amber vial contains 50 mg of cisplatin.

VEPESID® ℞

[vĕ′pĭ-sĭd]

(etoposide [VP-16-213])

INJECTION

This is the full text of the latest Official Package Circular dated December 1985 [3095 DIM-08].

> **WARNINGS**
>
> VePesid (etoposide) should be administered under the supervision of a qualified physician experienced in the use of cancer chemotherapeutic agents. Severe myelosuppression with resulting infection or bleeding may occur.

DESCRIPTION

VePesid (etoposide) (VP-16-213) is a semisynthetic derivative of podophyllotoxin used in the treatment of certain neoplastic diseases. It is 4′-Demethylepipodophyllotoxin 9-[4,6-0-(R)-ethylidene-β-D-glucopyranoside]. It is very soluble in methanol and chloroform, slightly soluble in ethanol and sparingly soluble in water and ether. It is made more miscible with water by means of organic solvents. It has a molecular weight of 588.58 and a molecular formula of $C_{29}H_{32}O_{13}$.

VePesid is administered by intravenous infusion. VePesid Injection is available in 100 mg (5 ml) and 100 mg (5 ml) sterile multiple dose vials. The pH of the clear yellow solution is 3 to 4.

Each ml contains 20 mg etoposide, 2 mg citric acid, 30 mg benzyl alcohol, 80 mg polysorbate 80/Tween 80, 650 mg polyethylene glycol 300, and 30.5 percent (v/v) alcohol.

The structural formula is:

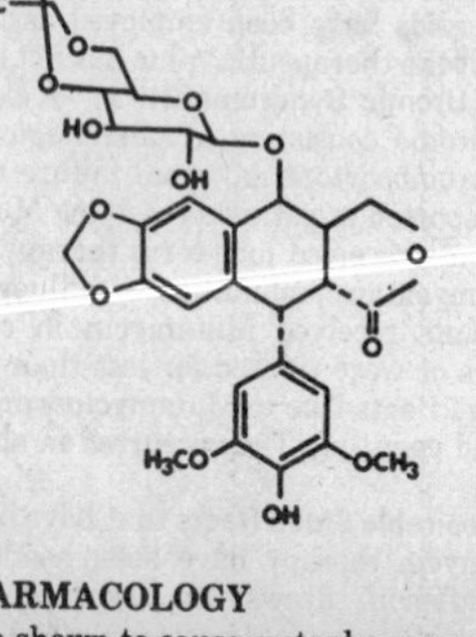

CLINICAL PHARMACOLOGY

VePesid has been shown to cause metaphase arrest in chick fibroblasts. Its main effect, however, appears to be at the G_2 portion of the cell cycle in mammalian cells. Two different dose-dependent responses are seen. At high concentrations

(10 μg/ml or more), lysis of cells entering mitosis is observed. At low concentrations (0.3 to 10μg/ml), cells are inhibited from entering prophase. It does not interfere with microtubular assembly. The predominant macromolecular effect of VePesid appears to be DNA synthesis inhibition.

Pharmacokinetics: In adult patients, VePesid is cleared from the plasma in a biphasic manner. The terminal half-life ($T\frac{1}{2}\beta$) is 7 hours with a range of 3 to 12 hours. The steady state volume of distribution is approximately 28% of body weight. Approximately 94% of the drug is bound to human serum proteins at etoposide concentrations of 10 μg/ml. The distribution of etoposide and metabolites into the CSF is low and variable. During the 72 hours after intravenous infusion of radioactive etoposide, 44 to 60% of the total radioactivity was recovered in the urine with 67% of the total amount as unchanged drug and the remainder as metabolites. Recovery in the feces ranges from less than 2 to 16% over 3 days.

In a limited number of children, VePesid administered in a dose of 200–250 mg/m^2 produced peak serum concentrations between 17 and 88 μg/ml and showed a terminal half-life ($T\frac{1}{2}\beta$) of 5.7±1.3 hours. Mean plasma clearance was 21.5 ml/min/m^2 and CSF concentrations 24 hours post-infusion ranged from less than 10 ng/ml to 45 μg/ml.

INDICATION AND USAGE

VePesid has been shown to be useful in the management of the following neoplasms:

Refractory Testicular Tumors—in combination therapy with other approved chemotherapeutic agents in patients with refractory testicular tumors who have already received appropriate surgical, chemotherapeutic and radiotherapeutic therapy.

CONTRAINDICATIONS

VePesid is contraindicated in patients who have demonstrated a previous hypersensitivity to it.

WARNINGS

Patients being treated with VePesid must be observed for myelosuppression carefully and frequently both during and after therapy. Dose limiting bone marrow suppression is the most significant toxicity associated with VePesid therapy. Therefore, the following studies should be obtained at the start of therapy and prior to each subsequent dose of VePesid: platelet count, hemoglobin, white blood cell count and differential. The occurrence of a platelet count below 50,000/mm^3 or an absolute neutrophil count below 500/mm^3 is an indication to withhold further therapy until the blood counts have sufficiently recovered.

Physicians should be aware of the possible occurrence of an anaphylactic reaction manifested by chills, fever, tachycardia, bronchospasm, dyspnea and hypotension. Treatment is symptomatic. The infusion should be terminated immediately, followed by the administration of pressor agents, corticosteroids, antihistamines, or volume expanders at the discretion of the physician.

VePesid should be given only by slow intravenous infusion (usually over a 30 to 60 minute period) since hypotension has been reported as a possible side effect of rapid intravenous injection.

Pregnancy: Pregnancy "Category D". VePesid can cause fetal harm when administered to a pregnant woman. VePesid has been shown to be teratogenic in mice and rats. There are no adequate and well-controlled studies in pregnant women. If this drug is used during pregnancy, or if the patient becomes pregnant while receiving this drug, the patient should be apprised of the potential hazard to the fetus. Women of childbearing potential should be advised to avoid becoming pregnant.

VePesid is teratogenic and embryocidal in rats and mice at doses of 1 to 3% of the recommended clinical dose based on body surface area.

VePesid was subjected to a teratology study in SPF rats at doses of 0.13, 0.4, 1.2 and 3.6 mg/kg/day administered intravenously on Days 6 to 15 of gestation. VePesid caused a dose-related maternal toxicity, embryotoxicity, and teratogenicity at dose levels of 0.4 mg/kg/day and higher. Embryonic resorptions were 90 and 100% at the 2 highest dosages. At 0.4 and 1.2 mg/kg, fetal weights were decreased and fetal abnormalities occurred including major skeletal abnormalities, exencephaly, encephalocele and anophthalmia. Even at the lowest dose tested, 0.13 mg/kg, a significant increase in retarded ossification was observed.

A study by Sieber, et. al. in Swiss-Albino mice given a single intraperitoneal injection of VePesid at dosages of 1, 1.5 and 2 mg/kg on Days 6, 7 or 8 of gestation disclosed dose-related embryotoxicity, cranial abnormalities and major skeletal malformations.

PRECAUTIONS

General: In all instances where the use of VePesid is considered for chemotherapy, the physician must evaluate the need and usefulness of the drug against the risk of adverse reactions. Most such adverse reactions are reversible if detected early. If severe reactions occur, the drug should be reduced in dosage or discontinued and appropriate corrective measures should be taken according to the clinical judgment of the physician. Reinstitution of VePesid therapy should be carried out with caution, and with adequate consideration of the further need for the drug and alertness as to possible recurrence of toxicity.

Laboratory Tests: Periodic complete blood counts should be done during the course of VePesid treatment. They should be performed prior to therapy and at appropriate periods during therapy. At least one determination should be done prior to each dose of VePesid.

Carcinogenesis, Mutagenesis, Impairment of Fertility: Carcinogenicity tests with VePesid have not been conducted in laboratory animals. Given its mechanism of action, it should be considered a possible carcinogen in humans.

VePesid induced aberrations in chromosome number and structure in embryonic murine cells.

Treatment of Swiss Albino mice with 1.5 mg/kg IP of VePesid on day 7 of gestation increased the incidence of intrauterine death and fetal malformations as well as significantly decreasing the average fetal body weights. Maternal weight gain was not affected.

Treatment of pregnant SPF rats with 1.2 mg/kg/day IV for 10 days of VePesid led to a prenatal mortality of 92%, and 50% of the implanting fetuses were abnormal.

Pregnancy: Pregnancy "Category D". See "WARNINGS" section.

Nursing Mothers: It is not known whether this drug is excreted in human milk. Because many drugs are excreted in human milk and because of the potential for serious adverse reactions in nursing infants from VePesid, a decision should be made whether to discontinue nursing or to discontinue the drug, taking into account the importance of the drug to the mother.

Pediatric Use: Safety and effectiveness in children have not been established.

ADVERSE REACTIONS

The following data on adverse reactions is based on intravenous administration of VePesid as a single agent on several different dose schedules for treatment of a wide variety of malignancies. The incidences of adverse reactions are derived from two different data bases—Bristol-sponsored studies comprised of a population of 148 patients and studies reported in the published literature comprised of a population of 1,393 patients.

In the paragraphs below, the incidence of adverse reactions is reported for each of the two data bases.

Hematological Toxicity: Myelotoxicity is most often dose limiting, with granulocyte nadirs occuring 7 to 14 days and platelet nadirs occurring 9 to 16 days after drug administration. Bone marrow recovery is usually complete by day 20, and no cumulative toxicity has been reported. Leukopenia was observed in 91% of patients in Bristol-sponsored studies and 60% of patients in the published literature. Severe leukopenia (less than 1,000 WBC/mm^3) was observed in 17% of patients in Bristol-sponsored studies and 7% of patients in the published literature. Thrombocytopenia was reported in 41% of patients in the Bristol-sponsored studies and 28% of patients in the published literature. Severe thrombocytopenia (less than 50,000 platelets/mm^3) was reported in 20% of patients in Bristol-sponsored studies and 4% of patients in the published literature.

Gastrointestinal Toxicity: Nausea and vomiting are the major gastrointestinal toxicities. The incidence was 32% in patients in Bristol-sponsored studies and 31% in patients in the published literature. Nausea and vomiting can usually be controlled with standard antiemetic therapy. Anorexia was reported in 10% and 13%, respectively, of patients in Bristol-sponsored studies and patients in the published literature. Diarrhea was reported in 1% of patients in Bristol-sponsored studies and 13% of patients in the published literature. Stomatitis was reported in 1% of patients in Bristol-sponsored studies but was not reported in the literature. Liver toxicity was not reported in Bristol-sponsored studies, but a 3% incidence was reported in the literature.

Alopecia: Reversible alopecia, sometimes progressing to total baldness, was observed in 8% of patients in Bristol-sponsored studies and 20% of patients in the published literature.

Hypotension: Temporary hypotension following rapid intravenous administration has been reported in 1% of patients in Bristol-sponsored studies and 2% of patients in the published literature. It has not been associated with cardiac toxicity or electrocardiographic changes. No delayed hypotension has been noted. To prevent this rare occurrence, it is recommended that VePesid be administered by slow intravenous infusion over a 30 to 60 minute period. If hypotension occurs, it usually responds to stopping the infusion and administering fluids or other supportive therapy as appropriate. When restarting the infusion, a slower administration rate should be used.

Allergic Reactions: Anaphylactic-like reactions characterized by chills, fever, tachycardia, bronchospasm, dyspnea and hypotension have been reported to occur in 0.7% of patients in Bristol-sponsored studies and 2% of patients in the published literature. These reactions have usually responded promptly to the cessation of the infusion and administration of pressor agents, corticosteroids, antihistamines or volume expanders as appropriate. One fatal acute reaction associated with bronchospasm has been reported.

Neurotoxicity: Peripheral neuropathy was reported in 0.7% of patients. Central nervous system toxicity (somnolence and fatigue) was reported in 3% of patients in Bristol-sponsored studies and none was reported in the published literature.

Other Toxicities: The following adverse reactions have been rarely reported: aftertaste, hypertension, rash and a single report of radiation recall dermatitis.

OVERDOSAGE

No proven antidotes have been established for VePesid overdosage.

DOSAGE AND ADMINISTRATION

The usual dose for VePesid is 50 to 100 mg/M^2/day, days 1 to 5 or 100 mg/M^2/day, days 1, 3 and 5 every 3 to 4 weeks in combination with other drugs approved for use in the disease to be treated. Dosage should be modified to take into account the myelosuppressive effects of other drugs in the combination or the effects of prior x-ray therapy or chemotherapy which may have compromised bone marrow reserve.

Administration Precautions: As with other potentially toxic compounds, caution should be exercised in handling and preparing the solution of VePesid. Skin reactions associated with accidental exposure to VePesid may occur. The use of gloves is recommended. If VePesid solution contacts the skin or mucosa, immediately wash the skin or mucosa thoroughly with soap and water.

Preparation for Intravenous Administration: VePesid Injection may be diluted with either 5% Dextrose Injection, USP or 0.9% Sodium Chloride Injection, USP to give a final concentration of 0.2 or 0.4 mg/ml. Hypotension following rapid intravenous administration has been reported, hence, it is recommended that the VePesid solution be administered over a 30 to 60 minute period. **VePesid SHOULD NOT BE GIVEN BY RAPID INTRAVENOUS PUSH.**

Parenteral drug products should be inspected visually for particulate matter and discoloration (see DESCRIPTION section) prior to administration whenever solution and container permit.

Stability: Unopened vials of VePesid Injection are stable for 24 months at room temperature (25°C). VePesid vials when diluted as recommended to a concentration of 0.2 or 0.4 mg/ml are stable for 96 and 48 hours, respectively, at room temperature (25°C) under normal room fluorescent light in both glass and plastic containers.

REFERENCFS

1. Recommendations for the Safe Handling of Parenteral Antineoplastic Drugs. NIH Publication No. 83-2621. For sale by the Superintendent of Documents, U.S. Government Printing Office, Washington, D.C. 20402.
2. AMA Council Report. Guidelines for Handling Parenteral Antineoplastics. JAMA, March 15, 1985.
3. National Study Commission on Cytotoxic Exposure—Recommendations for Handling Cytotoxic Agents. Available from Louis P. Jeffrey, Sc. D., Director of Pharmacy Services, Rhode Island Hospital, 593 Eddy Street, Providence, Rhode Island 02902.
4. Clinical Oncological Society of Australia: Guidelines and Recommendations for Safe Handling of Antineoplastic Agents. Med. J. Australia 1:426–428, 1983.
5. Jones, R. B., et. al. Safe Handling of Chemotherapeutic Agents: A Report from the Mount Sinai Medical Center. Ca—A Cancer Journal for Clinicians Sept./Oct., 258–263, 1983.
6. American Society of Hospital Pharmacists Technical Assistance Bulletin on Handling Cytotoxic Drugs in Hospitals Am. J. Hosp. Pharm. 42:131–137, 1985.

HOW SUPPLIED

VePesid (etoposide) Injection

NDC 0015-3095-20—100 mg/5 ml Multiple Dose Vial, 10's

For information on package sizes available, refer to the current price schedule.

Bristol-Myers Products

(Div. of Bristol-Myers Co.)
345 PARK AVENUE
NEW YORK, NY 10154

Arthritis Strength BUFFERIN®

[*bŭf'fĕr-ĭn*]

Analgesic

COMPOSITION

Active Ingredient: Each tablet contains Aspirin 7½ gr. (486 mg.) in a formulation buffered with Di-Alminate,® Bristol-Myers' brand of Aluminum Glycinate and Magnesium Carbonate. Also contains: Corn Starch, Corn Starch Pregelatinized.

ACTION AND USES

For the temporary relief from the minor aches and pains, stiffness, swelling and inflammation of arthritis and rheumatism. ARTHRITIS STRENGTH BUFFERIN also reduces pain and fever of colds and "flu" and provides fast, effective pain relief for: simple headache, lower back muscular aches from fatigue, sinusitis, neuralgia, neuritis, tooth extraction, muscle strain, athletic soreness, painful distress associated with normal menstrual periods.

CONTRAINDICATIONS

Hypersensitivity to salicylates.

CAUTION

If pain persists for more than 10 days or redness is present or in arthritic or rheumatic conditions affecting children under 12, consult physician immediately. Do not take without consulting physician if under medical care.

WARNING

Children and teenagers should not use this medicine for chicken pox or flu symptoms before a doctor is consulted about Reye syndrome, a rare but serious illness. KEEP THIS AND ALL MEDICINES OUT OF CHILDREN'S REACH. IN CASE OF ACCIDENTAL OVERDOSE, CONSULT A PHYSICIAN IMMEDIATELY. As with any drug, if you are pregnant or nursing a baby, seek the advice of a health professional before using this product.

ADMINISTRATION AND DOSAGE

Adults: Two tablets with water. Repeat after four hours if necessary. Do not exceed 8 tablets in any 24 hour period. If dizziness, impaired hearing or ringing in ear occurs, discontinue use. Not recommended for children.

OVERDOSE

(Symptoms and treatment) Typical of aspirin.

HOW SUPPLIED

Tablets in bottles of 40 and 100. Samples available upon request.

PRODUCT IDENTIFICATION

Plain white elongated tablet.

BUFFERIN® Analgesic

[*bŭf'fĕr-ĭn*]

COMPOSITION

Active Ingredient: Each tablet contains Aspirin 5 gr. (324 mg.), in a formulation buffered with Di-Alminate®, Bristol-Myers's brand of Aluminum Glycinate, and Magnesium Carbonate. Also Contains: Corn Starch, Corn Starch Pregelatinized.

ACTION AND USES

For relief of simple headache; and for temporary relief of: toothache, minor arthritic pain, the painful discomforts and fever of colds and "flu", menstrual cramps, and muscular aches from fatigue.

CONTRAINDICATIONS

Hypersensitivity to salicylates.

CAUTION

If pain persists for more than 10 days or redness is present or, in arthritic or rheumatic conditions affecting children under 12, consult physician immediately. Do not take without consulting physician if under medical care. Consult a dentist for toothache promptly.

WARNING

Children and teenagers should not use this medicine for chicken pox or flu symptoms before a doctor is consulted about Reye syndrome, a rare but serious illness. KEEP THIS AND ALL MEDICINES OUT OF CHILDREN'S REACH. IN CASE OF ACCIDENTAL OVERDOSE, CONSULT A PHYSICIAN IMMEDIATELY. As with any drug, if you are pregnant or nursing a baby, seek the advice of a health professional before using this product.

ADMINISTRATION AND DOSAGE

Adults: 2 tablets every four hours as needed. Do not exceed 12 tablets in 24 hours, unless directed by a physician. For children 6-12, one-half dose. Under 6, consult physician.

OVERDOSE

(Symptoms and treatment) Typical of aspirin.

PROFESSIONAL LABELING

BUFFERIN Tablets FOR MYOCARDIAL INFARCTION

(324 mg. aspirin in a formulation buffered with aluminum glycinate and magnesium carbonate)

INDICATION

Aspirin is indicated to reduce the risk of death and/or nonfatal myocardial infarction in patients with a previous infarction or unstable angina pectoris.

CLINICAL TRIALS

The indication is supported by the results of six, large, randomized multicenter, placebo-controlled studies[1–7] involving 10,816, predominantly male, post-myocardial infarction (MI) patients and one randomized placebo-controlled study of 1,266 men with unstable angina. Therapy with aspirin was begun at intervals after the onset of acute MI varying from less than 3 days to more than 5 years and continued for periods of from less than one year to four years. In the unstable angina study, treatment was started within 1 month after the onset of unstable angina and continued for 12 weeks and complicating conditions such as congestive heart failure were not included in the study.

Aspirin therapy in MI patients was associated with about a 20 percent reduction in the risk of subsequent death and/or nonfatal reinfarction, a median absolute decrease of 3 percent from the 12 to 22 percent event rates in the placebo groups. In the aspirin-treated unstable angina patients the reduction in risk was about 50 percent, a reduction in the event rate of 5% from the 10% rate in the placebo group over the 12 weeks of the study.

Daily dosage of aspirin in the post-myocardial infarction studies was 300 mg. in one study and 900 to 1500 mg. in five studies. A dose of 325 mg. was used in the study of unstable angina.

ADVERSE REACTIONS

Gastrointestinal Reactions: Doses of 1000 mg. per day of aspirin caused gastrointestinal symptoms and bleeding that in some cases were clinically significant. In the largest post-infarction study (The Aspirin Myocardial Infarction Study (AMIS) with 4,500 people), the percentage incidences of gastrointestinal symptoms for the aspirin (1000 mg. of a standard, solid-tablet formulation) and placebo-treated subjects, respectively, were: stomach pain (14.5%; 4.4%); heartburn (11.9%, 4.8%); nausea and/or vomiting (7.6%; 2.1%); hospitalization for gastrointestinal disorder (4.9%; 3.5%). In the AMIS and other trials, aspirin treated patients had increased rates of gross gastrointestinal bleeding. Symptoms and signs of gastrointestinal irritation were not significantly increased in subjects treated for unstable angina with buffered aspirin in solution.

CARDIOVASCULAR AND BIOCHEMICAL

In the AMIS trial, the dosage of 1000 mg. per day of aspirin was associated with small increases in systolic blood pressure (BP) (average 1.5 to 2.1 mm) and diastolic BP (0.5 to 0.6 mm), depending upon whether maximal or last available readings were used. Blood urea nitrogen and uric acid levels were also increased, but by less than 1.0 mg%. Subjects with marked hypertension or renal insufficiency had been excluded from the trial so that the clinical importance of these observations for such subjects or for any subjects treated over more prolonged periods is not known. It is recommended that patients placed on long-term aspirin treatment, even at doses of 300 mg. per day, be seen at regular intervals to assess changes in these measurements.

DOSAGE AND ADMINISTRATION

Although most of the studies used dosages exceeding 300 mg., two trials used only 300 mg. and pharmacologic data indicate that this dose inhibits platelet function fully. Therefore, 300 mg. or a conventional 325 mg. aspirin dose is a reasonable, routine dose that would minimize gastrointestinal adverse reactions.

REFERENCES

1. Elwood P.C., et al., "A Randomized Controlled Trial of Acetylsalicylic Acid in the Secondary Prevention of Mortality from Myocardial Infarction," British Medical Journal, 1:436–440, 1974. 2. The Coronary Drug Project Research Group, "Aspirin in Coronary Heart Disease," Journal of Chronic Disease, 29:625–642, 1976. 3. Breddin K, et al., "Secondary Prevention of Myocardial Infarction; Comparison of Acetylsalicylic Acid Phenprocoumon and Placebo," Homeostasis, 470:263–268, 1979. 4. Aspirin Myocardial Infarction Study Research Group, "A Randomized, Controlled Trial of Aspirin in Persons Recovered from Myocardial Infarction," Journal American Medical Association, 245:661–669, 1980. 5. Elwood P.C., and Sweetnam, P.M., "Aspirin and Secondary Mortality after Myocardial Infarction," Lancet, pp. 1313–1315, December 22–29, 1979. 6. The Persantine-Aspirin Reinfarction Study Research Group. "Persantine and Aspirin in Coronary Heart Disease," Circulation 62:449–460, 1980. 7. Lewis H.D., et al., "Protective Effects of Aspirin Against Acute Myocardial Infarction and Death in Men with Unstable Angina, Results of a Veterans Administration Cooperative Study," New England Journal of Medicine, 309:396–403, 1983.

HOW SUPPLIED

Tablets in bottles of 12, 36, 60, 100, 165, and 225. For hospital and clinical use: bottle—1,000; boxed 200x2 tablet foil packets. Samples available on request.

PRODUCT IDENTIFICATION MARK

Tablet is white with letter "B" on one surface.

Extra-Strength BUFFERIN®

[*bŭf'fĕr-ĭn*]

Analgesic

COMPOSITION

Active Ingredient: Each coated tablet contains aspirin 500 mg. Tablets are buffered with Di-Alminate®, Bristol-Myers' brand of Aluminum Glycinate and Magnesium Carbonate. Also Contains: Corn Starch, Corn Starch Pregelatinized.

ACTION AND USES

For relief of headaches, menstrual cramps, muscular aches, painful discomforts and fever of colds or flu, and temporary relief from toothache and the minor aches, pain and inflammation of arthritis and rheumatism.

CONTRAINDICATIONS

Hypersensitivity to salicylates.

CAUTION

If pain persists for more than 10 days, or redness is present, or in arthritic or rheumatic conditions affecting children under 12, consult a physician immediately. Do not take without consulting a physician if under medical care. Consult a dentist for toothache promptly.

WARNING

Children and teenagers should not use this medicine for chicken pox or flu symptoms before a doctor is consulted about Reye syndrome, a rare but serious illness. KEEP THIS AND ALL MEDICINES OUT OF CHILDREN'S REACH. IN CASE OF ACCIDENTAL OVERDOSE, CONSULT A PHYSICIAN IMMEDIATELY. As with any drug, if you are pregnant or nursing a baby, seek the advice of a health professional before using this product.

ADMINISTRATION AND DOSAGE

Adults: Tablets—2 every 4 hours as needed. Do not exceed 8 in 24 hours, or give to children 12 or under, unless directed by a physician.

OVERDOSE

(Symptoms and treatment) Typical of aspirin.

HOW SUPPLIED

Tablets in bottles of 30, 60 and 100. All sizes packaged in child resistant closures except 60's which size is not recommended for households with young children.

PRODUCT IDENTIFICATION MARK

White, elongated tablets with Red "ESB" imprinted on one side.

COMTREX®

[*cŏm'trĕx*]

Multi-Symptom Cold Reliever

COMPOSITION

Each tablet, fluid ounce (30 ml.), and caplet contains:

[See table on top next page].

ACTION AND USES

COMTREX contains a combination of ingredients including a non-aspirin analgesic, a decongestant, an antihistamine and a non-narcotic antitussive. COMTREX is of value in relieving the following cold symptoms when they occur together: nasal and sinus congestion, post nasal drip, coughing due to minor throat and bronchial irritation, fever, minor sore throat pain (systemically), headache, body aches and pain.

CONTRAINDICATIONS

Hypersensitivity to acetaminophen or antihistamines.

CAUTION

Do not take without consulting a physician if under medical care. Do not drive a car or operate machinery while taking this cold remedy as it may cause drowsiness.

WARNING

Keep this and all medicine out of children's reach. In case of accidental overdose, consult a physician immediately. Persistent cough may indicate the presence of a serious condition. Persons with a high fever or persistent cough, or with high blood pressure, diabetes, heart or thyroid disease, asthma, glaucoma or difficulty in urination due to enlargement of the prostate gland should not use this preparation unless directed by a physician. Do not use for more than 10 days unless directed by a physician. As with any drug, if you are pregnant or nursing a baby, seek the advice of a health professional before using this product.

ADMINISTRATION AND DOSAGE

Tablets or Caplets—Adults: 2 tablets every 4 hours as needed not to exceed 12 tablets in 24 hours. Children 6-12 years: ½ the adult dose. Under 6, consult a physician.

Liquid—Adults: 1 fluid ounce (30 ml.) every 4 hours as needed, not to exceed 6 fluid ounces (180 ml.) in 24 hours. Children 6-12 years: ½ the adult dose. Under 6, consult a physician.

Caplets—Adults 2 caplets every 4 hours as needed not to exceed 12 caplets in 24 hours. Children 6–12 years: ½ the adult dose. Under 6, consult a physician.

OVERDOSE

For overdose treatment information, consult a regional poison control center.

HOW SUPPLIED

Tablets in bottles of 24's, 50's, 100's. Caplets carded 16's and in bottles of 36's. Liquid in 6 oz. and 10 oz. plastic bottles. Samples available on request.

PRODUCT IDENTIFICATION MARK

Yellow tablet with letter "C" on one surface. Orange and Yellow caplets with and "Comtrex" on one side. Liquid is orange in color.

	COMTREX Per Tablet or Caplet	COMTREX Per Ounce
Acetaminophen:	325 mg.	650 mg.
Phenylpropanolamine HCl:	12.5 mg.	25 mg.
Chlorpheniramine Maleate:	2 mg.	4 mg.
Dextromethorphan HBr:	10 mg.	10 mg.
Also Contains:	Corn Starch	Alcohol (20% by volume)
	D&C Yellow No. 10 Lake	Citric Acid
	Erythorbic Acid	D&C Yellow No. 10
	FD&C Yellow No. 6 Lake	FD&C Red No. 40
	Magnesium Stearate	Flavors
	Methylparaben	Povidone
	Microcrystaline cellulose	Sodium Citrate
	Povidine	Sucrose
	Propylparaben	Water
May Also Contain:	Polysorbate 80	
	Silicone Dioxide	
	Wood Cellulose	

CONGESPIRIN® for Children Aspirin Free

[*cŏn "gĕs 'pir-in*]

Chewable Cold Tablets

COMPOSITION

Each tablet contains acetaminophen 81 mg. (1¼ grains), phenylephrine hydrochloride 1¼ mg. Also Contains: Calcium Stearate, Ethyl Cellulose, FD&C Yellow No. 6 Aluminum Lake, Flavor, Mannitol, Polyethylene, Saccharin, Calcium, Sucrose.

ACTION AND USES

A non-aspirin analgesic/nasal decongestant to temporarily reduce fever and relieve aches, pains and nasal congestion associated with colds and flu.

WARNINGS

KEEP THIS AND ALL MEDICATIONS OUT OF CHILDREN'S REACH. IN CASE OF ACCIDENTAL OVERDOSE, CONTACT A PHYSICIAN IMMEDIATELY.

CAUTION

If child is under medical care, do not administer without consulting physician. Do not exceed recommended dosage. Consult your physician if symptoms persist or if high blood pressure, heart disease, diabetes or thyroid disease is present. Do not administer for more than 10 days unless directed by physician.

DOSAGE AND ADMINISTRATION

Under 2, consult your physician.

2–3 years	2 tablets
4–5 years	3 tablets
6–8 years	4 tablets
9–10 years	5 tablets
11 years	6 tablets
12 years	8 tablets

Repeat dose in four hours if necessary. Do not give more than four doses per day unless prescribed by your physician.

OVERDOSE

For overdose treatment information consult a regional poison control center. See also: Congespirin for Children Aspirin Free Liquid Cold Medicine and Congespirin for Children Cough Syrup.

PRODUCT IDENTIFICATION

Scored orange tablet with "C" on one side.

HOW SUPPLIED

Tablets, in bottles of 24.

CONGESPIRIN® for Children

[*cŏn "gĕs 'pir-in*]

Cough Syrup

COMPOSITION

Each 5 ml teaspoon contains Dextromethorphan hydrobromide—5 mg. Also Contains: Benzoic Acid, Citric Acid, D&C Yellow #10, FD&C Red #40, Flavor, Sodium Citrate, Sorbitol, Sucrose, Water.

ACTIONS AND USES

Contains a non-narcotic antitussive comparable in potency to codeine, in an orange flavored syrup. Reduces coughs due to colds and to minor throat irritations.

WARNING

Do not administer without consulting a physician if child is under medical care. Persistent cough may indicate the presence of a serious condition. Children with a cough persisting for more than 10 days, with high fever, or with fever lasting more than 3 days should not be given this preparation unless directed by a physician. Do not administer to children under two years of age, except as directed by physician. KEEP THIS AND ALL MEDICINES OUT OF THE REACH OF CHILDREN.

ADMINISTRATION AND DOSAGE

Children 2–5, one teaspoon every 4 hours as needed. Do not exceed 6 teaspoons in 24 hours. Children 6–12, two teaspoons every 4 hours as needed. Do not exceed 12 teaspoons in 24 hours.

OVERDOSE

For overdose treatment information, consult a regional poison control center. See also: Congespirin for Children Aspirin Free Chewable Cold Tablets and Congespirin for Children Aspirin Free Liquid Cold Medicine.

HOW SUPPLIED

Available in 3 oz plastic bottles

PRODUCT IDENTIFICATION

Clear Orange Liquid

CONGESPRIN® for Children

[*con "ges 'pir-in*]

Aspirin Free Liquid Cold Medicine

COMPOSITION

Each 5 ml. teaspoon contains Acetaminophen 130 mg., Phenylpropanolamine Hydrochloride 6 ¼ mg., Aso Contains: Alcohol (10% by volume), Citric Acid, FD&C Red No. 40, Flavor, Methylparaben, Polyethylene Glycol, Povidone, Sodium Citrate, Sucrose, Water.

ACTION AND USES

A non-aspirin analgesic/nasal decongestant to temporarily reduce fever and relieve aches, pains and nasal congestion associated with cold and flu.

DOSAGE AND ADMINISTRATION

Children 3–5, 1 teaspoon every 3–4 hours.

Children 6–12, 2 teaspoons every 3–4 hours.

Children under 3 years use only as directed by your physician.

Do not give more than 4 doses a day unless directed by your physician.

CAUTION

If child is under medical care, do not administer without consulting physician.

WARNING

KEEP THIS AND ALL MEDICINES OUT OF CHILDREN'S REACH. IN CASE OF ACCIDENTAL OVERDOSAGE, CONTACT A PHYSICIAN IMMEDIATELY. Do not exceed recommended dosage. Consult your physician if symptoms persist or if high fever, high blood pressure, heart disease, diabetes or thyroid disease is present. Do not administer for more than 10 days unless directed by your physician.

OVERDOSE

For overdose treatment information, consult a regional poison control center. See also: Congespirin for Children Aspirin Free Chewable Cold Tablets and Congespirin for Children Cough Syrup.

HOW SUPPLIED

In 3 oz. plastic, unbreakable bottles.

PRODUCT IDENTIFICATION

Clear red liquid.

Extra-Strength DATRIL®

[*dā 'tril*]

Analgesic

COMPOSITION

Each tablet or caplet contains acetaminophen, 500 mg. Tablets Also Contain: Corn Starch, Stearic Acid.

May Also Contain: Croscamellose Sodium, Povidone, Silicon Dioxide, Sodium Lauryl Sulfate, Wood Cellulose.

ACTIONS AND USES

Extra-Strength DATRIL contains non-aspirin acetaminophen which is less likely to irritate the stomach than plain aspirin. Extra-Strength DATRIL is intended for the temporary relief of minor aches, pains, headaches and fever. For most persons with peptic ulcer Extra-Strength DATRIL may be used when taken as directed for recommended conditions.

CONTRAINDICATIONS

There have been rare reports of skin rash or glossitis attributed to acetaminophen. Discontinue use if a sensitivity reaction occurs. However, acetaminophen is usually well tolerated by aspirin-sensitive patients.

CAUTION

Severe or recurrent pain or high or continued fever may be indicative of serious illness. Under these conditions consult a physician. Do not take without consulting a physician if under medical care.

WARNING

Do not give to children 12 and under or use for more than 10 days unless directed by a physician. Keep this and all medicines out of reach of children. In case of accidental overdose contact a physician immediately. As with any drug, if you are pregnant or nursing a baby, seek the advice of a health professional before using this product.

DOSAGE

Adults: Two tablets or caplets. May be repeated in 4 hours if needed. Do not exceed 8 tablets or caplets in any 24 hour period.

OVERDOSE

MUCOMYST (acetylcysteine) As An Antidote For Acetaminophen Overdose)

ACTIONS

(Antidotal) Acetaminophen is rapidly absorbed from the upper gastrointestinal tract with peak plasma levels occurring between 30 and 60 minutes after therapeutic doses and usually within 4 hours following an overdose. The parent compound, which is nontoxic, is extensively metabolized in the liver to form principally the sulfate and glucuronide conjugates which are also nontoxic and are rapidly excreted in the urine. A small fraction of an ingested dose is metabolized in the liver by the cytochrome P-450 mixed function oxidase enzyme system to form a reactive, potentially toxic, intermediate metabolite which preferentially conjugates with hepatic glutathione to form the nontoxic cysteine and mercapturic acid derivatives which are then excreted by the kidney. Therapeutic doses of acetaminophen do not saturate the glucuronide and sulfate conjugation pathways and do not result in the formation of sufficient reactive metabolite to deplete glutathione stores. However, following ingestion of a large overdose (150 mg/kg or greater) the glucuronide and sulfate conjugation pathways are saturated resulting in a larger fraction of the drug being metabolized via the P-450 pathway. The increased formation of reactive metabolite may deplete the hepatic stores of glutathione with subse-

Continued on next page

Bristol-Myers Products—Cont.

quent binding of the metabolite to protein molecules within the hepatocyte resulting in cellular necrosis. Acetylcysteine has been shown to reduce the extent of liver injury following acetaminophen overdose.

Early symptoms following a potentially hepatotoxic overdose may include: nausea, vomiting, diaphoresis and general malaise. Clinical and laboratory evidence of hepatic toxicity may not be apparent until 48 to 72 hours postingestion. In adults and adolescents, regardless of the quantity of acetaminophen reported to have been ingested, administer MUCOMYST® acetylcysteine immediately. MUCOMYST acetylcysteine therapy should be initiated and continued for a full course of therapy. Its effectiveness depends on early administration, with benefit seen principally in patients treated within 16 hours of the overdose.

If acetaminophen plasma assay capability is not available, and the estimated acetaminophen ingestion exceeds 150 mg/kg, MUCOMYST acetylcysteine therapy should be initiated and continued for a full course of therapy.

For full prescribing information, refer to the MUCOMYST package insert. Do not await the results of assays for acetaminophen level before initiating treatment with MUCOMYST acetylcysteine. The following additional procedures are recommended: The stomach should be emptied promptly by lavage or by induction of emesis with syrup of ipecac. A serum acetaminophen assay should be obtained as early as possible, but no sooner than four hours following ingestion. Liver function studies should be obtained initially and repeated at 24-hour intervals.

For additional emergency information call your regional poison center or toll-free (1-800-525-6115) to the Rocky Mountain Poison Center for assistance in diagnosis and for directions in the use of MUCOMYST acetylcysteine as an antidote.

HOW SUPPLIED

Tablets in bottles of 30's, 60's and 100's. Caplets in bottles of 24's and 50's. Samples available on request.

PRODUCT IDENTIFICATION MARK

White tablet with DATRIL on one surface. White caplet with "Datril" embossed.

EXCEDRIN® Extra-Strength Analgesic

[ĕx ″cĕd ′rĭn]

COMPOSITION

Each tablet or caplet contains Acetaminophen 250 mg.; Aspirin 250 mg.; and Caffeine 65 mg. Tablets Also Contain: Microcrystalline Cellulose, Stearic Acid.

ACTION AND USES

Extra-Strength Excedrin is intended for the relief of pain from: headache, sinusitis, colds or 'flu', muscular aches and menstrual discomfort. Also recommended for temporary relief of toothaches and minor arthritic pains.

CONTRAINDICATIONS

Hypersensitivity to salicylates or acetaminophen.

CAUTION

If sinus or arthritis pain persists (for a week), or if skin redness is present, or in arthritic conditions affecting children under 12, consult physician immediately. Consult dentist for toothache promptly. Do not take without consulting physician if under medical care. Store at room temperature.

WARNING

Children and teenagers should not use this medicine for chicken pox or flu symptoms before a doctor is consulted about Reye syndrome, a rare but serious illness. Do not exceed 8 capsules in 24 hours or use for more than 10 days unless directed by physician, or give to children under 12. KEEP THIS AND ALL MEDICINES OUT OF CHILDREN'S REACH. IN CASE OF ACCIDENTAL OVERDOSE, CONTACT A PHYSICIAN IMMEDIATELY. As with any drug, if you are pregnant or nursing a baby, seek the advice of a health professional before using this product.

ADMINISTRATION AND DOSAGE

Tablets or Capsules—Individuals 12 and over, take 2 tablets or capsules every 4 hours as needed. Do not exceed 8 tablets or capsules in any 24 hour period.

HOW SUPPLIED

Bottles of 12, 30, 60, 100, 165, 225, and 375 tablets. Caplets in bottles of 24's, 50's and 80's. A metal tin of 12 tablets. All sizes packaged in child resistant closures except 100's (for tablets); 80's (for caplets) which are sizes not recommended for households with young children.

OVERDOSE

For overdose treatment information, consult a regional poison control center.

PRODUCT IDENTIFICATION MARK

White, circular tablet with letter "E" imprinted on both sides. White caplets with red logo.

EXCEDRIN P.M.®

[ĕx ″cĕd ′rĭn]

Analgesic Sleeping Aid

COMPOSITION

Each tablet contains Acetaminophen 500 mg. and Diphenhydramine citrate 38 mg. Also Contains: Corn Starch Pregelatinized, D&C Yellow No. 10, D&C Yellow No. 10 Aluminum Lake, FD&C Blue No. 1, FD&C Blue No. 1 Aluminum Lake, Magnesium Stearate, Methylparaben, Microcrystalline Cellulose, Povidone, Propylparaben, Stearic Acid.

ACTION AND USES

For the temporary relief of occasional headaches and minor aches and pains with accompanying sleeplessness. Also for fever with accompanying sleeplessness.

CONTRAINDICATIONS

Hypersensitivity to acetaminophen or antihistamines.

CAUTION

Do not drive a car or operate machinery while taking this medication. Do not take without consulting physician if under medical care.

WARNING

KEEP THIS AND ALL MEDICINES OUT OF CHILDREN'S REACH. IN CASE OF ACCIDENTAL OVERDOSE, CONTACT A PHYSICIAN IMMEDIATELY. Do not give to children under 12 years of age or use for more than 10 days unless directed by a physician. Consult your physician if symptoms persist or new ones occur or if fever persists more than 3 days (72 hours) or recurs or if sleeplessness persists continuously for more than two weeks. Insomnia may be a symptom of serious underlying medical illness. Take this product with caution if alcohol is being consumed. DO NOT TAKE THIS PRODUCT IF YOU HAVE ASTHMA, GLAUCOMA OR ENLARGEMENT OF THE PROSTATE GLAND EXCEPT UNDER THE ADVICE AND SUPERVISION OF A PHYSICIAN. As with any drug, if you are pregnant or nursing a baby, seek the advice of a health professional before using this product.

ADMINISTRATION AND DOSAGE

Adults take two tablets at bedtime or as directed by a physician. Do not exceed recommended dosage.

OVERDOSE

For overdose treatment information, consult a regional poison control center.

HOW SUPPLIED

Bottles of 10, 30, 50, and 80 tablets. All sizes packaged in child resistant closures except 50's, which is a size not recommended for households with young children.

PRODUCT IDENTIFICATION MARK

Blue/green circular tablet with letters "PM" imprinted on one side.

4-WAY® Cold Tablets

COMPOSITION

Each tablet contains aspirin 324 mg., phenylpropanolamine HCl 12 ½ mg., and chlorpheniramine maleate 2 mg. Also Contains: Corn Starch, Corn Starch Pregelatinized, D&C Red No. 30 Lake, Lactose.

ACTION AND USES

For temporary relief of minor aches and pains, fever, nasal congestion and runny nose as may occur in the common cold.

DOSAGE AND ADMINISTRATION

Adults—2 tablets every 4 hours, if needed. Do not exceed 8 tablets in 24 hours. Children 6–12 years—1 tablet every 4 hours. Do not exceed 4 tablets in 24 hours. Under age 6, consult a physician.

CAUTION

This preparation may cause drowsiness. Do not drive or operate machinery while taking this medication.

WARNING

Children and teenagers should not use this medicine for chicken pox or flu symptoms before a doctor is consulted about Reye syndrome, a rare but serious illness. Keep this and all medicines out of children's reach. In case of accidental overdose, consult a physician immediately. Do not exceed recommended dosage or use for more than 10 days unless directed by a physician. Individuals with high blood pressure, diabetes, heart or thyroid disease, asthma, glaucoma or difficulty in urination due to enlargement of the prostate gland should not use this preparation unless directed by a physician. Do not take without consulting a physician if under medical care. As with any drug, if you are pregnant or nursing a baby, seek the advice of a health professional before using this product.

OVERDOSE

For overdose treatment information, consult a regional poison control center.

HOW SUPPLIED

Bottles of 36's and 60's.

PRODUCT IDENTIFICATION MARK

Pink and White tablet with number "4" on one surface.

4-WAY® Nasal Spray

COMPOSITION

Phenylephrine hydrochloride 0.5%, naphazoline hydrochloride 0.05%, pyrilamine maleate 0.2%, in a buffered isotonic aqueous solution with thimerosal 0.005% added as a preservative. Also Contains: Benzalkonium Chloride, Poloxamer 188, Potassium Phosphate, Sodium Chloride, Sodium Phosphate, Water. Also available in a mentholated formula with the same active ingredients but this formulation also contains: Benzalkonium Chloride, Camphor, Eucalyptol, Menthol, Poloxamer 188, Polysorbate 80, Potassium Phosphate, Sodium Chloride, Sodium Phosphate, Water.

ACTION AND USES

For temporary relief of nasal congestion due to the common cold, sinusitis, hay fever or other upper respiratory allergies.

DOSAGE AND ADMINISTRATION

With head in a normal upright position, put atomizer tip into nostril. Squeeze atomizer with firm, quick pressure while inhaling. Adults-spray twice into each nostril. Children 6-12-spray once. Under 6-consult physician. Repeat in three hours, if needed.

WARNING

Overdosage in young children may cause marked sedation. Do not exceed recommended dosage because symptoms may occur such as burning, stinging, sneezing or increase of nasal discharge. Follow directions carefully. Do not use this product for more than 3 days. If symptoms persist, consult physician. The use of this dispenser by more than one person may spread infection. Keep out of children's reach.

Store at room temperature.

OVERDOSAGE

For overdose treatment information, consult a regional poison control center.

HOW SUPPLIED

Atomizers of ½ fluid ounce and 1 fluid ounce.

4-WAY® Long Acting Nasal Spray

COMPOSITION

Oxymetazoline Hydrochloride 0.05% in a buffered isotonic aqueous solution. Phenylmercuric Acetate 0.002% added as a preservative. **Also Contains:** Benzalkonium Chloride, Glycine, Sorbitol Water.

ACTION AND USES

Provides temporary relief of nasal congestion due to the common cold, sinusitis, hayfever or other upper respiratory allergies.

DOSAGE AND ADMINISTRATION

With head in a normal upright position, put atomizer tip into nostril. Squeeze atomizer with firm, quick pressure while inhaling. Adults: Spray 2 or 3 times in each nostril twice daily. For children under 12, consult physician.

WARNING

For adult use only. Do not give this product to children under 12 years except under the advice and supervision of a physician. Do not exceed recommended dosage because symptoms may occur such as burning, stinging, sneezing, or an increase of nasal discharge. Do not use this product for more than 3 days. If symptoms persist, consult a physician. The use of this dispenser by more than one person may spread infection.

OVERDOSAGE

For overdose treatment information, consult a regional poison control center.

KEEP OUT OF CHILDREN'S REACH.

HOW SUPPLIED

Atomizers of ½ fluid ounce.

NO DOZ® Tablets
[*nō 'dōz*]

COMPOSITION
Each tablet contains 100 mg. Caffeine. Also Contains: Flavors, Mannitol, Microcrystalline Cellulose, Stearic Acid, Sucrose.

ACTION AND USES
Helps restore mental alertness.

DOSAGE AND ADMINISTRATION
For Adults: 2 tablets initially, thereafter, 1 tablet every three hours should be sufficient.

CAUTION
Do not take without consulting physician if under medical care. No stimulant should be substituted for normal sleep in activities requiring physical alertness.

WARNING
KEEP THIS AND ALL MEDICINES OUT OF THE REACH OF CHILDREN. As with any drug, if you are pregnant or nursing a baby, seek the advice of a health professional before using this product.

OVERDOSE
Typical of caffeine.

HOW SUPPLIED
Carded 15's and 36's and bottles of 60's.

PRODUCT IDENTIFICATION MARK
A white tablet with No Doz on one side.

NUPRIN®
(ibuprofen)
Analgesic

WARNING
ASPIRIN SENSITIVE PATIENTS should not take this product if they have had a severe allergic reaction to aspirin, e.g.—asthma, swelling, shock or hives, because even though this product contains no aspirin or salicylates, cross-reactions may occur in patients allergic to aspirin.

COMPOSITION
Each tablet contains ibuprofen USP, 200 mg. **Other Ingredients:** Carnauba wax, cornstarch, D&C Yellow No. 10, FD&C Yellow No. 6, hydroxypropyl methylcellulose, propyleneglycol, silicon dioxide, stearic acid, titanium dioxide.

ACTION AND USES
For the temporary relief of minor aches and pains associated with the common cold, headache, toothache, muscular aches, backache, for the minor pain of arthritis, for the pain of menstrual cramps and for reduction of fever.

WARNINGS
The following warnings are stated on the Nuprin label: Do not take for pain for more than 10 days or for fever for more than 3 days unless directed by a doctor. If pain or fever persists or gets worse, if new symptoms occur, or if the painful area is red or swollen, consult a doctor. These could be signs of serious illness. If you are under a doctor's care for any serious condition, consult a doctor before taking this product. As with aspirin and acetaminophen, if you have any condition which requires you to take prescription drugs or if you have had any problems or serious side effects from taking any non-prescription pain reliever, do not take NUPRIN without first discussing it with your doctor. If you experience any symptoms which are unusual or seem unrelated to the condition for which you took ibuprofen, consult a doctor before taking any more of it. Although ibuprofen is indicated for the same conditions as aspirin and acetaminophen, it should not be taken with them except under a doctor's direction. Before using any drug, including NUPRIN, you should seek the advice of a health professional if you are pregnant or nursing a baby. IT IS ESPECIALLY IMPORTANT NOT TO USE IBUPROFEN DURING THE LAST 3 MONTHS OF PREGNANCY UNLESS SPECIFICALLY DIRECTED TO DO SO BY A DOCTOR BECAUSE IT MAY CAUSE PROBLEMS IN THE UNBORN CHILD OR COMPLICATIONS DURING DELIVERY. Keep this and all drugs out of the reach of children. In case of accidental overdose, seek professional assistance or contact a poison control center immediately.

CAUTION
Store at room temperature. Avoid excessive heat 40°C (104°F).

ADMINISTRATION AND DOSAGE
Directions. Adults: Take 1 tablet every 4 to 6 hours while symptoms persist. If pain or fever does not respond to 1 tablet, 2 tablets may be used but do not exceed 6 tablets in 24 hours, unless directed by a doctor. The smallest effective dose should be used. Take with food or milk if occasional and mild heartburn, upset stomach, or stomach pain occurs with use. Consult a doctor if these symptoms are more than mild or if they persist. Children: Do not give this product to children under 12 except under the advice and supervision of a doctor.

OVERDOSAGE
For overdose treatment information, consult a regional poison control center.

HOW SUPPLIED
Tablets in bottles of: Trial size 8, 24's, 50's, 100's and 150's.

PRODUCT IDENTIFICATION
Golden yellow round tablet with NUPRIN 200 printed on one side.
Manufactured by The Upjohn Company
Distributed by Bristol-Myers Company

PAZO® Hemorrhoid
Ointment/Suppositories

COMPOSITION
Ointment: Triolyte®, [Bristol-Myers brand of the combination of benzocaine (0.8%) and ephedrine sulphate (0.2%)]; zinc oxide (4.0%); camphor (2.18%). Also Contains: Lanolin, Petrolatum.
Suppositories (per suppository): Triolyte® [Bristol-Myers brand of the combination of benzocaine (15.44 mg) and ephedrine sulfate(3.86 mg)]; zinc oxide (77.2 mg); camphor (42.07 mg). Also Contains: Hydrogenated Vegetable Oil.

ACTION AND USES
Pazo helps shrink swelling of inflamed hemorrhoid tissue. Provides prompt, temporary relief of burning itch and pain in many cases.

ADMINISTRATION
Ointment—Apply Pazo well up in rectum night and morning, and after each bowel movement. Repeat as often during the day as may be necessary to maintain comfort. Continue for one week after symptoms subside. When applicator is used, lubricate applicator first with Pazo. Insert slowly, then simply press tube.
Suppositories—Remove foil and insert one Pazo suppository night and morning, and after each bowel movement. Repeat as often during the day as may be necessary to maintain comfort. Continue for one week after symptoms subside.

WARNING
If the underlying condition persists or recurs frequently, despite treatment, or if any bleeding or hard irreducible swelling is present, consult your physician.
Keep out of children's reach. Keep in a cool place.

HOW SUPPLIED
Ointment—1-ounce and 2-ounce tubes with plastic applicator.
Suppositories—Boxes of 12 and 24 wrapped in silver foil.

The Brown Pharmaceutical Company, Inc.
P.O. BOX 1529
COSTA MESA, CA 92628-1529

ANDROID–5® ℞
(Methyltestosterone Buccal Tablets U.S.P., 5 mg.)

ANDROID–10® ℞
(Methyltestosterone Tablets U.S.P., 10 mg.)

ANDROID–25® ℞
(Methyltestosterone Tablets U.S.P., 25 mg.)

DESCRIPTION
Methyltestosterone is an androgenic steroid which occurs as white or creamy white crystals or crystalline powder. The androgens are steroids that develop and maintain primary and secondary male sex characteristics.
Structural Formula and Chemical Name:

METHYLTESTOSTERONE

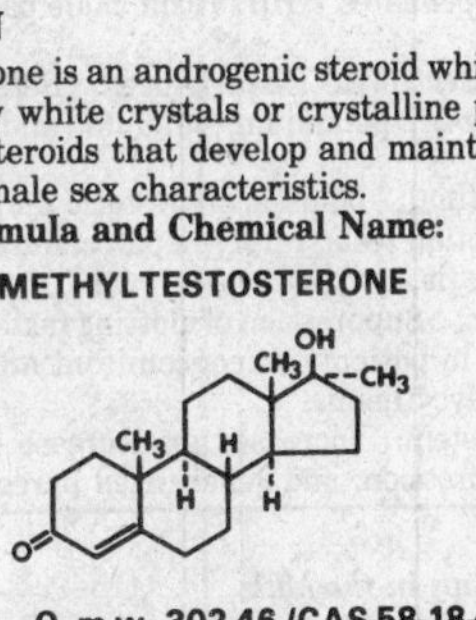

$C_{20}H_{30}O_2$m.w. 302.46 (CAS-58-18-4)
17β-Hydroxy-17-methylandrost-4-en-3-one

CLINICAL PHARMACOLOGY
Endogenous androgens are responsible for the normal growth and development of the male sex organs and for maintenance of secondary sex characteristics. These effects include the growth and maturation of prostate, seminal vesicles, penis, and scrotum; the development of male hair distribution, such as beard, pubic, chest and axillary hair; laryngeal enlargement, vocal chord thickening, alterations in body musculature, and fat distribution. Drugs in this class also cause retention of nitrogen, sodium, potassium, phosphorus, and decreased urinary excretion of calcium. Androgens have been reported to increase protein anabolism and decrease protein catabolism. Nitrogen balance is improved only when there is sufficient intake of calories and protein. Androgens are responsible for the growth spurt of adolescence and eventual termination of linear growth which is brought about by fusion of the epiphyseal growth centers. In children, exogenous androgens accelerate linear growth rates, but may cause a disproportionate advancement in bone maturation. Use over long periods may result in fusion of the epiphyseal growth centers and termination of growth process. Androgens have been reported to stimulate the production of red blood cells by enhancing the production of erythropoietic stimulating factor. During exogenous testosterone release is inhibited through feedback inhibition of pituitary luteinizing hormone (LH). At large doses of exogenous androgens, spermatogenesis may also be suppressed through feedback inhibition of pituitary follicle stimulating hormone (FSH).
There is a lack of substantial evidence that androgens are effective in fractures, surgery, convalescence, and functional uterine bleeding.

Pharmacokinetics
Testosterone given orally is metabolized by the gut and 44 percent is cleared by the liver in the first pass. Oral doses as high as 400 mg per day are needed to achieve clinically effective blood levels for full replacement therapy. The synthetic androgens (methyltestosterone) are less extensively metabolized by the liver and have longer half-lives. They are more suitable than testosterone for oral administration.
Testosterone in plasma is 98 percent bound to a specific testosterone-estradiol binding globulin, and about 2 percent is free. Generally, the amount of this sex-hormone binding globulin in the plasma will determine the distribution of testosterone between free and bound forms, and the free testosterone concentration will determine its half-life.
About 90 percent of a dose of testosterone is excreted in the urine as glucuronic and sulfuric acid conjugates of testosterone and its metabolites; about 6 percent of a dose is excreted in the feces, mostly in the unconjugated form. Inactivation of testosterone occurs primarily in the liver. Testosterone is metabolized to various 17-keto steroids through two different pathways. There are considerable variations of the half-life of testosterone as reported in the literature, ranging from 10 to 100 minutes.
In many tissues the activity of testosterone appears to depend on reduction to dihydrotestosterone, which binds to cytosol receptor proteins. The steroid-receptor complex is transported to the nucleous where it initiated transcription events and cellular changes related to androgen action.

INDICATIONS AND USAGE
1. Males
Androgens are indicated for replacement therapy in conditions associated with a deficiency or absence of endogenous testosterone:
a. Primary hypogonadism (congenital or acquired)-testicular failure due to cryptorchidism, bilateral torsion, orchitis, vanishing testis syndrome; or orchidectomy.
b. Hypogonadotropic hypogonadism (congenital or acquired)—idiopathic gonadotropin or LHRH deficiency, or pituitary-hypothalamic injury from tumors, trauma, or radiation.
If the above conditions occur prior to puberty, androgen replacement therapy will be needed during the adolescent years for development of secondary sexual characteristics. Prolonged androgen treatment will be required to maintain sexual characteristics in these and other males who develop testosterone deficiency after puberty.
c. Androgens may be used to stimulate puberty in carefully selected males with clearly delayed puberty. These patients usually have a familial pattern of delayed puberty that is not secondary to a pathological disorder; puberty is expected to occur spontaneously at a relatively late date. Brief treatment with conservative doses may occasionally be justified in these patients if they do not respond to psychological support. The potential adverse effect on bone maturation should be discussed with the patient and parents prior to androgen administration. An X-ray of the hand and wrist to determine bone age should be obtained every 6 months to assess the effect of treatment on the epiphyseal centers (see WARNINGS).
2. Females
Androgens may be used secondarily in women with advancing inoperable metastatic (skeletal) mammary cancer who are 1 to 5 years postmenopausal. Primary goals of therapy in these women include ablatio of the ovaries. Other methods of counteracting estrogen activity are adronalectomy, hypophysectomy, and/or antiestrogen therapy. This treatment has also been used in premenopausal women with breast cancer

Continued on next page

Brown—Cont.

who benefited from oophorectomy and are considered to have a hormone-responsive tumor. Judgment concerning adrogen therapy should be made by an oncologist with expertise in this field.

Androgens (including Methyltestosterone) have been used for the management of postpartum breast pain and engorgement.

CONTRAINDICATIONS

Androgens are contraindicated in men with carcinomas of the breast or with known or suspected carcinomas of the prostate, and in women who are or may become pregnant. When administered to pregnant women, androgens cause virilization of the external genitalia of the female fetus. This virilization includes clitoromegaly, abnormal vaginal development, and fusion of genital folds to form a scrotal-like structure. The degree of masculinization is related to the amount of drug given and the age of the fetus, and is most likely to occur in the female fetus when the drugs are given in the first trimester. If the patient becomes pregnant while taking these drugs, she should be apprised of the potential hazard to the fetus.

WARNINGS

In patients with breast cancer, androgen therapy may cause hypercalcemia by stimulating osteolysis. In this case, the drug should be discontinued.

Prolonged use of high doses of androgens have been associated with the development of peliosis hepatis and hepatic neoplasms including hepatocellular carcinoma. See PRECAUTIONS—Carcinogenesis). Peliosis hepatis can be life-threatening or fatal complication.

Cholestatic hepatitis and jaundice occur with 17-alpha-alkylandrogens at a relatively low dose. If cholestatic hepatitis with jaundice appears or if liver function tests become abnormal, the androgen should be discontinued and the etiology should be determined. Drug-induced jaundice is reversible when the medication is discontinued.

Geriatric patients treated with androgens may be at an increased risk for the development of prostatic hypertropy and prostatic carcinoma.

Edema with or without congestive heart failure may be a serious complication in patients with preexisting cardiac, renal, or hepatic disease. In addition to discontinuation of the drug, diuretic therapy may be required.

Gynecomastia frequently developes and occasionally persists in patients being treated for hypogonadism.

Androgen therapy should be used cautiously in healthy males with delayed puberty. The effect on bone maturation should be monitored by assessing bone age of the wrist and hand every 6 months. In children, androgen treatment may accelerate bone maturation without producing compensatory gain in linear growth. This adverse effect may result in compromised adult stature. The younger the child the greater the risk of compromising final mature height.

PRECAUTIONS

General

Women should be observed for signs of virilization (deepening of the voice, hirsutism, acne, clitoromegaly and menstrual irregularities). Discontinuation of drug therapy at the time of evidence of mild virilism is necessary to prevent irreversible virilization. Such virilization is usual following androgen use at high doses. A decision may be made by the patient and the physician that some virilization will be tolerated during treatment for breast carcinoma.

Information for the Patient

The physician should instruct patients to report any of the following side effects of androgens:

Adult or Adolescent Males: Too frequent or persistent erections of the penis.

Women: Hoarseness, acne, changes in menstrual periods, or more hair on the face.

All Patients: Any nausea, vomiting, changes in skin color or ankle swelling. Any male adolescent patient receiving androgens for delayed puberty should have bone development checked every six months.

Laboratory Tests

1. Women with disseminated breast carcinoma should have frequent determination of urine and serum calcium levels during the course of androgen therapy. (See WARNINGS).

2. Because of the hepatotoxicity associated with the use of 17-alpha-alkylated androgens, liver function tests should be obtained periodically.

3. Periodic (every 6 months) x-ray examinations of bone age should be made during treatment of prepubertal males to determine the rate of bone maturation and the effects of androgen therapy on the epiphyseal centers.

4. Hemoglobin and hematocrit should be checked periodically for polycythemia in patients who are receiving high doses of androgens.

Drug Interactions

1. Anticoagulants. C-17 substituted derivatives of testosterone, such as methandrostenolone, have been reported to decrease the anticoagulant requirements of patients receiving oral anticoagulants. Patients receiving anticoagulant therapy require close monitoring, especially when androgens are started or stopped.

2. Oxyphenbutazone. Concurrent administration of oxyphenbutazone and androgens may result in elevated serum levels of oxyphenbutazone.

3. Insulin. In diabetic patients the metabolic effects of androgens may decrease blood glucose and insulin requirements.

Drub/Laboratory Test Interferences

Androgens may decrease levels of thyroxine-binding globulin, resulting in decreased total T_4serum levels and increased resin uptake of T_3 and T_4. Free thyroid hormone levels remain unchanged, however, and there is no clinical evidence of thyroid dysfunction.

Carcinogenesis

Animal Data. Testosterone has been tested by subcutaneous injection and implantation in mice and rats. The implant induced cervical-uterine tumors in mice, which metastasized in some cases. There is suggestive evidence that injection of testosterone into some strains of female mice increases their susceptibility to hepatoma. Testosterone is also known to increase the number of tumors and decrease the degree of differention of chemically induced carcinomas of the liver in rats.

Human Data. There are rare reports of hepatocellular carcinoma in patients receiving long-term therapy with androgens in high doses. Withdrawal of the drugs did not lead to regression of the tumors in all cases.

Geriatric patients treated with androgens may be at an increased risk for the development of prostatic hypertrophy and prostatic carcinoma.

Nursing Mothers

It is not known whether androgens are excreted in human milk. Because many drugs are excreted in human milk and because of the potential for serious adverse reactions in nursing infants from androgens, a decision should be made whether to discontinue nursing or to discontinue the drug, taking into account the importance of the drug to the mother.

Pediatric Use

Androgen therapy should be used very cautiously in children and only by specialists who are aware of the adverse effects on bone maturation. Skeletal maturation must be monitored every six months by an x-ray of hand and wrist.

ADVERSE REACTIONS

Endocrine and Urogenital

Female. The most common side effects of androgen therapy are amenorrhea and other menstrual irregularities, inhibition of gonadotropin secretion, and virilization, including deepening of the voice and clitoral enlargement. The latter usually is not reversible after androgens are discontinued. When administered to a pregnant woman androgens cause virilization of external genitalia of the female fetus.

Male. Gynecomastia, and excessive frequency and duration of penile erections. Oligospermia may occur at high doses.

Skin and appendates: Hirsutism, male pattern of baldness, and acne.

Fluid and Electrolyte Disturbances: Retention of sodium, chloride, water, potassium, calcium, and inorganic phosphates.

Gastrointestinal: Nausea, cholestatic jaundice, alterations in liver function tests, rarely hepatocellular neoplasms and peliosis hepatis.

Hematologic: Suppression of clotting factors, II, V, VII, and X, bleeding in patients on concomitant anticoagulant therapy, and polycythemia.

Nervous System: Increased or decrease libido, headache, anxiety, depression, and generalized paresthesia.

Metabolic: Increased serum cholesterol.

OVERDOSAGE

There have been no reports of acute overdosage with the androgens.

DOSAGE AND ADMINISTRATION

The suggested dosage for androgens varies depending on the age, sex, and diagnosis of the individual patient. Dosage is adjusted according to the patient's response and the appearance of adverse reactions. See Table 1 for guidelines for replacement therapy in androgen-deficient males. Various dosage regimens have been used to induce pubertal changes in hypogonadal males: some experts have advocated lower dosages initially, gradually increasing the dose as puberty progresses, with or without a decrease to maintenance levels. Other experts emphasize that higher dosages are needed to induce pubertal changes and lower dosages can be used for maintenance after puberty. The chronological and skeletal ages must be taken into consideration, both in determining the initial dose and in adjusting the dose.

Dosages used in delayed puberty generally are in the lower ranges of those given in Table 1, and for a limited duration, for example 4 to 6 months.

Women with metastatic breast carcinoma must be followed closely because androgen therapy occasionally appears to accelerate the disease. Thus, many experts prefer to use the shorter acting androgen preparations rather than those with prolonged activity for treating breast carcinoma, particularly during the early stages of androgen therapy.

Guideline dosages of androgens for use in the palliative treatment of women with metastatic breast carcinoma are given in Table 2.

Suggested dosages of androgens for use in the prevention of postpartum breast pain and engorement are: methyltestosterone, buccal tablets 40 mg daily, or oral tablets 80 mg daily for 3 to 5 days after delivery.

[See table below].

HOW SUPPLIED

Android 5 mg Buccal Tablets are oblong white unscored tablets, imprinted BP 956, and are supplied in bottles of 60.

Android 10 mg Oral Tablets are square green unscored tablets, imprinted BP 958. and are supplied in bottles of 60.

Android 25 mg Oral Tablets are square yellow unscored tablets, imprinted BP 996, and are supplied in bottles of 60.

LITERATURE AVAILABLE

Samples.

Shown in Product Identification Section, page 406

ANDROID–F® ℞

(Fluoxymesterone Tablets U.S.P., 10mg.)

DESCRIPTION

Fluoxymesterone is an adrogenic steroid which occurs as white or creamy white crystals or crystalline powder. The androgens are steroids that develop and maintain primary and secondary male sex characteristics.

Structural Formula and Chemical Name:

FLUOXYMESTERONE

$C_{20}H_{29}FO_3$m.w.336.45 (CAS-76-43-7)

9-Fluoro-11β, 17β-dihydroxy-17-methylandrost-4-en-3-one

See preceding **Android** product information for **Clinical Pharmacology, Indications and Usage, Contraindications, Warnings, Precautions, Adverse Reactions,** and **Overdosage.**

DOSAGE AND ADMINISTRATION

The suggested dosage for androgens varies depending on the age, sex, and diagnosis of the individual patient. Dosage is adjusted according to the patient's response and the appearance of adverse reactions. See Table 1 for guidelines for replacement therapy in androgen-deficient males. Various dosage regimens have been used to induce pubertal changes in hypogonadal males: some experts have advocated lower dosages intially, gradually increasing the dose as puberty progresses, with or without a decrease to maintenance levels. Other experts emphasize that higher dosages are needed to induce pubertal changes and lower dosages can be used for maintenance after puberty. The chronological and skeletal ages must be taken into consideration, both in determining the initial dose and in adjusting the dose.

Dosages used in delayed puberty generally are in the lower ranges of those given in Table I, and for a limited duration, for example 4 to 6 months.

TABLE 1

Guidelines for Androgen Replacement Therapy in the Male

Drug	*Route*	*Dose*	*Frequency*
Methyltestosterone	Oral	10-50 mg	Daily
	Buccal	5-25 mg	Daily

TABLE 2

Guidelines for Androgen Therapy in Breast Carcinoma in Females

Drug	*Route*	*Dose*	*Frequency*
Methyltestosterone	Oral	50-200 mg	Daily
	Buccal	25-100 mg	Daily

Women with metastatic breast carcinoma must be followed closely because androgen therapy occasionally appears to accelerate the disease. Thus, many experts prefer to use the shorter acting androgen preparations rather than those with prolonged activity for treating breast carcinoma, particularly during the early stage of androgen therapy.
Guideline dosages of androgens for use in the palliative treatment of women with metastatic breast carcinoma are given Table 2.
Suggested dosages of androgens for use in the prevention of postpartum breast pain and engorgement are: Fluoxymesterone, 2.5 mg oral tablets starting shortly after delivery; thereafter, 5 to 10 mg daily, preferably in divided doses for 4 to 5 days.
[See table right].

TABLE I
Guidelines for Androgen Replacement Therapy in the Male

Drug	*Route*	*Dose*	*Frequency*
Fluoxymesterone	Oral	5–20 mg	Daily

TABLE 2
Guidelines for Androgen Therapy in Breast Carcinoma in Females

Drug	*Route*	*Dose*	*Frequency*
Fluoxymesterone	Oral	10–40 mg	Daily

HOW SUPPLIED

Android F (Fluoxymesterone 10 mg.) is supplied as a round white scored oral tablet, imprinted BP 998, and is supplied in bottles of 60.

LITERATURE AVAILABLE

Samples.
Shown in Product Identification Section, page 406

LIPO-NICIN®/100 mg. Tablets
LIPO-NICIN®/250 mg. Tablets

COMPOSITION

LIPO-NICIN®/100 mg.
Each blue tablet contains:

Nicotinic Acid	100 mg.
Niacinamide	75 mg.
Ascorbic Acid	150 mg.
Thiamine HCl (B-1)	25 mg.
Riboflavin (B-2)	2 mg.
Pyridoxine HCl (B-6)	10 mg.

LIPO-NICIN /250 mg.
Each yellow tablet contains:

Nicotinic Acid	250 mg.
Niacinamide	75 mg.
Ascorbic Acid	150 mg.
Thiamine HCl (B-1)	25 mg.
Riboflavin (B-2)	2 mg.
Pyridoxine HCl (B-6)	10 mg.

USES

Lipo-Nicin is used in all those conditions in which Niacin (Nicotinic Acid) supplementation is indicated.

SIDE EFFECTS

Temporary flushing with heat and itching, in some cases followed by sweating, nausea and abdominal cramps. This reaction is usually transient. Nausea caused by high acidity can be relieved by nonabsorbable antacid.

CAUTIONS

Lipo-Nicin should not be used by persons with a known sensitivity to Niacin (Nicotinic Acid) and by persons with arterial bleeding, glaucoma, severe diabetes, impaired Liver function, peptic ulcer, or by pregnant women.

ADMINISTRATION AND DOSAGE

LIPO-NICIN/100 mg.—1 to 5 tablets daily.
LIPO-NICIN/250 mg.—1 to 3 tablets daily.

AVAILABLE

Bottles of 100.

LITERATURE AVAILABLE

Samples.

Burroughs Wellcome Co.
3030 CORNWALLIS ROAD
RESEARCH TRIANGLE PARK, NC
27709

LITERATURE AVAILABLE: Folders, packaging inserts, file cards, films, slides, lecture guides, monographs, cassettes, videos and continuing education material.

ACTIFED® TABLETS, SYRUP, CAPSULES and 12-Hour Capsules
[*ăk 'tĭ-fĕd "*]

(See PDR For Nonprescription Drugs)
Shown in Product Identification Section, page 406

ACTIFED® With CODEINE ℞ Ⓒ
[*ak 'tĭ-fed*]
Cough Syrup

DESCRIPTION

Each 5 ml (1 teaspoonful) contains: codeine phosphate 10 mg (Warning—may be habit-forming), Actidil® (triprolidine hydrochloride) 1.25 mg, Sudafed® (pseudoephedrine hydrochloride) 30 mg and the inactive ingredients: alcohol 4.3%, sodium benzoate 0.1% and methylparaben 0.1% (added as preservatives), flavors, glycerin, and sorbitol. This medication is intended for oral administration.
Actifed with Codeine Cough Syrup has antitussive, antihistaminic and nasal decongestant effects. The components of Actifed with Codeine Cough Syrup have the following chemical names.
Codeine Phosphate, U.S.P.:
7,8-didehydro-4,5α-epoxy-3-methoxy-17-methyl-morphinan-6α-ol phosphate (1:1) (salt) hemihydrate
Triprolidine Hydrochloride Monohydrate:
(*E*)-2-[3-(1-pyrrolidinyl)-1-(*p-tolyl*)propenyl]pyridine monohydrochloride monohydrate
Pseudoephedrine Hydrochloride:
[*S*-(*R* *,*R* *)]-α-[1-(methylamino)ethyl]benzenemethanol hydrochloride

CLINICAL PHARMACOLOGY

Codeine: Codeine probably exerts its antitussive activity by depressing the medullary (brain) cough center, thereby raising its threshold for incoming cough impulses.
Codeine is readily absorbed from the gastrointestinal tract, with a therapeutic dose reaching peak antitussive effectiveness in about 2 hours and persisting for 4 to 6 hours. Codeine is rapidly distributed from blood to body tissues and taken up preferentially by parenchymatous organs such as liver, spleen and kidney. It passes the blood brain barrier and is found in fetal tissue and breast milk.
The drug is not bound by plasma proteins nor is it accumulated in body tissues. Codeine is metabolized in the liver to morphine and norcodeine, each representing about 10 percent of the administered codeine dose. About 90 percent of the dose is excreted within 24 hours, primarily through the kidneys. Urinary excretion products are free and glucuronide-conjugated codeine (about 70%), free and conjugated norcodeine (about 10%), free and conjugated morphine (about 10%), normorphine (under 4%) and hydrocodone ($<$ 1%). The remainder of the dose appears in the feces.
Triprolidine: Antihistamines such as triprolidine hydrochloride act as antagonists of the H_1 histamine receptor. Consequently, they prevent histamine from eliciting typical immediate hypersensitivity responses in the nose, eyes, lungs and skin.
Animal distribution studies have shown localization of triprolidine in lung, spleen and kidney tissue. Liver microsome studies have revealed the presence of several metabolites with an oxidized product of the toluene methyl group predominating.
Pseudoephedrine: Pseudoephedrine acts as an indirect sympathomimetic agent by stimulating sympathetic (adrenergic) nerve endings to release norepinephrine. Norepinephrine in turn stimulates alpha and beta receptors throughout the body. The action of pseudoephedrine hydrochloride is apparently more specific for the blood vessels of the upper respiratory tract and less specific for the blood vessels of the systemic circulation. The vasoconstriction elicited at these sites results in the shrinkage of swollen tissues in the sinuses and nasal passages.
Pseudoephedrine is rapidly and almost completely absorbed from the gastrointestinal tract. Considerable variation in half-life has been observed (from about 4½ to 10 hours), which is attributed to individual differences in absorption and excretion. Excretion rates are also altered by urine pH, increasing with acidification and decreasing with alkalinization. As a result, mean half-life falls to about 4 hours at pH 5 and increases to 12 to 13 hours at pH 8.
After administration of a 60 mg tablet, 87 to 96% of the pseudoephedrine is cleared from the body within 24 hours. The drug is distributed to body tissues and fluids, including fetal tissue, breast milk and the central nervous system (CNS). About 55 to 75% of an administered dose is excreted unchanged in the urine; the remainder is apparently metabolized in the liver to inactive compounds by N-demethylation, parahydroxylation and oxidative deamination.
The pharmacokinetic properties of codeine, triprolidine and pseudoephedrine from 10 ml of Actifed with Codeine Cough Syrup were investigated compared to a reference preparation of equal component doses in 18 healthy adults. The results of this study showed that Actifed with Codeine Cough Syrup and the reference preparation were bioequivalent.
Pharmacokinetic parameters for Actifed with Codeine Cough Syrup are as follows:
[See table below].

INDICATIONS AND USAGE

Actifed with Codeine Cough Syrup is indicated for temporary relief of coughs and upper respiratory symptoms, including nasal congestion, associated with allergy or the common cold.

CONTRAINDICATIONS

Actifed with Codeine Cough Syrup is contraindicated under the following conditions:
Use in Newborn or Premature Infants: This drug should *not* be used in newborn or premature infants.
Use in Lower Respiratory Disease: Antihistamines should *not* be used to treat lower respiratory tract symptoms, including asthma.
Hypersensitivity to: 1) codeine phosphate or other narcotics; 2) triprolidine hydrochloride or other antihistamines of similar chemical structure; or 3) sympathomimetic amines, including pseudoephedrine.
Sympathomimetic amines are contraindicated in patients with severe hypertension, severe coronary artery disease and in patients on monoamine oxidase (MAO) inhibitor therapy (see Drug Interaction Section).

WARNINGS

Actifed with Codeine Cough Syrup should be used with considerable caution in patients with increased intraocular pressure (narrow angle glaucoma), stenosing peptic ulcer, pyloroduodenal obstruction, symptomatic prostatic hypertrophy, bladder neck obstruction, hypertension, diabetes mellitus, ischemic heart disease, and hyperthyroidism.
In the presence of head injury or other intracranial lesions, the respiratory depressant effects of codeine and other narcotics may be markedly enhanced, as well as their capacity for elevating cerebrospinal fluid pressue.
Narcotics also produce other CNS depressant effects, such as drowsiness, that may further obscure the clinical course of patients with head injuries.
Codeine or other narcotics may obscure signs on which to judge the diagnosis or clinical course of patients with acute abdominal conditions.

PRECAUTIONS

General: Actifed with Codeine Cough Syrup should be prescribed with caution for certain special-risk patients, such as the eldery or debilitated, and for those with severe impair-

Parameter	Codeine*	Triprolidine†	Pseudoephedrine‡
Elimination Half Life (hr)	2.7 ± 0.4§	4.0 ± 2.2	5.5 ± 0.9
Time to Maximum Concentration (hr)	1.2 ± 0.5	1.8 ± 0.7	2.6 ± 1.0
Maximum Plasma Concentration (ng/ml)	44.8 ± 11.7	4.9 ± 1.8	189 ± 44
Area Under Plasma Curve from t = 0 to t = ∞ (ng/ml·hr)	226 ± 41	42.5 ± 34.0	1938 ± 440

* 20 mg Codeine Phosphate hemihydrate (equivalent to 14.7 mg free base)
† 2.5 mg Triprolidine HCl monohydrate (equivalent to 2.1 mg free base)
‡ 60 mg Pseudoephedrine HCl (equivalent to 49.1 mg free base)
§ Means + S.D.

Continued on next page

Burroughs Wellcome—Cont.

ment of renal or hepatic function, gallbladder disease or gallstones, respiratory impairment, cardiac arrhythmias, history of bronchial asthma, prostatic hypertrophy or urethral stricture, and in patients known to be taking other antitussive, antihistamine or decongestant medications. Patients' self-medication habits should be investigated to determine their use of such medications. Actifed with Codeine Cough Syrup is intended for short-term use only.

Information for Patients:

1. Patients should be warned about engaging in activities requiring mental alertness such as driving a car, operating dangerous machinery or hazardous appliances.
2. Patients with a history of glaucoma, peptic ulcer, urinary retention or pregnancy should be cautioned before starting Actifed.
3. Patients should be told not to take alcohol, sleeping pills, sedatives or tranquilizers while taking Actifed.
4. Antihistamines as in Actifed, may cause dizziness, drowsiness, dry mouth, blurred vision, weakness, nausea, headache or nervousness in some patients.
5. Patients should be told to store this medicine in a tightly closed container in a dry, cool place away from heat or direct sunlight and out of the reach of children.
6. **Nursing Mothers** refer to following section titled "Nursing Mothers."

Actifed with Codeine Cough Syrup should not be used by persons intolerant to sympathomimetics used for the relief of nasal congestion. Such drugs include ephedrine, epinephrine, phenylpropanolamine, and phenylephrine. Symptoms of intolerance include drowsiness, dizziness, weakness, difficulty in breathing, tenseness, muscle tremors or palpitations.

Codeine may be habit-forming when used over long periods or in high doses. Patients should take the drug only for as long, in the amounts, and as frequently as prescribed.

Drug Interactions: Actifed with Codeine Cough Syrup may **enhance** the effects of:

1. monoamine oxidase (MAO) inhibitors;
2. other narcotic analgesics, alcohol, general anesthetics, tranquilizers, sedative-hypnotics, surgical skeletal muscle relaxants, or other CNS depressants, by causing increased CNS depression.

Actifed with Codeine Cough Syrup may **diminish:**
the antihypertensive effects of guanethidine, bethanidine, methyldopa, and reserpine.

Drug/Laboratory Test Interactions:
Codeine: Narcotic administration may increase serum amylase levels.

Carcinogenesis, Mutagenesis, Impairment of Fertility: No adequate studies have been conducted in animals to determine whether the components of Actifed with Codeine Cough Syrup have a potential for carcinogenesis, mutagenesis or impairment of fertility.

Pregnancy: ***Teratogenic Effects:*** Pregnancy Category C. Animal reproduction studies have not been conducted with Actifed with Codeine Cough Syrup. It is also not known whether Actifed with Codeine Cough Syrup can cause fetal harm when administered to a pregnant woman or can affect reproduction capacity. Actifed with Codeine Cough Syrup should be given to a pregnant woman only if clearly needed. Teratology studies have been conducted with three of the ingredients of Actifed with Codeine Cough Syrup. Pseudoephedrine studies were conducted in rats at doses up to 150 times the human dose; triprolidine was studied in rats and rabbits at doses up to 125 times the human dose and codeine studies were conducted in rats and rabbits at doses up to 150 times the human dose. No evidence of teratogenic harm to the fetus was revealed in any of these studies. However, overt signs of toxicity were observed in the dams which received pseudoephedrine. This was reflected in reduced average weight and length and rate of skeletal ossification in their fetuses.

Nursing Mothers: The components of Actifed with Codeine Cough Syrup are excreted in breast milk in small amounts, but the significance of their effects on nursing infants is not known. Because of the potential for serious adverse reactions in nursing infants from maternal ingestion of Actifed with Codeine Cough Syrup, a decision should be made whether to discontinue nursing or to discontinue the drug, taking into account the importance of the drug to the mother.

Pediatric Use: As in adults, the combination of an antihistamine, sympathomimetic amine and codeine can elicit either mild stimulation or mild sedation in children. In infants and children particularly, the ingredients in this drug product in overdosage may produce hallucinations, convulsions and death. Symptoms of toxicity in children may include fixed dilated pupils, flushed face, dry mouth, fever, excitation, hallucinations, ataxia, incoordination, athetosis, tonic clonic convulsions and postictal depression, (see CONTRAINDICATIONS and OVERDOSAGE sections).

Use in Elderly (approximately 60 years or older): The ingredients in Actifed with Codeine Cough Syrup are more likely to cause adverse reactions in elderly patients.

ADVERSE REACTIONS

(The most frequent adverse reactions are underlined.)

General: <u>Dryness of mouth, dryness of nose, dryness of throat,</u> urticaria, drug rash, anaphylactic shock, photosensitivity, excessive perspiration and chills.

Cardiovascular System: Hypotension, headache, palpitations, tachycardia, extrasystoles.

Hematologic System: Hemolytic anemia, thrombocytopenia, agranulocytosis.

Nervous System: <u>Sedation, sleepiness, dizziness, disturbed coordination,</u> fatigue, confusion, restlessness, excitation, anxiety, nervousness, tremor, irritability, insomnia, euphoria, paresthesias, blurred vision, diplopia, vertigo, tinnitus, acute labyrinthitis, hysteria, neuritis, convulsions, CNS depression, hallucination.

G.I. System: Epigastric distress, anorexia, nausea, vomiting, diarrhea, constipation.

G.U. System: Urinary frequency, difficult urination, urinary retention, early menses.

Respiratory System: Thickening of bronchial secretions, tightness of chest and wheezing, nasal stuffiness, respiratory depression.

DRUG ABUSE AND DEPENDENCE

Like other medications containing a narcotic, Actifed with Codeine Cough Syrup is controlled by the Drug Enforcement Administration. It is classified under Schedule V.

Actifed with Codeine Cough Syrup can produce drug dependence of the morphine type, and therefore it has a potential for being abused. Psychic dependence, physical dependence and tolerance may develop on repeated administration.

The dependence liability of codeine has been found to be too small to permit a full definition of its characteristics. Studies indicate that addiction to codeine is extremely uncommon and requires very high parenteral doses.

When dependence on codeine occurs at therapeutic doses, it appears to require from one to two months to develop, and withdrawal symptoms are mild. Most patients on long-term oral codeine therapy show no signs of physical dependence upon abrupt withdrawal.

OVERDOSAGE

Since Actifed with Codeine Cough Syrup is comprised of three pharmacologically different compounds, it is difficult to predict the exact manifestation of symptoms in a given individual. Reaction to an overdosage of Actifed with Codeine Cough Syrup may vary from CNS depression to stimulation. A detailed description of symptoms which are likely to appear after ingestion of an excess of the individual components follows.

Overdosage with codeine can cause transient euphoria, drowsiness, dizziness, weariness, diminution of sensibility, loss of sensation, vomiting, transient excitement in children and occasionally in adult women, miosis progressing to nonreactive pinpoint pupils, itching sometimes with skin rashes and urticaria, and clammy skin with mottled cyanosis. In more severe cases, muscular relaxation with depressed or absent superficial and deep reflexes and a positive Babinski sign may appear. Marked slowing of the respiratory rate with inadequate pulmonary ventilation and consequent cyanosis may occur. Terminal signs include shock, pulmonary edema, hypostatic or aspiration pneumonia and respiratory arrest, with death occurring within 6–12 hours following ingestion.

Overdoses of antihistamines may cause hallucinations, convulsions, or possibly death, especially in infants and children. Antihistamines are more likely to cause dizziness, sedation, and hypotension in ederly patients.

Overdosage with triprolidine may produce reactions varying from depression to stimulation of the Central Nervous System (CNS); the latter is particularly likely in children. Atropine-like signs and symptoms (dry mouth, fixed dilated pupils, flushing, tachycardia, hallucinations, convulsions, urinary retention, cardiac arrthymias and coma) may occur.

Overdosage with pseudoephedrine can cause excessive CNS stimulation resulting in excitement, nervousness, anxiety, tremor, restlessness and insomnia. Other effects include tachycardia, hypertension, pallor, mydriasis, hyperglycemia and urinary retention. Severe overdosage may cause tachypnea or hyperpnea, hallucinations, convulsions, or delirium, but in some individuals there may be CNS depression with somnolence, stupor or respiratory depression. Arrhythmias (including ventricular fibrillation) may lead to hypotension and circulatory collapse. Severe hypokalemia can occur, probably due to compartmental shift rather than depletion of potassium. No organ damage or significant metabolic derangement is associated with pseudoephedrine overdosage.

The toxic plasma concentration of codeine is not known with certainty. Experimental production of mild to moderate CNS depression in healthy, nontolerant subjects occurs at plasma concentrations of 0.5–1.9 μg/ml when codeine is given by intravenous infusion. The single lethal dose of codeine in adults is estimated to be from 0.5 to 1.0 gram. It is also estimated that 5 mg/kg could be fatal in children.

The LD_{50} (single, oral dose) of triprolidine is 163 to 308 mg/kg in the mouse (depending upon strain) and 840 mg/kg in the rat.

Insufficient data are available to estimate the toxic and lethal doses of triprolidine in humans. No reports of acute poisoning with triprolidine have appeared.

The LD_{50} (single, oral dose) of pseudoephedrine is 726 mg/kg in the mouse, 2206 mg/kg in the rat and 1177 mg/kg in the rabbit. The toxic and lethal concentrations in human biologic fluids are not known. Excretion rates increase with urine acidification and decrease with alkalinization. Few reports of toxicity due to pseudoephedrine have been published and no case of fatal overdosage is known.

Therapy, if instituted within 4 hours of overdosage, is aimed at reducing further absorption of the drug. In the conscious patient, vomiting should be induced even though it may have occurred spontaneously. If vomiting cannot be induced, gastric lavage is indicated. Adequate precautions must be taken to protect against aspiration, especially in infants and children. Charcoal slurry or other suitable agents should be instilled into the stomach after vomiting or lavage. Saline cathartics or milk of magnesia may be of additional benefit. In the unconscious patient, the airway should be secured with a cuffed endotracheal tube before attempting to evacuate the gastric contents. Intensive supportive and nursing care is indicated, as for any comatose patient.

If breathing is significantly impaired, maintenance of adequate airway and mechanical support of respiration is the most effective means of providing adequate oxygenation.

Hypotension is an early sign of impending cardiovascular collapse and should be treated vigorously. Do not use CNS stimulants. Convulsions should be controlled by careful administration of diazepam or short-acting barbiturate, repeated as necessary. Physostigmine may be also considered for use in controlling centrally mediated convulsions.

Ice packs and cooling sponge baths, not alcohol, can aid in reducing the fever commonly seen in children.

For codeine, continuous stimulation that arouses, but does not exhaust, the patient is useful in preventing coma. Continuous or intermittent oxygen therapy is usually indicated, while Naloxone is useful as a codeine antidote. Close nursing care is essential.

Saline cathartics, such as Milk of Magnesia, help to dilute the concentration of the drugs in the bowel by drawing water into the gut, thereby hastening drug elimination.

Adrenergic receptor blocking agents are antidotes to pseudoephedrine. In practice, the most useful is the beta-blocker propranolol, which is indicated when there are signs of cardiac toxicity.

There are no specific antidotes to triprolidine. Histamine should not be given.

Pseudoephedrine and codeine are theoretically dialyzable, but the procedures have not been clinically established.

In severe cases of overdosage, it is essential to monitor both the heart (by electrocardiograph) and plasma electrolytes and to give intravenous potassium as indicated by these continuous controls. Vasopressors may be used to treat hypotension, and excessive CNS stimulation may be counteracted with parenteral diazepam. Stimulants should not be used.

DOSAGE AND ADMINISTRATION

DOSAGE SHOULD BE INDIVIDUALIZED ACCORDING TO THE NEEDS AND RESPONSE OF THE PATIENT.

Usual Dose:

	Teaspoonfuls (5 ml)	
Adults and children 12 years and older	2	every 4–6 hours
Children 6 to under 12 years	1	not to exceed 4 doses in a 24-hour period
Children 2 to under 6 years	½	

HOW SUPPLIED

Bottles of one pint (NDC-0081-0025-96), and one gallon (NDC-0081-0025-57).

Store at 15°–30°C (59°–86°F) and protect from light.

AEROSPORIN® ℞

[*air 'ō-spor "ĭn*]

brand Polymyxin B Sulfate

Sterile Powder

Polymyxin B Sulfate for Parenteral and/or Ophthalmic Administration

WARNING

CAUTION: **WHEN THIS DRUG IS GIVEN INTRAMUSCULARLY AND/OR INTRATHECALLY, IT SHOULD BE GIVEN ONLY TO HOSPITALIZED PATIENTS, SO AS TO PROVIDE CONSTANT SUPERVISION BY A PHYSICIAN.**

RENAL FUNCTION SHOULD BE CAREFULLY DETERMINED AND PATIENTS WITH RENAL DAMAGE AND

NITROGEN RETENTION SHOULD HAVE REDUCED DOSAGE. PATIENTS WITH NEPHROTOXICITY DUE TO POLYMYXIN B SULFATE USUALLY SHOW ALBUMINURIA, CELLULAR CASTS, AND AZOTEMIA. DIMINISHING URINE OUTPUT AND A RISING BUN ARE INDICATIONS FOR DISCONTINUING THERAPY WITH THIS DRUG.
NEUROTOXIC REACTIONS MAY BE MANIFESTED BY IRRITABILITY, WEAKNESS, DROWSINESS, ATAXIA, PERIORAL PARESTHESIA, NUMBNESS OF THE EXTREMITIES, AND BLURRING OF VISION. THESE ARE USUALLY ASSOCIATED WITH HIGH SERUM LEVELS FOUND IN PATIENTS WITH IMPAIRED RENAL FUNCTION AND/OR NEPHROTOXICITY. THE CONCURRENT USE OF OTHER NEPHROTOXIC AND NEUROTOXIC DRUGS, PARTICULARLY KANAMYCIN, STREPTOMYCIN, CEPHALORIDINE, PAROMOMYCIN, TOBRAMYCIN, POLYMYXIN E (COLISTIN), NEOMYCIN, GENTAMICIN, AND VIOMYCIN, SHOULD BE AVOIDED.
THE NEUROTOXICITY OF POLYMYXIN B SULFATE CAN RESULT IN RESPIRATORY PARALYSIS FROM NEUROMUSCULAR BLOCKADE, ESPECIALLY WHEN THE DRUG IS GIVEN SOON AFTER ANESTHESIA AND/OR MUSCLE RELAXANTS.
USAGE IN PREGNANCY: THE SAFETY OF THIS DRUG IN HUMAN PREGNANCY HAS NOT BEEN ESTABLISHED.

DESCRIPTION

Polymyxin B sulfate is one of a group of basic polypeptide antibiotics derived from *B polymyxa (B aerosporous).*
Aerosporin brand Sterile Polymyxin B Sulfate is in powder form suitable for preparation of sterile solutions for intramuscular, intravenous drip, intrathecal, or ophthalmic use. In the medical literature, dosages have frequently been given in terms of equivalent weight of pure polymyxin B base. Each milligram of pure polymyxin B base is equivalent to 10,000 units of polymyxin B and each microgram of pure polymyxin B base is equivalent to 10 units of polymyxin B.
Aqueous solutions of Aerosporin brand Polymyxin B Sulfate may be stored up to 12 months without significant loss of potency if kept under refrigeration. In the interest of safety, solutions for parenteral use should be stored under refrigeration and any unused portion should be discarded after 72 hours. Polymyxin B sulfate should not be stored in alkaline solutions since they are less stable.

ACTIONS

Aerosporin has a bactericidal action against almost all gram-negative bacilli except the *Proteus* group. Polymyxins increase the permeability of bacterial cell wall membranes. All gram-positive bacteria, fungi, and the gram-negative cocci, *N gonorrhoeae* and *N meningitidis*, are resistant.
Susceptibility plate testing: If the Kirby-Bauer method of disc susceptibility testing is used, a 300-unit polymyxin B disc should give a zone of over 11 mm when tested against a polymyxin B-susceptible bacterial strain.
Polymyxin B sulfate is not absorbed from the normal alimentary tract. Since the drug loses 50 percent of its activity in the presence of serum, active blood levels are low. Repeated injections may give a cumulative effect. Levels tend to be higher in infants and children. The drug is excreted slowly by the kidneys. Tissue diffusion is poor and the drug does not pass the blood brain barrier into the cerebrospinal fluid. In therapeutic dosage, polymyxin B sulfate causes some nephrotoxicity with tubule damage to a slight degree.

INDICATIONS

Acute Infections Caused by Susceptible Strains of *Pseudomonas aeruginosa.* Polymyxin B sulfate is a drug of choice in the treatment of infections of the urinary tract, meninges, and bloodstream caused by susceptible strains of *Ps aeruginosa.* It may also be used topically and subconjunctivally in the treatment of infections of the eye caused by susceptible strains of *Ps aeruginosa.*
It may be indicated in serious infections caused by susceptible strains of the following organisms, when less potentially toxic drugs are ineffective or contraindicated:
H. influenzae, specifically meningeal infections.
Escherichia coli, specifically urinary tract infections.
Aerobacter aerogenes, specifically bacteremia.
Klebsiella pneumoniae, specifically bacteremia.
Note. In Meningeal Infections, Polymyxin B Sulfate Should Be Administered Only by the Intrathecal Route.

CONTRAINDICATIONS

This drug is contraindicated in persons with a prior history of hypersensitivity reactions to the polymyxins.

PRECAUTIONS

See "Warning" box.
Baseline renal function should be done prior to therapy, with frequent monitoring of renal function and blood levels of the drug during parenteral therapy.
Avoid concurrent use of a curariform muscle relaxant and other neurotoxic drugs (ether, tubocurarine, succinylcholine, gallamine, decamethonium and sodium citrate) which may precipitate respiratory depression. If signs of respiratory paralysis appear, respiration should be assisted as required, and the drug discontinued.
As with other antibiotics, use of this drug may result in overgrowth of nonsusceptible organisms, including fungi. If superinfection occurs, appropriate therapy should be instituted.

ADVERSE REACTIONS

See "Warning" box.
Nephrotoxic reactions: Albuminuria, cylinduria, azotemia, and rising blood levels without any increase in dosage.
Neurotoxic reactions: Facial flushing, dizziness progressing to ataxia, drowsiness, peripheral paresthesias (circumoral and stocking-glove), apnea due to concurrent use of curariform muscle relaxants and other neurotoxic drugs or inadvertent overdosage, and signs of meningeal irritation with intrathecal administration, e.g., fever, headache, stiff neck and increased cell count and protein cerebrospinal fluid.
Other reactions occasionally reported: Drug fever, urticarial rash, pain (severe) at intramuscular injection sites, and thrombophlebitis at intravenous injection sites.

DOSAGE AND ADMINISTRATION

PARENTERAL:
Intravenous. Dissolve 500,000 units polymyxin B sulfate in 300-500 cc of 5 percent dextrose in water for continuous intravenous drip.
Adults and children. 15,000-25,000 units/kg body weight/day in individuals with normal kidney function. This amount should be reduced from 15,000 units/kg downward for individuals with kidney impairment. Infusions may be given every 12 hours; however, the total daily dose must not exceed 25,000 units/kg/day.
Infants. Infants with normal kidney function may receive up to 40,000 units/kg/day without adverse effects.
Intramuscular. Not recommended routinely because of severe pain at injection sites, particularly in infants and children. Dissolve 500,000 units polymyxin B sulfate in 2 cc sterile distilled water (Water for Injection, U.S.P.) or sterile physiologic saline (Sodium Chloride Injection, U.S.P.) or 1 percent procaine hydrochloride solution.
Adults and children. 25,000-30,000 units/kg/ day. This should be reduced in the presence of renal impairment. The dosage may be divided and given at either 4- or 6-hour intervals.
Infants. Infants with normal kidney function may receive up to 40,000 units/kg/day without adverse effects.
Note: Doses as high as 45,000 units/kg/day have been used in limited clinical studies in treating prematures and newborn infants for sepsis caused by *Ps aeruginosa.*
Intrathecal. A treatment of choice for *Ps aeruginosa* meningitis. Dissolve 500,000 units polymyxin B sulfate in 10 cc of sterile physiologic saline (Sodium Chloride Injection, U.S.P.) for 50,000 units per ml dosage unit.
Adults and children over 2 years of age. Dosage is 50,000 units once daily intrathecally for 3-4 days, then 50,000 units once every other day for at least 2 weeks after cultures of the cerebrospinal fluid are negative and sugar content has returned to normal.
Children under 2 years of age. 20,000 units once daily, intrathecally for 3-4 days or 25,000 units once every other day. Continue with a dose of 25,000 units once every other day for at least 2 weeks after cultures of the cerebrospinal fluid are negative and sugar content has returned to normal.
IN THE INTEREST OF SAFETY, SOLUTIONS FOR PARENTERAL USE SHOULD BE STORED UNDER REFRIGERATION, AND ANY UNUSED PORTIONS SHOULD BE DISCARDED AFTER 72 HOURS.

TOPICAL:
Ophthalmic. Dissolve 500,000 units polymyxin B sulfate in 20-50 cc sterile distilled water (Water for Injection, U.S.P.) or sterile physiologic saline (Sodium Chloride Injection, U.S.P.) for a 10,000-25,000 units per cc concentration.
For the treatment of *Ps aeruginosa* infections of the eye, a concentration of 0.1 percent to 0.25 percent (10,000 units to 25,000 units per cc) is administered 1-3 drops every hour, increasing the intervals as response indicates.
Subconjunctival injection of up to 10,000 units/day may be used for the treatment of *Ps aeruginosa* infections of the cornea and conjunctiva.
Note: Avoid total systemic and ophthalmic instillation over 25,000 units/kg/day.

HOW SUPPLIED

AEROSPORIN brand POLYMYXIN B SULFATE STERILE POWDER
500,000 units.
Rubber-stoppered glass vial with flip off cap.
Vial—VA NSN 6505-00-913-3124

ALKERAN® ℞

[*al-kur'an*]
(Melphalan)
2 mg Scored Tablets

WARNING: Melphalan is leukemogenic in humans.
Melphalan produces chromosomal aberrations *in vitro* and *in vivo* and therefore should be considered potentially mutagenic in humans.
Melphalan produces amenorrhea.

DESCRIPTION

Alkeran (melphalan), also known as L-phenylalanine mustard, phenylalanine mustard, L-PAM, or L-sarcolysin, is a phenylalanine derivative of nitrogen mustard. Alkeran is a bifunctional alkylating agent which is active against selective human neoplastic diseases. It is known chemically as 4-[bis(2-chloroethyl)amino]-*L* - phenylalanine.
Melphalan is the active L-isomer of the compound and was first synthesized in 1953 by Bergel and Stock; the D-isomer, known as medphalan, is less active against certain animal tumors, and the dose needed to produce effects on chromosomes is larger than that required with the L-isomer. The racemic (DL–) form is known as merphalan or sarcolysin. Melphalan is insoluble in water and has a pKa_1 of $\sim$ 2.1.
Alkeran (melphalan) is available in 2 mg scored tablets for oral administration. Each scored tablet contains 2 mg melphalan and the inactive ingredients lactose, magnesium stearate, potato starch, povidone, and sucrose.

CLINICAL PHARMACOLOGY

Alberts *et al*[1] found that plasma melphalan levels are highly variable after oral dosing, both with respect to the time of the first appearance of melphalan in plasma (range 0 to 336 minutes) and to the peak plasma concentration (range 0.166 to 3.741 μg/ml) achieved.[2] These results may be due to incomplete intestinal absorption, a variable "first pass" hepatic metabolism, or to rapid hydrolysis. Five patients were studied after both oral and intravenous dosing with 0.6 mg/kg as a single bolus dose by each route. The areas under the plasma concentration-time curves after oral administration averaged 61 ± 26% (± standard deviation; range 25 to 89%) of those following intravenous administration. In 18 patients given a single oral dose of 0.6 mg/kg of melphalan, the terminal plasma half-disappearance time of parent drug was 89.5 ± 50 minutes. The 24-hour urinary excretion of parent drug in these patients was 10 ± 4.5%, suggesting that renal clearance is not a major route of elimination of parent drug.
Tattersall *et al*,[3] using universally labeled ^{14}C-melphalan, found substantially less radioactivity in the urine of patients given the drug by mouth (30% of administered dose in nine days) than in the urine of those given it intravenously (35 to 65% in seven days). Following either oral or intravenous administration, the pattern of label recovery was similar, with the majority being recovered in the first 24 hours. Following oral administration, peak radioactivity occurred in plasma at two hours and then disappeared with a half-life of approximately 160 hours. In one patient where parent drug (rather than just radiolabel) was determined, the melphalan half-disappearance time was 67 minutes.[3]

INDICATIONS AND USAGE

Alkeran (melphalan) is indicated for the palliative treatment of multiple myeloma and for the palliation of non-resectable epithelial carcinoma of the ovary.

CONTRAINDICATIONS

Melphalan should not be used in patients whose disease has demonstrated a prior resistance to this agent. Patients who have demonstrated hypersensitivity to melphalan should not be given the drug.

WARNINGS

As with other nitrogen mustard drugs, excessive dosage will produce marked bone marrow depression. Frequent blood counts are essential to determine optimal dosage and to avoid toxicity. The drug should be discontinued or the dosage reduced upon evidence of depression of the bone marrow.
There are many reports of patients with multiple myeloma who have developed acute, non-lymphatic leukemia following therapy with alkylating agents (including melphalan). Evaluation of published reports strongly suggests that melphalan is leukemogenic in patients with multiple myeloma. The potential benefits from the drug and potential risk of carcinogenesis must be evaluated on an individual basis.
Pregnancy: "Pregnancy Category D." Melphalan may cause fetal harm when administered to a pregnant woman. Animal reproduction studies have not been conducted with melphalan. There are no adequate and well-controlled studies in pregnant women. If this drug is used during pregnancy, or if the patient becomes pregnant while taking this drug, the patient should be apprised of the potential hazard

Continued on next page

Burroughs Wellcome—Cont.

to the fetus. Women of childbearing potential should be advised to avoid becoming pregnant.

PRECAUTIONS

General: Melphalan should be used with extreme caution in patients whose bone marrow reserve may have been compromised by prior irradiation or chemotherapy, or whose marrow function is recovering from previous cytotoxic therapy. If the leukocyte count falls below 3,000/μl, or the platelet count below 100,000 μl, the drug should be discontinued until the peripheral blood cell counts have recovered.

A recommendation as to whether or not dosage reduction should be made routinely in patients with impaired creatinine clearance cannot be made because:

(a) There is considerable inherent patient-to-patient variability in the systemic availability of melphalan in patients with normal renal function.

(b) There is only a small amount of the administered dose that appears as parent drug in the urine of patients with normal renal function.

Patients with azotemia should be closely observed, however, in order to make dosage reductions, if required, at the earliest possible time.

Information for Patients: Patients should be informed that the major toxicities of melphalan are related to myelosuppression, hypersensitivity, gastrointestinal toxicity, pulmonary toxicity, infertility, and non-lymphocytic leukemia. Patients should never be allowed to take the drug without close medical supervision and should be advised to consult their physician if they experience skin rash, vasculitis, bleeding, fever, persistent cough, nausea, vomiting, amenorrhea, weight loss, or unusual lumps/masses. Women of childbearing potential should be advised to avoid becoming pregnant.

Laboratory Tests: Weekly examination of the blood should be made to determine hemoglobin levels, total and differential leukocyte counts, and platelet enumeration. Patients may develop symptoms of anemia if the hemoglobin falls below 9–10 gm/dl, and are at risk of severe infection if the absolute neutrophil count is below 1,000/mm^3, and may bleed if the platelet count falls below 50,000/mm^3.

Drug Interactions: There are no known drug/ drug interactions with melphalan.

Carcinogenesis, Mutagenesis, Impairment of Fertility: In an animal study to evaluate carcinogenesis, rats were given melphalan i.p. 3 times weekly for six months in doses ten to twenty times greater than the recommended dose in man. Fifty percent (50%) of the animals developed peritoneal sarcomas. Males and females developed lung tumors in excess of controls.[4] In a 39-week test melphalan produced a dose-related increase in lung tumors in mice.[5]

There are several reports of acute non-lymphocytic leukemia arising in patients with multiple myeloma and ovarian carcinoma following melphalan treatment.[6,7,8] In many instances, these patients also received other chemotherapeutic agents or some form of radiation therapy. The quantitation of the risk of melphalan-induction of leukemia or carcinoma in humans is not possible. Evaluation of published reports of leukemia developing in patients who have received melphalan (and other alkylating agents) suggests that the risk of leukemogenesis increases with both chronicity of treatment and large cumulative doses. However, it has proved impossible to find a cumulative dose below which there is no risk of the induction of secondary malignancy. The potential benefits from melphalan therapy must be weighed on an individual basis against the possible risk of the induction of a second malignancy.

Melphalan has been shown to cause chromatid or chromosome damage in man.[9] Melphalan causes suppression of ovarian function in pre-menopausal women, resulting in amenorrhea in a significant number of patients.[10,11]

Pregnancy: ***Teratogenic Effects:*** Pregnancy Category D: See WARNINGS section.

Nursing Mothers: It is not known whether this drug is excreted in human milk. Because many drugs are excreted in human milk and because of the potential for serious adverse reactions in nursing infants from melphalan, a decision should be made whether to discontinue nursing or to discontinue the drug, taking into account the importance of the drug to the mother.

Pediatric Use: The safety and effectiveness in children have not been established.

ADVERSE REACTIONS

Hematologic Effects: The most common side effect is bone marrow suppression.[12] Although bone marrow suppression frequently occurs, it is usually reversible if melphalan is withdrawn early enough. However, irreversible bone marrow failure has been reported.[13,14]

Gastrointestinal: Gastrointestinal disturbances such as nausea and vomiting, diarrhea and oral ulceration occur infrequently.

Miscellaneous: Other reported adverse reactions include: pulmonary fibrosis[15,16] and interstitial pneumonitis, skin hypersensitivity, vasculitis, alopecia, hemolytic anemia, and allergic reaction.

OVERDOSAGE

Immediate effects are likely to be vomiting, ulceration of the mouth, diarrhea and hemorrhage of the gastrointestinal tract. The main toxic effect is on the bone marrow, and there is no known antidote. The blood picture should be closely followed for three to six weeks. General supportive measures, together with appropriate blood transfusions and antibiotics, should be instituted if necessary. This drug is not removed from plasma to any significant degree by hemodialysis.[17]

The oral LD_{50} dose in mice is 21 mg/kg.

DOSAGE AND ADMINISTRATION

Multiple Myeloma: The usual oral dose is 6 mg (3 tablets) daily. The entire daily dose may be given at one time. It is adjusted, as required, on the basis of blood counts done at approximately weekly intervals. After two to three weeks of treatment, the drug should be discontinued for up to four weeks during which time the blood count should be followed carefully. When the white blood cell and platelet counts are rising, a maintenance dose of 2 mg daily may be instituted. Because of the patient-to-patient variation in melphalan plasma levels following oral administration of the drug, several investigators have recommended that melphalan dosage be cautiously escalated until some myelosuppression is observed, in order to assure that potentially therapeutic levels of the drug have been reached.[1,3]

Other dosage regimens have been used by various investigators. Osserman and Takatsuki have used an initial course of 10 mg/day for seven to ten days.[18,19] They report that maximal suppression of the leukocyte and platelet counts occurs within three to five weeks and recovery within four to eight weeks. Continuous maintenance therapy with 2 mg/day is instituted when the white blood cell count is greater than 4,000 and the platelet count is greater than 100,000. Dosage is adjusted to between 1 and 3 mg/day depending upon the hematological response. It is desirable to try to maintain a significant degree of bone marrow depression so as to keep the leukocyte count in the range of 3,000 to 3,500 cells/μl. Hoogstraten *et al* have started treatment with 0.15 mg/kg/day for seven days.[20] This is followed by a rest period of at least 14 days, but it may be as long as five to six weeks. Maintenance therapy is started when the white blood cell and platelet counts are rising. The maintenance dose is 0.05 mg/kg per day or less and is adjusted according to the blood count.

Available evidence suggests that about one third to one half of the patients with multiple myeloma show a favorable response to oral administration of the drug.

One study by Alexanian *et al* has shown that the use of melphalan in combination with prednisone significantly improves the percentage of patients with multiple myeloma who achieve palliation.[21] One regimen has been to administer courses of melphalan at 0.25 mg/kg/day for four consecutive days (or, 0.20 mg/kg/day for five consecutive days) for a total dose of 1 mg/kg per course. These four- to five-day courses are then repeated every four to six weeks if the granulocyte count and the platelet count have returned to normal levels.

It is to be emphasized that response may be very gradual over many months; it is important that repeated courses or continuous therapy be given since improvement may continue slowly over many months, and the maximum benefit may be missed if treatment is abandoned too soon.

In patients with moderate to severe renal impairment, currently available pharmacokinetic data does not justify an absolute recommendation on dosage reduction to those patients, but it may be prudent to use a reduced dose initially.[22,23]

Epithelial Ovarian Cancer: One commonly employed regimen for the treatment of ovarian carcinoma has been to administer melphalan at a dose of 0.2 mg/kg daily for five days as a single course. Courses are repeated every four to five weeks depending upon hematologic tolerance.[24,25]

HOW SUPPLIED

White, scored tablets containing 2 mg melphalan, imprinted with "ALKERAN" and "A2A"; in bottle of 50 (NDC-0081-0045-35).

Store at 15°–25°C (59°–77°F) in a dry place and protect from light.

REFERENCES

1. Alberts DS *et al:* Oral Melphalan Kinetics. *Clin Pharmacol Ther, 26* (6):737–745, 1979.
2. Alberts DS *et al:* Unpublished Data on File with Burroughs Wellcome Co., 1981.
3. Tattersall MHN *et al:* Pharmacokinetics of Melphalan Following Oral or Intravenous Administration in Patients with Malignant Disease. *Europ J Cancer, 11:* 507–513, 1977.
4. Weisburger JH *et al:* The Carcinogenic Properties of Some of the Principal Drugs used in Clinical Cancer Chemotherapy. *Recent Results Cancer Res, 52:* 1–17, 1975.
5. Shimkin MB *et al:* Bioassay of 29 Alkylating Chemicals by the Pulmonary-Tumor Response in Strain A Mice. *J Natl Cancer Inst, 36:* 915–935, 1966.
6. Meytes D, Seligsohn U and Ramot B: Multiple Myeloma with Terminal Erythroleukemia. *Acta Haemat, 55:* 358–362, 1976.
7. Reimer RR *et al:* Acute Leukemia after Alkylating-Agent Therapy of Ovarian Cancer. *N Engl J Med, 297(4):* 177–181, 1977.
8. Einhorn N *et al:* Acute Leukemia After Chemotherapy (Melphalan). *Cancer, 41:* 444–447, 1978.
9. Sharpe HB: Observations on the Effect of Therapy with Nitrogen Mustard or a Derivative on Chromosomes of Human Peripheral Blood Lymphocytes. *Cell Tissue Kinet, 4:* 501–504, 1971.
10. Rose DP and David TE: Ovarian Function in Patients Receiving Adjuvant Chemotherapy for Breast Cancer. *Lancet, 1:* 1174–1176, 1977.
11. Ahmann DL *et al:* Repeated Adjuvant Chemotherapy with Phenylalanine Mustard or 5-Fluorouracil, Cyclophosphamide and Prednisone With or Without Radiation, After Mastectomy for Breast Cancer. *Lancet, 1:* 893–896, 1978.
12. Speed DE *et al:* Melphalan in the Treatment of Myelomatosis. *Br Med J, 1:* 1664–1669, 1964.
13. Smith JP and Rutledge F: Chemotherapy in the Treatment of Cancer of the Ovary. *Am J Obstet Gynecol, 107:* 691–703, 1970.
14. Bergsagel DE *et al:* The Treatment of Plasma Cell Myeloma. *Adv Cancer Research, 10:* 311–359, 1967.
15. Taetle R, Dickman PS and Feldman PS. Pulmonary Histopathologic Changes Associated with Melphalan Therapy. *Cancer, 42:* 1239–1245, 1978.
16. Westerfield BT *et al:* Reversible Melphalan-Induced Lung Damage. *Am J Med, 68:* 767–771, 1980.
17. Pallante SL *et al:* Quantitation by Gas Chromatography-Chemical Ionization-Mass Spectrometry of Phenylalanine Mustard in Plasma of Patients. *Cancer Res, 40:* 2268–2272, 1980.
18. Osserman EF: Therapy of Plasma Cell Myeloma with Melphalan. *Proc Am Assoc Cancer Res, 4:* 50, 1963.
19. Osserman EF and Takatsuki K: Plasma Cell Myeloma: Gamma Globulin Synthesis and Structure. *Medicine, 42:* 357–384, 1963.
20. Hoogstraten B *et al:* Melphalan in Multiple Myeloma. *Blood, 30(1):* 74–83, 1967.
21. Alexanian R *et al:* Treatment for Multiple Myeloma. *JAMA, 208(9):* 1680–1685, 1969.
22. Alberts DS *et al:* Comparative Pharmokinetics of Chlorambucil and Melphalan in Man. *Recent Results Cancer Res, 74:* 124–131, 1980.
23. Alberts DS *et al:* Effect of Renal Dysfunction in Dogs on the Disposition and Marrow Toxicity of Melphalan. *Brit J Cancer, 43:* 330–334, 1981.
24. Smith JP and Rutledge FN: Chemotherapy in Advanced Ovarian Cancer. *Natl Cancer Inst Monogr, 42:* 141–143, 1975.
25. Young RC *et al:* Advanced Ovarian Adenocarcinoma. *N Engl J Med, 299(23):* 1261–1266, 1978.

Shown in Product Identification Section, page 406

ANECTINE® ℞

[*ă-nĕk'tēn*]

(Succinylcholine Chloride)

Injection, USP

ANECTINE® ℞

(Succinylcholine Chloride)

Sterile Powder Flo-Pack®

This drug should be used only by individuals familiar with its actions, characteristics and hazards.

DESCRIPTION

Anectine (succinylcholine chloride) is an ultra short-acting depolarizing-type, skeletal muscle relaxant for intravenous administration.

Succinylcholine chloride is a white, odorless, slightly bitter powder and very soluble in water. The drug is unstable in alkaline solutions but relatively stable in acid solutions, depending upon the concentration of the solution and the storage temperature. Solutions of succinylcholine chloride should be stored under refrigeration to preserve potency.

Anectine Injection is a sterile non-pyrogenic solution for intravenous injection, containing 20 mg succinylcholine chloride in each ml and made isotonic with sodium chloride. The pH is adjusted to 3.5 with hydrochloric acid. Methylparaben (0.1%) is added as a preservative. Anectine Flo-Pack is

a sterile powder, containing either 500 mg or 1000 mg of succinylcholine chloride in each vial.
The chemical name for succinylcholine chloride is 2,2'-[(1,4-dioxo-1,4-butanediyl)bis(oxy)]bis[*N,N,N*-trimethylethanaminium] dichloride.

CLINICAL PHARMACOLOGY

Succinylcholine is a depolarizing skeletal muscle relaxant. As does acetylcholine, it combines with the cholinergic receptors of the motor end plate to produce depolarization. This depolarization may be observed as fasciculations. Subsequent neuromuscular transmission is inhibited so long as adequate concentration of succinylcholine remains at the receptor site. Onset of flaccid paralysis is rapid (less than one minute after intravenous administration), and with single administration lasts approximately 4–6 minutes.
Succinylcholine is rapidly hydrolyzed by plasma pseudocholinesterase to succinylmonocholine (which possesses nondepolarizing muscle relaxant properties) and then more slowly to succinic acid and choline. About 10% of the drug is excreted unchanged in the urine. The paralysis following administration of succinylcholine is selective, initially involving consecutively the levator muscles of the face, muscles of the glottis and finally the intercostals and the diaphragm and all other skeletal muscles.
Succinylcholine has no direct action on the uterus or other smooth muscle structures. Because it is highly ionized and has low fat solubility, it does not readily cross the placenta.
Tachyphylaxis occurs with repeated administration.
When succinylcholine is given over a prolonged period of time, the characteristic depolarizing neuromuscular block (Phase I block) may change to a block with characteristics superficially resembling a non-depolarizing block (Phase II block). This may be associated with prolonged respiratory depression or apnea in patients who manifest the transition to Phase II block. When this diagnosis is confirmed by peripheral nerve stimulation, it may be reversed with anticholinesterase drugs such as neostigmine (See Precautions).
While succinylcholine has no direct effect on the myocardium, changes in rhythm may result from vagal stimulation, such as may result from surgical procedures (particularly in children) or from potassium-mediated alterations in electrical conductivity. These effects are enhanced by cyclopropane and halogenated anesthetics.
Succinylcholine causes a slight, transient increase in intraocular pressure immediately after its injection and during the fasciculation phase, and slight increases may persist after onset of complete paralysis. This suggests that the drug should not be used in the presence of open eye injuries.
As with other neuromuscular blockers, the potential for releasing histamine is present following succinylcholine administration. Serious histamine-mediated flushing, hypotension and bronchoconstriction are, however, uncommon in normal clinical usage.
Succinylcholine has no effect on consciousness, pain threshold or cerebration. It should be used only with adequate anesthesia.

INDICATIONS AND USAGE

Succinylcholine chloride is indicated as an adjunct to general anesthesia, to facilitate endotracheal intubation, and to provide skeletal muscle relaxation during surgery or mechanical ventilation.

CONTRAINDICATIONS

Succinylcholine is contraindicated for persons with genetically determined disorders of plasma pseudocholinesterase, personal or familial history of malignant hyperthermia, myopathies associated with elevated creatine phosphokinase (CPK) values, known hypersensitivity to the drug, acute narrow angle glaucoma, and penetrating eye injuries.

WARNINGS

Succinylcholine should be used only by those skilled in the management of artificial respiration and only when facilities are instantly available for endotracheal intubation and for providing adequate ventilation of the patient, including the administration of oxygen under positive pressure and the elimination of carbon dioxide. The clinician must be prepared to assist or control respiration.
Succinylcholine should not be mixed with short-acting barbiturates in the same syringe or administered simultaneously during intravenous infusion through the same needle. Solutions of succinylcholine have an acid pH, whereas those of barbiturates are alkaline. Depending upon the resultant pH of a mixture of solutions of these drugs, either free barbituric acid may be precipitated or succinylcholine hydrolyzed.
Succinylcholine administration has been associated with acute onset of fulminant hypermetabolism of skeletal muscle known as malignant hyperthermic crisis. This frequently presents as intractable spasm of the jaw muscles which may progress to generalized rigidity, increased oxygen demand, tachycardia, tachypnea and profound hyperpyrexia. Successful outcome depends on recognition of early signs, such as jaw muscle spasm, lack of laryngeal relaxation or generalized rigidity to initial administration of succinylcholine for endotracheal intubation, or failure of tachycardia to respond to deepening anesthesia. Skin mottling, rising temperature and coagulopathies occur late in the course of the hypermetabolic process. Recognition of the syndrome is a signal for discontinuance of anesthesia, attention to increased oxygen consumption, correction of metabolic acidosis, support of circulation, assurance of adequate urinary output and institution of measures to control rising temperature. Dantrolene sodium, intravenously, is recommended as an adjunct to supportive measures in the management of this problem. Consult literature references or the dantrolene prescribing information for additional information about the management of malignant hyperthermic crisis. Routine, continuous monitoring of temperature is recommended as an aid to early recognition of malignant hyperthermia.

PRECAUTIONS

General: Low levels or abnormal variants of pseudocholinesterase may be associated with prolonged respiratory depression or apnea following the use of succinylcholine. Low levels of pseudocholinesterase may occur in patients with the following conditions: burns, severe liver disease or cirrhosis, cancer, severe anemia, pregnancy, malnutrition, severe dehydration, collagen diseases, myxedema, and abnormal body temperature. Also, exposure to neurotoxic insecticides, antimalarial or anti-cancer drugs, monoamine oxidase inhibitors, contraceptive pills, pancuronium, chlorpromazine, ecothiopate iodide, or neostigmine may result in low levels of pseudocholinesterase. Succinylcholine should be administered with extreme care to such patients. If low pseudocholinesterase activity is suspected, a small test dose of from 5 to 10 mg of succinylcholine may be administered, or relaxation may be produced by the cautious administration of a 0.1% solution of the drug by intravenous drip. Apnea or prolonged muscle paralysis should be treated with controlled respiration.
Succinylcholine should be administered with great caution to patients recovering from severe trauma, those suffering from electrolyte imbalance, those receiving quinidine, and those who have been digitalized recently or who may have digitalis toxicity, because in these circumstances it may induce serious cardiac arrhythmias or cardiac arrest. Great caution should be observed also in patients with pre-existing hyperkalemia, those who are paraplegic, or have suffered extensive or severe burns, extensive denervation of skeletal muscle due to disease or injury of the central nervous system, or have degenerative or dystrophic neuromuscular disease, because such patients tend to become severely hyperkalemic when given succinylcholine.
When succinylcholine is given over a prolonged period of time, the characteristic depolarization block of the myoneural junction (Phase I block) may change to a block with characteristics superficially resembling a non-depolarizing block (Phase II block). Prolonged respiratory depression or apnea may be observed in patients manifesting this transition to Phase II block. The transition from Phase I to Phase II block has been reported in 7 of 7 patients studied under halothane anesthesia after an accumulated dose of 2 to 4 mg/kg succinylcholine (administered in repeated, divided doses). The onset of Phase II block coincided with the onset of tachyphylaxis and prolongation of spontaneous recovery. In another study, using balanced anesthesia (N_2O/O_2/narcotic-thiopental) and succinylcholine infusion, the transition was less abrupt, with great individual variability in the dose of succinylcholine required to produce Phase II block. Of 32 patients studied, 24 developed Phase II block. Tachyphylaxis was not associated with the transition to Phase II block, and 50% of the patients who developed Phase II block experienced prolonged recovery.
When Phase II block is suspected in cases of prolonged neuromuscular blockade, positive diagnosis should be made by peripheral nerve stimulation, prior to administration of any anticholinesterase drug. Reversal of Phase II block is a medical decision which must be made upon the basis of the individual clinical pharmacology and the experience and judgment of the physician. The presence of Phase II block is indicated by fade of responses to successive stimuli (preferably "train of four"). The use of anticholinesterase drugs to reverse Phase II block should be accompanied by appropriate doses of atropine to prevent disturbances of cardiac rhythm. After adequate reversal of Phase II block with an anticholinesterase agent, the patient should be continually observed for at least 1 hour for signs of return of muscle relaxation. Reversal should not be attempted unless: (1) a peripheral nerve stimulator is used to determine the presence of Phase II block (since anticholinesterase agents will potentiate succinylcholine-induced Phase I block), and (2) spontaneous recovery of muscle twitch has been observed for at least 20 minutes and has reached a plateau with further recovery proceeding slowly; this delay is to ensure complete hydrolysis of succinylcholine by pseudocholinesterase prior to administration of the anticholinesterase agent. Should the type of block be misdiagnosed, depolarization of the type initially induced by succinylcholine, that is depolarizing block, will be prolonged by an anticholinesterase agent.
Succinylcholine should be used with caution, if at all, during ocular surgery and in patients with glaucoma. The drug should be employed with caution in patients with fractures or muscle spasm because the initial muscle fasciculations may cause additional trauma.
Succinylcholine may increase intragastric pressure, which could result in regurgitation and possible aspiration of stomach contents.
Neuromuscular blockade may be prolonged in patients with hypokalemia or hypocalcemia.
Drug Interactions: Drugs which may enhance the neuromuscular blocking action of succinylcholine include: phenelzine, promazine, oxytocin, aprotinin, certain nonpenicillin antibiotics, quinidine, β-adrenergic blockers, procainamide, lidocaine, trimethaphan, lithium carbonate, magnesium salts, quinine, chloroquine, propanidid, diethylether, and isoflurane.
If other relaxants are to be used during the same procedure, the possibility of a synergistic or antagonistic effect should be considered.
Pregnancy: ***Teratogenic Effects:*** Pregnancy Category C. Animal reproduction studies have not been conducted with succinylcholine chloride. It is also not known whether succinylcholine can cause fetal harm when administered to a pregnant woman or can affect reproduction capacity. Succinylcholine should be given to a pregnant woman only if clearly needed.
Nonteratogenic Effects: Pseudocholinesterase levels are decreased by approximately 24% during pregnancy and for several days postpartum. Therefore, a higher proportion of patients may be expected to show sensitivity (prolonged apnea) to succinylcholine when pregnant than when nonpregnant.
Labor and Delivery: Succinylcholine is commonly used to provide muscle relaxation during delivery by caesarean section. While small amounts of succinylcholine are known to cross the placental barrier, under normal conditions the quantity of drug that enters fetal circulation after a single dose of 1 mg/kg to the mother will not endanger the fetus. However, since the amount of drug that crosses the placental barrier is dependent on the concentration gradient between the maternal and fetal circulations, residual neuromuscular blockade (apnea and flaccidity) may occur in the neonate after repeated high doses to, or in the presence of atypical pseudocholinesterase in, the mother.

ADVERSE REACTIONS

Adverse reactions consist primarily of an extension of the drug's pharmacological actions. It causes profound muscle relaxation resulting in respiratory depression to the point of apnea; this effect may be prolonged. Hypersensitivity to the drug may exist in rare instances. The following additional adverse reactions have been reported: cardiac arrest, malignant hyperthermia, arrhythmias, bradycardia, tachycardia, hypertension, hypotension, hyperkalemia, prolonged respiratory depression or apnea, increased intraocular pressure, muscle fasciculation, postoperative muscle pain, myoglobinemia, excessive salivation, and rash.

DOSAGE AND ADMINISTRATION

The dosage of succinylcholine is essentially individualized and its administration should always be determined by the clinician after careful assessment of the patient. To avoid distress to the patient, succinylcholine should not be administered before unconsciousness has been induced. Succinylcholine should not be mixed with short-acting barbiturates in the same syringe or administered simultaneously during intravenous infusion through the same needle.
For Short Surgical Procedures: The average dose for relaxation of short duration is 0.6 mg/kg (~2.0 ml) Anectine (succinylcholine chloride) Injection given intravenously. The optimum dose will vary among individuals and may be from 0.3 to 1.1 mg/kg for adults (1.0 to 4.0 ml). Following administration of doses in this range, relaxation develops in about 1 minute; maximum muscular paralysis may persist for about 2 minutes, after which recovery takes place within 4 to 6 minutes. However, very large doses may result in more prolonged apnea. An initial test dose of 0.1 mg/kg (~0.5 ml) may be used to determine the sensitivity of the patient and the individual recovery time.
For Long Surgical Procedures: The dosage of succinylcholine administered by infusion depends upon the duration of the surgical procedure and the need for muscle relaxation. The average rate for an adult ranges between 2.5 and 4.3 mg per minute.
Solutions containing from 0.1% to 0.2% (1 to 2 mg per ml) succinylcholine have commonly been used for continuous intravenous drip. Solutions of 0.1% or 0.2% may conveniently be prepared by adding 1 g succinylcholine (the contents of one Anectine Sterile Powder Flo-Pack unit containing 1 g succinylcholine chloride) respectively to 1,000 or 500 ml of sterile solution, such as sterile 5% dextrose solution or sterile isotonic saline solution. The more dilute solution (0.1% or 1 mg per ml) is probably preferable from the stand-

Continued on next page

Burroughs Wellcome—Cont.

point of ease of control of the rate of administration of the drug and, hence, of relaxation. This intravenous drip solution containing 1 mg per ml may be administered at a rate of 0.5 mg (0.5 ml) to 10 mg (10 ml) per minute to obtain the required amount of relaxation. The amount required per minute will depend upon the individual response as well as the degree of relaxation required. The 0.2% solution may be especially useful in those cases where it is desired to avoid overburdening the circulation with a large volume of fluid. It is recommended that neuromuscular function be carefully monitored with a peripheral nerve stimulator when using succinylcholine by infusion in order to avoid overdose, detect development of Phase II block, follow its rate of recovery, and assess the effects of reversing agents.
Solutions of succinylcholine must be used within 24 hours after preparation. Discard unused solutions.
Intermittent intravenous injections of succinylcholine may also be used to provide muscle relaxation for long procedures. An intravenous injection of 0.3 to 1.1 mg/kg may be given initially, followed, at appropriate intervals, by further injections of 0.04 to 0.07 mg/kg to maintain the degree of relaxation required.
Pediatric Use: For endotracheal intubation, the intravenous dose of succinylcholine is 2 mg/kg for infants and small children; for older children and adolescents the dose is 1 mg/kg.
Intravenous bolus administration of succinylcholine in infants or children may result in profound bradycardia or, rarely, asystole. As in adults, the incidence of bradycardia in children is higher following a second dose of succinylcholine. The occurrence of bradyarrhythmias may be reduced by pretreatment with atropine.
Intramuscular Use: If necessary, succinylcholine may be given intramuscularly to infants, older children or adults when a suitable vein is inaccessible. A dose of up to 3 to 4 mg/kg may be given, but not more than 150 mg total dose should be administered by this route. The onset of effect of succinylcholine given intramuscularly is usually observed in about 2 to 3 minutes.
Parenteral drug products should be inspected visually for particulate matter and discoloration prior to administration whenever solution and container permit.

HOW SUPPLIED

For immediate injection of single doses for short procedures:
Anectine® Injection, 20 mg succinylcholine chloride in each ml.
Multiple-dose vials of 10 ml.
Box of 12 vials (NDC-0081-0071-95).
Store in refrigerator at 2° to 8°C (36° to 46°F). The multi-dose vials are stable for up to 14 days at room temperature without significant loss of potency.
For preparation of intravenous drip solutions only:
Anectine® Flo-Pack®, 500 mg sterile succinylcholine chloride powder.
Box of 12 vials (NDC-0081-0085-15).
Anectine® Flo-Pack®, 1000 mg sterile succinylcholine chloride powder.
Box of 12 vials (NDC-0081-0086-15).
Anectine Flo-Pack does not require refrigeration. Store at 15° to 30°C (59° to 86°F). Solutions of succinylcholine must be used within 24 hours after preparation. Discard unused solutions.

CARDILATE® TABLETS ℞

[*kar′dĭ-lāt*]
(Erythrityl Tetranitrate)

DESCRIPTION

Cardilate (erythrityl tetranitrate) is an antianginal drug that belongs to the organic nitrate class of pharmaceutical agents. Erythrityl tetranitrate is soluble in alcohol, ether and glycerol, but insoluble in water. It has the empirical formula $C_4H_6N_4O_{12}$, molecular weight of 302.12 and melting point of 61°C.
Erythrityl tetranitrate is known chemically as *(R*S*)*-1,2,3,4-butanetetrol tetranitrate.
In the pure state, erythrityl tetranitrate will explode upon percussion, but properly diluted with lactose, as in Cardilate tablets, it is nonexplosive. Since it is a low melting solid, erythrityl tetranitrate does not evaporate from the Cardilate tablets.
Cardilate Oral/Sublingual Tablets contain either 5 or 10 mg erythrityl tetranitrate and the inactive ingredients lactose, magnesium stearate, and potato starch, with disintegration characteristics that permit sublingual or oral (swallowed) administration.

CLINICAL PHARMACOLOGY

Cardilate exerts its effects by relaxation of vascular smooth muscle.[1] The action is maximal on the post-capillary vessels, including the large veins. Venodilatation results in peripheral blood pooling, which decreases venous return to the heart, central venous pressure and pulmonary capillary wedge pressure (preload reduction).[2] Pulmonary arteriolar dilatation causes a reduction in pulmonary vascular resistance.[2] A decrease in systemic arterial pressure (afterload reduction) can also occur, but is usually less pronounced. Augmentation of cardiac output generally occurs in those patients with increased filling pressures and high resting systemic vascular resistance.[2]
Mechanism of Action: The inadequate myocardial oxygenation that precipitates angina can be corrected by: (1) increasing the supply of oxygen to ischemic myocardium through direct dilatation of the large coronary conductance vessels or (2) decreasing the myocardial oxygen demand secondary to a reduction of cardiac work (preload and afterload reduction).[3] The beneficial effect of Cardilate probably involves both mechanisms.
Pharmacokinetics and Metabolism: Cardilate is readily absorbed from the sublingual, buccal and gastrointestinal mucosae. The peak effect from a swallowed dose is diminished but of longer duration when compared to the sublingual route.[4] The biotransformation of Cardilate is thought to occur by reductive hydrolysis catalyzed by the hepatic enzyme glutathione-organic nitrate reductase.[3] Differences in response among various nitrates may relate to both intrinsic potency at cardiovascular sites, as well as factors related to pharmacokinetics and biotransformation.[5]
Time to onset of effect is approximately 5 minutes for the sublingual route and 15 to 30 minutes for swallowed tablets, with peak effect in 15 minutes and 60 minutes, respectively. Duration of action will vary, but vasodilatory effects have been demonstrated for up to 3 hours after sublingual administration[4,6] and for 6 hours after the oral (swallowed) route.[4]

INDICATIONS AND USAGE

Cardilate (Erythrityl Tetranitrate) is intended for the prophylaxis and long-term treatment of patients with frequent or recurrent anginal pain and reduced exercise tolerance associated with angina pectoris, rather than for the treatment of the acute attack of angina pectoris, since its onset is somewhat slower than that of nitroglycerin.

CONTRAINDICATIONS

Cardilate should not be administered to individuals with a known hypersensitivity or idiosyncratic reaction to organic nitrates.

WARNINGS

The use of nitrates in acute myocardial infarction or congestive heart failure should be undertaken only under close clinical observation and/or in conjunction with hemodynamic monitoring.

PRECAUTIONS

General: Cardilate should be used with caution in patients with severe liver or renal disease. Development of tolerance and cross-tolerance to the effects of erythrityl tetranitrate and other organic nitrates may occur. However, recent studies in patients with chronic heart failure[1] indicate that nitrates produce sustained beneficial hemodynamic effects.
Carcinogenesis, Mutagenesis, Impairment of Fertility: No long-term studies in animals have been performed.
Pregnancy: ***Teratogenic Effects.*** Pregnancy Category C. Animal reproduction studies have not been conducted with Cardilate. It is also not known whether Cardilate can cause fetal harm when administered to a pregnant woman or can affect reproduction capacity. Cardilate should be given to a pregnant woman only if clearly needed.
Nursing Mothers: It is not known whether this drug is excreted in human milk. Because many drugs are excreted in human milk, caution should be exercised when Cardilate is administered to a nursing woman.
Pediatric Use: Safety and effectiveness in children have not been established.

ADVERSE REACTIONS

The most frequent adverse reaction in patients treated with Cardilate is headache. Lowering the dose and the use of analgesics will help control headaches, which usually diminish or disappear as therapy is continued. Other adverse reactions occurring are the following: cutaneous vasodilatation with flushing, and transient episodes of dizziness and weakness, plus other signs of cerebral ischemia associated with postural hypotension. Occasional individuals exhibit marked sensitivity to the hypotensive effects of organic nitrates, and severe responses (e.g., nausea, vomiting, weakness, restlessness, pallor, perspiration and collapse) can occur even with the usual therapeutic dose. Alcohol may enhance this effect. Drug rash and/or exfoliative dermatitis may occasionally occur.

OVERDOSAGE

Accidental overdosage of Cardilate may result in severe hypotension and reflex tachycardia, which can be treated by laying the patient down and elevating the legs. If further treatment is required, the administration of intravenous fluids or other means of treating hypotension should be considered.

DOSAGE AND ADMINISTRATION

The Cardilate Oral/ Sublingual Tablet can be placed under the tongue or swallowed. Sublingual therapy may be initiated with a dose of 5 to 10 mg prior to each anticipated physical or emotional stress, and at bedtime for patients subject to nocturnal attacks of angina. The dose may be increased as needed.
If the patient is to swallow the tablet, therapy may be initiated with 10 mg before each meal, as well as mid-morning and mid-afternoon if needed, and at bedtime for patients subject to nocturnal attacks. The dose may be increased or decreased as needed.
Dosage titration up to 100 mg daily has been well tolerated, but temporary headache is more apt to occur with increasing doses. When headache occurs, the dose should be reduced for a few days. If headache is troublesome during adjustment of dosage, it may be effectively relieved with an analgesic.

HOW SUPPLIED

CARDILATE (Erythrityl Tetranitrate) ORAL/ SUBLINGUAL TABLETS (scored).

5 mg:	Bottles of 100 (NDC-0081-0166-55), Imprint "CARDILATE P2B" (round, white).
10 mg:	Bottles of 100 (NDC-0081-0168-55) and 1000 (NDC-0081-0168-75). Imprint "CARDILATE X7A" (square, white).

All tablets should be stored at 15°-25°C (59°- 77°F) in a dry place and dispensed in glass.

REFERENCES

1. Chatterjee K, Parmley WW: Vasodilator Therapy for Chronic Heart Failure. *Ann Rev Pharmacol Toxicol, 20*:475–512, 1980.
2. Goldberg S. Mann T, Grossman W: Nitrate Therapy of Heart Failure in Valvular Heart Disease. *Am J Med, 66*:161–66, 1978.
3. Needleman P, Johnson EM: Vasodilators and the Treatment of Angina. In: AG Gilman, LS Goodman, A Gilman, eds. The Pharmacological Basis of Therapeutics, 6th Edition, New York: Macmillan Publishing Co., Inc. 819–33, 1980.
4. Hannemann RE, Erb RJ, Stoltman WP, Bronson EC, Williams EJ, Long RA, Hull JH, Starbuck RR: Digital Plethysmograph for Assessing Erythrityl Tetranitrate Bioavailability. *Clin Pharmacol Ther, 29*:35–9, 1981.
5. Wastila WB, Namm DH, Maxwell RA: Comparison of the Vascular Effects of Several Organic Nitrates in Anesthetized Rats and Dogs after Intravenous and Intraportal Administration. Vascular Neuroeffector Mechanisms. 2nd Int. Symp., Odense. Basel: Karger Publishing Co. 216–25, 1975.
6. Haffty GB, Nakamura Y, Spodick DH, Long RA, Hull JH: Bioavailability of Organic Nitrates: a Comparison of Methods for Evaluating Plethysmographic Responses. *J Clin Pharmacol, 22*:117–124, 1982.

Shown in Product Identification Section, page 406

CORTISPORIN® CREAM ℞

[*kor′tĭ-spor″ĭn krēm*]
(Polymyxin B Sulfate-Neomycin Sulfate-Hydrocortisone Acetate)

DESCRIPTION

Cortisporin® Cream (polymyxin B sulfate-neomycin sulfate-hydrocortisone acetate) is a topical antibacterial cream. Each gram contains: Aerosporin® (polymyxin B sulfate) 10,000 units; neomycin sulfate equivalent to 3.5 mg neomycin base; and hydrocortisone acetate 5 mg (0.5%). The inactive ingredients are liquid petrolatum, white petrolatum, propylene glycol, polyoxyethylene polyoxypropylene compound, emulsifying wax, purified water, and 0.25% methylparaben added as a preservative. Sodium hydroxide or sulfuric acid may be added to adjust pH.
Polymyxin B sulfate is the sulfate salt of polymyxin B_1 and B_2, which are produced by the growth of *Bacillus polymyxa* (Prazmowski) Migula (Fam. Bacillaceae). It has a potency of not less than 6,000 polymyxin B units per mg, calculated on an anhydrous basis.
Neomycin sulfate is the sulfate salt of neomycin B and C, which are produced by the growth of *Streptomyces fradiae* Waksman (Fam. Streptomycetaceae). It has a potency equivalent of not less than 600 μg of neomycin standard per mg, calculated on an anhydrous basis.
Hydrocortisone acetate is the acetate ester of hydrocortisone, an anti-inflammatory hormone. Its chemical name is 21-(acetyloxy)-11β,17-dihydroxypregn-4-ene-3,20-dione.
The base is a smooth vanishing cream with a pH of approximately 5.0.

CLINICAL PHARMACOLOGY

Corticoids suppress the inflammatory response to a variety of agents and they may delay healing. Since corticoids may inhibit the body's defense mechanism against infection, a concomitant antimicrobial drug may be used when this inhi-

bition is considered to be clinically significant in a particular case.
The anti-infective components in the combination are included to provide action against specific organisms susceptible to them. Polymyxin B sulfate and neomycin sulfate together are considered active against the following microorganisms: *Staphylococcus aureus, Escherichia coli, Haemophilus influenzae, Klebsiella-Enterobacter* species, *Neisseria* species and *Pseudomonas aeruginosa.* The product does not provide adequate coverage against *Serratia marcescens* and streptococci, including *Streptococcus pneumoniae.*
The relative potency of corticosteroids depends on the molecular structure, concentration and release from the vehicle.
The acid pH helps restore normal cutaneous acidity. Owing to its excellent spreading and penetrating properties, the cream facilitates treatment of hairy and intertriginous areas. It may also be of value in selective cases where the lesions are moist.

INDICATIONS AND USAGE

For the treatment of corticosteroid-responsive dermatoses with secondary infection. It has not been demonstrated that this steroid-antibiotic combination provides greater benefit than the steroid component alone after 7 days of treatment (see WARNINGS section).

CONTRAINDICATIONS

Not for use in the eyes or in the external ear canal if the eardrum is perforated. This product is contraindicated in tuberculous, fungal or viral lesions of the skin (herpes simplex, vaccinia and varicella). This product is contraindicated in those individuals who have shown hypersensitivity to any of its components.

WARNINGS

Because of the concern of nephrotoxicity and ototoxicity associated with neomycin, this combination should not be used over a wide area or for extended periods of time.

PRECAUTIONS

General: As with any antibacterial preparation, prolonged use may result in overgrowth of nonsusceptible organisms, including fungi. Appropriate measures should be taken if this occurs. Use of steroids on infected areas should be supervised with care as anti-inflammatory steroids may encourage spread of infection. If this occurs, steroid therapy should be stopped and appropriate antibacterial drugs used. Generalized dermatological conditions may require systemic corticosteroid therapy.
Signs and symptoms of exogenous hyperadrenocorticism can occur with the use of topical corticosteroids, including adrenal suppression. Systemic absorption of topically applied steroids will be increased if extensive body surface areas are treated or if occlusive dressings are used. Under these circumstances, suitable precautions should be taken when long-term use is anticipated.
Information for Patients: If redness, irritation, swelling or pain persists or increases, discontinue use and notify physician. Do not use in the eyes.
Laboratory Tests: Systemic effects of excessive levels of hydrocortisone may include a reduction in the number of circulating eosinophils and a decrease in urinary excretion of 17-hydroxycorticosteroids.
Carcinogenesis, Mutagenesis, Impairment of Fertility: Long-term studies in animals (rats, rabbits, mice) showed no evidence of carcinogenicity attributable to oral administration of corticosteroids.
Pregnancy: ***Teratogenic Effects:*** Pregnancy Category C. Corticosteroids have been shown to be teratogenic in rabbits when applied topically at a concentration of 0.5% on days 6–18 of gestation and in mice when applied topically at a concentration of 15% on days 10–13 of gestation. There are no adequate and well controlled studies in pregnant women. Corticosteroids should be used during pregnancy only if the potential benefit justifies the potential risk to the fetus.
Nursing Mothers: Hydrocortisone acetate appears in human milk following oral administration of the drug. Since systemic absorption of hydrocortisone may occur when applied topically, caution should be exercised when Cortisporin Cream is used by a nursing woman.
Pediatric Use: Sufficient percutaneous absorption of hydrocortisone can occur in infants and children during prolonged use to cause cessation of growth, as well as other systemic signs and symptoms of hyperadrenocorticism.

ADVERSE REACTIONS

Neomycin occasionally causes skin sensitization. Ototoxicity and nephrotoxicity have also been reported (see WARNINGS section). Adverse reactions have occurred with topical use of antibiotic combinations including neomycin and polymyxin B. Exact incidence figures are not available since no denominator of treated patients is available. The reaction occurring most often is allergic sensitization. In one clinical study using a 20% neomycin patch, neomycin-induced allergic skin reactions occurred in two of 2,175 (0.09%) individuals in the general population.[1] In another study, the incidence was found to be approximately 1%.[2]
The following local adverse reactions have been reported with topical corticosteroids, especially under occlusive dressings: burning, itching, irritation, dryness, folliculitis, hypertrichosis, acneiform eruptions, hypopigmentation, perioral dermatitis, allergic contact dermatitis, maceration of the skin, secondary infection, skin atrophy, striae, and miliaria.
When steroid preparations are used for long periods of time in intertriginous areas or over extensive body areas, with or without occlusive non-permeable dressings, striae may occur; also there exists the possibility of systemic side effects when steroid preparations are used over large areas or for a long period of time.

DOSAGE AND ADMINISTRATION

A small quantity of the cream should be applied 2 to 4 times daily, as required. The cream should, if conditions permit, be gently rubbed into the affected areas.

HOW SUPPLIED

Tube of 7.5 g (NDC-0081-0185-98)
Store at 15°–30°C (59°–86°F).

REFERENCES

1. Leyden, JJ, Kligman AM: Contact dermatitis to neomycin sulfate. *JAMA* 1979;242(12):1276–1278.
2. Prystowsky SD, Allen AM, Smith RW, *et al:* Allergic contact hypersensitivity to nickel, neomycin, ethylenediamine, and benzocaine. *Arch Dermatol* 1979;115:959–962.

CORTISPORIN® OINTMENT ℞

[*kor 'tĭ-spor "ĭn*]
(Polymyxin B-Bacitracin-Neomycin-Hydrocortisone)

DESCRIPTION

Each gram contains:
Aerosporin® brand Polymyxin B Sulfate 5,000 units; bacitracin zinc 400 units; neomycin sulfate 5 mg (equivalent to 3.5 mg neomycin base); hydrocortisone 10 mg (1%); special white petrolatum qs.

ACTION

The ointment is useful wherever the anti-inflammatory and antipruritic action of hydrocortisone is indicated in conjunction with the bactericidal action of polymyxin B, neomycin, and bacitracin. For anti-inflammatory action, the naturally occurring adrenal corticosteroid hydrocortisone was selected.
The combination of Aerosporin brand Polymyxin B Sulfate with neomycin and bacitracin was selected because it most nearly meets the criteria for an ideal topical antibacterial preparation. The spectrum of action encompasses most pathogenic bacteria found topically, and the three antibiotics are bactericidal rather than bacteriostatic. When used topically, polymyxin B, neomycin and bacitracin are rarely irritating, and absorption from skin or mucous membrane is insignificant. The index of allergenicity of this combination has been shown over the years to be low. And finally, since these antibiotics are seldom used systemically, the patient is spared sensitization to those antibiotics which might later be required systemically.
Polymyxin B is one of a group of closely related substances produced by various strains of *Bacillus polymyxa.* Its activity is sharply restricted to gram-negative bacteria, including many strains of *Pseudomonas aeruginosa.*
Neomycin, isolated from *Streptomyces fradiae,* has antibacterial activity *in vitro* against a wide range of gram-negative and gram-positive organisms, with effectiveness against many strains of *Proteus.*
Bacitracin, an antibiotic substance derived from cultures of *Bacillus subtilis* (Tracy), exerts antibacterial action *in vitro* against a variety of gram-positive and a few gram-negative organisms.

INDICATIONS

For the treatment of corticosteroid-responsive dermatoses with secondary infection. It has not been demonstrated that this steroid-antibiotic combination provides better benefit than the steroid component alone after 7 days of treatment (see WARNINGS section).

CONTRAINDICATIONS

This product is contraindicated in those individuals who have shown hypersensitivity to any of its components. Do not use in the external ear canal if the eardrum is perforated.

WARNINGS

Because of the concern of nephrotoxicity and ototoxicity associated with neomycin, this combination product should not be used over a wide area or for extended periods of time.
When using neomycin-containing products to control secondary infection in the chronic dermatoses, such as chronic otitis externa or stasis dermatitis, it should be borne in mind that the skin in these conditions is more liable than is normal skin to become sensitized to many substances, including neomycin. The manifestation of sensitization to neomycin is usually a low grade reddening with swelling, dry scaling and itching; it may be manifest simply as a failure to heal. During long-term use of neomycin-containing products, periodic examination for such signs is advisable and the patient should be told to discontinue the product if they are observed. These symptoms regress quickly on withdrawing the medication. Neomycin-containing applications should be avoided for that patient thereafter.

PRECAUTIONS

As with any antibiotic preparation, prolonged use may result in the overgrowth of nonsusceptible organisms, including fungi. Appropriate measures should be taken if this occurs. Use of steroids on infected areas should be supervised with care as anti-inflammatory steroids may encourage spread of infection. If this occurs steroid therapy should be stopped and appropriate antibacterial drugs used. Generalized dermatological conditions may require systemic corticosteroid therapy. As the safety of topical steroid preparations during pregnancy has not been fully established, they should not be used unnecessarily, on extended areas, in large amounts, or for prolonged periods of time, in pregnancy.

ADVERSE REACTIONS

When steroid preparations are used for long periods of time in intertriginous areas or over extensive body areas, with or without occlusive non-permeable dressings, striae may occur; also there exists the possibility of systemic side effects when steroid preparations are used over larger areas or for a long period of time.
Neomycin is a not uncommon cutaneous sensitizer. Articles in the current literature indicate an increase in the prevalence of persons allergic to neomycin. Ototoxicity and nephrotoxicity have been reported (see Warnings section).

DOSAGE AND ADMINISTRATION

A thin film is applied 2 to 4 times daily. In chronic conditions, withdrawal of treatment is carried out by decreasing the frequency of application, until the ointment is applied as infrequently as once a week.

HOW SUPPLIED

Tube of ½ oz with applicator tip.

CORTISPORIN® OPHTHALMIC ℞

[*kor 'tĭ-spor 'ĭn*]
OINTMENT Sterile
(Polymyxin B Sulfate-Bacitracin Zinc-Neomycin Sulfate-Hydrocortisone)

DESCRIPTION

Cortisporin® Ophthalmic Ointment (polymyxin B sulfate-bacitracin zinc-neomycin sulfate-hydrocortisone) is a sterile antimicrobial and anti-inflammatory ointment for ophthalmic use. Each gram contains Aerosporin® (polymyxin B sulfate) 10,000 units, bacitracin zinc 400 units, neomycin sulfate equivalent to 3.5 mg neomycin base, hydrocortisone 10 mg (1%) and special white petrolatum, qs.
Polymyxin B sulfate is the sulfate salt of polymyxin B_1 and B_2 which are produced by the growth of *Bacillus polymyxa* (Prazmowski) Migula (Fam. Bacillaceae). It has a potency of not less than 6,000 Polymyxin B units per mg, calculated on an anhydrous basis.
Bacitracin zinc is the zinc salt of bacitracin, a mixture of related cyclic polypeptides (mainly bacitracin A) produced by the growth of an organism of the *licheniformis* group of *Bacillus subtilis* (Fam. Bacillaceae). It has a potency of not less than 40 bacitracin units per mg.
Neomycin sulfate is the sulfate salt of neomycin B and C, which are produced by the growth of *Streptomyces fradiae* Waksman (Fam. Streptomycetaceae). It has a potency equivalent of not less than 600 μg of neomycin standard per mg, calculated on an anhydrous basis.
Hydrocortisone, 11β, 17, 21-trihydroxypregn-4-ene-3, 20-dione, is an anti-inflammatory hormone.

CLINICAL PHARMACOLOGY

Corticoids suppress the inflammatory response to a variety of agents and they may delay healing. Since corticoids may inhibit the body's defense mechanism against infection, a concomitant antimicrobial drug may be used when this inhibition is considered to be clinically significant in a particular case.
The anti-infective components in the combination are included to provide action against specific organisms susceptible to them. Polymyxin B sulfate, bacitracin zinc and neomycin sulfate together are considered active against the following microorganisms: *Staphylococcus aureus,* streptococci, including *Streptococcus pneumoniae, Escherichia coli, Haemophilus influenzae, Klebsiella-Enterobacter* species, *Neisseria* species and *Pseudomonas aeruginosa.*
When used topically, polymyxin B, bacitracin and neomycin are rarely irritating, and absorption from the intact skin or mucous membrane is insignificant. The incidence of skin sensitization to this combination has been shown to be low on normal skin.[1,2] Since these antibiotics are seldom used sys-

Continued on next page

Burroughs Wellcome—Cont.

temically, the patient is spared sensitization to those antibiotics which might later be required systemically.
When a decision to administer both a corticoid and antimicrobials is made, the administration of such drugs in combination has the advantage of greater patient compliance and convenience, with the added assurance that the intended dosage of both drugs is administered, plus assured compatibility of ingredients when both types of drug are in the same formulation and, particularly, that the intended volume of each drug is delivered simultaneously, thereby avoiding dilution of either medication by successive applications.
The relative potency of corticosteroids depends on the molecular structure, concentration, and release from the vehicle.

INDICATIONS AND USAGE

For steroid-responsive inflammatory ocular conditions for which a corticosteroid is indicated and where bacterial infection or a risk of bacterial ocular infection exists.
Ocular steroids are indicated in inflammatory conditions of the palpebral and bulbar conjunctiva, cornea and anterior segment of the globe where the inherent risk of steroid use in certain infective conjunctivitides is accepted to obtain a diminution in edema and inflammation. They are also indicated in chronic anterior uveitis and corneal injury from chemical, radiation, or thermal burns, or penetration of foreign bodies.
The use of a combination drug with an anti-infective component is indicated where the risk of infection is high or where there is an expectation that potentially dangerous numbers of bacteria will be present in the eye.
The particular anti-infective drugs in this product are active against the following common bacterial eye pathogens: *Staphylococcus aureus*, streptococci, including *Streptococcus pneumoniae, Escherichia coli, Haemophilus influenzae, Klebsiella-Enterobacter* species, *Neisseria* species and *Pseudomonas aeruginosa.*
The product does not provide adequate coverage against *Serratia marcescens.*

CONTRAINDICATIONS

Epithelial herpes simplex keratitis (dendritic keratitis), vaccinia, varicella, and many other viral diseases of the cornea and conjunctiva. Mycobacterial infection of the eye. Fungal diseases of ocular structures. Hypersensitivity to a component of the medication. (Hypersensitivity to the antibiotic component occurs at a higher rate than for other components.)
The use of these combinations is always contraindicated after uncomplicated removal of a corneal foreign body.

WARNINGS

Prolonged use may result in glaucoma, with damage to the optic nerve, defects in visual acuity and fields of vision, and posterior subcapsular cataract formation. Prolonged use may suppress the host response and thus increase the hazard of secondary ocular infections. In those diseases causing thinning of the cornea or sclera, perforations have been known to occur with the use of topical steroids. In acute purulent conditions of the eye, steroids may mask infection or enhance existing infection. If these products are used for 10 days or longer, intraocular pressure should be routinely monitored even though it may be difficult in children and uncooperative patients.
Employment of steroid medication in the treatment of herpes simplex requires great caution.
Neomycin sulfate may cause cutaneous sensitization. A precise incidence of hypersensitivity reactions (primarily skin rash) due to topical neomycin is not known.
The manifestations of sensitization to neomycin are usually itching, reddening and edema of the conjunctiva and eyelid. It may be manifest simply as a failure to heal. During long-term use of neomycin-containing products, periodic examination for such signs is advisable, and the patient should be told to discontinue the product if they are observed. These symptoms subside quickly on withdrawing the medication. Neomycin-containing applications should be avoided for the patient thereafter.

PRECAUTIONS

General: The initial prescription and renewal of the medication order beyond 8 grams should be made by a physician only after examination of the patient with the aid of magnification, such as slit lamp biomicroscopy and, where appropriate, fluorescein staining.
The possibility of persistent fungal infections of the cornea should be considered after prolonged steroid dosing.
Allergic cross-reactions may occur which could prevent the use of any or all of the following antibiotics for the treatment of future infections: kanamycin, paromomycin, streptomycin, and possibly gentamicin.
Carcinogenesis, Mutagenesis, Impairment of Fertility: Long-term studies in animals (rats, rabbits, mice) showed no evidence of carcinogenicity attributable to oral administration of corticosteroids.
Pregnancy: ***Teratogenic Effects:*** Pregnancy Category C. Corticosteroids have been shown to be teratogenic in rabbits when applied topically at concentrations of 0.5% on days 6-18 of gestation and in mice when applied topically at a concentration of 15% on days 10-13 of gestation. There are no adequate and well-controlled studies in pregnant women. Corticosteroids should be used during pregnancy only if the potential benefit justifies the potential risk to the fetus.
Nursing Mothers: Hydrocortisone appears in human milk following oral administration of the drug. Since systemic absorption of hydrocortisone may occur when applied topically, caution should be exercised when Cortisporin Ophthalmic Ointment is used by a nursing woman.

ADVERSE REACTIONS

Adverse reactions have occurred with steroid/anti-infective combination drugs which can be attributed to the steroid component, the anti-infective component, or the combination. Reactions occurring most often from the presence of the anti-infective ingredient are localized hypersensitivity, including itching, swelling and conjunctival erythema. Local irritation on instillation has also been reported. Exact incidence figures are not available since no denominator of treated patients is available.
The reactions due to the steroid component in decreasing order of frequency are: elevation of introcular pressure (IOP) with possible development of glaucoma, and infrequent optic nerve damage; posterior subcapsular cataract formation; and delayed wound healing.
Secondary Infection: The development of secondary infection has occurred after use of combinations containing steroids and antimicrobials. Fungal infections of the cornea are particularly prone to develop coincidentally with long-term applications of steroid. The possibility of fungal invasion must be considered in any persistent corneal ulceration where steroid treatment has been used.
Secondary bacterial ocular infection following suppression of host responses also occurs.

DOSAGE AND ADMINISTRATION

Apply the ointment in the affected eye every 3 or 4 hours, depending on the severity of the condition.
Not more than 8 grams should be prescribed initally and the prescription should not be refilled without further evaluation as outlined in PRECAUTIONS above.

HOW SUPPLIED

Tube of 1/8 oz with ophthalmic tip (NDC-0081-0197-86).
Store at 15°–30°C (59°–86°F).
DoD NSN 6505-01-102-4303

References:

1. Leyden JJ and Kligman AM. Contact Dermatitis to Neomycin Sulfate *JAMA 242 (12)*:1276-1278, 1979.
2. Prystowsky SD, Allen AM, Smith RW, Nonomura JH, Odom RB and Akers WA. Allergic Contact Hypersensitivity to Nickel, Neomycin, Ethylenediamine, and Benzocaine. *Arch Dermatol 115* :959-962, 1979.

CORTISPORIN® ℞

[*kor'tĭ-spor"ĭn*]

OPHTHALMIC SUSPENSION Sterile

(Polymyxin B Sulfate-Neomycin Sulfate-Hydrocortisone)

DESCRIPTION

Cortisporin® Ophthalmic Suspension (polymyxin B sulfate-neomycin sulfate-hydrocortisone) is a sterile antimicrobial and anti-inflammatory suspension for ophthalmic use. Each ml contains: Aerosporin® (polymyxin B sulfate) 10,000 units, neomycin sulfate equivalent to 3.5 mg neomycin base and hydrocortisone 10 mg (1%). The vehicle contains thimerosal 0.001% (added as a preservative) and the inactive ingredients cetyl alcohol, glyceryl monostearate, mineral oil, polyoxyl 40 stearate, propylene gylcol and water for injection. Sulfuric acid may be added to adjust pH.
Polymyxin B sulfate is the sulfate salt of polymyxin B_1 and B_2, which are produced by the growth of *Bacillus polymyxa* (Prazmowski) Migula (fam. Bacillaceae). It has a potency of not less than 6,000 polymyxin B units per mg, calculated on an anhydrous basis.
Neomycin sulfate is the sulfate salt of neomycin B and C, which are produced by the growth of *Streptomyces fradiae* Waksman (Fam. Streptomycetaceae). It has a potency equivalent of not less than 600 μg of neomycin standard per mg, calculated on an anhydrous basis.
Hydrocortisone, 11β, 17, 21-trihydroxypregn-4-ene-3,20-dione, is an anti-inflammatory hormone.

CLINICAL PHARMACOLOGY

Corticoids suppress the inflammatory response to a variety of agents and they may delay healing. Since corticoids may inhibit the body's defense mechanism against infection, a concomitant antimicrobial drug may be used when this inhibition is considered to be clinically significant in a particular case.
The anti-infective components in the combination are included to provide action against specific organisms susceptible to them. Polymyxin B sulfate and neomycin sulfate together are considered active against the following microorganisms: *Staphylococcus aureus, Escherichia coli, Haemophilus influenzae, Klebsiella-Enterobacter* species, *Neisseria* species and *Pseudomonas aeruginosa.*
When used topically, polymyxin B and neomycin are rarely irritating, and absorption from the intact skin or mucous membrane is insignificant. The incidence of skin sensitization to this combination has been shown to be low on normal skin.[1,2] Since these antibiotics are seldom used systemically, the patient is spared sensitization to those antibiotics which might later be required systemically.
When a decision to administer both a corticoid and antimicrobials is made, the administration of such drugs in combination has the advantage of greater patient compliance and convenience, with the added assurance that the intended dosage of both drugs is administered, plus assured compatibility of ingredients when both types of drug are in the same formulation and, particularly, that the intended volume of each drug is delivered simultaneously, thereby avoiding dilution of either medication by successive instillations.
The relative potency of corticosteroids depends on the molecular structure, concentration, and release from the vehicle.

INDICATIONS AND USAGE

For steroid-responsive inflammatory ocular conditions for which a corticosteroid is indicated and where bacterial infection or a risk of bacterial ocular infection exists.
Ocular steroids are indicated in inflammatory conditions of the palpebral and bulbar conjunctiva, cornea and anterior segment of the globe where the inherent risk of steroid use in certain infective conjunctivitides is accepted to obtain a diminution in edema and inflammation. They are also indicated in chronic anterior uveitis and corneal injury from chemical, radiation, or thermal burns, or penetration of foreign bodies.
The use of a combination drug with an anti-infective component is indicated where the risk of infection is high or where there is an expectation that potentially dangerous numbers of bacteria will be present in the eye.
The particular anti-infective drugs in this product are active against the following common bacterial eye pathogens: *Staphylococcus aureus, Escherichia coli, Haemophilus influenzae, Klebsiella-Enterobacter* species, *Neisseria* species, and *Pseudomonas aeruginosa.*
The product does not provide adequate coverage against *Serratia marcescens* and streptococci, including *Streptococcus pneumoniae.*

CONTRAINDICATIONS

Epithelial herpes simplex keratitis (dendritic keratitis), vaccinia, varicella, and many other viral diseases of the cornea and conjunctiva. Mycobacterial infection of the eye. Fungal diseases of ocular structures. Hypersensitivity to a component of the medication. (Hypersensitivity to the antibiotic component occurs at a higher rate than for other components.)
The use of these combinations is always contraindicated after uncomplicated removal of a corneal foreign body.

WARNINGS

Prolonged use may result in glaucoma, with damage to the optic nerve, defects in visual acuity and fields of vision, and posterior subcapsular cataract formation. Prolonged use may suppress the host response and thus increase the hazard of secondary ocular infections. In those diseases causing thinning of the cornea or sclera, perforations have been known to occur with the use of topical steroids. In acute purulent conditions of the eye, steroids may mask infection or enhance existing infection. If these products are used for 10 days or longer, intraocular pressure should be routinely monitored even though it may be difficult in children and uncooperative patients.
Employment of steroid medication in the treatment of herpes simplex requires great caution.
Neomycin sulfate may cause cutaneous sensitization. A precise incidence of hypersensitivity reactions (primarily skin rash) due to topical neomycin is not known.
The manifestations of sensitization to neomycin are usually itching, reddening and edema of the conjunctiva and eyelid. It may be manifest simply as a failure to heal. During long-term use of neomycin-containing products, periodic examination for such signs is advisable, and the patient should be told to discontinue the product if they are observed. These symptoms subside quickly on withdrawing the medication. Neomycin-containing applications should be avoided for the patient thereafter.

PRECAUTIONS

General: The initial prescription and renewal of the medication order beyond 20 milliliters should be made by a physician only after examination of the patient with the aid of magnification, such as slit lamp biomicroscopy and, where appropriate, fluorescein staining.
The possibility of persistent fungal infections of the cornea should be considered after prolonged steroid dosing.
Allergic cross-reactions may occur which could prevent the use of any or all of the following antibiotics for the treatment

of future infections: kanamycin, paromomycin, streptomycin, and possibly gentamicin.

Carcinogenesis, Mutagenesis, Impairment of Fertility: Long-term studies in animals (rats, rabbits, mice) showed no evidence of carcinogenicity attributable to oral administration of corticosteroids.

Pregnancy: *Teratogenic Effects:* Pregnancy Category C. Corticosteroids have been shown to be teratogenic in rabbits when applied topically at concentrations of 0.5% on days 6–18 of gestation and in mice when applied topically at a concentration of 15% on days 10–13 of gestation. There are no adequate and well-controlled studies in pregnant women. Corticosteroids should be used during pregnancy only if the potential benefit justifies the potential risk to the fetus.

Nursing Mothers: Hydrocortisone appears in human milk following oral administration of the drug. Since systemic absorption of hydrocortisone may occur when applied topically, caution should be exercised when Cortisporin Ophthalmic Suspension is used by a nursing woman.

ADVERSE REACTIONS

Adverse reactions have occurred with steroid/anti-infective combination drugs which can be attributed to the steroid component, the anti-infective component, or the combination. Reactions occurring most often from the presence of the anti-infective ingredient are localized hypersensitivity, including itching, swelling and conjunctival erythema. Local irritation on instillation has also been reported. Exact incidence figures are not available since no denominator of treated patients is available.

The reactions due to the steroid component in decreasing order of frequency are: elevation of intraocular pressure (IOP) with possible development of glaucoma, and infrequent optic nerve damage; posterior subcapsular cataract formation; and delayed wound healing.

Secondary Infection: The development of secondary infection has occurred after use of combinations containing steroids and antimicrobials. Fungal infections of the cornea are particularly prone to develop coincidentally with long-term applications of steroid. The possibility of fungal invasion must be considered in any persistent corneal ulceration where steroid treatment has been used.

Secondary bacterial ocular infection following suppression of host responses also occurs.

DOSAGE AND ADMINISTRATION

One or two drops in the affected eye every 3 or 4 hours, depending on the severity of the condition. The suspension may be used more frequently if necessary.

Not more than 20 milliliters should be prescribed initially and the prescription should not be refilled without further evaluation as outlined in PRECAUTIONS above.

SHAKE WELL BEFORE USING.

HOW SUPPLIED

Plastic DROP DOSE® dispenser bottle of 7.5 ml (NDC-0081-0193-02).

Store at 15°–25°C (59°–77°F).

DOD NSN 6505-00-764-9042

REFERENCES

1. Leyden JJ and Kligman AM. Contact Dermatitis to Neomycin Sulfate. *JAMA 242 (12)*: 1276–1278, 1979.
2. Prystowsky SD, Allen AM, Smith RW, Nonomura JH, Odom RB and Akers WA. Allergic Contact Hypersensitivity to Nickel, Neomycin, Ethylenediamine, and Benzocaine. *Arch Dermatol 115*:959–962, 1979.

CORTISPORIN® OTIC SOLUTION ℞

[kor 'tĭ-spor "ĭn ō-tĭk]

Sterile

(Polymyxin B-Neomycin-Hydrocortisone)

DESCRIPTION

Each ml contains:

Aerosporin® (Polymyxin B Sulfate) ....10,000 Units

Neomycin sulfate ....5 mg

(equivalent to 3.5 mg neomycin base)

Hydrocortisone ....10 mg (1%)

The vehicle contains the inactive ingredients cupric sulfate, glycerin, hydrochloric acid, propylene glycol, water for injection and potassium metabisulfite (added as a preservative) 0.1%.

ACTION

Hydrocortisone, the naturally occurring adrenal corticosteroid, affords antiallergic, antipruritic and anti-inflammatory activity.

Polymyxin B is one of a group of closely related substances produced by various strains of *Bacillus polymyxa*. Its activity is sharply restricted to gram-negative bacteria, including many strains of *Pseudomonas aeruginosa*.

Neomycin, isolated from *Streptomyces fradiae*, has antibacterial activity *in vitro* against a wide range of gram-negative and gram-positive organisms, with effectiveness against many strains of *Proteus*.

INDICATIONS

For the treatment of superficial bacterial infections of the external auditory canal caused by organisms susceptible to the action of the antibiotics.

CONTRAINDICATIONS

This product is contraindicated in those individuals who have shown hypersensitivity to any of its components, and in herpes simplex, vaccinia and varicella.

WARNINGS

As with other antibiotic preparations, prolonged treatment may result in overgrowth of nonsusceptible organisms and fungi.

If the infection is not improved after one week, cultures and susceptibility tests should be repeated to verify the identity of the organism and to determine whether therapy should be changed.

When using neomycin-containing products to control secondary infection in the chronic dermatoses, such as chronic otitis externa, it should be borne in mind that the skin in these conditions is more liable than is normal skin to become sensitized to many substances, including neomycin. The manifestation of sensitization to neomycin is usually a low grade reddening with swelling, dry scaling and itching; it may be manifest simply as a failure to heal. During long-term use of neomycin-containing products, periodic examination for such signs is advisable and the patient should be told to discontinue the product if they are observed. These symptoms regress quickly on withdrawing the medication. Neomycin-containing applications should be avoided for that patient thereafter.

PRECAUTIONS

If sensitization or irritation occurs, medication should be discontinued promptly.

This drug should be used with care when the integrity of the tympanic membrane is in question because of the possibility of ototoxicity caused by neomycin.

Patients who prefer to warm the medication before using should be cautioned against heating the solution above body temperature, in order to avoid loss of potency.

Treatment should not be continued for longer than ten days.

Allergic cross-reactions may occur which could prevent the use of any or all of the following antibiotics for the treatment of future infections: kanamycin, paromomycin, streptomycin, and possibly gentamicin.

ADVERSE REACTIONS

Neomycin is a not uncommon cutaneous sensitizer. There are articles in the current literature that indicate an increase in the prevalence of persons sensitive to neomycin. Stinging and burning have been reported when this drug has gained access to the middle ear.

DOSAGE AND ADMINISTRATION

The external auditory canal should be thoroughly cleansed and dried with a sterile cotton applicator.

For adults, 4 drops of the solution should be instilled into the affected ear 3 or 4 times daily. For infants and children, 3 drops are suggested because of the smaller capacity of the ear canal.

The patient should lie with the affected ear upward and then the drops should be instilled. This position should be maintained for 5 minutes to facilitate penetration of the drops into the ear canal. Repeat, if necessary, for the opposite ear.

If preferred, a cotton wick may be inserted into the canal and then the cotton may be saturated with the solution. This wick should be kept moist by adding further solution every four hours. The wick should be replaced at least once every 24 hours.

The patient should be instructed to avoid contaminating the dropper with material from the ear, fingers, or other source. This caution is necessary if the sterility of the drops is to be preserved.

HOW SUPPLIED

Bottle of 10 ml with sterilized dropper.

10 ml—DoD & VA NSN 6505-01-014-1378

CORTISPORIN® OTIC SUSPENSION ℞

[kor 'tĭ-spor "ĭn ō-tĭk]

Sterile

(Polymyxin B-Neomycin-Hydrocortisone)

DESCRIPTION

Each ml contains: Aerosporin® (Polymyxin B Sulfate) 10,000 units, neomycin sulfate 5 mg (equivalent to 3.5 mg neomycin base), hydrocortisone 10 mg (1%). The vehicle contains the inactive ingredients cetyl alcohol, propylene glycol, polysorbate 80, water for injection and thimerosal (added as a preservative) 0.01%. Sulfuric acid may be added to adjust pH.

ACTION

Hydrocortisone, the naturally occurring adrenal corticosteroid, affords antiallergic, antipruritic and anti-inflammatory activity.

Polymyxin B is one of a group of closely related substances produced by various strains of *Bacillus polymyxa*. Its activity is sharply restricted to gram-negative bacteria, including many strains of *Pseudomonas aeruginosa*.

Neomycin, isolated from *Streptomyces fradiae*, has antibacterial activity *in vitro* against a wide range of gram-negative and gram-positive organisms, with effectiveness against many strains of *Proteus*.

INDICATIONS

For the treatment of superficial bacterial infections of the external auditory canal caused by organisms susceptible to the action of the antibiotics, and for the treatment of infections of mastoidectomy and fenestration cavities caused by organisms susceptible to the antibiotics.

CONTRAINDICATIONS

This product is contraindicated in those individuals who have shown hypersensitivity to any of its components, and in herpes simplex, vaccinia and varicella.

WARNINGS

As with other antibiotic preparations, prolonged treatment may result in overgrowth of nonsusceptible organisms and fungi.

If the infection is not improved after one week, cultures and susceptibility tests should be repeated to verify the identity of the organism and to determine whether therapy should be changed.

When using neomycin-containing products to control secondary infection in the chronic dermatoses, such as chronic otitis externa, it should be borne in mind that the skin in these conditions is more liable than is normal skin to become sensitized to many substances, including neomycin. The manifestation of sensitization to neomycin is usually a low grade reddening with swelling, dry scaling and itching; it may be manifest simply as a failure to heal. During long-term use of neomycin-containing products, periodic examination for such signs is advisable and the patient should be told to discontinue the product if they are observed. These symptoms regress quickly on withdrawing the medication. Neomycin-containing applications should be avoided for that patient thereafter.

PRECAUTIONS

If sensitization or irritation occurs, medication should be discontinued promptly.

This drug should be used with care in cases of perforated eardrum and in longstanding cases of chronic otitis media because of the possibility of ototoxicity caused by neomycin.

Patients who prefer to warm the medication before using should be cautioned against heating the solution above body temperature, in order to avoid loss of potency.

Treatment should not be continued for longer than ten days.

Allergic cross-reactions may occur which could prevent the use of any or all of the following antibiotics for the treatment of future infections: kanamycin, paromomycin, streptomycin, and possibly gentamicin.

ADVERSE REACTIONS

Neomycin is a not uncommon cutaneous sensitizer. There are articles in the current literature that indicate an increase in the prevalence of persons sensitive to neomycin.

DOSAGE AND ADMINISTRATION

The external auditory canal should be thoroughly cleansed and dried with a sterile cotton applicator.

For adults, 4 drops of the suspension should be instilled into the affected ear 3 or 4 times daily. For infants and children, 3 drops are suggested because of the smaller capacity of the ear canal.

The patient should lie with the affected ear upward and then the drops should be instilled. This position should be maintained for 5 minutes to facilitate penetration of the drops into the ear canal. Repeat, if necessary, for the opposite ear.

If preferred, a cotton wick may be inserted into the canal and then the cotton may be saturated with the suspension. This wick should be kept moist by adding further suspension every four hours. The wick should be replaced at least once every 24 hours.

The patient should be instructed to avoid contaminating the dropper with material from the ear, fingers, or other source. This caution is necessary if the sterility of the drops is to be preserved. SHAKE WELL BEFORE USING.

HOW SUPPLIED

Bottle of 10 ml with sterilized dropper.

10 ml DoD & VA NSN 6505-01-043-0230

Continued on next page

Burroughs Wellcome—Cont.

DARAPRIM® ℞
[*dair'ah-prĭm"*]
(Pyrimethamine)
25 mg Scored Tablets

DESCRIPTION

Daraprim (pyrimethamine) is an antimalarial available in tablet form for oral administration. Each scored tablet contains 25 mg pyrimethamine and the inactive ingredients corn and potato starch, lactose, and magnesium stearate.
Pyrimethamine is known chemically as 2, 4-diamino-5-(*p*-chlorophenyl)-6-ethylpyrimidine.

ACTIONS

Daraprim is a folic acid antagonist and the rationale for its therapeutic action is based on the differential requirement between host and parasite for nucleic acid precursors involved in growth. This activity is highly selective against plasmodia and *Toxoplasma gondii.*
Pyrimethamine possesses blood schizonticidal and some tissue schizonticidal activity against malaria parasites of man. However, its blood schizonticidal activity may be slower than that of 4-aminoquinoline compounds. It does not destroy gametocytes, but arrests sporogony in the mosquito.
The action of Daraprim against *Toxoplasma gondii* is greatly enhanced when used in conjunction with sulfonamides. This was demonstrated by Eyles and Coleman in the treatment of experimental toxoplasmosis in the mouse. Jacobs *et al* demonstrated that combination of the two drugs effectively prevented the development of severe uveitis in most rabbits following the inoculation of the anterior chamber of the eye with toxoplasma.

INDICATIONS

Daraprim (Pyrimethamine) is indicated for the chemoprophylaxis of malaria due to susceptible strains of plasmodia. Fast-acting schizonticides (chloroquine, amodiaquin, quinacrine or quinine) are indicated and preferable for the treatment of acute attacks. However, conjoint use of Daraprim will initiate *transmission control* and *suppressive cure.*
Daraprim is also indicated for the treatment of toxoplasmosis. For this purpose the drug should be used conjointly with a sulfonamide since synergism exists with this combination.

WARNINGS

The dosage of pyrimethamine required for the treatment of toxoplasmosis is 10 to 20 times the recommended antimalarial dosage and approaches the toxic level. If signs of folic or folinic acid deficiency develop (see Adverse Reactions) reduce the dosage or discontinue the drug according to the response of the patient. Folinic acid (leucovorin) may be administered in a dosage of 5 to 15 mg daily (orally, I.V. or I.M.) until normal hematopoiesis is restored.
Patients should be warned to keep Daraprim out of the reach of children since accidental ingestion has led to fatality.

USE IN PREGNANCY

Pyrimethamine, like other folic acid antagonists, may, in large doses, produce teratogenic effects in laboratory animals. The large doses required to treat toxoplasmosis should be used only after a definitive diagnosis of acute toxoplasmosis has been made, and the possibility of teratogenic effects from the drug has been carefully weighed against the possible risks of permanent damage to the fetus from the infection.
Concurrent administration of folinic acid is recommended when pyrimethamine is used for treatment of toxoplasmosis during pregnancy.

PRECAUTIONS

The recommended dosage for malaria suppression should not be exceeded. In patients receiving high dosage, as for the treatment of toxoplasmosis, semi-weekly blood counts, including platelet counts, should be made. In patients with convulsive disorders a small "starting" dose (for toxoplasmosis) is recommended to avoid the potential nervous system toxicity of pyrimethamine.

ADVERSE REACTIONS

With large doses, anorexia and vomiting may occur. Vomiting may be minimized by giving the medication with meals; it usually disappears promptly upon reduction of dosage. Also, large doses as used in toxoplasmosis may produce megaloblastic anemia, leukopenia, thrombocytopenia, pancytopenia and atrophic glossitis. Acute intoxication may follow the ingestion of an excessive amount of pyrimethamine; this may involve central nervous system stimulation including convulsions. In such cases a parenteral barbiturate may be indicated followed by folinic acid (leucovorin) (see Warnings).

DOSAGE AND ADMINISTRATION

For Chemoprophylaxis of Malaria: Adults and children over 10 years—25 mg (1 tablet) once weekly
Children 4 through 10 years—12.5 mg (½ tablet) once weekly
Infants and children under 4 years—6.25 mg (¼ tablet) once weekly
Regimens planned to include *suppressive cure* should be extended through any characteristic periods of early recrudescence and late relapse for at least 10 weeks in each case.
For Treatment of Acute Attacks: Daraprim is recommended in areas where only susceptible plasmodia exist. The drug is not recommended alone in the treatment of acute attacks of malaria in non-immune persons. Fast-acting schizonticides (chloroquine, amodiaquin, quinacrine or quinine) are indicated for treatment of acute attacks. However, conjoint Daraprim dosage of 25 mg daily for 2 days will initiate *transmission control* and *suppressive cure.* Should circumstances arise wherein Daraprim must be used alone in semi-immune persons, the adult dosage for an acute attack is 50 mg for 2 days; children 4 through 10 years old may be given 25 mg daily for 2 days. In any event, clinical cure should be followed by the once-weekly regimen described above.
For Toxoplasmosis: The dosage of Daraprim (Pyrimethamine) in the treatment of toxoplasmosis must be carefully adjusted so as to provide maximum therapeutic effect and a minimum of side effects. At the high dosage required, there is a marked variation in the tolerance to the drug. Young patients may tolerate higher doses than older individuals.
The adult *starting* dose is 50 to 75 mg of the drug daily, together with 1 to 4 g daily of a sulfonamide drug of the sulfapyrimidine type, e.g., sulfadiazine, triple-sulfa. This dosage is ordinarily continued for 1 to 3 weeks, depending on the response of the patient and his tolerance of the therapy. The dosage may then be reduced to about one-half that previously given for each drug and continued for an additional 4 to 5 weeks.
The pediatric dosage of Daraprim is 1 mg/kg per day divided into 2 equal daily doses; after 2 to 4 days this dose may be reduced to one-half and continued for approximately one month. The usual pediatric sulfonamide dosage is used in conjunction with Daraprim.

HOW SUPPLIED

White, scored tablets containing 25 mg pyrimethamine, imprinted with "DARAPRIM" and "A3A" in bottles of 100 (NDC-0081-0201-55).
Store at 15°-30°C (59°-86°F) in a dry place and protect from light.
100—DoD **NSN 6505-00-926-4765**
Shown in Product Identification Section, page 406

EMPIRIN®
[*ĭm'per-ĭn" or ĭmp'prĭn*]
ASPIRIN TABLETS
ASPIRIN—325 mg (5 grs)

(See PDR for Nonprescription Drugs)
Shown in Product Identification Section, page 406

EMPIRIN® with Codeine Tablets ℞Ⓒ
[*ĭm'per-ĭn with kō'dēn*]

DESCRIPTION

Empirin with Codeine is supplied in tablet form for oral administration. Each tablet contains aspirin (acetylsalicylic acid) 325 mg plus codeine phosphate in one of the following strengths: No. 2, 15 mg; No. 3, 30 mg and No. 4, 60 mg. (Warning—may be habit-forming), and the inactive ingredients colloidal silicon dioxide, microcrystalline cellulose, potato starch, and stearic acid.
Empirin with Codeine has analgesic, antipyretic and anti-inflammatory effects.

CLINICAL PHARMACOLOGY

Aspirin: The analgesic, anti-inflammatory and antipyretic effects of aspirin are believed to result from inhibition of the synthesis of certain prostaglandins. Aspirin interferes with clotting mechanisms primarily by diminishing platelet aggregation; at high doses prothrombin synthesis can be inhibited.
Aspirin in solution is rapidly absorbed from the stomach and from the upper small intestine. About 50 percent of an oral dose is absorbed in 30 minutes and peak plasma concentrations are reached in about 40 minutes. Higher than normal stomach pH or the presence of food slightly delays absorption.
Once absorbed, aspirin is mainly hydrolyzed to salicylic acid and distributed to all body tissues and fluids, including fetal tissue, breast milk and the central nervous system (CNS). Highest concentrations are found in plasma, liver, renal cortex, heart and lung.
From 50 to 80 percent of the salicylic acid and its metabolites in plasma are loosely bound to proteins. The plasma half-life of total salicylate is about 3.0 hours, with a 650 mg dose. Higher doses of aspirin cause increases in plasma salicylate half-life. Metabolism occurs primarily in the hepatocytes. The major metabolites are salicyluric acid (75%), the phenolic and acyl glucuronides of salicylate (15%), and gentisic and gentisuric acid (<1%).
Almost all of a therapeutic dose of aspirin is excreted through the kidneys, either as salicylic acid or the above mentioned metabolic products. Renal clearance of salicylates is greatly augmented by an alkaline urine, as is produced by concurrent administration of sodium bicarbonate or potassium citrate.
Toxic salicylate blood levels are usually above 30 mg/100 ml. The single lethal dose of aspirin in normal adults is approximately 25–30 g, but patients have recovered from much larger doses with appropriate treatment.
Codeine: Codeine probably exerts its analgesic effect through actions on opiate receptors in the CNS.
Codeine is readily absorbed from the gastrointestinal tract, and a therapeutic dose reaches peak analgesic effectiveness in about 2 hours and persists for 4 to 6 hours. Oral codeine (60 mg) given to healthy males has been shown to achieve peak blood levels of 0.016 mg/100 ml at approximately one hour post-dose. The codeine plasma half-life for a 60 mg oral dose is about 2.9 hours. Blood levels causing CNS depression begin at 0.05–0.19 mg/100 ml. The single lethal dose of codeine in adults is estimated to be approximately 0.5–1.0 g.
Codeine is rapidly distributed from blood to body tissues and taken up preferentially by parenchymatous organs such as liver, spleen and kidney. It passes the blood-brain barrier and is found in fetal tissue and breast milk.
The drug is not bound by plasma proteins nor is it accumulated in body tissues. Codeine is metabolized in liver to morphine and norcodeine, each representing about 10 percent of the administered dose of codeine. About 90 percent of the dose is excreted within 24 hours, primarily through the kidneys. Urinary excretion products are free and glucuronide-conjugated codeine (about 70%), free and conjugated norcodeine (about 10%), free and conjugated morphine (about 10%), normorphine (under 4%) and hydrocodone (<1%). The remainder of the dose appears in the feces.

INDICATIONS AND USAGE

Empirin with Codeine is indicated for the relief of mild, moderate, and moderate to severe pain.

CONTRAINDICATIONS

Empirin with Codeine is contraindicated under the following conditions:
(1) hypersensitivity or intolerance to aspirin or codeine,
(2) severe bleeding, disorders of coagulation or primary hemostasis, including hemophilia, hypoprothrombinemia, von Willebrand's disease, the thrombocytopenias, thrombasthenia and other ill-defined hereditary platelet dysfunctions, and well as such associated conditions as severe vitamin K deficiency and severe liver damage,
(3) anticoagulant therapy, and
(4) peptic ulcer, or other serious gastrointestinal lesions.

WARNINGS

Therapeutic doses of aspirin can cause anaphylactic shock and other severe allergic reactions. A history of allergy is often lacking.
Significant bleeding can result from aspirin therapy in patients with peptic ulcer or other gastrointestinal lesions, and in patients with bleeding disorders. Aspirin administered pre-operatively may prolong the bleeding time.
In the presence of head injury or other intracranial lesions, the respiratory depressant effects of codeine and other narcotics may be markedly enhanced, as well as their capacity for elevating cerebrospinal fluid pressure. Narcotics also produce other CNS depressant effects, such as drowsiness, that may further obscure the clinical course of patients with head injuries.
Codeine or other narcotics may obscure signs on which to judge the diagnosis or clinical course of patients with acute abdominal conditions.
Results from pilot epidemiologic studies suggest an association between aspirin and Reye Syndrome. Caution should be used in administering this product to children, including teenagers, with chicken pox or flu.

PRECAUTIONS

General: Empirin with Codeine should be prescribed with caution for certain special-risk patients such as the elderly or debilitated, and those with severe impairment of renal or hepatic function, gallbladder disease or gallstones, respiratory impairment, cardiac arrhythmias, inflammatory disorders of the gastrointestinal tract, hypothyroidism, Addison's disease, prostatic hypertrophy or urethral stricture, coagulation disorders, head injuries, or acute abdominal conditions.
Empirin with Codeine should not be prescribed for long-term therapy unless specifically indicated.
Precautions should be taken when administering salicylates to persons with known allergies. Hypersensitivity to aspirin is particularly likely in patients with nasal polyps, and relatively common in those with asthma.
Information for Patients: Empirin with Codeine may impair the mental and/or physical abilities required for the performance of potentially hazardous tasks such as driving a car or operating machinery. Such tasks should be avoided while taking Empirin with Codeine.

Alcohol and other CNS depressants may produce an additive CNS depression when taken with Empirin with Codeine, and should be avoided.
Codeine may be habit-forming when used over long periods or in high doses. Patients should take the drug only for as long as it is prescribed, in the amounts prescribed, and no more frequently than prescribed.
Laboratory Tests: Hypersensitivity to aspirin cannot be detected by skin testing or radioimmunoassay procedures.
The primary screening tests for detecting a bleeding tendency are platelet count, bleeding time, activated partial thromboplastin time and prothrombin time.
In patients with severe hepatic or renal disease, effects of therapy should be monitored with serial liver and/or renal function tests.
Drug Interactions: Empirin with Codeine may *enhance* the effects of:
(1) monoamine oxidase (MAO) inhibitors,
(2) oral anticoagulants, causing bleeding by inhibiting prothrombin formation in the liver and displacing anticoagulants from plasma protein binding sites,
(3) oral antidiabetic agents and insulin, causing hypoglycemia by contributing an additive effect, and by displacing the oral antidiabetic agents from secondary binding sites,
(4) 6-mercaptopurine and methotrexate, causing bone marrow toxicity and blood dyscrasias by displacing these drugs from secondary binding sites,
(5) penicillins and sulfonamides, increasing their blood levels by displacing these drugs from protein binding sites,
(6) non-steroidal anti-inflammatory agents, increasing the risk of peptic ulceration and bleeding by contributing additive effects,
(7) other narcotic analgesics, alcohol, general anesthetics, tranquilizers such as chlordiazepoxide, sedative-hypnotics, or other CNS depressants, causing increased CNS depression,
(8) corticosteroids, potentiating steroid anti-inflammatory effects by displacing steroids from protein binding sites. Aspirin intoxication may occur with corticosteroid withdrawal because steroids promote renal clearance of salicylates.

Empirin with Codeine may *diminish* the effects of:
(1) uricosuric agents such as probenecid and sulfinpyrazone, reducing their effectiveness in the treatment of gout. Aspirin competes with these agents for protein binding sites.

Aspirin and its metabolites may be caused to accumulate in the body, perhaps to toxic levels, by para-aminosalicylic acid, furosemide, and vitamin C.
Drug/Laboratory Test Interactions:
Aspirin: Aspirin may interfere with the following laboratory determinations in blood: serum amylase, fasting blood glucose, carbon dioxide, cholesterol, protein, protein bound iodine, uric acid, prothrombin time, bleeding time, and spectrophotometric detection of barbiturates. Aspirin may interfere with the following laboratory determinations in urine: glucose, 5-hydroxyindoleacetic acid, Gerhardt ketone, vanillylmandelic acid (VMA), protein, uric acid, and diacetic acid.
Codeine: Codeine may increase serum amylase levels.
Carcinogenesis, Mutagenesis, Impairment of Fertility: No adequate long-term studies have been conducted in animals to determine whether codeine has a potential for carcinogenesis, mutagenesis, or impairment of fertility.
Adequate long-term studies have been conducted in mice and rats with aspirin, alone or in combination with other drugs, in which no evidence of carcinogenesis was seen. No adequate studies have been conducted in animals to determine whether aspirin has a potential for mutagenesis or impairment of fertility.
Pregnancy: *Teratogenic Effects:* Pregnancy Category C. Animal reproduction studies have not been conducted with Empirin with Codeine. It is also not known whether Empirin with Codeine can cause fetal harm when administered to a pregnant woman or can affect reproduction capacity. Empirin with Codeine should be given to a pregnant woman only if clearly needed.
Reproductive studies in rats and mice have shown aspirin to be teratogenic and embryocidal at four to six times the human therapeutic dose. Studies in pregnant women, however, have not shown that aspirin increases the risk of abnormalities when administered during the first trimester of pregnancy. In controlled studies involving 41,337 pregnant women and their offspring, there was no evidence that aspirin taken during pregnancy caused stillbirth, neonatal death or reduced birthweight. In controlled studies of 50,282 pregnant women and their offspring, aspirin administration in moderate and heavy doses during the first four lunar months of pregnancy showed no teratogenic effect.
Reproduction studies have been performed in rabbits and rats at doses up to 150 times the human dose and have revealed no evidence of impaired fertility or harm to the fetus due to codeine.
Nonteratogenic Effects: Therapeutic doses of aspirin in pregnant women close to term may cause bleeding in mother, fetus, or neonate. During the last six months of pregnancy, regular use of aspirin in high doses may prolong pregnancy and delivery.
Labor and Delivery: Ingestion of aspirin prior to delivery may prolong delivery or lead to bleeding in the mother or neonate. Use of codeine during labor may lead to respiratory depression in the neonate.
Nursing Mothers: Aspirin and codeine are excreted in breast milk in small amounts, but the significance of their effects on nursing infants is not known. Because of the potential for serious adverse reactions in nursing infants from Empirin with Codeine, a decision should be made whether to discontinue nursing or to discontinue the drug, taking into account the importance of the drug to the mother.

ADVERSE REACTIONS

Codeine: The most frequently observed adverse reactions to codeine include light-headedness, dizziness, drowsiness, nausea, vomiting, constipation and depression of respiration. Less common reactions to codeine include euphoria, dysphoria, pruritis and skin rashes.
Aspirin: Mild aspirin intoxication (salicylism) can occur in response to chronic use of large doses. Manifestations include nausea, vomiting, hearing impairment, tinnitus, diminished vision, headache, dizziness, drowsiness, mental confusion, hyperpnea, hyperventilation, tachycardia, sweating and thirst.
Therapeutic doses of aspirin can induce mild or severe allergic reactions manifested by skin rashes, urticaria, angioedema, rhinorrhea, asthma, abdominal pain, nausea, vomiting, or anaphylactic shock. A history of allergy is often lacking, and allergic reactions may occur even in patients who have previously taken aspirin without any ill effects. Allergic reactions to aspirin are most likely to occur in patients with a history of allergic disease, especially in patients with nasal polyps or asthma.
Some patients are unable to take aspirin or other salicylates without developing nausea or vomiting. Occasional patients respond to aspirin (usually in large doses) with dyspepsia or heartburn, which may be accompanied by occult bleeding. Excessive bruising or bleeding is sometimes seen in patients with mild disorders of primary hemostasis who regularly use low doses of aspirin.
Prolonged use of aspirin can cause painless erosion of gastric mucosa, occult bleeding and, infrequently, iron-deficiency anemia. High doses of aspirin can exacerbate symptoms of peptic ulcer and, occasionally, cause extensive bleeding.
Excessive bleeding can follow injury or surgery in patients with or without known bleeding disorders who have taken therapeutic doses of aspirin within the preceding 10 days.
Hepatotoxicity has been reported in association with prolonged use of large doses of aspirin in patients with lupus erythematosus, rheumatoid arthritis and rheumatic disease.
Bone marrow depression, manifested by weakness, fatigue, or abnormal bruising or bleeding, has occasionally been reported.
In patients with glucose-6-phosphate dehydrogenase deficiency, aspirin can cause a mild degree of hemolytic anemia.
In hyperuricemic persons, low doses of aspirin may reduce the effectiveness of uricosuric therapy or precipitate an attack of gout.

DRUG ABUSE AND DEPENDENCE

Like other medications containing a narcotic analgesic, Empirin with Codeine is controlled by the Drug Enforcement Administration and is classified under Schedule III.
Empirin with Codeine can produce drug dependence of the morphine type; therefore, it has a potential for being abused. Psychic dependence, physical dependence and tolerance may develop on repeated administration.
The dependence liability of codeine has been found to be too small to permit a full definition of its characteristics. Studies indicate that addiction to codeine is extremely uncommon and requires very high parenteral doses.
When dependence on codeine occurs at therapeutic doses, it appears to require from one to two months to develop, and withdrawal symptoms are mild. Most patients on long-term oral codeine therapy show no signs of physical dependence upon abrupt withdrawal.

OVERDOSAGE

Severe intoxication, caused by overdose of Empirin with Codeine may produce: skin eruptions, dyspnea, vertigo, double vision, delusions, hallucinations, garbled speech, excitability, restlessness, delirium, constricted pupils, a positive Babinski sign, respiratory depression (slow and shallow breathing; Cheyne-Stokes respiration), cyanosis, clammy skin, muscle flaccidity, circulatory collapse, stupor and coma. In children, difficulty in hearing, tinnitus, dim vision, headache, dizziness, drowsiness, confusion, rapid breathing, sweating, thirst, nausea, vomiting, hyperpyrexia, dehydration and convulsions are prominent signs. The most severe manifestations from aspirin result from cardiovascular and respiratory insufficiency secondary to acid-base and electrolyte disturbances, complicated by hyperthermia and dehydration. The most severe manifestations from codeine are associated with respiratory depression.
Respiratory alkalosis is characteristic of the early phase of intoxication with aspirin while hyperventilation is occurring, but is quickly followed by metabolic acidosis in most people with severe intoxication. This occurs more readily in children. Hypoglycemia may occur in children who have taken large overdoses. Other laboratory findings associated with aspirin intoxication include ketonuria, hyponatremia, hypokalemia, and occasionally proteinuria. A slight rise in lactic dehydrogenase and hydroxybutyric dehydrogenase may occur.
Concentrations of aspirin in plasma above 30 mg/100 ml are associated with toxicity. (See Clinical Pharmacology section for information on factors influencing aspirin blood levels.) The single lethal dose of aspirin in adults is probably about 25–30 g, but is not known with certainty.
The toxic plasma concentration of codeine is not known with certainty. Experimental production of mild to moderate CNS depression in healthy, nontolerant subjects occurred at plasma concentrations of 0.05–0.19 mg/100 ml when codeine was given by intravenous infusion. The single lethal dose of codeine in adults is estimated to be from 0.5–1.0 g. It is also estimated that 5 mg/kg could be fatal in children. Hemodialysis and peritoneal dialysis can be performed to reduce the body aspirin content. Codeine is theoretically dialyzable but the procedure has not been clinically established.
Treatment of overdosage consists primarily of support of vital functions, management of codeine-induced respiratory depression, increasing salicylate elimination, and correcting the acid-base imbalance due primarily to salicylism.
In a comatose patient, primary attention should be given to establishment of adequate respiratory exchange through provisions of a patent airway and the institution of assisted or controlled ventilation. The narcotic antagonist naloxone is a specific antidote for respiratory depression which may result from overdose or unusual sensitivity to narcotics. Therefore, an appropriate dose of an antagonist should be administered, preferably by the intravenous route, simultaneously with efforts at respiratory resuscitation. Since the duration of action of Empirin with Codeine may exceed that of the antagonist, the patient should be kept under continued surveillance and repeated doses of the antagonist should be administered as needed to maintain adequate respiration. A narcotic antagonist should not be administered in the absence of clinically significant respiratory or cardiovascular depression.
Gastric emptying (Syrup of Ipecac) and/or lavage is recommended as soon as possible after ingestion, even if the patient has vomited spontaneously. (Apomorphine should not be used as an emetic for Empirin with Codeine, since it may potentiate hypotension and respiratory depression.) Administration of activated charcoal as a slurry is beneficial after lavage and/or emesis, if less than three hours have passed since ingestion. Charcoal adsorption should *not* be employed prior to emesis or lavage.
Severity of aspirin intoxication is determined by measuring the blood salicylate level. Acid-base status should be closely followed with serial blood gas and serum pH measurements. Fluid and electrolyte balance should also be regularly monitored.
A serum salicylate level of 30 mg/100 ml or higher indicates a need for enhanced salicylate excretion that can be achieved through body-fluid supplementation and urine alkalinization if renal function is normal. In mild intoxication, urine flow can be increased by forcing oral fluids and giving potassium citrate capsules. (DO NOT GIVE BICARBONATE BY MOUTH SINCE IT INCREASES THE RATE OF SALICYLATE ABSORPTION.)
In severe cases, hyperthermia and hypovolemia, as well as respiratory depression are the major immediate threats to life. Children should be sponged with tepid water. Replacement fluid should be administered intravenously and augmented with sufficient bicarbonate to correct acidosis, with monitoring of plasma electrolytes and pH, to promote alkaline diuresis of salicylate if renal function is normal. Complete control may also require infusion of glucose to control hypoglycemia.
Potassium deficiency may also be corrected through the infusion, once adequate urinary output is assured. Plasma or plasma expanders may be needed if fluid replacement is insufficient to maintain normal blood pressure or adequate urinary output.
In patients with renal insufficiency or in cases of life-threatening intoxication, dialysis is usually required. Peritoneal dialysis or exchange transfusion is indicated in infants and young children, and hemodialysis in older patients.
Oxygen, intravenous fluids, vasopressors and other supportive measures should be employed as needed.

DOSAGE AND ADMINISTRATION

Dosage is adjusted according to the severity of pain and the response of the patient. It may occasionally be necessary to exceed the usual dosage recommended below when pain is severe or the patient has become tolerant to the analgesic effect of codeine. Empirin with Codeine is given orally. The

Continued on next page

Burroughs Wellcome—Cont.

usual adult dose for Empirin with Codeine No. 2 and No. 3 is one or two tablets every four hours as required. The usual adult dose for Empirin with Codeine No. 4 is one tablet every four hours as required.
Empirin with Codeine should be taken with food or a full glass of milk or water to lessen gastric irritation.

HOW SUPPLIED

Empirin with Codeine No. 2, 15 mg: (white tablet imprinted with "EMPIRIN" and "2")

Bottle of 100	NDC 0081-0215-55
Bottle of 1000	NDC 0081-0215-75

Empirin with Codeine No. 3, 30 mg: (white tablet imprinted with "EMPIRIN" and "3")

Bottle of 100	NDC 0081-0220-55
	VA NSN 6505-00-959-4431
Bottle of 500	NDC 0081-0220-70
Bottle of 1000	NDC 0081-0220-75
	DoD NSN 6505-00-149-0116
Dispenserpak® of 25	NDC 0081-0220-25
	DoD NSN 6505-06-118-2347

Empirin with Codeine No. 4, 60 mg: (white tablet imprinted with "EMPIRIN" and "4")

Bottle of 100	NDC 0081-0225-55
Bottle of 500	NDC 0081-0225-70
Bottle of 1000	NDC 0081-0225-75
Dispenserpak® of 25	NDC 0081-0225-25

Store at 15°–30°C (59°–86°F) in a dry place and protect from light.

Shown in Product Identification Section, page 406

EMPRACET® with Codeine Phosphate ℞ ©III
[*ĭm 'prah-set "*]
30 mg, No. 3; 60 mg, No. 4

DESCRIPTION

Each Empracet with Codeine Phosphate tablet contains codeine phosphate* 30 mg in No. 3 and 60 mg in No. 4 (**WARNING:** May be habit-forming), acetaminophen 300 mg, and the inactive ingredients corn starch, dibasic calcium phosphate, FD&C Yellow No. 6 Lake, magnesium stearate, povidone, and stearic acid.
Acetaminophen occurs as a white, odorless crystalline powder, possessing a slightly bitter taste. Codeine is an alkaloid, obtained from opium or prepared from morphine by methylation. Codeine occurs as colorless or white crystals, effloresces slowly in dry air and is affected by light.

ACTIONS

Acetaminophen is a nonopiate, non-salicylate analgesic and antipyretic. Codeine is an opiate analgesic and antitussive. Codeine retains at least one-half of its analgesic activity when administered orally.

INDICATIONS

No. 3—for the relief of mild to moderate pain; No. 4—for the relief of moderate to moderately severe pain.

CONTRAINDICATIONS

Hypersensitivity to acetaminophen or codeine.

WARNINGS

Drug Dependence: Codeine can produce drug dependence of the morphine type, and therefore has the potential for being abused. Psychic dependence, physical dependence and tolerance may develop upon repeated administration of this drug and it should be prescribed and administered with the same degree of caution appropriate to the use of other oral narcotic medications. This acetaminophen and codeine dosage form is subject to the Federal Controlled Substances Act (Schedule III).

PRECAUTIONS

General:
Head injury and increased intracranial pressure: The respiratory depressant effects of narcotics and their capacity to elevate cerebrospinal fluid pressure may be markedly exaggerated in the presence of head injury, other intracranial lesions or a pre-existing increase in intracranial pressure. Furthermore, narcotics produce adverse reactions which may obscure the clinical course of patients with head injuries.
Acute abdominal conditions: The administration of products containing codeine or other narcotics may obscure the diagnosis or clinical course in patients with acute abdominal conditions.
Special risk patients: Acetaminophen with codeine should be given with caution to certain patients, such as the elderly or debilitated, and those with severe impairment of hepatic or renal function, hypothyroidism, Addison's disease, and prostatic hypertrophy or urethral stricture.
Information for Patients: Codeine may impair the mental and/or physical abilities required for the performance of potentially hazardous tasks such as driving a car or operating machinery. The patient taking this drug should be cautioned accordingly.
Drug Interactions: Patients receiving other narcotic analgesics, antipsychotics, antianxiety, or other CNS depressants (including alcohol) concomitantly with acetaminophen and codeine may exhibit additive CNS depression due to the codeine component. When such therapy is contemplated, the dose of one or both agents should be reduced.
The use of MAO inhibitors or tricyclic antidepressants with codeine preparations may increase the effect of either the antidepressant or codeine.
The concurrent use of anticholinergics with codeine may produce paralytic ileus.
Usage in Pregnancy: Safe use in pregnancy has not been established relative to possible adverse effects on fetal development. Therefore, acetaminophen and codeine should not be used in pregnant women unless, in the judgment of the physician, the potential benefits outweigh the possible hazards.
Nursing Mothers: It is not known whether the components of this drug are excreted in human milk. Because many drugs are excreted in human milk, caution should be exercised when acetaminophen and codeine is administered to a nursing woman.

ADVERSE REACTIONS

The most frequently observed adverse reactions include light-headedness, dizziness, sedation, shortness of breath, nausea and vomiting. These effects seem to be more prominent in ambulatory than in non-ambulatory patients, and some of these adverse reactions may be alleviated if the patient lies down.
Other adverse reactions include euphoria, dysphoria, constipation and pruritus. At higher doses, codeine has most of the disadvantages of morphine, including respiratory depression.

OVERDOSAGE

Acetaminophen:
Signs and Symptoms: Acetaminophen in massive overdosage may cause hepatic toxicity in some patients. In all cases of suspected overdose, immediately call your regional poison center or the Rocky Mountain Poison Center's toll-free number (800-525-6115) for assistance in diagnosis and for directions in the use of N-acetylcysteine as an antidote, a use currently restricted to investigational status.
In adults, hepatic toxicity has rarely been reported with acute overdoses of less than 10 grams and fatalities with less than 15 grams. Importantly, young children seem to be more resistant than adults to the hepatotoxic effect of an acetaminophen overdose. Despite this, the measures outlined below should be initiated in any adult or child suspected of having ingested an acetaminophen overdose.
Early symptoms following a potentially hepatotoxic overdose may include: nausea, vomiting, diaphoresis and general malaise. Clinical and laboratory evidence of hepatic toxicity may not be apparent until 48 to 72 hours post-ingestion.
Treatment: The stomach should be emptied promptly by lavage or by induction of emesis with syrup of ipecac. Patients' estimates of the quantity of a drug ingested are notoriously unreliable. Therefore, if an acetaminophen overdose is suspected, a serum acetaminophen assay should be obtained as early as possible, but no sooner than four hours following ingestion. Liver function studies should be obtained initially and repeated at 24-hour intervals.
The antidote, N-acetylcysteine, should be administered as early as possible, and within 16 hours of the overdose ingestion for optimal results. Following recovery, there are no residual, structural or functional hepatic abnormalities.
Codeine:
Signs and Symptoms: Serious overdose with codeine is characterized by respiratory depression (a decrease in respiratory rate and/or tidal volume. Cheyne-Stokes respiration, cyanosis), extreme somnolence progressing to stupor or coma, skeletal muscle flaccidity, cold and clammy skin, and sometimes bradycardia and hypotension. In severe overdosage, apnea, circulatory collapse, cardiac arrest, and death may occur.
Treatment: Primary attention should be given to the reestablishment of adequate respiratory exchange through provision of a patent airway and the institution of assisted or controlled ventilation. The narcotic antagonist naloxone is a specific antidote against respiratory depression which may result from overdosage or unusual sensitivity to narcotics, including codeine. Therefore, an appropriate dose of naloxone (see package insert) should be administered, preferably by the intravenous route, and simultaneously with efforts at respiratory resuscitation. Since the duration of action of codeine may exceed that of the antagonist, the patient should be kept under continued surveillance and repeated doses of the antagonist should be administered as needed to maintain adequate respiration.
An antagonist should not be administered in the absence of clinically significant respiratory or cardiovascular depression. Oxygen, intravenous fluids, vasopressors and other supportive measures should be employed as indicated.
Gastric emptying may be useful in removing unabsorbed drug.

DOSAGE AND ADMINISTRATION

Dosage should be adjusted according to severity of pain and response of the patient. However, it should be kept in mind that tolerance to codeine can develop with continued use and that the incidence of untoward effects is dose related. This product is inappropriate even in high doses for severe or intractable pain. Adult doses of codeine higher than 60 mg fail to give commensurate relief of pain, but merely prolong analgesia and are associated with an appreciably increased incidence of undesirable side effects. Equivalently high doses in children would have similar effects.
The usual adult dose of Empracet with Codeine phosphate 30 mg, No. 3 is one or two tablets every four hours, as required.
The usual adult dose of Empracet with Codeine phosphate 60 mg, No. 4 is one tablet every four hours, as required.

HOW SUPPLIED

Empracet® with Codeine phosphate 30 mg., No. 3, is available in tablets (peach) containing 30 mg codeine phosphate and 300 mg acetaminophen, imprinted with "EMPRACET 3". Bottles of 100, (NDC-0081-0315-55), 500 (NDC-0081-0315-70) and Dispenserpak® of 25 (NDC-0081-0315-25). Empracet® with Codeine Phosphate 60 mg, No. 4, is available in tablets (peach), containing 60 mg codeine phosphate and 300 mg acetaminophen, coded with "EMPRACET 4" and "L9B." Bottles of 100 (NDC-0081-0327-55) and 500 (NDC-0081-0327-70).

Shown in Product Identification Section, page 406

FEDRAZIL® TABLETS
[*fĕd 'rah-zĭl "*]

(See PDR For Nonprescription Drugs).

Shown in Product Identification Section, page 406

IMURAN® ℞
[*ĭm 'ū-ran "*]
(Azathioprine)
50 mg Scored Tablets

20 ml vial (as the sodium salt) for I.V. injection, equivalent to 100 mg Azathioprine sterile lyophilized material.

> **WARNING**
> Chronic immunosuppression with this purine antimetabolite increases *risk of neoplasia* in humans. Physicians using this drug should be very familiar with this risk as well as with the mutagenic potential to both men and women and with possible hematologic toxicities. See below under WARNINGS.

DESCRIPTION

Imuran (Azathioprine), an immunosuppressive antimetabolite, is available in tablet form for oral administration and 100 mg vials for intravenous injection. Each scored tablet contains 50 mg azathioprine and the inactive ingredients lactose, magnesium stearate, potato starch, povidone, and stearic acid. Each 100 mg vial contains azathioprine, as the sodium salt, equivalent to 100 mg azathioprine sterile lyophilized material and sodium hydroxide to adjust pH. Azathioprine is chemically 6-[(1-methyl-4-nitro-imidazol-5-yl)thio] purine. It is an imidazolyl derivative of 6-mercaptopurine (Purinethol®) and many of its biological effects are similar to those of the parent compound.
Azathioprine is insoluble in water, but may be dissolved with addition of one molar equivalent of alkali. The sodium salt of azathioprine is sufficiently soluble to make a 10 mg/ml water solution which is stable for 24 hours at 59° to 86°F (15° to 30°C). Azathioprine is stable in solution at neutral or acid pH but hydrolysis to mercaptopurine occurs in excess sodium hydroxide (0.1N), especially on warming. Conversion to mercaptopurine also occurs in the presence of sulfhydryl compounds such as cysteine, glutathione and hydrogen sulfide.

CLINICAL PHARMACOLOGY AND ACTIONS

Metabolism[1]: Azathioprine is well absorbed following oral administration. Maximum serum radioactivity occurs at one to two hours after oral ^{35}S-azathioprine and decays with a half-life of five hours. This is not an estimate of the half-life of azathioprine itself but is the decay rate for all ^{35}S-containing metabolites of the drug. Because of extensive metabolism, only a fraction of the radioactivity is present as azathioprine. Usual doses produce blood levels of azathioprine, and of mercaptopurine derived from it, which are low (<1 mcg/ml). Blood levels are of little predictive value for therapy since the magnitude and duration of clinical effects correlate with thiopurine nucleotide levels in tissues rather than with plasma drug levels. Azathioprine and mercaptopurine are moderately bound to serum proteins (30%) and are partially dialyzable.

Azathioprine is cleaved *in vivo* to mercaptopurine. Both compounds are rapidly eliminated from blood and are oxidized or methylated in erythrocytes and liver; no azathioprine or mercaptopurine is detectable in urine after eight hours. Conversion to inactive 6-thiouric acid by xanthine oxidase is an important degradative pathway, and the inhibition of this pathway in patients receiving allopurinol (Zyloprim®) is the basis for the azathioprine dosage reduction required in these patients (see DOSAGE AND ADMINISTRATION). Proportions of metabolites are different in individual patients, and this presumably accounts for variable magnitude and duration of drug effects. Renal clearance is probably not important in predicting biological effectiveness or toxicities, although dose reduction is practiced in patients with poor renal function.

Homograft Survival[1,2]: Summary information from transplant centers and registries indicates relatively universal use of Imuran with or without other immunosuppressive agents.[3,4,5] Although the use of azathioprine for inhibition of renal homograft rejection is well established, the mechanism(s) for this action are somewhat obscure. The drug suppresses hypersensitivities of the cell-mediated type and causes variable alterations in antibody production. Suppression of T-cell effects, including ablation of T-cell suppression, is dependent on the temporal relationship to antigenic stimulus or engraftment. This agent has little effect on established graft rejections or secondary responses.

Alterations in specific immune responses or immunologic functions in transplant recipients are difficult to relate specifically to immunosuppression by azathioprine. These patients have subnormal responses to vaccines, low numbers of T-cells, and abnormal phagocytosis by peripheral blood cells, but their mitogenic responses, serum immunoglobulins and secondary antibody responses are usually normal. Transplant recipients on azathioprine also receive corticosteroids and may be given antilymphocyte globulin; there are no known hazards or toxicities due to interactions of these agents.

Immunoinflammatory Response: Azathioprine suppresses disease manifestations as well as underlying pathology in animal models of auto-immune disease. For example, the severity of adjuvant arthritis is reduced by azathioprine.

The mechanisms whereby azathioprine affects auto-immune diseases are not known. Azathioprine is immunosuppressive, delayed hypersensitivity and cellular cytotoxicity tests being suppressed to a greater degree than are antibody responses. In the rat model of adjuvant arthritis, azathioprine has been shown to inhibit the lymph node hyperplasia which precedes the onset of the signs of the disease. Both the immunosuppressive and therapeutic effects in animal models are dose-related. Azathioprine is considered a slow acting drug and effects may persist after the drug has been discontinued.

INDICATIONS AND USAGE

Imuran is indicated as an adjunct for the prevention of rejection in renal homotransplantation. It is also indicated for the management of severe, active rheumatoid arthritis unresponsive to rest, aspirin or other nonsteroidal anti-inflammatory drugs, or to agents in the class of which gold is an example.

Renal Homotransplantation: Imuran is indicated as an adjunct for the prevention of rejection in renal homotransplantation. Experience with over 16,000 transplants shows a five-year patient survival of 35% to 55%, but this is dependent on donor, match for HLA antigens, anti-donor or anti B-cell alloantigen antibody and other variables. The effect of Imuran on these variables has not been tested in controlled trials.

Rheumatoid Arthritis[6,7]: Imuran is indicated only in adult patients meeting criteria for classic or definite rheumatoid arthritis as specified by the American Rheumatism Association[8]. Imuran should be restricted to patients with severe, active and erosive disease not responsive to conventional management including rest, aspirin or other non-steroidal drugs or to agents in the class of which gold is an example. Rest, physiotherapy and salicylates should be continued while Imuran is given, but it may be possible to reduce the dose of corticosteroids in patients on Imuran. The combined use of Imuran with gold, antimalarials or penicillamine has not been studied for either added benefit or unexpected adverse effects. The use of Imuran with these agents cannot be recommended.

CONTRAINDICATIONS

Imuran should not be given to patients who have shown hypersensitivity to the drug.

Imuran should not be used for treating rheumatoid arthritis in pregnant women.

Patients with rheumatoid arthritis previously treated with alkylating agents (cyclophosphamide, chlorambucil, melphalan or others) may have a prohibitive risk of neoplasia if treated with Imuran.

WARNINGS

Severe *leukopenia and/or thrombocytopenia* may occur in patients on Imuran. Macrocytic anemia and severe bone marrow depression may also occur. Hematologic toxicities are dose related and may be more severe in renal transplant patients whose homograft is undergoing rejection. It is suggested that patients on Imuran have complete blood counts, including platelet counts, weekly during the first month, twice monthly for the second and third months of treatment, then monthly or more frequently if dosage alterations or other therapy changes are necessary. Delayed hematologic suppression may occur. Prompt reduction in dosage or temporary withdrawal of the drug may be necessary if there is a rapid fall in, or persistently low leukocyte count or other evidence of bone marrow depression. Leukopenia does not correlate with therapeutic effect; therefore the dose should not be increased intentionally to lower the white blood cell count.

Serious infections are a constant hazard for patients on chronic immunosuppression, especially for homograft recipients. Fungal, viral, bacterial and protozoal infections may be fatal and should be treated vigorously. Reduction of azathioprine dosage and/or use of other drugs should be considered.

Imuran® is mutagenic in animals and humans, carcinogenic in animals, and may increase the patient's *risk of neoplasia.* Renal transplant patients are known to have an increased risk of malignancy, predominantly skin cancer and reticulum cell or lymphomatous tumors.[9] Information is available on the spontaneous neoplasia risk in Rheumatoid Arthritis[11], and on neoplasia following immunosuppressive therapy of other autoimmune diseases[12]. It has not been possible to define the precise risk of neoplasia due to Imuran[10], but the risk is lower for patients with rheumatoid arthritis than for transplant recipients. However, acute myelogenous leukemia as well as solid tumors have been reported in patients with rheumatoid arthritis who have received azathioprine. Data on neoplasia in patients receiving Imuran can be found under Adverse Reactions.

Pregnancy Warning[13]: Imuran should not be given during pregnancy without careful weighing of risk versus benefit. Whenever possible, use of Imuran in pregnant patients should be avoided.

Imuran has been shown to be mutagenic in both male and female animals. Chromosomal abnormalities have also been documented in patients; however, the abnormalities in humans were reversed upon discontinuance of the drug.[14]

Imuran is teratogenic in rodents. Transplacental transmission of azathioprine and its metabolites has been reported in man.[15] Limited immunologic and other abnormalities have occurred in some infants born of renal homograft recipients on Imuran. Benefit versus risk must be weighed carefully before use of Imuran in patients of reproductive potential. This drug should not be used for treating rheumatoid arthritis in pregnant women.

PRECAUTIONS

Patient information: Patients being started on Imuran should be informed of the necessity of periodic blood counts while they are receiving the drug and should be encouraged to report any unusual bleeding or bruising to their physician. They should be advised of the danger of infection while receiving Imuran and encouraged to report signs and symptoms of infection to their physician. Careful dosage instructions should be given to the patient, especially when Imuran is being administered in the presence of impaired renal function or concomitantly with allopurinol (see DOSAGE AND ADMINISTRATION). Patients should be advised of the potential risks of the use of Imuran during pregnancy and during the nursing period. The increased risk of neoplasia following Imuran therapy should be explained to the patient.

ADVERSE REACTIONS

The principal and potentially serious toxic effects of Imuran are hematologic and gastrointestinal. The risks of secondary infection and neoplasia are also important. The frequency and severity of adverse reactions depend on the dose and duration of Imuran as well as on the patient's underlying disease or concomitant therapies. The incidence of hematologic toxicities and neoplasia encountered in groups of renal homograft recipients is significantly higher than that in studies employing Imuran for rheumatoid arthritis. The relative incidences in clinical studies are summarized below:

Toxicity	*Renal Homograft*	*Rheumatoid Arthritis*
Leukopenia		
Any Degree	> 50%	28 %
< 2500/mm^3	16%	5.3%
Neoplasia		
Lymphoma	0.5%	
Others	2.8%	*

*18 reported cases; denominator unknown.

Hematologic: Leukopenia and/or thrombocytopenia are dose dependent and may occur late in the course of Imuran therapy. Dose reduction or temporary withdrawal allows reversal of these toxicities. Infection may occur as a secondary manifestation of bone marrow suppression or leukopenia, but the incidence of infection in renal homotransplantation is 30 to 60 times that in rheumatoid arthritis. Macrocytic anemia and/or bleeding have been reported in two patients on Imuran.

Gastrointestinal: Nausea and vomiting may occur within the first few months of Imuran therapy, and occurred in approximately 12% of 676 rheumatoid arthritis patients. The frequency of gastric disturbance can be reduced by administration of the drug in divided doses and/or after meals. Vomiting with abdominal pain may occur rarely with a hypersensitivity pancreatitis. Hepatotoxicity with elevated serum alkaline phosphatase and bilirubin is known to occur with thiopurines including Imuran and 6-mercaptopurine (Purinethol®). This toxic hepatitis with biliary stasis is known to occur in homograft recipients and has been generally reversible after interruption of Imuran. Hepatotoxicity has been uncommon in rheumatoid arthritis patients on Imuran (less than 1%).

Others: Additional side effects of low frequency have been reported. These include skin rashes (approximately 2%), alopecia, fever, arthralgias, diarrhea, steatorrhea and negative nitrogen balance (all less than 1%).

DOSAGE AND ADMINISTRATION

Renal Homotransplantation: The dose of Imuran required to prevent rejection and minimize toxicity will vary with individual patients; this necessitates careful management. Initial dose is usually 3 to 5 mg/kg daily, beginning at the time of transplant. Imuran is usually given as a single daily dose on the day of, and in a minority of cases one to three days before, transplantation. Imuran is often initiated with the intravenous administration of the sodium salt, with subsequent use of tablets (at the same dose level) after the postoperative period. Intravenous administration of the sodium salt is indicated only in patients unable to tolerate oral medications. Dose reduction to maintenance levels of 1 to 3 mg/kg daily is usually possible. The dose of Imuran should not be increased to toxic levels because of threatened rejection. Discontinuation may be necessary for severe hematologic or other toxicity, even if rejection of the homograft may be a consequence of drug withdrawal.

Rheumatoid Arthritis: Imuran is usually given on a daily basis. The initial dose should be approximately 1.0 mg/kg (50 to 100 mg) given as a single dose or on a twice daily schedule. The dose may be increased, beginning at six to eight weeks and thereafter by steps at four-week intervals, if there are no serious toxicities and if initial response is unsatisfactory. Dose increments should be 0.5 mg/kg daily, up to a maximum dose of 2.5 mg/kg/day. Therapeutic response occurs after several weeks of treatment, usually six to eight; an adequate trial should be a minimum of 12 weeks. Patients not improved after twelve weeks can be considered refractory. Imuran may be continued long-term in patients with clinical response, but patients should be monitored carefully, and gradual dosage reduction should be attempted to reduce risk of toxicities.

Maintenance therapy should be at the lowest effective dose, and the dose given can be lowered decrementally with changes of 0.5 mg/kg or approximately 25 mg daily every four weeks while other therapy is kept constant. The optimum duration of maintenance Imuran has not been determined. Imuran can be discontinued abruptly, but delayed effects are possible.

Use in Renal Dysfunction: Relatively oliguric patients, especially those with tubular necrosis in the immediate post-cadaveric transplant period, may have delayed clearance of Imuran or its metabolites, may be particularly sensitive to this drug and may require lower doses.

Use with Allopurinol (Zyloprim®): The principal pathway for detoxification of Imuran is inhibited by allopurinol (Zyloprim). Patients receiving Imuran and Zyloprim concomitantly should have a dose reduction of Imuran, to approximately $\frac{1}{3}$ to $\frac{1}{4}$ the usual dose.

Parenteral Administration: Add 10 ml of sterile Water for Injection, and swirl until a clear solution results. This solution is for intravenous use only; it has a pH of approximately 9.6, and it should be used within twenty-four hours. Further dilution into sterile saline or dextrose is usually made for infusion; the final volume depends on time for the infusion, usually 30-60 minutes but as short as 5 minutes and as long as 8 hours for the daily dose.

HOW SUPPLIED

50 mg oval-shaped, yellow, scored tablets imprinted with "IMURAN" and "50" on each tablet; bottle of 100. (NDC 0081-0597-55) **DoD & VA NSN 6505-00-119-9317**

20 ml vial (NDC-0081-0598-71) containing the equivalent of 100 mg azathioprine (as the sodium salt). The sterile, lyophilized sodium salt is yellow, and should be dissolved in sterile Water for Injection (see Parenteral Administration under DOSAGE AND ADMINISTRATION).

Continued on next page

Burroughs Wellcome—Cont.

REFERENCES

1. Elion, G.B. and G.H. Hitchings, "Azathioprine" in *Handbook of Experimental Pharmacology*, Vol. 38, ed. by Sartorelli and Johns, Springer Verlag, New York, 1975.
2. McIntosh, J., P. Hansen *et al.*, "Defective Immune and Phagocytic Functions in Uremia and Renal Transplantation," *Int. Arch. Allergy Appl. Immunol.*, 51:544–559, 1976.
3. Advisory Committee, Renal Transplant Registry, "The 12th Report of the Human Renal Transplant Registry," *JAMA*, 233:787–796, 1975.
4. McGeown, M., "Immunosuppression for Kidney Transplantation," *Lancet*, ii:310–312, 1973.
5. Simmons, R.L., E.J. Thompson *et al.*, "115 Patients with First Cadaver Kidney Transplants Followed Two to Seven and a Half Years," *Am. J. Med.*, 62:234–242, 1977.
6. Fye, K. and N. Talal, "Cytotoxic Drugs in the Treatment of Rheumatoid Arthritis," *Ration. Drug Ther.*, *9* (4): 1–5, 1975.
7. Davis, J.D., H.B. Muss, and R.A. Turner, "Cytotoxic Agents in the Treatment of Rheumatoid Arthritis," *South. Med. J.*, *71* (1): 58–64, 1978.
8. McEwen, C., "The Diagnosis and Differential Diagnosis of Rheumatoid Arthritis," *Arthritis and Allied Conditions*, Philadelphia, Lea and Febiger, pp. 403–418, 1972.
9. Hoover, R. and J.F. Fraumeni, "Risk of Cancer in Renal Transplant Recipients," *Lancet*, 2:55–57, 1973.
10. Sieber, S.M. and R.H. Adamson, "Toxicity of Antineoplastic Agents in Man," *Adv. Cancer Res.*, 22:57–155, 1975.
11. Lewis, R.B., C.W. Castor, R.E. Knisley, and G.C. Bole, "Frequency of Neoplasia in Systemic Lupus Erythematosus and Rheumatoid Arthritis," *Arthritis Rheum.*, *19* (6): 1256–1260, 1976.
12. Louie, S. and R.S. Schwartz, "Immunodeficiency and the Pathogenesis of Lymphoma and Leukemia," *Semin. Hematol.*, *15* (2): 117–138, 1978.
13. Tagatz, G.E. and R.L. Simmons, "Pregnancy After Renal Transplantation," *Ann. Intern. Med.*, 82:113–114, 1975 (Editorial).
14. Hunter, T., M.B. Urowitz, D.A. Gordon, H.A. Smythe and M.A. Ogryzlo, Azathioprine in Rheumatoid Arthritis. A Long-Term Follow-Up Study, Arthritis Rheum., *18* (1): 15–20, 1975.
15. Saarikoski, S. and M. Sepalla, Immunosuppressive During Pregnancy: Transmission of Azathioprine and its Metabolites from the Mother to the Fetus, Am. J. Obstet. Gynecol., *115* (8): 1100–1106, 1973.

Shown in Product Identification Section, page 407

KEMADRIN® ℞

[*kĕm 'ah-drĭn*]
(Procyclidine Hydrochloride)
5 mg Scored Tablets

DESCRIPTION

Kemadrin (Procyclidine Hydrochloride) is a synthetic antispasmodic compound of relatively low toxicity. It has been shown to be useful for the symptomatic treatment of parkinsonism (paralysis agitans) and extrapyramidal dysfunction caused by tranquilizer therapy. Procyclidine hydrochloride was developed at The Wellcome Research Laboratories as the most promising of a series of antiparkinsonism compounds produced by chemical modification of antihistamines. Procyclidine hydrochloride is a white crystalline substance which is soluble in water and almost tasteless. It is known chemically as α-cyclohexyl-α-phenyl-1-pyrrolidinepropanol hydrochloride.

Kemadrin® (Procyclidine Hydrochloride) is available in tablet form for oral administration. Each scored tablet contains 5 mg procyclidine hydrochloride and the inactive ingredients corn and potato starch, lactose, and magnesium stearate.

CLINICAL PHARMACOLOGY

Pharmacologic tests have shown that procyclidine hydrochloride has an atropine-like action and exerts an antispasmodic effect on smooth muscle. It is a potent mydriatic and inhibits salivation. It has no sympathetic ganglion blocking activity in doses as high as 4 mg/kg, as measured by the lack of inhibition of the response of the nictitating membrane to preganglionic electrical stimulation.

The intravenous LD_{50} in mice was about 60 mg/kg. Subcutaneously, doses of 300 mg/kg were not toxic. In dogs the intraperitoneal administration of procyclidine hydrochloride in doses of 5 mg/kg caused maximal dilation of the pupil and inhibition of salivation, but had no toxic action. When the dose was increased to 20 mg/kg the same symptoms occurred, and in addition there were tremors and ataxia lasting 4 to 5 hours. In one animal convulsions occurred which were controlled by pentobarbital. In all animals behavior returned to normal within 24 hours.

Chronic toxicity tests in rats showed that the compound caused only a very slight retardation in growth, and no change in the erythrocyte count or the histological appearance of the lungs, liver, spleen and kidney when as much as 10 mg/kg body weight was given subcutaneously daily for 9 weeks.

INDICATIONS

Kemadrin (Procyclidine Hydrochloride) is indicated in the treatment of parkinsonism including the postencephalitic, arteriosclerotic and idiopathic types. Partial control of the parkinsonism symptoms is the usual therapeutic accomplishment. Procyclidine hydrochloride is usually more efficacious in the relief of rigidity than tremor; but tremor, fatigue, weakness and sluggishness are frequently beneficially influenced. It can be substituted for all the previous medications in mild and moderate cases. For the control of more severe cases other drugs may be added to procyclidine therapy as indications warrant.

Clinical reports indicate that procyclidine often successfully relieves the symptoms of extrapyramidal dysfunction (dystonia, dyskinesia, akathisia and parkinsonism) which accompany the therapy of mental disorders with phenothiazine and rauwolfia compounds. In addition to minimizing the symptoms induced by tranquilizing drugs, the drug effectively controls sialorrhea resulting from neuroleptic medication. At the same time freedom from the side effects induced by tranquilizer drugs, as provided by the administration of procyclidine, permits a more sustained treatment of the patient's mental disorder.

Clinical results in the treatment of parkinsonism indicate that most patients experience subjective improvement characterized by a feeling of well-being and increased alertness, together with diminished salivation and a marked improvement in muscular coordination as demonstrated by objective tests of manual dexterity and by increased ability to carry out ordinary self-care activities. While the drug exerts a mild atropine-like action and therefore causes mydriasis, this may be kept minimal by careful adjustment of the daily dosage.

CONTRAINDICATIONS

Procyclidine hydrochloride should not be used in angle-closure glaucoma although simple type glaucomas do not appear to be adversely affected.

WARNINGS: Use in Children:

Safety and efficacy have not been established in the pediatric age group; therefore, the use of procyclidine hydrochloride in this age group requires that the potential benefits be weighed against the possible hazards to the child.

Pregnancy Warning: The safe use of this drug in pregnancy has not been established; therefore, the use of procyclidine hydrochloride in pregnancy, lactation or in women of childbearing age requires that the potential benefits be weighed against the possible hazards to the mother and child.

PRECAUTIONS

Conditions in which inhibition of the parasympathetic nervous system is undesirable such as tachycardia and urinary retention (such as may occur with marked prostatic hypertrophy) require special care in the administration of the drug. Hypotensive patients who receive the drug should be observed closely. Occasionally, particularly in older patients, mental confusion and disorientation may occur with the development of agitation, hallucinations and psychotic-like symptoms.

Patients with mental disorders occasionally experience a precipitation of a psychotic episode when the dosage of antiparkinsonism drugs is increased to treat the extrapyramidal side effects of phenothiazine and rauwolfia derivatives.

ADVERSE REACTIONS

Anticholinergic effects can be produced by therapeutic doses although these can frequently be minimized or eliminated by careful dosage. They include: dryness of the mouth, mydriasis, blurring of vision, giddiness, light headedness and gastrointestinal disturbances such as nausea, vomiting, epigastric distress and constipation. Occasionally an allergic reaction such as a skin rash may be encountered. Feelings of muscular weakness may occur. Acute suppurative parotitis as a complication of dry mouth has been reported.

DOSAGE AND ADMINISTRATION

For Parkinsonism: The dosage of the drug for the treatment of parkinsonism depends upon the age of the patient, the etiology of the disease, and individual responsiveness. Therefore, the dosage must remain flexible to permit adjustment to the individual tolerance and requirements of each patient. In general, younger and postencephalitic patients require and tolerate a somewhat higher dosage than older patients and those with arteriosclerosis.

For Patients Who Have Received No Other Therapy: The usual dose of procyclidine hydrochloride for initial treatment is 2.5 mg administered three times daily after meals. If well tolerated, this dose may be gradually increased to 5 mg three times a day and occasionally 5 mg given before retiring. In some cases smaller doses may be employed with good therapeutic results.

Occasionally a patient is encountered who cannot tolerate a bedtime dose of the drug. In such cases it may be desirable to adjust dosage so that the bedtime dose is omitted and the total daily requirement is administered in three equal daytime doses. It is best administered during or after meals to minimize the development of side reactions.

To Transfer Patients to Kemadrin (Procyclidine Hydrochloride) from Other Therapy: Patients who have been receiving other drugs may be transferred to procyclidine hydrochloride. This is accomplished gradually by substituting 2.5 mg three times a day for all or part of the original drug. The dose of procyclidine is then increased as required while that of the other drug is correspondingly omitted or decreased until complete replacement is achieved. The total daily dosage may then be adjusted to the level which produces maximum benefit.

For Drug-Induced Extrapyramidal Symptoms: For treatment of symptoms of extrapyramidal dysfunction induced by tranquilizer drugs during the therapy of mental disorders, the dosage of procyclidine hydrochloride will depend on the severity of side effects associated with tranquilizer administration. In general the larger the dosage of the tranquilizer the more severe will be the associated symptoms, including rigidity and tremors. Accordingly, the drug dosage should be adjusted to suit the needs of the individual patient and to provide maximum relief of the induced symptoms. A convenient method to establish the daily dosage of procyclidine is to begin with the administration of 2.5 mg three times daily. This may be increased by 2.5 mg daily increments until the patient obtains relief of symptoms. In most cases excellent results will be obtained with 10 to 20 mg daily.

HOW SUPPLIED

White, scored tablets containing 5 mg procyclidine hydrochloride imprinted with "KEMADRIN" and "S3A" in bottles of 100 (NDC 0081-0604-55). Store at 15°–30°C (59°–86°F) in a dry place.

Shown in Product Identification Section, page 407

LANOXICAPS® ℞

[*lă-nŏx 'ĭ-kăps "*]
(Digoxin Solution in Capsules)
50 μg (0.05 mg) I.D. Imprint A2C (red)
100 μg (0.1 mg) I.D. Imprint B2C (yellow)
200 μg (0.2 mg) I.D. Imprint C2C (green)

DESCRIPTION

Digoxin is one of the cardiac (or digitalis) glycosides, a closely related group of drugs having in common specific effects on the myocardium. These drugs are found in a number of plants. Digoxin is extracted from the leaves of *Digitalis lanata*. The term "digitalis" is used to designate the whole group. The glycosides are composed of two portions: a sugar and a cardenolide (hence "glycosides").

Digoxin has the molecular formula $C_{41}H_{64}O_{14}$, a molecular weight of 780.95 and melting and decomposition points above 235°C. The drug is practically insoluble in water and in ether; slightly soluble in diluted (50%) alcohol and in chloroform; and freely soluble in pyridine. Digoxin powder is composed of odorless white crystals.

Digoxin has the chemical name: 3β-[(O-2,6- dideoxy- β -D-*ribo* -hexopyranosyl- (1→4) -O -2,6- dideoxy- β -D-*ribo* -hexopyranosyl -(1→4)- 2,6-dideoxy-β-D-*ribo* -hexopyranosyl) oxy]-12β, 14-dihydroxy-5β-card-20(22)-enolide.

Lanoxicaps is a stable solution of digoxin enclosed within a soft gelatin capsule for oral use. Each capsule contains the labeled amount of digoxin USP dissolved in a solvent comprised of polyethylene glycol 400 USP, 8 percent ethyl alcohol, propylene glycol USP and purified water USP. Inactive ingredients in the capsule shell include FD&C Red No. 40 (0.05 mg Capsule), D&C Yellow No. 10 (0.1 mg and 0.2 mg Capsules), FD&C Blue No. 1 (0.2 mg Capsule), gelatin, glycerin, methylparaben and propylparaben (added as preservatives), purified water, and sorbitol. Capsules printed with edible ink.

CLINICAL PHARMACOLOGY

Mechanism of Action: The influence of digitalis glycosides on the myocardium is dose-related, and involves both a direct action on cardiac muscle and the specialized conduction system, and indirect actions on the cardiovascular system mediated by the autonomic nervous system. The indirect actions mediated by the autonomic nervous system involve a vagomimetic action, which is responsible for the effects of digitalis on the sino-atrial (SA) and atrioventricular (AV) nodes; and also a baroreceptor sensitization which results in increased carotid sinus nerve activity and enhanced sympathetic withdrawal for any given increment in mean arterial pressure. The pharmacologic consequences of these direct and indirect effects are: 1) an increase in the force and velocity of myocardial systolic contraction (positive inotropic ac-

LANOXICAPS PRODUCT	BIOAVAILABILITY	EQUIVALENT DOSES (IN MG)*		
Lanoxin® Tablet	60–80%	0.125	0.25	0.5
Lanoxin Elixir	70–85%	0.125	0.25	0.5
Lanoxin Injection/IM	70–85%	0.125	0.25	0.5
Lanoxin Injection/IV	100%	0.1	0.2	0.4
Lanoxicaps Capsules	90–100%	0.1	0.2	0.4

*1 mg = 1000 μg

tion); 2) a slowing of heart rate (negative chronotropic effect); and 3) decreased conduction velocity through the AV node. In higher doses, digitalis increases sympathetic outflow from the central nervous system (CNS) to both cardiac and peripheral sympathetic nerves. This increase in sympathetic activity may be an important factor in digitalis cardiac toxicity. Most of the extracardiac manifestations of digitalis toxicity are also mediated by the CNS.

Pharmacokinetics:

Absorption—Gastrointestinal absorption of digoxin is a passive process. Absorption of digoxin from Lanoxicaps capsules has been demonstrated to be 90 to 100% complete compared to an identical intravenous dose of digoxin. Conventional digoxin tablets are absorbed 60 to 80%. The enhanced absorption from Lanoxicaps compared to digoxin tablets and elixir is associated with reduced between-patient and within-patient variability in steady-state serum concentrations. The peak serum concentrations are higher than those observed after tablets. When digoxin tablets or capsules are taken after meals, the rate of absorption is slowed, but the total amount of digoxin absorbed is usually unchanged. When taken with meals high in bran fiber, however, the amount absorbed from an oral dose may be reduced. Comparisons of the systemic availability and equivalent doses for digoxin preparations are shown in the following table:
[See table above].

In some patients, orally administered digoxin is converted to cardioinactive reduction products (e.g., dihydrodigoxin) by colonic bacteria in the gut. Data suggest that one in ten patients treated with digoxin tablets will degrade 40% or more of the ingested dose. This phenomenon is minimized with Lanoxicaps because they are rapidly absorbed in the upper gastrointestinal tract.

Distribution—Following drug administration, a 6 to 8 hour distribution phase is observed. This is followed by a much more gradual serum concentration decline, which is dependent on digoxin elimination from the body. The peak height and slope of the early portion (absorption/distribution phases) of the serum concentration-time curve are dependent upon the route of administration and the absorption characteristics of the formulation. Clinical evidence indicates that the early high serum concentrations (particularly high for digoxin capsules) do not reflect the concentration of digoxin at its site of action, but that with chronic use, the steady-state post-distribution serum levels are in equilibrium with tissue levels and correlate with pharmacologic effects. In individual patients, these post-distribution serum concentrations are linearly related to maintenance dosage and may be useful in evaluating therapeutic and toxic effects (see Serum Digoxin Concentrations in DOSAGE AND ADMINISTRATION section).

Digoxin is concentrated in tissues and therefore has a large apparent volume of distribution. Digoxin crosses both the blood-brain barrier and the placenta. At delivery, serum digoxin concentration in the newborn is similar to the serum level in the mother. Approximately 20 to 25% of plasma digoxin is bound to protein. Serum digoxin concentrations are not significantly altered by large changes in fat tissue weight, so that its distribution space correlates best with lean (ideal) body weight, not total body weight.

Pharmacologic Response—The approximate times to onset of effect and to peak effect of all the Lanoxin and Lanoxicaps preparations are given in the following table:
[See table below].

Excretion—Elimination of digoxin follows first-order kinetics (that is, the quantity of digoxin eliminated at any time is proportional to the total body content). Following intravenous administration to normal subjects, 50 to 70% of a digoxin dose is excreted unchanged in the urine. Renal excretion of digoxin is proportional to glomerular filtration rate and is largely independent of urine flow. In subjects with normal renal function, digoxin has a half-life of 1.5 to 2.0 days. The half-life in anuric patients is prolonged to 4 to 6 days. Digoxin is not effectively removed from the body by dialysis, exchange transfusion or during cardiopulmonary by-pass because most of the drug is in tissue rather than circulating in the blood.

INDICATIONS AND USAGE

Heart Failure: The increased cardiac output resulting from the inotropic action of digoxin ameliorates the disturbances characteristic of heart failure (venous congestion, edema, dyspnea, orthopnea and cardiac asthma).

Digoxin is more effective in "low output" (pump) failure than in "high output" heart failure secondary to arteriovenous fistula, anemia, infection or hyperthyroidism.

Digoxin is usually continued after failure is controlled, unless some known precipitating factor is corrected. Studies have shown, however, that even though hemodynamic effects can be demonstrated in almost all patients, corresponding improvement in the signs and symptoms of heart failure is not necessarily apparent. Therefore, in patients in whom digoxin may be difficult to regulate, or in whom the risk of toxicity may be great (e.g., patients with unstable renal function or whose potassium levels tend to fluctuate) a cautious withdrawal of digoxin may be considered. If digoxin is discontinued, the patient should be regularly monitored for clinical evidence of recurrent heart failure.

Atrial Fibrillation: Digoxin reduces ventricular rate and thereby improves hemodynamics. Palpitation, precordial distress or weakness are relieved and concomitant congestive failure ameliorated. Digoxin should be continued in doses necessary to maintain the desired ventricular rate.

Atrial Flutter: Digoxin slows the heart and regular sinus rhythm may appear. Frequently the flutter is converted to atrial fibrillation with a controlled ventricular response. Digoxin treatment should be maintained if atrial fibrillation persists. (Electrical cardioversion is often the treatment of choice for atrial flutter. See discussion of cardioversion in PRECAUTIONS section.)

Paroxysmal Atrial Tachycardia (PAT): Digoxin may convert PAT to sinus rhythm by slowing conduction through the AV node. If heart failure has ensued or paroxysms recur frequently, digoxin should be continued. In infants, digoxin is usually continued for 3 to 6 months after a single episode of PAT to prevent recurrence.

CONTRAINDICATIONS

Digitalis glycosides are contraindicated in ventricular fibrillation.

In a given patient, an untoward effect requiring permanent discontinuation of other digitalis preparations usually constitutes a contraindication to digoxin. Hypersensitivity to digoxin itself is a contraindication to its use. Allergy to digoxin, though rare, does occur. It may not extend to all such preparations, and another digitalis glycoside may be tried with caution.

WARNINGS

Digitalis alone or with other drugs has been used in the treatment of obesity. This use of digoxin or other digitalis glycosides is unwarranted. Moreover, since they may cause potentially fatal arrhythmias or other adverse effects, the use of these drugs solely for the treatment of obesity is dangerous.

It is recommended that digoxin in soft capsules be administered in divided daily doses to minimize any potential adverse reactions, since peak serum digoxin concentrations resulting from the capsules are approximately twice those after bioequivalent tablet doses (400 μg of Lanoxicaps are bioequivalent to 500 μg of tablets). Studies are underway to determine if there are any increased risks associated with the higher peaks that occur with single daily dosing of soft gelatin capsules.

Anorexia, nausea, vomiting and arrhythmias may accompany heart failure or may be indications of digitalis intoxication. Clinical evaluation of the cause of these symptoms should be attempted before further digitalis administration. In such circumstances determination of the serum digoxin concentration may be an aid in deciding whether or not digitalis toxicity is likely to be present. If the possibility of digitalis intoxication cannot be excluded, cardiac glycosides should be temporarily withheld, if permitted by the clinical situation.

Patients with renal insufficiency require smaller than usual maintenance doses of digoxin (see DOSAGE AND ADMINISTRATION section).

Heart failure accompanying acute glomerulonephritis requires extreme care in digitalization. Relatively low loading and maintenance doses and concomitant use of antihypertensive drugs may be necessary and careful monitoring is essential. Digoxin should be discontinued as soon as possible.

Patients with severe carditis, such as carditis associated with rheumatic fever or viral myocarditis, are especially sensitive to digoxin-induced disturbances of rhythm.

Newborn infants display considerable variability in their tolerance to digoxin. Premature and immature infants are particularly sensitive, and dosage must not only be reduced but must be individualized according to their degree of maturity.

Note: Digitalis glycosides are an important cause of accidental poisoning in children.

PRECAUTIONS

General: Digoxin toxicity develops more frequently and lasts longer in patients with renal impairment because of the decreased excretion of digoxin. Therefore, it should be anticipated that dosage requirements will be decreased in patients with moderate to severe renal disease (see DOSAGE AND ADMINISTRATION section). Because of the prolonged half-life, a longer period of time is required to achieve an initial or new steady-state concentration in patients with renal impairment than in patients with normal renal function.

In patients with hypokalemia, toxicity may occur despite serum digoxin concentrations within the "normal range", because potassium depletion sensitizes the myocardium to digoxin. Therefore, it is desirable to maintain normal serum potassium levels in patients being treated with digoxin. Hypokalemia may result from diuretic, amphotericin B or corticosteroid therapy, and from dialysis or mechanical suction of gastrointestinal secretions. It may also accompany malnutrition, diarrhea, prolonged vomiting, old age and long-standing heart failure. In general, rapid changes in serum potassium or other electrolytes should be avoided, and intravenous treatment with potassium should be reserved for special circumstances as described below (see TREATMENT OF ARRHYTHMIAS PRODUCED BY OVERDOSAGE section).

Calcium, particularly when administered rapidly by the intravenous route, may produce serious arrhythmias in digitalized patients. Hypercalcemia from any cause predisposes the patient to digitalis toxicity. On the other hand, hypocalcemia can nullify the effects of digoxin in man; thus, digoxin may be ineffective until serum calcium is restored to normal. These interactions are related to the fact that calcium affects contractility and excitability of the heart in a manner similar to digoxin.

Hypomagnesemia may predispose to digitalis toxicity. If low magnesium levels are detected in a patient on digoxin, replacement therapy should be instituted.

Quinidine and verapamil cause a rise in serum digoxin concentration, with the implication that digitalis intoxication may result. This rise appears to be proportional to the dose. The effect is mediated by a reduction in the digoxin clearance and, in the case of quinidine, decreased volume of distribution as well. Due to considerable variability of these interactions, digoxin dosage should be carefully individualized when patients receive coadministered medications.

Certain antibiotics may increase digoxin absorption in patients who convert digoxin to inactive metabolites in the gut (see Pharmacokinetics portion of the CLINICAL PHARMACOLOGY section). Recent studies have shown that specific colonic bacteria in the lower gastrointestinal tract convert digoxin to cardioinactive reduction products, thereby reducing its bioavailability. Although inactivation of these bacteria by antibiotics is rapid, the serum digoxin concentration will rise at a rate consistent with the elimination half-life of digoxin. The magnitude of rise in serum digoxin concentration relates to the extent of bacterial inactivation, and may be as much as two-fold in some cases. This interaction is significantly reduced if digoxin is given as Lanoxicaps.

Patients with acute myocardial infarction or severe pulmonary disease may be unusually sensitive to digoxin-induced disturbances of rhythm.

Atrial arrhythmias associated with hypermetabolic states (e.g. hyperthyroidism) are particularly resistant to digoxin treatment. Large doses of digoxin are not recommended as the only treatment of these arrhythmias and care must be

LANOXICAPS PRODUCT	TIME TO ONSET OF EFFECT*	TIME TO PEAK EFFECT*
Lanoxin® Tablet	0.5–2 hours	2–6 hours
Lanoxin Elixir	0.5–2 hours	2–6 hours
Lanoxin Injection/IM	0.5–2 hours	2–6 hours
Lanoxin Injection/IV	5–30 minutes†	1–4 hours
Lanoxicaps Capsules	0.5–2 hours	2–6 hours

*Documented for ventricular response rate in atrial fibrillation, inotropic effect and electrocardiographic changes.
†Depending upon rate of infusion.

Continued on next page

Burroughs Wellcome—Cont.

taken to avoid toxicity if large doses of digoxin are required. In hypothyroidism, the digoxin requirements are reduced. Digoxin responses in patients with compensated thyroid disease are normal.

Reduction of digoxin dosage may be desirable prior to electrical cardioversion to avoid induction of ventricular arrhythmias, but the physician must consider the consequences of rapid increase in ventricular response to atrial fibrillation if digoxin is withheld 1 to 2 days prior to cardioversion. If there is a suspicion that digitalis toxicity exists, elective cardioversion should be delayed. If it is not prudent to delay cardioversion, the energy level selected should be minimal at first and carefully increased in an attempt to avoid precipitating ventricular arrhythmias.

Incomplete AV block, especially in patients with Stokes-Adams attacks, may progress to advanced or complete heart block if digoxin is given.

In some patients with sinus node disease (i.e. Sick Sinus Syndrome), digoxin may worsen sinus bradycardia or sino-atrial block.

In patients with Wolff-Parkinson-White Syndrome and atrial fibrillation, digoxin can enhance transmission of impulses through the accessory pathway. This effect may result in extremely rapid ventricular rates and even ventricular fibrillation.

Digoxin may worsen the outflow obstruction in patients with idiopathic hypertrophic subaortic stenosis (IHSS). Unless cardiac failure is severe, it is doubtful whether digoxin should be employed.

Patients with chronic constrictive pericarditis may fail to respond to digoxin. In addition, slowing of the heart rate by digoxin in some patients may further decrease cardiac output.

Patients with heart failure from amyloid heart disease or constrictive cardiomyopathies respond poorly to treatment with digoxin.

Digoxin is not indicated for the treatment of sinus tachycardia unless it is associated with heart failure.

Digoxin may produce false positive ST-T changes in the electrocardiogram during exercise testing.

Intramuscular injection of digoxin is extremely painful and offers no advantages unless other routes of administration are contraindicated.

Laboratory Tests: Patients receiving digoxin should have their serum electrolytes and renal function (BUN and/or serum creatinine) assessed periodically; the frequency of assessments will depend on the clinical setting. For discussion of serum digoxin concentrations, see DOSAGE AND ADMINISTRATION section.

Drug Interactions: Potassium-depleting *corticosteroids* and *diuretics* may be major contributing factors to digitalis toxicity. *Calcium,* particularly if administered rapidly by the intravenous route, may produce serious arrhythmias in digitalized patients. *Quinidine* and *verapamil* cause a rise in serum digoxin concentration, with the implication that digitalis intoxication may result. Certain *antibiotics* increase digoxin absorption in patients who inactivate digoxin by bacterial metabolism in the lower intestine, so that digitalis intoxication may result. *Propantheline* and *diphenoxylate,* by decreasing gut motility, may increase digoxin absorption. *Antacids, kaolin-pectin, sulfasalazine, neomycin, cholestyramine* and certain *anticancer drugs* may interfere with intestinal digoxin absorption, resulting in unexpectedly low serum concentrations. *Thyroid* administration to a digitalized, hypothyroid patient may increase the dose requirement of digoxin. Concomitant use of digoxin and *sympathomimetics* increases the risk of cardiac arrhythmias, because both enhance ectopic pacemaker activity. *Succinylcholine* may cause a sudden extrusion of potassium from muscle cells, and may thereby cause arrhythmias in digitalized patients. Although β adrenergic blockers or calcium channel blockers and digoxin may be useful in combination to control atrial fibrillation, their additive effects on AV node conduction can result in complete heart block.

Carcinogenesis, Mutagenesis, Impairment of Fertility: There have been no long-term studies performed in animals to evaluate carcinogenic potential.

Pregnancy: *Teratogenic Effects:* Pregnancy Category C. Animal reproduction studies have not been conducted with digoxin. It is also not known whether digoxin can cause fetal harm when administered to a pregnant woman or can affect reproduction capacity. Digoxin should be given to a pregnant woman only if clearly needed.

Nursing Mothers: Studies have shown that digoxin concentrations in the mother's serum and milk are similar. However, the estimated daily dose to a nursing infant will be far below the usual infant maintenance dose. Therefore, this amount should have no pharmacologic effect upon the infant. Nevertheless, caution should be exercised when digoxin is administered to a nursing woman.

ADVERSE REACTIONS

The frequency and severity of adverse reactions to digoxin depend on the dose and route of administration, as well as on the patient's underlying disease or concomitant therapies (see PRECAUTIONS section). The overall incidence of adverse reactions has been reported as 5 to 20%, with 15 to 20% of them being considered serious (one to four percent of patients receiving digoxin). Evidence suggests that the incidence of toxicity has decreased since the introduction of the serum digoxin assay and improved standardization of digoxin tablets. Cardiac toxicity accounts for about one-half, gastrointestinal disturbances for about one-fourth, and CNS and other toxicity for about one-fourth of these adverse reactions.

Adults:

Cardiac—Unifocal or multiform ventricular premature contractions, especially in bigeminal or trigeminal patterns, are the most common arrhythmias associated with digoxin toxicity in adults with heart disease. Ventricular tachycardia may result from digitalis toxicity. Atrioventricular (AV) dissociation, accelerated junctional (nodal) rhythm and atrial tachycardia with block are also common arrhythmias caused by digoxin overdosage.

Excessive slowing of the pulse is a clinical sign of digoxin overdosage. AV block (Wenckebach) of increasing degree may proceed to complete heart block.

Note: The electrocardiogram is fundamental in determining the presence and nature of these cardiac disturbances. Digoxin may also induce other changes in the ECG (e.g. PR prolongation, ST depression), which represent digoxin effect and may or may not be associated with digitalis toxicity.

Gastrointestinal—Anorexia, nausea, vomiting and, less commonly, diarrhea are common early symptoms of overdosage. However, uncontrolled heart failure may also produce such symptoms.

CNS—Visual disturbances (blurred or yellow vision), headache, weakness, apathy and psychosis can occur.

Other—Gynecomastia is occasionally observed.

Infants and Children: Toxicity differs from the adult in a number of respects. Anorexia, nausea, vomiting, diarrhea and CNS disturbances may be present but are rare as initial symptoms in infants. Cardiac arrhythmias are more reliable signs of toxicity. Digoxin in children may produce any arrhythmia. The most commonly encountered are conduction disturbances or supraventricular tachyarrhythmias, such as atrial tachycardia with or without block, and junctional (nodal) tachycardia. Ventricular arrhythmias are less common. Sinus bradycardia may also be a sign of impending digoxin intoxication, especially in infants, even in the absence of first degree heart block. Any arrhythmia or alteration in cardiac conduction that develops in a child taking digoxin should initially be assumed to be a consequence of digoxin intoxication.

Treatment of Arrhythmias Produced By Overdosage:

Adults: Digoxin should be discontinued until all signs of toxicity are gone. Discontinuation may be all that is necessary if toxic manifestations are not severe and appear only near the expected time for maximum effect of the drug.

Potassium salts are commonly used, particularly if hypokalemia is present. Potassium chloride in divided oral doses totaling 3 to 6 grams of the salt (40 to 80 mEq K +) for adults may be given provided renal function is adequate (see below for potassium recommendations in Infants and Children).

When correction of the arrhythmia is urgent and the serum potassium concentration is low or normal, potassium should be administered intravenously in 5% dextrose injection. For adults, a total of 40 to 80 mEq (diluted to a concentration of 40 mEq per 500 ml) may be given at a rate not exceeding 20 mEq per hour, or slower if limited by pain due to local irritation. Additional amounts may be given if the arrhythmia is uncontrolled and potassium well-tolerated. ECG monitoring should be performed to watch for any evidence of potassium toxicity (e.g. peaking of T waves) and to observe the effect on the arrhythmia. The infusion may be stopped when the desired effect is achieved.

Note: Potassium should not be used and may be dangerous in heart block due to digoxin, unless primarily related to supraventricular tachycardia.

Other agents that have been used for the treatment of digoxin intoxication include lidocaine, procainamide, propranolol and phenytoin, although use of the latter must be considered experimental. In advanced heart block, temporary ventricular pacing may be beneficial. Rapid reversal of potentially life-threatening digitalis intoxication unresponsive to other therapy has been reported* following intravenous administration of digoxin-specific (ovine) antibody fragments (Fab); this therapy should also be considered investigational at this time. (*New Engl J Med. 1982; *307*: 1357–1362.)

Infants and Children: See Adult section for general recommendations for the treatment of arrhythmias produced by overdosage and for cautions regarding the use of potassium.

If a potassium preparation is used to treat toxicity, it may be given orally in divided doses totaling 1 to 1.5 mEq K + per kilogram (kg) body weight (1 gram of potassium chloride contains 13.4 mEq K +).

When correction of the arrhythmia with potassium is urgent, approximately 0.5 mEq/kg of potassium per hour may be given intravenously, with careful ECG monitoring. The intravenous solution of potassium should be dilute enough to avoid local irritation; however, especially in infants, care must be taken to avoid intravenous fluid overload.

DOSAGE AND ADMINISTRATION

Recommended dosages are average values that may require considerable modification because of individual sensitivity or associated conditions. Diminished renal function is the most important factor requiring modification of recommended doses.

Due to the more complete absorption of digoxin from soft capsules, recommended oral doses are only 80 percent of those for Tablets, Elixir and I.M. Injection.

Because the significance of the higher peak serum concentrations associated with once daily capsules is not established, divided daily dosing is presently recommended for:

1. Infants and children under 10 years of age,
2. Patients requiring a daily dose of 300 μg (0.3 mg) or greater;
3. Patients with a previous history of digitalis toxicity;
4. Patients considered likely to become toxic;
5. Patients in whom compliance is not a problem.

Where compliance is considered a problem, single daily dosing may be appropriate.

In deciding the dose of digoxin, several factors must be considered:

1. The disease being treated. Atrial arrhythmias may require larger doses than heart failure.
2. The body weight of the patient. Doses should be calculated based upon lean or ideal body weight.
3. The patient's renal function, preferably evaluated on the basis of creatinine clearance.
4. Age is an important factor in infants and children.
5. Concomitant disease states, drugs or other factors likely to alter the expected clinical response to digoxin (see PRECAUTIONS and Drug Interactions sections).

Digitalization may be accomplished by either of two general approaches that vary in dosage and frequency of administration, but reach the same endpoint in terms of total amount of digoxin accumulated in the body.

1. Rapid digitalization may be achieved by administering a loading dose based upon projected body digoxin stores, then calculating the maintenance dose as a percentage of the loading dose.
2. More gradual digitalization may be obtained by beginning an appropriate maintenance dose, thus allowing digoxin body stores to accumulate slowly. Steady-state serum digoxin concentrations will be achieved in approximately 5 half-lives of the drug for the individual patient. Depending upon the patient's renal function, this will take between one and three weeks.

Adults:

Adults—Rapid Digitalization with a Loading Dose: Peak body digoxin stores of 8 to 12 μg/kg should provide therapeutic effect with minimum risk of toxicity in most patients with heart failure and normal sinus rhythm. Larger stores (10 to 15 μg/kg) are often required for adequate control of ventricular rate in patients with atrial flutter or fibrillation. Because of altered digoxin distribution and elimination, projected peak body stores for patients with renal insufficiency should be conservative (i.e. 6 to 10 μg/kg) [see PRECAUTIONS section].

The loading dose should be based on the projected peak body stores and administered in several portions, with roughly half the total given as the first dose. Additional fractions of this planned total dose may be given at 6 to 8 hour intervals, **with careful assessment of clinical response before each additional dose.**

If the patient's clinical response necessitates a change from the calculated dose of digoxin, then calculation of the maintenance dose should be based upon the amount actually given.

In previously undigitalized patients, a single initial Lanoxicaps dose of 400 to 600 μg (0.4 to 0.6 mg) usually produces a detectable effect in 0.5 to 2 hours that becomes maximal in 2 to 6 hours. Additional doses of 100 to 300 μg (0.1 to 0.3 mg) may be given cautiously at 6 to 8 hour intervals until clinical evidence of an adequate effect is noted.

The usual amount of Lanoxicaps that a 70 kg patient requires to achieve 8 to 15 μg/kg peak body stores is 600 to 1000 μg (0.6 to 1.0 mg).

Although peak body stores are mathematically related to loading doses and are utilized to calculate maintenance doses, they do not correlate with measured serum concentrations. This discrepancy is caused by digoxin distribution within the body during the first 6 to 8 hours following a dose. Serum concentrations drawn during this time are usually not interpretable.

The maintenance dose should be based upon the percentage of the peak body stores lost each day through elimination. The following formula has had wide clinical use:
[See formula right].
Ccr is creatinine clearance, corrected to 70 kg body weight or 1.73 m^2 body surface area. **For adults,** if only serum creatinine concentrations (Scr) are available, a Ccr (corrected to 70 kg body weight) may be estimated in men as (140 − Age)/Scr. For women, this result should be multiplied by 0.85.
Note: This equation cannot be used for estimating creatinine clearance in infants or children.
A common practice involves the use of Lanoxin® Injection to achieve rapid digitalization, with conversion to Lanoxicaps or Lanoxin Tablets for maintenance therapy. If patients are switched from IV to oral digoxin formulations, allowances must be made for differences in bioavailability when calculating maintenance dosages (see table, CLINICAL PHARMACOLOGY section).
Adults—Gradual Digitalization with a Maintenance Dose: The following table provides average Lanoxicaps daily maintenance dose requirements for patients with heart failure based upon lean body weight and renal function:
[See table below].
Example—based on the above table, a patient in heart failure with an estimated lean body weight of 70 kg and a Ccr of 60 ml/min, should be given 200 μg (0.2 mg) of Lanoxicaps per day, usually taken as a 100 μg (0.1 mg) capsule after the morning and evening meals. Steady-state serum concentrations should not be anticipated before 11 days.
Infants and Children: Digitalization must be individualized. Divided daily dosing is recommended for infants and young children. In these patients, where dosage adjustment is frequent and outside the fixed dosages available, Lanoxicaps may not be the formulation of choice. Children over 10 years of age require adult dosages in proportion to their body weight.
In the newborn period, renal clearance of digoxin is diminished and suitable dosage adjustments must be observed. This is especially pronounced in the premature infant. Beyond the immediate newborn period, children generally require proportionally larger doses than adults on the basis of body weight or body surface area.
Lanoxin® Injection Pediatric can be used to achieve rapid digitalization, with conversion to an oral Lanoxin formulation for maintenance therapy. If patients are switched from IV to oral digoxin tablets or elixir, allowances must be made for differences in bioavailability when calculating maintenance dosages (see bioavailability table in CLINICAL PHARMACOLOGY section and dosing table below).
Intramuscular injection of digoxin is extremely painful and offers no advantages unless other routes of administration are contraindicated.
Digitalizing and daily maintenance doses for each age group are given below and should provide therapeutic effect with minimum risk of toxicity in most patients with heart failure and normal sinus rhythm. Larger doses are often required for adequate control of ventricular rate in patients with atrial flutter or fibrillation.
The loading dose should be administered in several portions, with roughly half the total given as the first dose. Additional fractions of this planned total dose may be given at 6 to 8 hour intervals, **with careful assessment of clinical response before each additional dose.** If the patient's clinical response necessitates a change from the calculated dose of digoxin, then calculation of the maintenance dose should be based upon the amount actually given.
[See table on bottom next page].
More gradual digitalization can also be accomplished by beginning an appropriate maintenance dose. The range of percentages provided above can be used in calculating this dose for patients with normal renal function. In children with renal disease, digoxin dosing must be carefully titrated based upon desired clinical response.
Long-term use of digoxin is indicated in many children who have been digitalized for acute heart failure, unless the cause is transient. Children with severe congenital heart disease, even after surgery, may require digoxin for prolonged periods.

$$\text{Maintenance Dose} = \text{Peak Body Stores (i.e. Loading Dose)} \times \frac{\%\ \text{Daily Loss}}{100}$$

$$\text{Where: } \%\ \text{Daily Loss} = 14 + \text{Ccr}/5$$

It cannot be overemphasized that both the adult and pediatric dosage guidelines provided are based upon average patient response and substantial individual variation can be expected. Accordingly, ultimate dosage selection must be based upon clinical assessment of the patient.
Serum Digoxin Concentrations: Measurement of serum digoxin concentrations can be helpful to the clinician in determining the state of digitalization and in assigning certain probabilities to the likelihood of digoxin intoxication. Studies in adults considered adequately digitalized (without evidence of toxicity) show that about two-thirds of such patients have serum digoxin levels ranging from 0.8 to 2.0 ng/ml. Patients with atrial fibrillation or atrial flutter require and appear to tolerate higher levels than do patients with other indications. On the other hand, in adult patients with clinical evidence of digoxin toxicity, about two-thirds will have serum digoxin levels greater than 2.0 ng/ml. Thus, whereas levels less than 0.8 ng/ml are infrequently associated with toxicity, levels greater than 2.0 ng/ml are often associated with toxicity. Values in between are not very helpful in deciding whether a certain sign or symptom is more likely caused by digoxin toxicity or by something else. There are rare patients who are unable to tolerate digoxin even at serum concentrations below 0.8 ng/ml. Some researchers suggest that infants and young children tolerate slightly higher serum concentrations than do adults.
To allow adequate time for equilibration of digoxin between serum and tissue, **sampling of serum concentrations for clinical use should be at least 6 to 8 hours after the last dose,** regardless of the route of administration or formulation used. On a twice daily dosing schedule, there will be only minor differences in serum digoxin concentrations whether sampling is done at 8 or 12 hours after a dose. After a single daily dose, the concentration will be 10 to 25% lower when sampled at 24 versus 8 hours, depending upon the patient's renal function. Ideally, sampling for assessment of steady-state concentrations should be done just before the next dose.
If a discrepancy exists between the reported serum concentration and the observed clinical response, the clinician should consider the following possibilities:

1. Analytical problems in the assay procedure.
2. Inappropriate serum sampling time.
3. Administration of a digitalis glycoside other than digoxin.
4. Conditions (described in WARNINGS and PRECAUTIONS sections) causing an alteration in the sensitivity of the patient to digoxin.
5. The patient falls outside the norm in his response to or handling of digoxin. This decision should only be reached after exclusion of the other possibilities and generally should be confirmed by additional correlations of clinical observations with serum digoxin concentrations.

The serum concentration data should always be interpreted in the overall clinical context and an isolated serum concentration value should not be used alone as a basis for increasing or decreasing digoxin dosage.
Adjustment of Maintenance Dose in Previously Digitalized Patients: Lanoxicaps maintenance doses in individual patients on steady-state digoxin can be adjusted upward or downward in proportion to the ratio of the desired versus the measured serum concentration. For example, a patient at steady-state on 100 μg (0.1 mg) of Lanoxicaps per day with a measured serum concentration of 0.7 ng/ml, should have the dose increased to 200 μg (0.2 mg) per day to achieve a steady-state serum concentration of 1.4 ng/ml, **assuming the serum digoxin concentration measurement is correct, renal function remains stable during this time and the needed adjustment is not the result of a problem with compliance.**

Dosage Adjustment When Changing Preparations: The absolute bioavailability of the capsule formulation is greater than that of the standard tablets and very near that of the intravenous dosage form. As a result the doses recommended for Lanoxicaps capsules are the same as those for Lanoxin® Injection (see CLINICAL PHARMACOLOGY section). Adjustments in dosage will seldom be necessary when converting a patient from intravenous to Lanoxicaps formulation. The differences in bioavailability between injectable Lanoxin or Lanoxicaps, and Lanoxin Elixir Pediatric or Lanoxin Tablets must be considered when changing patients from one dosage form to another.
Lanoxin Injection and Lanoxicaps doses of 100 μg (0.1 mg) and 200 μg (0.2 mg) are approximately equivalent to 125 μg (0.125 mg) and 250 μg (0.25 mg) doses of Lanoxin Tablets and Elixir Pediatric (see table in CLINICAL PHARMACOLOGY section). Intramuscular injection of digoxin is extremely painful and offers no advantages unless other routes of administration are contraindicated.

HOW SUPPLIED

LANOXICAPS (DIGOXIN SOLUTION IN CAPSULES), 50 μg (0.05 mg): bottles of 100 (NDC-0081-0270-55). Imprint A2C (red).
LANOXICAPS (DIGOXIN SOLUTION IN CAPSULES), 100 μg (0.1 mg)* bottles of 100 (NDC 0081-0272-55); Unit Dose Pack of 100 (NDC 0081-0272-56); Unit of Use bottles of 30 (NDC-0081-0272-30). Imprint B2C (yellow).
LANOXICAPS (DIGOXIN SOLUTION IN CAPSULES), 200 μg (0.2 mg)* bottles of 100 (NDC-0081-0274-55); Unit Dose Pack of 100 (NDC 0081-0274-56); Unit of Use bottles of 30 (NDC-0081-0274-30). Imprint C2C (green).
Store at 15°–30°C (59°–86°F) in a dry place and protect from light.
Also Available:
LANOXIN® (DIGOXIN) TABLETS, Scored 125 μg (0.125 mg): Bottles of 100 and 1000; Unit Dose Pack of 1000; Unit of Use Bottles of 30. Imprinted with LANOXIN and Y3B (yellow).
LANOXIN (DIGOXIN) TABLETS, Scored 250 μg (0.25 mg): Bottles of 100, 1000 and 5000; Unit Dose Pack of 100; Unit of Use bottle of 30. Imprinted with LANOXIN and X3A (white).
LANOXIN (DIGOXIN) TABLETS Scored 500 μg (0.5 mg): Bottles of 100. Imprinted with LANOXIN and T9A (Green)
LANOXIN (DIGOXIN) ELIXIR PEDIATRIC, 50 μg (0.05 mg) per ml; bottle of 60 ml with calibrated dropper.
LANOXIN (DIGOXIN) INJECTION, 500 μg (0.5 mg) in 2 ml (250 μg [0.25 mg] per ml); boxes of 12 and 100 ampuls.
LANOXIN (DIGOXIN) INJECTION PEDIATRIC, 100 μg (0.1 mg) in 1 ml; box of 50 ampuls.
*U.S. Patent No. 0008750
Shown in Product Identification Section, page 407

LANOXIN® ℞
[*lă-nŏx 'in"*]
(Digoxin)
Tablets/Injections/Elixir Pediatric

DESCRIPTION

Digoxin is one of the cardiac (or digitalis) glycosides, a closely related group of drugs having in common specific effects on the myocardium. These drugs are found in a number of plants. Digoxin is extracted from the leaves of *Digitalis lanata.* The term "digitalis" is used to designate the whole group. The glycosides are composed of two portions: a sugar and a cardenolide (hence "glycosides").
Digoxin has the molecular formula $C_{41}H_{64}O_{14}$, a molecular weight of 780.95 and melting and decomposition points above 235°C. The drug is practically insoluble in water and in ether; slightly soluble in diluted (50%) alcohol and in chloroform; and freely soluble in pyridine. Digoxin powder is composed of odorless white crystals.
Digoxin has the chemical name: 3β-[(O- 2,6- dideoxy- β -D-*ribo* -hexopyranosyl -(1→4)- O-2,6- dideoxy- β -D-*ribo*-hexopyranosyl - (1→4)- 2,6-dideoxy-β-D-*ribo* -hexopyranosyl) oxy]-12β, 14-dihydroxy-5β-card-20(22)-enolide.
Lanoxin Tablets with 125μg (0.125 mg), 250 μg (0.25 mg) or 500 μg (0.5 mg) digoxin USP are intended for oral use. Each tablet contains the labeled amount of digoxin USP and the inactive ingredients: 0.125 mg tablet—corn and potato starch, D&C Yellow No. 10, FD&C Yellow No. 6, lactose, and magnesium stearate; 0.25 mg tablet—corn and potato starch, lactose, magnesium stearate, and stearic acid; 0.5 mg tablet—corn and potato starch, D&C Green No. 5 and Yellow No. 10, FD&C Red No. 40, lactose, magnesium stearate, and stearic acid.
Lanoxin (Digoxin) Injection and Injection Pediatric are sterile solutions of digoxin for intravenous or intramuscular

Continued on next page

Usual Lanoxicaps Daily Maintenance Dose Requirements (μg)
for Estimated Peak Body Stores of 10 μg/kg

Corrected Ccr (ml/min per 70 kg)	Lean Body Weight (kg/lbs) 50/110	60/132	70/154	80/176	90/198	100/220	Number of Days Before Steady-State Achieved
0	50	100	100	100	150	150	22
10	100	100	100	150	150	150	19
20	100	100	150	150	150	200	16
30	100	150	150	150	200	200	14
40	100	150	150	200	200	250	13
50	150	150	200	200	250	250	12
60	150	150	200	200	250	300	11
70	150	200	200	250	250	300	10
80	150	200	200	250	300	300	9
90	150	200	250	250	300	350	8
100	200	200	250	300	300	350	7

Burroughs Wellcome—Cont.

injection. The vehicle contains 40% propylene glycol and 10% alcohol. The injection is buffered to a pH of 6.8 to 7.2 with 0.3 percent sodium phosphate and 0.08 percent anhydrous citric acid. Each 2 ml ampul of Lanoxin Injection contains 500 μg (0.5 mg) digoxin [250 μg (0.25 mg) per ml]. Each 1 ml ampul of Lanoxin Injection Pediatric contains 100 μg (0.1 mg) digoxin. Dilution is not required.
Lanoxin Elixir Pediatric is a stable solution of digoxin specially formulated for oral use in infants and children. Each ml contains 50 μg (0.05 mg) digoxin USP. The lime-flavored elixir contains 10% alcohol and methylparaben 0.1% (added as a preservative), citric acid, D&C Green No. 5 and Yellow No. 10, flavor, propylene glycol, sodium phosphate, and sucrose. Each package is supplied with a specially calibrated dropper to facilitate the administration of accurate dosage even in premature infants. Starting at 0.2 ml, this 1 ml dropper is marked in divisions of 0.1 ml, each corresponding to 5 μg (0.005 mg) digoxin.

CLINICAL PHARMACOLOGY

Mechanism of Action:
The influence of digitalis glycosides on the myocardium is dose-related, and involves both a direct action on cardiac muscle and the specialized conduction system, and indirect actions on the cardiovascular system mediated by the autonomic nervous system. The indirect actions mediated by the autonomic nervous system involve a vagomimetic action, which is responsible for the effects of digitalis on the sinoatrial (SA) and atrioventricular (AV) nodes; and also a baroreceptor sensitization which results in increased carotid sinus nerve activity and enhanced sympathetic withdrawal for any given increment in mean arterial pressure. The pharmacologic consequences of these direct and indirect effects are: 1) an increase in the force and velocity of myocardial systolic contraction (positive inotropic action); 2) a slowing of heart rate (negative chronotropic effect); and 3) decreased conduction velocity through the AV node. In higher doses, digitalis increases sympathetic outflow from the central nervous system (CNS) to both cardiac and peripheral sympathetic nerves. This increase in sympathetic activity may be an important factor in digitalis cardiac toxicity. Most of the extracardiac manifestations of digitalis toxicity are also mediated by the CNS.

Pharmacokinetics:
Note: The following data are from studies performed in adults, unless otherwise stated.
Absorption—Gastrointestinal absorption of digoxin is a passive process. Absorption of digoxin from the Lanoxin® tablet formulation has been demonstrated to be 60 to 80% complete and absorption of digoxin from the Lanoxin® Elixir Pediatric formulation 70 to 85% complete compared to an identical intravenous dose of digoxin (absolute bioavailability). When digoxin elixir or tablets are taken after meals, the rate of absorption is slowed, but the total amount of digoxin absorbed is usually unchanged. When taken with meals high in bran fiber, however, the amount absorbed from an oral dose may be reduced. Comparison of the systemic availability and equivalent doses for digoxin preparations are shown in the following table.
[See table above].

PRODUCT	ABSOLUTE BIOAVAILABILITY	EQUIVALENT DOSES (IN MG*)		
Lanoxin Tablet	60–80%	0.125	0.25	0.5
Lanoxin Elixir	70–85%	0.125	0.25	0.5
Lanoxin Injection/IM	70–85%	0.125	0.25	0.5
Lanoxin Injection/IV	100%	0.1	0.2	0.4
Lanoxicaps Capsules	90–100%	0.1	0.2	0.4

*1 mg = 1000 μg

In some patients, orally administered digoxin is converted to cardioinactive reduction products (e.g., dihydrodigoxin) by colonic bacteria in the gut. Data suggest that one in ten patients treated with digoxin tablets will degrade 40% or more of the ingested dose.
Distribution—Following drug administration, a 6 to 8 hour distribution phase is observed. This is followed by a much more gradual serum concentration decline, which is dependent on digoxin elimination from the body. The peak height and slope of the early portion (absorption/distribution phases) of the serum concentration-time curve are dependent upon the route of administration and the absorption characteristics of the formulation. Clinical evidence indicates that the early high serum concentrations do not reflect the concentration of digoxin at its site of action, but that with chronic use, the steady-state post-distribution serum levels are in equilibrium with tissue levels and correlate with pharmacologic effects. In individual patients, these post-distribution serum concentrations are linearly related to maintenance dosage and may be useful in evaluating therapeutic and toxic effects (see Serum Digoxin Concentrations in DOSAGE AND ADMINISTRATION section).
Digoxin is concentrated in tissues and therefore has a large apparent volume of distribution. Digoxin crosses both the blood-brain barrier and the placenta. At delivery, serum digoxin concentration in the newborn is similar to the serum level in the mother. Approximately 20 to 25% of plasma digoxin is bound to protein. Serum digoxin concentrations are not significantly altered by large changes in fat tissue weight, so that its distribution space correlates best with lean (ideal) body weight, not total body weight.
Pharmacologic Response—The approximate times to onset of effect and to peak effect of all the Lanoxin® preparations are given in the following table:
[See table on next page].
Excretion—Elimination of digoxin follows first-order kinetics (that is, the quantity of digoxin eliminated at any time is proportional to the total body content). Following intravenous administration to normal subjects, 50 to 70% of a digoxin dose is excreted unchanged in the urine. Renal excretion of digoxin is proportional to glomerular filtration rate and is largely independent of urine flow. In subjects with normal renal function, digoxin has a half-life of 1.5 to 2.0 days. The half-life in anuric patients is prolonged to 4 to 6 days. Digoxin is not effectively removed from the body by dialysis, exchange transfusion or during cardiopulmonary by-pass because most of the drug is in tissue rather than circulating in the blood.

INDICATIONS AND USAGE

Heart Failure:
The increased cardiac output resulting from the inotropic action of digoxin ameliorates the disturbances characteristic of heart failure (venous congestion, edema, dyspnea, orthopnea and cardiac asthma).
Digoxin is more effective in "low output" (pump) failure than in "high output" heart failure secondary to arteriovenous fistula, anemia, infection or hyperthyroidism.
Digoxin is usually continued after failure is controlled, unless some known precipitating factor is corrected. Studies have shown, however, that even though hemodynamic effects can be demonstrated in almost all patients, corresponding improvement in the signs and symptoms of heart failure is not necessarily apparent. Therefore, in patients in whom digoxin may be difficult to regulate, or in whom the risk of toxicity may be great (e.g., patients with unstable renal function or whose potassium levels tend to flucututate) a cautious withdrawal of digoxin may be considered. If digoxin is discontinued, the patient should be regularly monitored for clinical evidence or recurrent heart failure.

Atrial Fibrillation:
Digoxin reduces ventricular rate and thereby improves hemodynamics. Palpitation, precordial distress or weakness are relieved and concomitant congestive failure ameliorated. Digoxin should be continued in doses necessary to maintain the desired ventricular rate.

Atrial Flutter:
Digoxin slows the heart and regular sinus rhythm may appear. Frequently the flutter is converted to atrial fibrillation with a controlled ventricular response. Digoxin treatment should be maintained if atrial fibrillation persists. (Electrical cardioversion is often the treatment of choice for atrial flutter. See discussion of cardioversion in PRECAUTIONS section.)

Paroxysmal Atrial Tachycardia (PAT):
Digoxin may convert PAT to sinus rhythm by slowing conduction through the AV node. If heart failure has ensued or paroxysms recur frequently, digoxin should be continued. In infants, digoxin is usually continued for 3 to 6 months after a single episode of PAT to prevent recurrence.

Usual Digitalizing and Maintenance Dosages for Lanoxicaps in Children with **Normal Renal Function Based on Lean Body Weight**

Age	Digitalizing* Dose (μg/kg)	**Daily** † Maintenance Dose (μg/kg)
2–5 Years	25–35	25–35% of the oral or IV
5–10 Years	15–30	loading dose ‡
Over 10 years	8–12	

*IV digitalizing doses are the same as Lanoxicaps digitalizing doses.
†Divided daily dosing is recommended for children under 10 years of age.
‡Projected or actual digitalizing dose providing desired clinical response.

CONTRAINDICATIONS

Digitalis glycosides are contraindicated in ventricular fibrillation.
In a given patient, an untoward effect requiring discontinuation of other digitalis preparations usually constitutes a contraindication to digoxin. Hypersensitivity to digoxin itself is a contraindication to its use. Allergy to digoxin, though rare, does occur. It may not extend to all such preparations, and another digitalis glycoside may be tried with caution.

WARNINGS

Digitalis alone or with other drugs has been used in the treatment of obesity. This use of digoxin or other digitalis glycosides is unwarranted. Moreover, since they may cause potentially fatal arrhythmias or other adverse effects, the use of these drugs solely for the treatment of obesity is dangerous.
Anorexia, nausea, vomiting and arrhythmias may accompany heart failure or may be indications of digitalis intoxication. Clinical evaluation of the cause of these symptoms should be attempted before further digitalis administration. In such circumstances determination of the serum digoxin concentration may be an aid in deciding whether or not digitalis toxicity is likely to be present. If the possibility of digitalis intoxication cannot be excluded, cardiac glycosides should be temporarily withheld, if permitted by the clinical situation.
Patients with renal insufficiency require smaller than usual maintenance doses of digoxin (see DOSAGE AND ADMINISTRATION section).
Heart failure accompanying acute glomerulonephritis requires extreme care in digitalization. Relatively low loading and maintenance doses and concomitant use of antihypertensive drugs may be necessary and careful monitoring is essential. Digoxin should be discontinued as soon as possible.
Patients with severe carditis, such as carditis associated with rheumatic fever or viral myocarditis, are especially sensitive to digoxin-induced disturbances of rhythm.
Newborn infants display considerable variability in their tolerance to digoxin. Premature and immature infants are particularly sensitive, and dosage must not only be reduced but must be individualized according to their degree of maturity.
Note: Digitalis glycosides are an important cause of accidental poisoning in children.

PRECAUTIONS

General:
Digoxin toxicity develops more frequently and lasts longer in patients with renal impairment because of the decreased excretion of digoxin. Therefore, it should be anticipated that dosage requirements will be decreased in patients with moderate to severe renal disease (see DOSAGE AND ADMINISTRATION section). Because of the prolonged half-life, a longer period of time is required to achieve an initial or new steady-state concentration in patients with renal impairment than in patients with normal renal function.
In patients with hypokalemia, toxicity may occur despite serum digoxin concentrations within the "normal range", because potassium depletion sensitizes the myocardium to digoxin. Therefore, it is desirable to maintain normal serum potassium levels in patients being treated with digoxin. Hypokalemia may result from diuretic, amphotericin B or corticosteroid therapy, and from dialysis or mechanical suction of gastrointestinal secretions. It may also accompany malnutrition, diarrhea, prolonged vomiting, old age and long-standing heart failure. In general, rapid changes in serum potassium or other electrolytes should be avoided, and intravenous treatment with potassium should be reserved for special circumstances as described below (see TREATMENT OF ARRHYTHMIAS PRODUCED BY OVERDOSAGE section).
Calcium, particularly when administered rapidly by the intravenous route, may produce serious arrhythmias in digitalized patients. Hypercalcemia from any cause predisposes the patient to digitalis toxicity. On the other hand, hypocalcemia can nullify the effects of digoxin in man; thus, digoxin may be ineffective until serum calcium is restored to normal. These interactions are related to the fact that calcium affects contractility and excitability of the heart in a manner similar to digoxin.
Hypomagnesemia may predispose to digitalis toxicity. If low magnesium levels are detected in a patient on digoxin, replacement therapy should be instituted.

Quinidine and verapamil cause a rise in serum digoxin concentration, with the implication that digitalis intoxication may result. This rise appears to be proportional to the dose. The effect is mediated by a reduction in the digoxin clearance and, in the case of quinidine, decreased volume of distribution as well. Due to the considerable variability of these interactions, digoxin dosage should be carefully individualized when patients receive coadministered medications.

Certain antibiotics may increase digoxin absorption in patients who convert digoxin to inactive metabolites in the gut (see Pharmacokinetics portion of the CLINICAL PHARMACOLOGY section). Recent studies have shown that specific colonic bacteria in the lower gastrointestinal tract convert digoxin to cardioinactive reduction products, thereby reducing its bioavailability. Although inactivation of these bacteria by antibiotics is rapid, the serum digoxin concentration will rise at a rate consistent with the elimination half-life of digoxin. The magnitude of rise in serum digoxin concentration relates to the extent of bacterial inactivation, and may be as much as two-fold in some cases. This interaction is significantly reduced if digoxin is given as Lanoxicaps.

Patients with acute myocardial infarction or severe pulmonary disease may be unusually sensitive to digoxin-induced disturbances of rhythm.

Atrial arrhythmias associated with hypermetabolic states (e.g. hyperthyroidism) are particularly resistant to digoxin treatment. Large doses of digoxin are not recommended as the only treatment of these arrhythmias and care must be taken to avoid toxicity if large doses of digoxin are required.

In hypothyroidism, the digoxin requirements are reduced. Digoxin responses in patients with compensated thyroid disease are normal.

Reduction of digoxin dosage may be desirable prior to electrical cardioversion to avoid induction of ventricular arrhythmias, but the physician must consider the consequences of rapid increase in ventricular response to atrial fibrillation if digoxin is withheld 1 to 2 days prior to cardioversion. If there is a suspicion that digitalis toxicity exists, elective cardioversion should be delayed. If it is not prudent to delay cardioversion, the energy level selected should be minimal at first and carefully increased in an attempt to avoid precipitating ventricular arrhythmias.

Incomplete AV block, especially in patients with Stokes-Adams attacks, may progress to advanced or complete heart block if digoxin is given.

In some patients with sinus node disease (i.e. Sick Sinus Syndrome), digoxin may worsen sinus bradycardia or sino-atrial block.

In patients with Wolff-Parkinson-White Syndrome and atrial fibrillation, digoxin can enhance transmission of impulses through the accessory pathway. This effect may result in extremely rapid ventricular rates and even ventricular fibrillation.

Digoxin may worsen the outflow obstruction in patients with idiopathic hypertrophic subaortic stenosis (IHSS). Unless cardiac failure is severe, it is doubtful whether digoxin should be employed.

Patients with chronic constrictive pericarditis may fail to respond to digoxin. In addition, slowing of the heart rate by digoxin in some patients may further decrease cardiac output.

Patients with heart failure from amyloid heart disease or constrictive cardiomyopathies respond poorly to treatment with digoxin.

Digoxin is not indicated for the treatment of sinus tachycardia unless it is associated with heart failure.

Digoxin may produce false positive ST-T changes in the electrocardiogram during exercise testing.

Intramuscular injection of digoxin is extremely painful and offers no advantages unless other routes of administration are contraindicated.

Laboratory Tests:

Patients receiving digoxin should have their serum electrolytes and renal function (BUN and /or serum creatinine) assessed periodically; the frequency of assessments will depend on the clinical setting. For discussion of serum digoxin concentrations, see DOSAGE AND ADMINISTRATION section.

Drug Interactions:

Potassium-depleting *corticosteroids* and *diuretics* may be major contributing factors to digitalis toxicity. *Calcium*, particularly if administered rapidly by the intravenous route, may produce serious arrhythmias in digitalized patients. *Quinidine* and *verapamil* cause a rise in serum digoxin concentration, with the implication that digitalis intoxication may result. Certain *antibiotics* increase digoxin absorption in patients who inactivate digoxin by bacterial metabolism in the lower intestine, so that digitalis intoxication may result. *Propantheline* and *diphenoxylate*, by decreasing gut motility, may increase digoxin absorption. *Antacids, kaolin-pectin, sulfasalazine, neomycin, cholestyramine* and certain *anticancer drugs* may interfere with intestinal digoxin absorption, resulting in unexpectedly low serum concentrations. *Thyroid* administration to a digitalized, hypothyroid patient may increase the dose requirement of digoxin. Concomitant use of digoxin and *sympathomimetics* increases the risk of cardiac arrhythmias because both enhance ectopic pacemaker activity. *Succinylcholine* may cause a sudden extrusion of potassium from muscle cells, and may thereby cause arrhythmias in digitalized patients. Although β adrenergic blockers or calcium channel blockers and digoxin may be useful in combination to control atrial fibrillation, their additive effects on AV node conduction can result in complete heart block.

PRODUCT	TIME TO ONSET OF EFFECT*	TIME TO PEAK EFFECT*
Lanoxin Tablet	0.5–2 hours	2–6 hours
Lanoxin Elixir	0.5–2 hours	2–6 hours
Lanoxin Injection/IM	0.5–2 hours	2–6 hours
Lanoxin Injection/IV	5–30 minutes†	1–4 hours
Lanoxicaps Capsules	0.5–2 hours	2–6 hours

*Documented for ventricular response rate in atrial fibrillation, inotropic effect and electrocardiographic changes.
†Depending upon rate of infusion.

Carcinogenesis, Mutagenesis, Impairment of Fertility:

There have been no long-term studies performed in animals to evaluate carcinogenic potential.

Pregnancy: *Teratogenic Effects:* Pregnancy Category C. Animal reproduction studies have not been conducted with digoxin. It is also not known whether digoxin can cause fetal harm when administered to a pregnant woman or can affect reproduction capacity. Digoxin should be given to a pregnant woman only if clearly needed.

Nursing Mothers:

Studies have shown that digoxin concentrations in the mother's serum and milk are similar. However, the estimated daily dose to a nursing infant will be far below the usual infant maintenance dose. Therefore, this amount should have no pharmacologic effect upon the infant. Nevertheless, caution should be exercised when digoxin is administered to a nursing woman.

ADVERSE REACTIONS

The frequency and severity of adverse reactions to digoxin depend on the dose and route of administration, as well as on the patient's underlying disease or concomitant therapies (see PRECAUTIONS section). The overall incidence of adverse reactions has been reported as 5 to 20%, with 15 to 20% of them being considered serious (one to four percent of patients receiving digoxin). Evidence suggests that the incidence of toxicity has decreased since the introduction of the serum digoxin assay and improved standardization of digoxin tablets. Cardiac toxicity accounts for about one-half, gastrointestinal disturbances for about one-fourth, and CNS and other toxicity for about one-fourth of these adverse reactions.

Adults:

Cardiac—Unifocal or multiform ventricular premature contractions, especially in bigeminal or trigeminal patterns, are the most common arrhythmias associated with digoxin toxicity in adults with heart disease.

Ventricular tachycardia may result from digitalis toxicity. Atrioventricular (AV) dissociation, accelerated junctional (nodal) rhythm and atrial tachycardia with block are also common arrhythmias caused by digoxin overdosage.

Excessive slowing of the pulse is a clinical sign of digoxin overdosage. AV block (Wenckebach) of increasing degree may proceed to complete heart block.

Note: The electrocardiogram is fundamental in determining the presence and nature of these cardiac disturbances. Digoxin may also induce other changes in the ECG (e.g. PR prolongation, ST depression), which represent digoxin effect and may or may not be associated with digitalis toxicity.

Gastrointestinal—Anorexia, nausea, vomiting and less commonly diarrhea are common early symptoms of overdosage. However, uncontrolled heart failure may also produce such symptoms.

CNS—Visual disturbances (blurred or yellow vision), headache, weakness, apathy and psychosis can occur.

Other—Gynecomastia is occasionally observed.

Infants and Children:

Toxicity differs from the adult in a number of respects. Anorexia, nausea, vomiting, diarrhea and CNS disturbances may be present but are rare as initial symptoms in infants. Cardiac arrhythmias are more reliable signs of toxicity. Digoxin in children may produce any arrhythmia.

Cardiac—Conduction disturbances or supraventricular tachyarrhythmias, such as atrioventricular (AV) block (Wenckebach), atrial tachycardia with or without block and junctional (nodal) tachycardia are the most common arrhythmias associated with digoxin toxicity in children. Ventricular arrhythmias, such as unifocal or multiform ventricular premature contractions, especially in bigeminal or trigeminal patterns, are less common. Ventricular tachycardia may result from digitalis toxicity. Sinus bradycardia may also be a sign of impending digoxin intoxication, especially in infants, even in the absence of first degree heart block. Any arrhythmias or alteration in cardiac conduction that develops in a child taking digoxin should initially be assumed to be a consequence of digoxin intoxication.

Note: The electrocardiogram is fundamental in determining the presence and nature of these cardiac disturbances. Digoxin may also induce other changes in the ECG (e.g. PR prolongation ST depression), which represent digoxin effect and may or may not be associated with digitalis toxicity.

Gastrointestinal—Anorexia, nausea, vomiting and diarrhea may be early symptoms of overdosage. However, uncontrolled heart failure may also produce such symptoms.

CNS—Visual disturbances (blurred or yellow vision), headache, weakness, apathy and psychosis can occur. These may be difficult to recognize in infants and children.

Other—Gynecomastia is occasionally observed.

Treatment of Arrhythmias Produced by Overdosage:

Adults:

Digoxin should be discontinued until all signs of toxicity are gone. Discontinuation may be all that is necessary if toxic manifestations are not severe and appear only near the expected time for maximum effect of the drug.

Potassium salts are commonly used, particularly if hypokalemia is present. Potassium chloride in divided oral doses totaling 3 to 6 grams of the salt (40 to 80 mEq K+) for adults may be given provided renal function is adequate (see below for potassium recommendations in Infants and Children).

When correction of the arrhythmia is urgent and the serum potassium concentration is low or normal, potassium should be administered intravenously in 5% dextrose injection. For adults, a total of 40 to 80 mEq (diluted to a concentration of 40 mEq per 500 ml) may be given at a rate not exceeding 20 mEq per hour, or slower if limited by pain due to local irritation. Additional amounts may be given if the arrhythmia is uncontrolled and potassium well-tolerated. ECG monitoring should be performed to watch for any evidence of potassium toxicity (e.g. peaking of T waves) and to observe the effect on the arrhythmia. The infusion may be stopped when the desired effect is achieved.

Note: Potassium should not be used and may be dangerous in heart block due to digoxin, unless primarily related to supraventricular tachycardia.

Other agents that have been used for the treatment of digoxin intoxication include lidocaine, procainamide, propranolol and phenytoin, although use of the latter must be considered experimental. In advanced heart block, temporary ventricular pacing may be beneficial. Rapid reversal of potentially life-threatening digitalis intoxication unresponsive to other therapy has been reported* following intravenous administration of digoxin-specific (ovine) antibody fragments (Fab); this therapy should also be considered investigational at this time. (*New Engl J Med, 1982; *307;* 1357-1362.)

Infants and Children:

See Adult section for general recommendations for the treatment of arrhythmias produced by overdosage and for cautions regarding the use of potassium.

If a potassium preparation is used to treat toxicity, it may be given orally in divided doses totaling 1 to 1.5 mEq K+ per kilogram (kg) body weight (1 gram of potassium chloride contains 13.4 mEq K+).

When correction of the arrhythmia with potassium is urgent, approximately 0.5 mEq/kg of potassium per hour may be given intravenously, with careful ECG monitoring. The intravenous solution of potassium should be dilute enough to avoid local irritation; however, especially in infants, care must be taken to avoid intravenous fluid overload.

DOSAGE AND ADMINISTRATION

Recommended dosages are average values that may require considerable modification because of individual sensitivity or associated conditions. Diminished renal function is the most important factor requiring modification of recommended doses.

Parenteral administration of digoxin should be used only when the need for rapid digitalization is urgent or when the drug cannot be taken orally. Intramuscular injection can lead to severe pain at the injection site, thus intravenous administration is preferred. If the drug must be administered by the intramuscular route, it should be injected deep into the muscle followed by massage. No more than 500 μg (2 ml) of Lanoxin Injection or 200 μg (2 ml) of Lanoxin Injection Pediatric should be injected into a single site.

Continued on next page

Burroughs Wellcome—Cont.

Lanoxin® Injection and Injection Pediatric can be administered undiluted or diluted with a 4-fold or greater volume of sterile water for injection, 0.9% sodium chloride injection or 5% dextrose injection. The use of less than a 4-fold volume of diluent could lead to precipitation of the digoxin. Immediate use of the diluted product is recommended.

If tuberculin syringes are used to measure very small doses, one must be aware of the problem of inadvertent overadministration of digoxin. The syringe should *not* be flushed with the parenteral solution after its contents are expelled into an indwelling vascular catheter.

Slow infusion of Lanoxin® Injection or Injection Pediatric is preferable to bolus administration. Rapid infusion of digitalis glycosides has been shown to cause systemic and coronary arteriolar constriction, which may be clinically undesirable. Caution is thus advised and Lanoxin Injection or Injection Pediatric should probably be administered over a period of 5 minutes or longer. Mixing of Lanoxin Injections with other drugs in the same container or simultaneous administration in the same intravenous line is not recommended.

In deciding the dose of digoxin, several factors must be considered:

1. The disease being treated. Atrial arrhythmias may require larger doses than heart failure.
2. The body weight of the patient. Doses should be calculated based upon lean or ideal body weight.
3. The patient's renal function, preferably evaluated on the basis of creatinine clearance.
4. Age is an important factor in infants and children.
5. Concomitant disease states, drugs or other factors likely to alter the expected clinical response to digoxin (see PRECAUTIONS and Drug Interactions sections).

Digitalization may be accomplished by either of two general approaches that vary in dosage and frequency of administration, but reach the same endpoint in terms of total amount of digoxin accumulated in the body.

1. Rapid digitalization may be achieved by administering a loading dose based upon projected peak body digoxin stores, then calculating the maintenance dose as a percentage of the loading dose.
2. More gradual digitalization may be obtained by beginning an appropriate maintenance dose, thus allowing digoxin body stores to accumulate slowly. Steady-state serum digoxin concentration will be achieved in approximately 5 half-lives of the drug for the individual patient. Depending upon the patient's renal function, this will take between one and three weeks.

Adults:

Adults—Rapid Digitalization with a Loading Dose. Peak body digoxin stores of 8 to 12 μg/kg should provide therapeutic effect with minimum risk of toxicity in most patients with heart failure and normal sinus rhythm. Larger stores (10 to 15 μg/kg) are often required for adequate control of ventricular rate in patients with atrial flutter or fibrillation. Because of altered digoxin distribution and elimination, projected peak body stores for patients with renal insufficiency should be conservative (i.e. 6 to 10 μg/kg) [see PRECAUTIONS section].

The loading dose should be based on the projected peak body stores and administered in several portions, with roughly half the total given as the first dose. Additional fractions of this planned total dose may be given at 4 to 8 hour intervals IV or 6 to 8 hour intervals orally, with **careful assessment of clinical response before each additional dose.**

If the patient's clinical response necessitates a change from the calculated dose of digoxin, then calculation of the maintenance dose should be based upon the amount actually given.

In previously undigitalized patients, a single initial intravenous Lanoxin® Injection dose of 400 to 600 μg (0.4 to 0.6 mg) usually produces a detectable effect in 5 to 30 minutes that becomes maximal in 1 to 4 hours. Additional doses of 100 to 300 μg (0.1 to 0.3 mg) may be given cautiously at 4 to 8 hour intervals until clinical evidence of an adequate effect is noted. The usual amount of Lanoxin Injection that a 70 kg patient requires to achieve 8 to 15 μg/kg peak body stores is 600 to 1000 μg (0.6 to 1.0 mg).

A single initial Lanoxin® Tablet or Elixir Pediatric dose of 500 to 750 μg (0.5 to 0.75 mg) usually produces a detectable effect in 0.5 to 2 hours that becomes maximal in 2 to 6 hours. Additional doses of 125 to 375 μg (0.125 to 0.375 mg) may be given cautiously at 6 to 8 hour intervals until clinical evidence of an adequate effect is noted. The usual amount of Lanoxin Tablets or Elixir that a 70 kg patient requires to achieve 8 to 15 μg/kg peak body stores is 750 to 1250 μg (0.75 to 1.25 mg).

Usual Lanoxin Daily Maintenance Dose Requirements (μg) For Estimated Peak Body Stores of 10 μg/kg

Corrected Ccr (ml/min per 70 kg)	Lean Body Weight (kg/lbs) 50/110	60/132	70/154	80/176	90/198	100/220	Number of Days Before Steady-State Achieved
0	63*†	125	125	125	188††	188	22
10	125	125	125	188	188	188	19
20	125	125	188	188	188	250	16
30	125	188	188	188	250	250	14
40	125	188	188	250	250	250	13
50	188	188	250	250	250	250	12
60	188	188	250	250	250	375	11
70	188	250	250	250	250	375	10
80	188	250	250	250	375	375	9
90	188	250	250	250	375	500	8
100	250	250	250	375	375	500	7

* 63 μg = 0.063 mg
† ½ of 125 μg tablet or 125 μg every other day
†† 1½ of 125 μg tablet.

Example—based on the above table, a patient in heart failure with an estimated lean body weight of 70 kg and a Ccr of 60 ml/min, should be given a 250 μg (0.25 mg) Lanoxin® Tablet each day, usually taken after the morning meal. Steady-state serum concentrations should not be anticipated before 11 days.

Although peak body stores are mathematically related to loading doses and are utilized to calculate maintenance doses, they do not correlate with measured serum concentrations. This discrepancy is caused by digoxin distribution within the body during the first 6 to 8 hours following a dose. Serum concentrations drawn during this time are usually not interpretable.

The maintenance dose should be based upon the percentage of the peak body stores lost each day through elimination. The following formula has had wide clinical use:

[See formula below].

Ccr is creatinine clearance, corrected to 70 kg body weight or 1.73 m^2 body surface area. *For adults,* if only serum creatinine concentrations (Scr) are available, a Ccr (corrected to 70 kg body weight) may be estimated in men as (140 – Age)/Scr. For women, this result should be multiplied by 0.85.

Note: This equation cannot be used for estimating creatinine clearance in infants or children.

A common practice involves the use of Lanoxin® Injection to achieve rapid digitalization, with conversion to Lanoxin Tablets or Lanoxicaps for maintenance therapy. If patients are switched from IV to oral digoxin formulations, allowances must be made for differences in bioavailability when calculating maintenance dosages (see table, CLINICAL PHARMACOLOGY section).

Adults—Gradual Digitalization with a Maintenance Dose: The following table provides average Lanoxin Tablet daily maintenance dose requirements for patients with heart failure based upon lean body weight and renal function:

[See table above].

Infants and Children:

Digitalization must be individualized. Divided daily dosing is recommended for infants and young children. Children over 10 years of age require adult dosages in proportion to their body weight.

In the newborn period, renal clearance of digoxin is diminished and suitable dosage adjustments must be observed. This is especially pronounced in the premature infant. Beyond the immediate newborn period, children generally require proportionally larger doses than adults on the basis of body weight or body surface area.

Infants and Children—Rapid Digitalization with a Loading Dose: Lanoxin Injection Pediatric can be used to achieve rapid digitalization, with conversion to an oral Lanoxin formulation for maintenance therapy. If patients are switched from IV to oral digoxin tablets or elixir, allowances must be made for differences in bioavailability when calculating maintenance dosages (see bioavailability table in CLINICAL PHARMACOLOGY section and dosing tables below).

Intramuscular injection of digoxin is extremely painful and offers no advantages unless other routes of administration are contraindicated.

Digitalizing and daily maintenance doses for each age group are given below and should provide therapeutic effect with minimum risk of toxicity in most patients with heart failure and normal sinus rhythm. Larger doses are often required for adequate control of ventricular rate in patients with atrial flutter or fibrillation.

The loading dose should be administered in several portions, with roughly half the total given as the first dose. Additional fractions of this planned total dose may be given at 6 to 8 hour intervals with Lanoxin Tablets or Elixir or at 4 to 8 hour intervals with Lanoxin Injection or Injection Pediatric **with careful assessment of clinical response before each additional dose.** If the patient's clinical response necessitates a change from the calculated dose of digoxin, then calculation of the maintenance dose should be based upon the amount actually given.

[See table on next page].

Infants and Children—Gradual Digitalization With A Maintenance Dose: More gradual digitalization can also be accomplished by beginning an appropriate maintenance dose. The range of percentages provided above can be used in calculating this dose for patients with normal renal function. In children with renal disease, digoxin dosing must be carefully titrated based upon clinical response.

Long-term use of digoxin is indicated in many children who have been digitalized for acute heart failure, unless the cause is transient. Children with severe congenital heart disease, even after surgery, may require digoxin for prolonged periods.

It cannot be overemphasized that both the adult and pediatric dosage guidelines provided are based upon average patient response and substantial individual variation can be expected. Accordingly, ultimate dosage selection must be based upon clinical assessment of the patient.

Serum Digoxin Concentrations:

Measurement of serum digoxin concentrations can be helpful to the clinician in determining the state of digitalization and in assigning certain probabilities to the likelihood of digoxin intoxication. Studies in adults considered adequately digitalized (without evidence of toxicity) show that about two-thirds of such patients have serum digoxin levels ranging from 0.8 to 2.0 ng/ml. Patients with atrial fibrillation or atrial flutter require and appear to tolerate higher levels than do patients with other indications. On the other hand, in adult patients with clinical evidence of digoxin toxicity, about two-thirds will have serum digoxin levels greater than 2.0 ng/ml. Thus, whereas levels less than 0.8 ng/ml are infrequently associated with toxicity, levels greater than 2.0 ng/ml are often associated with toxicity. Values in between are not very helpful in deciding whether a certain sign or symptom is more likely caused by digoxin toxicity or by something else. There are rare patients who are unable to tolerate digoxin even at serum concentrations below 0.8 ng/ml. Some researchers suggest that infants and young children tolerate slightly higher serum concentrations than do adults.

To allow adequate time for equilibration of digoxin between serum and tissue, **sampling of serum concentrations for clinical use should be at least 6 to 8 hours after the last dose,** regardless of the route of administration or formulation used. On a twice daily dosing schedule, there will be only minor differences in serum digoxin concentrations whether sampling is done at 8 or 12 hours after a dose. After a single daily dose, the concentration will be 10 to 25% lower when sampled at 24 versus 8 hours, depending upon the patient's renal function. Ideally, sampling for assessment of steady-state concentrations should be done just before the next dose.

If a discrepancy exists between the reported serum concentration and the observed clinical response, the clinician should consider the following possibilities:

1. Analytical problems in the assay procedure.
2. Inappropriate serum sampling time.
3. Administration of a digitalis glycoside other than digoxin.
4. Conditions (described in WARNINGS and PRECAUTIONS sections) causing an alteration in the sensitivity of the patient to digoxin.
5. The patient falls outside the norm in his response to or handling of digoxin. This decision should only be reached after exclusion of the other possibilities and generally should be confirmed by additional correla-

Lanoxin

$$\text{Maintenance Dose} = \text{Peak Body Stores (i.e. Loading Dose)} \times \frac{\%\ \text{Daily Loss}}{100}$$

$$\text{Where: } \%\ \text{Daily Loss} = 14 + \text{Ccr}/5$$

Usual Digitalizing and Maintenance Dosages for **Lanoxin® Tablets or Lanoxin® Elixir Pediatric** in Children with **Normal Renal Function Based on Lean Body Weight**

Age	Digitalizing* Dose (μg/kg)	*Daily* † Oral Maintenance Dose (μg/kg)
Premature	20–30	20–30% of *oral* loading dose††
Full-Term	25–35	25–35% of *oral* loading dose††
1–24 Months	35–60	
2–5 Years	30–40	
5–10 Years	20–35	
Over 10 years	10–15	

Usual Digitalizing and Maintenance Dosages for **Lanoxin® Injection or Lanoxin® Injection Pediatric** in Children with **Normal Renal Function Based on Lean Body Weight**

Age	Digitalizing* Dose (μg/kg)	*Daily* † IV Maintenance Dose (μg/kg)
Premature	15–25	20–30% of the IV loading dose††
Full-Term	20–30	25–35% of the IV loading dose††
1–24 Months	30–50	
2–5 Years	25–35	
5–10 Years	15–30	
Over 10 Years	8–12	

* IV digitalizing doses are 80% of oral digitalizing doses.
† Divided daily dosing is recommended for children under 10 years of age.
†† Projected or actual digitalizing dose providing clinical response.

tions of clinical observations with serum digoxin concentrations.

The serum concentration data should always be interpreted in the overall clinical context and an isolated serum concentration value should not be used alone as a basis for increasing or decreasing digoxin dosage.

Adjustment of Maintenance Dose in Previously Digitalized Patients:

Maintenance doses in individual patients on steady-state digoxin can be adjusted upward or downward in proportion to the ratio of the desired versus the measured serum concentration. For example, a patient at steady-state on 125 μg (0.125 mg) of Lanoxin Tablets per day with a measured serum concentration of 0.7 ng/ml, should have the dose increased to 250 μg (0.25 mg) per day to achieve a steady-state serum concentration of 1.4 ng/ml, **assuming the serum digoxin concentration measurement is correct, renal function remains stable during this time and the needed adjustment is not the result of a problem with compliance.**

Dosage Adjustment When Changing Preparations:

The difference in bioavailability between injectable Lanoxin or Lanoxicaps and Lanoxin Elixir Pediatric or Lanoxin Tablets must be considered when changing patients from one dosage form to another.

Lanoxin Injection and Lanoxicaps doses of 100 μg (0.1 mg) and 200 μg (0.2 mg) are approximately equivalent to 125 μg (0.125 mg) and 250 μg (0.25 mg) doses of Lanoxin Tablets and Elixir Pediatric (see table in CLINICAL PHARMACOLOGY section). Intramuscular injection of digoxin is extremely painful and offers no advantages unless other routes of administration are contraindicated.

HOW SUPPLIED

LANOXIN® (DIGOXIN) TABLETS, Scored 125 μg (0.125 mg): Bottles of 100 (NDC-0081-0242-55) and 1000 (NDC-0081-0242-75); Unit dose pack of 100 (NDC 0081-0242-56); Unit of Use bottles of 30 (NDC-0081-0242-30) **VA NSN** 6505-01-049-6807. Imprinted with LANOXIN and Y3B (yellow). Store at 15°-30°C (59°-86°F) in a dry place and protect from light.

LANOXIN (DIGOXIN) TABLETS, Scored 250 μg (0.25 mg): Bottles of 100 (NDC-0081-0249-55) **DoD NSN** 6505-00-116-7750. 1000 (NDC-0081-0249-75) **VA NSN** 6505-00-611-7898 and 5000 (NDC-0081-0249-80); Unit dose pack of 100 (10 x 10) (NDC-0081-0249-56) **DoD NSN** 6505-00-117-5689; Unit of Use bottles of 30 (NDC-0081-0249-30) **VA NSN** 6505-01-035-2104 and 100 (NDC-0081-0249-17). Imprinted with LANOXIN and X3A (white). Store at 15°-30°C (59°-86°F) in a dry place.

LANOXIN (DIGOXIN) TABLETS, Scored 500 μg (0.5 mg): Bottles of 100 (NDC-0081-0253-55). Imprinted with LANOXIN and T9A (green). Store at 15°-30°C (59°-86°F) in a dry place and protect from light.

LANOXIN (DIGOXIN) INJECTION, 500 μg (0.5 mg) in 2 ml [250 μg (0.25 mg) per ml]; boxes of 10 (NDC-0081-0260-10) **DoD NSN** 6505-00-531-7761 and 50 ampuls (NDC-0081-0260-35). Store at 15°-30°C (59°-86°F) and protect from light.

LANOXIN (DIGOXIN) INJECTION PEDIATRIC, 100 μg (0.1 mg) in 1 ml; box of 10 ampuls (NDC-0081-0262-10). Store at 15°-30°C (59°- 86°F) and protect from light.

LANOXIN (DIGOXIN) ELIXIR PEDIATRIC, 50 μg (0.05 mg) per ml; bottle of 60 ml with calibrated dropper (NDC-0081-0264-27) **DoD NSN** 6505-00-890-1726. Store at 15°-25°C (59°-77°F) and protect from light.

Tablets Shown in Product Identification Section, page 407

LEUKERAN® ℞
(Chlorambucil)
2 mg Sugar-coated Tablets

> **WARNING:** Leukeran (chlorambucil) can severely suppress bone marrow function. Chlorambucil is a carcinogen in humans. Chlorambucil is probably mutagenic and teratogenic in humans. Chlorambucil produces human infertility. See "WARNINGS" and "PRECAUTIONS" sections.

DESCRIPTION

Leukeran (chlorambucil) was first synthesized by Everett *et al.*[1] It is a bifunctional alkylating agent of the nitrogen mustard type that has been found active against selected human neoplastic diseases. Chlorambucil is known chemically as 4-[bis(2-chlorethyl)amino]benzenebutanoic acid.

Chlorambucil hydrolyzes in water and has a pKa of 5.8.

Leukeran (chlorambucil) is available in tablet form for oral administration. Each sugar-coated tablet contains 2 mg chlorambucil and the inactive ingredients corn and wheat starch, gum acacia, lactose, magnesium stearate, polysorbate 60, sucrose, and talc.

CLINICAL PHARMACOLOGY

Chlorambucil is rapidly and completely absorbed from the gastrointestinal tract. After single oral doses of 0.6–1.2 mg/kg, peak plasma chlorambucil levels are reached within one hour and the terminal half-life of the parent drug is estimated at 1.5 hours. Chlorambucil undergoes rapid metabolism to phenylacetic acid mustard, the major metabolite, and the combined chlorambucil and phenylacetic acid mustard urinary excretion is extremely low—less than 1% in 24 hours. The peak plasma levels of chlorambucil and phenylacetic acid mustard are similar, approximately 1 μg/ml; however, the metabolite's half-life is 1.6 times greater than the parent drug.[2,3]

Chlorambucil and its metabolites are extensively bound to plasma and tissue proteins. *In vitro,* chlorambucil is 99% bound to plasma proteins, specifically albumin.[4] Cerebrospinal fluid levels of chlorambucil have not been determined. Evidence of human teratogenicity suggests that the drug crosses the placenta.[5,6]

Chlorambucil is extensively metabolized in the liver primarily to phenylacetic acid mustard which has antineoplastic activity.[2,3] Chlorambucil and its major metabolite spontaneously degrade *in vivo* forming monohydroxy and dihydroxy derivatives.[2] After a single dose of radiolabeled chlorambucil (^{14}C) approximately 15% to 60% of the radioactivity appears in the urine after 24 hours. Again, less than 1% of the urinary radioactivity is in the form of chlorambucil or phenylacetic acid mustard.[2] In summary, the pharmacokinetic data suggest that oral chlorambucil undergoes rapid gastrointestinal absorption and plasma clearance and that it is almost completely metabolized, having extremely low urinary excretion.

INDICATIONS AND USAGE

Leukeran (chlorambucil) is indicated in the treatment of chronic lymphatic (lymphocytic) leukemia, malignant lymphomas including lymphosarcoma, giant follicular lymphoma and Hodgkin's disease. It is not curative in any of these disorders but may produce clinically useful palliation.

CONTRAINDICATIONS

Chlorambucil should not be used in patients whose disease has demonstrated a prior resistance to the agent. Patients who have demonstrated hypersensitivity to chlorambucil should not be given the drug.[7] There may be cross-hypersensitivity (skin rash) between chlorambucil and other alkylating agents.[8]

WARNINGS

Because of its carcinogenic properties, chlorambucil should not be given to patients with conditions other than chronic lymphatic leukemia or malignant lymphomas. Convulsions,[9] infertility,[10] leukemia[11,12] and secondary malignancies[13] have been observed when chlorambucil was employed in the therapy of malignant and non-malignant diseases.

There are many reports of acute leukemia arising with both malignant[15] and non-malignant[16] diseases following chlorambucil treatment. In many instances, these patients also received other chemotherapeutic agents or some form of radiation therapy. The quantitation of the risk of chlorambucil-induction of leukemia or carcinoma in humans is not possible.

Evaluation of published reports of leukemia developing in patients who have received chlorambucil (and other alkylating agents) suggests that the risk of leukemogenesis increases with both chronicity of treatment and large cumulative doses. However, it has proved impossible to define a cumulative dose below which there is no risk of the induction of secondary malignancy. The potential benefits from chlorambucil therapy must be weighed on an individual basis against the possible risk of the induction of a secondary malignancy.

Chlorambucil has been shown to cause chromatid or chromosome damage in man.[17,18] Both reversible and permanent sterility have been observed in both sexes receiving chlorambucil.

A high incidence of sterility has been documented when chlorambucil is administered to prepubertal and pubertal males.[19] Prolonged or permanent azoospermia has also been observed in adult males.[20] While most reports of gonadal dysfunction secondary to chlorambucil have related to males, the induction of amenorrhea in females with alkylating agents is well documented and chlorambucil is capable of producing amenorrhea. Autopsy studies of the ovaries from women with malignant lymphoma treated with combination chemotherapy including chlorambucil have shown varying degrees of fibrosis, vasculitis, and depletion of primordial follicles.[21,22]

Pregnancy: ***"Pregnancy Category D":*** Chlorambucil can cause fetal harm when administered to a pregnant woman. Unilateral renal agenesis has been observed in two offspring whose mothers received chlorambucil during the first trimester.[5,6] Urogenital malformations including absence of a kidney were found in fetuses of rats given chlorambucil.[14]

There are no adequate and well-controlled studies in pregnant women. If this drug is used during pregnancy, or if the patient becomes pregnant while taking this drug, the patient should be apprised of the potential hazard to the fetus. Women of childbearing potential should be advised to avoid becoming pregnant.

PRECAUTIONS

General: Many patients develop a slowly progressive lymphopenia during treatment. The lymphocyte count usually rapidly returns to normal levels upon completion of drug therapy. Most patients have some neutropenia after the third week of treatment and this may continue for up to ten days after the last dose. Subsequently, the neutrophil count usually rapidly returns to normal. Severe neutropenia appears to be related to dosage and usually occurs only in patients who have received a total dosage of 6.5 mg/kg or more in one course of therapy with continuous dosing. About one-quarter of all patients receiving the continuous-dose schedule, and one-third of those receiving this dosage in eight weeks or less may be expected to develop severe neutropenia.[23]

While it is not necessary to discontinue chlorambucil at the first evidence of a fall in neutrophil count, it must be remembered that the fall may continue for ten days after the last dose and that as the total dose approaches 6.5 mg/kg there is a risk of causing irreversible bone marrow damage. The dose of chlorambucil should be decreased if leukocyte or platelet counts fall below normal values and should be discontinued for more severe depression.

Continued on next page

Burroughs Wellcome—Cont.

Chlorambucil should **not** be given at full dosages before four weeks after a full course of radiation therapy or chemotherapy because of the vulnerability of the bone marrow to damage under these conditions. If the pretherapy leukocyte or platelet counts are depressed from bone marrow disease process prior to institution of therapy, the treatment should be instituted at a reduced dosage.
Persistently low neutrophil and platelet counts or peripheral lymphocytosis suggest bone marrow infiltration. If confirmed by bone marrow examination, the daily dosage of chlorambucil should not exceed 0.1 mg/kg. Chlorambucil appears to be relatively free from gastrointestinal side effects or other evidence of toxicity apart from the bone marrow depressant action. In humans, single oral doses of 20 mg or more may produce nausea and vomiting.
Information for Patients: Patients should be informed that the major toxicities of chlorambucil are related to hypersensitivity, drug fever, myelosuppression, hepatotoxicity, infertility, seizures, gastrointestinal toxicity, and secondary malignancies. Patients should never be allowed to take the drug without medical supervision and should consult their physician if they experience skin rash, bleeding, fever, jaundice, persistent cough, seizures, nausea, vomiting, amenorrhea, or unusual lumps/masses. Women of childbearing potential should be advised to avoid becoming pregnant.
Laboratory Tests: Patients must be followed carefully to avoid life-endangering damage to the bone marrow during treatment. Weekly examination of the blood should be made to determine hemoglobin levels, total and differential leukocyte counts, and quantitative platelet counts. Also, during the first 3 to 6 weeks of therapy, it is recommended that white blood cell counts be made 3 or 4 days after each of the weekly complete blood counts. Galton *et al* [23] have suggested that in following patients it is helpful to plot the blood counts on a chart at the same time that body weight, temperature, spleen size, etc., are recorded. It is considered dangerous to allow a patient to go more than two weeks without hematological and clinical examination during treatment.
Drug Interactions: There are no known drug/ drug interactions with chlorambucil.
Carcinogenesis, Mutagenesis, Impairment of Fertility: See WARNINGS section for information on carcinogenesis, mutagenesis and impairment of fertility.
Pregnancy: ***Teratogenic Effects:*** Pregnancy Category D: See WARNINGS section.
Nursing Mothers: It is not known whether this drug is excreted in human milk. Because many drugs are excreted in human milk and because of the potential for serious adverse reactions in nursing infants from chlorambucil, a decision should be made whether to discontinue nursing or to discontinue the drug, taking into account the importance of the drug to the mother.
Pediatric Use: The safety and effectiveness in children have not been established.

ADVERSE REACTIONS

Hematologic Effects: The most common side effect is bone marrow suppression.[24] Although bone marrow suppression frequently occurs, it is usually reversible if the chlorambucil is withdrawn early enough. However, irreversible bone marrow failure has been reported.[25,26]
Gastrointestinal: Gastrointestinal disturbances such as nausea and vomiting, diarrhea and oral ulceration occur infrequently.
Miscellaneous: Other reported adverse reactions include: pulmonary fibrosis, hepatotoxicity and jaundice, drug fever, skin hypersensitivity, peripheral neuropathy, interstitial pneumonia, sterile cystitis, infertility, leukemia and secondary malignancies (see WARNINGS). Seizures have occurred in children with nephrotic syndrome and dose-related focal fits have been reported in adults.[9,27]

OVERDOSAGE

Reversible pancytopenia was the main finding of inadvertent overdoses of chlorambucil.[28,29] Neurological toxicity ranging from agitated behavior and ataxia to multiple grand mal seizures has also occurred.[28,30] As there is no known antidote, the blood picture should be closely monitored and general supportive measures should be instituted, together with appropriate blood transfusions if necessary. Chlorambucil is not dialyzable.
Oral LD_{50} single doses in mice are 123 mg/kg. In rats, a single intraperitoneal dose of 12.5 mg/kg of chlorambucil produces typical nitrogen-mustard effects; these include atrophy of the intestinal mucous membrane and lymphoid tissues, severe lymphopenia becoming maximal in four days, anemia and thrombocytopenia. After this dose, the animals begin to recover within three days and appear normal in about a week although the bone marrow may not become completely normal for about three weeks. An intraperitoneal dose of 18.5 mg/kg kills about 50% of the rats with development of convulsions. As much as 50 mg/kg has been given orally to rats as a single dose, with recovery. Such a dose causes bradycardia, excessive salivation, hematuria, convulsions, and respiratory dysfunction.

DOSAGE AND ADMINISTRATION

The usual oral dosage is 0.1 to 0.2 mg/kg body weight daily for three to six weeks as required. This usually amounts to 4 to 10 mg a day for the average patient. The entire daily dose may be given at one time. These dosages are for initiation of therapy or for short courses of treatment. The dosage must be carefully adjusted according to the response of the patient and must be reduced as soon as there is an abrupt fall in the white blood cell count. Patients with Hodgkin's disease usually require 0.2 mg/kg daily whereas patients with other lymphomas or chronic lymphocytic leukemia usually require only 0.1 mg/kg daily. When lymphocytic infiltration of the bone marrow is present, or when the bone marrow is hypoplastic, the daily dose should not exceed 0.1 mg/kg (about 6 mg for the average patient).
Alternate schedules for the treatment of chronic lymphocytic leukemia employing intermittent, bi-weekly or once monthly pulse doses of chlorambucil have been reported.[31,32] Intermittent schedules of chlorambucil begin with an initial single dose of 0.4 mg/kg. Doses are generally increased by 0.1 mg/kg until control of lymphocytosis or toxicity is observed. Subsequent doses are modified to produce mild hematologic toxicity. It is felt that the response rate of chronic lymphocytic leukemia to the bi-weekly or once monthly schedule of chlorambucil administration is similar or better to that previously reported with daily administration and that hematologic toxicity was less than or equal to that encountered in studies using daily chlorambucil.
Radiation and cytotoxic drugs render the bone marrow more vulnerable to damage and chlorambucil should be used with particular caution within four weeks of a full course of radiation therapy or chemotherapy. However, small doses of palliative radiation over isolated foci remote from the bone marrow will not usually depress the neutrophil and platelet count. In these cases chlorambucil may be given in the customary dosage.
It is presently felt that short courses of treatment are safer than continuous maintenance therapy although both methods have been effective. It must be recognized that continuous therapy may give the appearance of "maintenance" in patients who are actually in remission and have no immediate need for further drug. If maintenance dosage is used, it should not exceed 0.1 mg/kg daily and may well be as low as 0.03 mg/kg daily. A typical maintenance dose is 2 mg to 4 mg daily, or less, depending on the status of the blood counts. It may, therefore, be desirable to withdraw the drug after maximal control has been achieved since intermittent therapy reinstituted at time of relapse may be as effective as continuous treatment.

HOW SUPPLIED

White sugar-coated tablet containing 2 mg chlorambucil; bottle of 50 (NDC-0081-0635-35).
Store at 15°-25°C (59°-77°F) in a dry place.

REFERENCES

1. Everett JL, Roberts JR, and Ross WCJ: Aryl-2-halogenoalkylamines. Part XII. Some Carboxylic Derivatives of NN-Di-2-chloroethylaniline. *J Chem Soc, 3:* 2386, 1953.
2. Alberts DS *et al:* Pharmacokinetics and Metabolism of Chlorambucil in Man: A Preliminary Report. *Cancer Treat Rev, 6* (Suppl.):9, 1979.
3. McLean A *et al:* Pharmacokinetics and Metabolism of Chlorambucil in Patients with Malignant Disease. *Cancer Treat Rev, 6* (Suppl.):33, 1979.
4. Ehrsson H *et al:* Degradation of Chlorambucil in Aqueous Solution - Influence of Human Albumin Binding. *J Pharm Pharmacol, 33:* 313, 1981.
5. Shotton D and Monie IW: Possible Teratogenic Effect of Chlorambucil on a Human Fetus. *JAMA, 186:* 74, 1963.
6. Steege JF and Caldwell DS: Renal Agenesis after First Trimester Exposure to Chlorambucil. *South Med J, 73:* 1414, 1980.
7. Knisley RE *et al:* Unusual Reaction to Chlorambucil in a Patient with Chronic Lymphocytic Leukemia. *Arch Dermatol, 104:* 77, 1971.
8. Weiss RB and Bruno S: Hypersensitivity Reactions to Cancer Chemotherapeutic Agents. *Ann Intern Med, 94:* 66, 1981.
9. Williams SA *et al:* Seizures: A Significant Side Effect of Chlorambucil Therapy in Children. *J Pediatr, 93:* 516, 1978.
10. Freckman HA *et al:* Chlorambucil-Prednisolone Therapy for Disseminated Breast Carcinoma. *JAMA 189:* 23, 1964.
11. Aymard JP *et al:* Acute Leukemia after Prolonged Chlorambucil Treatment for Non-Malignant Disease: A Report of a New Case and Literature Survey. *Acta Haematol* (Basel), *63:* 283, 1980.
12. Berk PD *et al:* Increased Incidence of Acute Leukemia in Polycythermia Vera Associated with Chlorambucil Therapy. *N Engl J Med, 304:* 441, 1981.
13. Lerner HJ: Acute Myelogenous Leukemia in Patients Receiving Chlorambucil as Long-Term Adjuvant Chemotherapy for Stage II Breast Cancer. *Cancer Treat Rep, 62:* 1135, 1978.
14. Monie IW: Chlorambucil-Induced Abnormalities of the Urogenital System of Rat Fetuses. *Anat Rec, 139:* 145–153, 1961.
15. Zarrabi MH *et al:* Chronic Lymphocytic Leukemia Terminating in Acute Leukemia. *Arch Intern Med, 137:* 1059, 1977.
16. Cameron S: Chlorambucil and Leukemia. *N Eng J Med, 296:* 1065, 1977.
17. Lawler SD and Lele KP: Chromosomal Damage Induced by Chlorambucil in Chronic Lymphocytic Leukemia. *Scand J.Hematol, 9:* 603, 1972.
18. Stevenson AC and Patel C: Effects of Chlorambucil on Human Chromosomes. *Mutat Res, 18:* 333, 1973.
19. Guesry P, Lenoir G, and Broyer M: Gonadal Effects of Chlorambucil Given to Prepubertal and Pubertal Boys for Nephrotic Syndrome. *J Pediatr, 92:* 299, 1978.
20. Richter, P *et al:* Effect of Chlorambucil on Spermatogenesis in the Human with Malignant Lymphoma. *Cancer, 25:* 1026, 1970.
21. Morgenfeld MC *et al:* Ovarian Lesions Due to Cytostatic Agents During the Treatment of Hodgkin's Disease. *Surg Gynecol Obstet, 134:* 826, 1972.
22. Sobrinho LG *et al:* Amenorrhea in Patients with Hodgkin's Disease Treated with Antineoplastic Agents. *Am J Obstet Gynecol, 109:* 135, 1971.
23. Galton DAG, Israels LG, Nabarro JDN, and Till M: Clinical Trials of p-(Di-2-chloroethylamino)-phenylbutyric Acid (CB 1348) in Malignant Lymphoma. *Brit Med J, 2:* 1172, 1955.
24. Moore GE *et al:* Effects of Chlorambucil (NSC-3088) in 374 Patients with Advanced Cancer. *Cancer Chemother Rep, (Part 1) 52:* 661 (1968).
25. Galton DAG *et al:* The Use of Chlorambucil and Steroids in the Treatment of Chronic Lymphocytic Leukemia. *Br J Haematol, 7:* 73, 1961.
26. Rudd P *et al:* Irreversible Bone Marrow Failure with Chlorambucil. *J Rheumatol, 2:* 421, 1975.
27. Naysmith A and Robson RH: Focal Fits During Chlorambucil Therapy. *Postgrad Med J, 55:* 806, 1979.
28. Green AA and Naiman JL: Chlorambucil Poisoning. *Am J. Dis Child, 116:* 190, 1968.
29. Enck RE and Bennett JM: Inadvertant Chlorambucil Overdose in Adults. *NY State J Med, 77:* 1480, 1977.
30. Wolfson S and Olney MB: Accidental Ingestion of a Toxic Dose of Chlorambucil: Report of a Case in a Child. *JAMA, 165:* 239, 1957.
31. Knospe WH *et al:* Bi-Weekly Chlorambucil Treatment of Chronic Lymphocytic Leukemia. *Cancer, 33:* 555, 1974.
32. Sawitsky A *et al:* Comparison of Daily Versus Intermittent Chlorambucil and Prednisone Therapy in the Treatment of Patients with Chronic Lymphocytic Leukemia. *Blood, 50:* 1049–1059, 1977.

Shown in Product Identification Section, page 407

MANTADIL® CREAM ℞

[măn'tah-dĭl"]

DESCRIPTION

Mantadil® Cream contains the antihistamine chlorcyclizine hydrochloride 2% and the corticosteroid hydrocortisone acetate 0.5%, with methylparaben 0.25% (added as a preservative) in a vanishing cream base. The inactive ingredients are liquid and white petrolatum, emulsifying wax and purified water.
Mantadil Cream is an ANTIPRURITIC-ANTI-INFLAMMATORY-ANESTHETIC for topical administration.
Chlorcyclizine hydrochloride is known chemically as 1-[(4-chlorophenyl) phenylmethyl]-4-methylpiperazine monohydrochloride.
Hydrocortisone acetate is the acetate ester of cortisol, known chemically as 21-(acetyloxy)-11β,17-dihydroxypregn-4-ene-3,20-dione.
The pH of this product is approximately 4.5.

CLINICAL PHARMACOLOGY

Chlorcyclizine hydrochloride is an H_1 histamine-receptor antagonist that will occupy receptor sites in effector cells to the exclusion of histamine. It blocks most of the effects of histamine mediated by H_1 receptors, including contraction of smooth muscle and increased capillary permeability. Absorption of chlorcyclizine hydrochloride into the skin is rapid following topical application, whereas systemic absorption from the skin is minimal. Chlorcyclizine hydrochloride prevents local edema and provides local anesthetic and antipruritic action in the skin.
Hydrocortisone acetate administered topically suppresses most inflammatory and allergic responses in the skin. Following topical application, it is absorbed rapidly into the skin, where it reduces local heat, redness, swelling, and tenderness. A small part of the dose applied to broken skin is absorbed systemically and metabolized by the liver.

INDICATIONS AND USAGE
Mantadil Cream is indicated for the treatment of pruritic skin eruptions and other dermatoses including: eczema (allergic, nuchal and nummular); dermatitis (atopic, lichenoid and seborrheic); contact dermatitis including poison ivy, poison oak and poison sumac; localized neurodermatitis; insect bites; sunburn; intertrigo; and anogenital pruritus.

CONTRAINDICATIONS
This preparation is contraindicated in patients who are hypersensitive to any of its components; in tuberculosis of the skin, vaccinia, varicella, and herpes simplex. As with other topical products containing hydrocortisone, the cream should not be used in bacterial infections of the skin unless antibacterial therapy is concomitant.
Not for ophthalmic use.

WARNINGS
Oral chlorcyclizine is teratogenic in animals. Long-term reproduction studies of topical chlorcyclizine have not been conducted in humans.

PRECAUTIONS
General: If signs of irritation develop with use of this cream, treatment should be discontinued and appropriate therapy instituted.
Any of the side effects reported following systemic use of corticosteroids, including adrenal suppression, may also occur following their topical use, especially in infants and children. Systemic absorption of topically applied steroids will be increased if extensive body surface areas are treated or if the occlusive technique is used. Under these circumstances, suitable precautions should be taken when long-term use is anticipated, particularly in infants and children.
Carcinogenesis, Mutagenesis, Impairment of Fertility: Oral chlorcyclizine is teratogenic in animals. Long-term reproduction studies of topical chlorcyclizine have not been conducted. It is poorly absorbed percutaneously.
Pregnancy: ***Teratogenic Effects:*** Pregnancy Category C. Animal reproduction studies have not been conducted with Mantadil Cream. It is also not known whether Mantadil Cream can cause fetal harm when administered to a pregnant woman or can affect reproduction capacity. Mantadil Cream should be given to a pregnant woman only if clearly needed.
Nursing Mothers: Hydrocortisone acetate appears in human milk following oral administration of the drug.
Caution should be exercised when hydrocortisone acetate is administered to a nursing woman.
It is not known whether chlorcyclizine hydrochloride is excreted in human milk. Because many drugs are excreted in human milk, caution should be exercised when chlorcyclizine hydrochloride is administered to a nursing woman.

ADVERSE REACTIONS
Allergic contact dermatitis may occur with topical application of chlorcyclizine hydrochloride. Systemic side effects have been reported after topical application of antihistamines to large areas of skin.
The following local adverse reactions have been reported with topical corticosteroids, especially under occlusive dressings: irritation, folliculitis, hypertrichosis, acneiform eruptions, hypopigmentation, allergic contact dermatitis, secondary infection, skin atrophy, striae and miliaria.

OVERDOSAGE
With continued application of topical corticosteroid on large areas of damaged skin and under occlusion, there is a remote possibility that sufficient absorption could occur to produce Cushing's syndrome. This is more likely in children.
Systemic toxicity following application of chlorcyclizine has never been reported.
The oral LD_{50} of chlorcyclizine hydrochloride in the mouse is 300 mg/kg.
The intraperitoneal LD_{50} of hydrocortisone acetate in the mouse is 2300 mg/kg.

DOSAGE AND ADMINISTRATION
Apply to the skin two to five times daily. If the condition of the skin will permit, the cream should be well rubbed in.

HOW SUPPLIED
Mantadil Cream (Chlorcyclizine hydrochloride 2% and hydrocortisone acetate 0.5%) is available in 15 gram tubes (**NDC**-0081-0650-94).
Store at 15°-30°C (59°-86°F).

MAREZINE® ℞
[*mair'uh-zēn"*]
(Cyclizine Lactate)
Injection
50 mg in 1 ml

DESCRIPTION
Chemically, cyclizine is N-benzhydryl-N′ methylpiperazine, and has a molecular weight of 266.4.
It is a white crystalline solid having a bitter taste, and is soluble in water and isotonic saline.
Marezine (Cyclizine Lactate) Injection is a sterile solution for INTRAMUSCULAR INJECTION ONLY.

Compatibility Table
Marezine (Cyclizine Lactate) Injection

Forms a clear solution with: (i.e., can be mixed with)	Is not compatible with: (requires separate injection)
Atropine sulfate	Oxytetracycline hydrochloride
Meperidine hydrochloride (Demerol)	Chlortetracycline hydrochloride
Morphine sulfate	Penicillin
Tetracycline hydrochloride	Any solution with pH of 6.8 or higher (this includes Pentothal sodium and other soluble barbiturates)
Streptomycin sulfate	
Pyridoxine hydrochloride*	
Codeine phosphate and sulfate	
Alphaprodine HCl (Nisentil)	
Scopolamine hydrobromide*	
Pantopon (Hydrochlorides of opium alkaloids)*	
Hydromorphone (Dilaudid)*	

*Administer within 4–10 minutes

ACTION
Marezine (Cyclizine Lactate) has antiemetic, anticholinergic and antihistaminic properties. It also reduces the sensitivity of the labyrinthine apparatus. The exact mechanism of action is unknown. In dogs the drug prevents emesis from intravenous threshold doses of apomorphine, but it is much less effective in blocking emesis from orally administered copper sulfate. These data suggest that the action is mediated through the chemoreceptive trigger zone.

INDICATIONS
For the treatment of nausea and vomiting of motion sickness when the oral route cannot be used.

CONTRAINDICATIONS
Marezine is contraindicated in individuals who have shown a previous hypersensitivity to the drug.

WARNINGS
Patients may become drowsy while taking Marezine and should be cautioned against engaging in activities requiring mental alertness, e.g., driving a car or operating heavy machinery or appliances.
Use in Children: Clinical studies establishing safety and efficacy in children have not been done; therefore, usage in this age group and nursing mothers cannot be recommended.
Use with CNS Depressants: May have additive effects with alcohol and other CNS depressants (hypnotics, sedatives, tranquilizers, antianxiety agents, etc.).

PRECAUTIONS
Because of its anticholinergic action, Marezine should be used with caution and appropriate monitoring in patients with glaucoma, obstructive disease of the gastrointestinal or genitourinary tract, and in elderly males with possible prostatic hypertrophy. Incipient glaucoma may be precipitated by anticholinergic drugs such as Marezine. The drug may have a hypotensive action. This may be confusing or dangerous in postoperative patients and should influence the decision on using the drug postoperatively.

ADVERSE REACTIONS
Urticaria, drug rash, dryness of mouth, nose and throat, drowsiness, restlessness, excitation, nervousness, insomnia, euphoria, anorexia, nausea, vomiting, diarrhea, constipation, hypotension, blurred vision, diplopia, vertigo, tinnitus, palpitation, tachycardia, urinary frequency, difficult urination, urinary retention, auditory and visual hallucinations have been reported, particularly when dosage recommendations are exceeded. Cholestatic jaundice has occurred in association with the use of Marezine.

DOSAGE AND ADMINISTRATION
Marezine (Cyclizine Lactate) Injection is administered INTRAMUSCULARLY. The usual dose is 1 ml (50 mg) every 4 to 6 hours as necessary.

OVERDOSAGE
Symptoms of Overdosage: Moderate overdosage may cause hyperexcitability alternating with drowsiness. Massive overdosage may cause convulsions; hallucinations; respiratory paralysis.
Treatment: Appropriate supportive and symptomatic treatment. Consider dialysis.
Caution: Do not use morphine or other respiratory depressants.
[See table above].

HOW SUPPLIED
MAREZINE® (CYCLIZINE LACTATE) INJECTION
50 mg in 1 ml
Boxes of 10 ampuls (NDC-0081-0663-10)
The injection should be stored in a cold place. It may develop a slight yellow tint if stored at room temperature for several months; however, it retains full potency.
Also Available:
MAREZINE® (CYCLIZINE HYDROCHLORIDE)
50 mg Scored TABLETS
Boxes of 12
Bottle of 100
Shown in Product Identification Section, page 407

MYLERAN® ℞
[*mī'lah-răn"*]
(Busulfan)
2 mg Scored Tablets

> ***Warnings:*** *Myleran ® (busulfan) is a potent drug. It should not be used unless a diagnosis of chronic myelogenous leukemia has been adequately established and the responsible physician is knowledgeable in assessing response to chemotherapy.*
> *Myleran (busulfan) can induce severe bone marrow hypoplasia. Reduce or discontinue the dosage immediately at the first sign of any unusual depression of bone marrow function as reflected by an abnormal decrease in any of the formed elements of the blood. A bone marrow examination should be performed if the bone marrow status is uncertain.*
> *SEE "WARNINGS" SECTION FOR INFORMATION REGARDING BUSULFAN-INDUCED LEUKEMOGENESIS IN HUMANS.*

DESCRIPTION
Myleran (busulfan) is a bifunctional alkylating agent. It is the most clinically useful member of a series of sulfonic acid esters of dihydric, straight chain, aliphatic alcohols synthesized by Haddow and Timmis at the Chester Beatty Research Institute.[1] Busulfan is known chemically as 1,4-butanediol dimethanesulfonate and has the following structural formula:

$$CH_3SO_2O(CH_2)_4OSO_2CH_3$$

Busulfan is *not* a structural analog of the nitrogen mustards. Myleran (busulfan) is available in tablet form for oral administration. Each scored tablet contains 2 mg busulfan and the inactive ingredients magnesium stearate and sodium chloride.
The activity of busulfan in chronic myelogenous leukemia was first reported by D.A.G. Galton in 1953.[2]

CLINICAL PHARMACOLOGY
No analytical method has been found which permits the quantitation of non-radiolabeled busulfan or its metabolites in biological tissues or plasma. All studies of the pharmacokinetics of busulfan in humans have employed radiolabeled drug using either sulfur-35 (labeling the "carrier" portion of the molecule) or carbon-14 or tritium in the alkane portion of the 4-carbon chain (labels in the "alkylating" portion of the molecule).
Studies with ^{35}S-busulfan.[3] Following the intravenous administration of a single therapeutic dose of ^{35}S-busulfan, there was rapid disappearance of radioactivity from the blood; 90 to 95% of the ^{35}S-label disappeared within three to five minutes after injection. Thereafter, a constant, low level of radioactivity (1 to 3% of the injected dose) was maintained during the subsequent forty-eight hour period of observation. Following the oral administration of ^{35}S-busulfan, there was a lag period of one-half to two hours prior to the detection of radioactivity in the blood. However, at four

Continued on next page

Burroughs Wellcome—Cont.

hours the (low) level of circulating radioactivity was comparable to that obtained following intravenous administration. After either oral or intravenous administration of ^{35}S-busulfan to humans, 45 to 60% of the radioactivity was recovered in the urine in the forty-eight hours after administration; the majority of the total urinary excretion occurred in the first twenty-four hours. In man, over 95% of the urinary sulfur-35 occurs as ^{35}S-methanesulfonic acid.

The fact that urinary recovery of sulfur-35 was equivalent, irrespective of whether the drug was given intravenously or orally, suggests virtually complete absorption by the oral route.

Studies with ^{14}C-busulfan.[3] Oral and intravenous administration of 1,4-^{14}C-busulfan showed the same rapid initial disappearance of plasma radioactivity with a subsequent low-level plateau as observed following the administration of ^{35}S-labeled drug. Cumulative radioactivity in the urine after forty-eight hours was 25 to 30% of the administered dose (contrasting with 45 to 60% for ^{35}S-busulfan) and suggests a slower excretion of the alkylating portion of the molecule and its metabolites than for the sulfonoxymethyl moieties. Regardless of the route of administration, 1,4-^{14}C-busulfan yielded a complex mixture of at least 12 radiolabeled metabolites in urine; the main metabolite being 3-hydroxytetrahydrothiophene-1, 1-dioxide.

Studies with ^{3}H-busulfan.[4] Human pharmacokinetic studies have been conducted employing busulfan labeled with tritium on the tetramethylene chain. These experiments confirmed a rapid initial clearance of the radioactivity from plasma, irrespective of whether the drug was given orally or intravenously, and showed a gradual accumulation of radioactivity in the plasma after repeated doses. Urinary excretion of less than 50% of the total dose given suggested a slow elimination of the metabolic products from the body.

There is no experience with the use of dialysis in an attempt to modify the clinical toxicity of busulfan. One technical difficulty would derive from the extremely poor water solubility of busulfan. Additionally, all studies of the metabolism of busulfan employing radiolabeled materials indicate rapid chemical reactivity of the parent compound with prolonged retention of some of the metabolites (particularly the metabolites arising from the "alkylating" portion of the molecule). The effectiveness of dialysis at removing significant quantities of unreacted drug would be expected to be minimal in such a situation.

No information is available regarding the penetration of busulfan into brain or cerebrospinal fluid.

BIOCHEMICAL PHARMACOLOGY

In aqueous media, busulfan undergoes a wide range of nucleophilic substitution reactions. While this chemical reactivity is relatively non-specific, alkylation of the DNA is felt to be an important biological mechanism for its cytotoxic effect.[5] Coliphage T7 exposed to busulfan was found to have the DNA crosslinked by intrastrand crosslinkages, but no interstrand linkages were found.

The metabolic fate of busulfan has been studied in rats and humans using ^{14}C- and ^{35}S-labeled materials.[3,6,7] In man,[3] as in the rat,[7] almost all of the radioactivity in ^{35}S-labeled busulfan is excreted in the urine in the form of ^{35}S-methanesulfonic acid. No unchanged drug was found in human urine,[3] although a small amount has been reported in rat urine.[7] Roberts and Warwick demonstrated that the formation of methanesulfonic acid *in vivo* in the rat is not due to a simple hydrolysis of busulfan to 1,4-butanediol, since only about 4% of 2,3-^{14}C-busulfan was excreted as carbon dioxide whereas 2,3-^{14}C-1,4-butanediol was converted almost exclusively to carbon dioxide.[6] The predominant reaction of busulfan in the rat is the alkylation of sulfhydryl groups (particularly cysteine and cysteine-containing compounds) to produce a cyclic sulfonium compound which is the precursor of the major urinary metabolite of the 4-carbon portion of the molecule, 3-hydroxytetrahydrothiophene-1, 1-dioxide.[6] This has been termed a "sulfur-stripping" action of busulfan and it may modify the function of certain sulfur-containing amino acids, polypeptides, and proteins; whether this action makes an important contribution to the cytotoxicity of busulfan is unknown.

The biochemical basis for acquired resistance to busulfan is largely a matter of speculation. Although altered transport of busulfan into the cell is one possibility, increased intracellular inactivation of the drug before it reaches the DNA is also possible. Experiments with other alkylating agents have shown that resistance to this class of compounds may reflect an acquired ability of the resistant cell to repair alkylation damage more effectively.[5]

INDICATIONS AND USAGE

Myleran® (busulfan) is indicated for the palliative treatment of chronic myelogenous (myeloid, myelocytic, granulocytic) leukemia. Although not curative, busulfan reduces the total granulocyte mass, relieves symptoms of the disease, and improves the clinical state of the patient. Approximately 90% of adults with previously untreated chronic myelogenous leukemia will obtain hematologic remission with regression or stabilization of organomegaly following the use of busulfan. It has been shown to be superior to splenic irradiation with respect to survival times and maintenance of hemoglobin levels, and to be equivalent to irradiation at controlling splenomegaly.[8]

It is not clear whether busulfan unequivocally prolongs the survival of responding patients beyond the 31 months experienced by an untreated group of historical controls.[9] Median survival figures of 31–42 months have been reported for several groups of patients treated with busulfan, but concurrent control groups of comparable, untreated patients are not available.[8,10,11,12] The median survival figures reported from different studies will be influenced by the percentage of "poor risk" patients initially entered into the particular study. Patients who are alive two years following the diagnosis of chronic myelogenous leukemia, and who have been treated during that period with busulfan, are estimated to have a mean annual mortality rate during the second to fifth year which is approximately two-thirds that of patients who received either no treatment, conventional x-ray or ^{32}P-irradiation, or chemotherapy with minimally active drugs.[13]

Busulfan is clearly less effective in patients with chronic myelogenous leukemia who lack the Philadelphia (Ph^{1}) chromosome.[14] Also, the so-called "juvenile" type of chronic myelogenous leukemia, typically occurring in young children and associated with the absence of a Philadelphia chromosome, responds poorly to busulfan.[15] The drug is of no benefit in patients whose chronic myelogenous leukemia has entered a "blastic" phase.

CONTRAINDICATIONS

Myleran® (busulfan) should not be used unless a diagnosis of chronic myelogenous leukemia has been adequately established and the responsible physician is knowledgeable in assessing response to chemotherapy.

Myleran should not be used in patients whose chronic myelogenous leukemia has demonstrated prior resistance to this drug.

Myleran is of no value in chronic lymphocytic leukemia, acute leukemia, or in the "blastic crisis" of chronic myelogenous leukemia.

WARNINGS

The most frequent, serious side effect of treatment with busulfan is the induction of bone marrow failure (which may or may not be anatomically hypoplastic) resulting in severe pancytopenia. The pancytopenia caused by busulfan may be more prolonged than that induced with other alkylating agents. It is generally felt that the usual cause of busulfan-induced pancytopenia is the failure to stop administration of the drug soon enough; individual idiosyncrasy to the drug does not seem to be an important factor. *Myleran should be used with extreme caution and exceptional vigilance in patients whose bone marrow reserve may have been compromised by prior irradiation or chemotherapy, or whose marrow function is recovering from previous cytotoxic therapy.* Although recovery from busulfan-induced pancytopenia may take from one month to two years, this complication is potentially reversible and the patient should be vigorously supported through any period of severe pancytopenia.[16]

A rare, important complication of busulfan therapy is the development of bronchopulmonary dysplasia with pulmonary fibrosis.[17] Symptoms have been reported to occur within eight months to ten years after initiation of therapy—the average duration of therapy being four years. The histologic findings associated with "busulfan lung" mimic those seen following pulmonary irradiation. Clinically, patients have reported the insidious onset of cough, dyspnea, and low-grade fever. Pulmonary function studies have revealed diminished diffusion capacity and decreased pulmonary compliance. It is important to exclude more common conditions (such as opportunistic infections or leukemic infiltration of the lungs) with appropriate diagnostic techniques. If measures such as sputum cultures, virologic studies, and exfoliative cytology fail to establish an etiology for the pulmonary infiltrates, lung biopsy may be necessary to establish the diagnosis. Treatment of established busulfan-induced pulmonary fibrosis is unsatisfactory; in most cases the patients have died within six months after the diagnosis was established. There is no specific therapy for this complication other than the immediate discontinuation of busulfan. The administration of corticosteroids has been suggested, but the results have not been impressive or uniformly successful.

Busulfan may cause cellular dysplasia in many organs in addition to the lung. Cytologic abnormalities characterized by giant, hyperchromatic nuclei have been reported in lymph nodes, pancreas, thyroid, adrenal glands, liver, and bone marrow. This cytologic dysplasia may be severe enough to cause difficulty in interpretation of exfoliative cytologic examinations from the lung, bladder, breast, and the uterine cervix.

In addition to the widespread epithelial dysplasia that has been observed during busulfan therapy, chromosome aberrations have been reported in cells from patients receiving busulfan.

Busulfan is mutagenic in mice and, possibly, in man.

A number of malignant tumors have been reported in patients on busulfan therapy and this drug may be a human carcinogen. Four cases of acute leukemia occurred among 243 patients treated with busulfan as adjuvant chemotherapy following surgical resection of bronchogenic carcinoma. All four cases were from a subgroup of 19 of these 243 patients who developed pancytopenia while taking busulfan five to eight years before leukemia became clinically apparent. These findings suggest that busulfan is leukemogenic, although its mode of action is uncertain.[18]

Busulfan may cause fetal harm when administered to a pregnant woman. Although there have been a number of cases reported where apparently normal children have been born after busulfan treatment during pregnancy,[19] one case has been cited where a malformed baby was delivered by a mother treated with busulfan. During the pregnancy that resulted in the malformed infant, the mother received x-ray therapy early in the first trimester, mercaptopurine until the third month, then busulfan until delivery.[20] In pregnant rats, busulfan produces sterility in both male and female offspring due to the absence of germinal cells in testes and ovaries.[21] Germinal cell aplasia or sterility in offspring of mothers receiving busulfan during pregnancy has not been reported in humans. If this drug is used during pregnancy or if the patient becomes pregnant while taking this drug, the patient should be apprised of the potential hazard to the fetus.

Ovarian suppression and amenorrhea with menopausal symptoms commonly occur during busulfan therapy in premenopausal patients. Busulfan interferes with spermatogenesis in experimental animals, and there have been clinical reports of sterility, azoospermia and testicular atrophy in male patients.

PRECAUTIONS

General: The most consistent, dose-related toxicity is bone marrow suppression. This may be manifest by anemia, leukopenia, thrombocytopenia, or any combination of these. It is imperative that patients be instructed to report promptly the development of fever, sore throat, signs of local infection, bleeding from any site, or symptoms suggestive of anemia. Any one of these findings may indicate busulfan toxicity; however, they may also indicate transformation of the disease to an acute "blastic" form. Since busulfan may have a delayed effect, it is important to withdraw the medication temporarily at the first sign of an abnormally large or exceptionally rapid fall in any of the formed elements of the blood. *Patients should never be allowed to take the drug without close medical supervision.*

Laboratory Tests: It is recommended that evaluation of the hemoglobin or hematocrit, total white blood cell count and differential count, and quantitative platelet count be obtained weekly while the patient is on busulfan therapy. In cases where the cause of fluctuation in the formed elements of the peripheral blood is obscure, bone marrow examination may be useful for evaluation of marrow status. A decision to increase, decrease, continue, or discontinue a given dose of busulfan must be based not only on the absolute hematologic values, but also on the rapidity with which changes are occurring. The dosage of busulfan may need to be reduced if this agent is combined with other drugs whose primary toxicity is myelosuppression. Occasional patients may be unusually sensitive to busulfan administered at standard dosage and suffer neutropenia or thrombocytopenia after a relatively short exposure to the drug. Busulfan should not be used where facilities for complete blood counts, including quantitative platelet counts, are not available at weekly (or more frequent) intervals.

Carcinogenesis, Mutagenesis, Impairment of Fertility: See "WARNINGS" section.

Pregnancy: ***Teratogenic effects:*** Pregnancy Category D. See "WARNINGS" section.

Non-Teratogenic effects: There have been reports in the literature of small infants being born after the mothers received busulfan during pregnancy, in particular, during the third trimester.[22] One case was reported where an infant had mild anemia and neutropenia at birth after busulfan was administered to the mother from the eighth week of pregnancy to term.[19]

Nursing Mothers: It is not known whether this drug is excreted in human milk. Because of the potential for tumorigenicity shown for Myleran (busulfan) in animal and human studies, a decision should be made whether to discontinue nursing or to discontinue the drug, taking into account the importance of the drug to the mother.

ADVERSE REACTIONS

Hematological Effects: The most frequent, serious, toxic effect of busulfan is myelosuppression resulting in leukopenia, thrombocytopenia, and anemia. Myelosuppression is most frequently the result of a failure to discontinue dosage in the face of an undetected decrease in leukocyte or platelet counts.[16]

Pulmonary: Interstitial pulmonary fibrosis has been reported rarely, but it is a clinically significant adverse effect when observed and calls for immediate discontinuation of further administration of the drug. The role of corticosteroids in arresting or reversing the fibrosis has been reported to be beneficial in some cases and without effect in others.[17]
Cardiac: One case of endocardial fibrosis has been reported in a 79-year-old woman who received a total dose of 7,200 mg of busulfan over a period of nine years for the management of chronic myelogenous leukemia.[23] At autopsy, she was found to have endocardial fibrosis of the left ventricle in addition to interstitial pulmonary fibrosis.
Ocular: Busulfan is capable of inducing cataracts in rats and there have been several reports indicating that this is a rare complication in humans. In the few cases reported in humans, cataracts have occurred only after prolonged administration of busulfan.[24]
Dermatologic: Hyperpigmentation is the most common adverse skin reaction and occurs in 5–10% of patients, particularly those with a dark complexion.
Metabolic: In a few cases, a clinical syndrome closely resembling adrenal insufficiency and characterized by weakness, severe fatigue, anorexia, weight loss, nausea and vomiting, and melanoderma has developed after prolonged busulfan therapy. The symptoms have sometimes been reversible when busulfan was withdrawn. Adrenal responsiveness to exogenously administered ACTH has usually been normal. However, pituitary function testing with metyrapone revealed a blunted urinary 17-hydroxycorticosteroid excretion in two patients.[25] Following the discontinuation of busulfan (which was associated with clinical improvement), rechallenge with metyrapone revealed normal pituitary-adrenal function.
Hyperuricemia and/or hyperuricosuria are not uncommon in patients with chronic myelogenous leukemia. Additional rapid destruction of granulocytes may accompany the initiation of chemotherapy and increase the urate pool. Adverse effects can be minimized by increased hydration, urine alkalinization, and the prophylactic administration of a xanthine oxidase inhibitor such as Zyloprim® (allopurinol).
Miscellaneous: Other reported adverse reactions include: urticaria, erythema multiforme, erythema nodosum, alopecia, porphyria cutanea tarda, excessive dryness and fragility of the skin with anhidrosis, dryness of the oral mucous membranes and cheilosis, gynecomastia, cholestatic jaundice, and myasthenia gravis. Most of these are single case reports, and in many a clear cause and effect relationship with busulfan has not been demonstrated.

OVERDOSAGE

There is no known antidote to busulfan. The principal toxic effect is on the bone marrow. Survival after a single 140 mg dose has been reported in an 18 kg, 4 year old child,[26] but hematologic toxicity is likely to be more profound with chronic overdosage. The hematologic status should be closely monitored and vigorous supportive measures instituted if necessary.

DOSAGE AND ADMINISTRATION

Busulfan is administered orally. The usual adult dose for *remission induction* is four to eight mg total dose, daily. Dosing on a weight basis (mg/kg) is the same for both children and adults, approximately 60 μg per kg of body weight or 1.8 mg per square meter of body surface, daily. Since the rate of fall of the leukocyte count is dose related, daily doses exceeding four mg per day should be reserved for patients with the most compelling symptoms; the greater the total daily dose, the greater is the possibility of inducing bone marrow aplasia.
A decrease in the leukocyte count is not usually seen during the first ten to fifteen days of treatment; the leukocyte count may actually increase during this period and it should not be interpreted as resistance to the drug, nor should the dose be increased.[27] Since the leukocyte count may continue to fall for more than one month after discontinuing the drug, it is important that busulfan be discontinued *prior* to the total leukocyte count falling into the normal range. When the total leukocyte count has declined to approximately 15,000/μl the drug should be withheld.
With a constant dose of busulfan, the total leukocyte count declines exponentially; a weekly plot of the leukocyte count on semilogarithmic graph paper aids in predicting the time when therapy should be discontinued.[28] With the recommended dose of busulfan, a normal leukocyte count is usually achieved in twelve to twenty weeks.
During remission, the patient is examined at monthly intervals and treatment resumed with the induction dosage when the total leukocyte count reaches approximately 50,000/μl. When remission is shorter than three months, maintenance therapy of 1 to 3 mg daily may be advisable in order to keep the hematological status under control and prevent rapid relapse.

HOW SUPPLIED

White, scored tablets containing 2 mg busulfan, imprinted with "MYLERAN" and "K2A" on each tablet; in bottle of 25 (NDC-0081-0713-25). Store at 15°-30°C (59°-86°F) in a dry place.

REFERENCES

1. Haddow, A., and Timmis, G.M.: Myleran in Chronic Myeloid Leukaemia; Chemical Constitution and Biological Action. Lancet *1*: 207–208, 1953.
2. Galton, D.A.G.: Myleran in Chronic Myeloid Leukaemia, Lancet *1*: 208–213, 1953.
3. Nadkarni, M.V., Trams, E.G., and Smith, P.K.: Preliminary Studies on the Distribution and Fate of TEM, TEPA, and Myleran in the Human. Cancer Res. *19*: 713–718, 1959.
4. Vodopick, H., Hamilton, H.E., Jackson, H.L., Peng, C.T., and Sheets, R.F.: Metabolic Fate of Tritiated Busulfan in Man. J. Lab. & Clin. Med. *73*: 266–276, 1969.
5. Fox, B.W.: Mechanism of Action of Methanesulfonates. In, *Antineoplastic and Immunosuppressive Agents,* Part II. (Edited by A.C. Sartorelli and D.G. Johns) Berlin, Springer-Verlag, 35–46, 1975.
6. Roberts, J.J., and Warwick, G.P.: The Mode of Action of Alkylating Agents—III. The Formation of 3-hydroxytetrahydrothiophene-1:1-dioxide from 1:4-dimethanesulphonyloxybutane (Myleran), S-β-L-alanyltetrahydrothio- phenium mesylate, tetrahydrothiophene and tetrahydrothiophene-1:1-dioxide in the Rat, Rabbit and Mouse, Biochem. Pharmacol. *6*: 217–227, 1961.
7. Peng, C.T.: Distribution and Metabolic Fate of S-35 Labeled Myleran (Busulfan) in Normal and Tumor Bearing Rats. J. Pharmac. Exp. Therap. *120*: 229–238, 1957.
8. Medical Research Council's Working Party for Therapeutic Trials in Leukemia: Chronic Granulocytic Leukaemia: Comparison of Radiotherapy and Busulphan Therapy, Brit. Med. J. *1*: 201–208, 1968.
9. Minot, G.R., Buckman, T.E., and Isaacs, R.: Chronic Myelogenous Leukemia: Age Incidence, Duration, and Benefit Derived From Irradiation, JAMA *82*: 1489–1494, 1924.
10. Haut, A., Abbott, W.S., Wintrobe, M.M., and Cartwright, G.E.: Busulfan in the Treatment of Chronic Myelocytic Leukemia. The Effect of Long Term Intermittent Therapy. Blood *17*: 1–19, 1961.
11. Monfardini, S., Gee, T., Fried J. and Clarkson, B.: Survival in Chronic Myelogenous Leukemia: Influence of Treatment and Extent of Disease at Diagnosis. Cancer *31*: 492–501, 1973.
12. Conrad, F.G.: Survival in Chronic Granulocytic Leukemia. Arch. Intern. Med. *131*: 684–685, 1973.
13. Sokal, J.E.: Evaluation of Survival Data for Chronic Myelocytic Leukemia. Am. J. Hematol. *1*: 493–500, 1976.
14. Ezdinli, E.Z., Sokal, J.E., Crosswhite, L., and Sandberg, A.A.: Philadelphia-Chromosome-Positive and -Negative Chronic Myelocytic Leukemia. Ann. Intern. Med. *72*: 175–182, 1970.
15. Smith, K.L., and Johnson, W.: Classification of Chronic Myelocytic Leukemia in Children. Cancer *34*: 670–679, 1974.
16. Stuart, J.J., Crocker, D.L., and Roberts, H.R.: Treatment of Busulfan-Induced Pancytopenia. Arch. Intern. Med. *136*: 1181–1183, 1976.
17. Sostman, H.D., Matthay, R.A., and Putman, C.E.: Cytotoxic Drug-Induced Lung Disease. Am. J. Med. *62*: 608–615, 1977.
18. Stott, H., Fox, W., Girling, D.J., Stephens, R.J., and Galton, D.A.G.: Acute Leukemia After Busulphan. Brit. Med. J. *2*: 1513–1517, 1977.
19. Dugdale, M. and Fort, A.T.: Busulfan Treatment of Leukemia During Pregnancy. Case Report and Review of the Literature. JAMA *199*: 131–133, 1967.
20. Diamond, I., Anderson, M.M. and McCreadie, S.R.: Transplacental Transmission of Busulfan (Myleran®) in a Mother with Leukemia. Pediatrics *25*: 85–90, 1960.
21. Bollag, W.: Cytostatica in der Schwangershaft, Schweiz. Med. Wochenschr. *84*: 393–395, 1954.
22. Boros, S.J. and Reynolds, J.W.: Intrauterine Growth Retardation Following Third-Trimester-Exposure to Busulfan. Am. J. Obstet. Gynecol. *129*: 111–112, 1977.
23. Weinberger, A., Pinkhas, J., Sandbank, U., Shaklai, M., and Vries, A. de: Endocardial Fibrosis Following Busulfan Treatment. JAMA *231*: 495, 1975.
24. Ravindranathan, M.P., Paul, V.J., and Kuriakose, E.T.: Cataract after Busulphan Treatment. Brit. Med. J. *1*: 218–219, 1972.
25. Vivacqua, R.J., Haurani, F.I., and Erslev, A.J.: "Selective", Pituitary Insufficiency Secondary to Busulfan. Ann. Intern. Med. *67*: 380–387, 1967.
26. Oliveira, H.P. de, Cruz, E., Fonseca, A. de S., and Medeiros, M.: Accidental Ingestion of a Toxic Dose of Myleran by a Child. Acta Haemat. (Basel) *29*: 249–255, 1963.
27. Stryckmans, P.A.: Current Concepts in Chronic Myelogenous Leukemia. Semin. Hematol. *11*: 101–139, 1974.
28. Galton, D.A.G.: Chemotherapy of Chronic Myelocytic Leukaemia. Semin. Hematol. *6*: 323–343, 1969.

Shown in Product Identification Section, page 407

NEOSPORIN® CREAM ℞

[*ne"o-spor'in*]

(See PDR For Nonprescription Drugs)

NEOSPORIN® G.U. IRRIGANT ℞

[*ne"o-spor'in*]

STERILE
(Neomycin Sulfate-Polymyxin B Sulfate Solution For Irrigation)
NOT FOR INJECTION

DESCRIPTION

Neosporin G.U. Irrigant is a concentrated sterile antibiotic solution to be diluted for urinary bladder irrigation. Each ml contains neomycin sulfate equivalent to 40 mg neomycin base, 200,000 units polymyxin B sulfate and water for injection. The 20-ml multiple-dose vial contains, in addition to the above, 1 mg methylparaben (0.1%) added as a preservative.
Neomycin sulfate, an antibiotic of the aminoglycoside group, is the sulfate salt of neomycin B and C produced by *Streptomyces fradiae.* It has a potency equivalent to not less than 600 μg of neomycin per mg.
Polymyxin B sulfate, a polypeptide antibiotic, is the sulfate salt of polymyxin B_1 and B_2 produced by the growth of *Bacillus polymyxa.* It has a potency of not less than 6,000 polymyxin B units per mg.

CLINICAL PHARMACOLOGY

After prophylactic irrigation of the intact urinary bladder, neomycin and polymyxin B are absorbed in clinically insignificant quantities. A neomycin serum level of 0.1 μg/ml was observed in three of 33 patients receiving the rinse solution. This level is well below that which has been associated with neomycin-induced toxicity.
When used topically, polymyxin B sulfate and neomycin are rarely irritating.
Microbiology: The prepared Neosporin G.U. Irrigant Sterile solution is bactericidal. The aminoglycosides act by inhibiting normal protein synthesis in susceptible microorganisms. Polymyxins increase the permeability of bacterial cell wall membranes. The solution is active *in vitro* against

Escherichia coli
Staphylococcus aureus
Haemophilus influenzae
Klebsiella and *Enterobacter* species
Neisseria species, and
Pseudomonas aeruginosa

It is not active *in vitro* against *Serratia marcescens* and streptococci.
Bacterial resistance may develop following the use of the antibiotics in the catheter-rinse solution.

INDICATIONS AND USAGE

Neosporin G.U. Irrigant is indicated for short-term use (up to 10 days) as a continuous irrigant or rinse in the urinary bladder of abacteriuric patients to help prevent bacteriuria and gram-negative rod septicemia associated with the use of indwelling catheters.
Since organisms gain entrance to the bladder by way of, through, and around the catheter, significant bacteriuria is induced by bacterial multiplication in the bladder urine, in the mucoid film often present between catheter and urethra, and in other sites. Urinary tract infection may result from the repeated presence in the urine of large numbers of pathogenic bacteria. The use of closed systems with indwelling catheters has been shown to reduce the risk of infection. A three-way closed catheter system with constant neomycin-polymyxin B bladder rinse is indicated to prevent the development of infection while using indwelling catheters.
If uropathogens are isolated, they should be identified and tested for susceptibility so that appropriate antimicrobial therapy for systemic use can be initiated.

CONTRAINDICATIONS

Hypersensitivity to neomycin, the polymyxins, or any ingredient in the solution is a contraindication to its use. A history of hypersensitivity or serious toxic reaction to an aminoglycoside may also contraindicate the use of any other aminoglycoside because of the known cross-sensitivity of patients to drugs of this class.

WARNINGS

PROPHYLACTIC BLADDER CARE WITH NEOSPORIN G.U. IRRIGANT STERILE SHOULD NOT BE GIVEN WHERE THERE IS A POSSIBILITY OF SYSTEMIC ABSORPTION. NEOSPORIN G.U. IRRIGANT STERILE SHOULD NOT BE USED FOR IRRIGATION OTHER THAN FOR THE URINARY BLADDER. Systemic absorption after topical application of neomycin to open wounds, burns, and granulating surfaces is significant and serum concentrations comparable to and often higher than those attained following oral and parenteral therapy have been

Continued on next page

reported. Absorption of neomycin from the denuded bladder surface has been reported.

However, the likelihood of toxicity following topical irrigation of the intact urinary bladder with Neosporin G.U. Irrigant Sterile is low since no appreciable amounts of these antibiotics enter the systemic circulation by this route if irrigation does not exceed ten days.

Neosporin G.U. Irrigant is intended for continuous prophylactic irrigation of the lumen of the intact urinary bladder of patients with indwelling catheters. Patients should be under constant supervision by a physician. Irrigation should be avoided in patients with defects in the bladder mucosa or bladder wall, such as vesical rupture, or in association with operative procedures on the bladder wall, because of the risk of toxicity due to systemic absorption following diffusion into absorptive tissues and spaces. When absorbed, neomycin and polymyxin B are nephrotoxic antibiotics, and the nephrotoxic potentials are additive. In addition, both antibiotics, when absorbed, are neurotoxins: neomycin can destroy fibers of the acoustic nerve causing permanent bilateral deafness; neomycin and polymyxin B are additive in their neuromuscular blocking effects, not only in terms of potency and duration but also in terms of characteristics of the blocks produced.

Aminoglycosides, when absorbed, can cause fetal harm when administered to a pregnant woman. Aminoglycoside antibiotics cross the placenta and there have been reports of total, irreversible, bilateral, congenital deafness in children whose mothers received streptomycin during pregnancy. Although serious side effects have not been reported in the treatment of pregnant women with other aminoglycosides, the potential for harm exists. If Neosporin G.U. Irrigant Sterile is used during pregnancy, the patient should be apprised of the potential hazard to the fetus (See PRECAUTIONS).

PRECAUTIONS

General: Ototoxicity, nephrotoxicity, and neuromuscular blockade may occur if Neosporin G.U. Irrigant ingredients are systemically absorbed (See WARNINGS). Absorption of neomycin from the denuded bladder surface has been reported. Patients with impaired renal function, infants, dehydrated patients, elderly patients, and patients receiving high doses of prolonged treatment are especially at risk for the development of toxicity.

Irrigation of the bladder with Neosporin G.U. Irrigant may result in overgrowth of nonsusceptible organisms, including fungi. Appropriate measures should be taken if this occurs. The safety and effectiveness of the preparation for use in the care of patients with recent lower urinary tract surgery have not been established. Urine specimens should be collected during prophylactic bladder care for urinalysis, culture, and susceptibility testing. Positive cultures suggest the presence of organisms which are resistant to the bladder rinse antibiotics.

Pregnancy: ***Teratogenic Effects:*** Pregnancy Category D. (See WARNINGS section).

ADVERSE REACTIONS

Neomycin occasionally causes skin sensitization when applied topically; however, topical application to mucus membranes rarely results in local or systemic hypersensitivity reactions.

Irritation of the urinary bladder mucosa has been reported. Signs of ototoxicity and nephrotoxicity have been reported following parenteral use of these drugs and following the oral and topical use of neomycin (See WARNINGS).

DOSAGE AND ADMINISTRATION

This preparation is specifically designed for use with "three-way" catheters or with other catheter systems permitting **continuous** irrigation of the urinary bladder. The usual irrigation dose is one 1-ml ampul a day for up to ten days.

Using strict aseptic techniques, the contents of one 1-ml ampul of Neosporin G.U. Irrigant Sterile (Neomycin Sulfate-Polymyxin B Sulfate Solution for Irrigation) should be added to a 1,000-ml container of isotonic saline solution. This container should then be connected to the inflow lumen of the "three-way" catheter which has been inserted with full aseptic precautions; use of a sterile lubricant is recommended during insertion of the catheter. The outflow lumen should be connected, via a sterile disposable plastic tube, to a disposable plastic collection bag. Stringent procedures, such as taping the inflow and outflow junction at the catheter, should be observed when necessary to insure the junctional integrity of the system.

For most patients, the inflow rate of the 1,000-ml saline solution of neomycin and polymyxin B should be adjusted to a slow drip to deliver about 1,000 ml every twenty-four hours. If the patient's urine output exceeds 2 liters per day, it is recommended that the inflow rate should be adjusted to deliver 2,000 ml of the solution in a twenty-four hour period. It is important that the rinse of the bladder be **continuous;** the inflow or rinse solution should not be interrupted for more than a few minutes.

Preparation of the irrigation solution should be performed with strict aseptic techniques. The prepared solution should be stored at 4°C, and should be used within 48 hours following preparation to reduce the risk of contamination with resistant microorganisms.

HOW SUPPLIED

1-ml ampuls, boxes of 10 (NDC-0081-0748-10) and 50 ampuls (NDC-0081-0748-35); 20-ml multi-dose vial (NDC-0081-0748-93).

Store at 2° to 8°C (36° to 46°F).

NEOSPORIN®

[*nē″ō-spor′ĭn*]

OINTMENT

(Polymyxin B-Bacitracin-Neomycin)

(See PDR For Nonprescription Drugs)

NEOSPORIN® ℞

[*nē″ō-spor′ĭn*]

OPHTHALMIC OINTMENT Sterile

(Polymyxin B Sulfate-Bacitracin Zinc-Neomycin Sulfate)

DESCRIPTION

Neosporin Ophthalmic Ointment (polymyxin B sulfate-bacitracin zinc-neomycin sulfate) is a sterile antimicrobial ointment for ophthalmic use. Each gram contains: Aerosporin® (polymyxin B sulfate) 10,000 units, bacitracin zinc 400 units, neomycin sulfate equivalent to 3.5 mg neomycin base and special white petrolatum, qs.

Polymyxin B sulfate is the sulfate salt of polymyxin B_1 and B_2 which are produced by the growth of *Bacillus polymyxa* (Prazmowski) Migula (Fam. Bacillaceae). It has a potency of not less than 6,000 polymyxin B units per mg, calculated on an anhydrous basis.

Bacitracin zinc is the zinc salt of bacitracin, a mixture of related cyclic polypeptides (mainly bacitracin A) produced by the growth of an organism of the *licheniformis* group of *Bacillus subtilis* (Fam. Bacillaceae). It has a potency of not less than 40 bacitracin units per mg. The precise formula is not known.

Neomycin sulfate is the sulfate salt of neomycin B and C, which are produced by the growth of *Streptomyces fradiae* Waksman (Fam. Streptomycetaceae). It has a potency equivalent of not less than 600 μg of neomycin standard per mg, calculated on an anhydrous basis.

CLINICAL PHARMACOLOGY

A wide range of antibacterial action is provided by the overlapping spectra of polymyxin B sulfate, bacitracin and neomycin. The spectrum of action encompasses most bacterial pathogens capable of causing external infections of the eye and its adnexa.

Polymyxin B is a bactericidal for a variety of gram negative organisms. It increases the permeability of the bacterial cell membrane by interacting with the phospholipid components of the membrane.

Bacitracin is bactericidal for a variety of gram-positive and gram-negative organisms. It interferes with bacterial cell wall synthesis by inhibition of the regeneration of phospholipid receptors involved in peptidoglycan synthesis.

Neomycin is bactericidal for many gram-positive and gram-negative organisms. It is an aminoglycoside antibiotic which inhibits protein synthesis by binding with ribosomal RNA and causing misreading of the bacterial genetic code.

When used topically, polymyxin B, bacitracin and neomycin are rarely irritating, and absorption from the intact skin or mucous membrane is insignificant. The incidence of skin sensitization to this combination has been shown to be low on normal skin.[1,2] Since these antibiotics are seldom used systemically, the patient is spared sensitization to those antibiotics which might later be required systemically.

Microbiology: Polymyxin B sulfate, bacitracin zinc and neomycin sulfate together are considered active against the following microorganisms: *Staphylococcus aureus*, streptococci, including *Streptococcus pneumoniae, Escherichia coli, Haemophilus influenzae, Klebsiella-Enterobacter* species, *Neisseria* species and *Pseudomonas aeruginosa*. The product does not provide adequate coverage against *Serratia marcescens*.

INDICATIONS AND USAGE

Neosporin Ophthalmic Ointment is indicated in the short-term treatment of superficial external ocular infections caused by organisms susceptible to one or more of the antibiotics contained therein.

CONTRAINDICATIONS

This product is contraindicated in those persons who have shown hypersensitivity to any of its components.

WARNINGS

The manifestations of sensitization to neomycin are usually itching, reddening and edema of the conjunctiva and eyelid. It may be manifest simply as a failure to heal. During long-term use of neomycin-containing products, periodic examination for such signs is advisable, and the patient should be told to discontinue the product if they are observed. These symptoms subside quickly on withdrawing the medication. Neomycin-containing applications should be avoided for the patient thereafter.

PRECAUTIONS

General: As with other antibiotic preparations, prolonged use may result in overgrowth of nonsusceptible organisms including fungi. Appropriate measures should be taken if this occurs.

Allergic cross-reactions may occur which could prevent the use of any or all of the following antibiotics for the treatment of future infections: kanamycin, paromomycin, streptomycin, and possibly gentamicin.

Information for Patients: If redness, irritation, swelling or pain persists or increases, discontinue use and contact your physician.

Avoid contaminating the applicator tip with material from the eye, fingers or other source. This caution is necessary if the sterility of the ointment is to be preserved.

ADVERSE REACTIONS

Neomycin Sulfate may cause cutaneous and conjunctival sensitization. A precise incidence of hypersensivity reactions (primarily skin rash) due to topical neomycin is not known.

DOSAGE AND ADMINISTRATION

Apply the ointment every 3 or 4 hours for 7 to 10 days, depending on the severity of the infection.

HOW SUPPLIED

Tube of ⅛ oz with ophthalmic tip. (NDC 0081-0732-86)

Store at 15°-30°C (59°-86°F).

⅛ oz. × 12—DoD NSN 6505-01-143-4644

REFERENCES

1. Leyden JJ, and Kligman AM. Contact Dermatitis to Neomycin Sulfate, *JAMA 242* (12): 1276–1278, 1979.
2. Prystowsky SD, Allen AM, Smith RW, Nonomura JH, Odom RB, and Akers WA. Allergic Contact Hypersensitivity to Nickle, Neomycin, Ethylenediamine, and Benzocaine. *Arch Dermatol 115:* 959–962, 1979.

NEOSPORIN® OPHTHALMIC SOLUTION Sterile ℞

[*nē′ō-spor′ĭn*]

(Polymyxin B Sulfate-Neomycin Sulfate-Gramicidin)

DESCRIPTION

Neosporin Ophthalmic Solution (polymyxin B sulfate-neomycin sulfate-gramicidin) is a sterile antimicrobial solution for ophthalmic use. Each ml contains: Aerosporin® (polymyxin B sulfate) 10,000 units, neomycin sulfate equivalent to 1.75 mg neomycin base and gramicidin 0.025 mg. The vehicle contains alcohol 0.5%, thimerosal 0.001% (added as a preservative) and the inactive ingredients propylene glycol, polyoxyethylene polyoxypropylene compound, sodium chloride and water for injection.

Polymyxin B sulfate is the sulfate salt of polymyxin B_1 and B_2 which are produced by the growth of *Bacillus polymyxa* (Prazmowski) Migula (Fam. Bacillaceae). It has a potency of not less than 6,000 polymyxin B units per mg, calculated on an anhydrous basis.

Neomycin sulfate is the sulfate salt of neomycin B and C, which are produced by the growth of *Streptomyces fradiae* Waksman (Fam. Streptomycetaceae). It has a potency equivalent of not less than 600 μg of neomycin standard per mg, calculated on an anhydrous basis.

Gramicidin (also called Gramicidin D) is a mixture of three pairs of antibacterial substances (Gramicidin A, B and C) produced by the growth of *Bacillus brevis* Dubos (Fam. Bacillaceae). It has a potency of not less than 900 μg of standard gramicidin per mg. The structural formulae are:

Gramicidin D

$$\overset{O}{\overset{\|}{HC}}\text{-X-Gly-Ala-}\underline{D}\text{-Leu-Ala-}\underline{D}\text{-Val-Val-}\underline{D}\text{-Val-Trp-}\underline{D}\text{-Leu-Y-}\underline{D}\text{-Leu-Trp-}\underline{D}\text{-Leu-Trp-}NHCH_2CH_2OH$$

	X	Y
Valine - gramicidin A	Val	Trp
Isoleucine - gramicidin A	Ileu	Trp
Valine - gramicidin B	Val	Phe
Isoleucine - gramicidin B	Ileu	Phe
Valine - gramicidin C	Val	Tyr
Isoleucine - gramicidin C	Ileu	Tyr

CLINICAL PHARMACOLOGY

A wide range of antibacterial action is provided by the overlapping spectra of polymyxin B sulfate, neomycin and gramicidin. The spectrum of action encompasses most bacterial pathogens capable of causing external infections of the eye and its adnexa.

Polymyxin B is bactericidal for a variety of gram-negative organisms. It increases the permeability of the bacterial cell membrane by interacting with the phospholipid components of the membrane.
Neomycin is bactericidal for many gram-positive and gram-negative organisms. It is an aminoglycoside antibiotic which inhibits protein synthesis by binding with ribosomal RNA and causing misreading of the bacterial genetic code.
Gramicidin is bactericidal for a variety of gram-positive organisms. It increases the permeability of the bacterial cell membrane to inorganic cations by forming a network of channels through the normal lipid bilayer of the membrane.
When used topically, polymyxin B, neomycin and gramicidin are rarely irritating, and absorption from the intact skin or mucous membrane is insignificant. The incidence of skin sensitization to this combination has been shown to be low on normal skin.[1,2] Since these antibiotics are seldom used systemically, the patient is spared sensitization to those antibiotics which might later be required systemically.

MICROBIOLOGY

Polymyxin B sulfate, neomycin sulfate and gramicidin together are considered active against the following microorganisms: *Staphylococcus aureus*, streptococci, including *Streptococcus pneumoniae*, *Escherichia coli*, *Haemophilus influenzae*, *Klebsiella-Enterobacter* species, *Neisseria* species and *Pseudomonas aeruginosa*. The product does not provide adequate coverage against *Serratia marcescens*.

INDICATIONS AND USAGE

Neosporin Ophthalmic Solution is indicated in the short-term treatment of superficial external ocular infections caused by organisms susceptible to one or more of the antibiotics contained therein.

CONTRAINDICATIONS

This product is contraindicated in those individuals who have shown hypersensitivity to any of its components.

WARNINGS

The manifestations of sensitization to neomycin are usually itching, reddening and edema of the conjunctiva and eyelid. It may be manifest simply as a failure to heal. During long-term use of neomycin-containing products, periodic examination for such signs is advisable, and the patient should be told to discontinue the product if they are observed. These symptoms subside quickly on withdrawing the medication. Neomycin-containing applications should be avoided for the patient thereafter.

PRECAUTIONS

General: As with other antibiotic preparations, prolonged use may result in overgrowth of nonsusceptible organisms including fungi. Appropriate measures should be taken if this occurs.
Allergic cross-reactions may occur which could prevent the use of any or all of the following antibiotics for the treatment of future infections: kanamycin, paromomycin, streptomycin, and possibly gentamicin.
Information for Patients: If redness, irritation, swelling or pain persists or increases, discontinue use and contact your physician.
Avoid contaminating the dropper with material from the eye, fingers, or other source. This caution is necessary if the sterility of the drops is to be preserved.

ADVERSE REACTIONS

Neomycin Sulfate may cause cutaneous and conjunctival sensitization. A precise incidence of hypersensitivity reactions (primarily skin rash) due to topical neomycin is not known.

DOSAGE AND ADMINISTRATION

The suggested dosage is one or two drops in the affected eye two to four times daily, or more frequently as required, for 7 to 10 days. In acute infections, initiate therapy with one or two drops every 15 to 30 minutes, reducing the frequency of instillation gradually as the infection is controlled.

HOW SUPPLIED

Drop Dose® of 10 ml (plastic dispenser bottle). (NDC-0081-0728-69)
Store at 15°–30°C (59°–86°F) and protect from light.
10 ml-DoD & VA NSN 6505-01-143-4643

REFERENCES

1. Leyden JJ, and Kligman AM. Contact Dermatitis to Neomycin Sulfate. JAMA *242* (12): 1276–1278, 1979.
2. Prystowsky SD, Allen AM, Smith RW, Nonomura JH, Odom RB and Akers WA, Allergic Contact Hypersensitivity to Nickel, Neomycin, Ethylenediamine, and Benzocaine. Arch Dermatol *115*: 959–962, 1979.

NIX™ ℞

[*niks*]
(Permethrin) 1%
Creme Rinse

DESCRIPTION

Nix™ (Permethrin) 1% Creme Rinse is a topical pediculicide and ovicide for the treatment of infestation with *Pediculus humanus* var. *capitis* (the head louse) and its nits (eggs). The product is a creme rinse, each gram containing Permethrin 10 mg (1%). Inactive ingredients are: stearalkonium chloride, hydrolyzed animal protein, cetyl alcohol, polyoxyethylene 10 cetyl ether, hydroxyethylcellulose, balsam canada, fragrance, citric acid, propylene glycol and FD&C Yellow No. 6. Also contains isopropyl alcohol 200 mg (20%) and added as preservatives, methylparaben 2 mg (0.2%), propylparaben 0.8 mg (0.08%) and imidazoldinyl urea 2 mg (0.2%).
Permethrin is a mixture of the *cis* and *trans* isomers of the synthetic pyrethroid (+-)-3-phenoxybenzyl 3-(2,2-dichlorovinyl)-2,2-dimethylcyclopropanecarboxylate (*cis:trans*/25:75). It is a yellow to light orange-brown low melting solid or viscous liquid. The molecular weight is 391.29.

CLINICAL PHARMACOLOGY

Permethrin is a synthetic pyrethroid, active against lice, ticks, mites, and fleas. It acts on the nerve cell membrane to disrupt the sodium channel current by which the polarization of the membrane is regulated. Delayed repolarization and paralysis of the pests are the consequences of this disturbance.
Permethrin is rapidly metabolized by ester hydrolysis to inactive metabolites which are excreted primarily in the urine. Although the amount of permethrin absorbed after a single application of the 1% Creme Rinse has not been determined precisely, preliminary data suggest it is less than 2% of the amount applied. Residual persistence of Nix is detectable on the hair for at least 10 days following a single application.

PEDICULICIDAL/OVICIDAL ACTIVITIES

In vitro data indicate that permethrin has pediculicidal and ovicidal activity against *Pediculus humanus* var. *capitis*. The high cure rate (97–99%) of Nix in patients with head lice demonstrated at 14 days following a single application is attributable to a combination of its pediculicidal and ovicidal activities and its residual persistence on the hair which may also prevent reinfestation.

INDICATIONS AND USAGE

Nix is indicated for the single-application treatment of infestation with *Pediculus humanus* var. *capitis* (the head louse) and its nits (eggs). Retreatment for recurrences is required in less than 1% of patients since the ovicidal activity may be supplemented by residual persistence in the hair. If live lice are observed after at least seven days following the initial application, a second application can be given.

CONTRAINDICATIONS

Nix is contraindicated in patients with known hypersensitivity to any of its components, to any synthetic pyrethroid or pyrethrin, or to chrysanthemums.

WARNING

If hypersensitivity to Nix occurs, discontinue use.

PRECAUTIONS

General: Head lice infestation is often accompanied by pruritus, erythema, and edema. Treatment with Nix may temporarily exacerbate these conditions.
Information for Patients: Patients with head lice should be advised that itching, redness, or swelling of the scalp may occur after application of Nix. If irritation persists, they should consult their physician. Nix is not irritating to the eyes; however, patients should be advised to avoid contact with eyes during application and to flush with water immediately if Nix gets in the eyes. In order to prevent accidental ingestion by children, the remaining contents of Nix should be discarded after use.
Combing of nits following treatment with Nix is not necessary for effective treatment. However, patients may do so for cosmetic or other reasons. The nits are easily combed from the hair treated with Nix after drying.
Carcinogenesis, Mutagenesis, Impairment of Fertility: Six carcinogenicity bioassays were evaluated with permethrin, three each in rats and mice. No tumorigencity was seen in the rat studies. However, species-specific increases in pulmonary adenomas, a common bengn tumor of mice of high spontaneous background incidence, were seen in the three mouse studies. In one of these studies there was an increased incidence of pulmonary alveolar-cell carcinomas and benign liver adenomas only in female mice when permethrin was given in their food at a concentration of 5000 ppm. Mutagenicity assays, which give useful correlative data for interpreting results from carcinogenicity bioassays in rodents, were negative. Permethrin showed no evidence of mutagenic potential in a battery of *in vitro* and *in vivo* genetic toxicity studies.
Permethrin did not have any adverse effect on reproductive function at a dose of 180 mg/kg/day orally in a three-generation rat study.
Pregnancy: ***Teratogenic Effects:*** Pregnancy Category B: Reproduction studies have been performed in mice, rats, and rabbits (200–400 mg/kg/day orally) and have revealed no evidence of impaired fertility or harm to the fetus due to permethrin. There are, however, no adequate and well controlled studies in pregnant women. Because animal reproduction studies are not always predictive of human response, this drug should be used during pregnancy only if clearly needed.
Nursing Mothers: It is not known whether this drug is excreted in human milk. Because many drugs are excreted in human milk and because of the evidence for tumorigenic potential of permethrin in animal studies, consideration should be given to discontinuing nursing temporarily or withholding the drug while the mother is nursing.
Pediatric Use: Nix is safe and effective in children two years of age and older. Safety and effectiveness in children less than two years of age have not been established.

ADVERSE REACTIONS

The most frequent adverse reaction to Nix is pruritus. This is usually a consequence of head lice infestation itself, but may be temporarily aggravated following treatment with Nix. 5.9% of patients in clinical studies experienced mild temporary itching; 3.4% experienced mild transient burning/stinging, tingling, numbness, or scalp discomfort; and 2.1% experienced mild transient erythema, edema, or rash of the scalp.

OVERDOSAGE

No instance of accidental ingestion of Nix has been reported. If ingested, gastric lavage and general supportive measures should be employed.

DOSAGE AND ADMINISTRATION

Adults and Children: Nix is intended for use after the hair has been washed with shampoo, rinsed with water and towel dried. Apply a sufficient volume of Nix to saturate the hair and scalp. Nix should remain on the hair for 10 minutes before being rinsed off with water. A single treatment is sufficient to eliminate head lice infestation. Combing of nits is not required for therapeutic efficacy, but may be done for cosmetic or other reasons.
SHAKE WELL BEFORE USING.

HOW SUPPLIED

Nix (Permethrin) 1% (wt./wt.) Creme Rinse is supplied in plastic squeeze bottles that contain 2 fl. oz. weighing 56 g. (NDC-0081-0780-81)
Store at 15°–25°C (59°–77°F).

POLYSPORIN® OINTMENT

[*pah″lĕ-spor′ĭn*]
(Polymyxin B-Bacitracin)

(See PDR For Nonprescription Drugs)

POLYSPORIN® OPHTHALMIC OINTMENT ℞

[*pah″lĕ-spor′ĭn*]
(Polymyxin B-Bacitracin)
Sterile

DESCRIPTION

Each gram contains:
Aerosporin® (Polymyxin B Sulfate) 10,000 units, bacitracin zinc 500 units, special white petrolatum qs.

ACTIONS

Polymyxin B attacks gram-negative bacilli, including virtually all strains of *Pseudomonas aeruginosa* and *H influenzae* species.
Bacitracin is active against most gram-positive bacilli and cocci, including hemolytic streptococci.

INDICATIONS

For the treatment of superficial ocular infections involving the conjunctiva and/or cornea caused by organisms susceptible to polymyxin B sulfate and bacitracin zinc.

CONTRAINDICATIONS

This product is contraindicated in those individuals who have shown hypersensitivity to any of its components.

WARNINGS

Ophthalmic ointments may retard corneal healing.

PRECAUTIONS

As with other antibiotic preparations, prolonged use may result in overgrowth of nonsusceptible organisms, including fungi. Appropriate measures should be taken if this occurs.

DOSAGE AND ADMINISTRATION

Apply the ointment every 3 or 4 hours, depending on the severity of the infection.

HOW SUPPLIED

Tube of ⅛ oz with ophthalmic tip. (NDC 0081-0797-86)

Continued on next page

Burroughs Wellcome—Cont.

PROLOPRIM® ℞
[*prō'lah-prĭm"*]
(Trimethoprim)
100 mg and 200 mg Scored Tablets

DESCRIPTION

Proloprim® (trimethoprim)* is a synthetic antibacterial, available in tablet form for oral administration. Each scored white tablet contains 100 mg trimethoprim and the inactive ingredients corn starch, lactose, magnesium stearate, and sodium starch glycolate. Each scored yellow tablet contains 200 mg trimethoprim and the inactive ingredients corn starch, D&C Yellow No. 10, magnesium stearate, and sodium starch glycolate. Trimethoprim is 2,4-diamino-5- (3,4,5,-trimethoxybenzyl) pyrimidine. It is a white to light yellow, odorless, bitter compound with a molecular weight of 290.3.

CLINICAL PHARMACOLOGY

Trimethoprim is rapidly absorbed following oral administration. Mean peak serum levels of approximately 1.0 mcg/ml occur 1 to 4 hours after oral administration of a single 100 mg dose. A single 200 mg dose will result in serum levels approximately twice as high. The half-life of trimethoprim is 8 to 10 hours.

Trimethoprim exists in the blood as free, protein-bound and metabolized forms. Approximately 44% of trimethoprim is protein-bound in the blood. The free form is considered to be the therapeutically active form. Excretion of trimethoprim is chiefly by the kidneys through glomerular filtration and tubular secretion. Urine concentrations of trimethoprim are considerably higher than are the concentrations in the blood.

Trimethoprim urine levels, after a single oral dose of 100 mg, ranged from 30 to 160 mcg/ml during the 0 to 4 hour period and declined to approximately 18 to 91 mcg/ml during the 8 to 24 hour period. A 200 mg single oral dose will result in trimethoprim urine levels twice as high. After oral administration, 50% to 60% of trimethoprim is excreted in the urine within 24 hours, approximately 80% of this being unmetabolized trimethoprim.

Microbiology: Proloprim blocks the production of tetrahydrofolic acid from dihydrofolic acid by binding to and reversibly inhibiting the enzyme dihydrofolate reductase. This binding is very much stronger for the bacterial enzyme than for the corresponding mammalian enzyme. Thus, Proloprim selectively interferes with bacterial biosynthesis of nucleic acids and proteins.

In vitro serial dilution tests have shown that the spectrum of antibacterial activity of Proloprim includes the common urinary tract pathogens with the exception of *Pseudomonas aeruginosa.*

REPRESENTATIVE MINIMUM INHIBITORY CONCENTRATIONS FOR TRIMETHOPRIM-SUSCEPTIBLE ORGANISMS

Bacteria	Trimethoprim MIC—mcg/ml (Range)
Escherichia coli	0.05–1.5
Proteus mirabilis	0.5 –1.5
Klebsiella pneumoniae	0.5 –5.0
Enterobacter species	0.5 –5.0
Staphylococcus species, coagulase-negative	0.15–5.0

The recommended quantitative disc susceptibility method[1,2] may be used for estimating the susceptibility of bacteria to Proloprim.

Reports from the laboratory giving results of the standardized test using the 5 mcg trimethoprim disc should be interpreted according to the following criteria:

Organisms producing zones of 16 mm or greater are classified as susceptible whereas those producing zones of 11 to 15 mm are classified as having intermediate susceptibility. A report from the laboratory of "Susceptible" to trimethoprim or "Intermediate" susceptibility to trimethoprim indicates that the infection is likely to respond when, as in uncomplicated urinary tract infections, effective therapy is dependent upon the urine concentration of trimethoprim.

Organisms producing zones of 10 mm or less are reported as resistant, indicating that other therapy should be selected.

Dilution methods for determining susceptibility are also used, and results are reported as the minimum drug concentration inhibiting microbial growth (MIC)[3].

If the MIC is 8 mcg per ml or less, the microorganism is considered "susceptible." If the MIC is 16 mcg per ml or greater the microorganism is considered "resistant."

Normal vaginal and fecal flora are the source of most pathogens causing urinary tract infections. It is therefore relevant to consider the suppressive effect of trimethoprim in these sites.

Concentrations of trimethoprim in vaginal secretions are consistently greater than those found simultaneously in the serum, being typically 1.6 times the concentration of simultaneously obtained serum samples. Sufficient trimethoprim is excreted in the feces to markedly reduce or eliminate trimethoprim susceptible organisms from the fecal flora.

The dominant fecal organisms *(non-Enterobacteriaceae), Bacteroides* spp. and *Lactobacillus* spp., are not susceptible to trimethoprim levels obtained with the recommended dosage.

INDICATIONS AND USAGE

For the treatment of initial episodes of uncomplicated urinary tract infections due to susceptible strains of the following organisms: *Escherichia coli, Proteus mirabilis, Klebsiella pneumoniae* and *Enterobacter* species and coagulase-negative *Staphylococcus* species, including *S. saprophyticus.*

Cultures and susceptibility tests should be performed to determine the susceptibility of the bacteria to trimethoprim. Therapy may be initiated prior to obtaining the results of these tests.

CONTRAINDICATIONS

Proloprim is contraindicated in individuals hypersensitive to trimethoprim and in those with documented megaloblastic anemia due to folate deficiency.

WARNINGS

Experience with trimethoprim alone is limited, but it has been reported rarely to interfere with hematopoiesis, especially when administered in large doses and/or for prolonged periods.

The presence of clinical signs such as sore throat, fever, pallor or purpura may be early indications of serious blood disorders. Complete blood counts should be obtained if any of these signs are noted in a patient receiving trimethoprim and the drug discontinued if a significant reduction in the count of any formed blood element is found.

PRECAUTIONS

General: Trimethoprim should be given with caution to patients with possible folate deficiency. Folates may be administered concomitantly without interfering with the antibacterial action of trimethoprim. Trimethoprim should also be given with caution to patients with impaired renal or hepatic function.

Pregnancy: *Teratogenic Effects:* Pregnancy Category C. Trimethoprim has been shown to be teratogenic in the rat when given in doses 40 times the human dose. In some rabbit studies, an overall increase in fetal loss (dead and resorbed and malformed conceptuses) was associated with doses 6 times the human therapeutic dose. While there are no large well-controlled studies on the use of trimethoprim in pregnant women, Brumfitt and Pursell[4] reported the outcome of 186 pregnancies during which the mother received either placebo or trimethoprim in combination with sulfamethoxazole. The incidence of congenital abnormalities was 4.5% (3 of 66) in those who received placebo and 3.3% (4 of 120) in those receiving trimethoprim plus sulfamethoxazole. There were no abnormalities in the 10 children whose mothers received the drug during the first trimester. In a separate survey, Brumfitt and Pursell also found no congenital abnormalities in 35 children whose mothers had received trimethoprim plus sulfamethoxazole at the time of conception or shortly thereafter.

Because trimethoprim may interfere with folic acid metabolism, Proloprim should be used during pregnancy only if the potential benefit justifies the potential risk to the fetus.

Nursing Mothers: Trimethoprim is excreted in human milk. Because trimethoprim may interfere with folic acid metabolism, caution should be exercised when Proloprim is administered to a nursing mother.

Pediatric Use: The safety of trimethoprim in infants under 2 months has not been demonstrated. The effectiveness of trimethoprim has not been established in children under 12 years of age.

ADVERSE REACTIONS

The adverse effects encountered most often with trimethoprim are rash and pruritus. Other adverse effects reported involved the gastrointestinal and hematopoietic systems.

Dermatologic Reactions: Rash, pruritus and exfoliative dermatitis. At the recommended dosage regimens of 100 mg b.i.d. or 200 mg q.d., each for 10 days, the incidence of rash is 2.9% to 6.7%. In clinical studies which employed high doses of Proloprim, an elevated incidence of rash was noted. These rashes were maculopapular, morbilliform, pruritic and generally mild to moderate, appearing 7 to 14 days after the initiation of therapy.

Gastrointestinal Reactions: Epigastric distress, nausea, vomiting, and glossitis.

Hematologic Reactions: Thrombocytopenia, leukopenia, neutropenia, megaloblastic anemia, and methemoglobinemia.

Miscellaneous Reactions: Fever, elevation of serum transaminases and bilirubin, and increases in BUN and serum creatinine levels.

OVERDOSAGE

Acute: Signs of acute overdosage with trimethoprim may appear following ingestion of 1 gram or more of the drug and include nausea, vomiting, dizziness, headaches, mental depression, confusion and bone marrow depression (SEE CHRONIC OVERDOSAGE). Treatment consists of gastric lavage and general supportive measures. Acidification of the urine will increase renal elimination of trimethoprim. Peritoneal dialysis is not effective and hemodialysis only moderately effective in eliminating the drug.

Chronic: Use of trimethoprim at high doses and/or for extended periods of time may cause bone marrow depression manifested as thrombocytopenia, leukopenia and/or megaloblastic anemia. If signs of bone marrow depression occur, trimethoprim should be discontinued and the patient should be given leucovorin, 3 to 6 mg intramuscularly daily for three days, or as required to restore normal hematopoiesis.

DOSAGE AND ADMINISTRATION

The usual oral adult dosage is 100 mg of Proloprim every 12 hours or 200 mg of Proloprim every 24 hours, each for 10 days.

The use of trimethoprim in patients with a creatinine clearance of less than 15 ml/min is not recommended. For patients with a creatinine clearance of 15 to 30 ml/min, the dose should be 50 mg every 12 hours. The effectiveness of trimethoprim has not been established in children under 12 years of age.

HOW SUPPLIED

100 mg (white) scored tablets, imprinted with "PROLOPRIM 09A"— bottle of 100 (NDC-0081-0820-55). Store at 15°- 30°C (59°–86°F) in a dry place. 200 mg (yellow) scored tablets, imprinted with "PROLOPRIM 200"—bottle of 100 (NDC-0081-0825-55). Store at 15°–30°C (59°–86°F) in a dry place and protect from light.

REFERENCES

1. Bauer AW, Kirby WMM, Sherris JC, Turck M: Antibiotic Susceptibility Testing by Standardized Single Disk Method. Am J Clin Path *45*: 493–496, 1966.
2. Approved Standard ASM-2 Performance Standards for Antimicrobial Disc Susceptibility Test: National Committee for Clinical Laboratory Standards, 771 East Lancaster Avenue, Villanova, Pennsylvania 19085.
3. Ericsson HM and Sherris JC: Antibiotic Sensitivity Testing. Report of an International Collaborative Study. Acta Pathologica et Microbiologica Scandinavica, Section B, Suppl. 217, 1971, pp. 1–90.
4. Brumfitt W and Pursell R: Trimethoprim/ Sulfamethoxazole in the Treatment of Bacteriuria in Women. J Inf Dis Suppl *128*: S657–S663, 1973.

*Mfd. under U.S. Pat. #3,956,327.

Shown in Product Identification Section, page 407

PURINETHOL® ℞
[*pur'ĭn-thawl'*]
(Mercaptopurine)
50 mg Scored Tablets

Caution: Purinethol*® *(mercaptopurine) is a potent drug. It should not be used unless a diagnosis of acute leukemia or chronic myelogenous leukemia has been adequately established and the responsible physician is knowledgeable in assessing response to chemotherapy.

DESCRIPTION

Purinethol® (mercaptopurine) (6-mercaptopurine) was synthesized and developed by Hitchings, Elion, and associates at the Wellcome Research Laboratories.[1] It is one of a large series of purine analogues which interfere with nucleic acid biosynthesis. Mercaptopurine, known chemically as 1,7 dihydro-6*H*-purine-6-thione monohydrate, is an analogue of the purine bases adenine and hypoxanthine.

Purinethol (mercaptopurine) is available in tablet form for oral administration. Each scored tablet contains 50 mg mercaptopurine and the inactive ingredients corn and potato starch, lactose, magnesium stearate, and stearic acid.

BIOCHEMICAL PHARMACOLOGY

Mercaptopurine competes with hypoxanthine and guanine for the enzyme hypoxanthine-guanine phosphoribosyltransferase (HGPRTase) and is itself converted to thioinosinic acid (TIMP). This intracellular nucleotide inhibits several reactions involving inosinic acid (IMP), including the conversion of IMP to xanthylic acid (XMP) and the conversion of IMP to adenylic acid (AMP) via adenylosuccinate (SAMP). In addition, 6-methylthioinosinate (MTIMP) is formed by the methylation of TIMP. Both TIMP and MTIMP have been reported to inhibit glutamine-5-phosphoribosylpyrophosphate amidotransferase, the first enzyme unique to the *de novo* pathway for purine ribonucleotide synthesis.[2]

Experiments indicate that radiolabeled mercaptopurine may be recovered from the DNA in the form of deoxythioguanosine.[3] Some mercaptopurine is converted to nucleotide derivatives of 6-thioguanine (6-TG) by the sequential actions of inosinate (IMP) dehydrogenase and xanthylate (XMP) aminase, converting TIMP to thioguanylic acid (TGMP).

Animal tumors that are resistant to mercaptopurine have lost the ability to convert mercaptopurine to TIMP. However, it is clear that resistance to mercaptopurine may be acquired by other means as well, particularly in human leukemias.

It is not known exactly which of any one or more of the biochemical effects of mercaptopurine and its metabolites are directly or predominantly responsible for cell death.[4]

The catabolism of mercaptopurine and its metabolites is complex. In man, after oral administration of ^{35}S-6-mercaptopurine, urine contains intact mercaptopurine, thiouric acid (formed by direct oxidation by xanthine oxidase, probably via 6-mercapto-8-hydroxypurine) and a number of 6-methylated thiopurines. The methylthiopurines yield appreciable amounts of inorganic sulfate.[2] The importance of the metabolism by xanthine oxidase relates to the fact that Zyloprim® (allopurinol) inhibits this enzyme and retards the catabolism of mercaptopurine and its active metabolites. A significant reduction in mercaptopurine dosage is mandatory if a potent xanthine oxidase inhibitor and Purinethol (mercaptopurine) are used simultaneously in a patient (see "WARNINGS").

CLINICAL PHARMACOLOGY

Clinical studies have shown that the absorption of an oral dose of mercaptopurine in man is incomplete and variable, averaging approximately 50% of the administered dose.[5] The factors influencing absorption are unknown. Intravenous administration of an investigational preparation of mercaptopurine revealed a plasma half-disappearance time of 21 minutes in children and 47 minutes in adults. The volume of distribution usually exceeded that of the total body water.[5]

Following the oral administration of ^{35}S-6-mercaptopurine in one subject, a total of 46% of the dose could be accounted for in the urine (as parent drug and metabolites) in the first 24 hours. Metabolites of mercaptopurine were found in urine within the first 2 hours after administration. Radioactivity (in the form of sulfate) could be found in the urine for weeks afterwards.[2]

There is negligible entry of mercaptopurine into cerebrospinal fluid.

Plasma protein binding averages 19% over the concentration range 10 to 50 micrograms per milliliter (a concentration only achieved by intravenous administration of mercaptopurine at doses exceeding 5 to 10 mg/kg).[5]

Monitoring plasma levels of mercaptopurine during therapy is of questionable value.[2] It is technically difficult to determine plasma concentrations which are seldom greater than 1 to 2 micrograms per milliliter after a therapeutic oral dose. More significantly, mercaptopurine enters rapidly into the anabolic and catabolic pathways for purines and the active intracellular metabolites have appreciably longer half-lives than the parent drug. The biochemical effects of a single dose of mercaptopurine are evident long after the parent drug has disappeared from plasma. Because of this rapid metabolism of mercaptopurine to active intracellular derivatives, hemodialysis would not be expected to appreciably reduce toxicity of the drug. There is no known pharmacologic antagonist to the biochemical actions of mercaptopurine *in vivo*.

INDICATIONS AND USAGE

Purinethol (mercaptopurine) is indicated for remission induction, remission consolidation, and maintenance therapy of the acute leukemias. The response to this agent depends upon the particular subclassification of the acute leukemia (lymphatic, myelogenous, undifferentiated, etc.) and the age of the patient (child or adult). Purinethol (mercaptopurine) is also indicated for the palliative treatment of chronic myelogenous (granulocytic) leukemia.

a) **Acute Lymphatic (Lymphocytic, Lymphoblastic) Leukemia:** Acute lymphatic leukemia occurring in children responds, in general, more favorably to mercaptopurine than the same disorder occuring in adults. Given as a single agent for remission induction, mercaptopurine induces complete remission in approximately 25% of children and 10% of adults. These results can be improved upon considerably by using multiple, carefully selected agents in combination. Reliance upon mercaptopurine alone is seldom justified. The duration of complete remission induced in children with acute lymphatic leukemia is so brief without the use of maintenance therapy that some form of drug therapy is considered essential following remission induction. Mercaptopurine, as a single agent, is capable of significantly prolonging complete remission duration in children; however, combination therapy with multiple agents has produced results superior to that achieved with mercaptopurine alone. The effectiveness of mercaptopurine in maintenance programs in adult acute lymphatic leukemia has not been established.

b) **Acute Myelogenous (and Acute Myelomonocytic) Leukemia:** As a single agent, mercaptopurine will induce complete remission in approximately 10% of children and adults with acute myelogenous leukemia or its subclassifications. These results are inferior to those achieved with combination chemotherapy employing optimum treatment schedules.

c) **Chronic Myelogenous (Granulocytic) Leukemia:** Mercaptopurine is one of several agents with demonstrated efficacy in the treatment of chronic myelogenous leukemia. Approximately 30 to 50% of patients with chronic myelogenous leukemia obtain an objective response to mercaptopurine. This is less than the 90% objective responses with busulfan, and, of these two agents, Myleran® (busulfan) is usually regarded as the preferred drug for initial therapy.

d) **Central Nervous System Leukemia:** Mercaptopurine is not effective for prophylaxis or treatment of central nervous system leukemia.

e) **Other Neoplasms:** Purinethol (mercaptopurine) is not effective in chronic lymphatic leukemia, the lymphomas (including Hodgkin's Disease), or solid tumors.

CONTRAINDICATIONS

Purinethol (mercaptopurine) should not be used unless a diagnosis of acute leukemia or chronic myelogenous leukemia has been adequately established and the responsible physician is knowledgeable in assessing response to chemotherapy.

Mercaptopurine should not be used in patients whose disease has demonstrated prior resistance to this drug. In animals and man there is usually complete cross-resistance between Purinethol (mercaptopurine) and Tabloid® brand thioguanine.

WARNINGS

a) **Bone Marrow Toxicity:** The most consistent, dose-related toxicity is bone marrow suppression. This may be manifest by anemia, leukopenia, thrombocytopenia, or any combination of these. Any of these findings may also indicate progression of the underlying disease. It is imperative that patients be instructed to report promptly the development of fever, sore throat, signs of local infection, bleeding from any site, or symptoms suggestive of anemia. Since mercaptopurine may have a delayed effect, it is important to withdraw the medication temporarily at the first sign of an abnormally large fall in any of the formed elements of the blood.

b) **Hepatotoxicity:**[6] Purinethol (mercaptopurine) is hepatotoxic in animals and man; deaths have been reported from hepatic necrosis. Hepatic injury can occur with any dosage, but seems to occur with greatest frequency when doses of 2.5 mg/kg/day are exceeded. The histologic pattern of mercaptopurine hepatotoxicity includes features of both intrahepatic cholestasis and parenchymal cell necrosis, either of which may predominate. It is not clear how much of the hepatic damage is due to direct toxicity from the drug and how much may be due to a hypersensitivity reaction. In some patients jaundice has cleared following withdrawal of mercaptopurine and reappeared with its reintroduction.

Published reports have cited widely varying incidences of overt hepatotoxicity; several reports have indicated that as many as 10 to 40% of patients with acute leukemia develop jaundice while receiving treatment with mercaptopurine. Usually, clinically detectable jaundice appears early in the course of treatment (one to two months). However, jaundice has been reported as early as one week and as late as eight years after the start of treatment with mercaptopurine.

Monitoring of serum transaminase levels, alkaline phosphatase, and bilirubin levels may allow early detection of hepatotoxicity. It is advisable to monitor these liver function tests at weekly intervals when first beginning therapy and at monthly intervals thereafter. Liver function tests may be advisable more frequently in patients who are receiving mercaptopurine with other hepatotoxic drugs or with known pre-existing liver disease.

The concomitant administration of mercaptopurine with other hepatotoxic agents requires especially careful clinical and biochemical monitoring of hepatic function. Combination therapy involving mercaptopurine with other drugs not felt to be hepatotoxic should nevertheless be approached with caution. The combination of mercaptopurine with doxorubicin (Adriamycin®) was reported to be hepatotoxic in 19 of 20 patients undergoing remission-induction therapy for leukemia resistant to previous therapy.

The hepatotoxicity has been associated in some cases with anorexia, diarrhea, jaundice, and ascites. Hepatic encephalopathy has occurred.

The onset of clinical jaundice, hepatomegaly, or anorexia with tenderness in the right hypochondrium are immediate indications for withholding mercaptopurine until the exact etiology can be identified. Likewise, any evidence of deterioration in liver function studies, toxic hepatitis, or biliary stasis should prompt discontinuation of the drug and lead to a search for an etiology of the hepatotoxicity.

c) **Interaction with Zyloprim® (Allopurinol): When allopurinol and mercaptopurine are administered concomitantly, it is imperative that the dose of mercaptopurine be reduced to one-third to one-quarter of the usual dose. Failure to observe this dosage reduction will result in a delayed catabolism of mercaptopurine and the strong likelihood of inducing severe toxicity.**

d) **Immunosuppression:** Mercaptopurine recipients may manifest decreased cellular hypersensitivities and impaired allograft rejection. Induction of immunity to infectious agents or vaccines will be subnormal in these patients; the degree of immunosuppression will depend on antigen dose and temporal relationship to drug. This drug effect is similar to that of Imuran® (azathioprine) and should be carefully considered with regard to intercurrent infections and risk of subsequent neoplasia.

e) **Mutagenesis and Carcinogenesis:** Purinethol (mercaptopurine) causes chromosomal aberrations in animals and man and induces dominant-lethal mutations in male mice. Carcinogenic potential exists in man, but the extent of the risk is unknown.

f) **Teratogenesis:** Mercaptopurine has embryopathic effects in rats. Women receiving mercaptopurine in the first trimester of pregnancy have an increased incidence of abortion; the risk of malformation in offspring surviving first trimester exposure is not accurately known. In a series of twenty-eight women receiving mercaptopurine after the first trimester of pregnancy, three mothers died undelivered, one delivered a stillborn child, and one aborted; there were no cases of macroscopically abnormal fetuses. Since such experience cannot exclude the possibility of fetal damage, mercaptopurine should be used during pregnancy only if the benefit clearly justifies the possible risk to the fetus, and particular caution should be given to the use of mercaptopurine in the first trimester of pregnancy.

g) **Effects on Fertility:** The effect of mercaptopurine on human fertility is unknown for either males or females.

PRECAUTIONS

The safe and effective use of Purinethol demands a thorough knowledge of the natural history of the condition being treated. For example, remission induction of adult acute leukemia virtually always necessitates the production of moderate to severe bone marrow hypoplasia. The degree of myelosuppression acceptable in this disease would not be desirable in the management of chronic granulocytic leukemia. After selection of an initial dosage schedule, therapy will frequently need to be modified depending upon the patient's response and manifestations of toxicity.

The most frequent, serious, toxic effect of mercaptopurine is myelosuppression resulting in leukopenia, thrombocytopenia, and anemia. These toxic effects are often unavoidable during the induction phase of adult acute leukemia if remission induction is to be successful. Whether or not these manifestations demand modification or cessation of dosage depends both upon the response of the underlying disease and a careful consideration of supportive facilities (granulocyte and platelet transfusions) which may be available. Life-threatening infections and bleeding have been observed as a consequence of mercaptopurine induced granulocytopenia and thrombocytopenia. Severe hematologic toxicity may require supportive therapy with platelet transfusions for bleeding, and antibiotics and granulocyte transfusions if sepsis is documented.

If it is not the intent to intentionally induce bone marrow hypoplasia, it is important to discontinue the drug temporarily at the first evidence of an abnormally large fall in white blood cell count, platelet count, or hemoglobin concentration. In many patients with severe depression of the formed elements of the blood due to mercaptopurine, the bone marrow appears hypoplastic on aspiration or biopsy, whereas in other cases it may appear normocellular. The qualitative changes in the erythroid elements toward the megaloblastic series, characteristically seen with the folic acid antagonists and some other antimetabolites, are not seen with this drug.

It is recommended that evaluation of the hemoglobin or hematocrit, total white blood cell count and differential count, and quantitative platelet count be obtained weekly while the patient is on mercaptopurine therapy. In cases where the cause of fluctuations in the formed elements in the peripheral blood is obscure, bone marrow examination may be useful for the evaluation of marrow status. The decision to increase, decrease, continue, or discontinue a given dosage of mercaptopurine must be based not only on the absolute hematologic values, but also upon the rapidity with which changes are occurring. In many instances, particularly during the induction phase of acute leukemia, complete blood counts will need to be done more frequently than once weekly in order to evaluate the effect of the therapy. The dosage of mercaptopurine may need to be reduced when this

Continued on next page

Burroughs Wellcome—Cont.

agent is combined with other drugs whose primary toxicity is myelosuppression.
It is probably advisable to start with smaller dosages in patients with impaired renal function, since the latter might result in slower elimination of the drug and a greater cumulative effect.
See "WARNINGS" section for information on immunosuppression, mutagenesis and carcinogenesis, teratogenesis, and effects on fertility.

ADVERSE REACTIONS

Intestinal ulceration has been reported.[8] Nausea, vomiting and anorexia are uncommon during initial administration, but they may occur during toxicity. Mild diarrhea and sprue-like symptoms have been noted occasionally, but it is difficult at present to attribute these to the medication. Oral lesions are rarely seen, and when they occur they resemble thrush rather than antifolic ulcerations.
Hyperuricemia frequently occurs in patients receiving mercaptopurine as a consequence of rapid cell lysis accompanying the antineoplastic effect. Adverse effects can be minimized by increased hydration, urine alkalinization, and the prophylactic administration of a xanthine oxidase inhibitor such as Zyloprim® (allopurinol). The dosage of mercaptopurine should be reduced to one-third to one-quarter of the usual dose if Zyloprim® (allopurinol) is given concurrently.

Drug fever has been very rarely reported with mercaptopurine. Before attributing fever to mercaptopurine, every attempt should be made to exclude more common causes of pyrexia, such as sepsis, in patients with acute leukemia.

OVERDOSAGE

There is no known pharmacologic antagonist of mercaptopurine. The drug should be discontinued immediately if unintended toxicity occurs during treatment. If a patient is seen immediately following an accidental overdosage of the drug, induced emesis may be useful. Hemodialysis is thought to be of marginal use due to the rapid intracellular incorporation of mercaptopurine into active metabolites with long persistence.

DOSAGE AND ADMINISTRATION

a) **Induction and Consolidation Therapy:** Purinethol (mercaptopurine) is administered orally. The dosage which will be tolerated or will be effective varies from patient-to-patient, and therefore careful titration is necessary to obtain the optimum therapeutic effect without incurring excessive, unintended toxicity. The usual initial dosage for children and adults is 2.5 mg/kg of body weight per day (100 to 200 mg in the average adult and 50 mg in an average 5-year-old child). Children with acute leukemia have tolerated this dose without difficulty in most cases; it may be continued daily for several weeks or more in some patients. If, after four weeks at this dosage, there is no clinical improvement and no definite evidence of leukocyte or platelet depression, the dosage may be increased up to 5 mg/kg daily.
A dosage of 2.5 mg/kg per day may result in a rapid fall in leukocyte count within 1 to 2 weeks in some adults with acute leukemia and high total leukocyte counts, as well as in certain adults with chronic myelocytic leukemia.
The total daily dosage may be given at one time. It is calculated to the nearest multiple of 25 mg. The dosage of mercaptopurine should be reduced to one-third to one-quarter of the usual dose if Zyloprim® (allopurinol) is given concurrently. Since the drug may have a delayed action, it should be discontinued at the first sign of an abnormally large or rapid fall in the leukocyte or platelet count. If subsequently the leukocyte count or platelet count remains constant for two or three days, or rises, treatment may be resumed.

b) **Maintenance Therapy:** If a complete hematologic remission is obtained with mercaptopurine, either alone or in combination with other agents, maintenance therapy should be considered. This is indicated in children with acute lymphatic leukemia. The use of mercaptopurine in maintenance schedules for adults with acute leukemia has not been established to be effective. If remission is achieved, maintenance doses will vary from patient-to-patient. A usual daily maintenance dose of mercaptopurine is 1.5 to 2.5 mg/kg/day as a single dose. It is to be emphasized that in children with acute lymphatic leukemia in remission, superior results have been obtained when mercaptopurine has been combined with other agents (most frequently with methotrexate) for remission maintenance. Mercaptopurine should rarely be relied upon as a single agent for the maintenance of remissions induced in acute leukemia.

HOW SUPPLIED

Off-white, scored tablets containing 50 mg mercaptopurine, imprinted with "PURINETHOL" and "04A" on each tablet; bottles of 25 (NDC-0081-0807-25) and 250 (NDC 0081-0807-65).

REFERENCES

1. New York Academy of Sciences: 6-mercaptopurine. ANN NY ACAD SCI *60*: 359–507 (1954).
2. Elion GB: Biochemistry and pharmacology of purine analogues. FED PROC *26*: 898–904 (1967).
3. Scannell JP, Hitchings GH: Thioguanine in deoxyribonucleic acid from tumors of 6-mercaptopurine-treated mice. PROC SOC EXP BIOL MED *122*: 627–629 (1966).
4. Paterson ARP, Tidd DM: 6-thiopurines. pp. 384–403. In: Sartorelli AC, Johns DG, ed. Antineoplastic and Immunosuppressive Agents, Part II, Berlin, Springer-Verlag, 1975.
5. Loo TL, Luce JK, Sullivan MP, Frei E: Clinical pharmacologic observations on 6-mercaptopurine and 6-methylthiopurine ribonucleoside. CLIN PHARMACOL THER *9*: 180–194 (1968).
6. Schein PS, Winokur SH: Immunosuppressive and cytotoxic chemotherapy: long-term complications. ANN INTERN MED *82*: 84–95 (1975).
7. Stern MH, Minow MD, Casey MD: Hepatotoxicity in patients treated with adriamycin and 6-mercaptopurine for refractory leukemia. AM J CLIN PATHOL *63*: 758–759 (1975).
8. Clark PA, Hsia YE, Huntsman RG: Toxic complications of treatment with 6-mercaptopurine. BR MED J *1*: 393–395 (1960).

Shown in Product Identification Section, page 407

SEPTRA® ℞

[sĕp 'trah]
I.V. INFUSION
(TRIMETHOPRIM AND SULFAMETHOXAZOLE)

DESCRIPTION

Septra I.V. Infusion (Trimethoprim and Sulfamethoxazole), a sterile solution for intravenous infusion only, is a synthetic antibacterial combination product. Each ml contains 16 mg trimethoprim* and 80 mg sulfamethoxazole compounded with 40% propylene glycol, 10% ethyl alcohol and 0.3% diethanolamine; 1% benzyl alcohol and 0.1% sodium metabisulfite added as preservatives, water for injection, and pH adjusted to approximately 10 with sodium hydroxide.

REPRESENTATIVE MINIMUM INHIBITORY CONCENTRATION VALUES FOR SEPTRA SUSCEPTIBLE ORGANISMS (MIC-μg/ml)

Bacteria	TMP Alone	SMX Alone	TMP/SMX (1:19) TMP	TMP/SMX (1:19) SMX
Escherichia coli	0.05–1.5	1.0–245	0.05–0.5	0.95–9.5
Proteus species (indole positive)	0.5–5.0	7.35–300	0.05–1.5	0.95–28.5
Morganella morganii	0.5–5.0	7.35–300	0.05–1.5	0.95–28.5
Proteus mirabilis	0.5–1.5	7.35–30	0.05–0.15	0.95–2.85
Klebsiella species	0.15–5.0	2.45–245	0.05–1.5	0.95–28.5
Enterobacter species	0.15–5.0	2.45–245	0.05–1.5	0.95–28.5
Haemophilus influenzae	0.15–1.5	2.85–95	0.015–0.15	0.285–2.85
Streptococcus pneumoniae	0.15–1.5	7.35–24.5	0.05–0.15	0.95–2.85
Shigella flexneri †	<0.01–0.04	<0.16–>320	<0.002–0.03	0.04–0.625
Shigella sonnei †	0.02–0.08	0.625–>320	0.004–0.06	0.08–1.25

TMP = Trimethoprim SMX = Sulfamethoxazole
†Rudoy RC, Nelson JD, Haltalin KC. *Antimicrobial Agents and Chemotherapy* 5:439-43, 1974.

*Trimethoprim is 2,4-diamino-5-(3,4,5-trimethoxybenzyl)-pyrimidine. It is a white to light yellow, odorless, bitter compound with a molecular weight of 290.3.
Sulfamethoxazole is N^1-(5-methyl-3-isoxazolyl)sulfanilamide. It is an almost white, odorless, tasteless compound with a molecular weight of 253.28.

CLINICAL PHARMACOLOGY

Following a one-hour intravenous infusion of a single dose of 160 mg trimethoprim and 800 mg sulfamethoxazole to 11 patients whose weight ranged from 105 lbs. to 165 lbs. (mean, 143 lbs.), the mean peak plasma concentrations of trimethoprim and sulfamethoxazole were 3.4 ± 0.3 μg/ml and 46.3 ± 2.7 μg/ml, respectively. Following repeated intravenous administration of the same dose at eight-hour intervals, the mean plasma concentrations just prior to and immediately after each infusion at steady state were 5.6 ± 0.6 μg/ml and 8.8 ± 0.9 μg/ml for trimethoprim and 70.6 ± 7.3 μg/ml and 105.6 ± 10.9 μg/ml for sulfamethoxazole. The mean plasma half-life was 11.3 ± 0.7 hours for trimethoprim and 12.8 ± 1.8 hours for sulfamethoxazole. All of these 11 patients had normal renal function and their ages ranged from 17 to 78 years (median, 60 years)[1].
Pharmacokinetic studies in children and adults suggest an age-dependent half-life of trimethoprim as indicated in the following table.[2]

Age (yrs.)	No. of Patients	Mean TMP Half-life (hours)
<1	2	7.67
1–10	9	5.49
10–20	5	8.19
20–63	6	12.82

Patients with severely impaired renal function exhibit an increase in the half-lives of both components requiring dosage regimen adjustment (see DOSAGE AND ADMINISTRATION section).
Both trimethoprim and sulfamethoxazole exist in the blood as unbound, protein-bound and metabolized forms; sulfamethoxazole also exists as the conjugated form. The metabolism of sulfamethoxazole occurs predominately by N_4-acetylation, although the glucuronide conjugate has been identified. The principal metabolites of trimethoprim are the 1- and 3- oxides and the 3'- and 4'-hydroxy derivatives. The free forms of trimethoprim and sulfamethoxazole are considered to be the therapeutically active forms. Approximately 44% of trimethoprim and 70% of sulfamethoxazole are bound to plasma proteins. The presence of 10 mg percent sulfamethoxazole in plasma decreases the protein binding of trimethoprim by an insignificant degree; trimethoprim does not influence the protein binding of sulfamethoxazole.
Excretion of trimethoprim and sulfamethoxazole is primarily by the kidneys through both glomerular filtration and tubular secretion. Urine concentrations of both trimethoprim and sulfamethoxazole are considerably higher than are the concentrations in the blood. The percent of dose excreted in urine over a 12-hour period following the intravenous administration of the first dose of 240 mg of trimethoprim and 1200 mg of sulfamethoxazole on day 1 ranged from 17% to 42.4% as free trimethoprim; 7% to 12.7% as free sulfamethoxazole; and 36.7% to 56% as total (free plus the N_4-acetylated metabolite) sulfamethoxazole. When administered together as Septra, neither trimethoprim nor sulfamethoxazole affects the urinary excretion pattern of the other.
Both trimethoprim and sulfamethoxazole distribute to sputum and vaginal fluid; trimethoprim also distributes to bronchial secretions and both pass the placental barrier and are excreted in breast milk.
Microbiology: Sulfamethoxazole inhibits bacterial synthesis of dihydrofolic acid by competing with *para*- aminobenzoic acid (PABA). Trimethoprim blocks the production of tetrahydrofolic acid from dihydrofolic acid by binding to and reversibly inhibiting the required enzyme, dihydrofolate reductase. Thus, Septra blocks two consecutive steps in the biosynthesis of nucleic acids and proteins essential to many bacteria.
In vitro studies have shown that bacterial resistance develops more slowly with Septra than with trimethoprim or sulfamethoxazole alone.
In vitro serial dilution tests have shown that the spectrum of antibacterial activity of Septra includes common bacterial pathogens with the exception of *Pseudomonas aeruginosa*. The following organisms are usually susceptible: *Escherichia coli, Klebsiella* species, *Enterobacter* species, *Morganella morganii, Proteus mirabilis,* indole-positive *Proteus* species, including *Proteus vulgaris, Haemophilus influenzae* (including ampicillin-resistant strains), *Streptococcus pneumoniae, Shigella flexneri* and *Shigella sonnei.* It should be noted, however, that there are little clinical data on the use of Septra I.V. Infusion in serious systemic infections due to *Haemophilus influenzae* and *Streptococcus pneumoniae.*
[See table left].
The recommended quantitative disc susceptibility method may be used for estimating the susceptibility of bacteria to Septra.[3,4] With this procedure, a report from the laboratory of "Susceptible to trimethoprim and sulfamethoxazole" indi-

cates that the infection is likely to respond to therapy with Septra. If the infection is confined to the urine, a report of "Intermediate susceptibility to trimethoprim and sulfamethoxazole" also indicates that the infection is likely to respond. A report of "Resistant to trimethoprim and sulfamethoxazole" indicates that the infection is unlikely to respond to therapy with Septra.

INDICATIONS AND USAGE

PNEUMOCYSTIS CARINII PNEUMONITIS: Septra I.V. Infusion is indicated in the treatment of *Pneumocystis carinii* pneumonitis in children and adults. (see PRECAUTIONS section)

SHIGELLOSIS: Septra I.V. Infusion is indicated in the treatment of enteritis caused by susceptible strains of *Shigella flexneri* and *Shigella sonnei* in children and adults.

URINARY TRACT INFECTIONS: Septra I.V. Infusion is indicated in the treatment of severe or complicated urinary tract infections due to susceptible strains of *Escherichia coli, Klebsiella* species, *Enterobacter* species, *Morganella morganii*, and *Proteus* species when oral administration of Septra is not feasible and when the organism is not susceptible to single agent antibacterials effective in the urinary tract.

Although appropriate culture and susceptibility studies should be performed, therapy may be started while awaiting the results of these studies.

CONTRAINDICATIONS

Hypersensitivity to trimethoprim or sulfonamides. Patients with documented megaloblastic anemia due to folate deficiency. Pregnancy at term and during the nursing period, because sulfonamides pass the placenta and are excreted in the milk and may cause kernicterus. Infants less than two months of age.

WARNINGS

FATALITIES ASSOCIATED WITH THE ADMINISTRATION OF SULFONAMIDES, ALTHOUGH RARE, HAVE OCCURRED DUE TO SEVERE REACTIONS, INCLUDING STEVENS-JOHNSON SYNDROME, TOXIC EPIDERMAL NECROLYSIS, FULMINANT HEPATIC NECROSIS, AGRANULOCYTOSIS, APLASTIC ANEMIA AND OTHER BLOOD DYSCRASIAS.

SEPTRA SHOULD BE DISCONTINUED AT THE FIRST APPEARANCE OF SKIN RASH OR ANY SIGN OF ADVERSE REACTION. Clinical signs, such as rash, sore throat, fever, pallor, purpura or jaundice may be early indications of serious reactions. In rare instances, a skin rash may be followed by more severe reactions, such as Stevens-Johnson syndrome, toxic epidermal necrolysis, hepatic necrosis or serious blood disorder. Complete blood counts should be done frequently in patients receiving sulfonamides.

SEPTRA SHOULD NOT BE USED IN THE TREATMENT OF STREPTOCOCCAL PHARYNGITIS. Clinical studies have documented that patients with group A β-hemolytic streptococcal tonsillopharyngitis have a greater incidence of bacteriologic failure when treated with Septra than do those patients treated with penicillin, as evidenced by failure to eradicate this organism from the tonsillopharyngeal area.

Contains sodium metabisulfite, a sulfite that may cause allergic-type reactions (e.g., hives, itching, wheezing, anaphylaxis) in certain susceptible persons. Although the overall presence of sulfite sensitivity in the general population is probably low, it is seen more frequently in asthmatics or in atopic nonasthmatic persons.

PRECAUTIONS

General: Septra should be given with caution to patients with impaired renal or hepatic function, to those with possible folate deficiency (e.g., the elderly, chronic alcoholics, patients receiving anticonvulsant therapy, patients with malabsorption syndrome, and patients in malnutrition states) and to those with severe allergy or bronchial asthma. In glucose-6-phosphate dehydrogenase-deficient individuals, hemolysis may occur. This reaction is frequently dose-related. Adequate fluid intake must be maintained in order to prevent crystalluria and stone formation.

Local irritation and inflammation due to extravascular infiltration of the infusion has been observed with Septra I.V. Infusion. If these occur the infusion should be discontinued and restarted at another site.

Use in the Elderly: There may be an increased risk of severe adverse reactions in elderly patients, particularly when complicating conditions exist, e.g., impaired kidney and/or liver function, or concomitant use of other drugs. Severe skin reactions, or generalized bone marrow suppression (see WARNINGS and ADVERSE REACTIONS sections) or a specific decrease in platelets (with or without purpura) are the most frequently reported severe adverse reactions in elderly patients. In those concurrently receiving certain diuretics, primarily thiazides, an increased incidence of thrombocytopenia with purpura has been reported. Appropriate dosage adjustments should be made for patients with impaired kidney function (see DOSAGE AND ADMINISTRATION section).

Use in the Treatment of *Pneumocystis carinii* Pneumonitis in Patients with Acquired Immunodeficiency Syndrome (AIDS): Because of their unique immune dysfunction, AIDS patients may not tolerate or respond to Septra in the same manner as non-AIDS patients. The incidence of side effects, particularly rash, fever, and leukopenia, with Septra therapy in AIDS patients who are being treated for *Pneumocystis carinii* pneumonitis has been reported to be greatly increased compared with the incidence normally associated with the use of Septra in non-AIDS patients.

Laboratory Tests: Appropriate culture and susceptibility studies should be performed before and throughout treatment. Complete blood counts should be done frequently in patients receiving Septra; if a significant reduction in the count of any formed blood element is noted, Septra should be discontinued. Urinalyses with careful microscopic examination and renal function tests should be performed during therapy, particularly for those patients with impaired renal function.

Drug Interactions: In elderly patients concurrently receiving certain diuretics, primarily thiazides, an increased incidence of thrombocytopenia with purpura has been reported.

It has been reported that Septra may prolong the prothrombin time in patients who are receiving the anticoagulant warfarin. This interaction should be kept in mind when Septra is given to patients already on anticoagulant therapy, and the coagulation time should be reassessed.

Septra may inhibit the hepatic metabolism of phenytoin. Septra, given at a common clinical dosage, increased the phenytoin half-life by 39% and decreased the phenytoin metabolic clearance rate by 27%. When administering these drugs concurrently, one should be alert for possible excessive phenytoin effect.

Sulfonamides can also displace methotrexate from plasma protein binding sites, thus increasing free methotrexate concentrations.

Drug/Laboratory Test Interactions: Septra, specifically the trimethoprim component, can interfere with a serum methotrexate assay as determined by the competitive binding protein technique (CBPA) when a bacterial dihydrofolate reductase is used as the binding protein. No interference occurs, however, if methotrexate is measured by a radioimmunoassay (RIA).

The presence of trimethoprim and sulfamethoxazole may also interfere with the Jaffé alkaline picrate reaction assay for creatinine resulting in over-estimations of about 10% in the range of normal values.

Carcinogenesis, Mutagenesis, Impairment of Fertility:

Carcinogenesis: Long-term studies in animals to evaluate carcinogenic potential have not been conducted with Septra I.V. Infusion.

Mutagenesis: Bacterial mutagenic studies have not been performed with sulfamethoxazole and trimethoprim in combination. Trimethoprim was demonstrated to be non-mutagenic in the Ames assay. No chromosomal damage was observed in human leukocytes cultured *in vitro* with sulfamethoxazole and trimethoprim alone or in combination; the concentrations used exceeded blood levels of these compounds following therapy with Septra. Observations of leukocytes obtained from patients treated with Septra revealed no chromosomal abnormalities.

Impairment of Fertility: Septra I.V. Infusion has not been studied in animals for evidence of impairment of fertility. However, studies in rats at oral dosages as high as 70 mg/kg trimethoprim plus 350 mg/kg sulfamethoxazole daily showed no adverse effects on fertility or general reproductive performance.

Pregnancy: *Teratogenic Effects:* Pregnancy Category C. In rats, oral doses of 533 mg/kg sulfamethoxazole or 200 mg/kg trimethoprim produced teratological effects manifested mainly as cleft palates. The highest dose which did not cause cleft palates in rats was 512 mg/kg sulfamethoxazole or 192 mg/kg trimethoprim when administered separately. In two studies in rats, no teratology was observed when 512 mg/kg of sulfamethoxazole was used in combination with 128 mg/kg of trimethoprim. In one study, however, cleft palates were observed in one litter out of 9 when 355 mg/kg of sulfamethoxazole was used in combination with 88 mg/kg of trimethoprim.

In some rabbit studies, an overall increase in fetal loss (dead and resorbed and malformed conceptuses) was associated with doses of trimethoprim 6 times the human therapeutic dose.

While there are no large, well-controlled studies on the use of trimethoprim and sulfamethoxazole in pregnant women. Brumfitt and Pursell[5], in a retrospective study, reported the outcome of 186 pregnancies during which the mother received either placebo or oral trimethoprim and sulfamethoxazole. The incidence of congenital abnormalities was 4.5% (3 of 66) in those who received placebo and 3.3% (4 of 120) in those receiving trimethoprim and sulfamethoxazole. There were no abnormalities in the 10 children whose mothers received the drug during the first trimester. In a separate survey, Brumfitt and Pursell also found no congenital abnormalities in 35 children whose mothers had received oral trimethoprim and sulfamethoxazole at the time of conception or shortly thereafter.

Because trimethoprim and sulfamethoxazole may interfere with folic acid metabolism, Septra I.V. Infusion should be used during pregnancy only if the potential benefit justifies the potential risk to the fetus.

Nonteratogenic Effects: See CONTRAINDICATIONS section.

Nursing Mothers: See CONTRAINDICATIONS section.

Pediatric Use: Septra I.V. Infusion is not recommended for infants younger than two months of age (see CONTRAINDICATIONS section).

ADVERSE REACTIONS

The most common adverse effects are gastrointestinal disturbances (nausea, vomiting, anorexia) and allergic skin reactions (such as rash and urticaria). **FATALITIES ASSOCIATED WITH THE ADMINISTRATION OF SULFONAMIDES, ALTHOUGH RARE, HAVE OCCURRED DUE TO SEVERE REACTIONS, INCLUDING STEVENS-JOHNSON SYNDROME, TOXIC EPIDERMAL NECROLYSIS, FULMINANT HEPATIC NECROSIS, AGRANULOCYTOSIS, APLASTIC ANEMIA AND OTHER BLOOD DYSCRASIAS (SEE WARNINGS SECTION).** Local reaction, pain and slight irritation on I.V. administration are infrequent. Thrombophlebitis has rarely been observed.

Hematologic: Agranulocytosis, aplastic anemia, thrombocytopenia, leukopenia, neutropenia, hemolytic anemia, megaloblastic anemia, hypoprothrombinemia, methemoglobinemia, eosinophilia.

Allergic Reactions: Stevens-Johnson syndrome, toxic epidermal necrolysis, anaphylaxis, allergic myocarditis, erythema multiforme, exfoliative dermatitis, angioedema, drug fever, chills, Henoch-Schoenlein purpura, serum sickness-like syndrome, generalized allergic reactions, generalized skin eruptions, conjunctival and scleral injection, photosensitivity, pruritus, urticaria and rash. In addition, periarteritis nodosa and systemic lupus erythematosus have been reported.

Gastrointestinal: Hepatitis including cholestatic jaundice and hepatic necrosis, elevation of serum transaminase and bilirubin, pseudomembranous enterocolitis, pancreatitis, stomatitis, glossitis, nausea, emesis, abdominal pain, diarrhea, anorexia.

Genitourinary: Renal failure, interstitial nephritis, BUN and serum creatinine elevation, toxic nephrosis with oliguria and anuria, and crystalluria.

Neurologic: Aseptic meningitis, convulsions, peripheral neuritis, ataxia, vertigo, tinnitus, headache.

Psychiatric: Hallucinations, depression, apathy, nervousness.

Endocrine: The sulfonamides bear certain chemical similarities to some goitrogens, diuretics (acetazolamide and the thiazides) and oral hypoglycemic agents. Cross-sensitivity may exist with these agents. Diuresis and hypoglycemia have occurred rarely in patients receiving sulfonamides.

Musculoskeletal: Arthralgia and myalgia.

Miscellaneous: Weakness, fatigue, insomnia.

OVERDOSAGE

Acute: Since there has been no extensive experience in humans with single doses of Septra I.V. Infusion in excess of 25 ml (400 mg trimethoprim and 2000 mg sulfamethoxazole), the maximum tolerated dose in humans is unknown. Signs and symptoms of overdosage reported with sulfonamides include anorexia, colic, nausea, vomiting, dizziness, headache, drowsiness and unconsciousness. Pyrexia, hematuria and crystalluria may be noted. Blood dyscrasias and jaundice are potential late manifestations of overdosage. Signs of acute overdosage with trimethoprim include nausea, vomiting, dizziness, headache, mental depression, confusion and bone marrow depression.

General principles of treatment include the administration of intravenous fluids if urine output is low and renal function is normal. Acidification of the urine will increase renal elimination of trimethoprim. The patient should be monitored with blood counts and appropriate blood chemistries, including electrolytes. If a significant blood dyscrasia or jaundice occurs, specific therapy should be instituted for these complications. Peritoneal dialysis is not effective and hemodialysis is only moderately effective in eliminating trimethoprim and sulfamethoxazole.

Chronic: Use of Septra I.V. Infusion at high doses and/or for extended periods of time may cause bone marrow depression manifested as thrombocytopenia, leukopenia, and/or megaloblastic anemia. If signs of bone marrow depression occur, the patient should be given leucovorin 5 to 15 mg daily until normal hematopoiesis is restored.

Animal Toxicity: The LD_{50} of Septra I.V. Infusion in mice is 700 mg/kg or 7.3 ml/kg; in rats and rabbits the LD_{50} is > 500 mg/kg or > 5.2 ml/kg. The vehicle produced the same LD_{50} in each of these species as the active drug.

The signs and symptoms noted in mice, rats and rabbits with Septra I.V. Infusion or its vehicle at the high I.V. doses used

Continued on next page

Burroughs Wellcome—Cont.

in acute toxicity studies included ataxia, decreased motor activity, loss of righting reflex, tremors or convulsions, and/or respiratory depression.

DOSAGE AND ADMINISTRATION

CONTRAINDICATED IN INFANTS LESS THAN TWO MONTHS OF AGE. CAUTION—SEPTRA I.V. INFUSION MUST BE DILUTED IN 5% DEXTROSE IN WATER SOLUTION PRIOR TO ADMINISTRATION. DO NOT MIX SEPTRA I.V. INFUSION WITH OTHER DRUGS OR SOLUTIONS. RAPID INFUSION OR BOLUS INJECTION MUST BE AVOIDED.

DOSAGE

Children and Adults:

PNEUMOCYSTIS CARINII PNEUMONITIS: Total daily dose is 15 to 20 mg/kg (based on the trimethoprim component) given in three to four equally divided doses every 6 or 8 hours for up to 14 days. One investigator noted that a total daily dose of 10 to 15 mg/kg was sufficient in 10 adult patients with normal renal function.[6]

SEVERE URINARY TRACT INFECTIONS AND SHIGELLOSIS: Total daily dose is 8 to 10 mg/kg (based on the trimethoprim component) given in two to four equally divided doses every 6, 8 or 12 hours for up to 14 days for severe urinary tract infections and 5 days for shigellosis. The maximum recommended daily dose is 60 ml per day.

For Patients with Impaired Renal Function: When renal function is impaired, a reduced dosage should be employed using the following table:

Creatinine Clearance (ml/min)	Recommended Dosage Regimen
Above 30	Use Standard Regimen
15–30	½ the Usual Regimen
Below 15	Use Not Recommended

Method of Preparation: Septra I.V. Infusion must be diluted. EACH 5 ML SHOULD BE ADDED TO 125 ML OF 5% DEXTROSE IN WATER. After diluting with 5% dextrose in water the solution should not be refrigerated and should be used within 6 hours. If a dilution of 5 ml per 100 ml of 5% dextrose in water is desired, it should be used within 4 hours. If upon visual inspection there is cloudiness or evidence of crystallization after mixing, the solution should be discarded and a fresh solution prepared.

Multiple Dose Vial: After initial entry into the vial, the remaining contents must be used within 48 hours.

The following infusion systems have been tested and found satisfactory: unit-dose glass containers; unit-dose polyvinyl chloride and polyolefin containers. No other systems have been tested and therefore no others can be recommended.

Dilution: EACH 5 ML OF SEPTRA I.V. INFUSION SHOULD BE ADDED TO 125 ML OF 5% DEXTROSE IN WATER.

***NOTE:* In those instances where fluid restriction is desirable,** each 5 ml may be added to 75 ml of 5% dextrose in water. Under these circumstances the solution should be mixed just prior to use and should be administered within two (2) hours. If upon visual inspection there is cloudiness or evidence of crystallization after mixing, the solution should be discarded and a fresh solution prepared.

DO NOT MIX SEPTRA I.V. INFUSION-5% DEXTROSE IN WATER WITH DRUGS OR SOLUTIONS IN THE SAME CONTAINER.

ADMINISTRATION

The solution should be given by intravenous infusion over a period of 60 to 90 minutes. Rapid infusion or bolus injections must be avoided. Septra I.V. Infusion should not be given intramuscularly.

HOW SUPPLIED

5 ml ampuls, containing 80 mg trimethoprim (16 mg/ml) and 400 mg sulfamethoxazole (80 mg/ml) for infusion with 5% dextrose in water. Boxes of 10 (NDC-0081-0856-10)

5 ml vials, containing 80 mg trimethoprim (16 mg/ml) and 400 mg sulfamethoxazole (80 mg/ml) for infusion with 5% dextrose in water. Box of 10. (NDC-0081-0856-44).

10 ml multiple dose vials, containing 160 mg trimethoprim (16 mg/ml) and 800 mg sulfamethoxazole (80 mg/ml) for infusion with 5% dextrose in water. Box of 10 (NDC-0081-0856-95)

20 ml multiple dose vial, containing 320 mg trimethoprim (16 mg/ml) and 1600 mg sulfamethoxazole (80 mg/ml) for infusion with 5% dextrose in water. Box of 1 (NDC-0081-0856-93)

STORE AT ROOM TEMPERATURE 15°–30°C (59°–86°F). DO NOT REFRIGERATE.

Also available in tablets containing 80 mg trimethoprim and 400 mg sulfamethoxazole (bottles of 100 and 500; unit dose pack of 100); DS (double strength) tablets containing 160 mg trimethoprim and 800 mg sulfamethoxazole (bottles of 100 and 250; unit dose pack of 100, and COMPLIANCE™ Pak of 20); and oral suspension containing 40 mg trimethoprim and 200 mg sulfamethoxazole in each 5 ml (bottle of 1 pint [473 ml]; Unit of Use: bottle of 100 ml with child-resistant cap).

REFERENCES

1. Grose WE, Bodey GP, Loo TL: Clinical Pharmacology of Intravenously Administered Trimethoprim-Sulfamethoxazole. *Antimicrob Agents Chemother 15:* 447–451, March 1979.
2. Siber GR, Gorham C, Durbin W, Lesko L, Levin MJ: Pharmacology of Intravenous Trimethoprim-Sulfamethoxazole in Children and Adults. Current Chemotherapy and Infectious Diseases, American Society for Microbiology, Washington, D.C., 1980, Vol. 1, pp. 691–692.
3. Bauer AW, Kirby WMM, Sherris JC, Turck M: Antibiotic Susceptibility Testing by Standardized Single Disk Method. *Am J Clin Path 45:* 493–496, April 1966.
4. Approved Standard ASM-2 Performance Standards for Antimicrobial Disc Susceptibility Test: National Committee for Clinical Laboratory Standards, 771 East Lancaster Avenue, Villanova, Pennsylvania 19085.
5. Brumfitt W and Pursell R: Trimethoprim/Sulfamethoxazole in the Treatment of Bacteriuria in Women. *J Infect Dis 128 (Suppl):* S657–S663, Nov. 1973.
6. Winston DJ, Lau WK, Gale RP, Young LS: Trimethoprim-Sulfamethoxazole for the Treatment of *Pneumocystis carinii* pneumonia. *Ann Int Med 92:* 762–769, June 1980.

*Mfd. under U.S. Patent No. 3,956,327

SEPTRA® TABLETS ℞

[sĕp'trah]

SEPTRA ® DS (Double Strength) TABLETS ℞

SEPTRA® SUSPENSION ℞

(TRIMETHOPRIM AND SULFAMETHOXAZOLE)

DESCRIPTION

Septra (Trimethoprim and Sulfamethoxazole) is a synthetic antibacterial combination product.

Each Septra Tablet contains 80 mg trimethoprim* and 400 mg sulfamethoxazole and the inactive ingredients docusate sodium, FD&C Red No. 40, magnesium stearate, povidone, and sodium starch glycolate.

Each Septra DS (double strength) Tablet contains 160 mg trimethoprim* and 800 mg sulfamethoxazole and the inactive ingredients docusate sodium, FD&C Red No. 40, magnesium stearate, povidone, and sodium starch glycolate.

Each teaspoonful (5 ml) of Septra Suspension contains 40 mg trimethoprim* and 200 mg sulfamethoxazole and the inactive ingredients alcohol 0.26%, methylparaben 0.1% and sodium benzoate 0.1% (added as preservatives), carboxymethylcellulose sodium, citric acid, FD&C Red No. 40 and Yellow No. 6, flavor, gvlycerin, microcrystalline cellulose, Polysorbate 80, saccharin, sodium, and sorbitol. Both tablet and suspension forms are for oral administration.

Trimethoprim is 2,4-diamino-5-(3,4,5-trimethoxybenzyl)-pyrimidine. It is a white to light yellow, odorless, bitter compound with a molecular weight of 290.3.

Sulfamethoxazole is N^1-(5-methyl-3-isoxazolyl)sulfanilamide. It is an almost white, odorless, tasteless compound with a molecular weight of 253.28.

CLINICAL PHARMACOLOGY

Septra is rapidly absorbed following oral administration. Both sulfamethoxazole and trimethoprim exist in the blood as unbound, protein-bound and metabolized forms; sulfamethoxazole also exists as the conjugated form. The metabolism of sulfamethoxazole occurs predominately by N_4-acetylation, although the glucuronide conjugate has been identified. The principal metabolites of trimethoprim are the 1- and 3-oxides and the 3'- and 4'-hydroxy derivatives. The free forms of sulfamethoxazole and trimethoprim are considered to be the therapeutically active forms. Approximately 44% of trimethoprim and 70% of sulfamethoxazole are bound to plasma proteins. The presence of 10 mg percent sulfamethoxazole in plasma decreases the protein binding of trimethoprim by an insignificant degree; trimethoprim does not influence the protein binding of sulfamethoxazole.

Peak blood levels for the individual components occur 1 to 4 hours after oral administration. The mean serum half-lives of sulfamethoxazole and trimethoprim are 10 and 8 to 10 hours, respectively. However, patients with severely impaired renal function exhibit an increase in the half-lives of both components, requiring dosage regimen adjustment (see DOSAGE AND ADMINISTRATION section). Detectable amounts of trimethoprim and sulfamethoxazole are present in the blood 24 hours after drug administration. During administration of 160 mg trimethoprim and 800 mg sulfamethoxazole *b.i.d.*, the mean steady state plasma concentration of trimethoprim was 1.72 μg/ml. The steady state minimal plasma levels of free and total sulfamethoxazole were 57.4 μg/ml and 68.0 μg/ml, respectively. These steady state levels were achieved after three days of drug administration[1].

Excretion of sulfamethoxazole and trimethoprim is primarily by the kidneys through both glomerular filtration and tubular secretion. Urine concentrations of both sulfamethoxazole and trimethoprim are considerably higher than are the concentrations in the blood. The average percentage of the dose recovered in urine from 0 to 72 hours after a single oral dose is 84.5% for total sulfonamide and 66.8% for free trimethoprim. Thirty percent of the total sulfonamide is excreted as free sulfamethoxazole, with the remaining as N_4-acetylated metabolite.[2] When administered together as Septra, neither sulfamethoxazole nor trimethoprim affects the urinary excretion pattern of the other.

Both trimethoprim and sulfamethoxazole distribute to sputum, vaginal fluid, and middle ear fluid; trimethoprim also distributes to bronchial secretion and both pass the placental barrier and are excreted in breast milk.

Microbiology: Sulfamethoxazole inhibits bacterial synthesis of dihydrofolic acid by competing with *para*-aminobenzoic acid (PABA). Trimethoprim blocks the production of tetrahydrofolic acid from dihydrofolic acid by binding to and reversibly inhibiting the required enzyme, dihydrofolate reductase. Thus, Septra blocks two consecutive steps in the biosynthesis of nucleic acids and proteins essential to many bacteria.

In vitro studies have shown that bacterial resistance develops more slowly with Septra than with either trimethoprim or sulfamethoxazole alone.

In vitro serial dilution tests have shown that the spectrum of antibacterial activity of Septra includes the common urinary tract pathogens with the exception of *Pseudomonas aeruginosa*. The following organisms are usually susceptible: *Escherichia coli, Klebsiella* species, *Enterobacter* species, *Morganella morganii, Proteus mirabilis* and indole-positive *Proteus* species including *Proteus vulgaris*.

The usual spectrum of antimicrobial activity of Septra includes bacterial pathogens isolated from middle ear exudate and from bronchial secretions: *Haemophilus influenzae*, including ampicillin-resistant strains, and *Streptococcus pneumoniae. Shigella flexneri* and *Shigella sonnei* are also usually susceptible.

[See table left].

The recommended quantitative disc susceptibility method may be used for estimating the susceptibility of bacteria to Septra.[3,4] With this procedure, a report from the laboratory of "Susceptible to trimethoprim and sulfamethoxazole" indicates that the infection is likely to respond to therapy with Septra. If the infection is confined to the urine, a report of "Intermediate susceptibility to trimethoprim and sulfamethoxazole" also indicates that the infection is likely to respond. A report of "Resistant to trimethoprim and sulfamethoxazole" indicates that the infection is unlikely to respond to therapy with Septra.

REPRESENTATIVE MINIMUM INHIBITORY CONCENTRATION VALUES FOR SEPTRA SUSCEPTIBLE ORGANISMS (MIC-μg/ml)

Bacteria	TMP Alone	SMX Alone	TMP/SMX (1:19) TMP	SMX
Escherichia coli	0.05–1.5	1.0–245	0.05–0.5	0.95–9.5
Proteus species (indole positive)	0.5–5.0	7.35–300	0.05–1.5	0.95–28.5
Morganella morganii	0.5–5.0	7.35–300	0.05–1.5	0.95–28.5
Proteus mirabilis	0.5–1.5	7.35–30	0.05–0.15	0.95–2.85
Klebsiella species	0.15–5.0	2.45–245	0.05–1.5	0.95–28.5
Enterobacter species	0.15–5.0	2.45–245	0.05–1.5	0.95–28.5
Haemophilus influenzae	0.15–1.5	2.85–95	0.015–0.15	0.285–2.85
Streptococcus pneumoniae	0.15–1.5	7.35–24.5	0.05–0.15	0.95–2.85
Shigella flexneri †	<0.01–0.04	<0.16–>320	<0.002–0.03	0.04–0.625
Shigella sonnei †	0.02–0.08	0.625–>320	0.004–0.06	0.08–1.25

TMP = Trimethoprim SMX = Sulfamethoxazole

†Rudoy RC, Nelson JD, Haltalin KC. *Antimicrobial Agents and Chemotherapy* 5:439-43, 1974.

INDICATIONS AND USAGE

URINARY TRACT INFECTIONS: For the treatment of urinary tract infections due to susceptible strains of the following organisms: *Escherichia coli*, *Klebsiella* species, *Enterobacter* species, *Morganella morganii*, *Proteus mirabilis*, and *Proteus vulgaris*. It is recommended that initial episodes of uncomplicated urinary tract infections be treated with a single effective antibacterial agent rather than the combination.

ACUTE OTITIS MEDIA: For the treatment of acute otitis media in children due to susceptible strains of *Streptococcus pneumoniae* or *Haemophilus influenzae* when in the judgment of the physician Septra offers some advantage over the use of other antimicrobial agents. To date, there are limited data on the safety of repeated use of Septra in children under two years of age. Septra is not indicated for prophylactic or prolonged administration in otitis media at any age.

ACUTE EXACERBATIONS OF CHRONIC BRONCHITIS IN ADULTS: For the treatment of acute exacerbations of chronic bronchitis due to susceptible strains of *Streptococcus pneumoniae* or *Haemophilus influenzae* when in the judgment of the physician, Septra offers some advantage over the use of a single antimicrobial agent.

SHIGELLOSIS: For the treatment of enteritis caused by susceptible strains of *Shigella flexneri* and *Shigella sonnei* when antibacterial therapy is indicated.

PNEUMOCYSTIS CARINII PNEUMONITIS: For the treatment of documented *Pneumocystis carinii* pneumonitis (see PRECAUTIONS section).

CONTRAINDICATIONS

Hypersensitivity to trimethoprim or sulfonamides. Patients with documented megaloblastic anemia due to folate deficiency. Pregnancy at term and during the nursing period, because sulfonamides pass the placenta and are excreted in the milk and may cause kernicterus. Infants less than two months of age.

WARNINGS

FATALITIES ASSOCIATED WITH THE ADMINISTRATION OF SULFONAMIDES, ALTHOUGH RARE, HAVE OCCURRED DUE TO SEVERE REACTIONS, INCLUDING STEVENS-JOHNSON SYNDROME, TOXIC EPIDERMAL NECROLYSIS, FULMINANT HEPATIC NECROSIS, AGRANULOCYTOSIS, APLASTIC ANEMIA AND OTHER BLOOD DYSCRASIAS.

SEPTRA SHOULD BE DISCONTINUED AT THE FIRST APPEARANCE OF SKIN RASH OR ANY SIGN OF ADVERSE REACTION. Clinical signs, such as rash, sore throat, fever, pallor, purpura or jaundice may be early indications of serious reactions. In rare instances a skin rash may be followed by more severe reactions, such as Stevens-Johnson syndrome, toxic epidermal necrolysis, hepatic necrosis or serious blood disorder. Complete blood counts should be done frequently in patients receiving sulfonamides.

SEPTRA SHOULD NOT BE USED IN THE TREATMENT OF STREPTOCOCCAL PHARYNGITIS. Clinical studies have documented that patients with group A β-hemolytic streptococcal tonsillopharyngitis have a greater incidence of bacteriologic failure when treated with Septra than do those patients treated with penicillin, as evidenced by failure to eradicate this organism from the tonsillopharyngeal area.

PRECAUTIONS

General: Septra should be given with caution to patients with impaired renal or hepatic function, to those with possible folate deficiency (e.g., the elderly, chronic alcoholics, patients receiving anticonvulsant therapy, patients with malabsorption syndrome, and patients in malnutrition states) and to those with severe allergy or bronchial asthma. In glucose-6-phosphate dehydrogenase-deficient individuals, hemolysis may occur. This reaction is frequently dose-related.

Use in the Elderly: There may be an increased risk of severe adverse reactions in elderly patients, particularly when complicating conditions exist, e.g., impaired kidney and/or liver function, or concomitant use of other drugs. Severe skin reactions, or generalized bone marrow suppression (see WARNINGS and ADVERSE REACTIONS sections) or a specific decrease in platelets (with or without purpura) are the most frequently reported severe adverse reactions in elderly patients. In those concurrently receiving certain diuretics, primarily thiazides, an increased incidence of thrombocytopenia with purpura has been reported. Appropriate dosage adjustments should be made for patients with impaired kidney function (see DOSAGE AND AMDINISTRATION section).

Use in the Treatment of *Pneumocystis carinii* Pneumonitis in Patients with Acquired Immunodeficiency Syndrome (AIDS): Because of their unique immune dysfunction, AIDS patients may not tolerate or respond to Septra in the same manner as non-AIDS patients. The incidence of side effects, particularly rash, fever, and leukopenia, with Septra therapy in AIDS patients who are being treated for *Pneumocystis carinii* pneumonitis has been reported to be greatly increased compared with the incidence normally associated with the use of Septra in non-AIDS patients.

Information for Patients: Patients should be instructed to maintain an adequate fluid intake in order to prevent crystalluria and stone formation.

Laboratory Tests: Complete blood counts should be done frequently in patients receiving Septra; if a significant reduction in the count of any formed blood element is noted, Septra should be discontinued. Urinalysis with careful microscopic examination and renal function tests should be performed during therapy, particularly for those patients with impaired renal function.

Drug Interactions: In elderly patients concurrently receiving certain diuretics, primarily thiazides, an increased incidence of thrombocytopenia with purpura has been reported. It has been reported that Septra may prolong the prothrombin time in patients who are receiving the anticoagulant warfarin. This interaction should be kept in mind when Septra is given to patients already on anticoagulant therapy, and the coagulation time should be reassessed.

Septra may inhibit the hepatic metabolism of phenytoin. Septra, given at a common clinical dosage, increased the phenytoin half-life by 39% and decreased the phenytoin metabolic clearance rate by 27%. When administering these drugs concurrently, one should be alert for possible excessive phenytoin effect. Sulfonamides can also displace methotrexate from plasma protein binding sites, thus increasing free methotrexate concentrations.

Drug/Laboratory Test Interactions: Septra, specifically the trimethoprim component, can interfere with a serum methotrexate assay as determined by the competitive binding protein technique (CBPA) when a bacterial dihydrofolate reductase is used as the binding protein. No interference occurs, however, if methotrexate is measured by a radioimmunoassay (RIA).

The presence of trimethoprim and sulfamethoxazole may also interfere with the Jaffé alkaline picrate reaction assay for creatinine resulting in over-estimations of about 10% in the range of normal values.

Carcinogenesis, Mutagenesis, Impairment of Fertility:

Carcinogenesis: Long-term studies in animals to evaluate carcinogenic potential have not been conducted with Septra.

Mutagenesis: Bacterial mutagenic studies have not been performed with sulfamethoxazole and trimethoprim in combination. Trimethoprim was demonstrated to be non-mutagenic in the Ames assay. No chromosomal damage was observed in human leukocytes cultured *in vitro* with sulfamethoxazole and trimethoprim alone or in combination; the concentrations used exceeded blood levels of these compounds following therapy with Septra. Observations of leukocytes obtained from patients treated with Septra revealed no chromosomal abnormalities.

Impairment of Fertility: No adverse effects on fertility or general reproductive performance were observed in rats given oral dosages as high as 70 mg/kg/day trimethoprim plus 350 mg/kg/day sulfamethoxazole.

Pregnancy: *Teratogenic Effects:* Pregnancy Category C. In rats, oral doses of 533 mg/kg sulfamethoxazole or 200 mg/kg trimethoprim produced teratological effects manifested mainly as cleft palates. The highest dose which did not cause cleft palates in rats was 512 mg/kg sulfamethoxazole or 192 mg/kg trimethoprim when administered separately. In two studies in rats, no teratology was observed when 512 mg/kg of sulfamethoxazole was used in combination with 128 mg/kg of trimethoprim. In one study, however, cleft palates were observed in one litter out of 9 when 355 mg/kg of sulfamethoxazole was used in combination with 88 mg/kg of trimethoprim.

In some rabbit studies, an overall increase in fetal loss (dead and resorbed and malformed conceptuses) was associated with doses of trimethoprim 6 times the human therapeutic dose.

While there are no large, well-controlled studies on the use of trimethoprim and sulfamethoxazole in pregnant women, Brumfitt and Pursell[5], in a retrospective study, reported the outcome of 186 pregnancies during which the mother received either placebo or trimethoprim and sulfamethoxazole. The incidence of congenital abnormalities was 4.5% (3 of 66) in those who received placebo and 3.3% (4 of 120) in those receiving trimethoprim and sulfamethoxazole. There were no abnormalities in the 10 children whose mothers received the drug during the first trimester. In a separate survey, Brumfitt and Pursell also found no congenital abnormalities in 35 children whose mothers had received oral trimethoprim and sulfamethoxazole at the time of conception or shortly thereafter.

Because trimethoprim and sulfamethoxazole may interfere with folic acid metabolism, Septra should be used during pregnancy only if the potential benefit justifies the potential risk to the fetus.

Nonteratogenic Effects: See CONTRAINDICATIONS section.

Nursing Mothers: See CONTRAINDICATIONS section.

Pediatric Use: Septra is not recommended for infants younger than two months of age (see INDICATIONS AND USAGE and CONTRAINDICATIONS sections).

ADVERSE REACTIONS

The most common adverse effects are gastrointestinal disturbances (nausea, vomiting, anorexia) and allergic skin reactions (such as rash and urticaria). **FATALITIES ASSOCIATED WITH THE ADMINISTRATION OF SULFONAMIDES, ALTHOUGH RARE, HAVE OCCURRED DUE TO SEVERE REACTIONS, INCLUDING STEVENS-JOHNSON SYNDROME, TOXIC EPIDERMAL NECROLYSIS, FULMINANT HEPATIC NECROSIS, AGRANULOCYTOSIS, APLASTIC ANEMIA AND OTHER BLOOD DYSCRASIAS (SEE WARNINGS SECTION).**

Hematologic: Agranulocytosis, aplastic anemia, thrombocytopenia, leukopenia, neutropenia, hemolytic anemia, megaloblastic anemia, hypoprothrombinemia, methemoglobinemia, eosinophilia.

Allergic Reactions: Stevens-Johnson syndrome, toxic epidermal necrolysis, anaphylaxis, allergic myocarditis, erythema multiforme, exfoliative dermatitis, angioedema, drug fever, chills, Henoch-Schoenlein purpura, serum sickness-like syndrome, generalized allergic reactions, generalized skin eruptions, photosensitivity, conjunctival and scleral injection, pruritus, urticaria and rash. In addition, periarteritis nodosa and systemic lupus erythematosus have been reported.

Gastrointestinal: Hepatitis including cholestatic jaundice and hepatic necrosis, elevation of serum transaminase and bilirubin, pseudomembranous enterocolitis, pancreatitis, stomatitis, glossitis, nausea, emesis, abdominal pain, diarrhea, anorexia.

Genitourinary: Renal failure, interstitial nephritis, BUN and serum creatinine elevation, toxic nephrosis with oliguria and anuria, and crystalluria.

Neurologic: Aseptic meningitis, convulsions, peripheral neuritis, ataxia, vertigo, tinnitus, headache.

Psychiatric: Hallucinations, depression, apathy, nervousness.

Endocrine: The sulfonamides bear certain chemical similarities to some goitrogens, diuretics (acetazolamide and the thiazides) and oral hypoglycemic agents. Cross-sensitivity may exist with these agents. Diuresis and hypoglycemia have occurred rarely in patients receiving sulfonamides.

Musculoskeletal: Arthralgia and myalgia.

Miscellaneous: Weakness, fatigue, insomnia.

OVERDOSAGE

Acute: The amount of a single dose of Septra that is either associated with symptoms of overdosage or is likely to be life-threatening has not been reported. Signs and symptoms of overdosage reported with sulfonamides include anorexia, colic, nausea, vomiting, dizziness, headache, drowsiness and unconsciousness. Pyrexia, hematuria and crystalluria may be noted. Blood dyscrasias and jaundice are potential late manifestations of overdosage. Signs of acute overdosage with trimethoprim include nausea, vomiting, dizziness, headache, mental depression, confusion and bone marrow depression.

General principles of treatment include the institution of gastric lavage or emesis; forcing oral fluids; and the administration of intravenous fluids if urine output is low and renal function is normal. Acidification of the urine will increase renal elimination of trimethoprim. The patient should be monitored with blood counts and appropriate blood chemistries, including electrolytes. If a significant blood dyscrasia or jaundice occurs, specific therapy should be instituted for these complications. Peritoneal dialysis is not effective and hemodialysis is only moderately effective in eliminating trimethoprim and sulfamethoxazole.

Chronic: Use of Septra at high doses and/or for extended periods of time may cause bone marrow depression manifested as thrombocytopenia, leukopenia and/or megaloblastic anemia. If signs of bone marrow depression occur, the patient should be given leucovorin 5 to 15 mg daily until normal hematopoiesis is restored.

DOSAGE AND ADMINISTRATION

Not recommended for use in infants less than two months of age.

URINARY TRACT INFECTIONS AND SHIGELLOSIS IN ADULTS AND CHILDREN AND ACUTE OTITIS MEDIA IN CHILDREN:

Adults: The usual adult dosage in the treatment of urinary tract infections is one Septra DS (double strength) tablet, two Septra tablets or four teaspoonfuls (20 ml) Septra Suspension every 12 hours for 10 to 14 days. An identical daily dosage is used for 5 days in the treatment of shigellosis.

Children: The recommended dose for children with urinary tract infections or acute otitis media is 8 mg/kg trimethoprim and 40 mg/kg sulfamethoxazole per 24 hours, given in two divided doses every 12 hours for 10 days. An identical daily dosage is used for 5 days in the treatment of shigellosis.

Continued on next page

Burroughs Wellcome—Cont.

The following table is a guideline for the attainment of this dosage:

Children: Two months of age or older

Weight lb	Weight kg	Dose—every 12 hours Teaspoonfuls	Dose—every 12 hours Tablets
22	10	1 (5 ml)	
44	20	2 (10 ml)	1
66	30	3 (15 ml)	1 ½
88	40	4 (20 ml)	2 (or 1 DS Tablet)

For patients with impaired renal function: When renal function is impaired, a reduced dosage should be employed using the following table:

Creatinine Clearance (ml/min)	Recommended Dosage Regimen
Above 30	Use Standard Regimen
15–30	½ the Usual Regimen
Below 15	Use Not Recommended

ACUTE EXACERBATIONS OF CHRONIC BRONCHITIS IN ADULTS: The usual adult dosage in the treatment of acute exacerbations of chronic bronchitis is one Septra DS (double strength) tablet, two Septra tablets or four teaspoonfuls (20 ml) Septra Suspension every 12 hours for 14 days.

PNEUMOCYSTIS CARINII PNEUMONITIS:

The recommended dosage for patients with documented *Pneumocystis carinii* pneumonitis is 20 mg/kg trimethoprim and 100 mg/kg sulfamethoxazole per 24 hours given in equally divided doses every 6 hours for 14 days. The following table is a guideline for the attainment of this dosage in children:

Weight lb	Weight kg	Dose—every 6 hours Teaspoonfuls	Dose—every 6 hours Tablets
18	8	1 (5 ml)	
35	16	2 (10 ml)	1
53	24	3 (15 ml)	1 ½
70	32	4 (20 ml)	2 (or 1 DS Tablet)

HOW SUPPLIED

TABLETS (pink, scored, round-shaped), containing 80 mg trimethoprim and 400 mg sulfamethoxazole—bottles of 100 (NDC-0081-0852-55) and 500 (NDC-0081-0852-70); unit dose pack of 100 (NDC-0081-0852-56). Imprint on tablets "SEPTRA" and "Y2B."

DS (DOUBLE STRENGTH) TABLETS (pink, scored, oval-shaped) containing 160 mg trimethoprim and 800 mg sulfamethoxazole-bottles of 100 (NDC-0081-0853-55) and 250 (NDC-0081-0853-65); unit dose pack of 100 (NDC-0081-0853-56) and COMPLIANCE™ Pak of 20 (NDC-0081-0853-20). Imprint on tablets "SEPTRA DS" and "O2C."

ORAL SUSPENSION (pink, cherry flavored) containing 40 mg trimethoprim and 200 mg sulfamethoxazole in each teaspoonful (5 ml) - bottle of 1 pint (473 ml) (NDC-0081-0855-96). Unit of Use: bottle of 100 ml with child-resistant cap (NDC-0081-0855-09).

Tablets should be stored at 15°–30°C (59°–86°F) in a dry place and protected from light.

Suspension should be stored at 15°–30°C (59°–86°F) and protected from light.

Also available:

SEPTRA I.V. Infusion: 5 ml ampul, containing 80 mg trimethoprim (16 mg/ml) and 400 mg sulfamethoxazole (80 mg/ml), box of 10; 10 ml multiple dose vial, containing 160 mg trimethoprim (16 mg/ml) and 800 mg sulfamethoxazole (80 mg/ml), box of 10; 20 ml multiple dose vial, containing 320 mg trimethoprim (16 mg/ml) and 1600 mg sulfamethoxazole (80 mg/ml), box of 1.

REFERENCES

1. Kremers P, Duvivier J and Heusghem C. Pharmacokinetic Studies of Co-Trimoxazole in Man after Single and Repeated Doses, *J. Clin Pharmacol 14:* 112–117, 1974.
2. Kaplan SA, *et al:* Pharmacokinetic Profile of Trimethoprim-Sulfamethoxazole in Man. *J Infect Dis 128:* S547–S554, November 1973.
3. Federal Register, *37:* 20527–20529, 1972.
4. Bauer AW, Kirby WMM, Sheriss JC, Turck M: Antibiotic Susceptibility Testing by Standardized Single Disk Method. *Am J Clin Path 45:* 493–496, April 1966.
5. Brumfitt W and Pursell R: Trimethoprim/Sulfamethoxazole in the Treatment of Bacteriuria in Women. *J Infect Dis 128 (Suppl):* S657–S663, November 1973.

*Mfd. under U.S. Patent No. 3,956,327
U.S. Patent No. 4,209,513 (Tablet)
Shown in Product Identification Section, page 407

SUDAFED® COUGH SYRUP

[*sū 'dah-fĕd"*]
Decongestant/Cough Suppressant/Expectorant

(See PDR For Nonprescription Drugs)

SUDAFED® TABLETS
CHILDREN'S SUDAFED® LIQUID

[*sū 'dah-fĕd"*]
(See PDR for Nonprescription Drugs)

SUDAFED® PLUS LIQUID/TABLETS

(See PDR For Nonprescription Drugs)
Shown in Product Identification Section, page 407

TABLOID® brand THIOGUANINE ℞

[*tab 'loid*]
40 mg Scored Tablets

CAUTION: Tabloid brand thioguanine is a potent drug. It should not be used unless a diagnosis of acute nonlymphocytic leukemia has been adequately established and the responsible physician is knowledgeable in assessing response to chemotherapy.

DESCRIPTION

Tabloid brand thioguanine was synthesized and developed by Hitchings, Elion and associates at the Wellcome Research Laboratories. It is one of a large series of purine analogues which interfere with nucleic acid biosynthesis, and has been found active against selective human neoplastic diseases.[1]

Thioguanine, known chemically as 2-amino-1,7-dihydro-6*H*-purine-6-thione, is an analogue of the nucleic acid constituent guanine, and is closely related structurally and functionally to Purinethol® (mercaptopurine).

Tabloid brand thioguanine is available in tablets for oral administration. Each scored tablet contains 40 mg thioguanine and the inactive ingredients gum acacia, lactose, magnesium stearate, potato starch, and stearic acid.

CLINICAL PHARMACOLOGY

Clinical studies have shown that the absorption of an oral dose of thioguanine in man is incomplete and variable, averaging approximately 30% of the administered dose (range: 14–46%).[2,3] Following oral administration of ^{35}S-6-thioguanine, total plasma radioactivity reached a maximum at eight hours and declined slowly thereafter. Parent drug represented only a very small fraction of the total plasma radioactivity at any time, being virtually undetectable throughout the period of measurements.

The oral administration of radiolabeled thioguanine revealed only trace quantities of parent drug in the urine. However, a methylated metabolite, 2-amino-6-methylthiopurine (MTG), appeared very early, rose to a maximum six to eight hours after drug administration, and was still being excreted after 12 to 22 hours. Radiolabeled sulfate appeared somewhat later than MTG but was the principal metabolite after eight hours. Thiouric acid and some unidentified products were found in the urine in small amounts.[3]

Intravenous administration of ^{35}S-6-thioguanine disclosed a median plasma half-disappearance time of 80 minutes (range: 25–240 minutes) when the compound was given in single doses of 65 to 300 mg/m^2. Although initial plasma levels of thioguanine did correlate with the dose level, there was no correlation between the plasma half-disappearance time and the dose.[2]

Thioguanine is incorporated into the DNA and the RNA of human bone marrow cells. Studies with intravenous ^{35}S-6-thioguanine have shown that the amount of thioguanine incorporated into nucleic acids is more than 100 times higher after five daily doses than after a single dose. With the 5-dose schedule, from one-half to virtually all of the guanine in the residual DNA was replaced by thioguanine.[2] Tissue distribution studies of ^{35}S-6-thioguanine in mice showed only traces of radioactivity in brain after oral administration. No measurements have been made of thioguanine concentrations in human cerebrospinal fluid, but observations on tissue distribution in animals, together with the lack of CNS penetration by the closely related compound, mercaptopurine, suggest that thioguanine does not reach therapeutic concentrations in the CSF.

Monitoring of plasma levels of thioguanine during therapy is of questionable value.[3] There is technical difficulty in determining plasma concentrations, which are seldom greater than 1 to 2 micrograms per ml after a therapeutic oral dose. More significantly, thioguanine enters rapidly into the anabolic and catabolic pathways for purines, and the active intracellular metabolites have appreciably longer half-lives than the parent drug. The biochemical effects of a single dose of thioguanine are evident long after the parent drug has disappeared from plasma. Because of this rapid metabolism of thioguanine to active intracellular derivatives, hemodialysis would not be expected to appreciably reduce toxicity of the drug.

Thioguanine competes with hypoxanthine and guanine for the enzyme hypoxanthine-guanine phosphoribosyltransferase (HGPRTase) and is itself converted to 6-thioguanylic acid (TGMP). This nucleotide reaches high intracellular concentrations at therapeutic doses. TGMP interferes at several points with the synthesis of guanine nucleotides. It inhibits *de novo* purine biosynthesis by pseudo-feedback inhibition of glutamine-5-phosphoribosylpyrophosphate amidotransferase—the first enzyme unique to the *de novo* pathway for purine ribonucleotide synthesis. TGMP also inhibits the conversion of inosinic acid (IMP) to xanthylic acid (XMP) by competition for the enzyme, IMP dehydrogenase. At one time TGMP was felt to be a significant inhibitor of ATP:GMP phosphotransferase (guanylate kinase),[4] but recent results have shown this not to be so.[5]

Thioguanylic acid is further converted to the di- and tri-phosphates, thioguanosine diphosphate (TGDP) and thioguanosine triphosphate (TGTP) (as well as their 2′-deoxyribosyl analogues) by the same enzymes which metabolize guanine nucleotides.[6] Thioguanine nucleotides are incorporated into both the RNA and the DNA by phosphodiester linkages[2] and it has been argued that incorporation of such fraudulent bases contributes to the cytotoxicity of thioguanine.

Thus, thioguanine has multiple metabolic effects and at present it is not possible to designate one major site of action. Its tumor inhibitory properties may be due to one or more of its effects on (a) feedback inhibition of *de novo* purine synthesis; (b) inhibition of purine nucleotide interconversions; or (c) incorporation into the DNA and the RNA. The net consequence of its actions is a sequential blockade of the synthesis and utilization of the purine nucleotides.[4,6,7]

The catabolism of thioguanine and its metabolites is complex and shows significant differences between man and the mouse.[2,3] In both humans and mice, after oral administration of ^{35}S-6-thioguanine, urine contains virtually no detectable intact thioguanine. While deamination and subsequent oxidation to thiouric acid occurs only to a small extent in man, it is the main pathway in mice. The product of deamination by guanase, 6-thioxanthine, is inactive, having negligible antitumor activity. This pathway of thioguanine inactivation is not dependent on the action of xanthine oxidase and an inhibitor of that enzyme (such as allopurinol), will not block the detoxification of thioguanine even though the inactive 6-thioxanthine is normally further oxidized by xanthine oxidase to thiouric acid before it is eliminated. In man, methylation of thioguanine is much more extensive than in the mouse. The product of methylation, 2-amino-6-methylthiopurine, is also substantially less active and less toxic than thioguanine and its formation is likewise unaffected by the presence of allopurinol. Appreciable amounts of inorganic sulfate are also found in both murine and human urine, presumably arising from further metabolism of the methylated derivatives.

In some animal tumors, resistance to the effect of thioguanine correlates with the loss of HGPRTase activity and the resulting inability to convert thioguanine to thioguanylic acid. However, other resistance mechanisms, such as increased catabolism of TGMP by a nonspecific phosphatase, may be operative. Although not invariable, it is usual to find cross-resistance between thioguanine and its close analogue, Purinethol® (mercaptopurine).

INDICATIONS AND USAGE

a) Acute Nonlymphocytic Leukemias: Tabloid brand thioguanine is indicated for remission induction, remission consolidation, and maintenance therapy of acute nonlymphocytic leukemias.[8,9] The response to this agent depends upon the age of the patient (younger patients faring better than older), and whether thioguanine is used in previously treated or previously untreated patients. Reliance upon thioguanine alone is seldom justified for initial remission induction of acute nonlymphocytic leukemias because combination chemotherapy including thioguanine results in more frequent remission induction and longer duration of remission than thioguanine alone.

b) Other Neoplasms: Tabloid brand thioguanine is not effective in chronic lymphocytic leukemia, Hodgkin's lymphoma, multiple myeloma, or solid tumors. Although thioguanine is one of several agents with activity in the treatment of the chronic phase of chronic myelogenous leukemia, more objective repsonses are observed with Myleran® (busulfan), and therefore busulfan is usually regarded as the preferred drug.

CONTRAINDICATIONS

Thioguanine should not be used in patients whose disease has demonstrated prior resistance to this drug. In animals and man, there is usually complete cross-resistance between Purinethol® (mercaptopurine) and Tabloid® brand thioguanine.

WARNINGS

SINCE DRUGS USED IN CANCER CHEMOTHERAPY ARE POTENTIALLY HAZARDOUS, IT IS RECOMMENDED THAT ONLY PHYSICIANS EXPERIENCED WITH THE RISKS OF THIOGUANINE AND KNOWLEDGEABLE IN THE NATURAL HISTORY OF ACUTE NONLYMPHOCYTIC LEUKEMIAS ADMINISTER THIS DRUG.

The most consistent, dose-related toxicity is bone marrow suppression. This may be manifest by anemia, leukopenia, thrombocytopenia, or any combination of these. Any one of these findings may also reflect progression of the underlying disease. Since thioguanine may have a delayed effect, it is important to withdraw the medication temporarily at the first sign of an abnormally large fall in any of the formed elements of the blood.

It is recommended that evaluation of the hemoglobin concentration or hematocrit; total white blood cell count and differential count; and quantitative platelet count be obtained frequently while the patient is on thioguanine therapy. In cases where the cause of fluctuations in the formed elements in the peripheral blood is obscure, bone marrow examination may be useful for the evaluation of marrow status. The decision to increase, decrease, continue or discontinue a given dosage of thioguanine must be based not only on the absolute hematologic values, but also upon the rapidity with which changes are occurring. In many instances, particularly during the induction phase of acute leukemia, complete blood counts will need to be done more frequently in order to evaluate the effect of the therapy. The dosage of thioguanine may need to be reduced when this agent is combined with other drugs whose primary toxicity is myelosuppression.

Myelosuppression is often unavoidable during the induction phase of adult acute nonlymphocytic leukemias if remission induction is to be successful. Whether or not this demands modification or cessation of dosage depends both upon the response of the underlying disease and a careful consideration of supportive facilities (granulocyte and platelet transfusions) which may be available. Life-threatening infections and bleeding have been observed as consequences of thioguanine-induced granulocytopenia and thrombocytopenia.

The effect of thioguanine on the immunocompetence of patients is unknown.

Pregnancy: ***"Pregnancy Category D":*** Drugs such as thioguanine are potential mutagens and teratogens. Thioguanine may cause fetal harm when administered to a pregnant woman. Thioguanine has been shown to be teratogenic in rats when given in doses five (5) times the human dose. When given to the rat on the 4th and 5th days of gestation, 13% of surviving placentas did not contain fetuses, and 19% of offspring were malformed or stunted. The malformations noted included generalized edema, cranial defects and general skeletal hypoplasia, hydrocephalus, ventral hernia, situs inversus, and incomplete development of the limbs.[10] There are no adequate and well-controlled studies in pregnant women. If this drug is used during pregnancy, or if the patient becomes pregnant while taking the drug, the patient should be apprised of the potential hazard to the fetus. Women of childbearing potential should be advised to avoid becoming pregnant.

PRECAUTIONS

General: Although the primary toxicity of thioguanine is myelosuppression, other toxicities have occasionally been observed, particularly when thioguanine is used in combination with other cancer chemotherapeutic agents.

A few cases of jaundice have been reported in patients with leukemia receiving thioguanine. Among these were two adult male patients and four children with acute myelogenous leukemia and an adult male with acute lymphocytic leukemia who developed veno-occlusive hepatic disease while receiving chemotherapy for their leukemia.[11,12] Six patients had received cytarabine prior to treatment with thioguanine, and some were receiving other chemotherapy in addition to thioguanine when they became symptomatic. While veno-occlusive hepatic disease has not been reported in patients treated with thioguanine alone, it is recommended that thioguanine be withheld if there is evidence of toxic hepatitis or biliary stasis, and that appropriate clinical and laboratory investigations be initiated to establish the etiology of the hepatic dysfunction. Deterioration in liver function studies during thioguanine therapy should prompt discontinuation of treatment and a search for an explanation of the hepatotoxicity.

Information For Patients: It is imperative that patients be instructed to report promptly the development of fever, sore throat, signs of local infection, bleeding from any site, or symptoms suggestive of anemia. Women of childbearing potential should be advised to avoid becoming pregnant.

Laboratory Tests: It is advisable to monitor liver function tests (serum transaminases, alkaline phosphatase, bilirubin) at weekly intervals when first beginning therapy and at monthly intervals thereafter. It may be advisable to perform liver function tests more frequently in patients with known pre-existing liver disease or in patients who are receiving thioguanine and other hepatotoxic drugs. Patients should be instructed to discontinue thioguanine immediately if clinical jaundice is detected. (See WARNINGS section).

Drug Interactions: There is usually complete cross-resistance between Purinethol® (mercaptopurine) and Tabloid® brand thioguanine.

Carcinogenesis, Mutagenesis, Impairment of Fertility: In view of its action on cellular DNA, thioguanine is potentially mutagenic and carcinogenic, and consideration should be given to the theoretical risk of carcinogenesis when thioguanine is administered. (See WARNINGS section)

Pregnancy: ***Teratogenic Effects:*** Pregnancy Category D. See WARNINGS section.

Nursing Mothers: It is not known whether this drug is excreted in human milk. Because of the potential for tumorigenicity shown for thioguanine, a decision should be made whether to discontinue nursing or to discontinue the drug, taking into account the importance of the drug to the mother.

ADVERSE REACTIONS

The most frequent adverse reaction to thioguanine is myelosuppression. The induction of complete remission of acute myelogenous leukemia usually requires combination chemotherapy in dosages which produce marrow hypoplasia.[13] Since consolidation and maintenance of remission are also effected by multiple drug regimens whose component agents cause myelosuppression, pancytopenia is observed in nearly all patients. Dosages and schedules must be adjusted to prevent life-threatening cytopenias whenever these adverse reactions are observed.

Hyperuricemia frequently occurs in patients receiving thioguanine as a consequence of rapid cell lysis accompanying the antineoplastic effect. Adverse effects can be minimized by increased hydration, urine alkalinization, and the prophylactic administration of a xanthine oxidase inhibitor such as Zyloprim® (allopurinol). Unlike Purinethol® (mercaptopurine) and Imuran® (azathioprine), thioguanine may be continued in the usual dosage when allopurinol is used conjointly to inhibit uric acid formation.

Less frequent adverse reactions include nausea, vomiting, anorexia and stomatitis. Liver enzyme and other liver function studies are occasionally abnormal. If jaundice, hepatomegaly or anorexia with tenderness in the right hypochondrium occurs, thioguanine should be withheld until the exact etiology can be determined. There have been reports of veno-occlusive liver disease occuring in patients who received combination chemotherapy including thioguanine.[11,12] Intestinal necrosis and perforation have been reported also in patients who received multiple drug chemotherapy including thioguanine.

OVERDOSAGE

Signs and symptoms of overdosage may be immediate, such as nausea, vomiting, malaise, hypertension and diaphoresis; or delayed, such as myelosuppression and azotemia.[14] It is not known whether thioguanine is dialyzable. Hemodialysis is thought to be of marginal use due to the rapid intracellular incorporation of thioguanine into active metabolites with long persistence. The oral LD_{50} of thioguanine was determined to be 823 mg/kg $\pm$ 50.73 mg/kg and 740 mg/kg $\pm$ 45.24 mg/kg for male and female rats respectively.[15] Symptoms of overdosage may occur after a single dose of as little as 2.0 to 3.0 mg/kg thioguanine. As much as 35 mg/kg has been given in a single oral dose with reversible myelosuppression observed. There is no known pharmacologic antagonist of thioguanine. The drug should be discontinued immediately if unintended toxicity occurs during treatment. Severe hematologic toxicity may require supportive therapy with platelet transfusions for bleeding, and granulocyte transfusions and antibiotics if sepsis is documented. If a patient is seen immediately following an accidental overdosage of the drug, it may be useful to induce emesis.

DOSAGE AND ADMINISTRATION

Tabloid brand thioguanine is administered orally. The dosage which will be tolerated and effective varies according to the stage and type of neoplastic process being treated. Because the usual therapies for adult and childhood acute nonlymphocytic leukemias involve the use of thioguanine with other agents in combination, physicians responsible for administering these therapies should be experienced in the use of cancer chemotherapy and in the chosen protocol.

Ninety-six (59%) of one hundred sixty-three children with previously untreated acute nonlymphocytic leukemia obtained complete remission with a multiple drug protocol including thioguanine, prednisone, cytarabine, cyclophosphamide, and vincristine. Remission was maintained with daily thioguanine, four-day pulses of cytarabine and cyclophosphamide, and a single dose of vincristine every 28 days. The median duration of remission was 11.5 months.[8]

Fifty-three percent of previously untreated adults with acute nonlymphocytic leukemias attained remission following use of the combination of thioguanine and cytarabine according to a protocol developed at The Memorial Sloan-Kettering Cancer Center. A median duration of remission of 8.8 months was achieved with the multiple drug maintenance regimen which included thioguanine.[9]

On those occasions when single agent chemotherapy with thioguanine may be appropriate, the usual initial dosage for children and adults is approximately 2 mg/kg of body weight per day. If, after four weeks on this dosage, there is no clinical improvement and no leukocyte or platelet depression, the dosage may be cautiously increased to 3 mg/kg per day. The total daily dose may be given at one time.

The dosage of thioguanine used does not depend on whether or not the patient is receiving Zyloprim® (allopurinol); **this is in contradistinction to the dosage reduction which is mandatory when Purinethol® (mercaptopurine) or IMURAN® (azathioprine) is given simultaneously with allopurinol.**

HOW SUPPLIED

Greenish-yellow, scored tablets containing 40 mg thioguanine, imprinted with "WELLCOME" and "U3B" on each tablet; in bottle of 25 (NDC-0081-0880-25). Store at 15°–25°C (59°–77°F) in a dry place.

REFERENCES

1. Hitchings GH, and Elion GB: The Chemistry and Biochemistry of Purine Analogs. *Ann NY Acad Sci 60:* 195–199, 1954.
2. LePage GA, and Whitecar JP Jr.: Pharmacology of 6-Thioguanine in Man. *Cancer Res 31:* 1627–1631, 1971.
3. Elion GB: Biochemistry and Pharmacology of Purine Analogues. *Fed Proc 26:* 898–904, 1967.
4. Miech RP, Parks RE, Jr., Anderson JH, Jr. and Sartorelli AC: An Hypothesis on the Mechanism of Action of 6-thioguanine. *Biochem Pharmacol 16:* 2222–2227, 1967.
5. Miller RL, Adamczyk DL, and Spector T: Reassessment of the Inter-Actions of Guanylate Kinase and 6-thioguanine 5′-phosphate. *Proc Am Assoc Cancer Res 18:* 6, 1977. *Abstract.*
6. Paterson ARP and Tidd DN: 6-Thiopurines. In: *Antineoplastic and Immunosuppressive Agents,* Part II. (Edited by AC Sartorelli and DG Johns.) Berlin, Springer-Verlag, 384–403, 1975.
7. Nelson JA, Carpenter JW, Rose LN, and Adamson DJ: Mechanisms of Action of 6-thioguanine, 6-mercaptopurine, and 8-azaguanine. *Cancer Res 35:* 2872–2878, 1975.
8. Chard RL, Finkelstein JZ, Sonley MJ, *et al.:* Increased Survival in Childhood Acute Nonlymphocytic Leukemia after Treatment with Prednisone, Cytosine Arabinoside, 6-thioguanine, Cyclophosphamide, and Oncovin (PATCO) Combination Chemotherapy. *Med Ped Oncol 4:* 263–273, 1978.
9. Mertelsmann R, Drapkin RL, Gee TS, *et al.:* Treatment of Acute Nonlymphocytic Leukemia in Adults. *Cancer 48:* 2136–2142, 1981.
10. Theiresch JB: Effect of 2-6 Diamino-purine (2-6 DP): 6 Chlorpurine (CIP) and Thioguanine (ThG) on Rat Litter *in utero. Proc Soc Exp Biol Med 94:* 40–43, 1957.
11. Griner PF, Elbadawi A, and Packman CH: Veno-Occlusive Disease of the Liver After Chemotherapy of Acute Leukemia. *Ann Inter Med 85:* 578–582, 1976.
12. Gill RA, Onstad GR, Cardamone, JM, *et al.:* Hepatic Veno-Occlusive Disease Caused by 6-thioguanine. *Ann Intern Med 96:* 58–60, 1982.
13. Clarkson B, Dowling MD, Gee TS, *et al.:* Treatment of Acute Leukemia in Adults. *Cancer 36:* 775–795, 1975.
14. Presant CA, Denes AE, Klein L, *et al.:* Phase I and Preliminary Phase II Observations of High-dose Intermittent 6-thioguanine. *Cancer Treat Rep 64(10–11):* 1109–1113, 1980.
15. Unpublished data on file with Burroughs Wellcome Co.

Shown in Product Identification Section, page 407

TRACRIUM® INJECTION ℞

[*trā ′krē ″um*]

(ATRACURIUM BESYLATE)

This drug should be used only by adequately trained individuals familiar with its actions, characteristics, and hazards.

DESCRIPTION

Tracrium (atracurium besylate) is an intermediate-duration, nondepolarizing, skeletal muscle relaxant for intravenous administration. Atracurium besylate is designated as 2,2′-[pentamethylenebis(oxycarbonylethylene)]-bis(1,2,3,4-tetrahydro-6,7-dimethoxy-2-methyl-1-veratrylisoquinolinium) dibenzenesulfonate. It has a molecular weight of 1243.49, and its molecular formula is $C_{53}H_{72}N_2O_{12}{\bullet}2C_6H_5O_3S$.

Atracurium besylate is a complex molecule containing four sites at which different stereochemical configurations can occur. The symmetry of the molecule, however, results in only ten, instead of sixteen, possible different isomers. The manufacture of atracurium besylate results in these isomers being produced in unequal amounts but with a consistent ratio. Those molecules in which the methyl group attached to the quaternary nitrogen projects on the opposite side to

Continued on next page

Burroughs Wellcome—Cont.

the adjacent substituted-benzyl moiety predominate by approximately 3:1.

Tracrium Injection is a sterile, non-pyrogenic aqueous solution. Each ml contains 10 mg atracurium besylate. The pH is adjusted to 3.25–3.65 with benzenesulfonic acid. The multiple dose vial contains 0.9% benzyl alcohol added as a preservative. Tracrium slowly loses potency with time at the rate of approximately 6% per *year* under refrigeration (5°C). Rate of loss in potency increases to approximately 5% per *month* at 25°C(77°F). Tracrium Injection should be stored under refrigeration at 2° to 8°C (36° to 46°F) to preserve potency.

CLINICAL PHARMACOLOGY

Tracrium is a nondepolarizing skeletal muscle relaxant. Nondepolarizing agents antagonize the neurotransmitter action of acetylcholine by binding competitively with cholinergic receptor sites on the motor end-plate. This antagonism is inhibited, and neuromuscular block reversed, by acetylcholinesterase inhibitors such as neostigmine, edrophonium, and pyridostigmine.

Tracrium can be used most advantageously if muscle twitch response to peripheral nerve stimulation is monitored to assess degree of muscle relaxation.

The duration of neuromuscular blockade produced by Tracrium is approximately one-third to one-half the duration of blockade by d-tubocurarine, metocurine, and pancuronium at initially equipotent doses. As with other nondepolarizing neuromuscular blockers, the time to onset of paralysis decreases and the duration of maximum effect increases with increasing Tracrium doses.

The ED_{95} (dose required to produce 95% suppression of the muscle twitch response with balanced anesthesia) has averaged 0.23 mg/kg (0.11 to 0.26 mg/kg in various studies). An initial Tracrium dose of 0.4 to 0.5 mg/kg generally produces maximum neuromuscular blockade within 3 to 5 minutes of injection, with good or excellent intubation conditions within 2 to 2.5 minutes in most patients. Recovery from neuromuscular blockade (under balanced anesthesia) can be expected to begin approximately 20 to 35 minutes after injection. Under balanced anesthesia, recovery to 25% of control is achieved approximately 35 to 45 minutes after injection, and recovery is usually 95% complete approximately 60–70 minutes after injection. The neuromuscular blocking action of Tracrium is enhanced in the presence of potent inhalation anesthetics. Isoflurane and enflurane increase the potency of Tracrium and prolong neuromuscular blockade by approximately 35%; however, halothane's potentiating effect (approximately 20%) is marginal (see DOSAGE AND ADMINISTRATION section).

Repeated administration of maintenance doses of Tracrium has no cumulative effect on the duration of neuromuscular blockade if recovery is allowed to begin prior to repeat dosing. Moreover, the time needed to recover from repeat doses does not change with additional doses. Repeat doses can therefore be administered at relatively regular intervals with predictable results. After an initial dose of 0.4 to 0.5 mg/kg under balanced anesthesia, the first maintenance dose (suggested maintenance dose is 0.08 to 0.10 mg/kg) is generally required within 20 to 45 minutes, and subsequent maintenance doses are usually required at approximately 15 to 25 minute intervals.

Once recovery from Tracrium's neuromuscular blocking effects begins, it proceeds more rapidly than recovery from d-tubocurarine, metocurine, and pancuronium. Regardless of Tracrium dose, the time from start of recovery (from complete block) to complete (95%) recovery is approximately 30 minutes under balanced anesthesia, and approximately 40 minutes under halothane, enflurane or isoflurane. Repeated doses have no cumulative effect on recovery rate.

Reversal of neuromuscular blockade produced by Tracrium can be achieved with an anticholinesterase agent such as neostigmine, edrophonium, or pyridostigmine, in conjunction with an anticholinergic agent such as atropine or glycopyrrolate. Under balanced anesthesia, reversal can usually be attempted approximately 20 to 35 minutes after an initial Tracrium dose of 0.4 to 0.5 mg/kg, or approximately 10 to 30 minutes after a 0.08 to 0.10 mg/kg maintenance dose, when recovery of muscle twitch has started. Complete reversal is usually attained within 8–10 minutes of the administration of reversing agents. Rare instances of breathing difficulties, possibly related to incomplete reversal, have been reported following attempted pharmacologic antagonism of Tracrium-induced neuromuscular blockade. As with other agents in this class, the tendency for residual neuromuscular block is increased if reversal is attempted at deep levels of blockade or if inadequate doses of reversal agents are employed.

The pharmacokinetics of Tracrium in man are essentially linear within the 0.3 to 0.6 mg/kg dose range. The elimination half-life is approximately 20 minutes. THE DURATION OF NEUROMUSCULAR BLOCKADE PRODUCED BY TRACRIUM DOES NOT CORRELATE WITH PLASMA PSEUDOCHOLINESTERASE LEVELS AND IS NOT ALTERED BY THE ABSENCE OF RENAL FUNCTION. This is consistent with the results of *in vitro* studies which have shown that Tracrium is inactivated in plasma via two nonoxidative pathways: ester hydrolysis, catalyzed by nonspecific esterases; and Hofmann elimination, a nonenzymatic chemical process which occurs at physiological pH. Some placental transfer occurs in humans.

Radiolabel studies demonstrated that Tracrium undergoes extensive degradation in cats, and that neither kidney nor liver plays a major role in its elimination. Biliary and urinary excretion were the major routes of excretion of radioactivity (totaling > 90% of the labeled dose within 7 hours of dosing), of which Tracrium represented only a minor fraction. The metabolites in bile and urine were similar, including products of Hofmann elimination and ester hydrolysis.

Tracrium is a less potent histamine releaser than d-tubocurarine or metocurine. Histamine release is minimal with initial Tracrium doses up to 0.5 mg/kg, and hemodynamic changes are minimal within the recommended dose range. A moderate histamine release and significant falls in blood pressure have been seen following 0.6 mg/kg of Tracrium. The histamine and hemodynamic responses were poorly correlated. The effects were generally short-lived and manageable, but the possibility of substantial histamine release in sensitive individuals or in patients in whom substantial histamine release would be especially hazardous (e.g., patients with significant cardiovascular disease) must be considered.

It is not known whether the prior use of other nondepolarizing neuromuscular blocking agents has any effect on the activity of Tracrium. The prior use of succinylcholine decreases by approximately 2 to 3 minutes the time to maximum blockade induced by Tracrium, and may increase the depth of blockade. Tracrium should be administered only after a patient recovers from succinylcholine-induced neuromuscular blockade.

INDICATIONS AND USAGE

Tracrium is indicated, as an adjunct to general anesthesia, to facilitate endotracheal intubation and to provide skeletal muscle relaxation during surgery or mechanical ventilation.

CONTRAINDICATIONS

Tracrium is contraindicated in patients known to have a hypersensitivity to it.

WARNINGS

TRACRIUM SHOULD BE USED ONLY BY THOSE SKILLED IN AIRWAY MANAGEMENT AND RESPIRATORY SUPPORT. EQUIPMENT AND PERSONNEL MUST BE IMMEDIATELY AVAILABLE FOR ENDOTRACHEAL INTUBATION AND SUPPORT OF VENTILATION, INCLUDING ADMINISTRATION OF POSITIVE PRESSURE OXYGEN. ADEQUACY OF RESPIRATION MUST BE ASSURED THROUGH ASSISTED OR CONTROLLED VENTILATION. ANTICHOLINESTERASE REVERSAL AGENTS SHOULD BE IMMEDIATELY AVAILABLE.

DO NOT GIVE TRACRIUM BY INTRAMUSCULAR ADMINISTRATION.

Tracrium has no known effect on consciousness, pain threshold, or cerebration. It should be used only with adequate anesthesia.

Tracrium Injection, which has an acid pH, should not be mixed with alkaline solutions (e.g., barbiturate solutions) in the same syringe or administered simultaneously during intravenous infusion through the same needle. Depending on the resultant pH of such mixtures, Tracrium may be inactivated and a free acid may be precipitated.

PRECAUTIONS

General: Although Tracrium is a less potent histamine releaser than d-tubocurarine or metocurine, the possibility of substantial histamine release in sensitive individuals must be considered. Special caution should be exercised in administering Tracrium to patients in whom substantial histamine release would be especially hazardous (e.g., patients with clinically significant cardiovascular disease) and in patients with any history (e.g., severe anaphylactoid reactions or asthma) suggesting a greater risk of histamine release. In these patients, the recommended initial Tracrium dose is lower (0.3 to 0.4 mg/kg) than for other patients and should be administered slowly or in divided doses over one minute.

Since Tracrium has no clinically significant effects on heart rate in the recommended dosage range, it will not counteract the bradycardia produced by many anesthetic agents or vagal stimulation. As a result, bradycardia during anesthesia may be more common with Tracrium than with other muscle relaxants.

Tracrium may have profound effects in patients with myasthenia gravis, Eaton-Lambert syndrome, or other neuromuscular diseases in which potentiation of nondepolarizing agents has been noted. The use of a peripheral nerve stimulator is especially important for assessing neuromuscular blockade in these patients. Similar precautions should be taken in patients with severe electrolyte disorders or carcinomatosis.

The safety of Tracrium has not been established in patients with bronchial asthma.

Drug Interactions: Drugs which may enhance the neuromuscular blocking action of Tracrium include: enflurane; isoflurane; halothane; certain antibiotics, especially the aminoglycosides and polymyxins; lithium; magnesium salts; procainamide; and quinidine.

If other muscle relaxants are used during the same procedure, the possibility of a synergistic or antagonist effect should be considered.

The prior administration of succinylcholine does not enhance the duration, but quickens the onset and may increase the depth of neuromuscular blockade induced by Tracrium. Tracrium should not be administered until a patient has recovered from succinylcholine-induced neuromuscular blockade.

Carcinogenesis, Mutagenesis, Impairment of Fertility: Carcinogenesis and fertility studies have not been performed. Atracurium was evaluated in a battery of three short term mutagenicity tests. It was non-mutagenic in both the Ames Salmonella assay at concentrations up to 1000 μg/plate, and in a rat bone marrow cytogenicity assay at up to paralyzing doses. A positive response was observed in the mouse lymphoma assay under conditions (80 and 100 μg/ml, in the absence of metabolic activation) which killed over 80% of the treated cells; there was no mutagenicity at 60 μg/ml and lower, concentrations which killed up to half of the treated cells. A far weaker response was observed in the presence of metabolic activation at concentrations (1200 μg/ml and higher) which also killed over 80% of the treated cells.

Mutagenicity testing is intended to stimulate chronic (years to lifetime) exposure in an effort to determine carcinogenicity. Thus, a single positive mutagenicity response for a drug used infrequently and/or briefly is of questionable clinical relevance.

Pregnancy: ***Teratogenic Effects:*** Pregnancy Category C. Tracrium has been shown to be potentially teratogenic in rabbits when given in doses up to approximately one-half the human dose. There are no adequate and well-controlled studies in pregnant women. Tracrium should be used during pregnancy only if the potential benefit justifies the potential risk to the fetus.

Tracrium was administered subcutaneously on days 6 through 18 of gestation to non-ventilated Dutch rabbits. Treatment groups were given either 0.15 mg/kg once daily or 0.10 mg/kg twice daily. Lethal respiratory distress occurred in two 0.15 mg/kg animals and in one 0.10 mg/kg animal, with transient respiratory distress or other evidence of neuromuscular blockade occurring in 10 of 19 and in 4 of 20 of the 0.15 mg/kg and 0.10 mg/kg animals, respectively. There was an increased incidence of certain spontaneously occurring visceral and skeletal anomalies or variations in one or both treated groups when compared to non-treated controls. The percentage of male fetuses was lower (41% vs. 51%) and the post-implantation losses were increased (15% vs. 8%) in the group given 0.15 mg/kg once daily when compared to the controls; the mean numbers of implants (6.5 vs. 4.4) and normal live fetuses (5.4 vs. 3.8) were greater in this group when compared to the control group.

Labor and Delivery: It is not known whether muscle relaxants administered during vaginal delivery have immediate or delayed adverse effects on the fetus or increase the likelihood that resuscitation of the newborn will be necessary. The possibility that forceps delivery will be necessary may increase.

Tracrium (0.3 mg/kg) has been administered to 26 pregnant women during delivery by cesarean section. No harmful effects were attributable to Tracrium in any of the newborn infants, although small amounts of Tracrium were shown to cross the placental barrier. The possibility of respiratory depression in the newborn infant should always be considered following cesarean section during which a neuromuscular blocking agent has been administered. In patients receiving magnesium sulfate, the reversal of neuromuscular blockade may be unsatisfactory and Tracrium dose should be lowered as indicated.

Nursing Mothers: It is not known whether this drug is excreted in human milk. Because many drugs are excreted in human milk, caution should be exercised when Tracrium is administered to a nursing woman.

Pediatric Use: Safety and effectiveness in children below the age of 1 month have not been established.

ADVERSE REACTIONS

Tracrium was well tolerated and produced few adverse reactions during extensive clinical trials. Most adverse reactions were suggestive of histamine release. In studies including 875 patients, Tracrium was discontinued in only one patient (who required treatment for bronchial secretions), and six other patients required treatment for adverse reactions attributable to Tracrium (wheezing in one, hypotension in five). Of the five patients who required treatment for hypotension, three had a history of significant cardiovascular disease. The overall incidence rate for clinically important adverse reactions, therefore, was 7/875 or 0.8%. The table

below includes all adverse reactions reported attributable to Tracrium during clinical trials with 875 patients.
[See table above].
Most adverse reactions were of little clinical significance unless they were associated with significant hemodynamic changes. The table below summarizes the incidences of substantial vital sign changes noted during Tracrium clinical trials with 530 patients, without cardiovascular disease, in whom these parameters were assessed.
[See table below].
Approximately one million patients received Tracrium during the first year following introduction to the U.S. market in December, 1983. Spontaneously reported adverse reactions were uncommon (approximately 0.02%). The following adverse reactions are among the most frequently reported, but there are insufficient data to support an estimate of their incidence:
Musculoskeletal: Inadequate block, prolonged block
Cardiovascular: Hypotension, vasodilatation (flushing), tachycardia, bradycardia
Respiratory: Dyspnea, bronchospasm, laryngospasm
Integumentary: Rash, urticaria, reaction at injection site

OVERDOSAGE

There has been limited experience with Tracrium overdosage. The possibility of iatrogenic overdosage can be minimized by carefully monitoring muscle twitch response to peripheral nerve stimulation. Excessive doses of Tracrium can be expected to produce enhanced pharmacological effects. Overdosage may increase the risk of histamine release and cardiovascular effects, especially hypotension. If cardiovascular support is necessary, this should include proper positioning, fluid administration, and the use of vasopressor agents if necessary. The patient's airway should be assured, with manual or mechanical ventilation maintained as necessary. A longer duration of neuromuscular blockade may result from overdosage and a peripheral nerve stimulator should be used to monitor recovery. Recovery may be facilitated by administration of an anticholinesterase reversing agent such as neostigmine, edrophonium, or pyridostigmine, in conjunction with an anticholinergic agent such as atropine or glycopyrrolate. The appropriate package inserts should be consulted for prescribing information.
Three pediatric patients (3 weeks, 4 and 5 months of age) unintentionally received doses of 0.8 mg/kg to 1.0 mg/kg of Tracrium. The time to 25% recovery (50 to 55 minutes) following these doses, which were 5 to 6 times the ED_{95} dose, was moderately longer than the corresponding time observed following doses 2.0 to 2.5 times the Tracrium ED_{95} dose in infants (22 to 36 minutes). Cardiovascular changes were minimal. Nonetheless the possibility of cardiovascular changes must be considered in the case of overdose.
An adult patient (17 years of age) unintentionally received an initial dose of 1.3 mg/kg of Tracrium. The time from injection to 25% recovery (83 minutes) was approximately twice that observed following maximum recommended doses in adults (35–45 minutes). The patient experienced moderate hemodynamic changes (13% increase in mean arterial pressure and 27% increase in heart rate) which persisted for 40 minutes and did not require treatment.
The intravenous LD_{50}'s determined in non-ventilated male and female albino mice and male Wistar rats were 1.9, 2.01 and 1.31 mg/kg, respectively. Deaths occurred within 2 minutes and were caused by respiratory paralysis. The subcutaneous LD_{50} determined in non-ventilated male Wistar rats was 282.8 mg/kg. Tremors, ptosis, loss of reflexes and respiratory failure preceded death which occurred 45–120 minutes after injection.

DOSAGE AND ADMINISTRATION

To avoid distress to the patient, Tracrium should not be administered before unconsciousness has been induced. Tracrium should not be mixed in the same syringe, or administered simultaneously through the same needle, with alkaline solutions (e.g., barbiturate solutions).
Tracrium should be administered intravenously. DO NOT GIVE TRACRIUM BY INTRAMUSCULAR ADMINISTRATION. Intramuscular administration of Tracrium may result in tissue irritation and there are no clinical data to support this route of administration.

PERCENT OF PATIENTS REPORTING ADVERSE REACTIONS

Adverse Reaction	Initial Tracrium Dose (mg/kg) 0.00-0.30 (n = 485)	0.31-0.50* (n = 366)	≥0.60 (n = 24)	Total (n = 875)
Skin Flush	1.0%	8.7%	29.2%	5.0%
Erythema	0.6%	0.5%	0%	0.6%
Itching	0.4%	0%	0%	0.2%
Wheezing/Bronchial Secretions	0.2%	0.3%	0%	0.2%
Hives	0.2%	0%	0%	0.1%

*Includes the recommended initial dosage range for most patients.

The use of a peripheral nerve stimulator to monitor muscle twitch suppression and recovery will permit the most advantageous use of Tracrium and minimize the possibility of overdosage.
Adults: A Tracrium dose of 0.4 to 0.5 mg/kg (1.7 to 2.2 times the ED_{95}), given as an intravenous bolus injection, is the recommended initial dose for most patients. With this dose, good or excellent conditions for nonemergency intubation can be expected in 2 to 2.5 minutes in most patients, with maximum neuromuscular blockade achieved approximately 3 to 5 minutes after injection. Clinically required neuromuscular blockade generally lasts 20 to 35 minutes under balanced anesthesia. Under balanced anesthesia, recovery to 25% of control is achieved approximately 35 to 45 minutes after injection, and recovery is usually 95% complete approximately 60 minutes after injection.
Tracrium is potentiated by isoflurane or enflurane anesthesia. The same initial Tracrium dose of 0.4 to 0.5 mg/kg may be used for intubation prior to administration of these inhalation agents; however, if Tracrium is first administered under steady state of isoflurane or enflurane, the initial Tracrium dose should be reduced by approximately one-third, i.e., to 0.25 to 0.35 mg/kg, to adjust for the potentiating effects of these anesthetic agents. With halothane, which has only a marginal (approximately 20%) potentiating effect on Tracrium, smaller dosage reductions may be considered.
Tracrium doses of 0.08 to 0.10 mg/kg are recommended for maintenance of neuromuscular blockade during prolonged surgical procedures. The first maintenance dose will generally be required 20 to 45 minutes after the initial Tracrium injection, but the need for maintenance doses should be determined by clinical criteria. Because Tracrium lacks cumulative effects, maintenance doses may be administered at relatively regular intervals for each patient, ranging approximately from 15 to 25 minutes under balanced anesthesia, slightly longer under isoflurane or enflurane. Higher Tracrium doses (up to 0.2 mg/kg) permit maintenance dosing at longer intervals.
Children and Infants: No Tracrium dosage adjustments are required for pediatric patients two years of age or older. A Tracrium dose of 0.3 to 0.4 mg/kg is recommended as the initial dose for infants (1 month to 2 years of age) under halothane anesthesia. Maintenance doses may be required with slightly greater frequency in infants and children than in adults.
Special Considerations: An initial Tracrium dose of 0.3 to 0.4 mg/kg, given slowly or in divided doses over one minute, is recommended for adults, children, or infants with significant cardiovascular disease and for adults, children, or infants with any history (e.g., severe anaphylactoid reactions or asthma) suggesting a greater risk of histamine release.
Dosage reductions must be considered also in patients with neuromuscular disease, severe electrolyte disorders, or carcinomatosis in which potentiation of neuromuscular blockade or difficulties with reversal have been demonstrated. There has been no clinical experience with Tracrium in these patients, and no specific dosage adjustments can be recommended. No Tracrium dosage adjustments are required for patients with renal disease.
An initial Tracrium dose of 0.3 to 0.4 mg/kg is recommended for adults following the use of succinylcholine for intubation under balanced anesthesia. Further reductions may be desirable with the use of potent inhalation anesthetics. The patient should be permitted to recover from the effects of succinylcholine prior to Tracrium administration. Insufficient data are available for recommendation of a specific initial Tracrium dose for administration following the use of succinylcholine in children and infants.
Parenteral drug products should be inspected visually for particulate matter and discoloration prior to administration, whenever solution and container permit.

HOW SUPPLIED

Tracrium Injection, 10 mg atracurium besylate in each ml.
5 ml ampuls (50 mg atracurium besylate per ampul). Box of 10 (NDC-0081-0940-10).
10 ml Multiple Dose Vial (100 mg atracurium besylate per vial). Box of 10 (NDC-0081-0940-95).
Store under refrigeration at 2° to 8°C (36° to 46°F); DO NOT FREEZE.
U.S. Patent No. 4179507

PERCENT OF PATIENTS SHOWING ≥30% VITAL SIGN CHANGES FOLLOWING ADMINISTRATION OF TRACRIUM

Vital Sign Change	Intial Tracrium Dose (mg/kg) 0.00-0.30 (n = 365)	0.31-0.50* (n = 144)	≥0.60 (n = 21)	Total (n = 530)
Mean Arterial Pressure				
Increase	1.9%	2.8%	0%	2.1%
Decrease	1.1%	2.1%	14.3%	1.9%
Heart Rate				
Increase	1.6%	2.8%	4.8%	2.1%
Decrease	0.8%	0%	0%	0.6%

*Includes the recommended initial dosage range for most patients.

VASOXYL® INJECTION ℞

[vāz″ox′ĭl]
(Methoxamine Hydrochloride)
20 mg in 1 ml

DESCRIPTION

Vasoxyl (methoxamine hydrochloride) Injection is a sterile solution for intravenous or intramuscular injection, made isotonic with sodium chloride. Each 1 ml ampul contains 20 mg methoxamine hydrochloride. Citric acid anhydrous 0.3% and sodium citrate 0.3% are added as buffers and potassium metabisulfite 0.1% is added as an antioxidant.
Methoxamine hydrochloride is a sympathomimetic amine. It has the empirical formula $C_{11}H_{17}NO_3 \cdot HCl$ and a molecular weight of 247.72. The drug is very soluble in water, soluble in ethanol, but practically insoluble in ether, benzene or chloroform. It is known chemically as α-(1-aminoethyl)-2,5-dimethoxybenzenemethanol hydrochloride.

CLINICAL PHARMACOLOGY

Vasoxyl is an alpha-receptor stimulant which produces a prompt and prolonged rise in blood pressure following parenteral administration. It is especially useful for maintaining blood pressure during operations under spinal anesthesia[1,2,3] and may also be safely used during general anesthesia. Vasoxyl does not increase the irritability of the cyclopropane-sensitized heart, making it useful during cyclopropane anesthesia.[4,5] Tachyphylaxis has not been a clinical problem.[1]
The major pharmaceutical effect of Vasoxyl is a potent, prolonged pressor action following parenteral administration. Vasoxyl differs from most other sympathomimetic amines both in animals[4,6,7] and in man[1,8] by having a predominantly peripheral action and lacking inotropic and chronotropic effects. Vasoxyl has less arrhythmogenic potential than other sympathomimetic amines and rarely causes ventricular tachycardia, fibrillation, or increased sinoatrial rate.[4] On occasion, a decrease in rate occurs as blood pressure increases,[1,9,10] apparently caused by a carotid sinus reflex. This bradycardia can be abolished by atropine.[9]
The pressor action appears to be due to peripheral vasoconstriction rather than a centrally mediated effect. Evidence for direct action of blood vessels is provided in part by the observation of intense constriction along the course of a vein into which Vasoxyl has been injected.[1] Vasoxyl also increases venous pressure.[8]
Following intravenous administration of Vasoxyl in dogs[11] and humans,[9,12] the peak pressor effect occurs within 0.5 to 2 minutes. In a group of human surgical patients,[13] the duration of the pressor effect following a single intravenous dose of 2 to 4 mg of Vasoxyl was 10 to 15 minutes. No clinical pharmacology studies are available concerning the onset and duration of action after administration of recommended intramuscular doses (10 to 15 mg). With administration of 10 to 40 mg Vasoxyl intramuscularly to patients, however, the peak effect occurs within 15 to 20 minutes, and the duration of action is approximately one and a half hours.[14]
Data from pharmacokinetic studies of Vasoxyl following either intravenous or intramuscular administration are not available.

Continued on next page

Burroughs Wellcome—Cont.

INDICATIONS AND USAGE

Vasoxyl is intended for supporting, restoring or maintaining blood pressure during anesthesia (including cyclopropane anesthesia). It can be used to terminate some episodes of supraventricular tachycardia.

CONTRAINDICATIONS

Vasoxyl is contraindicated in patients with severe hypertension, or in patients who are hypersensitive to methoxamine.

WARNINGS

The use of Vasoxyl in patients receiving monoamine oxidase inhibitors, tricyclic antidepressants or oxytocic agents such as vasopressin or certain ergot alkaloids may result in potentiation of the pressor effect (See "Drug Interactions" under PRECAUTIONS).

PRECAUTIONS

General: Vasoxyl, like other vasopressor agents, should be used with caution in patients with hyperthyroidism, bradycardia, partial heart block, myocardial disease, or severe arteriosclerosis. Caution should be exercised to avoid overdosage, preventing undesirable high blood pressure and/or bradycardia. Note: Bradycardia may be abolished with atropine (see OVERDOSAGE). Also, caution should be taken when Vasoxyl is used closely following the parenteral injection of ergot alkaloids to avoid an excessive rise in blood pressure.

Drug Interactions: The pressor effect of Vasoxyl may be markedly potentiated when Vasoxyl is used in conjunction with monoamine oxidase inhibitors, tricyclic antidepressants, vasopressin or ergot alkaloids such as ergotamine, ergonovine or methylergonovine. Therefore, when initiating pressor therapy in patients receiving these drugs the initial dose should be small and given with caution (see WARNINGS).

Drug/Laboratory Test Interactions: Vasoxyl may increase plasma cortisol and ACTH levels. Caution should be used when interpreting plasma cortisol and ACTH levels in a patient concurrently receiving Vasoxyl.[15,16]

Carcinogenesis, Mutagenesis, Impairment of Fertility: No long-term studies have been performed to evaluate the potential of Vasoxyl in these areas.

Pregnancy: *Teratogenic Effects:* Pregnancy Category C: Vasoxyl has been shown to decrease uterine blood flow, decrease fetal heart rate and adversely affect the fetal acid-base status in pregnant ewes and monkeys at doses comparable to those used in humans. There are no adequate and well-controlled studies in pregnant women. There has been one report of a fetal death; the mother received Vasoxyl concomitantly with several other drugs. A direct causal relationship to Vasoxyl was not established. Vasoxyl should be used during pregnancy only if the potential benefit justifies the potential risk to the fetus.

Vasoxyl (2.5 mg I.V., 1 to 3 times over a 45 min. period) given to 7 pregnant ewes showed a significant deterioration in fetal acid-base status as evidenced by hypoxia, hypercarbia and metabolic acidosis.[17] An inverse relationship between pressor response to Vasoxyl and uteroplacental blood flow has been shown in 16 pregnant ewes studied at doses ranging from 0.025 mg/kg to 0.2 mg/kg.[18] Uterine blood flow was decreased at all doses, but no significant change in fetal blood gas or acid-base status was demonstrated. Vasoxyl administration to 4 fetuses (50 mcg/kg/min for 60 min) and to 4 ewes (25 mcg/kg/min for 30 min) was associated with a decrease in fetal heart rate and uterine blood flow.[19] Nine monkeys studied at an average Vasoxyl dose of 1.3 mg/kg administered over 57 min showed a decrease in uterine blood flow and a possible association with fetal asphyxia.[20]

Labor and Delivery: If vasopressor drugs are used to correct hypotension or added to the local anesthetic solution during labor and delivery, some oxytocic drugs (vasopressin, ergotamine, ergonovine, methylergonovine) may cause severe persistent hypertension (see WARNINGS and "Drug Interactions" under PRECAUTIONS).

"Note": In pregnant animals, Vasoxyl has been shown to decrease uterine blood flow, possibly resulting in fetal asphyxia. Uterine hypertonus and fetal bradycardia may also be produced. (See ADVERSE REACTIONS and "Pregnancy" under PRECAUTIONS).

Nursing Mothers: It is not known whether this drug is excreted in human milk. Because many drugs are excreted in human milk, caution should be exercised when Vasoxyl is administered to a nursing woman.

Pediatric Use: Safety and effectiveness in children have not been established.

ADVERSE REACTIONS

The following adverse reactions have been observed, but there are insufficient data to support an estimate of their frequency:

Cardiovascular: Excessive blood pressure elevations particularly with high dosage, ventricular ectopic beats

Gastrointestinal: Nausea, vomiting (often projectile)

Central Nervous System: Headache (often severe), anxiety

Integumentary: Sweating, pilomotor response

Genitourinary: Uterine hypertonus, fetal bradycardia (see "Labor and Delivery" under PRECAUTIONS), urinary urgency

OVERDOSAGE

Overdosage of Vasoxyl may be manifested as an undesirable elevation in blood pressure and/or bradycardia. Should a clinically significant elevation of blood pressure occur that requires treatment, it may be immediately reversed with an alpha-adrenergic blocking agent (e.g. phentolamine). Bradycardia may be abolished by atropine.

DOSAGE AND ADMINISTRATION

Blood volume depletion should always be corrected before any vasopressor is administered. The usual intravenous dose of Vasoxyl for emergencies is 3 to 5 mg, injected slowly. Intravenous injection may be supplemented by intramuscular injections to provide a more prolonged effect. The usual intramuscular dose is 10 to 15 mg given shortly before or at the time of administering spinal anesthesia to prevent a fall in blood pressure. The tendency for the blood pressure to fall is greater with higher levels of spinal anesthesia, hence the dosage may be adjusted accordingly; 10 mg may be adequate at lower spinal levels while 15 to 20 mg may be required at high levels of spinal anesthesia. Repeated doses may be given if necessary, but time should be allowed for the previous dose to act (about 15 minutes, see CLINICAL PHARMACOLOGY). For cases of only moderate hypotension, 5 to 10 mg intramuscularly may be adequate.

For purposes of correcting a fall in blood pressure, an intramuscular injection of 10 to 15 mg of Vasoxyl may be given depending upon the degree of fall. In cases where the systolic pressure falls to 60 mmHg or less, or whenever an emergency exists, an intravenous injection of 3 to 5 mg Vasoxyl is indicated. This intravenous dose may be accompanied by 10 to 15 mg intramuscularly to provide more prolonged effect.

For termination of episodes of supraventricular tachycardia not responsive to other modes of therapy, the usual dose of Vasoxyl is 10 mg intravenously, administered by slow push (i.e 3 to 5 min).

Parenteral drug products should be inspected visually for particulate matter and discoloration prior to administration whenever solution and container permit.

HOW SUPPLIED

1 ml ampuls, containing 20 mg methoxamine hydrochloride. Box of 10 (NDC-0081-0957-10). Store at 15° to 30°C (59° to 86°F) and protect from light.

REFERENCES

1. King BD, Dripps RD: The use of methoxamine for maintenance of the circulation during spinal anesthesia. *Surg Gynecol Obstet* 1950;90:659–665.
2. Kistler EM, Ruben JE: Methoxamine in 1 percent procaine as a prophylactic vasopressor in spinal anesthesia. *Arch Surg* 1951;62:64–69.
3. Poe MF: Use of methoxamine hydrochloride as a pressor agent during spinal analgesia. *Anesthesiology* 1952;13:89–93.
4. Lahti RE, Brill IC, McCawley EL: The effect of methoxamine hydrochloride (Vasoxyl) on cardiac rhythm. *J Pharmacol Exp Ther* 1955;115:268–274.
5. Stutzman JW, Pettinga FL, Fruggiero EJ: Cardiac effects of methoxamine (β-[2,5-dimethoxy-phenyl]-β-hydroxyisopropylamine HCl) and desoxyephedrine during cyclopropane anesthesia. *J Pharmacol Exp Ther* 1949;97:385–387.
6. West JW, Faulk AT, Guzman SV: Comparative study of effects of levarterenol and methoxamine in shock associated with acute myocardial ischemia in dogs. *Circ Res* 1962;10:712–721.
7. Goldberg LI, Cotten M, Darby TD, Howell EV: Comparative heart contractile force effect of equipressor doses of several sympathomimetic amines. *J Pharmacol Exp Ther* 1953;108:177–185.
8. Aviado DM, Wnuck, AL: Mechanisms for cardiac slowing by methoxamine. *J Pharmacol Exp Ther* 1957;119:99–106.
9. Nathanson MH, Miller H: Clinical observations on a new epinephrin-like compound, methoxamine. *Am J Med Sci* 1952;223:270–279.
10. Stanfield, CA, Yu PN: Hemodynamic effects of methoxamine in mitral valve disease. *Circ Res* 1960;8:859–864.
11. Imai, S, Shigei T, Hashimoto K: Cardiac actions of methoxamine with special reference to its antagonist action to epinephrine. *Circ Res* 1961;9:552–560.
12. *The Extra Pharmacopoeia, Martindale* 28th Ed., Reynolds, JEF, ed., Pharmaceutical Press (London), pp.19.
13. Goldberg LI, Bloodwell RD, Braunwald E, *et al.* The direct effects of norepinephrine, epinephrine, and methoxamine on myocardial contractile force in man. *Circ* 1960;22:1125–1132.
14. Data on File, Burroughs Wellcome Co.
15. Laurian L, Oberman Z, Hoerner E, *et al.:* Low cortisol and growth hormone secretion in response to methoxamine administration in obese subjects. *Isr J Med Sci* 1977;13:477–481.
16. Nakai Y, Imura H, Yoshimi T, Matsukura S: Adrenergic control mechanism for acth secretion in man. *Acta Endocrinol* 1973; 74:263–270.
17. Shnider SM, DeLorimier AA, Asling JH, Morishima HO: Vasopressors in obstetrics. II. Fetal hazards of methoxamine administration during obstetric spinal anesthesia. *Am G Obstet Gynecol* 1970; 106:680–686.
18. Ralston DH, Shnider SM, DeLorimier AA: Effects of equipotent ephedrine, metaraminol, mephentermine and methoxamine on uterine blood flow in the pregnant ewe. *Anesthesiology* 1974;40:354–370.
19. Oakes GK, Ehrenkranz RA, Walker AM, *et al.:* Effect of α-adrenergic agonist and antagonist infusion on the umbilical and uterine circulations of pregnant sheep. *Biol Neonate* 1980;38:229–237.
20. Eng M, Berges PU, Ueland K, *et al.:* The effects of methoxamine and ephedrine in normotensive pregnant primates. *Anesthesiology* 1971;35:354–360.

VIROPTIC® OPHTHALMIC ℞
[*vī-rŏp 'tĭk"*]
SOLUTION, 1%
(trifluridine) Sterile

DESCRIPTION

Viroptic is the brand name for trifluridine (also known as trifluorothymidine, F_3TdR, F_3T), an antiviral drug for topical treatment of epithelial keratitis caused by Herpes simplex virus. The chemical name of trifluridine is 2′-deoxy-5-(trifluoromethyl)uridine.

Viroptic sterile ophthalmic solution contains 1% trifluridine in an aqueous solution with acetic acid and sodium acetate (buffers), sodium chloride, and thimerosal 0.001% (added as a preservative).

CLINICAL PHARMACOLOGY

Trifluridine is a fluorinated pyrimidine nucleoside with *in vitro* and *in vivo* activity against Herpes simplex virus, types 1 and 2 and vacciniavirus. Some strains of Adenovirus are also inhibited *in vitro.*

Trifluridine interferes with DNA synthesis in cultured mammalian cells. However, its antiviral mechanism of action is not completely known.

In vitro perfusion studies on excised rabbit corneas have shown that trifluridine penetrates the intact cornea as evidenced by recovery of parental drug and its major metabolite, 5-carboxy-2′-deoxyuridine, on the endothelial side of the cornea. Absence of the corneal epithelium enhances the penetration of trifluridine approximately two-fold.

Intraocular penetration of trifluridine occurs after topical instillation of Viroptic into human eyes. Decreased corneal integrity or stromal or uveal inflammation may enhance the penetration of trifluridine into the aqueous humor. Unlike the results of ocular penetration of trifluridine *in vitro*, 5-carboxy-2′-deoxyuridine was not found in detectable concentrations within the aqueous humor of the human eye.

Systemic absorption of trifluridine following therapeutic dosing with Viroptic appears to be negligible. No detectable concentrations of trifluridine or 5-carboxy-2′-deoxyuridine were found in the sera of adult healthy normal subjects who had Viroptic instilled into their eyes seven times daily for 14 consecutive days.

INDICATIONS AND USAGE

Viroptic (Trifluridine) Ophthalmic Solution, 1% is indicated for the treatment of primary keratoconjunctivitis and recurrent epithelial keratitis due to Herpes simplex virus, types 1 and 2. Viroptic is also effective in the treatment of epithelial keratitis that has not responded clinically to the topical administration of idoxuridine or when ocular toxicity or hypersensitivity to idoxuridine has occurred. In a smaller number of patients found to be resistant to topical vidarabine, Viroptic was also effective.

The clinical efficacy of Viroptic in the treatment of stromal keratitis and uveitis due to Herpes simplex virus or ophthalmic infections caused by vacciniavirus and Adenovirus has not been established by well-controlled clinical trials. Viroptic has not been shown to be effective in the prophylaxis of Herpes simplex virus keratoconjunctivitis and epithelial keratitis by well-controlled clinical trials. Viroptic is not effective against bacterial, fungal or chlamydial infections of the cornea or nonviral trophic lesions.

During controlled multicenter clinical trials, 92 of 97 (95%) patients (78 of 81 with dendritic and 14 of 16 with geographic ulcers) responded to Viroptic therapy as evidenced by complete corneal re-epithelialization within the 14 day therapy period. In these controlled studies, 56 of 75 (75%) patients (49 of 58 with dendritic and 7 of 17 with geographic ulcers) responded to idoxuridine therapy. The mean time to corneal re-epithelialization of dendritic ulcers (6 days) and geographic ulcers (7 days) was similar for both therapies. In other clinical studies, Viroptic was evaluated in the treatment of Herpes simplex virus keratitis in patients who were unresponsive or intolerant to the topical administration of idoxuridine or vidarabine. Viroptic was effective in 138 of 150 (92%) patients (109 of 114 with dendritic and 29 of 36 with geographic ulcers) as evidenced by corneal re-epithelialization. The mean time to corneal re-epithelialization was 6 days for patients with dendritic ulcers and 12 days for patients with geographic ulcers.

CONTRAINDICATIONS

Viroptic (Trifluridine) Ophthalmic Solution, 1%, is contraindicated for patients who develop hypersensitivity reactions or chemical intolerance to trifluridine.

WARNINGS

The recommended dosage and frequency of administration should not be exceeded (see Dosage and Administration).

PRECAUTIONS

General: Viroptic (Trifluridine) Ophthalmic Solution, 1% should be prescribed only for patients who have a clinical diagnosis of herpetic keratitis.

Viroptic may cause mild local irritation of the conjunctiva and cornea when instilled but these effects are usually transient.

Although documented *in vitro* viral resistance to trifluridine has not been reported following multiple exposure to Viroptic, the possibility exists of viral resistance development.

Drug Interactions: The following drugs have been administered topically to the eye and concurrently with Viroptic in a limited number of patients without apparent evidence of adverse interaction: antibiotics—chloramphenicol, erythromycin, polymyxin B sulfate, bacitracin, gentamicin sulfate, tetracycline HCl, sodium sulfacetamide, neomycin sulfate; steroids—dexamethasone, dexamethasone sodium phosphate, prednisolone acetate, prednisolone sodium phosphate, hydrocortisone, fluorometholone; and other ophthalmic drugs—atropine sulfate, scopolamine hydrobromide, naphazoline hydrochloride, cyclopentolate hydrochloride, homatropine hydrobromide, pilocarpine, 1-epinephrine hydrochloride, sodium chloride.

Carcinogenesis, Mutagenesis, Impairment of Fertility: ***Mutagenic Potential.*** Trifluridine has been shown to exert mutagenic, DNA damaging and cell transforming activities in various standard *in vitro* test systems, and clastogenic activity in *Vicia faba* cells.

Although the significance of these test results is not clear or fully understood, there exists the possibility that mutagenic agents may cause genetic damage in humans.

Oncogenic Potential. The oncogenic potential of trifluridine is unknown at this time. The oncogenic potential of trifluridine in rodents is being evaluated.

Pregnancy: The drug should not be prescribed for pregnant women unless the potential benefits outweigh the potential risks.

Teratogenic Potential: Kury and Crosby[1] found that trifluridine was teratogenic when injected directly into the yolk sac of developing chick embryos. Itoi *et al.*[2] found that topical application of 1% trifluridine ophthalmic solution to the eyes of rabbits on days 6–18 of pregnancy produced no teratogenic effects. Trifluridine was not teratogenic when given subcutaneously to rats at doses up to 5.0 mg/kg/day although drug induced fetal toxicity (delayed ossification of portions of the skeletal system) was observed at the 2.5 mg/kg/day dose level. Trifluridine was not teratogenic when given subcutaneously to rabbits at doses up to 5.0 mg/kg/day. Drug induced fetal toxicity (delayed ossification of portions of the skeletal system) was observed at the 2.5 mg/kg/day dose level. A 1.0 mg/kg/day dose was considered to be a no effect level in both rats and rabbits. Based upon these findings in animals, it is unlikely that Viroptic would cause embryonic or fetal damage if given in the recommended ophthalmic dosage to pregnant women. A safe dose, however, has not been established for the human embryo or fetus.

Nursing Mothers: It is unlikely that trifluridine is excreted in human milk after ophthalmic instillation of Viroptic because of the relatively small dosage ($\leq$5.0 mg/day), its dilution in body fluids and its extremely short half-life (approximately 12 minutes). The drug should not be prescribed for nursing mothers unless the potential benefits outweigh the potential risks.

ADVERSE REACTIONS

The most frequent adverse reactions reported during controlled clinical trials were mild, transient burning or stinging upon instillation (4.6%) and palpebral edema (2.8%). Other adverse reactions in decreasing order of reported frequency were superficial punctate keratopathy, epithelial keratopathy, hypersensitivity reaction, stromal edema, irritation, keratitis sicca, hyperemia, and increased intraocular pressure.

OVERDOSAGE

Overdosage by ocular instillation is unlikely because any excess solution should be quickly expelled from the conjunctival sac.

Acute overdosage by accidental oral ingestion of Viroptic has not occurred. However, should such ingestion occur, the 75 mg dosage of trifluridine in a 7.5 ml bottle of Viroptic is not likely to produce adverse effects. Single intravenous doses of 15–30 mg/kg/day in children and adults with neoplastic disease produce reversible bone marrow depression as the only potentially serious toxic effect and only after 3–5 courses of therapy.[3] The acute oral LD_{50} in the mouse and rat was 4379 mg/kg or higher.

DOSAGE AND ADMINISTRATION

Instill one drop of Viroptic Ophthalmic Solution, 1% onto the cornea of the affected eye every two hours while awake for a maximum daily dosage of nine drops until the corneal ulcer has completely re-epithelialized. Following re-epithelialization, treatment for an additional seven days of one drop every four hours while awake for a minimum daily dosage of five drops is recommended.

If there are no signs of improvement after seven days of therapy or complete re-epithelialization has not occurred after 14 days of therapy, other forms of therapy should be considered. Continuous administration of Viroptic for periods exceeding 21 days should be avoided because of potential ocular toxicity.

HOW SUPPLIED

Viroptic Opthalmic Solution, 1% is supplied as a sterile ophthalmic solution in a plastic Drop-Dose® dispenser bottle of 7.5 ml. (**NDC-0081-0968-02**)

Store under refrigeration 2° to 8°C (36° to 46°F)

Animal Pharmacology and Animal Toxicology: Corneal wound healing studies in rabbits showed that Viroptic did not significantly retard closure of epithelial wounds. However, mild toxic changes such as intracellular edema of the basal cell layer, mild thinning of the overlying epithelium and reduced strength of stromal wounds were observed.

Whereas instillation of Viroptic into rabbit eyes during a subchronic toxicity study produced some degree of corneal epithelial thinning, a 12-month chronic toxicity study in rabbits in which Viroptic was instilled into eyes in intermittent, multiple, full-therapy courses showed no drug related changes in the cornea.

DoD NSN 6505-01-142-8314

REFERENCES

1. Kury G and RJ Crosby: The teratogenic effect of 5-trifluoromethyl-2′-deoxyuridine in chicken embryos. *Toxicol Appl Pharmacol 11*(1):72–80, 1967.
2. Itoi M, Gefter JW, Kaneko N, Ishii Y, Ramer RM and Gasset AR: Teratogenicities of ophthalmic drugs. I. Antiviral ophthalmic drugs. *Arch Ophthalmol 93*(1):46–51, 1975.
3. Ansfield FJ and Ramirez G: Phase I and II Studies of 2′-deoxy-5-(trifluoromethyl)-uridine (NSC-75520). *Cancer Chemother Rep* (Pt. 1) *55*(2):205–208, 1971.

WELLCOVORIN® INJECTION ℞

[*wĕl "kō-vor 'ĭn*]

(Leucovorin Calcium)

DESCRIPTION

Wellcovorin® (leucovorin calcium) Injection, a sterile aqueous solution for intramuscular or intravenous administration, contains 5 mg leucovorin per ml, as the calcium salt of N-[*p* -[[(2-amino-5-formyl-1,4,5,6,7,8-hexahydro-4-oxo-6-pteridinyl)methyl]amino]benzoyl]-L-glutamic acid. This is the equivalent to 5.40 mg of anhydrous leucovorin calcium. The vehicle contains methylparaben 0.08% and propylparaben 0.02% added as preservatives; hydrochloric acid or sodium hydroxide q.s. to adjust the pH to approximately 7.8 and water for injection, q.s.

Leucovorin is a water soluble vitamin in the folate group; it is useful as an antidote to drugs which act as folic acid antagonists.

CLINICAL PHARMACOLOGY

Leucovorin is a mixture of the diastereoisomers of the 5-formyl derivative of tetrahydrofolic acid. The biologically active component of the mixture is the (-)-L-isomer, known as *Citrovorum factor*, or (-)-folinic acid. Leucovorin does *not* require reduction by the enzyme dihydrofolate reductase in order to participate in reactions utilizing folates as a source of "one-carbon" moieties. Following parenteral administration, leucovorin rapidly enters the general body pool of reduced folates[1]. The increase in plasma and serum folate activity (determined microbiologically with *Lactobacillus casei*) seen after parenteral administration of leucovorin is predominantly due to 5-methyl-tetrahydrofolate.[1,2,3,4,5]

Twenty normal men were given a single, intramuscular (gluteus maximus) 15 mg dose (7.5 mg/m^2) of leucovorin calcium and serum folate concentrations were assayed with *L casei.*[6]

Mean values observed ($\pm$ one standard error) were:[4]

a) Time to peak serum folate concentration: 0.71 $\pm$ .09 hrs.,
b) Peak serum folate concentration achieved: 241 $\pm$ 17 ng/ml,
c) Serum folate half-disappearance time: 3.7 hours.

Intragluteally administered leucovorin yielded areas under the serum folate concentration-time curves (AUC's) that were 8 percent less than an equal amount of leucovorin administered in the deltoid muscle, and 12% less than with an intravenous injection.

INDICATIONS AND USAGE

Wellcovorin (leucovorin calcium) Injection is indicated to diminish the toxicity and counteract the effect of inadvertently administered overdosages of folic acid antagonists. (See Warnings)

CONTRAINDICATIONS

Leucovorin is improper therapy for pernicious anemia and other megaloblastic anemias secondary to the lack of vitamin B_{12}. A hematologic remission may occur while neurologic manifestations remain progressive.

WARNINGS

In the treatment of accidental overdosage of folic acid antagonists, leucovorin should be administered as promptly as possible. As the time interval between antifolate administration (e.g. methotrexate) and leucovorin rescue increases, leucovorin's effectiveness in counteracting hematologic toxicity diminishes.

PRECAUTIONS

General: Following chemotherapy with folic acid antagonists, parenteral administration of leucovorin is preferable to oral dosing if there is a possibility that the patient may vomit and not absorb the leucovorin. In the presence of pernicious anemia a hematologic remission may occur while neurologic manifestations remain progressive.

Pregnancy: ***Teratogenic Effects:*** Pregnancy Category C. Animal reproduction studies have not been conducted with Wellcovorin. It is also not known whether Wellcovorin can cause fetal harm when administered to a pregnant woman or can affect reproduction capacity. Wellcovorin should be given to a pregnant woman only if clearly needed.

Nursing Mothers: It is not known whether this drug is excreted in human milk. Because many drugs are excreted in human milk, caution should be exercised when Wellcovorin is administered to a nursing mother.

ADVERSE REACTIONS

Allergic sensitization has been reported following both oral and parenteral administration of folic acid.

OVERDOSAGE

Excessive amounts of leucovorin may nullify the chemotherapeutic effect of folic acid antagonists.

DOSAGE AND ADMINISTRATION

Wellcovorin Injection is intended for intramuscular or intravenous injection. Leucovorin is a specific antidote for the hematopoietic toxicity of methotrexate and other strong inhibitors of the enzyme dihydrofolate reductase. Leucovorin rescue of high-dose methotrexate therapy is usally begun within 24 hours of administration. A conventional leucovorin rescue dosage schedule is 10 mg/m^2 I.M. or I.V. followed by 10 mg/m^2 orally every six hours for seventy-two hours. If, however, at 24 hours following methotrexate administration the serum creatinine is 50% or greater than the pretreatment serum creatinine, the leucovorin dose should be immediately increased to 100 mg/m^2 every three hours until the serum methotrexate level is below 5×10^{-8} M.[7,8]

The recommended dose of leucovorin to counteract hematologic toxicity from folic acid antagonists with less affinity for mammalian dihydrofolate reductase than methotrexate (i.e. trimethoprim, pyrimethamine) is a substantially less and 5 to 15 mg of leucovorin per day has been recommended by some investigators.[9,10,11]

HOW SUPPLIED

Wellcovorin® Injection is available in ampuls containing 5 mg leucovorin per ml, as a calcium salt.

1 ml amber ampuls, Box of 10 (NDC-0081-0633-49).

5 ml amber ampuls, Box of 10 (NDC-0081-0633-10).

Store at 15°–30°C (59°–86°F).

Also available in 5 mg tablets, bottles of 100, and in 25 mg tablets, bottles of 25.

REFERENCES

1. Nixon PF and Bertino JR: Effective Absorption and Utilization of Oral Formyltetrahydrofolate in Man. N Engl J Med *286* (4): 175–179, Jan. 27, 1972.
2. Baker H, Frank O, Feingold, S *et al* : The Fate of Orally and Parenterally Administered Folates. Am J Clin Nutr *17* :88–95, 1965.
3. Mehta BM, Gisolfi AL, Hutchison DJ, Nirenberg A, Kellick MG and Rosen G: Serum Distribution of Citrovorum Factor and 5-methyltetrahydrofolate Following

Continued on next page

Burroughs Wellcome—Cont.

Oral and I.M. Administration of Calcium Leucovorin in Normal Adults. Cancer Treat Rep *62* (3): 345–350, Mar. 1978.

4. Data on file, Medical Division, Burroughs Wellcome Co., Research Triangle Park, N.C. 27709, USA.
5. Whitehead VM, Pratt R, Viallet A and Cooper BA: Intestinal Conversion of Folinic Acid to 5-methyltetrahydrofolate in Man. Br J Haematol *22*: 63–72, 1972.
6. Herbert V: Asceptic Addition of *Lactobacillus casei* Assay of Folate Activity in Human Serum. J Clin Path *19*: 12–16, 1966.
7. Bleyer WA: The Clinical Pharmacology of Methotrexate. Cancer, *41* (1): 36–51, 1978.
8. Frei E, Blum RH, Pitman SW, *et al*: High Dose Methotrexate with Leucovorin Rescue: Rationale and Spectrum of Antitumor Activity. Am J Med, *68*: 370–376, 1980.
9. Golde DW, Bersch N, Quan SG: Trimethoprim and Sulphamethoxazole Inhibition of Haematopoiesis *in vitro*. Br J Haematol, *40* (3): 363–367, 1978.
10. Steinberg SE, Campbell CL, Rabinovitch PS, *et al*: The Effect of Trimethoprim/Sulfamethoxazole on Friend Erythroleukemia Cells. Blood, *55* (3): 501–504, 1980.
11. Mahmoud AAF and Warren KS: Algorithms in the Diagnosis and Management of Exotic Disease. XX. Toxoplasmosis. J Infect Dis, *135* (3): 493–496, 1977.

WELLCOVORIN® TABLETS ℞

[*wĕl"kō-vor'ĭn*]
(Leucovorin Calcium)

DESCRIPTION

Wellcovorin (leucovorin calcium) Tablets contain either 5 mg or 25 mg leucovorin as the calcium salt of N-[4-[[(2-amino-5-formyl-1, 4, 5, 6, 7, 8-hexahydro-4-oxo-6-pteridinyl)-methyl] amino]benzoyl]-L-glutamic acid and the inactive ingredients corn starch, FD&C Yellow No. 6 Lake (25 mg tablet only), lactose, povidone, and magnesium stearate. This is equivalent to 5.40 mg or 27.01 mg of anhydrous leucovorin calcium.

Leucovorin is a water soluble vitamin in the folate group; it is useful as an antidote to drugs which act as folic acid antagonists. These tablets are intended for oral administration only.

CLINICAL PHARMACOLOGY

Leucovorin is a mixture of the diastereoisomers of the 5-formyl derivative of tetrahydrofolic acid. The biologically active component of the mixture is the (-)-L-isomer, known as *Citrovorum factor*, or (-)-folinic acid. Leucovorin does *not* require reduction by the enzyme dihydrofolate reductase in order to participate in reactions utilizing folates as a source of "one-carbon" moieties. Following oral administration, leucovorin is rapidly absorbed and enters the general body pool of reduced folates.[1] The increase in plasma and serum folate activity (determined microbiologically with *Lactobacillus casei*) seen after oral administration of leucovorin is predominantly due to 5-methyltetrahydrofolate.[1,2,3,4,5]

Twenty normal men were given a single, oral 15 mg dose (7.5 mg/m^2) of leucovorin calcium and serum folate concentrations were assayed with *L casei*.[6] Mean values observed (± one standard error) were:[4]

a) Time to peak serum folate concentration: 1.72 ± 0.08 hrs.,
b) Peak serum folate concentration achieved: 268 ± 18 ng/ml,
c) Serum folate half-disappearance time: 3.5 hours.

Oral tablets yielded areas under the serum folate concentration-time curves (AUC's) that were 12% greater than equal amounts of leucovorin given intramuscularly and equal to the same amounts given intravenously.

INDICATIONS AND USAGE

Wellcovorin (leucovorin calcium) is indicated for the prophylaxis and treatment of undesired hematopoietic effects of folic acid antagonists (see WARNINGS).

CONTRAINDICATIONS

Leucovorin is improper therapy for pernicious anemia and other megaloblastic anemias secondary to the lack of vitamin B_{12}. A hematologic remission may occur while neurologic manifestations remain progressive.

WARNINGS

In the treatment of accidental overdosage of folic acid antagonists, leucovorin should be administered as promptly as possible. As the time interval between antifolate administration (e.g. methotrexate) and leucovorin rescue increases, leucovorin's effectiveness in counteracting hematologic toxicity diminishes.

PRECAUTIONS

General: Following chemotherapy with folic acid antagonists, parenteral administration of leucovorin is preferable to oral dosing if there is a possibility that the patient may vomit and not absorb the leucovorin. In the presence of pernicious anemia a hematologic remission may occur while neurologic manifestations remain progressive. Leucovorin has no effect on other toxicities of methotrexate, such as the nephrotoxicity resulting from drug precipitation in the kidney.

Drug Interactions: Folic acid in large amounts may counteract the antiepileptic effect of phenobarbital, phenytoin and primidone, and increase the frequency of seizures in susceptible children.

Pregnancy: ***Teratogenic Effects:*** Pregnancy Category C. Animal reproduction studies have not been conducted with Wellcovorin. It is also not known whether Wellcovorin can cause fetal harm when administered to a pregnant woman or can affect reproduction capacity. Wellcovorin should be given to a pregnant woman only if clearly needed.

Nursing Mothers: It is not known whether this drug is excreted in human milk. Because many drugs are excreted in human milk, caution should be exercised when Wellcovorin is administered to a nursing mother.

Pediatric Use: See "Drug Interactions".

ADVERSE REACTIONS

Allergic sensitization has been reported following both oral and parenteral administration of folic acid.

OVERDOSAGE

Excessive amounts of luecovorin may nullify the chemotherapeutic effect of folic acid antagonists.

DOSAGE AND ADMINISTRATION

Leucovorin is a specific antidote for the hematopoietic toxicity of methotrexate and other strong inhibitors of the enzyme dihydrofolate reductase. Leucovorin rescue must begin within 24 hours of antifolate administration. A conventional leucovorin rescue dosage schedule is 10 mg/m^2 orally or parenterally followed by 10 mg/m^2 orally every six hours for seventy-two hours. If, however, at 24 hours following methotrexate administration the serum creatinine is 50% or greater than the premethotrexate serum creatinine, the leucovorin dose should be immediately increased to 100 mg/m^2 every three hours until the serum methotrexate level is below 5×10^{-8} M.[7,8]

The recommended dose of leucovorin to counteract hematologic toxicity from folic acid antagonists with less affinity for mammalian dihydrofolate reductase than methotrexate (i.e. trimethoprim, pyrimethamine) is substantially less and 5 to 15 mg of leucovorin per day has been recommended by some investigators.[9,10,11]

HOW SUPPLIED

5 mg (off-white) tablets containing 5 mg leucovorin as the calcium salt imprinted with "WELLCOVORIN" and "R3C"; bottle of 100 (NDC-0081-0631-55).

25 mg (peach) scored tablets containing 25 mg leucovorin as the calcium salt imprinted with "WELLCOVORIN" and "T3C"; bottle of 25 (NDC-0081-0632-25).

Store at 15°–30°C (59°–86°F) in a dry place and protect from light and moisture.

REFERENCES

1. Nixon PF and Bertino JR; Effective Absorption and Utilization of Oral Formyltetrahydrofolate in Man. *N Engl J Med 286* (4):175–179, Jan. 27, 1972.
2. Ratanasthien K, Blair JA, Leeming RJ, Cooke WT and Melikian V: Folates in Human Serum. *J Clin Pathol 27*:875–879, 1974.
3. Mehta BM, Gisolfi AL, Hutchison DJ, Nirenberg A, Kellick MG and Rosen G: Serum Distribution of Citrovorum Factor and 5-methyltetrahydrofolate Following Oral and I.M. Administration of Calcium Leucovorin in Normal Adults. *Cancer Treat Rep 62* (3):345–350. Mar. 1978.
4. Data on file, Medical Division, Burroughs Wellcome Co., Research Triangle Park, N.C. 27709, USA.
5. Whitehead VM, Pratt R, Viallet A and Cooper BA: Intestinal Conversion of Folinic Acid to 5-methyltetrahydrofolate in Man. *Br J Haematol 22*:63–72, 1972.
6. Herbert V: Asceptic Addition for *Lactobacillus casei* Assay of Folate Activity in Human Serum. *J Clin Path 19*:12–16, 1966.
7. Bleyer WA: The Clinical Pharmacology of Methotrexate. *Cancer, 41* (1):36–51, 1978.
8. Frei E, Blum RH, Pitman SW, *et al:* High Dose Methotrexate with Leucovorin Rescue: Rationale and Spectrum of Antitumor Activity. *Am J Med, 68:* 370–376, 1980.
9. Golde DW, Bersch N, Quan SG: Trimethoprim and Sulphamethoxazole Inhibition of Haematopoiesis *in Vitro. Br J Haematol, 40* (3):363–367, 1978.
10. Steinberg SE, Campbell CL, Rabinovitch PS, *et al:* The Effect of Trimethoprim/Sulfamethoxazole on Friend Erythroleukemia Cells. *Blood, 55* (3):501–504, 1980.
11. Mahmoud AAF and Warren KS: Algorithms in the Diagnosis and Management of Exotic Disease. XX. Toxoplasmosis. *J Infect Dis, 135* (3):493–496, 1977.

Shown in Product Identification Section, page 407

ZOVIRAX® ℞

[*zō"vī'răx*]
(ACYCLOVIR)
CAPSULES

DESCRIPTION

Zovirax is the brand name for acyclovir, an antiviral drug. Zovirax Capsules are a formulation for oral administration. Each capsule of Zovirax contains 200 mg of acyclovir and the inactive ingredients corn starch, lactose, magnesium stearate, and sodium lauryl sulfate. Hard gelatin capsule contains FD&C Blue No. 2 and other ingredients. Printed with edible black ink.

The chemical name of acyclovir is 9-[(2-hydroxyethoxy)methyl]guanine.

Acyclovir is a white, crystalline powder with a molecular weight of 225 daltons, and a maximum solubility in water of 2.5 mg/ml at 37°C.

CLINICAL PHARMACOLOGY

Acyclovir is a synthetic acyclic purine nucleoside analogue with *in vitro* inhibitory activity against Herpes simplex types 1 and 2 (HSV-1 and HSV-2), varicella-zoster, Epstein-Barr and cytomegalovirus. In cell cultures, the inhibitory activity of acyclovir for Herpes simplex virus is highly selective. Cellular thymidine kinase does not effectively utilize acyclovir as a substrate. Herpes simplex virus-coded thymidine kinase, however, converts acyclovir into acyclovir monophosphate, a nucleotide analogue. The monophosphate is further converted into diphosphate by cellular guanylate kinase and into triphosphate by a number of cellular enzymes.[1] Acyclovir triphosphate interferes with Herpes simplex virus DNA polymerase and inhibits viral DNA replication. Acyclovir triphosphate also inhibits cellular α-DNA polymerase, but to a lesser degree. *In vitro,* acyclovir triphosphate can be incorporated into growing chains of DNA by viral DNA polymerase and to a much smaller extent by cellular α-DNA polymerase.[2] When incorporation occurs, the DNA chain is terminated.[3] Acyclovir is preferentially taken up and selectively converted to the active triphosphate form by herpes-virus-infected cells. Thus, acyclovir is much less toxic *in vitro* for normal uninfected cells because: 1) less is taken up; 2) less is converted to the active form; 3) cellular α-DNA polymerase is less sensitive to the effects of the active form.

Microbiology: The quantitative relationship between the *in vitro* susceptibility of Herpes simplex virus to acyclovir and the clinical response to therapy has not been established in man. Sensitivity results, expressed as the concentration of drug required to inhibit by 50% the growth of virus in a tissue culture ("ID_{50} value") vary greatly depending upon the particular assay used,[4] the cell type employed,[5] and the laboratory performing the test. Using a dye-uptake method in Vero cells,[6] which gives ID_{50} values approximately 5- to 10-fold higher than plaque reduction assays, 1417 isolates (553 HSV-1 and 864 HSV-2) from approximately 500 patients were examined over a 5-year period.[7] It must be emphasized that neither the patients nor the isolates were randomly selected and, therefore, do not represent the general population. Isolates obtained from patients who continued to shed virus during or after acyclovir therapy were selected for assay; a smaller number were examined from all patients in a given clinical study.

These assays found that 90% of HSV-1 isolates were sensitive to ≤0.9 μg/ml acyclovir and 50% of all isolates were sensitive to ≤0.2 μg/ml acyclovir. For HSV-2 isolates, 90% were sensitive to ≤2.2 μg/ml and 50% of all isolates were sensitive to ≤0.7 μg/ml of acyclovir. Isolates with significantly diminished sensitivity were found in 44 patients.

All of the less sensitive viruses obtained from patients to date have been the result of alterations in the thymidine kinase enzyme[8–13] and were not the result of changes in the viral DNA polymerase.

Pharmacokinetics: The pharmacokinetics of acyclovir after oral administration have been evaluated in 5 clinical studies involving 38 adult patients. In 14 immunocompromised patients with Herpes simplex or varicella zoster infection given Zovirax Capsules in doses of 200 or 400 mg every 4 hours, 6 times daily for 5 days, the bioavailability was estimated to be 15–20%. In this study, steady-state plasma levels were reached by the second day of dosing. Mean steady-state peak and trough concentrations following the 200 mg dose were 0.56 μg/ml (0.38 to 0.74 μg/ml) and 0.29 μg/ml (0.18 to 0.42 μg/ml), respectively, and following the 400 mg dose were 1.2 μg/ml (0.75 to 1.7 μg/ml) and 0.62 μg/ml (0.14 to 0.90 μg/ml). When 6 normal volunteers received 200 mg acyclovir as a solution every 4 hours, 5 times daily, similar

mean steady-state peak and trough concentrations (0.62 μg/ml and 0.30 μg/ml) were achieved.
A single oral dose bioavailability study in 23 normal volunteers showed that Zovirax Capsules 200 mg are bioequivalent to 200 mg acyclovir in aqueous solution. In another study in 6 volunteers, the influence of food on the absorption of acyclovir was not apparent.
Following oral administration of Zovirax Capsules 200 mg, the mean acyclovir plasma half-life in 14 patients with normal renal function was 3.3 hours. The mean renal excretion of unchanged drug accounts for 14.4% (8.6 to 19.8%) of the orally administered dose. The only urinary metabolite (identified by high performance liquid chromatography) is 9-[(carboxymethoxy)methyl]guanine.
The half-life and total body clearance of acyclovir are dependent on renal function. A dosage adjustment is recommended for patients with creatinine clearance ≤ 10 ml/min/1.73 m^2 (see DOSAGE AND ADMINISTRATION).

Orally administered acyclovir in pediatric and neonatal patients has not yet been fully studied.

INDICATIONS AND USAGE

Zovirax Capsules are indicated for the treatment of initial episodes and the management of recurrent episodes of genital herpes in certain patients.
The severity of disease is variable depending upon the immune status of the patient, the frequency and duration of episodes, and the degree of cutaneous or systemic involvement. These factors should determine patient management, which may include symptomatic support and counseling only, or the institution of specific therapy. The physical, emotional and psycho-social difficulties posed by herpes infections as well as the degree of debilitation, particularly in immunocompromised patients, are unique for each patient, and the physician should determine therapeutic alternatives based on his or her understanding of the individual patient's needs. Thus Zovirax Capsules are not appropriate in treating all genital herpes infections. The following guidelines may be useful in weighing the benefit/risk considerations in specific disease categories:

First Episodes (primary and nonprimary infections—commonly known as initial genital herpes):
Double-blind, placebo-controlled studies[14,15,16] have demonstrated that orally administered Zovirax significantly reduced the duration of acute infection (detection of virus in lesions by tissue culture) and lesion healing. The duration of pain and new lesion formation was decreased in some patient groups. The promptness of initiation of therapy and/or the patient's prior exposure to Herpes simplex virus may influence the degree of benefit from therapy. Patients with mild disease may derive less benefit than those with more severe episodes. In patients with extremely severe episodes, in which prostration, central nervous system involvement, urinary retention or inability to take oral medication require hospitalization and more aggressive management, therapy may be best initiated with intravenous Zovirax.

Recurrent Episodes:
Double-blind, placebo-controlled studies[13,17,18,19] in patients with frequent recurrences (6 or more episodes per year) have shown that Zovirax Capsules given for 4 to 6 months prevented or reduced the frequency and/or severity of recurrences in greater than 95% of patients. Clinical recurrences were prevented in 40 to 75% of patients. Some patients experienced increased severity of the first episode following cessation of therapy; the severity of subsequent episodes and the effect on the natural history of the disease are still under study.
The safety and efficacy of orally administered acyclovir in the suppression of frequent episodes of genital herpes have been established only for up to 6 months. Chronic suppressive therapy is most appropriate when, in the judgement of the physician, the benefits of such a regimen outweigh known or potential adverse effects. In general, Zovirax Capsules should not be used for the suppression of recurrent disease in mildly affected patients. Unanswered questions concerning the human relevance of *in vitro* mutagenicity studies and reproductive toxicity studies in animals given very high doses of acyclovir for short periods (see Carcinogenesis, Mutagenesis, Impairment of Fertility) should be borne in mind when designing long-term management for individual patients. Discussions of these issues with patients will provide them the opportunity to weigh the potential for toxicity against the severity of their disease. Thus, this regimen should be considered only for appropriate patients and only for six months until the results of ongoing studies allow a more precise evaluation of the benefit/risk assessment of prolonged therapy.
Limited studies[19,20] have shown that there are certain patients for whom intermittent short-term treatment of recurrent episodes is effective. This approach may be more appropriate than a suppressive regimen in patients with infrequent recurrences.
Immunocompromised patients with recurrent herpes infections can be treated with either intermittent or chronic suppressive therapy. Clinically significant resistance, although rare, is more likely to be seen with prolonged or repeated therapy in severely immunocompromised patients with active lesions.

Diagnosis:
The cutaneous vesicular lesions associated with Herpes simplex virus infections are often characteristic in appearance. However, other etiologic agents may cause similar lesions. Proof of herpesvirus infection rests on viral isolation and identification in tissue culture. Several other laboratory tests, however, can be used to establish presumptive evidence of herpesvirus infection. Smears prepared from lesion exudates or scrapings may be stained with Wright or Giemsa stains and examined for the presence of multinucleated giant cells (Tzanck preparation)[21]; this method is not specific for Herpes simplex virus infection. Smears may also be reacted in other test systems for herpes.

CONTRAINDICATIONS

Zovirax Capsules are contraindicated for patients who develop hypersensitivity or intolerance to the components of the formulation.

WARNINGS

Zovirax Capsules are intended for oral ingestion only.

PRECAUTIONS

General: Zovirax has caused decreased spermatogenesis at high doses in some animals and mutagenesis in some acute studies at high concentrations of drug (see PRECAUTIONS—Carcinogenesis, Mutagenesis, Impairment of Fertility). The recommended dosage and length of treatment should not be exceeded (see DOSAGE AND ADMINISTRATION).
Exposure of Herpes simplex isolates to acyclovir *in vitro* can lead to the emergence of less sensitive viruses. The possibility of the appearance of less sensitive viruses in man must be borne in mind when treating patients. The relationship between the *in vitro* sensitivity of Herpes simplex virus to acyclovir and clinical response to therapy has yet to be established (see CLINICAL PHARMACOLOGY—Microbiology).
Because of the possibility that less sensitive virus may be selected in patients who are receiving acyclovir, all patients should be advised to take particular care to avoid potential transmission of virus if active lesions are present while they are on therapy. In severely immunocompromised patients, the physician should be aware that prolonged or repeated courses of acyclovir may result in selection of resistant viruses which may not fully respond to continued acyclovir therapy.

Information for Patients: Educational material is being provided to pharmacists and other health care professionals to give to patients. It contains, in part, the following information:
Genital herpes is a sexually transmitted disease and patients should avoid intercourse when visible lesions are present because of the risk of infecting intimate partners. Zovirax Capsules are for oral ingestion only. Medication should not be shared with others. The prescribed dosage should not be exceeded. Zovirax Capsules do not eliminate latent viruses. Some patients experience increased severity of the first episode following cessation of therapy; the severity of subsequent episodes and the effect on the natural history of the disease are still under study.
There are still unanswered questions concerning reproductive/gonadal toxicity and mutagenesis; long-term studies are continuing. Decreased sperm production has been seen at high doses in some animals; preliminary analysis of a study using 400 mg or 1000 mg of Zovirax per day for six months in humans did not show similar findings. Chromosomal breaks were seen *in vitro* after brief exposure to high concentrations. Some other currently marketed medications also cause chromosomal breaks, and the significance of this finding is unknown.
Patients are instructed to consult with their physician if: they do not receive sufficient relief in the frequency and severity of their recurrences, they experience severe or troublesome adverse reactions, they become pregnant or intend to become pregnant, they intend to breastfeed while taking Zovirax Capsules, or they have any other questions.

Drug Interactions: Co-administration of probenecid with intravenous acyclovir has been shown to increase the mean half-life and the area under the concentration-time curve. Urinary excretion and renal clearance were correspondingly reduced.

Carcinogenesis, Mutagenesis, Impairment of Fertility: Acyclovir was tested in lifetime bioassays in rats and mice at single daily doses of 50, 150 and 450 mg/kg given by gavage. There was no statistically significant difference in the incidence of tumors between treated and control animals, nor did acyclovir shorten the latency of tumors. In 2 *in vitro* cell transformation assays, used to provide preliminary assessment of potential oncogenicity in advance of these more definitive life-time bioassays in rodents, conflicting results were obtained. Acyclovir was positive at the highest dose used in one system and the resulting morphologically transformed cells formed tumors when inoculated into immunosuppressed, syngeneic, weanling mice. Acyclovir was negative in another transformation system considered less sensitive.

In acute studies, there was an increase, not statistically significant, in the incidence of chromosomal damage at maximum tolerated parenteral doses of 100 mg/kg acyclovir in rats but not Chinese hamsters; higher doses of 500 and 1000 mg/kg were clastogenic in Chinese hamsters. In addition, no activity was found after 5 days dosing in a dominant lethal study in mice. In 6 of 11 microbial and mammalian cell assays, no evidence of mutagenicity was observed. At 3 loci in a Chinese hamster ovary cell line, the results were inconclusive. In 2 mammalian cell assays (human lymphocytes and L5178Y mouse lymphoma cells *in vitro*), positive responses for mutagenicity and chromosomal damage occurred, but only at concentrations at least 400 times the acyclovir plasma levels achieved in man.
Acyclovir has not been shown to impair fertility or reproduction in mice (450 mg/kg/day, p.o.) or in rats (25 mg/kg/day, s.c.). At 50 mg/kg/day s.c. in the rat, there was a statistically significant increase in post-implantation loss, but no concomitant decrease in litter size. In female rabbits treated subcutaneously with acyclovir subsequent to mating, there was a statistically significant decrease in implantation efficiency but no concomitant decrease in litter size at a dose of 50 mg/kg/day. No effect upon implantation efficiency was observed when the same dose was administered intravenously. In a rat peri- and postnatal study at 50 mg/kg/day s.c., there was a statistically significant decrease in the group mean numbers of corpora lutea, total implantation sites and life fetuses in the F_1 generation. Although not statistically significant, there was also a dose related decrease in group mean numbers of live fetuses and implantation sites at 12.5 mg/kg/day and 25 mg/kg/day, s.c. The intravenous administration of 100 mg/kg/day, a dose known to cause obstructive nephropathy in rabbits, caused a significant increase in fetal resorptions and a corresponding decrease in litter size. However, at a maximum tolerated intravenous dose of 50 mg/kg/day in rabbits, there were no drug-related reproductive effects.
Intraperitoneal doses of 320 or 80 mg/kg/day acyclovir given to rats for 1 and 6 months, respectively, caused testicular atrophy. Testicular atrophy was persistent through the 4-week postdose recovery phase after 320 mg/kg/day; some evidence of recovery of sperm production was evident 30 days postdose. Intravenous doses of 100 and 200 mg/kg/day acyclovir given to dogs for 31 days caused aspermatogenesis. Testicles were normal in dogs given 50 mg/kg/day i.v. for one month.

Pregnancy: ***Teratogenic Effects:*** Pregnancy Category C. Acyclovir was not teratogenic in the mouse (450 mg/kg/day, p.o.), rat (50 mg/kg/day, s.c.) or rabbit (50 mg/kg/day, s.c. and i.v.). There are no adequate and well-controlled studies in pregnant women. Acyclovir should not be used during pregnancy unless the potential benefit justifies the potential risk to the fetus. Although acyclovir was not teratogenic in animal studies, the drug's potential for causing chromosome breaks at high concentration should be taken into consideration in making this determination.

Nursing Mothers: It is not known whether this drug is excreted in human milk. Because many drugs are excreted in human milk, caution should be exercised when Zovirax is administered to a nursing woman. In nursing mothers, consideration should be given to not using acyclovir treatment or discontinuing breastfeeding.

Pediatric Use: Safety and effectiveness in children have not been established.

ADVERSE REACTIONS—Short-Term Administration

The most frequent adverse reactions reported during clinical trials of treatment with Zovirax Capsules were nausea and/or vomiting in 8 of 298 patient treatments (2.7%) and headache in 2 of 298 (0.6%). Nausea and/or vomiting occurred in 2 of 287 (0.7%) patients who received placebo.
Less frequent adverse reactions, each of which occurred in 1 of 298 patient treatments with Zovirax Capsules (0.3%), included diarrhea, dizziness, anorexia, fatigue, edema, skin rash, leg pain, inguinal adenopathy, medication taste and sore throat.

Long-Term Administration: The most frequent adverse reactions reported in clinical trials of continuous (up to 6 months) administration of Zovirax Capsules for the prevention of recurrences were headache in 33 of 251 Zovirax-treated patients (13.1%), diarrhea in 22 of 251 (8.8%), nausea and/or vomiting in 20 of 251 (8.0%), vertigo in 9 of 251 (3.6%), and arthralgia in 9 of 251 (3.6%). Of the control patients receiving either placebo or intermittent treatment of recurrences with Zovirax, headache was reported in 14 of 163 (8.6%), diarrhea in 7 of 163 (4.3%), and nausea and/or vomiting in 14 of 163 (8.6%).
Less frequent adverse reactions, each of which occurred in less than 3% of the 251 patients treated with Zovirax (see number of patients in parentheses), included skin rash (7), insomnia (4), fatigue (7), fever (4), palpitations (1), sore throat

Continued on next page

Burroughs Wellcome—Cont.

(2), superficial thrombophlebitis (1), muscle cramps (2), pars planitis (1), menstrual abnormality (4), acne (3), lymphadenopathy (2), irritability (1), accelerated hair loss (1), and depression (1).

OVERDOSAGE

No acute massive overdosage of Zovirax Capsules has been reported. Doses as high as 800 mg 6 times daily for 5 days have been administered to humans without acute untoward effects. This should not be construed as a recommended dosage for patients with more severe herpes. Peak plasma concentrations have reached 10.0 μg/ml.

Precipitation of acyclovir in renal tubules may occur when the solubility (2.5 mg/ml) in the intratubular fluid is exceeded. Renal lesions considered to be related to obstruction of renal tubules by precipitated drug crystals occurred in the following species: rats treated with i.v. and i.p. doses of 20 mg/kg/day for 21 and 31 days, respectively, and at s.c. doses of 100 mg/kg/day for 10 days; rabbits at s.c. and i.v. doses of 50 mg/kg/day for 13 days; and dogs at i.v. doses of 100 mg/kg/day for 31 days. A 6 hr hemodialysis results in a 60% decrease in plasma acyclovir concentration. Data concerning peritoneal dialysis are incomplete but indicate that this method may be significantly less efficient in removing acyclovir from the blood. In the event of acute renal failure and anuria, the patient may benefit from hemodialysis until renal function is restored (see DOSAGE AND ADMINISTRATION).

DOSAGE AND ADMINISTRATION

Treatment of initial genital herpes: One 200 mg capsule every 4 hours, while awake, for a total of 5 capsules daily for 10 days (total 50 capsules).

Chronic suppressive therapy for recurrent disease: One 200 mg capsule 3 times daily for up to 6 months. Some patients may require more drug, up to one 200 mg capsule 5 times daily for up to 6 months.

Intermittent Therapy: One 200 mg capsule every 4 hours, while awake, for a total of 5 capsules daily for 5 days (total 25 capsules). Therapy should be initiated at the earliest sign or symptom (prodrome) of recurrence.

Patients With Acute or Chronic Renal Impairment: Comprehensive pharmacokinetic studies have been completed following intravenous acyclovir infusions in patients with renal impairment. Based on these studies, a dosage adjustment is recommended for patients with creatinine clearance $\leq$10 ml/min/1.73 m^2. For these patients, a 200 mg dose every 12 hours is recommended.

HOW SUPPLIED

Zovirax Capsules (blue, opaque) containing 200 mg acyclovir and printed with "Wellcome ZOVIRAX 200"—Bottles of 100 (NDC-0081-0991-55), and unit dose pack of 100 (NDC-0081-0991-56).

Store at 15°-30°C (59°-86°F) and protect from light.

REFERENCES

1. Miller, W.H. and Miller, R.L. J. Biol. Chem. 255(15):7204–7207, 1980.
2. Furman, P.A. *et al.* J. Virol. 32(1):72–77, 1979.
3. Derse, D. *et al.* J. Biol. Chem. 256(22): 11447–11451, 1981.
4. Barry, D.W. and Blum, M.R. In: Recent Advances in Clinical Pharmacology. Turner P. and Shand, D.G. eds., 57–80, 1983.
5. DeClerq, E. Antimicrob. Agents Chemother. 21: 661–3, 1982.
6. McLaren, C., *et al.* Antiviral Res. 3: 223–34, 1983.
7. Barry, D.W. and Nusinoff-Lehrman, S. Pharmacological and Clinical Approaches to Herpes Viruses and Virus Chemotherapy. Oiso, Japan, September 10–13, 1984.
8. Dekker, C., *et al.* J. Antimicrob. Chemother. 12(B): 137–152, 1983.
9. Sibrack, C.D., *et al.* J. Infect. Dis. 146: 673–82, 1982.
10. Crumpacker, C.S., *et al.* N. Engl. J. Med. 306: 343–6, 1982.
11. Wade, J.C., *et al.* Ann. Int. Med. 96: 265–9, 1982.
12. Burns, W.H., *et al.* Lancet: 421–3, 1982.
13. Straus, S.E., *et al.* N. Engl. J. Med. 310: 1545–50, 1984.
14. Bryson, Y.J., *et al.* N. Engl. J. Med. 308(16): 916–921, 1983.
15. Mertz, G.J., *et al.* J.A.M.A. 252(9): 1147–1151, 1984.
16. Nilsen, A.E., *et al.* Lancet. 8298: 571–573, 1982.
17. Douglas, J.M. *et al.* N. Engl. J. Med. 310(24): 1551–1556, 1984.
18. Mindel, A., *et al.* Lancet: 8394: 57–59, 1984.
19. Data on File, Burroughs Wellcome Co.
20. Reichman, R.C., *et al.* J.A.M.A. 251(16) 2103–2107, 1984.
21. Naib, Z.M., *et al.* Cancer Res. 33:1452–1463, 1973.

U.S. Patent No. 4199574

Shown in Product Identification Section, page 407

ZOVIRAX® (Acyclovir) ℞

[*zō″vī′răx*]

Ointment 5%

DESCRIPTION

Zovirax is the brand name for acyclovir, an antiviral drug against herpes viruses. Zovirax Ointment 5% is a formulation for topical administration. Each gram of Zovirax Ointment 5% contains 50 mg of acyclovir in a polyethylene glycol (PEG) base.

The chemical name of acyclovir is 9-[(2-hydroxyethoxy)methyl]guanine.

Acyclovir is a white, crystalline powder with a molecular weight of 225 Daltons, and a maximum solubility in water of 1.3 mg/ml.

CLINICAL PHARMACOLOGY

Acyclovir is a synthetic acyclic purine nucleoside analogue with *in vitro* inhibitory activity against Herpes simplex types 1 and 2 (HSV-1 and HSV-2), varicella-zoster, Epstein-Barr and cytomegalovirus. In cell cultures, the inhibitory activity of acyclovir for Herpes simplex virus is highly selective. Cellular thymidine kinase does not effectively utilize acyclovir as a substrate. Herpes simplex virus-coded thymidine kinase, however, converts acyclovir into acyclovir monophosphate, a nucleotide. The monophosphate is further converted into diphosphate by cellular guanylate kinase and into triphosphate by a number of cellular enzymes.[1] Acyclovir triphosphate interferes with Herpes simplex virus DNA polymerase and inhibits viral DNA replication. Acyclovir triphosphate also inhibits cellular α-DNA polymerase but to a lesser degree. *In vitro*, acyclovir triphosphate can be incorporated into growing chains of DNA by viral DNA polymerase and to a much smaller extent by cellular α-DNA polymerase.[2] When incorporation occurs, the DNA chain is terminated.[3] Acyclovir is preferentially taken up and selectively converted to the active triphosphate form by herpesvirus-infected cells. Thus, acyclovir is much less toxic *in vitro* for normal uninfected cells because: 1) less is taken up; 2) less is converted to the active form; 3) cellular α-DNA polymerase is less sensitive to the effects of the active form.

The relationship between *in vitro* susceptibility of Herpes simplex virus to antiviral drugs and clinical response has not been established. The techniques and cell culture types used for determining *in vitro* susceptibility may influence the results obtained. Using a quantitative assay to determine the acyclovir concentration producing 50% inhibition of viral cytopathic effect (ID_{50}), 28 HSV-1 clinical isolates had a mean ID_{50} of 0.17 μg/ml and 32 HSV-2 clinical isolates had a mean ID_{50} of 0.46 μg/ml.* Results from other studies using different assays have yielded mean ID_{50} values for clinical HSV-1 isolates of 0.018, 0.03 and 0.043 μg/ml and for clinical HSV-2 isolates of 0.027, 0.36 and 0.03 μg/ml, respectively.[4,5,6]

Two clinical pharmacology studies were performed with Zovirax Ointment 5% in adult immunocompromised patients, at risk of developing mucocutaneous Herpes simplex virus infections or with localized varicella-zoster infections. These studies were designed to evaluate the dermal tolerance, systemic toxicity and percutaneous absorption of acyclovir.

In one of these studies, which included 16 inpatients, the complete ointment or its vehicle were randomly administered in a dose of 1 cm strips (25 mg acyclovir) four times a day for seven days to an intact skin surface area of 4.5 square inches. No local intolerance, systemic toxicity or contact dermatitis were observed. In addition, no drug was detected in blood and urine by radioimmunoassay (sensitivity, 0.01 μg/ml).

The other study included eleven patients with localized varicella-zoster. In this uncontrolled study, acyclovir was detected in the blood of 9 patients and in the urine of all patients tested. Acyclovir levels in plasma ranged from <0.01 to 0.28 μg/ml in eight patients with normal renal function, and from <0.01 to 0.78 μg/ml in one patient with impaired renal function. Acyclovir excreted in the urine ranged from <0.02 to 9.4 percent of the daily dose. Therefore, systemic absorption of acyclovir after topical application is minimal.

INDICATIONS AND USAGE

Zovirax (Acyclovir) Ointment 5% is indicated in the management of initial herpes genitalis and in limited nonlife-threatening mucocutaneous Herpes simplex virus infections in immunocompromised patients. In clinical trials of initial herpes genitalis, Zovirax Ointment 5% has shown a decrease in healing time and in some cases a decrease in duration of viral shedding and duration of pain. In studies in immunocompromised patients with mainly herpes labialis, there was a decrease in duration of viral shedding and a slight decrease in duration of pain.

By contrast, in studies of recurrent herpes genitalis and of herpes labialis in nonimmunocompromised patients, there was no evidence of clinical benefit; there was some decrease in duration of viral shedding.

Diagnosis: Whereas cutaneous lesions associated with Herpes simplex infections are often characteristic, the finding of multinucleated giant cells in smears prepared from lesion exudate or scrapings may assist in the diagnosis.[7] Positive cultures for Herpes simplex virus offer a reliable means for confirmation of the diagnosis. In genital herpes, appropriate examinations should be performed to rule out other sexually transmitted diseases.

CONTRAINDICATIONS

Zovirax Ointment 5% is contraindicated for patients who develop hypersensitivity or chemical intolerance to the components of the formulation.

WARNINGS

Zovirax Ointment 5% is intended for cutaneous use only and should not be used in the eye.

PRECAUTIONS

General: The recommended dosage, frequency of applications, and length of treatment should not be exceeded (see DOSAGE AND ADMINISTRATION). There exist no data which demonstrate that the use of Zovirax Ointment 5% will either prevent transmission of infection to other persons or prevent recurrent infections when applied in the absence of signs and symptoms. Zovirax Ointment 5% should not be used for the prevention of recurrent HSV infections. Although clinically significant viral resistance associated with the use of Zovirax Ointment 5% has not been observed, this possibility exists.

Drug Interactions: Clinical experience has identified no interactions resulting from topical or systemic administration of other drugs concomitantly with Zovirax Ointment 5%.

Carcinogenesis, Mutagenesis, Impairment of Fertility: Acyclovir was tested in lifetime bioassays in rats and mice at single daily doses of 50, 150 and 450 mg/kg/day given by gavage. These studies showed no statistically significant difference in the incidence of benign and malignant tumors produced in drug-treated as compared to control animals, nor did acyclovir induce the occurrence of tumors earlier in drug-treated animals as compared to controls. In 2 *in vitro* cell transformation assays, used to provide preliminary assessment of potential oncogenicity in advance of these more definitive lifetime bioassays in rodents, conflicting results were obtained. Acyclovir was positive at the highest dose used in one system and the resulting morphologically transformed cells formed tumors when inoculated into immunosuppressed, syngeneic, weanling mice. Acyclovir was negative in another transformation system.

No chromosome damage was observed at maximum tolerated parenteral doses of 100 mg/kg acyclovir in rats or Chinese hamsters; higher doses of 500 and 1000 mg/kg were clastogenic in Chinese hamsters. In addition, no activity was found in a dominant lethal study in mice. In 9 of 11 microbial and mammalian cell assays, no evidence of mutagenicity was observed. In 2 mammalian cell assays (human lymphocytes and L5178Y mouse lymphoma cells *in vitro*), positive response for mutagenicity and chromosomal damage occurred, but only at concentrations at least 1000 times the plasma levels achieved in man following topical application.

Acyclovir does not impair fertility or reproduction in mice at oral doses up to 450 mg/kg/day or in rats at subcutaneous doses up to 25 mg/kg/day. In rabbits given a high dose of acyclovir (50 mg/kg/day, s.c.), there was a statistically significant decrease in implantation efficiency.

Pregnancy: *Teratogenic Effects.* Pregnancy Category C. Acyclovir has been known to cause a statistically significant decrease in implantation efficiency in rabbits, when given at subcutaneous doses providing mean plasma levels of drug 2.2 times those expected from use in patients with normal renal function.

Reproduction studies were negative for impairment of fertility or harm to the fetus in mice given oral doses, and in rats given subcutaneous doses providing mean plasma levels of drug 84 times and 4 times (respectively) greater than those expected from use in patients with normal renal function.

Acyclovir was not teratogenic after subcutaneous administration of up to 50 mg/kg/day during the period of organogenesis in rats and rabbits; doses up to 450 mg/kg given daily by gavage to mice were not teratogenic. There are, however, no adequate and well-controlled studies in pregnant women. Acyclovir should be used during pregnancy only if the potential benefit justifies the potential risk to the fetus.

Nursing Mothers: It is not known whether this drug is excreted in human milk. Because many drugs are excreted in human milk, caution should be exercised when Zovirax is administered to a nursing woman.

ADVERSE REACTIONS

Because ulcerated genital lesions are characteristically tender and sensitive to any contact or manipulation, patients may experience discomfort upon application of ointment. In the controlled clinical trials, mild pain (including transient burning and stinging) was reported by 103 (28.3%) of 364 patients treated with acyclovir and by 115 (31.1%) of 370 patients treated with placebo; treatment was discontinued in 2 of these patients. Other local reactions among acyclovir-treated patients included pruritis in 15 (4.1%), rash in 1

(0.3%) and vulvitis in 1 (0.3%). Among the placebo-treated patients, pruritus was reported by 17 (4.6%) and rash by 1 (0.3%).
In all studies, there was no significant difference between the drug and placebo group in the rate or type of reported adverse reactions nor were there any differences in abnormal clinical laboratory findings.

OVERDOSAGE

Overdosage by topical application of Zovirax Ointment 5% is unlikely because of limited transcutaneous absorption (see Clinical Pharmacology).

DOSAGE AND ADMINISTRATION

Apply sufficient quantity to adequately cover all lesions every 3 hours 6 times per day for 7 days. The dose size per application will vary depending upon the total lesion area but should approximate a one-half inch ribbon of ointment per 4 square inches of surface area. A finger cot or rubber glove should be used when applying Zovirax to prevent autoinoculation of other body sites and transmission of infection to other persons. **Therapy should be initiated as early as possible following onset of signs and symptoms.**

HOW SUPPLIED

Zovirax Ointment 5% is supplied in 15 g tubes (NDC 0081-0993-94). Each gram contains 50 mg acyclovir in a polyethylene glycol base. Store at 15°-25°C (59°-77°F) in a dry place.
Animal Pharmacology And Animal Toxicology: Topical treatment of guinea pigs with 10% acyclovir in polyethylene glycol ointment for three weeks did not result in cutaneous irritation or systemic toxicity. Also, a wide variety of animal tests by parenteral routes demonstrated that acyclovir has a low order of toxicity.
Acyclovir did not cause dermal sensitization in guinea pigs.

REFERENCES

1. Miller WH and Miller RL. J Biol Chem *255* (15):7204–7207, 1980.
2. Furman PA et al. J Virol *32* (1):72–77, 1979.
3. Derse D et al. J Biol Chem *256* (22): 11447–11451, 1981.
4. Collins P and Bauer DJ. J Antimicrob Chemother *5* :431–436, 1979.
5. Crumpacker CS et al. Antimicrob Agents Chemother *15* :642–645, 1979.
6. De Clercq E et al. J Infect Dis *141* :563–574, 1980.
7. Naib ZM et al. Cancer Res *33* 1452–1463, 1973.
*Data on file at Burroughs Wellcome Co.

U.S. Patent No. 4199574

ZOVIRAX® Sterile Powder ℞

[zō″vī′răx]
(Acyclovir Sodium)
FOR INTRAVENOUS INFUSION ONLY

DESCRIPTION

Zovirax is the brand name for acyclovir, an antiviral drug active against herpesviruses. Zovirax Sterile Powder is a formulation for intravenous administration. Each vial of Zovirax Sterile Powder contains 549 mg of sterile lyophilized acyclovir sodium equivalent to 500 mg of acyclovir.
The chemical name of acyclovir sodium is 9-[(2-hydroxyethoxy)methyl]guanine sodium.
Acyclovir sodium is a white, crystalline powder with a molecular weight of 247 daltons, and a solubility in water exceeding 100 mg/ml. Recommended reconstitution with 10 ml diluent per vial yields 50 mg/ml acyclovir (pH approximately 11). Further dilution in any appropriate intravenous solution must be performed before infusion (see Method of Preparation). At physiologic pH, acyclovir exists as the unionized form with a molecular weight of 225 daltons and a maximum solubility of 2.5 mg/ml at 37°C.

CLINICAL PHARMACOLOGY

Acyclovir is a synthetic acyclic purine nucleoside analogue with *in vitro* and *in vivo* inhibitory activity against Herpes simplex, varicella-zoster, Epstein-Barr and cytomegalovirus. In cell cultures, the inhibitory activity of acyclovir for Herpes simplex virus is highly selective. Cellular thymidine kinase does not effectively utilize acyclovir as a substrate. Herpes simplex virus-coded thymidine kinase, however, converts acyclovir into acyclovir monophosphate, a nucleotide analogue. The monophosphate is further converted into diphosphate by cellular guanylate kinase and into triphosphate by a number of cellular enzymes.[1] Acyclovir triphosphate interferes with Herpes simplex virus DNA polymerase and inhibits viral DNA replication. Acyclovir triphosphate also inhibits cellular α-DNA polymerase but to a lesser degree. *In vitro*, acyclovir triphosphate can be incorporated into growing chains of DNA by viral DNA polymerase and to a much smaller extent by cellular α-DNA polymerase.[2] When incorporation occurs, the DNA chain is terminated.[3] Acyclovir is preferentially taken up and selectively converted to the active triphosphate form by herpesvirus-infected cells. Thus, acyclovir is much less toxic *in vitro* for normal uninfected cells because: 1) less is taken up; 2) less is converted to the active form; 3) cellular α-DNA polymerase is less sensitive to the effects of the active form.
The relationship between *in vitro* susceptibility of Herpes simplex virus to antiviral drugs and clinical response has not been established. The techniques and cell types used for determining *in vitro* susceptibility may influence the results obtained. With a quantitative assay to determine the acyclovir concentration producing 50% inhibition of viral cytopathic effect (ID_{50}), 28 HSV-1 clinical isolates had a mean ID_{50} of 0.17 μg/ml and 32 HSV-2 clinical isolates had a mean ID_{50} of 0.46 μg/ml. Results from other studies using different assays have yielded mean ID_{50} values for clinical HSV-1 isolates of 0.018, 0.03 and 0.043 μg/ml and for clinical HSV-2 isolates of 0.027, 0.36 and 0.03 μg/ml, respectively.[4,5,6]
Pharmacokinetics: The pharmacokinetics of acyclovir has been evaluated in 95 patients (9 studies). Results were obtained in adult patients with normal renal function during Phase I/II studies after single doses ranging from 0.5 to 15 mg/kg and after multiple doses ranging from 2.5 to 15 mg/kg every 8 hours. Pharmacokinetics was also determined in pediatric patients with normal renal function ranging in age from 1 to 17 years at doses of 250 mg/M^2 or 500 mg/M^2 every 8 hours. In these studies, dose-independent pharmacokinetics is observed in the range of 0.5 to 15 mg/kg. Proportionality between dose and plasma levels is seen after single doses or at steady state after multiple dosing.[7] When Zovirax was administered to adults at 5 mg/kg (approximately 250 mg/M^2) by 1-hr infusions every 8 hours, mean steady-state peak and trough concentrations of 9.8 μg/ml (5.5 to 13.8 μg/ml) and 0.7 μg/ml (0.2 to 1.0 μg/ml), respectively, were achieved. Similar concentrations are achieved in children over 1 year of age when doses of 250 mg/M^2 are given every 8 hours. Concentrations achieved in the cerebrospinal fluid are approximately 50% of plasma values. Plasma protein binding is relatively low (9% to 33%) and drug interactions involving binding site displacement are not anticipated.[7]
Renal excretion of unchanged drug by glomerular filtration and tubular secretion is the major route of acyclovir elimination accounting for 62 to 91% of the dose as determined by ^{14}C-labelled drug. The only major urinary metabolite detected is 9-carboxymethoxymethylguanine. This may account for up to 14.1% of the dose in patients with normal renal function. An insignificant amount of drug is recovered in feces and expired CO_2 and there is no evidence to suggest tissue retention.[7] However, postmortem examinations have shown that acyclovir is widely distributed in tissues and body fluids including brain, kidney, lung, liver, muscle, spleen, uterus, vaginal mucosa, vaginal secretions, cerebrospinal fluid and herpetic vesicular fluid.
In a Phase I study in 3 adult volunteers, 1 g of probenecid was administered orally prior to a single 1-hour 5 mg/kg intravenous infusion of acyclovir. The acyclovir half-life and area under the plasma concentration-time curve increased by 18 and 40%, respectively, compared to a control infusion of acyclovir without probenecid. The mean urinary excretion of acyclovir decreased from 79% to 69% of the dose indicating that probenecid can influence the renal excretion of acyclovir.[8]
The half-life and total body clearance of acyclovir is dependent on renal function as shown below.[7]

Creatinine Clearance (ml/min/1.73M²)	Half-Life (hr)	Total Body Clearance (ml/min/1.73M²)
> 80	2.5	327
50–80	3.0	248
15–50	3.5	190
0 (Anuric)	19.5	29

Zovirax was administered at a dose of 2.5 mg/kg to 6 adult patients with severe renal failure. The peak and trough plasma levels during the 47 hours preceding hemodialysis were 8.5 μg/ml and 0.7 μg/ml, respectively.
Consult DOSAGE AND ADMINISTRATION section for recommended adjustments in dosing based upon creatinine clearance.
The half-life and total body clearance of acyclovir in pediatric patients over 1 year of age is similar to those in adults with normal renal function (see DOSAGE AND ADMINISTRATION).

INDICATIONS AND USAGE

Zovirax Sterile Powder is indicated for the treatment of initial and recurrent mucosal and cutaneous Herpes simplex (HSV-1 and HSV-2) infections in immunocompromised adults and children. It is also indicated for severe initial clinical episodes of herpes genitalis in patients who are not immunocompromised.
These indications are based on the results of several double-blind, placebo-controlled studies which evaluated the drug's effect on virus excretion, complete healing of lesions, and relief of pain.

Herpes Simplex Infections in Immunocompromised Patients
A multicenter trial of Zovirax Sterile Powder at a dose of 250 mg/M^2 every 8 hours (750 mg/M^2/day) for 7 days was conducted in 97 immunocompromised patients with oro-facial, esophageal, genital and other localized infections (50 treated with Zovirax and 47 with placebo). Zovirax significantly decreased virus excretion, reduced pain, and promoted scabbing and rapid healing of lesions.[9,10,11]
Initial Episodes of Herpes Genitalis
A controlled trial was conducted in 28 patients with severe initial episodes of herpes genitalis with a Zovirax dosage of 5 mg/kg every 8 hours for 5 days (12 patients treated with Zovirax and 16 with placebo). Significant treatment effects were seen in elimination of virus from lesions and in reduction of healing times.[12]
In a similar study, 15 patients with initial episodes of genital herpes were treated with Zovirax 5 mg/kg every 8 hours for 5 days and 15 with placebo. Zovirax decreased the duration of viral excretion, new lesion formation, duration of vesicles and promoted more rapid healing of all lesions.[13]
Diagnosis
The use of appropriate laboratory diagnostic procedures will help to establish the etiologic diagnosis. Positive cultures for Herpes simplex virus offer a reliable means for confirmation of the diagnosis. In initial episodes of genital herpes, appropriate examinations should be performed to rule out other sexually transmitted diseases. Whereas cutaneous lesions associated with Herpes simplex infections are often characteristic, the finding of multinucleated giant cells in smears prepared from lesion exudate or scrapings may assist in the diagnosis.[14]

CONTRAINDICATIONS

Zovirax Sterile Powder is contraindicated for patients who develop hypersensitivity to the drug.

WARNINGS

Zovirax Sterile Powder is intended for intravenous infusion only, and should not be administered topically, intramuscularly, orally, subcutaneously, or in the eye. Intravenous infusions must be given over a period of at least 1 (one) hour to prevent renal tubular damage (see PRECAUTIONS and DOSAGE AND ADMINISTRATION).

PRECAUTIONS

General: The recommended dosage, frequency and length of treatment should not be exceeded (see DOSAGE AND ADMINISTRATION).

Although the aqueous solubility of acyclovir sodium (for infusion) is > 100 mg/ml, precipitation of acyclovir crystals in renal tubules can occur if the maximum solubility of free acyclovir (2.5 mg/ml at 37°C in water) is exceeded or if the drug is administered by bolus injection. This complication causes a rise in serum creatinine and blood urea nitrogen (BUN), and a decrease in renal creatinine clearance. Ensuing renal tubular damage can produce acute renal failure.

Abnormal renal function (decreased creatinine clearance) can occur as a result of acyclovir administration and depends on the state of the patient's hydration, other treatments, and the rate of drug administration. Bolus administration of the drug leads to a 10% incidence of renal dysfunction, while in controlled studies, infusion of 5 mg/kg (250 mg/M^2) over an hour was associated with a lower frequency—4.6%. Concomitant use of other nephrotoxic drugs, pre-existing renal disease, and dehydration make further renal impairment with acyclovir more likely. In most instances, alterations of renal function were transient and resolved spontaneously or with improvement of water and electrolyte balance, drug dosage adjustment or discontinuation of drug administration. However, in some instances, these changes may progress to acute renal failure.
Administration of Zovirax by intravenous infusion must be accompanied by adequate hydration. Since maximum urine concentration occurs within the first 2 hours following infusion, particular attention should be given to establishing sufficient urine flow during that period in order to prevent precipitation in renal tubules.
When dosage adjustments are required they should be based on estimated creatinine clearance (See DOSAGE AND ADMINISTRATION).
Approximately 1% of patients receiving intravenous acyclovir have manifested encephalopathic changes characterized by either lethargy, obtundation, tremors, confusion, hallucinations, agitation, seizures or coma. Zovirax should be used with caution in those patients who have underlying neurologic abnormalities and those with serious renal, hepatic, or electrolyte abnormalities or significant hypoxia. It should also be used with caution in patients who have manifested prior neurologic reactions to cytotoxic drugs or those receiving concomitant intrathecal methotrexate or interferon.
Exposure of HSV isolates to acyclovir *in vitro* can lead to the emergence of less sensitive viruses. These viruses usually are deficient in thymidine kinase (required for acyclovir activa-

Continued on next page

Burroughs Wellcome—Cont.

tion) and are less pathogenic in animals. Similar isolates have been observed in 6 severely immunocompromised patients during the course of controlled and uncontrolled studies of intravenously administered Zovirax. These occurred in patients with congenital severe combined immunodeficiencies or following bone marrow transplantation. The presence of these viruses was not associated with a worsening of clinical illness and, in some instances, the virus disappeared spontaneously. The possibility of the appearance of less sensitive viruses must be borne in mind when treating such patients. The relationship between the *in vitro* sensitivity of herpesviruses to acyclovir and clinical response to therapy has yet to be established.

Drug Interactions: Co-administration of probenecid with acyclovir has been shown to increase the mean half-life and the area under the concentration-time curve. Urinary excretion and renal clearance were correspondingly reduced. Clinical experience has identified no other significant interactions resulting from administration of other drugs concomitantly with Zovirax Sterile Powder.

Carcinogenesis, Mutagenesis, Impairment of Fertility: Acyclovir was tested in lifetime bioassays in rats and mice at single daily doses of 50, 150 and 450 mg/kg given by gavage. There was no statistically significant difference in the incidence of tumors between treated and control animals, nor did acyclovir appear to shorten the latency of tumors. In 2 *in vitro* cell transformation assays, used to provide preliminary assessment of potential oncogenicity in advance of these more definitive lifetime bioassays in rodents, conflicting results were obtained. Acyclovir was positive at the highest dose used in one system and the resulting morphologically transformed cells formed tumors when inoculated into immunosuppressed, syngeneic, weanling mice. Acyclovir was negative in another transformation system.

No chromosome damage was observed at maximum tolerated parenteral doses of 100 mg/kg acyclovir in rats or Chinese hamsters; higher doses of 500 and 1000 mg/kg were clastogenic in Chinese hamsters. In addition, no activity was found in a dominant lethal study in mice. In 9 of 11 microbial and mammalian cell assays, no evidence of mutagenicity was observed. In 2 mammalian cell assays (human lymphocytes and L5178Y mouse lymphoma cells *in vitro*), positive responses for mutagenicity and chromosomal damage occurred, but only at concentrations at least 25 times the acyclovir plasma levels achieved in man.

Acyclovir does not impair fertility or reproduction in mice at oral doses up to 450 mg/kg/day. In female rabbits treated subcutaneously with acyclovir subsequent to mating, there was a statistically significant decrease in implantation efficiency but no concomitant decrease in litter size at a dose of 50 mg/kg/day.

Pregnancy: Teratogenic Effects. Pregnancy Category C. Acyclovir was not teratogenic in the mouse (450 mg/kg/day, p.o.), rabbit (50 mg/kg/day, s.c.) or rat (50 mg/kg/day, s.c.).

Although maximum tolerated doses were tested in the teratology studies, the plasma levels obtained did not exaggerate maximum plasma levels that might occur with clinical use of intravenous acyclovir.

There have been no adequate and well-controlled studies in pregnant women. Acyclovir should be used during pregnancy only if the potential benefit justifies the potential risk to the fetus.

Nursing Mothers: It is not known whether this drug is excreted in human milk. Because many drugs are excreted in human milk, caution should be exercised when Zovirax is administered to a nursing woman.

ADVERSE REACTIONS

The most frequent adverse reactions reported during controlled clinical trials of Zovirax in 64 patients were inflammation or phlebitis at the injection site following infiltration of the I.V. fluid in 9 (14.0%), transient elevations of serum creatinine in 3 (4.7%), and rash or hives in 3 (4.7%). Less frequent adverse reactions were diaphoresis, hematuria, hypotension, headache and nausea, each of which occurred in 1 patient (1.6%). Of the 63 patients receiving placebo, 3 (4.8%) experienced inflammation/phlebitis and 3 (4.8%) experienced rash or itching. Hematuria and nausea were experienced by placebo recipients at the same frequency.

Among 51 immunocompromised patients, one, a bone marrow transplant recipient with pneumonitis, developed seizures, cerebral edema, coma and expired with changes consistent with cerebral anoxia on postmortem biopsy; another immunocompromised patient exhibited coarse tremor and clonus.

Additional adverse reactions were reported in uncontrolled trials. The most frequent adverse reaction was elevated serum creatinine. This occurred in 9.8 percent of patients, usually following rapid (less than 10 minutes) intranvenous infusion. Less frequent adverse experiences were thrombocytosis and jitters, each in 0.4% of patients.

Approximately 1% of patients receiving intravenous acyclovir have manifested encephalopathic changes characterized by either lethargy, obtundation, tremors, confusion, hallucinations, agitation, seizures or coma (see PRECAUTIONS).

OVERDOSAGE

Overdosage has been reported following administration of bolus injections, or inappropriately high doses, and in patients whose fluid and electrolyte balance was not properly monitored. This has resulted in elevations in BUN, serum creatinine and subsequent renal failure.

Precipitation of acyclovir in renal tubules may occur when the solubility (2.5 mg/ml) in the intratubular fluid is exceeded (see PRECAUTIONS). A six hour hemodialysis results in a 60% decrease in plasma acyclovir concentration. Data concerning peritoneal dialysis are incomplete but indicate that this method may be significantly less efficient in removing acyclovir from the blood. In the event of acute renal failure and anuria, the patient may benefit from hemodialysis until rena function is restored (see DOSAGE AND ADMINISTRATION).

DOSAGE AND ADMINISTRATION

CAUTION— RAPID OR BOLUS INTRAVENOUS AND INTRAMUSCULAR OR SUBCUTANEOUS INJECTION MUST BE AVOIDED.

Dosage: ***MUCOSAL AND CUTANEOUS HERPES SIMPLEX (HSV-1 and HSV-2) INFECTIONS IN IMMUNOCOMPROMISED PATIENTS***—5 mg/kg infused at a constant rate over 1 hour, every 8 hours (15 mg/kg/day) for 7 days in adult patients with normal renal function. In children under 12 years of age, more accurate dosing can be attained by infusing 250 mg/M^2 at a constant rate over 1 hour, every 8 hours (750 mg/M^2/day) for 7 days.

SEVERE INITIAL CLINICAL EPISODES OF HERPES GENITALIS—The same dose given above—administered for 5 days.

Therapy should be initiated as early as possible following onset of signs and symptoms.

PATIENTS WITH ACUTE OR CHRONIC RENAL IMPAIRMENT: Refer to DOSAGE AND ADMINISTRATION section for recommended doses, and adjust the dosing interval as indicated in the table below.

Creatinine Clearance (ml/min/1.73M^2)	Dose (mg/kg)	Dosing Interval (hours)
>50	5	8
25–50	5	12
10–25	5	24
0–10	2.5	24

Hemodialysis: For patients who require dialysis, the mean plasma half-life of acyclovir during hemodialysis is approximately 5 hours. This results in a 60% decrease in plasma concentrations following a 6 hour dialysis period. Therefore, the patient's dosing schedule should be adjusted so that a dose is administered after each dialysis.

Method of Preparation: Each 10 ml vial contains acyclovir sodium equivalent to 500 mg of acyclovir. The contents of the vial should be dissolved in 10 ml of sterile water for injection or bacteriostatic water for injection containing benzyl alcohol yielding a final concentration of 50 mg/ml of acyclovir (pH approximately 11). Shake the vial well to assure complete dissolution before measuring and transferring each individual dose. DO NOT USE BACTERIOSTATIC WATER FOR INJECTION CONTAINING PARABENS. It is incompatible with Zovirax Sterile Powder and may cause precipitation.

Administration: The calculated dose should then be removed and added to any appropriate intravenous solution at a volume selected for administration during each 1 hour infusion. Infusion concentrations of approximately 7 mg/ml or lower are recommended. In clinical studies, the average 70 kg adult received approximately 60 ml of fluid per dose. Higher concentrations (e.g., 10 mg/ml) may produce phlebitis or inflammation at the injection site upon inadvertent extravasation. Standard, commercially available electrolyte and glucose solutions are suitable for intravenous administration; biologic or colloidal fluids (e.g., blood products, protein solutions, etc.) are not recommended.

Once in solution in the vial at a concentration of 50 mg/ml, the drug should be used within 12 hours. Once diluted for administration, each dose should be used within 24 hours. Refrigeration of reconstituted solutions may result in formation of a precipitate which will redissolve at room temperature.

HOW SUPPLIED

ZOVIRAX Sterile Powder is supplied in 10 ml sterile vials, each containing acyclovir sodium equivalent to 500 mg of acyclovir, cartons of 5 (NDC 0081-0995-46) and 25 (NDC 0081-0995-95). Store at 15°–30°C (59°–86°F).

Also available: ZOVIRAX Ointment, 5% in 15 g tubes. Each gram contains 50 mg acyclovir in a polyethylene glycol base. U.S. Patent No. 4199574

References

1. W.H. Miller and R.L. Miller, J. Biol. Chem. *225* (15): 7204–7207, 1980.
2. P.A. Furman, *et al.*, J. Virol. *32* (1): 72–77, 1979.
3. D. Derse, *et al.*, J. Biol. Chem. *256* (22): 11447–11451, 1981.
4. P. Collins and D.J. Bauer. J. Antimicrob. Chemother. *5* :431–436, 1979.
5. C.S. Crumpacker, *et al.*, Antimicrob. Agents Chemother. *15* :642–645, 1979.
6. E. De Clercq. *et al.*, J. Infect. Dis. *141* :563–574, 1980.
7. M.R. Blum, *et al.*, Am. J. Med. *73* (1A): 186–192, Jul. 20, 1982.
8. O.L. Laskin, *et al.*, Antimicrob. Agents Chemother. *21* (5): 804–807, May 1982.
9. C.D. Mitchell, *et al.*, Lancet *1* (8235): 1389–1392, Jun. 27, 1981.
10. J.C. Wade, *et al.*, Ann. Intern. Med. *96* (3): 265–269, Mar. 1982.
11. J.D. Meyers, *et al.*, Am. J. Med. *73* (1A): 229–235, Jul. 20, 1982.
12. Data on file, Burroughs Wellcome Co.
13. A. Mindel, *et al.*, Lancet *1* (8274): 697–700, Mar. 27, 1982.
14. Z.M. Naib, *et al.*, Cancer Res. *33* :1452–1463, 1973.

ZYLOPRIM ® ℞

[*zī ′lō-prĭm*]
(ALLOPURINOL)
100 mg Scored Tablets and
300 mg Scored Tablets

DESCRIPTION

Zyloprim (Allopurinol) is known chemically as 1,5-dihydro-4*H* -pyrazolo- [3,4-*d*]pyrimidin-4-one. It is a xanthine oxidase inhibitor which is administered orally. Each scored white tablet contains 100 mg allopurinol and the inactive ingredients lactose, magnesium stearate, potato starch, and povidone. Each scored peach tablet contains 300 mg allopurinol and the inactive ingredients corn starch, FD&C Yellow No. 6 Lake, lactose, magnesium stearate, and povidone. Its solubility in water at 37°C is 80.0 mg/dl and is greater in an alkaline solution.

CLINICAL PHARMACOLOGY

Zyloprim (allopurinol) acts on purine catabolism, without disrupting the biosynthesis of purines. It reduces the production of uric acid by inhibiting the biochemical reactions immediately preceding its formation.

Zyloprim is a structural analogue of the natural purine base, hypoxanthine. It is an inhibitor of xanthine oxidase, the enzyme responsible for the conversion of hypoxanthine to xanthine and of xanthine to uric acid, the end product of purine metabolism in man. Zyloprim is metabolized to the corresponding xanthine analogue, oxipurinol (alloxanthine), which also is an inhibitor of xanthine oxidase.

It has been shown that reutilization of both hypoxanthine and xanthine for nucleotide and nucleic acid synthesis is markedly enhanced when their oxidations are inhibited by Zyloprim and oxipurinol. This reutilization does not disrupt normal nucleic acid anabolism, however, because feedback inhibition is an integral part of purine biosynthesis. As a result of xanthine oxidase inhibition, the serum concentration of hypoxanthine plus xanthine in patients receiving Zyloprim for treatment of hyperuricemia is usually in the range of 0.3 to 0.4 mg/dl compared to a normal level of approximately 0.15 mg/dl. A maximum of 0.9 mg/dl of these oxypurines has been reported when the serum urate was lowered to less than 2 mg/dl by high doses of Zyloprim. These values are far below the saturation levels at which point their precipitation would be expected to occur (above 7 mg/dl).

The renal clearance of hypoxanthine and xanthine is at least 10 times greater than that of uric acid. The increased xanthine and hypoxanthine in the urine have not been accompanied by problems of nephrolithiasis. Xanthine crystalluria has been reported in only three patients. Two of the patients had Lesch-Nyhan syndrome, which is characterized by excessive uric acid production combined with a deficiency of the enzyme, hypoxanthine-guanine phosphoribosyltransferase (HGPRTase). This enzyme is required for the conversion of hypoxanthine, xanthine, and guanine to their respective nucleotides. The third patient had lymphosarcoma and produced an extremely large amount of uric acid because of rapid cell lysis during chemotherapy.

Zyloprim is approximately 90% absorbed from the gastrointestinal tract. Peak plasma levels generally occur at 1.5 hours and 4.5 hours for Zyloprim and oxipurinol respectively, and after a single oral dose of 300 mg Zyloprim, maximum plasma levels of about 3 μg/ml of Zyloprim and 6.5 μg/ml of oxipurinol are produced.

Approximately 20% of the ingested Zyloprim is excreted in the feces. Because of its rapid oxidation to oxipurinol and a renal clearance rate approximately that of glomerular filtration rate, Zyloprim has a plasma half-life of about 1–2 hours. Oxipurinol, however, has a longer plasma half-life (approximately 15.0 hours) and therefore effective xanthine oxidase inhibition is maintained over a 24-hour period with single daily doses of Zyloprim. Whereas Zyloprim is cleared essentially by glomerular filtration, oxipurinol is reabsorbed in the kidney tubules in a manner similar to the reabsorption of uric acid.

The clearance of oxipurinol is increased by uricosuric drugs, and as a consequence, the addition of a uricosuric agent reduces to some degree the inhibition of xanthine oxidase by oxipurinol and increases to some degree the urinary excretion of uric acid. In practice, the net effect of such combined therapy may be useful in some patients in achieving minimum serum uric acid levels provided the total urinary uric acid load does not exceed the competence of the patient's renal function.

Hyperuricemia may be primary, as in gout, or secondary to diseases such as acute and chronic leukemia, polycythemia vera, multiple myeloma, and psoriasis. It may occur with the use of diuretic agents, during renal dialysis, in the presence of renal damage, during starvation or reducing diets and in the treatment of neoplastic disease where rapid resolution of tissue masses may occur. Asymptomatic hyperuricemia is not an indication for Zyloprim treatment (see INDICATIONS AND USAGE).

Gout is a metabolic disorder which is characterized by hyperuricemia and resultant deposition of monosodium urate in the tissues, particularly the joints and kidneys. The etiology of this hyperuricemia is the overproduction of uric acid in relation to the patient's ability to excrete it. If progressive deposition of urates is to be arrested or reversed, it is necessary to reduce the serum uric acid level below the saturation point to suppress urate precipitation.

Administration of Zyloprim generally results in a fall in both serum and urinary uric acid within two to three days. The degree of this decrease can be manipulated almost at will since it is dose-dependent. A week or more of treatment with Zyloprim may be required before its full effects are manifested; likewise, uric acid may return to pretreatment levels slowly (usually after a period of seven to ten days following cessation of therapy). This reflects primarily the accumulation and slow clearance of oxipurinol. In some patients a dramatic fall in urinary uric acid excretion may not occur, particularly in those with severe tophaceous gout. It has been postulated that this may be due to the mobilization of urate from tissue deposits as the serum uric acid level begins to fall.

Zyloprim's action differs from that of uricosuric agents, which lower the serum uric acid level by increasing urinary excretion of uric acid. Zyloprim reduces both the serum and urinary uric acid levels by inhibiting the formation of uric acid. The use of Zyloprim to block the formation of urates avoids the hazard of increased renal excretion of uric acid posed by uricosuric drugs.

Zyloprim can substantially reduce serum and urinary uric acid levels in previously refractory patients even in the presence of renal damage serious enough to render uricosuric drugs virtually ineffective. Salicylates may be given conjointly for their antirheumatic effect without compromising the action of Zyloprim. This is in contrast to the nullifying effect of salicylates on uricosuric drugs.

Zyloprim also inhibits the enzymatic oxidation of mercaptopurine, the sulfur-containing analogue of hypoxanthine, to 6-thiouric acid. This oxidation, which is catalyzed by xanthine oxidase, inactivates mercaptopurine. Hence, the inhibition of such oxidation by Zyloprim may result in as much as a 75% reduction in the therapeutic dose requirement of mercaptopurine when the two compounds are given together.

INDICATIONS AND USAGE

THIS IS NOT AN INNOCUOUS DRUG. IT IS NOT RECOMMENDED FOR THE TREATMENT OF ASYMPTOMATIC HYPERURICEMIA.

Zyloprim (allopurinol) reduces serum and urinary uric acid concentrations. Its use should be individualized for each patient and requires an understanding of its mode of action and pharmacokinetics (see CLINICAL PHARMACOLOGY, CONTRAINDICATIONS, WARNINGS and PRECAUTIONS).

Zyloprim is indicated in:

(1) the management of patients with signs and symptoms of primary or secondary gout (acute attacks, tophi, joint destruction, uric acid lithiasis and/or nephropathy).

(2) the management of patients with leukemia, lymphoma and malignancies who are receiving cancer therapy which causes elevations of serum and urinary uric acid levels. Zyloprim treatment should be discontinued when the potential for overproduction of uric acid is no longer present.

(3) the management of patients with recurrent calcium oxalate calculi whose daily uric acid excretion exceeds 800 mg/day in male patients and 750 mg/day in female patients. Therapy in such patients should be carefully assessed initially and reassessed periodically to determine in each case that treatment is beneficial and that the benefits outweigh the risks.

CONTRAINDICATIONS

Patients who have developed a severe reaction to Zyloprim (allopurinol) should not be restarted on the drug.

WARNINGS

ZYLOPRIM (ALLOPURINOL) SHOULD BE DISCONTINUED AT THE FIRST APPEARANCE OF SKIN RASH OR OTHER SIGNS WHICH MAY INDICATE AN ALLERGIC REACTION. In some instances a skin rash may be followed by more severe hypersensitivity reactions such as exfoliative, urticarial and purpuric lesions as well as Stevens-Johnson syndrome (erythema multiforme exudativum), and/or generalized vasculitis, irreversible hepatotoxicity and on rare occasions death.

In patients receiving Purinethol® (mercaptopurine) or Imuran® (azathioprine), the concomitant administration of 300–600 mg of Zyloprim per day will require a reduction in dose to approximately one-third to one-fourth of the usual dose of mercaptopurine or azathioprine. Subsequent adjustment of doses of mercaptopurine or azathioprine should be made on the basis of therapeutic response and the appearance of toxic effects (see CLINICAL PHARMACOLOGY).

A few cases of reversible clinical hepatotoxicity have been noted in patients taking Zyloprim, and in some patients asymptomatic rises in serum alkaline phosphatase or serum transaminase have been observed. If anorexia, weight loss or pruritus develop in patients on Zyloprim, evaluation of liver function should be part of their diagnostic workup. In patients with pre-existing liver disease, periodic liver function tests are recommended during the early stages of therapy.

Due to the occasional occurrence of drowsiness, patients should be alerted to the need for due precaution when engaging in activities where alertness is mandatory.

The occurrence of hypersensitivity reactions to Zyloprim may be increased in patients with decreased renal function receiving thiazides and Zyloprim concurrently. For this reason, in this clinical setting, such combinations should be administered with caution and patients should be observed closely.

PRECAUTIONS

General: An increase in acute attacks of gout has been reported during the early stages of Zyloprim (allopurinol) administration, even when normal or subnormal serum uric acid levels have been attained. Accordingly, maintenance doses of colchicine generally should be given prophylactically when Zyloprim is begun. In addition, it is recommended that the patient start with a low dose of Zyloprim (100 mg daily) and increase at weekly intervals by 100 mg until a serum uric acid level of 6 mg/dl or less is attained but without exceeding the maximum recommended dose (800 mg per day). The use of colchicine or anti-inflammatory agents may be required to suppress gouty attacks in some cases. The attacks usually become shorter and less severe after several months of therapy. The mobilization of urates from tissue deposits which cause fluctuations in the serum uric acid levels may be a possible explanation for these episodes. Even with adequate Zyloprim therapy, it may require several months to deplete the uric acid pool sufficiently to achieve control of the acute attacks.

A fluid intake sufficient to yield a daily urinary output of at least two liters and the maintenance of a neutral or, preferably, slightly alkaline urine are desirable to (1) avoid the theoretical possibility of formation of xanthine calculi under the influence of Zyloprim therapy and (2) help prevent renal precipitation of urates in patients receiving concomitant uricosuric agents.

Some patients with pre-existing renal disease or poor urate clearance have shown a rise in BUN during Zyloprim administration. Although the mechanism responsible for this has not been established, patients with impaired renal function should be carefully observed during the early stages of Zyloprim administration and dosage decreased or the drug withdrawn if increased abnormalities in renal function appear and persist.

Renal failure in association with Zyloprim administration has been observed among patients with hyperuricemia secondary to neoplastic diseases. Concurrent conditions such as multiple myeloma and congestive myocardial disease were present among those patients whose renal dysfunction increased after Zyloprim was begun. Renal failure is also frequently associated with gouty nephropathy and rarely with Zyloprim-associated hypersensitivity reactions. Albuminuria has been observed among patients who developed clinical gout following chronic glomerulonephritis and chronic pyelonephritis.

Patients with decreased renal function require lower doses of Zyloprim than those with normal renal function. Lower than recommended doses should be used to initiate therapy in any patients with decreased renal function and they should be observed closely during the early states of Zyloprim administration. In patients with severely impaired renal function or decreased urate clearance, the half-life of oxipurinol in the plasma is greatly prolonged. Therefore, a dose of 100 mg per day or 300 mg twice a week, or perhaps less, may be sufficient to maintain adequate xanthine oxidase inhibition to reduce serum urate levels.

Bone marrow depression has been reported in patients receiving Zyloprim, most of whom received concomitant drugs with the potential for causing this reaction. This has occurred as early as six weeks to as long as six years after the initiation of Zyloprim therapy. Rarely a patient may develop varying degrees of bone marrow depression, affecting one or more cell lines, while receiving Zyloprim alone.

Information for Patients: Patients should be informed of the following:

(1) They should be cautioned to discontinue Zyloprim (allopurinol) and to consult their physician immediately at the first sign of a skin rash, painful urination, blood in the urine, irritation of the eyes, or swelling of the lips or mouth. (2) They should be reminded to continue drug therapy prescribed for gouty attacks since optimal benefit of Zyloprim may be delayed for two to six weeks. (3) They should be encouraged to increase fluid intake during therapy to prevent renal stones. (4) If a single dose of Zyloprim is occasionally forgotton, there is no need to double the dose at the next scheduled time. (5) There may be certain risks associated with the concomitant use of Zyloprim and dicumarol, sulfinpyrazone, mercaptopurine, azathioprine, ampicillin, amoxicillin and thiazide diuretics, and they should follow the instructions of their physician. (6) Due to the occasional occurrence of drowsiness, patients should take precautions when engaging in activities where alertness is mandatory. (7) Patients may wish to take Zyloprim after meals to minimize gastric irritation.

Laboratory Tests: The correct dosage and schedule for maintaining the serum uric acid within the normal range is best determined by using the serum uric acid as an index.

In patients with pre-existing liver disease, periodic liver function tests are recommended during the early stages of therapy (see WARNINGS).

Zyloprim (allopurinol) and its primary active metabolite oxipurinol are eliminated by the kidneys; therefore, changes in renal function have a profound effect on dosage. In patients with decreased renal function or who have concurrent illnesses which can affect renal function such as hypertension and diabetes mellitus, periodic laboratory parameters of renal function, particularly BUN and serum creatinine or creatinine clearance, should be performed and the patient's Zyloprim dosage reassessed.

The prothrombin time should be reassessed periodically in the patients receiving dicumarol who are given Zyloprim.

Drug Interactions: In patients receiving Purinethol® (mercaptopurine) or Imuran® (azathioprine), the concomitant administration of 300-600 mg of Zyloprim (allopurinol) per day will require a reduction in dose to approximately one-third to one-fourth of the usual dose of mercaptopurine or azathioprine. Subsequent adjustment of doses of mercaptopurine or azathioprine should be made on the basis of therapeutic response and the appearance of toxic effects (see CLINICAL PHARMACOLOGY).

It has been reported that Zyloprim prolongs the half-life of the anticoagulant, dicumarol. The clinical basis of this drug interaction has not been established but should be noted when Zyloprim is given to patients already on dicumarol therapy.

Since the excretion of oxipurinol is similar to that of urate, uricosuric agents, which increase the excretion of urate, are also likely to increase the excretion of oxipurinol and thus lower the degree of inhibition of xanthine oxidase. The concomitant administration of uricosuric agents and Zyloprim has been associated with a decrease in the excretion of oxypurines (hypoxanthine and xanthine) and an increase in urinary uric acid excretion compared with that observed with Zyloprim alone. Although clinical evidence to date has not demonstrated renal precipitation of oxypurines in patients either on Zyloprim alone or in combination with uricosuric agents, the possibility should be kept in mind.

The reports that the concomitant use of Zyloprim and thiazide diuretics may contribute to the enhancement of allopurinol toxicity in some patients have been reviewed in an attempt to establish a cause-and-effect relationship and a mechanism of causation. Review of these case reports indicates that the patients were mainly receiving thiazide diuretics for hypertension and that tests to rule out decreased renal function secondary to hypertensive nephropathy were not often performed. In those patients in whom renal insufficiency was documented, however, the recommendation to lower the dose of Zyloprim was not followed. Although a causal mechanism and a cause-and-effect relationship have not been established, current evidence suggests that renal function should be monitored in patients on thiazide diuretics and Zyloprim even in the absence of renal failure, and dosage levels should be even more conservatively adjusted in those patients on such combined therapy if diminished renal function is detected.

Continued on next page

Burroughs Wellcome—Cont.

An increase in the frequency of skin rash has been reported among patients receiving ampicillin or amoxicillin concurrently with Zyloprim compared to patients who are not receiving both drugs. The cause of the reported association has not been established.
Enhanced bone marrow suppression by cyclophosphamide and other cytotoxic agents has been reported among patients with neoplastic disease, except leukemia, in the presence of Zyloprim. However, in a well-controlled study of patients with lymphoma on combination therapy, Zyloprim did not increase the marrow toxicity of patients treated with cyclophosphamide, doxorubicin, bleomycin, procarbazine and/or mechlorethamine.
Tolbutamide's conversion to inactive metabolites has been shown to be catalyzed by xanthine oxidase from rat liver. The clinical significance, if any, of these observations is unknown.
Chlorpropamide's plasma half-life may be prolonged by Zyloprim, since Zyloprim and chlorpropamide may compete for excretion in the renal tubule. The risk of hypoglycemia secondary to this mechanism may be increased if Zyloprim and chlorpropamide are given concomitantly in the presence of renal insufficiency.
Drug/Laboratory Test Interactions: Zyloprim (allopurinol) is not known to alter the accuracy of laboratory tests.
Pregnancy: *Teratogenic Effects:* Pregnancy Category C. Reproductive studies have been performed in rats and rabbits at doses up to twenty times the usual human dose (5 mg/kg/day), and it was concluded that there was no impaired fertility or harm to the fetus due to Zyloprim (allopurinol). There is a published report of a study in pregnant mice given 50 or 100 mg/kg allopurinol intraperitoneally on gestation days 10 or 13. There were increased numbers of dead fetuses in dams given 100 mg/kg allopurinol but not in those given 50 mg/kg. There were increased numbers of external malformations in fetuses at both doses of allopurinol on gestation day 10 and increased numbers of skeletal malformations in fetuses at both doses on gestation day 13. It cannot be determined whether this represented a fetal effect or an effect secondary to maternal toxicity. There are, however, no adequate or well-controlled studies in pregnant women. Because animal reproduction studies are not always predictive of human response, this drug should be used during pregnancy only if clearly needed.
Experience with Zyloprim during human pregnancy has been limited partly because women of reproductive age rarely require treatment with Zyloprim. There are two unpublished reports and one published paper of women giving birth to normal offspring after receiving Zyloprim during pregnancy.
Nursing Mothers: Zyloprim (allopurinol) and oxipurinol have been found in the milk of a mother who was receiving Zyloprim. Since the effect of Zyloprim on the nursing infant is unknown, caution should be exercised when Zyloprim is administered to a nursing woman.
Pediatric Use: Zyloprim (allopurinol) is rarely indicated for use in children with the exception of those with hyperuricemia secondary to malignancy or to certain rare inborn errors of purine metabolism (see INDICATIONS and DOSAGE AND ADMINISTRATION).

ADVERSE REACTIONS

Data upon which the following estimates of incidence of adverse reactions are made are derived from experiences reported in the literature, unpublished clinical trials and voluntary reports since marketing of Zyloprim (allopurinol) began. Past experience suggested that the most frequent event following the initiation of allopurinol treatment was an increase in acute attacks of gout (average 6% in early studies). An analysis of current usage suggests that the incidence of acute gouty attacks has diminished to less than 1%. The explanation for this decrease has not been determined but may be due in part to initiating therapy more gradually (see PRECAUTIONS and DOSAGE AND ADMINISTRATION).
The most frequent adverse reaction to Zyloprim is skin rash. Skin reactions can be severe and sometimes fatal. Therefore, treatment with Zyloprim should be discontinued immediately if a rash develops (see WARNINGS). Some patients with the most severe reaction also had fever, chills, arthralgias, cholestatic jaundice, eosinophilia and mild leukocytosis or leukopenia. Among 55 patients with gout treated with Zyloprim for 3 to 34 months (average greater than 1 year) and followed prospectively, Rundles observed that 3% of patients developed a type of drug reaction which was predominantly a pruritic maculopapular skin eruption, sometimes scaly or exfoliative. However, with current usage, skin reactions have been observed less frequently than 1%. The explanation for this decrease is not obvious. The incidence of skin rash may be increased in the presence of renal insufficiency. The frequency of skin rash among patients receiving ampicillin or amoxicillin concurrently with Zyloprim has been reported to be increased (see PRECAUTIONS).

Most Common Reactions*
Probably Causally Related

Gastrointestinal: diarrhea, nausea, alkaline phosphatase increase, SGOT/SGPT increase
Metabolic and Nutritional: acute attacks of gout
Skin and Appendages: rash, maculopapular rash
*Early clinical studies and incidence rates from early clinical experience with Zyloprim suggested that these adverse reactions were found to occur at a rate of greater than 1%. The most frequent event observed was acute attacks of gout following the initiation of therapy. Analyses of current usage suggest that the incidence of these adverse reactions is now less than 1%. The explanation for this decrease has not been determined, but it may be due to following recommended usage (See ADVERSE REACTIONS introduction, INDICATIONS, PRECAUTIONS and DOSAGE AND ADMINISTRATION).

Incidence Less Than 1%
Probably Causally Related

Body as a whole: ecchymosis, fever, headache
Cardiovascular: necrotizing angiitis, vasculitis
Gastrointestinal: hepatic necrosis, granulomatous hepatitis, hepatomegaly, hyperbilirubinemia, cholestatic jaundice, vomiting, intermittent abdominal pain, gastritis, dyspepsia
Hemic and Lymphatic: thrombocytopenia, eosinophilia, leukocytosis, leukopenia
Musculoskeletal: myopathy, arthralgias
Nervous: peripheral neuropathy, neuritis, paresthesia, somnolence
Repiratory: epistaxis
Skin and Appendages: erythema multiforme exudativum (Stevens-Johnson syndrome), toxic epidermal necrolysis (Lyell's syndrome), hypersensitivity vasculitis, purpura, vesicular bullous dermatitis, exfoliative dermatitis, eczematoid dermatitis, pruritus, urticaria, alopecia, onycholysis, lichen planus
Special Senses: taste loss/perversion
Urogenital: renal failure, uremia (see PRECAUTIONS)

Incidence Less Than 1%
Causal Relationship Unknown

Body as a whole: malaise
Cardiovascular: pericarditis, peripheral vascular disease, thrombophlebitis, bradycardia, vasodilation
Endocrine: infertility (male), hypercalcemia, gynecomastia (male)
Gastrointestinal: hemorrhagic pancreatitis, gastrointestinal bleeding, stomatitis, salivary gland swelling, hyperlipidemia, tongue edema, anorexia
Hemic and Lymphatic: aplastic anemia, agranulocytosis, eosinophilic fibrohistiocytic lesion of bone marrow, pancytopenia, prothrombin decrease, anemia, hemolytic anemia, reticulocytosis, lymphadenopathy, lymphocytosis
Musculoskeletal: myalgia
Nervous: optic neuritis, confusion, dizziness, vertigo, foot drop, decrease in libido, depression, amnesia, tinnitis, asthenia, insomnia
Respiratory: bronchospasm, asthma, pharyngitis, rhinitis
Skin and Appendages: furunculosis, facial edema, sweating, skin edema
Special Senses: cataracts, macular retinitis, iritis, conjunctivitis, amblyopia
Urogenital: nephritis, impotence, primary hematuria, albuminuria

OVERDOSAGE

Massive overdosing or acute poisoning by Zyloprim (allopurinol) has not been reported.
In mice the 50% lethal dose (LD_{50}) is 160 mg/kg given intraperitoneally (i.p.) with deaths delayed up to five days and 700 mg/kg orally (p.o.) (approximately 140 times the usual human dose) with deaths delayed up to three days. In rats the acute LD_{50} is 750 mg/kg i.p. and 6000 mg/kg p.o. (approximately 1200 times the human dose).
In the management of overdosage there is no specific antidote for Zyloprim. There has been no clinical experience in the management of a patient who has taken massive amounts of Zyloprim.
Both Zyloprim and oxipurinol are dialyzable; however, the usefulness of hemodialysis or peritoneal dialysis in the management of a Zyloprim overdose is unknown.

DOSAGE AND ADMINISTRATION

The dosage of Zyloprim (allopurinol) to accomplish full control of gout and to lower serum uric acid to normal or near-normal levels varies with the severity of the disease. The average is 200 to 300 mg per day for patients with mild gout and 400 to 600 mg per day for those with moderately severe tophaceous gout. The appropriate dosage may be administered in divided doses or as a single equivalent dose with the 300 mg tablet. Dosage requirements in excess of 300 mg should be administered in divided doses. The minimal effective dosage is 100 to 200 mg daily and the maximal recommended dosage is 800 mg daily. To reduce the possibility of flare-up of acute gouty attacks, it is recommended that the patient start with a low dose of Zyloprim (100 mg daily) and increase at weekly intervals by 100 mg until a serum uric acid level of 6 mg/dl or less is attained but without exceeding the maximal recommended dosage.
Normal serum urate levels are usually achieved in one to three weeks. The upper limit of normal is about 7 mg/dl for men and postmenopausal women and 6 mg/dl for premenopausal women. Too much reliance should not be placed on a single uric acid determination since, for technical reasons, estimation of uric acid may be difficult. By selecting the appropriate dosage and, in certain patients, using uricosuric agents concurrently, it is possible to reduce serum uric acid to normal or, if desired, to as low as 2 to 3 mg/dl and keep it there indefinitely.
While adjusting the dosage of Zyloprim in patients who are being treated with colchicine and/or anti-inflammatory agents, it is wise to continue the latter therapy until serum uric acid has been normalized and there has been freedom from acute gouty attacks for several months.
In transferring a patient from a uricosuric agent to Zyloprim, the dose of the uricosuric agent should be gradually reduced over a period of several weeks and the dose of Zyloprim gradually increased to the required dose needed to maintain a normal serum uric acid level.
It should also be noted that Zyloprim is generally better tolerated if taken following meals. A fluid intake sufficient to yield a daily urinary output of at least two liters and the maintenance of a neutral or, preferably, slightly alkaline urine are desirable.
Since Zyloprim and its metabolites are primarily eliminated only by the kidney, accumulation of the drug can occur in renal failure, and the dose of Zyloprim should consequently be reduced. With a creatinine clearance of 10 to 20 ml/min, a daily dosage of 200 mg of Zyloprim is suitable. When the creatinine clearance is less than 10 ml/min the daily dosage should not exceed 100 mg. With extreme renal impairment (creatinine clearance less than 3 ml/min) the interval between doses may also need to be lengthened.
The correct size and frequency of dosage for maintaining the serum uric acid just within the normal range is best determined by using the serum uric acid level as an index.
For the prevention of uric acid nephropathy during the vigorous therapy of neoplastic disease, treatment with 600 to 800 mg daily for two or three days is advisable together with a high fluid intake. Otherwise similar considerations to the above recommendations for treating patients with gout govern the regulation of dosage for maintenance purposes in secondary hyperuricemia.
The dose of Zyloprim recommended for management of recurrent calcium oxalate stones in hyperuricosuric patients is 200 to 300 mg/day in divided doses or as the single equivalent. This dose may be adjusted up or down depending upon the resultant control of the hyperuricosuria based upon subsequent 24 hour urinary urate determinations. Clinical experience suggests that patients with recurrent calcium oxalate stones may also benefit from dietary changes such as the reduction of animal protein, sodium, refined sugars, oxalate-rich foods, and excessive calcium intake as well as an increase in oral fluids and dietary fiber.
Children, 6 to 10 years of age, with secondary hyperuricemia associated with malignancies may be given 300 mg Zyloprim daily while those under 6 years are generally given 150 mg daily. The response is evaluated after approximately 48 hours of therapy and a dosage adjustment is made if necessary.

HOW SUPPLIED

100 mg (white) scored, flat cylindrical tablets imprinted with "ZYLOPRIM 100" on a raised hexagon.
Bottles of 100 (NDC 0081-0996-55) and 1000 (NDC 0081-0996-75) and Unit Dose Pack of 100 (NDC-0081-0996-56).
Store at 15° to 30°C (59° to 86°F) in a dry place.
300 mg (peach) scored, flat, cylindrical tablets imprinted with "ZYLOPRIM 300" on a raised hexagon.
Bottles of 30 (NDC 0081-0998-30), 100 (NDC 0081-0998-55) and 500 (NDC 0081-0998-70) and Unit Dose Pack of 100 (NDC 0081-0998-56). Store at 15° to 30°C (59° to 86°F) in a dry place and protect from light.

U.S. Patent No. 3,624,205 (Use Patent)

Shown in Product Identification Section, page 407

EDUCATIONAL MATERIAL

The following is a selected list of materials loaned free or available without charge to medical personnel, pharmacists, or patients. To order or obtain information regarding availability of continuing health-care education credit, contact your area Burroughs Wellcome Co. Representative or write: Burroughs Wellcome Co., Educational Services, 3030 Cornwallis Road, Research Triangle Park, NC 27709.

CONTINUING HEALTH-CARE EDUCATION MATERIAL AVAILABLE FROM BURROUGHS WELLCOME CO.

AAFP Annual Series
AAFP Monograph Series

Monographs in Urology Series
Wellcome Programs in Pharmacy
Wellcome Programs in Hospital Pharmacy
Video/Monograph Programs
- Calcium Oxalate Stones: Update on Diagnosis and Management
- Atracurium: First Year Report, Parts 1 and 2
- Second International Atracurium Symposium, Parts 1 and 2
- Atracurium Infusion Roundtable
- Sports Injuries of the Ankle
- Pitfalls in Digoxin Therapy
- Update on the Management of Recurrent Renal Stones
- Atracurium: Update on a New Intermediate-Acting Non-depolarizing Muscle Relaxant
- Atracurium: A Clinical Comprehensive
- New Perspectives in Anesthesia
- Atracurium in Clinical Use
- Otitis Externa: Handle with Care (for pharmacists)

Selected Monographs
- The Wellcome Atlas of Sexually Transmitted Diseases
- Outpatient and Home Chemotherapy

Collections of Symposia Presentations Covering the Following Medical Topics
- Therapeutic Workshop Modifying the Disease Process in Rheumatoid Arthritis
- Proceedings of a Symposium on Highlights on Neoplasia in Rheumatoid Arthritis
- Proceedings of a Symposium on Acyclovir
- Proceedings of a Symposium on Atracurium
- Proceedings of a Symposium on Antimicrobial Chemotherapy
- Digoxin Therapy

Medical Notes on the Following Disease States
- The Common Cold
- External Otitis
- Selected Skin Diseases
- Heart Failure
- Angina Pectoris
- Hyperuricemia
- Parkinsonism and Pseudoparkinsonism
- Medical Terminology

Learning Units—CE for Pharmacists/Nurses
- "Pathophysiology of Gout"
- "Virology—A Basic Science Learning Unit"
- "Virology and Herpetic Diseases"
- "Atracurium Learning Unit"—For Hospital Pharmacists
- Urinary Tract Infections Learning Unit
- Acute Otitis Media Learning Unit
- Acute Exacerbations of Chronic Bronchitis Learning Unit
- Intravenous Infusion Learning Unit
- Digoxin Learning Unit

Patient Instructions/Information
- "How to Administer Ear Drops" (English or Spanish)
- "Do You Have Arthritis?"
- "Treating Impetigo" (English or Spanish)
- Urinary Tract Infection
- Understanding Gout
- "Herpes Alert"—Public Service Pamphlet (English or Spanish)
- "Patient Instructions For Treating Genital Herpes" (English or Spanish)
- "Good News: It's Now Controllable"

C & M Pharmacal, Inc.
1519 E. EIGHT MILE ROAD
HAZEL PARK, MI 48030-2696

POD-BEN-25 (C&M) ℞
[*päd-bĕn-25*]
for the removal of warts (including condylomas)

DESCRIPTION
25% Podophyllin (Podophyllum Resin, Indian) in Tincture of Benzoin, USP.
NOTE: This entry does not represent full information regarding the use of this product. Write or call collect for full data: direct inquiry to Medical Information Dept.

HOW SUPPLIED
1 fl. oz. bottle (with data sheet). NDC 00398-0087-01.
NOTE: Pod-Ben-25 is available only from C&M and is to be used (applied) only by the doctor. It is not to be dispensed to the patient.

VERR–CANTH–C&M ℞
[*vĕr-kănth*]
for the removal of benign epithelial growths such as verruca vulgaris or molluscum contagiosum

DESCRIPTION
Cantharidin 0.7% in an adherent-film-forming base of ethylcellulose, cellosolve, collodion, castor oil, penederm (octylphenylpolyethylene glycol), acetone.
NOTE: This entry does not represent full information regarding the use of this product. Write or call collect for full data: direct inquiry to Medical Information Dept.

HOW SUPPLIED
7.5 cc bottle (with data sheet) NDC 00398-0085-75.
NOTE: Verr-Canth is available only from C&M and is to be used (applied) only by the doctor. It is not to be dispensed to the patient.

VERREX–C&M ℞
[*vĕr-rĕks*]
topically for the removal of benign epithelial growths such as common warts

DESCRIPTION
Salicylic acid 30.0%, podophyllin 10.0%, penederm 0.5% (octylphenylpolyethylene glycol) in an adherent-film-forming vehicle of ethylcellulose, cellosolve, collodion, castor oil, acetone.

CAUTION
Federal law prohibits dispensing without a prescription.
NOTE: This entry does not represent full information regarding the use of this product. Write or call collect for full data: direct inquiry to Medical Information Dept.

HOW SUPPLIED
7.5 cc bottle with thin-tipped applicator attached to inside of cap. NDC 00398-0080-75.

VERRUSOL–C&M ℞
[*vĕr 'yŭ-sol*]
for the removal of benign epithelial growths such as common warts

DESCRIPTION
Salicylic acid 30.0%, podophyllin 5.0%, cantharidin 1.0%, penederm 0.5% (octylphenylpolyethylene glycol) in an adherent-film-forming vehicle of ethylcellulose, cellosolve, collodion, castor oil, acetone.
NOTE: This entry does not represent full information regarding the use of this product. Write or call collect for full data: direct inquiry to Medical Information Dept.

HOW SUPPLIED
7.5 cc bottle (with data sheet). NDC 00398-0081-75.
NOTE: Verrusol is available only from C&M and is to be used (applied) only by the doctor. It is not to be dispensed to the patient.

Campbell Laboratories Inc.
300 EAST 51st STREET
P.O. BOX 812, F.D.R. STATION
NEW YORK, NY 10150

HERPECIN-L® Cold Sore Lip Balm OTC
[*her"puh-sin-el"*]

PRODUCT OVERVIEW

KEY FACTS
HERPECIN-L Lip Balm is a convenient, easy-to-use treatment for perioral herpes simplex (HSV-I) infections.

MAJOR USES
HERPECIN-L not only treats cold sores, sun and fever blisters, but with prophylactic use, its sunscreens also protect to help prevent them. Users report early use at the prodromal stages of an attack will often abort the lesions and prevent scabbing. Prescribe: Apply "early and often".

SAFETY INFORMATION
For topical use only. No contraindications. A rare sensitivity to pyridoxine or the sunscreen may occur.

PRESCRIBING INFORMATION

HERPECIN-L® Cold Sore Lip Balm OTC
[*her"puh-sin-el"*]

COMPOSITION
A soothing, emollient, cosmetically pleasant lip balm incorporating pyridoxine HCl; allantoin; the sunscreen, octyl p-(dimethylamino)-benzoate (Padimate O); and titanium dioxide in a balanced, acidic lipid system. (All ingredients appear on the package. Has no caines", antibiotics, phenol or camphor.) (NDC 38083-777-31)

ACTIONS AND USES
HERPECIN-L® relieves dryness and chapping by providing a lipid barrier to help restore normal moisture balance to labial tissues. The sunscreen is effective in 2900-3200 AU range while titanium dioxide helps to block, scatter and reflect the sun's rays.

ADMINISTRATION
(1) *Recurrent "cold sores, sun and fever blisters"*: Simply put, users report the sooner and more often applied, the better the results. Frequent sufferers report that with *prophylactic* use (B.I.D./P.R.N.), their attacks are fewer and less severe. Most recurrent herpes labialis patients are aware of the *prodromal* symptoms: tingling, itching, burning. At this stage, or if the lesion has already developed, HERPECIN-L should be applied liberally as often as convenient —at least *every hour* (qq. hor.). The prodrome will often persist and remind the patient to continue to reapply HERPECIN-L. (2) *Outdoor sun/winter protection:* Apply during and after exposure (and after swimming) and again at bedtime (h.s.). (3) *Dry, chapped lips:* Apply as needed.

NOTE
HERPECIN-L is for peri-oral use only; not for "canker sores" (aphthous stomatitis). Primary attacks, usually in children and young adults, are normally intra-oral and accompanied by foul breath, pain and fever. Lasting up to six weeks, they are resistant to most treatments. Adjunctive therapy for pain, fever and secondary infection may be indicated. Excessive chapping may be from mouth breathing.

ADVERSE REACTIONS
A few, rare instances of topical sensitivity to pyridoxine HCl (Vitamin B_6) and/or the sunscreen have been reported. Discontinue use if allergic reaction develops.

CONTRAINDICATIONS
HERPECIN-L does not contain any steroids. (Corticosteroids are normally contraindicated in *herpes* infections.)

HOW SUPPLIED
2.8 gm. swivel tubes. O.T.C.

SAMPLES AVAILABLE
Yes. (Request on your professional letterhead.)

The Carlton Corporation
(See Glenwood, Inc.)

Carnrick Laboratories, Inc.
65 HORSE HILL ROAD
CEDAR KNOLLS, NJ 07927

AMEN® ℞
[*ā 'men'*]
(medroxyprogesterone acetate tablet U.S.P. 10 mg)

CAUTION
Federal Law Prohibits Dispensing Without Prescription

WARNING:
THE USE OF PROGESTATIONAL AGENTS DURING THE FIRST FOUR MONTHS OF PREGNANCY IS NOT RECOMMENDED.
Progestational agents have been used beginning with the first trimester of pregnancy in an attempt to prevent habitual abortion or treat threatened abortion. There is no adequate evidence that such use is effective and there is evidence of potential harm to the fetus when such drugs are given during the first four months of pregnancy. Furthermore, in the vast majority of women, the cause of abortion is a defective ovum, which progestational agents could not be expected to influence. In addition, the use of progestational agents, with their uterine-relaxant properties, in patients with fertilized defective ova may cause a delay in spontaneous abortion. Therefore, the use of such drugs during the first four months of pregnancy is not recommended.
Several reports suggest an association between intrauterine exposure to female sex hormones and congenital anomalies, including congenital heart defects and limb reduction defects (Refs. 1-5). One study (Ref. 4) estimated a 4.7-fold increased risk of limb reduction defects in infants exposed in utero to sex hormones (oral contraceptives, hormone withdrawal test for pregnancy, or

Continued on next page

Carnrick—Cont.

attempted treatment for threatened abortion). Some of these exposures were very short and involved only a few days of treatment. The data suggest that the risk of limb reduction defects in exposed fetuses is somewhat less than 1 in 1,000.

If the patient is exposed to Amen® during the first four months of pregnancy or if she becomes pregnant while taking this drug, she should be apprised of the potential risks to the fetus.

DESCRIPTION

Amen® (medroxyprogesterone acetate U.S.P.) is a derivative of progesterone. It is a white to off-white, odorless crystalline powder, stable in air, melting between 200° and 210° C. It is freely soluble in chloroform, soluble in acetone and in dioxane, sparingly soluble in alcohol and in methanol, slightly soluble in ether, and insoluble in water.

The chemical name for medroxyprogesterone acetate is Pregn-4-ene-3,20-dione,17-(acetyloxy)-6- methyl-, (6α)-. The structural formula is:

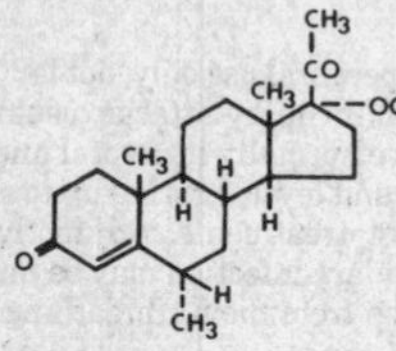

ACTIONS

Amen® (medroxyprogesterone acetate), administered orally in the recommended dose to women with adequate endogenous estrogen, transforms proliferative endometrium into secretory endometrium. Androgenic and anabolic effects have been noted, but the drug is apparently devoid of significant estrogenic activity.

INDICATIONS

Amen® (medroxyprogesterone acetate) is indicated in secondary amenorrhea and abnormal uterine bleeding due to hormonal imbalance in the absence of organic pathology, such as submucous fibroids or uterine cancer.

CONTRAINDICATIONS

1. Thrombophlebitis, thromboembolic disorders, cerebral apoplexy or patients with a past history of these conditions. **2.** Liver dysfunction or disease. **3.** Known or suspected malignancy of breast or genital organs. **4.** Undiagnosed vaginal bleeding. **5.** Missed abortion. **6.** As a diagnostic test for pregnancy. **7.** Known sensitivity to medroxyprogesterone acetate.

WARNINGS

1. The physician should be alert to the earliest manifestations of thrombotic disorders (thrombophlebitis, cerebrovascular disorders, pulmonary embolism, and retinal thrombosis). Should any of these occur or be suspected, the drug should be discontinued immediately.

2. Beagle dogs treated with medroxyprogesterone acetate developed mammary nodules, some of which were malignant. Although nodules occasionally appeared in control animals, they were intermittent in nature, whereas the nodules in the drug treated animals were larger, more numerous, persistent, and there were some breast malignancies with metastases, their significance with respect to humans has not been established.

3. Discontinue medication pending examination if there is sudden partial or complete loss of vision, or if there is sudden onset of proptosis, diplopia or migraine. If examination reveals papilledema, or retinal vascular lesions, medication should be withdrawn.

Detectable amounts of progestin have been identified in the milk of mothers receiving the drug. The effect of this on the nursing infant has not been determined. Masculinization of the female fetus has occurred when progestins have been used in pregnant women.

4. Retrospective studies of morbidity and mortality in Great Britain and studies of morbidity in the United States have shown a statistically significant association between thrombophlebitis, pulmonary embolism, and cerebral thrombosis and embolism and the use of oral contraceptives. There have been three principal studies in Great Britain[6–8] leading to this conclusion and one[9] in this country. The estimate of the relative risk of thromboembolism in the study by Vessey and Doll[8] was about sevenfold, while Sartwell and Associates[9] in the United States found a relative risk of 4.4, meaning that the users are several times as likely to undergo thromboembolic disease without evident cause as non-users. The American study also indicated that the risk did not persist after discontinuation of administration, and that it was not enhanced by long continued administration. The American study was not designed to evaluate a difference between products.

PRECAUTIONS

1. The pretreatment physical examination should include special reference to breast and pelvic organs, as well as Papanicolaou smear.

2. Because this drug may cause some degree of fluid retention, conditions which might be influenced by this factor, such as epilepsy, migraine, asthma, cardiac or renal dysfunction require careful observation.

3. In cases of breakthrough bleeding, as in all cases of irregular bleeding per vaginum, nonfunctional causes should be borne in mind. In cases of undiagnosed vaginal bleeding adequate diagnostic measures are indicated.

4. Patients who have a history of psychic depression should be carefully observed and the drug discontinued if the depression recurs to a serious degree.

5. Any possible influence of prolonged progestin therapy on pituitary, ovarian, adrenal, hepatic or uterine functions awaits further study.

6. A decrease in glucose tolerance has been observed in a small percentage of patients on estrogen-progestin combination drugs. The mechanism of this decrease is obscure. For this reason, diabetic patients should be carefully observed while receiving progestin therapy.

7. The age of the patient constitutes no absolute limiting factor although treatment with progestins may mask the onset of the climacteric.

8. The pathologist should be advised of progestin therapy when relevant specimens are submitted.

9. Because of the occasional occurence of thrombotic disorders, (thrombophlebitis, pulmonary embolism, retinal thrombosis, and cerebrovascular disorders) in patients taking estrogen-progestin combinations and since the mechanism is obscure, the physician should be alert to the earliest manifestation of these disorders.

10. Information for the patient. See text of Patient Information which is printed at the end of this insert.

ADVERSE REACTIONS

The following adverse reactions have been associated with the use of medroxyprogesterone acetate.

Breast: In a few instances, breast tenderness or galactorrhea have occurred.

Pregnancy: A few cases of clitoral hypertrophy have been reported in new born females, whose mothers received medroxyprogesterone acetate during pregnancy. Prolonged postpartum bleeding, postabortal bleeding and missed abortion have been reported. (See WARNING box for possible adverse effects on the fetus).

Psychic: An occasional patient has experienced nervousness, insomnia, somnolence, fatigue or dizziness.

Thromboembolic phenomena: Thromboembolic phenomena including thrombophlebitis and pulmonary embolism have been reported.

Skin and mucous membranes: Sensitivity reactions ranging from pruritus, urticaria, angioneurotic edema to generalized rash and anaphylaxis have occasionally been reported. Acne, alopecia, or hirsutism have been reported in a few cases.

Gastrointestinal: Rarely, nausea has been reported. Jaundice, including neonatal jaundice, has been noted in a few instances.

Miscellaneous: Rare cases of headache and hyperpyrexia have been reported. The following adverse reactions have been observed in women taking progestins including medroxyprogesterone acetate: breakthrough bleeding; spotting; change in menstrual flow; amenorrhea; edema; change in weight (increase or decrease); changes in cervical erosion and cervical secretions; cholestatic jaundice; rash (allergic) with and without pruritus; melasma or chloasma; mental depression.

A statistically significant association has been demonstrated between use of estrogen-progestin combination drugs and the following serious adverse reactions; thrombophlebitis, pulmonary embolism and cerebral thrombosis and embolism. For this reason patients on progestin therapy should be carefully observed.

Although available evidence is suggestive of an association, such a relationship has been neither confirmed nor refuted for the following serious adverse reactions: neuro-ocular lesions, e.g., retinal thrombosis and optic neuritis.

The following adverse reactions have been observed in patients receiving estrogen-progestin combination drugs; rise in blood pressure in susceptible individuals; premenstrual-like syndrome; changes in libido; changes in appetite; cystitis-like syndrome; headache; nervousness; dizziness; fatigue; backache; hirsutism; loss of scalp hair; erythema multiforme; erythema nodosum; hemorraghic eruption; itching. In view of these observations, patients on progestin therapy should be carefully observed.

Female fetal masculinization has been observed in patients receiving progestins. The following laboratory results may be altered by the use of estrogen-progestin combination drugs: Increased sulfobromophthalein and other hepatic function tests; Coagulation tests: increase in prothrombin factors VII, VIII, IX and X; Metyrapone test; Pregnanediol determination.

DOSAGE AND ADMINISTRATION

Secondary Amenorrhea—Amen®(medroxyprogesterone acetate) may be given in dosages of 5 to 10 mg daily for from 5 to 10 days. A dose for inducing an optimum secretory transformation of an endometrium that has been adequately primed with either endogenous or exogenous estrogen is 10 mg of Amen® daily for 10 days. In cases of secondary amenorrhea, therapy may be started at any time. Progestin withdrawal bleeding usually occurs within three to seven days after discontinuing therapy with Amen®.

Abnormal Uterine Bleeding Due to Hormonal Imbalance in the Absence of Organic Pathology—Beginning on the calculated 16th or 21st day of the menstrual cycle, 5 to 10 mg of Amen® may be given daily for from 5 to 10 days. To produce an optimum secretory transformation of an endometrium that has been adequately primed with either endogenous or exogenous estrogen, 10 mg of Amen® daily for 10 days beginning on the 16th day of the cycle is suggested. Progestin withdrawal bleeding usually occurs within three to seven days after discontinuing therapy with Amen®. Patients with a past history of recurrent episodes of abnormal uterine bleeding may benefit from planned menstrual cycling with Amen®.

REFERENCES

1. Gal, I., B. Kirman, and J. Stern, "Hormonal Pregnancy Tests and Congenital Malformation," Nature, 216:83, 1967.
2. Levy, E. P., A. Cohen, and F. C. Fraser, "Hormone Treatment During Pregnancy and Congenital Heart Defects," Lancet, 1:611, 1973.
3. Nora, J. and A. Nora, "Birth Defects and Oral Contraceptives," Lancet, 1:941, 1973.
4. Janerich, D. T., J. M. Piper, and D. M. Glebatis, "Oral Contraceptives and Congenital Limb-Reduction Defects," New England Journal of Medicine, 291:697, 1974.
5. Heinonen, O. P., D. Slone, R. R. Monson, E. B. Hook, and S. Shapiro, "Cardiovascular Birth Defects and Antenatal Exposure to Female Sex Hormones," New England Journal of Medicine, 296:67, 1977.
6. Royal College of General Practitioners; Oral Contraception and Thromboembolic Disease. J. Coll. Gen. Prac., 13:267–279, 1967.
7. Inman, W. H. W. and Vessey, M. P.: Investigation of Deaths From Pulmonary Coronary and Cerebral Thrombosis and Embolism in Women in Child-Bearing Age, Brit. Med. J., 2:193–199, 1968.
8. Vessey, M. P. and Doll, R.: Investigation of Relation Between Use of Oral Contraceptives and Thromboembolic Disease. A Further Report, Brit. Med. J., 2:651–657, 1969.
9. Sartwell, P. E., Masi, A. T., Arthes, G. R., Greene, R. R., and Smith, H. E.: Thromboembolism and Oral Contraceptives: An Epidemiological Case-Control Study, Am. J. Epidem., 90: 365–380, (Nov.) 1969.

Patient Information for Amen®—Warning for Women

There is an increased risk of birth defects in children whose mothers take this drug during the first four months of pregnancy.

Amen® is similar to the progesterone hormones naturally produced by the body. Progesterone and progesterone-like drugs are used to treat menstrual disorders, to test if the body is producing certain hormones, and to treat some forms of cancer in women.

They have been used as a test for pregnancy but such use is no longer considered safe because of possible damage to a developing baby. Also, more rapid methods for testing for pregnancy are now available. These drugs have also been used to prevent miscarriage in the first few months of pregnancy. No adequate evidence is available to show that they are effective for this purpose and there is evidence of an increased risk of birth defects, such as heart or limb defects, if these drugs are taken during the first four months of pregnancy. Furthermore, most cases of early miscarriage are due to causes which could not be helped by these drugs.

The exact risk of taking this drug early in pregnancy and having a baby with a birth defect is not known. However, one study found that babies born to women who had taken sex hormones (such as progesterone-like drugs) during the first three months of pregnancy were 4 to 5 times more likely to have abnormalities of the arms or legs than if their mothers had not taken such drugs. Some of these women had taken these drugs for only a few days. The chance that an infant whose mother had taken this drug will have this type of defect is about 1 in 1,000.

If you take Amen® and later find you were pregnant when you took it, be sure to discuss this with your doctor as soon as possible.

HOW SUPPLIED

Two-layered peach and white scored tablet with "C" on one side and "AMEN" on the other. Amen® tablets containing 10 mg. of medroxyprogesterone acetate U.S.P. are available in bottles of 50 (NDC 0086-0049-05) 100 (NDC 0086-0049-10) and 1000 (NDC 0086-0049-90).

The most recent revision of this labeling is April 1984.

Manufactured for Carnrick Laboratories, Inc.

Shown in Product Identification Section, page 407

BONTRIL® PDM Ⓒ III
[*bŏn'tril*]
(brand of phendimetrazine tartrate 35 mg. tablets)

HOW SUPPLIED
Three layered green, white and yellow tablets with 8648 on the scored side and the letter "C" on the other. Bontril® PDM tablets containing 35 mg. of phendimetrazine tartrate are available in bottles of 100 (NDC 0086-0048-10) and 1,000 (NDC 0086-0048-90).

CAUTION
Federal law prohibits dispensing without prescription.
See product insert for complete information.
Manufactured for Carnrick Laboratories, Inc.
Shown in Product Identification Section, page 407

BONTRIL® SLOW-RELEASE Ⓒ III
[*bŏn'tril*]
(brand of phendimetrazine tartrate slow-release capsules 105 mg

DESCRIPTION
Phendimetrazine tartrate, as the dextro isomer, has the chemical name of (+)-3,4-Dimethyl-2-phenylmorpholine Tartrate.
The structural formula is as follows:

M.W. 341

Phendimetrazine tartrate is a white, odorless powder with a bitter taste. It is soluble in water, methanol and ethanol.

ACTIONS
Phendimetrazine tartrate is a sympathomimetic amine with pharmacological activity similar to the prototype drugs of this class used in obesity, the amphetamines. Actions include central nervous system stimulation and elevation of blood pressure. Tachyphylaxis and tolerance have been demonstrated with all drugs of this class in which these phenomena have been looked for.
Drugs of this class used in obesity are commonly known as "anorectics" or "anorexigenics". It has not been established, however, that the action of such drugs in treating obesity is primarily one of appetite suppression. Other central nervous system actions or metabolic effects may be involved.
Adult obese subjects instructed in dietary management and treated with anorectic drugs lose more weight on the average than those treated with placebo and diet, as determined in relatively short term clinical trials.
The magnitude of increased weight loss of drug-treated patients over placebo-treated patients is only a fraction of a pound a week. The rate of weight loss is greatest in the first weeks of therapy for both drug and placebo subjects and tends to decrease in succeeding weeks. The possible origin of the increased weight loss due to the various drug effects is not established. The amount of weight loss associated with the use of an anorectic drug varies from trial to trial, and the increased weight loss appears to be related in part to variables other than the drug prescribed, such as the physician investigator, the population treated, and the diet prescribed. Studies do not permit conclusions as to the relative importance of the drug and non-drug factors on weight loss.
The natural history of obesity is measured in years, whereas the studies cited are restricted to a few weeks duration; thus, the total impact of drug-induced weight loss over that of diet alone must be considered clinically limited.
The active drug 105 mg of phendimetrazine tartrate in each capsule of this special slow-release dosage form approximates the action of three 35 mg non-time release doses taken at 4 hours intervals.
The major route of elimination is via the kidneys where most of the drug and metabolites are excreted. Some of the drug is metabolized to phenmetrazine and also phendimetrazine-N-oxide.
The average half-life of elimination when studied under controlled conditions is about 1.9 hours for the non-time and 9.8 hours for the slow-release dosage form. The absorption half-life of the drug from conventional non-time 35 mg phendimetrazine tablets is approximately the same. These data indicate that the slow-release product has a similar onset of action to the conventional non-time-release product and, in addition, has a prolonged therapeutic effect.

INDICATIONS
Phendimetrazine tartrate is indicated in the management of exogenous obesity as a short term adjunct (a few weeks) in a regimen of weight reduction based on caloric restriction. The limited usefulness of agents of this class (see ACTIONS) should be measured against possible risk factors inherent in their use such as those described below.

CONTRAINDICATIONS
Advanced arteriosclerosis, symptomatic cardiovascular disease, moderate and severe hypertension, hyperthyroidism, known hypersensitivity, or idiosyncrasy to the sympathomimetic amines. Agitated states. Patients with a history of drug abuse. Use in Patients taking other CNS stimulants including monoamine oxidase inhibitors.

WARNINGS
Tolerance to the anorectic effect usually develops within a few weeks. When this occurs, the recommended dose should not be exceeded in an attempt to increase the effect; rather, the drug should be discontinued.
Use of phendimetrazine within 14 days following the administration of monoamine oxidase inhibitors may result in a hypertensive crisis.
Abrupt cessation of administration following prolonged high dosage results in extreme fatigue and depression. Because of the effect on the central nervous system phendimetrazine tartrate may impair the ability of the patient to engage in potentially hazardous activities such as operating machinery or driving a motor vehicle; the patient should therefore be cautioned accordingly.

PRECAUTIONS
Caution is to be exercised in prescribing phendimetrazine for patients with even mild hypertension.
Insulin requirements in diabetes mellitus may be altered in association with the use of phendimetrazine and the concomitant dietary regimen.
Phendimetrazine may decrease the hypotensive effect of guanethidine.
The least amount feasible should be prescribed or dispensed at one time in order to minimize the possibility of overdosage.
Usage in Pregnancy: Safe use in pregnancy has not been established. Until more information is available, phendimetrazine tartrate should not be taken by women who are or may become pregnant unless, in the opinion of the physician, the potential benefits outweigh the possible hazards.
Usage in Children: Phendimetrazine tartrate is not recommended for use in children under 12 years of age.

ADVERSE REACTIONS
Cardiovascular: Palpitation, tachycardia, elevation of blood pressure.
Central Nervous System: Overstimulation, restlessness, dizziness, insomnia, tremor, headache, rarely psychotic episodes at recommended doses, agitation, flushing, sweating, blurring of vision.
Gastrointestinal: Dryness of the mouth, diarrhea, constipation, nausea, stomach pain.
Genitourinary: Changes in libido, urinary frequency, dysuria.

DRUG ABUSE AND DEPENDENCE
Controlled Substance: Phendimetrazine is a Schedule III controlled substance.
Dependence: Phendimetrazine Tartrate is related chemically and pharmacologically to the amphetamines. Amphetamines and related stimulant drugs have been extensively abused, and the possibility of abuse of phendimetrazine should be kept in mind when evaluating the desirability of including a drug as part of a weight reduction program.
Abuse of amphetamines and related drugs may be associated with intense psychological dependence and severe social dysfunction. There are reports of patients who have increased the dosage to many times that recommended. Abrupt cessation following prolonged high dosage administration results in extreme fatigue and mental depression; changes are also noted on the sleep EEG. Manifestations of chronic intoxication with anorectic drugs include severe dermatoses, marked insomnia, irritability, hyperactivity and personality changes. The most severe manifestation of chronic intoxications is psychosis, often clinically indistinguishable from schizophrenia.

OVERDOSAGE
Manifestations of acute overdosage may include restlessness, tremor, hyperreflexia, rapid respiration, confusion, assaultiveness, hallucinations, panic states.
Fatigue and depression usually follow the central stimulation.
Cardiovascular effects include arrhythmias, hypertension, or hypotension and circulatory collapse. Gastrointestinal symptoms include nausea, vomiting, diarrhea, and abdominal cramps. Poisoning may result in convulsions, coma, and death.
Management of acute intoxication is largely symptomatic and includes lavage and sedation with a barbiturate. Experience with hemodialysis or peritoneal dialysis is inadequate to permit recommendation in this regard.
Acidification of the urine increases phendimetrazine tartrate excretion.
Intravenous phentolamine (Regitine) has been suggested for possible acute, severe hypertension, if this complicates overdosage.

DOSAGE AND ADMINISTRATION
One Slow-Release Capsule (105 mg) in the morning, taken 30-60 minutes before the morning meal.
Phendimetrazine Tartrate is not recommended for use in children under twelve years of age.

HOW SUPPLIED
Phendimetrazine Slow-Release Capsules, 105 mg is supplied in bottles of 100 opaque green and clear yellow capsules, imprinted with the letter "C" and 8647. NDC # 0086-0047-10.
Store at controlled room temperature, 15°–30°C(59°–86°F).
The most recent revision of this labeling is Oct. 1984.

CAUTION
Federal law prohibits dispensing without prescription.
Manufactured for Carnrick Laboratories, Inc.
Shown in Product Identification Section, page 407

CAPITAL® and CODEINE
(acetaminophen and codeine)
Tablets Ⓒ III **Suspension** Ⓒ V

CAUTION
Federal law prohibits dispensing without prescription.

DESCRIPTION
Each CAPITAL® and CODEINE tablet contains:
Codeine Phosphate* 30 mg
***WARNING:** May be habit forming
Acetaminophen 325 mg
CAPITAL® and CODEINE suspension contains (in each 5ml):
Codeine Phosphate* 12 mg
***WARNING:** May be habit forming
Acetaminophen 120 mg

HOW SUPPLIED
CAPITAL® and CODEINE tablets: Pale blue scored tablet imprinted with 8644 and a sunburst on the scored side and the letter "C" on the other. Bottle of 100 tablets, NDC 0086-0044-10. Store at Controlled Room Temperature 15°–30°C (59°–86°F) in a dry place.
CAPTIAL® and CODEINE suspension: a pink, pleasantly flavored suspension—16 oz. bottles, NDC 0086-0046-16. Store at Controlled Room Temperature 15°–30°C (59°–86°F)
See product insert for complete information.
Manufactured for Carnrick Laboratories, Inc.
Shown in Product Identification Section, page 407

HYDROCET™ CAPSULES Ⓒ III

CAUTION
Federal law prohibits dispensing without prescription.

DESCRIPTION
Each Hydrocet™ capsule contains:
Acetaminophen, U.S.P. ....500 mg.
Hydrocodone Bitartrate, U.S.P. .... 5 mg.
(WARNING: May be habit forming.)
Acetaminophen is a nonopiate, non-salicylate analgesic and antipyretic which occurs as a white, odorless crystalline powder possessing a slightly bitter taste. It may be represented by the following structural formula:

HO–C_6H_4–NHCOCH$_3$

Hydrocodone bitartrate is an opioid analgesic and antitussive and occurs as fine, white crystals or as a crystalline powder. It is affected by light. The structural formula of hydrocodone bitartrate is:

$\cdot$ $2\frac{1}{2}H_2O$

CLINICAL PHARMACOLOGY
Hydrocodone is a semisynthetic narcotic analgesic and antitussive with multiple actions qualitatively similar to those of codeine. Most of these involve the central nervous system and smooth muscle. The precise mechanism of action of hy-

Continued on next page

Carnrick—Cont.

drocodone and other opiates is not known, although it is believed to relate to the existence of opiate receptors in the central nervous system. In addition to analgesia, narcotics may produce drowsiness, changes in mood, and mental clouding.

Radioimmunoassay techniques have recently been developed for the analysis of hydrocodone in human plasma. After a 10 mg oral dose of hydrocodone bitartrate, a mean peak serum drug level of 23.6 ng/ml and an elimination half-life of 3.8 hours were found.

The analgesic action of acetaminophen involves peripheral and central influences, but the specific mechanism is as yet undetermined. Antipyretic activity is mediated through hypothalamic heat regulating centers. Acetaminophen inhibits prostaglandin synthetase. Therapeutic doses of acetaminophen have negligible effects on the cardiovascular or respiratory systems; however, toxic doses may cause circulatory failure and rapid, shallow breathing. Acetaminophen is rapidly and almost completely absorbed from the gastrointestinal tract, producing maximum serum concentrations within 30 minutes to one hour. The plasma half-life in adults and children ranges from 0.90 hours to 3.25 hours with an average of approximately 2 hours. The drug distributes uniformly in most body fluids and is approximately 25% protein bound. Acetaminophen is conjugated in the liver, with less than 3% of the dose excreted unchanged in 24 hours. The primary metabolic pathway is conjugation to sulfate and glucuronide by-products. A minor oxidative pathway forms cysteine and mercapturic acid. These compounds are subsequently excreted by the kidneys into the urine.

INDICATIONS AND USAGE

For the relief of moderate to moderately severe pain.

CONTRAINDICATIONS

Hypersensitivity to acetaminophen or hydrocodone.

WARNINGS

Respiratory Depression: At high doses or in sensitive patients, hydrocodone may produce dose-related respiratory depression by acting directly on brain stem respiratory centers. Hydrocodone also affects centers that control respiratory rhythm, and may produce irregular and periodic breathing.

Head Injury and Increased Intracranial Pressure: The respiratory depressant effects of narcotics and their capacity to elevate cerebrospinal fluid pressure may be markedly exaggerated in the presence of head injury, other intracranial lesions or a preexisting increase in intracranial pressure. Furthermore, narcotics produce adverse reactions which may obscure the clinical course of patients with head injuries.

Acute Abdominal Conditions: The administration of narcotics may obscure the diagnosis or clinical course of patients with acute abdominal conditions.

PRECAUTIONS

Special Risk Patients: As with any narcotic analgesic agent, HYDROCET™ (Acetaminophen, USP 500 mg. and Hydrocodone Bitartrate, USP 5 mg.) should be used with caution in elderly or debilitated patients and those with severe impairment of hepatic or renal function, hypothyroidism, Addison's disease, prostatic hypertrophy or urethral stricture. The usual precautions should be observed and the possibility of respiratory depression should be kept in mind.

Information for Patients: HYDROCET™ (Acetaminophen, USP 500 mg. and Hydrocodone Bitartrate, USP 5 mg.) like all narcotics, may impair the mental and/or physical abilities required for the performance of potentially hazardous tasks such as driving a car or operating machinery; patients should be cautioned accordingly.

Cough Reflex: Hydrocodone suppresses the cough reflex; as with all narcotics, caution should be exercised when HYDROCET™ is used postoperatively and in patients with pulmonary disease.

Drug Interactions: Patients receiving other narcotic analgesics, antipsychotics, antianxiety agents, or other CNS depressants (including alcohol) concomitantly with HYDROCET™ may exhibit an additive CNS depression. When combined therapy is contemplated, the dose of one or both agents should be reduced.

The use of MAO inhibitors or tricyclic antidepressants with hydrocodone preparations may increase the effect of either the antidepressant or hydrocodone.

The concurrent use of anticholinergics with hydrocodone may produce paralytic ileus.

Usage In Pregnancy: Pregnancy Category C. Hydrocodone has been shown to be teratogenic in hamsters when given in doses 700 times the human dose. There are no adequate and well-controlled studies in pregnant women. HYDROCET™ should be used during pregnancy only if the potential benefit justifies the potential risk to the fetus.

Nonteratogenic Effects: Babies born to mothers who have been taking opioids regularly prior to delivery will be physically dependent. The withdrawal signs include irritability and excessive crying, tremors, hyperactive reflexes, increased respiratory rate, increased stools, sneezing, yawning, vomiting, and fever. The intensity of the syndrome does not always correlate with the duration of maternal opioid use or dose. There is no consensus on the best method of managing withdrawal. Chlorpromazine 0.7 to 1.0 mg/kg q6h, and paregoric 2 to 4 drops/kg q4h, have been used to treat withdrawal symptoms in infants. The duration of therapy is 4 to 28 days, with the dosage decreased as tolerated.

Labor and Delivery: As with all narcotics, administration of HYDROCET™ to the mother shortly before delivery may result in some degree of respiratory depression in the newborn, especially if higher doses are used.

Nursing Mothers: It is not known whether this drug is excreted in human milk. Because many drugs are excreted in human milk and because of the potential for serious adverse reactions in nursing infants from HYDROCET,™ (Acetaminophen, USP 500 mg. and Hydrocodone Bitartrate, USP 5 mg.) a decision should be made whether to discontinue nursing or to discontinue the drug, taking into account the importance of the drug to the mother.

Pediatric Use: Safety and effectiveness in children have not been established.

ADVERSE REACTIONS

Central Nervous System: Sedation, drowsiness, mental clouding, lethargy, impairment of mental and physical performance, anxiety, fear, dysphoria, dizziness, psychic dependence, mood changes.

Gastrointestinal System: Nausea and vomiting may occur; they are more frequent in ambulatory than in recumbent patients. The antiemetic phenothiazines are useful in suppressing these effects; however, some phenothiazine derivatives seem to be antianalgesic and to increase the amount of narcotic required to produce pain relief, while other phenothiazines reduce the amount of narcotic required to produce a given level of analgesia. Prolonged administration of HYDROCET™ may produce constipation.

Genitourinary System: Ureteral spasm, spasm of vesical sphincters and urinary retention have been reported.

Respiratory Depression: HYDROCET™ may produce dose-related respiratory depression by acting directly on brain stem respiratory centers. Hydrocodone also affects centers that control respiratory rhythm, and may produce irregular and periodic breathing. If significant respiratory depression occurs, it may be antagonized by the use of naloxone hydrochloride. Apply other supportive measures when indicated.

DRUG ABUSE AND DEPENDENCE

HYDROCET™ is subject to the Federal Controlled Substances Act (Schedule III). Psychic dependence, physical dependence, and tolerance may develop upon repeated administration of narcotics; therefore, HYDROCET™ should be prescribed and administered with caution. However, psychic dependence is unlikely to develop when HYDROCET™ is used for a short time for the treatment of pain. Physical dependence, the condition in which continued administration of the drug is required to prevent the appearance of a withdrawal syndrome, assumes clinically significant proportions only after several weeks of continued narcotic use, although some mild degree of physical dependence may develop after a few days of narcotic therapy. Tolerance, in which increasingly large doses are required in order to produce the same degree of analgesia, is manifested initially by a shortened duration of analgesic effect, and subsequently by decreases in the intensity of analgesia. The rate of development of tolerance varies among patients.

OVERDOSAGE

Acetaminophen:

Signs and Symptoms: Acetaminophen in massive overdosage may cause hepatic toxicity in some patients. In cases of suspected overdosage, you may wish to call your regional poison center for assistance in diagnosis and for directions in the use of N-acetylcysteine as an antidote.

In adults, hepatic toxicity has rarely been reported with acute overdoses of less than 10 grams and fatalities with less than 15 grams. Importantly, young children seem to be more resistant than adults to the hepatotoxic effect of an acetaminophen overdose. Despite this, the measures outlined below should be initiated in any adult or child suspected of having ingested an acetaminophen overdose.

Early symptoms following a potentially hepatotoxic overdose may include: nausea, vomiting, diaphoresis and general malaise. Clinical and laboratory evidence of hepatic toxicity may not be apparent until 48 to 72 hours post-ingestion.

Treatment: The stomach should be emptied promptly by lavage or by induction of emesis with syrup of ipecac. Patients' estimates of the quantity of a drug ingested are notoriously unreliable. Therefore, if an acetaminophen overdose is suspected, a serum acetaminophen assay should be obtained as early as possible, but no sooner than four hours following ingestion. Liver function studies should be obtained initially and repeated at 24-hour intervals.

The antidote, N-acetylcysteine, should be administered as early as possible, preferably within 16 hours of the overdose ingestion for optimal results, but in any case, within 24 hours. Following recovery, there are no residual, structural or functional hepatic abnormalities.

Hydrocodone:

Signs and Symptoms: Serious overdose with hydrocodone is characterized by respiratory depression (a decrease in respiratory rate and/or tidal volume. Cheyne-Stokes respiration, cyanosis), extreme somnolence progressing to stupor or coma, skeletal muscle flaccidity, cold and clammy skin, and sometimes bradycardia and hypotension. In severe overdosage, apnea, circulatory collapse, cardiac arrest and death may occur.

Treatment: Primary attention should be given to the reestablishment of adequate respiratory exchange through provision of a patent airway and the institution of assisted or controlled ventilation. The narcotic antagonist naloxone is a specific antidote against respiratory depression which may result from overdosage or unusual sensitivity to narcotics, including hydrocodone. Therefore, an appropriate dose of naloxone (see package insert) should be administered, preferably by the intravenous route, and simultaneously with efforts at respiratory resuscitation. Since the duration of action of hydrocodone may exceed that of the antagonist, the patient should be kept under continued surveillance and repeated doses of the antagonist should be administered as needed to maintain adequate respiration.

An antagonist should not be administered in the absence of clinically significant respiratory or cardiovascular depression. Oxygen, intravenous fluids, vasopressors and other supportive measures should be employed as indicated. Gastric emptying may be useful in removing unabsorbed drug.

DOSAGE AND ADMINISTRATION

Dosage should be adjusted according to the severity of the pain and the response of the patient. However, it should be kept in mind that tolerance to hydrocodone can develop with continued use and that the incidence of untoward effects is dose related.

The usual dose is one capsule every six hours as needed for pain. If necessary, this dose may be repeated at four hour intervals. In cases of more severe pain, two capsules every six hours (up to eight capsules in 24 hours) may be required.

HOW SUPPLIED

Blue and white, opaque capsules imprinted with the letter "C" and 8657.

Supplied in bottles of 100 capsules NDC 0086-0057-10 and Hospital Unit Dose Dispenser, Reverse Numbered—100 capsules (4 × 25 capsules) NDC 0086-0057-04.

Each capsule contains Acetaminophen. USP 500 mg., and Hydrocodone Bitartrate, USP 5 mg. (WARNING: MAY BE HABIT FORMING.)

Keep in tight, light resistant containers.

Store at controlled room temperature, 15°—30°C (59°—86°F).

The most recent revision of this labeling is May 1986.

Manufactured for Carnrick Laboratories, Inc.

Shown in Product Identification Section, page 407

MIDRIN® ℞

[mid'rin]

CAUTION

Federal law prohibits dispensing without prescription.

DESCRIPTION

Each red capsule with pink band contains Isometheptene Mucate 65 mg., Dichloralphenazone 100 mg., and Acetaminophen 325 mg.

Isometheptene Mucate is a white crystalline powder having a characteristic aromatic odor and bitter taste. It is an unsaturated aliphatic amine with sympathomimetic properties.

Dichloralphenazone is a white, microcrystalline powder, with slight odor and tastes saline at first, becoming acrid. It is a mild sedative.

Acetaminophen, a non-salicylate, occurs as a white, odorless, crystalline powder possessing a slightly bitter taste.

ACTIONS

Isometheptene Mucate, a sympathomimetic amine, acts by constricting dilated cranial and cerebral arterioles, thus reducing the stimuli that lead to vascular headaches. Dichloralphenazone, a mild sedative, reduces the patient's emotional reaction to the pain of both vascular and tension headaches. Acetaminophen raises the threshold to painful stimuli, thus exerting an analgesic effect against all types of headaches.

INDICATIONS

For relief of tension and vascular headaches.*

* Based on a review of this drug (isometheptene mucate) by the National Academy of Sciences-National Research Council and/or other information, FDA has classified the other indication as "Possibly" effective in the treatment of migraine headache. Final classification of the less-than-effective indication requires further investigation.

CONTRAINDICATIONS
Midrin is contraindicated in glaucoma and/or severe cases of renal disease, hypertension, organic heart disease, hepatic disease and in those patients who are on monoamine-oxidase (MAO) inhibitor therapy.

PRECAUTIONS
Caution should be observed in hypertension, peripheral vascular disease and after recent cardiovascular attacks.

ADVERSE REACTIONS
Transient dizziness and skin rash may appear in hypersensitive patients. This can usually be eliminated by reducing the dose.

DOSAGE AND ADMINISTRATION
FOR RELIEF OF MIGRAINE HEADACHE: The usual adult dosage is two capsules at once, followed by one capsule every hour until relieved, up to 5 capsules within a twelve hour period.
FOR RELIEF OF TENSION HEADACHE: The usual adult dosage is one or two capsules every four hours up to 8 capsules a day.

HOW SUPPLIED
Red capsules imprinted with pink band, the letter "C" and 86120. Bottles of 50 capsules, NDC 0086-0120-05. Bottles of 100 capsules, NDC 0086-0120-10. Store at controlled room temperature 15–30°C (59–86°F) in a dry place.
The most recent revision of this labeling is Dec. 1983.
Manufactured for Carnrick Laboratories, Inc.
Shown in Product Identification Section, page 407

NOLAHIST®
[nō'lă-hist]
(phenindamine tartrate)
ANTIHISTAMINE
Allergy/Cold Tablets

DESCRIPTION
Each dye-free NOLAHIST® tablet contains:

Phenindamine Tartrate	25 mg

INDICATIONS
Temporarily relieves runny nose, sneezing, itching of the nose or throat, and itchy, watery eyes due to hay fever or other upper respiratory allergies or allergic rhinitis. Temporarily relieves runny nose and sneezing associated with the common cold.

WARNINGS
May cause excitability especially in children. Do not take this product if you have asthma, glaucoma, emphysema, chronic pulmonary disease, shortness of breath, difficulty in breathing, or difficulty in urination due to enlargement of the prostate gland unless directed by a doctor. May cause drowsiness; alcohol may increase the drowsiness effect. Avoid alcoholic beverages while taking this product. Use caution when driving a motor vehicle or operating machinery. May cause nervousness and insomnia in some individuals. As with any drug, if you are pregnant or nursing a baby, seek the advice of a health professional before using this product. Keep this and all medication out of the reach of children. In case of accidental overdose, seek professional assistance or contact a Poison Control Center immediately.

DIRECTIONS
Adults: oral dosage is one tablet every 4 to 6 hours, not to exceed six tablets in 24 hours, or as directed by a doctor. Children 6 to under 12 years of age: oral dosage is one-half tablet every 4 to 6 hours, not to exceed 3 tablets in 24 hours, or as directed by a doctor. Children under 6 years of age: consult a doctor.

HOW SUPPLIED
White, capsule-shaped, scored tablet inscribed with 8652 on one side and C logo on the other side in bottles of 100. Each tablet contains phenindamine tartrate 25 mg. (NDC 0086-0052-10) Store at 15°–30°C (59°–86°F) and keep away from light.
Manufactured for Carnrick Laboratories, Inc.
Shown in Product Identification Section, page 407

NOLAMINE® ℞
[nō'lă-mēn']

DESCRIPTION
Each timed release tablet contains:

Phenindamine tartrate	24 mg
Chlorpheniramine maleate	4 mg
Phenylpropanolamine hydrochloride	50 mg

Formulated to provide 8 to 12 hours of continuous relief.

CAUTION
Federal law prohibits dispensing without prescription.

INDICATIONS
As a nasal decongestant associated with the common cold, sinusitis, hay fever and other allergies.

CONTRAINDICATIONS
Hypersensitivity to any of the components. Contraindicated in concurrent MAO inhibitor therapy.

SIDE EFFECTS
Nervousness, insomnia, tremors, dizziness and drowsiness may occur occasionally.

PRECAUTIONS
Antihistamines may cause drowsiness and should be used with caution in patients who operate motor vehicles or dangerous machinery. Use with caution in patients with hypertension, cardiovascular disease, diabetes or hyperthyroidism. This product should be used with caution in patients with prostatic hypertrophy or glaucoma.

DOSAGE
Usual adult dose: Orally, one tablet every 8 hours. In mild cases, one tablet every 10 to 12 hours.

HOW SUPPLIED
Pink, timed release tablets coded C 86204 in bottles of 100 (NDC 0086-0204-10) and 250 (NDC 0086-0204-25). Store at room temperature.
Manufactured for Carnrick Laboratories, Inc.
Shown in Product Identification Section, page 407

PHRENILIN® ℞
[fren'ĭ-lin]
and
PHRENILIN® FORTE ℞

CAUTION
Federal Law Prohibits Dispensing Without Prescription

DESCRIPTION
PHRENILIN®: Each PHRENILIN® tablet, an analgesic-sedative combination for oral administration contains: butalbital, USP 50 mg., (Warning—May be habit forming); acetaminophen, USP 325 mg.
PHRENILIN® FORTE: Each PHRENILIN® FORTE capsule, an analgesic-sedative combination for oral administration, contains: butalbital, USP 50 mg., (Warning—May be habit forming); acetaminophen, USP 650 mg.

Butalbital

Butalbital, 5-allyl-5-isobutyl-barbituric acid, a white odorless crystalline powder, is a short to intermediate acting barbiturate.

Acetaminophen

Acetaminophen, N-acetyl-p-amino-phenol, occurs as a white, odorless, crystalline powder, possessing a slightly bitter taste. Acetaminophen is a non-salicylate, non-narcotic analgesic, and antipyretic.

CLINICAL PHARMACOLOGY
Pharmacologically, Butalbital-Acetaminophen combines the analgesic properties of acetaminophen with the anxiolytic and muscle relaxant properties of butalbital.
Butalbital is a short to intermediate acting barbiturate which produces mild sedation. Barbiturates are capable of producing all levels of CNS mood alteration from excitation to mild sedation, to hypnosis, and deep coma. Overdosage can produce death.
Barbiturates depress the sensory cortex, decrease motor activity, alter cerebellar function, and produce drowsiness, sedation, and hypnosis. Barbiturates are respiratory depressants. The degree of respiratory depression is dependent on dose.
Barbiturates do not impair normal hepatic function, but have been shown to induce liver microsomal enzymes, thus increasing and/or altering the metabolism of barbiturates and other drugs.
Acetaminophen is a non-narcotic analgesic and antipyretic. Acetaminophen produces analgesia by elevation of the pain threshold and antipyresis through action on the hypothalamic heat-regulating center.

Pharmacokinetics: The onset and duration of action, which is related to the rate at which the barbiturates are redistributed throughout the body, varies among persons and in the same person from time to time. Butalbital has a duration of action from 3 to 6 hours.
Barbiturates are weak acids that are absorbed and rapidly distributed to all tissues and fluids with high concentrations in the brain, liver, and kidneys. The more lipid soluble the barbiturate, the more rapidly it penetrates all tissues of the body. Barbiturates are bound to plasma and tissue proteins to a varying degree with the degree of binding increasing directly as a function of lipid solubility.
Barbiturates are metabolized primarily by the hepatic microsomal enzyme system and the metabolic products are excreted in the urine, and less commonly, in the feces. The inactive metabolites of the barbiturates are excreted as conjugates of glucoronic acid.
Acetaminophen is rapidly and almost completely absorbed from the gastrointestinal tract, producing maximum serum concentrations within 30 minutes to one hour. The plasma half-life varies from one to four hours. Acetaminophen is relatively uniformly distributed throughout most body fluids and is approximately 25% protein bound. Approximately 90 to 95% of a dose is metabolized in the liver, primarily by conjugation with glucuronic acid, sulfuric acid, and cysteine. An intermediate metabolite is hepatotoxic. Excretion is renal; primarily as conjugates. About 3% of a dose may be excreted unchanged.

INDICATIONS AND USAGE
PHRENILIN® and PHRENILIN® FORTE are indicated for the relief of the symptom complex of tension (or muscle contraction) headache.

CONTRAINDICATIONS
Hypersensitivity to any of the components. Patients with porphyria.

WARNINGS
Acetaminophen in massive overdosage may cause hepatotoxicity in some patients. (See OVERDOSAGE.)
Habit Forming: Barbiturates may be habit forming. Tolerance, psychological and physical dependence may occur with continued use. (See DRUG ABUSE AND DEPENDENCE.) Abrupt cessation after prolonged use in the dependent person may result in withdrawal symptoms, including delirium, convulsions, and possibly death. Barbiturates should be withdrawn gradually from any patient known to be taking excessive dosage over long periods of time.
Acute or Chronic Pain: Caution should be exercised when barbiturates are administered to patients with acute or chronic pain, because paradoxical excitement could be induced or important symptoms could be masked.
Use in Pregnancy: (See PRECAUTIONS section.)
Synergistic Effects: The concomitant use of alcohol or other CNS depressants may produce additive CNS depressant effects.

PRECAUTIONS
General: Barbiturates may be habit forming. Tolerance and psychological and physical dependence may occur with continuing use. (See DRUG ABUSE AND DEPENDENCE.) Barbiturates should be administered with caution, if at all, to patients who are mentally depressed, have suicidal tendencies, or a history of drug abuse.
Elderly or debilitated patients may react to barbiturates with marked excitement, depression, and confusion. In some persons, barbiturates repeatedly produce excitement rather than depression.
In patients with hepatic damage, barbiturates should be administered with caution and initially in reduced doses. Barbiturates should not be administered to patients showing the premonitory signs of hepatic coma.
Use with caution in patients with severe renal function impairment.
Do not exceed recommended dosage. Excessive or prolonged use should be avoided.
Information for Patients: Practitioners should give the following information and instructions to patients receiving barbiturates.

1. The use of barbiturates carries with it an associated risk of psychological and/or physical dependence. The patient should be warned against increasing the dose of the drug without consulting a physician.
2. Barbiturates may impair mental and/or physical abilities required for the performance of potentially hazardous tasks (e.g., driving, operating machinery, etc.)
3. Alcohol should not be consumed while taking barbiturates. Concurrent use of the barbiturates with other CNS depressants (e.g., alcohol, narcotics, tranquilizers, and antihistamines) may result in additional CNS depressant effects.

Drug Interactions: The concomitant use of other central nervous system depressants, including other sedatives or hypnotics, antihistamines, tranquilizers, or alcohol, may

Continued on next page

Carnrick—Cont.

produce additive depressant effects. When such combined therapy is necessary, the dose of one or more agents may need to be reduced.

The presence of barbiturates decreases the effects of oral anticoagulants, griseofulvin, doxycycline, corticosteroids, and possibly phenytoin. Monoamine oxidase inhibitors (MAOI) prolong the effects of barbiturates.

Use in Pregnancy: Animal reproduction studies have not been conducted with PHRENILIN® or PHRENILIN® FORTE. It is also not known whether PHRENILIN® or PHRENILIN® FORTE can cause fetal harm when administered to a pregnant woman or can affect reproduction capacity.

BUTALBITAL:

First trimester: The teratogenic potential of butalbital has not been studied in either animals or humans. Although teratogenic effects with this combination medication have not been reported clinically, risk-benefit must be considered since other barbiturates have been shown to increase the risk of fetal abnormalities in humans. If this drug is used during pregnancy, or if the patient becomes pregnant while taking this drug, the patient should be apprised of the potential hazard to the fetus.

Third trimester: Use of barbiturates throughout the last trimester of pregnancy may cause physical dependence with resulting withdrawal symptoms (convulsions and hyperirritability) in the neonate. These withdrawal symptoms may occur up to 14 days after birth. (See DRUG ABUSE AND DEPENDENCE.) Also, one study in humans has shown that prenatal exposure to barbiturates may be associated with an increased incidence of brain tumors. In addition, use of barbiturates during pregnancy may be associated with neonatal hemorrhage due to reduction in levels of vitamin K-dependent clotting factors in the neonate.

Labor and delivery: Use of barbiturates just prior to or during delivery may cause respiratory depression in the neonate, especially the premature neonate, because of immature hepatic function.

ACETAMINOPHEN:

Problems in humans have not been documented; however, controlled studies have not been done. Risk-benefit must be considered since acetaminophen crosses the placenta.

Nursing Mothers:

BUTALBITAL

Barbiturates are excreted in breast milk; use by nursing mothers may cause CNS depression, bradycardia, or respiratory depression in the infant.

ACETAMINOPHEN

Problems in humans have not been documented; however, risk-benefit must be considered. Although peak concentrations of 10 to 15 mcg per ml have been measured in breast milk 1 to 2 hours following maternal ingestion of a single 650-mg dose, neither acetaminophen nor its metabolites were detected in the urine of the nursing infants. The half-life in breast milk is 1.35 to 3.5 hours.

Caution should be exercised when PHRENILIN® or PHRENILIN® FORTE is administered to a nursing woman.

Pediatric Use: Safety and effectiveness in children below the age of 12 have not been established.

ADVERSE REACTIONS

Drowsiness, dizziness, nausea, vomiting, constipation and skin rash may occur.

DRUG ABUSE AND DEPENDENCE

Barbiturates may be habit forming. Tolerance, psychological dependence, and physical dependence may occur especially following prolonged use of high doses of barbiturates.

The average daily dose for the barbiturate addict is usually about 1.5 grams. As tolerance to barbiturates develops, the amount needed to maintain the same level of intoxication increases; tolerance to a fatal dosage, however, does not increase more than two-fold. As this occurs, the margin between an intoxicating dosage and fatal dosage becomes smaller.

Symptoms of acute intoxication with barbiturates include unsteady gait, slurred speech, and sustained nystagmus. Mental signs of chronic intoxication include confusion, poor judgment, irritability, insomnia, and somatic complaints.

Symptoms of barbiturate dependence are similar to those of chronic alcoholism. If an individual appears to be intoxicated with alcohol to a degree that is radically disproportionate to the amount of alcohol in his or her blood the use of barbiturates should be suspected. The lethal dose of a barbiturate is far less if alcohol is also ingested.

The symptoms of barbiturate withdrawal can be severe and may cause death. Major withdrawal symptoms (convulsions and delirium) may occur within 16 hours and last up to 5 days after abrupt cessation of these drugs. Intensity of withdrawal symptoms gradually declines over a period of approximately 15 days. Individuals susceptible to barbiturate abuse and dependence include alcoholics and opiate abusers, as well as other sedative-hypnotic and amphetamine abusers.

Treatment of barbiturate dependence consists of cautious and gradual withdrawal of the drug. Barbiturate-dependent patients can be withdrawn by using a number of different withdrawal regimens. One method involves initiating treatment at the patient's regular dosage level and decreasing the daily dosage by 10 percent if tolerated by the patient.

OVERDOSAGE

BARBITURATES:

Signs and Symptoms: The toxic dose of barbiturates varies considerably. In general, an oral dose of 1 gram of most barbiturates produces serious poisoning in an adult. Death commonly occurs after 2 to 10 grams of ingested barbiturate. Barbiturate intoxication may be confused with alcoholism, bromide intoxication, and with various neurological disorders.

Acute overdosage with barbiturates is manifested by CNS and respiratory depression which may progress to Cheyne-Stokes respiration, areflexia, constriction of the pupils to a slight degree (though in severe poisoning they may show paralytic dilation), oliguria, tachycardia, hypotension, lowered body temperature, and coma. Typical shock syndrome (apnea, circulatory collapse, respiratory arrest, and death) may occur.

In extreme overdose, all electrical activity in the brain may cease, in which case a "flat" EEG normally equated with clinical death cannot be accepted. This effect is fully reversible unless hypoxic damage occurs. Consideration should be given to the possibility of barbiturate intoxication even in situations that appear to involve trauma.

Complications such as pneumonia, pulmonary edema, cardiac arrhythmias, congestive heart failure, and renal failure may occur. Uremia may increase CNS sensitivity to barbiturates if renal function is impaired. Differential diagnosis should include hypoglycemia, head trauma, cerebrovascular accidents, convulsive states, and diabetic coma.

Treatment: Treatment of barbiturate overdosage is mainly supportive and consists of the following:

1. Maintenance of an adequate airway, with assisted respiration and oxygen administration as necessary. 2. Monitoring of vital signs and fluid balance. 3. If the patient is conscious and has not lost the gag reflex, emesis may be induced with ipecac. Care should be taken to prevent pulmonary aspiration of vomitus. After completion of vomiting, 30 grams activated charcoal in a glass of water may be administered. 4. If emesis is contraindicated, gastric lavage may be performed with a cuffed endotracheal tube in place with the patient in the face down position. Activated charcoal may be left in the emptied stomach and a saline cathartic administered. 5. Fluid therapy and other standard treatment for shock, if needed. 6. If renal function is normal, forced diuresis may aid in the elimination of the barbiturate. Alkalinization of the urine increases renal excretion of some barbiturates. 7. Although not recommended as a routine procedure, hemodialysis may be used in severe barbiturate intoxications or if the patient is anuric or in shock. 8. Patient should be rolled from side to side every 30 minutes. 9. Antibiotics should be given if pneumonia is suspected. 10. Appropriate nursing care to prevent hypostatic pneumonia, decubiti, aspiration, and other complications of patients with altered states of consciousness.

ACETAMINOPHEN:

Signs and Symptoms: Acetaminophen in massive overdosage may cause hepatic toxicity in some patients. In all cases of suspected overdose, immediately call your regional poison center or the Rocky Mountain Poison Center's toll-free number (800-525-6115) for assistance in diagnosis and for directions in the use of N-acetylcysteine as an antidote, a use currently restricted to investigational status.

In adults, hepatic toxicity has rarely been reported with acute overdoses of less than 10 grams and fatalities with less than 15 grams. Importantly, young children seem to be more resistant than adults to the hepatotoxic effect of an acetaminophen overdose. Despite this, the measures outlined below should be initiated in any adult or child suspected of having ingested an acetaminophen overdose.

Early symptoms following a potentially hepatotoxic overdose may include: nausea, vomiting, diaphoresis, and general malaise. Clinical and laboratory evidence of hepatic toxicity may not be apparent until 48 to 72 hours post-ingestion.

Treatment: The stomach should be emptied promptly by lavage or by induction of emesis with syrup of ipecac. Patients' estimates of the quantity of a drug ingested are notoriously unreliable. Therefore, if an acetaminophen overdose is suspected, a serum acetaminophen assay should be obtained as early as possible, but no sooner than four hours following ingestion. Liver function studies should be obtained initially and repeated at 24-hour intervals.

The antidote, N-acetylcysteine, should be administered as early as possible, and within 16 hours of the overdose ingestion for optimal results. Following recovery, there are no residual, structural or functional hepatic abnormalities.

DOSAGE AND ADMINISTRATION

PHRENILIN®: One or two tablets every four hours. Total daily dosage should not exceed six tablets.

PHRENILIN® FORTE: One capsule every 4-6 hours. Total daily dosage should not exceed three capsules.

HOW SUPPLIED

PHRENILIN®: Pale violet scored tablets with the letter 'C' on one side and 8650 on the other, in bottles of 100 (NDC 0086-0050-10).

PHRENILIN® FORTE: Amethyst, opaque capsules imprinted with the letter 'C' and 8656, in bottles of 100 (NDC 0086-0056-10).

The most recent revision of this labeling is 11/82.

Manufactured for Carnrick Laboratories, Inc.

Shown in Product Identification Section, page 407

PHRENILIN® with CODEINE No. 3 Ⓒ

[fren'ĭ-lin]

CAUTION

Federal Law Prohibits Dispensing Without Prescription.

DESCRIPTION

Each capsule contains: butalbital, USP 50 mg. (Warning—May be habit forming), acetaminophen, USP 325 mg; and codeine phosphate, USP 30 mg, (Warning—May be habit forming).

HOW SUPPLIED

Amethyst and white, opaque capsules imprinted with the letter "C" and 8655. Supplied in bottles of 100 capsules NDC 0086-0055-10. Store at controlled room temperature, 15°–30°C (59°–86°F).

See package insert for prescribing information.

Manufactured for Carnrick Laboratories, Inc.

Shown in Product Identification Section, page 407

PROPAGEST®

(Phenylpropanolamine HCl)

NASAL DECONGESTANT TABLETS

DESCRIPTION

Each tablet contains:

Phenylpropanolamine HCl .... 25 mg.

INDICATIONS

For the temporary relief of nasal congestion associated with the common cold, sinusitis, hay fever or other upper respiratory allergies.

DOSAGE

Adult oral dosage is one tablet every 4 hours not to exceed 6 tablets in 24 hours. Children 6 to under 12 years oral dosage is one-half tablet every 4 hours not to exceed 3 tablets in 24 hours. For children under 6 years, there is no recommended dosage except under the advice and supervision of a doctor.

WARNINGS

Do not exceed recommended dosage because at higher doses nervousness, dizziness, sleeplessness, rapid pulse or high blood pressure may occur.

Do not take this product for more than 7 days. If symptoms do not improve or are accompanied by fever, consult a doctor.

Do not take this product if you have heart disease, high blood pressure, thyroid disease, diabetes, or difficulty in urination due to enlargement of the prostate gland unless directed by a doctor.

As with any drug, if you are pregnant or nursing a baby, seek the advice of a health professional before using this product.

Keep this and all medication out of the reach of children.

In case of accidental overdose, seek professional assistance or contact a Poison Control Center immediately.

Drug Interaction Precaution: Do not take this product if you are presently taking a prescription drug for high blood pressure or depression, without first consulting your doctor. Do not take this product concurrently with other medication except on the advice of a doctor.

TAMPER-RESISTANT PACKAGE FEATURE:

Bottle of 100—If printed outer wrap is broken or removed, do not purchase.

HOW SUPPLIED

White, oval, scored tablets with "C" logo containing 25 mg. phenylpropanolamine HCl in bottles of 100. (NDC 0086-0051-10). Keep tightly closed, away from light and store at room temperature.

Manufactured for Carnrick Laboratories, Inc.

Shown in Product Identification Section, page 407

SINULIN® (New Formulation)
Analgesic • Antihistamine • Decongestant

DESCRIPTION
NEW FORMULATION SINULIN contains acetaminophen, an analgesic and antipyretic that relieves pain, sinus headache and reduces fever; phenylpropanolamine HCl, a decongestant that promotes nasal drainage and relieves sinus pressure; and chlorpheniramine maleate, an antihistamine that helps control allergic symptoms.

ACTIVE INGREDIENTS
Each tablet contains: acetaminophen 650 mg. (650 mg. is a nonstandard strength of acetaminophen per tablet compared to the established standard of 325 mg. acetaminophen per tablet), chlorpheniramine maleate 4 mg., phenylpropanolamine HCl 25 mg.

INDICATIONS
For the temporary relief of nasal and sinus congestion, runny nose, sneezing, itching of the nose or throat, itchy watery eyes, headache and fever associated with the common cold, sinusitis, hay fever or other upper respiratory allergies.

WARNINGS
Do not exceed recommended dosage because severe liver damage may occur and at higher doses, nervousness, dizziness, sleeplessness, rapid pulse or high blood pressure may occur.
Adults should not take this product for more than 7 days. Children 6 to under 12 years of age should not take this product for more than 5 days. If fever persists for more than 3 days, or recurs, consult a doctor. If symptoms persist, do not improve, or new ones occur, consult a doctor.
Do not take this product if you have high blood pressure, heart disease, diabetes, thyroid disease, glaucoma, asthma, emphysema, chronic pulmonary disease, shortness of breath, difficulty in breathing, or difficulty in urination due to enlargement of the prostate gland, or if you are presently taking a prescription drug for high blood pressure or depression, unless directed by a doctor.
This product may cause drowsiness; alcohol may increase the drowsiness effect. Avoid alcoholic beverages while taking this product. Use caution when driving a motor vehicle or operating machinery. May cause excitability especially in children.
If a rare sensitivity reaction occurs, discontinue use and consult a doctor.
As with any drug, if you are pregnant or nursing a baby, seek the advice of a health professional before using this product.
Keep this and all medication out of the reach of children.
In case of accidental overdose, seek professional assistance or contact a Poison Control Center immediately.

DRUG INTERACTION PRECAUTION
Do not take this product if you are presently taking a prescription drug for high blood pressure or depression without first consulting your doctor. Do not take this product concurrently with other medication except on the advice of a doctor.

DIRECTIONS
Adults: oral dosage is one tablet every 4 to 6 hours, or as directed by a doctor. Do not exceed 6 tablets in 24 hours.
Children 6 to under 12 years of age: oral dosage is one-half tablet every 4 to 6 hours, or as directed by a doctor. Do not exceed 3 tablets in 24 hours.
Children under 6 years of age: do not use unless directed by a doctor.

TAMPER-RESISTANT PACKAGE FEATURE
Bottles of 20's & 100's—If printed outer wrap is broken or removed, do not purchase. Blisters—Each tablet in sealed unit; do not use if tablet seal is broken.

HOW SUPPLIED
Peach color, scored tablets inscribed with 8666 on one side and C logo on the other. Bottles of 20 (NDC 0086-0066-02), 7 boxes of 24 blisters (NDC 0086-0066-24), and Bottles of 100 (NDC 0086-0066-10). Store at controlled room temperature (59°–86°F). 9/86
Manufactured for Carnrick Laboratories, Inc.
Shown in Product Identification Section, page 407

SKELAXIN® ℞
brand of metaxalone

CAUTION
Federal law prohibits dispensing without prescription.

DESCRIPTION
Each pale rose, scored tablet contains: metaxalone, 400 mg. Skelaxin (metaxalone) has the following chemical structure and name:
5-[(3,4-dimethylphenoxy)methyl]-2 oxazolidinone
[See Chemical Formula at top of next column].

$$\text{(3,5-}(CH_3)_2C_6H_3)\text{–O–}CH_2\text{–}CH\text{–}CH_2\text{ (ring: O–C(=O)–NH)}$$

ACTIONS
The mechanism of action of metaxalone in humans has not been established, but may be due to general central nervous system depression. It has no direct action on the contractile mechanism of striated muscle, the motor end plate or the nerve fiber.

INDICATIONS
Skelaxin (metaxalone) is indicated as an adjunct to rest, physical therapy, and other measures for the relief of discomforts associated with acute, painful musculoskeletal conditions. The mode of action of this drug has not been clearly identified, but may be related to its sedative properties. Metaxalone does not directly relax tense skeletal muscles in man.

CONTRAINDICATIONS
Metaxalone is contraindicated in individuals who have shown hypersensitivity to the drug. Metaxalone should not be administered to patients with a known tendency to drug-induced, hemolytic, or other anemias. It is contraindicated in patients with significantly impaired renal or hepatic function.

PRECAUTIONS
Elevation in cephalin flocculation tests without concurrent changes in other liver function parameters have been noted. Hence, it is recommended that metaxalone be administered with great care to patients with pre-existing liver damage and that serial liver function studies be performed as required.
False-positive Benedict's tests, due to an unknown reducing substance, have been noted. A glucose-specific test will differentiate findings.
Pregnancy: Reproduction studies have been performed in rats and have revealed no evidence of impaired fertility or harm to the fetus due to metaxalone. Reactions reports from marketing experience have not revealed evidence of fetal injury, but such experience cannot exclude the possibility of infrequent or subtle damage to the human fetus. Safe use of metaxalone has not been established with regard to possible adverse effects upon fetal development. Therefore, metaxalone tablets should not be used in women who are or may become pregnant and particularly during early pregnancy unless in the judgment of the physician the potential benefits outweigh the possbile hazards.
Nursing Mothers: It is not known whether this drug is secreted in human milk. As a general rule, nursing should not be undertaken while a patient is on a drug since many drugs are excreted in human milk.
Pediatric Use: Safety and effectiveness in children 12 years of age and below have not been established.

ADVERSE REACTIONS
The most frequent reactions to metaxalone include nausea, vomiting, gastrointestinal upset, drowsiness, dizziness, headache, and nervousness or "irritability." Other adverse reactions are: hypersensitivity reaction, characterized by a light rash with or without pruritus; leukopenia; hemolytic anemia; jaundice.

DOSAGE
The recommended dose for adults and children over 12 years of age is two tablets (800 mg) three to four times a day.

MANAGEMENT OF OVERDOSAGE
Gastric lavage and supportive therapy as indicated. (When determining the LD_{50} in rats and mice, progressive sedation, hypnosis and finally respiratory failure were noted as the dosage increased. In dogs, no LD_{50} could be determined as the higher doses produced an emetic action in 15 to 30 minutes). No documented case of major toxicity has been reported.

HOW SUPPLIED
Skelaxin (metaxalone) is available as a 400 mg. pale rose tablet, inscribed with 8662 on the scored side and "C" on the other. Available in bottles of 100 (NDC 0086-0062-10).
Store at Controlled Room Temperature, between 15°C and 30°C (59°F and 86°F).
12/85
Manufactured for Carnrick Laboratories, Inc.
Shown in Product Identification Section, page 407

Center Laboratories
Division of EM Industries, Inc.
35 CHANNEL DRIVE
PORT WASHINGTON, NY 11050

EPIPEN®/EPIPEN® Jr. ℞
Epinephrine Auto-Injectors

BRIEF SUMMARY

DESCRIPTION
The EpiPen® device provides epinephrine for intramuscular auto-injection in a sterile solution prepared from epinephrine with the aid of hydrochloric acid in pyrogen-free water. **The EpiPen® Auto-Injector** contains 2 ml Epinephrine Injection 1:1,000 U.S.P., and is designed to deliver a single dose of 0.3 mg epinephrine. Each ml contains: Active: 1.00 mg epinephrine. Inactive: 6.0 mg sodium chloride, 1.67 mg sodium metabisulfite, and hydrochloric acid to adjust pH.
The EpiPen® Jr. Auto-Injector contains 2 ml Epinephrine Injection 1:2,000 U.S.P., and is designed to deliver a single dose of 0.15 mg epinephrine. Each ml contains: Active: 0.5 mg epinephrine. Inactive: 6.00 mg sodium chloride, 1.67 mg sodium metabisulfite, and hydrochloric acid to adjust pH.

CLINICAL PHARMACOLOGY
Epinephrine is a sympathomimetic drug, acting on both alpha and beta receptors. It is the drug of choice for the emergency treatment of severe allergic reactions (Type 1) to hymenoptera stings, foods, drugs and other allergens. The strong vasoconstrictor action of epinephrine acts quickly to counter vasodilation and resulting increased capillary permeability. By its effect on smooth muscle, epinephrine relaxes the bronchioles, thereby relieving wheezing and dyspnea. Its action also relieves angioedema or hives.

INDICATIONS AND USAGE
Epinephrine is indicated in the emergency treatment of severe allergic (anaphylaxis) to hymenoptera stings, foods, drugs and other allergens. The EpiPen® Auto-Injector is intended for immediate self-administration by individuals with a history of anaphylactic reactions. It is designed as emergency supportive therapy only and is not a replacement or substitute for subsequent medical or hospital care.

CONTRAINDICATIONS
Epinephrine is contraindicated in individuals with organic brain damage.

WARNINGS
Epinephrine is light sensitive and should be stored in the tube provided. **Store at room temperature (59°F–86°F). Do not refrigerate.** Before using, check to make sure solution in Auto-Injector is not brown in color. If it is discolored or contains a precipitate, do not use. Every effort should be made to avoid possible inadvertent intravascular administration through appropriate selection of an injection site such as the thigh. Do not inject into buttock.
Large doses or accidental intravenous injection of epinephrine may result in cerebral hemorrhage due to sharp rise in blood pressure. Rapidly acting vasodilators can counteract the marked pressor effects of epinephrine.
Epinephrine should be administered with extreme caution to patients who have developed degenerative heart disease. Use of epinephrine with drugs that sensitize the heart to arrhythmias is not recommended. Anginal pain may be induced by epinephrine in patients with coronary insufficiency.

PRECAUTIONS
The effects of epinephrine may be potentiated by tricyclic antidepressants; certain antihistamines, e.g., diphenhydramine, tripelennamine, d-chlorpheniramine, and sodium l-thyroxine.
Administer with caution to hyperthyroid individuals; psychoneurotic individuals, individuals with cardiovascular disease, hypertension, or diabetes, elderly individuals, pregnant women, and children under 30 kg (66 lbs.) body weight.

ADVERSE REACTIONS
Transient and minor side effects of epinephrine include palpitation, respiratory difficulty, pallor, dizziness, weakness, tremor, headache, throbbing, restlessness, tenseness, anxiety and fear.
Ventricular arrhythmias may follow administration of epinephrine.

DOSAGE AND ADMINISTRATION
Dosage in any specific patient should be based on body weight in addition to the patient's risk of anaphylaxis and ability to tolerate epinephrine. Usual Epinephrine adult dosage for allergic emergencies is 0.3 mg. Usual pediatric dose is 0.01 mg/kg body weight.
A physician who prescribes EpiPen® or EpiPen® Jr. should take appropriate steps to insure that his patient understands

Continued on next page

Center—Cont.

the indications and use of this device thoroughly. The physician should review with the patient, in detail, the package insert and operation of the Auto-Injector. Inject the delivered dose of the Auto-Injector intramuscularly into the anteriolateral aspect of the thigh. See package insert.

HOW SUPPLIED

Package containing one EpiPen® or EpiPen® Jr. Auto-Injector and in packages of six units. Training Device for patient instruction purposes also available.

Caution: Federal (U.S.A.) law prohibits dispensing without a prescription.

Central Pharmaceuticals, Inc.

120 EAST THIRD STREET
SEYMOUR, IN 47274

CODICLEAR DH SYRUP Ⓒ℞

[kō'dĭ-klēr"]

DESCRIPTION

A clear, colorless, sweet-tasting syrup which is alcohol-free, sugar-free and dye-free.

Each teaspoonful (5 ml.) contains:
Hydrocodone bitartrate ....5 mg.
(Warning - May be habit forming)
Potassium guaiacolsulfonate ....300 mg.

This product contains ingredients in the following classes: Antitussive, Expectorant.

CLINICAL PHARMACOLOGY

Hydrocodone bitartrate is a potent antitussive which causes suppression of the cough reflex by direct action on the cough center. Hydrocodone is approximately three times as potent as codeine on a weight basis and has a higher addiction potential also. Potassium guaiacolsulfonate has been used empirically for many decades as an expectorant.

INDICATIONS

For the temporary relief of dry, nonproductive cough due to colds, pertussis or influenza.

CONTRAINDICATIONS

Hypersensitivity to any of the ingredients.

WARNINGS

Hydrocodone can produce drug dependence and therefore has the potential for being abused. Codiclear DH should be prescribed and administered with the degree of caution appropriate for this type product.

PRECAUTIONS

General: The hydrocodone in this product may exhibit additive effects with other CNS depressants, including alcohol. Respiratory depression can be a real hazard so caution should be used, especially in patients with chronic obstructive pulmonary disease.

Information for Patients: The hydrocodone may cause drowsiness and ambulatory patients who operate machinery or motor vehicles should be cautioned accordingly.

Drug Interactions: Concommitant use of hydrocodone with alcohol and/or other CNS depressants may have an additive effect.

USAGE IN PREGNANCY

Pregnancy Category C. Hydrocodone has been shown to be teratogenic in hamsters when given in doses 700 times the human dose. There are no adequate and well-controlled studies in pregnant women. CODICLEAR DH Syrup should be used during pregnancy only if the potential benefit justifies the potential risk to the fetus.

ADVERSE REACTIONS

Adverse reactions include drowsiness, lassitude, nausea, giddiness, constipation, respiratory depression and addiction.

DRUG ABUSE AND DEPENDENCE

This product is a Schedule III Controlled Substance. Because of the hydrocodone content, some abuse might be expected. Psychic dependence, physical dependence and tolerance may develop upon repeated administration. It should be prescribed and administered with the degree of caution appropriate for this type product.

OVERDOSAGE

Symptoms of overdosage include respiratory depression, extreme somnolence progressing to stupor or coma, skeletal muscle flaccidity, cold and clammy skin and other symptoms common with narcotic overdosage.

Primary treatment consists of insuring adequate respiration through provision of a patent airway and the institution of assisted or controlled ventilation. Naloxone hydrochloride should be administered in small intravenous doses (consult specific product labeling before use). In addition, oxygen, intravenous fluids, vasopressors and other supportive measures should be employed as indicated. Gastric emptying may be useful in removing unabsorbed drug. Activated charcoal may also be of benefit.

DOSAGE AND ADMINISTRATION

Adults and older children–1 to 1½ teaspoonfuls; children, 6 to 12 years of age–½ to 1 teaspoonful; children, 3 to 6 years of age–¼ to ½ teaspoonful. These doses may be given four times daily as needed. Not recommended for children under 3 years of age.

HOW SUPPLIED

Bottles of 4 fl. oz.–NDC 0131-5034-64
Bottles of 1 pint–NDC 0131-5034-70

CODIMAL® DH Ⓒ℞

[kō'di-mahl"]

CODIMAL® DM
CODIMAL® PH Ⓒ
CODIMAL® EXPECTORANT

DESCRIPTION

Each teaspoonful (5 ml) of CODIMAL DH contains: Hydrocodone Bitartrate 1.66 mg. (Warning—May be habit forming); Phenylephrine Hydrochloride 5.0 mg.; Pyrilamine Maleate 8.33 mg.

Each teaspoonful (5 ml) of CODIMAL DM contains: Dextromethorphan hydrobromide 10 mg.; Phenylephrine hydrochloride 5 mg.; Pyrilamine maleate 8.33 mg.; Alcohol 4%. Sugar-free.

Each teaspoonful (5 ml) of CODIMAL PH contains: Codeine Phosphate 10 mg. (Warning —May be habit forming); Phenylephrine Hydrochloride 5 mg.; Pyrilamine Maleate 8.33 mg.

Each teaspoonful (5 ml) of CODIMAL EXPECTORANT contains: Phenylpropanolamine Hydrochloride 25 mg.; Guaifenesin 100 mg.

INDICATIONS AND USAGE

For temporary relief of cough due to the common cold or other upper respiratory infection or irritation.

CONTRAINDICATIONS

In persons with a known hypersensitivity to any of the ingredients.

PRECAUTIONS

Should be administered with extreme caution to patients with hypertension, heart disease, diabetes, thyroid disease or vascular disease, or those receiving MAO inhibitors. Codeine and its derivative, Hydrocodone Bitartrate, are narcotic agents and the usual precautions in their use should be observed, particularly in infants and elderly patients.

SIDE EFFECTS

Occasional drowsiness, blurred vision, palpitation, flushing, nervousness or gastrointestinal upsets.

WARNINGS

Patients should be instructed not to drive or operate machinery while taking the medication; and not to administer it to patients with a high fever or persistent cough unless so directed by a physician.

ADMINISTRATION AND DOSAGE

Codimal DH, Codimal DM and Codimal PH: Adults and older children—1 to 2 teaspoonfuls; children 6 to 12—1 teaspoonful; children 2 to 6—½ teaspoonful. These doses may be taken every 4 hours. Children 6 months to 2 years—¼ teaspoonful every 6 hours.

Codimal Expectorant: Adults and older children—1 teaspoonful; children, 6 to 12 years—½ teaspoonful; children, 2 to 6—¼ teaspoonful. This dose may be taken every four hours.

HOW SUPPLIED

Bottles of 4 ounces, pints and gallons. Codimal Expectorant not available in gallons.

CODIMAL®-L.A. CAPSULES ℞

[kō'di-mahl"]

DESCRIPTION

Each Timed Release Capsule contains:
Chlorpheniramine maleate ....8 mg.
Pseudoephedrine
hydrochloride ....120 mg.
in a specially prepared base to provide prolonged action.

HOW SUPPLIED

Bottle of 100 Capsules NDC 0131-4213-37
Bottle of 1000 Capsules NDC 0131-4213-43

Shown in Product Identification Section, page 407

CO-GESIC® TABLETS Ⓒ℞

[kō'je"zik]

DESCRIPTION

Each tablet contains:
Hydrocodone Bitartrate ....5 mg.
(WARNING—May be habit forming)
Acetaminophen ....500 mg.

This product is a narcotic analgesic.

INACTIVE INGREDIENTS

Magnesium Stearate, Microcrystalline Cellulose, Pregelatinized Starch and Sodium Starch Glycolate.

Acetaminophen is a nonopiate, non-salicylate analgesic and antipyretic which occurs as a white, odorless crystalline powder possessing a slightly bitter taste. Hydrocodone bitartrate is an opioid analgesic and antitussive and occurs as fine, white crystals or as a crystalline powder. It is affected by light.

CLINICAL PHARMACOLOGY

Hydrocodone is a semisynthetic narcotic analgesic and antitussive with multiple actions qualitatively similar to those of codeine. Most of these involve the central nervous system and smooth muscle. The precise mechanism of action of hydrocodone and other opiates is not known, although it is believed to relate to the existence of opiate receptors in the central nervous system. In addition to analgesia, narcotics may produce drowsiness, changes in mood and mental clouding.

Radioimmunoassay techniques have recently been developed for the analysis of hydrocodone in human plasma. After a 10 mg oral dose of hydrocodone bitartrate, a mean peak serum drug level of 23.6 ng/ml and an elimination half-life of 3.8 hours were found.

The analgesic action of acetaminophen involves peripheral and central influences, but the specific mechanism is as yet undetermined. Antipyretic activity is mediated through hypothalmic heat regulating centers. Acetaminophen inhibits prostaglandin synthetase. Therapeutic doses of acetaminophen have negligible effects on the cardiovascular or respiratory systems; however, toxic doses may cause circulatory failure and rapid, shallow breathing. Acetaminophen is rapidly and almost completely absorbed from the gastrointestinal tract, producing maximum serum concentrations within 30 minutes to one hour. The plasma half-life in adults and children ranges from 0.90 hours to 3.25 hours with an average of approximately 2 hours. The drug distributes uniformly in most body fluids and is approximately 25% protein bound. Acetaminophen is conjugated in the liver, with less than 3% of the dose excreted unchanged in 24 hours. The primary metabolic pathway is conjugation to sulfate and glucuronide by-products. A minor oxidative pathway forms cysteine and mercapturic acid. These compounds are subsequently excreted by the kidneys into the urine.

INDICATIONS AND USAGE

For the relief of moderate to moderately severe pain.

CONTRAINDICATIONS

Hypersensitivity to acetaminophen or hydrocodone.

WARNINGS

Respiratory Depression: At high doses or in sensitive patients, hydrocodone may produce dose-related respiratory depression by acting directly on brain stem respiratory centers. Hydrocodone also effects centers that control respiratory rhythm, and may produce irregular and periodic breathing.

Head Injury and Increased Intracranial Pressure: The respiratory depressant effects of narcotics and their capacity to elevate cerebrospinal fluid pressure may be markedly exaggerated in the presence of head injury, other intracranial lesions or a preexisting increase in intracranial pressure. Furthermore, narcotics produce adverse reactions which may obscure the clinical course of patients with head injuries.

Acute Abdominal Conditions: The administration of narcotics may obscure the diagnosis or clinical course of patients with acute abdominal conditions.

PRECAUTIONS

Special Risk Patients: As with any narcotic analgesic agent, CO-GESIC Tablets should be used with caution in elderly or debilitated patients and those with severe impairment of hepatic or renal function, hypothyroidism, Addison's disease, prostatic hypertrophy or urethral stricture. The usual precautions should be observed and the possibility of respiratory depression should be kept in mind.

Information for Patients: CO-GESIC Tablets, like all narcotics, may impair the mental and/or physical abilities required for the performance of potentially hazardous tasks such as driving a car or operating machinery; patients should be cautioned accordingly.

Cough Reflex: Hydrocodone suppresses the cough reflex; as with all narcotics, caution should be exercised when CO-GESIC Tablets are used postoperatively and in patients with pulmonary disease.

Drug Interactions: Patients receiving other narcotic analgesics, antipsychotics, antianxiety agents, or other CNS depressants (including alcohol) concomitantly with CO-GESIC Tablets may exhibit an additive CNS depression. When combined therapy is contemplated, the dose of one or both agents should be reduced.
The use of MAO inhibitors or tricyclic antidepressants with hydrocodone preparations may increase the effect of either the antidepressant or hydrocodone.
The concurrent use of anticholinergics with hydrocodone may produce paralytic ileus.
Usage in Pregnancy: Pregnancy Category C. Hydrocodone has been shown to be teratogenic in hamsters when given doses 700 times the human dose. There are no adequate and well-controlled studies in pregnant women. CO-GESIC Tablets should be used during pregnancy only if the potential benefit justifies the potential risk to the fetus.
Nonteratogenic Effects: Babies born to mothers who have been taking opioids regularly prior to delivery will be physically dependent. The withdrawal signs include irritability and excessive crying, tremors, hyperactive reflexes, increased respiratory rate, increased stools, sneezing, yawning, vomiting, and fever. The intensity of the syndrome does not always correlate with the duration of maternal opioid use or dose. There is no consensus on the best method of managing withdrawal. Chlorpromazine 0.7 to 1.0 mg/kg q6h, and paregoric 2 to 4 drops/kg q4h, have been used to treat withdrawal symptoms in infants. The duration of therapy is 4 to 28 days, with the dosage decreased as tolerated.
Labor and Delivery: As with all narcotics, administration of CO-GESIC Tablets to the mother shortly before delivery may result in some degree of respiratory depression in the newborn, especially if higher doses are used.
Nursing Mothers: It is not known whether this drug is excreted in human milk. Because many drugs are excreted in human milk and because of the potential for serious adverse reactions in nursing infants from CO-GESIC Tablets, a decision should be made whether to discontinue nursing or to discontinue the drug, taking into account the importance of the drug to the mother.
Pediatric Use: Safety and effectiveness in children have not been established.

ADVERSE REACTIONS

Central Nervous System: Sedation, drowsiness, mental clouding, lethargy, impairment of mental and physical performance, anxiety, fear, dysphoria, dizziness, psychic dependence, mood changes.
Gastrointestinal System: Nausea and vomiting may occur; they are more frequent in ambulatory than in recumbent patients. The antiemetic phenothiazines are useful in suppressing these effects; however, some phenothiazine derivatives seem to be antianalgesic and to increase the amount of narcotic required to produce pain relief, while other phenothiazines reduce the amount of narcotic required to produce a given level of analgesia. Prolonged administration of CO-GESIC Tablets may produce constipation.
Genitourinary System: Ureteral spasm, spasm of vesical sphincters and urinary retention have been reported.
Respiratory Depression: CO-GESIC Tablets may produce dose-related respiratory depression by acting directly on brain stem respiratory centers. Hydrocodone also affects centers that control respiratory rhythm, and may produce irregular and periodic breathing. If significant respiratory depression occurs, it may be antagonized by the use of naloxone hydrochloride. Apply other supportive measures when indicated.
Drug Abuse and Dependence: CO-GESIC Tablets are subject to the Federal Controlled Substance Act (Schedule III). Psychic dependence, physical dependence, and tolerance may develop upon repeated administration of narcotics; therefore CO-GESIC Tablets should be prescribed and administered with caution. However, psychic dependence is unlikely to develop when CO-GESIC Tablets are used for a short time for the treatment of pain.
Physical dependence, the condition in which continued administration of the drug is required to prevent the appearance of a withdrawal syndrome, assumes clinically significant proportions only after several weeks of continued narcotic use, although some mild degree of physical dependence may develop after a few days of narcotic therapy. Tolerance, in which increasingly large doses are required in order to produce the same degree of analgesia, is manifested initially by a shortened duration of analgesic effect, and subsequently by decreases in the intensity of analgesia. The rate of development of tolerance varies among patients.

OVERDOSAGE

Acetaminophen: Signs and Symptoms: Acetaminophen in massive overdosage may cause hepatic toxicity in some patients. In all cases of suspected overdose, immediately call your regional poison center for assistance in diagnosis and for directions in the use of an antidote.
In adults, hepatic toxicity has rarely been reported with acute overdoses of less than 10 grams and fatalities with less than 15 grams. Importantly, young children seem to be more resistant than adults to the hepatotoxic effect of an acetaminophen overdose. Despite this, the measures outlined below should be initiated in any adult or child suspected of having ingested an acetaminophen overdose.
Early symptoms following a potentially hepatotoxic overdose may include: nausea, vomiting, diaphoresis and general malaise. Clinical and laboratory evidence of hepatic toxicity may not be apparent until 48 to 72 hours post-ingestion.
Treatment: The stomach should be emptied promptly by lavage or by induction of emesis with syrup of ipecac. Patients' estimates of the quantity of a drug ingested are notoriously unreliable. Therefore, if an acetaminophen overdose is suspected, a serum acetaminophen assay should be obtained as early as possible, but no sooner than four hours following ingestion. Liver function studies should be obtained initially and repeated at 24-hour intervals.
The antidote, N-acetylcysteine, should be administered as early as possible, and within 16 hours of the overdose ingestion for optimal results, but in any case, within 24 hours. Following recovery, there are no residual, structural or functional hepatic abnormalities.
Hydrocodone: Signs and Symptoms: Serious overdose with hydrocodone is characterized by respiratory depression (a decrease in respiratory rate and/or tidal volume, Cheyne-Stokes respiration, cyanosis), extreme somnolence progressing to stupor or coma, skeletal muscle flaccidity, cold and clammy skin, and sometimes bradycardia and hypotension. In severe overdosage, apnea, circulatory collapse, cardiac arrest and death may occur.
Treatment: Primary attention should be given to the reestablishment of adequate respiratory exchange through provision of a patent airway and the institution of assisted or controlled ventilation. The narcotic antagonist naloxone is a specific antidote against respiratory depression which may result from overdosages or unusual sensitivity to narcotics, including hydrocodone. Therefore, an appropriate dose of naloxone (see package insert) should be administered, preferably by the intravenous route, and simultaneously with efforts at respiratory resuscitation. Since the duration of action of hydrocodone may exceed that of the antagonist, the patient should be kept under continued surveillance and repeated doses of the antagonist should be administered as needed to maintain adequate respiration.
An antagonist should not be administered in the absence of clinically significant respiratory or cardiovascular depression. Oxygen, intravenous fluids, vasopressors and other supportive measures should be employed as indicated.
Gastric emptying may be useful in removing unabsorbed drug.

DOSAGE AND ADMINISTRATION

Dosage should be adjusted according to the severity of the pain and the response of the patient. However, it should be kept in mind that tolerance to hydrocodone can develop with continued use and that the incidence of untoward effects is dose related.
The usual adult dose is one tablet every six hours as needed for pain. If necessary, this dose may be repeated at four hour intervals. In cases of more severe pain, two tablets every six hours (up to 8 tablets in 24 hours) may be required.

HOW SUPPLIED

Oval shaped white compressed tablet with 500 and 5 separated by bisect on one side and Central logo on the other.
Bottles of 100 tablets: NDC 0131-2104-37
Bottles of 500 tablets: NDC 0131-2104-41
Unit Dose—100 tablets: NDC 0131-2104-86
Shown in Product Identification Section, page 407

DIA-GESIC™ TABLETS Ⓒ℞

[di″ah-jē′zik]

DESCRIPTION

Each tablet contains:
Hydrocodone bitartrate .... 5 mg.
(WARNING—May be habit forming)
Aspirin .... 230 mg.
Acetaminophen .... 150 mg.
Caffeine .... 30 mg.

HOW SUPPLIED

Flat, truncated oval, bisected white tablets inscribed with the Central logo on one side and the number 31 and the score on the other side.
Bottles of 100 tablets—NDC 0131-2810-37
Bottles of 1000 tablets—NDC 0131-2810-43
Shown in Product Identification Section, page 407

MONO-GESIC® TABLETS ℞

[mon″o-je′zik]
(salsalate)
(salicylsalicylic acid)

DESCRIPTION

Mono-Gesic® (Salsalate) is a non-steroidal anti-inflammatory agent for oral administration. Chemically, salsalate (salicysalicylic acid or 2-hydroxy-benzoic acid 2-carboxyphenyl ester) is a dimer of salicylic acid.
Each oval, pink, film-coated tablet contains:
Salsalate (salicylsalicylic acid) .... 750 mg.
The ingredient in this product is of the following classes: non-steroidal anti-inflammatory agent, analgesic and antipyretic.

INACTIVE INGREDIENTS

Acetylated Monoglycerides, Alcohol, Castor Oil, Colloidal Silicon Dioxide, D & C Red #30, Ethyl Cellulose, Hydroxypropyl Cellulose, Hydroxypropyl Methylcellulose, Microcrystalline Cellulose, Polyethylene Glycol, Povidone, Shellac, Starch, Stearic Acid and Titanium Dioxide.

CLINICAL PHARMACOLOGY

Due to the poor solubility of salsalate in gastric fluid, most will pass through the stomach unhydrolyzed and unabsorbed. In the small intestine, it is partially hydrolyzed to two molecules of salicylic acid and rapidly absorbed both as the parent compound and as salicylic acid. A small proportion is excreted unchanged while the remainder is excreted as salicylic acid and its metabolites. Salsalate has a greater half-life of elimination than salicylic acid.
The mode of action of salsalate and other non-steroidal anti-inflammatory drugs is unresolved. It does, however, appear to be involved with the inhibition of prostaglandin synthesis. Unlike aspirin, salsalate has not been associated with reactions causing asthmatic attacks in susceptible people. Also, it is not known to effect the platelet adhesiveness involved in the clotting mechanism. Salsalate also does not cause the gastrointestinal blood loss common to other nonsteroidal anti-inflammatory agents.

INDICATIONS AND USAGE

MONO-GESIC is indicated for the temporary relief of symptoms of rheumatoid arthritis, osteoarthritis and related rheumatic disorders.

CONTRAINDICATIONS

Hypersensitivity to salsalate.

PRECAUTIONS

General: To avoid potentially toxic concentrations, the plasma salicylic acid levels should be monitored to maintain the therapeutically effective levels of 10 to 30 mg/100 ml. Changes in urinary pH can have significant effects on the plasma level of salsalate. Acidification can result in an increase in the plasma level resulting in toxicity while an increase in urinary pH will increase renal clearance and urinary excretion of salsalate, thus lowering plasma levels.
Information for Patients: Patients on long-term treatment should be warned not to take other salicylates. They should also be warned that if symptoms of overdosage, such as tinnitus, vertigo, headache, confusion, drowsiness, sweating, hyperventilation, vomiting or diarrhea appear, the drug should be stopped and physician notified.
Drug Interactions: Salicylates antagonize the uricosuric action of drugs used to treat gout. Salicylates will be additive to MONO-GESIC and could increase plasma concentrations to toxic levels. Drugs and foods that raise urine pH will increase renal clearance and urinary excretion of salicylic acid, thus lowering plasma levels; acidifying drugs or foods will decrease urinary excretion and increase plasma levels. Salicylates may competitively displace anticoagulant drugs from plasma protein binding sites and thereby predispose to systemic bleeding. Salicylates may enhance the hypoglycemic effect of oral antidiabetic drugs of the sulfonylurea class. Salicylate competes with a number of drugs for protein binding sites, notably penicillin, thiopental, thyroxine, triiodothyronine, phenytoin, sulfinpyrazone, naproxen, warfarin, methotrexate, and possibly corticosteroids.
Drug/Laboratory Test Interactions: Salicylate competes with thyroid hormone for binding to plasma proteins, which may be reflected in a depressed plasma T_4 value in some patients; thyroid function and basal metabolism are unaffected.
Carcinogenesis: No long-term animal studies have been performed with MONO-GESIC to evaluate its carcinogenic potential; however, several such studies using aspirin and other salicylates have failed to demonstrate any association of these agents with cancerous cell changes.
Use in Pregnancy: Pregnancy Category C: Salsalate and salicylic acid have been shown to be teratogenic and embryocidal in rats when given in doses four to five times the usual human dose. These effects were not observed at doses twice as great as the usual human dose. There are no adequate and

Continued on next page

Central—Cont.

well controlled studies in pregnant women. MONO-GESIC should be used during pregnancy only if the potential benefit justifies the potential risk to the fetus.

Labor and Delivery: There exists no adequate and well-controlled studies in pregnant women. Although adverse effects on mother or infant have not been reported with MONO-GESIC use during labor, caution is advised when anti-inflammatory dosage is involved. However, other salicylates have been associated with prolonged gestation and labor, maternal and neonatal bleeding sequelae, potentiation of narcotic and barbiturate effects (respiratory or cardiac arrest in the mother), delivery problems and stillbirth.

Nursing Mothers: It is not known whether salsalate per se is excreted in human milk; salicylic acid, the primary metabolite of MONO-GESIC, has been shown to appear in human milk in concentrations approximating the maternal blood level. Thus the infant of a mother on MONO-GESIC therapy might ingest in mother's milk 30 to 80% as much salicylate per kg body weight as the mother is taking. Accordingly, caution should be exercised when MONO-GESIC is administered to a nursing woman.

Pediatric Use: Not recommended for use in children.

WARNING

Drugs of this class, salicylates, have been reported to be associated with the development of Reye Syndrome in children and teenagers with chicken pox, influenza, and influenza-like infections.

ADVERSE REACTIONS

Adverse reactions are usually the result of overdosage and may include tinnitus and temporary hearing loss, vertigo, headache, confusion, drowsiness, sweating, hyperventilation, vomiting and diarrhea.

DRUG ABUSE AND DEPENDENCE

Drug abuse and dependence have not been reported with MONO-GESIC.

Overdosage: No deaths after overdosage have been reported for MONO-GESIC. Death has followed ingestion of 10 to 30 g of other salicylates in adults, but much larger amounts have been ingested without fatal outcome.

Symptoms: The usual symptoms of salicylism, tinnitus, vertigo, headache, confusion, drowsiness, sweating, hyperventilation, vomiting and diarrhea will occur. More severe intoxication will lead to disruption of electrolyte balance and blood pH, and hyperthermia and dehydration.

Treatment: Further absorption of MONO-GESIC from the G.I. tract should be prevented by emesis (syrup of ipecac) and, if necessary, by gastric lavage.

Fluid and electrolyte imbalance should be corrected by the administration of appropriate I.V. therapy. Adequate renal function should be maintained. Hemodialysis or peritoneal dialysis may be required in extreme cases.

DOSAGE AND ADMINISTRATION

Dosage should be adjusted according to the severity of the disease and the response of the patient. Response will be gradual and full benefits may not be evident for three to four days when plasma salicylate levels have achieved steady state.

The usual dosage is 3,000 mg. daily, given in divided doses, such as two tablets twice daily or one tablet four times daily.

HOW SUPPLIED

An oval, pink film coated tablet embossed with Central logo on one side and 750/mg on the other side.

Bottles of 100 tablets - NDC 0131-2164-37
Bottles of 500 tablets - NDC 0131-2164-41

Shown in Product Identification Section, page 407

NIFEREX® TABLETS/ELIXIR
[ni 'fer "ex]
NIFEREX®-150 CAPSULES
NIFEREX® with VITAMIN C TABLETS
(polysaccharide-iron complex)

DESCRIPTION

NIFEREX is a highly water-soluble complex of iron and a low molecular weight polysaccharide. Each NIFEREX-150 Capsule contains 150 mg. elemental iron. Each NIFEREX Film Coated Tablet and each NIFEREX with Vitamin C Chewable Tablet contains 50 mg. elemental iron. In addition, each NIFEREX with Vitamin C tablet contains Ascorbic acid, U.S.P., 100 mg. and Sodium ascorbate, 168.75 mg. Each 5 ml. (teaspoonful) NIFEREX Elixir contains 100 mg. elemental iron, alcohol 10% (sugar free).

ACTION AND USES

NIFEREX is an easily assimilated source of iron for treatment of uncomplicated iron deficiency anemia. Because NIFEREX is a polysaccharide bound iron complex, it is relatively nontoxic and there are relatively few, if any, of the gastrointestinal side effects associated with iron therapy, thus permitting full therapeutic dosage (150 to 300 mg. elemental iron daily) in a single dose if desirable. There is no staining of teeth and no metallic aftertaste.

INDICATIONS AND USAGE

For treatment of uncomplicated iron deficiency anemia.

CONTRAINDICATIONS

In patients with hemochromatosis and hemosiderosis, and in those with a known hypersensitivity to any of the ingredients.

ADMINISTRATION AND DOSAGE

ADULTS: One or two NIFEREX-150 Capsules daily, or one or two NIFEREX or NIFEREX with Vitamin C Tablets twice daily, *or* one to two teaspoonfuls NIFEREX Elixir daily. CHILDREN 6 to 12 years of age: One or two NIFEREX *or* one NIFEREX with Vitamin C Tablet daily, or one teaspoonful NIFEREX Elixir daily; Children 2 to 6 years of age: ½ teaspoonful NIFEREX Elixir daily. Children under 2 years: ¼ teaspoonful daily.

HOW SUPPLIED

NIFEREX-150 Capsules: Bottles of 100 and 1,000. NIFEREX Elixir: Bottles of 8 ounces. NIFEREX Tablets: Bottles of 100. NIFEREX with Vitamin C Chewable Tablets: Bottles of 50.

Shown in Product Identification Section, page 407

NIFEREX®-150 FORTE CAPSULES ℞
[ni 'fer "ex for 'ta]
NIFEREX® FORTE ELIXIR ℞

DESCRIPTION

Each capsule Niferex®-150 Forte contains:

Iron (Elemental) (as polysaccharide-iron complex)	150 mg.
Folic Acid	1 mg.
Vitamin B_{12}	25 mcg.

Each teaspoon (5 ml) Niferex® Forte Elixir contains:

Iron (Elemental) (as polysaccharide-iron complex)	100 mg.
Folic Acid	1 mg.
Vitamin B_{12}	25 mcg.
Alcohol	10%

Sugar-Free

HOW SUPPLIED

NIFEREX-150 FORTE CAPSULES

Bottle of 100	NDC 0131-4330-37
Bottle of 1000	NDC 0131-4330-43

NIFEREX FORTE ELIXIR

Bottle of 4 fl. oz.	NDC 0131-5065-64

Capsules Shown in Product Identification Section, page 407

NIFEREX®—PN TABLETS ℞
[ni 'fer "ex]

DESCRIPTION

Each film-coated tablet contains:

Iron (Elemental) (as polysaccharide-iron complex)	60 mg.
Folic acid	1 mg.
Ascorbic acid (as sodium ascorbate)	50 mg.
Cyanocobalamin (Vitamin B_{12})	3 mcg.
Vitamin A	4000 I.U.
Vitamin D_2	400 I.U.
Thiamine mononitrate	3 mg.
Riboflavin	3 mg.
Pyridoxine hydrochloride	2 mg.
Niacinamide	10 mg.
Calcium carbonate	312 mg.
Zinc sulfate USP (as 50 mg. dried zinc sulfate)	80 mg.

This product contains ingredients of the following therapeutic classes: vitamins and minerals.

INACTIVE INGREDIENTS

Acetylated Monoglycerides, Alcohol, Castor Oil, Corn Syrup, Ethyl Cellulose, F.D.&C. Blue #1 Lake, Ferric Chloride, Hydrogenated Vegetable Oil, Hydroxypropyl Cellulose, Hydroxypropyl Methylcellulose, Magnesium Stearate, Microcrystalline Cellulose, Polyethylene Glycol, Povidone, Shellac, Sodium Hydroxide, Sorbitol and Titanium Dioxide.

CLINICAL PHARMACOLOGY

This product is formulated to meet the needs of the pregnant or lactating patient with special consideration given to adequate amounts of hematopoietic factors, iron, folic acid and cyanocobalamin. Calcium (phosphorus-free) is also included in the formula to help supply the increased requirements of this mineral. The 60 mg. of elemental iron is available in the form of Niferex® (polysaccharide-iron complex). This form of iron is especially useful in the pregnant patient because, although it is absorbed as well as ferrous sulfate, it does not produce the gastrointestinal irritation commonly associated with iron salts. In addition, folic acid and cyanocobalamin in therapeutic amounts are included to prevent or treat the significant number of pregnant patients who develop megaloblastic anemia of pregnancy.

INDICATIONS AND USAGE

For the prevention and/or treatment of dietary vitamin and mineral deficiencies associated with pregnancy and lactation.

CONTRAINDICATIONS

Hypersensitivity to any of the ingredients.

WARNINGS

Folic acid alone is improper therapy in the treatment of pernicious anemia and other megaloblastic anemias where vitamin B_{12} is deficient.

PRECAUTIONS

Folic acid, especially in doses above 0.1 mg. daily may obscure pernicious anemia, in that hematologic remission may occur while neurological manifestations remain progressive.

ADVERSE REACTIONS

Allergic sensitization has been reported following both oral and parenteral administration of folic acid.

DOSAGE AND ADMINISTRATION

One tablet daily or as prescribed by a physician.

HOW SUPPLIED

Bottles of 100 tablets–NDC 0131-2209-37
Bottles of 1000 tablets–NDC 0131-2209-43

Shown in Product Identification Section, page 407

NIFEREX®-PN FORTE TABLETS ℞

DESCRIPTION

Each tablet contains:

Iron (Elemental) (as polysaccharide-iron complex)	60 mg.
Vitamin A acetate	5000 I.U.
Vitamin D (as ergocalciferol)	400 I.U.
Vitamin E (as dl-alpha-tocopheryl acetate)	30 I.U.
Vitamin C (ascorbic acid)	80 mg.
Folic acid	1 mg.
Thiamine (vitamin B_1) (as thiamine mononitrate)	3 mg.
Riboflavin (vitamin B_2)	3.4 mg.
Vitamin B_6 (as pyridoxine hydrochloride)	4 mg.
Niacinamide	20 mg.
Vitamin B_{12} (Cyanocobalamin)	12 mcg.
Calcium (as calcium carbonate)	250 mg.
Iodine (as potassium iodide)	0.2 mg.
Magnesium (as magnesium oxide)	10 mg.
Copper (as cupric oxide)	2 mg.
Zinc (as zinc sulfate)	25 mg.

HOW SUPPLIED

Bottles of 100 Tablets—NDC 0131-2309-37

Shown in Product Identification Section, page 407

PREDNICEN–M 21-Pak ℞
[pred 'nĭ-sĕn "]
(prednisone, 5 mg.)

HOW SUPPLIED

Each unit pack contains 21 × 5 mg. Prednisone, USP tablets. Also available in Bottles of 100: NDC 0131-2228-37, and Bottles of 1000: NDC 0131-2228-43.

SYNOPHYLATE® Elixir ℞
[sin-ah 'fil-āt "]
(theophylline sodium glycinate)
SYNOPHYLATE®-GG Tablets/Syrup ℞
(theophylline sodium glycinate and guaifenesin)

SYNOPHYLATE (theophylline sodium glycinate) Elixir contains per tbsp. (15 ml.): theophylline sodium glycinate, 330 mg. (equivalent to 150 mg. theophylline). Alcohol 20%. SYNOPHYLATE-GG Syrup or Tablets contain per tbsp. (15 ml.) or per tablet: theophylline sodium glycinate, 300 mg. (equivalent to 137 mg. theophylline); guaifenesin 100 mg. (Alcohol 10% in the syrup).

HOW SUPPLIED

SYNOPHYLATE ELIXIR

Pint	NDC 0131-5089-70

SYNOPHYLATE-GG TABLETS

100	NDC 0131-2253-37

SYNOPHYLATE-GG SYRUP

Pint	NDC 0131-5092-70
Gallon	NDC 0131-5092-72

THEOCLEAR® L.A.–260 CAPSULES ℞
[the 'ō-klēr"]
THEOCLEAR® L.A.–130 CAPSULES ℞
THEOCLEAR®–80 Syrup ℞
(theophylline anhydrous)

DESCRIPTION
THEOCLEAR L.A.-260 and **THEOCLEAR L.A.-130:** Each capsule contains 260 mg. or 130 mg. of theophylline anhydrous in a sustained release bead formulation.
THEOCLEAR-80: Each 15 ml. (1 tablespoonful) contains 80 mg. Anhydrous Theophylline as the active ingredient. Other ingredients are saccharin sodium; tartaric acid; benzoic acid; citric acid; sorbitol; glycerin; propylene glycol; artificial flavor and purified water. This formulation provides an alcohol-free, dye-free, and sugar-free vehicle containing no corn by-products.

HOW SUPPLIED
THEOCLEAR L.A.-260 CAPSULE
Bottle of 100 NDC 0131-4248-37
Bottle of 1000 NDC 0131-4248-43
THEOCLEAR L.A.-130 CAPSULE
Bottle of 100 NDC 0131-4247-37
THEOCLEAR-80 SYRUP
One Pint NDC 0131-5098-70
One Gallon NDC 0131-5098-72
Capsules shown in Product Identification Section, page 407

Cetylite Industries, Inc.
P.O. BOX CN6
9051 RIVER ROAD
PENNSAUKEN, NJ 08110

CETACAINE® ℞
[set 'a-cane"]
TOPICAL ANESTHETIC

A BRAND OF
Benzocaine 14.0%
Butyl Aminobenzoate 2.0%
Tetracaine Hydrochloride 2.0%
Benzalkonium Chloride 0.5%
Cetyl Dimethyl Ethyl
Ammonium Bromide 0.005%
In a bland water soluble base.

ACTION
Cetacaine produces anesthesia rapidly in approximately 30 seconds.

INDICATIONS
Cetacaine is a topical anesthetic indicated for the production of anesthesia of accessible mucous membrane.
Cetacaine Spray is indicated for use to control pain or gagging. Cetacaine in all forms is indicated for use to control pain.

DOSAGE AND ADMINISTRATION
Cetacaine Spray should be applied for approximately one second or less for normal anesthesia. Only limited quantity of Cetacaine is required for anesthesia and a spray in excess of 2 seconds is contraindicated. Average expulsion rate of residue from spray, at normal temperatures, is 200 mg. per second.
Tissue need not be dried prior to application of Cetacaine.
Cetacaine should be applied directly to the site where pain control is required.
Cetacaine Liquid or Cetacaine Ointment may be applied with a cotton pledget or directly to tissue. Cotton pledget should not be held in position for extended periods of time, since local reactions to benzoate topical anesthetics are related to the length of time of application.

ADVERSE REACTIONS
Although systemic reactions to Cetacaine have not been reported, local reactions to benzoate topical anesthetics may be associated with the condition of the mucous membrane treated and the length of time of application. Dehydration of the epithelium or an escharotic effect may result from prolonged contact. Allergic reactions are known to occur in some patients with preparations containing benzocaine.
Usage in Pregnancy: Safe use of Cetacaine has not been established with respect to possible adverse effects upon fetal development. Therefore Cetacaine should not be used during early pregnancy, unless in the judgment of a physician the potential benefits outweigh the unknown hazards.
Routine precaution for the use of any topical anesthetic should be observed when Cetacaine is used.

CONTRAINDICATIONS
Cetacaine is not for injection.
Do not use on the eyes.
To avoid excessive systemic absorption, Cetacaine should not be applied to large areas of denuded or inflamed tissue.
Cetacaine should not be administered to patients who are hypersensitive to any of its ingredients.
Individual dosage of tetracaine hydrochloride in excess of 20 mg. is contraindicated. Cetacaine should not be used under dentures or cotton rolls, as retention of the active ingredients under a denture or cotton roll could possibly cause an escharotic effect.
Jetco Cannula: The Jetco cannula for Cetacaine Spray is specially designed for accessibility and application of Cetacaine, at the required site of pain control.
The Jetco cannula is supplied in various sizes and shapes.
The Jetco cannula is inserted firmly onto the protruding plastic tubing on each bottle of Cetacaine Spray.
The Jetco cannula may be removed and re-inserted as many times as required for cleansing or sterilization.

PACKAGING AVAILABLE
Aerosol Spray 56 gm., including propellant.
Liquid 56 gm. bottle.
Ointment, flavored, 37 gram jar.
Hospital Gel, 29 grams in polyethylene tube.

CAUTION
Federal law prohibits dispensing Cetacaine without prescription.
Keep out of reach of children.

CETYLCIDE® SOLUTION
[see 'til-side"]

ACTIVE INGREDIENTS
Cetyl Dimethyl Ethyl
Ammonium Bromide 6.5%
Alkyl (50% C_{12}, 30% C_{14},
17% C_{16}, 3% C_{18}) Dimethyl
Benzyl Ammonium Chloride 6.5%
Isopropyl Alcohol 13.0%
Inert Ingredients 74.0%
Total Ingredients 100.0%
Formulation Contains Sodium Nitrite
An Instrument and Hard Surface Disinfectant, EPA Approved for Use in Hospitals and Dental/Medical Operatories.
In known hard water areas, use distilled water. Clean instruments thoroughly... rinse free of all soap before immersion, and allow them to remain in CETYLCIDE solution 15 minutes. Germicides containing a Quaternary Ammonium derivative should not be relied on to destroy spore forming organisms, Mycobacterium tuberculosis or the etiologic agent of viral hepatitis. Thus, instruments suspected of such contamination should be sterilized by heat. Needles, hypodermic syringes, corroded instruments or those with deep narrow crevices, as well as hinged or defective plated instruments should be sterilized by heat. To maintain disinfection, they may then be immersed in CETYLCIDE solution. Change solution periodically.

DIRECTIONS
PER GALLON: 1 oz. (30 ml) Cetylcide to one gallon (3.785 liters) tap water.
Dilution Directions For Use Against Pseudomonas Aeruginosa
PER GALLON: 2 oz. (60 ml) Cetylcide to one gallon (3.785 liters) tap water.
PER QUART: ½ oz. (15 ml) Cetylcide to one quart (946 ml) tap water.

STORAGE AND DISPOSAL
Do not reuse container.
Rinse thoroughly before discarding in trash.

INDICATIONS AND USES
CETYLCIDE... when diluted as directed, is a potent germicidal solution combining high bactericidal and bacteriostatic action against many kinds of pathogenic bacteria. CETYLCIDE is stable in both concentrated and diluted form. When diluted for use as directed, CETYLCIDE makes a RUST-INHIBITING • ODORLESS • COLORLESS, highly efficient germicidal solution for the chemical disinfection of ALL METAL, RUBBER AND PLASTIC SURGICAL AND DENTAL INSTRUMENTS AND APPLIANCES.

CAUTION
KEEP OUT OF REACH OF CHILDREN. HARMFUL IF SWALLOWED. CAUSES SEVERE EYE AND SKIN IRRITATION. DO NOT GET IN THE EYES OR ON SKIN. IN CASE OF EYE OR SKIN CONTACT, FLUSH WITH PLENTY OF WATER. FOR EYES, GET MEDICAL ATTENTION. AVOID CONTAMINATION OF FOOD.

HOW SUPPLIED
15 cc AMPULES, 32 OUNCE BOTTLES, AND 16 OUNCE BOTTLES.
EPA Reg. No. 3150-1
EPA Est. No. 3150-NJ-1 MADE IN U.S.A.

CIBA Consumer Pharmaceuticals
Division of CIBA-GEIGY Corporation
RARITAN PLAZA III
EDISON, NJ 08837

SLOW FE™
Slow Release Iron

DESCRIPTION
SLOW FE supplies ferrous sulfate, for the treatment of iron deficiency and iron deficiency anemia with a significant reduction in the incidence of common iron side effects. The wax matrix delivery system of SLOW FE is designed to maximize the release of ferrous sulfate in the duodenum and the jejunum where it is best tolerated and absorbed. SLOW FE is clinically shown to significantly reduce constipation, diarrhea and abdominal discomfort when compared to regular iron tablets and a leading capsule.

FORMULA
Each tablet contains 160 mg. dried ferrous sulfate USP, equivalent to 50 mg. elemental iron.

DOSAGE
ADULTS—one or two tablets daily or as recommended by a physician. A maximum of four tablets daily may be taken. CHILDREN—one tablet daily. Tablets must be swallowed whole.

WARNING
The treatment of any anemic condition should be under the advice and supervision of a physician. As oral iron products interfere with absorption of oral tetracycline antibiotics, these products should not be taken within two hours of each other. As with any drug, if you are pregnant or nursing a baby, seek the advice of a health professional before using this product.
Keep this and all medicines out of reach of children. In case of accidental overdose, contact your physician or poison control center immediately.
Tamper Resistant Packaging.

HOW SUPPLIED
Packages of 30 and 100.

Shown in Product Identification Section, page 407

The full prescribing information for each CIBA Consumer product is contained herein and is that in effect as of September 1, 1986.

Products are listed alphabetically in the
PINK SECTION.

Products are cross-indexed by product classifications in the
BLUE SECTION

Products are cross-indexed by generic and chemical names in the
YELLOW SECTION

CIBA Pharmaceutical Company

Division of CIBA-GEIGY Corporation
SUMMIT, NJ 07901

To provide a convenient and accurate means of identifying CIBA solid dosage form products, a code number has been imprinted on all tablets and capsules. To help you quickly identify a CIBA Tablet or Capsule by its code number, a numerical listing of codes (with corresponding product names) and an alphabetical listing of products (with corresponding codes and list numbers) have been compiled below.

CIBA Code #	ALPHABETICAL LISTING	List Number
	Antrenyl® bromide	
	oxyphenonium bromide	
15	TABLETS, 5 mg (white, scored)	
	100s	2410
	Anturane®	
	sulfinpyrazone USP	
41	TABLETS (white, single-scored) each containing 100 mg sulfinpyrazone USP	
	100s	1910
168	CAPSULES (green) each containing 200 mg sulfinpyrazone USP	
	100s	1920
	Apresazide®	
	hydralazine HCl and hydrochlorothiazide	
139	CAPSULES 25/25 (light blue and white opaque), each containing 25 mg hydralazine HCl and 25 mg hydrochlorothiazide	
	100s	3131
149	CAPSULES 50/50 (pink and white opaque), each containing 50 mg hydralazine HCl and 50 mg hydrochlorothiazide	
	100s	3132
159	CAPSULES 100/50 (pink flesh and white opaque), each containing 100 mg hydralazine HCl and 50 mg hydrochlorothiazide	
	100s	3133
	Apresoline® hydrochloride	
	hydralazine hydrochloride USP	
37	TABLETS, 10 mg (pale yellow, dry-coated)	
	100s	2629
	1000s	2627
	Consumer Pack	
	100s	2603
39	TABLETS, 25 mg (deep blue, dry-coated)	
	100s	2611
	500s	2613
	1000s	2615
	Accu-Pak® 100s	2647
	Consumer Pack	
	100s	2606
73	TABLETS, 50 mg (light blue, dry-coated)	
	100s	2619
	500s	2621
	1000s	2623
	Accu-Pak® 100s	2648
	Consumer Pack	
	100s	2643
101	TABLETS, 100 mg (peach, dry-coated)	
	100s	2638
	Apresoline®-Esidrix®	
	hydralazine hydrochloride and hydrochlorothiazide	
129	TABLETS (orange, dry-coated), each containing 25 mg hydralazine hydrochloride and 15 mg hydrochlorothiazide	
	100s	3120
	Cytadren®	
	aminoglutethamide USP	
24	TABLETS-250 mg (white, round, scored into quarters)	
	100s	2120
	Esidrix®	
	hydrochlorothiazide USP	
22	TABLETS, 25 mg (pink, scored)	
	100s	4310
	1000s	4313
	Accu-Pak®	
	100s	4312
	Consumer Pack	
	100s	4325
46	TABLETS, 50 mg (yellow, scored)	
	100s	4315
	1000s	4318
	Accu-Pak®	
	100s	4317
	Consumer Pack	
	30s	4328
	60s	4331
	100s	4330
192	TABLETS, 100 mg (blue, scored)	
	100s	4340
	Esimil®	
47	TABLETS (white, scored), each containing 10 mg guanethidine monosulfate USP and 25 mg hydrochlorothiazide USP	
	100s	4503
	Consumer Pack	
	100s	4512
	Ismelin® sulfate	
	guanethidine monosulfate	
49	TABLETS, 10 mg (pale yellow, scored)	
	100s	5010
	1000s	5012
	Consumer Pack	
	100s	5003
103	TABLETS, 25 mg (white, scored)	
	100s	5020
	1000s	5022
	Consumer Pack	
	100s	5026
	Lithobid®	
	lithium carbonate USP	
65	TABLETS, 300 mg (peach colored)	
	100s	0210
	1000s	0220
	Accu-Pak® 100s	0230
	Ludiomil®	
	maprotiline hydrochloride USP	
110	TABLETS, 25 mg (oval, dark orange, coated)	
	100s	1710
	Accu-Pak®	
	100s	1714
26	TABLETS, 50 mg (round, dark orange, coated)	
	100s	1720
	Accu-Pak®	
	100s	1721
135	TABLETS, 75 mg (oval, white, coated)	
	100s	1730
	Accu-Pak®	
	100s	1732
	Metandren®	
	methyltestosterone USP	
30	TABLETS, 10 mg (white, scored)	
	100s	1414
32	TABLETS, 25 mg (pale yellow, scored)	
	100s	1418
51	LINGUETS®, 5 mg (white)	
	100s	1432
64	LINGUETS®, 10 mg (yellow)	
	100s	1438
	Metopirone®	
	metyrapone USP	
130	TABLETS, 250 mg (white, scored)	
	18s	5403
	Rimactane®	
	rifampin USP	
154	CAPSULES, 300 mg (opaque scarlet and caramel)	
	30s	8903
	60s	8904
	100s	8901
	Rimactane®/INH Dual Pack	
	rifampin USP & isoniazid USP	
8912	Each Dual Pack contains two Rimactane 300-mg CAPSULES and one INH 300-mg TABLET	8912
	Ritalin® hydrochloride Ⓒ II	
	methylphenidate hydrochloride USP	
07	TABLETS, 5 mg (yellow)	
	100s	7410
	500s	7412
	1000s	7414
03	TABLETS, 10 mg (pale green, scored)	
	100s	7416
	500s	7418
	1000s	7420
	Accu-Pak® 100s	7415
34	TABLETS, 20 mg (pale yellow, scored)	
	100s	7422
	1000s	7426
	Ritalin-SR® Ⓒ II	
	methylphenidate hydrochloride sustained-release tablets	
16	TABLETS, 20 mg (round, white, scored)	
	100s	7442
	Ser-Ap-Es®	
71	TABLETS (light salmon pink, dry-coated), each containing 0.1 mg reserpine, 25 mg hydralazine hydrochloride and 15 mg hydrochlorothiazide	
	100s	6610
	1000s	6612
	Accu-Pak® 100s	6605
	Consumer Pack	
	100s	6617
	Serpasil®	
	reserpine USP	
35	TABLETS, 0.1 mg (white)	
	100s	7610
	1000s	7614
36	TABLETS, 0.25 mg (white, scored)	
	100s	7616
	500s	7618
	1000s	7620
	Consumer Pack	
	100s	7607
	Serpasil®-Apresoline®	
	reserpine and hydralazine hydrochloride	
40	TABLETS #1 (yellow, dry-coated), each containing 0.1 mg reserpine and 25 mg hydralazine hydrochloride	
	100s	7721
104	TABLETS #2 (yellow, dry-coated), each containing 0.2 mg reserpine and 50 mg hydralazine hydrochloride	
	100s	7709
	Serpasil®-Esidrix®	
	reserpine and hydrochlorothiazide	
13	TABLETS #1 (light orange), each containing 0.1 mg reserpine and 25 mg hydrochlorothiazide	
	100s	7010
	1000s	7012
97	TABLETS #2 (light orange), each containing 0.1 mg reserpine and 50 mg hydrochlorothiazide	
	100s	7020
	1000s	7022
	Slow-K®	
	potassium chloride USP	
165	TABLETS (pale orange, sugar-coated), each containing 8 mEq (600 mg) potassium chloride	
	100s	2807
	1000s	2811
	Accu-Pak®	
	100s	2817
	Consumer Pack	
	100s	2815
	[See table left].	
	Transderm Scōp®	
4345	Package of 3 cartons (4 discs per carton)	5921

Transderm-Nitro®
nitroglycerin

Code	Transderm-Nitro System Rated Release *in vivo*	Total Nitroglycerin in System	System Size	List No.	Carton Size
2025	2.5 mg/24 hr	12.5 mg	5 cm^2	2901	30 Systems
				2921	*100 Systems
2105	5 mg/24 hr	25 mg	10 cm^2	2903	30 Systems
				2923	*100 Systems
2110	10 mg/24 hr	50 mg	20 cm^2	2902	30 Systems
				2922	*100 Systems
2115	15 mg/24 hr	75 mg	30 cm^2	2904	30 Systems
				2924	*100 Systems

*Hospital Pack 100's

CIBA Code #	NUMERICAL LISTING
	Ritalin® hydrochloride Ⓒ II
	methylphenidate hydrochloride USP
03	TABLETS, 10 mg (pale green, scored)
07	TABLETS, 5 mg (yellow)
	Serpasil®-Esidrix®
	reserpine and hydrochlorothiazide
13	TABLETS #1 (light orange), each containing 0.1 mg reserpine and 25 mg hydrochlorothiazide

Antrenyl® bromide
oxyphenonium bromide
15 TABLETS, 5 mg (white, scored)
Ritalin-SR® Ⓒ
methylphenidate hydrochloride sustained-release tablets
16 TABLETS, 20 mg (round, white, scored)
Esidrix®
hydrochlorothiazide USP
22 TABLETS, 25 mg (pink, scored)
Cytadren®
aminoglutethamide
24 TABLETS, 250 mg (white, round, scored into quarters)
Ludiomil®
maprotiline hydrochloride USP
26 TABLETS, 50 mg (round, dark orange, coated)
Metandren®
methyltestosterone USP
30 TABLETS, 10 mg (white, scored)
Metandren®
methyltestosterone USP
32 TABLETS, 25 mg (pale yellow, scored)
Ritalin® hydrochloride Ⓒ
methylphenidate hydrochloride USP
34 TABLETS, 20 mg (pale yellow, scored)
Serpasil®
reserpine USP
35 TABLETS, 0.1 mg (white)
36 TABLETS, 0.25 mg (white, scored)
Apresoline® hydrochloride
hydralazine hydrochloride USP
37 TABLETS, 10 mg (pale yellow, dry- coated)
39 TABLETS, 25 mg (deep blue, dry- coated)
Serpasil®-Apresoline®
reserpine and hydralazine hydrochloride
40 TABLETS #1 (yellow, dry-coated), each containing 0.1 mg reserpine and 25 mg hydralazine hydrochloride
Anturane®
sulfinpyrazone USP
41 TABLETS (white, single-scored) each containing 100 mg sulfinpyrazone USP
Esidrix®
hydrochlorothiazide USP
46 TABLETS, 50 mg (yellow, scored)
Esimil®
47 TABLETS (white, scored), each containing 10 mg guanethidine monosulfate and 25 mg hydrochlorothiazide
Ismelin® sulfate
guanethidine monosulfate
49 TABLETS, 10 mg (pale yellow, scored)
Metandren®
methyltestosterone USP
51 LINGUETS®, 5 mg (white)
Metandren®
methyltestosterone USP
64 LINGUETS®, 10 mg (yellow)
Lithobid®
lithium carbonate
65 TABLETS, 300 mg (peach colored)
Ser-Ap-Es®
71 TABLETS (light salmon pink, dry- coated), each containing 0.1 mg reserpine, 25 mg hydralazine hydrochloride and 15 mg hydrochlorothiazide
Apresoline® hydrochloride
hydralazine hydrochloride USP
73 TABLETS, 50 mg (light blue, dry- coated)
Serpasil®-Esidrix®
reserpine and hydrochlorothiazide
97 TABLETS #2 (light orange), each containing 0.1 mg reserpine and 50 mg hydrochlorothiazide
Apresoline® hydrochloride
hydralazine hydrochloride USP
101 TABLETS, 100 mg (peach, dry- coated)
Ismelin® sulfate
guanethidine monosulfate
103 TABLETS, 25 mg (white, scored)
Serpasil®-Apresoline®
reserpine and hydralazine hydrochloride
104 TABLETS #2 (yellow, dry-coated), each containing 0.2 mg reserpine and 50 mg hydralazine hydrochloride
Ludiomil®
maprotiline hydrochloride USP
110 TABLETS, 25 mg (oval, dark orange coated)
Apresoline®-Esidrix®
hydralazine hydrochloride and hydrochlorothiazide
129 TABLETS (orange, dry-coated), each containing 25 mg hydralazine hydrochloride and 15 mg hydrochlorothiazide
Metopirone®
metyrapone USP
130 TABLETS, 250 mg (white, scored)
Ludiomil®
maprotiline hydrochloride USP
135 TABLETS, 75 mg (oval, white, coated)
Apresazide®
hydralazine HCl and hydrochlorothiazide
139 CAPSULES 25/25 (light blue and white opaque), each containing 25 mg hydralazine hydrochloride and 25 mg hydrochlorothiazide
149 CAPSULES 50/50 (pink and white opaque), each containing 50 mg hydralazine hydrochloride and 50 mg hydrochlorothiazide
Rimactane®
rifampin USP
154 CAPSULES, 300 mg (opaque scarlet and caramel)
Rimactane®/INH® Dual Pack
rifampin USP & isoniazid USP
8912 Each Dual Pack contains two Rimactane 300-mg CAPSULES and one INH 300-mg TABLET
Apresazide®
hydralazine HCl and hydrochlorothiazide
159 CAPSULES 100/50 (pink flesh and white opaque), each containing 100 mg hydralazine hydrochloride and 50 mg hydrochlorothiazide
Slow-K®
potassium chloride USP
165 TABLETS (buff colored, sugar- coated), each containing 8 mEq (600 mg) potassium chloride
Anturane®
sulfinpyrazone USP
168 CAPSULES (green) each containing 200 mg sulfinpyrazone USP
Esidrix®
hydrochlorothiazide USP
192 TABLETS, 100 mg (blue, scored)
Transderm-Nitro®
nitroglycerin

2025	2.5 mg	30 systems
		*100 systems
2105	5 mg	30 systems
		*100 systems
2110	10 mg	30 systems
		*100 systems
2115	15 mg	30 systems
		*100 systems

*Hospital Pack 100's

Transderm Scōp®
4345 Package of 3 cartons
(4 discs per carton)

ANTRENYL® bromide ℞

[*ann 'tre-nill*]
oxyphenonium bromide

DESCRIPTION

Antrenyl, a synthetic anticholinergic, is diethyl (2-hydroxyethyl) methylammonium *a*-phenylcyclohexane-glycolate bromide.

ACTIONS

The antisecretory and antispasmodic effects of Antrenyl result from antimuscarinic and ganglionic blocking activity. Recommended doses produce an inhibitory effect on gastric secretion and gastrointestinal motility through the antimuscarinic action and by blocking the stimulating effect of acetylcholine at parasympathetic nerve endings. CNS activity is generally lacking.

INDICATIONS

Peptic Ulcer, as adjunctive therapy.

CONTRAINDICATIONS

Glaucoma; obstructive uropathy (for example, bladder neck obstruction due to prostatic hypertrophy); obstructive disease of the gastrointestinal tract (as in achalasia, paralytic ileus, pyloroduodenal stenosis, etc.); intestinal atony of the elderly or debilitated patient; unstable cardiovascular status in acute hemorrhage; severe ulcerative colitis; toxic megacolon complicating ulcerative colitis; myasthenia gravis; hypersensitivity.

WARNINGS

In the presence of a high environmental temperature, heat prostration can occur with drug use (fever and heat stroke due to decreased sweating).

Diarrhea may be an early symptom of incomplete intestinal obstruction, especially in patients with ileostomy or colostomy. In this instance, treatment with Antrenyl would be inappropriate and possibly harmful.

Anticholinergics may produce drowsiness or blurred vision. Therefore, patients should be warned not to engage in activities requiring mental alertness (such as operating a motor vehicle or other machinery) or perform hazardous work while taking Antrenyl.

Usage in Pregnancy

The safe use of this drug in pregnant women or during lactation has not been established. Therefore, the benefits must be weighed against the potential hazards.

PRECAUTIONS

Give cautiously to patients with autonomic neuropathy; hepatic or renal disease; early evidence of ileus (as in peritonitis); ulcerative colitis (large doses may suppress intestinal motility to the point of producing a paralytic ileus and the use of anticholinergics may precipitate or aggravate the serious complication of toxic megacolon); hyperthyroidism; coronary heart disease; congestive heart failure; cardiac arrhythmias; hypertension; nonobstructing prostatic hypertrophy; hiatal hernia associated with reflux esophagitis, since anticholinergic drugs may aggravate this condition.

It should be noted that the use of anticholinergic drugs in the treatment of gastric ulcer may produce a delay in gastric emptying time and may complicate such therapy (antral stasis). Do not rely on the use of Antrenyl in the presence of biliary tract disease. Investigate any tachycardia before giving anticholinergic (atropine-like) drugs, since they may increase the heart rate.

With overdosage, a curare-like action may occur.

Use cautiously in debilitated patients with chronic lung disease, because reduction in bronchial secretions can lead to inspissation and formation of bronchial plugs. All anticholinergic agents should be used with caution in patients over 40 years of age because of the increased incidence of glaucoma in this age group.

ADVERSE REACTIONS

Anticholinergics produce certain effects which may be physiologic or toxic, depending upon the individual patient's response. The physician must delineate these.

Adverse reactions may include xerostomia; urinary hesitancy and retention; blurred vision; tachycardia; palpitations; mydriasis; dilatation of the pupil; cycloplegia; increased ocular tension; loss of taste; headaches; nervousness; drowsiness; weakness; dizziness; insomnia; nausea; vomiting; impotence; suppression of lactation; constipation; bloated feeling; severe allergic reaction or drug idiosyncrasies, including anaphylaxis, urticaria, and other dermal manifestation; some degree of mental confusion and/or excitement, especially in elderly persons.

Decreased sweating is another adverse reaction that may occur. It should be noted that adrenergic innervation of the eccrine sweat glands on the palms and soles make complete control of sweating impossible. An end point of complete anhidrosis cannot occur because large doses of drug would be required, and this would produce severe side effects from parasympathetic paralysis.

DOSAGE AND ADMINISTRATION

Average adult dosage is 10 mg (2 tablets) 4 times daily for several days. Dosage may then be reduced, depending on patient's response.

Not for use in children.

OVERDOSAGE

Treatment is the same as for atropine overdosage. Gastric lavage or, in the absence of coma, an emetic should be given, and activated charcoal slurry instilled into the stomach. If central nervous system excitation occurs, a short-acting barbiturate may be used. Avoid long-acting sedatives; the central depressive action of these agents may coincide with depression produced by oxyphenonium in later stages. Fever may be combated with ice bags, alcohol sponges, and other appropriate measures.

HOW SUPPLIED

Tablets, 5 mg (white, scored); bottles of 100.

C77-16 (3/77)

Shown in Product Identification Section, page 407

ANTURANE® ℞

[*ann 'too-rain*]
sulfinpyrazone USP
Tablets Capsules

DESCRIPTION

Anturane, sulfinpyrazone USP, is a uricosuric agent available as 100-mg tablets and 200-mg capsules for oral administration. Its chemical name is 1,2-diphenyl-4-[2-(phenylsulfinyl)ethyl]-3,5-pyrazolidinedione.

Sulfinpyrazone USP is a white to off-white powder practically insoluble in water and in solvent hexane, soluble in

Continued on next page

The full prescribing information for each CIBA drug is contained herein and is that in effect as of September 1, 1986

CIBA—Cont.

alcohol and in acetone, and sparingly soluble in dilute alkali. Its molecular weight is 404.48.

Inactive Ingredients. Anturane tablets: Colloidal silicon dioxide, gelatin, lactose, magnesium stearate, starch, stearic acid, and talc.

Anturane capsules: D&C Red No. 33, D&C Yellow No. 10, FD&C Blue No. 1, gelatin, lactose, magnesium stearate, silicon dioxide, sodium bisulfite, sodium lauryl sulfate, starch, stearic acid, talc, and titanium dioxide.

CLINICAL PHARMACOLOGY

Its pharmacologic activity is the potentiation of the urinary excretion of uric acid. It is useful for reducing the blood urate levels in patients with chronic tophaceous gout and acute intermittent gout, and for promoting the resorption of tophi.

INDICATIONS

Anturane is indicated for the treatment of:

1. Chronic gouty arthritis
2. Intermittent gouty arthritis

CONTRAINDICATIONS

Patients with an active peptic ulcer or symptoms of gastrointestinal inflammation or ulceration should not receive the drug.

The drug is contraindicated in patients with a history or the presence of:

1. Hypersensitivity to phenylbutazone or other pyrazoles
2. Blood dyscrasias

WARNINGS

Studies on the teratogenicity of pyrazole compounds in animals have yielded inconclusive results. Up to the present time, however, there have been no reported cases of human congenital malformation proved to be due to the use of the drug.

It is suggested that Anturane be used with caution in pregnant women, weighing the potential risks against the possible benefits.

PRECAUTIONS

As with all pyrazole compounds, patients receiving Anturane should be kept under close medical supervision and periodic blood counts are recommended. It may be administered with care to patients with a history of healed peptic ulcer.

Recent reports have indicated that Anturane potentiates the action of certain sulfonamides, such as sulfadiazine and sulfisoxazole. In addition, other pyrazole compounds (phenylbutazone) have been observed to potentiate the hypoglycemic sulfonylurea agents, as well as insulin. In view of these observations, it is suggested that Anturane be used with caution in conjunction with sulfa drugs, the sulfonylurea hypoglycemic agents and insulin.

Because Anturane is a potent uricosuric agent, it may precipitate urolithiasis and renal colic, especially in the initial stages of therapy. For this reason, an adequate fluid intake and alkalinization of the urine are recommended. In cases with significant renal impairment, periodic assessment of renal function is indicated. Occasional cases of renal failure have been reported; but a cause-and-effect relationship has not always been clearly established.

Salicylates antagonize the uricosuric action of Anturane and for this reason their concomitant use is contraindicated in gouty arthritis.

Anturane may accentuate the action of coumarin-type anticoagulants and further depress prothrombin activity when these medications are employed simultaneously.

NOTE

Anturane has minimal anti-inflammatory effect and is not intended for the relief of an acute attack of gout.

In the initial stages of therapy, because of the marked ability of Anturane to mobilize urates, acute attacks of gouty arthritis may be precipitated.

ADVERSE REACTIONS

The most frequently reported adverse reactions with Anturane have been upper gastrointestinal disturbances. In these patients it is advisable to administer the drug with food, milk, or antacids. Despite this precaution, Anturane may aggravate or reactivate peptic ulcer.

Rash has been reported. In most instances, this reaction did not necessitate discontinuance of therapy. In general, Anturane has not been observed to affect electrolyte balance.

Blood dyscrasias (anemia, leukopenia, agranulocytosis, thrombocytopenia and aplastic anemia) have rarely been reported. There has also been a published report associating Anturane, administered concomitantly with other drugs including colchicine, with leukemia following long-term treatment of patients with gout. However, the circumstances involved in the two cases reported are such that a cause-and-effect relationship to Anturane has not been clearly established.

OVERDOSAGE

Symptoms: Nausea, vomiting, diarrhea, epigastric pain, ataxia, labored respiration, convulsions, coma. Possible symptoms, seen after overdosage with other pyrazolone derivatives: anemia, jaundice, ulceration.

Treatment: No specific antidote. Induce emesis; gastric lavage; supportive treatment (intravenous glucose infusions, analeptics).

DOSAGE AND ADMINISTRATION

Initial: 200–400 mg daily in two divided doses, with meals or milk, gradually increasing when necessary to full maintenance dosage in one week.

Maintenance:

400 mg daily, given in two divided doses, as above. This dosage may be increased to 800 mg daily, if necessary, and may sometimes be reduced to as low as 200 mg daily after the blood urate level has been controlled. Treatment should be continued without interruption even in the presence of acute exacerbations, which can be concomitantly treated with phenylbutazone or colchicine. Patients previously controlled with other uricosuric therapy may be transferred to Anturane at full maintenance dosage.

HOW SUPPLIED

Tablets 100 mg—round, white, scored (imprinted CIBA 41)
Bottles of 100 ....NDC 0083-0041-30

Capsules 200 mg—green (imprinted Anturane 200 CIBA 168)
Bottles of 100 ....NDC 0083-0168-30

Dispense in tight container (USP).

C85-50 (Rev. 11/85)

Shown in Product Identification Section, page 407

APRESAZIDE® ℞

[*a-press 'a-zyde*]

hydralazine hydrochloride and hydrochlorothiazide Capsules

> **WARNING**
>
> This fixed-combination drug is not indicated for initial therapy of hypertension. Hypertension requires therapy titrated to the individual patient. If the fixed combination represents the dosage so determined, its use may be more convenient in patient management. The treatment of hypertension is not static but must be reevaluated as conditions in each patient warrant.

DESCRIPTION

Apresazide, hydralazine hydrochloride and hydrochlorothiazide, is an antihypertensive-diuretic combination available as capsules for oral administration. Apresazide capsules of 25/25 contain 25 mg of hydralazine hydrochloride USP and 25 mg of hydrochlorothiazide USP; capsules of 50/50 contain 50 mg of hydralazine hydrochloride USP and 50 mg of hydrochlorothiazide USP; and capsules of 100/50 contain 100 mg of hydralazine hydrochloride USP and 50 mg of hydrochlorothiazide USP.

Hydralazine hydrochloride is 1-hydrazinophthalazine monohydrochloride.

Hydralazine hydrochloride USP is a white to off-white, odorless crystalline powder. It is soluble in water, slightly soluble in alcohol, and very slightly soluble in ether. It melts at about 275°C, with decomposition, and has a molecular weight of 196.64.

Hydrochlorothiazide is 6-chloro-3,4-dihydro-2*H*-1,2,4-benzothiadiazine-7-sulfonamide 1,1-dioxide.

Hydrochlorothiazide USP is a white, or practically white, practically odorless crystalline powder. It is freely soluble in sodium hydroxide solution, in *n*-butylamine, and in dimethylformamide; sparingly soluble in methanol; slightly soluble in water; and insoluble in ether, in chloroform, and in dilute mineral acids. Its molecular weight is 297.73.

Inactive Ingredients: D&C Red No. 33 and D&C Yellow No. 10 (100/50 capsules only); FD&C Blue No. 1 and FD&C Red No. 3 (25/25 and 50/50 capsules only); gelatin; magnesium stearate; silicon dioxide; sodium bisulfite; sodium lauryl sulfate; starch; and titanium dioxide.

CLINICAL PHARMACOLOGY

Hydralazine

Although the precise mechanism of action of hydralazine is not fully understood, the major effects are on the cardiovascular system. Hydralazine apparently lowers blood pressure by exerting a peripheral vasodilating effect through a direct relaxation of vascular smooth muscle. Hydralazine, by altering cellular calcium metabolism, interferes with the calcium movements within the vascular smooth muscle that are responsible for initiating or maintaining the contractile state.

The peripheral vasodilating effect of hydralazine results in decreased arterial blood pressure (diastolic more than systolic); decreased peripheral vascular resistance; and an increased heart rate, stroke volume, and cardiac output. The preferential dilatation of arterioles, as compared to veins, minimizes postural hypotension and promotes the increase in cardiac output. Hydralazine usually increases renin activity in plasma, presumably as a result of increased secretion of renin by the renal juxtaglomerular cells in response to reflex sympathetic discharge. This increase in renin activity leads to the production of angiotension II, which then causes stimulation of aldosterone and consequent sodium reabsorption. Hydralazine also maintains or increases renal and cerebral blood flow.

Hydrochlorothiazide

Thiazides affect the renal tubular mechanism of electrolyte reabsorption. At maximal therapeutic dosage, all thiazides are approximately equal in their diuretic potency. Thiazides increase excretion of sodium and chloride in approximately equivalent amounts. Natriuresis causes a secondary loss of potassium.

The mechanism of the antihypertensive effect of thiazides is unknown. Thiazides do not affect normal blood pressure.

Pharmacokinetics

Hydralazine. Hydralazine is rapidly absorbed after oral administration, and peak plasma levels are reached at 1–2 hours. Plasma levels decline with a half-life of 3–7 hours. Binding to human plasma protein is 87%. Plasma levels of hydralazine vary widely among individuals. Hydralazine is subject to polymorphic acetylation; slow acetylators generally have higher plasma levels of hydralazine and require lower doses to maintain control of blood pressure. Hydralazine undergoes extensive hepatic metabolism; it is excreted mainly in the form of metabolites in the urine.

Administration of hydralazine with food results in higher levels of the drug in plasma.

Hydrochlorothiazide. Onset of action of thiazides occurs in 2 hours and the peak effect at about 4 hours. The action persists for approximately 6–12 hours. Hydrochlorothiazide is rapidly absorbed, as indicated by peak concentrations 1–2.5 hours after oral administration. Plasma levels of the drug are proportional to dose; the concentration in whole blood is 1.6–1.8 times higher than in plasma. Thiazides are eliminated rapidly by the kidney. After oral administration of 25- to 100-mg doses, 72–97% of the dose is excreted in the urine, indicating dose-independent absorption. Hydrochlorothiazide is eliminated from plasma in a biphasic fashion with a terminal half-life of 10–17 hours. Plasma protein binding is 67.9%. Plasma clearance is 15.9–30.0 L/hr; volume of distribution is 3.6–7.8 L/kg.

Gastrointestinal absorption of hydrochlorothiazide is enhanced when administered with food. Absorption is decreased in patients with congestive heart failure, and the pharmacokinetics are considerably different in these patients.

INDICATIONS AND USAGE

Hypertension (see boxed **WARNING**).

CONTRAINDICATIONS

Hydralazine

Hypersensitivity to hydralazine; coronary artery disease; mitral valvular rheumatic heart disease.

Hydrochlorothiazide

Anuria; hypersensitivity to this or other sulfonamide-derived drugs.

WARNINGS

Hydralazine

In a few patients hydralazine may produce a clinical picture simulating systemic lupus erythematosus including glomerulonephritis. In such patients hydralazine should be discontinued unless the benefit-to-risk determination requires continued antihypertensive therapy with this drug. Signs and symptoms usually regress when the drug is discontinued, but residua have been detected many years later. Long-term treatment with steroids may be necessary. (See **Precautions, Laboratory Tests.**)

Hydrochlorothiazide

Thiazides should be used with caution in patients with severe renal disease. In patients with renal disease, thiazides may precipitate azotemia. Cumulative effects of the drug may develop in patients with impaired renal function.

Thiazides should be used with caution in patients with impaired hepatic function or progressive liver disease, since minor alterations of fluid and electrolyte imbalance may precipitate hepatic coma.

Thiazides may add to or potentiate the action of other antihypertensive drugs. Potentiation occurs with ganglionic or peripheral adrenergic blocking drugs.

Sensitivity reactions are more likely to occur in patients with a history of allergy or bronchial asthma.

The possibility of exacerbation or activation of systemic lupus erythematosus has been reported.

PRECAUTIONS

General

Hydralazine. Myocardial stimulation produced by hydralazine can cause anginal attacks and ECG changes indicative of myocardial ischemia. The drug has been implicated in the production of myocardial infarction. It must, therefore, be used with caution in patients with suspected coronary artery disease.

The "hyperdynamic" circulation caused by hydralazine may accentuate specific cardiovascular inadequacies. For example, hydralazine may increase pulmonary artery pressure in patients with mitral valvular disease. The drug may reduce the pressor responses to epinephrine.

Postural hypotension may result from hydralazine but is less common than with ganglionic blocking agents. It should be used with caution in patients with cerebral vascular accidents.

In hypertensive patients with normal kidneys who are treated with hydralazine, there is evidence of increased renal blood flow and a maintenance of glomerular filtration rate. In some instances where control values were below normal, improved renal function has been noted after administration of hydralazine. However, as with any antihypertensive agent, hydralazine should be used with caution in patients with advanced renal damage.

Peripheral neuritis, evidenced by paresthesia, numbness, and tingling, has been observed. Published evidence suggests that hydralazine has an antipyridoxine effect and that pyridoxine should be added to the regimen if symptoms develop.

Hydrochlorothiazide. All patients receiving thiazide therapy should be observed for clinical signs of fluid or electrolyte imbalance, namely hyponatremia, hypochloremic alkalosis, and hypokalemia (see **Laboratory Tests** and **Drug/Drug Interactions**). Warning signs are dryness of mouth, thirst, weakness, lethargy, drowsiness, restlessness, muscle pains or cramps, muscular fatigue, hypotension, oliguria, tachycardia, and gastrointestinal disturbance, such as nausea or vomiting.

Hypokalemia may develop, especially in cases of brisk diuresis or severe cirrhosis.

Interference with adequate oral intake of electrolytes will also contribute to hypokalemia. Hypokalemia may be avoided or treated by the use of potassium supplements or foods with a high potassium content.

Any chloride deficit is generally mild and usually does not require specific treatment, except under extraordinary circumstances (as in liver disease or renal disease). Dilutional hyponatremia may occur in edematous patients in hot weather; appropriate therapy is water restriction, rather than administration of salt, except in rare instances when the hyponatremia is life-threatening. In cases of actual salt depletion, appropriate replacement is the therapy of choice.

Hyperuricemia may occur or frank gout may be precipitated in certain patients receiving thiazide therapy.

Latent diabetes may become manifest during thiazide administration (see **Drug/Drug Interactions**).

The antihypertensive effects of the drug may be enhanced in the postsympathectomy patient.

If progressive renal impairment becomes evident, withholding or discontinuing diuretic therapy should be considered.

Calcium excretion is decreased by thiazides. Pathological changes in the parathyroid gland with hypercalcemia and hypophosphatemia have been observed in a few patients on prolonged thiazide therapy. The common complications of hyperparathyroidism, such as renal lithiasis, bone resorption, and peptic ulceration, have not been seen.

Information for Patients

Patients should be informed of possible side effects and advised to take the medication regularly and continuously as directed.

Laboratory Tests

Hydralazine. Complete blood counts and antinuclear antibody titer determinations are indicated before and periodically during prolonged therapy with hydralazine even though the patient is asymptomatic. These studies are also indicated if the patient develops arthralgia, fever, chest pain, continued malaise, or other unexplained signs or symptoms. A positive antinuclear antibody titer requires that the physician carefully weigh the implications of the test results against the benefits to be derived from antihypertensive therapy with a combination drug containing hydralazine.

Blood dyscrasias, consisting of reduction in hemoglobin and red cell count, leukopenia, agranulocytosis, and purpura, have been reported. If such abnormalities develop, therapy should be discontinued.

Hydrochlorothiazide. Initial and periodic determinations of serum electrolytes to detect possible electrolyte imbalance should be performed at appropriate intervals.

Serum and urine electrolyte determinations are particularly important when the patient is vomiting excessively or receiving parenteral fluids.

Drug/Drug Interactions

Hydralazine. MAO inhibitors should be used with caution in patients receiving hydralazine.

When other potent parenteral antihypertensive drugs, such as diazoxide, are used in combination with hydralazine, patients should be continously observed for several hours for any excessive fall in blood pressure. Profound hypotensive episodes may occur when diazoxide injections and hydralazine are used concomitantly.

Hydrochlorothiazide. Hypokalemia can sensitize or exaggerate the response of the heart to the toxic effects of digitalis (e.g., increased ventricular irritability).

Hypokalemia may develop during concomitant use of steroids or ACTH.

Insulin requirements in diabetic patients may be increased, decreased, or unchanged.

Thiazides may decrease arterial responsiveness to norepinephrine, but not enough to preclude effectiveness of the pressor agent for therapeutic use.

Thiazides may increase the responsiveness to tubocurarine.

Lithium renal clearance is reduced by thiazides, increasing the risk of lithium toxicity.

Drug/Laboratory Test Interactions

Thiazides may decrease serum levels of protein-bound iodine without signs of thyroid disturbance. Apresazide should be discontinued before tests for parathyroid function are made (See **General, *Hydrochlorothiazide,*** Calcium excretion).

Carcinogenesis, Mutagenesis, Impairment of Fertility

Hydralazine. In a lifetime study in Swiss albino mice, there was a statistically significant increase in the incidence of lung tumors (adenomas and adenocarcinomas) of both male and female mice given hydralazine continuously in their drinking water at a dosage of about 250 mg/kg per day (about 80 times the maximum recommended human dose). In a 2-year carcinogenicity study of rats given hydralazine by gavage at dosages of 15, 30, and 60 mg/kg per day (approximately 5 to 20 times the recommended human daily dose), microscopic examination of the liver revealed a small, but statistically significant, increase in benign neoplastic nodules in male and female rats from the high-dose group and in female rats from the intermediate-dose group. Benign interstitial cell tumors of the testes were also significantly increased in male rats from the high-dose group. The tumors observed are common in aged rats, and a significantly increased incidence was not observed until 18 months of treatment. Hydralazine was shown to be mutagenic in three bacterial tester strains in the Ames test, both with and without metabolic activation, and elicited DNA repair both in the Pol A^+/A^- *E. coli* bacterial assay system and in cultured rat hepatocytes. (Evidence of DNA damage in the hepatocyte repair test is considered a strong indication of covalent binding, an established property of carcinogens and mutagens.) In tests with rabbit hepatocytes that exhibit an acetylator polymorphism like that of humans,hydralazine elicited DNA repair with only those hepatocytes having a slow rate of acetylation, suggesting that individuals who are rapid acetylators may have a diminished genotoxic liability. No increase in mutagenic potential was revealed in the mouse lymphoma assay, host-mediated assay, nucleus anomaly test, or dominant lethal test.

The extent to which these findings indicate a risk to man is uncertain. While long-term clinical observation has not suggested that human cancer is associated with hydralazine use, epidemiologic studies have so far been insufficient to arrive at any conclusions.

Hydrochlorothiazide. Long-term carcinogenicity studies in animals have not been conducted with hydrochlorothiazide.

Pregnancy Category C

Animal reproduction studies have not been conducted with Apresazide.

Animal studies indicate that hydralazine is teratogenic in mice at 20–30 times the maximum daily human dose of 200–300 mg and possibly in rabbits at 10–15 times the maximum daily human dose, but that it is nonteratogenic in rats. Teratogenic effects observed were cleft palate and malformations of facial and cranial bones. A reproduction study in rats receiving hydrochlorothiazide, 250 mg/kg daily, 62.5 times the maximum daily human dose, has revealed no evidence of impaired fertility or harm to the fetus.

There are no adequate and well-controlled studies of Apresazide in pregnant women. However, thiazides cross the placental barrier and appear in cord blood, and there is a risk of fetal or neonatal jaundice, thrombocytopenia, and possibly other adverse reactions that have occurred in adults. Apresazide should be used during pregnancy only if the potential benefit justifies the potential risk to the fetus.

Nursing Mothers

It is not known whether hydralazine is excreted in human milk. Thiazides are excreted in human milk. Because of the potential for serious adverse reactions in nursing infants, a decision should be made whether to discontinue nursing or to discontinue the drug, taking into account the importance of the drug to the mother.

Pediatric Use

Safety and effectiveness of the combination drug in children have not been established.

ADVERSE REACTIONS

Adverse reactions are usually reversible upon reduction of dosage or discontinuation of Apresazide. Whenever adverse reactions are moderate or severe, it may be necessary to discontinue the drug.

The following adverse reactions have been observed, but there has not been enough systematic collection of data to support an estimate of their frequency.

Hydralazine

Common

Headache, anorexia, nausea, vomiting, diarrhea, palpitations, tachycardia, angina pectoris.

Less Frequent

Digestive: Constipation, paralytic ileus.

Cardiovascular: Hypotension, paradoxical pressor response, edema.

Respiratory: Dyspnea.

Neurologic: Peripheral neuritis, evidenced by paresthesia, numbness, and tingling; dizziness; tremors; muscle cramps; psychotic reactions characterized by depression, disorientation, or anxiety.

Genitourinary: Difficulty in urination.

Hematologic: Blood dyscrasias, consisting of reduction in hemoglobin and red cell count, leukopenia, agranulocytosis, purpura; lymphadenopathy; splenomegaly.

Hypersensitive Reactions: Rash, urticaria, pruritus, fever, chills, arthralgia, eosinophilia, and, rarely, hepatitis.

Other: Nasal congestion, flushing, lacrimation, conjunctivitis.

Hydrochlorothiazide

Digestive: Anorexia, gastric irritation, nausea, vomiting, cramping, diarrhea, constipation, jaundice (intrahepatic cholestatic), pancreatitis, sialadenitis.

Cardiovascular: Orthostatic hypotension (may be potentiated by alcohol, barbiturates, or narcotics).

Neurologic: Dizziness, vertigo, paresthesia, headache, xanthopsia.

Hematologic: Leukopenia, agranulocytosis, thrombocytopenia, aplastic anemia.

Hypersensitive Reactions: Purpura, photosensitivity, rash, urticaria, necrotizing angiitis, Stevens-Johnson syndrome.

Other: Hyperglycemia, glycosuria, hyperuricemia, muscle spasm, weakness, restlessness, transient blurred vision.

OVERDOSAGE

Acute Toxicity

Oral LD_{50}'s in rats (mg/kg): hydralazine, 173 and 187; hydrochlorothiazide, 2750.

Signs and Symptoms

Hydralazine. Signs and symptoms of overdosage include hypotension, tachycardia, headache, and generalized skin flushing.

Complications can include myocardial ischemia and subsequent myocardial infarction, cardiac arrhythmia, and profound shock.

Hydrochlorothiazide. The most prominent feature of poisoning is acute loss of fluid and electrolytes.

Cardiovascular: Tachycardia, hypotension, shock.

Neuromuscular: Weakness, confusion, dizziness, cramps of the calf muscles, paresthesia, fatigue, impairment of consciousness.

Digestive: Nausea, vomiting, thirst.

Renal: Polyuria, oliguria, or anuria (due to hemoconcentration).

Laboratory Findings: Hypokalemia, hyponatremia, hypochloremia, alkalosis: increased BUN (especially in patients with renal insufficiency).

Combined Poisoning: Signs and symptoms may be aggravated or modified by concomitant intake of antihypertensive medication, barbiturates, curare, digitalis (hypokalemia), corticosteroids, narcotics, or alcohol.

Treatment

There is no specific antidote.

The gastric contents should be evacuated, taking adequate precautions against aspiration and for protection of the airway. An activated charcoal slurry may be instilled if conditions permit. Dialysis may not be effective for elimination of Apresazide because of its plasma protein binding (see **Clinical Pharmacology**).

These manipulations may have to be omitted or carried out after cardiovascular status has been stabilized, since they might precipitate cardiac arrhythmias or increase the depth of shock.

Support of the cardiovascular system is of primary importance in suspected hydralazine overdosage. Shock should be treated with plasma expanders. The patient's legs should be kept raised and lost fluid and electrolytes (potassium, sodium) should be replaced. If possible, vasopressors should not be given, but if a vasopressor is required, care should be taken not to precipitate or aggravate cardiac arrhythmia. Tachycardia responds to beta blockers. Digitalization may be necessary, and renal function should be monitored and supported as required.

DOSAGE AND ADMINISTRATION

Dosage should be determined by individual titration (see boxed **WARNING**).

Continued on next page

The full prescribing information for each CIBA drug is contained herein and is that in effect as of September 1, 1986

CIBA—Cont.

The usual dosage is one Apresazide capsule twice daily, the strength depending upon individual requirement following titration. For maintenance, the dosage should be adjusted to the lowest effective level.
When necessary, other antihypertensive agents such as sympathetic inhibitors may be added gradually in reduced dosages, and the effects should be watched carefully.

HOW SUPPLIED

Capsules 25/25—light blue and white opaque (imprinted APRESAZIDE® 25/25 CIBA 139)
25 mg of hydralazine hydrochloride and 25 mg of hydrochlorothiazide
Bottles of 100 .... NDC 0083-0139-30
Capsules 50/50—pink and white opaque (imprinted APRESAZIDE® 50/50 CIBA 149)
50 mg of hydralazine hydrochloride and 50 mg of hydrochlorothiazide
Bottles of 100 .... NDC 0083-0149-30
Capsules 100/50—flesh pink and white opaque (imprinted APRESAZIDE® 100/50 CIBA 159)
100 mg of hydralazine hydrochloride and 50 mg of hydrochlorothiazide
Bottles of 100 .... NDC 0083-0159-30
Do not store above 86°F.
Dispense in tight, light-resistant container (USP).
C85-23 (Rev. 8/85)
Shown in Product Identification Section, page 407

APRESOLINE® hydrochloride ℞

[*a-press 'oh-leen*]
hydralazine hydrochloride USP
Tablets

DESCRIPTION

Apresoline, hydralazine hydrochloride USP, is an antihypertensive, available as 10-, 25-, 50-, and 100-mg tablets for oral administration. Its chemical name is 1-hydrazinophthalazine monohydrochloride.
Hydralazine hydrochloride USP is a white to off-white, odorless crystalline powder. It is soluble in water, slightly soluble in alcohol, and very slightly soluble in ether. It melts at about 275°C, with decomposition, and has a molecular weight of 196.64. *Inactive Ingredients:* Acacia, D&C Yellow No. 10 (10-mg tablets), FD&C Blue No. 1 (25-mg and 50-mg tablets), FD&C Yellow No. 5 and FD&C Yellow No. 6 (100-mg tablets), lactose, magnesium stearate, mannitol, polyethylene glycol, sodium starch glycolate, starch and stearic acid.

CLINICAL PHARMACOLOGY

Although the precise mechanism of action of hydralazine is not fully understood, the major effects are on the cardiovascular system. Hydralazine apparently lowers blood pressure by exerting a peripheral vasodilating effect through a direct relaxation of vascular smooth muscle. Hydralazine, by altering cellular calcium metabolism, interferes with the calcium movements within the vascular smooth muscle that are responsible for initiating or maintaining the contractile state.
The peripheral vasodilating effect of hydralazine results in decreased arterial blood pressure (diastolic more than systolic); decreased peripheral vascular resistance; and an increased heart rate, stroke volume, and cardiac output. The preferential dilatation of arterioles, as compared to veins, minimizes postural hypotension and promotes the increase in cardiac output. Hydralazine usually increases renin activity in plasma, presumably as a result of increased secretion of renin by the renal juxtaglomerular cells in response to reflex sympathetic discharge. This increase in renin activity leads to the production of angiotensin II, which then causes stimulation of aldosterone and consequent sodium reabsorption. Hydralazine also maintains or increases renal and cerebral blood flow.
Hydralazine is rapidly absorbed after oral administration, and peak plasma levels are reached at 1–2 hours. Plasma levels of apparent hydralazine decline with a half-life of 3–7 hours. Binding to human plasma protein is 87%. Plasma levels of hydralazine vary widely among individuals. Hydralazine is subject to polymorphic acetylation; slow acetylators generally have higher plasma levels of hydralazine and require lower doses to maintain control of blood pressure. Hydralazine undergoes extensive hepatic metabolism; it is excreted mainly in the form of metabolites in the urine.

INDICATIONS AND USAGE

Essential hypertension, alone or as an adjunct.

CONTRAINDICATIONS

Hypersensitivity to hydralazine; coronary artery disease; mitral valvular rheumatic heart disease.

WARNINGS

In a few patients hydralazine may produce a clinical picture simulating systemic lupus erythematosus including glomerulonephritis. In such patients hydralazine should be discontinued unless the benefit-to-risk determination requires continued antihypertensive therapy with this drug. Symptoms and signs usually regress when the drug is discontinued but residua have been detected many years later. Long-term treatment with steroids may be necessary. (See **PRECAUTIONS, Laboratory Tests.**)

PRECAUTIONS

General: Myocardial stimulation produced by Apresoline can cause anginal attacks and ECG changes of myocardial ischemia. The drug has been implicated in the production of myocardial infarction. It must, therefore, be used with caution in patients with suspected coronary artery disease.
The "hyperdynamic" circulation caused by Apresoline may accentuate specific cardiovascular inadequacies. For example, Apresoline may increase pulmonary artery pressure in patients with mitral valvular disease. The drug may reduce the pressor responses to epinephrine. Postural hypotension may result from Apresoline but is less common than with ganglionic blocking agents. It should be used with caution in patients with cerebral vascular accidents.
In hypertensive patients wiith normal kidneys who are treated with Apresoline, there is evidence of increased renal blood flow and a maintenance of glomerular filtration rate. In some instances where control values were below normal, improved renal function has been noted after administration of Apresoline. However, as with any antihypertensive agent, Apresoline should be used with caution in patients with advanced renal damage.
Peripheral neuritis, evidenced by paresthesia, numbness, and tingling, has been observed. Published evidence suggests an antipyridoxine effect, and that pyridoxine should be added to the regimen if symptoms develop.
The Apresoline tablets (100 mg) contain FD&C Yellow No. 5 (tartrazine), which may cause allergic-type reactions (including bronchial asthma) in certain susceptible individuals. Although the overall incidence of FD&C Yellow No. 5 (tartrazine) sensitivity in the general population is low, it is frequently seen in patients who are also hypersensitive to aspirin.
Information for Patients: Patients should be informed of possible side effects and advised to take the medication regularly and continuously as directed.
Laboratory Tests: Complete blood counts and antinuclear antibody titer determinations are indicated before and periodically during prolonged therapy with hydralazine even though the patient is asymptomatic. These studies are also indicated if the patient develops arthralgia, fever, chest pain, continued malaise, or other unexplained signs or symptoms.
A positive antinuclear antibody titer requires that the physician carefully weigh the implications of the test results against the benefits to be derived from antihypertensive therapy with hydralazine.
Blood dyscrasias, consisting of reduction in hemoglobin and red cell count, leukopenia, agranulocytosis, and purpura, have been reported. If such abnormalities develop, therapy should be discontinued.
Drug/Drug Interactions: MAO inhibitors should be used with caution in patients receiving hydralazine.
When other potent parenteral antihypertensive drugs, such as diazoxide, are used in combination with hydralazine, patients should be continuously observed for several hours for any excessive fall in blood pressure. Profound hypotensive episodes may occur when diazoxide injection and Apresoline are used concomitantly.
Drug/Food Interactions: Administration of hydralazine with food results in higher plasma levels.
Carcinogensis, Mutagenesis, Impairment of Fertility: In a lifetime study in Swiss albino mice, there was a statistically significant increase in the incidence of lung tumors (adenomas and adenocarcinomas) of both male and female mice given hydralazine continuously in their drinking water at a dosage of about 250 mg/kg per day (about 80 times the maximum recommended human dose). In a 2-year carcinogenicity study of rats given hydralazine by gavage at dose levels of 15, 30, and 60 mg/kg/day (approximately 5 to 20 times the recommended human daily dosage), microscopic examination of the liver revealed a small, but statistically significant, increase in benign neoplastic nodules in male and female rats from the high-dose group and in female rats from the intermediate-dose group. Benign interstitial cell tumors of the testes were also significantly increased in male rats from the high-dose group. The tumors observed are common in aged rats and a significantly increased incidence was not observed until 18 months of treatment. Hydralazine was shown to be mutagenic in three bacterial tester strains in the Ames test, both with and without metabolic activation, and elicited DNA repair both in the Pol A^+/A^- *E. coli* bacterial assay system and in cultured rat hepatocytes. (Evidence of DNA damage in the hepatocyte repair test is considered a strong indication of covalent binding, an established property of carcinogens and mutagens.) In tests with rabbit hepatocytes that exhibit an acetylator polymorphism like that of humans, hydralazine elicited DNA repair with only those hepatocytes having a slow rate of acetylation, suggesting that individuals who are rapid acetylators may have a diminished genotoxic liability. No increase in mutagenic potential was revealed in the mouse lymphoma assay, host-mediated assay, nucleus anomaly test, or dominant lethal test.
The extent to which these findings indicate a risk to man is uncertain. While long-term clinical observation has not suggested that human cancer is associated with hydralazine use, epidemiologic studies have so far been insufficient to arrive at any conclusions.
Pregnancy Category C: Animal studies indicate that hydralazine is teratogenic in mice at 20–30 times the maximum daily human dose of 200–300 mg and possibly in rabbits at 10–15 times the maximum daily human dose, but that it is nonteratogenic in rats. Teratogenic effects observed were cleft palate and malformations of facial and cranial bones. There are no adequate and well-controlled studies in pregnant women. Although clinical experience does not include any positive evidence of adverse effects on the human fetus, hydralazine should be used during pregnancy only if the expected benefit justifies the potential risk to the fetus.
Nursing Mothers: It is not known whether this drug is excreted in human milk. Because many drugs are excreted in human milk, caution should be exercised when Apresoline is administered to a nursing woman.
Pediatric Use: Safety and effectiveness in children have not been established in controlled clinical trials, although there is experience with the use of Apresoline in children. The usual recommended oral starting dosage is 0.75 mg/kg of body weight daily in four divided doses. Dosage may be increased gradually over the next 3–4 weeks to a maximum of 7.5 mg/kg of 200 mg daily.

ADVERSE REACTIONS

Adverse reactions with Apresoline are usually reversible when dosage is reduced. However, in some cases it may be necessary to discontinue the drug.
The following adverse reactions have been observed, but there has not been enough systematic collection of data to support an estimate of their frequency.
Common: Headache, anorexia, nausea, vomiting, diarrhea, palpitations, tachycardia, angina pectoris.
Less Frequent: *Digestive:* constipation, paralytic ileus.
Cardiovascular: hypotension, paradoxical pressor response, edema.
Respiratory: dyspnea.
Neurologic: peripheral neuritis, evidenced by paresthesia, numbness, and tingling; dizziness; tremors; muscle cramps; psychotic reactions characterized by depression, disorientation, or anxiety.
Genitourinary: difficulty in urination.
Hematologic: blood dyscrasias, consisting of reduction in hemoglobin and red cell count, leukopenia, agranulocytosis, purpura; lymphadenopathy; splenomegaly.
Hypersensitive Reactions: rash, urticaria, pruritus, fever, chills, arthralgia, eosinophilia, and, rarely, hepatitis.
Other: nasal congestion, flushing, lacrimation, conjunctivitis.

OVERDOSAGE

Acute Toxicity: No deaths due to acute poisoning have been reported.
Highest known dose survived: adults, 10 g orally.
Oral LD_{50} in rats: 173 and 187 mg/kg.
Signs and Symptoms: Signs and symptoms of overdosage include hypotension, tachycardia, headache, and generalized skin flushing.
Complications can include myocardial ischemia and subsequent myocardial infarction, cardiac arrhythmia, and profound shock.
Treatment: There is no specific antidote.
The gastric contents should be evacuated, taking adequate precautions against aspiration and for protection of the airway. An activated charcoal slurry may be instilled if conditions permit. These manipulations may have to be omitted or carried out after cardiovascular status has been stabilized, since they might precipitate cardiac arrhythmias or increase the depth of shock.
Support of the cardiovascular system is of primary importance. Shock should be treated with plasma expanders. If possible, vasopressors should not be given, but if a vasopressor is required, care should be taken not to precipitate or aggravate cardiac arrhythmia. Tachycardia responds to beta blockers. Digitalization may be necessary, and renal function should be monitored and supported as required.
No experience has been reported with extracorporeal or peritoneal dialysis.

DOSAGE AND ADMINISTRATION

Initiate therapy in gradually increasing dosages; adjust according to individual response. Start with 10 mg four times daily for the first 2–4 days, increase to 25 mg four times daily for the balance of the first week. For the second and subsequent weeks, increase dosage to 50 mg four times daily. For maintenance, adjust dosage to the lowest effective levels.
The incidence of toxic reactions, particularly the L.E. cell syndrome, is high in the group of patients receiving large doses of Apresoline.

In a few resistant patients, up to 300 mg of Apresoline daily may be required for a significant antihypertensive effect. In such cases, a lower dosage of Apresoline combined with a thiazide and/or reserpine or a beta blocker may be considered. However, when combining therapy, individual titration is essential to ensure the lowest possible therapeutic dose of each drug.

HOW SUPPLIED

Tablets 10 mg—round, pale yellow, dry-coated (imprinted CIBA 37)
- Bottles of 100—NDC 0083-0037-30
- Bottles of 1000—NDC 0083-0037-40
- Consumer Pack—One Unit
- 12 bottles—100 tablets each—NDC 0083-0037-65

Tablets 25 mg—round, deep blue, dry-coated (imprinted CIBA 39)
- Bottles of 100—NDC 0083-0039-30
- Bottles of 500—NDC 0083-0039-35
- Bottles of 1000—NDC 0083-0039-40
- Consumer Pack—One Unit
- 12 bottles—100 tablets each—NDC 0083-0039-65
- Accu-Pak®—Unit Dose (blister pack)
- Box of 100 (strips of 10)—NDC 0083-0039-32

Tablets 50 mg—round, light blue, dry-coated (imprinted CIBA 73)
- Bottles of 100—NDC 0083-0073-30
- Bottles of 500—NDC 0083-0073-35
- Bottles of 1000—NDC 0083-0073-40
- Consumer Pack—One Unit
- 12 bottles—100 tablets each—NDC 0083-0073-65
- Accu-Pak®—Unit Dose (blister pack)
- Box of 100 (strips of 10)—NDC 0083-0073-32

Tablets 100 mg—round, peach, dry-coated (imprinted CIBA 101)
- Bottles of 100—NDC 0083-0101-30

Do not store above 86°F.
Dispense in tight, light-resistant container (USP).
C85-18 (Rev. 8/85)

Shown in Product Identification Section, page 407

APRESOLINE® hydrochloride ℞

[a-press 'oh-leen]
hydralazine hydrochloride USP
Parenteral

DESCRIPTION

Apresoline, hydralazine hydrochloride USP, is an antihypertensive available in 1-ml ampuls for intravenous and intramuscular administration. Each milliliter of the sterile, colorless solution contains hydralazine hydrochloride USP, 20 mg; methylparaben NF, 0.65 mg; propylparaben NF, 0.35 mg; propylene glycol USP, 103.6 mg. The pH of the solution is 3.4–4.0. Hydralazine hydrochloride is 1-hydrazinophthalazine monohydrochloride.
Hydralazine hydrochloride USP is a white to off-white, odorless crystalline powder. It is soluble in water, slightly soluble in alcohol, and very slightly soluble in ether. It melts at about 275°C, with decomposition, and has a molecular weight of 196.64.

CLINICAL PHARMACOLOGY

Although the precise mechanism of action of hydralazine is not fully understood, the major effects are on the cardiovascular system. Hydralazine apparently lowers blood pressure by exerting a peripheral vasodilating effect through a direct relaxation of vascular smooth muscle. Hydralazine, by altering cellular calcium metabolism, interferes with the calcium movements within the vascular smooth muscle that are responsible for initiating or maintaining the contractile state.
The peripheral vasodilating effect of hydralazine results in decreased arterial blood pressure (diastolic more than systolic); decreased peripheral vascular resistance; and an increased heart rate, stroke volume, and cardiac output. The preferential dilatation of arterioles, as compared to veins, minimizes postural hypotension and promotes the increase in cardiac output. Hydralazine usually increases renin activity in plasma, presumably as a result of increased secretion of renin by the renal juxtaglomerular cells in response to reflex sympathetic discharge. This increase in renin activity leads to the production of angiotensin II, which then causes stimulation of aldosterone and consequent sodium reabsorption. Hydralazine also maintains or increases renal and cerebral blood flow.
The average maximal decrease in blood pressure usually occurs 10–80 minutes after administration of parenteral Apresoline. No other pharamacokinetic data on parenteral Apresoline are available.

INDICATIONS AND USAGE

Severe essential hypertension when the drug cannot be given orally or when there is an urgent need to lower blood pressure.

CONTRAINDICATIONS

Hypersensitivity to hydralazine; coronary artery disease; mitral valvular rheumatic heart disease.

WARNINGS

In a few patients hydralazine may produce a clinical picture simulating systemic lupus erythematosus including glomerulonephritis. In such patients hydralazine should be discontinued unless the benefit-to-risk determination requires continued antihypertensive therapy with this drug. Symptoms and signs usually regress when the drug is discontinued but residua have been detected many years later. Long-term treatment with steroids may be necessary. (See **PRECAUTIONS, Laboratory Tests.**)

PRECAUTIONS

General: Myocardial stimulation produced by Apresoline can cause anginal attacks and ECG changes of myocardial ischemia. The drug has been implicated in the production of myocardial infarction. It must, therefore, be used with caution in patients with suspected coronary artery disease.
The "hyperdynamic" circulation caused by Apresoline may accentuate specific cardiovascular inadequacies. For example, Apresoline may increase pulmonary artery pressure in patients with mitral valvular disease. The drug may reduce the pressor responses to epinephrine. Postural hypotension may result from Apresoline but is less common than with ganglionic blocking agents. It should be used with caution in patients with cerebral vascular accidents.
In hypertensive patients with normal kidneys who are treated with Apresoline, there is evidence of increased renal blood flow and a maintenance of glomerular filtration rate. In some instances where control values were below normal, improved renal function has been noted after administration of Apresoline. However, as with any antihypertensive agent, Apresoline should be used with caution in patients with advanced renal damage.
Peripheral neuritis, evidenced by paresthesia, numbness, and tingling, has been observed. Published evidence suggests an antipyridoxine effect, and that pyridoxine should be added to the regimen if symptoms develop.
Laboratory Tests: Complete blood counts and antinuclear antibody titer determinations are indicated before and periodically during prolonged therapy with hydralazine even though the patient is asymptomatic. These studies are also indicated if the patient develops arthralgia, fever, chest pain, continued malaise, or other unexplained signs or symptoms.
A positive antinuclear antibody titer requires that the physician carefully weigh the implications of the test results against the benefits to be derived from antihypertensive therapy with hydralazine.
Blood dyscrasias, consisting of reduction in hemoglobin and red cell count, leukopenia, agranulocytosis, and purpura, have been reported. If such abnormalities develop, therapy should be discontinued.
Drug/Drug Interactions: MAO inhibitors should be used with caution in patients receiving hydralazine.
When other potent parenteral antihypertensive drugs, such as diazoxide, are used in combination with hydralazine, patients should be continuously observed for several hours for any excessive fall in blood pressure. Profound hypotensive episodes may occur when diazoxide injection and Apresoline are used concomitantly.
Carcinogenesis, Mutagenesis, Impairment of Fertility: In a lifetime study in Swiss albino mice, there was a statistically significant increase in the incidence of lung tumors (adenomas and adenocarcinomas) of both male and female mice given hydralazine continuously in their drinking water at a dosage of about 250 mg/kg per day (about 80 times the maximum recommended human dose). In a 2-year carcinogenicity study of rats given hydralazine by gavage at dose levels of 15, 30, and 60 mg/kg/day (approximately 5 to 20 times the recommended human daily dosage), microscopic examination of the liver revealed a small, but statistically significant, increase in benign neoplastic nodules in male and female rats from the high-dose group and in female rats from the intermediate-dose group. Benign interstitial cell tumors of the testes were also significantly increased in male rats from the high-dose group. The tumors observed are common in aged rats and a significantly increased incidence was not observed until 18 months of treatment. Hydralazine was shown to be mutagenic in three bacterial tester strains in the Ames test, both with and without metabolic activation, and elicited DNA repair both in the Pol A^+/A^- *E. coli* bacterial assay system and in cultured rat hepatocytes. (Evidence of DNA damage in the hepatocyte repair test is considered a strong indication of covalent binding, an established property of carcinogens and mutagens.) In tests with rabbit hepatocytes that exhibit an acetylator polymorphism like that of humans, hydralazine elicited DNA repair with only those hepatocytes having a slow rate of acetylation, suggesting that individuals who are rapid acetylators may have a diminished genotoxic liability. No increase in mutagenic potential was revealed in the mouse lymphoma assay, host-mediated assay, nucleus anomaly test, or dominant lethal test.
The extent to which these findings indicate a risk to man is uncertain. While long-term clinical observation has not suggested that human cancer is associated with hydralazine use, epidemiologic studies have so far been insufficient to arrive at any conclusions.
Pregnancy Category C: Animal studies indicate that hydralazine is teratogenic in mice at 20–30 times the maximum daily human dose of 200–300 mg and possibly in rabbits at 10–15 times the maximum daily human dose, but that it is nonteratogenic in rats. Teratogenic effects observed were cleft palate and malformations of facial and cranial bones. There are no adequate and well-controlled studies in pregnant women. Although clinical experience does not include any positive evidence of adverse effects on the human fetus, hydralazine should be used during pregnancy only if the expected benefit justifies the potential risk to the fetus.
Nursing Mothers: It is not known whether this drug is excreted in human milk. Because many drugs are excreted in human milk, caution should be exercised when Apresoline is administered to a nursing woman.
Pediatric Use: Safety and effectiveness in children have not been established in controlled clinical trials, although there is experience with the use of Apresoline in children. The usual recommended parenteral dosage, administered intramuscularly or intravenously, is 1.7–3.5 mg/kg of body weight daily, divided into four to six doses.

ADVERSE REACTIONS

Adverse reactions with Apresoline are usually reversible when dosage is reduced. However, in some cases it may be necessary to discontinue the drug.
The following adverse reactions have been observed, but there has not been enough systematic collection of data to support an estimate of their frequency.
Common: Headache, anorexia, nausea, vomiting, diarrhea, palpitations, tachycardia, angina pectoris.
Less Frequent: *Digestive:* constipation, paralytic ileus.
Cardiovascular: hypotension, paradoxical pressor response, edema.
Respiratory: dyspnea.
Neurologic: peripheral neuritis, evidenced by paresthesia, numbness, and tingling; dizziness; tremors; muscle cramps; psychotic reactions characterized by depression, disorientation, or anxiety.
Genitourinary: difficulty in urination.
Hematologic: blood dyscrasias, consisting of reduction in hemoglobin and red cell count, leukopenia, agranulocytosis, purpura; lymphadenopathy; splenomegaly.
Hypersensitive Reactions: rash, urticaria, pruritus, fever, chills, arthralgia, eosinophilia, and, rarely, hepatitis.
Other: nasal congestion, flushing, lacrimation, conjunctivitis.

OVERDOSAGE

Acute Toxicity: No deaths due to acute poisoning have been reported.
Highest known dose survived: adults, 10 g orally.
Oral LD_{50} in rats: 173 and 187 mg/kg.
Signs and Symptoms: Signs and symptoms of overdosage include hypotension, tachycardia, headache, and generalized skin flushing.
Complications can include myocardial ischemia and subsequent myocardial infarction, cardiac arrhythmia, and profound shock.
Treatment: There is no specific antidote.
Support of the cardiovascular system is of primary importance. Shock should be treated with plasma expanders. If possible, vasopressors should not be given, but if a vasopressor is required, care should be taken not to precipitate or aggravate cardiac arrhythmia. Tachycardia responds to beta blockers. Digitalization may be necessary, and renal function should be monitored and supported as required.
No experience has been reported with extracorporeal or peritoneal dialysis.

DOSAGE AND ADMINISTRATION

When there is urgent need, therapy in the hospitalized patient may be initiated intramuscularly or as a rapid intravenous bolus injection directly into the vein. Parenteral Apresoline should be used only when the drug cannot be given orally. The usual dose is 20–40 mg, repeated as necessary. Certain patients (especially those with marked renal damage) may require a lower dose. Blood pressure should be checked frequently. It may begin to fall within a few minutes after injection, with the average maximal decrease occurring in 10–80 minutes. In cases where there has been increased intracranial pressure, lowering the blood pressure may increase cerebral ischemia. Most patients can be transferred to oral Apresoline within 24–48 hours.

Continued on next page

The full prescribing information for each CIBA drug is contained herein and is that in effect as of September 1, 1986

CIBA—Cont.

The product should be used immediately after the ampul is opened. It should not be added to infusion solutions. Apresoline hydrochloride parenteral may discolor upon contact with metal; discolored solutions should be discarded. Parenteral drug products should be inspected visually for particulate matter and discoloration prior to administration, whenever solution and container permit.

HOW SUPPLIED

Ampuls 1 ml, containing 20 mg of hydralazine hydrochloride
Cartons of 5 ampuls—NDC 0083-2626-05
See **Dosage and Administration.**
Store between 59° and 86°F.
Dist. by:
CIBA Pharmaceutical Company
Division of CIBA-GEIGY Corporation
Summit, New Jersey 07901
C85-19 (Rev. 8/85)

APRESOLINE®-ESIDRIX® ℞

[*a-press 'oh-leen ess 'a-dricks*]
hydralazine hydrochloride and hydrochlorothiazide Combination Tablets

> **WARNING**
> This fixed-combination drug is not indicated for initial therapy of hypertension. Hypertension requires therapy titrated to the individual patient. If the fixed combination represents the dosage so determined, its use may be more convenient in patient management. The treatment of hypertension is not static but must be reevaluated as conditions in each patient warrant.

DESCRIPTION

Apresoline-Esidrix is an antihypertensive-diuretic combination, available as tablets containing hydralazine hydrochloride USP, 25 mg, and hydrochlorothiazide USP, 15 mg, for oral administration.
Hydralazine hydrochloride is 1-hydrazinophthalazine monohydrochloride.
Hydralazine hydrochloride USP is a white to off-white, odorless crystalline powder. It is soluble in water, slightly soluble in alcohol, and very slightly soluble in ether. It melts at about 275°C, with decomposition, and has a molecular weight of 196.64.
Hydrochlorothiazide is 6-chloro-3,4-dihydro-2*H*-1,2,4-benzothiadiazine-7-sulfonamide 1,1-dioxide.
Hydrochlorothiazide USP is a white, or practically white, practically odorless crystalline powder. It is slightly soluble in water; freely soluble in sodium hydroxide solution, in *n*-butylamine, and in dimethylformamide; sparingly soluble in methanol; and insoluble in ether, in chloroform, and in dilute mineral acids. Its molecular weight is 297.73.
Inactive Ingredients: Acacia, FD&C Yellow No. 6, lactose, polyethylene glycol, starch, stearic acid and sucrose.

CLINICAL PHARMACOLOGY

Hydralazine
Although the precise mechanism of action of hydralazine is not fully understood, the major effects are on the cardiovascular system. Hydralazine apparently lowers blood pressure by exerting a peripheral vasodilating effect through a direct relaxation of vascular smooth muscle. Hydralazine, by altering cellular calcium metabolism, interferes with the calcium movements within the vascular smooth muscle that are responsible for initiating or maintaining the contractile state.
The peripheral vasodilating effect of hydralazine results in decreased arterial blood pressure (diastolic more than systolic); decreased peripheral vascular resistance; and an increased heart rate, stroke volume, and cardiac output. The preferential dilatation of arterioles, as compared to veins, minimizes postural hypotension and promotes the increase in cardiac output. Hydralazine usually increases renin activity in plasma, presumably as a result of increased secretion of renin by the renal juxtaglomerular cells in response to reflex sympathetic discharge. This increase in renin activity leads to the production of angiotensin II, which then causes stimulation of aldosterone and consequent sodium reabsorption. Hydralazine also maintains or increases renal and cerebral blood flow.
Hydrochlorothiazide
Thiazides affect the renal tubular mechanism of electrolyte reabsorption. At maximal therapeutic dosage, all thiazides are approximately equal in their diuretic potency. Thiazides increase excretion of sodium and chloride in approximately equivalent amounts. Natriuresis causes a secondary loss of potassium.
The mechanism of the antihypertensive effect of thiazides is unknown. Thiazides do not affect normal blood pressure.
Pharmacokinetics
The Apresoline-Esidrix tablet is bioequivalent to Apresoline (hydralazine) and Esidrix (hydrochlorothiazide) tablets administered simultaneously.
Hydralazine: Hydralazine is rapidly absorbed after oral administration, and peak plasma levels are reached at 1–2 hours. Plasma levels decline with a half-life of 3–7 hours. Binding to human plasma protein is 87%. Plasma levels of hydralazine vary widely among individuals. Hydralazine is subject to polymorphic acetylation; slow acetylators generally have higher plasma levels of hydralazine and require lower doses to maintain control of blood pressure. Hydralazine undergoes extensive hepatic metabolism; it is excreted mainly in the form of metabolites in the urine.
Administration of hydralazine with food results in higher levels of the drug in plasma.
Hydrochlorothiazide: Onset of action of thiazides occurs in 2 hours and the peak effect at about 4 hours. The action persists for approximately 6–12 hours. Hydrochlorothiazide is rapidly absorbed, as indicated by peak concentrations 1–2.5 hours after oral administration. Plasma levels of the drug are proportional to dose; the concentration in whole blood is 1.6–1.8 times higher than in plasma. Thiazides are eliminated rapidly by the kidney. After oral administration of 25- to 100-mg doses, 72–97% of the dose is excreted in the urine, indicating dose-independent absorption. Hydrochlorothiazide is eliminated from plasma in a biphasic fashion with a terminal half-life of 10–17 hours. Plasma protein binding is 67.9%. Plasma clearance is 15.9–30.0 L/hr; volume of distribution is 3.6–7.8 L/kg.
Gastrointestinal absorption of hydrochlorothiazide is enhanced when administered with food. Absorption is decreased in patients with congestive heart failure, and the pharmacokinetics are considerably different in these patients.

INDICATIONS AND USAGE

Hypertension (see boxed **WARNING**).

CONTRAINDICATIONS

Hydralazine
Hypersensitivity to hydralazine; coronary artery disease; mitral valvular rheumatic heart disease.
Hydrochlorothiazide
Anuria; hypersensitivity to this or other sulfonamide-derived drugs.

WARNINGS

Hydralazine
In a few patients hydralazine may produce a clinical picture simulating systemic lupus erythematosus including glomerulonephritis. In such patients hydralazine should be discontinued unless the benefit-to-risk determination requires continued antihypertensive therapy with this drug. Signs and symptoms usually regress when the drug is discontinued, but residua have been detected many years later. Long-term treatment with steroids may be necessary. (See **PRECAUTIONS, Laboratory Tests.**)
Hydrochlorothiazide
Thiazides should be used with caution in patients with severe renal disease. In patients with renal disease, thiazides may precipitate azotemia. Cumulative effects of the drug may develop in patients with impaired renal function.
Thiazides should be used with caution in patients with impaired hepatic function or progressive liver disease, since minor alterations of fluid and electrolyte imbalance may precipitate hepatic coma.
Thiazides may add to or potentiate the action of other anithypertensive drugs. Potentiation occurs with ganglionic or peripheral adrenergic blocking drugs.
Sensitivity reactions are more likely to occur in patients with a history of allergy or bronchial asthma.
The possibility of exacerbation or activation of systemic lupus erythematosus has been reported.

PRECAUTIONS

General
Hydralazine: Myocardial stimulation produced by hydralazine can cause anginal attacks and ECG changes indicative of myocardial ischemia. The drug has been implicated in the production of myocardial infarction. It must, therefore, be used with caution in patients with suspected coronary artery disease.
The "hyperdynamic" circulation caused by hydralazine may accentuate specific cardiovascular inadequacies. For example, hydralazine may increase pulmonary artery pressure in patients with mitral valvular disease. The drug may reduce the pressor responses to epinephrine. Postural hypotension may result from hydralazine but is less common than with ganglionic blocking agents. It should be used with caution in patients with cerebral vascular accidents.
In hypertensive patients with normal kidneys who are treated with hydralazine, there is evidence of increased renal blood flow and a maintenance of glomerular filtration rate. In some instances where control values were below normal, improved renal function has been noted after administration of hydralazine. However, as with any antihypertensive agent, hydralazine should be used with caution in patients with advanced renal damage.
Peripheral neuritis, evidenced by paresthesia, numbness, and tingling, has been observed. Published evidence suggests that hydralazine has an antipyridoxine effect and that pyridoxine should be added to the regimen if symptoms develop.
Hydrochlorothiazide: All patients receiving thiazide therapy should be observed for clinical signs of fluid or electrolyte imbalance, namely hyponatremia, hypochloremic alkalosis, and hypokalemia (see **Laboratory Tests** and **Drug/Drug Interactions**). Warning signs are dryness of mouth, thirst, weakness, lethargy, drowsiness, restlessness, muscle pains or cramps, muscular fatigue, hypotension, oliguria, tachycardia, and gastrointestinal disturbance, such as nausea or vomiting.
Hypokalemia may develop, especially in cases of brisk diuresis or severe cirrhosis.
Interference with adequate oral intake of electrolytes will also contribute to hypokalemia. Hypokalemia may be avoided or treated by use of potassium supplements or foods with a high potassium content.
Any chloride deficit is generally mild and usually does not require specific treatment, except under extraordinary circumstances (as in liver disease or renal disease). Dilutional hyponatremia may occur in edematous patients in hot weather; appropriate therapy is water restriction, rather than administration of salt, except in rare instances when the hyponatremia is life-threatening. In cases of actual salt depletion, appropriate replacement is the therapy of choice.
Hyperuricemia may occur or frank gout may be precipitated in certain patients receiving thiazide therapy.
Latent diabetes may become manifest during thiazide administration (see **Drug/Drug Interactions**).
The antihypertensive effects of the drug may be enhanced in the postsympathectomy patient.
If progressive renal impairment becomes evident, withholding or discontinuing diuretic therapy should be considered.
Calcium excretion is decreased by thiazides. Pathological changes in the parathyroid gland with hypercalcemia and hypophosphatemia have been observed in a few patients on prolonged thiazide therapy. The common complications of hyperparathyroidism, such as renal lithiasis, bone resorption, and peptic ulceration, have not been seen.
Information for Patients: Patients should be informed of possible side effects and advised to take the medication regularly and continuously as directed.
Laboratory Tests
Hydralazine: Complete blood counts and antinuclear antibody titer determinations are indicated before and periodically during prolonged therapy with hydralazine even though the patient is asymptomatic. These studies are also indicated if the patient develops arthralgia, fever, chest pain, continued malaise, or other unexplained signs or symptoms.
A positive antinuclear antibody titer requires that the physician carefully weigh the implications of the test results against the benefits to be derived from antihypertensive therapy with a combination drug containing hydralazine.
Blood dyscrasias, consisting of reduction in hemoglobin and red cell count, leukopenia, agranulocytosis, and purpura, have been reported. If such abnormalities develop, therapy should be discontinued.
Hydrochlorothiazide: Initial and periodic determinations of serum electrolytes to detect possible electrolyte imbalance should be performed at appropriate intervals.
Serum and urine electrolyte determinations are particularly important when the patient is vomiting excessively or receiving parenteral fluids.
Drug/Drug Interactions
Hydralazine: MAO inhibitors should be used with caution in patients receiving hydralazine.
When other potent parenteral antihypertensive drugs, such as diazoxide, are used in combination with hydralazine, patients should be continuously observed for several hours for any excessive fall in blood pressure. Profound hypotensive episodes may occur when diazoxide injections and hydralazine are used concomitantly.
Hydrochlorothiazide: Hypokalemia can sensitize or exaggerate the response of the heart to the toxic effects of digitalis (e.g., increased ventricular irritability).
Hypokalemia may develop during concomitant use of steroids or ACTH.
Insulin requirements in diabetic patients may be increased, decreased, or unchanged.
Thiazides may decrease arterial responsiveness to norepinephrine, but not enough to preclude effectiveness of the pressor agent for therapeutic use.
Thiazides may increase the responsiveness to tubocurarine.
Lithium renal clearance is reduced by thiazides, increasing the risk of lithium toxicity.
Drug/Laboratory Test Interactions
Thiazides may decrease serum levels of protein-bound iodine without signs of thyroid disturbance. Apresoline-Esidrix should be discontinued before tests for parathyroid function are made (See **General, Hydrochlorothiazide,** Calcium excretion).

Carcinogenesis, Mutagenesis, Impairment of Fertility

Hydralazine: In a lifetime study in Swiss albino mice, there was a statistically significant increase in the incidence of lung tumors (adenomas and adenocarcinomas) of both male and female mice given hydralazine continuously in their drinking water at a dosage of about 250 mg/kg per day (about 80 times the maximum recommended human dose). In a 2-year carcinogenicity study of rats given hydralazine by gavage at dose levels of 15, 30, and 60 mg/kg/day (approximately 5 to 20 times the recommended human daily dosage), microscopic examination of the liver revealed a small, but statistically significant, increase in benign neoplastic nodules in male and female rats from the high-dose group and in female rats from the intermediate-dose group. Benign interstitial cell tumors of the testes were also significantly increased in male rats from the high-dose group. The tumors observed are common in aged rats and a significantly increased incidence was not observed until 18 months of treatment. Hydralazine was shown to be mutagenic in three bacterial tester strains in the Ames test, both with and without metabolic activation, and elicited DNA repair both in the Pol A^+/A^- *E. coli* bacterial assay system and in cultured rat hepatocytes. (Evidence of DNA damage in the hepatocyte repair test is considered a strong indication of covalent binding, an established property of carcinogens and mutagens.) In tests with rabbit hepatocytes that exhibit an acetylator polymorphism like that of humans, hydralazine elicited DNA repair with only those hepatocytes having a slow rate of acetylation, suggesting that individuals who are rapid acetylators may have a diminished genotoxic liability. No increase in mutagenic potential was revealed in the mouse lymphoma assay, host-mediated assay, nucleus anomaly test, or dominant lethal test.

The extent to which these findings indicate a risk to man is uncertain. While long-term clinical observation has not suggested that human cancer is associated with hydralazine use, epidemiologic studies have so far been insufficient to arrive at any conclusions.

Hydrochlorothiazide: Long-term carcinogenicity studies in animals have not been conducted with Esidrix.

Pregnancy Category C

Animal reproduction studies have not been conducted with Apresoline-Esidrix. Animal studies indicate that hydralazine is teratogenic in mice at 20–30 times the maximum daily human dose of 200–300 mg and possibly in rabbits at 10–15 times the maximum daily human dose, but that it is nonteratogenic in rats. Teratogenic effects observed were cleft palate and malformations of facial and cranial bones. A reproduction study in rats receiving hydrochlorothiazide, 250 mg/kg daily, 62.5 times the maximum daily human dose, has revealed no evidence of impaired fertility or harm to the fetus.

There are no adequate and well-controlled studies of Apresoline-Esidrix in pregnant women. However, thiazides cross the placental barrier and appear in cord blood, and there is a risk of fetal or neonatal jaundice, thrombocytopenia, and possibly other adverse reactions that have occurred in adults. Apresoline-Esidrix should be used during pregnancy only if the potential benefit justifies the potential risk to the fetus.

Nursing Mothers: It is not known whether hydralazine is excreted in human milk. Thiazides are excreted in human milk. Because of the potential for serious adverse reactions in nursing infants, a decision should be made whether to discontinue nursing or to discontinue the drug, taking into account the importance of the drug to the mother.

Pediatric Use: Safety and effectiveness of the combination drug in children have not been established.

ADVERSE REACTIONS

Adverse reactions are usually reversible upon reduction of dosage or discontinuation of Apresoline-Esidrix. Whenever adverse reactions are moderate or severe, it may be necessary to discontinue the drug.

The following adverse reactions have been observed, but there has not been enough systematic collection of data to support an estimate of their frequency.

Hydralazine

Common: Headache, anorexia, nausea, vomiting, diarrhea, palpitations, tachycardia, angina pectoris.

Less Frequent: *Digestive:* constipation, paralytic ileus.
Cardiovascular: hypotension, paradoxical pressor response, edema.
Respiratory: dyspnea.
Neurologic: peripheral neuritis, evidenced by paresthesia, numbness, and tingling; dizziness; tremors; muscle cramps; psychotic reactions characterized by depression, disorientation, or anxiety.
Genitourinary: difficulty in urination.
Hematologic: blood dyscrasias, consisting of reduction in hemoglobin and red cell count, leukopenia, agranulocytosis, purpura; lymphadenopathy; splenomegaly.
Hypersensitive Reactions: rash, urticaria, pruritus, fever, chills, arthralgia, eosinophilia, and, rarely, hepatitis.
Other: nasal congestion, flushing, lacrimation, conjunctivitis.

Hydrochlorothiazide: *Digestive:* anorexia, gastric irritation, nausea, vomiting, cramping, diarrhea, constipation, jaundice (intrahepatic cholestatic), pancreatitis, sialadenitis.
Cardiovascular: orthostatic hypotension (may be potentiated by alcohol, barbiturates, or narcotics).
Neurologic: dizziness, vertigo, paresthesia, headache, xanthopsia.
Hematologic: leukopenia, agranulocytosis, thrombocytopenia, aplastic anemia.
Hypersensitive Reactions: purpura, photosensitivity, rash, urticaria, necrotizing angiitis, Stevens-Johnson syndrome.
Other: hyperglycemia, glycosuria, hyperuricemia, muscle spasm, weakness, restlessness, transient blurred vision.

OVERDOSAGE

Acute Toxicity: No deaths due to acute poisoning with Apresoline-Esidrix have been reported.

Oral LD_{50}'s in rats (mg/kg): hydralazine, 173 and 187; hydrochlorothiazide, 2750.

Signs and Symptoms

Hydralazine: Signs and symptoms of overdosage include hypotension, tachycardia, headache, and generalized skin flushing.

Complications can include myocardial ischemia and subsequent myocardial infarction, cardiac arrhythmia, and profound shock.

Hydrochlorothiazide: The most prominent feature of poisoning is acute loss of fluid and electrolytes.
Cardiovascular: tachycardia, hypotension, shock.
Neuromuscular: weakness, confusion, dizziness, cramps of the calf muscles, paresthesia, fatigue, impairment of consciousness.
Digestive: nausea, vomiting, thirst.
Renal: polyuria, oliguria, or anuria (due to hemoconcentration).
Laboratory Findings: hypokalemia, hyponatremia, hypochloremia, alkalosis; increased BUN (especially in patients with renal insufficiency).
Combined Poisoning: Signs and symptoms may be aggravated or modified by concomitant intake of antihypertensive medication, barbiturates, curare, digitalis (hypokalemia), corticosteroids, narcotics, or alcohol.

Treatment: There is no specific antidote.

The gastric contents should be evacuated, taking adequate precautions against aspiration and for protection of the airway. An activated charcoal slurry may be instilled if conditions permit. Dialysis may not be effective for elimination of Apresoline-Esidrix because of its plasma protein binding (see **CLINICAL PHARMACOLOGY**).

These manipulations may have to be omitted or carried out after cardiovascular status has been stabilized, since they might precipitate cardiac arrhythmias or increase the depth of shock.

Support of the cardiovascular system is of primary importance in suspected hydralazine overdosage. Shock should be treated with plasma expanders. The patient's legs should be kept raised and lost fluid and electrolytes (potassium, sodium) should be replaced. If possible, vasopressors should not be given, but if a vasopressor is required, care should be taken not to precipitate or aggravate cardiac arrhythmia. Tachycardia responds to beta blockers. Digitalization may be necessary, and renal function should be monitored and supported as required.

DOSAGE AND ADMINISTRATION

Dosage should be determined by individual titration (see boxed **WARNING**).

The usual dosage is one tablet three times daily (maximal dosage is two tablets three times daily). For maintenance, dosage should be adjusted to the lowest effective level.

When necessary, other antihypertensives may be added gradually in reduced dosages. When the drug is given in conjunction with ganglionic blocking agents, dosage must be reduced by at least 50% and the effects should be watched carefully.

HOW SUPPLIED

Tablets—round, orange, dry-coated (imprinted CIBA 129) 25 mg of hydralazine hydrochloride and 15 mg of hydrochlorothiazide

Bottles of 100—NDC 0083-0129-30

Dispense in tight, light-resistant container (USP).

C85-20 (Rev. 8/85)

Shown in Product Identification Section, page 408

CORAMINE® ℞

[córe-a-meen]

nikethamide

Solution

DESCRIPTION

Coramine, nikethamide, is a central nervous system (CNS) stimulant, available as an aqueous solution (25% w/w) for oral administration. Nikethamide is N,N-diethyl-3-pyridinecarboxamide.

Nikethamide is a clear, colorless to pale yellow, somewhat viscous liquid that crystallizes in the cold and melts again as the temperature rises. It has a faint, characteristic, aromatic odor and a peculiar, bitter taste. Its solutions are clear and nearly colorless and have a faint amine-like odor. Nikethamide is miscible with water, with alcohol, and with ether. Its molecular weight is 178.24.

Inactive Ingredients: Citric acid and purified water.

CLINICAL PHARMACOLOGY

The mechanism of action of Coramine is unknown. Coramine stimulates the CNS at all levels of the cerebrospinal axis; it also acts as a respiratory and circulatory stimulant.

Coramine is absorbed from all routes of administration. Nikethamide is converted to nicotinamide and then excreted as n-methylnicotinamide.

Pharmacokinetic data in humans are not available.

INDICATIONS AND USAGE

Coramine is indicated for the treatment of CNS depression, respiratory depression, and circulatory failure, particularly when these are due to the effects of CNS depressant drugs.

CONTRAINDICATIONS

Coramine is contraindicated in patients with hypersensitivity to nikethamide or related compounds.

PRECAUTIONS

Carcinogenesis, Mutagenesis, Impairment of Fertility

Long-term carcinogenicity studies in animals have not been conducted with Coramine.

Pregnancy Category C

Animal reproduction studies have not been conducted with Coramine. It is also not known whether Coramine can cause fetal harm when administered to a pregnant woman or can affect reproduction capacity. Coramine should be given to a pregnant woman only if clearly needed.

Labor and Delivery

The effect of Coramine on labor and delivery or on the newborn is unknown.

Nursing Mothers

It is not known whether this drug is excreted in human milk. Because many drugs are excreted in human milk, caution should be exercised when Coramine is administered to a nursing woman.

Pediatric Use

Safety and effectiveness in children have not been established.

ADVERSE REACTIONS

The difference between the clinically effective dose and that producing side effects varies but is often small. The following side effects that have been reported may, in fact, be the result of overdosage.

The most common side effect is an unpleasant feeling or burning or itching, especially at the back of the nose. Occasionally, flushing or a subjective feeling of warmth, sneezing, coughing, sweating, nausea, vomiting, generalized restlessness, fearfulness, changing depth and frequency of respiration, tachycardia, elevated blood pressure, tics (especially facial), and convulsions have also been reported.

OVERDOSAGE

Acute Toxicity

The highest known dose survived is 6,250 mg orally (17-year-old woman).

Signs and Symptoms

Coughing, sneezing, hyperpnea, and muscle tremors can occur. Heart rate and blood pressure may increase, although probably not markedly. With severe overdosage, generalized muscle spasm and convulsive seizures can occur.

Treatment

Treatment is usually not required, except in severe overdosage. In such cases, a short-acting barbiturate is effective in controlling the generalized muscle spasm and convulsions that may be present.

Since the oral solution is rapidly absorbed, attempts to induce emesis or to perform gastric lavage are of little value and, in the presence of paroxysmal coughing or sneezing, could result in complications from aspiration.

DOSAGE AND ADMINISTRATION

Coramine is readily absorbed after oral administration.

Oral

For maintenance therapy, 3-5 ml of the oral solution may be given every 4-6 hours, when indicated.

HOW SUPPLIED

Available as 25% (by weight) aqueous solution.

Oral Solution

Bottles of 3 fluid ounces (approx. 90 ml) NDC 0083-3234-61

Store between 59°–86°F (15°–30°C).

Dispense in tight, light-resistant container (USP).

C85-47 (Rev. 11/85)

Continued on next page

The full prescribing information for each CIBA drug is contained herein and is that in effect as of September 1, 1986

CIBA—Cont.

CYTADREN® Tablets ℞
[*sight 'a-dren*]
aminoglutethimide tablets USP

DESCRIPTION

Cytadren, aminoglutethimide tablets USP, is an inhibitor of adrenocortical steroid synthesis, available as 250-mg tablets for oral administration. Its chemical name is 3-(4-aminophenyl)-3-ethyl-2, 6-piperidinedione.
Aminoglutethimide USP is a fine, white or creamy white, crystalline powder. It is very slightly soluble in water, and readily soluble in most organic solvents. It forms water-soluble salts with strong acids. Its molecular weight is 232.28.
*Inactive Ingredients.*Cellulose compounds, colloidal silicon dioxide, starch, stearic acid, and talc.

CLINICAL PHARMACOLOGY

Cytadren inhibits the enzymatic conversion of cholesterol to Δ^5-pregnenolone, resulting in a decrease in the production of adrenal glucocorticoids, mineralocorticoids, estrogens, and androgens.
Cytadren blocks several other steps in steroid synthesis, including the C-11, C-18, and C-21 hydroxylations and the hydroxylations required for the aromatization of androgens to estrogens, mediated through the binding of Cytadren to cytochrome P-450 complexes.
A decrease in adrenal secretion of cortisol is followed by an increased secretion of pituitary adrenocorticotropic hormone (ACTH), which will overcome the blockade of adrenocortical steroid synthesis by Cytadren. The compensatory increase in ACTH secretion can be suppressed by the simultaneous administration of hydrocortisone. Since Cytadren increases the rate of metabolism of dexamethasone but not that of hydrocortisone, the latter is preferred as the adrenal glucocorticoid replacement.
Although Cytadren inhibits the synthesis of thyroxine by the thyroid gland, the compensatory increase in thyroid-stimulating hormone (TSH) is frequently of sufficient magnitude to overcome the inhibition of thyroid synthesis due to Cytadren. In spite of an increase in TSH, Cytadren has not been associated with increased prolactin secretion.
Note: Cytadren was marketed previously as an anticonvulsant but was withdrawn from marketing for that indication in 1966 because of the effects on the adrenal gland.

Pharmacokinetics

Cytadren is rapidly and completely absorbed after oral administration. In 6 healthy male volunteers, maximum plasma levels of Cytadren averaged 5.9 μg/ml at a median of 1.5 hours after ingestion of two 250-mg tablets. The bioavailability of tablets is equivalent to equal doses given as a solution. After ingestion of a single oral dose, 34–54% is excreted in the urine as unchanged drug during the first 48 hours, and an additional fraction as the N-acetyl derivative.
The half-life of Cytadren in normal volunteers given single oral doses averaged 12.5 ± 1.6 hours.
Upon withdrawal of therapy with Cytadren, the ability of the adrenal glands to synthesize steroid returns, usually within 72 hours.

INDICATIONS AND USAGE

Cytadren is indicated for the suppression of adrenal function in selected patients with Cushing's syndrome. Morning levels of plasma cortisol in patients with adrenal carcinoma and ectopic ACTH-producing tumors were reduced on the average to about one half of the pretreatment levels, and in patients with adrenal hyperplasia to about two thirds of the pretreatment levels, during 1–3 months of therapy with Cytadren. Data available from the few patients with adrenal adenoma suggest similar reductions in plasma cortisol levels. Measurements of plasma cortisol showed reductions to at least 50% of baseline or to normal levels in one third or more of the patients studied, depending on diagnostic groups and time of measurement.
Because Cytadren does not affect the underlying disease process, it is used primarily as an interim measure until more definitive therapy such as surgery can be undertaken or in cases where such therapy is not appropriate. Only small numbers of patients have been treated for longer than 3 months. A decreased effect or "escape phenomenon" seems to occur more frequently in patients with pituitary-dependent Cushing's syndrome, probably because of increasing ACTH levels in response to decreasing glucocorticoid levels.
Cytadren should be used only in those patients who are responsive to treatment.

CONTRAINDICATIONS

Cytadren is contraindicated in those patients with serious forms, and/or severe manifestations, of hypersensitivity to glutethimide or aminoglutethimide.

WARNINGS

Cytadren may cause adrenocortical hypofunction, especially under conditions of stress, such as surgery, trauma, or acute illness. Patients should be carefully monitored and given hydrocortisone and mineralocorticoid supplements as indicated. Dexamethasone should not be used. (See **PRECAUTIONS, Drug Interactions.**)
Cytadren also may suppress aldosterone production by the adrenal cortex and may cause orthostatic or persistent hypotension. The blood pressure should be monitored in all patients at appropriate intervals. Patients should be advised of the possible occurrence of weakness and dizziness as symptoms of hypotension, and of measures to be taken should they occur.
The effects of Cytadren may be potentiated if it is taken in combination with alcohol.
Cytadren can cause fetal harm when administered to a pregnant woman. In the earlier experience with the drug in about 5000 patients, two cases of pseudohermaphroditism were reported in female infants whose mothers were treated with Cytadren and concomitant anticonvulsants. Normal pregnancies have also occurred in patients treated with Cytadren.
When administered to rats at doses ½ and 1¼ times the maximum daily human dose, Cytadren caused a decrease in fetal implantation, an increase in fetal deaths, and a variety of teratogenic effects. The compound also caused pseudohermaphroditism in rats treated with approximately 3 times the maximum daily human dose. If this drug must be used during pregnancy, or if the patient becomes pregnant while taking the drug, the patient should be apprised of the potential hazard to the fetus.

PRECAUTIONS

General

This drug should be administered only by physicians familiar with its use and hazards. Therapy should be initiated in a hospital. (See **DOSAGE AND ADMINISTRATION.**)

Information for Patients

Patients should be warned that drowsiness may occur and that they should not drive, operate potentially dangerous machinery, or engage in other activities that may become hazardous because of decreased alertness.
Patients should also be warned of the possibility of hypotension and its symptoms (see **WARNINGS**).

Laboratory Tests

Hypothyroidism may occur in association with Cytadren; hence, appropriate clinical observations should be made and laboratory studies of thyroid function performed as indicated. Supplementary thyroid hormone may be required.
Hematologic abnormalities in patients receiving Cytadren have been reported (see **ADVERSE REACTIONS**). Therefore, baseline hematologic studies should be performed, followed by periodic hematologic evaluation.
Since elevations in SGOT, alkaline phosphatase, and bilirubin have been reported, appropriate clinical observations and regular laboratory studies should be performed before and during therapy.
Serum electrolyte levels should be determined periodically.

Drug Interactions

Cytadren accelerates the metabolism of dexamethasone; therefore, if glucocorticoid replacement is needed, hydrocortisone should be prescribed.
Aminoglutethimide diminishes the effect of coumarin and warfarin.

Carcinogenesis, Mutagenesis, Impairment of Fertility

Long-term carcinogenicity studies in animals and mutagenicity studies have not been performed with Cytadren.
Cytadren affects fertility in female rats (see **WARNINGS**).
The relevance of these findings to humans is not known.

Pregnancy Category D

See **WARNINGS.**

Nursing Mothers

It is not known whether this drug is excreted in human milk. Because many drugs are excreted in human milk and because of the potential for serious adverse reactions in nursing infants from Cytadren, a decision should be made whether to discontinue nursing or to discontinue the drug, taking into account the importance of the drug to the mother.

Pediatric Use

Safety and effectiveness in children have not been established (see **CLINICAL STUDIES IN CHILDREN**).

ADVERSE REACTIONS

Untoward effects have been reported in about 2 out of 3 patients with Cushing's syndrome who were treated for 4 or more weeks with Cytadren as the only adrenocortical suppressant.
The most frequent and reversible side effects were drowsiness (approximately 1 in 3 patients), morbilliform skin rash (1 in 6 patients), nausea and anorexia (each approximately 1 in 8 patients), and dizziness (about 1 in 20 patients). The dizziness was possibly caused by lowered vascular resistance or orthostasis. These reactions often disappear spontaneously with continued therapy.

Other Effects Observed

Hematologic: Single instances of neutropenia, leukopenia (patient received concomitant *o,p'*-DDD), pancytopenia (patient received concomitant 5-fluorouracil), and agranulocytosis occurred in 4 of 27 patients with Cushing's syndrome caused by adrenal carcinoma who were treated for at least 4 weeks. In 1 patient with adrenal hyperplasia, hemoglobin levels and hematocrit decreased during the course of treatment with Cytadren. From the earlier experience with the drug used as an anticonvulsant in 1,214 patients, transient leukopenia was the only hematologic effect and was reported once; Coombs'-negative hemolytic anemia also occurred once. In approximately 300 patients with nonadrenal malignancy, 1 in 25 showed some degree of anemia, and 1 in 150 developed pancytopenia during treatment with Cytadren.
Endocrine: Adrenal insufficiency occurred in about 1 in 30 patients with Cushing's syndrome who were treated with Cytadren for 4 or more weeks. This insufficiency tended to involve glucocorticoids as well as mineralocorticoids. Hypothyroidism is occasionally associated with thyroid enlargement and may be detected or confirmed by measuring plasma levels of the thyroid hormone. Masculinization and hirsutism have occasionally occurred in females, as has precocious sexual development in males.
Central Nervous System: Headache was reported in about 1 in 20 patients.
Cardiovascular: Hypotension, occasionally orthostatic, occurred in 1 in 30 patients receiving Cytadren. Tachycardia occurred in 1 in 40 patients.
Gastrointestinal and Liver: Vomiting occurred in 1 in 30 patients. Isolated instances of abnormal findings on liver function tests were reported. Suspected hepatotoxicity occurred in less than 1 in 1000 patients.
Skin: In addition to rash (1 in 6 patients, and often reversible with continued therapy), pruritus was reported in 1 in 20 patients. These may be allergic or hypersensitive reactions. Urticaria has occurred rarely.
Miscellaneous: Fever was reported in several patients who were treated with Cytadren for less than 4 weeks; some of these patients also received other drugs. Myalgia occurred in 1 in 30 patients.

OVERDOSAGE

Acute Toxicity

No deaths due to overdosage with Cytadren have been reported.
The highest known doses that have been survived are 7 g (33-year-old woman) and 7.5–10.0 g (16-year-old girl).
Oral LD_{50}'s (mg/kg): rats, 1800; dogs, > 100. Intravenous LD_{50}'s (mg/kg): rats, 156; dogs > 100.

Signs and Symptoms

An acute overdose with Cytadren may reduce the production of steroids in the adrenal cortex to a degree that is clinically relevant. The following manifestations may be expected:
Respiratory Function: Respiratory depression, hyperventilation.
Cardiovascular System: Hypotension, hypovolemic shock due to dehydration.
Central Nervous System/Muscles: Somnolence, lethargy, coma, ataxia, dizziness, fatigue. (Extreme weakness has been reported with divided doses of 3 g daily).
Gastrointestinal System: Nausea, vomiting.
Renal Function: Loss of sodium and water.
Laboratory Findings: Hyponatremia, hypochloremia, hyperkalemia, hypoglycemia.
The signs and symptoms of acute overdosage with Cytadren may be aggravated or modified if alcohol, hypnotics, tranquilizers, or tricyclic antidepressants have been taken at the same time.

Treatment

Symptomatic treatment of overdosage is recommended.
Since aminoglutethimide and glutethimide are chemically related, measures that have been used in successfully removing glutethimide from the body might be useful in removing aminoglutethimide.
Gastric lavage and unspecified supportive treatment have been employed. Full consciousness following deep coma was regained 40 hours or less after ingestion of 3 or 4 g without lavage. No evidence of hematologic, renal, or hepatic effects was subsequently found.
Close monitoring should be provided, and appropriate measures taken to support vital functions, if necessary.
If deficiency of circulating glucocorticoid develops, an intravenous infusion of a soluble hydrocortisone preparation (100 mg of hydrocortisone sodium succinate in 500 ml of isotonic sodium chloride solution) and 50 ml of 40% glucose solution should be given within 3 hours. After the initial infusion is completed, an intravenous administration of hydrocortisone, 10 mg per hour, should be continued until the patient is able to take oral cortisone.
If hypovolemia or hypotension occurs, an intravenous administration of norepinephrine, 10 mg, in 500 ml of isotonic sodium chloride should be administered according to the patient's needs and response. After rehydration, 500 ml of plasma or blood should be given for maintenance of sufficient circulatory volume.
Dialysis may be considered in severe intoxication.

DOSAGE AND ADMINISTRATION

Adults

Treatment should be instituted in a hospital until a stable dosage regimen is achieved. Therapy should be initiated with 250 mg orally four times daily, preferably at 6-hour intervals. Adrenocortical response should be followed by careful monitoring of plasma cortisol levels until the desired level of suppression is achieved. If the level of cortisol suppression is inadequate, the dosage may be increased in increments of 250 mg daily at intervals of 1–2 weeks to a total daily dose of 2 g. Dose reduction or temporary discontinuation of therapy may be required in the event of adverse effects, including extreme drowsiness, severe skin rash, or excessively low cortisol levels. If a skin rash persists for longer than 5–8 days or becomes severe, the drug should be discontinued. It may be possible to reinstate therapy at a lower dosage following the disappearance of a mild or moderate rash. Mineralocorticoid replacement (e.g., fludrocortisone) may be necessary. If glucocorticoid replacement therapy is needed, 20–30 mg of hydrocortisone orally in the morning will replace endogenous secretion.

HOW SUPPLIED

Tablets 250 mg — white, round, scored into quarters (imprinted CIBA 24)

Bottles of 100 ....NDC 0083-0024-30

Protect from light.

Dispense in tight, light-resistant container (USP).

CLINICAL STUDIES IN CHILDREN

Clinical investigations included 9 patients aged 2½ to 16 years; 4 of these were aged 10 or less. Seven of the patients received other therapies (drugs or irradiation) either with Cytadren or within a short period before initiation of therapy with Cytadren. Diagnoses included 5 patients with adrenal carcinoma, 3 with adrenal hyperplasia, and 1 with ectopic ACTH-producing tumor. Duration of treatment ranged from 3 days to 6½ months. Dosages ranged from 0.375 g to 1.5 g daily. In general, smaller doses were used for younger patients; for example, a 2½-year-old received 0.5–0.75 g daily, a 3½-year-old received 0.5 g daily, and all others over 10 years of age received 0.75–1.5 g daily. Results are difficult to evaluate because of the concomitant therapy, duration of therapy, or inadequate laboratory documentation. Most patients did show decreases in plasma or urinary steroids at some time during treatment, but these may have been due to other therapeutic modalities or their combinations.

C85-51 (Rev. 11/85)

Shown in Product Identification Section, page 408

DESFERAL® mesylate ℞

[des 'fer-all]

deferoxamine mesylate USP

DESCRIPTION

Desferal, deferoxamine mesylate USP, is an iron-chelating agent, available in vials for intramuscular, subcutaneous, and intravenous administration. Each vial contains 500 mg of deferoxamine mesylate USP in sterile, lyophilized form. Deferoxamine mesylate is N-[5-[3-[(5-aminopentyl) hydroxycarbamoyl] propionamido]pentyl]-3-[[5-(N-hydroxyacetamido)pentyl]carbamoyl] propionohydroxamic acid monomethanesulfonate (salt).

Deferoxamine mesylate USP is a white to off-white powder. It is freely soluble in water and slightly soluble in methanol. Its molecular weight is 656.79.

ACTIONS

Desferal is a compound with a specific ability to chelate iron, forming a stable complex which prevents the iron from entering into further chemical reactions. This chelate is readily soluble in water and passes easily through the kidney, giving the urine a characteristic reddish color. Some is also excreted in the feces via the bile. Theoretically, 100 parts by weight of Desferal are capable of binding approximately 8.5 parts by weight of ferric iron. In studies thus far in man and animals, Desferal does not cause any demonstrable increase in the excretion of electrolytes and trace metals.

INDICATIONS

To facilitate the removal of iron in the treatment of acute iron intoxication and in chronic iron overload due to transfusion-dependent anemias.

ACUTE IRON INTOXICATION

Desferal is an adjunct to, and not a substitute for, standard measures generally used in treating acute iron intoxication which may include the following:

1. Induction of emesis with syrup of ipecac.
2. Gastric lavage.
3. Suction and maintenance of clear airway.
4. Control of shock with intravenous fluids, blood, oxygen, and vasopressors.
5. Correction of acidosis.

CHRONIC IRON OVERLOAD

Desferal can promote iron excretion in patients who have secondary iron overload from multiple transfusions (such as occur in some chronic anemias including thalassemia). One controlled study has found that long-term therapy with Desferal slows accumulation of hepatic iron and retards or eliminates progression of hepatic fibrosis.

Iron mobilization by Desferal is relatively poor in patients under the age of three with relatively small degrees of iron overload. The drug should ordinarily be withheld in such patients unless a demonstration of significant iron mobilization (eg, one mg of iron per day or more) can be demonstrated.

Desferal is not indicated for the treatment of primary hemochromatosis, since phlebotomy is the method of choice for removing excess iron in this indication.

CONTRAINDICATIONS

Desferal is contraindicated in patients with severe renal disease or anuria, since the drug and the chelate which it forms with iron are excreted primarily by the kidney.

WARNINGS

Rarely, cataracts have been observed in patients who received the drug over prolonged periods in the treatment of chronic iron storage diseases. Slit-lamp examinations performed in patients treated with Desferal for acute iron intoxication have not revealed cataracts. Slit-lamp examinations are recommended periodically in patients treated for chronic iron overload.

In addition, other ocular disturbances have been reported rarely during treatment with Desferal: decreased visual acuity; impaired peripheral, color, and night vision; and retinal pigmentary abnormalities. In most cases these disturbances were reversible upon cessation of treatment.

Usage in Pregnancy

Skeletal anomalies were noted in the fetuses of two animal species at doses just above those recommended for humans. Therefore, Desferal should not be administered to women of childbearing potential, particularly during early pregnancy, except when in the judgment of the physician the potential benefits outweigh the possible hazards.

PRECAUTIONS

Flushing of the skin, urticaria, hypotension, and even shock have occurred in a few patients when Desferal has been administered by rapid intravenous injection. To avoid these reactions, DESFERAL SHOULD BE GIVEN INTRAMUSCULARLY, OR BY SLOW SUBCUTANEOUS OR INTRAVENOUS INFUSION.

ADVERSE REACTIONS

Occasionally, pain and induration at the site of injection have been reported. Side effects reported in patients treated for acute iron intoxication include generalized erythema, urticaria, and hypotension, which occurred with rapid intravenous injection. Adverse effects reported in patients receiving long-term therapy for chronic iron storage diseases include allergic-type reactions (cutaneous wheal formation, generalized itching, rash, anaphylactic reaction), blurring of vision, dysuria, abdominal discomfort, diarrhea, leg cramps, tachycardia, and fever. Adverse effects reported in patients receiving subcutaneous therapy include localized pain, pruritus, erythema, skin irritation and swelling. These reactions might also occur in an occasional patient treated for acute iron intoxication.

DOSAGE AND ADMINISTRATION

Since little of the drug is absorbed when administered orally, it is necessary to administer Desferal parenterally to chelate the iron that has been absorbed.

ACUTE IRON INTOXICATION

Intramuscular Administration

Intramuscular administration is preferred and should be used for ALL PATIENTS NOT IN SHOCK.

Dose: One gm should be administered initially. This may be followed by 0.5 gm every four hours for two doses. Depending upon the clinical response, subsequent doses of 0.5 gm may be administered every four to twelve hours. The total amount administered should not exceed 6 gm in twenty-four hours.

Preparation of Solution for Intramuscular Administration: Dissolve the Desferal by adding 2 ml sterile water for injection to each vial. Make sure that the drug is completely dissolved and then withdraw the drug and administer intramuscularly.

Intravenous Administration

This route should be used ONLY FOR PATIENTS IN A STATE OF CARDIOVASCULAR COLLAPSE and then ONLY BY SLOW INFUSION. THE RATE OF INFUSION SHOULD NOT EXCEED 15 mg/kg/hour.

Dose: An initial dose of 1 gm should be administered at a rate NOT TO EXCEED 15 mg/kg/hour. This may be followed by 0.5 gm every four hours for two doses. Depending upon the clinical response, subsequent doses of 0.5 gm may be administered every four to twelve hours. The total amount administered should not exceed 6 gm in twenty-four hours.

As soon as the clinical condition of the patient permits, intravenous administration should be discontinued and the drug administered intramuscularly.

Preparation of Solution for Intravenous Administration: Dissolve the Desferal by adding 2 ml sterile water for injection to each vial. Make sure that the drug is completely dissolved and then withdraw the drug and add to physiologic saline, glucose in water, or Ringer's lactate solution and administer at a rate NOT TO EXCEED 15 mg/kg/hour.

CHRONIC IRON OVERLOAD

The more effective of the following two routes of administration must be individualized for each patient.

Intramuscular Administration: 0.5 to 1.0 gm daily administered intramuscularly. In addition, 2.0 gm should be administered intravenously with each unit of blood transfused. However, Desferal should be administered separately from blood. The rate of intravenous infusion must not exceed 15 mg/kg/hour.

Subcutaneous Administration: 1.0 gm to 2.0 gm (20–40 mg/kg/day) administered daily over 8 to 24 hours utilizing a small portable pump capable of providing continuous mini-infusion. The duration of infusion must be individualized. In some patients iron excretion will be as great after a short infusion of 8 to 12 hours as it is if the same dose is given over a 24-hour period.

Preparation of Solution for Subcutaneous Administration: Dissolve the Desferal by adding 2.0 ml sterile water to each vial. Make sure that the drug is completely dissolved and then withdraw the drug in syringe to be used for administration.

Note: Desferal reconstituted with sterile water may be stored under sterile conditions and protected from light at room temperature for not longer than one week.

Reconstituting Desferal in solvents or under conditions other than indicated may result in precipitation.

HOW SUPPLIED

Vials—each containing 500 mg of sterile, lyophilized deferoxamine mesylate

Cartons of 4 vials ....NDC 0083-3801-04

C85-37 (Rev. 11/85)

ESIDRIX® ℞

[ess 'a-dricks]

hydrochlorothiazide USP

DESCRIPTION

Esidrix, hydrochlorothiazide USP, is a diuretic and antihypertensive available as 25-mg, 50-mg, and 100-mg tablets for oral administration. Its chemical name is 6-chloro-3,4-dihydro-2*H*-1,2,4-benzothiadiazine-7-sulfonamide 1,1-dioxide.

Hydrochlorothiazide USP is a white, or practically white, practically odorless, crystalline powder. It is slightly soluble in water, freely soluble in sodium hydroxide solution, in *n*-butylamine and in dimethylformamide, sparingly soluble in methanol, and insoluble in ether, in chloroform, and in dilute mineral acids. Its molecular weight is 297.73.

Inactive ingredients: Colloidal silicon dioxide, D. & C. Yellow #10 (50 mg tablets), F. D. & C. Blue #1 (100 tablets), F. D. & C. Red #3 and F. D. & C. Yellow #6 (25 mg tablets), lactose, starch, stearic acid and sucrose.

CLINICAL PHARMACOLOGY

Thiazides affect the renal tubular mechanism of electrolyte reabsorption. At maximal therapeutic dosage all thiazides are approximately equal in their diuretic potency. Thiazides increase excretion of sodium and chloride in approximately equivalent amounts. Natriuresis causes a secondary loss of potassium.

The mechanism of the antihypertensive effect of thiazides is unknown. Thiazides do not affect normal blood pressure.

Onset of action of thiazides occurs in 2 hours and the peak effect at about 4 hours. Its action persists for approximately 6 to 12 hours. Thiazides are eliminated rapidly by the kidney.

INDICATIONS AND USAGE

Hypertension

In the management of hypertension either as the sole therapeutic agent or to enhance the effect of other antihypertensive drugs in the more severe forms of hypertension.

Edema

As adjunctive therapy in edema associated with congestive heart failure, hepatic cirrhosis, and corticosteroid and estrogen therapy.

Continued on next page

The full prescribing information for each CIBA drug is contained herein and is that in effect as of September 1, 1986

CIBA—Cont.

Esidrix has also been found useful in edema due to various forms of renal dysfunction, such as the nephrotic syndrome, acute glomerulonephritis, and chronic renal failure.

Usage in Pregnancy: The routine use of diuretics in an otherwise healthy woman is inappropriate and exposes mother and fetus to unnecessary hazard. Diuretics do not prevent development of toxemia of pregnancy, and there is no satisfactory evidence that they are useful in the treatment of developed toxemia.

Edema during pregnancy may arise from pathological causes or from the physiologic and mechanical consequences of pregnancy. Thiazides are indicated in pregnancy when edema is due to pathologic causes, just as they are in the absence of pregnancy (however, see PRECAUTIONS, **Pregnancy**). Dependent edema in pregnancy, resulting from restriction of venous return by the expanded uterus, is properly treated through elevation of the lower extremities and use of support hose; use of diuretics to lower intravascular volume in this case is illogical and unnecessary. There is hypervolemia during normal pregnancy which is not harmful to either the fetus or the mother (in the absence of cardiovascular disease) but which is associated with edema, including generalized edema, in the majority of pregnant women. If this edema produces discomfort, increased recumbency will often provide relief. In rare instances, this edema may cause extreme discomfort which is not relieved by rest. In these cases, a short course of diuretics may provide relief and may be appropriate.

CONTRAINDICATIONS

Anuria; hypersensitivity to this or other sulfonamide-derived drugs.

WARNINGS

Use with caution in severe renal disease. In patients with renal disease, thiazides may precipitate azotemia. Cumulative effects of the drug may develop in patients with impaired renal function.

Thiazides should be used with caution in patients with impaired hepatic function or progressive liver disease, since minor alterations of fluid and electrolyte imbalance may precipitate hepatic coma.

Thiazides may add to or potentiate the action of other antihypertensive drugs. Potentiation occurs with ganglionic or peripheral adrenergic blocking drugs.

Sensitivity reactions are more likely to occur in patients with a history of allergy or bronchial asthma.

The possibility of exacerbation or activation of systemic lupus erythematosus has been reported.

PRECAUTIONS

General

All patients receiving thiazide therapy should be observed for clinical signs of fluid or electrolyte imbalance: namely, hyponatremia, hypochloremic alkalosis, and hypokalemia (see **Laboratory Tests** and **Drug/Drug Interactions**). Warning signs are dryness of mouth, thirst, weakness, lethargy, drowsiness, restlessness, muscle pains or cramps, muscular fatigue, hypotension, oliguria, tachycardia, and gastrointestinal disturbance such as nausea or vomiting.

Hypokalemia may develop, especially with brisk diuresis or when severe cirrhosis is present.

Interference with adequate oral intake of electrolytes will also contribute to hypokalemia. Hypokalemia may be avoided or treated by use of potassium supplements or foods with a high potassium content.

Any chloride deficit is generally mild and usually does not require specific treatment except under extraordinary circumstances (as in liver disease or renal disease). Dilutional hyponatremia may occur in edematous patients in hot weather; appropriate therapy is water restriction rather than administration of salt, except in rare instances when the hyponatremia is life-threatening. In actual salt depletion, appropriate replacement is the therapy of choice.

Hyperuricemia may occur or frank gout may be precipitated in certain patients receiving thiazide therapy.

Latent diabetes may become manifest during thiazide administration (see **Drug/Drug Interactions**).

The antihypertensive effects of the drug may be enhanced in the postsympathectomy patient.

If progressive renal impairment becomes evident, withholding or discontinuing diuretic therapy should be considered.

Calcium excretion is decreased by thiazides. Pathological changes in the parathyroid gland with hypercalcemia and hypophosphatemia have been observed in a few patients on prolonged thiazide therapy. The common complications of hyperparathyroidism such as renal lithiasis, bone resorption, and peptic ulceration have not been seen.

Information for Patients

Patients should be informed of possible side effects and advised to take the medication regularly and continuously as directed.

Laboratory Tests

Initial and periodic determinations of serum electrolytes to detect possible electrolyte imbalance should be performed at appropriate intervals.

Serum and urine electrolyte determinations are particularly important when the patient is vomiting excessively or receiving parenteral fluids.

Drug/Drug Interactions

Hypokalemia can sensitize or exaggerate the response of the heart to the toxic effects of digitalis (e.g., increased ventricular irritability).

Hypokalemia may develop during concomitant use of steroids or ACTH.

Insulin requirements in diabetic patients may be increased, decreased, or unchanged.

Thiazides may decrease arterial responsiveness to norepinephrine. This diminution is not sufficient to preclude effectiveness of the pressor agent for therapeutic use.

Thiazide drugs may increase the responsiveness to tubocurarine.

Lithium renal clearance is reduced by thiazides, increasing the risk of lithium toxicity.

Drug/Laboratory Test Interactions

Thiazides may decrease serum PBI levels without signs of thyroid disturbance.

Thiazides should be discontinued before carrying out tests for parathyroid function (see **Precautions, General**, calcium excretion).

Carcinogenesis, Mutagenesis, Impairment of Fertility

Long-term carcinogenicity studies in animals have not been conducted with Esidrix. Esidrix does not appear to possess mutagenic properties nor to inhibit animal fertility.

Pregnancy Category B

A reproduction study in rats receiving hydrochlorothiazide, 250 mg/kg/day, 62.5 times the maximum daily human dosage, has revealed no evidence of impaired fertility or harm to the fetus. There are, however, no adequate and well-controlled studies of Esidrix in pregnant women. Because animal reproduction studies are not always predictive of human response, Esidrix should be used during pregnancy only if clearly needed.

Nonteratogenic Effects. Thiazides cross the placental barrier and appear in cord blood, and there is a risk of fetal or neonatal jaundice, thrombocytopenia, and possibly other adverse reactions that have occurred in adults.

Nursing Mothers

Thiazides are excreted in breast milk. Because of the potential for serious adverse reactions in nursing infants, a decision should be made whether to discontinue nursing or to discontinue Esidrix, taking into account the importance of the drug to the mother.

Pediatric Use

Safety and effectiveness in children have not been established.

ADVERSE REACTIONS

Adverse reactions are usually reversible upon reduction of dosage or discontinuation of Esidrix. Whenever adverse reactions are moderate or severe, it may be necessary to discontinue the drug.

The following adverse reactions have been observed, but there has not been enough systematic collection of data to support an estimate of their frequency. Consequently the reactions are categorized by organ systems and are listed in decreasing order of severity and not frequency.

Digestive: Pancreatitis, jaundice (intrahepatic cholestatic), sialadenitis, vomiting, diarrhea, cramping, nausea, gastric irritation, constipation, anorexia.

Cardiovascular: Orthostatic hypotension (may be potentiated by alcohol, barbiturates, or narcotics).

Neurologic: Vertigo, dizziness, transient blurred vision, headache, paresthesia, xanthopsia, weakness, restlessness.

Musculoskeletal: Muscle spasm.

Hematologic: Aplastic anemia, agranulocytosis, leukopenia, thrombocytopenia.

Metabolic: Hyperglycemia, glycosuria, hyperuricemia.

Hypersensitive Reactions: Necrotizing angiitis, Stevens-Johnson syndrome, purpura, urticaria, rash, photosensitivity.

OVERDOSAGE

Acute Toxicity

No deaths due to acute poisoning with Esidrix have been reported.

Highest known doses ingested: children, 500 mg (14-year-old girl); young children, 125 mg (2½-year-old child).

Oral LD_{50} in rats: >2750 mg/kg.

Signs and Symptoms

The most prominent feature of poisoning with Esidrix is acute loss of fluid and electrolytes.

Cardiovascular: Tachycardia, hypotension, shock.

Neuromuscular: Weakness, confusion, dizziness, cramps of the calf muscles, paresthesia, fatigue, impairment of consciousness.

Gastrointestinal: Nausea, vomiting, thirst.

Renal: Polyuria, oliguria or anuria (due to hemoconcentration).

Laboratory findings: Hypokalemia, hyponatremia, hypochloremia, alkalosis, increased BUN (especially in patients with renal insufficiency).

Combined poisoning: Signs and symptoms may be aggravated or modified by concomitant intake of antihypertensive medication, barbiturates, curare, digitalis (hypokalemia), corticosteroids, narcotics, or alcohol.

Treatment

There is no specific antidote.

Elimination of the drug: Induction of vomiting, gastric lavage.

Measures to reduce absorption: Activated charcoal.

Hypotension, shock: The patient's legs should be kept raised, and lost fluid and electrolytes (potassium, sodium) should be replaced.

Surveillance: Fluid and electrolyte balance (especially serum potassium) and renal function should be monitored until conditions become normal.

DOSAGE AND ADMINISTRATION

Therapy should be individualized according to patient response. Dosage should be titrated to gain maximal therapeutic response as well as the minimal dose possible to maintain that therapeutic response.

Adults

Hypertension

To Initiate Therapy: Usual dosage is 50–100 mg daily. May be given as a single dose every morning.

Maintenance: After a week dosage may be adjusted downward to as little as 25 mg a day, or upward. Rarely patients may require up to 200 mg daily in divided doses.

Combined Therapy: When necessary, other antihypertensive agents may be added cautiously. Since this drug potentiates the antihypertensive effect of other agents, such additions should be gradual. Dosages of ganglionic blockers in particular should be halved initially.

Edema

To Initiate Diuresis: 25 to 200 mg daily for several days, or until dry weight is attained.

Maintenance: 25 to 100 mg daily or intermittently depending on the patient's response. A few refractory patients may require up to 200 mg daily.

Infants and Children

The usual pediatric dosage is administered twice daily. The total daily dosage for infants up to 2 years of age: 12.5 to 37.5 mg; for children 2 to 12 years of age: 37.5 to 100 mg. Dosage should be based on body weight at the rate of 1 mg per pound, but infants below 6 months of age may require 1.5 mg per pound.

HOW SUPPLIED

Tablets 25 mg—round, pink, scored (imprinted CIBA 22)
- Bottles of 100 .... NDC 0083-0022-30
- Bottles of 1000 .... NDC 0083-0022-40

Consumer Pack—One Unit
- 12 bottles—100 tablets each .... NDC 0083-0022-65

Accu-Pak® Unit Dose (blister pack)
- Box of 100 (strips of 10) .... NDC 0083-0022-32

Tablets 50 mg—round, yellow, scored (imprinted CIBA 46)
- Bottles of 100 .... NDC 0083-0046-30
- Bottles of 1000 .... NDC 0083-0046-40

Consumer Pack—One Unit
- 12 bottles—30 tablets each .... NDC 0083-0046-82
- 12 bottles—60 tablets each .... NDC 0083-0046-73
- 12 bottles—100 tablets each .... NDC 0083-0046-65

Accu-Pak® Unit Dose (blister pack)
- Box of 100 (strips of 10) .... NDC 0083-0046-32

Tablets 100 mg—round, blue, scored (imprinted CIBA 192)
- Bottles of 100 .... NDC 0083-0192-30

Dispense in tight, light-resistant container (USP).

C85-65 (Rev. 11/85)

Shown in Product Identification Section, page 408

ESIMIL® ℞

[ess 'a-mill]

guanethidine monosulfate USP 10 mg
hydrochlorothiazide USP 25 mg
Combination Tablets

WARNING

This fixed-combination drug is not indicated for initial therapy of hypertension. Hypertension requires therapy titrated to the individual patient. If the fixed combination represents the dosage so determined, its use may be more convenient in patient management. The treatment of hypertension is not static, but must be reevaluated as conditions in each patient warrant.

DESCRIPTION

Esimil is an antihypertensive-diuretic combination, available as tablets for oral administration. Each tablet contains Ismelin (guanethidine monosulfate USP), 10 mg, and Esidrix (hydrochlorothiazide USP), 25 mg.

Guanethidine monosulfate is [2-(hexahydro-1(2*H*)-azocinyl) ethyl]guanidine sulfate 1:1.

Guanethidine monosulfate USP is a white to off-white crystalline powder with a molecular weight of 296.38. It is very soluble in water, sparingly soluble in alcohol and practically insoluble in chloroform.

Hydrochlorothiazide is 6-chloro-3,4-dihydro-2*H*-1,2,4-benzothiadiazine-7-sulfonamide 1,1-dioxide.

Hydrochlorothiazide USP is a white, or practically white, practically odorless crystalline powder. It is slightly soluble in water; freely soluble in sodium hydroxide solution, in *n*-butylamine, and in dimethylformamide; sparingly soluble in methanol; and insoluble in ether, in chloroform, and in dilute mineral acids. Its molecular weight is 297.73.

Inactive Ingredients: Colloidal silicon dioxide, lactose, starch, stearic acid, and sucrose.

CLINICAL PHARMACOLOGY

Guanethidine

Guanethidine acts at the sympathetic neuroeffector junction by inhibiting or interfering with the release and/or distribution of the chemical mediator (presumably the catecholamine norepinephrine), rather than acting at the effector cell by inhibiting the association of the transmitter with its receptors. In contrast to ganglionic blocking agents, guanethidine suppresses equally the responses mediated by alpha- and beta-adrenergic receptors but does not produce parasympathetic blockade. Since sympathetic blockade results in modest decreases in peripheral resistance and cardiac output, guanethidine lowers blood pressure in the supine position. It further reduces blood pressure by decreasing the degree of vasoconstriction that normally results from reflex sympathetic nervous activity upon assumption of the upright posture, thus reducing venous return and cardiac output more. The inhibition of sympathetic venoconstrictive mechanisms results in venous pooling of blood. Therefore, the effect of guanethidine is especially pronounced when the patient is standing. Both the systolic and diastolic pressures are reduced.

Other actions at the sympathetic nerve terminal include depletion of norepinephrine. Once it gains access to the neuron, guanethidine accumulates within the intraneuronal storage vesicles and causes depletion of norepinephrine stores within the nerve terminal. Prolonged oral administration of guanethidine produces a denervation sensitivity of the neuroeffector junction, probably resulting from the chronic reduction in norepinephrine released by the sympathetic nerve endings. Systemic responses to catecholamines released from the adrenal medulla are not prevented and may even be augmented as a result of this denervation sensitivity. A paradoxical hypertensive crisis may occur if guanethidine is given to patients with pheochromocytoma or if norepinephrine is given to a patient receiving the drug.

Due to its poor lipid solubility, guanethidine does not readily cross the blood-brain barrier. In contrast to most neural blocking agents, guanethidine does not appear to suppress plasma renin activity in many patients.

Pharmacokinetics

The pharmacokinetics of guanethidine are complex. The amount of drug in plasma and in urine is linearly related to dose, although large differences occur between individuals because of variation in absorption and metabolism. Adrenergic blockade occurs with a minimum concentration in plasma of 8 ng/ml; this concentration is achieved in different individuals with doses of 10–50 mg per day at steady state. Guanethidine is eliminated slowly because of extensive tissue binding. After chronic oral administration, the initial phase of elimination with a half-life of 1.5 days is followed by a second phase of elimination with a half-life of 4–8 days. The renal clearance of guanethidine is 56 ml/min. Guanethidine is converted by the liver to three metabolites, which are excreted in the urine. The metabolites are pharmacologically less active than guanethidine.

Hydrochlorothiazide

Thiazides affect the renal tubular mechanism of electrolyte reabsorption. At maximal therapeutic dosage, all thiazides are approximately equal in their diuretic potency. Thiazides increase excretion of sodium and chloride in approximately equivalent amounts. Natriuresis causes a secondary loss of potassium.

The mechanism of the antihypertensive effect of thiazides is unknown. Thiazides do not affect normal blood pressure.

Pharmacokinetics

The onset of action of thiazides occurs in 2 hours, and the peak effect at about 4 hours. The action persists for approximately 6–12 hours. Hydrochlorothiazide is rapidly absorbed, as indicated by peak plasma concentrations 1–2.5 hours after oral administration. Plasma levels of the drug are proportional to dose; the concentration in whole blood is 1.6–1.8 times higher than in plasma. Thiazides are eliminated rapidly by the kidney. After oral administration of 25- to 100-mg doses of hydrochlorothiazide, 72–97% of the dose is excreted in the urine, indicating dose-independent absorption. Hydrochlorothiazide is eliminated from plasma in a biphasic fashion with a terminal half-life of 10–17 hours. Plasma protein binding is 67.9%. Plasma clearance is 15.9–30.0 L/hr; volume of distribution is 3.6–7.8 L/kg.

Gastrointestinal absorption of hydrochlorothiazide is enhanced when administered with food. Absorption is decreased in patients with congestive heart failure, and the pharmacokinetics are considerably different in these patients.

INDICATIONS

Esimil is indicated for the treatment of hypertension (see boxed **WARNING**).

CONTRAINDICATIONS

Guanethidine

Known or suspected pheochromocytoma; hypersensitivity; frank congestive heart failure not due to hypertension; use of MAO inhibitors.

Hydrochlorothiazide

Anuria; hypersensitivity to this or other sulfonamide-derived drugs.

WARNINGS

Guanethidine and hydrochlorothiazide are potent drugs and their use can lead to disturbing and serious clinical problems. Physicians should be familiar with both drugs and their combination before prescribing, and patients should be warned not to deviate from instructions.

Guanethidine

> Orthostatic hypotension can occur frequently and patients should be properly instructed about this potential hazard. Fainting spells may occur unless the patient is forewarned to sit or lie down with the onset of dizziness or weakness. Postural hypotension is most marked in the morning and is accentuated by hot weather, alcohol, or exercise. Dizziness or weakness may be particularly bothersome during the initial period of dosage adjustment and with postural changes, such as arising in the morning. The potential occurrence of these symptoms may require alteration of previous daily activity. The patient should be cautioned to avoid sudden or prolonged standing or exercise while taking the drug.

Inhibition of ejaculation has been reported in animals (see **PRECAUTIONS, Carcinogenesis, Mutagenesis, Impairment of Fertility**) as well as in men given guanethidine. This effect, which results from the sympathetic blockade caused by the drug's action, is reversible after guanethidine has been discontinued for several weeks. The drug does not cause parasympathetic blockade, and erectile potency is usually retained during administration of guanethidine. The possible occurrence of inhibition of ejaculation should be kept in mind when considering the use of guanethidine in men of reproductive age.

If possible, therapy should be withdrawn 2 weeks prior to surgery to reduce the possibility of vascular collapse and cardiac arrest during anesthesia. If emergency surgery is indicated, preanesthetic and anesthetic agents should be administered cautiously in reduced dosage. Oxyg;en, atropine, vasopressors, and adequate solutions for volume replacement should be ready for immediate use to counteract vascular collapse in the surgical patient. Vasopressors should be used only with extreme caution, since guanethidine augments responsiveness to exogenously administered norepinephrine and vasopressors; specifically, blood pressure may rise and cardiac arrhythmias may be produced.

Hydrochlorothiazide

Thiazides should be used with caution in patients with severe renal disease. In patients with renal disease, thiazides may precipitate azotemia. Cumulative effects of the drug may develop in patients with impaired renal function.

Thiazides should be used with caution in patients with impaired hepatic function or progressive liver disease, since minor alterations of fluid and electrolyte imbalance may precipitate hepatic coma.

Thiazides may add to or potentiate the action of other antihypertensive drugs. Potentiation occurs with ganglionic or peripheral adrenergic blocking drugs.

Sensitivity reactions are more likely to occur in patients with a history of allergy or bronchial asthma.

The possibility of exacerbation or activation of systemic lupus erythematosus has been reported.

PRECAUTIONS

General

Guanethidine. Dosage requirements may be reduced in the presence of fever.

Special care should be exercised when treating patients with a history of bronchial asthma; asthmatic patients are more apt to be hypersensitive to catecholamine depletion, and their condition may be aggravated.

The effects of guanethidine are cumulative over long periods; initial doses should be small and increased gradually in small increments.

Guanethidine should be used very cautiously in hypertensive patients with: renal disease and nitrogen retention or rising BUN levels, since decreased blood pressure may further compromise renal function; coronary insufficiency or recent myocardial infarction; and cerebrovascular disease, especially with encephalopathy.

Guanethidine should not be given to patients with severe cardiac failure except with extreme caution, since guanethidine may interfere with the compensatory role of the adrenergic system in producing circulatory adjustment in patients with congestive heart failure.

Patients with incipient cardiac decompensation should be watched for weight gain or edema.

Guanethidine should be used cautiously in patients with a history of peptic ulcer or other chronic disorders that may be aggravated by a relative increase in parasympathetic tone.

Hydrochlorothiazide. All patients receiving thiazide therapy should be observed for clinical signs of fluid or electrolyte imbalance, namely hyponatremia, hypochloremic alkalosis, and hypokalemia (see **Laboratory Tests** and **Drug/Drug Interactions**). Warning signs are dryness of mouth, thirst, weakness, lethargy, drowsiness, restlessness, muscle pains or cramps, muscular fatigue, hypotension, oliguria, tachycardia, and gastrointestinal disturbance, such as nausea or vomiting.

Hypokalemia may develop, especially in cases of brisk diuresis or severe cirrhosis.

Interference with adequate oral intake of electrolytes will also contribute to hypokalemia. Hypokalemia may be avoided or treated by use of potassium supplements or foods with a high potassium content.

Any chloride deficit is generally mild and usually does not require specific treatment, except under extraordinary circumstances (as in liver disease or renal disease). Dilutional hyponatremia may occur in edematous patients in hot weather; appropriate therapy is water restriction, rather than administration of salt, except in rare instances when the hyponatremia is life-threatening. In cases of actual salt depletion, appropriate replacement is the therapy of choice.

Hyperuricemia may occur or frank gout may be precipitated in certain patients receiving thiazide therapy.

Latent diabetes may become manifest during thiazide administration (see **Drug/Drug Interactions**).

The antihypertensive effects of the drug may be enhanced in the postsympathectomy patient.

If progressive renal impairment becomes evident, withholding or discontinuing diuretic therapy should be considered.

Calcium excretion is decreased by thiazides. Pathological changes in the parathyroid gland with hypercalcemia and hypophosphatemia have been observed in a few patients on prolonged thiazide therapy. The common complications of hyperparathyroidism, such as renal lithiasis, bone resorption, and peptic ulceration, have not been seen.

Information for Patients

The patient should be advised to take this medication exactly as directed. If the patient misses a dose, he or she should be told to take only the next scheduled dose (without doubling it).

The patient should be advised to avoid sudden or prolonged standing or exercise and to arise slowly, especially in the morning, to reduce the orthostatic hypotensive effects of dizziness, lightheadedness, or fainting.

The patient should be cautioned about ingesting alcohol, since it aggravates the orthostatic hypotensive effects of guanethidine.

Male patients should be advised that guanethidine may interfere with ejaculation.

Laboratory Tests

Hydrochlorothiazide. Initial and periodic determinations of serum electrolytes to detect possible electrolyte imbalance should be performed at appropriate intervals.

Serum and urine electrolyte determinations are particularly important when the patient is vomiting excessively or receiving parenteral fluids.

Drug/Drug Interactions

Guanethidine. Concurrent use of guanethidine and rauwolfia derivatives may cause excessive postural hypotension, bradycardia, and mental depression.

Both digitalis and guanethidine slow the heart rate.

Amphetamine-like compounds, stimulants (e.g., ephedrine, methylphenidate), tricyclic antidepressants (e.g., amitriptyline, imipramine, desipramine) and other psychopharmacologic agents (e.g., phenothiazines and related compounds), as well as oral contraceptives, may reduce the hypotensive effect of guanethidine.

Continued on next page

The full prescribing information for each CIBA drug is contained herein and is that in effect as of September 1, 1986

CIBA—Cont.

MAO inhibitors should be discontinued for at least 1 week before starting therapy with guanethidine.

Hydrochlorothiazide. Hypokalemia can sensitize or exaggerate the response of the heart to the toxic effects of digitalis (e.g., increased ventricular irritability).

Hypokalemia may develop during concomitant use of steroids or ACTH.

Insulin requirements in diabetic patients may be increased, decreased, or unchanged.

Thiazides may decrease arterial responsiveness to norepinephrine, but not enough to preclude effectiveness of the pressor agent for therapeutic use.

Thiazides may increase the responsiveness to tubocurarine.

Lithium renal clearance is reduced by thiazides, increasing the risk of lithium toxicity.

Drug/Laboratory Test Interactions

Thiazides may decrease serum levels of protein-bound iodine without signs of thyroid disturbance. Esimil should be discontinued before tests for parathyroid function are made (see **General, Hydrochlorothiazide,** Calcium excretion).

Carcinogenesis, Mutagenesis, Impairment of Fertility

Long-term carcinogenicity studies in animals have not been conducted with Esimil.

While inhibition of sperm passage and accumulation of sperm debris have been reported in rats and rabbits after several weeks of administration of guanethidine, 5 or 10 mg/kg per day, subcutaneously or intraperitoneally, recovery of ejaculatory function and fertility has been demonstrated in rats given guanethidine intramuscularly, 25 mg/kg per day, for 8 weeks. Inhibition of ejaculation has also been reported in men (see **WARNINGS** and **ADVERSE REACTIONS**). This effect, which is attributable to the sympathetic blockade caused by the drug, is reversible several weeks after discontinuance of the drug.

Pregnancy Category B

A reproduction study performed in rats receiving doses at least 150 times the average daily human dose of Esimil has revealed no evidence of impaired fertility or harm to the fetus due to this drug.

There are no adequate and well-controlled studies of Esimil in pregnant women. Because animal reproduction studies are not always predictive of human response, this drug should be used during pregnancy only if clearly needed.

Nonteratogenic Effects. Thiazides cross the placental barrier and appear in cord blood, and there is a risk of fetal or neonatal jaundice, thrombocytopenia, and possibly other adverse reactions that have occurred in adults.

Nursing Mothers

Guanethidine is excreted in breast milk in very small quantity. Thiazides are also excreted in breast milk. Because of the potential for serious adverse reactions in nursing infants, a decision should be made whether to discontinue nursing or to discontinue Esimil, taking into account the importance of the drug to the mother.

Pediatric Use

Safety and effectiveness of the combination drug in children have not been established.

ADVERSE REACTIONS

Whenever adverse reactions are moderate or severe, it may be necessary to reduce the dosage of Esimil, discontinue the drug, or administer the individual active components, reducing the dosage of either quanethidine or hydrochlorothiazide.

The following adverse reactions have been observed, but there are not enough data to support an estimate of their frequency. Consequently the reactions are categorized by organ system and are listed in decreasing order of severity and not frequency.

Guanethidine

Digestive: Diarrhea, which may be severe at times and necessitate discontinuance of medication; vomiting; nausea; increased bowel movements; dry mouth; parotid tenderness.

Cardiovascular: Chest pains (angina); bradycardia; a tendency toward fluid retention and edema with occasional development of congestive heart failure.

Respiratory: Dyspnea; asthma in susceptible individuals; nasal congestion.

Neurologic: Syncope resulting from either postural or exertional hypotension; dizziness; blurred vision; muscle tremor; ptosis of the lids; mental depression; chest paresthesias; weakness; lassitude; fatigue.

Muscular: Myalgia.

Genitourinary: Rise in BUN; urinary incontinence; inhibition of ejaculation; nocturia.

Metabolic: Weight gain.

Skin and Appendages: Dermatitis; scalp hair loss.

Although a causal relationship has not been established, a few instances of blood dyscrasias (anemia, thrombocytopenia, and leukopenia) and of priapism or impotence have been reported.

Hydrochlorothiazide

Digestive: Pancreatitis, jaundice (intrahepatic cholestatic), sialadenitis, vomiting, diarrhea, cramping, nausea, gastric irritation, constipation, anorexia.

Cardiovascular: Orthostatic hypotension (may be potentiated by alcohol, barbiturates, or narcotics).

Neurologic: Vertigo, dizziness, transient blurred vision, headache, paresthesia, xanthopsia, weakness, restlessness.

Musculoskeletal: Muscle spasm.

Hematologic: Aplastic anemia, agranulocytosis, leukopenia, thrombocytopenia.

Metabolic: Hyperglycemia, glycosuria, hyperuricemia.

Hypersensitive Reactions: Necrotizing angitis, Stevens-Johnson syndrome, purpura, urticaria, rash, photosensitivity.

OVERDOSAGE

Acute Toxicity

No deaths due to acute poisoning with Esimil have been reported.

Oral LD_{50}'s in rats (mg/kg): guanethidine, 1262; hydrochlorothiazide, 2750.

Signs and Symptoms

Guanethidine. Postural hypotension (with dizziness, blurred vision, and possibly syncope when standing), shock, and bradycardia are most likely to occur; diarrhea (possibly severe), nausea, and vomiting may also occur. Unconsciousness is unlikely if adequate blood pressure and cerebral perfusion can be maintained by placing the patient in the supine position and by administering other treatment as required.

Hydrochlorothiazide. The most prominent feature of poisoning is acute loss of fluid and electrolytes.

Cardiovascular: Tachycardia, hypotension, shock.

Neuromuscular: Weakness, confusion, dizziness, cramps of the calf muscles, paresthesia, fatigue, impairment of consciousness.

Digestive: Nausea, vomiting, thirst.

Renal: Polyuria, oliguria, or anuria (due to hemoconcentration).

Laboratory Findings: Hypokalemia, hyponatremia, hypochloremia, alkalosis; increased BUN (especially in patients with renal insufficiency).

Combined Poisoning: Signs and symptoms may be aggravated or modified by concomitant intake of antihypertensive medication, barbiturates, digitalis (hypokalemia), corticosteroids, narcotics, or alcohol.

Treatment

There is no specific antidote.

The stomach contents should be evaculated. An activated charcoal slurry should be instilled and laxative given, if conditions permit.

If hypotension or shock occurs, the patient's legs should be kept raised, and lost fluid and electrolytes (potassium, sodium) should be replaced. Renal function should be monitored until conditions become normal.

In sinus bradycardia, atropine should be administered.

In previously normotensive patients, treatment has consisted essentially of restoring blood pressure and heart rate to normal by keeping the patient in the supine position. Normal homeostatic control usually returns gradually over a 72-hour period in these patients.

In previously hypertensive patients, particularly those with impaired cardiac reserve or other cardiovascular-renal disease, intensive treatment may be required to support vital functions and to control cardiac irregularities that might be present. The supine position must be maintained; if vasopressors are required, they must be used with extreme caution, since guanethidine may increase responsiveness, causing a rise in blood pressure and development of cardiac arrhythmias.

Diarrhea, if severe or persistent, should be treated with anticholinergic agents to reduce intestinal hypermotility, and hydration and electrolyte balance should be maintained.

Since guanethidine is excreted slowly, cardiovascular and renal function should be monitored for a few days.

DOSAGE AND ADMINISTRATION

Dosage should be determined by individual titration (see boxed **WARNING**).

The usual dosage of Esimil is two tablets daily. Depending upon the degree of hypertension, the patient should be started on the lowest possible dose (usually one tablet daily) and the dose gradually increased at weekly intervals until the desired response is obtained. Blood pressure should be recorded with the patient in the supine position and again after 10 minutes of standing. Dosage should be increased only if the standing blood pressure has not been reduced to desired levels. Dosage adjustment should be made at not less than weekly intervals; maximal dosage should not exceed four tablets daily. If additional effect is desirable, guanethidine tablets may be supplemented individually.

Before starting therapy with Esimil, at least 1 week should elapse after MAO inhibitors (see **CONTRAINDICATIONS**) or ganglionic blockers are discontinued.

When Esimil is to be substituted for other antihypertensive agents, the change should be made gradually. In general, dosage of the agent to be discontinued should be halved, and Esimil should be started at one tablet daily. This schedule should be followed for at least 1 week; then, dosage of the previous therapy may be halved again and the dosage of Esimil increased to two tablets daily. At the next weekly interval, the previously used drugs can generally be discontinued. The dosage of Esimil should be titrated at weekly intervals, as mentioned above.

Patients receiving more than 75 mg of guanethidine alone may do well on a smaller dose if also given hydrochlorothiazide. Because of the ratio of the combination, these patients are probably not candidates for Esimil.

HOW SUPPLIED

Tablets—round, white, scored (imprinted CIBA 47)
10 mg guanethidine monosulfate
25 mg hydrochlorothiazide
Bottles of 100 ....NDC 0083-0047-30
Consumer Pack—One Unit
12 bottles—
100 tablets each ....NDC 0083-0047-65

Dispense in tight container (USP) *C86-3 (Rev. 1/86)*

Shown in Product Identification Section, page 408

INH isoniazid USP ℞
Tablets

WARNING

Severe and sometimes fatal hepatitis associated with isoniazid therapy may occur and may develop even after many months of treatment. The risk of developing hepatitis is age related. Approximate case rates by age are: 0 per 1,000 for persons under 20 years of age, 3 per 1,000 for persons in the 20–34 year age group, 12 per 1,000 for persons in the 35–49 year age group, 23 per 1,000 for persons in the 50–64 year age group, and 8 per 1,000 for persons over 65 years of age. The risk of hepatitis is increased with daily consumption of alcohol. Precise data to provide a fatality rate for isoniazid-related hepatitis is not available; however, in a U.S. Public Health Service Surveillance Study of 13,838 persons taking isoniazid, there were 8 deaths among 174 cases of hepatitis.

Therefore, patients given isoniazid should be carefully monitored and interviewed at monthly intervals. Serum transaminase concentration becomes elevated in about 10–20 percent of patients, usually during the first few months of therapy but it can occur at any time. Usually enzyme levels return to normal despite continuance of drug but in some cases progressive liver dysfunction occurs. Patients should be instructed to report immediately any of the prodromal symptoms of hepatitis, such as fatigue, weakness, malaise, anorexia, nausea, or vomiting. If these symptoms appear or if signs suggestive of hepatic damage are detected, isoniazid should be discontinued promptly, since continued use of the drug in these cases has been reported to cause a more severe form of liver damage.

Patients with tuberculosis should be given appropriate treatment with alternative drugs. If isoniazid must be reinstituted, it should be reinstituted only after symptoms and laboratory abnormalities have cleared. The drug should be restarted in very small and gradually increasing doses and should be withdrawn immediately if there is any indication of recurrent liver involvement.

Preventive treatment should be deferred in persons with acute hepatic diseases.

DESCRIPTION

INH, isoniazid USP, is an antibiotic available as 300-mg tablets for oral administration. It is also available in Dual Packs of Rimactane® rifampin USP/INH containing one 300-mg tablet of INH and two 300-mg capsules of Rimactane. Isoniazid is isonicotinic acid hydrazide.

Isoniazid USP is a colorless or white crystalline powder or white crystals. It is odorless and slowly affected by exposure to air and light. It is freely soluble in water, sparingly soluble in alcohol, and slightly soluble in chloroform and in ether. Its molecular weight is 137.14.

Inactive Ingredients. Cellulose compounds, colloidal silicon dioxide, sodium starch glycolate, and stearic acid.

ACTIONS

Isoniazid acts against actively growing tubercle bacilli.

Within 1 to 2 hours after oral administration isoniazid produces peak blood levels which decline to 50% or less within 6 hours. It diffuses readily into all body fluids (cerebrospinal, pleural, and ascitic fluids), tissues, organs, and excreta (saliva, sputum, and feces). The drug also passes through the placental barrier and into milk in concentrations comparable to those in the plasma. From 50 to 70% of a dose of isoniazid is excreted in the urine in 24 hours.

Isoniazid is metabolized primarily by acetylation and dehydrazination. The rate of acetylation is genetically deter-

mined. Approximately 50% of Blacks and Caucasians are "slow inactivators" and the rest are rapid inactivators; the majority of Eskimos and Orientals are "rapid inactivators." The rate of acetylation does not significantly alter the effectiveness of isoniazid. However, slow acetylation may lead to higher blood levels of the drug, and thus an increase in toxic reactions.
Pyridoxine (B_6) deficiency is sometimes observed in adults with high doses of isoniazid and is considered probably due to its competition with pyridoxal phosphate for the enzyme apotryptophanase.

INDICATIONS

For all forms of tuberculosis in which organisms are susceptible.
For preventive therapy for the following groups, in order of priority:
1. Household members and other close associates of persons with recently diagnosed tuberculous disease.
2. Positive tuberculin skin test reactors with findings on the chest roentgenogram consistent with nonprogressive tuberculous disease, in whom there are neither positive bacteriologic findings nor a history of adequate chemotherapy.
3. Newly infected persons.
4. Positive tuberculin skin test reactors in the following special clinical situations: prolonged therapy with adrenocorticosteroids; immunosuppressive therapy; some hematologic and reticuloendothelial diseases, such as leukemia or Hodgkin's disease; diabetes mellitus; silicosis; after gastrectomy.
5. Other positive tuberculin reactors under 35 years of age.

The risk of hepatitis must be weighed against the risk of tuberculosis in positive tuberculin reactors over the age of 35. However, the use of isoniazid is recommended for those with the additional risk factors listed above (1–4) and on an individual basis in situations where there is likelihood of serious consequences to contacts who may become infected.

CONTRAINDICATIONS

Isoniazid is contraindicated in patients who develop severe hypersensitivity reactions, including drug-induced hepatitis.
Previous isoniazid-associated hepatic injury: severe adverse reactions to isoniazid, such as drug fever, chills, and arthritis; acute liver disease of any etiology.

WARNINGS

See the boxed warning.
Ophthalmologic examinations (including ophthalmoscopy) should be done *before* INH is started and periodically thereafter, even without occurrence of visual symptoms.

Carcinogenesis

Isoniazid has been reported to induce pulmonary tumors in a number of strains of mice.

Usage in Pregnancy and Lactation

It has been reported that in both rats and rabbits, isoniazid may exert an embryocidal effect when administered orally during pregnancy, although no isoniazid-related congenital anomalies have been found in reproduction studies in mammalian species (mice, rats, and rabbits). Isoniazid should be prescribed during pregnancy only when therapeutically necessary. The benefit of preventive therapy should be weighed against a possible risk to the fetus. Preventive treatment generally should be started after delivery because of the increased risk of tuberculosis for new mothers.
Since isoniazid is known to cross the placental barrier and to pass into maternal breast milk, neonates and breast-fed infants of isoniazid-treated mothers should be carefully observed for any evidence of adverse effects.

PRECAUTIONS

Use of isoniazid should be carefully monitored in the following:
1. Patients who are receiving phenytoin concurrently. Isoniazid may decrease the excretion of phenytoin or may enhance its effects. To avoid phenytoin intoxication, appropriate adjustment of the anticonvulsant should be made.
2. Daily users of alcohol. Daily ingestion of alcohol may be associated with a higher incidence of isoniazid hepatitis.
3. Patients with current chronic liver disease or severe renal dysfunction.

ADVERSE REACTIONS

The most frequent reactions are those affecting the nervous system and the liver.
Nervous system reactions: Peripheral neuropathy is the most common toxic effect. It is dose-related, occurs most often in the malnourished and in those predisposed to neuritis (*eg,* alcoholics and diabetics), and is usually preceded by paresthesias of the feet and hands. The incidence is higher in "slow inactivators."
Other neurotoxic effects, which are uncommon with conventional doses, are convulsions, toxic encephalopathy, optic neuritis and atrophy, memory impairment, and toxic psychosis.
Gastrointestinal reactions: Nausea, vomiting, epigastric distress.
Hepatic reactions: Elevated serum transaminases (SGOT; SGPT), bilirubinemia, bilirubinuria, jaundice and occasionally severe and sometimes fatal hepatitis. The common prodromal symptoms are anorexia, nausea, vomiting, fatigue, malaise, and weakness. Mild and transient elevation of serum transaminase levels, occurs in 10 to 20 percent of persons taking isoniazid. The abnormality usually occurs in the first 4 to 6 months of treatment but can occur at any time during therapy. In most instances, enzyme levels return to normal with no necessity to discontinue medication. In occasional instances, progressive liver damage occurs, with accompanying symptoms. In these cases, the drug should be discontinued immediately. The frequency of progressive liver damage increases with age. It is rare in persons under 20, but occurs in up to 2.3 percent of those over 50 years of age.
Hematologic reactions: Agranulocytosis; hemolytic, sideroblastic, or aplastic anemia; thrombocytopenia; and eosinophilia.
Hypersensitivity reactions: Fever, skin eruptions (morbilliform, maculopapular, purpuric, or exfoliative), lymphadenopathy and vasculitis.
Metabolic and endocrine reactions: Pyridoxine deficiency, pellagra, hyperglycemia, metabolic acidosis, and gynecomastia
Miscellaneous reactions: Rheumatic syndrome and systemic lupus erythematosus-like syndrome.

OVERDOSAGE

Signs and Symptoms

Isoniazid overdosage produces signs and symptoms within 30 minutes to 3 hours after ingestion. Nausea, vomiting, dizziness, slurring of speech, blurring of vision, and visual hallucinations (including bright colors and strange designs), are among the early manifestations. With marked overdosage, respiratory distress and CNS depression, progressing rapidly from stupor to profound coma, are to be expected, along with severe, intractable seizures. Severe metabolic acidosis, acetonuria, and hyperglycemia are typical laboratory findings.

Treatment

Untreated or inadequately treated cases of gross isoniazid overdosage can terminate fatally, but good response has been reported in most patients brought under adequate treatment within the first few hours after drug ingestion.
Secure the airway and establish adequate respiratory exchange. Gastric lavage within the first 2 to 3 hours is advised, but should not be attempted until convulsions are under control. To control convulsions administer I.V. short-acting barbiturates and I.V. pyridoxine (usually 1 mg/1mg isoniazid ingested).
Obtain blood samples for immediate determination of gases, electrolytes, BUN, glucose, etc.; type and crossmatch blood in preparation for possible hemodialysis.
Rapid control of metabolic acidosis is fundamental to management. Give I.V. sodium bicarbonate at once and repeat as needed, adjusting subsequent dosage on the basis of laboratory findings (*ie,* serum sodium, pH, etc.).
Forced osmotic diuresis must be started early and should be continued for some hours after clinical improvement to hasten renal clearance of drug and help prevent relapse; monitor fluid intake and output.
Hemodialysis is advised for severe cases; if this is not available, peritoneal dialysis can be used along with forced diuresis.
Along with measures based on initial and repeated determination of blood gases and other laboratory tests as needed, utilize meticulous respiratory and other intensive care to protect against hypoxia, hypotension, aspiration pneumonitis, etc.

DOSAGE AND ADMINISTRATION (See also INDICATIONS):

NOTE—For preventive therapy of tuberculous infection it is recommended that physicians be familiar with the joint recommendations of the American Thoracic Society, American Lung Association, and the Center for Disease Control, as published in the American Review of Respiratory Diseases Vol. 110, No. 3, September 1974, or CDC's Morbidity and Mortality Weekly Report, Vol. 24, No. 8, February 22, 1975.
For treatment of active tuberculosis: Isoniazid is used in conjunction with other effective antituberculous agents.
If the bacilli become resistant, therapy must be changed to agents to which the bacilli are susceptible.

Usual oral dosage

Adults: 5 mg/kg up to 300 mg daily in a single dose.
Infants and children: 10–20 mg/kg depending on severity of infection, (up to 300–500 mg daily) in a single dose.

For preventive therapy

Adults: 300 mg/day in a single dose.
Infants and children: 10 mg/kg (up to 300 mg daily) in a single dose.
Continuous administration of isoniazid for a sufficient period is an essential part of the regimen because relapse rates are higher if chemotherapy is stopped prematurely. In the treatment of tuberculosis, resistant organisms may multiply and the emergence of resistant organisms during the treatment may necessitate a change in the regimen.
Concomitant administration of pyridoxine (B_6) is recommended in the malnourished and in those predisposed to neuropathy (*eg,* alcoholics and diabetics).

HOW SUPPLIED

Tablets, 300 mg (white, scored); available as Rimactane® rifampin USP/INH Dual Pack containing 30 INH Tablets and 60 Rimactane 300-mg Capsules.
Protect from heat, light and moisture (Rimactane/INH Dual Pack).

C85-61 (Rev. 11/85)

ISMELIN® sulfate ℞

[*iz 'mel-lin*]
guanethidine monosulfate
Tablets

DESCRIPTION

Ismelin, guanethidine monosulfate, is an antihypertensive, available as tablets of 10 mg and 25 mg for oral administration. Each 10-mg and 25-mg tablet contains guanethidine monosulfate equivalent to 10 mg and 25 mg of guanethidine sulfate, USP. Its chemical name is [2-hexahydro-1(*2H*)-azocinyl)ethyl]guanidine sulfate 1:1.
Guanethidine monosulfate is a white to off-white crystalline powder with a molecular weight of 296.38. It is very soluble in water, sparingly soluble in alcohol, and practically insoluble in chloroform.

Inactive ingredients: Calcium stearate, colloidal silicon dioxide, D&C Yellow No. 10 (10-mg tablets), lactose, starch, stearic acid, and sucrose.

CLINICAL PHARMACOLOGY

Ismelin acts at the sympathetic neuroeffector junction by inhibiting or interfering with the release and/or distribution of the chemical mediator (presumably the catecholamine norepinephrine), rather than acting at the effector cell by inhibiting the association of the transmitter with its receptors. In contrast to ganglionic blocking agents, Ismelin suppresses equally the responses mediated by alpha- and beta-adrenergic receptors but does not produce parasympathetic blockade. Since sympathetic blockade results in modest decreases in peripheral resistance and cardiac output, Ismelin lowers blood pressure in the supine position. It further reduces blood pressure by decreasing the degree of vasoconstriction that normally results from reflex sympathetic nervous activity upon assumption of the upright posture, thus reducing venous return and cardiac output more. The inhibition of sympathetic venoconstrictive mechanisms results in venous pooling of blood. Therefore, the effect of Ismelin is especially pronounced when the patient is standing. Both the systolic and diastolic pressures are reduced.
Other actions at the sympathetic nerve terminal include depletion of norepinephrine. Once it gains access to the neuron, Ismelin accumulates within the intraneuronal storage vesicles and causes depletion of norepinephrine stores within the nerve terminal. Prolonged oral administration of Ismelin produces a denervation sensitivity of the neuroeffector junction, probably resulting from the chronic reduction in norepinephrine released by the sympathetic nerve endings. Systemic responses to catecholamines released from the adrenal medulla are not prevented and may even be augmented as a result of this denervation sensitivity. A paradoxical hypertensive crisis may occur if Ismelin is given to patients with pheochromocytoma or if norepinephrine is given to a patient receiving the drug.
Due to its poor lipid solubility, Ismelin does not readily cross the blood-brain barrier. In contrast to most neural blocking agents. Ismelin does not appear to suppress plasma renin activity in many patients.

Pharmacokinetics

The pharmacokinetics of Ismelin are complex. The amount of drug in plasma and in urine is linearly related to dose although large differences occur between individuals because of variation in absorption and metabolism. Adrenergic blockade occurs with a minimum concentration in plasma of 8 ng/ml; this concentration is achieved in different individuals with dosages of 10–50 mg day at steady state. Ismelin is eliminated slowly because of extensive tissue binding. After chronic oral administration, the initial phase of elimination with a half-life of 1.5 days is followed by a second phase of elimination with a half-life of 4–8 days. The renal clearance of Ismelin is 56 ml/min. Ismelin is converted by the liver to three metabolites, which are excreted in the urine. The metabolites are pharmacologically less active than Ismelin.

Continued on next page

The full prescribing information for each CIBA drug is contained herein and is that in effect as of September 1, 1986

CIBA—Cont.

INDICATIONS

Ismelin is indicated for the treatment of moderate and severe hypertension, either alone or as an adjunct, and for the treatment of renal hypertension, including that secondary to pyelonephritis, renal amyloidosis, and renal artery stenosis.

CONTRAINDICATIONS

Known or suspected pheochromocytoma, hypersensitivity; frank congestive heart failure not due to hypertension, use of monoamine oxidase (MAO) inhibitors.

WARNINGS

Ismelin is a potent drug and its use can lead to disturbing and serious clinical problems. Before prescribing, physicians should familiarize themselves with the details of its use and warn patients not to deviate from instructions.

> Orthostatic hypotension can occur frequently, and patients should be properly instructed about this potential hazard. Fainting spells may occur unless the patient is forewarned to sit or lie down with the onset of dizziness or weakness. Postural hypotension is most marked in the morning and is accentuated by hot weather, alcohol, or exercise. Dizziness or weakness may be particularly bothersome during the initial period of dosage adjustment and with postural changes, such as arising in the morning. The potential occurrence of these symptoms may require alteration of previous daily activity. The patient should be cautioned to avoid sudden or prolonged standing or exercise while taking the drug.

Inhibition of ejaculation has been reported in animals (see **PRECAUTIONS, Carcinogenesis, Mutagenesis, Impairment of Fertility**) as well as in men given Ismelin. This effect, which results from the sympathetic blockade caused by the drug's action, is reversible after Ismelin has been discontinued for several weeks. The drug does not cause parasympathetic blockade, and erectile potency is usually retained during administration of Ismelin. The possible occurrence of inhibition of ejaculation should be kept in mind when considering the use of guanethidine in men of reproductive age.

If possible, therapy should be withdrawn 2 weeks prior to surgery to reduce the possibility of vascular collapse and cardiac arrest during anesthesia. If emergency surgery is indicated, preanesthetic and anesthetic agents should be administered cautiously in reduced dosage. Oxygen, atropine, vasopressors, and adequate solutions for volume replacement should be ready for immediate use to counteract vascular collapse in the surgical patient. Vasopressors should be used only with extreme caution, since Ismelin augments responsiveness to exogenously administered norepinephrine and vasopressors; specifically, blood pressure may rise and cardiac arrhythmias may be produced.

PRECAUTIONS

General

Dosage requirements may be reduced in the presence of fever.

Special care should be exercised when treating patients with a history of bronchial asthma; asthmatic patients are more apt to be hypersensitive to catecholamine depletion, and their condition may be aggravated.

The effects of Ismelin are cumulative over long periods; initial doses should be small and increased gradually in small increments.

Ismelin should be used very cautiously in hypertensive patients with renal disease and nitrogen retention or rising BUN levels, since decreased blood pressure may further compromise renal function, coronary insufficiency or recent myocardial infarction; and cerebrovascular disease, especially with encephalopathy.

Ismelin should not be given to patients with severe cardiac failure except with extreme caution, since Ismelin may interfere with the compensatory role of the adrenergic system in producing circulatory adjustment in patients with congestive heart failure.

Patients with incipient cardiac decompensation should be watched for weight gain or edema, which may be averted by the concomitant administration of a thiazide.

Ismelin should be used cautiously in patients with a history of peptic ulcer or other chronic disorders that may be aggravated by a relative increase in parasympathetic tone.

Information for Patients

The patient should be advised to take Ismelin exactly as directed. If the patient misses a dose, he or she should be told to take only the next scheduled dose (without doubling it).

The patient should be advised to avoid sudden or prolonged standing or exercise and to arise slowly, especially in the morning, to reduce the orthostatic hypotensive effects of dizziness, lightheadedness, or fainting.

The patient should be cautioned about ingesting alcohol, since it aggravates the orthostatic hypotensive effects of Ismelin.

Male patients should be advised that guanethidine may interfere with ejaculation.

Drug Interactions

Concurrent use of Ismelin and rauwolfia derivatives may cause excessive postural hypotension, bradycardia, and mental depression.

Both digitalis and Ismelin slow the heart rate.

Thiazide diuretics enhance the antihypertensive action of Ismelin (see **DOSAGE AND ADMINISTRATION**)

Amphetamine-like compounds, stimulants (e.g., ephedrine, methylphenidate), tricylic antidepressants (e.g., amitriptyline, imipramine, desipramine) and other psychopharmacologic agents (e.g., phenothiazines and related compounds), as well as oral contraceptives, may reduce the hypotensive effect of Ismelin.

MAO inhibitors should be discontinued for at least 1 week before starting therapy with Ismelin.

Carcinogenesis, Mutagenesis, Impairment of Fertility

Long-term carcinogenicity studies in animals have not been conducted with Ismelin.

While inhibition of sperm passage and accumulation of sperm debris have been reported in rats and rabbits after several weeks of administration of Ismelin, 5 or 10 mg/kg per day, subcutaneously or intraperitoneally recovery of ejaculatory function and fertility has been demonstrated in rats given Ismelin intramuscularly, 25 mg/kg per day, for 8 weeks. Inhibition of ejaculation has also been reported in men (see **WARNINGS** and **ADVERSE REACTIONS**). This effect, which is attributable to the sympathetic blockade caused by the drug, is reversible several weeks after discontinuance of the drug.

Pregnancy Category C

Animal reproduction studies have not been conducted with Ismelin. It is also not known whether Ismelin can cause fetal harm when administered to a pregnant woman or can affect reproduction capacity. Ismelin should be given to a pregnant woman only if clearly needed.

Nursing Mothers

Ismelin is excreted in breast milk in very small quantity. Caution should be exercised when Ismelin is administered to a nursing woman.

Pediatric Use

Safety and effectiveness in children have not been established.

ADVERSE REACTIONS

The following adverse reactions have been observed, but there are not enough data to support an estimate of their frequency. Consequently the reactions are categorized by organ system and are listed in decreasing order of severity and not frequency.

Digestive: Diarrhea, which may be severe at times and necessitate discontinuance of medication; vomiting, nausea, increased bowel movements; dry mouth, parotid tenderness.

Cardiovascular: Chest pains (angina); bradycardia; a tendency toward fluid retention and edema with occasional development of congestive heart failure.

Respiratory: Dyspnea, asthma in susceptible individuals, nasal congestion.

Neurologic: Syncope resulting from either postural or exertional hypotension, dizziness, blurred vision, muscle tremor; ptosis of the lids; mental depression, chest paresthesias, weakness; lassitude, fatigue.

Muscular: Myalgia.

Genitourinary: Rise in BUN, urinary incontinence; inhibition of ejaculation, nocturia.

Metabolic: Weight gain.

Skin and Appendages: Dermatitis, scalp hair loss.

Although a causal relationship has not been established, a few instances of blood dycrasias (anemia, thrombocytopenia, and leukopenia) and of priapism or impotence have been reported.

OVERDOSAGE

Acute Toxicity

No deaths due to acute poisoning have been reported.

Oral LD_{50} in rats, 1262 mg kg.

Signs and Symptoms

Postural hypotension (with dizziness, blurred vision, and possibly syncope when standing), shock, and bradycardia are most likely to occur, diarrhea (possibly severe), nausea and vomiting may also occur. Unconsciousness is unlikely if adequate blood pressure and cerebral perfusion can be maintained by placing the patient in the supine position and by administering other treatment as required.

Treatment

There is no specific antidote.

Treatment should consist of gastric lavage. An activated charcoal slurry should be instilled and laxatives given, if conditions permit.

In sinus bradycardia, atropine should be administered.

In previously normotensive patients, treatment has consisted essentially of restoring blood pressure and heart rate to normal by keeping the patient in the supine position. Normal homeostatic control usually returns gradually over a 72-hour period in these patients.

In previously hypertensive patients, particularly those with impaired cardiac reserve or other cardiovascular-renal disease, intensive treatment may be required to support vital functions and to control cardiac irregularities that might be present. The supine position must be maintained; if vasopressors are required, they must be used with extreme caution, since Ismelin may increase responsiveness, causing a rise in blood pressure and development of cardiac arrhythmias.

Diarrhea, if severe or persistent, should be treated with anticholinergic agents to reduce intestinal hypermotility; hydration and electrolyte balance should be maintained.

Since Ismelin is excreted slowly, cardiovascular and renal function should be monitored for a few days.

DOSAGE AND ADMINISTRATION

Better control may be obtained, especially in the initial phases of treatment, if the patient can have his blood pressure recorded regularly at home.

Ambulatory Patients

Initial doses should be small (10 mg) and increased gradually, depending upon the patient's response. Ismelin has a long duration of action, therefore, dosage increases should not be made more often than every 5–7 days, unless the patient is hospitalized.

Blood pressure should be measured in the supine position, after standing for 10 minutes, and immediately after exercise if feasible. Dosage may be increased only if there has been no decrease in the standing blood pressure from previous levels. The average daily dose is 25–50 mg; only one dose a day is usually required.

Dosage Chart for Ambulatory Patients

Visits (Intervals of 5–7 Days)	*Daily Dose*
Visit 1 (Patient may be started on 10-mg tablets)	10 mg
Visit 2	20 mg
Visit 3 (Patient may be changed to 25-mg tablets whenever convenient)	30 mg (three 10-mg tablets) or 37.5 mg (one and one-half 25-mg tablets)
Visit 4	50 mg
Visit 5 and subsequent	Dosage may be increased by 12.5 mg or 25 mg if necessary

The dosage should be reduced in any of the following situations (1) normal supine pressure (2) excessive orthostatic fall in pressure (3) severe diarrhea.

Hospitalized Patients

Initial oral dose is 25–50 mg increased by 25 mg or 50 mg daily or every other day as indicated. This higher dosage is possible because hospitalized patients can be watched carefully. Unless absolutely impossible, the standing blood pressure should be measured regularly. Patients should not be discharged from the hospital until the effect of the drug on the standing blood pressure is known. Patients should be told about the possibility of orthostatic hypotension and warned not to get out of bed without help during the period of dosage adjustment.

Combination Therapy

Ismelin may be added gradually to thiazides and/or hydralazine. Thiazide diuretics enhance the effectiveness of Ismelin and may reduce the incidence of edema. When thiazide diuretics are added to the regimen in patients taking Ismelin, it is usually necessary to reduce the dosage of Ismelin. After control is established, the dosage of all drugs should be reduced to the lowest effective level.

Note: When Ismelin is replacing MAO inhibitors, at least 1 week should elapse before commencing treatment with Ismelin (see **CONTRAINDICATIONS**). If ganglionic blockers have not been discontinued before Ismelin is started, they should be gradually withdrawn to prevent a spiking blood pressure response during the transfer period.

HOW SUPPLIED

Tablets 10 mg—round, pale yellow, scored (imprinted CIBA 49)

Bottles of 100 .... NDC 0083-0049-30
Bottles of 1000 .... NDC 0083-0049-40
Consumer Pack—One Unit
 12 bottles—100 tablets each .... NDC 0083-0049-65

Tablets 25 mg—round, white, scored (imprinted CIBA 103)

Bottles of 100 .... NDC 0083-0103-30
Bottles of 1000 .... NDC 0083-0103-40
Consumer Pack—One Unit
 12 bottles—100 tablets each .... NDC 0083-0103-65

Dispense in tight container (USP)

C86-38
(Rev. 7/86)

Shown in Product Identification Section, page 408

LITHOBID® ℞
[lith 'oh-bidd]
lithium carbonate USP
slow-release tablets

CIBALITH-S® Syrup ℞
[see 'ba-lith-ess]
lithium citrate USP

> **WARNING**
> Lithium toxicity is closely related to serum lithium levels, and can occur at doses close to therapeutic levels. Facilities for prompt and accurate serum lithium determinations should be available before initiating therapy.

DESCRIPTION

Lithobid and **Cibalith-S** are two different forms of an antimanic medication for oral administration. Lithobid is a film-coated, slow-release, 300-mg lithium carbonate tablet. This slowly dissolving, film-coated tablet is designed to give lower serum lithium peaks than obtained with conventional oral lithium dosage forms.

Lithium carbonate USP is a white, granular, odorless powder, which is sparingly soluble in water and very slightly soluble in alcohol. It dissolves, with effervescence, in dilute mineral acids. Its molecular formula is Li_2CO_3, and its molecular weight is 73.89.

Cibalith-S is lithium citrate syrup containing 8mEq of lithium per 5 ml, equivalent to the amount in 300 mg of lithium carbonate.

Lithium citrate is prepared in solution from lithium hydroxide and citric acid in a ratio approximating di-lithium citrate.

Inactive Ingredients. Lithobid tablets 300 mg: Calcium stearate, carnauba wax, cellulose compounds, FD&C Blue No. 1 Aluminum Lake, FD&C Red No. 3 Aluminum Lake, FD&C Yellow No. 6 Aluminum Lake, povidone, propylene glycol, sodium chloride, sodium lauryl sulfate, sodium starch glycolate, sorbitol, and titanium dioxide.

Cibalith-S syrup. Citric acid, raspberry flavor, alcohol 0.3% v/v, purified water, sodium benzoate, sodium saccharin, and sorbitol.

INDICATIONS

Lithium is indicated in the treatment of manic episodes of manic-depressive illness. Maintenance therapy prevents or diminishes the intensity of subsequent episodes in those manic-depressive patients with a history of mania.

Typical symptoms of mania include pressure of speech, motor hyperactivity, reduced need for sleep, flight of ideas, grandiosity, elation, poor judgment, aggressiveness, and possibly hostility. When given to a patient experiencing a manic episode, lithium may produce a normalization of symptomatology within 1 to 3 weeks.

WARNINGS

Lithium should generally not be given to patients with significant renal or cardiovascular disease, severe debilitation or dehydration, or sodium depletion, and to patients receiving diuretics, since the risk of lithium toxicity is very high in such patients. If the psychiatric indication is life-threatening, and if such a patient fails to respond to other measures, lithium treatment may be undertaken with extreme caution, including daily serum lithium determinations and adjustment to the usually low doses ordinarily tolerated by these individuals. In such instances, hospitalization is a necessity.

Lithium toxicity is closely related to serum lithium levels, and can occur at doses close to therapeutic levels (see DOSAGE AND ADMINISTRATION).

Lithium therapy has been reported in some cases to be associated with morphologic changes in the kidneys. The relationship between such changes and renal function has not been established.

Outpatients and their families should be warned that the patient must discontinue lithium therapy and contact his physician if such clinical signs of lithium toxicity as diarrhea, vomiting, tremor, mild ataxia, drowsiness, or muscular weakness occur.

Lithium may prolong or potentiate the effects of neuromuscular blocking agents, such as decamethonium, pancuronium, and succinylcholine. Therefore, neuromuscular blocking agents should be given with caution to patients receiving lithium.

Lithium may impair mental and/or physical abilities. Caution patients about activities requiring alertness (*e.g.,* operating vehicles or machinery).

Combined use of haloperidol and lithium.

An encephalopathic syndrome (characterized by weakness, lethargy, fever, tremulousness and confusion, extrapyramidal symptoms, leucocytosis, elevated serum enzymes, BUN, and fasting blood sugar), followed by irreversible brain damage, has occurred in a few patients treated with lithium plus haloperidol. A causal relationship between these events and the concomitant administration of lithium and haloperidol has not been established. However, patients receiving such combined therapy should be monitored closely for early evidence of neurological toxicity, and treatment discontinued promptly if such signs appear. The possibility of similar adverse interactions with other antipsychotic medications exists. In addition, concurrent use of lithium with chlorpromazine and possibly other phenothiazines decreases serum chlorpromazine levels as much as 40%.

Concomitant administration of carbamezepine and lithium may increase the risk of neurotoxic side effects.

Aminophylline, caffeine, dyphylline, oxtriphylline, sodium bicarbonate, or theophylline used concurrently may decrease the therapeutic effect of lithium because of its increased urinary excretion.

Concurrent use of diuretics, especially thiazides, with lithium may provoke lithium toxicity due to reduced renal clearance.

Concurrent extended use of iodide preparations, especially potassium iodide, with lithium may produce hypothyroidism.

Usage in Pregnancy: Adverse effects on nidation in rats, embryo viability in mice, and metabolism *in vitro* of rat testis and human spermatozoa have been attributed to lithium, as have teratogenicity in submammalian species and cleft palates in mice. Studies in rats, rabbits and monkeys have shown no evidence of lithium-induced teratology.

There are lithium birth registries in the United States and elsewhere; however there are at the present time insufficient data to determine the effects of lithium on human fetuses. Therefore, at this point, lithium should not be used in pregnancy, especially the first trimester, unless in the opinion of the physician, the potential benefits outweigh the possible hazards.

Usage in Nursing Mothers:

Lithium is excreted in human milk. Nursing should not be undertaken during lithium therapy except in rare and unusual circumstances where, in the view of the physician, the potential benefits to the mother outweigh possible hazards to the child.

Usage in Children: Since information regarding the safety and effectiveness of lithium in children under 12 years of age is not available, its use in such patients is not recommended at this time.

PRECAUTIONS

The ability to tolerate lithium is greater during the acute manic phase and decreases when manic symptoms subside (see DOSAGE AND ADMINISTRATION).

The distribution space of lithium approximates that of total body water. Lithium is primarily excreted in urine with insignificant excretion in feces. Renal excretion of lithium is proportional to its plasma concentration. The half-elimination time of lithium is approximately 24 hours. Lithium decreases sodium reabsorption by the renal tubules which could lead to sodium depletion. Therefore, it is essential for the patient to maintain a normal diet, including salt, and an adequate fluid intake (2500–3000 ml) at least during the initial stabilization period. Decreased tolerance to lithium has been reported to ensue from protracted sweating or diarrhea and, if such occur, supplemental fluid and salt should be administered.

In addition to sweating and diarrhea, concomitant infection with elevated temperatures may also necessitate a temporary reduction or cessation of medication.

Previously existing underlying disorders do not necessarily constitute a contraindication to lithium treatment; where hypothyroidism exists, careful monitoring of thyroid function during lithium stabilization and maintenance allows for correction of changing thyroid parameters, if any, where hypothroidism occurs during lithium stabilization and maintenance, supplemental thyroid treatment may be used.

Indomethacin (50 mg t.i.d.) has been reported to increase steady-state plasma lithium levels from 30 to 59 percent. There is also some evidence that other nonsteroidal, anti-inflammatory agents may have a similar effect. When such combinations are used, increased monitoring of plasma lithium levels is recommended.

ADVERSE REACTIONS

Adverse reactions are seldom encountered at serum lithium levels below 1.5 mEq/l, except in the occasional patient sensitive to lithium. Mild-to-moderate toxic reactions may occur at levels from 1.5–2.5 mEq/l, and moderate-to-severe reactions may be seen at levels from 2.0–2.5 mEq/l, depending upon individual response to the drug.

Fine hand tremor, polyuria and mild thirst may occur during initial therapy for the acute manic phase, and may persist throughout treatment. Transient and mild nausea and general discomfort may also appear during the first few days of lithium administration.

These side effects are an inconvenience rather than a disabling condition, and usually subside with continued treatment or a temporary reduction or cessation of dosage. If persistent, a cessation of dosage is indicated.

Diarrhea, vomiting, drowsiness, muscular weakness and lack of coordination may be early signs of lithium intoxication, and can occur at lithium levels below 2.0 mEq/l. At higher levels, giddiness, ataxia, blurred vision, tinnitus and a large output of dilute urine may be seen. Serum lithium levels above 3.0 mEq/l may produce a complex clinical picture involving multiple organs and organ systems. Serum lithium levels should not be permitted to exceed 2.0 mEq/l during the acute treatment phase.

The following toxic reactions have been reported and appear to be related to serum lithium levels, including levels within the therapeutic range.

Neuromuscular: tremor, muscle hyperirritability (fasciculations, twitching, clonic movements of whole limbs), ataxia, choreoathetotic movements, hyperactive deep tendon reflexes.

Central Nervous System: blackout spells, epileptiform seizures, slurred speech, dizziness, vertigo, incontinence of urine or feces, somnolence, psychomotor retardation, restlessness, confusion, stupor, coma. Cases of pseudotumor cerebri (increased intracranial pressure and papilledema) have been reported with lithium use. If undetected, this condition may result in enlargement of the blind spot, constriction of visual fields, and eventual blindness due to optic atrophy. If this syndrome occurs, lithium should be discontinued if clinically possible.

Cardiovascular: cardiac arrhythmia, hypotension, peripheral circulatory collapse.

Gastrointestinal: anorexia, nausea, vomiting, diarrhea.

Genitourinary: albuminuria, oliguria, polyuria, glycosuria.

Dermatologic: drying and thinning of hair, anesthesia of skin, chronic folliculitis, xerosis cutis, alopecia, exacerbation of psoriasis.

Autonomic Nervous System: blurred vision, dry mouth.

Miscellaneous: fatigue, lethargy, tendency to sleep, dehydration, weight loss, transient scotomata.

Thyroid Abnormalities: euthyroid goiter and/or hypothyroidism (including myxedema) accompanied by lower T_3 and T_4.I_{131} iodine uptake may be elevated (See PRECAUTIONS). Paradoxically, rare cases of hyperthyroidism have been reported.

EEG Changes: diffuse slowing, widening of frequency spectrum, potentiation and disorganization of background rhythm.

EKG Changes: reversible flattening, isoelectricity or inversion of T-waves.

Miscellaneous reactions unrelated to dosage are: transient electroencephalographic and electrocardiographic changes, leucocytosis, headache, diffuse nontoxic goiter with or without hypothyroidism, transient hyperglycemia, generalized pruritus with or without rash, cutaneous ulcers, albuminuria, worsening of organic brain syndromes, excessive weight gain, edematous swelling of ankles or wrists, and thirst or polyuria, sometimes resembling diabetes insipidus and metallic taste.

A single report has been received of the development of painful discoloration of fingers and toes and coldness of the extremities within one day of the starting of treatment of lithium. The mechanism through which these symptoms (resembling Raynaud's Syndrome) developed is not known. Recovery followed discontinuance.

DOSAGE AND ADMINISTRATION

Acute Mania: Optimal patient response can usually be established and maintained with the following dosages:

Lithobid 900 mg b.i.d. or 600 mg t.i.d. (1800 mg per day)

Cibalith-S 10 ml (2 teaspoons) (16 mEq of lithium) t.i.d.

Such doses will normally produce an effective serum lithium level ranging between 1.0 and 1.5 mEq/l. Dosage must be individualized according to serum levels and clinical response. Regular monitoring of the patient's clinical state and of serum lithium levels is necessary. Serum levels should be determined twice per week during the acute phase, and until the serum level and clinical condition of the patient have been stabilized.

Long-Term Control: The desirable serum lithium levels are 0.6 to 1.2 mEq/l. Dosage will vary from one individual to another, but usually the following dosages will maintain this level:

Lithobid ....900 mg to 1200 mg per day given in two or three divided doses.

Cibalith-S ....5 ml (1 teaspoon) (8 mEq of lithium) t.i.d. or q.i.d.

Serum lithium levels in uncomplicated cases receiving maintenance therapy during remission should be monitored at least every two months. Patients abnormally sensitive to

Continued on next page

The full prescribing information for each CIBA drug is contained herein and is that in effect as of September 1, 1986

CIBA—Cont.

lithium may exhibit toxic signs at serum levels of 1.0 to 1.5 mEq/l. Elderly patients often respond to reduced dosage, and may exhibit signs of toxicity at serum levels ordinarily tolerated by other patients.

N.B.: Blood samples for serum lithium determinations should be drawn immediately prior to the next dose when lithium concentrations are relatively stable (i.e., 8–12 hours after previous dose). Total reliance must not be placed on serum levels alone. Accurate patient evaluation requires both clinical and laboratory analysis.

Lithobid slow-release tablets must be swallowed whole and never crushed or chewed.

OVERDOSAGE

The toxic levels for lithium are close to the therapeutic levels. It is therefore important that patients and their families be cautioned to watch for early toxic symptoms and to discontinue the drug and inform the physician should they occur. Toxic symptoms are listed in detail under ADVERSE REACTIONS.

Treatment: No specific antidote for lithium poisoning is known. Early symptoms of lithium toxicity can usually be treated by reduction or cessation of dosage of the drug and resumption of the treatment at a lower dose after 24 to 48 hours. In severe cases of lithium poisoning, the first and foremost goal of treatment consists of elimination of this ion from the patient.

Treatment is essentially the same as that used in barbiturate poisoning: 1) gastric lavage 2) correction of fluid and electrolyte imbalance and 3) regulation of kidney functioning. Urea, mannitol, and aminophylline all produce significant increases in lithium excretion. Hemodialysis is an effective and rapid means of removing the ion from the severely toxic patient. Infection prophylaxis, regular chest x-rays, and preservation of adequate respiration are essential.

HOW SUPPLIED

Lithobid, lithium carbonate

Tablets—slow-release 300 mg—peach-colored (imprinted CIBA 65)

Bottles of 100 .... NDC 0083-0065-30
Bottles of 1000 .... NDC 0083-0065-40

Accu-Pak® Unit Dose (blister pack)

Box of 100 (strips of 10) .... NDC 0083-0065-32

Store between 59°–86°F (15°–30°C).
Protect from moisture.

Cibalith-S, lithium citrate

Syrup—sugar-free, raspberry flavored, 8 mEq of lithium per 5 ml, equivalent to the amount in 300 mg of lithium carbonate.

Bottles of 480 ml .... NDC 0083-6565-76

Store between 59°–86°F (15°–30°C).
Dispense in tight container (USP).

Dist. by
CIBA Pharmaceutical Co.
Div. of CIBA-GEIGY Corp.
Summit, NJ 07901

C86-20 (Rev. 7/86)

Shown in Product Identification Section, page 408

LUDIOMIL® ℞

[*loó-dee-oh-mill*]
(maprotiline hydrochloride)
Tablets

DESCRIPTION

Ludiomil, maprotiline hydrochloride USP, is a tetracyclic antidepressant, available as 25-mg, 50-mg and 75-mg tablets for oral administration. Its chemical name is N-methyl-9,10-ethanoanthracene-9(10H)-propylamine hydrochloride.

Maprotiline hydrochloride USP is a fine, white to off-white, practically odorless crystalline powder. It is freely soluble in methanol and in chloroform, slightly soluble in water, and practically insoluble in isooctane. Its molecular weight is 313.87.

Inactive Ingredients. Calcium phosphate, cellulose compounds, colloidal silicon dioxide, FD&C Yellow No. 6 Lake (25-mg and 50-mg tablets), lactose, magnesium stearate, povidone, shellac, starch, stearic acid, talc, and titanium dioxide.

CLINICAL PHARMACOLOGY

The mechanism of action of Ludiomil is not precisely known. It does not act primarily by stimulation of the central nervous system and is not a monoamine oxidase inhibitor. The postulated mechanism of Ludiomil is that it acts primarily by potentiation of central adrenergic synapses by blocking reuptake of norepinephrine at nerve endings. This pharmacologic action is thought to be responsible for the drug's antidepressant and anxiolytic effects.

The mean time to peak is 12 hours. The half-life of elimination averages 51 hours.

Steady-state levels measured prior to the morning dose on a one-dosage regimen are summarized as follows:

Regimen	Average Minimum Concentration ng/ml	95% Confidence Limits ng/ml
50 mg x 3 daily	238	181–295

INDICATIONS AND USAGE

Ludiomil is indicated for the treatment of depressive illness in patients with depressive neurosis (dysthymic disorder) and manic-depressive illness, depressed type (major depressive disorder). Ludiomil is also effective for the relief of anxiety associated with depression.

CONTRAINDICATIONS

Ludiomil is contraindicated in patients hypersensitive to Ludiomil and in patients with known or suspected seizure disorders. It should not be given concomitantly with monoamine oxidase (MAO) inhibitors. A minimum of 14 days should be allowed to elapse after discontinuation of MAO inhibitors before treatment with Ludiomil is initiated. Effects should be monitored with gradual increase in dosage until optimum response is achieved. The drug is not recommended for use during the acute phase of myocardial infarction.

WARNINGS

Seizures have been associated with the use of Ludiomil. Most of the seizures have occurred in patients without a known history of seizures. However, in some of these cases, other confounding factors were present, including concomitant medications known to lower the seizure threshold, rapid escalation of the dosage of Ludiomil, and dosage that exceeded the recommended therapeutic range. The incidence of direct reports is less than 1/10 of 1%. The risk of seizures may be increased when Ludiomil is taken concomitantly with phenothiazines, when the dosage of benzodiazepines is rapidly tapered in patients receiving Ludiomil or when the recommended dosage of Ludiomil is exceeded. While a cause-and-effect relationship has not been established, the risk of seizures in patients treated with Ludiomil may be reduced by (1) initiating therapy at a low dosage, (2) maintaining the initial dosage for 2 weeks before raising it gradually in small increments as necessitated by the long half-life of Ludiomil (average 51 hours), and (3) keeping the dosage at the minimally effective level during maintenance therapy. (See **DOSAGE AND ADMINISTRATION.)**

Extreme caution should be used when this drug is given to:
—patients with a history of myocardial infarction;
—patients with a history or presence of cardiovascular disease because of the possibility of conduction defects, arrhythmias, myocardial infarction, strokes and tachycardia.

PRECAUTIONS

General: The possibility of suicide in seriously depressed patients is inherent in their illness and may persist until significant remission occurs. Therefore, patients must be carefully supervised during all phases of treatment with Ludiomil, and prescriptions should be written for the smallest number of tablets consistent with good patient management.

Hypomanic or manic episodes have been known to occur in some patients taking tricyclic antidepressant drugs, particularly in patients with cyclic disorders. Such occurrences have also been noted, rarely, with Ludiomil.

Prior to elective surgery, Ludiomil should be discontinued for as long as clinically feasible, since little is known about the interaction between Ludiomil and general anesthetics.

Ludiomil should be administered with caution in patients with increased intraocular pressure, history of urinary retention, or history of narrow-angle glaucoma because of the drug's anticholinergic properties.

Information for Patients: Patients should be warned of the association between seizures and the use of Ludiomil. Moreover, they should be informed that this association is enhanced in patients with a known history of seizures and in those patients who are taking certain other drugs. (See **WARNINGS.)**

Warn patients to exercise caution about potentially hazardous tasks, or operating automobiles or machinery since the drug may impair mental and/or physical abilities.

Ludiomil may enhance the response to alcohol, barbiturates, and other CNS depressants, requiring appropriate caution of administration.

Laboratory Tests: Ludiomil should be discontinued if there is evidence of pathological neutrophil depression. Leukocyte and differential counts should be performed in patients who develop fever and sore throat during therapy.

Drug Interactions: Close supervision and careful adjustment of dosage are required when administering Ludiomil concomitantly with anticholinergic or sympathomimetic drugs because of the possibility of additive atropine-like effects.

Concurrent administration of Ludiomil with electroshock therapy should be avoided because of the lack of experience in this area.

Caution should be exercised when administering Ludiomil to hyperthyroid patients or those on thyroid medication because of the possibility of enhanced potential for cardiovascular toxicity of Ludiomil.

Ludiomil should be used with caution in patients receiving guanethidine or similar agents since it may block the pharmacologic effects of these drugs.

The risk of seizures may be increased when Ludiomil is taken concomitantly with phenothiazines or when the dosage of benzodiazepines is rapidly tapered in patients receiving Ludiomil.

Because of the pharmacologic similarity of Ludiomil to the tricyclic antidepressants, the plasma concentration of Ludiomil may be increased when the drug is given concomitantly with cimetidine, as has occurred with tricyclic antidepressants. Adjustment of the dosage of Ludiomil may therefore be necessary in such cases both when cimetidine therapy is initiated and when it is discontinued.

(See **Information for Patients.)**

Carcinogenesis, Mutagenesis, Impairment of Fertility: Carcinogenicity and chronic toxicity studies have been conducted in laboratory rats and dogs. No drug- or dose-related occurrence of carcinogenesis was evident in rats receiving daily oral doses up to 60 mg/kg of Ludiomil for eighteen months or in dogs receiving daily oral doses up to 30 mg/kg of Ludiomil for one year. In addition, no evidence of mutagenic activity was found in offspring of female mice mated with males treated with up to 60 times the maximum daily human dose.

Pregnancy Category B: Reproduction studies have been performed in female laboratory rabbits, mice, and rats at doses up to 1.3, 7, and 9 times the maximum daily human dose respectively and have revealed no evidence of impaired fertility or harm to the fetus due to Ludiomil. There are, however, no adequate and well-controlled studies in pregnant women. Because animal reproduction studies are not always predictive of human response, this drug should be used during pregnancy only if clearly needed.

Labor and Delivery: Although the effect of Ludiomil on labor and delivery is unknown, caution should be exercised as with any drug with CNS depressant action.

Nursing Mothers: Ludiomil is excreted in breast milk. At steady state, the concentrations in milk correspond closely to the concentrations in whole blood. Caution should be exercised when Ludiomil is administered to a nursing woman.

Pediatric Use: Safety and effectiveness in children below the age of 18 have not been established.

ADVERSE REACTIONS

The following adverse reactions have been noted with Ludiomil and are generally similar to those observed with tricyclic antidepressants.

Cardiovascular: Rare occurrences of hypotension, hypertension, tachycardia, palpitation, arrhythmia, heart block, and syncope have been reported with Ludiomil.

Psychiatric: Nervousness (6%), anxiety (3%), insomnia (2%), and agitation (2%); rarely, confusional states (especially in the elderly), hallucinations, disorientation, delusions, restlessness, nightmares, hypomania, mania, exacerbation of psychosis, decrease in memory, and feelings of unreality.

Neurological: Drowsiness (16%), dizziness (8%), tremor (3%), and, rarely, numbness, tingling, motor hyperactivity, akathisia, seizures, EEG alterations, tinnitus, extrapyramidal symptoms, ataxia, and dysarthria.

Anticholinergic: Dry mouth (22%), constipation (6%), and blurred vision (4%); rarely, accommodation disturbances, mydriasis, urinary retention, and delayed micturition.

Allergic: Rare instances of skin rash, petechiae, itching, photosensitization, edema, and drug fever.

Gastrointestinal: Nausea (2%) and, rarely, vomiting, epigastric distress, diarrhea, bitter taste, abdominal cramps and dysphagia.

Endocrine: Rare instances of increased or decreased libido, impotence, and elevation or depression of blood sugar levels.

Other: Weakness and fatigue (4%) and headache (4%); rarely, altered liver function, jaundice, weight loss or gain, excessive perspiration, flushing, urinary frequency, increased salivation, nasal congestion and alopecia.

Note: Although there have been only isolated reports of the following adverse reactions with Ludiomil, its pharmacologic similarity to tricyclic antidepressants requires that each reaction be considered when administering Ludiomil.

—Bone marrow depression, including agranulocytosis, eosinophilia, purpura, and thrombocytopenia, myocardial infarction, stroke, peripheral neuropathy, sublingual adenitis, black tongue, stomatitis, paralytic ileus, gynecomastia in the male, breast enlargement and galactorrhea in the female, and testicular swelling.

OVERDOSAGE

Animal Oral LD_{50}: The oral LD_{50} of Ludiomil is 600–750 mg/kg in mice, 760–900 mg/kg in rats, > 1000 mg/kg in rabbits, > 300 mg/kg in cats, and > 30 mg/kg in dogs.

Signs and Symptoms: Data dealing with overdosage in humans are limited with only a few cases on record. Symptoms are drowsiness, tachycardia, ataxia, vomiting, cyanosis, hypotension, shock, restlessness, agitation, hyperpyrexia, muscle rigidity, athetoid movements, mydriasis, cardiac arrhythmias, impaired cardiac condition. In severe cases, loss of consciousness and generalized convulsions may occur. Since congestive heart failure has been seen with overdosages of tricyclic antidepressants, it should be considered with Ludiomil overdosage.

Treatment: There is no specific antidote. Induced emesis and gastric lavage are recommended. It may be helpful to leave the tube in the stomach with irrigation and continual aspiration of stomach contents possibly promoting more rapid elimination of the drug from the body. The room should be darkened, allowing only minimal external stimulation to reduce the tendency to convulsions.

Since it has been reported that physostigmine increases the risk of seizures, its use is not recommended in cases of overdosage with Ludiomil.

Hyperirritability and convulsions may be treated with carefully titrated parenteral barbiturates. Barbiturates should not be employed, however, if drugs that inhibit monoamine oxidase have also been taken by the patient in overdosage or in recent therapy. Similarly, barbiturates may induce respiratory depression, particularly in children. It is therefore advisable to have equipment available for artificial ventilation and resuscitation when barbiturates are employed. Paraldehyde may be used effectively in some children to counteract muscular hypertonus and convulsions with less likelihood of causing respiratory depression.

Shock (circulatory collapse) should be treated with supportive measures such as intravenous fluids, oxygen, and corticosteroids.

Hyperpyrexia should be controlled by whatever means available, including ice packs if necessary.

Signs of congestive heart failure may be satisfactorily treated by rapid digitalization.

Dialysis is of little value because of the low plasma concentration of this drug.

DOSAGE AND ADMINISTRATION

A single daily dose is an alternative to divided daily doses. Therapeutic effects are sometimes seen within 3 to 7 days, although as long as 2 to 3 weeks are usually necessary.

Initial Adult Dosage: An initial dosage of 75 mg daily is suggested for outpatients with mild-to-moderate depression. However, in some patients, particularly the elderly, an initial dosage of 25 mg daily may be used. Because of the long half-life of Ludiomil, the initial dosage should be maintained for two weeks. The dosage may then be increased gradually in 25-mg increments as required and tolerated. In most outpatients a maximum dose of 150 mg daily will result in therapeutic efficacy. It is recommended that this dose not be exceeded except in the most severely depressed patients. In such patients, dosage may be gradually increased to a maximum of 225 mg.

More severely depressed, hospitalized patients should be given an initial daily dose of 100 mg to 150 mg which may be gradually increased as required and tolerated. Most hospitalized patients with moderate-to-severe depression respond to a daily dosage of 150 mg although dosages as high as 225 mg may be required in some cases. Daily dosage of 225 mg should not be exceeded.

Elderly Patients: In general, lower dosages are recommended for patients over 60 years of age. Dosages of 50 mg to 75 mg daily are usually satisfactory as maintenance therapy for elderly patients who do not tolerate higher amounts.

Maintenance: Dosage during prolonged maintenance therapy should be kept at the lowest effective level. Dosage may be reduced to levels of 75 mg to 150 mg daily during such periods, with subsequent adjustment depending on therapeutic response.

HOW SUPPLIED

Tablets 25 mg—oval, dark orange, scored, coated (imprinted CIBA 110)

Bottle of 100....................NDC 0083-0110-30

Accu-Pak® Unit Dose (blister pack)

Box of 100 (strips of 10)....................NDC 0083-0110-32

Tablets 50 mg—round, dark orange, scored, coated (imprinted CIBA 26)

Bottle of 100....................NDC 0083-0026-30

Accu-Pak® Unit Dose (blister pack)

Box of 100 (strips of 10)....................NDC 0083-0026-32

Tablets 75 mg—oval, white, scored, coated (imprinted 135 CIBA)

Bottle of 100....................NDC 0083-0135-30

Accu-Pak® Unit Dose (blister pack)

Box of 100 (strips of 10)....................NDC 0083-0135-32

Dispense in tight container (USP).

C86-21 (Rev. 7/86)

Shown in Product Identification Section, page 408

METANDREN® ℞

[*meh-tan 'dren*]

(methyltestosterone USP)

Linguets® (buccal tablets)

Tablets

DESCRIPTION

Metandren, methyltestosterone USP, is a synthetic androgenic steroid available as 5-mg and 10-mg Linguets for absorption through the buccal mucosa and as 10-mg and 25-mg tablets for oral administration. Its chemical name is 17β-hydroxy-17-methylandrost-4-en-3-one.

Methyltestosterone USP occurs as white or creamy white, odorless, and slightly hygroscopic crystals or crystalline powder. It is practically insoluble in water, soluble in alcohol, in methanol, in ether, and in other organic solvents; and sparingly soluble in vegetable oils. Its molecular weight is 302.46.

Inactive Ingredients

Metandren Tablets: FD&C Yellow #5 (25-mg tablets), lactose, magnesium stearate, starch, sucrose, and talc.

Metandren Linguets: Acacia, FD&C Yellow #5 (10-mg linguets), lactose, magnesium stearate, mannitol, starch, sucrose, talc, and tragacanth.

CLINICAL PHARMACOLOGY

Endogenous androgens are responsible for the normal growth and development of the male sex organs and for maintenance of secondary sex characteristics. These effects include the growth and maturation of the prostate, seminal vesicles, penis, and scrotum; the development of male hair distribution, such as beard, pubic, chest, and axillary hair; laryngeal enlargement; vocal cord thickening; alterations in body musculature; and fat distribution. Drugs in this class also cause retention of nitrogen, sodium, potassium, and phosphorus, and decreased urinary excretion of calcium. Androgens have been reported to increase protein anabolism and decrease protein catabolism. Nitrogen balance is improved only when there is sufficient intake of calories and protein.

Androgens are responsible for the growth spurt of adolescence and for the eventual termination of linear growth, which is brought about by fusion of the epiphyseal growth centers. In children, exogenous androgens accelerate linear growth rates but may cause a disproportionate advancement in bone maturation. Use over long periods may result in fusion of the epiphyseal growth centers and termination of the growth process. Androgens have been reported to stimulate the production of red blood cells by enhancing the production of erythropoietic stimulating factor.

During exogenous administration of androgens, endogenous testosterone release is inhibited through feedback inhibition of pituitary luteinizing hormone (LH). At large doses of exogenous androgens, spermatogenesis may also be suppressed through feedback inhibition of pituitary follicle-stimulating hormone (FSH).

There is a lack of substantial evidence that androgens are effective in fractures, surgery, convalescence, and functional uterine bleeding.

Pharmacokinetics

Metandren is well absorbed, at a rate depending on the route of administration. Peak serum concentrations are attained about 1 hour after administration of a Linguet and about 2 hours after administration of a tablet.

The synthetic androgens, including methyltestosterone, are extensively metabolized by the liver, and they have a longer half-life than testosterone. They are more suitable than testosterone for oral administration.

After oral administration of a 10-mg tablet of Metandren in healthy human subjects, the serum concentration reaches a peak of about 30 ng/ml within 1–2 hours, then declines biphasically with half-lives of approximately 1 hour initially, changing to approximately 3.5 hours within 3–4 hours after dosage.

The bioavailability of Metandren Linguets approaches twice that of an equal dose of tablets, probably because the hepatic circulation is bypassed with sublingual administration.

About 10% of unchanged drug is recovered from the urine and feces. The major metabolic pathways of methyltestosterone are reduction of ring A, hydroxylation, and conjugation. The apparent elimination half-life averages 2.5–3 hours.

INDICATIONS AND USAGE

Males

Metandren is indicated for replacement therapy in conditions associated with a deficiency or absence of endogenous testosterone:

a. Primary hypogonadism—testicular failure due to cryptorchidism, bilateral torsion, orchitis, or vanishing testis syndrome; or orchidectomy.

b. Hypogonadotropic hypogonadism—idiopathic gonadotropin or LH-RH deficiency, or pituitary-hypothalamic injury from tumors, trauma, or radiation.

If the above conditions occur prior to puberty, androgen replacement therapy will be needed during the adolescent years for development of secondary sex characteristics. Prolonged androgen treatment will be required to maintain the sex characteristics in these males and in those who develop testosterone deficiency after puberty.

c. Metandren may be used to stimulate puberty in carefully selected males with clearly delayed puberty. These patients usually have a familial pattern of delayed puberty that is not secondary to a pathological disorder; puberty is expected to occur spontaneously at a relatively late date. Brief treatment with conservative doses may occasionally be justified in these patients if they do not respond to psychological support. The potential adverse effect on bone maturation should be discussed with the patient and his parents prior to androgen administration. An x-ray of the hand and wrist to determine bone age should be obtained every 6 months to assess the effect of treatment on the epiphyseal centers (see **WARNINGS** and **PRECAUTIONS, Pediatric Use**).

d. Metandren is indicated for the treatment of impotence and male climacteric symptoms, when these are secondary to androgen deficiency.

Females

Metandren may be used secondarily in women with advancing inoperable metastatic (skeletal) mammary cancer who are 1–5 years postmenopausal. Primary goals of therapy in these women include ablation of the ovaries. Other methods of counteracting estrogen activity are adrenalectomy, hypophysectomy, and antiestrogen therapy. Treatment with Metandren has also been used in premenopausal women with breast cancer who have benefited from oophorectomy and are considered to have a hormone-responsive tumor. Judgment concerning androgen therapy should be made by an oncologist with expertise in this field.

Metandren has been used for the management of postpartum breast pain and engorgement. There is no satisfactory evidence that this drug prevents or suppresses lactation.

CONTRAINDICATIONS

Metandren is contraindicated in men with carcinoma of the breast or with known or suspected carcinoma of the prostate, in women who are or may become pregnant, and in prepuberal males and females except those males with clearly delayed puberty as detailed in the **INDICATIONS AND USAGE** section, **Males,** c. When administered to pregnant women, androgens cause virilization of the external genitalia of the female fetus. This virilization includes clitoromegaly, abnormal vaginal development, and fusion of genital folds to form a scrotum-like structure. The degree of masculinization is related to the amount of drug given and the age of the fetus, and is most likely to occur in the female fetus when the drugs are given in the first trimester. If the patient becomes pregnant while taking these drugs, she should be apprised of the potential hazard to the fetus.

WARNINGS

In patients with breast cancer, androgen therapy may cause hypercalcemia by stimulating osteolysis. In this case, the drug should be discontinued.

Prolonged use of high doses of androgens has been associated with the development of peliosis hepatis and hepatic neoplasms including hepatocellular carcinoma (see **PRECAUTIONS, Carcinogenesis**). Peliosis hepatis can be a life-threatening or fatal complication.

Cholestatic hepatitis and jaundice occur with 17α-alkyl androgens at a relatively low dose. If cholestatic hepatitis with jaundice appears or if liver function tests become abnormal, the androgen should be discontinued and the etiology should be determined. Drug-induced jaundice is reversible when the medication is discontinued.

Geriatric patients treated with androgens may be at an increased risk for the development of prostatic hypertrophy, with resultant urinary obstruction, and prostatic carcinoma.

Males, especially the elderly, may become overly stimulated. Oligospermia and reduced ejaculatory volume may occur after prolonged administration or excessive dosage.

Edema with or without congestive heart failure may be a serious complication in patients with preexisting cardiac, renal, or hepatic disease. In addition to discontinuation of the drug, diuretic therapy may be required.

Gynecomastia frequently develops and occasionally persists in patients being treated for hypogonadism.

Hypersensitivity may occur.

Androgen therapy should be used cautiously in healthy males with delayed puberty. The effect on bone maturation should be monitored by assessing bone age of the wrist and hand every 6 months. In children, androgen treatment may accelerate bone maturation without producing compensatory gain in linear growth. This adverse effect may result in compromised adult stature. The younger the child, the greater the risk of compromising final mature height.

Women should be observed for signs of virilization (deepening of the voice, hirsutism, acne, clitorimegaly, and men-

Continued on next page

The full prescribing information for each CIBA drug is contained herein and is that in effect as of September 1, 1986

CIBA—Cont.

strual irregularities). Discontinuation of drug therapy at the time mild virilism becomes evident is necessary to prevent irreversible virilization. Some effects, such as voice changes, may not be reversible even when the drug is stopped. Such virilization is usual following androgen use at high doses. The physician should discuss with the patient being treated for breast carcinoma whether she is willing to tolerate this potential effect of the therapy.
In general, when any of these effects appear, androgen therapy should be stopped; if resumption of therapy is considered necessary, a lower dose should be utilized.

PRECAUTIONS

General
The Metandren Linguets® of 10 mg and tablets of 25 mg contain FD&C Yellow No. 5 (tartrazine), which may cause allergic-type reactions (including bronchial asthma) in certain susceptible individuals. Although the overall incidence of FD&C Yellow No. 5 (tartrazine) sensitivity in the general population is low, it is frequently seen in patients who are also hypersensitive to aspirin.

Information for Patients
The physician should instruct patients to report any of the following side effects of androgens:
Adult or Adolescent Males: Too frequent or persistent erections of the penis.
Females: Hoarseness, acne, changes in menstrual periods, or more hair on the face.
All Patients: Any nausea, vomiting, changes in skin color, or ankle swelling.

Laboratory Tests
Women with disseminated breast carcinoma should have frequent determinations of urine and serum calcium levels during the course of androgen therapy (see **WARNINGS**).
Because of the hepatotoxicity associated with the use of 17α-alkyl androgens, liver function tests should be obtained periodically.
Periodic (every 6 months) x-ray examinations of bone age should be made during treatment of prepubertal males to determine the rate of bone maturation and the effects of androgen therapy on the epiphyseal centers.
Hemoglobin and hematocrit should be checked periodically for polycythemia in patients who are receiving high doses of androgens.

Drug/Drug Interactions
Anticoagulants. C-17-substituted derivatives of testosterone, such as methandrostenolone, have been reported to decrease the anticoagulant requirements of patients receiving oral anticoagulants. Patients receiving oral anticoagulant therapy require close monitoring, especially when androgen therapy is started or stopped.
Oxyphenbutazone. Concurrent administration of oxyphenbutazone and androgens may result in elevated serum levels of oxyphenbutazone.
Insulin. In diabetic patients, the metabolic effects of androgens may decrease blood glucose levels and insulin requirements.

Drug/Laboratory Test Interactions
Androgens may decrease levels of thyroxine-binding globulin, resulting in decreased total T_4 serum levels and increased resin uptake of T_3 and T_4. Free-thyroid hormone levels remain unchanged, however, and there is no clinical evidence of thyroid dysfunction.

Carcinogenesis
Animal Data. No long-term carcinogenicity or reproduction studies in animals have been performed with Metandren. There is no information on mutagenesis. However, testosterone has been tested by subcutaneous injection and implantation in mice and rats. The implant induced cervical-uterine tumors in mice, which metastasized in some cases. There is suggestive evidence that injection of testosterone into some strains of female mice increases their susceptibility to hepatoma. Testosterone is also known to increase the number of tumors and decrease the degree of differentiation of chemically induced carcinomas of the liver in rats.
Human Data. There are rare reports of hepatocellular carcinoma in patients receiving long-term therapy with androgens in high doses. Withdrawal of the drugs did not lead to regression of the tumors in all cases.
Geriatric patients treated with androgens may be at an increased risk for the development of prostatic hypertrophy and prostatic carcinoma.

Pregnancy Category X
See **CONTRAINDICATIONS.**

Nursing Mothers
It is not known whether androgens are excreted in human milk. Because many drugs are excreted in human milk and because of the potential for serious adverse reactions in nursing infants from androgens, a decision should be made whether to discontinue nursing or to discontinue the drug, taking into account the importance of the drug to the mother.

Pediatric Use
Androgen therapy should be prescribed very cautiously for use in males with clearly delayed puberty and only by specialists who are aware of the adverse effects on bone maturation. Skeletal maturation must be monitored every 6 months by an x-ray of the hand and wrist (see **INDICATIONS AND USAGE** and **WARNINGS**).

ADVERSE REACTIONS

Endocrine and Urogenital: In females, the most common side effects are amenorrhea and other menstrual irregularities, inhibition of gonadotropin secretion, and virilization, including deepening of the voice and clitoral enlargement. The latter usually is not reversible after androgens are discontinued. When administered to a pregnant woman, androgens cause virilization of the external genitalia of the female fetus (see **CONTRAINDICATIONS**).
In males, gynecomastia and excessive frequency and duration of penile erections may occur. Oligospermia may occur at high dosages (see **CLINICAL PHARMACOLOGY**).
Skin and Appendages: Hirsutism, male pattern of baldness, acne, and hypersensitivity including skin manifestations.
Fluid and Electrolyte Disturbances: Retention of sodium, chloride, water, potassium, and inorganic phosphates; and hypercalcemia, especially in immobile patients and those with metastatic breast carcinoma.
Gastrointestinal: Nausea, cholestatic jaundice, alterations in liver functions; and, rarely, hepatocellular neoplasms and peliosis hepatis (see **WARNINGS**).
Hematologic: Suppresson of clotting factors II, V, VII, and X; bleeding in patients on concomitant anticoagulant therapy; and polycythemia.
Nervous System: Increased or decreased libido, headache, anxiety, depression, and generalized paresthesia.
Metabolic: Increased serum cholesterol.
Miscellaneous: Stomatitis with buccal preparations and, rarely, anaphylactoid reactions.

OVERDOSAGE

There have been no reports of acute overdosage with the androgens.

DOSAGE AND ADMINISTRATION

The suggested dosage for androgens varies, depending on the age, sex, and diagnosis of the individual patient. Dosage and duration of therapy are adjusted according to the patient's response and the appearance of adverse reactions. Suggested average daily dosages are given in the chart. Daily requirements are best administered in divided doses.
Note: Linguets have approximately twice the potency of the orally ingested hormone.

Males
Various dosage regimens have been used to induce pubertal changes in hypogonadal males. Some experts have advocated lower dosages initially, gradually increasing the dose as puberty progresses, with or without a decrease in maintenance levels. Other experts emphasize that higher dosages are needed to induce pubertal changes and that lower dosages can be used for maintenance after puberty. The chronological and skeletal ages must be taken into consideration, both in determining the initial dosage and in adjusting it.
Dosages used in delayed puberty generally are in the lower ranges of those given in the chart and are given for a limited duration, for example, 4–6 months.

Females
Women with metastatic breast carcinoma must be followed closely because androgen therapy occasionally appears to accelerate the disease.
Guideline dosages of androgens for use in the palliative treatment of women with metastatic breast carcinoma are also given in the chart.

INDICATION	AVERAGE DAILY DOSE	
Males	***Linguets***	***Tablets***
Hypogonadism	5–20 mg	10–40 mg
Male climacteric and male impotence	5–20 mg	10–40 mg
Cryptorchidism—postpubertal	15 mg	30 mg
Females		
Postpartum breast pain and engorgement (3–5 days)	40 mg	80 mg
Breast cancer	100 mg	200 mg

Administration of Linguets
Linguets should not be swallowed, since the hormone is meant to be absorbed through the mucous membranes. The Linguet should be placed in the upper or lower buccal pouch between the gum and cheek. The patient should avoid eating, drinking, chewing, or smoking while the Linguet is in place. Proper oral hygienic measures are particularly important after the use of Linguets.

HOW SUPPLIED

Linguets® 5 mg—capsule shaped, white (imprinted CIBA 51), for buccal administration
Bottles of 100 ....NDC 0083-0051-30
Linguets® 10 mg—capsule shaped, yellow (imprinted CIBA 64), for buccal administration
Bottles of 100 ....NDC 0083-0064-30
Tablets 10 mg—round, white, scored (imprinted CIBA 30)
Bottles of 100 ....NDC 0083-0030-30
Tablets 25 mg—round, yellow, scored (imprinted CIBA 32)
Bottles of 100 ....NDC 0083-0032-30
Dispense in tight, light-resistant container (USP).
C85-62 (Rev. 11/85)
Shown in Product Identification Section, page 408

METOPIRONE® ℞

[*met-oh-pie 'rone*]
metyrapone USP
Tablets
Diagnostic Test of Pituitary Adrenocorticotropic Function

DESCRIPTION

Metopirone, metyrapone USP, is an inhibitor of endogenous adrenal corticosteroid synthesis, available as 250-mg tablets for oral administration. Its chemical name is 2-methyl-1,2-di-3-pyridyl-1-propanone.
Metyrapone USP is a white to light amber, fine, crystalline powder, having a characteristic odor. It is sparingly soluble in water, and soluble in methanol and in chloroform. It forms water-soluble salts with acids. Its molecular weight is 226.28.
Inactive Ingredients. Calcium phosphate, colloidal silicon dioxide, gelatin, and magnesium stearate.

CLINICAL PHARMACOLOGY

The pharmacological effect of Metopirone is to reduce cortisol and corticosterone production by inhibiting the 11-β-hydroxylation reaction in the adrenal cortex. Removal of the strong inhibitory feedback mechanism exerted by cortisol results in an increase in adrenocorticotropic hormone (ACTH) production by the pituitary. With continued blockade of the enzymatic steps leading to production of cortisol and corticosterone, there is a marked increase in adrenocortical secretion of their immediate precursors, 11-deoxycortisol and desoxycorticosterone, which are weak suppressors of ACTH release, and a corresponding elevation of these steroids in the plasma and of their metabolites in the urine. These metabolites are readily determined by measuring urinary 17-hydroxycorticosteroids (17-OHCS) or 17-ketogenic steroids (17-KGS). Because of these actions. Metopirone is used as a diagnostic test, with urinary 17-OHCS measured as an index of pituitary ACTH responsiveness. Metopirone may also suppress biosynthesis of aldosterone, resulting in a mild natriuresis.
The response to Metopirone does not occur immediately. Following oral administration, peak steroid excretion occurs during the subsequent 24-hour period. Metopirone is absorbed rapidly and well when administered orally as prescribed. Plasma concentrations during the period of treatment are 0.5–1 μg/ml. The major biotransformation is reduction of the ketone to an alcohol and conjugation of metyrapone and reduced metyrapone to the corresponding glucuronides. The apparent half-life of elimination averages 1–2.5 hours. Within 2 days after initiation of treatment, about 40% of the administered dose is excreted in the urine, mostly in the form of glucuronides.

INDICATIONS AND USAGE

A diagnostic drug for testing hypothalamic-pituitary ACTH function.

CONTRAINDICATIONS

Adrenal cortical insufficiency, hypersensitivity to Metopirone.

WARNINGS

Metopirone may induce acute adrenal insufficiency in patients with reduced adrenal secretory capacity.

PRECAUTIONS

General
Ability of adrenals to respond to exogenous ACTH should be demonstrated before Metopirone is employed as a test. In the presence of hypo- or hyperthyroidism, response to the Metopirone test may be subnormal.

Laboratory Tests
See **INTERPRETATION.**

Drug Interactions
All corticosteroid therapy must be discontinued prior to and during testing with Metopirone.
The metabolism of Metopirone is accelerated by phenytoin; therefore, results of the test may be inaccurate in patients taking phenytoin within two weeks before. A subnormal response may occur in patients on estrogen therapy.

Carcinogenesis, Mutagenesis, Impairment of Fertility
Long-term carcinogenicity and reproduction studies in animals have not been conducted.

Pregnancy Category C
A subnormal response to Metopirone may occur in pregnant women. Animal reproduction studies have not been conducted with Metopirone. The Metopirone test was administered to 20 pregnant women in their second and third trimester of pregnancy and evidence was found that the fetal pitui-

tary responded to the enzymatic block. It is not known if Metopirone can affect reproduction capacity. Metopirone should be given to a pregnant woman only if clearly needed.

Nursing Mothers

It is not known whether this drug is excreted in human milk. Because many drugs are excreted in human milk, a decision should be made whether a woman undergoing the Metopirone test should discontinue nursing for the duration of the test.

Pediatric Use

See **DOSAGE AND ADMINISTRATION.**

ADVERSE REACTIONS

Gastrointestinal System: Nausea, abdominal discomfort
Central Nervous System: Headache, dizziness, sedation
Dermatologic System: Allergic rash
Hematologic System: Rarely, decreased white blood cell count or bone marrow depression.

OVERDOSAGE

Acute Toxicity

One case has been recorded in which a 6-year-old girl died after two doses of Metopirone, 2 g.

Oral LD_{50} in animals (mg/kg): rats, 521; maximum tolerated intravenous dose in one dog, 300.

Signs and Symptoms

The clinical picture of poisoning with Metopirone is characterized by gastrointestinal symptoms and by signs of acute adrenocortical insufficiency.

Cardiovascular System: Cardiac arrhythmias, hypotension, dehydration.

Nervous System and Muscles: Anxiety, confusion, weakness, impairment of consciousness.

Gastrointestinal System: Nausea, vomiting, epigastric pain, diarrhea.

Laboratory Findings: Hyponatremia, hypochloremia, hyperkalemia.

Combined Poisoning

In patients under treatment with insulin or oral antidiabetics, the signs and symptoms of acute poisoning with Metopirone may be aggravated or modified.

Treatment

There is no specific antidote. Besides general measures to eliminate the drug and reduce its absorption, a large dose of hydrocortisone should be administered at once, together with saline and glucose infusions.

Surveillance: For a few days blood pressure and fluid and electrolyte balance should be monitored.

DOSAGE AND ADMINISTRATION

Day 1: Control period—Collect 24-hour urine for measurement of 17-OHCS or 17-KGS.

Day 2: ACTH test to determine the ability of adrenals to respond—Standard ACTH test such as infusion of 50 units ACTH over 8 hours and measurement of 24-hour urinary steroids. If results indicate adequate response, the Metopirone test may proceed.

Day 3–4: Rest period.

Day 5: Administration of Metopirone:
Recommended with milk or snack.

Adults: 750 mg orally, every 4 hours for 6 doses. A single dose is approximately equivalent to 15 mg/kg.

Children: 15 mg/kg orally every 4 hours for 6 doses. A minimal single dose of 250 mg is recommended.

Day 6: After administration of Metopirone— Determination of 24-hour urinary steroids for effect.

INTERPRETATION

ACTH Test

The normal 24-hour urinary excretion of 17-OHCS ranges from 3 to 12 mg. Following continuous intravenous infusion of 50 units ACTH over a period of 8 hours, 17-OHCS excretion increases to 15 to 45 mg per 24 hours.

Metopirone

Normal response: In patients with a normally functioning pituitary, administration of Metopirone is followed by a two-to four-fold increase of 17-OHCS excretion or doubling of 17-KGS excretion.

Subnormal response: Subnormal response in patients without adrenal insufficiency is indicative of some degree of impairment of pituitary function, either panhypopituitarism or partial hypopituitarism (limited pituitary reserve).

1. *Panhypopituitarism* is readily diagnosed by the classical clinical and chemical evidences of hypogonadism, hypothyroidism, and hypoadrenocorticism. These patients usually have subnormal basal urinary steroid levels. Depending upon the duration of the disease and degree of adrenal atrophy, they may fail to respond to exogenous ACTH in the normal manner. Administration of Metopirone is not essential in the diagnosis, but if given, it will not induce an appreciable increase in urinary steroids.
2. *Partial hypopituitarism* or limited pituitary reserve is the more difficult diagnosis as these patients do not present the classical signs and symptoms of hypopituitarism. Measurements of target organ functions often are normal under basal conditions. The response to exogenous ACTH is usually normal, producing the expected rise of urinary steroids (17-OHCS or 17-KGS). The response, however, to Metopirone is *subnormal;* that is, no significant increase in 17-OHCS or 17-KGS excretion occurs.

This failure to respond to metyrapone may be interpreted as evidence of impaired pituitary-adrenal reserve. In view of the normal response to exogenous ACTH, the failure to respond to metyrapone is inferred to be related to a defect in the CNS-pituitary mechanisms which normally regulate ACTH secretions. Presumably the ACTH secreting mechanisms of these individuals are already working at their maximal rates to meet everyday conditions and possess limited "reserve" capacities to secrete additional ACTH either in response to stress or to decreased cortisol levels occurring as a result of metyrapone administration.

Subnormal response in patients with Cushing's syndrome is suggestive of either autonomous adrenal tumors that suppress the ACTH-releasing capacity of the pituitary or nonendocrine ACTH-secreting tumors.

Excessive response: An excessive excretion of 17-OHCS or 17-KGS after administration of Metopirone is suggestive of Cushing's syndrome associated with adrenal hyperplasia. These patients have an elevated excretion of urinary corticosteroids under basal conditions and will often, but not invariably, show a "supernormal" response to ACTH and also to Metopirone, excreting more than 35 mg per 24 hours of either 17-OHCS or 17-KGS.

HOW SUPPLIED

Tablets 250 mg—round, white, scored (imprinted CIBA 130)
Bottles of 18 .... NDC 0083-0130-11

Dispense in tight, light-resistant container (USP).

C86-6 (Rev. 3/86)

Shown in Product Identification Section, page 408

NUPERCAINAL®

[new-purr-cayne 'ull]
Anesthetic Ointment
Pain-Relief Cream

> **CAUTION**
>
> **Nupercainal** products are not for prolonged or extensive use and should never be applied in or near the eyes.
> **Consult labels before using.**
> **Keep this and all medications out of reach of children.**
> NUPERCAINAL SHOULD NOT BE SWALLOWED. SWALLOWING OR USE OF A LARGE QUANTITY IS HAZARDOUS, PARTICULARLY TO CHILDREN. CONSULT A PHYSICIAN OR POISON CONTROL CENTER IMMEDIATELY.

INDICATIONS

Nupercainal Ointment and Cream are fast-acting, long-lasting pain relievers that you can use for a number of painful skin conditions. **Nupercainal Anesthetic Ointment** is for hemorrhoids and for general use. **Nupercainal Pain-Relief Cream** is for general use only. The **Cream** is half as strong as the **Ointment.**

How to use Nupercainal Anesthetic Ointment (for general use). This soothing Ointment helps lubricate dry, inflamed skin and gives fast, temporary relief of pain and itching. It is recommended for sunburn, nonpoisonous insect bites, minor burns, cuts, and scratches. **DO NOT USE THIS PRODUCT IN OR NEAR YOUR EYES.**

Apply to affected areas gently. If necessary, cover with a light dressing for protection. Do not use more than 1 ounce of Ointment in a 24-hour period for an adult, do not use more than one-quarter of an ounce in a 24-hour period for a child. If irritation develops, discontinue use and consult your doctor.

How to use Nupercainal Anesthetic Ointment for fast, temporary relief of pain and itching due to hemorrhoids (also known as piles).

Remove cap from tube and set it aside. Attach the white plastic applicator to the tube. Squeeze the tube until you see the Ointment begin to come through the little holes in the applicator. Using your finger, lubricate the applicator with the Ointment. Now insert the entire applicator gently into the rectum. Give the tube a good squeeze to get enough Ointment into the rectum for comfort and lubrication. Remove applicator from rectum and wipe it clean. Apply additional Ointment to anal tissues to help relieve pain, burning, and itching. For best results use Ointment morning and night and after each bowel movement. After each use detach applicator, and wash it off with soap and water. Put cap back on tube before storing. In case of rectal bleeding, discontinue use and consult your doctor.

Pain-Relief Cream for general use. This Cream is particularly effective for fast, temporary relief of pain and itching associated with sunburn, cuts, scratches, minor burns and nonpoisonous insect bites. **DO NOT USE THIS PRODUCT IN OR NEAR YOUR EYES.** Apply liberally to affected area and rub in gently. This Cream is water-washable, so be sure to reapply after bathing, swimming or sweating. If irritation develops, discontinue use and consult your doctor.

Nupercainal Anesthetic Ointment contains 1% (one percent) dibucaine USP in a lubricant base. Available in tubes of 1 and 2 ounces.

Nupercainal Pain-Relief Cream contains 0.5% (one-half of one percent) dibucaine USP in a water-soluble base. Available in 1 1/2 ounce tubes.

Dibucaine USP is officially classified as a "topical anesthetic" and is one of the strongest and longest lasting of all pain relievers. It is not a narcotic.

Dist. by:
CIBA Pharmaceutical Co.
Division of CIBA-GEIGY Corp.
Summit, NJ 07901

C81-17 (5/81)

NUPERCAINAL®

[new-purr-cayne 'ull]
Suppositories

> **CAUTION**
>
> **Nupercainal Suppositories** are not for prolonged or extensive use. Contact with the eyes should be avoided.
> **Consult labels before using.**
> **Keep this and all medications out of reach of children.**
> NUPERCAINAL SUPPOSITORIES SHOULD NOT BE SWALLOWED. SWALLOWING CAN BE HAZARDOUS, PARTICULARLY TO CHILDREN. IN THE EVENT OF ACCIDENTAL SWALLOWING CONSULT A PHYSICIAN OR POISON CONTROL CENTER IMMEDIATELY.

INDICATIONS

Nupercainal Suppositories are for the temporary relief from itching, burning, and discomfort due to hemorrhoids or other anorectal disorders.

How to use Nupercainal Suppositories for hemorrhoids (also known as piles) or other anorectal disorders.

Tear off one suppository along the perforated line. Remove foil wrapper. Insert the suppository, rounded end first, well into the anus until you can feel it moving into your rectum. For best results, use one suppository after each bowel movement and as needed, but not to exceed 6 in a 24-hour period. Each suppository is sealed in its own foil packet to reduce danger of leakage when carried in pocket or purse. **To prevent melting, do not store above 86°F (30°C).**

Nupercainal Suppositories contain 2.4 gram cocoa butter, .25 gram zinc oxide, .1 gram bismuth subgallate, and acetone sodium bisulfite as preservative.

Dist. by:
CIBA Pharmaceutical Co.
Division of CIBA-GEIGY Corp.
Summit, New Jersey 07901

C82-56 (12/82)

PERCORTEN® acetate ℞

[per-core 'ten]
desoxycorticosterone acetate pellets USP
Pellets

DESCRIPTION

Percorten acetate, desoxycorticosterone acetate USP, is a mineralocorticoid hormone available as pellets for subcutaneous implantation in the infrascapular region.

Each pellet consists only of sterile, uniformly compressed, crystalline desoxycorticosterone acetate and weighs approximately 125 mg (the accurate weight of each pellet is stated on the label).

Desoxycorticosterone acetate is 21-hydroxy-4-pregnene-3,20-dione acetate.

Desoxycorticosterone acetate USP is an odorless, white or creamy white, crystalline powder. It is practically insoluble in water; slightly soluble in vegetable oils; and sparingly soluble in alcohol, in acetone, and in dioxane. It melts between 155°C and 161°C. Its molecular weight is 372.50.

CLINICAL PHARMACOLOGY

Percorten acetate is an adrenocortical hormone. In recommended doses, it acts as a mineralocorticoid and is devoid of glucocorticoid activity. It has more prolonged activity than the unesterified desoxycorticosterone because of the addition of the acetate radical.

The principal action of the mineralocorticoids is on the distal tubules of the kidney where the reabsorption of sodium ions from tubular fluid into the plasma is enhanced and urinary

Continued on next page

The full prescribing information for each CIBA drug is contained herein and is that in effect as of September 1, 1986

CIBA—Cont.

excretion of both potassium and hydrogen ion is increased. After several days of administration, intact or adrenal-ectomized subjects may "escape" from the sodium-retaining action of the drug and come into sodium balance. However, potassium continues to be excreted despite developing hypokalemia.

Desoxycorticosterone is unique among the corticosteroids in that it is ineffective when given orally. The sterile crystalline desoxycorticosterone acetate pellets, when implanted in the subcutaneous tissue, provide a repository for slow release of active drug over a period of 8–12 months. There is extensive, competitive, reversible plasma protein binding among the corticosteroids, with highest affinity for globulin. Metabolism is primarily oxidative, with metabolites excreted in the urine.

INDICATIONS AND USAGE

Percorten acetate is indicated as partial replacement therapy for primary and secondary adrenocortical insufficiency in Addison's disease and for the treatment of salt-losing adrenogenital syndrome.

CONTRAINDICATIONS

Percorten acetate is contraindicated in patients with hypersensitivity to desoxycorticosterone acetate, hypertension, congestive heart failure, or cardiac disease.

WARNINGS

Use of mineralocorticoids should be accompanied by adequate glucocorticoid therapy in adrenal insufficiency or the salt-losing form of the adrenogenital syndrome.

PRECAUTIONS

General

Patients receiving Percorten acetate should be watched for evidence of intercurrent infection. Should infection occur, appropriate anti-infective therapy should be initiated.

Since Percorten acetate is a potent adrenocortical preparation, which may produce side effects, patients should be closely watched. Patients with Addison's disease are more sensitive to the action of the hormone and may exhibit side effects to an exaggerated degree. Treatment should be stopped in the event of a significant increase in weight or blood pressure, or the development of edema or cardiac enlargement.

Sodium retention and the loss of potassium are accelerated by a high intake of sodium. Hence, it may be necessary to restrict the intake of sodium and increase that of potassium. Especially if edema occurs, dietary sodium restriction may be required.

Information For Patients

Patients should be clearly informed about the nature of their condition, the action of the hormone, and the possibility of unwanted side effects. A medical identification card should be carried during long-term therapy.

Laboratory Tests

Serum electrolyte determinations and blood pressure and weight measurements should be performed frequently; potassium supplementation may be necessary.

Only if absolutely necessary should a glucose tolerance test (particularly intravenous) be performed, as patients with Addison's disease tend to react with severe hypoglycemia within 3 hours, whether or not they are receiving desoxycorticosterone therapy.

Drug/Drug Interactions

Excessive potassium loss may result from the concomitant use of potassium-depleting diuretics such as thiazides. By induction of hepatic enzymes, concomitant use of drugs such as phenobarbital, phenytoin, or rifampin may increase the metabolism of corticosteroids. Adverse effects from cardiac glycosides may be enhanced by corticosteroids.

Drug/Laboratory Test Interactions

See **Laboratory Tests.**

Carcinogenesis, Mutagenesis, Impairment of Fertility

Long-term carcinogenicity studies in animals have not been performed with Percorten acetate.

Pregnancy Category C

Animal reproduction studies have not been conducted with Percorten acetate. It is also not known whether Percorten acetate can cause fetal harm when administered to a pregnant woman or can affect reproduction capacity. Percorten acetate should be given to a pregnant woman only if clearly needed. If it is necessary to give steroids to a pregnant woman, the newborn infant should be watched closely for signs of hypoadrenalism, and appropriate therapy instituted if such signs are present.

Nursing Mothers

Corticosteroids are excreted in breast milk. Caution should be exercised when Percorten acetate is administered to a nursing woman.

Pediatric Use

Safety and effectiveness in children have not been established.

ADVERSE REACTIONS

Cardiovascular: Generalized edema; hypertension and cardiac enlargement, especially if hypertension was present before the onset of adrenal insufficiency; cardiac arrhythmias.

Neurologic: Frontal or occipital headaches; extreme weakness of extremities with ascending paralysis secondary to low serum potassium.

Musculoskeletal: Arthralgia and tendon contractures.

Other: Hypersensitive reactions; rarely, irritation at the site of pellet implantation.

OVERDOSAGE

Acute Toxicity

No cases of acute overdosage with Percorten acetate have been reported.

Oral LD_{50} in rats is >1000 mg/kg.

Possible Signs and Symptoms

Since Percorten acetate is available only for infrascapular implantation, acute poisoning is most unlikely to occur. In the improbable event of such poisoning, however, the patient might develop clinical manifestations that represent extensions of its therapeutic effect, such as disturbances in fluid and electrolyte balance, hypokalemia, edema, hypertension, and cardiac insufficiency.

Treatment

There is no specific antidote.

In cases of acute poisoning, symptomatic treatment, together with measures to correct fluid and electrolyte imbalance, would be indicated.

In case of hypokalemia, digitalis should be used only with caution.

DOSAGE AND ADMINISTRATION

Mineralocorticoid therapy may not be necessary if the patient's condition can be controlled with adequate salt intake and glucocorticoid therapy.

If mineralocorticoid therapy is necessary, dosage must be chosen according to the severity of the disease and the response of the patient, and it should be accompanied by adequate amounts of glucocorticoid hormone.

Percorten acetate pellets should be implanted only after the optimal daily maintenance dose of desoxycorticosterone acetate in oil has been carefully determined. Implantation of a number of pellets not exactly calculated on the basis of the optimal daily maintenance dose by injection may lead to irreparable damage.

For determination of the ultimate optimal maintenance dose, several weeks are required. It is advisable, however, in order to eliminate the possibility of overdosage, that the patient be maintained on desoxycorticosterone acetate in oil for at least 2–3 months prior to pellet implantation.

Calculation of Pellet Requirement

One pellet is implanted for each 0.5 mg of the daily injected maintenance dose of desoxycorticosterone acetate in oil. For example, a patient with Addison's disease whose optimal daily maintenance requirement is 5 mg of desoxycorticosterone acetate in oil should receive a maximum of ten pellets.

Technique of Pellet Implantation

Pellets should be implanted only in a fully equipped operating room. Aseptic precautions and careful hemostasis are primary requirements for successful implantation.

The infrascapular region is the most suitable site for the implantation. Strict asepsis is observed. The operative field is prepared with iodine and alcohol, and the site of incision is anesthetized. A 2-to 4-cm transverse incision is made a few centimeters below the inferior angle of the scapula. A number of small pockets, determined by the number of pellets to be implanted, are prepared in the subcutaneous tissue by blunt dissection, radiating from the incision.

The pellets, which have been removed from the vial under sterile conditions and kept close at hand on a sterile towel, are placed in the pockets with forceps. The use of a nasal dilator, introduced into the opening of the pocket, permits placement of the pellet sufficiently far away from the incision. If the pellet is not placed a least 2 cm away from the incision, the chances are greatly increased that it may be extruded later. No pellet should be extruded spontaneously if implanted aseptically and sufficiently far away from the incision and if careful hemostasis is observed. It is a matter of technique and experience whether each single pellet pocket should be closed with an individual suture or whether the skin incision only should be closed with subcuticular sutures of fine black silk. As many as 15 pellets may be inserted through a single incision by this technique.

Observation After Implantation

The pellets are effective for an average period of 8–12 months. In case of infection, disease, or other stress, supplementary injections of desoxycorticosterone acetate in oil may be necessary until the patient has returned to the condition established when the pellets were implanted.

In a few instances, it has been necessary to remove pellets even though the maintenance dose was adequately determined prior to implantation. The occurrence of edema, excessive weight gain, and rise in blood pressure are signs of overdosage.

Reimplantation of Pellets

The effect of the implanted pellets fades after approximately 8–12 months. A gradual decrease in blood pressure and weight, increased fatigue, and loss of appetite are usually the first indications of this decrease in hormonal supply, and the patient must be carefully watched. It may be necessary to resume daily injections of desoxycorticosterone acetate in oil with slowly increasing doses. Over a period of 4–6 weeks, the maintenance requirement of desoxycorticosterone acetate in oil can be reestablished; from this dosage the number of new pellets to be implanted can be calculated. Under no circumstances should pellets be arbitrarily implanted on the basis of the initial assay, as the condition of the patient may have undergone a change in hormone requirement during the year.

HOW SUPPLIED

Pellets—White, oval—each consisting of approximately 125 mg of desoxycorticosterone acetate.

Cartons of 1 ....NDC 0083-2232-01

Dist. by:
CIBA Pharmaceutical Co.
Division of CIBA-GEIGY Corp.
Summit, NJ 07901

C83-33 (Rev. 7/83)

PERCORTEN® pivalate ℞

[purr-core 'ten]
desoxycorticosterone pivalate

Not USP, differs in pH range (5.0-8.5)
INTRAMUSCULAR REPOSITORY

DESCRIPTION

Percorten pivalate, a mineralocorticoid hormone and an analog of desoxycorticosterone, is 21-hydroxypregn-4-ene-3,20-dione pivalate.

ACTIONS

The chief effects of Percorten pivalate are on the metabolism of sodium, potassium, and water. When the drug is given to the adrenalectomized animal or to the patient with Addison's disease, there is decreased excretion of sodium accompanied by increased excretion of potassium; the concentration of sodium in the blood is thereby increased whereas that of potassium is decreased. There is a concomitant increase in the volume of blood and extracellular fluids, with a fall in hematocrit. Percorten pivalate has very little, if any, effect on carbohydrate metabolism and none on the number of circulating lymphocytes or eosinophiles.

INDICATIONS

As partial replacement therapy for primary and secondary adrenocortical insufficiency in Addison's disease and for treatment of salt-losing adrenogenital syndrome.

CONTRAINDICATIONS

Hypersensitivity to Percorten pivalate suspension or any of its ingredients. Patients with hypertension or cardiac disease.

WARNINGS

Since Percorten pivalate is potent and long-acting, do not administer more frequently than once per month.

Usage in Pregnancy

The safe use of this drug in pregnant women or during lactation has not been established. Therefore, the benefits must be weighed against the potential hazards.

PRECAUTIONS

Patients with Addison's disease are more sensitive to the action of the hormone and may exhibit side effects in an exaggerated degree.

Since Percorten pivalate is a potent adrenocortical preparation which may produce side effects, patients should be closely watched. Treatment should be stopped in the event of a significant increase in weight or blood pressure, or the development of edema or cardiac enlargement.

Sodium retention and the loss of potassium are accelerated by a high intake of sodium. Hence, it may be necessary to restrict intake of sodium and increase that of potassium.

Only if absolutely necessary should a glucose tolerance test (particularly intravenous) be performed, as addisonian patients with or without desoxycorticosterone therapy have the tendency to react with severe hypoglycemia within 3 hours.

ADVERSE REACTIONS

Like other adrenocortical hormones, Percorten pivalate may cause severe side effects if dosage is too high or prolonged. It may cause increased blood volume, edema, elevation of blood pressure, and enlargement of the heart shadow. In patients with essential hypertension or a tendency toward its development, a marked rise in blood pressure may follow administration of this drug.

Headache, arthralgia, weakness, ascending paralysis, low potassium syndrome, and hypersensitivity may occur.

On rare occasions, irritation at the site of injection has been reported.

DOSAGE AND ADMINISTRATION

In treating Addison's disease, Percorten pivalate should be used only in conjunction with other supplemental measures (*eg*, other hormonal agents, electrolytes, control of infection). At initiation of treatment, the daily requirement for maintenance therapy should be determined with desoxycorticosterone acetate in oil. For each mg of desoxycorticosterone acetate in oil, 1 ml (25 mg) Percorten pivalate suspension is to be injected intramuscularly through a 20-gauge needle into the upper outer quadrant of one or both buttocks.
The average dose is 25 to 100 mg every 4 weeks.

HOW SUPPLIED

Multiple-Dose Vials, 4 ml, each ml containing 25 mg desoxycorticosterone pivalate, 10.5 mg methylcellulose, 3 mg sodium carboxymethylcellulose, 1 mg polysorbate 80, and 8 mg sodium chloride with 0.002% thimerosal added as preservative in aqueous suspension.
Cartons of 1 ....NDC 0083-2222-01
For intramuscular use only.
Shake well before using.
Dist. by:
CIBA Pharmaceutical Co.
Division of CIBA-GEIGY Corp.
Summit, NJ 07921

C81-12 (2/81)

PRISCOLINE® hydrochloride ℞

[*priss 'coe-leen*]
tolazoline hydrochloride USP
Ampuls

DESCRIPTION

Priscoline, tolazoline hydrochloride USP, is a peripheral vasodilator available in ampuls for intravenous administration. Each milliliter of sterile, aqueous solution contains tolazoline hydrochloride USP, 25 mg; anhydrous chlorobutanol NF, 5 mg; tartaric acid ACS, 6.5 mg; and hydrous sodium citrate USP, 6.5 mg. Tolazoline hydrochloride is 4,5-dihydro-2-(phenylmethyl)-1*H*-imidazole monohydrochloride.
Tolazoline hydrochloride USP is a white to off-white crystalline powder. Its solutions are slightly acid to litmus. It is freely soluable in water and in alcohol. Its molecular weight is 196.68.

CLINICAL PHARMACOLOGY

Priscoline is a direct peripheral vasodilator with moderate competitive alpha-adrenergic blocking activity. It decreases peripheral resistance and increases venous capacitance. It has the following additional actions: (1) sympathomimetic, including cardiac stimulation; (2) parasympathomimetic, including gastrointestinal tract stimulation that is blocked by atropine; and (3) histamine-like, including stimulation of gastric secretion and peripheral vasodilatation. Priscoline given intravenously produces vasodilatation, primarily due to a direct effect on vascular smooth muscle, and cardiac stimulation; the blood pressure response depends on the relative contributions of the two effects. Priscoline usually reduces pulmonary arterial pressure and vascular resistance.
In neonates the half-life of Priscoline ranges from 3 to 10 hours.

INDICATIONS AND USAGE

Priscoline is indicated for the treatment of persistent pulmonary hypertension of the newborn ("persistent fetal circulation") when systemic arterial oxygenation cannot be satisfactorily maintained by usual supportive care (supplemental oxygen and/or mechanical ventilation).
Priscoline should be used in a highly supervised setting, where vital signs, oxygenation, acid-base status, fluid, and electrolytes can be monitored and maintained.

CONTRAINDICATIONS

Priscoline is contraindicated in patients with hypersensitivity to tolazoline.

WARNINGS

Priscoline stimulates gastric secretion and may activate stress ulcers. Through this mechanism, it can produce significant hypochloremic alkalosis. Pretreatment of infants with antacids may prevent gastrointestinal bleeding.
Patients should be observed closely for signs of systemic hypotension, and supportive therapy should be instituted if needed.
In patients with mitral stenosis, parenterally administered Priscoline may produce a rise or fall in pulmonary artery pressure and total pulmonary resistance; therefore, it must be used with caution in patients with known or suspected mitral stenosis.

PRECAUTIONS

General: The effects of Priscoline on pulmonary vessels may be pH dependent. Acidosis may decrease the effect of Priscoline.
Carcinogenesis, Mutagenesis, Impairment of Fertility: Long-term carcinogenicity studies in animals have not been performed with Priscoline.
Pregnancy Category C: Animal reproduction studies have not been conducted with Priscoline. It is also not known whether Priscoline can cause fetal harm when administered to a pregnant woman or can affect reproduction capacity. Priscoline should be given to a pregnant woman only if clearly needed.
Nursing Mothers: It is not known whether this drug is excreted in human milk. Because many drugs are excreted in human milk, caution should be exercised when Priscoline is administered to a nursing woman.

ADVERSE REACTIONS

The following adverse reactions have been observed, but there are insufficient data to support an estimate of their frequency:
Cardiovascular: Hypotension, tachycardia, cardiac arrhythmias, hypertension, pulmonary hemorrhage.
Digestive and Hepatic: Gastrointestinal hemorrhage, nausea, vomiting, diarrhea, hepatitis.
Skin: Flushing, increased pilomotor activity with tingling or chilliness, rash.
Hematologic: Thrombocytopenia, leukopenia.
Renal: Edema, oliguria, hematuria.

OVERDOSAGE

Acute Toxicity
Oral LD_{50}'s (mg/kg): mice, 400; rats, 1200.
Signs and Symptoms
Signs and symptoms of overdosage may include increased pilomotor activity, peripheral vasodilatation, skin flushing, and, in rare instances, hypotension and shock.
Treatment
In treating hypotension, it is most important to place the patient's head low and administer intravenous fluids. Epinephrine should not be used, since large doses of Priscoline may cause "epinephrine reversal" (further reduction in blood pressure, followed by an exaggerated rebound).

DOSAGE AND ADMINISTRATION

An initial dose of 1 to 2 mg/kg, via scalp vein, followed by an infusion of 1 to 2 mg/kg per hour have usually resulted in significant increases in arterial oxygen. There is very little experience with infusions lasting beyond 36 to 48 hours. Response, if it occurs, can be expected within 30 minutes after the initial dose.
Note: Parenteral drug products should be inspected visually for particulate matter and discoloration prior to administration, whenever solution and container permit.

HOW SUPPLIED

Ampuls—4 ml—each milliliter contains 25 mg of tolazoline hydrochloride.
Carton of 4 ampuls .... NDC 0083-6732-04
Store between 15° and 30°C (59°–86°F). Protect from light.

C85-26 (Rev. 3/85)

PRIVINE® hydrochloride

[*pri-veen '*]
naphazoline hydrochloride USP
0.05% Nasal Solution
0.05% Nasal Spray

CAUTION

Do not use Privine if you have glaucoma. Privine is an effective nasal decongestant **when you use it in the recommended dosage.** If you use too much, too long, or too often, Privine may be harmful to your nasal mucous membranes and cause burning, stinging, sneezing or an increased runny nose.
Do not use Privine by mouth.
Keep this and all medications out of the reach of children. Do not use Privine with children under 6 years of age, except with the advice and supervision of a doctor.
OVERDOSAGE IN YOUNG CHILDREN MAY CAUSE MARKED SEDATION AND IF SEVERE, EMERGENCY TREATMENT MAY BE NECESSARY.
IF NASAL STUFFINESS PERSISTS AFTER 3 DAYS OF TREATMENT, DISCONTINUE USE AND CONSULT A DOCTOR.
Privine is a nasal decongestant that comes in two forms: Nasal Solution (in a bottle with a dropper) and Nasal Spray (in a plastic squeeze bottle). Both are for prompt, and prolonged relief of nasal congestion due to common colds, sinusitis, hay fever, etc.
How to use Nasal Solution. Squeeze rubber bulb to fill dropper with proper amount of medication. For best results, tilt head as far back as possible and put two drops of solution into your right nostril. Then lean head forward, inhaling and turning your head to the left. Refill dropper by squeezing bulb. Now tilt head as far back as possible and put two drops of solution into your left nostril. Then lean head forward, inhaling, and turning your head to the right.
Use only 2 drops in each nostril. Do not repeat this dosage more than every 3 hours.
The Privine dropper bottle is designed to make administration of the proper dosage easy and to prevent accidental overdosage. Privine will not cause sleeplessness, so you may use it before going to bed.

IMPORTANT

After use, be sure to rinse the dropper with very hot water. This helps prevent contamination of the bottle with bacteria from nasal secretions. Use of the dispenser by more than one person may spread infection.

NOTE

Privine Nasal Solution may be used on contact with glass, plastic, stainless steel and specially treated metals used in atomizers. Do not let the solution come in contact with reactive metals, especially aluminum. If solution becomes discolored, it should be discarded.
How to use Nasal Spray. For best results do *not* shake the plastic squeeze bottle.
Remove cap. With head held upright, spray twice into each nostril. Squeeze the bottle sharply and firmly while sniffing through the nose.
For best results use every 4 to 6 hours. Do not use more often than every 3 hours.
Avoid overdosage. Follow directions for use carefully.
Privine Nasal Solution contains 0.05% naphazoline hydrochloride USP with benzalkonium chloride as a preservative. Available in bottles of .66 fl. oz. (20 ml) with dropper, and bottles of 16 fl. oz. (473 ml). Privine Nasal Spray contains 0.05% naphazoline hydrochloride USP with benzalkonium chloride as a preservative. Available in plastic squeeze bottles of ½ fl. oz. (15 ml).

C80-5 (1/80)

REGITINE® ℞

[*rej 'a-teen*]
phentolamine mesylate USP
Vials

DESCRIPTION

Regitine, phentolamine mesylate USP, is an antihypertensive, available in vials for intravenous and intramuscular administration. Each vial contains phentolamine mesylate USP, 5 mg, and mannitol USP, 25 mg, in sterile, lyophilized form.
Phentolamine mesylate is 4,5-dihydro-2-[N-(*m* -hydroxyphenyl)-N-(*p* -methylphenyl)aminomethyl]-1*H* -imidazole 1:1 methanesulfonate.
Phentolamine mesylate USP is a white or off-white, odorless crystalline powder with a molecular weight of 377.46. Its solutions are acid to litmus. It is freely soluble in water and in alcohol, and slightly soluble in chloroform. It melts at about 178°C.

CLINICAL PHARMACOLOGY

Regitine produces an alpha-adrenergic block of relatively short duration. It also has direct, but less marked, positive inotropic and chronotropic effects on cardiac muscle and vasodilator effects on vascular smooth muscle.
Regitine has a half-life in the blood of 19 minutes following intravenous administration. Approximately 13% of a single intravenous dose appears in the urine as unchanged drug.

INDICATIONS AND USAGE

Regitine is indicated for the prevention or control of hypertensive episodes that may occur in a patient with pheochromocytoma as a result of stress or manipulation during preoperative preparation and surgical excision.
Regitine is indicated for the prevention or treatment of dermal necrosis and sloughing following intravenous administration or extravasation of norepinephrine.
Regitine is also indicated for the diagnosis of pheochromocytoma by the Regitine blocking test.

CONTRAINDICATIONS

Myocardial infarction, history of myocardial infarction, coronary insufficiency, angina, or other evidence suggestive of coronary artery disease; hypersensitivity to phentolamine or related compounds.

WARNINGS

Myocardial infarction, cerebrovascular spasm, and cerebrovascular occlusion have been reported to occur following the administration of Regitine, usually in association with marked hypotensive episodes.
For screening tests in patients with hypertension, the generally available urinary assay of catecholamines or other biochemical assays have largely replaced the Regitine and other pharmacological tests for reasons of accuracy and safety. None of the chemical or pharmacological tests is in-

Continued on next page

The full prescribing information for each CIBA drug is contained herein and is that in effect as of September 1, 1986

CIBA—Cont.

fallible in the diagnosis of pheochromocytoma. The Regitine blocking test is not the procedure of choice and should be reserved for cases in which additional confirmatory evidence is necessary and the relative risks involved in conducting the test have been considered.

PRECAUTIONS

General

Tachycardia and cardiac arrhythmias may occur with the use of Regitine or other alpha-adrenergic blocking agents. When possible, administration of cardiac glycosides should be deferred until cardiac rhythm returns to normal.

Drug Interactions

See **DOSAGE AND ADMINISTRATION, Diagnosis of pheochromocytoma,** *Preparation.*

Carcinogenesis, Mutagenesis, Impairment of Fertility

Long-term carcinogenicity studies, mutagenicity studies, and fertility studies have not been conducted with Regitine.

Pregnancy Category C

Administration of Regitine to pregnant rats and mice at oral doses 24–30 times the usual daily human dose (based on a 60-kg human) resulted in slightly decreased growth and slight skeletal immaturity of the fetuses. Immaturity was manifested by increased incidence of incomplete or unossified calcanei and phalangeal nuclei of the hind limb and of incompletely ossified sternebrae. At oral doses 60 times the usual daily human dose (based on a 60-kg human), a slightly lower rate of implantation was found in the rat. Regitine did not affect embryonic or fetal development in the rabbit at oral doses 20 times the usual daily human dose (based on a 60-kg human). No teratogenic or embryotoxic effects were observed in the rat, mouse, or rabbit studies.

There are no adequate and well-controlled studies in pregnant women. Regitine should be used during pregnancy only if the potential benefit justifies the potential risk to the fetus.

Nursing Mothers

It is not known whether this drug is excreted in human milk. Because many drugs are excreted in human milk and because of the potential for serious adverse reactions in nursing infants from Regitine, a decision should be made whether to discontinue nursing or to discontinue the drug, taking into account the importance of the drug to the mother.

Pediatric Use

See **DOSAGE AND ADMINISTRATION.**

ADVERSE REACTIONS

Acute and prolonged hypotensive episodes, tachycardia, and cardiac arrhythmias have been reported. In addition, weakness, dizziness, flushing, orthostatic hypotension, nasal stuffiness, nausea, vomiting, and diarrhea may occur.

OVERDOSAGE

Acute Toxicity

No deaths due to acute poisoning with Regitine have been reported.

Oral LD_{50}'s (mg/kg): mice, 1000; rats, 1250.

Signs and Symptoms

Overdosage with Regitine is characterized chiefly by cardiovascular disturbances, such as arrhythmias, tachycardia, hypotension, and possibly shock. In addition, the following might occur: excitation, headache, sweating, pupillary contraction, visual disturbances; nausea, vomiting, diarrhea; hypoglycemia.

Treatment

There is no specific antidote.

A decrease in blood pressure to dangerous levels or other evidence of shocklike conditions should be treated vigorously and promptly. The patient's legs should be kept raised and a plasma expander should be administered. If necessary, intravenous infusion of norepinephrine, titrated to maintain blood pressure at the normotensive level, and all available supportive measures should be included. Epinephrine should not be used, since it may cause a paradoxical reduction in blood pressure.

DOSAGE AND ADMINISTRATION

The reconstituted solution should be used upon preparation and should not be stored.

Note: Parenteral drug products should be inspected visually for particulate matter and discoloration prior to administration, whenever solution and container permit.

1. Prevention or control of hypertensive episodes in the patient with pheochromocytoma.

For preoperative reduction of elevated blood pressure, 5 mg of Regitine (1 mg for children) is injected intravenously or intramuscularly 1 or 2 hours before surgery, and repeated if necessary.

During surgery, Regitine (5 mg for adults, 1 mg for children) is administered intravenously as indicated, to help prevent or control paroxysms of hypertension, tachycardia, respiratory depression, convulsions, or other effects of epinephrine intoxication. (Postoperatively, norepinephrine may be given to control the hypotension that commonly follows complete removal of a pheochromocytoma.)

2. Prevention or treatment of dermal necrosis and sloughing following intravenous administration or extravasation of norepinephrine.

For Prevention: 10 mg of Regitine is added to each liter of solution containing norepinephrine. The pressor effect of norepinephrine is not affected.

For Treatment: 5–10 mg of Regitine in 10 ml of saline is injected into the area of extravasation within 12 hours.

3. Diagnosis of pheochromocytoma—Regitine blocking test.

The test is most reliable in detecting pheochromocytoma in patients with sustained hypertension and least reliable in those with paroxysmal hypertension. False-positive tests may occur in patients with hypertension without pheochromocytoma.

a. Intravenous

Preparation

The **CONTRAINDICATIONS, WARNINGS,** and **PRECAUTIONS** sections should be reviewed. Sedatives, analgesics, and all other medications except those that might be deemed essential (such as digitalis and insulin) are withheld for at least 24 hours, and preferably 48–72 hours, prior to the test. Antihypertensive drugs are withheld until blood pressure returns to the untreated, hypertensive level. This test is not performed on a patient who is normotensive.

Procedure

The patient is kept at rest in the supine position throughout the test, preferably in a quiet, darkened room. Injection of Regitine is delayed until blood pressure is stabilized, as evidenced by blood pressure readings taken every 10 minutes for at least 30 minutes.

Five milligrams of Regitine is dissolved in 1 ml of Sterile Water for Injection. The dose for adults is 5 mg; for children, 1 mg.

The syringe needle is inserted into the vein, and injection is delayed until pressor response to venipuncture has subsided. Regitine is injected rapidly. Blood pressure is recorded immediately after injection, at 30-second intervals for the first 3 minutes, and at 60-second intervals for the next 7 minutes.

Interpretation

A positive response, suggestive of pheochromocytoma, is indicated when the blood pressure is reduced more than 35 mm Hg systolic and 25 mm Hg diastolic. A typical positive response is a reduction in pressure of 60 mm Hg systolic and 25 mm Hg diastolic. Usually, maximal effect is evident within 2 minutes after injection. A return to preinjection pressure commonly occurs within 15–30 minutes but may occur more rapidly.

If blood pressure decreases to a dangerous level, the patient should be treated as outlined under **OVERDOSAGE:**

A positive response should always be confirmed by other diagnostic procedures, preferably by measurement of urinary catecholamines or their metabolites.

A negative response is indicated when the blood pressure is elevated, unchanged, or reduced less than 35 mm Hg systolic and 25 mm Hg diastolic after injection of Regitine. A negative reponse to this test does not exclude the diagnosis of pheochromocytoma, especially in patients with paroxysmal hypertension in whom the incidence of false-negative responses is high.

b. Intramuscular

If the intramuscular test for pheochromocytoma is preferred, preparation is the same as for the intravenous test. Five milligrams of Regitine is then dissolved in 1 ml of Sterile Water for Injection. The dose for adults is 5 mg intramuscularly; for children, 3 mg. Blood pressure is recorded every 5 minutes for 30–45 minutes following injection. A positive response is indicated when the blood pressure is reduced 35 mm Hg systolic and 25 mm Hg diastolic, or more, within 20 minutes following injection.

HOW SUPPLIED

Vials —each containing 5 mg of phentolamine mesylate USP and 25 mg of mannitol USP, in lyophilized form

Cartons of 2 .... NDC 0083-6830-02
Cartons of 6 .... NDC 0083-6830-06

The reconstituted solution should be used upon preparation and should not be stored.

Store between 59° and 86°F.

Dist. by:
CIBA Pharmaceutical Co.
Division of CIBA-GEIGY Corp.
Summit, NJ 07901

C85-2 (Rev. 8/85)

RIMACTANE® ℞

[*re-mack 'tayne*]
rifampin USP

DESCRIPTION

Rimactane, rifampin USP , is a semisynthetic antibiotic derivative of rifamycin B, available as 300-mg capsules for oral administration. It is also available in Dual Packs containing two 300-mg capsules of Rimactane and one 300-mg tablet of INH®, isoniazid USP. Rimactane is 3-[[(4-methyl-1-piperazinyl)imino] methyl] rifamycin.

Rifampin USP is a red-brown crystalline powder. It is very slightly soluble in water, freely soluble in chloroform, and soluble in ethyl acetate and in methanol. Its molecular weight is 822.95.

Inactive ingredients: FD&C Blue No. 1, FD&C Red No. 3, FD&C Red No. 40, FD&C Yellow No. 6, gelatin, lactose, magnesium stearate, silicon dioxide, sodium lauryl sulfate, starch, talc, and titanium dioxide.

ACTIONS

Rimactane inhibits DNA-dependent RNA polymerase activity in susceptible cells. Specifically, it interacts with bacterial RNA polymerase but does not inhibit the mammalian enzyme. This is the mechanism of action by which Rimactane exerts its therapeutic effect. Rimactane cross resistance has only been shown with other rifamycins.

Peak blood levels in normal adults vary widely from individual to individual. Peak levels occur between 2 and 4 hours following the oral administration of a 600-mg dose. The average peak value is 7 mcg/ml; however, the peak level may vary from 4 to 32 mcg/ml.

In normal subjects the $T\frac{1}{2}$ (biological half-life) of Rimactane in blood is approximately 3 hours. Elimination occurs mainly through the bile and, to a much lesser extent, the urine.

INDICATIONS

Pulmonary Tuberculosis

In the initial treatment and in the retreatment of pulmonary tuberculosis, Rimactane must be used in conjunction with at least one other antituberculous drug.

Frequently used regimens have been the following:
- isoniazid and Rimactane
- ethambutol and Rimactane
- isoniazid, ethambutol, and Rimactane

Neisseria Meningitidis Carriers

Rimactane is indicated for the treatment of asymptomatic carriers of *N. meningitidis* to eliminate meningococci from the nasopharynx.

Rimactane is not indicated for the treatment of meningococcal infection.

To avoid the indiscriminate use of Rimactane, diagnostic laboratory procedures, including serotyping and susceptibility testing, should be performed to establish the carrier state and the correct treatment. In order to preserve the usefulness of Rimactane in the treatment of asymptomatic meningococcal carriers, it is recommended that the drug be reserved for situations in which the risk of meningococcal meningitis is high.

Both in the treatment of tuberculosis and in the treatment of meningococcal carriers, small numbers of resistant cells, present within large populations of susceptible cells, can rapidly become the predominating type. Since rapid emergence of resistance can occur, culture and susceptibility tests should be performed in the event of persistent positive cultures.

CONTRAINDICATIONS

A history of previous hypersensitivity reaction to any of the rifamycins.

WARNINGS

Rifampin has been shown to produce liver dysfunction. There have been fatalities associated with jaundice in patients with liver disease or receiving rifampin concomitantly with other hepatotoxic agents. Since an increased risk may exist for individuals with liver disease, benefits must be weighed carefully against the risk of further liver damage. Periodic liver function monitoring is mandatory.

The possibility of rapid emergence of resistant meningococci restricts the use of Rimactane to short-term treatment of the asymptomatic carrier state. Rimactane is not to be used for the treatment of meningococcal disease.

Several studies of tumorigenicity potential have been done in rodents. In one strain of mice known to be particularly susceptible to the spontaneous development of hepatomas, rifampin given at a level 2–10 times the maximum dosage used clinically, resulted in a significant increase in the occurrence of hepatomas in female mice of this strain after one year of administration. There was no evidence of tumorigenicity in the males of this strain, in males or females of another mouse strain, or rats.

Usage in Pregnancy: Although rifampin has been reported to cross the placental barrier and appear in cord blood, the effect of Rimactane, alone or in combination with other antituberculous drugs, on the human fetus is not known. An increase in congenital malformations, primarily spina bifida and cleft palate, has been reported in the offspring of rodents given oral doses of 150-250 mg/kg/day of rifampin during pregnancy.

The possible teratogenic potential in women capable of bearing children should be carefully weighed against the benefits of therapy.

PRECAUTIONS

Rimactane is not recommended for intermittent therapy; the patient should be cautioned against intentional or accidental interruption of the daily dosage regimen since rare renal hypersensitivity reactions have been reported when therapy was resumed in such cases.

Rifampin has been observed to increase the requirements for anticoagulant drugs of the coumarin type. The cause of this phenomenon is unknown. In patients receiving anticoagulants and rifampin concurrently, it is recommended that the prothrombin time be performed daily or as frequently as necessary to establish and maintain the required dose of anticoagulant.

Urine, feces, saliva, sputum, sweat, and tears may be colored red-orange by rifampin and its metabolites. Soft contact lenses may be permanently stained. Individuals to be treated should be made aware of these possibilities.

It has been reported that the reliability of oral contraceptives may be affected in some patients being treated for tuberculosis with rifampin in combination with at least one other antituberculous drug. In such cases, alternative contraceptive measures may need to be considered.

Rifampin has been reported to diminish the effects of concurrently administered methadone, oral hypoglycemics, corticosteroids, dapsone, digitalis preparations and to reduce the bioavailability and efficacy of verapamil. Appropriate dosage adjustments may be necessary if indicated by the patient's clinical condition.

When rifampin is taken in combination with PAS, decreased rifampin serum levels may result. Therefore, the drugs should be given at least 4 hours apart.

Therapeutic levels of rifampin have been shown to inhibit standard assays for serum folate and vitamin B_{12}. Alternative methods must be considered when determining folate and vitamin B_{12} concentrations in the presence of rifampin.

Since rifampin has been reported to cross the placental barrier and appear in cord blood, neonates of rifampin-treated mothers should be carefully observed for any evidence of adverse effects. Rifampin is excreted in breast milk.

ADVERSE REACTIONS

Gastrointestinal disturbances such as heartburn, epigastric distress, anorexia, nausea, vomiting, gas, cramps, and diarrhea have been noted in some patients. Rarely, pseudomembranous enterocolitis has been reported. Headache, drowsiness, fatigue, ataxia, dizziness, inability to concentrate, mental confusion, visual disturbances, muscular weakness, fever, pains in extremities, generalized numbness, and menstrual disturbances have also been noted.

Hypersensitivity reactions have been reported. Encountered occasionally have been pruritus, urticaria, rash, pemphigoid reaction, eosinophilia, sore mouth, sore tongue, and exudative conjunctivitis. Rarely, hepatitis or a shock-like syndrome with hepatic involvement and abnormal liver function tests have been reported. Transient abnormalities in liver function tests (eg, elevations in serum bilirubin, BSP, alkaline phosphatase, serum transaminases) have also been observed. The BSP test should be performed prior to the morning dose of rifampin to avoid false-positive results.

Thrombocytopenia, transient leukopenia, hemolytic anemia, and decreased hemoglobin have been observed. Thrombocytopenia has occurred when rifampin and ethambutol were administered concomitantly according to an intermittent dose schedule twice weekly and in high doses.

Elevations in BUN and serum uric acid have occurred. Rarely, hemolysis, hemoglobinuria, hematuria, renal insufficiency or acute renal failure have been reported and are generally considered to be hypersensitivity reactions. These have usually occurred during intermittent therapy or when treatment was resumed following intentional or accidental interruption of a daily dosage regimen and were reversible when rifampin was discontinued and appropriate therapy instituted.

Although rifampin has been reported to have an immunosuppressive effect in some animal experiments, available human data indicate that this has no clinical significance.

DOSAGE AND ADMINISTRATION

It is recommended that Rimactane be administered once daily, either one hour before or two hours after a meal.

Data are not available for determination of dosage for children under 5.

Pulmonary Tuberculosis

Adults: 600 mg (two 300-mg Capsules) in a single daily administration.

Children: 10 to 20 mg/kg, not to exceed 600 mg/day.

In the treatment of pulmonary tuberculosis, Rimactane must be used in conjunction with at least one other antituberculous agent. In general, therapy should be continued until bacterial conversion and maximal improvement have occurred.

Meningococcal Carriers

It is recommended that Rimactane be administered once daily for four consecutive days in the following doses:

Adults: 600 mg (two 300-mg Capsules) in a single daily administration.

Children: 10 to 20 mg/kg, not to exceed 600 mg/day.

Susceptibility Testing

Pulmonary Tuberculosis: Rifampin susceptibility powders are available for both direct and indirect methods of determining the susceptibility of strains of mycobacteria. The MIC's of susceptible clinical isolates when determined in 7H10 or other non-egg-containing media have ranged from 0.1 to 2 mcg/ml.

Meningococcal Carriers: Susceptibility discs containing 5 mcg rifampin are available for susceptibility testing of *N. meningitidis.*

Quantitative methods that require measurement of zone diameters give the most precise estimates of antibiotic susceptibility. One such procedure[1] has been recommended for use with discs for testing susceptibility to rifampin. Interpretations correlate zone diameters from the disc test with MIC (minimal inhibitory concentration) values for rifampin. A range of MIC's from 0.1 to 1 mcg/ml has been found *in vitro* for susceptible strains of *N. meningitidis.* With this procedure, a report from the laboratory of "resistant" indicates that the organism is not likely to be eradicated from the nasopharynx of asymptomatic carriers.

OVERDOSAGE

Signs and Symptoms

Nausea, vomiting, and increasing lethargy will probably occur within a short time after ingestion; actual unconsciousness may occur with severe hepatic involvement. Brownish-red or orange discoloration of the skin, urine, sweat, saliva, and feces is proportional to amount ingested.

Liver enlargement, possibly with tenderness, can develop within a few hours after severe overdosage and jaundice may develop rapidly. Hepatic involvement may be more marked in patients with prior impairment of hepatic function. Other physical findings remain essentially normal.

Direct and total bilirubin levels may increase rapidly with severe overdosage; hepatic enzyme levels may be affected, especially with prior impairment of hepatic function. A direct effect upon hemopoietic system, electrolyte levels, or acid-base balance is unlikely.

Treatment

Since nausea and vomiting are likely to be present, gastric lavage is probably preferable to induction of emesis. Activated charcoal slurry instilled into the stomach following evacuation of gastric contents can help absorb any remaining drug in G.I. tract. Antiemetic medication may be required to control severe nausea/vomiting.

Active diuresis (with measured intake and output) will help promote excretion of the drug. Bile drainage may be indicated in presence of serious impairment of hepatic function lasting more than 24–48 hours; under these circumstances, extracorporeal hemodialysis may be required.

In patients with previously adequate hepatic function, reversal of liver enlargement and impaired hepatic excretory function probably will be noted within 72 hours, with rapid return toward normal thereafter.

HOW SUPPLIED

Capsules 300 mg—opaque, scarlet, caramel (imprinted CIBA 154)

Bottles of 30 .... NDC 0083-0154-26
Bottles of 60 .... NDC 0083-0154-29
Bottles of 100 .... NDC 0083-0154-30

Keep tightly closed. Protect from heat and moisture.

Dispense in tight, light-resistant container (USP).

Also available—Rimactane®/INH® (isoniazid USP) Dual Pack. Each Dual Pack contains two Rimactane 300-mg capsules and one INH 300-mg tablet.

Cartons of 30 Dual Packs (60 Rimactane capsules and 30 INH tablets) .... NDC 0083-8912-23

Protect from heat and moisture.

REFERENCE

1. Bauer, A. W., Kirby, W. M. M., Sherris, J. C., and Turck, M. Antibiotic susceptibility testing by a standardized single disk method. *Am J Clin Path* 1966;45:493–496.

C85-43 (Rev. 11/85)

Shown in Product Identification Section, page 408

RITALIN® hydrochloride Ⓒ
[rit'ah-lin]
methylphenidate hydrochloride tablets USP

RITALIN-SR® Ⓒ
methylphenidate hydrochloride USP sustained-release tablets

DESCRIPTION

Ritalin, methylphenidate hydrochloride USP, is a mild central nervous system (CNS) stimulant, available as tablets of 5, 10, and 20 mg for oral administration; Ritalin-SR is available as sustained-release tablets of 20 mg for oral administration. Methylphenidate hydrochloride is methyl α-phenyl-2-piperidineacetate hydrochloride.

Methylphenidate hydrochloride USP is a white, odorless, fine crystalline powder. Its solutions are acid to litmus. It is freely soluble in water and in methanol, soluble in alcohol, and slightly soluble in chloroform and in acetone. Its molecular weight is 269.77.

Inactive Ingredients. Ritalin tablets: D&C Yellow No. 10 (5-mg and 20-mg tablets), FD&C Green No. 3 (10-mg tablets), lactose, magnesium stearate, polyethylene glycol, starch (5-mg and 10-mg tablets), sucrose, talc, and tragacanth (20-mg tablets).

Ritalin-SR tablets: Cellulose compounds, cetostearyl alcohol, lactose, magnesium stearate, mineral oil, povidone, titanium dioxide, and zein.

CLINICAL PHARMACOLOGY

Ritalin is a mild central nervous system stimulant.

The mode of action in man is not completely understood, but Ritalin presumably activates the brain stem arousal system and cortex to produce its stimulant effect.

There is neither specific evidence which clearly establishes the mechanism whereby Ritalin produces its mental and behavioral effects in children, nor conclusive evidence regarding how these effects relate to the condition of the central nervous system.

Ritalin in the SR tablets is more slowly but as extensively absorbed as in the regular tablets. Relative bioavailability of the SR tablet compared to the Ritalin tablet, measured by the urinary excretion of Ritalin major metabolite (α-phenyl-2-piperidine acetic acid) was 105% (49–168%) in children and 101% (85–152%) in adults. The time to peak rate in children was 4.7 hours (1.3–8.2 hours) for the SR tablets and 1.9 hours (0.3–4.4 hours) for the tablets. An average of 67% of SR tablet dose was excreted in children as compared to 86% in adults.

INDICATIONS

Attention Deficit Disorders, Narcolepsy

Attention Deficit Disorders (previously known as Minimal Brain Dysfunction in Children). Other terms being used to describe the behavioral syndrome below include: Hyperkinetic Child Syndrome, Minimal Brain Damage, Minimal Cerebral Dysfunction, Minor Cerebral Dysfunction.

Ritalin is indicated as an integral part of a total treatment program which typically includes other remedial measures (psychological, educational, social) for a stabilizing effect in children with a behavioral syndrome characterized by the following group of developmentally inappropriate symptoms: moderate-to-severe distractibility, short attention span, hyperactivity, emotional lability, and impulsivity. The diagnosis of this syndrome should not be made with finality when these symptoms are only of comparatively recent origin. Nonlocalizing (soft) neurological signs, learning disability, and abnormal EEG may or may not be present, and a diagnosis of central nervous system dysfunction may or may not be warranted.

Special Diagnostic Considerations

Specific etiology of this syndrome is unknown, and there is no single diagnostic test. Adequate diagnosis requires the use not only of medical but of special psychological, educational, and social resources.

Characteristics commonly reported include: chronic history of short attention span, distractibility, emotional lability, impulsivity, and moderate-to-severe hyperactivity; minor neurological signs and abnormal EEG. Learning may or may not be impaired. The diagnosis must be based upon a complete history and evaluation of the child and not solely on the presence of one or more of these characteristics.

Drug treatment is not indicated for all children with this syndrome. Stimulants are not intended for use in the child who exhibits symptoms secondary to environmental factors and/or primary psychiatric disorders, including psychosis. Appropriate educational placement is essential and psychosocial intervention is generally necessary. When remedial measures alone are insufficient, the decision to prescribe stimulant medication will depend upon the physician's assessment of the chronicity and severity of the child's symptoms.

CONTRAINDICATIONS

Marked anxiety, tension, and agitation are contraindications to Ritalin, since the drug may aggravate these symptoms. Ritalin is contraindicated also in patients known to be hypersensitive to the drug, in patients with glaucoma, and in patients with motor tics or with a family history or diagnosis of Tourette's syndrome.

WARNINGS

Ritalin should not be used in children under six years, since safety and efficacy in this age group have not been established.

Continued on next page

The full prescribing information for each CIBA drug is contained herein and is that in effect as of September 1, 1986

CIBA—Cont.

Sufficient data on safety and efficacy of long-term use of Ritalin in children are not yet available. Although a causal relationship has not been established, suppression of growth (*ie*, weight gain, and/or height) has been reported with the long-term use of stimulants in children. Therefore, patients requiring long-term therapy should be carefully monitored.
Ritalin should not be used for severe depression of either exogenous or endogenous origin. Clinical experience suggests that in psychotic children, administration of Ritalin may exacerbate symptoms of behavior disturbance and thought disorder.
Ritalin should not be used for the prevention or treatment of normal fatigue states.
There is some clinical evidence that Ritalin may lower the convulsive threshold in patients with prior history of seizures, with prior EEG abnormalities in absence of seizures, and, very rarely, in absence of history of seizures and no prior EEG evidence of seizures. Safe concomitant use of anticonvulsants and Ritalin has not been established. In the presence of seizures, the drug should be discontinued.
Use cautiously in patients with hypertension. Blood pressure should be monitored at appropriate intervals in all patients taking Ritalin, especially those with hypertension.
Symptoms of visual disturbances have been encountered in rare cases. Difficulties with accommodation and blurring of vision have been reported.

Drug Interactions
Ritalin may decrease the hypotensive effect of guanethidine. Use cautiously with pressor agents and MAO inhibitors.
Human pharmacologic studies have shown that Ritalin may inhibit the metabolism of coumarin anticoagulants, anticonvulsants (phenobarbital, diphenylhydantoin, primidone), phenylbutazone, and tricyclic antidepressants (imipramine, desipramine). Downward dosage adjustments of these drugs may be required when given concomitantly with Ritalin.

Usage in Pregnancy
Adequate animal reproduction studies to establish safe use of Ritalin during pregnancy have not been conducted. Therefore, until more information is available, Ritalin should not be prescribed for women of childbearing age unless, in the opinion of the physician, the potential benefits outweigh the possible risks.

Drug Dependence
Ritalin should be given cautiously to emotionally unstable patients, such as those with a history of drug dependence or alcoholism, because such patients may increase dosage on their own initiative.
Chronically abusive use can lead to marked tolerance and psychic dependence with varying degrees of abnormal behavior. Frank psychotic episodes can occur, especially with parenteral abuse. Careful supervision is required during drug withdrawal, since severe depression as well as the effects of chronic overactivity can be unmasked. Long-term follow-up may be required because of the patient's basic personality disturbances.

PRECAUTIONS

Patients with an element of agitation may react adversely; discontinue therapy if necessary.
Periodic CBC, differential, and platelet counts are advised during prolonged therapy.
Drug treatment is not indicated in all cases of this behavioral syndrome and should be considered only in light of the complete history and evaluation of the child. The decision to prescribe Ritalin should depend on the physician's assessment of the chronicity and severity of the child's symptoms and their appropriateness for his/her age. Prescription should not depend solely on the presence of one or more of the behavioral characteristics.
When these symptoms are associated with acute stress reactions, treatment with Ritalin is usually not indicated.
Long-term effects of Ritalin in children have not been well established.

ADVERSE REACTIONS

Nervousness and insomnia are the most common adverse reactions but are usually controlled by reducing dosage and omitting the drug in the afternoon or evening. Other reactions include hypersensitivity (including skin rash, urticaria, fever, arthralgia, exfoliative dermatitis, erythema multiforme with histopathological findings of necrotizing vasculitis, and thrombocytopenic purpura); anorexia; nausea; dizziness; palpitations; headache; dyskinesia; drowsiness; blood pressure and pulse changes, both up and down; tachycardia; angina; cardiac arrhythmia; abdominal pain; weight loss during prolonged therapy. There have been rare reports of Tourette's syndrome. Toxic psychosis has been reported. Although a definite causal relationship has not been established, the following have been reported in patients taking this drug: leukopenia and/or anemia; a few instances of scalp hair loss.
In children, loss of appetite, abdominal pain, weight loss during prolonged therapy, insomnia, and tachycardia may occur more frequently; however, any of the other adverse reactions listed above may also occur.

DOSAGE AND ADMINISTRATION

Dosage should be individualized according to the needs and responses of the patient.

Adults
Tablets: Administer in divided doses 2 or 3 times daily, preferably 30 to 45 minutes before meals. Average dosage is 20 to 30 mg daily. Some patients may require 40 to 60 mg daily. In others, 10 to 15 mg daily will be adequate. Patients who are unable to sleep if medication is taken late in the day should take the last dose before 6 p.m.
SR Tablets: Ritalin-SR tablets have a duration of action of approximately 8 hours. Therefore, Ritalin-SR tablets may be used in place of Ritalin tablets when the 8-hour dosage of Ritalin-SR corresponds to the titrated 8-hour dosage of Ritalin. Ritalin-SR tablets must be swallowed whole and never crushed or chewed.

Children (6 years and over)
Ritalin should be initiated in small doses, with gradual weekly increments. Daily dosage above 60 mg is not recommended.
If improvement is not observed after appropriate dosage adjustment over a one-month period, the drug should be discontinued.
Tablets: Start with 5 mg twice daily (before breakfast and lunch) with gradual increments of 5 to 10 mg weekly.
SR Tablets: Ritalin-SR tablets have a duration of action of approximately 8 hours. Therefore, Ritalin-SR tablets may be used in place of Ritalin tablets when the 8-hour dosage of Ritalin-SR corresponds to the titrated 8-hour dosage of Ritalin. Ritalin-SR tablets must be swallowed whole and never crushed or chewed.
If paradoxical aggravation of symptoms or other adverse effects occur, reduce dosage, or, if necessary, discontinue the drug.
Ritalin should be periodically discontinued to assess the child's condition. Improvement may be sustained when the drug is either temporarily or permanently discontinued.
Drug treatment should not and need not be indefinite and usually may be discontinued after puberty.

OVERDOSAGE

Signs and symptoms of acute overdosage, resulting principally from overstimulation of the central nervous system and from excessive sympathomimetic effects, may include the following: vomiting, agitation, tremors, hyperreflexia, muscle twitching, convulsions (may be followed by coma), euphoria, confusion, hallucinations, delirium, sweating, flushing, headache, hyperpyrexia, tachycardia, palpitations, cardiac arrhythmias, hypertension, mydriasis, and dryness of mucous membranes.
Treatment consists of appropriate supportive measures. The patient must be protected against self-injury and against external stimuli that would aggravate overstimulation already present. If signs and symptoms are not too severe and the patient is conscious, gastric contents may be evacuated by induction of emesis or gastric lavage. In the presence of severe intoxication, use a carefully titrated dosage of a *short-acting* barbiturate *before* performing gastric lavage.
Intensive care must be provided to maintain adequate circulation and respiratory exchange; external cooling procedures may be required for hyperpyrexia.
Efficacy of peritoneal dialysis or extracorporeal hemodialysis for Ritalin overdosage has not been established.

HOW SUPPLIED

Tablets 5 mg—round, yellow (imprinted CIBA 7)

Bottles of 100	NDC 0083-0007-30
Bottles of 500	NDC 0083-0007-35
Bottles of 1000	NDC 0083-0007-40

Tablets 10 mg —round, pale green, scored (imprinted CIBA 3)

Bottles of 100	NDC 0083-0003-30
Bottles of 500	NDC 0083-0003-35
Bottles of 1000	NDC 0083-0003-40
Accu-Pak® Unit Dose (blister pack) Box of 100 (strips of 10)	NDC 0083-0003-32

Tablets 20 mg—round, pale yellow, scored (imprinted CIBA 34)

Bottles of 100	NDC 0083-0034-30
Bottles of 1000	NDC 0083-0034-40

Protect from light.
Dispense in tight, light-resistant container (USP).
SR Tablets 20 mg—round, white, coated (imprinted CIBA 16)

Bottles of 100	NDC 0083-0016-30

Note: SR Tablets are color-additive free.
Do not store above 86°F (30°C). Protect from moisture.
Dispense in tight, light-resistant container (USP).
C85-55 (Rev.11/85)
Shown in Product Identification Section, page 408

SER-AP-ES® ℞

[*su-rapp 'ess*]
reserpine 0.1 mg
hydralazine hydrochloride 25 mg
hydrochlorothiazide 15 mg
Combination Tablets

WARNING
This fixed-combination drug is not indicated for initial therapy of hypertension. Hypertension requires therapy titrated to the individual patient. If the fixed combination represents the dosage so determined, its use may be more convenient in patient management. The treatment of hypertension is not static but must be reevaluated as conditions in each patient warrant.

DESCRIPTION

Ser-Ap-Es is an antihypertensive-diuretic combination, available as tablets for oral administration. Each tablet contains Serpasil (reserpine USP), 0.1 mg; Apresoline (hydralazine hydrochloride USP), 25 mg; and Esidrix (hydrochlorothiazide USP), 15 mg.
Reserpine is methyl 18β-hydroxy-11, 17α-dimethoxy-3β, 20α-yohimban-16β-carboxylate 3,4,5-trimethoxybenzoate (ester).
Reserpine USP, a pure crystalline alkaloid of rauwolfia, is a white or pale buff to slightly yellowish, odorless crystalline powder. It darkens slowly on exposure to light, but more rapidly when in solution. It is insoluble in water, freely soluble in acetic acid and in chloroform, slightly soluble in benzene, and very slightly soluble in alcohol and in ether. Its molecular weight is 608.69.
Hydralazine hydrochloride is 1-hydrazinophthalazine monohydrochloride.
Hydralazine hydrochloride USP is a white to off-white, odorless crystalline powder. It is soluble in water, slightly soluble in alcohol, and very slightly soluble in ether. It melts at about 275°C, with decomposition, and has a molecular weight of 196.64.
Hydrochlorothiazide is 6-chloro-3,4-dihydro-2*H*-1,2,4-benzothiadiazine-7-sulfonamide 1,1-dioxide.
Hydrochlorothiazide USP is a white, or practically white, practically odorless crystalline powder. It is slightly soluble in water; freely soluble in sodium hydroxide solution, in *n*-butylamine, and in dimethylformamide; sparingly soluble in methanol; and insoluble in ether, in chloroform, and in dilute mineral acids. Its molecular weight is 297.73.
Inactive ingredients: Acacia, FD&C Blue No. 1, FD&C Green No. 3, FD&C Red No. 40, FD&C Yellow No. 6, lactose, polyethylene glycol, starch, stearic acid and sucrose.

CLINICAL PHARMACOLOGY

Reserpine: Reserpine depletes stores of catecholamines and 5-hydroxytryptamine in many organs, including the brain and adrenal medulla. Most of its pharmacological effects have been attributed to this action. Depletion is slower and less complete in the adrenal medulla than in other tissues. The depression of sympathetic nerve function results in a decreased heart rate and a lowering of arterial blood pressure. The sedative and tranquilizing properties of reserpine are thought to be related to depletion of catecholamines and 5-hydroxytryptamine from the brain.
Reserpine, like other rauwolfia compounds, is characterized by slow onset of action and sustained effects. Both cardiovascular and central nervous system effects may persist for a period of time following withdrawal of the drug.
Mean maximum plasma levels of 1.54 ng/ml were attained after a median of 3.5 hours in six normal subjects receiving a single oral dose of four 0.25-mg Serpasil tablets. Bioavailability was approximately 50% of that of a corresponding intravenous dose. Plasma levels of reserpine after intravenous administration declined with a mean half-life of 33 hours. Reserpine is extensively bound (96%) to plasma proteins. No definitive studies on the human metabolism of reserpine have been made.
Hydralazine: Although the precise mechanism of action of hydralazine is not fully understood, the major effects are on the cardiovascular system. Hydralazine apparently lowers blood pressure by exerting a peripheral vasodilating effect through a direct relaxation of vascular smooth muscle. Hydralazine, by altering cellular calcium metabolism, interferes with the calcium movements within the vascular smooth muscle that are responsible for initiating or maintaining the contractile state.
The peripheral vasodilating effect of hydralazine results in decreased arterial blood pressure (diastolic more than systolic); decreased peripheral vascular resistance; and an increased heart rate, stroke volume, and cardiac output. The preferential dilatation of arterioles, as compared to veins, minimizes postural hypotension and promotes the increase in cardiac output. Hydralazine usually increases renin activity in plasma, presumably as a result of increased secretion of renin by the renal juxtaglomerular cells in response to

reflex sympathetic discharge. This increase in renin activity leads to the production of angiotensin II, which then causes stimulation of aldosterone and consequent sodium reabsorption. Hydralazine also maintains or increases renal and cerebral blood flow.
Hydralazine is rapidly absorbed after oral administration, and peak plasma levels are reached at 1–2 hours. Plasma levels decline with a half-life of 3–7 hours. Binding to human plasma protein is 87%. Plasma levels of hydralazine vary widely among individuals. Hydralazine is subject to polymorphic acetylation; slow acetylators generally have higher plasma levels of hydralazine and require lower doses to maintain control of blood pressure. Hydralazine undergoes extensive hepatic metabolism; it is excreted mainly in the form of metabolites in the urine.
Administration of hydralazine with food results in higher levels of the drug in plasma.
Hydrochlorothiazide: Thiazides affect the renal tubular mechanism of electrolyte reabsorption. At maximal therapeutic dosage, all thiazides are approximately equal in their diuretic potency. Thiazides increase excretion of sodium and chloride in approximately equivalent amounts. Natriuresis causes a secondary loss of potassium.
The mechanism of the antihypertensive effect of thiazides is unknown. Thiazides do not affect normal blood pressure.
The onset of action of thiazides occurs in 2 hours, and the peak effect at about 4 hours. The action persists for approximately 6–12 hours. Hydrochlorothiazide is rapidly absorbed, as indicated by peak plasma concentrations 1–2.5 hours after oral administration. Plasma levels of the drug are proportional to dose; the concentration in whole blood is 1.6–1.8 times higher than in plasma. Thiazides are eliminated rapidly by the kidney. After oral administration of 25- to 100-mg doses of hydrochlorothiazide, 72–97% of the dose is excreted in the urine, indicating dose-independent absorption. Hydrochlorothiazide is eliminated from plasma in a biphasic fashion with a terminal half-life of 10–17 hours. Plasma protein binding is 67.9%. Plasma clearance is 15.9–30.0 L/hr; volume of distribution is 3.6–7.8 L/kg.
Gastrointestinal absorption of hydrochlorothiazide is enhanced when administered with food. Absorption is decreased in patients with congestive heart failure, and the pharmacokinetics are considerably different in these patients.

INDICATIONS AND USAGE

Hypertension (see boxed **WARNING**).

CONTRAINDICATIONS

Reserpine: Hypersensitivity to reserpine; mental depression (especially with suicidal tendencies); active peptic ulcer, ulcerative colitis; patients receiving electroconvulsive therapy.
Hydralazine: Hypersensitivity to hydralazine; coronary artery disease; mitral valvular rheumatic heart disease.
Hydrochlorothiazide: Anuria; hypersensitivity to this or other sulfonamide-derived drugs.

WARNINGS

Reserpine: Extreme caution should be exercised in treating patients with a history of mental depression. The drug should be discontinued at the first sign of despondency, early morning insomnia, loss of appetite, impotence, or self-deprecation. Drug-induced depression may persist for several months after drug withdrawal and may be severe enough to result in suicide.
Hydralazine: In a few patients hydralazine may produce a clinical picture simulating systemic lupus erythematosus including glomerulonephritis. In such patients hydralazine should be discontinued unless the benefit-to-risk determination requires continued antihypertensive therapy with this drug. Signs and symptoms usually regress when the drug is discontinued, but residua have been detected many years later. Long-term treatment with steroids may be necessary. (See **PRECAUTIONS, Laboratory Tests.**)
Hydrochlorothiazide: Thiazides should be used with caution in patients with severe renal disease. In patients with renal disease, thiazides may precipitate azotemia. Cumulative effects of the drug may develop in patients with impaired renal function.
Thiazides should be used with caution in patients with impaired hepatic function or progressive liver disease, since minor alterations of fluid and electrolyte imbalance may precipitate hepatic coma.
Thiazides may add to or potentiate the action of other antihypertensive drugs. Potentiation occurs with ganglionic or peripheral adrenergic blocking drugs.
Sensitivity reactions are more likely to occur in patients with a history of allergy or bronchial asthma.
The possibility of exacerbation or activation of systemic lupus erythematosus has been reported.

PRECAUTIONS

General

Reserpine: Since reserpine increases gastrointestinal motility and secretion, it should be used cautiously in patients with a history of peptic ulcer, ulcerative colitis, or gallstones (biliary colic may be precipitated).
Caution should be exercised when treating hypertensive patients with renal insufficiency, since they adjust poorly to lowered blood pressure levels.
Preoperative withdrawal of reserpine does not assure that circulatory instability will not occur. It is important that the anesthesiologist be aware of the patient's drug intake and consider this in the overall management, since hypotension has occurred in patients receiving rauwolfia preparations. Anticholinergic and adrenergic drugs (e.g., metaraminol, norepinephrine) have been employed to treat adverse vagocirculatory effects.
Hydralazine: Myocardial stimulation produced by hydralazine can cause anginal attacks and ECG changes indicative of myocardial ischemia. The drug has been implicated in the production of myocardial infarction. It must, therefore, be used with caution in patients with suspected coronary artery disease.
The "hyperdynamic" circulation caused by hydralazine may accentuate specific cardiovascular inadequacies. For example, hydralazine may increase pulmonary artery pressure in patients with mitral valvular disease. The drug may reduce the pressor responses to epinephrine. Postural hypotension may result from hydralazine but is less common than with ganglionic blocking agents. It should be used with caution in patients with cerebral vascular accidents.
In hypertensive patients with normal kidneys who are treated with hydralazine, there is evidence of increased renal blood flow and a maintenance of glomerular filtration rate. In some instances where control values were below normal, improved renal function has been noted after administration of hydralazine. However, as with any antihypertensive agent, hydralazine should be used with caution in patients with advanced renal damage.
Peripheral neuritis, evidenced by paresthesia, numbness, and tingling, has been observed. Published evidence suggests that hydralazine has an antipyridoxine effect and that pyridoxine should be added to the regimen if symptoms develop.
Hydrochlorothiazide: All patients receiving thiazide therapy should be observed for clinical signs of fluid or electrolyte imbalance, namely hyponatremia, hypochloremic alkalosis, and hypokalemia (see **Laboratory Tests** and **Drug/Drug Interactions**). Warning signs are dryness of mouth, thirst, weakness, lethargy, drowsiness, restlessness, muscle pains or cramps, muscular fatigue, hypotension, oliguria, tachycardia, and gastrointestinal disturbance, such as nausea or vomiting.
Hypokalemia may develop, especially in cases of brisk diuresis or severe cirrhosis.
Interference with adequate oral intake of electrolytes will also contribute to hypokalemia. Hypokalemia may be avoided or treated by use of potassium supplements or foods with a high potassium content.
Any chloride deficit is generally mild and usually does not require specific treatment, except under extraordinary circumstances (as in liver disease or renal disease). Dilutional hyponatremia may occur in edematous patients in hot weather; appropriate therapy is water restriction, rather than administration of salt, except in rare instances when the hyponatremia is life-threatening. In cases of actual salt depletion, appropriate replacement is the therapy of choice.
Hyperuricemia may occur or frank gout may be precipitated in certain patients receiving thiazide therapy.
Latent diabetes may become manifest during thiazide administration (see **Drug/Drug Interactions**).
The antihypertensive effects of the drug may be enhanced in the postsympathectomy patient.
If progressive renal impairment becomes evident, withholding or discontinuing diuretic therapy should be considered.
Calcium excretion is decreased by thiazides. Pathological changes in the parathyroid gland with hypercalcemia and hypophosphatemia have been observed in a few patients on prolonged thiazide therapy. The common complications of hyperparathyroidism, such as renal lithiasis, bone resorption, and peptic ulceration, have not been seen.
Information for Patients: Patients should be informed of possible side effects and advised to take the medication regularly and continuously as directed.

Laboratory Tests

Hydralazine: Complete blood counts and antinuclear antibody titer determinations are indicated before and periodically during prolonged therapy with hydralazine even though the patient is asymptomatic. These studies are also indicated if the patient develops arthralgia, fever, chest pain, continued malaise, or other unexplained signs or symptoms.
A positive antinuclear antibody titer requires that the physician carefully weigh the implications of the test results against the benefits to be derived from antihypertensive therapy with a combination drug containing hydralazine.
Blood dyscrasias, consisting of reduction in hemoglobin and red cell count, leukopenia, agranulocytosis, and purpura, had been reported. If such abnormalities develop, therapy should be discontinued.
Hydrochlorothiazide: Initial and periodic determinations of serum electrolytes to detect possible electrolyte imbalance should be performed at appropriate intervals.
Serum and urine electrolyte determinations are particularly important when the patient is vomiting excessively or receiving parenteral fluids.

Drug/Drug Interactions

Reserpine: MAO inhibitors should be avoided or used with extreme caution.
Reserpine should be used cautiously with digitalis and quinidine, since cardiac arrhythmias have occurred with rauwolfia preparations.
Hydralazine: MAO inhibitors should be used with caution in patients receiving hydralazine.
When other potent parenteral antihypertensive drugs, such as diazoxide, are used in combination with hydralazine, patients should be continuously observed for several hours for any excessive fall in blood pressure. Profound hypotensive episodes may occur when diazoxide injections and hydralazine are used concomitantly.
Hydrochlorothiazide: Hypokalemia can sensitize or exaggerate the response of the heart to the toxic effects of digitalis (e.g., increased ventricular irritability).
Hypokalemia may develop during concomitant use of steroids or ACTH.
Insulin requirements in diabetic patients may be increased, decreased, or unchanged.
Thiazides may decrease arterial responsiveness to norepinephrine, but not enough to preclude effectiveness of the pressor agent for therapeutic use.
Thiazides may increase the responsiveness to tubocurarine.
Lithium renal clearance is reduced by thiazides, increasing the risk of lithium toxicity.
Drug/Laboratory Test Interactions: Thiazides may decrease serum levels of protein-bound iodine without signs of thyroid disturbance. Ser-Ap-Es should be discontinued before tests for parathyroid function are made (see **General, Hydrochlorothiazide,** Calcium excretion).

Carcinogenesis, Mutagenesis, Impairment of Fertility

Reserpine. *Animal Tumorigenicity:* Rodent studies have shown that reserpine is an animal tumorigen, causing an increased incidence of mammary fibroadenomas in female mice, malignant tumors of the seminal vesicles in male mice, and malignant adrenal medullary tumors in male rats. These findings arose in 2-year studies in which the drug was administered in the feed at concentrations of 5 and 10 ppm—about 100 to 300 times the usual human dose. The breast neoplasms are thought to be related to reserpine's prolactin-elevating effect. Several other prolactin-elevating drugs have also been associated with an increased incidence of mammary neoplasia in rodents.
The extent to which these findings indicate a risk to humans is uncertain. Tissue culture experiments show that about one third of human breast tumors are prolactin-dependent *in vitro*, a factor of considerable importance if the use of the drug is contemplated in a patient with previously detected breast cancer. The possibility of an increased risk of breast cancer in reserpine users has been studied extensively; however, no firm conclusion has emerged. Although a few epidemiologic studies have suggested a slightly increased risk (less than twofold in all studies except one) in women who have used reserpine, other studies of generally similar design have not confirmed this. Epidemiologic studies conducted using other drugs (neuroleptic agents) that, like reserpine, increase prolactin levels and therefore would be considered rodent mammary carcinogens have not shown an association between chronic administration of the drug and human mammary tumorigenesis. While long-term clinical observation has not suggested such an association, the available evidence is considered too limited to be conclusive at this time. An association of reserpine intake with pheochromocytoma or tumors of the seminal vesicles has not been explored.
Hydralazine: In a lifetime study in Swiss albino mice, there was a statistically significant increase in the incidence of lung tumors (adenomas and adenocarcinomas) of both male and female mice given hydralazine continuously in their drinking water at a dosage of about 250 mg/kg per day (about 80 times the maximum recommended human dose). In a 2-year carcinogenicity study of rats given hydralazine by gavage at dose levels of 15, 30, and 60 mg/kg/day (approximately 5 to 20 times the recommended human daily dosage), microscopic examination of the liver revealed a small, but statistically significant, increase in benign neoplastic nodules in male and female rats from the high-dose group and in female rats from the intermediate-dose group. Benign interstitial cell tumors of the testes were also significantly increased in male rats from the high-dose group. The tumors observed are common in aged rats and a significantly in-

Continued on next page

The full prescribing information for each CIBA drug is contained herein and is that in effect as of September 1, 1986

CIBA—Cont.

creased incidence was not observed until 18 months of treatment. Hydralazine was shown to be mutagenic in three bacterial tester strains in the Ames test, both with and without metabolic activation, and elicited DNA repair both in the Pol A^+/A^- *E. coli* bacterial assay system and in cultured rat hepatocytes. (Evidence of DNA damage in the hepatocyte repair test is considered a strong indication of covalent binding, an established property of carcinogens and mutagens.) In tests with rabbit hepatocytes that exhibit an acetylator polymorphism like that of humans, hydralazine elicited DNA repair with only those hepatocytes having a slow rate of acetylation, suggesting that individuals who are rapid acetylators may have a diminished genotoxic liability. No increase in mutagenic potential was revealed in the mouse lymphoma assay, host-mediated assay, nucleus anomaly test, or dominant lethal test.
The extent to which these findings indicate a risk to man is uncertain. While long-term clinical observation has not suggested that human cancer is associated with hydralazine use, epidemiologic studies have so far been insufficient to arrive at any conclusions.
Hydrochlorothiazide: Long-term carcinogenicity studies in animals have not been conducted with Esidrix.
Pregnancy Category C: Animal reproduction studies have not been conducted with Sep-Ap-Es. Reserpine administered parenterally has been shown to be teratogenic in rats at doses up to 2 mg/kg and to have an embryocidal effect in guinea pigs given dosages of 0.5 mg daily. Animal studies indicate that hydralazine is teratogenic in mice at 20–30 times the maximum daily human dose of 200–300 mg and possibly in rabbits at 10–15 times the maximum daily human dose, but that it is nonteratogenic in rats. Teratogenic effects observed were cleft palate and malformations of facial and cranial bones. A reproduction study in rats receiving hydrochlorothiazide, 250 mg/kg daily, 62.5 times the maximum daily human dose, has revealed no evidence of impaired fertility or harm to the fetus.
There are no adequate and well-controlled studies of Ser-Ap-Es in pregnant women. Ser-Ap-Es should be used during pregnancy only if the potential benefit justifies the potential risk to the fetus.
Nonteratogenic Effects: Reserpine crosses the placental barrier, and increased respiratory tract secretions, nasal congestion, cyanosis, and anorexia may occur in neonates of mothers treated with reserpine. Thiazides also cross the placental barrier and appear in cord blood, and there is a risk of fetal or neonatal jaundice, thrombocytopenia, and possibly other adverse reactions that have occurred in adults.
Nursing Mothers: Reserpine is excreted in maternal breast milk, and increased respiratory tract secretions, nasal congestion, cyanosis, and anorexia may occur in breast-fed infants. Thiazides are also excreted in breast milk. Because of the potential for serious adverse reactions in nursing infants and the potential for tumorigenicity shown for reserpine in animal studies, a decision should be made whether to discontinue nursing or to discontinue Ser-Ap-Es, taking into account the importance of the drug to the mother.
Pediatric Use: Safety and effectiveness of the combination drug in chilren have not been established.

ADVERSE REACTIONS

Adverse reactions are usually reversible upon reduction of dosage or discontinuation of Ser-Ap-Es. Whenever adverse reactions are moderate or severe, it may be necessary to discontinue the drug.
The following adverse reactions have been observed, but there has not been enough systematic collection of data to support an estimate of their frequency. Consequently the reactions are categorized by organ system and are listed in decreasing order of severity and not frequency.
Reserpine: The following have been observed with rauwolfia preparations:
Digestive: Vomiting, diarrhea, nausea, anorexia, dryness of mouth, hypersecretion.
Cardiovascular: Arrhythmias (particularly when used concurrently with digitalis or quinidine), syncope, angina-like symptoms, bradycardia, edema.
Respiratory: Dyspnea, epistaxis, nasal congestion.
Neurologic: Rare parkinsonian syndrome and other extrapyramidal tract symptoms; dizziness; headache; paradoxical anxiety; depression; nervousness; nightmares; dull sensorium; drowsiness.
Musculoskeletal: Muscular aches.
Genitourinary: Pseudolactation, impotence, dysuria, gynecomastia, decreased libido, breast engorgement.
Metabolic: Weight gain.
Special Senses: Deafness, optic atrophy, glaucoma, uveitis, conjunctival injection.
Hypersensitive Reactions: Purpura, rash, pruritus.
Hydralazine: *Digestive:* Hepatitis, paralytic ileus, vomiting, diarrhea, nausea, constipation, anorexia.
Cardiovascular: Angina pectoris, hypotension, paradoxical pressor response, tachycardia, palpitations, edema, flushing.
Respiratory: Dyspnea, nasal congestion.
Neurologic: Psychotic reactions characterized by depression, disorientation, or anxiety; peripheral neuritis, evidenced by paresthesia, numbness, and tingling; tremors; dizziness; headache.
Musculoskeletal: Muscle cramps, arthralgia.
Genitourinary: Difficulty in urination.
Hematologic: Blood dyscrasias, consisting of reduction in hemoglobin and red cell count, leukopenia, agranulocytosis; lymphadenopathy; splenomegaly; eosinophilia.
Special Senses: Conjunctivitis, lacrimation.
Hypersensitive Reactions: Purpura, fever, urticaria, rash, pruritus, chills.
Hydrochlorothiazide: *Digestive:* Pancreatitis, jaundice (intrahepatic cholestatic), sialadenitis, vomiting, diarrhea, cramping, nausea, gastric irritation, constipation, anorexia.
Cardiovascular: Orthostatic hypotension (may be potentiated by alcohol, barbiturates, or narcotics).
Neurologic: Vertigo, dizziness, transient blurred vision, headache, paresthesia, xanthopsia, weakness, restlessness.
Musculoskeletal: Muscle spasm.
Hematologic: Aplastic anemia, agranulocytosis, leukopenia, thrombocytopenia.
Metabolic: Hyperglycemia, glycosuria, hyperuricemia.
Hypersensitive Reactions: Necrotizing angiitis, Stevens-Johnson syndrome, purpura, urticaria, rash, photosensitivity.

OVERDOSAGE

Acute Toxocity: No deaths due to acute poisoning with Ser-Ap-Es have been reported.
Oral LD_{50}'s in animals (mg/kg): rats, 397; mice, 272.
Signs and Symptoms
Reserpine. The clinical picture of acute poisoning is characterized chiefly by signs and symptoms due to the reflex parasympathomimetic effect of reserpine.
Impairment of consciousness may occur and may range from drowsiness to coma, depending upon the severity of overdosage. Flushing of the skin, conjunctival injection, and pupillary constriction are to be expected. Hypotension, hypothermia, central respiratory depression, and bradycardia may develop in cases of severe overdosage. Increased salivary and gastric secretion and diarrhea may also occur.
Hydralazine. Signs and symptoms of overdosage include hypotension, tachycardia, headache, and generalized skin flushing.
Complications can include myocardial ischemia and subsequent myocardial infarction, cardiac arrhythmia, and profound shock.
Hydrochlorothiazide. The most prominent feature of poisoning is acute loss of fluid and electrolytes.
Cardiovascular: Tachycardia, hypotension, shock.
Neuromuscular: Weakness, confusion, dizziness, cramps of the calf muscles, paresthesia, fatigue, impairment of consciousness.
Digestive: Nausea, vomiting, thirst.
Renal: Polyuria, oliguria, or anuria (due to hemoconcentration).
Laboratory Findings: Hypokalemia, hyponatremia, hypochloremia, alkalosis; increased BUN (especially in patients with renal insufficiency).
Combined Poisoning: Signs and symptoms may be aggravated or modified by concomitant intake of antihypertensive medication, barbiturates, digitalis (hypokalemia), corticosteroids, narcotics, or alcohol.
Treatment: There is no specific antidote.
The gastric contents should be evacuated, taking adequate precautions against aspiration and for protection of the airway. An activated charcoal slurry may be instilled if conditions permit. Dialysis may not be effective for elimination of Ser-Ap-Es because of its plasma protein binding (see **CLINICAL PHARMACOLOGY**).
These manipulations may have to be omitted or carried out after cardiovascular status has been stabilized, since they might precipitate cardiac arrhythmias or increase the depth of shock.
If hypotension or shock occurs, the patient's legs should be kept raised and lost fluid and electrolytes (potassium, sodium) should be replaced.
Support of the cardiovascular system is of primary importance in suspected hydralazine overdosage. If possible, vasopressors should not be given, but if a vasopressor is required, care should be taken not to precipitate or aggravate cardiac arrhythmia. Tachycardia responds to beta blockers. Digitalization may be necessary.
If hypotension is severe enough to require treatment with a vasopressor, one having a direct action upon vascular smooth muscle (e.g., phenylephrine, levarterenol, metaraminol) should be used to treat the symptomatic effects of reserpine overdosage.
Fluid and electrolyte balance (especially serum potassium) and renal function should be monitored until conditions become normal. Since reserpine is long-acting, the patient should be observed carefully for at least 72 hours.

DOSAGE AND ADMINISTRATION

Dosage should be determined by individual titration (see boxed **WARNING**). The usual dosage is one to two tablets three times daily.
Since the antihypertensive effects of reserpine are not immediately apparent, maximal reduction in blood pressure from a given dosage may not occur for 2 weeks. For maintenance, dosage should be adjusted to the lowest requirement of the individual patient.
When necessary, more potent antihypertensives may be added gradually in dosages reduced by at least 50%; the effects should be carefully observed.

HOW SUPPLIED

Tablets—round, light-salmon pink, dry-coated (imprinted CIBA 71) 0.1 mg of reserpine, 25 mg of hydralazine hydrochloride, 15 mg of hydrochlorothiazide
Bottles of 100—NDC 0083-0071-30
Bottles of 1000—NDC 0083-0071-40
Consumer Pack—One Unit
12 bottles—100 tablets each—NDC 0083-0071-65
Accu-Pak® Unit Dose (blister pack)
Box of 100 (strips of 10)—NDC 0083-0071-32
Dispense in tight, light-resistant container (USP).
C85-21 (Rev. 8/85)
Shown in Product Identification Section, page 408

SERPASIL® ℞

[*sir'pah-sill*]
reserpine USP
Tablets

DESCRIPTION

Serpasil, reserpine USP, is an antihypertensive, available as 0.1-mg and 0.25-mg tablets for oral administration. Its chemical name is methyl 18β-hydroxy-11,17α-dimethoxy-3β,20α-yohimban-16β-carboxylate 3,4,5-trimethoxybenzoate (ester).
Reserpine USP, a pure crystalline alkaloid of rauwolfia, ia a white or pale buff to slightly yellowish, odorless crystalline powder. It darkens slowly on exposure to light, but more rapidly when in solution. It is insoluble in water, freely soluble in acetic acid and in chloroform, slightly soluble in benzene, and very slightly soluble in alcohol and in ether. Its molecular weight is 608.69.
Inactive Ingredients. Lactose, magnesium stearate, polyethylene glycol, starch, sucrose, talc, and tragacanth (0.1-mg tablets.)

CLINICAL PHARMACOLOGY

Serpasil depletes stores of catecholamines and 5-hydroxytryptamine in many organs, including the brain and adrenal medulla. Most of its pharmacological effects have been attributed to this action. Depletion is slower and less complete in the adrenal medulla than in other tissues.
The depression of sympathetic nerve function results in a decreased heart rate and a lowering of arterial blood pressure. The sedative and tranquilizing properties of Serpasil are thought to be related to depletion of catecholamines and 5-hydroxytryptamine from the brain.
Serpasil, like other rauwolfia compounds, is characterized by slow onset of action and sustained effects. Both cardiovascular and central nervous system effects may persist for a period of time following withdrawal of the drug.
Mean maximum plasma levels of 1.54 ng/ml were attained after a median of 3.5 hours in six normal subjects receiving a single oral dose of four 0.25-mg Serpasil tablets. Bioavailability was approximately 50% of that of a corresponding intravenous dose. Plasma levels of reserpine after intravenous administration declined with a mean half-life of 33 hours. Reserpine is extensively bound (96%) to plasma proteins. No definitive studies on the human metabolism of reserpine have been made.

INDICATIONS AND USAGE

Mild essential hypertension; also useful as adjunctive therapy with other antihypertensive agents in the more severe forms of hypertension; relief of symptoms in agitated psychotic states (e.g., schizophrenia), primarily in those individuals unable to tolerate phenothiazine derivatives or in those who also require antihypertensive medication.

CONTRAINDICATIONS

Known hypersensitivity, mental depression (especially with suicidal tendencies), active peptic ulcer, ulcerative colitis, and patients receiving electroconvulsive therapy.

WARNINGS

Extreme caution should be exercised in treating patients with a history of mental depression. Discontinue the drug at first sign of despondency, early morning insomnia, loss of appetite, impotence, or self-deprecation. Drug-induced depression may persist for several months after drug withdrawal and may be severe enough to result in suicide.

PRECAUTIONS

General

Since Serpasil increases gastrointestinal motility and secretion, it should be used cautiously in patients with a history of peptic ulcer, ulcerative colitis, or gallstones (biliary colic may be precipitated).

Caution should be exercised when treating hypertensive patients with renal insufficiency, since they adjust poorly to lowered blood pressure levels.

Preoperative withdrawal of reserpine does not assure that circulatory instability will not occur. It is important that the anesthesiologist be aware of the patient's drug intake and consider this in the overall management, since hypotension has occurred in patients receiving rauwolfia preprations. Anticholinergic and/or adrenergic drugs (e.g., metaraminol, norepinephrine) have been employed to treat adverse vagocirculatory effects.

Information for Patients

Patients should be informed of possible side effects and advised to take the medication regularly and continuously as directed.

Drug Interactions

MAO inhibitors should be avoided or used with extreme caution.

Serpasil should be used cautiously with digitalis and quinidine, since cardiac arrhythmias have occurred with rauwolfia preparations.

Concomitant use of Serpasil with other antihypertensive agents necessitates careful titration of dosage with each agent.

Carcinogenesis, Mutagenesis, Impairment of Fertility

Animal Tumorigenicity. Rodent studies have shown that reserpine is an animal tumorigen, causing an increased incidence of mammary fibroadenomas in female mice, malignant tumors of the seminal vesicles in male mice, and malignant adrenal medullary tumors in male rats. These findings arose in 2-year studies in which the drug was administered in the feed at concentrations of 5 and 10 ppm—about 100 to 300 times the usual human dose. The breast neoplasms are thought to be related to reserpine's prolactin-elevating effect. Several other prolactin-elevating drugs have also been associated with an increased incidence of mammary neoplasia in rodents.

The extent to which these findings indicate a risk to humans is uncertain. Tissue culture experiments show that about one third of human breast tumors are prolactin-dependent *in vitro*, a factor of considerable importance if the use of the drug is contemplated in a patient with previously detected breast cancer. The possibility of an increased risk of breast cancer in reserpine users has been studied extensively; however, no firm conclusion has emerged. Although a few epidemiologic studies have suggested a slightly increased risk (less than twofold in all studies except one) in women who have used reserpine, other studies of generally similar design have not confirmed this. Epidemiologic studies conducted using other drugs (neuroleptic agents) that, like reserpine, increase prolactin levels and therefore would be considered rodent mammary carcinogens have not shown an association between chronic administration of the drug and human mammary tumorigenesis. While long-term clinical observation has not suggested such an association, the available evidence is considered too limited to be conclusive at this time. An association of reserpine intake with pheochromocytoma or tumors of the seminal vesicles has not been explored.

Pregnancy Category C

Reserpine administered parenterally has been shown to be teratogenic in rats at doses up to 2 mg/kg and to have an embryocidal effect in guinea pigs given dosages of 0.5 mg daily.

There are no adequate and well-controlled studies of Serpasil in pregnant women. Serpasil should be used during pregnancy only if the potential benefit justifies the potential risk to the fetus.

Nonteratogenic Effects. Reserpine crosses the placental barrier, and increased respiratory tract secretions, nasal congestion, cyanosis, and anorexia may occur in neonates of reserpine-treated mothers.

Nursing Mothers

Reserpine is excreted in maternal breast milk, and increased respiratory tract secretions, nasal congestion, cyanosis, and anorexia may occur in breast-fed infants. Because of the potential for adverse reactions in nursing infants and the potential for tumorigenicity shown for reserpine in animal studies, a decision should be made whether to discontinue nursing or to discontinue the drug, taking into account the importance of the drug to the mother.

Pediatric Use

Safety and effectiveness in children have not been established by means of controlled clinical trials, although there is experience with the use of Serpasil in children. (See **DOSAGE AND ADMINISTRATION.**) Because of adverse effects such as emotional depression and lability, sedation, and stuffy nose, Serpasil is not usually recommended as a step-2 drug in the treatment of hypertension in children.

ADVERSE REACTIONS

The following adverse reactions have been observed with rauwolfia preparations, but there has not been enough systematic collection of data to support an estimate of their frequency. Consequently the reactions are categorized by organ system and are listed in decreasing order of severity and not frequency.

Digestive: Vomiting, diarrhea, nausea, anorexia, dryness of mouth, hypersecretion.

Cardiovascular: Arrhythmias (particularly when used concurrently with digitalis or quinidine), syncope, angina-like symptoms, bradycardia, edema.

Respiratory: Dyspnea, epistaxis, nasal congestion.

Neurologic: Rare parkinsonian syndrome and other extrapyramidal tract symptoms; dizziness; headache; paradoxical anxiety; depression; nervousness; nightmares; dull sensorium; drowsiness.

Musculoskeletal: Muscular aches.

Genitourinary: Pseudolactation, impotence, dysuria, gynecomastia, decreased libido, breast engorgement.

Metabolic: Weight gain.

Special Senses: Deafness, optic atrophy, glaucoma, uveitis, conjunctival injection.

Hypersensitive Reactions: Purpura, rash, pruritus.

OVERDOSAGE

Acute Toxicity

No deaths due to acute poisoning with reserpine have been reported.

Highest known doses survived: children, 1000 mg (age and sex not specified); young children, 200 mg (20-month-old boy).

Oral LD_{50}'s in animals (mg/kg): rat, 2993; mouse, 47 and 500.

Signs and Symptoms

The clinical picture of acute poisoning is characterized chiefly by signs and symptoms due to the reflex parasympathomimetic effect of reserpine.

Impairment of consciousness may occur and may range from drowsiness to coma, depending upon the severity of overdosage. Flushing of the skin, conjunctival injection, and pupillary constriction are to be expected. Hypotension, hypothermia, central respiratory depression, and bradycardia may develop in cases of severe overdosage. Increased salivary and gastric secretion and diarrhea may also occur.

Treatment

There is no specific antidote.

Stomach contents should be evacuated, taking adequate precautions against aspiration and for protection of the airway. Activated charcoal slurry should be instilled.

The effects of reserpine overdosage should be treated symptomatically. If hypotension is severe enough to require treatment with a vasopressor, one having a direct action upon vascular smooth muscle (e.g., phenylephrine, levarterenol, metaraminol) should be used. Since reserpine is long-acting, the patient should be observed carefully for at least 72 hours, and treatment administered as required.

DOSAGE AND ADMINISTRATION

Hypertension

In the average patient not receiving other antihypertensive agents, the usual initial dosage is 0.5 mg daily for 1 or 2 weeks. For maintenance, reduce to 0.1–0.25 mg daily. Higher dosages should be used cautiously, because occurrence of serious mental depression and other side effects may increase considerably.

Psychiatric Disorders

The usual initial dosage is 0.5 mg daily, but may range from 0.1 mg to 1.0 mg. Adjust dosage upward or downward according to the patient's response.

Children

Serpasil is not recommended for use in children (see **PRECAUTIONS, Pediatric Use**). If it is to be used in treating a child, the usual recommended starting dose is 20 μg/kg daily. The maximum recommended dose is 0.25 mg (total) daily.

HOW SUPPLIED

Tablets 0.1 mg—round, white (imprinted CIBA 35)
Bottles of 100 .... NDC 0083-0035-30
Bottles of 1000 .... NDC 0083-0035-40

Tablets 0.25 mg—round, white, scored (imprinted CIBA 36)
Bottles of 100 .... NDC 0083-0036-30
Bottles of 500 .... NDC 0083-0036-35
Bottles of 1000 .... NDC 0083-0036-40
Consumer Pack—One Unit
12 bottles—100 tablets each .... NDC 0083-0036-65

Protect from light.
Dispense in tight, light-resistant container (USP).

C85-64 (Rev. 11/85)

Shown in Product Identification Section, page 408

SERPASIL® ℞

[*sir 'pah-sill*]
reserpine USP
Parenteral Solution

Listed in USP, a Medicare designated compendium.

DESCRIPTION

Reserpine, a pure crystalline alkaloid of rauwolfia, is a white or pale buff to slightly yellowish crystalline powder which darkens slowly on exposure to light and is insoluble in water. Chemically, it is methyl-0-(3,4,5-trimethoxybenzoyl)-reserpate.

ACTIONS

Serpasil probably produces its antihypertensive effects through depletion of tissue stores of catecholamines (epinephrine and norepinephrine) from peripheral sites. This depression of sympathetic nerve function results in a decreased heart rate and a lowering of arterial blood pressure. In contrast, Serpasil's sedative and tranquilizing properties are thought to be related to depletion of 5-hydroxytryptamine from the brain.

Serpasil, like other rauwolfia compounds, is characterized by slow onset of action and sustained effects. Both cardiovascular and central nervous system effects may persist for a period of time following withdrawal of the drug.

INDICATIONS

Hypertensive emergencies, such as acute hypertensive encephalopathy, in which it is desired to reduce blood pressure rapidly; psychiatric conditions only to initiate treatment in those patients unable to accept oral medication or to control symptoms of extreme agitation.

CONTRAINDICATIONS

Known hypersensitivity, mental depression (especially with suicidal tendencies), active peptic ulcer, ulcerative colitis, and patients receiving electroconvulsive therapy.

WARNINGS

Extreme caution should be exercised in treating patients with a history of mental depression. Discontinue the drug at first sign of despondency, early morning insomnia, loss of appetite, impotence, or self-deprecation. Drug-induced depression may persist for several months after drug withdrawal and may be severe enough to result in suicide.

MAO inhibitors should be avoided or used with extreme caution.

Usage in Pregnancy

The safety of reserpine for use during pregnancy or lactation has not been established; therefore, the drug should be used in pregnant patients or in women of childbearing potential only when, in the judgment of the physician, it is essential to the welfare of the patient. Increased respiratory tract secretions, nasal congestion, cyanosis, and anorexia may occur in neonates and breast-fed infants of reserpine-treated mothers since reserpine crosses the placental barrier and also appears in maternal breast milk.

PRECAUTIONS

Since Serpasil increases gastrointestinal motility and secretion, it should be used cautiously in patients with a history of peptic ulcer, ulcerative colitis, or gallstones (biliary colic may be precipitated).

Caution should be exercised when treating hypertensive patients with renal insufficiency since they adjust poorly to lowered blood pressure levels.

Use Serpasil cautiously with digitalis and quinidine since cardiac arrhythmias have occurred with rauwolfia preparations.

Preoperative withdrawal of reserpine does not assure that circulatory instability will not occur. It is important that the anesthesiologist be aware of the patient's drug intake and consider this in the overall management, since hypotension has occurred in patients receiving rauwolfia preparations. Anticholinergic and/or adrenergic drugs (*eg*, metaraminol, norepinephrine) have been employed to treat adverse vagocirculatory effects.

Animal tumorigenicity: Rodent studies have shown that reserpine is an animal tumorigen, causing an increased incidence of mammary fibroadenomas in female mice, malignant tumors of the seminal vesicles in male mice, and malignant adrenal medullary tumors in male rats. These findings arose in 2-year studies in which the drug was administered in the feed at concentrations of 5 and 10 ppm—about 100 to 300 times the usual human dose. The breast neoplasms are thought to be related to reserpine's prolactin-elevating effect. Several other prolactin-elevating drugs have also been associated with an increased incidence of mammary neoplasia in rodents.

Continued on next page

The full prescribing information for each CIBA drug is contained herein and is that in effect as of September 1, 1986

CIBA—Cont.

The extent to which these findings indicate a risk to humans is uncertain. Tissue culture experiments show that about one-third of human breast tumors are prolactin-dependent *in vitro*, a factor of considerable importance if the use of the drug is contemplated in a patient with previously detected breast cancer. The possibility of an increased risk of breast cancer in reserpine users has been studied extensively, however, no firm conclusion has emerged. Although a few epidemiologic studies have suggested a slightly increased risk (less than twofold in all studies except one) in women who have used reserpine, other studies of generally similar design have not confirmed this. Epidemiologic studies conducted using other drugs (neuroleptic agents) that, like reserpine, increase prolactin levels and therefore would be considered rodent mammary carcinogens, have not shown an association between chronic administration of the drug and human mammary tumorigenesis. While long-term clinical observation has not suggested such an association, the available evidence is considered too limited to be conclusive at this time. An association of reserpine intake with pheochromocytoma or tumors of the seminal vesicles has not been explored.

ADVERSE REACTIONS

Rauwolfia preparations have caused gastrointestinal reactions including hypersecretion, nausea, vomiting, anorexia, and diarrhea; cardiovascular reactions including angina-like symptoms, arrhythmias (particularly when used concurrently with digitalis or quinidine), bradycardia; central nervous system reactions including drowsiness, depression, nervousness, paradoxical anxiety, nightmares, rare parkinsonian syndrome and other extrapyramidal tract symptoms, and CNS sensitization manifested by dull sensorium, deafness, glaucoma, uveitis, and optic atrophy. Nasal congestion is a frequent occurrence. Pruritus, rash, dryness of mouth, dizziness, headache, dyspnea, syncope, epistaxis, purpura and other hematologic reactions, impotence or decreased libido, dysuria, muscular aches, conjunctival injection, weight gain, breast engorgement, pseudolactation, and gynecomastia have been reported. These reactions are usually reversible and usually disappear after the drug is discontinued.

Water retention with edema in patients with hypertensive vascular disease may occur rarely, but the condition generally clears with cessation of therapy or with the administration of a diuretic agent.

DOSAGE AND ADMINISTRATION

Serpasil may be administered intramuscularly in the short-term treatment of hypertensive crises. Because of the varying responsiveness, a titration procedure should be used. An initial dose of 0.5 to 1 mg intramuscularly is followed at intervals of 3 hours, if necessary, by doses of 2 and 4 mg until the blood pressure falls to the desired level. If the 4-mg dose is ineffective, other antihypertensive agents should be used. An initial dose larger than 0.5 mg may induce severe hypotension, particularly in patients with cerebral hemorrhage.

Serpasil may be administered intramuscularly in psychiatric emergencies to initiate treatment in those patients unable to accept oral medication or to control extreme agitation. The usual dose is from 2.5 mg to 5.0 mg, following a small initial dose to test patient responsiveness.

Concomitant use of Serpasil with ganglionic blocking agents, guanethidine, veratrum, hydralazine, methyldopa, chlorthalidone, or thiazides necessitates careful titration of dosage with each agent.

OVERDOSAGE

Signs and Symptoms

Impairment of consciousness may occur and may range from drowsiness to coma, depending upon the severity of overdosage. Flushing of the skin, conjunctival injection, and pupillary constriction are to be expected. Hypotension, hypothermia, central respiratory depression, and bradycardia may develop in cases of severe overdosage. Diarrhea may also occur.

Treatment

Hypotension is likely to require major therapeutic attention. If a vasopressor is necessary, use one having a direct action upon vascular smooth muscle (*eg*, phenylephrine, levarterenol, metaraminol).

If bradycardia becomes marked, especially with cardiac arrhythmia, consider use of vagal blocking agents along with other appropriate measures.

Treat other effects of reserpine overdosage symptomatically. Since reserpine is long-acting, observe the patient carefully for at least 72 hours, administering treatment as required.

HOW SUPPLIED

Parenteral Solution: Each ml contains 2.5 mg reserpine, 0.1 ml dimethylacetamide, 10 mg adipic acid, 0.1 mg versene, 0.01 ml benzyl alcohol, 0.05 ml polyethylene glycol, 0.5 mg ascorbic acid, and 0.1 mg sodium sulfite in water. *Ampuls*, 2 ml; cartons of 5.

C83-25 (Rev. 9/83)

SERPASIL®–APRESOLINE® ℞

[*sir 'pah-sill a-press 'oh-leen*]

reserpine and hydralazine hydrochloride
Combination Tablets

> **WARNING**
> This fixed-combination drug is not indicated for initial therapy of hypertension. Hypertension requires therapy titrated to the individual patient. If the fixed combination represents the dosage so determined, its use may be more convenient in patient management. The treatment of hypertension is not static but must be reevaluated as conditions in each patient warrant.

DESCRIPTION

Serpasil-Apresoline is an antihypertensive combination, available as tablets for oral administration. Tablets #1 contain reserpine USP, 0.1 mg, and hydralazine hydrochloride USP, 25 mg; tablets #2 contain reserpine USP, 0.2 mg, and hydralazine hydrochloride USP, 50 mg.

Reserpine is methyl 18β-hydroxy-11,17α-dimethoxy-3β, 20α-yohimban-16β-carboxylate, 3,4,5-trimethoxybenzoate (ester).

Reserpine USP, a pure crystalline alkaloid of rauwolfia, is a white or pale buff to slightly yellowish, odorless crystalline powder. It darkens slowly on exposure to light, but more rapidly when in solution. It is insoluble in water, freely soluble in acetic acid and in chloroform, slightly soluble in benzene, and very slightly soluble in alcohol and in ether. Its molecular weight is 608.69.

Hydralazine hydrochloride is 1-hydrazinophthalazine monohydrochloride.

Hydralazine hydrochloride USP is a white to off-white, odorless crystalline powder. It is soluble in water, slightly soluble in alcohol, and very slightly soluble in ether. It melts at about 275°C, with decomposition, and has a molecular weight of 196.64.

Inactive Ingredients: FD&C Yellow No. 5, lactose, magnesium stearate, polyethylene glycol, starch, sucrose, talc and tragacanth.

CLINICAL PHARMACOLOGY

Reserpine

Reserpine depletes stores of catecholamines and 5-hydroxytryptamine in many organs, including the brain and adrenal medulla. Most of its pharmacological effects have been attributed to this action. Depletion is slower and less complete in the adrenal medulla than in other tissues.

The depression of sympathetic nerve function results in a decreased heart rate and a lowering of arterial blood pressure. The sedative and tranquilizing properties of reserpine are thought to be related to depletion of catecholamines and 5-hydroxytryptamine from the brain.

Reserpine, like other rauwolfia compounds, is characterized by slow onset of action and sustained effects. Both cardiovascular and central nervous system effects may persist for a period of time following withdrawal of the drug.

Mean maximum plasma levels of 1.54 ng/ml were attained after a median of 3.5 hours in six normal subjects receiving a single oral dose of four 0.25-mg Serpasil tablets. Bioavailability was approximately 50% of that of a corresponding intravenous dose. Plasma levels of reserpine after intravenous administration declined with a mean half-life of 33 hours. Reserpine is extensively bound (96%) to plasma proteins. No definitive studies on the human metabolism of reserpine have been made.

Hydralazine

Although the precise mechanism of action of hydralazine is not fully understood, the major effects are on the cardiovascular system. Hydralazine apparently lowers blood pressure by exerting a peripheral vasodilating effect through a direct relaxation of vascular smooth muscle. Hydralazine, by altering cellular calcium metabolism, interferes with the calcium movements within the vascular smooth muscle that are responsible for initiating or maintaining the contractile state.

The peripheral vasodilating effect of hydralazine results in decreased arterial blood pressure (diastolic more than systolic); decreased peripheral vascular resistance; and an increased heart rate, stroke volume, and cardiac output. The preferential dilatation of arterioles, as compared to veins, minimizes postural hypotension and promotes the increase in cardiac output. Hydralazine usually increases renin activity in plasma, presumably as a result of increased secretion of renin by the renal juxtaglomerular cells in response to reflex sympathetic discharge. This increase in renin activity leads to the production of angiotensin II, which then causes stimulation of aldosterone and consequent sodium reabsorption. Hydralazine also maintains or increases renal and cerebral blood flow.

Hydralazine is rapidly absorbed after oral administration, and peak plasma levels are reached at 1–2 hours. Plasma levels decline with a half-life of 3–7 hours. Binding to human plasma protein is 87%. Plasma levels of hydralazine vary widely among individuals. Hydralazine is subject to polymorphic acetylation; slow acetylators generally have higher plasma levels of hydralazine and require lower doses to maintain control of blood pressure. Hydralazine undergoes extensive hepatic metabolism; it is excreted mainly in the form of metabolites in the urine.

Administration of hydralazine with food results in higher levels of the drug in plasma.

INDICATIONS AND USAGE

Hypertension (see boxed **WARNING**).

CONTRAINDICATIONS

Reserpine

Hypersensitivity to reserpine; mental depression (especially with suicidal tendencies); active peptic ulcer, ulcerative colitis; patients receiving electroconvulsive therapy.

Hydralazine

Hypersensitivity to hydralazine; coronary artery disease; mitral valvular rheumatic heart disease.

WARNINGS

Reserpine

Extreme caution should be exercised in treating patients with a history of mental depression. The drug should be discontinued at the first sign of despondency, early morning insomnia, loss of appetite, impotence, or self-deprecation. Drug-induced depression may persist for several months after drug withdrawal and may be severe enough to result in suicide.

Hydralazine

In a few patients hydralazine may produce a clinical picture stimulating systemic lupus erythematosus including glomerulonephritis. In such patients hydralazine should be discontinued unless the benefit-to-risk determination requires continued antihypertensive therapy with this drug. Signs and symptoms usually regress when the drug is discontinued, but residua have been detected many years later. Long-term treatment with steroids may be necessary. (See **PRECAUTIONS, Laboratory Tests.**)

PRECAUTIONS

General

The Serpasil-Apresoline tablets (#1 and #2) contain FD&C Yellow No. 5 (tartrazine) which may cause allergic-type reactions (including bronchial asthma) in certain susceptible individuals. Although the overall incidence of FD&C Yellow No. 5 (tartrazine) sensitivity in the general population is low, it is frequently seen in patients who also have aspirin hypersensitivity.

Reserpine. Since reserpine increases gastrointestinal motility and secretion, it should be used cautiously in patients with a history of peptic ulcer, ulcerative colitis, or gallstones (biliary colic may be precipitated).

Caution should be exercised when treating hypertensive patients with renal insufficiency, since they adjust poorly to lowered blood pressure levels.

Preoperative withdrawal of reserpine does not assure that circulatory instability will not occur. It is important that the anesthesiologist be aware of the patient's drug intake and consider this in the overall management, since hypotension has occurred in patients receiving rauwolfia preparations. Anticholinergic and adrenergic drugs (e.g., metaraminol, norepinephrine) have been employed to treat adverse vagocirculatory effects.

Hydralazine. Myocardial stimulation produced by hydralazine can cause anginal attacks and ECG changes indicative of myocardial ischemia. The drug has been implicated in the production of myocardial infarction. It must, therefore, be used with caution in patients with suspected coronary artery disease.

The "hyperdynamic" circulation caused by hydralazine may accentuate specific cardiovascular inadequacies. For example, hydralazine may increase pulmonary artery pressure in patients with mitral valvular disease. The drug may reduce the pressor response to epinephrine. Postural hypotension may result from hydralazine but is less common than with ganglionic blocking agents. It should be used with caution in patients with cerebral vascular accidents.

In hypertensive patients with normal kidneys who are treated with hydralazine, there is evidence of increased renal blood flow and a maintenance of glomerular filtration rate. In some instances where control values were below normal, improved renal function has been noted after administration of hydralazine. However, as with any antihypertensive agent, hydralazine should be used with caution in patients with advanced renal damage.

Peripheral neuritis, evidenced by paresthesia, numbness, and tingling, has been observed. Published evidence suggests that hydralazine has an antipyridoxine effect and that pyridoxine should be added to the regimen if symptoms develop.

Information for Patients

Patients should be informed of possible side effects and advised to take the medication regularly and continously as directed.

Laboratory Tests

Hydralazine. Complete blood counts and antinuclear antibody titer determinations are indicated before and periodi-

cally during prolonged therapy with hydralazine even though the patient is asymptomatic. These studies are also indicated if the patient develops arthralgia, fever, chest pain, continued malaise, or other unexplained signs or symptoms.
A positive antinuclear antibody titer requires that the physician carefully weigh the implications of the test results against the benefits to be derived from antihypertensive therapy with a combination drug containing hydralazine.
Blood dyscrasias, consisting of reduction in hemoglobin and red cell count, leukopenia, agranulocytosis, and purpura, have been reported. If such abnormalities develop, therapy should be discontinued.

Drug Interactions
MAO inhibitors should be avoided or used with extreme caution.
Reserpine should be used cautiously with digitalis and quinidine, since cardiac arrhythmias have occurred with rauwolfia preparations.
When other potent parenteral antihypertensive drugs, such as diazoxide, are used in combination with hydralazine, patients should be continuously observed for several hours for any excessive fall in blood pressure. Profound hypotensive episodes may occur when diazoxide injection and hydralazine are used concomitantly.

Carcinogenesis, Mutagenesis, Impairment of Fertility
Reserpine. *Animal Tumorigenicity:* Rodent studies have shown that reserpine is an animal tumorigen, causing an increased incidence of mammary fibroadenomas in female mice, malignant tumors of the seminal vesicles in male mice, and malignant adrenal medullary tumors in male rats. These findings arose in 2-year studies in which the drug was administered in the feed at concentrations of 5 and 10 ppm—about 100 to 300 times the usual human dose. The breast neoplasms are thought to be related to reserpine's prolactin-elevating effect. Several other prolactin-elevating drugs have also been associated with an increased incidence of mammary neoplasia in rodents.
The extent to which these findings indicate a risk to humans is uncertain. Tissue culture experiments show that about one third of human breast tumors are prolactin-dependent *in vitro*, a factor of considerable importance if the use of the drug is contemplated in a patient with previously detected breast cancer. The possibility of an increased risk of breast cancer in reserpine users has been studied extensively; however, no firm conclusion has emerged. Although a few epidemiologic studies have suggested a slightly increased risk (less than twofold in all studies except one) in women who have used reserpine, other studies of generally similar design have not confirmed this. Epidemiologic studies conducted using other drugs (neuroleptic agents) that, like reserpine, increase prolactin levels and therefore would be considered rodent mammary carcinogens, have not shown an association between chronic administration of the drug and human mammary tumorigenesis. While long-term clinical observation has not suggested such an association, the available evidence is considered too limited to be conclusive at this time. An association of reserpine intake with pheochromocytoma or tumors of the seminal vesicles has not been explored.
Hydralazine. In a lifetime study in Swiss albino mice, there was a statistically significant increase in the incidence of lung tumors (adenomas and adenocarcinomas) of both male and female mice given hydralazine continuously in their drinking water at a dosage of about 250 mg/kg per day (about 80 times the maximum recommended human dose). In a 2-year carcinogenicity study of rats given hydralazine by gavage at dose levels of 15, 30, and 60 mg/kg/day (approximately 5 to 20 times the recommended human daily dosage), microscopic examination of the liver revealed a small, but statistically significant, increase in benign neoplastic nodules in male and female rats from the high-dose group and in female rats from the intermediate-dose group. Benign interstitial cell tumors of the testes were also significantly increased in male rats from the high-dose group. The tumors observed are common in aged rats and a significantly increased incidence was not observed until 18 months of treatment. Hydralazine was shown to be mutagenic in three bacterial tester strains in the Ames test, both with and without metabolic activation, and elicited DNA repair both in the Pol A^+/A^- *E. coli* bacterial assay system and in cultured rat hepatocytes. (Evidence of DNA damage in the hepatocyte repair test is considered a strong indication of covalent binding, an established property of carcinogens and mutagens.) In tests with rabbit hepatocytes that exhibit an acetylator polymorphism like that of humans, hydralazine elicited DNA repair with only those hepatocytes having a slow rate of acetylation, suggesting that individuals who are rapid acetylators may have a diminished genotoxic liability. No increase in mutagenic potential was revealed in the mouse lymphoma assay, host-mediated assay, nucleus anomaly test, or dominant lethal test.
The extent to which these findings indicate a risk to man is uncertain. While long-term clinical observation has not suggested that human cancer is associated with hydralazine use, epidemiologic studies have so far been insufficient to arrive at any conclusions.

Pregnancy Category C
Animal reproduction studies have not been conducted with Serpasil-Apresoline. Reserpine administered parenterally has been shown to be teratogenic in rats at doses up to 2 mg/kg and to have an embryocidal effect in guinea pigs given dosages of 0.5 mg daily. Animal studies indicate that hydralazine is teratogenic in mice at 20–30 times the maximum daily human dose of 200–300 mg and possibly in rabbits at 10–15 times the maximum daily human dose, but that it is nonteratogenic in rats. Teratogenic effects observed were cleft palate and malformations of facial and cranial bones. There are no adequate and well-controlled studies of Serpasil-Apresoline in pregnant women. Serpasil-Apresoline should be used during pregnancy only if the potential benefit justifies the potential risk to the fetus.
Nonteratogenic Effects. Reserpine crosses the placental barrier, and increased respiratory tract secretions, nasal congestion, cyanosis, and anorexia may occur in neonates of mothers treated with reserpine.

Nursing Mothers
Reserpine is excreted in maternal breast milk, and increased respiratory tract secretions, nasal congestion, cyanosis, and anorexia may occur in breast-fed infants. Because of the potential for serious adverse reactions in nursing infants and the potential for tumorigenicity shown for reserpine in animal studies, a decision should be made whether to discontinue nursing or to discontinue Serpasil-Apresoline, taking into account the importance of the drug to the mother.

Pediatric Use
Safety and effectiveness of the combination drug in children have not been established.

ADVERSE REACTIONS

Adverse reactions are usually reversible upon reduction of dosage or discontinuation of Serpasil-Apresoline. Whenever adverse reactions are moderate or severe, it may be necessary to discontinue the drug.
The following adverse reactions have been observed, but there has not been enough systematic collection of data to support an estimate of their frequency. Consequently the reactions are categorized by organ system and are listed in decreasing order of severity and not frequency.

Reserpine
The following have been observed with rauwolfia preparations:
Digestive: Vomiting, diarrhea, nausea, anorexia, dryness of mouth, hypersecretion.
Cardiovascular: Arrhythmias (particularly when used concurrently with digitalis or quinidine), syncope, angina-like symptoms, bradycardia, edema.
Respiratory: Dyspnea, epistaxis, nasal congestion.
Neurologic: Rare parkinsonian syndrome and other extrapyramidal tract symptoms; dizziness; headache; paradoxical anxiety; depression; nervousness; nightmares; dull sensorium; drowsiness.
Musculoskeletal: Muscular aches.
Genitourinary: Pseudolactation, impotence, dysuria, gynecomastia, decreased libido, breast engorgement.
Metabolic: Weight gain.
Special Senses: Deafness, optic atrophy, glaucoma, uveitis, conjunctival injection.
Hypersensitive Reactions: Purpura, rash, pruritus.

Hydralazine
Digestive: Hepatitis, paralytic ileus, vomiting, diarrhea, nausea, constipation, anorexia.
Cardiovascular: Angina pectoris, hypotension, paradoxical pressor response, tachycardia, palpitations, edema, flushing.
Respiratory: Dyspnea, nasal congestion.
Neurologic: Psychotic reactions characterized by depression, disorientation, or anxiety; peripheral neuritis, evidenced by paresthesia, numbness, and tingling; tremors; dizziness; headache.
Musculoskeletal: Muscle cramps, arthralgia.
Genitourinary: Difficulty in urination.
Hematologic: Blood dyscrasias, consisting of reduction in hemoglobin and red cell count, leukopenia, agranulocytosis, lymphadenopathy; splenomegaly; eosinophilia.
Special Senses: Conjunctivitis, lacrimation.
Hypersensitive Reactions: Purpura, fever, urticaria, rash, pruritus, chills.

OVERDOSAGE

Acute Toxicity
No deaths due to acute poisoning with Serpasil-Apresoline have been reported.
Oral LD_{50}'s in animals (mg/kg): rats, 261; mice, 218.

Signs and Symptoms
Reserpine. The clinical picture of acute poisoning is characterized chiefly by signs and symptoms due to the reflex parasympathomimetic effect of reserpine.
Impairment of consciousness may occur and may range from drowsiness to coma, depending upon the severity of overdosage. Flushing of the skin, conjunctival injection, and pupillary constriction are to be expected. Hypotension, hypothermia, central respiratory depression, and bradycardia may develop in cases of severe overdosage. Increased salivary and gastric secretion and diarrhea may also occur.
Hydralazine: Signs and symptoms of overdosage include hypotension, tachycardia, headache, and generalized skin flushing.
Complications can include myocardial ischemia and subsequent myocardial infarction, cardiac arrhythmia, and profound shock.

Treatment
There is no specific antidote.
The gastric contents should be evacuated, taking adequate precautions against aspiration and for protection of the airway. An activated charcoal slurry may be instilled if conditions permit. Dialysis may not be effective for elimination of Serpasil-Aspresoline because of its plasma protein binding (see **CLINICAL PHARMACOLOGY**).
These manipulations may have to be omitted or carried out after cardiovascular status has been stabilized, since they might precipitate cardiac arrhythmias or increase the depth of shock.
Support of the cardiovascular system is of primary importance in suspected hydralazine overdosage. Shock should be treated with plasma expanders. If possible, vasopressors should not be given, but if a vasopressor is required, care should be taken not to precipitate or aggravate cardiac arrhythmia. A vasopressor having direct action upon vascular smooth muscle (e.g., phenylephrine, levarterenol, metaraminol) should be used to treat the symptomatic effects of reserpine overdosage. Tachycardia responds to beta blockers. Digitalization may be necessary, and renal function should be monitored and supported as required. Since reserpine is long-acting, the patient should be observed carefully for at least 72 hours.

DOSAGE AND ADMINISTRATION

Dosage should be determined by individual titration (see boxed **WARNING**).
Step 1. Therapy should be started with reserpine alone, at an average dosage of 0.5 mg daily and continued for at least 1 week. If results prove satisfactory—as they will in many cases—no other medication is required. For maintenance, the dosage should be reduced to 0.25 mg, or less, daily.
Step 2. Should more than the therapeutic action of reserpine be indicated, therapy with one Serpasil-Apresoline tablet #2 (resperine, 0.2 mg/hydralazine hydrochloride, 50 mg) four times daily should be initiated.
When reduction of dosage is indicated, one Serpasil-Apresoline tablet #1 (reserpine, 0.1 mg/hydralazine hydrochloride, 25 mg) four times daily should be used.
Side effects associated with hydralazine (headache, tachycardia, palpitations) are seldom encountered when the patient has been "primed" with reserpine before combination therapy is begun. Should side effects appear, however, reduction of dosage to one tablet #1 two to four times daily for a few days will usually alleviate them.
In cases where further individualization of dosage is necessary, the adjustment may be made by increasing or decreasing the dosage of reserpine and/or hydralazine.
For maintenance, daily dosage of hydralazine should probably not exceed 200 mg, nor should the dosage of reserpine exceed 1 mg.

Patients on Hydralazine
Patients already on this drug may be given a combination tablet as required. With the addition of reserpine, it is usually possible to reduce the dose of hydralazine.

HOW SUPPLIED

Tablets #1—round, yellow, dry-coated (imprinted CIBA 40)
0.1 mg reserpine, 25 mg hydralazine hydrochloride
Bottles of 100 .... NDC 0083-0040-30
Tablets #2—round, yellow, dry-coated (imprinted CIBA 104)
0.2 mg reserpine, 50 mg hydralazine hydrochloride
Bottles of 100 .... NDC 0083-0104-30
Dispense in tight, light-resistant container (USP).
C85-22 (Rev. 8/85)
Shown in Product Identification Section, page 408

SERPASIL®–ESIDRIX® ℞
[sir 'pah-sill ess 'ah-dricks]
reserpine and hydrochlorothiazide
Combination Tablets

> **WARNING**
> This fixed-combination drug is not indicated for initial therapy of hypertension. Hypertension requires therapy titrated to the individual patient. If the fixed combi-

Continued on next page

The full prescribing information for each CIBA drug is contained herein and is that in effect as of September 1, 1986

CIBA—Cont.

nation represents the dosage so determined, its use may be more convenient in patient management. The treatment of hypertension is not static but must be reevaluated as conditions in each patient warrant.

DESCRIPTION

Serpasil-Esidrix is an antihypertensive-diuretic combination, available as tablets for oral administration. Tablets #1 contain reserpine USP, 0.1 mg, and hydrochlorothiazide USP, 25 mg; tablets #2 contain reserpine USP, 0.1 mg, and hydrochlorothiazide USP, 50 mg.

Reserpine is methyl 18β-hydroxy-11,17α-dimethoxy-3β, 20α-yohimban-16β-carboxylate 3,4,5-trimethoxybenzoate (ester).

Reserpine USP, a pure crystalline alkaloid of rauwolfia, is a white or pale buff to slightly yellowish, odorless crystalline powder. It darkens slowly on exposure to light, but more rapidly when in solution. It is insoluble in water, freely soluble in acetic acid and in chloroform, slightly soluble in benzene, and very slightly soluble in alcohol and in ether. Its molecular weight is 608.69.

Hydrochlorothiazide is 6-chloro-3,4-dihydro-2*H*-1,2,4-benzothiadiazine-7-sulfonamide 1,1-dioxide.

Hydrochlorothiazide USP is a white, or practically white, practically odorless crystalline powder. It is slightly soluble in water; freely soluble in sodium hydroxide solution, in *n*-butylamine, and in dimethylformamide; sparingly soluble in methanol; and insoluble in ether, in chloroform, and in dilute mineral acids. Its molecular weight is 297.73.

Inactive ingredients: FD&C Yellow No. 5, FD&C Yellow No. 6, lactose, magnesium stearate, starch and sucrose.

CLINICAL PHARMACOLOGY

Reserpine: Reserpine depletes stores of catecholamines and 5-hydroxytryptamine in many organs, including the brain and adrenal medulla. Most of its pharmacological effects have been attributed to this action. Depletion is slower and less complete in the adrenal medulla than in other tissues. The depression of sympathetic nerve function results in a decreased heart rate and a lowering of arterial blood pressure. The sedative and tranquilizing properties of reserpine are thought to be related to depletion of catecholamines and 5-hydroxytryptamine from the brain.

Reserpine, like other rauwolfia compounds, is characterized by slow onset of action and sustained effects. Both cardiovascular and central nervous system effects may persist for a period of time following withdrawal of the drug.

Mean maximum plasma levels of 1.54 ng/ml were attained after a median of 3.5 hours in six normal subjects receiving a single oral dose of four 0.25-mg Serpasil tablets. Bioavailability was approximately 50% of that of a corresponding intravenous dose. Plasma levels of reserpine after intravenous administration declined with a mean half-life of 33 hours. Reserpine is extensively bound (96%) to plasma proteins. No definitive studies on the human metabolism of reserpine have been made.

Hydrochlorothiazide: Thiazides affect the renal tubular mechanism of electrolyte reabsorption. At maximal therapeutic dosage, all thiazides are approximately equal in their diuretic potency. Thiazides increase excretion of sodium and chloride in approximately equivalent amounts. Natriuresis causes a secondary loss of potassium.

The mechanism of the antihypertensive effect of thiazides is unknown. Thiazides do not affect normal blood pressure.

The onset of action of thiazides occurs in 2 hours and the peak effect at about 4 hours. The action persists for approximately 6–12 hours. Hydrochlorothiazide is rapidly absorbed, as indicated by peak plasma concentrations 1–2.5 hours after oral administration. Plasma levels of the drug are proportional to dose; the concentration in whole blood is 1.6–1.8 times higher than in plasma. Thiazides are eliminated rapidly by the kidney. After oral administration of 25- to 100-mg doses, 72–97% of the dose is excreted in the urine, indicating dose-independent absorption. Hydrochlorothiazide is eliminated from plasma in a biphasic fashion, with a terminal half-life of 10–17 hours. Plasma protein binding is 67.9%. Plasma clearance is 15.9–30.0 L/hr; volume of distribution is 3.6–7.8 L/kg.

Gastrointestinal absorption of hydrochlorothiazide is enhanced when administered with food. Absorption is decreased in patients with congestive heart failure, and the pharmacokinetics are considerably different in these patients.

INDICATIONS AND USAGE

Hypertension (see boxed **WARNING**).

CONTRAINDICATIONS

Reserpine: Hypersensitivity to reserpine; mental depression (especially with suicidal tendencies); active peptic ulcer, ulcerative colitis; patients receiving electroconvulsive therapy.

Hydrochlorothiazide: Anuria; hypersensitivity to this or other sulfonamide-derived drugs.

WARNINGS

Reserpine: Extreme caution should be exercised in treating patients with a history of mental depression. The drug should be discontinued at the first sign of despondency, early morning insomnia, loss of appetite, impotence, or self-deprecation. Drug-induced depression may persist for several months after drug withdrawal and may be severe enough to result in suicide.

Hydrochlorothiazide: Thiazides should be used with caution in patients with severe renal disease. In patients with renal disease, thiazides may precipitate azotemia. Cumulative effects of the drug may develop in patients with impaired renal function.

Thiazides should be used with caution in patients with impaired hepatic function or progressive liver disease, since minor alterations of fluid and electrolyte imbalance may precipitate hepatic coma.

Thiazides may add to or potentiate the action of other antihypertensive drugs. Potentiation occurs with ganglionic or peripheral adrenergic blocking drugs.

Sensitivity reactions are more likely to occur in patients with a history of allergy or bronchial asthma.

The possibility of exacerbation or activation of systemic lupus erythmatosus has been reported.

PRECAUTIONS

General

The Serpasil-Esidrix tablets (#1 and #2) contain FD&C Yellow No. 5 (tartrazine) which may cause allergic-type reactions (including bronchial asthma) in certain susceptible individuals. Although the overall incidence of FD&C Yellow No. 5 (tartrazine) sensitivity in the general population is low, it is frequently seen in patients who also have aspirin hypersensitivity.

Reserpine: Since reserpine increases gastrointestinal motility and secretion, it should be used cautiously in patients with a history of peptic ulcer, ulcerative colitis, or gallstones (biliary colic may be precipitated).

Caution should be exercised when treating hypertensive patients with renal insufficiency, since they adjust poorly to lowered blood pressure levels.

Preoperative withdrawal of reserpine does not assure that circulatory instability will not occur. It is important that the anesthesiologist be aware of the patient's drug intake and consider this in the overall management, since hypotension has occurred in patients receiving rauwolfia preparations. Anticholinergic and adrenergic drugs (e.g., metaraminol, norepinephrine) have been employed to treat adverse vagocirculatory effects.

Hydrochlorothiazide: All patients receiving thiazide therapy should be observed for clinical signs of fluid or electrolyte imbalance, namely hyponatremia, hypochloremic alkalosis, and hypokalemia (see **Laboratory Tests** and **Drug/Drug Interactions**). Warning signs are dryness of mouth, thirst, weakness, lethargy, drowsiness, restlessness, muscle pains or cramps, muscular fatigue, hypotension, oliguria, tachycardia, and gastrointestinal disturbance, such as nausea or vomiting.

Hypokalemia may develop, especially in cases of brisk diuresis or severe cirrhosis.

Interference with adequate oral intake of electrolytes will also contribute to hypokalemia. Hypokalemia may be avoided or treated by use of potassium supplements or foods with a high potassium content.

Any chloride deficit is generally mild and usually does not require specific treatment, except under extraordinary circumstances (as in liver disease or renal disease). Dilutional hyponatremia may occur in edematous patients in hot weather; appropriate therapy is water restriction, rather than administration of salt, except in rare instances when the hyponatremia is life-threatening. In cases of actual salt depletion, appropriate replacement is the therapy of choice.

Hyperuricemia may occur or frank gout may be precipitated in certain patients receiving thiazide therapy.

Latent diabetes may become manifest during thiazide administration (see **Drug/Drug Interactions**).

The antihypertensive effects of the drug may be enhanced in the postsympathectomy patient.

If progressive renal impairment becomes evident, withholding or discontinuing diuretic therapy should be considered.

Calcium excretion is decreased by thiazides. Pathological changes in the parathyroid gland with hypercalcemia and hypophosphatemia have been observed in a few patients on prolonged thiazide therapy. The common complications of hyperparathyroidism, such as renal lithiasis, bone resorption, and peptic ulceration, have not been seen.

Information for Patients: Patients should be informed of possible side effects and advised to take the medication regularly and continously as directed.

Laboratory Tests

Hydrochlorothiazide: Initial and periodic determinations of serum electrolytes to detect possible electrolyte imbalance should be performed at appropriate intervals.

Serum and urine electrolyte determinations are particularly important when the patient is vomiting excessively or receiving parenteral fluids.

Drug/Drug Interactions

Reserpine: MAO inhibitors should be avoided or used with extreme caution.

Reserpine should be used cautiously with digitalis and quinidine, since cardiac arrhythmias have occurred with rauwolfia preparations.

Hydrochlorothiazide: Hypokalemia can sensitize or exaggerate the response of the heart to the toxic effects of digitalis (e.g., increased ventricular irritability).

Hypokalemia may develop during concomitant use of steroids or ACTH.

Insulin requirements in diabetic patients may be increased, decreased, or unchanged.

Thiazides may decrease arterial responsiveness to norepinephrine, but not enough to preclude effectiveness of the pressor agent for therapeutic use.

Thiazides may increase the responsiveness to tubocurarine.

Lithium renal clearance is reduced by thiazides, increasing the risk of lithium toxicity.

Drug/Laboratory Test Interactions: Thiazides may decrease serum levels of protein-bound iodine without signs of thyroid disturbance. Serpasil-Esidrix should be discontinued before carrying out tests for parathyroid function (see **General, Hydrochlorothiazide,** Calcium excretion).

Carcinogenesis, Mutagenesis, Impairment of Fertility

Reserpine. Animal Tumorigenicity: Rodent studies have shown that reserpine is an animal tumorigen, causing an increased incidence of mammary fibroadenomas in female mice, malignant tumors of the seminal vesicles in male mice, and malignant adrenal medullary tumors in male rats. These findings arose in 2-year studies in which the drug was administered in the feed at concentrations of 5 and 10 ppm—about 100 to 300 times the usual human dose. The breast neoplasms are thought to be related to reserpine's prolactin-elevating effect. Several other prolactin-elevating drugs have also been associated with an increased incidence of mammary neoplasia in rodents.

The extent to which these findings indicate a risk to humans is uncertain. Tissue culture experiments show that about one third of human breast tumors are prolactin-dependent *in vitro,* a factor of considerable importance if the use of the drug is contemplated in a patient with previously detected breast cancer. The possibility of an increased risk of breast cancer in reserpine users has been studied extensively; however, no firm conclusion has emerged. Although a few epidemiologic studies have suggested a slightly increased risk (less than twofold in all studies except one) in women who have used reserpine, other studies of generally similar design have not confirmed this. Epidemiologic studies conducted using other drugs (neuroleptic agents) that, like reserpine, increase prolactin levels and therefore would be considered rodent mammary carcinogens, have not shown an association between chronic administration of the drug and human mammary tumorigenesis. While long-term clinical observation has not suggested such an association, the available evidence is considered too limited to be conclusive at this time. An association of reserpine intake with pheochromocytoma or tumors of the seminal vesicles has not been explored.

Hydrochlorothiazide: Long-term carcinogenicity studies in animals have not been conducted with Esidrix.

Pregnancy Category C: Animal reproduction studies have not been conducted with Serpasil-Esidrix. Reserpine administered parenterally has been shown to be teratogenic in rats at doses up to 2 mg/kg and to have an embryocidal effect in guinea pigs given dosages of 0.5 mg daily. A reproduction study in rats receiving hydrochlorothiazide, 250 mg/kg daily, 62.5 times the maximum daily human dose, has revealed no evidence of impaired fertility or harm to the fetus. There are no adequate and well-controlled studies of Serpasil-Esidrix in pregnant women. Serpasil-Esidrix should be used during pregnancy only if the potential benefit justifies the potential risk to the fetus.

Nonteratogenic Effects. Reserpine crosses the placental barrier, and increased respiratory tract secretions, nasal congestion, cyanosis, and anorexia may occur in neonates of mothers treated with reserpine. Thiazides also cross the placental barrier and appear in cord blood, and there is a risk of fetal or neonatal jaundice, thrombocytopenia, and possibly other adverse reactions that have occurred in adults.

Nursing Mothers: Reserpine is excreted in maternal breast milk, and increased respiratory tract secretions, nasal congestion, cyanosis, and anorexia may occur in breast-fed infants. Thiazides are also excreted in breast milk. Because of the potential for serious adverse reactions in nursing infants and the potential for tumorigenicity shown for reserpine in animal studies, a decision should be made whether to discontinue nursing or to discontinue Serpasil-Esidrix, taking into account the importance of the drug to the mother.

Pediatric Use: Safety and effectiveness of the combination drug in children have not been established.

ADVERSE REACTIONS
Adverse reactions are usually reversible upon reduction of dosage or discontinuation of Serpasil-Esidrix. Whenever adverse reactions are moderate or severe, it may be necessary to discontinue the drug.
The following adverse reactions have been observed, but there has not been enough systematic collection of data to support an estimate of their frequency. Consequently the reactions are categorized by organ systems and are listed in decreasing order of severity and not frequency.
Reserpine: The following have been observed with rauwolfia preparations:
Digestive: Vomiting, diarrhea, nausea, anorexia, dryness of mouth, hypersecretion.
Cardiovascular: Arrhythmias (particularly when used concurrently with digitalis or quinidine), syncope, angina-like symptoms, bradycardia, edema.
Respiratory: Dyspnea, epistaxis, nasal congestion.
Neurologic: Rare parkinsonian syndrome and other extrapyramidal tract symptoms; dizziness; headache; paradoxical anxiety; depression; nervousness; nightmares; dull sensorium; drowsiness.
Musculoskeletal: Muscular aches.
Genitourinary: Pseudolactation, impotence, dysuria, gynecomastia, decreased libido, breast engorgement.
Metabolic: Weight gain.
Special Senses: Deafness, optic atrophy, glaucoma, uveitis, conjunctival injection.
Hypersensitive Reactions: Purpura, rash, pruritus.
Hydrochlorothiazide: *Digestive:* Pancreatitis, jaundice (intrahepatic cholestatic), sialadenitis, vomiting, diarrhea, cramping, nausea, gastric irritation, constipation, anorexia.
Cardiovascular: Orthostatic hypotension (may be potentiated by alcohol, barbiturates, or narcotics).
Neurologic: Vertigo, dizziness, transient blurred vision, headache, paresthesia, xanthopsia, weakness, restlessness.
Musculoskeletal: Muscle spasm.
Hematologic: Aplastic anemia, agranulocytosis, leukopenia, thrombocytopenia.
Metabolic: Hyperglycemia, glycosuria, hyperuricemia.
Hypersensitive Reactions: Necrotizing angiitis, Stevens-Johnson syndrome, purpura, urticaria, rash, photosensitivity.

OVERDOSAGE
Acute Toxicity: No deaths due to acute poisoning with the combination drug have been reported.
Oral LD_{50}'s in animals (mg/kg): (reserpine) rats, 2993; mice, 47 and 500; (hydrochlorothiazide) rats, 2750.
Signs and Symptoms:
Reserpine. The clinical picture of acute poisoning is characterized chiefly by signs and symptoms due to the reflex parasympathomimetic effect of reserpine.
Impairment of consciousness may occur and may range from drowsiness to coma, depending upon the severity of overdosage. Flushing of the skin, conjunctival injection, and pupillary constriction are to be expected. Hypotension, hypothermia, central respiratory depression, and bradycardia may develop in cases of severe overdosage. Increased salivary and gastric secretion and diarrhea may also occur.
Hydrochlorothiazide. The most prominent feature of poisoning is acute loss of fluid and electrolytes.
Cardiovascular: Tachycardia, hypotension, shock.
Neuromuscular: Weakness, confusion, dizziness, cramps of the calf muscles, paresthesia, fatigue, impairment of consciousness.
Digestive: Nausea, vomiting, thirst.
Renal: Polyuria, oliguria, or anuria (due to hemoconcentration).
Laboratory Findings: Hypokalemia, hyponatremia, hypochloremia, alkalosis; increased BUN (especially in patients with renal insufficiency).
Combined Poisoning: Signs and symptoms may be aggravated or modified by concomitant intake of antihypertensive medication, barbiturates, curare, digitalis (hypokalemia), corticosteroids, narcotics, or alcohol.
Treatment: There is no specific antidote.
Stomach contents should be evacuated, taking adequate precautions against aspiration and for protection of the airway. An activated charcoal slurry should be instilled if conditions permit. Dialysis may not be effective for elimination of Serpasil-Esidrix because of its plasma protein binding (see **CLINICAL PHARMACOLOGY**).
The effects of reserpine overdosage should be treated symptomatically. If hypotension or shock occurs, the patient's legs should be kept raised and lost fluid and electrolytes (potassium, sodium) should be replaced. If hypotension is severe enough to require treatment with a vasopressor, one having a direct action upon vascular smooth muscle (e.g., phenylephrine, levarterenol, metaraminol) should be used.
Fluid and electrolyte balance (especially serum potassium) and renal function should be monitored until conditions become normal. Since reserpine is long-acting, the patient should be observed carefully for at least 72 hours.

DOSAGE AND ADMINISTRATION
Dosage should be determined by individual titration (see boxed **WARNING**).
The usual dosage is two Serpasil-Esidrix #2 Tablets daily in single or divided doses. For patients requiring less hydrochlorothiazide, Serpasil- Esidrix #1 Tablets should be substituted.
Since the antihypertensive effects of reserpine are not immediately apparent, maximal reduction in blood pressure from a given dosage may not occur for 2 weeks. For maintenance, dosage should be reduced to the lowest effective level; as little as one tablet daily may suffice.
When necessary, more potent antihypertensive agents may be added gradually in reduced dosages. The effects should be watched carefully.

HOW SUPPLIED
Tablets #1—round, light orange (imprinted CIBA 13) 0.1 mg of reserpine, 25 mg of hydrochlorothiazide
Bottles of 100—NDC 0083-0013-30
Bottles of 1000—NDC 0083-0013-40
Tablets #2—round, light orange (imprinted CIBA 97) 0.1 mg reserpine, 50 mg hydrochlorothiazide
Bottles of 100—NDC 0083-0097-30
Bottles of 1000—NDC 0083-0097-40
Protect from light.
Dispense in tight, light-resistant container (USP).
C85-33 (Rev. 9/85)

Shown in Product Identification Section, page 408

SLOW-K® ℞
[*sloe-kay*]
potassium chloride USP
slow-release tablets

DESCRIPTION
Slow-K, potassium chloride USP, is a sugar-coated (not enteric-coated) tablet for oral administration, containing 600 mg of potassium chloride (equivalent to 8 mEq) in a wax matrix. This formulation is intended to provide a controlled release of potassium from the matrix to minimize the likelihood of producing high, localized concentrations of potassium within the gastrointestinal tract.
Slow-K is an electrolyte replenisher. Its chemical name is potassium chloride, and its structural formula is KCl. Potassium chloride USP is a white, granular powder or colorless crystals. It is odorless and has a saline taste. Its solutions are neutral to litmus. It is freely soluble in water and insoluble in alcohol.
Inactive Ingredients. Acacia, cetostearyl alcohol, gelatin, iron oxide, magnesium stearate, polyvinylpyrrolidone, parabens, sodium benzoate, starch, sucrose, talc, and titanium dioxide.

CLINICAL PHARMACOLOGY
The potassium ion is the principal intracellular cation of most body tissues. Potassium ions participate in a number of essential physiological processes, including the maintenance of intracellular tonicity, the transmission of nerve impulses, the contraction of cardiac, skeletal, and smooth muscle, and the maintenance of normal renal function.
In adults normal plasma potassium concentration is 3.5–5.0 mEq/L.
Potassium depletion may occur whenever the rate of potassium loss through renal excretion and/or loss from the gastrointestinal tract exceeds the rate of potassium intake. Such depletion usually develops slowly as a consequence of prolonged therapy with oral diuretics, primary or secondary hyperaldosteronism, diabetic ketoacidosis, severe diarrhea, or inadequate replacement of potassium in patients on prolonged parenteral nutrition. Potassium depletion due to these causes is usually accompanied by a concomitant deficiency of chloride and is manifested by hypokalemia and metabolic alkalosis. Potassium depletion may produce weakness, fatigue, disturbances of cardiac rhythm (primarily ectopic beats), prominent U-waves in the electrocardiogram, and in advanced cases flaccid paralysis and/or impaired ability to concentrate urine.
Potassium depletion associated with metabolic alkalosis is managed by correcting the fundamental causes of the deficiency whenever possible and administering supplemental potassium chloride, in the form of high potassium food or potassium chloride solution or tablets.
In rare circumstances (*e.g.,* patients with renal tubular acidosis) potassium depletion may be associated with metabolic acidosis and hyperchloremia. In such patients potassium replacement should be accomplished with potassium salts other than the chloride, such as potassium bicarbonate, potassium citrate, or potassium acetate.
The potassium chloride in Slow-K is completely absorbed before it leaves the small intestine. The wax matrix is not absorbed and is excreted in the feces; in some instances the empty matrices may be noticeable in the stool. When the bioavailability of the potassium ion from Slow-K is compared to that of a true solution the extent of absorption is similar.
The slow-release properties of Slow-K are demonstrated by the finding that a significant increase in time is required for renal excretion of the first 50% of the Slow-K dose as compared to the solution.
Increased urinary potassium excretion is first observed 1 hour after administration of Slow-K, reaches a peak at 4 hours, and extends up to 8 hours. Mean daily steady-state plasma levels of potassium following daily administration of Slow-K cannot be distinguished from those following administration of a potassium chloride solution or from control plasma levels of potassium ion.

INDICATIONS AND USAGE
BECAUSE OF REPORTS OF INTESTINAL AND GASTRIC ULCERATION AND BLEEDING WITH SLOW-RELEASE POTASSIUM CHLORIDE PREPARATIONS, THESE DRUGS SHOULD BE RESERVED FOR THOSE PATIENTS WHO CANNOT TOLERATE OR REFUSE TO TAKE LIQUID OR EFFERVESCENT POTASSIUM PREPARATIONS OR FOR PATIENTS IN WHOM THERE IS A PROBLEM OF COMPLIANCE WITH THESE PREPARATIONS.
1. For therapeutic use in patients with hypokalemia with or without metabolic alkalosis; in digitalis intoxication and in patients with hypokalemic familial periodic paralysis.
2. For prevention of potassium depletion when the dietary intake of potassium is inadequate in the following conditions: patients receiving digitalis and diuretics for congestive heart failure; hepatic cirrhosis with ascites; states of aldosterone excess with normal renal function; potassium-losing nephropathy; and certain diarrheal states.
3. The use of potassium salts in patients receiving diuretics for uncomplicated essential hypertension is often unnecessary when such patients have a normal dietary pattern. Serum potassium should be checked periodically, however, and, if hypokalemia occurs, dietary supplementation with potassium-containing foods may be adequate to control milder cases. In more severe cases supplementation with potassium salts may be indicated.

CONTRAINDICATIONS
Potassium supplements are contraindicated in patients with hyperkalemia, since a further increase in serum potassium concentration in such patients can produce cardiac arrest. Hyperkalemia may complicate any of the following conditions: chronic renal failure, systemic acidosis such as diabetic acidosis, acute dehydration, extensive tissue breakdown as in severe burns, adrenal insufficiency, or the administration of a potassium-sparing diuretic (*e.g.,* spironolactone, triamterene). (See OVERDOSAGE.)
All solid dosage forms of potassium supplements are contraindicated in any patient in whom there is cause for arrest or delay in tablet passage through the gastrointestinal tract. In these instances, potassium supplementation should be with a liquid preparation. Wax-matrix potassium chloride preparations have produced esophageal ulceration in certain cardiac patients with esophageal compression due to an enlarged left atrium.

WARNINGS
Hyperkalemia (See **OVERDOSAGE**)
In patients with impaired mechanisms for excreting potassium, the administration of potassium salts can produce hyperkalemia and cardiac arrest. This occurs most commonly in patients given potassium by the intravenous route but may also occur in patients given potassium orally. Potentially fatal hyperkalemia can develop rapidly and be asymptomatic.
The use of potassium salts in patients with chronic renal disease, or any other condition which impairs potassium excretion, requires particularly careful monitoring of the serum potassium concentration and appropriate dosage adjustment.
Interaction with Potassium-Sparing Diuretics
Hypokalemia should not be treated by the concomitant administration of potassium salts and a potassium-sparing diuretic (*e.g.,* spironolactone or triamterene), since the simultaneous administration of these agents can produce severe hyperkalemia.
Gastrointestinal lesions
Potassium chloride tablets have produced stenotic and/or ulcerative lesions of the small bowel and deaths. These lesions are caused by a high localized concentration of potassium ion in the region of a rapidly dissolving tablet, which injures the bowel wall and thereby produces obstruction, hemorrhage, or perforation. Slow-K is a wax-matrix tablet formulated to provide a controlled rate of release of potassium chloride and thus to minimize the possibility of a high local concentration of potassium ion near the bowel wall. While the reported frequency of small-bowel lesions is much

Continued on next page

The full prescribing information for each CIBA drug is contained herein and is that in effect as of September 1, 1986

CIBA—Cont.

less with wax-matrix tablets (less than one per 100,000 patient-years) than with enteric-coated potassium chloride tablets (40–50 per 100,000 patient-years) cases associated with wax-matrix tablets have been reported both in foreign countries and in the United States. In addition, perhaps because the wax-matrix preparations are not enteric-coated and release potassium in the stomach, there have been reports of upper gastrointestinal bleeding associated with these products. The total number of gastrointestinal lesions remains approximately one per 100,000 patient-years. Slow-K should be discontinued immediately and the possibility of bowel obstruction or perforation considered if severe vomiting, abdominal pain, distention, or gastrointestinal bleeding occurs.

Metabolic acidosis

Hypokalemia in patients with metabolic *acidosis* should be treated with an alkalinizing potassium salt such as potassium bicarbonate, potassium citrate, or potassium acetate.

PRECAUTIONS

General: The diagnosis of potassium depletion is ordinarily made by demonstrating hypokalemia in a patient with a clinical history suggesting some cause for potassium depletion. In interpreting the serum potassium level, the physician should bear in mind that acute alkalosis *per se* can produce hypokalemia in the absence of a deficit in total body potassium, while acute acidosis *per se* can increase the serum potassium concentration into the normal range even in the presence of a reduced total body potassium.

Information for Patients

Physicians should consider reminding the patient of the following:

To take each dose without crushing, chewing, or sucking the tablets.

To take this medicine only as directed. This is especially important if the patient is also taking both diuretics and digitalis preparations.

To check with the physician if there is trouble swallowing tablets or if the tablets seem to stick in the throat.

To check with the doctor at once if tarry stools or other evidence of gastrointestinal bleeding is noticed.

Laboratory Tests

Regular serum potassium determinations are recommended. In addition, during the treatment of potassium depletion, careful attention should be paid to acid-base balance, other serum electrolyte levels, the electrocardiogram, and the clinical status of the patient, particularly in the presence of cardiac disease, renal disease, or acidosis.

Drug Interactions

Potassium-sparing diuretics: see WARNINGS

Carcinogenesis, Mutagenesis, Impairment of Fertility

Long-term carcinogenicity studies in animals have not been performed.

Pregnancy Category C

Animal reproduction studies have not been conducted with Slow-K. It is also not known whether Slow-K can cause fetal harm when administered to a pregnant woman or can affect reproduction capacity. Slow-K should be given to a pregnant woman only if clearly needed.

Nursing Mothers

The normal potassium ion content of human milk is about 13 mEq/L. It is not known if Slow-K has an effect on this content. Caution should be exercised when Slow-K is administered to a nursing woman.

Pediatric Use

Safety and effectiveness in children have not been established.

ADVERSE REACTIONS

One of the most severe adverse effects is hyperkalemia (see **CONTRAINDICATIONS, WARNINGS** and **OVERDOSAGE**). There also have been reports of upper and lower gastrointestinal conditions including obstruction, bleeding, ulceration and perforation (see **CONTRAINDICATIONS** and **WARNINGS**); other factors known to be associated with such conditions were present in many of these patients.

The most common adverse reactions to oral potassium sales are nausea, vomiting, abdominal discomfort, and diarrhea. These symptoms are due to irritation of the gastrointestinal tract and are best managed by diluting the preparation further, taking the dose with meals, or reducing the dose.

Skin rash has been reported rarely.

OVERDOSAGE

The administration of oral potassium salts to persons with normal excretory mechanisms for potassium rarely causes serious hyperkalemia. However, if excretory mechanisms are impaired or if potassium is administered too rapidly intravenously, potentially fatal hyperkalemia can result (see **CONTRAINDICATIONS** and **WARNINGS**). It is important to recognize that hyperkalemia is usually asymptomatic and may be manifested only by an increased serum potassium concentration (6.5–8.0 mEq/L) and characteristic electrocardiographic changes (peaking of T waves, loss of P wave, depression of ST segment, and prolongation of the QT interval). Late manifestations include muscle paralysis and cardiovascular collapse from cardiac arrest (9–12 mEq/L).

Treatment measures for hyperkalemia include the following: (1) elimination of foods and medications containing potassium and of potassium-sparing diuretics; (2) intravenous administration of 300 to 500 ml/hr of 10% dextrose solution containing 10–20 units of insulin per 1,000 ml; (3) correction of acidosis, if present, with intravenous sodium bicarbonate; (4) use of exchange resins, hemodialysis, or peritoneal dialysis.

In treating hyperkalemia in patients who have been stabilized on digitalis, too rapid a lowering of the serum potassium concentration can produce digitalis toxicity.

DOSAGE AND ADMINISTRATION

The usual dietary intake of potassium by the average adult is 40–80 mEq per day. Potassium depletion sufficient to cause hypokalemia usually requires the loss of 200 or more mEq of potassium from the total body store. Dosage must be adjusted to the individual needs of each patient but is typically in the range of 20 mEq per day for the prevention of hypokalemia to 40–100 mEq or more per day for the treatment of potassium depletion. Large numbers of tablets should be given in divided doses.

NOTE:

Slow-K slow-release tablets must be swallowed whole and never crushed, chewed, or sucked.

HOW SUPPLIED

Tablets 600 mg potassium chloride (equiv. to 8 mEq)
—round, buff colored, sugar-coated (imprinted CIBA 165)

Bottles of 100 ....NDC 0083-0165-30
Bottles of 1000 ....NDC 0083-0165-40
Consumer Pack—One Unit
(12 Bottles—100 tablets each) ....NDC 0083-0165-65
Accu-Pak® Unit Dose (Blister pack)
Box of 100 (strips of 10) ....NDC 0083-0165-32

Do not store above 86°F (30°C). Protect from moisture. Protect from light.

Dispense in tight, light-resistant container (USP).

Dist. by:
CIBA Pharmaceutical Co.
Division of CIBA-GEIGY Corp.
Summit, NJ 07901

C85-39 (Rev. 7/86)

Shown in Product Identification Section, page 408

TRANSDERM-NITRO® ℞

[*trans 'derm nye 'trow*]
nitroglycerin
Transdermal Therapeutic System

DESCRIPTION

Transderm-Nitro (nitroglycerin) transdermal therapeutic system is a flat unit designed to provide controlled release of nitroglycerin through a semipermeable membrane continuously for 24 hours following application to intact skin. Nitroglycerin (glyceryl trinitrate) is a prompt-acting vasodilator for the relief and prevention of anginal attacks. Systems are rated to release *in vivo* 2.5, 5, 10 and 15 mg nitroglycerin over 24 hours and are in sizes of 5, 10, 20 and 30 cm^2 respectively. One-fifth of the total nitroglycerin in the system is delivered transdermally to the patient over 24 hours; the remainder serves as the reservoir to release the drug and remains in the system. The rated release of drug is dependent upon the area of the system; 0.5 mg nitroglycerin is delivered *in vivo* for every cm^2 of system size.

The Transderm-Nitro system comprises four layers as shown below. Proceeding from the visible surface towards the surface attached to the skin, these layers are: 1) a tan-colored backing layer (aluminized plastic) that is impermeable to nitroglycerin; 2) a drug reservoir containing nitroglycerin adsorbed on lactose, colloidal silicon dioxide, and silicone medical fluid; 3) an ethylene/vinyl acetate copolymer membrane that is permeable to nitroglycerin; and 4) a layer of hypoallergenic silicone adhesive. Prior to use, a protective peel strip is removed from the adhesive surface.

Cross section of the system:

Backing
Drug Reservoir
Semipermeable Membrane
Adhesive
Protective Peel Strip

ACTIONS

When the Transderm-Nitro system is applied to the skin, nitroglycerin is absorbed continuously through the skin into the systemic circulation. This results in active drug reaching the target organs (heart, extremities) before being inactivated by the liver. Nitroglycerin is a smooth muscle relaxant with vascular effects manifested predominantly by venous dilatation and pooling. The major beneficial effect of nitroglycerin in angina pectoris is a reduction in myocardial oxygen consumption secondary to vascular smooth muscle relaxation and consequent reduced cardiac preload and afterload. In recent years there has been an increasing recognition of a direct vasodilator effect of nitroglycerin on the coronary vessels.

In healthy volunteers transdermal absorption of nitroglycerin from a nitroglycerin system occurred in a continuous and well-controlled manner for a minimum of 24 hours. Steady-state plasma levels are attained within 2 hours after application, and continue for the duration of wearing the system. Precise definition of "therapeutic plasma level" is not known at this time. Plasma levels of nitroglycerin fall to approximately one-half the steady-state values 1 hour after system removal and are undetectable after 2 hours.

The amount of nitroglycerin released (2.5 mg, 5 mg, 10 mg, or 15 mg per 24 hours) represents the mean release rate of nitroglycerin from the system as determined from healthy volunteers, and hence, the amount potentially available for absorption through the skin. Absorption will vary among individuals.

INDICATIONS AND USAGE

This drug product has been conditionally approved by the FDA for the prevention and treatment of angina pectoris due to coronary artery disease. The conditional approval reflects a determination that the drug may be marketed while further investigation of its effectiveness is undertaken. A final evaluation of the effectiveness of the product will be announced by the FDA.

CONTRAINDICATIONS

Intolerance of organic nitrate drugs, marked anemia, increased intraocular pressure or increased intracranial pressure.

WARNINGS

In patients with acute myocardial infarction or congestive heart failure, Transderm-Nitro system should be used under careful clinical and/or hemodynamic monitoring.

In terminating treatment of anginal patients, both the dosage and frequency of application must be gradually reduced over a period of 4 to 6 weeks to prevent sudden withdrawal reactions, which are characteristic of all vasodilators in the nitroglycerin class.

Transdermal nitroglycerin systems should be removed before attempting defibrillation or cardioversion because of the potential for altered electrical conductivity which may enhance the possibility of arcing, a phenomenon associated with the use of defibrillators.

PRECAUTIONS

Symptoms of hypotension, such as faintness, weakness or dizziness, particularly orthostatic hypotension may be due to overdosage. When these symptoms occur, the dosage should be reduced or use of the product discontinued.

Transderm-Nitro system is not intended for immediate relief of anginal attacks. For this purpose occasional use of the sublingual preparations may be necessary.

ADVERSE REACTIONS

Transient headaches are the most common side effect, especially when higher doses of the drug are used. These headaches should be treated with mild analgesics while Transderm-Nitro therapy is continued. When such headaches are unresponsive to treatment, the nitroglycerin dosage should be reduced or use of the product discontinued.

Adverse reactions reported less frequently include hypotension, increased heart rate, faintness, flushing, dizziness, nausea and vomiting. These symptoms are attributable to the known pharmacologic effects of nitroglycerin, but may be symptoms of overdosage. When they persist the dose should be reduced or use of the product discontinued. In some patients, dermatitis may occur.

DOSAGE AND ADMINISTRATION

Therapy should be initiated with application of one Transderm-Nitro 5 system to the desired area of skin. Many patients prefer the chest; if hair is likely to interfere with system adhesion or removal, it can be clipped prior to placement of the system. Each system is designed to remain in place for 24 hours, and each successive application should be to a different skin area. Transderm-Nitro system should not be applied to the distal parts of the extremities.

The usual dosage is one Transderm-Nitro 5 system every 24 hours. Some patients, however, may require the Transderm-Nitro 10 system. If a single Transderm-Nitro 5 system fails to provide adequate clinical response, the patient should be instructed to remove it and apply either two Transderm-Nitro 5 systems or one Transderm-Nitro 10 system. More systems may be added as indicated by continued careful monitoring of clinical response. The Transderm-Nitro 2.5 system is useful principally for decreasing the dosage gradually, though it may provide adequate therapy for some patients when used alone.

The optimal dosage should be selected based upon the clinical response, side effects, and the effects of therapy upon blood pressure. The greatest attainable decrease in resting

blood pressure that is not associated with clinical symptoms of hypotension especially during orthostasis indicates the optimal dosage. To decrease adverse reactions, the size and/or number of systems should be tailored to the individual patient's needs.
Do not store above 86°F (30°C).
Patient Instructions For Applications: A patient leaflet is supplied with the systems.

HOW SUPPLIED
[See table right].
Dist. by **CIBA Pharmaceutical Company**
Division of CIBA-GEIGY Corporation
Summit, New Jersey 07901
C85-35 (Rev. 11/85)

How to use

TRANSDERM-NITRO®
nitroglycerin
for the prevention of angina

Transderm-Nitro is easy to use—it has a clear plastic backing, and a special adhesive that keeps the system firmly in place for 24 hours.

Where to place Transderm-Nitro
Select any area of skin on the body, EXCEPT the extremities below the knee or elbow. The chest is the preferred site. The area should be clean, dry, and hairless. If hair is likely to interfere with system adhesion or removal, it can be clipped, but not shaved. Take care to avoid areas with cuts or irritations. Do NOT apply the system immediately after showering or bathing. It is best to wait until you are certain the skin is completely dry.

How to apply Transderm-Nitro® nitroglycerin

1. Open the package by tearing at the indicated indentations. Carefully pick up the system lengthwise with the tab up, and the clear plastic backing facing you. You should be able to see the white cream containing nitroglycerin. (On very rare occasions, you may find a system without any white medication in it. Do not use it. Simply apply another system.)

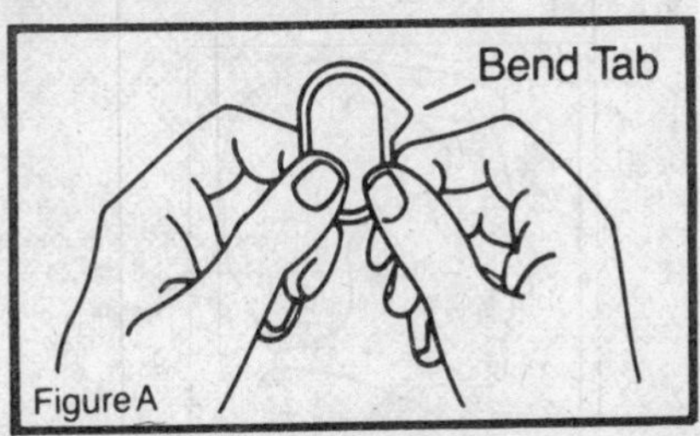

Figure A

2. Firmly bend tab forward with thumb (Figure A). With both thumbs, begin to remove the clear plastic backing from the system at the tab (Figure B). Do not touch the inside of the exposed system, because the adhesive covers the entire surface.

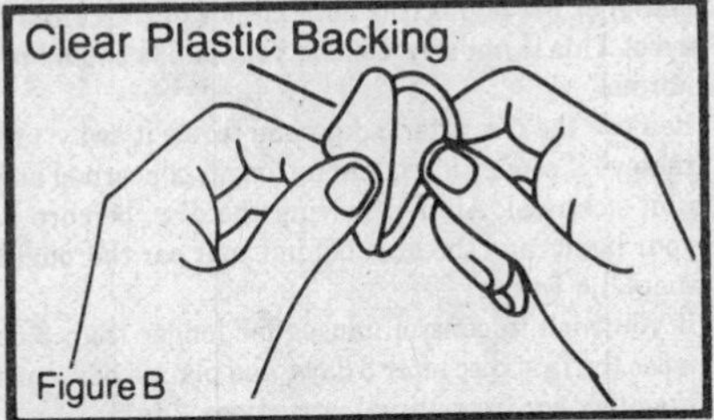

Figure B

3. Continue to remove the clear plastic backing slowly along the length of the system, allowing the system to rest on the outside of your fingers (Figure C).

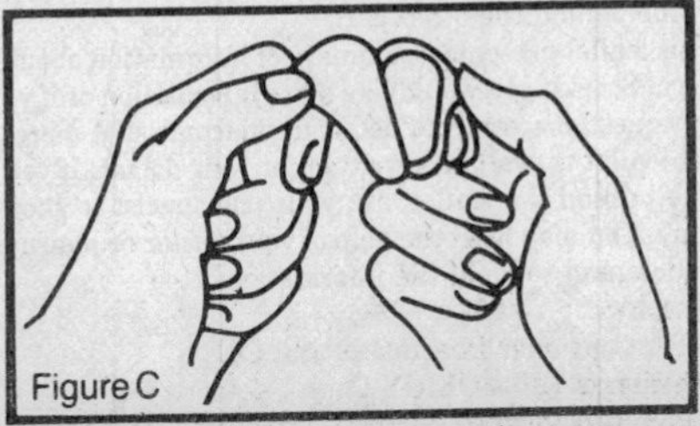
Figure C

4. Place the exposed, adhesive side of the system on the chosen skin site. Press firmly in place with the palm of your hand (Figure D). Once the system is in place, do not test the adhesion by pulling on it.

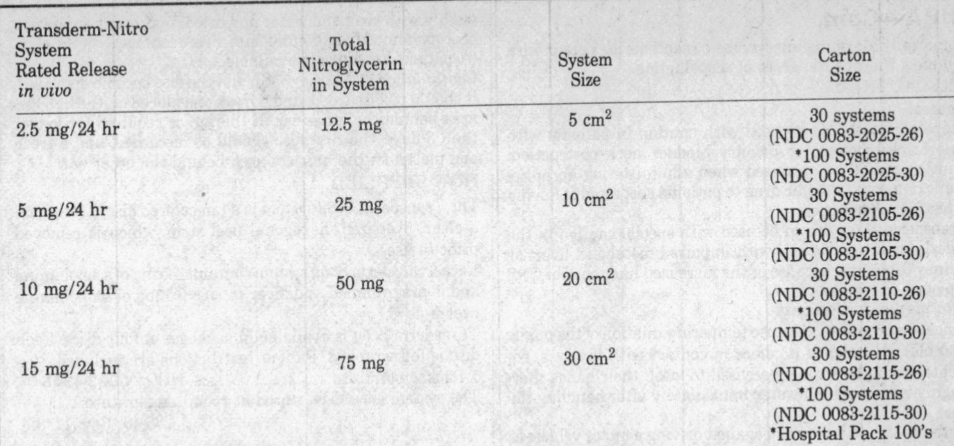

Transderm-Nitro System Rated Release *in vivo*	Total Nitroglycerin in System	System Size	Carton Size
2.5 mg/24 hr	12.5 mg	5 cm²	30 systems (NDC 0083-2025-26) *100 Systems (NDC 0083-2025-30)
5 mg/24 hr	25 mg	10 cm²	30 Systems (NDC 0083-2105-26) *100 Systems (NDC 0083-2105-30)
10 mg/24 hr	50 mg	20 cm²	30 Systems (NDC 0083-2110-26) *100 Systems (NDC 0083-2110-30)
15 mg/24 hr	75 mg	30 cm²	30 Systems (NDC 0083-2115-26) *100 Systems (NDC 0083-2115-30)

*Hospital Pack 100's

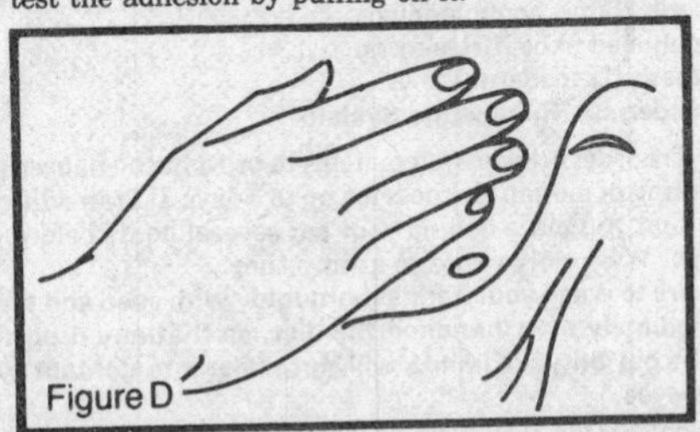
Figure D

5. Remove and discard the system after 24 hours. Place a new system on a different skin site, following steps 1–4.

Please note:
Contact with water, as in bathing, swimming, or showering will not affect the system. In the unlikely event that a system falls off, discard it and put a new one on a different skin site.

PRECAUTIONS
The most common side effect is headaches, which often decreases as therapy is continued, but may require treatment with a mild analgesic. Although uncommon, faintness, flushing, and dizziness may occur, especially when suddenly rising from the recumbent (lying horizontal) position. If these symptoms occur, remove the system and notify your physician.
Skin irritation may occur. If it persists, consult your physician.
Keep these systems and all drugs out of the reach of children.
Important: Your doctor may decide to increase or decrease the size of the system, or prescribe a combination of systems, to suit your particular needs. The dose may vary depending on your individual response to the system.
DO NOT STORE ABOVE 86°F (30°C).
Dist. by:
CIBA Pharmaceutical Co.
Div. of CIBA-GEIGY Corp.
Summit, NJ 07901
C85-36 (Rev. 11/85)

Shown in Product Identification Section, page 408

TRANSDERM SCŌP® ℞
[*trans-derm scōpe*]
scopolamine
(formerly Transderm-V)

Transdermal Therapeutic System

Programmed delivery *in vivo* of 0.5 mg of scopolamine over 3 days

This product is now marketed by CIBA Consumer Pharmaceutical Company, Division of CIBA-GEIGY Corporation.

DESCRIPTION
The Transderm Scōp system is a circular flat disc designed for continuous release of scopolamine following application to an area of intact skin on the head, behind the ear. Clinical evaluation has demonstrated that the system provides effective antiemetic and antinauseant actions when tested against motion-sickness stimuli in adults.
The Transderm Scōp system is a film 0.2 mm thick and 2.5cm², with four layers. Proceeding from the visible surface towards the surface attached to the skin, these layers are: (1) a backing layer of tan-colored, aluminized, polyester film; (2) a drug reservoir of scopolamine, mineral oil, and polyisobutylene; (3) a microporous polypropylene membrane that controls the rate of delivery of scopolamine from the system to the skin surface; and (4) an adhesive formulation of mineral oil, polyisobutylene, and scopolamine. A protective peel strip of siliconized polyester, which covers the adhesive layer, is removed before the system is used. The inactive components, mineral oil (12.4 mg) and polyisobutylene (11.4 mg), are not released from the system.

Cross section of the system:

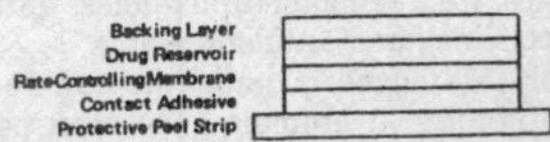

Release-Rate Concept: The Transderm Scōp system contains 1.5 mg of scopolamine. The system is programmed to deliver 0.5 mg of scopolamine at an approximately constant rate to the systemic circulation over the 3-day lifetime of the system. An initial priming dose of scopolamine, released from the adhesive layer of the system, saturates the skin binding sites and rapidly brings the plasma concentration of scopolamine to the required steady-state level. A continuous controlled release of scopolamine, which flows from the drug reservoir through the rate-controlling membrane, maintains the plasma level constant.

CLINICAL PHARMACOLOGY
The sole active agent of Transderm Scōp is scopolamine, a belladonna alkaloid with well-known pharmacological properties. The drug has a long history of oral and parenteral use for central anticholinergic activity, including prophylaxis of motion sickness. The mechanism of action of scopolamine in the central nervous system (CNS) is not definitely known but may include anticholinergic effects. The ability of scopolamine to prevent motion-induced nausea is believed to be associated with inhibition of vestibular input to the CNS, which results in inhibition of the vomiting reflex. In addition, scopolamine may have a direct action on the vomiting center within the reticular formation of the brain stem. Applied to the postauricular skin, Transderm Scōp provides for a gradual release of scopolamine from an adhesive matrix of mineral oil and polyisobutylene.

INDICATIONS AND USAGE
Transderm Scōp is indicated for prevention of nausea and vomiting associated with motion sickness in adults. The disc should be applied only to skin in the postauricular area.
Clinical Results: Transderm Scōp provides antiemetic protection within several hours following application of the disc behind the ear. In 195 adult subjects of different racial origins who participated in clinical efficacy studies at sea or in a controlled motion environment, there was a 75% reduction in the incidence of motion-induced nausea and vomiting. Transderm Scōp provided significantly greater protection than that obtained with oral dimenhydrinate.

CONTRAINDICATIONS
Transderm Scōp should not be used in patients with known hypersensitivity to scopolamine or any of the components of the adhesive matrix making up the therapeutic system, or in patients with glaucoma.

WARNINGS
Transderm Scōp should not be used in children and should be used with special caution in the elderly. See **PRECAUTIONS.**
Since drowsiness, disorientation, and confusion may occur with the use of scopolamine, patients should be warned of the possibility and cautioned against engaging in activities that require mental alertness, such as driving a motor vehicle or operating dangerous machinery.

Continued on next page

The full prescribing information for each CIBA drug is contained herein and is that in effect as of September 1, 1986

CIBA—Cont.

Potentially alarming idiosyncratic reactions may occur with ordinary therapeutic doses of scopolamine.

PRECAUTIONS

General

Scopolamine should be used with caution in patients with pyloric obstruction, or urinary bladder neck obstruction. Caution should be exercised when administering an antiemetic or antimuscarinic drug to patients suspected of having intestinal obstruction.

Transderm Scōp should be used with special caution in the elderly or in individuals with impaired metabolic, liver, or kidney functions, because of the increased likelihood of CNS effects.

Information for Patients

Since scopolamine can cause temporary dilation of the pupils and blurred vision if it comes in contact with the eyes, patients should be strongly advised to wash their hands thoroughly with soap and water immediately after handling the disc.

Patients should be warned against driving a motor vehicle or operating dangerous machinery. A patient brochure is available.

Drug Interactions

Scopolamine should be used with care in patients taking drugs, including alcohol, capable of causing CNS effects. Special attention should be given to drugs having anticholinergic properties, e.g., belladonna alkaloids, antihistamines (including meclizine), and antidepressants.

Carcinogenesis, Mutagenesis, Impairment of Fertility

No long-term studies in animals have been performed to evaluate carcinogenic potential.

Fertility studies were performed in female rats and revealed no evidence of impaired fertility or harm to the fetus due to scopolamine hydrobromide administered by daily subcutaneous injection. In the highest-dose group (plasma level approximately 500 times the level achieved in humans using a transdermal system), reduced maternal body weights were observed.

Pregnancy Category C

Teratogenic studies were performed in pregnant rats and rabbits with scopolamine hydrobromide administered by daily intravenous injection. No adverse effects were recorded in the rats. In the rabbits, the highest dose (plasma level approximately 100 times the level achieved in humans using a transdermal system) of drug administered had a marginal embryotoxic effect.

Transderm Scōp should be used during pregnancy only if the anticipated benefit justifies the potential risk to the fetus.

Nursing Mothers

It is not known whether scopolamine is excreted in human milk. Because many drugs are excreted in human milk, caution should be exercised when Transderm Scōp is administered to a nursing woman.

Pediatric Use

Children are particularly susceptible to the side effects of belladonna alkaloids. Transderm Scōp should not be used in children because it is not known whether this system will release an amount of scopolamine that could produce serious adverse effects in children.

ADVERSE REACTIONS

The most frequent adverse reaction to Transderm Scōp is dryness of the mouth. This occurs in about two thirds of the people. A less frequent adverse reaction is drowsiness, which occurs in less than one sixth of the people. Transient impairment of eye accommodation, including blurred vision and dilation of the pupils, is also observed.

The following adverse reactions have also been reported on infrequent occasions during the use of Transderm Scōp: disorientation; memory disturbances; dizziness; restlessness; hallucinations; confusion; difficulty urinating; rashes and erythema; acute narrow-angle glaucoma; and dry, itchy, or red eyes. *Drug Withdrawal:* Symptoms including dizziness, nausea, vomiting, headache and disturbances of equilibrium have been reported in a few patients following discontinuation of the use of the Transderm Scōp System. These symptoms have occurred most often in patients who have used the Systems for more than three days.

OVERDOSAGE

Overdosage with scopolamine may cause disorientation, memory disturbances, dizziness, restlessness, hallucinations, or confusion. Should these symptoms occur, the Transderm Scōp disc should be immediately removed. Appropriate parasympathomimetic therapy should be initiated if these symptoms are severe.

DOSAGE AND ADMINISTRATION

Initiation of Therapy: One Transderm Scōp disc (programmed to deliver 0.5 mg of scopolamine over 3 days) should be applied to the hairless area behind one ear at least 4 hours before the antiemetic effect is required. Only one disc should be worn at any time.

Handling: After the disc is applied on dry skin behind the ear, the hands should be washed thoroughly with soap and water and dried. Upon removal of the disc, it should be discarded, and the hands and application site washed thoroughly with soap and water and dried, to prevent any traces of scopolamine from coming into direct contact with the eyes. (A patient brochure is available.)

Continuation of Therapy: Should the disc become displaced, it should be discarded, and a fresh one placed on the hairless area behind the other ear. If therapy is required for longer than 3 days, the first disc should be discarded, and a fresh one placed on the hairless area behind the other ear.

HOW SUPPLIED

The Transderm Scōp system is a tan-colored disc, 2.5 cm^2, on a clear, oversized, hexagonal peel strip, which is removed prior to use.

Each Transderm Scōp system contains 1.5 mg of scopolamine and is programmed to deliver *in vivo* 0.5 mg of scopolamine over 3 days.

Transderm Scōp is available in packages of four discs. Each disc is foil wrapped. Patient instructions are included.

1 Package (4 discs) ....NDC **0083-4345-04**

The system should be stored at room temperature.

C85-40 (Rev. 11/85)

Information for the Patient About—

TRANSDERM SCŌP®

Generic Name: scopolamine, pronounced skoe-POL-a-meen (formerly Transderm-V) Transdermal Therapeutic System

The Transderm Scōp system helps to prevent the nausea and vomiting of motion sickness for up to 3 days. It is an adhesive disc that you place behind your ear several hours before you travel. Wear only one disc at any time.

Be sure to wash your hands thoroughly with soap and water immediately after handling the disc, so that any drug that might get on your hands will not come into contact with your eyes.

Avoid drinking alcohol while using Transderm Scōp. Also, be careful about driving or operating any machinery while using the system because the drug might make you drowsy.

TRANSDERM SCŌP SHOULD NOT BE USED IN CHILDREN AND SHOULD BE USED WITH SPECIAL CAUTION IN THE ELDERLY.

How the Transderm Scōp System Works

A group of nerve fibers deep inside the ear helps people keep their balance. For some people, the motion of ships, airplanes, trains, automobiles, and buses increases the activity of these nerve fibers. This increased activity causes the *dizziness, nausea, and vomiting* of motion sickness. People may have one, some, or all of these symptoms.

Transderm Scōp contains the drug scopolamine, which helps reduce the activity of the nerve fibers in the inner ear. When a Transderm Scōp disc is placed on the skin behind one of the ears, scopolamine passes through the skin and into the bloodstream. One disc may be kept in place for 3 days if needed.

PRECAUTIONS

Before using Transderm Scōp be sure to tell your doctor if you—

- Are pregnant or nursing (or planning to become pregnant)
- Have glaucoma (increased pressure in the eyeball)
- Have (or have had) any metabolic, liver, or kidney disease
- Have any obstructions of the stomach or intestine
- Have trouble urinating or any bladder obstruction
- Have any skin allergy or have had a skin reaction such as a rash or redness to any drug, especially scopolamine, or chemical or food substance.

Any of these conditions could make Transderm Scōp unsuitable for you. Also tell your doctor if you are taking any other medicines.

Transderm Scōp should not be used in children. The safety of its use in children has not been determined. Children and the elderly may be particularly sensitive to the effects of scopolamine.

Side Effects: The most common side effect experienced by people using Transderm Scōp is dryness of the mouth. This occurs in about two thirds of the people. A less frequent side effect is drowsiness, which occurs in less than one sixth of the people. Temporary blurring of vision and dilation (widening) of the pupils may occur, especially if the drug is on your hands and comes in contact with the eyes. On infrequent occasions, disorientation, memory disturbances, dizziness, restlessness, hallucinations, confusion, difficulty urinating, skin rashes or redness, and dry, itchy, or red eyes have been reported. If these effects do occur, remove the disc and call your doctor. Since drowsiness, disorientation, and confusion may occur with the use of scopolamine, be careful driving or operating any dangerous machinery, especially when you first start using the drug system.

Drug Withdrawal: Symptoms including dizziness, nausea, vomiting, headache and disturbances of equilibrium have been reported in a few people following discontinuation of the Transderm Scōp System. These symptoms have occurred most often in people who have used the Systems for more than three days. We recommend that you consult your doctor if these symptoms occur.

How to Use Transderm Scōp

Transderm Scōp may be kept at room temperature until you are ready to use it.

1. Plan to apply one Transderm Scōp disc at least 4 hours before you need it. **Wear only one disc at any time.**
2. Select a hairless area of skin behind one ear, taking care to avoid any cuts or irritations. Wipe the area with a clean, dry tissue.
3. Peel the package open and remove the disc (Figure 1).

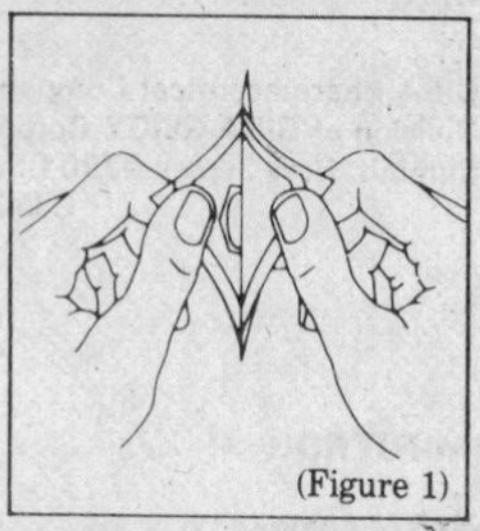

(Figure 1)

4. Remove the clear plastic six-sided backing from the round system. Try not to touch the adhesive surface on the disc with your hands (Figure 2).

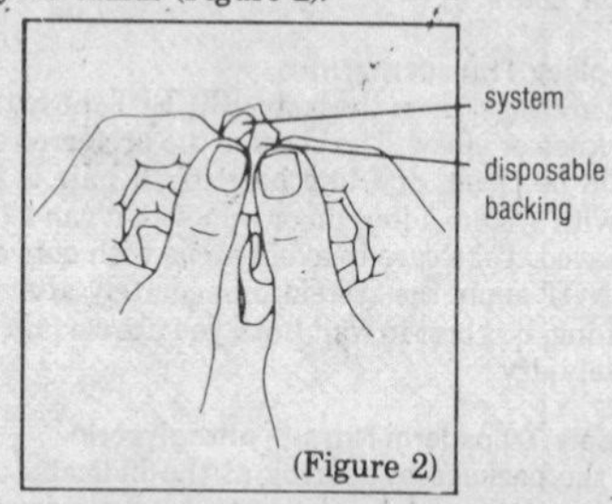

(Figure 2)

5. Firmly apply the adhesive surface (metallic side) to the dry area of skin behind the ear so that the tan-colored side is showing (Figure 3). Make good contact, especially around the edge. Once you have placed the disc behind your ear, do not move it for as long as you want to use it (up to 3 days).

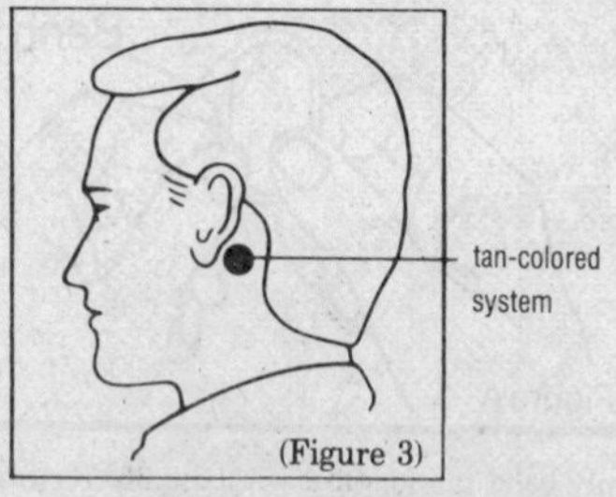

(Figure 3)

6. ***Important:*** **After the disc is in place, be sure to wash your hands thoroughly with soap and water to remove any scopolamine. If this drug were to contact your eyes, it could cause temporary blurring of vision and dilation (widening) of the pupils (the dark circles in the center of your eyes). This is not serious, and your pupils should return to normal.**
7. Remove the disc after 3 days and throw it away. (You may remove it sooner if you are no longer concerned about motion sickness). After removing the disc, be sure to wash your hands and the area behind your ear thoroughly with soap and water.
8. If you wish to control nausea for longer than 3 days, *remove* the first disc after 3 days, and place a new one *behind the other ear,* repeating instructions 2 to 7.
9. Keep the disc dry, if possible, to prevent it from falling off. Limited contact with water, however, as in bathing or swimming, will not affect the system. In the unlikely event that the disc falls off, throw it away and put a new one behind the other ear.

This leaflet presents a summary of information about Transderm Scōp. If you would like more information or if you have any questions, ask your doctor or pharmacist. A more technical leaflet is available, written for your doctor. If you would like to read the leaflet, ask your pharmacist to show you a copy. You may need the help of your doctor or pharmacist to understand some of the information.

Dist. by:
CIBA Consumer Pharmaceutical Co.
Division of CIBA-GEIGY Corp.
Summit, NJ 07901

C85-41 (Rev. 11/85)

Shown in Product Identification Section, page 408

VIOFORM®
[*vye-oh-form*]
(clioquinol USP)
Antifungal/Antibacterial Ointment and Cream

Listed in USP, a Medicare designated compendium.

DESCRIPTION
Vioform is 5-chloro-7-iodo-8-quinolinol—an effective antifungal and antibacterial agent—available as 3% *Ointment* and 3% *Cream.*

Indications and Directions For Use:
A soothing antifungal and antibacterial preparation for the treatment of inflamed conditions of the skin, such as eczema, athlete's foot and other fungal infections.
Apply to the affected area 2 or 3 times a day or use as directed by physician.
Do not use in children under 2 years of age.

CAUTION
May prove irritating to sensitized skin in rare cases. If this should occur, discontinue treatment and consult physician. May stain.
KEEP OUT OF REACH OF CHILDREN.

HOW SUPPLIED
Ointment, 3% clioquinol in a petrolatum base; tubes of 1 ounce.
Cream, 3% clioquinol in a water-washable base; tubes of 1 ounce.
Do not store above 86°F.
C86-8 (Rev. 2/86)

VIOFORM®-HYDROCORTISONE ℞
[*vye-oh-form*]
(clioquinol USP and hydrocortisone USP)

DESCRIPTION
Vioform-Hydrocortisone, a topical compound for dermatologic use, combines the antifungal and antibacterial actions of clioquinol and the anti-inflammatory and antipruritic effects of hydrocortisone to provide broad control of acute and chronic dermatoses. It is available as *Cream, Ointment,* or *Lotion* containing 3% clioquinol and 1% hydrocortisone and as *Mild Cream* and *Mild Ointment* containing 3% clioquinol and 0.5% hydrocortisone.
Vioform is 5-chloro-7-iodo-8-quinolinol.
Hydrocortisone is 11β,17,21-trihydroxypregn-4-ene,3,20-dione.

ACTIONS
In vitro studies have demonstrated that Vioform effectively inhibits the growth of various mycotic organisms such as Microsporons, Trichophytons, and Candida albicans and gram positive cocci such as staphylococci and enterococci. The role of steroids in alleviating the inflammation and pruritus associated with many dermatoses has been well established.

INDICATIONS
Based on a review of this drug by the National Academy of Sciences-National Research Council and/or other information, FDA has classified the indications as follows:
"Possibly" effective: Contact or atopic dermatitis; impetiginized eczema; nummular eczema; infantile eczema; endogenous chronic infectious dermatitis; stasis dermatitis; pyoderma; nuchal eczema and chronic eczematoid otitis externa; acne urticata; localized or disseminated neurodermatitis; lichen simplex chronicus; anogenital pruritus (vulvae, scroti, ani); folliculitis; bacterial dermatoses; mycotic dermatoses such as tinea (capitis, cruris, corporis, pedis); moniliasis; intertrigo.
Final classification of the less-than-effective indications requires further investigation.

CONTRAINDICATIONS
Hypersensitivity to Vioform-Hydrocortisone, or any of its ingredients or related compounds; lesions of the eye; tuberculosis of the skin; most viral skin lesions (including herpes simplex, vaccinia, and varicella).
Vioform should not be used in children under 2 years of age.

WARNINGS
This product is not for ophthalmic use.
In the presence of systemic infections, appropriate systemic antibiotics should be used.
Usage in Pregnancy: Although topical steroids have not been reported to have an adverse effect on pregnancy, the safety of their use in pregnant women has not been absolutely established. In laboratory animals, increases in incidence of fetal abnormalities have been associated with exposure of gestating females to topical corticosteroids, in some cases at rather low dosage levels. Therefore, drugs of this class should not be used extensively on pregnant patients in large amounts or for prolonged periods of time.

PRECAUTIONS
May prove irritating to sensitized skin in rare cases. If irritation occurs, discontinue therapy. Staining of skin and fabrics may occur. Additionally, there are rare reports of discoloration of hair and nails.
Signs and symptoms of systemic toxicity, electrolyte imbalance, or adrenal suppression have not been reported with Vioform-Hydrocortisone. Nevertheless, the possibility of suppression of the pituitary-adrenal axis during therapy should be kept in mind, especially when the drug is used under occlusive dressings, for a prolonged period, or for treating extensive cutaneous areas since significant absorption of corticosteroid may occur under these conditions, particularly in children and infants.
Vioform may be absorbed through the skin and interfere with thyroid function tests. If such tests are contemplated, wait at least one month between discontinuation of therapy and performance of these tests. The ferric chloride test for phenylketonuria (PKU) can yield a false-positive result if Vioform is present in the diaper or urine.
Prolonged use may result in overgrowth of nonsusceptible organisms requiring appropriate therapy.

ADVERSE REACTIONS
There have been a few reports of rash and hypersensitivity. The following local adverse reactions have been reported with topical corticosteroids, especially under occlusive dressings: burning; itching; irritation; dryness; folliculitis; hypertrichosis; acneiform eruptions; hypopigmentation; perioral dermatitis; allergic contact dermatitis; maceration of the skin; secondary infection; skin atrophy; striae; miliaria. Discontinue therapy if any untoward reaction occurs.

DOSAGE AND ADMINISTRATION
Apply a thin layer to the affected parts 3 or 4 times daily. The *Cream,* because of its slight drying effect, is primarily useful for moist, weeping lesions; the *Lotion* is particularly suitable for application behind the ears and in intertriginous areas of the body; the *Ointment* is best used for dry lesions accompanied by thickening and scaling of the skin.
The *Mild Cream* and *Mild Ointment* should be used when treating lesions involving extensive body areas or less severe dermatoses.

HOW SUPPLIED
Cream, 3% clioquinol and 1% hydrocortisone in a water-washable base containing stearyl alcohol, cetyl alcohol, stearic acid, petrolatum, sodium lauryl sulfate, and glycerin in water; tubes of 5 and 20 Gm.
Ointment, 3% clioquinol and 1% hydrocortisone in a petrolatum base; tubes of 20 Gm.
Lotion, 3% clioquinol and 1% hydrocortisone in a water-washable base containing stearic acid, cetyl alcohol, lanolin, propylene glycol, sorbitan trioleate, polysorbate 60, triethanolamine, methylparaben, propylparaben, and perfume Flora in water; plastic squeeze bottles of 15 ml.
Mild Cream, 3% clioquinol and 0.5% hydrocortisone in a water-washable base containing stearyl alcohol, cetyl alcohol, stearic acid, petrolatum, sodium lauryl sulfate, and glycerin in water; tubes of ½ and 1 ounce.
Mild Ointment, 3% clioquinol and 0.5% hydrocortisone in a petrolatum base; tubes of 1 ounce.
Do not store above 86°F.
C86-9 (Rev. 2/86)

Colgate-Hoyt Laboratories
(Formerly Hoyt Laboratories)
Division of Colgate-Palmolive Co.
1 COLGATE WAY
CANTON, MA 02021 U.S.A.

LURIDE® Drops ℞
brand of Sodium Fluoride

DESCRIPTION
Each ml. (18 drops) contains 2.25 mg fluoride ion (F^-) from 4.97 mg sodium fluoride (NaF), approximately 0.125 mg F per drop. For use as a dental caries preventive in children. Sugar-free. Saccharin-free.

CLINICAL PHARMACOLOGY
Sodium fluoride acts systemically (before tooth eruption) and topically (post-eruption) by increasing tooth resistance to acid dissolution, by promoting remineralization, and by inhibiting the cariogenic microbial process.

INDICATIONS AND USAGE
It has been established that ingestion of fluoridated drinking water (1 ppm F) during the period of tooth development results in a significant decrease in the incidence of dental caries.[1] LURIDE Drops was developed to provide systemic fluoride for use as a supplement in infants and children from birth to age 3 and older, living in areas where the drinking water fluoride level does not exceed 0.7 ppm.

CONTRAINDICATIONS
Do not use in areas where the drinking water exceeds 0.7 ppm F.

WARNINGS
See "Contraindications" above. As in the case of all medications, keep out of reach of children.

PRECAUTIONS
See "Overdosage" section below. Incompatibility of fluoride with dairy foods has been reported due to formation of calcium fluoride which is poorly absorbed.

ADVERSE REACTIONS
Allergic rash and other idiosyncrasies have been rarely reported.

OVERDOSAGE
Prolonged daily ingestion of excessive fluoride will result in varying degrees of dental fluorosis. (The total amount of sodium fluoride in a bottle of 30 ml LURIDE Drops (67.5 mg F) conforms with the recommendations of the American Dental Association for the maximum to be dispensed at one time for safety purposes.)

DOSAGE[2] AND ADMINISTRATION
Invert bottle vertically for proper drop delivery.

F-Content of Drinking Water	Daily Dosage: Birth to Age 2	Age 2–3	Age 3–12
<0.3 ppm	2 drops	4 drops	8 drops
0.3–0.7 ppm	One-half above dosage.		
>0.7 ppm	Fluoride supplements contraindicated.		

LURIDE Drops may be administered orally undiluted or mixed with fluids.

HOW SUPPLIED
Squeeze-bottles of 30 ml. (peach flavor—NDC#0126-0003-31)

CAUTION
Federal (U.S.A.) law prohibits dispensing without prescription.

REFERENCES
1. *Accepted Dental Therapeutics,* Ed. 40, American Dental Association, Chicago, 1984, p. 399–402.
2. Ibid., p. 401; American Academy of Pediatrics, Pediatrics 63:150–152, 1979.

LURIDE® Lozi-Tabs® Tablets ℞
brand of Sodium Fluoride
Full-strength 1.0 mg F
Luride-SF (no artificial flavor or color) 1.0 mg F
Half-strength 0.5 mg F
Quarter-strength 0.25 mg F

DESCRIPTION
LURIDE® brand of sodium fluoride Lozi-Tabs® brand of lozenge/chewable tablets for use as a dental caries preventive in children. Sugar-free. Saccharin-free.
Each LURIDE 1.0 mg F tablet (full-strength) contains 1.0 mg fluoride (F) from 2.2 mg sodium fluoride (NaF).
Each LURIDE-SF 1.0 mg F tablet (SF for Special Formula: no artificial color or flavor) contains 1.0 mg F from 2.2 mg NaF.
Each LURIDE 0.5 mg F tablet (half-strength) contains 0.5 mg F from 1.1 mg NaF.
Each Luride 0.25 mg F tablet (quarter-strength) contains 0.25 mg F from 0.55 mg NaF.

CLINICAL PHARMACOLOGY
Sodium fluoride acts systemically (before tooth eruption) and topically (post-eruption) by increasing tooth resistance to acid dissolution, by promoting remineralization, and by inhibiting the cariogenic microbial process.

INDICATIONS AND USAGE
It is well established that ingestion of fluoridated drinking water (1 ppm F) during the period of tooth development results in a significant decrease in the incidence of dental caries.[1] LURIDE tablets were developed to provide fluoride for children living in areas where the water fluoride level is 0.7 ppm or less.

CONTRAINDICATIONS
LURIDE and LURIDE-SF 1.0 mg F tablets are contraindicated when the F-content of drinking water is 0.3 ppm or more and should not be administered to children under age 3. LURIDE 0.5 mg F and .25 mg F tablets are contraindicated when the F-content of drinking water exceeds 0.7 ppm.

Continued on next page

Colgate-Hoyt—Cont.

WARNINGS

Do not use LURIDE or LURIDE-SF 1.0 mg F tablets for children under age 3, nor in areas where the F-content of the drinking water is 0.3 ppm or more. Do not use LURIDE 0.5 mg F or LURIDE 0.25 mg F in areas where the F-content of the drinking water is more than 0.7 ppm. As in the case of all medications, keep out of reach of children.

PRECAUTIONS

See "Overdosage" section below. Incompatibility of fluoride with dairy foods has been reported due to formation of calcium fluoride which is poorly absorbed.

ADVERSE REACTIONS

Allergic rash and other idiosyncrasies have been rarely reported.

OVERDOSAGE

Prolonged daily ingestion of excessive fluoride will result in varying degrees of dental fluorosis. (The total amount of sodium fluoride in a bottle of 120 LURIDE tablets (all strengths) conforms with the recommendations of the American Dental Association for the maximum to be dispensed at one time for safety purposes.)

DOSAGE[2] AND ADMINISTRATION

F-Content of Drinking Water	Daily Dosage (F ion) Birth to Age 2	Age 2–3	Age 3–12
<0.3 ppm	0.25 mg	0.5 mg	1.0 mg.
0.3–0.7 ppm	One-half above dosages.		
>0.7 ppm	Fluoride supplements contraindicated.		

One tablet daily, to be dissolved in the mouth or chewed before swallowing, preferably at bedtime after brushing teeth.

HOW SUPPLIED

[See table below].

CAUTION

Federal (U.S.A.) law prohibits dispensing without prescription.

REFERENCES

1. *Accepted Dental Therapeutics*, Ed. 40, American Dental Association, Chicago, 1984, p. 399–402.
2. Ibid., p. 401; American Academy of Pediatrics, Pediatrics 63:150–152, 1979

Shown in Product Identification Section, page 408

ORABASE® HCA ℞
Oral Paste

DESCRIPTION

ORABASE® HCA is an adrenocorticoid topical dental paste for application to the oral mucosa. Each gram contains hydrocortisone acetate 5mg (0.5%) in a paste vehicle containing pectin, gelatin, sodium carboxymethylcellulose dispersed in a plasticized hydrocarbon gel composed of 5% polyethylene in mineral oil, flavored with imitation vanilla.
Hydrocortisone acetate is also known as cortisol acetate. Structural formula: Pregn-4-ene-3,20-dione,21-(acetyloxy)-11,17 dihydroxy-, (11β)-.

CLINICAL PHARMACOLOGY

Hydrocortisone acetate is a natural corticosteroid and possesses properties of an anti-inflammatory, antipruritic, and vasoconstrictive nature. The paste acts as an adhesive vehicle for applying the active medication to oral tissues. The protective action of the adhesive vehicle may serve to reduce oral irritation.
The mechanism of anti-inflammatory activity of the topical corticosteroids is unclear. Various laboratory methods, including vasoconstrictor assays, are used to compare and predict potencies and/or clinical efficacies of the topical corticosteroids. There is some evidence to suggest that a recognizable correlation exists between vasoconstrictor potency and therapeutic efficacy in man.
Once absorbed, topical corticosteroids are handled through pharmacokinetic pathways similar to systemically administered corticosteroids. Corticosteroids are bound to plasma proteins in varying degrees. Corticosteroids are metabolized primarily in the liver and are then excreted by the kidneys. Some of the topical corticosteroids and their metabolites are also excreted into the bile.

INDICATIONS AND USAGE

Indicated for adjunctive treatment and for temporary relief of symptoms associated with oral inflammatory lesions and ulcerative lesions resulting from trauma.

CONTRAINDICATIONS

Topical corticosteroids are contraindicated in those patients with a history of hypersensitivity to any of the components of the preparation.

PRECAUTIONS

General: Systemic absorption of topical corticosteroids has produced reversible hypothalamic-pituitary-adrenal (HPA) axis suppression, manifestations of Cushing's syndrome, hyperglycemia, and glucosuria in some patients. Conditions which augment systemic absorption include the application of the more potent steroids, use over large surface areas, and prolonged use.
Therefore, patients receiving a large dose of a potent topical steroid applied to a large surface area should be evaluated periodically for evidence of HPA axis suppression by using the urinary free cortisol and ACTH stimulation tests. If HPA axis suppression is noted, an attempt should be made to withdraw the drug or to reduce the frequency of application.
Recovery of HPA axis function is generally prompt and complete upon discontinuation of the drug. Infrequently, signs and symptoms of steroid withdrawal may occur, requiring supplemental systemic corticosteroids.
Children may absorb proportionally larger amounts of topical corticosteroids and thus be more susceptible to systemic toxicity (See PRECAUTIONS-Pediatric Use).
If irritation develops, topical corticosteroids should be discontinued and appropriate therapy instituted.
In the presence of infections, the use of an appropriate antifungal or antibacterial agent should be instituted. If a favorable response does not occur promptly, the corticosteroid should be discontinued until the infection has been adequately controlled.
Information for the Patient: Patients using topical corticosteroids should receive the following information and instructions:

1. This medication is to be used as directed by the dentist or physician. Avoid contact with the eyes.
2. Patients should be advised not to use this medication for any disorder other than for which it was prescribed.
3. The treated area should not be bandaged or otherwise covered or wrapped as to be occlusive unless directed by the dentist or physician.
4. Patients should report any signs of local adverse reactions especially under occlusive dressing.

Laboratory Tests: The following tests may be helpful in evaluating the HPA axis suppression:
Urinary free cortisol test
ACTH stimulation test
Carcinogenesis, Mutagenesis, and Impairment of Fertility: Long-term animal studies have not been performed to evaluate the carcinogenic potential or the affect on fertility of topical corticosteroids.
Studies to determine mutagenicity with hydrocortisone have revealed negative results.
Pregnancy Category C: Corticosteroids are generally teratogenic in laboratory animals when administered systemically at relatively low dosage levels. The more potent corticosteroids have been shown to be teratogenic after dermal application in laboratory animals. There are no adequate and well-controlled studies in pregnant women on teratogenic effects from topically applied corticosteroids. Therefore, topical corticosteroids should be used during pregnancy only if the potential benefit justifies the potential risk to the fetus. Drugs of this class should not be used extensively on pregnant patients, in large amounts, or for prolonged periods of time.
Nursing Mothers: It is not known whether topical administration of corticosteroids could result in sufficient systemic absorption to produce detectable quantities in breast milk. Systemically administered corticosteroids are secreted into breast milk in quantities not likely to have a deleterious effect on the infant. Nevertheless, caution should be exercised when topical corticosteroids are administered to a nursing woman.
Pediatric Use: Pediatric patients may demonstrate greater susceptibility to topical corticosteroid-induced HPA axis suppression and Cushing's syndrome than mature patients.
Hypothalamic-pituitary-adrenal (HPA) axis suppression, Cushing's syndrome, and intracranial hypertension have been reported in children receiving topical corticosteroids. Manifestations of adrenal suppression in children include linear growth retardation, delayed weight gain, low plasma cortisol levels, and absence of response to ACTH stimulation. Manifestations of intracranial hypertension include bulging fontanelles, headaches, and bilateral papilledema.
Adminstration of topical corticosteroids to children should be limited to the least amount compatible with an effective therapeutic regimen. Chronic corticosteroid therapy may interfere with the growth and development of children.

ADVERSE REACTIONS

The following local adverse reactions are reported infrequently with topical corticosteroids. These reactions are listed in an approximate decreasing order of occurrence:
Burning
Itching
Irritation
Dryness
Hypopigmentation
Perioral dermatitis
Allergic contact dermatitis
Secondary infection
Striae
Miliaria

OVERDOSAGE

Topically applied corticosteroids can be absorbed in sufficient amounts to produce systemic effects (See PRECAUTIONS).

DOSAGE AND ADMINISTRATION

Dab, *do not rub*, on the lesion until the paste adheres. (Rubbing this preparation on lesions may result in a granular, gritty sensation.) After application, a smooth, slippery film develops.
Usual adult dose: Topical, to the oral mucous membrane, 2 or 3 times a day following meals and at bedtime.
Usual pediatric dose: Dosage has not been established.

HOW SUPPLIED

Net weight 5 Gm. tubes (NDC#0126-0101-45) and 0.75 Gm. patient starter packets in boxes of 100 (NDC#0126-0101-01).

CAUTION

Federal (U.S.A.) law prohibits dispensing without a prescription.

Keep Out of Reach of Children

LURIDE

Strength (F ion)	Tablets per Bottle	Flavor	NDC Number 0126-
1.0mg F (full strength)	120	cherry	0006-21
		assorted(1)	0143-21
		SF(2)	0007-21
	1000*	cherry	0006-10
		assorted(1)	0143-10
	5000*	cherry	0006-51
0.5mg F (half-strength)	120	grape	0014-21
	1200*	grape	0014-81
0.25mg F (quarter-strength)	120	vanilla	0186-21

* FOR DISPENSING ONLY (1) cherry, orange, lemon, lime (2) Special Formula: no artificial flavor or coloring

PHOS-FLUR® Oral Rinse/Supplement ℞
brand of Acidulated Phosphate Fluoride

DESCRIPTION

Each teaspoonful (5 ml) contains 1.0 mg fluoride ion (F^-) from 2.2 mg sodium fluoride (NaF), in a 0.1 Molar phosphate solution at pH 4, for use as a dental caries preventive in children. Cherry, orange, lime–sugar and saccharin free. Cinnamon–contains saccharin but is sugar free.

CLINICAL PHARMACOLOGY

Sodium fluoride acts systemically (before tooth eruption) and topically (post-eruption) by increasing tooth resistance to acid dissolution, by promoting remineralization, and by inhibiting the cariogenic microbial process. Acidulation provides greater topical fluoride uptake by dental enamel than neutral solutions.[1] Phosphate protects enamel from demineralization by the acidulated formulation (common ion effect).[1]

INDICATIONS AND USAGE

It has been well established that ingestion of fluoridated drinking water (1 ppm F) during the period of tooth development results in a significant decrease in the incidence of dental caries.[2] PHOS-FLUR was developed to provide topical and systemic fluoride for use as a rinse/supplement (rinse-and-swallow) in children age 3 and older living in areas where the water fluoride level does not exceed 0.7 ppm. Where the drinking water contains more than 0.7 ppm F, PHOS-FLUR provides benefits as a topical fluoride dental rinse only (rinse-and-expectorate) for children age 6 and older.[3] Pioneering clinical studies on PHOS-FLUR were published by Frankl et al.[4] and Aasenden et al,[5] in 1972.

CONTRAINDICATIONS

DO NOT SWALLOW in areas where the F-content of drinking water exceeds 0.7 ppm, nor in children under age 3.

WARNINGS

Do not use as a rinse in children under age 6. Do not use as a supplement in children under age 3, nor in areas where the drinking water exceeds 0.7 ppm F. As in the case of all medications, keep out of reach of children.

PRECAUTIONS

See "Overdosage" section below. Incompatibility of systemic fluoride with dairy foods has been reported due to formation of calcium fluoride which is poorly absorbed.

ADVERSE REACTIONS

Allergic reactions and other idiosyncrasies have been rarely reported.

OVERDOSAGE

Prolonged daily ingestion of excessive fluoride will result in varying degrees of dental fluorosis. (The total amount of sodium fluoride in a bottle of 500ml PHOS-FLUR Rinse/Supplement conforms to the recommendations of the American Dental Association for the maximum to be dispensed at one time for safety purposes).

DOSAGE AND ADMINISTRATION

As A Daily Dental Rinse—Children age 6 and over, preferably at bedtime after thoroughly brushing the teeth, rinse one teaspoonful (5 ml) or two teaspoonfuls (10 ml) vigorously around and between teeth for one minute, then expectorate.
As A Daily Supplement—Children age 3 and over, in areas where the drinking water contains less than 0.3 ppm F, rinse one teaspoonful (5 ml) as above and swallow. When drinking water contains 0.3 to 0.7 ppm F, inclusive, reduce dosage to ½ teaspoonful.

HOW SUPPLIED

Bottles of	Flavors	NDC# 0126
250 ml	cherry	0129-99
500 ml	cherry	0129-46
	cinnamon	0126-46
	lime	0017-46
	orange	0128-46
1 gallon	cherry	0129-28

CAUTION

Federal (U.S.A.) law prohibits dispensing without prescription.

REFERENCES

[1]F. Brudevold et al. Arch. Oral Biol. 8:167–177, 1963. [2]Accepted Dental Therapeutics, American Dental Association, Chicago, 1984, p. 399–402. [3]Ibid., p. 399–402. [4]S.N. Frankl, S. Fleisch, and R. P. Diodati. J.A.D.A. 85:882–886, 1972. [5]R. Aasenden, P.F. DePaola, and F. Brudevold. Arch. Oral Biol. 17:1705–1714, 1972.

POINT-TWO® Dental Rinse ℞
brand of Sodium Fluoride

DESCRIPTION

0.2% sodium fluoride (NaF) in a mint-flavored, neutral aqueous solution containing 6% alcohol. For weekly use as a caries preventive in children.

CLINICAL PHARMACOLOGY

Topical application of sodium fluoride increases tooth resistance to acid dissolution, promotes remineralization, and inhibits the cariogenic microbial process.

INDICATIONS AND USAGE

It has been established that weekly rinsing with a neutral 0.2% sodium fluoride solution protects against dental caries in children.[1] POINT-TWO Rinse was developed to provide a ready-to-use, flavored preparation for convenient administration and favorable compliance.

CONTRAINDICATIONS

None. (May be used whether drinking water is fluoridated or not, since **topical** fluoride cannot produce fluorosis).

WARNINGS

DO NOT SWALLOW. Do not use in children under age 6, since younger children frequently cannot perform the rinse process without significant swallowing. As in the case of all medications, keep out of reach of children.

PRECAUTIONS

Not for systemic use. (Each 5 ml contains 5 mg fluoride ion).

ADVERSE REACTIONS

In patients with mucositis, gingival tissues may be hypersensitive to flavor or alcohol present in formulation.

OVERDOSAGE

In the event a dose is accidentally swallowed, nausea and/or vomiting may result (treat with milk or antacids).

DOSAGE AND ADMINISTRATION[2]

Children age 6 to 12, one teaspoonful (5 ml); over age 12, 2 teaspoonfuls (10 ml). Once a week, preferably at bedtime after thoroughly brushing the teeth, rinse vigorously around and between the teeth for one minute, then expectorate. DO NOT SWALLOW. For maximum benefit, do not eat, drink, or rinse mouth for at least 30 minutes afterwards.

HOW SUPPLIED

Bottles of 8 fl. oz. with child-resistant closure.
(Mint—NDC #0126-0178-99)
Gallon (with pump dispenser) (Mint—NDC #0126-0178-28)

CAUTION

Federal (U.S.A.) law prohibits dispensing without prescription.

REFERENCES

[1]Accepted Dental Therapeutics, Ed. 40, American Dental Association, Chicago, 1984, p. 404–405. [2]Ibid. p. 405.

PREVIDENT® Brush-On Gel ℞
brand of Neutral Sodium Fluoride

DESCRIPTION

Self-topical neutral fluoride containing 1.1% sodium fluoride for use as a dental caries preventive in children and adults. This prescription product is not a dentifrice.

CLINICAL PHARMACOLOGY

Frequent topical applications to the teeth with preparations having a relatively high fluoride content increase tooth resistance to acid dissolution and enhance penetration of the fluoride ion into tooth enamel.

INDICATIONS AND USAGE

It is well established that 1.1% sodium fluoride is safe and extraordinarily effective as a caries preventive when applied frequently with mouthpiece applicators[1-4]. PreviDent Brush-On Gel in a squeeze-tube is a particularly convenient dosage form which permits the application of a thin ribbon of gel onto a toothbrush as well as a mouthpiece tray.

CONTRAINDICATIONS

None (May be used in areas where drinking water is fluoridated or not, because topical fluoride cannot produce fluorosis).

WARNINGS

As with all medications, keep out of reach of children. Use in children under age 6 requires special supervision to prevent repeated swallowing of gel which could cause dental fluorosis.

OVERDOSE

Accidental ingestion of a usual treatment dose (1-2 mgF) is not harmful.

DOSAGE AND ADMINISTRATION

Adults and children 6 years of age and older. Apply daily a thin ribbon of gel to the teeth with a toothbrush or mouth-trays, for at least one minute preferably at bedtime, after brushing with toothpaste. After use, expectorate gel and rinse mouth thoroughly.

HOW SUPPLIED

2 oz plastic tubes and 0.8 oz plastic tubes.
2 oz Fresh mint flavor—NDC #0126-0088-02
Cool lime flavor—NDC #0126-0089-02
Very berry flavor—NDC #0126-0288-02
Fruit sherbet flavor—NDC #0126-0289-02
0.8 oz Very berry flavor—NDC #0126-0288-82
Fruit sherbet flavor—NDC #0126-0289-82
Fresh mint flavor—NDC #0126-0088-82

CAUTION

Federal (U.S.A.) law prohibits dispensing without prescription.

REFERENCES

1. Accepted Dental Therapeutics, Ed. 40, ADA, Chicago, p. 405–407, 1984.
2. Englander HR, Keyes PH and Gestwicki M: JADA 75:638–644, 1967.
3. Englander HR et al: JADA 78:783–787, 1969.
4. Englander HR et al: JADA 82:354–358, 1971.

THERA-FLUR® Topical Gel-Drops ℞
brand of Acidulated Phosphate Fluoride

THERA-FLUR®-N Topical Gel-Drops ℞
brand of Neutral Sodium Fluoride

DESCRIPTION

THERA-FLUR (acidulated) gel-drops contains 0.5% fluoride ion (F^-) from 1.1% sodium fluoride (NaF) in a lime-flavored aqueous solution containing 0.1 Molar phosphate at pH 4.5. THERA-FLUR-N (neutral) also contains 0.5% (F^-) from 1.1% NaF, but with no acid phosphate, nor artificial flavor or color, at neutral pH. For daily self-topical use as a dental caries preventive.

CLINICAL PHARMACOLOGY

Frequent topical applications to the teeth with preparations having a relatively high fluoride content increase tooth resistance to acid dissolution and enhance penetration of the fluoride ion into tooth enamel.

INDICATIONS AND USAGE

It is well established that 1.1% sodium fluoride is a safe and effective caries preventive when applied frequently with mouthpiece applicators.[1] Pioneering clinical studies with THERA-FLUR and THERA-FLUR-N Gel-Drops in schoolchildren were conducted by Englander et al.[2,3,4]
Both neutral and acidulated phosphate fluoride gels have been effective in controlling rampant dental decay which frequently follows xerostomia-producing radiotherapy of tumors in the head and neck region.[5,6]

CONTRAINDICATIONS

None (May be used in areas where drinking water is fluoridated or not, because **topical** fluoride cannot produce fluorosis).

WARNINGS

As with all medications, keep out of reach of children.

PRECAUTIONS

Laboratory tests indicate that use of acidulated fluoride may cause dulling of porcelain and ceramic restorations. Therefore, THERA-FLUR-N (neutral) is recommended for this type of patient.

ADVERSE REACTIONS

In patients with mucositis, gingival tissues may be hypersensitive to the acidity of THERA-FLUR, but will tolerate THERA-FLUR-N (neutral).

OVERDOSAGE

Accidental ingestion of a usual treatment dose (2–4 mg F) is not harmful.

DOSAGE AND ADMINISTRATION

Age 6 and older. For daily use with applicators supplied by the dentist.[2] Apply 4 to 8 drops as required to cover inner surface of each applicator. Spread gel-drops with tip of bottle. Place applicators over upper and lower teeth at the same time. Bite down lightly for 6 minutes. Remove applicators and rinse mouth. Clean applicators with cold water.

HOW SUPPLIED

24 ml and 60 ml plastic squeeze bottles.

		NDC# 0126-
THERA-FLUR (lime flavor)	24ml	0048-54
	60ml	0048-02
THERA-FLUR-N (no artificial flavor or color)	24ml	0196-54
	60ml	0196-02

CAUTION

Federal (U.S.A.) law prohibits dispensing without prescription.

REFERENCES

[1]Accepted Dental Therapeutics, Ed.40, American Dental Association, Chicago, 1984, p. 405–407. [2]H. R. Englander, P. H. Keyes, and M. Gestwicki. J.A.D.A. 75:638–644, 1967. [3]H. R. Englander et al. J.A.D.A. 78:783–787, 1969. [4]H. R. Englander et al. J.A.D.A. 82:354–358, 1971. [5]E. Johansen and T. O. Olsen in "Continuing Evaluation of the Use of Fluorides" (AAAS Selected Symposium 11), Westview Press, Boulder, CO, 1979, p.66. [6]S. Dreizen et al. J. Dent. Res. 56:99–104, 1977.

Connaught Laboratories, Inc.
SWIFTWATER, PA 18370

Full product and prescribing information is contained in the package insert.

DIPHTHERIA ANTITOXIN, USP ℞
(Purified, Concentrated Globulin—EQUINE)

HOW SUPPLIED
20,000 unit vial.

DIPHTHERIA AND TETANUS TOXOIDS ADSORBED USP ℞
(For Pediatric Use) (DT)

HOW SUPPLIED
5 ml vial.

DIPHTHERIA AND TETANUS TOXOIDS AND PERTUSSIS VACCINE ADSORBED USP ℞
(For Pediatric Use) (DTP)

HOW SUPPLIED
7.5 ml vial.

HibVAX™ ℞
(Haemophilus b Polysaccharide Vaccine)

HOW SUPPLIED
1 dose vial with 0.6 ml diluent pkg. of 5; 5 dose vial with 3 ml diluent; 10 dose vial with 6 ml diluent.

MENOMUNE®—A/C/Y/W-135 ℞
(Meningococcal Polysaccharide Vaccine, Groups A,C,Y and W-135 Combined) (Freeze-Dried)

HOW SUPPLIED
10 dose vial with 6 ml diluent (needle and syringe administration); 50 dose vial with 27.5 ml diluent (jet injector administration only).

MSTA™ ℞
(Mumps Skin Test Antigen USP) Standardized to 40 CFU per ml. (not for diagnosis of immunity to mumps)

HOW SUPPLIED
1 ml vial (10 tests).

TETANUS AND DIPHTHERIA TOXOIDS ADSORBED FOR ADULT USE USP ℞

HOW SUPPLIED
5 ml vial.

TETANUS TOXOID ADSORBED USP ℞

HOW SUPPLIED
5 ml vial.

TETANUS TOXOID USP ℞
("Fluid" or "Plain")

HOW SUPPLIED
7.5 ml vial.

YF-VAX® (Yellow Fever Vaccine) ℞
(Live, 17D Virus, Avian Leukosis-Free, Stabilized) (Freeze-Dried)

HOW SUPPLIED
1 dose vial with 0.6 ml diluent pkg. of 5; 5 dose vial with 3 ml diluent.

The following products are manufactured by Connaught Laboratories, Ltd., Canada. Full product and prescribing information is contained in the package insert.

POLIOVIRUS VACCINE INACTIVATED ℞
(For the Prevention of Poliomyelitis [Salk Type])

HOW SUPPLIED
1 ml ampul, package of 5; 10 ml vial.

TUBERSOL® ℞
Tuberculin Purified Protein Derivative (Mantoux) (PPD)

HOW SUPPLIED
1 U.S. Unit (TU) per test dose (0.1 ml), 10 test vial; 5 U.S. Units (TU) per test dose (0.1 ml), 10 test and 50 test vials; 250 U.S. Units (TU) per test dose (0.1 ml), 10 test vial.

Cook-Waite Laboratories, Inc.
90 PARK AVENUE
NEW YORK, NEW YORK 10016

CARBOCAINE® ℞
hydrochloride 3% Injection (mepivacaine hydrochloride injection, USP)

CARBOCAINE® ℞
hydrochloride 2% with NEO-COBEFRIN® 1:20,000 Injection (mepivacaine hydrochloride and levonordefrin injection, USP)

THESE SOLUTIONS ARE INTENDED FOR DENTAL USE ONLY.

DESCRIPTION
Carbocaine hydrochloride (mepivacaine hydrochloride), a tertiary amine used as a local anesthetic, is 1-methyl-2′, 6′-pipecoloxylidide monohydrochloride with the following structural formula:

It is a white, crystalline, odorless powder soluble in water, but very resistant to both acid and alkaline hydrolysis.
Neo-Cobefrin (levonordefrin), a sympathomimetic amine used as a vasoconstrictor in local anesthetic solutions, is (—)-α-(1-Aminoethyl)-3, 4-dihydroxybenzyl alcohol with the following structural formula:

It is a white or buff-colored crystalline solid, freely soluble in aqueous solutions of mineral acids, but practically insoluble in water.
DENTAL CARTRIDGES MAY NOT BE AUTOCLAVED.
CARBOCAINE hydrochloride 3% Injection and CARBOCAINE hydrochloride 2% with Neo-Cobefrin 1:20.000 Injection are sterile solutions for injection.

COMPOSITION	CARTRIDGE	
Each ml contains:	2%	3%
mepivacaine hydrochloride	20.0 mg	30.0 mg
levonordefrin	0.05 mg	—
sodium chloride	4.0 mg	3.0 mg
acetone sodium bisulfite not more than	2.0 mg	—
water for injection qs ad	1.0 ml	1.0 ml

The pH of the 2% cartridge solution is adjusted between 3.3 and 5.5 with NaOH or HCl.
The pH of the 3% cartridge solution is adjusted between 4.5 and 6.8 with NaOH or HCl.

CLINICAL PHARMACOLOGY
CARBOCAINE stabilizes the neuronal membrane and prevents the initiation and transmission of nerve impulses, thereby effecting local anesthesia.
CARBOCAINE is rapidly metabolized, with only a small percentage of the anesthetic (5 to 10 per cent) being excreted unchanged in the urine. CARBOCAINE, because of its amide structure, is not detoxified by the circulating plasma esterases. The liver is the principal site of metabolism, with over 50 per cent of the administered dose being excreted into the bile as metabolites. Most of the metabolized mepivacaine is probably resorbed in the intestine and then excreted into the urine since only a small percentage is found in the feces. The principal route of excretion is via the kidney. Most of the anesthetic and its metabolites are eliminated within 30 hours. It has been shown that hydroxylation and N-demethylation, which are detoxification reactions, play important roles in the metabolism of the anesthetic. Three metabolites of mepivacaine have been identified from adult humans: two phenols, which are excreted almost exclusively as their glucuronide conjugates, and the N-demethylated compound (2′,6′-pipecoloxylidide).
The onset of action is rapid (30 to 120 seconds in the upper jaw; 1 to 4 minutes in the lower jaw) and CARBOCAINE hydrochloride 3% without vasoconstrictor will ordinarily provide operating anesthesia of 20 minutes in the upper jaw and 40 minutes in the lower jaw.
CARBOCAINE hydrochloride 2% with Neo-Cobefrin 1:20,000 provides anesthesia of longer duration for more prolonged procedures, 1 hour to 2.5 hours in the upper jaw and 2.5 hours to 5.5 hours in the lower jaw.
CARBOCAINE does not ordinarily produce irritation or tissue damage.
Neo-Cobefrin is a sympathomimetic amine used as a vasoconstrictor in local anesthetic solutions. It has pharmacologic activity similar to that of epinephrine but it is more stable than epinephrine. In equal concentrations, Neo-Cobefrin is less potent than epinephrine in raising blood pressure, and as a vasoconstrictor.

INDICATIONS AND USAGE
CARBOCAINE is indicated for production of local anesthesia for dental procedures by infiltration or nerve block in adults and children.

CONTRAINDICATIONS
Mepivacaine is contraindicated in patients with a known hypersensitivity to amide type local anesthetics.

WARNINGS
RESUSCITATIVE EQUIPMENT AND DRUGS SHOULD BE IMMEDIATELY AVAILABLE. (See Adverse Reactions).
Reactions resulting in fatality have occurred on rare occasions with the use of local anesthetics, even in the absence of a history of hypersensitivity.
Fatalities may occur with use of local anesthetics in the head and neck region as the result of retrograde arterial flow to vital CNS areas even when maximum recommended doses are observed. The practitioner should be alert to early evidences of alteration in sensorium or vital signs.
The solution which contains a vasoconstrictor should be used with extreme caution for patients whose medical history and physical evaluation suggest the existence of hypertension, arteriosclerotic heart disease, cerebral vascular insufficiency, heart block, thyrotoxicosis and diabetes, etc.

PRECAUTIONS
The safety and effectiveness of mepivacaine depend upon proper dosage, correct technique, adequate precautions, and readiness for emergencies.
The lowest dose that results in effective anesthesia should be used to avoid high plasma levels and possible adverse effects. Injection of repeated doses of mepivacaine may cause significant increase in blood levels with each repeated dose due to slow accumulation of the drug or its metabolites, or due to slower metabolic degradation than normal.
Tolerance varies with the status of the patient. Debilitated, elderly patients, acutely ill patients, and children should be given reduced doses commensurate with their weight and physical status.
Mepivacaine should be used with caution in patients with a history of severe disturbances of cardiac rhythm or heart block.
INJECTIONS SHOULD ALWAYS BE MADE SLOWLY WITH ASPIRATION TO AVOID INTRAVASCULAR INJECTION AND THEREFORE SYSTEMIC REACTION TO BOTH LOCAL ANESTHETIC AND VASOCONSTRICTOR.
If sedatives are employed to reduce patient apprehension, use reduced doses, since local anesthetic agents, like sedatives, are central nervous system depressants which in combination may have an additive effect. Young children should be given minimal doses of each agent.
Changes in sensorium such as excitation, disorientation, drowsiness, may be early indications of a high blood level of the drug and may occur following inadvertent intravascular administration or rapid absorption of mepivacaine.
Local anesthetic procedures should be used with caution when there is inflammation and/or sepsis in the region of the proposed injection.
Information for Patients: The patient should be cautioned against loss of sensation and possibility of biting trauma should the patient attempt to eat or chew gum prior to return of sensation.

Drug Interactions: The solution which contains a vasoconstrictor, should also be used with extreme caution in patients receiving drugs known to produce blood pressure alterations (i.e., MAO inhibitors, tricyclic anti-depressants, phenothiazines, etc.) as either sustained hypotension or hypertension may occur.

Solutions containing a vasoconstrictor should be used cautiously in the presence of diseases which may adversely affect the patient's cardiovascular system. Serious cardiac arrhythmias may occur if preparations containing a vasoconstrictor are employed in patients during or following the administration of potent inhalation anesthetics.

Mepivacaine SHOULD BE USED WITH CAUTION IN PATIENTS WITH KNOWN DRUG ALLERGIES AND SENSITIVITIES. A thorough history of the patient's prior experience with mepivacaine or other local anesthetics as well as concomitant or recent drug use should be taken (see Contraindications). Patients allergic to methylparaben or para-aminobenzoic acid derivatives (procaine, tetracaine, benzocaine, etc.) have not shown cross-sensitivity to agents of the amide type such as mepivacaine. Since mepivacaine is metabolized in the liver and excreted by the kidneys, it should be used cautiously in patients with liver and renal disease.

Carcinogenesis, Mutagenesis, Impairment of Fertility: Studies of CARBOCAINE hydrochloride in animals to evaluate the carcinogenic and mutagenic potential or the effect on fertility have not been conducted.

Pregnancy Category C: Animal reproduction studies have not been conducted with this solution. It is also not known whether this solution can cause fetal harm when administered to a pregnant woman or can effect reproduction capacity. This solution should be given to a pregnant woman only if clearly needed.

Nursing Mothers: It is not known whether this drug is excreted in human milk. Because many drugs are excreted in human milk, caution should be exercised when this solution is administered to a nursing woman.

Pediatric Use: Great care must be exercised in adhering to safe concentrations and dosages for pedodontic administration (see Dosage and Administration).

ADVERSE REACTIONS

Systemic adverse reactions involving the central nervous system and the cardiovascular system usually result from high plasma levels due to excessive dosage, rapid absorption, or inadvertent intravascular injection.

A small number of reactions may result from hypersensitivity, idiosyncrasy or diminished tolerance to normal dosage on the part of the patient.

Reactions involving the *central nervous system* are characterized by excitation and/or depression. Nervousness, dizziness, blurred vision, or tremors may occur followed by drowsiness, convulsions, unconsciousness, and possibly respiratory arrest. Since excitement may be transient or absent, the first manifestations may be drowsiness merging into unconsciousness and respiratory arrest.

Cardiovascular reactions are depressant. They may be the result of direct drug effect or more commonly in dental practice, the result of vasovagal reaction, particularly if the patient is in the sitting position. Failure to recognize premonitory signs such as sweating, feeling of faintness, changes in pulse or sensorium may result in progressive cerebral hypoxia and seizure or serious cardiovascular catastrophe. Management consists of placing the patient in the recumbent position and administration of oxygen. Vasoactive drugs such as ephedrine or methoxamine may be administered intravenously.

Allergic reactions are rare and may occur as a result of sensitivity to the local anesthetic and are characterized by cutaneous lesions of delayed onset or urticaria, edema and other manifestations of allergy. The detection of sensitivity by skin testing is of limited value. As with other local anesthetics, anaphylactoid reactions to CARBOCAINE have occurred rarely. The reaction may be abrupt and severe and is not usually dose related.

OVERDOSAGE

Treatment of a patient with toxic manifestations consists of assuring and maintaining a patent airway and supporting ventilation (respiration) as required. This usually will be sufficient in the management of most reactions. Should a convulsion persist despite ventilatory therapy, small increments of anticonvulsive agents may be given intravenously, such as benzodiazepine (e.g., diazepam) or ultrashort-acting barbiturates (e.g., thiopental or thiamylal) or short-acting barbiturate (e.g., pentobarbital or secobarbital). Cardiovascular depression may require circulatory assistance with intravenous fluids and/or vasopressor (e.g., ephedrine) as dictated by the clinical situation. Allergic reactions should be managed by conventional means.

IV and SC LD_{50}s in mice for CARBOCAINE hydrochloride 3% are 33 and 258 mg/kg respectively. The acute IV and SC LD_{50}s in mice for CARBOCAINE hydrochloride 2% with Neo-Cobefrin 1:20.000 are 30 and 184 mg/kg respectively.

DOSAGE AND ADMINISTRATION

As with all local anesthetics, the dose varies and depends upon the area to be anesthetized, the vascularity of the tissues, individual tolerance and the technique of anesthesia. The lowest dose needed to provide effective anesthesia should be administered. For specific techniques and procedures refer to standard dental manuals and textbooks.

For infiltration and block injections in the upper or lower jaw, the average dose of 1 cartridge will usually suffice.

Each cartridge contains 1.8 ml (36 mg of 2% or 54 mg of 3%). Five cartridges (180 mg of the 2% solution or 270 mg of the 3% solution) are usually adequate to effect anesthesia of the entire oral cavity. Whenever a larger dose seems to be necessary for an extensive procedure, the maximum dose should be calculated according to that patient's weight. A dose of up to 3 mg per pound of body weight may be administered. At any single dental sitting the total dose for all injected sites should not exceed 400 mg in adults.

The maximum pediatric dose should be *carefully calculated* and should not exceed 5 cartridges (180 mg of the 2% solution [67.5 lbs.] and 270 mg of the 3% solution [101.25 lbs.]). The maximum pediatric dose should be calculated as:

Maximum Dose for Children =

$$\frac{\text{Child's Weight (lbs.)}}{150} \times \text{Maximum Recommended Dose for Adults (400 mg)}$$

When using CARBOCAINE for infiltration or regional block anesthesia, injection should always be made slowly and with frequent aspiration.

Any unused portion of a cartridge should be discarded.

Parenteral drug products should be inspected visually for particulate matter and discoloration prior to administration, whenever solution and container permit.

DISINFECTION OF CARTRIDGES

As in the case of any cartridge, the diaphragm should be disinfected before needle puncture. The diaphragm should be thoroughly swabbed with either pure 91% isopropyl alcohol or 70% ethyl alcohol, USP just prior to use. Many commercially available alcohol solutions contain ingredients which are injurious to container components, and therefore, should not be used. Cartridges should not be immersed in any solution.

HOW SUPPLIED

Both formulas are available in 1.8 ml cartridges, containers of 50, to fit the Carpule® Aspirator.

The 2% solution should be stored at controlled room temperature, between 15° and 30° C (59° and 86° F).

2% solution	Code 0101	NDC 0961-0010-04
3% solution	Code 0201	NDC 0961-0020-04

Marketed by:
COOK-WAITE LABORATORIES, INC.
Mfg. by Sterling Drug Inc.
New York, N.Y. 10016
CARBOCAINE and Neo-Cobefrin
are the registered trademarks
of Sterling Drug Inc.

For full prescribing information on the medical use of CARBOCAINE, see Winthrop-Breon Laboratories product listing in this publication.

MARCAINE® hydrochloride 0.5% ℞
with epinephrine 1:200,000 (as bitartrate)
brand of bupivacaine and epinephrine injection, USP
THIS SOLUTION IS INTENDED FOR DENTAL USE

DESCRIPTION

Bupivacaine hydrochloride is 1-butyl-2′, 6′-pipecoloxylidide hydrochloride, a white crystalline powder that is freely soluble in 95 per cent ethanol, soluble in water, and slightly soluble in chloroform or acetone. It has the following structural formula:

$(CH_2)_3CH_3$ — N — CONH — CH_3, CH_3 · HCl

Epinephrine is (-)-3,4-Dihydroxy-α-[(methylamino)methyl] benzyl alcohol. It has the following structural formula:

HO, HO — C(OH)(H) — CH_2NHCH_3

MARCAINE is available in a sterile isotonic solution with epinephrine (as bitartrate) 1:200,000. Solutions of MARCAINE containing epinephrine may not be autoclaved.

MARCAINE is related chemically and pharmacologically to the aminoacyl local anesthetics. It is a homologue of mepivacaine and is chemically related to lidocaine. All three of these anesthetics contain an amide linkage between the aromatic nucleus and the amino or piperidine group. They differ in this respect from the procaine-type local anesthetics, which have an ester linkage.

CLINICAL PHARMACOLOGY

MARCAINE stabilizes the neuronal membrane and prevents the initiation and transmission of nerve impulses, thereby effecting local anesthesia.

The onset of action following dental injections is usually 2 to 10 minutes and anesthesia may last two or three times longer than lidocaine and mepivacaine for dental use, in many patients up to 7 hours. The duration of anesthetic effect is prolonged by the addition of epinephrine 1:200,000.

It has also been noted that there is a period of analgesia that persists after the return of sensation, during which time the need for strong analgesic is reduced.

After injection of MARCAINE for caudal, epidural or peripheral nerve block in man, peak levels of MARCAINE In the blood are reached in 30 to 45 minutes, followed by a decline to insignificant levels during the next three to six hours. Because of its amide structure, MARCAINE is not detoxified by plasma esterases but is detoxified, via conjugation with glucuronic acid, in the liver. When administered in recommended doses and concentrations, MARCAINE does not ordinarily produce irritation or tissue damage, and does not cause methemoglobinemia.

Systemic absorption of local anesthetics produces effects on the cardiovascular and central nervous systems (CNS). At blood concentrations achieved with normal therapeutic doses, changes in cardiac conduction, excitability, refractoriness, contractility, and peripheral vascular resistance are minimal. However, toxic blood concentrations depress cardiac conduction and excitability, which may lead to atrioventricular block, ventricular arrhythmias, and cardiac arrest, sometimes resulting in fatalities. In addition, myocardial contractility is depressed and peripheral vasodilation occurs, leading to decreased cardiac output and arterial blood pressure. Recent clinical reports and animal research suggest that these cardiovascular changes are more likely to occur after unintended intravascular injection of bupivacaine. Therefore, incremental dosing is necessary.

Following systemic absorption, local anesthetics can produce central nervous system stimulation, depression, or both. Apparent central stimulation is manifested as restlessness, tremors and shivering progressing to convulsions, followed by depression and coma progressing ultimately to respiratory arrest. However, the local anesthetics have a primary depressant effect on the medulla and on higher centers. The depressed stage may occur without a prior excited state.

INDICATIONS AND USAGE

MARCAINE is indicated for the production of local anesthesia for dental procedures by infiltration injection or nerve block in adults.

MARCAINE is not recommended for children.

CONTRAINDICATION

MARCAINE is contraindicated in patients with a known hypersensitivity to it or to any local anesthetic agent of the amide type or to other components of MARCAINE solutions.

WARNINGS

LOCAL ANESTHETICS SHOULD BE EMPLOYED ONLY BY CLINICIANS WHO ARE WELL VERSED IN DIAGNOSIS AND MANAGEMENT OF DOSE-RELATED TOXICITY AND OTHER ACUTE EMERGENCIES WHICH MIGHT ARISE FROM THE BLOCK TO BE EMPLOYED, AND THEN ONLY AFTER INSURING THE *IMMEDIATE* AVAILABILITY OF OXYGEN, OTHER RESUSCITATIVE DRUGS, CARDIOPULMONARY RESUSCITATIVE EQUIPMENT, AND THE PERSONNEL RESOURCES NEEDED FOR PROPER MANAGEMENT OF TOXIC REACTIONS AND RELATED EMERGENCIES. (See also ADVERSE REACTIONS and PRECAUTIONS.) DELAY IN PROPER MANAGEMENT OF DOSE-RELATED TOXICITY, UNDERVENTILATION FROM ANY CAUSE, AND/OR ALTERED SENSITIVITY MAY LEAD TO THE DEVELOPMENT OF ACIDOSIS, CARDIAC ARREST AND, POSSIBLY, DEATH.

Small doses of local anesthetics injected into the head and neck area, as small as nine to eighteen milligrams, may produce adverse reactions similar to systemic toxicity seen with unintentional intravascular injections of larger doses. Confusion, convulsions, respiratory depression, and/or respiratory arrest, cardiovascular stimulation or depression and cardiac arrest have been reported. Reactions resulting in fatalities have occurred on rare occasions. In a few cases,

Continued on next page

Cook-Waite—Cont.

resuscitation has been difficult or impossible despite apparently adequate preparation and appropriate management. These reactions may be due to intra-arterial injection of the local anesthetic with retrograde flow to the cerebral circulation. Patients receiving these blocks should have their circulation and respiration monitored and be constantly observed. Resuscitative equipment and personnel for treating adverse reactions should be immediately available. Dosage recommendations should not be exceeded (See DOSAGE AND ADMINISTRATION).

It is essential that aspiration for blood or cerebrospinal fluid (where applicable) be done prior to injecting any local anesthetic, both the original dose and all subsequent doses, to avoid intravascular injection. However, a negative aspiration does *not* ensure against an intravascular injection.

Reactions resulting in fatality have occurred on rare occasions with the use of local anesthetics, even in the absence of a history of hypersensitivity.

This solution which contains a vasoconstrictor should be used with extreme caution for patients whose medical history and physical evaluation suggest the existence of hypertension, arteriosclerotic heart disease, cerebral vascular insufficiency, heart block, thyrotoxicosis and diabetes, etc., as well as patients receiving drugs likely to produce alterations in blood pressure.

MARCAINE with epinephrine 1:200,000 or other vasopressors should not be used concomitantly with ergot-type oxytocic drugs, because a severe persistent hypertension may occur. Likewise, solutions of MARCAINE containing a vasoconstrictor, such as epinephrine, should be used with extreme caution in patients receiving monoamine oxidase inhibitors (MAOI) or antidepressants of the triptyline or imipramine types, because severe prolonged hypertension may result.

Until further experience is gained in children younger than 12 years, administration of MARCAINE in this age group is not recommended.

PRECAUTIONS

The safety and effectiveness of local anesthetics depend upon proper dosage, correct technique, adequate precautions, and readiness for emergencies.

The lowest dosage that gives effective anesthesia should be used in order to avoid high plasma levels and serious systemic side effects. Injection of repeated doses of MARCAINE may cause significant increase in blood levels with each additional dose, due to accumulation of the drug or its metabolites or due to slow metabolic degradation. Tolerance varies with the status of the patient. Debilitated, elderly patients and acutely ill patients should be given reduced doses commensurate with age and physical condition.

Because of the long duration of anesthesia, when MARCAINE 0.5% with epinephrine is used for dental injections, patients should be cautioned about the possibility of inadvertent trauma to tongue, lips, and buccal mucosa and advised not to chew solid foods or test the anesthetized area by biting or probing.

Changes in sensorium such as excitation, disorientation, drowsiness, may be early indications of a high blood level of the drug and may occur following inadvertent intravascular administration or rapid absorption of MARCAINE.

Solutions containing a vasoconstrictor should be used cautiously in areas with limited blood supply, in the presence of diseases that may adversely affect the patient's cardiovascular system, or in patients with peripheral vascular disease.

Caution is advised in administration of repeat doses of MARCAINE to patients with severe liver disease.

Local anesthetic procedures should be used with caution when there is inflammation and/or sepsis in the region of the proposed injection.

Drug Interactions: See WARNINGS concerning solutions containing a vasoconstrictor.

If sedatives are employed to reduce patient apprehension, use reduced doses, since local anesthetic agents, like sedatives, are central nervous system depressants which in combination may have an additive effect.

MARCAINE should be used cautiously in persons with known drug allergies or sensitivities, particularly to the amide-type local anesthetics.

Serious dose-related cardiac arrhythmias may occur if preparations containing a vasoconstrictor such as epinephrine are employed in patients during or following the administration of chloroform, halothane, cyclopropane, trichloroethylene, or other related agents. In deciding whether to use these products concurrently in the same patient, the combined action of both agents upon the myocardium, the concentration and volume of vasoconstrictor used, and the time since injection, when applicable, should be taken into account.

INFORMATION FOR PATIENTS: When appropriate, the dentist should discuss information including adverse reactions in the package insert for MARCAINE.

Clinically Significant Drug Interactions: The administration of local anesthetic solutions containing epinephrine or norepinephrine to patients receiving monoamine oxidase inhibitors or tricyclic antidepressants may produce severe, prolonged hypertension. Concurrent use of these agents should generally be avoided. In situations when concurrent therapy is necessary, careful patient monitoring is essential. Concurrent administration of vasopressor drugs and of ergot-type oxytocic drugs may cause severe, persistent hypertension or cerebrovascular accidents.

Phenothiazines and butyrophenones may reduce or reverse the pressor effect of epinephrine.

Carcinogenesis, Mutagenesis, Impairment of Fertility: Long-term studies in animals of most local anesthetics including bupivacaine to evaluate the carcinogenic potential have not been conducted. Mutagenic potential or the effect on fertility has not been determined. There is no evidence from human data that MARCAINE may be carcinogenic or mutagenic or that it impairs fertility.

Pregnancy Category C: Decreased pup survival in rats and an embryocidal effect in rabbits have been observed when bupivacaine hydrochloride was administered to these species in doses comparable to nine and five times respectively the maximum recommended daily human dose (400 mg). There are no adequate and well-controlled studies in pregnant women of the effect of bupivacaine on the developing fetus. Bupivacaine hydrochloride should be used during pregnancy only if the potential benefit justifies the potential risk to the fetus. This does not exclude the use of MARCAINE at term for obstetrical anesthesia or analgesia.

Nursing Mothers: It is not known whether local anesthetic drugs are excreted in human milk. Because many drugs are excreted in human milk, caution should be exercised when local anesthetics are administered to a nursing woman.

Pediatric Use: Until further experience is gained in children younger than 12 years, administration of MARCAINE in this age group is not recommended.

ADVERSE REACTIONS

Reactions to MARCAINE are characteristic of those associated with other amide-type local anesthetics. A major cause of adverse reactions to this group of drugs is excessive plasma levels, which may be due to overdosage, inadvertent intravascular injection, or slow metabolic degradation.

Excessive plasma levels of the amide-type local anesthetics cause systemic reactions involving the central nervous system and the cardiovascular system. The *central nervous system effects* are characterized by excitation or depression. The first manifestation may be nervousness, dizziness, blurred vision, or tremors, followed by drowsiness, convulsions, unconsciousness, and possibly respiratory arrest. Since excitement may be transient or absent, the first manifestation may be drowsiness, sometimes merging into unconsciousness and respiratory arrest. Other central nervous system effects may be nausea, vomiting, chills, constriction of the pupils, or tinnitus. The *cardiovascular manifestations* of excessive plasma levels may include depression of the myocardium, blood pressure changes (usually hypotension), and cardiac arrest. *Allergic reactions,* which may be due to hypersensitivity, idiosyncrasy, or diminished tolerance, are characterized by cutaneous lesions (e.g., urticaria), edema, and other manifestations of allergy. Detection of sensitivity by skin testing is of doubtful value.

Treatment of Reactions: Toxic effects of local anesthetics require symptomatic treatment: there is no specific cure. The dentist should be prepared to maintain an airway and to support ventilation with oxygen and assisted or controlled respiration as required. Supportive treatment of the cardiovascular system includes intravenous fluids and, when appropriate, vasopressors (preferably those that stimulate the myocardium). Convulsions may be controlled with oxygen and intravenous administration, in small increments, of a barbiturate, as follows: preferably, an ultrashort-acting barbiturate such as thiopental or thiamylal; if this is not available, a short-acting barbiturate (e.g. secobarbital or pentobarbital) or diazepam. Intravenous barbiturates or anticonvulsant agents should only be administered by those familiar with their use.

DOSAGE AND ADMINISTRATION

As with all local anesthetics, the dosage varies and depends upon the area to be anesthetized, the vascularity of the tissues, the number of neuronal segments to be blocked, individual tolerance, and the technique of anesthesia. The lowest dosage needed to provide effective anesthesia should be administered. For specific techniques and procedures refer to standard textbooks.

The 0.5% concentration wth epinephrine is recommended for infiltration and block injection in the maxillary and mandibular area when a longer duration of local anesthetic action is desired, such as for oral surgical procedures generally associated with significant postoperative pain. The average dose of 1.8 ml (9 mg) per injection site will usually suffice; an occasional second dose of 1.8 ml (9 mg) may be used if necessary to produce adequate anesthesia after making allowance for 2 to 10 minutes onset time (see Clinical Pharmacology). The lowest effective dose should be employed and time should be allowed between injections; it is recommended that the total dose for all injection sites, *spread out* over a single dental sitting, should not ordinarily exceed 90 mg for a healthy adult patient (ten 1.8 ml injections of 0.5% MARCAINE with epinephrine). Injections should be made slowly and with frequent aspirations. Until further experience is gained, MARCAINE in dentistry is not recommended for children younger than 12 years.

Parenteral drug products should be inspected visually for particulate matter and discoloration prior to administration, whenever solution and container permit.

HOW SUPPLIED

Store at controlled room temperature, between 15° and 30°C (59° and 86°F).

0.5% MARCAINE hydrochloride with epinephrine 1:200,000 (as bitartrate)—Sterile isotonic solutions containing sodium chloride. Each 1 ml contains 5 mg bupivacaine hydrochloride and 0.0091 mg epinephrine bitartrate, with 0.5 mg sodium metabisulfite, 0.001 ml monothioglycerol, and 2 mg ascorbic acid as antioxidants, 0.0017 ml 60% sodium lactate buffer, and 0.1 mg edetate calcium disodium as stabilizer. The pH of these solutions is adjusted with sodium hydroxide or hydrochloric acid. Solutions of MARCAINE that contain epinephrine should not be autoclaved and should be protected from light. Do not use if solution is discolored or contains a precipitate.

This solution is available in 1.8 ml cartridges, containers of 50, to fit the Carpule® Aspirator.

Code 6301 **NDC** 0961-1230-50

Marketed by
Cook-Waite Laboratories, Inc.
Mfg. by Sterling Drug Inc.
New York, NY 10016

MARCAINE is the registered trademark of Sterling Drug Inc.

For full prescribing information on the medical use of Marcaine, see Winthrop-Breon Laboratories product listing in this publication.

CooperVision Ophthalmic Products

SAN JOSE, CA 95134
(Representing CooperVision Pharmaceuticals Inc., San Germán, Puerto Rico, and CooperVision Optics Division, CooperVision Inc.)

OPHTHALMIC PRODUCTS

For information on CooperVision Ophthalmic Products prescription and OTC ophthalmic products, consult the Physicians' Desk Reference For Ophthalmology. For literature, service items or sample material, contact your CooperVision Ophthalmic Products representative. See a complete listing of products in the Manufacturers' Index section of this book.

Cutter Biological

Div. Miles Laboratories, Inc.
2200 POWELL STREET
EMERYVILLE, CA 94662

GAMASTAN® ℞
[găm 'as-tan "]
Immune Globulin (Human) U.S.P.

2 ml., 10 ml. vials.

IMMUNE GLOBULIN INTRAVENOUS (HUMAN) 5% (in 10% Maltose), pH 4.25 ℞
GAMIMUNE® N
[gam 'i-mūne " n]

DESCRIPTION

Immune Globulin Intravenous (Human) 5% (in 10% Maltose), pH 4.25—Gamimune® N is a sterile 4.5–5.5% solution of human protein stabilized with 9–11% maltose; it contains no preservative. Each milliliter (mL) contains approximately 50 mg of protein, not less than 98% of which has the electrophoretic mobility of gamma globulin. Not less than 90% of the gamma globulin is monomer. Also present are traces of IgA and of IgM. The distribution of IgG subclasses is similar to that found in normal serum. Gamimune N has a buffer capacity of 16.5 mEq/L of solution (~0.3 mEq/g of protein).

The calculated osmolality is 309 milliosmoles per kilogram of solvent (water) and the calculated osmolarity is 278 milliosmoles per liter of solution.
The product is made by cold ethanol fractionation of large pools of human plasma; each individual unit of plasma used in the pool has been tested and found nonreactive for hepatitis B surface antigen (HBsAg) by an FDA approved method. The immunoglobulin is isolated from Cohn Effluent III by diafiltration and ultrafiltration. The protein has not been chemically modified other than in the adjustment of the pH of the solution to 4.0–4.5.[1] Isotonicity is achieved by the addition of maltose. The product is intended for intravenous administration.

CLINICAL PHARMACOLOGY

Gamimune N supplies a broad spectrum of opsonic and neutralizing igG antibodies for the prevention or attenuation of a wide variety of infectious diseases. As Gamimune N is administered intravenously, essentially 100% of the infused IgG antibodies are immediately available in the recipient's circulation.[2] A relatively rapid fall in serum IgG level in the first week post-infusion is to be expected; this decrease averages 40% of the peak level achieved immediately post-infusion and is mainly due to the equilibration of IgG between the plasma and the extravascular space.[2,10,11,14] The *in vivo* half-life of Gamimune N equals or exceeds the three week half-life reported for IgG in the literature, but individual patient variation in half-life has been observed.[2] Thus, this variable as well as the amount of immune globulin administered per dose is important in determining the frequency of administration of the drug for each individual patient.
The intravenous administration of solutions of maltose has been studied by several investigators.[4–8] Healthy subjects tolerated the infusions well, and no adverse effects were observed at a rate of 0.25 g maltose/kg body weight per hour.[5] In safety studies conducted by Cutter Biological, infusions of 10% maltose administered at 0.27–0.62 g maltose/kg per hour[6] to normal subjects produced either mild side effects (e.g., headache) or no adverse reaction.[2] Following intravenous administrations of maltose, maltose was detected in the peripheral blood; there was a dose-dependent excretion of maltose and glucose in the urine and a mild diuretic effect.[2] These alterations were well tolerated without significant adverse effects.[2] The highest recommended infusion rate, 0.08 mL/kg body weight per minute (see DOSAGE AND ADMINISTRATION), is equivalent to 0.48 g maltose/kg body weight per hour.
The buffer capacity of Immune Globulin Intravenous (Human) 5% (in 10% Maltose), pH 4.25—Gamimune® N is 16.5 mEq/L (~0.3 mEq/g protein); a dose of 150–400 mg/kg (3–8 mL/kg) body weight therefore represents an acid load of 0.0495-0.1320 mEq/kg body weight. The total buffering capacity of whole blood in a normal individual is 45–50 mEq/L of blood, or 3.6 mEq/kg body weight.[9] Thus, the acid load delivered in the largest dose of Gamimune N would be neutralized by the buffering capacity of whole blood alone, even if the dose were infused instantaneously. (An infusion usually lasts several hours.)
In Phase I human studies, no change in arterial blood pH measurements was detected following the intravenous administration of Gamimune N at a dose of 150 mg/kg body weight;[2] following a dose of 400 mg/kg body weight in 37 patients, there were no clinically important differences in mean venous pH or bicarbonate measurements in patients who received Gamimune N compared with those who received a chemically modified intravenous immunoglobulin preparation with a pH of 6.8.[2]
In patients with limited or compromised acid-base compensatory mechanisms, consideration should be given to the effect of the additional acid load Gamimune N might present.

INDICATIONS AND USAGE

Immunodeficiency Syndromes: Gamimune N is indicated for the maintenance treatment of patients who are unable to produce sufficient amounts of IgG antibodies. Usage of Gamimune N may be preferred to that of intramuscular immunoglobulin preparations, especially in patients who require an immediate increase in intravascular immunoglobulin levels, in patients with a small muscle mass, and in patients with bleeding tendencies in whom intramuscular injections are contraindicated. It may be used in disease states such as congenital agammaglobulinemia (e.g., X-linked agammaglobulinemia), common variable hypogammaglobulinemia, X-linked immunodeficiency with hyper IgM and in severe combined immunodeficiency.[3,12–15]
Idiopathic Thrombocytopenic Purpura (ITP): Investigations in both children and adults have shown that Gamimune N may initiate a therapeutic increase in the platelet count.[2] In clinical studies of Gamimune N, five of six (83.3%) children and 10 of 16 (62.5%) adults with acute or chronic ITP demonstrated clinically significant increments in the platelet count during or following an initial treatment course with Gamimune N at a dose of 400 mg/kg body weight daily for five days. The duration of the platelet rise following treatment of ITP with Gamimune N was variable, ranging from several days up to 12 months or more. Several ITP patients demonstrated continuing responsiveness over many months to intermittent Gamimune N 400 mg/kg body weight single dose maintenance courses. Two of three children with acute ITP treated with Gamimune N rapidly went into complete remission. However, childhood ITP may respond spontaneously without treatment. Four patients with refractory ITP were able to undergo major surgical procedures as a result of the rapid rise in platelet count associated with Gamimune N treatment.
In addition, one patient with severe thrombocytopenia due to post-transfusion purpura (PL^{A1} alloimmune antibody with platelet anti PL^{A1} specificity) also responded to treatment with Gammimune N, at a dose of 400 mg/kg body weight daily for 5 days; there was a rapid rise in the platelet count commencing on the third day of treatment.[2]
It is presently not possible to predict which patients with ITP will respond to therapy, although the increase in platelet counts in children seems to be better than that of adults. In clinical situations in which a rapid rise in platelet count is needed to control bleeding or to allow a patient with ITP to undergo surgery, administration of Immune Globulin Intravenous (Human) 5% (in 10% Maltose), pH 4.25—Gamimune® N should be considered; in patients in whom a response is achieved, the rise of platelets is generally rapid (within 1–5 days), transient (most often lasting from several days to several weeks) and should not be considered curative. In some patients who relapse, a maintenance dose of Gamimune N administered every several weeks may be of benefit once the platelet count decreases to clinically hazardous levels (see DOSAGE AND ADMINISTRATION).

CONTRAINDICATIONS

Gamimune N is contraindicated in individuals who are known to have had an anaphylactic or severe systemic response to Immune Globulin (Human). Individuals with selective IgA deficiencies who have known antibody agains IgA (anti-IgA antibody) should not receive Gamimune N since these patients may experience severe reactions to the IgA which may be present.[13]

WARNINGS

Gamimune N should be administered only intravenously as the intramuscular and subcutaneous routes have not been evaluated.
Gamimune N may, on rare occasions, cause a precipitous fall in blood pressure and a clinical picture of anaphylaxis, even when the patient is not known to be sensitive to immune globulin preparations. These reactions may be related to the rate of infusion. Accordingly, the infusion rate given under DOSAGE AND ADMINISTRATION should be closely followed at least until the physician has had sufficient experience with a given patient. The patient's vital signs should be monitored continuously and careful observation made for any symptoms throughout the entire infusion. Epinephrine should be available for the treatment of an acute anaphylactic reaction.

PRECAUTIONS

General: Any vial that has been entered should be used promptly. Partially used vials should be discarded. Do not use if turbid. Solution which has been frozen should not be used.
Drug Interactions: If dilution is required, Gamimune N may be diluted with 5% dextrose in water (D5/W). No other drug interactions or compatibilities have been evaluated. It is recommended that infusion of Gamimune N be given by a separate line, by itself, without mixing with other intravenous fluids or medications the patient might be receiving.
Pregnancy Category C: Animal reproduction studies have not been conducted with Gamimune N. It is not known whether Gamimune N can cause fetal harm when administered to a pregnant woman or can affect reproduction capacity. Gamimune N should be given to a pregnant woman only if clearly needed.

ADVERSE REACTIONS

In a study of 37 patients with immunodeficiency syndromes receiving Gamimune N at a monthly dose of 400 mg/kg body weight, reactions were seen in 5.2% of the infusions of Gamimune N. Symptoms reported with Gamimune N included malaise, a feeling of faintness, fever, chills, headache, nausea, vomiting, chest tightness, dyspnea and chest, back or hip pain. In addition, mild erythema following infiltration of Immune Globulin Intravenous (Human) 5% (in 10% Maltose), pH 4.25—Gamimune® N at the infusion site was reported in some cases.
In further studies of Gamimune N in the treatment of both adult and pediatric patients with ITP, systemic reactions were noted in only 4 of 154 (2.6%) infusions, and all but one occurred at rates of infusion greater than 0.04 mL/kg body weight per minute. The symptoms reported included chest tightness, a sense of tachycardia (pulse was 84 beats per minute), and a burning sensation in the head; these symptoms were all mild and transient. Erythema, pain, phlebitis, or exzematous reactions at the infusion site were also reported following infusion of Gamimune N to adult ITP patients. These reactions occurred in 11.6% of the infusions of Gamimune N and in 43.8% of the adult ITP population. No pediatric patients experienced localized reactions at the infusion site.
In the studies undertaken to date, other types of reactions have not been reported with Gamimune N. It may be, however, that adverse effects will be similar to those previously reported with intravenous and intramuscular immunoglobulin administration. Potential reactions, therefore, may also include anxiety, flushing, wheezing, abdominal cramps, myalgias, arthralgia, and dizziness; rash has been reported only rarely. Reactions to intravenous immunoglobulin tend to be related to the rate of infusion.
True anaphylactic reactions to Gamimune N may occur in recipients with documented prior histories of severe allergic reactions to Intramuscular immunoglobulin, but some patients may tolerate cuatiously administered intravenous immunoglobulin without adverse effects.[2,16] Very rarely an anaphylactoid reaction may occur in patients with no prior history of severe allergic reactions to either intramuscular or intravenous immunoglobulin.[2]

Dosage and Administration:

Immunodeficiency Syndromes: The usual dosage of Gamimune N for prophylaxis in immunodeficiency syndromes is 100–200 mg/kg (2–4 mL/kg) of body weight administered approximately once a month by intravenous infusion. If the clinical response is inadequate, or the level of IgG achieved in the circulation response is felt to be insufficient, the dosage may be given more frequently or increased as high as 400 mg/kg (8 mL/kg) body weight.
Idiopathic Thrombocytopenic Purpura: An increase in platelet count has been observed in children and some adults with acute or chronic ITP receiving Gamimune N, 400 mg/kg body weight daily for five days. A response usually occurs within several days and is maintained for a variable period of time. In general a response is seen less often in adults than in children. In patients who have shown a response, a maintenance dose of Gamimune N of 400 mg/kg body weight administered as a single dose every several weeks may be of benefit once the platelet count decreases to clinically hazardous levels.
Investigations indicate that Gamimune N is well-tolerated and less likely to produce side effects when infused at the indicated rate. It is recommended that Gamimune N be infused by itself at a rate of 0.01 to 0.02 mL/kg body weight per minute for 30 minutes; if well tolerated, the rate may be gradually increased to a maximun of 0.08 mL/kg body weight per minute. If side effects occur, the rate may be reduced or the infusion interrupted until symptoms subside. The infusion may then be resumed at the rate which is comfortable for the patient.
Parenteral drug products should be inspected visually for particulate matter and discoloration prior to administration, whenever solution and container permit.

HOW SUPPLIED

Immune Globulin Intravenous (Human) 5% (In 10% Maltose), pH 4.25—Gamimune® is supplied in 10, 50, and 100 mL single dose vials. The 10 mL vial contains 0.5 g protein, the 50 mL vial contains 2.5 g protein, and the 100 mL vial contains 5.0 g protein.

STORAGE

Store at 2–8° C (35–46° F). Do not freeze. Do not use after expiration date.

CAUTION

U.S. federal law prohibits dispensing without a prescription.
Limited Warranty: A number of factors beyond our control could reduce the efficacy of this product or even result in an ill effect following its use. These include improper storage and handling of the product after it leaves our hands, diagnosis, dosage, method of amdinistration, and biological differences in individual patients. Because of these factors, it is important that this product be stored properly and that the directions be followed carefully during use.
The foregoing statement is made in lieu of any other warranty, express or implied, including any warranty of merchantability or fitness. Representatives of the Company are not authorized to vary the terms of this warranty or the contents of any printed labeling for this product except by printed notice from the Company's Berkeley office. The prescriber and user of this product must accept the terms hereof.

REFERENCES

1. Tenold RA, Inventor; Cutter Laboratories, assignee. Intravenously injectable immune serum globulin. U.S. Patent 4,396,608 August 2, 1983.
2. Data on file at Cutter Biological.
3. Ochs HD, Buckley RH, Pirofsky B, *et al:* Safety and patient acceptability of intravenous immune globulin in 10% maltose. *Lancet* 2(8205):1158–9, 1980.

Continued on next page

Cutter—Cont.

4. Berg G. Matzkies F: Wirkung von Maltose nach Intravenoser Dauerinfusion auf den Stoffwechsel. *Z Ernahrungswiss* 15:255-62, 1976.
5. Forster H. Hoos I, Boecker S: Versuche mit Probanded zur parenteralen Verwertung von Maltose. *Z Ernahrungswiss* 15(3):284-93, 1976.
6. Finke C. Reinauer H: Utilization of maltose and oligosaccharides after intravenous infusion in man. *Nutr Metab* 21(Suppl 1):115/7, 1977.
7. Young EA, Drumond A, Cioletti L, *et al:* Metabolism of continuously infused intravenous maltose. *Clin Res* 25(3):543A, 1977.
8. Soroff HS, Hansen LM, Sasvary D, *et al:* Clinical pharmacology and metabolism of maltose in normal human volunteers. *Clin Res* 26(3):286A, 1978.
9. Guyton AC: *Textbook of Medical Physiology,* 5th ed. Philadelphia, W.B. Saunders Company, 1976, pp 499-500.
10. Pirofsky B, Campbell SM, Montanaro A: Individual patient variation in the kinetics of intravenous immunoglobulin administration. *J Clin Immunol* 2 (2):7S-14S, 1982.
11. Pirofsky B: Intravenous immune globulin therapy in hypogammaglobulinemia. *Amer J Med* 76 (3A):53-60, 1984.
12. Nolte MT, Pirofsky B, Gerritz GA, *et al:* Intravenous immunoglobulin therapy for antibody deficiency. *Clin Exp Immunol* 336:237-43, 1979.
13. Buckley RH: Immunoglobulin replacement therapy: indications and contraindications for use and variable IgG levels achieved. In: Alving BM (ed.): *Immunoglobulins: characteristics and uses of intravenous preparations.* Washington,D.C., U.S. Government Printing Office (1980), pp 3-8.
14. Pirofsky B, Anderson CJ, Bardana EJ Jr.: Therapeutic and deterimental effects of intravenous immunoglobulin therapy. In: Alving BM (ed.): *Immunoglobulins: characteristics and uses of intravenous prepations.* Washington, D.C., U.S. Government Printing Office (1980), pp 15-22.
15. Ochs HD: Intravenous immunoglobulin therapy of patients with primary immunodeficiency syndromes: efficacy and safety of a new modified immune globulin preparation. In: Alving BM (ed.): *Immunoglobulins: characteristics and uses of intravenous preparations.* Washington, D.C., U.S. Government Printing Office (1980), pp 9-14.
16. Peerless AG, Stiehm ER: Intravenous gammaglobulin for reaction to intramuscular preparation. *Lancet* 2(8347):461, 1983.

14-7640-001
(Issued March 1986)

HYPERAB® ℞
[*hī'per-ab"*]
(Rabies Immune Globulin—Human)
2 ml. (300 IU) pediatric vial
10 ml. (1500 IU) adult vial

HYPERHEP® ℞
[*hī'per-hep"*]
(Hepatitis B Immune Globulin—Human)
1 ml., 5 ml. vials

HYPER-TET® ℞
[*hī'per-tet"*]
(Tetanus Immune Globulin—Human U.S.P.)
250 units vial or prefilled disposable syringe

HypRho®-D Mini-Dose ℞
[*hī"prō-d'*]
Rh_o(D) Immune Globulin (Human)

DESCRIPTION
Rh_o(D) Immune Globulin (Human)—HypRho®-D Mini-Dose—is a sterile solution of immune globulin containing antibodies to Rh_o(D) which is for intramuscular injection only. It is prepared from human venous plasma collected from carefully screened donors. It contains 15–18% protein stabilized with 0.21–0.32 M glycine and preserved with 80–120 μg/mL thimerosal (a mercury derivative), as measured by mercury assay. The pH is adjusted with sodium carbonate.
One dose of HypRho-D Mini-Dose contains not less than one-sixth the quantity of Rh_o(D) antibody contained in one standard dose of Rh_o(D) Immune Globulin (Human), USP and it will suppress the immunizing potential of 2.5 mL of Rh_o(D) positive packed red blood cells or the equivalent of whole blood (5 mL). The quantity of Rh_o(D) antibody in HypRho-D Mini-Dose is not less than one-sixth of that contained in 1 mL of the U.S. Food and Drug Administration Reference Rh_o(D) Immune Globulin (Human).
Each individual unit of plasma used in the manufacturing of this product has been tested and found nonreactive for hepatitis B surface antigen (HBsAg) by an FDA approved method. No instances of transmission of hepatitis have been reported from the use of human immune globulin prepared by the fractionation methods employed at Cutter (Biological) Laboratories.

CLINICAL PHARMACOLOGY
Rh sensitization may occur in nonsensitized Rh_o(D) negative women following transplacental hemorrhage resulting from spontaneous or induced abortions.[1–2] The risk of sensitization is higher in women undergoing induced abortions than in those aborting spontaneously.[1–3]
HypRho-D Mini-Dose is used to prevent the formation of anti-Rh_o(D) antibody in Rh_o(D) negative women who are exposed to the Rh_o(D) antigen at the time of spontaneous or induced abortion (up to 12 weeks gestation).[3–5] HypRho-D Mini-Dose suppresses the stimulation of active immunity by Rh_o(D) positive fetal erythrocytes that may enter the maternal circulation at the time of termination of the pregnancy.
The amount of anti-Rh_o(D) in HypRho-D Mini-Dose has been shown to effectively prevent maternal isosensitization to the Rh_o(D) antigens following spontaneous or induced abortion occurring up to the 12th week of gestation.[6–8] After the 12th week of gestation, a standard dose of Rh_o(D) Immune Globulin (Human), USP—HypRho®-D is indicated.

INDICATIONS AND USAGE
Rh_o(D) Immune Globulin (Human)—HypRho®-D Mini-Dose is recommended to prevent the isoimmunization of Rh_o(D) negative women at the time of spontaneous or induced abortion of up to 12 weeks gestation provided the following criteria are met:
1. The mother must be Rh_o(D) negative and must not already be sensitized to the Rh_o(D) antigen.
2. The father is not known to be Rh_o(D) negative.
3. Gestation is not more than 12 weeks at termination.

Note: Rh_o(D) Immune Globulin (Human) prophylaxis is not indicated if the fetus or father can be determined to be Rh negative. If the Rh status of the fetus is unknown, the fetus must be assumed to be Rh_o(D) positive, and HypRho-D Mini-Dose should be administered to the mother.
FOR ABORTIONS OR MISCARRIAGES OCCURRING AFTER 12 WEEKS GESTATION, A STANDARD DOSE OF RH_O(D) IMMUNE GLOBULIN (HUMAN), USP IS INDICATED.
HypRho-D Mini-Dose should be administered within three hours or as soon as possible after spontaneous passage or surgical removal of the products of conception. However, if HypRho-D Mini-Dose is not given within this time period, consideration should still be given to its administration since clinical studies in male volunteers have demonstrated the effectiveness of Rh_o(D) Immune Globulin (Human), USP in preventing isoimmunization as long as 72 hours after infusion of Rh_o(D) positive red cells.[9]

CONTRAINDICATIONS
None known.

WARNINGS
NEVER ADMINISTER HYPRHO-D MINI-DOSE INTRAVENOUSLY. INJECT ONLY INTRAMUSCULARLY. ADMINISTER ONLY TO WOMEN POST-ABORTION OR POST-MISCARRIAGE OF UP TO 12 WEEKS GESTATION.
HypRho-D Mini-Dose should be given with caution to patients with a history of prior systemic allergic reactions following the administration of human immune globulin preparations or in patients who are known to have had an allergic response to thimerosal.
The attending physician who wishes to administer HypRho-D Mini-Dose to persons with isolated immunoglobulin A (IgA) deficiency must weigh the benefits of immunization against the potential risks of hypersensitivity reactions. Such persons have increased potential for developing antibodies to IgA and could have anaphylactic reactions to subsequent administration of blood products that contain IgA.
As with all preparations administered by the intramuscular route, bleeding complications may be encountered in patients with thrombocytopenia or other bleeding disorders.

PRECAUTIONS
General
Although systemic reactions to immunoglobulin preparations are rare, epinephrine should be available for treatment of acute anaphylactic symptoms.
Drug Interactions
Other antibodies in the Rh_o(D) Immune Globulin (Human) —HypRho®-D Mini-Dose preparation may interfere with the response to live vaccines such as measles, mumps, polio or rubella. Therefore, immunization with live vaccines should not be given within three months after HypRho-D Mini-Dose administration.
Pregnancy Category C
Animal reproduction studies have not been conducted with HypRho-D Mini-Dose. It is also not known whether HypRho-D Mini-Dose can cause fetal harm when administered to a pregnant woman or can affect reproduction capacity.
It should be again noted, however, that HypRho-D Mini-Dose is **not** indicated for use during pregnancy and it should be administered only post-abortion or post-miscarriage.

ADVERSE REACTIONS
Reactions to HypRho-D Mini-Dose are infrequent in Rh_o(D) negative individuals and consist primarily of slight soreness at the site of injection and slight temperature elevation. While sensitization to repeated injections of human globulin is extremely rare, it has occurred.

DOSAGE AND ADMINISTRATION
One syringe of HypRho-D Mini-Dose provides sufficient antibody to prevent Rh sensitization to 2.5 mL Rh_o(D) positive packed red cells or the equivalent (5 mL) of whole blood. This dose is sufficient to provide protection against maternal Rh sensitization for women undergoing spontaneous or induced abortion of up to 12 weeks gestation.
HypRho-D Mini-Dose should be administered within three hours or as soon as possible following spontaneous or induced abortion. If prompt administration is not possible, HypRho-D Mini-Dose should be given within 72 hours following termination of the pregnancy.
Parenteral drug products should be inspected visually for particulate matter and discoloration prior to administration, whenever solution and container permit.

HOW SUPPLIED
Each HypRho-D Mini-Dose package contains:
Ten single dose prefilled syringes of HypRho-D Mini-Dose, a package insert giving directions for use, and patient identification cards.

STORAGE
Store at 2°–8°C (35°–46°F). Do not freeze.

CAUTION
U.S. Federal law prohibits dispensing without prescription.

LIMITED WARRANTY
A number of factors beyond our control could reduce the efficacy of this product or even result in an ill effect following its use. These include improper storage and handling of the product after it leaves our hands, diagnosis, dosage, method of administration, and biological differences in individual patients. Because of these factors, it is important that this product be stored properly and that the directions be followed carefully during use.
The foregoing statement is made in lieu of any other warranty, express or implied, including any warranty of merchantability or fitness. Representatives of the Company are not authorized to vary the terms of this warranty or the contents of any printed labeling for this product except by printed notice from the Company's Berkeley office. The prescriber and user of this product must accept the terms hereof.

REFERENCES
1. Queenan JT, Shah S, Kubarych SF, *et al:* Role of induced abortion in rhesus immunisation. *Lancet* 1(7704): 815–7, 1971.
2. Goldman JA, Eckerling B: Prevention of Rh immunization after abortion with anti-Rh_o(D)-immunoglobulin. *Obstet Gynecol* 40(3):366–70, 1972.
3. The selective use of Rh_o(D) immune globulin (RhIG). *ACOG Tech Bull* 61, 1981.
4. Prevention of Rh sensitization. *WHO Tech Rep Ser* 468, 1971.
5. Recommendation of the Public Health Service Advisory Committee on Immunization Practices: Rh immune globulin. *Morbid Mortal Wkly Rep* 21(15):126–7, 1972.
6. Stewart FH, Burnhill MS, Bozorgi N: Reduced dose of Rh immunoglobulin following first trimester pregnancy termination. *Obstet Gynecol* 51(3):318–22, 1978.
7. McMaster conference on prevention of Rh immunization, 28-30 September, 1977. *Vox Sang* 36(1):50–64, 1979.
8. Simonovits I: Efficiency of anti-D IgG prevention after induced abortion. *Vox Sang* 26(4):361–7, 1974.
9. Freda VJ, Gorman JG, Pollack W: Prevention of Rh-hemolytic disease with Rh-immune globulin. *Am J Obstet Gynecol* 128(4):456–60, 1977.

14-7621-052
(Rev Oct 1985)

HypRho®-D ℞

[hī″prō-d′]
Rh$_o$(D) Immune Globulin (Human)

DESCRIPTION

Rh$_o$(D) Immune Globulin (Human)—HypRho®-D is a sterile solution of immune globulin containing antibodies to Rh$_o$(D) which is intended for intramuscular injection. It contains 15–18% protein stabilized with 0.21–0.32 M glycine and is preserved with 80–120 μg/mL thimerosal (a mercury derivative), as measured by mercury assay. The pH is adjusted with sodium carbonate. The potency is equal to or greater than that of the U.S. Food and Drug Administration Reference Rh$_o$(D) Immune Globulin (Human). Each single dose vial or syringe contains sufficient anti-RH$_o$(D) (approximately 300 μg*) to effectively suppress the immunizing potential of 15 mL of Rh$_o$(D) positive red blood cells.[2–4]

This product has been prepared from large pools of human venous plasma. Each individual unit of plasma has been tested and found nonreactive for hepatitis B surface antigen (HBsAg) using an FDA approved method. No instances of transmission of hepatitis have been reported from the use of human immune globulin prepared by the fractionation methods employed at Cutter Biological.

*A full dose of Rh$_o$(D) Immune Globulin (Human) has traditionally been referred to as a "300 μg" dose and this usage is employed here for convenience in terminology. **It should not be construed as the actual anti-D content.** Each full dose of RH$_o$(D) Immune Globulin (Human) must contain at least as much anti-D as 1mL of the U.S. Reference Rh$_o$(D) Immune Globulin (Human). Studies performed at the FDA have shown that the U.S. Reference contains 820 international units (IU) of anti-D per mL. When the conversion factor determined for the International (WHO) Reference Preparation[1] is used, 820 IU per mL is equivalent to 164 μg per mL of anti-D.

CLINICAL PHARMACOLOGY

HypRho-D is used to prevent isoimmunization in the Rh$_o$(D) negative individual exposed to Rh$_o$(D) positive blood as the result of a fetomaternal hemorrhage occurring during a delivery of an Rh$_o$(D) positive infant, abortion (either spontaneous or induced), or following amniocentesis or abdominal trauma. Similarly, immunization resulting in the production of anti-Rh$_o$(D) following transfusion of Rh positive red cells to an Rh$_o$(D) negative recipient may be prevented by administering Rh$_o$(D) Immune Globulin (Human).[5,6]

Rh hemolytic disease of the newborn is the result of the active immunization of an Rh$_o$(D) negative mother by Rh$_o$(D) positive red cells entering the maternal circulation during a previous delivery, abortion, amniocentesis, abdominal trauma, or as a result of red cell transfusion.[7,8] HypRho-D acts by suppressing the immune response of Rh$_o$(D) negative individuals to Rh$_o$(D) positive red blood cells. The mechanism of action of HypRho-D is not fully understood.

The administration of Rh$_o$(D) Immune Globulin (Human) within 72 hours of a full-term delivery of an Rh$_o$(D) positive infant by an Rh$_o$(D) negative mother reduces the incidence of Rh isoimmunization from 12–13% to 1–2%. The 1–2% treatment failures are probably due to isoimmunization occurring during the latter part of pregnancy or following delivery.[10] Bowman, *et al*,[11] have reported that the incidence of isoimmunization can be further reduced from approximately 1.6% to less than 0.1% by administering Rh$_o$(D) Immune Globulin in two doses, one antenatal at 28 weeks gestation and another following delivery.

INDICATIONS AND USAGE

Pregnancy and Other Obstetric Conditions

Rh$_o$(D) Immune Globulin (Human)—HypRho-D is recommended for the prevention of Rh hemolytic disease of the newborn by its administration to the Rh$_o$(D) negative mother within 72 hours after birth of an Rh$_o$(D) positive infant,[12] providing the following criteria are met:

1. The mother must be Rh$_o$(D) negative, and must not already be sensitized to the Rh$_o$(D) factor.
2. Her child must be Rh$_o$(D) positive, and should have a negative direct antiglobulin test (see PRECAUTIONS).

If HypRho-D is administered antepartum, it is essential that the mother receive another dose of HypRho-D after delivery of an Rh$_o$(D) positive infant.

If the father can be determined to be Rh$_o$(D) negative, HypRho-D need not be given.

HypRho-D should be administered within 72 hours to all nonimmunized Rh$_o$(D) negative women who have underdone spontaneous or induced abortion, following ruptured tubal pregnancy, amniocentesis or abdominal trauma unless the blood group of the fetus or the father is known to be Rh$_o$(D) negative.[7,8] If the fetal blood group cannot be determined, one must assume that it is Rh$_o$(D) positive,[2] and HypRho-D should be administered to the mother.

Transfusion

HypRho-D may be used to prevent isoimmunization in Rh$_o$(D) negative individuals who have been transfused with Rh$_o$(D) positive red blood cells or blood components containing red blood cells.[5,13]

CONTRAINDICATIONS

None known.

WARNINGS

NEVER ADMINISTER HypRho-D INTRAVENOUSLY. INJECT ONLY INTRAMUSCULARLY. NEVER ADMINISTER TO THE NEONATE.

Rh$_o$(D) Immune Globulin (Human) should be given with caution to patients with a history of prior systemic allergic reactions following the administration of human immunoglobulin preparations or to patients who are known to have had an allergic respose to thimerosal.

The attending physician who wishes to administer Rh$_o$(D) Immune Globulin (Human) to persons with isolated immunoglobulin A (IgA) deficiency must weigh the benefits of immunization against the potential risks of hypersensitivity reactions. Such persons have increased potential for developing antibodies to IgA and could have anaphylactic reactions to subsequent administration of blood products that contain IgA.

As with all preparations administered by the intramuscular route, bleeding complications may be encountered in patients with thrombocytopenia or other bleeding disorders.

PRECAUTIONS

General

A large fetomaternal hemorrhage late in pregnancy or following delivery may cause a weak mixed field positive D^u test result. If there is any doubt about the mother's Rh type, she should be given RH$_o$(D) Immune Globulin (Human). A screening test to detect fetal red blood cells may be helpful in such cases.

If more than 15 mL of D positive fetal red blood cells are present in the mother's circulation, more than a single dose of Rh$_o$(D) Immune Globulin (Human)—HypRho®-D is required. Failure to recognize this may result in the administration of an inadequate dose.

Although systemic reactions to human immunoglobulin preparations are rare, epinephrine should be available for treatment of acute anaphylactic reactions.

Drug Interactions

Other antibodies in the Rh$_o$(D) Immune Globulin (Human) preparation may interfere with the response to live vaccines such as measles, mumps, polio or rubella. Therefore, immunization with live vaccines should not be given within three months after Rh$_o$(D) Immune Globulin (Human) administration.

Drug/Laboratory Interactions

Babies born of women given Rh$_o$(D) Immune Globulin (Human) antepartum may have a weekly positive direct antiglobulin test at birth.

Passively acquired anti-Rh$_o$(D) may be detected in maternal serum if antibody screening tests are performed subsequent to antepartum or post partum administration of Rh$_o$(D) Immune Globulin (Human).

Pregnancy Category C

Animal reproduction studies have not been conducted with HypRho-D. It is also not known whether HypRho-D can cause fetal harm when administered to a pregnant woman or can affect reproduction capacity. HypRho-D should be given to a pregnant woman only if clearly needed.

ADVERSE REACTIONS

Reactions to Rh$_o$(D) Immune Globulin (Human) are infrequent in Rh$_o$(D) negative individuals and consist primarily of slight soreness at the site of injection and slight temperature elevation. While sensitization to repeated injections of human immune globulin is extremely rare, it has occurred. Elevated bilirubin levels have been reported in some individuals receiving multiple doses of Rh$_o$(D) Immune Globulin (Human) following mismatched tranfusions. This is believed to be due to a relatively rapid rate of foreign red cell destruction.

DOSAGE AND ADMINISTRATION

Pregnancy and Other Obstetric Conditions

1. For postpartum prophylaxis, administer one vial or syringe of HypRho-D (300 μg*), preferably within 72 hours of delivery. Although a lesser degree of protection is afforded if Rh antibody is administered beyond the 72-hour period, HypRho-D may still be given.[7,14] Full-term deliveries can vary in their dosage requirements depending on the magnitude of the fetomaternal hemorrhage. One 300 μg* vial or syringe of HypRho-D provides sufficient antibody to prevent Rh sensitization if the volume of red blood cells that has entered the circulation is 15 mL or less.[2–4] In instances where a large (greater than 30 mL of whole blood or 15 mL red blood cells) fetomaternal hemorrhage is suspected, a fetal red cell count by an approved laboratory technique (e.g., modified Kleihauer-Betke acid elution stain technique) should be performed to determine the dosage of immune globulin required.[8,15] The red blood cell volume of the calculated fetomaternal hemorrhage is divided by 15 mL to obtain the number of vials or syringes of Rh$_o$(D) Immune Globulin (Human)—HypRho®-D for administration.[3,8,13] If more than 15 mL of red cells is suspected or if the dose calculation results in a fraction, administer the next higher whole number of vials or syringes (e.g., if 1.4, give 2 vials or syringes).
2. For antenatal prophylaxis, one 300 μg* vial or syringe of HypRho(D) is administered at approximately 28 weeks gestation. This must be followed by another 300 μg* dose, preferably within 72 hours following delivery, if the infant is Rh positive.
3. Following threatened abortion at any stage of gestation with continuation of pregnancy, it is recommended that 300 μg* of HypRho-D be given. If more than 15 mL of red cells is suspected due to fetomaternal hemorrhage, the same dose modification in #1 above applies.
4. Following miscarriage, abortion, or termination of ectopic pregnancy at or beyond 13 weeks gestation, it is recommended that 300 μg* of HypRho-D be given. If more than 15 mL of red blood cells is suspected due to fetomaternal hemorrhage, the same dose modification in #1 above applies. If pregnancy is terminated prior to 13 weeks gestation, a single dose of Mini-Dose Rh$_o$(D) (approximately 50 μg*) may be used instead of HypRho-D.
5. Following amniocentesis at either 15 to 18 weeks gestation or during the third trimester, or following abdominal trauma in the second or third trimester, it is recommended that 300 μg* of HypRho-D be administered. If there is a fetomaternal hemorrhage in excess of 15 mL of red cells, the same dose modification in #1 applies.

If abdominal trauma, amniocentesis, or other adverse event requires the administration of HypRho-D at 13 to 18 weeks gestation, another 300 μg* dose should be given at 26 to 28 weeks. To maintain protection throughout pregnancy, the level of passively acquired anti-Rh$_o$(D) should not be allowed to fall below the level required to prevent an immune response to Rh positive red cells. The half life of lgG is 23 to 26 days. In any case, a dose of HypRho-D should be given within 72 hours after delivery if the baby is Rh positive. If delivery occurs within three weeks after the last dose, the postpartum dose may be withheld unless there is a femomaternal hemorrhage in excess of 15 mL of red blood cells.[16]

*See footnote under DESCRIPTION.

Transfusion

In the case of a transfusion of Rh$_o$(D) positive red cells to an Rh$_o$(D) negative recipient, the volume of Rh positive whole blood administered is multiplied by the hematocrit of the donor unit giving the volume of red blood cells transfused. The volume of red blood cells is divided by 15 mL which provides the number of vials or syringes of HypRho-D to be administered.

If the dose calculated results in a fraction, the next higher whole number of vials or syringes should be administered (e.g., if 1.4, give 2 vials or 2 syringes). HypRho-D should be administered within 72 hours after an incompatible transfusion, but preferably as soon as possible.

Injection Procedure

DO NOT INJECT INTRAVENOUSLY. DO NOT INJECT NEONATE.

A. Single Vial or Syringe Dose
   INJECT ENTIRE CONTENTS OF THE VIAL OR SYRINGE INTO THE INDIVIDUAL INTRAMUSCULARLY.
B. Multiple Vial or Syringe Dose
   1. Calculate the number of vials or syringes of Rh$_o$(D) Immune Globulin (Human)—HypRho®-D to be given (See Dosage section above).
   2. The total volume of HypRho-D can be given in divided doses at different sites at one time or the total dose may be divided and injected at intervals, provided the total dosage is given within 72 hours of the fetomaternal hemorrhage or transfusion. USING STERILE TECHNIQUE, INJECT THE ENTIRE CONTENTS OF THE CALCULATED NUMBER OF VIALS OR SYRINGES INTRAMUSCULARLY INTO THE PATIENT.

Parenteral drug products should be inspected visually for particulate matter and discoloration prior to administration, whenever solution and container permit.

HOW SUPPLIED

HypRho-D is available in vials and in syringes as follows:

Product Code	Contents
621-10	Ten single dose vials of HypRho-D. Package insert giving directions for use and patient identification cards.
621-15	One single dose vial of HypRho-D. Package insert giving directions for use, an injection form and a patient identification card.
621-22	Ten single dose syringes of HypRho-D. Package insert giving directions for use, patient identification cards, and patient information booklets.
621-05	Five single dose syringes of HypRho-D. Package insert giving directions for use, patient identification cards, and patient information booklets.

Continued on next page

Cutter—Cont.

STORAGE

Store at 2–8°C (35–46°F). Do not freeze.

CAUTION

U.S. Federal law prohibits dispensing without a prescription.

LIMITED WARRANTY

A number of factors beyond our control could reduce the efficacy of this product or even result in an ill effect following its use. These include improper storage and handling of the product after it leaves our hands, diagnosis, dosage, method of administration, and biological differences in individual patients. Because of these factors, it is important that this product be stored properly and that the directions be followed carefully during use.

The foregoing statement is made in lieu of any other warranty, express or implied, including any warranty of merchantability or fitness.

Representatives of the Company are not authorized to vary the terms of this warranty or the contents of any printed labeling for this product except by printed notice from the Company's Berkeley office. The prescriber and user of this product must accept the terms hereof.

REFERENCES

1. Gunson HH, Bowell PJ, Kirkwood TBL: Collaborative study to recalibrate the International Reference Preparation of Anti-D Immunoglobulin. *J Clin Pathol* 33:249–53, 1980.
2. Rh_o(D) immune globulin (human). *Med Lett Drugs Ther* 16(1):3–4, 1974.
3. Pollack W, Ascari WQ, Kochesky RJ, *et al:* Studies on Rh prophylaxis I. Relationship between doses of anti-Rh and size of antigenic stimulus. *Transfusion* 11(6):333–9, 1971.
4. Unpublished data in files of Cutter Biological.
5. Pollack W, Asceri WQ, Crispen JF, *et al:* Studies on Rh prophylaxis. II. Rh immune prophylaxis after transfusion with Rh-positive blood. *Transfusion* 11 (6):340–4, 1971.
6. Keith LG, Houser GH: Anti-Rh immune globulin after a massive transfusion accident. *Transfusion* 11(3):176, 1971.
7. The selective use of Rh_o(D) Immune Globulin (RHIG). *ACOG Tech Bull* 61, 1981.
8. Current uses of Rh_o immune globulin and detection of antibodies. *ACOG Tech Bull* 35, 1976.
9. Pollack W: Rh hemolytic disease of the newborn; its cause and prevention. *Prog Clin Biol Res* 70:185–203, 1981.
10. Bowman JM, Chown B, Lewis M, *et al:* Rh isoimmunization during pregnancy: antenatal prophylaxis. *Can Med Assoc J* 118(6):623–7, 1978.
11. Bowman JM, Pollock JM: Antenatal prophylaxis of Rh isommunization: 28-weeks-gestation service program. *Can Med Assoc J* 118(6):627–30, 1978.
12. Ascari WQ, Allen AE, Baker WJ, et al: Rh-o(D) immune globulin (human): evaluation in women at risk of Rh immunization. *JAMA* 205(1): 1–4, 1968.
13. Prevention of Rh sensitization, *WHO Tech Rep Ser* 468:25, 1971.
14. Samson D. Mollison PL: Effect on primary Rh immunization of delayed administration of anti-Rh. *Immunology* 28:349–57, 175.
15. Finn R, Harper DT, Stallings, SA, et al: Transplacental hemorrhage. *Transfusion* 3(2):114–24, 1963.
16. Garraty G (ed): Hemolytic disease of the newborn. Arlington, VA, American Association of Blood Banks, 78, 1984.

14-7621-000
(Rev Oct 1985)

KOĀTE®-HT ℞

[*kō'ate*]

Antihemophilic Factor (Human)
(Factor VIII, AHF, AHG)

A heat-treated, stable, purified dried concentrate of human Antihemophilic Factor.

250 AHF units, approx., with 10 ml. Sterile Water for Injection, U.S.P., sterile filter needle, and transfer needle.
500 AHF units, approx., with 20 ml. Sterile Water for Injection, U.S.P., sterile filter needle, and transfer needle.
1000 AHF units, approx., with 40 ml Sterile Water for Injection, U.S.P., sterile filter needle, and transfer needle.
1500 AHF units, approx., with 40 ml. Sterile Water for Injection, U.S.P., sterile filter needle, and transfer needle.

KONYNE®–HT ℞

[*kō'nine-HT*]

(Factor IX Complex-Human-Heat Treated)

500 unit vial, approx., with 20 ml sterile water for Injection, U.S.P., sterile filter needle, and transfer needle.
1000 unit vial, approx., with 40 ml sterile water for Injection, U.S.P., sterile filter needle, and transfer needle.

PLAGUE VACCINE, U.S.P. ℞

20 ml. vials

Danbury Pharmacal, Inc.

131 WEST STREET
P.O. BOX 296
DANBURY, CT 06810

PRODUCT IDENTIFICATION CODE

Danbury Prescription Capsules and Tablets are identified with a symbol DAN and the NDC Product Number. Controlled Substance Products are identified with the Danbury NDC Number 591-followed by a letter identifying the product.

To quickly identify a product, a compilation of most of Danbury's products is listed below in alphabetical order with corresponding product codes.

NDC# 0591-	PRODUCT	IMPRINT
5430	Acetazolamide, 250 mg	U: DAN L: 5430
5543	Allopurinol Tablets, 100 mg	U: DAN L: 5543
5544	Allopurinol Tablets, 300 mg	U: DAN L: 5544
5370	Bethanechol Chloride Tablets, 5 mg	U: DAN L: 5370
5369	Bethanechol Chloride Tablets, 10 mg	U: DAN L: 5369
5402	Bethanechol Chloride Tablets, 25 mg	U: DAN L: 5402
5515	Bethanechol Chloride Tablets, 50 mg	U: DAN L: 5515
5519	Butalbital and Acetaminophen Tablets, 50 mg/325 mg	591-F
5513	Carisoprodol Tablets, 350 mg	U: DAN L: 5513
5548	Chloroquine Phosphate Tablets, 250 mg	U: DAN L: 5548
5549	Chloroquine Phosphate Tablets, 500 mg	U: DAN L: 5549
5444	Chlorothiazide Tablets, 250 mg	U: DAN L: 5444
5579	Chlorpropamide Tablets, 100 mg	U: DAN L: 5579
5455	Chlorpropamide Tablets, 250 mg	U: DAN L: 5455
5507	Chlorthalidone Tablets, 25 mg	U: DAN L: 5507
5518	Chlorthalidone Tablets, 50 mg	U: DAN L: 5518
5495	Chlorzoxazone Tablets, 250 mg	U: DAN L: 5495
5509	Chlorzoxazone with ÁPAP Tablets, 250 mg	U: DAN L: 5509
5609	Clonidine HCl Tablets, 0.1 mg	U: DAN L: 5609
5612	Clonidine HCl Tablets, 0.2 mg	U: DAN L: 5612
5613	Clonidine HCl Tablets, 0.3 mg	U: DAN L: 5613
0944	Colchicine Tablets, 0.6 mg	U: DAN L: 944
5325	Col-Probenecid Tablets, 0.5 mg/500 mg	U: DAN L: 5325
5484	Cyproheptadine HCl Tablets, 4 mg	U: DAN L: 5484
5309	Dicyclomine HCl Capsules, 10 mg	DAN/ 5309
5383	Dicyclomine HCl Tablets, 20 mg	U: DAN L: 5383
5002	Diphenhydramine HCl Capsules, 25 mg	DAN/ 5002
5003	Diphenhydramine HCl Capsules, 50 mg	DAN/ 5003
5510	Dipyridamole Tablets, 25 mg	U: DAN L: 5510
5511	Dipyridamole Tablets, 50 mg	U: DAN L: 5511
5512	Dipyridamole Tablets, 75 mg	U: DAN L: 5512
5560	Disopyramide Phosphate Capsules (Equivalent to 100 mg Disopyramide)	DAN/ 5560
5561	Disopyramide Phosphate Capsules (Equivalent to 150 mg Disopyramide)	DAN/ 5561
5376	Disulfiram Tablets, 250 mg	U: DAN L: 5376
5368	Disulfiram Tablets, 500 mg	U: DAN L: 5368
5535	Doxycycline Hyclate Capsules (Equivalent to 50 mg Doxycycline)	DAN/ 5535
5440	Doxycycline Hyclate Capsules (Equivalent to 100 mg Doxycycline)	DAN/ 5440
5553	Doxycycline Hyclate Tablets (Equivalent to 100 mg Doxycycline)	U: DAN L: 5553
5504	Ergoloid Mesylates Oral Tablets 1.0 mg	U: DAN L: 5504
5502	Ergoloid Mesylates Sublingual Tablets, 0.5 mg	U: DAN L: 5502
5501	Ergoloid Mesylates Sublingual Tablets, 1.0 mg	U: DAN L: 5501
5479	Erythromycin Estolate Capsules, 250 mg	DAN/ 5479
5216	Folic Acid Tablets, 1.0 mg	U: DAN L: 5216
5576	Furosemide Tablets, 20 mg	U: DAN L: 5576
5575	Furosemide Tablets, 40 mg	U: DAN L: 5575
5493	Glycopyrrolate Tablets, 1 mg	U: DAN L: 5493
5494	Glycopyrrolate Tablets, 2 mg	U: DAN L: 5494
5050	Hydralazine HCl Tablets, 25 mg	U: DAN L: 5050
5055	Hydralazine HCl Tablets, 50 mg	U: DAN L: 5055
5428	Hydrochlorothiazide, Hydralazine HCl, Reserpine Tablets, 15 mg, 25 mg 0.1 mg	U: DAN L: 5428
5406	Hydrochlorothiazide/ Reserpine Tablets, 25 mg/0.125 mg	U: DAN L: 5406
5407	Hydrochlorothiazide/ Reserpine Tablets, 50 mg/0.125 mg	U: DAN L: 5407
5345	Hydrochlorothiazide Tablets, 50 mg	U: DAN L: 5345
5183	Hydrocortisone Tablets, 20 mg	U: DAN L: 5183
5522	Hydroxyzine Hydrochloride Tablets, 10 mg	U: DAN L: 5522
5523	Hydroxyzine Hydrochloride Tablets, 25 mg	U: DAN L: 5523
5565	Hydroxyzine Hydrochloride Tablets, 50 mg	U: DAN L: 5565
5532	Hydroxyzine Pamoate Capsules (Equivalent to 50 mg Hydroxyzine HCl)	DAN/ 5532
5537	Hydroxyzine Pamoate Capsules (Equivalent to 100 mg Hydroxyzine HCl)	DAN/ 5537
5585	Ibuprofen Tablets, 200 mg	U: DAN L: 5585
5584	Ibuprofen Tablets, 400 mg	U: DAN L: 5584
5586	Ibuprofen Tablets, 600 mg	U: DAN L:5586
0528	Isoniazid Tablets, 50 mg	U: DAN L: 528
0525	Isoniazid Tablets, 100 mg	U: DAN L: 525
0526	Isoniazid Tablets, 300 mg	U: DAN L: 526
5374	Isosorbide Dinitrate Oral Tablets, 5 mg	U: DAN L: 5374
5373	Isosorbide Dinitrate Oral Tablets, 10 mg	U: DAN L: 5373
5387	Isosorbide Dinitrate Sublingual Tablets, 2.5 mg	U: DAN L: 5387
5385	Isosorbide Dinitrate Sublingual Tablets, 5 mg	U: DAN L: 5385
5400	Isoxsuprine HCl Tablets, 10 mg	U: 10 L: DAN/

5401	Isoxsuprine HCl Tablets, 20 mg	5400 U: 20 L: DAN/ 5401
5381	Methocarbamol Tablets, 500 mg	U: DAN L: 5381
5382	Methocarbamol Tablets, 750 mg	U: DAN L: 5382
5588	Methyldopa Tablets, 250 mg	U: DAN L:5588
5587	Methyldopa Tablets, 500 mg	U: DAN L:5587
5589	Metoclopramide HCl Tablets, (Equivalent to 10 mg Metoclopramide base)	U: DAN L: 5589
5540	Metronidazole Tablets, 250 mg	U: DAN L: 5540
5552	Metronidazole Tablets, 500 mg	U: DAN L: 5552
5342	Nylidrin HCl Tablets, 6 mg	U: DAN L: 5342
5390	Nylidrin HCl Tablets, 12 mg	U: DAN L: 5390
0938	Papaverine HCl Tablets, 100 mg	U: DAN L: 938
5196	Papaverine HCl T.D. Capsules, 150 mg	DAN/ 5196
5521	Phenylbutazone Tablets, 100 mg	U: DAN L: 5521
5059	Prednisolone Tablets, 5 mg	U: DAN L: 5059
5052	Prednisone Tablets, 5 mg	U: DAN L: 5052
5442	Prednisone Tablets, 10 mg	U: DAN L: 5442
5443	Prednisone Tablets, 20 mg	U: DAN L: 5443
5490	Prednisone Tablets, 50 mg	U: DAN L: 5490
5321	Primidone Tablets, 250 mg	U: DAN L: 5321
5347	Probenecid Tablets, 500 mg	U: DAN L: 5347
5026	Procainamide HCl Capsules, 250 mg	DAN/ 5026
5350	Procainamide HCl Capsules, 375 mg	DAN/ 5350
5333	Procainamide HCl Capsules, 500 mg	DAN/ 5333
5562	Procainamide HCl S.R. Tablets, 250 mg	U: DAN L: 5562
5563	Procainamide HCl S.R. Tablets, 500 mg	U: DAN L: 5563
5564	Procainamide HCl S.R. Tablets, 750 mg	U: DAN L: 5564
5257	Propantheline Bromide Tablets, 15 mg	DAN/ 5257
5554	Propranolol HCl Tablets, 10 mg	U: DAN L: 5554
5555	Propranolol HCl Tablets, 20 mg	U: DAN L: 5555
5556	Propranolol HCl Tablets, 40 mg	U: DAN L: 5556
5623	Propranolol HCl Tablets, 60 mg	U: DAN L: 5623
5557	Propranolol HCl Tablets, 80 mg	U: DAN L: 5557
5635	Propranolol HCl Tablets, 90 mg	U: DAN L: 5635
5204	Pseudoephedrine HCl Tablets, 60 mg	U: DAN L: 5204
5516	Quindan Tablets (Quinine Sulfate Tablets, 260 mg)	DAN/ 5516
5538	Quinidine Gluconate Sustained Action Tablets, 324 mg	U: DAN L: 5538
5453	Quinidine Sulfate Tablets, 100 mg	U: DAN L: 5453
5438	Quinidine Sulfate Tablets, 200 mg	U: DAN L: 5438
5454	Quinidine Sulfate Tablets, 300 mg	U: DAN L: 5454
5496	Spironolactone/Hydro-chlorothiazide Tablets, 25 mg/25 mg	U: DAN L: 5496
5546	Sulfamethoxazole 400 mg with Trimethoprim 80 mg Tablets	U: DAN L: 5546
5547	Sulfamethoxazole 800 mg with Trimethoprim 160 mg Tablets (Double Strength)	U: DAN L: 5547
5503	Sulfasalazine Tablets, 500 mg	DAN/ 5503
5514	Sulfinpyrazone Tablets, 100 mg	U: DAN L: 5514
5162	Tetracycline HCl Capsules, 250 mg	DAN/ 5162
5520	Tetracycline HCl Capsules, 500 mg	DAN/ 5520
5481	Theofedral Tablets	U: DAN L: 5481
5566	Thioridazine HCl Tablets, 10 mg	U: DAN L: 5566
5572	Thioridazine HCl Tablets, 15 mg	U: DAN L: 5572
5542	Thioridazine HCl Tablets, 25 mg	U: DAN L: 5542
5568	Thioridazine HCl Tablets, 50 mg	U: DAN L: 5568
5569	Thioridazine HCl Tablets, 100 mg	U: DAN L: 5569
5580	Thioridazine HCl Tablets, 150 mg	U: DAN L: 5580
5581	Thioridazine HCl Tablets, 200 mg	U: DAN L: 5581
5591	Tolazamide Tablets, 100 mg	U: DAN L: 5591
5582	Tolazamide Tablets, 250 mg	U: DAN L: 5582
5590	Tolazamide Tablets, 500 mg	U: DAN L: 5590
5508	Tolbutamide Tablets, 500 mg	U: DAN L: 5508
5388	Triamcinolone Tablets, 4 mg	U: DAN L: 5388
5335	Trihexyphenidyl HCl Tablets, 2 mg	U: DAN L: 5335
5337	Trihexyphenidyl HCl Tablets, 5 mg	U: DAN L: 5337
5571	Trimethoprim Tablets 100 mg	U: DAN L: 5571
5058	Tripelennamine HCl Tablets, 50 mg	U: DAN L: 5058
5434	Tripodrine Tablets	U: DAN L: 5434
5601	Verapamil HCl Tablets, 80 mg	U: DAN L: 5601
5602	Verapamil HCl Tablets, 120 mg	U: DAN L: 5602

CONTROLLED SUBSTANCE PRODUCTS

NDC#	SCHEDULE#	PRODUCT	IMPRINT
5621	C-IV	Diazepam Tablets, 2 mg	U: DAN/5621 L: 2
5619	C-IV	Diazepam Tablets, 5 mg	U: DAN/5619 L: 5
5620	C-IV	Diazepam Tablets, 10 mg	U: DAN/5620 L: 10
5614	C-IV	Flurazepam HCl Capsules, 15 mg	DAN/ 5614
5616	C-IV	Flurazepam HCl Capsules, 30 mg	DAN/ 5615
5625	C-IV	Lorazepam Tablets, 0.5 mg	U: DAN/5625 L: 0.5
5624	C-IV	Lorazepam Tablets, 1 mg	U: DAN/5624 L: 1
5622	C-IV	Lorazepam Tablets, 2 mg	U: DAN/5622 L: 2
5238	C-IV	Meprobamate Tablets, 400 mg	591-A
5239	C-IV	Meprobamate Tablets, 200 mg	591-B
5069	C-IV	Phenobarbital Tablets, 1/4 gr.	591-C
5180	C-IV	Phenobarbital Tablets, 1/2 gr.	591-D
5073	C-IV	Phenobarbital Tablets, 1/8 gr.	591-E
5366	C-III	Glutethimide Tablets, 500 mg	591-J
5346	C-IV	Phenobarbital Tablets, 1 ½ gr.	591-O
5476	C-IV	Phenobarbital Tablets, 30 mg	591-T
5478	C-IV	Phenobarbital Tablets, 60 mg	591-V

Products are cross-indexed by generic and chemical names in the **YELLOW SECTION**

Delmont Laboratories, Inc.
P.O. BOX AA
SWARTHMORE, PA 19081

STAPHAGE LYSATE (SPL)® ℞
[staf'faj lī'sāt]
BACTERIAL ANTIGEN MADE FROM STAPHYLOCOCCUS

DESCRIPTION

STAPHAGE LYSATE (SPL)® is a whole culture vaccine, in solution, of two strains of lysed *Staphylococcus aureus*, Serologic Types I & III, specially selected for their broad antigenic spectrum.

HOW SUPPLIED

1-ml ampules, boxes of 10 (NDC 48532-0299-2), for subcutaneous, aerosol, topical, and oral use; 10-ml multiple-dose vials (NDC 48532-0299-1) for aerosol, topical, and oral use.

For complete prescribing information and literature, please write, or call (215) 543-3365 or 543-2747.

Dermik Laboratories, Inc.
790 PENLLYN PIKE
BLUE BELL, PA 19422

ANTHRA-DERM® Ointment ℞
[anthra-derm]
(anthralin) 1%, ½%, ¼%, $^1/_{10}$%
FOR TOPICAL USE ONLY

DESCRIPTION

Each gram of Anthra-Derm® (anthralin) Ointment $^1/_{10}$%, ¼%, ½% and 1.0% contains 1 mg, 2.5 mg, 5 mg and 10 mg, respectively, of anthralin in a base consisting of mineral oil and white petrolatum. Anthralin is an anti-psoriatic agent with cytostatic, irritant and weak antimicrobial properties.

CLINICAL PHARMACOLOGY

Although the exact mechanism of anthralin's activity is unknown, there is experimental evidence that anthralin binds DNA, inhibiting synthesis of nucleic protein, and thus reduces mitotic activity.

Absorption in man has not been determined. However, based on a study in piglets it would appear to be quite low.

INDICATIONS AND USAGE

For the topical treatment of psoriasis.

CONTRAINDICATIONS

Anthra-Derm® (anthralin) Ointment is contraindicated in patients with acute psoriasis or where inflammation is present, and in those patients with a history of hypersensitivity to any of the ingredients.

WARNINGS

Although no renal, hepatic or hematologic abnormalities have been reported as a result of topical application of Anthra-Derm® (anthralin) Ointment, caution is advised in patients with renal disease. Patients with renal disease and those having extensive and prolonged applications should have periodic urine tests for albuminuria. Discontinue use if sensitivity reactions occur.

PRECAUTIONS

General: When redness is observed on adjacent normal skin, reduce frequency of application. For external use only. Do not apply to face, genitalia or intertriginous areas. Wash hands thoroughly and carefully after using. Keep out of the reach of children. Anthralin is a tumor-promoting agent in 2-stage carcinogenesis on mouse skin. However, there have not been any reports of such effects in humans at the usual dosages.

Pregnancy: Pregnancy Category C. Animal reproduction studies have not been conducted with anthralin. It is also not known whether anthralin can cause fetal harm when administered to a pregnant woman or can affect reproduction capacity. Anthra-Derm® Ointment should be given to a pregnant woman only if clearly needed.

Nursing mothers: It is not known whether this drug is excreted in human milk. Because many drugs are excreted in human milk and because of the potential for tumorigenicity shown for anthralin in animal studies, a decision should be made whether to discontinue nursing or to discontinue the drug, taking into account the importance of the drug to the mother.

Pediatric use: Safety and effectiveness in children have not been established.

Continued on next page

Dermik—Cont.

ADVERSE REACTIONS

Irritation of normal skin is the most frequently reported adverse reaction. Anthra-Derm® may stain skin, hair, or fabrics.

DOSAGE AND ADMINISTRATION

The usual dosage regimen begins with the lowest concentration (1/10%) and is gradually increased until the desired effect is obtained. Apply in a thin layer to affected areas once or twice daily, or as directed by a physician.

HOW SUPPLIED

Anthra-Derm® (anthralin) Ointment 1/10% (NDC 0066-0010-15), 1/4% (NDC 0066-0025-15), 1/2% (NDC 0066-0050-15) and 1.0% (NDC-0066-0100-15) is available in 1.5 oz (42.5 g) tubes.

5 BENZAGEL® ℞
[ben-za-jel]
(5% benzoyl peroxide) and
10 BENZAGEL® ℞
(10% benzoyl peroxide)
MICROGEL™ FORMULA
Acne Gels

DESCRIPTION

Each gram of 5 Benzagel® and 10 Benzagel® contains 50 mg and 100 mg respectively, of benzoyl peroxide in a gel vehicle of purified water, carbomer 940, sodium hydroxide, docusate sodium, fragrance and alcohol 14%.
Benzoyl peroxide is an antibacterial and keratolytic agent.

CLINICAL PHARMACOLOGY

Benzoyl peroxide is an antibacterial agent which has been shown to be effective against *Propionibacterium acnes.* This action is believed to be responsible for its usefulness in acne. One study in the rhesus monkey demonstrated a percutaneous absorption of about 1.8 μg per cm^2 of benzoyl peroxide or 45% of the applied dose in a 24-hour period. The absorbed benzoyl peroxide was completely converted in the skin to benzoic acid.

INDICATION AND USAGE

5 & 10 Benzagel® may be used alone topically for mild to moderate acne and as an adjunct in acne treatment regimens which might include retinoic acid products, systemic antibiotics, and/or sulfur and salicylic acid-containing preparations. The active ingredient, benzoyl peroxide, exerts a desquamative and antibacterial action. It provides mild peeling and keratolytic activity.

CONTRAINDICATIONS

Benzagel® should not be used by patients having known sensitivity to benzoyl peroxide or any of its components.

WARNINGS

If itching, redness, burning, swelling or undue dryness occurs, discontinue use.

PRECAUTIONS

For external use only. Not for ophthalmic use. Keep away from eyes and mucosae. Very fair individuals should begin with a single application at bedtime allowing overnight medication. May bleach colored fabrics. Keep this and all medications out of the reach of children.
Carcinogenesis, Mutagenesis and Impairment of Fertility—Long-term studies in animals have not been performed to evaluate carcinogenic potential.
Pregnancy Category C—Animal reproduction studies have not been conducted with benzoyl peroxide. It is also not known whether benzoyl peroxide can cause fetal harm when administered to a pregnant woman or can affect reproduction capacity. Benzoyl peroxide should be given to a pregnant woman only if clearly needed.
Nursing Mothers—It is not known whether this drug is excreted in human milk. Because many drugs are excreted in human milk, caution should be exercised when benzoyl peroxide is administered to a nursing woman.
Pediatric Use: Safety and effectiveness in children under the age of 12 have not been established.

ADVERSE REACTIONS

Irritation and contact dermatitis are the most frequent side reactions to benzoyl peroxide.

DOSAGE AND ADMINISTRATION

Wash and dry affected areas prior to application. Apply sparingly one or more times daily.

HOW SUPPLIED

5 & 10 Benzagel® are available in 1.5 oz (42.5 g) and 3 oz (85 g) plastic tubes; 5 Benzagel® contains 50 mg benzoyl peroxide per gram and 10 Benzagel® contains 100 mg benzoyl peroxide per gram.
5-Benzagel 1.5 oz NDC 0066-0430-15
5-Benzagel 3.0 oz NDC 0066-0430-30
10-Benzagel 1.5 oz NDC 0066-0431-15
10 Benzagel 3.0 oz NDC 0066-0431-30

BENZAMYCIN® Topical Gel ℞
[ben 'za-mi "sin]
(erythromycin—benzoyl peroxide)

Reconstitute Before Dispensing

DESCRIPTION

Each gram of Benzamycin® (erythromycin—benzoyl peroxide) topical gel contains, as dispensed, 30 mg (3%) of erythromycin and 50 mg (5%) of benzoyl peroxide in a gel vehicle of purified water, carbomer 940, alcohol 22%, sodium hydroxide, docusate sodium and fragrance.
Erythromycin ($C_{37}H_{67}NO_{13}$) is produced by a strain of *Streptomyces erythraeus* and belongs to the macrolide group of antibiotics.
Benzoyl peroxide ($C_{14}H_{10}O_4$), is an antibacterial and keratolytic agent.

CLINICAL PHARMACOLOGY

Erythromycin is a bacteriostatic macrolide antibiotic, but may be bactericidal in high concentrations. Although the mechanism by which erythromycin acts in reducing inflammatory lesions of acne vulgaris is unknown, it is presumably due to its antibiotic action. Antagonism has been demonstrated between clindamycin and erythromycin.
Benzoyl peroxide is an antibacterial agent which has been shown to be effective against *Propionibacterium acnes,* an anaerobe found in sebaceous follicles and comedones. The antibacterial action of benzoyl peroxide is believed to be due to the release of active oxygen. Benzoyl peroxide has a keratolytic and desquamative effect which may also contribute to its efficacy.
Benzoyl peroxide has been shown to be absorbed by the skin where it is converted to benzoic acid.

INDICATIONS AND USAGE

Benzamycin® Topical Gel is indicated for the topical control of acne vulgaris.

CONTRAINDICATIONS

Benzamycin® Topical Gel is contraindicated in those patients with a history of hypersensitivity to erythromycin, benzoyl peroxide or any of the other listed ingredients.

PRECAUTIONS

General—For external use only. Not for ophthalmic use. Avoid contact with eyes and mucous membranes. Concomitant topical acne therapy should be used with caution because a possible cumulative irritancy effect may occur, especially with peeling, desquamating or abrasive agents. If severe irritation develops, discontinue use and institute appropriate therapy.
The use of antibiotic agents may be associated with the overgrowth of antibiotic-resistant organisms. If this occurs, administration of this drug should be discontinued and appropriate measures taken.
Information for Patients—Patients using Benzamycin® Topical Gel should receive the following information and instructions:

1. Benzamycin® Topical Gel is for external use only. Avoid contact with the eyes and mucous membranes.
2. Patients should not use any other topical acne preparation unless otherwise directed by physician.
3. Benzamycin® Topical Gel may bleach hair or colored fabric.
4. If excessive irritation or dryness should occur, patient should discontinue medication and consult physician.
5. Discard product after 3 months and obtain fresh material.

Carcinogenesis, Mutagenesis and Impairment of Fertility: Long-term studies in animals have not been performed to evaluate carcinogenic potential or the effect on fertility.
Pregnancy Category C: Animal reproduction studies have not been conducted with Benzamycin® Topical Gel. It is also not known whether Benzamycin® Topical Gel can cause fetal harm when administered to a pregnant woman or can affect reproduction capacity. Benzamycin® Topical Gel should be given to a pregnant woman only if clearly needed.
Nursing Mothers: It is not known whether this drug is excreted in human milk. Because many drugs are excreted in human milk, caution should be exercised when Benzamycin® Topical Gel is administered to a nursing woman.
Pediatric Use: Safety and effectiveness in children under the age of 12 have not been established.

ADVERSE REACTIONS

Adverse reactions which may occur include dryness, erythema and pruritus. Of a total of 153 patients treated with Benzamycin® Topical Gel during clinical trials, 4 patients experienced adverse reactions, of whom three experienced dryness and one an urticarial reaction which responded well to symptomatic treatment.

DOSAGE AND ADMINISTRATION

Benzamycin® Topical Gel should be applied twice daily, morning and evening, or as directed by physician, to affected areas after the skin is thoroughly washed, rinsed with warm water and gently patted dry.
How Supplied and Dispensing Information: Benzamycin® Topical Gel is supplied in a package containing 20 g of benzoyl peroxide gel and a plastic vial containing 0.8 g of erythromycin powder. Prior to dispensing, add 3 mL of ethyl alcohol (to the mark) to vial and shake well to dissolve erythromycin. Add this solution to gel and stir until homogeneous in appearance (1–1½ minutes). Benzamycin® Topical Gel should then be stored under refrigeration. Place a 3-month expiration date on the label.
Benzamycin® Topical Gel (NDC 0066-0510-23), as dispensed, is 23.3 g net weight.
Note: *Prior* to reconstitution, store at room temperature. *After* reconstitution, store in a cold place, preferably in a refrigerator. Do not freeze. Keep tightly closed. Keep out of the reach of children.
U.S. Patent Nos. 4,387,107 and 4,497,794. Other Patents Pending.

DURRAX™ Tablets ℞
[Door-ax]
(hydroxyzine HCl)

DESCRIPTION

Durrax™, hydroxyzine hydrochloride, has the chemical name of Ethanol, 2-[2-[4-[(4-chlorophenyl) phenylmethyl]-1-piperazinyl]-ethoxy]-,dihydrochloride.
Inactive ingredients: lactose, microcrystalline cellulose, sodium starch glycolate, stearic acid, magnesium stearate, silica, hydroxypropyl cellulose, talc, confectioner's sugar, corn starch, sucrose, FD&C Blue No. 1, carnauba wax, white wax and other ingredients.
Hydroxyzine hydrochloride occurs as a white, odorless powder which is very soluble in water.

CLINICAL PHARMACOLOGY

Hydroxyzine hydrochloride is unrelated chemically to phenothiazine, reserpine, meprobamate or the benzodiazepines. Hydroxyzine is not a cortical depressant, but its action may be due to a suppression of activity in certain key regions of the subcortical area of the central nervous system.
Primary skeletal muscle relaxation has been demonstrated experimentally. Bronchodilator activity, and antihistaminic and analgesic effects have been demonstrated experimentally and confirmed clinically. An antiemetic effect, both by the apomorphine test and the veriloid test, has been demonstrated.
Pharmacological and clinical studies indicate that hydroxyzine, in therapeutic dosage, does not increase gastric secretion or acidity and in most cases has mild antisecretory activity.
Hydroxyzine hydrochloride is rapidly absorbed in the gastrointestinal tract and its effects are usually noted within 15 to 30 minutes after oral administration.

INDICATIONS

For symptomatic relief of anxiety and tension associated with psychoneurosis and as an adjunct in organic disease states in which anxiety is manifested.
Useful in the management of pruritus due to allergic conditions such as chronic urticaria and atopic and contact dermatoses and in histamine-mediated pruritus.
As a sedative when used as a premedication and following general anesthesia. Hydroxyzine may potentiate meperidine and barbiturates, so their use in pre-anesthetic adjunctive therapy should be modified on an individual basis. Atropine and other belladonna alkaloids are not affected by the drug. Hydroxyzine is not known to interfere with the action of digitalis in any way and it may be used concurrently with this agent.
The effectiveness of hydroxyzine as an anti-anxiety agent for long-term use, that is more than 4 months, has not been assessed by systematic clinical studies. The physician should reassess periodically the usefulness of the drug for the individual patient.

CONTRAINDICATIONS

Hydroxyzine, when administered to the pregnant mouse, rat, and rabbit induced fetal abnormalities in the rat and mouse at doses substantially above the human therapeutic range. Clinical data in human beings are inadequate to establish safety in early pregnancy. Until such data are available, hydroxyzine is contraindicated in early pregnancy.
Hydroxyzine hydrochloride is contraindicated for patients who have shown a previous hypersensitivity to it.

PRECAUTIONS

The potentiating action of hydroxyzine must be considered when the drug is used in conjunction with central nervous system depressants. Therefore, when central nervous system depressants are administered concomitantly with hydroxyzine their dosage should be reduced.

Since drowsiness may occur with use of this drug, patients should be warned of this possibility and cautioned against driving a car or operating dangerous machinery while taking hydroxyzine. Patients should also be advised against the simultaneous use of other CNS depressant drugs, and cautioned that the effect of alcohol may be increased.
Nursing Mothers: It is not known whether this drug is excreted in human milk. Since many drugs are so excreted, hydroxyzine should not be given to nursing mothers.

ADVERSE REACTIONS

Side effects reported with the administration of hydroxyzine are usually mild and transitory in nature.
Anticholinergic: Dry mouth.
Central Nervous System: Drowsiness is usually transitory and may disappear in a few days of continued therapy or upon reduction of the dose. Involuntary motor activity including rare instances of tremor and convulsions have been reported, usually with doses considerably higher than those recommended. Clinically significant respiratory depression has not been reported at recommended doses.

OVERDOSAGE

The most common manifestation of hydroxyzine overdosage is hypersedation. As in the management of overdosage with any drug, it should be borne in mind that multiple agents may have been taken.
If vomiting has not occurred spontaneously, it should be induced. Immediate gastric lavage is also recommended. General supportive care, including frequent monitoring of the vital signs and close observation of the patient, is indicated. Hypotension, though unlikely, may be controlled with intravenous fluids and norepinephrine or metaraminol. Do not use epinephrine as hydroxyzine counteracts its pressor action. Caffeine and Sodium Benzoate Injection, U.S.P. may be used to counteract central nervous system depressant effects.
There is no specific antidote. It is doubtful that hemodialysis would be of any value in the treatment of overdosage with hydroxyzine. However, if other agents such as barbiturates have been ingested concomitantly, hemodialysis may be indicated. There is no practical method to quantitate hydroxyzine in body fluids or tissue after its ingestion or administration.

DOSAGE AND ADMINISTRATION

For symptomatic relief of anxiety and tension associated with psychoneurosis and as an adjunct in organic disease states in which anxiety is manifested: Adults, 50–100 mg q.i.d.; children under 6 years, 50 mg daily in divided doses; children over 6 years, 50–100 mg daily in divided doses.
For use in the management of pruritus due to allergic conditions such as chronic urticaria and atopic and contact dermatoses and in histamine-mediated pruritus: Adults, 25 mg t.i.d. or q.i.d.; children under 6 years, 50 mg daily in divided doses; children over 6 years, 50–100 mg daily in divided doses.
As a sedative when used as a premedication and following general anesthesia: 50–100 mg for adults, and 0.6 mg/kg of body weight in children.
When treatment is initiated by the intramuscular route of administration, subsequent doses may be administered orally.
As with all potent medication, the dosage should be adjusted according to the patient's response to therapy.
Store below 86°F (30°C) and dispense in tight, light-resistant container as defined in the U.S.P.

HOW SUPPLIED

10 mg—light lavender colored, coated tablets in bottles of 100 (NDC 0066-0044-68); 25 mg—dark lavender colored, coated tablets in bottles of 100 (NDC 0066-0045-68).
Manufactured by Par Pharmaceutical, Inc.
Upper Saddle River, NJ 07458
FOR
DERMIK LABORATORIES, INC.
Fort Washington, PA 19034

FLORONE® ℞

[flōr-ōhn]
(brand of diflorasone diacetate cream and diflorasone diacetate ointment 0.05%)
Not For Ophthalmic Use

DESCRIPTION

Each gram of FLORONE Cream and FLORONE Ointment contains 0.5 mg diflorasone diacetate in a cream or ointment base.
Chemically, diflorasone diacetate is: 6α, 9α-difluoro-11β, 17,21-trihydroxy-16β-methylpregna-1,4-diene-3,20-dione 17,21 diacetate.
FLORONE Cream contains diflorasone diacetate in an emulsified and hydrophilic cream base consisting of propylene glycol, stearic acid, polysorbate 60, sorbitan monostearate and monooleate, sorbic acid, citric acid and water. The corticosteroid is formulated as a solution in the vehicle using 15 percent propylene glycol to optimize drug delivery.
FLORONE Ointment contains diflorasone diacetate in an emollient, occlusive base consisting of polyoxypropylene 15-stearyl ether, stearic acid, lanolin alcohol and white petrolatum.

CLINICAL PHARMACOLOGY

Topical corticosteroids share anti-inflammatory, antipruritic and vasoconstrictive actions.
The mechanism of anti-inflammatory activity of the topical corticosteroids is unclear. Various laboratory methods, including vasoconstrictor assays, are used to compare and predict potencies and/or clinical efficacies of the topical corticosteroids. There is some evidence to suggest that a recognizable correlation exists between vasoconstrictor potency and therapeutic efficacy in man.
Pharmacokinetics: The extent of percutaneous absorption of topical corticosteroids is determined by many factors including the vehicle, the integrity of the epidermal barrier and the use of occlusive dressings.
Topical corticosteroids can be absorbed from normal intact skin. Inflammation and/or other disease processes in the skin increase percutaneous absorption. Occlusive dressings substantially increase the percutaneous absorption of topical corticosteroids. Thus, occlusive dressings may be a valuable therapeutic adjunct for treatment of resistant dermatoses. (See DOSAGE AND ADMINISTRATION).
Once absorbed through the skin, topical corticosteroids are handled through pharmacokinetic pathways similar to systemically administered corticosteroids. Corticosteroids are bound to plasma proteins in varying degrees. They are metabolized primarily in the liver and are then excreted by the kidneys. Some of the topical corticosteroids and their metabolites are also excreted into the bile.

INDICATIONS AND USAGE

Topical corticosteroids are indicated for relief of the inflammatory and pruritic manifestations of corticosteroid-responsive dermatoses.

CONTRAINDICATIONS

Topical steroids are contraindicated in those patients with a history of hypersensitivity to any of the components of the preparation.

PRECAUTIONS

General:
Systemic absorption of topical corticosteroids has produced reversible hypothalamic-pituitary-adrenal (HPA) axis suppression, manifestations of Cushing's syndrome, hyperglycemia, and glucosuria in some patients.
Conditions which augment systemic absorption include the application of the more potent steroids, use over large surface areas, prolonged use, and the addition of occlusive dressings.
Therefore, patients receiving a large dose of a potent topical steroid applied to a large surface area or under an occlusive dressing should be evaluated periodically for evidence of HPA axis suppression by using the urinary free cortisol and ACTH stimulation tests. If HPA axis suppression is noted, an attempt should be made to withdraw the drug, to reduce the frequency of application, or to substitute a less potent steroid.
Recovery of HPA axis function is generally prompt and complete upon discontinuation of the drug. Infrequently, signs and symptoms of steroid withdrawal may occur, requiring supplemental systemic corticosteroids.
Children may absorb proportionally larger amounts of topical corticosteroids and thus be more susceptible to systemic toxicity. (See PRECAUTIONS—Pediatric Use)
If irritation develops, topical corticosteroids should be discontinued and appropriate therapy instituted.
In the presence of dermatological infections, the use of an appropriate antifungal or antibacterial agent should be instituted. If a favorable response does not occur promptly, the corticosteroid should be discontinued until the infection has been adequately controlled.
Information for the Patient: Patients using topical corticosteroids should receive the following information and instructions:

1. This medication is to be used as directed by the physician. It is for external use only. Avoid contact with the eyes.
2. Patients should be advised not to use this medication for any disorder other than for which it was prescribed.
3. The treated skin area should not be bandaged or otherwise covered or wrapped as to be occlusive unless directed by the physician.
4. Patients should report any signs of local adverse reactions especially under occlusive dressing.
5. Parents of pediatric patients should be advised not to use tight-fitting diapers or plastic pants on a child being treated in the diaper area, as these garments may constitute occlusive dressings.

Laboratory Tests: The following tests may be helpful in evaluating the HPA axis suppression:
Urinary free cortisol test
ACTH stimulation test
Carcinogenesis, Mutagenesis, and Impairment of Fertility: Long-term animal studies have not been performed to evaluate the carcinogenic potential or the effect on fertility of topical corticosteroids.
Studies to determine mutagenicity with prednisolone and hydrocortisone have revealed negative results.
Pregnancy Category C: Corticosteroids are generally teratogenic in laboratory animals when administered systemically at relatively low dosage levels. The more potent corticosteroids have been shown to be teratogenic after dermal application in laboratory animals. There are no adequate and well-controlled studies in pregnant women on teratogenic effects from topically applied corticosteroids. Therefore, topical corticosteroids should be used during pregnancy only if the potential benefit justifies the potential risk to the fetus. Drugs of this class should not be used extensively on pregnant patients, in large amounts, or for prolonged periods of time.
Nursing Mothers: It is not known whether topical administration of corticosteroids could result in sufficient systemic absorption to produce detectable quantities in breast milk. Systemically administered corticosteroids are secreted into breast milk in quantities **not** likely to have a deleterious effect on the infant. Nevertheless, caution should be exercised when topical corticosteroids are administered to a nursing woman.
Pediatric Use *Pediatric patients may demonstrate greater susceptibility to topical corticosteroid-induced HPA axis suppression and Cushing's syndrome than mature patients because of a larger skin surface area to body weight ratio.*
Hypothalamic-pituitary-adrenal (HPA) axis suppression, Cushing's syndrome, and intracranial hypertension have been reported in children receiving topical corticosteroids. Manifestations of adrenal suppression in children include linear growth retardation, delayed weight gain, low plasma cortisol levels, and absence of response to ACTH stimulation. Manifestations of intracranial hypertension include bulging fontanelles, headaches, and bilateral papilledema.
Administration of topical corticosteroids to children should be limited to the least amount compatible with an effective therapeutic regimen. Chronic corticosteroid therapy may interfere with the growth and development of children.

ADVERSE REACTIONS

The following local adverse reactions have been reported with topical corticosteroids, but may occur more frequently with the use of occlusive dressings. These reactions are listed in an approximate decreasing order of occurrence:

1. Burning
2. Itching
3. Irritation
4. Dryness
5. Folliculitis
6. Hypertrichosis
7. Acneiform eruptions
8. Hypopigmentation
9. Perioral dermatitis
10. Allergic contact dermatitis
11. Maceration of the skin
12. Secondary infection
13. Skin atrophy
14. Striae
15. Miliaria

OVERDOSAGE

Topically applied corticosteroids can be absorbed in sufficient amounts to produce systemic effects (See PRECAUTIONS).

DOSAGE AND ADMINISTRATION

Topical corticosteroids are generally applied to the affected area as a thin film from one to four times daily depending on the severity of the condition.
Occlusive dressings may be used for the management of psoriasis or recalcitrant conditions.
If an infection develops, the use of occlusive dressings should be discontinued and appropriate antimicrobial therapy instituted.

HOW SUPPLIED

FLORONE Cream is available as follows:
15 gram tube NDC 0066-0074-17
30 gram tube NDC 0066-0074-31
60 gram tube NDC 0066-0074-60
FLORONE Ointment is available as follows:
15 gram tube NDC 0066-0075-17
30 gram tube NDC 0066-0075-31
60 gram tube NDC 0066-0075-60

Continued on next page

Dermik—Cont.

HYTONE® Cream, Lotion and Ointment ℞
[*hi-tōne*]
(hydrocortisone)

DESCRIPTION

Cream —Each gram of 1% and 2½% Cream contains 10 mg or 25 mg, respectively, of hydrocortisone in a water-washable base of purified water, propylene glycol, glyceryl monostearate SE, cholesterol and related sterols, isopropyl myristate, polysorbate 60, cetyl alcohol, sorbitan monostearate, polyoxyl 40 stearate and sorbic acid.
Lotion —Each ml of 1% and 2½% Lotion contains 10 mg or 25 mg, respectively, of hydrocortisone in a vehicle consisting of carbomer 940, propylene glycol, polysorbate 40, propylene glycol stearate, cholesterol and related sterols, isopropyl myristate, sorbitan palmitate, cetyl alcohol, triethanolamine, sorbic acid, simethicone and purified water.
Ointment —Each gram of 1% and 2½% contains 10 mg or 25 mg, respectively, of hydrocortisone in a topical emollient base of mineral oil, white petrolatum and sorbitan sesquioleate.
Chemically, hydrocortisone is 11, 17, 21-trihydroxypregn-4-ene 3, 20-dione.
The topical corticosteroids including hydrocortisone, constitute a class of primarily synthetic steroids used as anti-inflammatory and antipruritic agents.

CLINICAL PHARMACOLOGY

Topical corticosteroids share anti-inflammatory, antipruritic and vasoconstrictive actions. The mechanism of anti-inflammatory activity of the topical corticosteroids is unclear. Various laboratory methods, including vasoconstrictor assays, are used to compare and predict potencies and/or clinical efficacies of the topical corticosteroids. There is some evidence to suggest that a recognizable correlation exists between vasoconstrictor potency and therapeutic efficacy in man.

Pharmacokinetics
The extent of percutaneous absorption of topical corticosteroids is determined by many factors including the vehicle, the integrity of the epidermal barrier, and the use of occlusive dressings.
Topical corticosteroids can be absorbed from normal intact skin. Inflammation and/or other disease processes in the skin increase percutaneous absorption. Occlusive dressings substantially increase the percutaneous absorption of topical corticosteroids. Thus, occlusive dressings may be a valuable therapeutic adjunct for treatment of resistant dermatoses.
(See *DOSAGE AND ADMINISTRATION.*)
Once absorbed through the skin, topical corticosteroids are handled through pharmacokinetic pathways similar to systemically administered corticosteroids. Corticosteroids are bound to plasma proteins in varying degrees. Corticosteroids are metabolized primarily in the liver and are then excreted by the kidneys. Some of the topical corticosteroids and their metabolites are also excreted into the bile.

INDICATIONS AND USAGE

Topical corticosteroids are indicated for the relief of the inflammatory and pruritic manifestations of corticosteroid-responsive dermatoses.

CONTRAINDICATIONS

Topical corticosteroids are contraindicated in those patients with a history of hypersensitivity to any of the components of the preparation.

PRECAUTIONS

General — Systemic absorption of topical corticosteroids has produced reversible hypothalamic-pituitary-adrenal (HPA) axis suppression, manifestations of Cushing's syndrome, hyperglycemia, and glucosuria in some patients.
Conditions which augment systemic absorption include the application of the more potent steroids, use over large surface areas, prolonged use, and the addition of occlusive dressings.
Therefore, patients receiving a large dose of a potent topical steroid applied to a large surface area or under an occlusive dressing should be evaluated periodically for evidence of HPA axis suppression by using the urinary free cortisol and ACTH stimulation tests. If HPA axis suppression is noted, an attempt should be made to withdraw the drug, to reduce the frequency of application, or to substitute a less potent steroid.
Recovery of HPA axis function is generally prompt and complete upon discontinuation of the drug. Infrequently, signs and symptoms of steroid withdrawal may occur, requiring supplemental systemic corticosteroids.
Children may absorb proportionally larger amounts of topical corticosteroids and thus be more susceptible to systemic toxicity (See PRECAUTIONS—Pediatric Use).
If irritation develops, topical corticosteroids should be discontinued and appropriate therapy instituted.
In the presence of dermatological infections, the use of an appropriate antifungal or antibacterial agent should be instituted. If a favorable response does not occur promptly, the corticosteroid should be discontinued until the infection has been adequately controlled.

Information for the Patient — Patients using topical corticosteroids should receive the following information and instructions:

1. This medication is to be used as directed by the physician. It is for external use only. Avoid contact with the eyes.
2. Patients should be advised not to use this medication for any disorder other than for which it was prescribed.
3. The treated skin area should not be bandaged or otherwise covered or wrapped as to be occlusive unless directed by the physician.
4. Patients should report any signs of local adverse reactions, especially under occlusive dressing.
5. Parents of pediatric patients should be advised not to use tight-fitting diapers or plastic pants on a child being treated in the diaper area, as these garments may constitute occlusive dressings.

Laboratory Tests — The following tests may be helpful in evaluating the HPA axis suppression:
Urinary free cortisol test
ACTH stimulation test

Carcinogenesis, Mutagenesis, and Impairment of Fertility — Long-term animal studies have not been performed to evaluate the carcinogenic potential or the effect on fertility of topical corticosteroids.
Studies to determine mutagenicity with prednisolone and hydrocortisone have revealed negative results.

Pregnancy Category C — Corticosteroids are generally teratogenic in laboratory animals when administered systemically at relatively low dosage levels. The more potent corticosteroids have been shown to be teratogenic after dermal application in laboratory animals. There are no adequate and well-controlled studies in pregnant women on teratogenic effects from topically applied corticosteroids. Therefore, topical corticosteroids should be used during pregnancy only if the potential benefit justifies the potential risk to the fetus. Drugs of this class should not be used extensively on pregnant patients, in large amounts, or for prolonged periods of time.

Nursing Mothers — It is not known whether topical administration of corticosteroids could result in sufficient systemic absorption to produce detectable quantities in breast milk. Systemically administered corticosteroids are secreted into breast milk in quantities *not* likely to have a deleterious effect on the infant. Nevertheless, caution should be exercised when topical corticosteroids are administered to a nursing woman.

Pediatric Use —*Pediatric patients may demonstrate greater susceptibility to topical corticosteroid-induced HPA axis suppression and Cushing's syndrome than mature patients because of a larger skin surface area to body weight ratio.*
Hypothalamic-pituitary-adrenal (HPA) axis suppression, Cushing's syndrome, and intracranial hypertension have been reported in children receiving topical corticosteroids. Manifestations of adrenal suppression in children include linear growth retardation, delayed weight gain, low plasma cortisol levels, and absence of response to ACTH stimulation. Manifestations of intracranial hypertension include bulging fontanelles, headaches, and bilateral papilledema.
Administration of topical corticosteroids to children should be limited to the least amount compatible with an effective therapeutic regimen. Chronic corticosteroid therapy may interfere with the growth and development of children.

ADVERSE REACTIONS

The following local adverse reactions are reported infrequently with topical corticosteroids, but may occur more frequently with the use of occlusive dressings. These reactions are listed in an approximate decreasing order of occurrence:

Burning	Perioral dermatitis
Itching	Allergic contact dermatitis
Irritation	Maceration of the skin
Dryness	Secondary infection
Folliculitis	Skin atrophy
Hypertrichosis	Striae
Acneiform eruptions	Miliaria
Hypopigmentation	

OVERDOSAGE

Topically applied corticosteroids can be absorbed in sufficient amounts to produce systemic effects (See PRECAUTIONS).

DOSAGE AND ADMINISTRATION

Topical corticosteroids are generally applied to the affected area as a thin film from two to four times daily depending on the severity of the condition. Occlusive dressings may be used for the management of psoriasis or recalcitrant conditions.
If an infection develops, the use of occlusive dressings should be discontinued and appropriate antimicrobial therapy instituted.

HOW SUPPLIED

Cream —2½% - tube 1 oz NDC 0066-0095-01; 1% - tube 1 oz NDC 0066-0083-01 and jar 4 oz NDC 0066-0083-04; ½% - tube 1 oz (OTC) NDC 0066-0182-01.
Lotion —2½% - bottle 2 fl oz NDC 0066-0098-02; 1% - bottle 4 fl oz NDC 0066-0090-04.
Ointment —2 ½% - tube 1 oz NDC 0066-0085-01; 1% - tube 1 oz NDC 0066-0087-01 and jar 4 oz NDC 0066-0087-04.

SULFACET-R® Acne Lotion ℞
[*sul-fa-set*]
(sodium sulfacetamide 10% and sulfur 5%)

DESCRIPTION

Each gram of Sulfacet-R® Acne Lotion (sodium sulfacetamide 10% and sulfur 5%) as dispensed, contains 100 mg of sodium sulfacetamide and 50 mg of sulfur in a flesh-tinted lotion of purified water, alkylaryl sulfonic acid salts, hydroxyethylcellulose, propylene glycol, xanthan gum, lauric myristic diethanolamide, polyoxyethylene laurate, butylparaben, methylparaben, silicone emulsion, talc, zinc oxide, titanium dioxide, attapulgite, iron oxides, pH buffers and 2-bromo-2-nitropropane-1, 3-diol.
Sodium sulfacetamide is a sulfonamide with antibacterial activity while sulfur acts as a keratolytic agent. Chemically sodium sulfacetamide is N′-[(4-aminophenyl)sulfonyl]-acetamide, monosodium salt, monohydrate.

CLINICAL PHARMACOLOGY

The most widely accepted mechanism of action of sulfonamides is the Woods-Fildes theory which is based on the fact that sulfonamides act as competitive antagonists to para-aminobenzoic acid (PABA), an essential component for bacterial growth. While absorption through intact skin has not been determined, sodium sulfacetamide is readily absorbed from the gastrointestinal tract when taken orally and excreted in the urine, largely unchanged. The biological half-life has variously been reported as 7 to 12.8 hours.
The exact mode of action of sulfur in the treatment of acne is unknown, but it has been reported that it inhibits the growth of *p. acnes* and the formation of free fatty acids.

INDICATIONS

Sulfacet-R® is indicated in the topical control of acne vulgaris, acne rosacea and seborrheic dermatitis.

CONTRAINDICATIONS

Sulfacet-R® Acne Lotion is contraindicated for use by patients having known hypersensitivity to sulfonamides, sulfur, or any other component of this preparation. Sulfacet-R® Acne Lotion is not to be used by patients with kidney disease.

WARNINGS

Although rare, sensitivity to sodium sulfacetamide may occur. Therefore, caution and careful supervision should be observed when prescribing this drug for patients who may be prone to hypersensitivity to topical sulfonamides. Systemic toxic reactions such as agranulocytosis, acute hemolytic anemia, purpura hemorrhagica, drug fever, jaundice and contact dermatitis indicate hypersensitivity to sulfonamides. Particular caution should be employed if areas of denuded or abraded skin are involved.

PRECAUTIONS

General—if irritation develops, use of the product should be discontinued and appropriate therapy instituted. For external use only. Keep away from eyes. Patients should be carefully observed for possible local irritation or sensitization during long-term therapy. The object of this therapy is to achieve desquamation without irritation, but sodium sulfacetamide and sulfur can cause reddening and scaling of epidermis. These side effects are not unusual in the treatment of acne vulgaris, but patients should be cautioned about the possibility. Keep out of the reach of children.

Carcinogenesis, Mutagenesis and Impairment of Fertility—Long-term studies in animals have not been performed to evaluate carcinogenic potential.

Pregnancy—Pregnancy Category C. Animal reproduction studies have not been conducted with Sulfacet-R® Acne Lotion. It is also not known whether Sulfacet-R® Acne Lotion can cause fetal harm when administered to a pregnant woman or can affect reproduction capacity. Sulfacet-R® Acne Lotion should be given to a pregnant woman only if clearly needed.

Nursing Mothers—It is not known whether sodium sulfacetamide is excreted in the human milk following topical use of Sulfacet-R® Acne Lotion. However, small amounts of orally administered sulfonamides have been reported to be eliminated in human milk. In view of this and because many drugs are excreted in human milk, caution should be exer-

cised when Sulfacet-R® Acne Lotion is administered to a nursing woman.
Pediatric Use—Safety and effectiveness in children under the age of 12 have not been established.

ADVERSE REACTIONS
Although rare, sodium sulfacetamide may cause local irritation.

DOSAGE AND ADMINISTRATION
Shake well before using. Apply a thin film to affected areas with light massaging to blend in each application 1 to 3 times daily. Each package contains a Dermik Color Blender™ which enables the patient to alter the basic shade of the lotion so that it matches the skin color exactly.
(Important to the Pharmacist—At the time of dispensing, add contents of vial* to the bottle.
Shake well and/or stir with a glass rod to ensure uniform dispersion. Place expiration date of four (4) months on bottle label.)
*Sulfa-Pak™ vial contains 2.1 grams of sodium sulfacetamide.

HOW SUPPLIED
25g bottles
NDC 0066-0028-25

VANOXIDE-HC® Acne Lotion ℞
[*van-ox-īd*]
(Clear)

DESCRIPTION
Each gram of Vanoxide-HC® Lotion contains, as dispensed, 50 mg benzoyl peroxide, and 5 mg hydrocortisone, incorporated in a water-washable lotion of purified water, calcium phosphate, propylene glycol, caprylic/capric triglyceride, propylene glycol monostearate, laneth-10 acetate, decyl oleate, polysorbate 20, cetyl alcohol, mineral oil, lanolin alcohol, sodium phosphate, sodium biphosphate, stearyl heptanoate, hydroxyethylcellulose, tetrasodium EDTA, cyclohexanediamine tetraacetic acid, propylparaben, methylparaben, vegetable oil, monoglyceride citrate, silica, simethicone, BHT, sodium hydroxide, BHA, propyl gallate, FD&C colors.

CLINICAL PHARMACOLOGY
Benzoyl peroxide is an antibacterial agent which has been shown to be effective against *Propionibacterium acnes.* This action is believed to be largely responsible for its usefulness. In addition, benzoyl peroxide exerts a desquamative and keratolytic action. One study in the rhesus monkey demonstrated a percutaneous absorption of about 1.8 μg per cm^2 of benzoyl peroxide or 45% of the applied dose in a 24-hour period. The absorbed benzoyl peroxide was completely converted in the skin to benzoic acid.
Topical steroids are primarily effective because of their anti-inflammatory, antipruritic and vasoconstrictive actions.

INDICATIONS AND USAGE
Treatment of acne vulgaris and oily skin.

CONTRAINDICATIONS
Vanoxide-HC® Lotion is contraindicated in individuals having known sensitivity to benzoyl peroxide, hydrocortisone or any of the components of the product. Topical steroids are contraindicated in viral diseases of the skin, such as varicella or vaccinia.

WARNINGS
If itching, redness, swelling or undue dryness occurs, discontinue use.

PRECAUTIONS
For external use only. Keep away from the eyes and mucosae. Very fair individuals should begin with a single application at bedtime allowing overnight medication. May bleach colored fabrics.
Carcinogenesis, Mutagenesis, Impairment of Fertility—Long-term studies in animals have not been performed to evaluate carcinogenic potential.
Pregnancy, Category C—Animal reproduction studies have not been conducted with Vanoxide-HC® Lotion. It is not known whether Vanoxide-HC® Lotion can cause fetal harm when administered to a pregnant woman or can affect reproduction capacity. Vanoxide-HC® Lotion should be given to a pregnant woman only if clearly needed.
Nursing Mothers—It is not known whether this drug is excreted in human milk. Because many drugs are excreted in human milk, caution should be exercised when Vanoxide-HC® Lotion is administered to a nursing woman.
Pediatric Use—Safety and effectiveness in children under the age of 12 have not been established.

ADVERSE REACTIONS
Irritation and contact dermatitis are the most frequent side reactions to benzoyl peroxide. Although 0.5% hydrocortisone is considered safe, the following adverse reactions have been reported with topical corticosteroids, especially under occlusive dressings: burning, itching, irritation, dryness, folliculitis, hypertrichosis, acneform eruptions, hypopigmentation, perioral dermatitis, allergic contact dermatitis, maceration of the skin, secondary infection, skin atrophy, striae, miliaria.

DOSAGE AND ADMINISTRATION
Shake well before using. Apply a thin film 1 to 3 times daily with gentle massaging to blend with skin, or as directed by physician.

HOW SUPPLIED
Bottles, 25 grams net weight as dispensed. Package contains a bottle of lotion base and a Benzie-Pak™ vial containing a mixture of benzoyl peroxide, 35%, and calcium phosphate, 64%, silica 1%. Net weight of vial is 3.8 grams.
To the Pharmacist—At the time of dispensing, add contents of Benzie-Pak™ to the lotion in the bottle. Shake well and /or stir with glass rod to ensure uniform dispersion. Place expiration date of three (3) months on bottle label.

VLEMASQUE®
[*vle-mask*]
(6% sulfurated lime topical solution)

DESCRIPTION
Contains sulfurated lime topical solution 6%, S.D. alcohol 7% in a drying clay mask.

INDICATION
For the treatment of acne.

DIRECTIONS
Daily, apply generous layer over entire face and neck, or as directed by physician. Avoid eyes, nostrils and lips. Leave on for 20-25 minutes. Remove with lukewarm water, using a gentle circular motion. Pat dry.

WARNINGS
Keep away from eyes. In case of contact, flush eyes thoroughly. For external use only. If any irritation appears, stop treatment immediately and consult physician.

HOW SUPPLIED
4 oz jars

VYTONE® CREAM ℞
[*vī-tone*]
(hydrocortisone-iodoquinol)

DESCRIPTION
Each gram of Vytone® Cream ½% and 1% contains 5 mg or 10 mg of hydrocortisone, respectively, and 10 mg of iodoquinol in a greaseless base of purified water, propylene glycol, glyceryl monostearate SE, cholesterol and related sterols, isopropyl myristate, polysorbate 60, cetyl alcohol, sorbitan monostearate, polyoxyl 40 stearate, sorbic acid, and polysorbate 20.
Chemically, hydrocortisone is 11, 17, 21-trihydroxypregn-4-ene-3, 20-dione and iodoquinol, 5,7-diiodo-8-quinolinol.
Hydrocortisone is an anti-inflammatory and antipruritic agent, while iodoquinol is an antifungal and antibacterial agent.

CLINICAL PHARMACOLOGY
Hydrocortisone has anti-inflammatory, antipruritic and vasoconstrictor properties. The mechanism of anti-inflammatory activity is unclear. There is some evidence to suggest that a recognizable correlation exists between vasoconstrictor potency and therapeutic efficacy in man.
Iodoquinol has both antifungal and antibacterial properties.
Pharmacokinetics
The extent of percutaneous absorption of topical corticosteroids is determined by many factors including vehicle, the integrity of the epidermal barrier, and the use of occlusive dressings.
Hydrocortisone can be absorbed from normal intact skin. Inflammation and/or other inflammatory disease processes in the skin increase percutaneous absorption. Occlusive dressings substantially increase the percutaneous absorption of topical corticosteroids.
Once absorbed through the skin, hydrocortisone is metabolized in the liver and most body tissues to hydrogenated and degraded forms such as tetrahydrocortisone and tetrahydrocortisol. These are excreted in the urine, mainly conjugated as glucuronides, together with a very small proportion of unchanged hydrocortisone.
There are no data available regarding the percutaneous absorption of iodoquinol; however, following oral administration, 3–5% of the dose was recovered in the urine as a glucuronide.

INDICATIONS AND USAGE
Based on a review of a related drug by the National Research Council and subsequent FDA classification for that drug, the indications are as follows:
"Possibly" Effective: Contact or atopic dermatitis; impetiginized eczema; nummular eczema; infantile eczema; endogenous chronic infectious dermatitis; stasis dermatitis; pyoderma; nuchal eczema and chronic eczematoid otitis externa; acne urticata; localized or disseminated neurodermatitis; lichen simplex chronicus; anogenital pruritus (vulvae, scroti, ani); folliculitis, bacterial dermatoses; mycotic dermatoses such as tinea (capitis, cruris, corporis, pedis); moniliasis, intertrigo.
Final classification of the less-than-effective indications requires further investigation.

CONTRAINDICATIONS
Vytone® Cream is contraindicated in those patients with a history of hypersensitivity to hydrocortisone, iodoquinol or any other components of the preparation.

WARNINGS AND PRECAUTIONS
For external use only. Keep away from eyes. If irritation develops, the use of Vytone® Cream should be discontinued and appropriate therapy instituted. Staining of the skin and fabrics may occur. If extensive areas are treated or if the occlusive technique is used, the possibility exists of increased systemic absorption of the corticosteroid, and suitable precautions should be taken. Children may absorb proportionally larger amounts of topical corticosteroids and thus be more susceptible to systemic toxicity. Parents of pediatric patients should be advised not to use tight-fitting diapers or plastic pants on a child being treated in the diaper area, as these garments may constitute occlusive dressings. Iodoquinol may be absorbed through the skin and interfere with thyroid function tests. If such tests are contemplated, wait at least one month after discontinuance of therapy to perform these tests. The ferric chloride test for phenylketonuria (PKU) can yield a false positive result if iodoquinol is present in the diaper or urine.
Prolonged use may result in overgrowth of non-susceptible organisms requiring appropriate therapy. Keep out of reach of children.
Carcinogenesis, Mutagenesis and Impairment of Fertility: Long-term animal studies have not been performed to evaluate the carcinogenic potential or the effect on fertility of hydrocortisone or iodoquinol.
In vitro studies to determine mutagenicity with hydrocortisone have revealed negative results. Mutagenicity studies have not been conducted with iodoquinol.
Pregnancy Category C: Animal reproduction studies have not been conducted with Vytone® Cream. It is not known whether Vytone® Cream can cause fetal harm when administered to a pregnant woman or can affect reproductive capacity. Vytone® Cream should be given to a pregnant woman only if clearly needed.
Nursing Mothers: It is not known whether this drug is excreted in human milk. Because many drugs are excreted in human milk, caution should be exercised when Vytone® Cream is administered to a nursing woman.
Pediatric Use: Safety and effectiveness in children under the age of 12 have not been established.

ADVERSE REACTIONS
The following local adverse reactions are reported infrequently with topical corticosteroids. These reactions are listed in an approximate decreasing order of occurrence.

Burning	Perioral dermatitis
Itching	Allergic contact dermatitis
Irritation	Maceration of the skin
Dryness	Secondary infection
Folliculitis	Skin atrophy
Hypertrichosis	Striae
Acneiform eruptions	Miliaria
Hypopigmentation	

DOSAGE AND ADMINISTRATION
Apply to affected area 3 to 4 times daily in accordance with physician's directions.

HOW SUPPLIED
½%-Tube 1 oz NDC 0066-0049-01,
1%-Tube 1 oz NDC 0066-0051-01

ZETAR® EMULSION (Coal Tar) ℞
[*zē-tar*]

DESCRIPTION
Zetar® Emulsion, coal tar, is a liquid for topical application, following dilution in aqueous media. Each ml contains 300 mg whole coal tar in polysorbates. It is a topical anti-eczematic. The complete chemical composition of coal tar has not been ascertained; components are grouped into six categories: aromatic hydrocarbons, acidic phenolic compounds, cyclic nitrogen compounds, organic sulfur compounds, nonacidic phenolics and nonbasic nitrogen compounds.

Continued on next page

Dermik—Cont.

CLINICAL PHARMACOLOGY

There is no confirmed scientific evidence as to the clinical pharmacologic effects of coal tar. Its actions in humans have been reported in the literature as antiseptic, antipruritic, antiparasitic, antifungal, antibacterial, keratoplastic and antiacanthotic. Vasoconstrictive activity of coal tar has also been reported.

INDICATIONS AND USAGE

Zetar® Emulsion is indicated for the relief of symptoms associated with generalized, persistent dermatoses such as psoriasis, eczema, atopic dermatitis and seborrheic dermatitis.

CONTRAINDICATIONS

Not to be used on open or infected lesions.

WARNINGS

Application of coal tar may elicit a pustular eruption or a cyst (epidermal) like reaction.

Patients who have previously exhibited sensitivity to tars must be under careful and continuous supervision by the physician.

PRECAUTIONS

For external (topical) use only. Keep away from the eyes. When used in the bath, add lukewarm water (not hot water). For 72 hours following treatment with coal tar, patients should avoid exposure to either direct sunlight or sunlamps (ultra-violet A and/or B) unless directed by physician, as this drug may photoactivate the skin. Prior to exposure to sunlight, completely remove all tar from skin. Sensitization or dermatitis may occur after prolonged use. If irritation develops or increases, discontinue use and consult physician. Keep out of the reach of children.

While no known drug interactions have been reported pertaining to the clinical use of this drug in patients, the concomitant use of drugs with phototoxic and/or photoactivating potential is not recommended (i.e. tetracyclines, psoralens, topical retinoic acid).

Carcinogenesis—Coal tar applied to the skin of mice resulted in an increase in epidermal carcinomas. Painting rabbit ears with coal tar appears to increase self-limiting keratoacanthomas. To date, existing reports do not suggest an increased incidence of skin cancer in psoriatics treated with coal tar.

Pregnancy Category C—Animal reproduction studies have not been conducted with Zetar® Emulsion (coal tar). It is also not known whether Zetar® Emulsion can cause fetal harm when administered to a pregnant woman or can affect reproduction capacity. Zetar® Emulsion should be given to a pregnant woman only if clearly needed.

Nursing Mothers—It is not known whether this drug is excreted in human milk. Because of the tumorigenicity shown for coal tar in animal studies, a decision should be made whether to discontinue nursing or to discontinue the drug, taking into account the importance of the drug to the mother.

ADVERSE REACTIONS

Application of coal tar may result in superficial folliculitis. Patients hypersensitive to coal tar may exhibit a pustular or keratocystic response.

DOSAGE AND ADMINISTRATION

Add 3 to 5 teaspoonfuls of Zetar® Emulsion to a bath of lukewarm water. This is mixed throughout the bath. The patient immerses in the bath for 15 to 20 minutes. The interval recommended between dosing is from once-a-day to once every third day, and usual duration of treatment is 30 to 45 days.

If the physician decides to administer supplemental ultraviolet irradiation (Goeckerman treatment) to the patient (ultraviolet B; A or A/B), this may be accomplished between 2 and 72 hours. A determination of minimal erythemal dosage (MED) should be made for each patient; initial irradiation should be suberythemal, not to exceed MED.

Compounding: Zetar® Emulsion (coal tar) may be utilized in compounding prescriptions in aqueous based vehicles requiring coal tar. Each ml of Zetar® Emulsion contains 300 mg whole coal tar.

HOW SUPPLIED

Zetar® Emulsion (coal tar) is available in 6 fl oz (177 ml) plastic bottles. The strength of the preparation is 300 mg coal tar/mL.

SHAKE WELL before each use. No special handling or storage conditions are required.

ZETAR® SHAMPOO
[zē-tar]

DESCRIPTION

WHOLE Coal Tar (as Zetar®) 1.0% in a golden foam shampoo which produces soft, fluffy abundant lather.

ACTIONS AND INDICATIONS

Antiseptic, antibacterial, antiseborrheic. Loosens and softens scales and crusts. Indicated in psoriasis, seborrhea, dandruff, cradle-cap and other oily, itchy conditions of the body and scalp.

CONTRAINDICATIONS

Acute inflammation, open or infected lesions.

PRECAUTIONS

If undue skin irritation develops or increases, discontinue use and consult physician. In rare instances, temporary discoloration of blond, bleached, or tinted hair may occur. Avoid contact with eyes.

DOSAGE AND ADMINISTRATION

Massage into moistened scalp. Rinse. Repeat; leave on 5 minutes. Rinse thoroughly.

HOW SUPPLIED

6 oz plastic bottles.

Dista Products Company
Division of Eli Lilly and Company
LILLY CORPORATE CENTER
INDIANAPOLIS, IN 46285

LEGEND

Hyporets®—*Disposable Syringes, Dista*
Identi-Code®—*Formula Identification Code, Dista*
Identi-Dose®—*Unit Dose Medication, Dista*
Pulvules®—*Filled Gelatin Capsules, Dista*
℞Pak—*Prescription Package, Dista*
Traypak™—*Multivial Carton, Dista*

IDENTI-CODE® Index

Illustrations of examples of products bearing Identi-Code® appear in the Product Identification Section.

Identi-Code® Product Name

C03-C22 (Coated Tablets)

C03 Ilotycin®
Composition (Each Enteric-Coated Tablet): Erythromycin, USP, 250 mg

C19 Mi-Cebrin®
Composition (Each Coated Tablet): Thiamine (vitamin B_1), 10 mg; riboflavin (vitamin B_2), 5 mg; pyridoxine (vitamin B_6), 1.7 mg; pantothenic acid, 10 mg; niacinamide, 30 mg; vitamin B_{12} (activity equivalent), 3 mcg; ascorbic acid (vitamin C), 100 mg; *dl*-alpha tocopheryl acetate (vitamin E), 5.5 IU (5.5 mg); vitamin A, 10,000 IU (3 mg); vitamin D, 400 IU (10 mcg); contains also (approximately): iron (as ferrous sulfate), 15 mg; copper (as the sulfate), 1 mg; iodine (as potassium iodide), 0.15 mg; manganese (as the glycerophosphate), 1 mg; magnesium (as the hydroxide), 5 mg; zinc (as the chloride), 1.5 mg

C20 Mi-Cebrin T®
Composition (Each Coated Tablet): Thiamine mononitrate (vitamin B_1), 15 mg; riboflavin (vitamin B_2), 10 mg; pyridoxine hydrochloride (vitamin B_6), 2 mg; pantothenic acid (as calcium pantothenate), 10 mg; niacinamide, 100 mg; vitamin B_{12} (activity equivalent), 7.5 mcg; ascorbic acid (vitamin C), 150 mg; *dl*-alpha tocopheryl acetate (vitamin E), 5.5 IU (5.5 mg); vitamin A, 10,000 IU (3 mg); vitamin D, 400 IU (10 mcg); contains also (approximately): iron (as ferrous sulfate), 15 mg; copper (as the sulfate), 1 mg; iodine (as potassium iodide), 0.15 mg; manganese (as the glycerophosphate), 1 mg; magnesium (as the hydroxide), 5 mg; zinc (as the chloride), 1.5 mg

C22 Becotin®-T
Composition (Each Coated Tablet): Thiamine mononitrate (vitamin B_1), 15 mg; riboflavin (vitamin B_2), 10 mg; pyridoxine hydrochloride (vitamin B_6), 5 mg; niacinamide, 100 mg; pantothenic acid (as calcium pantothenate), 20 mg; vitamin B_{12} (activity equivalent), 4 mcg; ascorbic acid (vitamin C) (as sodium ascorbate), 300 mg

---

F62-H77 (Pulvules®)

F62 Becotin®
Composition (Each Pulvule®): Thi- amine hydrochloride (vitamin B_1), 10 mg; riboflavin (vitamin B_2), 10 mg; pyridoxine (vitamin B_6), 4.1 mg; niacinamide, 50 mg; pantothenic acid, 25 mg; vitamin B_{12} (activity equivalent), 1 mcg

F77 Becotin® with Vitamin C
Composition (Each Pulvule®): Thi- amine hydrochloride (vitamin B_1), 10 mg; riboflavin (vitamin B_2), 10 mg; pyridoxine (vitamin B_6), 4.1 mg; niacinamide, 50 mg; pantothenic acid, 25 mg; vitamin B_{12} (activity equivalent), 1 mcg; ascorbic acid (vitamin C), 150 mg

3055 Cinobac®
Composition (Each Pulvule®): Cinoxacin, USP, 250 mg

3056 Cinobac®
Composition (Each Pulvule®): Cinoxacin, USP, 500 mg

3122 Co-Pyronil 2®, Pediatric
Composition (Each Pulvule®): chlorpheniramine maleate, 2 mg; pseudoephedrine hydrochloride, 30 mg

3123 Co-Pyronil 2®
Composition (Each Pulvule®): chlorpheniramine maleate, 4 mg; pseudoephedrine hydrochloride, 60 mg

---

H07 Ilosone®
Composition (Each Pulvule®): Erythromycin Estolate, USP, 125 mg (equiv. to erythromycin)

H09 Ilosone®
Composition (Each Pulvule®): Erythromycin Estolate, USP, 250 mg (equiv. to erythromycin)

H69 Keflex®
Composition (Each Pulvule®): Cephalexin, USP, 250 mg

H71 Keflex®
Composition (Each Pulvule®): Cephalexin, USP, 500 mg

ⒸH74 Valmid®
Composition (Each Pulvule®): Ethinamate, USP, 500 mg

H76 Nalfon® 200
Composition (Each Pulvule®): Fenoprofen Calcium, USP, 200 mg (equiv. to fenoprofen)

H77 Nalfon®
Composition (Each Pulvule®): Fenoprofen Calcium, USP, 300 mg (equiv. to fenoprofen)

U05-U60 (Compressed Tablets)

U05 Ilosone® Chewable
Composition (Each Compressed Tablet): Erythromycin Estolate, USP, 125 mg (equiv. to erythromycin)

U25 Ilosone® Chewable
Composition (Each Compressed Tablet): Erythromycin Estolate, USP, 250 mg (equiv. to erythromycin)

U26 Ilosone®
Composition (Each Compressed Tablet): Erythromycin Estolate, USP, 500 mg (equiv. to erythromycin)

U59 Nalfon®
Composition (Each Compressed Tablet): Fenoprofen Calcium, USP, 600 mg (equiv. to fenoprofen)

U60 Keflex®
Composition (Each Compressed Tablet): Cephalexin, 1 g

W03-W68 (Miscellaneous)

W03 Ilosone®, for Oral Suspension
Composition (When Mixed as Directed): Each 5 ml contain erythromycin estolate equivalent to 125 mg erythromycin (USP).

W14 Cordran® Tape
Composition: Flurandrenolide, USP, 4 mcg/sq cm

W15 Ilosone® Liquid, Oral Suspension
Composition: Each 5 ml contain erythromycin estolate equivalent to 125 mg erythromycin (USP).

W17 Ilosone® Liquid, Oral Suspension
Composition: Each 5 ml contain erythromycin estolate equivalent to 250 mg erythromycin (USP).

W18 Ilosone® Ready-Mixed Drops
Composition: Each ml contains erythromycin estolate equivalent to 100 mg erythromycin (USP).

W21 Keflex®, for Oral Suspension
Composition (When Mixed as Directed): Each 5 ml contain 125 mg cephalexin (USP).

W22 Keflex®, for Pediatric Drops
Composition (When Mixed as Directed): Each ml contains 100 mg cephalexin (USP).

W68 Keflex®, for Oral Suspension
Composition (When Mixed as Directed): Each 5 ml contain 250 mg cephalexin (USP).

UNIT-DOSE PACKAGING

Identi-Dose® (unit dose medication, Dista) Closed-circuit control of medication from pharmacy to nurse to patient and return. Simplifies counting and dispensing whether in single-unit or prescription-size quantities. Fits into any dispensing system for ready identification and legibility, better inventory control, protection from contamination, easier handling and recording under Medicare, prevention of drug loss through pilferage or spilling, better control of Federal Controlled Substances, and less chance of medication errors. The following products are available through normal channels of supply:

Identi-Dose®

Pulvules®

No.
325 Becotin® with Vitamin C
375 Ilosone®, 250 mg
402 Keflex®, 250 mg
403 Keflex®, 500 mg

Tablets

No.
1790 Mi-Cebrin®
1807 Mi-Cebrin T®
1810 Becotin®-T
1896 Keflex®, 1 g

Miscellaneous

No.
M-201 Keflex®, for Oral Suspension, 125 mg/5 ml
M-202 Keflex®, for Oral Suspension, 250 mg/5 ml

Shown in Product Identification Section, page 408

CINOBAC® ℞
[sĭn´ō-băk]
(cinoxacin)
Capsules, USP

DESCRIPTION
Cinobac® (cinoxacin, Dista) is a synthetic antimicrobial agent for oral administration. It is 1-ethyl-1,4-dihydro-4-oxo-[1,3] dioxolo[4,5-g]cinnoline-3-carboxylic acid and occurs as white or very light-yellow needle-shaped crystals. Cinobac is available as 250 and 500-mg Pulvules®. These Pulvules also contain D&C Yellow No. 10, FD&C Blue No. 1, FD&C Red No. 3, FD&C Yellow No. 6, gelatin, starch, titanium dioxide, and other inactive ingredients. Examples of other antibacterial drugs in this class are nalidixic acid and oxolinic acid.

CLINICAL PHARMACOLOGY
Cinoxacin is rapidly absorbed after oral administration. A 500-mg dose produced a peak serum concentration of 15 mcg/ml, which declined to approximately 1 to 2 mcg/ml six hours after administration, as determined by fluorometric assay. A 500-mg dose produced an average urine concentration of approximately 300 mcg/ml during the first four hours and approximately 100 mcg/ml during the second four-hour period. These urine concentrations are many times greater than the minimum inhibitory concentration (MIC) of cinoxacin for most gram-negative organisms commonly found in urinary tract infections.
Ninety-seven percent of a 500-mg oral dose of radiolabeled cinoxacin was recovered in the urine within 24 hours, 60 percent of which was present as unaltered cinoxacin and the remainder as inactive metabolic products.
The presence of food did not affect the total absorption of cinoxacin. Peak serum concentrations were reduced, but the 24-hour urinary recovery of antibacterial activity was unaltered. The mean serum half-life is 1.5 hours.
Microbiology—Cinoxacin has in vitro activity against a wide variety of aerobic gram-negative bacilli, particularly strains of *Enterobacteriaceae*. In vitro tests demonstrate that cinoxacin is bactericidal. The mode of action has been shown to be inhibition of bacterial DNA replication. It is active within the range of urinary pH.
Cinoxacin is active against most strains of the following organisms: *Escherichia coli, Klebsiella* species, *Enterobacter* species (including *E. aerogenes, E. cloacae,* and *E. hafniae*), *Proteus mirabilis,* and *P. vulgaris.*
Cinoxacin is not active against *Pseudomonas,* enterococci, or staphylococci. Cross-resistance with drugs in this class (nalidixic acid and oxolinic acid) has been demonstrated. Bacterial resistance to cinoxacin has been reported in less than 4 percent of patients treated with recommended doses; however, bacterial resistance to cinoxacin has not been shown to be transferable via R-factor.
Susceptibility Tests—Quantitative methods give the most precise estimates of susceptibility to antibacterial drugs. For purposes of judging susceptibility of bacterial isolates to cinoxacin, minimum inhibitory concentration and disc test breakpoints were established on the basis of (1) human drug bioavailability studies and (2) test results obtained with normally susceptible strains compared with results from resistant strains. The breakpoints have been verified by comparison with results of the clinical trials with cinoxacin.
One quantitative method, a standardized disc test, has been recommended.* Reports from the laboratory giving results of the standardized test using the 100-mcg cinoxacin disc should be interpreted according to the following criteria:

Organisms producing zones of 19 mm or greater are classified as susceptible, whereas those producing zones of 15 to 18 mm are classified as having intermediate susceptibility. Organisms in either of these categories are likely to respond to therapy if the infection is confined to the urinary tract.

Organisms producing zones of 14 mm or less are reported as resistant, indicating that other therapy should be selected.

Certain strains of *Enterobacteriaceae* exhibit heterogeneity of resistance to cinoxacin. These strains produce isolated colonies within the inhibition zone. When such strains are encountered, the clear inhibition zone should be measured *within* the isolated colonies.
Dilution methods for determining susceptibility are also used, and results are reported as the minimum drug concentration inhibiting microbial growth (MIC).

If the MIC is 16 mcg/ml or less, the microorganism is considered "susceptible"; if greater than 16 mcg/ml and less than 64 mcg/ml, it is "intermediate"; and it is "resistant" if the MIC is 64 mcg/ml or greater.

* Approved Standard ASM-2 Performance Standards for Antimicrobial Disc Susceptibility Tests; National Committee for Clinical Laboratory Standards, 771 East Lancaster Avenue, Villanova, Pennsylvania 19085.

INDICATIONS AND USAGE
Cinobac® (cinoxacin, Dista) is indicated for the treatment of initial and recurrent urinary tract infections in adults caused by the following susceptible microorganisms: *E. coli, P. mirabilis, P. vulgaris, Klebsiella pneumoniae* and *Klebsiella* species, and *Enterobacter* species.
In vitro susceptibility testing should be performed prior to administration of the drug and, when clinically indicated, during treatment.

CONTRAINDICATION
Cinobac® (cinoxacin, Dista) is contraindicated in patients with a history of hypersensitivity to cinoxacin.

WARNINGS
The use of cinoxacin in prepubertal children and during pregnancy is not recommended. The oral administration of a single 250-mg/kg dose of cinoxacin caused lameness in immature dogs. Histologic examination of the weight-bearing joints of these dogs revealed permanent lesions of the cartilage. Related drugs (e.g., nalidixic acid, oxolinic acid) also produce erosions of the cartilage in weight-bearing joints and other signs of arthropathy in immature animals of various species.

PRECAUTIONS
General—Since Cinobac® (cinoxacin, Dista) is eliminated primarily by the kidney, the usual dosage should be lower in patients with reduced renal function (*see* Dosage and Administration). Administration of Cinobac is not recommended for anuric patients.
Cinobac should be used with caution in patients with a history of hepatic disease.
Pregnancy—Pregnancy Category B—Reproduction studies have been performed in rats and rabbits at doses up to ten times the daily human dose and have revealed no evidence of impaired fertility or harm to the fetus due to cinoxacin. There are, however, no adequate and well-controlled studies in pregnant women. **Since cinoxacin, like other drugs in its class, causes arthropathy in immature animals, its use during pregnancy is not recommended (*see* Warnings).**
Nursing Mothers—It is not known whether cinoxacin is excreted in human milk. Because other drugs in this class are excreted in human milk and because of the potential for serious adverse reactions from cinoxacin in nursing infants, a decision should be made to discontinue nursing or to discontinue the drug, taking into account the importance of the drug to the mother.
Pediatric Use—Cinoxacin is not recommended for use in prepubertal children (*see* Warnings).

ADVERSE REACTIONS
In clinical studies in 1118 patients, the following adverse effects were considered related to cinoxacin therapy:

Gastrointestinal—Nausea was reported most commonly and occurred in less than 3 in 100 patients. Other side effects, occurring less frequently (1 in 100), were anorexia, vomiting, abdominal cramps, and diarrhea.

Central Nervous System—The most frequent side effects were headache and dizziness, reported by 1 in 100 patients. Other adverse reactions possibly related to Cinobac® (cinoxacin, Dista) include insomnia, tingling sensation, perineal burning, photophobia, and tinnitus, and these were reported by less than 1 in 100 patients.

Hypersensitivity—Rash, urticaria, pruritus, and edema were reported by less than 3 in 100 patients. Rare cases of anaphylactoid reactions.

Hematologic—Rare reports of thrombocytopenia.

Laboratory values that were reported to be abnormal were, in order of frequency, BUN (1 in 100) and SGOT, SGPT, serum creatinine, and alkaline phosphatase (each less than 1 in 100).

Although not observed in the 1118 patients treated with cinoxacin, the following side effects have been reported for other drugs in the same pharmacologically active and chemically related class: restlessness, nervousness, overbrightness of lights, change in color perception, difficulty in focusing, decrease in visual acuity, double vision, abdominal pain, weakness, constipation, angioedema, erythema and bullae, feelings of disorientation or agitation or acute anxiety, palpitation, soreness of the gums, drowsiness, joint stiffness, swelling of the extremities, metallic taste, toxic psychosis or convulsions (rare), reduction in hematocrit/hemoglobin, and eosinophilia.
All adverse reactions observed with drugs in this class were reversible.

DOSAGE AND ADMINISTRATION
The usual adult dosage for the treatment of urinary tract infections is 1 g daily, administered orally in two or four divided doses (500 mg b.i.d. or 250 mg q.i.d.) for seven to 14 days. Although susceptible organisms may be eradicated within a few days after therapy has begun, the full treatment course is recommended.
Impaired Renal Function—When renal function is impaired, a reduced dosage must be employed. After an initial dose of 500 mg, a maintenance dosage schedule should be used (*see* table).

MAINTENANCE DOSAGE GUIDE FOR PATIENTS WITH RENAL IMPAIRMENT

Creatinine Clearance ($ml/min./1.73\ m^2$)	Renal Function	Dosage
>80	Normal	500 mg b.i.d.
80–50	Mild Impairment	250 mg t.i.d.
50–20	Moderate Impairment	250 mg b.i.d.
<20	Marked Impairment	250 mg q.d.

Administration of Cinobac® (cinoxacin, Dista) to anuric patients is not recommended.
When only serum creatinine is available, the following formula (based on sex, weight, and age of the patient) may be used to convert this value into creatinine clearance. The serum creatinine should represent a steady state of renal function.

Males: $\frac{\text{Weight (kg)} \times (140 - \text{age})}{72 \times \text{serum creatinine}}$

Females: 0.9 x male value

HOW SUPPLIED
Pulvules:
250 mg, orange and green (No. 3055)—40 (NDC 0777-3055-40).
500 mg, orange and green (No. 3056)—50 (NDC 0777-3056-50).

ANIMAL PHARMACOLOGY
Crystalluria, sometimes associated with secondary urinary tract pathology, occurs in laboratory animals treated orally with cinoxacin. In the rhesus monkey, crystalluria (without urinary tract pathology) has been noted at doses as low as 50 mg/kg/day (lowest dose tested). Cinoxacin-related crystalluria has not been observed in humans receiving twice the recommended daily dosage.

Continued on next page

Dista—Cont.

Cinoxacin and related drugs have been shown to cause arthropathy in immature animals of most species tested (*see* Warnings).
Some drugs of this class have been shown to have oculotoxic potential. Cinoxacin administered to cats at high dosages (200 mg/kg/day) resulted in retinal degeneration and other ocular changes. The dog appeared to be somewhat resistant to these effects, but high dosages (500 mg/kg/day) resulted in mild retinal atrophy. No cinoxacin-related ocular changes were noted in the rabbit, rat, or monkey or in human studies. (In one of the studies in the monkey, cinoxacin was administered for one year at ten times the recommended clinical dose.)

[080585]

Shown in Product Identification Section, page 408

CORDRAN® and CORDRAN® SP ℞

[*kôr'drăn and kôr'drăn ĕs pē*]
(flurandrenolide) USP

DESCRIPTION

Cordran® (Flurandrenolide, USP, Dista) is a potent corticosteroid intended for topical use. It occurs as white to off-white, fluffy, crystalline powder and is odorless. Cordran is practically insoluble in water and in ether. One g dissolves in 72 ml of alcohol and in 10 ml of chloroform. The molecular weight of Cordran is 436.52.
The chemical name of Cordran is 6α-fluoro-16α -hydroxyhydrocortisone-16, 17 -acetonide; its empirical formula is $C_{24}H_{33}FO_6$.
Each g of Cream Cordran® SP (Flurandrenolide Cream, USP, Dista) contains 0.5 mg (0.05 percent) or 0.25 mg (0.025 percent) flurandrenolide in an emulsified base composed of cetyl alcohol, citric acid, mineral oil, polyoxyl 40 stearate, propylene glycol, sodium citrate, stearic acid, and purified water.
Each g of Ointment Cordran® (Flurandrenolide Ointment, USP, Dista) contains 0.5 mg (0.05 percent) or 0.25 mg (0.025 percent) flurandrenolide in a base composed of white wax, cetyl alcohol, sorbitan sesquioleate, and white petrolatum.
Each ml of Lotion Cordran® (Flurandrenolide Lotion, USP, Dista) contains 0.5 mg (0.05 percent) flurandrenolide in an oil-in-water emulsion base composed of glycerin, cetyl alcohol, stearic acid, glyceryl monostearate, mineral oil, polyoxyl 40 stearate, menthol, benzyl alcohol, and purified water.

CLINICAL PHARMACOLOGY

Cordran® (flurandrenolide, Dista) is primarily effective because of its anti-inflammatory, antipruritic, and vasoconstrictive actions.
The mechanism of the anti-inflammatory effect of topical corticosteroids is not completely understood. Various laboratory methods, including vasoconstrictor assays, are used to compare and predict potencies and/or clinical efficacies of the topical corticosteroids. There is some evidence to suggest that a recognizable correlation exists between vasoconstrictor potency and therapeutic efficacy in man. Corticosteroids with anti-inflammatory activity may stabilize cellular and lysosomal membranes. There is also the suggestion that the effect on the membranes of lysosomes prevents the release of proteolytic enzymes and, thus, plays a part in reducing inflammation.
Evaporation of water from the lotion vehicle produces a cooling effect which is often desirable in the treatment of acutely inflamed or weeping lesions.
Pharmacokinetics —The extent of percutaneous absorption of topical corticosteroids is determined by many factors, including the vehicle, the integrity of the epidermal barrier, and the use of occlusive dressings.
Topical corticosteroids can be absorbed from normal intact skin. Inflammation and/or other disease processes in the skin increase percutaneous absorption. Occlusive dressings substantially increase the percutaneous absorption of topical corticosteroids. Thus, occlusive dressings may be a valuable therapeutic adjunct for treatment of resistant dermatoses. *See* Dosage and Administration.
Once absorbed through the skin, topical corticosteroids are handled through pharmacokinetic pathways similar to those of systemically administered corticosteroids. Corticosteroids are bound to plasma proteins in varying degrees. Corticosteroids are metabolized primarily in the liver and then excreted in the kidneys. Some of the topical corticosteroids and their metabolites are also excreted into the bile.

INDICATIONS AND USAGE

Cordran® (flurandrenolide, Dista) is indicated for the relief of the inflammatory and pruritic manifestations of corticosteroid-responsive dermatoses.

CONTRAINDICATIONS

Topical corticosteroids are contraindicated in patients with a history of hypersensitivity to any of the components of these preparations.

PRECAUTIONS

General Precautions —Systemic absorption of topical corticosteroids has produced reversible hypothalamic-pituitary-adrenal (HPA) axis suppression, manifestations of Cushing's syndrome, hyperglycemia, and glucosuria in some patients. Conditions which augment systemic absorption include application of the more potent steroids, use over large surface areas, prolonged use, and the addition of occlusive dressings. Therefore, patients receiving a large dose of a potent topical steroid applied to a large surface area or under an occlusive dressing should be evaluated periodically for evidence of HPA axis suppression by using urinary-free cortisol and ACTH stimulation tests. If HPA axis suppression is noted, an attempt should be made to withdraw the drug, to reduce the frequency of application, or to substitute a less potent steroid.
Recovery of HPA axis function is generally prompt and complete upon discontinuation of the drug. Infrequently, signs and symptoms of steroid withdrawal may occur, so that supplemental systemic corticosteroids are required.
Children may absorb proportionately larger amounts of topical corticosteroids and thus be more susceptible to systemic toxicity *See* Precautions—Usage in Children.
If irritation develops, topical corticosteroids should be discontinued and appropriate therapy instituted.
In the presence of dermatologic infections, the use of an appropriate antifungal or antibacterial agent should be instituted. If a favorable response does not occur promptly, Cordran® (flurandrenolide, Dista) should be discontinued until the infection has been adequately controlled.
Information for the Patient —Patients using topical corticosteroids should receive the following information and instructions.

1. This medication is to be used as directed by the physician. It is for external use only. Avoid contact with the eyes.
2. Patients should be advised not to use this medication for any disorder other than that for which it was prescribed.
3. The treated skin area should not be bandaged or otherwise covered or wrapped in order to be occlusive unless the patient is directed to do so by the physician.
4. Patients should report any signs of local adverse reactions, especially under occlusive dressing.
5. Parents of pediatric patients should be advised not to use tight-fitting diapers or plastic pants on a child being treated in the diaper area, because these garments may constitute occlusive dressings.

Laboratory Tests —The following tests may be helpful in evaluating the HPA axis suppression:
Urinary-free cortisol test
ACTH stimulation test
Carcinogenesis, Mutagenesis, and Impairment of Fertility —Long-term animal studies have not been performed to evaluate the carcinogenic potential or the effect on fertility of topical corticosteroids.
Studies to determine mutagenicity with prednisolone and hydrocortisone have revealed negative results.
Usage in Pregnancy—Pregnancy Category C —Corticosteroids are generally teratogenic in laboratory animals when administered systemically at relatively low dosage levels. The more potent corticosteroids have been shown to be teratogenic after dermal application in laboratory animals. There are no adequate and well-controlled studies in pregnant women on teratogenic effects from topically applied corticosteroids. Therefore, topical corticosteroids should be used during pregnancy only if the potential benefit justifies the potential risk to the fetus. Drugs of this class should not be used extensively on pregnant patients or in large amounts or for prolonged periods of time.
Nursing Mothers —It is not known whether topical administration of corticosteroids could result in sufficient systemic absorption to produce detectable quantities in breast milk. Systemically administered corticosteroids are secreted into breast milk in quantities *not* likely to have a deleterious effect on the infant. Nevertheless, caution should be exercised when topical corticosteroids are administered to a nursing woman.
Usage in Children —Pediatric patients may demonstrate greater susceptibility to topical corticosteroid-induced HPA axis suppression and Cushing's syndrome than do mature patients because of a larger skin surface area to body weight ratio.
Hypothalamic-pituitary-adrenal (HPA) axis suppression, Cushing's syndrome, and intracranial hypertension have been reported in children receiving topical corticosteroids. Manifestations of adrenal suppression in children include linear growth retardation, delayed weight gain, low plasma cortisol levels, and absence of response to ACTH stimulation. Manifestations of intracranial hypertension include bulging fontanelles, headaches, and bilateral papilledema.
Administration of topical corticosteroids to children should be limited to the least amount compatible with an effective therapeutic regimen. Chronic corticosteroid therapy may interfere with the growth and development of children.

ADVERSE REACTIONS

The following local adverse reactions are reported infrequently with topical corticosteroids but may occur more frequently with the use of occlusive dressings. These reactions are listed in an approximate decreasing order of occurrence:
Burning
Itching
Irritation
Dryness
Folliculitis
Hypertrichosis
Acneiform eruptions
Hypopigmentation
Perioral dermatitis
Allergic contact dermatitis
Maceration of the skin
Secondary infection
Skin atrophy
Striae
Miliaria

OVERDOSAGE

Topically applied corticosteroids can be absorbed in sufficient amounts to produce systemic effects (*See* Precautions).

DOSAGE AND ADMINISTRATION

For moist lesions, a small quantity of the cream or lotion should be rubbed gently into the affected areas two or three times a day. For dry, scaly lesions, the ointment is applied as a thin film to affected areas two or three times daily.
Occlusive dressings may be used for the management of psoriasis or recalcitrant conditions.
If an infection develops, the use of occlusive dressings should be discontinued and appropriate antimicrobial therapy instituted.
Topical corticosteroids are generally applied to the affected area as a thin film one to four times daily, depending on the severity of the condition.

Use with Occlusive Dressings

The technique of occlusive dressings (for management of psoriasis and other persistent dermatoses) is as follows:
1. Remove as much as possible of the superficial scaling before applying Cream Cordran® SP (flurandrenolide, Dista) or Ointment or Lotion Cordran. Soaking in a bath will help soften the scales and permit easier removal by brushing, picking, or rubbing.
2. Rub Cream Cordran SP or Ointment or Lotion Cordran thoroughly into the affected areas.
3. Cover with an occlusive plastic film, such as polyethylene, Saran Wrap™, or Handi-Wrap®. (When Cream Cordran SP or Lotion Cordran is used, added moisture may be provided by placing a slightly dampened cloth or gauze over the lesion before the plastic film is applied.)
4. Seal the edges to adjacent normal skin with tape or hold in place by a gauze wrapping.
5. For convenience, the patient may remove the dressing during the day. The dressing should then be reapplied each night.
6. For daytime therapy, the condition may be treated by rubbing Cream Cordran SP or Ointment or Lotion Cordran sparingly into the affected areas.
7. In more resistant cases, leaving the dressing in place for three to four days at a time may result in a better response.
8. Thin polyethylene gloves are suitable for treatment of the hands and fingers; plastic garment bags may be utilized for treating lesions on the trunk or buttocks. A tight shower cap is useful in treating lesions on the scalp.

Occlusive Dressings Have the Following Advantages —1. Percutaneous penetration of the corticosteroid is enhanced.
2. Medication is concentrated on the areas of skin where it is most needed.
3. This method of administration frequently is more effective in very resistant dermatoses than is the conventional application of Cordran® (flurandrenolide, Dista).
Precautions to Be Observed in Therapy with Occlusive Dressings —Treatment should be continued for at least a few days after clearing of the lesions. If it is stopped too soon, a relapse may occur. Reinstitution of treatment frequently will cause remission.
Because of the increased hazard of secondary infection from resistant strains of staphylococci among hospitalized patients, it is suggested that the use of occlusive plastic films for corticosteroid therapy in such cases be restricted.
Generally, occlusive dressings should not be used on weeping, or exudative, lesions.
When large areas of the body are covered, thermal homeostasis may be impaired. If elevation of body temperature occurs, use of the occlusive dressing should be discontinued.
Rarely, a patient may develop miliaria, folliculitis, or a sensitivity to either the particular dressing material or a combination of Cordran® (flurandrenolide, Dista) and the occlusive dressing. If miliaria or folliculitis occurs, use of the oc-

clusive dressing should be discontinued. Treatment by inunction with a corticosteroid such as Cordran may be continued. If the sensitivity is caused by the particular material of the dressing, substitution of a different material may be tried.

Warnings—Some plastic films are readily flammable. Patients should be cautioned against the use of any such material.

When plastic films are used on infants and children, the persons caring for the patients must be reminded of the danger of suffocation if the plastic material accidentally covers the face.

HOW SUPPLIED

(℞) *Cordran® (Flurandrenolide, USP), 0.05%, Lotion No. M-128,* in 15-ml (NDC 0777-2352-47) and 60-ml (NDC 0777-2352-97) plastic squeeze bottles. *Avoid freezing.*

(℞) *Cordran® (Flurandrenolide, USP), 0.025%, Ointment No. 79,* in 30-g (NDC 0777-1824-67) and 60-g (NDC 0777-1824-97) tubes and in 225-g (NDC 0777-1824-88) jars.

(℞) *Cordran® (Flurandrenolide, USP), 0.05%, Ointment No. 85,* in 15-g (NDC 0777-1826-47), 30-g (NDC 0777-1826-67), and 60-g (NDC 0777-1826-97) tubes and in 225-g (NDC 0777-1826-88) jars.

(℞) *Cordran® SP (Flurandrenolide, USP), 0.025%, Cream No. 9,* in 30-g (NDC 0777-6034-67) and 60-g (NDC 0777-6034-97) tubes and in 225-g (NDC 0777-6034-88) jars.

(℞) *Cordran® SP (Flurandrenolide, USP), 0.05%, Cream No. 11,* in 15-g (NDC 0777-6035-47), 30-g (NDC 0777-6035-67), and 60-g (NDC 0777-6035-97) tubes and in 225-g (NDC 0777-6035-88) jars.

Cream No. 11, 0.05%—15 g—6505-00-890-1554; 60 g—6505-00-728-2623; 225 g—6505-00-728-2624
Lotion No. M-128, 0.05%—15 ml—6505-00-926-9110
Ointment No. 85, 0.05%—15 g—6505-00-728-2626

[050283]

CORDRAN®-N ℞

[*kôr'drăn ĕn*]
(neomycin sulfate with flurandrenolide)
USP

DESCRIPTION

Cordran® (Flurandrenolide, USP, Dista) is a potent corticosteroid intended for topical use. The chemical formula of Cordran is 6α-fluoro-16α-hydroxyhydrocortisone 16,17-acetonide.

Each g of Cordran-N cream contains 0.5 mg (0.05 percent) flurandrenolide and 5 mg neomycin sulfate (equivalent to 3.5 mg neomycin base) in a base composed of stearic acid, cetyl alcohol, mineral oil, polyoxyl 40 stearate, ethylparaben, glycerin, and purified water.

Each g of Cordran-N ointment contains 0.5 mg (0.05 percent) flurandrenolide and 5 mg neomycin sulfate (equivalent to 3.5 mg neomycin base) in a base composed of white wax, cetyl alcohol, sorbitan sesquioleate, and white petrolatum.

ACTIONS

Cordran® (flurandrenolide, Dista) is primarily effective because of its anti-inflammatory, antipruritic, and vasoconstrictive actions.

The addition of neomycin broadens the usefulness of Cordran so that dermatoses complicated by actual skin infections may be treated more effectively and with safety.

INDICATIONS

For the treatment of corticosteroid-responsive dermatoses with secondary infection. It has not been demonstrated that this steroid antibiotic combination provides greater benefit than the steroid component alone after seven days of treatment (*see* Warning section).

CONTRAINDICATIONS

Topical corticosteroids are contraindicated in patients with a history of hypersensitivity to any of the components of these preparations.

WARNING

Because of the concern of nephrotoxicity and ototoxicity associated with neomycin, this combination product should not be used over a wide area or for extended periods of time.

PRECAUTIONS

If irritation develops, the product should be discontinued and appropriate therapy instituted.

Patients with superficial fungus or yeast infections should be treated with additional appropriate methods and observed frequently.

Prolonged use of neomycin preparations may result in the overgrowth of nonsusceptible organisms. If this occurs, appropriate measures should be taken.

There are articles in the current medical literature that indicate an increase in the prevalence of persons who are sensitive to neomycin.

If extensive areas are treated or if the occlusive technique is used, there will be increased systemic absorption of the corticosteroid, and suitable precautions should be taken, particularly in children and infants.

Although topical corticosteroids have not been reported to have an adverse effect on human pregnancy, the safety of their use on pregnant women has not been absolutely established. In laboratory animals, increases in incidence of fetal abnormalities have been associated with exposure of gestating females to topical corticosteroids, in some cases at rather low dosage levels. Therefore, drugs of this class should not be used extensively, in large amounts, or for prolonged periods of time on pregnant patients.

These products are not for ophthalmic use.

ADVERSE REACTIONS

The following local adverse reactions have been reported with topical corticosteroid formulations:

- Acneform eruptions
- Allergic contact dermatitis
- Burning
- Dryness
- Folliculitis
- Hypertrichosis
- Hypopigmentation
- Irritation
- Itching
- Perioral dermatitis

The following may occur more frequently with occlusive dressings:

- Maceration of the skin
- Miliaria
- Secondary infection
- Skin atrophy
- Striae

Topical neomycin has been reported to cause allergic contact dermatitis, ototoxicity, and nephrotoxicity.

DOSAGE AND ADMINISTRATION

For moist lesions, a small quantity of the cream should be rubbed gently into the affected areas two or three times a day. For dry, scaly lesions, the ointment is applied as a thin film to affected areas two or three times daily.

Use with Occlusive Dressings—See under Cordran and Cordran SP.

HOW SUPPLIED

(℞) *Cordran ®-N (Neomycin Sulfate with Flurandrenolide, USP), Cream No. 12,* in 15 (NDC 0777-1884-47), 30 (NDC 0777-1884-67), and 60-g (NDC 0777-1884-97) tubes.

(℞) *Cordran ®-N (Neomycin Sulfate with Flurandrenolide, USP), Ointment No. 86,* in 15 (NDC 0777-1827-47), 30 (NDC 0777-1827-67), and 60-g (NDC 0777-1827-97) tubes.

[011085]

CORDRAN® TAPE ℞

[*kôr'drăn tāp*]
(flurandrenolide tape)
USP

DESCRIPTION

Cordran Tape is a transparent, inconspicuous, plastic surgical tape, impervious to moisture. It contains Cordran® (flurandrenolide, Dista), a potent corticosteroid for topical use. *See also under* Cordran® and Cordran SP.

Each square centimeter contains 4 mcg of flurandrenolide uniformly distributed in the adhesive layer. The tape is made of a thin, matte-finish polyethylene film which is slightly elastic and highly flexible.

The adhesive is a synthetic copolymer of acrylate ester and acrylic acid which is free from substances of plant origin. The pressure-sensitive adhesive surface is covered with a protective paper liner to permit handling and trimming before application.

CLINICAL PHARMACOLOGY

Cordran® (flurandrenolide, Dista) is primarily effective because of its anti-inflammatory, antipruritic, and vasoconstrictive actions.

See also under Cordran and Cordran SP.

The tape serves as both a vehicle and an occlusive dressing. Retention of insensible perspiration by the tape results in hydration of the stratum corneum and improved diffusion of the medication. The skin is protected from scratching, rubbing, desiccation, and chemical irritation. The tape acts as a mechanical splint to fissured skin. Since it prevents removal of the medication by washing or the rubbing action of clothing, the tape formulation provides a sustained action.

Pharmacokinetics —See under Cordran and Cordran SP.

INDICATIONS AND USAGE

For relief of the inflammatory and pruritic manifestations of corticosteroid-responsive dermatoses, particularly dry, scaling localized lesions.

CONTRAINDICATIONS

Topical corticosteroids are contraindicated in patients with a history of hypersensitivity to any of the components of this preparation.

Use of Cordran® Tape (flurandrenolide tape, Dista) is not recommended for lesions exuding serum or in intertriginous areas.

PRECAUTIONS, ADVERSE REACTIONS, and OVERDOSAGE

See under Cordran and Cordran SP.

DOSAGE AND ADMINISTRATION

Occlusive dressings may be used for the management of psoriasis or recalcitrant conditions.

If an infection develops, the use of occlusive dressings should be discontinued and appropriate antimicrobial therapy instituted.

Replacement of the tape every 12 hours produces the lowest incidence of adverse reactions, but it may be left in place for 24 hours if it is well tolerated and adheres satisfactorily. When necessary, the tape may be used at night only and removed during the day.

If ends of the tape loosen prematurely, they may be trimmed off and replaced with fresh tape.

The directions given below are included on a separate package insert for the patient to follow unless otherwise instructed by the physician.

Application of Cordran Tape

IMPORTANT: Skin should be clean and dry before tape is applied. Tape should always be cut, never torn.

DIRECTIONS FOR USE:

1. Prepare skin as directed by your physician or as follows: Gently clean the area to be covered to remove scales, crusts, dried exudates, and any previously used ointments or creams. A germicidal soap or cleanser should be used to prevent the development of odor under the tape. Shave or clip the hair in the treatment area to allow good contact with the skin and comfortable removal. If shower or tub baths are to be taken, they should be completed before the tape is applied. The skin should be dry before application of the tape.
2. Remove tape from package and cut a piece slightly larger than area to be covered. Round off corners.
3. Pull white paper from transparent tape. Be careful that tape does not stick to itself.
4. Apply tape, keeping skin smooth; press tape into place.

REPLACEMENT OF TAPE:

Unless instructed otherwise by your physician, replace tape after 12 hours. Cleanse skin and allow it to dry for one hour before applying new tape.

IF IRRITATION OR INFECTION DEVELOPS, REMOVE TAPE AND CONSULT PHYSICIAN.

HOW SUPPLIED

(℞) *Cordran® Tape (Flurandrenolide Tape, USP), M-170, W14,** 4 mcg flurandrenolide/sq cm, in Small Rolls 24 inches long and 3 inches wide (60 cm x 7.5 cm) (NDC 0777-2314-24) and in Large Rolls 80 inches long and 3 inches wide (200 cm x 7.5 cm) (NDC 0777-2314-28), in single packages.

Directions for the patient are included in each package.

[062182]

Cordran Tape is manufactured by Minnesota Mining and Mfg. Co., St. Paul, Minnesota 55101, for Dista Products Company.

M-170—Cordran Tape, 80 in × 3 in—6505-00-168-6813

*Identi-Code® symbol.

ILOSONE® ℞

[*ī-lō-sōn*]
(erythromycin estolate)
USP

WARNING

Hepatic dysfunction with or without jaundice has occurred, chiefly in adults, in association with erythromycin estolate administration. It may be accompanied by malaise, nausea, vomiting, abdominal colic, and fever. In some instances, severe abdominal pain may simulate an abdominal surgical emergency.

If the above findings occur, discontinue Ilosone® (erythromycin estolate, Dista) promptly.

Ilosone is contraindicated for patients with a known history of sensitivity to this drug and for those with preexisting liver disease.

DESCRIPTION

Erythromycin is produced by a strain of *Streptomyces erythraeus* and belongs to the macrolide group of antibiotics. It is basic and readily forms salts with acids. The base, the stea-

Continued on next page

Dista—Cont.

rate salt, and the esters are poorly soluble in water and are suitable for oral administration.

Ilosone® (erythromycin estolate, Dista) is the lauryl sulfate salt of the propionyl ester of erythromycin.

The Pulvules® and chewable tablets contain 125 mg or 250 mg erythromycin estolate, and the tablets contain 500 mg erythromycin estolate. They may contain any or all of the following: cellulose, citric acid, D&C Red No. 30, D&C Yellow No. 10, FD&C Red No. 3, FD&C Red No. 40, FD&C Yellow No. 6, flavors, gelatin, iron oxides, magnesium stearate, mannitol, mineral oil, povidone, saccharin, silica gel, sodium chloride, sodium citrate, starch, stearic acid, sucrose, talc, titanium dioxide, and other inactive ingredients.

The suspensions contain 125 mg or 250 mg/5ml of erythromycin estolate. The drops contain 5 mg/drop or erythromycin estolate. The suspensions and drops may contain any or all of the following: butylparaben, carboxymethylcellulose, cellulose, citric acid, edetate calcium disodium, FD&C Red No. 40, FD&C Yellow No. 6, flavors, methylparaben, propylparaben, saccharin, silicone, sodium chloride, sodium citrate, sodium lauryl sulfate, sucrose, and water.

ACTIONS

Erythromycin inhibits protein synthesis without affecting nucleic acid synthesis. Some strains of *Haemophilus influenzae* and staphylococci have demonstrated resistance to erythromycin. Some strains of *H. influenzae* that are resistant in vitro to erythromycin alone are susceptible to erythromycin and sulfonamides used concomitantly.

Culture and susceptibility testing should be done. If the Bauer-Kirby method of disc susceptibility testing is used, a 15-mcg erythromycin disc should give a zone diameter of at least 18 mm when tested against an erythromycin-susceptible organism.

Orally administered erythromycin estolate is readily and reliably absorbed. Because of acid stability, serum levels are comparable whether the estolate is taken in the fasting state or after food. After a single 250-mg dose, blood concentrations average 0.29, 1.2, and 1.2 mcg/ml respectively at two, four, and six hours. Following a 500-mg dose, blood concentrations average 3, 1.9, and 0.7 mcg/ml respectively at two, six, and 12 hours.

After oral administration, serum antibiotic levels consist of erythromycin base and propionyl erythromycin ester. The propionyl ester continuously hydrolyzes to the base form of erythromycin to maintain an equilibrium ratio of approximately 20 percent base and 80 percent ester in the serum.

After absorption, erythromycin diffuses readily into most body fluids. In the absence of meningeal inflammation, low concentrations are normally achieved in the spinal fluid, but passage of the drug across the blood-brain barrier increases in meningitis. In the presence of normal hepatic function, erythromycin is concentrated in the liver and excreted in the bile; the effect of hepatic dysfunction on excretion of erythromycin by the liver into the bile is not known. After oral administration, less than 5 percent of the administered dose can be recovered as the active form in the urine.

Erythromycin crosses the placental barrier, but fetal plasma levels are low.

INDICATIONS

Streptococcus pyogenes (Group A Beta-Hemolytic)—Upper and lower respiratory tract, skin, and soft-tissue infections of mild to moderate severity.

Injectable penicillin G benzathine is considered by the American Heart Association to be the drug of choice in the treatment and prevention of streptococcal pharyngitis and in long-term prophylaxis of rheumatic fever.

When oral medication is preferred for treating the above-mentioned conditions, penicillin G or V or erythromycin is the alternate drug of choice.

The importance of the patient's strict adherence to the prescribed dosage regimen must be stressed when oral medication is given. A therapeutic dose should be administered for at least ten days.

Alpha-Hemolytic Streptococci (Viridans Group) —Although no controlled clinical efficacy trials have been conducted, oral erythromycin has been suggested by the American Heart Association and American Dental Association for use in a regimen for prophylaxis against bacterial endocarditis in patients hypersensitive to penicillin who have congenital heart disease or rheumatic or other acquired valvular heart disease when they undergo dental procedures and surgical procedures of the upper respiratory tract.[1] Erythromycin is not suitable for such prophylaxis prior to genitourinary or gastrointestinal tract surgery.

Note: When selecting antibiotics for the prevention of bacterial endocarditis, the physician or dentist should read the full joint statement of the American Heart Association and the American Dental Association.[1]

Staphylococcus aureus —Acute infections of skin and soft tissue which are mild to moderately severe. Resistance may develop during treatment.

S. (Diplococcus) pneumoniae —Infections of the upper respiratory tract (e.g., otitis media, pharyngitis) and lower respiratory tract (e.g., pneumonia) of mild to moderate severity.

Mycoplasma pneumoniae (Eaton Agent, PPLO) —In the treatment of respiratory tract infections due to this organism.

H. influenzae —May be used concomitantly with adequate doses of sulfonamides in treating upper respiratory tract infections of mild to moderate severity. Not all strains of this organism are susceptible at the erythromycin concentrations ordinarily achieved (see appropriate sulfonamide labeling for prescribing information).

Treponema pallidum —Erythromycin is an alternate choice of treatment for primary syphilis in penicillin-allergic patients. In primary syphilis, spinal-fluid examinations should be done before treatment and as part of follow-up after therapy.

Corynebacterium diphtheriae —As an adjunct to antitoxin, to prevent establishment of carriers, and to eradicate the organism in carriers.

C. minutissimum —In the treatment of erythrasma.

Entamoeba histolytica —In the treatment of intestinal amebiasis only. Extraenteric amebiasis requires treatment with other agents.

Listeria monocytogenes —Infections due to this organism.

Bordetella pertussis —Erythromycin is effective in eliminating the organism from the nasopharynx of infected individuals, rendering them noninfectious. Some clinical studies suggest that erythromycin may be helpful in the prophylaxis of pertussis in exposed susceptible individuals.

Legionnaires' Disease —Although no controlled clinical efficacy studies have been conducted, in vitro and limited preliminary clinical data suggest that erythromycin may be effective in treating Legionnaires' disease.

Chlamydia trachomatis —Erythromycins are indicated for treatment of the following infections caused by *C. trachomatis:* conjunctivitis of the newborn, pneumonia of infancy, urogenital infections during pregnancy (*see* Warnings). When tetracyclines are contraindicated or not tolerated, erythromycin is indicated for the treatment of adults with uncomplicated urethral, endocervical, or rectal infections due to *C. trachomatis.*[2]

CONTRAINDICATION

Erythromycin is contraindicated in patients with known hypersensitivity to this antibiotic.

WARNINGS

(*See* Warning box above.) The administration of erythromycin estolate has been associated with the infrequent occurrence of cholestatic hepatitis. Laboratory findings have been characterized by abnormal hepatic function test values, peripheral eosinophilia, and leukocytosis. Symptoms may include malaise, nausea, vomiting, abdominal cramps, and fever. Jaundice may or may not be present. In some instances, severe abdominal pain may simulate the pain of biliary colic, pancreatitis, perforated ulcer, or an acute abdominal surgical problem. In other instances, clinical symptoms and results of liver function tests have resembled findings in extrahepatic obstructive jaundice.

Initial symptoms have developed in some cases after a few days of treatment but generally have followed one or two weeks of continuous therapy. Symptoms reappear promptly, usually within 48 hours after the drug is readministered to sensitive patients. The syndrome seems to result from a form of sensitization, occurs chiefly in adults, and has been reversible when medication is discontinued.

Pseudomembranous colitis has been reported with virtually all broad-spectrum antibiotics (including macrolides, semisynthetic penicillins, and cephalosporins); therefore, it is important to consider its diagnosis in patients who develop diarrhea in association with the use of antibiotics. Such colitis may range in severity from mild to life-threatening.

Treatment with broad-spectrum antibiotics alters the normal flora of the colon and may permit overgrowth of clostridia. Studies indicate that a toxin produced by *Clostridium difficile* is one primary cause of antibiotic-associated colitis.

Mild cases of pseudomembraneous colitis usually respond to drug discontinuance alone. In moderate to severe cases, management should include sigmoidoscopy, appropriate bacteriologic studies, and fluid, electrolyte, and protein supplementation. When the colitis does not improve after the drug has been discontinued, or when it is severe, oral vancomycin is the drug of choice for antibiotic-associated pseudomembranous colitis produced by *C. difficile.* Other causes of colitis should be ruled out.

Usage in Pregnancy —Safety of this drug for use during pregnancy has not been established.

Therefore, the physician should consider carefully the benefits and risks of use of this drug during pregnancy.

PRECAUTIONS

Since erythromycin is excreted principally by the liver, caution should be exercised in administering the antibiotic to patients with impaired hepatic function.

Surgical procedures should be performed when indicated.

Drug Interactions —The use of erythromycin in patients who are receiving high doses of theophylline may be associated with an increase in serum theophylline levels and potential theophylline toxicity. In case of theophylline toxicity and/or elevated serum theophylline levels, the dose of theophylline should be reduced while the patient is receiving concomitant erythromycin therapy.

There have been reports of excessive prolongation of prothrombin times in patients receiving erythromycin concurrently with chronic warfarin therapy. Such patients, particularly the elderly who generally exhibit slower warfarin clearance, may be at risk for developing bleeding due to this interaction. In patients receiving erythromycin during chronic treatment with warfarin, prothrombin times should be monitored closely and warfarin dosage adjusted accordingly.

ADVERSE REACTIONS

The most frequent side effects of erythromycin preparations are gastrointestinal (e.g., abdominal cramping and discomfort) and are dose related. Nausea, vomiting, and diarrhea occur infrequently with usual oral doses.

During prolonged or repeated therapy, there is a possibility of overgrowth of nonsusceptible bacteria or fungi. If such infections arise, the drug should be discontinued and appropriate therapy instituted.

Mild allergic reactions, such as urticaria and other skin rashes, have occurred. Serious allergic reactions, including anaphylaxis, have been reported.

There have been isolated reports of reversible hearing loss occurring chiefly in patients with renal insufficiency and in patients receiving high doses of erythromycin.

DOSAGE AND ADMINISTRATION

Adults —The usual dosage is 250 mg every six hours. This may be increased up to 4 g or more/day according to the severity of the infection.

Children —Age, weight, and severity of the infection are important factors in determining the proper dosage. The usual regimen is 30 to 50 mg/kg/day in divided doses. For more severe infections, this dosage may be doubled.

If administration is desired on a twice-a-day schedule in either adults or children, one-half of the total daily dose may be given every 12 hours.

Twice-a-day dosing is not recommended when doses larger than 1 g daily are administered.

Streptococcal Infections —For the treatment of streptococcal pharyngitis and tonsillitis, the usual dosage range is 20 to 50 mg/kg/day in divided doses.

Body Weight	Total Daily Dose
10 kg or less (less than 25 lb)	250 mg
11–18 kg (25–40 lb)	375 mg
18–25 kg (40–55 lb)	500 mg
25–36 kg (55–80 lb)	750 mg
36 kg or more (more than 80 lb)	1000 mg (adult dose)

In the treatment of group A beta-hemolytic streptococcal infections, a therapeutic dosage of erythromycin should be administered for at least ten days. In continuous prophylaxis of streptococcal infections in persons with a history of rheumatic heart disease, the dosage is 250 mg twice a day.

For prophylaxis against bacterial endocarditis[1] in penicillin-allergic patients with congenital heart disease or rheumatic or other acquired valvular heart disease when undergoing dental procedures or surgical procedures of the upper respiratory tract, the dosage schedule for adults is 1 g (20 mg/kg for children) orally one hour before the procedure and then 500 mg (10 mg/kg for children) orally six hours later.

Primary Syphilis —A regimen of 20 g of erythromycin estolate in divided doses over a period of ten days has been shown to be effective in the treatment of primary syphilis.

Dysenteric Amebiasis —Dosage for adults is 250 mg four times daily for ten to 14 days; for children, 30 to 50 mg/kg/day in divided doses for ten to 14 days.

Pertussis —Although optimum dosage and duration have not been established, the dosage of erythromycin utilized in reported clinical studies was 40 to 50 mg/kg/day, given in divided doses for five to 14 days.

Legionnaires' Disease —Although optimum doses have not been established, doses utilized in reported clinical data were those recommended above (1 to 4 g erythromycin estolate daily in divided doses).

Conjunctivitis of the Newborn Caused by C. trachomatis —Oral erythromycin suspension, 50 mg/kg/day in four divided doses for at least two weeks.[2]

Pneumonia of Infancy Caused by C. trachomatis —Although the optimum duration of therapy has not been established, the recommended therapy is oral erythromycin suspension, 50 mg/kg/day in four divided doses for at least three weeks.[2]

Urogenital Infections During Pregnancy Due to C. trachomatis—Although the optimum dose and duration of therapy have not been established, the suggested treatment is erythromycin, 500 mg orally four times a day for at least seven days. For women who cannot tolerate this regimen, a decreased dose of 250 mg orally four times a day should be used for at least 14 days.[2]

For adults with uncomplicated urethral, endocervical, or rectal infections caused by *C. trachomatis* in whom tetracyclines are contraindicated or not tolerated: 500 mg orally four times a day for at least seven days.[2]

REFERENCES

1. American Heart Association: Prevention of Bacterial Endocarditis, Circulation, *70*:1123A, 1984.

2. Sexually Transmitted Diseases Treatment Guidelines 1982. Centers for Disease Control, Morbidity and Mortality Weekly Report, U.S. Department of Health and Human Services, Atlanta, *31*:355, 1982.

HOW SUPPLIED

(℞) *Pulvules Ilosone® (Erythromycin Estolate Capsules, USP): No. 375, H09,** 250 mg (equivalent to erythromycin) (No. 0, Ivory Opaque Body, Red Opaque Cap), in bottles of 24 (NDC 0777-0809-24) and 100 (NDC 0777-0809-02) and in 10 strips of 10 individually labeled blisters each containing 1 Pulvule (ID100) (NDC 0777-0809-33).

(℞) *Tablets Ilosone® (Erythromycin Estolate Tablets, USP), No. 1863, U26,** 500 mg (equivalent to erythromycin), Specially Coated, Light-Pink (capsule-shaped, scored), in bottles of 50 (NDC 0777-2126-50).

(℞) *Tablets Ilosone® Chewable (Erythromycin Estolate Tablets, USP), No. 1834, U05,** 125 mg (equivalent to erythromycin), Light-Pink, in bottles of 50 (NDC 0777-2105-50); *No. 1865, U25,** 250 mg (equivalent to erythromycin), Light-Pink, in bottles of 50 (NDC 0777-2125-50).

(℞) *Ilosone® Liquid (Erythromycin Estolate Oral Suspension, USP), M-148, W15,** in 100-ml (NDC 0777-2315-48) and 16-fl-oz (NDC 0777-2315-05) bottles.

Each 5 ml contain erythromycin estolate equivalent to 125 mg erythromycin in an orange-flavored vehicle. *Shake well before using. Refrigerate to maintain optimum taste.*

(℞) *Ilosone® Liquid (Erythromycin Estolate Oral Suspension, USP), M-153, W17,** in 100-ml bottles (NDC 0777-2317-48) and 16-fl-oz (NDC 0777-2317-05) bottles.

Each 5 ml contain erythromycin estolate equivalent to 250 mg erythromycin in a cherry-flavored vehicle. *Shake well before using. Refrigerate to maintain optimum taste.*

(℞) *Ilosone® Ready-Mixed Drops (Erythromycin Estolate Oral Suspension, USP), M-159, W18,** in 10-ml bottles (NDC 0777-2318-37).

Each package consists of a bottle containing erythromycin estolate equivalent to 1 g erythromycin in a pleasantly flavored vehicle and a special dropper calibrated at approximately 25 mg and 50 mg.

Each ml contains erythromycin estolate equivalent to 100 mg erythromycin. *Shake well before using. Refrigerate to maintain optimum taste.*

[032086]

Shown in Product Identification Section, page 408

*Identi-Code® symbol.

ILOTYCIN® ℞

[ī-lō-tī′sĭn]
(erythromycin)
Ophthalmic Ointment, USP

DESCRIPTION

Ilotycin® (erythromycin, Dista) is a wide-range antibiotic discovered in the research laboratories of Eli Lilly and Company and produced from a strain of *Streptomyces erythraeus.* The special sterile ophthalmic ointment base, containing mineral oil and white petrolatum, flows freely over the conjunctiva.

INDICATIONS

For the treatment of superficial ocular infections involving the conjunctiva and/or cornea caused by organisms susceptible to Ilotycin® (erythromycin, Dista).

For prophylaxis of ophthalmia neonatorum due to *Neisseria gonorrhoeae* or *Chlamydia trachomatis.* The Centers for Disease Control (U.S.P.H.S.) and the Committee on Drugs, the Committee on Fetus and Newborn, and the Committee on Infectious Diseases of the American Academy of Pediatrics recommend 1 percent silver nitrate solution in single-dose ampoules or single-use tubes of an ophthalmic ointment containing 0.5 percent erythromycin or 1 percent tetracycline as "effective and acceptable regimens for prophylaxis of gonococcal ophthalmia neonatorum."[1] (For infants born to mothers with clinically apparent gonorrhea, intravenous or intramuscular injections of aqueous crystalline penicillin G should be given: a single dose of 50,000 units for term infants or 20,000 units for infants of low birth weight. Topical prophylaxis alone is inadequate for these infants.[1]) Ophthalmic Ointment Ilotycin also has been effective for prevention of neonatal conjunctivitis due to *C. trachomatis,*[2] a condition that may develop one to several weeks after delivery in infants of mothers whose birth canals harbor the organism.

CONTRAINDICATION

This drug is contraindicated in patients with a history of hypersensitivity to erythromycin.

PRECAUTIONS

The use of antimicrobial agents may be associated with the overgrowth of antibiotic-resistant organisms; in such a case, antibiotic administration should be stopped and appropriate measures taken.

ADVERSE REACTIONS

As with any other medicament intended for topical use, there is always the possibility that sensitivity reactions will occur in certain individuals. If such reactions develop, the medication should be discontinued. Eye irritation has been infrequently reported.

DOSAGE AND ADMINISTRATION

In the treatment of external ocular infections, Ophthalmic Ointment Ilotycin® (erythromycin, Dista) should be applied directly to the infected structure one or more times daily, depending on the severity of the infection.

For prophylaxis of neonatal gonococcal or chlamydial conjunctivitis, a ribbon of ointment approximately 0.5 to 1 cm in length should be instilled into each conjunctival sac. The ointment should not be flushed from the eye following instillation. A new tube should be used for each infant. Infants born by cesarean section as well as those delivered by the vaginal route should receive prophylaxis.

REFERENCES

1. American Academy of Pediatrics: Prophylaxis and Treatment of Neonatal Gonococcal Infections, Pediatrics, *65:* 1047, 1980.

2. Hammerschlag, M. R., *et al.:* Erythromycin Ointment for Ocular Prophylaxis of Neonatal Chlamydial Infection, J.A.M.A., *244:* 2291, 1980.

HOW SUPPLIED

(℞) *Sterile Ophthalmic Ointment No. 52, Ilotycin® (Erythromycin Ophthalmic Ointment, USP),* 5 mg/g, in ⅛-oz tamper-proof tubes (NDC 0777-1863-17) and 1-g plastic containers (ID24) (NDC 0777-1863-52). *Store at controlled room temperature, 15° to 30°C (59° to 86°F).*

[102085]

ILOTYCIN® ℞

[ī-lō-tī′sĭn]
(erythromycin)
Tablets, USP
(Enteric-Coated)

DESCRIPTION

Erythromycin is produced by a strain of *Streptomyces erythraeus* and belongs to the macrolide group of antibiotics. It is basic and readily forms salts with acids. The base, the stearate salt, and the esters are poorly soluble in water and are suitable for oral administration.

Tablets Ilotycin® (erythromycin, Dista) are specially coated to protect the contents from the inactivating effect of gastric acid and to permit efficient absorption of the antibiotic in the small intestine.

Each enteric-coated tablet contains 250 mg erythromycin. Each tablet also contains carboxymethyl cellulose, cellulose, dibasic calcium phosphate, hydroxypropyl cellulose, iron oxide, magnesium stearate, stearic acid, silicon dioxide, titanium dioxide, and other inactive ingredients.

ACTIONS

Erythromycin inhibits protein synthesis without affecting nucleic acid synthesis. Some strains of *Haemophilus influenzae* and staphylococci have demonstrated resistance to erythromycin. Some strains of *H. influenzae* that are resistant in vitro to erythromycin alone are susceptible to erythromycin and sulfonamides used concomitantly. Culture and susceptibility testing should be done. If the Bauer-Kirby method of disc susceptibility testing is used, a 15-mcg erythromycin disc should give a zone diameter of at least 18 mm when tested against an erythromycin-susceptible organism.

Tablets Ilotycin® (erythromycin, Dista) are well absorbed and may be given without regard to meals.

After absorption, erythromycin diffuses readily into most body fluids. In the absence of meningeal inflammation, low concentrations are normally achieved in the spinal fluid, but passage of the drug across the blood-brain barrier increases in meningitis. In the presence of normal hepatic function, erythromycin is concentrated in the liver and excreted in the bile; the effect of hepatic dysfunction on excretion of erythromycin by the liver into the bile is not known. After oral administration, less than 5 percent of the administered dose can be recovered as the active form in the urine.

Erythromycin crosses the placental barrier, but fetal plasma levels are low.

INDICATIONS

Streptococcus pyogenes (Group A Beta-Hemolytic)—Upper and lower respiratory tract, skin, and soft-tissue infections of mild to moderate severity.

Injectable penicillin G benzathine is considered by the American Heart Association to be the drug of choice in the treatment and prevention of streptococcal pharyngitis and in long-term prophylaxis of rheumatic fever.

When oral medication is preferred for treating the above-mentioned conditions, penicillin G or V or erythromycin is the alternate drug of choice.

The importance of the patient's strict adherence to the prescribed dosage regimen must be stressed when oral medication is given. A therapeutic dose should be administered for at least ten days.

Alpha-Hemolytic Streptococci (Viridans Group) —Although no controlled clinical efficacy trials have been conducted, oral erythromycin has been suggested by the American Heart Association and American Dental Association for use in a regimen for prophylaxis against bacterial endocarditis in patients hypersensitive to penicillin who have congenital heart disease or rheumatic or other acquired valvular heart disease when they undergo dental procedures and surgical procedures of the upper respiratory tract.[1] Erythromycin is not suitable for such prophylaxis prior to genitourinary or gastrointestinal tract surgery.

Note: When selecting antibiotics for the prevention of bacterial endocarditis, the physician or dentist should read the full joint statement of the American Heart Association and the American Dental Association.[1]

Staphylococcus aureus —Acute infections of skin and soft tissue which are mild to moderately severe. Resistance may develop during treatment.

S. (Diplococcus) pneumoniae —Infections of the upper respiratory tract (e.g., otitis media, pharyngitis) and lower respiratory tract (e.g., pneumonia) of mild to moderate severity.

Mycoplasma pneumoniae (Eaton Agent, PPLO) —In the treatment of respiratory tract infections due to this organism.

H. influenzae —May be used concomitantly with adequate doses of sulfonamides in treating upper respiratory tract infections of mild to moderate severity. Not all strains of this organism are susceptible at the erythromycin concentrations ordinarily achieved (see appropriate sulfonamide labeling for prescribing information).

Treponema pallidum —Erythromycin is an alternate choice of treatment for primary syphilis in penicillin-allergic patients. In primary syphilis, spinal-fluid examinations should be done before treatment and as part of follow-up after therapy.

Corynebacterium diphtheriae —As an adjunct to antitoxin, to prevent establishment of carriers, and to eradicate the organism in carriers.

C. minutissimum —In the treatment of erythrasma.

Entamoeba histolytica —In the treatment of intestinal amebiasis only. Extraenteric amebiasis requires treatment with other agents.

Listeria monocytogenes —Infections due to this organism.

Neisseria gonorrhoeae —In female patients with a history of sensitivity to penicillin, a parenteral erythromycin (such as the gluceptate) may be administered in conjunction with an oral erythromycin as alternate therapy in acute pelvic inflammatory disease caused by *N. gonorrhoeae.* In the treatment of gonorrhea, patients suspected of having concomitant syphilis should have microscopic examinations (by immunofluorescence or darkfield) before receiving erythromycin and monthly serologic tests for a minimum of four months.

Bordetella pertussis —Erythromycin is effective in eliminating the organism from the nasopharynx of infected individuals and in rendering them noninfectious. Some clinical studies suggest that erythromycin may be helpful in the prophylaxis of pertussis in exposed susceptible individuals.

Legionnaires' Disease —Although no controlled clinical efficacy studies have been conducted, in vitro and limited preliminary clinical data suggest that erythromycin may be effective in treating Legionnaires' disease.

Chlamydia trachomatis —Erythromycins are indicated for treatment of the following infections caused by *C. trachomatis:* conjunctivitis of the newborn, pneumonia of infancy, urogenital infections during pregnancy (*see* Warning). When tetracyclines are contraindicated or not tolerated, erythromycin is indicated for the treatment of adults with uncomplicated urethral, endocervical, or rectal infections due to *C. trachomatis.*[2]

CONTRAINDICATION

Erythromycin is contraindicated in patients with known hypersensitivity to this antibiotic.

WARNINGS

Usage in Pregnancy —Safety of this drug for use during pregnancy has not been established. Therefore, the physician should consider carefully the benefits and risks of the use of this drug during pregnancy.

Continued on next page

Dista—Cont.

Pseudomembranous colitis has been reported with virtually all broad-spectrum antibiotics (including macrolides, semisynthetic penicillins, and cephalosporins); therefore, it is important to consider its diagnosis in patients who develop diarrhea in association with the use of antibiotics. Such colitis may range in severity from mild to life-threatening.
Treatment with broad-spectrum antibiotics alters the normal flora of the colon and may permit overgrowth of clostridia. Studies indicate that a toxin produced by *Clostridium difficile* is one primary cause of antibiotic-associated colitis.
Mild cases of pseudomembranous colitis usually respond to drug discontinuance alone. In moderate to severe cases, management should include sigmoidoscopy, appropriate bacteriologic studies, and fluid, electrolyte, and protein supplementation. When the colitis does not improve after the drug has been discontinued, or when it is severe, oral vancomycin is the drug of choice for antibiotic-associated pseudomembranous colitis produced by *C. difficile*. Other causes of colitis should be ruled out.

PRECAUTIONS

Surgical procedures should be performed when indicated.
Since erythromycin is excreted principally by the liver, caution should be exercised in administering the antibiotic to patients with impaired hepatic function. There have been reports of hepatic dysfunction, with or without jaundice, occurring in patients taking oral erythromycin products.
Drug Interactions —The use of erythromycin in patients who are receiving high doses of theophylline may be associated with an increase in serum theophylline levels and potential theophylline toxicity. In case of theophylline toxicity and/or elevated serum theophylline levels, the dose of theophylline should be reduced while the patient is receiving concomitant erythromycin therapy.
There have been reports of excessive prolongation of prothrombin times in patients receiving erythromycin concurrently with chronic warfarin therapy. Such patients, particularly the elderly who generally exhibit slower warfarin clearance, may be at risk for developing bleeding due to this interaction. In patients receiving erythromycin during chronic treatment with warfarin, prothrombin times should be monitored closely and warfarin dosage adjusted accordingly.

ADVERSE REACTIONS

The most frequent side effects of erythromycin preparations are gastrointestinal (e.g., abdominal cramping and discomfort) and are dose related. Nausea, vomiting, and diarrhea occur infrequently with usual oral doses.
During prolonged or repeated therapy, there is a possibility of overgrowth of nonsusceptible bacteria or fungi. If such infections arise, the drug should be discontinued and appropriate therapy instituted.
Mild allergic reactions, such as urticaria and other skin rashes, have occurred. Serious allergic reactions, including anaphylaxis, have been reported.
There have been isolated reports of reversible hearing loss occurring chiefly in patients with renal insufficiency and in patients receiving high doses of erythromycin.

DOSAGE AND ADMINISTRATION

Tablets Ilotycin® (erythromycin, Dista) are well absorbed whether given immediately after meals or between meals on an empty stomach.
Adults —The usual dosage is 250 mg every six hours. This may be increased up to 4 g or more/day according to the severity of the infection.
Children —Age, weight, and severity of the infection are important factors in determining the proper dosage. The usual regimen is 30 to 50 mg/kg/day in divided doses. For more severe infections, this dosage may be doubled.
If administration is desired on a twice-a-day schedule in either adults or children, one-half of the total daily dose may be given every 12 hours.
Streptococcal Infections —In the treatment of group A beta-hemolytic streptococcal infections, a therapeutic dosage of erythromycin should be administered for at least ten days. In continuous prophylaxis of streptococcal infections in persons with a history of rheumatic heart disease, the dosage is 250 mg twice a day.
For prophylaxis against bacterial endocarditis[1] in patients with congenital heart disease or rheumatic or other acquired valvular heart disease when undergoing dental procedures or surgical procedures of the upper respiratory tract, the dosage schedule for adults is 1 g (20 mg/kg for children) orally one and one-half to two hours before the procedure and then 500 mg (10 mg/kg for children) orally every six hours for eight doses.
Primary Syphilis —30 to 40 g given in divided doses over a period of ten to 15 days.
Acute Pelvic Inflammatory Disease Caused by N. gonorrhoeae—Ilotycin® Gluceptate (Sterile Erythromycin Gluceptate, USP, Dista), 500 mg intravenously every six hours for at least three days, followed by Ilotycin, 250 mg every six hours for seven days.
Dysenteric Amebiasis —250 mg four times daily for ten to 14 days for adults; 30 to 50 mg/kg/day in divided doses for ten to 14 days for children.
Pertussis —Although optimum dosage and duration of treatment have not been established, the dosage of erythromycin utilized in reported clinical studies was 40 to 50 mg/kg/day, given in divided doses for five to 14 days.
Legionnaires' Disease —Although optimum doses have not been established, doses utilized in reported clinical data were those recommended above (1 to 4 g erythromycin base daily in divided doses).
Conjunctivitis of the Newborn Caused by C. trachomatis —Oral erythromycin suspension, 50 mg/kg/day in four divided doses for at least two weeks.[2]
Pneumonia of Infancy Caused by C. trachomatis —Although the optimum duration of therapy has not been established, the recommended therapy is oral erythromycin suspension, 50 mg/kg/day in four divided doses for at least three weeks.[2]
Urogenital Infections during Pregnancy Due to C. trachomatis —Although the optimum dose and duration of therapy have not been established, the suggested treatment is erythromycin, 500 mg orally four times a day for at least seven days. For women who cannot tolerate this regimen, a decreased dose of 250 mg orally four times a day should be used for at least 14 days.[2]
For adults with uncomplicated urethral, endocervical, or rectal infections caused by *C. trachomatis* in whom tetracyclines are contraindicated or not tolerated: 500 mg orally four times a day for at least seven days.[2]

REFERENCES

1. American Heart Association: Prevention of Bacterial Endocarditis, Circulation, *70:* 1123A, 1984.
2. Sexually Transmitted Diseases Treatment Guidelines 1982. Centers for Disease Control, Morbidity and Mortality Weekly Report, U.S. Department of Health and Human Services, Atlanta, *31* (Supplement):355, 1982.

HOW SUPPLIED

(℞) *Tablets No. 23, Ilotycin® (Erythromycin Tablets, USP) (Enteric-Coated), C03,** 250 mg, Orange, in bottles of 24 (NDC 0777-0303-24), 100 (NDC 0777-0303-02), and 500 (NDC 0777-0303-03).

[080585]

---

*Identi-Code® symbol.

ILOTYCIN® GLUCEPTATE ℞

[ĭ-lō-tĭ'sĭn gloo-sĕp'tāt]
(erythromycin gluceptate)
Sterile, USP
IntraVenous

DESCRIPTION

Erythromycin is produced by a strain of *Streptomyces erythraeus* and belongs to the macrolide group of antibiotics. It is basic and readily forms salts with acids.

ACTIONS

Erythromycin inhibits protein synthesis without affecting nucleic acid synthesis. Some strains of *Haemophilus influenzae* and staphylococci have demonstrated resistance to erythromycin. Culture and susceptibility testing should be done. If the Bauer-Kirby method of disc susceptibility testing is used, a 15-mcg erythromycin disc should give a zone diameter of at least 18 mm when tested against an erythromycin-susceptible organism.
Intravenous injection of 200 mg of erythromycin produces peak serum levels of 3 to 4 mcg/ml at one hour and 0.5 mcg/ml at six hours.
Erythromycin diffuses readily into the body fluids. Only low concentrations are normally achieved in the spinal fluid, but passage of the drug across the blood-brain barrier increases in meningitis. In the presence of normal hepatic function, erythromycin is concentrated in the liver and excreted in the bile; the effect of hepatic dysfunction on excretion of erythromycin by the liver into the bile is not known. From 12 to 15 percent of intravenously administered erythromycin is excreted in active form in the urine.
Erythromycin crosses the placental barrier, but fetal plasma levels are low.

INDICATIONS

Streptococcus pyogenes (Group A Beta-Hemolytic)—Upper and lower respiratory tract, skin, and soft-tissue infections of mild to moderate severity.
Injectable penicillin G benzathine is considered by the American Heart Association to be the drug of choice in the treatment and prevention of streptococcal pharyngitis and in long-term prophylaxis of rheumatic fever.
Staphylococcus aureus —Acute infections of skin and soft tissue which are mild to moderately severe. Resistance may develop during treatment.
S. (Diplococcus) pneumoniae —Infections of the upper respiratory tract (e.g., otitis media, pharyngitis) and lower respiratory tract (e.g., pneumonia) of mild to moderate severity.
Mycoplasma pneumoniae (Eaton Agent, PPLO) —In the treatment of respiratory tract infections due to this organism.
H. influenzae —May be used concomitantly with adequate doses of sulfonamides in treating upper respiratory tract infections of mild to moderate severity. Not all strains of this organism are susceptible at the erythromycin concentrations ordinarily achieved (see appropriate sulfonamide labeling for prescribing information).
Corynebacterium diphtheriae —As an adjunct to antitoxin.
Listeria monocytogenes —Infections due to this organism.
Neisseria gonorrhoeae —In female patients with a history of sensitivity to penicillin, a parenteral erythromycin (such as the gluceptate) may be administered in conjunction with an oral erythromycin as alternate therapy in acute pelvic inflammatory disease caused by *N. gonorrhoeae*. In the treatment of gonorrhea, patients suspected of having concomitant syphilis should have microscopic examinations (by immunofluorescence or darkfield) before receiving erythromycin and monthly serologic tests for a minimum of four months.
Legionnaires' Disease —Although no controlled clinical efficacy studies have been conducted, in vitro and limited preliminary clinical data suggest that erythromycin may be effective in treating Legionnaires' disease.

CONTRAINDICATION

Intravenous erythromycin is contraindicated in patients with known hypersensitivity to this antibiotic.

WARNING

Usage in Pregnancy —Safety of this drug for use during pregnancy has not been established.
Pseudomembranous colitis has been reported with virtually all broad-spectrum antibiotics (including macrolides, semisynthetic penicillins, and cephalosporins); therefore, it is important to consider its diagnosis in patients who develop diarrhea in association with the use of antibiotics. Such colitis may range in severity from mild to life-threatening.
Treatment with broad-spectrum antibiotics alters the normal flora of the colon and may permit overgrowth of clostridia. Studies indicate that a toxin produced by *Clostridium difficile* is one primary cause of antibiotic-associated colitis.
Mild cases of pseudomembranous colitis usually respond to drug discontinuance alone. In moderate to severe cases, management should include sigmoidoscopy, appropriate bacteriologic studies, and fluid, electrolyte, and protein supplementation. When the colitis does not improve after the drug has been discontinued, or when it is severe, oral vancomycin is the drug of choice for antibiotic-associated pseudomembranous colitis produced by *C. difficile*. Other causes of colitis should be ruled out.

PRECAUTIONS

Surgical procedures should be performed when indicated.
Side effects following the use of intravenous erythromycin are rare. Occasional venous irritation has been encountered, but if the injection is given slowly, in dilute solution, preferably by continuous intravenous infusion over 20 to 60 minutes, pain and vessel trauma are minimized.
Since erythromycin is excreted principally by the liver, caution should be exercised in administering the antibiotic to patients with impaired hepatic function.
Drug Interactions —The use of erythromycin in patients who are receiving high doses of theophylline may be associated with an increase in serum theophylline levels and potential theophylline toxicity. In case of theophylline toxicity and/or elevated serum theophylline levels, the dose of theophylline should be reduced while the patient is receiving concomitant erythromycin therapy.
There have been reports of excessive prolongation of prothrombin times in patients receiving erythromycin concurrently with chronic warfarin therapy. Such patients, particularly the elderly who generally exhibit slower warfarin clearance, may be at risk for developing bleeding due to this interaction. In patients receiving erythromycin during chronic treatment with warfarin, prothrombin times should be monitored closely and warfarin dosage adjusted accordingly.

ADVERSE REACTIONS

Allergic reactions, ranging from urticaria and mild skin eruptions to anaphylaxis, have occurred with intravenously administered erythromycin.
During prolonged or repeated therapy, there is a possibility of overgrowth of nonsusceptible bacteria or fungi. If such infections arise, the drug should be discontinued and appropriate therapy instituted.
Variations in liver function have been observed following daily doses at high levels or after prolonged therapy. Hepatic function tests should be performed when such therapy is given.
Reversible hearing loss associated with the intravenous infusion of 4 g or more/day of erythromycin has been reported rarely.

DOSAGE AND ADMINISTRATION

Prepare the initial solution of Ilotycin® Gluceptate (erythromycin gluceptate, Dista) by (1) adding at least 10 ml of Sterile Water for Injection to the 250 or 500-mg vial or at least 20 ml of Sterile Water for Injection to the 1-g vial of Ilotycin Gluceptate and (2) shaking the vial until all of the drug is dissolved.

It is important that the product be diluted only with Sterile Water for Injection without preservatives.

After reconstitution, the sterile solutions should be stored in a refrigerator and used within seven days.

When all of the drug is dissolved, the solution may then be added to 0.9% Sodium Chloride Injection or to 5% Dextrose in Water to give 1 g/liter for slow, continuous infusion. IV fluid admixtures with a pH below 5.5 tend to lose potency rapidly. Therefore, such solutions should be administered completely within four hours after dilution.

If the period of administration is prolonged, the pH of the infusion fluid should be buffered to neutrality with a sterile agent such as Neut® (Sodium Bicarbonate 4% Additive Solution, Abbott) or Buff™ (Phosphate-Carbonate Buffer, Travenol). For administration of the antibiotic in 500 or 1000 ml of 5% Dextrose in Water, add one ampoule full-strength Buff or 5 ml of Neut; for administration of the antibiotic in the same volumes of 0.9% Sodium Chloride Injection, add one ampoule half-strength Buff or 5 ml of Neut. These solutions should be completely administered within 24 hours after dilution.

If the medication is to be given in 100 to 250 ml of fluid by a volume control set such as Metriset® (McGaw), Volu-Trole® "B" (Cutter), Soluset® (Abbott), or Buretrol® (Baxter-Travenol), the IV fluid should be buffered in its primary container before being added to the volumetric administration set.

If the medication is to be given by intermittent injection, one-fourth of the total daily dose can be given in 20 to 60 minutes by slow intravenous injection of 250 to 500 mg in 100 to 250 ml of 0.9% Sodium Chloride Injection or 5% Dextrose in Water. Injection should be sufficiently slow to avoid pain along the vein.

The recommended IV dosage for severe infections in adults and children is 15 to 20 mg/kg of body weight/day. Higher doses (up to 4 g/day) may be given in very severe infections. Continuous infusion is preferable, but administration in divided doses at intervals of no more than every six hours is also effective.

For treatment of acute pelvic inflammatory disease caused by *N. gonorrhoeae*, administer 500 mg Ilotycin Gluceptate intravenously every six hours for at least three days, followed by 250 mg Ilotycin® (Erythromycin Tablets, USP, Dista) every six hours for seven days.

Patients receiving intravenous erythromycin should be changed to the oral dosage form as soon as possible.

For Treatment of Legionnaires' Disease—Although optimum doses have not been established, doses utilized in reported clinical data were those recommended above (1 to 4 g daily in divided doses).

HOW SUPPLIED

(℞) *Vials Ilotycin® Gluceptate (Sterile Erythromycin Gluceptate, USP), IV,* rubber-stoppered (Dry Powder): *No. 524,* 250 mg (equivalent to erythromycin), 30-ml size (NDC 0777-1404-01); *No. 538,* 500 mg (equivalent to erythromycin), 30-ml size (NDC 0777-1409-01); and *No. 646,* 1 g (equivalent to erythromycin), 30-ml size (NDC 0777-1441-01), in singles (10 per carton).

[022585]

KEFLEX® ℞

[kĕf′lĕks]
(cephalexin)
USP

DESCRIPTION

Keflex® (cephalexin, Dista) is a semisynthetic cephalosporin antibiotic intended for oral administration. It is 7-(D-α-amino-α-phenylacetamido) - 3 - methyl - 3 - cephem - 4 - carboxylic acid, monohydrate.

The nucleus of cephalexin is related to that of other cephalosporin antibiotics. The compound is a zwitterion; i.e., the molecule contains both a basic and an acidic group. The isoelectric point of cephalexin in water is approximately 4.5 to 5.

The crystalline form of cephalexin which is available is a monohydrate. It is a white crystalline solid having a bitter taste. Solubility in water is low at room temperature; 1 or 2 mg/ml may be dissolved readily, but higher concentrations are obtained with increasing difficulty.

The cephalosporins differ from penicillins in the structure of the bicyclic ring system. Cephalexin has a D-phenylglycyl group as substituent at the 7-amino position and an unsubstituted methyl group at the 3-position.

Each Pulvule® contains cephalexin monohydrate equivalent to 250 mg or 500 mg of cephalexin. Each tablet contains cephalexin monohydrate equivalent to 1 g of cephalexin. The Pulvules and tablets may contain any or all of the following: cellulose, D & C Yellow No. 10, F D & C Blue No. 1, F D & C Blue No. 2, F D & C Yellow No. 6, gelatin, magnesium stearate, povidone, silicone, starch, titanium dioxide, and other inactive ingredients.

After mixing, each 5 ml of Keflex, for Oral Suspension, will contain cephalexin monohydrate equivalent to 125 mg or 250 mg of cephalexin. The pediatric drops contain 100 mg/ml. The suspension and drops may contain any or all of the following: D & C Yellow No. 10, F D & C Red No. 40, F D & C Yellow No. 6, flavors, methylcellulose, silicone, sodium lauryl sulfate, and sucrose.

CLINICAL PHARMACOLOGY

Human Pharmacology—Keflex® (cephalexin, Dista) is acid stable and may be given without regard to meals. It is rapidly absorbed after oral administration. Following doses of 250 mg, 500 mg, and 1 g, average peak serum levels of approximately 9, 18, and 32 mcg/ml respectively were obtained at one hour. Measurable levels were present six hours after administration. Cephalexin is excreted in the urine by glomerular filtration and tubular secretion. Studies showed that over 90 percent of the drug was excreted unchanged in the urine within eight hours. During this period, peak urine concentrations following the 250-mg, 500-mg, and 1-g doses were approximately 1000, 2200, and 5000 mcg/ml respectively.

Microbiology—In vitro tests demonstrate that the cephalosporins are bactericidal because of their inhibition of cell-wall synthesis. Keflex is active against the following organisms in vitro:

- Beta-hemolytic streptococci
- Staphylococci, including coagulase-positive, coagulase-negative, and penicillinase-producing strains
- *Streptococcus (Diplococcus) pneumoniae*
- *Escherichia coli*
- *Proteus mirabilis*
- *Klebsiella* sp.
- *Haemophilus influenzae*
- *Neisseria catarrhalis*

Note—Most strains of enterococci (*S. faecalis*) and a few strains of staphylococci are resistant to Keflex. It is not active against most strains of *Enterobacter* sp., *P. morganii,* and *P. vulgaris.* It has no activity against *Pseudomonas* or *Herellea* species. When tested by in vitro methods, staphylococci exhibit cross-resistance between Keflex and methicillin-type antibiotics.

Disc Susceptibility Tests—Quantitative methods that require measurement of zone diameters give the most precise estimates of antibiotic susceptibility. One such procedure (*Am. J. Clin. Pathol., 45:* 493, 1966; *Federal Register, 39:* 19182–19184, 1974) has been recommended for use with discs for testing susceptibility to cephalothin. Interpretations correlate zone diameters of the disc test with MIC values for Keflex. With this procedure, a report from the laboratory of "resistant" indicates that the infecting organism is not likely to respond to therapy. A report of "intermediate susceptibility" suggests that the organism would be susceptible if the infection is confined to the urine, in which high antibiotic levels can be obtained, or if high dosage is used in other types of infection.

INDICATIONS AND USAGE

Keflex® (cephalexin, Dista) is indicated for the treatment of the following infections when caused by susceptible strains of the designated microorganisms:

- Respiratory tract infections caused by *S. pneumoniae* and group A beta-hemolytic streptococci (Penicillin is the usual drug of choice in the treatment and prevention of streptococcal infections, including the prophylaxis of rheumatic fever. Keflex is generally effective in the eradication of streptococci from the nasopharynx; however, substantial data establishing the efficacy of Keflex in the subsequent prevention of rheumatic fever are not available at present.)
- Otitis media due to *S. pneumoniae, H. influenzae,* staphylococci, streptococci, and *N. catarrhalis*
- Skin and skin-structure infections caused by staphylococci and/or streptococci
- Bone infections caused by staphylococci and/or *P. mirabilis*
- Genitourinary tract infections, including acute prostatitis, caused by *E. coli, P. mirabilis,* and *Klebsiella* sp.

Note—Culture and susceptibility tests should be initiated prior to and during therapy. Renal function studies should be performed when indicated.

CONTRAINDICATION

Keflex® (cephalexin, Dista) is contraindicated in patients with known allergy to the cephalosporin group of antibiotics.

WARNINGS

BEFORE CEPHALEXIN THERAPY IS INSTITUTED, CAREFUL INQUIRY SHOULD BE MADE CONCERNING PREVIOUS HYPERSENSITIVITY REACTIONS TO CEPHALOSPORINS AND PENICILLIN. CEPHALOSPORIN C DERIVATIVES SHOULD BE GIVEN CAUTIOUSLY TO PENICILLIN-SENSITIVE PATIENTS.

SERIOUS ACUTE HYPERSENSITIVITY REACTIONS MAY REQUIRE EPINEPHRINE AND OTHER EMERGENCY MEASURES.

There is some clinical and laboratory evidence of partial cross-allergenicity of the penicillins and the cephalosporins. Patients have been reported to have had severe reactions (including anaphylaxis) to both drugs.

Any patient who has demonstrated some form of allergy, particularly to drugs, should receive antibiotics cautiously. No exception should be made with regard to Keflex® (cephalexin, Dista).

Pseudomembranous colitis has been reported with virtually all broad-spectrum antibiotics (including macrolides, semisynthetic penicillins, and cephalosporins); therefore, it is important to consider its diagnosis in patients who develop diarrhea in association with the use of antibiotics. Such colitis may range in severity from mild to life-threatening.

Treatment with broad-spectrum antibiotics alters the normal flora of the colon and may permit overgrowth of clostridia. Studies indicate that a toxin produced by *Clostridium difficile* is one primary cause of antibiotic-associated colitis.

Mild cases of pseudomembranous colitis usually respond to drug discontinuance alone. In moderate to severe cases, management should include sigmoidoscopy, appropriate bacteriologic studies, and fluid, electrolyte, and protein supplementation. When the colitis does not improve after the drug has been discontinued, or when it is severe, oral vancomycin is the drug of choice for antibiotic-associated pseudomembranous colitis produced by *C. difficile.* Other causes of colitis should be ruled out.

Usage in Pregnancy—Safety of this product for use during pregnancy has not been established.

PRECAUTIONS

General Precautions—Patients should be followed carefully so that any side effects or unusual manifestations of drug idiosyncrasy may be detected. If an allergic reaction to Keflex® (cephalexin, Dista) occurs, the drug should be discontinued and the patient treated with the usual agents (e.g., epinephrine or other pressor amines, antihistamines, or corticosteroids).

Prolonged use of Keflex may result in the overgrowth of nonsusceptible organisms. Careful observation of the patient is essential. If superinfection occurs during therapy, appropriate measures should be taken.

Positive direct Coombs' tests have been reported during treatment with the cephalosporin antibiotics. In hematologic studies or in transfusion cross-matching procedures when antiglobulin tests are performed on the minor side or in Coombs' testing of newborns whose mothers have received cephalosporin antibiotics before parturition, it should be recognized that a positive Coombs' test may be due to the drug.

Keflex should be administered with caution in the presence of markedly impaired renal function. Under such conditions, careful clinical observation and laboratory studies should be made because safe dosage may be lower than that usually recommended.

Indicated surgical procedures should be performed in conjunction with antibiotic therapy.

As a result of administration of Keflex, a false-positive reaction for glucose in the urine may occur. This has been observed with Benedict's and Fehling's solutions and also with Clinitest® tablets but not with Tes-Tape® (Glucose Enzymatic Test Strip, USP, Lilly).

Broad-spectrum antibiotics should be prescribed with caution in individuals with a history of gastrointestinal disease, particularly colitis.

Usage in Pregnancy—*Pregnancy Category B*—The daily oral administration of cephalexin to rats in doses of 250 or 500 mg/kg prior to and during pregnancy, or to rats and mice during the period of organogenesis only, had no adverse effect on fertility, fetal viability, fetal weight, or litter size. Note that the safety of cephalexin during pregnancy in humans has not been established.

Cephalexin showed no enhanced toxicity in weanling and newborn rats as compared with adult animals. Nevertheless, because the studies in humans cannot rule out the possibility of harm, Keflex should be used during pregnancy only if clearly needed.

Nursing Mothers—The excretion of cephalexin in the milk increased up to four hours after a 500-mg dose; the drug reached a maximum level of 4 mcg/ml, then decreased gradually, and had disappeared eight hours after administration. Caution should be exercised when Keflex is administered to a nursing woman.

ADVERSE REACTIONS

Gastrointestinal—Symptoms of pseudomembranous colitis may appear either during or after antibiotic treatment. Nausea and vomiting have been reported rarely. The most frequent side effect has been diarrhea. It was very rarely severe enough to warrant cessation of therapy. Dyspepsia and abdominal pain have also occurred. As with some penicillins

Continued on next page

Dista—Cont.

and some other cephalosporins, transient hepatitis and cholestatic jaundice have been reported rarely.
Hypersensitivity—Allergies (in the form of rash, urticaria, and angioedema) have been observed. These reactions usually subsided upon discontinuation of the drug. Anaphylaxis has also been reported.
Other reactions have included genital and anal pruritus, genital moniliasis, vaginitis and vaginal discharge, dizziness, fatigue, and headache. Eosinophilia, neutropenia, and slight elevations in SGOT and SGPT have been reported.

DOSAGE AND ADMINISTRATION

Keflex® (cephalexin, Dista) is administered orally.
Adults—The adult dosage ranges from 1 to 4 g daily in divided doses. The usual adult dose is 250 mg every six hours. For the following infections, a dosage of 500 mg may be administered every 12 hours: streptococcal pharyngitis, skin and skin-structure infections, and uncomplicated cystitis in patients over 15 years of age. Cystitis therapy should be continued for seven to 14 days. For more severe infections or those caused by less susceptible organisms, larger doses may be needed. If daily doses of Keflex greater than 4 g are required, parenteral cephalosporins, in appropriate doses, should be considered.
Children—The usual recommended daily dosage for children is 25 to 50 mg/kg in divided doses. For streptococcal pharyngitis in patients over one year of age and for skin and skin-structure infections, the total daily dose may be divided and administered every 12 hours.
[See table below].
In severe infections, the dosage may be doubled.
In the therapy of otitis media, clinical studies have shown that a dosage of 75 to 100 mg/kg/day in four divided doses is required.
In the treatment of beta-hemolytic streptococcal infections, a therapeutic dosage of Keflex should be administered for at least ten days.

HOW SUPPLIED

(℞) *For Oral Suspension, Kef- lex ® (Cephalexin for Oral Suspension, USP), M-201, W21,* in 60 (NDC 0777-2321-97), 100 (NDC 0777-2321-48), and 200-ml-size (NDC 0777-2321-89) packages and in unit-dose bottles of 100 (ID100) (NDC 0777-2321-33).
Each 60-ml-size package contains 1.5 g cephalexin in a dry, pleasantly flavored mixture. At the time of dispensing, add 36 ml of water in *two* portions to the dry mixture in the bottle. Shake well after each addition.
Each 100-ml-size package contains 2.5 g cephalexin in a dry, pleasantly flavored mixture. At the time of dispensing, add 60 ml of water in *two* portions to the dry mixture in the bottle. Shake well after each addition.
Each 200-ml-size package contains 5 g cephalexin in a dry, pleasantly flavored mixture. At the time of dispensing, add 120 ml of water in *two* portions to the dry mixture in the bottle. Shake well after each addition.
When mixed as directed, each 5 ml (approximately 1 teaspoonful) will contain 125 mg cephalexin. After mixing, store in a refrigerator. The mixture may be kept for 14 days without significant loss of potency. *Shake well before using. Keep tightly closed.*
(℞) *For Oral Suspension, Keflex ® (Cephalexin for Oral Suspension, USP), M-202, W68,** in 100 (NDC 0777-2368-48) and 200-ml-size (NDC 0777-2368-89) packages and in unit-dose bottles of 100 (ID100) (NDC 0777-2368-33).
Each 100-ml-size package contains 5 g cephalexin in a dry, pleasantly flavored mixture. At the time of dispensing, add 60 ml of water in *two* portions to the dry mixture in the bottle. Shake well after each addition.
Each 200-ml-size package contains 10 g cephalexin in a dry, pleasantly flavored mixture. At the time of dispensing, add 124 ml of water in *two* portions to the dry mixture in the bottle. Shake well after each addition.
When mixed as directed, each 5 ml (approximately 1 teaspoonful) will contain 250 mg cephalexin. After mixing, store in a refrigerator. The mixture may be kept for 14 days without significant loss of potency. *Shake well before using. Keep tightly closed.*
(℞) *For Pediatric Drops, Keflex ® (Cephalexin for Oral Suspension, USP), M-204, W22,** in 10-ml-size packages (NDC 0777-2322-37).
This package contains 1 g cephalexin in a dry, pleasantly flavored mixture and a special dropper calibrated at approximately 25 and 50 mg.
At the time of dispensing, add 5.5 ml of water to the dry mixture in the bottle. Close with original bottle cap and shake promptly until all of the powder is in suspension. Remove detachable portion of bottle label but leave white tab affixed.
When mixed as directed, each ml will contain 100 mg cephalexin. After being mixed, the suspension may be kept in a refrigerator for 14 days without significant loss of potency. *Shake well before using. Keep tightly closed.*
(℞) *Pulvules ® Keflex ® (Cephalexin Capsules, USP): No. 402, H69,** 250 mg (No. 0, White Opaque Body, Dark-Green Opaque Cap), and *No. 403, H71,** 500 mg (No. 0, Light-Green Opaque Body, Dark-Green Opaque Cap), in bottles of 20 (NDC 0777-0869-20 and 0871-20) and 100 (NDC 0777-0869-02 and 0871-02) and in 10 strips of 10 individually labeled blisters each containing 1 Pulvule (ID100) (NDC 0777-0869-33 and 0871-33).
(℞) *Tablets No. 1896, Keflex ® (Cephalexin Tablets, USP), U60,** 1 g, Green (capsule-shaped), in bottles of 24 (NDC 0777-2160-24) and in 10 strips of 10 individually labeled blisters each containing 1 tablet (ID100) (NDC 0777-2160-33).
[031786]

Pulvules No. 402, 250 mg—100's—6505-00-165-6545; ID100's—6505-00-197-9200
Pulvules No. 403, 500 mg—100's—6505-00-183-8543; ID100's—6505-00-171-1213
M-201—For Oral Suspension—100-ml size—6505-00-009-1833

Shown in Product Identification Section, page 408

* Identi-Code® symbol.

NALFON® ℞
[*năl'fŏn*]
NALFON® 200
(fenoprofen calcium)
USP

DESCRIPTION

Nalfon® (fenoprofen calcium, Dista) is a nonsteroidal, anti-inflammatory, antiarthritic drug. Pulvules® and Tablets Nalfon contain fenoprofen calcium as the dihydrate in an amount equivalent to 200 mg or 300 mg (Pulvules) or 600 mg (Tablets) of fenoprofen. Each Pulvule and tablet may also contain any or all of the following: amberlite, calcium phosphate, cellulose, D & C Yellow No. 10, F D & C Yellow No. 6, gelatin, iron oxide, magnesium stearate, silicone, starch, stearic acid, titanium dioxide, and other inactive ingredients. Chemically, Nalfon is an arylacetic acid derivative.
Nalfon is a white crystalline powder, soluble in alcohol (95%) to the extent of approximately 15 mg/ml at 25°C, slightly soluble in water, and insoluble in benzene.
The pK_a of Nalfon is 4.5 at 25°C.

CLINICAL PHARMACOLOGY

Nalfon® (fenoprofen calcium, Dista) is a nonsteroidal, anti-inflammatory, antiarthritic drug that also prossesses analgesic and antipyretic activities. Its exact mode of action is unknown, but it is thought that prostaglandin synthetase inhibition is involved. Nalfon has been shown to inhibit prostaglandin synthetase isolated from bovine seminal vesicles.
Reproduction studies in rats have shown Nalfon to be associated with prolonged labor and difficult parturition when given during late pregnancy. Evidence suggests that this may be due to decreased uterine contractility resulting from the inhibition of prostaglandin synthesis. Its action is not mediated through the adrenal gland.
Fenoprofen shows anti-inflammatory effects in rodents by inhibiting the development of redness and edema in acute inflammatory conditions and by reducing soft-tissue swelling and bone damage associated with chronic inflammation. It exhibits analgesic activity in rodents by inhibiting the writhing response caused by the introduction of an irritant into the peritoneal cavities of mice and by elevating pain thresholds to pressure in edematous hindpaws of rats. In rats made febrile by the subcutaneous administration of brewer's yeast, fenoprofen produces antipyretic action. These effects are characteristic of nonsteroidal, anti-inflammatory, antipyretic, analgesic drugs.
The results in humans confirmed the anti-inflammatory and analgesic actions found in animals. The emergence and degree of erythemic response were measured in adult male volunteers exposed to ultraviolet irradiation. The effects of Nalfon, aspirin, and indomethacin were compared separately with those of a placebo. All three drugs demonstrated antierythemic activity.
In patients with rheumatoid arthritis, the anti-inflammatory action of Nalfon has been evidenced by relief of pain; by increase in grip strength; by reductions in joint swelling, duration of morning stiffness, and disease activity (as assessed by both the investigator and the patient); and by increased mobility (a decrease in the number of joints having limited motion).
The use of Nalfon® (fenoprofen calcium, Dista) in combination with gold salts or corticosteroids has been studied in patients with rheumatoid arthritis. The studies, however, were inadequate in demonstrating whether further improvement is obtained by adding Nalfon to maintenance therapy with gold salts or steroids. Whether or not Nalfon, used in conjunction with partially effective doses of a corticosteroid, has a "steroid-sparing" effect is unknown.
In patients with osteoarthritis, the anti-inflammatory and analgesic effects of Nalfon have been demonstrated by reduction in tenderness on pressure; relief of pain with motion and at rest; reductions in night pain, stiffness, swelling, and overall disease activity (as assessed by both the patient and the investigator); and increased range of motion in involved joints.
In patients with rheumatoid arthritis and osteoarthritis, clinical studies have shown Nalfon to be comparable to aspirin in controlling the aforementioned measures of disease activity, but mild gastrointestinal adverse reactions (nausea, dyspepsia) and tinnitus occurred less frequently than in aspirin-treated patients. It is not known whether Nalfon causes less peptic ulceration than does aspirin.
In patients with pain, the analgesic action of Nalfon has produced a reduction in pain intensity, an increase in pain relief, improvement in total analgesia scores, and a sustained analgesic effect.
Under fasting conditions, Nalfon is rapidly absorbed, and peak plasma levels of 50 mcg/ml are achieved within two hours after oral administration of 600-mg doses. Good dose proportionality was observed between 200-mg and 600-mg doses in fasting male volunteers. The plasma half-life is approximately three hours. About 90% of a single oral dose is eliminated within 24 hours as fenoprofen glucuronide and 4'-hydroxyfenoprofen glucuronide, the major urinary metabolites of fenoprofen. Fenoprofen is highly bound (99%) to albumin.
The concomitant administration of antacid (containing both aluminum and magnesium hydroxide) does not interfere with absorption of Nalfon.
There is less suppression of collagen-induced platelet aggregation with single doses of Nalfon than there is with aspirin.

INDICATIONS AND USAGE

Nalfon® (fenoprofen calcium, Dista) is indicated for relief of the signs and symptoms of rheumatoid arthritis and osteoarthritis. It is recommended for the treatment of acute flares and exacerbations and for the long-term management of these diseases.
Nalfon is also indicated for the relief of mild to moderate pain.
Controlled trials are currently in progress to establish the safety and efficacy of Nalfon in children.

CONTRAINDICATIONS

Nalfon® (fenoprofen calcium, Dista) is contraindicated in patients who have shown hypersensitivity to it.
The drug should not be administered to patients with a history of significantly impaired renal function.
Nalfon should not be given to patients in whom aspirin and other nonsteroidal anti-inflammatory drugs induce the symptoms of asthma, rhinitis, or urticaria, because cross-sensitivity to these drugs occurs in a high proportion of such patients.

WARNINGS

Nalfon® (fenoprofen calcium, Dista) should be given under close supervision to patients with a history of upper gastrointestinal tract disease and only after the Adverse Reactions section has been consulted. Gastrointestinal bleeding, sometimes severe (with fatalities having been reported), may occur in patients receiving Nalfon as with other nonsteroidal anti-inflammatory drugs.
If Nalfon must be given to patients with an active peptic ulcer, the patient should be on a vigorous anti-ulcer treatment regimen and under close supervision for signs of ulcer perforation or severe gastrointestinal bleeding.
Since Nalfon has been marketed, there have been reports of genitourinary tract problems in patients taking it. The most frequently reported problems have been episodes of dysuria, cystitis, hematuria, interstitial nephritis, and the nephrotic syndrome. This syndrome may be preceded by the appearance of fever, rash, arthralgia, oliguria, and azotemia and may progress to anuria. There may also be substantial pro-

Keflex Suspension

Child's Weight	125 mg/5 ml	250 mg/5 ml
10 kg (22 lb)	½ to 1 tsp q.i.d.	¼ to ½ tsp q.i.d.
20 kg (44 lb)	1 to 2 tsp q.i.d.	½ to 1 tsp q.i.d.
40 kg (88 lb)	2 to 4 tsp q.i.d.	1 to 2 tsp q.i.d.
	or	
Child's Weight	125 mg/5 ml	250 mg/5 ml
10 kg (22 lb)	1 to 2 tsp b.i.d.	½ to 1 tsp. b.i.d.
20 kg (44 lb)	2 to 4 tsp b.i.d.	1 to 2 tsp b.i.d.
40 kg (88 lb)	4 to 8 tsp b.i.d.	2 to 4 tsp b.i.d.

teinuria, and, on renal biopsy, electron microscopy has shown foot process fusion and T-lymphocyte infiltration in the renal interstitium. Early recognition of the syndrome and withdrawal of the drug have been followed by rapid recovery. Administration of steroids and the use of dialysis have also been included in the treatment. Because a syndrome with some of these characteristics has also been reported with other nonsteroidal anti-inflammatory drugs, it is recommended that patients who have had these reactions with other such drugs not be treated with Nalfon. In patients with possibly compromised renal function, periodic renal function examinations should be done.

PRECAUTIONS

General—Renal Effects—There have been reports of acute interstitial nephritis and nephrotic syndrome (*see* Contraindications and Warnings).

A second form of renal toxicity has been seen in patients with prerenal conditions leading to a reduction in renal blood flow or blood volume, where the renal prostaglandins have a supportive role in the maintenance of renal perfusion. In these patients, administration of an NSAID may cause a dose-dependent reduction in prostaglandin formation and may precipitate overt renal decompensation. Patients at greatest risk of this reaction are those with impaired renal function, heart failure, liver dysfunction, those taking diuretics, and the elderly. Discontinuation of NSAID therapy is typically followed by recovery to the pretreatment state.

Since Nalfon is eliminated primarily by the kidneys, patients with possibly compromised renal function should be closely monitored; a lower daily dosage should be anticipated to avoid excessive drug accumulation.

In chronic studies in rats, high doses of Nalfon®(fenoprofen calcium, Dista) caused elevation of serum transaminase and hepatocellular hypertrophy. In clinical trials, some patients developed elevation of serum transaminase, LDH, and alkaline phosphatase that persisted for some months and usually, but not always, declined despite continuation of the drug. The significance of this is unknown. It is recommended, therefore, that Nalfon be discontinued if any significant liver abnormalities occur.

As with other nonsteroidal anti-inflammatory drugs, borderline elevations of one or more liver tests may occur in up to 15 percent of patients. These abnormalities may progress, may remain essentially unchanged, or may be transient with continued therapy. The SGPT (ALT) test is probably the most sensitive indicator of liver dysfunction. Meaningful (three times the upper limit of normal) elevations of SGPT or SGOT (AST) occurred in controlled clinical trials in less than 1 percent of patients. A patient with symptoms and/or signs suggesting liver dysfunction, or in whom an abnormal liver test has occurred, should be evaluated for evidence of the development of more severe hepatic reaction while on therapy with Nalfon. Severe hepatic reactions, including jaundice and cases of fatal hepatitis, have been reported with Nalfon as with other nonsteroidal anti-inflammatory drugs. Although such reactions are rare, if abnormal liver tests persist or worsen, if clinical signs and symptoms consistent with liver disease develop, or if systemic manifestations occur (e.g., eosinophilia, rash, etc.), Nalfon should be discontinued.

Safe use of Nalfon during pregnancy and lactation has not been established; therefore, administration to pregnant patients and nursing mothers is not recommended. Reproduction studies have been performed in rats and rabbits. When fenoprofen was given to rats during pregnancy and continued to the time of labor, parturition was prolonged. Similar results have been found with other nonsteroidal anti-inflammatory drugs that inhibit prostaglandin synthetase.

In patients receiving Nalfon and a steroid concomitantly, any reduction in steroid dosage should be gradual in order to avoid the possible complications of sudden steroid withdrawal.

Patients with initial low hemoglobin values who are receiving long-term therapy with Nalfon should have a hemoglobin determination at reasonable intervals.

Peripheral edema has been observed in some patients taking Nalfon; therefore, Nalfon should be used with caution in patients with compromised cardiac function or hypertension. The possibility of renal involvement should be considered.

Studies to date have not shown changes in the eyes attributable to the administration of Nalfon. However, adverse ocular effects have been observed with other anti-inflammatory drugs. Eye examinations, therefore, should be performed if visual disturbances occur in patients taking Nalfon.

Caution should be exercised by patients whose activities require alertness if they experience central-nervous-system side effects from Nalfon.

Since the safety of Nalfon has not been established in patients with impaired hearing, these patients should have periodic tests of auditory function during chronic therapy with Nalfon.

Nalfon decreases platelet aggregation and may prolong bleeding time. Patients who may be adversely affected by prolongation of the bleeding time should be carefully observed when Nalfon is administered.

DRUG INTERACTIONS

The coadministration of aspirin decreases the biologic half-life of fenoprofen because of an increase in metabolic clearance that results in a greater amount of hydroxylated fenoprofen in the urine. Although the mechanism of interaction between fenoprofen and aspirin is not totally known, enzyme induction and displacement of fenoprofen from plasma albumin binding sites are possibilities. Because Nalfon® (fenoprofen calcium, Dista) has not been shown to produce any additional effect beyond that obtained with aspirin alone and because aspirin increases the rate of excretion of Nalfon, the concomitant use of Nalfon and salicylates is not recommended.

Chronic administration of phenobarbital, a known enzyme inducer, may be associated with a decrease in the plasma half-life of fenoprofen. When phenobarbital is added or withdrawn, dosage adjustment of Nalfon may be required.

In vitro studies have shown that fenoprofen, because of its affinity for albumin, may displace from their binding sites other drugs which are also albumin bound, and this may lead to drug interaction. Theoretically, fenoprofen could likewise be displaced. Patients receiving hydantoin, sulfonamides, or sulfonylureas should be observed for increased activity of these drugs and, therefore, signs of toxicity to these drugs. In patients receiving coumarin-type anticoagulants, the addition of Nalfon to therapy could prolong the prothrombin time. Patients receiving both drugs should be under careful observation.

ADVERSE REACTIONS

During clinical studies for rheumatoid arthritis or osteoarthritis, complaints were compiled from a checklist of potential adverse reactions, from which the following data emerged. These encompass observations in 3391 patients, including 188 observed for at least 52 weeks. During short-term studies for analgesia, the incidence of adverse reactions was markedly lower than that seen in longer-term studies.

INCIDENCE GREATER THAN 1%

Probable Causal Relationship

Digestive System—During clinical trials with Nalfon® (fenoprofen calcium, Dista), the most common adverse reactions were gastrointestinal in nature and occurred in about 14% of patients. In descending order of frequency, these reactions included dyspepsia,* constipation,* nausea,* vomiting,* abdominal pain, anorexia, occult blood in the stool, diarrhea, flatulence, and dry mouth.

The drug was discontinued because of adverse gastrointestinal reactions in less than 2% of patients.

Nervous System—The most frequent adverse neurologic reactions were headache and somnolence, which occurred in about 15% of patients. Dizziness,* tremor, confusion, and insomnia were noted less frequently.

Nalfon was discontinued in less than 0.5% of patients because of these side effects.

Skin and Appendages—Pruritus,* rash, increased sweating, and urticaria.

Nalfon was discontinued in about 1% of patients because of an adverse effect related to the skin.

Special Senses—Tinnitus, blurred vision, and decreased hearing.

Nalfon was discontinued in less than 0.5% of patients because of adverse effects related to the special senses.

Cardiovascular—Palpitations* and tachycardia.

Nalfon was discontinued in about 0.5% of patients because of adverse cardiovascular reactions.

Miscellaneous—Nervousness,* asthenia,* dyspnea, fatigue, and malaise.

* Reactions in 3% to 9% of patients treated with Nalfon. (Those reactions occurring in less than 3% of the patients are unmarked.)

INCIDENCE LESS THAN 1%

Probable Causal Relationship

The following adverse reactions, occurring in less than 1% of patients, were reported in controlled clinical trials and through voluntary reports since Nalfon® (fenoprofen calcium, Dista) was initially marketed. The probability of a causal relationship exists between Nalfon and these adverse reactions:

Digestive System—Gastritis, peptic ulcer with/without perforation, and/or gastrointestinal hemorrhage. Increases in alkaline phosphatase, LDH, and SGOT, jaundice, and cholestatic hepatitis were observed (*see* Precautions).

Genitourinary Tract—Dysuria, cystitis, hematuria, oliguria, azotemia, anuria, interstitial nephritis, nephrosis, and papillary necrosis (*see* Warnings).

Hematologic—Purpura, bruising, hemorrhage, thrombocytopenia, hemolytic anemia, aplastic anemia, agranulocytosis, and pancytopenia.

Miscellaneous—Peripheral edema and anaphylaxis.

INCIDENCE LESS THAN 1%

Causal Relationship Unknown

Other reactions have been reported but occurred in circumstances in which a causal relationship could not be established. However, with these rarely reported reactions, the possibility of such a relationship cannot be excluded. Therefore, these observations are listed to alert the physician.

Skin and Appendages—Stevens-Johnson syndrome, angioneurotic edema, exfoliative dermatitis, and alopecia.

Digestive System—Aphthous ulcerations of the buccal mucosa, metallic taste, and pancreatitis.

Cardiovascular—Atrial fibrillation, pulmonary edema, electrocardiographic changes, and supraventricular tachycardia.

Nervous System—Depression, disorientation, seizures, and trigeminal neuralgia.

Special Senses—Burning tongue, diplopia, and optic neuritis.

Miscellaneous—Personality change, lymphadenopathy, mastodynia, and fever.

OVERDOSAGE

No specific information is available on the treatment of overdosage with Nalfon® (fenoprofen calcium, Dista). If it should occur, standard procedures to evacuate gastric contents and to support vital functions should be employed. Since Nalfon is acidic and is excreted in the urine, it may be beneficial to administer alkali and charcoal and induce diuresis. Furosemide did not lower blood levels.

DOSAGE AND ADMINISTRATION

Analgesia—For the treatment of mild to moderate pain, the recommended dosage is 200 mg every four to six hours, as needed.

Rheumatoid Arthritis and Osteoarthritis—The suggested dosage is 300 to 600 mg three or four times a day. The dose should be tailored to the needs of the patient and may be increased or decreased depending on the severity of the symptoms. Dosage adjustments may be made after initiation of drug therapy or during exacerbations of the disease. Total daily dosage should not exceed 3200 mg.

If gastrointestinal complaints occur, Nalfon® (fenoprofen calcium, Dista) may be administered with meals or with milk. Although the total amount absorbed is not affected, peak blood levels are delayed and diminished.

Patients with rheumatoid arthritis generally seem to require larger doses of Nalfon than do those with osteoarthritis. The smallest dose that yields acceptable control should be employed.

Although improvement may be seen in a few days in many patients, an additional two to three weeks may be required to gauge the full benefits of therapy.

HOW SUPPLIED

(℞) *Pulvules Nalfon ® 200 (Fenoprofen Calcium Capsules, USP): No. 415, H76,* * 200 mg (equivalent to fenoprofen) (No. 1, White Opaque Body, Ocher Opaque Cap), in an ℞Pak of 100 (NDC 0777-0876-02). All ℞Paks have safety closures.

(℞) *Pulvules Nalfon, No. 416, H77,* * 300 mg (equivalent to fenoprofen) (No. 0, Yellow Opaque Body, Ocher Opaque Cap), in an ℞Pak of 100 (NDC 0777-0877-02) and in bottles of 500 (NDC 0777-0877-03).

(℞) *Tablets Nalfon ® (Fenoprofen Calcium Tablets, USP), No. 1900, U59,** 600 mg (equivalent to fenoprofen), Yellow (paracapsule-shaped, scored), in an ℞Pak of 100 (NDC 0777-2159-02) and in bottles of 500 (NDC 0777-2159-03). All ℞Paks have safety closures.

[062885]

Shown in Product Identification Section, page 408

* Identi-Code® symbol.

VALMID® ©

[*văl'mĭd*]

(ethinamate)

Capsules, USP

DESCRIPTION

Valmid® (ethinamate, Dista) is 1-ethinyl-cyclohexyl-carbamate. It is a nonirritating, colorless, faintly bitter, stable crystalline powder with a melting point of 96°-98° C. Valmid is relatively insoluble in water but quite soluble in many alcohols and oils.

Each Pulvule® contains 500 mg ethinamate. These Pulvules also contains F D & C Blue No. 1, F D & C Red No. 3, gelatin, silicone, sodium bicarbonate, sodium carboxymethyl starch, sodium lauryl sulfate, titanium dioxide, and other inactive ingredients.

Valmid is a hypnotic agent for oral administration. Its site and mechanism of action are unknown.

Continued on next page

Dista—Cont.

CLINICAL PHARMACOLOGY
Valmid® (ethinamate, Dista) is rapidly absorbed after oral administration. Following a single oral dose of 1 g, peak plasma levels are reached in approximately 36 minutes and decline to negligible values over the next eight hours. Approximately 36 percent of the administered dose appears in the urine within 24 hours. The effect of multiple doses and prolonged administration on pharmacodynamics and pharmacokinetics is not known.

INDICATIONS AND USAGE
Valmid® (ethinamate, Dista) is a short-acting hypnotic. It has not been sufficiently well studied with currently available sleep laboratory techniques to delimit its value in specific types of insomnia. Valmid is best used for limited periods. Should insomnia persist, drug-free intervals of one week or more should elapse before re-treatment is considered. Attempts should be made to find alternative nondrug therapy for chronic insomnia. The prolonged administration of Valmid is not recommended, since it has not been shown to be effective for a period of more than seven days.

CONTRAINDICATION
Valmid® (ethinamate, Dista) is contraindicated in patients with known hypersensitivity to the drug.

WARNINGS
Patients receiving Valmid® (ethinamate, Dista) should be cautioned about possible additive effects when it is taken in combination with alcohol or other CNS depressants. Patients should be cautioned against becoming involved in hazardous occupations requiring complete mental alertness, such as operating machines or driving a motor vehicle, shortly after ingestion of the drug.

PRECAUTIONS
Drug Interactions—If Valmid® (ethinamate, Dista) is to be administered in combination with other drugs known to have a hypnotic or CNS-depressant effect, consideration should be given to the potential additive effects.
Carcinogenesis—Long-term studies in animals have *not* been performed to evaluate carcinogenic potential.
Usage in Pregnancy—Pregnancy Category C—Animal reproduction studies have not been conducted with Valmid. It is also not known whether the drug can cause fetal harm when administered to a pregnant woman or can affect reproduction capacity. Valmid should be given to a pregnant woman only if clearly needed.
Nursing Mothers—It is not known whether this drug is excreted in human milk. Because many drugs are excreted in human milk, caution should be exercised when Valmid is administered to a nursing woman.
Usage in Children—Safety and effectiveness in children below the age of 15 years have not been established.

ADVERSE REACTIONS
Rare cases of thrombocytopenic purpura and drug idiosyncrasy with fever have been reported. Paradoxical excitement in children, mild gastrointestinal symptoms, and skin rashes have occurred after the use of Valmid® (ethinamate, Dista).

DRUG ABUSE AND DEPENDENCE
Controlled Substance—Valmid® (ethinamate, Dista) is a Schedule IV drug.
Dependence—Drug dependence characterized by both a psychologic and a physical dependence has occurred when Valmid has been taken at higher than recommended doses for prolonged intervals. It is, therefore, desirable to exercise caution in administering Valmid to individuals who are addiction-prone and to those whose history suggests that they may increase dosage on their own initiative. It is advisable to limit repeated prescriptions without adequate medical supervision.
In the event that an individual has established dependence on Valmid, withdrawal must be accomplished with extreme care. Abrupt withdrawal may cause a typical abstinence syndrome accompanied by convulsions. Withdrawal may be accomplished by hospitalizing the patient and reducing the addictive daily dose at a rate of 500 to 1000 mg every two or three days. Psychiatric follow-up is indicated.

OVERDOSAGE
In suicidal overdosage, CNS and respiratory depression should be treated in the same manner as barbiturate intoxication. Valmid® (ethinamate, Dista) is dialyzable.

DOSAGE AND ADMINISTRATION
For insomnia, 1 or 2 Pulvules (500 mg or 1 g) of Valmid® (ethinamate, Dista) should be taken 20 minutes before retiring.
Special Patient Population—Since the risk of oversedation, dizziness, confusion, and/or ataxia substantially increases with the administration of large doses of sedatives and hypnotics in the elderly and debilitated, it is recommended that a single 500-mg Pulvule be the dose given to such individuals. Should this dose prove to be ineffective, clinical judgment must weigh the risk of increasing the dosage against the potential hazards mentioned above.

HOW SUPPLIED
(Ⓒ) *Pulvules No. 399, Valmid ® (Ethinamate Capsules, USP), H74,** 500 mg (No. 0, Light-Blue Opaque Body, Blue Opaque Cap), in bottles of 100 (NDC 0777-0874-02). [050985]
Shown in Product Identification Section, page 408

*Identi-Code® symbol.

Dorsey Laboratories
Division of Sandoz, Inc.
LINCOLN, NE 68501

ACID MANTLE® CREME OTC
[*ă'sid-mănt'l*]

DESCRIPTION
A greaseless, water-miscible preparation containing buffered aluminum acetate. Other ingredients: aluminum sulfate, calcium acetate, cetearyl alcohol, glycerin, light mineral oil, methylparaben, purified water, sodium lauryl sulfate, synthetic beeswax, white petrolatum, white potato dextrin. May also contain: ammonium hydroxide, citric acid.

INDICATIONS
A vehicle for compatible topical drugs. Restores and maintains protective acidity of the skin. Provides relief from mild skin irritation due to exposure to soaps, detergents, chemicals, alkalis. Aids in the treatment of diaper rash, acne, eczema and dry, rough, scaly skin from varied causes.

APPLICATION
Apply several times daily, especially after wet work.

CAUTION
Limited compatibility and stability with Vitamin A, neomycin and water-soluble antibiotics. For external use only. Not for ophthalmic use.

HOW SUPPLIED
1 oz tubes; 4 oz and 1 lb jars.

CAMA® ARTHRITIS PAIN RELIEVER OTC
[*kă'măh*]

(See PDR For Nonprescription Drugs)

DORCOL® CHILDREN'S COUGH SYRUP OTC
[*door'call*]

DESCRIPTION
Each teaspoonful (5 ml) of DORCOL Children's Cough Syrup contains: pseudoephedrine hydrochloride 15 mg, guaifenesin 50 mg and dextromethorphan hydrobromide 5 mg. Other ingredients: benzoic acid, Blue 1, edetate disodium, flavors, glycerin, propylene glycol, purified water, Red 40, sodium hydroxide, sucrose, tartaric acid.

INDICATIONS
Provides prompt relief of cough and nasal congestion due to the common cold. Reduces swelling of the nasal passages, decreases cough and helps loosen phlegm and bronchial secretions to rid the bronchial passageways of bothersome mucus.

CONTRAINDICATIONS
Hypersensitivity to any of the ingredients. The use of sympathomimetic agents such as pseudoephedrine hydrochloride is contraindicated in patients with severe hypertension, severe coronary artery disease or in those taking monoamine oxidase inhibitors.

PRECAUTIONS:
Exercise prescribing caution in patients with persistent or chronic cough such as occurs with chronic bronchitis or bronchial asthma or with cough that is accompanied by excessive secretions. Use with caution in patients with hypertension, hyperthyroidism, cardiovascular disease, diabetes mellitus, elevated intraocular pressure, prostatic hypertrophy or impaired hepatic function.

ADVERSE REACTIONS
Mild CNS stimulation, gastrointestinal upsets, headache, drowsiness or dizziness may occur.

DOSAGE AND ADMINISTRATION
Bottle label dosage reads:
By age: Children 2 to under 6 years:
1 teaspoonful every 4 hours
Children 6 to under 12 years: 2 teaspoonfuls every 4 hours
By weight: Children 25 to 45 pounds:
1 teaspoonful every 4 hours
Children 46 to 85 pounds: 2 teaspoonfuls every 4 hours
Children under 2 years—consult physician.
Unless directed by a physician, do not exceed 4 doses in 24 hours.
The suggested dosage for pediatric patients 3 months to under 12 months of age is 3 drops per kilogram of body weight administered every 4 hours. The suggested dosage for patients 12 months to under 24 months of age is 7 drops (0.2 ml) per kilogram of body weight administered every 4 hours. A maximum of 4 doses per 24 hours is recommended.

HOW SUPPLIED
DORCOL Children's Cough Syrup (grape colored), in 4 fl oz and 8 fl oz plastic bottles with tamper- evident band around child-resistant cap.

DORCOL® CHILDREN'S DECONGESTANT LIQUID OTC
[*door'call*]

DESCRIPTION
Each teaspoonful (5 ml) of DORCOL Children's Decongestant Liquid contains pseudoephedrine hydrochloride 15 mg. Other ingredients: benzoic acid, edetate disodium, flavors, purified water, sodium hydroxide, sorbitol, sucrose, Yellow 6, Yellow 10.

INDICATIONS
Provides temporary relief of nasal congestion due to the common cold, hay fever or other upper respiratory allergies, or associated with sinusitis. Reduces swelling of nasal passages to restore freer breathing through the nose. Promotes nasal and sinus drainage; relieves sinus pressure.

CONTRAINDICATIONS
Hypersensitivity to any of the components. The use of sympathomimetic agents such as pseudoephedrine hydrochloride is contraindicated in patients with severe hypertension, severe coronary artery disease or in those taking monoamine oxidase inhibitors.

PRECAUTIONS
Exercise prescribing caution in patients with hypertension, cardiovascular disease, diabetes mellitus, hyperthyroidism, elevated intraocular pressure or prostatic hypertrophy.

ADVERSE REACTIONS
Mild CNS stimulation or dizziness may occur. Headache and drowsiness have been reported. Large doses may cause lightheadedness, nausea and/or vomiting.

DOSAGE AND ADMINISTRATION
Bottle label dosage reads:
By age:
Children 2 to under 6 years:
1 teaspoonful every 4 to 6 hours
Children 6 years: 2 teaspoonfuls every 4 to 6 hours
By weight:
Children 25 to 45 pounds
1 teaspoonful every 4 to 6 hours
Children 46 to 85 pounds
2 teaspoonfuls every 4 to 6 hours
Children under 2 years—consult physician.
Unless directed by a physician, do not exceed 4 doses in 24 hours.
The suggested dosage for pediatric patients 3 months to under 12 months of age is 3 drops per kilogram of body weight every 4 to 6 hours. The suggested dosage for patients 12 months to under 24 months of age is 7 drops (0.2 ml) per kilogram of body weight every 4 to 6 hours. A maximum of 4 doses per 24 hours is recommended.

HOW SUPPLIED
DORCOL Children's Decongestant Liquid (pale orange), in 4 fl oz bottles with tamper-evident band around child-resistant cap.

DORCOL® CHILDREN'S FEVER & PAIN REDUCER OTC
[*door'call*]

DESCRIPTION
Each teaspoonful (5 ml) of DORCOL Children's Fever & Pain Reducer contains acetaminophen 160 mg. Other ingredients: benzoic acid, edetate disodium, flavors, glycerin, polyethylene glycol, purified water, Red 40, sodium chloride, sucrose.

INDICATIONS
Provides analgesic/antipyretic action for infants and children with conditions requiring relief of pain or reduction of fever.

CONTRAINDICATIONS
Hypersensitivity to any of the ingredients. Repeated administration of acetaminophen is contraindicated in patients with anemia or renal or hepatic disease.

PRECAUTIONS
Acetaminophen is relatively nontoxic in therapeutic doses. However, it should be used with caution in patients with preexisting anemia, since cyanosis may not be apparent despite very high levels of methemoglobin.

ADVERSE REACTIONS
Acetaminophen has rarely been found to produce any side effects. Sensitivity reactions have been reported.

DOSAGE AND ADMINISTRATION
Bottle label dosage reads:
Children under 2 years—consult physician.
By age:

Children 2 to under 4 years:	1 teaspoonful
Children 4 to under 6 years:	1½ teaspoonfuls
Children 6 years of age:	2 teaspoonfuls

By weight:

Children 25 to 35 pounds:	1 teaspoonful
Children 36 to 45 pounds:	1½ teaspoonfuls
Children 46 to 60 pounds:	2 teaspoonfuls

Give every 4 hours while symptoms persist or as directed by a physician. Unless directed by a physician, do not exceed 5 doses in 24 hours.
The suggested dosage for pediatric patients 3 months to under 12 months of age is 3 drops per kilogram of body weight. The suggested dosage for patients 12 months to under 24 months of age is 7 drops (0.2 ml) per kilogram of body weight. Give dose every 4 hours while symptoms persist. A maximum of 5 doses per 24 hours is recommended.

HOW SUPPLIED
DORCOL Children's Fever & Pain Reducer (red), in 4 fl oz bottles with tamper-evident band around child-resistant cap.

DORCOL® CHILDREN'S LIQUID COLD FORMULA OTC
[door'call]

DESCRIPTION
Each teaspoonful (5 ml) of DORCOL Children's Liquid Cold Formula contains pseudoephedrine hydrochloride 15 mg and chlorpheniramine maleate 1 mg. Other ingredients: benzoic acid, Blue 1, flavors, purified water, Red 40, sorbitol, sucrose, Yellow 10. May also contain sodium hydroxide.

INDICATIONS
Provides temporary relief of nasal congestion, sneezing and rhinorrhea due to the common cold, hay fever or other upper respiratory allergies, or associated with sinusitis. Reduces swelling of nasal passages and restores freer breathing through the nose. Promotes nasal and sinus drainage; relieves sinus pressure.

CONTRAINDICATIONS
Hypersensitivity to any of the ingredients. The use of sympathomimetic agents such as pseudoephedrine hydrochloride is contraindicated in patients with severe hypertension, severe coronary artery disease or in those taking monoamine oxidase inhibitors. Antihistamines such as chlorpheniramine maleate should not be administered to premature or newborn infants or be used to treat lower respiratory tract symptoms.

PRECAUTIONS
Exercise prescribing caution in patients with hypertension, cardiovascular disease, diabetes mellitus, hyperthyroidism, elevated intraocular pressure, prostatic hypertrophy, bladder neck obstruction or chronic pulmonary disease.

ADVERSE REACTIONS
Mild CNS stimulation, drowsiness, blurred vision, dry mouth, tachycardia, dizziness, gastrointestinal upset may occur occasionally. May produce thickening of bronchial secretions.

DOSAGE AND ADMINISTRATION
Bottle label dosage reads:
Children under 6 years—consult physician.
By age:
Children 6 to under 12 years:
2 teaspoonfuls every 4 to 6 hours
By weight:
Children 45 to 85 pounds:
2 teaspoonfuls every 4 to 6 hours
Unless directed by a physician, do not exceed 4 doses in 24 hours.
The suggested dosage for pediatric patients 3 months to under 12 months of age is 2 drops per kilogram of body weight every 4 to 6 hours. The suggested dosage for patients 12 months to under 24 months of age is 5 drops (0.2 ml) per kilogram of body weight every 4 to 6 hours. The suggested dosage for patients 2 years to under 6 years is 1 teaspoonful every 4 to 6 hours. A maximum of 4 doses per 24 hours is recommended.

HOW SUPPLIED
DORCOL Children's Liquid Cold Formula (light brown), in 4 fl oz bottles with tamper-evident band around child-resistant cap.

KANULASE® TABLETS OTC
[căn'ū-lāce]

DESCRIPTION
Each KANULASE Tablet contains: Dorase® (cellulase) standardized to 9 mg; pancreatin (equivalent to the following enzyme activities: lipase 1000 USP units, amylase 1000 USP units; protease 12,000 USP units); glutamic acid hydrochloride 200 mg; ox bile extract 100 mg; pepsin 150 mg. Other ingredients: alginic acid, colloidal silicon dioxide, flavor, lactose, magnesium stearate, methylcellulose, methylparaben, microcrystalline cellulose, pharmaceutical glaze, polyethylene glycol, polysorbate 20, povidone, Red 30, starch, stearic acid, talc, titanium dioxide.

INDICATIONS
For relief of discomforts of intestinal gas such as belching, bloating and flatulence.

CONTRAINDICATIONS
Hypersensitivity to any of the ingredients.

PRECAUTIONS
KANULASE contains glutamic acid hydrochloride which is not usually given to patients with peptic ulcer. Use with caution in pregnant and nursing women.

DOSAGE AND ADMINISTRATION
Adults—1 or 2 tablets, swallowed whole, with meals. If looseness of stools occurs, decrease the dosage.

HOW SUPPLIED
KANULASE Tablets (pink), in bottles of 50.

TRIAMINIC® ALLERGY TABLETS OTC
[trī"ah-mĭn'ĭc]

(See PDR For Nonprescription Drugs)

TRIAMINIC® CHEWABLES OTC
[trī"ah-mĭn'ĭc]

(See PDR For Nonprescription Drugs)

TRIAMINIC® COLD SYRUP OTC
[trī"ah-mĭn'ĭc]

DESCRIPTION
Each teaspoonful (5 ml) of TRIAMINIC Cold Syrup contains phenylpropanolamine hydrochloride 12.5 mg and chlorpheniramine maleate 2 mg in a nonalcoholic vehicle. Other ingredients: benzoic acid, edetate disodium, flavors, purified water, sodium hydroxide, sorbitol, sucrose, Yellow 6.

INDICATIONS
Provides temporary relief of nasal congestion, runny nose and sneezing that may occur with the common cold or with hay fever or other upper respiratory allergies. Relieves itching of the nose or throat and itchy, watery eyes.

CONTRAINDICATIONS
Hypersensitivity to any of the ingredients. The use of sympathomimetic agents such as phenylpropanolamine hydrochloride is contraindicated in patients with severe hypertension, severe coronary artery disease or in those taking monoamine oxidase inhibitors. Antihistamines such as chlorpheniramine maleate should not be administered to premature or newborn infants or be used to treat lower respiratory tract symptoms.

PRECAUTIONS
Exercise prescribing caution in patients with hypertension, cardiovascular disease, diabetes mellitus, hyperthyroidism, elevated intraocular pressure, prostatic hypertrophy, bladder neck obstruction or chronic pulmonary disease. Alcoholic beverages and other CNS depressants may potentiate the sedative effects of antihistamines. Use with caution in pregnant and nursing women.

ADVERSE REACTIONS
Mild CNS stimulation, drowsiness, blurred vision, dry mouth, tachycardia, dizziness, gastrointestinal upset may occur occasionally. May produce thickening of bronchial secretions.

DOSAGE AND ADMINISTRATION
Bottle label dosage reads: Adults—2 teaspoonfuls every 4 hours. Children 6–12 years—1 teaspoonful every 4 hours. Children under 6 years—consult physician.
The suggested dosage for pediatric patients 3 months to under 12 months of age is 1 drop per kilogram of body weight administered every 4 hours. The suggested dosage for patients 12 months to under 24 months of age is 3 drops per kilogram of body weight administered every 4 hours. The suggested dosage for patients 2 to under 6 years is ½ teaspoonful every 4 hours.

HOW SUPPLIED
TRIAMINIC Cold Syrup (orange), in 4 fl oz and 8 fl oz plastic bottles with tamper-evident band around child-resistant cap.

TRIAMINIC® COLD TABLETS OTC
[trī"ah-mĭn'ĭc]

DESCRIPTION
Each TRIAMINIC Cold Tablet contains phenylpropanolamine hydrochloride 12.5 mg and chlorpheniramine maleate 2 mg. Other ingredients: calcium stearate, colloidal silicon dioxide, flavor, lactose, methylcellulose, methylparaben, microcrystalline cellulose, polyethylene glycol, povidone, Red 40, saccharin sodium, starch, titanium dioxide, Yellow 6.

INDICATIONS
For the temporary relief of nasal congestion, runny nose and sneezing that may occur with the common cold or with hay fever or other upper respiratory allergies. Promotes nasal and sinus drainage.

CONTRAINDICATIONS
Hypersensitivity to any of the ingredients. The use of sympathomimetic agents such as phenylpropanolamine hydrochloride is contraindicated in patients with severe hypertension, severe coronary artery disease or in those taking monoamine oxidase inhibitors. Antihistamines such as chlorpheniramine maleate should not be used to treat lower respiratory tract symptoms.

PRECAUTIONS
Exercise prescribing caution in patients with hypertension, cardiovascular disease, diabetes mellitus, hyperthyroidism, elevated intraocular pressure, prostatic hypertrophy, bladder neck obstruction or chronic pulmonary disease. Alcoholic beverages and other CNS depressants may potentiate the sedative effects of antihistamines. Use with caution in pregnant and nursing women.

ADVERSE REACTIONS
Mild CNS stimulation, drowsiness, blurred vision, dry mouth, tachycardia, dizziness or gastrointestinal upset may occur. May produce thickening of bronchial secretions.

DOSAGE AND ADMINISTRATION
Adults — 2 tablets every 4 hours. Children 6-12 years — 1 tablet every 4 hours.

HOW SUPPLIED
TRIAMINIC Cold Tablets (orange), imprinted "DORSEY" on one side, "TRIAMINIC" on the other, in blister packs of 24.

TRIAMINIC® EXPECTORANT OTC
[trī"ah-mĭn'ĭc]

DESCRIPTION
Each teaspoonful (5 ml) of TRIAMINIC Expectorant contains phenylpropanolamine hydrochloride 12.5 mg and guaifenesin 100 mg. Other ingredients: alcohol (5%), benzoic acid, edetate disodium, flavors, purified water, saccharin, saccharin sodium, sodium hydroxide, sorbitol, sucrose, Yellow 6, Yellow 10.

INDICATIONS
Provides prompt relief of cough and nasal congestion due to the common cold. The expectorant component helps loosen bronchial secretions and rid the bronchial passageways of bothersome mucus. The decongestant and expectorant are provided in an antihistamine-free formula.

CONTRAINDICATIONS
Hypersensitivity to any of the ingredients. The use of sympathomimetic agents such as phenylpropanolamine hydrochloride is contraindicated in patients with severe hypertension, severe coronary artery disease or in those taking monoamine oxidase inhibitors.

PRECAUTIONS
Exercise prescribing caution in patients with persistent or chronic cough such as occurs with chronic bronchitis or bronchial asthma. Use with caution in patients with hypertension, hyperthyroidism, cardiovascular disease or diabetes mellitus. Use with caution in pregnant and nursing women.

ADVERSE REACTIONS
Mild CNS stimulation, drowsiness, headache or gastrointestinal upsets may occur.

DOSAGE AND ADMINISTRATION
Bottle label dosage reads: Adults—2 teaspoonfuls every 4 hours. Children 6–12 years—1 teaspoonful every 4 hours.

Continued on next page

Dorsey Labs.—Cont.

Children 2–6 years—½ teaspoonful every 4 hours. Children under 2 years—consult physician.
The suggested dosage for pediatric patients 3 months to under 12 months of age is 2 drops per kilogram of body weight administered every 4 hours. The suggested dosage for patients 12 months to under 24 months of age is 3 drops per kilogram of body weight administered every 4 hours.

HOW SUPPLIED
TRIAMINIC Expectorant (yellow), in 4 fl oz and 8 fl oz plastic bottles with tamper-evident band around child-resistant cap.

TRIAMINIC® EXPECTORANT DH Ⓒ III
[trī″ah-mĭn′ĭc]

DESCRIPTION
Each teaspoonful (5 ml) of TRIAMINIC Expectorant DH contains: hydrocodone bitartrate 1.67 mg (Warning: May be habit forming), phenylpropanolamine hydrochloride 12.5 mg, pheniramine maleate 6.25 mg, pyrilamine maleate 6.25 mg, and guaifenesin 100 mg. Other ingredients: alcohol (5%), benzoic acid, Blue 1, flavors, purified water, saccharin sodium, sorbitol, sucrose, Yellow 6, Yellow 10.
Phenylpropanolamine hydrochloride, a sympathomimetic drug, is structurally related to ephedrine and amphetamine.
Pheniramine maleate is an antihistamine of the alkylamine class while pyrilamine maleate belongs to the ethylenediamine class.
The expectorant component is guaifenesin (3-(o-methoxyphenoxy)-1,2- propanediol) which helps loosen and thus clear the bronchial passageways of bothersome, thickened mucus.
The antitussive component, hydrocodone, is 7,8 dihydrocodeinone, a derivative of codeine.

CLINICAL PHARMACOLOGY
Phenylpropanolamine presumably acts on α-adrenergic receptors in the mucosa of the respiratory tract producing vasoconstriction which results in shrinkage of swollen mucous membranes, reduction of tissue hyperemia, edema and nasal congestion, and an increase in nasal airway patency.
Antihistamines competitively act as H_1 receptor antagonists of histamine. They exhibit anticholinergic (drying) and sedative side effects. There are several classes of antihistamines which vary with respect to potency, dosage and the relative incidence of side effects. Antihistamines inhibit the effects of histamine on capillary permeability and on vascular, bronchial and many other types of smooth muscle.
By increasing respiratory tract fluid, guaifenesin reduces the viscosity of tenacious secretions and acts as an expectorant. The drug is effective in productive as well as nonproductive cough, but is of particular value in dry, nonproductive cough which tends to injure the mucous membranes of the air passages.
Hydrocodone is a centrally acting narcotic antitussive providing cough relief for up to 6 hours.

INDICATIONS
For relief of troublesome cough, nasal congestion and postnasal drip associated with colds, nasal allergies, sinusitis, and rhinitis. Also effective for relief of severe, prolonged or refractory cough associated with other respiratory disorders. For the relief of symptoms associated with allergic rhinitis such as sneezing, rhinorrhea, pruritus and lacrimation.

CONTRAINDICATIONS
TRIAMINIC Expectorant DH is contraindicated in patients exhibiting hypersensitivity to any of the ingredients. Antihistamines are contraindicated in patients receiving monoamine oxidase inhibitors since these agents may prolong and intensify the anticholinergic effects of antihistamines (see Drug Interactions). Antihistamines *should not* be used to treat lower respiratory tract symptoms or be given to premature or newborn infants. Sympathomimetic agents such as phenylpropanolamine are contraindicated in patients with severe hypertension, severe coronary artery disease and in those taking monoamine oxidase inhibitors. Narcotic analgesics are contraindicated in patients with acute respiratory depression. Continuous dosage over an extended period is generally contraindicated since hydrocodone can cause addiction.
Nursing Mothers: Because of the higher risk of antihistamines for premature and newborn infants, antihistamine therapy is contraindicated in nursing mothers.

WARNINGS
TRIAMINIC Expectorant DH can produce drug dependence, and therefore has the potential for abuse.
Sympathomimetic agents should be used with caution in patients with hypertension, hyperthyroidism, diabetes mellitus and cardiovascular disease. Antihistamines should be used with caution in patients with narrow angle glaucoma, stenosing peptic ulcer, pyloroduodenal obstruction, symptomatic prostatic hypertrophy, bladder neck obstruction or chronic pulmonary disease. Narcotic analgesics should be used with caution in patients with chronic respiratory impairment, cardiac arrhythmias, history of convulsions, history of drug dependence, gallbladder disease or impaired renal or hepatic function.
Use in the Elderly (Approximately 60 Years or Older): Antihistamines are more likely to cause dizziness, sedation and hypotension in elderly patients. Overdosage of sympathomimetic agents in this age group may cause hallucinations, convulsions, CNS depression or death. Geriatric patients may be more susceptible to the effects of hydrocodone, especially the respiratory depressant effects.

PRECAUTIONS
General: Use with caution in patients with hypertension, hyperthyroidism, diabetes mellitus, cardiovascular disease, bronchial asthma, increased intraocular pressure (see WARNINGS). Before prescribing medication to suppress or modify cough, it is important to ascertain that the underlying cause of cough is identified, that modification of cough does not increase the risk of clinical complications, and that appropriate therapy for the primary disease is provided.
Information for Patients: Patients should be informed of the potential for sedation or drowsiness and cautioned about engaging in activities requiring mental alertness such as driving or operating machinery. The concomitant consumption of alcoholic beverages or other sedative drugs should be avoided.
Drug Interactions:
(1) Monoamine oxidase inhibitors: MAO inhibitors may prolong and intensify the anticholinergic effects of antihistamines and potentiate the pressor effects of sympathomimetics.
(2) Alcohol and CNS depressants: These agents potentiate the sedative effects of antihistamines and hydrocodone. The CNS and respiratory depressant effects of some opioids may be exaggerated and prolonged by phenothiazines, alcohol, CNS depressants, MAO inhibitors, and tricyclic antidepressants; the mechanism of this supra-additive effect is not fully understood, but may involve alterations in the rate of metabolic transformation of the opioid or alterations in neurotransmitters involved in opioid actions.
(3) Certain antihypertensives: Sympathomimetics may reduce the antihypertensive effects of methyldopa, mecamylamine, reserpine and veratrum alkaloids.

Drug/Laboratory Test Interactions: Guaifenesin or its metabolites may cause color interference with the VMA test for catechols. It may also falsely elevate the level of urinary 5HIAA in certain serotonin metabolite chemical tests because of color interference.
Carcinogenesis, Mutagenesis, Impairment of Fertility: No data are available on the long-term potential for carcinogenicity, mutagenicity or impairment of fertility in animals or humans.
Pregnancy: *Pregnancy Category C*— Animal reproduction studies have not been conducted. Safe use in pregnancy has not been established relative to possible adverse effects on fetal development. Therefore, this product should not be used in pregnant patients unless, in the judgement of the physician, the potential benefits outweigh possible hazards.
Nursing Mothers: See CONTRAINDICATIONS.
Pediatric Use: TRIAMINIC Expectorant DH is intended for administration to children 1 to 12 years of age (see DOSAGE AND ADMINISTRATION). It is important to note the variability of response infants and small children exhibit to antihistamines and sympathomimetics. As in adults, the combination of an antihistamine and sympathomimetic can elicit either mild stimulation or mild sedation in children. In the young child, mild stimulation is the response most frequently seen. In infants and children, overdosage of antihistamines may cause hallucinations, convulsions or death. Pediatric patients may be more susceptible to the effects of hydrocodone, especially the respiratory depressant effects.

ADVERSE REACTIONS
The most frequent adverse reactions are underlined.
(1) General: urticaria, drug rash, anaphylactic shock, photosensitivity, excessive perspiration, chills, dryness of mouth, nose and throat.
(2) Cardiovascular System: hypotension, headache, palpitations, tachycardia, extrasystoles.
(3) Hematologic System: hemolytic anemia, thrombocytopenia, agranulocytosis.
(4) Nervous System: <u>sedation</u>, <u>sleepiness</u>, <u>dizziness</u>, <u>disturbed coordination</u>, fatigue, confusion, restlessness, excitation, nervousness, tremor, irritability, insomnia, euphoria, paresthesias, blurred vision, diplopia, vertigo, tinnitus, acute labyrinthitis, hysteria, neuritis, convulsions, CNS depression, hallucinations.
(5) GI System: <u>epigastric distress</u>, anorexia, nausea, vomiting, diarrhea, <u>constipation</u>.
(6) GU System: urinary frequency, difficult urination, urinary retention, early menses.
(7) Respiratory System: thickening of bronchial secretions, tightness of chest and wheezing, nasal stuffiness.

DRUG ABUSE AND DEPENDENCE: Tolerance and physical dependence may occur following prolonged administration of hydrocodone.

OVERDOSAGE
Symptoms: The triad of coma, pinpoint pupils, and depressed respiration strongly suggest hydrocodone poisoning. Serious overdose with TRIAMINIC Expectorant DH may be characterized by respiratory depression, extreme somnolence progressing to stupor or coma, convulsions, skeletal muscle flaccidity, cold and clammy skin, and sometimes bradycardia and hypotension. In severe overdosage, apnea, circulatory collapse, cardiac arrest and death may occur. In the presence of fever and dehydration excitation may occur in children.
Treatment of Overdosage: Primary attention should be given to the reestablishment of adequate respiratory exchange through provision of patent airway and the institution of assisted or controlled ventilation. The narcotic antagonists naloxone and levallorphan are specific antidotes against respiratory depression which may result from overdosage or unusual sensitivity to narcotics, including hydrocodone. An appropriate dose of one of these antagonists should be administered, preferably by the intravenous route, simultaneously with efforts at respiratory resuscitation. The fact that an opioid antagonist may precipitate withdrawal symptoms in patients who are physically dependent on hydrocodone must be kept in mind and dosage titrated accordingly. Since the duration of action of hydrocodone may exceed that of the antagonist, the patient should be kept under continued surveillance and repeated doses of the antagonist should be administered as needed to maintain adequate respiration. Oxygen, intravenous fluids, vasopressors and other supportive measures should be employed as indicated, including treatment for anticholinergic drug intoxication. Gastric emptying may be useful in removing unabsorbed drug. Activated charcoal may be of benefit.

DOSAGE AND ADMINISTRATION
Adults—2 teaspoonfuls every 4 hours; children 6 to 12—1 teaspoonful every 4 hours; children 1 to 6—1/2 teaspoonful every 4 hours.

HOW SUPPLIED
TRIAMINIC Expectorant DH (green), in pint bottles. Store at room temperature. TRIAMINIC Expectorant DH is a Schedule III controlled substance.

TRIAMINIC® EXPECTORANT WITH CODEINE Ⓒ V
[trī″ah-mĭn′ĭc]

DESCRIPTION
Each teaspoonful (5 ml) of TRIAMINIC Expectorant with Codeine contains: codeine phosphate 10 mg (Warning: May be habit forming), phenylpropanolamine hydrochloride 12.5 mg, and guaifenesin 100 mg. Other ingredients: alcohol (5%), benzoic acid, Blue 1, flavors, purified water, saccharin sodium, sorbitol, sucrose. Yellow 10.

INDICATIONS
For use in providing temporary relief of coughs and nasal congestion due to the common cold, when the antitussive properties of codeine are desired. The expectorant component helps loosen bronchial secretions. The ingredients are provided in an antihistamine-free formula.

CONTRAINDICATIONS
Hypersensitivity to any of the ingredients. The use of sympathomimetic agents such as phenylpropanolamine hydrochloride is contraindicated in those patients with severe hypertension, severe coronary artery disease or in those taking monoamine oxidase inhibitors. Continuous dosage over an extended period is generally contraindicated since codeine phosphate may cause addiction.

PRECAUTIONS
Exercise prescribing caution in patients with persistent or chronic cough such as occurs with chronic bronchitis, bronchial asthma, or emphysema. Use with caution in patients with hypertension, hyperthyroidism, cardiovascular disease, diabetes mellitus, chronic pulmonary disease or shortness of breath. Exercise caution in prescribing this product to children taking other drugs. Pediatric and geriatric patients may be more susceptible to the effects of codeine, especially the respiratory depressant effects. Tolerance and physical dependence may occur following prolonged administration. Use with caution in pregnant and nursing women.

ADVERSE REACTIONS
Nausea, vomiting, constipation, dizziness, sedation or mild CNS stimulation may occur.

DOSAGE AND ADMINISTRATION
Bottle label dosage reads: Adults—2 teaspoonfuls every 4 hours. Children 6 to 12 years—1 teaspoonful every 4 hours. Children 2 to 6 years—½ teaspoonful every 4 hours. Children under 2 years—consult physician.

The suggested dosage in pediatric patients 3 months to 2 years of age is 2 drops per kilogram of body weight administered every 4 hours.

HOW SUPPLIED

TRIAMINIC Expectorant with Codeine (green), in pint bottles. TRIAMINIC Expectorant with Codeine is a Schedule V controlled substance.

TRIAMINIC® TR TABLETS ℞

[trī″ah mĭn′ĭc]

(Timed Release)

DESCRIPTION

Each TRIAMINIC TR Tablet (Timed Release) contains: phenylpropanolamine hydrochloride 50 mg, pheniramine maleate 25 mg, and pyrilamine maleate 25 mg. Other ingredients: acacia, colloidal silicon dioxide, lactose, magnesium stearate, methylcellulose, methylparaben, pharmaceutical glaze, polyethylene glycol, povidone, starch, stearic acid, sucrose, talc, titanium dioxide, Yellow 6, Yellow 10.

This product combines the nasal decongestant properties of phenylpropanolamine hydrochloride with the antihistaminic activities of pheniramine maleate and pyrilamine maleate.

Phenylpropanolamine hydrochloride, a sympathomimetic drug, is structurally related to ephedrine and amphetamine. Pheniramine maleate is an antihistamine of the alkylamine class while pyrilamine maleate belongs to the ethylenediamine class.

CLINICAL PHARMACOLOGY

Phenylpropanolamine presumably acts on α-adrenergic receptors in the mucosa of the respiratory tract producing vasoconstriction which results in shrinkage of swollen mucous membranes, reduction of tissue hyperemia, edema and nasal congestion, and an increase in nasal airway patency. Antihistamines competitively act as H_1 receptor antagonists of histamine. They exhibit anticholinergic (drying) and sedative side effects. There are several classes of antihistamines which vary with respect to potency, dosage and the relative incidence of side effects. Antihistamines inhibit the effects of histamine on capillary permeability and on vascular, bronchial and many other types of smooth muscle.

INDICATIONS AND USAGE

For relief from such symptoms as nasal congestion and postnasal drip associated with colds, allergies, sinusitis and rhinitis. Also for the relief of symptoms associated with allergic rhinitis such as sneezing, rhinorrhea, pruritus and lacrimation.

CONTRAINDICATIONS

TRIAMINIC TR Tablets are contraindicated in patients exhibiting hypersensitivity to any of the ingredients. Antihistamines are contraindicated in patients receiving monoamine oxidase inhibitors since these agents may prolong and intensify the anticholinergic effects of antihistamines (see Drug Interactions). Antihistamines should not be used to treat lower respiratory tract symptoms. Sympathomimetic agents such as phenylpropanolamine are contraindicated in patients with severe hypertension, severe coronary artery disease and in those taking monoamine oxidase inhibitors.

Nursing Mothers: Because of the higher risk of antihistamines for premature or newborn infants, antihistamine therapy is contraindicated in nursing mothers.

WARNINGS

Sympathomimetic agents should be used with caution in patients with hypertension, hyperthyroidism, diabetes mellitus and cardiovascular disease. Antihistamines should be used with caution in patients with narrow angle glaucoma, stenosing peptic ulcer, pyloroduodenal obstruction, symptomatic prostatic hypertrophy, bladder neck obstruction or chronic pulmonary disease.

Use In The Elderly (approximately 60 years or older): Antihistamines are more likely to cause dizziness, sedation and hypertension in elderly patients. Overdosage of sympathomimetic agents in this age group may cause hallucinations, convulsions, CNS depression or death.

PRECAUTIONS

General: See WARNINGS.

Information For Patients: Patients should be informed of the potential for sedation or drowsiness and cautioned about driving or operating machinery. The concomitant consumption of alcoholic beverages or other sedative drugs should be avoided.

Drug Interactions:

(1) Monoamine oxidase inhibitors: MAO inhibitors may prolong and intensify the anticholinergic effects of antihistamines and potentiate the pressor effects of sympathomimetics.

(2) Alcohol and CNS depressants: These agents potentiate the sedative effects of antihistamines.

(3) Certain antihypertensives: Sympathomimetics may reduce the antihypertensive effects of methyldopa, mecamylamine, reserpine and veratrum alkaloids.

Carcinogenesis, Mutagenesis, Impairment Of Fertility: No data are available on the long-term potential for carcinogenicity, mutagenicity or impairment of fertility in animals or humans.

Pregnancy: ***Pregnancy Category C***—Animal reproduction studies have not been conducted. Safe use in pregnancy has not been established relative to possible adverse effects on fetal development. Therefore, TRIAMINIC TR Tablets should not be used in pregnant patients unless, in the judgment of the physician, the potential benefits outweigh possible hazards.

Nursing Mothers: See CONTRAINDICATIONS.

ADVERSE REACTIONS

The most frequent adverse reactions are underlined.

(1) *General:* urticaria, drug rash, anaphylactic shock, photosensitivity, excessive perspiration, chills, dryness of mouth, nose and throat.

(2) *Cardiovascular System:* hypotension, headache, palpitations, tachycardia, extrasystoles.

(3) *Hematologic System:* hemolytic anemia, thrombocytopenia, agranulocytosis.

(4) *Nervous System:* sedation, sleepiness, dizziness, disturbed coordination, fatigue, confusion, restlessness, excitation, nervousness, tremor, irritability, insomnia, euphoria, paresthesias, blurred vision, diplopia, vertigo, tinnitus, acute labyrinthitis, hysteria, neuritis, convulsions, CNS depression, hallucinations.

(5) *GI System:* epigastic distress, anorexia, nausea, vomiting, diarrhea, constipation.

(6) *GU System:* urinary frequency, difficult urination, urinary retention, early menses.

(7) *Respiratory System:* thickening of bronchial secretions, tightness of chest and wheezing, nasal stuffiness.

OVERDOSAGE

TRIAMINIC TR Tablets overdosage reactions may vary from central nervous system depression to stimulation. Stimulation is particularly likely in children. Atropine-like signs and symptoms—dry mouth; fixed, dilated pupils; flushing—and gastrointestinal symptoms may also occur.

If vomiting has not occurred spontaneously, the conscious patient should be induced to vomit. This is best done by having the patient drink a glass of water or milk after which they should be made to gag. Precautions against aspiration must be taken, especially in infants and children.

If vomiting is unsuccessful, gastric lavage is indicated within 3 hours after ingestion, and even later if large amounts of milk or cream were given beforehand. Isotonic and ½ isotonic saline is the lavage solution of choice.

Saline cathartics, such as milk of magnesia, by osmosis draw water into the bowel and therefore are valuable for their action in rapid dilution of bowel content.

Stimulants should *not* be used. Vasopressors may be used to treat hypotension.

DOSAGE AND ADMINISTRATION

TRIAMINIC TR Tablets (Timed Release): Adults and children over 12 years—1 tablet swallowed whole, in the morning, midafternoon and before retiring.

HOW SUPPLIED

TRIAMINIC TR Tablets (Timed Release) (yellow, round, film-coated, imprinted "DORSEY" on one side and "TRIAMINIC TR" on the other), in bottles of 100 and 250.

TRIAMINIC® ORAL INFANT DROPS ℞

[trī″ah-mĭn′ĭc]

DESCRIPTION

Each ml of TRIAMINIC Oral Infant Drops contains: phenylpropanolamine hydrochloride 20 mg, pheniramine maleate 10 mg, and pyrilamine maleate 10 mg. Other ingredients: benzoic acid, flavor, glycerin, purified water, Red 33, saccharin sodium, sorbitol, sucrose, Yellow 6.

This product combines the nasal decongestant properties of phenylpropanolamine hydrochloride with the antihistaminic activities of pheniramine maleate and pyrilamine maleate.

Phenylpropanolamine hydrochloride, a sympathomimetic drug, is structurally related to ephedrine and amphetamine. Pheniramine maleate is an antihistamine of the alkylamine class while pyrilamine maleate belongs to the ethylenediamine class.

CLINICAL PHARMACOLOGY

Phenylpropanolamine presumably acts on α-adrenergic receptors in the mucosa of the respiratory tract producing vasoconstriction which results in shrinkage of swollen mucous membranes, reduction of tissue hyperemia, edema and nasal congestion, and an increase in nasal airway patency. Antihistamines competitively act as H_1 receptor antagonists of histamine. They exhibit anticholinergic (drying) and sedative side effects. There are several classes of antihistamines which vary with respect to potency, dosage and the relative incidence of side effects. Antihistamines inhibit the effects of histamine on capillary permeability and on vascular, bronchial and many other types of smooth muscle.

INDICATIONS AND USAGE

For relief from such symptoms as nasal congestion and postnasal drip associated with colds, allergies, sinusitis and rhinitis. Also for relief of symptoms associated with allergic rhinitis such as sneezing, rhinorrhea, pruritus and lacrimation.

CONTRAINDICATIONS

TRIAMINIC Oral Infant Drops are contraindicated in patients exhibiting hypersensitivity to any of the ingredients. Antihistamines are contraindicated in patients receiving monoamine oxidase inhibitors since these agents may prolong and intensify the anticholinergic and CNS depressant effects of antihistamines (see Drug Interactions). Antihistamines should not be used to treat lower respiratory tract symptoms or be given to premature or newborn infants. Sympathomimetic agents such as phenylpropanolamine are contraindicated in patients with severe hypertension, severe coronary artery disease and in those taking monoamine oxidase inhibitors.

WARNINGS

Sympathomimetic agents should be used with caution in patients with hypertension, hyperthyroidism, diabetes mellitus and cardiovascular disease. Antihistamines should be used with caution in patients with narrow angle glaucoma, stenosing peptic ulcer, pyloroduodenal obstruction, symptomatic prostatic hypertrophy, bladder neck obstruction or chronic pulmonary disease.

PRECAUTIONS

General: see WARNINGS.

Information For Patients: Mothers should be informed of the potential for sedation or drowsiness. When prescribing antihistamine preparations, patients should be cautioned against mechanical activity requiring alertness.

Drug Interactions:

(1) Monoamine oxidase inhibitors: MAO inhibitors prolong and intensify the anticholinergic effects of antihistamines and potentiate the pressor effects of sympathomimetics.

(2) Alcohol and CNS depressants: These agents potentiate the sedative effects of antihistamines.

(3) Certain antihypertensives: Sympathomimetics may reduce the antihypertensive effects of methyldopa, mecamylamine, reserpine and veratrum alkaloids.

Carcinogenesis, Mutagenesis, Impairment Of Fertility: No data are available on the long-term potential for carcinogenicity, mutagenicity or impairment of fertility in animals or humans.

Pediatric Use: TRIAMINIC Oral Infant Drops have been formulated to provide safe and effective symptomatic relief for infants and small children. Precise dosage (on a body weight basis) is facilitated through the use of the plastic squeeze bottle with attached dropper tip (see DOSAGE AND ADMINISTRATION). It is important to note the variability of response infants and small children exhibit to antihistamines and sympathomimetics. As in adults, the combination of an antihistamine and sympathomimetic can elicit either mild stimulation or mild sedation in children. In the young child, mild stimulation is the response most frequently seen. In infants and children, overdosage of antihistamines may cause hallucinations, convulsions or death.

ADVERSE REACTIONS

The most frequent adverse reactions are underlined.

(1) *General:* urticaria, drug rash, anaphylactic shock, photosensitivity, excessive perspiration, chills, dryness of mouth, nose, and throat.

(2) *Cardiovascular System:* hypotension, headache, palpitations, tachycardia, extrasystoles.

(3) *Hematologic System:* hemolytic anemia, thrombocytopenia, agranulocytosis.

(4) *Nervous System:* sedation, sleepiness, dizziness, disturbed coordination, fatigue, confusion, restlessness, excitation, nervousness, tremor, irritability, insomnia, euphoria, paresthesias, blurred vision, diplopia, vertigo, tinnitus, acute labyrinthitis, hysteria, neuritis, convulsions, CNS depression, hallucinations.

(5) *GI System:* epigastic distress, anorexia, nausea, vomiting, diarrhea, constipation.

(6) *GU System:* urinary frequency, difficult urination, urinary retention.

(7) *Respiratory System:* thickening of bronchial secretions, tightness of chest and wheezing, nasal stuffiness.

OVERDOSAGE

TRIAMINIC product overdosage reactions may vary from central nervous system depression to stimulation. Stimulation is particularly likely in children. Atropine-like signs

Continued on next page

Dorsey Labs.—Cont.

and symptoms—dry mouth; fixed, dilated pupils; flushing—and gastrointestinal symptoms may also occur.

If vomiting has not occurred spontaneously, the conscious patient should be induced to vomit. This is best done by having the patient drink a glass of water or milk after which they should be made to gag. Precautions against aspiration must be taken, especially in infants and children.

If vomiting is unsuccessful, gastric lavage is indicated within 3 hours after ingestion, and even later if large amounts of milk or cream were given beforehand. Isotonic and ½ isotonic saline is the lavage solution of choice.

Saline cathartics, such as milk of magnesia, draw water by osmosis into the bowel and therefore are valuable for their action in rapid dilution of bowel content.

Stimulants should *not* be used. Vasopressors may be used to treat hypotension.

DOSAGE AND ADMINISTRATION

1 drop per 2 pounds of body weight administered orally 4 times daily. The prescribed number of drops may be put directly into child's mouth or on a spoon for administration.

HOW SUPPLIED

TRIAMINIC Oral Infant Drops, in 15 ml plastic squeeze bottles which deliver approximately 24 drops per ml. Store TRIAMINIC Oral Infant Drops at room temperature.

TRIAMINIC-DM® COUGH FORMULA OTC

[trī″ah-mĭn′ĭc]

DESCRIPTION

Each teaspoonful (5 ml) of TRIAMINIC-DM Cough Formula contains phenylpropanolamine hydrochloride 12.5 mg and dextromethorphan hydrobromide 10 mg in a nonalcoholic vehicle. Other ingredients: benzoic acid, Blue 1, flavors, propylene glycol, purified water, Red 40, sodium chloride, sorbitol, sucrose.

INDICATIONS

Provides relief of cough due to minor throat and bronchial irritation as may occur with the common cold or inhaled irritants. Promotes nasal and sinus drainage. The decongestant and antitussive are provided in an antihistamine-free formula.

CONTRAINDICATIONS

Hypersensitivity to any of the ingredients. The use of sympathomimetic agents such as phenylpropanolamine hydrochloride is contraindicated in patients with severe hypertension, severe coronary artery disease or in those taking monoamine oxidase inhibitors.

PRECAUTIONS

Exercise prescribing caution in patients with persistent or chronic cough such as occurs with chronic bronchitis, bronchial asthma or emphysema. Use with caution in patients with hypertension, hyperthyroidism, cardiovascular disease or diabetes mellitus. Use with caution in pregnant and nursing women.

ADVERSE REACTIONS

Mild CNS stimulation, dizziness, headache or gastrointestinal upsets may occur.

DOSAGE AND ADMINISTRATION

Bottle label dosage reads: Adults—2 teaspoonfuls every 4 hours. Children 6–12 years—1 teaspoonful every 4 hours. Children 2–6 years—½ teaspoonful every 4 hours. Children under 2 years—consult physician.

The suggested dosage for pediatric patients 3 months to under 12 months of age is 1 drop per kilogram of body weight administered every 4 hours. The suggested dosage for patients 12 months to under 24 months of age is 3 drops per kilogram of body weight administered every 4 hours.

HOW SUPPLIED

TRIAMINIC-DM Cough Formula (dark red), in 4 fl oz and 8 fl oz plastic bottles with tamper-evident band around child-resistant cap.

TRIAMINIC-12® TABLETS OTC

[trī″ah-mĭn′ĭc]

DESCRIPTION

Each TRIAMINIC-12 Tablet contains phenylpropanolamine hydrochloride 75 mg and chlorpheniramine maleate 12 mg. Other ingredients: acetylated monoglycerides, carnauba wax, colloidal silicon dioxide, ethylcellulose, lactose, hydroxypropyl methylcellulose, Red 30, stearic acid, titanium dioxide, Yellow 6. TRIAMINIC-12 Tablets contain the nasal decongestant, phenylpropanolamine, and the antihistamine, chlorpheniramine, in a formulation providing 12 hours of symptomatic relief.

INDICATIONS

For the temporary relief of nasal congestion due to the common cold, hay fever or other upper respiratory allergies and associated with sinusitis. Helps decongest sinus openings, sinus passages; promotes nasal and/or sinus drainage; temporarily restores freer breathing through the nose.

For temporary relief of running nose, sneezing, itching of the nose or throat and itchy and watery eyes as may occur in allergic rhinitis (such as hay fever).

DOSAGE

Adults and children over 12 years of age—1 tablet swallowed whole every 12 hours.

NOTE: The nonactive portion of the tablet that supplies the active ingredients may occasionally appear in the stool as a soft mass.

WARNINGS

This product is not recommended for use in children under 12 years of age. Use with caution in patients with high blood pressure, heart disease, diabetes, thyroid disease, asthma, glaucoma or difficulty in urination due to enlargement of the prostate gland. Do not exceed the recommended dosage because at higher doses nervousness, dizziness, or sleeplessness may occur. This preparation may cause drowsiness; this preparation may cause excitability, especially in children.

CAUTION

Patients should be advised to avoid driving a motor vehicle or operating heavy machinery. Patients should also be advised to avoid alcoholic beverages while taking this product. Use with caution in pregnant and nursing women.

DRUG INTERACTION PRECAUTION

Use with caution in patients presently taking a prescription antihypertensive or antidepressant drug containing a monoamine oxidase inhibitor.

HOW SUPPLIED

TRIAMINIC-12 Tablets (orange), imprinted "DORSEY" on one side, "TRIAMINIC 12" on the other, in blister packs of 10 and 20.

TRIAMINICIN® TABLETS OTC

[trī″ah-mĭn′ĭ-sĭn]

(See PDR For Nonprescription Drugs)

TRIAMINICOL® MULTI-SYMPTOM COLD SYRUP OTC

[trī″ah-mĭn′ĭ-call]

DESCRIPTION

Each teaspoonful (5 ml) of TRIAMINICOL Multi-Symptom Cold Syrup contains: phenylpropanolamine hydrochloride 12.5 mg, chlorpheniramine maleate 2 mg, and dextromethorphan hydrobromide 10 mg, in a palatable nonalcoholic vehicle. Other ingredients: benzoic acid, flavors, propylene glycol, purified water, Red 40, saccharin sodium, sodium chloride, sorbitol, sucrose.

INDICATIONS

Provides relief of runny nose, nasal congestion and sneezing that may occur with the common cold. Suppresses cough due to minor throat and bronchial irritation. Promotes nasal and sinus drainage.

CONTRAINDICATIONS

Hypersensitivity to any of the ingredients. The use of sympathomimetic agents such as phenylpropanolamine hydrochloride is contraindicated in patients with severe hypertension, severe coronary artery disease and in those taking monoamine oxidase inhibitors. Antihistamines should not be administered to premature or newborn infants or be used to treat lower respiratory tract symptoms.

PRECAUTIONS

Exercise prescribing caution in patients with hypertension, cardiovascular disease, diabetes mellitus, hyperthyroidism, elevated intraocular pressure, prostatic hypertrophy, bladder neck obstruction or chronic pulmonary disease. Use caution in patients with persistent or chronic cough such as occurs with chronic bronchitis, bronchial asthma or emphysema. Alcoholic beverages and other CNS depressants may potentiate the sedative effects of antihistamines. Use with caution in pregnant and nursing women.

ADVERSE REACTIONS

Mild CNS stimulation, drowsiness, blurred vision, dry mouth, tachycardia, dizziness or gastrointestinal upset may occur. May produce thickening of bronchial secretions. May cause excitability, especially in children.

DOSAGE AND ADMINISTRATION

Bottle label dosage reads: Adults—2 teaspoonfuls every 4 hours. Children 6–12 years—1 teaspoonful every 4 hours. Children under 6 years—consult physician.

The suggested dosage for pediatric patients 3 months to under 12 months of age is 1 drop per kilogram of body weight administered every 4 hours. The suggested dosage for patients 12 months to under 24 months of age is 3 drops per kilogram of body weight administered every 4 hours. The suggested dosage for children 2 to under 6 years is ½ teaspoonful every 4 hours.

HOW SUPPLIED

TRIAMINICOL Multi-Symptom Cold Syrup (red), in 4 fl oz and 8 fl oz plastic bottles with tamper-evident band around child-resistant cap.

TRIAMINICOL® MULTI-SYMPTOM COLD TABLETS OTC

[trī″ah-mĭn′ĭ-call]

DESCRIPTION

Each TRIAMINICOL Multi-Symptom Cold Tablet contains: phenylpropanolamine hydrochloride 12.5 mg, chlorpheniramine maleate 2 mg, and dextromethorphan hydrobromide 10 mg. Other ingredients: calcium stearate, colloidal silicon dioxide, flavors, lactose, methylcellulose, methylparaben, microcrystalline cellulose, polyethylene glycol, povidone, Red 40, saccharin sodium, starch, titanium dioxide.

INDICATIONS

Provides relief of runny nose, nasal congestion and sneezing that may occur with the common cold. Suppresses cough due to minor throat and bronchial irritation. Promotes nasal and sinus drainage.

CONTRAINDICATIONS

Hypersensitivity to any of the ingredients. The use of sympathomimetic agents such as phenylpropanolamine hydrochloride is contraindicated in patients with severe hypertension, severe coronary artery disease and in those taking monoamine oxidase inhibitors. Antihistamines should not be administered to premature or newborn infants or be used to treat lower respiratory tract symptoms.

PRECAUTIONS

Exercise prescribing caution in patients with hypertension, cardiovascular disease, diabetes mellitus, hyperthyroidism, elevated intraocular pressure, prostatic hypertrophy, bladder neck obstruction or chronic pulmonary disease. Use with caution in patients with persistent or chronic cough such as occurs with chronic bronchitis, bronchial asthma or emphysema. Alcoholic beverages and other CNS depressants may potentiate the sedative effects of antihistamines. Use with caution in pregnant and nursing women.

ADVERSE REACTIONS

Mild CNS stimulation, drowsiness, blurred vision, dry mouth, tachycardia, dizziness or gastrointestinal upset may occur. May produce thickening of bronchial secretions.

DOSAGE AND ADMINISTRATION

Adults—2 tablets every 4 hours. Children 6–12 years—1 tablet every 4 hours.

HOW SUPPLIED

TRIAMINICOL Multi-Symptom Cold Tablets (cherry pink), imprinted "DORSEY" on one side, "TRIAMINICOL" on the other, in blister packs of 24.

TUSSAGESIC® TABLETS OTC

[tuss″ah-gee′zĭk]

(See PDR For Nonprescription Drugs)

URSINUS® INLAY-TABS® OTC

[yer-sī′nus]

(See PDR For Nonprescription Drugs)

Dorsey Pharmaceuticals

FOR DORSEY PRESCRIPTION PRODUCTS, PLEASE SEE SANDOZ PHARMACEUTICALS CORPORATION LISTING.

Du Pont Pharmaceuticals

E.I. duPont de Nemours & Co. (Inc.)
WILMINGTON, DE 19898

COUMADIN® ℞

[ku 'ma-din]
(crystalline warfarin sodium, U.S.P.)*

DESCRIPTION

COUMADIN (crystalline warfarin sodium), a prothrombinopenic anticoagulant, is chemically crystalline sodium warfarin isopropanol clathrate. The crystallization of warfarin sodium virtually eliminates trace impurities present in amorphous warfarin sodium, thus achieving a crystalline product of the highest purity. Warfarin* is the coined generic name for 3-(α-Acetonylbenzyl)-4-hydroxycoumarin. On a dose-for-dose basis, COUMADIN (crystalline warfarin sodium) is therapeutically equivalent to amorphous warfarin sodium.

COUMADIN® Tablets also contain:

All strengths:	Lactose, starch and other ingredients
2 mg:	FD&C Blue 2 and FD&C Red 40
2½ mg:	FD&C Yellow 6
5 mg:	FD&C Red 3 and FD&C Yellow 6
7½ mg:	D&C Yellow 10 and FD&C Yellow 6
10 mg:	Dye Free

ACTIONS

COUMADIN and other coumarin anticoagulants act by depressing synthesis in the liver of several factors which are known to be active in the coagulation mechanisms in a variety of diseases characterized by thromboembolic phenomena. The resultant **in vivo** effect is a sequential depression of Factors VII, IX, X and II. The degree of depression is dependent upon the dosage administered. Anticoagulants have no direct effect on an established thrombus, nor do they reverse ischemic tissue damage. However, once a thrombosis has occurred, anticoagulant treatment aims to prevent further extension of the formed clot and prevents secondary thromboembolic complications which may result in serious and possible fatal sequelae.

After oral administration, absorption is essentially complete, and maximal plasma concentrations are reached in 1 to 9 hours. Approximately 97% is bound to albumin within the plasma. COUMADIN usually induces hypoprothrombinemia in 36 to 72 hours, and its duration of action may persist for 4 to 5 days, thus producing a smooth, long lasting response curve. Little is known of the metabolic pathways involved in the biotransformation of oral anticoagulants in man. However, their metabolites appear to be eliminated principally in the urine.

INDICATIONS

COUMADIN is indicated for the prophylaxis and treatment of venous thrombosis and its extension, the treatment of atrial fibrillation with embolization, the prophylaxis and treatment of pulmonary embolism, and as an adjunct in the treatment of coronary occulsion.

CONTRAINDICATIONS

Anticoagulation is contraindicated in any localized or general physical condition or personal circumstance in which the hazard of hemorrhage might be greater than its potential clinical benefits, such as:

Pregnancy—COUMADIN is contraindicated in pregnancy because the drug passes through the placental barrier and may cause fatal hemorrhage to the fetus in utero. Furthermore, there have been reports of birth malformations in children born to mothers who have been treated with warfarin during pregnancy. Women of childbearing potential who are candidates for anticoagulant therapy should be carefully evaluated and the indications critically reviewed with the patient. If the patient becomes pregnant while taking this drug, she should be apprised of the potential risks to the fetus, and the possibility of termination of the pregnancy should be discussed in light of those risks.

Hemorrhagic tendencies or blood dyscrasias.

Recent or contemplated surgery of: (1) central nervous system; (2) eye; (3) traumatic surgery resulting in large open surfaces.

Bleeding tendencies associated with active ulceration or overt bleeding of: (1) gastrointestinal, genitourinary or respiratory tracts; (2) cerebrovascular hemorrhage; (3) aneurysms—cerebral, dissecting aorta; (4) pericarditis and pericardial effusions; (5) subacute bacterial endocarditis.

Threatened abortion, eclampsia and preeclampsia.

Inadequate laboratory facilities or unsupervised senility, alcoholism, psychosis; or lack of patient cooperation.

Spinal puncture and other diagnostic or therapeutic procedures with potential for uncontrollable bleeding.

Miscellaneous: major regional, lumbar block anesthesia and malignant hypertension.

WARNINGS

The most serious risks associated with anticoagulant therapy with sodium warfarin are hemorrhage in any tissue or organ and, less frequently, necrosis and/or gangrene of skin and other tissues. The risk of hemorrhage is related to the level of intensity and the duration of anticoagulant therapy. Hemorrhage and necrosis have in some cases been reported to result in death or permanent disability. Necrosis appears to be associated with local thrombosis and usually appears within a few days of the start of anticoagulant therapy. In severe cases of necrosis, treatment through debridement or amputation of the affected tissue, limb, breast or penis has been reported. Careful diagnosis is required to determine whether necrosis is caused by an underlying disease. Warfarin therapy should be discontinued when warfarin is suspected to be the cause of developing necrosis and heparin therapy may be considered for anticoagulation. Although various treatments have been attempted, no treatment for necrosis has been considered uniformly effective. See below for information on predisposing conditions. These and other risks associated with anticoagulant therapy must be weighed against the risk of thrombosis or embolization in untreated cases.

Warfarin sodium is a potent drug with a half-life of 2½ days; therefore its effects may become more pronounced as daily maintenance doses overlap. It cannot be emphasized too strongly that treatment of each patient is a highly individualized matter. Dosage should be controlled by periodic determinations of prothrombin time or other suitable coagulation tests. Determinations of whole blood clotting and bleeding times are not effective measures for control of therapy. Heparin prolongs the one-stage prothrombin time. Therefore, to obtain a valid prothrombin time when heparin and COUMADIN (crystalline warfarin sodium) are given together, a period of at least 5 hours should elapse after the last intravenous dose and 24 hours after the last subcutaneous dose of heparin, before blood is drawn.

Caution should be observed when COUMADIN is administered in any situation or in the presence of any predisposing condition where added risk of hemorrhage or necrosis is present.

Administration of anticoagulants in the following conditions will be based upon clinical judgment in which the risks of anticoagulant therapy are weighed against the risk of thrombosis or embolization in untreated cases. The following may be associated with these increased risks:

Lactation—coumarins may pass into the milk of mothers and cause a prothrombinopenic state in the nursing infant.

Severe to moderate hepatic or renal insufficiency.

Infectious diseases or disturbances of intestinal flora—sprue, antibiotic therapy.

Trauma which may result in internal bleeding.

Surgery or trauma resulting in large exposed raw surfaces.

Indwelling catheters.

Severe to moderate hypertension.

Known or suspected hereditary, familial or clinical deficiency in protein C—This condition, which should be suspected if there is a history of recurrent episodes of thromboembolic disorders in the patient or in the family, has been associated with an increased risk of developing necrosis following warfarin administration. Skin necrosis may occur in the absence of protein C deficiency. It has been reported that initiation of anticoagulation therapy with heparin for 4 to 5 days before initiation of therapy with COUMADIN may minimize the incidence of this reaction. Warfarin therapy should be discontinued when warfarin is suspected to be the cause of developing necrosis and heparin therapy may be considered for anticoagulation.

Miscellaneous: polycythemia vera, vasculitis, severe diabetes, severe allergic and anaphylactic disorders.

Patients with congestive heart failure may become more sensitive to COUMADIN, thereby requiring more frequent laboratory monitoring, and reduced doses of COUMADIN.

Concurrent use of anticoagulants with streptokinase or urokinase is not recommended and may be hazardous. (Please note recommendations accompanying these preparations.)

Abrupt cessation of anticoagulant therapy is not generally recommended; taper dose gradually over 3 to 4 weeks.

PRECAUTIONS

Periodic determination of prothrombin time or other suitable coagulation test is essential.

Numerous factors, alone or in combination, including travel, changes in diet, environment, physical state and medication may influence response of the patient to anticoagulants. It is generally good practice to monitor the patient's response with additional prothrombin time determinations in the period immediately after discharge from the hospital, and whenever other medications are initiated, discontinued or taken haphazardly. The following factors are listed for your reference; however, other factors may also affect the prothrombin response.

The following factors, alone or in combination, may be responsible for increased prothrombin time response:

ENDOGENOUS FACTORS: Carcinoma; collagen disease; congestive heart failure; diarrhea; elevated temperature; hepatic disorders—infectious hepatitis, hyperthyroidism; jaundice; poor nutritional state; vitamin K deficiency—steatorrhea.

EXOGENOUS FACTORS: Alcohol†; allopurinol; aminosalicylic acid; amiodarone; anabolic steroids; antibiotics; bromelains; chloral hydrate†; chlorpropamide; chymotrypsin; cimetidine; cinchophen; clofibrate; COUMADIN overdosage; dextran; dextrothyroxine; diazoxide; dietary deficiencies; diflunisal; diuretics†; disulfiram; drugs affecting blood elements; ethacrynic acid; fenoprofen; glucagon; hepatotoxic drugs; ibuprofen; indomethacin; influenza virus vaccine; inhalation anesthetics; mefenamic acid; methyldopa; methylphenidate; metronidazole; miconazole; monoamine oxidase inhibitors; nalidixic acid: naproxen; oxolinic acid; oxyphenbutazone; pentoxifylline; phenylbutazone; phenyramidol; phenytoin; prolonged hot weather; prolonged narcotics; pyrazolones; quinidine; quinine; ranitidine†; salicylates; sulfinpyrazone; sulfonamides, long acting; sulindac; thyroid drugs; tolbutamide; triclofos sodium; trimethoprim/sulfamethoxazole; unreliable prothrombin time determinations.

†Increased and decreased prothrombin time responses have been reported.

The following factors, alone or in combination, may be responsible for decreased prothrombin time response:

ENDOGENOUS FACTORS: Edema; hereditary resistance to coumarin therapy; hyperlipemia; hypothyroidism.

EXOGENOUS FACTORS: Adrenocortical steroids; alcohol†; antacids; antihistamines; barbiturates; carbamazepine; chloral hydrate†; chlordiazepoxide; cholestyramine; COUMADIN underdosage; diet high in vitamin K; diuretics†; ethchlorvynol; glutethimide; griseofulvin; haloperidol; meprobamate; oral contraceptives; paraldehyde; primidone; ranitidine†; rifampin; unreliable prothrombin time determinations; vitamin C.

† Increased and decreased prothrombin time responses have been reported.

A patient may be exposed to a combination of the above factors, some of which may increase and some decrease his sensitivity to COUMADIN (crystalline warfarin sodium). Because the net effect on his prothrombin time response may be unpredictable under these circumstances, more frequent laboratory monitoring is advisable.

Drugs not yet shown to interact or not to interact with coumarins are best regarded with suspicion, and when their administration is started or stopped, the prothrombin time should be determined more often than usual.

Coumarins also affect the action of other drugs. Hypoglycemic agents (chlorpropamide and tolbutamide) and anticonvulsants (phenytoin and phenobarbital) may accumulate in the body as a result of interference with either their metabolism or excretion.

ADVERSE REACTIONS

Potential adverse reactions to COUMADIN (crystalline warfarin sodium) may include:

- Hemorrhage from any tissue or organ. This is a consequence of the anticoagulant effect. The signs and symptoms will vary according to the location and degree or extent of the bleeding. Therefore, the possibility of hemorrhage should be considered in evaluating the condition of any anticoagulated patient with complaints which do not indicate an obvious diagnosis. Bleeding during anticoagulant therapy does not always correlate with prothrombin activity. (See TREATMENT FOR OVERDOSAGE.)
  Bleeding which occurs when the prothrombin time is within the therapeutic range warrants diagnostic investigation since it may unmask a previously unsuspected lesion, e.g. tumor, ulcer, etc.
- Necrosis of skin and other tissues. (See WARNINGS.)
- Other adverse reactions are infrequent and consist of alopecia, urticaria, dermatitis, fever, nausea, diarrhea, abdominal cramping, a syndrome called "purple toes," and hypersensitivity reactions.
- Priapism has been associated with anticoagulant administration, however, a causal relationship has not been established.

DOSAGE AND LABORATORY CONTROL

The aim of anticoagulant therapy is to impede the coagulation or clotting mechanism to such an extent that thrombosis will not occur, but at the same time avoiding such extensive impairment as might produce spontaneous bleeding. Effective therapeutic levels with minimal complications can best be achieved in cooperative and well-instructed patients, who keep the doctor informed of their status between visits. COUMADIN patient aids are available to physicians on request.

Continued on next page

DuPont—Cont.

The administration and dosage of COUMADIN must be individualized for each patient according to the particular patient's sensitivity to the drug as indicated by the prothrombin time. The prothrombin time reflects the depression of vitamin K dependent Factors VII, X and II. These factors, in addition to Factor IX, are affected by coumarin anticoagulants. There are several modifications of the Quick one-stage prothrombin time and the physician should become familiar with the specific method used in his laboratory.
Administration of COUMADIN should be gauged according to prothrombin time determinations by a suitable method. The blood prothrombin time should usually be determined daily after the administration of the initial dose until prothrombin time results stabilize in the therapeutic range. Intervals between subsequent prothrombin time determinations should be based upon the physician's judgment of the patient's reliability and response to warfarin in order to maintain the individual within the therapeutic range. Acceptable intervals for prothrombin time determinations have usually fallen within the range of one to four weeks. Satisfactory levels for maintenance of therapeutic anticoagulation are 1½ to 2½ times the normal prothrombin time (e.g. 18 to 30 seconds, with a control of 12 seconds).
Induction—Induction may be initiated with 10 to 15 mg daily and thereafter (usually 2 or 3 days) adjusted according to prothrombin time response. The basis for this no-loading dose regimen is that the depression of Factors II, IX, and X is not accelerated by the administration of a loading dose. Avoidance of a large priming dose may minimize the possibility of excessive increases in prothrombin time.
Alternatively, 40 to 60 mg for average adult or 20 to 30 mg for elderly and/or debilitated patients for one dose only administered orally, intravenously, or intramuscularly.
Maintenance—Most patients are satisfactorily maintained at a dose of 2 to 10 mg daily. Flexibility of dosage is provided by breaking scored tablets in half. The individual dose and interval should be gauged by the patient's prothrombin response.
Duration of therapy—The duration of therapy in each patient should be individualized. In general, anticoagulant therapy should be continued until the danger of thrombosis and embolism has passed.
Treatment during dentistry and surgery—The management of patients who undergo dental and surgical procedures requires close liaison between attending physicians, surgeons and dentists. Interruption of anticoagulant therapy may precipitate thromboembolism, and conversely, if anticoagulants are maintained at full doses, some patients may hemorrhage excessively. If it is elected to administer anticoagulants prior to, during, or immediately following dental or surgical procedures, it is recommended that the dosage of COUMADIN (crystalline warfarin sodium) be adjusted to maintain the prothrombin time at approximately 1½ to 2½ times the control level. The operative site should be sufficiently limited to permit the effective use of local procedures for hemostasis including absorbable hemostatic agents, sutures, and pressure dressings if necessary. Under these conditions dental and surgical procedures may be performed without undue risk of hemorrhage.
COUMADIN with Heparin—Since a delay intervenes between the administration of the initial dose and the therapeutic prolongation of prothrombin time, it may be advisable in emergency situations to administer sodium heparin initially along with COUMADIN. The initial dose of heparin and injectable COUMADIN may be administered together in the same syringe.
It should be noted that heparin may affect the prothrombin time, and therefore, when patients are receiving both heparin and COUMADIN, the blood sample for prothrombin time determination should be drawn just prior to the next heparin dosage, at least 5 hours after the last intravenous injection or 24 hours after the last subcutaneous injection.
Treatment For Overdosage: Excessive prothrombinopenia, with or without bleeding, is readily controlled by discontinuing COUMADIN (crystalline warfarin sodium), and if necessary, the oral or parenteral administration of vitamin K_1. The appearance of microscopic hematuria, excessive menstrual bleeding, melena, petechiae or oozing from nicks made while shaving are early manifestations of hypoprothrombinemia beyond a safe and satisfactory level.
In excessive prothrombinopenia with mild or no bleeding, omission of one or more doses of COUMADIN may suffice; and if necessary, small doses of vitamin K_1 orally, 2½ to 10 mg will usually correct the problem.
If minor bleeding persists, or progresses to frank bleeding, vitamin K_1 in doses of 5 to 25 mg may be given parenterally. (Please note recommendations accompanying vitamin K preparations prior to use.)
Fresh whole blood transfusions should be considered in cases of severe bleeding or prothrombinopenic states unresponsive to vitamin K_1.
Resumption of COUMADIN administration reverses the effect of vitamin K_1, and a therapeutic hypoprothrombinemia level can again be obtained.

SUPPLIED

Tablets: COUMADIN (crystalline warfarin sodium, USP). For oral use, single scored, imprinted numerically in bottles with potencies and colors as follows:
[See table below].
Also available in Military Depot:
2 mg. NSN 6505-00-982-4230
5 mg. NSN 6505-00-982-4229
In VA Depot:
2 mg. NSN 6505-00-982-4230A
5 mg. NSN 6505-00-982-4229B
Also available in Hospital Unit-Dose blister package of 100:
2 mg NDC 0056-0170-75
2½ mg NDC 0056-0171-75
5 mg NDC 0056-0172-75
7½ NDC 0056-0173-75
10 mg NDC 0056-0174-75
Also available in Military Depot:
5 mg NSN 6505-00-149-0317
In VA Depot:
5 mg. NSN 6505-00-149-0317A
Injection: Available as single injection units of amorphous warfarin sodium lyophilized for intravenous or intramuscular use in a box of 6 units (NDC 0056-0330-06) for use immediately after reconstitution.
50 mg: Unit consists of 1 vial, 50 mg; sodium chloride, 10 mg; thimerosal, 0.2 mg. pH is adjusted with sodium hydroxide, accompanied by a 2 ml ampul Sterile Water for Injection. Sterile Water for Injection contains no antimicrobial or other substance, and it is not suitable for intravascular injection without first having been made approximately isotonic by the addition of a suitable solute. Use only for reconstitution of the lyophilized product.

---

* Present as crystalline sodium warfarin isopropanol clathrate.

Injection manufactured by Lypho-Med, Inc., Chicago, Illinois 60651 for Du Pont Pharmaceuticals.
COUMADIN® is a Registered U.S. Trademark of E.I. du Pont de Nemours & Co. (Inc.)
6136-8 Rev. March, 1986
Shown in Product Identification Section, page 408

COUMADIN

	100's	1000's
2 mg lavender	NDC 0056-0170-70	NDC 0056-0170-90
2½ mg orange	NDC 0056-0171-70	NDC 0056-0171-90
5 mg peach	NDC 0056-0172-70	NDC 0056-0172-90
7½ mg yellow	NDC 0056-0173-70	
10 mg white	NDC 0056-0174-70	

HYCODAN® Ⓒ

[*hī-kō-dan*]
Tablets and Syrup

DESCRIPTION

Each HYCODAN® Tablet or teaspoonful (5 ml) contains:
Hydrocodone bitartrate U.S.P. .... 5 mg
WARNING: May be habit forming
Homatropine methylbromide U.S.P. .... 1.5 mg
Hydrocodone is 7, 8-dihydrocodeinone, a derivative of codeine.
HYCODAN® Tablets also contain: calcium phosphate dibasic, colloidal silicon dioxide, lactose, magnesium stearate, starch and stearic acid. HYCODAN® Syrup: caramel coloring, FD&C Red 40, liquid sugar, methylparaben, propylparaben, sorbitol solution and wild cherry imitation flavor.

HYCODAN® DOSAGE AND ADMINISTRATION
Usual Dosage

	TABLETS		SYRUP teaspoonful (5 ml)	
	Initial dose	Maximum single dose	Initial dose	Maximum single dose
Adults	1	3	1 tsp.	3 tsps.
Children				
over 12 years	1	2	1 tsp.	2 tsps.
2 to 12 years	½	1	½ tsp.	1 tsp.
under 2 years	¼	¼	¼ tsp.	¼ tsp.

ACTIONS

Hydrocodone is a centrally acting narcotic antitussive providing cough relief for up to 6 hours.

INDICATIONS

Based on a review of this drug by the National Academy of Sciences-National Research Council and/or other information, FDA has classified HYCODAN® Tablets and Syrup as follows:
"Probably" effective: for the symptomatic relief of cough.
Final classification of this "probably" effective indication requires further investigation.

CONTRAINDICATIONS

HYCODAN® should not be used in patients with glaucoma or hypersensitivity to hydrocodone or homatropine methylbromide.

WARNINGS

HYCODAN® should be prescribed and administered with the same degree of caution appropriate for the use of other oral narcotic-containing medications since it can produce drug dependence and, therefore, has the potential for abuse. Patients should be warned not to drive a car or operate machinery if they become drowsy or show impaired mental and/or physical abilities while taking HYCODAN®. Patients receiving narcotic analgesics, phenothiazines, other tranquilizers, sedative-hypnotics or other central nervous system depressants (including alcohol) concomitantly with HYCODAN® may exhibit an additive central nervous system depression. When such combined therapy is contemplated, the dose of one or both agents should be reduced.

PRECAUTIONS

Before prescribing medication to suppress or modify cough, it is important to ascertain that the underlying cause of cough is identified, that modification of cough does not increase the risk of clinical or physiologic complications, and that appropriate therapy for the primary disease is provided.

ADVERSE REACTIONS

Adverse reactions when they occur include sedation, nausea, vomiting and constipation.

DOSAGE AND ADMINISTRATION

HYCODAN® should be taken after meals and at bedtime, with food, not less than 4 hours apart. Treatment should be started with the suggested initial dose and subsequent doses adjusted if required.
[See table above].

DRUG INTERACTIONS

The central nervous system depressant effects of HYCODAN® may be additive with that of other central nervous system depressants. See WARNINGS.

MANAGEMENT OF OVERDOSAGE

Signs and Symptoms: Serious overdose with HYCODAN® may be characterized by respiratory depression, extreme somnolence progressing to stupor or coma, skeletal muscle flaccidity, cold and clammy skin, and sometimes bradycardia and hypotension. In severe overdosage, apnea, circulatory collapse, cardiac arrest and death may occur. The ingestion of very large amounts of HYCODAN® may, in addition, result in acute homatropine intoxication.
Treatment: Primary attention should be given to the reestablishment of adequate respiratory exchange through provision of a patent airway and the institution of assisted or controlled ventilation. The narcotic antagonist naloxone hydrochloride (NARCAN®) is a specific antidote against respiratory depression which may result from overdosage or unusual sensitivity to narcotics including hydrocodone. Therefore, an appropriate dose of naloxone hydrochloride should be administered, (usual initial adult dose: 0.4 mg–2 mg) preferably by the intravenous route and simultaneously with efforts at respiratory resuscitation. Since the duration of action of hydrocodone may exceed that of the antagonist, the patient should be kept under continued surveillance and repeated doses of the antagonist should be administered as needed to maintain adequate respiration.

Oxygen, intravenous fluids, vasopressors and other supportive measures should be employed as indicated, including treatment for anticholinergic drug intoxication.
Gastric emptying may be useful in removing unabsorbed drug. Activated charcoal may be of benefit.

HOW SUPPLIED

As white, scored tablets available in

Bottles of 100	NDC 0056-0042-70
Bottles of 500	NDC 0056-0042-85

As a red-colored, wild cherry flavored syrup available in

Bottles of one pint	NDC 0056-0234-16
Bottles of one gallon	NDC 0056-0234-82

Oral prescription where permitted by State law.
Store at controlled room temperature (59°-86°F, 15°-30°C).
HYCODAN® is a Registered U.S. Trademark of E.I. du Pont de Nemours & Co. (Inc.) NARCAN® is a Registered U.S. Trademark of Du Pont Pharmaceuticals, Inc.
6014-14

Shown in Product Identification Section, page 408

HYCOMINE® Ⓒ

[*hī-ko-mēn*]
Pediatric Syrup

HYCOMINE® Ⓒ

Syrup

DESCRIPTION

Hycomine® contains hydrocodone (dihydrocodeinone) bitartrate, a semi-synthetic centrally-acting narcotic antitussive and phenylpropanolamine hydrochloride, a sympathomimetic amine decongestant for oral administration.

	Hycomine® Pediatric Syrup	Hycomine® Syrup
Each teaspoonful (5 ml) contains:		
Hydrocodone bitartrate, U.S.P. WARNING: May be habit forming	2.5 mg	5 mg
Phenylpropanolamine hydrochloride, U.S.P.	12.5 mg	25 mg.

Also, HYCOMINE®, both strengths, contain: artificial cherry flavor, glycerin, methylparaben, propylparaben, saccharin sodium, and sorbitol solution. HYCOMINE® Pediatric Syrup contains: D&C Yellow 10 and FD&C Green 3. HYCOMINE® Syrup: FD&C Red 40 and FD&C Yellow 6.

CLINICAL PHARMACOLOGY

Clinical trials have proven hydrocodone bitartrate to be an effective antitussive agent which is pharmacologically 2 to 8 times as potent as codeine. At equi-effective doses, its sedative action is greater than codeine. The precise mechanism of action of hydrocodone and other opiates is not known, however, hydrocodone is believed to act by directly depressing the cough center. In excessive doses, hydrocodone, like other opium derivatives, will depress respiration. The effects of hydrocodone in therapeutic doses on the cardiovascular system is insignificant. The constipation effects of hydrocodone are much weaker than that of morphine and no stronger than that of codeine. Hydrocodone can produce miosis, euphoria, physical and psychological dependence. At therapeutic antitussive doses, it does exert analgesic effects. Following a 10 mg oral dose of hydrocodone administered to five adult male subjects, the mean peak concentration was 23.6 ± 5.2 ng/ml. Maximum serum levels were achieved at 1.3 ± 0.3 hours and the half-life was determined to be 3.8 ± 0.3 hours. Hydrocodone exhibits a complex pattern of metabolism including O-demethylation, N-demethylation and 6-keto reduction to the corresponding 6-α- and 6-β-hydroxymetabolites.
Phenylpropanolamine effects its vasoconstrictor activity by releasing noradrenaline from sympathetic nerve endings, and from direct stimulation of α-adrenoreceptors in blood vessels.

INDICATIONS AND USAGE

Hycomine® is indicated for the symptomatic relief of cough and nasal congestion.

CONTRAINDICATIONS

Hycomine® is contraindicated in patients hypersensitive to hydrocodone or phenylpropanolamine, and in patients on concurrent MAO inhibitor therapy. Patients known to be hypersensitive to other opioids or sympathomimetic amines may exhibit cross sensitivity to Hycomine®. Phenylpropanolamine is contraindicated in patients with heart disease, hypertension, diabetes or hyperthyroidism. Hydrocodone is contraindicated in the presence of an intracranial lesion associated with increased intracranial pressure; and whenever ventilatory function is depressed.

WARNINGS

May be habit forming. Hydrocodone can produce drug dependence of the morphine type and, therefore, has the potential for being abused. Psychic dependence, physical dependence and tolerance may develop upon repeated administration of Hycomine® and it should be prescribed and administered with the same degree of caution appropriate to the use of other narcotic drugs (See DRUG ABUSE AND DEPENDENCE).
Respiratory Depression: Hycomine® produces dose-related respiratory depression by directly acting on brain stem respiratory centers. If respiratory depression occurs, it may be antagonized by the use of Narcan® (naloxone hydrochloride) and other supportive measures when indicated.
Head Injury and Increased Intracranial Pressure: The respiratory depression properties of narcotics and their capacity to elevate cerebrospinal fluid pressure may be markedly exaggerated in the presence of head injury, other intracranial lesions or a preexisting increase in intracranial pressure. Furthermore, narcotics produce adverse reactions which may obscure the clinical course of patients with head injuries.
Acute Abdominal Conditions: The administration of Hycomine® or other narcotics may obscure the diagnosis or clinical course of patients with acute abdominal conditions.
Phenylpropanolamine: Hypertensive crises can occur with concurrent use of phenylpropanolamine and monoamine oxidase (MAO) inhibitors, indomethacin or with beta-blockers and methyldopa.
If a hypertensive crisis occurs, these drugs should be discontinued immediately and therapy to lower blood pressure should be instituted immediately. Fever should be managed by means of external cooling.

PRECAUTIONS

Before prescribing medication to suppress or modify cough, it is important to ascertain that the underlying cause of cough is identified, that modification of cough does not increase the risk of clinical or physiologic complications, and that appropriate therapy for the primary disease is provided.
Usage in Ambulatory Patients: Hydrocodone, like all narcotics, may impair the mental and/or physical abilities required for the performance of potentially hazardous tasks such as driving a car or operating machinery; phenylpropanolamine may produce a rapid pulse, dizziness or palpitations; patients should be cautioned accordingly.
Drug Interactions: Patients receiving other narcotic analgesics, general anesthetics, phenothiazines, other tranquilizers, sedative-hypnotics or other CNS depressants (including alcohol) concomitantly with hydrocodone may exhibit an additive CNS depression. When such combined therapy is contemplated, the dose of one or both agents should be reduced. The use of phenylpropanolamine with other sympathomimetic amines and MAO inhibitors may produce an additive elevation of blood pressure (See WARNINGS).
Carcinogenesis, Mutagenesis, Impairment of Fertility: Carcinogenicity, mutagenicity and reproduction studies have not been conducted with Hycomine®.
Usage in Pregnancy: Pregnancy Category C: Animal reproduction studies have not been conducted with Hycomine®. It is also not known whether Hycomine® can cause fetal harm when administered to a pregnant woman or can affect reproductive capacity. Hycomine® should be given to a pregnant woman only if clearly needed.
Nonteratogenic Effects: Babies born to mothers who have been taking opioids regularly prior to delivery will be physically dependent. The withdrawal signs include irritability and excessive crying, tremors, hyperactive reflexes, increased respiratory rate, increased stools, sneezing, yawning, vomiting and fever. The intensity of the syndrome does not always correlate with the duration of maternal opioid use or dose. There is no consensus on the best method of managing withdrawal. Chlorpromazine 0.7–1.0 mg/kg q 6 h, phenobarbital 2 mg/kg q 6 h, and paregoric 2–4 drops/kg q 4 h, have been used to treat withdrawal symptoms in infants. The duration of therapy is 4 to 28 days, with the dosages decreased as tolerated.
Nursing Mothers: It is not known whether this drug is excreted in human milk. Because many drugs are excreted in human milk and because of the potential for serious adverse reactions in nursing infants from Hycomine®, a decision should be made whether to discontinue nursing or discontinue the drug, taking into account the importance of the drug to the mother.
Usage in Patients Below the Age of 6 Years: Safety and effectiveness in this group have not been established.

ADVERSE REACTIONS

Respiratory System: Hydrocodone produces dose-related respiratory depression by acting directly on brain stem respiratory centers.
Cardiovascular System: Hypertension, postural hypotension, tachycardia and palpitations.
Genitourinary System: Ureteral spasm, spasm of vesical sphincters and urinary retention have been reported with opiates.
Central Nervous System: Sedation, drowsiness, mental clouding, lethargy, impairment of mental and physical performance, anxiety, fear, dysphoria, dizziness, psychic dependence, mood changes and blurred vision.
Gastrointestinal System: Nausea and vomiting occur more frequently in ambulatory than in recumbent patients.

DRUG ABUSE AND DEPENDENCE

Special care should be exercised in prescribing hydrocodone for emotionally unstable patients and for those with a history of drug misuse. Such patients should be closely supervised when long-term therapy is contemplated.
Hycomine® is a Schedule III narcotic. Psychic dependence, physical dependence, and tolerance may develop upon repeated administration of narcotics; therefore, Hycomine® should always be prescribed and administered with caution. Physical dependence is the condition in which continued administration of the drug is required to prevent the appearance of a withdrawal syndrome.
Patients physically dependent on opioids will develop an abstinence syndrome upon abrupt discontinuation of the opioid or following the administration of a narcotic antagonist. The character and severity of the withdrawal symptoms are related to the degree of physical dependence. Manifestations of opioid withdrawal are similar to but milder than that of morphine and include lacrimation, rhinorrhea, yawning, sweating, restlessness, dilated pupils, anorexia, gooseflesh, irritability and tremor. In more severe forms, nausea vomiting, intestinal spasm and diarrhea, increased heart rate and blood pressure, chills, and pains in bones and muscles of the back and extremities may occur. Peak effects will usually be apparent at 48 to 72 hours.
Treatment of withdrawal is usually managed by providing sufficient quantities of an opioid to suppress severe withdrawal symptoms and then gradually reducing the dose of opioid over a period of several days.

OVERDOSAGE

Signs and Symptoms: Serious overdosage with Hycomine® is characterized by respiratory depression (a decrease in respiratory rate and/or tidal volume, Cheyne-Stokes respiration, cyanosis), extreme somnolence progressing to stupor or coma, skeletal muscle flaccidity, cold and clammy skin, and sometimes bradycardia and hypotension. In severe overdosage apnea, circulatory collapse, cardiac arrest, and death may occur.
The signs and symptoms of overdosage of the individual components of Hycomine® may be modified in varying degrees by the presence of other active ingredients. Overdosage with phenylpropanolamine alone may result in tremor, restlessness, increased motor activity, agitation and hallucinations.
Treatment: Primary attention should be given to the reestablishment of adequate respiratory exchange through provision of a patent airway and the institution of assisted or controlled ventilation. The narcotic antagonist naloxone hydrochloride (NARCAN®) is a specific antidote against respiratory depression which may result from overdosage or unusual sensitivity to narcotics including hydrocodone. Therefore, an appropriate dose of naloxone hydrochloride should be administered (Usual initial dose: 0.4 mg–2 mg; usual initial child dose: 0.01 mg/kg body weight. For further information see NARCAN® full prescribing information.) preferably by the intravenous route, simultaneously with efforts at respiratory resuscitation. Since the duration of action of hydrocodone may exceed that of the antagonist, the patient should be kept under continued surveillance and repeated doses of the antagonist should be administered as needed to maintain adequate respiration. Oxygen, intravenous fluids, vasopressors and other supportive measures should be employed as indicated.
Gastric emptying may be useful in removing unabsorbed drug. Activated charcoal may be of benefit.

DOSAGE AND ADMINISTRATION

Usual Dosage:

	Hycomine® Pediatric Syrup	Hycomine® Syrup
Adults	—	1 tsp. (5 ml)
Children		
6 to 12 years	1 tsp. (5 ml)	—

After meals and at bedtime, not less than 4 hours apart (not to exceed 6 teaspoonfuls in a 24 hour period).

HOW SUPPLIED

Hycomine® Syrup is available as an orange-colored, fruit-flavored syrup in bottles as follows:
One Pint: NDC 0056-0246-16
One Gallon: NDC 0056-0246-82
Hycomine® Pediatric Syrup is available as a green-colored, fruit-flavored syrup in bottles as follows:
One Pint: NDC 0056-0247-16
Store at controlled room temperature (59°-86°F, 15°-30°C).
Oral prescription where permitted by state law.
Hycomine® is a Registered U.S. Trademark of E. I. du Pont de Nemours & Co. (Inc.)
Narcan® is a Registered U.S. Trademark of Du Pont Pharmaceuticals, Inc.
6153-2 July, 1985

Continued on next page

DuPont—Cont.

HYCOMINE® COMPOUND

[*hī-ko-mēn kom 'pound*]

DESCRIPTION

HYCOMINE Compound tablets contain hydrocodone (dihydrocodeinone) bitartrate, a semi-synthetic centrally-acting narcotic antitussive; chlorpheniramine maleate, an antihistamine; phenylephrine hydrochloride, a sympathomimetic amine decongestant; acetaminophen, an analgesic/antipyretic; and caffeine, a centrally-acting stimulant; for oral administration.

Each HYCOMINE Compound tablet contains:

Hydrocodone bitartrate U.S.P.	5 mg
WARNING: May be habit forming	
Chlorpheniramine maleate U.S.P.	2 mg
Phenylephrine hydrochloride U.S.P.	10 mg
Acetaminophen U.S.P.	250 mg
Caffeine, Anhydrous, U.S.P.	30 mg

HYCOMINE Compound tablets also contain: cherry flavor, colloidal silicon dioxide, FD&C Red 40, magnesium stearate, microcrystalline cellulose, povidone and starch.

CLINICAL PHARMACOLOGY

Clinical trials have proven hydrocodone bitartrate to be an effective antitussive agent which is pharmacologically 2 to 8 times as potent as codeine. At equi-effective doses, its sedative action is greater than codeine. The precise mechanism of action of hydrocodone and other opiates is not known, however, hydrocodone is believed to act by directly depressing the cough center. In excessive doses hydrocodone, like other opium derivatives, will depress respiration. The effects of hydrocodone in therapeutic doses on the cardiovascular system is insignificant. The constipation effects of hydrocodone are much weaker than that of morphine and no stronger than that of codeine. Hydrocodone can produce miosis, euphoria, physical and psychological dependence. At therapeutic antitussive doses, it does exert analgesic effects. Following a 10 mg oral dose of hydrocodone administered to five adult male human subjects, the mean peak concentration was 23.6 ± 5.2 ng/ml. Maximum serum levels were achieved at 1.3 ± 0.3 hours and the half-life was determined to be 3.8 ± 0.3 hours. Hydrocodone exhibits a complex pattern of metabolism including O-demethylation, N-demethylation and 6-keto reduction to the corresponding 6-α- and 6-β-hydroxymetabolites.

Chlorpheniramine maleate is a competitive H_1-receptor histamine blocking drug, thereby counteracting the effects of histamine release associated with allergic manifestations of upper respiratory tract inflammatory disorders. H_1-blocking drugs inhibit the actions of histamine on smooth muscle, capillary permeability, and can both stimulate and depress the central nervous system. Phenylephrine hydrochloride effects its vasoconstrictor activity by releasing noradrenaline from sympathetic nerve endings, and from direct stimulation of α-adrenoreceptors in blood vessels. Acetaminophen is an antipyretic and peripherally acting analgesic. Caffeine is a central nervous system stimulant.

INDICATIONS AND USAGE

HYCOMINE Compound is indicated for the symptomatic relief of cough, nasal congestion, and discomfort associated with upper respiratory tract infections.

CONTRAINDICATIONS

HYCOMINE Compound is contraindicated in patients hypersensitive to any component of the drug, and concurrent MAO inhibitor therapy. Patients known to be hypersensitive to other opioids, antihistamines, or sympathomimetic amines may exhibit cross sensitivity with HYCOMINE Compound. Phenylephrine is contraindicated in patients with heart disease, hypertension, diabetes or hyperthyroidism. Hydrocodone is contraindicated in the presence of an intracranial lesion associated with increased intracranial pressure; and whenever ventilatory function is depressed.

WARNINGS

May be habit forming. Hydrocodone can produce drug dependence of the morphine type and therefore has the potential for being abused. Psychic dependence, physical dependence and tolerance may develop upon repeated administration of HYCOMINE Compound and it should be prescribed and administered with the same degree of caution appropriate to the use of other narcotic drugs. (See DRUG ABUSE AND DEPENDENCE).

Respiratory Depression: HYCOMINE Compound produces dose-related respiratory depression by directly acting on brain stem respiratory centers. If respiratory depression occurs, it may be antagonized by the use of NARCAN® (naloxone hydrochloride) and other supportive measures when indicated.

Head Injury and Increased Intracranial Pressure: The respiratory depressant properties of narcotics and their capacity to elevate cerebrospinal fluid pressure may be markedly exaggerated in the presence of head injury, other intracranial lesions or a pre-existing increase in intracranial pressure. Furthermore, narcotics produce adverse reactions which may obscure the clinical course of patients with head injuries.

Acute abdominal conditions: The administration of HYCOMINE Compound or other narcotics may obscure the diagnosis or clinical course of patients with acute abdominal conditions.

Phenylephrine: Hypersensitive crises can occur with concurrent use of phenylephrine and monoamine oxidase (MAO) inhibitors, indomethacin or with beta-blockers and methyldopa.

If a hypertensive crisis occurs these drugs should be discontinued immediately and therapy to lower blood pressure should be instituted immediately. Fever should be managed by means of external cooling.

Chlorpheniramine: Antihistamines may produce drowsiness or excitation, particularly in children and elderly patients.

PRECAUTIONS

Before prescribing medication to suppress or modify cough, it is important to ascertain that the underlying cause of cough is identified, that modification of cough does not increase the risk of clinical or physiologic complications, and that appropriate therapy for the primary disease is provided.

Usage in Ambulatory Patients: Hydrocodone, like all narcotics, and antihistamines such as chlorpheniramine maleate, may impair the mental and/or physical abilities required for the performance of potentially hazardous tasks such as driving a car or operating machinery; phenylephrine may produce a rapid pulse, dizziness or palpitations; patients should be cautioned accordingly.

Drug Interactions: Patients receiving other narcotic analgesics, general anesthetics, phenothiazines, other tranquilizers, sedative-hypnotics or other CNS depressants (including alcohol) concomitantly with hydrocodone may exhibit an additive CNS depression. When such combined therapy is contemplated, the dose of one or both agents should be reduced. The use of phenylephrine with other sympathomimetic amines and MAO inhibitors may produce an additive elevation of blood pressure. MAO inhibitors may prolong the anticholinergic effects of antihistamines. (See WARNINGS).

Carcinogenesis, mutagenesis, impairment of fertility: Carcinogenicity, mutagenicity, and reproduction studies have not been conducted with HYCOMINE Compound.

Usage in Pregnancy: Pregnancy Category C. Animal reproduction studies have not been conducted with HYCOMINE Compound. It is also not known whether HYCOMINE Compound can cause fetal harm when administered to a pregnant woman or can affect reproductive capacity. HYCOMINE Compound should be given to a pregnant woman only if clearly needed.

Nonteratogenic effects: Babies born to mothers who have been taking opioids regularly prior to delivery will be physically dependent. The withdrawal signs include irritability and excessive crying, tremors, hyperactive reflexes, increased respiratory rate, increased stools, sneezing, yawning, vomiting and fever. The intensity of the syndrome does not always correlate with the duration of maternal opioid use or dose. Chlorpromazine 0.7–1.0 mg/kg q 6 h, phenobarbital 2 mg/kg q 6 h, and paregoric 2–4 drops/kg q 4 h, have been used to treat withdrawal symptoms in infants. The duration of therapy is 4 to 28 days, with the dosages decreased as tolerated.

Nursing mothers: It is not known whether this drug is excreted in human milk. Because many drugs are excreted in human milk and because of the potential for serious adverse reactions in nursing infants from HYCOMINE Compound, a decision should be made whether to discontinue nursing or discontinue the drug, taking into account the importance of the drug to the mother.

Pediatric use: Safety and effectiveness in children below the age of 2 years have not been established.

ADVERSE REACTIONS

Respiratory System: Hydrocodone produces dose-related respiratory depression by acting directly on brain stem respiratory centers.

Cardiovascular System: Hypertension, postural hypotension, tachycardia and palpitations.

Genitourinary System: Ureteral spasm, spasm of vesical sphincters and urinary retention have been reported with opiates.

Central Nervous System: Sedation, drowsiness, mental clouding, lethargy, impairment of mental and physical performance, anxiety, fear, dysphoria, dizziness, psychic dependence, mood changes, and blurred vision.

Gastrointestinal System: Nausea and vomiting occur more frequently in ambulatory than in recumbent patients.

DRUG ABUSE AND DEPENDENCE

Special care should be exercised in prescribing hydrocodone for emotionally unstable patients and for those with a history of drug misuse. Such patients should be closely supervised when long-term therapy is contemplated.

HYCOMINE Compound is a Schedule III narcotic. Psychic dependence, physical dependence, and tolerance may develop upon repeated administration of narcotics; therefore, HYCOMINE Compound should always be prescribed and administered with caution. Physical dependence is the condition in which continued administration of the drug is required to prevent the appearance of a withdrawal syndrome. Patients physically dependent on opioids will develop an abstinence syndrome upon abrupt discontinuation of the opioid or following the administration of a narcotic antagonist. The character and severity of the withdrawal symptoms are related to the degree of physical dependence. Manifestations of opioid withdrawal are similar to but milder than that of morphine and include lacrimation, rhinorrhea, yawning, sweating, restlessness, dilated pupils, anorexia, gooseflesh, irritability and tremor. In more severe forms, nausea, vomiting, intestinal spasms and diarrhea, increased heart rate and blood pressure, chills, and pains in bones and muscles of the back and extremities may occur. Peak effects will usually be apparent at 48 to 72 hours.

Treatment of withdrawal is usually managed by providing sufficient quantities of an opioid to suppress **severe** withdrawal symptoms and then gradually reducing the dose of opioid over a period of several days.

OVERDOSAGE

The signs and symptoms of overdosage of the individual components of HYCOMINE Compound may be modified in varying degrees by the presence of other active ingredients.

Signs and Symptoms: Serious overdosage with hydrocodone is characterized by respiratory depression (a decrease in respiratory rate and/or tidal volume. Cheyne-Stokes respiration, cyanosis), extreme somnolence progressing to stupor or coma, skeletal muscle flaccidity, cold and clammy skin, and sometimes bradycardia and hypotension. In severe overdosage apnea, circulatory collapse, cardiac arrest, and death may occur. The ingestion of large amounts of acetaminophen may produce hepatic toxicity.

The signs and symptoms of overdosage of the individual components of HYCOMINE Compound may be modified in varying degrees by the presence of other active ingredients. Overdosage with phenylephrine alone may result in tremor, restlessness, increased motor activity, agitation and hallucinations.

Treatment: Primary attention should be given to the reestablishment of adequate respiratory exchange through provision of a patent airway and the institution of assisted or controlled ventilation. The narcotic antagonist naloxone hydrochloride (NARCAN®) is a specific antidote against respiratory depression which may result from overdosage or unusual sensitivity to narcotics including hydrocodone. Therefore, an appropriate dose of naloxone hydrochloride should be administered (usual initial adult dose: 0.4 mg–2 mg; usual initial child dose is 0.01 mg/kg body weight. For further information see NARCAN® full prescribing information) preferably by the intravenous route, simultaneously with efforts at respiratory resuscitation. Since the duration of action of hydrocodone may exceed that of the antagonist, the patient should be kept under continued surveillance and repeated doses of the antagonist should be administered as needed to maintain adequate respiration. Oxygen, intravenous fluids, vasopressors and other supportive measures should be employed as indicated.

Gastric emptying may be useful in removing unabsorbed drug. Activated charcoal may be of benefit.

Treatment of acute acetaminophen overdosage is purely symptomatic.

DOSAGE AND ADMINISTRATION

Usual dosage, not less than 4 hours apart:

Adults:	1 tablet 4 times a day
Children:	6 to 12 years: ½ tablet 4 times a day
Children:	2 to 6 years: ½ tablet twice daily

HOW SUPPLIED

HYCOMINE® Compound is available as a coral pink, scored tablet in bottles as follows:

Bottles of 100	NDC 0056-0048-70
Bottles of 500	NDC 0056-0048-85

Store at controlled room temperature (59°–86° F, 15°–30° C)

Oral prescription where permitted by State Law.

HYCOMINE® is a Registered U.S. Trademark of E. I. du Pont de Nemours & Co. (Inc.)

NARCAN® is a Registered U.S. Trademark of Du Pont Pharmaceuticals, Inc.

6015-10

HYCOTUSS®

[*hī-kō-tus*]

Expectorant

DESCRIPTION

HYCOTUSS Expectorant Syrup contains hydrocodone (dihydrocodeinone) bitartrate, a semi-synthetic centrally-acting narcotic antitussive and guaifenesin, an expectorant for oral administration.

Each teaspoonful (5 ml) contains:
Hydrocodone bitartrate U.S.P. .... 5 mg
WARNING: May be habit forming
Guaifenesin U.S.P. .... 100 mg
Alcohol U.S.P. .... 10% v/v

HYCOTUSS Expectorant Syrup also contains: artificial butterscotch flavor, FD&C Red 40, FD&C Yellow 6, glycerin, liquid sugar, methylparaben, propylparaben, saccharin sodium, and sorbitol solution.

CLINICAL PHARMACOLOGY

Clinical trials have proven hydrocodone bitartrate to be an effective antitussive agent which is pharmacologically 2 to 8 times as potent as codeine. At equi-effective doses, its sedative action is greater than codeine. The precise mechanism of action of hydrocodone and other opiates is not known, however, hydrocodone is believed to act by directly depressing the cough center. In excessive doses hydrocodone, like other opium derivatives, can depress respiration. The effects of hydrocodone in therapeutic doses on the cardiovascular system is insignificant. The constipation effects of hydrocodone are much weaker than that of morphine and no stronger than that of codeine. Hydrocodone can produce miosis, euphoria, physical and psychological dependence. At therapeutic antitussive doses, it does exert analgesic effects. Following a 10 mg oral dose of hydrocodone administered to five male human subjects, the mean peak concentration was 23.6 $\pm$ 5.2 ng/ml. Maximum serum levels were achieved at 1.3 $\pm$ 0.3 hours and half-life was determined to be 3.8 $\pm$ 0.3 hours. Hydrocodone exhibits a complex pattern of metabolism including O-demethylation, N-demethylation and 6-keto reduction to the corresponding 6-α- and 6-β-hydroxymetabolites.

The exact mechanism of action is not established but guaifenesin is believed to act by stimulating receptors in the gastric mucosa that initiates a reflex secretion of respiratory tract fluid, thereby increasing the volume and decreasing the viscosity of bronchial secretions. Studies with guaifenesin indicate that it is rapidly absorbed from the gastrointestinal tract and has a half-life of one hour.

INDICATIONS AND USAGE

HYCOTUSS Expectorant is indicated for the symptomatic relief of irritating non-productive cough associated with upper and lower respiratory tract congestion.

CONTRAINDICATIONS

HYCOTUSS Expectorant is contraindicated in patients hypersensitive to hydrocodone or guaifenesin. Patients known to be hypersensitive to other opioids may exhibit cross sensitivity to HYCOTUSS Expectorant. Hydrocodone is contraindicated in the presence of an intracranial lesion associated with increased intracranial pressure; and whenever ventilatory function is depressed.

WARNINGS

May be habit forming. Hydrocodone can produce drug dependence of the morphine type and therefore has the potential for being abused. Psychic dependence, physical dependence and tolerance may develop upon repeated administration of HYCOTUSS Expectorant and it should be prescribed and administered with the same degree of caution appropriate to the use of other narcotic drugs (See DRUG ABUSE AND DEPENDENCE).

Respiratory Depression: HYCOTUSS Expectorant produces dose-related respiratory depression by directly acting on the brain stem respiratory centers. If respiratory depression occurs, it may be antagonized by the use of NARCAN® (naloxone hydrochloride) and other supportive measures when indicated.

Head Injury and Increased Intracranial Pressure: The respiratory depressant properties of narcotics and their capacity to elevate cerebrospinal fluid pressure may be markedly exaggerated in the presence of head injury, other intracranial lesions or a pre-existing increase in intracranial pressure. Furthermore, narcotics produce adverse reactions which may obscure the clinical course of patients with head injuries.

Acute Abdominal Conditions: The administration of HYCOTUSS Expectorant or other opioids may obscure the diagnosis or clinical course of patients with acute abdominal conditions.

PRECAUTIONS

Before prescribing medication to suppress or modify cough, it is important to ascertain that the underlying cause of cough is identified, that modification of cough does not increase the risk of clinical or physiologic complications, and that appropriate therapy for the primary disease is provided.

Usage in Ambulatory Patients: Hydrocodone, like all narcotics, may impair the mental and/ or physical abilities required for the performance of potentially hazardous tasks such as driving a car or operating machinery, and patients should be warned accordingly.

Drug Interactions: Patients receiving other narcotic analgesics, general anesthetics, phenothiazines, other tranquilizers, sedative hypnotics or other CNS depressants (including alcohol) concomitantly with hydrocodone may exhibit an additive CNS depression. When such combined therapy is contemplated, the dose of one or both agents should be reduced. (See WARNINGS).

Laboratory Interactions: The metabolite of guaifenesin has been found to produce an apparent increase in urinary 5-hydroxyindoleacetic acid, and guaifenesin therefore may interfere with the interpretation of this test for the diagnosis of carcinoid syndrome. Guaifenesin administration should be discontinued 24 hours prior to the collection of urine specimens for the determination of 5-hydroxyindoleacetic acid.

Carcinogenesis, mutagenesis, impairment of fertility: Carcinogenicity, mutagenicity and reproduction studies have not been conducted with HYCOTUSS Expectorant.

Usage in Pregnancy: Pregnancy Category C. Animal reproduction studies have not been conducted with HYCOTUSS Expectorant. It is also not known whether HYCOTUSS Expectorant can cause fetal harm when administered to a pregnant woman or can affect reproductive capacity. HYCOTUSS Expectorant should be given to a pregnant woman only if clearly needed.

Nonteratogenic effects: Babies born to mothers who have been taking opioids regularly prior to delivery will be physically dependent. The withdrawal signs include irritability and excessive crying, tremors, hyperactive reflexes, increased respiratory rate, increased stools, sneezing, yawning, vomiting and fever. The intensity of the syndrome does not always correlate with the duration of maternal opioid use or dose. There is no consensus on the best method of managing withdrawal. Chlorpromazine 0.7–1.0 mg/kg q 6 h, phenobarbital 2 mg/kg q 6 h, and paregoric 2–4 drops/kg q 4 h, have been used to treat withdrawal symptoms in infants. The duration of therapy is 4 to 28 days, with the dosages decreased as tolerated.

Nursing mothers: It is not known whether this drug is excreted in human milk. Because many drugs are excreted in human milk and because of the potential for serious adverse reactions in nursing infants from HYCOTUSS Expectorant, a decision should be made whether to discontinue nursing or discontinue the drug, taking into account the importance of the drug to the mother.

ADVERSE REACTIONS

Respiratory System: Hydrocodone produces dose-related respiratory depression by acting directly on brain stem respiratory centers.

Cardiovascular System: Hypertension, postural hypotension and palpitations.

Genitourinary System: Ureteral spasm, spasm of vesical sphincters and urinary retention have been reported with opiates.

Central Nervous System: Sedation, drowsiness, mental clouding, lethargy, impairment of mental and physical performance, anxiety, fear, dysphoria, dizziness, psychic dependence, mood changes and blurred vision.

Gastrointestinal System: Nausea and vomiting occur more frequently in ambulatory than in recumbent patients.

DRUG ABUSE AND DEPENDENCE

Special care should be exercised in prescribing hydrocodone for emotionally unstable patients and for those with a history of drug misuse. Such patients should be closely supervised when long-term therapy is contemplated.

HYCOTUSS Expectorant is a Schedule III narcotic. Psychic dependence, physical dependence and tolerance may develop upon repeated administration of narcotics; therefore, HYCOTUSS Expectorant should always be prescribed and administered with caution. Physical dependence is the condition in which continued administration of the drug is required to prevent the appearance of a withdrawal syndrome.

Patients physically dependent on opioids will develop an abstinence syndrome upon abrupt discontinuation of the opioid or following the administration of a narcotic antagonist. The character and severity of the withdrawal symptoms are related to the degree of physical dependence. Manifestations of opioid withdrawal are similar to but milder than that of morphine and include lacrimation, rhinorrhea, yawning, sweating, restlessness, dilated pupils, anorexia, gooseflesh, irritability and tremor. In more severe forms, nausea, vomiting, intestinal spasm and diarrhea, increased heart rate and blood pressure, chills, and pains in bones and muscles of the back and extremities may occur. Peak effects will usually be apparent at 48 to 72 hours.

Treatment of withdrawal is usually managed by providing sufficient quantities of an opioid to suppress **severe** withdrawal symptoms and then gradually reducing the dose of opioid over a period of several days.

OVERDOSAGE

Signs and Symptoms: Serious overdosage with HYCOTUSS Expectorant is characterized by respiratory depression (a decrease in respiratory rate and/or tidal volume, Cheyne-Stokes respiration, cyanosis), extreme somnolence progressing to stupor or coma, skeletal muscle flaccidity, cold and clammy skin, and sometimes bradycardia and hypotension. In severe overdosage apnea, circulatory collapse, cardiac arrest, and death may occur.

Treatment: Primary attention should be given to the reestablishment of adequate respiratory exchange through provision of a patent airway and the institution of assisted or controlled ventilation. The narcotic antagonist naloxone hydrochloride (NARCAN®) is a specific antidote against respiratory depression which may result from overdosage or unusual sensitivity to narcotics including hydrocodone. Therefore, an appropriate dose of naloxone hydrochloride should be administered (usual initial adult dose: 0.4 mg–2 mg. For further information see NARCAN® full prescribing information) preferably by the intravenous route, simultaneously with efforts at respiratory resuscitation. Since the duration of action of hydrocodone may exceed that of the antagonist, the patient should be kept under continued surveillance and repeated doses of the antagonist should be administered as needed to maintain adequate respiration. Oxygen, intravenous fluids, vasopressors and other supportive measures should be employed as indicated.

Gastric emptying may be useful in removing unabsorbed drug. Activated charcoal may be of benefit.

DOSAGE AND ADMINISTRATION

Usual Adult Dose: One teaspoonful (5 ml) after meals and at bedtime, not less than 4 hours apart (not to exceed 6 teaspoonsful in a 24 hour period). Treatment should be initiated with one teaspoonful and subsequent doses, up to a maximum single dose of 3 teaspoonsful, adjusted if required.

Usual Children's Dose:

Over 12 years: Initial dose 1 teaspoonful; maximum single dose, 2 teaspoonsful.

2 to 12 years: Initial dose ½ teaspoonful; maximum single dose, 1 teaspoonful.

Under 2 years: Dosage should be calculated as Hydrocodone, 0.3 mg/kg/24 hours, divided into four equal doses.

HOW SUPPLIED

HYCOTUSS Expectorant is available as an orange-colored, butterscotch flavored syrup in bottles as follows:

One pint: NDC 0056-0235-16

Store at controlled room temperature (59°–86° F, 15°–30° C).

Oral prescription as permitted by State Law.

HYCOTUSS® is a Registered U.S. Trademark of E.I. du Pont de Nemours & Co. (Inc.)

NARCAN® is a Registered U.S. Trademark of Du Pont Pharmaceuticals, Inc.

6131-4

MOBAN® ℞

[mō'ban]

(molindone hydrochloride)

DESCRIPTION

MOBAN (molindone hydrochloride) is a dihydroindolone compound which is not structurally related to the phenothiazines, the butyrophenones or the thioxanthenes.

MOBAN is 3-ethyl-6, 7-dihydro-2-methyl-5-(morpholinomethyl) indol-4 (5*H*)-one hydrochloride. It is a white crystalline powder, freely soluble in water and alcohol and has a molecular weight of 312.67.

MOBAN Tablets also contain:

All strengths: calcium sulfate, lactose, magnesium stearate, microcrystalline cellulose and povidone.

5 mg: alginic acid, colloidal silicon dioxide and FD&C Yellow 6.

10 mg: alginic acid, colloidal silicon dioxide, FD&C Blue 2 and FD&C Red 40.

25 mg: alginic acid, colloidal silicon dioxide, D&C Yellow 10, FD&C Blue 2, and FD&C Yellow 6.

50 mg: FD&C Blue 2 and starch.

100 mg: FD&C Blue 2, FD&C Yellow 6 and sodium starch glycolate.

MOBAN Concentrate contains: alcohol, artificial cherry flavor, artificial cover flavor, edetate disodium, glycerin, liquid sugar, methylparaben, propylparaben, sodium metabisulfite, sorbitol solution, and hydrochloric acid reagent grade for pH adjustment.

O N–CH₂ … O … CH₂–CH₃ · HCl … CH₃ … N H

ACTIONS

MOBAN (molindone hydrochloride) has a pharmacological profile in laboratory animals which predominantly resembles that of major tranquilizers causing reduction of spontaneous locomotion and aggressiveness, suppression of a conditioned response and antagonism of the bizarre stereotyped behavior and hyperactivity induced by amphetamines. In addition, MOBAN antagonizes the depression caused by the tranquilizing agent tetrabenazine.

Continued on next page

DuPont—Cont.

In human clinical studies tranquilization is achieved in the absence of muscle relaxing or incoordinating effects. Based on EEG studies, MOBAN exerts its effect on the ascending reticular activating system.
Human metabolic studies show MOBAN (molindone hydrochloride) to be rapidly absorbed and metabolized when given orally. Unmetabolized drug reached a peak blood level at 1.5 hours. Pharmacological effect from a single oral dose persists for 24-36 hours. There are 36 recognized metabolites with less than 2-3% unmetabolized MOBAN being excreted in urine and feces.

INDICATIONS

MOBAN is indicated for the management of the manifestations of psychotic disorders. The antipsychotic efficacy of MOBAN was established in clinical studies which enrolled newly hospitalized and chronically hospitalized, acutely ill, schizophrenic patients as subjects.

CONTRAINDICATIONS

MOBAN (molindone hydrochloride) is contraindicated in severe central nervous system depression (alcohol, barbiturates, narcotics, etc.) or comatose states, and in patients with known hypersensitivity to the drug.

WARNINGS

Tardive Dyskinesia: Tardive dyskinesia, a syndrome consisting of potentially irreversible, involuntary, dyskinetic movements may develop in patients treated with neuroleptic (antipsychotic) drugs. Although the prevalence of the syndrome appears to be highest among the elderly, especially elderly women, it is impossible to rely upon prevalence estimates to predict, at the inception of neuroleptic treatment, which patients are likely to develop the syndrome. Whether neuroleptic drug products differ in their potential to cause tardive dyskinesia is unknown.
Both the risk of developing the syndrome and the likelihood that it will become irreversible are believed to increase as the duration of treatment and the total cumulative dose of neuroleptic drugs administered to the patient increase. However, the syndrome can develop, although much less commonly, after relatively brief treatment periods at low doses.
There is no known treatment for established cases of tardive dyskinesia, although the syndrome may remit, partially or completely, if neuroleptic treatment is withdrawn. Neuroleptic treatment, itself, however, may suppress (or partially suppress) the signs and symptoms of the syndrome and thereby may possibly mask the underlying disease process. The effect that symptomatic suppression has upon the long-term course of the syndrome is unknown.
Given these considerations, neuroleptics should be prescribed in a manner that is most likely to minimize the occurrence of tardive dyskinesia. Chronic neuroleptic treatment should generally be reserved for patients who suffer from a chronic illness that, 1) is known to respond to neuroleptic drugs, and 2) for whom alternative, equally effective, but potentially less harmful treatments are *not* available or appropriate. In patients who do require chronic treatment, the smallest dose and the shortest duration of treatment producing a satisfactory clinical response should be sought. The need for continued treatment should be reassessed periodically.
If signs and symptoms of tardive dyskinesia appear in a patient on neuroleptics, drug discontinuation should be considered. However, some patients may require treatment despite the presence of the syndrome.
(For further information about the description of tardive dyskinesia and its clinical detection, please refer to the section on Adverse Reactions.)

Usage in Pregnancy: Studies in pregnant patients have not been carried out. Reproduction studies have been performed in the following animals:

Pregnant Rats oral dose—

no adverse effect	20 mg/kg/day—10 days
no adverse effect	40 mg/kg/day—10 days

Pregnant Mice oral dose—

slight increase resorptions	20 mg/kg/day—10 days
slight increase resorptions	40 mg/kg/day—10 days

Pregnant Rabbits oral dose—

no adverse effect	5 mg/kg/day—12 days
no adverse effect	10 mg/kg/day—12 days
no adverse effect	20 mg/kg/day—12 days

Animal reproductive studies have not demonstrated a teratogenic potential. The anticipated benefits must be weighed against the unknown risks to the fetus if used in pregnant patients.

Nursing Mothers: Data are not available on the content of MOBAN (molindone hydrochloride) in the milk of nursing mothers:

Usage in Children: Use of MOBAN (molindone hydrochloride) in children below the age of twelve years is not recommended because safe and effective conditions for its usage have not been established.

MOBAN has not been shown effective in the management of behavioral complications in patients with mental retardation.

SULFITES SENSITIVITY

MOBAN Concentrate contains sodium metabisulfite, a sulfite that may cause allergic-type reactions (e.g. hives, itching, wheezing, anaphylaxis) in certain susceptible persons. Although the overall prevalence of sulfite sensitivity in the general population is probably low, it is seen more frequently in asthmatics or in atopic nonasthmatic persons.

PRECAUTIONS

Some patients receiving MOBAN (molindone hydrochloride) may note drowsiness initially and they should be advised against activities requiring mental alertness until their response to the drug has been established.
Increased activity has been noted in patients receiving MOBAN. Caution should be exercised where increased activity may be harmful.
MOBAN does not lower the seizure threshold in experimental animals to the degree noted with more sedating antipsychotic drugs. However, in humans convulsive seizures have been reported in a few instances.
The physician should be aware that this tablet preparation contains calcium sulfate as an excipient and that calcium ions may interfere with the absorption of preparations containing phenytoin sodium and tetracyclines.
MOBAN has an antiemetic effect in animals. A similar effect may occur in humans and may obscure signs of intestinal obstruction or brain tumor.
Neuroleptic drugs elevate prolactin levels; the elevation persists during chronic administration. Tissue culture experiments indicate that approximately one-third of human breast cancers are prolactin dependent in vitro, a factor of potential importance if the prescription of these drugs is contemplated in a patient with a previously detected breast cancer. Although disturbances such as galactorrhea, amenorrhea, gynecomastia, and impotence have been reported, the clinical significance of elevated serum prolactin levels is unknown for most patients. An increase in mammary neoplasms has been found in rodents after chronic administration of neuroleptic drugs. Neither clinical studies nor epidemiologic studies conducted to date, however, have shown an association between chronic administration of these drugs and mammary tumorigenesis; the available evidence is considered too limited to be conclusive at this time.

ADVERSE REACTIONS

CNS Effects

The most frequently occurring effect is initial drowsiness that generally subsides with continued usage of the drug or lowering of the dose.
Noted less frequently were depression, hyperactivity and euphoria.

Neurological

Extrapyramidal Reactions

Extrapyramidal reactions noted below may occur in susceptible individuals and are usually reversible with appropriate management.

Akathisia

Motor restlessness may occur early.

Parkinson Syndrome

Akinesia, characterized by rigidity, immobility and reduction of voluntary movements and tremor, have been observed. Occurrence is less frequent than akathisia.

Dystonic Syndrome

Prolonged abnormal contractions of muscle groups occur infrequently. These symptoms may be managed by the addition of a synthetic antiparkinson agent (other than L-dopa), small doses of sedative drugs, and/or reduction in dosage.

Tardive Dyskinesia

Neuroleptic drugs are known to cause a syndrome of dyskinetic movements commonly referred to as tardive dyskinesia. The movements may appear during treatment or upon withdrawal of treatment and may be either reversible or irreversible (i.e., persistent) upon cessation of further neuroleptic administration.
The syndrome is known to have a variable latency for development and the duration of the latency cannot be determined reliably. It is thus wise to assume that any neuroleptic agent has the capacity to induce the syndrome and act accordingly until sufficient data has been collected to settle the issue definitively for a specific drug product. In the case of neuroleptics known to produce the irreversible syndrome, the following has been observed:
Tardive dyskinesia has appeared in some patients on long-term therapy and has also appeared after drug therapy has been discontinued. The risk appears to be greater in elderly patients on high-dose therapy, especially females. The symptoms are persistent and in some patients appear to be irreversible. The syndrome is characterized by rhythmical involuntary movements of the tongue, face, mouth or jaw (e.g., protrusion of tongue, puffing of cheeks, puckering of mouth, chewing movements). There may be involuntary movements of extremities.
There is no known effective treatment of tardive dyskinesia; antiparkinsonism agents usually do not alleviate the symptoms of this syndrome. It is suggested that all antipsychotic agents be discontinued if these symptoms appear. Should it be necessary to reinstitute treatment, or increase the dosage of the agent, or switch to a different antipsychotic agent, the syndrome may be masked. It has been reported that fine vermicular movements of the tongue may be an early sign of the syndrome and if the medication is stopped at that time the syndrome may not develop (See WARNINGS).

Autonomic Nervous System

Occasionally blurring of vision, tachycardia, nausea, dry mouth and salivation have been reported. Urinary retention and constipation may occur particularly if anticholinergic drugs are used to treat extrapyramidal symptoms.

Laboratory Tests

There have been rare reports of leucopenia and leucocytosis. If such reactions occur, treatment with MOBAN may continue if clinical symptoms are absent. Alterations of blood glucose, B.U.N., and red blood cells have not been considered clinically significant.

Metabolic and Endrocrine Effects

Alteration of thyroid function has not been significant. Amenorrhea has been reported infrequently. Resumption of menses in previously amenorrheic women has been reported. Initially heavy menses may occur. Galactorrhea and gynecomastia have been reported infrequently. Increase in libido has been noted in some patients. Impotence has not been reported. Although both weight gain and weight loss have been in the direction of normal or ideal weight, excessive weight gain has not occurred with MOBAN.

Hepatic Effects

There have been rare reports of clinically significant alterations in liver function in association with MOBAN use.

Cardiovascular

Rare, transient, non-specific T wave changes have been reported on E.K.G. Association with a clinical syndrome has not been established. Rarely has significant hypotension been reported.

Ophthalmological

Lens opacities and pigmentary retinopathy have not been reported where patients have received MOBAN (molindone hydrochloride). In some patients, phenothiazine induced lenticular opacities have resolved following discontinuation of the phenothiazine while continuing therapy with MOBAN.

Skin

Early, non-specific skin rash, probably of allergic origin, has occasionally been reported. Skin pigmentation has not been seen with MOBAN usage alone.
MOBAN (molindone hydrochloride) has certain pharmacological similarities to other antipsychotic agents. Because adverse reactions are often extensions of the pharmacological activity of a drug, all of the known pharmacological effects associated with other antipsychotic drugs should be kept in mind when MOBAN is used. Upon abrupt withdrawal after prolonged high dosage an abstinence syndrome has not been noted.

DOSAGE AND ADMINISTRATION

Initial and maintenance doses of MOBAN (molindone hydrochloride) should be individualized.

Initial Dosage Schedule

The usual starting dosage is 50-75 mg/day.

- Increase to 100 mg/day in 3 or 4 days.
- Based on severity of symptomatology, dosage may be titrated up or down depending on individual patient response.
- An increase to 225 mg/day may be required in patients with severe symptomatology.

Elderly and debilitated patients should be started on lower dosage.

Maintenance Dosage Schedule

1. Mild-5 mg-15 mg three or four times a day.
2. Moderate-10 mg-25 mg three or four times a day.
3. Severe-225 mg/day may be required.

DRUG INTERACTIONS

Potentiation of drugs administered concurrently with MOBAN (molindone hydrochloride) has not been reported. Additionally, animal studies have not shown increased toxicity when MOBAN is given concurrently with representative members of three classes of drugs (i.e., barbiturates, chloral hydrate and antiparkinson drugs).

MANAGEMENT OF OVERDOSAGE

Symptomatic, supportive therapy should be the rule.
Gastric lavage is indicated for the reduction of absorption of MOBAN (molindone hydrochloride) which is freely soluble in water.
Since the adsorption of MOBAN (molindone hydrochloride) by activated charcoal has not been determined, the use of this antidote must be considered of theoretical value.
Emesis in a comatose patient is contraindicated. Additionally, while the emetic effect of apomorphine is blocked by MOBAN in animals, this blocking effect has not been determined in humans.

A significant increase in the rate of removal of unmetabolized MOBAN from the body by forced diuresis, peritoneal or renal dialysis would not be expected. (Only 2% of a single ingested dose of MOBAN is excreted unmetabolized in the urine). However, poor response of the patient may justify use of these procedures.
While the use of laxatives or enemas might be based on general principles, the amount of unmetabolized MOBAN in feces is less than 1%. Extrapyramidal symptoms have responded to the use of diphenhydramine (Benadryl*), Amantadine HCL (Symmetrel®) and the synthetic anticholinergic antiparkinson agents, (i.e., Artane*, Cogentin*, Akineton*).

HOW SUPPLIED

As tablets in bottles of 100 with potencies and colors as follows:

5 mg orange	NDC 0056-0072-70
10 mg lavender	NDC 0056-0073-70
25 mg light green	NDC 0056-0074-70
50 mg blue	NDC 0056-0076-70
100 mg tan	NDC 0056-0077-70

As a concentrate containing 20 mg molindone hydrochloride per ml in 4 oz. (120 ml) bottles, NDC 0056-0460-04.
Store at controlled room temperature (59°–86°F, 15°–30°C).
* Benadryl-Trademark, Parke Davis and Co.
* Artane-Trademark, Lederle Laboratories
* Cogentin-Trademark, Merck Sharp & Dohme
* Akineton-Trademark, Knoll Pharmaceutical Co.
* Symmetrel-Trademark of E. I. du Pont de Nemours & Co. (Inc.)

MOBAN® is a registered U.S. Trademark of E.I. du Pont de Nemours & Co. (Inc.)

6145-8/Rev. May 1986

Shown in Product Identification Section, page 408

NARCAN® INJECTION ℞

[nar'kan]
(naloxone hydrochloride)
Narcotic Antagonist

DESCRIPTION

NARCAN (naloxone hydrochloride), a narcotic antagonist, is a synthetic congener of oxymorphone. In structure it differs from oxymorphone in that the methyl group on the nitrogen atom is replaced by an allyl group.
Naloxone hydrochloride occurs as a white to slightly off-white powder, and is soluble in water, in dilute acids, and in strong alkali; slightly soluble in alcohol; practically insoluble in ether and in chloroform.
NARCAN injection is available as a sterile solution for intravenous, intramuscular and subcutaneous administration in three concentrations, 0.02 mg, 0.4 mg and 1.0 mg of naloxone hydrochloride per ml. One ml of the 0.02 mg and 0.4 mg strengths contains 8.6 mg of sodium chloride. One ml of the 1.0 mg strength contains 8.35 mg of sodium chloride. One ml of all strengths also contains 2.0 mg of methylparaben and propylparaben as preservatives in a ratio of 9 to 1. pH is adjusted to 3.5 ± 0.5 with hydrochloric acid.
NARCAN injection is also available in a paraben-free formulation in two concentrations: 0.02 mg and 0.4 mg of naloxone hydrochloride per ml. One ml of each strength contains 9.0 mg of sodium chloride. pH is adjusted to 3.5 ± 0.5 with hydrochloric acid.

CLINICAL PHARMACOLOGY

NARCAN (naloxone hydrochloride) prevents or reverses the effects of opioids including respiratory depression, sedation and hypotension. Also, it can reverse the psychotomimetic and dysphoric effects of agonist-antagonists such as pentazocine.
NARCAN (naloxone hydrochloride) is an essentially pure narcotic antagonist, i.e., it does not possess the "agonistic" or morphine-like properties characteristic of other narcotic antagonists; NARCAN does not produce respiratory depression, psychotomimetic effects or pupillary constriction. In the absence of narcotics or agonistic effects of other narcotic antagonists it exhibits essentially no pharmacologic activity. NARCAN has not been shown to produce tolerance nor to cause physical or psychological dependence.
In the presence of physical dependence on narcotics NARCAN will produce withdrawal symptoms.
Mechanisms of Action: While the mechanism of action of NARCAN is not fully understood, the preponderance of evidence suggests that NARCAN antagonizes the opioid effects by competing for the same receptor sites.
When NARCAN is administered intravenously the onset of action is generally apparent within two minutes; the onset of action is only slightly less rapid when it is administered subcutaneously or intramuscularly. The duration of action is dependent upon the dose and route of administration of NARCAN. Intramuscular administration produces a more prolonged effect than intravenous administration. The requirement for repeat doses of NARCAN, however, will also be dependent upon the amount, type and route of administration of the narcotic being antagonized.
Following parenteral administration NARCAN is rapidly distributed in the body. It is metabolized in the liver, primarily by glucuronide conjugation and excreted in urine. In one study the serum half-life in adults ranged from 30 to 81 minutes (mean 64 ± 12 minutes). In a neonatal study the mean plasma half-life was observed to be 3.1 ± 0.5 hours.

INDICATIONS AND USAGE

NARCAN is indicated for the complete or partial reversal of narcotic depression, including respiratory depression, induced by opioids including natural and synthetic narcotics, propoxyphene, methadone and the narcotic-antagonist analgesics: nalbuphine, pentazocine and butorphanol. NARCAN is also indicated for the diagnosis of suspected acute opioid overdosage.

CONTRAINDICATIONS

NARCAN is contraindicated in patients known to be hypersensitive to it.

WARNINGS

NARCAN should be administered cautiously to persons including newborns of mothers who are known or suspected to be physically dependent on opioids. In such cases an abrupt and complete reversal of narcotic effects may precipitate an acute abstinence syndrome.
The patient who has satisfactorily responded to NARCAN should be kept under continued surveillance and repeated doses of NARCAN should be administered, as necessary, since the duration of action of some narcotics may exceed that of NARCAN.
NARCAN is not effective against respiratory depression due to non-opioid drugs.

PRECAUTIONS

In addition to NARCAN, other resuscitative measures such as maintenance of a free airway, artificial ventilation, cardiac massage, and vasopressor agents should be available and employed when necessary to counteract acute narcotic poisoning.
Several instances of hypotension, hypertension, ventricular tachycardia and fibrillation, and pulmonary edema have been reported. These have occurred in postoperative patients most of whom had pre-existing cardiovascular disorders or received other drugs which may have similar adverse cardiovascular effects. Although a direct cause and effect relationship has not been established, NARCAN should be used with caution in patients with pre-existing cardiac disease or patients who have received potentially cardiotoxic drugs.
Carcinogenesis, Mutagenesis, Impairment of Fertility: Carcinogenicity and mutagenicity studies have not been performed with NARCAN. Reproductive studies in mice and rats demonstrated no impairment of fertility.
Use in Pregnancy: Pregnancy Catagory B: Reproduction studies performed in mice and rats at doses up to 1,000 times the human dose, revealed no evidence of impaired fertility or harm to the fetus due to NARCAN. There are, however, no adequate and well controlled studies in pregnant women. Because animal reproduction studies are not always predictive of human response, NARCAN should be used during pregnancy only if clearly needed.
Nursing Mothers: It is not known whether NARCAN is excreted in human milk. Because many drugs are excreted in human milk, caution should be exercised when NARCAN is administered to a nursing woman.

ADVERSE REACTIONS

Abrupt reversal of narcotic depression may result in nausea, vomiting, sweating, tachycardia, increased blood pressure, and tremulousness. In postoperative patients, larger than necessary dosage of NARCAN may result in significant reversal of analgesia, and in excitement. Hypotension, hypertension, ventricular tachycardia and fibrillation, and pulmonary edema have been associated with the use of NARCAN postoperatively (see PRECAUTIONS & USAGE IN ADULTS-POSTOPERATIVE NARCOTIC DEPRESSION). Seizures have been reported to occur infrequently after the administration of naloxone; however, a causal relationship has not been established.

OVERDOSAGE

There is no clinical experience with NARCAN overdosage in humans.
In the mouse and rat the intravenous LD_{50} is 150 ± 5 mg/kg and 109 ± 4 mg/kg respectively. In acute subcutaneous toxicity studies in newborn rats the LD_{50} (95% CL) is 260 (228-296) mg/kg. Subcutaneous injection of 100 mg/kg/day in rats for 3 weeks produced only transient salivation and partial ptosis following injection: no toxic effects were seen at 10 mg/kg/day for 3 weeks.

DOSAGE AND ADMINISTRATION

NARCAN (naloxone hydrochloride) may be administered intravenously, intramuscularly, or subcutaneously. The most rapid onset of action is achieved by intravenous administration and it is recommended in emergency situations.
Since the duration of action of some narcotics may exceed that of NARCAN the patient should be kept under continued surveillance and repeated doses of NARCAN should be administered, as necessary.
Intravenous Infusion: NARCAN may be diluted for intravenous infusion in normal saline or 5% dextrose solutions. The addition of 2 mg of NARCAN in 500 ml of either solution provides a concentration of 0.004 mg/ml. Mixtures should be used within 24 hours. After 24 hours, the remaining unused solution must be discarded. The rate of administration should be titrated in accordance with the patient's response.
Parenteral drug products should be inspected visually for particulate matter and discoloration prior to administration whenever solution and container permit. NARCAN should not be mixed with preparations containing bisulfite, metabisulfite, long-chain or high molecular weight anions, or any solution having an alkaline pH. No drug or chemical agent should be added to NARCAN unless its effect on the chemical and physical stability of the solution has first been established.

Usage in Adults:

Narcotic Overdose—Known or Suspected: An initial dose of 0.4 mg to 2 mg of NARCAN may be administered intravenously. If the desired degree of counteraction and improvement in respiratory functions is not obtained, it may be repeated at 2 to 3 minute intervals. If no response is observed after 10 mg of NARCAN have been administered, the diagnosis of narcotic induced or partial narcotic induced toxicity should be questioned. Intramuscular or subcutaneous administration may be necessary if the intravenous route is not available.
Postoperative Narcotic Depression: For the partial reversal of narcotic depression following the use of narcotics during surgery, smaller doses of NARCAN are usually sufficient. The dose of NARCAN should be titrated according to the patient's response. For the initial reversal of respiratory depression, NARCAN should be injected in increments of 0.1 to 0.2 mg intravenously at two to three minute intervals to the desired degree of reversal i.e. adequate ventilation and alertness without significant pain or discomfort. Larger than necessary dosage of NARCAN may result in significant reversal of analgesia and increase in blood pressure. Similarly, too rapid reversal may induce nausea, vomiting, sweating or circulatory stress.
Repeat doses of NARCAN may be required within one to two hour intervals depending upon the amount, type (i.e., short or long acting) and time interval since last administration of narcotic. Supplemental intramuscular doses have been shown to produce a longer lasting effect.

USAGE IN CHILDREN

Narcotic Overdose—Known or Suspected: The usual initial dose in children is 0.01 mg/kg body weight given I.V. If this dose does not result in the desired degree of clinical improvement, a subsequent dose of 0.1 mg/kg body weight may be administered. If an I.V. route of administration is not available, NARCAN may be administered I.M. or S.C. in divided doses. If necessary, NARCAN can be diluted with sterile water for injection.
Postoperative Narcotic Depression: Follow the recommendations and cautions under **Adult Postoperative Depression**. For the initial reversal of respiratory depression NARCAN should be injected in increments of 0.005 mg to 0.01 mg intravenously at two to three minute intervals to the desired degree of reversal.

Usage in Neonates:

Narcotic-Induced Depression: The usual initial dose is 0.01 mg/kg body weight administered I.V., I.M., or S.C. This dose may be repeated in accordance with adult administration guidelines for postoperative narcotic depression.

HOW SUPPLIED

NARCAN (naloxone hydrochloride) for intravenous, intramuscular and subcutaneous administration is available as:

0.4 mg/ml	1 ml ampul-box of 10	NDC 0590-0365-10
	1 ml disposable prefilled syringe-box of 10	NDC 0590-0365-15
	10 ml vial-box of 1	NDC 0590-0365-05
0.4 mg/ml (paraben-free)	1 ml ampul-box of 10	NDC 0590-0358-10
1.0 mg/ml	1 ml ampul-box of 10	NDC 0590-0368-09
1.0 mg/ml	2 ml ampul-box of 10	NDC 0590-0368-10
1.0 mg/ml	10 ml vial-box of 1	NDC 0590-0368-05
0.02 mg/ml	2 ml ampul-box of 10	NDC 0590-0367-10
0.02 mg/ml (paraben-free)	2 ml ampul-box of 10	NDC 0590-0359-10

Store at controlled room temperature (59°–86°F, 15°–30°C).

6108-7/Rev., Feb. 1986

Shown in Product Identification Section, page 408

Continued on next page

DuPont—Cont.

NUBAIN® ℞
[*nū 'bān*]
(nalbuphine hydrochloride)

DESCRIPTION
NUBAIN® (nalbuphine hydrochloride) is a synthetic narcotic agonist-antagonist analgesic of the phenanthrene series. It is chemically related to both the widely used narcotic antagonist, naloxone, and the potent narcotic analgesic, oxymorphone.
Nalbuphine hydrochloride is (-)-17-(cyclobutylmethyl)-4, 5α-epoxymorphinan-3,6α, 14-triol, hydrochloride.
NUBAIN® is available in two concentrations, 10 mg and 20 mg of nalbuphine hydrochloride per ml. Both strengths contain 0.94% sodium citrate hydrous, 1.26% citric acid anhydrous, 0.1% sodium metabisulfite, and 0.2% of a 9:1 mixture of methylparaben and propylparaben as preservatives; pH is adjusted, if necessary, with hydrochloric acid. The 10 mg/ml strength contains 0.1% sodium chloride.

ACTIONS
NUBAIN is a potent analgesic. Its analgesic potency is essentially equivalent to that of morphine on a milligram basis. Its onset of action occurs within 2 to 3 minutes after intravenous administration, and in less than 15 minutes following subcutaneous or intramuscular injection. The plasma half-life of nalbuphine is 5 hours and in clinical studies the duration of analgesic activity has been reported to range from 3 to 6 hours.
The narcotic antagonist activity of NUBAIN is one-fourth as potent as nalorphine and 10 times that of pentazocine.

INDICATIONS
For the relief of moderate to severe pain. NUBAIN can also be used for preoperative analgesia, as a supplement to surgical anesthesia, and for obstetrical analgesia during labor.

CONTRAINDICATIONS
NUBAIN should not be administered to patients who are hypersensitive to it.

WARNINGS
Drug Dependence NUBAIN has been shown to have a low abuse potential which is approximate to that of pentazocine. When compared with drugs which are not mixed agonist-antagonists, it has been reported that nalbuphine's potential for abuse would be less than that of codeine and propoxyphene. Psychological and physical dependence and tolerance may follow the abuse or misuse of nalbuphine. Therefore, caution should be observed in prescribing it for emotionally unstable patients, or for individuals with a history of narcotic abuse. Such patients should be closely supervised when long-term therapy is contemplated.
Care should be taken to avoid increases in dosage or frequency of administration which in susceptible individuals might result in physical dependence.
Abrupt discontinuation of NUBAIN following prolonged use has been followed by symptoms of narcotic withdrawal, i.e., abdominal cramps, nausea and vomiting, rhinorrhea, lacrimation, restlessness, anxiety, elevated temperature and piloerection.
Use in Ambulatory Patients NUBAIN may impair the mental or physical abilities required for the performance of potentially dangerous tasks such as driving a car or operating machinery. Therefore, NUBAIN should be administered with caution to ambulatory patients who should be warned to avoid such hazards.
Use in Emergency Procedures Maintain patient under observation until recovered from NUBAIN effects that would affect driving or other potentially dangerous tasks.
Use in Children Clinical experience to support administration to patients under 18 years is not available at present.
Use in Pregnancy (other than labor) Safe use of NUBAIN in pregnancy has not been established. Although animal reproductive studies have not revealed teratogenic or embryotoxic effects, nalbuphine should only be administered to pregnant women when, in the judgment of the physician, the potential benefits outweigh the possible hazards.
Use During Labor and Delivery NUBAIN can produce respiratory depression in the neonate. It should be used with caution in women delivering premature infants.
Head Injury and Increased Intracranial Pressure The possible respiratory depressant effects and the potential of potent analgesics to elevate cerebrospinal fluid pressure (resulting from vasodilation following CO_2 retention) may be markedly exaggerated in the presence of head injury, intracranial lesions or a pre-existing increase in intracranial pressure. Furthermore, potent analgesics can produce effects which may obscure the clinical course of patients with head injuries. Therefore, NUBAIN should be used in these circumstances only when essential, and then should be administered with extreme caution.
Interaction With Other Central Nervous System Depressants Although NUBAIN possesses narcotic antagonist activity, there is evidence that in nondependent patients it will not antagonize a narcotic analgesic administered just before, concurrently, or just after an injection of NUBAIN. Therefore, patients receiving a narcotic analgesic, general anesthetics, phenothiazines, or other tranquilizers, sedatives, hypnotics, or other CNS depressants (including alcohol) concomitantly with NUBAIN may exhibit an additive effect. When such combined therapy is contemplated, the dose of one or both agents should be reduced.
Sulfites Sensitivity: NUBAIN contains sodium metabisulfite, a sulfite that may cause allergic-type reactions (e.g. hives, itching, wheezing, anaphylaxis) in certain susceptible persons. Although the overall prevalence of sulfite sensitivity in the general population is probably low, it is seen more frequently in asthmatics or in atopic nonasthmatic persons.

PRECAUTIONS
Impaired Respiration At the usual adult dose of 10 mg/70 kg, NUBAIN causes some respiratory depression approximately equal to that produced by equal doses of morphine. However, in contrast to morphine, respiratory depression is not appreciably increased with higher doses of NUBAIN. Respiratory depression induced by NUBAIN can be reversed by NARCAN® (naloxone hydrochloride) when indicated. NUBAIN should be administered with caution at low doses to patients with impaired respiration (e.g., from other medication, uremia, bronchial asthma, severe infection, cyanosis or respiratory obstructions).
Impaired Renal or Hepatic Function Because NUBAIN is metabolized in the liver and excreted by the kidneys, patients with renal or liver dysfunction may over-react to customary doses. Therefore, in these individuals, NUBAIN should be used with caution and administered in reduced amounts.
Myocardial Infarction As with all potent analgesics, NUBAIN should be used with caution in patients with myocardial infarction who have nausea or vomiting.
Biliary Tract Surgery As with all narcotic analgesics, NUBAIN should be used with caution in patients about to undergo surgery of the biliary tract since it may cause spasm of the sphincter of Oddi.

ADVERSE REACTIONS
The most frequent adverse reaction in 1066 patients treated with NUBAIN is sedation 381(36%).
Less frequent reactions are: sweaty/clammy 99(9%), nausea/vomiting 68(6%), dizziness/ vertigo 58(5%), dry mouth 44(4%), and headache 27(3%).
Other adverse reactions which may occur (reported incidence of 1% or less) are:
CNS Effects nervousness, depression, restlessness, crying, euphoria, floating, hostility, unusual dreams, confusion, faintness, hallucinations, dysphoria, feeling of heaviness, numbness, tingling, unreality. The incidence of psychotomimetic effects, such as unreality, depersonalization, delusions, dysphoria and hallucinations has been shown to be less than that which occurs with pentazocine.
Cardiovascular Hypertension, hypotension, bradycardia, tachycardia.
Gastrointestinal Cramps, dyspepsia, bitter taste.
Respiration Depression, dyspnea, asthma.
Dermatological Itching, burning, urticaria.
Miscellaneous Speech difficulty, urinary urgency, blurred vision, flushing and warmth.

DOSAGE AND ADMINISTRATION
The usual recommended adult dose is 10 mg for a 70 kg individual, administered subcutaneously, intramuscularly or intravenously; this dose may be repeated every 3 to 6 hours as necessary. Dosage should be adjusted according to the severity of the pain, physical status of the patient, and other medications which the patient may be receiving. (See Interaction with Other Central Nervous System Depressants under WARNINGS). In non-tolerant individuals, the recommended single maximum dose is 20 mg, with a maximum total daily dose of 160 mg.
Patients Dependent on Narcotics Patients who have been taking narcotics chronically may experience withdrawal symptoms upon the administration of NUBAIN. If unduly troublesome, narcotic withdrawal symptoms can be controlled by the slow intravenous administration of small increments of morphine, until relief occurs. If the previous analgesic was morphine, meperidine, codeine, or other narcotic with similar duration of activity, one-fourth of the anticipated dose of NUBAIN can be administered initially and the patient observed for signs of withdrawal, i.e., abdominal cramps, nausea and vomiting, lacrimation, rhinorrhea, anxiety, restlessness, elevation of temperature or piloerection. If untoward symptoms do not occur, progressively larger doses may be tried at appropriate intervals until the desired level of analgesia is obtained with NUBAIN.
Management of Overdosage The immediate intravenous administration of NARCAN® (naloxone hydrochloride) is a specific antidote. Oxygen, intravenous fluids, vasopressors and other supportive measures should be used as indicated.
The administration of single doses of 72 mg of NUBAIN subcutaneously to eight normal subjects has been reported to have resulted primarily in symptoms of sleepiness and mild dysphoria.

HOW SUPPLIED
NUBAIN® (nalbuphine hydrochloride) injection for intramuscular, subcutaneous, or intravenous use is available in:
NDC 0590-0385-10
10 mg/ml, 1 ml ampuls (box of 10)
NDC 0590-0386-01
10 mg/ml, 10 ml vial (box of 1)
NDC 0590-0396-10
20 mg/ml, 1 ml ampuls (box of 10)
NDC 0590-0396-15
20 mg/ml, 1 ml disposable pre-filled syringes (box of 10)
NDC 0590-0399-01
20 mg/ml, 10 ml vials (box of 1)
Also available in Military Depot:
10 mg/ml, 1 ml box of 10
NSN 6505-01-115-9852
10 mg/ml, 10 ml box of 1
NSN 6505-01-117-9690
Store At Controlled Room Temperature (59°–86°F, 15°–30°C).
NUBAIN is a Registered U.S. Trademark of E.I. du Pont de Nemours & Co. (Inc.)
NARCAN® is a Registered U.S. Trademark of DuPont Pharmaceuticals, Inc.
6109-6 Rev. April 1986
Shown in Product Identification Section, page 409

NUMORPHAN® Ⓒ II
[*nū-mor 'fan*]
(oxymorphone hydrochloride)
injection

DESCRIPTION
NUMORPHAN® (oxymorphone hydrochloride), a semisynthetic narcotic substitute for morphine, is a potent analgesic.
NUMORPHAN is 4,5α-Epoxy-3, 14-dihydroxy-17-methylmorphinan-6-one hydrochloride.
Oxymorphone hydrochloride occurs as a white or slightly off-white, odorless powder, sparingly soluble in alcohol and ether, but freely soluble in water.
NUMORPHAN injection is available in two concentrations, 1.0 mg and 1.5 mg of oxymorphone hydrochloride per ml. Both strengths contain sodium chloride 0.8%; with methylparaben 0.18%, propylparaben 0.02% and sodium dithionite 0.1%, as preservatives. pH is adjusted with sodium hydroxide.

ACTIONS
NUMORPHAN (oxymorphone hydrochloride) is a potent narcotic analgesic. Administered parenterally, one mg of NUMORPHAN is approximately equivalent in analgesic activity to 10 mg of morphine sulfate.
The onset of action is rapid; initial effects are usually perceived within 5 to 10 minutes. Its duration of action is approximately 3 to 6 hours.
NUMORPHAN produces mild sedation and causes little depression of the cough reflex. These properties make it particularly useful in postoperative patients.

INDICATIONS
NUMORPHAN (oxymorphone hydrochloride) is indicated for the relief of moderate to severe pain. This drug is also indicated parenterally for preoperative medication, for support of anesthesia, for obstetrical analgesia, and for relief of anxiety in patients with dyspnea associated with acute left ventricular failure and pulmonary edema.

CONTRAINDICATIONS
Safe use of NUMORPHAN (oxymorphone hydrochloride) in children under 12 years of age has not been established. This drug should not be used in patients known to be hypersensitive to morphine analogs.

WARNINGS
May be habit forming. As with other narcotic drugs, tolerance and addiction may develop. The addicting potential of the drug appears to be about the same as for morphine. Like other narcotic-containing medications, NUMORPHAN is subject to the Federal Controlled Substances Act.
Interaction with other central nervous system depressants: Patients receiving other narcotic analgesics, general anesthetics, phenothiazines, other tranquilizers, sedatives, hypnotics or other CNS depressants (including alcohol) concomitantly with NUMORPHAN may exhibit an additive CNS depression. When such combined therapy is contemplated, the dose of one or both agents should be reduced.
Safe use in pregnancy has not been established (relative to possible adverse effects on fetal development). As with other analgesics, the use of NUMORPHAN (oxymorphone hydrochloride) in pregnancy, in nursing mothers, or in women of child-bearing potential requires that the possible benefits of the drug be weighed against the possible hazards to the mother and the child.

PRECAUTIONS

The same care and caution should be taken when administering NUMORPHAN (oxymorphone hydrochloride) as when other potent narcotic analgesics are used. It should be borne in mind that some respiratory depression may occur as with all potent narcotics especially when other analgesic and/or anesthetic drugs with depressant action have been given shortly before administration of NUMORPHAN.

The respiratory depressant effects of narcotics and their capacity to elevate cerebrospinal fluid pressure may be markedly exaggerated in the presence of head injury, other intracranial lesions or a pre-existing increase in intracranial pressure. Furthermore narcotics produce adverse reactions which may obscure the clinical course of patients with head injuries.

As with other analgesics, caution must also be exercised in elderly and debilitated patients and in patients who are known to be sensitive to central nervous system depressants, such as those with cardiovascular, pulmonary, or hepatic disease, in hypothyroidism (myxedema), acute alcoholism, delirium tremens, convulsive disorders, bronchial asthma and kyphoscoliosis. Debilitated and elderly patients and those with severe liver diseases should receive smaller doses of NUMORPHAN.

ADVERSE REACTIONS

As with all potent narcotic analgesics, possible side effects include drowsiness, nausea, vomiting, miosis, itching, dysphoria, light-headedness, and headache. Respiratory depression may occur with oxymorphone as with other narcotics.

DOSAGE AND ADMINISTRATION

Usual Adult Dosage of NUMORPHAN (oxymorphone hydrochloride) Injection: Subcutaneous or intramuscular administration: initially 1 mg to 1.5 mg, repeated every 4 to 6 hours as needed. Intravenous: 0.5 mg initially. In nondebilitated patients the dose can be cautiously increased until satisfactory pain relief is obtained. For analgesia during labor 0.5 mg to 1 mg intramuscularly is recommended.

MANAGEMENT OF OVERDOSAGE

Signs and Symptoms: Serious overdosage with NUMORPHAN is characterized by respiratory depression (a decrease in respiratory rate and/or tidal volume, Cheyne-Stokes respiration, cyanosis), extreme somnolence progressing to stupor or coma, skeletal muscle flaccidity, cold and clammy skin, and sometimes bradycardia and hypotension. In severe overdosage, apnea, circulatory collapse, cardiac arrest and death may occur.

Treatment: Primary attention should be given to the reestablishment of adequate respiratory exchange through provision of a patent airway and the institution of assisted or controlled ventilation. The narcotic antagonist naloxone hydrochloride (NARCAN®) is a specific antidote against respiratory depression which may result from overdosage or unusual sensitivity to narcotics including oxymorphone. Therefore, an appropriate dose of naloxone hydrochloride should be administered (usual initial adult dose: 0.4–2 mg) preferably by the intravenous route and simultaneously with efforts at respiratory resuscitation. Since the duration of action of oxymorphone may exceed that of the antagonist, the patient should be kept under continued surveillance and repeated doses of the antagonist should be administered as needed to maintain adequate respiration.

Oxygen, intravenous fluids, vasopressors and other supportive measures should be employed as indicated.

HOW SUPPLIED

For Injection: DEA Order Form Required

1 mg/ml 1 ml ampuls (box of 10)
NDC 0590-0370-10

1.5 mg/ml 1 ml ampuls (box of 10)
NDC 0590-0373-10

10 ml multiple dose vial (box of 1)
NDC 0590-0374-01

Numorphan® is a Registered U.S. Trademark of E.I. du Pont de Nemours & Co. (Inc.)

NARCAN® is a Registered U.S. Trademark of DuPont Pharmaceuticals, Inc.

6110-3

NUMORPHAN® Ⓒ℞

(oxymorphone hydrochloride)
RECTAL SUPPOSITORIES
Narcotic
Analgesic

DESCRIPTION

NUMORPHAN (oxymorphone hydrochloride), a semi-synthetic narcotic substitute for morphine, is a potent analgesic. 4,5α-Epoxy-3, 14-dihydroxy-17-methylmorphinan-6-one hydrochloride

Oxymorphone hydrochloride occurs as a white or slightly off-white, odorless powder, sparingly soluble in alcohol and ether, but freely soluble in water.

The NUMORPHAN rectal suppository is available in a concentration of 5 mg of oxymorphone hydrochloride in a base consisting of polyethylene glycol 1000 and polyethylene glycol 3350.

ACTIONS

NUMORPHAN (oxymorphone hydrochloride) is a potent narcotic analgesic. Administered parenterally, one mg of NUMORPHAN is approximately equivalent in analgesic activity to 10 mg of morphine sulfate.

The onset of action of parenterally administered NUMORPHAN is rapid; initial effects are usually perceived within 5 to 10 minutes. Its duration of action is approximately 3 to 6 hours.

NUMORPHAN produces mild sedation and causes little depression of the cough reflex. These properties make it particularly useful in postoperative patients.

INDICATIONS

For the relief of moderate to severe pain.

CONTRAINDICATIONS

Safe use of NUMORPHAN (oxymorphone hydrochloride) in children under 12 years of age has not been established. This drug should not be used in patients known to be hypersensitive to morphine analogs.

WARNINGS

May be habit forming. As with other narcotic drugs, tolerance and addiction may develop. The addicting potential of the drug appears to be about the same as for morphine. Like other narcotic-containing medications, NUMORPHAN is subject to the Federal Controlled Substances Act.

Interaction with other central nervous system depressants: Patients receiving other narcotic analgesics, general anesthetics, phenothiazines, other tranquilizers, sedatives, hypnotics or other CNS depressants (including alcohol) concomitantly with NUMORPHAN may exhibit an additive CNS depression. When such combined therapy is contemplated, the dose of one or both agents should be reduced.

Safe use in pregnancy has not been established (relative to possible adverse effects on fetal development). As with other potent analgesics the use of NUMORPHAN (oxymorphone hydrochloride) in pregnancy, in nursing mothers, or in women of child-bearing potential requires that the possible benefits of the drug be weighed against the possible hazards to the mother and child.

PRECAUTIONS

The same care and caution should be taken when administering NUMORPHAN (oxymorphone hydrochloride) as when other potent narcotic analgesics are used. It should be borne in mind that some respiratory depression may occur as with all potent narcotics especially when other analgesic and/or anesthetic drugs with depressant action have been given shortly before administration of NUMORPHAN.

The respiratory depressant effects of narcotics and their capacity to elevate cerebrospinal fluid pressure may be markedly exaggerated in the presence of head injury, other intracranial lesions or a pre-existing increase in intracranial pressure. Furthermore, narcotics produce adverse reactions which may obscure the clinical course of patients with head injuries.

As with other analgesics, caution must also be exercised in elderly and debilitated patients and in patients who are known to be sensitive to central nervous system depressants, such as those with cardiovascular, pulmonary, or hepatic disease, in hypothyroidism (myxedema), acute alcoholism, delirium tremens, convulsive disorders, bronchial asthma and kyphoscoliosis. Debilitated and elderly patients and those with severe liver diseases should receive smaller doses of NUMORPHAN.

ADVERSE REACTIONS

As with all potent narcotic analgesics, possible side effects include drowsiness, nausea, vomiting, miosis, itching, dysphoria, light-headedness, and headache. Respiratory depression may occur with oxymorphone as with other narcotics.

DOSAGE AND ADMINISTRATION

Usual Adult Dosage of NUMORPHAN (oxymorphone hydrochloride) Rectal Suppositories: One suppository, 5 mg, every 4 to 6 hours. In nondebilitated patients the dose can be cautiously increased until satisfactory pain relief is obtained.

MANAGEMENT OF OVERDOSAGE

Signs and Symptoms: Serious overdosage with NUMORPHAN is characterized by respiratory depression, (a decrease in respiratory rate and/or tidal volume, Cheyne-Stokes respiration, cyanosis), extreme somnolence progressing to stupor or coma, skeletal muscle flaccidity, cold and clammy skin, and sometimes bradycardia and hypotension. In severe overdosage, apnea, circulatory collapse, cardiac arrest and death may occur.

Treatment: Primary attention should be given to the reestablishment of adequate respiratory exchange through provision of a patent airway and the institution of assisted or controlled ventilation. The narcotic antagonist naloxone hydrochloride (NARCAN®) is a specific antidote against respiratory depression which may result from overdosage or unusual sensitivity to narcotics including oxymorphone. Therefore, an appropriate dose of naloxone hydrochloride should be administered (usual initial adult dose: 0.4 mg-2 mg) preferably by the intravenous route and simultaneously with efforts at respiratory resuscitation. Since the duration of action of oxymorphone may exceed that of the antagonist, the patient should be kept under continued surveillance and repeated doses of the antagonist should be administered as needed to maintain adequate respiration.

Oxygen, intravenous fluids, vasopressors and other supportive measures should be employed as indicated.

HOW SUPPLIED

Rectal Suppositories: DEA Order Form Required
5 mg, wrapped in gold foil, box of 6
Store under refrigeration (35°–46°F, 2°–8°C).

NUMORPHAN® is a Registered U.S. Trademark of E.I. du Pont de Nemours & Co. (Inc.)

NARCAN® is a Registered U.S. Trademark of Du Pont Pharmaceuticals, Inc.

6111-2/Rev. July, 1985

Shown in Product Identification Section, page 409

†PERCOCET® Ⓒ

[perk 'o-set]

DESCRIPTION

Each tablet of PERCOCET® contains:

Oxycodone hydrochloride .... 5 mg
WARNING: May be habit forming
Acetaminophen U.S.P. .... 325 mg

PERCOCET Tablets also contain: microcrystalline cellulose, povidone, starch, stearic acid and other ingredients.

Acetaminophen occurs as a white, odorless crystalline powder, possessing a slightly bitter taste.

The oxycodone component is 14-hydroxydihydrocodeinone, a white, odorless crystalline powder having a saline, bitter taste. It is derived from the opium alkaloid thebaine, and may be represented by the following structural formula:

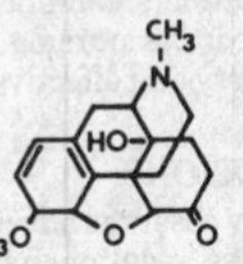

ACTIONS

The principal ingredient, oxycodone, is a semisynthetic narcotic analgesic with multiple actions qualitatively similar to those of morphine; the most prominent of these involve the central nervous system and organs composed of smooth muscle. The principal actions of therapeutic value of the oxycodone in PERCOCET are analgesia and sedation.

Oxycodone is similar to codeine and methadone in that it retains at least one-half of its analgesic activity when administered orally.

Acetaminophen is a non-opiate, non-salicylate analgesic and antipyretic.

INDICATIONS AND USAGE

PERCOCET is indicated for the relief of moderate to moderately severe pain.

CONTRAINDICATIONS

PERCOCET should not be administered to patients who are hypersensitive to oxycodone or acetaminophen.

WARNINGS

Drug Dependence: Oxycodone can produce drug dependence of the morphine type and, therefore, has the potential for being abused. Psychic dependence, physical dependence and tolerance may develop upon repeated administration of PERCOCET, and it should be prescribed and administered with the same degree of caution appropriate to the use of other oral narcotic-containing medications. Like other narcotic-containing medications, PERCOCET is subject to the Federal Controlled Substances Act (Schedule II).

PRECAUTIONS

General

Head Injury and Increased Intracranial Pressure: The respiratory depressant effects of narcotics and their capacity to elevate cerebrospinal fluid pressure may be markedly exaggerated in the presence of head injury, other intracranial lesions or a pre-existing increase in intracranial pressure. Furthermore, narcotics produce adverse reactions which may obscure the clinical course of patients with head injuries.

Acute Abdominal Conditions: The administration of PERCOCET or other narcotics may obscure the diagnosis or clinical course in patients with acute abdominal conditions.

Continued on next page

DuPont—Cont.

Special Risk Patients: PERCOCET should be given with caution to certain patients such as the elderly or debilitated, and those with severe impairment of hepatic or renal function, hypothyroidism, Addison's disease, and prostatic hypertrophy or urethral stricture.
Information for Patients: Oxycodone may impair the mental and or physical abilities for the performance of potentially hazardous tasks such as driving a car or operating machinery. The patient using PERCOCET should be cautioned accordingly.
Drug Interactions: Patients receiving other narcotic analgesics, general anesthetics, phenothiazines, other tranquilizers, sedative-hypnotics or other CNS depressants (including alcohol) concomitantly with PERCOCET may exhibit an additive CNS depression. When such combined therapy is contemplated, the dose of one or both agents should be reduced.
The use of MAO inhibitors or tricyclic antidepressants with oxycodone preparations may increase the effect of either the antidepressant or oxycodone.
The concurrent use of anticholinergics with narcotics may produce paralytic ileus.
Usage In Pregnancy: Pregnancy Category C: Animal reproductive studies have not been conducted with PERCOCET. It is also not known whether PERCOCET can cause fetal harm when administered to a pregnant woman or can affect reproductive capacity. PERCOCET should not be given to a pregnant woman unless in the judgment of the physician, the potential benefits outweigh the possible hazards.
Nonteratogenic Effects: Use of narcotics during pregnancy may produce physical dependence in the neonate.
Labor and Delivery: As with all narcotics, administration of PERCOCET to the mother shortly before delivery may result in some degree of respiratory depression in the newborn and the mother, especially if higher doses are used.
Nursing Mothers: It is not known whether PERCOCET is excreted in human milk. Because many drugs are excreted in human milk, caution should be exercised when PERCOCET is administered to a nursing woman.
Pediatric Use: Safety and effectiveness in children have not been established.

ADVERSE REACTIONS

The most frequently observed adverse reactions include light headedness, dizziness, sedation, nausea and vomiting. These effects seem to be more prominent in ambulatory than in nonambulatory patients, and some of these adverse reactions may be alleviated if the patient lies down.
Other adverse reactions include euphoria, dysphoria, constipation, skin rash and pruritus.
At higher doses, oxycodone has most of the disadvantages of morphine including respiratory depression.

OVERDOSAGE

Acetaminophen

Signs and Symptoms: Acetaminophen in massive overdosage may cause hepatic toxicity in some patients. In all cases of suspected overdose, immediately call your regional poison center or the Rocky Mountain Poison Center's toll-free number (800-525-6115) for assistance in diagnosis and for directions in the use of N-acetylcysteine as an antidote, a use currently restricted to investigational status.
In adults, hepatic toxicity has rarely been reported with acute overdoses of less than 10 grams and fatalities with less than 15 grams. Importantly, young children seem to be more resistant than adults to the hepatotoxic effect of an acetaminophen overdose. Despite this, the measures outlined below should be initiated in any adult or child suspected of having ingested an acetaminophen overdose.
Early symptoms following a potentially hepatotoxic overdose may include: nausea, vomiting, diaphoresis and general malaise. Clinical and laboratory evidence of hepatic toxicity may not be apparent until 48 to 72 hours post-ingestion.
Treatment: The stomach should be emptied promptly by lavage or by induction of emesis with syrup of ipecac. Patient's estimates of the quantity of a drug ingested are notoriously unreliable. Therefore, if an acetaminophen overdose is suspected, a serum acetaminophen assay should be obtained as early as possible, but no sooner than four hours following ingestion. Liver function studies should be obtained initially and repeated at 24-hour intervals.
The antidote, N-acetylcysteine, should be administered as early as possible, and within 16 hours of the overdose ingestions for optimal results. Following recovery, there are no residual, structural, or functional hepatic abnormalities.

Oxycodone

Signs and Symptoms: Serious overdose with oxycodone is characterized by respiratory depression (a decrease in respiratory rate and or tidal volume, Cheyne-Stokes respiration, cyanosis), extreme somnolence progressing to stupor or coma, skeletal muscle flaccidity, cold and clammy skin, and sometimes bradycardia and hypotension. In severe overdosage, apnea, circulatory collapse, cardiac arrest and death may occur.
Treatment: Primary attention should be given to the reestablishment of adequate respiratory exchange through provision of a patent airway and the institution of assisted or controlled ventilation. The narcotic antagonist naloxone hydrochloride (Narcan®) is a specific antidote against respiratory depression which may result from overdosage or unusual sensitivity to narcotics, including oxycodone. Therefore, an appropriate dose of naloxone hydrochloride (usual initial adult dose 0.4 mg to 2 mg) should be administered preferably by the intravenous route, and simultaneously with efforts at respiratory resuscitation (see package insert). Since the duration of action of oxycodone may exceed that of the antagonist, the patient should be kept under continued surveillance and repeated doses of the antagonist should be administered as needed to maintain adequate respiration.
An antagonist should not be administered in the absence of clinically significant respiratory or cardiovascular depression. Oxygen, intravenous fluids, vasopressors and other supportive measures should be employed as indicated.
Gastric emptying may be useful in removing unabsorbed drug.

DOSAGE AND ADMINISTRATION

Dosage should be adjusted according to the severity of the pain and the response of the patient. It may occasionally be necessary to exceed the usual dosage recommended below in cases of more severe pain or in those patients who have become tolerant to the analgesic effect of narcotics. PERCOCET is given orally. The usual adult dose is one tablet every 6 hours as needed for pain.

HOW SUPPLIED

PERCOCET, supplied as a white tablet, with one face scored and inscribed PERCOCET, and the other inscribed with Du Pont name is available in:

Bottles of 100	NDC 0060-0127-70
Bottles of 500	NDC 0060-0127-85
Hospital blister pack of 25 (in units of 250 and 1000 tablets)	NDC 0060-0127-25

Store at controlled room temperature (59°–86°F, 15°–30°C).
DEA Order Form Required
† PERCOCET® is a Registered Trademark of DuPont Pharmaceuticals Caribe, Inc. NARCAN® is a Registered U.S. Trademark of DuPont Pharmaceuticals, Inc.

6090-5 Rev. July 1985

Shown in Product Identification Section, page 409

†PERCODAN® Ⓒ

[perk'o-dan]

†PERCODAN®–DEMI

Tablets

DESCRIPTION

Each tablet of PERCODAN® contains:
Oxycodone hydrochloride .... 4.50 mg
WARNING: May be habit forming
Oxycodone terephthalate .... 0.38 mg
WARNING: May be habit forming
Aspirin, U.S.P. .... 325 mg
PERCODAN Tablets also contain: D&C Yellow 10, FD&C Yellow 6, microcrystalline cellulose and starch.
Each tablet of PERCODAN®-Demi contains:
Oxycodone hydrochloride .... 2.25 mg
WARNING: May be habit forming
Oxycodone terephthalate .... 0.19 mg
WARNING: May be habit forming
Aspirin, U.S.P. .... 325 mg
PERCODAN-Demi Tablets also contain: FD&C Blue 2, FD&C Red 3, microcrystalline cellulose and starch.
The oxycodone component is 14-hydroxydihydrocodeinone, a white odorless crystalline powder which is derived from the opium alkaloid, thebaine.

ACTIONS

The principal ingredient, oxycodone, is a semisynthetic narcotic analgesic with multiple actions qualitatively similar to those of morphine; the most prominent of these involve the central nervous system and organs composed of smooth muscle. The principal actions of therapeutic value of the oxycodone in PERCODAN® and PERCODAN®-Demi are analgesia and sedation.
Oxycodone is similar to codeine and methadone in that it retains at least one half of its analgesic activity when administered orally.
PERCODAN® and PERCODAN®-Demi also contain the non-narcotic antipyretic-analgesic, aspirin.

INDICATIONS

For the relief of moderate to moderately severe pain.

CONTRAINDICATIONS

Hypersensitivity to oxycodone or aspirin.

WARNINGS

Drug Dependence: Oxycodone can produce drug dependence of the morphine type and, therefore, has the potential for being abused. Psychic dependence, physical dependence and tolerance may develop upon repeated administration of PERCODAN® and PERCODAN®-Demi, and it should be prescribed and administered with the same degree of caution appropriate to the use of other oral narcotic-containing medications. Like other narcotic-containing medications, PERCODAN® and PERCODAN®-Demi are subject to the Federal Controlled Substances Act.
Usage in ambulatory patients: Oxycodone may impair the mental and/or physical abilities required for the performance of potentially hazardous tasks such as driving a car or operating machinery. The patient using PERCODAN® and PERCODAN®-Demi should be cautioned accordingly.
Interaction with other central nervous system depressants:-
Patients receiving other narcotic analgesics, general anesthetics, phenothiazines, other tranquilizers, sedative-hypnotics or other CNS depressants (including alcohol) concomitantly with PERCODAN® and PERCODAN®-Demi may exhibit an additive CNS depression. When such combined therapy is contemplated, the dose of one or both agents should be reduced.
Usage in pregnancy: Safe use in pregnancy has not been established relative to possible adverse effects on fetal development. Therefore, PERCODAN® and PERCODAN®-Demi should not be used in pregnant women unless, in the judgment of the physician, the potential benefits outweigh the possible hazards.
Usage in children: PERCODAN® should not be administered to children. PERCODAN®-Demi, containing half the amount of oxycodone, can be considered. (See Dosage and Administration for PERCODAN®-Demi).
Reye Syndrome is a rare but serious disease which can follow flu or chicken pox in children and teenagers. While the cause of Reye Syndrome is unknown, some reports claim aspirin (or salicylates) may increase the risk of developing this disease.
Salicylates should be used with caution in the presence of peptic ulcer or coagulation abnormalities.

PRECAUTIONS

Head injury and increased intracranial pressure: The respiratory depressant effects of narcotics and their capacity to elevate cerebrospinal fluid pressure may be markedly exaggerated in the presence of head injury, other intracranial lesions or a pre-existing increase in intracranial pressure. Furthermore, narcotics produce adverse reactions which may obscure the clinical course of patients with head injuries.
Acute abdominal conditions: The administration of PERCODAN® and PERCODAN®-Demi or other narcotics may obscure the diagnosis or clinical course in patients with acute abdominal conditions.
Special risk patients: PERCODAN® and PERCODAN®-Demi should be given with caution to certain patients such as the elderly or debilitated, and those with severe impairment of hepatic or renal function, hypothyroidism, Addison's disease, and prostatic hypertrophy or urethral stricture.

ADVERSE REACTIONS

The most frequently observed adverse reactions include light headedness, dizziness, sedation, nausea and vomiting. These effects seem to be more prominent in ambulatory than in nonambulatory patients, and some of these adverse reactions may be alleviated if the patient lies down.
Other adverse reactions include euphoria, dysphoria, constipation and pruritus.

DOSAGE AND ADMINISTRATION

Dosage should be adjusted according to the severity of the pain and the response of the patient. It may occasionally be necessary to exceed the usual dosage recommended below in cases of more severe pain or in those patients who have become tolerant to the analgesic effect of narcotics. PERCODAN® and PERCODAN®-Demi are given orally.
PERCODAN®: The usual adult dose is one tablet every 6 hours as needed for pain.
PERCODAN®-Demi: Adults—One or two tablets every six hours. Children 12 years and older—One-half tablet every six hours. Children 6 to 12 years—One-quarter tablet every six hours. PERCODAN®-Demi is not indicated for children under 6 years of age.

DRUG INTERACTIONS

The CNS depressant effects of PERCODAN® and PERCODAN®-Demi may be additive with that of other CNS depressants. See WARNINGS.
Aspirin may enhance the effect of anticoagulants and inhibit the uricosuric effects of uricosuric agents.

MANAGEMENT OF OVERDOSAGE

Signs and Symptoms: Serious overdose with PERCODAN® or PERCODAN®-Demi is characterized by respiratory depression (a decrease in respiratory rate and/or tidal volume, Cheyne-Stokes respiration, cyanosis), extreme somnolence progressing to stupor or coma, skeletal muscle flaccidity, cold and clammy skin, and sometimes bradycardia and hypotension. In severe overdosage, apnea, circulatory collapse, cardiac arrest and death may occur. The ingestion of very large amounts of PERCODAN® or PERCODAN®-Demi may, in addition, result in acute salicylate intoxication.

Treatment: Primary attention should be given to the reestablishment of adequate respiratory exchange through provision of a patent airway and the institution of assisted or controlled ventilation. The narcotic antagonist naloxone hydrochloride (NARCAN®) is a specific antidote against respiratory depression which may result from overdosage or unusual sensitivity to narcotics, including oxycodone. Therefore, an appropriate dose of naloxone hydrochloride should be administered (usual adult dose: 0.4 mg–2 mg) preferably by the intravenous route, simultaneously with efforts at respiratory resuscitation. Since the duration of action of oxycodone may exceed that of the antagonist, the patient should be kept under continued surveillance and repeated doses of the antagonist should be administered as needed to maintain adequate respiration.
Oxygen, intravenous fluids, vasopressors and other supportive measures should be employed as indicated.
Gastric emptying may be useful in removing unabsorbed drug.

HOW SUPPLIED

Percodan®—As yellow, scored tablets, available in:

Bottles of 100	NDC 0060-0135-70
Bottles of 500	NDC 0060-0135-85
Bottles of 1000	NDC 0060-0135-90
Hospital blister pack of 25 (available in units of 250 and 1000)	NDC 0060-0135-65

Also available in Military Depot:
Btl's of 100 NSN 6505-01-030-9493
Blister Pack (250) NSN 6505-01-030-9492
Percodan®-Demi—As pink, scored tablets available in:

Bottles of 100	NDC 0060-0136-70

"Store At Controlled Room Temperature (59°–86°F, 15°–30°C)."
DEA Order Form Required

PERCODAN is a registered U.S. trademark of DuPont Pharmaceuticals Caribe, Inc.
†Products of DuPont Pharmaceuticals Caribe, Inc.
6117-4/6118-4
NARCAN is a Registered U.S. Trademark of DuPont Pharmaceuticals, Inc.

Shown in Product Identification Section, page 409

SYMMETREL® ℞

[sim'e-trel"]
(amantadine hydrochloride)

DESCRIPTION

SYMMETREL is designated generically as amantadine hydrochloride and chemically as 1-adamantanamine hydrochloride.
Amantadine hydrochloride is a stable white or nearly white crystalline powder, freely soluble in water and soluble in alcohol and in chloroform.
Amantadine hydrochloride has pharmacological actions as both an anti-Parkinson and an antiviral drug.
SYMMETREL is available in capsules and syrup.
SYMMETREL capsules contain: FD&C Red 40, gelatin, glycerin, hydrogenated vegetable oil, lecithin, methylparaben, propylparaben, soybean oil, titanium dioxide, vegetable shortening, and yellow wax.
SYMMETREL syrup contains: artificial raspberry flavor, citric acid, methylparaben, propylparaben, and sorbitol solution.

CLINICAL PHARMACOLOGY

SYMMETREL is readily absorbed, is not metabolized, and is excreted unchanged in the urine.
After oral administration of a single dose of 100 mg. maximum blood levels are reached, based on the mean time of the peak urinary excretion rate, in approximately 4 hours; the peak excretion rate is approximately 5 mg/hr; the mean half-life of the excretion rate approximates 15 hours.
The mechanism of action of SYMMETREL in the treatment of Parkinson's disease and drug-induced extrapyramidal reactions is not known. It has been shown to cause an increase in dopamine release in the animal brain. The drug does not possess anticholinergic activity in animal tests at doses similar to those used clinically. The antiviral activity of SYMMETREL against influenza A virus is not completely understood. The mode of action of SYMMETREL appears to be the prevention of the release of infectious viral nucleic acid into the host cell. SYMMETREL does not appear to interfere with the immunogenicity of inactivated influenza A virus vaccine.

INDICATIONS AND USAGE

Parkinson's Disease/ Syndrome and Drug-Induced Extrapyramidal Reactions: SYMMETREL is indicated in the treatment of idiopathic Parkinson's disease (Paralysis Agitans), postencephalitic parkinsonism, drug-induced extrapyramidal reactions, and symptomatic parkinsonism which may follow injury to the nervous system by carbon monoxide intoxication. It is indicated in those elderly patients believed to develop parkinsonism in association with cerebral arteriosclerosis. In the treatment of Parkinson's disease, SYMMETREL is less effective than levodopa, (-)-3-(3, 4-dihydroxyphenyl)-L-alanine, and its efficacy in comparison with the anticholinergic antiparkinson drugs has not yet been established. Although anticholinergic type side effects have been noted with SYMMETREL when used in patients with drug-induced extrapyramidal reactions, there is a lower incidence of these side effects than that observed with anticholinergic antiparkinson drugs.

Influenza A Virus Respiratory Tract Illness: SYMMETREL (amantadine hydrochloride) is indicated in the prevention and treatment of respiratory tract illness caused by influenza A virus strains. SYMMETREL should be considered especially for high risk patients, close household or hospital ward contacts of index cases and patients with severe influenza A virus illness. In the prophylaxis of influenza due to A virus strains, early immunization as periodically recommended by the Public Health Service Advisory Committee on Immunization Practices is the method of choice. When early immunization is not feasible, or when the vaccine is contraindicated or not available, SYMMETREL can be used for chemoprophylaxis against influenza A virus illness. Because SYMMETREL does not appear to suppress antibody response, it can be used chemoprophylactically in conjunction with inactivated influenza A virus vaccine until protective antibody responses develop. There is no clinical evidence that this drug has efficacy in the prophylaxis or treatment of viral respiratory tract illnesses other than those caused by influenza A virus strains.

CONTRAINDICATIONS

SYMMETREL is contraindicated in patients with known hypersensitivity to the drug.

WARNINGS

Patients with a history of epilepsy or other "seizures" should be observed closely for possible increased seizure activity.
Patients with a history of congestive heart failure or peripheral edema should be followed closely as there are patients who developed congestive heart failure while receiving SYMMETREL.
Patients with Parkinson's disease improving on SYMMETREL should resume normal activities gradually and cautiously, consistent with other medical considerations, such as the presence of osteoporosis or phlebothrombosis.
Patients receiving SYMMETREL who note central nervous system effects or blurring of vision should be cautioned against driving or working in situations where alertness is important.

PRECAUTIONS

SYMMETREL (amantadine hydrochloride) should not be discontinued abruptly since a few patients with Parkinson's disease experienced a parkinsonian crisis, i.e., a sudden marked clinical deterioration, when this medication was suddenly stopped. The dose of anticholinergic drugs or of SYMMETREL should be reduced if atropine-like effects appear when these drugs are used concurrently.
The dose of SYMMETREL may need careful adjustment in patients with renal impairment, congestive heart failure, peripheral edema, or orthostatic hypotension. Since SYMMETREL is not metabolized and is mainly excreted in the urine, it may accumulate when renal function is inadequate.
Care should be exercised when administering SYMMETREL to patients with liver disease, a history of recurrent eczematoid rash, or to patients with psychosis or severe psychoneurosis not controlled by chemotherapeutic agents. Careful observation is required when SYMMETREL is administered concurrently with central nervous system stimulants.
No long-term studies in animals have been performed to evaluate the carcinogenic potential of SYMMETREL.
The mutagenic potential of the drug has not yet been determined in experimental systems.

Pregnancy Category C: SYMMETREL (amantadine hydrochloride) has been shown to be embryotoxic and teratogenic in rats at 50 mg/kg/day, about 12 times the recommended human dose, but not at 37 mg/kg/day. Embryotoxic and teratogenic drug effects were not seen in rabbits which received up to 25 times the recommended human dose. There are no adequate and well-controlled studies in pregnant women. SYMMETREL should be used during pregnancy only if the potential benefit justifies the potential risk to the embryo or the fetus.

Nursing Mothers: SYMMETREL is excreted in human milk. Caution should be exercised when SYMMETREL is administered to a nursing woman.

Pediatric Use: The safety and efficacy of SYMMETREL in newborn infants, and infants below the age of 1 year have not been established.

ADVERSE REACTIONS

The most frequently occurring serious adverse reactions are depression, congestive heart failure, orthostatic hypotensive episodes, psychosis, and urinary retention. Rarely convulsions, leukopenia, and neutropenia have been reported.
Other adverse reactions of a less serious nature which have been observed are the following: hallucinations, confusion, anxiety and irritability, anorexia, nausea, and constipation; ataxia and dizziness (lightheadedness); livedo reticularis and peripheral edema. Adverse reactions observed less frequently are the following: vomiting; dry mouth; headache; dyspnea; fatigue, insomnia, and a sense of weakness. Infrequently, skin rash, slurred speech, and visual disturbances have been observed. Rarely eczematoid dermatitis and oculogyric episodes have been reported.

OVERDOSAGE

There is no specific antidote. However, slowly administered intravenous physostigmine in 1 and 2 mg doses in an adult[1] at 1 to 2 hour intervals and 0.5 mg doses in a child[2] at 5 to 10 minute intervals up to a maximum of 2 mg/hour have been reported to be effective in the control of central nervous system toxicity caused by amantadine hydrochloride. For acute overdosing, general supportive measures should be employed along with immediate gastric lavage or induction of emesis. Fluids should be forced, and if necessary, given intravenously. The pH of the urine has been reported to influence the excretion rate of SYMMETREL. Since the excretion rate of SYMMETREL increases rapidly when the urine is acidic, the administration of urine acidifying drugs may increase the elimination of the drug from the body. The blood pressure, pulse, respiration and temperature should be monitored. The patient should be observed for hyperactivity and convulsions; if required, sedation, and anticonvulsant therapy should be administered. The patient should be observed for the possible development of arrhythmias and hypotension, if required, appropriate antiarrhythmic and antihypotensive therapy should be given. The blood electrolytes, urine pH and urinary output should be monitored. If there is no record of recent voiding, catheterization should be done. The possibility of multiple drug ingestion by the patient should be considered.

[1]D.F. Casey, N. Engl. J. Med. 298:516, 1978.
[2]C.D. Berkowitz, J. Pediatr. 95:144, 1979.

DOSAGE AND ADMINISTRATION

Dosage for Parkinsonism:

Adult: The usual dose of SYMMETREL (amantadine hydrochloride) is 100 mg twice a day when used alone. SYMMETREL has an onset of action usually within 48 hours.
The initial dose of SYMMETREL is 100 mg daily for patients with serious associated medical illnesses or who are receiving high doses of other antiparkinson drugs. After one to several weeks at 100 mg once daily, the dose may be increased to 100 mg twice daily, if necessary.
Occasionally, patients whose responses are not optimal with SYMMETREL at 200 mg daily may benefit from an increase up to 400 mg daily in divided doses. However, such patients should be supervised closely by their physicians.
Patients initially deriving benefit from SYMMETREL not uncommonly experience a fall-off of effectiveness after a few months. Benefit may be regained by increasing the dose to 300 mg daily. Alternatively, temporary discontinuation of SYMMETREL for several weeks, followed by reinitiation of the drug, may result in regaining benefit in some patients. A decision to use other antiparkinson drugs may be necessary.

Dosage for Concomitant Therapy

Some patients who do not respond to anticholinergic antiparkinson drugs may respond to SYMMETREL. When SYMMETREL or anticholinergic antiparkinson drugs are each used with marginal benefit, concomitant use may produce additional benefit.
When SYMMETREL and levodopa are initiated concurrently, the patient can exhibit rapid therapeutic benefits. SYMMETREL should be held constant at 100 mg daily or twice daily while the daily dose of levodopa is gradually increased to optimal benefit.
When SYMMETREL is added to optimal well-tolerated doses of levodopa, additional benefit may result, including smoothing out the fluctuations in improvement which sometimes occur in patients on levodopa alone. Patients who require a reduction in their usual dose of levodopa because of development of side effects may possibly regain lost benefit with the addition of SYMMETREL.

Dosage for Drug-induced Extrapyramidal Reactions:

Adult: The usual dose of SYMMETREL (amantadine hydrochloride) is 100 mg twice a day. Occasionally, patients whose responses are not optimal with SYMMETREL at 200 mg daily may benefit from an increase up to 300 mg daily in divided doses.

Dosage for Prophylaxis and Treatment of Influenza A Virus Respiratory Tract Illness:

Adult: The adult daily dosage of SYMMETREL (amantadine hydrochloride) is 200 mg; two 100 mg capsules (or four

Continued on next page

DuPont—Cont.

teaspoonfuls of syrup) as a single daily dose, or the daily dosage may be split into one capsule of 100 mg (or two teaspoonfuls of syrup) twice a day. If central nervous system effects develop on once-a-day dosage, a split dosage schedule may reduce such complaints.
Children: 1 yr.–9 yrs. of age: The total daily dose should be calculated on the basis of 2 to 4 mg/lb/day (4.4 to 8.8 mg/kg/day), but not to exceed 150 mg per day.
9 yrs.–12 yrs. of age: The total daily dose is 200 mg given as one capsule of 100 mg (or two teaspoonfuls of syrup) twice a day.
Prophylactic dosing should be started in anticipation of contact or as soon as possible after contact with individuals with influenza A virus respiratory illness. SYMMETREL should be continued daily for at least 10 days following a known exposure. If SYMMETREL is used chemoprophylactically in conjunction with inactivated influenza A virus vaccine until protective antibody responses develop, then it should be administered for 2 to 3 weeks after the vaccine has been given. When inactivated influenza A virus vaccine is unavailable or contraindicated, SYMMETREL should be administered for up to 90 days in case of possible repeated and unknown exposures. Treatment of influenza A virus illness should be started as soon as possible after onset of symptoms and should be continued for 24 to 48 hours after the disappearance of symptoms.

HOW SUPPLIED

SYMMETREL (amantadine hydrochloride) is available as capsules (each red, soft gelatin capsule contains 100 mg amantadine hydrochloride) in

Bottles of 100 NDC 0056-0105-70
Bottles of 500 NDC 0056-0105-85
Hospital Unit-Dose blister package of 100 NDC 0056-0105-75

As a syrup (each 5 ml [1 teaspoonful] contains 50 mg amantadine hydrochloride) in 16 oz. (480 ml) bottles NDC 0056-0205-16.
Also available in Military Depot:
Btl's of 100 NSN 6505-00-148-4624
In VA Depot:
Btls. of 100 NSN 6505-00-148-4624A
Store at controlled room temperature (59°–86°F, 15°–30°C).
SYMMETREL is a Registered U.S. Trademark of E.I. duPont de Nemours & Co. (Inc.)
Capsules manufactured by
R.P. Scherer-North America,
St. Petersburg, Florida 33702
For DuPont Pharmaceuticals
6043-16

Shown in Product Identification Section, page 409

TESSALON® ℞

[tes 'a-lon ″]
(benzonatate USP)

DESCRIPTION

TESSALON®, a nonnarcotic oral antitussive agent, is 2, 5, 8, 11, 14, 17, 20, 23, 26-nonaoxaoctacosan-28-yl p-(butylamino) benzoate.

$CH_3(CH_2)_2CH_2NH$—⟨benzene ring⟩—$COOCH_2CH_2(OCH_2CH_2)_{11}OCH_3$

Each TESSALON Perle contains:
Benzonatate, USP .... 100 mg
TESSALON Perles also contain: D&C Yellow 10, gelatin, glycerin, methylparaben and propylparaben.

CLINICAL PHARMACOLOGY

TESSALON acts peripherally by anesthetizing the stretch receptors located in the respiratory passages, lungs, and pleura by dampening their activity and thereby reducing the cough reflex at its source. It begins to act within 15 to 20 minutes and its effect lasts for 3 to 8 hours. TESSALON has no inhibitory effect on the respiratory center in recommended dosage.

INDICATIONS AND USAGE

TESSALON is indicated for the symptomatic relief of cough.

CONTRAINDICATIONS

Hypersensitivity to benzonatate or related compounds.

PRECAUTIONS

Information for patients: Release of TESSALON from the perle in the mouth can produce a temporary local anesthesia of the oral mucosa and choking could occur. Therefore, the perles should be swallowed without chewing.
Usage in Pregnancy: Pregnancy Category C. Animal reproduction studies have not been conducted with TESSALON. It is also not known whether TESSALON can cause fetal harm when administered to a pregnant woman or can affect reproduction capacity. TESSALON should be given to a pregnant woman only if clearly needed.
Nursing mothers: It is not known whether this drug is excreted in human milk. Because many drugs are excreted in human milk caution should be exercised when TESSALON is administered to a nursing woman.
Carcinogenesis, mutagenesis, impairment of fertility: Carcinogenicity, mutagenicity, and reproduction studies have not been conducted with TESSALON.

ADVERSE REACTIONS

Sedation, headache, mild dizziness, pruritus and skin eruptions, nasal congestion, constipation, nausea, gastrointestinal upset, sensation of burning in the eyes, a vague "chilly" sensation, numbness in the chest, and hypersensitivity have been reported.

OVERDOSAGE

No clinically significant cases have been reported, to our knowledge. The drug is chemically related to tetracaine and other topical anesthetics and shares various aspects of their pharmacology and toxicology. Drugs of this type are generally well absorbed after ingestion.
Signs and Symptoms
If perles are chewed or dissolved in the mouth, oropharyngeal anesthesia will develop rapidly. CNS stimulation may cause restlessness and tremors which may proceed to clonic convulsions followed by profound CNS depression.
Treatment
Evacuate gastric contents and administer copious amounts of activated charcoal slurry. Even in the conscious patient, cough and gag reflexes may be so depressed as to necessitate special attention to protection against aspiration of gastric contents and orally administered materials.
Convulsions should be treated with a short-acting barbiturate given intravenously and carefully titrated for the smallest effective dosage.
Intensive support of respiration and cardiovascular-renal function is an essential feature of the treatment of severe intoxication from overdosage.
Do not use CNS stimulants.

DOSAGE AND ADMINISTRATION

Adults and Children over 10: Usual dose is one 100 mg perle t.i.d. as required. If necessary, up to 6 perles daily may be given.

HOW SUPPLIED

Perles, 100 mg (yellow); bottles of 100 NDC 0056-0010-70.
Store at controlled room temperature (59°–86°F, 15°–30°C).
Manufactured by
R.P. Scherer-North America
St. Petersburg, Florida 33702
for
DuPont Pharmaceuticals
E.I. duPont de Nemours & Co. (Inc.)
Wilmington, Delaware 19898

6075-12/Rev. Feb, 1985

Shown in Product Identification Section, page 409

TREXAN™ ℞

[treks 'an]
(naltrexone hydrochloride)

DESCRIPTION

TREXAN (naltrexone hydrochloride), an opioid antagonist, is a synthetic congener of oxymorphone, and is technically, therefore, a thebaine derivative. However, it has no opioid agonist properties. Naltrexone differs in structure from oxymorphone in that the methyl group on the nitrogen atom is replaced by a cyclopropylmethyl group. TREXAN (naltrexone hydrochloride) is also related to the potent opioid antagonist, naloxone, or n-allylnoroxymorphone (NARCAN®).
TREXAN (naltrexone hydrochloride) is a white, crystalline compound. The hydrochloride salt is soluble to the extent of about 100 mg/cc. TREXAN is available in scored tablets containing 50 mg of naltrexone hydrochloride.
TREXAN Tablets also contain: alginic acid, FD&C Yellow 6, microcrystalline cellulose, stearic acid, and sugar.

CLINICAL PHARMACOLOGY

Pharmacodynamic actions: TREXAN (naltrexone hydrochloride) is a pure opioid antagonist. It markedly attenuates or completely blocks, reversibly, the subjective effects of intravenously administered opioids. [In this context, the term opioid is used to describe 1) classic morphine-like agonists and 2) analgesics possessing agonist and antagonist activity (e.g., butorphanol, nalbuphine and pentazocine).]
When co-administered with morphine, on a chronic basis, TREXAN blocks the physical dependence to morphine and presumably other opioids.
TREXAN has few, if any, intrinsic actions besides its opioid blocking properties. However, it does produce some pupillary constriction, by an unknown mechanism.
The administration of TREXAN is not associated with the development of tolerance or dependence.
In subjects physically dependent on opioids, TREXAN will precipitate withdrawal symptomatology.
Clinical studies indicate that 50 mg of TREXAN will block the pharmacologic effects of 25 mg of intravenously administered heroin for periods as long as 24 hours. Other data suggest that doubling the dose of TREXAN provides blockade for 48 hours, and tripling the dose of TREXAN provides blockade for about 72 hours.
While the mechanism of action is not fully understood, the preponderance of evidence suggests that TREXAN blocks the effects of opioids by competitive binding (i.e., analogous to competitive inhibition of enzymes) at opioid receptors. This makes the blockade produced potentially surmountable.
Bioavailability/Pharmacokinetics: Following oral administration, TREXAN (naltrexone hydrochloride) is subject to extensive "first pass" hepatic metabolism (its major route of elimination) with approximately 95% of the absorbed drug being converted to several metabolites. The major metabolite, 6-β-naltrexol, like TREXAN, is believed to be a pure antagonist and may contribute to the pharmacological blockade of opioid receptors. A minor metabolite is 2-hydroxy-3-methoxy-6-β-naltrexol. TREXAN and its metabolites are also conjugated to form additional metabolic products. TREXAN and its metabolites are excreted primarily by the kidney, with fecal excretion being a minor elimination pathway. The urinary excretion of unchanged TREXAN accounts for less than 1% of an oral dose; urinary excretion of unchanged and conjugated 6-β-naltrexol accounts for approximately 38% of an oral dose. The pharmacokinetic profile of TREXAN suggests that TREXAN and its metabolites undergo enterohepatic recycling.
Following the administration of 50 mg TREXAN tablets to 24 healthy adult male volunteers, the C_{max} for TREXAN and its major metabolite, 6-β-naltrexol were 8.6 ng/ml and 99.3 ng/ml, respectively. The maximum concentration (C_{max}), area under the curve (AUC), and amount excreted in the urine for both TREXAN and 6-β-naltrexol increased proportionally as the amount of TREXAN administered increased from 50 mg to 200 mg. The time to maximum concentration (T_{max}) is one hour for both TREXAN and 6-β-naltrexol. The mean elimination half-life (T-½) values for TREXAN and 6-β-naltrexol are 3.9 hours and 12.9 hours, respectively. The mean elimination half-life (T-½) and time to maximum concentration (T_{max}) for TREXAN and 6-β-naltrexol are independent of dose. TREXAN does not accumulate during chronic dosing. As predicted by its longer half-life, plasma levels of 6-β-naltrexol increase by 40% during chronic TREXAN dosing.
The total body clearance of TREXAN is 1.5 L/min, which approximates liver blood flow, and suggests TREXAN is a highly extracted compound. A renal clearance of 127 ml/min for TREXAN suggests it is solely cleared by glomerular filtration. A renal clearance of 283 ml/min for 6-β-naltrexol suggests an additional renal tubular secretory mechanism. The volume of distribution for TREXAN following intravenous administration is estimated to be 1350 liters. In vitro tests with human plasma show TREXAN to be 21% bound to plasma protein over the therapeutic dose range.
In a relative bioavailability study in 24 healthy adult male volunteers, TREXAN tablets were found to be bioequivalent to TREXAN syrup; no differences were observed for C_{max}, AUC, and urinary excretion. As expected, the time to maximum concentration (T_{max}) occurred slightly earlier for the syrup (0.6 hours) than for the tablet (1.0 hr).

INDICATIONS AND USAGE

TREXAN (naltrexone hydrochloride) is indicated to provide blockade of the pharmacologic effects of exogenously administered opioids as an adjunct to the maintenance of the opioid free-state in detoxified formerly opioid-dependent individuals.
There are no data that demonstrate an unequivocally beneficial effect of TREXAN on rates of recidivism among detoxified, formerly opioid-dependent individuals.

CONTRAINDICATIONS

TREXAN is contraindicated in:
1) Patients receiving opioid analgesics.
2) Opioid dependent patients.
3) Patients in acute opioid withdrawal (see WARNINGS).
4) Any individual who has failed to pass the NARCAN challenge. (See DOSAGE AND ADMINISTRATION section)
5) Any individual who has a positive urine screen for opioids.
6) Any individual with a history of sensitivity to TREXAN (naltrexone hydrochloride). It is not known if there is any cross-sensitivity with naloxone or other phenanthrene containing opioids.
7) Any individual with acute hepatitis or liver failure.

WARNINGS

Hepatotoxicity:

TREXAN has the capacity to cause dose related hepatocellular injury.

Prior to making a decision to initiate treatment with TREXAN, the physician should establish whether the patient has subclinical liver injury or disease. (See PRECAUTIONS; Laboratory Tests). TREXAN is contraindicated in acute hepatitis or liver failure, but its use even in patients with evidence of less severe liver disease or a history of recent liver disease must be carefully considered in light of its hepatotoxic potential.

The evidence that identified TREXAN as a hepatotoxin was not obtained in studies involving its use at the doses recommended for opiate blockade, where the changes in serum levels of liver enzymes seen were similar to those present at baseline in the study population. However, the margin of separation between the apparently safe and the hepatotoxic doses appears to be only five-fold or less.

Evidence of TREXAN's hepatotoxic potential is derived primarily from a placebo controlled study in which TREXAN was administered to obese subjects at a dose approximately five-fold that recommended for the blockade of opiate receptors (300 mg per day). In the study, 5 of 26 TREXAN recipients developed elevations of serum transaminases (i.e., peak SGPT values ranging from a low of 121 to a high of 532; or 3 to 19 times their baseline values) after three to eight weeks of treatment. Although the patients involved were generally clinically asymptomatic and the transaminase levels of all patients on whom follow-up was obtained returned to (or toward) baseline values in a matter of weeks, the lack of any transaminase elevations of similar magnitude in any of the 24 placebo patients in the same study is persuasive evidence that TREXAN is a direct (i.e., not an idiosyncratic) hepatoxin. This conclusion is also supported by evidence from other placebo controlled studies in which exposure to TREXAN at doses from one to two-fold the amount recommended for opiate blockade consistently produced more numerous and more significant elevations of serum transaminases than did placebo, and reports of transaminase elevations in 3 of 9 patients with Alzheimer's Disease who received TREXAN (up to 300 mg/day) for 5 to 8 weeks in a open clinical trial.

Unintended Precipitation of Abstinence: To prevent occurrence of an acute abstinence syndrome, or exacerbation of a pre-existing sub-clinical abstinence syndrome, patients should remain opioid-free for a minimum of 7–10 days before starting TREXAN. Since the absence of an opioid drug in the urine is often not sufficient proof that a patient is opioid-free, a NARCAN challenge should be employed to exclude the possibility of precipitating a withdrawal reaction following administration of TREXAN. The NARCAN challenge test is described in the DOSAGE AND ADMINISTRATION section.

While TREXAN is a potent antagonist with a prolonged pharmacologic effect (24 to 72 hours), the blockade produced by TREXAN is surmountable. This is useful in patients who may require analgesia, but poses a potential risk to individuals who attempt, on their own, to overcome the blockade by administering large amounts of exogenous opioids. Indeed, any attempt by a patient to overcome the antagonism by taking opioids is very dangerous and may lead to a fatal overdose. Injury may arise because the plasma concentration of exogenous opioids attained immediately following their acute administration may be sufficient to overcome the competitive receptor blockade. As a consequence, the patient may be in immediate danger of suffering life endangering opioid intoxication (e.g., respiratory arrest, circulatory collapse). Also, lesser amounts of exogenous opioids may prove dangerous if they are taken in a manner (i.e. relatively long after the last dose of naltrexone) and in an amount so that they persist in the body longer than effective concentrations of naltrexone and its metabolites. Patients should be told of the serious consequences of surmounting the opiate blockade. See Information for Patients section.

PRECAUTIONS

General:

Actions Suggested When Reversal of TREXAN Blockade is Required: In an emergency situation requiring analgesia which can only be achieved with opioids, the amount of opioid required may be greater than usual, and the resulting respiratory depression may be deeper and more prolonged. No methods to reverse overdose have been established by controlled clinical trials; therefore in such circumstances, a rapidly acting analgesic which minimizes respiratory depression is preferred. The amount of analgesic administered should be titrated to the needs of the patient.

Additionally, non-receptor mediated actions may occur (e.g., facial swelling, itching, generalized erythema presumably due to histamine release).

Irrespective of the drug chosen to reverse TREXAN (naltrexone hydrochloride) blockade, the patient should be monitored closely by appropriately trained personnel in a hospital setting.

Actions Suggested When Withdrawal is Accidentally Precipitated With TREXAN: Severe opioid withdrawal syndromes precipated by the accidental ingestion of TREXAN have been reported in opioid-dependent individuals. Symptoms of withdrawal have usually appeared within five minutes of ingestion of TREXAN and have lasted for up to 48 hours. Mental status changes including confusion, somnolence and visual hallucinations have occurred. Significant fluid losses from vomiting and diarrhea have required intravenous fluid administration. In all cases patients were closely monitored and therapy tailored to meet individual requirements.

Interference With the Action of Narcotic Containing Drug Product: Patients taking TREXAN may not benefit from opioid containing medicines, such as cough and cold preparations, antidiarrheal preparations, and opioid analgesics. Where a non-opioid containing alternative is available, it should be used.

Information for Patients: It is suggested that the prescribing physician relate the following information to patients being treated with TREXAN:

You have been prescribed TREXAN (naltrexone hydrochloride) as part of the comprehensive treatment for your drug dependence. You should carry identification to alert medical personnel to the fact that you are taking TREXAN. A TREXAN medication card may be obtained from your physician and can be used for this purpose. Carrying the identification card should help to ensure that you can obtain adequate treatment in an emergency. If you require medical treatment be sure to tell the treating physician that you are receiving TREXAN therapy.

You should take TREXAN as directed by your physician. If you attempt to self-administer heroin or any other opiate drug, in small doses, you will not perceive any effect. Most important, however, if you attempt to self-administer large doses of heroin or any other narcotic, you may die or sustain serious injury, including coma.

Laboratory tests: Tests designed to detect hepatic injury should be obtained prior to initiation of TREXAN therapy and periodically thereafter. (See "WARNINGS" section on Hepatotoxicity).

Periodic testing of all patients after initiation of treatment is critical if the occurrence of TREXAN induced liver damage is to be detected at the earliest possible time. Evaluations, using appropriate batteries of tests to detect liver injury are recommended on a monthly basis during the first six months of use; thereafter, clinical judgment about the frequency of monitoring must be relied upon.

Laboratory tests which may be used for the separation and detection of morphine, methadone or quinine in the urine and with which TREXAN does not interfere include thin-layer, gas-liquid, and high pressure liquid chromatographic methods.

Carcinogenesis, Mutagenesis and Impairment of Fertility:

Carcinogenesis: In a two-year carcinogenicity study in rats, there were small increases in the numbers of mesotheliomas in males, and tumors of vascular origin in both sexes. The number of tumors were within the range seen in historical control groups, except for the vascular tumors in females, where the 4% incidence exceeded the historical maximum of 2%.

Mutagenesis: A total of twenty-two distinct tests were performed using bacterial, mammalian, and tissue culture systems. All tests were negative except for weakly positive findings in the Drosophila recessive lethal assay and non-specific DNA repair tests with *E. coli*. The significance of these findings is undetermined.

Impairment of Fertility: TREXAN (100 mg/kg, approximately 140 times the human therapeutic dose) caused a significant increase in pseudopregnancy in the rat. A decrease in the pregnancy rate of mated female rats also occurred. The relevance of these observations to human fertility is not known.

Pregnancy: Category C. TREXAN has been shown to have an embryocidal effect in the rat and rabbit when given in doses approximately 140 times the human therapeutic dose. This effect was demonstrated in rats dosed with TREXAN (100 mg/kg) prior to and throughout gestation, and rabbits treated with 60 mg/kg of TREXAN during the period of organogenesis.

There are no adequate and well-controlled studies in pregnant women. TREXAN should be used in pregnancy only when the potential benefit justifies the potential risk to the fetus.

LABOR AND DELIVERY

Whether or not TREXAN affects the duration of labor and delivery is unknown.

NURSING MOTHERS

Whether or not TREXAN is excreted in human milk is unknown. Because many drugs are excreted in human milk, caution should be exercised when TREXAN is administered to a nursing mother.

PEDIATRIC USE

The safe use of TREXAN in subjects younger than 18 years old has not been established.

ADVERSE REACTIONS

While extensive clinical studies evaluating the use of TREXAN in detoxified, formerly opioid dependent individuals failed to identify any single, serious untoward risk of TREXAN use, placebo controlled studies employing up to five-fold higher doses of TREXAN (up to 300 mg per day) than that recommended for use in opiate receptor blockade have shown that TREXAN causes hepatocellular injury in a substantial proportion of patients exposed at this higher dose. (See WARNINGS and PRECAUTIONS: Laboratory Tests).

Aside from this finding, however, available evidence does not incriminate TREXAN, used at any dose, as a cause of any other serious untoward event for the patient who is "opioid free." It is critical to recognize that TREXAN can precipitate or exacerbate abstinence signs and symptoms in any individual who is not completely free of exogenous opioids.

TREXAN used at the doses recommended to produce opiate receptor blockade does *not* appear to be the cause of any of the numerous adverse events and abnormal laboratory findings, *including liver function abnormalities*, that were observed in the course of the clinical trials that enrolled individuals with a history of both alcohol and substance abuse. In the one placebo controlled trial intended to assess the effects of opiate receptor blockade on drug abuse recidivism, observed untoward events and laboratory abnormalities occurred with nearly equal frequency among placebo and TREXAN recipients. In all open studies, the untoward events observed (e.g., lymphocytosis, transaminase elevations, GI disturbances) were findings that would be anticipated in any similar population not treated with naltrexone. Supporting this judgment, many of the abnormalities detected during the course of the clinical trials were present at baseline, and in some instances, baseline abnormalities, including transaminase elevations, improved or returned to normal during the course of treatment with naltrexone.

In summary, among opioid free individuals, TREXAN administration at the recommended dose has not been associated with a predictable profile of serious adverse or untoward events. However, as mentioned above, among individuals using opioids, TREXAN may cause serious reactions (see CONTRAINDICATIONS, WARNINGS, DOSAGE AND ADMINISTRATION).

Events other than hepatocellular injury reported during clinical testing:

The following adverse reactions have been reported both at baseline and during the TREXAN medication period at an incidence rate of more than 10%:

Difficulty sleeping, anxiety, nervousness, abdominal pain/-cramps, nausea and/or vomiting, low energy, joint and muscle pain, and headache.

The incidence was less than 10% for:

Loss of appetite, diarrhea, constipation, increased thirst, increased energy, feeling down, irritability, dizziness, skin rash, delayed ejaculation, decreased potency, and chills.

The following events occurred in less than 1% of subjects:

Respiratory: nasal congestion, itching, rhinorrhea, sneezing, sore throat, excess mucus or phlegm, sinus trouble, heavy breathing, hoarseness, cough, shortness of breath.

Cardiovascular: nose bleeds, phlebitis, edema, increased blood pressure, non-specific ECG changes, palpitations, tachycardia.

Gastrointestinal: excessive gas, hemorrhoids, diarrhea, ulcer.

Musculoskeletal: painful shoulders, legs or knees; tremors, twitching.

Genitourinary: increased frequency of or discomfort during urination; increased or decreased sexual interest.

Dermatologic: oily skin, pruritus, acne, athlete's foot, cold sores, alopecia.

Psychiatric: depression, paranoia; fatigue, restlessness, confusion, disorientation, hallucinations, nightmares, bad dreams.

Special senses: eyes-blurred, burning, light sensitive, swollen, aching, strained; ears "clogged", aching, tinnitus.

General: increased appetite, weight loss, weight gain, yawning, drowsiness, fever, dry mouth, head "pounding", inguinal pain, swollen glands, "side" pains, cold feet, "hot spells."

Laboratory tests: With the exception of liver test abnormalities in investigator studies (See WARNINGS, PRECAUTIONS, etc.), results of laboratory tests, like adverse reaction reports, have not shown consistent patterns of abnormalities that can be attributed to treatment with TREXAN.

In the trials evaluating TREXAN for the blockade of opiate receptors, abnormal liver function tests and lymphocytosis were the two most common categories of abnormalities reported. As noted earlier, these abnormalities are common among populations of parenteral opioid users and alcoholics. As is the case with the untoward events described above, a large proportion of patients had abnormal laboratory tests at baseline, further supporting the conclusion that the abnormalities observed are not attributable to TREXAN.

Continued on next page

DuPont—Cont.

Idiopathic thrombocytopenic purpura was reported in one patient who may have been sensitized to TREXAN in a previous course of treatment with TREXAN. The condition cleared without sequelae after discontinuation of TREXAN and corticosteroid treatment.

DRUG ABUSE AND DEPENDENCE

TREXAN is a pure opioid antagonist. It does not lead to physical or psychological dependence. Tolerance to the opioid antagonist effect is not known to occur.

OVERDOSAGE

There is no clinical experience with TREXAN overdosage in humans. In one study, subjects who received 800 mg daily TREXAN for up to one week showed no evidence of toxicity.
In the mouse, rat and guinea pig, the oral LD_{50}s were 1,100 $\pm$ 96 mg/kg; 1,450 $\pm$ 265 mg/kg; and 1,490 $\pm$ 102 mg/kg, respectively.
In acute toxicity studies in the mouse, rat, and dog, cause of death was due to clonic-tonic convulsions and/or respiratory failure.

TREATMENT OF OVERDOSAGE

Consideration should be given to contacting a poison control center for the most up-to-date information.
In view of the lack of actual experience in the treatment of TREXAN overdose, patients should be treated symptomatically in a closely supervised environment.

DOSAGE AND ADMINISTRATION

Induction of TREXAN Therapy: DO NOT ATTEMPT TREATMENT UNTIL NARCAN CHALLENGE IS NEGATIVE (see below). Initiate treatment with TREXAN using the following guidelines:

1. Treatment should not be attempted until the patient has remained opioid-free for 7–10 days. Self-reporting of abstinence from opioids should be verified by analysis of the patient's urine for absence of opioids. The patient should not be manifesting withdrawal signs or reporting withdrawal symptoms.
2. A NARCAN challenge test (see below) should be administered to the patient. If signs of opioid withdrawal are still observed following NARCAN challenge, treatment with TREXAN should not be attempted. The NARCAN challenge can be repeated in 24 hours.
3. Treatment should be initiated carefully, slowly increasing the dose of TREXAN administered. This can be accomplished by administration of 25 mg of TREXAN initially. The patient should be observed for 1 hour. If no withdrawal signs occur, the patient may be given the rest of the daily dose.

NARCAN Challenge Test: The NARCAN challenge test should *not* be performed in a patient showing clinical signs or symptoms of opioid withdrawal, or in a patient whose urine contains opioids.
The NARCAN challenge test may be administered by either the intravenous or subcutaneous routes.
Intravenous challenge: Following appropriate screening of the patient, 0.8 mg of NARCAN should be drawn into a sterile syringe. If the intravenous route of administration is selected, 0.2 mg of NARCAN should be injected, and while the needle is still in the patient's vein, the patient should be observed for 30 seconds for evidence of withdrawal signs or symptoms. If there is no evidence of withdrawal, the remaining 0.6 mg of NARCAN should be injected, and the patient observed for an additional period of 20 minutes for signs and symptoms of withdrawal.
Subcutaneous challenge: If the subcutaneous route is selected, 0.8 mg should be administered subcutaneously, and the patient observed for signs and symptoms of withdrawal for 45 minutes.
Conditions and technique for observation of patient: During the appropriate period of observation, the patient's vital signs should be monitored and the patient should be monitored for signs of withdrawal. It is also important to question the patient carefully. The signs and symptoms of opioid withdrawal include, but are not limited to, the following:
WITHDRAWAL SIGNS: stuffiness or running nose, tearing, yawning, sweating, tremor, vomiting or piloerection.
WITHDRAWAL SYMPTOMS: feeling of temperature change, joint or bone and muscle pain, abdominal cramps, skin crawling, etc.
Interpretation of the Challenge: Warning: the elicitation of the enumerated signs or symptoms indicates a potential risk for the subject, and TREXAN should not be administered. If no signs or symptoms of withdrawal are observed, elicited, or reported, TREXAN MAY BE ADMINISTERED. If there is any doubt in the observer's mind that the patient is not in an opioid-free state, or is in continuing withdrawal, NARCAN should be readministered as follows:
Confirmatory rechallenge (if necessary): 1.6 mg of NARCAN should be injected intravenously and the patient again observed for signs and symptoms of withdrawal. If none are present, TREXAN may be administered. If signs and symptoms of withdrawal are present, administration of TREXAN should be delayed until repeated NARCAN challenge indicates the patient is no longer at risk.
Maintenance Treatment: Once the patient has been started on TREXAN, 50 mg every 24 hours will produce adequate clinical blockade of the actions of parenterally administered opioids (i.e., this dose will block the effects of a 25 mg intravenous heroin challenge). A flexible approach to a dosing regimen may be employed. Thus, patients may receive 50 mg of TREXAN every weekday with a 100 mg dose on Saturday or patients may receive 100 mg every other day, or 150 mg every third day. While the degree of opioid blockade may be somewhat reduced by using higher doses at longer dosing intervals, improved patient compliance may result from dosing every 48–72 hours.
Several of the clinical studies reported in the literature have employed the following dosing regimen: 100 mg on Monday, 100 mg on Wednesday, and 150 mg on Friday. This dosing schedule appeared to be acceptable to many TREXAN patients successfully maintaining their opioid free state.

HOW SUPPLIED

TREXAN tablets are available in 50 mg round tablets, scored imprinted with DuPont on one side and TREXAN on the other. Bottles of 50 tablets (NDC 0056-0080-50).
Additional medical information may be obtained from Du Pont Pharmaceuticals by calling 1-800-441-9861. In Delaware, call 302-992-3273. For medical emergencies, call 1-212-340-4494 or your Regional Poison Control Center.
NARCAN® is a Registered U.S. Trademark of Du Pont Pharmaceuticals, Inc.
TREXAN™ is a U.S. Trademark of E.I. du Pont de Nemours & Co. (Inc.).

6162-1/Rev. July, 1985

Shown in Product Identification Section, page 409

VALPIN® 50 ℞

[val 'pin]
anisotropine methylbromide 50 mg

DESCRIPTION

VALPIN® 50 is anisotropine methylbromide, a quaternary ammonium salt which differs chemically from atropine and most other anticholinergics in the substitution of an aliphatic for an aromatic side chain in the acid moiety of the ester.
Chemically, VALPIN® 50 is 2-propyl pentanoyl tropinium methylbromide. Its stability both to acid and alkaline hydrolysis minimizes inactivation.
VALPIN 50 Tablets also contain: colloidal silicon dioxide, FD&C Blue 2, FD&C Yellow 6, magnesium stearate, microcrystalline cellulose, starch, stearic acid and sugar.

ACTIONS

VALPIN® 50 inhibits gastric acid secretion and reduces gastrointestinal motility.

INDICATIONS

For use as adjunctive therapy in the treatment of peptic ulcer.
AS WITH ALL ANTICHOLINERGICS, IT SHOULD BE NOTED THAT AT THE PRESENT TIME THERE IS LACK OF CONCURRENCE AS TO THEIR VALUE IN THE TREATMENT OF GASTRIC ULCER. IT HAS NOT BEEN SHOWN CONCLUSIVELY WHETHER ANTICHOLINERGIC DRUGS AID IN THE HEALING OF A PEPTIC ULCER, DECREASE THE RATE OF RECURRENCES OR PREVENT COMPLICATION.

CONTRAINDICATIONS

Glaucoma; obstructive uropathy (for example, bladder neck obstruction due to prostatic hypertrophy); obstructive disease of the gastrointestinal tract (as in achalasia, pyloroduodenal stenosis, etc.); paralytic ileus, intestinal atony of the elderly or debilitated patient; unstable cardiovascular status in acute hemorrhage; severe ulcerative colitis; toxic megacolon complicating ulcerative colitis; myasthenia gravis.

WARNINGS

Use in Pregnancy Since the safety of these preparations in pregnancy, lactation or in women of child-bearing age has not been established, use of the drugs in such patients requires that the potential benefits of the drug be weighed against possible hazards to the mother and child.
In the presence of a high environmental temperature, heat prostration can occur with drug use (fever and heat stroke due to decreased sweating).
Diarrhea may be an early symptom of incomplete intestinal obstruction, especially in patients with ileostomy or colostomy. In this instance treatment with this drug would be inappropriate and possibly harmful.
VALPIN® 50 may produce drowsiness or blurred vision. In this event, the patient should be warned not to engage in activities requiring mental alertness such as operating a motor vehicle or other machinery or perform hazardous work while taking this drug.

PRECAUTIONS

Use with caution in patients with:
- —Autonomic neuropathy.
- —Hepatic or renal disease.
- —Ulcerative colitis—large doses may suppress intestinal motility to the point of producing a paralytic ileus and the use of this drug may precipitate or aggravate the serious complication of toxic megacolon.
- —Hyperthyroidism, coronary heart disease, congestive heart failure, cardiac arrhythmias, hypertension and non-obstructing prostatic hypertrophy.
- —Hiatal hernia associated with reflux esophagitis since anticholinergic drugs may aggravate this condition.

It should be noted that the use of anticholinergic drugs in the treatment of gastric ulcer may produce a delay in gastric emptying time and may complicate such therapy (antral stasis).
Do not rely on the use of the drug in the presence of complication of biliary tract disease.
Investigate any tachycardia before giving anticholinergic (atropine-like) drugs since they may increase the heart rate. With overdosage, a curare-like action may occur.

ADVERSE REACTIONS

Anticholinergic drugs produce certain effects which may be physiologic or toxic depending upon the individual patient's response. The physician must delineate these.
Adverse reactions may include xerostomia; urinary hesitancy and retention; blurred vision and tachycardia; palpitations; mydriasis; cycloplegia; increased ocular tension; loss of taste; headaches; nervousness; drowsiness; weakness; dizziness; insomnia; nausea; vomiting; impotence; suppression of lactation; constipation; bloated feeling; severe allergic reaction or drug idiosyncrasies including anaphylaxis; urticaria and other dermal manifestations; some degree of mental confusion and/or excitement especially in elderly persons.
Decreased sweating is another adverse reaction that may occur.

DOSAGE AND ADMINISTRATION

To be effective dosage must be titrated to individual patient needs. Usual adult dosage—VALPIN® 50 mg tablet; one tablet 3 times daily.

MANAGEMENT OF OVERDOSAGE

While overdosage intoxication with anisotropine methylbromide has not been reported, theoretically it could occur since anisotropine methylbromide is an anticholinergic drug. When anticholinergic drugs are taken in sufficient overdose to produce severe symptoms, prompt treatment should be instituted. If the drug has been taken orally, gastric lavage and other measures to limit intestinal absorption should be initiated without delay. Physostigmine administered parenterally may be necessary for treatment of the serious manifestations of intoxication. Additionally, symptomatic therapy, including oxygen, sedatives, and control of hyperthermia may be necessary.

HOW SUPPLIED

VALPIN® 50: 50 mg anisotropine methylbromide in each scored, beige tablet.
Bottles of 100 tablets NDC 0056-0161-70
Store at controlled room temperature (59°–86°F, 15°–30°C).
Animal Pharmacology and Toxicology: VALPIN® 50 (anisotropine methylbromide) is a relatively non-toxic drug. In dogs, mice, rats and guinea pigs both acute toxic and chronic toxic dose-levels are at many times in excess of the clinically useful range.
Both **in vitro** and oral **in vivo** data in mice and rats indicate that VALPIN® 50 (anisotropine methylbromide) is at least 2 or 3 times as potent as homatropine methylbromide in antispasmodic action while it is less than two-thirds as active in mydriatic effect. It has less than one-fiftieth of the mydriatic activity of atropine sulfate. In inhibition of salivary flow, VALPIN® 50 (anisotropine methylbromide) is one-fifth as active as homatropine methylbromide and only one-hundredth as active as atropine sulfate. This pharmacologic profile is consistent with relative specificity of action on the gastrointestinal smooth muscle and the lesser tendency to produce side effects.
VALPIN® is a registered U.S. trademark of E.I. duPont de Nemours & Co. (Inc.)
6083-9

ZYDONE™ Ⓒ III

[zī"dōn']
Capsules

DESCRIPTION

Each ZYDONE capsule contains:

Acetaminophen	500 mg
Hydrocodone bitartrate*	5 mg

*WARNING: May be habit forming
Acetaminophen is a nonopiate, non-salicylate analgesic and antipyretic which occurs as a white, odorless crystalline pow-

der, possessing a slightly bitter taste. Hydrocodone bitartrate is an opioid analgesic and antitussive and occurs as fine, white crystals or as a crystalline powder. It is affected by light.

CLINICAL PHARMACOLOGY

Hydrocodone is a semisynthetic narcotic analgesic and antitussive with multiple actions qualitatively similar to those of codeine. Most of these involve the central nervous system and smooth muscle. The precise mechanism of action of hydrocodone and other opiates is not known, although it is believed to relate to the existence of opiate receptors in the central nervous system. In addition to analgesia, narcotics may produce drowsiness, changes in mood and mental clouding. Radioimmunoassay techniques have recently been developed for the analysis of hydrocodone in human plasma. After a 10 mg oral dose of hydrocodone bitartrate, a mean peak serum drug level of 23.6 ng/ml and an elimination half-life of 3.8 hours were found. The analgesic action of acetaminophen involves peripheral and central influences, but the specific mechanism is as yet undetermined. Antipyretic activity is mediated through hypothalamic heat regulating centers. Acetaminophen inhibits prostaglandin synthetase. Therapeutic doses of acetaminophen have negligible effects on the cardiovascular or respiratory systems; however, toxic doses may cause circulatory failure and rapid, shallow breathing. Acetaminophen is rapidly and almost completely absorbed from the gastrointestinal tract, producing maximum serum concentrations within 30 minutes to one hour. The plasma half-life in adults and children ranges from 0.90 hours to 3.25 hours with an average of approximately 2 hours. The drug distributes uniformly in most body fluids and is approximately 25% protein bound. Acetaminophen is conjugated in the liver, with less than 3% of the dose excreted unchanged in 24 hours. The primary metabolic pathway is conjugation to sulfate and glucuronide by-products. A minor oxidative pathway forms cysteine and mercapturic acid. These compounds are subsequently excreted by the kidneys into the urine.

INDICATIONS AND USAGE

For the relief of moderate to moderately severe pain.

CONTRAINDICATIONS

Hypersensitivity to acetaminophen or hydrocodone.

WARNINGS

Respiratory Depression: At high doses or in sensitive patients, hydrocodone may produce dose-related respiratory depression by acting directly on brain stem respiratory centers. Hydrocodone also affects centers that control respiratory rhythm, and may produce irregular and periodic breathing.

Head Injury and Increased Intracranial Pressure: The respiratory depressant effects of narcotics and their capacity to elevate cerebrospinal fluid pressure may be markedly exaggerated in the presence of head injury, other intracranial lesions or a preexisting increase in intracranial pressure. Furthermore, narcotics produce adverse reactions which may obscure the clinical course of patients with head injuries.

Acute Abdominal Conditions: The administration of narcotics may obscure the diagnosis or clinical course of patients with acute abdominal conditions.

PRECAUTIONS

Special Risk Patients: As with any narcotic analgesic agent, ZYDONE Capsules should be used with caution in elderly or debilitated patients and those with severe impairment of hepatic or renal function, hypothyroidism, Addison's disease, prostatic hypertrophy or urethral stricture. The usual precautions should be observed and the possibility of respiratory depression should be kept in mind.

Information for Patients: ZYDONE Capsules, like all narcotics, may impair the mental and/or physical abilities required for the performance of potentially hazardous tasks such as driving a car or operating machinery; patients should be cautioned accordingly.

Cough Reflex: Hydrocodone suppresses the cough reflex; as with all narcotics, caution should be exercised when ZYDONE Capsules are used postoperatively and in patients with pulmonary disease.

Drug Interactions: Patients receiving other narcotic analgesics, antipsychotics, antianxiety agents, or other CNS depressants (including alcohol) concomitantly with ZYDONE Capsules may exhibit an additive CNS depression. When combined therapy is contemplated, the dose of one or both agents should be reduced.

The use of MAO inhibitors or tricyclic antidepressants with hydrocodone preparations may increase the effect of either the antidepressant or hydrocodone.

The concurrent use of anticholinergics with hydrocodone may produce paralytic ileus.

Usage in Pregnancy: Pregnancy Category C. Hydrocodone has been shown to be teratogenic in hamsters when given in doses 700 times the human dose. There are no adequate and well-controlled studies in pregnant women. ZYDONE Capsules should be used during pregnancy only if the potential benefit justifies the potential risk to the fetus.

Nonteratogenic Effects: Babies born to mothers who have been taking opioids regularly prior to delivery will be physically dependent. The withdrawal signs include irritability and excessive crying, tremors, hyperactive reflexes, increased respiratory rate, increased stools, sneezing, yawning, vomiting, and fever. The intensity of the syndrome does not always correlate with the duration of maternal opioid use or dose. There is no consensus on the best method of managing withdrawal. Chlorpromazine 0.7 to 1.0 mg/kg q6h, and paregoric 2 to 4 drops/kg q4h, have been used to treat withdrawal symptoms in infants. The duration of therapy is 4 to 28 days, with the dosage decreased as tolerated.

Labor and Delivery: As with all narcotics, administration of ZYDONE Capsules to the mother shortly before delivery may result in some degree of respiratory depression in the newborn, especially if higher doses are used.

Nursing Mothers: It is not known whether this drug is excreted in human milk. Because many drugs are excreted in human milk and because of the potential for serious adverse reactions in nursing infants from ZYDONE Capsules, a decision should be made whether to discontinue nursing or to discontinue the drug, taking into account the importance of the drug to the mother.

Pediatric Use: Safety and effectiveness in children have not been established.

ADVERSE REACTIONS

Central Nervous System: Sedation, drowsiness, mental clouding, lethargy, impairment of mental and physical performance, anxiety, fear, dysphoria, dizziness, psychic dependence, mood changes.

Gastrointestinal System: Nausea and vomiting may occur; they are more frequent in ambulatory than in recumbent patients. The antiemetic phenothiazines are useful in suppressing these effects; however, some phenothiazine derivatives seem to be antianalgesic and to increase the amount of narcotic required to produce pain relief, while other phenothiazines reduce the amount of narcotic required to produce a given level of analgesia. Prolonged administration of ZYDONE Capsules may produce constipation.

Genitourinary System: Ureteral spasm, spasm of vesical sphincters and urinary retention have been reported.

Respiratory Depression: ZYDONE Capsules may produce dose-related respiratory depression by acting directly on brain stem respiratory centers. Hydrocodone also affects centers that control respiratory rhythm, and may produce irregular and periodic breathing. If significant respiratory depression occurs, it may be antagonized by the use of naloxone hydrochloride. Apply other supportive measures when indicated.

DRUG ABUSE AND DEPENDENCE

ZYDONE Capsules are subject to the Federal Controlled Substance Act (Schedule III). Psychic dependence, physical dependence, and tolerance may develop upon repeated administration of narcotics; therefore, ZYDONE Capsules should be prescribed and administered with caution. However, psychic dependence is unlikely to develop when ZYDONE Capsules are used for a short time for the treatment of pain.

Physical dependence, the condition in which continued administration of the drug is required to prevent the appearance of a withdrawal syndrome, assumes clinically significant proportions only after several weeks of continued narcotic use, although some mild degree of physical dependence may develop after a few days of narcotic therapy. Tolerance, in which increasingly large doses are required in order to produce the same degree of analgesia, is manifested initially by a shortened duration of analgesic effect, and subsequently by decreases in the intensity of analgesia. The rate of development of tolerance varies among patients.

OVERDOSAGE

Acetaminophen

Signs and Symptoms: Acetaminophen in massive overdosage may cause hepatic toxicity in some patients. In cases of suspected overdosage, you may wish to call your regional poison center for assistance in diagnosis and for directions in the use of N-acetylcysteine as an antidote. In adults, hepatic toxicity has rarely been reported with acute overdoses of less than 10 grams and fatalities with less than 15 grams. Importantly, young children seem to be more resistant than adults to the hepatotoxic effect of an acetaminophen overdose. Despite this, the measures outlined below should be initiated in any adult or child suspected of having ingested an acetaminophen overdose.

Early symptoms following a potentially hepatotoxic overdose may include: nausea, vomiting, diaphoresis and general malaise. Clinical and laboratory evidence of hepatic toxicity may not be apparent until 48 to 72 hours postingestion.

Treatment: The stomach should be emptied promptly by lavage or by induction of emesis with syrup of ipecac. Patients' estimates of the quantity of a drug ingested are notoriously unreliable. Therefore, if an acetaminophen overdose is suspected, a serum acetaminophen assay should be obtained as early as possible, but no sooner than four hours following ingestion. Liver function studies should be obtained initially and repeated at 24-hour intervals. The antidote, N-acetylcysteine, should be administered as early as possible, preferably within 16 hours of the overdose ingestion for optimal results, but in any case, within 24 hours. Following recovery, there are no residual, structural or functional hepatic abnormalities.

Hydrocodone

Signs and Symptoms: Serious overdose with hydrocodone is characterized by respiratory depression (a decrease in respiratory rate and/or tidal volume, Cheyne-Stokes respiration, cyanosis), extreme somnolence progressing to stupor or coma, skeletal muscle flaccidity, cold and clammy skin, and sometimes bradycardia and hypotension. In severe overdosage, apnea, circulatory collapse, cardiac arrest and death may occur.

Treatment: Primary attention should be given to the reestablishment of adequate respiratory exchange through provision of a patent airway and the institution of assisted or controlled ventilation. The narcotic antagonist naloxone is a specific antidote against respiratory depression which may result from overdosage or unusual sensitivity to narcotics, including hydrocodone. Therefore, an appropriate dose of naloxone (see package insert) should be administered, preferably by the intravenous route, and simultaneously with efforts at respiratory resuscitation. Since the duration of action of hydrocodone may exceed that of the antagonist, the patient should be kept under continued surveillance and repeated doses of the antagonist should be administered as needed to maintain adequate respiration. An antagonist should not be administered in the absence of clinically significant respiratory or cardiovascular depression. Oxygen, intravenous fluids, vasopressors and other supportive measures should be employed as indicated. Gastric emptying may be useful in removing unabsorbed drug.

DOSAGE AND ADMINISTRATION

Dosage should be adjusted according to the severity of the pain and the response of the patient. However, it should be kept in mind that tolerance to hydrocodone can develop with continued use and that the incidence of untoward effects is dose related.

The usual dose is one capsule every six hours as needed for pain. If necessary, this dose may be repeated at four-hour intervals. In cases of more severe pain, two capsules every six hours (up to 8 capsules in 24 hours) may be required.

HOW SUPPLIED

White hard gelatin capsule with red band. Capsule is imprinted in red, DU PONT ZYDONE. Bottles of 100: NDC 0056-0091-70

CAUTION

Federal law prohibits dispensing without prescription.

STORAGE

Store at controlled room temperature 59°–86°F, 15°–30°C.

Manufactured by
D.M. Graham Laboratories, Inc., Hobart, New York 13788
for
DuPont Pharmaceuticals
E.I. duPont de Nemours & Co. (Inc.)
Wilmington, Delaware 19898

ZYDONE™ is a U.S. Trademark of E.I. duPont de Nemours & Co. (Inc.)

6173/Jan. 1986

Shown in Product Identification Section, page 409

EDUCATIONAL MATERIAL

COUMADIN ®

Books/Booklets/Brochures

"COUMADIN Patient Aid." This patient aid kit is designed to increase patient compliance and understanding of COUMADIN therapy. The kit includes an easy-to-understand patient guide, a dosing calendar, and a wallet card. No charge to physicians, pharmacists, patients, and others involved with the management of patients on COUMADIN.

Guide to Anticoagulant Therapy Series

"Guide to Anticoagulant Therapy #1: Management of Heparin & Warfarin" by Joseph S. Alpert, MD, and J. Dennis Mull, MD. Includes guidelines on initiation of heparin, conversion to warfarin, warfarin maintenance, potential complications, and case histories.

"Guide to Anticoagulant Therapy #2: Counseling and Follow-up" by Joseph A. Alpert, MD, and J. Dennis Mull, MD. Comprehensive guide to managing patients on anticoagulant therapy.

"Guide to Antithrombotic Therapy #3: Anticoagulant and Antiplatelet Drugs" by James E. Dalen, MD. Discusses the appropriate uses of and differences between

Continued on next page

DuPont—Cont.

anticoagulant and antiplatelet drugs. The Guide to Anticoagulant series is available to physicians, pharmacists, and other healthcare professionals at no charge.

Films/Slides/Video

"Pulmonary Embolism Film Series." This three-part series on the diagnosis, treatment, and prevention of pulmonary embolism is available for loan to physicians, pharmacists, and other healthcare professionals in 3/4" videotape or 16mm film.

"Helping Yourself... The Control of Blood Clotting." A patient education film designed to increase the comfort level of the new patient on COUMADIN is available for loan to physicians, pharmacists, and other healthcare professionals in 3/4" videotape or 16mm film.

Pictures/Charts

"COUMADIN Drug Interaction Chart." A 8½" × 11" chart highlighting the drugs which can increase or decrease the effects of COUMADIN is available at no charge to physicians, pharmacists, and other healthcare professionals.

"COUMADIN Conversion Chart." This 8½" × 11" flow chart demonstrates visually how to convert patients from heparin to COUMADIN therapy. No charge to physicians, pharmacists, and other healthcare professionals.

"COUMADIN Patient Anticoagulant Record Charts." These packs of 8½" × 11" charts provide a convenient way to record patient prothrombin times and COUMADIN doses. Available at no charge to physicians, pharmacists, and other healthcare professionals involved with the management of patients on COUMADIN therapy.

Samples for HYCODAN® (hydrocodone bitartrate), HYCOMINE®, HYCOTUSS®:

Samples are available through your local Du Pont Pharmaceuticals Representative or by writing Du Pont Pharmaceuticals, E. I. du Pont de Nemours & Co. (Inc.), Wilmington, DE 19898.

MOBAN®

Samples of MOBAN (molindone HCl) are available in 10 mg, 25 mg and 50 mg dosage forms. Please contact your local Du Pont Pharmaceuticals representative or write Du Pont Pharmaceuticals, E. I. du Pont de Nemours & Co. (Inc.), Wilmington, DE 19898.

PERCODAN®/PERCOCET®

Books/Booklets

"Mediguide to Pain." Booklet includes original articles and literature summaries on pain research and management. No charge publication. Write Du Pont Pharmaceuticals.

Films/Videos (Permission to duplicate, at users expense, for educational purposes may be granted in response to written request to Du Pont Pharmaceuticals.)

Pain Update #1
"Practical Concepts on the Management of Pain"
Provides practicing physicians with information on advances in neuroscience and management strategies for common pain problems. Features medical experts from University of Washington School of Medicine. 16mm film; 3/4 in. videotape. 15 min.

Pain Update #2
"Treating Acute Pain Effectively"
Describes basic principles of treating acute pain to reduce risk of chronicity. Features medical experts from University of Washington School of Medicine. 16 mm film; 3/4 in. videotape. 15 min.

Pain Update #3
"Postoperative Pain Management—A discussion with John Bonica"
Presents physiology of postoperative pain and current treatment strategies. Features leading expert of pain management at the University of Washington School of Medicine. 16 mm film; 3/4 in. videotape. 15 min.

Pain Update #4
"Individualizing Cancer Pain Management"
Explains why an individualized approach is essential for effective cancer pain management. Features medical experts explaining their techniques to physicians at Baltimore County General Hospital. 16mm film; 3/4 in. videotape. 15 min.

SYMMETREL®

Two films on Parkinson's disease, produced by Du Pont, are available by contacting the United Parkinson Foundation, 360 W. Superior St., Chicago, IL 60610. (312) 664-2344.

#1 "Moment-to-Moment: Living with Parkinson's." This award winning program is intended for viewing by both heatlhcare professionals and patients. It follows two patients with PD as they describe how they have coped with the special challenge of this disorder. Time: 25 min.

#2 "Heart of the Matter." Intended for viewing by healthcare professionals, primarily nurses, this program features Stanley Fahn, M.D., and Susan Bowar-Ferres, RN, MS, as they discuss care of PD patients with student nurses. Time: 25 min.

#3 "Drug-Induced Extrapyramidal Movement Disorders." Available at no charge directly from Du Pont, this program features Richard L. Borison, M.D., Ph.D., discussing diagnosis, neurochemical causes and pharmacologic control. Time: 20 min

Samples for SYMMETREL® (amantadine HCl):

Samples are available through your local Du Pont Pharmaceuticals Representative or by writing Du Pont Pharmaceuticals, E. I. du Pont de Nemours & Co. (Inc.), Wilmington, DE 19898

Samples for TESSALON® (benzonatate NF):

Samples are available through your local Du Pont Pharmaceuticals Representative or by writing Du Pont Pharmaceuticals, E. I. du Pont de Nemours & Co. (Inc.), Wilmington, DE 19898

TREXAN™ (naltrexone HCl)

Books/Booklets

"TREXAN™ in Opioid Addiction." Forward by Charles P. O'Brien, M.D., Ph.D. A comprehensive Monograph. No Charge. 1985. 56 pages.

"TREXAN™: A Pharmacologic Adjunct for the Detoxified Opioid Addict." Herbert D. Kleber, M.D. Yale University. No Charge. 1984. 16 pages.

"TREXAN™ in Outpatient Practice: Representative Protocol." Adapted from H. M. Ginzburg, M.D., MPH. NIDA Treatment Research Report. No Charge. 1984. 2 pages.

"TREXAN™: Information for the Criminal Justice and Corrections Professional." No Charge. 1985. 11 pages.

Films/Videos

Films (available on loan with permission to copy)

"Expanding Your Treatment Options." Interview with Susan F. Neshin, M.D., and Cynthia W. Clark, R.N., discussing use of TREXAN™ from the counselor's perspective. 30 min.

"TREXAN™: A New Approach to the Management of Opioid Dependence." Satellite Teleconference with Charles P. O'Brien, M.D., Ph.D., Forest Tennant, Jr., M.D., and Cynthia W. Clark, R.N. 30 min.

"TREXAN™: The Road to Recovery." Three patients treated with TREXAN™ discuss their experience with the therapy. Excellent viewing for prospective patients. 54 min.

Patient Materials

Patient-Family Guide. "TREXAN™, An Aid for the Recovering Narcotic-Addict." No Charge.
Medical Alert Card. No Charge.

ZYDONE™

Books/Booklets

"Mediguide to Pain." Booklet includes original articles and literature summaries on pain research and management. No charge publication. Write Du Pont Pharmaceuticals.

Films/Videos (Permission to duplicate, at users expense, for educational purposes may be granted in response to written request to Du Pont Pharmaceuticals.)

Pain Update #1
"Practical Concepts on the Management of Pain"
Provides practicing physicians with information on advances in neuroscience and management strategies for common pain problems. Features medical experts from University of Washington School of Medicine. 16mm film; 3/4 in. videotape. 15 min.

Pain Update #2
"Treating Acute Pain Effectively"
Describes basic principles of treating acute pain to reduce risk of chronicity. Features medical experts from University of Washington School of Medicine. 16mm film; 3/4 in. videotape. 15 min.

Pain Update #3
"Postoperative Pain Management—A Discussion with John Bonica"
Presents physiology of postoperative pain and current treatment strategies. Features leading expert of pain management at the University of Washington School of Medicine. 16mm film; 3/4 in. videotape. 15 min.

Pain Update #4
"Individualizing Cancer Pain Management"
Explains why an individualized approach is essential for effective cancer pain management. Features medical experts explaining their techniques to physicians at Baltimore County General Hospital. 16mm film; 3/4 in. videotape. 15 min.

Products are cross-indexed by generic and chemical names in the **YELLOW SECTION**

Dura Pharmaceuticals, Inc.

P.O. BOX 28331
SAN DIEGO, CA 92128

DURA-GEST™

DESCRIPTION

Each Dura-Gest gray and white capsule for oral administration contains:

phenylephrine hydrochloride	5 mg.
phenylpropanolamine hydrochloride	45 mg.
guaifenesin	200 mg.

HOW SUPPLIED

DURA-GEST gray and white capsules are imprinted with DURA-GEST and 51479005.
NDC 51479-005-01 Bottle of 100
NDC 51479-005-05 Bottle of 500
Dispense in tight containers as defined in USP/NF.
Store between 15°-30°C (59°-86°F).
Dispense in child resistant containers.

DURA-TAP/PD™ CAPSULES ℞

DESCRIPTION

Each timed release capsule contains:

Brompheniramine Maleate	6 mg.
Phenylephrine Hydrochloride	10 mg.
Phenylpropanolamine Hydrochloride	10 mg.

in specially prepared base to provide prolonged action.

HOW SUPPLIED

Dura-Tap/PD™ capsules are supplied in bottles of 100. NDC 51479-004-01. Dispense in tight, light resistant container. Store between (59°-86°F).

DURA-VENT™ CAPSULES ℞

DESCRIPTION

Each continuous release blue and clear capsule imprinted "Dura-Vent™" contains:

Phenylpropanolamine Hydrochloride	75 mg
Guaifenesin (immediate release)	400 mg

in a special base to provide a prolonged therapeutic effect.

HOW SUPPLIED

Dura-Vent™ capsules are supplied in bottles of 100. NDC 51479-001-01. Dispense in tight, light resistant container. Store between (59°-86°F).

DURA-VENT™/A CAPSULES ℞

DESCRIPTION

Each continuous release clear capsule imprinted "Dura-Vent™/A" contains:

Phenylpropanolamine Hydrochloride	75 mg.
Chlorpheniramine Maleate	10 mg.

in a specially prepared base to provide prolonged action.

HOW SUPPLIED

Dura-Vent™/A capsules are supplied in bottles of 100. NDC 51479-002-01. Dispense in tight, light resistant container. Store between (59°-86°F).

DURA-VENT™/DA CAPSULES ℞

DESCRIPTION

Each brown and clear capsule contains:

Chlorpheniramine Maleate	8 mg.
Phenylephrine Hydrochloride	20 mg.
Methscopolamine Nitrate	2.5 mg.

in a specially prepared base to provide prolonged action.

HOW SUPPLIED

Dura-Vent™/DA capsules are supplied in bottles of 100. NDC 51479-003-01. Dispense in tight light resistant container. Store between (59°-86°F).

Products are listed alphabetically in the **PINK SECTION.**

Eaton Laboratories
See NORWICH EATON PHARMACEUTICALS, INC.

Edwards Pharmacal, Inc.
100 EAST HALE
OSCEOLA, AR 72370-9990

BLANEX® Capsules ℞

DESCRIPTION
Each capsule contains:
Chlorzoxazone .... 250 mg.
Acetaminophen .... 300 mg.

HOW SUPPLIED
Capsules in bottles of 100 (NDC 0485-0031-01). Dispense in tight, light-resistant container.

PRODUCT IDENTIFICATION MARK
Both ends of red capsule imprinted "Blanex" in white.

C-SPAN® Capsules OTC

Each capsule contains:
Ascorbic Acid .... 500 mg.
(In special timed-release base)

PRODUCT IDENTIFICATION MARK
Each end of the orange and clear capsule is imprinted "C-Span" in black.

DOXY-CAPS ℞

DESCRIPTION
Each light blue Doxy-Cap capsule contains:
Doxycycline Hyclate .... 100 mg.

HOW SUPPLIED
Doxy-Caps are supplied in bottles of 50's (NDC #0485-0041-50).

ECEE PLUS Tablets OTC

Each tablet contains:
Vitamin E .... 200 I.U.
(d-alpha tolopheryl and succinate .... 165 mg.
Ascorbic Acid .... 100 mg.
Magnesium sulfate .... 70 mg.
(as 50 mg. of dried magnesium sulfate)
Zinc Sulfate .... 80 mg.
(as 50 mg. of dried zinc sulfate)

HOW SUPPLIED
Each orange, film-coated capsule-shaped tablet is bottled in 100's. (NDC-0485-0023-01).

E.P. MYCIN Capsules ℞

DESCRIPTION
Each yellow E.P. Mycin capsule contains:
Oxytetracycline Hydrochloride .... 250 mg.

HOW SUPPLIED
E.P. Mycin Capsules are supplied in bottles of 100's (NDC #0485-0036-01).

PRODUCT IDENTIFICATION MARK
Each yellow E.P. Mycin capsule is imprinted R-278 in black.

E-TAPP Elixir ℞

DESCRIPTION
Each 5 ml. of grape flavored E-Tapp Elixir contains:
Brompheniramine Maleate .... 4 mg.
Phenylephrine HCL .... 5 mg.
Phenylpropanolamine HCL .... 5 mg.
Alcohol 2.3%

HOW SUPPLIED
Pints (NDC 0485-0048-16).

HYDROGESIC Capsules Ⓒ℞

DESCRIPTION
Each capsule contains:
Hydrocodone Bitartrate .... 5 mg.
(may be habit forming)
Acetaminophen .... 500 mg.

HOW SUPPLIED
Hydrogesic Capsules are supplied in bottles of 100's (NDC-0485-0050-01).

NICO-VERT® Capsules ℞

DESCRIPTION
Each capsule contains:
Dimenhydrinate .... 50 mg.

HOW SUPPLIED
Bottles of 100 orange and black imprinted capsules (NDC 0485-0047-01). Dispense in tight, light-resistant container.

PRODUCT IDENTIFICATION MARK
Each half of the orange and black capsule is imprinted "Nico-Vert" in white.

RYMED® Capsules

DESCRIPTION
Each maroon and white capsule contains:
Pseudophedrine HCL .... 30 mg.
Guaifenesin .... 250 mg.

HOW SUPPLIED
Each maroon and white capsule supplied in bottles of 100 capsules. Keep in tight, light-resistant container. (NDC 0485-0043-01).

PRODUCT IDENTIFICATION MARK
One half imprinted "Rymed" in black, one half imprinted with Edwards logo.

RYMED®-JR. Capsules ℞

DESCRIPTION
Each capsule contains:
Guaifenesin .... 100 mg.
Phenylpropanolamine HCL .... 22.5 mg.
Phenylephrine HCL .... 2.5 mg.

HOW SUPPLIED
Bottles of 100 (NDC 0485-0030-01).

PRODUCT IDENTIFICATION MARK
Each orange capsule is imprinted "Rymed-Jr" on both sides.

RYMED® Liquid ℞

DESCRIPTION
Each 5 cc contains:
Guaifenesin .... 250 mg.
Pseudoephedrine HCL .... 30 mg.
Alcohol 5%

HOW SUPPLIED
Rymed Liquid is supplied in pints (NDC 0485-0044-16).

RYMED®-TR Tablets ℞

DESCRIPTION
Each tablet contains:
Guaifenesin .... 400 mg
Pseudoephedrine HCL .... 75 mg.

HOW SUPPLIED
Rymed TR Tablets are supplied in bottles of 100's (NDC-0485-0045-01).

SENILEZOL Elixir ℞

DESCRIPTION
Each 30cc (2 tablespoonfuls) of elixir contain:
Thiamine Hydrochloride (B_1) .... 2.50 mg.
Riboflavin (B_2) .... 2.50 mg.
Dexpanthenol .... 5.00 mg.
Niacin .... 10.0 mg.
Cyanocobalamin (B_{12}) .... 5.0 mcg.
Pyridoxine Hydrochloride (B_6) .... 1.0 mg.
Ferric Pyrophosphate .... 20.0 mg.
Alcohol 15.0%

HOW SUPPLIED
Senilezol Elixir is supplied in bottles of 1 pint (473 ml.), NDC 0485-0038-01.

SLYN-LL® Capsules Ⓒ℞

DESCRIPTION
Each capsule contains:
Phendimetrazine Tartrate .... 105 mg.

HOW SUPPLIED
Slyn-LL is a brown and clear capsule supplied in bottles of 100 (NDC 0485-0033-01).

PRODUCT IDENTIFICATION MARK
Each brown & clear Slyn-LL capsule is imprinted "RPC" in black.

UROGESIC® Tablets ℞

DESCRIPTION
Each tablet contains:
Phenazopyridine HCl .... 100 mg.

HOW SUPPLIED
UROGESIC, a red, sugar-coated tablet is packaged in bottles of 100 (NDC 0485-0046-01).

Elder Pharmaceuticals Inc.
A subsidiary of the ICN Pharmaceuticals, Inc. Group
ICN PLAZA
3300 HYLAND AVENUE
COSTA MESA, CA 92626

BENOQUIN® ℞
[ben'ō-kwin]
(Monobenzone USP 20% Cream)

Federal (U.S.A.) law prohibits dispensing without prescription.

DESCRIPTION
Each gram of Benoquin Cream contains 200 mg of monobenzone, USP, in a water-washable base consisting of purified water, cetyl alcohol, propylene glycol, sodium lauryl sulfate and beeswax.

CLINICAL PHARMACOLOGY
The mechanism of action of Benoquin is not fully understood. Denton et al.[1] suggested that Benoquin may be converted to hydroquinone, which they found to inhibit the enzymatic oxidation of tyrosine to DOPA.
Iijima and Watanabe[2] suggested a direct action on tyrosinase.
Another suggestion by Denton and his group was that Benoquin acts as an anti-oxidant to prevent SH-group oxidation so that more SH groups are available to inhibit tyrosinase.
The primary role of inflammation in the depigmentation process was studied by Becker and Spencer[3] who suggested that increased cell permeability allows Benoquin to enter the melanocyte to form an antigenic substance which attached to the melanin granule enters the dermis where antibodies are produced, remote positive patch-testing may result.

INDICATIONS AND USAGE
Benoquin Cream is indicated for final depigmentation in extensive vitiligo.
Benoquin Cream is not recommended for freckling, hyperpigmentation due to photosensitization following use of certain perfumes (berlock dermatitis), melasma (chloasma) of pregnancy, and hyperpigmentation following inflammation of the skin. Benoquin Cream is of no value in the treatment of cafe-au-lait spots, pigmented nevi, malignant melanoma, or pigment resulting from pigments other than melanin, including bile, silver, and artificial pigments.

CONTRAINDICATIONS
Prior history of sensitivity or allergic reaction to this product or any of its ingredients. The safety of topical monobenzone use during pregnancy or in children (12 years and under) has not been established.

WARNINGS
A. Benoquin Cream is a potent depigmenting agent, not a mild cosmetic bleach. Do not use except for final depigmentation in extensive vitiligo.
B. Keep this and all medication out of the reach of children. In case of accidental ingestion, call a physician or a poison control center immediately.

PRECAUTIONS
See Warnings.
A. Pregnancy Category C. Animal reproduction studies have not been conducted with topical monobenzone. It is also not known whether monobenzone can cause fetal

Continued on next page

Elder—Cont.

harm when used topically on a pregnant woman or affect reproductive capacity. It is not known to what degree, if any, topical monobenzone is absorbed systemically. Topical monobenzone should be used in pregnant women only when clearly indicated.

B. Nursing mothers. It is not known whether topical monobenzone is absorbed or excreted in human milk. Caution is advised when topical monobenzone is used by a nursing mother.

C. Pediatric usage. Safety and effectiveness in children below the age of 12 years have not been established.

ADVERSE REACTIONS

Occasional irritation, a burning sensation, or dermatitis may occur in which case medication should be discontinued and the physician notified immediately.

DOSAGE AND ADMINISTRATION

Benoquin should be applied to the pigmented area and rubbed in well two or three times daily or as directed by physician. There is no recommended dosage for children under 12 years of age except under the advice and supervision of a physician.

NOTE

Depigmentation is usually observed after one to four months of therapy. If satisfactory results have not been obtained within four months, treatment should be discontinued.

HOW SUPPLIED

BENOQUIN Cream, 20% in 1¼ oz. tubes (NDC 0163-0380-34).

BENOQUIN Cream should be stored at room temperature (15-30°C) (59-86°F)

ELDOPAQUE Forte® 4% Cream ℞

[él-do-pāk" for'tā]

(Hydroquinone USP, 4%)

Skin Bleaching Cream With SunBlock

CAUTION: FEDERAL LAW (U.S.A.) PROHIBITS DISPENSING WITHOUT A PRESCRIPTION.

FOR EXTERNAL USE ONLY

DESCRIPTION

Each gram of Eldopaque Forte 4% Cream contains 40 mg of hydroquinone in a tinted sunblocking base of water, stearic acid, talc, PEG-40 stearate, PEG-25 propylene glycol stearate, propylene glycol, glyceryl stearate, iron oxides, mineral oil, squalane, disodium EDTA, sodium metabisulfite, and potassium sorbate.

CLINICAL PHARMACOLOGY

Topical application of hydroquinone produces a reversible depigmentation of the skin by inhibition of the enzymatic oxidation of tyrosine to 3, 4-dihydroxyphenylalanine (dopa) and suppression of other melanocyte metabolic processes. Exposure to sunlight or ultraviolet light will cause repigmentation which may be prevented by the sunblocking agents contained in Eldopaque Forte.

INDICATIONS AND USAGE

Eldopaque Forte 4% Cream is indicated for the gradual bleaching of hyperpigmented skin conditions such as chloasma, melasma, freckles, senile lentigines, and other unwanted areas of melanin hyperpigmentation.

CONTRAINDICATIONS

Prior history of sensitivity or allergic reaction to this product or any of its ingredients. The safety of topical hydroquinone use during pregnancy or in children (12 years and under) has not been established.

WARNINGS

A. CAUTION: Hydroquinone is a skin bleaching agent which may produce unwanted cosmetic effects if not used as directed. The physician should be familiar with the contents of this insert before prescribing or dispensing this medication.

B. Test for skin sensitivity before using Eldopaque Forte 4% Cream by applying a small amount to an unbroken patch of skin and check in 24 hours. Minor redness is not a contraindication, but where there is itching or vesicle formation or excessive inflammatory response, further treatment is not advised. Close patient supervision is recommended.

Contact with the eyes should be avoided. If no bleaching or lightening effect is noted after 2 months of treatment use, Eldopaque Forte 4% Cream should be discontinued. Eldopaque Forte 4% Cream is formulated for use as a skin bleaching agent and should not be used for the prevention of sunburn.

C. Sunscreen use is an essential aspect of hydroquinone therapy because even minimal sunlight exposure sustains melanocytic activity. The sunscreens in Eldopaque Forte 4% Cream provide the necessary sun protection during skin bleaching therapy. After clearing and during maintenance therapy, sun exposure should be avoided on bleached skin by application of a sunscreen or sunblock agent, or protective clothing to prevent repigmentation.

D. Keep this and all medications out of the reach of children. In case of accidental ingestion, call a physician or a poison control center immediately.

PRECAUTIONS

SEE WARNINGS.

A. Pregnancy Category C. Animal reproduction studies have not been conducted with topical hydroquinone. It is also not known whether hydroquinone can cause fetal harm when used topically on a pregnant woman or affect reproductive capacity. It is not known to what degree, if any, topical hydroquinone is absorbed systemically. Topical hydroquinone should be used in women only when clearly indicated.

B. Nursing mothers. It is not known whether topical hydroquinone is absorbed or excreted in human milk. Caution is advised when topical hydroquinone is used by a nursing mother.

C. Pediatric usage. Safety and effectiveness in children below the age of 12 years have not been established.

ADVERSE REACTIONS

No systemic adverse reactions have been reported. Occasional hypersensitivity (localized contact dermatitis) may occur in which case the medication should be discontinued and the physician notified immediately.

OVERDOSAGE

There have been no systemic reactions from the use of topical hydroquinone or the sunblockers in Eldopaque Forte 4% Cream. However, treatment should be limited to relatively small areas of the body at one time since some patients experience a transient skin reddening and a mild burning sensation which does not preclude treatment.

DRUG DOSAGE AND ADMINISTRATION

A thin application of Eldopaque Forte 4% Cream should be applied to the affected area twice daily or as directed by a physician. Do not rub in. There is no recommendation for children under 12 years of age except under the advice and supervision of a physician.

HOW SUPPLIED

Eldopaque Forte 4% Cream is available as follows:

Size	NDC Number
0.5 ounce tube (15 grams)	0163-0395-35
1.0 ounce tube (30 grams)	0163-0395-31

Available without prescription for maintenance therapy: Eldopaque® (2% Hydroquinone) in ½ ounce (NDC 0163-0518-35) and 1 ounce (NDC 0163-0518-31) tubes.

Eldopaque Forte 4% Cream should be stored at room temperature (15-30°C) (59-86°F).

ELDOQUIN Forte® 4% Cream ℞

[el'-dō-kwin" for'tā]

(Hydroquinone USP, 4%)

Skin Bleaching Cream

CAUTION: FEDERAL LAW (U.S.A.) PROHIBITS DISPENSING WITHOUT A PRESCRIPTION.

FOR EXTERNAL USE ONLY

DESCRIPTION

Each gram of Eldoquin Forte contains 40 mg of hydroquinone in a vanishing cream base of purified water, stearic acid, propylene glycol, poloxyl 40 stearate, propylene glycol monostearate, glyceryl monostearate, mineral oil, squalane, propylparaben and sodium metabisulfite.

CLINICAL PHARMACOLOGY

Topical application of hydroquinone produces a reversible depigmentation of the skin by inhibition of the enzymatic oxidation of tyrosine to 3, 4-dihydroxyphenylalanine (dopa) and suppression of the other melanocyte metabolic processes. Exposure to sunlight or ultraviolet light will cause repigmentation of the bleached areas.

INDICATIONS AND USAGE

Eldoquin Forte 4% Cream is indicated for the gradual bleaching of hyperpigmented skin conditions such as chloasma, melasma, freckles, senile lentigines, and other unwanted areas of melanin hyperpigmentation. It is intended for night-time use only since it contains no sunblocking agents. For daytime usage, Solaquin Forte™ 4% Cream or Eldopaque Forte® 4% Cream should be prescribed.

CONTRAINDICATIONS

Prior history of sensitivity or allergic reaction to this product or any of its ingredients. The safety of topical hydroquinone use during pregnancy or in children (12 years and under) has not been established.

WARNINGS

A. CAUTION: Hydroquinone is a skin bleaching agent which may produce unwanted cosmetic effects if not used as directed. The physician should be familiar with the contents of this insert before prescribing or dispensing this medication.

B. Test for skin sensitivity before using Eldoquin Forte 4% Cream by applying a small amount to an unbroken patch of skin and check in 24 hours. Minor redness is not a contraindication, but where there is itching or vesicle formation or excessive inflammatory response, further treatment is not advised. Close patient supervision is recommended.

Contact with the eyes should be avoided. If no bleaching or lightening effect is noted after 2 months of treatment, the medication should be discontinued.

C. There are no sunblocking or sunscreening agents in Eldoquin Forte 4% Cream and since minimal sunlight exposure may reverse the bleaching effect of this preparation, it should be used only at night or on areas of the body covered by protective clothing. During the daytime, sunblocking or broad spectrum sunscreen preparations or protective clothing should be used to prevent the bleached areas from repigmentation. For daytime bleaching of unwanted pigmented areas, the use of Solaquin Forte™ 4% Cream or Eldopaque Forte® 4% Cream should be considered.

D. Keep this and all medication out of the reach of children. In case of accidental ingestion, call a physician or a poison control center immediately.

PRECAUTIONS

SEE WARNINGS.

A. Pregnancy Category C. Animal reproduction studies have not been conducted with topical hydroquinone. It is also not known whether hydroquinone can cause fetal harm when used topically on a pregnant woman or affect reproductive capacity. It is not known to what degree, if any, topical hydroquinone is absorbed systemically. Topical hydroquinone should be used in women only when clearly indicated.

B. Nursing mothers. It is not known whether topical hydroquinone is absorbed or excreted in human milk. Caution is advised when topical hydroquinone is used by a nursing mother.

C. Pediatric usage. Safety and effectiveness in children below the age of 12 years have not been established.

ADVERSE REACTIONS

No systemic adverse reactions have been reported. Occasional hypersensitivity (localized contact dermatitis) may occur in which case the medication should be discontinued and the physician notified immediately.

OVERDOSAGE

There have been no systemic reactions from the use of topical hydroquinone in Eldoquin Forte 4% Cream. However, treatment should be limited to relatively small areas of the body at one time since some patients experience a transient skin reddening and a mild burning sensation which does not preclude treatment.

DRUG DOSAGE AND ADMINISTRATION

Eldoquin Forte 4% Cream should be applied to the affected area and rubbed in well twice daily or as directed by a physician. There is no recommended dosage for children under 12 years of age except under the advice and supervision of a physician.

HOW SUPPLIED

ELDOQUIN FORTE 4% Cream is available as follows:

Size	NDC Number
0.5 ounce tube (15 grams)	0163-0394-35
1.0 ounce tube (30 grams)	0163-0394-31

Available without prescription for maintenance therapy: Eldoquin® (2% Hydroquinone) in ½ ounce (NDC 0163-0382-35) and 1 ounce tubes (NDC 0163-0382-31); Eldoquin Lotion (2% Hydroquinone) in ½ ounce bottles (NDC 0163-0423-35).

Eldoquin Forte 4% Cream should be stored at room temperature (15–30°C) (59–86°F).

FOTOTAR® CREAM

[fōtō'tar]

2% Coal Tar USP

(Equivalent to 10% Coal Tar Solution, USP)

Therapeutic Coal Tar Cream

FOR EXTERNAL USE ONLY

DESCRIPTION

Fototar® Cream contains Eldotar® (equivalent to 2% Coal Tar USP), in an emollient moisturizing cream base containing purified water, white petrolatum, mineral oil, microcrystalline cellulose, PEG 8, stearyl alcohol, glyceryl stearate PEG 100 stearate blend, coceth 6, imidazolidinyl urea, methylparaben, and propylparaben.

CLINICAL PHARMACOLOGY

The mechanism of action of coal tar products is largely unknown. Coal tars have antiseptic qualities, because they contain many substituted phenols. Coal tars also act as mild irritants and have a keratoplastic and antipruritic action. Coal tars have a photosensitizing effect and have been used for years with sunlight or ultraviolet (UV) radiation (Goeckerman Therapy) for the treatment of psoriasis. Coal tars have been successfully used in the treatment of seborrhea, eczema, psoriasis, lichen simplex chronicus, and other chronic skin diseases with lichenification. Pharmaceutical compounding of the crude coal tars has not lessened their therapeutic effectiveness and has increased patient acceptability.

INDICATIONS

Fototar is indicated in chronic skin disorders that are responsive to coal tars such as psoriasis, infantile and atopic eczema, seborrhea, lichen simplex chronicus, and other chronic skin disorders exhibiting lichenification. Fototar is useful in the Goeckerman program (tars plus UV radiation) in the treatment of psoriasis or other conditions responding to this combined therapy.

CONTRAINDICATIONS

A. Fototar is contraindicated in patients with a history of sensitivity to this product or with a history of sensitivity to coal tar products.
B. Fototar should not be used on patients who have a disease characterized by photosensitivity such as lupus erythematosus or allergy to sunlight.

WARNINGS

A. Fototar should not be applied to inflamed or broken skin except on the advice of a physician.
B. Since Fototar is photosensitizing, care must be exercised in exposing the areas of application to excessive UV or sunlight for 24 hours. In the Goeckerman treatment of psoriasis or other skin conditions, care must be taken against overexposure of the areas of application during therapeutic UV radiation or subsequent to such treatment because serious burns may result. Sunscreening or sunblocking agents or protective clothing for at least 24 hours after treatment is recommended to protect the treated areas against additional UV exposure from sunlight.
C. Fototar contains a coal tar derivative. Coal tar preparations should not be used in patients with an exacerbation of psoriasis since this may precipitate total body exfoliation.
D. In psoriatic patients receiving Goeckerman therapy, care should be taken that Fototar application and/or subsequent sunlight exposure be avoided over normal skin since this may cause the appearance of new psoriatic lesions in areas of skin trauma (Koebner Phenomenon).
E. Contact with the eyes should be avoided.
F. Staining of clothing may occur which is normally removed by standard laundry methods. Use on the scalp may cause temporary staining of light colored hair.

PRECAUTIONS

A. Patients should be advised of the photosensitizing effect of Fototar.
B. Laboratory tests—none required.
C. Carcinogenesis. Skin cancer following the use of Fototar has not been seen. The use of crude coal tar combined with UV radiation in the production of skin cancer has been studied with conflicting results. Stern, et al, 1980, estimated an increased risk for such cancer in patients with high exposure to tar and ultraviolet radiation compared with those lacking high exposure. They recommended continued surveillance for tumors among psoriatic patients who receive long-term tar and/or UV radiation therapy. However, Pittelkow, et al, 1981, did a 25 year follow-up study on patients receiving combined crude coal tar and UV radiation for psoriasis at the Mayo Clinic and found the incidence of skin cancer not appreciably increased above the expected incidence for the general population, and concluded that this combined regimen (Goeckerman) could be used with minimal risk for skin cancer in the treatment of psoriasis.
D. Pregnancy Category C. Animal reproduction studies have not been conducted with Fototar. It is not known whether Fototar can cause fetal harm when administered to a pregnant woman or can affect reproductive capacity. Fototar should be given to a pregnant woman only if clearly indicated.
E. Nursing Mothers. The absorption of Fototar in nursing mothers has not been studied and caution should be exercised when Fototar is administered to a nursing woman.
F. Pediatric Use. Safety and effectiveness of Fototar in children have not been established.

ADVERSE REACTIONS

A. SEE WARNINGS
B. Chemical folliculitis has been observed in areas of skin which have received long term coal tar applications. This phenomenon has not been observed with the use of Fototar, but its possibility should be borne in mind. This reaction normally clears if coal tar is discontinued or frequency of application reduced.

OVERDOSAGE

A. SEE WARNINGS about use on normal skin.
B. If Fototar is accidentally ingested, call a physician or a poison control center for instructions.

DOSAGE AND ADMINISTRATION

Fototar should be rubbed in the desired area well prior to UV radiation. After several minutes, the excess cream remaining on the skin can be patted with paper tissues to remove the excess.

HOW SUPPLIED

Fototar is supplied in 3.0 ounce (90 gm) tubes (NDC 0163-0373-03) and in 1-lb. (453.6 gm) jars (NDC 0163-0373-05).
Fototar Cream should be stored at room temperature (15–30°C) (59–86°F).

FOTOTAR® STIK ℞

[fōtō 'tar stik]
(Coal Tar USP, 6.25%)
Therapeutic Coal Tar Stick
FOR EXTERNAL USE ONLY

CAUTION: FEDERAL (U.S.A.) LAW PROHIBITS DISPENSING WITHOUT A PRESCRIPTION.

DESCRIPTION

Each gram of Fototar Stik 6.25% contains 62.5 mg of Eldotar® (equivalent to 50 mg of Coal Tar, USP) in a hydrophilic wax base containing methyl gluceth-20 sesquistearate, C_{18-36} acid triglyceride, methyl sesquistearate, C_{18-36} acid glycol ester, steareth 2, and polysorbate 80.

CLINICAL PHARMACOLOGY

The mechanism of action of coal tar products is largely unknown. Coal tars have antiseptic qualities because they contain many substituted phenols. Coal tars also act as mild irritants and have a keratoplastic and antipruritic action. Coal tars have a photosensitizing effect and have been used for years with sunlight or ultraviolet (UV) radiation (Goeckerman Therapy) for the treatment of psoriasis. Coal tars have been successfully used in the treatment of seborrhea, eczema, psoriasis, lichen simplex chronicus, and other chronic skin diseases with lichenification. Pharmaceutical compounding of the crude coal tars has not lessened their therapeutic effectiveness and has increased patient acceptability.

INDICATIONS

Fototar Stik is indicated in chronic skin disorders that are responsive to coal tars such as psoriasis, infantile and atopic eczema, seborrhea, lichen simplex chronicus, and other chronic skin disorders exhibiting lichenification. Fototar Stik is useful in the Goeckerman program (tars plus UV radiation) in the treatment of psoriasis or other conditions responding to this combined therapy.

CONTRAINDICATIONS

A. Fototar Stik is contraindicated in patients with a history of sensitivity to this product or with a history of sensitivity to coal tar products.
B. Fototar Stik should not be used on patients who have a disease characterized by photosensitivity such as lupus erythematosus or allergy to sunlight.

WARNINGS

A. Fototar Stik should not be applied to inflamed or broken skin except on the advice of a physician.
B. Since Fototar Stik is photosensitizing, care must be exercised in exposing the areas of application to excessive UV or sunlight for 24 hours. In the Goeckerman treatment of psoriasis or other skin conditions, care must be taken against overexposure of the areas of application during therapeutic UV radiation or subsequent to such treatment because serious burns may result. Sunscreening or sunblocking agents or protective clothing for at least 24 hours after treatment is recommended to protect the treated areas against additional UV exposure from sunlight.
C. Fototar Stik contains a coal tar derivative. Coal tar preparations should not be used in patients with an exacerbation of psoriasis since this may precipitate total body exfoliation.
D. In psoriatic patients receiving Goeckerman therapy, care should be taken that Fototar Stik application and /or subsequent sunlight exposure be avoided over normal skin since this may cause the appearance of new psoriatic lesions in areas of skin trauma (Koebner Phenomenon).
E. Contact with the eyes should be avoided.
F. Staining of clothing may occur which is normally removed by standard laundry methods. Use on the scalp may cause temporary staining of light colored hair.

PRECAUTIONS

A. Patients should be advised of the photosensitizing effect of Fototar Stik.
B. Laboratory tests - none required.
C. Carcinogenesis. Skin cancer following the use of Fototar Stik has not been seen. The use of crude coal tar combined with UV radiation in the production of skin cancer has been studied with conflicting results. Stern, et al, 1980, estimated an increased risk for such cancer in patients with high exposure to tar and ultraviolet radiation compared with those lacking high exposure. They recommended continued surveillance for tumors among psoriatic patients who receive long-term tar and/or UV radiation therapy. However, Pittelkow, et al, 1981, did a 25 year follow-up study on patients receiving combined crude coal tar and UV radiation for psoriasis at the Mayo Clinic and found the incidence of skin cancer not appreciably increased above the expected incidence for the general population, and concluded that this combined regimen (Goeckerman) could be used with minimal risk for skin cancer in the treatment of psoriasis.
D. Pregnancy Category C. Animal reproduction studies have not been conducted with Fototar Stik. It is not known whether Fototar Stik can cause fetal harm when administered to a pregnant woman or can affect reproductive capacity. Fototar Stik should be given to a pregnant woman only if clearly indicated.
E. Nursing Mothers. The absorption of Fototar Stik in nursing mothers has not been studied and caution should be exercised when Fototar Stik is administered to a nursing woman.
F. Pediatric Use. Safety and effectiveness of Fototar Stik in children have not been established.

ADVERSE REACTIONS

A. SEE WARNINGS
B. Chemical folliculitis has been observed in areas of skin which have received long term coal tar applications. This phenomenon has not been observed with the use of Fototar Stik, but its possibility should be borne in mind. This reaction normally clears if coal tar is discontinued or frequency of application reduced.

OVERDOSAGE

A. SEE WARNINGS about use on normal skin.
B. If Fototar Stik is accidentally ingested, call a physician or a poison control center for instructions.

DOSAGE AND ADMINISTRATION

Fototar Stik should be applied on the desired area well prior to UV radiation.

HOW SUPPLIED

Fototar Stik (NDC 0163-0522-35) is supplied in 0.5 ounce (15 gram) plastic stick applicator container.
Fototar Stik should be stored at room temperature (15–30°C) (59–86°F).

OXSORALEN® CAPSULES ℞

[ox'-sore"a-len]
(Methoxsalen USP, 10 mg)

CAUTION: FEDERAL LAW PROHIBITS DISPENSING WITHOUT PRESCRIPTION.
CAUTION: METHOXSALEN IS A POTENT DRUG. READ ENTIRE BROCHURE BEFORE PRESCRIBING OR DISPENSING THIS MEDICATION.

> Methoxsalen with UV radiation should be used only by physicians who have special competence in the diagnosis and treatment of psoriasis and vitiligo and who have special training and experience in photochemotherapy. Psoralen and ultraviolet radiation therapy should be under constant supervision of such a physician. For the treatment of patients with psoriasis, photochemotherapy should be restricted to patients with severe, recalcitrant, disabling psoriasis which is not adequately responsive to other forms of therapy, and only when the diagnosis has been supported by biopsy. Because of the possibilities of ocular damage, aging of the skin, and skin cancer (including melanoma), the patient should be fully informed by the physician of the risks inherent in this therapy.

DESCRIPTION

Oxsoralen (Methoxsalen, 8-Methoxypsoralen) Capsules, 10 mg. Methoxsalen is a naturally occuring photoactive substance found in the seeds of the Ammi majus (Umbelliferae) plant. It belongs to a group of compounds known as psoralens, or furocoumarins. The chemical name of methoxsalen is 9-methoxy-7H-furo[3,2-g][1]-benzopyran-7-one.

Continued on next page

Elder—Cont.

CLINICAL PHARMACOLOGY

The combination treatment regimen of psoralen (P) and ultraviolet radiation of 320-400 nm wavelength commonly referred to as UVA is known by the acronym, PUVA. Skin reactivity to UVA (320-400 nm) radiation is markedly enhanced by the ingestion of methoxsalen. The drug reaches its maximum bioavailability 1½-3 hours after oral administration and may last for up to 8 hours (Pathak et al, 1974). Methoxsalen is reversibly bound to serum albumen and is also preferentially taken up by epidermal cells (Artuc et al, 1979). At a dose which is six times larger than that used in humans, it induces mixed function oxidases in the liver of mice (Mandula et al, 1978). In both mice and man, methoxsalen is rapidly metabolized. Approximately 95% of the drug is excreted as a series of metabolites in the urine within 24 hours (Pathak et al, 1977).

The exact mechanism of action of methoxsalen with the epidermal melanocytes and keratinocytes is not known. The best known biochemical reaction of methoxsalen is with DNA. Methoxsalen, upon photoactivation, conjugates and forms covalent bonds with DNA which leads to the formation of both monofunctional (addition to a single strand of DNA) and bifunctional adducts (crosslinking of psoralen to both strands of DNA)(Dall'Acqua et al, 1971; Cole, 1970; Musajo et al, 1974; Dall'Acqua et al, 1979). Reactions with proteins have also been described (Yoshikawa et al, 1979).

Methoxsalen acts as a photosensitizer. Administration of the drug and subsequent exposure to UVA can lead to cell injury. Orally administered methoxsalen reaches the skin via the blood and UVA penetrates well into the skin. If sufficient cell injury occurs in the skin, an inflammatory reaction occurs. The most obvious manifestation of this reaction is delayed erythema, which may not begin for several hours and peaks at 48-72 hours. The inflammation is followed, over several days to weeks, by repair which is manifested by increased melanization of the epidermis and thickening of the stratum corneum. The mechanisms of therapy are not known. In the treatment of vitiligo, it has been suggested that melanocytes in the hair follicle are stimulated to move up the follicle and to repopulate the epidermis (Ortonne et al, 1979). In the treatment of psoriasis, the mechanism is most often assumed to be DNA photodamage and resulting decrease in cell proliferation but other vascular, leukocyte, or cell regulatory mechanisms may also be playing some role. Psoriasis is a hyperproliferative disorder and other agents known to be therapeutic for psoriasis are known to inhibit DNA synthesis.

INDICATIONS AND USAGE

A. Photochemotherapy (methoxsalen with long wave UVA radiation) is indicated for the symptomatic control of severe, recalcitrant, disabling psoriasis not adequately responsive to other forms of therapy and when the diagnosis has been supported by biopsy. Photochemotherapy is intended to be administered only in conjunction with a schedule of controlled doses of long wave ultraviolet radiation.

B. Photochemotherapy (methoxsalen with long wave ultraviolet radiation) is indicated for the repigmentation of idiopathic vitiligo.

CONTRAINDICATIONS

A. Patients exhibiting idiosyncratic reactions to psoralen compounds.

B. Patients possessing a specific history of light sensitive disease states should not initiate methoxsalen therapy. Diseases associated with photosensitivity include lupus erythematosus, porphyria cutanea tarda, erythropoietic protoporphyria, variegate porphyria, xeroderma pigmentosum, and albinism.

C. Patients exhibiting melanoma or possessing a history of melanoma.

D. Patients exhibiting invasive squamous cell carcinomas.

E. Patients with aphakia, because of the significantly increased risk of retinal damage due to the absence of lenses.

WARNINGS—General:

A. Skin Burning: Serious burns from either UVA or sunlight (even through window glass) can result if the recommended dosage of the drug and/or exposure schedules are not maintained.

B. Carcinogenicity.

1. ANIMAL STUDIES: Topical or intraperitoneal methoxsalen has been reported to be a potent photocarcinogen in albino mice and hairless mice. However, methoxsalen given by the oral route to albino mice or by any route in pigmented mice is considerably less phototoxic or carcinogenic (Hakim et al, 1960; Pathak et al, 1959).

2. HUMAN STUDIES: A prospective study of 1380 patients over 5 years revealed an approximately nine-fold increase in risks of squamous cell carcinoma among PUVA treated patients. (Stern et al, 1979 and Stern et al, 1980) This increase in risk appears greatest among patients who are fair skinned or had pre-PUVA exposure to 1) prolonged tar and UVB treatment, 2) ionizing radiation, or 3) arsenic.

In addition, an approximately two-fold increase in the risk of basal cell carcinoma was noted in this study. Roenigk et al, 1980 studied 690 patients for up to 4 years and found no increase in the risk of non-melanoma skin cancer. However, patients in this cohort had significantly less exposure to PUVA than in the Stern et al study. After 5 years, two of 1380 patients in the Stern et al PUVA study have developed malignant melanoma. In addition, more than 1/5 of patients in this cohort have developed macular pigmented lesions on the buttocks. While there is no evidence that an increased risk of melanoma exists in PUVA treated patients, these observations indicate the need for continued evaluation of melanoma risk in PUVA treated patients.

In a study in Indian patients treated for 4 years for vitiligo, 12 percent developed keratoses, but not cancer, in the depigmented, vitiliginous areas (Mosher, 1980). Clinically, the keratoses were keratotic papules, actinic keratosis-like macules, nonscaling dome-shaped papules, and lichenoid porokeratotic-like papules.

C. Cataractogenicity:

1. ANIMAL STUDIES: Exposure to large doses of UVA causes cataracts in animals, and this effect is enhanced by the administration of methoxsalen (Cloud et al, 1960; Cloud et al, 1961; Freeman et al, 1969).

2. HUMAN STUDIES: It has been found that the concentration of methoxsalen in the lens is proportional to the serum level. If the lens is exposed to UVA during the time methoxsalen is present in the lens, photochemical action may lead to irreversible binding of methoxsalen to proteins and the DNA components of the lens (Lerman et al, 1980). However, if the lens is shielded from UVA, the methoxsalen will diffuse out of the lens in a 24 hour period. Patients should be told emphatically to wear UVA-absorbing, wrap-around sunglasses for the twenty-four (24) hour period following ingestion of methoxsalen, whether exposed to direct or indirect sunlight in the open or through a window glass.

Among patients using proper eye protection, there is no evidence for a significantly increased risk of cataracts in association with PUVA therapy. Thirty-five of 1380 patients have developed cataracts in the five years since their first PUVA treatment. This incidence is comparable to that expected in a population of this size and age distribution. No relationship between PUVA dose and cataract risk in this group has been noted.

D. Actinic Degeneration: Exposure to sunlight and/or ultraviolet radiation may result in "premature aging" of the skin.

E. Basal Cell Carcinomas: Patients exhibiting multiple basal cell carcinomas or having a history of basal cell carcinomas should be diligently observed and treated.

F. Radiation Therapy: Patients having a history of previous x-ray therapy or grenz ray therapy should be diligently observed for signs of carcinoma.

G. Arsenic Therapy: Patients having a history of previous arsenic therapy should be diligently observed for signs of carcinoma.

H. Hepatic Diseases: Patients with hepatic insufficiency should be treated with caution since hepatic biotransformation is necessary for drug urinary excretion.

I. Cardiac Diseases: Patients with cardiac diseases or others who may be unable to tolerate prolonged standing or exposure to heat stress should not be treated in a vertical UVA chamber.

J. Total Dosage: The total cumulative dose of UVA that can be given over long periods of time with safety has not as yet been established.

K. Concomitant Therapy: Special care should be exercised in treating patients who are receiving concomitant therapy (either topically or systemically) with known photosensitizing agents such as anthralin, coal tar or coal tar derivatives, griseofulvin, phenothiazines, nalidixic acid, halogenated salicylanilides (bacteriostatic soaps), sulfonamides, tetracyclines, thiazides and certain organic staining dyes such as methylene blue, toluidine blue, rose bengal, and methyl orange.

PRECAUTIONS

This product contains FD&C Yellow No. 5 (tartrazine) as a color additive which may cause allergic-type reactions (including bronchial asthma) in certain susceptible individuals. Although the overall incidence of FD&C Yellow #5 (tartrazine) sensitivity is low it is frequently seen in patients who also have aspirin hypersensitivity.

A. General-Applicable To Both Vitiligo and Psoriasis Treatment

1. BEFORE METHOXSALEN INGESTION
Patients must not sunbathe during the 24 hours prior to methoxsalen ingestion and UV exposure. The presence of a sunburn may prevent an accurate evaluation of the patient's response to photochemotherapy.

2. AFTER METHOXSALEN INGESTION
a. UVA-absorbing wrap-around sunglasses should be worn during daylight for 24 hours after methoxsalen ingestion. The protective eyewear must be designed to prevent entry of stray radiation to the eyes, including that which may enter from the sides of the eyewear. The protective eyewear is used to prevent the irreversible binding of methoxsalen to the proteins and DNA components of the lens. Cataracts form when enough of the binding occurs. Visual discrimination should be permitted by the eyewear for patient well-being and comfort.
b. Patients must avoid sun exposure, even through window glass or cloud cover, for at least 8 hours after methoxsalen ingestion. If sun exposure cannot be avoided, the patient should wear protective devices such as a hat and gloves, and/or apply sunscreens which contain ingredients that filter out UVA radiation (e.g. sunscreens containing benzophenone and/or PABA esters which exhibit a sun protective factor equal to or greater than 15). These chemical sunscreens should be applied to all areas that might be exposed to the sun (including lips). Sunscreens should not be applied to areas affected by psoriasis until after the patient has been treated in the UVA chamber.

3. DURING PUVA THERAPY
a. Total UVA-absorbing/blocking goggles mechanically designed to give maximal ocular protection must be worn. Failure to do so may increase the risk of cataract formation. A reliable radiometer can be used to verify elimination of UVA transmission through the goggles.
b. Abdominal skin, breasts, genitalia, and other sensitive areas should be protected for approximately 1/3 of the initial exposure time until tanning occurs.
c. Unless affected by disease, male genitalia should be shielded.

4. AFTER COMBINED METHOXSALEN/ UVA THERAPY
a. UVA-absorbing wrap-around sunglasses should be worn during the daylight for 24 hours after combined methoxsalen/UVA therapy.
b. Patients should not sunbathe for 48 hours after therapy. Erythema and/or burning due to photochemotherapy and sunburn due to sun exposure are additive.

5. VITILIGO THERAPY
a. The dosage of methoxsalen should not be increased above 0.6 mg/kg since overdosage may result in serious burning of the skin.
b. Eye and skin sun protection as described in the Precautions-General section should be observed.

B. Information For Patients: See Patient Package Insert.

C. Laboratory Tests:

1. Patients should have an ophthalmologic examination prior to start of therapy, and thence yearly.
2. Patients should have the following tests prior to the start of therapy and should be retested 6-12 months subsequently. Additional tests at more extended time periods should be conducted as clinically indicated.
   a. Complete Blood Count (Hemoglobin or Hematocrit; White Blood Count-if abnormal, a differential count).
   b. Anti-nuclear Antibodies.
   c. Liver Function Tests.
   d. Renal Function Tests (Creatinine or Blood Urea Nitrogen).

D. Drug Interactions: See Warnings Section.

E. Carcinogenesis: See Warnings Section.

F. Pregnancy:
Pregnancy Category C. Animal reproduction studies have not been conducted with methoxsalen. It is also not known whether methoxsalen can cause fetal harm when administered to a pregnant woman or can affect reproduction capacity. Methoxsalen should be given to a pregnant woman only if clearly needed.

G. Nursing Mothers:
It is not known whether this drug is excreted in human milk. Because many drugs are excreted in human milk, caution should be exercised when methoxsalen is administered to a nursing woman.

H. Pediatric Use:
Safety in children has not been established. Potential hazards of long-term therapy include the possibilities of carcinogenicity and cataractogenicity as described in the Warnings Section as well as the probability of actinic degeneration which is also described in the Warnings Section.

ADVERSE REACTIONS

A. Methoxsalen
The most commonly reported side effect of methoxsalen alone is nausea, which occurs with approximately 10% of all patients. This effect may be minimized or avoided by instructing the patient to take methoxsalen with milk or food, or to divide the dose into two portions, taken approximately one-half hour apart. Other effects include nervousness, insomnia, and psychological depression.

B. Combined Methoxsalen/UVA Therapy

1. PRURITUS: This adverse reaction occurs with approximately 10% of all patients. In most cases, pruritus can be

alleviated with frequent application of bland emollients or other topical agents; severe pruritus may require systemic treatment. If pruritus is unresponsive to these measures, shield pruritic areas from further UVA exposure until the condition resolves. If intractable pruritus is generalized, UVA treatment should be discontinued until the pruritus disappears.

2. ERYTHEMA: Mild, transient erythema at 24-48 hours after PUVA therapy is an expected reaction and indicates that a therapeutic interaction between methoxsalen and UVA occurred. Any area showing moderate erythema (greater than Grade 2—See Table 1 for grades of erythema) should be shielded during subsequent UVA exposures until the erythema has resolved. Erythema greater than Grade 2 which appears within 24 hours after UVA treatment may signal a potentially severe burn. Erythema may become progressively worse over the next 24 hours, since the peak erythemal reaction characteristically occurs 48 hours or later after methoxsalen ingestion. The patient should be protected from further UVA exposures and sunlight, and should be monitored closely.

3. IMPORTANT DIFFERENCES BETWEEN PUVA ERYTHEMA AND SUNBURN: PUVA-induced inflammation differs from sunburn or UVB phototherapy in several ways. The *in situ* depth of photochemistry is deeper within the tissue because UVA is transmitted further into the skin. The DNA lesions induced by PUVA are very different from UV-induced thymine dimers and may lead to a DNA crosslink. This DNA lesion may be more problematic to the cell because crosslinks are more lethal and psoralen-DNA photoproducts may be "new" or unfamiliar substrates for DNA repair enzymes. DNA synthesis is also suppressed longer after PUVA. The time course of delayed erythema is different with PUVA and may not involve the usual mediators seen in sunburn. PUVA-induced redness may be just beginning at 24 hours, when UVB erythema has already passed its peak. The erythema dose-response curve is also steeper for PUVA. Compared to equally erythemogenic doses of UVB, the histologic alterations induced by PUVA show more dermal vessel damage and longer duration of epidermal and dermal abnormalities.

4. OTHER ADVERSE REACTIONS: Those reported include edema, dizziness, headache, malaise, depression, hypopigmentation, vesiculation and bullae formation, non-specific rash, herpes simplex, miliaria, urticaria, folliculitis, gastrointestinal disturbances, cutaneous tenderness, leg cramps, hypotension, and extension of psoriasis.

OVERDOSAGE

In the event of methoxsalen overdosage, induce emesis and keep the patient in a darkened room for at least 24 hours. Emesis is beneficial only within the first 2 to 3 hours after ingestion of methoxsalen, since maximum blood levels are reached by this time.

DRUG DOSAGE & ADMINISTRATION

A. Vitiligo Therapy

1. DRUG DOSAGE: Two capsules (10 mg each) in one dose taken with milk or in food two to four hours before ultraviolet light exposure.

2. LIGHT EXPOSURE: The exposure time to sunlight should comply with the following guide:

	Basic Skin Color		
	Light	Medium	Dark
Initial Exposure	15 min	20 min	25 min
Second Exposure	20 min	25 min	30 min
Third Exposure	25 min	30 min	35 min
Fourth Exposure	30 min	35 min	40 min

Subsequent Exposure: Gradually increase exposure based on erythema and tenderness of the amelanotic skin.

Therapy should be on alternate days and never two consecutive days.

B. Psoriasis Therapy

1. DRUG DOSAGE-INITIAL THERAPY: The methoxsalen capsules should be taken two hours before UVA exposure with some food or milk according to the following table:

Patient's Weight		Dose
(kg.)	(lbs.)	(mg.)
<30	<65	10
30-50	65-100	20
51-65	101-145	30
66-80	146-175	40
81-90	176-200	50
91-115	201-250	60
>115	>250	70

Additional drug dosage directions are as follows:

a. Weight Change: In the event that the weight of a patient changes during treatment such that he/she falls into an adjacent weight range/dose category, no change in the dose of methoxsalen is usually required. If, in the physician's opinion, however, a weight change is sufficiently great to modify the drug dose, then an adjustment in the time of exposure to UVA should be made.

b. Dose/Week: The number of doses per week of methoxsalen capsules will be determined by the patient's schedule of UVA exposures. In no case should treatments be given more often than once every other day because the full extent of phototoxic reactions may not be evident until 48 hours after each exposure.

c. Dosage Increase: Dosage may be increased by 10 mg. after the fifteenth treatment under the conditions outlined in the section titled PUVA Treatment Protocol, part B)4)b).

UVA Radiation Source Specifications & Information:

A. Irradiance Uniformity

The following specifications should be met with the window of the detector held in a vertical plane:

1. Vertical variation: For readings taken at any point along the vertical center axis of the chamber (to within 15 cm from the top and bottom), the lowest reading should not be less than 70 percent of the highest reading.

2. Horizontal variation: Throughout any specific horizontal plane, the lowest reading must be at least 80 percent of the highest reading, excluding the peripheral 3 cm of the patient treatment space.

B. Patient Safety Features

The following safety features should be present: (1) Protection from electrical hazard: All units should be grounded and conform to applicable electrical codes. The patient or operator should not be able to touch any live electrical parts. There should be ground fault protection. (2) Protective shielding of lamps: The patient should not be able to come in contact with the bare lamps. In the event of lamp breakage, the patient should not be exposed to broken lamp components. (3) Hand rails and hand holds: Appropriate supports should be available to the patient. (4) Patient viewing window: A window which blocks UV should be provided for viewing the patient during treatment. (5) Door and latches: Patients should be able to open the door from the inside with only slight pressure to the door. (6) Non-skid floor: The floor should be of a non-skid nature. (7) Thermoregulation: Sufficient air flow should be provided for patient safety and comfort, limiting temperature within the UVA radiator cabinet to approximately less than 100°F. (8) Timer: The irradiator should be equipped with an automatic timer which terminates the exposure at the conclusion of a pre-set time interval. (9) Patient alarm device: An alarm device within the UVA irradiator chamber should be accessible to the patient for emergency activation. (10) Danger label: The unit should have a label prominently displayed which reads as follows: Danger-Ultraviolet radiation-Follow your physicians instructions-Failure to use protective eyewear may result in eye injury.

C. UVA Exposure Dosimetry Measurements:

The maximum radiant exposure or irradiance (within ± 15 percent) of UVA (320-400 nm) delivered to the patient should be determined by using an appropriate radiometer calibrated to be read in Joules/cm^2 or mW/cm^2. In the absence of a standard measuring technique approved by the National Bureau of Standards, the system should use a detector corrected to a cosine spatial response. The use and recalibration frequency of such a radiometer for a specific UVA irradiator chamber should be specified by the manufacturer because the UVA dose (exposure) is determined by the design of the irradiator, the number of lamps, and the age of the lamps. If irradiance is measured, the radiometer reading in mW/cm^2 is used to calculate the exposure time in minutes to deliver the required UVA dose in Joules/cm^2 to a patient in the UVA irradiator cabinet. The equation is:

$$\text{Exposure Time in Minutes} = \frac{\text{Desired UVA Dose (J/cm}^2\text{)}}{0.06 \times \text{Irradiance (mW/cm}^2\text{)}}$$

Overexposure due to human error should be minimized by using an accurate automatic timing device, which is set by the operator and controlled by energizing and de-energizing the UVA irradiator lamp. The timing device calibration interval should be specified by the manufacturer. Safety systems should be included to minimize the possibility of delivering a UVA exposure which exceeds the prescribed dose, in the event that the timer of radiometer should malfunction.

D. UVA Spectral Output Distribution

The spectral distributions of the lamps should meet the following specifications:

Wavelength band (nanometers)	Output[1]
<310	<1
310 to 320	1 to 3
320 to 330	4 to 8
330 to 340	11 to 17
340 to 350	18 to 25
350 to 360	19 to 28
360 to 370	15 to 23
370 to 380	8 to 12
380 to 390	3 to 7
390 to 400	1 to 3

[1]As a percentage of total irradiance between 320 and 400 nanometers.

PUVA Treatment Protocol:

A. Initial Exposure: The initial UVA exposure radiation level and corresponding time of exposure is determined by the patient's skin characteristics for sun burning and tanning as follows:

[See table above].

OXSORALEN Skin Type	History	Recommended Joules/cm^2
I	Always burn, never tan (Patients with erythrodermic psoriasis are to be classed as Type I for determination of UVA dosage.)	0.5 J/cm^2
II	Always burn, but sometimes tan	1.0 J/cm^2
III	Sometimes burn, but always tan	1.5 J/cm^2
IV	Never burn, always tan	2.0 J/cm^2
	Physician Examination	
V*	Moderately pigmented	2.5 J/cm^2
VI*	Blacks	3.0 J/cm^2

[*Patients with natural pigmentation of these types should be classified into a lower skin type category if the sunburning history so indicates.]

B. Clearing Phase: Specific recommendations for patient treatment are as follows:

1. SKIN TYPES I, II, and III. Patients with skin types I, II, and III may be treated 2 or 3 times per week. UVA exposure may be held constant or increased by up to 1.0 Joule/cm^2 at each treatment, according to the patient's response. If erythema occurs, however, do not increase exposure time until erythema resolves. The severity and extent of the patient's erythema may be used to determine whether the next exposure should be shortened, omitted, or maintained at the previous dosage. See Adverse Reactions section for additional information.

2. SKIN TYPES IV, V, and VI. Patients with skin types IV, V, and VI may be treated 2 or 3 times per week. UVA exposure may be held constant or increased by up to 1.5 Joules/cm^2 at each treatment unless erythema occurs. If erythema occurs, follow instructions outlined above in the procedures for patients with skin types I, II, and III.

3. ERYTHRODERMIC PSORIASIS. Patients with erythrodermic psoriasis should be treated with special attention because pre-existing erythema may obscure observations of possible treatment-related phototoxic erythema. These patients may be treated 2 or 3 times per week, as a Type I patient.

4. MISCELLANEOUS SITUATIONS:

a. If there is no response after a total of 10 treatments, the exposure of UVA energy may be increased by an additional 0.5-1.0 Joules/cm^2 above the prior incremental increases for each treatment. (Example: a patient whose exposure dosage is being increased by 1.0 Joule/cm^2 may now have all subsequent doses increased by 1.5-2.0 Joules/cm^2.)

b. If there is no response, or only minimal response, after 15 treatments, the dosage of methoxsalen may be increased by 10 mg. (a one-time increase in dosage). This increased dosage may be continued for the remainder of the course of treatment but should not be exceeded.

c. If a patient misses a treatment, the UVA exposure time of the next treatment should not be increased. If more than one treatment is missed, reduce the exposure by 0.5 Joule/cm^2 for each treatment missed.

d. If the lower extremities are not responding as well as the rest of the body and do not show erythema, cover all other body areas and give 25 percent of the present exposure dose as an additional exposure to the lower extremities. This additional exposure to the lower extremities should be terminated if erythema develops on these areas.

e. Non-responsive psoriasis: If a patient's generalized psoriasis is not responding, or if the condition appears to be worsening during treatment, the possibility of a generalized phototoxic reaction should be considered. This may be confirmed by the improvement of the condition following temporary discontinuance of this therapy for two weeks. If no improvement occurs during

Continued on next page

Elder—Cont.

the interruption of treatment, this patient may be considered a treatment failure.

C. Alternative Exposure Schedule:

As an alternative to increasing the UVA exposure at each treatment, the following schedule may be followed; this schedule may reduce the total number of Joules/cm^2 received by the patient over the entire course of therapy.

1. Incremental increases in UVA exposure for all patients may range from 0.5 to 1.5 Joules/cm^2, according to the patient's response to therapy.
2. Once Grade 2 clearing (see Table 2) has been reached and the patient is progressing adequately, UVA dosage is held constant. The dosage is maintained until Grade 4 clearing is reached.
3. If the rate of clearing significantly decreases, exposure dosage may be increased at each treatment (0.1-1.5 Joules/cm^2) until Grade 3 clearing and a satisfactory progress rate is attained. The UVA exposure will be held constant again until Grade 4 clearing is attained. These increases may be used also if the rate of clearing significantly decreases between Grade 3 and Grade 4 response. However, the possibility of a phototoxic reaction should be considered; see Non-responsive Psoriasis, above.
4. In summary, this schedule raises slightly the increments (Joules/cm^2) of UVA dosage, but limits these increases to those periods when the patient is not responding adequately. Otherwise, the UVA exposure is held at the lowest effective dose.

D. Maintenance Phase:

The goal of maintenance treatment is to keep the patient symptom-free as possible with the least amount of UVA exposure.

1. SCHEDULE OF EXPOSURES: When patients have achieved 95 percent clearing, or Grade 4 response (Table 2), they may be placed on the following maintenance schedules (M_1-M_4), in sequence. It is recommended that each maintenance schedule be adhered to for at least 2 treatments (unless erythema or psoriatic flare occurs, in which case see (2a) and (2b) below).

Maintenance Schedules
M_1–once/week
M_2–once/2 weeks
M_3–once/3 weeks
M_4–p.r.n. (i.e. for flares)

2. LENGTH OF EXPOSURE: The UVA exposure for the first maintenance treatment of any schedule (except M_4 as noted below) is the same as that of the patient's last treatment under the previous schedule. For skin types I-IV, however, it is recommended that the maximum UVA dosage during maintenance treatments not exceed the following:

Skin Type	Joules/cm^2/treatment
I	12
II	14
III	18
IV	22

If the patient develops erythema or new lesions of psoriasis, proceed as follows:

a. Erythema: During maintenance therapy, the patient's tan and threshold dose for erythema may gradually decrease. If maintenance treatments produce significant erythema, the exposure to UVA should be decreased by 25 percent until further treatments no longer produce erythema.

b. Psoriasis: If the patient develops new areas of psoriasis during maintenance therapy (but still is classified as having a Grade 4 response), the exposure to UVA may be increased by 0.5-1.5 Joules/cm^2 at each treatment; this is appropriate for all types of patients. These increases are continued until the psoriasis is brought under control and the patient is again clear. The exposure being administered when this clearing is reached should be used for further maintenance treatment.

3. FLARES DURING MAINTENANCE: If the patient flares during maintenance treatment (i.e., develops psoriasis on more than 5 percent of the originally involved areas of the body) his maintenance treatment schedule may be changed to the preceding maintenance or clearing schedule. The patient may be kept on his schedule until again 95 percent clear. If the original maintenance treatment schedule is unable to control the psoriasis, the schedule may be changed to a more frequent regimen. If a flare occurs less than 6 weeks after the last treatment, 25 percent of the maximum exposure received during the clearing phase may be used and proceed with the clearing schedule previously followed for this patient. (At 95 percent clearing follow regular maintenance until the optimum maintenance schedule is determined for the patient.) If more than 6 weeks have elapsed since the last treatment was given, treat patients as if they were beginning therapy insofar as exposure dosages are concerned, since their threshold for erythema may have decreased.

Table 1.—Grades of Erythema

Grade	Erythema Level
0	No erythema
1	Minimally perceptible erythema— faint pink
2	Marked erythema but with no edema
3	Fiery erythema with edema
4	Fiery erythema with edema and blistering

[See table below].

HOW SUPPLIED

Oxsoralen Capsules, each containing 10 mg. of methoxsalen packaged in amber glass bottles are available as follows:

Unit Count	NDC Number
30	NDC 0163-0600-30
100	NDC 0163-0600-01

Oxsoralen should be stored at room temperature (15–30°C) (59–86°F).

Shown in Product Identification Section, page 409

OXSORALEN

Table 2.—Response to Therapy

Grade	Criteria	Percent Improvement (compared to original extent of disease)
−1	Psoriasis worse	0
0	No change	0
1	Minimal improvement—slightly less scale and/or erythema	5-20
2	Definite improvement—partial flattening of all plaque—less scaling and less erythema	20-50
3	Considerable improvement—nearly complete flattening of all plaque but borders of plaque still palpable	50-95
4	Clearing; complete flattening of plaque including borders; plaque may be outlined by pigmentation	95

OXSORALEN® LOTION 1% ℞

[ox 'sore "a-len]

(methoxsalen USP, 1%)

CAUTION: FEDERAL (U.S.A.) LAW PROHIBITS DISPENSING WITHOUT A PRESCRIPTION.

CAUTION: METHOXSALEN LOTION IS A POTENT TOPICAL DRUG. READ ENTIRE BROCHURE BEFORE PRESCRIBING OR USING THIS MEDICATION.

WARNING: METHOXSALEN LOTION IS A POTENT DRUG CAPABLE OF PRODUCING SEVERE BURNS IF IMPROPERLY USED. IT SHOULD BE APPLIED ONLY BY A PHYSICIAN UNDER CONTROLLED CONDITIONS FOR LIGHT EXPOSURE AND SUBSEQUENT LIGHT SHIELDING. THIS PREPARATION SHOULD NEVER BE DISPENSED TO A PATIENT.

DESCRIPTION

Each ml. of Oxsoralen Lotion contains 10 mg. methoxsalen in an inert vehicle containing alcohol (71% v/v), propylene glycol, acetone, and purified water.

Methoxsalen is a naturally occurring substance found in the seeds of the Ammi majus (Umbelliferae) plant; it belongs to a group of compounds known as psoralens or furocoumarins. The chemical name of methoxsalen is 9-methoxy-7H-furo(3, 2g) (1)-benzopyran-7-one. It has the following structure:

OCH_3

CLINICAL PHARMACOLOGY

The exact mechanism of action of methoxsalen with the epidermal melanocytes and keratinocytes is not known. Psoralens given orally are preferentially taken up by epidermal cells (Artuc et al, 1979). The best known biochemical reaction of methoxsalen is with DNA. Methoxsalen, upon photoactivation, conjugates and forms covalent bonds with DNA which leads to the formation of both monofunctional (addition to a single strand of DNA) and bifunctional adducts (crosslinking of psoralen to both strands of DNA) (Dall'Acqua et al, 1971). Reactions with proteins have also been described (Yoshikawa et al, 1979).

Methoxsalen acts as a photosensitizer. Topical application of this drug and subsequent exposure to UVA, whether artificial or sunlight, can cause cell injury. If sufficient cell injury occurs in the skin an inflammatory reaction will result. The most obvious manifestation of this reaction is delayed erythema which may not begin for several hours and may not peak for 2 to 3 days or longer. It is crucial to realize that the length of time the skin remains sensitized or when the maximum erythema will occur is quite variable from person to person. The erythematous reaction is followed over several days or weeks by repair which is manifested by increased melanization of the epidermis and thickening of the stratum corneum. The exact mechanics are unknown but it has been suggested melanocytes in the hair follicles are stimulated to move up the follicle and to repopulate the epidermis. (Ortonne, et al, 1979)

INDICATIONS AND USAGE

As a topical repigmenting agent in vitiligo in conjunction with controlled doses of ultraviolet A (320–400 nm) or sunlight.

CONTRAINDICATIONS

A. Patients exhibiting idiosyncratic reactions to psoralen compounds or a history of sensitivity reactions to them.
B. Patients exhibiting melanoma or with a history of melanoma.
C. Patients exhibiting invasive skin carcinoma generally.
D. Patients with photosensitivity diseases such as porphyria, acute lupus erythematosus, xeroderma pigmentosum, etc.
E. Children under 12 since clinical studies to determine the efficacy and safety of treatment in this age group have not been done.

WARNINGS

A. **Skin Burns**

Serious skin burns from either UVA or sunlight (even through window glass) can result if recommended exposure schedule is exceeded and/or protective covering or sunscreens are not used. The blistering of the skin sometimes encountered after UVA exposure generally heals without complication or scarring. (Farrington Daniels, Jr, M.D., personal communication). Suitable covering of the area of application or a topical sunblock should follow the therapeutic UVA exposure.

B. **Carcinogenicity**

1. Animal Studies. Topical methoxsalen has been reported to be a potent photocarcinogen in certain strains of mice. (Pathak et al 1959).
2. Human Studies. None of our clinical investigators reported skin cancers as a complication of topical treatment for vitiligo. However, it is recommended that caution be exercised when the patient is fair-skinned or has a history of prior coal tar UVA treatment, or has had ionizing radiation or taken arsenical compounds. Such patients who subsequently have oral psoralen—UVA treatment (PUVA) are at increased risk for developing skin cancer.

C. **Concomitant Therapy**

Special care should be exercised in treating patients who are receiving concomitant therapy (either topically or systemically) with known photosensitizing agents such as anthralin, coal tar or coal tar derivatives, griseofulvin, phenothiazines, nalidixic acid, halogenated salicylanilides (bacteriostatic soaps), sulfonamides, tetracyclines, thiazides, and certain organic staining dyes such as methylene blue, toluidine blue, rose bengal, and methyl orange.

PRECAUTIONS

A. This product should be applied only in small well defined lesions and preferably on lesions which can be protected by clothing or a sunscreen from subsequent exposure to radiant UVA. If this product is used to treat vitiligo of face or hands, be very emphatic when instructing patient to keep the treated areas protected from light by use of protective clothing or sunscreening agents. The area of application may be highly photosensitive for several days and may result in severe burn injury if exposed to additional UVA or sunlight.
B. CARCINOGENESIS: See Warning Section
C. Pregnancy Category C. Animal reproduction studies have not been conducted with topical methoxsalen. It is also not known whether methoxsalen can cause fetal harm when used topically on a pregnant woman or affect reproductive capacity. It is not known to what degree, if any, topical methoxsalen is absorbed systemically. Topical methoxsalen should be used in pregnant women only when clearly indicated.
D. Nursing Mothers. It is not known whether topical methoxsalen is absorbed or excreted in human milk. Caution is advised when topical methoxsalen is used in a nursing mother.
E. Pediatric Usage. Safety and effectiveness in children below the age of 12 years have not been established.

ADVERSE REACTIONS

Systemic adverse reactions have not been reported. The most common adverse reaction is severe burns of the treated area from overexposure to UVA, including sunlight. TREATMENT MUST BE INDIVIDUALIZED. Minor blistering of the skin is not a contraindication to further treatment and generally heals without incident. Treatment would be the standard for burn therapy. Since 1953, many studies have demonstrated the safety and effectiveness of topical methoxsalen and UVA for the treatment of vitiligo when used as directed. (Lerner, A.B., et al, 1953) (Fitzpatrick, T.B., et al, 1966) (Fulton, James F. et al, 1969)

OVERDOSAGE

This does not apply to topical usage. In the unlikely event that the lotion is ingested, standard procedures for poisoning should be followed, including gastric lavage. Protection from UVA or daylight for hours or days would also be necessary and the patient kept in a darkened room.

ADMINISTRATION

The OXSORALEN® Lotion is applied to a well-defined area of vitiligo by the physician and the area is then exposed to a suitable source of UVA. Initial exposure time should be conservative and not exceed that which is predicted to be one-half the minimal erythema dose. Treatment intervals should be regulated by the erythema response; generally once a week is recommended or less often depending on the results. The hands and fingers of the person applying the medication should be protected by gloves or finger cots to avoid photosensitization and possible burns.

Pigmentation may begin after a few weeks but significant repigmentation may require up to 6 to 9 months of treatment. Periodic re-treatment may be necessary to retain all of the new pigment. Idiopathic vitiligo is reversible but not equally reversible in every patient. Treatment must be individualized. Repigmentation will vary in completeness, time of onset, and duration. Repigmentation occurs more rapidly in fleshy areas such as face, abdomen, and buttocks and less rapidly over less fleshy areas such as the dorsum of the hands or feet.

HOW SUPPLIED

Oxsoralen Lotion containing 1% methoxsalen (8-methoxypsoralen) packaged in 1 ounce (30 ml) amber glass bottles (NDC 0163-0402-31).

Oxsoralen Lotion 1% should be stored at room temperature (15–30°C) (59–86°F).

RVP® OINTMENT
(Red Petrolatum-ELDER)

COMPOSITION

Red petrolatum, paraben and lanolin-free sunscreen. Now improved with 2.5% surfactants for easier application and easier removal with soap and water.

ACTION AND USE

Topical sunscreen. Absorbs erythemal spectrum through 340 nanometers, but allows the tanning rays to pass. RVP gives sun protection and sun tanning when applied before sun exposure in the thinnest possible film.

Resists water and perspiration; safe around the eyes and on the lips.

HOW SUPPLIED

2 ounce tube (NDC 0163-0384-02).

RVP should be stored at room temperature (15–30°C) (59–86°F).

RVPaba® LIP STICK
5% ParaAminobenzoic Acid (PABA) + Red Petrolatum (RVP)

ACTIONS AND USES

RVPaba LIP STICK is a topical sunscreen and protectant for lips and small areas of exposed dermis. ParaAminobenzoic Acid (Paba) in Red Petrolatum (RVP) absorbs burning UV in a wide spectrum. Protects against sunburn, windburn and chapping winter or summer. RVPaba LIP STICK contains no perfumes or colors.

DOSAGE AND ADMINISTRATION

Apply to lips and other sensitive areas of the face and hands before exposure to the sun. Reapply as needed.

CAUTION

Individuals sensitive to Paba should not use RVPaba LIP STICK.

SUPPLY

1/7 oz. lipstick tubes (NDC 0163-0505-41).

Military—Cold Climate Stock #6508-00-116-1479. Hot Climate Stock #6508-00-116-1473.

RVPaba should be stored at room temperature (15–30°C) (59–86°F).

RVPaque® OINTMENT
[r-v-pāk']
(Physical Sunscreen)

COMPOSITION

Red petrolatum, zinc oxide, and 2-ethoxyethyl p-methoxycinnamate in a greaseless, water-resistant base.

ACTIONS AND USES

Unlike chemical sunscreens, RVPaque functions by reflecting instead of absorbing incident solar radiation. It therefore provides a significant barrier to a wide range of solar wavelengths including visible light. Tinted to blend with most skin tones.

INDICATIONS

RVPaque provides extra sun protection in any condition in which ultraviolet and visible light are contraindicated. It may be used adjunctively with depigmenting and skin bleaching agents.

TO USE

Apply in a uniformly thin film which is visible to areas requiring exclusion of light. Reapply if removed by abrasion.

CONTRAINDICATIONS

None reported; discontinue use if reaction develops.

HOW SUPPLIED

½ ounce (NDC 0163-0397-35) and 1¼ ounce tubes (NDC 0163-0397-34).

RVPaque should be stored at room temperature (15–30°C) (59–86°F).

SOLAQUIN FORTE® 4% Cream ℞
[sōl'a-kwin" for'tā]
(HYDROQUINONE USP, 4%)
Skin Bleaching Cream with Sunscreens

CAUTION: FEDERAL (U.S.A.) LAW PROHIBITS DISPENSING WITHOUT PRESCRIPTION.
FOR EXTERNAL USE ONLY.

DESCRIPTION

Each gram of Solaquin Forte contains 40 mg hydroquinone, 50 mg ethyl dihydroxypropyl-p-aminobenzoate, 30 mg dioxybenzone USP and 20 mg oxybenzone USP in a vanishing cream base of purified water, glyceryl monostearate, octyldodecyl stearoyl stearate, glyceryl dilaurate, quaternium-26, coceth-6, stearyl alcohol, diethylaminoethyl stearate, dimethicone, polysorbate-80, lactic acid, ascorbic acid, hydroxyethylcellulose, quaternium-14, myristylkonium chloride, disodium EDTA, and sodium metabisulfite.

CLINICAL PHARMACOLOGY

Topical application of hydroquinone produces a reversible depigmentation of the skin by inhibition of the enzymatic oxidation of tyrosine to 3, 4-dihy- droxyphenylalanine (dopa) and suppression of other melanocyte metabolic processes. Exposure to sunlight or ultraviolet light will cause repigmentation which may be prevented by the broad spectrum sunscreen agents contained in Solaquin Forte.

INDICATIONS AND USAGE

Solaquin Forte 4% Cream is indicated for the gradual bleaching of hyperpigmented skin conditions such as chloasma, melasma, freckles, senile lentigines, and other unwanted areas of melanin hyperpigmentation.

CONTRAINDICATIONS

Prior history of sensitivity or allergic reaction to this product or any of its ingredients. The safety of topical hydroquinone use during pregnancy or in children (12 years and under) has not been established.

WARNINGS

A. CAUTION: Hydroquinone is a skin bleaching agent which may produce unwanted cosmetic effects if not used as directed. The physician should be familiar with the contents of this insert before prescribing or dispensing this medication.
B. Test for skin sensitivity before using Solaquin Forte 4% Cream by applying a small amount to an unbroken patch of skin and check in 24 hours. Minor redness is not a contraindication, but where there is itching or vesicle formation or excessive inflammatory response further treatment is not advised. Close patient supervision is recommended. Contact with the eyes should be avoided. If no bleaching or lightening effect is noted after 2 months of treatment use, Solaquin Forte 4% Cream should be discontinued. Solaquin Forte 4% Cream is formulated for use as a skin bleaching agent and should not be used for the prevention of sunburn.
C. Sunscreen use is an essential aspect of hydroquinone therapy because even minimal sunlight exposure sustains melanocytic activity. The sunscreens in Solaquin Forte 4% Cream provide the necessary sun protection during skin bleaching therapy. After clearing and during maintenance therapy, sun exposure should be avoided on bleached skin by application of a sunscreen or sunblock agent or protective clothing to prevent repigmentation.
D. Keep this and all medication out of the reach of children. In case of accidental ingestion, call a physician or a poison control center immediately.

PRECAUTIONS

SEE WARNINGS.

A. Pregnancy Category C. Animal reproduction studies have not been conducted with topical hydroquinone. It is also not known whether hydroquinone can cause fetal harm when used topically on a pregnant woman or affect reproductive capacity. It is not known to what degree, if any, topical hydroquinone is absorbed systemically. Topical hydroquinone should be used in pregnant women only when clearly indicated.
B. Nursing mothers. It is not known whether topical hydroquinone is absorbed or excreted in human milk. Caution is advised when topical hydroquinone is used by a nursing mother.
C. Pediatric usage. Safety and effectiveness in children below the age of 12 years have not been established.

ADVERSE REACTIONS

No systemic adverse reactions have been reported. Occasional hypersensitivity (localized contact dermatitis) may occur in which case the medication should be discontinued and the physician notified immediately.

OVERDOSAGE

There have been no systemic reactions from the use of topical hydroquinone in Solaquin Forte. However, treatment should be limited to relatively small areas of the body at one time since some patients experience a transient skin reddening and a mild burning sensation which does not preclude treatment.

DRUG DOSAGE AND ADMINISTRATION

Solaquin Forte 4% Cream should be applied to the affected area and rubbed in well twice daily or as directed by a physician. There is no recommended dosage for children under 12 years of age except under the advice and supervision of a physician.

HOW SUPPLIED

SOLAQUIN FORTE 4% Cream is available as follows:

Size	NDC Number
0.5 ounce tube (15 grams)	0163-0396-35
1.0 ounce tube (30 grams)	0163-0396-31

Available without prescription for maintenance therapy: Solaquin (2% Hydroquinone) in 1 ounce tubes (NDC 0163-0372-31).

Solaquin Forte 4% Cream should be stored at room temperature (15–30°C) (59–86°F).

SOLAQUIN FORTE® 4% GEL ℞
[sōl'a-kwin for'tā]
(Hydroquinone USP, 4%)
Skin Bleaching Gel with Sunscreens

CAUTION: FEDERAL (U.S.A.) LAW PROHIBITS DISPENSING WITHOUT A PRESCRIPTION.
FOR EXTERNAL USE ONLY

DESCRIPTION

Each gram of Solaquin Forte 4% Gel contains 40 mg of Hydroquinone, 50 mg Ethyl Dihydroxypropyl-p-aminobenzoate and 30 mg Dioxybenzone in a hydroalcoholic base of alcohol, purified water, propylene glycol, tetrahydroxypropyl ethylenediamine, carbomer 940, disodium EDTA and sodium metabisulfite.

CLINICAL PHARMACOLOGY

Topical application of hydroquinone produces a reversible depigmentation of the skin by inhibition of the enzymatic oxidation of tyrosine to 3,4-dihydroxyphenylalanine (dopa) and suppression of other melanocyte metabolic processes. Exposure to sunlight or ultraviolet light will cause repigmentation which may be prevented by the broad spectrum sunscreen agents contained in Solaquin Forte 4% Gel.

INDICATIONS AND USAGE

Solaquin Forte 4% Gel is indicated for the gradual bleaching of hyperpigmented skin conditions such as chloasma, melasma, freckles, senile lentigines and other unwanted areas of melanin hyperpigmentation.

CONTRAINDICATIONS

Prior history of sensitivity or allergic reaction to this product or any of its ingredients. The safety of topical hydroquinone use during pregnancy or in children (12 years and under) has not been established.

Continued on next page

Elder—Cont.

WARNINGS

A. CAUTION: Hydroquinone is a skin bleaching agent which may produce unwanted cosmetic effects if not used as directed. The physician should be familiar with the contents of this insert before prescribing or dispensing this medication.

B. Test for skin sensitivity before using Solaquin Forte 4% Gel by applying a small amount to an unbroken patch of skin and check in 24 hours. Minor redness is not a contraindication, but where there is itching or vesicle formation or excessive inflammatory response further treatment is not advised. Close patient supervision is recommended. Contact with the eyes should be avoided. If no bleaching or lightening effect is noted after 2 months of treatment use, Solaquin Forte 4% Gel should be discontinued. Solaquin Forte 4% Gel is formulated for use as a skin bleaching agent and should not be used for the prevention of sunburn.

C. Sunscreen use is an essential aspect of hydroquinone therapy because even minimal sunlight sustains melanocytic activity. The sunscreens in Solaquin Forte 4% Gel provide the necessary sun protection during skin bleaching therapy. After clearing and during maintenance therapy, sun exposure should be avoided on bleached skin by application of a sunscreen or sunblock agent or protective clothing to prevent repigmentation.

D. Keep this and all medication out of the reach of children. In case of accidental ingestion, call a physician or a poison control center immediately.

PRECAUTIONS

SEE WARNINGS

A. Pregnancy Category C. Animal reproduction studies have not been conducted with topical hydroquinone. It is also not known whether hydroquinone can cause fetal harm when used topically on a pregnant woman or affect reproductive capacity. It is not known to what degree, if any, topical hydroquinone is absorbed systemically. Topical hydroquinone should be used in pregnant women only when clearly indicated.

B. Nursing mothers. It is not known whether topical hydroquinone is absorbed or excreted in human milk. Caution is advised when topical hydroquinone is used by a nursing mother.

C. Pediatric usage. Safety and effectiveness in children below the age of 12 years have not been established.

ADVERSE REACTIONS

No systemic adverse reactions have been reported. Occasional hypersensitivity (localized contact dermatitis) may occur in which case the medication should be discontinued and the physician notified immediately.

OVERDOSAGE

There have been no systemic reactions from the use of topical hydroquinone in Solaquin Forte 4% Gel. However, treatment should be limited to relatively small areas of the body at one time since some patients experience a transient skin reddening and a mild burning sensation which does not preclude treatment.

DRUG DOSAGE AND ADMINISTRATION

Solaquin Forte 4% Gel should be applied to the affected area and rubbed in well twice daily or as directed by a physician. There is no recommended dosage for children under 12 years of age except under the advice and supervision of a physician.

HOW SUPPLIED

SOLAQUIN FORTE 4% Gel is available as follows:

Size	NDC Number
0.5 ounce tube (15 grams)	0163-0523-35
1.0 ounce tube (30 grams)	0163-0523-31

Solaquin Forte 4% Gel should be stored at room temperature (15–30°C) (59–86°F).

TRISORALEN® TABLETS ℞

[*trī'sore"a-len*]

(Trioxsalen USP, 5 mg)

To facilitate repigmentation in vitiligo, increase tolerance to solar exposure and enhance pigmentation.

Caution: *THIS IS A POTENT DRUG.*

CAUTION

Federal (U.S.A.) law prohibits dispensing without prescription.

DESCRIPTION

Trisoralen Tablets 5 mg.

TRISORALEN (trioxsalen) is the first synthetic psoralen compound made available to the medical profession. It possesses greater activity than Methoxsalen, yet the LD 50 of (trioxsalen) is six times that of Methoxsalen.

Contains color additives including FD&C Yellow No. 5 (Tartrazine).

ACTIONS

Pigment formation with TRISORALEN.

The normal pigmentation of the skin is due to melanin which is produced in the cytoplasm of the melanocytes located in the basal layers of the epidermis at its junction with the dermis. Melanin is formed by the oxidation of tyrosine to DOPA (Dihydroxyphenylalanine) with tyrosinase as catalyst. This enzymatic reaction, however, must be activated by radiant energy in the form of ultraviolet light, preferably between 2900 and 3800 angstroms (black light).

The exact mechanism of the action of psoralens in the process of melanogenesis is not known. One group of investigators feel that the psoralens have a specific effect on the epidermis or, more specifically, on the melanocytes. Another group feels that the primary response to the psoralens is an inflammatory one and that the process of melanogenesis is secondary.

INDICATIONS

TRISORALEN taken approximately two hours before measured periods of exposure to ultraviolet facilitates:

1. Repigmentation of idiopathic vitiligo. Repigmentation, not equally reversible in every patient, will vary in completeness, time of onset, and duration. The rate of completeness of pigmentation with respect to locations of lesions, occurs more rapidly on fleshy regions, such as the face, abdomen, and buttocks, and less rapidly over bony areas such as the dorsum of the hands and feet. Repigmentation may begin after a few weeks; however, significant results may take as long as six to nine months, and repigmentation, at the optimum level, may, in some cases, require maintenance dosage to retain the new pigment. If follicular repigmentation is not apparent after three months of daily treatment, treatment should be discontinued as a failure.

2. Increasing tolerance to sunlight. In blond persons and those with fair complexions who suffer painful reactions when exposed to sunlight, TRISORALEN aids in increasing resistance to solar damage. Certain persons who are allergic to sunlight or exhibit sun sensitivity may be benefited by the protective action of TRISORALEN. In albinism, TRISORALEN will increase the tolerance of the skin to sunlight, although no pigment is formed. This protective action seems to be related to the thickening of the horny layer and retention of melanin which produces a thickened melanized stratum corneum and formation of a stratum lucidum.

3. Enhancing pigmentation. The use of TRISORALEN accelerates pigmentation only when the administration of the drug is followed by exposure of the skin to sunlight or ultraviolet irradiation. The increase in pigmentation is not immediate but occurs gradually within a few days of repeated exposure and may become equivalent in a degree to that achieved by a full summer of sun exposure. Since sufficient pigment will have been formed within two weeks of continuous therapy, the use of TRISORALEN should not be continued beyond this period. Pigmentation can be maintained by periodic exposure to sunlight.

CONTRAINDICATIONS

In those diseases associated with photosensitivity, such as porphyria, acute lupus erythematosus, or leukoderma of infectious origin. To date, the safety of this drug in young persons (12 and under), has not been established and is, therefore contraindicated. No preparation with any photosensitizing capacity, internal or external should be used concomitantly with TRISORALEN therapy.

WARNINGS

TRISORALEN IS A POTENT DRUG.

Read entire brochure before prescribing or dispensing this medication. The dosage of this medication should not be increased.

The dosage of TRISORALEN and exposure time should not be increased. Overdosage and/or overexposure may result in serious burning and blistering. When used to increase tolerance to sunlight or accelerate tanning, TRISORALEN total dosage should not exceed 28 tablets, taken in daily single doses of two tablets on a continuous or interrupted regimen. To prevent harmful effects, the physician should carefully instruct the patient to adhere to the prescribed dosage schedule and procedure.

PRECAUTIONS

Accidental Overdosage:

If an overdose of TRISORALEN or ultraviolet light has been taken, emesis should be encouraged. The individual should be kept in a darkened room for eight hours or until cutaneous reactions subside. The treatment for severe reactions resulting from overdosage or over-exposure should follow accepted procedures for treatment of severe burns. There have not been any clinical reports or tests to verify that more severe reactions may result from the concomitant ingestion of furocoumarin-containing food while on TRISORALEN therapy; but the physician should warn the patient that taking limes, figs, parsley, parsnips, mustard, carrots and celery, might be dangerous.

This product contains FD&C Yellow No. 5 (Tartrazine) as a color additive, which may cause allergic-type reactions (including bronchial asthma) in certain susceptible individuals. Although the overall incidence of FD&C Yellow No. 5 (Tartrazine) sensitivity is low, it is frequently seen in patients who also have aspirin hypersensitivity.

ADVERSE REACTIONS AND SIDE EFFECTS

Severe burns can result from excessive sunlight or sun lamp ultraviolet exposure.

Occasionally, there may occur gastric discomfort; to minimize this gastric effect, the tablets may be taken with milk or after a meal. Some patients who are unable to tolerate 10 mg. will tolerate 5 mg. This dosage produces the same therapeutic effect but more slowly.

DOSAGE

(Adults and children over 12 years of age)

VITILIGO: Two tablets daily, taken two to four hours before measured periods of ultraviolet exposure or fluorescent black light. (See suggested sun exposure guide.)

To increase tolerance to sunlight and/or enhance pigmentation: Two tablets daily, taken two hours before measured periods of exposure to sun or ultraviolet irradiation. Not to be continued for longer than 14 days. The dosage should NOT be increased, as severe burning may occur. (See suggested sun exposure guide.)

SUGGESTED SUN EXPOSURE GUIDE

The exposure time to sunlight should be limited according to the following plan:

	Basic Skin Color	
	Light	Medium
Initial Exposure	15 min.	20 min.
Second Exposure	20 min.	25 min.
Third Exposure	25 min.	30 min.
Fourth Exposure	30 min.	35 min.
Subsequent Exposure:	Gradually increase exposure based on erythema and tenderness.	

Sunglasses should be worn during exposure and the lips protected with a light-screening lipstick.

SUN-LAMP EXPOSURE: Should be initiated according to directions of the sun-lamp manufacturer.

HOW SUPPLIED

TRISORALEN Tablets 5 mg. in bottles of 28 (NDC 0163-0303-28) and 100 (NDC 0163-0303-01).

Military—TRIOXSALEN Tablets 5 mg. stock # 6505-00-560-7022.

Trisoralen should be stored at room temperature (15–30°C) (59–86°F).

Shown in Product Identification Section, page 409

VITADYE® LOTION

[*vīta 'dī*]

(Cosmetic Cover for hypopigmented skin)

COMPOSITION

Dihydroxyacetone (5%), water, isopropyl alcohol, acetone, sodium metabisulfite, disodium edetate. FD&C yellow #5, FD&C red #40, FD&C blue #1.

USE

To cover light colored or white patches of skin. For external use only.

ADMINISTRATION

Use the applicator and apply Vitadye to affected skin areas as often as necessary. To obtain darker shades repeated applications may be necessary. Allow previous applications to dry before reapplying.

Concomitant Therapy: Vitadye transmits most UVA radiation so it can be used concurrently with psoralens in vitiligo therapy.

PRECAUTION

If rash or irritation of the skin develops, discontinue use and contact a physician. Avoid contact with the eyes. Avoid flame. VITADYE will stain, avoid contact with clothing until dry.

WARNING

Keep this and all drugs out of the reach of children. In case of accidental ingestion, seek professional assistance or contact a poison control center immediately. Avoid open flame.

HOW SUPPLIED

Vitadye is available in ½ fluid ounce (NDC 0163-0413-35) and 2 fluid ounce (NDC 0163-0413-02) packages.

Vitadye should be stored at room temperature (15–30°C) (59–86°F).

Elkins-Sinn, Inc.

A subsidiary of A. H. Robins Company
2 ESTERBROOK LANE
CHERRY HILL, NJ 08003-4099

Elkins-Sinn's DOSETTE® line offers a broad spectrum of injectable products in a variety of unit-of-use containers—DOSETTE vials, DOSETTE ampuls, and DOSETTE syringes. Easily adaptable to any hospital pharmacy set-up, the DOSETTE system combines easily identifiable, clearly printed product labeling with space-conserving packaging. Each DOSETTE container is characterized by product name and strength in large, bold-faced type, important usage and storage data, lot identification number, and expiration date. Elkins-Sinn also produces a vast number of multiple dose vials. Listed below are some major ESI products. For a complete catalog and price list, direct inquiries to Marketing Services. For specific product information, direct inquiries to the Professional Services Department.

DOSETTE® SYRINGES

Dexamethasone Sodium Phosphate Injection, USP
4 mg/1 ml
10 mg/1ml
Diazepam Injection, USP
5 mg/1 mL
10 mg/2 mL
Gentamicin Sulfate Injection, USP
60 mg/1.5 ml
80 mg/2 ml
Hydroxyzine Hydrochloride Intramuscular Injection
25 mg/1 ml
50 mg/1 ml
100 mg/2 ml

DOSETTE® VIALS

Aminophylline Injection, USP
250 mg/10 ml
500 mg/20 ml
Atropine Sulfate Injection, USP
400 mcg/1ml (0.4 mg, 1/150 gr)
1.0 mg/1 ml
1.2 mg/1 ml
Bretylium Tosylate Injection
500 mg/10 mL
Codeine Phosphate Injection, USP
30 mg/1 ml
60 mg/1 ml
Cyanocobalamin Injection, USP (Vit. B-12)
1 mg/1 ml (1000 mcg)
Dexamethasone Sodium Phosphate Injection, USP
4 mg/1 ml
10 mg/1 ml
Dexpanthenol Injection
500 mg/2 ml
Dextrose Injection, USP
50%-50 ml
Diazepam Injection, USP
5 mg/1 mL
10 mg/2 mL
Diphenhydramine Hydrochloride Injection, USP
50 mg/1 ml
Dopamine Hydrochloride Injection
200 mg/5 ml
400 mg/5 ml
Doxycycline Hyclate for Injection, USP
100 mg
200 mg
Furosemide Injection, USP
20 mg/2 ml
40 mg/4 ml
100 mg/10 ml
Gentamicin Sulfate Injection, USP
20 mg/2 ml (Pediatric)
80 mg/2 ml
Heparin Sodium Injection, USP
1000 USP units/ml-1 ml and 2 ml
5000 USP units/1 ml
10,000 USP units/1 ml
Hep-Lock U/P (Preservative-Free Heparin Lock Flush Solution, USP)
10 USP units/1ml
100 USP units/1ml
Hep-Lock® (Heparin Lock Flush Solution, USP)
10 USP units/ml-1ml and 2 ml
100 USP units/ml-1ml and 2 ml
Hydromorphone Hydrochloride Injection, USP
2 mg/1 ml
Hydroxyzine Hydrochloride Intramuscular Injection
25 mg/1 ml
50 mg/1 ml
75 mg/1.5 ml
100 mg/2 ml
Lidocaine Hydrochloride Injection, USP
1%-2 ml
2%-2 ml
Lidocaine Hydrochloride Injection, USP (Preservative-free)
1%-5 ml
2%-5 ml
Lidocaine Hydrochloride Injection for Intravenous Use in Cardiac Arrhythmias
50 mg/5 ml
100 mg/5 ml
1 gram/25 ml
2 grams/50 ml
Meperidine Hydrochloride Injection, USP
25 mg/1 ml
50 mg/1 ml
75 mg/1 ml
100 mg/1 ml
Mineral Oil, Sterile Light
10 ml
30 ml
Morphine Sulfate Injection, USP
5 mg/1 ml (1/12 gr)
8 mg/1 ml (1/8 gr)
10 mg/1 ml (1/6 gr)
15 mg/1 ml (1/4 gr)
Naloxone Hydrochloride Injection, USP
400 mcg/1 ml (0.4 mg)
Pentobarbital Sodium Injection, USP
100 mg/2 ml
Phenobarbital Sodium Injection, USP
65 mg/1 ml
130 mg/1 ml
Phenytoin Sodium Injection, USP
100 mg/2 ml
250 mg/5 ml
Scopolamine Hydrobromide Injection, USP
400 mcg/1 ml (0.4 mg, 1/150 gr)
Sodium Chloride Injection, USP (Preservative-free)
0.9%-2 ml
Sodium Nitroprusside (Sterile), USP
50 mg
Thiamine Hydrochloride Injection, USP
100 mg/1 ml
Vials, Sterile Empty
2 ml

DOSETTE® AMPULS

Aminophylline Injection, USP
250 mg/10 ml
500 mg/20 ml
Atropine Sulfate Injection, USP
400 mcg/1 ml (0.4 mg, 1/150 gr)
400 mcg/0.5 ml (0.4 mg, 1/150 gr)
Bretylium Tosylate Injection
500 mg/10 mL
Calcium Chloride Injection, USP
10% 1 gram/10 mL
Calcium Gluconate Injection, USP
10% 1 gram/10 mL
Chlorpromazine Hydrochloride Injection, USP
25 mg/1 ml
50 mg/2 ml
Cyanocobalamin Injection, USP (Vit. B-12)
1 mg/1 ml (1000 mcg)
Diazepam Injection, USP
10 mg/2 mL
Digoxin Injection, USP
0.5 mg/2 ml
Dopamine Hydrochloride Injection
200 mg/5 ml
400 mg/5 ml
Duramorph® (morphine sulfate injection, USP) Preservative-Free
5 mg/10 ml
10 mg/10 ml
Epinephrine Injection, USP
1 mg/1 ml (1:1000)
Fentanyl Citrate Injection, USP
100 mcg/2 ml
250 mcg/5 ml
500 mcg/10 ml
1 mg/20 ml
Furosemide Injection, USP
20 mg/2 ml
40 mg/4 ml
100 mg/10 ml
Isoproterenol Hydrochloride Injection, USP
1 mg/5 ml (1:5000)
Magnesium Sulfate Injection, USP
50% 1 gram/2 ml
Meperidine Hydrochloride Injection, USP
25 mg/1 ml
50 mg/1 ml
75 mg/1 ml
100 mg/1 ml
Methylene Blue Injection, USP
1%-10 ml
Morphine Sulfate Injection, USP
8 mg/1 ml (1/8 gr)
10 mg/1 ml (1/6 gr)
15 mg/1 ml (1/4 gr)
Naloxone Hydrochloride Injection, USP
400 mcg/1 ml (0.4 mg)
Paraldehyde Sterile, USP
5 ml
Phenytoin Sodium Injection, USP
100 mg/2 ml
250 mg/5 ml
Potassium Chloride Injection, USP
20 mEq/10 ml
40 mEq/20 ml
Prochlorperazine Edisylate Injection, USP
10 mg/2 ml
Promethazine Hydrochloride Injection, USP
25 mg/1 ml
50 mg/1 ml
Sodium Chloride Injection, USP (Preservative-free)
0.9%-5 ml
0.9%-10 ml
Sotradecol® (Sodium Tetradecyl Sulfate)
1%-2 ml
3%-2 ml
Water for Injection, Sterile, USP (Preservative-free)
5 ml
10 ml

MULTIPLE DOSE VIALS

Aminocaproic Acid Injection, USP
250 mg/ml-20 ml
Atropine Sulfate Injection, USP
400 mcg/ml (0.4 mg, 1/150 gr)-20 ml
Chlorpromazine Hydrochloride Injection, USP
25 mg/ml-10 ml
Cyanocobalamin Injection, USP (Vit. B-12)
1 mg/ml (1000 mcg)-10 ml and 30 ml
Dexamethasone Sodium Phosphate Injection, USP
4 mg/ml-5 ml and 25 ml
10 mg/ml-10 ml
Diazepam Injection, USP
5 mg/mL-10 mL
Erythromycin Lactobionate for Injection, USP
500 mg
1 gram
500 mg Piggyback
Gentamicin Sulfate Injection, USP
40 mg/ml-20 ml
Heparin Sodium Injection, USP
1000 USP units/ml-10 ml and 30 ml
5000 USP units/ml-10 ml
10,000 USP units/ml-4 ml
Hep-Lock® (Heparin Lock Flush Solution, USP)
10 USP units/ml-10 ml and 30 ml
100 USP units/ml-10 ml and 30 ml
Hydrocortisone Sodium Succinate For Injection, USP
100 mg
250 mg
500 mg
1000 mg (1 gram)
Hydroxyzine Hydrochloride Intramuscular Injection
50 mg/ml-10 ml
Lidocaine Hydrochloride Injection, USP
1%-30 ml and 50 ml
2%-30 ml and 50 ml
Lidocaine Hydrochloride and Epinephrine 1:100,000 Injection, USP
1%-30 ml
2%-30 ml
Methylprednisolone Sodium Succinate for Injection, USP
40 mg
125 mg
500 mg
1000 mg (1 gram)
Morphine Sulfate Injection, USP
10 mg/mL-10 mL
15 mg/mL-20 mL
Naloxone Hydrochloride Injection, USP
400 mcg/1 mL (0.4 mg)—10 mL
Neostigmine Methylsulfate Injection, USP
1:1000 (1 mg/1 ml)-10 ml
Potassium Chloride Injection, USP
2 mEq/ml-30 ml
Procaine Hydrochloride Injection, USP
1%-30 ml
2%-30 ml
Sodium Chloride Injection, Bacteriostatic, USP
0.9%-30 ml

Continued on next page

Elkins-Sinn—Cont.

Vials, Sterile Empty
- 2 ml
- 5 ml
- 10 ml
- 30 ml

Water for Injection, Bacteriostatic, USP
- 30 ml

PIGGYBACK VIALS

Erythromycin Lactobionate for Injection, USP
- 500 mg

Metronidazole Redi Infusion™ (Preservative-Free, Single Use)
- 500 mg/100 mL (With IV set)
- 500 mg/100 mL (w/o IV set)

DURAMORPH® Ⓒ
[dūr″a′mŏrf]
(morphine sulfate injection, USP)
Preservative-Free

PRODUCT OVERVIEW

KEY FACTS

Preservative-free DURAMORPH® is a sterile, pyrogen-free, isobaric solution free of antioxidants, preservatives or other potentially neurotoxic additives, and is intended for intravenous, epidural or intrathecal administration as a narcotic analgesic.

MAJOR USES

DURAMORPH® is used for the management of pain not responsive to non-narcotic analgesics. Administered epidurally or intrathecally, it provides pain relief for extended periods without attendant loss of motor, sensory or sympathetic function.

SAFETY INFORMATION

The most serious side effect is respiratory depression. When administered epidurally or intrathecally, patient monitoring should be continued for at least 24 hours after each dose since delayed respiratory depression may occur.

PRESCRIBING INFORMATION

DURAMORPH® Ⓒ
[dūr″a′mŏrf]
(morphine sulfate injection, USP)
Preservative-Free

DESCRIPTION

Morphine is the most important alkaloid of opium and is a phenanthrene derivative. It is available as the sulfate, having the following structural formula:

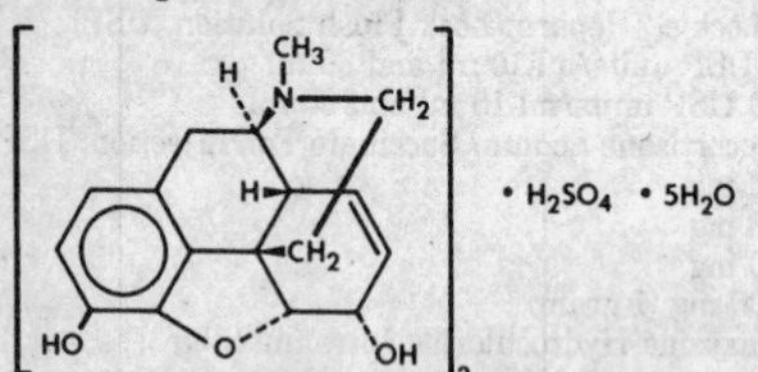

7,8 Didehydro-4,5-epoxy-17-methyl-(5α,6α)-morphinan-3,6-diol sulfate (2:1) (salt), pentahydrate

Preservative-free DURAMORPH® (Morphine Sulfate Injection, USP) is a sterile, pyrogen-free, isobaric solution free of antioxidants, preservatives or other potentially neurotoxic additives, and is intended for intravenous, epidural or intrathecal administration as a narcotic analgesic. Each milliliter contains morphine sulfate 0.5 mg or 1 mg (Warning: May Be Habit Forming) and sodium chloride 9 mg in Water for Injection. pH range is 2.5–6.0. Ampuls are sealed under nitrogen. Each Dosette® ampul is intended for SINGLE USE ONLY. Discard any unused portion. DO NOT AUTOCLAVE.

CLINICAL PHARMACOLOGY

Morphine exerts its primary effects on the central nervous system and organs containing smooth muscle. Pharmacologic effects include analgesia, drowsiness, alteration in mood (euphoria), reduction in body temperature (at low doses), dose-related depression of respiration, interference with adrenocortical response to stress (at high doses), reduction in peripheral resistance with little or no effect on cardiac index and miosis.

Morphine, as other opioids, acts as an agonist interacting with stereospecific and saturable binding sites/receptors in the brain, spinal cord and other tissues. These sites have been classified as μ receptors and are widely distributed throughout the central nervous system being present in highest concentration in the limbic system (frontal and temporal cortex, amygdala and hippocampus), thalamus, striatum, hypothalamus, midbrain and laminae I, II, IV and V of the dorsal horn in the spinal cord. It has been postulated that exogenously administered morphine exerts its analgesic effect, in part, by altering the central release of neurotransmitter from afferent nerves sensitive to noxious stimuli. Peripheral threshold or responsiveness to noxious stimuli is unaffected leaving monosynaptic reflexes such as the patellar or the Achilles tendon reflex intact.

Autonomic reflexes are not affected by epidural or intrathecal morphine, however morphine exerts spasmogenic effects on the gastrointestinal tract that result in decreased peristaltic activity.

Central nervous system effects of intravenously administered morphine sulfate are influenced by ability to cross the blood-brain barrier.

The delay in the onset of analgesia following epidural or intrathecal injection may be attributed to its relatively poor lipid solubility (i.e., an oil/water partition coefficient of 1.42), and its slow access to the receptor sites. The hydrophilic character of morphine may also explain its retention in the CNS and its slow release into the systemic circulation, resulting in a prolonged effect.

Nausea and vomiting may be prominent and are thought to be the result of central stimulation of the chemoreceptor trigger zone. Histamine release is common; allergic manifestations of urticaria and, rarely, anaphylaxis may occur. Bronchoconstriction may occur either as an idiosyncratic reaction or from large dosages.

Approximately one-third of intravenous morphine is bound to plasma proteins. Free morphine is rapidly redistributed in parenchymatous tissues. The major metabolic pathway is through conjugation with glucuronic acid in the liver. Elimination half-life is approximately 1.5 to 2 hours in healthy volunteers. For intravenously administered morphine, 90% is excreted in the urine within 24 hours and traces are detectable in urine up to 48 hours. About 7-10% of administered morphine eventually appears in the feces as conjugated morphine.

Peak serum levels following epidural or intrathecal administration of DURAMORPH® are reached within 30 minutes in most subjects and decline to very low levels during the next 2 to 4 hours. The onset of action occurs in 15 to 60 minutes following epidural administration or intrathecal administration; analgesia may last up to 24 hours. Due to this extended duration of action, sustained pain relief can be provided with lower daily doses (by these two routes) than are usually required with intravenous or intramuscular morphine administration.

INDICATIONS AND USAGE

Preservative-free DURAMORPH® is a systemic narcotic analgesic for administration by the intravenous, epidural or intrathecal routes. It is used for the management of pain not responsive to non-narcotic analgesics. Morphine sulfate, administered epidurally or intrathecally, provides pain relief for extended periods without attendant loss of motor, sensory or sympathetic function.

CONTRAINDICATIONS

DURAMORPH® is contraindicated in those medical conditions which would preclude the administration of opioids by the intravenous route—allergy to morphine or other opiates, acute bronchial asthma, upper airway obstruction.

Administration of morphine by the epidural or intrathecal route is contraindicated in the presence of infection at the injection site, anticoagulant therapy, bleeding diathesis, parenterally administered corticosteroids within a two week period or other concomitant drug therapy or medical condition which would contraindicate the technique of epidural or intrathecal analgesia.

WARNINGS

DURAMORPH® administration should be limited to use by those familiar with the management of respiratory depression, and in the case of epidural or intrathecal administration, familiar with the techniques and patient management problems associated with epidural or intrathecal drug administration. Because epidural administration has been associated with lessened potential for immediate or late adverse effects than intrathecal administration, the epidural route should be used whenever possible. Rapid intravenous administration may result in chest wall rigidity. FACILITIES WHERE DURAMORPH® IS ADMINISTERED MUST BE EQUIPPED WITH RESUSCITATIVE EQUIPMENT, OXYGEN, NALOXONE INJECTION, AND OTHER RESUSCITATIVE DRUGS. WHEN THE EPIDURAL OR INTRATHECAL ROUTE OF ADMINISTRATION IS EMPLOYED, PATIENTS MUST BE OBSERVED IN A FULLY EQUIPPED AND STAFFED ENVIRONMENT FOR AT LEAST 24 HOURS.

SEVERE RESPIRATORY DEPRESSION UP TO 24 HOURS FOLLOWING EPIDURAL OR INTRATHECAL ADMINISTRATION HAS BEEN REPORTED.

Morphine sulfate may be habit forming. (See Drug Abuse and Dependence section.)

PRECAUTIONS

GENERAL

Preservative-free DURAMORPH® (Morphine Sulfate Injection, USP) should be administered with extreme caution in aged or debilitated patients, in the presence of increased intracranial/intraocular pressure and in patients with head injury. Pupillary changes (miosis) may obscure the course of intracranial pathology. Care is urged in patients who have a decreased respiratory reserve (e.g., emphysema, severe obesity, kyphoscoliosis).

Seizures may result from high doses. Patients with known seizure disorders should be carefully observed for evidence of morphine-induced seizure activity.

It is recommended that administration of DURAMORPH® by the epidural or intrathecal routes be limited to the lumbar area. Intrathecal use has been associated with a higher incidence of respiratory depression than epidural use.

Smooth muscle hypertonicity may result in biliary colic, difficulty in urination and possible urinary retention requiring catheterization. Consideration should be given to risks inherent in urethral catheterization, e.g., sepsis, when epidural or intrathecal administration is considered, especially in the perioperative period.

Elimination half-life may be prolonged in patients with reduced metabolic rates and with hepatic or renal dysfunction. Hence, care should be exercised in administering morphine in these conditions, particularly with repeated dosing.

Patients with reduced circulating blood volume, impaired myocardial function or on sympatholytic drugs should be observed carefully for orthostatic hypotension, particularly in transport.

Patients with chronic obstructive pulmonary disease and patients with acute asthmatic attack may develop acute respiratory failure with administration of morphine. Use in these patients should be reserved for those whose conditions require endotracheal intubation and respiratory support or control of ventilation.

DRUG INTERACTIONS

Depressant effects of morphine are potentiated by either concomitant administration or in the presence of other CNS depressants such as alcohol, sedatives, antihistaminics or psychotropic drugs (e.g., MAO inhibitors, phenothiazines, butyrophenones and tricyclic antidepressants). Premedication or intra-anesthetic use of neuroleptics with morphine may increase the risk of respiratory depression.

CARCINOGENESIS, MUTAGENESIS, IMPAIRMENT OF FERTILITY

Studies of morphine sulfate in animals to evaluate the carcinogenic and mutagenic potential or the effect on fertility have not been conducted.

PREGNANCY

Teratogenic effects—Pregnancy Category C. Animal reproduction studies have not been conducted with morphine. It is also not known whether morphine sulfate can cause fetal harm when administered to a pregnant woman or can affect reproduction capacity. Morphine sulfate should be given to a pregnant woman only if clearly needed.

Nonteratogenic effects. Infants born from mothers who have been taking morphine chronically may exhibit withdrawal symptoms.

LABOR AND DELIVERY

Intravenous morphine readily passes into the fetal circulation and may result in respiratory depression in the neonate. Naloxone and resuscitative equipment should be available for reversal of narcotic-induced respiratory depression in the neonate. In addition, intravenous morphine may reduce the strength, duration and frequency of uterine contraction resulting in prolonged labor.

Epidurally and *intrathecally* administered morphine readily passes into the fetal circulation and may result in respiratory depression of the neonate. Controlled clinical studies have shown that *epidural* administration has little or no effect on the relief of pain.

However, studies have suggested that in most cases 0.2 to 1 mg of morphine *intrathecally* provides adequate pain relief with little effect on the duration of first stage labor. The second stage labor, though, may be prolonged if the parturient is not encouraged to bear down. A continuous intravenous infusion of naloxone, 0.6 mg/hr, for 24 hours after intrathecal injection may be employed to reduce the incidence of potential side effects.

NURSING MOTHERS

Morphine is excreted in maternal milk. Effect on the nursing infant is not known.

PEDIATRIC USE

Safety and effectiveness in children have not been established.

ADVERSE REACTIONS

The most serious side effect is respiratory depression. Because of delay in maximum CNS effect with intravenously administered drug (30 min), rapid administration may result in overdosing. Bolus administration by the epidural or intrathecal route may result in early respiratory depression due to direct venous redistribution of morphine to the respiratory centers in the brain. Late (up to 24 hours) onset of acute respiratory depression has been reported with administration by the epidural or intrathecal route and is believed to be the result of rostral spread. Reports of respiratory depression following intrathecal administration have been more frequent, but the dosage used in most of these cases has been considerably higher than that recommended. This depression may be severe and could require intervention (see Warnings and Overdosage sections). Even without clinical evidence of ventilatory inadequacy, a diminished CO_2 ventilation response may be noted for up to 22 hours following epidural or intrathecal administration.

While low doses of intravenously administered morphine have little effect on cardiovascular stability, high doses are excitatory, resulting from sympathetic hyperactivity and increase in circulating catecholamines. Excitation of the central nervous system resulting in convulsions may accompany high doses of morphine given intravenously. Dysphoric reactions may occur and toxic psychoses have been reported.

Epidural or intrathecal administration is accompanied by a high incidence of pruritus which is dose related but not confined to site of administration. Nausea and vomiting are frequently seen in patients following morphine administration. Urinary retention which may persist for 10-20 hours following single epidural or intrathecal administration has been reported in approximately 90% of males. Incidence is somewhat lower in females. Patients may require catheterization (see Precautions). Pruritus, nausea/vomiting and urinary retention frequently can be alleviated by the intravenous administration of low doses of naloxone (0.2 mg).

Tolerance and dependence to chronically administered morphine, by whatever route, is known to occur (see Drug Abuse and Dependence section).

Miscellaneous side effects include constipation, headache, anxiety, depression of cough reflex, interference with thermal regulation and oliguria. Evidence of histamine release such as urticaria, wheals and/or local tissue irritation may occur.

In general, side effects are amenable to reversal by narcotic antagonists. NALOXONE INJECTION AND RESUSCITATIVE EQUIPMENT SHOULD BE IMMEDIATELY AVAILABLE FOR ADMINISTRATION IN CASE OF LIFE-THREATENING OR INTOLERABLE SIDE EFFECTS.

DRUG ABUSE AND DEPENDENCE

CONTROLLED SUBSTANCE

Morphine sulfate is a Schedule II substance under the Drug Enforcement Administration classification.

ABUSE

Morphine has recognized abuse and dependence potential.

DEPENDENCE

Cerebral and spinal receptors may develop tolerance/dependence independently, as a function of local dosage. Care must be taken to avert withdrawal in those patients who have been maintained on parenteral/oral narcotics when epidural or intrathecal administration is considered. Withdrawal may occur following chronic epidural or intrathecal administration, as well as the development of tolerance to morphine by these routes. (See nonteratogenic effects under Pregnancy.)

OVERDOSAGE

Overdosage is characterized by respiratory depression with or without concomitant CNS depression. Since respiratory arrest may result either through direct depression of the respiratory center or as the result of hypoxia, primary attention should be given to the establishment of adequate respiratory exchange through provision of a patent airway and institution of assisted or controlled ventilation. The narcotic antagonist, naloxone, is a specific antidote. Naloxone (usually 0.4 mg) should be administered intravenously, simultaneously with respiratory resuscitation. *As the duration of effect of naloxone is considerably shorter than that of epidural or intrathecal morphine, repeated administration may be necessary.* Patients should be closely observed for evidence of renarcotization. *Note: Respiratory depression may be delayed in onset up to 24 hours* following epidural or intrathecal administration. In painful conditions, reversal of narcotic effect may result in acute onset of pain and release of catecholamines. Careful administration of naloxone may permit reversal of side effects without affecting analgesia. Parenteral administration of narcotics in patients receiving epidural or intrathecal morphine may result in overdosage.

DOSAGE AND ADMINISTRATION

Preservative-free DURAMORPH® (Morphine Sulfate Injection, USP) is intended for intravenous, epidural or intrathecal administration.

INTRAVENOUS ADMINISTRATION

Dosage: The initial dose of morphine should be 2 mg to 10 mg/70 kg of body weight. Patients under the age of 18; no information available.

EPIDURAL ADMINISTRATION

DURAMORPH® SHOULD BE ADMINISTERED EPIDURALLY ONLY BY PHYSICIANS EXPERIENCED IN THE TECHNIQUES OF EPIDURAL ADMINISTRATION AND WHO ARE THOROUGHLY FAMILIAR WITH THE LABELING. IT SHOULD BE ADMINISTERED ONLY IN SETTINGS WHERE ADEQUATE PATIENT MONITORING IS POSSIBLE. RESUSCITATIVE EQUIPMENT AND A SPECIFIC ANTAGONIST (NALOXONE INJECTION) SHOULD BE IMMEDIATELY AVAILABLE FOR THE MANAGEMENT OF RESPIRATORY DEPRESSION AS WELL AS COMPLICATIONS WHICH MIGHT RESULT FROM INADVERTENT INTRATHECAL OR INTRAVASCULAR INJECTION. [NOTE: INTRATHECAL DOSAGE IS USUALLY 1/10 THAT OF EPIDURAL DOSAGE.] **PATIENT MONITORING SHOULD BE CONTINUED FOR AT LEAST 24 HOURS AFTER EACH DOSE, SINCE DELAYED RESPIRATORY DEPRESSION MAY OCCUR.**

Proper placement of a needle or catheter in the epidural space should be verified before DURAMORPH® is injected. Acceptable techniques for verifying proper placement include: a) aspiration to check for absence of blood or cerebrospinal fluid, or b) administration of 5 mL (3 mL in obstetric patients) of 1.5% UNPRESERVED Lidocaine and Epinephrine (1:200,000) Injection and then observe the patient for lack of tachycardia (this indicates that vascular injection has *not* been made) and lack of sudden onset of segmental anesthesia (this indicates that intrathecal injection has *not* been made.)

Epidural Adult Dosage: Initial injection of 5 mg in the lumbar region may provide satisfactory pain relief for up to 24 hours. If adequate pain relief is not achieved within one hour, careful administration of incremental doses of 1 to 2 mg at intervals sufficient to assess effectiveness may be given. No more than 10 mg/24 hr should be administered.

Thoracic administration has been shown to dramatically increase the incidence of early and late respiratory depression even at doses of 1 to 2 mg.

For continuous infusion an initial dose of 2 to 4 mg/24 hours is recommended. Further doses of 1 to 2 mg may be given if pain relief is not achieved initially.

Aged or debilitated patients—Administer with extreme caution (see Precautions section). Doses of less than 5 mg may provide satisfactory pain relief for up to 24 hours.

Epidural Pediatric Use: No information on use in pediatric patients is available.

INTRATHECAL ADMINISTRATION

NOTE: INTRATHECAL DOSAGE IS USUALLY 1/10 THAT OF EPIDURAL DOSAGE.

DURAMORPH® SHOULD BE ADMINISTERED INTRATHECALLY ONLY BY PHYSICIANS EXPERIENCED IN THE TECHNIQUES OF INTRATHECAL ADMINISTRATION AND WHO ARE THOROUGHLY FAMILIAR WITH THE LABELING. IT SHOULD BE ADMINISTERED ONLY IN SETTINGS WHERE ADEQUATE PATIENT MONITORING IS POSSIBLE. RESUSCITATIVE EQUIPMENT AND A SPECIFIC ANTAGONIST (NALOXONE INJECTION) SHOULD BE IMMEDIATELY AVAILABLE FOR THE MANAGEMENT OF RESPIRATORY DEPRESSION AS WELL AS COMPLICATIONS WHICH MIGHT RESULT FROM INADVERTENT INTRAVASCULAR INJECTION. **PATIENT MONITORING SHOULD BE CONTINUED FOR AT LEAST 24 HOURS AFTER EACH DOSE, SINCE DELAYED RESPIRATORY DEPRESSION MAY OCCUR.** RESPIRATORY DEPRESSION (BOTH EARLY AND LATE ONSET) HAS OCCURRED MORE FREQUENTLY FOLLOWING INTRATHECAL ADMINISTRATION.

Intrathecal Adult Dosage: A single injection of 0.2 to 1 mg may provide satisfactory pain relief for up to 24 hours. (CAUTION: THIS IS ONLY 0.4 TO 2 ML OF THE 5 MG/10 ML AMPUL OR 0.2 TO 1 ML OF THE 10 MG/10 ML AMPUL OF DURAMORPH®.) DO NOT INJECT INTRATHECALLY MORE THAN 2 ML OF THE 5 MG/10 ML AMPUL OR 1 ML OF THE 10 MG/10 ML AMPUL. USE IN THE LUMBAR AREA ONLY IS RECOMMENDED. Repeated intrathecal injections of DURAMORPH® are not recommended. A constant intravenous infusion of naloxone, 0.6 mg/hr, for 24 hours after intrathecal injection may be used to reduce the incidence of potential side effects.

Aged or debilitated patients—Administer with extreme caution (see Precautions section). A lower dosage is usually satisfactory.

Repeat Dosage: If pain recurs, alternative routes of administration should be considered, since experience with repeated doses of morphine by the intrathecal route is limited.

Intrathecal Pediatric Use: No information on use in pediatric patients is available.

Parenteral drug products should be inspected for particulate matter and discoloration prior to administration, whenever solution and container permit.

HOW SUPPLIED

Amber Dosette® ampuls for intravenous, epidural and intrathecal administration.

5 mg/10 mL (0.5 mg/mL) packaged in 10s (NDC 0641-1113-33)

10 mg/10 mL (1 mg/1 mL) packaged in 10s (NDC 0641-1115-33)

STORAGE

Protect from light. Store in carton at controlled room temperature, 15° to 30°C (59° to 86°F) until ready to use. DURAMORPH® contains no preservative. DISCARD ANY UNUSED PORTION. DO NOT AUTOCLAVE.

SOTRADECOL® ℞

[sō 'trah "de 'kol "]
(Sodium Tetradecyl Sulfate)
For Intravenous Use Only

PRODUCT OVERVIEW

KEY FACTS

Sotradecol is a mild sclerosing agent which acts by irritation of the vein intimal endothelium.

MAJOR USES

Sotradecol is indicated in the treatment of small uncomplicated varicose veins of the lower extremities. The benefit-to-risk ratio should be considered in selected patients who are great surgical risks due to conditions such as old age.

SAFTEY INFORMATION

Sotradecol is contraindicated in acute superficial thrombophlebitis; underlying arterial disease; varicosities caused by abdominal and pelvic tumors, uncontrolled diabetes mellitus, thyrotoxicosis, tuberculosis, neoplasms, asthma, sepsis, blood dyscrasias, acute respiratory or skin diseases; and any condition which causes the patient to be bedridden. Do not use if precipitated.

PRESCRIBING INFORMATION

SOTRADECOL® ℞

[sō 'trah "de 'kol "]
(Sodium Tetradecyl Sulfate)
For Intravenous Use Only

DESCRIPTION

Sotradecol (sodium tetradecyl sulfate) Injection is a sterile solution containing in each ml sodium tetradecyl sulfate 10 mg (1%) or 30 mg (3%) in Water for Injection with 0.02 ml benzyl alcohol and buffered with dibasic sodium phosphate. pH is adjusted to 7–8.1 with monobasic sodium phosphate or sodium hydroxide.

ACTIONS

The product is a mild sclerosing agent which acts by irritation of the vein intimal endothelium.

INDICATIONS

Indicated in the treatment of small uncomplicated varicose veins of the lower extremities.

The benefit-to-risk ratio should be considered in selected patients who are great surgical risks due to conditions such as old age.

CONTRAINDICATIONS

Contraindicated in acute superficial thrombophlebitis; underlying arterial disease; varicosities caused by abdominal and pelvic tumors, uncontrolled diabetes mellitus, thyrotoxicosis, tuberculosis, neoplasms, asthma, sepsis, blood dyscrasias, acute respiratory or skin diseases; and any condition which causes the patient to be bedridden. Do not use if precipitated.

WARNINGS

Sotradecol (sodium tetradecyl sulfate) should be used in pregnant women only when clearly needed. See Precautions.

PRECAUTIONS

For varicosities, sclerotherapy should not be undertaken if tests such as the Trendelenberg and Perthes, and angiography show significant valvular or deep venous incompetence.

The physician should bear in mind the fact that injection necrosis may result from direct injection of sclerosing agents.

The drug should be administered by physicians who are familiar with an acceptable injection technique. Because of the danger of extension of thrombosis into the deep venous system, thorough pre-injection evaluation for valvular competency should be carried out, and slow injections with a small amount (not over 2 ml) of the preparation should be injected into the varicosity. In particular, deep venous patency must be determined by angiography and/or the Perthes test before sclerotherapy is undertaken.

No well controlled studies have been performed on patients taking anti-ovulatory agents. The physician must use judgment and evaluate any patient taking anti-ovulatory drugs prior to initiating treatment with Sotradecol (sodium tetradecyl sulfate). See Adverse Reactions.

Continued on next page

Elkins-Sinn—Cont.

Pregnancy category C. Adequate reproduction studies have not been performed in animals to determine whether this drug affects fertility in males or females, has teratogenic potential, or has other adverse effects on the fetus. There are no well-controlled studies in pregnant women, but investigational and marketing experience does not include any positive evidence of adverse effects on the fetus. Although there is no clearly defined risk, such experience cannot exclude the possibility of infrequent or subtle damage to the human fetus.

ADVERSE REACTIONS
Post-operative complication of sloughing may occur. A permanent discoloration, usually small and hardly noticeable may occur at the site of injection, and may be objectionable from a cosmetic viewpoint. Allergic reactions have been reported. Therefore, as a precaution against anaphylactic shock, it is recommended that an injection of 0.5 ml of the product into a varicosity be followed by observance of the patient for several hours before a larger injection is administered. The possibility of an anaphylactic reaction should be kept in mind, and the physician should be prepared to treat it appropriately. In extreme emergencies, 0.25 ml of a 1:1000 solution of epinephrine (0.25 mg) intravenously should be used and side reactions controlled with antihistamines.
One death has been reported in a patient who received Sotradecol (sodium tetradecyl sulfate) and who had been receiving an anti-ovulatory agent. Another death (fatal pulmonary embolism) has been reported in a 36-year-old female treated with sodium tetradecyl **acetate** and who was **not** taking oral contraceptives.

DOSAGE AND ADMINISTRATION
For intravenous use only. Do not use if precipitated. The strength of solution required depends on the size and degree of varicosity. In general, the 3% solution will be found most useful, with the 1% solution preferred for small varicosities. The dosage should be kept small, using 0.5 to 2 ml for each injection, and the maximum single treatment should not exceed 10 ml.
Literature describing various current techniques of administration is available upon request from the Professional Services Department.

HOW SUPPLIED
1% — 2 ml Dosette® Ampuls, 5's — #341514 (NDC 0641-1514-34)
3% — 2 ml Dosette® Ampuls, 5's — #341516 (NDC 0641-1516-34)
CAUTION: Federal law prohibits dispensing without prescription

Ethitek Pharmaceuticals Company
8104 N. LAWNDALE AVENUE
SKOKIE, IL 60076

MOCTANIN™ ℞
[mok 'ta-nin]
(monooctanoin)

PRODUCT OVERVIEW

KEY FACTS
Moctanin™ is a semisynthetic esterfied glycerol, intended for perfusion of the common bile duct for cholesterol stone dissolution. It is supplied in glass bottles containing 120 ml of sterile, clear, viscous liquid, ready for use, with disposable bottle hanger.

MAJOR USES
Moctanin is indicated as a solubilizing agent for cholesterol (radiolucent) gallstones retained in the biliary tract following cholecystectomy. It is administered as a continuous perfusion through a catheter inserted directly into the common bile duct generally via a T-tube or through a nasobiliary tube. Due to the product's viscosity a pressure infusion device is recommended. Daily dose is approximately 120 ml (1 bottle) at rate of 5 ml/hour.

SAFETY INFORMATION
It is essential to utilize an overflow manometer, or similar means to assure that perfusion pressure does not exceed 15 cm H_2O, in the biliary tract.
Moctanin is intended for biliary tract perfusion only and is not for parenteral use. It is contraindicated in patients with clinical jaundice, significant biliary tract infection or with a history of recent duodenal ulcer or jejunitis. Patients with impaired liver function may experience metabolic acidosis with Moctanin perfusion. Abominal pain or distress and nausea and/or vomiting were the most common side effects reported by patients receiving Moctanin therapy.

PRESCRIBING INFORMATION

MOCTANIN™ ℞
[mok 'ta-nin]
(monooctanoin)

DESCRIPTION
MOCTANIN™ (MONOOCTANOIN) is a semisynthetic esterified glycerol. The mixed mono-diglyceride has the following approximate composition:

Glyceryl-1-mono-octanoate	80–85%
Glyceryl-1-mono-decanoate	10–15%
Glyceryl-1-2-di-octanoate	
Free Glycerol	max. 2.5%

with the basic structural formula

$$\begin{array}{l} CH_2\text{-}OH \\ CH\text{-}OH \\ CH_2\text{-}OOR \end{array}$$

MOCTANIN™ is clear, viscous, sterile liquid intended for perfusion of the common bile duct for cholesterol stone dissolution.

CLINICAL PHARMACOLOGY
MOCTANIN™ (monooctanoin) has been shown, *in vitro*, to have 2.5 times greater dissolution capacity for cholesterol gallstones (about 120 mg cholesterol/ml of MOCTANIN™) than does sodium cholate.
MOCTANIN™ is readily hydrolyzed by pancreatic and other digestive lipases. The liberated fatty acids are excreted or absorbed and metabolized in a normal fashion.
MOCTANIN™ is irritating to the gastrointestinal and biliary tracts in animals and man. The degree of irritation is related to perfusion pressure and rate. Such irritation was found to be reversible and disappeared 2–7 days after therapy was completed.
In several animal species, perfusions of MOCTANIN™ into the biliary tract were associated with inflammation of the common bile duct and gastric mucosa. Administration to dogs via a Heidenhain pouch resulted in a disruption of the ionic mucosal barrier, similar to that seen with bile acid reflux. Direct injection of low doses of MOCTANIN™ into the left hepatic lobe of rat livers produced fibrotic areas with hyalinized, necrotic centers, and at a higher dose 9 out of 10 rats died of hemorrhagic pneumonitis within 30 minutes of the injection.
In man, biopsies from the gastric antrum, duodenum and bile ducts have shown diffuse erythema in the antral and duodenal mucosa. Ulceration or irritation of the common bile duct mucosa has also been observed on endoscopic examination. Duodenal erosion, inflammatory cell infiltration and localized inflammation have been reported. In one patient, multiple duodenal ulcerations adjacent to the infusion catheter were observed. No mucosal abnormalities were seen one month after discontinuation of therapy.

INDICATIONS AND USAGE
MOCTANIN™ is indicated as a solubilizing agent for cholesterol (radiolucent) gallstones retained in the biliary tract following cholecystectomy, when other means of removing cholesterol stones retained in the common bile duct have failed or cannot be undertaken.
Treatment results in complete stone dissolution about one-third of the time and in reduction in stone size in approximately another one-third of patients. When reduced in size these stones may pass spontaneously or may be more susceptible to physical extraction. Complete dissolution is much more likely when there is a single stone (almost 50%) than when there are multiple stones (about 20%). For unclear reasons, complete dissolution is uncommon in diabetic patients (about 10%).

CONTRAINDICATIONS
MOCTANIN™ should not be used in patients with clinical jaundice, significant biliary tract infection or with a history of recent duodenal ulcer or jejunitis.

WARNING
MOCTANIN™ IS INTENDED FOR BILIARY TRACT PERFUSION ONLY AND IS NOT FOR PARENTERAL USE.
Pressure of the infusion should be kept below 15 cm of H_2O. (See Dosage and Administration.)
MOCTANIN™ has been shown to be irritating to the gastrointestinal and biliary tracts of animals and humans. The irritation seems closely related to perfusion pressure and rate of administration; both should be closely monitored. (See Dosage and Administration.) Ascending cholangitis has been reported with MOCTANIN™ therapy, possibly related to some form of obstruction in the common bile duct. If fever, anorexia, chills, leucocytosis, severe right upper quadrant abdominal pain or jaundice occur, discontinue treatment.

PRECAUTIONS
Patients should have routine liver function tests since those with impaired function may experience metabolic acidosis during MOCTANIN™ perfusion.

Carcinogenesis, Mutagenesis, Impairment of Fertility:
No data available.

PREGNANCY
TERATOGENIC EFFECTS: Pregnancy Category C. Animal reproduction studies have not been conducted with MOCTANIN™. It is also not known whether MOCTANIN™ can cause fetal harm when administered to a pregnant woman or can affect reproduction capacity.
MOCTANIN™ should be given to a pregnant woman only if clearly needed.

NURSING MOTHERS
It is not known whether this drug is excreted in human milk. Because many drugs are excreted in human milk, caution should be exercised when MOCTANIN™ is administered to a nursing woman.

PEDIATRIC USE
Safety and effectiveness in children have not been established.

ADVERSE REACTIONS
Abdominal pain or distress and nausea and/or vomiting were the most common side effects reported by patients receiving MOCTANIN™ therapy.
Irritation of the duodenal mucosa during perfusion has been observed by endoscopy. This was found to be reversible and disappeared 2–7 days after MOCTANIN™ therapy was completed.
The adverse reaction incidences listed in the following tables are based on observations of 326 patients (274 U.S. and 52 foreign) treated with MOCTANIN™. The reactions are arranged in order of decreasing frequency.

ADVERSE REACTIONS OCCURRING IN MORE THAN 1% OF MOCTANIN™ TREATED PATIENTS
N=326

Reactions	No. of Reactions	Frequency (%)
Gastrointestinal		
Pain	139	43
Nausea	104	32
Emesis	65	20
Diarrhea	63	19
Discomfort	24	7.3
Fever	19	6.3
Anorexia	10	3.0
Loose Stool	5	1.5
Indigestion	4	1.2

ADVERSE REACTIONS OCCURRING IN LESS THAN 1% OF MOCTANIN™ TREATED PATIENTS
N=326

Reaction	No. of Reactions	Frequency (%)
Gastrointestinal		
Burning Epigastrium	1	0.3
Increased Drainage from Fistula	1	0.3
Hepatic		
Increased Serum Amylase	2	0.6
Bile Shock	1	0.3
Hematological		
Persistent Leucopenia	1	0.3
Electrolyte		
Hypokalemia	1	0.3
Other		
Intolerance	2	0.6
Pruritus	3	0.9
Chills	1	0.3
Fatigue/Lethargy	3	0.9
Depression	1	0.3
Diaphoresis	1	0.3
Headache	1	0.3
Allergic Reaction	1	0.3

The following table identifies those reactions which were considered severe enough to discontinue therapy.

REASONS FOR PATIENT DISCONTINUATION
N=326

Reason	No. of Patients
Severe and/or immediate gastrointestinal side effects	25
Pt. refused further Rx.	4
No reason given.	2
Stone impacted, obstructive jaundice.	2
Bile shock, diaphoresis.	1
Allergic reaction.	1
Pressure > 15 cm.	1
Liver function enzymes elevated.	1
Pt. had cerebrovascular accident.	1
Pt. with sepsis, CHF, and renal failure died after 24 hr perfusion.	1

Overall, 251 (77%) of the MOCTANIN™ treated patients had side effects: 134 (41%) had multiple side effects. Most of these were mild gastrointestinal symptoms. Some were tolerated, some abated with reduced perfusion rate and discontinuation during meals. Side effects and other events caused discontinuation in 41 (12.5%) of the 326 patients.

Also reported in literature are one death apparently due to acute pancreatitis and cholangitis, and one patient with hematemesis from multiple duodenal ulcerations. A patient with lupus erythematosus developed upper right quadrant abdominal pain, dyspnea and hypotension with hyperventilation. The symptoms abated when the drug administration was discontinued.

DOSAGE AND ADMINISTRATION

MOCTANIN™ (monooctanoin) is administered as a continuous perfusion through a catheter inserted directly into the common bile duct generally via a T-tube or through a nasobiliary tube placed endoscopically.

IT IS ESSENTIAL TO HAVE AN OVERFLOW MANOMETER, OR SIMILAR MEANS TO ASSURE THAT PERFUSION PRESSURE DOES NOT EXEED 15 cm H_2O, IN BILIARY TRACT.

Manometer may be connected directly to T-tube or nasobiliary tube and should be securely positioned at an appropriate height to assure measurement of pressure in the biliary tract.

Perfusion should be at a rate of not more than 3.0 to 5.0 ml/hour at a pressure of 10 cm H_2O to minimize gastrointestinal and/or biliary tract irritation. Administration may be interrupted during meals.

MOCTANIN™ MUST NOT BE ADMINISTERED INTRAVENOUSLY OR INTRAMUSCULARLY.

MOCTANIN™ should be warmed to 70–80°F prior to being perfused and care should be taken that the temperature of the perfusate does not fall below 65°F during administration. When stored at temperatures below 59°F, MOCTANIN™may form a semi-solid. Warming to 70–80°F will completely reliquify.

Stones must be radiolucent and readily accessible to the perfusate. If recently removed stones are available they should be analyzed for composition or incubated in MOCTANIN™ at body temperature with stirring. If analysis shows the stone to be other than cholesterol or if no dissolution is observed after 72 hours incubation, MOCTANIN™ therapy should not be instituted or should be discontinued.

Average duration of perfusion of MOCTANIN™ is 9.4 days. If, after 10 days, endoscopy or x-ray shows neither elimination nor reduction in size of stones therapy should be discontinued.

HOW SUPPLIED

MOCTANIN™ (47679-399-18) is supplied in glass bottles containing 120 ml of sterile liquid, ready to use, with disposable bottle hanger.

Store at controlled room temperature (59–86°F; 15–30°C)

Distributed by: Ethitek Pharmaceuticals, Co.
Skokie, Illinois 60076

Rev. 4/86

EDUCATIONAL MATERIAL

Videos

Gallstone Dissolution Therapy—A New Era

General review of medical techniques used to treat common duct gallstones. Also, discussion of dissolution of gallstones using Moctanin™ including indications, adverse reactions, proper set-up and administration techniques.

Available on loan without charge to interested hospitals and medical professionals.

Everett Laboratories, Inc.
76 FRANKLIN STREET
EAST ORANGE, NEW JERSEY 07017

FLORVITE Chewable Tablets 0.5 mg & 1 mg ℞
Children's Vitamins + Fluoride

SUPPLIED

Multiflavored chewable tablets in bottles of 100 and 1000.

FLORVITE Drops 0.25 mg & 0.5 mg ℞
Children's Vitamins + Fluoride

SUPPLIED

Bottles of 50 ml.

FLORVITE + IRON Chewable Tablets 1 mg ℞
Children's Vitamins + Iron + Fluoride

SUPPLIED

Grape flavored chewable tablets in bottles of 100.

FLORVITE + IRON Drops ℞
Children's Vitamins-Iron-Fluoride

SUPPLIED

Bottles of 50 ml.

REPAN Tablets ℞

EACH TABLET CONTAINS

Butalbital 50 mg.
(Warning: May be habit forming.), Caffeine (Anhydrus) 40 mg., Acetaminophen 325 mg.

SUPPLIED

Bottles of 100 tablets imprinted EVERETT and 162.

STROVITE PLUS Tablets ℞
Therapeutic Multivitamin Mineral Supplement

SUPPLIED

Bottles of 100.

TUSSAFED DROPS & SYRUP
Antitussive-Decongestant-Antihistamine

Each dropperful (A) & each teaspoonful (B) contains:

	A	B
Dextromethorphan	4 mg	15 mg
Pseudoephedrine	25 mg	60 mg
Carbinoxamine	2 mg	4 mg

VITAFOL Tablets ℞
Vitamins, Minerals, Iron, Folic Acid Supplement

SUPPLIED

Bottles of 100 and 1000 pink film coated tablets.

ZE CAPS Soft Gel Capsules OTC

EACH CAPSULE CONTAINS

Zinc Gluconate 75 mg., Vitamin E 200 I.U.

SUPPLIED

Bottles of 60 sugar and salt free capsules.

Ferndale Laboratories, Inc.
780 W. EIGHT MILE ROAD
FERNDALE, MI 48220

ANALPRAM-HC CREAM ℞
Rectal Cream

DESCRIPTION

Contains Hydrocortisone acetate 1% and Pramoxine HCl 1% in a washable, nongreasy base containing stearic acid, cetyl alcohol, aquaphor, isopropyl palmitate, polyoxyl 40 stearate, propylene glycol, potassium sorbate 0.1%, sorbic acid 0.1%, trieth anolamine lauryl sulfate and water.

ACTIONS

Hydrocortisone acetate is a corticosteroid. Topically, it is primarily effective because of its anti-inflammatory, antipruritic and vaso-constrictive actions. Pramoxine hydrochloride is a topical anesthetic which provides temporary relief from itching and pain.

INDICATIONS AND USAGE

Topical corticosteroids are indicated for the relief of the inflammatory and pruritic manifestations of corticosteroid-responsive dermatoses of the anal region.

CONTRAINDICATIONS

Topical steroids are contraindicated in viral diseases of the skin, such as varicella and vaccinia. Topical steroids are contraindicated in those patients with a history of hypersensitivity to any of the components of the preparation. Topical steroids should not be used when circulation is markedly impaired.

PRECAUTIONS

If irritation develops, the product should be discontinued and appropriate therapy instituted. In the presence of an infection, the use of appropriate antifungal or antibacterial agents should be instituted. If a favorable response does not occur promptly, the corticosteroid should be discontinued until the infection has been adequately controlled. If extensive areas are treated or if the occlusive technique is used, the possibility exists of increased systemic absorption of the corticosteroid and suitable precautions should be taken. The product is not for ophthalmic use.

WARNINGS

USAGE IN PREGNANCY: Although topical steroids have not been reported to have an adverse effect on the fetus, the safety of their use in pregnant females has not absolutely been established. Therefore, they should not be used extensively on pregnant patients, or in large amounts, or for prolonged periods of time.

CAUTION

Federal law prohibits despensing without prescription.

ADVERSE REACTIONS

The following local adverse reactions have been reported with topical corticosteroids, especially under occlusive dressings.

Burning, Itching, Irritation, Dryness, Folliculitis, Hypertrichosis, Acneiform eruptions, Hypopigmentation, Perioral dermatitis, Allergic Contact Dermatitis, Maceration of the skin, Secondary infection, Skin atrophy, Striae, and Miliaria.

DOSAGE AND ADMINISTRATION

Apply to affected area 3 or 4 times daily.

HOW SUPPLIED

ANALPRAM-HC Cream is supplied in a 1 oz. tube with six (6) rectal applicators.

AQUAPHYLLIN SYRUP ℞
(Theophylline, anhydrous 80 mg/15 ml)
Dye-Free, Alcohol-free and saccharin-free.

ACTIONS AND USES

Theophylline is most effective in relaxing smooth muscles of bronchi, particularly if there is bronchial constriction, as in asthma. AQUAPHYLLIN is indicated for relief of acute bronchial asthma and for reversible bronchospasm associated with chronic asthma, bronchitis and emphysema.

DOSAGE AND ADMINISTRATION

AQUAPHYLLIN SYRUP:

Severe Asthma Attack: Adults—75 ml (5 tablespoonfuls). Children—One ml per kg. body weight, Do not repeat within six hours.

Maintenance 24-Hour Therapy: Adults for first six doses—45 ml (3 tablespoonfuls) upon every 6–8 hours, then 30 ml (2 tablespoonfuls) doses every 6–8 hours.

Children 3 to 5 mg. of theophylline per kg. body weight every 6–8 hours. It is recommended that dosage increases be based on serum theophylline determinations, particularly when exceeding the usual dosage range.

ADVERSE EFFECTS

Nausea, vomiting, epigastric or substernal pain, palpitation, headache, dizziness may occur.

HOW SUPPLIED

Liquid: Pints, gallons and unit dose vials.

KRONOFED-A® Kronocaps ℞
Dye-Free
Decongestant plus Antihistamine

Each sustained release, white and clear capsule contains:

Pseudoephedrine HCl .... 120 mg
Chlorpheniramine Maleate .... 8 mg

KRONOFED-A-JR® Kronocaps ℞
Dye-Free
Decongestant plus Antihistamine

Each sustained release, white and clear capsule contains:

Pseudoephedrine HCl .... 60 mg
Chlorpheniramine Maleate .... 4 mg

INDICATIONS

For temporary relief of upper respiratory and nasal congestion associated with the common cold, hay fever and allergies, sinusitis and vasomotor and allergic rhinitis.

CONTRAINDICATIONS

Severe hypertension or severe cardiac disease. Sensitivity to antihistamines or sympathomimetic agents.

PRECAUTIONS

Use with caution in patients with hyperthyroidism. Patients susceptible to the soporific effects of chlorpheniramine should be warned against driving or operating of machinery which requires complete mental alertness.

DOSAGE

Kronofed-A Capsules: Adults and children over 12 years of age—1 capsule every 12 hours. **Kronofed-A-JR** Capsules: Children 6–12 years of age—1 capsule every 12 hours. Adults 1 or 2 capsules every 12 hours.

HOW SUPPLIED

Bottles of 100 and 500 Capsules.

Continued on next page

Ferndale—Cont.

PRAMOSONE® CREAM, LOTION AND OINTMENT ℞

DESCRIPTION

Pramosone Cream: Contains Hydrocortisone acetate 0.5%, 1% or 2.5% and Pramoxine HCl 1% in a hydrophilic base containing stearic acid, cetyl alcohol, aquaphor, isopropyl palmitate, polyoxyl 40 stearate, propylene glycol, potassium sorbate 0.1%, sorbic acid 0.1%, triethanolamine lauryl sulfate and water.

Pramosone Lotion: Contains Hydrocortisone acetate 0.5%, 1% or 2.5% and Pramoxine HCl 1% in a base containing forlan-L, cetyl alcohol, stearic acid, di-isopropyl adipate, polyoxyl 40 stearate, silicon, triethanolamine, glycerine, polyvinylpyrolidone, potassium sorbate 0.1%, sorbic acid 0.1% and water.

Pramosone Ointment: Contains Hydrocortisone acetate 1% or 2.5% and Pramoxine HC1 1% in an emollient ointment base containing Sorbitan sesquioleate, Water, Aquaphor and White petrolatum.

ACTIONS

Hydrocortisone acetate is a corticosteroid. Topically, it is primarily effective because of its anti-inflammatory, antipruritic and vaso-constrictive actions. Pramoxine hydrochloride is a topical anesthetic which provides temporary relief from itching and pain.

INDICATIONS AND USAGE

Topical corticosteroids are indicated for the relief of the inflammatory and pruritic manifestations of corticosteroid-responsive dermatoses.

CONTRAINDICATIONS

Topical steroids are contraindicated in viral diseases of the skin, such as varicella and vaccinia. Topical steroids are contraindicated in those patients with a history of hypersensitivity to any of the components of the preparation. Topical steroids should not be used when circulation is markedly impaired.

PRECAUTIONS

If irritation develops, the product should be discontinued and appropriate therapy instituted. In the presence of an infection, the use of appropriate antifungal or antibacterial agents should be instituted. If a favorable response does not occur promptly, the corticosteroid should be discontinued until the infection has been adequately controlled. If extensive areas are treated or if the occlusive technique is used, the possibility exists of increased systemic absorption of the corticosteroid and suitable precautions should be taken. The product is not for opthalmic use.

WARNINGS

USAGE IN PREGNANCY: Although topical steroids have not been reported to have an adverse effect on the fetus, the safety of their use in pregnant females has not absolutely been established. Therefore, they should not be used extensively on pregnant patients, or in large amounts, or for prolonged periods of time.

CAUTION

Federal law prohibits despensing without prescription.

ADVERSE REACTIONS

The following local adverse reactions have been reported with topical corticosteroids, especially under occlusive dressings.

Burning, Itching, Irritation, Dryness, Folliculitis, Hypertrichosis, Acneiform eruptions, Hypopigmentation, Perioral dermatitis, Allergic Contact Dermatitis, Maceration of the skin, Secondary infection, Skin atrophy, Striae, and Miliaria.

DOSAGE AND ADMINISTRATION

Apply to affected area 3 or 4 times daily.

HOW SUPPLIED

CREAM: ½%, 1% or 2½% in 1 oz. tubes, 4 oz. jars and lb. jars. LOTION: ½% or 1% in 2 fl. oz., 4 fl. oz. and 8 fl. oz. dispenser bottles. 2½% in 2 fl. oz. dispenser bottles. OINTMENT: 1% or 2½% in 1 oz. tubes, 4 oz. jars and lb. jars.

PRAX® CREAM AND LOTION*
(Pramoxine HCl 1% in an emollient hydrophilic base)

AVAILABLE

CREAM: 1 oz. tubes, 4 oz. jars and lb. jars. LOTION: 15 mL., 120 mL., and 240 mL. dispenser bottles.

*Additional information available upon request.

The Fielding Company

2384 CENTERLINE INDUSTRIAL DRIVE
ST. LOUIS, MO 63146

GERIMED® Tablets

DESCRIPTION

A multivitamin-multimineral supplement useful as adjunctive therapy in osteoporosis. Provides a balanced ratio of calcium and phosphorus (2.8 to 1) with adequate Vitamin D for proper absorption.

Each tablet contains:		U.S. RDA
Dibasic Calcium Phosphate	600 mg.	*
Calcium Carbonate	500 mg.	*
Vitamin A	5000 I. U.	100%
Vitamin D	400 I. U.	100%
Vitamin E	30 I. U.	100%
Vitamin C	120 mg.	200%
Thiamine B_2	3 mg.	200%
Riboflavin B_2	3 mg.	176%
Niacinamide	25 mg.	100%
Pyridoxine B_6	2 mg.	100%
Vitamin B_{12}	6 mcg.	100%
Magnesium	50 mg.	11%
Zinc	15 mg.	100%

*Total Calcium	370 mg.	37%
*Total Phosphorus	130 mg.	13%
Calcium/Phosphorus ratio 2.8 - 1		

DOSAGE

One tablet daily, or as prescribed by the physician.

HOW SUPPLIED

Bottle of 60 tablets.
NDC 0421-0080-60

IROSPAN® Tablets/Capsules

Each tablet or capsule contains:	
Ferrous Sulfate (exsic.)	200 mg.
Ascorbic Acid (Vit. C)	150 mg.

DESCRIPTION

Irospan is a unique presentation of sustained release ferrous sulfate and ascorbic acid. Irospan is of particular value during pregnancy and lactation providing excellent tolerance and absorption.

DOSAGE

One tablet or capsule daily or as prescribed by the physician.

HOW SUPPLIED

Irospan Tablets—bottles of 100.
Irospan Capsules—bottles of 60.

METRIC® 21 ℞
(metronidazole)

DESCRIPTION

An antiprotozoal and antibacterial agent for use in the treatment of trichomoniasis in both the female and male patient.

DOSAGE

Metric 21 (250 mg) one tablet three times a day for seven days. The seven day course of treatment appears to provide a higher cure rate than the one day treatment regimen.

HOW SUPPLIED

Metric 21 (250 mg) in bottles of 100.
NDC 0421-8282-01

NESTABS® FA TABLETS ℞
Prenatal Tablets

DESCRIPTION

East tablet contains:			U.S. RDA
Vitamin A	8000	Units	100%
Vitamin D	400	Units	100%
Vitamin E	30	Units	100%
Vitamin C	120	mg.	200%
Folic Acid	1	mg.	125%
Thiamine	3	mg.	176%
Riboflavin	3	mg.	125%
Niacinamide	20	mg.	100%
Pyridoxine	3	mg.	120%
Vitamin B12	8	mcg.	100%
Calcium Carbonate	500	mg.	15%
Iodine	150	mcg.	100%
Ferrous Fumarate	110	mg.	200%
Zinc	15	mg.	100%

A comprehensive vitamin-mineral supplement expressly formulated for use during pregnancy and lactation.

DOSAGE

One tablet daily, or as prescribed by the physician.

PRECAUTION

Folic acid may obscure pernicious anemia in that hematologic remission can occur while neurological manifestations remain progressive.

HOW SUPPLIED

Bottles of 100 tablets.
NDC 0421-1594-01

Fisons Corporation

Pharmaceutical Division
TWO PRESTON COURT
BEDFORD, MA 01730

In addition to the products described in this section, Fisons also distributes the following products. On these and all Fisons products, information may be obtained by addressing Fisons Corporation, 2 Preston Court, Bedford, MA 01730.

BACID® CAPSULES OTC
lactobacillus acidophilus

ERGOMAR® SUBLINGUAL TABLETS ℞
ergotamine tartrate
2.0 mg sublingual tablet

KONDREMUL® OTC
KONDREMUL® with CASCARA
KONDREMUL® with PHENOLPHTHALEIN
mineral oil microemulsion

NEO-CULTOL® OTC
refined mineral oil, jelly, chocolate flavored

PERSISTIN® OTC
salicylsalicylic acid - 7 ½ gr
aspirin - 2 ½ gr

PROFERDEX™ ℞
iron dextran injection, USP
complex of ferric hydroxide
and dextran in a 0.9% sodium
chloride solution.

VAPO-ISO® ℞
isoproterenol HCl
solution 0.5% (1:200)

VAPONEFRIN® SOLUTION OTC
(racepinephrine)

VITRON-C® OTC
ferrous fumarate - 200 mg
ascorbic acid - 125 mg

VITRON-C PLUS® OTC
ferrous fumarate - 400 mg
ascorbic acid - 250 mg

INTAL® Capsules ℞
(cromolyn sodium for inhalation, USP)
For Inhalation Only
For Use With The SPINHALER®
TURBO-INHALER

INTAL® Nebulizer Solution ℞
(cromolyn sodium inhalation, USP)
For Inhalation Use Only—Not for Injection

DESCRIPTION

Chemically, cromolyn sodium is the disodium salt of 1,3-bis (2-carboxychromon-5-yloxy)-2-hydroxypropane.
Please see package insert for complete instructions.

INTAL® Inhaler ℞
[in'tă]
(cromolyn sodium inhalation aerosol)

DESCRIPTION

The active ingredient of INTAL Inhaler is cromolyn sodium. Cromolyn sodium is the disodium salt of 1,3 bis (2-carboxychromon-5-yloxy)-2-hydroxypropane. Cromolyn sodium has a molecular weight of 512.34. Cromolyn sodium is soluble in water.

The molecular structure of cromolyn sodium is:

NaOOC … COONa
OH
O-CH₂-CH-CH₂-O

INTAL Inhaler is a metered dose aerosol unit for oral inhalation containing micronized cromolyn sodium, sorbitan triole-

ate with dichlorotetrafluoroethane and dichlorodifluoromethane as propellants. Each metered spray delivers to the patient approximately 800 mcg of cromolyn sodium. Each 8.1 g canister delivers at least 112 metered sprays (56 doses); each 14.2 g canister delivers at least 200 metered sprays (100 doses).
Pharmacological Category: Mast cell stabilizer/antiallergic.
Therapeutic Category: Prophylactic antiasthmatic; reduces bronchial hyperreactivity.

CLINICAL PHARMACOLOGY

In vitro and *in vivo* animal studies have shown that cromolyn sodium inhibits sensitized mast cell degranulation which occurs after exposure to specific antigens. Cromolyn sodium acts by inhibiting the release of mediators from mast cells. Studies show that cromolyn sodium indirectly blocks calcium ions from entering the mast cell, thereby preventing mediator release.
Cromolyn sodium inhibits both the immediate and non-immediate bronchoconstrictive reactions to inhaled antigen. Cromolyn sodium also attenuates bronchospasm caused by exercise, toluene diisocyanate, aspirin, cold air, sulfur dioxide and environmental pollutants, at least in some patients.
Cromolyn sodium has no intrinsic bronchodilator, antihistaminic or anti-inflammatory activity.
After administration of cromolyn sodium capsules by inhalation, approximately 8% of the total dose administered is absorbed and rapidly excreted unchanged, approximately equally divided between urine and bile. The remainder of the dose is either exhaled or deposited in the oropharynx, swallowed, and excreted via the alimentary tract.

INDICATIONS AND USAGE

INTAL Inhaler is a prophylactic agent indicated in the management of patients with bronchial asthma.
In patients whose symptoms are sufficiently frequent to require a continuous program of medication, INTAL Inhaler is given by inhalation on a regular daily basis (see Dosage and Administration). The effect of INTAL Inhaler is usually evident after several weeks of treatment, although some patients show an almost immediate response.
If improvement occurs, it will ordinarily occur within the first 4 weeks of administration as manifested by a decrease in the severity of clinical symptoms of asthma, or in the need for concomitant therapy, or both.
In patients who develop acute bronchoconstriction in response to exposure to exercise, toluene diisocyanate, environmental pollutants, known antigens, etc., INTAL Inhaler should be used shortly before exposure to the precipitating factor, i.e., within 10–15 minutes but not more than 60 minutes (see Dosage and Administration). INTAL Inhaler may be effective in relieving bronchospasm in some, but not all, patients with exercise induced bronchospasm.

CONTRAINDICATIONS

INTAL Inhaler is contraindicated in those patients who have shown hypersensitivity to cromolyn sodium or other components.

WARNINGS

INTAL Inhaler has no role in the treatment of an acute attack of asthma, especially status asthmaticus. Severe anaphylactic reactions can occur after cromolyn sodium administration. The recommended dosage should be decreased in patients with decreased renal or hepatic function. INTAL Inhaler should be discontinued if the patient develops eosinophilic pneumonia (or pulmonary infiltrates with eosinophilia). Because of the propellants in this preparation, it should be used with caution in patients with coronary artery disease or a history of cardiac arrhythmias.

PRECAUTIONS

General: In view of the biliary and renal routes of excretion for cromolyn sodium, consideration should be given to decreasing the dosage or discontinuing the administration of the drug in patients with impaired renal or hepatic function.
Occasionally, patients may experience cough and/or bronchospasm following cromolyn sodium inhalation. At times, patients who develop bronchospasm may not be able to continue administration despite prior bronchodilator administration. Rarely, very severe bronchospasm has been encountered.
Carcinogenesis, Mutagenesis, Impairment of Fertility: Long term studies in mice (12 months intraperitoneal treatment followed by 6 months observation), hamsters (12 months intraperitoneal treatment followed by 12 months observation), and rats (18 months subcutaneous treatment) showed no neoplastic effect of cromolyn sodium.
No evidence of chromosomal damage or cytotoxicity was obtained in various mutagenesis studies.
No evidence of impaired fertility was shown in laboratory animal reproduction studies.
Pregnancy: Pregnancy Category B. Reproduction studies with cromolyn sodium administered parenterally to pregnant mice, rats, and rabbits in doses up to 338 times the human clinical doses produced no evidence of fetal malformations. Adverse fetal effects (increased resorptions and decreased fetal weight) were noted only at the very high parenteral doses that produced maternal toxicity. There are, however, no adequate and well-controlled studies in pregnant women. Because animal reproduction studies are not always predictive of human response, this drug should be used during pregnancy only if clearly needed.
Drug Interaction During Pregnancy: Cromolyn sodium and isoproterenol were studied following subcutaneous injections in pregnant mice. Cromolyn sodium alone in doses of 60 to 540 mg/kg (38 to 338 times the human dose) did not cause significant increases in resorptions or major malformations. Isoproterenol alone at a dose of 2.7 mg/kg (90 times the human dose) increased both resorptions and malformations. The addition of cromolyn sodium (338 times the human dose) to isoproterenol (90 times the human dose) appears to have increased the incidence of both resorptions and malformations.
Nursing Mothers: It is not known whether this drug is excreted in human milk, therefore, caution should be exercised when INTAL Inhaler is administered to a nursing woman and the attending physician must make a benefit/risk assessment in regard to its use in this situation.
Pediatric Use: Safety and effectiveness in children below the age of 5 years have not been established. For young children unable to utilize the Inhaler, INTAL Nebulizer Solution (cromolyn sodium inhalation, USP) is recommended. Because of the possibility that adverse effects of this drug could become apparent only after many years, a benefit/risk consideration of the long-term use of INTAL Inhaler is particularly important in pediatric patients.

ADVERSE REACTIONS

In controlled clinical studies of INTAL Inhaler, the most frequently reported adverse reactions attributed to cromolyn sodium treatment were: throat irritation or dryness, bad taste, cough, wheeze, and nausea.
The most frequently reported adverse reactions attributed to other forms of cromolyn sodium (on the basis of reoccurrence following readministration) involve the respiratory tract and are: bronchospasm [sometimes severe, associated with a precipitous fall in pulmonary function (FEV_1)], cough, laryngeal edema (rare), nasal congestion (sometimes severe), pharyngeal irritation and wheezing.
Adverse reactions which occur infrequently and are associated with administration of the drug are: anaphylaxis, angioedema, dizziness, dysuria and urinary frequency, joint swelling and pain, lacrimation, nausea and headache, rash, swollen parotid gland, urticaria, pulmonary infiltrates with eosinophilia, substernal burning, and myopathy.
The following adverse reactions have been reported as rare events and it is unclear whether they are attributable to the drug: anemia, exfoliative dermatitis, hemoptysis, hoarseness, myalgia, nephrosis, periarteritic vasculitis, pericarditis, peripheral neuritis, photodermatitis, sneezing, drowsiness, nasal itching, nasal bleeding, nasal burning, serum sickness, stomach ache, polymyositis, vertigo, and liver disease.

OVERDOSAGE

No action other than medical observation should be necessary.

DOSAGE AND ADMINISTRATION

For management of bronchial asthma in adults and children (5 years of age and over) who are able to use the Inhaler, the usual starting dosage is two metered sprays inhaled four times daily at regular intervals. This dose should not be exceeded. Not all patients will respond to the recommended dose and there is evidence to suggest, at least in younger patients, that a lower dose may provide efficacy.
Patients with chronic asthma should be advised that the effect of INTAL Inhaler therapy is dependent upon its administration at regular intervals, as directed. INTAL Inhaler should be introduced into the patient's therapeutic regimen when the acute episode has been controlled, the airway has been cleared and the patient is able to inhale adequately.
For the prevention of acute bronchospasm which follows exercise, exposure to cold dry air or environmental agents, the usual dose is inhalation of two metered dose sprays shortly, i.e., 10–15 minutes but not more than 60 minutes, before exposure to the precipitating factor.
INTAL INHALER THERAPY IN RELATION TO OTHER TREATMENTS FOR ASTHMA: Non-steroidal agents: INTAL Inhaler should be **added** to the patient's existing treatment regimen (e.g., bronchodilators). When a clinical response to INTAL Inhaler is evident, usually within two to four weeks, and if the asthma is under good control, an attempt may be made to decrease concomitant medication usage gradually.
If concomitant medications are eliminated or required on no more than a prn basis, the frequency of administration of INTAL Inhaler may be titrated downward to the lowest level consistent with the desired effect. The usual decrease is from four to three to two inhalations of two sprays per day. It is important that the dosage be reduced gradually to avoid exacerbation of asthma. It is emphasized that in patients whose dosage has been titrated to fewer than four inhalations per day, an increase in the dosage of INTAL Inhaler and the introduction of, or increase in, symptomatic medications may be needed if the patient's clinical condition deteriorates.
Corticosteroids: In patients chronically receiving corticosteroids for the management of bronchial asthma, the dosage should be maintained following the introduction of INTAL Inhaler. If the patient improves, an attempt to decrease corticosteroids should be made. Even if the corticosteroid-dependent patient fails to show symptomatic improvement following INTAL Inhaler administration, the potential to reduce corticosteroids may nonetheless be present. Thus, gradual tapering of corticosteroid dosage may be attempted. It is important that the dose be reduced slowly, maintaining close supervision of the patient to avoid an exacerbation of asthma.
It should be borne in mind that prolonged corticosteroid therapy frequently causes an impairment in the activity of the hypothalamo-pituitary-adrenal axis and a reduction in the size of the adrenal cortex. A potentially critical degree of impairment or insufficiency may persist asymptomatically for some time even after gradual discontinuation of adrenocortical steroids. Therefore, if a patient is subjected to significant stress, such as a severe asthmatic attack, surgery, trauma or severe illness while being treated or within one year (occasionally up to two years) after corticosteroid treatment has been terminated, consideration should be given to reinstituting corticosteroid therapy. When respiratory function is impaired, as may occur in severe exacerbation of asthma, a temporary increase in the amount of corticosteroids may be required to regain control of the patient's asthma.
It is particularly important that great care be exercised if for any reason cromolyn sodium is withdrawn in cases where its use has permitted a reduction in the maintenance dose of corticosteroids. In such cases, continued close supervision of the patient is essential since there may be sudden reappearance of severe manifestations of asthma which will require immediate therapy and possible reintroduction of corticosteroids.

HOW SUPPLIED

INTAL Inhaler, 8.1 g or 14.2 g canister, box of one. Supplied with inhalation adapter and patient instructions.

NDC 0585-0675-01	14.2 g canister
NDC 0585-0675-02	8.1 g canister

Store between 2°–30°C (36°–86°F). Contents under pressure. Do not puncture or incinerate. Keep out of the reach of children.

CAUTION

Federal law prohibits dispensing without prescription.
Manufactured for:
FISONS CORPORATION
BEDFORD, MA 01730 U.S.A.
By:
Riker Laboratories
One Morley Street
Loughborough, England LE11 1EP

Issued 12/85
Made in England FC7518
®Registered Trademark of Fisons plc

ISOCLOR® Timesule® OTC
[īs 'ō-klŏr]
Capsules

DESCRIPTION

Each sustained-action Timesule capsule contains 8 mg chlorpheniramine maleate and 120 mg pseudoephedrine HCl in a special form providing a prolonged therapeutic effect.

INDICATIONS

For temporary relief of upper respiratory and nasal congestion associated with the common cold, hay fever and allergies, sinusitis, and vasomotor and allergic rhinitis.

CONTRAINDICATIONS

Severe hypertension or severe cardiac disease. Sensitivity to antihistamines or sympathomimetic agents.

PRECAUTIONS

Use with caution in patients with hyperthyroidism. Patients susceptible to the soporific effects of chlorpheniramine should be warned against driving or operating machinery which requires complete mental alertness.

DOSAGE

Adults—1 Timesule capsule every 12 hrs.

SUPPLIED

Bottles of 100 and 500.
Isoclor® and Timesule® are registered trademarks of American Hospital Supply Corporation
Distributed by FISONS CORPORATION
Bedford, MA 01730

Continued on next page

Fisons—Cont.

NASALCROM® NASAL SOLUTION ℞

[*nāz 'ŭl-krōm "*]

(cromolyn sodium nasal solution, USP)

DESCRIPTION

Each milliliter of NASALCROM® Nasal Solution (cromolyn sodium nasal solution, USP) contains 40 mg cromolyn sodium in purified water with benzalkonium chloride 0.01% and EDTA (disodium edetate) 0.01% added to stabilize and to provide antimicrobial protection for the solution. NASALCROM possesses a natural pH of 4.5–6.5 and negligible titratable acidity. Chemically, cromolyn sodium is the disodium salt of 1,3-bis(2-carboxychromon-5-yloxy)-2-hydroxypropane.

The molecular structure is:

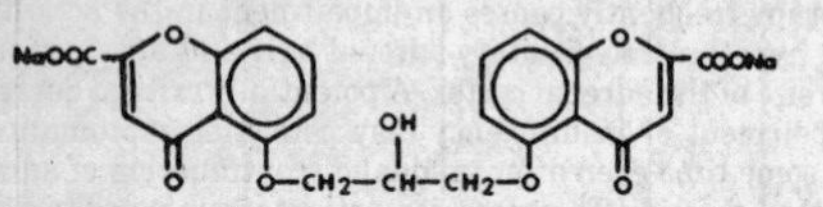

Pharmacologic Category: Mast cell stabilizer/ antiallergic.
Therapeutic Category: Antiallergic.

After priming the delivery system for NASALCROM, each actuation of the unit delivers a metered spray containing 5.2 mg of cromolyn sodium. The contents of one nasal spray bottle delivers at least 100 sprays.

CLINICAL PHARMACOLOGY

In vitro and *in vivo* animal studies have shown that cromolyn sodium inhibits the degranulation of sensitized mast cells which occurs after exposure to specific antigens. Cromolyn sodium inhibits the release of histamine and SRS-A (the slow-reacting substance of anaphylaxis). Rhinitis induced by the inhalation of specific antigens can be inhibited to varying degrees by pretreatment with NASALCROM.

Another activity demonstrated *in vitro* is the capacity of cromolyn sodium to inhibit the degranulation of non-sensitized rat mast cells by phospholipase A and the subsequent release of chemical mediators. An additional *in vitro* study showed that cromolyn sodium did not inhibit the enzymatic activity of released phospholipase A on its specific substrate.

Cromolyn sodium has no intrinsic bronchodilator, antihistaminic or anti-inflammatory activity.

Cromolyn sodium is poorly absorbed from the gastrointestinal tract. After instillation of NASALCROM, less than 7% of the total dose administered is absorbed and is rapidly excreted unchanged in the bile and urine. The remainder of the dose is expelled from the nose, or swallowed and excreted via the alimentary tract.

INDICATIONS

NASALCROM is indicated for the prevention and treatment of the symptoms of allergic rhinitis.

CONTRAINDICATIONS

NASALCROM is contraindicated in those patients who have shown hypersensitivity to any of the ingredients.

PRECAUTIONS

General: Some patients may experience transient nasal stinging and/or sneezing immediately following instillation of NASALCROM. Except in rare occurrences, these experiences have not caused discontinuation of therapy.

In view of the biliary and renal routes of excretion for cromolyn sodium, consideration should be given to decreasing the dosage or discontinuing the administration of the drug in patients with impaired renal or hepatic function.

Carcinogenesis, Mutagenesis, and Impairment of Fertility: Long term studies in mice (12 months intraperitoneal treatment followed by 6 months observation), hamsters (12 months intraperitoneal treatment followed by 12 months observation), and rats (18 months subcutaneous treatment) showed no neoplastic effect of cromolyn sodium.

No evidence of chromosomal damage or cytotoxicity was obtained in various mutagenesis studies.

No evidence of impaired fertility was shown in laboratory animal reproduction studies.

Pregnancy: Pregnancy Category B. Reproduction studies with cromolyn sodium administered parenterally to pregnant mice, rats, and rabbits in doses up to 338 times the human clinical doses produced no evidence of fetal malformations. Adverse fetal effects (increased resorptions and decreased fetal weight) were noted only at the very high parenteral doses that produced maternal toxicity. There are, however, no adequate and well-controlled studies in pregnant women. Because animal reproduction studies are not always predictive of human response, this drug should be used during pregnancy only if clearly needed.

Drug Interaction During Pregnancy: Cromolyn sodium and isoproterenol were studied following subcutaneous injections in pregnant mice. Cromolyn sodium alone in doses of 60 to 540 mg/kg (38 to 338 times the human dose) did not cause significant increases in resorptions or major malformations. Isoproterenol alone at a dose of 2.7 mg/kg (90 times the human dose) increased both resorptions and malformations. The addition of cromolyn sodium (338 times the human dose) to isoproterenol (90 times the human dose) appears to have increased the incidence of both resorptions and malformations.

Nursing Mothers: It is not known whether this drug is excreted in human milk. Because many drugs are excreted in human milk, caution should be exercised when NASALCROM is administered to a nursing woman.

Pediatric Use: Safety and effectiveness in children below the age of 6 years have not been established.

ADVERSE REACTIONS

The most frequent adverse reactions occurring in the 430 patients included in the clinical trials with NASALCROM were sneezing (1 in 10 patients), nasal stinging (1 in 20), nasal burning (1 in 25), and nasal irritation (1 in 40). Headaches and bad taste were reported in about 1 in 50 patients. Epistaxis, postnasal drip, and rash were reported in less than one percent of the patients. One patient in the clinical trials developed anaphylaxis.

Adverse reactions which have occurred in the use of other cromolyn sodium formulations for inhalation include angioedema, joint pain and swelling, urticaria, cough, and wheezing. Other reactions reported rarely are serum sickness, periarteritic vasculitis, polymyositis, pericarditis, photodermatitis, exfoliative dermatitis, peripheral neuritis, and nephrosis.

DOSAGE AND ADMINISTRATION

The dose for adults and children 6 years and older is one spray in each nostril 3–4 times daily at regular intervals. If needed, this dose may be increased to one spray to each nostril 6 times daily. The patient should be instructed to clear the nasal passages before administering the spray and should inhale through the nose during administration.

In the management of seasonal (pollenotic) rhinitis, and for prevention of rhinitis caused by exposure to other types of specific inhalant allergens, treatment with NASALCROM will be more effective if started prior to expected contact with the offending allergen. Treatment should be continued throughout the period of exposure, i.e., until the pollen season is over or until exposure to the offending allergen is terminated.

In the management of perennial allergic rhinitis, the effects of treatment with NASALCROM may become apparent only after two to four weeks of treatment. The concomitant use of antihistamine and/or nasal decongestant may be necessary during the initial phase of treatment, but the need for this type of medication should diminish and may be eliminated when the full benefit of NASALCROM is achieved.

HOW SUPPLIED

Each 13 ml NASALCROM Nasal Solution (cromolyn sodium, nasal solution, USP) spray bottle contains 520 mg (40 mg/ml) of cromolyn sodium and is to be used with the Nasalmatic® metered spray device. The Nasalmatic device consists of a pump unit, plastic case and a patient leaflet of instructions. The cleaning of this device is not recommended. The pump device should be replaced at six month intervals. NASALCROM should be stored at controlled room temperature (15°–30°C).

NDC 0585-0671-02	Complete pack (13 ml bottle, metered spray device)
NDC 0585-0671-01	Refill (13 ml bottle)

Caution: Federal law prohibits dispensing without prescription.

Rev.3/85
FC7102C

OPTICROM® 4%

[*op 'ti-krōm*]

(cromolyn sodium ophthalmic solution, USP)
Ophthalmic Solution

DESCRIPTION

Each milliliter of OPTICROM 4% Ophthalmic Solution (cromolyn sodium ophthalmic solution, USP) contains 40 mg cromolyn sodium in purified water with 0.01% benzalkonium chloride to preserve and 0.1% EDTA (edetate disodium, USP) to stabilize the solution. OPTICROM is a clear, colorless, sterile solution with a pH of 4.0–7.0. It is intended for topical administration to the eye.

Chemically, cromolyn sodium is the disodium salt of 1,3-bis(2-carboxychromon-5-yloxy)-2-hydroxypropane. Its chemical structure is:

[See Chemical Formula at top of next column].

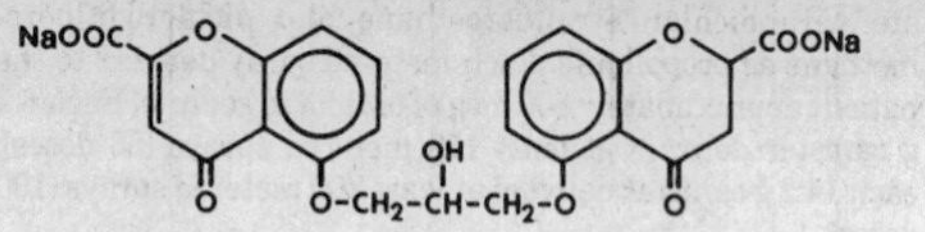

Pharmacologic Category: Mast cell stabilizer
Therapeutic Category: Antiallergic

CLINICAL PHARMACOLOGY

In vitro and *in vivo* animal studies have shown that cromolyn sodium inhibits the degranulation of sensitized mast cells which occurs after exposure to specific antigens. Cromolyn sodium acts by inhibiting the release of histamine and SRS-A (slow-reacting substance of anaphylaxis) from the mast cell.

Another activity demonstrated *in vitro* is the capacity of cromolyn sodium to inhibit the degranulation of non-sensitized rat mast cells by phospholipase A and the subsequent release of chemical mediators. Another study showed that cromolyn sodium did not inhibit the enzymatic activity of released phospholipase A on its specific substrate.

Cromolyn sodium has no intrinsic vasoconstrictor, antihistaminic or anti-inflammatory activity.

Cromolyn sodium is poorly absorbed. When multiple doses of cromolyn sodium ophthalmic solution are instilled into normal rabbit eyes, less than 0.07% of the administered dose of cromolyn sodium is absorbed into the systemic circulation (presumably by way of the eye, nasal passages, buccal cavity and gastrointestinal tract). Trace amounts (less than 0.01%) of the cromolyn sodium dose penetrate into the aqueous humor and clearance from this chamber is virtually complete within 24 hours after treatment is stopped.

In normal volunteers, analysis of drug excretion indicates that approximately 0.03% of cromolyn sodium is absorbed following administration to the eye.

A study on corneal epithelial wound healing in albino rabbits failed to demonstrate any significant difference in the rate of corneal re-epithelialization between cromolyn sodium ophthalmic solution, sterile saline solution, no treatment and an ophthalmic corticosteroid.

INDICATIONS AND USAGE

OPTICROM is indicated in the treatment of certain allergic ocular disorders referred to by the terms vernal keratoconjunctivitis, vernal conjunctivitis, giant papillary conjunctivitis, vernal keratitis, and allergic keratoconjunctivitis. The etiologic factors are unknown, but common airborne allergens and contact lenses have been implicated[1].

Symptomatic response to therapy (decreased itching, tearing, redness, and discharge) is usually evident within a few days, but longer treatment for up to six weeks is sometimes required. Once symptomatic improvement has been established, therapy should be continued for as long as needed to sustain improvement.

If required, corticosteroids may be used concomitantly with OPTICROM.

Users of soft (hydrophilic) contact lenses should refrain from wearing lenses while under treatment with OPTICROM (see **Contraindications**). Wear can be resumed within a few hours after discontinuation of the drug.

CONTRAINDICATIONS

OPTICROM is contraindicated in those patients who have shown hypersensitivity to cromolyn sodium or to any of the other ingredients.

As with all ophthalmic preparations containing benzalkonium chloride, patients are advised not to wear soft contact lenses during treatment with OPTICROM.

PRECAUTIONS

General: Patients may experience a transient stinging or burning sensation following application of OPTICROM.

The recommended frequency of administration should not be exceeded. The dose for adults and children is 1–2 drops in each eye 4–6 times a day at regular intervals.

Carcinogenesis, Mutagenesis, and Impairment of Fertility: Long term studies in mice (12 months intraperitoneal treatment followed by six months observation), hamsters (12 months intraperitoneal treatment followed by 12 months observation), and rats (18 months subcutaneous treatment) showed no neoplastic effect of cromolyn sodium.

No evidence of chromosomal damage or cytotoxicity was obtained in various mutagenesis studies.

No evidence of impaired fertility was shown in laboratory animal reproduction studies.

Pregnancy: Pregnancy Category B. Reproduction studies with cromolyn sodium administered parenterally to pregnant mice, rats and rabbits in doses up to 338 times the human clinical doses produced no evidence of fetal malformations. Adverse fetal effects (increased resorption and decreased fetal weight) were noted only at the very high parenteral doses that produced maternal toxicity. There are, however, no adequate and well controlled studies in pregnant women. Because animal reproduction studies are not always predictive of human response, this drug should be used during pregnancy only if clearly needed.

Nursing Mothers: It is not known whether this drug is excreted in human milk. Because many drugs are excreted in human milk, caution should be exercised when OPTICROM is administered to a nursing woman.

Pediatric Use: Safety and effectiveness in children below the age of 4 years have not been established.

ADVERSE REACTIONS

The most frequently reported adverse reaction attributed to the use of OPTICROM, on the basis of reoccurrence following readministration, is transient ocular stinging or burning upon instillation.

The following adverse reactions have been reported as infrequent events. It is unclear whether they are attributable to the drug: conjunctival injection, watery eyes, itchy eyes, dryness around the eye, puffy eyes, eye irritation, styes.

DOSAGE AND ADMINISTRATION

The dose for adults and children is 1–2 drops in each eye 4–6 times a day at regular intervals. One drop contains approximately 1.6 mg cromolyn sodium.

Patients should be advised that the effect of OPTICROM therapy is dependent upon its administration at regular intervals, as directed.

HOW SUPPLIED

OPTICROM is supplied as 10 ml of solution in an opaque polyethylene eye drop bottle.

NDC 0585-0680-01 10 ml bottle

Keep tightly closed and out of the reach of children. Store below 30°C (86°F) and protect from direct sunlight.

CAUTION

Federal law prohibits dispensing without prescription.

REFERENCE

[1]Allansmith MR, Abelson MB. Ocular Allergies. In: The Cornea, ed. by G. Smolin, RA Thoft. Little, Brown and Co., Boston/Toronto, 1983; 231–43.

FC 8003A
Revised 11/85

PEDIAPRED ™ ℞

[pēd 'ē-uh-pred]
(prednisolone sodium phosphate, USP)
ORAL LIQUID

DESCRIPTION

PEDIAPRED Oral Liquid is a dye free, colorless to light straw colored, raspberry flavored solution. Each 5 ml (teaspoonful) of PEDIAPRED contains 6.70 mg prednisolone sodium phosphate (5.00 mg prednisolone base) in a palatable, aqueous vehicle.

Prednisolone sodium phosphate occurs as white or slightly yellow, friable granules or powder. It is freely soluble in water, soluble in methanol, slightly soluble in alcohol and in chloroform; and very slightly soluble in acetone and in dioxane. The chemical name of prednisolone sodium phosphate is pregna-1,4-diene-3,20-dione,11,17-dihydroxy-21-(phosphonooxy)-, disodium salt, (11β)-. Its chemical structure is:

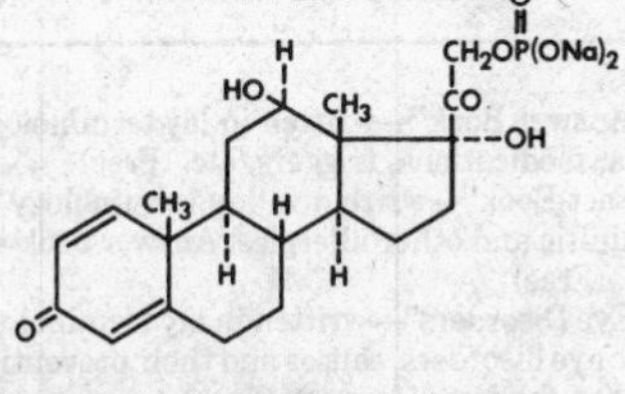

Pharmacological Category: Glucocorticoid

CLINICAL PHARMACOLOGY

Prednisolone is a synthetic adrenocortical steroid drug with predominantly glucocorticoid properties. Some of these properties reproduce the physiological actions of endogenous glucocorticosteroids, but others do not necessarily reflect any of the adrenal hormones' normal functions; they are seen only after administration of large therapeutic doses of the drug. The pharmacological effects of prednisolone which are due to its glucocorticoid properties include: promotion of gluconeogenesis; increased deposition of glycogen in the liver; inhibition of the utilization of glucose; anti-insulin activity; increased catabolism of protein; increased lipolysis; stimulation of fat synthesis and storage; increased glomerular filtration rate and resulting increase in urinary excretion of urate (creatinine excretion remains unchanged); and increased calcium excretion.

Depressed production of eosinophils and lymphocytes occurs, but erythropoiesis and production of polymorphonuclear leukocytes are stimulated. Anti-inflammatory processes (edema, fibrin deposition, capillary dilatation, migration of leukocytes and phagocytosis) and the later stages of wound healing (capillary proliferation, deposition of collagen, cicatrization) are inhibited. Prednisolone can stimulate secretion of various components of gastric juice. Stimulation of the production of corticotropin may lead to suppression of endogenous corticosteroids. Prednisolone has slight mineralocorticoid activity, whereby entry of sodium into cells and loss of intracellular potassium is stimulated. This is particularly evident in the kidney, where rapid ion exchange leads to sodium retention and hypertension.

Prednisolone is rapidly and well absorbed from the gastrointestinal tract following oral administration. PEDIAPRED Oral Liquid produces a 20% higher peak plasma level of prednisolone which occurs approximately 15 minutes earlier than the peak seen with tablet formulations. Prednisolone is 70–90% protein-bound in the plasma and it is eliminated from the plasma with a half-life of 2 to 4 hours. It is metabolized mainly in the liver and excreted in the urine as sulfate and glucuronide conjugates.

INDICATIONS AND USAGE

PEDIAPRED Oral Liquid is indicated in the following conditions:

1. **Endocrine Disorders**
   Primary or secondary adrenocortical insufficiency (hydrocortisone or cortisone is the first choice; synthetic analogs may be used in conjunction with mineralocorticoids where applicable; in infancy mineralocorticoid supplementation is of particular importance); congenital adrenal hyperplasia; hypercalcemia associated with cancer; nonsuppurative thyroiditis
2. **Rheumatic Disorders**
   As adjunctive therapy for short term administration (to tide the patient over an acute episode or exacerbation) in: psoriatic arthritis; rheumatoid arthritis, including juvenile rheumatoid arthritis (selected cases may require low dose maintenance therapy); ankylosing spondylitis; acute and subacute bursitis; acute nonspecific tenosynovitis; acute gouty arthritis; post-traumatic osteoarthritis; synovitis of osteoarthritis; epicondylitis
3. **Collagen Diseases**
   During an exacerbation or as maintenance therapy in selected cases of: systemic lupus erythematosus; systemic dermatomyositis (polymyositis); acute rheumatic carditis
4. **Dermatologic Diseases**
   Pemphigus; bullous dermatitis herpetiformis; severe erythema multiforme (Stevens-Johnson syndrome); exfoliative dermatitis; mycosis fungoides; severe psoriasis; severe seborrheic dermatitis
5. **Allergic States**
   Control of severe or incapacitating allergic conditions intractable to adequate trials of conventional treatment in: seasonal or perennial allergic rhinitis; bronchial asthma; contact dermatitis; atopic dermatitis; serum sickness; drug hypersensitivity reactions
6. **Ophthalmic Diseases**
   Severe acute and chronic allergic and inflammatory processes involving the eye and its adnexa such as: allergic conjunctivitis; keratitis; allergic corneal marginal ulcers; herpes zoster ophthalmicus; iritis and iridocyclitis; chorioretinitis; anterior segment inflammation; diffuse posterior uveitis and choroiditis; optic neuritis; sympathetic ophthalmia
7. **Respiratory Diseases**
   Symptomatic sarcoidosis; Loeffler's syndrome not manageable by other means; berylliosis; fulminating or disseminated pulmonary tuberculosis when used concurrently with appropriate antituberculous chemotherapy; aspiration pneumonitis
8. **Hematologic Disorders**
   Idiopathic thrombocytopenic purpura in adults; secondary thrombocytopenia in adults; acquired (autoimmune) hemolytic anemia; Erythroblastopenia (RBC anemia); congenital (erythroid) hypoplastic anemia
9. **Neoplastic Diseases**
   For palliative management of: leukemias and lymphomas in adults; acute leukemia of childhood
10. **Edematous States**
    To induce a diuresis or remission of proteinuria in the nephrotic syndrome, without uremia, of the idiopathic type or that due to lupus erythematosus.
11. **Gastrointestinal Diseases**
    To tide the patient over a critical period of the disease in: ulcerative colitis; regional enteritis
12. **Nervous System**
    Acute exacerbations of multiple sclerosis
13. **Miscellaneous**
    Tuberculous meningitis with subarachnoid block or impending block when used concurrently with appropriate antituberculous chemotherapy; trichinosis with neurologic or myocardial involvement

CONTRAINDICATIONS

Systemic fungal infections.

WARNINGS

In patients on corticosteroid therapy subjected to unusual stress, increased dosage of rapidly acting corticosteroids before, during and after the stressful situation is indicated.

Corticosteroids may mask some signs of infection, and new infections may appear during their use. There may be decreased resistance and inability to localize infection when corticosteroids are used.

Prolonged use of corticosteroids may produce posterior subcapsular cataracts, glaucoma with possible damage to the optic nerves, and may enhance the establishment of secondary ocular infections due to fungi or viruses.

Average and large doses of hydrocortisone or cortisone can cause elevation of blood pressure, salt and water retention, and increased excretion of potassium. These effects are less likely to occur with the synthetic derivatives except when used in large doses. Dietary salt restriction and potassium supplementation may be necessary. All corticosteroids increase calcium excretion. **While on corticosteroid therapy patients should not be vaccinated against smallpox. Other immunization procedures should not be undertaken in patients who are on corticosteroids, especially on high doses, because of possible hazards of neurological complications and a lack of antibody response.**

The use of prednisolone in active tuberculosis should be restricted to those cases of fulminating or disseminated tuberculosis in which the corticosteroid is used for the management of the disease in conjunction with an appropriate antituberculous regimen.

If corticosteroids are indicated in patients with latent tuberculosis or tuberculin reactivity, close observation is necessary as reactivation of the disease may occur. During prolonged corticosteroid therapy these patients should receive chemoprophylaxis.

PRECAUTIONS

General: Drug-induced secondary adrenocortical insufficiency may be minimized by gradual reduction of dosage. This type of relative insufficiency may persist for months after discontinuation of therapy; therefore, in any situation of stress occurring during that period, hormone therapy should be reinstituted. Since mineralocorticoid secretion may be impaired, salt and/or a mineralocorticoid should be administered concurrently.

There is an enhanced effect of corticosteroids in patients with hypothyroidism and in those with cirrhosis.

Corticosteroids should be used cautiously in patients with ocular herpes simplex because of possible corneal perforation.

The lowest possible dose of corticosteroid should be used to control the condition under treatment, and when reduction in dosage is possible, the reduction should be gradual.

Psychic derangements may appear when corticosteroids are used, ranging from euphoria, insomnia, mood swings, personality changes, and severe depression, to frank psychotic manifestations. Also, existing emotional instability or psychotic tendencies may be aggravated by corticosteroids.

Aspirin should be used cautiously in conjunction with corticosteroids in hypoprothrombinemia.

Steroids should be used with caution in nonspecific ulcerative colitis, if there is a probability of impending perforation, abscess or other pyogenic infection; diverticulitis; fresh intestinal anastomoses; active or latent peptic ulcer; renal insufficiency; hypertension; osteoporosis; and myasthenia gravis.

Growth and development of infants and children on prolonged corticosteroid therapy should be carefully observed.

Although controlled clinical trials have shown corticosteroids to be effective in speeding the resolution of acute exacerbations of multiple sclerosis, they do not show that they affect the ultimate outcome or natural history of the disease. The studies do show that relatively high doses of corticosteroids are necessary to demonstrate a significant effect. (See DOSAGE AND ADMINISTRATION.)

Since complications of treatment with glucocorticoids are dependent on the size of the dose and the duration of treatment, a risk/benefit decision must be made in each individual case as to dose and duration of treatment and as to whether daily or intermittent therapy should be used.

Information for Patients: Patients should be warned not to discontinue the use of PEDIAPRED abruptly or without medical supervision, to advise any medical attendants that they are taking PEDIAPRED and to seek medical advice at once should they develop fever or other signs of infection.

Drug Interactions: Drugs such as barbiturates which induce hepatic microsomal drug metabolizing enzyme activity may enhance metabolism of prednisolone and require that the dosage of PEDIAPRED be increased.

Pregnancy: Pregnancy Category C—Prednisolone has been shown to be teratogenic in many species when given in doses equivalent to the human dose. There are no adequate and well controlled studies in pregnant women. PEDIAPRED should be used during pregnancy only if the potential benefit justifies the potential risk to the fetus. Animal studies in which prednisolone has been given to pregnant mice, rats and rabbits have yielded an increased incidence of cleft palate in the offspring.

Continued on next page

Fisons—Cont.

Nursing Mothers: Prednisolone is excreted in breast milk, but only to a small (less than 1% of the administered dose) and probably clinically insignificant extent. Caution should be exercised when PEDIAPRED is administered to a nursing woman.

ADVERSE REACTIONS

Fluid and Electrolyte Disturbances
Sodium retention; fluid retention; congestive heart failure in susceptible patients; potassium loss; hypokalemic alkalosis; hypertension

Musculoskeletal
Muscle weakness; steroid myopathy; loss of muscle mass; osteoporosis; vertebral compression fractures; aseptic necrosis of femoral and humeral heads; pathologic fracture of long bones

Gastrointestinal
Peptic ulcer with possible perforation and hemorrhage; pancreatitis; abdominal distention; ulcerative esophagitis

Dermatologic
Impaired wound healing; thin fragile skin; petechiae and ecchymoses; facial erythema; increased sweating; may suppress reactions to skin tests

Metabolic
Negative nitrogen balance due to protein catabolism

Neurological
Convulsions; increased intracranial pressure with papilledema (pseudotumor cerebri) usually after treatment; vertigo; headache

Endocrine
Menstrual irregularities; development of cushingoid state; secondary adrenocortical and pituitary unresponsiveness, particularly in times of stress, as in trauma, surgery or illness; suppression of growth in children; decreased carbohydrate tolerance; manifestations of latent diabetes mellitus; increased requirements for insulin or oral hypoglycemic agents in diabetes.

Ophthalmic
Posterior subcapsular cataracts; increased intraocular pressure; glaucoma; exophthalmos

OVERDOSAGE

The effects of accidental ingestion of large quantities of prednisolone over a very short period of time have not been reported, but prolonged use of the drug can produce mental symptoms, moon face, abnormal fat deposits, fluid retention, excessive appetite, weight gain, hypertrichosis, acne, striae, ecchymosis, increased sweating, pigmentation, dry scaly skin, thinning scalp hair, increased blood pressure, tachycardia, thrombophlebitis, decreased resistance to infection, negative nitrogen balance with delayed bone and wound healing, headache, weakness, menstrual disorders, accentuated menopausal symptoms, neuropathy, fractures, osteoporosis, peptic ulcer, decreased glucose tolerance, hypokalemia, and adrenal insufficiency. Hepatomegaly and abdominal distention have been observed in children.

Treatment of acute overdosage is by immediate gastric lavage or emesis. For chronic overdosage in the face of severe disease requiring continuous steroid therapy the dosage of prednisolone may be reduced only temporarily, or alternate day treatment may be introduced.

DOSAGE AND ADMINISTRATION

The initial dosage of PEDIAPRED may vary from 5 ml to 60 ml (5 to 60 mg prednisolone base) per day depending on the specific disease entity being treated. In situations of less severity lower doses will generally suffice while in selected patients higher initial doses may be required. The initial dosage should be maintained or adjusted until a satisfactory response is noted. If after a reasonable period of time there is a lack of satisfactory clinical response, PEDIAPRED should be discontinued and the patient transferred to other appropriate therapy. **IT SHOULD BE EMPHASIZED THAT DOSAGE REQUIREMENTS ARE VARIABLE AND MUST BE INDIVIDUALIZED ON THE BASIS OF THE DISEASE UNDER TREATMENT AND THE RESPONSE OF THE PATIENT.**

After a favorable response is noted, the proper maintenance dosage should be determined by decreasing the initial drug dosage in small decrements at appropriate time intervals until the lowest dosage which will maintain an adequate clinical response is reached. It should be kept in mind that constant monitoring is needed in regard to drug dosage. Included in the situations which may make dosage adjustments necessary are changes in clinical status secondary to remissions or exacerbations in the disease process, the patient's individual drug responsiveness, and the effect of patient exposure to stressful situations not directly related to the disease entity under treatment; in this latter situation it may be necessary to increase the dosage of PEDIAPRED for a period of time consistent with the patient's condition. If after long term therapy the drug is to be stopped, it is recommended that it be withdrawn gradually rather than abruptly.

In the treatment of acute exacerbations of multiple sclerosis daily doses of 200 mg of prednisolone for a week followed by 80 mg every other day or 4 to 8 mg dexamethasone every other day for one month have been shown to be effective.

For the purpose of comparison, the following is the equivalent milligram dosage of the various glucocorticoids: cortisone, 25; hydrocortisone, 20; prednisolone, 5; prednisone, 5; methylprednisolone, 4; triamcinolone, 4; paramethasone, 2; betamethasone, 0.75; dexamethasone, 0.75. These dose relationships apply only to oral or intravenous administration of these compounds. When these substances or their derivatives are injected intramuscularly or into joint spaces, their relative properties may be greatly altered.

HOW SUPPLIED

PEDIAPRED Oral Liquid is a colorless to light straw colored solution containing 6.70 mg prednisolone sodium phosphate (5.00 mg prednisolone base) per 5 ml (teaspoonful).

NDC 0585-2250-01 4 Fl. oz bottle

Store at room temperature. Do not refrigerate. Keep tightly closed and out of the reach of children.

CAUTION

Federal law prohibits dispensing without prescription.

FISONS CORPORATION
BEDFORD, MA 01730 U.S.A.

Revised 1/86
FC2286

SOMOPHYLLIN® ℞

[*sōm "ăh-fĭ-lĭn*]
Oral Liquid

SOMOPHYLLIN®-DF ℞

Oral Liquid
(aminophylline oral solution)

DESCRIPTION

Somophyllin Oral Liquid contains aminophylline, USP, calculated on the anhydrous basis, a xanthine bronchodilator which occurs as a soluble complex containing about 86% anhydrous theophylline and about 14.25% ethylenediamine. Aminophylline occurs as white or slightly yellowish granules or powder, having a slight ammoniacal odor and bitter taste. Somophyllin Oral Liquid is a red, raspberry flavored solution. Somophyllin-DF Oral Liquid is a dye free, colorless to light straw colored, raspberry flavored solution. Each 5 ml (teaspoonful) contains aminophylline 105 mg (equivalent to 90 mg anhydrous theophylline) in a palatable, aqueous vehicle.

Each 15 ml (tablespoonful) contains aminophylline 315 mg (equivalent to 270 mg anhydrous theophylline).

Theophylline is the active ingredient.

The chemical name of aminophylline is 1*H*-Purine-2,6-dione,3,7-dihydro-1,3-dimethyl-, compd. with 1,2-ethanediamine (2:1). Its chemical structure is:

INDICATIONS

For relief and/or prevention of symptoms from asthma and reversible bronchospasm associated with chronic bronchitis and emphysema.

CONTRAINDICATIONS

This product is contraindicated in individuals who have shown hypersensitivity to its components, including ethylenediamine.

ADVERSE REACTIONS

The most consistent adverse reactions are usually due to overdose and are:

1. **Gastrointestinal:** nausea, vomiting, epigastric pain, hematemesis, diarrhea.
2. **Central nervous system:** headaches, irritability, restlessness, insomnia, reflex hyperexcitability, muscle twitching, clonic and tonic generalized convulsions.
3. **Cardiovascular:** palpitation, tachycardia, extrasystoles, flushing, hypotension, circulatory failure, ventricular arrhythmias.
4. **Respiratory:** tachypnea.
5. **Renal:** albuminuria, increased excretion of renal tubular and red blood cells, potentiation of diuresis.
6. **Others:** hyperglycemia and inappropriate ADH syndrome; rash (consider ethylenediamine).

OVERDOSAGE

Management: If potential oral overdose is established and seizure has not occurred:

A. Induce vomiting.
B. Administer a cathartic (this is particularly important if sustained release preparations have been taken).
C. Administer activated charcoal.

If patient is having a seizure:

A. Establish an airway.
B. Administer oxygen.
C. Treat the seizure with intravenous diazepam, 0.1 to 0.3 mg/kg up to 10 mg.
D. Monitor vital signs, maintain blood pressure and provide adequate hydration.

Post-seizure coma:

A. Maintain airway and oxygenation.
B. If a result of oral medication, follow above recommendations to prevent absorption of the drug, but intubation and lavage will have to be performed instead of inducing emesis, and the cathartic and charcoal will need to be introduced via a large bore gastric lavage tube.
C. Continue to provide full supportive care and adequate hydration while waiting for drug to be metabolized. In general, the drug is metabolized sufficiently rapidly so as not to warrant consideration of dialysis, however, if serum levels exceed 50 mcg/ml, charcoal hemoperfusion may be indicated.

HOW SUPPLIED

Somophyllin Oral Liquid is a red colored solution containing 105 mg aminophylline per 5 ml (equivalent to 90 mg anhydrous theophylline).

NDC 0585-2218-80 8 Fl. oz. bottle
NDC 0585-2218-82 32 Fl. oz. bottle

Somophyllin-DF Oral Liquid is a colorless to light straw colored solution containing 105 mg aminophylline per 5 ml (equivalent to 90 mg anhydrous theophylline).

NDC 0585-0218-84 8 Fl. oz. bottle

CAUTION

Federal law prohibits dispensing without prescription. Keep tightly closed and out of the reach of children.

FISONS CORPORATION
BEDFORD, MA 01730 U.S.A.

Revised 1/86
FC1787I

ADDITIONAL SOMOPHYLLIN® PRODUCTS ARE:

Somophyllin® Rectal Solution ℞
(aminophylline enema, USP)

Somophyllin®-T Capsules ℞
(theophylline capsules)

Somophyllin®-CRT Capsules ℞
(theophylline controlled release capsules)
100 mg, 200 mg, 250 mg, 300 mg

Please see package inserts for full prescribing information.

EDUCATIONAL MATERIAL

Booklets:
"Asthma Answer Book"—written in lay terminology outlining asthma, medications, triggers, etc. (Free)
"Allergy Fact Book"—written in lay terminology outlining allergic rhinitis and other allergies. Answer book about Nasalcrom®. (Free)
"Allergic Eye Disorders"—written in lay terminology outlining allergic eye disorders, causes and their prevention. (Free)
Monographs—for Nasalcrom®. (Free)
Monograph—for Opticrom®. (Free)

Pictures—Charts:
Instructional Wall Charts—for Intal® via Spinhaler®, Intal® Nebulizer Solution and Intal® Inhaler. (Free)

Samples:
Intal®, Intal® Inhaler, Spinhaler® Demo Kit, Intal® Nebulizer Solution, Nasalcrom® Sample Pack, Opticrom® Sample Pack, Somophyllin®-Oral Liquid and -DF (dye free) Oral Liquid, Isoclor® Timesule® Capsules, and Liquid. Available in limited quantities.

Products are cross-indexed
by product classifications
in the
BLUE SECTION

C. B. Fleet Co., Inc.

4615 MURRAY PL.
LYNCHBURG, VA. 24502-2235

FLEET® BABYLAX® OTC

ACTIVE INGREDIENT

Glycerin (USP)

INDICATIONS

For temporary relief of constipation in young children. Children under 1 year old, consult physician.

ACTIONS

This product generally produces a bowel movement in ¼ to 1 hour. The exact mode of action of glycerin administered rectally as a laxative is not known. It has been suggested that glycerin causes dehydration of exposed tissues to produce an irritant effect which results in a laxative response.

WARNINGS

For rectal use only. Glycerin administered rectally may produce rectal discomfort or a burning sensation in some individuals. If use results in unusual pain or side effects, consult a physician.

GENERAL LAXATIVE WARNINGS

Do not use a laxative product when nausea, vomiting or abdominal pain are present unless directed by a physician. If you have noticed a sudden change in bowel habits that persists over two weeks, consult a physician before using a laxative. Laxative products should not be used longer than one week except under a physician's advice. Frequent or prolonged use of laxatives may result in dependence. Rectal bleeding or failure to have a bowel movement after use of a laxative may indicate a serious condition; discontinue use and consult a physician. Keep this and all drugs out of the reach of children. In case of accidental ingestion, seek professional assistance or contact a Poison Control Center immediately.

DOSAGE AND ADMINISTRATION

Children under 1 year old: consult physician. Children 1–6 years of age: 1 rectal applicator containing 4 ml. of glycerin as needed or as directed by physician. Hold unit upright. Remove protective shield and discard. With steady pressure, gently insert stem with tip pointing toward navel. Squeeze unit until nearly all liquid is expelled. Remove tip from rectum. Note: A small amount of liquid will remain in unit. Store and use at room temperature.

HOW SUPPLIED

Six 4 ml. rectal applicators per package.

IS THIS PRODUCT OTC

Yes.

FLEET® BISACODYL ENEMA OTC
(bisacodyl U.S.P.)

COMPOSITION

Each 30 ml (delivered dose) contains 10 mg. of bisacodyl, U.S.P. suspended in an aqueous medium. The FLEET® Bisacodyl Enema unit, with a 2-inch prelubricated Comfortip®, contains 1¼ fl. oz. of enema suspension in a ready-to-use plastic squeeze bottle. Designed for quick, convenient administration by nurse or patient according to instructions. Disposable after single use.

ACTION AND USES

FLEET® Bisacodyl Enema is a contact laxative acting directly on the colonic mucosa to produce peristalsis. FLEET® Bisacodyl Enema actually produces peristalsis and evacuation of the large intestine by stimulating sensory nerve endings in the colonic mucosa to produce parasympathetic reflexes. FLEET® Bisacodyl Enema is very effective usually producing an evacuation within 15 minutes to 1 hour. FLEET® Bisacodyl Enema may be used whenever a laxative or enema is indicated. It is useful as a laxative for occasional relief of constipation, in bowel cleansing in preparation before X-ray and endoscopic examination.

WARNINGS

Do not use a laxative product when nausea, vomiting, or abdominal pain is present unless directed by a physician. If you have noticed a sudden change in bowel habits that persists over a period of 2 weeks, consult a physician before using a laxative. Rectal bleeding or failure to have a bowel movement after use of a laxative may indicate a serious condition. Discontinue use and consult a physician. Laxative products should not be used longer than 1 week unless directed by a physician. Frequent or prolonged use of a laxative may result in dependence. Keep this and all drugs out of the reach of children. In case of accidental ingestion, seek professional assistance or contact a Poison Control Center immediately.

DOSAGE AND ADMINISTRATION

Adults—one unit or as directed by a physician. **Precaution:** Do not administer to children under 2 years of age. **Administration:** Preferred position—Lying on left side with left knee slightly bent and the right leg drawn up, or knee-chest position. Rubber diaphragm at base of tube prevents accidental leakage and assures controlled flow of the enema solution. May be used at room temperature.

PROFESSIONAL ADMINISTRATION

See FLEET® Ready-to-Use Enema.

HOW SUPPLIED

FLEET® Bisacodyl Enema is supplied in 1¼ fl. oz. ready-to-use squeeze bottle.

IS THIS PRODUCT OTC

Yes.

LITERATURE AVAILABLE

Professional literature mailed on request.

FLEET® ENEMA OTC

COMPOSITION

Each 118 ml (delivered dose) contains 19 g. sodium biphosphate and 7 g. sodium phosphate. The FLEET® Enema unit, with a 2-inch, pre-lubricated Comfortip®, contains 4½ fl. oz. of enema solution in a hand-size plastic squeeze bottle. Designed for quick, convenient administration by nurse or patient according to instructions. Disposable after single use.

ACTION AND USES

FLEET Enema is useful as a laxative in the relief of constipation, and as a bowel evacuant for a variety of diagnostic, surgical, and therapeutic indications. Used as directed, FLEET Enema provides thorough yet safe cleansing action and induces complete emptying of the left colon usually within 2 to 15 minutes without pain or spasm. FLEET Enema may be used for the occasional relief of constipation; as a routine enema; for cleansing of the colon in preparation for rectal examination; preoperative cleansing and general postoperative care; to help relieve fecal or barium impaction.

GENERAL LAXATIVE WARNINGS

Do not use laxative products when nausea, vomiting, or abdominal pain is present. If you notice a sudden change in bowel habits that persists over a period of 2 weeks, consult a physician. Rectal bleeding or failure to have a bowel movement after use of a laxative may indicate a serious condition. Discontinue use and consult a physician. Laxative products should not be used longer than 1 week unless directed by a physician. Frequent or prolonged use of a laxative may result in dependence. Keep this and all drugs out of the reach of children. In case of accidental ingestion, seek professional assistance or contact a Poison Control Center immediately.

PROFESSIONAL USE WARNINGS

Do not use in patients with congenital megacolon or congestive heart failure as hypernatremic dehydration may occur. Use with caution in patients with impaired renal function or where colostomy exists, as hypocalcemia, hyperphosphatemia, hypernatremia and acidosis may occur. Since FLEET® Ready-To-Use Enema contains sodium phosphate and sodium biphosphate, there is a risk of acute elevation of sodium concentration in the serum and consequent dehydration, particularly in children with megacolon. Additional fluids by mouth are recommended where appropriate (Fonkalsrud, E. and Keen, J.: "Hypernatremic Dehydration Hypertonic Enemas in Congenital Megacolon," *JAMA* 199:584–586, 1967. Zumoff, B. and Hellman, L.: "Rectal Absorption of Sodium from Hypertonic Sodium Phosphate Solutions," data on file, C. B. Fleet Company, Inc. Gilman, A., Goodman, L., Gilman, A., eds., *The Pharmacological Basis of Therapeutics*, Sixth Edition, 1980, p. 1005.) In addition, elevated levels of serum phosphates and decreased levels of serum calcium have been reported in patients with renal disease (and with prolonged use). (McConnell, T. H., "Fatal Hypocalcemia from Phosphate Absorption from Laxative Preparation," *JAMA*, 216:147–148, 1971.) If any of these complications occur following administration of Fleet® Ready-To-Use Enema, immediate corrective action should be taken to restore electrolyte balance with appropriate fluid replacements. Calcium and phosphorous levels should be carefully monitored.

PRECAUTIONS

DO NOT ADMINISTER TO CHILDREN UNDER 2 YEARS OF AGE.

ADMINISTRATION AND DOSAGE

Preferred position: Lying on left side with left knee slightly bent and the right leg drawn up, or knee-chest position. Dosage: Adults, 4 fl. oz. Rubber diaphragm at base of tube prevents accidental leakage and assures controlled flow of the enema solution. May be used at room temperature. Each 118 ml. (delivered dose) contains 4.4 g. sodium.

PROFESSIONAL DOSAGE AND ADMINISTRATION

Fleet® Ready-To-Use Enema should not be used in children under 2 years of age. In those cases where complications are reported, infants and young children are often involved. Fleet® Ready-To-Use Enema for Children should be used with caution in children of any age. Careful consideration of the use of enemas in general in children is recommended. The adult size enema should not be used in children under 12 years of age. For children 2 to 12 years of age, use Fleet® Ready-To-Use Enema for Children, which contains a dosage of one-half the adult size enema. For children less than 2 years of age, Fleet® Glycerin Suppositories for Children should be used.

Proper and safe use of Fleet® Ready-To-Use Enema also requires that the product be administered according to the Directions for Use. Health care professionals should remember, when administering the product, to *gently* insert the enema into the rectum with steady pressure with the tip pointing toward the navel. Care during insertion is necessary due to lack of sensory innervation of the rectum. Once inserted, squeeze the bottle until nearly all the liquid is expelled. If resistance is encountered on insertion of the nozzle or in administering the solution, the procedure should be discontinued. Forcing the enema can result in perforation and/or abrasion of the rectum.

HOW SUPPLIED

FLEET® Enema is supplied in a 4½ fl. oz. ready-to-use squeeze bottle. Pediatric size, 2¼ fl. oz.

IS THIS PRODUCT OTC

Yes.

LITERATURE AVAILABLE

Professional literature mailed on request.

FLEET® MINERAL OIL ENEMA OTC

COMPOSITION

The FLEET Mineral Oil Enema unit, with a 2-inch, prelubricated Comfortip®, contains 4½ fl.oz. (133 ml.) mineral oil USP in a hand-size plastic squeeze bottle.

ACTION AND INDICATIONS

Serves to soften and lubricate hard stools, easing their passage without irritating the mucosa. Results approximate a normal bowel movement in that only the rectum, sigmoid, and part or all of the descending colon are evacuated. Indicated for relief of fecal impaction; valuable in relief of constipation when straining must be avoided (in hypertension, coronary occlusion, proctologic procedures, postoperative care); for removal of barium sulfate residues from the colon after barium administration for GI series or outlining the left atrium; to obtain the laxative benefits of mineral oil while avoiding possible untoward effects of oral administration such as (1) interference with intestinal absorption of fat-soluble vitamins A, D, E and K and other nutrients (2) danger of systemic absorption (3) possible risk of lipid pneumonia due to aspiration.

WARNINGS

Do not use laxative products when nausea, vomiting, abdominal pain is present unless directed by a physician. If you have noticed a sudden change in bowel habits that persists over a period of 2 weeks, consult a physician. Rectal bleeding or failure to have a bowel movement after use of a laxative may indicate a serious condition. Discontinue use and consult a physician. Laxative products should not be used longer than 1 week unless directed by a physician. Frequent and prolonged use of enemas may result in dependence. Keep this and all drugs out of the reach of children. In case of accidental ingestion, seek professional assistance or contact a Poison Control Center immediately.

PRECAUTIONS

DO NOT ADMINISTER TO CHILDREN UNDER 2 YEARS OF AGE.

ADMINISTRATION AND DOSAGE

For rectal administration only. Ready-to-use unit permits easy, rapid administration by physician, nurse, or patient; disposable after single use.

PROFESSIONAL DOSAGE AND ADMINISTRATION

Fleet® Ready-To-Use Mineral Oil Enema should not be used in children under 2 years of age. Fleet® Ready-To-Use Mineral Oil Enema should be used with caution in children of any age. Careful consideration of the use of enemas in general in children is recommended.

Proper and safe use of Fleet® Ready-To-Use Mineral Oil Enema also requires that the product be administered according to the Directions for Use. Health care professionals should remember, when administering the product, to gently insert the enema into the rectum with steady pressure with the tip pointing toward the naval. Care during insertion is necessary due to lack of sensory innervation of the rectum.

Continued on next page

Fleet—Cont.

Once inserted, squeeze the bottle until nearly all the liquid is expelled. If resistance is encountered on insertion of the nozzle or in administering the solution, the procedure should be discontinued. Forcing the enema can result in perforation and/or abrasion of the rectum.

HOW SUPPLIED

FLEET Mineral Oil Enema is supplied in 4½ fl.oz. ready-to-use squeeze bottle.

IS THIS PRODUCT OTC

Yes.

FLEET® PHOSPHO®-SODA OTC

Buffered Laxative

COMPOSITION

Each 100 ml. of regular or flavored PHOSPHO-SODA contains 48 g. sodium biphosphate and 18 g. sodium phosphate in a stable, buffered aqueous solution.

INDICATIONS

For relief of occasional constipation or for preparing the colon for x-ray or other endoscopic examination.

ACTION AND USES

Versatile in action as a gentle laxative or purgative, according to dosage. This product produces a bowel movement in ½ to 6 hours.

CONTRAINDICATIONS

DO NOT USE THIS PRODUCT IF YOU HAVE KIDNEY DISEASE UNLESS DIRECTED BY A PHYSICIAN.

PROFESSIONAL USE WARNINGS

Do not use in patients with congenital megacolon or congestive heart failure, as hypernatremic dehydration may occur. Use with caution in patients with impaired renal function as hypocalcemia, hyperphosphatemia, hypernatremia and acidosis may occur. Since FLEET® Phospho®-Soda contains sodium phosphate and sodium biphosphate, there is a risk of acute elevation of sodium concentration in the serum and consequent dehydration, particularly in children with megacolon. Additional fluids by mouth are recommended where appropriate. (Fonkalsrud, E. and Keen, J.: "Hypernatremic Dehydration Hypertonic Enemas in Congenital Megacolon," *JAMA* 199:584–586, 1967. Zumoff, B. and Hellman, L.: "Rectal Absorption of Sodium from Hypertonic Sodium Phosphate Solutions," data on file, C. B. Fleet Company, Inc. Gilman, A., Goodman, L., Gilman, A., eds., *The Pharmacological Basis of Therapeutics,* Sixth Edition, 1980, p. 1005.) In addition, elevated levels of serum phosphates and decreased levels of serum calcium have been reported in patients with renal disease (and with prolonged use). (McConnell, T. H., "Fatal Hypocalcemia from Phosphate Absorption from Laxative Preparation," *JAMA,* 216:147–148, 1971.) If any of these complications occurs following administration of Fleet® Phospho®-Soda, immediate corrective action should be taken to restore electrolyte balance with appropriate fluid replacements. Calcium and phosphorous levels should be carefully monitored.

GENERAL LAXATIVE WARNINGS

Do not use a laxative product when nausea, vomiting, or abdominal pain is present unless directed by a physician. If you have noticed a sudden change in bowel habits that persists over a period of 2 weeks, consult a physician before using a laxative. Rectal bleeding or failure to have a bowel movement may indicate a serious condition. Discontinue use and consult a physician. Laxative products should not be used longer than 1 week unless directed by a physician. Frequent or prolonged use of a laxative may result in dependence on laxatives. Keep this and all drugs out of the reach of children. In case of accidental overdose or ingestion, seek professional assistance or contact a Poison Control Center immediately.

ADMINISTRATION AND DOSAGE

Mix required dose with one-half glass cold clear liquid and follow with a full glass of water, preferably on arising or at least 30 minutes before a meal, or at bedtime for overnight action.

As a laxative: 4 teaspoonfuls, diluted as directed.
As a purgative: 8 teaspoonfuls, diluted as directed.
Children: One half the adult dose for children 10 years old or older; one quarter the adult dose for children between 5 and 10 years of age. DO NOT GIVE TO CHILDREN UNDER 5 YEARS OF AGE.

Each recommended dose (4 teaspoonfuls) contains 96.4 meq. sodium.

HOW SUPPLIED

Regular or Flavored, in bottles of 3 and 8 fl. oz.; 1½ fl. oz. size for hospitals.

IS THIS PRODUCT OTC

Yes.

FLEET® PREP KITS OTC

Bowel Evacuant

DESCRIPTION

FLEET® Prep Kit No. 1 contains:

1. FLEET® Phospho®-Soda—1½ fl. oz. Ingredients: Each teaspoonful (5 ml) contains : Active Ingredients: Sodium Biphosphate 2.4 Gm. and Sodium Phosphate 0.9 Gm.
2. FLEET® Bisacodyl—4 laxative tablets. Ingredients: Each enteric-coated tablet contains Bisacodyl, USP, 5 mg.
3. FLEET® Bisacodyl—1 laxative suppository. Ingredients: Bisacodyl, USP, 10 mg.
4. 1 Patient Instruction Sheet.

FLEET® Prep Kit No. 2 contains:

1. FLEET® Phospho®-Soda—1½ fl. oz.
2. FLEET® Bisacodyl—4 tablets.
3. FLEET® Bagenema—1. Ingredients: Liquid castile soap ⅔ fl. oz.
4. 1 Patient Instruction Sheet.

FLEET® Prep Kit No. 3 contains:

1. FLEET® Phospho®-Soda—1½ fl. oz.
2. FLEET® Bisacodyl—4 tablets.
3. FLEET® Bisacodyl Enema—1 laxative enema. Ingredients: 1–30 ml. dose containing 10 mg. of Bisacodyl.
4. 1 Patient Instruction Sheet.

FLEET® Prep Kit No. 4 contains:

1. FLEET® Flavored Castor Oil Emulsion-1½ fl. oz. Ingredients: Each tablespoonful (15 ml.) contains: Active Ingredients: Castor Oil U.S.P. 10 ml.
2. FLEET® Bisacodyl—4 tablets.
3. FLEET® Bisacodyl—1 suppository.
4. 1 Patient Instruction Sheet.

FLEET® Prep Kit No. 5 contains:

1. FLEET® Flavored Castor Oil Emulsion-1½ fl. oz.
2. FLEET® Bisacodyl—4 tablets.
3. FLEET® Bagenema—1.
4. 1 Patient Instruction Sheet.

FLEET® Prep Kit No. 6 contains:

1. FLEET® Flavored Castor Oil Emulsion-1½ fl. oz.
2. FLEET® Bisacodyl—4 tablets.
3. FLEET® Bisacodyl Enema—30 ml.
4. 1 Patient Instruction Sheet.

ACTIONS

Bowel Cleansing System

INDICATIONS

For use as part of a bowel cleansing regiment in preparation of the colon for radiology (prior to barium enemas or I.V.P.'s), surgery, and many proctologic and colonoscopic procedures.

WARNINGS

Each recommended dose ((1½ fl. oz.) (45 ml)) of Phospho®-Soda contains 216.9 milli-equivalents (meq) of sodium. Persons on a low salt diet should consult a health professional before use.

Castor oil affects the small intestine, and regular use may cause excessive loss of water and body salts which can have debilitating effects.

GENERAL LAXATIVE WARNINGS

Do not use a laxative product when nausea, vomiting, or abdominal pain is present unless directed by a physician. If you have noticed a sudden change in bowel habits that persists over a period of 2 weeks, consult a doctor before using a laxative. Rectal bleeding or failure to have a bowel movement may indicate a serious condition. Discontinue use and consult a physician. Laxative products should not be used longer than 1 week unless directed by a physician. Frequent or prolonged use of a laxative may result in dependence on laxatives. Keep this and all drugs out of the reach of children. In case of accidental overdose or ingestion, seek professional assistance or contact a Poison Control Center immediately.

PROFESSIONAL USE WARNINGS

Do not use in patients with congenital megacolon or congestive heart failure as hypernatremic dehydration may occur. Use with caution in patients with impaired renal function or where colostomy exists as hypocalcemia, hyperphosphatemia, hypernatremia and acidosis may occur. Since FLEET® Phospho®-Soda contains sodium phosphate and sodium biphosphate, there is a risk of acute elevation of sodium concentration in the serum and consequent dehydration, particularly in children with megacolon. Additional fluids by mouth are recommended where appropriate. (Fonkalsrud, E. and Keen, J.: "Hypernatremic Dehydration Hypertonic Enemas in Congenital Megacolon," *JAMA* 199:584–586, 1967. Zumoff, B. and Hellman, L.: "Rectal Absorption of Sodium from Hypertonic Sodium Phosphate Solutions," data on file, C. B. Fleet Company, Inc. Gilman, A., Goodman, L., Gilman, A., eds., *The Pharmacological Basis of Therapeutics,* Sixth Edition, 1980, p. 1005.) In addition, elevated levels of serum phosphates and decreased levels of serum calcium have been reported in patients with renal disease (and with prolonged use). (McConnell, T. H., "Fatal Hypocalcemia from Phosphate Absorption from Laxative Preparation," *JAMA,* 216:147–148, 1971.) If any of these complications occur following administration of FLEET® Phospho®-Soda, immediate corrective action should be taken to restore electrolyte balance with appropriate fluid replacements. Calcium and phosphorous levels should be carefully monitored.

THESE KITS SHOULD NOT BE USED BY PATIENTS UNDER 2 YEARS OF AGE.

DOSAGE AND ADMINISTRATION

SEE PATIENT INSTRUCTION SHEET FOR 12, 24, AND 48 HOUR PREPARATION SCHEDULE IN EACH KIT.

HOW SUPPLIED

See "Description" for contents of each kit.

Shipping Unit: 48 FLEET® Prep Kits per carton.

For full prescribing information on specific products, see individual listings (FLEET® Phospho®-Soda, FLEET® Bisacodyl Enema and FLEET® Flavored Castor Oil Emulsion).

IS THIS PRODUCT OTC

Yes.

LITERATURE AVAILABLE

Yes.

FLEET® FLAVORED CASTOR OIL EMULSION OTC

(Stimulant Laxative)

INGREDIENTS

Each tablespoonful (15 ml.) contains:
Inactive Ingredients: Water, flavoring, emulsifying agents, propylene glycol, sodium benzoate, citric acid and sodium saccharin.

ACTIVE INGREDIENTS

Castor Oil U.S.P. 10 ml.

INDICATIONS

For the occasional relief of constipation and preparation of the colon for x-ray and endoscopic examination. (See FLEET® Prep Kit listings.)

ACTIONS

Works directly on the small intestine to promote bowel movement. This product usually produces a bowel movement in 6 to 12 hours.

WARNINGS

Do not use laxative products when nausea, vomiting or abdominal pain is present unless directed by a physician. If you have noticed a sudden change in bowel habits that persists over a period of 2 weeks, consult a physician before using a laxative. Laxative products should not be used longer than 1 week unless directed by a physician. Frequent or prolonged use of a laxative may result in a dependence on laxatives. Rectal bleeding or failure to have a bowel movement may indicate a serious condition. Discontinue use and consult a physician. Castor oil affects the small intestine and regular use may cause excessive loss of water and body salts, which can have a debilitating effect. Keep this and all drugs out of the reach of children. In case of accidental overdose, seek professional assistance or contact a Poison Control Center immediately.

DOSAGE AND ADMINISTRATION

Adults: Purgative: 6 tablespoonfuls (90 ml). Laxative: 3 tablespoonfuls (45 ml.) Children 2 to 12 years: 1 tablespoonful (15 ml.) Children up to 2 years: up to 1 teaspoonful (5 ml.) or as directed by a physician. For best results, take on an empty stomach. Follow with one full glass of cool water. May be chilled to enhance taste.

HOW SUPPLIED

Bottles of 1½ and 3 fl. oz.

IS THIS PRODUCT OTC

Yes.

FLEET® RELIEF OTC

Anesthetic Hemorrhoidal Ointment

ACTIVE INGREDIENT

Pramoxine Hydrochloride 1%

INDICATIONS

For the temporary relief of itching, burning and pain associated with hemorrhoids or other anorectal disorders.

ACTIONS
Pramoxine hydrochloride is a topical anesthetic proven to be safe and effective in clinical tests. Delivered in a water soluble base that is greaseless, stainless, and odorless, it begins to work immediately to relieve hemorrhoidal discomforts.

WARNING
In case of bleeding, consult a physician promptly. Certain persons can develop allergic reactions to ingredients in this product. If the symptom being treated does not subside or redness, irritation, swelling, pain, itching or other symptoms develop or increase, within 7 days, discontinue use and consult a physician. Do not exceed recommended daily dosage except under the supervision of a physician. If introduction of this product into the rectum causes additional pain, stop use and consult physician promptly. As with any drug, if you are pregnant or nursing a baby, seek the advice of a health professional before using this product. The safety of this product has not been established for use by pregnant women or nursing mothers. Keep this and all drugs out of the reach of children. In case of accidental ingestion, seek professional assistance or contact a Poison Control Center immediately.

DOSAGE AND ADMINISTRATION
When practical, wash the anorectal area with mild soap and warm water and rinse off all soap before application of this product. Disposable Pre-filled Applicator—Remove protective cap and gently insert prelubricated stem into the rectum. Squeeze gently until applicator is empty. Remove and discard unit. Use one unit as needed each morning and night and after bowel movements. Do not exceed 5 applications in 24 hours. Tube—Apply Fleet Relief Ointment generously to the affected area up to 5 times daily. If accompanying applicator is used, attach to tube and lubricate with small amount of ointment. Insert gently into rectum and squeeze tube. Cleanse applicator after each use.

HOW SUPPLIED
Six 4 ml. rectal applicators per package or single one ounce tube with applicator.

IS THIS PRODUCT OTC
Yes.

SUMMER'S EVE® MEDICATED DOUCHE — OTC

ACTIVE INGREDIENT
Povidone-iodine provided as a 0.23 percent solution when packet and sanitized fluid are mixed.

INDICATIONS
For temporary relief of minor vaginal irritation and itching. Clinically effective in a program of treatment for vaginal moniliasis, vaginales vaginitis and non-specific vaginitis due to Candida albicans, Trichomonas vaginalis, and Gardnerella vaginalis.

ACTIONS
Povidone-iodine is an effective broad spectrum anti-microbial agent used in treatment of both gram negative and gram positive bacteria, fungi, yeast, and protozoa.

WARNINGS
DOUCHING DOES NOT PREVENT PREGNANCY. Do not use during pregnancy or if nursing a baby except with the approval of a physician. If douching results in pain, soreness, itching, excessive dryness, or irritation, stop douching. If symptoms persist consult a physician. If minor irritation has not improved after 1 week of use, consult a physician. Women with iodine sensitivity should not use this product. The use of iodine as a douche may cause a transient rise of serum protein-bound iodine. Keep this and all drugs out of the reach of children. In case of accidental ingestion, seek professional assistance or contact a Poison Control Center immediately.

DOSAGE AND ADMINISTRATION
Dosage is contained in a single-unit concentrate packet to be added to 4.5 fluid ounces of sanitized solution supplied in a disposable unit. Remove the sanitary overwrap. Unscrew nozzle cap. Carefully open medicated packet and pour contents into bottle. Screw nozzle cap back on to bottle. Swirl gently to assure complete mixing. Pull up the flexible nozzle until it clicks and locks, and Summer's Eve® Medicated Douche is ready to use. After use, the unit is discarded. Use once daily for seven days even if symptoms disappear.

HOW SUPPLIED
4.5 fluid ounce single pack with one 0.14 fluid ounce medicated packet or twin pack containing two 4.5 fluid ounce units and two 0.14 fluid ounce packets.

IS THIS PRODUCT OTC
Yes.

Fleming & Company

1600 FENPARK DR.
FENTON, MO 63026

AEROLATE SR & JR & III Capsules ℞
(theophylline, anhydrous T.D.)

AEROLATE LIQUID
(theophylline, anhydrous)

COMPOSITION
Contains theophylline 4 grs. (260 mg) as SR, 2 grs (130 mg) as JR, 1 gr. as III (65 mg), in red/clear capsules. Liquid has 150 mg theophylline/15cc in a non-sugar, non-alcoholic, non-saccharin tangerine flavored base.

ACTION AND USES
Timed action pellets by-pass stomach to prevent gastric upset. Bronchodilation is achieved through bowel absorption only. Liquid is for the acute attack primarily.

ADMINISTRATION AND DOSAGE
One capsule every 12 hours. Every 8 hours in severe attacks. Liquid—adults—40 ml (2.5 tablespoonfuls) for acute attack. Children—0.25 ml/lb. Maintainance therapy—adults—for the first 6 doses, 25 ml (1.5 tablespoonfuls) before breakfast, at 3 p.m., at bedtime. Then 15 ml doses at above times. Children—0.15ml/lb. at these times, then 0.1ml/lb per dose.

SIDE EFFECTS
Nausea, vomiting, epigastric or substernal pain, palpitation, headache, dizziness may occur.

HOW SUPPLIED
Capsules in bottles of 100 and 1000.
Liquid in pints and gallons.

CONGESS SR & JR Capsules ℞
Expectorant/Decongestant T.D.

COMPOSITION
Contains guaifenesin 250 mgs/pseudoephedrine 120 mgs as SR; guaifenesin 125 mgs/pseudoephedrine 60 mgs as JR in blue/pink capsules.

ACTION AND USES
To loosen mucus plugs in upper respiratory tract and congestion in acute pulmonary disorders, and in coughing. Nasal decongestion and alleviation of bronchospasm is also achieved up to 12 hrs. that accompany most coughs, especially during the nocturnal period.

INDICATIONS
Nasal congestion, sinusitis, acute aerotitis media, bronchial asthma, serous otitis media, and symptoms of the common cold.

DOSAGE
Adults and children over 12 yrs. one SR capsule every 12 hrs. Under 12 yrs. one JR capsule as prescribed by physician.

PRECAUTION AND SIDE EFFECTS
Use with care in severe hypertension, heart disease, hyperthyroidism, diabetes. Low grade sensitivity to drugs may be experienced.

CONTRAINDICATIONS
Glaucoma, prostatic hypertrophy, patients receiving MAO inhibitors.

HOW SUPPLIED
Plastic bottles of 100 and 1000 capsules.

EXTENDRYL ℞
T.D. Capsules SR & JR, Syrup and Tablets

Each timed action SR capsule contains phenylephrine HCl 20 mg; methscopolamine nitrate 2.5 mg; chlorpheniramine maleate 8 mg. The JR potency is exactly half-strength. Green/red color for both. Each 5 cc of root beer flavored syrup and tablet contains: phenylephrine HCl 10 mg; methscopolamine nitrate 1.25 mg; chlorpheniramine maleate 2 mg.

ACTION AND USES
Antihistaminic-decongestant for relief of respiratory congestion; allergic rhinitis; allergic skin reactions of urticaria and angioedema.

ADMINISTRATION AND DOSAGE
Capsules—one every 12 hrs of the SR for adults; one JR every 12 hrs for children 6–12 yrs. Syrup-two teaspoonfuls every 4 hrs for adults; children 1 teaspoonful every 4 hrs. Tablets —adults two and children one every 4 hrs. Do not exceed 4 doses in 24 hrs.
Children under 6 yrs. as recommended by a physician.

PRECAUTIONS
Withdraw therapy if drowsiness occurs. Patients are cautioned against driving or operating mechanical devices.

CONTRAINDICATIONS
Glaucoma, cardiac disease, hyperthyroidism and hypertension.

HOW SUPPLIED
Capsules and tablets in bottles of 100 and 1000. Syrup in pints and gallons.

MARBLEN
(calcium and magnesium carbonates)
ANTACID SUSPENSIONS AND TABLET

(See PDR For Nonprescription Drugs)

NEPHROCAPS ℞
Dialysis Vitamin Supplement

DESCRIPTION
Each black oval gelatin 'liquid' capsule provides: Thiamin 1.5 mg; Riboflavin 1.7 mg; Niacin 20 mg; Pantothenic acid 5 mg; Biotin 150 mcg; Cyanocobalamin 6 mcg; Pyridoxin 10 mg; Ascorbic acid 100 mg and Folic acid 1.0 mg.

INDICATIONS
The wasting syndrome in chronic renal failure; uremia; impaired metabolic functions of the kidney.

DOSAGE
One capsule daily. On dialysis days, one Nephrocap must be taken after treatment.

SUPPLIED
Plastic bottles of 100 only.

NEPHROX SUSPENSION
(aluminum hydroxide)
Antacid Suspension

(See PDR For Nonprescription Drugs)

NICOTINEX Elixir
nicotinic acid

(See PDR For Nonprescription Drugs)

OCEAN-A/S Nasal Spray

COMPOSITION
Each 45ml bottle contains 0.893mg atropine sulfate.

ACTION AND USES
For 'post nasal drip'; snoring due to mucus formation; smokers cough due to irritants.

ADMINISTRATION AND DOSAGE
Two sprays in each nostril t.i.d. & h.s. for 'p.n.d.' and cough; two sprays at 7 p.m. and h.s. for snoring.

HOW SUPPLIED
20cc bottles only.

OCEAN MIST
(buffered isotonic saline)

(See PDR For Nonprescription Drugs)

PIMA Syrup ℞
(potassium iodide)

COMPOSITION
Contains KI 5 grs./tsp., in a black raspberry flavored base.

ACTION AND USES
An expectorant in the symptomatic treatment of chronic pulmonary diseases where tenacious mucus complicates the problem, including bronchial asthma, bronchitis and pulmonary emphysema.

ADMINISTRATION AND DOSAGE
Children—one half to one tsp. and adults one or two tsp. every 4-6 hours.

SIDE EFFECTS
May include gastrointestinal upset, metallic taste, minor skin eruptions, nausea, vomiting and epigastric pain. Therapy should be withdrawn.

Continued on next page

Fleming—Cont.

PRECAUTIONS
In patients sensitive to iodides, in hyperthyroidism, and in rare cases iodine-induced goiter may occur.

HOW SUPPLIED
Plastic pints and gallons.

PURGE
(flavored castor oil)

(See PDR For Nonprescription Drugs)

RUM-K ℞
(potassium chloride 15% conc.)

DESCRIPTION
Each 10 ml. contains 1.5 Gm. potassium chloride (20 mEq) in a butter/rum synthetic flavored base that is alcohol and sugar free.

INDICATIONS
Hypokalemic-hypochloremic alkalosis; digitalis toxicity; hypokalemia prevention secondary to corticosteroid or diuretic administration.

CONTRAINDICATIONS
Impaired renal function, untreated Addison's Disease, acute dehydration, heat cramps, hyperkalemia.

PRECAUTIONS
Do not use in patients with low urinary output or renal decompensation. Potassium replacements vary and should be individualized. Patients should be checked frequently, ECG and plasma K^+ levels should be made. High serum concentrations of K^+ cause death thru cardiac depression, arrhythmias or arrest. Use with caution in cardiac disease.

ADVERSE REACTIONS
Vomiting, nausea, abdominal discomfort, diarrhea may occur. Symptoms and signs of potassium overdose include paresthesias of extremities, flaccid paralysis, listlessness, fall in blood pressure, weakness and heaviness of the legs, cardiac arrhythmias and heart block. Hyperkalemia may cause ECG changes as disappearance of the P wave, widening and slurring of QRS complex, changes of the S-T segment, tall peaked T waves.

DOSAGE AND ADMINISTRATION
Adults—two teaspoonsful (10ml) in 4–6 oz water 2 to 4 times daily after meals to supply 40–80 mEq of elemental potassium and chloride. Larger doses may be required and administered under close supervision due to possible potassium intoxication or saline laxative effect.

HOW SUPPLIED
2 oz; 4 oz; pints and gallons.

S-P-T ℞
(Pork thyroid "liquid" capsules USP)

COMPOSITION
S-P-T is prepared by special process from cleaned, fresh pork thyroid glands, deprived of connective tissue, defatted and suspended in soy bean oil and encapsulated in gelatin for greater oral absorption. The active hormones (T4 and T3) are available in their natural state in a ratio of approximately 2.5:1, as in humans, to insure therapeutic availability. Capsules are standardized by USP method for iodine content and also biologically to insure 100% metabolic potency.

ACTION
To increase metabolic rate of body tissues. S-P-T is replacement therapy for diminished or absent thyroid function. Effect develops slowly and is fully reached in 10—14 days per grain increase in most instances.

INDICATIONS
As replacement therapy in hypothyroidism, cretinism, myxedema, and after surgery following complete thyroidectomy.

CONTRAINDICATIONS
In thyrotoxicosis, angina pectoris, myocardial infarction and hypertension unless complicated by hypothyroidism, and uncorrected adrenal insufficiency.

PRECAUTION AND SIDE EFFECTS
Overdosage may cause tachycardia, angina pectoris, diarrhea, nervousness, sweating, headache and increased pulse action. In most cases, reduction of dosage overcomes side effects.

DOSAGE AND ADMINISTRATION
Patients should be titrated starting at lower levels and increasing by 1 gr every 2 weeks until mild thyromimetic effects are noted. Then lower the dose to the level at which the patient felt best, as patients vary widely as to thyroid need.

WARNINGS
Drugs with thyroid hormone activity, alone or together with other therapeutic agents, have been used for the treatment of obesity. In euthyroid patients, doses within the range of daily hormonal requirements are ineffective for weight reduction. Larger doses may produce serious or even life-threatening manifestations of toxicity, particularly when given in association with sympathomimetic amines such as those used for their anorectic effects.

HOW SUPPLIED
As 1 gr (green); 2 gr (brown); 3 gr (red); 5 gr (black) gelatin sealed capsules in bottles of 100 and 1000.

Flint
Division of Travenol Laboratories, Inc.
ONE BAXTER PKWY.
DEERFIELD, IL 60015

CHOLOXIN® ℞
[*kō"lŏcks'ĭn*]
(Dextrothyroxine Sodium Tablets, USP) Flint

DESCRIPTION
CHOLOXIN (dextrothyroxine sodium) is the sodium salt of the dextrorotatory isomer of thyroxine. It is chemically described as D-3,5,3',5'-tetraiodothyronine sodium salt.

CLINICAL PHARMACOLOGY
The predominant effect of CHOLOXIN (dextrothyroxine sodium) is the reduction of serum cholesterol levels in hyperlipidemic patients. Beta lipoprotein and triglyceride fractions may also be reduced from previously elevated levels. Available evidence indicates that CHOLOXIN (dextrothyroxine sodium) stimulates the liver to increase catabolism and excretion of cholesterol and its degradation products via the biliary route into the feces. Cholesterol synthesis is not inhibited and abnormal metabolic end-products do not accumulate in the blood.

INDICATION AND USAGE
For treatment of hyperlipidemia in patients with no known heart disease.
This is not an innocuous drug. Strict attention should be paid to the indications and contraindications.
CHOLOXIN (dextrothyroxine sodium) is an antilipidemic agent used as an adjunct to diet and other measures for the reduction of elevated serum cholesterol (low density lipoproteins) in euthyroid patients with no known evidence of organic heart disease.
It has not been clearly established whether the drug-induced lowering of serum cholesterol or lipid levels has a detrimental, beneficial, or no effect on the morbidity or mortality due to atherosclerosis or coronary heart disease. Several years will be required before current investigations will yield an answer to this question.

CONTRAINDICATIONS
The administration of CHOLOXIN (dextrothyroxine sodium) to euthyroid patients with one or more of the following conditions is contraindicated:

1. Known organic heart disease, including angina pectoris; history of myocardial infarction; cardiac arrhythmia or tachycardia, either active or in patients with demonstrated propensity for arrhythmias; rheumatic heart disease; history of congestive heart failure; and decompensated or borderline compensated cardiac status.
2. Hypertensive states (other than mild, labile systolic hypertension).
3. Advanced liver or kidney disease.
4. Pregnancy.
5. Nursing mothers.
6. History of iodism.

WARNINGS

Drugs with thyroid hormone activity, alone or together with other therapeutic agents, have been used for the treatment of obesity. In euthyroid patients, doses within the range of daily hormonal requirements are ineffective for weight reduction. Larger doses may produce serious or even life threatening manifestations of toxicity, particularly when given in association with sympathomimetic amines such as those used for their anorectic effects.

CHOLOXIN (dextrothyroxine sodium) may potentiate the effects of anticoagulants on prothrombin time. Reductions of anticoagulant dosage by as much as 30% have been required in some patients. Consequently, the dosage of anticoagulants should be reduced by one-third upon initiation of CHOLOXIN (dextrothyroxine sodium) therapy and the dosage subsequently readjusted on the basis of prothrombin time. The prothrombin time of patients receiving anticoagulant therapy concomitantly with CHOLOXIN (dextrothyroxine sodium) therapy should be observed as frequently as necessary, at least weekly during the first few weeks of treatment.
In the surgical patient, it is wise to consider withdrawal of the drug two weeks prior to surgery if the use of anticoagulants during surgery is contemplated.
Special consideration must be given to the dosage of other thyroid medications used concomitantly with CHOLOXIN (dextrothyroxine sodium). As with all thyroactive drugs, hypothyroid patients are more sensitive than euthyroid patients to a given dose of dextrothyroxine sodium.
The injection of epinephrine into patients with coronary artery disease may precipitate an episode of coronary insufficiency. This condition may be enhanced in patients receiving thyroid analogues. These phenomena should be kept in mind when catecholamine injections are required in dextrothyroxine sodium-treated patients with coronary artery disease.
Since the possibility of precipitating cardiac arrhythmias during surgery may be greater in patients treated with thyroid hormones, it may be wise to discontinue CHOLOXIN (dextrothyroxine sodium) in euthyroid patients at least two weeks prior to an elective operation. During emergency surgery in euthyroid patients, the patients should be carefully observed.
There are reports that dextrothyroxine sodium in diabetic patients is capable of increasing blood sugar levels with a resultant increase in requirements of insulin or oral hypoglycemic agents. Special attention should be paid to parameters necessary for good control of the diabetic state in dextrothyroxine sodium-treated subjects and to dosage requirements of insulin or other antidiabetic drugs. If dextrothyroxine sodium is later withdrawn from patients who had required a dosage increase of insulin or oral hypoglycemic agents during its administration, the dosage of antidiabetic drugs should be reduced and adjusted to maintain good control of the diabetic state.
When impaired liver and/or kidney function are present, the advantages of CHOLOXIN (dextrothyroxine sodium) therapy must be weighed against the possibility of deleterious results.

PRECAUTIONS
It is expected that patients on CHOLOXIN (dextrothyroxine sodium) therapy will show increased serum thyroxine levels. These increased serum thyroxine values are evidence of absorption and transport of the drug, and should NOT be interpreted as evidence of hypermetabolism; therefore, they may not be used to determine the effective dose of dextrothyroxine sodium. Thyroxine values in the range of 10 to 25 mcg% in dextrothyroxine sodium-treated patients are common.
If signs or symptoms of iodism develop during dextrothyroxine sodium therapy, the drug should be discontinued.
A few children with familial hypercholesterolemia have been treated with CHOLOXIN (dextrothyroxine sodium) for periods of one year or longer with no adverse effects on growth. However, it is recommended that the drug be continued in patients in this age group only if a significant serum cholesterol-lowering effect is observed.
The 2 mg and 6 mg tablets of CHOLOXIN (dextrothyroxine sodium) contain FD&C Yellow No. 5 (tartrazine) which may cause allergic-type reactions (including bronchial asthma) in certain susceptible individuals. Although the overall incidence of FD&C Yellow No. 5 (tartrazine) sensitivity in the general population is low, it is frequently seen in patients who also have aspirin hypersensitivity.
Usage in Women of Childbearing Age: Women of childbearing age with familial hypercholesterolemia or hyperlipemia should not be deprived of the use of this drug; it can be given to those patients exercising strict birth control procedures. Since pregnancy may occur despite the use of birth control procedures, administration of CHOLOXIN (dextrothyroxine sodium) to women of this age group should be undertaken only after weighing the possible risk to the fetus against the possible benefits to the mother. Teratogenic studies in two animal species have resulted in no abnormalities in the offspring.

ADVERSE REACTIONS
The side effects attributed to CHOLOXIN (dextrothyroxine sodium) therapy are, for the most part, due to increased metabolism, and may be minimized by following the recommended dosage schedule. Adverse effects are least commonly seen in euthyroid patients with no signs or symptoms of organic heart disease.
In the absence of known organic heart disease, some cardiac changes may be precipitated during dextrothyroxine sodium

therapy. Angina pectoris, extrasystoles, ectopic beats, supraventricular tachycardia, ECG evidence of ischemic myocardial changes and increase in heart size have all been observed. Myocardial infarctions, both fatal and nonfatal, have occurred, but these are not unexpected in untreated patients in the age groups studied. It is not known whether any of these infarcts were drug related.

Changes in clinical status that may be related to the metabolic action of the drug include the development of insomnia, nervousness, palpitations, tremors, loss of weight, lid lag, sweating, flushing, hyperthermia, hair loss, diuresis, and menstrual irregularities. Gastrointestinal complaints during therapy have included dyspepsia, nausea and vomiting, constipation, diarrhea, and decrease in appetite.

Other side effects reported to be associated with dextrothyroxine sodium therapy include the development of headache, changes in libido (increase or decrease), hoarseness, tinnitus, dizziness, peripheral edema, malaise, tiredness, visual disturbances, psychic changes, paresthesia, muscle pain, and various bizarre subjective complaints. Skin rashes, including a few which appeared to be due to iodism, and itching have been attributed to dextrothyroxine sodium by some investigators. Gallstones have been discovered in occasional dextrothyroxine sodium-treated patients and cholestatic jaundice has occurred in one patient, although its relationship to dextrothyroxine sodium therapy was not established. In several instances, the previously existing conditions of the patient appeared to continue or progress during the administration of dextrothyroxine sodium. A worsening of peripheral vascular disease, sensorium, exophthalmos and retinopathy have been reported.

Dextrothyroxine sodium potentiates the effects of anticoagulants on prothrombin time, thus indicating a decrease in the dosage requirements of the anticoagulants. On the other hand, dosage requirements of antidiabetic drugs have been reported to be increased during dextrothyroxine sodium therapy (see WARNINGS section).

DOSAGE AND ADMINISTRATION

For **adult** euthyroid hypercholesterolemic patients, the recommended maintenance dose of CHOLOXIN (dextrothyroxine sodium) is 4 to 8 mg per day. The initial dose should be 1 to 2 mg daily, to be increased in 1 to 2 mg increments at intervals of not less than one month to a maximal level of 4 to 8 mg daily.

For **pediatric** hypercholesterolemic patients, the recommended maintenance dose of CHOLOXIN (dextrothyroxine sodium) is approximately 0.1 mg (100 mcg) per kilogram. The initial dosage should be approximately 0.05 mg (50 mcg) per kilogram daily, increased at not more than 0.05 mg (50 mcg) per kilogram increments at monthly intervals. The recommended maximal dose is 4 mg daily.

If signs or symptoms of cardiac disease develop during the treatment period, the drug should be withdrawn.

HOW SUPPLIED

CHOLOXIN (dextrothyroxine sodium) Tablets are supplied as scored, color-coded tablets in 4 concentrations: 1 mg-orange... 2 mg-yellow... 4 mg-white... 6 mg-green.

LITERATURE AVAILABLE

Upon request.

Shown in Product Identification Section, page 409

FLINT SSD™ ℞
(1% Silver Sulfadiazine Cream)

DESCRIPTION

Flint SSD™ (1% Silver Sulfadiazine Cream) is a topical antibacterial preparation which has as its active antimicrobial ingredient silver sulfadiazine. The active moiety is contained within an opaque, white, water-miscible cream base.

Each 1000 grams of Flint SSD™ Cream contains 10 grams of silver sulfadiazine. The cream base contains White Petrolatum, USP; Stearyl Alcohol, NF; Isopropyl Myristate, NF; Sorbitan Monooleate, NF; Polyoxyl 40 Stearate, NF; Propylene Glycol, USP; and Purified Water, USP; with 0.3% Methylparaben, NF, as a preservative.

Silver sulfadiazine has an empirical formula of $C_{10}H_9AgN_4O_2S$, molecular weight of 357.14, and structural formula as shown:

H_2N–(benzene ring)–SO_2N(Ag)–(pyrimidine ring, N, N)

CLINICAL PHARMACOLOGY

Flint SSD™ Cream has demonstrated *in vitro* antimicrobial activity against actual clinical burn wound isolates. Representative organisms included numerous strains of gram-negative and gram-positive bacteria and yeasts. *In vitro* test results evaluating the antimicrobial effectiveness of silver sulfadiazine are summarized in Table 1. All microorganisms analyzed for susceptibility are isolates from burn patients obtained nationwide.

[See table above].

TABLE 1
NUMBER OF SENSITIVE BURN ISOLATED STRAINS/
TOTAL BURN ISOLATED STRAINS TESTED

Genus & Species	CONCENTRATION OF SILVER SULFADIAZINE 62.5 mcg/ml	125 mcg/ml
Pseudomonas aeruginosa	46/54	50/54
Pseudomonas cepacia	2/3	2/3
Pseudomonas species	2/3	2/3
Enterobacter cloacae	6/14	6/14
Enterobacter aerogenes	4/6	4/6
Enterobacter agglomerans	1/1	1/1
Klebsiella pneumoniae	4/4	4/4
Klebsiella species	1/3	1/3
Escherichia coli	11/15	11/15
Serratia liquifaciens	3/3	3/3
Serratia marcescens	6/6	6/6
Serratia rubidae	2/2	2/2
Serratia species	0/1	1/1
Proteus mirabilis	8/8	8/8
Proteus morganii	8/9	8/9
Proteus rettgeri	1/1	1/1
Proteus vulgaris	3/4	4/4
Providencia species	3/3	3/3
Citrobacter diversus	0/2	0/2
Shigella species	1/2	1/2
Acinetobacter anitratum	2/2	2/2
Aeromonas hydrophilia	3/3	3/3
Arizona hinshawii	1/1	1/1
Alcaligenes faecalis	2/2	2/2
Staphylococcus aureus	7/7	7/7
Streptococcus Group D (including *Enterococcus*)	17/18	18/18
Bacillus species	0/1	1/1
Candida albicans	1/3	3/3
Candida species	0/1	1/1

Flint SSD™ (1% Silver Sulfadiazine Cream) exerts its principal antimicrobial effect at the level of the cell membrane and cell wall. The mechanism and site of action differ from sodium sulfadiazine and silver nitrate. *In vitro* analysis has demonstrated that the bactericidal activity exerted by Flint SSD™ (1% Silver Sulfadiazine Cream) is superior to sulfadiazine alone.

Flint SSD™ Cream may be especially applicable to the treatment of pediatric burn patients, because it is not a carbonic anhydrase inhibitor. There have been no reports of acidosis attributable to treatment with Flint SSD™ Cream.

INDICATIONS AND USAGE

Flint SSD™ Cream is a topical antibacterial preparation which is indicated as an adjunct to currently accepted principles of burn wound care, for the prevention and treatment of burn wound sepsis in patients with partial and full thickness burns.

CONTRAINDICATIONS

Since sulfonamide derivatives are known to increase the possibility of kernicterus[1], Flint SSD™ Cream should not be used in pregnant women approaching or at term, premature infants, or neonates less than two months of age.

WARNINGS

Flint SSD™ Cream should be administered with caution to patients with a history of hypersensitivity to silver sulfadiazine. It is not known whether prior sensitivity to other sulfonamides will precipitate an allergic response to Flint SSD™ Cream.

Should manifestation of allergic response to Flint SSD™ Cream be observed, continuation of therapy must be weighed against the potential hazards of the particular allergic reaction.

While Flint SSD™ Cream is exerting a bacteriostatic effect on the burn wound, fungal proliferation in and below the eschar may occur. However, the incidence of clincially reported fungal superinfection is low.

Flint SSD™ Cream should be used with caution in patients with a history of glucose-6-phosphate dehydrogenase deficiency, as hemolysis may occur.

When treatment with Flint SSD™ Cream involves prolonged administration and /or large burn surfaces, considerable amounts of silver sulfadiazine are absorbed. Serum sulfa concentrations may approach adult therapeutic levels (8-12 mg%).

In extensively burned patients, serum sulfa concentrations and renal function should be closely monitored, and urine should be analyzed for presence of sulfa crystals.

PRECAUTIONS

Following administration of Flint SSD™ (1% Silver Sulfadiazine Cream), absorption of sulfadiazine has been reported. In addition, small amounts of silver are absorbed over the course of repeated application of Flint SSD™ Cream. Impairment of hepatic and renal functions which results in diminished excretion of drug constituents may lead to accumulation of silver and sulfadiazine moieties. In the presence of hepatic and/or renal dysfunction, the therapeutic benefits of continued silver sulfadiazine administration must be assessed in light of the possibility of accumulation of by-products.

When utilizing topical enzymatic preparations for debridement of partial and full thickness burn wounds, concomitant or alternating topical antimicrobial therapy must be employed.

Pregnancy Category C. Animal reproduction studies have not been conducted with Flint SSD™ Cream. It is also not known whether Flint SSD™ Cream can cause fetal harm when administered to a pregnant woman or can affect reproduction capacity. Flint SSD™ Cream should be given to a pregnant woman only if clearly needed. To date, there are no reports in the medical literature which associate Flint SSD™ Cream therapy with adverse effects on the fetus or reproductive capacity.

Flint SSD™ Cream should be administered to pregnant women only when the physician decides that the potentially life-saving benefits of silver sulfadiazine therapy in the larger burn (extent greater than 20% body surface area) outweigh possible hazard to the fetus.

There is no evidence that topical application of Flint SSD™ Cream results in excretion of any of its constituents in human milk. However, since all sulfonamide derivatives are known to increase the possibility of kernicterus, caution should be exercised when Flint SSD™ Cream is administered to nursing women.

ADVERSE REACTIONS

Several cases of transient leukopenia have been reported in patients receiving silver sulfadiazine therapy. Leukopenia associated with silver sulfadiazine administration is primarily characterized by decreased neutrophil count. Maximal white blood cell depression occurs within two to four days of initiation of therapy. Rebound to normal leukocyte levels follows onset within two to three days. Recovery is not influenced by continuation of silver sulfadiazine therapy. This reaction has been reported to occur in approximately one in twenty patients.[6,7]

A low incidence of other adverse reactions has been reported. These include burning sensation, rashes and pruritus, and rarely, interstitial nephritis.

It is often difficult to differentiate topical reactions which are precipitated by Flint SSD™ (1% Silver Sulfadiazine Cream) from those resulting from routine burn wound effects, or caused by hypersensitivity to other therapeutic agents being administered concurrently to the patient.

During the treatment of burns over large body surfaces (greater than 20% body surface area), significant amounts of silver sulfadiazine are systemically absorbed. Therefore, it is possible that any adverse reactions associated with sulfonamides may occur.

DOSAGE AND ADMINISTRATION

In the patients with a major burn, evaluation of airway and fluid replacement needs should precede treatment of the burn wound. After appropriate resuscitative measures are

Continued on next page

Flint—Cont.

instituted, the burn wound is evaluated for extent and depth, and an appropriate treatment regimen is instituted.
Flinit SSD™ Cream should be applied to a thickness of at least 1/16 inch, to selected burned surfaces once or twice daily.
It is recommended that a protocol for management of the burn wound using accepted principles and techniques of debridement be followed. Flint SSD™ Cream should be applied with sterile gloves.
Flint SSD™ Cream will provide antimicrobial protection when used with either open treatment or occlusive dressing regimens. When treating patients utilizing the open method, care must be taken to promptly reapply Flint SSD™ Cream whenever it is removed by patient movement.
Daily hydrotherapy facilitates debridement of loosened eschar and removal of accumulated debris. Flint SSD™ Cream should be reapplied immediately after hydrotherapy.
Treatment of burns with topical antimicrobial agents has been reported to allow spontaneous healing of deep partial thickness burn wounds, by preventing bacterial proliferation which could otherwise cause conversion to full thickness loss. However, delayed separation of eschar associated with the use of topical antimicrobial agents such as Flint SSD™ Cream may require definitive surgical treatment of the eschar.
should be applied continually until either spontaneous healing or grafting of the burn wound is achieved.
In order to avoid the possibility of infection, Flint SSD™ Cream should not be withdrawn from the therapeutic regimen until definitive wound closure is accomplished, unless there is a significant adverse reaction to the drug.

HOW SUPPLIED

Flint SSD™ (1% Silver Sulfadiazine Cream) is supplied in plastic jars containing 50, 400 and 1000 grams.
Store between 15°–30° C (59°–86° F).

References:

1. **AMA Drug Evaluations**, Fourth Edition: Chapter 77, Sulfonamides and related compounds. 1980, p 1305.
2. Delaveau P, Freidrich-Noue P: Cutaneous absorption and urinary elimination of silver sulfadiazine compounds used in the treatment of burns. **Therapy 32**:563-572, 1977.
3. Dimick AR: Experience with the use of proteolytic enzyme (Travase®) in burn patients. **J Trauma 17**:948-955, 1977.
4. Fox CL Jr: Silver Sulfadiazine - A new topical therapy for Pseudomonas in burns. Therapy of Pseudomonas infection in burns. **Arch Surg 96**:184-188, 1968.
5. Fox CL, Modak SM: Mechanism of silver sulfadiazine action of burn wound infections. **Antimicrobial Agents for Chemotherapy 5**:582-588, 1974.
6. Harrison HN: Pharmacology of sulfadiazine silver - its attachment to burned human and rat skin and studies of gastrointestinal absorption and extension. **Arch Surg 114**:281-285, 1979.
7. Jarret F, Ellerbe S, Demling R: Acute leukopenia during topical burn therapy with silver sulfadiazine. **Amer J Surg 135**:818-819, 1978.
8. Kiker RG, Carvajal HF, Mlcak RP, Larson DL: A controlled study of the effects of silver sulfadiazine on white blood cell counts in burned children. **J Trauma 17**:835-836, 1977.
9. Krizek TJ: Emergency nonsurgical escharotomy in the burned extremity. **Ortho Rev**, July 1975, p 53-55.
10. Pennisi VR, Abril F, Cappozzi A: The combined efficacy of Travase and silver sulphadiazine in the acute burn. **Burns 2**:169-172, 1976.
11. Rodeheaver G: Proteolytic enzymes as adjuncts to antimicrobial prophylaxis of contaminated wounds. **Amer J Surg 129**:537-544, 1975.

Literature Available: Upon request.
Shown in Product Identification Section, page 409

SYNTHROID® ℞

[sĭn'throid]
(Levothyroxine Sodium, USP) Flint
Synthroid Tablets—for oral administration
Synthroid Injection—for parenteral administration after reconstitution

DESCRIPTION

SYNTHROID (levothyroxine sodium) **Tablets** and SYNTHROID **Injection** contain synthetic crystalline levothyroxine sodium (L-thyroxine). L-thyroxine is the principal hormone secreted by the normal thyroid gland.
Pharmacologic Category: SYNTHROID (levothyroxine sodium) **Tablets**, taken orally, provide hormone that is absorbed readily from the gastrointestinal tract. SYNTHROID **Injection** is effective by any parenteral route. Following absorption, the synthetic L-thyroxine provided by SYNTHROID (levothyroxine sodium) products cannot be distinguished from L-thyroxine that is secreted endogenously. Each is bound to the same serum proteins forming a reservoir of circulating L-thyroxine.
Both SYNTHROID (levothyroxine sodium) products will provide L- thyroxine (T_4) as a substrate for physiologic deiodination to L-triiodothyronine (T_3). Therefore, patients taking properly adjusted doses of both SYNTHROID (levothyroxine sodium) products will demonstrate normal blood levels of L- triiodothyronine even when the thyroid gland has been removed surgically or destroyed by radioiodine. Administration of levothyroxine sodium alone will result in complete physiologic thyroid replacement.

INDICATIONS AND USAGE

SYNTHROID (levothyroxine sodium) products serve as specific replacement therapy for reduced or absent thyroid function of any etiology. SYNTHROID (levothyroxine sodium) **Injection** can be used intravenously whenever a rapid onset of effect is critical, and either intravenously or intramuscularly in hypothyroid patients whenever the oral route is precluded for long periods of time.

CONTRAINDICATIONS

There are no absolute contraindications to SYNTHROID (levothyroxine sodium) therapy. Relative contraindications include acute myocardial infarction, uncorrected adrenal insufficiency and thyrotoxicosis (see WARNINGS).

WARNINGS

> Drugs with thyroid hormone activity, alone or together with other therapeutic agents, have been used for the treatment of obesity. In euthyroid patients, doses within the range of daily hormonal requirements are ineffective for weight reduction. Larger doses may produce serious or even life threatening manifestations of toxicity, particularly when given in association with sympathomimetic amines such as those used for their anorectic effects.

Patients with cardiovascular diseases warrant particularly close attention during the restoration of normal thyroid function by any thyroid drug. In such cases, low initial dosage increased slowly by small increments is indicated. Occasionally, the cardiovascular capacity of the patient is so compromised that the metabolic demands of the normal thyroid state cannot be met. Clinical judgment will then dictate a less-than-complete restoration of thyroid status.
Endocrine disorders such as diabetes mellitus, adrenal insufficiency (Addison's disease), hypopituitarism and diabetes insipidus are characterized by signs and symptoms which may be diminished in severity or obscured by hypothyroidism. SYNTHROID (levothyroxine sodium) therapy for such patients may aggravate the intensity of previously obscured symptoms and require appropriate adjustment of therapeutic measures directed at these concomitant disorders.
Thyroid replacement may potentiate the effects of anticoagulants. Patients on anticoagulant therapy should have frequent prothrombin determinations when instituting thyroid replacement to gauge the need to reduce anticoagulant dosage.

PRECAUTIONS

Overdosage with any thyroid drug may produce the signs and symptoms of thyrotoxicosis, but resistance to such factitious thyrotoxicosis is the general rule. With SYNTHROID (levothyroxine sodium) **Tablets**, the relatively slow onset of action minimizes the risk of overdose but close observation in the weeks following institution of a dosage regimen is advised. Treatment of thyroid hyperactivity induced by oral medication is confined to interruption of therapy for a week, followed by reinstitution of daily therapy at an appropriately reduced dosage.
Close observation of the patient following the administration of SYNTHROID (levothyroxine sodium) **Injection** is advised, and appropriate adjustment of repeated dosage is recommended.
The 100 mcg (0.1 mg) and 300 mcg (0.3 mg) tablets of SYNTHROID (levothyroxine sodium) contain FD&C Yellow No. 5 (tartrazine) which may cause allergic-type reactions (including bronchial asthma) in certain susceptible individuals. Although the overall incidence of FD&C Yellow No. 5 (tartrazine) sensitivity in the general population is low, it is frequently seen in patients who also have aspirin hypersensitivity.

ADVERSE REACTIONS

Adverse reactions are due to overdose and are those of induced hyperthyroidism.

DOSAGE AND ADMINISTRATION

For most adults, a final dosage of 100 mcg. (0.1 mg.) to 200 mcg. (0.2 mg.) of SYNTHROID (levothyroxine sodium) **Tablets** daily will provide adequate thyroid replacement, and only occasionally will patients require larger doses. Failure to respond adequately to a daily oral intake of 400 mcg. (0.4 mg.) or more is rare and should prompt reconsideration of the diagnosis of hypothyroidism, special investigation of the patient in terms of malabsorption of L-thyroxine from the gastrointestinal tract or evaluation of patient compliance to therapy.
The concomitant appearance of other diseases, especially cardiovascular diseases, usually dictates a replacement regimen with initial doses smaller than 100 mcg. (0.1 mg.) per day.
In otherwise healthy adults with relatively recent onset of hypothyroidism, full replacement doses of 150 mcg. (0.15 mg.) or 200 mcg. (0.2 mg.) have been instituted immediately without untoward effect and with good therapeutic response. General experience, however, favors a more cautious approach in view of the possible presence of subclinical disorders of the cardiovascular system or other endocrinopathies.
The age and general physicial condition of the patient and the severity and duration of hypothyroid symptoms determine the starting dosage and the rate of incremental dosage increase leading to a final maintenance dosage. In the elderly patient with long standing disease, evidence of myxedematous infiltration and symptomatic, functional or electrocardiographic evidence of cardiovascular dysfunction, the starting dose may be as little as 25 mcg. (0.025 mg.) per day. Further incremental increases of 25 mcg. (0.025 mg.) per day may be instituted at three to four week intervals depending on patient response. Conversely, otherwise healthy adults may be started at higher daily doses and raised to a full replacement dose in two to three weeks. Clearly it is the physician's judgment of the severity of the disease and close observation of patient response which determine the rate and extent of dosage increase.
Appropriate laboratory tests are beneficial in monitoring thyroid replacement therapy. Although measurements of normal blood levels of thyroxine in patients on oral replacement regimens frequently coincide with clinical impressions of normal thyroid status, higher than normal levels occur occasionally and should not be considered evidence of overdosage per se. In all cases, clinical impressions of the well-being of the patient take precedence over laboratory determinations of appropriate individual dosage.
In infants and children, there is a great urgency to achieve full thyroid replacement because of the critical importance of thyroid hormone in sustaining growth and maturation. Despite the smaller body size, the dosage needed to sustain a full rate of growth, development and general thriving is higher in the child than in the adult.
The recommended daily replacement dosage of levothyroxine sodium in childhood is: 0-1 years: 9 mcg/kg; 1-5 years: 6 mcg/kg; 6-10 years: 4 mcg/kg; 11-20 years: 3 mcg/kg. Dose is administered once daily only. Optimal maintenance levels should be adjusted individually to obtain normal serum T_3, T_4, free T_4 index and Thyroid Stimulating Hormone (TSH) values after several weeks of therapy for hypothyroidism. The patient's clinical status is most important and some patients may be clinically euthyroid with individual laboratory values that are not within normal range (i.e. elevated total T_4 with normal T_3). An exception may be seen in congenital hypothyroidism where elevated serum TSH values may persist for the first 2-3 years of life despite normalization of free T_4 measurements. In such cases, it generally is recommended that maintenance of normal serum free T_4 values alone should be considered therapeutically sufficient.
In myxedema coma or stupor, without concomitant severe heart disease, 200 to 500 mcg. of SYNTHROID (levothyroxine sodium) **Injection** may be administered intravenously as a solution containing 100 mcg./ml. DO NOT ADD TO OTHER INTRAVENOUS FLUIDS. Although the patient may show evidence of increased responsivity within six to eight hours, full therapeutic effect may not be evident until the following day. An additional 100 to 300 mcg. or more may be given on the second day if evidence of significant and progressive improvement has not occurred. Like the oral dosage form, SYNTHROID (levothyroxine sodium) **Injection** produces a predictable increase in the reservoir level of hormone with a seven day half-life. This usually precludes the need for multiple injections but continued daily administration of lesser amounts parenterally should be maintained until the patient is fully capable of accepting a daily oral dose. A daily maintenance dose of 50 to 100 mcg parenterally should suffice to maintain the euthyroid state, once established.
In the presence of concomitant heart disease, the sudden administration of such large doses of L-thyroxine intravenously is clearly not without its cardiovascular risks. Under such circumstances, intravenous therapy should not be undertaken without weighing the alternative risks of the myxedema coma and the cardiovascular disease. Clinical judgment in this situation may dictate smaller intravenous doses of SYNTHROID (levothyroxine sodium) **Injection**.
SYNTHROID (levothyroxine sodium) **Injection** by intravenous or intramuscular routes can be substituted for the oral dosage form when ingestion of SYNTHROID (levothyroxine sodium) **Tablets** is precluded for long periods of time. The initial parenteral dosage should be approximately one half of the previously established oral dosage of levothyroxine sodium tablets. Close observation of the patient, with individual adjustment of the dosage as needed, is recommended.

HOW SUPPLIED

SYNTHROID (levothyroxine sodium) **Tablets** are supplied as scored, color-coded potency-marked tablets in 8 strengths: 25 mcg. (0.025 mg.)—orange . . . 50 mcg. (0.05 mg.)—white . . . 75 mcg. (0.075 mg)—violet . . . 100 mcg. (0.1 mg.)—yellow . . . 125 mcg. (0.125 mg)—brown . . . 150 mcg. (0.15 mg.)—blue . . . 200 mcg. (0.2 mg.)—pink . . . 300 mcg. (0.3 mg.)—green.

SYNTHROID (levothyroxine sodium) **Injection** is lyophilized in the final container with 10 mg Mannitol, USP and 0.7 mg tribasic sodium phosphate anhydrous. pH may be adjusted with sodium hydroxide. It is supplied in color-coded 10 ml vials in 2 strengths: 200 mcg—gray. . . 500 mcg—yellow.

DIRECTIONS FOR RECONSTITUTION

Reconstitute the lyophilized levothyroxine sodium by aseptically adding 5 ml. of 0.9% Sodium Chloride Injection, USP or Bacteriostatic Sodium Chloride Injection, USP with Benzyl Alcohol, only. Shake vial to insure complete mixing. **Use immediately** after reconstitution. Do not add to other intravenous fluids. Discard any unused portion.

LITERATURE AVAILABLE

Upon request.

Shown in Product Identification Section, page 409

TRAVASE® OINTMENT ℞

[trăv 'āz]

(Sutilains Ointment, USP)

DESCRIPTION

TRAVASE Ointment (Sutilains Ointment, USP) is a sterile preparation of proteolytic enzymes, elaborated by **Bacillus subtilis,** in a hydrophobic ointment base consisting of 95% white petrolatum and 5% polyethylene. One gram of ointment contains approximately 82,000 casein units* of proteolytic activity.

*A casein unit is the amount of enzyme required to produce the same optical density at 275 mμ as that of a solution of 1.5 mcg. tyrosine/ml. after the enzyme has been incubated with 35 mg. of casein at 37° C. for one minute.

ACTION

TRAVASE Ointment selectively digests necrotic soft tissues by proteolytic action. It dissolves and facilitates the removal of necrotic tissues and purulent exudates that otherwise impair formation of granulation tissue and delay wound healing.

At body temperatures these proteolytic enzymes have optimal activity in the pH range from 6.0 to 6.8.

INDICATIONS

For wound debridement—TRAVASE Ointment is indicated as an adjunct to established methods of wound care for biochemical debridement of the following lesions:

- Second and third degree burns,
- Decubitus ulcers,
- Incisional, traumatic, and pyogenic wounds,
- Ulcers secondary to peripheral vascular disease.

CONTRAINDICATIONS

Application of TRAVASE Ointment is contraindicated in the following conditions:

- Wounds communicating with major body cavities,
- Wounds containing exposed major nerves or nervous tissue,
- Fungating neoplastic ulcers,
- Wounds in women of child-bearing potential— because of lack of laboratory evidence of effects of TRAVASE Ointment upon the developing fetus.

WARNING

Do not permit TRAVASE Ointment to come into contact with the eyes. In treatment of burns or lesions about the head or neck, should the ointment inadvertently come into contact with the eyes, the eyes should be immediately rinsed with copious amounts of water, preferably sterile.

PRECAUTIONS

A moist environment is essential to optimal activity of the enzyme. Enzyme activity may also be impaired by certain agents. **In vitro**, several detergents and antiseptics (benzalkonium chloride, hexachlorophene, iodine, and nitrofurazone) may render the substrate indifferent to the action of the enzyme. Compounds such as thimerosal, containing metallic ions, interfere directly with enzyme activity to a slight degree, whereas neomycin, sulfamylon, streptomycin, and penicillin do not affect enzyme activity. In cases where adjunctive topical therapy has been used and no dissolution of slough occurs after treatment with TRAVASE Ointment for 24 to 48 hours, further application, because of interference by the adjunctive agents, is unlikely to be rewarding.

In cases where there is existent or threatening invasive infection, appropriate systemic antibiotic therapy should be instituted concurrently.

Although there have been no reports of systemic allergic reaction to TRAVASE Ointment in humans, studies have shown that there may be an antibody response in humans to absorbed enzyme material.

ADVERSE REACTIONS

Adverse reactions consist of mild, transient pain, paresthesias, bleeding and transient dermatitis. Pain usually can be controlled by administration of mild analgesics. Side effects severe enough to warrant discontinuation of therapy occasionally have occurred.

If bleeding or dermatitis occurs as a result of the application of TRAVASE Ointment, therapy should be discontinued. No systemic toxicity has been observed as a result of the topical application of TRAVASE Ointment.

DOSAGE AND ADMINISTRATION

STRICT ADHERENCE TO THE FOLLOWING IS REQUIRED FOR EFFECTIVE RESULTS OF TREATMENT

1. Thoroughly cleanse and irrigate wound area with sodium chloride or water solutions. Wound MUST be cleansed of antiseptics or heavy-metal antibacterials which may denature enzyme or alter substrate characteristics (e.g., hexachlorophene, silver nitrate, benzalkonium chloride, nitrofurazone).
2. Thoroughly moisten wound area either through tubbing, showering, or wet soaks (e.g., sodium chloride or water solutions).
3. Apply TRAVASE Ointment in a thin layer assuring intimate contact with necrotic tissue and complete wound coverage extending to ¼ to ½ inch beyond the area to be debrided.
4. Apply loose moist dressings.
5. Repeat entire procedure 3 to 4 times per day for best results.

HOW SUPPLIED

TRAVASE Ointment (Sutilains Ointment, USP) is supplied sterile in one-half ounce (14.2 g) tubes. Each gram contains 82,000 casein units of proteolytic activity in a hydrophobic ointment base.

The ointment must be refrigerated at 2° to 8° C (35° to 46° F).

Shown in Product Identification Section, page 409

EDUCATIONAL MATERIAL

Booklet-Pamphlet

"Thyroid Today" various authors, publication issued 4 times per year. Publication provides information written by physicians for physicians concerning thyroid disease diagnosis and treatment. Free to Physicians and Pharmacists.

"A Closer Look at Your Thyroid" patient publication on hypothyroidism. Free to Physicians and Pharmacists.

Samples

Provide physicians with professional supply of Synthroid® (Levothyroxine Sodium, USP) when written prescription is included. (Allow 8 wks. delivery.) Strengths include 0.025 mg., 0.05 mg., 0.1 mg., 0.125 mg, 0.150 mg, 0.2 mg, 0.3 mg in unit size of 100 tablets per bottle. Only 2 samples per order.

Educational Programs

FLINT offers a modular series of educational programs on thyroid disease free to registered pharmacists.

Fluoritab Corporation

P.O. BOX 381
FLINT, MICHIGAN 48501-0381

FLUORITAB® ℞

[floor 'a tab]

sodium fluoride (Active Ingredient)

COMPOSITION

Sodium fluoride	2.2 mg.
Inert organic filler	75.8 mg.

Each tablet contains 1 mg. of fluorine (as fluoride ion)

ACTION AND USES

FLUORITAB dietary fluoride products are straight fluoride and contain no other active ingredients. They are to provide optimum fluoride where water supplies are deficient in fluorine. Dietary fluoride is beneficial in providing teeth that are more resistant to decay. Fluorine combines with calcium to form the apatite molecule of teeth and bone to form fluorapatite crystals.

ADMINISTRATION AND DOSAGE

FLUORITAB dietary fluoride can be given in baby formulas, or in any liquid. They can be swallowed quickly, or permitted to remain in the mouth to dissolve, which may provide surface benefit to tooth enamel. Fluoride must be taken on a continued basis throughout the period of tooth formation to be fully effective.

Dosage should provide the child with ½ mg. per day from birth to 3 years of age and 1 mg. per day from 3 years of age up.

Water supplies with 0.2 parts per million or less require supplementing with ½ mg. and 1 mg. dosage per day for children under and over 3, respectively. Water supplies with 0.2 to 0.6 parts per million require ¼ mg. and ½ mg. dosage per day for children under 3 and over 3 respectively.

SIDE EFFECTS

Excess fluoride is to be avoided, as it may cause dental fluorosis (mottling of the teeth).

PRECAUTIONS

Where water with 0.7 P.P.M. of fluoride is used, dietary fluoride ought not be used.

CONTRAINDICATIONS

None.

OVERDOSAGE

(Symptoms and Treatment): The total contents of our safety limited packages can be taken without any effect.

HOW SUPPLIED

FLUORITAB TABLETS are supplied in bottles of 100, scored, easily divided 1.2 grain tablets, 1 mg. fluorine per tablet. FLUORITAB LIQUID is supplied in 19 cc. (480 drop) (.25 mg. fluorine per drop) polyethelene squeeze type dropper bottles.

PRODUCT IDENTIFICATION MARK(S)

FLUORITAB products have the "FLUORITAB" name on all packages.

REMARKS

FLUORITAB dietary fluoride was the first dietary fluoride product given A.D.A. acceptance (July, 1958). We adhere rigidly to their recommendation of restricting our package size to their safety admonition: *Never* to sell packages containing more than 264 mg. of sodium fluoride.

LITERATURE AVAILABLE

Educational folders and prescription instructions will be sent free, on request.

Forest Pharmaceuticals, Inc.

(Subsidiary of Forest Laboratories, Inc.)
2510 METRO BLVD.
ST. LOUIS MO 63043

AEROBID® ℞

(flunisolide)
Inhaler system
For oral inhalation only

DESCRIPTION

Flunisolide, the active component of **AeroBid** Inhaler System, is an anti-inflammatory steroid having the chemical name 6α-fluoro-11β, 16α, 17, 21-tetrahydroxypregna-1, 4-diene-3, 20-dione cyclic-16, 17-acetal with acetone. It has the following structure:

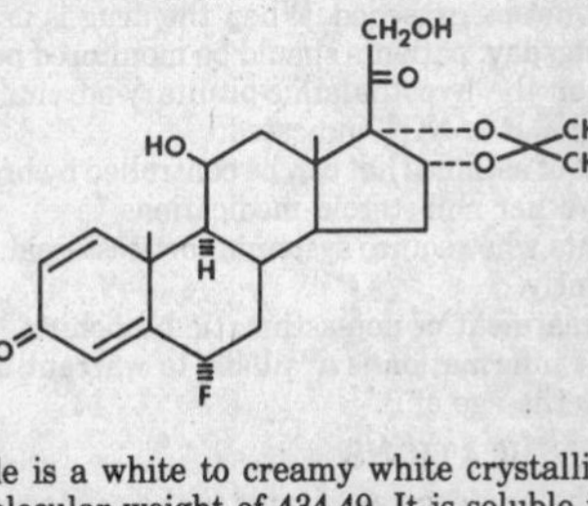

Flunisolide is a white to creamy white crystalline powder with a molecular weight of 434.49. It is soluble in acetone, sparingly soluble in chloroform, slightly soluble in methanol, and practically insoluble in water. It has a melting point of about 245°C.

AeroBid Inhaler is delivered in a metered-dose aerosol system containing a microcrystalline suspension of flunisolide as the hemihydrate in propellants (trichloromonofluoromethane, dichlorodifluoromethane and dichlorotetrafluoroethane) with sorbitan trioleate as a dispersing agent. Each activation delivers approximately 250 mcg of flunisolide to the patient. One **AeroBid** Inhaler System is designed to deliver at least 100 metered inhalations.

CLINICAL PHARMACOLOGY

Flunisolide has demonstrated marked anti-inflammatory and anti-allergic activity in classical test systems. It is a corticosteroid that is several hundred times more potent in animal anti-inflammatory assays than the cortisol standard. The molar dose of each activation of flunisolide in this prepa-

Continued on next page

Forest Pharmaceuticals—Cont.

ration is approximately 2½ to 7 times that of comparable inhaled corticosteroid products marketed for the same indication. The dose of flunisolide delivered per activation in this preparation is 10 times that per activation of Nasalide® (flunisolide) nasal solution. Clinical studies have shown therapeutic activity on bronchial mucosa with minimal evidence of systemic activity at recommended doses.

After oral inhalation of 1 mg flunisolide, total systemic availability was 40%. The flunisolide that is swallowed is rapidly and extensively converted to the 6β-OH metabolite and to water-soluble conjugates during the first pass through the liver. This offers a metabolic explanation for the low systemic activity of oral flunisolide itself since the metabolite has low corticosteroid potency (on the order of the cortisol standard). The inhaled flunisolide absorbed through the bronchial tree is converted to the same metabolites. Repeated inhalation of 2.0 mg of flunisolide per day (the maximum recommended dose) for 14 days did not show accumulation of the drug in plasma. The plasma half-life of flunisolide is approximately 1.8 hours.

The following observations relevant to systemic absorption were made in clinical studies. In one uncontrolled study a statistically significant decrease in responsiveness to metyrapone was noted in 15 adult steroid-independent patients treated with 2.0 mg of flunisolide per day (the maximum recommended dose) for 3 months. A small but statistically significant drop in eosinophils from 11.5% to 7.4% of total circulating leucocytes was noted in another study in children who were not taking oral corticosteroids simultaneously. A 5% incidence of menstrual disturbances was reported during open studies, in which there were no control groups for comparison.

Aerosol administration of flunisolide 2.0 mg twice daily for one week to 6 healthy male subjects revealed neither suppression of adrenal function as measured by early morning cortisol levels nor impairment of HPA axis function as determined by insulin hypoglycemia tests.

Controlled clinical studies have included over 500 patients with asthma, among them 150 children age 6 and over. More than 120 patients have been treated in open trials for two years or more. No significant adrenal suppression attributed to flunisolide was seen in these studies.

Significant decreases of systemic steroid dosages have been possible in flunisolide-treated patients. Asthma patients have had further symptomatic improvement with flunisolide treatment even while reducing concomitant medication.

INDICATIONS AND USAGE

AeroBid Inhaler is indicated only for patients who require chronic treatment with corticosteroids for control of the symptoms of bronchial asthma. Such patients would include those already receiving systemic corticosteroids, and selected patients who are inadequately controlled on a non-steroid regimen and in whom steroid therapy has been withheld because of concern over potential adverse effects.

As with any topically applied medication, flunisolide is absorbed through the mucous membrane and is systemically available. For these reasons, **AeroBid** Inhaler should be used with caution for initial therapy and the recommended dosage should not be exceeded. When the drug is used chronically at 2 mg/day, patients should be monitored periodically for effects on the hypothalamic-pituitary-adrenal axis.

AeroBid Inhaler is NOT indicated:

1. For relief of asthma that can be controlled by bronchodilators and other non-steroid medications.
2. In patients who require systemic corticosteroid treatment infrequently.
3. In the treatment of non-asthmatic bronchitis.

Insufficient information is available to warrant use in children under the age of 6.

CONTRAINDICATIONS

AeroBid Inhaler is contraindicated in the primary treatment of status asthmaticus or other acute episodes of asthma where intensive measures are required. Hypersensitivity to any of the ingredients of this preparation contraindicates its use.

WARNINGS

Particular care is needed in patients who are transferred from systemically active corticosteroids to **AeroBid** Inhaler because deaths due to adrenal insufficiency have occurred in asthmatic patients during and after transfer from systemic corticosteroids to aerosol corticosteroids. After withdrawal from systemic corticosteroids, a number of months are required for recovery of hypothalamic-pituitary-adrenal (HPA) function. During this period of HPA suppression, patients may exhibit signs and symptoms of adrenal insufficiency when exposed to trauma, surgery or infections, particularly gastroenteritis. Although **AeroBid** Inhaler may provide control of asthmatic symptoms during these episodes, it does NOT provide the systemic steroid that is necessary for coping with these emergencies.

During periods of stress or a severe asthmatic attack, patients who have been withdrawn from systemic corticosteroids should be instructed to resume systemic steroids (in large doses) immediately and to contact their physician for further instruction. These patients should also be instructed to carry a warning card indicating that they may need supplementary systemic steroids during periods of stress or a severe asthma attack. To assess the risk of adrenal insufficiency in emergency situations, routine tests of adrenal cortical function, including measurement of early morning resting cortisol levels, should be performed periodically in all patients. An early morning resting cortisol level may be accepted as normal if it falls at or near the normal mean level.

Localized infections with *Candida albicans* or *Aspergillus niger* have occurred in the mouth and pharynx and occasionally in the larynx. Positive cultures for oral *Candida* may be present in up to 34% of patients. Although the frequency of clinically apparent infection is considerably lower, these infections may require treatment with appropriate antifungal therapy or discontinuance of treatment with **AeroBid** inhaler.

AeroBid Inhaler is not to be regarded as a bronchodilator and is not indicated for rapid relief of bronchospasm.

Patients should be instructed to contact their physician immediately when episodes of asthma that are not responsive to bronchodilators occur during the course of treatment. During such episodes, patients may require therapy with systemic corticosteroids.

There is no evidence that control of asthma can be achieved by administration of the drug in amounts greater than the recommended doses, which appear to be the therapeutic equivalent of approximately 10 mg/day of oral prednisone.

Theoretically, the use of inhaled corticosteroids with alternate day prednisone systemic treatment should be accompanied by more HPA suppression than a therapeutically equivalent regimen of either alone.

Transfer of patients from systemic steroid therapy to **AeroBid** Inhaler may unmask allergic conditions previously suppressed by the systemic steroid therapy, e.g., rhinitis, conjunctivitis, and eczema.

PRECAUTIONS

General: Because of the relatively high molar dose of flunisolide per activation in this preparation, and because of the evidence suggesting higher levels of systemic absorption with flunisolide than with other comparable inhaled corticosteroids (see CLINICAL PHARMACOLOGY section), patients treated with **AeroBid** should be observed carefully for any evidence of systemic corticosteroid effect, including suppression of bone growth in children. Particular care should be taken in observing patients post-operatively or during periods of stress for evidence of a decrease in adrenal function. During withdrawal from oral steroids, some patients may experience symptoms of systemically active steroid withdrawal, e.g., joint and/or muscular pain, lassitude and depression, despite maintenance or even improvement of respiratory function (See DOSAGE AND ADMINISTRATION for details).

In responsive patients, flunisolide may permit control of asthmatic symptoms without suppression of HPA function. Since flunisolide is absorbed into the circulation and can be systemically active, the beneficial effects of **AeroBid** Inhaler in minimizing or preventing HPA dysfunction may be expected only when recommended dosages are not exceeded.

The long-term effects of the drug in human subjects are still unknown. In particular, the local effects of the agent on developmental or immunologic processes in the mouth, pharynx, trachea, and lung are unknown. There is also no information about the possible long-term systemic effects of the agent.

The potential effects of the drug on acute, recurrent, or chronic pulmonary infections, including active or quiescent tuberculosis, are not known. Similarly, the potential effects of long-term administration of the drug on lung or other tissues are unknown.

Pulmonary infiltrates with eosinophilia may occur in patients on **AeroBid** Inhaler therapy. Although it is possible that in some patients this state may become manifest because of systemic steroid withdrawal when inhalational steroids are administered, a causative role for the drug and/or its vehicle cannot be ruled out.

Information for Patients

There is no evidence that better control of asthma can be achieved by the administration of **AeroBid** Inhaler in amounts greater than the recommended doses; higher doses may induce adrenal suppression.

Since the relief from **AeroBid** Inhaler depends on its regular use and on proper inhalation technique, patients must be instructed to take inhalations at regular intervals. They should also be instructed in the correct method of use (See Patient instruction Leaflet).

Patients receiving bronchodilators by inhalation should be advised to use the bronchodilator before **AeroBid** Inhaler in order to enhance penetration of flunisolide into the bronchial tree. After use of an aerosol bronchodilator, several minutes should elapse before using the **AeroBid** Inhaler.

Patients whose systemic corticosteroids have been reduced or withdrawn should be instructed to carry a warning card indicating that they may need supplemental systemic steroids during periods of stress or a severe asthmatic attack that is not responsive to bronchodilators.

An illustrated leaflet of patient instructions for proper use accompanies each **AeroBid** Inhaler System.

CONTENTS UNDER PRESSURE

Do not puncture. Do not use or store near heat or open flame. Exposure to temperatures above 120°F (49°C) may cause container to explode. Never throw container into fire or incinerator. Keep out of reach of children.

Carcinogenesis: A 22-month study was conducted in Swiss derived mice to evaluate the carcinogenic potential of the drug. There was an increase in the incidence of pulmonary adenomas within the range of adenomas previously reported in the literature for untreated or control Swiss derived mice. An additional study is being conducted in a species with a lower incidence of spontaneous pulmonary tumors.

Impairment of Fertility: Female rats receiving high doses of flunisolide (200 mcg/kg/day) showed some evidence of impaired fertility. Reproductive performance in the low (8 mcg/kg/day) and mid-dose (40 mcg/kg/day) groups was comparable to controls.

Pregnancy: Pregnancy Category C. As with other corticosteroids, flunisolide has been shown to be teratogenic in rabbits and rats at doses of 40 and 200 mcg/kg/day respsectively. It was also fetotoxic in these animal reproductive studies. There are no adequate and well-controlled studies in pregnant women. Flunisolide should be used during pregnancy only if the potential benefit justifies the potential risk to the fetus.

Nursing Mothers: It is not known whether this drug is excreted in human milk. Because other corticosteroids are excreted in human milk, caution should be exercised when flunisolide is administered to nursing women.

ADVERSE REACTIONS

Adverse events reported in controlled clinical trials and long-term open studies in 514 patients treated with **AeroBid** are described below. Of those patients, 463 were treated for 3 months or longer, 407 for 6 months or longer, 287 for 1 year or longer, and 122 for 2 years or longer.

Musculoskeletal reactions were reported in 35% of steroid-dependent patients in whom the dose of oral steroid was being tapered. This is a well-known effect of steroid withdrawal.

Incidence 10% or greater:

Gastrointestinal: diarrhea (10%), nausea and/or vomiting (25%), upset stomach (10%)
General: flu (10%)
Mouth and Throat: sore throat (20%)
Nervous system: headache (25%)
Respiratory: cold symptoms (15%), nasal congestion (15%), upper respiratory infection (25%)
Special Senses: unpleasant taste (10%)

Incidence 3–9%

Cardiovascular: palpitations
Gastrointestinal: abdominal pain, heartburn
General: chest pain, decreased appetite, edema, fever
Mouth and Throat: *Candida* infection
Nervous System: dizziness, irritability, nervousness, shakiness
Reproductive: menstrual disturbances
Respiratory: chest congestion, cough*, hoarseness, rhinitis, runny nose, sinus congestion, sinus drainage, sinus infection, sinusitis, sneezing, sputum, wheezing*
Skin: eczema, itching (pruritus), rash
Special Senses: ear infection, loss of smell or taste

Incidence 1–3%

General: chills, increased appetite and weight gain, malaise, peripheral edema, sweating, weakness
Cardiovascular: hypertension, tachycardia
Gastrointestinal: constipation, dyspepsia, gas
Hemic/Lymph: capillary fragility, enlarged lymph nodes
Mouth and Throat: dry throat, glossitis, mouth irritation, pharyngitis, phlegm, throat irritation
Nervous System: anxiety, depression, faintness, fatigue, hyperactivity, hypoactivity, insomnia, moodiness, numbness, vertigo
Respiratory: bronchitis, chest tightness*, dyspnea, epistaxis, head stuffiness, laryngitis, nasal irritation, pleurisy, pneumonia, sinus discomfort
Skin: acne, hives, or urticaria
Special Senses: blurred vision, earache, eye discomfort, eye infection

Incidence less than 1%, judged by investigators as possibly or probably drug related: abdominal fullness, shortness of breath.

*The incidences as shown of cough, wheezing, and chest tightness were judged by investigators to be possibly or probably drug-related. In placebo-controlled trials, the *overall* incidences of these adverse events (regardless of investigators' judgment of drug relationship) were similar for drug and placebo-treated groups. They may be related to the vehicle or delivery system.

DOSAGE AND ADMINISTRATION

The **AeroBid** Inhaler System is for oral inhalation only.

Adults: The recommended starting dose is 2 inhalations twice daily morning and evening for a total daily dose of 1 mg. The maximum daily dose should not exceed 4 inhalations twice a day for a total daily dose of 2 mg. When the drug is used chronically at 2 mg/day, patients should be monitored periodically for effects on the hypothalamic-pituitary-adrenal axis.

Children: For children 6–15 years of age, two inhalations may be administered twice daily for a total daily dose of 1 mg. Higher doses have not been studied. Insufficient information is available to warrant use in children under age 6. With chronic use, children should be monitored for growth as well as for effects on the HPA axis.

Rinsing the mouth after inhalation is advised. Patients receiving bronchodilators by inhalation should be advised to use the bronchodilator before **AeroBid** Inhaler in order to enhance penetration of flunisolide into the bronchial tree. After use of an aerosol bronchodilator, several minutes should elapse before use of the **AeroBid** inhaler to reduce the potential toxicity from the inhaled fluorocarbon propellants in the two aerosols.

Different considerations must be given to the following groups of patients in order to obtain the full therapeutic benefit of **AeroBid** Inhaler.

Patients not receiving systemic steroids: The use of **AeroBid** Inhaler is straightforward in patients who are inadequately controlled with non-steroid medications but in whom systemic steroid therapy has been withheld because of concern over potential adverse reactions. In patients who respond to the drug, an improvement in pulmonary function is usually apparent within one to four weeks after the start of treatment.

Patients receiving systemic steroids: In those patients dependent on systemic steroids, transfer to **AeroBid** and subsequent management may be more difficult because recovery from impaired adrenal function is usually slow. Such suppression has been known to last for up to 12 months. Clinical studies, however, have demonstrated that **AeroBid** may be effective in the management of these asthmatic patients and may permit replacement or significant reduction in the dosage of systemic corticosteroids.

Inhaled corticosteroids generally are not recommended for chronic use with alternate day prednisone regimens (see WARNINGS).

The patient's asthma should be reasonably stable before treatment with **AeroBid** Inhaler is started. Initially, the aerosol should be used concurrently with the patient's usual maintenance dose of systemic steroid. After approximately one week, gradual withdrawal of the systemic steroid is started by reducing the daily or alternate daily dose. The next reduction is made after an interval of one or two weeks, depending on the response of the patient. Generally, these decrements should not exceed 2.5 mg of prednisone or its equivalent. A slow rate of withdrawal cannot be overemphasized. During withdrawal, some patients may experience symptoms of systemically active steroid withdrawal, e.g., joint and/or muscular pain, lassitude and depression, despite maintenance or even improvement of respiratory function. Such patients should be encouraged to continue with the Inhaler but should be watched carefully for objective signs of adrenal insufficiency, such as hypotension and weight loss. If evidence of adrenal insufficiency occurs, the systemic steroid dose should be boosted temporarily and thereafter further withdrawal should continue more slowly. *During periods of stress or a severe asthma attack, transfer patients will require supplementary treatment with systemic steroids.* Exacerbations of asthma that occur during the course of treatment with **AeroBid** Inhaler should be treated with a short course of systemic steroid that is gradually tapered as these symptoms subside. There is no evidence that control of asthma can be achieved by administration of the drug in amounts greater than the recommended doses.

HOW SUPPLIED

AeroBid (flunisolide) Inhaler System is available in canisters of 100 metered inhalations.

Caution: FEDERAL LAW PROHIBITS DISPENSING WITHOUT PRESCRIPTION.

Shown in Product Identification Section, page 409

AMBENYL® Cough Syrup ℂ ℞

[*ăm 'bĕn-ĭl*]

DESCRIPTION

Each 5 ml of AMBENYL Cough Syrup contains:

Codeine phosphate (Warning—May be habit-forming) .... 10 mg
Bromodiphenhydramine hydrochloride .... 12.5 mg
Alcohol, 5%

Chemically, codeine phosphate is morphinan-6-ol,7,8-didehydro-4,5-epoxy -3- methoxy-17-methyl-,(5α,6α)-, phosphate (1:1)(salt),hemihydrate and bromodiphenhydramine hydrochloride is ethanamine,2-[(4-bromophenyl) phenylmethoxy]-N,N-dimethyl-, hydrochloride.

AMBENYL Cough Syrup is for oral administration.

CLINICAL PHARMACOLOGY

AMBENYL is a combination of an antihistaminic agent, along with a well-recognized agent exhibiting antitussive properties.

INDICATIONS AND USAGE

AMBENYL is indicated for relief of upper respiratory symptoms and coughs associated with allergies or the common cold.

CONTRAINDICATIONS

Use in Newborn or Premature Infants: This drug should *not* be used in newborn or premature infants.

Use in Nursing Mothers: Because of the higher risk of antihistamines for infants generally and for newborns and prematures in particular, antihistamine therapy is contraindicated in nursing mothers.

Use in Lower Respiratory Disease: Antihistamines *should NOT* be used to treat lower respiratory tract symptoms including asthma.

Antihistamines are also contraindicated in the following conditions: Hypersensivity to bromodiphenhydramine and other antihistamines of similar chemical structures.

Monoamine oxidase inhibitor therapy (see Drug Interactions section).

WARNINGS

Antihistamines should be used with considerable caution in patients with:

Narrow angle glaucoma
Stenosing peptic ulcer
Pyloroduodenal obstruction
Symptomatic prostatic hypertrophy
Bladder neck obstruction

Use in Children: In infants and children, especially, antihistamines in *overdosage* may cause hallucinations, convulsions or death. As in adults, antihistamines may diminish mental alertness in children. In the young child, particularly, they may produce excitation.

Use in Pregnancy: Experience with this drug in pregnant women is inadequate to determine whether there exists a potential for harm to the developing fetus.

Use With CNS Depressants: AMBENYL Cough Syrup has additive effects with alcohol and other CNS depressants (hypnotics, sedatives, tranquilizers, etc).

Use in Activities Requiring Mental Alertness: Patients should be warned about engaging in activities requiring mental alertness such as driving a car or operating appliances, machinery, etc.

Use in the Elderly (approximately 60 years or older): Antihistamines are more likely to cause dizziness, sedation, and hypotension in elderly patients.

PRECAUTIONS

Bromodiphenhydramine has an atropine-like action and, therefore, should be used with caution in patients with:

History of bronchial asthma
Increased intraocular pressure
Hyperthyroidism
Cardiovascular disease
Hypertension

Drug Interactions: Codeine may potentiate the effects of other narcotics, general anesthetics, tranquilizers, sedatives and hypnotics, tricyclic antidepressants, MAO inhibitors, alcohol, and other CNS depressants.

ADVERSE REACTIONS

The following side effects may occur in patients taking AMBENYL:

drowsiness
confusion
nervousness
restlessness
nausea
vomiting
diarrhea
blurring of vision
diplopia
difficulty in urination
constipation
tightness of the chest and wheezing
tingling, heaviness, weakness of hands
nasal stuffiness
vertigo
palpitation
headache
insomnia
urticaria
drug rash
photosensitivity
hemolytic anemia
hypotension
epigastric distress
thickening of bronchial secretions
dryness of mouth, nose, and throat

DRUG ABUSE AND DEPENDENCE

Codeine can produce drug dependence of the morphine type and, therefore, has the potential for being abused. Psychic dependence, physical dependence, and tolerance may develop upon repeated administration of this drug, and it should be prescribed and administered with the same degree of caution appropriate to the user of other oral narcotic-containing medications. Like other narcotic-containing medications, the drug is subject to the Federal Controlled Substances Act.

OVERDOSAGE

Antihistamine overdosage reactions may vary from central nervous system depression to stimulation. Stimulation is particularly likely in children. Atropine-like signs and symptoms—dry mouth; fixed dilated pupils; flushing; and gastrointestinal symptoms may also occur.

If vomiting has not occurred spontaneously, the patient should be induced to vomit. This is best done by having him drink a glass of water or milk after which he should be made to gag. Precautions against aspiration must be taken, especially in infants and children.

If vomiting is unsucessful, gastric lavage is indicated within three hours after ingestion and even later if large amounts of milk or cream were given beforehand. Isotonic and ½ isotonic saline solution of choice.

Saline cathartics, as milk of magnesia, by osmosis draw water into the bowel, and therefore, are valuable for their action in rapid dilution of bowel content.

Stimulants should *not* be used.

Vasopressors may be used to treat hypotension.

DOSAGE AND ADMINISTRATION

DOSAGE SHOULD BE INDIVIDUALIZED ACCORDING TO THE NEEDS AND THE RESPONSE OF THE PATIENT.

Adults—one or two teaspoonfuls every four to six hours, not to exceed 12 teaspoonfuls in 24 hours. Children (total intake of codeine phosphate should not exceed 1 mg/kg/24 hours) —Six to under 12 years of age—one-half to one teaspoonful every six hours.

Not recommended for use in children under 6 years of age.

HOW SUPPLIED

AMBENYL Cough Syrup is red and is supplied in 4-fl-oz (NDC 0456-0681-04), 1-pt (NDC 0456-0681-16), and 1-gal (NDC 0456-0681-28) bottles. Store at controlled room temperature (59°–86°F).

Issued 1/84

AMBENYL®-D OTC

[*ăm 'bĕ-nĭl*]

Decongestant Cough Formula

Antitussive-Expectorant-Nasal Decongestant

Two teaspoonfuls (10 ml) contain the following active ingredients:

Guaifenesin (glyceryl guaiacolate) .... 200 mg
Pseudoephedrine hydrochloride .... 60 mg
Dextromethorphan hydrobromide .... 30 mg

Also contains 9.5% alcohol, citric acid, FD&C Blue #1, FD&C Red #40, flavors, glycerin, menthol, methylparaben, saccharin sodium, sodium chloride, sorbitol solution, sucrose, and water.

INDICATIONS

AMBENYL®-D is for temporary relief of nasal congestion due to the common cold or associated with sinusitis, helps loosen phlegm, calms cough impulses without narcotics, and temporarily helps you cough less.

DIRECTIONS FOR USE

Adult Dose (12 years and over)—Two teaspoonfuls every six hours. Child Dose (6–12 years)—One teaspoonful every six hours. (2–6 years)—One-half teaspoonful every six hours. No more than four doses per day.

WARNINGS

Do not give this product to children under two years except under the advice and supervision of a physician. Do not take this product for persistent or chronic cough such as occurs with smoking, asthma, or emphysema, or where cough is accompanied by excessive secretions, except under the advice and supervision of a physician.

Do not exceed recommended dosage because at higher doses nervousness, dizziness, or sleeplessness may occur.

CAUTION

A persistent cough may be a sign of a serious condition. If cough persists for more than one week, tends to recur, or is accompanied by a high fever, rash, or persistent headache, consult a physician.

Continued on next page

Forest Pharmaceuticals—Cont.

If symptoms do not improve within seven days or are accompanied by a high fever, consult a physician before continuing use. Do not take this product if you have high blood pressure, heart disease, diabetes, or thyroid disease, except under the advice and supervision of a physician.
If pregnant or nursing a baby, consult your physician or pharmacist before using this product.

DRUG INTERACTION PRECAUTION

Do not take this product if you are presently taking a prescription antihypertensive or antidepressant drug containing a monoamine oxidase inhibitor except under the advice and supervision of a physician.
Store at a controlled room temperature (59°–86°F).
Keep this and all drugs out of reach of children.
In case of accidental overdose, seek professional assistance or contact a poison control center immediately.

HOW SUPPLIED

AMBENYL-D Decongestant Cough Formula is supplied in a 4-fl-oz bottle (NDC 0456-0682-04).

Issued 5/85

ANTILIRIUM ℞
(physostigmine salicylate)

DESCRIPTION

ANTILIRIUM (Physostigmine Salicylate) is a derivative of the Calabar bean, and its active moiety, physostigmine, is also known as eserine.
It is soluble in water and a 0.5% aqueous solution has a pH of 5.8.
ANTILIRIUM Injection is available in 2 ml ampuls, each ml containing 1 mg of Physostigmine Salicylate in a vehicle composed of sodium bisulfite 0.1%, benzyl alcohol 2.0% as a preservative in water for injection.

CLINICAL PHARMACOLOGY

ANTILIRIUM is a reversible anticholinesterase which effectively increases the concentration of acetylcholine at the sites of cholinergic transmission. The action of acetylcholine is normally very transient because of its hydrolysis by the enzyme, acetylcholinesterase. ANTILIRIUM inhibits the destructive action of acetylcholinesterase and thereby prolongs and exaggerates the effect of the acetylcholine.
ANTILIRIUM contains a tertiary amine and easily penetrates the blood brain barrier, while an anticholinesterase, such as neostigmine, which has a quaternary ammonium ion is not capable of crossing the barrier. ANTILIRIUM can reverse both central and peripheral anticholinergia. The anticholinergic syndrome has both central and peripheral signs and symptoms. Central toxic effects include anxiety, delirium, disorientation, hallucinations, hyper-activity and seizures. Severe poisoning may produce coma, medullary paralysis and death. Peripheral toxicity is characterized by tachycardia, hyperpyrexia, mydriasis, vasodilatation, urinary retention, diminution of gastrointestinal motility, decrease of secretion in salivary and sweat glands, and loss of secretions in the pharynx, bronchi, and nasal passages.
Dramatic reversal of the effects of anticholinergic symptoms can be expected in minutes after the intravenous administration of ANTILIRIUM, if the diagnosis is correct and the patient has not suffered anoxia or other insult. The duration of action of ANTILIRIUM is relatively short, approx. 45 to 60 minutes.
Numerous drugs and some plants produce the anticholinergic syndrome either directly or as a side effect; this undesirable or potentially dangerous phenomenon may be brought about by either therapeutic doses or overdoses of the drugs. Such drugs include among others, atropine, other derivatives of the belladonna alkaloids, tricyclic antidepressants, phenothiazines, and antihistamines.

INDICATIONS AND USAGES

To reverse the effect upon the central nervous system, caused by clinical or toxic dosages of drugs capable of producing the anticholinergic syndrome.

CONTRAINDICATIONS

ANTILIRIUM should not be used in the presence of asthma, gangrene, diabetes, cardiovascular disease, mechanical obstruction of the intestine or urogenital tract or any vagotonic state, and in patients receiving choline esters or depolarizing neuromuscular blocking agents (decamethonium succinylcholine).
For post-anesthesia, the concomitant use of atropine with the physostigmine salicylate is not recommended, since the atropine antagonizes the action of physostigmine.

WARNINGS

If excessive symptoms of salivation, emesis, urination and defecation occur, the use of ANTILIRIUM should be terminated. If excessive sweating or nausea occur, the dosage should be reduced.
Intravenous administration should be a slow, controlled rate, no more than 1 mg per minute (see dosage). Rapid administration can cause bradycardia, hypersalivation leading to respiratory difficulties and possible convulsions.
An overdosage of ANTILIRIUM can cause a cholinergic crisis.

PRECAUTIONS

Because of the possibility of hypersensitivity in an occasional patient, atropine sulfate injection should always be at hand since it is an antagonist and antidote for physostigmine.

USAGE IN PREGNANCY

Safe use in pregnancy and lactation has not been established; therefore, use in pregnant women, nursing mothers or women who may become pregnant requires that possible benefits be weighed against possible hazards to mother and child.

ADVERSE REACTIONS

Nausea, vomiting and salivation; can be offset by reducing dosage. Bradycardia and convulsions, if intravenous administration is too rapid. See DOSAGE AND ADMINISTRATION.

OVERDOSAGE

Can cause a cholinergic crisis. Appropriate antidote is atropine sulfate.

DOSAGE AND ADMINISTRATION

Post Anesthesia Care: 0.5 to 1.0 mg intramuscularly or intravenously. INTRAVENOUS ADMINISTRATION SHOULD BE AT A SLOW CONTROLLED RATE OF NO MORE THAN 1 MG PER MINUTE. Dosage may be repeated at intervals of 10 to 30 minutes if desired patient response is not obtained.
Overdosages of Drugs That Cause Anticholinergia: 2.0 mg intramuscularly or INTRAVENOUSLY AT SLOW CONTROLLED RATE (SEE ABOVE). Dosage may be repeated if life threatening signs, such as arrhythmia, convulsions or coma occurs.
Pediatric Dosage: Recommended dosage is .02 mg/kg, intramuscularly or by slow intravenous injection, no more than 0.5 mg per minute. If the toxic effects persist, and there is no sign of cholinergic effects, the dosage may be repeated at 5 to 10 minute intervals until a therapeutic effect is obtained or a maximum dose of 2 mg is attained.
IN ALL CASES OF POISONING, THE USUAL SUPPORTIVE MEASURES SHOULD BE UNDERTAKEN.

HOW SUPPLIED

Ampuls, 2 ml packed 12 per box, 1 mg per ml. NDC-0456-1037-12.

CAUTION

Federal law prohibits dispensing without prescription.

BANALG® HOSPITAL STRENGTH ARTHRITIC PAIN RELIEVER BANALG® LINIMENT

(See PDR For Nonprescription Drugs)

BANCAP HC® CAPSULES Ⓒ℞

DESCRIPTION

Each hard gelatin capsule contains:
Hydrocodone Bitartrate ....5 mg
(WARNING: May be habit forming)
Acetaminophen ....500 mg
Acetaminophen is a nonopiate, non-salicylate analgesic and antipyretic which occurs as a white, odorless crystalline powder possessing a slightly bitter taste. Hydrocodone bitartrate is an opioid analgesic and antitussive and occurs as fine, white crystals or as a crystalline powder. It is affected by light.

CLINICAL PHARMACOLOGY

Hydrocodone is a semisynthetic narcotic analgesic and antitussive with multiple actions qualitatively similar to those of codeine. Most of these involve the central nervous system and smooth muscle. The precise mechanism of action of hydrocodone and other opiates is not known, although it is believed to relate to the existence of opiate receptors in the central nervous system. In additon to analgesia, narcotics may produce drowsiness, changes in mood and mental clouding.
Radioimmunoassay techniques have recently been developed for the analysis of hydrocodone in human plasma. After a 10 mg oral dose of hydrocodone bitartrate, a mean peak serum drug level of 23.6 ng/ml and an elimination half-life of 3.8 hours were found.
The analgesic action of acetaminophen involves peripheral and central influences, but the specific mechanism is as yet undetermined. Antipyretic activity is mediated through hypothalamic heat regulating centers. Acetaminophen inhibits prostaglandin synthetase. Therapeutic doses of acetaminophen have negligible effects on the cardiovascular or respiratory systems; however, toxic doses may cause circulatory failure and rapid, shallow breathing. Acetaminophen is rapidly and almost completely absorbed from the gastrointestinal tract, producing maximum serum concentrations within 30 minutes to one hour. The plasma half-life in adults and children ranges from 0.90 hours to 3.25 hours with an average of approximately 2 hours. The drug distributes uniformly in most body fluids and is approximately 25% protein bound. Acetaminophen is conjugated in the liver, with less than 3% of the dose excreted unchanged in 24 hours. The primary metabolic pathway is conjugation to sulfate and glucuronide by-products. A minor oxidative pathway forms cysteine and mercapturic acid. These compounds are subsequently excreted by the kidneys into the urine.

INDICATIONS AND USAGE

For the relief of moderate to moderately severe pain.

CONTRAINDICATIONS

Hypersensitivity to acetaminophen or hydrocodone.

WARNINGS

Respiratory Depression: At high doses or in sensitive patients, hydrocodone may produce dose-related respiratory depression by acting directly on brain stem respiratory centers. Hydrocodone also affects centers that control respiratory rhythm, and may produce irregular and periodic breathing.
Head Injury and Increased Intracranial Pressure: The respiratory depressant effects of narcotics and their capacity to elevate cerebrospinal fluid pressure may be markedly exaggerated in the presence of head injury, other intracranial lesions or a preexisting increase in intracranial pressure. Furthermore, narcotics produce adverse reactions which may obscure the clinical course of patients with head injuries.
Acute Abdominal Conditions: The administration of narcotics may obscure the diagnosis or clinical course of patients with acute abdominal conditions.

PRECAUTIONS

Special Risk Patients: As with any narcotic analgesic agent, BANCAP HC Capsules should be used with caution in elderly or debilitated patients and those with severe impairment of hepatic or renal function, hypothyroidism, Addison's disease, prostatic hypertrophy or urethral stricture. The usual precautions should be observed and the possibility of respiratory depression should be kept in mind.
Information for Patients: BANCAP HC Capsules like all narcotics, may impair the mental and/or physical abilities required for the performance of potentially hazardous tasks such as driving a car or operating machinery; patients should be cautioned accordingly.
Cough Reflex: Hydrocodone suppresses the cough reflex; as with all narcotics, caution should be exercised when BANCAP HC Capsules are used postoperatively and in patients with pulmonary disease.
Drug Interactions: Patients receiving other narcotic analgesics, antipsychotics, antianxiety agents, or other CNS depressants (including alcohol) concomitantly with BANCAP HC Capsules may exhibit an additive CNS depression. When combined therapy is contemplated, the dose of one or both agents should be reduced.
The use of MAO inhibitors or tricyclic antidepressants with hydrocodone preparations may increase the effect of either the antidepressant or hydrocodone.
The concurrent use of anticholinergics with hydrocodone may produce paralytic ileus.
Usage in Pregnancy: Pregnancy Category C. Hydrocodone has been shown to be teratogenic in hamsters when given in doses 700 times the human dose. There are no adequate and well-controlled studies in pregnant women. BANCAP HC Capsules should be used during pregnancy only if the potential benefit justifies the potential risk to the fetus.
Nonteratogenic Effects: Babies born to mothers who have been taking opioids regularly prior to delivery will be physically dependent. The withdrawal signs include irritability and excessive crying, tremors, hyperactive reflexes, increased respiratory rate, increased stools, sneezing, yawning, vomiting, and fever. The intensity of the syndrome does not always correlate with the duration of maternal opioid use or dose. There is no consensus on the best method of managing withdrawal. Chlorpromazine 0.7 to 1.0 mg/kg q6h, and paregoric 2 to 4 drops/kg q4h, have been used to treat withdrawal symptoms in infants. The duration of therapy is 4 to 28 days, with the dosage decreased as tolerated.
Labor and Delivery: As with all narcotics, administration of BANCAP HC Capsules to the mother shortly before delivery may result in some degree of respiratory depression in the newborn, especially if higher doses are used.
Nursing Mothers: It is not known whether this drug is excreted in human milk. Because many drugs are excreted in human milk and because of the potential for serious adverse reactions in nursing infants from BANCAP HC Capsules, a decision should be made whether to discontinue nursing or to discontinue the drug, taking into account the importance of the drug to the mother.

Pediatric Use: Safety and effectiveness in children have not been established.

ADVERSE REACTIONS

Central Nervous System: Sedation, drowsiness, mental clouding, lethargy, impairment of mental and physical performance, anxiety, fear, dysphoria, dizziness, psychic dependence, mood changes.

Gastrointestinal System: Nausea and vomiting may occur; they are more frequent in ambulatory than in recumbent patients. The antiemetic phenothiazines are useful in suppressing these effects; however, some phenothiazine derivatives seem to be antianalgesic and to increase the amount of narcotic required to produce pain relief, while other phenothiazines reduce the amount of narcotic required to produce a given level of analgesia. Prolonged administration of BANCAP HC Capsules may produce constipation.

Genitourinary System: Ureteral spasm, spasm of vesical sphincters and urinary retention have been reported.

Respiratory Depression: BANCAP HC Capsules may produce dose-related respiratory depression by acting directly on brain stem respiratory centers. Hydrocodone also affects centers that control respiratory rhythm, and may produce irregular and periodic breathing. If significant respiratory depression occurs, it may be antagonized by the use of naloxone hydrochloride. Apply other supportive measures when indicated.

Drug Abuse and Dependence: BANCAP HC Capsules are subject to the Federal Controlled Substances Act (Schedule III). Psychic dependence, physical dependence, and tolerance may develop upon repeated administration of narcotics; therefore, BANCAP HC Capsules should be prescribed and administered with caution. However, psychic dependence is unlikely to develop when BANCAP HC Capsules are used for a short time for the treatment of pain.

Physical dependence, the condition in which continued administration of the drug is required to prevent the appearance of a withdrawal syndrome, assumes clinically significant proportions only after several weeks of continued narcotic use, although some mild degree of physical dependence may develop after a few days of narcotic therapy. Tolerance, in which increasingly large doses are required in order to produce the same degree of analgesia, is manifested initially by a shortened duration of analgesic effect, and subsequently by decreases in the intensity of analgesia. The rate of development of tolerance varies among patients.

OVERDOSAGE

Acetaminophen: Signs and Symptoms: Acetaminophen in massive overdosage may cause hepatic toxicity in some patients. In all cases of suspected overdose, immediately call your regional poison center or the Rocky Mountain Poison Center's toll-free number (800-525-6115) for assistance in diagnosis and for directions in the use of N-acetylcysteine as an antidote, a use currently restricted to investigational status.

In adults, hepatic toxicity has rarely been reported with acute overdoses of less than 10 grams and fatalities with less than 15 grams. Importantly, young children seem to be more resistant than adults to the hepatotoxic effect of an acetaminophen overdose. Despite this, the measures outlined below should be initiated in any adult or child suspected of having ingested an acetaminophen overdose.

Early symptoms following a potentially hepatotoxic overdose may include: nausea, vomiting, diaphoresis and general malaise. Clinical and laboratory evidence of hepatic toxicity may not be apparent until 48 to 72 hours post-ingestion.

Treatment: The stomach should be emptied promptly by lavage or by induction of emesis with syrup of ipecac. Patients' estimates of the quantity of a drug ingested are notoriously unreliable. Therefore, if an acetaminophen overdose is suspected, a serum acetaminophen assay should be obtained as early as possible, but no sooner than four hours following ingestion. Liver function studies should be obtained initially and repeated at 24-hour intervals.

The antidote, N-acetylcysteine, should be administered as early as possible, and within 16 hours of the overdose ingestion for optimal results. Following recovery, there are no residual, structural or functional hepatic abnormalities.

Hydrocodone: Signs and Symptoms: Serious overdose with hydrocodone is characterized by respiratory depression (a decrease in respiratory rate and Cortidal volume, Cheyne-Stokes respiration, cyanosis), extreme somnolence progressing to stupor or coma, skeletal muscle flaccidity, cold and clammy skin, and sometimes bradycardia and hypotension. In severe overdosage, apnea, circulatory collapse, cardiac arrest and death may occur.

Treatment: Primary attention should be given to the reestablishment of adequate respiratory exchange through provision of a patent airway and the institution of assisted or controlled ventilation. The narcotic antagonist, naloxone is a specific antidote against respiratory depression which may result from overdosage or unusual sensitivity to narcotics, including hydrocodone. Therefore, an appropriate dose of naloxone should be administered, preferably by the intravenous route, and simultaneously with efforts at respiratory resuscitation. Since the duration of action of hydrocodone may exceed that of the antagonist, the patient should be kept under continued surveillance and repeated doses of the antagonist should be administered as needed to maintain adequate respiration.

An antagonist should not be administered in the absence of clinically significant respiratory or cardiovascular depression. Oxygen, intravenous fluids, vasopressors and other supportive measures should be employed as indicated. Gastric emptying may be useful in removing unabsorbed drug.

DOSAGE AND ADMINISTRATION

Dosage should be adjusted according to the severity of the pain and the response of the patient. However, it should be kept in mind that tolerance to hydrocodone can develop with continued use and that the incidence of untoward effects is dose related.

The usual dose is one capsule every six hours as needed for pain. If necessary, this dose may be repeated at four hour intervals. In cases of more severe pain, two capsules every six hours (up to 8 capsules in 24 hours) may be required.

HOW SUPPLIED

Black and red capsules imprinted FOREST 610.
Bottles of 100—NDC 0456-0610-01
Bottles of 500—NDC 0456-0610-02
Unit Dose of 100 (4 × 25) NDC 0456-0610-63

Caution: Federal law prohibits dispensing without prescription.

Revised: APRIL 1985

Shown in Product Identification Section, page 409

DALALONE D.P.® INJECTION ℞

(Dexamethasone acetate suspension)
Equivalent to Dexamethasone 16 mg/ml

NOT FOR INTRAVENOUS OR INTRALESIONAL USE
FOR INTRAMUSCULAR, INTRA-ARTICULAR AND SOFT TISSUE USE

DESCRIPTION

Dexamethasone acetate, a synthetic adrenocortical steroid, is a white to practically white, odorless powder. It is a practically insoluble ester of dexamethasone.

It has a molecular weight of 434.5 and its empirical formula is $C_{24}H_{31}FO_6$.

Dexamethasone Acetate suspension is a sterile white suspension that settles on standing, but is easily resuspended by mild shaking.

Each ml. contains: Dexamethasone Acetate equivalent to Dexamethasone 16 mg., Sodium Chloride 6.67 mg., Creatinine 5 mg., Edetate Disodium 0.5 mg., Carboxymethylcellulose Sodium 5 mg., Polysorbate 80 - 0.75 mg. Benzyl Alcohol 9 mg., Sodium Bisulfite 1 mg. as preservatives in Water for Injection q.s. Sodium Hydroxide to adjust pH.

CLINICAL PHARMACOLOGY

Dexamethasone Acetate suspension is a long-acting, repository adrenocorticosteroid preparation with a prompt onset of action. It is suitable for intramuscular or local injection, but not when an immediate effect of short duration is desired.

Naturally occurring glucocorticoids (hydrocortisone and cortisone), which also have salt-retaining properties, are used as replacement therapy in adrenocortical deficiency states. Their synthetic analogs, including dexamethasone, are primarily used for their potent anti-inflammatory effects in disorders of many organ systems.

Glucocorticoids cause profound and varied metabolic effects. In addition, they modify the body's immune responses to diverse stimuli.

At equipotent anti-inflammatory doses, dexamethasone almost completely lacks the sodium-retaining property of hydrocortisone.

INDICATIONS AND USAGE

A. Intramuscular administration. When oral therapy is not feasible and the strength, dosage form, and route of administration of the drug reasonably lend the preparation to the treatment of the condition, those products labeled for intramuscular use are indicated as follows:

1. Endocrine disorders

Primary or secondary adrenocortical insufficiency (hydrocortisone or cortisone is the drug of choice; synthetic analogs may be used in conjunction with mineralocorticoids where applicable; in infancy, mineralocorticoid supplementation is of particular importance).

Acute adrenocortical insufficiency (hydrocortisone or cortisone is the drug of choice; mineralocorticoid supplementation may be necessary, particularly when synthetic analogs are used).

Preoperatively and in the event of serious trauma or illness, in patients with known adrenal insufficiency or when adrenocortical reserve is doubtful.

Shock unresponsive to conventional therapy if adrenocortical insufficiency exists or is suspected.

Congenital adrenal hyperplasia.

Nonsuppurative thyroiditis.

Hypercalcemia associated with cancer.

2. Rheumatic disorders

As adjunctive therapy for short-term administration (to tide the patient over an acute episode or exacerbation) in:

Post-traumatic osteoarthritis
Synovitis of osteoarthritis
Rheumatoid arthritis, including juvenile rheumatoid arthritis (selected cases may require low-dose maintenance therapy).
Acute and subacute bursitis
Epicondylitis
Acute nonspecific tenosynovitis
Acute gouty arthritis
Psoriatic arthritis
Ankylosing spondylitis

3. Collagen diseases

During an exacerbation or as maintenance therapy in selected cases of:

Systemic lupus erythematosus
Acute rheumatic carditis

4. Dermatologic diseases

Pemphigus
Severe erythema multiforme (Stevens-Johnson syndrome)
Exfoliative dermatitis
Bullous dermatitis herpetiformis
Severe seborrheic dermatitis
Severe psoriasis
Mycosis fungoides.

5. Allergic states

Control of severe or incapacitating allergic conditions intractable to adequate trials of conventional treatment in:

Bronchial asthma
Contact dermatitis
Atopic dermatitis
Serum sickness
Seasonal or perennial allergic rhinitis
Drug hypersensitivity reactions
Urticarial transfusion reactions
Acute noninfectious laryngeal edema (epinephrine is the drug of first choice).

6. Ophthalmic diseases

Severe acute and chronic allergic and inflammatory processes involving the eye, such as:

Herpes zoster ophthalmicus
Iritis, Iridocyclitis
Chorioretinitis
Diffuse posterior uveitis and choroiditis
Optic neuritis
Sympathetic ophthalmia
Anterior segment inflammation
Allergic conjunctivitis
Allergic corneal marginal ulcers

7. Gastrointestinal diseases

To tide the patient over a critical period of disease in:

Ulcerative colitis—(Systemic therapy)
Regional enteritis—(Systemic therapy)

8. Respiratory diseases

Symptomatic sarcoidosis
Berylliosis
Fulminating or disseminated pulmonary tuberculosis when used concurrently with appropriate antituberculous chemotherapy.
Loeffler's syndrome not manageable by other means.
Aspiration pneumonitis.

9. Hematologic disorders

Acquired (autoimmune) hemolytic anemia
Idiopathic thrombocytopenic purpura in adults (I.V. only; I.M. administration is contraindicated)
Secondary thrombocytopenia in adults
Erythroblastopenia (RBC anemia)
Congenital (erythroid) hypoplastic anemia.

10. Neoplastic diseases

For palliative management of leukemias and lymphomas in adults
Acute leukemia of childhood.

11. Edematous state

To induce diuresis or remission of proteinuria in the nephrotic syndrome without uremia, of the idiopathic type, or that due to lupus erythematosus.

12. Miscellaneous

Tuberculous meningitis with subarachnoid block or impending block when used concurrently with appropriate antituberculous chemotherapy.
Trichinosis with neurologic or myocardial involvement
Diagnostic testing of adrenocortical hyperfunction.

B. By intra-articular or soft tissue injection as adjunctive therapy for short-term administration (to tide the patient over an acute episode of exacerbation) in:

Synovitis of osteoarthritis
Rheumatoid arthritis
Acute and subacute bursitis

Continued on next page

Forest Pharmaceuticals—Cont.

Acute gouty arthritis
Epicondylitis
Acute nonspecific tenosynovitis
Post-traumatic osteoarthritis

CONTRAINDICATION

Systemic fungal infections.

WARNINGS

DO NOT INJECT INTRAVENOUSLY. In patients on corticosteroid therapy subjected to any unusual stress, increased dosage of rapidly acting corticosteroids before, during, and after the stressful situation is indicated.

Corticosteroids may mask some signs of infection, and new infections may appear during their use. There may be decreased resistance and inability to localize infection when corticosteroids are used.

Prolonged use of corticosteroids may produce posterior subcapsular cataracts, glaucoma with possible damage to the optic nerves, and may enhance the establishment of secondary ocular infections due to fungi or viruses.

Usage in pregnancy. Since adequate human reproduction studies have not been done with corticosteroids, the use of these drugs in pregnancy, nursing mothers, or women of childbearing potential requires that the possible benefits of the drug be weighed against the potential hazards to the mother and embryo or fetus. Infants born of mothers who have received substantial doses of corticosteroids during pregnancy should be carefully observed for signs of hypoadrenalism.

Average and large doses of cortisone or hydrocortisone can cause elevation of blood pressure, salt and water retention, and increased excretion of potassium. These effects are less likely to occur with the synthetic derivatives except when used in large doses. Dietary salt restriction and potassium supplementation may be necessary. All corticosteroids increase calcium excretion.

While on corticosteroid therapy patients should not be vaccinated against smallpox. Other immunization procedures should not be undertaken in patients who are on corticosteroids, especially in high doses, because of possible hazards of neurologic complications and lack of antibody response.

If corticosteroids are indicated in patients with latent tuberculosis or tuberculin reactivity, close observation is necessary as reactivation of the disease may occur. During prolonged corticosteroid therapy, these patients should receive chemoprophylaxis.

Because rare instances of anaphylactoid reactions have occurred in patients receiving parenteral corticosteroid therapy, appropriate precautionary measures should be taken prior to administration, especially when the patient has a history of allergy to any drug.

Corticosteroids may suppress reaction to skin tests.

Repository adrenocorticosteroid preparations may cause atrophy at the site of injection. To minimize the likelihood and/or severity of atrophy, do not inject subcutaneously, avoid injection into the deltoid muscle, and avoid repeated intramuscular injections into the same site if possible.

Dosage in children under 12 has not been established.

PRECAUTIONS

Dexamethasone Acetate suspension is not recommended as initial therapy in acute, life-threatening situations.

This product, like many other steroid formulations, is sensitive to heat. Therefore, it should not be autoclaved when it is desirable to sterilize the exterior of the vial.

Drug-induced secondary adrenocortical insufficiency may be minimized by gradual reduction of dosage. This type of relative insufficiency may persist for months after discontinuation of therapy; therefore, in any situation of stress occurring during that period, hormone therapy should be reinstituted. If the patient is receiving steroids already, the dosage may have to be increased. Since mineralocorticoid secretion may be impaired, salt and/or a mineralocorticoid should be administered concurrently.

There is an enhanced effect of corticosteroids in patients with hypothyroidism and in those with cirrhosis.

Corticosteroids should be used cautiously in patients with ocular herpes simplex for fear of corneal ulceration and perforation.

Psychic derangements may appear when corticosteroids are used, ranging from euphoria, insomnia, mood swings, personality changes, and severe depression to frank psychotic manifestations. Also, existing emotional instability or psychotic tendencies may be aggravated by corticosteroids.

Aspirin should be used cautiously in conjunction with corticosteroids in hypoprothrombinemia.

Steroids should be used with caution in nonspecific ulcerative colitis, if there is a probability of impending perforation, abscess or other pyogenic infection, also in diverticulitis, fresh intestinal anastomoses, active or latent peptic ulcer, renal insufficiency, hypertension, osteoporosis, and myasthenia gravis. Fat embolism has been reported as a possible complication of hypercortisonism.

An ulcer regimen including an antacid should be considered as a prophylactic measure during prolonged therapy.

Growth and development of infants and children on prolonged corticosteroid therapy should be carefully followed.

Steroids may increase or decrease motility and number of spermatozoa in some patients.

Since phenytoin, phenobarbital, ephedrine and rifampin may alter cortisol metabolism, glucocorticoid dosage adjustments may be required when any of these substances is started or stopped.

The prothrombin time should be checked frequently in patients who are receiving corticosteroids and coumarin anticoagulants at the same time because of reports that corticosteroids have altered the response to these anticoagulants. There are some reports of potentiation; others of inhibition.

Intra-articular injection of a corticosteroid may produce systemic as well as local effects.

Appropriate examination of any joint fluid present is necessary to exclude a septic process.

A marked increase in pain accompanied by local swelling, further restriction of joint motion, fever, and malaise are suggestive of septic arthritis. If this complication occurs and the diagnosis of sepsis is confirmed, appropriate antimicrobial therapy should be instituted.

Local injection of a steroid into an infected site is to be avoided.

Corticosteroids should not be injected into unstable joints.

Patients should be impressed strongly with the importance of not over-using joints in which symptomatic benefit has been obtained as long as the inflammatory process remains active.

ADVERSE REACTIONS

Fluid and electrolyte disturbances:
Sodium retention
Fluid retention
Congestive heart failure in susceptible patients
Potassium loss
Hypokalemic alkalosis
Hypertension
Hypotensive or shock-like reaction

Musculoskeletal:
Muscle weakness
Steroid myopathy
Loss of muscle mass
Osteoporosis
Vertebral compression fractures
Aseptic necrosis of femoral and humeral heads
Pathologic fracture of long bones

Gastrointestinal:
Peptic ulcer with possible subsequent perforation and hemorrhage
Pancreatitis
Abdominal distention
Ulcerative esophagitis

Dermatologic:
Impaired wound healing
Thin fragile skin
Petechiae and ecchymoses
Erythema
Increased sweating
Other cutaneous reactions

Neurologic:
Convulsions
Increased intracranial pressure with papilledema (pseudotumor cerebri) usually after treatment
Vertigo
Headache

Endocrine:
Menstrual irregularities
Development of cushingoid state
Suppression of growth in children
Secondary adrenocortical and pituitary unresponsiveness, particularly in times of stress, as in trauma, surgery or illness
Decreased carbohydrate tolerance
Manifestations of latent diabetes mellitus
Increased requirements for insulin or oral hypoglycemic agents in diabetics

Ophthalmic:
Posterior subcapsular cataracts
Increased intraocular pressure
Glaucoma
Exophthalmos

Metabolic:
Negative nitrogen balance due to protein catabolism

Other:
Hypersensitivity
Thromboembolism
Weight gain
Increased appetite
Nausea
Malaise

The following **additional** adverse reactions are related to parenteral corticosteroid therapy:

Rare instances of blindness associated with intralesional therapy around the face and head
Hyperpigmentation or hypopigmentation
Subcutaneous and cutaneous atrophy
Sterile abscess
Postinjection flare (following intra-articular use)
Charcot-like arthropathy
Scarring
Induration
Inflammation
Paresthesia
Ecchymosis
Delayed pain or soreness
Muscle twitching, ataxia, hiccups, and nystagmus have been reported in low incidence after injection of Dexamethasone Acetate suspension

DRUG ABUSE AND DEPENDENCE

(See WARNINGS section).

OVERDOSAGE

(See ADVERSE REACTION section).

DOSAGE AND ADMINISTRATION

Dosage Requirements Are Variable and Must Be Individualized on the Basis of the Disease Under Treatment and the Response of the Patient.

Dosage in children under 12 has not been established.

Intramuscular Injection

Dosage ranges from 0.5 to 1 ml., equivalent to 8 to 16 mg. of dexamethasone. If further treatment is needed, dosage may be repeated at intervals of 1 to 3 weeks.

Intra-articular and Soft Tissue Injection

The dose varies, depending on the location and the severity of inflammation. The usual dose is 0.25 to 1 ml., equivalent to 4 to 16 mg. of dexamethasone. If further treatment is needed, dosage may be repeated at intervals of 1 to 3 weeks.

PROTECT FROM LIGHT, STORE AT CONTROLLED ROOM TEMPERATURE 59°–86° F. (15°–30° C). DO NOT PERMIT TO FREEZE. SENSITIVE TO HEAT—DO NOT AUTOCLAVE.

CAUTION: Federal law prohibits dispensing without prescription.

Literature Revised: **May 1982**

HOW SUPPLIED

5ML multiple dose vial, NDC 0456-1097-05. 1ML single dose vial, box of 5 NDC 0456-1097-41.

DALCAINE INJECTION ℞

Each ml. contains:
Lidocaine HCl 2% without preservative

HOW SUPPLIED

5 ml. unit dose vial (box of 6).
NDC 0456-1099-05.

DURAPHYL™ ℞

(anhydrous theophylline)
Theophylline Controlled Release Tablets

DESCRIPTION

Theophylline anhydrous, a xanthine bronchodilator, is a white odorless, crystalline powder having a bitter taste. Theophylline has the following structural formula:

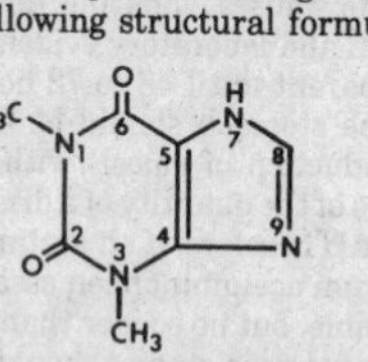

1H-Purine-2,6-dione,3,7-dihydro-1,3-dimethyl

Duraphyl Tablets are available as a controlled release formulation containing 100 mg, 200 mg and 300 mg of anhydrous theophylline.

CLINICAL PHARMACOLOGY

Theophylline directly relaxes the smooth muscle of the bronchial airways and pulmonary blood vessels, thus acting mainly as a bronchodilator and smooth muscle relaxant. The drug also produces other actions typical of the xanthine derivatives: Coronary vasodilator, cardiac stimulant, diuretic, cerebral stimulant, and skeletal muscle stimulant. The actions of theophylline may be mediated through inhibition of phosphodiesterase and a resultant increase in intracellular cyclic AMP. *In vitro,* theophylline has been shown to act synergistically with beta agonists that increase intracellular cyclic AMP through the stimulation of adenyl cyclase, but synergism has not been demonstrated in the patient studies. More data are needed to determine if theophylline and beta agonists have a clinically important additive effect *in vivo.* Apparently, no development of tolerance occurs with chronic use of theophylline.

Pharmacokinetics: The half life of theophylline is influenced by a number of known variables. It is prolonged in patients suffering from chronic alcoholism, impaired hepatic or renal function, congestive heart failure, and in patients receiving macrolide antibiotics and cimetidine. Older adults (over age 55) and patients with chronic obstructive pulmonary disease, with or without cor pulmonale, may also have much slower clearance rates. For such patients, the theophylline half-life may exceed 24 hours.

Newborns and neonates have extremely slow clearance rates compared to older infants (over 6 months), and children, and may also have a theophylline half-life of over 24 hours. High fever for prolonged periods may also reduce the rate of theophylline elimination.

THEOPHYLLINE ELIMINATION CHARACTERISTICS

	Theophylline Clearance Rates (mean±S.D.)	Half-life Average (mean±S.D.)
Children (over 6 months of age)	1.45 ± 0.58 ml/kg/min	3.7 ±1.1 hrs
Adult non-smokers uncomplicated asthma	0.65 ± 0.19 ml/kg/min	8.7 ± 2.2 hrs

The half-life of theophylline in smokers (1 to 2 packs/day) averages 4–5 hours, much shorter than the half-life in non-smokers (average 7–9 hours). The increase in theophylline clearance caused by smoking is probably the result of induction of drug-metabolizing enzymes that do not readily normalize after cessation of smoking. It appears that between 3 months and 2 years may be necessary for normalization of the effect of smoking on theophylline pharmacokinetics.

Pharmacokinetic Studies: The three strengths of Duraphyl tablets are made from the same formulation mix and the weights of the 100, 200 and 300 mg tablets are essentially proportional to each other.

A single dose three way crossover study was conducted in 18 normal subjects. Subjects were fasted for 10 to 12 hours before and for 4 additional hours after dosing. All subjects received a single 300 mg tablet, two 200 mg tablets and three 100 mg tablets with intervening washout periods. Mean peak theophylline serum levels for the 100 mg, 200 mg (normalized to an equivalent 300 mg dose) and 300 mg tablets were 3.8 plus or minus 0.9 mcg/ml, 3.9 plus or minus 1.4 mcg/ml and 3.4 plus or minus 0.9 mcg/ml, respectively. The peak serum level varied from subject to subject, occurring from 3 to 12 hours after dosing. However 80% of the subjects had serum levels of at least 75% of the maximum value between 5 and 8 hours after dosing. Therefore, blood samples taken 5 and 8 hours should reference the peak serum level for most subjects.

A multiple dose, five day study was conducted with 18 normal subjects given 300 mg twice daily. For this group, theophylline half-lives after dosing with a liquid preparation were determined to be between 5.5 and 11.0 hours (mean 7.7 plus or minus 1.6 hours). On the fifth day, after steady state had been established, the AM dose was administered after a twelve hour fast which continued for 4 hours after dosing. Mean Cmax and Cmin levels were determined to be 8.3 plus or minus 1.4 mcg/ml and 5.3 plus or minus 1.3 mcg/ml, respectively, while the average percent fluctuation (Cmax minus Cmin/Cmin ×100) was 57%. Complete bioavailability was exhibited when compared to an immediate release product.

INDICATIONS

For relief and/or prevention of symptoms from asthma and reversible bronchospasm associated with chronic bronchitis and emphysema.

CONTRAINDICATIONS

Duraphyl is contraindicated in individuals who have shown hypersensitivity to its components.

WARNINGS

Status asthmatics should be considered a medical emergency and is defined as that degree of bronchospasm which is not rapidly responsive to usual doses of conventional bronchodilators. Optimal therapy for such patients frequently requires both *additional medication*, parenterally administered and *close monitoring*, preferably in an intensive care setting.

Although increasing the dose of theophylline may bring about relief, such treatment may be associated with toxicity. The likelihood of such toxicity developing increases significantly when the serum theophylline concentration exceeds 20 mcg/ml. Therefore, determination of serum theophylline levels is recommended to assure maximal benefit without excessive risk.

Serum levels above 20 mcg/ml are rarely found after appropriate administration of the recommended doses. However, in individuals in whom theophylline plasma clearance is reduced *for any reason*, even conventional doses may result in increased serum levels and potential toxicity. Reduced theophylline clearance has been documented in the following readily identifiable groups: 1) patients with impaired renal or liver function; 2) patients over 55 years of age, particularly males and those with chronic lung disease; 3) those with cardiac failure from any cause; 4) neonates; and 5) those taking certain drugs (macrolide antibiotics and cimetidine). Decreased clearance of theophylline may be associated with either influenza immunization or active infection with influenza.

Reduction of dosage and laboratory monitoring is especially appropriate in the above individuals.

Less serious signs of theophylline toxicity, i.e, nausea and restlessness, may appear in up to 50% of patients. Unfortunately however, serious side effects such as ventricular arrhythmias, convulsions, or even death may appear as the first sign of toxicity without any previous warning. Stated differently, *serious toxicity is not reliably preceded by less severe side effects.*

Many patients who require theophylline may exhibit tachycardia due to their underlying disease process so that the cause/effect relationship to elevated serum theophylline concentrations may not be appreciated.

Theophylline products may cause dysrhythmia and/or worsen pre-existing arrhythmias and any significant change in rate and/or rhythm warrants monitoring and further investigation.

The occurrence of arrhythmias and sudden death (with histological evidence of necrosis of the myocardium) has been recorded in laboratory animals (minipigs, rodents and dogs) when theophylline and beta agonists were administered concomitantly, although not when either was administered alone. The significance of these findings when applied to human usage is currently unknown.

PRECAUTIONS

General: Theophylline half-life is shorter in smokers than in non-smokers. Therefore, smokers may require larger or more frequent doses. Morphine and curare should be used with caution in patients with airway obstruction as they may suppress respiration and stimulate histamine release. Alternative drugs should be used when possible. Duraphyl should not be administered concurrently with other xanthine medications. Use with caution in patients with severe cardiac disease, severe hypoxemia, hypertension, hyperthyroidism, acute myocardial injury, cor pulmonale, congestive heart failure, liver disease, in the elderly (especially males) and in neonates. In particular, great caution should be used in giving Duraphyl to patients with congestive heart failure. Frequently such patients have markedly prolonged theophylline serum levels with theophylline persisting in serum for long periods following discontination of the drug.

Theophylline preparations should be used cautiously in patients with history of peptic ulcer, since they may occasionally act as a local irritant to the G.I. tract; gastrointestinal symptoms, however, are more commonly centrally mediated and associated with serum drug concentrations over 20 mcg/ml.

Information for Patients: The physician should reinforce the importance of taking only the prescribed dose and time interval between doses. Duraphyl tablets should not be chewed or crushed. The patient should alert the physician if symptoms should occur repeatedly, especially near the end of a dosing interval.

Drug Interactions:

Drug: Toxic synergism with ephedrine has been documented and may occur with some other sympathomimetic bronchodilators. In addition, the following drug interactions have been demonstrated:

DRUG	EFFECT
Lithium Carbonate	Increased excretion of Lithium Carbonate
Propranolol	Antagonism of Propranolol effect
Cimetidine	Increased theophylline blood levels
Troleandomycin, erythromycin	Increased theophylline blood levels

Drug-Food: Duraphyl has not been adequately studied to determine whether its bioavailability is altered when it is given with food.

Available data suggest that drug administration at the time of food ingestion may influence the absorption characteristics of some or all theophylline controlled-release products resulting in serum values different from those found after administration in the fasting state.

A drug-food effect, if any, would likely have its greatest clinical significance when high theophylline serum levels are being maintained and/or when large single doses (greater than 13 mg/kg or 900 mg) of a controlled-release theophylline product are given. The influence of the type and amount of food on performance of controlled-release theophylline products is under study at this time.

Drug-Laboratory Tests Interactions: When plasma levels of theophylline are measured by spectrophotometric methods. Coffee, tea, cola beverages, chocolate, and acetaminophen contribute falsely high values.

Carcinogenesis, Mutagenesis, and Impairment of Fertility: Long-term animal studies have not been performed to evaluate the carcinogenic potential, mutagenic potential or the effect on fertility of xanthine compounds.

Pregnancy: Category C—Animal reproduction studies have not been conducted with theophylline. It is not known whether theophylline can cause fetal harm when administered to a pregnant woman or affect reproduction capacity. Duraphyl should be given to a pregnant woman only if clearly needed.

Nursing Mothers: It has been reported that theophylline distributes readily into breast milk and may cause adverse effects in the infant. Caution must be used if prescribing xanthines to a mother who is nursing, taking into account the risk-benefit of this therapy.

Pediatric Use: The safety and effectiveness of Duraphyl in children under 6 years of age has not been established.

ADVERSE REACTIONS

The most consistent adverse reactions are usually due to overdose and are:

1. ***Gastrointestinal:*** nausea, vomiting, epigastric pain, hematemesis, diarrhea.
2. ***Central nervous system:*** headaches, irritability, restlessness, insomnia, reflex hyperexcitability, muscle twitching, clonic and tonic generalized convulsions.
3. ***Cardiovascular:*** Palpitation, tachycardia, extraystoles, flushing hypotension, circulatory failure, ventricular arrhythmias.
4. ***Respiratory:*** tachypnea.
5. ***Renal:*** Albuminuria, increased excretion of renal tubular and red blood cells, potentiation of diuresis.
6. ***Others:*** hyperglycemia and inappropriate ADH Syndrome; rash.

OVERDOSAGE

Management: If potential overdose is established and seizure has not occurred.

a. Induce vomiting.
b. Administer a cathartic (this is particularly important if sustained release preparations have been taken).
c. Administer activated charcoal.

If patient is having a seizure:

a. Establish an airway.
b. Administer oxygen.
c. Treat the seizure with intravenous diazepam, 0.1 to 0.3 mg/kg up to 10 mg.
d. Monitor vital signs, maintain blood pressure and provide adequate hydration.

Post Seizure Coma:

a. Maintain airway and oxygenation.
b. In addition to the above recommendations to prevent absorption of the drug, intubation and lavage will have to be performed instead of inducing emesis, and the carthatic and charcoal will need to be introduced via a large bore gastric lavage tube.
c. Continue to provide full supportive care and adequate hydration while waiting for drug to be metabolized. In general, the drug is metabolized sufficiently rapid so as not to warrant consideration of dialysis, however, if serum levels exceed 50 mcg/ml, charcoal hemoperfusion may be indicated.

DOSAGE AND ADMINISTRATION

Duraphyl has not been adequately studied for its bioavailability when administered with food (see **PRECAUTIONS, Drug-Food Interactions**). For most patients, the *effective use* of theophylline, i.e., associated with optimal likelihood of benefit combined with minimal risk of toxicity is considered to occur when serum levels are maintained between 10 and 20 mcg/ml. Levels above 20 mcg/ml may produce toxicity, and in a small number of patients, toxicity may even be seen with serum levels between 15–20 mcg/ml, particularly during initiation of therapy.

There is considerable variation from patient to patient in the dosage of theophylline required to achieve and maintain therapeutic and safe levels, primarily due to variable rates of elimination. Therefore, it is essential that not only must dosage be individualized, but titration and monitoring of serum levels be utilized where available. When serum concentration cannot be obtained, restriction of dosage to the amounts and intervals recommended in the guidelines listed below becomes essential. Dosage should be calculated on the basis of lean (ideal) body weight where mg/kg doses are presented. Theophylline does not distribute into fatty tissue.

Duraphyl tablets (controlled release) are recommended for chronic or long term management and prevention of symptoms, *and not for use in treating acute symptoms* of asthma and reversible bronchospasm.

Dosage guidelines are approximations only and the wide range of theophylline clearance between individuals (particularly those with concomitant disease) makes indiscriminate usage hazardous.

As a practical consideration, it is not always possible to obtain serum level determinations. Under such conditions, restriction of the daily dose (in otherwise healthy adults) to not greater than 13 mg/kg/day (or 900 mg, whichever is less), of anhydrous theophylline in divided doses will result

Continued on next page

Forest Pharmaceuticals—Cont.

in relatively few patients exceeding serum levels of 20 mg/ml and the resultant risk of toxicity.

INITIATING THERAPY

1) **Acute Symptoms:** Duraphyl is not intended for patients experiencing an acute episode of bronchospasm (associated with asthma, chronic bronchitis, or emphysema). Such patients require *rapid* relief of symptoms and should be treated with an immediate-release or intravenous theophylline preparation (or other bronchodilators) and not with controlled release products.
2) **Chronic Therapy:** It is recommended that appropriate dosage be established using either an immediate or sustained release xanthine preparation of unit strength sufficiently small to allow flexibility in incremental dose titration. Slow clinical titration is generally preferred to help assure acceptance and safety of the medication. If the 24 hour dose corresponds to that which can be delivered by Duraphyl, the patient can then usually be switched to Duraphyl tablets by administering one-half of the 24 hour dose at 12 hour intervals.

However, certain patients, such as the young, smokers, and some nonsmoking adults are likely to metabolize theophylline rapidly and require dosing at 8 hour intervals. Such patients can generally be identified as having through serum concentrations lower than desired or repeatedly exhibiting symptoms near the end of a dosing interval.

Maximum Dose of Theophylline Where the Serum Concentration is Not Measured: Not to exceed the following:

Age	
<9 years	24 mg/kg/day
9–12 years	20 mg/kg/day
12–16 years	18 mg/kg/day
>16 years	13 mg/kg/day OR 900 mg (whichever is less)

WARNING: DO NOT ATTEMPT TO MAINTAIN ANY DOSE THAT IS NOT TOLERATED

Measurement of Serum Theophylline Concentration During Chronic Therapy with Duraphyl: If the above maximum doses are to be maintained or exceeded, serum theophylline measurement is recommended. The serum sample should be obtained at the time of peak absorption (approximately 4 hours after dosing). It is important that the patient will have missed ***no*** doses during the previous 48 hours and that dosing intervals will have been reasonably typical with no added doses during that period of time. DOSAGE ADJUSTMENT BASED ON SERUM THEOPHYLLINE MEASUREMENTS WHEN THESE INSTRUCTIONS HAVE NOT BEEN FOLLOWED MAY RESULT IN RECOMMENDATIONS THAT PREVENT RISK OF TOXICITY OR INADEQUATE DOSING TO THE PATIENT.

Final Adjustment of Dosage: Dosage adjustment after serum theophylline measurement.
[See table below].

Caution should be exercised for younger children who cannot complain of minor side effects. Older adults, those with cor pulmonale, congestive heart failure and/or liver disease, may have unusually low dosage requirements, and thus may experience toxicity at the maximum dosage recommended above.

It is important that no patient be maintained on any dosage that is not tolerated. Patients instructed to increase dosage according to the above schedule should be told not to take a subsequent dose if apparent side effects occur and to resume therapy at a lower dose once adverse effects have disappeared.

HOW SUPPLIED

Duraphyl (Theophylline Anhydrous) is available as 100 mg. 200 mg. and 300 mg. controlled release tablets having the following identification characteristics:

Duraphyl 300 mg: capsule shaped, white, scored tablets, imp. McNeil, 427/300. Available in bottles of 100 (NDC 0456-0634-01).

Duraphyl 200 mg: capsule shaped, white, bisected tablets, imp. McNeil, 426/200. Available in bottles of 100 (NDC 0456-0633-01).

Duraphyl 100 mg: round concave, white, bisected tablets, imp. McNeil, 425/100. Available in bottles of 100 (NDC 0456-0632-01)

STORAGE

Store at controlled room temperature 15°–30°C (59°–86°F). Dispense in tight containers.

CAUTION

Federal law prohibits dispensing without prescription.

Revised January 1985

If serum theophylline is:		Directions:
Within normal limits	10 to 20 mcg/ml	Maintain dosage if tolerated. Recheck serum theophylline concentrations at 6–12 month intervals.*
Too high	20 to 25 mcg/ml	Decrease doses by about 10%. Recheck serum theophylline concentrations at 6–12 month intervals.*
	25 to 30 mcg/ml	Skip next dose and decrease subsequent doses by about 25%.
	Over 30 mcg/ml	Skip next 2 doses and decrease subsequent doses by 50%. Recheck serum theophylline.
Too low	7.5 to 10 mcg/ml	Increase dose by about 25%.** Recheck serum theophylline concentrations at 6–12 month intervals.*
	5 to 7.5 mcg/ml	Increase dose by about 25% to the nearest dose increment and recheck serum theophylline for guidance in further dosage adjustment (another increase will probably be needed, but this provides a safety check).

*Finer adjustments in dosage may be needed for some patients.
**Dividing the daily dose into 3 doses administered at 8 hour intervals may be indicated if symptoms occur repeatedly at the end of a dosing interval.
From the Journal of Respiratory Disease 2(7):16, 1981

ELIXOPHYLLIN® ℞
[*ē″lĭx′off′fĭl-ĭn*]
(theophylline anhydrous)
Capsules

ELIXOPHYLLIN® SR ℞
(theophylline anhydrous)
Capsules

ELIXOPHYLLIN® ℞
(theophylline anhydrous)
Elixir

DESCRIPTION

Elixophyllin® (theophylline anhydrous) Capsules
100 mg capsule—Each off-white, dye-free soft gelatin Elixophyllin® Capsule contains 100 mg anhydrous theophylline in a suspension of polyethylene glycol.
200 mg capsule—Each off-white, dye-free soft gelatin Elixophyllin® Capsule contains 200 mg anhydrous theophylline in a suspension of polyethylene glycol.

Elixophyllin® (theophylline anhydrous) SR Capsules
Elixophyllin® SR Capsules are designed to provide a prolonged therapeutic effect.
125 mg capsule—Each white, opaque, dye-free capsule contains 125 mg anhydrous theophylline.
250 mg capsule—Each clear, dye-free capsule contains 250 mg anhydrous theophylline.

Elixophyllin® (theophylline anhydrous) Elixir
Each 15 mL (tablespoonful) of Elixophyllin® Elixir contains 80 mg anhydrous theophylline and 20% alcohol in a palatable aromatic base.

Theophylline (1H-purine-2,6-dione, 3,7-dihydro-1,3-dimethyl), a xanthine bronchodilator, is a white, odorless, crystalline powder having a bitter taste and is represented by the following structural formula:

CLINICAL PHARMACOLOGY

Theophylline directly relaxes the smooth muscle of the bronchial airways and pulmonary blood vessels, thus acting mainly as a bronchodilator and smooth muscle relaxant. The drug also produces other actions typical of xanthine derivatives: coronary vasodilation, cardiac stimulation, diuresis, cerebral stimulation and skeletal muscle stimulation. The actions of theophylline may be mediated through inhibition of phosphodiesterase and a resultant increase in intracellular cyclic AMP. In vivo studies indicate that xanthines improve the contractile properties of the diaphragm in normal human subjects.

In vitro theophylline has been shown to act synergistically with beta agonists that increase intracellular cyclic AMP through the stimulation of adenyl cyclase, but synergism has not been demonstrated in patient studies. More data are needed to determine if theophylline and beta agonists have clinically important additive effects in vivo.

Apparently, tolerance does not develop with chronic use of theophylline.

Pharmacokinetics: The half-life of theophylline is influenced by a number of known variables. It is prolonged in patients suffering from chronic alcoholism, impaired hepatic or renal function, congestive heart failure, and in patients receiving macrolide antibiotics or cimetidine. Older adults (over age 55) and patients with chronic obstructive pulmonary disease, with or without cor pulmonale, may also have much slower clearance rates. For such patients, the theophylline half-life may exceed 24 hours.

Newborns and neonates have extremely slow clearance rates compared with older infants (over 6 months) and children, and may also have a theophylline half-life of over 24 hours. High fever for prolonged periods may also reduce the rate of theophylline elimination in adults as well as children.

THEOPHYLLINE ELIMINATION CHARACTERISTICS

	Theophylline Clearance Rates (mean±SD)	Half-life Average (mean±SD)
Children (over 6 months of age)	1.45 ± 0.58 mL/kg/min	3.7 ± 1.1 hr
Adult nonsmokers (uncomplicated asthma)	0.65 ± 0.19 mL/kg/min	8.7 ± 2.2 hr

The half-life of theophylline in smokers (1 to 2 packs/day) averages 4 to 5 hours, much shorter than the half-life in nonsmokers (which averages 7 to 9 hours). The increase in theophylline clearance caused by smoking is probably the result of induction of drug-metabolizing enzymes that do not readily normalize after cessation of smoking. It appears that three months to two years may be necessary for normalization of the effect of smoking on theophylline pharmacokinetics.

INDICATIONS

For relief and/or prevention of symptoms of asthma and reversible bronchospasm associated with chronic bronchitis and emphysema.

CONTRAINDICATIONS

This product is contraindicated in individuals who have shown hypersensitivity to any of its components.

WARNINGS

Status asthmaticus should be considered a medical emergency and is that degree of bronchospasm which is not rapidly responsive to usual doses of conventional bronchodilators. Optimal therapy for such patients frequently requires both *additional medication,* parenterally administered, and *close monitoring,* preferably in an intensive care setting.

Although increasing the dose of theophylline may bring about relief, such treatment may be associated with toxicity. The likelihood of such toxicity developing increases significantly when the serum theophylline concentration exceeds 20 μg/mL. Therefore, determination of serum theophylline levels is recommended to assure maximum benefit without excessive risk.

Serum levels above 20 μg/mL are rarely found after appropriate administration of the recommended doses. However, in individuals in whom theophylline plasma clearance is reduced *for any reason,* even conventional doses may result in increased serum levels and potential toxicity. Reduced theophylline clearance has been documented in the following readily identifiable groups: 1) patients with impaired renal or liver function; 2) patients over 55 years of age, particularly males, and those with chronic lung disease; 3) patients with cardiac failure from any cause; 4) neonates and 5) those patients taking certain drugs (macrolide antibiotics or cimetidine). Decreased clearance of theophylline may be associated with either influenza immunization or active infection with influenza. Reduction of dosage and laboratory monitoring is especially appropriate in the above individuals.

Less serious signs of theophylline toxicity (eg, nausea and restlessness) may appear in up to 50% of patients. Unfortunately however, serious side effects (such as ventricular arrhythmias, convulsions or even death) may appear as the first sign of toxicity without any previous warning. *Serious toxicity is not reliably preceded by less severe side effects.*

Many patients who require theophylline may exhibit tachycardia due to their underlying disease process so that the cause/effect relationship to elevated serum theophylline concentrations may not be appreciated.

Theophylline products may cause arrhythmia and/or worsen preexisting arrhythmias. Any significant change in rate and/or rhythm warrants monitoring and further investigation.

PRECAUTIONS

General: Theophylline half-life is shorter in smokers than in nonsmokers. Therefore, smokers may require larger or more frequent doses. Theophylline should not be administered concurrently with other xanthine medications. Use with caution in patients with severe cardiac disease, severe hypoxemia, hypertension, hyperthyroidism, acute myocardial injury, cor pulmonale, congestive heart failure, liver disease, in the elderly (especially males) and in neonates. In particular, great caution should be used in giving theophylline to patients with congestive heart failure. Frequently, such patients have markedly prolonged theophylline serum levels, with theophylline persisting in the serum for long periods following discontinuation of the drug.

Use theophylline cautiously in a patient with a history of peptic ulcer. Theophylline may occasionally act as a local irritant to the GI tract, although gastrointestinal symptoms are more commonly centrally mediated and are associated with serum drug concentrations exceeding 20 μg/mL.

Information for Patients: The physician should reinforce the importance of taking only the prescribed dose and only at the prescribed time interval between doses.

Drug Interactions: Toxic synergism with ephedrine has been documented and may occur with some other sympathomimetic bronchodilators. In addition, the following drug interactions have been demonstrated:

DRUG	EFFECT
Aminophylline with lithium carbonate	Increased excretion of lithium carbonate
Aminophylline with propranolol	Antagonism of propranolol effect
Theophylline with cimetidine	Increased theophylline blood levels
Theophylline with troleandomycin, erythromycin	Increased theophylline blood levels

Drug-Laboratory Test Interactions: When plasma levels of theophylline are measured by spectrophotometric methods, coffee, tea, cola beverages, chocolate and acetaminophen contribute to falsely high values.

Carcinogenesis, Mutagenesis and Impairment of Fertility: Long-term animal studies have not been performed to evaluate the carcinogenic potential, mutagenic potential or the effect on fertility of xanthine compounds.

Pregnancy: Category C—Animal reproduction studies have not been conducted with theophylline. It is not known whether theophylline can cause fetal harm when administered to a pregnant woman or whether it can affect reproductive capacity. Xanthines should be given to a pregnant woman only if clearly indicated.

Nursing Mothers: It has been reported that theophylline distributes readily into breast milk and may cause adverse effects in the infant. Caution must be used if prescribing xanthines to a nursing mother, taking into account the risk-benefit of this therapy.

Pediatric Use: This drug is not recommended for infants under 6 months of age because of their marked variation in theophylline metabolism. The use of Elixophyllin® SR capsules is not recommended for children under 6 years of age.

ADVERSE REACTIONS

The most consistent adverse reactions are due to overdose and are:

1. **Gastrointestinal:** nausea, vomiting, epigastric pain, hematemesis, diarrhea.
2. **Central nervous system:** headaches, irritability, restlessness, insomnia, reflex hyperexcitability, muscle twitching, clonic and tonic generalized convulsions.
3. **Cardiovascular:** palpitations, tachycardia, extrasystoles, flushing, hypotension, circulatory failure, ventricular arrhythmias.
4. **Respiratory:** tachypnea.
5. **Renal:** albuminuria, increased excretion of renal tubular and red blood cells, potentiation of diuresis.
6. **Others:** hyperglycemia, inappropriate ADH secretion, rash

OVERDOSAGE

Management:

If potential oral overdose is established and seizure has not occurred:

a. Induce vomiting.
b. Administer a cathartic (this is particularly important if a sustained-release preparation has been taken).
c. Administer activated charcoal.

If patient is having a seizure:

a. Establish an airway.
b. Administer oxygen.
c. Treat the seizure with intravenous diazepam, 0.1 to 0.3 mg/kg up to 10 mg.
d. Monitor vital signs, maintain blood pressure and provide adequate hydration.

Postseizure Coma:

a. Maintain airway and oxygenation.
b. If a result of oral medication, follow above recommendations to prevent absorption of the drug; however, intubation and lavage will have to be performed instead of inducing emesis. Any cathartic or charcoal will need to be introduced via a large bore gastric lavage tube.
c. Continue to provide full supportive care and adequate hydration while waiting for the drug to be metabolized. In general, the drug is rapidly metabolized and does not warrant consideration of dialysis. However, if serum levels exceed 50 μg/mL, charcoal hemoperfusion may be indicated.

Elixophyllin® Elixir and Elixophyllin® Capsules

	Oral Loading:	Followed by:	Maintenance:
1. Children 6 months to 9 years	6 mg/kg	4 mg/kg q4h × 3 doses	4 mg/kg q6h
2. Children 9-16 years and young adult smokers	6 mg/kg	3 mg/kg q4h × 3 doses	3 mg/kg q6h
3. Otherwise healthy nonsmoking adults	6 mg/kg	3 mg/kg q6h × 2 doses	3 mg/kg q8h
4. Older patients and patients with cor pulmonale	6 mg/kg	2 mg/kg q6h × 2 doses	2 mg/kg q8h
5. Patients with congestive heart failure	6 mg/kg	2 mg/kg q8h × 2 doses	1–2 mg/kg q12h

DOSAGE AND ADMINISTRATION

For most patients, *effective use* of theophylline, ie, use associated with optimal likelihood of benefit combined with minimal risk of toxicity, is considered to occur when serum levels are maintained between 10 and 20 μg/mL. Levels above 20 μg/mL may produce toxicity. In a small number of patients, toxicity may even be seen with serum levels between 15 and 20 μg/mL, particularly during initiation of therapy.

There is considerable variation among patients in the dosage required to achieve and maintain safe and therapeutic levels, primarily due to variable rates of elimination. Therefore, it is not only essential to individualize the dosage but also to titrate and monitor serum levels when possible. When serum concentration cannot be obtained, restriction of dosage to the amounts and intervals recommended in the guidelines listed below becomes essential. Dosage should be calculated on the basis of lean (ideal) body weight wherever mg/kg doses are presented. Theophylline does not distribute into fatty tissue.

Frequency of Dosing: When immediate-release products with rapid absorption (such as Elixophyllin® Capsules and Elixophyllin® Elixir) are used, dosing to maintain serum levels generally requires administration every 6 hours. This is particularly true in children, but dosing intervals up to 8 hours may be satisfactory in adults, since they eliminate the drug at a slower rate. Some children and adults having rapid clearance rates (eg, half-lives of under 6 hours) require higher than average doses and may benefit from and be more effectively controlled during chronic therapy when given Elixophyllin® SR Capsules, since this provides longer dosing intervals and/or less fluctuation in serum concentration between dosing.

Elixophyllin® SR Capsules provide a prolonged therapeutic effect and should be used for chronic or long-term use, not for initial treatment in a patient with acute symptoms. It is recommended that the appropriate dosage be established using an immediate-release preparation (such as Elixophyllin® Elixir or Elixophyllin® Capsules). Slow clinical titration is generally preferred to help assure medication acceptance and safety. If the total daily dose can be given by using a sustained-release product, the patient can usually be switched to Elixophyllin® SR Capsules. The total daily dose should be divided and administered at 12 hour intervals. However, certain patients, such as the young, smokers and some nonsmoking adults, are likely to metabolize theophylline rapidly and require dosing at 8-hour intervals. Such patients can generally be identified as having trough serum concentrations lower than desired or repeatedly exhibit symptoms near the end of the dosing interval.

Dosage guidelines are only approximations. The wide range of theophylline clearance among individuals (particularly those with concomitant disease) makes indiscriminate usage hazardous.

As a practical consideration, it is not always possible to determine serum levels. Under such conditions, the daily dosage (in otherwise healthy adults) should not be greater than 16 mg/kg/day of anhydrous theophylline taken in divided doses. This will result in relatively few patients exceeding a serum level of 20 μg/mL and the resultant risk of toxicity.

Dosage Guidelines:

I. Acute Symptoms of Asthma Requiring Rapid Theophyllinization:

A. Patients not currently receiving theophylline products. Dosage recommendations are for anhydrous theophylline.

[See table above].

B. Patients currently receiving theophylline products:

When possible, determine the time, amount, dosage form and route of administration of the patient's last dose.

The loading dose for theophylline is based on the principle that each 0.5 mg/kg of theophylline administered as a loading dose will result in a 1.0 μg/mL increase in serum theophylline concentration. Ideally, the loading dose should be deferred if a serum theophylline concentration can be obtained rapidly.

If this is not possible, the clinician must exercise judgment in selecting a dose based on the potential for benefit and risk. When there is sufficient respiratory distress to warrant a small risk, then 2.5 mg/kg of theophylline administered in rapidly absorbed form is likely to increase serum concentration by approximately 5 μg/mL. If the patient is not experiencing theophylline toxicity, this is unlikely to result in dangerous adverse effects.

After modifying the loading dose for this group of patients, the maintenance dosage recommendations are the same as those described above.

II. Chronic Therapy

Theophylline administration is a treatment of first choice for the management of chronic asthma (to prevent symptoms and maintain patent airways). Slow titration is generally preferred to assure safety and medication acceptance.

Initial Dose: 16 mg/kg/24 hr or 400 mg/24 hr (whichever is less) of anhydrous theophylline in divided doses at 6- or 8-hour intervals.

Increasing Dose: The above dosage may be increased in approximately 25% increments at 2- to 3-day intervals, so long as the drug is tolerated, and until the maximum dose indicated in Section III (below) is reached.

III. Maximum Theophylline Dose When Serum Concentration is Not Measured:

WARNING: DO NOT ATTEMPT TO MAINTAIN ANY DOSE THAT IS NOT TOLERATED.

	Not to exceed the following:
Age <9 years	24 mg/kg/day
Age 9–12 years	20 mg/kg/day
Age 12–16 years	18 mg/kg/day
Age >16 years	13 mg/kg/day *OR* 900 mg (*WHICHEVER IS LESS*)

Note: Use ideal body weight for obese patients

IV. Measurement of Serum Theophylline Concentrations During Chronic Therapy:

If the above maximum doses are to be maintained or exceeded, serum theophylline measurement is recommended. The serum sample should be obtained at the time of peak absorption: 1 to 2 hours after administration for immediate-release products, and 4 hours after administration for most sustained-release formulations. It is important that the patient has not missed any doses during the previous 48 hours and that dosing intervals have been reasonably typical with no added doses during that period. IF THESE INSTRUCTIONS HAVE NOT BEEN FOLLOWED, DOSAGE ADJUSTMENT BASED ON SERUM THEOPHYLLINE MEASUREMENTS MAY RESULT IN RECOMMENDATIONS THAT PRESENT RISK OF TOXICITY TO THE PATIENT.

V. Final Adjustment of Dosage:

[See Table I on next page].

[1] From the J Resp Dis, 1981; 2(7):16

Caution should be exercised in younger children who cannot complain of minor side effects. Older adults, and those with cor pulmonale, congestive heart failure and/or liver disease may have unusually low dosage requirements and thus may experience toxicity at the maximal dosage recommended above.

It is important that no patient be maintained on any dosage that is not tolerated. In instructing patients to increase dosage according to the above schedule, they should be instructed not to take a subsequent dose if apparent side effects occur and to resume therapy at a lower dose after adverse effects have disappeared.

Continued on next page

Forest Pharmaceuticals—Cont.

Table I—Dosage adjustment after serum theophylline measurement[1]

Elixophyllin® Elixir, Elixophyllin® Capsules and Elixophyllin® SR Capsules

If serum theophylline is:		Directions:
Within normal limits	10 to 20 μg/mL	Maintain dosage, if tolerated. Recheck serum theophylline concentration at 6- to 12-month intervals.*
Too high	20 to 25 μg/mL	Decrease doses by about 10%. Recheck serum theophylline concentration at 6- to 12-month intervals.*
	25 to 30 μg/mL	Skip next dose and decrease subsequent doses by about 25%. Recheck serum theophylline.
	Over 30 μg/mL	Skip next 2 doses and decrease subsequent doses by about 50%. Recheck serum theophylline.
Too low	7.5 to 10 μg/mL	Increase dose by about 25%.** Recheck serum theophylline concentration at 6- to 12-month intervals.*
	5 to 7.5 μg/mL	Increase dose by about 25% to the nearest dose increment and recheck serum theophylline for guidance in further dosage adjustment. Another increase will probably be needed, but this provides a safety check.

* Finer adjustments in dosage may be needed for some patients

**The total daily dose may need to be administered at more frequent intervals if symptoms occur repeatedly at the end of a dosing interval.

HOW SUPPLIED

Elixophyllin® Capsules

100 mg Capsules
Bottles of 100 ....NDC 0456-0642-01
200 mg Capsules
Bottles of 100 ....NDC 0456-0643-01
Bottles of 500 ....NDC 0456-0643-02
Unit Dose Boxes of 100 ....NDC 0456-0643-63

Store at controlled room temperature. Avoid excessive heat.

Elixophyllin® SR Capsules

125 mg Capsules
Bottles of 100 ....NDC 0456-0646-01
Bottles of 1000 ....NDC 0456-0646-00
Unit Dose Boxes of 100 ....NDC 0456-0646-63
250 mg Capsules
Bottles of 100 ....NDC 0456-0647-01
Bottles of 1000 ....NDC 0456-0647-00
Unit Dose Boxes of 100 ....NDC 0456-0647-63

Store at controlled room temperature.

Elixophyllin® Elixir

Bottles of:
473 mL ....NDC 0456-0644-16
946 mL ....NDC 0456-0644-32
3785 mL ....NDC 0456-0644-28

Store at controlled room temperature.

ELIXOPHYLLIN®-GG ℞

[ē″lĭx-off′fĭl-ĭn gēē-gēē]

(theophylline anhydrous - guaifenesin)
ORAL LIQUID

DESCRIPTION

Each 15 mL (tablespoonful) of Elixophyllin®-GG Oral Liquid contains 100 mg anhydrous theophylline and 100 mg guaifenesin (glyceryl guaiacolate) in a clear, colorless cherry-berry flavored, non-alcoholic liquid. Elixophyllin®-GG Oral Liquid does not contain sugar or dye.

(Please refer to Elixophyllin® [theophylline anhydrous] Elixir for complete information on theophylline.)

CLINICAL PHARMACOLOGY

Guaifenesin (glyceryl guaiacolate) exerts its expectorant action by reducing the viscosity of bronchial secretions, thereby increasing the efficiency of the cough reflex and of ciliary action in removing accumulated secretions from the trachea and bronchi. Unlike many other expectorants, guaifenesin rarely causes gastric irritation.

INDICATIONS

For relief and/or prevention of symptoms of asthma and reversible bronchospasm associated with chronic bronchitis and emphysema.

PRECAUTIONS

Drug-Laboratory Test Interactions—Guaifenesin has been shown to produce a color interference with certain clinical laboratory determinations of 5-hydroxyindoleacetic acid (5-HIAA) and vanillylmandelic acid (VMA).

HOW SUPPLIED

Elixophyllin®-GG Oral Liquid in bottles of:
237 mL ....NDC 0456-0648-08
473 mL ....NDC 0456-0648-16

Store at controlled room temperature.

ELIXOPHYLLIN-KI® ℞

(brand of theophylline anhydrous and potassium iodide)
Elixir

DESCRIPTION

Each 15 ml (tablespoonful) of ELIXOPHYLLIN-KI® (brand of theophylline anhydrous and potassium iodide) Elixir contains 80 mg anhydrous theophylline and 130 mg potassium iodide.

Theophylline, a xanthine bronchodilator, is a white, odorless, crystalline powder having a bitter taste. Potassium iodide is either colorless or white cubical crystals, or a white powder. Theophylline is represented by the following structural formula:

ANYDROUS THEOPHYLLINE

ELIXOPHYLLIN-KI® Elixir also contains the following inactive ingredients; alcohol 10%, anise oil, citric acid, coloring agent, flavoring agents, glycerin, saccharin sodium, sodium bisulfite, sucrose and water.

CLINICAL PHARMACOLOGY

Theophylline directly relaxes the smooth muscle of the bronchial airways and pulmonary blood vessels, thus acting mainly as a bronchodilator and smooth muscle relaxant. The drug also produces other actions typical of the xanthine derivatives: cornary vasodilation, cardiac stimulation, diuresis, cerebral stimulation, and skeletal muscle stimulation. The actions of theophylline may be mediated through inhibition of phosphodiesterase and a resultant increase in intracellular cyclic AMP. *In vivo* studies indicate that xanthine improve the contractile properties of the diaphragm in normal human subjects.

In vitro, theophylline has been shown to act synergistically with beta agonists that increase intracellular cyclic AMP through the stimulation of adenyl cyclase, but synergism has not been demonstrated in patient studies. More data are needed to determine if theophylline and beta agonists have a clinically important additive effect *in vivo.*

Apparently, tolerance does not develop with chronic use of theophylline.

Potassium iodide acts as an expectorant by liquifying tenacious bronchial secretions.

Pharmacokinetics:

The half-life of theophylline is influenced by a number of known variables. It is prolonged in patients suffering from chronic alcoholism, impaired hepatic or renal function, congestive heart failure, and in patients receiving macrolide antibiotics or cimetidine. Adults over age 55 and patients with chronic obstructive pulmonary disease, with or without cor pulmonale, may also have much slower clearance rates. For such patients, the theophylline half-life may exceed 24 hours.

High fever for prolonged periods may also reduce the rate of theophylline elimination in adults as well as children.

THEOPHYLLINE ELIMINATION CHARACTERISTICS

	Theophylline Clearance Rates (mean ± S.D.)	Half-life Average (mean ± S.D.)
Children	1.45 ± 0.58 ml/kg/min	3.7 ± 1.1 hr
Adult non-smokers with uncomplicated asthma	0.65 ± 0.19 ml/kg/min	8.7 ± 2.2 hr

The half-life of theophylline in smokers (1 to 2 packs/day) averages 4 to 5 hours, much shorter than the half-life in non-smokers which averages 7 to 9 hours. The increase in theophylline clearance caused by smoking is probably the result of induction of drug-metabolizing enzymes that do not readily normalize after cessation of smoking. It appears that 3 months to 2 years may be necessary for normalization of theophylline pharmacokinetics following cessation of smoking.

INDICATIONS

For excessive tenacious mucus in chronic asthma, severe chronic and allergic bronchitis and chronic pulmonary emphysema.

WARNINGS

Status asthmaticus should be considered a medical emergency and is that degree of bronchospasm which is not rapidly responsive to usual doses of conventional bronchodilators. Optimal therapy for such patients frequently requires both *additional medication,* parenterally administered, and *close monitoring,* preferably in an intensive care setting.

Although increasing the dose of theophylline may bring about relief, such treatment may be associated with toxicity. The likelihood of such toxicity developing increases significantly when the serum theophylline concentration exceeds 20 μg/ml. Therefore, determination of serum theophylline levels is recommended to assure maximum benefit without excessive risk.

Serum levels above 20 μg/ml are rarely found after appropriate administration of the recommended doses. However, in individuals in whom theophylline plasma clearance is reduced *for any reason,* even conventional doses may result in increased serum levels and potential toxicity. Reduced theophylline clearance has been documented in the following readily identifiable groups: 1) patients with impaired renal or liver function; 2) patients over 55 years of age, particularly males and those with chronic lung disease; 3) those with cardiac failure from any cause; and 4) those patients taking certain drugs (macrolide antibiotics or cimetidine). Decreased clearance of theophylline may be associated with either influenza immunization or active infection with influenza.

Reduction of dosage and laboratory monitoring is especially appropriate in the above individuals.

Less serious signs of theophylline toxicity, ie, nausea and restlessness, may appear in up to 50% of patients. Unfortunately, serious side effects such as ventricular arrhythmias, convulsions or even death may appear as the first sign of toxicity without any previous warning. Stated differently *serious toxicity is not reliably preceded by less severe side effects.*

Many patients who require theophylline may exhibit tachycardia due to their underlying disease process so that the cause/effect relationship to elevated serum theophylline concentrations may not be appreciated.

Theophylline products may cause arrhythmia and/or worsen pre-existing arrhythmias. Any significant change in cardiac rate and/or rhythm warrants monitoring and further investigation.

Potassium iodide can cause fetal harm when administered to a pregnant woman. Because of the possible development of fetal goiter, if this drug is used during pregnancy or if the patient becomes pregnant while taking it, the patient should be apprised of the potential hazard to the fetus.

PRECAUTIONS

General:

Theophylline half-life is shorter in smokers than in nonsmokers. Therefore, smokers may require larger or more frequent doses. Theophylline should not be administered concurrently with other xanthine medications. Use with caution in patients with severe cardiac disease, severe hypoxemia, hypertension, hyperthyroidism, acute myocardial injury, cor pulmonale, congestive heart failure, liver disease, and in the elderly (especially males). In particular, great caution should be used in giving theophylline to patients with congestive heart failure. Frequently, such patients have markedly prolonged theophylline serum levels with theophylline persisting in the serum for long periods following discontinuation of the drug.

Use theophylline cautiously in patients with history of peptic ulcer. Theophylline may occasionally act as a local irritant to the G.I. tract although gastrointestinal symptoms are more commonly centrally mediated and are associated with serum drug concentrations over 20 μg/ml.

Occasionally, persons are markedly sensitive to iodides and care should be used in administering ELIXOPHYLLIN-KI® Elixir for the first time. Caution is recommended in patients sensitive to iodides and in patients receiving potassium sparing diuretics or potassium supplements.

Information for Patients:

The physician should reinforce the importance of taking only the prescribed dose and the time interval between doses. If necessary, taking the drug with food will help avoid local irritation of the G.I. tract.

Drug Interactions:

Toxic synergism with ephedrine has been documented and may occur with some other sympathomimetic bronchodilators. In addition, the following drug interactions have been demonstrated:

DRUG	EFFECT
Aminophylline with lithium carbonate	Increased excretion of lithium carbonate
Aminophylline with propanolol	Antagonism of propanolol effect
Theophylline with cimetidine	Increased theophylline blood levels
Theophylline with troleandomycin, erythromycin	Increased theophyllin blood levels
Potassium iodide with lithium carbonate	Increased hypothyroid and goitrogenic effect

Drug—Laboratory Test Interactions:

Theophylline—When plasma levels of theophylline are measured by spectrophotometric methods, coffee, tea, cola beverages, chocolate, and acetaminophen contribute to falsely high values.

Potassium Iodide—Thyroid function tests may be altered by iodides. As with any potassium containing medication, the potential for developing hyperkalemia is increased.

Carcinogenesis, Mutagenesis, and Impairment of Fertility:

Long-term animal studies have not been performed to evaluate the carcinogenic potential, mutagenic potential, or the effect on fertility of xanthine compounds.

Pregnancy:

Category D—see WARNINGS.

Nursing Mothers:

It has been reported that theophylline distributes readily into breast milk and may cause adverse effects in the infant. Since iodides are also secreted in human milk, caution must be used when prescribing ELIXOPHYLLIN-KI® Elixir to a nursing mother, taking into account the risk-benefit of this therapy.

Usage in Children:

Since safety and effectiveness in children have not been established it is recommended that ELIXOPHYLLIN-KI® Elixir not be used in children under 12 years of age.

ADVERSE REACTIONS

Theophylline—The most consistent adverse reactions are due to overdose and are:

1. ***Gastrointestinal:*** nausea, vomiting, epigastric pain, hematemesis, diarrhea.
2. ***Central nervous system:*** headaches, irritability, restlessness, insomnia, reflex hyperexcitability, muscle twitching, clonic and tonic generalized convulsions.
3. ***Cardiovascular:*** palpitations, tachycardia, extrasystoles, flushing, hypotension, circulatory failure, ventricular arrhythmias.
4. ***Respiratory:*** tachypnea.
5. ***Renal:*** albuminuria, increased excretion of renal tubular and red blood cells, potentiation of diuresis.
6. ***Others:*** hyperglycemia, inappropriate ADH secretion, rash.

Potassium Iodide—Thyroid adenoma, goiter and myxedema are possible side effects of potassium iodide.

Hypersensitivity to iodides may be manifested by angioneurotic edema, cutaneous and mucosal hemorrhages, and symptoms resembling serum sickness, such as fever, arthralgia, lymph node enlargement and eosinophilia.

Iodism or chronic iodine poisoning may occur during prolonged treatment. The symptoms of iodism include: a metallic taste, soreness of the mouth, increased salivation, coryza, sneezing and swelling of the eyelids. There may be a severe headache, productive cough, pulmonary edema and swelling and tenderness of the salivary glands. Acneform skin lesions are seen in the seborrheic areas. Severe and sometimes fatal skin eruptions may develop. Gastric disturbance and diarrhea are common. If iodism appears, the drug should be withdrawn and the patient given appropriate supportive therapy.

OVERDOSAGE

Management:

If potential oral overdose is established and seizure has not occurred.:

A. Induce vomiting
B. Administer a cathartic.
C. Administer activated charcoal.

If patient is having a seizure:

A. Establish an airway.
B. Administer oxygen.
C. Treat the seizure with intravenous diazepam, 0.1 to 0.3 mg/kg up to 10 mg.
D. Monitor vital signs, maintain blood pressure and provide adequate hydration.

Postseizure Coma:

A. Maintain airway and oxygenation.
B. If a result of oral medication, follow above recommendations to prevent absorption of the drug, but intubation and lavage should be performed instead of inducing emesis, and the cathartic and charcoal will need to be introduced via a large bore gastric lavage tube.
C. Continue to provide full supportive care and adequate hydration while waiting for the drug to be metabolized. In general, the drug is rapidly metabolized so as not to warrant consideration of dialysis. However, if serum levels exceed 50 μg/ml, charcoal hemoperfusion may be indicated.

DOSAGE AND ADMINISTRATION

For most patients, *effective use* of theophylline, ie, associated with optimal likelihood of benefit combined with minimal risk of toxicity, is considered to occur when serum levels are maintained between 10 and 20 μg/ml. Levels above 20 μg/ml may produce toxicity, and in a small number of patients, toxicity may even be seen with serum levels between 15 and 20 μg/ml, particularly during initiation of therapy. Periodic and carefully controlled monitoring of theophylline serum levels is highly recommended.

If gastrointestinal irritation is experienced the medication may be taken with or after meals. Although absorption may be slowed, it is still complete.

It is important that no patient be maintained on any dosage that is not tolerated.

Usual dose in chronic asthma:

Children: Ages 12 and over—0.2 ml per pound of body weight, t.i.d.

Adults: 30 ml (2 tablespoonfuls) t.i.d.

HOW SUPPLIED

ELIXOPHYLLIN-KI® Elixir is a clear yellowish amber solution with an anise aroma. Each tablespoonful (15 ml) contains 80 mg anhydrous theophylline and 130 mg potassium iodide.

ELIXOPHYLLIN-KI® Elixir is available in bottles of:

237 ml ....NDC 0456-0645-08

RECOMMENDED STORAGE

Product should be stored at controlled room temperature 15°–30°C (59°–86°F).

Dispense in tight container.

ESGIC® ℞

[es'*jik*]

Tablets and Capsules

DESCRIPTION

Each ESGIC tablet or capsule for oral administration contains:

Butalbital* (isobutylallylbarbituric acid)	50 mg.
*Warning: May be habit forming	
Acetaminophen	325 mg.
Caffeine	40 mg.

Butalbital, 5-allyl-5-isobutyl-barbituric acid, a white, odorless crystalline powder having a slightly bitter taste, is an intermediate-acting barbiturate. Its structure is as follows:

$CH_2{=}CHCH_2$, $(CH_3)_2CHCH_2$ [structural formula]

$C_{11}H_{16}N_2O_3$
M.W. 224.26

Acetaminophen, N-acetyl-p-aminophenol, occurs as a white, odorless, crystalline powder, possessing a slightly bitter taste. Acetaminophen is a non-salicylate, non-narcotic analgesic, and antipyretic. Caffeine, 1,3,7-trimethylxanthine, is a white crystalline, glistening substance soluble in water to the extent of 1:50.

CLINICAL PHARMACOLOGY

Pharmacologically, ESGIC combines the analgesic properties of acetaminophen-caffeine with the anxiolytic and muscle relaxant properties of butalbital (isobutyl-allylbarbituric acid). Acetaminophen may be used safely by most persons sensitive to aspirin.

INDICATIONS

ESGIC is indicated for the relief of the symptom complex of stress (or muscle contraction) headache.

CONTRAINDICATIONS

Hypersensitivity to acetaminophen, caffeine, or barbiturates. Patients with porphyria.

PRECAUTIONS

1. **General:** Barbiturates should be administered with caution, if at all, to patients who are mentally depressed, have suicidal tendencies, or a history of drug abuse.
Elderly or debilitated patients may react to barbiturates with marked excitement, depression, and confusion. In some persons, barbiturates repeatedly produce excitement rather than depression.
2. **Information for the Patient:** Practitioners should give the following information and instructions to patients receiving barbiturates.
   1. The use of barbiturates carries with it an associated risk of psychological and/or physical dependence. The patient should be warned against increasing the dose of the drug without consulting a physician.
   2. Barbiturates may impair mental and/or physical abilities required for the performance of potentially hazardous tasks (e.g., driving, operating machinery, etc.).
   3. Alcohol should not be consumed while taking barbiturates. Concurrent use of the barbiturates with other CNS depressants (e.g., alcohol, narcotics, tranquilizers, and antihistamines) may result in additional CNS depressant effects.
3. **Drug Interactions:** Patients receiving narcotic analgesics, antipsychotics, antianxiety agents, or other CNS depressants (including alcohol) concomitantly with ESGIC may exhibit additive CNS depressant effects.

DRUGS	EFFECT
Butalbital with coumarin anticoagulants	Decreased effect of anticoagulant because of increased metabolism resulting from enzyme induction
Butalbital with tricyclic antidepressants	Decreased blood levels of the antidepressant

4. **Usage in Pregnancy:** Adequate studies have not been performed in animals to determine whether this drug affects fertility in males or females, has teratogenic potential or has other adverse effects on the fetus. There are no well-controlled studies in pregnant women. Although there is no clearly defined risk, one cannot exclude the possibility of infrequent or subtle damage to the human fetus. ESGIC should be used in pregnant women only when clearly needed.
5. **Nursing Mothers:** The effects of ESGIC on infants of nursing mothers are not known. Barbiturates are excreted in the breast milk of nursing mothers. The serum levels in infants are believed to be insignificant with therapeutic doses.
6. **Pediatric Use:** Safety and effectiveness in children below the age of 12 have not been established.

ADVERSE REACTIONS

The most frequent adverse reactions are drowsiness and dizziness. Less frequent adverse reactions are lightheadedness and nausea. Mental confusion or depression can occur due to intolerance or overdosage of butalbital.

DRUG ABUSE AND DEPENDENCE

Prolonged use of barbiturates can produce drug dependence, characterized by psychic dependence and tolerance. The abuse liability of ESGIC is similar to that of other barbiturate-containing drug combinations. Caution should be exercised when prescribing medication for patients with a known propensity for taking excessive quantities of drugs, which is not uncommon in patients with chronic stress headache.

OVERDOSAGE

The toxic effects of acute overdosage of ESGIC are attributable mainly to its barbiturate component, and, to a lesser extent, acetaminophen. Because toxic effects of caffeine occur in very high dosages only, the possibility of significant caffeine toxicity from ESGIC overdosage is unlikely.

Barbiturate Poisoning:

Symptoms: Drowsiness, confusion, coma; respiratory depression; hypotension; shock.

Treatment:

1. Maintenance of an adequate airway, with assisted respiration and oxygen administration as necessary.
2. Monitoring of vital signs and fluid balance.
3. If the patient is conscious and has not lost the gag reflex, emesis may be induced with ipecac. Care should be taken to prevent pulmonary aspiration of vomitus. After completion of vomiting, 30 grams activated charcoal in a glass of water may be administered.
4. If emesis is contraindicated, gastric lavage may be performed with a cuffed endotracheal tube in place with the patient in the face down position. Activated charcoal may be left in the emptied stomach and a saline cathartic administered.
5. Fluid therapy and other standard treatment for shock, if needed.
6. If renal function is normal, forced diuresis may aid in the elimination of the barbiturate. Alkalinization of the urine increases renal excretion of some barbiturates.
7. Although not recommended as a routine procedure, hemodialysis may be used in severe barbiturate intoxications or if the patient is anuric or in shock.

Continued on next page

Forest Pharmaceuticals—Cont.

Acetaminophen Poisoning:

Symptoms: Acetaminophen in massive overdosage may cause hepatic toxicity in some patients. In all cases of suspected overdose, immediately call your regional poison center or The Rocky Mountain Poison Center's toll-free number (800-525-6115) for assistance in diagnosis and for directions in the use of N-acetylcysteine as an antidote, a use currently restricted to investigational status.

In adults, hepatic toxicity has rarely been reported with acute overdoses of less than 10 grams and fatalities with less than 15 grams. Importantly, young children seem to be more resistant than adults to the hepatotoxic effect of an acetaminophen overdose.

Early symptoms following a potentially hepatotoxic overdose may include: nausea, vomiting, diaphoresis and general malaise. Clinical and laboratory evidence of hepatic toxicity may not be apparent until 48 to 72 hours post-ingestion.

Treatment: The stomach should be emptied promptly by lavage or by induction of emesis with syrup of ipecac. Patients' estimates of the quantity of a drug ingested are notoriously unreliable. Therefore, if an acetaminophen overdose is suspected, a serum acetaminophen assay should be obtained as early as possible, but no sooner than four hours following ingestion. Liver function studies should be obtained initially and repeated at 24-hour intervals.

The antidote, N-acetylcysteine, should be administered as early as possible, and within 16 hours of the overdose ingestion for optimal results. Following recovery, there are no residual, structural or functional hepatic abnormalities.

DOSAGE AND ADMINISTRATION

Oral: One or two tablets or capsules every four hours as needed. Do not exceed six tablets or capsules per day.

HOW SUPPLIED

ESGIC Tablets: White round, compressed tablet imprinted with GL logo on one side and 535-11 on the opposite side. Supplied in bottles of 100 tablets.

ESGIC Capsules: White, opaque capsules imprinted with GL logo and 535-12 in black print. Supplied in bottles of 100 capsules.

Shown in Product Identification Section, page 409

FEOSTAT Tablets OTC
FEOSTAT Suspension
FEOSTAT Drops
(Ferrous Fumarate)

FEOSTAT Tablets

Each chocolate-flavored chewable tablet contains:

Ferrous fumarate .... 100 mg.
(Elemental iron .... 33 mg.)

FEOSTAT Suspension

Each 5 cc. (teaspoonful) contains:

Ferrous fumarate .... 100 mg.
(Elemental iron .... 33 mg.)

FEOSTAT Drops

Each 12 drops (0.6 cc.) contains:

Ferrous fumarate .... 45 mg.
(Elemental iron .... 15 mg.)

HOW SUPPLIED

Suspension: 8 ounce bottle; NDC-0456-0373-08.
Drops: 2 ounce bottle; NDC-0456-0374-21.
Tablets:
Bottle of 100, NDC-0456-372-01.
Bottle of 1000, NDC-0456-372-00.

IODO-NIACIN® TABLETS ℞

DESCRIPTION

Each controlled action tablet contains:

Potassium Iodide .... 135 mg
Niacinamide Hydroiodide .... 25 mg

HOW SUPPLIED

Bottles of 100, NDC 0456-0295-01
Bottles of 500, NDC 0456-0295-02.

KAY CIEL® ℞
[*kā 'sēēl*"]
(potassium chloride)
Oral Solution 10%

KAY CIEL® ℞
(potassium chloride)
Powder

DESCRIPTION

ORAL SOLUTION—

Each 15 ml (tablespoonful) contains 1.5 g (20 mEq) potassium chloride in a palatable base.

KAY CIEL® Oral Solution also contains the following inactive ingredients; alcohol 4%, coloring agent, flavoring agent, methylparaben, propylparaben, saccharin sodium and water. Contains no sugar.

POWDER—

Each packet contains 1.5 g (20 mEq) potassium chloride. KAY CIEL® Powder also contains the following inactive ingredients; coloring agents, flavoring agent and saccharin sodium. Contains no sugar.

INDICATIONS

Treatment and prevention of potassium deficiency occurring especially during thiazide diuretic or corticosteroid therapy, digitalis intoxication, low dietary intake of potassium, or as a result of excessive vomiting and diarrhea and for correction of associated hypochloremic alkalosis.

CONTRAINDICATIONS

Impaired renal function, untreated Addison's Disease, dehydration, heat cramps and hyperkalemia.

WARNINGS

Do not use excessively.

PRECAUTIONS

Administer with caution and adjust to requirements of individual patient. Patient should be checked frequently, periodic ECG recorded and/or plasma potassium levels determined. Use with caution in patients with cardiac disease. In hypokalemic states, attention should be directed toward correction of frequently associated hypochloremic alkalosis. ***PATIENTS SHOULD BE CAUTIONED TO ADHERE TO DILUTION INSTRUCTIONS TO ASSURE AGAINST GASTROINTESTINAL INJURY.***

ADVERSE REACTIONS

Potassium intoxication indicated by listlessness, mental confusion, paresthesia of the extremities, weakness of the legs, flaccid paralysis, fall in blood pressure, cardiac depression, arrhythmias, arrest and heartblock. Vomiting, nausea, abdominal discomfort and diarrhea may occur.

DOSAGE AND ADMINISTRATION

Oral Solution—One tablespoonful (15 ml supplying 20 mEq) ***diluted*** in 4 ounces cold water or fruit juice twice daily (preferably after a meal), or as directed by physician.

Powder—Contents of 1 packet dissolved in 4 ounces cold water or fruit juice twice daily (preferably after a meal), or as directed by physician.

OVERDOSAGE

In case of excessive use resulting in hyperkalemia or potassium intoxication, discontinue use of potassium chloride and/or take other steps to lower serum levels if indicated.

HOW SUPPLIED

Oral Solution in bottles of:

118 ml .... NDC 0456-0661-04
473 ml .... NDC 0456-0661-16
3785 ml .... NDC 0456-0661-28

Powder in boxes of:

30 packets .... NDC 0456-0662-70
100 packets .... NDC 0456-0662-71

Revised 4-86
mfd by
Berlex Laboratories, Inc.
Wayne, NJ 07470

mfd for
FOREST PHARMACEUTICALS, INC.
SUBSIDIARY OF FOREST LABORATORIES
ST. LOUIS, MISSOURI 63043

OXYMYCIN INJECTION ℞

Each ml. contains:

Oxytetracycline .... 50 mg.

HOW SUPPLIED

10 ml. multiple dose vial; NDC 0456-0920-10.

PEDAMETH® CAPSULE ℞
PEDAMETH® LIQUID ℞
(racemethionine)

COMPOSITION

CAPSULES—200 mg. racemethionine.
LIQUID—75 mg. racemethionine per 5 cc. (teaspoon) in a fruit flavored base.

HOW SUPPLIED

PEDAMETH® (racemethionine) is available in 200 mg. Capsules in bottles of 50 (NDC 0456-0355-50) and 500 (NDC 0456-0355-02) and as 75 mg. per 5 ml. Liquid in bottles of 16 fluid ounces (NDC 0456-1039-16).

PYOCIDIN-OTIC® ℞
[*pī"ō-cĭ 'dĭn ō 'tĭk*"]
(polymyxin B-hydrocortisone)
Sterile Otic Solution

DESCRIPTION

Each ml contains 10,000 USP units of polymyxin B sulfate and 5 mg hydrocortisone in a vehicle containing propylene glycol and water. Sodium hydroxide or hydrochloric acid may have been added to adjust pH.

ACTIONS

Polymyxin B sulfate is effective against the gram-negative *Pseudomonas aeruginosa*, one of the most resistant microorganisms commonly causing otitis externa. The addition of hydrocortisone to the antibiotic affords an anti-inflammatory effect and relief against allergic manifestations and reduces the possibility of sensitivity and tissue reaction.

INDICATIONS

For the treatment of superficial bacterial infections of the external auditory canal caused by organisms susceptible to the action of the antibiotic.

CONTRAINDICATIONS

This product is contraindicated in those individuals who have shown hypersensitivity to any of its components, and in herpes simplex, vaccinia and varicella.

WARNINGS

As with other antibiotic preparations, prolonged treatment may result in overgrowth of nonsusceptible organisms and fungi.

If the infection is not improved after one week, cultures and susceptibility tests should be repeated to verify the identity of the organism and to determine whether therapy should be changed.

Patients who prefer to warm the medication before using should be cautioned against heating the solution above body temperature, in order to avoid loss of potency.

PRECAUTIONS

If sensitization or irritation occurs, medication should be discontinued promptly.

DOSAGE AND ADMINISTRATION

The external auditory canal should be thoroughly cleaned and dried with a sterile cotton applicator.

For adults, 4 drops of the solution should be instilled into the affected ear 3 or 4 times daily. For infants and children, 3 drops are suggested because of the smaller capacity of the ear canal.

The patient should lie with the affected ear upward and then the drops should be instilled. This position should be maintained for 5 minutes to facilitate penetration of the drops into the ear canal. Repeat, if necessary, for the opposite ear.

If preferred, a cotton wick may be inserted into the canal and then the cotton may be saturated with the solution. This wick should be kept moist by adding further solution every four hours. The wick should be replaced at least once every 24 hours.

HOW SUPPLIED

10 ml bottle with sterile dropper
NDC 0456-0663-10

RECOMMENDED STORAGE

Product should be stored at controlled room temperature 15°–30°C (59°–86°F).

SUS-PHRINE® ℞
[*sŭs 'frĭn*"]
(epinephrine)
1:200 Aqueous Suspension for Subcutaneous Injection

DESCRIPTION

Each ml of Sus-Phrine® (brand of epinephrine) Suspension contains 5 mg epinephrine in a sterile aqueous vehicle containing ascorbic acid 10 mg and thioglycolic acid 6.6 mg (as sodium salts), phenol 5 mg and glycerin (USP) 325 mg. Sodium hydroxide is added to adjust the pH. Approximately 80% of the total epinephrine is in suspension.

CLINICAL PHARMACOLOGY

Sus-Phrine® Suspension (epinephrine) acts at both the alpha and beta receptor sites. Beta stimulation provides bronchodilator action by relaxing bronchial muscle. Alpha stimulation increases vital capacity by relieving congestion of the bronchial mucosa and by constricting pulmonary vessels.
Sus-Phrine® Suspension provides both rapid and sustained epinephrine activity. The rapid action is due to the epinephrine in solution, while the sustained activity is due to the crystalline epinephrine free base in suspension.

INDICATIONS

For the symptomatic treatment of bronchial asthma, and reversible bronchospasm associated with chronic bronchitis and emphysema.

CONTRAINDICATIONS

Hypersensitivity to any of the components.
Narrow angle glaucoma, shock, cerebral arteriosclerosis and organic heart disease. Epinephrine is also contraindicated during general anesthesia with halogenated hydrocarbons or cyclopropane, and in local anesthesia of certain areas, e.g., fingers, toes, because of the danger of vasoconstriction producing sloughing of tissue, and in labor because the drug may delay the second stage.

WARNINGS

SUS-PHRINE SUSPENSION SHOULD NOT BE EMPLOYED TO CORRECT DRUG INDUCED HYPOTENSION.
Administer with caution to elderly people; those with cardiovascular disease, diabetes, hypertension or hyperthyroidism; in psychoneurotic individuals and in pregnancy. Administer with extreme caution to patients with long-standing bronchial asthma and emphysema who have developed degenerative heart disease.
Cardiac arrhythmias may follow administration of epinephrine.
Anginal pain may be induced when coronary insufficiency is present.

PRECAUTIONS

DO NOT USE IF PRODUCT IS DISCOLORED. Discoloration indicates the oxidation of epinephrine and possible loss of potency.
Use of Sus-Phrine® Suspension with digitalis, mercurial diuretics or other drugs that sensitize the heart to arrhythmias is not recommended.
Sus-Phrine® Suspension should not be administered concomitantly with other sympathomimetic agents, since their combined effects on the cardiovascular system may be deleterious to the patient.
The effects of epinephrine may be potentiated by tricyclic antidepressants; sodium l-thyroxine, and certain antihistamines (eg, diphenhydramine, tripelennamine or chlorpheniramine).

ADVERSE REACTIONS

In some individuals, restlessness, anxiety, headache, tremor, weakness, dizziness, pallor, respiratory difficulties, palpitation, nausea and vomiting may occur. These reactions may be exaggerated in hyperthyroidism. Occlusion of the central retinal artery and shock have also been reported.
Also, urticaria, wheal and hemorrhage at the site of injection may occur. Repeated injections at the same site may result in necrosis from vascular constriction.
Tolerance to epinephrine may occur with prolonged use.

OVERDOSAGE

Overdosage or inadvertent intravenous injection may cause cerebrovascular hemorrhage resulting from the sharp rise in blood pressure. Fatalities may also result from pulmonary edema because of peripheral constriction and cardiac stimulation produced. Rapidly acting vasodilators such as nitrites, or alpha blocking agents may counteract the marked pressor effects. Cardiac arrhythmias may be countered by administering rapidly acting antiarrhythmic or beta blocking agents.

DOSAGE AND ADMINISTRATION

NOTE: INJECT SUBCUTANEOUSLY.

It is suggested that Sus-Phrine® Suspension be administered with a tuberculin syringe and a 26 gauge, ½ inch needle.
A small initial test dose may be administered subcutaneously as a possible aid in determining patient sensitivity to epinephrine.
Site of injection should be varied to avoid necrosis at the site of injection.
Each time before withdrawing Sus-Phrine® Suspension into syringe, shake vial or ampul thoroughly to disperse particles and obtain a uniform suspension. Inject promptly subcutaneously to avoid settling of suspension in the syringe.
Adults:
Adult dosage range is 0.1 to 0.3 mL depending on patient response.
Subsequent doses should be administered only when necessary and not more frequently than every six hours.
Infants 1 month to 2 years and Children 2 to 12 years:
Pediatric dose is 0.005 mL/kg (2.2 lb) body weight injected subcutaneously.
FOR CHILDREN 30 kg OR LESS MAXIMUM SINGLE DOSE IS 0.15 ml.
Subsequent doses should be administered only when necessary and not more frequently than every six hours.

CLINICAL STUDIES

Controlled studies comparing the effectiveness of Sus-Phrine® Suspension 1:200 and an aqueous solution of epinephrine 1:1000 were conducted in both pediatric and adult asthmatics. The studies demonstrated rapid bronchodilator activity following administration of either Sus-Phrine® Suspension or epinephrine 1:1000; however during the 6 hour study period, a greater improvement in FEV_1 and $FEF_{25-75\%}$ was observed 4 to 6 hours subsequent to Sus-Phrine® Suspension administration. Improvement in Wright Peak Expiratory Flow Rate was greater for Sus-Phrine® Suspension than epinephrine 1:1000 3 to 8 hours following administration (10 hour study duration).

HOW SUPPLIED

In boxes of:
12 × 0.3 ml ampuls....NDC 0456-0664-12
25 × 0.3 ml ampuls....NDC 0456-0664-34
5.0 ml multiple dose vial....NDC 0456-0664-05
Store under refrigeration. Do not freeze. Do not expose to temperature above 30° C (86°F).

Shown in Product Identification Section, page 409

E. Fougera & Company

a Division of Altana Inc.
60 BAYLIS ROAD
MELVILLE, NY 11747

NDC 0168	PRODUCT		
	Atropine Sulfate Ophthalmic Ointment, U.S.P. 1% (Rx)		
0065-38			⅛ oz. tube
	Bacitracin Ointment U.S.P. 500 units per g		
0011-09		1 gross	1/32 oz. foilpac
0011-35			½ oz. tube
0011-31			1 oz. tube
0011-04			4 oz. tube
0011-16			1 lb. jar
	Bacitracin Ophthalmic Ointment U.S.P. (Rx)		
0026-38			⅛ oz. tube
	Bacitracin-Neomycin-Polymyxin Ointment		
0012-09		1 gross	1/32 oz. foilpac
0012-35			½ oz. tube
0012-31			1 oz. tube
	Bacitracin-Neomycin-Polymyxin Ophthalmic Ointment (Rx)		
0027-38			⅛ oz. tube
	Bacitracin Zinc-Polymyxin B Sulfate Ointment		
0021-35			½ oz. tube
0021-31			1 oz. tube
	Betamethasone Dipropionate Cream, U.S.P. 0.05% (Rx)		
0055-15			15 g tube
0055-46			45 g tube
	Betamethasone Dipropionate Ointment, U.S.P. 0.05% (Rx)		
0056-15			15 g tube
0056-46			45 g tube
	Betamethasone Dipropionate Lotion, U.S.P. 0.05% (Rx)		
0057-60			60 ml bottle
	Betamethasone Valerate Cream, U.S.P. 0.1% (Rx)		
0040-15			15 g tube
0040-46			45 g tube
	Betamethasone Valerate Ointment, U.S.P. 0.1% (Rx)		
0033-15			15 g tube
0033-46			45 g tube
	Betamethasone Valerate Lotion, U.S.P. 0.1% (Rx)		
0041-60			60 ml bottle
	Boric Acid Ophthalmic Ointment 5%		
0066-38			⅛ oz. tube
	Dibucaine Ointment, U.S.P. 1%		
0046-31			1 oz. tube
	Efodine® Ointment (Povidone-Iodine)		
0090-09		1 gross	1/32 oz. foilpac
0090-31			1 oz. tube
0090-16			1 lb. jar
	Erythromycin Ophthalmic Ointment U.S.P. (Rx)		
0070-38			⅛ oz. tube
	Fluocinolone Acetonide Cream, U.S.P. 0.01% (Rx)		
0058-15			15 g tube
0058-60			60 g tube
	Fluocinolone Acetonide Topical Solution, U.S.P. 0.01% (Rx)		
0059-60			60 ml bottle
	Fluocinolone Acetonide Cream, U.S.P. 0.025% (Rx)		
0060-15			15 g tube
0060-60			60 g tube
	Fluocinolone Acetonide Ointment, U.S.P. 0.025% (Rx)		
0064-15			15 g tube
0064-60			60 g tube
	Gentamicin Sulfate Cream, U.S.P. 0.1% (Rx)		
0071-15			15 g tube
	Gentamicin Sulfate Ointment, U.S.P. 0.1% (Rx)		
0078-15			15 g tube
	Hydrocortisone Cream, U.S.P. 0.5%		
0014-31			1 oz. tube
	Hydrocortisone Ointment, U.S.P. 0.5%		
0016-31			1 oz. tube
	Hydrocortisone Cream, U.S.P. 1% (Rx)		
0015-29			20 g tube
0015-31			1 oz. tube
0015-04			4 oz. jar
0015-16			1 lb. jar
	Hydrocortisone Ointment, U.S.P. 1% (Rx)		
0020-31			1 oz. tube
0020-16			1 lb. jar
	Hydrocortisone Cream, USP 2.5% (Rx)		
0080-31			30 g tube
	Ichthammol Ointment, U.S.P. 10%		
0048-31			1 oz. tube
	Ichthammol Ointment 20%		
0049-31			1 oz. tube
	Iodochlorhydroxyquin 3% with Hydrocortisone 1% Cream (Rx)		
0022-29			20 g tube
	Lanolin U.S.P.		
0051-31			1 oz. tube
0051-16			1 lb. jar
	Lidocaine Ointment, U.S.P. 5% (Rx)		
0204-37			1¼ oz. tube
	Nitroglycerin Ointment 2% (Rx)		
0038-30			30 g tube
0038-60			60 g tube
	Nystatin Cream U.S.P. (Rx) 100,000 u/g		
0054-15			15 g tube
0054-30			30 g tube
	Nystatin Ointment U.S.P. (Rx) 100,000 u/g		
0007-15			15 g tube
	Nystatin Oral Suspension U.S.P. (Rx) 100,000 u/ml		
0037-60			60 ml bottle
0037-03		box of 100	5 ml bottle
	Nystatin Vaginal Tablets U.S.P. (Rx) 100,000 Units		
0031-15			box of 15
0031-30			box of 30
	Nystatin-Triamcinolone Acetonide Cream (Rx)		
0081-15			15 g tube
0081-30			30 g tube
0081-60			60 g tube
	Nystatin-Triamcinolone Acetonide Ointment (Rx)		
0089-15			15 g tube
0089-30			30 g tube
0089-60			60 g tube
	Petrolatum (White) U.S.P.		
0053-45		1 gross	5 g foilpac
0053-21			1 oz. tube
0053-31	Hospital Pak	1 gross	1 oz. tube
0053-16			1 lb. jar
	Petrolatum (White) Ophthalmic Ointment		
0053-38			⅛ oz. tube
	Polysorb® Hydrate Cream		
0217-02			2 oz. tube
0217-16			16 oz. jar

Continued on next page

Fougera—Cont.

Code		
	Sulfacetamide Sodium Ophthalmic Ointment (*Rx*)	
0079-38		⅛ oz. tube
	Surgilube® Surgical Lubricant	
0205-43	1 gross	3 g foilpac
0205-45	1 gross	5 g foilpac
0205-55	1 gross	5 g tube
0205-02	1 dozen	2 oz. tube
0205-36	1 dozen	4¼ oz. tube
	Swim Ear®	
7931-91	1 dozen	1 oz. bottle
	Tolnaftate Cream 1% (Antifungal Cream)	
0008-15		15 g tube
	Tolnaftate Solution 1% (Antifungal Solution)	
0009-10		10 ml bottle
	Triamcinolone Acetonide Cream, U.S.P. 0.025% (*Rx*)	
0003-15		15 g tube
0003-80		80 g tube
	Triamcinolone Acetonide Ointment, U.S.P. 0.025% (*Rx*)	
0005-80		80 g tube
	Triamcinolone Acetonide Cream, U.S.P. 0.1% (*Rx*)	
0004-15		15 g tube
0004-80		80 g tube
0004-16		1 lb. jar
	Triamcinolone Acetonide Ointment, U.S.P. 0.1% (*Rx*)	
0006-15		15 g tube
0006-80		80 g tube
	Triamcinolone Acetonide Cream, U.S.P. 0.5% (*Rx*)	
0002-15		15 g tube
	Triple Sulfa Vaginal Cream (*Rx*)	
0018-33	(Sulfathiazole 3.42%, Sulfacetamide 2.86%, Sulfabenzamide 3.7% and Urea 0.64%)	2¾ oz. tube w/applicator
	Vitamin A + Vitamin D Ointment	
0035-45	1 gross	5 g foilpac
0035-01		2 oz. tube
0035-02	Hospital Pak 6 dozen	2 oz. tube
0035-04		4 oz. tube
0035-16		1 lb. jar
	Whitfield's Ointment	
0061-31	(Benzoic & Salicylic Acid Ointment U.S.P.)	1 oz. tube
	Yellow Mercuric Oxide Ophthalmic Ointment 1%	
0075-38		⅛ oz. tube
	Yellow Mercuric Oxide Ophthalmic Ointment 2%	
0076-38		⅛ oz. tube
	Zinc Oxide Ointment U.S.P.	
0062-31		1 oz. tube
0062-02		2 oz. tube
0062-16		1 lb. jar

GELIPERM® ℞
[*jel-e-perm'*]
Wound Management System

DESCRIPTION

GELIPERM is an inert hydrogel formulation composed of sterile water bound by a polyacrylamide/agar network. The GELIPERM Wound Management System is available as GELIPERM WET, a smooth transparent moist gel sheet and GELIPERM GRANULATE which is supplied in tubes.

CHARACTERISTICS

GELIPERM WET Sheets and GELIPERM GRANULATE are both sterile, non-toxic, non-allergenic, and non-adherent. GELIPERM WET Sheet allows for easy monitoring, relatively painless and non-traumatic dressing changes and aids in protection against infection. GELIPERM GRANULATE has a gel-like consistency and can thus adapt itself to the shape and depth of uneven wounds.

INDICATIONS

GELIPERM is indicated in the management of partial thickness skin wounds and ulcerations such as decubitus ulcers, donor sites, 1st and 2nd degree burns, and skin trauma. It is also indicated in cases where allergic reactions to other wound dressings and external applications have occurred. Side effects or interactions have not been reported.

CONTRAINDICATIONS

GELIPERM WET and GELIPERM GRANULATE should not be used for the following conditions: necrotising ulcerations in which anerobic infection is suspected, dry necroses, third degree burns, and full thickness burns.

WARNING

Highly infected wounds should be treated in combination with antimicrobial agents. For external use only. Keep out of reach of children.

HOW SUPPLIED

GELIPERM WET: 6 sheets (10.4 × 4.8 in.) per pack
NDC 0168-2111-66
GELIPERM GRANULATE: 6 tubes per pack
NDC 0168-2110-20—20 g tube
NDC 0168-2110-50—50 g tube

CAUTION

Federal law restricts this device to sale by or on the order of a physician.

GEIGY Pharmaceuticals

Division of CIBA-GEIGY Corporation
ARDSLEY, NY 10502

GY-CODE® INDEX

Geigy Pharmaceuticals has established a Drug Identity Code System entitled GY-CODE. This system affords a convenient and accurate means of uniquely identifying each Geigy solid dosage form on which the GY-CODE number and the name "Geigy" appear. The GY-CODE number also appears as part of the National Drug Code number.

GY-CODE NUMBER	PROD. DESCRIPTION		NATIONAL DRUG CODE
14	**Butazolidin® Tablets**		
	phenylbutazone USP	100 mg	
	Red, film-coated tablets		
	100's		0028-0014-01
	1000's		0028-0014-10
	100's Unit Dose Pkg.		0028-0014-61
20	**Tofranil-PM® Capsules**		
	imipramine pamoate	75 mg	
	Coral-colored capsules		
	30's		0028-0020-26
	100's		0028-0020-01
	1000's		0028-0020-10
	100's Unit Dose Pkg.		0028-0020-61
22	**Tofranil-PM® Capsules**		
	imipramine pamoate	150 mg	
	Coral-colored capsules		
	30's		0028-0022-26
	100's		0028-0022-01
	100's Unit Dose Pkg.		0028-0022-61
23	**Lioresal® Tablets**		
	baclofen	10 mg	
	White, oval, scored tablets		
	100's		0028-0023-01
	100's Unit Dose Pkg.		0028-0023-61
32	**Tofranil® Tablets**		
	imipramine hydrochloride USP	10 mg	
	Triangular, coral-colored, coated tablets		
	100's		0028-0032-01
	1000's		0028-0032-10
33	**Lioresal® Tablets**		
	baclofen	20 mg	
	White, capsule shaped, scored tablets		
	100's		0028-0033-01
	100's Unit Dose Pkg.		0028-0033-61
40	**Tofranil-PM® Capsules**		
	imipramine pamoate	100 mg	
	Dark yellow/coral-colored capsules		
	30's		0028-0040-26
	100's		0028-0040-01
42	**Constant-T® Tablets**		
	theophylline (anhydrous)	200 mg	
	Light pink, oval, scored tablets		
	100's		0028-0042-01
	100's Unit Dose Pkg.		0028-0042-61
	Gy-Pak® 60's		
	One Unit (12 × 60)		0028-0042-73
	Six Units (72 × 60)		0028-0042-73
44	**Butazolidin® Capsules**		
	phenylbutazone USP	100 mg	
	Orange/white capsules		
	100's		0028-0044-01
	1000's		0028-0044-10
	100's Unit Dose Pkg.		0028-0044-61
	Gy-Pak® 100's		
	One Unit (12 × 100)		0028-0044-65
	Six Units (72 × 100)		0028-0044-65
45	**Tofranil-PM® Capsules**		
	imipramine pamoate	125 mg	
	Light yellow/coral-colored capsules		
	30's		0028-0045-26
	100's		0028-0045-01
48	**PBZ-SR® Tablets**		
	tripelennamine hydrochloride	100 mg	
	Lavender-colored tablets		
	100's		0028-0048-01
51	**Lopressor® Tablets**		
	metoprolol tartrate	50 mg	
	Light red, capsule-shaped, scored tablets		
	100's		0028-0051-01
	1000's		0028-0051-10
	100's Unit Dose Pkg.		0028-0051-61
	Gy-Pak® 60's		
	One Unit (12 × 60)		0028-0051-73
	Six Units (72 × 60)		0028-0051-73
	Gy-Pak® 100's		
	One Unit (12 × 100)		0028-0051-65
	Six Units (72 × 100)		0028-0051-65
52	**Tegretol® Chewable Tablets**		
	carbamazepine USP	100 mg	
	Round, red-speckled, pink, single-scored tablets		
	100's		0028-0052-01
	100's Unit Dose Pkg.		0028-0052-61
57	**Constant-T® Tablets**		
	theophylline (anhydrous)	300 mg	
	Light blue, oval, scored tablets		
	100's		0028-0057-01
	100's Unit Dose Pkg.		0028-0057-61
	Gy-Pak® 60's		
	One Unit (12 × 60)		0028-0057-73
	Six Units (72 × 60)		0028-0057-73
67	**Tegretol® Tablets**		
	carbamazepine USP	200 mg	
	White, single-scored tablets		
	100's		0028-0067-01
	1000's		0028-0067-10
	100's Unit Dose Pkg.		0028-0067-61
	Gy-Pak® 100's		
	One Unit (12 × 100)		0028-0067-65
	Six Units (72 × 100)		0028-0067-65
71	**Lopressor® Tablets**		
	metoprolol tartrate	100 mg	
	Light blue, capsule-shaped, scored tablets		
	100's		0028-0071-01
	1000's		0028-0071-10
	100's Unit Dose Pkg.		0028-0071-61
	Gy-Pak® 60's		
	One Unit (12 × 60)		0028-0071-73
	Six Units (72 × 60)		0028-0071-73
	Gy-Pak® 100's		
	One Unit (12 × 100)		0028-0071-65
	Six Units (72 × 100)		0028-0071-65
72	**Brethine® Tablets**		
	terbutaline sulfate USP	2.5 mg	
	Oval, white, scored tablets		
	100's		0028-0072-01
	1000's		0028-0072-10
	100's Unit Dose Pkg.		0028-0072-61
	Gy-Pak® 90's		
	One Unit (12 × 90)		0028-0072-90
	Six Units (72 × 90)		0028-0072-90
	Gy-Pak® 100's		
	One Unit (12 × 100)		0028-0072-65
	Six Units (72 × 100)		0028-0072-65
105	**Brethine® Tablets**		
	terbutaline sulfate USP	5 mg	
	Round, scored, white tablets		
	100's		0028-0105-01
	1000's		0028-0105-10
	100's Unit Dose Pkg.		0028-0105-61
	Gy-Pak® 90's		
	One Unit (12 × 90)		0028-0105-90
	Six Units (72 × 90)		0028-0105-90
	Gy-Pak® 100's		
	One unit (12 × 100)		0028-0105-65
	Six units (72 × 100)		0028-0105-65
111	**PBZ® Tablets**		
	tripelennamine hydrochloride USP	25 mg	
	Round, white, scored tablets		
	100's		0028-0111-01
117	**PBZ® Tablets**		
	tripelennamine hydrochloride USP	50 mg	
	Round, white, scored tablets		
	100's		0028-0117-01
	1000's		0028-0117-10
136	**Tofranil® Tablets**		
	imipramine hydrochloride USP	50 mg	
	Coral-colored (white Geigy imprint) coated tablets		
	100's		0028-0136-01
	1000's		0028-0136-10
	100's Unit Dose Pkg.		0028-0136-61

Gy-Pak® 100's	
One unit (12 × 100)	0028-0136-65
Six units (72 × 100)	0028-0136-65
140 Tofranil® Tablets	
imipramine hydrochloride USP	25 mg
Coral-colored (black Geigy imprint) coated tablets	
100's	0028-0140-01
1000's	0028-0140-10
100's Unit Dose Pkg.	0028-0140-61
Gy-Pak® 100's	
One unit (12 × 100)	0028-0140-65
Six units (72 × 100)	0028-0140-65
6114 Otrivin® Nasal Drops (0.1%)	
xylometazoline hydrochloride USP	
20 ml.	0028-6114-58
6116 Otrivin® Pediatric (0.05%)	
xylometazoline hydrochloride USP	
20 ml.	0028-6116-58
6118 Otrivin® Spray (0.1%)	
xylometazoline hydrochloride USP	
15 ml.	0028-6118-57
6925 PBZ® Elixir	
Per 5-ml. teaspoon:	
tripelennamine citrate USP	37.5 mg
(equivalent to 25 mg tripelennamine hydrochloride)	
473 ml.	0028-6925-16
6946 PBZ® Antihistamine Cream	
tripelennamine hydrochloride	
Cream 2% (water-washable base)	
1 oz.	0028-6946-76

BRETHAIRE® ℞

[breth-air´]
terbutaline sulfate USP inhaler
Bronchodilator Aerosol
For Oral Inhalation Only

DESCRIPTION

The active ingredient of Brethaire is terbutaline sulfate USP, α-[(*tert*-butylamino)methyl]-3,5-dihydroxybenzyl alcohol sulfate (2:1) (salt), a relatively selective beta$_2$-adrenergic bronchodilator.

Terbutaline sulfate USP is a white to gray-white crystalline powder. It is odorless or has a faint odor of acetic acid. It is soluble in water and in 0.1N hydrochloric acid, slightly soluble in methanol, and insoluble in chloroform. Its molecular weight is 548.65.

Brethaire is a metered-dose dispenser containing micronized terbutaline sulfate in a suspension of the following composition:

	7.5-ml (10.5-g) Canister
terbutaline sulfate USP	0.075 g
sorbitan trioleate	0.105 g
trichloromonofluoromethane NF	2.58 g
dichlorotetrafluoroethane NF	2.58 g
dichlorodifluoromethane NF	5.16 g

Each actuation delivers 0.20 mg of terbutaline sulfate from the mouthpiece (0.25 mg valve delivery). Each canister provides about 300 inhalations.

CLINICAL PHARMACOLOGY

Brethaire is a beta-adrenergic-receptor agonist that has been shown by *in vitro* and *in vivo* studies in animals to exert a preferential effect on beta$_2$-adrenergic receptors such as those located in bronchial smooth muscle. However, controlled clinical studies in patients who were administered the drug have not revealed a preferential beta$_2$-adrenergic effect.

It has been postulated that beta-adrenergic agonists produce many of their pharmacologic effects by activation of adenyl cyclase, the enzyme that catalyzes the conversion of adenosine triphosphate to cyclic adenosine monophosphate.

Terbutaline sulfate by inhaler has been shown in controlled clinical studies to relieve bronchospasm associated with chronic obstructive pulmonary disease such as asthma, chronic bronchitis, and emphysema. This action was manifested by a clinically significant improvement in pulmonary function as demonstrated by an increase in FEV$_1$ of 15% or more in some patients. Terbutaline sulfate by inhaler also produced clinically significant increases in peak expiratory flow rates and instantaneous flow rates at 75, 50, and 25% of vital capacity. There were also clinically significant reductions in functional residual capacity, residual volume, and airway resistance in some patients. Clinically significant improvement in pulmonary function occurred within 5 to 30 minutes in most patients after administration of the drug. The response was well established by 5 minutes and the maximal effect usually occurred between 1 and 2 hours in most patients. Significant bronchodilator activity has been observed to persist for 3 to 4 hours after dosing in many patients in 3-month repetitive-dose studies. With continued administration of Brethaire, the duration of effectiveness decreases in most patients.

INDICATIONS AND USAGE

Brethaire is indicated for the relief of bronchospasm in patients with reversible obstructive airway disease.

In controlled clinical trials the onset of improvement in pulmonary function was within 5 to 30 minutes. These studies also showed that maximum improvement in pulmonary function occurred at 120 minutes following two inhalations of Brethaire and that clinically significant improvement (i.e., 15% increase in FEV$_1$/predicted FEV$_1$) generally continued for 3 to 4 hours in most patients. In some studies there was a significant decrease in improvement of pulmonary function noted with continued administration of terbutaline sulfate aerosol. Continued effectiveness of Brethaire was demonstrated over a 14-week period in some patients in these clinical trials. Some patients with asthma, in single-dose studies only, have shown a therapeutic response that was still apparent at 6 hours.

CONTRAINDICATIONS

Brethaire is contraindicated in patients with a history of hypersensitivity to any of its components.

WARNINGS

As with other adrenergic aerosols, the potential for paradoxical bronchospasm should be kept in mind. If it occurs, the preparation should be discontinued immediately and alternative therapy instituted.

Fatalities have been reported in association with excessive use of inhaled sympathomimetic drugs. The exact cause of death is unknown.

The contents of Brethaire are under pressure. Do not puncture the container. Do not use or store it near heat or open flame. Exposure to temperatures above 120°F may cause bursting. Never throw the container into a fire or incinerator. Keep it out of children's reach.

PRECAUTIONS

General: Terbutaline sulfate is a sympathomimetic amine and, as such, should be used with caution in patients with cardiovascular disorders, including coronary insufficiency and hypertension, in patients with hyperthyroidism or diabetes mellitus, and in patients who are unusually responsive to sympathomimetic amines.

Large doses of intravenous terbutaline sulfate have been reported to aggravate preexisting diabetes and ketoacidosis.

Aerosol terbutaline sulfate is not indicated for tocolysis.

Although there have been no reports concerning the use of aerosol terbutaline sulfate during labor and delivery, it has been reported that high doses of terbutaline sulfate administered intravenously inhibit uterine contractions. Although this effect is extremely unlikely as a consequence of aerosol use, it should be kept in mind.

Information for Patients: The action of Brethaire may last up to 6 hours, and therefore, it should not be used more frequently than recommended. Patients should not increase the number or frequency of doses without consulting the physician. If symptoms get worse, patients should consult their physician promptly. While taking Brethaire, patients should not take other inhaled medicines that have not been prescribed by the physician.

See illustrated **Instructions for Patients.**

Drug Interactions: Other sympathomimetic aerosol bronchodilators or epinephrine should not be used concomitantly with terbutaline sulfate. Terbutaline sulfate should be administered with caution to patients being treated with monoamine oxidase inhibitors or tricyclic antidepressants, since the action of terbutaline sulfate on the vascular system may be potentiated.

Beta-receptor-blocking agents and terbutaline sulfate inhibit the effect of each other.

Carcinogenesis, Mutagenesis, Impairment of Fertility: A 2-year oral carcinogenesis bioassay of terbutaline sulfate (50, 500, 1000, and 2000 mg/kg, corresponding to 1042, 10,417, 20,833, and 41,667 times the recommended daily adult dose) in Sprague-Dawley rats revealed drug-related changes in the female genital system. Female rats showed drug-related increases in leiomyomas of the mesovarium: 3 (5%) at 50 mg/kg, 17 (28%) at 500 mg/kg, 21 (35%) at 1000 mg/kg, and 23 (38%) at 2000 mg/kg, which were significant at the three highest levels. None occurred in female controls. The incidence of ovarian cysts was significantly elevated at all dose levels except at 2000 mg/kg, and hyperplasia of the mesovarium was increased significantly at 500 and 2000 mg/kg.

A 21-month oral (feeding) study of terbutaline sulfate (5, 50, and 200 mg/kg, corresponding to 104, 1042, and 4167 times the recommended daily adult dose) in the mouse revealed no evidence of carcinogenicity.

Studies of terbutaline sulfate have not been conducted to determine mutagenic potential.

A Segment 1 oral reproduction study of terbutaline sulfate (up to 50 mg/kg corresponding to 1042 times the maximum clinical dose) in the rat revealed no adverse effects on fertility.

Pregnancy Category B: Reproduction studies have been performed in rats and rabbits at doses up to 1042 times the human dose and have revealed no evidence of impaired fertility or harm to the fetus due to terbutaline sulfate. There are, however, no adequate and well-controlled studies in pregnant women. Because animal reproduction studies are not always predictive of human response, this drug should be used during pregnancy only if clearly needed. For use in labor and delivery, see **Precautions, General.**

Nursing Mothers: It is not known whether this drug is excreted in human milk. Because many drugs are excreted in human milk, caution should be exercised when terbutaline sulfate is administered to a nursing woman.

Pediatric Use: Safety and effectiveness in children below the age of 12 years have not been established.

ADVERSE REACTIONS

The adverse reactions of terbutaline sulfate are similar to those of other sympathomimetic agents. A 14-week double-blind study compared terbutaline sulfate and isoproterenol aerosols in 259 asthmatic patients. The results of this study showed that the incidence of cardiovascular effects was as follows: palpitations, none with terbutaline and fewer than 5 per 100 with isoproterenol; tachycardia, about 3 per 100 with terbutaline and about 2 per 100 with isoproterenol; and increased blood pressure, fewer than 1 per 100 with terbutaline and about 2 per 100 with isoproterenol. In the same study, both drugs caused headache and nausea or digestive disorder in fewer than 10 patients per 100, tremor or nervousness in fewer than 5 patients per 100, and drowsiness in fewer than 5 patients per 100. About 4% of patients receiving terbutaline and about 1% of patients receiving isoproterenol had dysrhythmias. In addition, terbutaline sulfate, like other sympathomimetic agents, can cause adverse reactions such as angina, dyspnea and wheezing, vomiting, vertigo, central stimulation, insomnia, unusual taste, and drying or irritation of the oropharynx. Significantly more patients experienced dyspnea or wheezing, or both, after terbutaline than after isoproterenol administration. ECG changes such as sinus pause, atrial premature beats, AV block, ventricular premature beats, ST-T-wave depression, T-wave inversion, sinus bradycardia, and atrial escape beat with aberrant conduction were described after terbutaline administration. ECG changes were similar in frequency after isoproterenol administration.

OVERDOSAGE

Overdosage experience is limited. Excessive adrenergic-receptor stimulation may augment the signs and symptoms listed under **ADVERSE REACTIONS** and may be accompanied by other adrenergic effects. In the case of terbutaline overdosage, the patient should be treated symptomatically for the sympathomimetic overdosage with careful consideration given to the appropriateness of any chosen therapy and to the possible effect on the patient's underlying disease state.

DOSAGE AND ADMINISTRATION

The usual dosage for adults and children 12 years and older is two inhalations separated by a 60-second interval, repeated every 4 to 6 hours. Dosing should not be repeated more often than every 4 to 6 hours. The use of Brethaire can be continued as medically indicated to control recurring bouts of bronchospasm. During this time most patients gain optimal benefit from regular use of the inhaler. Safe usage for periods extending over several years has been documented.

If a previously effective dosage regimen fails to provide the usual relief, medical advice should be sought immediately, as this is often a sign of seriously worsening asthma, which would require reassessment of therapy.

HOW SUPPLIED

Brethaire contains 75 mg of terbutaline sulfate as a micronized powder in an inert propellant. This is sufficient medication for about 300 actuations. Each actuation delivers approximately 0.20 mg of terbutaline sulfate from the mouthpiece (0.25 mg valve delivery).

Brethaire canister with mouthpiece, 7.5 ml (10.5 g) .... NDC 0028-5557-88

Brethaire canister refill, 7.5 ml (10.5 g) .... NDC 0028-5557-87

Do not store above 86°F.
Dispense with enclosed instructions for use.
Federal law prohibits dispensing without a prescription.
U.S. Patent No. 3,937,838

C85-67 (11/85)

Dist. by:
GEIGY Pharmaceuticals
Division of CIBA-GEIGY Corporation
Ardsley, New York 10502

Continued on next page

The full prescribing information for each GEIGY drug is contained herein and is that in effect as of September 1, 1986

Geigy—Cont.

BRETHANCER® ℞
[*breth-anc 'er*]
spacer-inhaler

The Brethancer spacer-inhaler is recommended for patients with difficulty coordinating conventional aerosol inhalers, so those patients may derive greater therapeutic benefit from their medication.
Although aerosol medications offer patients the benefits of rapidity of action, many patients have difficulty coordinating inhalation with aerosol activation. With Brethancer, the patient no longer requires this coordination but can inhale the aerosolized drug from the spacer tube after the canister is activated.
Unlike other devices designed to aid in the proper use of aerosol medications, Brethancer is compact and easy to carry in its closed form. The Brethancer has three interlocking and telescoping plastic components which, when extended, assist in improving the use of aerosol medications. Opening the device is accomplished in one motion, which simplifies use by the patient. As an additional feature, the breathing hole is closed when the Brethancer is telescoped, which prevents foreign matter from entering the unit.
The Brethancer unit will accommodate any of several currently available prescription aerosol bronchodilator medications.
The patient's inhalation technique should be checked regularly. See the patient package insert for operating instructions.
Mfd by: Perlos, Finland
Dist. by: GEIGY Pharmaceuticals
Division of CIBA-GEIGY Corporation
Ardsley, New York 10502

C85-8 (Rev. 1/85)

BRETHINE® ℞
[*breth-een '*]
terbutaline sulfate USP
Tablets of 5 mg
Tablets of 2.5 mg

DESCRIPTION

Brethine, terbutaline sulfate USP, is a bronchodilator available as tablets of 2.5 mg (2.05 mg of the free base) and 5 mg (4.1 mg of the free base) for oral administration. Terbutaline sulfate is α [(*tert*-Butylamino) methyl]-3,5 dihydroxybenzyl alcohol sulfate (2:1) (salt).
Terbutaline sulfate USP is a white to gray-white crystalline powder. It is odorless or has a faint odor of acetic acid. It is soluble in water and in 0.1N hydrochloric acid, slightly soluble in methanol, and insoluble in chloroform. Its molecular weight is 548.65.
Inactive Ingredients. Cellulose compounds, lactose, magnesium stearate, povidone, and starch.

ACTIONS

Brethine is a β-adrenergic receptor agonist which has been shown by *in vitro* and *in vivo* pharmacological studies in animals to exert a preferential effect on β_2-adrenergic receptors such as those located in bronchial smooth muscle. Controlled clinical studies in patients who were administered the drug orally have revealed proportionally greater changes in pulmonary function parameters than in heart rate or blood pressure. While this *suggests* a relative preference for the β_2 receptor in man, the usual cardiovascular effects commonly associated with sympathomimetic agents were also observed with Brethine.
Brethine has been shown in controlled clinical studies to relieve bronchospasm in chronic obstructive pulmonary disease.
This action is manifested by a clinically significant increase in pulmonary function as demonstrated by an increase of 15% or more in FEV_1 and in $FEF_{25\text{-}75\%}$. Following administration of Brethine tablets, a measurable change in flow rate is usually observed in 30 minutes, and a clinically significant improvement in pulmonary function occurs at 60–120 minutes. The maximum effect usually occurs within 120-180 minutes. Brethine also produces a clinically significant decrease in airway and pulmonary resistance which persists for at least four hours or longer. Significant bronchodilator action, as measured by various pulmonary function determinations (airway resistance, $FEF_{25\text{-}75\%}$, or PEFR), has been demonstrated in some studies for periods up to eight hours.
Clinical studies were conducted in which the effectiveness of Brethine was evaluated in comparison with ephedrine over periods up to three months. Both drugs continued to produce significant improvement in pulmonary function throughout this period of treatment.

INDICATIONS

Brethine is indicated as a bronchodilator for bronchial asthma and for reversible bronchospasm which may occur in association with bronchitis and emphysema.

CONTRAINDICATIONS

Brethine is contraindicated when there is known hypersensitivity to sympathomimetic amines.

WARNINGS

Usage in Pregnancy: Animal reproductive studies have been negative with respect to adverse effects on fetal development. The safe use of Brethine has not, however, been established in human pregnancy. As with any medication, the use of the drug in pregnancy, lactation, or women of childbearing potential requires that the expected therapeutic benefit of the drug be weighed against its possible hazards to the mother or child.
Usage in Pediatrics: Brethine tablets are not presently recommended for children below the age of 12 years due to insufficient clinical data in this pediatric group.

PRECAUTIONS

Brethine should be used with caution in patients with diabetes, hypertension, hyperthyroidism, and a history of seizures. Large doses of intravenous terbutaline sulfate have been reported to aggravate preexisting diabetes and ketoacidosis.
As with other sympathomimetic bronchodilator agents, Brethine should be administered cautiously to cardiac patients, especially those with associated arrhythmias.
The concomitant use of Brethine with other sympathomimetic agents is not recommended, since their combined effect on the cardiovascular system may be deleterious to the patient. However, this does not preclude the use of an aerosol bronchodilator of the adrenergic stimulant type for the relief of an acute bronchospasm in patients receiving chronic oral Brethine therapy.
Terbutaline sulfate is not indicated for tocolysis. Serious adverse reactions may occur following administration of parenteral terbutaline sulfate to women in labor. In the mother, these include increased heart rate, transient hyperglycemia, transient hypokalemia, and possibly pulmonary edema. Increased fetal heart rate and neonatal hypoglycemia may occur as a result of maternal parenteral administration.

ADVERSE REACTIONS

Commonly observed side effects include nervousness and tremor. Other reported reactions include headache, increased heart rate, palpitations, drowsiness, nausea, vomiting, sweating, and muscle cramps. These reactions are generally transient in nature and usually do not require treatment. The frequency of these side effects appears to diminish with continued therapy. In general, all the side effects observed are characteristic of those commonly seen with sympathomimetic amines.

DOSAGE AND ADMINISTRATION

The usual oral dose of Brethine for adults is 5 mg administered at approximately six-hour intervals, three times daily, during the hours the patient is usually awake. If side effects are particularly disturbing, the dose may be reduced to 2.5 mg three times daily, and still provide a clinically significant improvement in pulmonary function. A dose of 2.5 mg, three times daily, also is recommended for children in the 12- to 15-year group. Brethine is not recommended at present for use in children below the age of 12 years. In adults, a total dose of 15 mg should not be exceeded in a 24-hour period. In children, a total dose of 7.5 mg should not be exceeded in a 24-hour period.

OVERDOSAGE

Overdosage experience is limited. Excessive beta-adrenergic receptor stimulation may augment the signs or symptoms listed under **ADVERSE REACTIONS** and they may be accompanied by other adrenergic effects. Treat the alert patient who has taken excessive oral medication by emptying the stomach by means of induced emesis, followed by gastric lavage. In the unconscious patient, secure the airway with a cuffed endotracheal tube before beginning lavage (do not induce emesis). Instillation of activated charcoal slurry may help reduce absorption of terbutaline sulfate. Maintain adequate respiratory exchange. Provide cardiac and respiratory support as needed. Continue observation until symptom-free.

HOW SUPPLIED

Tablets 2.5 mg—oval, white, scored (imprinted Geigy 72)
Bottles of 100 .... NDC 0028-0072-01
Bottles of 1000 .... NDC 0028-0072-10
Gy-Pak®—One Unit
12 bottles—100 tablets each .... NDC 0028-0072-65
Unit Dose (blister pack)
Box of 100 (strips of 10) .... NDC 0028-0072-61
Tablets 5 mg—round, white, scored (imprinted Geigy 105)
Bottles of 100 .... NDC 0028-0105-01
Bottles of 1000 .... NDC 0028-0105-10
Gy-Pak®—one Unit
12 bottles—100 tablets each .... NDC 0028-0105-65
Unit Dose (blister pack)
Box of 100 (strips of 10) .... NDC 0028-0105-61
Store at controlled room temperature 59°-86°F (15°-30°C).
Dispense in tight, light-resistant container (USP).

C85-56 (Rev. 11/85)

Shown in Product Identification Section, page 409

BRETHINE® ℞
[*breth-een '*]
terbutaline sulfate USP
Ampuls
A sterile aqueous solution for subcutaneous injection.

DESCRIPTION

Brethine, terbutaline sulfate USP, is a bronchodilator available as a sterile aqueous solution in ampuls, for subcutaneous administration. Each milliliter of solution contains 1 mg of terbutaline sulfate USP (0.82 mg of the free base); sodium chloride ACS, for isotonicity; and hydrochloric acid ACS, for pH adjustment (3.0–5.0). Terbutaline sulfate is α-[(*tert*-Butylamino) methyl]-3,5-dihydroxybenzyl alcohol sulfate (2:1) (salt).
Terbutaline sulfate USP is a white to gray-white crystalline powder. It is odorless or has a faint odor of acetic acid. It is soluble in water and in 0.1N hydrochloric acid, slightly soluble in methanol, and insoluble in chloroform. Its molecular weight is 548.65.

ACTIONS

Brethine is a β-adrenergic receptor agonist which has been shown by *in vitro* and *in vivo* pharmacological studies in animals to exert a preferential effect on β_2-adrenergic receptors such as those located in bronchial smooth muscle. However, controlled clinical studies in patients who were administered the drug subcutaneously have not revealed a preferential β_2 adrenergic effect.
Brethine has been shown in controlled clinical studies to relieve acute bronchospasm in acute and chronic obstructive pulmonary disease, resulting in a clinically significant increase in pulmonary flow rates, e.g., an increase of 15% or greater in FEV_1. Following administration of 0.25 mg of subcutaneous Brethine, a measurable change in flow rate is usually observed within five minutes, and a clinically significant increase in FEV_1 occurs by 15 minutes following the injection. The maximum effect usually occurs within 30–60 minutes and clinically significant bronchodilator activity has been observed to persist for 90 minutes to four hours. The duration of clinically significant improvement is comparable to that found with equimilligram doses of epinephrine.

INDICATIONS

Brethine is indicated as a bronchodilator for bronchial asthma and for reversible bronchospasm which may occur in association with bronchitis and emphysema.

CONTRAINDICATIONS

Brethine is contraindicated when there is known hypersensitivity to sympathomimetic amines.

PRECAUTIONS

Brethine should be used with caution in patients with diabetes, hypertension, hyperthyroidism, and a history of seizures.
Large doses of intravenous terbutaline sulfate have been reported to aggravate preexisting diabetes and ketoacidosis.
As with other sympathomimetic bronchodilator agents, Brethine should be administered cautiously to cardiac patients, especially those with associated arrhythmias.
The concomitant use of Brethine with other sympathomimetic agents is not recommended, since their combined effect on the cardiovascular system may be deleterious to the patient.
Preparation of Other Dosage Forms: Use of the subcutaneous injection for preparation of other dosage forms, i.e., I.V. infusion, is inappropriate. Sterility and accurate dosing cannot be assured if the ampuls are not used in accordance with **DOSAGE AND ADMINISTRATION.**
Carcinogenesis, Mutagenesis, Impairment of Fertility: An 18-month oral (feeding) carcinogenicity study of terbutaline (5, 50, and 200 mg/kg, corresponding to 500x, 5000x, and 20,000x the clinical subcutaneous dose) in NMRI strain mice revealed no drug-related tumorigenicity. Mutagenicity and fertility studies were not performed.
Pregnancy Category B: Reproduction studies have been performed in mice and rats at doses up to 1,000 times the human dose and have revealed no evidence of impaired fertility or harm to the fetus due to terbutaline. There are, however, no adequate and well-controlled studies in pregnant women. Because animal reproduction studies are not always predictive of human response, this drug should be used during pregnancy only if clearly needed.
Usage in Labor and Delivery: Terbutaline sulfate is not indicated for tocolysis. Serious adverse reactions may occur

following administration of parenteral terbulatine sulfate to women in labor. In the mother, these include increased heart rate, transient hyperglycemia, transient hypokalemia, and possibly pulmonary edema. Increased fetal heart rate and neonatal hypoglycemia may occur as a result of maternal parenteral administration.

Pediatric Use: Studies are in progress to define the safe and effective dose of Brethine in children. Therefore, until such studies are completed and evaluated, Brethine is not recommended for use in pediatrics.

ADVERSE REACTIONS

Commonly observed side effects include increases in heart rate, nervousness, tremor, palpitations and dizziness. These occur more frequently at doses in excess of 0.25 mg. Other reported reactions include headache, nausea, vomiting, anxiety, and muscle cramps. These reactions are transient in nature and usually do not require treatment. In general, all side effects are characteristic of those commonly seen with sympathomimetic amines such as epinephrine.

DOSAGE AND ADMINISTRATION

The usual subcutaneous dose of Brethine is 0.25 mg injected into the lateral deltöid area. If significant clinical improvement does not occur by 15–30 minutes, a second dose of 0.25 mg may be administered. A total dose of 0.5 mg should not be exceeded within a four-hour period. If a patient fails to respond to a second 0.25-mg dose of Brethine within 15–30 minutes, other therapeutic measures should be considered.

OVERDOSAGE

Overdosage experience is limited. Excessive beta-adrenergic receptor stimulation may augment the signs or symptoms listed under **ADVERSE REACTIONS** and they may be accompanied by other adrenergic effects. In the case of subcutaneous injectable terbutaline overdosage, the patient should be treated symptomatically under guidelines for sympathomimetic overdosage.

HOW SUPPLIED

Ampuls 1mg/ml—each 2-ml ampul contains 1 mg of Brethine in 1 ml of solution; 0.25 ml of solution will provide the usual clinical dose of 0.25 mg. Ampuls are expiration-dated.

Box of 10 ampuls ....NDC 0028-7507-23
Box of 100 ampuls ....NDC 0028-7507-01

Store at controlled room temperature 59–86°F (15°–30°C). Protect from light by storing ampuls in original carton until dispensed. Do not use if solution is discolored.
U.S. Patent No. 3,937,838

C85-66 (Rev. 11/85)

BUTAZOLIDIN® ℞

[bew-ta-zahl 'eh-dinn]
phenylbutazone USP
Tablets
Capsules

Because of the increased risk of agranulocytosis and aplastic anemia (see **ADVERSE REACTIONS**), Butazolidin is not recommended as initial therapy for any of its indications. It should be used only after other nonsteroidal anti-inflammatory drugs have been tried and found unsatisfactory. Butazolidin cannot be considered a simple analgesic and should never be administered casually. If it is used, the following cautions should be observed:

1. Therapy should not be initiated until a careful detailed history is taken and complete physical and laboratory examinations, including an examination of red cells, white cells and platelets, have been made. These examinations should be repeated if any signs or symptoms suggesting blood dyscrasia appear.
2. Patients should be told to discontinue use of the drug and report to the physician immediately any sign of:
   a. Fever, sore throat, or lesions in the mouth (symptoms of blood dyscrasia);
   b. Dyspepsia, epigastric pain; symptoms of anemia; unusual bleeding or bruising; black or tarry stools, or other evidence of intestinal ulceration;
   c. Skin rashes;
   d. Significant weight gain or edema.
3. The risk of aplastic anemia is greater in women, in the elderly of both sexes, and with chronic therapy, but even short-term exposure of healthy young persons can result in fatal aplastic anemia.
4. A trial period of 1 week of therapy is considered adequate to determine the therapeutic effect of the drug. In the absence of a favorable response, therapy should be discontinued.
   a. In patients 60 years and over, the drug should be restricted to short-term treatment periods only—if possible, 1 week maximum.
5. If long-term treatment is necessary, the lowest possible effective dose should be used, and patients should be adequately warned (see **Information for Patients**) and closely monitored.

DESCRIPTION

Butazolidin, phenylbutazone USP, is a nonsteroidal, anti-inflammatory agent, available as 100-mg tablets and capsules for oral administration. Phenylbutazone is 4-butyl-1,2-diphenyl-3,5-pyrazolidinedione.

Phenylbutazone USP is a white to off-white, odorless crystalline powder. It is very slightly soluble in water; freely soluble in acetone and in ether; soluble in alcohol. Its molecular weight is 308.38.

Butazolidin is closely related chemically and pharmacologically, including toxic effects, to the pyrazole compounds aminopyrine and antipyrine.

Inactive Ingredients (Butazolidin Tablets 100 mg); cellulose compounds, D&C Red No. 7 Lake, D&C Yellow No. 10 Aluminum Lake, magnesium stearate, starch and titanium dioxide.

(Butazolidin Capsules 100 mg): D&C Yellow No. 10, FD&C Red No. 3, gelatin, magnesium stearate, silicon dioxide, sodium bisulfite, sodium lauryl sulfate, starch and titanium dioxide.

CLINICAL PHARMACOLOGY

Butazolidin is a nonsalicylate, nonsteroidal, anti-inflammatory drug. It has anti-inflammatory, antipyretic, analgesic and mild uricosuric properties that produce symptomatic relief but do not alter the disease process.

The exact mechanism of the anti-inflammatory effects of Butazolidin has not been elucidated, but clinical pharmacology studies have shown that Butazolidin inhibits certain factors believed to be involved in the inflammatory process. These processes are (1) prostaglandin synthesis; (2) leukocyte migration; (3) release and activity of lysosomal enzymes.

Pharmacokinetics: Butazolidin is rapidly absorbed after oral administration and distributed partially into an extravascular compartment, with about one third remaining in plasma. About 98% of the drug in plasma is bound to albumin.

After administration of single 100-, 300-, and 600-mg doses, the mean elimination half-life is approximately 77 (54–99) hours ($n = 6$). There is a linear relationship between dose and area-under-the-curve.

After the administration of three 100-mg tablets, a peak plasma concentration of 43.3 mg/L is attained within 2.5 ± 1.4 hours. Elimination half-lives corresponding to the apparent elimination rate constant in each subject do not differ greatly for the first and last doses administered.

The pharmacokinetics of single doses of Butazolidin can be described by a two-compartment open model. Steady-state plasma concentrations of phenylbutazone are about four times higher than the peak concentration after the first single dose.

Steady-state plasma concentrations of the major, active metabolite, oxyphenbutazone, are about 50% of those of phenylbutazone. Less than 2% of the dose appears in the urine as oxyphenbutazone.

At steady state, 61% of ^{14}C-labelled Butazolidin can be recovered from the urine and 27% from the feces. However, only about 1% of total urinary radioactivity is eliminated in the urine as unchanged drug. The sum of nonconjugated urinary metabolites (oxyphenbutazone, γ-hydroxyphenylbutazone, p,γ-dihydroxyphenylbutazone) and phenylbutazone itself amounts to only about 10%. About 40% of the drug (total urinary radioactivity) is excreted in the urine as the C-4 glucuronide of phenylbutazone and an additional 12% is the C-4 glucuronide of γ-hydroxyphenylbutazone.

INDICATIONS AND USAGE

Butazolidin is indicated for the relief of symptoms associated with the following conditions, but only after other therapeutic measures, including other nonsteroidal, anti-inflammatory drugs, have been tried and found unsatisfactory: active ankylosing spondylitis, acute gouty arthritis, active rheumatoid arthritis, and acute attacks of degenerative joint disease of the hips and knees.

CONTRAINDICATIONS

Butazolidin is contraindicated in patients with a hypersensitivity to phenylbutazone or oxyphenbutazone, and in patients who have a bronchospastic reaction to aspirin or other nonsteroidal anti-inflammatory drugs.

WARNINGS

Hematologic: Butazolidin can cause aplastic anemia and agranulocytosis (see **ADVERSE REACTIONS**).

If patients develop any signs or symptoms suggesting a blood cell dyscrasia, then an examination of red cells, white cells, and platelets should be performed. If there is any significant change in the total leukocyte count, relative decrease in granulocytes, appearance of immature forms, or fall in hematocrit or platelet count, treatment with this drug should be discontinued immediately and a complete hematologic investigation should be made. Hematologic toxicity may occur shortly after initiation of therapy or after prolonged treatment; it may develop abruptly or gradually and may become apparent days or weeks after cessation of therapy. It is manifested by the appearance of anemia, leukopenia, thrombocytopenia, or clinically significant hemorrhagic diathesis.

Gastrointestinal: Peptic ulceration, reactivation of latent peptic ulcer, perforation, and gastrointestinal bleeding, sometimes severe, have been reported with the use of Butazolidin (see **ADVERSE REACTIONS,** *Gastrointestinal*).

Hepatic: As with other nonsteroidal anti-inflammatory drugs, borderline elevations of values measured by one or more liver tests may occur in up to 15% of patients. These abnormalities may progress, may remain essentially unchanged, or may be transient with continued therapy. The SGPT (ALT) test is probably the most sensitive indicator of liver dysfunction. Meaningful elevations (three times the upper limit of normal) of SGPT or SGOT (AST) have occurred in controlled clinical trials in less than 1% of patients. A patient with symptoms and/or signs suggesting liver dysfunction, or in whom abnormal liver test results have occurred, should be evaluated for evidence of the development of more severe hepatic reactions while on therapy with Butazolidin. Severe hepatic reactions, including jaundice and cases of fatal hepatitis, have been reported with Butazolidin as with other nonsteroidal anti-inflammatory drugs. Although such reactions are rare, if abnormal liver tests persist or worsen, if clinical signs and symptoms consistent with liver disease develop, or if systemic manifestations (eosinophilia, rash, etc.) occur, therapy with Butazolidin should be discontinued.

Respiratory: Like other drugs that inhibit prostaglandin synthetase activity, such as aspirin and sulfinpyrazone, Butazolidin may precipitate acute episodes of asthmatic attacks in patients with asthma (see **CONTRAINDICATIONS**).

PRECAUTIONS

General: Because serious adverse reactions or aggravation of existing medical problems can occur and have been reported, Butazolidin should be used with caution in patients with incipient cardiac failure; blood dyscrasias; pancreatitis; parotitis; stomatitis; polymyalgia rheumatica; temporal arteritis; severe renal, cardiac and hepatic disease; and in patients with a history of peptic ulcer disease or with symptoms of gastrointestinal inflammation or active ulceration.

Renal Effects: As with other nonsteroidal anti-inflammatory drugs, long-term administration of phenylbutazone to animals has resulted in renal papillary necrosis and other abnormal renal pathology. In humans, there have been reports of acute interstitial nephritis with hematuria, proteinuria, and occasionally nephrotic syndrome.

A second form of renal toxicity has been seen in patients with prerenal conditions leading to a reduction in renal blood flow or blood volume, where the renal prostaglandins have a supportive role in the maintenance of renal perfusion. In these patients, administration of an NSAID may cause a dose-dependent reduction in prostaglandin formation and may precipitate overt renal decompensation. Patients at greatest risk of this reaction are those with impaired renal function, heart failure, liver dysfunction, those taking diuretics, and the elderly. Discontinuation of NSAID therapy is typically followed by recovery to the pretreatment state.

Patients with significantly impaired renal function should be closely monitored; a lower daily dose should be anticipated to avoid excessive drug accumulation.

Patients reporting visual disturbances while receiving the drug should discontinue treatment and have an ophthalmologic examination, because ophthalmic adverse reactions have been reported (see **ADVERSE REACTIONS,** *Special Senses*).

Butazolidin increases sodium retention. As with other nonsteroidal anti-inflammatory drugs, Butazolidin should be used with caution in patients with whom fluid retention would aggravate an underlying condition such as severe cardiac or renal disease.

From age 40 on, the possibility of adverse reactions increases, and therefore Butazolidin should be used with commensurately greater care in these patients.

Information for Patients: Patients should be warned not to exceed the recommended dosage, since this may lead to toxic effects.

Patients should be told to discontinue use of the drug and report to the physician immediately any sign of fever, sore throat, or lesions in the mouth (symptoms of blood dyscrasia); dyspepsia, epigastric pain; symptoms of anemia; unusual bleeding or bruising; black or tarry stools, or other evidence of intestinal ulceration; skin rashes; or significant weight gain or edema.

Continued on next page

The full prescribing information for each GEIGY drug is contained herein and is that in effect as of September 1, 1986

Geigy—Cont.

Laboratory Tests: Therapy should not be initiated until a careful detailed history is taken and complete physical and laboratory examinations, including an examination of red cells, white cells, and platelets, have been made. These examinations should also be made if any signs or symptoms appear suggesting depression of the formed blood elements.

Drug/Drug Interactions (see **CONTRAINDICATIONS.**)
Butazolidin competitively displaces other drugs, e.g., other anti-inflammatory agents, oral anticoagulants, oral antidiabetics, sulfonamides, sodium valproate, and phenytoin, from serum-binding sites. The activity, duration of effect, and toxicity of the displaced drugs may thus be increased. Butazolidin accentuates the prothrombin depression produced by coumarin-type anticoagulants. When administered alone, Butazolidin does not affect prothrombin activity.
Butazolidin may induce the hepatic microsomal metabolism of dicoumarol, amidopyrine, digitoxin, hexobarbital, and cortisone. Conversely, it may inhibit the metabolism of phenytoin.
Concomitant administration of phenylbutazone and phenytoin may result in increased serum levels of phenytoin which could lead to increased phenytoin toxicity.
Inducers of hepatic microsomal enzymes, e.g., barbiturates, promethazine, chlorpheniramine, rifampin, and corticosteroids (prednisone), may decrease the half-life of Butazolidin.
The effects of methotrexate, insulin, antidiabetic and sulfonamide drugs may be potentiated by Butazolidin. Butazolidin increases the serum concentration of lithium by increasing tubular reabsorption, and it reduces the renal clearance of sulfonylureas.
Methylphenidate is reported to prolong the half-life of Butazolidin and to increase the serum level of oxyphenbutazone.
Cholestyramine reduces the enteral absorption of Butazolidin.

Drug/Laboratory Test Interactions: Butazolidin reduces iodine uptake by the thyroid and may interfere with laboratory tests of thyroid function. (Thyroid hyperplasia, goiters, and hypothyroidism have also been reported; see **ADVERSE REACTIONS.**)

Carcinogenesis, Mutagenesis, Impairment of Fertility
Long-term carcinogenicity studies in animals have not been performed with Butazolidin.
An increased incidence of chromosome anomalies has been reported in cultured leukocyte cells from patients receiving therapeutic doses of phenylbutazone. In other similar studies in humans and horses, results were inconclusive or negative. In Chinese-hamster fibroblast cells *in vitro*, chromosome aberrations were induced at a concentration of phenylbutazone exceeding 20 times the human plasma level of 43 mg/L. In mice, Chinese hamsters, and rats given up to 33 times the maximum daily human dose of phenylbutazone, no evidence of mutagenic activity or adverse effects on fertility was found. Phenylbutazone was not mutagenic in bacteria or fungi.

Pregnancy Category C: Reproduction studies in rats and rabbits given Butazolidin in oral doses up to 16 times the maximum daily human dose have revealed no evidence of teratogenicity due to Butazolidin. However, slightly reduced litter sizes were observed after oral or subcutaneous administration of phenylbutazone to pregnant rats or rabbits; an increase in stillbirths and a reduced survival of offspring were observed after oral administration of 3.5 times the maximum daily human dose of phenylbutazone to rats during late pregnancy and lactation.
There are no adequate and well-controlled studies in pregnant women. However, Butazolidin may appear in cord blood. Butazolidin should be used during pregnancy only if the potential benefit justifies the potential risk to the fetus.

Nursing Mothers: Butazolidin is excreted in breast milk in small quantity. Because of the potential for serious adverse reactions in nursing infants from Butazolidin, a decision should be made whether to discontinue nursing or to discontinue use of the drug, taking into account the importance of the drug to the mother.

Pediatric Use: Safety and effectiveness in children 14 years of age or younger have not been established.

ADVERSE REACTIONS

Aplastic anemia and agranulocytosis are the most serious adverse reactions that have been reported with use of Butazolidin. An incidence of 2.2 deaths from aplastic anemia and agranulocytosis per 100,000 exposures to Butazolidin was reported by Inman, in a review of all deaths in England and Wales from October 1974 through September 1975 in which aplastic anemia or agranulocytosis was considered a primary or contributing cause of death. The study found an increased risk with long-term use and use in elderly patients, especially women, with a rate of 6.5 deaths per 100,000 elderly women (over age 65). These data, while generated under conditions of use which differ from those presently recommended in the United States, indicate the need for careful consideration in any contemplated long-term use or use in the elderly.

The following adverse reactions have been reported with phenylbutazone and oxyphenbutazone:

Incidence Greater Than 1%
Gastrointestinal (see **WARNINGS**): Abdominal discomfort and distress*; nausea; dyspepsia, including indigestion and heartburn.
Dermatologic: Rash.
Cardiovascular/Fluid and Electrolyte: Edema, water retention.*

Incidence Less Than 1%—(Causal Relationship Probable)
Hematologic (see **WARNINGS**): Aplastic anemia; agranulocytosis; bone marrow depression; thrombocytopenia; pancytopenia; leukopenia; anemia; hemolytic anemia.
Gastrointestinal (see **WARNINGS**): Vomiting; abdominal distention with flatulence; constipation; diarrhea; esophagitis; gastritis; salivary gland enlargement; stomatitis, sometimes with ulceration; ulceration and perforation of the intestinal tract, including acute and reactivated peptic ulcer; anemia due to occult gastrointestinal bleeding, hepatitis.
Hypersensitive Reactions: Urticaria; anaphylactic shock; arthralgia; fever; vasculitis; Lyell's syndrome; serum sickness; Stevens-Johnson syndrome; activation of systemic lupus erythematosus; aggravation of temporal arteritis.
Dermatologic: Pruritus; erythema nodosum; erythema multiforme; nonthrombocytopenic purpura.
Cardiovascular/Fluid and Electrolyte: Sodium and chloride retention; fluid retention and plasma dilution; congestive heart failure; metabolic acidosis; respiratory alkalosis; hypertension; pericarditis; interstitial myocarditis.
Renal: Hematuria; proteinuria; ureteral obstruction with uric acid crystals; anuria; glomerulonephritis; acute tubular necrosis; cortical necrosis; renal stones; nephrotic syndrome; impaired renal function and renal failure; interstitial nephritis.
Central Nervous System: Headache; drowsiness; agitation; confusional states and lethargy; tremors; numbness; weakness.
Endocrine-Metabolic: Hyperglycemia.
Special Senses, Otic: Hearing loss; tinnitus.

Incidence Less Than 1%—(Causal Relationship Unknown)
Hematologic: Leukemia. (There have been reports associating phenylbutazone with leukemia. However, the circumstances involved in these reports are such that a causal relationship to the drug has not been clearly established.)
Special Senses, Ocular (see **PRECAUTIONS, General**): Blurred vision; optic neuritis; toxic amblyopia; scotomata; retinal detachment; retinal hemorrhage; oculomotor palsy.
Endocrine-Metabolic: Thyroid hyperplasia; goiters associated with hyperthyroidism and hypothyroidism (see **PRECAUTIONS, Drug/Laboratory Test Interactions**); pancreatitis.

OVERDOSAGE

Acute Toxicity: The lowest known lethal doses are 14 g (45-year-old man) and 2 g (3-year-old child). The highest known doses that have been survived are 40 g (20-year-old man) and 5 g (3-year-old boy). Oral LD_{50}'s (mg/kg): mice, 650; rats, 364; guinea pigs, 1220.

Signs and Symptoms: The first signs and symptoms, referable chiefly to the stomach and the nervous system, appear 1 to 2 hours after ingestion of the overdose in children and somewhat later in adults.
The signs and symptoms of phenylbutazone poisoning can be summarized as follows:

Mild poisoning
- Nausea, abdominal pain, drowsiness

Severe poisoning
- Early onset
  - Upper abdominal pain, nausea, vomiting, hematemesis, diarrhea, restlessness, dizziness, agitation, hallucinations, psychosis, coma, convulsions (more prevalent in children), hyperpyrexia, electrolyte disturbances, hyperventilation, alkalosis or acidosis, respiratory arrest, hypotension, hypertension, cyanosis.
- Late onset (2–7 days)
  - Acute renal failure, edema, hematuria, oliguria, abnormal laboratory test results, jaundice, electrocardiographic abnormalities, cardiac arrest, blood dyscrasias (anemia, thrombocytopenia, leukopenia, leukocytosis, hypoprothrombinemia).

Abnormalities evident on laboratory tests after overdosage may include respiratory or metabolic acidosis, impaired hepatic or renal function, and abnormalities of formed blood elements.

Treatment: There is no specific antidote.
In the alert patient, the stomach should be emptied promptly by induced emesis followed by lavage. In the obtunded patient, the airway should be secured with a cuffed endotracheal tube before lavage; emesis should not be induced. Adequate respiratory exchange should be maintained; respiratory stimulants should not be used. Shock should be treated with appropriate supportive measures. Seizures should be controlled with intravenous diazepam or short-acting barbiturates. Hemoperfusion has been used as an adjunct to supportive therapy in cases with poor prognosis.

DOSAGE AND ADMINISTRATION

Butazolidin should be used at the smallest effective dosage that provides rapid relief of severe symptoms. If a favorable symptomatic response to treatment is not obtained after 1 week, use of the drug should be discontinued. When a favorable therapeutic response has been obtained, the dosage should be reduced and the therapy discontinued as soon as possible.
In elderly patients (60 years and over), every effort should be made to discontinue therapy on, or as soon as possible after, the seventh day, because of the increased risk of severe or fatal toxic reactions in this age group.
The drug should be taken with milk or with meals so that the possibility of gastric upset will be minimized.
In selecting the appropriate dosage, the physician should consider the patient's age, weight, general health, and any other factors that may influence the patient's response to the drug.

Rheumatoid Arthritis, Ankylosing Spondylitis, and Acute Attacks of Degenerative Joint Disease:
Initial Dosage: The initial daily dosage in adult patients is 300–600 mg in three to four divided doses. Maximum therapeutic response is usually obtained with a total daily dose of 400 mg. A trial period of 1 week of therapy is considered adequate to determine the therapeutic effect of the drug; in the absence of a favorable response, therapy should be discontinued.
Maintenance Dosage: When improvement is obtained, the dosage should be promptly decreased to the minimum effective level necessary to maintain relief and not exceeding 400 mg daily, because of the possibility of cumulative toxicity. A satisfactory clinical response may be obtained with daily doses as low as 100–200 mg.

Acute Gouty Arthritis: Satisfactory results may be obtained after an initial dose of 400 mg followed by doses of 100 mg every 4 hours. The articular inflammation usually subsides within 4 days. Treatment should not be continued longer than 1 week.

HOW SUPPLIED

Tablets 100 mg—round, red, film-coated (imprinted Geigy 14)
Bottles of 100 .... NDC 0028-0014-01
Bottles of 1000 .... NDC 0028-0014-10
Unit Dose (blister pack)
Box of 100 (strips of 10) .... NDC 0028-0014-61

Capsules 100 mg—orange and white (imprinted Geigy 44 on one portion and Butazolidin® 100 mg on the other portion)
Bottles of 100 .... NDC 0028-0044-01
Bottles of 1000 .... NDC 0028-0044-10
Gy-Pak®—One Unit
12 bottles .... NDC 0028-0044-65
(100 capsules each)
Unit Dose (blister pack)
Box of 100 (strips of 10) .... NDC 0028-0044-61

Dispense in tight, light-resistant container (USP).
*Reactions occurring in 3–9% of patients.
C85-52 (Rev. 8/85)

Shown in Product Identification Section, page 409

CONSTANT-T® ℞

[*kahn-stant 'tee'*]
theophylline (anhydrous) USP
Sustained-Action Tablets
Tablets
200 mg
300 mg

DESCRIPTION

Constant-T, theophylline (anhydrous) USP, is a xanthine bronchodilator available as sustained-action tablets of 200 mg and 300 mg for oral administration. Its chemical name is 3,7-Dihydro-1,3-dimethyl-.1*H*-purine-2.6-dione.
Theophylline (anhydrous) USP is a white, odorless crystalline powder having a bitter taste. It is stable in air. It is freely soluble in solutions of alkali hydroxides and in ammonia; sparingly soluble in alcohol, in chloroform, and in ether; and slightly soluble in water but more soluble in hot water. Its molecular weight is 180.17.
Inactive Ingredients. Cellulose compound, FD&C Blue No. 1 (300-mg tablets), FD&C Red No. 3 (200-mg tablets), lactose, magnesium stearate, povidone, and stearic acid.

ACTIONS

The pharmacologic actions of Constant-T are as a bronchodilator, pulmonary vasodilator and smooth muscle relaxant, since the drug directly relaxes the smooth muscle of the bronchial airways and pulmonary blood vessels. Theophylline also possesses other actions typical of the xanthine derivatives: coronary vasodilator, diuretic, cardiac stimulant, cerebral stimulant and skeletal muscle stimulant. The actions of theophylline may be mediated through inhibition of phosphodiesterase and a resultant increase in intracellular cyclic AMP which could mediate smooth muscle relax-

ation. No development of tolerance appears to occur with chronic use of theophylline.
The half-life is shortened with cigarette smoking and prolonged in alcoholism, reduced hepatic or renal function, congestive heart failure, and in patients receiving certain antibiotics (see **Drug Interactions**). High fever for prolonged periods may decrease theophylline elimination. Children over six months of age have rapid clearances with average half-lives of approximately 3–5 hours. Newborn infants have extremely slow clearances and half-lives exceeding 24 hours. Older adults with chronic obstructive pulmonary disease, any patients with cor pulmonale or other causes of heart failure, and patients with liver pathology may have much lower clearances with half-lives that exceed 24 hours. The half-life of theophylline in smokers (1–2 packs per day) averages 4–5 hours; the half-life in nonsmokers averages 7–9 hours.
In single-dose studies, adjusting the data to dosing equivalent to 8 mg/kg body weight, Constant-T produced mean peak theophylline blood levels of 9.1 ± 0.7 μg/ml at 5.0 ± 1.2 hours with the 200-mg dosage form, and 9.8 ± 0.9 μg/ml at 4.6 ± 0.9 hours with the 300-mg dosage form. In a multidose, steady-state, 5-day study, Constant-T achieved constant intrasubject theophylline levels with an average peak-trough difference of only 3.4 μg/ml. This is indicative of smooth and stable maintenance therapeutic theophylline levels throughout a 12-hour dosing interval.

INDICATIONS

Symptomatic relief and/or prevention of asthma and reversible bronchospasm associated with chronic bronchitis and emphysema.

CONTRAINDICATIONS

Constant-T is contraindicated in individuals who have shown hypersensitivity to any of its components or to xanthine derivatives.

WARNINGS

Excessive theophylline doses may be associated with toxicity; serum theophylline levels should be monitored to assure maximum benefit with minimum risk. Incidence of toxicity increases at serum levels greater than 20 μg/ml. High blood levels of theophylline resulting from conventional doses are correlated with clinical manifestations of toxicity in: patients with lowered body plasma clearances; patients with liver dysfunction or chronic obstructive lung disease, and patients who are older than 55 years of age, particularly males. There are often no early signs of less serious theophylline toxicity such as nausea and restlessness, which may appear in up to 50% of patients prior to onset of convulsions. Ventricular arrhythmias or seizures may be the first signs of toxicity. Many patients who have higher theophylline serum levels exhibit a tachycardia. Theophylline products may worsen preexisting arrhythmias.
Usage in Pregnancy: Safe use in pregnancy has not been established relative to possible adverse effects on fetal development, but neither have adverse effects on fetal development been established. This is, unfortunately, true for most antiasthmatic medications. Therefore, use of theophylline in pregnant women should be balanced against the risk of uncontrolled asthma.

PRECAUTIONS

CONSTANT-T TABLETS SHOULD NOT BE CHEWED OR CRUSHED. Theophylline should not be administered concurrently with other xanthine medications. It should be used with caution in patients with severe cardiac disease, severe hypoxemia, hypertension, hyperthyroidism, acute myocardial injury, cor pulmonale, congestive heart failure, liver disease and in the elderly, particularly males, and in neonates. Great caution should be used in giving theophylline to patients in congestive heart failure since these patients show markedly prolonged theophylline blood level curves. Use theophylline cautiously in patients with history of peptic ulcer. Theophylline may occasionally act as a local irritant to GI tract although gastrointestinal symptoms are more commonly central and associated with high serum concentrations above 20 μg/ml.

ADVERSE REACTIONS

The most consistent adverse reactions are usually due to overdose and are:
Gastrointestinal: Nausea, vomiting, epigastric pain, hematemesis, diarrhea.
Central Nervous System: Headaches, irritability, restlessness, insomnia, reflex hyperexcitability, muscle twitching, clonic and tonic generalized convulsions.
Cardiovascular: Palpitation, tachycardia, extrasystoles, flushing, hypotension, circulatory failure, life-threatening ventricular arrhythmias.
Respiratory: Tachypnea.
Renal: Albuminuria, increased excretion of renal tubular cells and red blood cells; potentiation of diuresis.
Others: Hyperglycemia and inappropriate ADH syndrome.

Drug/Drug Interactions:

Drug	*Effect*
Theophylline with Furosemide	Increased Diuresis
Theophylline with Hexamethonium	Decreased Chronotropic Effect
Theophylline with Reserpine	Tachycardia
Theophylline with Cyclamycin (TAO), Erythromycin, or Lincomycin	Increased Theophylline Blood Levels

Drug/Food Interactions:
Constant-T has not been adequately studied to determine whether its bioavailability is altered when it is given with food.
Available data suggest that drug administration at the time of food ingestion may influence the absorption characteristics of some or all theophylline controlled-release products resulting in serum values different from those found after administration in the fasting state.
A drug-food effect, if any, would likely have its greatest clinical significance when high theophylline serum levels are being maintained and/or when large single doses (greater than 13 mg/kg or 900 mg) of a controlled-release theophylline product are given. The influence of the type and amount of food on performance of controlled-release theophylline products is under study at this time.

OVERDOSAGE

Management:

A. If potential oral overdose is established and seizure has not occurred:
   1) Induce vomiting.
   2) Administer a cathartic (this is particularly important if sustained-release preparations have been taken).
   3) Administer activated charcoal.

B. If patient is having a seizure:
   1) Establish an airway.
   2) Administer 0_2.
   3) Treat the seizure with intravenous diazepam, 0.1 to 0.3 mg/kg up to 10 mg.
   4) Monitor vital signs, maintain blood pressure and provide adequate hydration.

C. Postseizure coma:
   1) Maintain airway and oxygenation.
   2) If a result of oral medication, follow above recommendations to prevent absorption of the drug, but intubation and lavage will have to be performed instead of inducing emesis, and the cathartic and charcoal will need to be introduced via a large-bore gastric lavage tube.
   3) Continue to provide full supportive care and adequate hydration while waiting for drug to be metabolized. In general, the drug is metabolized sufficiently rapidly so as to not warrant consideration of dialysis.

DOSAGE AND ADMINISTRATION

Therapeutic serum levels associated with optimal likelihood for benefit and minimal risk of toxicity are considered to be between 10 and 20 μg/ml. There is a great variation from patient to patient in dosage needed in order to achieve a therapeutic blood level due to variable rates of elimination. Because of this wide variation from patient to patient, and the relatively narrow therapeutic range, dosage must be individualized. Constant-T has not been adequately studied for its bioavailability when administered with food. (see **PRECAUTIONS, Drug/Food Interactions**).
THE AVERAGE INITIAL CHILDREN'S (15 to 20 kg) DOSE IS ONE-HALF OF A CONSTANT-T 200-mg TABLET q12h.
THE AVERAGE INITIAL CHILDREN'S (20 to 25 kg) DOSE IS ONE-HALF (150 mg) OF A CONSTANT-T 300-mg TABLET q12h.
THE AVERAGE INITIAL ADULT AND CHILDREN'S (OVER 25 kg) DOSE IS ONE CONSTANT-T 200-mg TABLET q12h.
If the desired response is not achieved with the above AVERAGE INITIAL DOSAGE recommendations, and there are no adverse reactions, the dose may be increased, after 3 days, to the following MAXIMUM DOSE WITHOUT MEASUREMENT OF SERUM CONCENTRATION.

MAXIMUM DOSE WITHOUT MEASUREMENT OF SERUM CONCENTRATION

	Dose Per Interval
Children (15–20 kg)	150 mg q12h
Children (20–25 kg)	200 mg q12h
Children (25–35 kg)	250 mg q12h
Adults and Children (over 35 kg)	300 mg q12h

If increased dose is not tolerated because of headaches or stomach upset (nausea, vomiting, diarrhea, etc.), decrease dose to AVERAGE INITIAL DOSE. If tolerated, the dose may be increased, after 3 days, to the following MINIMUM DOSE REQUIRING MEASUREMENT OF SERUM CONCENTRATION.

MINIMUM DOSE REQUIRING MEASUREMENT OF SERUM CONCENTRATION

	Dose Per Interval
Children (15–20 kg)	200 mg q12h
Children (20–30 kg)	250 mg q12h
Children (30–35 kg)	300 mg q12h
Children (35–40 kg)	350 mg q12h
Adults and Children (over 40 kg)	400 mg q12h

CHECK SERUM CONCENTRATION BETWEEN 3 AND 8 HOURS AFTER A DOSE WHEN NONE HAVE BEEN MISSED OR ADDED FOR AT LEAST 3 DAYS.
If serum theophylline concentration is between 10 and 20 μg/ml, maintain dose, if tolerated. RECHECK SERUM THEOPHYLLINE CONCENTRATION AT 6- TO 12-MONTH INTERVALS.*
* Finer adjustments in dosage may be needed for some patients.
Take the following action if the serum theophylline concentration is too high.
20 to 25 μg/ml—Decrease dose by 50 mg q12h.
25 to 30 μg/ml—Skip next dose and decrease subsequent doses by 25% to the nearest 50 mg q12h.
Over 30 μg/ml—Skip next 2 doses and decrease subsequent doses by 50% to nearest 50 mg q12h. RECHECK SERUM THEOPHYLLINE CONCENTRATION.
Take the following action if the serum theophylline concentration is too low.
7.5 to 10 μg/ml—Increase dose by 25% to the nearest 50 mg.†
5 to 7.5 μg/ml—Increase dose by 25% to the nearest 50 mg and RECHECK SERUM THEOPHYLLINE FOR GUIDANCE IN FURTHER DOSAGE ADJUSTMENT.
† Dividing the daily dosage into 3 doses administered at 8-hour intervals may be indicated if symptoms occur repeatedly at the end of a dosing interval.
DOSAGE ADJUSTMENT, BASED ON SERUM THEOPHYLLINE CONCENTRATION MEASUREMENTS WHEN THESE INSTRUCTIONS HAVE NOT BEEN FOLLOWED, MAY RESULT IN RECOMMENDATIONS THAT PRESENT RISK OF TOXICITY TO THE PATIENT.

HOW SUPPLIED

Sustained-Action Tablets 200 mg—light pink, oval, scored (imprinted Geigy 42)
Bottles of 100 ....NDC 0028-0042-01
Unit Dose (blister pack)
Box of 100 (strips of 10) ....NDC 0028-0042-61
Sustained-Action Tablets 300 mg—light blue, oval, scored (imprinted Geigy 57)
Bottles of 100 ....NDC 0028-0057-01
Unit Dose (blister pack)
Box of 100 (strips of 10) ....NDC 0028-0057-61
Do not store above 86°F (30°C). Protect from moisture.
Dispense in tight, light-resistant container (USP).
C85-57 (Rev. 11/85)

Dist. by:
GEIGY Pharmaceuticals
Div. of CIBA-GEIGY Corp.
Ardsley, New York 10502
Shown in Product Identification Section, page 409

LIORESAL® **10 mg ℞**
[lye-oar 'eh-sal]
baclofen USP
Muscle Relaxant, Antispastic **20 mg ℞**

DESCRIPTION

Lioresal, baclofen USP, is a muscle relaxant and antispastic, available as 10-mg and 20-mg tablets for oral administration. Its chemical name is 4-amino-3-(4-chlorophenyl) butanoic acid.
Baclofen USP is a white to off-white, odorless or practically odorless crystalline powder, with a molecular weight of 213.66. It is slightly soluble in water, very slightly soluble in methanol, and insoluble in chloroform.
Inactive Ingredients. Cellulose compounds, magnesium stearate, povidone, and starch.

ACTIONS

The precise mechanism of action of Lioresal is not fully known. Lioresal is capable of inhibiting both monosynaptic and polysynaptic reflexes at the spinal level, possibly by hyperpolarization of afferent terminals, although actions at supraspinal sites may also occur and contribute to its clinical effect. Although Lioresal is an analog of the putative inhibi-

Continued on next page

The full prescribing information for each GEIGY drug is contained herein and is that in effect as of September 1, 1986

Geigy—Cont.

tory neurotransmitter gamma-aminobutyric acid (GABA), there is no conclusive evidence that actions on GABA systems are involved in the production of its clinical effects. In studies with animals, Lioresal has been shown to have general CNS depressant properties as indicated by the production of sedation with tolerance, somnolence, ataxia, and respiratory and cardiovascular depression. Lioresal is rapidly and extensively absorbed and eliminated. Absorption may be dose-dependent, being reduced with increasing doses. Lioresal is excreted primarily by the kidney in unchanged form and there is relatively large intersubject variation in absorption and/or elimination.

INDICATIONS

Lioresal is useful for the alleviation of signs and symptoms of spasticity resulting from multiple sclerosis, particularly for the relief of flexor spasms and concomitant pain, clonus, and muscular rigidity.

Patients should have reversible spasticity so that Lioresal treatment will aid in restoring residual function.

Lioresal may also be of some value in patients with spinal cord injuries and other spinal cord diseases.

Lioresal is not indicated in the treatment of skeletal muscle spasm resulting from rheumatic disorders.

The efficacy of Lioresal in stroke, cerebral palsy, and Parkinson's disease has not been established and, therefore, it is not recommended for these conditions.

CONTRAINDICATIONS

Hypersensitivity to baclofen.

WARNINGS

a. *Abrupt Drug Withdrawal:* Hallucinations and seizures have occurred on abrupt withdrawal of Lioresal. Therefore, except for serious adverse reactions, the dose should be reduced slowly when the drug is discontinued.

b. *Impaired Renal Function:* Because Lioresal is primarily excreted unchanged through the kidneys, it should be given with caution, and it may be necessary to reduce the dosage.

c. *Stroke:* Lioresal has not significantly benefited patients with stroke. These patients have also shown poor tolerability to the drug.

d. *Pregnancy:* Lioresal has been shown to increase the incidence of omphaloceles (ventral hernias) in fetuses of rats given approximately 13 times the maximum dose recommended for human use, at a dose which caused significant reductions in food intake and weight gain in dams. This abnormality was not seen in mice or rabbits. There was also an increased incidence of incomplete sternebral ossification in fetuses of rats given approximately 13 times the maximum recommended human dose, and an increased incidence of unossified phalangeal nuclei of forelimbs and hindlimbs in fetuses of rabbits given approximately 7 times the maximum recommended human dose. In mice, no teratogenic effects were observed, although reductions in mean fetal weight with consequent delays in skeletal ossification were present when dams were given 17 or 34 times the human daily dose. There are no studies in pregnant women. Lioresal should be used during pregnancy only if the benefit clearly justifies the potential risk to the fetus.

PRECAUTIONS

Safe use of Lioresal in children under age 12 has not been established, and it is, therefore, not recommended for use in children.

Because of the possibility of sedation, patients should be cautioned regarding the operation of automobiles or other dangerous machinery, and activities made hazardous by decreased alertness. Patients should also be cautioned that the central nervous system effects of Lioresal may be additive to those of alcohol and other CNS depressants.

Lioresal should be used with caution where spasticity is utilized to sustain upright posture and balance in locomotion or whenever spasticity is utilized to obtain increased function.

In patients with epilepsy, the clinical state and electroencephalogram should be monitored at regular intervals, since deterioration in seizure control and EEG have been reported occasionally in patients taking Lioresal.

It is not known whether this drug is excreted in human milk. As a general rule, nursing should not be undertaken while a patient is on a drug since many drugs are excreted in human milk.

A dose-related increase in incidence of ovarian cysts and a less marked increase in enlarged and /or hemorrhagic adrenal glands was observed in female rats treated chronically with Lioresal.

Ovarian cysts have been found by palpation in about 4% of the multiple sclerosis patients that were treated with Lioresal for up to one year. In most cases these cysts disappeared spontaneously while patients continued to receive the drug. Ovarian cysts are estimated to occur spontaneously in approximately 1% to 5% of the normal female population.

ADVERSE REACTIONS

The most common is transient drowsiness (10–63%). In one controlled study of 175 patients, transient drowsiness was observed in 63% of those receiving Lioresal compared to 36% of those in the placebo group. Other common adverse reactions are dizziness (5–15%), weakness (5–15%) and fatigue (2–4%). Others reported:

Neuropsychiatric: Confusion (1–11%), headache (4–8%), insomnia (2–7%); and, rarely, euphoria, excitement, depression, hallucinations, paresthesia, muscle pain, tinnitus, slurred speech, coordination disorder, tremor, rigidity, dystonia, ataxia, blurred vision, nystagmus, strabismus, miosis, mydriasis, diplopia, dysarthria, epileptic seizure.

Cardiovascular: Hypotension (0–9%). Rare instances of dyspnea, palpitation, chest pain, syncope.

Gastrointestinal: Nausea (4–12%), constipation (2–6%); and, rarely, dry mouth, anorexia, taste disorder, abdominal pain, vomiting, diarrhea, and positive test for occult blood in stool.

Genitourinary: Urinary frequency (2–6%); and, rarely, enuresis, urinary retention, dysuria, impotence, inability to ejaculate, nocturia, hematuria.

Other: Instances of rash, pruritus, ankle edema, excessive perspiration, weight gain, nasal congestion.

Some of the CNS and genitourinary symptoms may be related to the underlying disease rather than to drug therapy.

The following laboratory tests have been found to be abnormal in a few patients receiving Lioresal: increased SGOT, elevated alkaline phosphatase, and elevation of blood sugar.

OVERDOSAGE

Signs and Symptoms: Vomiting, muscular hypotonia, drowsiness, accommodation disorders, coma, respiratory depression, and seizures.

Treatment: In the alert patient, empty the stomach promptly by induced emesis followed by lavage. In the obtunded patient, secure the airway with a cuffed endotracheal tube before beginning lavage (do not induce emesis). Maintain adequate respiratory exchange, do not use respiratory stimulants.

DOSAGE AND ADMINISTRATION

The determination of optimal dosage requires individual titration. Start therapy at a low dosage and increase gradually until optimum effect is achieved (usually between 40–80 mg daily).

The following dosage titration schedule is suggested:

5 mg t.i.d. for 3 days
10 mg t.i.d. for 3 days
15 mg t.i.d. for 3 days
20 mg t.i.d. for 3 days

Thereafter additional increases may be necessary but the total daily dose should not exceed a maximum of 80 mg daily (20 mg q.i.d.).

The lowest dose compatible with an optimal response is recommended. If benefits are not evident after a reasonable trial period, patients should be slowly withdrawn from the drug (see **Warnings** *Abrupt Drug Withdrawal*).

HOW SUPPLIED

Tablets 10 mg —oval, white, scored (imprinted GEIGY 23)
Bottles of 100 ....NDC 0028-0023-01
Unit Dose (blister pack)
Box of 100 (strips of 10) ....NDC 0028-0023-61

Tablets 20 mg —capsule shaped, white, scored (imprinted GEIGY 33)
Bottles of 100 ....NDC 0028-0033-01
Unit Dose (blister pack)
Box of 100 (strips of 10) NDC 0028-0033-61

Do not store above 86°F (30°C).
Dispense in tight container (USP).

C86-29 (Rev. 7/86)

Shown in Product Identification Section, page 409

LOPRESSOR® ℞
metoprolol tartrate USP
Tablets
Ampuls
Prefilled syringes

DESCRIPTION

Lopressor, metoprolol tartrate, is a selective $beta_1$-adrenoreceptor blocking agent, available as 50- and 100-mg tablets for oral administration and in 5-ml ampuls or 5-ml prefilled syringes for intravenous administration. Each ampul or prefilled syringe contains a sterile solution of metoprolol tartrate USP, 5 mg, and sodium chloride USP, 45 mg. Metoprolol tartrate is 1-(isopropylamino)-3-[*p*-(2-methoxyethyl) phenoxyl]-2-propanol (2:1) *dextro*-tartrate salt.

Metoprolol tartrate is a white, practically odorless, crystalline powder with a molecular weight of 684.82. It is very soluble in water; freely soluble in methylene chloride, in chloroform, and in alcohol; slightly soluble in acetone; and insoluble in ether.

Inactive Ingredients: Cellulose compounds, colloidal silicon dioxide, D&C Red No. 30 aluminum lake (50-mg tablets), FD&C Blue No. 2 aluminum lake (100-mg tablets), lactose, magnesium stearate, polyethylene glycol, propylene glycol, povidone, sodium starch glycolate, talc, and titanium dioxide.

CLINICAL PHARMACOLOGY

Lopressor is a beta-adrenergic receptor blocking agent. *In vitro* and *in vivo* animal studies have shown that it has a preferential effect on $beta_1$ adrenoreceptors, chiefly located in cardiac muscle. This preferential effect is not absolute, however, and at higher doses, Lopressor also inhibits $beta_2$ adrenoreceptors, chiefly located in the bronchial and vascular musculature.

Clinical pharmacology studies have confirmed the beta-blocking activity of metoprolol in man, as shown by (1) reduction in heart rate and cardiac output at rest and upon exercise, (2) reduction of systolic blood pressure upon exercise, (3) inhibition of isoproterenol-induced tachycardia, and (4) reduction of reflex orthostatic tachycardia.

Relative $beta_1$ selectivity has been confirmed by the following: (1) In normal subjects, Lopressor is unable to reverse the $beta_2$-mediated vasodilating effects of epinephrine. This contrasts with the effect of nonselective ($beta_1$ plus $beta_2$) beta blockers, which completely reverse the vasodilating effects of epinephrine. (2) In asthmatic patients, Lopressor reduces FEV_1 and FVC significantly less than a nonselective beta blocker, propranolol, at equivalent $beta_1$-receptor blocking doses.

Lopressor has no intrinsic sympathomimetic activity, and membrane-stabilizing activity is detectable only at doses much greater than required for beta blockade. Lopressor crosses the blood-brain barrier and has been reported in the CSF in a concentration 78% of the simultaneous plasma concentration. Animal and human experiments indicate that Lopressor slows the sinus rate and decreases AV nodal conduction.

In controlled clinical studies, Lopressor has been shown to be an effective antihypertensive agent when used alone or as concomitant therapy with thiazide-type diuretics, at dosages of 100–450 mg daily. In controlled, comparative, clinical studies, Lopressor has been shown to be as effective an antihypertensive agent as propranolol, methyldopa, and thiazide-type diuretics, and to be equally effective in supine and standing positions.

The mechanism of the antihypertensive effects of beta-blocking agents has not been elucidated. However, several possible mechanisms have been proposed: (1) competitive antagonism of catecholamines at peripheral (especially cardiac) adrenergic neuron sites, leading to decreased cardiac output; (2) a central effect leading to reduced sympathetic outflow to the periphery; and (3) suppression of renin activity.

By blocking catecholamine-induced increases in heart rate, in velocity and extent of myocardial contraction, and in blood pressure, Lopressor reduces the oxygen requirements of the heart at any given level of effort, thus making it useful in the long-term management of angina pectoris. However, in patients with heart failure, beta-adrenergic blockade may increase oxygen requirements by increasing left ventricular fiber length and end-diastolic pressure.

Although beta-adrenergic receptor blockade is useful in the treatment of angina and hypertension, there are situations in which sympathetic stimulation is vital. In patients with severely damaged hearts, adequate ventricular function may depend on sympathetic drive. In the presence of AV block, beta blockade may prevent the necessary facilitating effect of sympathetic activity on conduction. $Beta_2$-adrenergic blockade results in passive bronchial constriction by interfering with endogenous adrenergic bronchodilator activity in patients subject to bronchospasm and may also interfere with exogenous bronchodilators in such patients.

In controlled clinical trials, Lopressor, administered two or four times daily, has been shown to be an effective antianginal agent, reducing the number of angina attacks and increasing exercise tolerance. The dosage used in these studies ranged from 100 to 400 mg daily. A controlled, comparative, clinical trial showed that Lopressor was indistinguishable from propranolol in the treatment of angina pectoris.

In a large (1,395 patients randomized), double-blind, placebo-controlled clinical study, Lopressor was shown to reduce 3-month mortality by 36% in patients with suspected or definite myocardial infarction.

Patients were randomized and treated as soon as possible after their arrival in the hospital, once their clinical condition had stabilized and their hemodynamic status had been carefully evaluated. Subjects were ineligible if they had hypotension, bradycardia, peripheral signs of shock, and/or more than minimal basal rales as signs of congestive heart failure. Initial treatment consisted of intravenous followed by oral administration of Lopressor or placebo, given in a coronary care or comparable unit. Oral maintenance therapy with Lopressor or placebo was then continued for 3 months. After this double-blind period, all patients were given Lopressor and followed up to 1 year.

The median delay from the onset of symptoms to the initiation of therapy was 8 hours in both the Lopressor and placebo treatment groups. Among patients treated with Lopressor, there were comparable reductions in 3-month mortality for those treated early (≤ 8 hours) and those in whom treatment was started later. Significant reductions in the incidence of ventricular fibrillation and in chest pain following initial intravenous therapy were also observed with Lopressor and were independent of the interval between onset of symptoms and initiation of therapy.

The precise mechanism of action of Lopressor in patients with suspected or definite myocardial infarction is not known.

In this study, patients treated with metoprolol received the drug both very early (intravenously) and during a subsequent 3-month period, while placebo patients received no beta-blocker treatment for this period. The study thus was able to show a benefit from the overall metoprolol regimen but cannot separate the benefit of very early intravenous treatment from the benefit of later beta-blocker therapy. Nonetheless, because the overall regimen showed a clear beneficial effect on survival without evidence of an early adverse effect on survival, one acceptable dosage regimen is the precise regimen used in the trial. Because the specific benefit of very early treatment remains to be defined however, it is also reasonable to administer the drug orally to patients at a later time as is recommended for certain other beta blockers.

Pharmacokinetics

In man, absorption of Lopressor is rapid and complete. Plasma levels following oral administration, however, approximate 50% of levels following intravenous administration, indicating about 50% first-pass metabolism.

Plasma levels achieved are highly variable after oral administration. Only a small fraction of the drug (about 12%) is bound to human serum albumin. Elimination is mainly by biotransformation in the liver, and the plasma half-life ranges from approximately 3 to 7 hours. Less than 5% of an oral dose of Lopressor is recovered unchanged in the urine; the rest is excreted by the kidneys as metabolites that appear to have no clinical significance. The systemic availability and half-life of Lopressor in patients with renal failure do not differ to a clinically significant degree from those in normal subjects. Consequently, no reduction in dosage is usually needed in patients with chronic renal failure.

Significant beta-blocking effect (as measured by reduction of exercise heart rate) occurs within 1 hour after oral administration, and its duration is dose-related. For example, a 50% reduction of the maximum registered effect after single oral doses of 20, 50, and 100 mg occurred at 3.3, 5.0, and 6.4 hours, respectively, in normal subjects. After repeated oral dosages of 100 mg twice daily, a significant reduction in exercise systolic blood pressure was evident at 12 hours.

Following intravenous administration of Lopressor, the urinary recovery of unchanged drug is approximately 10%. When the drug was infused over a 10-minute period, in normal volunteers, maximum beta blockade was achieved at approximately 20 minutes. Doses of 5 mg and 15 mg yielded a maximal reduction in exercise-induced heart rate of approximately 10% and 15%, respectively. The effect on exercise heart rate decreased linearly with time at the same rate for both doses, and disappeared at approximately 5 hours and 8 hours for the 5-mg and 15-mg doses, respectively.

Equivalent maximal beta-blocking effect is achieved with oral and intravenous doses in the ratio of approximately 2.5:1.

There is a linear relationship between the log of plasma levels and reduction of exercise heart rate. However, antihypertensive activity does not appear to be related to plasma levels. Because of variable plasma levels attained with a given dose and lack of a consistent relationship of antihypertensive activity to dose, selection of proper dosage requires individual titration.

In several studies of patients with acute myocardial infarction, intravenous followed by oral administration of Lopressor caused a reduction in heart rate, systolic blood pressure, and cardiac output. Stroke volume, diastolic blood pressure, and pulmonary artery end diastolic pressure remained unchanged.

In patients with angina pectoris, plasma concentration measured at 1 hour is linearly related to the oral dose within the range of 50 to 400 mg. Exercise heart rate and systolic blood pressure are reduced in relation to the logarithm of the oral dose of metoprolol. The increase in exercise capacity and the reduction in left ventricular ischemia are also significantly related to the logarithm of the oral dose.

INDICATIONS AND USAGE

Hypertension

Lopressor tablets are indicated for the treatment of hypertension. They may be used alone or in combination with other antihypertensive agents.

Angina Pectoris

Lopressor is indicated in the long-term treatment of angina pectoris.

Myocardial Infarction

Lopressor ampuls, prefilled syringes and tablets are indicated in the treatment of hemodynamically stable patients with definite or suspected acute myocardial infarction to reduce cardiovascular mortality. Treatment with intravenous Lopressor can be initiated as soon as the patient's clinical condition allows (see **DOSAGE AND ADMINISTRATION, CONTRAINDICATIONS,** and **WARNINGS**). Alternatively, treatment can begin within 3 to 10 days of the acute event (see **DOSAGE AND ADMINISTRATION**).

CONTRAINDICATIONS

Hypertension and Angina

Lopressor is contraindicated in sinus bradycardia, heart block greater than first degree, cardiogenic shock, and overt cardiac failure (see **WARNINGS**).

Myocardial Infarction

Lopressor is contraindicated in patients with a heart rate < 45 beats/min; second- and third-degree heart block; significant first-degree heart block (P-R interval ≥ 0.24 sec); systolic blood pressure < 100 mmHg; or moderate-to-severe cardiac failure (see **WARNINGS**).

WARNINGS

Hypertension and Angina

Cardiac Failure: Sympathetic stimulation is a vital component supporting circulatory function in congestive heart failure, and beta blockade carries the potential hazard of further depressing myocardial contractility and precipitating more severe failure. In hypertensive and angina patients who have congestive heart failure controlled by digitalis and diuretics, Lopressor should be administered cautiously. Both digitalis and Lopressor slow AV conduction.

In Patients Without a History of Cardiac Failure: Continued depression of the myocardium with beta-blocking agents over a period of time can, in some cases, lead to cardiac failure. At the first sign or symptom of impending cardiac failure, patients should be fully digitalized and/or given a diuretic. The response should be observed closely. If cardiac failure continues, despite adequate digitalization and diuretic therapy, Lopressor should be withdrawn.

Ischemic Heart Disease: Following abrupt cessation of therapy with certain beta-blocking agents, exacerbations of angina pectoris and, in some cases, myocardial infarction have occurred. When discontinuing chronically administered Lopressor, particularly in patients with ischemic heart disease, the dosage should be gradually reduced over a period of 1–2 weeks and the patient should be carefully monitored. If angina markedly worsens or acute coronary insufficiency develops, Lopressor administration should be reinstated promptly, at least temporarily, and other measures appropriate for the management of unstable angina should be taken. Patients should be warned against interruption or discontinuation of therapy without the physician's advice. Because coronary artery disease is common and may be unrecognized, it may be prudent not to discontinue Lopressor therapy abruptly even in patients treated only for hypertension.

Bronchospastic Diseases: **PATIENTS WITH BRONCHOSPASTIC DISEASES SHOULD, IN GENERAL, NOT RECEIVE BETA-BLOCKERS. Because of its relative $beta_1$ selectivity, however, Lopressor may be used with caution in patients with bronchospastic disease who do not respond to, or cannot tolerate, other antihypertensive treatment. Since $beta_1$ selectivity is not absolute, a $beta_2$-stimulating agent should be administered concomitantly, and the lowest possible dose of Lopressor should be used. In these circumstances it would be prudent initially to administer Lopressor in smaller doses three times daily, instead of larger doses two times daily, to avoid the higher plasma levels associated with the longer dosing interval. (See DOSAGE AND ADMINISTRATION.)**

Major Surgery: The necessity or desirability of withdrawing beta-blocking therapy prior to major surgery is controversial; the impaired ability of the heart to respond to reflex adrenergic stimuli may augment the risks of general anesthesia and surgical procedures.

Lopressor, like other beta blockers, is a competitive inhibitor of beta-receptor agonists, and its effects can be reversed by administration of such agents, e.g., dobutamine or isoproterenol. However, such patients may be subject to protracted severe hypotension. Difficulty in restarting and maintaining the heart beat has also been reported with beta blockers.

Diabetes and Hypoglycemia: Lopressor should be used with caution in diabetic patients if a beta-blocking agent is required. Beta blockers may mask tachycardia occurring with hypoglycemia, but other manifestations such as dizziness and sweating may not be significantly affected.

Thyrotoxicosis: Beta-adrenergic blockade may mask certain clinical signs (e.g., tachycardia) of hyperthyroidism. Patients suspected of developing thyrotoxicosis should be managed carefully to avoid abrupt withdrawal of beta blockade, which might precipitate a thyroid storm.

Myocardial Infarction

Cardiac Failure: Sympathetic stimulation is a vital component supporting circulatory function, and beta blockade carries the potential hazard of depressing myocardial contractility and precipitating or exacerbating minimal cardiac failure.

During treatment with Lopressor, the hemodynamic status of the patient should be carefully monitored. If heart failure occurs or persists despite appropriate treatment, Lopressor should be discontinued.

Bradycardia: Lopressor produces a decrease in sinus heart rate in most patients; this decrease is greatest among patients with high initial heart rates and least among patients with low initial heart rates. Acute myocardial infarction (particularly inferior infarction) may in itself produce significant lowering of the sinus rate. If the sinus rate decreases to < 40 beats/min, particularly if associated with evidence of lowered cardiac output, atropine (0.25–0.5 mg) should be administered intravenously. If treatment with atropine is not successful, Lopressor should be discontinued, and cautious administration of isoproterenol or installation of a cardiac pacemaker should be considered.

AV Block: Lopressor slows AV conduction and may produce significant first- (P-R interval ≥ 0.26 sec), second-, or third-degree heart block. Acute myocardial infarction also produces heart block.

If heart block occurs, Lopressor should be discontinued and atropine (0.25–0.5 mg) should be administered intravenously. If treatment with atropine is not successful, cautious administration of isoproterenol or installation of a cardiac pacemaker should be considered.

Hypotension: If hypotension (systolic blood pressure ≤ 90 mmHg) occurs, Lopressor should be discontinued, and the hemodynamic status of the patient and the extent of myocardial damage carefully assessed. Invasive monitoring of central venous, pulmonary capillary wedge, and arterial pressures may be required. Appropriate therapy with fluids, positive inotropic agents, balloon counterpulsation, or other treatment modalities should be instituted. If hypotension is associated with sinus bradycardia or AV block, treatment should be directed at reversing these (see above).

Bronchospastic Diseases: **PATIENTS WITH BRONCHOSPASTIC DISEASES SHOULD, IN GENERAL, NOT RECEIVE BETA BLOCKERS. Because of its relative $beta_1$ selectivity, Lopressor may be used with extreme caution in patients with bronchospastic disease. Because it is unknown to what extent $beta_2$-stimulating agents may exacerbate myocardial ischemia and the extent of infarction, these agents should *not* be used prophylactically. If bronchospasm not related to congestive heart failure occurs, Lopressor should be discontinued. A theophylline derivative or a $beta_2$ agonist may be administered cautiously, depending on the clinical condition of the patient. Both theophylline derivatives and $beta_2$ agonists may produce serious cardiac arrhythmias.**

PRECAUTIONS

General

Lopressor should be used with caution in patients with impaired hepatic function.

Information for Patients

Patients should be advised to take Lopressor regularly and continuously, as directed, with or immediately following meals. If a dose should be missed, the patient should take only the next scheduled dose (without doubling it). Patients should not discontinue Lopressor without consulting the physician.

Patients should be advised (1) to avoid operating automobiles and machinery or engaging in other tasks requiring alertness until the patient's response to therapy with Lopressor has been determined; (2) to contact the physician if any difficulty in breathing occurs; (3) to inform the physician or dentist before any type of surgery that he or she is taking Lopressor.

Laboratory Tests

Clinical laboratory findings may include elevated levels of serum transaminase, alkaline phosphatase, and lactate dehydrogenase.

Drug Interactions

Catecholamine-depleting drugs (e.g., reserpine) may have an additive effect when given with beta-blocking agents. Patients treated with Lopressor plus a catecholamine depletor should therefore be closely observed for evidence of hypotension or marked bradycardia, which may produce vertigo, syncope, or postural hypotension.

Carcinogenesis, Mutagenesis, Impairment of Fertility

Long-term studies in animals have been conducted to evaluate carcinogenic potential. In 2-year studies in rats at three oral dosage levels of up to 800 mg/kg per day, there was no increase in the development of spontaneously occurring be-

Continued on next page

The full prescribing information for each GEIGY drug is contained herein and is that in effect as of September 1, 1986

Geigy—Cont.

nign or malignant neoplasms of any type. The only histologic changes that appeared to be drug related were an increased incidence of generally mild focal accumulation of foamy macrophages in pulmonary alveoli and a slight increase in biliary hyperplasia. Neither finding represents symptoms of a known disease entity in man. In a 21-month study in Swiss albino mice at three oral dosage levels of up to 750 mg/kg per day, benign lung tumors (small adenomas) occurred more frequently in female mice receiving the highest dose than in untreated control animals. There was no increase in malignant or total (benign plus malignant) lung tumors, nor in the overall incidence of tumors or malignant tumors. This 21-month study was repeated in CD-1 mice, and no statistically or biologically significant differences were observed between treated and control mice of either sex for any type of tumor.
All mutagenicity tests performed (a dominant lethal study in mice, chromosome studies in somatic cells, a Salmonella/mammalian-microsome mutagenicity test, and a nucleus anomaly test in somatic interphase nuclei) were negative.
No evidence of impaired fertility due to Lopressor was observed in a study performed in rats at doses up to 55.5 times the maximum daily human dose of 450 mg.

Pregnancy Category C
Lopressor has been shown to increase postimplantation loss and decrease neonatal survival in rats at doses up to 55.5 times the maximum daily human dose of 450 mg. Distribution studies in mice confirm exposure of the fetus when Lopressor is administered to the pregnant animal. These studies have revealed no evidence of impaired fertility or teratogenicity. There are no adequate and well-controlled studies in pregnant women. Because animal reproduction studies are not always predictive of human response, this drug should be used during pregnancy only if clearly needed.

Nursing Mothers
Lopressor is excreted in breast milk in very small quantity. An infant consuming 1 liter of breast milk daily would receive a dose of less than 1 mg of the drug. Caution should be exercised when Lopressor is administered to a nursing woman.

Pediatric Use
Safety and effectiveness in children have not been established.

ADVERSE REACTIONS

Hypertension and Angina
Most adverse effects have been mild and transient.
Central Nervous System: Tiredness and dizziness have occurred in about 10 of 100 patients. Depression has been reported in about 5 of 100 patients. Mental confusion and short-term memory loss have been reported. Headache, nightmares, and insomnia have also been reported.
Cardiovascular: Shortness of breath and bradycardia have occurred in approximately 3 of 100 patients. Cold extremities; arterial insufficiency, usually of the Raynaud type; palpitations; congestive heart failure; peripheral edema; and hypotension have been reported in about 1 of 100 patients. (See **CONTRAINDICATIONS, WARNINGS,** and **PRECAUTIONS.**)
Respiratory: Wheezing (bronchospasm) and dyspnea have been reported in about 1 of 100 patients (see **WARNINGS**).
Gastrointestinal: Diarrhea has occurred in about 5 of 100 patients. Nausea, dry mouth, gastric pain, constipation, flatulence, and heartburn have been reported in about 1 of 100 patients.
Hypersensitive Reactions: Pruritus or rash have occurred in about 5 of 100 patients. Worsening of psoriasis has also been reported
Miscellaneous: Peyronie's disease has been reported in fewer than 1 of 100,000 patients. Musculoskeletal pain, blurred vision, and tinnitus have also been reported.
There have been rare reports of reversible alopecia, agranulocytosis, and dry eyes. Discontinuation of the drug should be considered if any such reaction is not otherwise explicable.
The oculomucocutaneous syndrome associated with the beta blocker practolol has not been reported with Lopressor.

Myocardial Infarction
Central Nervous System: Tiredness has been reported in about 1 of 100 patients. Vertigo, sleep disturbances, hallucinations, headache, dizziness, visual disturbances, confusion, and reduced libido have also been reported, but a drug relationship is not clear.
Cardiovascular: In the randomized comparison of Lopressor and placebo described in the **CLINICAL PHARMACOLOGY** section, the following adverse reactions were reported:

	Lopressor	Placebo
Hypotension (systolic BP < 90 mmHg)	27.4%	23.2%
Bradycardia (heart rate < 40 beats/min)	15.9%	6.7%
Second- or third-degree heart block	4.7%	4.7%
First-degree heart block (P-R ≥ 0.26 sec)	5.3%	1.9%
Heart failure	27.5%	29.6%

Respiratory: Dyspnea of pulmonary origin has been reported in fewer than 1 of 100 patients.
Gastrointestinal: Nausea and abdominal pain have been reported in fewer than 1 of 100 patients.
Dermatologic: Rash and worsened psoriasis have been reported, but a drug relationship is not clear.
Miscellaneous: Unstable diabetes and claudication have been reported, but a drug relationship is not clear.

Potential Adverse Reactions
A variety of adverse reactions not listed above have been reported with other beta-adrenergic blocking agents and should be considered potential adverse reactions to Lopressor.
Central Nervous System: Reversible mental depression progressing to catatonia; an acute reversible syndrome characterized by disorientation for time and place, short-term memory loss, emotional lability, slightly clouded sensorium, and decreased performance on neuropsychometrics.
Cardiovascular: Intensification of AV block (See **CONTRAINDICATIONS**).
Hematologic: Agranulocytosis, nonthrombocytopenic purpura, thrombocytopenic purpura.
Hypersensitive Reactions: Fever combined with aching and sore throat, laryngospasm, and respiratory distress.

OVERDOSAGE

Acute Toxicity
Several cases of overdosage have been reported, some leading to death.
Oral LD_{50}'s (mg/kg): mice, 1158–2460; rats, 3090–4670.

Signs and Symptoms
Potential signs and symptoms associated with overdosage with Lopressor are bradycardia, hypotension, bronchospasm, and cardiac failure.

Treatment
There is no specific antidote.
In general, patients with acute or recent myocardial infarction may be more hemodynamically unstable than other patients and should be treated accordingly (see **WARNINGS, Myocardial Infarction**).
On the basis of the pharmacologic actions of Lopressor, the following general measures should be employed:
Elimination of the Drug: Gastric lavage should be performed.
Bradycardia: Atropine should be administered. If there is no response to vagal blockade, isoproterenol should be administered cautiously.
Hypotension: A vasopressor should be administered, e.g., levarterenol or dopamine.
Bronchospasm: A $beta_2$-stimulating agent and/or a theophylline derivative should be administered.
Cardiac Failure: A digitalis glycoside and diuretic should be administered. In shock resulting from inadequate cardiac contractility, administration of dobutamine, isoproterenol, or glucagon may be considered.

DOSAGE AND ADMINISTRATION

Hypertension
The dosage of Lopressor should be individualized. Lopressor should be taken with or immediately following meals.
The usual initial dosage is 100 mg daily in single or divided doses, whether used alone or added to a diuretic. The dosage may be increased at weekly (or longer) intervals until optimum blood pressure reduction is achieved. In general, the maximum effect of any given dosage level will be apparent after 1 week of therapy. The effective dosage range is 100 to 450 mg per day. Dosages above 450 mg per day have not been studied. While once-daily dosing is effective and can maintain a reduction in blood pressure throughout the day, lower doses (especially 100 mg) may not maintain a full effect at the end of the 24-hour period, and larger or more frequent daily doses may be required. This can be evaluated by measuring blood pressure near the end of the dosing interval to determine whether satisfactory control is being maintained throughout the day. $Beta_1$ selectivity diminishes as the dose of Lopressor is increased.

Angina Pectoris
The dosage of Lopressor should be individualized. Lopressor should be taken with or immediately following meals.
The usual initial dosage is 100 mg daily, given in two divided doses. The dosage may be gradually increased at weekly intervals until optimum clincial response has been obtained or there is pronounced slowing of the heart rate. The effective dosage range is 100 to 400 mg per day. Dosages above 400 mg per day have not been studied. If treatment is to be discontinued, the dosage should be reduced gradually over a period of 1–2 weeks. (See **WARNINGS.**)

Myocardial Infarction
Early Treatment: During the early phase of definite or suspected acute myocardial infarction, treatment with Lopressor can be initiated as soon as possible after the patient's arrival in the hospital. Such treatment should be initiated in a coronary care or similar unit immediately after the patient's hemodynamic condition has stabilized.
Treatment in this early phase should begin with the intravenous administration of three bolus injections of 5 mg of Lopressor each; the injections should be given at approximately 2-minute intervals. During the intravenous administration of Lopressor, blood pressure, heart rate, and electrocardiogram should be carefully monitored.
In patients who tolerate the full intravenous dose (15 mg), Lopressor tablets, 50 mg every 6 hours, should be initiated 15 minutes after the last intravenous dose and continued for 48 hours. Thereafter, patients should receive a maintenance dosage of 100 mg twice daily (see ***Late Treatment*** below).
Patients who appear not to tolerate the full intravenous dose should be started on Lopressor tablets either 25 mg or 50 mg every 6 hours (depending on the degree of intolerance) 15 minutes after the last intravenous dose or as soon as their clinical condition allows. In patients with severe intolerance, treatment with Lopressor should be discontinued (see **WARNINGS**).
Late Treatment: Patients with contraindications to treatment during the early phase of suspected or definite myocardial infarction, patients who appear not to tolerate the full early treatment, and patients in whom the physician wishes to delay therapy for any other reason should be started on Lopressor tablets, 100 mg twice daily, as soon as their clinical condition allows. Therapy should be continued for at least 3 months. Although the efficacy of Lopressor beyond 3 months has not been conclusively established, data from studies with other beta blockers suggest that treatment should be continued for 1–3 years.
Note: **Parenteral drug products should be inspected visually for particulate matter and discoloration prior to administration, whenever solution and container permit.**

HOW SUPPLIED

Tablets 50 mg—capsule-shaped, biconvex, pink, scored (imprinted GEIGY on one side and 51 twice on the scored side)

Bottles of 100	NDC 0028-0051-01
Bottles of 1000	NDC 0028-0051-10
Gy-Pak®—One Unit	
12 bottles—60 tablets each	NDC 0028-0051-73
12 bottles—100 tablets each	NDC 0028-0051-65
Unit Dose (blister pack)	
Box of 100 (strips of 10)	NDC 0028-0051-61

Tablets 100 mg—capsule-shaped, biconvex, light blue, scored (imprinted GEIGY on one side and 71 twice on the scored side)

Bottles of 100	NDC 0028-0071-01
Bottles of 1000	NDC 0028-0071-10
Gy-Pak®—One Unit	
12 bottles—60 tablets each	NDC 0028-0071-73
12 bottles—100 tablets each	NDC 0028-0071-65
Unit Dose (blister pack)	
Box of 100 (strips of 10)	NDC 0028-0071-61

Store at controlled room temperature and protect from moisture.
Dispense in tight, light-resistant container (USP).
Ampuls 5 ml—each containing 5 mg of metoprolol tartrate
Box of 12 ampuls .... NDC 0028-4201-12
Protect from light.
Prefilled Syringes 5 ml—each containing 5 mg of metoprolol tartrate
Box of 12 syringes .... NDC 0028-4202-12
Protect from light.

C86-36 (Rev. 6/86)

Shown in Product Identification Section, page 409

LOPRESSOR HCT® ℞

metoprolol tartrate USP and hydrochlorothiazide USP
50/25 Tablets
100/25 Tablets
100/50 Tablets
Beta Blocker/Diuretic Antihypertensive

DESCRIPTION

Lopressor HCT has the antihypertensive effect of Lopressor®, metoprolol tartrate, a selective $beta_1$-adrenoreceptor blocking agent, and the antihypertensive and diuretic actions of hydrochlorothiazide. It is available as tablets for oral administration. The 50/25 tablets contain 50 mg of metoprolol tartrate USP and 25 mg of hydrochlorothiazide USP; the 100/25 tablets contain 100 mg of metoprolol tartrate USP and 25 mg of hydrochlorothiazide USP; and the 100/50 tablets contain 100 mg of metoprolol tartrate USP and 50 mg of hydrochlorothiazide USP.
Metoprolol tartrate is 1-isopropylamino-3-[*p*-(2-methoxyethyl)phenoxy]-2-propanol 2:1 *dextro*-tartrate salt.
Metoprolol tartrate is a white, practically odorless, crystalline powder with a molecular weight of 684.82. It is readily soluble in chloroform, in methylene chloride, and in water; soluble in ethanol; and sparingly soluble in acetone.
Hydrochlorothiazide is 6-chloro-3,4-dihydro-2*H*-1,2,4-benzothiadiazine-7-sulfonamide, 1,1-dioxide.
Hydrochlorothiazide USP is a white, or practically white, practically odorless, crystalline powder. It is freely soluble in sodium hydroxide solution, in *n*-butylamine, and in dime-

thylformamide; sparingly soluble in methanol; slightly soluble in water; and insoluble in ether, in chloroform, and in dilute mineral acids. Its molecular weight is 297.73.

Inactive Ingredients: Cellulose compounds, colloidal silicon dioxide, D&C Yellow No. 10 (100/50-mg tablets), FD&C Blue No. 1 (50/25-mg tablets), FD&C Red No. 3 and FD&C Yellow No. 6 (100/25-mg tablets), lactose, magnesium stearate, povidone, sodium starch glycolate, starch, stearic acid, and sucrose.

CLINICAL PHARMACOLOGY

Lopressor

Lopressor is a beta-adrenergic receptor blocking agent. *In vitro* and *in vivo* animal studies have shown that it has a preferential effect on $beta_1$ adrenoreceptors, chiefly located in cardiac muscle. This preferential effect is not absolute, however, and at higher doses. Lopressor also inhibits $beta_2$ adrenoreceptors, chiefly located in the bronchial and vascular musculature.

Clinical pharmacology studies have confirmed the beta-blocking activity of metoprolol in man, as shown by (1) reduction in heart rate and cardiac output at rest and upon exercise, (2) reduction of systolic blood pressure upon exercise, (3) inhibition of isoproterenol-induced tachycardia, and (4) reduction of reflex orthostatic tachycardia.

Relative $beta_1$ selectivity has been confirmed by the following: (1) in normal subjects, Lopressor is unable to reverse the $beta_2$-mediated vasodilating effects of epinephrine. This contrasts with the effect of nonselective ($beta_1$ plus $beta_2$) beta blockers, which completely reverse the vasodilating effects of epinephrine. (2) In asthmatic patients, Lopressor reduces FEV_1 and FVC significantly less than a nonselective beta blocker, propranolol at equivalent $beta_1$-receptor blocking doses.

Lopressor has no intrinsic sympathomimetic activity and only weak membrane-stabilizing activity. Lopressor crosses the blood-brain barrier and has been reported in the CSF in a concentration 78% of the simultaneous plasma concentration. Animal and human experiments indicate that Lopressor slows the sinus rate and decreases AV nodal conduction.

In controlled clinical studies, Lopressor has been shown to be an effective antihypertensive agent when used alone or as concomitant therapy with thiazide-type diuretics, at dosages of 100–450 mg daily. In controlled, comparative, clinical studies. Lopressor has been shown to be as effective an antihypertensive agent as propranolol, methyldopa, and thiazide-type diuretics, and to be equally effective in supine and standing positions.

The mechanism of the antihypertensive effects of beta-blocking agents has not been elucidated. However, several possible mechanisms have been proposed: (1) competitive antagonism of catecholamines at peripheral (especially cardiac) adrenergic neuron sites, leading to decreased cardiac output; (2) a central effect leading to reduced sympathetic outflow to the periphery; and (3) suppression of renin activity.

In man, absorption of Lopressor is rapid and complete. Plasma levels following oral administration, however, approximate 50% of levels following intravenous administration, indicating about 50% first-pass metabolism. Plasma levels achieved are highly variable after oral administration. Only a small fraction of the drug (about 12%) is bound to human serum albumin. Elimination is mainly by biotransformation in the liver, and the plasma half-life ranges from approximately 3 to 7 hours. Less than 5% of an oral dose of Lopressor is recovered unchanged in the urine; the rest is excreted by the kidneys as metabolites that appear to have no clinical significance. The systemic availability and half-life of Lopressor in patients with renal failure do not differ to a clinically significant degree from those in normal subjects. Conequently, no reduction in dosage is usually needed in patients with chronic renal failure.

Significant beta-blocking effect (as measured by reduction of exercise heart rate) occurs within 1 hour after oral administration, and its duration is dose-related. For example, a 50% reduction of the maximum registered effect after single oral doses of 20, 50, and 100 mg occurred at 3.3, 5.0, and 6.4 hours, respectively, in normal subjects. After repeated oral dosages of 100 mg twice daily, a significant reduction in exercise systolic blood pressure was evident at 12 hours.

There is a linear relationship between the log of plasma levels and reduction of exercise heart rate. However, antihypertensive activity does not appear to be related to plasma levels. Because of variable plasma levels attained with a given dose and lack of a consistent relationship of antihypertensive activity to dose, selection of proper dosage requires individual titration.

Hydrochlorothiazide

Thiazides affect the renal tubular mechanism of electrolyte reabsorption. At maximal therapeutic dosage, all thiazides are approximately equal in their diuretic potency. Thiazides increase excretion of sodium and chloride in approximately equivalent amounts. Natriuresis causes a secondary loss of potassium.

The mechanism of the antihypertensive effect of thiazides is unknown. Thiazides do not affect normal blood pressure.

The onset of action of thiazides occurs in 2 hours and the peak effect at about 4 hours. The action persists for approximately 6–12 hours. Hydrochlorothiazide is rapidly absorbed, as indicated by peak plasma concentrations 1–2.5 hours after oral administration. Plasma levels of the drug are proportional to dose; the concentration in whole blood is 1.6–1.8 times higher than in plasma. Thiazides are eliminated rapidly by the kidney. After oral administration of 25- to 100-mg doses, 72–97% of the dose is excreted in the urine, indicating dose-independent absorption. Hydrochlorothiazide is eliminated from plasma in a biphasic fashion with a terminal half-life of 10–17 hours. Plasma protein binding is 67.9%. Plasma clearance is 15.9–30.0 L/hr; volume of distribution is 3.6–7.8 L/kg.

Gastrointestinal absorption of hydrochlorothiazide is enhanced when administered with food. Absorption is decreased in patients with congestive heart failure, and the pharmacokinetics are considerably different in these patients.

INDICATIONS AND USAGE

Lopressor HCT is indicated for the management of hypertension.

This fixed-combination drug is not indicated for initial therapy of hypertension. If the fixed combination represents the dose titrated to the individual patient's needs, therapy with the fixed combination may be more convenient than with the separate components.

CONTRAINDICATIONS

Lopressor

Lopressor is contraindicated in sinus bradycardia, heart block greater than first degree, cardiogenic shock, and overt cardiac failure (see WARNINGS).

Hydrochlorothiazide

Hydrochlorothiazide is contraindicated in patients with anuria or hypersensitivity to this or other sulfonamide-derived drugs (see WARNINGS).

WARNINGS

Lopressor

Cardiac Failure. Sympathetic stimulation is a vital component supporting circulatory function in congestive heart failure, and beta blockade carries the potential hazard of further depressing myocardial contractility and precipitating more severe failure. In hypertensive patients who have congestive heart failure controlled by digitalis and diuretics, Lopressor should be administered cautiously. Both digitalis and Lopressor slow AV conduction.

In Patients Without a History of Cardiac Failure. Continued depression of the myocardium with beta-blocking agents over a period of time can, in some cases, lead to cardiac failure. At the first sign or symptom of impending cardiac failure, patients should be fully digitalized and/or given a diuretic. The response should be observed closely. If cardiac failure continues, despite adequate digitalization and diuretic therapy, Lopressor should be withdrawn.

Ischemic Heart Disease. Following abrupt cessation of therapy with certain beta-blocking agents, exacerbations of angina pectoris and, in some cases, myocardial infarction have been reported. Even in the absence of overt angina pectoris, when discontinuing therapy, Lopressor should not be withdrawn abruptly, and patients should be cautioned against interruption of therapy without the physician's advice (see PRECAUTIONS, Information for Patients).

Bronchospastic Diseases. **PATIENTS WITH BRONCHOSPASTIC DISEASES SHOULD, IN GENERAL, NOT RECEIVE BETA BLOCKERS. Because of its relative $beta_1$ selectivity, however, Lopressor may be used with caution in patients with bronchospastic disease who do not respond to, or cannot tolerate, other antihypertensive treatment. Since $beta_1$ selectivity is not absolute, a $beta_2$-stimulating agent should be administered concomitantly, and the lowest possible dose of Lopressor should be used. In these circumstances it would be prudent initially to administer Lopressor in smaller doses three times daily, instead of larger doses two times daily, to avoid the higher plasma levels associated with the longer dosing interval. (See DOSAGE AND ADMINISTRATION.)**

Major Surgery. The necessity or desirability of withdrawing beta-blocking therapy prior to major surgery is controversial; the impaired ability of the heart to respond to reflex adrenergic stimuli may augment the risks of general anesthesia and surgical procedures.

Lopressor, like other beta blockers, is a competitive inhibitor of beta-receptor agonists, and its effects can be reversed by administration of such agents, e.g., dobutamine or isoproterenol. However, such patients may be subject to protracted severe hypotension. Difficulty in restarting and maintaining the heart beat has also been reported with beta blockers.

Diabetes and Hypoglycemia. Lopressor should be used with caution in diabetic patients if a beta-blocking agent is required. Beta blockers may mask tachycardia occurring with hypoglycemia, but other manifestations such as dizziness and sweating may not be significantly affected. Selective beta blockers do not potentiate insulin-induced hypoglycemia and, unlike nonselective beta blockers, do not delay recovery of blood glucose to normal levels.

Thyrotoxicosis. Beta-adrenergic blockade may mask certain clinical signs (e.g., tachycardia) or hyperthyroidism. Patients suspected of developing thyrotoxicosis should be managed carefully to avoid abrupt withdrawal of beta blockade, which might precipitate a thyroid storm.

Hydrochlorothiazide

Thiazides should be used with caution in patients with severe renal disease. In patients with renal disease, thiazides may precipitate azotemia. Cumulative effects of the drug may develop in patients with impaired renal function.

Thiazides should be used with caution in patients with impaired hepatic function or progressive liver disease, since minor alterations of fluid and electrolyte imbalance may precipitate hepatic coma.

Thiazides may add to or potentiate the action of other antihypertensive drugs. Potentiation occurs with ganglionic or peripheral adrenergic blocking drugs.

Sensitivity reactions are more likely to occur in patients with a history of allergy or bronchial asthma.

The possibility of exacerbation or activation of systemic lupus erythematosus has been reported.

PRECAUTIONS

General

Lopressor. Lopressor should be used with caution in patients with impaired hepatic function.

Hydrochlorothiazide. All patients receiving thiazide therapy should be observed for clinical signs of fluid or electrolyte imbalance, namely hyponatremia, hypochloremic alkalosis, and hypokalemia (see Laboratory Tests and Drug/Drug Interactions). Warning signs are dryness of mouth, thirst, weakness, lethargy, drowsiness, restlessness, muscle pains or cramps, muscular fatigue, hypotension, oliguria, tachycardia, and gastrointestinal disturbance, such as nausea or vomiting.

Hypokalemia may develop, especially in cases of brisk diuresis or severe cirrhosis.

Interference with adequate oral intake of electrolytes will also contribute to hypokalemia. Hypokalemia may be avoided or treated by the use of potassium supplements or foods with a high potassium content.

Any chloride deficit is generally mild and usually does not require specific treatment, except under extraordinary circumstances (as in liver disease or renal disease). Dilutional hyponatremia may occur in edematous patients in hot weather; appropriate therapy is water restriction, rather than administration of salt, except in rare instances when the hyponatremia is life-threatening. In cases of actual salt depletion, appropriate replacement is the therapy of choice.

Hyperuricemia may occur or frank gout may be precipitated in certain patients receiving thiazide therapy.

Latent diabetes may become manifest during thiazide administration (see Drug/Drug Interactions).

The antihypertensive effects of the drug may be enhanced in the postsympathectomy patient.

If progressive renal impairment becomes evident, withholding or discontinuing diuretic therapy should be considered.

Calcium excretion is decreased by thiazides. Pathological changes in the parathyroid gland with hypercalcemia and hypophosphatemia have been observed in a few patients on prolonged thiazide therapy. The common complications of hyperparathyroidism, such as renal lithiasis, bone resorption, and peptic ulceration, have not been seen.

Information for Patients

Patients should be advised to take Lopressor HCT regularly and continuously, as directed, with or immediately following meals. If a dose should be missed, the patient should take only the next scheduled dose (without doubling it). Patients should not discontinue Lopressor HCT without consulting the physician.

Patients should be advised (1) to avoid operating automobiles and machinery or engaging in other tasks requiring alertness until the patient's response to therapy with Lopressor has been determined: (2) to contact the physician if any difficulty in breathing occurs: (3) to inform the physician or dentist before any type of surgery that he or she is taking Lopressor HCT.

Laboratory Tests

Lopressor. Clinical laboratory findings may include elevated levels of serum transaminase, alkaline phosphatase, and lactate dehydrogenase.

Hydrochlorothiazide. Initial and periodic determinations of serum electrolytes to detect possible electrolyte imbalance should be performed at appropriate intervals.

Serum and urine electrolyte determinations are particularly important when the patient is vomiting excessively or receiving parenteral fluids.

Continued on next page

The full prescribing information for each GEIGY drug is contained herein and is that in effect as of September 1, 1986

Geigy—Cont.

Drug/Drug Interactions

Lopressor. Catecholamine-depleting drugs (e.g., reserpine) may have an additive effect when given with beta-blocking agents. Patients treated with Lopressor plus a catecholamine depletor should therefore be closely observed for evidence of hypotension or marked bradycardia, which may produce vertigo, syncope, or postural hypotension.

Hydrochlorothiazide. Hypokalemia can sensitize or exaggerate the response of the heart to the toxic effects of digitalis (e.g., increased ventricular irritability).

Hypokalemia may develop during concomitant use of steroids or ACTH.

Insulin requirements in diabetic patients may be increased, decreased, or unchanged.

Thiazides may decrease arterial responsiveness to norepinephrine, but not enough to preclude effectiveness of the pressor agent for therapeutic use.

Thiazides may increase the responsiveness to tubocurarine.

Lithium renal clearance is reduced by thiazides, increasing the risk of lithium toxicity.

Drug/Laboratory Test Interactions

Hydrochlorothiazide. Thiazides may decrease serum levels of protein-bound iodine without signs of thyroid disturbance. Thiazides should be discontinued before tests for parathyroid function are made. (See General, *Hydrochlorothiazide,* Calcium excretion.)

Carcinogenesis, Mutagenesis, Impairment of Fertility

Lopressor. Long-term studies in animals have been conducted to evaluate carcinogenic potential. In 2-year studies in rats at three oral dosage levels of up to 800 mg/kg per day, there was no increase in the development of spontaneously occurring benign or malignant neoplasms of any type. The only histologic changes that appeared to be drug related were an increased incidence of generally mild focal accumulation of foamy macrophages in pulmonary alveoli and a slight increase in biliary hyperplasia. Neither finding represents symptoms of a known disease entity in man. In a 21-month study in Swiss albino mice at three oral dosage levels of up to 750 mg/kg per day, benign lung tumors (small adenomas) occurred more frequently in female mice receiving the highest dose than in untreated control animals. There was no increase in malignant or total (benign plus malignant) lung tumors, nor in the overall incidence of tumors or malignant tumors. This 21-month study was repreated in CD-1 mice, and no statistically or biologically significant differences were observed between treated and control mice of either sex for any type of tumor.

All mutagenicity tests performed (a dominant lethal study in mice, chromosome studies in somatic cells, a *Salmonella* / mammalian-microsome mutagenicity test, and a nucleus anomaly test in somatic interphase nuclei) were negative.

No evidence of impaired fertility due to Lopressor was observed in a study performed in rats at doses up to 55.5 times the maximum daily human dose of 450 mg.

Hydrochlorothiazide. Long-term carcinogenicity studies in animals have not been conducted.

Pregnancy Category C

Lopressor has been shown to increase postimplantation loss and decrease neonatal survival in rats at doses up to 55.5 times the maximum daily human dose of 450 mg. Distribution studies in mice confirm exposure of the fetus when Lopressor is administered to the pregnant animal. These studies have revealed no evidence of impaired fertility or teratogenicity.

A reproduction study with hydrochlorothiazide has been performed in rats at doses 62.5 times the maximum daily human dose and has revealed no evidence of impaired fertility or teratogenicity due to hydrochlorothiazide.

There are, however, no adequate and well-controlled studies in pregnant women with Lopressor HCT. Because animal reproduction studies are not always predictive of human response, this drug should be used during pregnancy only if clearly needed.

Nonteratogenic Effects. Thiazides cross the placental barrier and appear in cord blood, and there is a risk of fetal or neonatal jaundice, thrombocytopenia, and possibly other adverse reactions that have occurred in adults.

Nursing Mothers

Lopressor is excreted in breast milk in very small quantity. An infant consuming 1 liter of breast milk daily would receive a dose of metoprolol of less than 1 mg. Thiazides are also excreted in breast milk. If the use of Lopressor HCT is deemed essential, the patient should stop nursing.

Pediatric Use

Safely and effectiveness in children have not been established.

ADVERSE REACTIONS

Lopressor HCT

The following adverse reactions were reported in controlled clinical studies of the combination of Lopressor and hydrochlorothiazide.

Body as a Whole: Fatigue or lethargy and flu syndrome have each been reported in about 10 in 100 patients.

Nervous System: Dizziness or vertigo, drowsiness or somnolence, and headache have each occurred in about 10 in 100 patients. Nightmare has occurred in 1 in 100 patients.

Cardiovascular: Bradycardia has occurred in about 6 in 100 patients.

Decreased exercise tolerance and dyspnea have each occurred in about 1 of 100 patients.

Digestive: Diarrhea, digestive disorder, dry mouth, nausea or vomiting, and constipation have each occurred in about 1 in 100 patients.

Metabolic and Nutritional: Hypokalemia has occurred in fewer than 10 in 100 patients. Edema, gout, and anorexia have each occurred in 1 in 100 patients.

Special Senses: Blurred vision, tinnitus, and earache have each been reported in 1 in 100 patients.

Skin: Sweating and purpura have each occurred in 1 in 100 patients.

Urogenital: Impotence has occurred in 1 in 100 patients.

Musculoskeletal: Muscle pain has occurred in 1 in 100 patients.

Lopressor

Most adverse effects have been mild and transient.

Central Nervous System: Tiredness and dizziness have occurred in about 10 of 100 patients. Depression has been reported in about 5 of 100 patients. Mental confusion and short-term memory loss have been reported. Headache, nightmares, and insomnia have also been reported, but a drug relationship is not clear.

Cardiovascular: Shortness of breath and bradycardia have occurred in approximately 3 of 100 patients. Cold extremities; arterial insufficiency, usually of the Raynaud type; palpitations; and congestive heart failure have been reported. (See CONTRAINDICATIONS, WARNINGS, and PRECAUTIONS.)

Respiratory: Wheezing (bronchospasm) has been reported in fewer than 1 of 100 patients (see WARNINGS).

Gastrointestinal: Diarrhea has occurred in about 5 of 100 patients. Nausea, gastric pain, constipation, flatulence, and heartburn have been reported in 1 of 100, or fewer, patients.

Hypersensitive Reactions: Pruritus has occurred in fewer than 1 of 100 patients. Rash has been reported.

Miscellaneous: Peyronie's disease has been reported in fewer than 1 of 100,000 patients. Alopecia has been reported.

The oculomucocutaneous syndrome associated with the beta blocker practolol has not been reported with Lopressor.

Potential Adverse Reactions

A variety of adverse reactions not listed above have been reported with other beta-adrenergic blocking agents and should be considered potential adverse reactions to Lopressor.

Central Nervous System: Reversible mental depression progressing to catatonia; visual disturbances; hallucinations; an acute reversible syndrome characterized by disorientation for time and place, short-term memory loss, emotional lability, slightly clouded sensorium, and decreased performance on neuropsychometrics.

Cardiovascular: Intensification of AV block (see CONTRAINDICATIONS).

Hematologic: Agranulocytosis, nonthrombocytopenic purpura, thrombocytopenic purpura.

Hypersensitive Reactions: Fever combined with aching and sore throat, laryngospasm, and respiratory distress.

Hydrochlorothiazide

Gastrointestinal: Anorexia, gastric irritation, nausea, vomiting, cramping, diarrhea, constipation, jaundice (intrahepatic cholestatic), pancreatitis, sialadenitis.

Cardiovascular: Orthostatic hypotension (may be potentiated by alcohol, barbiturates, or narcotics).

Neurologic: Dizziness, vertigo, paresthesia, headache, xanthopsia.

Hematologic: Leukopenia, agranulocytosis, thrombocytopenia, aplastic anemia.

Hypersensitive Reactions: Purpura, photosensitivity, rash, urticaria, necrotizing angiitis, Stevens-Johnson syndrome, other hypersensitive reactions.

Other: Hyperglycemia, glycosuria, hyperuricemia, muscle spasm, weakness, restlessness, transient blurred vision.

OVERDOSAGE

Acute Toxicity

Several cases of overdosage with Lopressor have been reported, some leading to death. No deaths have been reported with hydrochlorothiazide.

Oral LD_{50}'s (mg/kg): mice, 1158 (Lopressor); rats, 3090 (Lopressor), 2750 (hydrochlorothiazide).

Signs and Symptoms

Lopressor. Potential signs and symptoms associated with overdosage with Lopressor are bradycardia, hypotension, bronchospasm, and cardiac failure.

Hydrochlorothiazide. The most prominent feature of poisoning is acute loss of fluid and electrolytes.

Cardiovascular: Tachycardia, hypotension, shock.

Neuromuscular: Weakness, confusion, dizziness, cramps of the calf muscles, paresthesia, fatigue, impairment of consciousness.

Digestive: Nausea, vomiting, thirst.

Renal: Polyuria, oliguria, or anuria (due to hemoconcentration).

Laboratory Findings: Hypokalemia, hyponatremia, hypochloremia, alkalosis; increased BUN (especially in patients with renal insufficiency).

Combined Poisoning: Signs and symptoms may be aggravated or modified by concomitant intake of antihypertensive medication, barbiturates, curare, digitalis (hypokalemia), corticosteroids, narcotics, or alcohol.

Treatment

There is no specific antidote.

On the basis of the pharmacologic actions of Lopressor and hydrochlorothiazide, the following general measures should be employed:

Elimination of the Drug: Inducement of vomiting, gastric lavage, and activated charcoal.

Bradycardia: Atropine should be administered. If there is no response to vagal blockade, isoproterenol should be administered cautiously.

Hypotension: The patient's legs should be elevated, and lost fluid and electrolytes (potassium, sodium) should be replaced. A vasopressor should be administered, e.g., levarterenol or dopamine.

Bronchospasm: A $beta_2$-stimulating agent and/or a theophylline derivative should be administered.

Cardiac Failure: A digitalis glycoside and diuretic should be administered. In shock resulting from inadequate cardiac contractility, administration of dobutamine, isorproterenol, or glucagon may be considered.

Surveillance: Fluid and electrolyte balance (especially serum potassium) and renal function should be monitored until conditions become normal.

DOSAGE AND ADMINISTRATION

Dosage should be determined by individual titration (see INDICATIONS AND USAGE).

Hydrochlorothiazide is usually given at a dosage of 25 to 100 mg per day. The usual initial dosage of Lopressor is 100 mg daily in single or divided doses. Dosage may be increased gradually until optimum blood pressure control is achieved. The effective dosage range is 100 to 450 mg per day. While once-daily dosing is effective and can maintain a reduction in blood pressure throughout the day, lower doses (especially 100 mg) may not maintain a full effect at the end of the 24-hour period, and larger or more frequent daily doses may be required. This can be evaluated by measuring blood pressure near the end of the dosing interval to determine whether satisfactory control is being maintained throughout the day. $Beta_1$ selectivity diminishes as dosage of Lopressor is increased.

The following dosage schedule may be used to administer from 100 to 200 mg of Lopressor per day and from 25 to 50 mg of hydrochlorothiazide per day:

Lopressor HCT	***Dosage***
Tablets of 50/25	2 tablets per day in single or divided doses
Tablets of 100/25	1 to 2 tablets per day in single or divided doses
Tablets of 100/50	1 tablet per day in single or divided doses

Dosing regimens that exceed 50 mg of hydrochlorothiazide per day are not recommended. When necessary, another antihypertensive agent may be added gradually, beginning with 50% of the usual recommended starting dose to avoid an excessive fall in blood pressure.

HOW SUPPLIED

Tablets 50/25 —capsule-shaped, white and blue, scored (imprinted Geigy on one side and 35 twice on the scored side) 50 mg of metoprolol tartrate and 25 mg of hydrochlorothiazide

Bottles of 100 .... NDC 0028-0035-01

Tablets 100/25 —capsule-shaped, white and pink, scored (imprinted Geigy on one side and 53 twice on the scored side) 100 mg of metoprolol tartrate and 25 mg of hydrochlorothiazide

Bottles of 100 .... NDC 0028-0053-01

Tablets 100/50 —capsule-shaped, white and yellow, scored (imprinted Geigy on one side and 73 twice on the scored side) 100 mg of metoprolol tartrate and 50 mg of hydrochlorothiazide

Bottles of 100 .... NDC 0028-0073-01

Store between 59°–86°F (15°–30°C). Protect from moisture.

Dispense in tight, light-resistant container (USP).

C85-45 (Rev. 11/85)

Shown in Product Identification Section, page 409

OTRIVIN®
[oh'trah-vinn]
xylometazoline hydrochloride USP
Nasal Spray and Nasal Drops 0.1%
Pediatric Nasal Drops 0.05%

One application provides rapid and long-lasting relief of nasal congestion for up to 10 hours.
Quickly clears stuffy noses due to common cold, sinusitis, hay fever.
Nasal congestion can make life miserable—you can't breathe, smell, taste, or sleep comfortably. That is why Otrivin is so helpful. It clears away that stuffy feeling, usually within 5 to 10 minutes, and your head feels clear for hours.
Otrivin has been prescribed by doctors for many years. Here is how you use it:
Nasal Spray 0.1%—Spray 2 to 3 times into each nostril every 8–10 hours. With head upright, squeeze sharply and firmly while inhaling (sniffing) through the nose.
Nasal Drops 0.1%—for adults and children 12 years and older. Put 2 or 3 drops into each nostril every 8 to 10 hours. Tilt head as far back as possible. Immediately bend head forward toward knees, hold for a few seconds, then return to upright position.
Do not give Nasal Spray 0.1% or Nasal Drops 0.1% to children under 12 years except under the advice and supervision of a physician.
Pediatric Nasal Drops 0.05%—for children 2 to 12 years of age. Put 2 to 3 drops into each nostril every 8 to 10 hours. Tilt head as far back as possible. Immediately bend head forward toward knees, hold a few seconds, then return to upright position.
Do not give this product to children under 2 years except under the advice and supervision of a physician.
Otrivin Nasal Spray/Nasal Drops are available in unbreakable plastic spray package of ½ fl oz (15 ml) and in plastic dropper bottle of .66 fl oz (20 ml).
Otrivin Pediatric Nasal Drops
Available in plastic dropper bottle of .66 fl oz (20 ml).

WARNINGS

Do not exceed recommended dosage, because symptoms such as burning, stinging, sneezing, or increase of nasal discharge may occur. Do not use this product for more than 3 days. If symptoms persist, consult a physician. The use of this dispenser by more than one person may cause infection.
Keep this and all medicines out of the reach of children. In case of accidental ingestion, seek professional assistance or contact a Poison Control Center immediately.
C80-47 (8/80)

PBZ-SR® ℞
tripelennamine HCl
sustained-release tablets
Tablets of 100 mg

DESCRIPTION

PBZ-SR, tripelennamine hydrochloride USP, is an antihistamine for oral administration available as 100-mg *sustained-release tablets* that provide a gradual and prolonged release of drug from the wax matrix.
Tripelennamine hydrochloride is 2-[Benzyl[2-(dimethylamino)ethyl]amino]pyridine monohydrochloride.
Tripelennamine hydrochloride USP is a white, crystalline powder. Its solutions are practically neutral to litmus. It is freely soluble in water, in alcohol, and in chloroform; slightly soluble in acetone; and insoluble in benzene, in ether, and in ethyl acetate. Its molecular weight is 291.82.
Inactive ingredients: Cellulose compounds, cetostearyl alcohol, D&C Red No. 30 lake, FD&C Blue No. 2 lake, magnesium stearate, mineral oil, titanium dioxide and zein.

ACTIONS

Antihistamines are competitive antagonists of histamine, which also produce central nervous system effects (both stimulant and depressant) and peripheral anticholinergic, atropine-like effects (e.g., drying).

INDICATIONS

Perennial and seasonal allergic rhinitis; vasomotor rhinitis; allergic conjunctivitis due to inhalant allergens and foods; mild, uncomplicated allergic skin manifestations of urticaria and angioedema; amelioration of allergic reactions to blood or plasma; dermographism; anaphylactic reactions as adjunctive therapy to epinephrine and other standard measures after the acute manifestations have been controlled.

CONTRAINDICATIONS

PBZ-SR should not be used in premature infants, neonates, or nursing mothers; patients receiving MAO inhibitors; patients with narrow-angle glaucoma, stenosing peptic ulcer, symptomatic prostatic hypertrophy, bladder neck obstruction, pyloroduodenal obstruction, lower respiratory tract symptoms (including asthma), or hypersensitivity to tripelennamine or related compounds.

WARNINGS

Antihistamines often produce drowsiness and may reduce mental alertness in children and adults. Patients should be warned about engaging in activities requiring mental alertness (e.g., driving a car, operating machinery or hazardous appliances). In elderly patients, approximately 60 years or older, antihistamines are more likely to cause dizziness, sedation and hypotension.
Patients should be warned that the central nervous system effects of PBZ-SR may be additive with those of alcohol and other CNS depressants (e.g., hypnotics, sedatives, tranquilizers, antianxiety agents).
Antihistamines may produce excitation, particularly in children.

USAGE IN PREGNANCY

Although no tripelennamine-related teratogenic potential or other adverse effects on the fetus have been observed in limited animal reproduction studies, the safe use of this drug in pregnancy or during lactation has not been established. Therefore, the drug should not be used during pregnancy or lactation unless, in the judgment of the physician, the expected benefits outweigh the potential hazards.

USAGE IN CHILDREN

In infants and children particularly, antihistamines in overdosage may produce hallucinations, convulsions and/or death.

PRECAUTIONS

PBZ-SR, like other antihistamines, has atropine-like, anticholinergic activity and should be used with caution in patients with increased intraocular pressure, hyperthyroidism, cardiovascular disease, hypertension, or history of bronchial asthma.

ADVERSE REACTIONS

The most frequent adverse reactions to antihistamines are sedation or drowsiness; sleepiness; dryness of the mouth, nose, and throat; thickening of bronchial secretions; dizziness; disturbed coordination; epigastric distress.
Other adverse reactions which may occur are: fatigue; chills; confusion; restlessness; excitation; hysteria; nervousness; irritability; insomnia; euphoria; anorexia; nausea; vomiting; diarrhea; constipation; hypotension; tightness in the chest; wheezing; blurred vision; diplopia; vertigo; tinnitus; convulsions; headache; palpitations; tachycardia; extrasystoles; nasal stuffiness; urinary frequency; difficult urination; urinary retention; leukopenia; hemolytic anemia; thrombocytopenia; agranulocytosis; aplastic anemia; allergic or hypersensitivity reactions, including drug rash, urticaria, anaphylactic shock, and photosensitivity. Although the following may have been reported to occur in association with some antihistamines, they have not been known to result from the use of PBZ-SR: excessive perspiration, tremor, paresthesias, acute labyrinthitis, neuritis and early menses.

DOSAGE AND ADMINISTRATION

Dosage should be individualized according to the needs and response of the patient.
Adults: One 100-mg PBZ-SR Tablet in the morning and one in the evening is generally adequate. In difficult cases, one 100-mg PBZ-SR Tablet every 8 hours may be required.
Children: PBZ-SR Tablets are not intended for use in children.
Note: PBZ-SR sustained-release tablets must be swallowed whole and never crushed or chewed.

OVERDOSAGE

Signs and Symptoms: The greatest danger from acute overdosage with antihistamines is their central nervous system effects which produce depression and/or stimulation.
In children, stimulation predominates initially in a syndrome which may include excitement, hallucinations, ataxia, incoordination, athetosis, and convulsions followed by postictal depression. Dry mouth, fixed dilated pupils, flushing of the face, and fever are common and resemble the syndrome of atropine poisoning.
In adults, CNS depression (i.e., drowsiness, coma) is more common. CNS stimulation is rare; fever and flushing are uncommon.
In both children and adults, there can be a terminal deepening of coma and cardiovascular collapse; death can occur, especially in infants and children.
Treatment: There is no specific therapy for acute overdosage with antihistamines. General symptomatic and supportive measures should be instituted promptly and maintained for as long as necessary.
In the conscious patient, vomiting should be induced even though it may have occurred spontaneously. If vomiting cannot be induced, gastric lavage is indicated. Adequate precautions must be taken to protect against aspiration, especially in infants and children. Charcoal slurry or other suitable agent should be instilled into the stomach after vomiting or lavage. Saline cathartics or milk of magnesia may be of additional benefit.
In the unconscious patient, the airway should be secured with a cuffed endotracheal tube before attempting to evacuate the gastric contents. Intensive supportive and nursing care is indicated, as for any comatose patient.
If breathing is significantly impaired, maintenance of an adequate airway and mechanical support of respiration is the safest and most effective means of providing for adequate oxygenation of tissues to prevent hypoxia (especially brain hypoxia during convulsions).
Hypotension is an early sign of impending cardiovascular collapse and should be treated vigorously. Although general supportive measures are important, specific treatment with intravenous infusion of a vasopressor (e.g., levarterenol bitartrate) titrated to maintain adequate blood pressure is also necessary.
Do *not* use CNS stimulants.
Convulsions should be controlled by careful titration of a short-acting barbiturate, repeated as necessary.
Ice packs and cooling sponge baths can aid in reducing the fever commonly seen in children.

HOW SUPPLIED

PBZ-SR Tablets (sustained-release) 100 mg—round, lavender (imprinted Geigy 48)
Bottles of 100 ....NDC 0028-0048-01
Do not store above 86°F (30°C). Protect from moisture.
Dispense in tight container (USP).
C85-58 (Rev. 11/85)

Shown in Product Identification Section, page 409

PBZ® ℞
tripelennamine hydrochloride
Tablets USP
tripelennamine citrate Elixir USP

Listed in USP, a Medicare designated compendium.

DESCRIPTION

PBZ, an antihistamine for oral administration, is available as tripelennamine hydrochoride USP, and tripelennamine citrate USP. PBZ *tablets* contain 25 mg and 50 mg of the hydrochoride salt. PBZ *elixir* contains 37.5 mg of the citrate salt per 5 ml. Tripelennamine hydrochloride is 2-]Benzyl[2-(dimethylamino)ethyl]amino]pyridine monohydrochloride.
Tripelennamine hydrochloride USP is a white, crystalline powder. Its solutions are practically neutral to litmus. It is freely soluble in water, in alcohol, and in chloroform; slightly soluble in acetone; and insoluble in benzene, in ether, and in ethyl acetate. Its molecular weight is 291.82.
Tripelennamine citrate is 2-[Benzyl[2-(dimethylamino) ethyl]amino]pyridine citrate (1:1).
Tripelennamine citrate USP is a white, crystalline powder. It solutions are acid to litmus. It is freely soluble in water and in alcohol, very slightly soluble in ether, and practically insoluble in benzene and in chloroform. It melts at about 107°C and has a molecular weight of 447.49.
Inactive ingredients (PBZ Tablets 25 mg): Lactose, magnesium stearate, polyethylene glycol, starch, sucrose and talc.
(PBZ Tablets 50 mg): Acacia, lactose, magnesium stearate, polyethylene glycol, talc and tragacanth.
(PBZ citrate Elixir): Alcohol (12% [v/v/]), D&C Green No. 5, flavoring, glycerin, purified water and sucrose.

ACTIONS

Antihistamines are competitive antagonists of histamine, which also produce central nervous system effects (both stimulant and depressant) and peripheral anticholinergic, atropine-like effects (e.g., drying).

INDICATIONS

Perennial and seasonal allergic rhinitis; vasomotor rhinitis; allergic conjunctivitis due to inhalant allergens and foods; mild, uncomplicated allergic skin manifestations of urticaria and angioedema; amelioration of allergic reactions to blood or plasma; dermographism; anaphylactic reactions as adjunctive therapy to epinephrine and other standard measures after the acute manifestations have been controlled.

CONTRAINDICATIONS

PBZ should not be used in premature infants, neonates, or nursing mothers; patients receiving MAO inhibitors; patients with narrow-angle glaucoma, stenosing peptic ulcer, symptomatic prostatic hypertrophy, bladder neck obstruction, pyloroduodenal obstruction, lower respiratory tract symptoms (including asthma), or hypersensitivity to tripelennamine or related compounds.

WARNINGS

Antihistamines often produce drowsiness and may reduce mental alertness in children and adults. Patients should be warned about engaging in activities requiring mental alertness (e.g., driving a car, operating machinery or hazardous

Continued on next page

The full prescribing information for each GEIGY drug is contained herein and is that in effect as of September 1, 1986

Geigy—Cont.

appliances). In elderly patients, approximately 60 years or older, antihistamines are more likely to cause dizziness, sedation and hypotension.

Patients should be warned that the central nervous system effects of PBZ may be additive with those of alcohol and other CNS depressants (e.g., hypnotics, sedatives, tranquilizers, antianxiety agents).

Antihistamines may produce excitation, particularly in children.

Usage in Pregnancy

Although no tripelennamine-related teratogenic potential or other adverse effects on the fetus have been observed in limited animal reproduction studies, the safe use of this drug in pregnancy or during lactation has not been established. Therefore, the drug should not be used during pregnancy or lactation unless, in the judgment of the physician, the expected benefits outweigh the potential hazards.

Usage in Children

In infants and children particularly, antihistamines in overdosage may produce hallucinations, convulsions and/or death.

PRECAUTIONS

PBZ, like other antihistamines, has atropine-like, anticholinergic activity and should be used with caution in patients with increased intraocular pressure, hyperthyroidism, cardiovascular disease, hypertension, or history of bronchial asthma.

ADVERSE REACTIONS

The most frequent adverse reactions to antihistamines are sedation or drowsiness; sleepiness; dryness of the mouth, nose, and throat; thickening of bronchial secretions; dizziness; disturbed coordination; epigastric distress.

Other adverse reactions which may occur are: fatigue; chills; confusion; restlessness; excitation; hysteria; nervousness; irritability; insomnia; euphoria; anorexia; nausea; vomiting; diarrhea; constipation; hypotension; tightness in the chest; wheezing; blurred vision; diplopia; vertigo; tinnitus; convulsions; headache; palpitations; tachycardia; extrasystoles; nasal stuffiness; urinary frequency; difficult urination; urinary retention; leukopenia; hemolytic anemia; thrombocytopenia; agranulocytosis; aplastic anemia; allergic or hypersensitivity reactions, including drug rash, urticaria, anaphylactic shock, and photosensitivity. Although the following may have been reported to occur in association with some antihistamines, they have not been known to result from the use of PBZ: excessive perspiration, tremor, paresthesias, acute labyrinthitis, neuritis and early menses.

DOSAGE AND ADMINISTRATION

Dosage should be individualized.

Usual Adult Dose: 25 to 50 mg every four to six hours. As little as 25 mg may control symptoms, but as much as 600 mg daily may be given in divided doses, if necessary.

Children and Infants: 5 mg/kg/24 hours or 150 mg/m²/24 hours divided into four to six doses. Do not exceed maximum total dose of 300 mg/24 hours.

Note: Recommended dosages are based on the hydrochloride salt; each ml of Elixir (tripelennamine citrate) is equivalent to 5 mg tripelennamine hydrochloride.

OVERDOSAGE

Signs and Symptoms

The greatest danger from acute overdosage with antihistamines is their central nervous system effects which produce depression and/or stimulation.

In children, stimulation predominates initially in a syndrome which may include excitement, hallucinations, ataxia, incoordination, athetosis, and convulsions followed by postictal depression. Dry mouth, fixed dilated pupils, flushing of the face, and fever are common and resemble the syndrome of atropine poisoning. In adults, CNS depression (i.e., drowsiness, coma) is more common. CNS stimulation is rare; fever and flushing are uncommon.

In both children and adults, there can be a terminal deepening of coma and cardiovascular collapse; death can occur, especially in infants and children.

Treatment

There is no specific therapy for acute overdosage with antihistamines. General symptomatic and supportive measures should be instituted promptly and maintained for as long as necessary.

In the conscious patient, vomiting should be induced even though it may have occurred spontaneously. If vomiting cannot be induced, gastric lavage is indicated. Adequate precautions must be taken to protect against aspiration, especially in infants and children. Charcoal slurry or other suitable agent should be instilled into the stomach after vomiting or lavage. Saline cathartics or milk of magnesia may be of additional benefit.

In the unconscious patient, the airway should be secured with a cuffed endotracheal tube before attempting to evacuate the gastric contents. Intensive supportive and nursing care is indicated, as for any comatose patient.

If breathing is significantly impaired, maintenance of an adequate airway and mechanical support of respiration is the safest and most effective means of providing for adequate oxygenation of tissues to prevent hypoxia (especially brain hypoxia during convulsions).

Hypotension is an early sign of impending cardiovascular collapse and should be treated vigorously. Although general supportive measures are important, specific treatment with intravenous infusion of a vasopressor (e.g., levarterenol bitartrate) titrated to maintain adequate blood pressure may be necessary.

Do *not* use CNS stimulants.

Convulsions should be controlled by careful titration of a short-acting barbiturate, repeated as necessary.

Ice packs and cooling sponge baths can aid in reducing the fever commonly seen in children.

HOW SUPPLIED

Tablets 25 mg—round, white to off-white, biconvex (scored on one side and imprinted Geigy 111 on the other side)

Bottles of 100 ....NDC 0028-0111-01

Tablets 50 mg—round, white to off-white, biconvex (scored on one side and imprinted Geigy 117 on the other side)

Bottles of 100 ....NDC 0028-0117-01
Bottles of 1000 ....NDC 0028-0117-10

Elixir—green, cinnamon-flavored—37.5 mg tripelennamine citrate USP (equivalent to 25 mg tripelennamine hydrochloride) per 5 ml

Bottles of 473 ml..NDC 0028-6925-16

Dispense in tight, light-resistant container.

C85-53 (Rev. 8/85)

Shown in Product Identification Section, page 409

TEGRETOL® ℞

[teg′rit-tall]

carbamazepine USP

Chewable Tablets of 100 mg—red-speckled, pink

Tablets of 200 mg—pink

WARNING

SERIOUS AND SOMETIMES FATAL ABNORMALITIES OF BLOOD CELLS (APLASTIC ANEMIA, AGRANULOCYTOSIS, THROMBOCYTOPENIA, AND LEUKOPENIA) HAVE BEEN REPORTED FOLLOWING TREATMENT WITH TEGRETOL, CARBAMAZEPINE.

EARLY DETECTION OF HEMATOLOGIC CHANGE IS IMPORTANT SINCE, IN SOME PATIENTS, APLASTIC ANEMIA IS REVERSIBLE.

COMPLETE PRETREATMENT BLOOD COUNTS, INCLUDING PLATELET AND POSSIBLY RETICULOCYTE AND SERUM IRON, SHOULD BE OBTAINED. ANY SIGNIFICANT ABNORMALITIES SHOULD RULE OUT USE OF THE DRUG. THESE SAME TESTS SHOULD BE REPEATED AT FREQUENT INTERVALS, POSSIBLY WEEKLY DURING THE FIRST THREE MONTHS OF THERAPY AND MONTHLY THEREAFTER FOR AT LEAST TWO TO THREE YEARS. THE DRUG SHOULD BE STOPPED IF ANY EVIDENCE OF BONE MARROW DEPRESSION DEVELOPS.

PATIENTS SHOULD BE MADE AWARE OF THE EARLY TOXIC SIGNS AND SYMPTOMS OF A POTENTIAL HEMATOLOGIC PROBLEM, SUCH AS FEVER, SORE THROAT, ULCERS IN THE MOUTH, EASY BRUISING, PETECHIAL OR PURPURIC HEMORRHAGE, AND SHOULD BE ADVISED TO DISCONTINUE THE DRUG AND TO REPORT TO THE PHYSICIAN IMMEDIATELY IF ANY SUCH SIGNS OR SYMPTOMS APPEAR.

This drug is not a simple analgesic and should not be used for the relief of trivial aches or pains. Treatment of epilepsy should be restricted to those classifications listed under "INDICATIONS AND USAGE."

Before prescribing Tegretol, the physician should be thoroughly familiar with the details of this prescribing information, particularly regarding use with other drugs, especially those which accentuate toxicity potential.

DESCRIPTION

Tegretol, carbamazepine USP, is an anticonvulsant and specific analgesic for trigeminal neuralgia, available as chewable tablets of 100 mg and tablets of 200 mg for oral administration. Its chemical name is 5H-dibenz[b,f]azepine-5-carboxamide.

Carbamazepine USP is a white to off-white powder, practically insoluble in water and soluble in alcohol and in acetone. Its molecular weight is 236.27.

Inactive Ingredients: Colloidal silicon dioxide, FD&C Red No. 3 (chewable tablets only), FD&C Red No. 40 (200-mg tablet only), flavoring (chewable tablets only), gelatin, glycerin, magnesium stearate, sodium starch glycolate (chewable tablets only), starch, stearic acid, and sucrose (chewable tablets only).

CLINICAL PHARMACOLOGY

In controlled clinical trials, Tegretol has been shown to be effective in the treatment of psychomotor and grand mal seizures, as well as trigeminal neuralgia.

It has demonstrated anticonvulsant properties in rats and mice with electrically and chemically induced seizures. It appears to act by reducing polysynaptic responses and blocking the posttetanic potentiation. Tegretol greatly reduces or abolishes pain induced by stimulation of the infraorbital nerve in cats and rats. It depresses thalamic potential and bulbar and polysynaptic reflexes, including the linguomandibular reflex in cats. Tegretol is chemically unrelated to other anticonvulsants or other drugs used to control the pain of trigeminal neuralgia. The mechanism of action remains unknown.

Tegretol tablets are adequately absorbed after oral administration at a slower rate than a solution, thus avoiding undesirably high peak concentrations. Tegretol in blood is 76% bound to plasma proteins. Plasma levels of Tegretol are variable and may range from 0.5–25 μg/ml, with no apparent relationship to the daily intake of the drug. Usual adult therapeutic levels are between 4 and 12 μg/ml. Following oral administration, serum levels peak at 4 to 5 hours. The CSF/serum ratio is 0.22, similar to the 22% unbound Tegretol in serum. Because Tegretol may induce its own metabolism, the half-life is also variable. Initial half-life values range from 25–65 hours, with 12–17 hours on repeated doses. Tegretol is metabolized in the liver. After oral administration of ^{14}C-carbamazepine, 72% of the administered radioactivity was found in the urine and 28% in the feces. This urinary radioactivity was composed largely of hydroxylated and conjugated metabolites, with only 3% of unchanged Tegretol. Transplacental passage of Tegretol is rapid (30 to 60 minutes), and the drug is accumulated in fetal tissues, with higher levels found in liver and kidney than in brain and lungs.

INDICATIONS AND USAGE

Epilepsy: Tegretol is indicated for the following conditions in patients who have not responded satisfactorily to treatment with other agents such as phenytoin, phenobarbital, or primidone:

1. Partial seizures with complex symptomatology (psychomotor, temporal lobe). Patients with these seizures appear to show greater improvement than those with other types.
2. Generalized tonic-clonic seizures (grand mal).
3. Mixed seizure patterns which include the above, or other partial or generalized seizures.

Absence seizures (petit mal) do not appear to be controlled by Tegretol (see **PRECAUTIONS General**).

Because of the necessity for frequent laboratory evaluation for potentially serious side effects, Tegretol is not recommended as the drug of first choice in seizure disorders. It should be reserved for patients whose seizures are difficult to control or patients experiencing marked side effects (e.g., excessive sedation).

Trigeminal Neuralgia: Tegretol is indicated in the treatment of the pain associated with true trigeminal neuralgia. Beneficial results have also been reported in glossopharyngeal neuralgia.

CONTRAINDICATIONS

Tegretol should not be used in patients with a history of previous bone marrow depression, hypersensitivity to the drug, or known sensitivity to any of the tricyclic compounds, such as amitriptyline, desipramine, imipramine, protriptyline, nortriptyline, etc. Likewise, on theoretical grounds its use with monoamine oxidase inhibitors is not recommended. Before administration of Tegretol, MAO inhibitors should be discontinued for a minimum of fourteen days, or longer if the clinical situation permits.

WARNINGS

The drug should be discontinued if evidence of significant bone marrow depression occurs, as follows:

1)	Erythrocytes	less than 4,000,000/cu mm
	Hematocrit	less than 32%
	Hemoglobin	less than 11 gm/100 ml
2)	Leukocytes	less than 4000/cu mm
3)	Platelets	less than 100,000/cu mm
4)	Reticulocytes	less than 0.3% (20,000/cu mm)
5)	Serum iron	greater than 150 μg/100 ml

Patients with a history of adverse hematologic reaction to any drug may be particularly at risk.

Severe dermatologic reactions including toxic epidermal necrolysis (Lyell's syndrome) and Stevens-Johnson syndrome, have been reported with Tegretol. These reactions have been extremely rare. However, a few fatalities have been reported.

Tegretol has shown mild anticholinergic activity; therefore, patients with increased intraocular pressure should be closely observed during therapy.

Because of the relationship of the drug to other tricyclic compounds, the possibility of activation of a latent psychosis and, in elderly patients, of confusion or agitation should be borne in mind.

PRECAUTIONS

General: Before initiating therapy, a detailed history and physical examination should be made.

Tegretol should be used with caution in patients with a mixed seizure disorder that includes atypical absence seizures, since in these patients Tegretol has been associated with increased frequency of generalized convulsions (see **INDICATIONS AND USAGE**).

Therapy should be prescribed only after critical benefit-to-risk appraisal in patients with a history of cardiac, hepatic or renal damage, adverse hematologic reaction to other drugs, or interrupted courses of therapy with Tegretol.

Information for Patients: Since dizziness and drowsiness may occur, patients should be cautioned about the hazards of operating machinery or automobiles or engaging in other potentially dangerous tasks.

Laboratory Tests: Complete pretreatment blood counts, including platelets and possibly reticulocytes and serum iron, should be obtained. Any significant abnormalities should rule out use of the drug. These same tests should be repeated at frequent intervals, possibly weekly, during the first three months of therapy and monthly thereafter for at least two to three years.

Baseline and periodic evaluations of liver function, particularly in patients with a history of liver disease, must be performed during treatment with this drug since liver damage may occur. The drug should be discontinued immediately in cases of aggravated liver dysfunction or active liver disease.

Baseline and periodic eye examinations, including slit-lamp, funduscopy and tonometry, are recommended since many phenothiazines and related drugs have been shown to cause eye changes.

Baseline and periodic complete urinalysis and BUN determinations are recommended for patients treated with this agent because of observed renal dysfunction.

Monitoring of blood levels (see **CLINICAL PHARMACOLOGY**) has increased the efficacy and safety of anticonvulsants. This monitoring may be particularly useful in cases of dramatic increase in seizure frequency and for verification of compliance. In addition, measurement of drug serum levels may aid in determining the cause of toxicity when more than one medication is being used.

Thyroid function tests have been reported to show decreased values with Tegretol administered alone.

Drug Interactions: The simultaneous administration of phenobarbital, phenytoin, or primidone, or a combination of two, produces a marked lowering of serum levels of Tegretol. The half-lives of phenytoin, warfarin, doxycycline, and theophylline were significantly shortened when administered concurrently with Tegretol. Haloperidol serum levels may be reduced when the drug is administered with Tegretol. The doses of these drugs may therefore have to be increased when Tegretol is added to the therapeutic regime.

Concomitant administration of Tegretol with erythromycin, cimetidine, propoxyphene, isoniazid or calcium channel blockers has been reported to result in elevated plasma levels of carbamazepine resulting in toxicity in some cases. Also, concomitant administration of carbamazepine and lithium may increase the risk of neurotoxic side effects.

Alterations of thyroid function have been reported in combination therapy with other anticonvulsant medications.

Breakthrough bleeding has been reported among patients receiving concomitant oral contraceptives and their reliability may be adversely affected.

Carcinogenicity, Mutagenesis, Impairment of Fertility: Carbamazepine, when administered to Sprague-Dawley rats for two years in the diet at doses of 25, 75, and 250 mg/kg/day, resulted in a dose-related increase in the incidence of hepatocellular tumors in females and of benign interstitial cell adenomas in the testes of males.

Carbamazepine must, therefore, be considered to be carcinogenic in Sprague-Dawley rats. Bacterial and mammalian mutagenicity studies using carbamazepine produced negative results. The significance of these findings relative to the use of carbamazepine in humans is, at present, unknown.

Pregnancy Category C: Tegretol has been shown to have adverse effects in reproduction studies in rats when given orally in dosages 10–25 times the maximum human daily dosage of 1200 mg. In rat teratology studies, 2 of 135 offspring showed kinked ribs at 250 mg/kg and 4 of 119 offspring at 650 mg/kg showed other anomalies (cleft palate, 1; talipes, 1; anophthalmos, 2). In reproduction studies in rats, nursing offspring demonstrated a lack of weight gain and an unkempt appearance at a maternal dosage level of 200 mg/kg.

There are no adequate and well-controlled studies in pregnant women. Tegretol should be used during pregnancy only if the potential benefit justifies the potential risk to the fetus.

It is important to note that anticonvulsant drugs should not be discontinued in patients in whom the drug is administered to prevent major seizures because of the strong possibility of precipitating status epilepticus with attendant hypoxia and threat to life. In individual cases where the severity and frequency of the seizure disorder are such that removal of medication does not pose a serious threat to the patient, discontinuation of the drug may be considered prior to and during pregnancy, although it cannot be said with any confidence that even minor seizures do not pose some hazard to the developing embryo or fetus.

Labor and Delivery: The effect of Tegretol on human labor and delivery is unknown.

Nursing Mothers: During lactation, concentration of Tegretol in milk is approximately 60% of the maternal plasma concentration.

Because of the potential for serious adverse reactions in nursing infants from carbamazepine, a decision should be made whether to discontinue nursing or to discontinue the drug, taking into account the importance of the drug to the mother.

Pediatric Use: Safety and effectiveness in children below the age of 6 years have not been established.

ADVERSE REACTIONS

If adverse reactions are of such severity that the drug must be discontinued, the physician must be aware that abrupt discontinuation of any anticonvulsant drug in a responsive epileptic patient may lead to seizures or even status epilepticus with its life-threatening hazards.

The most severe adverse reactions have been observed in the hemopoietic system (see boxed **WARNING**), the skin and the cardiovascular system.

The most frequently observed adverse reactions, particularly during the initial phases of therapy, are dizziness, drowsiness, unsteadiness, nausea, and vomiting. To minimize the possibility of such reactions, therapy should be initiated at the low dosage recommended.

The following additional adverse reactions have been reported:

Hemopoietic System: Aplastic anemia, agranulocytosis, thrombocytopenia, leukopenia, leukocytosis, eosinophilia.

Skin: Pruritic and erythematous rashes, urticaria, toxic epidermal necrolysis (Lyell's syndrome) (see **WARNINGS**), Stevens-Johnson syndrome (see **WARNINGS**), photosensitivity reactions, alterations in skin pigmentation, exfoliative dermatitis, erythema multiforme and nodosum, purpura, aggravation of disseminated lupus erythematosus, alopecia, and diaphoresis. In certain cases, discontinuation of therapy may be necessary.

Cardiovascular System: Congestive heart failure, edema, aggravation of hypertension, hypotension, syncope and collapse, aggravation of coronary artery disease, arrhythmias and AV block, primary thrombophlebitis, recurrence of thrombophlebitis, and adenopathy or lymphadenopathy.

Some of these cardiovascular complications have resulted in fatalities. Myocardial infarction has been associated with other tricyclic compounds.

Liver: Abnormalities in liver function tests, cholestatic and hepatocellular jaundice, hepatitis.

Respiratory System: Pulmonary hypersensitivity characterized by fever, dyspnea, pneumonitis or pneumonia.

Genitourinary System: Urinary frequency, acute urinary retention, oliguria with elevated blood pressure, azotemia, renal failure, and impotence. Albuminuria, glycosuria, elevated BUN and microscopic deposits in the urine have also been reported.

Testicular atrophy occurred in rats receiving Tegretol orally from 4 to 52 weeks at dosage levels of 50 to 400 mg/kg/day. Additionally, rats receiving Tegretol in the diet for two years at dosage levels of 25, 75, and 250 mg/kg/day had a dose-related incidence of testicular atrophy and aspermatogenesis. In dogs, it produced a brownish discoloration, presumably a metabolite, in the urinary bladder at dosage levels of 50 mg/kg and higher. Relevance of these findings to humans is unknown.

Nervous System: Dizziness, drowsiness, disturbances of coordination, confusion, headache, fatigue, blurred vision, visual hallucinations, transient diplopia, oculomotor disturbances, nystagmus, speech disturbances, abnormal involuntary movements, peripheral neuritis and paresthesias, depression with agitation, talkativeness, tinnitus, and hyperacusis.

There have been reports of associated paralysis and other symptoms of cerebral arterial insufficiency, but the exact relationship of these reactions to the drug has not been established.

Digestive System: Nausea, vomiting, gastric distress and abdominal pain, diarrhea, constipation, anorexia, and dryness of the mouth and pharynx, including glossitis and stomatitis.

Eyes: Scattered, punctate, cortical lens opacities, as well as conjunctivitis have been reported. Although a direct causal relationship has not been established, many phenothiazines and related drugs have been shown to cause eye changes.

Musculoskeletal System: Aching joints and muscles and leg cramps.

Metabolism: Fever and chills. Inappropriate antidiuretic hormone (ADH) secretion syndrome has been reported.

DRUG ABUSE AND DEPENDENCE

No evidence of abuse potential has been associated with Tegretol, nor is there evidence of psychological or physical dependence in humans.

OVERDOSAGE

Acute Toxicity: Lowest known lethal dose: adults, >60 g (39-year-old man).

Highest known doses survived: adults, 30 g (31-year-old woman); children, 10 g (6-year-old boy); small children, 5 g (3-year-old girl).

Oral LD_{50} in animals (mg/kg); mice, 1100–3750; rats, 3850–4025; rabbits, 1500–2680; guinea pigs, 920.

Signs and Symptoms:

The first signs and symptoms appear after 1–3 hours. Neuromuscular disturbances are the most prominent. Cardiovascular disorders are generally milder, and severe cardiac complications occur only when very high doses (>60 g) have been ingested.

Respiration: Irregular breathing, respiratory depression.

Cardiovascular System: Tachycardia, hypotension or hypertension, shock, conduction disorders.

Nervous System and Muscles: Impairment of consciousness ranging in severity to deep coma. Convulsions, especially in small children. Motor restlessness, muscular twitching, tremor, athetoid movements, opisthotonos, ataxia, drowsiness, dizziness, mydriasis, nystagmus, adiadochokinesia, ballism, psychomotor disturbances, dysmetria. Initial hyperreflexia, followed by hyporeflexia.

Gastrointestinal Tract: Nausea, vomiting.

Kidneys and Bladder: Anuria or oliguria, urinary retention.

Laboratory Findings: Isolated instances of overdosage have included leukocytosis, reduced leukocyte count, glycosuria and acetonuria. EEG may show dysrhythmias.

Combined Poisoning: When alcohol, tricyclic antidepressants, barbiturates or hydantoins are taken at the same time, the signs and symptoms of acute poisoning with Tegretol may be aggravated or modified.

Treatment:

The prognosis in cases of severe poisoning is critically dependent upon prompt elimination of the drug, which may be achieved by inducing vomiting, irrigating the stomach, and by taking appropriate steps to diminish absorption. If these measures cannot be implemented without risk on the spot, the patient should be transferred at once to a hospital, while ensuring that vital functions are safeguarded. There is no specific antidote.

Elimination of the Drug: Induction of vomiting.

Gastric lavage. Even when more than 4 hours have elapsed following ingestion of the drug, the stomach should be repeatedly irrigated, especially if the patient has also consumed alcohol.

Measures to Reduce Absorption: Activated charcoal, laxatives.

Measures to Accelerate Elimination: Forced diuresis.

Dialysis is indicated only in severe poisoning associated with renal failure. Replacement transfusion is indicated in severe poisoning in small children.

Respiratory Depression: Keep the airways free; resort, if necessary, to endotracheal intubation, artificial respiration, and administration of oxygen.

Hypotension, Shock: Keep the patient's legs raised and administer a plasma expander. If blood pressure fails to rise despite measures taken to increase plasma volume, use of vasoactive substances should be considered.

Convulsions: Diazepam or barbiturates.

Warning: Diazepam or barbiturates may aggravate respiratory depression (especially in children), hypotension, and coma. However, barbiturates should not be used if drugs that inhibit monoamine oxidase have also been taken by the patient either in overdosage or in recent therapy (within one week).

Surveillance: Respiration, cardiac function (ECG monitoring), blood pressure, body temperature, pupillary reflexes, and kidney and bladder function should be monitored for several days.

Treatment of Blood Count Abnormalities: If evidence of bone marrow depression develops, the following recommendations are suggested: 1) stop the drug, (2) perform daily CBC, platelet and reticulocyte counts, (3) do a bone marrow

Continued on next page

Geigy—Cont.

aspiration and trephine biopsy immediately and repeat with sufficient frequency to monitor recovery.
Special periodic studies might be helpful as follows: (1) white cell and platelet antibodies, (2) ^{59}Fe—ferrokinetic studies, (3) peripheral blood cell typing, (4) cytogenetic studies on marrow and peripheral blood, (5) bone marrow culture studies for colony-forming units, (6) hemoglobin electrophoresis for A_2 and F hemoglobin, and (7) serum folic acid and B_{12} levels.
A fully developed aplastic anemia will require appropriate, intensive monitoring and therapy, for which specialized consultation should be sought.

DOSAGE AND ADMINISTRATION

Monitoring of blood levels has increased the efficacy and safety of anticonvulsants (see **PRECAUTIONS Laboratory Tests**). Dosage should be adjusted to the needs of the individual patient. A low initial daily dosage with a gradual increase is advised. As soon as adequate control is achieved, the dosage may be reduced very gradually to the minimum effective level. Tablets should be taken with meals.

Epilepsy (see **INDICATIONS AND USAGE**)
Adults and children over 12 years of age—Initial: 200 mg b.i.d. Increase at weekly intervals by adding up to 200 mg per day using a t.i.d. or q.i.d. regimen until the best response is obtained. Dosage should generally not exceed 1000 mg daily in children 12 to 15 years of age, and 1200 mg daily in patients above 15 years of age. Doses up to 1600 mg daily have been used in adults in rare instances. ***Maintenance:*** Adjust dosage to the minimum effective level, usually 800–1200 mg daily.
Children 6–12 years of age—Initial: 100 mg b.i.d. Increase at weekly intervals by adding 100 mg per day using a t.i.d. or q.i.d. regimen until the best response is obtained. Dosage should generally not exceed 1000 mg. ***Maintenance:*** Adjust dosage to the minimum effective level, usually 400–800 mg daily.
Combination Therapy: Tegretol may be used alone or with other anticonvulsants. When added to existing anticonvulsant therapy, the drug should be added gradually while the other anticonvulsants are maintained or gradually decreased, except phenytoin, which may have to be increased. (see **PRECAUTIONS Drug Interactions**).

Trigeminal Neuralgia (see **INDICATIONS AND USAGE**)
Initial: 100 mg b.i.d. on the first day for a total daily dose of 200 mg. This daily dose may be increased by up to 200 mg a day using increments of 100 mg every 12 hours only as needed to achieve freedom from pain. Do not exceed 1200 mg daily.
Maintenance: Control of pain can be maintained in most patients with 400 mg to 800 mg daily. However, some patients may be maintained on as little as 200 mg daily, while others may require as much as 1200 mg daily. At least once every 3 months throughout the treatment period, attempts should be made to reduce the dose to the minimum effective level or even to discontinue the drug.

HOW SUPPLIED

Chewable Tablets 100 mg—round, red-speckled, pink, single-scored (imprinted Tegretol on one side and 52 twice on the scored side)
Bottles of 100 .... NDC 0028-0052-01
Unit Dose (blister pack)
Box of 100
(strips of 10) .... NDC 0028-0052-61
Tablets 200 mg—capsule-shaped, pink, single-scored (imprinted Tegretol on one side and 27 twice on the scored side)
Bottles of 100 .... NDC 0028-0027-01
Bottles of 1000 .... NDC 0028-0027-10
Gy-Pak®—One Unit
12 bottles—100 tablets each .... NDC 0028-0027-65
Unit Dose (blister pack)
Box of 100
(strips of 10) .... NDC 0028-0027-61
Protect from moisture.
Dispense in tight container (USP).

C86-33 (Rev. 6/86)

Shown in Product Identification Section, page 409

TOFRANIL® ℞

[toe-fray'nill]
imipramine hydrochloride USP
Ampuls, 2 cc
For intramuscular administration

Each 2 cc ampul contains: imipramine hydrochloride USP, 25 mg; ascorbic acid, 2 mg; sodium bisulfite, 1 mg; sodium sulfite, anhydrous, 1 mg

DESCRIPTION

Tofranil, imipramine hydrochloride USP, the original tricyclic antidepressant, is a member of the dibenzazepine group of compounds. It is designated 5-[3-(Dimethylamino)propyl]-10, 11-dihydro- 5H-dibenz[b,f] azepine Monohydrochloride.
Imipramine hydrochloride USP is a white to off-white, odorless, or practically odorless crystalline powder. It is freely soluble in water and in alcohol, soluble in acetone, and insoluble in ether and in benzene. Its molecular weight is 316.87.

CLINICAL PHARMACOLOGY

The mechanism of action of Tofranil is not definitely known. However, it does not act primarily by stimulation of the central nervous system. The clinical effect is hypothesized as being due to potentiation of adrenergic synapses by blocking uptake of norepinephrine at nerve endings.

INDICATIONS

Depression: For the relief of symptoms of depression. Endogenous depression is more likely to be alleviated than other depressive states. One to three weeks of treatment may be needed before optimal therapeutic effects are evident.

CONTRAINDICATIONS

The concomitant use of monoamine oxidase inhibiting compounds is contraindicated. Hyperpyretic crises or severe convulsive seizures may occur in patients receiving such combinations. The potentiation of adverse effects can be serious, or even fatal. When it is desired to substitute Tofranil in patients receiving a monoamine oxidase inhibitor, as long an interval should elapse as the clinical situation will allow, with a minimum of 14 days. Initial dosage should be low and increases should be gradual and cautiously prescribed.
The drug is contraindicated during the acute recovery period after a myocardial infarction. Patients with a known hypersensitivity to this compound should not be given the drug. The possibility of cross-sensitivity to other dibenzazepine compounds should be kept in mind.

WARNINGS

Children: A dose of 2.5 mg/kg/day of imipramine hydrochloride should not be exceeded in childhood. ECG changes of unknown significance have been reported in pediatric patients with doses twice this amount.
Extreme caution should be used when this drug is given to:
patients with cardiovascular disease because of the possibility of conduction defects, arrhythmias, congestive heart failure, myocardial infarction, strokes and tachycardia. These patients require cardiac surveillance at all dosage levels of the drug;
patients with increased intraocular pressure, history of urinary retention, or history of narrow-angle glaucoma because of the drug's anticholinergic properties;
hyperthyroid patients or those on thyroid medication because of the possibility of cardiovascular toxicity;
patients with a history of seizure disorder because this drug has been shown to lower the seizure threshold;
patients receiving guanethidine, clonidine, or similar agents, since imipramine hydrochloride may block the pharmacologic effects of these drugs;
patients receiving methylphenidate hydrochloride. Since methylphenidate hydrochloride may inhibit the metabolism of imipramine hydrochloride, downward dosage adjustment of imipramine hydrochloride may be required when given concomitantly with methylphenidate hydrochloride.
Tofranil may enhance the CNS depressant effects of alcohol. Therefore, it should be borne in mind that the dangers inherent in a suicide attempt or accidental overdosage with the drug may be increased for the patient who uses excessive amounts of alcohol. (See **PRECAUTIONS.**)
Since imipramine hydrochloride may impair the mental and/or physical abilities required for the performance of potentially hazardous tasks, such as operating an automobile or machinery, the patient should be cautioned accordingly.

PRECAUTIONS

An ECG recording should be taken prior to the initiation of larger-than-usual doses of imipramine hydrochloride and at appropriate intervals thereafter until steady state is achieved. (Patients with any evidence of cardiovascular disease require cardiac surveillance at all dosage levels of the drug. See **WARNINGS.**) Elderly patients and patients with cardiac disease or a prior history of cardiac disease are at special risk of developing the cardiac abnormalities associated with the use of imipramine hydrochloride.
It should be kept in mind that the possibility of suicide in seriously depressed patients is inherent in the illness and may persist until significant remission occurs. Such patients should be carefully supervised during the early phase of treatment with imipramine hydrochloride, and may require hospitalization. Prescriptions should be written for the smallest amount feasible.
Hypomanic or manic episodes may occur, particularly in patients with cyclic disorders.
Such reactions may necessitate discontinuation of the drug. If needed, imipramine hydrochloride may be resumed in lower dosage when these episodes are relieved.
Administration of a tranquilizer may be useful in controlling such episodes.
An activation of the psychosis may occasionally be observed in schizophrenic patients and may require reduction of dosage and the addition of a phenothiazine.
Concurrent administration of imipramine hydrochloride with electroshock therapy may increase the hazards; such treatment should be limited to those patients for whom it is essential, since there is limited clinical experience.
Usage During Pregnancy and Lactation:
Animal reproduction studies have yielded inconclusive results. (See also **Animal Pharmacology & Toxicology.**)
There have been no well-controlled studies conducted with pregnant women to determine the effect of imipramine hydrochloride on the fetus. However, there have been clinical reports of congenital malformations associated with the use of the drug. Although a causal relationship between these effects and the drug could not be established, the possibility of fetal risk from the maternal ingestion of imipramine hydrochloride cannot be excluded. Therefore, imipramine hydrochloride should be used in women who are or might become pregnant only if the clinical condition clearly justifies potential risk to the fetus.
Limited data suggest that imipramine hydrochloride is likely to be excreted in human breast milk. As a general rule, a woman taking a drug should not nurse since the possibility exists that the drug may be excreted in breast milk and be harmful to the child.
Usage in Children: The effectiveness of the drug in children for conditions other than nocturnal enuresis given orally has not been established.
Patients should be warned that imipramine hydrochloride may enhance the CNS depressant effects of alcohol. (See **WARNINGS.**)
Imipramine hydrochloride should be used with caution in patients with significantly impaired renal or hepatic function.
Patients who develop a fever and a sore throat during therapy with imipramine hydrochloride should have leukocyte and differential blood counts performed. Imipramine hydrochloride should be discontinued if there is evidence of pathological neutrophil depression.
Prior to elective surgery, imipramine hydrochloride should be discontinued for as long as the clinical situation will allow.
In occasional susceptible patients or in those receiving anticholinergic drugs (including antiparkinsonism agents) in addition, the atropine-like effects may become more pronounced (e.g., paralytic ileus).
Close supervision and careful adjustment of dosage is required when imipramine hydrochloride is administered concomitantly with anticholinergic drugs.
Avoid the use of preparations, such as decongestants and local anesthetics, which contain any sympathomimetic amine (e.g., epinephrine, norepinephrine), since it has been reported that tricyclic antidepressants can potentiate the effects of catecholamines.
Caution should be exercised when imipramine hydrochloride is used with agents that lower blood pressure.
Imipramine hydrochloride may potentiate the effects of CNS depressant drugs.
The plasma concentration of imipramine may increase when the drug is given concomitantly with cimetidine, and adjustment of the dosage of imipramine may therefore be necessary both when cimetidine therapy is initiated and when it is discontinued.
Patients taking imipramine hydrochloride should avoid excessive exposure to sunlight since there have been reports of photosensitization.
Both elevation and lowering of blood sugar levels have been reported with imipramine hydrochloride use.

ADVERSE REACTIONS

Note: Although the listing which follows includes a few adverse reactions which have not been reported with this specific drug, the pharmacological similarities among the tricyclic antidepressant drugs require that each of the reactions be considered when imipramine is administered.
Cardiovascular: Orthostatic hypotension, hypertension, tachycardia, palpitation, myocardial infarction, arrhythmias, heart block, ECG changes, precipitation of congestive heart failure, stroke.
Psychiatric: Confusional states (especially in the elderly) with hallucinations, disorientation, delusions; anxiety, restlessness, agitation; insomnia and nightmares; hypomania; exacerbation of psychosis.
Neurological: Numbness, tingling, paresthesias of extremities; incoordination, ataxia, tremors; peripheral neuropathy; extrapyramidal symptoms; seizures, alterations in EEG patterns; tinnitus.
Anticholinergic: Dry mouth, and, rarely, associated sublingual adenitis; blurred vision, disturbances of accommodation, mydriasis; constipation, paralytic ileus; urinary retention, delayed micturition, dilation of the urinary tract.
Allergic: Skin rash, petechiae, urticaria, itching, photosensitization; edema (general or of face and tongue); drug fever; cross-sensitivity with desipramine.

Hematologic: Bone marrow depression including agranulocytosis; eosinophilia; purpura; thrombocytopenia.
Gastrointestinal: Nausea and vomiting, anorexia, epigastric distress, diarrhea; peculiar taste, stomatitis, abdominal cramps, black tongue.
Endocrine: Gynecomastia in the male; breast enlargement and galactorrhea in the female; increased or decreased libido, impotence; testicular swelling; elevation or depression of blood sugar levels; inappropriate antidiuretic hormone (ADH) secretion syndrome.
Other: Jaundice (simulating obstructive); altered liver function; weight gain or loss; perspiration; flushing; urinary frequency; drowsiness; dizziness, weakness and fatigue; headache; parotid swelling; alopecia; proneness to falling.
Withdrawal Symptoms: Though not indicative of addiction, abrupt cessation of treatment after prolonged therapy may produce nausea, headache and malaise.

DOSAGE AND ADMINISTRATION

Initially, up to 100 mg/day intramuscularly in divided doses. Parenteral administration should be used only for starting therapy in patients unable or unwilling to use oral medication. The oral form should supplant the injectable as soon as possible.
Lower dosages are recommended for elderly patients and adolescents. Lower dosages are also recommended for outpatients as compared to hospitalized patients who will be under close supervision. Dosage should be initiated at a low level and increased gradually, noting carefully the clinical response and any evidence of intolerance. Following remission, oral maintenance medication may be required for a longer period of time, at the lowest dose that will maintain remission.

OVERDOSAGE

Children have been reported to be more sensitive than adults to an acute overdosage of imipramine hydrochloride. An acute overdose of any amount in infants or young children, especially, must be considered serious and potentially fatal.
Signs and Symptoms: These may vary in severity depending upon factors such as the amount of drug absorbed, the age of the patient, and the interval between drug ingestion and the start of treatment. Blood and urine levels of imipramine may not reflect the severity of poisoning; they have chiefly a qualitative rather than quantitative value, and are unreliable indicators in the clinical management of the patient.
CNS abnormalities may include drowsiness, stupor, coma, ataxia, restlessness, agitation, hyperactive reflexes, muscle rigidity, athetoid and choreiform movements, and convulsions.
Cardiac abnormalities may include arrhythmia, tachycardia, ECG evidence of impaired conduction, and signs of congestive failure.
Respiratory depression, cyanosis, hypotension, shock, vomiting, hyperpyrexia, mydriasis, and diaphoresis may also be present.
Treatment: Because CNS involvement, respiratory depression and cardiac arrhythmia can occur suddenly, hospitalization and close observation are necessary, even when the amount ingested is thought to be small or the initial degree of intoxication appears slight or moderate. All patients with ECG abnormalities should have continuous cardiac monitoring for at least 72 hours and be closely observed until well after cardiac status has returned to normal; relapses may occur after apparent recovery.
The *slow* intravenous administration of physostigmine salicylate has been reported to reverse most of the cardiovascular and CNS effects of overdosage with tricyclic antidepressants. In adults, 1 to 3 mg has been reported to be effective. In children, start with 0.5 mg and repeat at 5-minute intervals to determine the minimum effective dose; do not exceed 2 mg. Because of the short duration of action of physostigmine, repeat the effective dose at 30- to 60-minute intervals, as necessary. Avoid rapid injection to reduce the possibility of physostigmine-induced convulsions.
In the alert patient, empty the stomach promptly by induced emesis followed by lavage. In the obtunded patient, secure the airway with a cuffed endotracheal tube before beginning lavage (do not induce emesis). Continue lavage for 24 hours or longer, depending on the apparent severity of intoxication. Use normal or half-normal saline to avoid water intoxication, especially in children. Instillation of activated charcoal slurry may help reduce absorption of imipramine.
Minimize external stimulation to reduce the tendency to convulsions. If anticonvulsants are necessary, diazepam, short-acting barbiturates, paraldehyde or methocarbamol may be useful. Do not use barbiturates if MAO inhibitors have been taken recently.
Maintain adequate respiratory exchange. Do not use respiratory stimulants.
Shock should be treated with supportive measures, such as intravenous fluids, oxygen and corticosteroids. Digitalis may increase conduction abnormalities and further irritate an already sensitized myocardium. If congestive heart failure necessitates rapid digitalization, particular care must be exercised.
Hyperpyrexia should be controlled by whatever external means are available, including ice packs and cooling sponge baths, if necessary.
Hemodialysis, peritoneal dialysis, exchange transfusions and forced diuresis have been generally reported as ineffective because of the rapid fixation of imipramine in tissues. Blood and urine levels of imipramine may not correlate with the degree of intoxication, and are unreliable indicators in the clinical management of the patient.

HOW SUPPLIED

Ampuls 2 ml—For intramuscular administration only
25 mg imipramine hydrochloride, 2 mg ascorbic acid, 1 mg sodium bisulfite, 1 mg sodium sulfite
Boxes of 10 ....NDC 0028-0065-23
Note: Upon storage, minute crystals may form in some ampuls. This has no influence on the therapeutic efficacy of the preparation, and the crystals redissolve when the affected ampuls are immersed in hot tap water for 1 minute.

Animal Pharmacology & Toxicology:
A. *Acute:* Oral LD_{50} ranges are as follows:

Rat	355 to 682 mg/kg
Dog	100 to 215 mg/kg

Depending on the dosage in both species, toxic signs proceeded progressively from depression, irregular respiration and ataxia to convulsions and death.
B. *Reproduction/Teratogenic:* The overall evaluation may be summed up in the following manner:
Oral: Independent studies in three species (rat, mouse and rabbit) revealed that when Tofranil is administered orally in doses up to approximately 2½ times the maximum human dose in the first 2 species and up to 25 times the maximum human dose in the third species, the drug is essentially free from teratogenic potential. In the three species studied, only one instance of fetal abnormality occurred (in the rabbit) and in that study there was likewise an abnormality in the control group. However, evidence does exist from the rat studies that some systemic and embryotoxic potential is demonstrable. This is manifested by reduced litter size, a slight increase in the stillborn rate and a reduction in the mean birth weight.
Parenteral: In contradistinction to the oral data, Tofranil does exhibit a slight but definite teratogenic potential when administered by the subcutaneous route. Drug effects on both the mother and fetus in the rabbit are manifested in higher resorption rates and decrease in mean fetal birth weights, while teratogenic findings occurred at a level of 5 times the maximum human dose. In the mouse, teratogenicity occurred at 1½ and 6½ times the maximum human dose, but no teratogenic effects were seen at levels 3 times the maximum human dose. Thus, in the mouse, the findings are equivocal.

C85-68 (Rev. 11/85)

Dist. by:
GEIGY Pharmaceuticals
Division of CIBA-GEIGY Corporation
Ardsley, New York 10502

TOFRANIL®

℞

[toe-fray'nill]
imipramine hydrochloride USP
Tablets of 10 mg
Tablets of 25 mg
Tablets of 50 mg
For oral administration

DESCRIPTION

Tofranil, imipramine hydrochloride USP, the original tricyclic antidepressant, is a member of the dibenzazepine group of compounds. It is designated 5-[3-(Dimethylamino)propyl]-10, 11-dihydro-5H-dibenz[b,f] azepine monohydrochloride.
Imipramine hydrocloride USP is a white to off-white, odorless, or practically odorless crystalline powder. It is freely soluble in water and in alcohol, soluble in acetone, and insoluble in ether and in benzene. Its molecular weight is 316.87.
Inactive Ingredients. Calcium phosphate, cellulose compounds, docusate sodium, iron oxides, magnesium stearate, polyethylene glycol, povidone, sodium starch glycolate, sucrose, talc and titanium dioxide.

CLINICAL PHARMACOLOGY

The mechanism of action of Tofranil is not definitely known. However, it does not act primarily by stimulation of the central nervous system. The clinical effect is hypothesized as being due to potentiation of adrenergic synapses by blocking uptake of norepinephrine at nerve endings. The mode of action of the drug in controlling childhood enuresis is thought to be apart from its antidepressant effect.

INDICATIONS

Depression: For the relief of symptoms of depression. Endogenous depression is more likely to be alleviated than other depressive states. One to three weeks of treatment may be needed before optimal therapeutic effects are evident.
Childhood Enuresis: May be useful as temporary adjunctive therapy in reducing enuresis in children aged 6 years and older, after possible organic causes have been excluded by appropriate tests. In patients having daytime symptoms of frequency and urgency, examination should include voiding cystourethrography and cystoscopy, as necessary. The effectiveness of treatment may decrease with continued drug administration.

CONTRAINDICATIONS

The concomitant use of monoamine oxidase inhibiting compounds is contraindicated. Hyperpyretic crises or severe convulsive seizures may occur in patients receiving such combinations. The potentiation of adverse effects can be serious, or even fatal. When it is desired to substitute Tofranil in patients receiving a monoamine oxidase inhibitor, as long an interval should elapse as the clinical situation will allow, with a minimum of 14 days. Initial dosage should be low and increases should be gradual and cautiously prescribed.
The drug is contraindicated during the acute recovery period after a myocardial infarction. Patients with a known hypersensitivity to this compound should not be given the drug. The possibility of cross-sensitivity to other dibenzazepine compounds should be kept in mind.

WARNINGS

Children: A dose of 2.5 mg/kg/day of Tofranil should not be exceeded in childhood. ECG changes of unknown significance have been reported in pediatric patients with doses twice this amount.
Extreme caution should be used when this drug is given to:
patients with cardiovascular disease because of the possibility of conduction defects, arrhythmias, congestive heart failure, myocardial infarction, strokes and tachycardia. These patients require cardiac surveillance at all dosage levels of the drug;
patients with increased intraocular pressure, history of urinary retention, or history of narrow-angle glaucoma because of the drug's anticholinergic properties;
hyperthyroid patients or those on thyroid medication because of the possibility of cardiovascular toxicity;
patients with a history of seizure disorder because this drug has been shown to lower the seizure threshold;
patients receiving guanethidine, clonidine, or similar agents, since Tofranil may block the pharmacologic effects of these drugs;
patients receiving methylphenidate hydrochloride. Since methylphenidate hydrochloride may inhibit the metabolism of Tofranil, downward dosage adjustment of imipramine hydrochloride may be required when given concomitantly with methylphenidate hydrochloride.
Tofranil may enhance the CNS depressant effects of alcohol. Therefore, it should be borne in mind that the dangers inherent in a suicide attempt or accidental overdosage with the drug may be increased for the patient who uses excessive amounts of alcohol. (See **PRECAUTIONS.**)
Since Tofranil may impair the mental and/or physical abilities required for the performance of potentially hazardous tasks, such as operating an automobile or machinery, the patient should be cautioned accordingly.

PRECAUTIONS

An ECG recording should be taken prior to the initiation of larger-than-usual doses of Tofranil and at appropriate intervals thereafter until steady state is achieved. (Patients with any evidence of cardiovascular disease require cardiac surveillance at all dosage levels of the drug. See **Warnings.**) Elderly patients and patients with cardiac disease or a prior history of cardiac disease are at special risk of developing the cardiac abnormalities associated with the use of Tofranil.
It should be kept in mind that the possibility of suicide in seriously depressed patients is inherent in the illness and may persist until significant remission occurs. Such patients should be carefully supervised during the early phase of treatment with Tofranil, and may require hospitalization. Prescriptions should be written for the smallest amount feasible.
Hypomanic or manic episodes may occur, particularly in patients with cyclic disorders. Such reactions may necessitate discontinuation of the drug. If needed, Tofranil may be resumed in lower dosage when these episodes are relieved. Administration of a tranquilizer may be useful in controlling such episodes.
An activation of the psychosis may occasionally be observed in schizophrenic patients and may require reduction of dosage and the addition of a phenothiazine.
Concurrent administration of Tofranil with electroshock therapy may increase the hazards; such treatment should be limited to those patients for whom it is essential, since there is limited clinical experience.

Continued on next page

The full prescribing information for each GEIGY drug is contained herein and is that in effect as of September 1, 1986

Geigy—Cont.

Usage During Pregnancy and Lactation:
Animal reproduction studies have yielded inconclusive results. (See also **Animal Pharmacology & Toxicology.**)
There have been no well-controlled studies conducted with pregnant women to determine the effect of Tofranil on the fetus. However, there have been clinical reports of congenital malformations associated with the use of the drug. Although a causal relationship between these effects and the drug could not be established, the possibility of fetal risk from the maternal ingestion of Tofranil cannot be excluded. Therefore, Tofranil should be used in women who are or might become pregnant only if the clinical condition clearly justifies potential risk to the fetus.
Limited data suggest that Tofranil is likely to be excreted in human breast milk. As a general rule, a woman taking a drug should not nurse since the possibility exists that the drug may be excreted in breast milk and be harmful to the child.
Usage in Children: The effectiveness of the drug in children for conditions other than nocturnal enuresis has not been established.
The safety and effectiveness of the drug as temporary adjunctive therapy for nocturnal enuresis in children less than 6 years of age has not been established.
The safety of the drug for long-term, chronic use as adjunctive therapy for nocturnal enuresis in children 6 years of age or older has not been established; consideration should be given to instituting a drug-free period following an adequate therapeutic trial with a favorable response.
A dose of 2.5 mg/kg/day should not be exceeded in childhood. ECG changes of unknown significance have been reported in pediatric patients with doses twice this amount.
Patients should be warned that Tofranil may enhance the CNS depressant effects of alcohol. (See **WARNINGS.**)
Tofranil should be used with caution in patients with significantly impaired renal or hepatic function.
Patients who develop a fever and a sore throat during therapy with Tofranil should have leukocyte and differential blood counts performed. Tofranil should be discontinued if there is evidence of pathological neutrophil depression.
Prior to elective surgery, Tofranil should be discontinued for as long as the clinical situation will allow.
In occasional susceptible patients or in those receiving anticholinergic drugs (including antiparkinsonism agents) in addition, the atropine-like effects may become more pronounced (e.g., paralytic ileus).
Close supervision and careful adjustment of dosage is required when Tofranil is administered concomitantly with anticholinergic drugs.
Avoid the use of preparations, such as decongestants and local anesthetics, which contain any sympathomimetic amine (e.g., epinephrine, norepinephrine), since it has been reported that tricyclic antidepressants can potentiate the effects of catecholamines.
Caution should be exercised when Tofranil is used with agents that lower blood pressure.
Tofranil may potentiate the effects of CNS depressant drugs.
The plasma concentration of Tofranil may increase when the drug is given concomitantly with cimetidine, and adjustment of the dosage of Tofranil may therefore be necessary both when cimetidine therapy is initiated and when it is discontinued.
Patients taking Tofranil should avoid excessive exposure to sunlight since there have been reports of photosensitization.
Both elevation and lowering of blood sugar levels have been reported with Tofranil use.

ADVERSE REACTIONS

Note: Although the listing which follows includes a few adverse reactions which have not been reported with this specific drug, the pharmacological similarities among the tricyclic antidepressant drugs require that each of the reactions be considered when Tofranil is administered.
Cardiovascular: Orthostatic hypotension, hypertension, tachycardia, palpitation, myocardial infarction, arrhythmias, heart block, ECG changes, precipitation of congestive heart failure, stroke.
Psychiatric: Confusional states (especially in the elderly) with hallucinations, disorientation, delusions; anxiety, restlessness, agitation; insomnia and nightmares; hypomania; exacerbation of psychosis.
Neurological: Numbness, tingling, paresthesias of extremities; incoordination, ataxia, tremors; peripheral neuropathy; extrapyramidal symptoms; seizures, alterations in EEG patterns; tinnitus.
Anticholinergic: Dry mouth, and, rarely, associated sublingual adenitis; blurred vision, disturbances of accommodation, mydriasis; constipation, paralytic ileus; urinary retention, delayed micturition, dilation of the urinary tract.
Allergic: Skin rash, petechiae, urticaria, itching, photosensitization; edema (general or of face and tongue); drug fever; cross-sensitivity with desipramine.
Hematologic: Bone marrow depression including agranulocytosis; eosinophilia; purpura; thrombocytopenia.
Gastrointestinal: Nausea and vomiting, anorexia, epigastric distress, diarrhea; peculiar taste, stomatitis, abdominal cramps, black tongue.
Endocrine: Gynecomastia in the male; breast enlargement and galactorrhea in the female; increased or decreased libido, impotence; testicular swelling; elevation or depression of blood sugar levels; inappropriate antidiuretic hormone (ADH) secretion syndrome.
Other: Jaundice (simulating obstructive); altered liver function; weight gain or loss; perspiration; flushing; urinary frequency; drowsiness; dizziness, weakness and fatigue; headache; parotid swelling; alopecia; proneness to falling.
Withdrawal Symptoms: Though not indicative of addiction, abrupt cessation of treatment after prolonged therapy may produce nausea, headache and malaise.
Note: In enuretic children treated with imipramine hydrochloride the most common adverse reactions have been nervousness, sleep disorders, tiredness, and mild gastrointestinal disturbances. These usually disappear during continued drug administration or when dosage is decreased. Other reactions which have been reported include constipation, convulsions, anxiety, emotional instability, syncope, and collapse. All of the adverse reactions reported with adult use should be considered.

DOSAGE AND ADMINISTRATION

Depression: Lower dosages are recommended for elderly patients and adolescents. Lower dosages are also recommended for outpatients as compared to hospitalized patients who will be under close supervision. Dosage should be initiated at a low level and increased gradually, noting carefully the clinical response and any evidence of intolerance. Following remission, maintenance medication may be required for a longer period of time, at the lowest dose that will maintain remission.
Usual Adult Dose:
Hospitalized patients— Initially, 100 mg/day in divided doses gradually increased to 200 mg/day as required. If no response after two weeks, increase to 250–300 mg/day.
Outpatients—Initially, 75 mg/day increased to 150 mg/day. Dosages over 200 mg/day are not recommended. Maintenance, 50–150 mg/day.
Adolescent and geriatric patients—Initially, 30–40 mg/day; it is generally not necessary to exceed 100 mg/day.
Childhood Enuresis: Initially, an oral dose of 25 mg/day should be tried in children aged 6 and older. Medication should be given one hour before bedtime. If a satisfactory response does not occur within one week, increase the dose to 50 mg nightly in children under 12 years; children over 12 may receive up to 75 mg nightly. A daily dose greater than 75 mg does not enhance efficacy and tends to increase side effects. Evidence suggests that in early night bedwetters, the drug is more effective given earlier and in divided amounts, i.e., 25 mg in midafternoon, repeated at bedtime. Consideration should be given to instituting a drug-free period following an adequate therapeutic trial with a favorable response. Dosage should be tapered off gradually rather than abruptly discontinued; this may reduce the tendency to relapse. Children who relapse when the drug is discontinued do not always respond to a subsequent course of treatment.
A dose of 2.5 mg/kg/day should not be exceeded. ECG changes of unknown significance have been reported in pediatric patients with doses twice this amount.
The safety and effectiveness of Tofranil as temporary adjunctive therapy for nocturnal enuresis in children less than 6 years of age has not been established.

OVERDOSAGE

Children have been reported to be more sensitive than adults to an acute overdosage of imipramine hydrochloride. An acute overdose of any amount in infants or young children, especially, must be considered serious and potentially fatal.
Signs and Symptoms: These may vary in severity depending upon factors such as the amount of drug absorbed, the age of the patient, and the interval between drug ingestion and the start of treatment. Blood and urine levels of Tofranil may not reflect the severity of poisoning; they have chiefly a qualitative rather than quantitative value, and are unreliable indicators in the clinical management of the patient.
CNS abnormalities may include drowsiness, stupor, coma, ataxia, restlessness, agitation, hyperactive reflexes, muscle rigidity, athetoid and choreiform movements, and convulsions.
Cardiac abnormalities may include arrhythmia, tachycardia, ECG evidence of impaired conduction, and signs of congestive failure.
Respiratory depression, cyanosis, hypotension, shock, vomiting, hyperpyrexia, mydriasis, and diaphoresis may also be present.
Treatment: Because CNS involvement, respiratory depression and cardiac arrhythmia can occur suddenly, hospitalization and close observation are necessary, even when the amount ingested is thought to be small or the initial degree of intoxication appears slight or moderate. All patients with ECG abnormalities should have continuous cardiac monitoring for at least 72 hours and be closely observed until well after cardiac status has returned to normal; relapses may occur after apparent recovery.
The *slow* intravenous administration of physostigmine salicylate has been reported to reverse most of the cardiovascular and CNS effects of overdosage with tricyclic antidepressants. In adults, 1 to 3 mg has been reported to be effective. In children, start with 0.5 mg and repeat at 5-minute intervals to determine the minimum effective dose; do not exceed 2 mg. Because of the short duration of action of physostigmine, repeat the effective dose at 30- to 60-minute intervals, as necessary. Avoid rapid injection to reduce the possibility of physostigmine-induced convulsions.
In the alert patient, empty the stomach promptly by induced emesis followed by lavage. In the obtunded patient, secure the airway with a cuffed endotracheal tube before beginning lavage (do not induce emesis). Continue lavage for 24 hours or longer, depending on the apparent severity of intoxication. Use normal or half-normal saline to avoid water intoxication, especially in children. Instillation of activated charcoal slurry may help reduce absorption of imipramine.
Minimize external stimulation to reduce the tendency to convulsions. If anticonvulsants are necessary, diazepam, short-acting barbiturates, paraldehyde or methocarbamol may be useful.
Do not use barbiturates if MAO inhibitors have been taken recently.
Maintain adequate respiratory exchange. Do not use respiratory stimulants.
Shock should be treated with supportive measures, such as intravenous fluids, oxygen and corticosteroids. Digitalis may increase conduction abnormalities and further irritate an already sensitized myocardium. If congestive heart failure necessitates rapid digitalization, particular care must be exercised.
Hyperpyrexia should be controlled by whatever external means are available, including ice packs and cooling sponge baths, if necessary.
Hemodialysis, peritoneal dialysis, exchange transfusions and forced diuresis have been generally reported as ineffective because of the rapid fixation of Tofranil in tissues. Blood and urine levels of Tofranil may not correlate with the degree of intoxication, and are unreliable indicators in the clinical management of the patient.

HOW SUPPLIED

Tablets 10 mg — triangular, coral, sugar-coated (imprinted black Geigy 32)
Bottles of 100 ....NDC 0028-0032-01
Bottles of 1000 ....NDC 0028-0032-10

Tablets 25 mg — round, biconvex, coral, sugar-coated (imprinted black Geigy 140)
Bottles of 100 ....NDC 0028-0140-01
Bottles of 1000 ....NDC 0028-0140-10
Gy-Pak®—One Unit
12 bottles - 100 tablets each
............NDC 0028-0140-65
Unit Dose (blister pack)
Box of 100 (strips of 10)
............NDC 0028-0140-61

Tablets 50 mg — round, biconvex, coral, sugar-coated (imprinted black Geigy 136)
Bottles of 100 ....NDC 0028-0136-01
Bottles of 1000 ....NDC 0028-0136-10
Gy-Pak®—One Unit
12 bottles - 100 tablets each
............NDC 0028-0136-65
Unit Dose (blister pack)
Box of 100 (strips of 10)
............NDC 0028-0136-61

Store at controlled room temperature 15°–30°C (59°–86°F).
Dispense in tight container (USP).

ANIMAL PHARMACOLOGY & TOXICOLOGY

A. *Acute:* Oral LD_{50} ranges are as follows:

Rat	355 to 682 mg/kg
Dog	100 to 215 mg/kg

Depending on the dosage in both species, toxic signs proceeded progressively from depression, irregular respiration and ataxia to convulsions and death.

B. *Reproduction/Teratogenic:* The overall evaluation may be summed up in the following manner:
Oral: Independent studies in three species (rat, mouse and rabbit) revealed that when Tofranil is administered orally in doses up to approximately 2½ times the maximum human dose in the first 2 species and up to 25 times the maximum human dose in the third species, the drug is essentially free from teratogenic potential. In the three species studied, only one instance of fetal abnormality occurred (in the rabbit) and in that study there was likewise an abnormality in the control group. However, evidence does exist from the rat studies

that some systemic and embryotoxic potential is demonstrable. This is manifested by reduced litter size, a slight increase in the stillborn rate and a reduction in the mean birth weight.

C85-59 (Rev. 11/85)

Shown in Product Identification Section, page 409

For full prescribing information on Enuresis, please refer to Tofranil® imipramine hydrochloride USP, on page 964.

TOFRANIL-PM® ℞

[toe-fray'nill]

imipramine pamoate

Capsules of 75 mg

Capsules of 100 mg

Capsules of 125 mg

Capsules of 150 mg

For oral administration

Each 75-mg capsule contains imipramine pamoate equivalent to 75 mg of imipramine hydrochloride.
Each 100-mg capsule contains imipramine pamoate equivalent to 100 mg of imipramine hydrochloride.
Each 125-mg capsule contains imipramine pamoate equivalent to 125 mg of imipramine hydrochloride.
Each 150-mg capsule contains imipramine pamoate equivalent to 150 mg of imipramine hydrochloride.

DESCRIPTION

Tofranil-PM, imipramine pamoate, is a tricyclic antidepressant, available as capsules for oral administration. The 75-, 100-, 125-, and 150-mg capsules contain imipramine pamoate equivalent to 75, 100, 125, and 150 mg of imipramine hydrochloride.
Imipramine pamoate is 5-(3-[dimethylamino)propyl]-10, 11-dihydro-5H-dibenz[b,f] azepine 4,4′-methylenebis-(3-hydroxy-2-naphthoate) (2:1).
Imipramine pamoate is a fine, yellow, tasteless and odorless powder. It is soluble in ethanol, in acetone, in ether, in chloroform and in carbon tetrachloride, and is insoluble in water. Its molecular weight is 949.21.
Inactive Ingredients. Edetate calcium disodium, FD&C Blue No. 1, FD&C Red No. 3, FD&C Yellow No. 5 (100-mg and 125-mg capsules), FD&C Yellow No. 6, gelatin, magnesium stearate, parabens, sodium lauryl sulfate, sodium propionate, starch, talc, and titanium dioxide.

CLINICAL PHARMACOLOGY

The mechanism of action of imipramine is not definitely known. However, it does not act primarily by stimulation of the central nervous system. The clinical effect is hypothesized as being due to potentiation of adrenergic synapses by blocking uptake of norepinephrine at nerve endings.

INDICATIONS

For the relief of symptoms of depression. Endogenous depression is more likely to be alleviated than other depressive states. One to three weeks of treatment may be needed before optimal therapeutic effects are evident.

CONTRAINDICATIONS

The concomitant use of monoamine oxidase inhibiting compounds is contraindicated. Hyperpyretic crises or severe convulsive seizures may occur in patients receiving such combinations. The potentiation of adverse effects can be serious, or even fatal. When it is desired to substitute Tofranil-PM in patients receiving a monoamine oxidase inhibitor, as long an interval should elapse as the clinical situation will allow, with a minimum of 14 days. Initial dosage should be low and increases should be gradual and cautiously prescribed.
The drug is contraindicated during the acute recovery period after a myocardial infarction. Patients with a known hypersensitivity to this compound should not be given the drug. The possibility of cross-sensitivity to other dibenzazepine compounds should be kept in mind.

WARNINGS

Extreme caution should be used when this drug is given to:
patients with cardiovascular disease because of the possibility of conduction defects, arrhythmias, congestive heart failure, myocardial infarction, strokes and tachycardia. These patients require cardiac surveillance at all dosage levels of the drug;
patients with increased intraocular pressure, history of urinary retention, or history of narrow-angle glaucoma because of the drug's anticholinergic properties;
hyperthyroid patients or those on thyroid medication because of the possibility of cardiovascular toxicity;
patients with a history of seizure disorder because this drug has been shown to lower the seizure threshold;
patients receiving guanethidine, clonidine, or similar agents, since imipramine pamoate may block the pharmacologic effects of these drugs;
patients receiving methylphenidate hydrochloride. Since methylphenidate hydrochloride may inhibit the metabolism of imipramine pamoate, downward dosage adjustment of imipramine pamoate may be required when given concomitantly with methylphenidate hydrochloride.
Since imipramine pamoate may impair the mental and/or physical abilities required for the performance of potentially hazardous tasks, such as operating an automobile or machinery, the patient should be cautioned accordingly.
Tofranil-PM may enhance the CNS depressant effects of alcohol. Therefore, it should be borne in mind that the dangers inherent in a suicide attempt or accidental overdosage with the drug may be increased for the patient who uses excessive amounts of alcohol. (See **PRECAUTIONS.**)
Usage in Children: Tofranil-PM should not be used in children of any age because of the increased potential for acute overdosage due to the high unit potency (75 mg, 100 mg, 125 mg and 150 mg). Each capsule contains imipramine pamoate equivalent to 75 mg, 100 mg, 125 mg or 150 mg imipramine hydrochloride.

PRECAUTIONS

An ECG recording should be taken prior to the initiation of larger-than-usual doses of imipramine pamoate and at appropriate intervals thereafter until steady state is achieved. (Patients with any evidence of cardiovascular disease require cardiac surveillance at all dosage levels of the drug. See **WARNINGS.**) Elderly patients and patients with cardiac disease or a prior history of cardiac disease are at special risk of developing the cardiac abnormalities associated with the use of imipramine pamoate. It should be kept in mind that the possibility of suicide in seriously depressed patients is inherent in the illness and may persist until significant remission occurs. Such patients should be carefully supervised during the early phase of treatment with imipramine pamoate and may require hospitalization. Prescriptions should be written for the smallest amount feasible.
Hypomanic or manic episodes may occur, particularly in patients with cyclic disorders. Such reactions may necessitate discontinuation of the drug. If needed, imipramine pamoate may be resumed in lower dosage when these episodes are relieved. Administration of a tranquilizer may be useful in controlling such episodes.
An activation of the psychosis may occasionally be observed in schizophrenic patients and may require reduction of dosage and the addition of a phenothiazine.
Concurrent administration of imipramine pamoate with electroshock therapy may increase the hazards; such treatment should be limited to those patients for whom it is essential, since there is limited clinical experience.
Usage During Pregnancy and Lactation:
Animal reproduction studies have yielded inconclusive results. (See also **ANIMAL PHARMACOLOGY & TOXICOLOGY.**)
There have been no well-controlled studies conducted with pregnant women to determine the effect of imipramine on the fetus. However, there have been clinical reports of congenital malformations associated with the use of the drug. Although a causal relationship between these effects and the drug could not be established, the possibility of fetal risk from the maternal ingestion of imipramine cannot be excluded. Therefore, imipramine should be used in women who are or might become pregnant only if the clinical condition clearly justifies potential risk to the fetus.
Limited data suggest that imipramine is likely to be excreted in human breast milk. As a general rule, a woman taking a drug should not nurse since the possibility exists that the drug may be excreted in breast milk and be harmful to the child.
Patients should be warned that imipramine pamoate may enhance the CNS depressant effects of alcohol. (See **WARNINGS.**)
Imipramine pamoate should be used with caution in patients with significantly impaired renal or hepatic function.
Patients who develop a fever and a sore throat during therapy with imipramine pamoate should have leukocyte and differential blood counts performed. Imipramine pamoate should be discontinued if there is evidence of pathological neutrophil depression.
Prior to elective surgery, imipramine pamoate should be discontinued for as long as the clinical situation will allow.
In occasional susceptible patients or in those receiving anticholinergic drugs (including antiparkinsonism agents) in addition, the atropine-like effects may become more pronounced (e.g., paralytic ileus). Close supervision and careful adjustment of dosage is required when imipramine pamoate is administered concomitantly with anticholinergic drugs.
Avoid the use of preparations, such as decongestants and local anesthetics, which contain any sympathomimetic amine (e.g., epinephrine, norepinephrine), since it has been reported that tricyclic antidepressants can potentiate the effects of catecholamines.
Caution should be exercised when imipramine pamoate is used with agents that lower blood pressure.
Imipramine pamoate may potentiate the effects of CNS depressant drugs.
The plasma concentration of imipramine may increase when the drug is given concomitantly with cimetidine, and adjustment of the dosage of imipramine may therefore be necessary both when cimetidine therapy is initiated and when it is discontinued.
Patients taking imipramine pamoate should avoid excessive exposure to sunlight since there have been reports of photosensitization.
Both elevation and lowering of blood sugar levels have been reported with imipramine pamoate use.
The Tofranil-PM capsules (100 and 125 mg) contain FD&C Yellow No. 5 (tartrazine) which may cause allergic-type reactions (including bronchial asthma) in certain susceptible individuals. Although the overall incidence of FD&C Yellow No. 5 (tartrazine) sensitivity in the general population is low, it is frequently seen in patients who also have aspirin hypersensitivity.

ADVERSE REACTIONS

Note: Although the listing which follows includes a few adverse reactions which have not been reported with this specific drug, the pharmacological similarities among the tricyclic antidepressant drugs require that each of the reactions be considered when imipramine is administered.
Cardiovascular: Orthostatic hypotension, hypertension, tachycardia, palpitation, myocardial infarction, arrhythmias, heart block, ECG changes, precipitation of congestive heart failure, stroke.
Psychiatric: Confusional states (especially in the elderly) with hallucinations, disorientation, delusions; anxiety, restlessness, agitation; insomnia and nightmares; hypomania; exacerbation of psychosis.
Neurological: Numbness, tingling, paresthesias of extremities; incoordination, ataxia, tremors; peripheral neuropathy; extrapyramidal symptoms; seizures, alterations in EEG patterns; tinnitus.
Anticholinergic: Dry mouth, and, rarely, associated sublingual adenitis; blurred vision, disturbances of accommodation, mydriasis; constipation, paralytic ileus; urinary retention, delayed micturition, dilation of the urinary tract.
Allergic: Skin rash, petechiae, urticaria, itching, photosensitization; edema (general or of face and tongue); drug fever; cross-sensitivity with desipramine.
Hematologic: Bone marrow depression including agranulocytosis; eosinophilia; purpura; thrombocytopenia.
Gastrointestinal: Nausea and vomiting, anorexia, epigastric distress, diarrhea; peculiar taste, stomatitis, abdominal cramps, black tongue.
Endocrine: Gynecomastia in the male; breast enlargement and galactorrhea in the female; increased or decreased libido, impotence; testicular swelling; elevation or depression of blood sugar levels; inappropriate antidiuretic hormone (ADH) secretion syndrome.
Other: Jaundice (simulating obstructive); altered liver function; weight gain or loss; perspiration; flushing; urinary frequency; drowsiness, dizziness, weakness and fatigue; headache; parotid swelling; alopecia; proneness to falling.
Withdrawal Symptoms: Though not indicative of addiction, abrupt cessation of treatment after prolonged therapy may produce nausea, headache and malaise.

DOSAGE AND ADMINISTRATION

The following recommended dosages for Tofranil-PM should be modified as necessary by the clinical response and any evidence of intolerance.
Initial Adult Dosage:
Outpatients—Therapy should be initiated at 75 mg/day. Dosage may be increased to 150 mg/day which is the dose level at which optimum response is usually obtained. If necessary, dosage may be increased to 200 mg/day.
Dosage higher than 75 mg/day may also be administered on a once-a-day basis after the optimum dosage and tolerance have been determined. The daily dosage may be given at bedtime. In some patients it may be necessary to employ a divided-dose schedule.

Continued on next page

The full prescribing information for each GEIGY drug is contained herein and is that in effect as of September 1, 1986

Geigy—Cont.

As with all tricyclics, the antidepressant effect of imipramine may not be evident for one to three weeks in some patients.

Hospitalized Patients—Therapy should be initiated at 100–150 mg/day and may be increased to 200 mg/day. If there is no response after two weeks, dosage should be increased to 250–300 mg/day.

Dosage higher than 150 mg/day may also be administered on a once-a-day basis after the optimum dosage and tolerance have been determined. The daily dosage may be given at bedtime. In some patients it may be necessary to employ a divided-dose schedule.

As with all tricyclics, the antidepressant effect of imipramine may not be evident for one to three weeks in some patients.

Adult Maintenance Dosage: Following remission, maintenance medication may be required for a longer period of time at the lowest dose that will maintain remission after which the dosage should gradually be decreased.

The usual maintenance dosage is 75–150 mg/day. The total daily dosage can be administered on a once-a-day basis, preferably at bedtime. In some patients it may be necessary to employ a divided-dose schedule.

In cases of relapse due to premature withdrawal of the drug, the effective dosage of imipramine should be reinstituted.

Adolescent and Geriatric Patients: Therapy in these age groups should be initiated with Tofranil®, brand of imipramine hydrochloride, tablets at a total daily dosage of 25–50 mg, since Tofranil-PM capsules are not available in these strengths. Dosage may be increased according to response and tolerance, but it is generally unnecessary to exceed 100 mg/day in these patients. Tofranil-PM capsules may be used when total daily dosage is established at 75 mg or higher. The total daily dosage can be administered on a once-a-day basis, preferably at bedtime. In some patients it may be necessary to employ a divided-dose schedule.

As with all tricyclics, the antidepressant effect of imipramine may not be evident for one to three weeks in some patients.

Adolescent and geriatric patients can usually be maintained at lower dosage. Following remission, maintenance medication may be required for a longer period of time at the lowest dose that will maintain remission after which the dosage should gradually be decreased.

The total daily maintenance dosage can be administered on a once-a-day basis, preferably at bedtime. In some patients it may be necessary to employ a divided-dose schedule.

In cases of relapse due to premature withdrawal of the drug, the effective dosage of imipramine should be reinstituted.

OVERDOSAGE

Children have been reported to be more sensitive than adults to an acute overdosage of imipramine pamoate. An acute overdose of any amount in infants or young children, especially, must be considered serious and potentially fatal.

Signs and Symptoms: These may vary in severity depending upon factors such as the amount of drug absorbed, the age of the patient, and the interval between drug ingestion and the start of treatment. Blood and urine levels of imipramine may not reflect the severity of poisoning; they have chiefly a qualitative rather than a quantitative value, and are unreliable indicators in the clinical management of the patient.

CNS abnormalities may include drowsiness, stupor, coma, ataxia, restlessness, agitation, hyperactive reflexes, muscle rigidity, athetoid and choreiform movements, and convulsions.

Cardiac abnormalities may include arrhythmia, tachycardia, ECG evidence of impaired conduction, and signs of congestive failure.

Respiratory depression, cyanosis, hypotension, shock, vomiting, hyperpyrexia, mydriasis, and diaphoresis may also be present.

Treatment: Because CNS involvement, respiratory depression and cardiac arrhythmia can occur suddenly, hospitalization and close observation are necessary, even when the amount ingested is thought to be small or the initial degree of intoxication appears slight or moderate. All patients with ECG abnormalities should have continuous cardiac monitoring for at least 72 hours and be closely observed until well after cardiac status has returned to normal; relapses may occur after apparent recovery.

The *slow* intravenous administration of physostigmine salicylate has been reported to reverse most of the cardiovascular and CNS effects of overdosage with tricyclic antidepressants. In adults, 1 to 3 mg has been reported to be effective. In children, start with 0.5 mg and repeat at 5-minute intervals to determine the minimum effective dose; do not exceed 2 mg. Because of the short duration of action of physostigmine, repeat the effective dose at 30- to 60-minute intervals, as necessary. Avoid rapid injection to reduce the possibility of physostigmine-induced convulsions.

In the alert patient, empty the stomach promptly by induced emesis followed by lavage. In the obtunded patient, secure the airway with a cuffed endotracheal tube before beginning lavage (do not induce emesis). Continue lavage for 24 hours or longer, depending on the apparent severity of intoxication. Use normal or half-normal saline to avoid water intoxication, especially in children. Instillation of activated charcoal slurry may help reduce absorption of imipramine.

Minimize external stimulation to reduce the tendency to convulsions. If anticonvulsants are necessary, diazepam, short-acting barbiturates, paraldehyde or methocarbamol may be useful. Do not use barbiturates if MAO inhibitors have been taken recently.

Maintain adequate respiratory exchange. Do not use respiratory stimulants.

Shock should be treated with supportive measures, such as intravenous fluids, oxygen and corticosteroids. Digitalis may increase conduction abnormalities and further irritate an already sensitized myocardium. If congestive heart failure necessitates rapid digitalization, particular care must be exercised.

Hyperpyrexia should be controlled by whatever external means are available, including ice packs and cooling sponge baths, if necessary.

Hemodialysis, peritoneal dialysis, exchange transfusions and forced diuresis have been generally reported as ineffective because of the rapid fixation of imipramine in tissues. Blood and urine levels of imipramine may not correlate with the degree of intoxication, and are unreliable indicators in the clinical management of the patient.

HOW SUPPLIED

Capsules 75 mg — coral (imprinted Geigy 20) equivalent to 75 mg imipramine hydrochloride

Bottles of 30 ....NDC 0028-0020-26
Bottles of 100 ....NDC 0028-0020-01
Bottles of 1000 ....NDC 0028-0020-10
Unit Dose (blister pack)
Box of 100 (strips of 10)
....NDC 0028-0020-61

Capsules 100 mg — dark yellow/coral (imprinted Geigy 40) equivalent to 100 mg imipramine hydrochloride

Bottles of 30 ....NDC 0028-0040-26
Bottles of 100 ....NDC 0028-0040-01

Capsules 125 mg — light yellow/coral (imprinted Geigy 45) equivalent to 125 mg imipramine hydrochloride

Bottles of 30 ....NDC 0028-0045-26
Bottles of 100 ....NDC 0028-0045-01

Capsules 150 mg — coral (imprinted Geigy 22) equivalent to 150 mg imipramine hydrochloride

Bottles of 30 ....NDC 0028-0022-26
Bottles of 100 ....NDC 0028-0022-01
Unit Dose (blister pack)
Box of 100 (strips of 10)
....NDC 0028-0022-61

Do not store above 86°F (30°C).
Dispense in tight container (USP).

ANIMAL PHARMACOLOGY & TOXICOLOGY

A. *Acute:* Oral LD_{50}:

Mouse	2185 mg/kg
Rat (F)	1142 mg/kg
(M)	1807 mg/kg
Rabbit	1016 mg/kg
Dog	693 mg/kg (Emesis ED_{50})

B. *Subacute:*

Two three-month studies in dogs gave evidence of an adverse drug effect on the testes, but only at the highest dose level employed, i.e., 90 mg/kg (10 times the maximum human dose). Depending on the histological section of the testes examined, the findings consisted of a range of degenerative changes up to and including complete atrophy of the seminiferous tubules, with spermatogenesis usually arrested.

Human studies show no definitive effect on sperm count, sperm motility, sperm morphology or volume of ejaculate.

Rat

One three-month study was done in rats at dosage levels comparable to those of the dog studies. No adverse drug effect on the testes was noted in this study, as confirmed by histological examination.

C. *Reproduction/Teratogenic:*

Oral: Imipramine pamoate was fed to male and female albino rats for 28 weeks through two breeding cycles at dose levels of 15 mg/kg/day and 40 mg/kg/day (equivalent to 2½ and 7 times the maximum human dose). No abnormalities which could be related to drug administration were noted in gross inspection. Autopsies performed on pups from the second breeding likewise revealed no pathological changes in organs or tissues; however, a decrease in mean litter size from both matings was noted in the drug-treated groups and significant growth suppression occurred in the nursing pups of both sexes in the high group as well as in the females of the low-level group. Finally, the lactation index (pups weaned divided by number left to nurse) was significantly lower in the second litter of the high-level group.

C86-32 (Rev. 7/86)

Shown in Product Identification Section, page 409

GenDerm Corporation
425 HUEHL ROAD
NORTHBROOK, IL 60062

OCCLUSAL® ℞
[*ō-kloo'sal*]
(Salicylic Acid, U.S.P., 17%)

DESCRIPTION

Occlusal is a topical preparation containing 17% Salicylic Acid, U.S.P., in a polyacrylic vehicle containing butyl acetate, ethyl acetate, 20% isopropyl alcohol, toluene, nitrocellulose, dibutyl phthalate, polyester, camphor, acrylates copolymer and benzophenone-1. The pharmacologic activity of Occlusal is generally attributed to the keratolytic action of Salicylic Acid. The structural formula of Salicylic Acid is:

COOH
OH

CLINICAL PHARMACOLOGY

Although the exact mode of action of Salicylic Acid in the treatment of warts is not known, its activity appears to be associated with its keratolytic action which results in mechanical removal of epidermal cells infected with wart viruses.

INDICATIONS AND USAGE

Occlusal is indicated in the treatment and removal of common warts and plantar warts.

CONTRAINDICATIONS

Occlusal should not be used by diabetics or patients with impaired blood circulation. Occlusal should not be used on moles, birthmarks, unusual warts with hair growing from them, or warts on the face.

PRECAUTIONS

Occlusal is for external use only. Do not permit Occlusal to contact eyes or mucous membranes. If contact with eyes or mucous membranes occurs, immediately flush with water for 15 minutes. Occlusal should not be allowed to contact normal skin surrounding wart. Treatment should be discontinued if excessive irritation occurs. Occlusal is flammable and should be kept away from fire or flame. Keep bottle tightly capped when not in use.

ADVERSE REACTIONS

A localized irritant reaction may occur if Occlusal is applied to the normal skin surrounding the wart. Any irritation may normally be controlled by temporarily discontinuing use of Occlusal, and by applying the medication only to the wart site when treatment is resumed.

DOSAGE AND ADMINISTRATION

Prior to application of Occlusal, soak wart in warm water for five minutes. Remove any loosened tissue by gently rubbing with a brush, wash cloth, or emery board. Dry thoroughly. Using the brush applicator supplied, apply twice to affected area, allowing the first application to dry before applying the second. Treatment should be once a day and should continue as directed by physician. Be careful not to apply to surrounding skin.

Clinically visible improvement will normally occur during the first two to four weeks of therapy. Maximum resolution may be expected after six to twelve weeks of drug use.

HOW SUPPLIED

½ fl. oz. bottle with brush applicator, (NDC 52761-121-15). See Precautions section for special handling and storage conditions.

PENTRAX®
[*pen'trax*]
Tar Shampoo with Fractar®

DESCRIPTION

Pentrax Tar Shampoo contains 8.75% Fractar (equal to 4.3% crude coal tar), a standardized tar extract, a blend of highly concentrated detergents, and conditioning agents. Spectrophotometric standardization, based on hydrocarbon analysis, assures uniform therapeutic activity from batch to batch. Pentrax Tar Shampoo does not contain parabens or other preservatives. Pentrax Tar Shampoo contains the highest concentration of coal tar currently available. Fractar consists of the desirable crude coal tar fractions without undesirable residues. It has excellent lathering qualities and leaves hair clean and manageable.

ACTION AND INDICATIONS

Coal tar helps correct abnormalities of keratinization by decreasing epidermal proliferation and dermal infiltration. Pentrax Tar Shampoo is indicated for the adjunctive, topical management of dandruff, seborrheic dermatitis, psoriasis and subacute and chronic eczematous dermatoses of the scalp. Pentrax relieves itching, irritation and scaling of the scalp.

WARNINGS

FOR EXTERNAL USE ONLY. Avoid contact with the eyes —if this happens, rinse thoroughly with water. If condition worsens or does not improve after regular use of this product as directed, consult your physician. Do not use on children under 2 years of age except as directed by your physician. Use caution in exposing skin to sunlight after applying this product. It may increase your tendency to sunburn for up to 24 hours after application. Do not use this product in or around the rectum or in the genital area or groin except on the advice of your physician. Keep this and all drugs out of the reach of children.

DIRECTIONS

Apply Pentrax Tar Shampoo to wet hair; massage, adding water liberally to produce lather. Rinse. Reapply. Second lather may be allowed to remain up to 10 minutes. Rinse. Use 2–3 times weekly or as directed by your physician.

HOW SUPPLIED

4 fl. oz. plastic bottle (NDC 52761-665-04) and
8 fl. oz. plastic bottle (NDC 52761-665-08)

PRAMEGEL®

[pram 'eh-gel]

Emollient Antipruritic Gel

DESCRIPTION

PrameGel contains pramoxine hydrochloride 1% and menthol 0.5% in a cosmetically elegant emollient gel base.

INDICATIONS

PrameGel provides prompt temporary relief of itching associated with mild eczemas (including poison ivy and poison oak), insect bites, heat rash, sunburn, and other pruritic skin conditions, as well as for external anal itching.

WARNINGS

FOR EXTERNAL USE ONLY. Avoid contact with the eyes. If itching worsens or if symptoms persist for more than 7 days, advise your physician. Keep this and all drugs out of the reach of children.

DIRECTIONS

Adults and children 2 years of age or older: Apply PrameGel liberally to affected area 3 to 4 times daily or as directed by physician. Children 2 year and younger: Apply as directed by physician.

HOW SUPPLIED

4 fl. oz. bottle (NDC 52761-395-04).

SALAC®

[sal 'ak]

Acne Medication-Cleanser

DESCRIPTION

SalAc is an acne medication-cleanser containing 2% salicylic acid in a surfactant blend.

INDICATIONS

For the management of acne. Helps prevent new comedones papules, and pustules.

WARNINGS

For External Use Only. Keep Cleanser Out of Eyes. Keep Out of Reach of Children. Using other topical acne medications at the same time or immediately following use of this product may increase skin dryness or irritation. If this occurs, only one medication should be used unless directed otherwise by physician.

DIRECTIONS

Wash affected area 2–3 times daily. Amount delivered by a single pump stroke is generally adequate for cleansing. Lather with warm water, massage into skin, rinse, and dry. Container will provide approximately 350 washings when used as directed.

HOW SUPPLIED

6 fl. oz. bottle with pump dispenser (NDC 52761-077-06).

TEXACORT® ℞

[tex 'ah-cort]

(Hydrocortisone, U.S.P.)

DESCRIPTION

Texacort Scalp Lotion contains hydrocortisone as the active corticosteroid having the chemical formula of pregn-4-one 3, 20-dione, 11, 17, 21-trihydroxy, (11β)

Each milliliter of 1.0% Lotion contains 10 mg/ml of hydrocortisone in specially formulated vehicle containing S.D. alcohol (33%), propylene glycol, polysorbate 20 and purified water preserved with benzalkonium chloride.

CLINICAL PHARMACOLOGY

Topical corticosteroids share anti-inflammatory, anti-pruritic and vasoconstrictive actions. The mechanisms of anti-inflammatory activity of the topical corticosteroids is unclear. Various laboratory methods, including vasoconstrictor assays are used to compare and predict potencies and/or clinical efficacies of the topical corticosteroids. There is some evidence to suggest that a recognizable correlation exists between vasoconstrictor potency and therapeutic efficacy in man.

Pharmacokinetics: The extent of percutaneous absorption of topical corticosteroids is determined by many factors including the vehicle, the integrity of the epidermal barrier, and the use of occlusive dressings.

Topical corticosteroids can be absorbed from normal intact skin. Inflammation and/or other disease processes in the skin increase percutaneous absorption. Occlusive dressing substantially increase the pecutaneous absorption of topical corticosteroids. Thus occlusive dressings may be a valuable therapeutic adjunct for treatment of resistant dermatoses. (See DOSAGE AND ADMINISTRATION.)

Once absorbed through the skin, topical corticosteroids are handled through pharmacokinetic pathways similar to systemically administered corticosteroids. Corticosteroids are metabolized primarily in the liver and are then excreted by the kidneys. Some of the topical corticosteroids and their metabolites are also excreted into the bile.

MEDICATIONS AND USAGE

Topical corticosteroids are indicated for the relief of the inflammatory and pruritic manifestations of corticosteroid-responsive dermatoses.

CONTRAINDICATIONS

Topical corticosteroids are contraindicated in those patients with a history of hypersensitivity to any of the components of the preparation.

PRECAUTIONS

General: Systemic absorption of topical corticosteroids has produced reversible hypothalamic pituitary adrenal (HPA) axis suppression, manifestations of Cushing's syndrome, hyperglycemia, and glucosuria in some patients.

Conditions which augment systemic absorption include the application of the more potent steroids, use over large surface areas, prolonged use and the addition of occlusive dressings.

Therefore, patients receiving a large dose of a potent topical steroid applied to a large surface area or under an occlusive dressing should be evaluated periodically for evidence of HPA axis suppression by using the urinary free cortisol and ACTH stimulation tests. If HPA axis suppression is noted, an attempt should be made to withdraw the drug, to reduce the frequency of application, or to substitute a less potent steroid.

Recovery of HPA axis function is generally prompt and complete upon discontinuation of the drug. Infrequently, signs and symptoms of steroid withdrawal may occur, requiring supplemental systemic corticosteroids.

Children may absorb proportionally larger amounts of topical corticosteroids and thus be more susceptible to systemic toxicity (See PRECAUTIONS Pediatric Use)

If irritation develops, topical corticosteroids should be discontinued and appropriate therapy instituted.

In the presence of dermatological infections, the use of an appropriate antifungal or antibacterial agent should be instituted. If a favorable response does not occur promptly, the corticosteroid should be discontinued until the infection has been adequately controlled.

Information for the Patient: Patients using topical corticosteroids should receive the following information and instructions.

1. This medication is to be used as directed by the physician. It is for external use only. Avoid contact with the eyes.
2. Patients should be advised not to use this medication for any disorder other than for which it was prescribed.
3. The treated skin area should not be bandaged or otherwise covered or wrapped as to be occlusive unless directed by the physician.
4. Patients should report any signs of local adverse reactions especially under occlusive dressing.
5. Parents of pediatric patients should be advised not to use tight fitting diapers or plastic pants on a child being treated in the diaper area, as these garments may constitute occlusive dressings.

Laboratory Tests: The following tests may be helpful in evaluating the HPA axis suppression:

Urinary free cortisol test
ACTH stimulation test

Carcinogenesis, Mutagenesis, and Impairment of Fertility: Long-term animal studies have not been performed to evaluate the carcinogenic potential on the effect on fertility of topical corticosteroids.

Studies to determine mutagenicity with prednisolone and hydrocortisone have revealed negative results.

Pregnancy Category C: Corticosteroids are generally teratogenic in laboratory animals when administered systemically at relatively low dosage levels. The more potent corticosteroids have been shown to be teratogenic after dermal application in laboratory animals. There are no adequate and well-controlled studies in pregnant women on teratogenic effects from topically applied corticosteroids. Therefore, topical corticosteroids should be used during pregnancy only if the potential benefit justifies the potential risk to the fetus. Drugs of this class should not be used extensively on pregnant patients, in large amounts, or for prolonged periods of time.

Nursing Mothers: It is not known whether topical administration of corticosteroids could result in sufficient systemic absorption to produce detectable quantities in breast milk. Systemically administered corticosteroids are secreted into breast milk in quantities *not* likely to have a deleterious effect on the infant. Nevertheless, caution should be exercised when topical corticosteroids are administered to a nursing woman.

Pediatric Use: *Pediatric patients may demonstrate greater susceptibility to topical corticosteroid-induced HPA axis suppression and Cushing's syndrome than mature patients because of a larger skin surface area to body weight ratio.*

Hypothalamic-pituitary-adrenal (HPA) axis suppression, Cushing's syndrome, and intracranial hypertension have been reported in children receiving topical corticosteroids. Manifestations of adrenal suppression in children include linear growth retardation, delayed weight gain, low plasma cortisol levels, and absence of response to ACTH stimulation. Manifestations of intracranial hypertension include bulging fontanelles, headaches, and bilateral papilledema.

Administration of topical corticosteroids to children should be limited to the least amount compatible with an effective therapeutic regimen. Chronic corticosteroid therapy may interfere with the growth and development of children.

ADVERSE REACTIONS

The following local adverse reactions are reported infrequently with topical corticosteroids, but may occur more frequently with the use of occlusive dressings. These reactions are listed in an approximate decreasing order of occurrence:

Burning
Itching
Irritation
Dryness
Folliculitis
Hypertrichosis
Acneiform eruptions
Hypopigmentation
Perioral dermatitis
Allergic contact dermatitis
Maceration of the skin
Secondary infection
Skin Atrophy
Striae
Miliaria

OVERDOSAGE

Topically applied corticosteroids can be absorbed in sufficient amounts to produce systemic effects. (See PRECAUTIONS.)

DOSAGE AND ADMINISTRATION

Topical corticosteroids are generally applied to the affected areas as a thin film from three to four times daily depending on the severity of the condition.

Occlusive dressings may be used for the management of psoriasis or recalcitrant conditions.

If an infection develops, the use of occlusive dressings should be discontinued and appropriate antimicrobial therapy instituted.

HOW SUPPLIED

1 fl. oz. bottle with dropper (NDC 52761-247-01)
Store between 59°–86°F (15°–30°C).

Continued on next page

GenDerm—Cont.

ZOSTRIX™
[*zos 'trix*]
Topical Analgesic Cream

DESCRIPTION
Zostrix cream contains capsaicin .025% in an emollient base. Capsaicin is a natural chemical derived from plants of the Solanaceae family with the chemical name trans-8-methyl-N-vanillyl-6-nonenamide. Capsaicin is a white crystalline powder with a molecular weight of 305.4. It is practically insoluble in water but very soluble in alcohol, ether, and chloroform.

ACTION AND INDICATIONS
Although the precise mechanism of action of capsaicin is not fully understood, current evidence suggests that capsaicin renders skin insensitive to pain by depleting and preventing reaccumulation of substance P in peripheral sensory neurons. Substance P is thought to be the principal chemomediator of pain impulses from the periphery to the central nervous system.
Zostrix cream is indicated for relief of the pain (neuralgia) which may accompany or follow Herpes Zoster infections.

WARNINGS
For external use only. Avoid getting in eyes or on broken or irritated skin. Do not bandage tightly. If condition worsens, or if symptoms persist for more than 14 days or clear up and occur again within a few days, discontinue use of this product and consult your physician. Keep this and all drugs out of the reach of children.

DIRECTIONS
Adults and children 2 years of age or older: Apply Zostrix to affected area not more than 3 or 4 times daily. Zostrix may cause transient burning on application. This burning is observed more frequently when application schedules of less than 3 or 4 times daily are utilized. After Zostrix is applied with the fingers, the hands should be washed immediately afterwards.

HOW SUPPLIED
45g. tubes (NDC 52761-552-45)
U.S. Patents No. 4486450, 5536404

Genentech, Inc.
460 POINT SAN BRUNO BLVD.
SOUTH SAN FRANCISCO, CA 94080

PROTROPIN®   ℞
(somatrem for injection)

DESCRIPTION
Protropin is the Genentech trademark for somatrem, a polypeptide hormone which is of recombinant DNA origin. Protropin has 192 amino acid residues and a molecular weight of about 22,000 daltons. The product contains the identical sequence of 191 amino acids constituting pituitary-derived human growth hormone plus an additional amino acid, methionine, on the N-terminus of the molecule. Protropin growth hormone is synthesized in a special laboratory strain of **E. coli** bacteria which has been modified by the addition of the gene for human growth hormone production.
Protropin growth hormone, a sterile, white, lyophilized powder, is intended for intramuscular administration after reconstitution with Bacteriostatic Water for Injection, USP (Benzyl Alcohol Preserved).
The quantitative composition of the lyophilized drug per vial is:

Somatrem 5.0 mg (approximately 10 IU)
Mannitol 40.0 mg
Sodium Phosphates 1.7 mg
(Monobasic Sodium Phosphate 0.1 mg and Dibasic Sodium Phosphate 1.6 mg)

Phosphoric acid may be used for pH adjustment.
Protropin growth hormone is a highly purified preparation. Biological potency is determined by measuring the increase in body weight induced in hypophysectomized rats.
Bacteriostatic Water for Injection, USP (Benzyl Alcohol Preserved) is a sterile water for injection packaged in a multiple dose vial. It contains an antimicrobial preservative. Each mL contains 0.9 percent benzyl alcohol. The pH is 4.5–7.0.

CLINICAL PHARMACOLOGY
Linear Growth: The primary and most intensively studied action of Protropin (somatrem for injection) is the stimulation of linear growth. This effect is demonstrated in patients lacking adequate endogenous growth hormone production.
In vitro, preclinical, and clinical testing has demonstrated that Protropin growth hormone is therapeutically equivalent to somatropin (human growth hormone, pituitary origin). Short term clinical studies in normal adults show equivalent pharmacokinetics. Treatment of growth hormone deficient children with Protropin growth hormone results in an increase in growth rate and somatomedin-C levels similar to that seen with somatropin therapy.
Other actions that have been demonstrated for Protropin (somatrem for injection) and/or somatropin include:

A. Tissue Growth

1. Skeletal Growth. Protropin (somatrem for injection) stimulates skeletal growth in patients with growth hormone deficiency. The measurable increase in body length after administration of somatropin results from its effect on the epiphyseal growth plates of long bones. Studies **in vitro** have shown that the incorporation of sulfate into proteoglycans is not due to a direct effect of somatropin, but rather is accomplished by a mediator called somatomedin-C. Somatomedin-C is low in the serum of growth hormone deficient children but increases during treatment with Protropin.

2. Cell Growth. It has been shown that the total number of skeletal muscle cells is markedly decreased in short-stature children lacking endogenous growth hormone compared with normal children. Treatment with somatropin results in an increase in both the number and the size of muscle cells.

3. Organ Growth. Somatropin influences the size of internal organs and it also increases red cell mass.

B. Protein Metabolism
Linear growth is facilitated in part by increased cellular protein synthesis. This is reflected by nitrogen retention as demonstrated by a decline in urinary nitrogen excretion and blood urea nitrogen following the initiation of somatropin therapy. Treatment with Protropin (somatrem for injection) results in a similar decline in blood urea nitrogen.

C. Carbohydrate Metabolism
Both somatropin and Protropin (somatrem for injection) have been found to influence carbohydrate metabolism. It is recognized that children with hypopituitarism sometimes experience fasting hypoglycemia. In normal healthy subjects, large doses of Protropin growth hormone may impair glucose tolerance. Administration of either somatropin or Protropin to normal adults resulted in an increase in serum insulin levels. Although the precise mechanism by which somatropin and Protropin induce insulin resistance is presently not known, it is attributed to a decrease in insulin sensitivity. An increase in serum glucose levels is observed during treatment with somatropin.

D. Lipid Metabolism
In growth hormone deficient subjects long term administration of somatropin often results in a general reduction in body fat stores. Acute administration of somatropin to humans results in lipid mobilization. Nonesterified fatty acids increase in plasma within two hours of somatropin administration.

E. Mineral Metabolism
The retention of total body potassium and phosphorus which is induced by somatropin administration is thought to be due to cell growth. Sodium retention also occurs.
Serum levels of inorganic phosphate increase in patients with growth hormone deficiency after somatropin or Protropin (somatrem for injection) therapy due to metabolic activity associated with bone growth as well as increased tubular reabsorption of phosphate by the kidney. Serum calcium is not significantly altered in patients treated with either somatropin or Protropin.
Although calcium excretion in the urine is increased, there is a simultaneous increase in calcium absorption from the intestine.

F. Connective Tissue Metabolism
Somatropin stimulates the synthesis of chondroitin sulfate and collagen as well as the urinary excretion of hydroxyproline.

INDICATIONS AND USAGE
Protropin (somatrem for injection) is indicated only for the long term treatment of children who have growth failure due to a lack of adequate endogenous growth hormone secretion. Other etiologies of short stature should be excluded.

CONTRAINDICATIONS
Protropin (somatrem for injection) should not be used in subjects with closed epiphyses.
Protropin growth hormone should not be used when there is evidence of any progression of underlying intracranial lesion. Intracranial lesions must be inactive and antitumor therapy complete prior to instituting therapy. Protropin growth hormone should be discontinued if there is evidence of recurrent tumor growth.
Protropin growth hormone, when reconstituted with Bacteriostatic Water for Injection, USP (Benzyl Alcohol Preserved) should not be used in patients with a known sensitivity to benzyl alcohol.

WARNINGS
Benzyl alcohol as a preservative in Bacteriostatic Water for Injection has been associated with toxicity in newborns. When administering Protropin to newborns, reconstitute with Water for Injection, USP. USE ONLY ONE DOSE PER VIAL AND DISCARD THE UNUSED PORTION.

PRECAUTIONS
Protropin (somatrem for injection) should be used only by physicians experienced in the diagnosis and management of patients with pituitary growth hormone deficiency.
Patients with growth hormone deficiency secondary to an intracranial lesion should be examined frequently for progression or recurrence of the underlying disease process.
Because Protropin may induce a state of insulin resistance, patients should be observed for evidence of glucose intolerance.
Concomitant glucocorticoid therapy may inhibit the growth promoting effect of Protropin growth hormone. Patients with coexisting ACTH deficiency should have their glucocorticoid replacement dose carefully adjusted to avoid an inhibitory effect on growth.
Hypothyroidism may develop during Protropin treatment. Untreated hypothyroidism prevents optimal response to Protropin growth hormone. Therefore, patients should have periodic thyroid function tests and should be treated with thyroid hormone when indicated.
Slipped capital femoral epiphysis may occur more frequently in patients with endocrine disorders. Physicians and parents should be alert to the development of a limp or complaints of hip or knee pain in Protropin-treated patients.
As for any protein, a systemic allergic reaction may occur. See WARNINGS for use of Bacteriostatic Water for Injection, USP (Benzyl Alcohol Preserved) in newborns.

ADVERSE REACTIONS
A. Protropin (somatrem for injection)

Approximately 30 percent of all Protropin treated patients developed persistent antibodies to growth hormone.
In patients who had been previously treated with pituitary-derived growth hormone, one of twenty-two subjects developed persistent antibodies to growth hormone in response to Protropin therapy.
In children not previously treated with any exogenous growth hormone approximately 40 percent developed persistent antibodies to growth hormone.
In general, the growth hormone antibodies are not neutralizing and do not interfere with the growth response to Protropin growth hormone. One of eighty-four subjects treated with Protropin growth hormone for 6 to 36 months developed antibodies associated with high binding capacities and failed to respond to treatment with Protropin growth hormone.
In addition to an evaluation of compliance with treatment program and thyroid status, testing for antibodies to human growth hormone should be carried out in any patient who fails to respond to therapy.
Additional short term immunologic and renal function studies were carried out in a group of patients after approximately two years of treatment to detect other potential adverse effects of antibodies to growth hormone. The antibody was determined to be of the IgG class; no antibodies to growth hormone of the IgE class were detected. Testing included immune complex determination, measurement of total hemolytic complement and specific complement components, and immunochemical analyses. No adverse effects of growth hormone antibody formation were observed.
These findings are supported by a toxicity study conducted in a primate model in which a similar antibody response to growth hormone was observed. Protropin (somatrem for injection), administered to monkeys by intramuscular injection at doses of 125 and 625 μg/kg t.i.w. was compared to pituitary-human growth hormone at the same doses and with placebo over a period of 90 days. Most monkeys treated with high-dose Protropin growth hormone developed persistent antibodies at week four. There were no biologically significant drug related changes in standard laboratory variables. Histopathologic examination of the kidney and other selected organs (pituitary, lungs, liver and pancreas) showed no treatment related toxicity. There was no evidence of immune complexes or immune complex toxicity when the kidney was also examined for the presence of immune complexes and possible toxic effects of immune complexes by immunohistochemistry and electron microscopy.

B. Bacteriostatic Water for Injection, USP (Benzyl Alcohol Preserved)

Toxicity in newborns has been associated with benzyl alcohol as a preservative (see WARNINGS).

OVERDOSAGE
The recommended dosage of up to 0.1 mg (0.2 IU) per kg body weight three times per week should not be exceeded due to the potential risk of side effects.

DOSAGE AND ADMINISTRATION

The Protropin (somatrem for injection) dosage must be individualized for each patient. A dosage and schedule of up to 0.1 mg/kg (0.2 IU/kg) body weight administered three times per week (t.i.w.) by intramuscular injection is recommended. After the dose has been determined, reconstitute each 5 mg vial with 1–5 mL of Bacteriostatic Water for Injection, USP (Benzyl Alcohol Preserved) only. For use in newborns see WARNINGS. The pH of Protropin after reconstitution is approximately 7.8.

To prepare the Protropin solution, inject the Bacteriostatic Water for Injection, USP (Benzyl Alcohol Preserved) into the vial of Protropin growth hormone, aiming the stream of liquid against the glass wall. Then swirl the product vial with a **GENTLE** rotary motion until the contents are completely dissolved. **DO NOT SHAKE.** Because Protropin growth hormone is a protein, shaking can result in a cloudy solution. Immediately after reconstitution, the Protropin solution should be clear. Occassionally, after refrigeration, you may notice that small colorless particles of protein are present in the Protropin solution. This is not unusual for proteins like Protropin growth hormone. If the solution is cloudy immediately after reconstitution or refrigeration the contents **MUST NOT** be injected. Before and after injections the septum of the vial should be wiped with an antiseptic solution to prevent contamination of the contents after repeated needle insertions. It is recommended that Protropin growth hormone be administered using sterile, disposable syringes and needles. The syringes should be of small enough volume that the prescribed dose can be drawn from the vial with reasonable accuracy. The needle should be of sufficient length (usually 1 inch or more) to ensure that the injection reaches the muscular layer.

STORAGE

Protropin (somatrem for injection), before and after reconstitution with Bacteriostatic Water for Injection, USP (Benzyl Alcohol Preserved), must be stored at 2° to 8°C/36° to 46°F (refrigerator).

Reconstituted vials should be used within seven days after reconstitution.

Avoid freezing the reconstituted vial of Protropin growth hormone and the Bacteriostatic Water for Injection, USP (Benzyl Alcohol Preserved).

Expiration dates are stated on the labels.

HOW SUPPLIED

Protropin (somatrem for injection) is supplied as 5 mg (approximately 10 IU) of lyophilized, sterile somatrem per vial. There are two vials of Protropin (somatrem for injection) and one 10 mL multiple dose vial of Bacteriostatic Water for Injection, USP (Benzyl Alcohol Preserved) per carton.
NDC 50242-015-02.

Protropin (somatrem for injection) Manufactured by:
Genentech, Inc.
460 Point San Bruno Boulevard
South San Francisco, CA 94080
Bacteriostatic Water for Injection, USP (Benzyl Alcohol Preserved) Manufactured for:
Genentech, Inc.
G40053-R2
Revised Oct. 1985

Geriatric Pharm. Corp.
1249 NORTH FRANKLIN PLACE
MILWAUKEE, WI 53202

B-C-BID™ CAPSULES
B Complex with Vitamin C
SUSTAINED RELEASE
BY MICRODIALYSIS DIFFUSION

COMPOSITION

Each capsule contains: Vitamin B-1 15 mg., Vitamin B-2 10 mg., Vitamin B-6 5 mg., Niacinamide 50 mg., Calcium Pantothenate 10 mg., Vitamin C 300 mg., and Vitamin B-12 (Cyanocobalamin) 5 mcg.

Medication is released at a smooth, continuous, predictable rate dependent only upon the presence of fluid in the G.I. tract, and not dependent on pH and other variables. *No regurgitation; no after-taste.*

On b.i.d. dosage, this smooth, continuous release of B-C-BID's essential vitamins frees your patient from the "peak and valley" effect of ordinary capsules or tablets.

DOSAGE

For continuous 24 hour therapy, one capsule after breakfast and one after supper.

SUPPLIED

Bottles of 30, 100, and 500. (NDC #249-1153-01,-02 and -03)

BILEZYME™ ℞
[bī'le zīm]
Bile Acids and Digestive Enzymes

COMPOSITION

Each BILEZYME tablet contains 30 mg. of Gerilase (Standardized Amylolytic Enzyme derived from Aspergillus oryzae), 6 mg. of Geriprotase (Standardized Proteolytic Enzyme derived from Carica papaya), 200 mg. Dehydrocholic Acid (a choleretic) and 50 mg. Desoxycholic Acid (a cholagogue). Not enteric coated.

SUPPLIED

Bottles of 42, 100 and 500. (NDC #249-1110-01, -02, and 03)

CAL-BID™
Calcium Supplement with Vitamin C and D Added

COMPOSITION

Each tablet contains:	Quantity:	% USRDA:
Vitamin C (ascorbic acid)	100 mg.	167
Vitamin D	125 IU	31.25
Calcium Carbonate*	625 mg.	25

(*equivalent to 250 mg. elemental Calcium)

SUPPLIED

As bottles of 100 and 500. (NDC #249-1168-01, -02 and -03)

CAL-PLUS™ TABLETS
High Potency Calcium Supplement

COMPOSITION

Each tablet contains Calcium Carbonate, 1500 mg. (equivalent to 600 mg. elemental Calcium or 60% USRDA).

SUPPLIED

As bottles of 100 and 500 (NDC #249-1170-01, -02 and -03).

CEVI-BID™ Capsules (500 mg. Vitamin C)
SUSTAINED RELEASE
BY MICRO-DIALYSIS DIFFUSION

COMPOSITION

Each CEVI-BID capsule contains 500 mg. Vitamin C.

ACTION AND USES

For treatment of Vitamin C deficiency. CEVI-BID maintains optimal blood levels of Vitamin C around the clock on b.i.d. dosage, and avoids "peak and valley" effects of ordinary Vitamin C tablets. Medication is released at a smooth, continuous, predictable rate dependent only upon the presence of fluid in the G.I. tract and independent of pH or other variables.

DOSAGE

For continuous 24 hour therapy, one capsule after breakfast and one after supper.

SUPPLIED

Bottles of 30, 100 and 500. (NDC #249-1161-01, -02 and -03)

CEVI-FER™ CAPSULES ℞
Hematinic with 300 mg Vitamin C
SUSTAINED RELEASE BY
MICRO-DIALYSIS DIFFUSION

COMPOSITION

CEVI-FER capsules contain *Ferrous Fumarate 60 mg. (Equivalent to 20 mg. elemental iron), *Ascorbic Acid 300 mg., Folic Acid 1 mg.

*Prepared in a special base for prolonged therapeutic effect. Ferrous fumarate and ascorbic acid are released at a smooth, continuous, predictable rate dependent only upon the presence of fluid in the G.I. tract; not dependent on the variable digestive processes.

INDICATIONS

Cevi-Fer Capsules is a high potency formulation of Iron, Ascorbic Acid, and Folic Acid and is intended for use as:

1) intensive therapy for the acute and/or severe iron deficiency anemia where a high intake of elemental iron is required.
2) a maintenance hematinic for those patients needing a daily iron supplement to maintain normal hemoglobin levels.
3) prevention of concomitant folic acid deficiency in adults.
4) especially indicated in geriatric patients who are on special diets or suffer from nutritional anemias.
5) folic acid is effective in the treatment of megaloblastic anemias due to a deficiency of folic acid (as may be seen in tropical or nontropical sprue) and in anemias of nutritional origin, pregnancy, infancy, or childhood.

ACTIONS AND USES

The Ferrous form of iron is better absorbed and utilized than the ferric form. Absorption of iron can occur along the entire length of the alimentary tract, but is greatest in the duodenum and becomes progressively less distal.

The stomach being acid, keeps the iron salts in Ferrous state. Reducing agents such as Ascorbic Acid increase iron absorption.

In Cevi-Fer's special sustained release pattern, Ferrous Fumerate and the Ascorbic Acid will be released over a 12 hour period.

The advantage of having Ferrous Fumarate present in a Sustained Release pellet formulation is that it provides high levels of elemental iron with a low incidence of gastric distress.

300 mg. of Sustained Release Ascorbic Acid serves to maintain the iron in a more absorbable Ferrous state.

Studies have found that large doses of Ascorbic Acid tend to enhance iron absorption.

CONTRAINDICATIONS

Folic acid, (pteroylglutamic acid), is contraindicated in patients with untreated and uncomplicated pernicious anemia, and in those with anaphylactic sensitivity to folic acid. Iron therapy is contraindicated in patients with hemachromatosis, iron storage disease or the potential for iron storage disease due to chronic hemolytic anemia (e.g., inherited anomalies of hemoglobin structure or synthesis and/or red cell enzyme deficiencies, etc.), pyridoxine responsive anemia, or cirrhosis of the liver.

WARNINGS

Pernicious anemia should be ruled out before starting treatment. While folic acid corrects the blood picture of pernicious anemia, it does not ameliorate the attendant neurologic involvement.

Resistance to treatment may be due to depressed hematopoiesis, alcoholism, the presence of antimetabolic drugs and to deficiencies of vitamins.

Iron deficiency anemia may be due to occult blood loss, the cause of which should be determined and treated appropriately. Prolonged therapeutic use of iron salts may produce iron storage disease.

PRECAUTIONS

Folic acid in doses above 0.1 mg. daily may obscure pernicious anemia, in that hematologic remission may occur while neurological manifestations remain progressive.

Folic acid (pteroylglutamic acid) microbiological blood assays are invalidated by the administration of most antibiotics, methotrexate, and pyrimethamine. Folic acid is not effective in reversing the toxic effects of methotrexate. Folinic acid (5-formyl-5,6,7,8-tetrahydrofolic acid) must be used in this situation. Black tarry stools may be due to either occult G.I. bleeding or iron therapy, or both.

ADVERSE REACTIONS

Allergic sensitivity reactions and gastrointestinal disturbances may occur.

DOSAGE AND ADMINISTRATION

One capsule after breakfast and supper for two weeks in severe anemias, then one capsule a day. Not to be administered to children under 12 years of age.

OVERDOSAGE

The average human lethal dose of iron is about 200 to 250 mg. iron/kg. body weight. In the case of a 4 kg. infant, this is about 800 mg. iron or about (2) grams anhydrous ferrous sulfate or ferrous fumarate.

WARNING

Keep out of the reach of children. In case of accidental overdose, seek professional assistance or contact a poison control center immediately. Protect from heat and moisture.

HOW SUPPLIED

Available in bottles of 30 and 100 capsules. (NDC #'s 249-1166-01 and -02)

CAUTION

Federal law prohibits dispensing without a prescription.

GERITONIC™ LIQUID
Elixir with Vitamin B Complex and Iron

COMPOSITION

Each teaspoonful (5 cc.) contains:		
Iron (from Ferric Ammonium Citrate)	35	mg.
Thiamine Hydrochloride (Vitamin B-1)	1	mg.
Riboflavin (Vitamin B-2)	1	mg.

Continued on next page

Geriatric Pharm.—Cont.

Niacinamide	10	mg.
Vitamin B-12 (Cyanacobalamin)	3	mcg.
Pyridoxine Hydrochloride (Vitamin B-6)	0.1	mg.
Magnesium (from Magnesium Sulfate)	1	mg.
Manganese (from Manganese Sulfate)	0.5	mg.
Calcium (from Calcium Glycerophosphate)	10	mg.
Phosphorus (from Calcium Glycerophosphate)	8	mg.
Potassium (from Potassium Sulfate)	1	mg.
Alcohol (by volume)	20	%

In a base of Yeast Concentrate and Liver Fraction 1

SUPPLIED

8 ounce bottles and gallon bottles (NDC# 249-1118-01 and -02)

GUSTASE®
Gastrointestinal Enzyme Tablets

COMPOSITION

Each GUSTASE tablet contains GERILASE (standardized amylolytic enzyme) 30 mg., GERIPROTASE (standardized proteolytic enzyme) 6 mg., GERICELLULASE (standardized cellulolytic enzyme) 2 mg. Not enteric coated.

SUPPLIED

Bottles of 42, 100 and 500. (NDC #249-1120-01, -02 and -03).

GUSTASE PLUS™ ℞
Gastrointestinal Enzyme Tablets with Phenobarbital

COMPOSITION

Each GUSTASE PLUS tablet contains Phenobarbital, 8 mg.; Homatrophine Methylbromide, 2.5 mg.; Gerilase (standardized amylolytic enzyme) 30 mg.; Geriprotase (standardized proteolytic enzyme) 6 mg.; Gericellulase (standardized cellulytic enzyme) 2 mg. Not enteric coated.

SUPPLIED

Bottles of 42, 100 and 500. (NDC #249-1121-01, -02, -03).

ISO-BID® CAPSULES 40 mg. ℞
SUSTAINED RELEASE BY MICRO-DIALYSIS DIFFUSION

COMPOSITION

Each ISO-BID SUSTAINED-MEDICATION CAPSULE contains 40 mg. Isosorbide Dinitrate. Medication is released at a smooth, continuous, predictable rate dependent only upon the presence of fluid in the G.I. tract; not dependent on the variable digestive processes.

SUPPLIED

Bottles of 30, 100, and 500. (NDC #249-1164-01, -02 and -03).

EDUCATIONAL MATERIAL

Brochures and samples available on all Geriatric Phamaceutical Products.

Important Notice

Before prescribing or administering any product described in PHYSICIANS' DESK REFERENCE always consult the PDR Supplement for possible new or revised information

Gilbert Laboratories
(Affiliate of Forest Pharmaceuticals, Inc.)
2510 METRO BLVD.
ST. LOUIS, MO 63043

ESGIC product information is listed under Forest Pharmaceuticals, Inc.

Glaxo Inc.
FIVE MOORE DRIVE
RESEARCH TRIANGLE PARK, NC 27709

B C G VACCINE, USP ℞
For Intradermal Use Only
Freeze-Dried

DESCRIPTION

BCG Vaccine, USP, is a standardized preparation of a dried living culture of the bacillus Calmette-Guerin (BCG) strain of *Mycobacterium bovis* for use in immunization against tuberculosis by the intradermal route. It is prepared from a Glaxo culture of the Danish 1077 substrain of BCG. The organisms are harvested, suspended in a medium consisting of suitable concentrations of dextran, glucose, and Triton WR 1339 (tyloxapol), and then freeze-dried to give a product free from microorganisms other than BCG. This vaccine, when reconstituted as directed, contains not less than eight million and not more than 26 million colony-forming units per ml.

CLINICAL PHARMACOLOGY

BCG Vaccine induces active immunity to tuberculosis.

It appears that BCG vaccination does not prevent the establishment of infection in exposed subjects but does limit the multiplication and dissemination of the bacilli and the development of lesions following infection.[1]

The immunity to tuberculosis induced by BCG Vaccine is only relative and is not permanent or entirely predictable. There is no animal test for potency of BCG Vaccine known to correlate directly with protective efficacy in man; however, tuberculin skin test conversion and TB case rates serve as indirect indicators of immunity. When the Danish substrain was administered to 13,598 people in a 20-year controlled clinical trial, an average protective efficacy case rate of 77% was reported.[2] However, the protective efficacy case rate was 84% during the first five years and only 59% ten to 15 years postvaccination. A reliable assessment of efficacy in the last five years was not possible. In studies with other BCG substrains, a strikingly wide range of 0% to 80% of protective efficacy was observed.[3] Published works indicate a high skin test conversion rate (greater than 90% of BCG vaccinees) with the Glaxo freeze-dried BCG Vaccine.[4] Immunity may persist despite a negative skin test developing over time.[2]

After proper intradermal injection of the immunizing dose, the initial skin lesion usually appears within seven to ten days. The normal lesion consists of a small red papule at the site of injection; it reaches its maxium diameter of approximately 8 mm after about five weeks. The top of the papule scales and dries, and the whole lesion gradually shrinks to a smooth or scaly, pink or bluish scar approximately three months after vaccination and becomes a smooth or pitted white scar in approximately six months.

Vaccinated persons normally become tuberculin-positive (Mantoux test) after a period of eight weeks has elapsed, but sometimes up to 14 weeks are needed.

A tuberculin test should be conducted two to three months after vaccination. Successful inoculation as determined by a positive skin test conversion almost always develops after the first vaccination if it is administered properly. If the test is negative, the vaccination should be repeated.

INDICATIONS AND USAGE

BCG Vaccine is indicated for the prevention of tuberculosis. The Immunization Practices Advisory Committee of the US Public Health Service has made the following specific recommendations[5] for the use of BCG Vaccine.

1. BCG vaccination should be seriously considered for persons who are tuberculin skin test-negative and are repeatedly exposed to persistently untreated or ineffectively treated sputum-positive pulmonary tuberculosis.
2. BCG vaccination should be considered for well-defined communities or groups if an excessive rate of new infections can be demonstrated and the usual surveillance and treatment programs have failed or have been shown not to be applicable. Such groups might exist among the socially disaffiliated and those without a regular source of health care, possibly including some alcoholics, drug addicts, and migrants. Groups such as health workers who may be at particular risk of exposure to unrecognized pulmonary tuberculosis should, where possible, be kept under surveillance for evidence of newly acquired tuberculosis infection. It must be recognized that only the occurrence of new infections reflects whether transmission is actually occurring.

CONTRAINDICATIONS

BCG Vaccine is contraindicated in tuberculin-positive individuals, burn patients, and individuals known to have a serious hypersensitivity to it. BCG Vaccine should not be given to persons with impaired immune response, particularly impaired cell-mediated immune mechanisms such as occurs with certain congenital immunodeficiency states, lymphoreticular malignancies, sarcoidosis, or when immunologic response has been suppressed with corticosteroids, alkylating agents, antimetabolites, or radiation.

WARNINGS

BCG vaccination has been associated with adverse reactions, including severe or prolonged ulceration at the vaccination site, lymphadenitis, osteomyelitis, disseminated BCG infection, and death. Systemic treatment with antitubercular chemotherapy (such as isoniazid, rifampin, or streptomycin) should be given where generalized infection with BCG is suspected. In cases of severe local reactions with abscess formation, aspiration should be carried out.

There has been the occasional report of an anaphylactic reaction after BCG Vaccine. In keeping with good medical practice, epinephrine should be available.

PRECAUTIONS

General: Although chronic diseases involving the skin are not contraindications, individuals with such conditions should be vaccinated in a healthy area of skin.

BCG vaccination is not normally undertaken without prior determination that the patient is nonreactive to a tuberculin skin test. The individual to be vaccinated should first be tuberculin-tested by a suitable method. A Mantoux test at 5 TU of Tuberculin PPD (Purified Protein Derivative) is suitable. If this test is negative, the person may be vaccinated immediately. The test should be performed within the six week period preceding vaccination. The protection from tuberculosis afforded by BCG vaccination is only relative and is not permanent or entirely predictable. If the tuberculin test again becomes negative and the risk of infection continues, BCG vaccination may need to be repeated.

A separate, heat-sterilized syringe and needle or a sterile disposable unit should be used for each individual patient to prevent possible transmission of homologous serum hepatitis virus and other infectious agents from one person to another.

Tuberculosis in Vaccinated Persons: Since full, lasting protection from BCG vaccination cannot be assured, tuberculosis should be included in the differential diagnosis of any tuberculosis-like illness in a BCG vaccinee.

A positive tuberculin skin test in a former BCG vaccinee might reflect active infection and lost immunoprotection, so additional clinical tests should be performed for a proper differential diagnosis of overt tuberculous disease. The American Thoracic Society considers a reaction of 10 mm or more to a 5-TU PPD Mantoux test significant regardless of prior BCG immunization history.[6] Persons with significant reactions should receive chest roentgenographic examinations.[7]

Drug Interactions: BCG Vaccine will not be effective if given during treatment with isoniazid, rifampin, streptomycin, or other drugs that inhibit multiplication of BCG.

BCG Vaccine may be given at the same time as oral poliomyelitis vaccine. With other live vaccines it is preferable to allow an interval of three weeks between administration of BCG and the other vaccine, but the interval can be reduced to ten days if a longer period is not available.

In general, vaccines containing toxoids or killed organisms should be given at least seven days before or ten days after BCG Vaccine. However, diphtheria/tetanus vaccine has been given at the same time as BCG Vaccine (but in the other arm) with satisfactory results.[8]

Pregnancy: ***Teratogenic Effects: Pregnancy Category C:*** Animal reproduction studies have not been conducted with BCG Vaccine. It is also not known whether BCG Vaccine can cause fetal harm when administered to a pregnant woman or can affect reproduction capacity. BCG Vaccine should be avoided during pregnancy unless there is an excessive risk of unavoidable exposure to infective tuberculosis.

ADVERSE REACTIONS

The BCG strain used by Glaxo has proved to be associated with a very low incidence of adverse reactions.

However, BCG vaccination has been associated with adverse reactions, including severe or prolonged ulceration at the vaccination site, lymphadenitis, osteomyelitis, disseminated BCG infection, and death.

The reported frequency of complications, mostly from other countries, has varied greatly depending on the substrain of BCG used and on the extent of the surveillance effort. For example, the occurrence of ulceration and lymphadenitis has been reported to range from 1% to 10%, depending on the vaccine, the dosage, and the age of vaccinees. Osteomyelitis has been noted in one per one million vaccinees, although recent information indicates that the rate may be as high as

five per 100,000 in newborns. Disseminated BCG infection and death are very rare; they range from one to ten per ten million vaccinees and occur almost exclusively in children with impaired immune response.
Autoinoculation ulcers are seen occasionally. Abscesses in the skin at the site of inoculation may occur from secondary infection. Rarely, abscesses may develop in the regional lymph nodes draining the site of the BCG vaccination.
Most local reactions are excessive hypersensitivity responses not related to BCG infections. These should be treated with a local corticosteroid and, perhaps, with a broad spectrum antibacterial agent. Granulomas appearing approximately four to six weeks following the vaccination have been reported at the site of the injection. They may result from application of irritating dressings to a normal BCG reaction or may occur occasionally as an idiosyncrasy. Such granulomas may persist for variable periods of time and may have a keloid scar after final healing. Rarely, persistent lupus reactions of the skin that required treatment have been reported. For these, isoniazid in a daily dose of 4 mg/kg of body weight taken for three months has been recommended.
One case of histiocytoma at the vaccination site required excision.[9]
Transient urticaria has been observed, and there have been occasional reports of anaphylaxis, erythema nodosum, and erythema multiforme following BCG vaccination.
Very large doses of BCG given by other than intradermal routes have resulted in rare anecdotal reports of Guillain-Barre syndrome and of aplastic anemia.

OVERDOSAGE

If gross overdosage occurs, and there is reason to suspect the development of a more generalized infection with BCG, systemic treatment with isoniazid or any other suitable antituberculous drug should be given.

DOSAGE AND ADMINISTRATION

Preparation of Vaccine: Using appropriate aseptic technique, add 1 ml of Sterile Water for Injection, USP to each 1-ml size multi-dose ampule of vaccine. Allow to stand for approximately one minute. Avoid shaking, since this results in foaming. The process of withdrawing the solution from the ampule will yield a homogeneous suspension.
Parenteral drug products should be inspected visually for particulate matter and discoloration before administration whenever solution and container permit.
After the vaccine has been prepared, the immunizing dose of 0.1 ml is given by **intradermal** injection using a 26 or 27 gauge needle. Subcutaneous injection must be avoided. For infants under 3 months of age the recommended dose is 0.05 ml. The recommended vaccination site is the arm, over the insertion of the deltoid muscle.
Following reconstitution, the liquid vaccine should be used immediately and any material remaining should be discarded, preferably incinerated or treated with a disinfectant such as strong hypochlorite solution.
The vaccine must not be contaminated with any antiseptic or detergent. If alcohol is used to swab the skin, it must be allowed to evaporate before the vaccine is injected.
Vaccinees should be advised to leave the vaccinated lesion open to the air and keep it dry and clean to facilitate healing. A tuberculin test should be conducted two to three months after vaccination. If the test is negative, the vaccination should be repeated.
Interpretation of Tuberculin Test: After BCG vaccination it is usually not possible to distinguish between a tuberculin reaction caused by virulent suprainfection and a reaction resulting from persistent postvaccination sensitivity. Therefore, caution is advised in attributing a positive skin test to BCG (except in the immediate postvaccination period), especially if the vaccinee has recently been exposed to infective tuberculosis.
Measles and rubella infection can cause tuberculin-positive patients to revert temporarily to tuberculin-negative.

HOW SUPPLIED

BCG Vaccine, USP is supplied in individually boxed 1-ml multi-dose ampules (NDC 0173-0339-65).
This vaccine, when reconstituted as directed, contains not less than eight million and not more than 26 million colony-forming units per ml when measured using a method appropriate to the vaccine being examined.[10]
Before use, store at a uniform temperature between 2° and 8°C (36° and 46°F), preferably at the lower limit. This vaccine contains live bacteria and should be protected against exposure to light.

REFERENCES

1. Sutherland I, Lindgren I: The protective effect of BCG vaccination as indicated by autopsy studies. *Tubercle* 1979;60:225–231.
2. Hart PD, Sutherland I: BCG and vole bacillus vaccines in the prevention of tuberculosis in adolescence and early adult life. *Br Med J* 1977;2:293–295.
3. Biological products; bacterial vaccines and toxoids; implementation of efficacy review; proposed rule (21 CFR 610). *Federal Register* 1985;50(December 13); 51002–51117.
4. Dawodu AH: Tuberculin conversion following BCG vaccination in preterm infants. *Acta Paediatr Scand* 1985;74:564–567.
5. US Dept. of Health, Education, and Welfare: BCG vaccines. *MMWR* 1979;28:241–244.
6. American Thoracic Society: BCG vaccines for tuberculosis. *Am Rev Resp Dis* 1975;112:478–480.
7. Farer LS: Prior BCG vaccination and PPD skin test. *JAMA* 1983;250:3106.
8. Galbraith NS, Crosby G, Barnes JM, et al: Simultaneous immunization with B.C.G., diphtheria-tetanus, and oral poliomyelitis vaccines in children aged 13–14. *Br Med J* 1971;2:193–197.
9. Hartston W: Uncommon skin reactions after BCG vaccination. *Tubercle* 1959;40:265–270.
10. Wright D, Muggleton PW, Griffiths MI: Evaluation of the stability of dried BCG Vaccine. *Tubercle* 1972;53:92–99.

BECLOVENT® Oral Inhaler ℞

[*bek 'lo-vent"*]
(beclomethasone dipropionate, USP)
For Oral Inhalation Only

DESCRIPTION

Beclomethasone dipropionate, USP, the active component of BECLOVENT® (beclomethasone dipropionate) Oral Inhaler, is an anti-inflammatory steroid having the chemical name 9-chloro - 11β, 17, 21 - trihydroxy - 16β-methylpregna-1, 4 - diene - 3, 20 - dione 17, 21 - dipropionate.
BECLOVENT Oral Inhaler is a metered-dose aerosol unit containing a microcrystalline suspension of beclomethasone dipropionate-trichloromonofluoromethane clathrate in a mixture of propellants (trichloromonofluoromethane and dichlorodifluoromethane) with oleic acid. Each canister contains beclomethasone dipropionate–trichloromonofluoromethane clathrate having a molecular proportion of beclomethasone dipropionate to trichloromonofluoromethane between 3:1 and 3:2. Each actuation delivers from the mouthpiece a quantity of clathrate equivalent to 42 mcg of beclomethasone dipropionate, USP. The contents of one canister provide at least 200 oral inhalations.

CLINICAL PHARMACOLOGY

Beclomethasone 17, 21-dipropionate is a diester of beclomethasone, a synthetic corticosteroid which is chemically related to betamethasone. Beclomethasone differs from betamethasone in having a chlorine at the 9-alpha position in place of a fluorine. Animal studies showed that beclomethasone dipropionate has potent anti-inflammatory activity. When beclomethasone dipropionate was administered systemically to mice, the anti-inflammatory activity was accompanied by other features typical of glucocorticoid action, including thymic involution, liver glycogen deposition, and pituitary-adrenal suppression. However, after systemic administration to rats, the anti-inflammatory action was associated with little or no effect on other tests of glucocorticoid activity.
Beclomethasone dipropionate is sparingly soluble and is poorly mobilized from subcutaneous or intramuscular injection sites. However, systemic absorption occurs after all routes of administration. When given to animals in the form of an aerosolized suspension of the trichloromonofluoromethane clathrate, the drug is deposited in the mouth and nasal passages, the trachea and principal bronchi, and the lung; a considerable portion of the drug is also swallowed. Absorption occurs rapidly from all respiratory and gastrointestinal tissues, as indicated by the rapid clearance of radioactively labeled drug from local tissues and appearance of tracer in the circulation. There is no evidence of tissue storage of beclomethasone dipropionate or its metabolites. Lung slices can metabolize beclomethasone dipropionate rapidly to beclomethasone 17-monopropionate and more slowly to free beclomethasone (which has very weak anti-inflammatory activity). However, irrespective of the route of administration (injection, oral, or aerosol), the principal route of excretion of the drug and its metabolites is the feces. Less than 10% of the drug and its metabolites is excreted in the urine. In humans, 12% to 15% of an orally administered dose of beclomethasone dipropionate was excreted in the urine as both conjugated and free metabolites of the drug.
The mechanisms responsible for the anti-inflammatory action of beclomethasone dipropionate are unknown. The precise mechanism of the aerosolized drug's action in the lung is also unknown.

INDICATIONS AND USAGE

BECLOVENT® (beclomethasone dipropionate) Oral Inhaler is indicated only for patients who require chronic treatment with corticosteroids for control of the symptoms of bronchial asthma. Such patients would include those already receiving systemic corticosteroids, and selected patients who are inadequately controlled on a nonsteroid regimen and in whom steroid therapy has been withheld because of concern over potential adverse effects.
BECLOVENT Oral Inhaler is NOT indicated:
1. For relief of asthma which can be controlled by bronchodilators and other nonsteroid medications.
2. In patients who require systemic corticosteroid treatment infrequently.
3. In the treatment of nonasthmatic bronchitis.

CONTRAINDICATIONS

BECLOVENT® Oral Inhaler is contraindicated in the primary treatment of status asthmaticus or other acute episodes of asthma where intensive measures are required.
Hypersensitivity to any of the ingredients of this preparation contraindicates its use.

WARNINGS

Particular care is needed in patients who are transferred from systemically active corticosteroids to BECLOVENT® Oral Inhaler because <u>deaths due to adrenal insufficiency have occurred in asthmatic patients during and after transfer from systemic corticosteroids to aerosol beclomethasone dipropionate</u>. After withdrawal from systemic corticosteroids, a number of months are required for recovery of hypothalamic-pituitary-adrenal (HPA) function. During this period of HPA suppression, patients may exhibit signs and symptoms of adrenal insufficiency when exposed to trauma, surgery or infections, particularly gastroenteritis. Although BECLOVENT Oral Inhaler may provide control of asthmatic symptoms during these episodes, it does NOT provide the systemic steroid which is necessary for coping with these emergencies.
During periods of stress or a severe asthmatic attack, patients who have been withdrawn from systemic corticosteroids should be instructed to resume systemic steroids (in large doses) immediately and to contact their physician for further instruction. These patients should also be instructed to carry a warning card indicating that they may need supplementary systemic steroids during periods of stress or a severe asthma attack. To assess the risk of adrenal insufficiency in emergency situations, routine tests of adrenal cortical function, including measurement of early morning resting cortisol levels, should be performed periodically in all patients. An early morning resting cortisol level may be accepted as normal only if it falls at or near the normal mean level.

Localized infections with *Candida albicans* or *Aspergillus niger* have occurred frequently in the mouth and pharynx and occasionally in the larynx. Positive cultures for oral *Candida* may be present in up to 75% of patients. Although the frequency of clinically apparent infection is considerably lower, these infections may require treatment with appropriate antifungal therapy or discontinuance of treatment with BECLOVENT Oral Inhaler.
BECLOVENT Oral Inhaler is not to be regarded as a bronchodilator and is not indicated for rapid relief of bronchospasm.
Patients should be instructed to contact their physician immediately when episodes of asthma which are not responsive to bronchodilators occur during the course of treatment with BECLOVENT (beclomethasone dipropionate) Oral Inhaler. During such episodes, patients may require therapy with systemic corticosteroids.
There is no evidence that control of asthma can be achieved by the administration of BECLOVENT Oral Inhaler in amounts greater than the recommended doses.
Transfer of patients from systemic steroid therapy to BECLOVENT Oral Inhaler may unmask allergic conditions previously suppressed by the systemic steroid therapy, eg, rhinitis, conjunctivitis, and eczema.

PRECAUTIONS

During withdrawal from oral steroids, some patients may experience symptoms of systemically active steroid withdrawal, eg, joint and/or muscular pain, lassitude, and depression, despite maintenance or even improvement of respiratory function (see **DOSAGE AND ADMINISTRATION**).
In responsive patients, beclomethasone dipropionate may permit control of asthmatic symptoms without suppression of HPA function, as discussed below (see **CLINICAL STUDIES**). Since beclomethasone dipropionate is absorbed into the circulation and can be systemically active, the beneficial effects of BECLOVENT® Oral Inhaler in minimizing or preventing HPA dysfunction may be expected only when recommended dosages are not exceeded.
The long-term effects of beclomethasone dipropionate in human subjects are still unknown. In particular, the local effects of the agent on developmental or immunologic processes in the mouth, pharynx, trachea, and lung are unknown. There is also no information about the possible long-term systemic effects of the agent.

Continued on next page

Glaxo—Cont.

The potential effects of BECLOVENT Oral Inhaler on acute, recurrent, or chronic pulmonary infections, including active or quiescent tuberculosis, are not known. Similarly, the potential effects of long-term administration of the drug on lung or other tissues are unknown.
Pulmonary infiltrates with eosinophilia may occur in patients on BECLOVENT Oral Inhaler therapy. Although it is possible that in some patients this state may become manifest because of systemic steroid withdrawal when inhalational steroids are administered, a causative role for beclomethasone dipropionate and/or its vehicle cannot be ruled out.
Pregnancy: ***Teratogenic Effects:*** Glucocorticoids are known teratogens in rodent species and beclomethasone dipropionate is no exception.
Teratology studies were done in rats, mice, and rabbits treated with subcutaneous beclomethasone dipropionate. Beclomethasone dipropionate was found to produce fetal resorption, cleft palate, agnathia, microstomia, absence of tongue, delayed ossification, and partial agenesis of the thymus. Well-controlled trials relating to fetal risk in humans are not available. Glucocorticoids are secreted in human milk. It is not known whether beclomethasone dipropionate would be secreted in human milk, but it is safe to assume that it is likely. The use of beclomethasone dipropionate in pregnancy, nursing mothers, or women of childbearing potential requires that the possible benefits of the drug be weighed against the potential hazards to the mother, embryo, or fetus. Infants born of mothers who have received substantial doses of corticosteroids during pregnancy should be carefully observed for hypoadrenalism.

ADVERSE REACTIONS

Deaths due to adrenal insufficiency have occurred in asthmatic patients during and after transfer from systemic corticosteroids to aerosol beclomethasone dipropionate (see **WARNINGS**).
Suppression of HPA function (reduction of early morning plasma cortisol levels) has been reported in adult patients who received 1,600-mcg daily doses of BECLOVENT® (beclomethasone dipropionate) Oral Inhaler for one month. A few patients on BECLOVENT Oral Inhaler have complained of hoarseness or dry mouth.
Rare cases of immediate and delayed hypersensitivity reactions, including urticaria, angioedema, rash, and bronchospasm, have been reported after the use of beclomethasone oral or intranasal inhalers.

DOSAGE AND ADMINISTRATION

Adults and Children 12 Years of Age and Older: The usual dosage is two inhalations (84 mcg) given three or four times a day. In patients with severe asthma, it is advisable to start with 12 to 16 inhalations a day and adjust the dosage downward according to the response of the patient. The maximal daily intake should not exceed 20 inhalations, 840 mcg (0.84 mg), in adults.
Children 6 to 12 Years of Age: The usual dosage is one or two inhalations (42 to 84 mcg) given three or four times a day according to the response of the patient. The maximal daily intake should not exceed ten inhalations, 420 mcg (0.42 mg), in children 6 to 12 years of age. Insufficient clinical data exist with respect to the administration of BECLOVENT® Oral Inhaler in children below the age of 6.
Rinsing the mouth after inhalation is advised.
Patients receiving bronchodilators by inhalation should be advised to use the bronchodilator before BECLOVENT Oral Inhaler in order to enhance penetration of beclomethasone dipropionate into the bronchial tree. After use of an aerosol bronchodilator, several minutes should elapse before use of the BECLOVENT Oral Inhaler to reduce the potential toxicity from the inhaled fluorocarbon propellants in the two aerosols.
Different considerations must be given to the following groups of patients in order to obtain the full therapeutic benefit of BECLOVENT Oral Inhaler.
Patients Not Receiving Systemic Steroids: The use of BECLOVENT Oral Inhaler is straightforward in patients who are inadequately controlled with nonsteroid medications but in whom systemic steroid therapy has been withheld because of concern over potential adverse reactions. In patients who respond to BECLOVENT Oral Inhaler, an improvement in pulmonary function is usually apparent within one to four weeks after the start of BECLOVENT Oral Inhaler.
Patients Receiving Systemic Steroids: In those patients dependent on systemic steroids, transfer to BECLOVENT Oral Inhaler and subsequent management may be more difficult because recovery from impaired adrenal function is usually slow. Such suppression has been known to last for up to 12 months. Clinical studies, however, have demonstrated that BECLOVENT Oral Inhaler may be effective in the management of these asthmatic patients and may permit replacement or significant reduction in the dosage of systemic corticosteroids.
The patient's asthma should be reasonably stable before treatment with BECLOVENT Oral Inhaler is started. Initially, the aerosol should be used concurrently with the patient's usual maintenance dose of systemic steroid. After approximately one week, gradual withdrawal of the systemic steroid is started by reducing the daily or alternate-daily dose. The next reduction is made after an interval of one or two weeks, depending on the response of the patient. Generally, these decrements should not exceed 2.5 mg of prednisone or its equivalent. A slow rate of withdrawal cannot be overemphasized. During withdrawal, some patients may experience symptoms of systemically active steroid withdrawal, eg, joint and/or muscular pain, lassitude, and depression, despite maintenance or even improvement of respiratory function. Such patients should be encouraged to continue with the inhaler but should be watched carefully for objective signs of adrenal insufficiency such as hypotension and weight loss. If evidence of adrenal insufficiency occurs, the systemic steroid dose should be boosted temporarily and thereafter further withdrawal should continue more slowly. During periods of stress or a severe asthma attack, transfer patients will require supplementary treatment with systemic steroids. Exacerbations of asthma which occur during the course of treatment with BECLOVENT (beclomethasone dipropionate) Oral Inhaler should be treated with a short course of systemic steroid which is gradually tapered as these symptoms subside. There is no evidence that control of asthma can be achieved by administration of BECLOVENT Oral Inhaler in amounts greater than the recommended doses.
Directions For Use: Illustrated Patient's Instructions for Use accompany each package of BECLOVENT Oral Inhaler.
CONTENTS UNDER PRESSURE. Do not puncture. Do not use or store near heat or open flame. Exposure to temperatures above 120°F may cause bursting. Never throw container into fire or incinerator. Keep out of reach of children.

HOW SUPPLIED

BECLOVENT® Oral Inhaler is supplied in a 16.8-g canister with oral adapter and patient's instructions (NDC 0173-0312-88). BECLOVENT Oral Inhaler Refill is supplied in a 16.8-g canister only with patient's instructions (NDC 0173-0312-98).

ANIMAL PHARMACOLOGY AND TOXICOLOGY

Studies in a number of animal species, including rats, rabbits, and dogs, have shown no unusual toxicity during acute experiments. However, the effects of beclomethasone dipropionate in producing signs of glucocorticoid excess during chronic administration by various routes were dose-related.

CLINICAL STUDIES

The effects of beclomethasone dipropionate on HPA function have been evaluated in adult volunteers. There was no suppression of early morning plasma cortisol concentrations when beclomethasone dipropionate was administered in a dose of 1,000 mcg/day for one month as an aerosol or for three days by intramuscular injection. However, partial suppression of plasma cortisol concentration was observed when beclomethasone dipropionate was administered in doses of 2,000 mcg/day either intramuscularly or by aerosol. Immediate suppression of plasma cortisol concentrations was observed after single doses of 4,000 mcg of beclomethasone dipropionate.
In one study the effects of beclomethasone dipropionate on HPA function were examined in patients with asthma. There was no change in basal early morning plasma cortisol concentrations or in the cortisol responses to tetracosactrin (ACTH 1:24) stimulation after daily administration of 400, 800, or 1,200 mcg of beclomethasone dipropionate for 28 days. After daily administration of 1,600 mcg each day for 28 days, there was slight reduction in basal cortisol concentrations and a statistically significant ($p < .01$) reduction in plasma cortisol responses to tetracosactrin stimulation. The effects of a more prolonged period of beclomethasone dipropionate administration on HPA function have not been evaluated. However, a number of investigators have noted that when systemic corticosteroid therapy in asthmatic subjects can be replaced with recommended doses of beclomethasone dipropionate, there is gradual recovery of endogenous cortisol concentrations to the normal range. There is still no documented evidence of recovery from other adverse systemic corticosteroid-induced reactions during prolonged therapy of patients with beclomethasone dipropionate.
Clinical experience has shown that some patients with bronchial asthma who require corticosteroid therapy for control of symptoms can be partially or completely withdrawn from systemic corticosteroids if therapy with beclomethasone dipropionate aerosol is substituted. Beclomethasone dipropionate aerosol is not effective for all patients with bronchial asthma or at all stages of the disease in a given patient.
The early clinical experience has revealed several new problems that may be associated with the use of beclomethasone dipropionate by inhalation for treatment of patients with bronchial asthma.

1. There is a risk of adrenal insufficiency when patients are transferred from systemic corticosteroids to aerosol beclomethasone dipropionate. Although the aerosol may provide adequate control of asthma during the transfer period, it does not provide the systemic steroid which is needed during acute stress situations. Deaths due to adrenal insufficiency have occurred in asthmatic patients during and after transfer from systemic corticosteroids to aerosol beclomethasone dipropionate (see **WARNINGS**).
2. Transfer of patients from systemic steroid therapy to beclomethasone dipropionate aerosol may unmask allergic conditions that were previously controlled by the systemic steroid therapy, eg, rhinitis, conjunctivitis, and eczema.
3. Localized infections with *Candida albicans* or *Aspergillus niger* have occurred frequently in the mouth and pharynx and occasionally in the larynx. It has been reported that up to 75% of the patients who receive prolonged treatment with beclomethasone dipropionate have positive oral cultures for *Candida albicans*. The incidence of clinically apparent infection is considerably lower but may require therapy with appropriate antifungal agents or discontinuation of treatment with beclomethasone dipropionate aerosol.

The long-term effects of beclomethasone dipropionate in human subjects are still unknown. In particular, the local effects of the agent on developmental or immunologic processes in the mouth, pharynx, trachea, and lung are unknown. There is also no information about the possible long-term systemic effects of the agent. The possible relevance of the data in animal studies to results in human subjects cannot be evaluated.

Shown in Product Identification Section, page 410

BECONASE® Nasal Inhaler ℞

[*bek'ō-nāz"*]
(beclomethasone dipropionate, USP)
For Nasal Inhalation Only

DESCRIPTION

Beclomethasone dipropionate, USP, the active component of BECONASE® Nasal Inhaler, is an anti-inflammatory steroid having the chemical name, 9-Chloro-11β, 17, 21-trihydroxy-16β-methylpregna-1, 4-diene-3, 20-dione 17,21-dipropionate.
Beclomethasone dipropionate is a white to creamy-white, odorless powder with a molecular weight of 521.25. It is very slightly soluble in water, very soluble in chloroform, and freely soluble in acetone and in alcohol.
BECONASE Nasal Inhaler is a metered-dose aerosol unit containing a microcrystalline suspension of beclomethasone dipropionate-trichloromonofluoromethane clathrate in a mixture of propellants (trichloromonofluoromethane and dichlorodifluoromethane) with oleic acid. Each canister contains beclomethasone dipropionate-trichloromonofluoromethane clathrate having a molecular proportion of beclomethasone dipropionate to trichloromonofluoromethane between 3:1 and 3:2. Each actuation delivers from the nasal adapter a quantity of clathrate equivalent to 42 mcg of beclomethasone dipropionate, USP. The contents of one canister provide at least 200 metered doses.

CLINICAL PHARMACOLOGY

Beclomethasone 17,21-dipropionate is a diester of beclomethasone, a synthetic corticosteroid which is chemically related to betamethasone. Beclomethasone differs from betamethasone in having a chlorine at the 9-alpha position in place of a fluorine. Animal studies showed that beclomethasone dipropionate has potent glucocorticoid and weak mineralocorticoid activity.
The mechanisms for the anti-inflammatory action of beclomethasone dipropionate are unknown. The precise mechanism of the aerosolized drug's action in the nose is also unknown. Biopsies of nasal mucosa obtained during clinical studies showed no histopathologic changes when beclomethasone dipropionate was administered intranasally.
The effects of beclomethasone dipropionate on hypothalamic-pituitary-adrenal (HPA) function have been evaluated in adult volunteers by other routes of administration. Studies are currently being undertaken with beclomethasone dipropionate by the intranasal route that may demonstrate that there is more or that there is less absorption by this route of administration. There was no suppression of early morning plasma cortisol concentrations when beclomethasone dipropionate was administered in a dose of 1,000 mcg/day for one month as an oral aerosol or for three days by intramuscular injection. However, partial suppression of plasma cortisol concentration was observed when beclomethasone dipropionate was administered in doses of 2,000 mcg/day either by oral aerosol or intramuscular injection. Immediate suppression of plasma cortisol concentrations was observed after single doses of 4,000 mcg of beclomethasone dipropionate. Suppression of HPA function (reduction of early morning plasma cortisol levels) has been reported in adult patients who received 1,600-mcg daily doses of oral beclomethasone dipropionate for one month. In clinical studies

using beclomethasone dipropionate intranasally, there was no evidence of adrenal insufficiency.

Beclomethasone dipropionate is sparingly soluble. When given by nasal inhalation in the form of an aerosolized suspension, the drug is deposited primarily in the nasal passages. A portion of the drug is swallowed. Absorption occurs rapidly from all respiratory and gastrointestinal tissues. There is no evidence of tissue storage of beclomethasone dipropionate or its metabolites. In vitro studies have shown that tissue other than the liver (lung slices) can rapidly metabolize beclomethasone dipropionate to beclomethasone 17-monopropionate and more slowly to free beclomethasone (which has very weak anti-inflammatory activity). However, irrespective of the route of entry, the principal route of excretion of the drug and its metabolites is the feces. In humans, 12% to 15% of an orally administered dose of beclomethasone dipropionate is excreted in the urine as both conjugated and free metabolites of the drug. The half-life of beclomethasone dipropionate in humans is approximately 15 hours.

Studies have shown that the degree of binding to plasma proteins is 87%.

INDICATIONS AND USAGE

BECONASE® Nasal Inhaler is indicated for the relief of the symptoms of seasonal or perennial rhinitis in those cases poorly responsive to conventional treatment.

BECONASE Nasal Inhaler is also indicated for the prevention of recurrence of nasal polyps responsive to conventional treatment.

Clinical studies in patients with seasonal or perennial rhinitis have shown that improvement is usually apparent within a few days. However, symptomatic relief may not occur in some patients for as long as two weeks. Although systemic effects are minimal at recommended doses, BECONASE Nasal Inhaler should not be continued beyond three weeks in the absence of significant symptomatic improvement. BECONASE Nasal Inhaler should not be used in the presence of untreated localized infection involving the nasal mucosa.

Clinical studies have shown that treatment of the symptoms associated with nasal polyps may have to be continued for several weeks or more before a therapeutic result can be fully assessed. Recurrence of symptoms due to polyps can occur after stopping treatment, depending on the severity of the disease.

CONTRAINDICATIONS

Hypersensitivity to any of the ingredients of this preparation contraindicates its use.

WARNINGS

The replacement of a systemic corticosteroid with BECONASE® Nasal Inhaler can be accompanied by signs of adrenal insufficiency.

Careful attention must be given when patients previously treated for prolonged periods with systemic corticosteroids are transferred to BECONASE Nasal Inhaler. This is particularly important in those patients who have associated asthma or other clinical conditions where too rapid a decrease in systemic corticosteroids may cause a severe exacerbation of their symptoms.

Studies have shown that the combined administration of alternate-day prednisone systemic treatment and orally inhaled beclomethasone increases the likelihood of HPA suppression compared to a therapeutic dose of either one alone. Therefore, BECONASE Nasal Inhaler treatment should be used with caution in patients already on alternate-day prednisone regimens for any disease.

PRECAUTIONS

General: During withdrawal from oral steroids, some patients may experience symptoms of withdrawal, eg, joint and/or muscular pain, lassitude, and depression.

In clinical studies with beclomethasone dipropionate administered intranasally, the development of localized infections of the nose and pharynx with *Candida albicans* has occurred only rarely. When such an infection develops, it may require treatment with appropriate local therapy or discontinuance of treatment with BECONASE® Nasal Inhaler.

Beclomethasone dipropionate is absorbed into the circulation. Use of excessive doses of BECONASE Nasal Inhaler may suppress HPA function.

BECONASE Nasal Inhaler should be used with caution, if at all, in patients with active or quiescent tuberculous infections of the respiratory tract; untreated fungal, bacterial, or systemic viral infections; or ocular herpes simplex.

For BECONASE Nasal Inhaler to be effective in the treatment of nasal polyps, the aerosol must be able to enter the nose. Therefore, treatment of nasal polyps with BECONASE Nasal Inhaler should be considered adjunctive therapy to surgical removal and/or the use of other medications which will permit effective penetration of BECONASE Nasal Inhaler into the nose. Nasal polyps may recur after any form of treatment.

As with any long-term treatment, patients using BECONASE Nasal Inhaler over several months or longer should be examined periodically for possible changes in the nasal mucosa.

Because of the inhibitory effect of corticosteroids on wound healing, patients who have experienced recent nasal septal ulcers, nasal surgery, or trauma should not use a nasal corticosteroid until healing has occurred.

Although systemic effects have been minimal with recommended doses, this potential increases with excessive doses. Therefore, larger than recommended doses should be avoided.

Information for Patients: Patients should use BECONASE Nasal Inhaler at regular intervals since its effectiveness depends on its regular use. The patient should take the medication as directed. It is not acutely effective and the prescribed dosage should not be increased. Instead, nasal vasoconstrictors or oral antihistamines may be needed until the effects of BECONASE Nasal Inhaler are fully manifested. One to two weeks may pass before full relief is obtained. The patient should contact the doctor if symptoms do not improve, or if the condition worsens, or if sneezing or nasal irritation occurs. For the proper use of this unit and to attain maximum improvement, the patient should read and follow the accompanying patient's instructions carefully.

Carcinogenesis, Mutagenesis, Impairment of Fertility: Treatment of rats for a total of 95 weeks, 13 weeks by inhalation and 82 weeks by the oral route, resulted in no evidence of carcinogenic activity. Mutagenic studies have not been performed.

Impairment of fertility, as evidenced by inhibition of the estrous cycle in dogs, was observed following treatment by the oral route. No inhibition of the estrous cycle in dogs was seen following treatment with beclomethasone dipropionate by the inhalation route.

Pregnancy: ***Teratogenic Effects: Pregnancy Category C:*** Like other corticoids, parenteral (subcutaneous) beclomethasone dipropionate has been shown to be teratogenic and embryocidal in the mouse and rabbit when given in doses approximately ten times the human dose. In these studies, beclomethasone was found to produce fetal resorption, cleft palate, agnathia, microstomia, absence of tongue, delayed ossification, and agenesis of the thymus. No teratogenic or embryocidal effects have been seen in the rat when beclomethasone dipropionate was administered by inhalation at ten times the human dose or orally at 1,000 times the human dose. There are no adequate and well-controlled studies in pregnant women. Beclomethasone dipropionate should be used during pregnancy only if the potential benefit justifies the potential risk to the fetus.

Nonteratogenic Effects: Hypoadrenalism may occur in infants born of mothers receiving corticosteroids during pregnancy. Such infants should be carefully observed.

Nursing Mothers: It is not known whether beclomethasone dipropionate is excreted in human milk. Because other corticosteroids are excreted in human milk, caution should be exercised when BECONASE Nasal Inhaler is administered to nursing women.

Pediatric Use: Safety and effectiveness in children below 12 years of age have not been established.

ADVERSE REACTIONS

In general, side effects in clinical studies have been primarily associated with the nasal mucous membranes.

Sensations of irritation and burning in the nose (11 per 100 patients) following the use of BECONASE® Nasal Inhaler have been reported. Also, occasional sneezing attacks (10 per 100 patients) have occurred immediately following the use of the intranasal inhaler.

Localized infections of the nose and pharynx with *Candida albicans* have occurred rarely (see **PRECAUTIONS**).

Less than 2 per 100 patients reported transient episodes of bloody discharge from the nose.

Ulceration of the nasal mucosa has been reported rarely.

Extremely rare instances of nasal septum perforation have been reported following the intranasal application of aerosolized corticosteroids.

Rare cases of immediate and delayed hypersensitivity reactions, including urticaria, angioedema, rash, and bronchospasm, have been reported following the oral and intranasal inhalation of beclomethasone.

Systemic corticosteroid side effects were not reported during the controlled clinical trials. If recommended doses are exceeded, however, or if individuals are particularly sensitive, symptoms of hypercorticism, ie, Cushing's syndrome, could occur.

DOSAGE AND ADMINISTRATION

Adults and Children 12 Years of Age and Older: The usual dosage is one inhalation (42 mcg) in each nostril two to four times a day (total dose 168 to 336 mcg/day). Patients can often be maintained on a maximum dose of one inhalation in each nostril three times a day (252 mcg/day).

The therapeutic effects of corticosteroids on seasonal or perennial rhinitis or on nasal polyps are not immediate. This should be explained to the patient in advance in order to ensure cooperation and continuation of treatment with the prescribed dosage regimen.

BECONASE Nasal Inhaler is *not* recommended for children below 12 years of age.

In the presence of excessive nasal mucus secretion or edema of the nasal mucosa, the drug may fail to reach the site of intended action. In such cases it is advisable to use a nasal vasoconstrictor during the first two to three days of BECONASE Nasal Inhaler therapy.

Directions for Use: Illustrated **Patient's Instructions for Use** accompany each package of BECONASE Nasal Inhaler.

CONTENTS UNDER PRESSURE. Do not puncture. Do not use or store near heat or open flame. Exposure to temperatures above 120°F may cause bursting. Never throw container into fire or incinerator. Keep out of reach of children.

OVERDOSAGE

When used at excessive doses, systemic corticosteroid effects such as hypercorticism and adrenal suppression may appear. If such symptoms appear, the dosage should be decreased. The oral LD_{50} of beclomethasone dipropionate is greater than 1 g/kg in rodents. One canister of BECONASE® Nasal Inhaler contains 8.4 mg of beclomethasone dipropionate; therefore, acute overdosage is unlikely.

HOW SUPPLIED

BECONASE® Nasal Inhaler is supplied in a 16.8-g canister with nasal adapter and patient's instructions (NDC 0173-0336-88).

Store between 2° and 30°C (36° and 86°F).

Shown in Product Identification Section, page 410

CORTICAINE® Cream ℞

[*kort 'ah-kān"*]

DESCRIPTION

CORTICAINE® Cream contains hydrocortisone acetate 0.5% and dibucaine 0.5% in a washable, non-greasy, mentholated, cream base composed of esters of mixed saturated fatty acids, stearyl alcohol, glycerin, polysorbate 40, BHA, BHT, disodium EDTA, and purified water with methylparaben and propylparaben as preservatives. CORTICAINE Cream is an anti-inflammatory and local anesthetic cream for topical and intrarectal use.

CLINICAL PHARMACOLOGY

Hydrocortisone acetate is a corticosteroid that acts to reduce swelling, itching, hyperemia, and other manifestations of inflammation, regardless of the cause. Dibucaine, an amide-type local anesthetic, provides relief from pain, itching, and burning by reversibly blocking nerve conduction when applied topically. Because dibucaine is an amide, it can often be used in patients sensitive to ester-type local anesthetics such as procaine and tetracaine. The base has a soothing, lubricant action.

INDICATIONS AND USAGE

CORTICAINE® Cream is indicated for the relief of the inflammatory manifestations of corticosteroid-responsive dermatoses. When combined with other recognized therapeutic measures, it is recommended for the symptomatic relief of itching, pain, and irritation of certain anorectal, anogenital, and dermatological conditions. On the skin, it offers symptomatic relief in atopic dermatitis, sumac or ivy dermatitis, mild sunburn, minor burns, insect bites, prickly heat, eczema, discomfort after anal surgery, diaper rash, and intertrigo. When introduced into the rectum, it helps to relieve the itching, pain, and inflammation of internal hemorrhoids, as well as the anorectal discomfort of associated conditions such as proctitis, papillitis, and cryptitis. When applied perianally, it can provide symptomatic relief from pruritus ani and external hemorrhoids.

CONTRAINDICATIONS

CORTICAINE® Cream is contraindicated in patients with local tuberculosis and fungal and viral infections. Topical steroids and local anesthetics are contraindicated in those patients with a history of hypersensitivity to any of the components of these preparations. CORTICAINE Cream is not recommended for use in such diseases as pemphigus and discoid lupus erythematosus.

PRECAUTIONS

General: Avoid use in the eyes. Do not apply to extensive areas for prolonged periods or with occlusive dressings as there may be increased systemic absorption of the ingredients. If irritation develops, CORTICAINE® Cream should be discontinued and appropriate therapy instituted. In the presence of a secondary bacterial infection, the use of an appropriate antibacterial agent should be instituted; if a favorable response does not occur promptly, this preparation should be discontinued until the infection has been adequately controlled. CORTICAINE Cream should not be used rectally without adequate proctologic examination and should not be used with anorectal fistulas and abscesses.

Usage in Pregnancy: Although topical steroids have not been reported to have an adverse effect on human preg-

Continued on next page

Glaxo—Cont.

nancy, the safety of their use in pregnant women has not been absolutely established. In laboratory animals, increases in the incidence of fetal abnormalities have been associated with exposure of gestating females to topical corticosteroids, in some cases at rather low dosage levels. Therefore, drugs of this class should not be used extensively on pregnant patients in large amounts or for prolonged periods of time.

ADVERSE REACTIONS

The following local adverse reactions have been reported with topical corticosteroids, especially under occlusive dressings: burning sensations, itching, irritation, dryness, folliculitis, hypertrichosis, acneiform eruptions, hypopigmentation, perioral dermatitis, allergic contact dermatitis, maceration of the skin, secondary infection, skin atrophy, striae, and miliaria.

DOSAGE AND ADMINISTRATION

For Rectal Use: Cleanse the rectal area and dry thoroughly before use. Attach plastic applicator to tube and squeeze tube lightly to fill applicator with cream. Lubricate applicator with cream, then gently insert into rectum and squeeze tube again lightly to extrude a similar applicator dose of cream into the rectum. CORTICAINE® Cream can also be applied topically to irritated anorectal tissues. Use morning and evening and after each bowel movement. The recommended duration of treatment is two to six days.

For Topical Use: Apply to affected areas of the skin two to four times daily. The recommended duration of treatment is two weeks.

HOW SUPPLIED

CORTICAINE® Cream (hydrocortisone acetate 0.5% and dibucaine 0.5%) is supplied in a 1-oz tube with a rectal applicator (NDC 0173-0358-72).

Keep container well closed and store between 15° and 30° C (59° and 86° F).

Shown in Product Identification Section, page 410

ETHATAB® Tablets ℞

[eth' ah-tab]

(ethaverine hydrochloride)

DESCRIPTION

Each ETHATAB® tablet contains ethaverine hydrochloride 100 mg, D&C Yellow No. 10, FD&C Yellow No. 6, and other ingredients.

ACTION

ETHATAB® acts directly on the smooth muscle cells, without involving the autonomic nervous system or its receptors. It produces smooth muscle relaxation, particularly where spasm exists, affecting the larger blood vessels, especially systemic, peripheral and pulmonary vessels, smooth muscle of the intestines, biliary tree, and ureters.

INDICATIONS AND USAGE

In peripheral and cerebral vascular insufficiency associated with arterial spasm; also useful as a smooth muscle spasmolytic in spastic conditions of the gastrointestinal and genitourinary tracts.

CONTRAINDICATIONS

The use of ETHATAB® is contraindicated in the presence of complete atrioventricular dissociation.

PRECAUTIONS

As with vasodilators, ETHATAB® should be administered with caution to patients with glaucoma. The safety of ethaverine hydrochloride during pregnancy or lactation has not been established; therefore, it should not be used in pregnant women or in women of childbearing age unless, in the judgment of the physician, its use is deemed essential to the welfare of the patient.

ADVERSE REACTIONS

Even though the incidence of adverse reactions as reported in the literature is very low, it is possible for a patient to evidence nausea, anorexia, abdominal distress, dryness of the throat, hypotension, malaise, lassitude, drowsiness, flushing, sweating, vertigo, respiratory depression, cardiac depression, cardiac arrhythmia, and headache. If these adverse reactions occur, reduce dosage or discontinue medication.

DOSAGE AND ADMINISTRATION

In mild or moderate disease, the usual dosage for adults is one tablet three times a day. In more difficult cases, dosage may be increased to two tablets three times a day. It is most effective given early in the course of the vascular disorder. Because of the chronic nature of the disease, long-term therapy is required.

HOW SUPPLIED

ETHATAB® (ethaverine hydrochloride) Tablets, yellow, oval, scored tablets, engraved with "Glaxo" and "281"; bottles of 100 (NDC 0173-0281-43) and 500 (NDC 0173-0281-44) and unit dose packs of 100 (NDC 0173-0281-47).

FORTAZ® ℞

[for' taz]

(ceftazidime for injection, Glaxo)

For Intravenous or Intramuscular Use

DESCRIPTION

Ceftazidime is a semisynthetic, broad-spectrum, beta-lactam antibiotic for parenteral administration. It is the pentahydrate of Pyridinium, 1-[[7-[[(2-amino-4-thiazolyl)[(1-carboxy-1-methylethoxy)imino]acetyl]-amino]-2-carboxy -8- oxo-5-thia -1- azabicyclo[4.2.0]oct-2-en-3-yl]methyl]-, hydroxide, inner salt, [6R-[6α,7β(Z)]]. It has the following structure:

FORTAZ® is a sterile, dry, powdered mixture of ceftazidime pentahydrate and sodium carbonate. The sodium carbonate at a concentration of 118 mg/g of ceftazidime activity has been admixed to facilitate dissolution. The total sodium content of the mixture is approximately 54 mg (2.3 mEq)/g of ceftazidime activity. Solutions of FORTAZ range in color from light yellow to amber, depending upon the diluent and volume used. The pH of freshly constituted solutions usually ranges from 5 to 8.

CLINICAL PHARMACOLOGY

After intravenous administration of 500-mg and 1-g doses of ceftazidime over five minutes to normal adult male volunteers, mean peak serum concentrations of 45 and 90 mcg/ml, respectively, were achieved. After intravenous infusion of 500-mg, 1-g, and 2-g doses of ceftazidime over 20 to 30 minutes to normal adult male volunteers, mean peak serum concentrations of 42, 69, and 170 mcg/ml, respectively, were achieved. The average serum concentrations following intravenous infusion of 500-mg, 1-g, and 2-g doses to these volunteers over an eight-hour interval are given in **Table 1**.

Table 2: Ceftazidime Concentrations in Body Tissues and Fluids

Tissue or Fluid	Dose/ Route	No. Patients	Time of Sample Post-dose	Average Tissue or Fluid Level (mcg/ml or mcg/g)
Urine	500 mg IM	6	0–2 hrs	2,100.0
	2 g IV	6	0–2 hrs	12,000.0
Bile	2 g IV	3	90 min	36.4
Synovial fluid	2 g IV	13	2 hrs	25.6
Peritoneal fluid	2 g IV	8	2 hrs	48.6
Sputum	1 g IV	8	1 hr	9.0
Cerebrospinal fluid	2 g q8h IV	5	120 min	9.8
(inflamed meninges)	2 g q8h IV	6	180 min	9.4
Aqueous humor	2 g IV	13	1–3 hrs	11.0
Blister fluid	1 g IV	7	2–3 hrs	19.7
Lymphatic fluid	1 g IV	7	2–3 hrs	23.4
Bone	2 g IV	8	0.67 hr	31.1
Heart muscle	2 g IV	35	30–280 min	12.7
Skin	2 g IV	22	30–180 min	6.6
Skeletal muscle	2 g IV	35	30–280 min	9.4
Myometrium	2 g IV	31	1–2 hrs	18.7

Table 1

Ceftazidime IV Dosage	Serum Concentrations (mcg/ml) 0.5 hr	1 hr	2 hrs	4 hrs	8 hrs
500 mg	42	25	12	6	2
1 g	60	39	23	11	3
2 g	129	75	42	13	5

The absorption and elimination of ceftazidime were directly proportional to the size of the dose. The half-life following intravenous administration was approximately 1.9 hours. Less than 10% of ceftazidime was protein bound. The degree of protein binding was independent of concentration. There was no evidence of accumulation of ceftazidime in the serum in individuals with normal renal function following multiple intravenous doses of 1 and 2 g every eight hours for ten days.

Following intramuscular administration of 500-mg and 1-g doses of ceftazidime to normal adult volunteers, the mean peak serum concentrations were 17 and 39 mcg/ml, respectively, at approximately one hour. Serum concentrations remained above 4 mcg/ml for six and eight hours after the intramuscular administration of 500-mg and 1-g doses, respectively. The half-life of ceftazidime in these volunteers was approximately two hours.

The presence of hepatic dysfunction had no effect on the pharmacokinetics of ceftazidime in individuals administered 2 g intravenously every eight hours for five days. Therefore, a dosage adjustment from the normal recommended dosage is not required for patients with hepatic dysfunction, provided renal function is not impaired.

Approximately 80% to 90% of an intramuscular or intravenous dose of ceftazidime is excreted unchanged by the kidneys over a 24-hour period. After the intravenous administration of single 500-mg or 1-g doses, approximately 50% of the dose appeared in the urine in the first two hours. An additional 20% was excreted between two and four hours after dosing, and approximately another 12% of the dose appeared in the urine between four and eight hours later. The elimination of ceftazidime by the kidneys resulted in high, therapeutic concentrations in the urine.

The mean renal clearance of ceftazidime was approximately 100 ml/min. The calculated plasma clearance of approximately 115 ml/min indicated nearly complete elimination of ceftazidime by the renal route. Administration of probenecid prior to dosing had no effect on the elimination kinetics of ceftazidime. This suggested that ceftazidime is eliminated by glomerular filtration and is not actively secreted by renal tubular mechanisms.

Since ceftazidime is eliminated almost solely by the kidneys, its serum half-life is significantly prolonged in patients with impaired renal function. Consequently, dosage adjustments in such patients as described in the **DOSAGE AND ADMINISTRATION** section are suggested.

Therapeutic concentrations of ceftazidime are achieved in the following body tissues and fluids.

[See table below].

Microbiology: Ceftazidime is bactericidal in action, exerting its effect by inhibition of enzymes responsible for cell-wall synthesis. A wide range of gram-negative organisms is susceptible to ceftazidime in vitro, including strains resistant to gentamicin and other aminoglycosides. In addition, ceftazidime has been shown to be active against gram-positive organisms. It is highly stable to most clinically important beta-lactamases, plasmid or chromosomal, which are produced by both gram-negative and gram-positive organisms, and consequently is active against many strains resistant to ampicillin and other cephalosporins.

Ceftazidime has been shown to be active against the following organisms both in vitro and in clinical infections (see **INDICATIONS AND USAGE**).

Aerobes, Gram-Negative: *Pseudomonas* sp including *Pseudomonas aeruginosa*); *Klebsiella* sp (including *Klebsiella pneumoniae*); *Proteus mirabilis; Proteus vulgaris; Escherichia coli; Enterobacter* sp, including *Enterobacter cloacae* and *Enterobacter aerogenes; Citrobacter* sp, including *Citrobacter freundii* and *Citrobacter diversus; Serratia* sp; *Haemophilus influenzae*, including ampicillin-resistant strains; and *Neisseria meningitidis.*

Aerobes, Gram-Positive: *Staphylococcus aureus*, including penicillinase- and non-penicillinase-producing strains; *Streptococcus pyogenes* (group A beta-hemolytic streptococci); *Streptococcus agalactiae* (group B streptococci); and *Streptococcus pneumoniae.*

Anaerobes: *Bacteroides* sp (NOTE: many strains of *Bacteroides fragilis* are resistant).

Ceftazidime has also been shown to demonstrate in vitro activity against the following microorganisms, although its clinical significance is not known: *Staphylococcus epidermidis; Morganella morganii* (formerly *Proteus morganii*); *Providencia* sp (including *Providencia rettgeri*, formerly *Proteus rettgeri*); *Acinetobacter* sp; *Salmonella* sp; *Clostridium* sp (not including *Clostridium difficile*); *Peptococcus* sp; *Peptostrepto-*

coccus sp; *Neisseria gonorrhoeae; Haemophilus parainfluenzae; Yersinia enterocolitica;* and *Shigella* sp.
Ceftazidime and the aminoglycosides have been shown to be synergistic in vitro against *P aeruginosa* and the enterobacteriaceae. Ceftazidime and carbenicillin have also been shown to be synergistic in vitro against *P aeruginosa.*
Ceftazidime is not active in vitro against methicillin-resistant staphylococci; *Streptococcus faecalis* and many other enterococci; *Listeria monocytogenes; Campylobacter* species; or *C difficile.*
Susceptibility Tests: ***Diffusion Techniques:*** Quantitative methods that require measurement of zone diameters give an estimate of antibiotic susceptibility. One such procedure[1–3] has been recommended for use with disks to test susceptibility to ceftazidime.
Reports from the laboratory giving results of the standard single-disk susceptibility test with a 30-mcg ceftazidime disk should be interpreted according to the following criteria:
Susceptible organisms produce zones of 18 mm or greater, indicating that the test organism is likely to respond to therapy.
Organisms that produce zones of 15 to 17 mm are expected to be susceptible if high dosage is used or if the infection is confined to tissues and fluids (eg, urine) in which high antibiotic levels are attained.
Resistant organisms produce zones of 14 mm or less, indicating that other therapy should be selected.
Organisms should be tested with the ceftazidime disk, since ceftazidime has been shown by in vitro tests to be active against certain strains found resistant when other beta-lactam disks are used.
Standardized procedures require the use of laboratory control organisms. The 30-mcg ceftazidime disk should give zone diameters between 25 and 32 mm for *E coli* ATCC 25922. For *P aeruginosa* ATCC 27853, the zone diameters should be between 22 and 29 mm. For *S aureus* ATCC 25923, the zone diameters should be between 16 and 20 mm.
Dilution Techniques: In other susceptibility testing procedures, eg, ICS agar dilution or the equivalent, a bacterial isolate may be considered susceptible if the MIC value for ceftazidime is not more than 16 mcg/ml. Organisms are considered resistant to ceftazidime if the MIC is equal to or greater than 64 mcg/ml. Organisms having an MIC value of less than 64 mcg/ml but greater than 16 mcg/ml are expected to be susceptible if high dosage is used or if the infection is confined to tissues and fluids (eg, urine) in which high antibiotic levels are attained.
As with standard diffusion methods, dilution procedures require the use of laboratory control organisms. Standard ceftazidime powder should give MIC values in the range of 4 to 16 mcg/ml for *S aureus* ATCC 25923. For E *coli* ATCC 25922, the MIC range should be between 0.125 and 0.5 mcg/ml. For *P aeruginosa* ATCC 27853, the MIC range should be between 0.5 and 2 mcg/ml.

INDICATIONS AND USAGE

FORTAZ® (ceftazidime for injection, Glaxo) is indicated for the treatment of patients with infections caused by susceptible strains of the designated organisms in the following diseases:

1. **Lower Respiratory Tract Infections,** including pneumonia, caused by *P aeruginosa* and other *Pseudomonas* sp; *H influenzae,* including ampicillin-resistant strains; *Klebsiella* sp; *Enterobacter* sp; *P mirabilis; E coli; Serratia* sp; *Citrobacter* sp; *S pneumoniae;* and *S aureus* (methicillin-susceptible strains).
2. **Skin and Skin Structure Infections** caused by *P aeruginosa; Klebsiella* sp; *E coli; Proteus* sp, including *P mirabilis* and indole-positive *Proteus; Enterobacter* sp; *Serratia* sp; *S aureus* (methicillin-susceptible strains); and *S pyogenes* (group A beta-hemolytic streptococci).
3. **Urinary Tract Infections,** both complicated and uncomplicated, caused by *P aeruginosa; Enterobacter* sp; *Proteus* sp, including *P mirabilis* and indole-positive *Proteus; Klebsiella* species; and *E coli.*
4. **Bacterial Septicemia,** caused by *P aeruginosa; Klebsiella* sp; *H influenzae; E coli; Serratia* sp; *S pneumoniae;* and *S aureus* (methicillin-susceptible strains).
5. **Bone and Joint Infections** caused by *P aeruginosa; Klebsiella* sp; *Enterobacter* sp; and *S aureus* (methicillin-susceptible strains).
6. **Gynecological Infections,** including endometritis, pelvic cellulitis, and other infections of the female genital tract caused by *E coli.*
7. **Intra-abdominal Infections,** including peritonitis caused by *E coli, Klebsiella* species, and *S aureus* (methicillin-susceptible strains) and polymicrobial infections caused by aerobic and anaerobic organisms and *Bacteroides* sp (many strains of *B fragilis* are resistant).
8. **Central Nervous System Infections,** including meningitis, caused by *H influenzae* and *Neisseria meningitidis.* FORTAZ has also been used successfully in a limited number of cases of meningitis due to *P aeruginosa* and *S pneumoniae.*

Specimens for bacterial cultures should be obtained prior to therapy in order to isolate and identify causative organisms and to determine their susceptibility to ceftazidime. Therapy may be instituted before results of susceptibility studies are known; however, once these results become available, the antibiotic treatment should be adjusted accordingly.
FORTAZ may be used alone in cases of confirmed or suspected sepsis. FORTAZ has been used successfully in clinical trials as empiric therapy in cases where various concomitant therapies with other antibiotics have been used.
FORTAZ may also be used concomitantly with other antibiotics, such as aminoglycosides, vancomycin, and clindamycin, in severe and life-threatening infections, and in the immunocompromised patient. When such concomitant treatment is appropriate, prescribing information in the labeling for the other anitibiotics should be followed. The dose depends on the severity of the infection and the patient's condition.

CONTRAINDICATIONS

FORTAZ® is contraindicated in patients who have shown hypersensitivity to ceftazidime or the cephalosporin group of antibiotics.

WARNINGS

BEFORE THERAPY WITH FORTAZ® IS INSTITUTED, CAREFUL INQUIRY SHOULD BE MADE TO DETERMINE WHETHER THE PATIENT HAS HAD PREVIOUS HYPERSENSITIVITY REACTIONS TO CEFTAZIDIME, CEPHALOSPORINS, PENICILLINS, OR OTHER DRUGS. ANTIBIOTICS SHOULD BE ADMINISTERED WITH CAUTION TO ANY PATIENT WHO HAS DEMONSTRATED SOME FORM OF ALLERGY, PARTICULARLY TO DRUGS. THIS PRODUCT SHOULD BE GIVEN WITH CAUTION TO PATIENTS WITH TYPE 1 HYPERSENSITIVITY REACTIONS TO PENICILLIN. IF AN ALLERGIC REACTION TO FORTAZ OCCURS, DISCONTINUE TREATMENT WITH THE DRUG. SERIOUS ACUTE HYPERSENSITIVITY REACTIONS MAY REQUIRE EPINEPHRINE AND OTHER EMERGENCY MEASURES.
Pseudomembranous colitis has been reported with the use of cephalosporins (and other broad-spectrum antibiotics); therefore, it is important to consider its diagnosis in patients who develop diarrhea in association with antibiotic use.
Treatment with broad-spectrum antibiotics alters normal flora of the colon and may permit overgrowth of clostridia. Studies indicate a toxin produced by *C difficile* is one primary cause of antibiotic-associated colitis.
Mild cases of colitis may respond to drug discontinuance alone. Moderate to severe cases should be managed with fluid, electrolyte, and protein supplementation as indicated. When the colitis is not relieved by drug discontinuance or when it is severe, oral vancomycin is the treatment of choice for antibiotic-associated pseudomembranous colitis produced by *C difficile.* Other causes of colitis should also be considered.

PRECAUTIONS

FORTAZ® has not been shown to be nephrotoxic; however, because high and prolonged serum antibiotic concentrations can occur from usual doses in patients with transient or persistent reduction of urinary output because of renal insufficiency, the total daily dosage should be reduced when ceftazidime is administered to such patients (see **DOSAGE AND ADMINISTRATION**). Continued dosage should be determined by degree of renal impairment, severity of infection, and susceptibility of the causative organisms.
As with other antibiotics, prolonged use of FORTAZ (ceftazidime for injection, Glaxo) may result in overgrowth of nonsusceptible organisms. Repeated evaluation of the patient's condition is essential. If superinfection occurs during therapy, appropriate measures should be taken.
FORTAZ should be prescribed with caution in individuals with a history of gastrointestinal disease, particularly colitis.
Drug Interactions: Nephrotoxicity has been reported following concomitant administration of cephalosporins with aminoglycoside antibiotics or potent diuretics such as furosemide. Renal function should be carefully monitored, especially if higher dosages of the aminoglycosides are to be administered or if therapy is prolonged, because of the potential nephrotoxicity and ototoxicity of aminoglycosidic antibiotics. Nephrotoxicity and ototoxicity were not noted when FORTAZ was given alone in clinical trials.
Carcinogenesis, Mutagenesis, Impairment of Fertility: Long-term studies in animals have not been performed to evaluate carcinogenic potential. However, a mouse Micronucleus test and an Ames test were both negative for mutagenic effects.
Pregnancy: ***Teratogenic Effects: Pregnancy Category B:*** Reproduction studies have been performed in mice and rats at doses up to 40 times the human dose and have revealed no evidence of impaired fertility or harm to the fetus due to FORTAZ. There are, however, no adequate and well-controlled studies in pregnant women. Because animal reproduction studies are not always predictive of human response, this drug should be used during pregnancy only if clearly needed.
Nursing Mothers: Ceftazidime is excreted in human milk in low concentrations. Caution should be exercised when FORTAZ is administered to a nursing woman.

ADVERSE REACTIONS

FORTAZ® is generally well tolerated. The incidence of adverse reactions associated with the administration of FORTAZ was low in clinical trials. The most common were local reactions following intravenous injection and allergic and gastrointestinal reactions. Other adverse reactions were encountered infrequently. No disulfiram-like reactions were reported.
The following adverse effects from clinical trials were considered to be either related to ceftazidime therapy or were of uncertain etiology:
Local Effects, reported in less than 2% of patients, were phlebitis and inflammation at the site of injection (1 in 69 patients).
Hypersensitivity Reactions, reported in 2% of patients, were pruritus, rash, and fever. Immediate hypersensitivity reactions occurred in 1 in 285 patients.
Gastrointestinal Symptoms, reported in less than 2% of patients, were diarrhea (1 in 78), nausea (1 in 156), vomiting (1 in 500), and abdominal pain (1 in 416).
Less Frequent Adverse Events (less than 1%) were candidiasis, vaginitis, and central nervous system events which included headache, dizziness, and paresthesia.
Laboratory Test Changes noted during FORTAZ clinical trials were transient and included: eosinophilia (1 in 13), positive Coombs' test without hemolysis (1 in 23), thrombocytosis (1 in 45), and slight elevations in one or more of the hepatic enzymes, SGOT (1 in 16), SGPT (1 in 15), LDH (1 in 18), GGT (1 in 19), and alkaline phosphatase (1 in 23). As with some other cephalosporins, transient elevations of blood urea, blood urea nitrogen, and/or serum creatinine were observed occasionally. Transient leukopenia, neutropenia, thrombocytopenia, and lymphocytosis were seen very rarely.

DOSAGE AND ADMINISTRATION

Dosage: The usual adult dosage is 1 g administered intravenously or intramuscularly every eight to 12 hours. The dosage and route should be determined by the susceptibility of the causative organisms, the severity of infection, and the condition and renal function of the patient.
The guidelines for dosage of FORTAZ® are listed in **Table 3.** The following dosage schedule is recommended.
[See table on bottom next page].
Impaired Hepatic Function: No adjustment in dosage is required for patients with hepatic dysfunction.
Impaired Renal Function: Ceftazidime is excreted by the kidneys, almost exclusively by glomerular filtration.
Therefore, in patients with impaired renal function (GFR <50 ml/min), it is recommended that the dosage of ceftazidime be reduced to compensate for its slower excretion. In patients with suspected renal insufficiency, an initial loading dose of 1 g of ceftazidime may be given. An estimate of GFR should be made to determine the appropriate maintenance dose. The recommended dosage is presented in **Table 4.**

Table 4: Recommended Maintenance Doses of FORTAZ in Renal Insufficiency

Creatinine Clearance (ml/min)	Recommended Unit Dose of Ceftazidime	Frequency of Dosing
50–31	1 g	q12h
30–16	1 g	q24h
15–6	500 mg	q24h
<5	500 mg	q48h

When only serum creatinine is available, the following formula (Cockcroft's equation)[4] may be used to estimate creatinine clearance. The serum creatinine should represent a steady state of renal function:

Males:

$$\text{Creatinine clearance (ml/min)} = \frac{\text{Weight (kg)} \times (140 - \text{age})}{72 \times \text{serum creatinine (mg/dl)}}$$

Females:
0.85 × above value

In patients with severe infections who would normally receive 6 g of ceftazidime daily were it not for renal insufficiency, the unit dose given in the table above may be increased by 50% or the dosing frequency increased appropriately. Further dosing should be determined by therapeutic monitoring, severity of the infection, and susceptibility of the causative organism.
In children as for adults, the creatinine clearance should be adjusted for body surface area or lean body mass and the dosing frequency reduced in cases of renal insufficiency.
In patients undergoing hemodialysis, a loading dose of 1 g is recommended, followed by 1 g after each hemodialysis period.
FORTAZ can also be used in patients undergoing intraperitoneal dialysis (IPD) and continuous ambulatory peritoneal dialysis (CAPD). In such patients, a loading dose of 1 g of cef-

Continued on next page

Glaxo—Cont.

tazidime may be given, followed by 500 mg every 24 hours. In addition to intravenous use, FORTAZ (ceftazidime for injection, Glaxo) can be incorporated in the dialysis fluid at a concentration of 250 mg for 2 L of dialysis fluid.

Note: Generally FORTAZ should be continued for two days after the signs and symptoms of infection have disappeared, but in complicated infections longer therapy may be required.

Administration: FORTAZ may be given intravenously or by deep intramuscular injection into a large muscle mass such as the upper outer quadrant of the gluteus maximus or lateral part of the thigh.

Intramuscular Administration: For intramuscular administration, FORTAZ should be constituted with one of the following diluents: Sterile Water for Injection, Bacteriostatic Water for Injection, or 0.5% or 1% Lidocaine Hydrochloride Injection. Refer to **Table 5.**

Intravenous Administration: The IV route is preferable for patients with bacterial septicemia, bacterial meningitis, peritonitis, or other severe or life-threatening infections, or for patients who may be poor risks because of lowered resistance resulting from such debilitating conditions as malnutrition, trauma, surgery, diabetes, heart failure, or malignancy, particularly if shock is present or pending.

For direct intermittent intravenous administration, constitute FORTAZ as directed in **Table 5** with Sterile Water for Injection. Slowly inject directly into the vein over a period of three to five minutes or give through the tubing of an administration set while the patient is also receiving one of the compatible intravenous fluids (see **COMPATIBILITY AND STABILITY**).

For intravenous infusion, constitute the 1- or 2-g Infusion Pack with 100 ml Sterile Water for Injection or one of the compatible intravenous fluids listed under the **COMPATIBILITY AND STABILITY** section. Alternatively, constitute the 500-mg, 1-g, or 2-g vial and add an appropriate quantity of the resulting solution to an IV container with one of the compatible intravenous fluids.

Intermittent intravenous infusion with a Y-type administration set can be accomplished with compatible solutions. However, during infusion of a solution containing ceftazidime, it is desirable to discontinue the other solution.

[See table above].

All vials of FORTAZ as supplied are under reduced pressure. When FORTAZ is dissolved, carbon dioxide is released and a positive pressure develops. For ease of use please follow the recommended techniques of constitution described on the detachable **Instructions for Constitution** section of the package insert.

Solutions of FORTAZ, like those of most beta-lactam antibiotics, should not be added to solutions of aminoglycoside antibiotics because of potential interaction.

However, if concurrent therapy with FORTAZ and an aminoglycoside is indicated, each of these antibiotics can be administered separately to the same patient.

COMPATIBILITY AND STABILITY

Intramuscular: FORTAZ®, when constituted as directed with Sterile Water for Injection, Bacteriostatic Water for Injection, or 0.5% or 1% Lidocaine Hydrochloride Injection, maintains satisfactory potency for 24 hours at room temperature or for seven days under refrigeration. Solutions in Sterile Water for Injection that are frozen immediately after constitution in the original container are stable for three months when stored at −20°C. Once thawed, solutions should not be refrozen. Thawed solutions may be stored for up to eight hours at room temperature or for four days in a refrigerator.

Intravenous: FORTAZ, when constituted as directed with Sterile Water for Injection, maintains satisfactory potency for 24 hours at room temperature or for seven days under refrigeration. Solutions in Sterile Water for Injection in the infusion vial or in 0.9% Sodium Chloride Injection in Viaflex® small volume containers that are frozen immediately after constitution are stable for six months when stored at −20°C. For these large volumes where it may be necessary to warm the frozen product (to a maximum of 40°C), care should be taken to avoid heating after thawing is complete. Once thawed, solutions should not be refrozen. Thawed solutions may be stored for up to 24 hours at room temperature or for seven days in a refrigerator. More concentrated solutions in Sterile Water for Injection in the original container that are frozen immediately after constitution are stable for three months when stored at -20°C. Once thawed, solutions should not be refrozen. Thawed solutions may be stored for up to eight hours at room temperature or for four days in a refrigerator.

FORTAZ is compatible with the more commonly used intravenous infusion fluids. Solutions at concentrations between 1 and 40 mg/ml in 0.9% Sodium Chloride Injection, M/6 Sodium Lactate Injection, 5% Dextrose Injection, 5% Dextrose and 0.225% Sodium Chloride Injection, 5% Dextrose and 0.45% Sodium Chloride Injection, 5% Dextrose and 0.9% Sodium Chloride Injection, and 10% Dextrose Injection, or at concentrations between 1 and 20 mg/ml in Ringer's Injection, USP; Lactated Ringer's Injection, USP; 10% Invert Sugar in Water for Injection; and Normosol® M in 5% Dextrose Injection may be stored for up to 24 hours at room temperature or seven days if refrigerated.

FORTAZ is less stable in Sodium Bicarbonate Injection than in other intravenous fluids. It is not recommended as a diluent. Solutions of FORTAZ in 5% Dextrose and 0.9% Sodium Chloride Injection are stable for at least six hours at room temperature in plastic tubing, drip chambers, and volume control devices of common intravenous infusion sets.

Ceftazidime at a concentration of 4 mg/ml has been found compatible for 24 hours at room temperature or seven days under refrigeration in 0.9% Sodium Chloride Injection when admixed with: Cefuroxime sodium (Zinacef®) 3 mg/ml; Heparin 10 U/ml or 50 U/ml; or Potassium Chloride 10 for 40 mEq/L.

Note: Parenteral drug products should be inspected visually for particulate matter prior to administration wherever solution and container permit.

As with other cephalosporins, FORTAZ powder as well as solutions tend to darken depending on storage conditions; within the stated recommendations, however, product potency is not adversely affected.

HOW SUPPLIED

FORTAZ® in the dry state should be stored at controlled room temperature, 15° to 30°C (59° to 86°F), and protected from light. FORTAZ is a dry, white to off-white powder supplied in vials and infusion packs as follows:

NDC 0173-0377-31 500-mg* Vials (Tray of 25)
NDC 0173-0378-35 1-g* Vials (Tray of 25)
NDC 0173-0379-34 2-g* Vials (Tray of 10)
NDC 0173-0380-32 1-g* Infusion Pack (Tray of 10)
NDC 0173-0381-32 2-g* Infusion Pack (Tray of 10)
NDC 0173-0382-37 6-g* Pharmacy Bulk Package (Tray of 6)

*Equivalent to anhydrous ceftazidime.

REFERENCES: 1. Bauer AW, Kirby WMM, Sherris JC, et al: Antibiotic susceptibility testing by a standardized single disc method. *Am J Clin Pathol* 1966;45:493. 2. National Committee for Clinical Laboratory Standards, Approved Standard: Performance Standards for Antimicrobial Disc Susceptibility Tests (M2-A3), December, 1984. 3. Standardized disc susceptibility test. *Federal Register* 1974;39(May 30):19182-19184 4. Cockcroft DW, Gault MH: Prediction of creatinine clearance from serum creatinine. *Nephron* 1976;16:31-41.

Shown in Product Identification Section, page 410

Table 5: Preparation of FORTAZ Solutions

Size	Amount of Diluent to be Added (ml)	Approximate Available Volume (ml)	Approximate Ceftazidime Concentration (mg/ml)
Intramuscular			
500-mg vial	1.5	1.8	280
1-g vial	3.0	3.6	280
Intravenous			
500-mg vial	5.0	5.3	100
1-g vial	10.0	10.6	100
2-g vial	10.0	11.2	180
Infusion Pack			
1-g vial	100*	100	10
2-g vial	100*	100	20
Pharmacy Bulk Package			
6-g vial	26.0	30	200

* **Note:** Addition should be in two stages (see **Instructions for Constitution** in the package insert).

Table 3: Recommended Dosage Schedule

	Dose	Frequency
Adults		
Usual recommended dose	**1 g IV or IM**	**q8-12h**
Uncomplicated urinary tract infections	250 mg IV or IM	q12h
Bone and joint infections	2 g IV	q12h
Complicated urinary tract infections	500 mg IV or IM	q8-12h
Uncomplicated pneumonia; mild skin and skin structure infections	500 mg–1 g IV or IM	q8h
Serious gynecological and intra-abdominal infections	2 g IV	q8h
Meningitis	2 g IV	q8h
Very severe life-threatening infections, especially in immunocompromised patients	2 g IV	q8h
Pseudomonal lung infections in patients with cystic fibrosis with normal renal function*	30–50 mg/kg IV to a maximum of 6 g/day	q8h
Neonates (0–4 weeks)	30 mg/kg IV	q12h
Infants and children (1 month–12 years)	30–50 mg/kg IV to a maximum of 6 g/day†	q8h

* Although clinical improvement has been shown, bacteriological cures cannot be expected in patients with chronic respiratory disease and cystic fibrosis.

† The higher dose should be reserved for immunocompromised children or children with cystic fibrosis or meningitis.

SEFFIN® ℞

[sef'in]
Cephalothin Sodium for Injection, USP Neutral

DESCRIPTION

SEFFIN® (cephalothin sodium for injection, USP, Glaxo) Neutral is a semisynthetic cephalosporin antibiotic for parenteral use. It is the sodium salt of 7-(thiophene-2-acetamido) cephalosporanic acid. Sodium bicarbonate has been added to result in constituted solutions having a pH ranging between 6 and 8.5. The total sodium content is approximately 63 mg (2.8 mEq sodium ion) per gram of SEFFIN.

Cephalothin is synthesized by the reaction of thiophene-2-acetic acid with 7-aminocephalosporanic acid. Cephalosporin C, which is produced by the fungus *Cephalosporium*, supplies cephalosporanic acid nucleus.

Cephalothin is a white to off-white crystalline solid which is stable in the dry state and moderately soluble in distilled water (250 to 300 mg/ml).

SEFFIN, Neutral contains 30 mg of sodium bicarbonate per gram of cephalothin. Free cephalothin acid does not form within the pH range of the constituted solutions, and the stability and freezability are thereby enhanced.

The molecular weight of cephalothin sodium is 418.4. The chemical structure is as follows:

[See Chemical Formula at top of next column].

CLINCIAL PHARMACOLOGY

Human Pharmacology: SEFFIN® is a broad-spectrum antibiotic for parenteral administration. After intramuscular administration of a 500-mg dose to normal volunteers, the average peak serum antibiotic level was 10 mcg/ml at one-half hour; with a 1-g dose, the average was about 20 mcg/ml. Following a single 1-g intravenous dose of SEFFIN, blood levels have been about 30 mcg/ml at 15 minutes, have ranged from 3 to 12 mcg at one hour, and have declined to about 1 mcg at four hours. With continuous infusion at the rate of 500 mg/hour, levels have been from 14 to 20 mcg/ml of serum. Dosages of 2 g given intravenously over a 30-minute period have produced serum concentrations of 80 to 100 mcg/ml one-half hour after the infusion; levels ranged from 10 to 40 mcg/ml at one hour and from 3 to 6 mcg/ml at two hours and were not assayable after five hours.

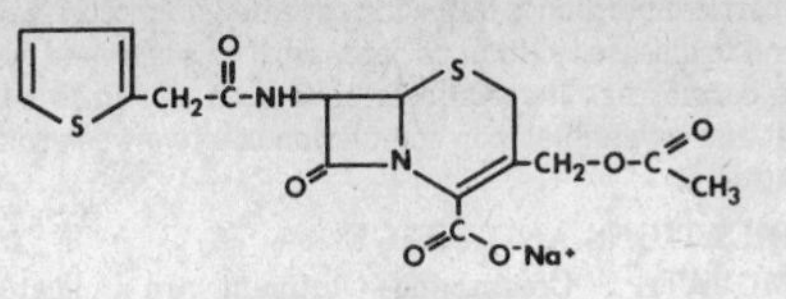

Sixty to 70 percent of an intramuscular dose is excreted by the kidneys in the first six hours; this results in high urine levels, eg, 800 mcg/ml of urine after a 500-mg dose and 2,500 mcg/ml following 1 g. Probenecid slows tubular excretion and almost doubles peak blood levels.

Spinal fluid levels have ranged from 0.4 to 1.4 mcg/ml in a child and from 0.15 to 5 mcg/ml in adults with meningeal inflammatory states. The antibiotic passes readily into other body fluids, eg, pleural, joint, and ascitic fluids. Studies of amniotic fluid and cord blood show prompt transfer of SEFFIN across the placenta.

Peak maternal levels were reached between 31 and 45 minutes after injection of single 1-g intramuscular doses of cephalothin; peak levels occurred in infants about 15 minutes later. Plasma levels in the infants were much lower than those in the mothers.

Secondary aqueous humor levels have averaged 0.5 mcg/ml 30 minutes after a single 1-g intravenous dose. The antibiotic has been detected in bile.

Microbiology: The in vitro bactericidal action of cephalothin results from inhibition of cell-wall synthesis.

SEFFIN is usually active against the following organisms in vitro: beta-hemolytic and other streptococci (many strains of enterococci, eg, *Streptococcus faecalis,* are relatively resistant); staphylococci, including coagulase-positive, coagulase-negative, and penicillinase-producing strains; *Streptococcus (Diplococcus) pneumoniae; Haemophilus influenzae; Escherichia coli* and other coliform bacteria; *Klebsiella* sp; *Proteus mirabilis; Salmonella* sp; and *Shigella* sp.

Pseudomonas sp organisms are resistant to SEFFIN, as are most indole-producing *Proteus* sp and motile *Enterobacter* sp.

Susceptibility Tests: If the Bauer-Kirby-Sherris-Turck method of disk susceptibility testing[1-2] is used, a disk containing 30 mcg of cephalothin should give a zone of over 17 mm when tested against a cephalothin-susceptible bacterial strain and a zone of over 14 mm with an organism of intermediate susceptibility.

INDICATIONS AND USAGE

SEFFIN® is indicated for the treatment of serious infections caused by susceptible strains of the designated microorganisms in the diseases listed below. Culture and susceptibility studies should be performed. Therapy may be instituted before results of susceptibility studies are obtained.

1. **Respiratory Tract Infections** caused by *S pneumoniae,* staphylococci (penicillinase- and non-penicillinase-producing), group A beta-hemolytic streptococci, *Klebsiella* sp, and *H influenzae.*
2. **Skin and Soft-Tissue Infections,** including peritonitis, caused by staphylococci (penicillinase- and non-penicillinase-producing), group A beta-hemolytic streptococci, *E coli, P mirabilis,* and *Klebsiella* sp.
3. **Genitourinary Tract Infections** caused by *E coli, P mirabilis,* and *Klebsiella* sp.
4. **Septicemia,** including endocarditis, caused by *S pneumoniae,* staphylococci (penicillinase- and non-penicillinase-producing), group A beta-hemolytic streptococci, *Streptococcus viridans, E coli, P mirabilis,* and *Klebsiella* sp.
5. **Gastrointestinal Infections** caused by *Salmonella* sp and *Shigella* sp.
6. **Meningitis** caused by *S pneumoniae,* group A beta-hemolytic streptococci, and staphylococci (penicillinase- and non-penicillinase-producing).

Note: Inasmuch as only low levels of SEFFIN are found in the cerebrospinal fluid, the drug is not reliable in the treatment of meningitis and cannot be recommended for that purpose. SEFFIN has, however, proved to be effective in a number of cases of meningitis and may be considered for unusual circumstances in which other, more reliably effective antibiotics cannot be used.

7. **Bone and Joint Infections** caused by staphylococci (penicillinase- and non-penicillinase-producing).

The prophylactic administration of SEFFIN (cephalothin sodium for injection, USP) Neutral preoperatively, intraoperatively, and postoperatively may reduce the incidence of certain postoperative infections in patients undergoing surgical procedures (eg, vaginal hysterectomy) that are classified as contaminated or potentially contaminated.

The perioperative use of SEFFIN may also be effective in surgical patients in whom infection at the operative site would present a serious risk, eg, during open heart surgery and prosthetic arthroplasty.

The prophylactic administration of SEFFIN should be discontinued within a 24-hour period after the surgical procedure. If there are signs of infection, specimens for culture should be obtained for the identification of the causative organism so that appropriate therapy may be instituted (see **Dosage and Administration**).

Note: If the susceptibility tests show that the causative organism is resistant to SEFFIN, other appropriate antibiotic therapy should be instituted.

CONTRAINDICATIONS

SEFFIN® is contraindicated in persons who have shown hypersensitivity to cephalosporin antibiotics.

WARNINGS

BEFORE THERAPY WITH SEFFIN® IS INSTITUTED, CAREFUL INQUIRY SHOULD BE MADE CONCERNING PREVIOUS HYPERSENSITIVITY REACTIONS TO CEPHALOSPORINS AND PENICILLIN. CEPHALOSPORIN C DERIVATIVES SHOULD BE GIVEN CAUTIOUSLY TO PENICILLIN-SENSITIVE PATIENTS. SERIOUS ACUTE HYPERSENSITIVITY REACTIONS MAY REQUIRE EPINEPHRINE AND OTHER EMERGENCY MEASURES.

There is some clinical and laboratory evidence of partial cross-allergenicity of the penicillins and the cephalosporins. Patients have reported severe reactions (including anaphylaxis) to both drugs.

Any patient who has demonstrated some form of allergy, particularly to drugs, should receive antibiotics cautiously and then only when absolutely necessary. No exceptions should be made with regard to SEFFIN.

Pseudomembranous colitis has been reported with the use of cephalosporins (and other broad-spectrum antibiotics); therefore, it is important to consider its diagnosis in patients who develop diarrhea in association with antibiotic use. Such colitis may range in severity from mild to life-threatening.

Treatment with broad-spectrum antibiotics alters normal flora of the colon and may permit overgrowth of clostridia. Studies indicate a toxin produced by *C difficile* is one primary cause of antibiotic-associated colitis.

Mild cases of pseudomembranous colitis may respond to drug discontinuance alone. In moderate to severe cases, management should include sigmoidoscopy, appropriate bacteriologic studies, and fluid, electrolyte, and protein supplementation. When the colitis is not relieved by drug discontinuance or when it is severe, oral vancomycin is the treatment of choice for antibiotic-associated pseudomembranous colitis produced by *C difficile.* Other causes of colitis should be ruled out.

PRECAUTIONS

General: Patients should be followed carefully so that any side effects or unusual manifestations or drug idiosyncrasy may be detected. If an allergic reaction to SEFFIN® occurs, the drug should be discontinued and the patient treated with the usual agents (eg, epinephrine or other pressor amines, antihistamines, or corticosteroids).

Although SEFFIN rarely produces alteration in kidney function, evaluation of renal status is recommended, especially in seriously ill patients receiving maximum doses. Patients with impaired renal function should be placed on the dosage schedule recommended under **DOSAGE AND ADMINISTRATION.** Usual doses in such individuals may result in excessive serum concentrations.

When intravenous doses of cephalothin larger than 6 g daily are given by infusion for periods longer than three days, they may be associated with thrombophlebitis, and the veins may have to be alternated. The addition of 10 to 25 mg of hydrocortisone to intravenous solutions containing 4 to 6 g of cephalothin may reduce the incidence of thrombophlebitis. The use of small IV needles in the larger available veins may be preferred.

Prolonged use of SEFFIN may result in the overgrowth of nonsusceptible organisms. Constant observation of the patient is essential. If superinfection occurs during therapy, appropriate measures should be taken.

A false-positive reaction for glucose in the urine may occur with Benedict's or Fehling's solution or with Clinitest® tablets but not with Tes-Tape® (Glucose Enzymatic Test Strip, USP, Lilly).

An increased incidence of nephrotoxicity has been reported following concomitant administration of cephalosporins and aminoglycoside antibiotics.

Prescribe broad-spectrum antibiotics with caution in individuals with a history of gastrointestinal disease, particularly colitis.

Pregnancy: ***Teratogenic Effects: Pregnancy Category B:*** Reproduction studies have been performed in rabbits given doses of 200 mg/kg and have revealed no evidence of impaired fertility or harm to the fetus due to SEFFIN. There are, however, no adequate and well-controlled studies in pregnant women. Because animal reproduction studies are not always predictive of human response, this drug should be used during pregnancy only if clearly needed.

Nursing Mothers: Caution should be exercised when SEFFIN® (cephalothin sodium for injection, USP, Glaxo) Neutral is administered to a nursing woman.

ADVERSE REACTIONS

Hypersensitivity: Maculopapular rash, urticaria, reactions resembling serum sickness, and anaphylaxis have been reported. Eosinophilia and drug fever have been observed to be associated with other allergic reactions. These reactions are most likely to occur in patients with a history of allergy, particularly to penicillin.

Blood: Neutropenia, thrombocytopenia, and hemolytic anemia have been reported. Some individuals, particularly those with azotemia, have developed positive direct Coombs' tests during cephalothin therapy.

Liver: Transient rise in SGOT and alkaline phosphatase has been noted.

Kidney: Rise in BUN and decreased creatinine clearance have been reported, particularly in patients with prior renal impairment. The role of SEFFIN® in renal changes is difficult to assess because other factors predisposing to prerenal azotemia or to acute renal failure usually have been present.

Local Reactions: Pain, induration, tenderness, and elevation of temperature have been reported following repeated intramuscular injections. Thrombophlebitis has occurred and is usually associated with daily doses of more than 6 g given by infusion for longer than three days.

Gastrointestinal: Symptoms of pseudomembranous colitis may appear either during or after antibiotic treatment. Nausea and vomiting have been reported rarely.

DOSAGE AND ADMINISTRATION

Adults: The usual dosage range is 500 mg to 1 g of cephalothin every four to six hours. A dosage of 500 mg every six hours is adequate in uncomplicated pneumonia, furunculosis with cellulitis, and most urinary tract infections. In severe infections, this may be increased by giving the injections every four hours or, when the desired response is not obtained, by raising the dose to 1 g. In life-threatening infections, doses up to 2 g every four hours may be required.

For perioperative prophylactic use to prevent postoperative infections in contaminated or potentially contaminated surgery in adults, the following doses are recommended: 1 to 2 g administered IV just prior to surgery (approximately one-half to one hour before the initial incision); 1 to 2 g during surgery (administration modified according to the duration of the operative procedure); and 1 to 2 g every six hours postoperatively for 24 hours.

In children, 20 to 30 mg/kg may be given at the times designated above.

Since SEFFIN® (cephalothin sodium for injection, USP) Neutral has a serum half-life of 30 to 50 minutes, it is important that the preoperative dose be given just prior to the start of surgery so that adequate antibiotic levels are present in the serum and tissues at the time of initial surgical incision and that SEFFIN be administered, if necessary, at appropriate intervals during surgery to provide sufficient levels of the antibiotic at the anticipated moments of greatest exposure to infective organisms.

When renal function is reduced, an intravenous loading dose of 1 to 2 g may be given. The continued dosage schedule should be determined by degree of renal impairment, severity of infection, and susceptibility of the causative organism. The maximum doses administered should be based on the following recommendations.

Dosage of SEFFIN
When Renal Function is Impaired

Status of Renal Function	Maximum Adult Dosage (Maintenance)
Mild impairment (C_{cr} = 80–50 ml/min)	2.0 g q6h
Moderate impairment (C_{cr} = 50–25 ml/min)	1.5 g q6h
Severe impairment (C_{cr} = 25–10 ml/min)	1.0 g q6h
Marked impairment (C_{cr} = 10–2 ml/min)	0.5 g q6h
Essentially no function (C_{cr} = <2 ml/min)	0.5 g q8h

Infants and Children: The dosage should be proportionately less in accordance with age, weight, and severity of infection. Daily administration of 100 mg/kg (80 to 160 mg/kg or 40 to

Continued on next page

Glaxo—Cont.

80 mg/lb) in divided doses has been found effective for most infections susceptible to SEFFIN.

Antibiotic therapy in beta-hemolytic streptococcal infections should continue for at least 10 days. In staphylococcal infections, surgical procedures such as incision and drainage should be carried out in all cases when indicated.

SEFFIN may be given intravenously or by deep intramuscular injection into a large muscle mass, such as the gluteus or lateral aspect of the thigh, to minimize pain and induration.

Intramuscular Administration: Each gram of cephalothin should be diluted with 4 ml of Sterile Water for Injection. If the vial contents do not completely dissolve, an additional small amount of diluent (eg, 0.2 to 0.4 ml) may be added and the contents warmed slightly.

Intravenous Administration: The intravenous route may be preferable for patients with bacteremia, septicemia, or other severe or life-threatening infections who may be poor risks because of lowered resistance resulting from such debilitating conditions as malnutrition, trauma, surgery, diabetes, heart failure, or malignancy, particularly if shock is present or impending. For these infections in patients with normal renal function, the intravenous dosage is 4 to 12 g of cephalothin daily. In conditions such as septicemia, 6 to 8 g/day may be given intravenously for several days at the beginning of therapy; then, depending on the clinical response and laboratory findings, the dosage may gradually be reduced.

For patients who are to receive cephalothin intravenously, it is convenient to use the 1-or 2-g 100-ml-size vial (see **PRECAUTIONS**).

For intermittent intravenous administration, a solution containing 1 g of cephalothin in 10 ml of diluent may be slowly injected directly into the vein over a period of three to five minutes or may be given through the tubing when the patient is receiving parenteral solutions.

Intermittent intravenous infusion with a Y-type administration set can also be accomplished while bulk intravenous solutions are being infused. However, it is desirable to discontinue the other solution during infusion of the solution containing SEFFIN. When this technique is employed, careful attention should be paid to the volume of the solution containing SEFFIN so that the calculated dose will be infused.

For continuous intravenous infusion, 1 or 2 g of cephalothin diluted and well mixed with at least 10 ml of Sterile Water for Injection may be added to an IV bottle containing one of the following intravenous solutions: Acetated Ringer's Injection, 5% Dextrose Injection, 5% Dextrose in Lactated Ringer's Injection, Ionosol® B in D5-W, Isolyte® M with 5% Dextrose, Lactated Ringer's Injection, Normosol®-M in D5-W, Plasma-Lyte® Injection, Plasma-Lyte®-M Injection in 5% Dextrose, Ringer's Injection, or 0.9% Sodium Chloride Injection. The choice of solution and the volume to be employed are dictated by fluid and electrolyte management.

Intraperitoneal Administration: In peritoneal dialysis procedures, cephalothin has been added to dialysis fluid in concentrations up to 6 mg/100 ml and instilled into the peritoneal space throughout an entire dialysis (16 to 30 hours). Careful assay procedures have shown that 44% of the administered drug was absorbed into the bloodstream. Serum levels of 10 mcg/ml were reported, with no evidence of accumulation and no untoward local or systemic reactions.

The intraperitoneal administration of solutions containing 0.1% to 4.0% SEFFIN® (cephalothin sodium for injection, USP) Neutral in saline has been used in treating patients with peritonitis or contaminated peritoneal cavities. (The total daily dosage of SEFFIN should take into account the amount given by the intraperitoneal route.)

Stability: While stored under **refrigeration,** the solution has a satisfactory potency for 96 hours after constitution. Solutions may precipitate; they can be redissolved by being warmed to room temperature with constant agitation. Kept at **room temperature,** solutions for intramuscular injection should be given within 12 hours after being mixed. Intravenous infusions should be started within 12 hours and completed within 24 hours. For prolonged infusions, replace with a freshly prepared solution at least every 24 hours.

The concentrated solution will darken, especially at room temperature. Slight discoloration of the solution is permissible.

Solutions of SEFFIN in Sterile Water for Injection, 5% Dextrose Injection, or 0.9% Sodium Chloride Injection that are frozen immediately after constitution in the original container are stable for as long as 12 weeks when stored at −20° C. **If the product is warmed, care should be taken to avoid heating it after the thawing is complete. Once thawed, the solution should not be refrozen.**

HOW SUPPLIED

SEFFIN® (cephalothin sodium for injection, USP) Neutral is supplied in rubber-stoppered vials, infusion bottles, and pharmacy bulk packages.

NDC 0173-0366-31 1-g* Vials (Tray of 25)
NDC 0173-0368-35 2-g* Vials (Tray of 25)
NDC 0173-0367-32 1-g* 100-ml Infusion Pack (Tray of 10)
NDC 0173-0369-32 2-g* 100-ml Infusion Pack (Tray of 10)
NDC 0173-0370-37 10-g* 100-ml Pharmacy Bulk Package (Tray of 6)

*Equivalent to cephalothin.

References: 1. Bauer AW, Kirby WMM, Sherris JC, et al: Antibiotic susceptibility testing by a standardized single disc method. *Am J Clin Pathol* 1966; 45:493.
2. Standardized disc susceptibility test. *Federal Register* 1974; 39 (May 30): 19182-19184.

TEMOVATE™ ℞

[*tim'ō-vāt"*]
(clobetasol propionate)
Cream, 0.05%
Ointment, 0.05%
(potency expressed as clobetasol propionate)

For Dermatological Use Only—
Not for Ophthalmic Use.

DESCRIPTION

TEMOVATE™ Cream and Ointment contain the active compound clobetasol propionate, a synthetic corticosteroid, for topical dermatologic use. Clobetasol, an analog of prednisolone, has a high degree of glucocorticoid activity and a slight degree of mineralocorticoid activity.

Chemically, clobetasol propionate is 21-chloro-9-fluoro-11β, 17-dihydroxy-16β-methylpregna-1, 4-diene-3, 20-dione, 17-propionate, with the empirical formula $C_{25}H_{32}ClFO_5$, a molecular weight of 467, and the following structural formula:

Clobetasol propionate is a white to cream-colored crystalline powder insoluble in water.

TEMOVATE Cream contains clobetasol propionate 0.5 mg/g in a cream base of propylene glycol, glyceryl monostearate, cetostearyl alcohol, glyceryl stearate, PEG 100 stearate, white wax, chlorocresol, sodium citrate, citric acid monohydrate, and purified water.

TEMOVATE Ointment contains clobetasol propionate 0.5 mg/g in a base of propylene glycol, sorbitan sesquioleate, and white petrolatum.

CLINICAL PHARMACOLOGY

The corticosteroids are a class of compounds comprising steroid hormones that are secreted by the adrenal cortex and their synthetic analogs. In pharmacologic doses, corticosteroids are used primarily for their anti-inflammatory and/or immunosuppressive effects. Topical corticosteroids, such as clobetasol propionate, are effective in the treatment of corticosteroid-responsive dermatoses primarily because of their anti-inflammatory, antipruritic, and vasoconstrictive actions. However, while the physiologic, pharmacologic, and clinical effects of the corticosteroids are well known, the exact mechanisms of their actions in each disease are uncertain.

Clobetasol propionate, a corticosteroid, has been shown to have topical (dermatologic) and systemic pharmacologic and metabolic effects characteristic of this class of drugs.

Pharmacokinetics: The extent of percutaneous absorption of topical corticosteroids, including clobetasol propionate, is determined by many factors, including the vehicle, the integrity of the epidermal barrier, and the use of occlusive dressings (see **DOSAGE AND ADMINISTRATION**).

As with all topical corticosteroids, clobetasol propionate can be absorbed from normal intact skin. Inflammation and/or other disease processes in the skin may increase percutaneous absorption. Occlusive dressings substantially increase the percutaneous absorption of topical corticosteroids (see **DOSAGE AND ADMINISTRATION**).

Once absorbed through the skin, topical corticosteroids enter pharmacokinetic pathways similar to systemically administered corticosteroids. Corticosteroids are bound to plasma proteins in varying degrees. Corticosteroids are metabolized primarily in the liver and are then excreted by the kidneys. Some of the topical corticosteroids, including clobetasol propionate and its metabolites, are also excreted into the bile.

TEMOVATE™ (clobetasol propionate) Cream and Ointment have been shown to depress the plasma levels of adrenal cortical hormones following repeated nonocclusive application to diseased skin in patients with psoriasis and eczematous dermatitis. These effects have been shown to be transient and reversible upon completion of a two-week course of treatment.

INDICATIONS AND USAGE

TEMOVATE™ Cream and Ointment are indicated for short-term treatment of inflammatory and pruritic manifestations of moderate to severe corticosteroid-responsive dermatoses. Treatment beyond two weeks is not recommended, and the total dosage should not exceed 50 g per week because of the potential for the drug to suppress the hypothalamic-pituitary-adrenal (HPA) axis.

These products are not recommended for use in children under 12 years of age.

CONTRAINDICATIONS

TEMOVATE™ Cream and Ointment are contraindicated in patients who are hypersensitive to clobetasol propionate, to other corticosteroids, or to any ingredient in these preparations.

PRECAUTIONS

General: TEMOVATE™ is a highly potent topical corticosteroid that has been shown to suppress the HPA axis at doses as low as 2 g per day. Systemic absorption of topical corticosteroids has resulted in reversible HPA axis suppression, manifestations of Cushing's syndrome, hyperglycemia, and glucosuria in some patients.

Conditions which augment systemic absorption include the application of the more potent corticosteroids, use over large surface areas, prolonged use, and the addition of occlusive dressings. Therefore, patients receiving a large dose of a potent topical steroid applied to a large surface area should be evaluated periodically for evidence of HPA axis suppression by using the urinary free cortisol and ACTH stimulation tests. If HPA axis suppression is noted, an attempt should be made to withdraw the drug, to reduce the frequency of application, or to substitute a less potent steroid.

Recovery of HPA axis function is generally prompt and complete upon discontinuation of the drug. Infrequently, signs and symptoms of steroid withdrawal may occur, requiring supplemental systemic corticosteroids.

Children may absorb proportionally large amounts of topical corticosteroids and thus be more susceptible to systemic toxicity (see **PRECAUTIONS: Pediatric Use**).

If irritation develops, topical corticosteroids should be discontinued and appropriate therapy instituted.

In the presence of dermatological infections, the use of an appropriate antifungal or antibacterial agent should be instituted. If a favorable response does not occur promptly, the corticosteroid should be discontinued until the infection has been adequately controlled.

Certain areas of the body, such as the face, groin, and axillae, are more prone to atrophic changes than other areas of the body following treatment with corticosteroids. Frequent observation of the patient is important if these areas are to be treated.

As with other potent topical corticosteroids, TEMOVATE™ (clobetasol propionate) Cream and Ointment should not be used in the treatment of rosacea and perioral dermatitis. Topical corticosteroids in general should not be used in the treatment of acne.

Information for Patients: Patients using TEMOVATE should receive the following information and instructions:

1. This medication is to be used as directed by the physician and should not be used longer than the prescribed time period. It is for external use only. Avoid contact with the eyes.
2. This medication should not be used for any disorder other than that for which it was prescribed.
3. The treated skin area should not be bandaged or otherwise covered or wrapped so as to be occlusive.
4. Any signs of local adverse reactions should be reported to your physician.

Laboratory Tests: The following tests may be helpful in evaluating HPA axis suppression:
Urinary free cortisol test
ACTH stimulation test

Carcinogenesis, Mutagenesis, Impairment of Fertility: Long-term animal studies have not been performed to evaluate the carcinogenic potential or the effect on fertility of topically applied corticosteroids.

Studies to determine mutagenicity with prednisolone have revealed negative results.

Pregnancy: *Teratogenic Effects: Pregnancy Category C:* Corticosteroids are generally teratogenic in laboratory animals when administered systemically at relatively low dosage levels. The more potent corticosteroids have been shown to be teratogenic in animals after dermal application. Clobetasol propionate has not been tested for teratogenicity by this route; however, it appears to be fairly well absorbed percutaneously, and when administered subcutaneously, it proved to be a relatively potent teratogen in both the rabbit and the mouse.

There are no adequate and well-controlled studies of the teratogenic effects of topically applied corticosteroids in pregnant women. Therefore, topical corticosteroids should be used during pregnancy only if the potential benefit justifies the potential risk to the fetus. Drugs of this class should not be used extensively on pregnant patients in large amounts or for prolonged periods of time.

Nursing Mothers: It is not known whether topical administration of corticosteroids could result in sufficient systemic absorption to produce detectable quantities in breast milk. Systemically administered corticosteroids are secreted into breast milk in quantities not likely to have a deleterious effect on the infant. Nevertheless, caution should be exercised when topical corticosteroids are prescribed for a nursing woman.

Pediatric Use: Use of TEMOVATE Cream and Ointment in children under 12 years of age is not recommended.

Pediatric patients may demonstrate greater susceptibility to topical corticosteroid-induced HPA axis suppression and Cushing's syndrome than mature patients because of a large skin surface area-to-body weight ratio.

HPA axis suppression, Cushing's syndrome, and intracranial hypertension have been reported in children receiving topical corticosteroids. Manifestations of adrenal suppression in children include linear growth retardation, delayed weight gain, low plasma cortisol levels, and absence of response to ACTH stimulation. Manifestations of intracranial hypertension include bulging fontanelles, headaches, and bilateral papilledema.

ADVERSE REACTIONS

TEMOVATE™ (clobetasol propionate) Cream and Ointment are generally well tolerated when used for two-week treatment periods.

The most frequent adverse reactions reported for TEMOVATE Cream have been local and have included burning sensation in 4 of 421 patients and stinging sensation in 3 of 421 patients. Less frequent adverse reactions were itching, skin atrophy, and cracking and fissuring of the skin, which occurred in 1 of 421 patients.

The most frequent adverse events reported for TEMOVATE Ointment have been local and have included burning sensation, irritation, and itching. These occurred in 2 of 366 patients. Less frequent adverse reactions were stinging, cracking, erythema, folliculitis, numbness of fingers, skin atrophy, and telangiectasia, which occurred in 1 of 366 patients.

The following local adverse reactions are reported infrequently when topical corticosteroids are used as recommended. These reactions are listed in an approximately decreasing order of occurrence: burning, itching, irritation, dryness, folliculitis, hypertrichosis, acneiform eruptions, hypopigmentation, perioral dermatitis, allergic contact dermatitis, maceration of the skin, secondary infection, skin atrophy, striae, and miliaria. Systemic absorption of topical corticosteroids has produced reversible HPA axis suppression, manifestations of Cushing's syndrome, hyperglycemia, and glucosuria in some patients. In rare instances, treatment (or withdrawal of treatment) of psoriasis with corticosteroids is thought to have provoked the pustular form of the disease.

OVERDOSAGE

Topically applied TEMOVATE™ can be absorbed in sufficient amounts to produce systemic effects (see **PRECAUTIONS**).

DOSAGE AND ADMINISTRATION

A thin layer of TEMOVATE™ Cream and Ointment should be applied with gentle rubbing to the affected skin areas twice daily, once in the morning and once at night.

TEMOVATE Cream and Ointment are potent; therefore, **treatment must be limited to 14 days, and amounts greater than 50 g per week should not be used.**

TEMOVATE Cream and Ointment are not to be used with occlusive dressings.

HOW SUPPLIED

TEMOVATE™ Cream, 0.05% is supplied in 15-g (NDC 0173-0375-73) and 30-g (NDC 0173-0375-72) tubes. TEMOVATE™ Ointment, 0.05% is supplied in 15-g (NDC 0173-0376-73) and 30-g (NDC 0173-0376-72) tubes.

Store between 15° and 30°C (59° and 86°F). TEMOVATE Cream should not be refrigerated.

Shown in Product Identification Section, page 410

THEOBID® and THEOBID® JR. DURACAP® ℞

[thē'ō-bid]
(theophylline, anhydrous)
(SUSTAINED RELEASE)

DESCRIPTION

Each sustained release capsule contains the labeled amount of theophylline anhydrous in a sustained release bead formulation. Each capsule also contains the inactive ingredients benzyl alcohol, butylparaben, edetate calcium disodium, FD&C Blue No. 1, FC&C Red No. 3 (THEOBID JR. only), gelatin, methylparaben, pharmaceutical glaze, propylparaben, sodium lauryl sulfate, sodium propionate, starch, sucrose, titanium dioxide, and other ingredients.

THEOBID® DURACAP® (theophylline, anhydrous) has been formulated to provide serum levels when administered every 12 hours.

Theophylline anhydrous, a xanthine bronchodilator, is a white, odorless, crystalline powder having a bitter taste. It has the chemical formula of : $C_7H_8N_4O_2$.

CLINICAL PHARMACOLOGY

Theophylline directly relaxes the smooth muscle of the bronchial airways and pulmonary blood vessels, thus acting mainly as a bronchodilator and smooth muscle relaxant. The drug also possesses other actions typical of the xanthine derivatives: coronary vasodilator, diuretic, cardiac stimulant, cerebral stimulant, and skeletal muscle stimulant. The actions of theophylline may be mediated through inhibition of phosphodiesterase and a resultant increase in intracellular cyclic AMP.

In vitro, theophylline has been shown to react synergistically with beta-agonists that increase intracellular cyclic AMP through the stimulation of adenyl cyclase, but synergism has not been demonstrated in patient studies and more data are needed to determine if theophylline and beta-agonists have a clinically important additive effect in vivo.

Apparently, no development of tolerance occurs with chronic use of theophylline.

Pharmacokinetics: The half-life of theophylline is influenced by a number of known variables. It is prolonged in patients suffering from chronic alcoholism, impaired hepatic or renal function, congestive heart failure, and in patients receiving macrolide antibiotics and cimetidine. Older adults (over age 55) and patients with chronic obstructive pulmonary disease, with or without cor pulmonale, may also have much slower clearance rates. For such patients, the theophylline half-life may exceed 24 hours.

Newborns and neonates have extremely slow clearance rates compared to older infants (over 6 months) and children, and may also have a theophylline half-life of over 24 hours. High fever for prolonged periods may also reduce the rate of theophylline elimination.

Theophylline Elimination Characteristics

	Theophylline Clearance Rates (mean±S.D.)	Half-life Average (mean±S.D.)
Children (over 6 months of age)	1.45±0.58 ml/kg/min	3.7±1.1 hrs
Adult Nonsmokers with Uncomplicated Asthma	0.65±0.19 ml/kg/min	8.7±2.2 hrs

The half-life of theophylline in smokers (one to two packs/-day) averages four to five hours among various studies, much shorter than the half-life in nonsmokers, which averages about seven to nine hours. The increase in theophylline clearance caused by smoking is probably the result of induction of drug-metabolizing enzymes that do not readily normalize after cessation of smoking. It appears that between three months and two years may be necessary for normalization of the effect of smoking on theophylline pharmacokinetics.

In a single-dose study using ten healthy males, with initial fasting of ten hours before dosing and two hours after dosing, THEOBID® dosed at 520 mg produced a mean peak theophylline serum level of 10.17 ± 1.01 mcg/ml (mean ± S.D.) at 5.2 ± 1 hour (mean ± S.D.) after administration.

In a multiple-dose crossover study of 18 healthy nonsmoking males fasting for ten hours prior to initial dosing and two hours after dosing, THEOBID dosed at 390 mg (mean, 4.8 mg/kg) every 12 hours for five consecutive days produced areas under the curve equivalent to immediate release aminophylline tablets dosed as 300 mg (mean, 3.2 mg/kg) at eight hours for the same time period.

INDICATIONS AND USAGE

For relief and/or prevention of symptoms from asthma and reversible bronchospasm associated with chronic bronchitis and emphysema.

CONTRAINDICATIONS

This product is contraindicated in individuals who have shown hypersensitivity to any of its components.

WARNINGS

Status asthmaticus should be considered a medical emergency and is defined as that degree of bronchospasm which is not rapidly responsive to usual doses of conventional bronchodilators. Optimal therapy for such patients frequently requires both **additional medication**, parenterally administered, and **close monitoring**, preferably in an intensive care setting.

Although increasing the dose of theophylline may bring about relief, such treatment may be associated with toxicity. The likelihood of such toxicity developing increases significantly when the serum theophylline concentration exceeds 20 mcg/ml. Therefore, determination of serum theophylline levels is recommended to assure maximal benefit without excessive risk.

Serum levels above 20 mcg/ml are rarely found after appropriate administration of the recommended doses. However, in individuals in whom theophylline plasma clearance is reduced **for any reason**, even conventional doses may result in increased serum levels and potential toxicity. Reduced theophylline clearance has been documented in the following readily identifiable groups: 1) patients with impaired renal or liver function; 2) patients over 55 years of age, particularly males and those with chronic lung disease; 3) those with cardiac failure from any cause; 4) neonates; and 5) those patients taking certain drugs (macrolide antibiotics and cimetidine). Decreased clearance of theophylline may be associated with either influenza immunization or active infection with influenza.

Reduction of dosage and laboratory monitoring is especially appropriate in the above individuals.

Less serious signs of theophylline toxicity, ie, nausea and restlessness, may appear in up to 50% of patients. Unfortunately, however, serious side effects such as ventricular arrhythmias, convulsions, or even death may appear as the first sign of toxicity without any previous warning. Stated differently, **serious toxicity is not reliably preceded by less severe side effects.**

Many patients who require theophylline may exhibit tachycardia due to their underlying disease process so that the cause/effect relationship to elevated serum theophylline concentrations may not be appreciated.

Theophylline products may cause dysrhythmia and/or worsen pre-existing arrhythmias, and any significant change in rate and/or rhythm warrants monitoring and further investigation.

The occurrence of arrhythmias and sudden death (with histological evidence of necrosis of the myocardium) has been recorded in laboratory animals (minipigs, rodents, and dogs) when theophylline and beta-agonists were administered concomitantly, although not when either was administered alone. The significance of these findings when applied to human usage is currently unknown.

PRECAUTIONS

General: Theophylline half-life is shorter in smokers than in nonsmokers. Therefore, smokers may require larger or more frequent doses. Morphine and curare should be used with caution in patients with airway obstruction as they may suppress respiration and stimulate histamine release. Alternative drugs should be used when possible. Theophylline should not be administered concurrently with other xanthine medications. Use with caution in patients with severe cardiac disease, severe hypoxemia, hypertension, hyperthyroidism, acute myocardial injury, cor pulmonale, congestive heart failure, and liver disease; in the elderly (especially males); and in neonates. In particular, great caution should be used in giving theophylline to patients with congestive heart failure. Frequently, such patients have markedly prolonged theophylline serum levels with theophylline persisting in serum for long periods following discontinuation of the drug.

Use theophylline cautiously in patients with history of peptic ulcer. Theophylline may occasionally act as a local irritant to the G.I. tract, although gastrointestinal symptoms are more commonly centrally mediated and associated with serum concentrations over 20 mcg/ml.

Information for Patients: The physician should reinforce the importance of taking only the prescribed dose and time interval between doses. The patient should alert the physician if symptoms occur repeatedly, especially near the end of a dosing interval.

Drug Interactions: ***Drug/Drug:*** Toxic synergism with ephedrine has been documented and may occur with some other sympathomimetic bronchodilators. In addition, the following drug interactions have been demonstrated:

DRUG	EFFECT
Aminophylline with lithium carbonate	Increased excretion of lithium carbonate
Aminophylline with propranolol	Antagonism of propranolol effect
Theophylline with cimetidine	Increased theophylline blood levels
Theophylline with troleandomycin, erythromycin	Increased theophylline blood levels

Drug/Food: THEOBID® has not been adequately studied to determine whether its bioavailability is altered when it is given with food.

Available data suggest that drug administration at the time of food ingestion may influence the absorption characteristics of some or all theophylline controlled-release products resulting in serum values different from those found after administration in the fasting state.

A drug/food effect, if any, would likely have its greatest clinical significance when high theophylline serum levels are

Continued on next page

Glaxo—Cont.

being maintained and/or when large single doses (greater than 13 mg/kg or 900 mg) of a controlled-release theophylline product are given. The influence of the type and amount of food on performance of controlled-release theophylline products is under study at this time.

Drug/Laboratory Test Interactions: When plasma levels of theophylline are measured by spectrophotometric methods, coffee, tea, cola beverages, chocolate, and acetaminophen contribute to falsely high values.

Carcinogenesis, Mutagenesis, Impairment of Fertility: Long-term studies have not been performed to evaluate the carcinogenic potential, mutagenic potential, or the effect on fertility of xanthine compounds.

Pregnancy: ***Teratogenic Effects: Pregnancy Category C:*** Animal studies have not been conducted with theophylline. It is not known whether theophylline can cause fetal harm when administered to a pregnant woman or can affect reproduction capacity. Xanthines should be given to a pregnant woman only if clearly needed.

Nursing Mothers: It has been reported that theophylline distributes readily into breast milk and may cause adverse effects in the infant. Caution must be used if prescribing xanthines to a mother who is nursing, taking into account the risk-benefit of this therapy.

Pediatric Use: Safety and effectiveness in children under 6 years of age have not been established with this product.

ADVERSE REACTIONS

The most consistent adverse reactions are usually due to overdose and are:

1. **Gastrointestinal:** nausea, vomiting, epigastric pain, hematemesis, and diarrhea.
2. **Central Nervous System:** headaches, irritability, restlessness, insomnia, reflex hyperexcitability, muscle twitching, and clonic and tonic generalized convulsions.
3. **Cardiovascular:** palpitation, tachycardia, extrasystoles, flushing, hypotension, circulatory failure, and ventricular arrhythmias.
4. **Respiratory:** tachypnea.
5. **Renal:** albuminuria, increased excretion of renal tubular cells and red blood cells, and potentiation of diuresis.
6. **Others:** hyperglycemia, inappropriate ADH syndrome, and rash.

OVERDOSAGE

Management: If potential oral overdose is established and seizure has not occurred:

A. Induce vomiting.
B. Administer a cathartic (this is particularly important if sustained-release preparations have been taken).
C. Administer activated charcoal.

If patient is having a seizure:

A. Establish an airway.
B. Administer oxygen.
C. Treat the seizure with intravenous diazepam, 0.1 to 0.3 mg/kg up to 10 mg.
D. Monitor vital signs, maintain blood pressure, and provide adequate hydration.

Post-Seizure Coma:

A. Maintain airway and oxygenation.
B. If a result of oral medication, follow above recommendations to prevent absorption of the drug, but intubation and lavage will have to be performed instead of inducing emesis, and the cathartic and charcoal will need to be introduced via a large bore gastric lavage tube.
C. Continue to provide full supportive care and adequate hydration while waiting for drug to be metabolized. In general, the drug is metabolized sufficiently rapidly so as not to warrant consideration of dialysis; however, if serum levels exceed 50 mcg/ml, charcoal hemoperfusion may be indicated.

DOSAGE AND ADMINISTRATION

THEOBID® DURACAP® has not been adequately studied for its bioavailability when administered with food (see **PRECAUTIONS, *Drug/Food*** Interactions).

For most patients, **effective use** of theophylline, ie, associated with optimal likelihood of benefit combined with minimal risk of toxicity, is considered to occur when serum levels are maintained between 10 and 20 mcg/ml. Levels above 20 mcg/ml may produce toxicity, and in a small number of patients, toxicity may even be seen with serum levels between 15 and 20 mcg/ml, particularly during initiation of therapy.

There is considerable variation from patient to patient in the dosage required to achieve and maintain therapeutic and safe levels, primarily due to variable rates of elimination. Therefore, it is essential that not only must dosage be individualized, but titration and monitoring of serum levels be utilized where available. When serum concentrations cannot be obtained, restriction of dosage to the amounts and intervals recommended in the guidelines listed below becomes essential. Dosage should be calculated on the basis of lean (ideal) body weight where mg/kg doses are presented. Theophylline does not distribute into fatty tissue.

Frequency of Dosing: When immediate release products with rapid absorption (such as tablets or liquid) are used, dosing to maintain serum levels generally requires administration every six hours. This is particularly true in children, but dosing intervals up to eight hours may be satisfactory in adults since they eliminate the drug at a slower rate. Some children, and adults requiring higher than average doses (those having rapid rates of clearance, eg, half-lives of under six hours), may benefit and be more effectively controlled during chronic therapy when given products with sustained-release characteristics, since these provide longer dosing intervals and/or less fluctuation in serum concentration between dosing. Those sustained-release preparations which provide flexibility in dosage through formulations of varying strengths are also helpful in controlling serum levels.

Dosage guidelines are approximations only, and the wide range of theophylline clearance between individuals (particularly those with concomitant disease) makes indiscriminate usage hazardous.

As a practical consideration, it is not always possible to obtain serum level determinations. Under such conditions, restriction of the daily dose (in otherwise healthy adults) to not greater than 16 mg/kg/day (of anhydrous theophylline) in divided doses will result in relatively few patients exceeding serum levels of 20 mcg/ml and the resultant risk of toxicity.

Dosage Guidelines: ***Acute Symptoms:*** THEOBID is not intended for patients experiencing an acute episode of bronchospasm (associated with asthma, chronic bronchitis, or emphysema). Such patients require **rapid** relief of symptoms and should be treated with an immediate-release or intravenous theophylline preparation (or other bronchodilators) and not with controlled-release products.

Chronic Therapy: It is recommended that the appropriate dosage be established using an immediate-release preparation. Slow clinical titration is generally preferred to help assure acceptance and safety of the medication.

Then, if the 24-hour dose can be given using THEOBID, the patient can usually be switched to THEOBID, giving one half of the daily dose at 12-hour intervals. However, certain patients, such as the young, smokers, and some nonsmoking adults, are more likely to metabolize theophylline more rapidly and require dosing at eight-hour intervals. Such patients can generally be identified as having trough serum concentrations lower than desired or repeatedly exhibiting symptoms near the end of a dosing interval.

Maximum Dose of Theophylline Where the Serum Concentration is Not Measured: **WARNING: DO NOT ATTEMPT TO MAINTAIN ANY DOSE THAT IS NOT TOLERATED.**

Not to exceed the following:

Age < 9 years	24 mg/kg/day
Age 9–12 years	20 mg/kg/day
Age 12–16 years	18 mg/kg/day
Age > 16 years	13 mg/kg/day **OR** 900 mg **(WHICHEVER IS LESS)**

Measurement of Serum Theophylline Concentrations During Chronic Therapy: If the above maximum doses are to be maintained or exceeded, serum theophylline measurement is recommended. The serum sample should be obtained at the time of peak absorption, one to two hours after administration for immediate-release products and **four hours after dosing for sustained-release formulations.** It is important that the patient will have missed no doses during the previous 48 hours and that dosing intervals will have been reasonably typical with no added doses during that period of time. DOSAGE ADJUSTMENT BASED ON SERUM THEOPHYLLINE MEASUREMENTS WHEN THESE INSTRUCTIONS HAVE NOT BEEN FOLLOWED MAY RESULT IN RECOMMENDATIONS THAT PRESENT RISK OF TOXICITY TO THE PATIENT.

[See table below].

Caution should be exercised for younger children who cannot complain of minor side effects. Older adults, those with cor pulmonale, congestive heart failure, and/or liver disease, may have unusually low dosage requirements and thus may experience toxicity at the maximal dosage recommended above.

It is important that no patient be maintained on any dosage that is not tolerated. In instructing patients to increase dosage according to the schedule above, they should be instructed not to take a subsequent dose if apparent side effects occur and to resume therapy at a lower dose once adverse effects have disappeared.

HOW SUPPLIED

THEOBID® DURACAP® capsules, blue and clear, 260-mg capsules, imprinted with "Glaxo 268", are supplied in bottles of 60 (NDC 0173-0268-12) and 500 (NDC 0173-0268-14).

The two-tone blue THEOBID® JR. DURACAP® 130-mg capsules, imprinted with "Glaxo 295", are supplied in bottles of 60 (NDC 0173-0295-12).

Caution: Federal law prohibits dispensing without prescription.

Store and dispense in tight containers as defined in USP/NF with a child-resistant closure. Store between 15° and 30° C (59° and 86°F).

REFERENCE

1. Weinberger M, Hendeles L: Practical guide to using theophylline. *J Resp Dis* 1981; 2:12–27.

Shown in Product Identification Section, page 410

Final Adjustment of Dosage:[1]
Dosage Adjustment After Serum Theophylline Measurement

If serum theophylline is:		**Directions:**
Within normal limits	10 to 20 mcg/ml	Maintain dosage if tolerated. Recheck serum theophylline concentration at 6- to 12-month intervals.*
Too high	20 to 25 mcg/ml	Decrease doses by about 10%. Recheck serum theophylline concentration at 6- to 12-month intervals.*
	25 to 30 mcg/ml	Skip next dose and decrease subsequent doses by about 25%.
	Over 30 mcg/ml	Skip next two doses and decrease subsequent doses by 50%. Recheck serum theophylline.
Too low	7.5 to 10 mcg/ml	Increase dose by about 25%.† Recheck serum theophylline concentration at 6- to 12-month intervals.*
	5 to 7.5 mcg/ml	Increase dose by about 25% to the nearest dose increment and recheck serum theophylline for guidance in further dosage adjustment (another increase will probably be needed, but this provides a safety check).

* Finer adjustments in dosage may be needed for some patients.
† Dividing the daily dose into three doses administered at eight-hour intervals may be indicated if symptoms occur repeatedly at the end of a dosing interval.

TRANDATE® Injection ℞

[*tran'dāt*]
(labetalol hydrochloride)

DESCRIPTION

TRANDATE® (labetalol HCl) is an adrenergic receptor blocking agent that has both selective $alpha_1$- and nonselective beta-adrenergic receptor blocking actions in a single substance.

Labetalol HCl is 5-[1-hydroxy-2-[(1-methyl-3-phenylpropyl) amino]ethyl]salicylamide monohydrochloride, and it has the following structure:

Labetalol HCl has the empirical formula $C_{19}H_{24}N_2O_3 \cdot HCl$ and a molecular weight of 364.9. It has two asymmetric centers and therefore exists as a molecular complex of two diastereoisomeric pairs.

Labetalol HCl is a white or off-white crystalline powder, soluble in water.

TRANDATE Injection is a clear, colorless to light yellow aqueous sterile isotonic solution for intravenous injection. It has a pH range of 3 to 4. Each ml contains 5 mg labetalol HCl, 45 mg anhydrous dextrose, 0.1 mg edetate disodium; 0.8 mg methylparaben and 0.1 mg propylparaben as preservatives; and citric acid monohydrate and sodium hydroxide, as necessary, to bring the solution into the pH range.

CLINICAL PHARMACOLOGY

TRANDATE® combines both selective, competitive $alpha_1$-adrenergic blocking and nonselective, competitive beta-adrenergic blocking activity in a single substance. In man, the ratios of alpha- to beta-blockade have been estimated to be approximately 1:3 to 1:7 following oral and intravenous administration, respectively. Beta$_2$-agonist activity has been demonstrated in animals with minimal beta$_1$-agonist (ISA) activity detected. In animals, at doses greater than those required for alpha- or beta-adrenergic blockade, a membrane stabilizing effect has been demonstrated.

Pharmacodynamics: The capacity of labetalol HCl to block alpha receptors in man has been demonstrated by attenuation of the pressor effect of phenylephrine and by a significant reduction of the pressor response caused by immersing the hand in ice-cold water ("cold-pressor test"). Labetalol HCl's beta$_1$-receptor blockade in man was demonstrated by a small decrease in the resting heart rate, attenuation of tachycardia produced by isoproterenol or exercise, and by attenuation of the reflex tachycardia to the hypotension produced by amyl nitrite. Beta$_2$-receptor blockade was demonstrated by inhibition of the isoproterenol-induced fall in diastolic blood pressure. Both the alpha- and beta-blocking actions of orally administered labetalol HCl contribute to a decrease in blood pressure in hypertensive patients. Labetalol HCl consistently, in dose-related fashion, blunted increases in exercise-induced blood pressure and heart rate and in their double product. The pulmonary circulation during exercise was not affected by labetalol HCl dosing.

Single oral doses of labetalol HCl administered in patients with coronary artery disease had no significant effect on sinus rate, intraventricular conduction, or QRS duration. The AV conduction time was modestly prolonged in two of seven patients. In another study, intravenous labetalol HCl slightly prolonged AV nodal conduction time and atrial effective refractory period with only small changes in heart rate. The effects on AV nodal refractoriness were inconsistent.

Labetalol HCl produces dose-related falls in blood pressure without reflex tachycardia and without significant reduction in heart rate, presumably through a mixture of its alpha-blocking and beta-blocking effects. Hemodynamic effects are variable, with small, nonsignificant changes in cardiac output seen in some studies but not others and small decreases in total peripheral resistance. Elevated plasma renins are reduced.

Doses of labetalol HCl that controlled hypertension did not affect renal function in mildly to severely hypertensive patients with normal renal function.

Due to the alpha$_1$-receptor blocking activity of labetalol HCl, blood pressure is lowered more in the standing than in the supine position, and symptoms of postural hypotension can occur. During dosing with intravenous labetalol HCl, the contribution of the postural component should be considered when positioning the patient for treatment, and the patient should not be allowed to move to an erect position unmonitored until his ability to do so is established.

In a clinical pharmacologic study in severe hypertensives, an initial 0.25-mg/kg injection of labetalol HCl administered to patients in the supine position decreased blood pressure by an average of 11/7 mmHg. Additional injections of 0.5 mg/kg at 15-minute intervals up to a total cumulative dose of 1.75 mg/kg of labetalol HCl caused further dose-related decreases in blood pressure. Some patients required cumulative doses of up to 3.25 mg/kg. The maximal effect of each dose level occurred within five minutes. Following discontinuation of intravenous treatment with labetalol HCl, the blood pressure rose gradually and progressively, approaching pretreatment baseline values within an average of 16 to 18 hours in the majority of patients.

Similar results were obtained in the treatment of patients with severe hypertension who required urgent blood pressure reduction with an initial dose of 20 mg (which corresponds to 0.25 mg/kg for an 80-kg patient) followed by additional doses of either 40 or 80 mg at ten-minute intervals to achieve the desired effect or up to a cumulative dose of 300 mg.

Labetalol HCl administered as a continuous intravenous infusion, with a mean dose of 136 mg (27 to 300 mg) over a period of two to three hours (mean of two hours and 39 minutes) lowered the blood pressure by an average of 60/35 mmHg.

Exacerbation of angina and, in some cases, myocardial infarction and ventricular dysrhythmias have been reported after abrupt discontinuation of therapy with beta-adrenergic blocking agents in patients with coronary artery disease. Abrupt withdrawal of these agents in patients without coronary artery disease has resulted in transient symptoms, including tremulousness, sweating, palpitation, headache, and malaise. Several mechanisms have been proposed to explain these phenomena, among them increased sensitivity to catecholamines because of increased numbers of beta receptors. Although beta-adrenergic receptor blockade is useful in the treatment of angina and hypertension, there are also situations in which sympathetic stimulation is vital. For example, in patients with severely damaged hearts, adequate ventricular function may depend on sympathetic drive. Beta-adrenergic blockade may worsen AV block by preventing the necessary facilitating effects of sympathetic activity on conduction. Beta$_2$-adrenergic blockade results in passive bronchial constriction by interfering with endogenous adrenergic bronchodilator activity in patients subject to bronchospasm, and it may also interfere with exogenous bronchodilators in such patients.

Pharmacokinetics and Metabolism: Following intravenous infusion of labetalol, the elimination half-life is about 5.5 hours and the total body clearance is approximately 33 ml/min/kg. The plasma half-life of labetalol following oral administration is about six to eight hours. In patients with decreased hepatic or renal function, the elimination half-life of labetalol is not altered; however, the relative bioavailability in hepatically impaired patients is increased due to decreased "first-pass" metabolism.

The metabolism of labetalol is mainly through conjugation to glucuronide metabolites. The metabolites are present in plasma and are excreted in the urine and, via the bile, into the feces. Approximately 55% to 60% of a dose appears in the urine as conjugates or unchanged labetalol within the first 24 hours of dosing.

Labetalol has been shown to cross the placental barrier in humans. Only negligible amounts of the drug crossed the blood-brain barrier in animal studies. Labetalol is approximately 50% protein bound. Neither hemodialysis nor peritoneal dialysis removes a significant amount of labetalol HCl from the general circulation (<1%).

INDICATIONS AND USAGE

TRANDATE® Injection is indicated for control of blood pressure in severe hypertension.

CONTRAINDICATIONS

TRANDATE® Injection is contraindicated in bronchial asthma, overt cardiac failure, greater-than-first-degree heart block, cardiogenic shock, and severe bradycardia (see **WARNINGS**).

WARNINGS

Cardiac Failure: Sympathetic stimulation is a vital component supporting circulatory function in congestive heart failure. Beta-blockade carries a potential hazard of further depressing myocardial contractility and precipitating more severe failure. Although beta-blockers should be avoided in overt congestive heart failure, if necessary labetalol HCl can be used with caution in patients with a history of heart failure who are well compensated. Congestive heart failure has been observed in patients receiving labetalol HCl. Labetalol HCl does not abolish the inotropic action of digitalis on heart muscle.

In Patients Without a History of Cardiac Failure: In patients with latent cardiac insufficiency, continued depression of the myocardium with beta-blocking agents over a period of time can, in some cases, lead to cardiac failure. At the first sign or symptom of impending cardiac failure, patients should be fully digitalized and/or be given a diuretic, and the response should be observed closely. If cardiac failure continues despite adequate digitalization and diuretic, TRANDATE® therapy should be withdrawn (gradually, if possible).

Ischemic Heart Disease: Angina pectoris has not been reported upon labetalol HCl discontinuation. However, following abrupt cessation of therapy with some beta-blocking agents in patients with coronary artery disease, exacerbations of angina pectoris and, in some cases, myocardial infarction have been reported. Therefore, such patients should be cautioned against interruption of therapy without the physician's advice. Even in the absence of overt angina pectoris, when discontinuation of TRANDATE is planned, the patient should be carefully observed and should be advised to limit physical activity. If angina markedly worsens or acute coronary insufficiency develops, TRANDATE administration should be reinstituted promptly, at least temporarily, and other measures appropriate for the management of unstable angina should be taken.

Nonallergic Bronchospasm (eg, Chronic Bronchitis and Emphysema): Since TRANDATE Injection at the usual intravenous therapeutic doses has not been studied in patients with nonallergic bronchospastic disease, it should not be used in such patients.

Pheochromocytoma: Intravenous labetalol HCl has been shown to be effective in lowering blood pressure and relieving symptoms in patients with pheochromocytoma; higher than usual doses may be required. However, paradoxical hypertensive responses have been reported in a few patients with this tunor; therefore, use caution when administering labetalol HCl to patients with pheochromocytoma.

Diabetes Mellitus and Hypoglycemia: Beta-adrenergic blockade may prevent the appearance of premonitory signs and symptoms (eg, tachycardia) of acute hypoglycemia. This is especially important with labile diabetics. Beta-blockade also reduces the release of insulin in response to hyperglycemia; it may therefore be necessary to adjust the dose of antidiabetic drugs.

Major Surgery: The necessity or desirability of withdrawing beta-blocking therapy prior to major surgery is controversial. Protracted severe hypotension and difficulty in restarting or maintaining a heartbeat have been reported with beta-blockers. The effect of labetalol HCl's alpha-adrenergic activity has not been evaluated in this setting.

A synergism between labetalol HCl and halothane anesthesia has been shown (see **Drug Interactions** under **PRECAUTIONS**).

Rapid Decreases of Blood Pressure: Caution must be observed when reducing severely elevated blood pressure. Although such findings have not been reported with intravenous labetalol HCl, a number of adverse reactions, including cerebral infarction, optic nerve infarction, angina, and ischemic changes in the electrocardiogram, have been reported with other agents when severely elevated blood pressure was reduced over time courses of several hours to as long as one or two days. The desired blood pressure lowering should therefore be achieved over as long a period of time as is compatible with the patient's status.

PRECAUTIONS

General: ***Impaired Hepatic Function:*** TRANDATE® Injection should be used with caution in patients with impaired hepatic function since metabolism of the drug may be diminished.

Hypotension: Symptomatic postural hypotension (incidence, 58%) is likely to occur if patients are tilted or allowed to assume the upright position within three hours of receiving TRANDATE Injection. Therefore, the patient's ability to tolerate an upright position should be established before permitting any ambulation.

Jaundice or Hepatic Dysfunction: On rare occasions, oral labetalol HCl has been associated with jaundice (both hepatic and cholestatic). It is therefore recommended that treatment with labetalol HCl be stopped immediately should a patient develop jaundice or laboratory evidence of liver injury. Both have been shown to be reversible on stopping therapy.

Information for Patients: The following information is intended to aid in the safe and effective use of this medication. It is not a disclosure of all possible adverse or intended effects. During and immediately following (for up to three hours) TRANDATE Injection, the patient should remain supine. Subsequently, the patient should be advised on how to proceed gradually to become ambulatory and should be observed at the time of first ambulation.

When the patient is started on TRANDATE® (labetalol hydrochloride) Tablets following adequate control of blood pressure with TRANDATE Injection, appropriate directions for titration of dosage should be provided (see **DOSAGE AND ADMINISTRATION**).

As with all drugs with beta-blocking activity, certain advice to patients being treated with labetalol HCl is warranted. While no incident of the abrupt withdrawal phenomenon (exacerbation of angina pectoris) has been reported with labetalol HCl, dosing with TRANDATE Tablets should not be interrupted or discontinued without the physician's advice. Patients being treated with TRANDATE Tablets should consult a physician at any sign of impending cardiac failure. Also, transient scalp tingling may occur, usually when treatment with TRANDATE Tablets is initiated (see **ADVERSE REACTIONS**).

Laboratory Tests: Routine laboratory tests are ordinarily not required before or after intravenous labetalol HCl. In patients with concomitant illnesses, such as impaired renal function, appropriate tests should be done to monitor these conditions.

Drug Interactions: Since TRANDATE Injection may be administered to patients already being treated with other medications, including other antihypertensive agents, careful monitoring of these patients is necessary to detect and treat promptly any undesired effect from concomitant administration.

In one survey, 2.3% of patients taking labetalol HCl orally in combination with tricyclic antidepressants experienced tremor as compared to 0.7% reported to occur with labetalol HCl alone. The contribution of each of the treatments to this adverse reaction is unknown, but the possibility of a drug interaction cannot be excluded.

Drugs possessing beta-blocking properties can blunt the bronchodilator effect of beta-receptor agonist drugs in patients with bronchospasm; therefore, doses greater than the normal antiasthmatic dose of beta-agonist bronchodilator drugs may be required.

Cimetidine has been shown to increase the bioavailability of labetalol HCl administered orally. Since this could be explained either by enhanced absorption or by an alteration of hepatic metabolism of labetalol HCl, special care should be used in establishing the dose required for blood pressure control in such patients.

Synergism has been shown between halothane anesthesia and intravenously administered labetalol HCl. During controlled hypotensive anesthesia using labetalol HCl in association with halothane, high concentrations (3% or above) of halothane should not be used because the degree of hypotension will be increased and because of the possibility of a large reduction in cardiac output and an increase in central venous pressure. The anesthesiologist should be informed when a patient is receiving labetalol HCl.

Continued on next page

Glaxo—Cont.

Labetalol HCl blunts the reflex tachycardia produced by nitroglycerin without preventing its hypotensive effect. If labetalol HCl is used with nitroglycerin in patients with angina pectoris, additional antihypertensive effects may occur.

Drug/Laboratory Test Interactions: The presence of a metabolite of labetalol in the urine may result in falsely increased levels of urinary catecholamines when measured by a nonspecific trihydroxyindole (THI) reaction. In screening patients suspected of having a pheochromocytoma and being treated with labetalol HCl, specific radioenzymatic or high performance liquid chromatography assay techniques should be used to determine levels of catecholamines or their metabolites.

Carcinogenesis, Mutagenesis, Impairment of Fertility: Long-term oral dosing studies with labetalol HCl for 18 months in mice and for two years in rats showed no evidence of carcinogenesis. Studies with labetalol HCl using dominant lethal assays in rats and mice and exposing microorganisms according to modified Ames tests showed no evidence of mutagenesis.

Pregnancy: ***Teratogenic Effects: Pregnancy Category C:*** Teratogenic studies have been performed with labetalol in rats and rabbits at oral doses up to approximately six and four times the maximum recommended human dose (MRHD), respectively. No reproducible evidence of fetal malformations was observed. Increased fetal resorptions were seen in both species at doses approximating the MRHD. There are no adequate and well-controlled studies in pregnant women. Labetalol should be used during pregnancy only if the potential benefit justifies the potential risk to the fetus.

Nonteratogenic Effects: Infants of mothers who were treated with labetalol HCl for hypertension during pregnancy did not appear to be adversely affected by the drug. Oral administration of labetalol to rats during late gestation through weaning at doses of two to four times the MRHD caused a decrease in neonatal survival.

Labor and Delivery: Labetalol HCl given to pregnant women with hypertension did not appear to affect the usual course of labor and delivery.

Nursing Mothers: Small amounts of labetalol (approximately 0.004% of the maternal dose) are excreted in human milk. Caution should be exercised when TRANDATE Injection is administered to a nursing woman.

Pediatric Use: Safety and effectiveness in children have not been established.

ADVERSE REACTIONS

TRANDATE® Injection is usually well tolerated. Most adverse effects have been mild and transient and, in controlled trials involving 92 patients, did not require labetalol HCl withdrawal. Symptomatic postural hypotension (incidence, 58%) is likely to occur if patients are tilted or allowed to assume the upright position within three hours of receiving TRANDATE Injection. Moderate hypotension occurred in 1 of 100 patients while supine. Increased sweating was noted in 4 of 100 patients, and flushing occurred in 1 of 100 patients.

The following also were reported with TRANDATE Injection with the incidence per 100 patients as noted:

Cardiovascular System: Ventricular arrhythmia in 1.

Central and Peripheral Nervous Systems: Dizziness in 9; tingling of the scalp/skin in 7; and hypoesthesia (numbness) and vertigo in 1 each.

Gastrointestinal System: Nausea in 13; vomiting in 4; and dyspepsia and taste distortion in 1 each.

Metabolic Disorders: Transient increases in blood urea nitrogen and serum creatinine levels occurred in 8 of 100 patients; these were associated with drops in blood pressure, generally in patients with prior renal insufficiency.

Psychiatric Disorders: Somnolence/yawning in 3.

Respiratory System: Wheezing in 1.

Skin: Pruritus in 1.

The incidence of adverse reactions depends upon the dose of labetalol HCl. The largest experience is with oral labetalol HCl (see **TRANDATE Tablets Product Information** for details). Certain of the side effects increased with increasing oral dose, as shown in the table below that depicts the entire US therapeutic trials data base for adverse reactions that are probably or possibly dose-related.

[See table below].

Labetalol HCl Daily Dose (mg)	**200**	**300**	**400**	**600**	**800**	**900**	**1200**	**1600**	**2400**
Number of Patients	522	181	606	608	503	117	411	242	175
Dizziness (%)	2	3	3	3	5	1	9	13	16
Fatigue	2	1	4	4	5	3	7	6	10
Nausea	<1	0	1	2	4	0	7	11	19
Vomiting	0	0	<1	<1	<1	0	1	2	3
Dyspepsia	1	0	2	1	1	0	2	2	4
Paresthesias	2	0	2	2	1	1	2	5	5
Nasal Stuffiness	1	1	2	2	2	2	4	5	6
Ejaculation Failure	0	2	1	2	3	0	4	3	5
Impotence	1	1	1	1	2	4	3	4	3
Edema	1	0	1	1	1	0	1	2	2

The oculomucocutaneous syndrome associated with the beta-blocker practolol has not been reported with labetalol HCl during investigational use and extensive foreign marketing experience.

Clinical Laboratory Tests: Among patients dosed with TRANDATE Tablets, there have been reversible increases of serum transaminases in 4% of patients tested and, more rarely, reversible increases in blood urea.

OVERDOSAGE

Overdosage with TRANDATE® Injection causes excessive hypotension that is posture sensitive and, sometimes, excessive bradycardia. Patients should be placed supine and their legs raised if necessary to improve the blood supply to the brain. If overdosage with labetalol HCl follows oral ingestion, gastric lavage or pharmacologically induced emesis (using syrup of ipecac) may be useful for removal of the drug shortly after ingestion. The following additional measures should be employed if necessary: **Excessive bradycardia**—administer atropine or epinephrine. **Cardiac failure**—administer a digitalis glycoside and a diuretic. Dopamine or dobutamine may also be useful. **Hypotension**—administer vasopressors, eg, norepinephrine. There is pharmacological evidence that norepinephrine may be the drug of choice. **Bronchospasm**—administer epinephrine and/or an aerosolized beta$_2$-agonist. **Seizures**—administer diazepam.

In severe beta-blocker overdose resulting in hypotension and/or bradycardia, glucagon has been shown to be effective when administered in large doses (5 to 10 mg rapidly over 30 seconds, followed by continuous infusion of 5 mg/hr that can be reduced as the patient improves).

Neither hemodialysis nor peritoneal dialysis removes a significant amount of labetalol from the general circulation (<1%).

The oral LD_{50} value of labetalol HCl in the mouse is approximately 600 mg/kg and in the rat is greater than 2 g/kg. The intravenous LD_{50} in these species is 50 to 60 mg/kg.

DOSAGE AND ADMINISTRATION

TRANDATE® Injection is intended for intravenous use in hospitalized patients. DOSAGE MUST BE INDIVIDUALIZED depending upon the severity of hypertension and the response of the patient during dosing.

Patients should always be kept in a supine position during the period of intravenous drug administration. A substantial fall in blood pressure on standing should be expected in these patients. The patient's ability to tolerate an upright position should be established before permitting any ambulation, such as using toilet facilities.

Either of two methods of administration of TRANDATE Injection may be used: a) repeated intravenous injection, or b) slow continuous infusion.

Repeated Intravenous Injection: Initially, TRANDATE Injection should be given in a 20-mg dose (which corresponds to 0.25 mg/kg for an 80-kg patient) by slow intravenous injection over a two-minute period.

Immediately before the injection and at five and ten minutes after injection, supine blood pressure should be measured to evaluate response. Additional injections of 40 or 80 mg can be given at ten-minute intervals until a desired supine blood pressure is achieved or a total of 300 mg of labetalol HCl has been injected. The maximum effect usually occurs within five minutes of each injection.

Slow Continuous Infusion: TRANDATE Injection is prepared for continuous intravenous infusion by diluting the vial contents with commonly used intravenous fluids (see below). Examples of two methods of preparing the infusion solution are:

Add 40 ml of TRANDATE Injection to 160 ml of a commonly used intravenous fluid such that the resultant 200 ml of solution contains 200 mg of labetalol HCl, 1 mg/ml. The diluted solution should be administered at a rate of 2 ml/min to deliver 2 mg/min.

Alternatively, add 40 ml of TRANDATE Injection to 250 ml of a commonly used intravenous fluid. The resultant solution will contain 200 mg of labetalol HCl, approximately 2 mg/3 ml. The diluted solution should be administered at a rate of 3 ml/min to deliver approximately 2 mg/min.

The rate of infusion of the diluted solution may be adjusted according to the blood pressure response, at the discretion of the physician. To facilitate a desired rate of infusion, the diluted solution can be infused using a controlled administration mechanism, eg, graduated burette or mechanically driven infusion pump.

Since the half-life of labetalol is five to eight hours, steady-state blood levels (in the face of a constant rate of infusion) would not be reached during the usual infusion time period. The infusion should be continued until a satisfactory response is obtained and should then be stopped and oral labetalol HCl started (see below). The effective intravenous dose is usually in the range of 50 to 200 mg. A total dose of up to 300 mg may be required in some patients.

Blood Pressure Monitoring: The blood pressure should be monitored during and after completion of the infusion or intravenous injection. Rapid or excessive falls in either systolic or diastolic blood pressure during intravenous treatment should be avoided. In patients with excessive systolic hypertension, the decrease in systolic pressure should be used as an indicator of effectiveness in addition to the response of the diastolic pressure.

Initiation of Dosing with TRANDATE Tablets: Subsequent oral dosing with TRANDATE Tablets should begin when it has been established that the supine diastolic blood pressure has begun to rise. The recommended initial dose is 200 mg, followed in six to 12 hours by an additional dose of 200 or 400 mg, depending on the blood pressure response. Thereafter, **inpatient titration with TRANDATE Tablets** may proceed as follows:

Inpatient Titration Instructions

Regimen	Daily Dose*
200 mg bid	400 mg
400 mg bid	800 mg
800 mg bid	1,600 mg
1,200 mg bid	2,400 mg

* If needed, the total daily dose may be given in three divided doses.

The dosage of TRANDATE Tablets used in the hospital may be increased at one-day intervals to achieve the desired blood pressure reduction.

For subsequent outpatient titration or maintenance dosing, see **DOSAGE AND ADMINISTRATION** in the **TRANDATE Tablets Product Information** for additional recommendations.

Compatibility with Commonly Used Intravenous Fluids: Parenteral drug products should be inspected visually for particulate matter and discoloration prior to administration whenever solution and container permit.

TRANDATE Injection was tested for compatibility with commonly used intravenous fluids at final concentrations of 1.25 to 3.75 mg of labetalol HCl per ml of the mixture. TRANDATE Injection was found to be compatible with and stable (for 24 hours refrigerated or at room temperature) in mixtures with the following solutions: Ringer's Injection, USP; Lactated Ringer's Injection, USP; 5% Dextrose and Ringer's Injection; 5% Lactated Ringer's and 5% Dextrose Injection; 5% Dextrose Injection, USP; 0.9% Sodium Chloride Injection, USP; 5% Dextrose and 0.2% Sodium Chloride Injection, USP; 2.5% Dextrose and 0.45% Sodium Chloride Injection, USP; 5% Dextrose and 0.9% Sodium Chloride Injection, USP; and 5% Dextrose and 0.33% Sodium Chloride Injection, USP.

TRANDATE Injection was NOT compatible with 5% Sodium Bicarbonate Injection, USP.

HOW SUPPLIED

TRANDATE® Injection, 5 mg/ml, is supplied in
20-ml (100-mg) vials, box of one (NDC 0173-0350-58), and
40-ml (200-mg) vials, box of one (NDC 0173-0350-57).

Store between 2° and 30°C (36° and 86°F). Do not freeze. Protect from light.

Shown in Product Identification Section, page 410

TRANDATE® Tablets ℞

[*tran'dāt*]

(labetalol hydrochloride)

DESCRIPTION

TRANDATE® (labetalol HCl) is an adrenergic receptor blocking agent that has both selective alpha$_1$- and nonselective beta-adrenergic receptor blocking actions in a single substance.

Labetalol HCl is 5-[1-hydroxy-2-[(1-methyl-3-phenylpropyl)amino]ethyl]salicylamide monohydrochloride, and it has the following structure:

[See Chemical Formula at top of next column].

Labetalol HCl has the empirical formula $C_{19}H_{24}N_2O_3 \cdot HCl$ and a molecular weight of 364.9. It has two asymmetric cen-

$CONH_2$ OH • HCl
$-CH_2CH_2CHNHCH_2CH$ CH_3 OH

ters and therefore exists as a molecular complex of two diastereoisomeric pairs.
Labetalol HCl is a white or off-white crystalline powder, soluble in water.
TRANDATE Tablets contain 100, 200, or 300 mg of labetalol HCl and are taken orally. Each tablet also contains the inactive ingredients corn starch, hydroxypropyl methylcellulose, lactose, magnesium stearate, methyl hydroxybenzoate, pregelatinized corn starch, propyl hydroxybenzoate, and other ingredients.

CLINICAL PHARMACOLOGY

TRANDATE® combines both selective, competitive $alpha_1$-adrenergic blocking and nonselective, competitive beta-adrenergic blocking activity in a single substance. In man, the ratios of alpha- to beta- blockade have been estimated to be approximately 1:3 and 1:7 following oral and intravenous administration, respectively. $Beta_2$-agonist activity has been demonstrated in animals with minimal $beta_1$-agonist (ISA) activity detected. In animals, at doses greater than those required for alpha- or beta-adrenergic blockade, a membrane stabilizing effect has been demonstrated.

Pharmacodynamics: The capacity of labetalol HCl to block alpha receptors in man has been demonstrated by attenuation of the pressor effect of phenylephrine and by a significant reduction of the pressor response caused by immersing the hand in ice-cold water ("cold-pressor test"). Labetalol HCl's $beta_1$-receptor blockade in man was demonstrated by a small decrease in the resting heart rate, attenuation of tachycardia produced by isoproterenol or exercise, and by attenuation of the reflex tachycardia to the hypotension produced by amyl nitrite. $Beta_2$-receptor blockade was demonstrated by inhibition of the isoproterenol-induced fall in diastolic blood pressure. Both the alpha- and beta-blocking actions of orally administered labetalol HCl contribute to a decrease in blood pressure in hypertensive patients. Labetalol HCl consistently, in dose-related fashion, blunted increases in exercise-induced blood pressure and heart rate, and in their double product. The pulmonary circulation during exercise was not affected by labetalol HCl dosing.
Single oral doses of labetalol HCl administered in patients with coronary artery disease had no significant effect on sinus rate, intraventricular conduction, or QRS duration. The AV conduction time was modestly prolonged in two of seven patients. In another study, intravenous labetalol HCl slightly prolonged AV nodal conduction time and atrial effective refractory period with only small changes in heart rate. The effects on AV nodal refractoriness were inconsistent.
Labetalol HCl produces dose-related falls in blood pressure without reflex tachycardia and without significant reduction in heart rate, presumably through a mixture of its alpha-blocking and beta-blocking effects. Hemodynamic effects are variable, with small, nonsignificant changes in cardiac output seen in some studies but not others and small decreases in total peripheral resistance. Elevated plasma renins are reduced.
Doses of labetalol HCl that controlled hypertension did not affect renal function in mildly to severely hypertensive patients with normal renal function.
Due to the $alpha_1$-receptor blocking activity of labetalol HCl, blood pressure is lowered more in the standing than in the supine position, and symptoms of postural hypotension (2%), including rare instances of syncope, can occur. Following oral administration, when postural hypotension has occurred, it has been transient and is uncommon when the recommended starting dose and titration increments are closely followed (see **DOSAGE AND ADMINISTRATION**). Symptomatic postural hypotension is most likely to occur two to four hours after a dose, especially following the use of large initial doses or upon large changes in dose.
The peak effects of single oral doses of labetalol HCl occur within two to four hours. The duration of effect depends upon dose, lasting at least eight hours following single oral doses of 100 mg and more than 12 hours following single oral doses of 300 mg. The maximum, steady-state blood pressure response upon oral, twice-a-day dosing occurs within 24 to 72 hours.
The antihypertensive effect of labetalol has a linear correlation with the logarithm of labetalol plasma concentration, and there is also a linear correlation between the reduction in exercise-induced tachycardia occurring at two hours after oral administration of labetalol HCl and the logarithm of the plasma concentration.
About 70% of the maximum beta-blocking effect is present for five hours after the administration of a single oral dose of 400 mg with suggestion that about 40% remains at eight hours.
The antianginal efficacy of labetalol HCl has not been studied. In 37 patients with hypertension and coronary artery disease, labetalol HCl did not increase the incidence or severity of angina attacks.
Exacerbation of angina and, in some cases, myocardial infarction and ventricular dysrhythmias have been reported after abrupt discontinuation of therapy with beta-adrenergic blocking agents in patients with coronary artery disease. Abrupt withdrawal of these agents in patients without coronary artery disease has resulted in transient symptoms, including tremulousness, sweating, palpitation, headache, and malaise. Several mechanisms have been proposed to explain these phenomena, among them increased sensitivity to catecholamines because of increased numbers of beta receptors.
Although beta-adrenergic receptor blockade is useful in the treatment of angina and hypertension, there are also situations in which sympathetic stimulation is vital. For example, in patients with severely damaged hearts, adequate ventricular function may depend on sympathetic drive. Beta-adrenergic blockade may worsen AV block by preventing the necessary facilitating effects of sympathetic activity on conduction. $Beta_2$-adrenergic blockade results in passive bronchial constriction by interfering with endogenous adrenergic bronchodilator activity in patients subject to bronchospasm, and it may also interfere with exogenous bronchodilators in such patients.

Pharmacokinetics and Metabolism: Labetalol HCl is completely absorbed from the gastrointestinal tract with peak plasma levels occurring one to two hours after oral administration. The relative bioavailability of labetalol HCl tablets compared to an oral solution is 100%. The absolute bioavailability (fraction of drug reaching systemic circulation) of labetalol when compared to an intravenous infusion is 25%; this is due to extensive "first-pass" metabolism. Despite "first-pass" metabolism there is a linear relationship between oral doses of 100 to 3,000 mg and peak plasma levels. The absolute bioavailability of labetalol is increased when administered with food.
The plasma half-life of labetalol following oral administration is about six to eight hours. Steady-state plasma levels of labetalol during repetitive dosing are reached by about the third day of dosing. In patients with decreased hepatic or renal function, the elimination half-life of labetalol is not altered; however, the relative bioavailability in hepatically impaired patients is increased due to decreased "first-pass" metabolism.
The metabolism of labetalol is mainly through conjugation to glucuronide metabolites. These metabolites are present in plasma and are excreted in the urine and, via the bile, into the feces. Approximately 55% to 60% of a dose appears in the urine as conjugates or unchanged labetalol within the first 24 hours of dosing.
Labetalol has been shown to cross the placental barrier in humans. Only negligible amounts of the drug crossed the blood-brain barrier in animal studies. Labetalol is approximately 50% protein bound. Neither hemodialysis nor peritoneal dialysis removes a significant amount of labetalol HCl from the general circulation (<1%).

INDICATIONS AND USAGE

TRANDATE® (labetalol HCl) Tablets are indicated in the management of hypertension. TRANDATE Tablets may be used alone or in combination with other antihypertensive agents, especially thiazide and loop diuretics.

CONTRAINDICATIONS

TRANDATE® Tablets are contraindicated in bronchial asthma, overt cardiac failure, greater-than-first-degree heart block, cardiogenic shock, and severe bradycardia (see **WARNINGS**).

WARNINGS

Cardiac Failure: Sympathetic stimulation is a vital component supporting circulatory function in congestive heart failure. Beta-blockade carries a potential hazard of further depressing myocardial contractility and precipitating more severe failure. Although beta-blockers should be avoided in overt congestive heart failure, if necessary labetalol HCl can be used with caution in patients with a history of heart failure who are well-compensated. Congestive heart failure has been observed in patients receiving labetalol HCl. Labetalol HCl does not abolish the inotropic action of digitalis on heart muscle.

In Patients Without a History of Cardiac Failure: In patients with latent cardiac insufficiency, continued depression of the myocardium with beta-blocking agents over a period of time can, in some cases, lead to cardiac failure. At the first sign or symptom of impending cardiac failure, patients should be fully digitalized and/or be given a diuretic, and the response should be observed closely. If cardiac failure continues despite adequate digitalization and diuretic, TRANDATE® (labetalol HCl) therapy should be withdrawn (gradually, if possible).

Exacerbation of Ischemic Heart Disease Following Abrupt Withdrawal: Angina pectoris has not been reported upon labetalol HCl discontinuation. However, hypersensitivity to catecholamines has been observed in patients withdrawn from beta-blocker therapy; exacerbation of angina and, in some cases, myocardial infarction have occurred after *abrupt* discontinuation of such therapy. When discontinuing chronically administered TRANDATE, particularly in patients with ischemic heart disease, the dosage should be gradually reduced over a period of one to two weeks and the patient should be carefully monitored. If angina markedly worsens or acute coronary insufficiency develops, TRANDATE administration should be reinstituted promptly, at least temporarily, and other measures appropriate for the management of unstable angina should be taken. Patients should be warned against interruption or discontinuation of therapy without the physician's advice. Because coronary artery disease is common and may be unrecognized, it may be prudent not to discontinue TRANDATE therapy abruptly even in patients treated only for hypertension.

Nonallergic Bronchospasm (eg, Chronic Bronchitis and Emphysema): Patients with bronchospastic disease should, in general, not receive beta-blockers. TRANDATE may be used with caution, however, in patients who do not respond to, or cannot tolerate, other antihypertensive agents. It is prudent, if TRANDATE is used, to use the smallest effective dose, so that inhibition of endogenous or exogenous beta-agonists is minimized.

Pheochromocytoma: Labetalol HCl has been shown to be effective in lowering the blood pressure and relieving symptoms in patients with pheochromocytoma. However, paradoxical hypertensive responses have been reported in a few patients with this tumor; therefore, use caution when administering labetalol HCl to patients with pheochromocytoma.

Diabetes Mellitus and Hypoglycemia: Beta-adrenergic blockade may prevent the appearance of premonitory signs and symptoms (eg, tachycardia) of acute hypoglycemia. This is especially important with labile diabetics. Beta-blockade also reduces the release of insulin in response to hyperglycemia; it may therefore be necessary to adjust the dose of antidiabetic drugs.

Major Surgery: The necessity or desirability of withdrawing beta-blocking therapy prior to major surgery is controversial. Protracted severe hypotension and difficulty in restarting or maintaining a heart beat have been reported with beta-blockers. The effect of labetalol HCl's alpha-adrenergic activity has not been evaluated in this setting.
A synergism between labetalol HCl and halothane anesthesia has been shown (see **Drug Interactions under PRECAUTIONS**).

PRECAUTIONS

General: ***Impaired Hepatic Function:*** TRANDATE® Tablets should be used with caution in patients with impaired hepatic function since metabolism of the drug may be diminished.

Jaundice or Hepatic Dysfunction: On rare occasions, labetalol HCl has been associated with jaundice (both hepatic and cholestatic). It is therefore recommended that treatment with labetalol HCl be stopped immediately should a patient develop jaundice or laboratory evidence of liver injury. Both have been shown to be reversible on stopping therapy.

Information for Patients: As with all drugs with beta-blocking activity, certain advice to patients being treated with labetalol HCl is warranted. This information is intended to aid in the safe and effective use of this medication. It is not a disclosure of all possible adverse or intended effects. While no incidence of the abrupt withdrawal phenomenon (exacerbation of angina pectoris) has been reported with labetalol HCl, dosing with TRANDATE Tablets should not be interrupted or discontinued without a physician's advice. Patients being treated with TRANDATE Tablets should consult a physician at any sign of impending cardiac failure. Also, transient scalp tingling may occur, usually when treatment with TRANDATE Tablets is initiated (see **ADVERSE REACTIONS**).

Laboratory Tests: As with any new drug given over prolonged periods, laboratory parameters should be observed over regular intervals. In patients with concomitant illnesses, such as impaired renal function, appropriate tests should be done to monitor these conditions.

Drug Interactions: In one survey, 2.3% of patients taking labetalol HCl in combination with tricyclic antidepressants experienced tremor as compared to 0.7% reported to occur with labetalol HCl alone. The contribution of each of the treatments to this adverse reaction is unknown, but the possibility of a drug interaction cannot be excluded.
Drugs possessing beta-blocking properties can blunt the bronchodilator effect of beta-receptor agonist drugs in patients with bronchospasm; therefore, doses greater than the normal antiasthmatic dose of beta-agonist bronchodilator drugs may be required.
Cimetidine has been shown to increase the bioavailability of labetalol HCl. Since this could be explained either by enhanced absorption or by an alteration of hepatic metabolism of labetalol HCl, special care should be used in establishing the dose required for blood pressure control in such patients.

Continued on next page

Glaxo—Cont.

Synergism has been shown between halothane anesthesia and intravenously administered labetalol HCl. During controlled hypotensive anesthesia using labetalol HCl in association with halothane, high concentrations (3% or above) of halothane should not be used because the degree of hypotension will be increased and because of the possibility of a large reduction in cardiac output and an increase in central venous pressure. The anesthesiologist should be informed when a patient is receiving labetalol HCl.

Labetalol HCl blunts the reflex tachycardia produced by nitroglycerin without preventing its hypotensive effect. If labetalol HCl is used with nitroglycerin in patients with angina pectoris, additional antihypertensive effects may occur.

Drug/Laboratory Test Interactions: The presence of a metabolite of labetalol in the urine may result in falsely increased levels of urinary catecholamines when measured by a nonspecific trihydroxyindole (THI) reaction. In screening patients suspected of having a pheochromocytoma and being treated with labetalol HCl, specific radioenzymatic or high performance liquid chromatography assay techniques should be used to determine levels of catecholamines or their metabolites.

Carcinogenesis, Mutagenesis, Impairment of Fertility: Long-term oral dosing studies with labetalol HCl for 18 months in mice and for two years in rats showed no evidence of carcinogenesis. Studies with labetalol HCl using dominant lethal assays in rats and mice and exposing microorganisms according to modified Ames tests showed no evidence of mutagenesis.

Pregnancy: ***Teratogenic Effects: Pregnancy Category C:*** Teratogenic studies have been performed with labetalol in rats and rabbits at oral doses up to approximately six and four times the maximum recommended human dose (MRHD), respectively. No reproducible evidence of fetal malformations was observed. Increased fetal resorptions were seen in both species at doses approximating the MRHD. There are no adequate and well-controlled studies in pregnant women. Labetalol should be used during pregnancy only if the potential benefit justifies the potential risk to the fetus.

Nonteratogenic Effects: Infants of mothers who were treated with labetalol HCl during pregnancy did not appear to be adversely affected by the drug. Oral administration of labetalol to rats during late gestation through weaning at doses of two to four times the MRHD caused a decrease in neonatal survival.

Labor and Delivery: Labetalol HCl given to pregnant women with hypertension did not appear to affect the usual course of labor and delivery.

Nursing Mothers: Small amounts of labetalol (approximately 0.004% of the maternal dose) are excreted in human milk. Caution should be exercised when TRANDATE (labetalol HCl) Tablets are administered to a nursing mother.

Labetalol HCl Daily Dose (mg)	200	300	400	600	800	900	1200	1600	2400
Number of Patients	522	181	606	608	503	117	411	242	175
Dizziness (%)	2	3	3	3	5	1	9	13	16
Fatigue	2	1	4	4	5	3	7	6	10
Nausea	<1	0	1	2	4	0	7	11	19
Vomiting	0	0	<1	<1	<1	0	1	2	3
Dyspepsia	1	0	2	1	1	0	2	2	4
Paresthesias	2	0	2	2	1	1	2	5	5
Nasal Stuffiness	1	1	2	2	2	2	4	5	6
Ejaculation Failure	0	2	1	2	3	0	4	3	5
Impotence	1	1	1	1	2	4	3	4	3
Edema	1	0	1	1	1	0	1	2	2

Pediatric Use: Safety and effectiveness in children have not been established.

ADVERSE REACTIONS

Most adverse effects are mild, transient, and occur early in the course of treatment. In controlled clinical trials of three to four months' duration, discontinuation of TRANDATE® Tablets due to one or more adverse effects was required in 7% of all patients. In these same trials, beta-blocker control agents led to discontinuation in 8% to 10% of patients, and a centrally acting alpha-agonist in 30% of patients.

The incidence rates of adverse reactions listed in the following table were derived from multicenter, controlled clinical trials comparing labetalol HCl, placebo, metoprolol, and propranolol over treatment periods of three and four months. Where the frequency of adverse effects for labetalol HCl and placebo is similar, causal relationship is uncertain. The rates are based on adverse reactions considered probably drug-related by the investigator. If all reports are considered, the rates are somewhat higher (eg, dizziness 20%, nausea 14%, fatigue 11%), but the overall conclusions are unchanged.

[See table below].

The adverse effects were reported spontaneously and are representative of the incidence of adverse effects that may be observed in a properly selected hypertensive patient population, ie, a group excluding patients with bronchospastic disease, overt congestive heart failure, or other contraindications to beta-blocker therapy.

Clinical trials also included studies utilizing daily doses up to 2,400 mg in more severely hypertensive patients. Certain of the side effects increased with increasing dose, as shown in the table below that depicts the entire US therapeutic trials data base for adverse reactions that are clearly or possibly dose-related.

[See table above].

In addition, a number of other less common adverse events have been reported in clinical trials or the literature:

Cardiovascular: Postural hypotension, including rarely, syncope.

Central and Peripheral Nervous Systems: Paresthesias, most frequently described as scalp tingling. In most cases, it was mild, transient, and usually occurred at the beginning of treatment.

Collagen Disorders: Systemic lupus erythematosus; positive antinuclear factor (ANF).

Eyes: Dry eyes.

Immunological System: Antimitochondrial antibodies.

Liver and Biliary System: Cholestasis with or without jaundice.

Musculoskeletal System: Muscle cramps; toxic myopathy.

Respiratory System: Bronchospasm.

Skin and Appendages: Rashes of various types, such as generalized maculopapular, lichenoid, urticarial, bullous lichen planus, psoriaform, and facial erythema; Peyronie's disease; reversible alopecia.

Urinary System: Difficulty in micturition, including acute urinary bladder retention.

Following approval for marketing in the United Kingdom, a monitored release survey involving approximately 6,800 patients was conducted for further safety and efficacy evaluation of this product. Results of this survey indicate that the type, severity, and incidence of adverse effects were comparable to those cited above.

Potential Adverse Effects: In addition, other adverse effects not listed above have been reported with other beta-adrenergic blocking agents.

Central Nervous System: Reversible mental depression progressing to catatonia, an acute reversible syndrome characterized by disorientation for time and place, short-term memory loss, emotional lability, slightly clouded sensorium, and decreased performance or neuropsychometrics.

Cardiovascular: Intensification of AV block (see **CONTRAINDICATIONS**).

Allergic: Fever combined with aching and sore throat; laryngospasm; respiratory distress.

Hematologic: Agranulocytosis; thrombocytopenic or nonthrombocytopenic purpura.

Gastrointestinal: Mesenteric artery thrombosis; ischemic colitis.

The oculomucocutaneous syndrome associated with the beta-blocker practolol has not been reported with labetalol HCl.

Clinical Laboratory Tests: There have been reversible increases of serum transaminases in 4% of patients treated with labetalol HCl and tested, and more rarely, reversible increases in blood urea.

OVERDOSAGE

Overdosage with TRANDATE® (labetalol HCl) Tablets causes excessive hypotension that is posture sensitive, and sometimes, excessive bradycardia. Patients should be placed supine and their legs raised if necessary to improve the blood supply to the brain. If overdosage with labetalol HCl follows oral ingestion, gastric lavage or pharmacologically induced emesis (using syrup of ipecac) may be useful for removal of the drug shortly after ingestion. The following additional measures should be employed if necessary: **Excessive bradycardia**—administer atropine or epinephrine. **Cardiac failure**—administer a digitalis glycoside and a diuretic. Dopamine or dobutamine may also be useful. **Hypotension**—administer vasopressors, eg, norepinephine. There is pharmacological evidence that norepinephrine may be the drug of choice. **Bronchospasm**—administer epinephrine and/or an aerosolized $beta_2$-agonist. **Seizures**—administer diazepam.

In severe beta-blocker overdose resulting in hypotension and/or bradycardia, glucagon has been shown to be effective when administered in large doses (5 to 10 mg rapidly over 30 seconds, followed by continuous infusion of 5 mg/hr that can be reduced as the patient improves).

Neither hemodialysis nor peritoneal dialysis removes a significant amount of labetalol HCl from the general circulation (<1%).

The oral LD_{50} value of labetalol HCl in the mouse is approximately 600 mg/kg and in the rat is greater than 2 g/kg. The intravenous LD_{50} in these species is 50 to 60 mg/kg.

DOSAGE AND ADMINISTRATION

DOSAGE MUST BE INDIVIDUALIZED. The recommended *initial* dose is 100 mg *twice* daily whether used alone or added

	Labetalol HCl (N=227) %	Placebo (N=98) %	Propranolol (N=84) %	Metoprolol (N=49) %
Body as a whole				
fatigue	5	0	12	12
asthenia	1	1	1	0
headache	2	1	1	2
Gastrointestinal				
nausea	6	1	1	2
vomiting	<1	0	0	0
dyspepsia	3	1	1	0
abdominal pain	0	0	1	2
diarrhea	<1	0	2	0
taste distortion	1	0	0	0
Central and Peripheral Nervous Systems				
dizziness	11	3	4	4
paresthesias	<1	0	0	0
drowsiness	<1	2	2	2
Autonomic Nervous System				
nasal stuffiness	3	0	0	0
ejaculation failure	2	0	0	0
impotence	1	0	1	3
increased sweating	<1	0	0	0
Cardiovascular				
edema	1	0	0	0
postural hypotension	1	0	0	0
bradycardia	0	0	5	12
Respiratory				
dyspnea	2	0	1	2
Skin				
rash	1	0	0	0
Special Senses				
vision abnormality	1	0	0	0
vertigo	2	1	0	0

to a diuretic regimen. After two or three days, using standing blood pressure as an indicator, dosage may be titrated in increments of 100 mg bid every two or three days. The usual *maintenance* dosage of labetalol HCl is between 200 and 400 mg *twice* daily.
Since the full antihypertensive effect of labetalol HCl is usually seen within the first one to three hours of the initial dose or dose increment, the assurance of a lack of an exaggerated hypotensive response can be clinically established in the office setting. The antihypertensive effects of continued dosing can be measured at subsequent visits, approximately 12 hours after a dose, to determine whether further titration is necessary.
Patients with severe hypertension may require from 1,200 to 2,400 mg per day, with or without thiazide diuretics. Should side effects (principally nausea or dizziness) occur with these doses administered bid, the same total daily dose administered tid may improve tolerability and facilitate further titration. Titration increments should not exceed 200 mg bid.
When a diuretic is added, an additive antihypertensive effect can be expected. In some cases this may necessitate a labetalol HCl dosage adjustment. As with most antihypertensive drugs, optimal dosages of TRANDATE® Tablets are usually lower in patients also receiving a diuretic.
When transferring patients from other antihypertensive drugs, TRANDATE Tablets should be introduced as recommended and the dosage of the existing therapy progressively decreased.

HOW SUPPLIED

TRANDATE® Tablets, 100 mg, light orange, round, scored, film-coated tablets engraved on one side with "TRANDATE 100 GLAXO," bottles of 100 (NDC 0173-0346-43) and 500 (NDC 0173-0346-44) and unit dose packs of 100 tablets (NDC 0173-0346-47).
TRANDATE Tablets, 200 mg, white, round, scored, film-coated tablets engraved on one side with "TRANDATE 200 GLAXO," bottles of 100 (NDC 0173-0347-43) and 500 (NDC 0173-0347-44) and unit dose packs of 100 tablets (NDC 0173-0347-47).
TRANDATE Tablets, 300 mg, peach, round, scored, film-coated tablets engraved on one side with "TRANDATE 300 GLAXO," bottles of 100 (NDC 0173-0348-43) and 500 (NDC 0173-0348-44) and unit dose packs of 100 tablets (NDC 0173-0348-47).
TRANDATE Tablets should be stored between 2° and 30°C (36° and 86°F).
TRANDATE Tablets in the unit dose boxes should be protected from excessive moisture.

Shown in Product Identification Section, page 410

TRINSICON® ℞

[tren 'sa-kon]
Hematinic Concentrate
With Intrinsic Factor

A Highly Potent Oral Antianemia Preparation

DESCRIPTION

Each capsule contains:

Special liver-stomach concentrate (containing intrinsic factor)	240 mg
Vitamin B_{12} (activity equivalent)	15 mcg
Iron, elemental (as ferrous fumarate)	110 mg
Ascorbic acid (Vitamin C)	75 mg
Folic acid	0.5 mg

with other factors of Vitamin B complex present in the liver-stomach concentrate.
Each capsule also contains FD&C Blue No. 1, FD&C Red No. 3, FD&C Red No. 40, FD&C Yellow No. 6, gelatin, silicone fluid, starch, and titanium dioxide.

CLINICAL PHARMACOLOGY

Vitamin B_{12} with Intrinsic Factor: When secretion of intrinsic factor in gastric juice is inadequate or absent (eg, in Addisonian pernicious anemia or after gastrectomy), vitamin B_{12} in physiologic doses is absorbed poorly, if at all. The resulting deficiency of vitamin B_{12} leads to the clinical manifestations of pernicious anemia. Similar megaloblastic anemias may develop in fish tapeworm *(Diphyllobothrium latum)* infection or after a surgically created small-bowel blind loop; in these situations, treatment requires freeing the host of the parasites or bacteria which appear to compete for the available vitamin B_{12}. Strict vegetarianism and malabsorption syndromes may also lead to vitamin B_{12} deficiency. In the latter case, parenteral therapy, or oral therapy with so-called massive doses of vitamin B_{12}, may be necessary for adequate treatment of the patient.
Potency of intrinsic factor concentrates is determined physiologically, ie, by their use in patients with pernicious anemia. The liver-stomach concentrate with intrinsic factor and the vitamin B_{12} contained in two TRINSICON capsules provide 1½ times the minimum amount of therapeutic agent which, when given daily in an uncomplicated case of pernicious anemia, will produce a satisfactory reticulocyte response and relief of anemia and symptoms.
Concentrates of intrinsic factor derived from hog gastric, pyloric, and duodenal mucosa have been used successfully in patients who lack intrinsic factor. For example, Fouts et al maintained patients with pernicious anemia in clinical remission with oral therapy (liver extracts or intrinsic factor concentrate with vitamin B_{12}) for as long as 29 years.
After total gastrectomy, Ficarra found multifactor preparations taken orally to be "just as effective in maintaining blood levels as any medication that has to be administered parenterally." His study was based on 24 patients who had survived for five years after total gastrectomy for cancer and who had been taking two TRINSICON capsules daily.
Folic Acid: Folic acid deficiency is the immediate cause of most, if not all, cases of nutritional megaloblastic anemia and of the megaloblastic anemias of pregnancy and infancy; usually, it is also at least partially responsible for the megaloblastic anemias of malabsorption syndromes, eg, tropical and nontropical sprue.
It is apparent that in vitamin B_{12} deficiency (eg, pernicious anemia), lack of this vitamin results in impaired utilization of folic acid. There are other evidences of the close folic acid-vitamin B_{12} interrelationship: (1) B_{12} influences the storage, absorption, and utilization of folic acid, and (2), as a deficiency of B_{12} progresses, the requirement for folic acid increases. However, folic acid does not change the requirement for vitamin B_{12}.
Iron: A very common anemia is that due to iron deficiency. In most cases, the response to iron salts is prompt, safe, and predictable. Within limits, the response is quicker and more certain to large doses of iron than to small doses.
Each TRINSICON capsule furnishes 110 mg of elemental iron (as ferrous fumarate) to provide a maximum response.
Ascorbic Acid: Vitamin C plays a role in anemia therapy. It augments the conversion of folic acid to its active form, folinic acid. In addition, ascorbic acid promotes the reduction of ferric iron in food to the more readily absorbed ferrous form. Severe and prolonged vitamin C deficiency is associated with an anemia which is usually hypochromic but occasionally megaloblastic in type.

INDICATIONS AND USAGE

TRINSICON® (hematinic concentrate with intrinsic factor) is a multifactor preparation effective in the treatment of anemias that respond to oral hematinics, including pernicious anemia and other megaloblastic anemias and also iron-deficiency anemia. Therapeutic quantities of hematopoietic factors that are known to be important are present in the recommended daily dose.

CONTRAINDICATIONS

Hemochromatosis and hemosiderosis are contraindications to iron therapy.

PRECAUTIONS

General: Anemia is a manifestation that requires appropriate investigation to determine its cause or causes.
Folic acid *alone* is unwarranted in the treatment of pure vitamin B_{12} deficiency states, such as pernicious anemia. Folic acid may obscure pernicious anemia in that the blood picture may revert to normal while neurological manifestations remain progressive.
As with all preparations containing intrinsic factor, resistance may develop in some cases of pernicious anemia to the potentiation of absorption of physiologic doses of vitamin B_{12}. If resistance occurs, parenteral therapy or oral therapy with so-called massive doses of vitamin B_{12} may be necessary for adequate treatment of the patient. No single regimen fits all cases, and the status of the patient observed in follow-up is the final criterion for adequacy of therapy. Periodic clinical and laboratory studies are considered essential and are recommended.
Pregnancy: *Pregnancy Category C:* Animal reproduction studies have not been conducted with TRINSICON. It is also not known whether TRINSICON can cause fetal harm when administered to a pregnant woman or can affect reproduction capacity. TRINSICON should be given to a pregnant woman only if clearly needed.
Nursing Mothers: It is not known whether this drug is excreted in human milk. Because many drugs are excreted in human milk, caution should be exercised when TRINSICON is administered to a nursing woman.
Usage in Children: Safety and effectiveness in children below the age of 10 have not been established.

ADVERSE REACTIONS

Rarely, iron in therapeutic doses produces gastrointestinal reactions, such as diarrhea or constipation. Reducing the dose and administering it with meals will minimize these effects in the iron-sensitive patient.
In extremely rare instances, skin rash suggesting allergy has been noted following the oral administration of liver-stomach material. Allergic sensitization has been reported following both oral and parenteral administration of folic acid.

OVERDOSAGE

Symptoms: Those of iron intoxication, which may include pallor and cyanosis, vomiting, hematemesis, diarrhea, melena, shock, drowsiness, and coma.
Treatment: For specific therapy, exchange transfusion and chelating agents. For general management, gastric and rectal lavage with sodium bicarbonate solution or milk, administration of intravenous fluids and electrolytes, and use of oxygen.

DOSAGE AND ADMINISTRATION

One capsule twice a day. (Two capsules daily produce a standard response in the average uncomplicated case of pernicious anemia.)

HOW SUPPLIED

Capsules, dark pink and dark red (No. 2). Bottles of 60 (NDC 0173-0364-22), bottles of 500 (NDC 0173-0364-24), and unit dose packs of 100 capsules (NDC 0173-0364-27).

Shown in Product Identification Section, page 410

VENTOLIN® Inhaler ℞

[vent 'ō-lin]
(albuterol)
Bronchodilator Aerosol
For Oral Inhalation Only

DESCRIPTION

The active component of VENTOLIN® Inhaler is albuterol (α^1-[(*tert*-butylamino) methyl] - 4- hydroxy-*m*-xylene-α, α'-diol), a relatively selective beta$_2$-adrenergic bronchodilator having the chemical structure:

HOCH$_2$
HO– [benzene ring] –CHCH$_2$NHC(CH$_3$)$_3$
OH

Albuterol is the official generic name in the United States. The international generic name for the drug is salbutamol. The molecular weight of albuterol is 239.3, and the empirical formula is $C_{13}H_{21}NO_3$. Albuterol is a white to off-white crystalline solid. It is soluble in ethanol, sparingly soluble in water, and very soluble in chloroform.
VENTOLIN Inhaler is a metered-dose aerosol unit for oral inhalation. It contains a microcrystalline suspension of albuterol in propellants (trichloromonofluoromethane and dichlorodifluoromethane) with oleic acid. Each actuation delivers from the mouthpiece 90 mcg of albuterol. Each canister provides at least 200 inhalations.

CLINICAL PHARMACOLOGY

The prime action of beta-adrenergic drugs is to stimulate adenyl cyclase, the enzyme that catalyzes the formation of cyclic-3′, 5′-adenosine monophosphate (cyclic AMP) from adenosine triphosphate (ATP). The cyclic AMP thus formed mediates the cellular responses. By virtue of its relatively selective action on beta$_2$-adrenoceptors, albuterol relaxes smooth muscle of the bronchi and uterus and the vascular supply to skeletal muscle, but may have less cardiac stimulant effects than isoproterenol.
Albuterol is longer acting than isoproterenol by any route of administration in most patients because it is not a substrate for the cellular uptake processes for catecholamines nor for catechol-*O*-methyl transferase.
Because of its gradual absorption from the bronchi, systemic levels of albuterol are low after inhalation of recommended doses. Studies undertaken with four subjects administered tritiated albuterol resulted in maximum plasma concentrations occurring within two to four hours. Due to the sensitivity of the assay method, the metabolic rate and half-life of elimination of albuterol in plasma could not be determined. However, urinary excretion provided data indicating that albuterol has an elimination half-life of 3.8 hours. Approximately 72% of the inhaled dose is excreted within 24 hours in the urine, and consists of 28% of unchanged drug and 44% as metabolite.
Results of animal studies show that albuterol does not pass the blood-brain barrier.
The effects of rising doses of albuterol and isoproterenol aerosols were studied in volunteers and asthmatic patients. Results in normal volunteers indicated that albuterol is one half to one quarter as active as isoproterenol in producing increases in heart rate. In asthmatic patients similar cardiovascular differentiation between the two drugs was also seen.

INDICATIONS AND USAGE

VENTOLIN® (albuterol) Inhaler is indicated for the relief of bronchospasm in patients with reversible obstructive airway disease and for the prevention of exercise-induced bronchospasm.

Continued on next page

Glaxo—Cont.

In controlled clinical trials, the onset of improvement in pulmonary function was within 15 minutes, as determined by both maximum midexpiratory flow rate (MMEF) and forced expiratory volume in one second (FEV_1). MMEF measurements also showed that near maximum improvement in pulmonary function generally occurs within 60 to 90 minutes following two inhalations of albuterol and that clinically significant improvement generally continues for three to four hours in most patients. In clinical trials, some patients with asthma showed a therapeutic response (defined by maintaining FEV_1 values 15% or more above baseline) that was still apparent at six hours. Continued effectiveness of albuterol was demonstrated over a 13-week period in these same trials.
In clinical studies, two inhalations of albuterol taken approximately 15 minutes before exercise prevented exercise-induced bronchospasm, as demonstrated by the maintenance of FEV_1 within 80% of baseline values in the majority of patients. One of these studies also evaluated the duration of the prophylactic effect to repeated exercise challenges, which was evident at four hours in the majority of patients and at six hours in approximately one third of the patients.

CONTRAINDICATIONS

VENTOLIN® Inhaler is contraindicated in patients with a history of hypersensitivity to any of its components.

WARNINGS

As with other adrenergic aerosols, the potential for paradoxical bronchospasm should be kept in mind. If it occurs, the preparation should be discontinued immediately and alternative therapy instituted.
Fatalities have been reported in association with excessive use of inhaled sympathomimetic drugs. The exact cause of death is unknown, but cardiac arrest following the unexpected development of a severe acute asthmatic crisis and subsequent hypoxia is suspected.
The contents of VENTOLIN® Inhaler are under pressure. Do not puncture. Do not use or store near heat or open flame. Exposure to temperatures above 120°F may cause bursting. Never throw container into fire or incinerator. Keep out of reach of children.

PRECAUTIONS

Although it has less effect on the cardiovascular system than isoproterenol at recommended dosages, albuterol is a sympathomimetic amine and as such should be used with caution in patients with cardiovascular disorders, including coronary insufficiency and hypertension, in patients with hyperthyroidism or diabetes mellitus, and in patients who are unusually responsive to sympathomimetic amines.
Large doses of intravenous albuterol have been reported to aggravate pre-existing diabetes and ketoacidosis. The relevance of this observation to the use of VENTOLIN® Inhaler is unknown, since the aerosol dose is much lower than the doses given intravenously.
Although there have been no reports concerning the use of VENTOLIN Inhaler during labor and delivery, it has been reported that high doses of albuterol administered intravenously inhibit uterine contractions. Although this effect is extremely unlikely as a consequence of aerosol use, it should be kept in mind.
Information For Patients: The action of VENTOLIN Inhaler may last up to six hours, and therefore it should not be used more frequently than recommended. Do not increase the number or frequency of doses without medical consultation. If symptoms get worse, medical consultation should be sought promptly. While taking VENTOLIN Inhaler, other inhaled medicines should not be used unless prescribed.
See illustrated **Patient's Instructions For Use.**
Drug Interactions: Other sympathomimetic aerosol bronchodilators or epinephrine should not be used concomitantly with albuterol.
Albuterol should be administered with caution to patients being treated with monoamine oxidase inhibitors or tricyclic antidepressants because the action of albuterol on the vascular system may be potentiated.
Beta-receptor blocking agents and albuterol inhibit the effect of each other.
Carcinogenesis, Mutagenesis, Impairment of Fertility: In a two-year study in the rat, albuterol sulfate caused a significant dose-related increase in the incidence of benign leiomyomas of the mesovarium at doses corresponding to 111, 555, and 2,800 times the maximum human inhalational dose. The relevance of these findings to humans is not known. An 18-month study in mice revealed no evidence of tumorigenicity. Studies with albuterol revealed no evidence of mutagenesis. Reproduction studies in rats revealed no evidence of impaired fertility.
Pregnancy: ***Teratogenic Effects: Pregnancy Category C:*** Albuterol has been shown to be teratogenic in mice when given in doses corresponding to 14 times the human dose. There are no adequate and well-controlled studies in pregnant women. Albuterol should be used during pregnancy only if the potential benefit justifies the potential risk to the fetus. A reproduction study in CD-1 mice with albuterol (0.025, 0.25, and 2.5 mg/kg, corresponding to 1.4, 14, and 140 times the maximum human inhalational dose) showed cleft palate formation in 5 of 111 (4.5%) fetuses at 0.25 mg/kg and in 10 of 108 (9.3%) fetuses at 2.5 mg/kg. None was observed at 0.025 mg/kg. Cleft palate also occurred in 22 of 72 (30.5%) fetuses treated with 2.5 mg/kg isoproterenol (positive control). A reproduction study in Stride Dutch rabbits revealed cranioschisis in 7 of 19 (37%) fetuses at 50 mg/kg, corresponding to 2,800 times the maximum human inhalational dose.
Nursing Mothers: It is not known whether this drug is excreted in human milk. Because of the potential for tumorigenicity shown for albuterol in animal studies, a decision should be made whether to discontinue nursing or to discontinue the drug, taking into account the importance of the drug to the mother.
Pediatric Use: Safety and effectiveness in children below 12 years of age have not been established.

ADVERSE REACTIONS

The adverse reactions to albuterol are similar in nature to reactions to other sympathomimetic agents, although the incidence of certain cardiovascular effects is less with albuterol. A 13-week double-blind study compared albuterol and isoproterenol aerosols in 147 asthmatic patients. The results of this study showed that the incidence of cardiovascular effects was: palpitations, less than 10 per 100 with albuterol and less than 15 per 100 with isoproterenol; tachycardia, 10 per 100 with both albuterol and isoproterenol; and increased blood pressure, less than 5 per 100 with albuterol and isoproterenol. In the same study, both drugs caused tremor or nausea in less than 15 patients per 100, and dizziness or heartburn in less than 5 per 100 patients. Nervousness occurred in less than 10 per 100 patients receiving albuterol and in less than 15 per 100 patients receiving isoproterenol.
Rare cases of urticaria, angioedema, rash, bronchospasm, and oropharyngeal edema have been reported after the use of inhaled albuterol.
In addition, albuterol, like other sympathomimetic agents, can cause adverse reactions such as hypertension, angina, vomiting, vertigo, central nervous system stimulation, insomnia, headache, unusual taste, and drying or irritation of the oropharynx.

OVERDOSAGE

Exaggeration of the effects listed in **ADVERSE REACTIONS** can occur. Anginal pain and hypertension may result.
The oral LD_{50} in male and female rats and mice was greater than 2,000 mg/kg. The aerosol LD_{50} could not be determined.
Dialysis is not appropriate treatment for overdosage of VENTOLIN® (albuterol) Inhaler. The judicious use of a cardioselective beta-receptor blocker, such as a metoprolol tartrate, is suggested, bearing in mind the danger of inducing an asthmatic attack.

DOSAGE AND ADMINISTRATION

The usual dosage for adults and children 12 years and older is two inhalations repeated every four to six hours; in some patients, one inhalation every four hours may be sufficient. More frequent administration or a larger number of inhalations is not recommended. The use of VENTOLIN® Inhaler can be continued as medically indicated to control recurring bouts of bronchospasm. During this time most patients gain optimal benefit from regular use of the inhaler. Safe usage for periods extending over several years has been documented.
If a previously effective dosage regimen fails to provide the usual relief, medical advice should be sought immediately as this is often a sign of seriously worsening asthma that would require reassessment of therapy.
Exercise-Induced Bronchospasm Prevention: The usual dosage for adults and children 12 years and older is two inhalations 15 minutes prior to exercise.
For treatment, see above.

HOW SUPPLIED

VENTOLIN® Inhaler, 17-g canister, box of one. Each actuation delivers 90 mcg of albuterol from the mouthpiece. It is supplied with an oral adapter and patient's instructions (NDC 0173-0321-88). Also available, VENTOLIN Inhaler Refill, 17-g canister only with patient's instructions (NDC 0173-0321-98).
Store between 15° and 30°C (59° and 86°F).
Shake well before using.
Shown in Product Identification Section, page 410

VENTOLIN® Syrup ℞

[vent'ō-lin]
(albuterol sulfate)

DESCRIPTION

VENTOLIN® Syrup contains albuterol sulfate, a relatively selective $beta_2$-adrenergic bronchodilator. Albuterol sulfate has the chemical name α^1- [(*tert*-butylamino) methyl]-4-hydroxy-*m*-xylene-α,α'- diol sulfate (2:1) (salt), and the following chemical structure:

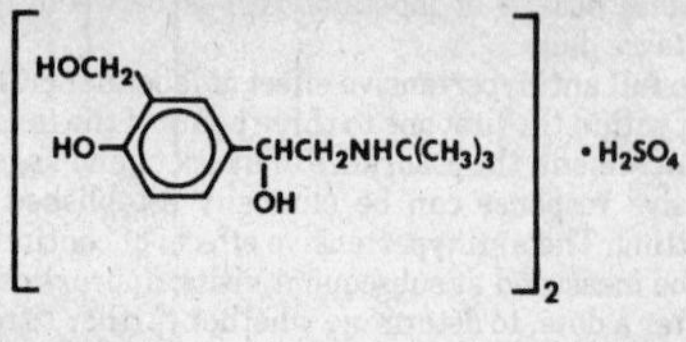

Albuterol sulfate has a molecular weight of 576.7 and the empirical formula $(C_{13}H_{21}NO_3)_2 \cdot H_2SO_4$. Albuterol sulfate is a white crystalline powder, soluble in water and slightly soluble in ethanol.
The international generic name for albuterol base is salbutamol.
VENTOLIN Syrup contains 2 mg of albuterol as 2.4 mg of albuterol sulfate in each teaspoonful (5 ml).
The inactive ingredients for VENTOLIN Syrup include citric acid monohydrate, FD&C Yellow No. 6, hydroxypropyl methylcellulose, saccharin sodium, sodium benzoate, sodium citrate, strawberry flavor, and purified water.

CLINICAL PHARMACOLOGY

The prime action of beta-adrenergic drugs is to stimulate adenyl cyclase, the enzyme that catalyzes the formation of cyclic-3′, 5′-adenosine monophosphate (cyclic AMP) from adenosine triphosphate (ATP). The cyclic AMP thus formed mediates the cellular responses. Based on pharmacologic studies in animals, albuterol appears to exert direct and preferential action on $beta_2$-adrenoceptors, including those of the bronchial tree and uterus, and may have less cardiac stimulant effect than isoproterenol when given in the usual recommended dose.
Albuterol is longer acting than isoproterenol in most patients by any route of administration because it is not a substrate for the cellular uptake processes for catecholamines nor for catechol-*0*-methyl transferase.
Albuterol is rapidly absorbed after oral administration of 10 ml of VENTOLIN® Syrup (4 mg of albuterol) in normal volunteers. Maximum plasma albuterol concentrations of about 18 ng/ml are achieved within two hours, and the drug is eliminated with a half-life of about five hours.
In other studies, the analysis of urine samples of patients given 8 mg of tritiated albuterol orally showed that 76% of the dose was excreted over three days, with the majority of the dose being excreted within the first 24 hours. Sixty percent of this radioactivity was shown to be the metabolite. Feces collected over this period contained 4% of the administered dose.
Animal studies show that albuterol does not pass the blood-brain barrier.

INDICATIONS AND USAGE

VENTOLIN® Syrup is indicated for the relief of bronchospasm in adults and children 2 years of age and older with reversible obstructive airway disease.
In controlled clinical trials in patients with asthma, the onset of improvement in pulmonary function, as measured by maximum midexpiratory flow rate (MMEF) and forced expiratory volume in one second (FEV_1), was within 30 minutes after a dose of VENTOLIN Syrup. Peak improvement of pulmonary function occurred between two and three hours. In a controlled clinical trial involving 55 children, clinically significant improvement (defined as maintaining a 15% or more increase in FEV_1 and a 20% or more increase in MMEF over baseline values) continued to be recorded up to six hours. No decrease in the effectiveness was reported in one uncontrolled study of 32 children who took VENTOLIN Syrup for a three-month period.

CONTRAINDICATIONS

VENTOLIN® Syrup is contraindicated in patients with a history of hypersensitivity to any of its components.

PRECAUTIONS

General: Although albuterol *usually* has minimal effects on the $beta_1$-adrenoceptors of the cardiovascular system at the recommended dosage, *occasionally* the usual cardiovascular and CNS stimulatory effects common to all sympathomimetic agents have been seen with patients treated with albuterol, necessitating discontinuation. Therefore, albuterol should be used with caution in patients with cardiovascular disorders, including coronary insufficiency and hypertension, in patients with hyperthyroidism or diabetes mellitus, and in patients who are unusually responsive to sympathomimetic amines.
Large doses of intravenous albuterol have been reported to aggravate pre-existing diabetes mellitus and ketoacidosis. Additionally, albuterol and other beta-agonists, when given intravenously, may cause a decrease in serum potassium, possibly through intracellular shunting. The decrease is usually transient, not requiring supplementation. The relevance of these observations to the use of VENTOLIN® Syrup is unknown.

Information for Patients: The action of VENTOLIN Syrup may last up to six hours, and therefore it should not be taken more frequently than recommended. Do not increase the dose or frequency of medication without medical consultation. If symptoms get worse, medical consultation should be sought promptly.

Drug Interactions: The concomitant use of VENTOLIN Syrup and other oral sympathomimetic agents is not recommended since such combined use may lead to deleterious cardiovascular effects. This recommendation does not preclude the judicious use of an aerosol bronchodilator of the adrenergic stimulant type in patients receiving VENTOLIN Syrup. Such concomitant use, however, should be individualized and not given on a routine basis. If regular coadministration is required, then alternative therapy should be considered.

Albuterol should be administered with extreme caution to patients being treated with monoamine oxidase inhibitors or tricyclic antidepressants because the action of albuterol on the vascular system may be potentiated.

Beta-receptor blocking agents and albuterol inhibit the effect of each other.

Carcinogenesis, Mutagenesis, Impairment of Fertility: Albuterol sulfate, like other agents in its class, caused a significant dose-related increase in the incidence of benign leiomyomas of the mesovarium in a two-year study in the rat, at doses corresponding to 2, 9, and 46 times the maximum human (child weighing 21 kg) oral dose. In another study this effect was blocked by the coadministration of propranolol. The relevance of these findings to humans is not known. An 18-month study in mice and a lifetime study in hamsters revealed no evidence of tumorigenicity. Studies with albuterol revealed no evidence of mutagenesis. Reproduction studies in rats revealed no evidence of impaired fertility.

Pregnancy: ***Teratogenic Effects: Pregnancy Category C:*** Albuterol has been shown to be teratogenic in mice when given subcutaneously in doses corresponding to 0.2 times the maximum human (child weighing 21 kg) oral dose.

There are no adequate and well-controlled studies in pregnant women. Albuterol should be used during pregnancy only if the potential benefit justifies the potential risk to the fetus. A reproduction study in CD-1 mice with albuterol showed cleft palate formation in 5 of 111 (4.5%) fetuses at 0.25 mg/kg and in 10 of 108 (9.3%) fetuses at 2.5 mg/kg. None was observed at 0.025 mg/kg. Cleft palate also occurred in 22 of 72 (30.5%) fetuses treated with 2.5 mg/kg isoproterenol (positive control). A reproduction study in Stride Dutch rabbits revealed cranioschisis in 7 of 19 (37%) fetuses at 50 mg/kg, corresponding to 46 times the maximum human (child weighing 21 kg) oral dose of albuterol sulfate.

Labor and Delivery: Oral albuterol has been shown to delay preterm labor in some reports. There are presently no well-controlled studies which demonstrate that it will stop preterm labor or prevent labor at term. Therefore, cautious use of VENTOLIN Syrup is required in pregnant patients when given for relief of bronchospasm so as to avoid interference with uterine contractility. Use in such patients should be restricted to those patients in whom the benefits clearly outweigh the risks.

Nursing Mothers: It is not known whether this drug is excreted in human milk. Because of the potential for tumorigenicity shown for albuterol in animal studies, a decision should be made whether to discontinue nursing or to discontinue the drug, taking into account the importance of the drug to the mother.

Pediatric Use: Safety and effectiveness in children below 2 years of age have not yet been adequately demonstrated.

ADVERSE REACTIONS

The adverse reactions to albuterol are similar in nature to reactions to other sympathomimetic agents. The most frequent adverse reactions to VENTOLIN® Syrup in adults and older children were tremor, 10 of 100 patients, and nervousness and shakiness, each in 9 of 100 patients. Other reported adverse reactions were headache, 4 of 100 patients; dizziness and increased appetite, each in 3 of 100 patients; hyperactivity and excitement, each in 2 of 100 patients; tachycardia, epistaxis, and sleeplessness, each in 1 of 100 patients. The following adverse effects each occurred in less than 1 of 100 patients: muscle spasm, disturbed sleep, epigastric pain, cough, palpitations, stomachache, irritable behavior, dilated pupils, sweating, chest pain, and weakness.

In young children 2 to 6 years of age, some adverse reactions were noted more frequently than in adults and older children. Excitement was noted in approximately 20% of patients and nervousness in 15%. Hyperkinesia occurred in 4% of patients, with isomnia, tachycardia, and gastrointestinal symptoms in 2% each. Anorexia, emotional lability, pallor, fatigue, and conjunctivitis were seen in 1%.

In addition, albuterol, like other sympathomimetic agents, can cause adverse reactions such as hypertension, angina, vomiting, vertigo, central nervous system stimulation, unusual taste, and drying or irritation of the oropharynx.

The reactions are generally transient in nature, and it is usually not necessary to discontinue treatment with VENTOLIN® Syrup. In selected cases, however, dosage may be reduced temporarily; after the reaction has subsided, dosage should be increased in small increments to the optimal dosage.

OVERDOSAGE

Manifestations of overdosage include anginal pain, hypertension, hypokalemia, and exaggeration of the effects listed in **ADVERSE REACTIONS.**

The oral LD_{50} in rats and mice was greater than 2,000 mg/kg.

Dialysis is not appropriate treatment for overdosage of VENTOLIN® Syrup. The judicious use of a cardioselective beta-receptor blocker, such as metoprolol tartrate, is suggested, bearing in mind the danger of inducing an asthmatic attack.

DOSAGE AND ADMINISTRATION

The following dosages of VENTOLIN® Syrup are expressed in terms of albuterol base.

Usual Dosage: The usual starting dosage for adults and children over age 14 is 2 mg (1 teaspoonful) or 4 mg (2 teaspoonfuls) three or four times a day.

The usual starting dosage for children 6 to 14 years of age is 2 mg (1 teaspoonful) three or four times a day.

For children 2 to 6 years of age, dosing should be initiated at 0.1 mg/kg of body weight three times a day. This starting dosage should not exceed 2 mg (1 teaspoonful) three times a day.

Dosage Adjustment: For adults and children over age 14, a dosage above 4 mg four times a day should be used only when the patient fails to respond. If a favorable response does not occur, the dosage may be cautiously increased stepwise, but not to exceed 8 mg four times a day.

For children from 6 to 14 years of age who fail to respond to the initial starting dosage of 2 mg four times a day, the dosage may be cautiously increased stepwise, but not to exceed 24 mg per day (given in divided doses).

For children 2 to 6 years of age who do not respond satisfactorily to the initial dosage, the dose may be increased stepwise to 0.2 mg/kg of body weight three times a day, but not to exceed maximum of 4 mg (2 teaspoonfuls) given three times a day.

Elderly Patients and Those Sensitive to Beta-adrenergic Stimulators:

The initial dosage should be restricted to 2 mg three or four times a day and individually adjusted thereafter.

HOW SUPPLIED

VENTOLIN® Syrup, a clear, orange-yellow liquid with a strawberry flavor, contains 2 mg of albuterol as the sulfate per 5 ml in bottles of 16 fluid ounces (one pint) (NDC 0173-0351-54).

Store between 2° and 30°C (36° and 86°F).

Shown in Product Identification Section, page 410

VENTOLIN® Tablets ℞

[*vent'ō-lin*]

(albuterol sulfate)

DESCRIPTION

VENTOLIN® Tablets contain albuterol sulfate, a relatively selective $beta_2$-adrenergic bronchodilator. Albuterol sulfate has the chemical name α^1-[(*tert*-butylamino)methyl]-4-hydroxy-*m*-xylene-α,α'-diol sulfate (2:1)(salt).

Albuterol sulfate has a molecular weight of 576.7 and the empirical formula $(C_{13}H_{21}NO_3)_2 \cdot H_2SO_4$. Albuterol sulfate is a white crystalline powder, soluble in water and slightly soluble in ethanol.

The international generic name for albuterol base is salbutamol.

Each VENTOLIN tablet contains 2 or 4 mg of albuterol as 2.4 or 4.8 mg of albuterol sulfate, respectively. Each tablet also contains the inactive ingredients corn starch, lactose, and magnesium stearate.

CLINICAL PHARMACOLOGY

The prime action of beta-adrenergic drugs is to stimulate adenyl cyclase, the enzyme that catalyzes the formation of cyclic-3′,5′-adenosine monophosphate (cyclic AMP) from adenosine triphosphate (ATP). The cyclic AMP thus formed mediates the cellular responses. Based on pharmacologic studies in animals, albuterol appears to exert direct and preferential action on $beta_2$ -adrenoceptors, including those of the bronchial tree and uterus, and may have less cardiac stimulant effect than isoproterenol when given in the usual recommended dose.

Albuterol is longer acting than isoproterenol in most patients by any route of administration because it is not a substrate for the cellular uptake processes for catecholamines nor for catechol-*O*-methyl transferase.

Albuterol is rapidly absorbed after oral administration of 4-mg VENTOLIN® Tablets in normal volunteers. Maximum plasma albuterol concentrations of about 18 ng/ml are achieved within two hours, and the drug is eliminated with a half-life of about five hours. In other studies, the analysis of urine samples of patients given 8 mg of tritiated albuterol orally showed that 76% of the dose was excreted over three days, with the majority of the dose being excreted within the first 24 hours. Sixty percent of this radioactivity was shown to be the metabolite. Feces collected over this period contained 4% of the administered dose.

Animal studies show that albuterol does not pass the blood-brain barrier.

INDICATIONS AND USAGE

VENTOLIN® Tablets are indicated for the relief of bronchospasm in patients with reversible obstructive airway disease.

In controlled clinical trials in patients with asthma, the onset of improvement in pulmonary function, as measured by maximum midexpiratory flow rate (MMEF), was noted within 30 minutes after a dose of VENTOLIN Tablets, with peak improvement occurring between two and three hours. In controlled clinical trials in which measurements were conducted for six hours, significant clinical improvement in pulmonary function (defined as maintaining a 15% or more increase in forced expiratory volume in one second [FEV_1] and a 20% or more increase in MMEF over baseline values) was observed in 60% of patients at four hours and in 40% at six hours. In other single-dose, controlled clinical trials, clinically significant improvement was observed in at least 40% of the patients at eight hours. No decrease in the effectiveness of VENTOLIN Tablets has been reported in patients who received long-term treatment with the drug in uncontrolled studies for periods up to six months.

CONTRAINDICATIONS

VENTOLIN® Tablets are contraindicated in patients with a history of hypersensitivity to any of their components.

PRECAUTIONS

General: Although albuterol usually has minimal effects on the $beta_1$-adrenoceptors of the cardiovascular system at the recommended dosage, occasionally the usual cardiovascular and CNS stimulatory effects common to all sympathomimetic agents have been seen with patients treated with albuterol, necessitating discontinuation. Therefore, albuterol should be used with caution in patients with cardiovascular disorders, including coronary insufficiency and hypertension, in patients with hyperthyroidism or diabetes mellitus, and in patients who are unusually responsive to sympathomimetic amines.

Large doses of intravenous albuterol have been reported to aggravate pre-existing diabetes mellitus and ketoacidosis. Additionally, albuterol and other beta-agonists, when given intravenously, may cause a decrease in serum potassium, possibly through intracellular shunting. The decrease is usually transient, not requiring supplementation. The relevance of these observations to the use of VENTOLIN® Tablets is unknown.

Information for Patients: The action of VENTOLIN Tablets may last for eight hours or longer, and therefore they should not be taken more frequently than recommended. Do not increase the dose or frequency of medication without medical consultation. If symptoms get worse, medical consultation should be sought promptly.

Drug Interactions: The concomitant use of VENTOLIN Tablets and other oral sympathomimetic agents is not recommended since such combined use may lead to deleterious cardiovascular effects. This recommendation does not preclude the judicious use of an aerosol bronchodilator of the adrenergic stimulant type in patients receiving VENTOLIN Tablets. Such concomitant use, however, should be individualized and not given on a routine basis. If regular coadministration is required, then alternative therapy should be considered.

Albuterol should be administered with extreme caution to patients being treated with monoamine oxidase inhibitors or tricyclic antidepressants because the action of albuterol on the vascular system may be potentiated.

Beta-receptor blocking agents and albuterol inhibit the effect of each other.

Carcinogenesis, Mutagenesis, Impairment of Fertility: Albuterol sulfate, like other agents in its class, caused a significant dose-related increase in the incidence of benign leiomyomas of the mesovarium in a two-year study in the rat, at doses corresponding to 3, 16, and 78 times the maximum human oral dose. In another study this effect was blocked by the coadministration of propranolol. The relevance of these findings to humans is not known. An 18-month study in mice and a lifetime study in hamsters revealed no evidence of tumorigenicity. Studies with albuterol revealed no evidence of mutagenesis. Reproduction studies in rats revealed no evidence of impaired fertility.

Pregnancy: ***Teratogenic Effects: Pregnancy Category C:*** Albuterol has been shown to be teratogenic in mice when given subcutaneously in doses corresponding to 0.4 times the maximum human oral dose. There are no adequate and well-controlled studies in pregnant women. Albuterol should be used during pregnancy only if the potential benefit justifies the potential risk to the fetus. A reproduction study in CD-1

Continued on next page

Glaxo—Cont.

mice with albuterol showed cleft palate formation in 5 of 111 (4.5%) fetuses at 0.25 mg/kg and in 10 of 108 (9.3%) fetuses at 2.5 mg/kg. None was observed at 0.025 mg/kg. Cleft palate also occurred in 22 of 72 (30.5%) fetuses treated with 2.5 mg/kg isoproterenol (positive control). A reproduction study in Stride Dutch rabbits revealed cranioschisis in 7 of 19 (37%) fetuses at 50 mg/kg, corresponding to 78 times the maximum human oral dose of albuterol.

Labor and Delivery: Oral albuterol has been shown to delay preterm labor in some reports. There are presently no well-controlled studies which demonstrate that it will stop preterm labor or prevent labor at term. Therefore, cautious use of VENTOLIN Tablets is required in pregnant patients when given for relief of bronchospasm so as to avoid interference with uterine contractibility.

Nursing Mothers: It it not known whether this drug is excreted in human milk. Because of the potential for tumorigenicity shown for albuterol in animal studies, a decision should be made whether to discontinue nursing or to discontinue the drug, taking into account the importance of the drug to the mother.

Pediatric Use: Safety and effectiveness in children below 6 years of age have not been established.

ADVERSE REACTIONS

The adverse reactions to albuterol are similar in nature to those to other sympathomimetic agents. The most frequent adverse reactions to VENTOLIN® Tablets were nervousness and tremor, with each occurring in approximately 20 of 100 patients. Other reported reactions were headache, 7 of 100 patients; tachycardia and palpitations, 5 of 100 patients; muscle cramps, 3 of 100 patients; and insomnia, nausea, weakness, and dizziness, each in 2 of 100 patients. Drowsiness, flushing, restlessness, irritability, chest discomfort, and difficulty in micturition each occurred in less than 1 of 100 patients.

In addition, albuterol, like other sympathomimetic agents, can cause adverse reactions such as hypertension, angina, vomiting, vertigo, central nervous system stimulation, unusual taste, and drying or irritation of the oropharynx.

The reactions are generally transient in nature, and it is usually not necessary to discontinue treatment with VENTOLIN Tablets. In selected cases, however, dosage may be reduced temporarily; after the reaction has subsided, dosage should be increased in small increments to the optimal dosage.

OVERDOSAGE

Manifestations of overdosage include anginal pain, hypertension, hypokalemia, and exaggeration of the effects listed in **ADVERSE REACTIONS.**

The oral LD_{50} in rats and mice was greater than 2,000 mg/kg.

Dialysis is not appropriate treatment for overdosage of VENTOLIN® Tablets. The judicious use of a cardioselective beta-receptor blocker, such as metoprolol tartrate, is suggested, bearing in mind the danger of inducing an asthmatic attack.

DOSAGE AND ADMINISTRATION

The following dosages of VENTOLIN® Tablets are expressed in terms of albuterol base.

Usual Dosage: The usual starting dosage for children 6 to 12 years of age is 2 mg three or four times a day.

The usual starting dosage for adults and children 12 years and older is 2 or 4 mg three or four times a day.

Dosage Adjustment: For children from 6 to 12 years of age who fail to respond to the initial starting dosage of 2 mg four times a day, the dosage may be cautiously increased stepwise, but not to exceed 24 mg per day (given in divided doses). For adults and children 12 years and older, a dosage above 4 mg four times a day should be used only when the patient fails to respond. If a favorable response does not occur with the 4-mg initial dosage, it should be cautiously increased stepwise up to a maximum of 8 mg four times a day as tolerated.

Elderly Patients and Those Sensitive to Beta-adrenergic Stimulators: An initial dosage of 2 mg three or four times a day is recommended for elderly patients and for those with a history of unusual sensitivity to beta-adrenergic stimulators. If adequate bronchodilatation is not obtained, dosage may be increased gradually to as much as 8 mg three or four times a day.

The total daily dose should not exceed 32 mg in adults and children 12 years and older.

HOW SUPPLIED

VENTOLIN® Tablets, 2 mg of albuterol as the sulfate, are white, round, compressed tablets impressed with the product name (VENTOLIN) and the number 2 on one side and scored on the other with "GLAXO" impressed on each side of the score in bottles of 100 (NDC 0173-0341-43) and 500 (NDC 0173-0341-44).

VENTOLIN® Tablets, 4 mg of albuterol as the sulfate, are white, round, compressed tablets impressed with the product name (VENTOLIN) and the number 4 on one side and scored on the other with "GLAXO" impressed on each side of the score in bottles of 100 (NDC 0173-0342-43) and 500 (NDC 0173-0342-44).

Store between 2° and 30°C (36° and 86°F).

Shown in Product Identification Section, page 410

VICON-C® Capsules

[vi'kon]

(Therapeutic Vitamins and Minerals)

COMPOSITION

Each yellow and orange capsule contains:

Ascorbic acid	300 mg
Niacinamide	100 mg
Zinc sulfate, USP*	80 mg
Magnesium sulfate, USP†	70 mg
Thiamine mononitrate	20 mg
d-Calcium pantothenate	20 mg
Riboflavin	10 mg
Pyridoxine hydrochloride	5 mg

* As 50 mg of dried zinc sulfate.

† As 35 mg of anhydrous magnesium sulfate.

INDICATIONS AND USAGE

VICON-C® is indicated in the treatment of patients with deficiencies of, or increased requirements for, Vitamin C, B-Complex vitamins, zinc, and/or magnesium. The components of VICON-C have important roles in nutrition, tissue growth and repair, and the prevention of hemorrhage. Tissue injury resulting from trauma, burns, or surgery may rapidly deplete the body stores of Vitamin C, the B-Complex vitamins, and zinc. Patients maintained on parenteral fluids for extended periods or patients with burns, wounds, or diarrhea often develop deficiencies of Vitamin C, the B-Complex vitamins, and zinc.

VICON-C is recommended for deficiencies or the prevention of deficiencies of Vitamin C, the B-Complex vitamins, magnesium, and/or zinc in conditions such as febrile diseases, chronic or acute infections, burns, fractures, surgery, toxic conditions, physiologic stress, alcoholism, pregnancy, lactation, geriatrics, gastritis, peptic ulcer, colitis, and in conditions involving special diets and weight-reduction diets. It is also recommended in dentistry for these deficiencies in conditions such as herpetic stomatitis, aphthous stomatitis, cheilosis, herpangina, gingivitis, and states involving oral surgery.

DOSAGE AND ADMINISTRATION

One capsule two or three times daily or as directed by a physician for treatment of deficiencies.

HOW SUPPLIED

Bottles of 60 (NDC 0173-0273-22) and 500 (NDC 0173-0273-24) capsules and unit dose pack of 100 capsules (NDC 0173-0273-27).

Shown in Product Identification Section, page 410

VICON® PLUS Capsules

[vi'kon]

(Therapeutic Vitamins and Minerals)

COMPOSITION

Each red and beige capsule contains:

Vitamin A	4,000 IU
Vitamin E	50 IU
Ascorbic acid	150 mg
Zinc sulfate, USP*	80 mg
Magnesium sulfate, USP†	70 mg
Niacinamide	25 mg
Thiamine mononitrate	10 mg
d-Calcium pantothenate	10 mg
Riboflavin	5 mg
Manganese chloride	4 mg
Pyridoxine hydrochloride	2 mg

* As 50 mg of dried zinc sulfate.

† As 35 mg of anhydrous magnesium sulfate.

VICON® PLUS is an extended range vitamin-mineral supplement formulated to aid patient recovery by helping to meet increased nutritional demands.

INDICATIONS AND USAGE

For nutritional supplementation of the patient undergoing physiologic stress due to surgery, burns, trauma, febrile illnesses, or poor nutrition.

DOSAGE AND ADMINISTRATION

One capsule twice daily or as prescribed by a physician for treatment of deficiencies. Dosage should not exceed eight capsules daily due to the possible toxicity of large doses of vitamin A.

HOW SUPPLIED

Bottles of 60 capsules (NDC 0173-0305-22).

Shown in Product Identification Section, page 410

VICON FORTE® Capsules ℞

[vi'kon for'ta]

(Therapeutic Vitamins-Minerals)

DESCRIPTION

Each black and orange VICON FORTE® capsule for oral administration contains:

Vitamin A	8,000 IU
Vitamin E	50 IU
Ascorbic acid	150 mg
Zinc sulfate, USP*	80 mg
Magnesium sulfate, USP†	70 mg
Niacinamide	25 mg
Thiamine mononitrate	10 mg
d-Calcium pantothenate	10 mg
Riboflavin	5 mg
Manganese chloride	4 mg
Pyridoxine hydrochloride	2 mg
Folic acid	1 mg
Vitamin B_{12}(Cyanocobalamin)	10 mcg

*As 50 mg of dried zinc sulfate.

†As 35 mg of anhydrous magnesium sulfate.

Each capsule also contains FD&C Blue No. 1, FD&C Red No. 40, FD&C Yellow No. 6, gelatin, lactose, magnesium stearate, sodium proprionate, and titanium dioxide.

INDICATIONS AND USAGE

VICON FORTE® is indicated for the treatment and/or prevention of vitamin and mineral deficiencies associated with restricted diets, improper food intake, alcoholism, and decreased absorption. VICON FORTE is also indicated in patients with increased requirements for vitamins and minerals due to chronic disease, infection, and burns and in persons using alcohol to excess. Preoperative and postoperative use of VICON FORTE can provide the increased amounts of vitamins and minerals necessary for optimal recovery from the stress of surgery.

CONTRAINDICATIONS

None known.

PRECAUTIONS

General: Folic acid in doses above 0.1 mg daily may obscure pernicious anemia in that hematologic remission can occur while neurological manifestations remain progressive.

DOSAGE AND ADMINISTRATION

One capsule daily or as directed by physician.

HOW SUPPLIED

Orange and black capsules imprinted with "Glaxo" and "316" in bottles of 60 (NDC 0173-0316-22) and 500 (NDC 0173-0316-24) and in unit dose packs of 100 (NDC 0173-0316-27).

Dispense in tight, light-resistant containers as defined in the USP/NF.

Shown in Product Identification Section, page 410

VI-ZAC® Capsules

[vi'zak]

(Therapeutic Vitamin-Mineral)

COMPOSITION

Each orange capsule contains:

Vitamin A	5,000 IU
Ascorbic acid	500 mg
Vitamin E	50 IU
Zinc sulfate, USP*	80 mg

*As 50 mg of dried zinc sulfate.

INDICATIONS AND USAGE

VI-ZAC® is indicated in the treatment of patients with deficiencies of, or increased requirements for, Vitamins A, C, and E and zinc. The VI-ZAC formulation is a limited vitamin-mineral formulation designed to meet special needs. It is particularly indicated where there is no requirement for supplemental amounts of the B-Complex vitamins and their attendant appetite stimulation. The formulation is also designed for patients who cannot tolerate magnesium supplements but do need supplemental amounts of zinc.

PRECAUTIONS

Although rarely encountered, vitamin A in large doses daily for several months or longer may cause toxicity.

DOSAGE AND ADMINISTRATION

One or two capsules daily or as directed by the physician for the treatment of deficiencies.

HOW SUPPLIED

Bottles of 60 (NDC 0173-0292-22).

Shown in Product Identification Section, page 410

ZANTAC® Injection ℞

[*zan 'tak*]

(ranitidine hydrochloride)

DESCRIPTION

The active ingredient in ZANTAC® Injection, ranitidine hydrochloride, is a histamine H_2-receptor antagonist. Chemically, it is N[2-[[[5-[(dimethylamino)-methyl]-2-furanyl]methyl]-thio]ethyl]-N'-methyl-2-nitro-1,1-ethenediamine, hydrochloride. It has the following structure:

$(CH_3)_2NCH_2$–[furan]–$CH_2SCH_2CH_2NH$–C(=$CHNO_2$)–$NHCH_3$ · HCl

The empirical formula is $C_{13}H_{22}N_4O_3S.HCl$, representing a molecular weight of 350.87.

Ranitidine hydrochloride is a white to pale yellow granular substance which is soluble in water.

ZANTAC Injection is a clear, colorless to yellow liquid that tends to darken slightly without adversely affecting potency. The pH of the injection solution is 6.7 to 7.3.

Sterile Injection for IM or IV Administration: ***Single-Dose Vials: 2 ml (25 mg/ml):*** Each 1 ml of aqueous solution contains ranitidine 25 mg (as the hydrochloride); phenol 5 mg as preservative; and 0.96 mg monobasic potassium phosphate and 2.4 mg dibasic sodium phosphate as buffers.

Multi-dose Vials: 10 ml (25 mg/ml): Each 1 ml of aqueous solution contains ranitidine 25 mg (as the hydrochloride); phenol 5 mg as preservative; and 0.96 mg monobasic potassium phosphate and 2.4 mg dibasic sodium phosphate as buffers.

CLINICAL PHARMACOLOGY

ZANTAC® (ranitidine hydrochloride) is a competitive, reversible inhibitor of the action of histamine at the histamine H_2-receptors, including receptors on the gastric cells. ZANTAC does not lower serum Ca^{++} in hypercalcemic states. ZANTAC is not an anticholinergic agent.

Antisecretory Activity:

1. Effects on Acid Secretion: ZANTAC Injection inhibits basal gastric acid secretion as well as gastric acid secretion stimulated by betazole and pentagastrin, as shown in the table above:

Effect of IV ZANTAC on Gastric Acid Secretion

	Time after Dose, hrs.	% Inhibition of Gastric Acid Output by IV Dose, mg 20 mg	60 mg	100 mg
Betazole	Up to 2	93	99	99
Pentagastrin	Up to 3	47	66	77

In a group of ten known hypersecretors, ranitidine plasma levels of 71, 180, and 376 ng/ml inhibited basal acid secretion by 76%, 90%, and 99.5%, respectively.

It appears that basal- and betazole-stimulated secretions are most sensitive to inhibition by ZANTAC, while pentagastrin-stimulated secretion is more difficult to suppress.

2. Effects on Other Gastrointestinal Secretions:

Pepsin: ZANTAC does not affect pepsin secretion. Total pepsin output is reduced in proportion to the decrease in volume of gastric juice.

Intrinsic Factor: ZANTAC has no significant effect on pentagastrin-stimulated intrinsic factor secretion.

Serum Gastrin: ZANTAC has little or no effect on fasting or postprandial serum gastrin.

Other Pharmacological Actions:

a. Gastric bacterial flora—increase in nitrate-reducing organisms, significance not known.
b. Prolactin levels—no effect in recommended oral or IV dosage, but small, transient dose-related increases in serum prolactin have been reported after IV bolus injections of 100 mg or more.
c. Other pituitary hormones—no effect on serum gonadotropins, TSH, or GH. Possible impairment of vasopressin release.
d. No change in cortisol, aldosterone, androgen, or estrogen levels.
e. No antiandrogenic action.
f. No effect on count, motility, or morphology of sperm.

Pharmacokinetics: Serum concentrations necessary to inhibit 50% of stimulated gastric acid secretion are estimated to be 36 to 94 ng/ml. Following single intravenous or intramuscular 50-mg doses, serum concentrations of ZANTAC are in this range for six to eight hours.

Following intravenous injection, approximately 70% of the dose is recovered in the urine as unchanged drug. Renal clearance averages 530 ml/min, with a total clearance of 760 ml/min. The volume of distribution is 1.4 L/kg, and the elimination half-life is 2 to 2.5 hours.

Four patients with clinically significant renal function impairment (creatinine clearance 25 to 35 ml/min) administered 50 mg of ranitidine IV had an average plasma half-life of 4.8 hours, a ranitidine clearance of 29 ml/min, and a volume of distribution of 1.76 L/kg. In general, these parameters appear to be altered in proportion to creatinine clearance (see **Dosage and Administration**).

ZANTAC is absorbed very rapidly after intramuscular injection. Mean peak levels of 576 ng/ml occur within 15 minutes or less following a 50-mg intramuscular dose. Absorption from intramuscular sites is virtually complete, with a bioavailability of 90% to 100% compared with intravenous administration. Following oral administration, the relative bioavailability of ZANTAC Tablets is 50%.

In man, the N-oxide is the principal metabolite in the urine; however, this amounts to less than 4% of the dose. Other metabolites are the S-oxide (1%) and the desmethyl ranitidine (1%). The remainder of the administered dose is found in the stool.

Studies in patients with hepatic dysfunction (compensated cirrhosis) indicate that there are minor, but clinically insignificant, alterations in ranitidine half-life, distribution, clearance, and bioavailability.

Serum protein binding averages 15%.

Clinical Trials: ***Duodenal Ulcer:*** In a multicenter, double-blind, controlled US study of endoscopically diagnosed duodenal ulcers, earlier healing was seen in the patients treated with oral ZANTAC as shown below:

[See table below].

	Oral ZANTAC* Number Entered	Oral ZANTAC* Healed/Evaluable	Oral Placebo* Number Entered	Oral Placebo* Healed/Evaluable
Outpatients				
Week 2	195	69/182 (38%)†	188	31/164 (19%)
Week 4		137/187 (73%)†		76/168 (45%)

*All patients were permitted prn antacids for relief of pain

†p < 0.0001

In these studies, patients treated with oral ZANTAC reported a reduction in both daytime and nocturnal pain, and they also consumed less antacid than the placebo-treated patients.

[See table on bottom next page].

Pathological Hypersecretory Conditions (such as Zollinger-Ellison Syndrome): ZANTAC inhibits gastric acid secretion and reduces occurrence of diarrhea, anorexia, and pain in patients with pathological hypersecretion associated with Zollinger-Ellison syndrome, systemic mastocytosis, and other pathological hypersecretory conditions (eg, postoperative, "short-gut" syndrome, idiopathic). Use of oral ZANTAC was followed by healing of ulcers in 8 of 19 (42%) patients who were intractable to previous therapy.

INDICATIONS AND USAGE

ZANTAC (ranitidine hydrochloride) Injection is indicated in some hospitalized patients with pathological hypersecretory conditions or intractable duodenal ulcers, or as an alternative to the oral dosage form for short-term use in patients who are unable to take oral medication.

CONTRAINDICATIONS

ZANTAC® Injection is contraindicated for patients known to have hypersensitivity to the drug.

PRECAUTIONS

General: 1. Symptomatic response to ZANTAC® therapy does not preclude the presence of gastric malignancy.

2. Since ZANTAC is excreted primarily by the kidney, dosage should be adjusted in patients with impaired renal function (see **Dosage and Administration**). Caution should be observed in patients with hepatic dysfunction since ZANTAC is metabolized in the liver.

3. In controlled studies in normal volunteers, elevations in SGPT have been observed when H_2-antagonists have been administered intravenously at greater than recommended doses for five days or longer. Therefore, it seems prudent in patients receiving IV ranitidine at doses greater than or equal to 100 mg qid for periods of five days or longer to monitor SGPT daily (from day 5) for the remainder of IV therapy.

Laboratory Tests: False-positive tests for urine protein with Multistix® may occur during ZANTAC therapy, and therefore testing with sulfosalicylic acid is recommended.

Drug Interactions: Although ZANTAC has been reported to bind weakly to cytochrome P-450 in vitro, recommended doses of the drug do not inhibit the action of the cytochrome P-450-linked oxygenase enzymes in the liver. However, there have been isolated reports of drug interactions which suggest that ZANTAC may affect the bioavailability of certain drugs by some mechanism as yet unidentified (eg, a pH-dependent effect on absorption or a change in volume of distribution).

Carcinogenesis, Mutagenesis, Impairment of Fertility: There is no indication of tumorigenic or carcinogenic effects in lifespan studies in mice and rats at oral doses up to 2,000 mg/kg/day.

Ranitidine was not mutagenic in standard bacterial tests (*Salmonella, E coli*) for mutagenicity at concentrations up to the maximum recommended for these assays.

In a dominant lethal assay, a single oral dose of 1,000 mg/kg to male rats was without effect on the outcome of two matings per week for the next nine weeks.

Pregnancy: ***Teratogenic Effects: Pregnancy Category B:*** Reproduction studies have been performed in rats and rabbits at oral doses up to 160 times the human oral dose and have revealed no evidence of impaired fertility or harm to the fetus due to ZANTAC. There are, however, no adequate and well-controlled studies in pregnant women. Because animal reproduction studies are not always predictive of human response, this drug should be used during pregnancy only if clearly needed.

Nursing Mothers: ZANTAC is secreted in human milk. Caution should be exercised when ZANTAC is administered to a nursing mother.

Pediatric Use: Safety and effectiveness in children have not been established.

Use in Elderly Patients: Ulcer healing rates in elderly patients (65 to 82 years of age) treated with oral ZANTAC were no different from those in younger age groups. The incidence rates for adverse events and laboratory abnormalities were also not different from those seen in other age groups.

ADVERSE REACTIONS

Transient pain at the site of intramuscular injection has been reported. Transient local burning or itching has been reported with intravenous administration of ZANTAC®.

The following have been reported as events in clinical trials or in the routine management of patients treated with oral ZANTAC. The relationship to ZANTAC therapy has been unclear in many cases. Headache, sometimes severe, seeems to be related to ZANTAC administration.

Central Nervous System: Rarely, malaise, dizziness, somnolence, insomnia, and vertigo. Rare cases of reversible mental confusion, agitation, depression, and hallucinations have been reported, predominantly in severely ill elderly patients.

Cardiovascular: Rare reports of tachycardia, bradycardia, and premature ventricular beats.

Gastrointestinal: Constipation, diarrhea, nausea/vomiting, and abdominal discomfort/pain.

Hepatic: In normal volunteers, SGPT values were increased to at least twice the pretreatment levels in 6 of 12 subjects receiving 100 mg qid IV for seven days, and in 4 of 24 subjects receiving 50 mg qid for five days. With oral administration there have been occasional reports of reversible hepatitis, hepatocellular or hepatocanalicular or mixed, with or without jaundice.

Musculoskeletal: Rare reports of arthralgias.

Hematologic: Rare reports of reversible leukopenia, granulocytopenia, thrombocytopenia, and pancytopenia.

Endocrine: Controlled studies in animals and man have shown no stimulation of any pituitary hormone by ZANTAC and no antiandrogenic activity, and cimetidine-induced gynecomastia and impotence in hypersecretory patients have resolved when ZANTAC has been substituted. However, occasional cases of gynecomastia, impotence, and loss of libido have been reported in male patients receiving ZANTAC, but the incidence did not differ from that in the general population.

Integumental: Rash and, rarely, alopecia.

Other: Rare cases of hypersensitivity reactions (eg, bronchospasm, fever, rash, eosinophilia) and small increases in serum creatinine.

OVERDOSAGE

There is no experience to date with deliberate overdosage. Clinical monitoring and supportive therapy should be employed.

Studies in dogs receiving doses of ZANTAC® in excess of 225 mg/kg/day have shown muscular tremors, vomiting, and rapid respiration. Single oral doses of 1,000 mg/kg in mice and rats were not lethal. Intravenous LD_{50} values in rat and mouse were 83 and 77 mg/kg, respectively.

Continued on next page

Glaxo—Cont.

DOSAGE AND ADMINISTRATION

Parenteral Administration: In some hospitalized patients with pathological hypersecretory conditions or intractable duodenal ulcers, or in patients who are unable to take oral medication, ZANTAC ® may be administered parenterally according to the following recommendations:

Intramuscular Injection: 50 mg (2 ml) every six to eight hours. (No dilution necessary.)

Intravenous Injection: 50 mg (2 ml) every six to eight hours. Dilute ZANTAC Injection, 50 mg, in 0.9% Sodium Chloride Injection or other compatible IV solution (see **Stability of ZANTAC Injection**) to a total volume of 20 ml and inject over a period of not less than five minutes.

Intermittent Intravenous Infusion: 50 mg (2 ml) every six to eight hours. Dilute ZANTAC Injection, 50 mg, in 100 ml of 5% Dextrose Injection or other compatible IV solution (see **Stability of ZANTAC Injection**) and infuse over 15 to 20 minutes. In some patients it may be necessary to increase dosage. When this is necessary, the increases should be made by more frequent administration of a 50-mg dose, but generally should not exceed 400 mg per day.

Dosage Adjustment for Patients with Impaired Renal Function: On the basis of experience with a group of subjects with severely impaired renal function treated with ZANTAC, the recommended dosage in patients with a creatinine clearance less than 50 ml/min is 50 mg every 18 to 24 hours. Should the patient's condition require, the frequency of dosing may be increased to every 12 hours or even further with caution. Hemodialysis reduces the level of circulating ranitidine. Ideally, the dosage schedule should be adjusted so that the timing of a scheduled dose coincides with the end of hemodialysis.

Stability of ZANTAC Injection: ZANTAC Injection is stable for 48 hours at room temperature when added to or diluted with most commonly used intravenous solutions, eg, 0.9% Sodium Chloride Injection, 5% Dextrose Injection, 10% Dextrose Injection, Lactated Ringer's Solution, or 5% Sodium Bicarbonate Injection.

Note: Parenteral drug products should be inspected visually for particulate matter and discoloration prior to administration wherever solution and container permit.

HOW SUPPLIED

ZANTAC® Injection, 25 mg/ml, is available in 2-ml single dose vials in boxes of 10 (NDC 0173-0362-38) and in 10-ml multi-dose vials (NDC 0173-0363-39).

Store below 30°C (86°F). Protect from light.

Shown in Product Identification Section, page 410

ZANTAC® 150 Tablets ℞
[zan'tak]
(ranitidine hydrochloride)
ZANTAC® 300 Tablets
(ranitidine hydrochloride)

DESCRIPTION

The active ingredient in ZANTAC® 150 and ZANTAC® 300 Tablets, ranitidine hydrochloride, is a histamine H_2-receptor antagonist. Chemically it is N[2-[[[5-[(dimethylamino)methyl]-2-furanyl]methyl]thio]ethyl]-N'-methyl -2- nitro-1,1-ethenediamine, hydrochloride.

The empirical formula is $C_{13}H_{22}N_4O_3S \cdot HCl$, representing a molecular weight of 350.87.

Ranitidine hydrochloride is a white to pale yellow granular substance that is soluble in water. It has a slightly bitter taste and sulfur-like odor.

Each ZANTAC 150 tablet for oral administration contains 168 mg of ranitidine hydrochloride equivalent to 150 mg ranitidine. Each tablet also contains the inactive ingredients hydroxypropyl methylcellulose, magnesium stearate, microcrystalline cellulose, and titanium dioxide.

Each ZANTAC 300 tablet for oral administration contains 336 mg of ranitidine hydrochloride equivalent to 300 mg of ranitidine. Each tablet also contains the inactive ingredients croscarmellose sodium, D&C Yellow No. 10, hydroxypropyl methylcellulose, magnesium stearate, microcrystalline cellulose, and titanium dioxide.

CLINICAL PHARMACOLOGY

ZANTAC® (ranitidine hydrochloride) is a competitive, reversible inhibitor of the action of histamine at the histamine H_2-receptors, including receptors on the gastric cells. ZANTAC does not lower serum Ca^{++} in hypercalcemic states. ZANTAC is not an anticholinergic agent.

Effect of Oral ZANTAC on Gastric Acid Secretion

	Time After Dose, hrs.	% Inhibition of Gastric Acid Output by Dose, mg			
		75–80	100	150	200
Basal	Up to 4		99	95	
Nocturnal	Up to 13	95	96	92	
Betazole	Up to 3		97	99	
Pentagastrin	Up to 5	58	72	72	80
Meal	Up to 3		73	79	95

Antisecretory Activity: ***1. Effects on Acid Secretion:*** ZANTAC inhibits both daytime and nocturnal basal gastric acid secretions as well as gastric acid secretion stimulated by food, betazole, and pentagastrin, as shown in the table above:

It appears that basal-, nocturnal-, and betazole-stimulated secretions are most sensitive to inhibition by ZANTAC, responding almost completely to doses of 100 mg or less, while pentagastrin- and food-stimulated secretions are more difficult to suppress.

2. Effects on Other Gastrointestinal Secretions:

Pepsin: Oral ZANTAC 150 mg did not affect pepsin secretion. Total pepsin output was reduced in proportion to the decrease in volume of gastric juice.

Intrinsic Factor: Oral ZANTAC 150 mg had no significant effect on pentagastrin-stimulated intrinsic factor secretion.

Serum Gastrin: ZANTAC has little or no effect on fasting or postprandial serum gastrin.

Other Pharmacological Actions:

a. Gastric bacterial flora—increase in nitrate-reducing organisms, significance not known.

b. Prolactin levels—no effect in recommended oral or IV dosage, but small, transient dose-related increases in serum prolactin have been reported after IV bolus injections of 100 mg or more.

c. Other pituitary hormones—no effect on serum gonadotropins, TSH, or GH. Possible impairment of vasopressin release.

d. No change in cortisol, aldosterone, androgen, or estrogen levels.

e. No antiandrogenic action.

f. No effect on count, motility, or morphology of sperm.

Pharmacokinetics: ZANTAC is 50% absorbed after oral administration, compared to an IV injection with mean peak levels of 440 to 545 ng/ml occurring at two to three hours after a 150-mg dose. The elimination half-life is 2.5 to 3 hours.

Absorption is not significantly impaired by the administration of food or antacids. Propantheline slightly delays and increases peak blood levels of ZANTAC, probably by delaying gastric emptying and transit time. In one study, simultaneous administration of high-potency antacid (150 m mol) in fasting subjects has been reported to decrease the absorption of ZANTAC.

Serum concentrations necessary to inhibit 50% of stimulated gastric acid secretion are estimated to be 36 to 94 ng/ml. Following a single oral dose of 150 mg, serum concentrations of ZANTAC are in this range up to 12 hours. However, blood levels bear no consistent relationship to dose or degree of acid inhibition.

The principal route of excretion is the urine, with approximately 30% of the orally administered dose collected in the urine as unchanged drug in 24 hours. Renal clearance is about 410 ml/min, indicating active tubular excretion. Four patients with clinically significant renal function impairment (creatinine clearance 25 to 35 ml/min) administered 50 mg of ranitidine IV had an average plasma half-life of 4.8 hours, a ranitidine clearance of 29 ml/min, and a volume of distribution of 1.76 L/kg. In general, these parameters appear to be altered in proportion to creatinine clearance (see **DOSAGE AND ADMINISTRATION**).

In man, the N-oxide is the principal metabolite in the urine; however, this amounts to less than 4% of the dose. Other metabolites are the S-oxide (1%) and the desmethyl ranitidine (1%). The remainder of the administered dose is found in the stool. Studies in patients with hepatic dysfunction (compensated cirrhosis) indicate that there are minor, but clinically insignificant, alterations in ranitidine half-life, distribution, clearance, and bioavailability.

The volume of distribution is about 1.4 L/kg. Serum protein binding averages 15%.

Clinical Trials: ***Active Duodenal Ulcer:*** In a multicenter, double-blind, controlled US study of endoscopically diagnosed duodenal ulcers, earlier healing was seen in the patients treated with ZANTAC as shown in Table I.

[See table on next page].

In these studies patients treated with ZANTAC reported a reduction in both daytime and nocturnal pain, and they also consumed less antacid than the placebo-treated patients.

[See table on bottom next page].

Foreign studies have shown that patients heal equally well with 150 mg bid and 300 mg hs (85% vs 84%, respectively) during a usual four-week course of therapy. If patients require extended therapy of eight weeks, the healing rate may be higher for 150 mg bid as compared to 300 mg hs (92% vs 87%, respectively).

Studies have been limited to short-term treatment of acute duodenal ulcer. Patients whose ulcers healed during therapy had recurrences of ulcers at the usual rates. There have been no systematic studies to evaluate whether continued treatment with ZANTAC alters recurrence rates.

Maintenance Therapy in Duodenal Ulcer: Ranitidine has been found to be effective as maintenance therapy for patients following healing of acute duodenal ulcers. In two independent, double-blind, multicenter, controlled trials, the number of duodenal ulcers observed was significantly less in patients treated with ZANTAC (150 mg hs) than in patients treated with placebo over a 12-month period.

Duodenal Ulcer Prevalence

Double-blind, Multicenter, Placebo-controlled Trials

Multicenter Trial	Drug	Duodenal Ulcer Prevalence 0–4 Months	0–8 Months	0–12 Months	No. Patients
USA	RAN	20%*	24%*	35%*	138
	PLC	44%	54%	59%	139
Foreign	RAN	12%*	21%*	28%*	174
	PLC	56%	64%	68%	165

% = Life-Table estimate
* = $p<0.05$ (ZANTAC vs comparator)
RAN = Ranitidine (ZANTAC)
PLC = Placebo

As with other H_2-antagonists, the factors responsible for the significant reduction in the prevalence of duodenal ulcers include prevention of recurrence of ulcers, more rapid healing of ulcers that may occur during maintenance therapy, or both.

Gastric Ulcer: In a multicenter, double-blind, controlled US study of endoscopically diagnosed gastric ulcers, earlier healing was seen in the patients treated with ZANTAC as shown below:

	ZANTAC*		Placebo*	
	Number Entered	Healed/ Evaluable	Number Entered	Healed/ Evaluable
Outpatients				
Week 2	92	16/83 (19%)	94	10/83 (12%)
Week 6		50/73 (68%)†		35/69 (51%)

* All patients were permitted prn antacids for relief of pain.
† = 0.009

In this multicenter trial, significantly more patients treated with ZANTAC became pain-free during therapy.

Pathological Hypersecretory Conditions (such as Zollinger-Ellison Syndrome): ZANTAC inhibits gastric acid secretion and reduces occurrence of diarrhea, anorexia, and pain in patients with pathological hypersecretion associated with Zollinger-Ellison syndrome, systemic mastocytosis, and other pathological hypersecretory conditions (eg, postoperative, "short-gut" syndrome, idiopathic). Use of oral ZANTAC was followed by healing of ulcers in 8 of 19 (42%) patients who were intractable to previous therapy.

Gastroesophageal Reflux Disease (GERD): In two multicenter, double-blind, placebo-controlled, six-week trials performed in the United States and Europe, ZANTAC was more effective than placebo for the relief of heartburn and other

Mean Daily Doses of Antacid

	Ulcer Healed	Ulcer Not Healed
Oral ZANTAC	0.06	0.71
Oral Placebo	0.71	1.43

symptoms associated with GERD. Ranitidine-treated patients consumed significantly less antacid than did placebo-treated patients.

The US trial indicated that ZANTAC significantly reduced the frequency of heartburn attacks and severity of heartburn pain within one to two weeks after starting therapy. The improvement was maintained throughout the six-week trial period. Moreover, patient response rates demonstrated that the effect on heartburn extends through both the day and night time periods.

In patients with endoscopically verified reflux esophagitis prior to treatment, those treated with ZANTAC had a somewhat higher incidence of healing at six weeks than did placebo-treated patients.

INDICATIONS AND USAGE

ZANTAC® (ranitidine hydrochloride) is indicated in:

1. Short-term treatment of active duodenal ulcer. Most patients heal within four weeks. Studies available to date have not assessed the safety of ranitidine in uncomplicated duodenal ulcer for periods of more than eight weeks.
2. Maintenance therapy for duodenal ulcer patients at reduced dosage after healing of acute ulcers. No placebo-controlled comparative studies have been carried out for periods of longer than one year.
3. The treatment of pathological hypersecretory conditions (eg, Zollinger-Ellison syndrome and systemic mastocytosis).
4. Short-term treatment of active, benign gastric ulcer. Most patients heal within six weeks and the usefulness of further treatment has not been demonstrated. Studies available to date have not assessed the safety of ranitidine in uncomplicated, benign gastric ulcer for periods of more than six weeks.
5. Treatment of gastroesophageal reflux disease. Symptomatic relief commonly occurs within one or two weeks after starting therapy. Therapy for longer than six weeks has not been studied.

In active duodenal ulcer; active, benign gastric ulcer; hypersecretory states; and GERD, concomitant antacids should be given as needed for relief of pain.

CONTRAINDICATIONS

ZANTAC® is contraindicated for patients known to have hypersensitivity to the drug.

PRECAUTIONS

General: 1. Symptomatic response to ZANTAC® therapy does not preclude the presence of gastric malignancy.

2. Since ZANTAC is excreted primarily by the kidney, dosage should be adjusted in patients with impaired renal function (see **DOSAGE AND ADMINISTRATION**). Caution should be observed in patients with hepatic dysfunction since ZANTAC is metabolized in the liver.

Laboratory Tests: False-positive tests for urine protein with Multistix® may occur during ZANTAC therapy, and therefore testing with sulfosalicylic acid is recommended.

Drug Interactions: Although ZANTAC has been reported to bind weakly to cytochrome P-450 in vitro, recommended doses of the drug do not inhibit the action of the cytochrome P-450-linked oxygenase enzymes in the liver. However, there have been isolated reports of drug interactions which suggest that ZANTAC may affect the bioavailability of certain drugs by some mechanism as yet unidentified (eg, a pH-dependent effect on absorption or a change in volume of distribution).

Carcinogenesis, Mutagenesis, Impairment of Fertility: There was no indication of tumorigenic or carcinogenic effects in lifespan studies in mice and rats at doses up to 2,000 mg/kg/day.

Ranitidine was not mutagenic in standard bacterial tests *(Salmonella, E coli)* for mutagenicity at concentrations up to the maximum recommended for these assays.

In a dominant lethal assay, a single oral dose of 1,000 mg/kg to male rats was without effect on the outcome of two matings per week for the next nine weeks.

Pregnancy: ***Teratogenic Effects: Pregnancy Category B:*** Reproduction studies have been performed in rats and rabbits at doses up to 160 times the human dose and have revealed no evidence of impaired fertility or harm to the fetus due to ZANTAC. There are, however, no adequate and well-controlled studies in pregnant women. Because animal reproduction studies are not always predictive of human response, this drug should be used during pregnancy only if clearly needed.

Nursing Mothers: ZANTAC is secreted in human milk. Caution should be exercised when ZANTAC is administered to a nursing mother.

Pediatric Use: Safety and effectiveness in children have not been established.

Table I

	ZANTAC*		Placebo*	
	Number Entered	Healed/ Evaluable	Number Entered	Healed/ Evaluable
Outpatients				
Week 2	195	69/182 (38%)†	188	31/164 (19%)
Week 4		137/187 (73%)†		76/168 (45%)

*All patients were permitted prn antacids for relief of pain. †p < 0.0001

Use in Elderly Patients: Ulcer healing rates in elderly patients (65 to 82 years of age) were no different from those in younger age groups. The incidence rates for adverse events and laboratory abnormalities were also not different from those seen in other age groups.

ADVERSE REACTIONS

The following have been reported as events in clinical trials or in the routine management of patients treated with ZANTAC®. The relationship to ZANTAC therapy has been unclear in many cases. Headache, sometimes severe, seems to be related to ZANTAC administration.

Central Nervous System: Rarely, malaise, dizziness, somnolence, insomnia, and vertigo. Rare cases of reversible mental confusion, agitation, depression, and hallucinations have been reported, predominantly in severely ill elderly patients.

Cardiovascular: Rare reports of tachycardia, bradycardia, and premature ventricular beats.

Gastrointestinal: Constipation, diarrhea, nausea/vomiting, and abdominal discomfort/pain.

Hepatic: In normal volunteers, SGPT values were increased to at least twice the pretreatment levels in 6 of 12 subjects receiving 100 mg qid IV for seven days, and in 4 of 24 subjects receiving 50 mg qid IV for five days. With oral administration there have been occasional reports of reversible hepatitis, hepatocellular or hepatocanalicular or mixed, with or without jaundice.

Musculoskeletal: Rare reports of arthralgias.

Hematologic: Rare reports of reversible leukopenia, granulocytopenia, thrombocytopenia, and pancytopenia.

Endocrine: Controlled studies in animals and man have shown no stimulation of any pituitary hormone by ZANTAC and no antiandrogenic activity, and cimetidine-induced gynecomastia and impotence in hypersecretory patients have resolved when ZANTAC has been substituted. However, occasional cases of gynecomastia, impotence, and loss of libido have been reported in male patients receiving ZANTAC, but the incidence did not differ from that in the general population.

Integumental: Rash, including rare cases suggestive of mild erythema multiforme, and, rarely, alopecia.

Other: Rare cases of hypersensitivity reactions (eg, bronchospasm, fever, rash, eosinophilia) and small increases in serum creatinine.

OVERDOSAGE

There is no experience to date with deliberate overdosage. The usual measures to remove unabsorbed material from the gastrointestinal tract, clinical monitoring, and supportive therapy should be employed.

Studies in dogs receiving doses of ZANTAC® in excess of 225 mg/kg/day have shown muscular tremors, vomiting, and rapid respiration. Single oral doses of 1,000 mg/kg in mice and rats were not lethal. Intravenous LD_{50} values in rat and mouse were 83 and 77 mg/kg, respectively.

DOSAGE AND ADMINISTRATION

Active Duodenal Ulcer: The current recommended adult oral dosage of ZANTAC® for duodenal ulcer is 150 mg twice daily. An alternate dosage of 300 mg once daily at bedtime can be used for patients in whom dosing convenience is important. The advantages of one treatment regimen compared to the other in a particular patient population have yet to be demonstrated (see **Clinical Trials: *Active Duodenal Ulcer***). Smaller doses have been shown to be equally effective in inhibiting gastric acid secretion in US studies, and several foreign trials have shown that 100 mg bid is as effective as the 150-mg dose.

Antacid should be given as needed for relief of pain (see **Pharmacokinetics** under **CLINICAL PHARMACOLOGY**).

Maintenance Therapy: The current recommended adult oral dosage is 150 mg at bedtime.

Pathological Hypersecretory Conditions (such as Zollinger-Ellison Syndrome): The current recommended adult oral dosage is 150 mg twice a day. In some patients it may be necessary to administer ZANTAC 150-mg doses more frequently. Doses should be adjusted to individual patient needs, and should continue as long as clinically indicated. Doses up to 6 g/day have been employed in patients with severe disease.

Benign Gastric Ulcer: The current recommended adult oral dosage is 150 mg twice a day.

GERD: The current recommended adult oral dosage is 150 mg twice a day.

Dosage Adjustment for Patients with Impaired Renal Function: On the basis of experience with a group of subjects with severely impaired renal function treated with ZANTAC, the recommended dosage in patients with a creatinine clearance less than 50 ml/min is 150 mg every 24 hours. Should the patient's condition require, the frequency of dosing may be increased to every 12 hours or even further with caution. Hemodialysis reduces the level of circulating ranitidine. Ideally, the dosage schedule should be adjusted so that the timing of a scheduled dose coincides with the end of hemodialysis.

HOW SUPPLIED

ZANTAC® 150 Tablets (ranitidine hydrochloride equivalent to 150 mg of ranitidine) are white tablets embossed with "ZANTAC 150" on one side and "Glaxo" on the other. They are available in bottles of 60 tablets (NDC 0173-0344-42) and unit dose packs of 100 tablets (NDC 0173-0344-47).

ZANTAC® 300 Tablets (ranitidine hydrochloride equivalent to 300 mg ranitidine) are yellow, capsule-shaped tablets embossed with "ZANTAC 300" on one side and "Glaxo" on the other. They are available in bottles of 30 (NDC 0173-0393-40) and unit dose packs of 100 tablets (NDC 0173-0393-47).

Store between 15° and 30°C (59° and 86°F) in a dry place. Protect from light. Replace cap securely after each opening.

Shown in Product Identification Section, page 410

Table II

	Mean Daily Doses of Antacid	
	Ulcer Healed	Ulcer Not Healed
Oral ZANTAC	0.06	0.71
Oral Placebo	0.71	1.43

ZINACEF® ℞

[zin'ah-sef]

(sterile cefuroxime sodium)

DESCRIPTION

ZINACEF® (sterile cefuroxime sodium, Glaxo) is a semisynthetic, broad-spectrum cephalosporin antibiotic for parenteral administration. It is the sodium salt of (6R, 7R)-3-carbamoyloxymethyl-7-[Z-2-methoxyimino-2-(fur-2-yl) acetamido]ceph-3-em-4-carboxylate. ZINACEF contains approximately 54.2 mg (2.4 mEq) of sodium per gram of cefuroxime activity. Solutions of ZINACEF range from light yellow to amber, depending on the concentration and diluent used. The pH of freshly constituted solutions usually ranges from 6 to 8.5.

Structural Formula:

CLINICAL PHARMACOLOGY

After intramuscular injection of a 750-mg dose of cefuroxime to normal volunteers, the mean peak serum concentration was 27 mcg/ml. The peak occurred at approximately 45 minutes (range, 15 to 60 minutes). Following intravenous doses of 750 mg and 1.5 g, serum concentrations were approximately 50 and 100 mcg/ml, respectively, at 15 minutes. Therapeutic serum concentrations of approximately 2 mcg/ml or more were maintained for 5.3 hours and 8 hours or more, respectively. There was no evidence of accumulation of cefuroxime in the serum following intravenous administration of 1.5-g doses every eight hours to normal volunteers. The serum half-life after either intramuscular or intravenous injections is approximately 80 minutes.

Approximately 89% of a dose of cefuroxime is excreted by the kidneys over an eight-hour period, resulting in high urinary concentrations.

Following the intramuscular administration of a 750-mg single dose, urinary concentrations averaged 1,300 mcg/ml during the first eight hours. Intravenous doses of 750 mg and 1.5 g produced urinary levels averaging 1,150 and 2,500 mcg/ml, respectively, during the first eight-hour period.

Continued on next page

Glaxo—Cont.

The concomitant oral administration of probenecid with cefuroxime slows tubular secretion, decreases renal clearance by approximately 40%, increases the peak serum level by approximately 30%, and increases the serum half-life by approximately 30%. ZINACEF® is detectable in therapeutic concentrations in pleural fluid, joint fluid, bile, sputum, bone, cerebrospinal fluid (in patients with meningitis), and aqueous humor.

Cefuroxime is approximately 50% bound to serum protein.

Microbiology: Cefuroxime has in vitro activity against a wide range of gram-positive and gram-negative organisms, and it is highly stable in the presence of beta-lactamases of certain gram-negative bacteria. The bactericidal action of cefuroxime results from inhibition of cell-wall synthesis. Cefuroxime is usually active against the following organisms in vitro.

Aerobes, Gram-Negative: *Haemophilus influenzae* (including ampicillin-resistant strains); *Haemophilus parainfluenzae; Neisseria gonorrhoeae* (including penicillinase- and non-penicillinase-producing strains); *Neisseria meningitidis; Escherichia coli; Klebsiella* sp (including *Klebsiella pneumoniae*); *Enterobacter* sp; *Citrobacter* sp; *Salmonella* sp; *Shigella* sp; *Proteus mirabilis; Proteus inconstans* (formerly *Providencia*); *Providencia rettgeri* (formerly *Proteus rettgeri*); *Morganella morganii* (formerly *Proteus morganii*).

Some strains of *M morganii, Enterobacter cloacae* and *Citrobacter* sp have been shown by in vitro tests to be resistant to cefuroxime and other cephalosporins.

Aerobes, Gram-Positive: *Staphylococcus aureus* (including penicillinase- and non-penicillinase-producing strains); *Staphylococcus epidermidis; Streptococcus pyogenes* (and other streptococci); and *Streptococcus pneumoniae* (formerly *Diplococcus pneumoniae*).

Certain strains of enterococci, eg, *Streptococcus faecalis,* are resistant.

Anaerobes: Gram-positive and gram-negative cocci (including *Peptococcus* and *Peptostreptococcus* sp); gram-positive bacilli (including *Clostridium* sp); gram-negative bacilli (including *Bacteroides* and *Fusobacterium* sp). Most strains of *Bacteroides fragilis* are resistant.

Pseudomonas and *Campylobacter* sp, *Acinetobacter calcoaceticus* (formerly *Mima* and *Herellea* sp) and most strains of *Serratia* and *Proteus vulgaris* are resistant to cephalosporins. Methicillin-resistant staphylococci, *Clostridium difficile,* and *Listeria monocytogenes* are resistant to cefuroxime.

Susceptibility Tests: ***Diffusion Techniques:*** Quantitative methods that require measurement of zone diameters give an estimate of antibiotic susceptibility. One such procedure[1–3] has been recommended for use with disks to test susceptibility to cefuroxime. Interpretation involves correlation of the diameters obtained in the disk test with minimum inhibitory concentration (MIC) values for cefuroxime.

Reports from the laboratory giving results of the standard single-disk susceptibility test using a 30-mcg cefuroxime disk should be interpreted according to the following criteria:

Susceptible organisms produce zone sizes of 18 mm or greater, indicating that the test organism is likely to respond to therapy.

Organisms that produce zones of 15 to 17 mm are expected to be susceptible if high dosage is used or if the infection is confined to tissues and fluids (eg, urine) in which high antibiotic levels are attained.

Resistant organisms produce zones of 14 mm or less, indicating that other therapy should be selected.

For gram-positive isolates, the test can be performed with either the cephalosporin-class disk (30 mcg of cephalothin) or the cefuroxime disk (30 mcg of cefuroxime), and a zone of 18 mm or greater indicates a cefuroxime-susceptible organism.

Gram-negative organisms should be tested with the cefuroxime disk (using the above criteria), since cefuroxime has been shown by in vitro tests to have activity against certain strains of enterobacteriaceae found resistant when tested with the cephalosporin-class disk. Gram-negative organisms having zones of less than 18 mm around the cephalothin disk are not necessarily of intermediate susceptibility or resistant to cefuroxime.

The cefuroxime disk should not be used for testing susceptibility to other cephalosporins.

Standardized procedures require the use of laboratory control organisms. The 30-mcg cefuroxime disk should give zone diameters between 27 and 35 mm for *S aureus* ATCC 25923. For *E coli* ATCC 25922, the zone diameters should be between 20 and 26 mm.

Dilution Techniques: A bacterial isolate may be considered susceptible if the MIC value for cefuroxime is not more than 16 mcg/ml. Organisms are considered resistant if the MIC is greater than 32 mcg/ml.

As with standard diffusion methods, dilution procedures require the use of laboratory control organisms. Standard cefuroxime powder should give MIC values in the range of 0.5 and 2 mcg/ml for *S aureus* ATCC 25923. For *E coli* ATCC 25922, the MIC range should be between 2 and 8 mcg/ml.

INDICATIONS AND USAGE

ZINACEF® is indicated for the treatment of patients with infections caused by susceptible strains of the designated microorganisms in the following diseases:

1. **Lower Respiratory Tract Infections,** including pneumonia caused by *S pneumoniae* (formerly *D pneumoniae*), *H influenzae* (including ampicillin-resistant strains), *Klebsiella* sp, *S aureus* (penicillinase- and non-penicillinase-producing), *S pyogenes,* and *E coli.*
2. **Urinary Tract Infections** caused by *E coli* and *Klebsiella* sp.
3. **Skin and Skin Structure Infections** caused by *S aureus* (penicillinase- and non-penicillinase-producing), *S pyogenes, E coli, Klebsiella* sp, and *Enterobacter* sp.
4. **Septicemia** caused by *S aureus* (penicillinase- and non-penicillinase-producing), *S pneumoniae, E coli, H influenzae* (including ampicillin-resistant strains), and *Klebsiella* sp.
5. **Meningitis** caused by *S pneumoniae, H influenzae* (including ampicillin-resistant strains), *N meningitidis,* and *S aureus* (penicillinase- and non-penicillinase-producing).
6. **Gonorrhea:** Uncomplicated and disseminated gonococcal infections due to *N gonorrhoeae* (penicillinase- and non-penicillinase-producing strains) in both males and females.
7. **Bone and Joint Infections** caused by *S aureus* (including penicillinase- and non-penicillinase-producing strains).

Clinical microbiological studies in skin and skin structure infections frequently reveal the growth of susceptible strains of both aerobic and anaerobic organisms. ZINACEF (sterile cefuroxime sodium, Glaxo) has been used successfully in these mixed infections in which several organisms have been isolated. Appropriate cultures and susceptibility studies should be performed to determine the susceptibility of the causative organisms to ZINACEF.

Therapy may be started while awaiting the results of these studies; however, once these results become available, the antibiotic treatment should be adjusted accordingly. In certain cases of confirmed or suspected gram-positive or gram-negative sepsis or in patients with other serious infections in which the causative organism has not been identified, ZINACEF may be used concomitantly with an aminoglycoside (see **Precautions).** The recommended doses of both antibiotics may be given depending on the severity of the infection and the patient's condition.

Prevention: The preoperative prophylactic administration of ZINACEF may prevent the growth of susceptible disease-causing bacteria and thereby may reduce the incidence of certain postoperative infections in patients undergoing surgical procedures (eg, vaginal hysterectomy) that are classified as clean-contaminated or potentially contaminated procedures. Effective prophylactic use of antibiotics in surgery depends on the time of administration. ZINACEF should usually be given one-half to one hour before the operation to allow sufficient time to achieve effective antibiotic concentrations in the wound tissues during the procedure. The dose should be repeated intraoperatively if the surgical procedure is lengthy.

Prophylactic administration is usually not required after the surgical procedure ends and should be stopped within 24 hours. In the majority of surgical procedures, continuing prophylactic administration of any antibiotic does not reduce the incidence of subsequent infections but will increase the possibility of adverse reactions and the development of bacterial resistance.

The perioperative use of ZINACEF has also been effective during open heart surgery for surgical patients in whom infections at the operative site would present a serious risk. For these patients it is recommended that ZINACEF therapy be continued for at least 48 hours after the surgical procedure ends. If an infection is present, specimens for culture should be obtained for the identification of the causative organism and appropriate antimicrobial therapy should be instituted.

CONTRAINDICATIONS

ZINACEF® is contraindicated in patients with known allergy to the cephalosporin group of antibiotics.

WARNINGS

BEFORE THERAPY WITH ZINACEF® IS INSTITUTED, CAREFUL INQUIRY SHOULD BE MADE TO DETERMINE WHETHER THE PATIENT HAS HAD PREVIOUS HYPERSENSITIVITY REACTIONS TO CEPHALOSPORINS, PENICILLINS, OR OTHER DRUGS. THIS PRODUCT SHOULD BE GIVEN CAUTIOUSLY TO PENICILLIN-SENSITIVE PATIENTS. ANTIBIOTICS SHOULD BE ADMINISTERED WITH CAUTION TO ANY PATIENT WHO HAS DEMONSTRATED SOME FORM OF ALLERGY, PARTICULARLY TO DRUGS. IF AN ALLERGIC REACTION TO ZINACEF OCCURS, DISCONTINUE THE DRUG. SERIOUS ACUTE HYPERSENSITIVITY REACTIONS MAY REQUIRE EPINEPHRINE AND OTHER EMERGENCY MEASURES.

Pseudomembranous colitis has been reported with the use of cephalosporins (and other broad-spectrum antibiotics); therefore, it is important to consider its diagnosis in patients who develop diarrhea in association with antibiotic use.

Treatment with broad-spectrum antibiotics alters normal flora of the colon and may permit overgrowth of clostridia. Studies indicate a toxin produced by *C difficile* is one primary cause of antibiotic-associated colitis. Cholestyramine and colestipol resins have been shown to bind the toxin in vitro.

Mild cases of colitis may respond to drug discontinuance alone. Moderate to severe cases should be managed with fluid, electrolyte, and protein supplementation as indicated.

When the colitis is not relieved by drug discontinuance or when it is severe, oral vancomycin is the treatment of choice for antibiotic-associated pseudomembranous colitis produced by *C difficile.* Other causes of colitis should also be considered.

PRECAUTIONS

Although ZINACEF® rarely produces alterations in kidney function, evaluation of renal status during therapy is recommended, especially in seriously ill patients receiving the maximum doses. Cephalosporins should be given with caution to patients receiving concurrent treatment with potent diuretics as these regimens are suspected of adversely affecting renal function.

The total daily dose of ZINACEF should be reduced in patients with transient or persistent renal insufficiency (see **DOSAGE AND ADMINISTRATION**), because high and prolonged serum antibiotic concentrations can occur in such individuals from usual doses.

As with other antibiotics, prolonged use of ZINACEF may result in overgrowth of nonsusceptible organisms. Careful observation of the patient is essential. If superinfection occurs during therapy, appropriate measures should be taken.

Broad-spectrum antibiotics should be prescribed with caution in individuals with a history of gastrointestinal disease, particularly colitis.

Nephrotoxicity has been reported following concomitant administration of aminoglycoside antibiotics and cephalosporins.

Interference with Laboratory Tests: A false-positive reaction for glucose in the urine may occur with copper reduction tests (Benedict's or Fehling's solution or with Clinitest® tablets), but not with enzyme-based tests for glycosuria (eg, Tes-Tape®). As a false-negative result may occur in the ferricyanide test, it is recommended that either the glucose oxidase or hexokinase method be used to determine blood plasma glucose levels in patients receiving ZINACEF.

Cefuroxime does not interfere with the assay of serum and urine creatinine by the alkaline picrate method.

Carcinogenesis, Mutagenesis, Impairment of Fertility: Although no long-term studies in animals have been performed to evaluate carcinogenic potential, no mutagenic potential of cefuroxime was found in standard laboratory tests.

Reproductive studies revealed no impairment of fertility in animals.

Pregnancy: ***Teratogenic Effects: Pregnancy Category B:*** Reproduction studies have been performed in mice and rabbits at doses up to 60 times the human dose and have revealed no evidence of impaired fertility or harm to the fetus due to cefuroxime. There are, however, no adequate and well-controlled studies in pregnant women. Because animal reproduction studies are not always predictive of human response, this drug should be used during pregnancy only if clearly needed.

Nursing Mothers: Since ZINACEF is excreted in human milk, caution should be exercised when ZINACEF is administered to a nursing woman.

Pediatric Use: Safety and effectiveness in children below 3 months of age have not been established. Accumulation of other members of the cephalosporin class in newborn infants (with resulting prolongation of drug half-life) has been reported.

ADVERSE REACTIONS

ZINACEF® is generally well tolerated. The most common adverse effects have been local reactions following intravenous administration. Other adverse reactions have been encountered only rarely.

Local Reactions: Thrombophlebitis has occurred with intravenous administration in 1 in 60 patients.

Gastrointestinal: Gastrointestinal symptoms occurred in 1 in 150 patients and included diarrhea (1 in 220 patients) and nausea (1 in 440 patients). Symptoms of pseudomembranous colitis can appear during or after antibiotic treatment.

Hypersensitivity Reactions: Hypersensitivity reactions have been reported in less than 1% of the patients treated with ZINACEF and include rash (1 in 125). Pruritus, urticaria, and positive Coombs' test each occurred in less than 1 in 250 patients.

Blood: A decrease in hemoglobin and hematocrit has been observed in 1 in 10 patients and transient eosinophilia in 1 in 14 patients. Less common reactions seen were transient neutropenia (less than 1 in 100 patients) and leukopenia (1 in 750 patients). A similar pattern and incidence was seen with other cephalosporins used in controlled studies.

Hepatic: Transient rise in SGOT and SGPT (1 in 25 patients), alkaline phosphatase (1 in 50 patients), LDH (1 in 75 patients), and bilirubin (1 in 500 patients) levels has been noted.

Kidney: Elevations in serum creatinine and/or blood urea nitrogen and a decreased creatinine clearance have been observed, but their relationship to cefuroxime is unknown.

DOSAGE AND ADMINISTRATION

Dosage: ***Adults:*** The usual adult dosage range for ZINACEF® is 750 mg to 1.5 g every eight hours, usually for five to ten days. In uncomplicated urinary tract infections, skin and skin structure infections, disseminated gonococcal infections, and uncomplicated pneumonia, a 750-mg dose every eight hours is recommended. In severe or complicated infections, a 1.5-g dose every eight hours is recommended.
In bone and joint infections, a 1.5-g dose every eight hours is recommended. In clinical trials, surgical intervention was performed when indicated as an adjunct to ZINACEF therapy. A course of oral antibiotics was administered when appropriate following the completion of parenteral administration of ZINACEF.
In life-threatening infections or infections due to less susceptible organisms, 1.5 g every six hours may be required. In bacterial meningitis, the dose should not exceed 3 g every eight hours. The recommended dose for uncomplicated gonococcal infection is 1.5 g given intramuscularly as a single dose at two different sites together with 1 g of oral probenecid. For preventive use for clean-contaminated or potentially contaminated surgical procedures, a 1.5-g dose administered intravenously just prior to surgery (approximately one-half to one hour before the initial incision) is recommended. Thereafter, give 750 mg intravenously or intramuscularly every eight hours when the procedure is prolonged.
For preventive use during open heart surgery, a 1.5-g dose administered intravenously at the induction of anesthesia and every 12 hours thereafter for a total of 6 g is recommended.

Impaired Renal Function: A reduced dosage must be employed when renal function is impaired. Dosage should be determined by the degree of renal impairment and the susceptibility of the causative organism (see **Table 1**).

Table 1: Dosage of ZINACEF in Adults with Reduced Renal Function

Creatinine Clearance (ml/min)	Dose	Frequency
>20	750 mg–1.5 g	q8h
10–20	750 mg	q12h
<10	750 mg	q24h*

* Since ZINACEF is dialyzable, patients on hemodialysis should be given a further dose at the end of the dialysis.

When only serum creatinine is available, the following formula[4] (based on sex, weight, and age of the patient) may be used to convert this value into creatinine clearance. The serum creatinine should represent a steady state of renal function.

Males: $\frac{\text{Weight (kg)} \times (140\text{—age})}{72 \times \text{serum creatinine (mg/dl)}}$

Females: 0.85 × above value

Note: As with antibiotic therapy in general, administration of ZINACEF should be continued for a minimum of 48 to 72 hours after the patient becomes asymptomatic or after evidence of bacterial eradication has been obtained; a minimum of ten days of treatment is recommended in infections caused by *S pyogenes* in order to guard against the risk of rheumatic fever or glomerulonephritis; frequent bacteriologic and clinical appraisal is necessary during therapy of chronic urinary tract infection and may be required for several months after therapy has been completed; persistent infections may require treatment for several weeks; and doses smaller than those indicated above should not be used. In staphylococcal and other infections involving a collection of pus, surgical drainage should be carried out where indicated.

Infants and Children Above 3 Months of Age: Administration of 50 to 100 mg/kg/day in equally divided doses, every six to eight hours, has been successful for most infections susceptible to cefuroxime. The higher dose of 100 mg/kg/day (not to exceed the maximum adult dose) should be used for the more severe or serious infections.
In bone and joint infections, 150 mg/kg/day (not to exceed the maximum adult dose) is recommended in equally divided doses every eight hours. In clinical trials a course of oral antibiotics was administered to children following the completion of parenteral administration of ZINACEF.
In cases of bacterial meningitis, larger doses of ZINACEF are recommended, 200 to 240 mg/kg/day intravenously in divided doses every six to eight hours.

Table 2: Preparation of Solution and Suspension

Strength	Amount of Diluent to be Added (ml)	Volume to be Withdrawn	Approximate Cefuroxime Concentration (mg/ml)
750-mg Vial	3.0 (IM)	Total*	220.0
750-mg Vial	8.0 (IV)	Total	90.0
1.5-g Vial	16.0 (IV)	Total	90.0
750-mg Infusion Pack	100.0 (IV)	—	7.5
1.5-g Infusion Pack	100.0 (IV)	—	15.0
7.5-g Pharmacy Bulk Package	77.0 (IV)	Amount needed+	95.0

***Note:** ZINACEF is a suspension at IM concentrations.
+8 ml of solution contains 750 mg of cefuroxime; 16 ml of solution contains 1.5 g of cefuroxime.

In children with renal insufficiency, the frequency of dosage should be modified consistent with the recommendations for adults.

Preparation of Solution and Suspension: The directions for preparing ZINACEF for both intravenous and intramuscular use are summarized in **Table 2.**

For Intramuscular Use: Each 750-mg vial of ZINACEF should be constituted with 3 ml of Sterile Water for Injection. Shake gently to disperse and withdraw completely the resulting suspension for injection.

For Intravenous Use: Each 750-mg vial should be constituted with 8 ml of Sterile Water for Injection. Withdraw completely the resulting solution for injection.
Each 1.5-g vial should be constituted with 16 ml of Sterile Water for Injection and the solution should be completely withdrawn for injection.
The 7.5-g Pharmacy Bulk vial should be constituted with 77 ml of Sterile Water for Injection; each 8 ml of the resulting solution contains 750 mg of cefuroxime.
Each 750-mg and 1.5-g infusion pack should be constituted with 100 ml of Sterile Water for Injection, 5% Dextrose Injection, 0.9% Sodium Chloride Injection, or any of the solutions listed under the **Intravenous** portion of the **COMPATIBILITY AND STABILITY** SECTION.
[See table above].

Administration: After constitution, ZINACEF may be given intravenously or by deep intramuscular injection into a large muscle mass (such as the gluteus or lateral part of the thigh). Prior to injecting intramuscularly, aspiration is necessary to avoid inadvertent injection into a blood vessel.

Intravenous Administration: The intravenous route may be preferable for patients with bacterial septicemia or other severe or life-threatening infections or for patients who may be poor risks because of lowered resistance, particularly if shock is present or impending.

For direct intermittent intravenous administration, slowly inject the solution into a vein over a period of three to five minutes or give it through the tubing system by which the patient is also receiving other intravenous solutions.

For intermittent intravenous infusion with a Y-type administration set, dosing can be accomplished through the tubing system by which the patient may be receiving other intravenous solutions. However, during infusion of the solution containing ZINACEF, it is advisable to temporarily discontinue administration of any other solutions at the same site.

For continuous intravenous infusion, a solution of ZINACEF may be added to an intravenous bottle containing one of the following fluids: 0.9% Sodium Chloride Injection; 5% Dextrose Injection; 10% Dextrose Injection; 5% Dextrose and 0.9% Sodium Chloride Injection; 5% Dextrose and 0.45% Sodium Chloride Injection; or M/6 Sodium Lactate Injection.
Solutions of ZINACEF, like those of most beta-lactam antibiotics, should not be added to solutions of aminoglycoside antibiotics because of potential interaction.
However, if concurrent therapy with ZINACEF and an aminoglycoside is indicated, each of these antibiotics can be administered separately to the same patient.

COMPATIBILITY AND STABILITY

Intramuscular: When constituted as directed with Sterile Water for Injection, suspensions of ZINACEF® for intramuscular injection maintain satisfactory potency for 24 hours at room temperature and for 48 hours under refrigeration (5°C).
After the periods mentioned above any unused suspensions should be discarded.

Intravenous: When the 750-mg, 1.5-g, and 7.5-g Pharmacy Bulk vials are constituted as directed with Sterile Water for Injection, the ZINACEF solutions for intravenous administration maintain satisfactory potency for 24 hours at room temperature and for 48 hours under refrigeration (5°C). More dilute solutions, such as 750 mg or 1.5 g plus 100 ml of Sterile Water for Injection, 5% Dextrose Injection, or 0.9% Sodium Chloride Injection, maintain satisfactory potency for 24 hours at room temperature and for seven days under refrigeration.
These solutions may be further diluted to concentrations of between 1 and 30 mg/ml in the following solutions and will lose not more than 10% activity for 24 hours at room temperature or for at least seven days under refrigeration: 0.9% Sodium Chloride Injection; M/6 Sodium Lactate Injection; Ringer's Injection, USP; Lactated Ringer's Injection, USP; 5% Dextrose and 0.9% Sodium Chloride Injection; 5% Dextrose Injection; 5% Dextrose and 0.45% Sodium Chloride Injection; 5% Dextrose and 0.225% Sodium Chloride Injection; 10% Dextrose Injection; and 10% Invert Sugar in Water for Injection.
Unused solutions should be discarded after the time periods mentioned above.
ZINACEF has also been found compatible for 24 hours at room temperature when admixed in intravenous infusion with Heparin (10 and 50 U/ml) in 0.9% Sodium Chloride Injection and Potassium Chloride (10 and 40 mEq/L) in 0.9% Sodium Chloride Injection.

Frozen Stability: Constitute the 750-mg or 1.5-g vial as directed for IV administration in **Table 2.** Immediately withdraw the total contents and add to a Travenol Viaflex® Mini-bag™ containing 50 or 100 ml of 0.9% Sodium Chloride Injection or 5% Dextrose Injection and freeze. Frozen solutions are stable for six months when stored at −20°C. Frozen solutions should be thawed at room temperature and not refrozen. Thawed solutions may be stored for 24 hours at room temperature or seven days in a refrigerator.

Note: Parenteral drug products should be inspected visually for particulate matter and discoloration prior to administration whenever solution and container permit.
As with other cephalosporins, however, ZINACEF powder as well as solutions and suspensions tend to darken, depending on storage conditions, without adversely affecting product potency.

HOW SUPPLIED

ZINACEF® is a dry, white to off-white powder supplied in vials and infusion bottles.
Each vial contains cefuroxime sodium equivalent to 750 mg or 1.5 g of cefuroxime. ZINACEF in the dry state should be stored at controlled room temperature, 15° to 30° C (59° to 86°F), and protected from light.
NDC 0173-0352-30 750-mg Vials (10 singles)
NDC 0173-0352-31 750-mg Vials (Tray of 25)
NDC 0173-0354-34 1.5-g Vials (10 singles)
NDC 0173-0354-35 1.5-g Vials (Tray of 25)
NDC 0173-0353-32 750-mg Infusion Pack (Tray of 10)
NDC 0173-0356-32 1.5-g Infusion Pack (Tray of 10)
NDC 0173-0400-00 7.5-g Pharmacy Bulk Package (Tray of 6)

REFERENCES

1. Bauer AW, Kirby WMM, Sherris JC, et al: Antibiotic susceptibility testing by a standardized single disc method. *Am J Clin Pathol* 1966;45:493.
2. National Committee for Clinical Laboratory Standards, Approved Standard: Performance Standards for Antimicrobial Disc Susceptibility Tests (M2-A3), December, 1984.
3. Standardized disc susceptibility test. *Federal Register* 1974;39(May 30):19182–19184.
4. Cockcroft DW, Gault MH: Prediction of creatinine clearance from serum creatinine. *Nephron* 1976;16:31–41.

Shown in Product Identification Section, page 410

EDUCATIONAL MATERIAL

Booklets:
"Living With Hypertension"—A patient oriented booklet explains hypertension and is designed to enhance compliance. Free to physicians and pharmacists.
Samples:
Trandate® samples available upon request.

Glenbrook Laboratories
Division of Sterling Drug Inc.
90 PARK AVENUE
NEW YORK, NY 10016

BAYER® CHILDREN'S CHEWABLE ASPIRIN
Aspirin (Acetylsalicylic Acid)

COMPOSITION
Bayer Children's Chewable Aspirin-Aspirin 1¼ grains (81 mg) per orange flavored chewable tablet.

ACTIONS AND USES
Analgesic, antipyretic, anti-inflammatory. For relief of headache: painful discomfort and fever of colds, sore throats; muscular aches and pains; temporary relief of minor pains of arthritis, rheumatism, bursitis, lumbago, sciatica; toothache, teething pains, and pain following dental procedures; neuralgia and neuritic pain; functional menstrual pain; sleeplessness when caused by minor painful discomforts; painful discomfort and fever accompanying immunizations.

WARNINGS
Children and teenagers should not use this medicine for chicken pox or flu symptoms before a doctor is consulted about Reye Syndrome, a rare but serious illness. Keep this and all drugs out of the reach of children. In case of accidental overdose, seek professional assistance or contact a poison control center immediately. As with any drug, if you are pregnant or nursing a baby, seek the advice of a health professional before using this product.

ADMINISTRATION AND DOSAGE
The following dosages are those provided in the packaging, as appropriate for self-medication.
Children's Dose: To be administered only under adult supervision. For children under 3 consult physician.

Age (Years)	Weight (Lbs.)	Dosage
Under 3 consult a physician		
3 up to 4	32 to 35	2 tablets
4 up to 6	36 to 45	3 tablets
6 up to 9	46 to 65	4 tablets
9 up to 11	66 to 76	5 tablets
11 up to 12	77 to 83	6 tablets
12 and over	84 and over	8 tablets

indicated dosage may be repeated every four hours up to but not more than five times a day. Larger dosage may be prescribed by a physician.
Ways to Administer: CHEW then follow with a half glass of water, milk or fruit juice.
SWALLOW WHOLE with a half a glass of water, milk or fruit juice.
DISSOLVE ON TONGUE follow with a half a glass of water, milk or fruit juice.
DISSOLVE TABLET in a little water, milk or fruit juice and drink the solution.
CRUSHED in a teaspoonful of water—followed with part of a glass of water.
HOW SUPPLIED: Bayer Children's Chewable Aspirin 1¼ grains (81 mg)—
NDC 12843-131-05, bottle of 36 tablets with child resistant safety closure.
Samples available on request.
Shown in Product Identification Section, page 410

GENUINE BAYER® ASPIRIN
Aspirin (Acetylsalicylic Acid)

COMPOSITION
Bayer-Aspirin—Aspirin 5 grains (325 mg) contains a thin, inert, methyl-cellulose coating for easier swallowing. This is not an enteric coating and does not alter the onset of action of Genuine Bayer Aspirin.

ACTIONS AND USES
Analgesic, antipyretic, anti-inflammatory, antiplatelet. For relief of headache; painful discomfort and fever of colds and flu; sore throats; muscular aches and pains; temporary relief of minor pains of arthritis, rheumatism, bursitis, lumbago, sciatica; toothache, teething pains, and pain following dental procedures; neuralgia and neuritic pain; functional menstrual pain; sleeplessness when caused by minor painful discomfort; paintful discomfort and fever accompanying immunizations.

CAUTION
If pain persists for more than 10 days, or redness is present, or in conditions affecting children under 12 years of age, consult a physician immediately.

WARNINGS
Children and teenagers should not use this medicine for chicken pox or flu symptoms before a doctor is consulted about Reye Syndrome, a rare but serious illness. Keep this and all drugs out of the reach of children. In case of accidental overdose, seek professional assistance or contact a poison control center immediately. As with any drug, if you are pregnant or nursing a baby, seek the advice of a health professional before using this product.

ADMINISTRATION AND DOSAGE
The following dosages are those provided in the packaging, as appropriate for self-medication. Larger or more frequent dosage may be necessary as appropriate to the condition or needs of the patient.
The methyl-cellulose coating makes Genuine Bayer Aspirin particularly appropriate for those who must take frequent doses of aspirin and for those who have difficulty in swallowing uncoated tabelts.
Genuine Bayer Aspirin-5 grain (325 mg) tablets.
Usual Adult Dose: One or two tablets with water. May be repeated every four hours as necessary up to 12 tablets a day.
For Antiplatelet Use:
In recurrent TIA's
Larger dosage may be prescribed per physician.

INDICATION
There is evidence that aspirin is safe and effective for reducing the risk of stroke in those males with recurrent transient ischemic attacks.
There is no evidence that aspirin is effective in reducing CUA's in women, or is of benefit after CUA has occurred. Patients presenting with signs and symptoms of TIA's should have a complete medical and neurologic evaluation. Consideration should be given to other disorders which resemble TIA's.
It is important to evaluate and treat, if appropriate, other diseases associated with TIA's and stroke, such as hypertension and diabetes.
DOSAGE: The recommended dosage for this new indication is 1,300 mg/day (650 mg twice/day or 325 mg four times a day).

PRECAUTIONS
A complete medical and neurologic evaluation should be performed on the male patient with recurrent TIA prior to instituting antiplatelet therapy with aspirin. The differential diagnosis should include consideration of disorders that resemble TIA's. An assessment of the presence and need for treatment of other diseases associated with TIA's or stroke, such as diabetes and hypertension, should be made.

IN MI PROPHYLAXIS

INDICATION
Aspirin is indicated to reduce the risk of death and/or nonfatal myocardial infarction in patients with a previous infarction or unstable angina pectoris.

CLINICAL TRIALS
The indication is supported by the results of six, large, randomized multicenter, placebo-controlled studies[1–7] involving 10.816, predominantly male, post-myocardial infarction (MI) patients and one randomized placebo-controlled study of 1.266 men with unstable angina. Therapy with aspirin was begun at intervals after the onset of acute MI varying from less than 3 days to more than 5 years and continued for periods from less than one year to four years. In the unstable angina study, treatment was started within 1 month after the onset of unstable angina and continued for 12 weeks and complicating conditions such as congestive heart failure were not included in the study.
Aspirin therapy in MI patients was associated with about a 20 percent reduction in the risk of subsequent death and or non-fatal reinfarction, a median absolute decrease of 3 percent from the 12 to 22 percent event rates in the placebo groups. In aspirin-treated unstable angina patients the reduction in risk was about 50 percent, a reduction in event rate of 5 percent from the 10 percent rate in the placebo group over the 12 weeks of the study.
Daily dosage of aspirin in the post-myocardial infarction studies was 300 mg in one study and 900—1500 mg in five studies. A dose of 325 mg was used in the study of unstable angina.

ADVERSE REACTIONS
Gastrointestinal reactions: Doses of 1000 mg per day of aspirin caused gastrointestinal symptoms and bleeding that in some cases were clinically significant in the largest post-infarction study (the Aspirin Myocardial Infarction Study (AMIS) trial with 4.500 people), the percentage incidences of gastrointestinal symptoms for the aspirin (1000 mg of a standard, solid-tablet formulation) and placebo-treated subjects, respectively, were stomach pain (14 3%, 4.4%); heartburn (11.9%, 4.3%); nausea and/or vomiting (7.3%, 2.1%) hospitalization for GI disorder (4.9%, 3.3%). In the AMIS and other trials, aspirin treated patients had increased rates of gross gastrointestinal bleeding. Symptoms and signs of gastrointestinal irritation were not significantly increased in subjects treated for unstable angina with buffered aspirin in solution.

CARDIOVASCULAR AND BIOCHEMICAL
In the AMIS trial, the dosage of 1000 mg per day of aspirin was associated with small increases in systolic blood pressure (BP) (average 1.5 to 2.1 mm) and diastolic BP (0.5 to 0.6 mm), depending upon whether maximal or last available readings were used. Blood urea nitrogen and uric acid levels were also increased, but by less than 1.0 mg%. Subjects with marked hypertension or renal insufficiency had been excluded from the trial so that the clinical importance of these observations for such periods or for any subjects treated over more prolonged periods is not known. It is recommended that patients placed on long-term aspirin treatment, even at doses of 300 mg per day, be seen at regular intervals to assess changes in these measurements.

SODIUM IN BUFFERED ASPIRIN FOR SOLUTION FORMULATIONS
One tablet daily of buffered aspirin in solution adds 553 mg of sodium to that in the diet and may not be tolerated by patients with active sodium-retaining states such as congestive heart or renal failure. This amount of sodium adds about 30 percent to the 70 to 90 meq intake suggested as appropriate for dietary treatment of essential hypertension in the 1984 Report of the Joint National Committee on Detection, Evaluation, and Treatment of High Blood Pressure.

DOSAGE AND ADMINISTRATION
Although most of the studies used dosages exceeding 300 mg, two trials used only 300 mg, daily and pharmacologic data indicate that this dose inhibits platelet function fully. Therefore, 300 mg or a conventional 325 mg aspirin dose, daily is a reasonable routine dose that would minimize gastrointestinal adverse reactions. This use of aspirin applies to both solid, oral dosage forms (buffered and plain aspirin) and buffered aspirin in solution.

HOW SUPPLIED
Genuine Bayer Aspirin 5 grains (325 mg)—
NDC 12843-101-10, packs of 12 tablets
NDC 12843-101-11, bottles of 24 tablets
NDC 12843-101-17, bottles of 50 tablets
NDC 12843-101-12, bottles of 100 tablets
NDC 12843-101-20, bottles of 200 tablets
NDC 12843-101-13, bottles of 300 tablets
Child resistant safety closures on 12's, 24's, 50's, 200's, 300's. Bottle of 100's available without safety closure for households without small children.
Samples available on request.
Shown in Product Identification Section, page 410

MAXIMUM BAYER® ASPIRIN
Aspirin (Acetylsalicylic Acid)

COMPOSITION
Maximum Bayer Aspirin — Aspirin 500 mg (7.7 grains) contains a thin, inert, methylcellulose coating for easier swallowing. This is not an enteric coating and does not alter the onset of action of Bayer Aspirin.

ACTIONS AND USES
Analgesic, antipyretic, anti-inflammatory. For relief of headache; painful discomfort and fever of colds and flu; sore throats; muscular aches and pains, temporary relief of minor pains of arthritis, rheumatism, bursitis, lumbago, sciatica, toothache, teething pains, and pain following dental prodecures; neuralgia and neurtic pain; functional menstrual pain; sleeplessness when caused by minor painful discomfors; painful discomfort and fever accompanying immunizations.

CAUTION
If pain persists for more than 10 days or redness is present, or in conditions affecting children under 12 years of age, consult a physician immediately.

WARNINGS
Children and teenagers should not use this medicine for chicken pox or flu symptons before a doctor is consulted about Reye Syndrome, a rare but serious illness. Keep this and all drugs out of the reach of children. In case of accidental overdose, seek professional assistance or conact a poison control center immediately. As with any drugs, if you are pregnant or nursing a baby, seek the advice of a health professional before using this product.

ADMINISTRATION AND DOSAGE
The following dosages are those provided on the packaging, as appropriate for self-medication. Larger or more frequent dosage may be necessary as appropriate to the condition or needs of the patient.
The methyl-cellulose coating makes Maximum Bayer Aspirin particularly appropriate for those who must take frequent doses of aspirin and for those who have difficulty in swallowing uncoated tablets.
Maximum Bayer Aspirin — 500 mg (7.7 grains) tablets.
Usual Adult Dose: One or two tablets with water. May be repeated every four hours as necessary up to 8 tablets a day.

HOW SUPPLIED
Maximum Bayer Aspirin 500 mg (7.7 grains)
NDC 12843-161-51 tube of 10 tablets
NDC-12843-161-53 bottles of 30 tablets

NDC-12483-161-56 bottles of 60 tablets
NDC-12843-161-58 bottles of 100 tablets
Child-resistant safety closures on 10's, 30's and 100's. Bottle of 60's available without safety closure for households without small children.
Samples available on request.

Shown in Product Identification Section, page 410

8 HOUR BAYER® TIMED-RELEASE ASPIRIN
(aspirin)

DESCRIPTION
Each oblong white scored tablet contains 10 grains (650 mg) of aspirin in microencapsulation form.

INDICATIONS
8 Hour Bayer Timed-Release Aspirin is indicated for the temporary relief of low grade pain amenable to relief with salicylates, such as in rheumatoid arthritis, osteoarthritis, spondylitis, bursitis and other forms of rheumatism, as well as in many common musculoskeletal disorders. It possesses the same advantages for other types of prolonged aches and pains, such as minor injuries, dental pain and dysmenorrhea. Its long-lasting effectiveness should also make it valuable as an analgesic in simple headache, colds, grippe, flu and other similar conditions in which aspirin is indicated for symptomatic relief, either by itself or as an adjunct to specific therapy.

CAUTION
If pain persists for more than 10 days, or redness is present, or in conditions affecting children under 12 years, consult a physician immediately.

WARNINGS
Children and teenagers should not use this medicine for chicken pox or flu symptoms before a doctor is consulted about Reye Syndrome, a rare but serious illness. Keep this and all drugs out of the reach of children. In case of accidental overdose, seek professional assistance or contact a poison control center immediately. As with any drug, if you are pregnant or nursing a baby, seek the advice of a health professional before using this product.

ADMINISTRATION AND DOSAGE
Two 8 Hour Bayer Timed-Release Aspirin tablets q. 8 h. provide effective long-lasting pain relief. This two-tablet (20 grain or 1300 mg) dose of timed-release aspirin promptly produces salicylate blood levels greater than those achieved by a 10-grain (650 mg) dose of regular aspirin, and in the second 4 hour period produces a salicylate blood level curve which approximates that of two successive 10-grain (650 mg) doses of regular aspirin at 4 hour intervals. The 10-grain (650 mg) scored 8 Hour Bayer Timed-Release Aspirin tablets permit administration of aspirin in multiples of 5 grains (325 mg) allowing individualization of dosage to meet the specific needs of the patient. For the convenience of patients on a regular aspirin dosage schedule, two 10-grain (650 mg) 8 Hour Bayer Timed-Release Aspirin tablets may be administered with water every 8 hours. Whenever necessary, two tablets (20 grains or 1300 mg) should be given before retiring to provide effective analgesic and anti-inflammatory action—for relief of pain throughout the night and lessening of stiffness upon arising. Do not exceed 6 tablets in 24 hours. 8 Hour Bayer Timed-Release Aspirin has been made in a special capsule-shaped tablet to permit easy swallowing. However, for patients who do have difficulty, 8 Hour Bayer Timed-Release Aspirin tablets may be gently crumbled in the mouth and swallowed with water without loss of timed-release effect. There is no bitter "aspirin" taste. For children under 12, per physician.

SIDE EFFECTS
Side effects encountered with regular aspirin may be encountered with 8 Hour Bayer Timed-Release Aspirin. Tinnitus and dizziness are the ones most frequently encountered.

CONTRAINDICATIONS AND PRECAUTIONS
8 Hour Bayer Timed-Release Aspirin is contraindicated in patients with marked aspirin hypersensitivity, and should be given with extreme caution to any patient with a history of adverse reaction to salicylates. It may cautiously be tried in patients intolerant to aspirin because of gastric irritation, but the usual precautions for any form of aspirin should be observed in patients with gastric ulcers, bleeding tendencies, asthma, or hypoprothrombinemia.

SUPPLIED

Tablets in Bottle of 30's	NDC-12843-191-72
Tablets in Bottle of 72's	NDC-12843-191-74
Tablets in Bottle of 125's	NDC-12843-191-76

All sizes packaged in child-resistant safety closure except 72's which is a size recommended for households without young children.
Samples available upon request.

Shown in Product Identification Section, page 410

MIDOL®
Original Formula

COMPOSITION
Each Caplet® contains Aspirin 454 mg (7 grains); Cinnamedrine Hydrochloride 14.9 mg; Caffeine 32.4 mg.

ACTION AND USES
Analgesic, antispasmodic. For fast relief of functional menstrual pain, pain of cramps, irritability; headache, aches from swelling, and the irritability associated with premenstrual tension; headache, and low backache associated with menstruation. Inhibits the body's production of prostaglandins, known to be a major cause of menstrual cramps.

WARNINGS
Children and teenagers should not use this medicine for chicken pox or flu symptoms before a doctor is consulted about Reye Syndrome, a rare but serious illness. Keep this and all drugs out of the reach of children. In case of accidental overdose, seek professional assistance or contact a poison control center immediately. As with any drug, if you are pregnant or nursing a baby, seek the advice of a health professional before using this product.

Usage Adult Dosage: Two Caplets with water. Repeat two Caplets every four hours as needed, up to eight Caplets per day.

HOW SUPPLIED
White, capsule-shaped Caplets.
NDC-12843-151-29, professional dispenser, 250 2-Caplet Packets
NDC-12843-151-02, sample size bottle of 6 Caplets
NDC-12843-151-34, bottle of 12 Caplets
NDC-12843-151-36, bottles of 30 Caplets
NDC-12843-151-38, bottles of 60 Caplets
Child-resistant safety closures on bottles of 60 Caplets.
Samples Supplied: Available upon request.

Shown in Product Identification Section, page 410

MAXIMUM STRENGTH MIDOL® PMS

COMPOSITION
Each capsule contains: Acetaminophen 500 mg; Pamabrom 25 mg; Pyrilamine Maleate 15 mg.

ACTION AND USES
Relieves the symptoms of Premenstrual Syndrome. For fast relief from premenstrual tension, irritability, bloating, water-weight gain, pain of cramps, backache and headache.

USUAL ADULT DOSAGE
Two capsules with water. Repeat two capsules every four hours as needed, up to eight capsules per day.

CAUTION
If drowsiness occurs, do not drive or operate machinery.

WARNINGS
Keep this and all drugs out of the reach of children. In case of accidental overdose, seek professional assistance or contact a poison control center immediately. As with any drug, if you are pregnant or nursing a baby, seek the advice of a health professional before using this product.

HOW SUPPLIED
Red and white capsules.
NDC 12843-153-42 bottles of 8 capsules
NDC 12843-153-43 bottles of 16 capsules
NDC 12843-153-44 bottles of 32 capsules
Samples Supplied: Available upon request.

Shown in Product Identification Section, page 410

MAXIMUM STRENGTH MIDOL® FOR PAIN OF CRAMPS

COMPOSITION
Each Caplet® Contains: Aspirin 500 mg, Cinnamedrine Hydrochloride 14.9 mg, Caffeine 32.4 mg.

ACTION AND USES
Analgesic, antispasmodic. For fast relief of pain of cramps, functional menstrual pain, headache, backache, leg aches, aches from swelling. Inhibits the body's production of prostaglandins, known to be a major cause of menstrual cramps.

WARNINGS
Children and teenagers should not use this medicine for chicken pox or flu symptoms before a doctor is consulted about Reye Syndrome, a rare but serious illness. Keep this and all drugs out of the reach of children. In case of accidental overdose, seek professional assistance or contact a poison control center immediately. As with any drug, if you are pregnant or nursing a baby, seek the advice of a health professional before using this product.

Usual Adult Dosage:
Two Caplets with water. Repeat two Caplets every four hours as needed, up to eight Caplets per day.

HOW SUPPLIED
White capsule shaped Caplets
NDC 12843-152-48 bottles of 8 Caplets
NDC 12843-152-49 bottles of 16 Caplets
NDC 12843-152-50 bottles of 32 Caplets
Samples Supplied: Available upon request.

Shown in Product Identification Section, page 410

CHILDREN'S PANADOL®
Acetaminophen Chewable Tablets, Liquid, Drops

DESCRIPTION
Each Children's PANADOL Chewable Tablet contains 80 mg acetaminophen in a fruit flavored sugar free tablet. Children's PANADOL Acetaminophen Liquid is fruit flavored, red in color, and is alcohol free and sugar free and aspirin-free. Each ½ teaspoon contains 80 mg of acetaminophen. Infant's PANADOL Drops are fruit flavored, red in color, and are alcohol free, sugar free and aspirin free. Each 0.8 ml (one calibrated dropper full) contains 80 mg acetaminophen.

ACTIONS AND INDICATIONS
Acetaminophen, the active ingredient in PANADOL, is the analgesic/ antipyretic most widely recommended by pediatricians for fast, effective relief of children's fevers. It also relieves the aches and pains of colds and flu, earaches, (otitis media) headaches, teething, immunizations, tonsillectomy, and childhood illnesses.
Children's PANADOL Tablets, Liquid, and Drops are aspirin free and contain no alcohol or sugar. The pleasant tasting formulations are not likely to upset or irritate children's stomachs.

USUAL DOSAGE
Dosing is based on single doses in the range of 10–15 mg/kg body weight. Doses may be repeated every four hours up to 4 or 5 times daily, but not to exceed 5 doses in 24 hours. The package labeling states that for children under 2 years to "consult a physician".
Children's PANADOL Chewable Tablets: Children under 2 yrs., under 24 lbs., contact a physician. 2–3 yrs., 24–35 lbs., 2 tablets; 4–5 yrs., 36–47 lbs., 3 tablets; 6–8 yrs., 48–59 lbs., 4 tablets; 9–10 yrs., 60–71 lbs., 5 tablets; 11–12 yrs., 72–95 lbs., 6 tablets. Dosage may be repeated every four hours, no more than 5 times in 24 hours.
Children's PANADOL Liquid: (a special 3 teaspoon cup for accurate measurement is provided) Under 2 yrs., under 24 lbs. consult a physician; 2–3 yrs., 24–35 lbs., 1 teaspoonful; 4–5 yrs., 36–47 lbs., 1½ teaspoonfuls; 6–8 yrs., 48–59 lbs., 2 teaspoonfuls; 9–10 yrs., 60–71 lbs., 2½ teaspoonfuls; 11–12 yrs., 72–95 lbs., 3 teaspoonfuls. Repeat every 4 hours up to 5 times in a 24 hour period. Children's PANADOL Liquid may be administered alone or mixed with formula, milk, juice, cereal, etc.
Infant's PANADOL Drops: Under 2 yrs., under 24 lbs., consult a physician; 2–3 yrs., 24–35 lbs., 2 dropperfuls (1.6 ml); 4–5 yrs., 36–47 lbs., 3 dropperfuls (2.4 ml); 6–8 yrs., 48–59 lbs., 4 dropperfuls (3.2 ml). May be repeated every 4 hours, up to 5 times in a 24 hour period.

WARNING
Since Children's PANADOL Acetaminophen Chewable Tablets, Liquid, and Drops are available without a prescription as an analgesic/ antipyretic, the following appears on the package labels: "WARNING: Do not take this product for more than 5 days. If symptoms persist or new ones occur, consult a physician. If fever persists for more than 3 days, or recurs, consult a physician. Keep this and all drugs out of the reach of children. In case of accidental overdose, seek professional assistance or contact a poison control center immediately. High fever, severe or persistent sore throat, headache, nausea, or vomiting may be serious; consult a physician."
Tamper Resistant: Children's PANADOL Acetaminophen Chewable Tablets packaging provides tamper resistant features on both the outer carton and bottle. The following copy appears on the end flaps of this carton—"Purchase only if carton end flaps are sealed." The following copy appears on the bottle—"Use only if printed seal under cap is intact." Children's PANADOL Liquid and Drops provide tamper resistant features on the bottle—"Purchase only if carton overwrap and red tear tape are intact."

HOW SUPPLIED
Chewable Tablets (colored pink and scored)—bottles of 30. Liquid (colored red)— bottles of 2 fl. oz. and 4 fl. oz. Drops (colored red)— bottles of ½ oz. (15 ml).
All packages listed above have child resistant safety caps and tamper resistant features.

Shown in Product Identification Section, page 410

Continued on next page

Glenbrook—Cont.

MAXIMUM STRENGTH
PANADOL®
Tablets, Capsules and Caplets

DESCRIPTION
Each Maximum Strength PANADOL micro-thin coated Tablet, Caplet and sonically-sealed Capsule contains acetaminophen 500 mg.

ACTIONS
PANADOL acetaminophen has been clinically proven as a fast, effective analgesic (pain reliever) and antipyretic (fever reducer). PANADOL acetaminophen is a non-aspirin product designed to provide relief without stomach upset. Its patented micro-thin coating makes each 500 mg. tablet or caplet easy to swallow.

INDICATIONS
For the temporary relief from pain of headaches, colds or flu, sinusitis, backaches, muscle aches, and menstrual discomfort. Also to reduce fever and for temporary relief of minor arthritis pain and headache.

PRECAUTIONS
If a rare sensitivity reaction occurs, the drug should be stopped. PANADOL acetaminophen has rarely been found to produce any side effects. It is usually well tolerated by aspirin sensitive patients.
Severe recurrent pain or high continued fever may indicate a serious condition. Under these circumstances consult a physician.

WARNING
As with other products available without prescription, the following appears on the label of PANADOL acetaminophen: "Do not give to children under 12 or use for more than 10 days unless directed by a physician. Keep this and all drugs out of the reach of children. In case of accidental overdose, seek professional assistance or contact a poison control center immediately. As with any drug, if you are pregnant or nursing a baby, seek the advice of a health professional before using this product.

USUAL DOSAGE
Adults: Two tablets or capsules every 4 hours as needed. Do not exceed 8 tablets or capsules in 24 hours.

OVERDOSAGE
In massive overdosage acetaminophen may cause hepatic toxicity in some patients. Clinical and laboratory evidence of overdosage may be delayed up to 7 days. Under circumstances of suspected overdose, contact your regional poison control center immediately.

HOW SUPPLIED
Tablets and Caplets (white, micro-thin coated, imprinted "PANADOL" and "500"). Tablets packaged in tamper-evident bottles of 10, 30, 60, and 100. Caplets packaged in tamper-evident bottles of 24, 50. Capsules (white, imprinted "PANADOL" and "500") packaged in tamper-evident bottles of 24, 50, and 75.
Shown in Product Identification Section, page 410

PHILLIPS' LAXCAPS

COMPOSITION
A combination of phenolphthalein (90 mg) and Docusate Sodium (83 mg) per gelatin capsule.

INDICATIONS
For relief of occasional constipation (irregularity.)

ACTION
Phenolphthalein is a stimulant laxative which increases the peristaltic activity of the intestine. Docusate Sodium is a stool softener which allows easier passage of the stool. This product generally produces bowel movement in 6 to 12 hours.

ADMINISTRATION AND DOSAGE
Adults and children 12 and over take one (1) or two (2) capsules daily with a full glass (8 ounce) of liquid, or as directed by a physician. For children under 12, consult your physician.

WARNINGS
Do not take any laxative if abdominal pain, nausea, vomiting, change in bowel habits persisting for over 2 weeks, rectal bleeding or kidney disease are present. Laxative products should not be used for a period longer than one week, unless directed by a physician. If there is a failure to have a bowel movement after use, discontinue and consult your doctor. If a skin rash appears do not take this or any other preparation which contains phenolphthalein. Keep this and all drugs out of the reach of children. In case of accidental overdose, seek professional assistance or contact a Poison Control Center immediately. As with any drug, if you are pregnant or nursing a baby, seek the advice of a health professional before using this product.

HOW SUPPLIED
Blister packs for safety of:
8's NDC 12843-384-18
24's NDC 12843-384-19
48's NDC 12843-384-20
Shown in Product Identification Section, page 411

PHILLIPS'® MILK OF MAGNESIA

COMPOSITION
A suspension of magnesium hydroxide in purified water meeting all USP specifications. Phillips' Milk of Magnesia contains 405 mg per teaspoon (5 ml) of Magnesium Hydroxide.

INDICATIONS
For relief of occasional constipation (irregularity) relief of acid indigestion, sour stomach and heartburn.

ACTION AT LAXATIVE DOSAGE:
Phillips' Milk of Magnesia is a mild saline laxative which acts by drawing water into the gut, increasing intraluminal pressure, and increasing intestinal motility. This product generally produces bowel movement in ½ to 6 hours.
At Antacid Dosage: Philips' Milk of Magnesia is an effective acid neutralizer.

ADMINISTRATION AND DOSAGE
As a laxative, adults and children 12 years and older, 2–4 tbsp; children 6–11, 1–2 tbsp.; children 2–5, 1–3 tsp. followed by a full glass (8 oz.) of liquid. Children under 2, consult a physician.
As an antacid, 1–3 tsps with a little water up to four times a day, or as directed by your physician.

WARNINGS
Do not take any laxative if abdominal pain, nausea, vomiting, change in bowel habits persisting for over 2 weeks, rectal bleeding, or kidney disease are present. Do not take more than the maximum daily dose in a twenty four hour period or use the maximum dosage of this product for more than two weeks except under the advice and supervision of a physician. If there is a failure to have a bowel movement after use, discontinue and consult a doctor. Keep this and all drugs out of the reach of children. In case of accidental overdose, seek professional assistance or contact a poison control center immediately.

HOW SUPPLIED
Phillips' Milk of Magnesia is available in regular and mint flavor in bottles of:
Regular
4 fl. oz. NDC 12843-353-01, 12 fl. oz. NDC 12843-353-02, 26 fl. oz. NDC 12843-353-03
Mint
4 fl. oz. NDC 12843-363-04, 12 fl. oz. NDC 12843-363-05 26 fl. oz. NDC 12843-363-06
Also available in tablet form.
Shown in Product Identification Section, page 411

PHILLIPS'® MILK OF MAGNESIA TABLETS

COMPOSITION
Each Tablet contains 311 mg of Magnesium Hydroxide.

INDICATIONS
For relief of acid indigestion, sour stomach, heartburn and occasional constipation (irregularity).

ACTIONS
At Laxative Dosage: Phillips' Milk of Magnesia Tablets offer the same mild saline laxative ingredient as liquid Phillips' Milk of Magnesia in a convenient, chewable tablet form. It acts by drawing water into the gut, increasing intraluminal pressure, and increasing intestinal motility. This product generally produces bowel movement in ½ to 6 hours.
At Antacid Dosage: Phillips' Milk of Magnesia Tablets are effective acid neutralizers.

ADMINISTRATION AND DOSAGE
As an Antacid, adults chew thoroughly 2 to 4 tablets up to 4 times a day. Children 7 to 14 years, 1 tablet up to 4 times a day or as directed by a physician.
As a laxative, adults and children 12 years of age and older chew thoroughly 6 to 8 tablets. Children 6 to 11, 3 to 4 tablets; children 2 to 5, 1 to 2 tablets, preferably before bedtime and follow with a full glass (8 oz.) of liquid. Children under 2, consult a physician.

WARNINGS
Do not take any laxative if abdominal pain, nausea, vomiting, change in bowel habits persisting for over 2 weeks, rectal bleeding, or kidney disease are present. Do not take more than the maximum daily dose in a twenty-four hour period or use the maximum dosage of this product for more than two weeks except under the advice and supervision of a physician. If there is a failure to have a bowel movement after use, discontinue and consult a doctor. Keep this and all drugs out of the reach of children. In case of accidental overdose, seek professional assistance or contact a poison control center immediately.
Shown in Product Identification Section, page 411

VANQUISH®

COMPOSITION
Each Caplet contains aspirin 227 mg, acetaminophen 194 mg, caffeine 33 mg, dried aluminum hydroxide gel 25 mg; magnesium hydroxide 50 mg.

ACTION AND USES
A buffered analgesic, antipyretic for relief of headache; muscular aches and pains; neuralgia and neuritic pain; pain following dental procedures; for painful discomforts and fever of colds and flu; functional menstrual pain, headache and pain due to cramps; temporary relief from minor pains of arthritis, rheumatism, bursitis, lumbago, sciatica.

WARNINGS
Children and teenagers should not use this medicine for chicken pox or flu symptoms before a doctor is consulted about Reye Syndrome, a rare but serious illness. Keep this and all drugs out of the reach of children. In case of accidental overdose, seek professional assistance or contact a poison control center immediately. As with any drug, if you are pregnant or nursing a baby, seek the advice of a health professional before using this product.

USUAL ADULT DOSAGE
Two caplets with water. May be repeated every four hours if necessary up to 12 tablets per day. Larger or more frequent doses may be prescribed by physician if necessary.

CONTRAINDICATIONS
Hypersensitivity to salicylates.
(To be used with caution during anticoagulant therapy or in asthmatic patients.)

HOW SUPPLIED
White, capsule-shaped Caplets in bottles of:
15 Caplets NDC 12843-171-42
30 Caplets NDC 12843-171-44
60 Caplets NDC 12843-171-46
100 Caplets NDC 12843-171-48

Glenwood, Inc.
83 N. SUMMIT STREET
TENAFLY, NJ 07670

CALPHOSAN® ℞
(calcium glycerophosphate/calcium lactate)
calcium/phosphorus solution in metabolic disorders involving low calcium

COMPOSITION
CALPHOSAN is a specially processed solution containing calcium glycerophosphate and calcium lactate. CALPHOSAN is isotonic, with a pH of about 7 or somewhat above. (Other calcium solutions are usually quite acid, with pH values of 4.5 to 5.5). Each 10 ml. CALPHOSAN contains calcium glycerophosphate 50 mg. and calcium lactate 50 mg. in a physiological solution of sodium chloride, with 0.25% phenol as a preservative.

ADVANTAGES
Intramuscular injections of CALPHOSAN raise blood serum calcium levels, do not raise the calcium levels above normal. Of conspicuous importance, intramuscular injections of CALPHOSAN are without pain, inflammatory reactions or sloughing.

INDICATIONS
Wherever calcium is indicated or in conditions associated with hypocalcemia.

ADMINISTRATION
One or two 10 ml. injections of CALPHOSAN each week for the first four or five weeks, and on a when-needed basis thereafter, is usually sufficient to raise blood calcium levels.

USE IN PREGNANCY
Safety for use in pregnancy or during Lactation has not been established.

CONTRAINDICATIONS
Hypercalcemia; and in view of the fact that hypercalcemia is associated with sarcoidosis and bone metastasis of neoplastic processes, it should not be used in those conditions. As there is a similarity in the actions of calcium and digitalis on the

contractility and excitability of the heart muscle, CALPHOSAN is contraindicated in fully digitalized patients. **Do not use intramuscularly in infants and young children.**

AVAILABILITY

10 ml. ampuls in boxes of 10's—NDC 0516-0060-70 and 60 ml. multiple dose vials—NDC 0516-0060-60.

MYOTONACHOL™ ℞
Bethanechol Chloride—Oral USP

HOW SUPPLIED

Myotonachol.
10 mg. tablets, flat, NDC 0516-0021-01 in bottles of 100s.
25 mg. tablets, flat, NDC 0516-0022-01 in bottles of 100s.

POTABA® ℞
Systemic ANTIFIBROSIS THERAPY

FORMULA

POTABA is chemically Aminobenzoate Potassium, U.S.P.

INDICATIONS

Based on a review of this drug by the National Academy of Sciences-National Research Council and/or other information, FDA has classified the indications as follows:

"Possibly" effective: Potassium aminobenzoate is possibly effective in the treatment of scleroderma, dermatomyositis, morphea, linear scleroderma, pemphigus, and Peyronie's disease.

Final classification of the less-than-effective indications requires further investigation.

ADVANTAGES

POTABA offers a means of treatment of serious and often chronic entities involving fibrosis and nonsuppurative inflammation.

PHARMACOLOGY

P-Aminobenzoate is considered a member of the vitamin B complex. Small amounts are found in cereal, eggs, milk and meats. Detectable amounts are normally present in human blood, spinal fluid, urine, and sweat. PABA is a component of several biologically important systems, and it participates in a number of fundamental biological processes. It has been suggested that the antifibrosis action of POTABA is due to its mediation of increased oxygen uptake at the tissue level. Fibrosis is believed to occur from either too much serotonin or too little monoamine oxidase activity over a period of time. Monoamine oxidase requires an adequate supply of oxygen to function properly. By increasing oxygen supply at the tissue level POTABA may enhance MAO activity and prevent or bring about regression of fibrosis.

CLINICAL USES

PEYRONIE'S DISEASE: 21 patients with Peyronie's disease were placed on POTABA therapy for periods ranging from 3 months to 2 years. Pain disappeared from 16 of 16 cases in which it had been present. There was objective improvement in penile deformity in 10 of 17 patients, and decrease in plaque size in 16 of 21. The authors suggest that this medication offers no hazard of further local injury as may result from other therapy. There were no significant untoward effects encountered on long term POTABA therapy.

SCLERODERMA: Of 135 patients with diffuse systemic sclerosis treated with POTABA every patient but one has shown softening of the involved skin if treatment has been continued for 3 months or longer. The responses have been reported in a number of publications. The treatment program consists of systemic antifibrosis therapy with POTABA, physical therapy, including deep breathing exercises and dynamic traction splints where indicated, and bethanechol chloride (MYOTONACHOL, Glenwood) for relief of dysphagia as well as small doses of reserpine for amelioration of Raynaud's phenomena.

DERMATOMYOSITIS: Five patients with scleroderma and 2 with dermatomyositis were treated with POTABA. There was striking clinical improvement in each patient. Doses of 15-20 grams per day were well tolerated, and patients were easily able to take these doses.

MORPHEA and LINEAR SCLERODERMA: All 14 patients with localized forms of scleroderma placed on long-term POTABA treatment showed softening of the sclerotic component of their disorder. Treatment is particularly indicated in patients where persistent compressive sclerosis may contribute even greater disfigurement or functional embarrassment from secondary pressure atrophy.

DOSAGE AND ADMINISTRATION

The average adult daily dose of POTABA is 12 grams, usually given in four to six divided doses. Tablets and capsules 0.5 gram are given at the rate of 4 tablets or capsules 6 times daily, or 6 given four times daily, usually with meals, and at bed-time with a snack. Tablets must be dissolved in an adequate amount of liquid to prevent gastrointestinal upset.

POTABA Envules contain 2 grams pure drug each, and constitute the individual average dose. 6 Envules are given for a total of 12 grams POTABA daily.

POTABA Powder is used to prepare solutions, which are kept refrigerated, but for no longer than one week. 100 grams POTABA powder make 1 quart of 10% solution when dissolved in potable tap water. Children are given 1 gram POTABA daily in divided doses for each 10 lbs. of body weight.

SIDE EFFECTS

Anorexia, nausea, fever and rash have occurred infrequently and subside with omission of the drug. Often, desensitization can be accomplished and treatment resumed.

USAGE IN PREGNANCY

Safety for use in pregnancy or during lactation has not been established.

PRECAUTIONS

Should anorexia or nausea occur, therapy is interrupted until the patient is eating normally again. This permits prompt subsidence of symptoms and also avoids the possible development of hypoglycemia. Give cautiously to patients with renal disease. If a hypersensitivity reaction should occur, POTABA should be stopped.

CONTRAINDICATIONS

POTABA should not be administered to patients taking sulfonamides.

HOW SUPPLIED

POTABA Capsules 0.5 gm. in 250's and 1,000's; POTABA Envules 2.0 gm. in boxes of 50's; POTABA Powder, pure, in 100 gm. and 1 lb.; POTABA Tablets 0.5 gm. in 100's and 1,000's.

Shown in Product Identification Section, page 411

PRIMER® Unna Boot

COMPOSITION

Zinc Oxide, Acacia, Glycerin, Castor Oil and White Petrolatum. No preservatives.

ACTIONS AND USES

Treatment of venous insufficiency conditions such as stasis ulcers.

ADMINISTRATION AND DOSAGE

The combination of PRIMER and TENSOPLAST elastic adhesive bandage produces a flexible cast boot. Apply the PRIMER over the entire lower leg, starting immediately behind the toes and continue up to the knee. Apply the elastic bandage over the PRIMER using firm evenly distributed pressure. Continue bandaging until the PRIMER is completely covered. The treatment is ambulatory and the patient should be encouraged to walk as much as possible. Change bandage at least once a week for the first two or three weeks, then every two or three weeks until healing is complete.

PRECAUTIONS

If skin sensitivity or irritation develops discontinue use and consult a physician.

HOW SUPPLIED

3½" × 10 yards—Unna Boot-List. No. 300-1
NDC 0516-1410-30

RENOQUID® ℞
(Sulfacytine)

HOW SUPPLIED

Renoquid 250 mg tablets, NDC 0516-0081-01 in bottles of 100's.

YODOXIN® ℞
210 mg. & 650 mg. Tablets
(IODOQUINOL TABLETS U.S.P.)

DESCRIPTION

Iodoquinol is of a light yellowish to tan color, nearly odorless and stable in air. The compound is practically insoluble in water, and sparingly soluble in most other solvents. It contains 64 per cent organically bound iodine.

ACTION

Iodoquinol is amebicidal against Entamoeba histolytica and is considered effective against the trophozoite and cyst forms.

INDICATIONS

Iodoquinol is used in the treatment of intestinal amebiasis.

CONTRAINDICATIONS

Known hypersensitivity to iodine and 8-hydroxyquinolines. Contraindicated in patients with hepatic damage.

WARNINGS

Optic neuritis, optic atrophy, and peripheral neuropathy have been reported following prolonged high dosage therapy with halogenated 8-hydroxyquinolines. Long term use of this drug should be avoided.

USE IN PREGNANCY

Safety for use in pregnancy or during lactation has not been established.

PRECAUTIONS

Iodoquinol should be used with caution in patients with thyroid disease.

Protein-bound serum iodine levels may be increased during treatment with iodoquinol and therefore interfere with certain thyroid function tests. These effects may persist for as long as six months after discontinuation of therapy. Discontinue the drug if hypersensitivity reactions occur.

ADVERSE REACTIONS

Skin: various forms of skin eruptions (acneiform papular and pustular; bullae; vegetating of tuberous iododerma), urticaria and pruritus. Gastrointestinal: nausea, vomiting, abdominal cramps, diarrhea, and pruritus ani.

Fever, chills, headache, vertigo and enlargement of thyroid have been reported. Optic neuritis, optic atrophy and peripheral neuropathy have been reported in association with prolonged high-dosage 8-hydroxyquinoline therapy.

DOSAGE AND ADMINISTRATION

Usual adult dose: (210 mg. each) 3 tablets three times daily, after meals for 20 days. Children 6 to 12 years: (210 mg. each) 2 tablets, t.i.d. Children under 6: (210 mg. each) one tablet per 15 pounds of body weight. Usual adult dose: (650 mg. each) one tablet three times a day for twenty days, to be taken after meals. Children (650 mg. each): For twenty days, 40 mg. per Kg. of body weight daily divided into 3 doses, not to exceed 1.95 grams in 24 hours, for 20 days.

HOW SUPPLIED

YODOXIN Tablets—210 mg.
NDC-0516-0092-01 Bottle of 100
NDC-0516-0092-10 Bottle of 1000
YODOXIN Tablets—650 mg.
NDC-0516-0093-01 Bottle of 100
NDC-0516-0093-10 Bottle of 1000

STORAGE

Store at Controlled Room Temperature 15–30°C. (59–86°F.)

CAUTION

Federal law prohibits dispensing without prescription.

Distributed by:
GLENWOOD INC.
Tenafly, New Jersey 07670

Shown in Product Identification Section, page 411

Gray Pharmaceutical Co.
100 CONNECTICUT AVENUE
NORWALK, CT 06856

X-PREP® LIQUID
[*ĕx 'prep*]
(standardized extract of senna fruit)

ACTION AND USES

An easy-to-administer, palatable, highly effective bowel evacuant for the preparation of the intestinal tract prior to G.I. and urological radiography as well as colonoscopy, sigmoidoscopy and other diagnostic bowel procedures. In addition, X-PREP Liquid may be used for preparation of the bowel prior to elective colon surgery. Permits excellent visualization without residual oil droplets. X-PREP Liquid is fully prepared in a single dose container—all the patient has to do is drink the contents of one small bottle (2½ fl. oz.). Good patient cooperation is ensured because of highly pleasant taste. Predictable effectiveness helps reduce or eliminate the need for enemas prior to radiography.

CONTRAINDICATIONS

Acute surgical abdomen.

CAUTION

In diabetic patients, the physician should be aware of the sugar content of X-PREP Liquid (50 grams per 2½ fl. oz. dose).

Continued on next page

Gray—Cont.

ADVERSE REACTIONS
As with all potent purgatives, some patients may experience abdominal discomfort and nausea; vomiting is rare.

ADMINISTRATION AND DOSAGE
For adults: Entire contents of X-PREP Liquid bottle should be taken between 2:00 and 4:00 p.m. on the day prior to diagnostic procedure or elective colon surgery. Patients should be advised to expect a thorough, strong bowel action to begin approximately six hours later. After X-PREP Liquid is taken, diet should be confined to clear fluids.
X-PREP Liquid has proved to be effective following the above regimen. However, at physician's discretion, X-PREP Liquid may be given in divided doses, particularly to elderly or debilitated patients. The following split dosage regimens are equally effective: (1) One-half (½) of the contents of the bottle is taken at bedtime two days prior to diagnostic procedure. On day prior to examination, remaining contents of bottle is taken, also at bedtime. OR (2) On the day prior to examination, one-half (½) contents of bottle is taken at noon and the remaining one-half (½) at 4:00 p.m.
Some physicians prefer the hydration method, with 24-hour liquid diet and consumption of several extra glasses of water during this period, prior to the administration of X-PREP Liquid. Morning enema is optional. X-PREP Liquid may be successfully combined with adjunctive laxative suppositories or citrate of magnesia

HOW SUPPLIED
2½ fl. oz. bottles (alcohol 7% by volume), each providing a single, complete adult dose.
Also Available—Two X-PREP® Bowel Evacuant Kits.
Kit #1 contains: Two SENOKOT-S® Tablets (standardized senna concentrate and docusate sodium), one bottle of X-PREP Liquid 2½ fl. oz., and one RECTOLAX® Suppository (bisacodyl 10 mg), plus easy-to-follow patient instructions for hydration, clear liquid diet, and the correct time-sequence for administering the above laxatives.
Kit #2 contains: One dose CITRALAX® Granules 1.06 oz. (effervescent citrate/sulfate of magnesia), one bottle of X-PREP Liquid 2½ fl. oz., and one RECTOLAX Suppository (bisacodyl 10 mg), plus easy-to-follow patient instructions.

Guardian Chemical
a division of United-Guardian, Inc.
P.O. Box 2500
SMITHTOWN, N.Y. 11787

CLORPACTIN® WCS-90
[klor-pak 'tin]
(brand of sodium oxychlorosene)

COMPOSITION
Stabilized organic derivative of hypochlorous acid. A white, water soluble powder with a characteristic smell of hypochlorous acid. Active chlorine derived from calcium hypochlorite: 3–4%.

ACTION AND USES
For use as a topical antiseptic for treating localized infections, particularly when resistant organisms are present. Complete spectrum (bacteria, fungi, viruses, mold, yeast and spores); effective in cases of antibiotic resistance; nontoxic and non-allergenic in use concentrations.

ADMINISTRATION AND DOSAGE
Applied by irrigation, instillations, spray, soaks or wet compresses, preferably thoroughly cleansing with gravity flow irrigation or syringe to provide copious quantities of fresh solution to remove the organic wastes and debris from the site of the involvement. Also for preoperative skin preparation and postoperative protection. Generally applied as the 0.4% solution in water, or isotonic saline, but as the 0.1% to 0.2% in Urology and Ophthalmology.

CONTRAINDICATIONS
The use of this product is contraindicated where the site of the infection is not exposed to the direct contact with the solution. Not for systemic use.

HOW SUPPLIED
In boxes containing 5 x 2 gram bottles.

LUBRASEPTIC® JELLY
[loo-bra "sep 'tik]

COMPOSITION
Active ingredients: Aryl phenols, as phenyl phenol 0.1%, Alkyl phenols, as amyl phenol 0.02%, in water miscible form as an acid complex. Phenyl mercuric nitrate 0.007%.

USES
For urethral instillation, prior to insertion of cystoscopes or sounds; for urethral dilations in the case of strictures. For proctologic use, in cases of hemorrhoids, or for post-hemorrhoidectomies, to provide increased comfort between and during the passage of stools. For endotracheal intubation. For use whenever a sterile water soluble lubricant is required: on cystoscopes and proctoscopes, in urological, rectal, and vaginal examinations or for use as a sterile dressing on burns, abrasions, and decubitus ulcers (bedsores).

PRECAUTIONS AND SIDE EFFECTS
No serious side effects or contraindications are known. Urethral instillation, in some individuals, may cause a temporary burning or stinging sensation but this usually disappears in several minutes. Excessive pressure should be avoided when instilling where strictures may exist.

HOW SUPPLIED
In boxes containing 24 sterile packets each with a 10 gram "bellows" shaped tube of jelly and a urethral Dispostip.

pHos-pHaid® ℞
[fos 'fād]
(brand of urinary acidifier)

COMPOSITION
Each 0.5 Gm. tablet contains ammonium biphosphate, 190 mg., sodium biphosphate, 200 mg., and sodium acid pyrophosphate, 110 mg. pH: approximately 4.5. Sodium content: less than one grain per tablet.

ACTION AND USES
pHos-pHaid is a highly effective urinary acidifier which, in conjunction with an acid ash diet, can decrease the urinary pH to a 5–5.5 level. Useful in increasing the solubility of calcium in the urine to assist in preventing formation of calculi in the urinary tract.

ADMINISTRATION AND DOSAGE
In conjunction with an acidifying diet, the recommended dosage is two 0.5 Gm. tablets, followed by a glass of water, t.i.d. Occasionally, higher dosage is required and may be employed when necessary.

SIDE EFFECTS
Occasional hyperacidity, particularly where gastritis or ulceration exists, and/or occasional nausea have been observed in some patients on a high dosage level. This may be decreased or eliminated by the use of the Enteric-Coated tablets. Excessive doses may also act as a saline cathartic and cause diarrhea. In such cases dosage should be decreased until the symptoms disappear. In cases of severe or extensive renal damage, pHos-pHaid should be administered with caution.

HOW SUPPLIED
In color-coded tablets, either regular or Enteric- Coated.

Size	*Type*	*Packaged*	*Color*
0.5 Gm.	Reg.	90 & 500	Blue
0.5 Gm.	Ent.-Coat	90 & 500	Orange
0.25 Gm.	Reg.	150	Pink
0.25 Gm.	Ent.-Coat	150	Green

LITERATURE AVAILABLE
Literature on pHospHaid and Acid Ash Diet Sheets are available to physicians on request.

RENACIDIN® ℞
[ren "a-sē 'din]

COMPOSITION
Active Ingredients (in a 300 gram bottle): Citric acid, anhydrous, 156–171 grams; D-gluconic acid (primarily as the lactone), 21–30 grams. Inert Ingredients: Purified magnesium hydroxycarbonate, 75–87 grams; Magnesium Acid Citrate ($MgHC_6H_5O_7$), 9–15 grams; Calcium (as the carbonate), 2–6 grams; Water, combined and free, 17–21 grams.

ACTION AND USES
For use in preparing solutions for irrigating indwelling urethral catheters and the urinary bladder in order to dissolve or prevent formation of calcifications.

ADMINISTRATION AND DOSAGE
As a 10% solution (sterile) in distilled water. Irrigation is carried out with 1-2 ounces, b.i.d. or t.i.d. by means of a small, sterile, rubber syringe.

SIDE EFFECTS
Only occasionally will a patient complain of some temporary pain or burning sensation from this procedure, in which case use of the solution should be discontinued.

CONTRAINDICATIONS
It is contraindicated for therapy or preventive therapy above the ureteral-vesical junction; therefore it is contraindicated for ureteral catheters, nephrostomy or pyelostomy tubes or renal lavage for dissolving calculi. Contraindicated for biliary calculi.

HOW SUPPLIED
In bottles containing 300 grams; also in boxes containing six 25 gram bottles.

W. E. Hauck, Inc.
P.O. BOX 1065
ROSWELL, GA 30075

BESTA® CAPSULES OTC
(Therapeutic Vitamins and Minerals)

SUPPLIED
Bottles of 100.

CHLORAFED H.S. TIMECELLES* ℞

COMPOSITION
Chlorpheniramine Maleate 4 mg.; Pseudoephedrine HCl 60 mg.
* In special time release beads.

SUPPLIED
Bottles of 100.

CHLORAFED LIQUID OTC
(Corn, Dye, Alcohol, Sugar Free)

COMPOSITION
Each 5 ml. of liquid contains: Chlorpheniramine Maleate 2 mg.; Pseudoephedrine HCl 30 mg.

SUPPLIED
4 oz. and pints.

CHLORAFED TIMECELLES* ℞

COMPOSITION
Chlorpheniramine Maleate 8 mg.; Pseudoephedrine HCl-120 mg.;
*In special time release beads.

SUPPLIED
Bottles of 100 and 500

DOLACET CAPSULES ℞ Ⓒ III

COMPOSITION
Each imprinted capsule contains Hydrocodone Bitartrate 5 mg. and Acetaminophen 500 mg.

SUPPLIED
Imprinted capsules in bottles of 100 and 500.

ENTUSS TABLETS and LIQUID Ⓒ III ℞
(Sugar, Alcohol, Corn, Tartrazine Free)

COMPOSITION
Each tablet contains: Hydrocodone Bitartrate 5 mg., Guaifenesin 300 mg. Each 5 ml. of liquid contains: Hydrocodone Bitartrate 5 mg. Potassium Guaiacolsulfonate 300 mg.

SUPPLIED
Tablets—bottles of 100. Liquid—4 oz. and pints

ENTUSS-D LIQUID and TABLETS Ⓒ III ℞
Sugar, Dye, Corn, Alcohol Free

COMPOSITION
Each tablet or teaspoonful contains Hydrocodone Bitartrate 5 mg., Guaifenesin 300 mg. and Pseudoephedrine Hydrochloride 30 mg.

SUPPLIED
Imprinted Tablets—Bottles of 100. Liquid—16 oz. bottles.

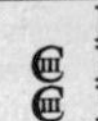

G–1® CAPSULES ℞
G–2® CAPSULES ℞
G–3® CAPSULES ℞

COMPOSITION
Each G-1 Capsule contains: Acetaminophen 500 mg., Butalbital 50 mg., Caffeine 40 mg. Each G-2 Capsule contains: Acetamionphen 500 mg., Butalbital 50 mg., Codeine PO_4 15 mg. Each G-3 Capsule contains: Acetaminophen 500 mg., Butalbital 50 mg., Codeine PO_4 30 mg.

SUPPLIED
Bottles of 100.

HISTOR-D® TIMECELLES* ℞

COMPOSITION
Chlorpheniramine Maleate 8 mg.; Phenylephrine 20 mg.; Methscopolamine Nitrate 2.5 mg.
*In special time release beads.

SUPPLIED
Bottles of 100 and 500.

ISOTRATE TIMECELLES ℞
(Isosorbide Dinitrate)

COMPOSITION
Each Timecelle contains: 40 mg. Isosorbide Dinitrate in a microdialysis release base which lasts for 12 hours.

SUPPLIED
Bottles of 100 and 500.

OTIC–H.C. EAR DROPS ℞

COMPOSITION
Each ml. contains: Chloroxylenol 1 mg., Hydrocortisone 10 mg., Pramoxine 10 mg., in a non-aqueous Propylene Glycol vehicle with Acetic Acid and Benzalkonium Chloride.

SUPPLIED
10 ml. dropper tip bottle.

SINUFED TIMECELLES ℞

COMPOSITION
Each imprinted capsule contains Pseudoephedrine hydrochloride 60 mg. in a special base to provide for prolonged action and Guaifenesin 300 mg. designed for immediate release for rapid action.

SUPPLIED
Imprinted capsules in bottles of 100.

WEHLESS–105 TIMECELLES ℞

COMPOSITION
Each capsule contains: Phendimetrazine Tartrate 105 mg. in a sustained release base which lasts for 10 hours. Black and clear capsule imprinted WEHLESS T.C. 105 mg.

SUPPLIED
Bottles of 100.

Herbert Laboratories
Dermatology Division of Allergan Pharmaceuticals, Inc.
2525 DUPONT DRIVE
IRVINE, CA 92715

AEROSEB–DEX® ℞
(dexamethasone)
Topical Aerosol Spray

DESCRIPTION
The topical corticosteroids constitute a class of primarily synthetic steroids used as anti-inflammatory and antipruritic agents.
Chemical Name: Pregna-1, 4-diene-3, 20-dione, 9-fluoro-11, 17, 21-trihydroxy-16-methyl-, (11β, 16α)-.
Contains:
dexamethasone 0.01%
alcohol 65.1%
with: isopropyl myristate and propellant (butane).
Each 1 second of spray dispenses approximately 0.02 mg of dexamethasone.

CLINICAL PHARMACOLOGY
Topical corticosteroids share anti-inflammatory, antipruritic and vasoconstrictive actions.
The mechanism of anti-inflammatory activity of the topical corticosteroids is unclear. Various laboratory methods, including vasoconstrictor assays, are used to compare and predict potencies and/or clinical efficacies of the topical corticosteroids. There is some evidence to suggest that a recognizable correlation exists between vasoconstrictor potency and therapeutic efficacy in man.
Pharmacokinetics: The extent of percutaneous absorption of topical corticosteroids is determined by many factors, including the vehicle, the integrity of the epidermal barrier and the use of occlusive dressings.
Topical corticosteroids can be absorbed from normal intact skin. Inflammation and/or other disease processes in the skin increase percutaneous absorption. Occlusive dressings substantially increase the percutaneous absorption of topical corticosteroids. Thus, occlusive dressings may be a valuable therapeutic adjunct for treatment of resistant dermatoses (see DOSAGE AND ADMINISTRATION).
Once absorbed through the skin, topical corticosteroids are handled through pharmacokinetic pathways similar to systemically-administered corticosteroids. Corticosteroids are bound to plasma proteins in varying degrees. Corticosteroids are metabolized primarily in the liver and are then excreted by the kidneys. Some of the topical corticosteroids and their metabolites are also excreted into the bile.

INDICATIONS AND USAGE
Topical corticosteroids are indicated for the relief of the inflammatory and pruritic manifestations of corticosteroid-responsive dermatoses. Aeroseb-Dex is particularly useful in treating conditions of the scalp such as seborrheic dermatitis.

CONTRAINDICATIONS
Topical corticosteroids are contraindicated in those patients with a history of hypersensitivity to any of the components of the preparation.

PRECAUTIONS
General: Systemic absorption of topical corticosteroids has produced reversible hypothalamic-pituitary-adrenal (HPA) axis suppression, manifestations of Cushing's syndrome, hyperglycemia and glucosuria in some patients.
Conditions which augment systemic absorption include the application of more potent steroids, use over large surface areas, prolonged use and the addition of occlusive dressings.
Therefore, patients receiving a large dose of a potent topical steroid applied to a large surface area or under an occlusive dressing should be evaluated periodically for evidence of HPA axis suppression by using the urinary-free cortisol and ACTH stimulation tests. If HPA axis suppression is noted, an attempt should be made to withdraw the drug, to reduce the frequency of application, or to substitute a less potent steroid.
Recovery of HPA axis function is generally prompt and complete upon discontinuation of the drug. Infrequently, signs and symptoms of steroid withdrawal may occur, requiring supplemental systemic corticosteroids.
Children may absorb proportionally larger amounts of topical corticosteroids and thus be more susceptible to systemic toxicity (see PRECAUTIONS—Pediatric Use).
This medication contains alcohol. It may produce irritation or burning sensations in open lesions. If irritation develops, topical corticosteroids should be discontinued and appropriate therapy instituted.
In the presence of dermatological infections, the use of an appropriate antifungal or antibacterial agent should be instituted. If a favorable response does not occur promptly, the corticosteroid should be discontinued until the infection has been adequately controlled.
Information for the Patient: Patients using topical corticosteroids should receive the following information and instructions:
1. This medication is to be used as directed by the physician. It is for external use only. Avoid contact with the eyes. When used about the face, the eyes should be covered and inhalation of the spray should be avoided.
2. Patients should be advised not to use this medication for any disorder other than for which it was prescribed.
3. The treated skin area should not be bandaged or otherwise covered or wrapped as to be occlusive unless directed by the physician.
4. Patients should report any signs of local adverse reactions, especially under occlusive dressing.
5. Parents of pediatric patients should be advised not to use tight-fitting diapers or plastic pants on a child being treated in the diaper area, as these garments may constitute occlusive dressings.

Laboratory Tests: The urinary-free cortisol test and the ACTH stimulation test may be helpful in evaluating the HPA axis suppression.
Carcinogenesis, Mutagenesis, Impairment of Fertility: Long-term animal studies have not been performed to evaluate the carcinogenic potential or the effect of topical corticosteroids on fertility.
Studies to determine mutagenicity with prednisolone and hydrocortisone have revealed negative results.
Pregnancy Category C: Corticosteroids are generally teratogenic in laboratory animals when administered systemically at relatively low dosage levels. The more potent corticosteroids have been shown to be teratogenic after dermal application in laboratory animals. There are no adequate and well-controlled studies in pregnant women on teratogenic effects from topically applied corticosteroids. Therefore, topical corticosteroids should be used during pregnancy only if the potential benefit justifies the potential risk to the fetus. Drugs of this class should not be used extensively on pregnant patients, in large amounts, or for prolonged periods of time.
Nursing Mothers: It is not known whether topical administration of corticosteroids could result in sufficient systemic absorption to produce detectable quantities in breast milk. Systemically administered corticosteroids are secreted into breast milk in quantities not likely to have a deleterious effect on the infant. Nevertheless, caution should be exercised when topical corticosteroids are administered to a nursing woman.
Pediatric Use: Pediatric patients may demonstrate greater susceptibility to topical corticosteroid-induced HPA axis suppression and Cushing's syndrome than mature patients because of a larger skin surface area to body weight ratio.
Hypothalamic-pituitary-adrenal (HPA) axis suppression, Cushing's syndrome and intracranial hypertension have been reported in children receiving topical corticosteroids. Manifestations of adrenal suppression in children include linear growth retardation, delayed weight gain, low plasma cortisol levels and absence of response to ACTH stimulation. Manifestations of intracranial hypertension include bulging fontanelles, headaches and bilateral papilledema.
Administration of topical corticosteroids to children should be limited to the least amount compatible with an effective therapeutic regimen. Chronic corticosteroid therapy may interfere with the growth and development of children.

ADVERSE REACTIONS
The following local adverse reactions are reported infrequently with topical corticosteroids, but may occur more frequently with the use of occlusive dressings. These reactions are listed in an approximate decreasing order of occurrence:

Burning	Perioral dermatitis
Itching	Allergic contact dermatitis
Irritation	
Dryness	Maceration of the skin
Folliculitis	Secondary infection
Hypertrichosis	Skin atrophy
Acneiform eruptions	Striae
Hypopigmentation	Miliaria

OVERDOSAGE
Topically applied corticosteroids can be absorbed in sufficient amounts to produce systemic effects (see PRECAUTIONS).

DOSAGE AND ADMINISTRATION
Aeroseb-Dex® (dexamethasone) should be applied to the affected area two or three times daily depending on the severity of the condition.
Occlusive dressings may be used for management of psoriasis or recalcitrant conditions.
If an infection develops, the use of occlusive dressings should be discontinued and appropriate antimicrobial therapy instituted.
For use on the scalp: Apply to dry scalp after shampoo. Shake well before spraying.
1. Hold aerosol upright. Slide applicator tube under the hair so that it touches scalp. Spray while moving tube to all affected areas, keeping tube under hair and in contact with scalp throughout treatment. Spraying should take 1 to 2 seconds.
2. If some areas of the scalp are not covered adequately, they may be "spot" sprayed by sliding applicator tube through hair to touch scalp— press and immediately release spray button.
3. It is unnecessary to massage medication into the scalp.
4. Be sure that the tip of the applicator tube stops at the hairline so that forehead and eyes are not sprayed.

For other dermatoses: Remove applicator tube. Shake well before spraying. Hold the can upright, approximately six inches from the area to be treated. Spray each four-inch square of affected area for one or two seconds, two or three times a day.
Note: For best results and to avoid wasting medication, it is important to follow the application instructions carefully (application instructions appear on the carton; however, it is preferable that the physician demonstrate the proper application method to the patient).

Continued on next page

Herbert—Cont.

CAUTION

Flammable. Do not spray near flame or heated surfaces. If medication accidentally gets in the eyes, wash thoroughly with water and contact physician immediately. Keep out of the reach of children. Contents under pressure. Do not puncture, incinerate, or expose to temperatures above 120°F.

HOW SUPPLIED

In a 58 g aerosol with applicator tube.* On prescription only.
*U.S. Patent 3,730,182

AEROSEB-HC® ℞
(hydrocortisone)
Topical Aerosol Spray

DESCRIPTION

The topical corticosteroids constitute a class of primarily synthetic steroids used as anti-inflammatory and antipruritic agents.

Chemical Name: Pregn-4-ene-3, 20-dione, 11, 17, 21, trihydroxy-, (11β)-.

Contains:
hydrocortisone 0.5%
alcohol 64.6%
with: isopropyl myristate and propellant (butane).
Each 1 second of spray dispenses approximately 1 mg of hydrocortisone.

CLINICAL PHARMACOLOGY

Topical corticosteroids share anti-inflammatory, antipruritic and vasoconstrictive actions.

The mechanism of anti-inflammatory activity of the topical corticosteroids is unclear. Various laboratory methods, including vasoconstrictor assays, are used to compare and predict potencies and/or clinical efficacies of the topical corticosteroids. There is some evidence to suggest that a recognizable correlation exists between vasoconstrictor potency and therapeutic efficacy in man.

Pharmacokinetics: The extent of percutaneous absorption of topical corticosteroids is determined by many factors, including the vehicle, the integrity of the epidermal barrier and the use of occlusive dressings.

Topical corticosteroids can be absorbed from normal intact skin. Inflammation and/or other disease processes in the skin increase percutaneous absorption. Occlusive dressings substantially increase the percutaneous absorption of topical corticosteroids. Thus, occlusive dressings may be a valuable therapeutic adjunct for treatment of resistant dermatoses (see DOSAGE AND ADMINISTRATION).

Once absorbed through the skin, topical corticosteroids are handled through pharmacokinetic pathways similar to systemically-administered corticosteroids. Corticosteroids are bound to plasma proteins in varying degrees. Corticosteroids are metabolized primarily in the liver and are then excreted by the kidneys. Some of the topical corticosteroids and their metabolites are also excreted into the bile.

INDICATIONS AND USAGE

Topical corticosteroids are indicated for the relief of the inflammatory and pruritic manifestations of corticosteroid-responsive dermatoses. Aeroseb-HC is particularly useful in treating conditions of the scalp such as seborrheic dermatitis.

CONTRAINDICATIONS

Topical corticosteroids are contraindicated in those patients with a history of hypersensitivity to any of the components of the preparation.

PRECAUTIONS

General: Systemic absorption of topical corticosteroids has produced reversible hypothalamic-pituitary-adrenal (HPA) axis suppression, manifestations of Cushing's syndrome, hyperglycemia and glucosuria in some patients.

Conditions which augment systemic absorption include the application of more potent steroids, use over large surface areas, prolonged use and the addition of occlusive dressings.

Therefore, patients receiving a large dose of a potent topical steroid applied to a large surface area or under an occlusive dressing should be evaluated periodically for evidence of HPA axis suppression by using the urinary-free cortisol and ACTH stimulation tests. If HPA axis suppression is noted, an attempt should be made to withdraw the drug, to reduce the frequency of application, or to substitute a less potent steroid.

Recovery of HPA axis function is generally prompt and complete upon discontinuation of the drug. Infrequently, signs and symptoms of steroid withdrawal may occur, requiring supplemental systemic corticosteroids.

Children may absorb proportionally larger amounts of topical corticosteroids and thus be more susceptible to systemic toxicity (see PRECAUTIONS - Pediatric Use).

This medication contains alcohol. It may produce irritation or burning sensations in open lesions. If irritation develops, topical corticosteroids should be discontinued and appropriate therapy instituted.

In the presence of dermatological infections, the use of an appropriate antifungal or antibacterial agent should be instituted. If a favorable response does not occur promptly, the corticosteroid should be discontinued until the infection has been adequately controlled.

Information for the Patient: Patients using topical corticosteroids should receive the following information and instructions:

1. This medication is to be used as directed by the physician. It is for external use only. Avoid contact with the eyes. When used about the face, the eyes should be covered and inhalation of the spray should be avoided.
2. Patients should be advised not to use this medication for any disorder other than for which it was prescribed.
3. The treated skin area should not be bandaged or otherwise covered or wrapped as to be occlusive unless directed by the physician.
4. Patients should report any signs of local adverse reactions, especially under occlusive dressing.
5. Parents of pediatric patients should be advised not to use tight-fitting diapers or plastic pants on a child being treated in the diaper area, as these garments may constitute occlusive dressings.

Laboratory Tests: The urinary-free cortisol test and the ACTH stimulation test may be helpful in evaluating the HPA axis suppression.

Carcinogenesis, Mutagenesis, Impairment of Fertility: Long-term animal studies have not been performed to evaluate the carcinogenic potential or the effect of topical corticosteroids on fertility.

Studies to determine mutagenicity with prednisolone and hydrocortisone have revealed negative results.

Pregnancy Category C: Corticosteroids are generally teratogenic in laboratory animals when administered systemically at relatively low dosage levels. The more potent corticosteroids have been shown to be teratogenic after dermal application in laboratory animals. There are no adequate and well-controlled studies in pregnant women on teratogenic effects from topically applied corticosteroids. Therefore, topical corticosteroids should be used during pregnancy only if the potential benefit justifies the potential risk to the fetus. Drugs of this class should not be used extensively on pregnant patients, in large amounts, or for prolonged periods of time.

Nursing Mothers: It is not known whether topical administration of corticosteroids could result in sufficient systemic absorption to produce detectable quantities in breast milk. Systemically administered corticosteroids are secreted into breast milk in quantities not likely to have a deleterious effect on the infant. Nevertheless, caution should be exercised when topical corticosteroids are administered to a nursing woman.

Pediatric Use: Pediatric patients may demonstrate greater susceptibility to topical corticosteroid-induced HPA axis suppression and Cushing's syndrome than mature patients because of a larger skin surface area to body weight ratio.

Hypothalamic-pituitary-adrenal (HPA) axis suppression, Cushing's syndrome and intracranial hypertension have been reported in children receiving topical corticosteroids. Manifestations of adrenal suppression in children include linear growth retardation, delayed weight gain, low plasma cortisol levels and absence of response to ACTH stimulation. Manifestations of intracranial hypertension include bulging fontanelles, headaches and bilateral papilledema.

Administration of topical corticosteroids to children should be limited to the least amount compatible with an effective therapeutic regimen. Chronic corticosteroid therapy may interfere with the growth and development of children.

ADVERSE REACTIONS

The following local adverse reactions are reported infrequently with topical corticosteroids, but may occur more frequently with the use of occlusive dressings. These reactions are listed in an approximate decreasing order of occurrence:

Burning	Perioral dermatitis
Itching	Allergic contact dermatitis
Irritation	Maceration of the skin
Dryness	Secondary infection
Folliculitis	Skin atrophy
Hypertrichosis	Striae
Acneiform eruptions	Miliaria
Hypopigmentation	

OVERDOSAGE

Topically applied corticosteroids can be absorbed in sufficient amounts to produce systemic effects (see PRECAUTIONS).

DOSAGE AND ADMINISTRATION

Aeroseb-HC® (hydrocortisone) should be applied to the affected area two or three times daily depending on the severity of the condition.

Occlusive dressings may be used for management of psoriasis or recalcitrant conditions.

If an infection develops, the use of occlusive dressings should be discontinued and appropriate antimicrobial therapy instituted.

For use on the scalp: Apply to dry scalp after shampoo. Shake well before spraying.

1. Hold aerosol upright. Slide applicator tube under the hair so that it touches scalp. Spray while moving tube to all affected areas, keeping tube under hair and in contact with scalp throughout treatment. Spraying should take 1 to 2 seconds.
2. If some areas of the scalp are not covered adequately, they may be "spot" sprayed by sliding applicator tube through hair to touch scalp— press and immediately release spray button.
3. It is unnecessary to massage medication into the scalp.
4. Be sure that the tip of the applicator tube stops at the hairline so that forehead and eyes are not sprayed.

For other dermatoses: Remove applicator tube. Shake well before spraying. Hold the can upright, approximately six inches from the area to be treated. Spray each four-inch square of affected area for one or two seconds, two or three times a day.

Note: For best results and to avoid wasting medication, it is important to follow the application instructions carefully (application instructions appear on the carton; however, it is preferable that the physician demonstrate the proper application method to the patient).

CAUTION

Flammable. Do not spray near flame or heated surfaces. If medication accidentally gets in the eyes, wash thoroughly with water and contact physician immediately. Keep out of the reach of children. Contents under pressure. Do not puncture, incinerate, or expose to temperatures above 120°F.

HOW SUPPLIED

In a 58 g aerosol with applicator tube.* On prescription only.
*U.S. Patent 3,730,182

AQUACARE®
Dry Skin Cream, 2% Urea

(See 1987 PDR For Nonprescription Drugs)

AQUACARE®
Dry Skin Lotion

(See 1987 PDR For Nonprescription Drugs)

AQUACARE/HP®
Dry Skin Cream and Lotion, 10% Urea

(See 1987 PDR For Nonprescription Drugs)

AQUATAR®
Therapeutic Tar Gel

(See 1987 PDR For Nonprescription Drugs)

BLUBORO® Powder
Astringent Soaking Solution

(See 1987 PDR For Nonprescription Drugs)

CLEAR BY DESIGN®
Acne Skin Medication

(See 1987 PDR For Nonprescription Drugs)

DANEX®
Protein Enriched Dandruff Shampoo

(See 1987 PDR For Nonprescription Drugs)

ERYMAX® ℞
(erythromycin) 2% Topical Solution, USP

DESCRIPTION

Erythromycin is an antibiotic produced from a strain of **Streptomyces erythraeus.** It is basic and readily forms salts with acids.

Contains: erythromycin .... 2% (20 mg/mL)
with: SD Alcohol 40-2 (66%), propylene glycol, and citric acid.

ACTION

Although the mechanism by which Erymax Topical Solution acts in reducing inflammatory lesions of acne vulgaris is unknown, it is presumably due to its antibiotic action.

INDICATIONS
Erymax Topical Solution is indicated for the topical control of acne vulgaris.

CONTRAINDICATIONS
Erymax Topical Solution is contraindicated in persons who have shown hypersensitivity to erythromycin or any of the other listed ingredients.

WARNING
The safe use of Erymax Topical Solution during pregnancy or lactation has not been established.

PRECAUTIONS
General: The use of antibiotic agents may be associated with the overgrowth of antibiotic-resistant organisms. If this occurs, administration of this drug should be discontinued and appropriate measures taken.
Information for patients: Erymax Topical Solution is for external use only and should be kept away from the eyes, nose, mouth and other mucous membranes. Concomitant topical acne therapy should be used with caution because a cumulative irritancy effect may occur, especially with the use of peeling, desquamating or abrasive agents.
Carcinogenesis, Mutagenesis, Impairment of Fertility: Long-term animal studies to evaluate carcinogenic potential, mutagenicity or the effect on fertility of erythromycin have not been performed.
Pregnancy: Pregnancy Category C: Animal reproduction studies have not been conducted with erythromycin. It is also not known whether erythromycin can cause fetal harm when administered to a pregnant woman or can affect reproduction capacity. Erythromycin should be given to a pregnant woman only if clearly needed.
Nursing Mothers: Erythromycin is excreted in breast milk. Caution should be exercised when erythromycin is administered to a nursing woman.

ADVERSE REACTIONS
Adverse conditions reported include dryness, tenderness, pruritus, desquamation, erythema, oiliness, and burning sensation. Irritation of the eyes has also been reported. A case of generalized urticarial reaction, possibly related to the drug, which required the use of systemic steroid therapy, has been reported.

DOSAGE AND ADMINISTRATION
Erymax Topical Solution should be applied to the affected area(s) each morning and evening after the skin is thoroughly washed with warm water and soap and patted dry. Use enough solution to thoroughly wet the affected area(s). The hands should be washed after application.
When using the Dab-O-Matic applicator (accompanying the 2 fl oz size only) to apply Erymax Topical Solution, it should be moistened first by holding the bottle upside down and pressing once on the applicator surface with a clean finger. Then Erymax can be applied with the applicator to the affected area(s) using a dabbing motion. The bottle should be closed tightly after each use.

HOW SUPPLIED
Erymax® Topical Solution, USP is supplied in a 2 fl oz plastic bottle with optional Dab-O-Matic applicator and a 4 fl oz plastic bottle:
2 fl oz (59 mL)—NDC 0023-0540-02
4 fl oz (118 mL)—NDC 0023-0540-04
Note: Store in tight, light-resistant container at controlled room temperature (59°–86°F).

CAUTION
Federal law prohibits dispensing without prescription.

EXSEL® ℞
(selenium sulfide) 2.5%
Lotion

DESCRIPTION
Exsel (selenium sulfide) Lotion is an antiseborrheic and antifungal preparation for dermatological use. Selenium sulfide has the formula SeS_2 and a molecular weight of 143.08.
Contains:
selenium sulfide 2.5%
with: edetate disodium; bentonite; sodium dodecylbenzene sulfonate; sodium C14-16 olefin sulfonate; glyceryl ricinoleate; dimethicone copolyol; titanium dioxide; citric acid monohydrate; sodium phosphate monobasic, monohydrate; fragrance; and purified water.

CLINICAL PHARMACOLOGY
Selenium sulfide appears to have a cytostatic effect on cells of the epidermis and follicular epithelium, thus reducing corneocyte production.

INDICATIONS AND USAGE
Selenium sulfide is indicated in the treatment of seborrheic dermatitis of the scalp, including dandruff, and for the treatment of tinea versicolor.

CONTRAINDICATIONS
This product should not be used by patients who are allergic to any of its components.

WARNING
Chemical conjunctivitis may result if this preparation comes in contact with the eyes.

PRECAUTIONS
General: This product should be used with caution when acute inflammation or exudation is present as an increase in absorption may occur. When applied to the body for treatment of tinea versicolor, Exsel may produce skin irritation especially in the genital area and where skin folds occur. These areas should be thoroughly rinsed after application.
Information for Patients: Application to the skin or scalp may produce skin irritation or sensitization. If sensitivity reactions occur, use should be discontinued. May be irritating to mucous membranes of the eyes and contact with this area should be avoided.
Carcinogenesis: Studies in mice using dermal application of 25% and 50% solutions of 2.5% selenium sulfide lotion over an 88-week period indicated no carcinogenic effects.
Pregnancy Category C: Animal reproduction studies have not been conducted with selenium sulfide. It is not known whether selenium sulfide can cause fetal harm when administered to a pregnant woman or can affect reproduction capacity. Under ordinary circumstances, Exsel should not be used for treatment of tinea versicolor in pregnant women.
Pediatric Use: Safety and effectiveness in children have not been established.

ADVERSE REACTIONS
In decreasing order of severity: Skin irritation; occasional reports of increase in amount of normal hair loss; discoloration of hair (can be avoided or minimized by thorough rinsing of hair after treatment). As with other shampoos, oiliness or dryness of the hair and scalp may occur.

OVERDOSAGE
Accidental Oral Ingestion: There have been no documented reports of serious toxicity in humans resulting from acute ingestion of selenium sulfide lotion. However, acute toxicity studies in animals suggest the ingestion of large amounts could result in potential human toxicity. For this reason, evacuation of the stomach contents should be considered in case of acute oral ingestion.

DOSAGE AND ADMINISTRATION
SHAKE WELL BEFORE USING. Keep tightly closed. Remove jewelry before use.
For the treatment of dandruff or seborrheic dermatitis of the scalp:
1. Massage about 1 or 2 teaspoonsful of the medicated shampoo into the wet scalp. Avoid contact with eyes.
2. Allow product to remain on the scalp for 2 to 3 minutes.
3. Rinse scalp thoroughly.
4. Repeat application and rinse thoroughly.
5. After treatment, wash hands well.
6. Repeat treatments as directed by physician.

For the usual case, two applications each week for two weeks will afford control. After this, the lotion may be used at less frequent intervals—weekly, every two weeks, or even every 3 or 4 weeks in some cases. The preparation should not be applied more frequently than required to maintain control of symptoms.
For the treatment of tinea versicolor:
1. Apply a sufficient amount of lotion to cover affected areas of the body. Avoid contact with the eyes or genital region.
2. Lather well.
3. Allow product to remain on the skin for 10 minutes.
4. Rinse thoroughly in the shower.
5. After treatment, wash hands well.
6. Follow this procedure once daily for seven successive days.

Additional courses of treatment should be employed only in cases of persistence or recurrence of infection.

HOW SUPPLIED
In 4 oz plastic bottles. On prescription only. Protect from heat. For external use only. Keep out of the reach of children. NDC 0023-0817-99

FLUONID® ℞
(fluocinolone acetonide)
Cream 0.025%
Ointment 0.025%
Topical Solution 0.01%

DESCRIPTION
The topical corticosteroids constitute a class of primarily synthetic steroids used as anti-inflammatory and antipruritic agents.
Chemical Name: Pregna-1, 4-diene-3, 20-dione, 6,9-difluoro-11,21-dihydroxy-16,17-[(1-methylethylidene)-bis(oxy)]-, (6α, 11β,16α)-.
Fluonid Cream contains:
fluocinolone acetonide 0.025%
with: methylparaben, propylparaben, stearic acid, propylene glycol, sorbitan monostearate, sorbitan monooleate, polyoxyethylene sorbitan monostearate, citric acid and purified water.
Fluonid Ointment contains:
fluocinolone acetonide 0.025%
in white petrolatum.
Fluonid Topical Solution contains:
fluocinolone acetonide 0.01%
with: propylene glycol and citric acid.

CLINICAL PHARMACOLOGY
Topical corticosteroids share anti-inflammatory, antipruritic and vasoconstrictive actions.
The mechanism of anti-inflammatory activity of the topical corticosteroids is unclear. Various laboratory methods, including vasoconstrictor assays, are used to compare and predict potencies and/or clinical efficacies of the topical corticosteroids. There is some evidence to suggest that a recognizable correlation exists between vasoconstrictor potency and therapeutic efficacy in man.
Pharmacokinetics: The extent of percutaneous absorption of topical corticosteroids is determined by many factors, including the vehicle, the integrity of the epidermal barrier and the use of occlusive dressings.
Topical corticosteroids can be absorbed from normal intact skin. Inflammation and/or other disease processes in the skin increase percutaneous absorption. Occlusive dressings substantially increase the percutaneous absorption of topical corticosteroids. Thus, occlusive dressings may be a valuable therapeutic adjunct for treatment of resistant dermatoses (see DOSAGE AND ADMINISTRATION).
Once absorbed through the skin, topical corticosteroids are handled through pharmacokinetic pathways similar to systemically-administered corticosteroids. Corticosteroids are bound to plasma proteins in varying degrees. Corticosteroids are metabolized primarily in the liver and are then excreted by the kidneys. Some of the topical corticosteroids and their metabolites are also excreted into the bile.

INDICATIONS AND USAGE
Topical corticosteroids are indicated for the relief of the inflammatory and pruritic manifestations of corticosteroid-responsive dermatoses. Fluonid Cream 0.025% is useful in corticosteroid-responsive dermatoses that require a mid-potency corticosteroid.
Fluonid Ointment 0.025% is useful in such conditions as atopic dermatitis where an emollient effect is desired.
Fluonid Topical Solution 0.01% is useful in hairy sites such as the scalp, particularly in treating seborrheic dermatitis.

CONTRAINDICATIONS
Topical corticosteroids are contraindicated in those patients with a history of hypersensitivity to any of the components of the preparation.

PRECAUTIONS
General: Systemic absorption of topical corticosteroids has produced reversible hypothalamic-pituitary-adrenal (HPA) axis suppression, manifestations of Cushing's syndrome, hyperglycemia and glucosuria in some patients.
Conditions which augment systemic absorption include the application of more potent steroids, use over large surface areas, prolonged use and the addition of occlusive dressings.
Therefore, patients receiving a large dose of a potent topical steroid applied to a large surface area or under an occlusive dressing should be evaluated periodically for evidence of HPA axis suppression by using the urinary-free cortisol and ACTH stimulation tests. If HPA axis suppression is noted, an attempt should be made to withdraw the drug, to reduce the frequency of application, or to substitute a less potent steroid.
Recovery of HPA axis function is generally prompt and complete upon discontinuation of the drug. Infrequently, signs and symptoms of steroid withdrawal may occur, requiring supplemental systemic corticosteroids.
Children may absorb proportionally larger amounts of topical corticosteroids and thus be more susceptible to systemic toxicity (see PRECAUTIONS—Pediatric Use).
If irritation develops, topical corticosteroids should be discontinued and appropriate therapy instituted.
In the presence of dermatological infections, the use of an appropriate antifungal or antibacterial agent should be instituted. If a favorable response does not occur promptly, the corticosteroid should be discontinued until the infection has been adequately controlled.
Information for the Patient: Patients using topical corticosteroids should receive the following information and instructions:
1. This medication is to be used as directed by the physician. It is for external use only. Avoid contact with the eyes.
2. Patients should be advised not to use this medication for any disorder other than for which it was prescribed.

Continued on next page

Herbert—Cont.

3. The treated skin area should not be bandaged or otherwise covered or wrapped as to be occlusive unless directed by the physician.
4. Patients should report any signs of local adverse reactions, especially under occlusive dressing.
5. Parents of pediatric patients should be advised not to use tight-fitting diapers or plastic pants on a child being treated in the diaper area, as these garments may constitute occlusive dressings.

Laboratory Tests: The urinary-free cortisol test and the ACTH stimulation test may be helpful in evaluating the HPA axis suppression.

Carcinogenesis, Mutagenesis, Impairment of Fertility: Long-term animal studies have not been performed to evaluate the carcinogenic potential or the effect of topical corticosteroids on fertility.

Studies to determine mutagenicity with prednisolone and hydrocortisone have revealed negative results.

Pregnancy Category C: Corticosteroids are generally teratogenic in laboratory animals when administered systemically at relatively low dosage levels. The more potent corticosteroids have been shown to be teratogenic after dermal application in laboratory animals. There are no adequate and well-controlled studies in pregnant women on teratogenic effects from topically applied corticosteroids. Therefore, topical corticosteroids should be used during pregnancy only if the potential benefit justifies the potential risk to the fetus. Drugs of this class should not be used extensively on pregnant patients, in large amounts, or for prolonged periods of time.

Nursing Mothers: It is not known whether topical administration of corticosteroids could result in sufficient systemic absorption to produce detectable quantities in breast milk. Systemically administered corticosteroids are secreted into breast milk in quantities not likely to have a deleterious effect on the infant. Nevertheless, caution should be exercised when topical corticosteroids are administered to a nursing woman.

Pediatric Use: Pediatric patients may demonstrate greater susceptibility to topical corticosteroid-induced HPA axis suppression and Cushing's syndrome than mature patients because of a larger skin surface area to body weight ratio.

Hypothalamic-pituitary-adrenal (HPA) axis suppression, Cushing's syndrome and intracranial hypertension have been reported in children receiving topical corticosteroids. Manifestations of adrenal suppression in children include linear growth retardation, delayed weight gain, low plasma cortisol levels and absence of response to ACTH stimulation. Manifestations of intracranial hypertension include bulging fontanelles, headaches and bilateral papilledema.

Administration of topical corticosteroids to children should be limited to the least amount compatible with an effective therapeutic regimen. Chronic corticosteroid therapy may interfere with the growth and development of children.

ADVERSE REACTIONS

The following adverse reactions are reported infrequently with topical corticosteroids, but may occur more frequently with the use of occlusive dressings. These reactions are listed in an approximate decreasing order of occurrence:

Burning	Perioral dermatitis
Itching	Allergic contact dermatitis
Irritation	Maceration of the skin
Dryness	Secondary infection
Folliculitis	Skin atrophy
Hypertrichosis	Striae
Acneiform eruptions	Miliaria
Hypopigmentation	

OVERDOSAGE

Topically applied corticosteroids can be absorbed in sufficient amounts to produce systemic effects (see PRECAUTIONS).

DOSAGE AND ADMINISTRATION

Fluonid® (fluocinolone acetonide) Cream 0.025% should be applied to the affected area three to four times daily depending on the severity of the condition.

Fluonid® Cream 0.025% may be used over long periods of time in specific conditions when deemed necessary. The cream should be massaged in gently and thoroughly until it disappears. Fluonid Ointment 0.025% should be applied to the affected area two to three times daily depending on the severity of the condition. Where an emollient effect is desired, as in atopic dermatitis, Fluonid Ointment 0.025% may be preferred. Fluonid Topical Solution 0.01% should be applied to the affected area two to four times daily depending on the severity of the condition.

Fluonid Topical Solution should be applied directly on the lesion, taking note that small quantities are adequate. It should be rubbed in thoroughly but gently at each application. In hairy sites, the hair should be parted to allow direct contact with the lesion.

In some cases treated with Fluonid Topical Solution, it has been observed that saprophytic or low-grade infections may clear spontaneously as the skin recovers its integrity under the influence of Fluonid Topical Solution alone. This may be partially attributed to the inherent antimicrobial activity of the solution base, propylene glycol.

Occlusive dressings may be used for the management of psoriasis or recalcitrant conditions.

If an infection develops, the use of occlusive dressings should be discontinued and appropriate antimicrobial therapy instituted.

HOW SUPPLIED

Fluonid (fluocinolone acetonide)

Cream 0.025%—15 g and 60 g collapsible tubes. 15 g NDC 0023-0873-15; 60 g NDC 0023-0873-60.

Ointment 0.025%—15 g and 60 g collapsible tubes. 15 g NDC 0023-0876-15; 60 g NDC 0023-0876-60.

Topical Solution 0.01%—20 mL and 60 mL plastic squeeze bottles. 20 mL NDC 0023-0878-20; 60 mL NDC 0023-0878-60.

These preparations are available on prescription only.

Note: Store solution at room temperature. Protect from freezing. Store cream and ointment at controlled room temperature (59°-86°F).

FLUOROPLEX® ℞

(fluorouracil)
1% Topical Cream
and 1% Topical Solution

DESCRIPTION

Fluoroplex (fluorouracil) 1% Topical Cream and 1% Topical Solution are antineoplastic/antimetabolite products for dermatological use. Fluorouracil has the empirical formula $C_4H_3FN_2O_2$ and a molecular weight of 130.08. The pH is approximately 8.5 for Fluoroplex Topical Cream and 9.2 for Fluoroplex Topical Solution.

Chemical Name

2,4(1H,3H)-Pyrimidinedione, 5-fluoro-.

Fluoroplex 1% Topical Cream contains:

fluorouracil 1.0%

with: benzyl alcohol, emulsifying wax, mineral oil, isopropyl myristate, sodium hydroxide and purified water.

Fluoroplex 1% Topical Solution contains:

fluorouracil 1.0%

with: propylene glycol, sodium hydroxide and/or hydrochloric acid to adjust the pH, and purified water.

CLINICAL PHARMACOLOGY

There is evidence that fluorouracil (or its metabolites) blocks the methylation reaction of deoxyuridylic acid to thymidylic acid. In this fashion, fluorouracil interferes with the synthesis of deoxyribonucleic acid (DNA) and to a lesser extent inhibits the formation of ribonucleic acid (RNA).

INDICATIONS AND USAGE

Fluoroplex is indicated for the topical treatment of multiple actinic (solar) keratoses.

CONTRAINDICATIONS

These products should not be used by patients who are allergic to any of their components.

WARNINGS

There exists the potential for a delayed hypersensitivity reaction to 5-fluorouracil. Patch testing to prove hypersensitivity may be inconclusive.[1]

If an occlusive dressing is used, there may be an increase in the incidence of inflammatory reactions in the adjacent normal skin.

The patient should avoid prolonged exposure to sunlight or other forms of ultraviolet irradiation during treatment with Fluoroplex, as the intensity of the reaction may be increased.

PRECAUTIONS

General: To rule out the presence of a frank neoplasm, a biopsy should be made of those areas failing to respond to treatment or recurring after treatment.

Information for patients: The medication should be applied with care near the eyes, nose and mouth. Excessive reaction in these areas may occur due to irritation from accumulation of drug.

The reaction to Fluoroplex in treated areas may be unsightly during therapy, and, in some cases, for several weeks following cessation of therapy.

Carcinogenesis, mutagenesis, impairment of fertility: No studies have been conducted in animals or in humans to evaluate the potential of these effects.

Pregnancy Category C: Fluorouracil has been shown to be teratogenic in mice and rats when injected intraperitoneally in doses of 20 mg/Kg and above on day 9, 10, 11, 12, or 13 of gestation. There are no adequate and well-controlled studies in pregnant women. Fluorouracil should be used during pregnancy only if the potential benefit justifies the potential risk to the fetus.

Nursing Mothers: It is not known whether this drug is excreted in human milk. Because many drugs are excreted in human milk, caution should be exercised when fluorouracil is administered to a nursing woman.

Pediatric use: Safety and effectiveness in children have not been established.

ADVERSE REACTIONS

Pain, pruritus, burning, irritation, inflammation, allergic contact dermatitis and telangiectasia have been reported. Occasionally, hyperpigmentation and scarring have also been reported.

OVERDOSAGE

Ordinarily, overdosage will not cause acute problems. If Fluoroplex accidentally comes in contact with the eye(s), flush the eye(s) with water or normal saline. If Fluoroplex is accidentally ingested, induce emesis and gastric lavage. Administer symptomatic and supportive care as needed.

DOSAGE AND ADMINISTRATION

The patient should be instructed to apply sufficient medication to cover the entire face or other affected areas.

Apply medication twice daily with nonmetallic applicator or fingertips and wash hands afterwards. A treatment period of 2-6 weeks is usually required.

Increasing the frequency of application and a longer period of administration with Fluoroplex® may be required on areas other than the head and neck.

When Fluoroplex is applied to keratotic skin, a response occurs with the following sequence: erythema, usually followed by scaling, tenderness, erosion, ulceration, necrosis and re-epithelization. When the inflammatory reaction reaches the erosion, ulceration and necrosis stages, the use of the drug should be terminated. Responses may sometimes occur in areas which appear clinically normal. These may be sites of subclinical actinic (solar) keratoses which the medication is affecting.

HOW SUPPLIED

Fluoroplex (fluorouracil) 1% Topical Solution is available in 30 mL plastic dropper bottles (NDC 0023-0810-30). On prescription only. Fluoroplex (fluorouracil) 1% Topical Cream is available in 30 g tubes (NDC 0023-0812-30). On prescription only.

Avoid freezing.

Store at controlled room temperature (59°-86°F).

Reference:

1. Epstein E. Testing for 5-fluorouracil allergy: patch and intradermal tests. Contact Dermatitis 1984; 10:311.

Gris-PEG® ℞

(griseofulvin ultramicrosize)
Tablets, USP
125 mg; 250 mg

DESCRIPTION

Gris-PEG Tablets contain ultramicrosize crystals of griseofulvin, an antibiotic derived from a species of *Penicillium.*

Each Gris-PEG Tablet contains:

griseofulvin ultramicrosize .... 125 mg

with: lactose; magnesium stearate; methylcellulose; methylparaben; polyethylene glycol 400 and 8000; polyvinylpolypyrrolidone; polyvinylpyrrolidone; silicon dioxide, colloidal; and titanium dioxide,

or

griseofulvin ultramicrosize .... 250 mg

with: magnesium stearate; methylcellulose; methylparaben; polyethylene glycol 400 and 8000; polyvinylpyrrolidone; silicon dioxide, colloidal; sodium lauryl sulfate; and titanium dioxide.

ACTION

Microbiology—Griseofulvin is fungistatic with *in vitro* activity against various species of *Microsporum, Epidermophyton* and *Trichophyton.* It has no effect on bacteria or other genera of fungi.

Human Pharmacology—Following oral administration, griseofulvin is deposited in the keratin precursor cells and has a greater affinity for diseased tissue. The drug is tightly bound to the new keratin which becomes highly resistant to fungal invasions.

The efficiency of gastrointestinal absorption of ultramicrocrystalline griseofulvin is approximately one and one-half times that of the conventional microsize griseofulvin. This factor permits the oral intake of two-thirds as much ultramicrocrystalline griseofulvin as the microsize form. However, there is currently no evidence that this lower dose confers any significant clinical differences with regard to safety and/or efficacy.

INDICATIONS

Gris-PEG (griseofulvin ultramicrosize) is indicated for the treatment of the following ringworm infections: tinea corporis (ringworm of the body). tinea pedis (athlete's foot), tinea cruris (ringworm of the groin and thigh), tinea barbae (barber's itch), tinea capitis (ringworm of the scalp), and tinea unguium (onychomycosis, ringworm of the nails), when caused by one or more of the following genera of fungi: *Tri-*

chophyton rubrum, Trichophyton tonsurans, Trichophyton mentagrophytes, Trichophyton interdigitalis, Trichophyton verrucosum, Trichophyton megnini, Trichophyton gallinae, Trichophyton crateriform, Trichophyton sulphureum, Trichophyton schoenleini, Microsporum audouini, Microsporum canis, Microsporum gypseum and *Epidermophyton floccosum.* Note: Prior to therapy, the type of fungi responsible for the infection should be identified. The use of the drug is not justified in minor or trivial infections which will respond to topical agents alone. Griseofulvin is *not* effective in the following: bacterial infections, candidiasis (moniliasis), histoplasmosis, actinomycosis, sporotrichosis, chromoblastomycosis, coccidioidomycosis, North American blastomycosis, cryptococcosis (torulosis), tinea versicolor and nocardiosis.

CONTRAINDICATIONS

This drug is contraindicated in patients with porphyria or hepatocellular failure and in individuals with a history of hypersensitivity to griseofulvin.

WARNINGS

Prophylactic Usage—Safety and efficacy of griseofulvin for prophylaxis of fungal infections has not been established. *Animal Toxicology*—Chronic feeding of griseofulvin, at levels ranging from 0.5%–2.5% of the diet resulted in the development of liver tumors in several strains of mice, particularly in males. Smaller particle sizes result in an enhanced effect. Lower oral dosage levels have not been tested. Subcutaneous administration of relatively small doses of griseofulvin once a week during the first three weeks of life has also been reported to induce hepatomata in mice. Thyroid tumors, mostly adenomas but some carcinomas, have been reported in male rats receiving griseofulvin at levels of 2.0%, 1.0% and 0.2% of the diet, and in female rats receiving the two higher dose levels. Although studies in other animal species have not yielded evidence of tumorigenicity, these studies were not of adequate design to form a basis for conclusion in this regard. In subacute toxicity studies, orally administered griseofulvin produced hepatocellular necrosis in mice, but this has not been seen in other species. Disturbances in porphyrin metabolism have been reported in griseofulvin-treated laboratory animals. Griseofulvin has been reported to have a colchicine-like effect on mitosis and cocarcinogenicity with methylcholanthrene in cutaneous tumor induction in laboratory animals. *Usage in Pregnancy*—The safety of this drug during pregnancy has not been established. *Animal Reproduction Studies*—It has been reported in the literature that griseofulvin was found to be embryotoxic and teratogenic on oral administration to pregnant rats. Pups with abnormalities have been reported in the litters of a few bitches treated with griseofulvin. Suppression of spermatogenesis has been reported to occur in rats, but investigation in man failed to confirm this.

PRECAUTIONS

Patients on prolonged therapy with any potent medication should be under close observation. Periodic monitoring of organ system function, including renal, hepatic and hematopoietic, should be done. Since griseofulvin is derived from species of *Penicillium,* the possibility of cross-sensitivity with penicillin exists; however, known penicillin-sensitive patients have been treated without difficulty. Since a photosensitivity reaction is occasionally associated with griseofulvin therapy, patients should be warned to avoid exposure to intense natural or artificial sunlight. Lupus erythematosus or lupus-like syndromes have been reported in patients receiving griseofulvin. Griseofulvin decreases the activity of warfarin-type anticoagulants so that patients receiving these drugs concomitantly may require dosage adjustment of the anticoagulant during and after griseofulvin therapy. Barbiturates usually depress griseofulvin activity and concomitant administration may require a dosage adjustment of the antifungal agent. There have been reports in the literature of possible interactions between griseofulvin and oral contraceptives. The effect of alcohol may be potentiated by griseofulvin, producing such effects as tachycardia and flush.

ADVERSE REACTIONS

When adverse reactions occur, they are most commonly of the hypersensitivity type such as skin rashes, urticaria, and rarely, angioneurotic edema, and may necessitate withdrawal of therapy and appropriate countermeasures. Paresthesias of the hands and feet have been reported rarely after extended therapy. Other side effects reported occasionally are oral thrush, nausea, vomiting, epigastric distress, diarrhea, headache, fatigue, dizziness, insomnia, mental confusion, and impairment of performance of routine activities. Proteinuria and leukopenia have been reported rarely. Administration of the drug should be discontinued if granulocytopenia occurs. When rare, serious reactions occur with griseofulvin, they are usually associated with high dosages, long periods of therapy or both.

DOSAGE AND ADMINISTRATION

Accurate diagnosis of the infecting organism is essential. Identification should be made either by direct microscopic examination of a mounting of infected tissue in a solution of potassium hydroxide or by culture on an appropriate medium. Medication must be continued until the infecting organism is completely eradicated as indicated by appropriate clinical or laboratory examination. Representative treatment periods are tinea capitis, 4 to 6 weeks; tinea corporis, 2 to 4 weeks; tinea pedis, 4 to 8 weeks; tinea unguium—depending on rate of growth—fingernails, at least 4 months; toenails, at least 6 months.

General measures in regard to hygiene should be observed to control sources of infection or reinfection. Concomitant use of appropriate topical agents is usually required, particularly in treatment of tinea pedis. In some forms of athlete's foot, yeasts and bacteria may be involved as well as fungi. Griseofulvin will not eradicate the bacterial or monilial infection.

Adults: Daily administration of 375 mg (as a single dose or in divided doses) will give a satisfactory response in most patients with tinea corporis, tinea cruris and tinea capitis. For those fungal infections more difficult to eradicate, such as tinea pedis and tinea unguium, a divided dose of 750 mg is recommended.

Children: Approximately 3.3 mg per pound of body weight per day of ultramicrosize griseofulvin is an effective dose for most children. On this basis, the following dosage schedule is suggested: Children weighing 35–60 pounds—125 mg to 187.5 mg daily. Children weighing over 60 pounds—187.5 mg to 375 mg daily. Children 2 years of age and younger—dosage has not been established.

Clinical experience with griseofulvin in children with tinea capitis indicates that a single daily dose is effective. Clinical relapse will occur if the medication is not continued until the infecting organism is eradicated.

HOW SUPPLIED

Gris-PEG® (griseofulvin ultramicrosize) Tablets, 125 mg, white, scored, elliptical-shaped, embossed "Gris-PEG" on one side and "125" on the other. Gris-PEG (griseofulvin ultramicrosize) Tablets, 250 mg, white, scored, capsule-shaped, embossed "Gris-PEG" on one side and "250" on the other. The 125 mg strength is available in bottles of 100 and 500 (NDC 0023-0763-04 and NDC 0023-0763-99, respectively). The 250 mg strength is available in bottles of 100 and 500 (NDC 0023-0773-04 and NDC 0023-0773-50, respectively). Both strengths are film-coated.

Storage: Store Gris-PEG® (griseofulvin ultramicrosize) tablets at controlled room temperature 15°–30°C (59°–86°F) in tight, light-resistant containers.

CAUTION

Federal law prohibits dispensing without prescription.

MAXIFLOR® ℞

(diflorasone diacetate)
Cream, USP, 0.05%
Ointment, USP, 0.05%

DESCRIPTION

Each gram of MAXIFLOR Cream and MAXIFLOR Ointment contains 0.5 mg diflorasone diacetate, USP, in a cream or ointment base.

Chemically, diflorasone diacetate is: 6α,9-Difluoro-11β, 17, 21-trihydroxy-16β-methylpregna-1, 4-diene-3,20-dione 17,21-diacetate.

MAXIFLOR Cream contains diflorasone diacetate, USP, in an emulsified and hydrophilic cream base consisting of propylene glycol, stearic acid, polysorbate 60, sorbitan monostearate and monooleate, sorbic acid, citric acid and water. The corticosteroid is formulated as a solution in the vehicle using 15 percent propylene glycol to optimize drug delivery.

MAXIFLOR Ointment contains diflorasone diacetate, USP, in an emollient, occlusive base consisting of polyoxypropylene 15-stearyl ether, stearic acid, lanolin alcohol and white petrolatum.

CLINICAL PHARMACOLOGY

Topical corticosteroids share anti-inflammatory, antipruritic and vasoconstrictive actions.

The mechanism of anti-inflammatory activity of the topical corticosteroids is unclear. Various laboratory methods, including vasoconstrictor assays, are used to compare and predict potencies and/or clinical efficacies of the topical corticosteroids. There is some evidence to suggest that a recognizable correlation exists between vasoconstrictor potency and therapeutic efficacy in man.

Pharmacokinetics

The extent of percutaneous absorption of topical corticosteroids is determined by many factors including the vehicle, the integrity of the epidermal barrier, and the use of occlusive dressings.

Topical corticosteroids can be absorbed from normal intact skin. Inflammation and/or other disease processes in the skin increase percutaneous absorption. Occlusive dressings substantially increase the percutaneous absorption of topical corticosteroids. Thus, occlusive dressings may be a valuable therapeutic adjunct for treatment of resistant dermatoses. (See DOSAGE AND ADMINISTRATION.)

Once absorbed through the skin, topical corticosteroids are handled through pharmacokinetic pathways similar to systemically-administered corticosteroids. Corticosteroids are bound to plasma proteins in varying degrees. They are metabolized primarily in the liver and are then excreted by the kidneys. Some of the topical corticosteroids and their metabolites are also excreted into the bile.

INDICATIONS AND USAGE

Topical corticosteroids are indicated for relief of the inflammatory and pruritic manifestations of corticosteroid-responsive dermatoses.

CONTRAINDICATIONS

Topical steroids are contraindicated in those patients with a history of hypersensitivity to any of the components of the preparation.

PRECAUTIONS

Not For Ophthalmic Use

General

Systemic absorption of topical corticosteroids has produced reversible hypothalamic-pituitary-adrenal (HPA) axis suppression, manifestations of Cushing's syndrome, hyperglycemia, and glucosuria in some patients.

Conditions which augment systemic absorption include the application of the more potent steroids, use over large surface areas, prolonged use, and the addition of occlusive dressings.

Therefore, patients receiving a large dose of a potent topical steroid applied to a large surface area or under an occlusive dressing should be evaluated periodically for evidence of HPA axis suppression by using the urinary-free cortisol and ACTH stimulation tests. If HPA axis suppression is noted, an attempt should be made to withdraw the drug, to reduce the frequency of application, or to substitute a less potent steroid.

Recovery of HPA axis function is generally prompt and complete upon discontinuation of the drug. Infrequently, signs and symptoms of steroid withdrawal may occur, requiring supplemental systemic corticosteroids.

Children may absorb proportionally larger amounts of topical corticosteroids and thus be more susceptible to systemic toxicity. (See PRECAUTIONS—Pediatric Use.)

If irritation develops, topical corticosteroids should be discontinued and appropriate therapy instituted.

In the presence of dermatological infections, the use of an appropriate antifungal or antibacterial agent should be instituted. If a favorable response does not occur promptly, the corticosteroid should be discontinued until the infection has been adequately controlled.

Information for the Patient

Patients using topical corticosteroids should receive the following information and instructions:

1. This medication is to be used as directed by the physician. It is for external use only. Avoid contact with the eyes.
2. Patients should be advised not to use this medication for any disorder other than for which it was prescribed.
3. The treated skin area should not be bandaged or otherwise covered or wrapped as to be occlusive unless directed by the physician.
4. Patients should report any signs of local adverse reactions, especially under occlusive dressing.
5. Parents of pediatric patients should be advised not to use tight-fitting diapers or plastic pants on a child being treated in the diaper area, as these garments may constitute occlusive dressings.

Laboratory Tests

The following tests may be helpful in evaluating the HPA axis suppression:

Urinary-free cortisol test
ACTH stimulation test

Carcinogenesis, Mutagenesis, and Impairment of Fertility

Long-term animal studies have not been performed to evaluate the carcinogenic potential or the effect of topical corticosteroids on fertility.

Studies to determine mutagenicity with prednisolone and hydrocortisone have revealed negative results.

Pregnancy Category C

Corticosteroids are generally teratogenic in laboratory animals when administered systemically at relatively low dosage levels. The more potent corticosteroids have been shown to be teratogenic after dermal application in laboratory animals. There are no adequate and well-controlled studies in pregnant women on teratogenic effects from topically applied corticosteroids. Therefore, topical corticosteroids should be used during pregnancy only if the potential benefit justifies the potential risk to the fetus. Drugs of this class should not be used extensively on pregnant patients, in large amounts, or for prolonged periods of time.

Nursing Mothers

It is not known whether topical administration of corticosteroids could result in sufficient systemic absorption to produce detectable quantities in breast milk. Systemically-administered corticosteroids are secreted into breast milk in

Continued on next page

Herbert—Cont.

quantities *not* likely to have a deleterious effect on the infant. Nevertheless, caution should be exercised when topical corticosteroids are administered to a nursing woman.

Pediatric Use

Pediatric patients may demonstrate greater susceptibility to topical corticosteroid-induced HPA axis suppression and Cushing's syndrome than mature patients because of a larger skin surface area to body weight ratio.

Hypothalamic-pituitary-adrenal (HPA) axis suppression, Cushing's syndrome, and intracranial hypertension have been reported in children receiving topical corticosteroids. Manifestations of adrenal suppression in children include linear growth retardation, delayed weight gain, low plasma cortisol levels, and absence of response to ACTH stimulation. Manifestations of intracranial hypertension include bulging fontanelles, headaches, and bilateral papilledema.

Administration of topical corticosteroids to children should be limited to the least amount compatible with an effective therapeutic regimen. Chronic corticosteroid therapy may interfere with the growth and development of children.

ADVERSE REACTIONS

The following local adverse reactions have been reported with topical corticosteroids, but may occur more frequently with the use of occlusive dressings. These reactions are listed in an approximate decreasing order of occurrence:

Burning	Perioral dermatitis
Itching	Allergic contact dermatitis
Irritation	Maceration of the skin
Dryness	Secondary infection
Folliculitis	Skin atrophy
Hypertrichosis	Striae
Acneiform eruptions	Miliaria
Hypopigmentation	

OVERDOSAGE

Topically applied corticosteroids can be absorbed in sufficient amounts to produce systemic effects. (See PRECAUTIONS.)

DOSAGE AND ADMINISTRATION

Topical corticosteroids are generally applied to the affected area as a thin film from one to four times daily depending on the severity of the condition.

Occlusive dressings may be used for the management of psoriasis or recalcitrant conditions.

If an infection develops, the use of occlusive dressings should be discontinued and appropriate antimicrobial therapy instituted.

HOW SUPPLIED

MAXIFLOR® (diflorasone diacetate) Cream, USP, 0.05% is available in collapsible tubes in the following sizes:

15 gram NDC 0023-0766-15
30 gram NDC 0023-0766-30
60 gram NDC 0023-0766-60

MAXIFLOR® (diflorasone diacetate) Ointment, USP, 0.05% is available in collapsible tubes in the following sizes:

15 gram NDC 0023-0770-15
30 gram NDC 0023-0770-30
60 gram NDC 0023-0770-60

Store at controlled room temperature 15°-30°C (59°-86°F).

CAUTION

Federal law prohibits dispensing without prescription.

PENECORT® ℞

(hydrocortisone)
Cream, USP, 1% and 2.5%
Ointment, USP, 2.5%
Topical Solution 1%

DESCRIPTION

The topical corticosteroids constitute a class of primarily synthetic steroids used as anti-inflammatory and anti-pruritic agents.

Chemical Name: Pregn-4-ene-3,20-dione, 11,17,21, trihydroxy-,(11β)-.

PENECORT Cream contains:

hydrocortisone, USP 1%, 2.5%

with: benzyl alcohol; petrolatum; stearyl alcohol; propylene glycol; isopropyl myristate; polyoxyl 40 stearate; carbomer 934; sodium lauryl sulfate; edetate disodium; sodium hydroxide to adjust the pH; and purified water.

PENECORT Ointment contains:

hydrocortisone, USP 2.5%

in a white petrolatum base.

PENECORT Topical Solution contains:

hydrocortisone, USP 1%

with: alcohol (57%); propylene glycol; benzyl alcohol; and purified water.

CLINICAL PHARMACOLOGY

Topical corticosteroids share anti-inflammatory, antipruritic and vasoconstrictive actions.

The mechanism of anti-inflammatory activity of the topical corticosteroids is unclear. Various laboratory methods, including vasoconstrictor assays, are used to compare and predict potencies and/or clinical efficacies of the topical corticosteroids. There is some evidence to suggest that a recognizable correlation exists between vasoconstrictor potency and therapeutic efficacy in man.

Pharmacokinetics: The extent of percutaneous absorption of topical corticosteroids is determined by many factors, including the vehicle, the integrity of the epidermal barrier and the use of occlusive dressings.

Topical corticosteroids can be absorbed from normal intact skin. Inflammation and/or other disease processes in the skin increase percutaneous absorption. Occlusive dressings substantially increase the percutaneous absorption of topical corticosteroids. Thus, occlusive dressings may be a valuable therapeutic adjunct for treatment of resistant dermatoses. (See DOSAGE AND ADMINISTRATION.)

Once absorbed through the skin, topical corticosteroids are handled through pharmacokinetic pathways similar to systemically-administered corticosteroids. Corticosteroids are bound to plasma proteins in varying degrees. Corticosteroids are metabolized primarily in the liver and are then excreted by the kidneys. Some of the topical corticosteroids and their metabolites are also excreted into the bile.

INDICATIONS AND USAGE

Topical corticosteroids are indicated for the relief of the inflammatory and pruritic manifestations of corticosteroid-responsive dermatoses.

CONTRAINDICATIONS

Topical corticosteroids are contraindicated in those patients with a history of hypersensitivity to any of the components of the preparation.

PRECAUTIONS

General: Systemic absorption of topical corticosteroids has produced reversible hypothalamic-pituitary-adrenal (HPA) axis suppression, manifestations of Cushing's syndrome, hyperglycemia and glucosuria in some patients. Conditions which augment systemic absorption include the application of more potent steroids, use over large surface areas, prolonged use and the addition of occlusive dressings.

If HPA axis suppression is noted (by using the urinary-free cortisol and ACTH stimulation tests), an attempt should be made to withdraw the drug or to reduce the frequency of application.

Recovery of HPA axis function is generally prompt and complete upon discontinuation of the drug. Infrequently, signs and symptoms of steroid withdrawal may occur, requiring supplemental systemic corticosteroids.

Children may absorb proportionally larger amounts of topical corticosteroids and thus be more susceptible to systemic toxicity. (See PRECAUTIONS—Pediatric Use.)

If irritation develops, topical corticosteroids should be discontinued and appropriate therapy instituted.

In the presence of dermatological infections, the use of an appropriate antifungal or antibacterial agent should be instituted. If a favorable response does not occur promptly, the corticosteroid should be discontinued until the infection has been adequately controlled.

Information for the Patient: Patients using topical corticosteroids should receive the following information and instructions:

1. This medication is to be used as directed by the physician. It is for external use only. Avoid contact with the eyes.
2. Patients should be advised not to use this medication for any disorder other than for which it was prescribed.
3. The treated skin area should not be bandaged or otherwise covered or wrapped as to be occlusive unless directed by the physician.
4. Patients should report any signs of local adverse reactions, especially under occlusive dressing.
5. Parents of pediatric patients should be advised not to use tight-fitting diapers or plastic pants on a child being treated in the diaper area, as these garments may constitute occlusive dressings.

Laboratory Tests: The urinary-free cortisol test and the ACTH stimulation test may be helpful in evaluating the HPA axis suppression.

Carcinogenesis, Mutagenesis, Impairment of Fertility: Long-term animal studies have not been performed to evaluate the carcinogenic potential or the effect of topical corticosteroids on fertility.

Studies to determine mutagenicity with hydrocortisone have revealed negative results.

Pregnancy Category C: Corticosteroids are generally teratogenic in laboratory animals when administered systemically at relatively low dosage levels. The more potent corticosteroids have been shown to be teratogenic after dermal application in laboratory animals. There are no adequate and well-controlled studies in pregnant women on teratogenic effects from topically applied corticosteroids. Therefore, topical corticosteroids should be used during pregnancy only if the potential benefit justifies the potential risk to the fetus. Drugs of this class should not be used extensively on pregnant patients, in large amounts, or for prolonged periods of time.

Nursing Mothers: It is not known whether topical administration of corticosteroids could result in sufficient systemic absorption to produce detectable quantities in breast milk. Systemically administered corticosteroids are secreted into breast milk in quantities *not* likely to have a deleterious effect on the infant. Nevertheless, caution should be exercised when topical corticosteroids are administered to a nursing woman.

Pediatric Use: Pediatric patients may demonstrate greater susceptibility to topical corticosteroid-induced HPA axis suppression and Cushing's syndrome than mature patients because of a larger skin surface area to body weight ratio.

Hypothalamic-pituitary-adrenal (HPA) axis suppression, Cushing's syndrome and intracranial hypertension have been reported in children receiving topical corticosteroids. Manifestations of adrenal suppression in children include linear growth retardation, delayed weight gain, low plasma cortisol levels and absence of response to ACTH stimulation. Manifestations of intracranial hypertension include bulging fontanelles, headaches and bilateral papilledema.

Administration of topical corticosteroids to children should be limited to the least amount compatible with an effective therapeutic regimen. Chronic corticosteroid therapy may interfere with the growth and development of children.

ADVERSE REACTIONS

The following local adverse reactions are reported infrequently with topical corticosteroids, but may occur more frequently with the use of occlusive dressings. These reactions are listed in an approximate decreasing order of occurrence:

Burning	Perioral dermatitis
Itching	Allergic contact dermatitis
Irritation	Maceration of the skin
Dryness	Secondary infection
Folliculitis	Skin atrophy
Hypertrichosis	Striae
Acneiform eruptions	Miliaria
Hypopigmentation	

OVERDOSAGE

Topically applied corticosteroids can be absorbed in sufficient amounts to produce systemic effects. (See PRECAUTIONS.)

DOSAGE AND ADMINISTRATION

PENECORT® (hydrocortisone) 1% and 2.5% should be applied to the affected area two to four times daily, depending on the severity of the condition.

Occlusive dressings may be used for the management of psoriasis or recalcitrant conditions. If an infection develops, the use of occlusive dressings should be discontinued and appropriate antimicrobial therapy instituted.

HOW SUPPLIED

PENECORT® (hydrocortisone):

Cream, USP, 1%—30 g and 60 g collapsible tubes: 30 g NDC 0023-0510-30; 60 g NDC 0023-0510-60

Cream, USP, 2.5%—30 g collapsible tubes: NDC 0023-0550-30

Ointment, USP, 2.5%—30 g collapsible tubes: NDC 0023-0552-30

Topical Solution 1%—30 mL and 60 mL plastic bottles: 30 mL NDC 0023-0889-30; 60 mL NDC 0023-0889-60

Store away from heat. Protect cream from freezing.

These preparations are available on prescription only.

TEMARIL® ℞

(trimeprazine tartrate)
Tablets, Syrup and Spansule® capsules
(sustained release capsules)

DESCRIPTION

'Temaril', available as trimeprazine tartrate, a phenothiazine derivative is 10-[3-(dimethylamino)-2-methylpropyl]-phenothiazine tartrate.

Trimeprazine tartrate is a white to off-white odorless, crystalline powder readily soluble in water.

Tablets—Each round, gray, coated tablet is imprinted HL and T41 and contains trimeprazine tartrate equivalent to 2.5 mg of trimeprazine. Inactive ingredients consist of acacia, calcium sulfate, FD&C Yellow No. 6, gelatin, iron oxide, mineral oil, starch, stearic acid, sucrose, talc, titanium dioxide and trace amounts of other inactive ingredients.

Syrup—Each 5 ml (one teaspoonful) of clear, red, raspberry/strawberry flavored liquid contains trimeprazine tartrate equivalent to 2.5 mg of trimeprazine, and alcohol, 5.7%. Inactive ingredients consist of citric acid, FD&C Green No. 3,

FD&C Red No. 40, flavors, glycerin, saccharin sodium, sodium benzoate, sucrose and water.

Spansule® sustained release capsules—Each 'Spansule' sustained release capsule is so prepared that an initial dose is released promptly and the remaining medication is released gradually over a prolonged period. Each capsule, with opaque gray cap and natural body, is imprinted HL and T50 and contains trimeprazine tartrate equivalent to 5 mg of trimeprazine. Inactive ingredients consist of benzyl alcohol, cetylpyridinium chloride, FD&C Green No. 3, FD&C Red No. 40, FD&C Yellow No. 6, gelatin, glyceryl distearate, glyceryl monostearate, iron oxide, sodium lauryl sulfate, starch, sucrose, titanium dioxide, wax and trace amounts of other inactive ingredients.

ACTIONS

Temaril (trimeprazine tartrate), a phenothiazine, possesses antipruritic and antihistaminic properties with anticholinergic (drying) and sedative side effects.

INDICATIONS

Treatment of pruritic symptoms in urticaria. Relief of pruritic symptoms in a variety of allergic and non-allergic conditions including atopic dermatitis, neurodermatitis, contact dermatitis, pityriasis rosea, poison ivy dermatitis, eczematous dermatitis, pruritus ani and vulvae, and drug rash.

CONTRAINDICATIONS

Temaril (trimeprazine tartrate) is contraindicated: in comatose patients; in patients who have received large amounts of central nervous system depressants (alcohol, barbiturates, narcotics, etc.); in patients with bone marrow depression; in patients who have demonstrated an idiosyncrasy or hypersensitivity to 'Temaril' or other phenothiazines; in newborn or premature children; and in nursing mothers. It should not be used in children who are acutely ill and/or dehydrated, as there is an increased susceptibility to dystonias in such patients.

WARNINGS

Temaril® (trimeprazine tartrate) may impair the mental and/ or physical ability required for the performance of potentially hazardous tasks, such as driving a vehicle or operating machinery. Similarly, it may impair mental alertness in children. The concomitant use of alcohol or other central nervous system depressants may have an additive effect. Patients should be warned accordingly.

'Temaril' should be used with extreme caution in patients with:

- Asthmatic attack
- Narrow-angle glaucoma
- Prostatic hypertrophy
- Stenosing peptic ulcer
- Pyloroduodenal obstruction
- Bladder neck obstruction
- Patients receiving monoamine oxidase inhibitors

Usage in Pregnancy: The safe use of 'Temaril' has not been established with respect to the possible adverse effects upon fetal development. Therefore, it should not be used in women of childbearing potential. Jaundice and prolonged extrapyramidal symptoms have been reported in infants whose mothers received phenothiazines during pregnancy.

Usage in Children: 'Temaril' should be used with caution in children who have a history of sleep apnea or a family history of sudden infant death syndrome (SIDS). It should also be used with caution in young children, in whom it may cause excitation.

Overdosage may produce hallucinations, convulsions and sudden death.

Usage in Elderly Patients (60 years or older): Elderly patients are more prone to develop the following side effects from phenothiazines:

- Hypotension
- Syncope
- Toxic confusional states
- Extrapyramidal symptoms' especially parkinsonism
- Excessive sedation

PRECAUTIONS

Temaril (trimeprazine tartrate) may significantly affect the actions of other drugs. It may increase, prolong or intensify the sedative action of central nervous system depressants such as anesthetics, barbiturates or alcohol. When 'Temaril' is administered concomitantly the dose of a narcotic or barbiturate should be reduced to ¼ or ½ the usual amount. In the patient with pain, receiving treatment with narcotics, excessive amounts of 'Temaril' may lead to restlessness and motor hyperactivity. 'Temaril' can block and even reverse the usual pressor effect of epinephrine.

'Temaril' should be used cautiously in persons with acute or chronic respiratory impairment, particularly children, as it may suppress the cough reflex.

This drug should be used cautiously in persons with cardiovascular disease, impairment of liver function, or those with a history of ulcer disease.

Since Temaril® (trimeprazine tartrate) has a slight antiemetic action, it may obscure signs of intestinal obstruction, brain tumor, or overdosage of txoic drugs.

Phenothiazines have been shown to elevate prolactin levels; the elevation persists during chronic administration. Tissue culture experiments indicate that approximately one-third of human breast cancers are prolactin-dependent in vitro, a factor of potential importance if the prescribing of these drugs is contemplated in a patient with a previously detected breast cancer. Although disturbances such as galactorrhea, amenorrhea, gynecomastia, and impotence have been reported, the clinical significance of elevated serum prolactin levels is unknown for most patients. An increase in mammary neoplasms has been found in rodents after chronic administration of neuroleptic drugs. Neither clinical nor epidemiologic studies conducted to date, however, have shown an association between chronic administration of these drugs and mammary tumorigenesis; the available evidence is considered too limited to be conclusive at this time.

Drugs which lower the seizure threshold, including phenothiazine derivatives, should not be used with 'Amipaque'.•

As with other phenothiazine derivatives, 'Temaril' should be discontinued at least 48 hours before myelography, should not be resumed for at least 24 hours postprocedure, and should not be used for the control of nausea and vomiting occurring either prior to myelography or postprocedure.

ADVERSE REACTIONS

Temaril (trimeprazine tartrate) may produce adverse reactions attributable to both phenothiazines and antihistamines.

Note: Not all of the following adverse reactions have been reported with Temaril (trimeprazine tartrate); however, pharmacological similarities among the phenothiazine derivatives require that each be considered when 'Temaril' is administered. There have been occasional reports of sudden death in patients receiving phenothiazine derivatives chronically.

C.N.S. Effects: Drowsiness is the most common C.N.S. effect of this drug. Extrapyramidal reactions (opisthotonos, dystonia, akathisia, dyskinesia, parkinsonism) occur, particularly with high doses. (See Overdosage section for management of extrapyramidal symptoms). Hyperreflexia has been reported in the newborn when a phenothiazine was used during pregnancy. Other reported reactions include dizziness, headache, lassitude, tinnitus, incoordination, fatigue, blurred vision, euphoria, diplopia, nervousness, insomnia, tremors and grand mal seizures, excitation, catatonic-like states, neuritis and hysteria, oculogyric crises, disturbing dreams/nightmares, pseudoschizophrenia, and intensification and prolongation of the action of C.N.S. depressants (opiates, analgesics, antihistamines, barbiturates, alcohol), atropine, heat, organophosphorus insecticides.

Cardiovascular Effects: Postural hypotension is the most common cardiovascular effect of phenothiazines. Reflex tachycardia may be seen. Bradycardia, faintness, dizziness and cardiac arrest have been reported. ECG changes, including blunting of T waves and prolongation of the Q-T interval, may be seen.

Gastrointestinal: Anorexia, nausea, vomiting, epigastric distress, diarrhea, constipation, and dry mouth may occur. Increased appetite and weight gain have also been reported.

Genitourinary: Urinary frequency and dysuria, urinary retention, early menses, induced lactation, gynecomastia, decreased libido, inhibition of ejaculation and false positive pregnancy tests have been reported.

Respiratory: Thickening of bronchial secretions, tightness of the chest, wheezing and nasal stuffiness may occur.

Allergic Reactions: These include urticaria, dermatitis, asthma, laryngeal edema, angioneurotic edema, photosensitivity, lupus erythematosus-like syndrome and anaphylactoid reactions.

Other Reported Reactions: Leukopenia, agranulocytosis, pancytopenia, hemolytic anemia, elevation of plasma cholesterol levels and thrombocytopenic purpura have been reported. Jaundice of the obstructive type has also been reported, it is usually reversible but chronic jaundice has been reported. Erythema, peripheral edema, and stomatitis have been reported. High or prolonged glucose tolerance curves, glycosuria, elevated spinal fluid proteins and reversed epinephrine effects may also occur.

Rare occurrences of neuroleptic malignant syndrome (NMS) have been reported in patients receiving phenothiazines. This syndrome is comprised of the symptom complex of hyperthermia, altered consciousness, muscular rigidity and autonomic dysfunction and is potentially fatal.

Long-Term Therapy Considerations: After prolonged phenothiazine administration at high dosage, pigmentation of the skin has occurred, chiefly in the exposed areas. Ocular changes consist of the appearance of lenticular and corneal opacities, epithelial keratopathies and pigmentary retinopathy. Vision may be impaired.

DOSAGE AND ADMINISTRATION

Tablets and Syrup:

Adults: Usual dosage is 2.5 mg q.i.d.

Children over three years: Usual dosage is 2.5 mg h.s., or t.i.d. if needed.

Children 6 months to 3 years: Usual dosage is 1.25 mg (½ teaspoonful of syrup) h.s., or t.i.d. if needed.

'Spansule' capsules:

Adults: Usual daily dosage is 1 capsule q12h.

Children over 6 years of age: 1 capsule daily.

This product form is not recommended for children under 6 years of age. Use tablets or syrup for their dosage flexibility.

Because some side effects appear to be dose-related, it is important to use the lowest effective dosage.

DRUG INTERACTIONS

MAO inhibitors and thiazide diuretics prolong and intensify the anticholinergic effects of Temaril (trimeprazine tartrate). Combined use of MAO inhibitors and phenothiazines may result in hypertension and extrapyramidal reactions.

Narcotics: The C.N.S. depressant and analgesic effects of narcotics are potentiated by phenothiazines.

The following drugs may result in potentiation of phenothiazine effects:

- Oral contraceptives
- Progesterone
- Reserpine
- Nylidrin hydrochloride

MANAGEMENT OF OVERDOSAGE

Signs and symptoms of Temaril® (trimeprazine tartrate) overdosage range from mild depression of the central nervous system and cardiovascular system to profound hypotension, respiratory depression and unconsciousness. Stimulation may be evident, especially in children and geriatric patients. Atropine-like signs and symptoms—dry mouth, fixed, dilated pupils, flushing, etc.—as well as gastrointestinal symptoms may occur. The treatment of overdosage is essentially symptomatic and supportive. Early gastric lavage may be beneficial. **Do not administer emetics or attempt to induce vomiting because a dystonic reaction of the head or neck might result in aspiration of vomitus.** Extrapyramidal symptoms may be treated with anti-parkinsonism drugs, barbiturates, or 'Benadryl'.†

Avoid analeptics, which may cause convulsions. Severe hypotension usually responds to the administration of levarterenol or phenylephrine. EPINEPHRINE SHOULD NOT BE USED, since its use in a patient with partial adrenergic blockade may further lower the blood pressure. Additional measures include oxygen and intravenous fluids. Limited experience with dialysis indicates that it is not helpful.

Special note on 'Spansule' capsules—Since much of the 'Spansule' capsule medication is coated for gradual release, therapy directed at reversing the effects of the ingested drug and at supporting the patient should be continued for as long as overdosage symptoms remain. Saline cathartics are useful for hastening evacuation of pellets that have not already released medication.

HOW SUPPLIED

Tablets—2.5 mg in bottles of 100 and 1000; Single Unit Packages of 100 (intended for institutional use only).

Syrup—2.5 mg/5 mL (teaspoonful) and alcohol 5.7%, in 4 fl oz bottles.

'Spansule' capsules—5 mg in bottles of 50; Single Unit Packages of 100 (intended for institutional use only).

---

† Trademark Reg. U.S. Pat. Off.: 'Benadryl' for diphenhydramine hydrochloride, Parke-Davis.

• Trademark Reg. U.S. Pat. Off.: 'Amipaque' for metrizamide, distributed by Winthrop-Breon Laboratories.

VANSEB® Cream and Lotion
Dandruff Shampoo

(See 1987 PDR For Nonprescription Drugs)

VANSEB–T® Cream and Lotion
Tar Dandruff Shampoo

(See 1987 PDR For Nonprescription Drugs)

Dow B. Hickam, Inc.

P.O. BOX 2006
SUGAR LAND, TX 77487-2006

GRANULEX ℞

COMPOSITION

Each 0.82 cc. of medication delivered to the wound site contains Trypsin crystallized 0.1 mg., Balsam Peru 72.5 mg., Castor Oil 650.0 mg., and an emulsifier.

ACTION

Trypsin is intended for debridement of eschar and other necrotic tissue. It appears that in many instances removal of wound debris strengthens humoral defense mechanisms sufficiently to retard proliferation of local pathogens. Balsam Peru is an effective capillary bed stimulant used to increase circulation in the wound site area. Also, Balsam Peru has a mildly bactericidal action. Castor Oil is used to improve epithelialization by reducing premature epithelial desiccation and cornification. Also, it can act as a protective covering and aids in the reduction of pain.

INDICATIONS

For the treatment of decubitus ulcers, varicose ulcers, debridement of eschar, dehiscent wounds and sunburn.

USES

Granulex is in aerosol form which can be important to healing. It must be remembered, healing starts with a thin sheath of epithelium no more than a cell or two thick. Any rough movement or trauma can quickly destroy the healing tissue. Aerosols have the advantage of eliminating all extraneous physical contact with the wound. Granulex is easy to apply and quickly reduces odor frequently accompanying a decubitus ulcer. The wound may be left open or a wet bandage may be applied. As a suggestion; keep in mind wounds heal poorly in the presence of hemoglobin or zinc deficiency.

WARNING

Do not spray on fresh arterial clots. Avoid spraying in eyes. Flammable, do not expose to fire or open flame. Contents under pressure. Do not puncture or incinerate. Do not store at temperature above 120°F. Keep out of reach of children. Use only as directed. Intentional misuse by deliberately concentrating and inhaling the contents can be harmful or fatal.

DOSAGE

Apply a minimum of twice daily or as often as necessary. Shake well, press the aerosol valve and coat the wound rapidly but not excessively.

HOW SUPPLIED

2 oz. Aerosol NDC 0514-0001-01
4 oz. Aerosol NDC 0514-0001-02

High Chemical Co.

Div. Day & Frick, Inc.
1760 N. HOWARD ST.
PHILADELPHIA, PA 19122

SARAPIN ℞
[sarah 'pin]

COMPOSITION

An aqueous distillate of Sarracenia purpurea, pitcher plant, prepared for parenteral administration.

ACTION AND USES

Local injection therapy for the relief of pain of neuro-muscular or neuralgic origin.

ADMINISTRATION AND DOSAGE

Paravertebral nerve injection—2 to 10 cc. Local neuromuscular infiltration—5 to 10 cc.

SIDE EFFECTS

None.

PRECAUTIONS

Non-toxic.

CONTRAINDICATIONS

Local inflammation.

HOW SUPPLIED

One dozen 10 cc. ampuls and 50 cc. multi-dose vials.

LITERATURE AVAILABLE

Booklet "SARAPIN, Injection Technique in Pain Control."

Hoechst-Roussel Pharmaceuticals Inc.

SOMERVILLE, NJ 08876

A/T/S® ℞
(erythromycin)
2% Acne Topical Solution

DESCRIPTION

A/T/S® (erythromycin) is an antibiotic produced from a strain of *Streptomyces erythraeus*. It is basic and readily forms salts with acids. Each mL of A/T/S (erythromycin) topical solution contains 20 mg of erythromycin base in a vehicle consisting of alcohol USP (66%), propylene glycol USP, and citric acid USP to adjust pH.

ACTIONS

Although the mechanism by which A/T/S (erythromycin) acts in reducing inflammatory lesions of acne vulgaris is unknown, it is presumably due to its antibiotic action.

INDICATIONS

A/T/S (erythromycin) is indicated for the topical control of acne vulgaris.

CONTRAINDICATIONS

A/T/S (erythromycin) is contraindicated in persons who have shown hypersensitivity to any of its ingredients.

WARNING

The safe use of A/T/S (erythromycin) during pregnancy or lactation has not been established.

PRECAUTIONS

General: The use of antibiotic agents may be associated with the overgrowth of antibiotic-resistant organisms. If this occurs, administration of the drug should be discontinued and appropriate measures taken.

Information for Patients: A/T/S® is for external use only and should be kept away from the eyes, nose, mouth, and other mucous membranes. Concomitant topical acne therapy should be used with caution because a cumulative irritant effect may occur, especially with the use of peeling, desquamating, or abrasive agents.

Carcinogenesis, Mutagenesis, Impairment of Fertility: Long-term animal studies to evaluate carcinogenic potential, mutagenicity, or the effect on fertility of erythromycin have not been performed.

Pregnancy: Pregnancy Category C. Animal reproduction studies have not been conducted with erythromycin. It is also not known whether erythromycin can cause fetal harm when administered to a pregnant woman or can affect reproduction capacity. Erythromycin should be given to a pregnant woman only if clearly needed.

Nursing Mothers: Erythromycin is excreted in breast milk. Caution should be exercised when erythromycin is administered to a nursing woman.

ADVERSE REACTIONS

Adverse conditions reported with the use of erythromycin topical solutions include dryness, tenderness, pruritis, desquamation, erythema, oiliness, and burning sensation. Irritation of the eyes has also been reported. A case of generalized urticarial reaction, possibly related to the drug, which required the use of systemic steroid therapy has been reported.

Of a total of 90 patients exposed to A/T/S® during clinical effectiveness studies, 17 experienced some type of adverse effect. These included dry skin, scaly skin, pruritus, irritation of the eye, and burning sensation.

DOSAGE AND ADMINISTRATION

A/T/S® (erythromycin) Topical Solution should be applied to the affected area twice a day after the skin is thoroughly washed with warm water and soap and patted dry. Moisten the applicator or a pad with A/T/S®, then rub over the affected area. Acne lesions on the face, neck, shoulder, chest, and back may be treated in this manner.

HOW SUPPLIED

A/T/S® 2% Acne Topical Solution—60 mL
Store at controlled room temperature 59°-86°F (15°-30°C).
716000-4/86

Shown in Product Identification Section, page 411

CLAFORAN® ℞
[klăf'or-an]
(cefotaxime sodium)*
Sterile and Injection

DESCRIPTION

Sterile Claforan® (cefotaxime sodium) is a semisynthetic, broad spectrum cephalosporin antibiotic for parenteral administration. It is the sodium salt of 7-[2-(2-amino-4-thiazolyl) glyoxylamido]-3-(hydroxymethyl)-8-oxo-5-thia-1-azabicyclo [4.2.0] oct-2-ene-2-carboxylate 7^2-(Z)-(O-methyloxime), acetate (ester). Claforan contains approximately 50.5 mg (2.2 mEq) of sodium per gram of cefotaxime activity. Solutions of Claforan range from very pale yellow to light amber depending on the concentration and the diluent used. The pH of the injectable solutions usually ranges from 5.0 to 7.5. Claforan is supplied as a dry powder in vials, infusion bottles, pharmacy bulk package bottles, and as a frozen, premixed injection in a buffered diluent solution in plastic containers. Claforan, equivalent to 1 gram and 2 grams cefotaxime, is supplied as frozen, premixed injections in plastic containers in 5% dextrose (containing dextrose hydrous, USP). The injections are buffered with sodium citrate hydrous, USP. The pH is adjusted with hydrochloric acid and may be adjusted with sodium hydroxide. The plastic container is fabricated from a specially formulated polyvinyl chloride. Solutions in contact with the plastic container can leach out certain of its chemical components in very small amounts within the expiration period, e.g., di-2-ethylhexyl phthalate (DEHP), up to 5 parts per million. However, the safety of the plastic has been confirmed in tests in animals according to USP biological tests for plastic containers as well as by tissue culture toxicity studies.

CLINICAL PHARMACOLOGY

Following IM administration of a single 500 mg or 1 g dose of Claforan to normal volunteers, mean peak serum concentrations of 11.7 and 20.5 μg/mL respectively were attained within 30 minutes and declined with an elimination half-life of approximately 1 hour. There was a dose-dependent increase in serum levels after the IV administration of 500 mg, 1 g and 2 g of Claforan (38.9, 101.7, and 214.4 μg/mL respectively) without alteration in the elimination half-life. There is no evidence of accumulation following repetitive IV infusion of 1 g doses every 6 hours for 14 days as there are no alterations of serum or renal clearance. About 60% of the administered dose was recovered from urine during the first 6 hours following the start of the infusion.

Approximately 20–36% of an intravenously administered dose of ^{14}C-cefotaxime is excreted by the kidney as unchanged cefotaxime and 15–25% as the desacetyl derivative, the major metabolite. The desacetyl metabolite has been shown to contribute to the bactericidal activity. Two other urinary metabolites (M_2 and M_3) account for about 20–25%. They lack bactericidal activity.

A single 50 mg/kg dose of Claforan was administered as an intravenous infusion over a 10- to 15-minute period to 29 newborn infants grouped according to birth weight and age. The mean half-life of cefotaxime in infants with lower birth weights ($\leq$ 1500 grams), regardless of age, was longer (4.6 hours) than the mean half-life (3.4 hours) in infants whose birth weight was greater than 1500 grams. Mean serum clearance was also smaller in the lower birth weight infants. Although the differences in mean half-life values are statistically significant for weight, they are not clinically important. Therefore, dosage should be based solely on age. (See **Dosage and Administration** section.)

Additionally, no disulfiram-like reactions were reported in a study conducted in 22 healthy volunteers administered Claforan and ethanol.

Microbiology

The bactericidal activity of cefotaxime sodium results from inhibition of cell wall synthesis. Cefotaxime sodium has *in vitro* activity against a wide range of gram-positive and gram-negative organisms. Claforan has a high degree of stability in the presence of beta-lactamases, both penicillinases and cephalosporinases, of gram-negative and gram-positive bacteria. Cefotaxime sodium has been shown to be a potent inhibitor of β-lactamases produced by certain gram-negative bacteria. Cefotaxime sodium is usually active against the following microorganisms both *in vitro* and in clinical infections (see **Indications and Usage**).

Aerobes, Gram-positive: *Staphylococcus aureus*, including penicillinase and non-penicillinase producing strains, *Staphylococcus epidermidis*, *Streptococcus pyogenes* (Group A beta-hemolytic streptococci), *Streptococcus agalactiae* (Group B streptococci), (NOTE: Most strains of enterococci, e.g., *S. faecalis* are resistant), *Streptococcus pneumoniae* (formerly *Diplococcus pneumoniae*).

Aerobes, Gram-negative: *Citrobacter* species, *Enterobacter* species, *Escherichia coli*, *Haemophilus influenzae* (including ampicillin-resistant *H. influenzae*), *Klebsiella* species (including *K. pneumoniae*), *Neisseria gonorrhoeae* (including penicillinase and non-penicillinase producing strains), *Neisseria meningitidis*, *Proteus mirabilis*, *Proteus vulgaris*, *Morganella morganii*, *Providencia rettgeri*, *Serratia* species.

NOTE: Many strains of the above organisms that are multiply resistant to other antibiotics, e.g., penicillins, cephalosporins, and aminoglycosides, are susceptible to cefotaxime sodium.

Cefotaxime sodium is active against some strains of *Pseudomonas aeruginosa*.

Anaerobes: *Bacteroides* species, including some strains of *B. fragilis*, *Clostridium* species (NOTE: Most strains of *C. difficile* are resistant), *Peptococcus* species, *Peptostreptococcus* species.

Cefotaxime sodium is highly stable *in vitro* to four of the five major classes of β-lactamases described by Richmond et al., including type IIIa (TEM) which is produced by many gram-negative bacteria. The drug is also stable to β-lactamase (penicillinase) produced by staphylococci. In addition, cefotaxime sodium shows high affinity for penicillin-binding proteins in the cell wall, including PBP, Ib and III.

Cefotaxime sodium also demonstrates *in vitro* activity against the following microorganisms although clinical significance is unknown: *Salmonella* species (including *S. typhi*), *Providencia* species, and *Shigella* species.

Cefotaxime sodium and aminoglycosides have been shown to be synergistic *in vitro* against some strains of *Pseudomonas aeruginosa.*

Susceptibility Tests

Quantitative methods that require measurement of zone diameters give the most precise estimate of antibiotic susceptibility. One such procedure[1] has been recommended for use with discs to test susceptibility to cefotaxime sodium. Interpretation involves correlation of the diameters obtained in the disc test with minimum inhibitory concentration (MIC) values for cefotaxime sodium.

Reports from the laboratory giving results of the standardized single-disc susceptibility test using a 30-μg cefotaxime sodium disc should be interpreted according to the following criteria:

Susceptible organisms produce zones of 20 mm or greater, indicating that the tested organism is likely to respond to therapy.

Organisms that produce zones of 15 to 19 mm are expected to be susceptible if high dosage is used or if the infection is confined to tissues and fluids (e.g., urine) in which high antibiotic levels are attained.

Resistant organisms produce zones of 14 mm or less, indicating that other therapy should be selected.

Organisms should be tested with the cefotaxime sodium disc, since cefotaxime sodium has been shown by *in vitro* tests to be active against certain strains found resistant when other beta lactam discs are used. The cefotaxime sodium disc should not be used for testing susceptibility to other cephalosporins. Organisms having zones of less than 18 mm around the cephalothin disc are not necessarily of intermediate susceptibility or resistant to cefotaxime sodium.

A bacterial isolate may be considered susceptible if the MIC value for cefotaxime sodium is not more than 16 μg/mL. Organisms are considered resistant to cefotaxime sodium if the MIC is equal to or greater than 64 μg/mL. Organisms having an MIC value of less than 64 μg/mL but greater than 16μg/mL are expected to be susceptible if high dosage is used or if the infection is confined to tissues and fluids (e.g., urine) in which high antibiotic levels are attained.

INDICATIONS AND USAGE

Treatment

Claforan is indicated for the treatment of patients with serious infections caused by susceptible strains of the designated microorganisms in the diseases listed below.

(1) **Lower respiratory tract infections,** including pneumonia, caused by *Streptococcus pneumoniae* (formerly *Diplococcus pneumoniae*), *Streptococcus pyogenes* (Group A streptococci) and other streptococci (excluding enterococci, e.g., *Streptococcus faecalis*), *Staphylococcus aureus* (penicillinase and non-penicillinase producing), *Escherichia coli, Klebsiella* species, *Haemophilus influenzae* (including ampicillin resistant strains), *Proteus mirabilis, Serratia marcescens,* and *Enterobacter* species.

(2) **Genitourinary infections.** Urinary tract infections caused by *Enterococcus* species, *Staphylococcus epidermidis, Staphylococcus aureus* (penicillinase and non-penicillinase producing), *Citrobacter* species, *Enterobacter* species, *Escherichia coli, Klebsiella* species, *Proteus mirabilis, Proteus vulgaris, Morganella morganii, Providencia rettgeri,* and *Serratia marcescens.* Also, uncomplicated gonorrhea of single or multiple sites caused by *Neisseria gonorrhoeae,* including penicillinase producing strains.

(3) **Gynecologic infections,** including pelvic inflammatory disease, endometritis and pelvic cellulitis caused by *Staphylococcus epidermidis, Streptococcus* species, *Enterococcus* species, *Escherichia coli, Proteus mirabilis, Bacteroides* species (including *B. fragilis*), *Clostridium* species, and anaerobic cocci (including *Peptostreptococcus* species and *Peptococcus* species).

(4) **Bacteremia/Septicemia** caused by *Escherichia coli, Klebsiella* species, and *Serratia marcescens.*

(5) **Skin and skin structure infections** caused by *Staphylococcus aureus* (penicillinase and non-penicillinase producing), *Staphylococcus epidermidis, Streptococcus pyogenes* (Group A streptococci) and other streptococci, *Enterococcus* species, *Escherichia coli, Enterobacter* species, *Klebsiella* species, *Proteus mirabilis, Proteus vulgaris, Morganella morganii, Providencia rettgeri, Pseudomonas* species, *Serratia marcescens, Bacteroides* species, and anaerobic cocci (including *Peptostreptococcus* species and *Peptococcus* species).

(6) **Intra-abdominal infections** including peritonitis caused by *Escherichia coli, Klebsiella* species, *Bacteroides* species, and anaerobic cocci (including *Peptostreptococcus* species and *Peptococcus species*).

(7) **Bone and/or joint infections** caused by *Staphylococcus aureus* (penicillinase and non-penicillinase producing strains).

(8) **Central nervous system infections,** e.g. meningitis and ventriculitis, caused by *Neisseria meningitidis, Haemophilus influenzae, Streptococcus pneumoniae, Klebsiella pneumoniae,* and *Escherichia coli.*

Although many strains of enterococci (e.g., *S. faecalis*) and *Pseudomonas* species are resistant to cefotaxime sodium *in vitro,* Claforan has been used successfully in treating patients with infections caused by susceptible organisms.

Specimens for bacteriologic culture should be obtained prior to therapy in order to isolate and identify causative organisms and to determine their susceptibilities to Claforan. Therapy may be instituted before results of susceptibility studies are known; however, once these results become available, the antibiotic treatment should be adjusted accordingly.

In certain cases of confirmed or suspected gram-positive or gram-negative sepsis or in patients with other serious infections in which the causative organism has not been identified, Claforan may be used concomitantly with an aminoglycoside. The dosage recommended in the labeling of both antibiotics may be given and depends on the severity of the infection and the patient's condition. Renal function should be carefully monitored, especially if higher dosages of the aminoglycosides are to be administered or if therapy is prolonged, because of the potential nephrotoxicity and ototoxicity of aminoglycoside antibiotics. Some β-lactam antibiotics also have a certain degree of nephrotoxicity. Although, to date, this has not been noted when Claforan was given alone, it is possible that nephrotoxicity may be potentiated if Claforan is used concomitantly with an aminoglycoside.

Prevention

The administration of Claforan preoperatively may reduce the incidence of certain infections in patients undergoing elective surgical procedures (e.g. abdominal or vaginal hysterectomy, gastrointestinal and genitourinary tract surgery) that may be classified as contaminated or potentially contaminated.

In patients undergoing cesarean section, intraoperative (after clamping the umbilical cord) and postoperative use of Claforan may also reduce the incidence of certain postoperative infections. See **Dosage and Administration** section.

Effective use for elective surgery depends on the time of administration. To achieve effective tissue levels, Claforan should be given ½ to 1½ hours before surgery. See **Dosage and Administration** section.

For patients undergoing gastrointestinal surgery, preoperative bowel preparation by mechanical cleansing as well as with a non-absorbable antibiotic (e.g., neomycin) is recommended.

If there are signs of infection, specimens for culture should be obtained for identification of the causative organism so that appropriate therapy may be instituted.

CONTRAINDICATIONS

Claforan is contraindicated in patients who have shown hypersensitivity to cefotaxime sodium or the cephalosporin group of antibiotics.

WARNINGS

BEFORE THERAPY WITH CLAFORAN IS INSTITUTED, CAREFUL INQUIRY SHOULD BE MADE TO DETERMINE WHETHER THE PATIENT HAS HAD PREVIOUS HYPERSENSITIVITY REACTIONS TO CEFOTAXIME SODIUM, CEPHALOSPORINS, PENICILLINS, OR OTHER DRUGS. THIS PRODUCT SHOULD BE GIVEN WITH CAUTION TO PATIENTS WITH TYPE 1 HYPERSENSITIVITY REACTIONS TO PENICILLIN. ANTIBIOTICS SHOULD BE ADMINISTERED WITH CAUTION TO ANY PATIENT WHO HAS DEMONSTRATED SOME FORM OF ALLERGY, PARTICULARLY TO DRUGS. IF AN ALLERGIC REACTION TO CLAFORAN OCCURS, DISCONTINUE TREATMENT WITH THE DRUG. SERIOUS HYPERSENSITIVITY REACTIONS MAY REQUIRE EPINEPHRINE AND OTHER EMERGENCY MEASURES.

Pseudomembranous colitis has been reported with the use of cephalosporins (and other broad spectrum antibiotics); therefore, it is important to consider its diagnosis in patients who develop diarrhea in association with antibiotic use.

Treatment with broad spectrum antibiotics alters normal flora of the colon and may permit overgrowth of Clostridia. Studies indicate a toxin produced by *Clostridium difficile* is one primary cause of antibiotic-associated colitis. Cholestyramine and colestipol resins have been shown to bind the toxin *in vitro.*

Mild cases of colitis may respond to drug discontinuance alone.

Moderate to severe cases should be managed with fluid, electrolyte, and protein supplementation as indicated.

When the colitis is not relieved by drug discontinuance or when it is severe, oral vancomycin is the treatment of choice for antibiotic-associated pseudomembranous colitis produced by *C. difficile.* Other causes of colitis should also be considered.

PRECAUTIONS

Claforan® (cefotaxime sodium) should be prescribed with caution in individuals with a history of gastrointestinal disease, particularly colitis.

Claforan has not been shown to be nephrotoxic; however, because high and prolonged serum antibiotic concentrations can occur from usual doses in patients with transient or persistent reduction of urinary output because of renal insufficiency, the total daily dosage should be reduced when Claforan is administered to such patients. Continued dosage should be determined by degree of renal impairment, severity of infection, and susceptibility of the causative organism.

Although there is no clinical evidence supporting the necessity of changing the dosage of cefotaxime sodium in patients with even profound renal dysfunction, it is suggested that, until further data are obtained, the dose of cefotaxime sodium be halved in patients with estimated creatinine clearances of less than 20 mL/min/1.73 m².

When only serum creatinine is available, the following formula[2] (based on sex, weight, and age of the patient) may be used to convert this value into creatinine clearance. The serum creatinine should represent a steady state of renal function.

$$\text{Males} \quad \frac{\text{Weight (kg)} \times (140 - \text{age})}{72 \times \text{serum creatinine}}$$

$$\text{Females} \quad 0.85 \times \text{above value}$$

As with other antibiotics, prolonged use of Claforan may result in overgrowth of nonsusceptible organisms. Repeated evaluation of the patient's condition is essential. If superinfection occurs during therapy, appropriate measures should be taken.

Drug Interactions: Increased nephrotoxicity has been reported following concomitant administration of cephalosporins and aminoglycoside antibiotics.

Carcinogenesis, Mutagenesis: Long-term studies in animals have not been performed to evaluate carcinogenic potential. Mutagenic tests included a micronucleus and an Ames test. Both tests were negative for mutagenic effects.

Pregnancy (Category B): Reproduction studies have been performed in mice and rats at doses up to 30 times the usual human dose and have revealed no evidence of impaired fertility or harm to the fetus because of cefotaxime sodium. However, there are no well-controlled studies in pregnant women. Because animal reproductive studies are not always predictive of human response, this drug should be used during pregnancy only if clearly needed.

Nonteratogenic Effects: Use of the drug in women of childbearing potential requires that the anticipated benefit be weighed against the possible risks.

In perinatal and postnatal studies with rats, the pups in the group given 1200 mg/kg of Claforan were significantly lighter in weight at birth and remained smaller than pups in the control group during the 21 days of nursing.

Nursing Mothers: Claforan is excreted in human milk in low concentrations. Caution should be exercised when Claforan is administered to a nursing woman.

ADVERSE REACTIONS

Claforan is generally well tolerated. The most common adverse reactions have been local reactions following IM or IV injection. Other adverse reactions have been encountered infrequently.

The most frequent adverse reactions (greater than 1%) are:

Local (4.7%) - Injection site inflammation with IV administration. Pain, induration, and tenderness after IM injection.

Hypersensitivity (1.8%) - Rash, pruritus, and fever.

Gastrointestinal (1.7%) - Colitis, diarrhea, nausea, and vomiting.

Symptoms of pseudomembranous colitis can appear during or after antibiotic treatment.

Nausea and vomiting have been reported rarely.

Less frequent adverse reactions (less than 1%) are:

Hemic and Lymphatic System - Granulocytopenia, transient leukopenia, eosinophilia, neutropenia and thrombocytopenia have been reported. Some individuals have developed positive direct Coombs Tests during treatment with the cephalosporin antibiotics.

Genitourinary System - Moniliasis, vaginitis.

Central Nervous System - Headache.

Liver - Transient elevations in SGOT, SGPT, serum LDH, and serum alkaline phosphatase levels have been reported.

Kidney - As with some other cephalosporins, transient elevations of BUN have been occasionally observed with Claforan.

Continued on next page

Hoechst-Roussel—Cont.

DOSAGE AND ADMINISTRATION

Adults

Dosage and route of administration should be determined by susceptibility of the causative organisms, severity of the infection, and the condition of the patient (see table for dosage guideline). Claforan may be administered IM or IV after reconstitution. Premixed Claforan Injection is intended for IV administration after thawing. The maximum daily dosage should not exceed 12 grams.
[See table below].

To prevent postoperative infection in contaminated or potentially contaminated surgery, the recommended dose is a single 1 gram IM or IV administered 30 to 90 minutes prior to start of surgery.

Cesarean Section Patients

The first dose of 1 gram is administered intravenously as soon as the umbilical cord is clamped. The second and third doses should be given as 1 gram intravenously or intramuscularly at 6 and 12 hours after the first dose.

Neonates, Infants and Children

The following dosage schedule is recommended:
Neonates (birth to 1 month):

0–1 week of age	50 mg/kg IV q 12 h
1–4 weeks of age	50 mg/kg IV q 8 h

It is not necessary to differentiate between premature and normal-gestational age infants.

Infants and Children (1 month to 12 years): For body weights less than 50 kg, the recommended daily dose is 50 to 180 mg/kg IM or IV of body weight divided into four to six equal doses. The higher dosages should be used for more severe or serious infections, including meningitis. For body weights 50 kg or more, the usual adult dosage should be used; the maximum daily dosage should not exceed 12 grams.

Impaired Renal Function - see **Precautions** section.

NOTE: As with antibiotic therapy in general, administration of Claforan should be continued for a minimum of 48 to 72 hours after the patient defervesces or after evidence of bacterial eradication has been obtained; a minimum of 10 days of treatment is recommended for infections caused by Group A beta-hemolytic streptococci in order to guard against the risk of rheumatic fever or glomerulonephritis; frequent bacteriologic and clinical appraisal is necessary during therapy of chronic urinary tract infection and may be required for several months after therapy has been completed; persistent infections may require treatment of several weeks and doses smaller than those indicated above should not be used.

PREPARATION OF CLAFORAN STERILE

Claforan for IM or IV administration should be reconstituted as follows:

Strength	Diluent (mL)	Withdrawable Volume (mL)	Approximate Concentration (mg/mL)
1g vial (IM)	3	3.4	300
2g vial (IM)	5	6.0	330
1g vial (IV)	10	10.4	95
2g vial (IV)	10	11.0	180
1g infusion	50–100	50–100	20–10
2g infusion	50–100	50–100	40–20
10g bottle	47	52.0	200
10g bottle	97	102.0	100

Shake to dissolve; inspect for particulate matter and discoloration prior to use. Solutions of Claforan range from light yellow to amber, depending on concentration, diluent used, and length and condition of storage.

For intramuscular use: Reconstitute VIALS with Sterile Water for Injection or Bacteriostatic Water for Injection as described above.

For intravenous use: Reconstitute VIALS with at least 10 mL of Sterile Water for Injection. Reconstitute INFUSION BOTTLES with 50 or 100 mL of 0.9% Sodium Chloride Injection or 5% Dextrose Injection. For other diluents, see **COMPATIBILITY and STABILITY** section.

Pharmacy Bulk Package: Reconstitute with 47 mL of diluent for an approximate concentration of 200 mg/mL or 97 mL of diluent for an approximate concentration of 100 mg/mL. Stock solutions may be further diluted for IV infusion with diluents as listed in **COMPATIBILITY and STABILITY** section.

NOTE: Solutions of Claforan must not be admixed with aminoglycoside solutions. If Claforan and aminoglycosides are to be administered to the same patient, they must be administered separately and not as mixed injection.

A SOLUTION OF 1 G CLAFORAN IN 14 ML OF STERILE WATER FOR INJECTION IS ISOTONIC.

IM Administration: As with all IM preparations, Claforan should be injected well within the body of a relatively large muscle such as the upper outer quadrant of the buttock (i.e., gluteus maximus); aspiration is necessary to avoid inadvertent injection into a blood vessel. Individual IM doses of 2 grams may be given if the dose is divided and is administered in different intramuscular sites.

IV Administration: The IV route is preferable for patients with bacteremia, bacterial septicemia, peritonitis, meningitis, or other severe or life-threatening infections, or for patients who may be poor risks because of lowered resistance resulting from such debilitating conditions as malnutrition, trauma, surgery, diabetes, heart failure, or malignancy, particularly if shock is present or impending.

For intermittent IV administration, a solution containing 1 gram or 2 grams in 10 mL of Sterile Water for Injection can be injected over a period of three to five minutes. With an infusion system, it may also be given over a longer period of time through the tubing system by which the patient may be receiving other IV solutions. However, during infusion of the solution containing Claforan, it is advisable to discontinue temporarily the administration of other solutions at the same site.

For the administration of higher doses by continuous IV infusion, a solution of Claforan may be added to IV bottles containing the solutions discussed below.

Preparation of Premixed Claforan Injection in Plastic Container

Premixed Claforan Injection may be used directly after thawing at room temperature. Solutions range from very pale yellow to light amber. After thawing, check for minute leaks by squeezing bag firmly and inspect for particulate matter, discoloration and solution clarity. Discard if leaks are found or seal is not intact. Additives should not be introduced into this solution.

Use sterile equipment.

WARNING: Do not use plastic containers in series connections. Such use could result in air embolism due to residual air being drawn from the primary container before administration of the fluid from the secondary container is complete.

Preparation for administration:

1. Suspend container from eyelet support.
2. Remove plastic protector from outlet port at bottom of container.
3. Attach administration set. Refer to complete directions accompanying set.

After thawing, premixed Claforan Injection, 1 gram and 2 grams in 50 mL plastic containers may be used for continuous or intermittent intravenous infusion.

COMPATIBILITY AND STABILITY

Solutions of Claforan Sterile reconstituted as described above (**Preparation of Claforan Sterile**) maintain satisfactory potency for 24 hours at room temperature (at or below 22°C), 10 days under refrigeration (at or below 5°C), and for at least 13 weeks frozen. Solutions may be stored in disposable glass or plastic syringes for 24 hours at room temperature (at or below 22°C), 5 days under refrigeration (at or below 5°C), and 13 weeks frozen.

Reconstituted solutions may be further diluted up to 1000 mL with the following solutions and maintain satisfactory potency for 24 hours at room temperature (at or below 22°C), and at least 5 days under refrigeration (at or below 5°C); 0.9% Sodium Chloride Injection; 5 or 10% Dextrose Injection; 5% Dextrose and 0.9% Sodium Chloride Injection; 5% Dextrose and 0.45% Sodium Chloride Injection; 5% Dextrose and 0.2% Sodium Chloride Injection; Lactated Ringers Solution; Sodium Lactate Injection (M/6); 10% Invert Sugar Injection, FREAMINE® II Injection.

Solutions of Claforan Sterile reconstituted in 0.9% Sodium Chloride Injection or 5% Dextrose Injection in Viaflex® plastic containers maintain satisfactory potency for 24 hours at room temperature (at or below 22°C), 5 days under refrigeration (at or below 5°C) and 13 weeks frozen.

NOTE: Claforan solutions exhibit maximum stability in the pH 5–7 range. Solutions of Claforan should not be prepared with diluents having a pH above 7.5, such as Sodium Bicarbonate Injection.

Claforan supplied as premixed, frozen injection is stable for the expiration dating period as indicated on the label. Thawed solutions of premixed Claforan Injection in plastic containers are stable for 24 hours at room temperature (at or below 22°C) or for 10 days under refrigeration (at or below 5°C).

Frozen samples should not be heated but should be thawed at room temperature before use. After the periods mentioned above, any unused solutions or frozen material should be discarded. DO NOT REFREEZE.

HOW SUPPLIED

Sterile Claforan is a dry off-white to pale yellow crystalline powder supplied in vials and bottles containing cefotaxime sodium as follows:

1 gram cefotaxime free acid equivalent in vials (NDC 0039 0018 01) and in infusion bottles (NDC 0039 0018 02)
2 gram cefotaxime free acid equivalent in vials (NDC 0039 0019 01) and in infusion bottles (NDC 0039 0019 02)
10 gram cefotaxime free acid equivalent in pharmacy bulk package bottles (NDC 0039 0020 01)

NOTE: Claforan in the dry state should be stored below 30°C. The dry material as well as solutions tend to darken depending on storage conditions and should be protected from elevated temperatures and excessive light.

Premixed Claforan Injection is supplied as a frozen, sterile, nonpyrogenic solution in 50 mL single dose plastic containers as follows:

1 gram cefotaxime free acid equivalent in 5% dextrose solution (NDC 0039 0043 50) 2B3518
2 grams cefotaxime free acid equivalent in 5% dextrose solution (NDC 0039 0044 50) 2B3519

NOTE: Premixed Claforan Injection in the frozen state should not be stored above −20°C.

Claforan Injection supplied as a frozen, sterile, nonpyrogenic solution in plastic containers is manufactured for Hoechst-Roussel Pharmaceuticals Inc., by Travenol Laboratories, Inc., Deerfield, IL 60015.

References:

1) Bauer, A.W.; Kirby, W.M.M.; Sherris, J.C.; and Turck, M.: Antibiotic Susceptibility Testing by a Standardized Single Disk Method, Am. J. Clin. Pathol., 45:493, 1966; Standardized Disc Susceptibility Test, Federal Register, 39:19182-4, 1974. National Committee for Clinical Laboratory Standards, Approved Standard: ASM-2, Performance Standards for Antimicrobial Disc Susceptibility Tests, July, 1975.
2) Cockcroft, D.W. and Gault, M.H.: Prediction of Creatinine Clearance from Serum Creatinine. Nephron 16:31-41, 1976.

CLAFORAN® REG TM ROUSSEL-UCLAF
VIAFLEX® REG TM BAXTER TRAVENOL LABS, INC.
71789T-9/85
*U.S. Patent 4,152,432

GUIDELINES FOR DOSAGE OF CLAFORAN

Type of Infection	Daily Dose (grams)	Frequency and Route
Gonorrhea	1	1 gram IM (single dose)
Uncomplicated infections	2	1 gram every 12 hours IM or IV
Moderate to severe infections	3–6	1–2 grams every 8 hours IM or IV
Infections commonly needing antibiotics in higher dosage (e.g., septicemia)	6–8	2 grams every 6–8 hours IV
Life-threatening infections	up to 12	2 grams every 4 hours IV

DIAβETA® ℞

(glyburide)*

Tablets 1.25, 2.5 and 5.0 mg

DESCRIPTION

Diaβeta® (glyburide) is an oral blood-glucose-lowering drug of the sulfonylurea class. It is a white, crystalline compound, formulated as tablets of 1.25 mg, 2.5 mg, and 5.0 mg strengths for oral administration.

Chemically, Diaβeta® (glyburide) is identified as 1-[[p-[2-(5-chloro-O-anisamido)ethyl] phenyl] -sulfonyl] -3-cyclohexylurea.

The molecular weight is 493.99. The aqueous solubility of Diaβeta® (glyburide) increases with pH as a result of salt formation.

CLINICAL PHARMACOLOGY

Diaβeta® (glyburide) appears to lower the blood glucose acutely by stimulating the release of insulin from the pancreas, an effect dependent upon functioning beta cells in the pancreatic islets. The mechanism by which Diaβeta® (glyburide) lowers blood glucose during long-term administration has not been clearly established.

With chronic administration in Type II diabetic patients, the blood glucose lowering effect persists despite a gradual decline in the insulin secretory response to the drug. Extrapancreatic effects may play a part in the mechanism of action of oral sulfonylurea hypoglycemic drugs.

In addition to its blood glucose lowering actions, Diaβeta® (glyburide) produces a mild diuresis by enhancement of renal free water clearance. Clinical experience to date indicates an extremely low incidence of disulfiram-like reactions in patients while taking Diaβeta® (glyburide).

Pharmacokinetics

Single-dose studies with Diaβeta® (glyburide) in normal subjects demonstrate significant absorption within one hour, peak drug levels at about four hours, and low but detectable levels at twenty-four hours. Mean serum levels of glyburide, as reflected by areas under the serum concentration-time curve, increase in proportion to corresponding increases in dose. Multiple-dose studies with Diaβeta® (glyburide) in diabetic patients demonstrate drug level concentration-time curves similar to single-dose studies, indicating no build-up of drug in tissue depots. The decrease of glyburide in the serum of normal healthy individuals is biphasic, the terminal half-life being about 10 hours. In single-dose studies in fasting normal subjects, the degree and duration of blood glucose lowering is proportional to the dose administered and to the area under the drug level concentration-time curve. The blood glucose lowering effect persists for 24 hours following single morning doses in non-fasting diabetic patients. Under conditions of repeated administration in diabetic patients, however, there is no reliable correlation between blood drug levels and fasting blood glucose levels. A one-year study of diabetic patients treated with Diaβeta® (glyburide) showed no reliable correlation between administered dose and serum drug level.

The major metabolite of Diaβeta® (glyburide) is the 4-trans-hydroxy derivative. A second metabolite, the 3-cis-hydroxy derivative, also occurs. These metabolites contribute no significant hypoglycemic action since they are only weakly active (1/400th and 1/40th, respectively, as glyburide) in rabbits.

Diaβeta® (glyburide) is excreted as metabolites in the bile and urine, approximately 50% by each route. This dual excretory pathway is qualitatively different from that of other sulfonylureas, which are excreted primarily in the urine.

Sulfonylurea drugs are extensively bound to serum proteins. Displacement from protein binding sites by other drugs may lead to enhanced hypoglycemic action. *In vitro*, the protein binding exhibited by Diaβeta® (glyburide) is predominantly non-ionic, whereas that of other sulfonylureas (chlorpropamide, tolbutamide, tolazamide) is predominantly ionic. Acidic drugs such as phenylbutazone, warfarin, and salicylates displace the ionic-binding sulfonylureas from serum proteins to a far greater extent than the non-ionic binding Diaβeta® (glyburide). It has not been shown that this difference in protein binding will result in fewer drug-drug interactions with Diaβeta® (glyburide) in clinical use.

INDICATIONS AND USAGE

Diaβeta® (glyburide) is indicated as an adjunct to diet to lower the blood glucose in patients with non-insulin-dependent diabetes mellitus (Type II) whose hyperglycemia cannot be controlled by diet alone.

In initiating treatment for non-insulin-dependent diabetes, diet should be emphasized as the primary form of treatment. Caloric restriction and weight loss are essential in the obese diabetic patient. Proper dietary management alone may be effective in controlling the blood glucose and symptoms of hyperglycemia. The importance of regular physical activity should also be stressed, and cardiovascular risk factors should be identified and corrective measures taken where possible.

If this treatment program fails to reduce symptoms and/or blood glucose, the use of an oral sulfonylurea or insulin should be considered. Use of Diaβeta® (glyburide) must be viewed by both the physician and patient as a treatment in addition to diet, and not as a substitute for diet or as a convenient mechanism for avoiding dietary restraint. Furthermore, loss of blood glucose control on diet alone may be transient, thus requiring only short-term administration of Diaβeta® (glyburide).

During maintenance programs, Diaβeta® (glyburide) should be discontinued if satisfactory lowering of blood glucose is no longer achieved. Judgments should be based on regular clinical and laboratory evaluations.

In considering the use of Diaβeta® (glyburide) in asymptomatic patients, it should be recognized that controlling the blood glucose in non-insulin dependent diabetes has not been definitely established to be effective in preventing the long-term cardiovascular or neural complications of diabetes.

CONTRAINDICATIONS

Diaβeta® (glyburide) is contraindicated in patients with:

1. Known hypersensitivity to the drug.
2. Diabetic ketoacidosis, with or without coma. This condition should be treated with insulin.

WARNINGS:

SPECIAL WARNING ON INCREASED RISK OF CARDIOVASCULAR MORTALITY

The administration of oral hypoglycemic drugs has been reported to be associated with increased cardiovascular mortality as compared to treatment with diet alone or diet plus insulin. This warning is based on the study conducted by the University Group Diabetes Program (UGDP), a long-term prospective clinical trial designed to evaluate the effectiveness of glucose-lowering drugs in preventing or delaying vascular complications in patients with non-insulin-dependent diabetes. The study involved 823 patients who were randomly assigned to one of four treatment groups (Diabetes, 19 (supp. 2): 747-830, 1970).

UDGP reported that patients treated for 5 to 8 years with diet plus a fixed dose of tolbutamide (1.5 grams per day) had a rate of cardiovascular mortality approximately 2½ times that of patients treated with diet alone. A significant increase in total mortality was not observed, but the use of tolbutamide was discontinued based on the increase in cardiovascular mortality, thus limiting the opportunity for the study to show an increase in overall mortality. Despite controversy regarding the interpretation of these results, the findings of the UGDP study provide an adequate basis for this warning. The patient should be informed of the potential risks and advantages of Diaβeta® (glyburide) and of alternative modes of therapy.

Although only one drug in the sulfonylurea class (tolbutamide) was included in this study, it is prudent from a safety standpoint to consider that this warning may also apply to other oral hypoglycemic drugs in this class, in view of their close similarities in mode of action and chemical structure.

PRECAUTIONS

General

Hypoglycemia: All sulfonylurea drugs are capable of producing severe hypoglycemia. Proper patient selection, dosage, and instructions are important to avoid hypoglycemic episodes. Renal or hepatic insufficiency may cause elevated blood levels of Diaβeta® (glyburide) and the latter may also diminish gluconeogenic capacity, both of which increase the risk of serious hypoglycemic reactions. Elderly, debilitated or malnourished patients, and those with adrenal or pituitary insufficiency are particularly susceptible to the hypoglycemic action of glucose-lowering drugs. Hypoglycemia may be difficult to recognize in the elderly, and in people who are taking beta-adrenergic blocking drugs. Hypoglycemia is more likely to occur when caloric intake is deficient, after severe or prolonged exercise, when alcohol is ingested, or when more than one glucose-lowering drug is used.

Loss of control of blood glucose: When a patient stabilized on any diabetic regimen is exposed to stress such as fever, trauma, infection, or surgery, a loss of control may occur. At such times, it may be necessary to discontinue Diaβeta® (glyburide) and administer insulin.

The effectiveness of any oral hypoglycemic drug, including Diaβeta® (glyburide), in lowering blood glucose to a desired level decreases in many patients over a period of time, which may be due to progression of the severity of the diabetes or to diminished responsiveness to the drug. This phenomenon is known as secondary failure, to distinguish it from primary failure in which the drug is ineffective in an individual patient when first given.

Information for Patients

Patients should be informed of the potential risks and advantages of Diaβeta® (glyburide) and of alternative modes of therapy. They should also be informed about the importance of adherence to dietary instructions, of a regular exercise program, and of regular testing of urine and/or blood glucose.

The risks of hypoglycemia, its symptoms and treatment, and conditions that predispose to its development should be explained to patients and responsible family members. Primary and secondary failure should also be explained.

Laboratory Tests

Blood and urine glucose should be monitored periodically. Measurement of glycosylated hemoglobin may be useful.

Drug Interactions

The hypoglycemic action of sulfonylureas may be potentiated by certain drugs including nonsteroidal anti-inflammatory agents and other drugs that are highly protein bound, salicylates, sulfonamides, chloramphenicol, probenecid, coumarins, monoamine oxidase inhibitors, and beta adrenergic blocking agents. When such drugs are administered to a patient receiving Diaβeta® (glyburide), the patient should be observed closely for hypoglycemia. When such drugs are withdrawn from a patient receiving Diaβeta® (glyburide), the patient should be observed closely for loss of control.

Certain drugs tend to produce hyperglycemia and may lead to loss of control. These drugs include the thiazides and other diuretics, corticosteroids, phenothiazines, thyroid products, estrogens, oral contraceptives, phenytoin, nicotinic acid, sympathomimetics, calcium channel blocking drugs, and isoniazid. When such drugs are administered to a patient receiving Diaβeta® (glyburide), the patient should be closely observed for loss of control. When such drugs are withdrawn from a patient receiving Diaβeta® (glyburide), the patient should be observed closely for hypoglycemia.

A potential interaction between oral miconazole and oral hypoglycemic agents leading to severe hypoglycemia has been reported. Whether this interaction also occurs with the intravenous, topical or vaginal preparations of miconazole is not known.

Carcinogenesis, Mutagenesis, and Impairment of Fertility

Diaβeta® (glyburide) is non-mutagenic when studied in the Salmonella microsome test (Ames test) and in the DNA damage/alkaline elution assay. Studies in rats at doses up to 300 mg/kg/day for 18 months showed no carcinogenic effects.

Pregnancy

Teratogenic Effects: Pregnancy Category B

Reproduction studies have been performed in rats and rabbits at doses up to 500 times the human dose and have revealed no evidence of impaired fertility or harm to the fetus due to Diaβeta®(glyburide). There are, however, no adequate and well controlled studies in pregnant women. Because animal reproduction studies are not always predictive of human response, this drug should be used during pregnancy only if clearly needed.

Because recent information suggests that abnormal blood glucose levels during pregnancy are associated with a higher incidence of congenital abnormalities, many experts recommend that insulin be used during pregnancy to maintain blood glucose levels as close to normal as possible.

Nonteratogenic Effects

Prolonged severe hypoglycemia (4 to 10 days) has been reported in neonates born to mothers who were receiving a sulfonylurea drug at the time of delivery. This had been reported more frequently with the use of agents with prolonged half-lives. If Diaβeta® (glyburide) is used during pregnancy, it should be discontinued at least two weeks before the expected delivery date.

Nursing Mothers

Although it is not known whether Diaβeta® (glyburide) is excreted in human milk, some sulfonylureas are known to be excreted in human milk. Because the potential for hypoglycemia in nursing infants may exist, a decision should be made whether to discontinue nursing or to discontinue administering the drug, taking into account the importance of the drug to the mother. If Diaβeta® (glyburide) is discontinued and if diet alone is inadequate for controlling blood glucose, insulin therapy should be considered.

Pediatric Use: Safety and effectiveness in children have not been established.

ADVERSE REACTIONS

Hypoglycemia: See **Precautions** and **Overdosage** Sections.

Gastrointestinal Reactions: Cholestatic jaundice may occur rarely; Diaβeta® (glyburide) should be discontinued if this occurs. Gastrointestinal disturbances, e.g., nausea, epigastric fullness, and heartburn, are the most common reactions and occur in 1.8% of treated patients. They tend to be dose-related and may disappear when dosage is reduced.

Dermatologic Reactions: Allergic skin reactions, e.g., pruritus, erythema, urticaria, and morbilliform or maculopapular eruptions, occur in 1.5% of treated patients. These may be transient and may disappear despite continued use of Diaβeta® (glyburide); if skin reactions persist, the drug should be discontinued.

Porphyria cutanea tarda and photosensitivity reactions have been reported with sulfonylureas.

Hematologic Reactions: Leukopenia, agranulocytosis, thrombocytopenia, hemolytic anemia, aplastic anemia, and pancytopenia have been reported with sulfonylureas.

Metabolic Reactions: Hepatic porphyria reactions have been reported with sulfonylureas; however, these have not been reported with Diaβeta® (glyburide). Disulfiram-like reactions have been reported very rarely with Diaβeta® (glyburide).

OVERDOSAGE

Overdosage of sulfonylureas, including Diaβeta® (glyburide), can produce hypoglycemia. Mild hypoglycemic symptoms without loss of consciousness or neurologic findings should be treated aggressively with oral glucose and adjustments in drug dosage and/or meal patterns. Close monitoring should continue until the physician is assured that the patient is out of danger. Severe hypoglycemic reactions with coma, seizure, or other neurological impairment occur infrequently, but constitute medical emergencies requiring immediate hospitalization. If hypoglycemic coma is diagnosed or suspected, the patient should be given a rapid intravenous injection of concentrated (50%) glucose solution. This should be followed by a continuous infusion of a more dilute (10%) glucose solution at a rate that will maintain the blood glucose at a level above 100 mg/dL. Patients should be closely monitored for a minimum of 24 to 48 hours, since hypoglycemia may recur after apparent clinical recovery.

DOSAGE AND ADMINISTRATION

There is no fixed dosage regimen for the management of diabetes mellitus with Diaβeta® (glyburide) or any other hypoglycemic agent. In addition to the usual monitoring of urinary glucose, the patient's blood glucose must also be monitored periodically to determine the minimum effective dose for the patient; to detect primary failure, i.e., inadequate lowering of blood glucose at the maximum recommended dose of medication; and to detect secondary failure, i.e., loss of adequate blood glucose lowering response after an initial period of effectiveness. Glycosylated hemoglobin levels may also be of value in monitoring the patient's response to therapy.

Continued on next page

Hoechst-Roussel—Cont.

Short-term administration of Diaβeta® (glyburide) may be sufficient during periods of transient loss of control in patients usually controlled well on diet.

1. **Usual Starting Dose**
   The usual starting dose of Diaβeta® (glyburide) as initial therapy is 2.5–5 mg daily, administered with breakfast or the first main meal. Those patients who may be more sensitive to hypoglycemic drugs should be started at 1.25 mg daily. (See **Precautions** Section for patients at increased risk). Failure to follow an appropriate dosage regimen may precipitate hypoglycemia. Patients who do not adhere to their prescribed dietary and drug regimen are more prone to exhibit unsatisfactory response to therapy.
   Transfer of patients from other oral antidiabetic regimens to Diaβeta® (glyburide) should be done conservatively and the initial daily dose should be 2.5 to 5 mg. When transferring patients from oral hypoglycemic agents other than chlorpropamide to Diaβeta® (glyburide), no transition period and no initial or priming dose is necessary. When transferring patients from chlorpropamide, particular care should be exercised during the first two weeks because the prolonged retention of chlorpropamide in the body and subsequent overlapping drug effects may provoke hypoglycemia.
   Some Type II diabetic patients being treated with insulin may respond satisfactorily to Diaβeta® (glyburide). If the insulin dose is less than 20 units daily, substitution of Diaβeta® (glyburide) 2.5 to 5 mg as a single daily dose may be tried. If the insulin dose is between 20 and 40 units daily, the patient may be placed directly on Diaβeta® (glyburide) 5 mg daily as a single dose. If the insulin dose is more than 40 units daily, a transition period is required for conversion to Diaβeta® (glyburide). In these patients, insulin dosage is decreased by 50% and Diaβeta® (glyburide) 5 mg daily is started. Please refer to Usual Maintenance Dose for further explanation.
2. **Usual Maintenance Dose**
   The usual maintenance dose is in the range of 1.25 to 20 mg daily, which may be given as a single dose or in divided doses (See Dosage Interval Section). Dosage increases should be made in increments of no more than 2.5 mg at weekly intervals based upon the patient's blood glucose response.
   No exact dosage relationship exists between Diaβeta® (glyburide) and the other oral hypoglycemic agents. Although patients may be transferred from the maximum dose of other sulfonylureas, the maximum starting dose of 5 mg of Diaβeta® (glyburide) should be observed. A maintenance dose of 5 mg Diaβeta® (glyburide) provides approximately the same degree of blood glucose control as 250 to 375 mg chlorpropamide, 250 to 375 mg tolazamide, 500 to 750 mg acetohexamide, or 1000 to 1500 mg tolbutamide.
   When transferring patients receiving more than 40 units of insulin daily, they may be started on a daily dose of Diaβeta® (glyburide) 5 mg concomitantly with a 50% reduction in insulin dose. Progressive withdrawal of insulin and increase of Diaβeta® (glyburide) in increments of 1.25 to 2.5 mg every 2 to 10 days is then carried out. During this conversion period when both insulin and Diaβeta® (glyburide) are being used, hypoglycemia may rarely occur. During insulin withdrawal, patients should test their urine for glucose and acetone at least three times daily and report results to their physician. The appearance of persistent acetonuria with glycosuria indicates that the patient is a Type I diabetic who requires insulin therapy.
3. **Maximum Dose**
   Daily doses of more than 20 mg are not recommended.
4. **Dosage Interval**
   Once-a-day therapy is usually satisfactory, based upon usual meal patterns and a 10 hour half-life of Diaβeta® (glyburide). Some patients, particularly those receiving more than 10 mg daily, may have a more satisfactory response with twice-a-day dosage.

In elderly patients, debilitated or malnourished patients, and patients with impaired renal or hepatic function, the initial and maintenance dosing should be conservative to avoid hypoglycemic reactions. (See **Precautions** Section.)

HOW SUPPLIED

Diaβeta® (glyburide) tablets are supplied as white, oblong, monogrammed, scored tablets of 1.25 mg in bottles of 50 (NDC 0039-0050-05); pink, oblong, monogrammed, scored tablets of 2.5 mg in bottles of 100 (NDC 0039-0051-10) and Unit Dose Cartons of 100 (NDC 0039-0051-11); and light green, oblong, monogrammed, scored tablets of 5 mg in bottles of 100 (NDC 0039-0052-10) and 500 (NDC 0039-0052-50), and in Unit Dose Cartons of 100 (NDC 0039-0052-11).

Store at controlled room temperature (59°–86°F).
Dispense in well-closed containers with safety closures.
Caution: Federal law prohibits dispensing without a prescription.

*U.S. Patents 3,454,635 and 3,507,954 75100-6/86

Shown in Product Identification Section, page 411

DOXIDAN®

[dox 'i-dan"]

(See PDR For Nonprescription Drugs)
Shown in Product Identification Section, page 411

FESTAL® II

[fes 'tal]

(See PDR For Nonprescription Drugs)
Shown in Product Identification Section, page 411

FESTALAN® ℞

[fes' tah-lan"]

DESCRIPTION

Festalan® tablets contain the active ingredients: lipase 6,000 USP units, amylase 30,000 USP units, protease 20,000 USP units, atropine methyl nitrate 1 mg, and the following inactive ingredients: acacia NF, calcium carbonate USP, castor oil USP, cellulose acetate phthalate NF, D&C Yellow #6, D&C Yellow #10, flavors, gelatin NF, microcrystalline cellulose NF, povidone USP, sodium benzoate, sodium chloride USP, sucrose NF, talc USP, titanium dioxide USP.

The enzymes Lipase, Amylase and Protease in Festalan® are obtained from porcine pancreas. Although allergic reactions to the animal protein in this preparation occur only rarely, these enzymes should be used cautiously in patients with known sensitivity.

CLINICAL PHARMACOLOGY

Pharmacologic and biochemical effects of Lipase, Amylase and Protease are limited to their actions upon the contents of the gastrointestinal tract. None of these enzymes are known to exert systemic pharmacologic effects after oral administration.

Atropine, atropine methyl nitrate and related belladonna alkaloids block the parasympathomimetic (muscarinic) effects of acetylcholine. These drugs are variously known as anticholinergic, parasympatholytic or antispasmodic agents. They act distally on parasympathetic nerve endings to inhibit the action of acetylcholine on smooth muscle, exocrine glands and the heart. Atropine does not block transmission at the neuromuscular junction of skeletal muscle. Atropine is readily absorbed from the gastrointestinal tract and crosses the blood-brain barrier. Most is excreted in the urine within the first 12 hours.

It reduces both motility and secretory activity of the gastrointestinal system. Atropine does not cause CNS depression at usual oral clinical doses, but may decrease heart rate slightly without changing blood pressure. Most of the pharmacologic effects reported with atropine and its analogs are attributable to its cholinergic blockade of parasympathetic effectors.

INDICATIONS AND USAGE

Festalan® is indicated for the treatment of functional gastrointestinal disorders involving disturbed motor function, hypermotility and spasticity as in patients with irritable colon syndrome. Atropine methyl nitrate reduces gastrointestinal tone and spasm. The enzyme content is helpful in reducing symptoms of postprandial intestinal distress in conditions involving digestive enzyme insufficiency.

CONTRAINDICATIONS

Festalan® should not be used in patients with glaucoma, reflux esophagitis (gastric retention), prostate hypertrophy, pyloric obstruction, obstruction of the bladder neck, congestive heart failure with tachycardia and achalasia (cardiospasm). Festalan® should not be given to patients sensitive to protein of porcine origin or to atropine.

WARNINGS

Serious adverse reactions to atropine usually occur at higher doses and are extensions of known pharmacologic effects such as signs of CNS stimulation followed by depression, orthostatic hypotension and respiratory arrest. Children are more susceptible to the toxic effects than adults.

PRECAUTIONS

General: Festalan® should be used with caution in patients with cardiac disease. Patients using Festalan® should be warned of signs of atropine intoxication, particularly with doses exceeding the usual recommended dose. These may include dry mouth, difficulty with speech and swallowing and marked thirst. Vision may be blurred and skin may feel hot, dry and flushed. Usage of the drug should be discontinued and a physician consulted if any of the above symptoms appear.

Drug Interactions: Antacids may interfere with absorption of atropine and should not be given with this drug.

Pregnancy: Pregnancy Category C. Animal reproduction studies have not been conducted with Festalan®. It is also not known whether Festalan® can cause fetal harm when administered to a pregnant woman or can effect reproduction capacity. Festalan® should be given to a pregnant woman only if clearly needed.

Atropine has negligible effects on the human uterus and the fetus is not adversely affected nor is respiration of the newborn depressed.*

Nursing Mothers: Traces of atropine are found in human milk. Caution should be observed when Festalan® is administered to a nursing woman.

Pediatric Use: The safety and effectiveness of Festalan® in children have not been established. See WARNINGS section.

ADVERSE REACTIONS

Adverse reactions associated with Festalan® may be of two main types: those due to allergic manifestations to pork proteins and those due to pharmacologic properties of atropine methyl nitrate. Allergic reactions occur only rarely and patients with known sensitivity should not be treated with Festalan®.

The most frequent adverse reactions seen after atropine are primarily due to the anticholinergic effects on various organs and systems. Dryness of the mouth, anhidrosis, mydriasis, cycloplegia, tachycardia (sometimes preceded by slowing), constipation, dysuria, and acute urinary retention may occur at clinical doses. At higher doses, marked dryness of the mouth, thirst, cardiac acceleration, blurring of vision, and speech difficulties may be encountered. Larger doses produce more marked development of symptoms, including CNS stimulation.

OVERDOSAGE

Symptoms of overdosage with atropine may comprise signs of CNS stimulation followed by depression, orthostatic hypotension and respiratory arrest. Children are more susceptible to the toxic effects than adults. Overdosage with atropine should be treated by gastric lavage to limit absorption. Physostigmine is an antidote for atropine poisoning and 1 to 4 mg (0.5 to 1.0 mg in children) may be given by slow intravenous injection to reduce or abolish delirium and coma caused by large doses of atropine. Phenothiazines should not be used for treatment of overdosage.

DOSAGE AND ADMINISTRATION

Usual adult dose is one or two tablets with each meal. Pediatric dosage has not been established.

HOW SUPPLIED

Festalan® is available in bottles of 100 and 1,000 orange, enteric-coated tablets. Store at controlled room temperature—59° to 86°F.

REFERENCE

*Goodman and Gilman, *The Pharmacological Basis of Therapeutics*, 1980, 6th Edition, p. 126.

77301-3/85

Shown in Product Identification Section, page 411

LASIX® ℞

[la' siks]
(furosemide)
Oral Solution
Tablets/Injection
Diuretic

WARNING

Lasix (furosemide) is a potent diuretic which, if given in excessive amounts, can lead to a profound diuresis with water and electrolyte depletion. Therefore, careful medical supervision is required, and dose and dose schedule have to be adjusted to the individual patient's needs. (See under "DOSAGE AND ADMINISTRATION.")

DESCRIPTION

Lasix (furosemide) is an anthranilic acid derivative. Chemically, it is 4-chloro-N-furfuryl-5-sulfamoylanthranilic acid.

Lasix® (furosemide) tablets for oral administration contain furosemide as the active ingredient and the following inactive ingredients: lactose USP, magnesium stearate NF, starch NF and talc USP.

Lasix® (furosemide) Oral Solution contains furosemide as the active ingredient and the following inactive ingredients: alcohol USP 11.5%, D&C Yellow #10, FD&C Yellow #6, flavors, glycerin USP, parabens NF, purified water USP, sodium hydroxide NF, and sorbitol NF. Lasix® (furosemide) Oral Solution 10 mg/mL is an orange flavored liquid for oral administration. Furosemide is a white to off-white odorless crystalline powder. It is practically insoluble in water, sparingly soluble in alcohol, freely soluble in dilute alkali solutions and insoluble in dilute acids.

ACTIONS

Investigations into the mode of action of Lasix (furosemide) have utilized micropuncture studies in rats, stop flow experiments in dogs, and various clearance studies in both humans and experimental animals. It has been demonstrated that Lasix (furosemide) inhibits primarily the reabsorption of sodium and chloride not only in the proximal and distal tubules but also in the loop of Henle. The high degree of efficacy is largely due to this unique site of action. The action on the distal tubule is independent of any inhibitory effect on carbonic anhydrase and aldosterone.

The onset of diuresis following oral administration is within 1 hour. The peak effect occurs within the first or second hour. The duration of diuretic effect is 6 to 8 hours.

The onset of diuresis following intravenous administration is within 5 minutes and somewhat later after intramuscular administration. The peak effect occurs within the first half hour. The duration of diuretic effect is approximately 2 hours.

INDICATIONS

Edema—Lasix (furosemide) is indicated for the treatment of edema associated with congestive heart failure, cirrhosis of the liver, and renal disease, including the nephrotic syndrome. Lasix (furosemide) is particularly useful when an agent with greater diuretic potential than that of those commonly employed is desired.

Parenteral therapy should be reserved for patients unable to take oral medication or for patients in emergency clinical situations.

Lasix (furosemide) Injection is also indicated as adjunctive therapy in acute pulmonary edema. The intravenous administration of Lasix (furosemide) is indicated when a rapid onset of diuresis is desired, eg, in acute pulmonary edema.

If gastrointestinal absorption is impaired or oral medication is not practical for any reason, Lasix (furosemide) is indicated by the intravenous or intramuscular route. Parenteral use should be replaced with oral Lasix (furosemide) as soon as practical.

Hypertension—Oral Lasix (furosemide) may be used for the treatment of hypertension alone or in combination with other antihypertensive agents. Hypertensive patients who cannot be adequately controlled with thiazides will probably also not be adequately controlled with Lasix (furosemide) alone.

CONTRAINDICATIONS

Lasix (furosemide) is contraindicated in anuria. It is contraindicated in patients with a history of hypersensitivity to this compound.

WARNINGS

Excessive diuresis may result in dehydration and reduction in blood volume with circulatory collapse and with the possibility of vascular thrombosis and embolism, particularly in elderly patients. Excessive loss of potassium in patients receiving digitalis glycosides may precipitate digitalis toxicity. Care should also be exercised in patients receiving potassium-depleting steroids.

Frequent serum electrolyte, CO_2, and BUN determinations should be performed during the first few months of therapy and periodically thereafter, and abnormalities corrected or the drug temporarily withdrawn.

In patients with hepatic cirrhosis and ascites, initiation of therapy with Lasix (furosemide) is best carried out in the hospital. In hepatic coma and in states of electrolyte depletion, therapy should not be instituted until the basic condition is improved. Sudden alterations of fluid and electrolyte balance in patients with cirrhosis may precipitate hepatic coma; therefore, strict observation is necessary during the period of diuresis. Supplemental potassium chloride and, if required, an aldosterone antagonist are helpful in preventing hypokalemia and metabolic alkalosis.

If increasing azotemia and oliguria occur during treatment of severe progressive renal disease, the drug should be discontinued.

As with many other drugs, patients should be observed regularly for the possible occurrence of blood dyscrasias, liver damage, or other idiosyncratic reactions.

Patients with known sulfonamide sensitivity may show allergic reactions to Lasix (furosemide).

Lasix (furosemide) may add to or potentiate the therapeutic effect of other antihypertensive drugs. Potentiation occurs with ganglionic or peripheral adrenergic blocking drugs.

The possibility exists of exacerbation or activation of systemic lupus erythematosus.

Lasix (furosemide) appears in breast milk. If use of the drug is deemed essential, the patient should stop nursing.

Parenterally administered Lasix (furosemide) may increase the ototoxic potential of aminoglycoside antibiotics. Especially in the presence of impaired renal function, the use of parenterally administered Lasix (furosemide) in patients to whom aminoglycoside antibiotics are also being given should be avoided, except in life-threatening situations.

When parenteral use of Lasix (furosemide) precedes its oral use, it should be kept in mind that cases of tinnitus and reversible hearing impairment have been reported. There have also been some reports of cases in which irreversible hearing impairment occurred. Usually, ototoxicity has been reported when Lasix (furosemide) was injected rapidly in patients with severe impairment of renal function at doses exceeding several times the usual recommended dose and in whom other drugs known to be ototoxic were given. If the physician elects to use high dose parenteral therapy in patients with severely impaired renal function, controlled intravenous infusion is advisable [for adults, an infusion rate not exceeding 4 mg Lasix (furosemide) per minute has been used].

PRECAUTIONS

As with any effective diuretic, electrolyte depletion may occur during therapy with Lasix (furosemide), especially in patients receiving higher doses and a restricted salt intake. Periodic determinations of serum electrolytes to detect possible imbalance should be performed at appropriate intervals.

All patients receiving Lasix (furosemide) therapy should be observed for signs of fluid or electrolyte imbalance: namely, hyponatremia, hypochloremic alkalosis, and hypokalemia. Serum and urine electrolyte determinations are particularly important when the patient is vomiting excessively or receiving parenteral fluids. Medications such as digitalis may also influence serum electrolytes. Warning signs, irrespective of cause, are: dryness of mouth, thirst, weakness, lethargy, drowsiness, restlessness, muscle pains or cramps, muscular fatigue, hypotension, oliguria, tachycardia, arrhythmia, and gastrointestinal disturbances such as nausea and vomiting.

Hypokalemia may develop with Lasix (furosemide) as with any other potent diuretic, especially with brisk diuresis, when cirrhosis is present, or during concomitant use of corticosteroids or ACTH.

Interference with adequate oral electrolyte intake will also contribute to hypokalemia. Digitalis therapy may exaggerate metabolic effects of hypokalemia, especially with reference to myocardial activity.

Asymptomatic hyperuricemia can occur and gout may rarely be precipitated.

When higher doses of Lasix® (furosemide) Oral Solution are given, the sorbitol present in the vehicle may cause diarrhea (especially in children).

Periodic checks on urine and blood glucose should be made in diabetics and even those suspected of latent diabetes when receiving Lasix (furosemide). Increases in blood glucose and alterations in glucose tolerance tests with abnormalities of the fasting and 2-hour postprandial sugar have been observed, and rare cases of precipitation of diabetes mellitus have been reported.

Lasix (furosemide) may lower serum calcium levels, and rare cases of tetany have been reported. Accordingly, periodic serum calcium levels should be obtained.

Reversible elevations of BUN may be seen. These have been observed in association with dehydration, which should be avoided, particularly in patients with renal insufficiency.

Patients receiving high doses of salicylates, as in rheumatic disease, in conjunction with Lasix (furosemide) may experience salicylate toxicity at lower doses because of competitive renal excretory sites.

Lasix (furosemide) has a tendency to antagonize the skeletal muscle relaxing effect of tubocurarine and may potentiate the action of succinylcholine.

Lithium generally should not be given with diuretics because they reduce its renal clearance and add a high risk of lithium toxicity.

It has been reported in the literature that diuretics such as furosemide may enhance the nephrotoxicity of cephaloridine. Therefore, Lasix (furosemide) and cephaloridine should not be administered simultaneously.

Lasix (furosemide) may decrease arterial responsiveness to norepinephrine. This diminution is not sufficient to preclude effectiveness of the pressor agent for therapeutic use.

It has been reported in the literature that coadministration of indomethacin may reduce the natriuretic and antihypertensive effects of Lasix (furosemide) in some patients. This effect has been attributed to inhibition of prostaglandin synthesis by indomethacin. Indomethacin may also affect plasma renin levels and aldosterone excretion; this should be borne in mind when a renin profile is evaluated in hypertensive patients. Patients receiving both indomethacin and Lasix (furosemide) should be observed closely to determine if the desired diuretic and/or antihypertensive effect of Lasix (furosemide) is achieved.

Renal calcifications (from barely visible on x-ray to staghorn) have occurred in some severely premature infants treated with intravenous Lasix® (furosemide) for edema due to patent ductus arteriosus and hyaline membrane disease. The concurrent use of chlorothiazide has been reported to decrease hypercalciuria and to dissolve some calculi.

Pregnancy

Pregnancy Category C. Furosemide has been shown to cause unexplained maternal deaths and abortions in rabbits at 2, 4 and 8 times the human dose. There are no adequate and well-controlled studies in pregnant women. Furosemide should be used during pregnancy only if the potential benefit justifies the potential risk to the fetus.

The effects of furosemide on embryonic and fetal development and on pregnant dams were studied in mice, rats and rabbits.

Furosemide caused unexplained maternal deaths and abortions in the rabbit when 50 mg/kg (4 times the maximal recommended human dose of 600 mg per day) was administered between days 12 and 17 of gestation. In a previous study the lowest dose of only 25 mg/kg (2 times the maximal recommended human dose of 600 mg per day) caused maternal deaths and abortions. In a third study, none of the pregnant rabbits survived a dose of 100 mg/kg. Data from the above studies indicate fetal lethality that can precede maternal deaths.

The results of the mouse study and one of the three rabbit studies also showed an increased incidence of hydronephrosis (distention of the renal pelvis and, in some cases, of the ureters) in fetuses derived from treated dams as compared to the incidence in fetuses from the control group.

ADVERSE REACTIONS

Gastrointestinal System Reactions

1. anorexia
2. oral and gastric irritation
3. nausea
4. vomiting
5. cramping
6. diarrhea
7. constipation
8. jaundice (intrahepatic cholestatic jaundice)
9. pancreatitis

Central Nervous System Reactions

1. dizziness
2. vertigo
3. paresthesias
4. headache
5. xanthopsia
6. blurred vision
7. tinnitus and hearing loss

Hematologic Reactions

1. anemia
2. leukopenia
3. agranulocytosis (rare)
4. thrombocytopenia
5. aplastic anemia (rare)

Dermatologic—Hypersensitivity Reactions

1. purpura
2. photosensitivity
3. rash
4. urticaria
5. necrotizing angiitis (vasculitis, cutaneous vasculitis)
6. exfoliative dermatitis
7. erythema multiforme
8. pruritus

Cardiovascular Reaction

Orthostatic hypotension may occur and be aggravated by alcohol, barbiturates, or narcotics.

Other

1. hyperglycemia
2. glycosuria
3. hyperuricemia
4. muscle spasm
5. weakness
6. restlessness
7. urinary bladder spasm
8. thrombophlebitis
9. transient pain at the injection site following intramuscular injection

Whenever adverse reactions are moderate or severe, Lasix (furosemide) dosage should be reduced or therapy withdrawn.

DOSAGE AND ADMINISTRATION

Oral Administration

Edema—Therapy should be individualized according to patient response. This therapy should be titrated to gain maximal therapeutic response as well as the minimal dose possible to maintain that therapeutic response.

ADULTS—The usual initial daily dose of oral Lasix (furosemide) is 20 to 80 mg given as a single dose. Ordinarily a prompt diuresis ensues. Depending on the patient's response, a second dose can be administered 6 to 8 hours later. If the diuretic response to a single dose of 20 to 80 mg is not satisfactory, increase this dose by increments of 20 or 40 mg not sooner than 6 to 8 hours after the previous dose until the desired diuretic effect has been obtained. This individually determined single dose should then be given once or twice daily (eg, at 8:00 a.m. and 2:00 p.m.). The dose of Lasix (furosemide) may be carefully titrated up to 600 mg/day in those patients with severe clinical edematous states.

The mobilization of edema may be most efficiently and safely accomplished by utilizing an intermittent dosage schedule in which the diuretic is given for 2 to 4 consecutive days each week.

When doses exceeding 80 mg/day are given for prolonged periods, careful clinical and laboratory observations are particularly advisable.

INFANTS AND CHILDREN—The usual initial dose of oral Lasix (furosemide) in infants and children is 2 mg/kg body weight, given as a single dose. If the diuretic response is not satisfactory after the initial dose, dose may be increased by 1 or 2 mg/kg no sooner than 6 to 8 hours after the previous dose. Doses greater than 6 mg/kg body weight are not recommended.

For maintenance therapy in infants and children, the dose should be adjusted to the minimum effective level.

Hypertension—Therapy should be individualized according to the patient's response. This therapy should be titrated to gain maximal therapeutic response as well as the minimal dose possible to maintain that therapeutic response.

Continued on next page

Hoechst-Roussel—Cont.

ADULTS—The usual initial daily dose of Lasix (furosemide) for antihypertensive therapy is 80 mg, usually divided into 40 mg twice a day. Dosage should then be adjusted according to response. If the patient does not respond, add other antihypertensive agents.

Careful observations for changes in blood pressure must be made when this compound is used with other antihypertensive drugs, especially during initial therapy. The dosage of other agents must be reduced by at least 50 percent as soon as Lasix (furosemide) is added to the regimen, to prevent excessive drop in blood pressure. As the blood pressure falls under the potentiating effect of Lasix (furosemide), a further reduction in dosage or even discontinuation of other antihypertensive drugs may be necessary.

Parenteral Administration

ADULTS—Parenteral therapy should be reserved for patients for whom oral medication is not practical or in emergency situations where prompt diuresis is desired. Parenteral therapy should be replaced by oral therapy as soon as this is practical for continued mobilization of edema.

Edema—The usual initial dose of Lasix (furosemide) is 20 to 40 mg given as a single dose, injected intramuscularly or intravenously. The intravenous injection should be given slowly (1 to 2 minutes). Ordinarily, a prompt diuresis ensues. Depending on the patient's response, a second dose can be administered 2 hours after the first dose or later.

If the diuretic response with a single dose of 20 to 40 mg is not satisfactory, increase this dose by increments of 20 mg not sooner than 2 hours after the previous dose until the desired diuretic effect has been obtained. This individually determined single dose should then be given once or twice daily.

If the physician elects to use high dose parenteral therapy it should be administered as a controlled infusion at a rate not exceeding 4 mg/min. Lasix (furosemide) Injection is a mildly buffered alkaline solution which should not be mixed with acidic solutions of pH below 5.5. To prepare infusion solutions, isotonic saline and lactated Ringer's injection and 5% dextrose injection have been used after pH has been adjusted when necessary.

Therapy should be individualized according to patient response. This therapy should be titrated to gain maximal therapeutic response as well as the minimal dose possible to maintain that therapeutic response. Close medical supervision is necessary.

Acute Pulmonary Edema—The usual initial dose of Lasix (furosemide) is 40 mg injected intravenously. The injection should be given slowly (1 to 2 minutes). If 40 mg Lasix (furosemide) does not produce a satisfactory response within 1 hour the dose may be increased to 80 mg given intravenously (over 1 to 2 minutes).

If deemed necessary, additional therapy (eg, digitalis, oxygen) can be administered concomitantly.

INFANTS AND CHILDREN—Parenteral therapy should be reserved for patients for whom oral medication is not practical or in emergency situations where prompt diuresis is desired. Parenteral therapy should be replaced by oral therapy as soon as this is practical for continued mobilization of edema.

The usual initial dose of Lasix (furosemide) Injection (intravenously or intramuscularly) in infants and children is 1 mg/kg body weight and should be given slowly under close medical supervision. If the diuretic response after the initial dose is not satisfactory, dosage may be increased by 1 mg/kg not sooner than 2 hours after the previous dose, until the desired diuretic effect has been obtained. Doses greater than 6 mg/kg body weight are not recommended.

HOW SUPPLIED

Lasix (furosemide) Tablets are supplied as white, round, monogrammed, scored tablets of 40 mg in amber bottles of 100, 500, and 1,000; unit dose 100s (20 strips of 5); and Unit of Use trays of 12 × 100, 25 × 30 and 25 × 60; white, oval, monogrammed tablets of 20 mg in amber bottles of 100, 500 and 1000, and unit dose 100s (10 strips of 10); and white, round, monogrammed, facetted-edge scored tablets of 80 mg in amber bottles of 50 and 500, and unit dose 100s (20 strips of 5).

***Note:* Dispense in well-closed, light-resistant containers. Exposure to light may cause slight discoloration. Discolored tablets should not be dispensed.**

Lasix (furosemide) Oral Solution is supplied as an orange-flavored liquid containing furosemide 10 mg/mL in bottles of 60 mL (accompanied by graduated dropper) and bottles of 120 mL (accompanied by graduated dispensing spoon). The alcohol content is 11.5%.

***Note:* Store at controlled room temperature (59° -86°F). Dispense in light-resistant containers. Discard opened bottle after 60 days.**

Lasix (furosemide) Injection is supplied as a sterile solution in 2 mL amber ampuls, boxes of 5 and 50; 4 mL amber ampuls, boxes of 5 and 25; 10 mL amber ampuls, boxes of 5 and 25; 2 mL prefilled syringes, boxes of 5; 4 mL prefilled syringes, boxes of 5; and 10 mL prefilled syringes, boxes of 5; 2mL, 4mL and 10mL single-use vials in cartons of 25. Each mL contains 10 mg furosemide. Syringes supplied with 22 gauge × 1¼"needle.

***Note:* Store at controlled room temperature. (59°-86°F). Do not use if solution is discolored. Protect syringes from light. Do not remove syringes from individual package until time of use.**

Edition 5/86

Shown in Product Identification Section, page 411

LOPROX® ℞

[lo' prahks]

(ciclopirox olamine) Cream 1%

DESCRIPTION

Loprox® (ciclopirox olamine) Cream 1% is for topical use. Each gram of Loprox® (ciclopirox olamine) Cream 1% contains 10 mg ciclopirox olamine in a water miscible vanishing cream base consisting of purified water USP, 2-octyldodecanol, mineral oil USP, stearyl alcohol NF, cetyl alcohol NF, cocamide DEA, polysorbate 60 NF, myristyl alcohol NF, sorbitan monostearate NF, lactic acid USP, and benzyl alcohol NF (1%) as preservative.

Loprox® (ciclopirox olamine) Cream contains a synthetic broad-spectrum, antifungal agent ciclopirox olamine. The chemical name is 6-cyclohexyl-1-hydroxy-4-methyl-2(1*H*)-pyridone, 2-aminoethanol salt.

Loprox® (ciclopirox olamine) Cream 1% has a pH of 7.

CLINICAL PHARMACOLOGY

Ciclopirox olamine is a broad-spectrum, antifungal agent that inhibits the growth of pathogenic dermatophytes, yeasts, and *Malassezia furfur*. Ciclopirox olamine exhibits fungicidal activity *in vitro* against isolates of *Trichophyton rubrum, Trichophyton mentagrophytes, Epidermophyton floccosum, Microsporum canis,* and *Candida albicans.*

Pharmacokinetic studies in men with tagged 1% ciclopirox olamine solution in polyethylene glycol 400 showed an average of 1.3% absorption of the dose when it was applied topically to 750 cm^2 on the back followed by occlusion for 6 hours. The biological half-life was 1.7 hours and excretion occurred via the kidney. Two days after application only 0.01% of the dose applied could be found in the urine. Fecal excretion was negligible.

Penetration studies in human cadaverous skin from the back, with Loprox® (ciclopirox olamine) Cream 1% with tagged ciclopirox olamine showed the presence of 0.8 to 1.6% of the dose in stratum corneum 1.5 to 6 hours after application. The levels in the dermis were still 10 to 15 times above the minimum inhibitory concentrations.

Autoradiographic studies with human cadaverous skin showed that ciclopirox olamine penetrates into the hair and through the epidermis and hair follicles into the sebaceous glands and dermis, while a portion of the drug remains in the stratum corneum.

Draize Human Sensitization Assay, 21-Day Cumulative Irritancy study, Phototoxicity study, and Photo-Draize study conducted in a total of 142 healthy male subjects showed no contact sensitization of the delayed hypersensitivity type, no irritation, no phototoxicity, and no photo-contact sensitization due to Loprox® (ciclopirox olamine) Cream 1%.

INDICATIONS AND USAGE

Loprox® (ciclopirox olamine) Cream 1% is indicated for the topical treatment of the following dermal infections: tinea pedis, tinea cruris and tinea corporis due to *Trichophyton rubrum, Trichophyton mentagrophytes, Epidermophyton floccosum,* and *Microsporum canis;* candidiasis (moniliasis) due to *Candida albicans;* and tinea (pityriasis) versicolor due to *Malassezia furfur.*

CONTRAINDICATIONS

Loprox® (ciclopirox olamine) Cream 1% is contraindicated in individuals who have shown hypersensitivity to any of its components.

WARNINGS

General: Loprox® (ciclopirox olamine) Cream 1% is not for ophthalmic use.

PRECAUTIONS

If a reaction suggesting sensitivity or chemical irritation should occur with the use of Loprox® (ciclopirox olamine) Cream 1%, treatment should be discontinued and appropriate therapy instituted.

Information for patients—

The patient should be told to:

1. Use the medication for the full treatment time even though symptoms may have improved and notify the physician if there is no improvement after four weeks.
2. Inform the physician if the area of application shows signs of increased irritation (redness, itching, burning, blistering, swelling, oozing) indicative of possible sensitization.
3. Avoid the use of occlusive wrappings or dressings.

Carcinogenesis, mutagenesis, impairment of fertility:

A carcinogenicity study in female mice dosed cutaneously twice per week for 50 weeks followed by a 6-month drug-free observation period prior to necropsy revealed no evidence of tumors at the application site. Several mutagenic tests indicated no potential for mutagenesis.

Pregnancy Category B:

Reproduction studies have been performed in the mouse, rat, rabbit, and monkey, (via various routes of administration) at doses 10 times or more the topical human dose and have revealed no significant evidence of impaired fertility or harm to the fetus due to ciclopirox olamine. There are, however, no adequate or well-controlled studies in pregnant women. Because animal reproduction studies are not always predictive of human response this drug should be used during pregnancy only if clearly needed.

Nursing mothers:

It is not known whether this drug is excreted in human milk. Because many drugs are excreted in human milk, caution should be exercised when Loprox® (ciclopirox olamine) Cream 1% is administered to a nursing woman.

Pediatric use:

Safety and effectiveness in children below the age of 10 years have not been established.

ADVERSE REACTIONS

In all controlled clinical studies with 514 patients using Loprox® (ciclopirox olamine) Cream 1% and in 296 patients using the vehicle cream, the incidence of adverse reactions was low. This included pruritus at the site of application in one patient and worsening of the clinical signs and symptoms in another patient using ciclopirox olamine cream 1% and burning in one patient and worsening of the clinical signs and symptoms in another patient using the vehicle cream.

DOSAGE AND ADMINISTRATION

Gently massage Loprox® (ciclopirox olamine) Cream 1% into the affected and surrounding skin areas twice daily, in the morning and evening. Clinical improvement with relief of pruritus and other symptoms usually occurs within the first week of treatment. If a patient shows no clinical improvement after four weeks of treatment with Loprox® (ciclopirox olamine) Cream 1%, the diagnosis should be redetermined. Patients with tinea versicolor usually exhibit clinical and mycological clearing after two weeks of treatment.

HOW SUPPLIED

Loprox® (ciclopirox olamine) Cream 1% is supplied in 15 gram, 30 gram and 90 gram tubes.

Store at controlled room temperature (59°- 86°F).

Loprox® REG TM HOECHST AG

70900-7/85

Shown in Product Identification Section, page 411

STREPTASE® ℞

[strep' tās]

(streptokinase)

DESCRIPTION

Streptase® (streptokinase) is a sterile, purified preparation of a bacterial protein elaborated by group C β-hemolytic streptococci. It is supplied as a lyophilized white powder containing 25 mg cross-linked gelatin polypeptides, 25 mg sodium L-glutamate and 100 mg Normal Serum Albumin (Human) as stabilizers for intravenous and intracoronary administration.

CLINICAL PHARMACOLOGY

Streptase® (streptokinase) acts with plasminogen to produce an "activator complex" that converts plasminogen to the proteolytic enzyme plasmin. Plasmin degrades fibrin clots as well as fibrinogen and other plasma proteins (1). Intravenous infusion of streptokinase is followed by increased fibrinolytic activity. This hyperfibrinolytic effect disappears within a few hours after discontinuation, but a prolonged thrombin time, especially with prolonged administration, may persist for up to 24 hours due to a decrease in plasma levels of fibrinogen and an increase in the amount of circulating fibrin(ogen) degradation products (FDP). The thrombin time will usually decrease to less than two times normal control value within 4 hours.

INDICATIONS AND USAGE

STREPTASE® (STREPTOKINASE) IS INDICATED FOR THE LYSIS OF THROMBI IN SEVERAL CONDITIONS. THE ROUTE (METHOD) OF ADMINISTRATION, DURATION, AND DOSAGE VARY WITH EACH CONDITION (SEE DOSAGE AND ADMINISTRATION).

Pulmonary Embolism

With Streptase® (streptokinase) therapy, angiographic, lung scan and/or hemodynamic improvement is more rapid and complete than with heparin therapy (2-4).

Streptase® (streptokinase) is indicated in adults for:

- the lysis of acute pulmonary emboli, involving obstruction of blood flow to a lobe or multiple segments (5), or
- the lysis of pulmonary emboli accompanied by unstable hemodynamics, i.e., failure to maintain blood pressure without supportive measures.

The diagnosis should be confirmed by objective means, such as pulmonary angiography via an upper extremity vein, or noninvasive procedures such as lung scanning.

Deep Vein Thrombosis

Streptase® (streptokinase) is indicated in adults for lysis of acute, extensive thrombi of the deep veins, such as those involving the popliteal and more proximal vessels. Diagnosis should be confirmed by objective means, preferably ascending venography. Studies have demonstrated better salvage of valvular function and prevention of postphlebitic syndrome by streptokinase plus heparin than by heparin alone (6-8).

Should pulmonary embolism or recurrent pulmonary embolism occur during streptokinase therapy, the originally planned course of treatment should be completed in an attempt to lyse these emboli. While pulmonary embolism may occasionally occur during Streptase® (streptokinase) treatment of deep vein thrombosis, the incidence is no greater than when patients are treated with heparin alone (4,9-11).

Arterial Thrombosis and Embolism

Streptase® (streptokinase) is indicated in adults for the lysis of acute arterial thrombi and for the lysis of arterial emboli (12-14). However, the use of Streptase® (streptokinase) in arterial emboli originating from the left side of the heart (e.g., in mitral stenosis accompanied by atrial fibrillation) should be avoided due to the danger of new embolic phenomena, including those to cerebral vessels.

Arteriovenous Cannulae Occlusion

Streptase® (streptokinase) is indicated for clearing of totally or partially occluded arteriovenous cannulae as an alternative to surgical revision when acceptable flow cannot otherwise be achieved (15).

Coronary Artery Thrombosis

Streptase® (streptokinase) has been reported to lyse acute thrombi obstructing coronary arteries, associated with evolving transmural myocardial infarction. Diagnosis of acute myocardial infarction has been confirmed, and the site of coronary thrombosis identified by selective coronary angiography (16,17). Other studies (18-24) have demonstrated that (a) a thrombus is present in approximately 90% of patients evaluated within four hours of onset of symptoms; (b) when compared to concurrent or historical controls, the majority of patients who received intracoronary streptokinase within 6 hours of onset of symptoms, showed a more immediate recanalization (within a few minutes vs hours/days) of the involved vessel.

IT HAS NOT BEEN ESTABLISHED THAT INTRACORONARY ADMINISTRATION OF STREPTOKINASE DURING EVOLVING TRANSMURAL MYOCARDIAL INFARCTION RESULTS IN SALVAGE OF MYOCARDIAL TISSUE, NOR THAT IT REDUCES MORTALITY. CONTROLLED STUDIES ADDRESSING THESE PARAMETERS ARE IN PROGRESS (25) AND UNTIL COMPLETED, THOSE PATIENTS WHO MIGHT BENEFIT FROM THIS THERAPY CANNOT BE DEFINED.

CONTRAINDICATIONS

Because thrombolytic therapy increases the risk of bleeding, Streptase® (streptokinase) is contraindicated in the following situations:

- active internal bleeding
- recent (within 2 months) cerebrovascular accident, intracranial or intraspinal surgery (see **Warnings**)
- intracranial neoplasm

WARNINGS

Bleeding

The aim of Streptase® (streptokinase) therapy is the production of sufficient amounts of plasmin for the lysis of intravascular deposits of fibrin; however, fibrin deposits which provide hemostasis, for example, at sites of needle punctures, are also lysed and bleeding from such sites may occur.

Intramuscular injections and nonessential handling of the patient must be avoided during treatment with Streptase® (streptokinase). Venipunctures should be performed carefully and as infrequently as possible.

Should an arterial puncture be necessary during intravenous therapy, upper extremity vessels are preferable. Pressure should be applied for at least 30 minutes, a pressure dressing applied and the puncture site checked frequently for evidence of bleeding.

When internal bleeding occurs, it may be more difficult to manage than that which occurs with conventional anticoagulant therapy.

In the following conditions the risks of therapy may be increased and should be weighed against the anticipated benefits.

- Recent (within 10 days) major surgery, obstetrical delivery, organ biopsy, previous puncture of noncompressible vessels
- Recent serious gastrointestinal bleeding (within 10 days)
- Recent trauma including cardiopulmonary resuscitation
- Severe, uncontrolled arterial hypertension
- High likelihood of left heart thrombus, e.g., mitral stenosis with atrial fibrillation
- Subacute bacterial endocarditis
- Hemostatic defects including those secondary to severe hepatic or renal disease
- Pregnancy
- Cerebrovascular disease
- Diabetic hemorrhagic retinopathy
- Prior severe allergic reaction to streptokinase
- Septic thrombophlebitis or occluded AV cannula at seriously infected site
- Any other condition in which bleeding constitutes a significant hazard or would be particularly difficult to manage because of its location.

Should serious spontaneous bleeding (not controllable by local pressure) occur, the infusion of Streptase® (streptokinase) should be terminated immediately and treatment instituted as described under **Adverse Reactions.**

Use of Anticoagulants

Concurrent use of anticoagulants with intravenous administration of Streptase® (streptokinase) is not recommended. However, concurrent use of heparin may be required during intracoronary administration of Streptase® (streptokinase). Clinical studies with concurrent use of heparin and lower Streptase® (streptokinase) dosages employed during intracoronary administration have demonstrated no tendency toward increased bleeding that would not be attributable to the procedure or Streptase® (streptokinase) alone. Nevertheless, careful monitoring for excessive bleeding is advised.

Arrhythmias

Rapid lysis of coronary thrombi has been reported occasionally to cause reperfusion atrial or ventricular dysrhythmias requiring immediate treatment. During studies, careful monitoring for arrhythmia was maintained during and immediately following intracoronary administration of Streptase® (streptokinase).

PRECAUTIONS

General:

Non-cardiogenic pulmonary edema has been reported rarely in patients treated with streptokinase. The risk of this appears greatest in patients who have large myocardial infarctions and are undergoing thrombolytic therapy by the intracoronary route.

Use in Pregnancy and Children

Safety and effectiveness of Streptase® (streptokinase) therapy in children and during pregnancy has not been established. Therefore, treatment of such patients is not recommended.

Drug Interactions

The interaction of Streptase® (streptokinase) with other drugs has not been studied. Drugs that alter platelet function should not be used during therapy. Common examples are: aspirin, indomethacin, and phenylbutazone (6).

Patient Monitoring

Before commencing thrombolytic therapy, it is desirable to obtain a thrombin time (TT), activated partial thromboplastin time (APTT), prothrombin time (PT), hematocrit and platelet count to obtain hemostatic status of the patient.

Intracoronary Artery Infusion

During studies, laboratory monitoring of hemostatic parameters during intracoronary artery infusion showed minimal changes, if any. Heparin was continued during therapy or instituted following therapy and monitored accordingly.

Intravenous Infusion

If heparin has been given, it should be discontinued and the TT or APTT should be less than twice the normal control value before thrombolytic therapy is started.

During the infusion, decreases in the plasminogen and fibrinogen level and an increase in the level of FDP (the latter two serving to prolong the clotting times of coagulation tests) will generally confirm the existence of a lytic state. Therefore, therapy can be monitored by performing the TT or PT, approximately 4 hours after initiation of therapy.

Following the infusion, **before (re)instituting heparin,** the TT should be less than twice the normal control value.

ADVERSE REACTIONS

The following adverse reactions have been frequently associated with intravenous therapy but may also occur with intracoronary artery infusion:

Bleeding

Minor bleeding occurs often with thrombolytic therapy mainly at invaded or disturbed sites. When lytic therapy is continued while local measures are used to control minor bleeding, do **not** reduce the dose as this will increase lytic activity since more plasminogen will be available for conversion to plasmin. Severe internal bleeding involving gastrointestinal, genitourinary, retroperitoneal or intracerebral sites, may occur. Several fatalities due to cerebral and other serious internal hemorrhage have occurred during intravenous thrombolytic therapy.

Should uncontrollable bleeding occur, Streptase® (streptokinase) infusion should be discontinued and, if necessary, blood loss and reversal of the bleeding tendency can be effectively managed with whole blood (fresh blood preferable), packed red blood cells and cryoprecipitate or fresh frozen plasma. Although the use of aminocaproic acid (ACA, AMICAR®) in humans as an antidote for streptokinase has not been documented, it may be considered in an emergency situation.

Allergic Reactions

Reactions attributed to possible anaphylaxis have been observed rarely in patients treated with Streptase® (streptokinase) intravenously. These ranged in severity from minor breathing difficulty to bronchospasm, periorbital swelling or angioneurotic edema. Other milder allergic effects such as urticaria, itching, flushing, nausea, headache and musculoskeletal pain have also been observed.

Mild or moderate reactions may be managed with concomitant antihistamine and/or corticosteroid therapy. Severe allergic reactions require immediate discontinuation of Streptase® (streptokinase), with adrenergics, antihistamines, or corticosteroids administered intravenously as required.

Fever

Although Streptase® (streptokinase) is nonpyrogenic in standard animal tests, approximately one-third of patients treated with Streptase® (streptokinase) intravenously have shown increases in body temperature of ≥ 1.5°F. Symptomatic treatment is usually sufficient to alleviate discomfort. The use of acetaminophen rather than aspirin is recommended.

DOSAGE AND ADMINISTRATION

A. Lysis of Coronary Artery Thrombi (18-23)

During clinical studies, Streptase® (streptokinase) was administered selectively into the thrombosed coronary artery via coronary catheter placed by the Judkins or Sones Technique. When administered within 6 hours of onset of symptoms of acute transmural myocardial infarction, at a bolus dose averaging 20,000 IU and a maintenance dose averaging 2,000 IU/min for 60 minutes, greater than 75% of occlusions were opened in less than 1 hour.

B. Treatment of Deep Vein Thrombosis, Pulmonary or Arterial Embolism or Arterial Thrombosis (26,27)

Streptokinase treatment should be instituted as soon as possible after onset of thrombotic event, preferably no later than seven days after onset. Any delay in instituting lytic therapy to evaluate the effect of heparin therapy decreases the potential for optimal efficacy (28). Reconstituted streptokinase solution may alter drop size which will influence the accuracy of drop counting infusion devices, either manually or instrument controlled. Use of volumetric or syringe infusion pumps is recommended.

Loading Dose

Since human exposure to streptococci is common, antibodies to streptokinase (streptokinase resistance) are found normally. Thus, a loading dose of Streptase® (streptokinase) sufficient to neutralize the resistance is required. A dose of 250,000 IU Streptase® (streptokinase) infused into a peripheral vein over 30 minutes has been found appropriate in over 90% of patients.

Maintenance Dose*

A maintenance dose infusion of 100,000 IU/hr is given following the loading dose. Administer this maintenance dose for 24 hours for the treatment of pulmonary embolism (up to 72 hours if concurrent deep vein thrombosis is suspected), 24-72 hours for the treatment of arterial thrombosis and arterial embolism, and 72 hours for the treatment of deep vein thrombosis.

If the thrombin time or any other parameter of lysis after 4 hours of therapy is less than approximately 1½ times the normal control value, discontinue Streptase® (streptokinase) as excessive resistance to streptokinase is present.

*A variable dosage of Streptase® (streptokinase) and frequent laboratory monitoring were recommended in the past (29). However, since experience shows that these do not increase the efficacy or safety of Streptase® (streptokinase) therapy, they are no longer recommended.

Anticoagulation after Terminating Intravenous Streptokinase Treatment

At the end of Streptase® (streptokinase) therapy, treatment with heparin by continuous intravenous infusion is recommended to prevent recurrent thrombosis (3). Heparin treatment (without a loading dose) should not begin until the thrombin time has decreased to **less than twice** the normal control value (approximately 3 to 4 hours). (See manufacturer's prescribing information for proper use of heparin.) This should be followed by oral anticoagulation in the conventional manner.

C. Treatment of Arteriovenous Cannula Occlusion:

1. Before Treatment:
   Before using Streptase® (streptokinase), an attempt should be made to clear the cannula by careful syringe technique, using heparinized saline solution. If adequate flow is not reestablished, Streptase® (streptokinase) may be employed. Allow the effect of any pretreatment anticoagulants to diminish.
2. Streptase® (streptokinase) Administration:
   Instill 250,000 IU Streptase® (streptokinase) in 2 mL intravenous solution into each occluded limb of the

Continued on next page

Hoechst-Roussel—Cont.

cannula slowly. Clamp off cannula limb(s) for 2 hours. Observe the patient closely for possible adverse effects.

3. After Treatment:
   Aspirate contents of infused cannula limb(s), flush with saline, reconnect cannula.

RECONSTITUTION AND DILUTION

For Intracoronary Artery and Intravenous Administration
Slight flocculation (described as thin translucent fibers) of reconstituted Streptase® (streptokinase) occurred occasionally during clinical trials but did not interfere with safe use of the solution. Do not add any other medication to the container of Streptase® (streptokinase).
The following reconstitution and dilution procedure will minimize flocculation:

1. Slowly add 5 mL Sodium Chloride Injection, USP or Dextrose (5%) Injection, USP, directing it at the side of the vacuum packed vial rather than into the Streptase® (streptokinase).
2. Roll and tilt the vial gently to reconstitute. **Avoid shaking.** (Shaking may cause foaming and/or increase flocculation.)
3. Further dilute the entire reconstituted contents of the vial slowly and carefully to a total volume of approximately 45 mL (see Table 1). Avoid shaking and agitation on dilution. (If necessary, total volume may be increased to a maximum of 500 mL with the infusion pump rate in Table 1 increased accordingly. To facilitate setting the infusion pump rate, a total volume of 45 mL, or multiple thereof, is recommended.)
4. The solution may be filtered through a 0.22 μm or a 0.45 μm filter.
5. Solutions containing **large amounts** of flocculation should be discarded.
6. If not used soon after reconstitution, store Streptase® (streptokinase) at 2-4°C. Discard reconstituted drug if not administered within 24 hours.

[See table below].

For Use in Arteriovenous Cannulae
Slowly reconstitute the contents of 250,000 IU Streptase® (streptokinase) vacuum packed vial with 2 mL Sodium Chloride Injection, USP or Dextrose (5%) Injection, USP.

HOW SUPPLIED

Streptase® (streptokinase) is supplied as a lyophilized white powder in 6.5 mL vials (in packages of 10) with color-coded labels corresponding to the amount of purified Streptase® (streptokinase) in each vial as follows:
green-250,000 IU blue-750,000 IU
Store unopened vials at controlled room temperature (15-30°C).

References:

1. McNicol, G.P.: The fibrinolytic system. Postgrad Med J 49 (Suppl): 10-2, 1973.
2. Brogden, R.N., Speight, T.M., Avery, G.S.: Streptokinase: A review of its clinical pharmacology, mechanism of action and therapeutic uses. Drugs 5:357-445, 1973.
3. Fratantoni, J.C., Ness, P., Simon, T.L.: Thrombolytic therapy: Current status. N Engl J Med 293:1073-8, 1975.
4. Urokinase Pulmonary Embolism Study Group: Urokinase-streptokinase embolism trial. JAMA 229:1606-13, 1974.
5. Sharma, G.V.R.K., Burleson, V.A., Sasahara, A.A.: Effect of thrombolytic therapy on pulmonary-capillary blood volume in patients with pulmonary embolism. N Engl J Med 303:842-5, 1980.
6. Common, H.H., Seaman, A.J., Rosch, J., et al: Deep vein thrombosis treated with streptokinase or heparin. Follow-up of a randomized study. Angiology 27:645-54, 1976.
7. Marder, V.J., Soulen, R.L., Atichartakarn, V., et al: Quantitative venographic assessment of deep vein thrombosis in the evaluation of streptokinase and heparin therapy. J Lab Clin Med 89:1018-29, 1977.
8. Johansson, L., Nylander, G., Hedner, U., et al: Comparison of streptokinase with heparin: Late results in the treatment of deep venous thrombosis. Acta Med Scand 206:93-8, 1979.
9. Urokinase pulmonary embolism trial study group: A urokinase pulmonary embolism trial. A national cooperative study. Circulation 47 (Suppl II): 1-108, 1973.
10. Arnesen, H., Heilo, A., Jakobsen, E., et al: A prospective study of streptokinase and heparin in the treatment of venous thrombosis. Acta Med Scand 203: 457-463, 1978.
11. Elliot, M. S., Immelman, E. J., Jeffery, P., et al: A comparative randomized trial of heparin versus streptokinase in the treatment of acute proximal venous thrombosis. An interim report of a prospective trial. Br J Surg 66: 838-843, 1979.
12. Dotter, C.T., Rosch, J., Seaman, A.J., et al: Streptokinase treatment of thromboembolic disease. Radiology 102:283-90, 1972.
13. Persson, A.V., Thompson, J.E., Patman, R.D.: Acute arterial occlusions. Vasc Surg 11:359-63, 1977.
14. Reichle, F.A., Rao, N.A., Chang, K.H., et al: Thrombolysis of acute or subacute nonembolic arterial thrombosis. J Surg Res 22:202-208, 1977.
15. Data on File for Arteriovenous Cannulae Occlusion. Hoechst-Roussel Pharmaceuticals Inc.
16. Mathey, D.G., Kuck, K.H., Tilsner, V., et al: Nonsurgical coronary artery recanalization in acute transmural myocardial infarction. Circulation 63: 489-97, 1981.
17. Rentrop, P., Blanke H., Karsch, K.R., et al: Selective intracoronary thrombolysis in acute myocardial infarction and unstable angina pectoris. Circulation 63: 307-17, 1981.
18. Cowley, M.J., Hastillo, A., Vetrovec, G.W., et al: Effects of intracoronary streptokinase in acute myocardial infarction. Am Heart J 102:1149-1158, 1981.
19. Mathey, D.G., Rodewald, G., Rentrop, P., et al: Intracoronary streptokinase thrombolytic recanalization and subsequent surgical bypass of remaining atherosclerotic stenosis in acute myocardial infarction: Complimentary combined approach effecting reduced infarct size, preventing reinfarction, and improving left ventricular function. Am Heart J 102:1194-1201, 1981.
20. Merx, W., Doerr, R., Rentrop, P., et al: Evaluation of the effectiveness of intracoronary streptokinase infusion in acute myocardial infarction: Postprocedure management and hospital course in 204 patients. Am Heart J 102:1181-1187, 1981.
21. Reduto, L.A., Freund, G.C., Gaeta, J.M., et al: Coronary artery reperfusion in acute myocardial infarction: Beneficial effects of intracoronary streptokinase on left ventricular salvage and performance. Am Heart J 102:1168-1177, 1981.
22. Rentrop, K.P., Karsch, K.R., Blanke H., et al: Changes in left ventricular function after intracoronary streptokinase infusion in clinically evolving myocardial infarction. Am Heart J 102:1188-1193, 1981.
23. Rutsch, W., Schartl, M., Mathey, D., et al: Percutaneous transluminal coronary recanalization: Procedure, results and acute complications. Am Heart J 102:1178-1180, 1981.
24. De Wood, M.A.; Spores J; Notske R; et al: Prevalence of total coronary occlusion during the early hours of transmural myocardial infarction. New Eng J. Med 303:897-902, 1980.
25. Workshop on Limitations of Infarct Size with Thrombolytic Agents. NIH, Bethesda, Maryland, 1981.
26. Marder, V.J.: The use of thrombolytic agents: Choice of patient, drug administration, laboratory monitoring. Ann Intern Med 90:802-8, 1979.
27. Bell, W.R., Meek, A.G.: Guidelines for the use of thrombolytic agents. N Eng J Med 301:1266-70, 1979.
28. Sherry, S., Bell, W.R., Duckert, F.H., et al: Thrombolytic Therapy in Thrombosis: A National Institutes of Health Consensus Development Conference. Ann Intern Med 93:141-4, 1980.
29. Porter, J.M., Seaman, A.J., Common, H.H., et al: Comparison of heparin and streptokinase in the treatment of venous thrombosis. Am Surg 40:511-19, 1975.

78500-1/84

TABLE I
Suggested Dilutions and Infusion Rates

Streptase® (streptokinase) Dosage/Infusion Rate	Streptase® (streptokinase) Vial Content Needed	Total Volume of Solution (mL)	Infusion Pump Rate
I. Intracoronary Artery Administration			
A. Bolus Injection 20,000 IU	1 vial, 250,000 IU*	125	Inject 10 mL
B. Maintenance Dose 2,000 IU/min			60 mL per hour
*sufficient for Bolus Injection and Maintenance Dose			
II. Intravenous Administration			
A. Loading Dose 250,000 IU/30 min	a) 1 vial, 250,000 IU	45	90 mL per hour for 30 min
	or		
	b) 1 vial, 750,000 IU	45	30 mL per hour for 30 min
B. Maintenance Dose 100,000 IU/hr	1 vial, 750,000 IU	45**	6 mL per hour

** If necessary, total volume may be increased, in increments of 45 mL, to a maximum of 500 mL with the infusion pump rate increased accordingly. The total volume of 45 mL or multiple thereof is recommended.

SURFAK®

[ser' fak]
(docusate calcium USP)

(See PDR For Nonprescription Drugs)
Shown in Product Identification Section, page 411

TOPICORT® ℞

[top' i-kort"]
(desoximetasone)
EMOLLIENT CREAM 0.25%

TOPICORT® LP

(desoximetasone)
EMOLLIENT CREAM 0.05%

TOPICORT® GEL

(desoximetasone) 0.05%

TOPICORT® OINTMENT

(desoximetasone) 0.25%

DESCRIPTION

Topicort® (desoximetasone) Emollient Cream 0.25%, Topicort® LP (desoximetasone) Emollient Cream 0.05%, Topicort® Gel (desoximetasone) 0.05%, and Topicort® Ointment (desoximetasone) 0.25% contain the active synthetic corticosteroid desoximetasone. The topical corticosteroids constitute a class of primarily synthetic steroids used as anti-inflammatory and anti-pruritic agents. Each gram of Topicort® (desoximetasone) Emollient Cream 0.25% contains 2.5 mg of desoximetasone in an emollient cream consisting of isopropyl myristate, cetylstearyl alcohol, white petrolatum, mineral oil, lanolin alcohol and purified water.

Each gram of Topicort® LP (desoximetasone) Emollient Cream 0.05% contains 0.5 mg of desoximetasone in an emollient cream consisting of isopropyl myristate, cetylstearyl alcohol, white petrolatum, mineral oil, lanolin alcohol, edetate disodium, lactic acid and purified water.

Each gram of Topicort® Gel (desoximetasone) 0.05% contains 0.5 mg desoximetasone in a gel consisting of purified water, SD alcohol 40 (20% w/w), isopropyl myristate, carbomer 940, trolamine, edetate disodium and docusate sodium.

Each gram of Topicort® Ointment (desoximetasone) 0.25% contains 2.5 mg of desoximetasone in a base of propylene glycol, sorbitan sesquioleate, fatty alcohol citrate, fatty acid pentaerythritol ester, beeswax, aluminum stearate, citric acid, butylated hydroxyanisole and white petrolatum.

The chemical name of desoximetasone is Pregna-1, 4-diene-3, 20-dione, 9-fluoro-11, 21-dihydroxy-16-methyl-, (11β,16α)-.

Desoximetasone has the empirical formula $C_{22}H_{29}FO_4$ and a molecular weight of 376.47. The CAS Registry Number is 382-67-2.

CLINICAL PHARMACOLOGY

Topical corticosteroids share anti-inflammatory, anti-pruritic and vasoconstrictive actions.

The mechanism of anti-inflammatory activity of the topical corticosteroids is unclear. Various laboratory methods, including vasoconstrictor assays, are used to compare and predict potencies and/or clinical efficacies of the topical corticosteroids. There is some evidence to suggest that a recognizable correlation exists between vasoconstrictor potency and therapeutic efficacy in man.

Pharmacokinetics
The extent of percutaneous absorption of topical corticosteroids is determined by many factors including the vehicle, the integrity of the epidermal barrier, and the use of occlusive dressings.

Topical corticosteroids can be absorbed from normal intact skin. Inflammation and/or other disease processes in the skin increase percutaneous absorption. Occlusive dressings substantially increase the percutaneous absorption of topical corticosteroids. Thus, occlusive dressings may be a valuable therapeutic adjunct for treatment of resistant dermatoses.

Once absorbed through the skin, topical corticosteroids are handled through pharmacokinetic pathways similar to systemically administered corticosteroids. Corticosteroids are bound to plasma proteins in varying degrees. Corticosteroids are metabolized primarily in the liver and are then excreted

by the kidneys. Some of the topical corticosteroids and their metabolites are also excreted into the bile.
Pharmacokinetic studies in men with Topicort® (desoximetasone) Emollient Cream 0.25% with tagged desoximetasone showed a total of 5.2% ± 2.9% excretion in urine (4.1% ± 2.3%) and feces (1.1% ± 0.6%) and no detectable level (limit of sensitivity: 0.005 μg/mL) in the blood when it was applied topically on the back followed by occlusion for 24 hours. Seven days after application, no further radioactivity was detected in urine or feces. The half-life of the material was 15 ± 2 hours (for urine) and 17 ± 2 hours (for feces) between the third and fifth trial day.
Pharmacokinetic studies in men with Topicort® Ointment (desoximetasone) 0.25% with tagged desoximetasone showed no detectable level (limit of sensitivity: 0.003 μg/mL) in 1 subject and 0.004 and 0.006 μg/mL in the remaining 2 subjects in the blood when it was applied topically on the back followed by occlusion for 24 hours. The extent of absorption for the ointment was 7% based on radioactivity recovered from urine and feces. Seven days after application, no further radioactivity was detected in urine or feces.
Studies with other similarly structured steroids have shown that predominant metabolite reaction occurs through conjugation to form the glucuronide and sulfate ester.

INDICATIONS AND USAGE

Topicort® (desoximetasone) Emollient Cream 0.25%, Topicort® LP (desoximetasone) Emollient Cream 0.05%, Topicort® Gel (desoximetasone) 0.05% and Topicort® Ointment (desoximetasone) 0.25% are indicated for the relief of the inflammatory and pruritic manifestations of corticosteroid-responsive dermatoses.

CONTRAINDICATIONS

Topical corticosteroids are contraindicated in those patients with a history of hypersensitivity to any of the components of the preparation.

PRECAUTIONS

General

Systemic absorption of topical corticosteroids has produced reversible hypothalamic-pituitary-adrenal (HPA) axis suppression, manifestations of Cushing's syndrome, hyperglycemia, and glucosuria in some patients.
Conditions which augment systemic absorption include the application of the more potent steroids, use over large surface areas, prolonged use, and the addition of occlusive dressings.
Therefore, patients receiving a large dose of a potent topical steroid applied to a large surface area or under an occlusive dressing should be evaluated periodically for evidence of HPA axis suppression by using the urinary free cortisol and ACTH stimulation tests. If HPA axis suppression is noted, an attempt should be made to withdraw the drug, to reduce the frequency of application, or to substitute a less potent steroid.
Recovery of HPA axis function is generally prompt and complete upon discontinuation of the drug. Infrequently, signs and symptoms of steroid withdrawal may occur, requiring supplemental systemic corticosteroids.
Children may absorb proportionally larger amounts of topical corticosteroids and thus be more susceptible to systemic toxicity (See **Precautions—Pediatric Use**)
If irritation develops, topical corticosteroids should be discontinued and appropriate therapy instituted.
In the presence of dermatological infections, the use of an appropriate antifungal or antibacterial agent should be instituted. If a favorable response does not occur promptly, the corticosteroid should be discontinued until the infection has been adequately controlled.

Information for the Patient

Patients using topical corticosteroids should receive the following information and instructions:

1. This medication is to be used as directed by the physician. It is for external use only. Avoid contact with the eyes.
2. Patients should be advised not to use this medication for any disorder other than for which it was prescribed.
3. The treated skin area should not be bandaged or otherwise covered or wrapped as to be occlusive unless directed by the physician.
4. Patients should report any signs of local adverse reactions especially under occlusive dressing.
5. Parents of pediatric patients should be advised not to use tight-fitting diapers or plastic pants on a child being treated in the diaper area, as these garments may constitute occlusive dressings.

Laboratory Tests

The following tests may be helpful in evaluating the HPA axis suppression:
Urinary free cortisol test
ACTH stimulation test

Carcinogenesis, Mutagenesis, and Impairment of Fertility

Long-term animal studies have not been performed to evaluate the carcinogenic potential or the effect on fertility of topical corticosteroids.
Studies to determine mutagenicity with prednisolone and hydrocortisone have revealed negative results.

Pregnancy Category C

Corticosteroids are generally teratogenic in laboratory animals when administered systemically at relatively low dosage levels. The more potent corticosteroids have been shown to be teratogenic after dermal application in laboratory animals.
Desoximetasone has been shown to be teratogenic and embryotoxic in mice, rats, and rabbits when given by subcutaneous or dermal routes of administration in doses 3 to 30 times the human dose of Topicort® (desoximetasone) Emollient Cream 0.25% and Topicort® Ointment (desoximetasone) 0.25%, or 15 to 150 times the human dose of Topicort® LP (desoximetasone) Emollient Cream 0.05% and Topicort® Gel (desoximetasone) 0.05%.
There are no adequate and well-controlled studies in pregnant women on teratogenic effects from topically applied corticosteroids. Therefore, Topicort® (desoximetasone) Emollient Cream 0.25%, Topicort® LP (desoximetasone) Emollient Cream 0.05%, Topicort® Gel (desoximetasone) 0.05% and Topicort® Ointment (desoximetasone) 0.25% should be used during pregnancy only if the potential benefit justifies the potential risk to the fetus. Drugs of this class should not be used extensively on pregnant patients, in large amounts, or for prolonged periods of time.

Nursing Mothers

It is not known whether topical administration of corticosteroids could result in sufficient systemic absorption to produce detectable quantities in breast milk. Systemically administered corticosteroids are secreted into breast milk in quantities not likely to have a deleterious effect on the infant. Nevertheless, caution should be exercised when topical corticosteroids are administered to a nursing woman.

Pediatric Use

Pediatric patients may demonstrate greater susceptibility to topical corticosteroid-induced HPA axis suppression and Cushing's syndrome than mature patients because of a larger skin surface area to body weight ratio.
Hypothalamic-pituitary-adrenal (HPA) axis suppression, Cushing's syndrome, and intracranial hypertension have been reported in children receiving topical corticosteroids. Manifestations of adrenal suppression in children include linear growth retardation, delayed weight gain, low plasma cortisol levels, and absence of response to ACTH stimulation. Manifestations of intracranial hypertension include bulging fontanelles, headaches, and bilateral papilledema.
Administration of topical corticosteroids to children should be limited to the least amount compatible with an effective therapeutic regimen. Chronic corticosteroid therapy may interfere with the growth and development of children. The safety and effectiveness of Topicort® Ointment (desoximetasone) 0.25% in children below the age of 10 have not been established.

ADVERSE REACTIONS

The following local adverse reactions are reported infrequently with topical corticosteroids, but may occur more frequently with the use of occlusive dressings. These reactions are listed in an approximate decreasing order of occurrence:

Burning	Perioral dermatitis
Itching	Allergic contact dermatitis
Irritation	Maceration of the skin
Dryness	Secondary infection
Folliculitis	Skin Atrophy
Hypertrichosis	Striae
Acneiform eruptions	Miliaria
Hypopigmentation	

In controlled clinical studies the incidence of adverse reactions was low (0.8%) for Topicort® (desoximetasone) Emollient Cream 0.25% and included burning, folliculitis and folliculo-pustular lesions. The incidence of adverse reactions was also 0.8% for Topicort® LP (desoximetasone) Emollient Cream 0.05% and included pruritus, erythema, vesiculation and burning sensation. In controlled clinical studies the incidence of adverse reactions was low (0.3%) for Topicort® Ointment (desoximetasone) 0.25% and consisted of development of comedones at the site of application.

OVERDOSAGE

Topically applied corticosteroids can be absorbed in sufficient amounts to produce systemic effects (See **Precautions**).

DOSAGE AND ADMINISTRATION

Apply a thin film of Topicort® (desoximetasone) Emollient Cream 0.25%, Topicort® LP (desoximetasone) Emollient Cream 0.05%, Topicort® Gel (desoximetasone) 0.05% or Topicort® Ointment (desoximetasone) 0.25% to the affected skin areas twice daily. Rub in gently.

HOW SUPPLIED

Topicort® (desoximetasone) Emollient Cream 0.25% is supplied in 15 gram, 60 gram, and 4 ounce tubes.
Topicort® LP (desoximetasone) Emollient Cream 0.05% is supplied in 15 gram and 60 gram tubes.
Topicort® Gel (desoximetasone) 0.05% is supplied in 15 gram and 60 gram tubes.
Topicort® Ointment (desoximetasone) 0.25% is supplied in 15 gram and 60 gram tubes.
Store at controlled room temperature (59°-86°F).
Topicort® REG TM Roussel Uclaf
Edition 6/85

Shown in Product Identification Section, page 411

TRENTAL® ℞

(pentoxifylline)*
Tablets, 400 mg

DESCRIPTION

Trental® (pentoxifylline) tablets for oral administration contain 400 mg of the active drug and the following inactive ingredients: benzyl alcohol NF, FD&C Red #3, hydroxypropyl methylcellulose USP, magnesium stearate NF, polyethylene glycol NF, povidone USP, talc USP, titanium dioxide USP, and other ingredients in a controlled-release formulation. Trental® (pentoxifylline) is a trisubstituted xanthine derivative designated chemically as 1-(5-oxohexyl)-3, 7-dimethylxanthine that, unlike theophylline, is a hemorheologic agent, i.e. an agent that affects blood viscosity. Pentoxifylline is soluble in water and ethanol, and sparingly soluble in toluene.

CLINICAL PHARMACOLOGY

Mode of Action

Pentoxifylline and its metabolites improve the flow properties of blood by decreasing its viscosity. In patients with chronic peripheral arterial disease, this increases blood flow to the affected microcirculation and enhances tissue oxygenation. The precise mode of action of pentoxifylline and the sequence of events leading to clinical improvement are still to be defined. Pentoxifylline administration has been shown to produce dose related hemorheologic effects, lowering blood viscosity, and improving erythrocyte flexibility. Tissue oxygen levels have been shown to be significantly increased by therapeutic doses of pentoxifylline in patients with peripheral arterial disease.

Pharmacokinetics and Metabolism

After oral administration in aqueous solution pentoxifylline is almost completely absorbed. It undergoes a first-pass effect and the various metabolites appear in plasma very soon after dosing. Peak plasma levels of the parent compound and its metabolites are reached within 1 hour. The major metabolites are Metabolite I (1-[5-hydroxyhexyl]-3,7-dimethylxanthine) and Metabolite V (1-[3-carboxypropyl]-3,-7-dimethylxanthine), and plasma levels of these metabolites are 5 and 8 times greater, respectively, than pentoxifylline.
Following oral administration of aqueous solutions containing 100 to 400 mg of pentoxifylline, the pharmacokinetics of the parent compound and Metabolite I are dose-related and not proportional (non-linear), with half-life and area under the blood-level time curve (AUC) increasing with dose. The elimination kinetics of Metabolite V are not dose-dependent. The apparent plasma half-life of pentoxifylline varies from 0.4 to 0.8 hours and the apparent plasma half-lives of its metabolites vary from 1 to 1.6 hours. There is no evidence of accumulation or enzyme induction (Cytochrome P_{450}) following multiple oral doses.
Excretion is almost totally urinary; the main biotransformation product is Metabolite V. Essentially no parent drug is found in the urine. Despite large variations in plasma levels of parent compound and its metabolites, the urinary recovery of Metabolite V is consistent and shows dose proportionality. Less than 4% of the administered dose is recovered in feces. Food intake shortly before dosing delays absorption of an immediate release dosage form but does not affect total absorption. The pharmacokinetics and metabolism of Trental® (pentoxifylline) have not been studied in patients with renal and/or hepatic dysfunction, but AUC was increased and elimination rate decreased in an older population (60–68 years) compared to younger individuals (22–30 years).
After administration of the 400 mg controlled-release Trental® (pentoxifylline) tablet, plasma levels of the parent compound and its metabolites reach their maximum within 2 to 4 hours and remain constant over an extended period of time. The controlled release of pentoxifylline from the tablet eliminates peaks and troughs in plasma levels for improved gastrointestinal tolerance.

INDICATIONS AND USAGE

Trental® (pentoxifylline) is indicated for the treatment of patients with intermittent claudication on the basis of chronic occlusive arterial disease of the limbs. Trental® (pentoxifylline) can improve function and symptoms but is not intended to replace more definitive therapy, such as surgical bypass, or removal of arterial obstructions when treating peripheral vascular disease.

Continued on next page

Hoechst-Roussel—Cont.

CONTRAINDICATIONS

Trental® (pentoxifylline) should not be used in patients who have previously exhibited intolerance to this product or methylxanthines such as caffeine, theophylline, and theobromine.

PRECAUTIONS

General: Patients with chronic occlusive arterial disease of the limbs frequently show other manifestations of arteriosclerotic disease. Trental® (pentoxifylline) has been used safely for treatment of peripheral arterial disease in patients with concurrent coronary artery and cerebrovascular diseases, but there have been occasional reports of angina, hypotension, and arrhythmia. Controlled trials do not show that Trental® (pentoxifylline) causes such adverse effects more often than placebo, but, as it is a methylxanthine derivative, it is possible some individuals will experience such responses.

Drug Interactions: Although a causal relationship has not been established, there have been reports of bleeding and/or prolonged prothrombin time in patients treated with Trental® (pentoxifylline) with and without anticoagulants or platelet aggregation inhibitors. Patients on warfarin should have more frequent monitoring of prothrombin times, while patients with other risk factors complicated by hemorrhage (e.g., recent surgery, peptic ulceration) should have periodic examinations for bleeding including hematocrit and/or hemoglobin. Trental® (pentoxifylline) has been used concurrently with antihypertensive drugs, beta blockers, digitalis, diuretics, antidiabetic agents, and antiarrhythmics, without observed problems. Small decreases in blood pressure have been observed in some patients treated with Trental® (pentoxifylline); periodic systemic blood pressure monitoring is recommended for patients receiving concomitant antihypertensive therapy. If indicated, dosage of the antihypertensive agents should be reduced.

Carcinogenesis, Mutagenesis and Impairment of Fertility: Long-term studies of the carcinogenic potential of pentoxifylline were conducted in mice and rats by dietary administration of the drug at doses up to approximately 24 times (570 mg/kg) the maximum recommended human daily dose (MRHD) of 24 mg/kg for 18 months in mice and 18 months in rats with an additional 6 months without drug exposure in the latter. No carcinogenic potential for pentoxifylline was noted in the mouse study. In the rat study, there was a statistically significant increase in benign mammary fibroadenomas in females in the high dose group (24 × MRHD). The relevance of this finding to human use is uncertain since this was only a marginal statistically significant increase for a tumor that is common in aged rats. Pentoxifylline was devoid of mutagenic activity in various strains of *Salmonella* (Ames test) when tested in the presence and absence of metabolic activation.

Pregnancy: Category C. Teratogenic studies have been performed in rats and rabbits at oral doses up to about 25 and 10 times the maximum recommended human daily dose (MRHD) of 24 mg/kg, respectively. No evidence of fetal malformation was observed. Increased resorption was seen in rats at 25 times MRHD. There are, however, no adequate and well controlled studies in pregnant women. Because animal reproduction studies are not always predictive of human response. Trental® (pentoxifylline) should be used during pregnancy only if clearly needed.

Nursing Mothers: Pentoxifylline and its metabolites are excreted in human milk. Because of the potential for tumorigenicity shown for pentoxifylline in rats, a decision should be made whether to discontinue nursing or discontinue the drug, taking into account the importance of the drug to the mother.

Pediatric Use: Safety and effectiveness in children below the age of 18 years have not been established.

ADVERSE REACTIONS

Clinical trials were conducted using either controlled-release Trental® (pentoxifylline) tablets for up to 60 weeks or immediate-release Trental® (pentoxifylline) capsules for up to 24 weeks. Dosage ranges in the tablet studies were 400 mg bid to tid and in the capsule studies, 200–400 mg tid.

The table summarizes the incidence (in percent) of adverse reactions considered drug related, as well as the numbers of patients who received controlled-release Trental® (pentoxifylline) tablets, immediate-release Trental® (pentoxifylline) capsules, or the corresponding placebos. The incidence of adverse reactions was higher in the capsule studies (where dose related increases were seen in digestive and nervous system side effects) than in the tablet studies. Studies with the capsule include domestic experience, whereas studies with the controlled-release tablets were conducted outside the U.S. The table indicates that in the tablet studies few patients discontinued because of adverse effects.

[See table below].

Trental® (pentoxifylline) has been marketed in Europe and elsewhere since 1972. In addition to the above symptoms, the following have been reported spontaneously since marketing or occurred in other clinical trials with an incidence of less than 1%; the causal relationship was uncertain: Cardiovascular—dyspnea, edema, hypotension; Digestive—anorexia, cholecystitis, constipation, dry mouth/thirst; Nervous—anxiety, confusion; Respiratory—epistaxis, flu-like symptoms, laryngitis, nasal congestion; Skin and Appendages—brittle fingernails, pruritus, rash, urticaria; Special Senses—blurred vision, conjunctivitis, earache, scotoma; and Miscellaneous—bad taste, excessive salivation, leukopenia, malaise, sore throat/swollen neck glands, weight change.

A few rare events have been reported spontaneously worldwide since marketing in 1972. Although they occurred under circumstances in which a causal relationship with pentoxifylline could not be established, they are listed to serve as information for physicians: Cardiovascular—angina, arrhythmia, tachycardia; Digestive—hepatitis, jaundice; and Hemic and Lymphatic—decreased serum fibrinogen, pancytopenia, purpura, thrombocytopenia.

OVERDOSAGE

Overdosage with Trental® (pentoxifylline) has been reported in children and adults. Symptoms appear to be dose related. A report from a poison control center on 44 patients taking overdoses of enteric-coated pentoxifylline tablets noted that symptoms usually occurred 4–5 hours after ingestion and lasted about 12 hours. The highest amount ingested was 80 mg/kg; flushing, hypotension, convulsions, somnolence, loss of consciousness, fever, and agitation occurred. All patients recovered.

In addition to symptomatic treatment and gastric lavage, special attention must be given to supporting respiration, maintaining systemic blood pressure, and controlling convulsions. Activated charcoal has been used to adsorb pentoxifylline in patients who have overdosed.

DOSAGE AND ADMINISTRATION

The usual dosage of Trental® (pentoxifylline) in controlled-release tablet form is one tablet (400 mg) three times a day with meals.

While the effect of Trental® (pentoxifylline) may be seen within 2 to 4 weeks, it is recommended that treatment be continued for at least 8 weeks. Efficacy has been demonstrated in double-blind clinical studies of 6 months duration.

Digestive and central nervous system side effects are dose related. if patients develop these side effects it is recommended that the dosage be lowered to one tablet twice a day (800 mg/day). If side effects persist at this lower dosage, the administration of Trental® (pentoxifylline) should be discontinued.

HOW SUPPLIED

Trental® (pentoxifylline) is available for oral administration as 400 mg pink film-coated oblong tablets imprinted Trental®; supplied in Unit of Use bottles of 100 (NDC 0039-0078-10) and Unit Dose packs of 100 (NDC 0039-0078-11).

Store at controlled room temperature (59°–86°F).

Dispense in well closed, light resistant containers.

*U.S. Patents 3,737,433 and 4,189,469 77800-11/85

Shown in Product Identification Section, page 411

INCIDENCE (%) OF SIDE EFFECTS

	Controlled-Release Tablets		Immediate-Release Capsules	
	Trental®	Placebo	Trental®	Placebo
(Numbers of Patients at Risk)	(321)	(128)	(177)	(138)
Discontinued for Side Effect	3.1	0	9.6	7.2
CARDIOVASCULAR SYSTEM				
Angina/Chest pain	0.3	—	1.1	2.2
Arrhythmia/Palpitation	—	—	1.7	0.7
Flushing	—	—	2.3	0.7
DIGESTIVE SYSTEM				
Abdominal Discomfort	—	—	4.0	1.4
Belching/Flatus/Bloating	0.6	—	9.0	3.6
Diarrhea	—	—	3.4	2.9
Dyspepsia	2.8	4.7	9.6	2.9
Nausea	2.2	0.8	28.8	8.7
Vomiting	1.2	—	4.5	0.7
NERVOUS SYSTEM				
Agitation/Nervousness	—	—	1.7	0.7
Dizziness	1.9	3.1	11.9	4.3
Drowsiness	—	—	1.1	5.8
Headache	1.2	1.6	6.2	5.8
Insomnia	—	—	2.3	2.2
Tremor	0.3	0.8	—	—
Blurred Vision	—	—	2.3	1.4

Hollister-Stier

Division of Miles Laboratories, Inc.
400 MORGAN LANE
WEST HAVEN, CT 06516

Emergency
ANA-KIT® ℞
INSECT STING TREATMENT KIT

DESCRIPTION

Epinephrine Injection, USP, (1:1000), contained in a sterile, 1 ml syringe, designed to deliver 2 doses of 0.3 ml each. Product is intended for subcutaneous or intramuscular use.

Each ml of Epinephrine Injection, USP, (1:1000) contains 1 mg epinephrine as the hydrochloride, 8.5 mg sodium chloride, not more than 5 mg chlorobutanol (chloral derivative) and 1.5 mg sodium bisulfite.

Epinephrine is a sympathomimetic catecholamine. Its naturally occurring levo isomer, which is twenty times as active as the *d* isomer, is now obtained in pure form by separation from the synthetically produced racemate.

Chemically, epinephrine is β-(3,4-dihydroxyphenyl)-α-methylaminoethanol with the following structure:

Chlo-Amine® Chlorpheniramine Maleate Tablets, USP., 4 chewable tablets, each containing 2 mg chlorpheniramine maleate, for oral administration. Chlorpheniramine maleate is an antihistamine having the chemical name γ-(4-chlorophenyl)-N,N-dimethyl-2-pyridinepropanamine, (Z)-2-butenedioate(1:1) with the following structure:

DEVICES: 2 sterile pads containing isopropyl alcohol 70% by volume. One tourniquet.

CLINICAL PHARMACOLOGY

EPINEPHRINE: The most valuable drug for the emergency treatment of severe allergic reactions is epinephrine. The vasoconstrictor effect of epinephrine on the capillary directly antagonizes the generalized vasodilation produced by histamine. Epinephrine reverses the increased permeability of dilated capillaries to plasma. The shock of severe allergic reactions is due to the loss of circulating blood volume by pooling in the dilated capillary beds and loss of plasma into the tissues. Epinephrine quickly restores circulating blood volume and blood pressure by constricting the capillary bed. The itching during episodes of hives or angioedema is promptly relieved by epinephrine. Epinephrine is a powerful relaxer of the smooth muscle of the bronchioles, stomach, intestine, pregnant uterus and urinary bladder wall. The bronchospasm, wheezing and dyspnea of the acute allergic reactions are relieved. Where abdominal cramping, defecation or involuntary urination have occurred during severe allergic attacks, epinephrine rapidly produces relief. Subcutaneously or intramuscularly administered epinephrine has a rapid onset and short duration of action. Subcutaneous administration during asthmatic attacks may produce bronchodilation within 5 to 10 minutes, and maximal effects may occur within 20 minutes.

CHLO-AMINE: Chlo-Amine is an effective agent in nullifying the characteristic effects of histamine and is especially valuable in the prophylaxis and relief of many allergic symptoms. It is readily absorbed from the intestinal tract and released into the tissues from the bloodstream. This action is both prompt and sustained. Elimination of the drug is such that there is a low incidence of side effects.

INDICATIONS AND USAGE

HOLLISTER-STIER Allergic Emergency Kit (Ana-Kit®) is indicated for use by insect sting sensitive patients should they encounter severe symptoms when away from home or out of reach of immediate attention by a doctor or hospital. Sensitive patients who are stung by one of the stinging insects, primarily of the Hymenoptera order (bees, wasps, hornets, yellow jackets, or bumble bees), may present a syndrome of human anaphylactic shock that is different from typical allergic symptoms. Within minutes after the sting, the patient experiences apprehension, faintness, flushing followed by paleness, tachycardia, thready pulse, a fall in blood pressure, unobtainable pulse and blood pressure, and visual changes. Occasionally, unconsciousness, convulsions, abominal cramps and involuntary voiding or defecation may occur. If the patient survives the shock, there is rapid recovery and in an hour or so he may feel perfectly well. In many episodes of severe allergic reactions, the symptoms of anaphylaxis and typical allergic symptoms may be intermixed. Occasionally the typical allergic symptoms of urticaria, rhinitis and asthma may appear during or after the initial shock phase of anaphylaxis.

CONTRAINDICATIONS

EPINEPHRINE: Epinephrine must not be given intra-arterially as marked vasoconstriction may result in gangrene. **This unit is not intended for intravenous use.** Further dilution would be necessary and is not practical with this emergency syringe. Use is probably contraindicated in patients with hypertension, diabetes, hyperthyroidism, and coronary artery disease. Epinephrine should not be administered concomitantly with other sympathomimetic agents, since the effects are additive and may be detrimental to the patient.

CHLO-AMINE: No known contraindications.

WARNINGS

EPINEPHRINE: Overdosage or accidental intravenous administration of conventional subcutaneous doses may induce severe or fatal hypertension, or cerebrovascular hemorrhage. Fatalities may also occur from pulmonary edema resulting from peripheral constriction and cardiac stimulation. The marked pressor effects may be counteracted by use of rapidly acting vasodilators, such as the nitrites and alpha-adrenergic blockers.

Deaths have been reported in asthmatics treated with epinephrine following the use of isoproterenol or orciprenaline. Epinephrine must be administered with great caution, if at all, in patients with cardiac arrhythmias, coronary artery or organic heart disease, and hypertension. In patients with coronary insufficiency or ischemic heart disease, epinephrine may precipitate or aggravate angina pectoris as well as produce potentially fatal ventricular arrhythmias. Epinephrine should be administered only with great caution to elderly patients, those with diabetes mellitus, hyperthyroidism or psychoneurotic disorders; also to those with long-standing bronchial asthma or emphysema if such individuals may also have degenerative heart disease, and to pregnant women (see "Pregnancy").

CHLO-AMINE®: Chlorpheniramine maleate should be used with extreme caution in patients with stenosing peptic ulcer, pyloroduodenal obstruction, prostatic hypertrophy, or bladder neck obstruction. These compounds have an atropine-like action and therefore should be used with caution in patients with a history of increased intraocular pressure, cardiovascular disease, or hypertension.

PRECAUTIONS

GENERAL: Hollister-Stier Ana-Kit® is not intended to be a substitute for medical attention or hospital care. The kit is designed to be compact and easy to carry, and to provide emergency treatment when medical care is not immediately available. Highly sensitive individuals should have the kit readily available at all times. Because of its small size it can be carried by outdoor sportsmen, golfers, gardeners, or any sensitive individual who may be exposed to stinging insects (wasps, hornets, yellow jackets or bees). The drugs in the Ana-Kit®, when used as directed immediately following a sting, may prove life-saving. Certain changes in the emergency instructions and in the kit itself may be made by the doctor according to the needs of the patient. IN ALL CASES THE PHYSICIAN SHOULD INSTRUCT THE PATIENT IN USE OF THE SYRINGE AND THE OTHER DRUGS AND DEVICES.

The effects of epinephrine may be potentiated by **tricyclic antidepressants,** sodium levothyroxine, and certain antihistamines, notably chlorpheniramine, tripeiennamine, and diphenhydramine.

Carcinogenesis, Mutagenesis, Impairment of Fertility: There are no data from either animal or human studies regarding the carcinogenicity or mutagenicity of epinephrine or Chlo-Amine, and no studies have been conducted to determine their potential for the impairment of fertility.

Pregnancy: Teratogenic Effects. Pregnancy Category C—Epinephrine has been shown to be teratogenic in rats and hamsters at dose levels hundreds of times as high as the maximal human dose. Although there are no adequate or well-controlled studies in pregnant women, epinephrine crosses the placenta and its use during pregnancy may cause anoxia in the fetus. Epinephrine should be used in pregnancy only if the potential benefit justifies the potential risk to the fetus.

Pediatric Use: Administer Epinephrine or Chlo-Amine with caution to infants and children (see "Dosage and Aministration"). Syncope has occurred following the administration of epinephrine to asthmatic children.

INFORMATION FOR PATIENTS: Complete patient information, including dosage, directions for proper administration, and precautions, can be found at the end of the package insert, as well as inside each Anakit® kit.

ADVERSE REACTIONS

EPINEPHRINE: Adverse reactions include transient, moderate anxiety, apprehensiveness, restlessness, tremor, weakness, dizziness, sweating, palpitations, pallor, nausea and vomiting, headache, and respiratory difficulties. These symptoms occur in some persons receiving therapeutic doses of epinephrine, but are more likely to occur, or to occur in exaggerated form, in those with hypertension or hyperthyroidism. Excessive doses cause acute hypertension and cardiac arrhythmias.

CHLO-AMINE: Drowsiness, dizziness, blurred vision, dry mouth and gastrointestinal upsets may occur. Patients should not drive or operate machinery after taking the drug. Large doses produce central nervous system depression and occasionally tremors or convulsions. Reports of hematological disorders are rare.

OVERDOSAGE

EPINEPHRINE: Epinephrine is rapidly inactivated in the body, and treatment is primarily supportive. If necessary, pressor effects may be counteracted by rapidly acting vasodilators or alpha-adrenergic blocking drugs. If prolonged hypotension follows such measures, it may be necessary to administer another pressor drug, such as levarterenol.

If an epinephrine overdose induces pulmonary edema that interferes with respiration, treatment consists of a rapidly acting alpha-adrenergic blocking drug such as phentolamine and/or intermittent positive-pressure respiration.

Epinephrine overdosage can also cause transient bradycardia followed by tachycardia, and these may be accompanied by potentially fatal cardiac arrhythmias. Ventricular premature contractions may appear within one minute after injection and may be followed by multilocal ventricular tachycardia (prefibrillation rhythm). Subsidence of the ventricular effects may be followed by atrial tachycardia and occasionally by atrioventricular block. Treatment of arrhythmias consists of administration of beta-adrenergic blocking drug such as propranolol.

Overdosage sometimes also results in extreme pallor and coldness of the skin, metabolic acidosis, and kidney failure. Suitable corrective measures must be taken.

CHLO-AMINE: Overdose symptoms may be sedation, apnea, cardiovascular collapse to stimulation, insomnia, hallucinations, tremors or convulsions. Also there may be dizziness, tinnitus, ataxia, blurred vision, hypotension, dry mouth, flushing, and abdominal symptoms.

Treatment—The patient should be induced to vomit, preferably with ipecac syrup—and large amounts of water. Prevent aspiration of vomitus. Gastric lavage may be necessary using activated charcoal and saline. Hyperosmotic cathartics such as Milk of Magnesia may hasten elimination of residual cling. Vasopressors can be used to correct hypotension. Diazepam may be used to control seizures. Hyperpyrexia can be treated with cool sponges or a hypothermic blanket.

DOSAGE AND ADMINISTRATION

The physician who prescribes the Ana-Kit® should review the package insert in detail with the patient. This review should include the proper use of the 2-dose epinephrine syringe to insure that subcutaneous or intramuscular injections are given into the deltoid region of the arm or the anteriolateral aspect of the thigh. See also the PATIENT DIRECTIONS FOR USE.

EPINEPHRINE: For subcutaneous or intramuscular injection only.

Adults and children over 12 years: 0.3 ml; 6–12 years: 0.2 ml; 2–6 years: 0.15 ml; Infants to 2 years: 0.05 to 0.1 ml.

When syringe is properly set up, as directed in the Patient Instruction Sheet, a 0.3 ml dose is administered when plunger is pushed until it stops. Syringe barrel has 0.1 ml graduations so that smaller doses can be measured. (Operation of syringe is explained in the Patient Directions For Use section at the end of this package insert.)

If after 10 minutes from the first injection symptoms are not noticeably improved, administer a second dose of epinephrine from the syringe.

CHLO-AMINE: Tablets are chewable antihistamines. Adults and children over 12 years: 4 tablets; children 6–12 years: 2 tablets; children under 6 years: 1 tablet.

HOW SUPPLIED

EMERGENCY ANA-KIT® INSECT STING TREATMENT KIT CONTAINS:

SYRINGE: One sterile syringe containing 1 ml Epinephrine Injection, USP, (1:1000). Syringe delivers two 0.3 ml doses.

TABLETS: Four 2 mg chewable Chlo-Amine® tablets, Chlorpheniramine Maleate Tablets, USP.

DEVICES: Two sterile pads containing 70% isopropyl alcohol (by volume) and 1 tourniquet.

STORE IN DARK AT ROOM TEMPERATURE

CAUTION: U.S. Federal Law Prohibits Dispensing Without Prescription.

Distributed by:
Hollister-Stier
Division of Miles Laboratories, Inc.
Spokane, WA 99207

PATIENT DIRECTIONS FOR USE

***Emergency* ANA-KIT® Insect Sting Treatment Kit**

(Please read entire direction sheet before an emergency arises.)

The Ana-Kit®, as prescribed by a physician, is to be used by patients who are highly allergic to the stings of bees, wasps, hornets, yellow jackets, or bumble bees.

IN THE EVENT OF AN INSECT STING PRODUCING A LIFE THREATENING SITUATION, FOLLOW THESE STEPS IMMEDIATELY TO ADMINISTER THE EPINEPHRINE.

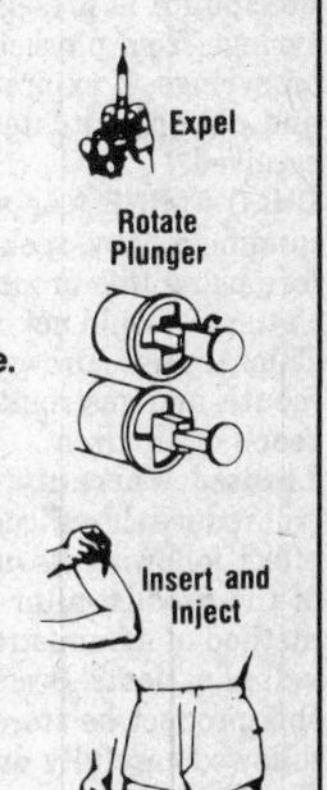

1. **Remove red rubber needle cover. Hold syringe upright and push plunger to expel air and excess epinephrine (plunger will stop).**
2. **Rotate rectangular plunger ¼ turn to the right. Plunger will align with slot in barrel of syringe. Wipe injection site with alcohol swab.**
3. **Insert needle straight into arm or thigh as illustrated.**
4. **Push plunger until it stops. Syringe will inject a 0.3 ml dose for adults and children over 12 years.**
   Children: Syringe barrel has 0.1 ml graduations so that smaller doses can be measured. Administer to infants to 2 years: 0.05 to 0.1 ml; 2–6 years: 0.15 ml; and 6–12 years: 0.2 ml.

ONCE THE INITIAL EPINEPHRINE INJECTION HAS BEEN ADMINISTERED, FOLLOW THESE ADDITIONAL STEPS.

1. CONTACT PHYSICIAN, IF POSSIBLE.
2. REMOVE STINGER if left in the skin with fingernails. (DO NOT push, pinch or squeeze, or further imbed the stinger into the skin as this may cause further venom to be injected.)

3. APPLY TOURNIQUET, if stung on the arm or leg, between the sting and the body. (If the sting is elsewhere—on the neck, face, or body, for example—proceed immediately to STEP 5.)

Apply Tourniquet

4. TIGHTEN TOURNIQUET. To tighten, pull on the end of ONE STRING. Then, at least every ten minutes, loosen the tourniquet by pulling on the small metal ring.
5. CHEW AND SWALLOW CHLO-AMINE TABLETS. For adults and children over 12 years, take 4 tablets; children 6–12 years take 2 tablets; children under 6 years take 1 tablet. These tablets are chewable antihistamine which is generally tolerated.

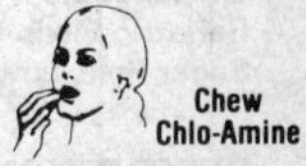

6. PREPARE SYRINGE FOR A POSSIBLE SECOND INJECTION. Turn the rectangular plunger ¼ turn to the right to line up with rectangular slot in the syringe. (A slight wiggling may aid the turning and alignment of the plunger.)
7. THE SECOND INJECTION. If after 10 minutes from the first injection symptoms are not noticeably improved, a second injection is required.

Continued on next page

Hollister-Stier—Cont.

Cleanse skin area with alcohol swab and make second injection as in STEPS 3 and 4 for the first epinephrine injection. (A small amount of epinephrine will remain in syringe after the second dose and cannot be expelled.)

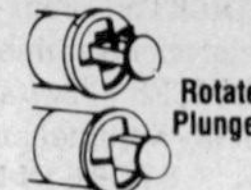

8. APPLY ICE PACKS IF AVAILABLE TO STUNG AREA.
9. KEEP PATIENT WARM AND AVOID EXERTION.

PRECAUTIONS

EPINEPHRINE: For subcutaneous or intramuscular injection only. **Not intended for intravenous use.**
Epinephrine is light sensitive and should be stored in box provided. STORE AT ROOM TEMPERATURE. Do not try to force air out of the syringe until you are ready to use the epinephrine. This may rupture the seal and allow the epinephrine solution to contact the metal promoting deterioration.
Never remove rubber protector over needle until ready to use syringe as this may cause needle and contents to become contaminated. Any epinephrine solution in contact with the needle may cause rusting of the metal.
Periodically check contents of the syringe. If discoloration or precipitate is present, DO NOT USE. Obtain replacement syringe from physician. Periodically check expiration date on syringe. If expiration date is near, re-order new syringe and discard outdated syringe after new syringe has been received.
CHLO-AMINE: As with any drug, if you are pregnant or nursing a baby, seek the advice of a health professional before using this product.
Patients should not drive or operate machinery after taking Chlo-Amine. Drowsiness, dizziness, blurred vision, dry mouth and gastrointestinal upsets may occur. Keep out of reach of children.
Limited Warranty: A number of factors beyond our control reduce the efficacy of this product or even result in an ill effect following its use. These include storage and handling of the product after it leaves our hands, diagnosis, dosage, method of administration and biological differences in individual patients. Because of these factors, it is important that this product be stored properly and that the directions be followed carefully during use.
The foregoing statement is made in lieu of any other warranty, express or implied, including any warranty of merchantability or fitness. Representatives of the Company are not authorized to vary the terms of this warranty or the contents of any printed labeling for this product except by printed notice from the Company's Spokane, WA office. The prescriber and user of this product must accept the terms hereof.

Distributed by:
Hollister-Stier
Division of Miles Laboratories, Inc.
Spokane, WA 99207

Anakit 471107 M10 5/85
CR. Ref. 471108 MO1

Hoyt Laboratories
See Colgate-Hoyt Laboratories

Huffman Laboratories
7356 N.W. 35TH TERRACE
MIAMI, FL 33122

GEROBION ℞
Geriatric Elixir
Sugar Free, Low Sodium

DESCRIPTION
GEROBION is a hematinic, mineral and folic acid combination for oral administration.
Each 15 mL (tablespoon) contains:

Pantothenic Acid	3.3mg
Niacinamide	13.3mg
Vitamin B-6	1.3mg
Vitamin B-12	4mcg
Folic Acid	0.33mg
Iron	12.0mg
Zinc	5.3mg
Manganese	1.3mg
Alcohol	13 percent

In a flavored, sugar-free base containing less than 0.1 mg sodium per 5 mL.

Active ingredients: dexpanthenol, niacinamide, pyridoxine hydrochloride, cyanocobalamin, folic acid, ferric ammonium citrate, zinc acetate diphosphate, manganese chloride.

CLINICAL PHARMACOLOGY
Oral iron is absorbed most efficiently when it is administered between meals. Conventional iron preparations, however, frequently cause gastric irritation when taken on an empty stomach.
Iron is found in the body principally as hemoglobin. Storage in the form of ferritin occurs in the liver, spleen, and bone marrow. Concentrations of plasma iron and the total iron-binding capacity of plasma vary greatly in different physiological conditions and disease states.
Large amounts of ascorbic acid administered orally with ferric ammonium citrate have been shown to enhance iron absorption. Apparently this is due to the ability of ascorbic acid to prevent the oxidation of ferrous iron to the less effectively absorbed ferric form.
Folic acid and iron are absorbed in the proximal small intestine, particularly the duodenum. Folic acid is absorbed maximally and rapidly at this site, and iron is absorbed in a decending gradient from the duodenum distally.
After absorption folic acid is rapidly converted into its metabolically active forms. Approximately two-thirds is bound to plasma protein. Half of the folic acid stored in the body is found in the liver. Folic acid is also concentrated in spinal fluid. Except for the folates ingested in liver, yeast, and egg yolk, the percentage of absorption of food folates averages about 10%.
The vitamins in GEROBION are absorbed by the active transport process. B-vitamins are rapidly eliminated and therefore are not stored in the body.
Dexpanthenol is absorbed readily from the gastrointestinal tract and distributed to all body tissues.

INDICATIONS AND USAGE
GEROBION is indicated for the treatment of iron deficiency and prevention of concomitant folic acid deficiency in non-pregnant adults. GEROBION is also indicated in prenancy for the prevention and treatment of iron deficiency and to supply a maintenance dosage of folic acid.
GEROBION is indicated in non-pregnant adults for the treatment of iron deficiency and prevention of concomitant folic acid deficiency where there is an associated deficient intake or increased need for vitamins. GEROBION is also indicated in pregnancy for the prevention and treatment of iron deficiency where there is a concomitant deficient intake or increased need for vitamins (including folic acid).

CONTRAINDICATIONS
GEROBION is contraindicated in patients with pernicious anemia.
GEROBION is also contraindicated in the rare instance of hypersensitivity to folic acid.

WARNINGS
Folic acid alone is improper therapy in the treatment of pernicious anemia and other magaloblastic anemias where vitamin B_{12} is deficient.

PRECAUTIONS
Where anemia exists, its nature should be established and underlying causes determined.
GEROBION contains 0.33 mg of folic acid per 15 mL (tablespoon). Folic acid especially in doses above 0.1 mg daily may obscure pernicious anemia, in that hematologic remission may occur while neurological manifestations remain progressive. Concomitant parenteral therapy with vitamin B_{12} may be necessary in patients with deficiency of vitamin B_{12}.
Pernicious anemia is rare in women of childbearing age, and the likelihood of its occurrence along with pregnancy is reduced by the impairment of fertility associated with vitamin B_{12} deficiency.
Like other oral iron preparations, GEROBION should be stored out of reach of children to guard against accidental iron poisoning (see Overdoseage).
Laboratory Tests: In older patients and those with conditions tending to lead to vitamin B_{12} depletion, serum B_{12} levels should be regularly assessed during treatment with GEROBION.
Drug Interactions: Absorption of iron is inhibited by *magnesium trisilicate* and *antacids containing carbonates.*
Ferric ammonium citrate may interfere with the absorption of *tetracyclines.*
The antiparkinsonism effects of *levodopa* may be reversed by pyridoxine.
Iron absorption is inhibited by the ingestion of eggs or milk.
Carcinogenesis: Adequate data is not available on long-term potential for carcinogenesis in animals or humans.
Pregnancy: Pregnancy Category A. Studies in pregnant women have not shown that GEROBION increases the risk of fetal abnormalities if administered during pregnancy. If this drug is used during pregnancy, the possibility of fetal harm appears remote. Because studies cannot rule out the possibility of harm, however, GEROBION should be used during pregnancy only if clearly needed.
Nursing Mothers: Folic acid, ascorbic acid, and B-vitamins are excreted in breast milk.

ADVERSE REACTIONS
Gastric intolerance to iron. If such should occur, GEROBION may be taken after a meal. Allergic sensitization has been reported following both oral and parenteral administration of folic acid.

OVERDOSAGE
Increased capillary permeability, reduced plasma volume, increased cardiac output, and sudden cardiovascular collapse may occur in acute iron intoxication. In overdosage, efforts should be made to hasten the elimination of the iron ingested. An emetic should be administered as soon as possible, followed by gastric lavage if indicated. Immediately following emesis, a large dose of a saline cathartic should be used to speed passage through the intestinal tract.

DOSAGE AND ADMINSTRATION
GEROBION is administered orally and may be taken on an empty stomach.
Adults: For treatment of iron deficiency and prevention of folic acid deficiency, the recommended dose is 15 mL (one tablespoonful) daily.
Pregnant Adults: For prevention and treatment of iron deficiency and to supply a maintenance dosage of folic acid, the recommended dose is 15 mL (one tablespoonful) daily.

HOW SUPPLIED
GEROBION Geriatric Elixir is available in 16 fluid ounce (473 mL) containers.
Keep tightly closed and protect from light.
Store at controlled room temperature 15°–30°C (59°–86°F).
Dispense in tight, light-resistant container as described in official compendia.

CAUTION
Federal law prohibits dispensing without prescription.

3/86

Hyland Therapeutics Division
Travenol Laboratories, Inc.
444 W. GLENOAKS BLVD.
GLENDALE, CA 91202

AUTOPLEX® ℞
Anti-Inhibitor Coagulant Complex, Dried

Supplied in single dose 30 ml vials (Hyland Factor VIII correctional activity is stated on label of each vial) with sterile diluent and needles for reconstitution and withdrawal.

BUMINATE® 5% ℞
Albumin (Human),
USP, 5% Solution

Supplied as a 5% solution in 250 ml and 500 ml bottles. For use with intravenous administration set.

BUMINATE® 25% ℞
Albumin (Human),
USP, 25% Solution

Supplied as a 25% solution in 20 ml, 50 ml, and 100 ml vials. For use with intravenous administration set.

Immune Globulin ℞
Intravenous (Human)
GAMMAGARD®
[gam 'ah-gard]

This prescribing information is based on approved labelling in effect June 30, 1986.

DESCRIPTION
Immune Globulin Intravenous (Human), GAMMAGARD®* is a sterile, dried, highly purified preparation of immunoglobulin which is derived from the cold ethanol fractionation process and is further purified using ultrafiltration and ion exchange adsorption. When reconstituted with the appropriate volume of diluent, this preparation contains approximately 50 mg of protein per mL, of which at least 90% is gamma globulin. The reconstituted product contains approximately 1% sodium chloride, not more than 20 mg/mL glucose, not more than 0.2 g/dL PEG, and 0.3 M glycine as a stabilizing agent. It has a pH of 6.8 ± 0.4.
The manufacturing process for Immune Globulin Intravenous (Human), GAMMAGARD, isolates gamma globulin without additional chemical or enzymatic modification and the Fc portion is maintained intact. Immune Globulin Intravenous (Human), GAMMAGARD contains all the immunoglobulin G antibody activities which are present in the donor population. On the average, the distribution of IgG sub-

classes present in this product is the same as is present in normal plasma.[1] Immune Globulin Intravenous (Human), GAMMAGARD contains only trace amounts of IgM and IgA. Immune Globulin Intravenous (Human), GAMMAGARD contains no preservative.

This product has been prepared from large pools of human plasma which was taken only from plasma units found to have normal levels of alanine aminotransferase (ALT). Each unit of plasma used in the manufacture of this product has been found to be nonreactive for HBsAg and HTLV-III antibody by FDA approved tests.

CLINICAL PHARMACOLOGY

Immune Globulin Intravenous (Human), GAMMAGARD contains a broad spectrum of IgG antibodies against bacterial and viral agents that are capable of opsonization and neutralization of microbes and toxins.

Peak levels of IgG are reached immediately after infusion of Immune Globulin Intravenous (Human), GAMMAGARD. It has been shown that IgG is distributed relatively rapidly between plasma and extravascular fluid until approximately half of the total body pool is partitioned in the extravascular space. A rapid initial drop in serum levels is, therefore, to be expected.[2]

As a class, IgG survives longer *in vivo* than other serum proteins.[2,3] Studies show that the half-life of Immune Globulin Intravenous (Human), GAMMAGARD is approximately 24 days. These findings are consistent with reports of a 21 to 25 day half-life for IgG.[2,3,4] The half-life of IgG can vary considerably from person to person, however. In particular, high concentrations of IgG and hypermetabolism associated with fever and infection have been seen to coincide with a shortened half-life of IgG.[2,3,4,5]

INDICATIONS AND USAGE

Antibody Deficiency

Immune Globulin Intravenous (Human), GAMMAGARD is efficacious in the treatment of primary immunodeficient states in which severe impairment of antibody forming capacity has been shown, such as: congenital aggammaglobulinemias, common variable immunodeficiency, Wiskott-Aldrich syndrome, and severe combined immunodeficiencies.[4,5]

Immune Globulin Intravenous (Human), GAMMAGARD is especially useful when high levels or rapid elevation of circulating gamma globulins are desired or when intramuscular injections are contraindicated.

CONTRAINDICATIONS

None known.

WARNINGS

Immune Globulin Intravenous (Human), GAMMAGARD should only be administered intravenously. Other routes of administration have not been evaluated.

Immune Globulin Intravenous (Human), GAMMAGARD contains very low quantities of IgA (not more than 10 μg/mL) and although no instances of anaphylaxis associated with the use of this product have been observed during the clinical trials, such reactions have been observed with other immunoglobulin products.[5,6] Immune Globulin Intravenous (Human), GAMMAGARD should be given with caution to patients with antibodies to IgA or selective IgA deficiencies.

PRECAUTIONS

Drug Interaction

Admixtures of Immune Globulin Intravenous (Human), GAMMAGARD with other drugs have not been evaluated. It is recommended that Immune Globulin Intravenous (Human), GAMMAGARD be administered separately from other drugs or medication which the patient may be receiving.

Pregnancy Category C

Animal reproduction studies have not been conducted with Immune Globulin Intravenous (Human), GAMMAGARD. It is also not known whether Immune Globulin Intravenous (Human), GAMMAGARD can cause fetal harm when administered to a pregnant woman or can affect reproduction capacity. Immune Globulin Intravenous (Human), GAMMAGARD should be given to a pregnant woman only if clearly needed.

ADVERSE REACTIONS

The incidence of untoward reactions to Immune Globulin Intravenous (Human), GAMMAGARD is low, although various minor reactions, such as headache, fatigue, chills, backache, light-headedness, fever and nausea may occasionally occur. The incidence of these reactions during the clinical trials was less than 6%. Slowing or stopping the infusion usually allows the symptoms to disappear promptly.

Immediate anaphylactic and hypersensitivity reactions due to previous sensitization, although they have not been observed during the clinical trials, are a possibility. Epinephrine should be available for treatment of any acute anaphylactoid reaction. (See WARNINGS.)

DOSAGE AND ADMINISTRATION

Antibody Deficiency

For patients with primary immunodeficiencies, monthly doses of at least 100 mg/kg are recommended. Initially, patients may receive 200–400 mg/kg. As there are significant differences in the half-life of IgG among patients with primary immunodeficiencies, the frequency and amount of immunoglobulin therapy may vary from patient to patient. The proper amount can be determined by monitoring clinical response and/or the serum IgG levels before each dose, to ensure that they do not drop below 500 mg/dL.

Reconstitution: Use Aseptic Technic

1. NOTE: RECONSTITUTE IMMEDIATELY BEFORE USE.
2. Warm Sterile Water for Injection, USP (diluent) and Immune Globulin Intravenous (Human), GAMMAGARD (dried concentrate) to room temperature.
3. Remove caps from concentrate and diluent bottles to expose central portion of rubber stoppers.
4. Cleanse stoppers with germicidal solution.
5. Remove protective covering from the spike at one end of the transfer device (Fig. 1).

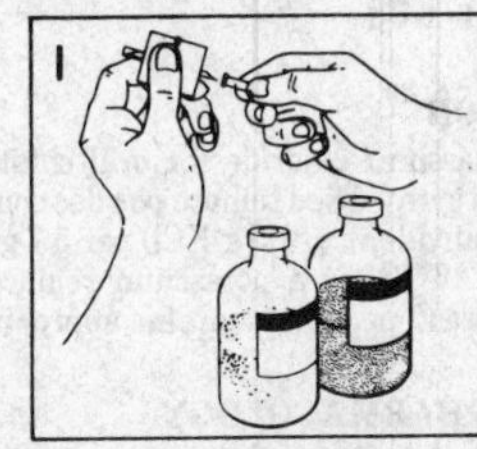

6. Place the diluent bottle on a flat surface and, while holding the bottle to prevent slipping, insert the spike of the transfer device perpendicularly through the center of the bottle stopper. Press down firmly so that the transfer device fits snugly against the shoulder of the diluent bottle (Fig. 2). A slight twist at the end of the downward push helps ensure a snug fit.

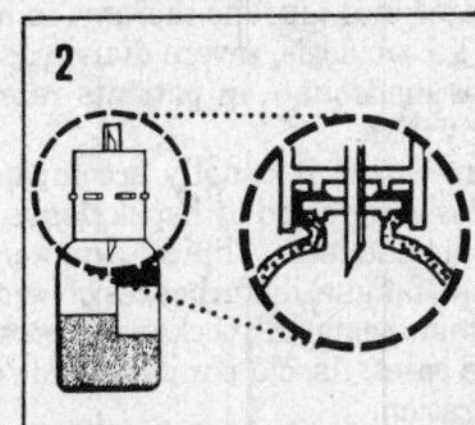

7. Remove the protective covering from the other end of the transfer device. Hold diluent bottle to prevent slipping. Invert concentrate bottle and press firmly onto the transfer device until the shoulder of the concentrate bottle fits snugly against the transfer device.
8. Invert both bottles while connected by the transfer device. Diluent will flow into the concentrate bottle (Fig. 3). When diluent transfer is complete, remove empty diluent bottle and transfer device from concentrate bottle. Discard transfer device after single use.

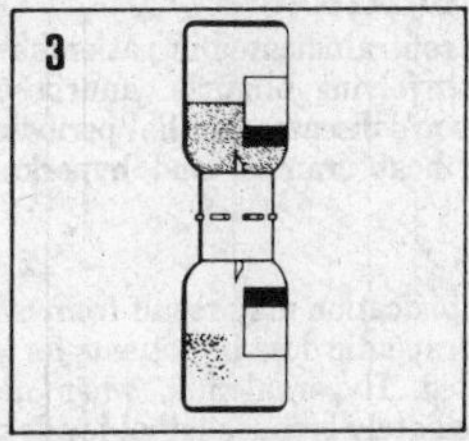

9. Thoroughly wet dried material by tilting or inverting and gently rotating the bottle (Fig. 4). DO NOT SHAKE. AVOID FOAMING.

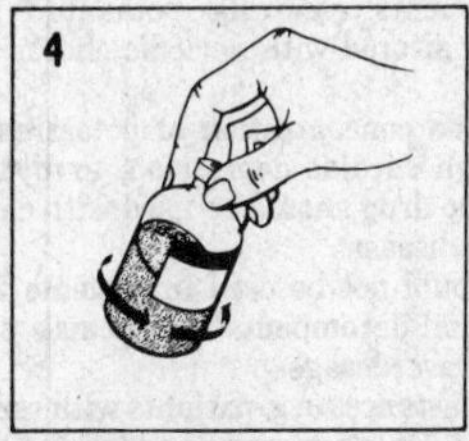

10. Repeat gentle rotation at 5 minute intervals as long as undissolved product is observed.

Rate of Administration

It is recommended that initially a rate of 0.5 mL/kg/Hr be used. If infusion at this rate causes the patient no distress, the administration rate may be gradually increased but should not exceed 4 mL/kg/Hr.

A rate of administration which is too rapid may cause flushing and changes in pulse rate and blood pressure. Slowing or stopping the infusion usually allows the symptoms to disappear promptly.

Administration

Immune Globulin Intravenous (Human), GAMMAGARD should be administered as soon after reconstitution as possible. Administration should not begin more than 2 hours after reconstitution.

The reconstituted material should be at room temperature during administration.

Parenteral drug products should be inspected visually for particulate matter and discoloration prior to administration, whenever solution and container permit.

Follow directions for use which accompany the administration set. If a Hyland set is not used, make sure the administration set contains an adequate filter.

HOW SUPPLIED

Immune Globulin Intravenous (Human), GAMMAGARD is supplied in either 2.5 g or 5.0 g single use vials. Each vial of Immune Globulin Intravenous (Human), GAMMAGARD is furnished with a suitable volume of Sterile Water for Injection, USP, a transfer device and an administration set which contains an integral airway and a 15 micron filter.

STORAGE

Immune Globulin Intravenous (Human), GAMMAGARD should be stored under ordinary refrigeration, (2 to 8°C, 36 to 46°F). Freezing should be avoided to prevent the diluent bottle from breaking.

REFERENCES

1. Unpublished data in the files of Travenol Laboratories, Inc.
2. Waldmann TA, Storber W: Metabolism of Immunoglobulins. **Prog Allergy 13:** 1–110, 1969
3. Morell A, Riesen W: Structure, function and catabolism of immunoglobulins in **Immunohemotherapy.** Nydegger UE (ed), London, Academic Press, 1981, pp 17–26
4. Stiehm ER: Standard and special human immune serum globulin as therapeutic agents. **Pediatrics 63:** 301–319, 1979
5. Buckley RH: Immunoglobulin replacement therapy: indications and contraindications for use and variable IgG levels achieved in **Immunoglobulins: Characteristics and Use of Intravenous Preparations.** Alving BM, Finlayson JS (eds), Washington, DC, U.S. Department of Health and Human Services, 1979, pp 3–8 .
6. Burks AW, Sampson HA, Buckley RH: Anaphylactic reactions following gamma-globulin administration in patients with hypogammaglobulinemia: detection if IgE antibodies to IgA. Submitted for publication.

U.S. License No. 140

30-35-01-300B | Revised February 1986

*Manufactured under U.S. Patent No. 4,439,421

HEMOFIL® T ℞

Antihemophilic Factor (Human), Factor VIII, AHF, AHG
Method Four, Dried, Heat Treated

Supplied in single dose 10 ml, 20 ml, and 30 ml vials (AHF activity is stated on label of each vial) with sterile diluent, a double-ended needle for reconstitution, and a filter spike for withdrawal.

PROPLEX® SX-T ℞

Factor IX Complex
Heat Treated

Supplied in single dose 30 ml vials (Factor IX activity is stated on label of each vial) with sterile diluent and needles for reconstitution and withdrawal.

PROPLEX® T ℞

[pro 'plex]
Factor IX Complex, Heat Treated

Supplied in single dose 30 ml vials (Factor IX and Factor VII content are stated on the label of each vial) with sterile diluent and needles for reconstitution and withdrawal.

PROTENATE® 5% ℞

Plasma Protein Fraction (Human), USP, 5% Solution

Supplied as a 5% solution in 250 ml and 500 ml bottles. For use with intravenous administration set.

Hynson, Westcott & Dunning Products

BBL Microbiology Systems
Division of Becton Dickinson and Company
P.O. BOX 243
COCKEYSVILLE, MD 21030

BAL IN OIL AMPULES ℞
(Dimercaprol Injection, USP)

DESCRIPTION

Dimercaprol (2,3-dimercapto-1-propanol) is a colorless or almost colorless liquid, having a disagreeable, mercaptan-like odor. Each 1 ml sterile BAL in Oil contains 100 mg Dimercaprol in 200 mg benzyl benzoate and 700 mg peanut oil. The slight sediment which may be noticed in some ampules develops during sterilization. It is not an indication that the solution is deteriorating.

ACTION

Dimercaprol promotes the excretion of arsenic, gold and mercury in cases of poisoning. It is also used in combination with Edetate Calcium Disodium Injection, USP to promote the excretion of lead.

INDICATIONS

BAL in Oil (Dimercaprol Injection, USP) is indicated in the treatment of arsenic, gold and mercury poisoning. It is indicated in acute lead poisoning when used concomitantly with Edetate Calcium Disodium Injection, USP.
Dimercaprol Injection, USP is effective for use in acute poisoning by mercury salts if therapy is begun within one or two hours following ingestion. It is not very effective for chronic mercury poisoning.
Dimercaprol Injection, USP is of questionable value in poisoning caused by other heavy metals such as antimony and bismuth. It should not be used in iron, cadmium, or selenium poisoning because the resulting dimercaprol-metal complexes are more toxic than the metal alone, especially to the kidneys.

CONTRAINDICATIONS

BAL in Oil is contraindicated in most instances of hepatic insufficiency with the exception of postarsenical jaundice. The drug should be discontinued or used only with extreme caution if acute renal insufficiency develops during therapy.

WARNINGS

There may be local pain at the site of the injection. A reaction apparently peculiar to children is fever which may persist during therapy. It occurs in approximately 30% of children. A transient reduction of the percentage of polymorphonuclear leukocytes may also be observed.

PRECAUTIONS

Because the dimercaprol-metal complex breaks down easily in an acid medium, production of an alkaline urine affords protection to the kidney during therapy. Medicinal iron should not be administered to patients under therapy with BAL. Data is not available regarding the use of dimercaprol during pregnancy and it should not be used unless judged by the physician to be necessary in the treatment of life threatening acute poisoning.

ADVERSE REACTIONS

One of the most consistent responses to Dimercaprol Injection, USP is a rise in blood pressure accompanied by tachycardia. This rise is roughly proportional to the dose administered. Doses larger than those recommended may cause other transitory signs and symptoms in approximate order of frequency as follows: (1) nausea and, in some instances, vomiting; (2) headache; (3) a burning sensation in the lips, mouth and throat; (4) a feeling of constriction, even pain, in the throat, chest, or hands; (5) conjunctivitis, lacrimation, blepharal spasm, rhinorrhea, and salivation; (6) tingling of the hands; (7) a burning sensation in the penis; (8) sweating of the forehead, hands and other areas; (9) abdominal pain; and (10) occasional appearance of painful sterile abscesses. Many of the above symptoms are accompanied by a feeling of anxiety, weakness, and unrest and often are relieved by administration of an antihistamine.

DOSAGE AND ADMINISTRATION

By deep intramuscular injection only. For mild arsenic or gold poisoning, 2.5 mg/kg of body weight four times daily for two days, two times on the third day, and once daily thereafter for ten days; for severe arsenic or gold poisoning, 3 mg/kg every four hours for two days, four times on the third day, then twice daily thereafter for ten days. For mercury poisoning, 5 mg/kg initially, followed by 2.5 mg/kg one or two times daily for ten days. For acute lead encephalopathy 4 mg/kg body weight is given alone in the first dose and thereafter at four hour intervals in combination with Edetate Calcium Disodium Injection, USP administered at a separate site. For less severe poisoning the dose can be reduced to 3 mg/kg after the first dose. Treatment is maintained for two to seven days depending on clinical response. Successful treatment depends on beginning injections at the earliest possible moment and on the use of adequate amounts at frequent intervals. Other supportive measures should always be used in conjunction with BAL in Oil therapy.

HOW SUPPLIED

3 ml (100 mg/ml, ampules, box of 10, NDC 0011-8341-09).

LACTINEX® TABLETS AND GRANULES

(See PDR For Nonprescription Drugs)

ICN Pharmaceuticals, Inc.

ICN PLAZA
3300 HYLAND AVENUE
COSTA MESA, CA 92626

KATO® ℞
[kay'tō]
(potassium chloride for oral solution)
20 mEq. (1.5 g. KCl)

DESCRIPTION

KATO® (potassium chloride for oral solution) is a pleasantly flavored spray-dried tomato powder containing 20 mEq potassium (equivalent to 1.5 g KCl) per 5.7-grams of powder (one dose). KATO® is a potassium replacement product. Each daily dose (2 packets) contains approximately 0.5 mEq sodium.

CLINICAL PHARMACOLOGY

As the principal intracellular cation of most body tissues, potassium is instrumental in physiological processes such as maintenance of intracellular tonicity, contractility of cardiac, skeletal, and smooth muscles, maintenance of renal function, and transmission of nervous impulses.
Potassium depletion may occur when potassium intake is insufficient to compensate for potassium loss from the G.I. tract or via renal excretion. Such loss may slowly develop during prolonged oral diuretic therapy, in hyperaldosteronism, diabetic ketoacidosis, severe diarrhea, or where potassium intake is inadequate in patients receiving prolonged parenteral nutrition.
The potassium deficit is usually accompanied by chloride depletion and is manifested by hypokalemia and a hypochloremic metabolic alkalosis. Clinical symptoms and signs include weakness, fatigue, disturbances of cardiac rhythmicity (primarily ectopic beats), EKG changes (prominent U waves) and, in severe cases, flaccid paralysis and /or impaired urinary concentration.
Potassium chloride is therefore regarded as the appropriate potassium salt for use in correcting potassium depletion states associated with metabolic alkalosis.

INDICATIONS AND USAGE

KATO® is indicated for the treatment or prevention of potassium deficit, particularly when accompanied by hypochloremic alkalosis in conjunction with thiazide diuretic therapy, in digitalis intoxication, or as a result of long-term corticosteroid therapy, low dietary intake of potassium, or excessive vomiting or diarrhea.

CONTRAINDICATION

Potassium is contraindicated in patients with: severe renal impairment involving oliguria, anuria or azotemia; untreated Addison's disease; familial periodic paralysis; acute dehydration; heat cramps; and hyperkalemia from any cause.

WARNINGS

Potassium intoxication may result from overdosage or from the usual therapeutic dose in patients for whom the drug is contraindicated. Hyperkalemia, when detected, must be treated immediately because lethal levels can be reached in a few hours. (See Overdosage for treatment of hyperkalemia).

PRECAUTIONS

General: Patients receiving potassium supplementation should be monitored with periodic checks of plasma potassium levels.
A high plasma concentration of potassium ion may cause death through cardiac depression, arrhythmias or arrest. Therefore, the drug should be used with caution in patients with cardiac disease.
The drug should not be used in patients with low urinary output or renal decompensation because of the heightened likelihood of overdosage.
In rare circumstances (e.g. patients with renal tubular acidosis) potassium depletion may be associated with a hyperchloremic metabolic acidosis. In such patients, potassium depletion is appropriately corrected using potassium salts other than the chloride.
As with other concentrated potassium supplements. KATO® must be reconstituted with the proper amount of water (2 oz. for 1 packet) to avoid the possibility of gastrointestinal irritation.

DRUG INTERACTIONS

Concomitant administration of potassium chloride and a potassium-sparing diuretic (e.g. aldosterone antagonists or triamterene) can lead to severe hyperkalemia.

ADVERSE REACTIONS

Adverse reactions are related to the gastrointestinal system. Vomiting, diarrhea, nausea and abdominal discomfort may occur.

OVERDOSAGE

The symptoms and signs of potassium intoxication include paresthesias of the extremities, flaccid paralysis, listlessness, mental confusion, weakness and heaviness of the legs, fall in blood pressure, cardiac arrhythmias and heart block. Hyperkalemia may be associated with the following electrocardiographic abnormalities: disappearance of the P wave, widening and slurring of QRS complex, changes of the S-T segment and tall peaked T waves.
The drug is dialyzable.
Treatment of hyperkalemia includes: 1. Elimination of potassium-containing foods and medicaments. 2. Dextrose solution 10% or 25% containing 10 units of crystalline insulin per 20 g dextrose, given i.v. with a dose of 300 cc to 500 cc in an hour. 3. Adsorption and exchange of potassium using sodium or ammonium cycle cation exchange resin, orally or as retention enema. 4. Hemodialysis or peritonial dialysis.
Warning: Digitalis toxicity can be precipitated by lowering the plasma potassium concentration too rapidly in digitalized patients.

DOSAGE AND ADMINISTRATION

The usual adult dose is 1 packet of KATO® (20 mEq potassium) mixed with 2 ounces of cold water twice daily. If possible it should stand for 15 minutes to allow the tomato powder to absorb moisture. The preparation should be taken with meals, if convenient. If not, drink ½ glass of water immediately after taking the medication. Larger doses may be required, but should be administered under close supervision because of the possibility of potassium intoxication.
The appropriate dosage of potassium for pediatric use may be calculated from the adult dosage according to relative total body weight.

HOW SUPPLIED

KATO® is available in cartons of 30 (NDC 0187-0112-03) and 120 (NDC 0187-0112-12) 5.7-gram unit dose packets (20 mEq potassium each). Store away from heat.
02-112-30 Rev. 6/85

TESTRED® ℞
brand of Methyltestosterone Capsules USP, 10 mg.

DESCRIPTION

The androgens are steroids that develop and maintain primary and secondary male sex characteristics. Methyltestosterone, a synthetic derivative of testosterone, is an androgenic preparation given by the oral route in a capsule form. Each capsule contains 10 mg. of USP Methyltestosterone, which has the following formula:

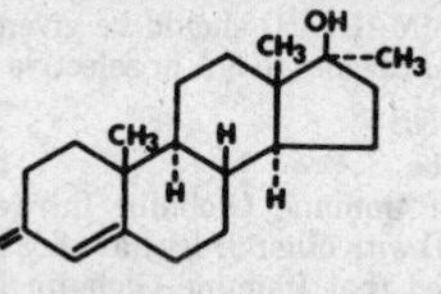

Methyltestosterone occurs as white or creamy white crystals or powder, which is soluble in various organic solvents but is practically insoluble in water.

CLINICAL PHARMACOLOGY

Endogenous androgens are responsible for the normal growth and development of the male sex organs and for maintenance of secondary sex characteristics. These effects include the growth and maturation of prostate, seminal vesicles, penis, and scrotum; the development of male hair distribution, such as beard, pubic, chest, and axillary hair; laryngeal enlargement, vocal chord thickening, alterations in body musculature, and fat distribution. Drugs in this class also cause retention of nitrogen, sodium, potassium, phosphorus, and decreased urinary excretion of calcium. Androgens have been reported to increase protein anabolism and decrease protein catabolism. Nitrogen balance is improved only when there is sufficient intake of calories and protein.
Androgens are responsible for the growth spurt of adolescence and for the eventual termination of linear growth which is brought about by fusion of the epiphyseal growth centers. In children, exogenous androgens accelerate linear growth rates, but may cause a disproportionate advancement in bone maturation. Use over long periods may result in fusion of the epiphyseal growth centers and termination of growth process. Androgens have been reported to stimu-

late the production of red blood cells by enhancing the production of erythropoietic stimulating factor.

During exogenous administration of androgens, endogenous testosterone release is inhibited through feedback inhibition of pituitary luteinizing hormone (LH). At large doses of exogenous androgens, spermatogenesis may also be suppressed through feedback inhibition of pituitary follicle stimulating hormone (FSH).

There is a lack of substantial evidence that androgens are effective in fractures, surgery, convalescence and functional uterine bleeding.

Pharmacokinetics

Testosterone given orally is metabolized by the gut and 44 percent is cleared by the liver in the first pass. Oral doses as high as 400 mg. per day are needed to achieve clinically effective blood levels for full replacement therapy. The synthetic androgen methyltestosterone is less extensively metabolized by the liver and has a longer half-life. It is more suitable than testosterone for oral administration.

Testosterone in plasma is 98 percent bound to a specific testosterone-estradiol binding globulin, and about 2 percent is free. Generally, the amount of this sex-hormone binding globulin in the plasma will determine the distribution of testosterone between free and bound forms, and the free testosterone concentration will determine its half-life.

About 90 percent of a dose of testosterone is excreted in the urine as glucuronic and sulfuric acid conjugates of testosterone and its metabolites; about 6 percent of a dose is excreted in the feces, mostly in the unconjugated form. Inactivation of testosterone occurs primarily in the liver. Testosterone is metabolized to various 17-keto steroids through two different pathways. There are considerable variations of the half-life of testosterone ranging from 10 to 100 minutes.

In many tissues the activity of testosterone appears to depend on reduction to dihydrotestosterone, which binds to cytosol receptor proteins. The steroid-receptor complex is transported to the nucleus where it initiates transcription events and cellular changes related to androgen action.

INDICATION AND USAGE

1. Males

Androgens are indicated for replacement therapy in conditions associated with a deficiency or absence of endogenous testosterone;

a. Primary hypogonadism (congenital or acquired)—testicular failure due to cryptorchidism, bilateral torsion, orchitis, vanishing testis syndrome; or orchidectomy.

b. Hypogonadotropic hypogonadism (congenital or acquired)—idiopathic gonadotropin or LHRH deficiency, or pituitary-hypothalamic injury from tumors, trauma, or radiation.

If the above conditions occur prior to puberty, androgen therapy will be needed during the adolescent years for development of secondary sexual characteristics. Prolonged androgen treatment will be required to maintain sexual characteristics in these and other males who develop testosterone deficiency after puberty.

c. Androgens may be used to stimulate puberty in carefully selected males with clearly delayed puberty. These patients usually have a familial pattern of delayed puberty that is not secondary to a pathological disorder; puberty is expected to occur spontaneously at a relatively late date. Brief treatment with conservative doses may occasionally be justified to these patients if they do not respond to psychological support. The potential adverse effect on bone maturation should be discussed with the patient and parents prior to androgen adminstration. An X-ray of the hand and wrist to determine bone age should be obtained every 6 months to assess the effect of treatment on the epiphyseal centers (see WARNINGS).

2. Females

Androgens may be used secondarily in women with advancing inoperable metastatic (skeletal) mammary cancer who are 1 to 5 years postmenopausal. Primary goals of therapy in these women include ablation of the ovaries. Other methods of counteracting estrogen activity are adrenalectomy, hypophysectomy, and/or antiestrogen therapy. This treatment has also been used in premenopausal women with breast cancer who have benefited from oophorectomy and are considered to have a hormone-responsive tumor. Judgment concerning androgen therapy should be made by an oncologist with expertise in this field.

Methyltestosterone has been used for the management of postpartum breast pain and engorgement.

CONTRAINDICATIONS

Androgens are contraindicated in men with carcinomas of the breast or with known or suspected carcinomas of the prostate, and in women who are or may become pregnant. When administered to pregnant women, androgens cause virilization of the external genitalia of the female fetus. This virilization includes clitoromegaly, abnormal vaginal development, and fusion of genital folds to form a scrotal-like structure. The degree of masculinization is related to the amount of drug given and the age of the fetus, and is most likely to occur in the female fetus when the drugs are given in the first trimester. If the patient becomes pregnant while taking these drugs, she should be apprised of the potential hazard to the fetus.

WARNINGS

In patients with breast cancer, androgen therapy may cause hypercalcemia by stimulating osteolysis. In the case, the drug should be discontinued.

Prolonged use of high doses of androgens has been associated with the development of peliosis hepatis and hepatic neoplasms including hepatocellular carcinoma. (See PRECAUTIONS-Carcinogenesis). Peliosis hepatis can be a life-threatening or fatal complication.

Cholestatic hepatitis and jaundice occur with 17-alpha-alkylandrogens at a relatively low dose. If cholestatic hepatitis with jaundice appears or if liver function tests become abnormal, the androgen should be discontinued and the etiology should be determined. Drug-induced jaundice is reversible when the medication is discontinued.

Geriatric patients treated with androgens may be at an increased risk for the development of prostatic hypertrophy and prostatic carcinoma. Edema with or without congestive heart failure may be a serious complication in patients with preexisting cardiac, renal, or hepatic disease. In addition to discontinuation of the drug, diuretic therapy may be required.

Gynecomastia frequently develops and occasionally persists in patients being treated for hypogonadism.

Androgen therapy should be used cautiously in healthy males with delayed puberty. The effect on bone maturation should be monitored by assessing bone age of the wrist and hand every 6 months. In children, androgen treatment may accelerate bone maturation without producing compensatory gain in linear growth.

These adverse effects may result in compromised adult stature. The younger the child the greater the risk of compromising final mature height.

PRECAUTIONS

General

Women should be observed for signs of virilization (deepening of the voice, hirsutism, acne, clitoromegaly and menstrual irregularities). Discontinuation of drug therapy at the time of evidence of mild virilism is necessary to prevent irreversible virilization. Such virilization is usual following androgen use at high doses. A decision may be made by the patient and the physician that some virilization will be tolerated during treatment for breast carcinoma.

Information for the Patient

The physician should instruct patients to report any of the following side effects of androgens:

Adult or Adolescent Males:	Too frequent or persistent erections of the penis.
Women:	Hoarseness, acne, changes in menstrual periods, or more hair on the face.
All Patients:	Any nausea, vomiting, changes in skin color or ankle swelling.

Laboratory Tests

1. Women with disseminated breast carcinoma should have frequent determination of urine and serum calcium levels during the course of androgen therapy. (See WARNINGS).
2. Because of the hepatotoxicity associated with the use of 17-alpha-alkylated androgens, liver function tests should be obtained periodically.
3. Periodic (every 6 months) x-ray examinations of bone age should be made during treatment of prepubertal males to determine the rate of bone maturation and the effects of androgen therapy on the epiphyseal centers.
4. Hemoglobin and hematocrit should be checked periodically for polycythemia in patients who are receiving high doses of androgens.

Drug Interactions

1. **Anticoagulants:** C-17 substituted derivatives of testosterone, such as methandrostenolone, have been reported to decrease the anticoagulant requirements of patients receiving oral anticoagulants. Patients receiving oral anticoagulant therapy require close monitoring, especially when androgens are started or stopped.
2. **Oxyphenbutazone:** Concurrent administration of oxyphenbutazone and androgens may result in elevated serum levels of oxyphenbutazone.
3. **Insulin:** In diabetic patients the metabolic effects of androgens may decrease blood glucose and insulin requirements.

Drug/Laboratory Test Interferences

Androgens may decrease levels of thyroxine-binding globulin, resulting in decreased total T4 serum levels and increased resin uptake of T3 and T4. Free thyroid hormone levels remain unchanged, however, and there is no clinical evidence of thyroid dysfunction.

Carcinogenesis

Animal Data

Testosterone has been tested by subcutaneous injection and implantation in mice and rats. The implant induced cervical-uterine tumors in mice, which metastasized in some cases. There is suggestive evidence that injection of testosterone into some strains of female mice increases their susceptibility to hepatoma. Testosterone is also known to increase the number of tumors and decrease the degree of differentiation of chemically induced carcinomas of the liver in rats.

Human Data

There are rare reports of hepatocellular carcinoma in patients receiving long-term therapy with androgens in high doses. Withdrawal of the drugs did not lead to regression of the tumors in all cases.

Geriatric patients treated with androgens may be at an increased risk for the development of prostatic hypertrophy and prostatic carcinoma.

Pregnancy

Teratogenic effects. Pregnancy Category X (See CONTRAINDICATIONS).

Nursing Mothers

It is not known whether androgens are excreted in human milk. Because many drugs are excreted in human milk and because of the potential for serious adverse reactions in nursing infants from androgens, a decision should be made whether to discontinue nursing or to discontinue the drug, taking into account the importance of the drug to the mother.

Pediatric Use

Androgen therapy should be used very cautiously in children and only by specialists who are aware of the adverse effects on bone maturation. Skeletal maturation must be monitored every six months by an x-ray of hand and wrist (See INDICATIONS AND USAGE and WARNINGS).

ADVERSE REACTIONS

Endocrine and Urogenital

Female: The most common side effects of androgen therapy are amenorrhea and other menstrual irregularities, inhibition of gonadotropin secretion, and virilization, including deepening of the voice and clitoral enlargement. The latter usually is not reversible after androgens are discontinued. When administered to a pregnant woman androgens cause virilization of external genitalia of the female fetus.

Male: Gynecomastia, and excessive frequency and duration of penile erections. Oligospermia may occur at high dosages (see CLINICAL PHARMACOLOGY).

Skin and appendages: Hirsutism, male pattern of baldness, and acne.

Fluid and Electrolyte Disturbances: Retention of sodium, chloride, water, potassium, calcium, and inorganic phosphates.

Gastrointestinal: Nausea, cholestatic jaundice, alterations in liver function tests, rarely hepatocellular neoplasms and peliosis hepatis (see WARNINGS).

Hematologic: Suppression of clotting factors II, V, VII, and X, bleeding in patients on concomitant anticoagulant therapy, and polycythemia.

Nervous System: Increased or decreased libido, headache, anxiety, depression, and generalized paresthesia.

Metabolic: Increased serum cholesterol.

Miscellaneous: Inflammation and pain at the site of intramuscular injection or subcutaneous implantation of testosterone containing pellets, stomatitis with buccal preparation, and rarely anaphylactoid reactions.

OVERDOSAGE

There have been no reports of acute overdosage with the androgens.

DOSAGE AND ADMINISTRATION

Androgens are administered as oral capsules. The suggested dosage for androgens varies depending on the age, sex, and diagnosis of the individual patient. Dosage is adjusted according to the patient's response and the appearance of adverse reactions. Replacement therapy in androgen-deficient males is 10–50 mg. of methyltestosterone daily. Various dosage regimens have been used to induce pubertal changes in hypogonadal males; some experts have advocated lower dosages initially, gradually increasing the dose as puberty progresses, with or without a decrease to maintenance levels. Other experts emphasize that higher dosages are needed to induce pubertal changes and lower dosages can be used for maintenance after puberty. The chronological and skeletal ages must be taken into consideration, both in determining the initial dose and in adjusting the dose.

Doses used in delayed puberty generally are in the range of 10 mg. of methyltestosterone daily, and for a limited duration, for example, 4 to 6 months.

Suggested dosages of oral methyltestosterone for use in the prevention of postpartum breast pain and engorgement is 80 mg. daily for 3 to 5 days after delivery.

Women with metastatic breast carcinoma must be followed closely because androgen therapy occasionally appears to

Continued on next page

ICN Pharmaceuticals—Cont.

accelerate the disease. Thus, many experts prefer to use the shorter acting androgen preparations rather than those with prolonged activity for treating breast carcinoma. The dosage of methyltestosterone for androgen therapy in breast carcinoma in females is from 50–200 mg. daily.

HOW SUPPLIED

Red capsules branded on both sections ICN 0901 containing 10 mg. of methyltestosterone in bottles of 100, 500, and 1000.
CAUTION: Federal (U.S.A.) law prohibits dispensing without prescription.

Revision February 1983

Shown in Product Identification Section, page 411

TESTRED® CYPIONATE 200 ℞

brand of Testosterone Cypionate Injection
200 mg./ml.
FOR INTRAMUSCULAR USE ONLY

DESCRIPTION

Testosterone Cypionate Injection is a sterile solution of Testosterone Cypionate for intramuscular use. Testosterone Cypionate ($C_{27}H_{40}O_3$) MW 412.59 is a white or creamy white, crystalline powder, is odorless or has a slight odor.
It is insoluble in water, freely soluble in alcohol and ether and soluble in vegetable oil. Its structural formula is:

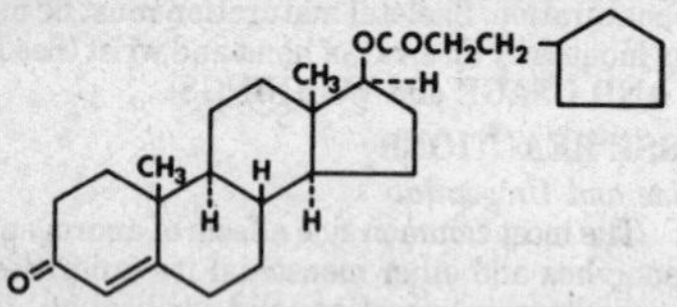

AVAILABLE AS: Sterile Testosterone Injection 200 mg. per ml. in multiple dose vials of 10 ml. Each ml. contains: Testosterone Cypionate 200 mg., Benzyl Benzoate 20%, Benzyl Alcohol 0.9% as preservative in Cottonseed Oil.
Androgens are derivatives of cyclopentano-perhydrophenanthrene. Endogenous androgens are C-19 steroids with a side chain at C-17, and with two angular methyl groups. Testosterone is the primary endogenous androgen.

CLINICAL PHARMACOLOGY

Endogenous androgens are responsible for the normal growth and development of the male sex organs and for maintenance of secondary sex characteristics. These effects include the growth and maturation of prostate, seminal vesicles, penis, and scrotum; the development of male hair distribution, such as beard, pubic, chest, and axillary hair; laryngeal enlargement, vocal chord thickening, alterations in body musculature, and fat distribution. Drugs in this class also cause retention of nitrogen, sodium, potassium, phosphorus, and decreased urinary excretion of calcium. Androgens have been reported to increase protein anabolism and decrease protein catabolism. Nitrogen balance is improved only when there is sufficient intake of calories and protein.
Androgens are responsible for the growth spurt of adolescence and for the eventual termination of linear growth which is brought about by fusion of the epiphyseal growth centers. In children, exogenous androgens accelerate linear growth rates, but may cause a disproportionate advancement in bone maturation. Use over long periods may result in fusion of the epiphyseal growth centers and termination of growth process. Androgens have been reported to stimulate the production of red blood cells by enhancing the production of erythropoietic stimulating factor.
During exogenous administration of androgens, endogenous testosterone release is inhibited through feedback inhibition of pituitary luteinizing hormone (LH). At large doses of exogenous androgens, spermatogenesis may also be suppressed through feedback inhibition of pituitary follicle stimulating hormone (FSH).
There is a lack of substantial evidence that androgens are effective in fractures, surgery, convalescence, and functional uterine bleeding.
Testosterone Cypionate is intended for androgen therapy, particularly when prolonged action is desirable. Following a single intramuscular injection, the androgenic effect is sustained over a period of about 4 weeks. This continuous flow of hormone is thought to resemble closely the endogenous production of testosterone.
Testosterone Cypionate is primarily used for its protein anabolic effect and its catabolic inhibiting effect on tissue. Nitrogen balance is improved with anabolic agents but only when there is sufficient intake of calories and protein. Whether this positive nitrogen balance is of primary benefit in the utilization of protein-building dietary substances has not been established.

Pharmacokinetics:
Testosterone esters are less polar than free testosterone. Testosterone esters in oil injected intramuscularly are absorbed slowly from the lipid phase; thus, testosterone cypionate and enanthate can be given at intervals of two to four weeks. Suspensions of testosterone or its esters in aqueous media may cause local irritation and the rate of absorption is not always uniform.
Testosterone in plasma is 98 percent bound to a specific testosterone-estradiol binding globulin, and about 2 percent is free. Generally, the amount of this sex-hormone binding globulin in the plasma will determine the distribution of testosterone between free and bound forms, and the free testosterone concentration will determine its half-life.
About 90 percent of a dose of testosterone is excreted in the urine as glucuronic and sulfuric acid conjugates of testosterone and its metabolites; about 6 percent of a dose is excreted in the feces, mostly in the unconjugated form. Inactivation of testosterone occurs primarily in the liver. Testosterone is metabolized to various 17-keto steroids through two different pathways. There are considerable variations of the half-life of testosterone as reported in the literature, ranging from 10 to 100 minutes.
In many tissues the activity of testosterone appears to depend on reduction to dihydrotestosterone, which binds to cytosol receptor proteins. The steroid-receptor complex is transported to the nucleus where it initiates transcription events and cellular changes related to androgen action.

INDICATIONS AND USAGE

1. Males: Androgens are indicated for replacement therapy in conditions associated with a deficiency or absence of endogenous testosterone;
a. Primary hypogonadism (congenital or acquired)—testicular failure due to cryptorchidism, bilateral torsion, orchitis, vanishing testis syndrome; or orchidectomy.
b. Hypogonadotropic hypogonadism (congenital or acquired)—idiopathic gonadotropin or LHRH deficiency, or pituitary-hypothalamic injury from tumors, trauma, or radiation.
If the above conditions occur prior to puberty, androgen replacement therapy will be needed during the adolescent years for development of secondary sexual characteristics. Prolonged androgen treatment will be required to maintain sexual characteristics in these and other males who develop testosterone deficiency after puberty.
c. Androgens may be used to stimulate puberty in carefully selected males with clearly delayed puberty. These patients usually have a familial pattern of delayed puberty that is not secondary to a pathological disorder; puberty is expected to occur spontaneously at a relatively late date. Brief treatment with conservative doses may occasionally be justified in these patients if they do not respond to psychological support. The potential adverse effect on bone maturation should be discussed with the patient and parents prior to androgen administration. An X-ray of the hand and wrist to determine bone age should be obtained every 6 months to assess the effect of treatment on the epiphyseal centers (see WARNINGS).

2. Females: Androgens may be used secondarily in women with advancing inoperable metastatic (skeletal) mammary cancer who are 1 to 5 years postmenopausal. Primary goals of therapy in these women include ablation of the ovaries. Other methods of counteracting estrogen activity are adrenalectomy, hypophysectomy, and/or antiestrogen therapy. This treatment has also been used in premenopausal women with breast cancer who have benefited from oophorectomy and are considered to have a hormone-responsive tumor. Judgment concerning androgen therapy should be made by an oncologist with expertise in this field.

CONTRAINDICATIONS

Androgens are contraindicated in men with carcinomas of the breast or with known or suspected carcinomas of the prostate, and in women who are or may become pregnant. When administered to pregnant women, androgens cause virilization of the external genitalia of the femal fetus. This virilization includes clitoromegaly, abnormal vaginal development, and fusion of genital folds to form a scrotal-like structure. The degree of masculinization is related to the amount of drug given and the age of the fetus, and is most likely to occur in the female fetus when the drugs are given in the first trimester. If the patient becomes pregnant while taking these drugs, she should be apprised of the potential hazard to the fetus.
Androgens are also contraindicated in patients with nephrosis or the nephrotic phase of nephritis.
Hypersensitivity to any of the components of the product.

WARNINGS

In patients with breast cancer, androgen therapy may cause hyercalcemia by stimulating osteolysis. In this case, the drug should be discontinued.
Prolonged use of high doses of androgens has been associated with the development of peliosis hepatis and hepatic neoplasms including hepatocellular carcinoma (See PRECAUTION—Carcinogenesis). Peliosis hepatis can be a life-threatening or fatal complication.
Cholestatic hepatitis and jaundice occur with 17-alpha-alkylandrogens at a relatively low dose. If cholestatic hepatitis with jaundice appears or if liver function tests become abnormal, the androgen should be discontinued and the etiology should be determined. Drug-induced jaundice is reversible when the medication is discontinued.
Geriatric patients treated with androgens may be at an increased risk for the development of prostatic hypertrophy and protastatic carcinoma. Edema with or without congestive heart failure may be a serious complication in patients with preexisting cardiac, renal, or hepatic disease. In addition to discontinuation of the drug, diuretic therapy may be required.
Gynecomastia frequently develops and occasionally persists in patients being treated for hypogonadism.
Androgen therapy should be used cautiously in healthy males with delayed puberty. The effect on bone maturation should be monitored by assessing bone age of the wrist and hand every six months. In children, androgen treatment may accelerate bone maturation without producing compensatory gain in linear growth.
This adverse effect may result in compromised adult stature. The younger the child the greater the risk of compromising final mature height.

PRECAUTIONS

General: Women should be observed for signs of virilization (deepening of the voice, hirsutism, acne, clitoromegaly and menstrual irregularities). Discontinuation of drug therapy at the time of evidence of mild virilism is necessary to prevent irreversible virilization. Such virilization is usual following androgen use at high doses. A decision may be made by the patient and the physician that some virilization will be tolerated during treatment for breast carcinoma.
Information for the Patient: The physician should instruct patients to report any of the following side effects of androgens:

Adult or Adolescent Males: Too frequent or persistent erections of the penis.
Women: Hoarseness, acne, changes in menstrual periods, or more hair on the face.
All Patients: Any nausea, vomiting, changes in skin color or ankle swelling.
Any male adolescent patient receiving androgens for delayed puberty should have bone development checked every six months.

Laboratory Tests:

1. Women with disseminated breast carcinoma should have frequent determination of urine and serum calcium levels during the course of androgen therapy (See WARNINGS).
2. Because of the hepatotoxicity associated with the use of 17-alpha-alkylated androgens, liver function tests should be obtained periodically.
3. Periodic (every 6 months) x-ray examinations of bone age should be made during treatment of prepubertal males to determine the rate of bone maturation and the effects of androgen therapy on the epiphyseal centers.
4. Hemoglobin and hematocrit should be checked periodically for polycythemia in patients who are receiving high doses of androgens.

Drug Interactions:

1. Anticoagulants. C-17 substituted derivatives of testosterone, such as methandrostenolone, have been reported to decrease the anticoagulant requirements of patients receiving oral anticoagulants. Patients receiving oral anticoagulant therapy require close monitoring, especially when androgens are started or stopped.
2. Oxyphenbutazone. Concurrent administration of oxyphenbutazone and androgens may result in elevated serum levels of oxyphenbutazone.
3. Insulin. In diabetic patients the metabolic effects of androgens may decrease blood glucose and insulin requirements.

Drug/Laboratory Interferences:
Androgens may decrease levels of thyroxine-binding globulin, resulting in decreased total T^4 serum levels and increased resin uptake of T^3 and T^4. Free thyroid hormone levels remain unchanged, however, and there is no clinical evidence of thyroid dysfunction.
Carcinogenesis:
Animal Data: Testosterone has been tested by subcutaneous injection and implantation in mice and rats. The implant induced cervical-uterine tumors in mice, which metastasized in some cases. There is suggestive evidence that injection of testosterone into some strains of female mice increases their susceptibility to hepatoma. Testosterone is also known to increase the number of tumors and decrease the degree of differentiation of chemically induced carcinomas of the liver in rats.
Human Data: There are rare reports of hepatocellular carcinoma in patients receiving long-term therapy with androgens in high doses. Withdrawal of the drugs did not lead to regression of the tumors in all cases.

Geriatric patients treated with androgens may be at an increased risk for the development of prostatic hypertrophy and prostatic carcinoma.

Pregnancy:

Teratogenic Effects. Pregnancy Category X (See CONTRAINDICATIONS).

Nursing Mothers:

It is not known whether androgens are excreted in human milk. Because many drugs are excreted in human milk and because of the potential for serious adverse reactions in nursing infants from androgens, a decision should be made whether to discontinue nursing or to discontinue the drug, taking into account the importance of the drug to the mother.

Pediatric Use:

Androgen therapy should be used very cautiously in children and only by specialists who are aware of the adverse effects on bone maturation. Skeletal maturation must be monitored every six months by an x-ray of hand and wrist (See INDICATIONS AND USAGE and WARNINGS).

ADVERSE REACTIONS

Endocrine and Urogenital:

Female: The most common side effects of androgen therapy are amenorrhea and other menstrual irregularities, inhibition of gonadotropin secretion, and virilization, including deepening of the voice and clitoral enlargement. The latter usually is not reversible after androgens are discontinued. When administered to a pregnant woman androgens cause virilization of external genitalia of the female fetus.

Male: Gynecomastia, and excessive frequency and duration of penile erections. Oligospermia may occur at high dosages (see CLINICAL PHARMACOLOGY).

Skin and appendages: Hirsutism, male pattern of baldness, and acne.

Fluid and Electrolyte Disturbances: Retention of sodium, chloride, water, potassium, calcium, and inorganic phosphates.

Gastrointestinal: Nausea, cholestatic jaundice, alterations in liver function tests, rarely hepatocellular neoplasms and peliosis hepatitis (see WARNINGS).

Hematologic: Suppression of clotting factors II, V, VII, and X, bleeding in patients of concomitant anticoagulant therapy, and polycythemia.

Nervous System: Increased or decreased libido, headache, anxiety, depression, and generalized paresthesia.

Metabolic: Increased serum cholesterol.

Miscellaneous: Inflammation and pain at the site of intramuscular injection or subcutaneous implantation of testosterone containing pellets, stomatitis with buccal preparations, and rarely anaphylactoid reactions.

OVERDOSAGE

There have been no reports of acute overdosage with the androgens.

DOSAGE AND ADMINISTRATION

Androgens should not be given intravenously. Intramuscular injections should be given deep in the gluteal muscle.

The suggested dosage for androgens varies depending on the age, sex, and diagnosis of the individual patient. Dosage is adjusted according to the patient's response and the appearance of adverse reactions. Various dosage regimens have been used to induce pubertal changes in hypogonadal males; some experts have advocated lower dosages initially, gradually increasing the dose as puberty progresses, with or without a decrease to maintenance levels. Other experts emphasize that higher dosages are needed to induce pubertal changes and lower dosages can be used for maintenance after puberty.

For androgen replacement therapy in the male, the recommended dosage is 50–400 mg. every 2 to 4 weeks. For androgen therapy in breast carcinomas in females, the recommended dosage is 200–400 mg. every 2 to 4 weeks.

When properly given, injections of Testosterone Cypionate are well tolerated. Care should be taken to inject the preparation deeply into the gluteal muscle following the usual precautions for intramuscular administration. In general, total doses above 400 mg. per month are not required because of the prolonged action of the preparation. Injections more frequently than every two weeks are rarely indicated.

NOTE: Use of a wet needle or wet syringe may cause the solution to become cloudy; however, this does not affect the potency of the material.

The chronological and skeletal ages must be taken into consideration, both in determining the initial dose and in adjusting the dose.

Dosages used in delayed puberty generally are in the lower ranges and for a limited duration, for example, 4 to 6 months.

Women with metastatic breast carcinoma must be followed closely because androgen therapy occasionally appears to accelerate the disease. Thus, may experts prefer to use the shorter acting androgen preparations rather than those with prolonged activity for treating breast carcinoma, particularly during the early stages of androgen therapy.

Parenteral drug products should be inspected visually for particulate matter and discoloration prior to administration, whenever the solution and container permit.

HOW SUPPLIED

Multiple dose vials of 10 ml. containing Testosterone Cypionate 200 mg. per ml. (NDC 0187-0200-10).

Store at room temperature 15°–30°C (59°–86°F).

PROTECT FROM LIGHT

Storage at low temperatures may produce crystal formation. If present, dissolve by warming to 85°F and shaking vial.

CAUTION

Federal law prohibits dispensing without prescription.

Literature Revised: April 1985

Shown in Product Identification Section, page 411

VIRAZOLE™ ℞

[vira 'zahl']

(Ribavirin)

lyophilized for aerosol administration

WARNING:

RIBAVIRIN AEROSOL SHOULD NOT BE USED FOR INFANTS REQUIRING ASSISTED VENTILATION BECAUSE PRECIPITATION OF THE DRUG IN THE RESPIRATORY EQUIPMENT MAY INTERFERE WITH SAFE AND EFFECTIVE VENTILATION OF THE PATIENT. Conditions for safe use with a ventilator are still in development.

Deterioration of respiratory function has been associated with ribavirin use in infants, and in adults with chronic obstructive lung disease or asthma. Respiratory function should be carefully monitored during treatment. If initiation of ribavirin aerosol treatment appears to produce sudden deterioration of respiratory function, treatment should be stopped and re-instituted only with extreme caution and continuous monitoring.

Although ribavirin is not indicated in adults, the physician should be aware that it is teratogenic in animals (see CONTRAINDICATIONS).

DESCRIPTION

Virazole® (ribavirin) Aerosol, an antiviral drug, is a sterile, lyophilized powder to be reconstituted for aerosol administration. Each 100 ml glass vial contains 6 grams of ribavirin, and when reconstituted to the recommended volume of 300 ml with sterile water for injection or sterile water for inhalation (no preservatives added), will contain 20 mg/ml ribavirin, pH approximately 5.5. Aerosolization is to be carried out in a SPAG-2 nebulizer only.

Ribavirin is 1-beta-D-ribofuranosyl-1,2,4-triazole-3-carboxamide, with the following structural formula:

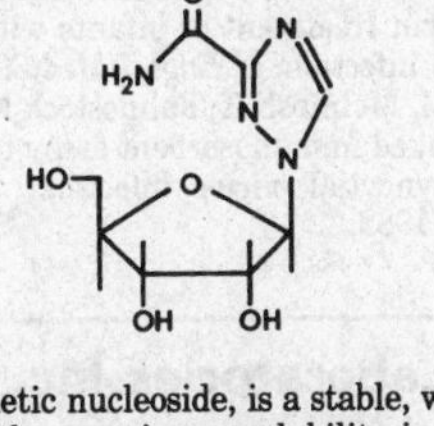

Ribavirin, a synthetic nucleoside, is a stable, white, crystalline compound with a maximum solubility in water of 142 mg/ml at 25°C and with only a slight solubility in ethanol. The empirical formula is $C_8H_{12}N_4O_5$ and the molecular weight is 244.2 Daltons.

CLINICAL PHARMACOLOGY

Antiviral effects: Ribavirin has antiviral inhibitory activity *in vitro* against respiratory syncytial virus,[1] influenza virus, and herpes simplex virus. Ribavirin is also active against respiratory syncytial virus (RSV) in experimentally infected cotton rats.[2]

In cell cultures, the inhibitory activity of ribavirin for RSV is selective. The mechanism of action is unknown. Reversal of the *in vitro* antiviral activity by guanosine or xanthosine suggests ribavirin may act as an analogue of these cellular metabolites.

Immunologic effects: Neutralizing antibody responses to RSV were decreased in ribavirin treated compared to placebo treated infants.[3] The clinical significance of this observation is unknown. In rats, ribavirin resulted in lymphoid atrophy of thymus, spleen, and lymph nodes. Humoral immunity was reduced in guinea pigs and ferrets. Cellular immunity was also mildly depressed in animal studies.

Microbiology: Several clinical isolates of RSV were evaluated for ribavirin susceptibility by plaque reduction in tissue culture. Plaques were reduced 85–98% by 16μg/ml; however, plaque reduction varies with the test system. The clinical significance of these data is unknown.

Pharmacokinetics: Assay for ribavirin in human materials is by a radioimmunoassay which detects ribavirin and at least one metabolite.

Ribavirin administered by aerosol is absorbed systemically. Four pediatric patients inhaling ribavirin aerosol administered by face mask for 2.5 hours each day for 3 days had plasma concentrations ranging from 0.44 to 1.55 μM, with a mean concentration of 0.76 μM. The plasma half-life was reported to be 9.5 hours. Three pediatric patients inhaling ribavirin aerosol administered by face mask or mist tent for 20 hours each day for 5 days had plasma concentrations ranging from 1.5 to 14.3 μM, with a mean concentration of 6.8 μM.

It is likely that the concentration of ribavirin in respiratory tract secretions is much higher than plasma concentrations in view of the route of administration.

The bioavailability of ribavirin aerosol is unknown and may depend on the mode of aerosol delivery. After aerosol treatment, peak plasma concentrations are less than the concentration that reduced RSV plaque formation in tissue culture by 85 to 98%. After aerosol treatment, respiratory tract secretions are likely to contain ribavirin in concentrations many fold higher than those required to reduce plaque formation. However, RSV is an intracellular virus and serum concentrations may better reflect intracellular concentrations in the respiratory tract than respiratory secretion concentrations.

In man, rats, and rhesus monkeys, accumulation of ribavirin and/or metabolites in the red blood cells has been noted, plateauing in red cells in man in about 4 days and gradually declining with an apparent half-life of 40 days. The extent of accumulation of ribavirin following inhalation therapy is not well defined.

INDICATIONS AND USAGE

Ribavirin aerosol is indicated in the treatment of carefully selected hospitalized infants and young children with severe lower respiratory tract infections due to respiratory syncytial virus (RSV). In two placebo controlled trials in infants hospitalized with RSV lower respiratory tract infection, ribavirin aerosol treatment had a therapeutic effect, as judged by the reduction by treatment day 3 of severity of clinical manifestations of disease.[3,4] Virus titers in respiratory secretions were also significantly reduced with ribavirin in one of these studies.[4]

Only severe RSV lower respiratory tract infection is to be treated with ribavirin aerosol. The vast majority of infants and children with RSV infection have no lower respiratory tract disease or have disease that is mild, self-limited, and does not require hospitalization or antiviral treatment. Many children with mild lower respiratory tract involvement will require shorter hospitalization than would be required for a full course of ribavirin aerosol (3 to 7 days) and should not be treated with the drug. Thus the decision to treat with ribavirin aerosol should be based on the severity of the RSV infection.

The presence of an underlying condition such as prematurity or cardiopulmonary disease may increase the severity of the infection and its risk to the patient. High risk infants and young children with these underlying conditions may benefit from ribavirin treatment, although efficacy has been evaluated in only a small number of such patients.

Ribavirin aerosol treatment must be accompanied by and does not replace standard supportive respiratory and fluid management for infants and children with severe respiratory tract infection.

Diagnosis: RSV infection should be documented by a rapid diagnostic method such as demonstration of viral antigen in respiratory tract secretions by immunofluorescence[3,4] or ELISA[5] before or during the first 24 hours of treatment. Ribavirin aerosol is indicated only for lower respiratory tract infection due to RSV. Treatment may be initiated while awaiting rapid diagnostic test results. However, treatment should not be continued without documentation of RSV infection.

CONTRAINDICATIONS

Ribavirin is contraindicated in women or girls who are or may become pregnant during exposure to the drug. Ribavirin may cause fetal harm and respiratory syncytial virus infection is self-limited in this population. Ribavirin is not completely cleared from human blood even four weeks after administration. Although there are no pertinent human data, ribavirin has been found to be teratogenic and/or embryolethal in nearly all species in which it has been tested. Teratogenicity was evident after a single oral dose of 2.5 mg/kg in the hamster and after daily oral doses of 10 mg/kg in the rat. Malformations of skull, palate, eye, jaw, skeleton, and gastrointestinal tract were noted in animal studies. Survival of fetuses and offspring was reduced. The drug causes embryolethality in the rabbit at daily oral dose levels as low as 1 mg/kg.

Continued on next page

ICN Pharmaceuticals—Cont.

WARNINGS

Ribavirin administered by aerosol produced cardiac lesions in mice and rats after 30 and 36 mg/kg, respectively, for 4 weeks, and after oral administration in monkeys at 120 and rats at 154 to 200 mg/kg for 1 to 6 months. Ribavirin aerosol administered to developing ferrets at 60 mg/kg for 10 or 30 days resulted in inflammatory and possibly emphysematous changes in the lungs. Proliferative changes were seen at 131 mg/kg for 30 days. The significance of these findings to human administration is unknown.

Ribavirin lyophilized in 6 gram vials in intended for use as an aerosol only.

PRECAUTIONS

General: Patients with lower respiratory tract infection due to respiratory syncytial virus require optimum monitoring and attention to respiratory and fluid status.

Drug Interactions: Interactions of ribavirin with other drugs such as digoxin, bronchodilators, other antiviral agents, antibiotics, or anti-metabolites has not been evaluated. Interference by ribavirin with laboratory tests has not been evaluated.

Carcinogenesis, mutagenesis, impairment of fertility: Ribavirin induces cell transformation in an *in vitro* mammalian system (Balb/C 3T3 cell line). However, *in vivo* carcinogenicity studies are incomplete. Results thus far, though inconclusive, suggest that chronic feeding of ribavirin to rats at dose levels in the range of 16–60 mg/kg body weight can induce benign mammary, pancreatic, pituitary and adrenal tumors. Ribavirin is mutagenic to mammalian (L5178Y) cells in culture. Results of microbial mutagenicity assays and a dominant lethal assay (mouse) were negative.

Ribavirin causes testicular lesions (tubular atrophy) in adult rats at oral dose levels as low as 16 mg/kg/day (lower doses not tested), but fertility of ribavirin-treated animals (male or female) has not been adequately investigated.

Pregnancy: Teratogenic Effects: Pregnancy Category X. See "CONTRAINDICATIONS" section.

Nursing Mothers: Use of ribavirin aerosol in nursing mothers is not indicated because RSV infection is self-limited in this population. Ribavirin is toxic to lactating animals and their offspring. It is not known whether the drug is excreted in human milk.

ADVERSE REACTIONS

Approximately 200 patients have been treated with ribavirin aerosol in controlled or uncontrolled clinical studies.

Pulmonary function significantly deteriorated during ribavirin aerosol treatment in six of six adults with chronic obstructive lung disease and in four of six asthmatic adults. Dyspnea and chest soreness were also reported in the latter group. Minor abnormalities in pulmonary function were also seen in healthy adult volunteers.

Several serious adverse events occurred in severely ill infants with life-threatening underlying diseases, many of whom required assisted ventilation. The role of ribavirin aerosol in these events is indeterminate. The following events were associated with ribavirin use:

Pulmonary: Worsening of respiratory status, bacterial pneumonia, pneumothorax, apnea, and ventilator dependence.

Cardiovascular: Cardiac arrest, hypotension, and digitalis toxicity.

There were 7 deaths during or shortly after treatment with ribavirin aerosol. No death was attributed to ribavirin aerosol by the investigators.

Some subjects requiring assisted ventilation have experienced serious difficulties, which may jeopardize adequate ventilation and gas exchange. Precipitation of drug within the ventilatory apparatus, including the endotracheal tube, has resulted in increased positive end expiratory pressure and increased positive inspiratory pressure. Accumulation of fluid in tubing ("rain out") has also been noted.

Although anemia has not been reported with use of the aerosol, it occurs frequently with oral and intravenous ribavirin, and most infants treated with the aerosol have not been evaluated 1 to 2 weeks post-treatment when anemia is likely to occur. Reticulocytosis has been reported with aerosol use.

Rash and conjunctivitis have been associated with the use of ribavirin aerosol.

Overdosage: No overdosage with ribavirin by aerosol administration has been reported in the human. The LD_{50} in mice is 2 gm orally. Hypoactivity and gastrointestinal symptoms occurred. In man, ribavirin is sequestered in red blood cells for weeks after dosing.

DOSAGE AND ADMINISTRATION

Before use, read thoroughly the Viratek Small Particle Aerosol Generator (SPAG) Model SPAG-2 Operation's Manual for small particle aerosol generator operating instructions.

Treatment was effective when instituted within the first 3 days of respiratory syncytial virus lower tract infection.[3] Treatment early in the course of severe lower respiratory tract infection may be necessary to achieve efficacy.

Treatment is carried out for 12–18 hours per day for at least 3 and no more than 7 days, and is part of a total treatment program. The aerosol is delivered to an infant oxygen hood from the SPAG-2 aerosol generator. Administration by face mask or oxygen tent may be necessary if a hood cannot be employed (see SPAG-2 manual). However, the volume of distribution and condensation area are larger in a tent and efficacy of this method of administering the drug has been evaluated in only a small number of patients. Ribavirin aerosol is not to be administered with any other aerosol generating device or together with other aerosolized medications. Ribavirin aerosol should not be used for patients requiring simultaneous assisted ventilation (see Boxed Warnings).

Virazole is supplied as 6 grams of lyophilized drug per 100 ml vial for aerosol administration only. By sterile technique, solubilize drug with sterile USP water for injection or inhalation in the 100 ml vial. Transfer to the clean, sterilized 500 ml wide-mouth Erlenmeyer flask (SPAG-2 Reservoir) and further dilute to a final volume of 300 ml with sterile USP water for injection or inhalation. The final concentration should be 20 mg/ml. **Important:** This water should not have had any antimicrobial agent or other substance added. The solution should be inspected visually for particulate matter and discoloration prior to administration. Solutions that have been placed in the SPAG-2 unit should be discarded at least every 24 hours and when the liquid level is low before adding newly reconstituted solutions.

Using the recommended drug concentration of 20 mg/ml ribavirin as the starting solution in the drug reservoir of the SPAG unit, the average aerosol concentration for a 12 hour period would be 190 micrograms/liter (0.19 mg/l) of air.

HOW SUPPLIED

Virazole (ribavirin) Aerosol is supplied in 100 ml glass vials with 6 grams of sterile, lyophilized drug which is to be reconstituted with 300 ml sterile water for injection or sterile water for inhalation (no preservatives added) and administered only by a small particle aerosol generator (SPAG-2). Vials containing the lyophilized drug powder should be stored in a dry place at 15–25°C (59–78°F). Reconstituted solutions may be stored, under sterile conditions, at room temperature (20–30°C, 68–86°F) for 24 hours. Solutions which have been placed in the SPAG-2 unit should be discarded at least every 24 hours.

REFERENCES

1. Hruska JF, Bernstein JM, Douglas Jr., RG, and Hall CB. Effects of ribavirin on respiratory syncytial virus in vitro. *Antimicrob Agents Chemother* 17:770–775, 1, 1980.
2. Hruska JF, Morrow PE, Suffin SC, and Douglas Jr., RG. *In vitro* inhibition of respiratory syncytial virus by ribavirin. *Antimicrob Agents Chemother* 21:125–130, 1982.
3. Taber LH, Knight V, Gilbert BE, McClung HW et al. Ribavirin aerosol treatment of bronchiolitis associated with respiratory tract infection in infants. *Pediatrics* 72:613–618, 1983.
4. Hall CB, McBride JT, Walsh EE, Bell DM et al. Aerosolized ribavirin treatment of infants with respiratory syncytial viral infection. *N Engl J Med* 308:1443–7, 1983.
5. Hendry RM, McIntosh K, Fahnestock ML, and Pierik LT. Enzyme-linked immunosorbent assay for detection of respiratory syncytial virus infection. *J Clin Microbiol* 16:329–33, 1982.

Ives Laboratories Inc.

Ives products may now be found in the Product Information Section for Wyeth Laboratories.

Important Notice

Before prescribing or administering any product described in PHYSICIANS' DESK REFERENCE always consult the PDR Supplement for possible new or revised information

Jacobus Pharmaceutical Co., Inc.

37 CLEVELAND LANE
P.O. BOX 5290
PRINCETON, NJ 08540

DAPSONE USP ℞
[*dap'sōne*]
25 mg. & 100 mg.

PRODUCT OVERVIEW

KEY FACTS

Dapsone is a sulfone for the primary treatment of Dermatitis herpetiformis and an antibacterial drug for susceptible cases of leprosy.

MAJOR USES

Dapsone is used to control the dermatologic symptoms of Dermatitis herpetiformis. Dapsone is used alone or in combination with other anti-leprosy drugs for leprosy.

SAFETY INFORMATION

Dapsone is contraindicated in patients with Dapsone hypersensitivity. Complete blood counts and laboratory monitoring should be done frequently. See labeling.

PRODUCT INFORMATION

DAPSONE USP ℞
[*dap'sōne*]
25 mg. & 100 mg.

DESCRIPTION

Dapsone-USP, 4–4′ diaminodiphenylsulfone (DDS) is a primary treatment for Dermatitis herpetiformis. It is an antibacterial drug for susceptible cases of leprosy. It is a white, odorless crystalline powder, practically insoluble in water and insoluble in fixed and vegetable oils.

Dapsone is issued on prescription in tablets of 25 and 100 mg. for oral use.

NH_2–[benzene ring]–SO_2–[benzene ring]–NH_2

CLINICAL PHARMACOLOGY

Actions: The mechanism of action in Dermatitis herpetiformis has not been established. By the kinetic method in mice, Dapsone is bactericidal as well as bacteriostatic against *Mycobacterium leprae.*

Absorption and Excretion: Dapsone, when given orally, is rapidly and almost completely absorbed. About 85 percent of the daily intake is recoverable from the urine mainly in the form of water-soluble metabolites. Excretion of the drug is slow and a constant blood level can be maintained with the usual dosage.

Blood Levels: Detected a few minutes after ingestion, the drug reaches peak concentration in 4–8 hours. Daily administration for at least eight days is necessary to achieve a plateau level. With doses of 200 mg. daily, this level averaged 2.3 μg/ml with a range of 0.1–7.0 μg/ml. The half-life in the plasma in different individuals varies from ten hours to fifty hours and averages twenty-eight hours. Repeat tests in the same individual are constant. Daily administration (50–100 mg.) in leprosy patients will provide blood levels in excess of the usual minimum inhibitory concentration even for patients with a short Dapsone half-life.

INDICATIONS AND USAGE

Dermatitis herpetiformis (D.H.) All forms of leprosy except for cases of proven Dapsone resistance.

CONTRAINDICATION

Hypersensitivity to Dapsone and/or its derivatives.

WARNINGS

The patient should be warned to respond to the presence of clinical signs such as sore throat, fever, pallor, purpura or jaundice. Deaths associated with the administration of Dapsone have been reported from agranulocytosis, aplastic anemia and other blood dyscrasias. Complete blood counts should be done frequently in patients receiving Dapsone. The FDA Dermatology Advisory Committee recommended that, when feasible counts should be done weekly for the first month, monthly for six months and semi-annually thereafter. If a significant reduction in leucocytes, platelets or hemopoiesis is noted, Dapsone should be discontinued and the patient followed intensively. Folic acid antagonists have similar effects and may increase the incidence of hematologic reactions; if co-administered with Dapsone the patient should be monitored more frequently. Patients on weekly Pyrimethamine and Dapsone have developed agranulocytosis during the second and third month of therapy.

Severe anemia should be treated prior to initiation of therapy and hemoglobin monitored. Hemolysis and methemoglobin may be poorly tolerated by patients with severe cardiopulmonary disease.

Carcinogenesis, mutagenesis: Dapsone has been found carcinogenic (sarcomagenic) for male rats and female mice causing mesenchymal tumors in the spleen and peritoneum, and thyroid carcinoma in female rats. Dapsone is not mutagenic with or without microsomal activation in *S. typhimurium* tester strains 1535, 1537, 1538, 98, or 100.
Cutaneous reactions, especially bullous, include exfoliative dermatitis and are probably one of the most serious, though rare, complications of sulfone therapy. They are directly due to drug sensitization. Such reactions include toxic erythema, erythema multiforme, toxic epidermal necrolysis, morbilliform and scariatiniform reactions, urticaria and erythema nodosum. If new or toxic dermatologic reactions occur, sulfone therapy must be promptly discontinued and appropriate therapy instituted.
Leprosy reactional states, including cutaneous, are not hypersensitivity reactions to Dapsone and do not require discontinuation. See special section.

PRECAUTIONS

General: Hemolysis and Heinz body formation may be exaggerated in individuals with a glucose-6-phosphate dehydrogenase (G6PD) deficiency, or methemoglobin reductase deficiency, or hemoglobin M. This reaction is frequently dose-related. Dapsone should be given with caution to these patients or if the patient is exposed to other agents or conditions such as infection or diabetic ketosis capable of producing hemolysis. Drugs or chemicals which have produced significant hemolysis in G6PD or methemoglobin reductase deficient patients include Dapsone, sulfamilamide, nitrite, aniline, phenylhydrazine, napthalene, niridazole, nitrofurantoin and 8-amino-antimalarials such as primaquine.
Toxic hepatitis and cholestatic jaundice have been reported early in therapy. Hyperbilirubinemia may occur more often in G6PD deficient patients. When feasible, baseline and subsequent monitoring of liver function is recommended. If abnormal, Dapsone should be discontinued until the source of the abnormality is established.
Drug Interactions: Rifampin lowers Dapsone levels 7 to 10-fold by accelerating plasma clearance; in leprosy this reduction has not required a change in dosage.
Folic acid antagonists such as pyrimethamine may increase the likelihood of hematologic reactions.
Pregnancy Category C: Animal reproduction studies have not been conducted with Dapsone. Extensive, but uncontrolled experience and two published surveys on the use of Dapsone in pregnant women have not shown that Dapsone increases the risk of fetal abnormalities if administered during all trimesters of pregnancy or can affect reproduction capacity. Because of the lack of animal studies or controlled human experience, Dapsone should be given to a pregnant woman only if clearly needed. In general, for leprosy, USPHS at Carville recommends maintenance of Dapsone. Dapsone has been important for the management of some pregnant D.H. patients.
Nursing Mothers: Dapsone is excreted in breast milk in substantial amounts. Hemolytic reactions can occur in neonates. See section on hemolysis. Because of the potential for tumorgenicity shown for Dapsone in animal studies a decision should be made whether to discontinue nursing or discontinue the drug taking into account the importance of the drug to the mother.
Pediatric Use: Children are treated on the same schedule as adults but with correspondingly smaller doses. Dapsone is generally not considered to have an effect on the later growth, development and functional development of the child.

ADVERSE REACTIONS

In addition to the warnings listed above, the following syndromes and serious reactions have been reported in patients on Dapsone.
Hematologic Effects: Dose-related hemolysis is the most common adverse effect and is seen in patients with or without G6PD deficiency. Almost all patients demonstrate the inter-related changes of a loss of 1–2g of HB, an increase in the reticulocytes (2–12%), a shortened red cell life span and a rise in methemoglobin. G6PD deficient patients have greater responses.
Nervous System Effects: Peripheral neuropathy is a definite but unusual complication of Dapsone therapy in non-leprosy patients. Motor loss is predominent. If muscle weakness appears, Dapsone should be withdrawn. Recovery on withdrawal is usually substantially complete. The mechanism of recovery is reportedly by axonal regeneration. Some recovered patients have tolerated retreatment at reduced dosage. In leprosy this complication may be difficult to distinguish from a leprosy reactional state.
Body As A Whole: In addition to the warnings and adverse effects reported above, additional adverse reactions include: nausea, vomiting, abdominal pains, vertigo, blurred vision, tinnitus, insomnia, fever, headache, psychosis, phototoxicity, tachycardia, albuminuria, the nephrotic syndrome, hypoalbuminemia without proteinuria, renal papillary necrosis, male infertility, drug-induced Lupus erythematosus and an infectious mononucleosis-like syndrome. In general, with the exception of the complications of severe anoxia from overdosage (retinal and optic nerve damage, etc.) these adverse reactions have regressed off drug.

OVERDOSAGE

Nausea, vomiting, hyper-excitability can appear a few minutes up to 24 hours after ingestion or an overdose. Methemoglobin induced depression, convulsions and severe cyanosis requires prompt treatment. In normal and methemoglobin reductase deficient patients, methylene blue, 1–2 mg/kg of body weight, given slowly intravenously is the treatment of choice. The effect is complete in 30 minutes, but may have to be repeated if methemoglobin reaccumulates. For non-emergencies, if treatment is needed, methylene blue may be given orally in doses of 3–5 mg/kg every 4–6 hours.
Methylene blue reduction depends on G6PD and should not be given to fully expressed G6PD deficient patients.

DOSAGE AND ADMINISTRATION

Dermatitis herpetiformis: The dosage should be individually titrated starting in adults with 50 mg. daily and correspondingly smaller doses in children. If full control is not achieved within the range of 50–300 mg. daily, higher doses may be tried. Dosage should be reduced to a minimum maintenance level as soon as possible. In responsive patients there is a prompt reduction in pruritus followed by clearance of skin lesions. There is no effect on the gastro-intestinal component of the disease.
Dapsone levels are influenced by acetylation rates. Patients with high acetylation rates, or who are receiving treatment affecting acetylation may require an adjustment in dosage.
A strict gluten free diet is an option for the patient to elect, permitting many to reduce or eliminate the need for Dapsone; the average time for dosage reduction is 8 months with a range of 4 months to 2½ years and for dosage elimination 29 months with a range of 6 months to 9 years.
Leprosy: In order to reduce secondary Dapsone resistance, the WHO Expert Committee on Leprosy and the USPHS at Carville, LA, recommend that Dapsone should be commenced in combination with one or more anti-leprosy drugs. In the multi-drug program Dapsone should be maintained at the full dosage of 100 mg. daily without interruption (with correspondingly smaller doses for children) and provided to all patients who have sensitive organisms with new or recrudescent disease or who have not yet completed a two year course of Dapsone monotherapy. For advice and other drugs, the USPHS at Carville, LA, (504-642-7771) should be contacted. Before using other drugs consult appropriate product labeling.
In bacteriologically negative tuberculoid and indeterminate disease, the recommendation is the coadministration of Dapsone 100 mg. daily with six months of Rifampin 600 mg. daily. Under WHO, daily Rifampin may be replaced by 600 mg. Rifampin monthly, if supervised. The Dapsone is continued until all signs of clinical activity are controlled—usually after an additional six months. Then Dapsone should be continued for an additional three years for tuberculoid and indeterminate patients and for five years for borderline tuberculoid patients.
In lepromatous and borderline lepromatous patients, the recommendation is the coadministration of Dapsone 100 mg. daily with two years of Rifampin 600 mg. daily. Under WHO, daily Rifampin may be replaced by 600 mg. Rifampin monthly, if supervised. One may elect the concurrent administration of a third anti-leprosy drug, usually either Clofazamine 50–100mg. daily or Ethionamide 250–500 mg. daily. Dapsone 100mg. daily is continued 3–10 years until all signs of clinical activity are controlled with skin scrapings and biopsies negative for one year. Dapsone should then be continued for an additional 10 years for borderline patients and for life for lepromatous patients.
Secondary Dapsone resistance should be suspected whenever a lepromatous or borderline lepromatous patient receiving Dapsone treatment relapses clinically and bacteriologically, solid staining bacilli being found in the smears taken from the new active lesions. If such cases show no response to regular and supervised Dapsone therapy within three to six months or good compliance for the past 3–6 months can be assured, Dapsone resistance should be considered confirmed clinically. Determination of drug sensitivity using the mouse footpad method is recommended and, after prior arrangement, is available without charge from the USPHS, Carville, LA. Patients with proven Dapsone resistance should be treated with other drugs.
Leprosy Reactional States: Abrupt changes in clinical activity occur in leprosy with any effective treatment and are known as reactional states. The majority can be classified into two groups.
The "Reversal" reaction (Type 1) may occur in borderline or tuberculoid leprosy patients often soon after chemotherapy is started. The mechanism is presumed to result from a reduction in the antigenic load: the patient is able to mount an enhanced delayed hypersensitivity response to residual infection leading to swelling ("Reversal") of existing skin and nerve lesions. If severe, or if neuritis is present, large doses of steroids should always be used. If severe, the patient should be hospitalized. In general anti-leprosy treatment is continued and therapy to suppress the reaction is indicated such as analgesics, steroids, or surgical decompression of swollen nerve trunks. USPHS at Carville, LA should be contacted for advice in management.
Erythema nodosum leprosum (ENL) (lepromatous lepra reaction) (Type 2 reaction) occurs mainly in lepromatous patients and small numbers of borderline patients. Approximately 50% of treated patients show this reaction in the first year. The principal clinical features are fever and tender erythematous skin nodules sometimes associated with malaise, neuritis, orchitis, albuminuria, joint swelling, iritis, epistaxis or depression. Skin lesions can become pustular and/or ulcerate. Histologically there is a vasculitis with an intense polymorphonuclear infiltrate. Elevated circulating immune complexes are considered to be the mechanism of the reaction. If severe, patients should be hospitalized. In general, anti-leprosy treatment is continued. Analgesics, steroids, and other agents available from USPHS, Carville, LA, are used to suppress the reaction.

HOW SUPPLIED

Rx: 25 mg. and 100 mg. white scored tablets in light resistant, child proof bottles of 100 (25 mg.—NDC 49938-102-01 Coded Jacobus 102) and 100 mg.—NDC 49938-101-01 Coded Jacobus 101).
Distributed by: Jacobus Pharmaceutical Co., Inc., P.O. Box 5290, Princeton, NJ 08540
Manufactured by: Reid-Rowell, Inc. Baudette, MN 56623.
5E June 85

Jamol Laboratories Inc.

13 ACKERMAN AVENUE
EMERSON, NEW JERSEY 07630

PONARIS

Nasal Mucosal Emollient

COMPOSITION

Essential oils of cajeput, eucalyptus, and peppermint in a specially prepared iodized cottonseed oil. (Total Iodine 0.6%) Assimilable hence NON-lipoid potential.

INDICATIONS AND USES

Nasal emollient, for relief of nasal congestion due to colds, nasal irritations, atrophic rhinitis, (dry inflamed nasal passages), nasal mucosal encrustations and allergy manifestations.
Also nasal intubations and sterile gauze impregnated for epistaxis packing.

ADMINISTRATION AND DOSAGE

3 to 4 drops in each nostril 3 to 4 times daily. May be used in a compressed air nebulizer or a DeVilbiss nebulizer No. 33 or 40.
Childrens Dosage: As directed by physician.

HOW SUPPLIED

One ounce bottle with dropper.

ROMA-NOL

ACTIVE INGREDIENT

An iodine solution for external use having none of the toxic, escharotic, or precipitating nature of usual iodine preparations.

INDICATIONS

For all skin and some mucous membrane infections.

ACTIONS

By the J-R process the iodine is highly subdivided thus making **Roma-nol** the highest form of a water soluble iodine. The color density is increased by its high solubility. Hospital studies have proven unusual penetration qualities.

DOSAGE AND ADMINISTRATION

The first 2 or 3 applications of **Roma-nol** act more like cleansers, the iodine color slowly disappearing as it combines with the infected organic matter, pus, mucous, etc. With the additional applications 2 to 4 times more, the impurities being eliminated, the iodine stain will remain. The infected parts have received the full compatible treatment with **Roma-nol** ending the treatment.

HOW SUPPLIED

Bottles of 30 cc. each.

Products are cross-indexed by generic and chemical names in the **YELLOW SECTION**

Janssen Pharmaceutica Inc.
40 KINGSBRIDGE ROAD
PISCATAWAY, NJ 08854

IMODIUM® ℞
(loperamide HCl) Capsules
(loperamide HCl) Liquid

DESCRIPTION

IMODIUM (loperamide hydrochloride), 4-(p-chlorophenyl)-4-hydroxy-N, N-dimethyl- α,α-diphenyl-1-piperidinebutyramide monohydrochloride, is a synthetic antidiarrheal for oral use.

IMODIUM is available in 2 mg capsules and as a liquid containing 1 mg/5 ml.

CLINICAL PHARMACOLOGY

In vitro and animal studies show that IMODIUM acts by slowing intestinal motility and by affecting water and electrolyte movement through the bowel. IMODIUM inhibits peristaltic activity by a direct effect on the circular and longitudinal muscles of the intestinal wall.

In man, IMODIUM prolongs the transit time of the intestinal contents. It reduces the daily fecal volume, increases the viscosity and bulk density, and diminishes the loss of fluid and electrolytes. Tolerance to the antidiarrheal effect has not been observed.

Clinical studies have indicated that the apparent elimination half-life of loperamide in man is 10.8 hours with a range of 9.1–14.4 hours. Plasma levels of unchanged drug remain below 2 nanograms per ml after the intake of a 2 mg capsule of IMODIUM. Plasma levels are highest approximately five hours after administration of the capsule and 2.5 hours after the liquid. The peak plasma levels of loperamide were similar for both formulations. Of the total excreted in urine and feces, most of the administered drug was excreted in feces.

In those patients in whom biochemical and hematological parameters were monitored during clinical trials, no trends toward abnormality during IMODIUM therapy were noted. Similarly, urinalyses, EKG and clinical ophthalmological examinations did not show trends toward abnormality.

INDICATIONS AND USAGE

IMODIUM is indicated for the control and symptomatic relief of acute nonspecific diarrhea and of chronic diarrhea associated with inflammatory bowel disease. IMODIUM is also indicated for reducing the volume of discharge from ileostomies.

CONTRAINDICATIONS

IMODIUM is contraindicated in patients with known hypersensitivity to the drug and in those in whom constipation must be avoided.

WARNINGS

IMODIUM should not be used in the case of acute dysentery, which is characterized by blood in stools and elevated temperatures.

Fluid and electrolyte depletion may occur in patients who have diarrhea. The use of IMODIUM does not preclude the administration of appropriate fluid and electrolyte therapy.

In some patients with acute ulcerative colitis, and in pseudomembranous colitis associated with broad-spectrum antibiotics, agents which inhibit intestinal motility or delay intestinal transit time have been reported to induce toxic megacolon. IMODIUM therapy should be discontinued promptly if abdominal distention occurs or if other untoward symptoms develop in patients with acute ulcerative colitis.

IMODIUM should be used with special caution in young children because of the greater variability of response in this age group. Dehydration, particularly in younger children, may further influence the variability of response to IMODIUM.

PRECAUTIONS

General: In acute diarrhea, if clinical improvement is not observed in 48 hours, the administration of IMODIUM should be discontinued.

Patients with hepatic dysfunction should be monitored closely for signs of CNS toxicity because of the apparent large first pass biotransformation.

Information for Patients: Patients should be advised to check with their physician if their diarrhea doesn't stop after a few days or if they develop a fever.

Drug Interactions: There was no evidence in clinical trials of drug interactions with concurrent medications.

Carcinogenesis, mutagenesis, impairment of fertility: In an 18-month rat study with doses up to 133 times the maximum human dose (on a mg/kg basis), there was no evidence of carcinogenesis. Mutagenicity studies were not conducted. Reproduction studies in rats indicated that high doses (150–200 times the human dose) could cause marked female infertility and reduced male fertility.

Pregnancy
Teratogenic Effects
Pregnancy Category B: Reproduction studies in rats and rabbits have revealed no evidence of impaired fertility or harm to the fetus at doses up to 30 times the human dose. Higher doses impaired the survival of mothers and nursing young. The studies offered no evidence of teratogenic activity. There are, however, no adequate and well controlled studies in pregnant women. Because animal reproduction studies are not always predictive of human response, this drug should be used during pregnancy only if clearly needed.

Nursing Mothers: It is not known whether this drug is excreted in human milk. Because many drugs are excreted in human milk, caution should be exercised when IMODIUM is administered to a nursing woman.

Pediatric Use: See the "Warnings" Section for information on the greater variability of response in this age group.

In case of accidental overdosage of IMODIUM by children, see "OVERDOSAGE" Section for suggested treatment.

ADVERSE REACTIONS

The adverse effects reported during clinical investigations of IMODIUM are difficult to distinguish from symptoms associated with the diarrheal syndrome. Adverse experiences recorded during clinical studies with IMODIUM were generally of a minor and self-limiting nature. They were more commonly observed during the treatment of chronic diarrhea.

The following patient complaints have been reported and are listed in decreasing order of frequency with the exception of hypersensitivity reactions which is listed first since it may be the most serious.

- Hypersensitivity reactions (including skin rash) have been reported with IMODIUM use.
- Abdominal pain, distention or discomfort
- Nausea and vomiting
- Constipation
- Tiredness
- Drowsiness or dizziness
- Dry mouth

DRUG ABUSE AND DEPENDENCE

Abuse: A specific clinical study designed to assess the abuse potential of loperamide at high doses resulted in a finding of extremely low abuse potential. Additionally, after years of extensive use there has been no evidence of abuse or dependence.

Dependence: Physical dependence to IMODIUM in humans has not been observed. However, studies in morphine-dependent monkeys demonstrated that loperamide hydrochloride at doses above those recommended for humans prevented signs of morphine withdrawal. However, in humans, the naloxone challenge pupil test, which when positive indicates opiate-like effects, performed after a single high dose, or after more than two years of therapeutic use of IMODIUM, was negative. Orally administered IMODIUM (loperamide formulated with magnesium stearate) is both highly insoluble and penetrates the CNS poorly.

OVERDOSAGE

Animal pharmacological and toxicological data indicate that overdosage in man may result in constipation, CNS depression and gastrointestinal irritation. Clinical trials have demonstrated that a slurry of activated charcoal administered promptly after ingestion of loperamide hydrochloride can reduce the amount of drug which is absorbed into the systemic circulation by as much as ninefold. If vomiting occurs spontaneously upon ingestion, a slurry of 100 gms of activated charcoal should be administered orally as soon as fluids can be retained.

If vomiting has not occurred, gastric lavage should be performed followed by administration of 100 gms of the activated charcoal slurry through the gastric tube. In the event of overdosage, patients should be monitored for signs of CNS depression for at least 24 hours. Children may be more sensitive to central nervous system effects than adults. If CNS depression is observed, naloxone may be administered. If responsive to naloxone, vital signs must be monitored carefully for recurrence of symptoms of drug overdose for at least 24 hours after the last dose of naloxone.

In view of the prolonged action of loperamide and the short duration (one to three hours) of naloxone, the patient must be monitored closely and treated repeatedly with naloxone as indicated. Since relatively little drug is excreted in the urine, forced diuresis is not expected to be effective for IMODIUM overdosage.

In clinical trials an adult who took three 20 mg doses within a 24 hour period was nauseated after the second dose and vomited after the third dose. In studies designed to examine the potential for side effects, intentional ingestion of up to 60 mg of loperamide hydrochloride in a single dose to healthy subjects resulted in no significant adverse effects.

DOSAGE AND ADMINISTRATION

(1 teaspoonful = 1 mg.; 1 capsule = 2 mg.)

Acute diarrhea

Adults: The recommended initial dose is two IMODIUM Capsules or four teaspoonfuls of IMODIUM Liquid (4 mg) followed by one capsule or two teaspoonfuls of liquid (2 mg) after each unformed stool. Daily dosage should not exceed eight capsules or sixteen teaspoonfuls of liquid (16 mg). Clinical improvement is usually observed within 48 hours.

Children: IMODIUM use is not recommended for children under 2 years of age. In children 2 to 5 years of age (20 kg or less), IMODIUM Liquid should be used; for ages 6 to 12, either IMODIUM Liquid or Capsules may be used. For children 2 to 12 years of age, the following schedule for capsules or liquid will usually fulfill initial dosage requirements:

Recommended First Day Dosage Schedule

Two to five years: (13 to 20 kg)	1 mg t.i.d. (3 mg daily dose) (1 teaspoonful t.i.d.)
Five to eight years: (20 to 30 kg)	2 mg b.i.d. (4 mg daily dose) (2 teaspoonfuls or 1 capsule b.i.d.)
Eight to twelve years: (greater than 30 kg)	2 mg t.i.d. (6 mg daily dose) (2 teaspoonfuls or 1 capsule t.i.d.)

Recommended Subsequent Daily Dosage

Following the first treatment day, it is recommended that subsequent IMODIUM doses (1 mg/10 kg body weight) be administered only after a loose stool. Total daily dosage should not exceed recommended dosages for the first day.

Chronic Diarrhea

Children: Although IMODIUM has been studied in a limited number of children with chronic diarrhea, the therapeutic dose for the treatment of chronic diarrhea in a pediatric population has not been established.

Adults: The recommended initial dose is two IMODIUM Capsules or four teaspoonfuls of IMODIUM Liquid (4 mg) followed by one capsule or two teaspoonfuls of liquid (2 mg) after each unformed stool until diarrhea is controlled, after which the dosage of IMODIUM should be reduced to meet individual requirements. When the optimal daily dosage has been established, this amount may then be administered as a single dose or in divided doses.

The average daily maintenance dosage in clinical trials was 4 to 8 mg (two to four capsules or four to eight teaspoonfuls of liquid). A dosage of 16 mg (eight capsules or sixteen teaspoonfuls of liquid) was rarely exceeded. If clinical improvement is not observed after treatment with 16 mg per day for at least 10 days, symptoms are unlikely to be controlled by further administration. IMODIUM administration may be continued if diarrhea cannot be adequately controlled with diet or specific treatment.

HOW SUPPLIED

Liquid—containing 1 mg loperamide hydrochloride per 5 ml. Bottles of 4 oz.

Capsules—each capsule contains 2 mg of loperamide hydrochloride. The capsules have a light green body and a dark green cap with "JANSSEN" imprinted on one segment and "IMODIUM" on the other segment. IMODIUM capsules are supplied in bottles of 100 and 500 and in blister packs of 10 × 10 capsules.

NDC 50458-410-04
(4 oz. Liquid)
NDC 50458-400-01
(10 × 10 capsules—blister)
NDC 50458-400-10
(100 capsules)
NDC 50458-400-50
(500 capsules)

Date: Dec. 1984, July 1985

CAUTION: FEDERAL LAW PROHIBITS DISPENSING WITHOUT A PRESCRIPTION

An original product of
JANSSEN PHARMACEUTICA, n.v.
B-2340 Beerse
Belgium
JANSSEN PHARMACEUTICA INC.
Piscataway
New Jersey 08854
Printed in USA
U.S. Patent 3,714,159

TRAVELERS' DIARRHEA BIBLIOGRAPHY

Traveler's Diarrhea: *NIH Consensus Development Conference Statement.* US Dept of Health and Human Services 1985;5(8).

Consensus Conference: Travelers' diarrhea. *JAMA* 1985;253(18):2700–2704.

Farthing MJ: Travelers' diarrhea. *Physician Assistant* 1985;9:57–66.

Steffen R, et al: Epidemiology of diarrhea in travelers. *JAMA* 1983;249(9):1176–1180.

Loosli J, et al: Etiology of acute infectious diarrhea in a highly industrialized area of Switzerland. *Gastroenterology* 1985;88:75–79.
DuPont HL: Using OTC drugs for acute diarrhea. *PA Drug Update*, May 1983, pp 39–49.
Ericsson CD: Travelers' diarrhea: Precautions, prophylaxis, and treatment. *Consultant* 1984;102(2):260–261.
DuPont HL, et al: Chemotherapy and chemoprophylaxis of travelers' diarrhea, editorial. *Ann Int Med* 1985;102:260–261.
DuPont HL, et al: Symptomatic treatment of diarrhea with bismuth subsalicylate among students attending a Mexican university. *Gastroenterology* 1977;73(4)(pt 1):715–718.
DuPont HL, et al: Prevention of travelers' diarrhea (emporiatric enteritis) *JAMA* 1980;243(3):237–241.
Graham DY, et al: Double-blind comparison of bismuth subsalicylate and placebo in the prevention and treatment of enterotoxigenic *Escherichia coli* induced diarrhea in volunteers. *Gastroenterology* 1983;85:1017–1022.
DuPont HL, et al: Treatment of travelers' diarrhea with trimethoprim/sulfamethoxazole and with trimethoprim alone. *N Engl J Med* 1982;307(14):841–844.
DuPont HL, et al: Prevention of travelers' diarrhea with trimethoprim-sulfamethoxazole and trimethoprim alone. *Gastroenterology* 1983;84(1):75–80.
Sack RB, et al: Prophylactic doxycycline for travelers' diarrhea. *Gastroenterology* 1979;76(6):1368–1373.
Ericsson CD, et al: Efficacy of bicozamycin in preventing traveler's diarrhea. *Gastroenterology* 1985;88:473–477.
DuPont HL, et al: Adverse effect of lomotil therapy in shigellosis. *JAMA* 1973;226(13):1525–1528.
Hamdi I, et al: Toddler diarrhoea: Observations on the effects of aspirin and loperamide. *J Pediatr Gastroenterol Nutr* 1985;4(3):362–365.
Levine MM: *Escherichia coli* infections, editorial. *N Engl J Med* 1985;313(7):445–447.
Mathewson JJ, et al: A newly recognized cause of travelers' diarrhea: Enteroadherent *Escherichia coli*. *J Infect Dis* 1985;151(3):471–475.
Johnson PC, et al: Comparison of loperamide to bismuth subsalicylate for the treatment of travelers' diarrhea, abstracted. *Gastroenterology* 1984;86(5(pt 2):1126.
Lipicky RJ: Letter of approval removing caution against use of Imodium in acute diarrhea, US Dept of Health and Human Services, November 1, 1985.
Gorbach SL: Travelers' diarrhea, editorial. *N Engl J Med* 1982;307(14):881–883.
Amery W, et al: A multicentre double-blind study in acute diarrhoea comparing loperamide (R 18553) with two common antidiarrhoeal agents and a placebo. *Curr Ther Res* 1975;17(3):263–270.
Ericsson CD, et al: Influence of subsalicylate bismuth on absorption of doxycycline. *JAMA* 1982;247(16):2266–2267.
Cornett JWD, et al: A double-blind comparative evaluation of loperamide versus diphenoxylate with atropine in acute diarrhea. *Curr Ther Res* 1977;21(5):629–637.
McIntyre RV: Letter to the editor. Prevention of travelers' diarrhea *JAMA* 1980;244(13):1435–1436.
DuPont HL: Nonfluid therapy and selected chemoprophylaxis of acute diarrhea. *Am J Med* 1985;78(suppl 6B):81–90.
Johnson PC: Comparison of loperamide with bismuth subsalicylate for the treatment of acute travelers' diarrhea. *JAMA* 1986;255(6):757–760.

Shown in Product Identification Section, page 411

INAPSINE® ℞
[*in-ăp-sēn*]
(droperidol) Injection
FOR INTRAVENOUS OR INTRAMUSCULAR USE ONLY

DESCRIPTION

INAPSINE (droperidol) is a neuroleptic (tranquilizer) agent available in ampoules and vials. Each milliliter contains 2.5 mg. of droperidol in an aqueous solution adjusted to pH 3.4 ± 0.4 with lactic acid. INAPSINE In 10 ml multidose vials also contains 1.8 mg of methylparaben and 0.2 mg propylparaben. Droperidol is chemically identified as 1-(1-[3-(p-flourobenzoyl) propyl]-1,2,3,6-tetrahydro-4-pyridyl)-2-benzimidazolinone with a molecular weight of 379.43.
INAPSINE is a sterile, non-pyrogenic aqueous solution for intravenous or intramuscular injection.

CLINICAL PHARMACOLOGY

INAPSINE (droperidol) produces marked tranquilization and sedation. It allays apprehension and provides a state of mental detachment and indifference while maintaining a state of reflex alertness. INAPSINE produces an antiemetic effect as evidenced by the antagonism of apomorphine in dogs. It lowers the incidence of nausea and vomiting during surgical procedures and provides antiemetic protection in the postoperative period.
INAPSINE potentiates other CNS depressants. It produces mild alpha-adrenergic blockade, peripheral vascular dilatation and reduction of the pressor effect of epinephrine. It can produce hypotension and decreased peripheral vascular resistance and may decrease pulmonary arterial pressure (particularly if it is abnormally high). It may reduce the incidence of epinephrine-induced arrhythmias but it does not prevent other cardiac arrhythmias.
The onset of action of single intramuscular and intravenous doses is from three to ten minutes following administration, although the peak effect may not be apparent for up to thirty minutes. The duration of the tranquilizing and sedative effects generally is two to four hours, although alteration of alertness may persist for as long as twelve hours.

INDICATIONS AND USAGE

INAPSINE (droperidol) is indicated:
- to produce tranquilization and to reduce the incidence of nausea and vomiting in surgical and diagnostic procedures.
- for premedication, induction, and as an adjunct in the maintenance of general and regional anesthesia.
- in neuroleptanalgesia in which INAPSINE is given concurrently with an opioid analgesic, such as SUBLIMAZE (fentanyl citrate) Injection, to aid in producing tranquility and decreasing anxiety and pain.

CONTRAINDICATIONS

INAPSINE (droperidol) is contraindicated in patients with known hypersensitivity to the drug.

WARNINGS

FLUIDS AND OTHER COUNTERMEASURES TO MANAGE HYPOTENSION SHOULD BE READILY AVAILABLE.
As with other CNS depressant drugs, patients who have received INAPSINE (droperidol) should have appropriate surveillance.
It is recommended that opioids, when required, initially be used in reduced doses.

PRECAUTIONS

General: The initial dose of INAPSINE (droperidol) should be appropriately reduced in elderly, debilitated and other poor-risk patients. The effect of the initial dose should be considered in determining incremental doses.
Certain forms of conduction anesthesia, such as spinal anesthesia and some peridural anesthetics, can alter respiration by blocking intercostal nerves and can cause peripheral vasodilatation and hypotension because of sympathetic blockade. Through other mechanisms (see CLINICAL PHARMACOLOGY), INAPSINE can also alter circulation. Therefore, when INAPSINE is used to supplement these forms of anesthesia, the anesthetist should be familiar with the physiological alterations involved, and be prepared to manage them in the patients elected for these forms of anesthesia.
If hypotension occurs, the possibility of hypovolemia should be considered and managed with appropriate parenteral fluid therapy. Repositioning the patient to improve venous return to the heart should be considered when operative conditions permit. It should be noted that in spinal and peridural anesthesia, tilting the patient into a head-down position may result in a higher level of anesthesia than is desirable, as well as impair venous return to the heart. Care should be exercised in moving and positioning of patients because of a possibility of orthostatic hypotension. If volume expansion with fluids plus these other countermeasures do not correct the hypotension, then the administration of pressor agents other than epinephrine should be considered. Epinephrine may paradoxically decrease the blood pressure in patients treated with INAPSINE due to the alpha-adrenergic blocking action of INAPSINE.
Since INAPSINE may decrease pulmonary arterial pressure, this fact should be considered by those who conduct diagnostic or surgical procedures where interpretation of pulmonary arterial pressure measurements might determine final management of the patient.
Vital signs should be monitored routinely.
When the EEG is used for postoperative monitoring, it may be found that the EEG pattern returns to normal slowly.
Impaired Hepatic or Renal Function: INAPSINE should be administered with caution to patients with liver and kidney dysfunction because of the importance of these organs in the metabolism and excretion of drugs.
Drug Interactions: Other CNS depressant drugs (e.g. barbiturates, tranquilizers, opioids and general anesthetics) have additive or potentiating effects with INAPSINE. When patients have received such drugs, the dose of INAPSINE required will be less than usual. Following the administration of INAPSINE, the dose of other CNS depressant drugs should be reduced.
Carcinogenesis, Mutagenesis, Impairment of Fertility: No carcinogenicity studies have been carried out with INAPSINE. The micronucleus test in female rats revealed no mutagenic effects in single oral doses as high as 160 mg/kg. An oral study in rats (Segment I) revealed no impairment of fertility in either male or females at 0.63, 2.5 and 10 mg/kg doses (approximately 2, 9 and 36 times maximum recommended human iv/im dosage).
Pregnancy—Category C: INAPSINE administered intravenously has been shown to cause a slight increase in mortality of the newborn rat at 4.4 times the upper human dose. At 44 times the upper human dose, mortality rate was comparable to that for control animals. Following intramuscular administration, increased mortality of the offspring at 1.8 times the upper human dose is attributed to CNS depression in the dams who neglected to remove placentae from their offspring. INAPSINE has not been shown to be terotogenic in animals. There are no adequate and well-controlled studies in pregnant women. INAPSINE should be used during pregnancy only if the potential benefit justifies the potential risk to the fetus.
Labor and Delivery: There are insufficient data to support the use of INAPSINE in labor and delivery. Therefore, such use is not recommended.
Nursing Mothers: It is not known whether INAPSINE is excreted in human milk. Because many drugs are excreted in human milk, caution should be exercised when INAPSINE is administered to a nursing mother.
Pediatric Use: The safety of INAPSINE in children younger than two years of age has not been established.

ADVERSE REACTIONS

The most common adverse reactions reported to occur with INAPSINE (droperidol) are mild to moderate hypotension and tachycardia, but these effects usually subside without treatment. If hypotension occurs and is severe or persists, the possibility of hypovolemia should be considered and managed with appropriate parenteral fluid therapy. Postoperative drowsiness is also frequently reported.
Extrapyramidal symptoms (dystonia, akathisia, and oculogyric crisis) have been observed following administration of INAPSINE. Restlessness, hyperactivity and anxiety which can be either the result of inadequate dosage of INAPSINE or a part of the symptom complex of akathisia may occur. When extrapyramidal symptoms occur, they can usually be controlled with antiparkinson agents.
Other adverse reactions that have been reported are dizziness, chills and/or shivering, laryngospasm, bronchospasm and postoperative hallucinatory episodes (sometimes associated with transient periods of mental depression).
Elevated blood pressure, with or without pre-existing hypertension, has been reported following administration of INAPSINE combined with SUBLIMAZE (fentanyl citrate) or other parenteral analgesics. This might be due to unexplained alterations in sympathetic activity following large doses; however, it is also frequently attributed to anesthetic or surgical stimulation during light anesthesia.

OVERDOSAGE

Manifestations: The manifestations of INAPSINE (droperidol) overdosage are an extension of its pharmacologic actions.
Treatment: In the presence of hypoventilation or apnea, oxygen should be administered and respiration should be assisted or controlled as indicated. A patent airway must be maintained; an oropharyngeal airway or endotracheal tube might be indicated. The patient should be carefully observed for 24 hours; body warmth and adequate fluid intake should be maintained. If hypotension occurs and is severe or persists, the possibility of hypovolemia should be considered and managed with appropriate parenteral fluid therapy. (See PRECAUTIONS).
The intravenous LD_{50} of INAPSINE is 20–43 mg/kg in mice; 30 mg/kg in rats; 25 mg/kg in dogs and 11–13 mg/kg in rabbits. The intramuscular LD_{50} of INAPSINE is 195 mg/kg in mice; 104–110 mg/kg in rats; 97 mg/kg in rabbits and 200 mg/kg in guinea pigs.

DOSAGE AND ADMINISTRATION

Dosage should be individualized. Some of the factors to be considered in determining the dose are age, body weight, physical status, underlying pathological condition, use of other drugs, type of anesthesia to be used, and the surgical procedure involved.
Vital signs should be monitored routinely.

Usual Adult Dosage

I. **Premedication**—(to be appropriately modified in the elderly debilitated and those who have received other depressant drugs) 2.5 to 10 mg (1 to 4 ml) may be administered intramuscularly 30 to 60 minutes preoperatively.

II. **Adjunct to General Anesthesia**—
Induction—2.5 mg (1 ml) per 20 to 25 pounds may be administered (usually intravenously) along with an analgesic and/or general anesthetic. Smaller doses may be adequate. The total amount of INAPSINE (droperidol) administered should be titrated to obtain the desired effect based on the individual patient's response.
Maintenance—1.25 to 2.5 mg (0.5 to 1 ml) usually intravenously.

III. **Use without a general anesthetic in diagnostic procedures**—Administer the usual I.M. premedication 2.5 to 10 mg (1 to 4 ml) 30 to 60 minutes before the procedure. Ad-

Continued on next page

Janssen—Cont.

ditional 1.25 to 2.5 mg (0.5 to 1 ml) amounts of INAPSINE may be administered, usually intravenously.

NOTE: When INAPSINE is used in certain procedures, such as bronchoscopy, appropriate topical anesthesia is still necessary.

IV. **Adjunct to regional anesthesia**—2.5 to 5 mg (1 to 2 ml) may be administered intramuscularly or slowly intravenously when additional sedation is required.

Usual Children's Dosage

For children two to 12 years of age, a reduced dose as low as 1.0 to 1.5 mg (0.4 to 0.6 ml) per 20 to 25 pounds is recommended for premedication or for induction of anesthesia.

See WARNINGS and PRECAUTIONS for use of INAPSINE with other CNS depressants and in patients with altered response.

Parenteral drug products should be inspected visually for particulate matter and discoloration prior to administration, whenever solution and container permit. If such abnormalities are observed, the drug should not be administered.

HOW SUPPLIED

INAPSINE (droperidol) Injection is available as:

NDC 50458-010-02, 2.5 mg/ml, 2 ml ampoules in packages of 10

NDC 50458-010-05, 2.5 mg/ml, 5 ml ampoules in packages of 10

NDC 50458-010-10, 2.5 mg/ml, 10 ml multiple-dose vials in packages of 10.

PROTECT FROM LIGHT. STORE AT ROOM TEMPERATURE 15°C–30°C (59°F–86°F).

Manufactured by TAYLOR PHARMACAL CO. for JANSSEN PHARMACEUTICA INC.
Piscataway, NJ 08854
U.S. Patent No. 3,161,645
Revised June 1980, July 1986.

INNOVAR® INJECTION ℂ℞

[ĭn 'nō-văr]

FOR INTRAVENOUS OR INTRAMUSCULAR USE ONLY

> The two components of INNOVAR Injection, fentanyl citrate and droperidol, have different pharmacologic actions. Before administering INNOVAR Injection, the user should become familiar with the special properties of each drug, particularly the widely differing durations of action.

DESCRIPTION

INNOVAR is a potent opioid analgesic (fentanyl citrate) and a neuroleptic (tranquilizer) agent (droperidol). Each milliliter contains (in a 1:50 ratio) fentanyl citrate equivalent to 50 ug of fentanyl base and 2.5 mg of droperidol in a solution adjusted to pH 3.5 ± 0.3 with lactic acid.

INNOVAR is a sterile, preservative free aqueous solution for intravenous or intramuscular injection.

CLINICAL PHARMACOLOGY

INNOVAR (fentanyl citrate/droperidol) is a combination drug containing an opioid analgesic, fentanyl citrate, and a neuroleptic (major tranquilizer), droperidol. The combined effect, sometimes referred to as neuroleptanalgesia, is characterized by general quiescence, reduced motor activity, and profound analgesia; complete loss of consciousness usually does not occur from use of INNOVAR Injection alone. The incidence of early postoperative pain and emesis may be reduced.

A. Fentanyl citrate is an opioid analgesic. A dose of 100 ug (0.1 mg) (2.0 ml), is approximately equivalent in analgesic activity to 10 mg of morphine or 75 mg of meperidine. The principal actions of therapeutic value are analgesia and sedation. Alterations in respiratory rate and alveolar ventilation, associated with opioid analgesics, may last longer than the analgesic effect. As the dose of opioid is increased, the decrease in pulmonary exchange becomes greater. Large doses may produce apnea. Fentanyl citrate appears to have less emetic activity than either morphine or meperidine. Histamine assays and skin wheal testing in man indicate that clinically significant histamine release rarely occurs with fentanyl citrate. Assays in man show no clinically significant histamine release in dosages up to 50 ug/kg (0.05 mg/kg) (1 ml/kg).

The pharmacokinetics of fentanyl citrate can be described as a three-compartment model, with a distribution time of 1.7 minutes, redistribution of 13 minutes and a terminal elimination half life of 219 minutes. The volume of distribution for fentanyl citrate is 4 L/kg.

Fentanyl citrate plasma protein binding capacity increases with increasing ionization of the drug. Alterations in pH may affect its distribution between plasma and the central nervous system. It accumulates in skeletal muscle and fat, and is released slowly into the blood. Fentanyl citrate, which is primarily transformed in the liver, demonstrates a high first pass clearance and releases approximately 75% of an intravenous dose in urine, mostly as metabolites with less than 10% representing the unchanged drug. Approximately 9% of the dose is recovered in the feces, primarily as metabolites.

The onset of action of fentanyl citrate is almost immediate when the drug is given intravenously; however, the maximal analgesic and respiratory depressant effect may not be noted for several minutes. The usual duration of action of the analgesic effect is 30 to 60 minutes after a single intravenous dose of up to 100 ug (0.1 mg) (2.0 ml). Following intramuscular administration, the onset of action is from seven to eight minutes, and the duration of action is one to two hours. As with longer acting opioid analgesics, the duration of the respiratory depressant effect of fentanyl citrate may be longer than the analgesic effect. The following observations have been reported concerning altered respiratory response to CO_2 stimulation following administration of fentanyl citrate to man:

1. DIMINISHED SENSITIVITY TO CO_2 STIMULATION MAY PERSIST LONGER THAN DEPRESSION OF RESPIRATORY RATE. [Altered sensitivity to CO_2 stimulation has been demonstrated for up to four hours following a single dose of 600 ug (0.6 mg) (12 ml) fentanyl citrate to healthy volunteers.] Fentanyl citrate frequently slows the respiratory rate, duration and degree of respiratory depression being dose related.
2. The peak respiratory depressant effect of a single intravenous dose of fentanyl citrate is noted 5 to 15 minutes following injection. See also WARNINGS and PRECAUTIONS concerning respiratory depression.

B. Droperidol produces marked tranquilization and sedation. Droperidol allays apprehension and provides a state of mental detachment and indifference while maintaining a state of reflex alertness.

Droperidol also produces an antiemetic effect as evidenced by the antagonism of apomorphine in dogs. It lowers the incidence of nausea and vomiting during surgical procedures and provides antiemetic protection in the postoperative period.

Droperidol potentiates other CNS depressants. It produces mild alpha-adrenergic blockade, peripheral vascular dilatation and reduction of the pressor effect of epinephrine. It can produce hypotension and decreased peripheral vascular resistance and may decrease pulmonary arterial pressure (particularly if it is abnormally high.) It may reduce the incidence of epinephrine-induced arrhythmias, but does not prevent other cardiac arrhythmias.

The onset of action of single intramuscular and intravenous doses of droperidol is from three to ten minutes following administration, although the peak effect may not be apparent for up to thirty minutes. The duration of the tranquilizing and sedative effects generally is two to four hours, although alteration of consciousness may persist for as long as twelve hours. This is in contrast to the much shorter duration of fentanyl citrate.

INDICATIONS AND USAGE

INNOVAR (fentanyl citrate/droperidol) is indicated to produce tranquilization and analgesia for surgical and diagnostic procedures. It may be used as an anesthetic premedication, as an adjunct to the induction of anesthesia, and as an adjunct in the maintenance of general and regional anesthesia. If the supplementation of analgesia is necessary, SUBLIMAZE (fentanyl citrate) alone rather than the combination drug, INNOVAR, should usually be used, see DOSAGE AND ADMINISTRATION Section.

CONTRAINDICATIONS

INNOVAR (fentanyl citrate/droperidol) is contraindicated in patients with known hypersensitivity to either component.

WARNINGS

INNOVAR (fentanyl citrate/droperidol) SHOULD BE ADMINISTERED ONLY BY PERSONS SPECIFICALLY TRAINED IN THE USE OF INTRAVENOUS ANESTHETICS AND MANAGEMENT OF THE RESPIRATORY EFFECTS OF POTENT OPIOIDS.

AN OPIOID ANTAGONIST, RESUSCITATIVE AND INTUBATION EQUIPMENT AND OXYGEN SHOULD BE READILY AVAILABLE.

See also discussion of opioid antagonists in PRECAUTIONS and OVERDOSAGE Sections.

FLUIDS AND OTHER COUNTERMEASURES TO MANAGE HYPOTENSION SHOULD ALSO BE AVAILABLE.

The respiratory depressant effect of opioids persists longer than the measured analgesic effect. When used with INNOVAR, the total dose of all opioid analgesics administered should be considered by the practitioner before ordering opioid analgesics during recovery from anesthesia. It is recommended that opioids, when required, be used in reduced doses initially, as low as ¼ to ⅓ those usually recommended.

INNOVAR may cause muscle rigidity, particularly involving the muscles of respiration. This effect is due to the fentanyl citrate component and is related to the dose and speed of injection. Its incidence can be reduced by the use of slow intravenous injection. Once the effect occurs, it is managed by the use of assisted or controlled respiration and, if necessary, by a neuromuscular blocking agent compatible with the patient's condition.

Head Injuries and Increased Intracranial Pressure: INNOVAR should be used with caution in patients who may be particularly susceptible to respiratory depression such as comatose patients who may have a head injury or a brain tumor. In addition, INNOVAR may obscure the clinical course of patients with head injury.

PRECAUTIONS

General: The initial dose of INNOVAR (fentanyl citrate/droperidol) should be appropriately reduced in elderly, debilitated and other poor-risk patients. The effect of the initial dose should be considered in determining incremental doses.

Certain forms of conduction anesthesia, such as spinal anesthesia and some peridural anesthetics, can alter respiration by blocking intercostal nerves and can cause peripheral vasodilation and hypotension because of sympathetic blockade. Through other mechanisms (see CLINICAL PHARMACOLOGY) fentanyl citrate and droperidol can also depress respiration and blood pressure. Therefore, when INNOVAR is used to supplement these forms of anesthesia, the anesthetist should be familiar with the physiological alterations involved, and be prepared to manage them in the patients selected for these forms of anesthesia.

The droperidol component of INNOVAR may decrease pulmonary arterial pressure. This fact should be considered by those who conduct diagnostic or surgical procedures where interpretation of pulmonary arterial pressure measurements might determine final management of the patient.

Vital signs should be monitored routinely.

When the EEG is used for postoperative monitoring, it may be found that the EEG pattern returns to normal slowly.

Hypotension: If hypotension occurs, the possibility of hypovolemia should be considered and managed with appropriate parenteral fluid therapy. Repositioning the patient to improve venous return to the heart should be considered when operative conditions permit. It should be noted that in spinal and peridural anesthesia, tilting the patient into a head down position may result in a higher level of anesthesia than is desirable, as well as impair venous return to the heart. Care should be exercised in the moving and positioning of patients because of a possibility of orthostatic hypotension. If volume expansion with fluids plus these other countermeasures do not correct the hypotension, then the administration of pressor agents other than epinephrine should be considered. Epinephrine may paradoxically decrease the blood pressure in patients treated with INNOVAR due to the alpha-adrenergic blocking action of droperidol.

Impaired Respiration: INNOVAR and SUBLIMAZE (fentanyl citrate) should be used with caution in patients with chronic obstructive pulmonary disease, patients with decreased respiratory reserve and others with potentially compromised ventilation. In such patients opioids may additionally decrease respiratory drive and increase airway resistance. During anesthesia, this can be managed by assisted or controlled respiration. Respiratory depression caused by opioid analgesics can be reversed by opioid antagonists. Appropriate surveillance should be maintained because the duration of respiratory depression of doses of fentanyl citrate (as SUBLIMAZE (fentanyl citrate) or INNOVAR) employed during anesthesia may be longer than the duration of the opioid antagonist action. Consult individual prescribing information (levallorphan, nalorphine and naloxone) before employing opioid antagonists.

Impaired Hepatic or Renal Function: INNOVAR should be administered with caution to patients with liver and kidney dysfunction because of the importance of these organs in the metabolism and excretion of drugs.

Cardiovascular Effects: The fentanyl citrate component may produce bradycardia, which may be treated with atropine. INNOVAR should be used with caution in patients with cardiac bradyarrhythmias.

Drug Interactions: Other CNS depressant drugs (e.g. barbiturates, tranquilizers, opioids and general anesthetics) have additive or potentiating effects with INNOVAR. When patients have received such drugs, the dose of INNOVAR required will be less than usual. Following the administration of INNOVAR, the dose of other CNS depressant drugs should be reduced.

Carcinogenesis, Mutagenesis, Impairment of Fertility: No carcinogenicity studies have been conducted with INNOVAR or its components, SUBLIMAZE and INAPSINE. A subcutaneous study of INNOVAR in female rats revealed no impairment of fertility at doses 9 times the upper human dose. An intravenous study revealed no effects on fertility at 2 times the upper human dose (highest dosage level tested).

Pregnancy — Category C: INNOVAR had no embryotoxic effects in rats at intravenous doses approximately 2 times the upper human dose. A subcutaneous study of INNOVAR in female rats showed increased fetal resorptions at 18 times the upper human dose. No teratogenic effects were revealed at 36 times the upper human dose. In rabbits, increased resorptions and decreased litter size were found at intravenous doses approximately 2 times the upper human dose. Maternal mortality occurred at 7 times the upper human dose.

INNOVAR has not been shown to be teratogenic in animals. There are no adequate and well-controlled studies in pregnant women. INNOVAR should be used during pregnancy only if the potential benefit justifies the potential risk to the fetus.

Labor and Delivery: There are insufficient data to support the use of INNOVAR in labor and delivery. Therefore, such use is not recommended.

Nursing Mothers: It is not known whether fentanyl citrate or droperidol are excreted in human milk. Because many drugs are excreted in human milk, caution should be exercised when INNOVAR is administered to a nursing woman.

Pediatric Use: The safety and efficacy of INNOVAR in children under two years of age has not been established.

ADVERSE REACTIONS

The most common serious adverse reactions reported to occur with INNOVAR (fentanyl citrate/droperidol) are respiratory depression, apnea, muscular rigidity and hypotension; if these remain untreated, respiratory arrest, circulatory depression or cardiac arrest could occur.

Extrapyramidal symptoms (dystonia, akathisia and oculogyric crisis) have been observed following administration of INNOVAR. Restlessness, hyperactivity and anxiety which can be either the result of inadequate tranquilization or part of the symptom complex of akathisia may occur. When extrapyramidal symptoms occur, they can usually be controlled with anti-Parkinson agents.

Elevated blood pressure, with and without pre-existing hypertension, has been reported following administration of INNOVAR. This might be due to unexplained alterations of sympathetic activity following large doses; however, it is also frequently attributed to anesthetic or surgical stimulation during light anesthesia.

Postoperative drowsiness is also frequently reported.

Other adverse reactions that have been reported are dizziness, chills and/or shivering, twitching, blurred vision, laryngospasm, brochospasm, bradycardia, tachycardia, nausea and emesis, diaphoresis, emergence delirium, and postoperative hallucinatory episodes (sometimes associated with transient periods of mental depression).

DRUG ABUSE AND DEPENDENCE

The fentanyl citrate component of INNOVAR (fentanyl citrate/droperidol) is a Schedule II opioid that can produce drug dependence of the morphine type and, therefore, has the potential for being abused.

OVERDOSAGE

Manifestations: The manifestations of INNOVAR (fentanyl citrate/droperidol) overdosage are an extension of its pharmacologic actions.

Treatment: In the presence of hypoventilation or apnea, oxygen should be administered and respiration should be assisted or controlled as indicated. A patent airway must be maintained; an oropharyngeal airway or endotracheal tube might be indicated. If depressed respiration is associated with muscular rigidity, an intravenous neuromuscular blocking agent might be required to facilitate assisted or controlled respiration. The patient should be carefully observed for 24 hours; body warmth and adequate fluid intake should be maintained. If hypotension occurs and is severe or persists, the possibility of hypovolemia should be considered and managed with appropriate parenteral fluid therapy (See PRECAUTIONS). A specific opioid antagonist such as nalorphine, levallorphan or naloxone should be available for use as indicated to manage respiratory depression caused by the opioid component fentanyl citrate. This does not preclude the use of more immediate countermeasures. The duration of respiratory depression following overdosage of fentanyl citrate may be longer than the duration of opioid antagonist action. Consult the package inserts of the individual opioid antagonists for details about use.

The LD_{50} values after intravenous administration were 4.1–5.27 mg/kg for the rat and the rabbit and 17 mg/kg or more for the mouse and the dog. After intramuscular administration LD_{50} determinations were 6.7–14.5 mg/kg for the rabbit and 75 mg/kg for the mouse.

DOSAGE AND ADMINISTRATION

Dosage should be individualized. Some of the factors to be considered in determining dose are age, body weight, physical status, underlying pathological condition, use of other drugs, the type of anesthesia to be used and the surgical procedure involved.

Vital signs should be monitored routinely.

Most patients who have received INNOVAR (fentanyl citrate/droperidol) do not require opioid analgesics during the immediate postoperative period. It is recommended that opioid analgesics, when required, be used initially in reduced doses, as low as 1/4 to 1/3 those usually recommended.

USUAL ADULT DOSAGE:

I. **Premedication**—(to be appropriately modified in the elderly, debilitated and those who have received other depressant drugs)—0.5 to 2.0 ml may be administered **intramuscularly** 45 to 60 minutes prior to surgery with or without atropine.

II. **Adjunct to General Anesthesia—**
Induction—1 ml per 20 to 25 pounds of body weight may be slowly administered intravenously. Smaller doses may be adequate.
The total amount of INNOVAR administered should be carefully titrated to obtain the desired effect based on the individual patient's response.
There are several methods of administration of INNOVAR Injection for induction of anesthesia.
  A. Intravenous injection—To allow for the variable needs of patients INNOVAR may be administered intravenously in fractional parts of the calculated dose. With the onset of somnolence, the general anesthetic may be administered.
  B. Intravenous drip—10 ml of INNOVAR are added to 250 ml of 5% dextrose in water and the drip given rapidly until the onset of somnolence. At that time, the drip may be either slowed or stopped and the general anesthetic administered.
Maintenance—INNOVAR is not indicated as the sole agent for the maintenance of surgical anesthesia. It is customarily used in combination with other measures such as nitrous oxide-oxygen, other inhalation anesthetics and/or topical or regional anesthesia.
To prevent the possibility of excessive accumulation of the relatively long-acting droperidol component, SUBLIMAZE (fentanyl citrate) alone should be used in increments of 25 to 50 ug (0.025 to 0.05 mg) (0.5 to 1.0 ml) for the maintenance of analgesia in patients initially given INNOVAR as an adjunct to general anesthesia. (See SUBLIMAZE (fentanyl citrate) package insert for additional prescribing information.) However, in prolonged operations, additional 0.5 to 1.0 ml amounts of INNOVAR may be administered with caution intravenously if changes in the patient's condition indicate lightening of tranquilization and analgesia.

III. **Use Without a General Anesthetic in Diagnostic Procedures**—Administer the usual intramuscular premedication (0.5 to 2.0 ml) 45 to 60 minutes before the procedure. To prevent the possibility of excessive accumulation of the relatively long-acting droperidol component, SUBLIMAZE (fentanyl citrate) alone should be used in increments of 25 to 50 ug (0.025 to 0.05 mg) (0.5 to 1.0 ml) for the maintenance of analgesia in patients initially given INNOVAR Injection. See SUBLIMAZE (fentanyl citrate) package insert for additional information. However, in prolonged operations, additional 0.5 to 1.0 ml amounts of INNOVAR may be administered with caution intravenously if changes in the patient's condition indicate lightening of tranquilization and analgesia.
Note: When INNOVAR is used in certain procedures such as bronchoscopy, appropriate topical anesthesia is still necessary.

IV. **Adjunct to Regional Anesthesia**—1 to 2 ml may be administered intramuscularly or slowly intravenously when additional sedation and analgesia are required.

USUAL CHILDREN'S DOSAGE:

For premedication and as an adjunct to general anesthesia in children over 2 years of age (see PRECAUTIONS):

I. **Premedication**—0.25 ml per 20 lbs. body weight administered *intramuscularly* 45 to 60 minutes prior to surgery with or without atropine.

II. **Adjunct to General Anesthesia**—The total combined dose for induction and maintenance averages 0.5 ml per 20 lbs. body weight. Following induction with INNOVAR Injection, SUBLIMAZE (fentanyl citrate) alone in a dose of 1/4 to 1/3 that recommended in the adult dosage section should usually be used when indicated to avoid the possibility of excessive accumulation of droperidol. However, in prolonged operations, additional increments of INNOVAR may be administered with caution when changes in the patient's condition indicate lightening of tranquilization and analgesia.

See WARNINGS and PRECAUTIONS for use of INNOVAR with other CNS depressants, and in patients with altered response.

Parenteral drug products should be inspected visually for particulate matter and discoloration prior to administration, whenever solution and container permit. If such abnormalities are observed, the drug should not be administered.

HOW SUPPLIED

INNOVAR (fentanyl citrate/droperidol) Injection is available as:

NDC 50458-020-02, 2 ml ampoules in packages of 10
NDC 50458-020-05, 5 ml ampoules in packages of 10
containing fentanyl citrate equivalent to 50 ug/ml of fentanyl base and 2.5 mg/ml of droperidol.

(FOR INTRAVENOUS USE BY HOSPITAL PERSONNEL SPECIFICALLY TRAINED IN THE USE OF OPIOID ANALGESICS.)

PROTECT FROM LIGHT. STORE AT ROOM TEMPERATURE 15°–30°C (59°–86°F).

JANSSEN PHARMACEUTICA INC.
Piscataway, NJ 08854
U.S. Patent No. 3,141,823
March 1980. Revised April, 1986.

MONISTAT i.v.™ ℞

[mŏn-ĭ-stăt]
(miconazole)
10mg/ml sterile solution for intravenous infusion

DESCRIPTION

MONISTAT i.v., (miconazole), 1-{2-(2,4-dichlorophenyl)-2-[(2,4-dichlorophenyl)methoxyl]ethyl}-1H-imidazole, is a synthetic antifungal supplied as a sterile solution for intravenous infusion. Each ml of this solution contains 10 mg of miconazole with 0.115 ml PEG 40 castor oil, 1.0 mg lactic acid USP, 0.5 mg methylparaben USP, 0.05 mg propylparaben USP in water for injection. Miconazole i.v. is a clear colorless to slightly yellow solution having a pH of 3.7 to 5.7.

CLINICAL PHARMACOLOGY

MONISTAT i.v. is rapidly metabolized in the liver and about 14% to 22% of the administered dose is excreted in the urine, mainly as inactive metabolites. The pharmacokinetic profile fits a three compartment open model with the following biologic half life: 0.4, 2.1, and 24.1 hours for each phase respectively. The pharmacokinetic profile of MONISTAT i.v. is unaltered in patients with renal insufficiency, including those patients on hemodialysis. The in vitro antifungal activity of MONISTAT i.v. is very broad. Clinical efficacy has been demonstrated in patients with the following species of fungi: *Coccidioides immitis, Candida albicans, Cryptococcus neoformans, Petriellidium boydii (Allescheria boydii),* and *Paracoccidioides brasiliensis.*

Recommended doses of MONISTAT i.v. produce serum concentrations of drug which exceed the in vitro MIC values for the fungal species noted above. Doses above 9 mg/kg of MONISTAT i.v. produce peak blood levels above 1μg/ml in most cases. The drug penetrates into joints.

INDICATIONS

MONISTAT i.v. is indicated for the treatment of the following severe systemic fungal infections: coccidioidomycosis, candidiasis, cryptococcosis, petriellidiosis (allescheriosis), paracoccidioidomycosis, and for the treatment of chronic mucocutaneous candidiasis.

However, in the treatment of fungal meningitis and urinary bladder infections an intravenous infusion alone is inadequate. It must be supplemented with intrathecal administration and bladder irrigation. Appropriate diagnostic procedures should be followed and MIC's should be determined.

MONISTAT i.v. should not be used to treat common trivial forms of fungal diseases.

CONTRAINDICATIONS

MONISTAT i.v. is contraindicated in those patients who have shown hypersensitivity to it.

WARNINGS

Rapid injection of undiluted MONISTAT i.v. may produce transient tachycardia or arrhythmia.

PRECAUTIONS

Before a treatment course of MONISTAT i.v. is started, the physician should make sure that the patient is not hypersensitive to the drug product. MONISTAT i.v. should be given by intravenous infusion. The treatment should be started under stringent conditions of hospitalization but subsequently may be given to suitable patients under ambulatory conditions with close clinical monitoring. It is recommended that an initial dose of 200 mg be given with the physician in attendance. It is also recommended that clinical laboratory monitoring including hemoglobin, hematocrit, electrolytes and lipids be performed.

It should be borne in mind that systemic fungal mycoses may be complications of chronic underlying conditions which in themselves may require appropriate measures.

Since Petriellidium boydii is difficult to histologically distinguish from species of Aspergillus, it is strongly recommended that cultures be grown.

Pregnancy: Reproductive studies with MONISTAT i.v. in rats and rabbits revealed no evidence of impaired fertility or harm to the fetus. There are no data, however, on the use of the drug in pregnant women.

Continued on next page

Janssen—Cont.

Children: Since the safety of miconazole i.v. in children under one year of age has not been extensively studied, its benefits in this age group must be weighed against the possible risks involved.

ADVERSE REACTIONS

Adverse reactions which have been observed with MONISTAT i.v. therapy include phlebitis, pruritus, rash, nausea, vomiting, febrile reactions, drowsiness, diarrhea, anorexia and flushes. In the U.S. studies, 29% of 209 patients studied had phlebitis, 21% pruritus, 18% nausea, 10% fever and chills, 9% rash, and 7% emesis. Transient decreases in hematocrit and serum sodium values have been observed following infusion of MONISTAT i.v.

Thrombocytopenia has also been reported. No serious renal or hepatic toxicity has been reported. If pruritus and skin rashes are severe, discontinuation of treatment may be necessary. Nausea and vomiting can be mitigated with antihistaminic or antiemetic drugs given prior to MONISTAT i.v. infusion, or by reducing the dose, slowing the rate of infusion, or avoiding administration at mealtime.

Aggregation of erythrocytes or rouleau formation on blood smears has been reported. Hyperlipemia has occurred in patients and is reported to be due to the vehicle, Cremophor EL (PEG 40 castor oil).

DRUG INTERACTIONS

Drugs containing cremophor type vehicles are known to cause electrophoretic abnormalities of the lipoprotein. These effects are reversible upon discontinuation of treatment but are usually not an indication that treatment should be discontinued.

Interaction with the coumarin drugs resulting in an enhancement of the anticoagulant effect has also been reported. In cases of simultaneous treatment with MONISTAT i.v. and coumarin drugs, the anticoagulant effect should be carefully titrated since reductions of the anticoagulant doses may be indicated.

A potential interaction between oral miconazole and oral hypoglycemic agents leading to severe hypoglycemia has been reported.

Since concomitant administration of rifampin and ketoconazole (an imidazole) reduces the blood levels of the latter, the concurrent administration of MONISTAT i.v. (an imidazole) and rifampin should be avoided.

Ketoconazole (an imidazole) increases the blood level of cyclosporin A; therefore, there is the possibility of a similar drug interaction involving cyclosporin A and MONISTAT i.v. (an imidazole). Blood levels of cyclosporin A should be monitored if the two drugs are given concomitantly.

Since concomitant administration of ketoconazole (an imidazole) with phenytoin may alter the metabolism of one or both of the drugs, it is also suggested that when MONISTAT i.v., (an imidazole) is used concurrently with phenytoin, consideration be given to the advisability of monitoring plasma levels of both drugs.

DOSAGE AND ADMINISTRATION

Dosage

Adults: The doses may vary with the diagnosis and with the infective agent, from 200 to 1200 mg per infusion. The following daily doses, which may be divided over 3 infusions, are recommended:

[See table below].

Repeated courses may be necessitated by relapse or reinfection.

Children: A total daily dose of about 20 to 40 mg/kg is generally adequate. However, a dose of 15 mg/kg body weight per infusion should not be exceeded.

Administration

MONISTAT i.v. should be diluted by adding at least 200 ml of diluent. The diluent of choice is 0.9% sodium chloride or alternatively Dextrose 5% injectable solution. The intravenous infusion should be given over a period of 30 to 60 minutes.

Generally, treatment should be continued until all clinical and laboratory tests no longer indicate that active fungal infection is present. Inadequate periods of treatment may yield poor response and lead to early recurrence of clinical symptoms. The dosing intervals and sites and the duration of treatment vary from patient to patient and depend on the causative organism.

Other Modes of Administration:

Intrathecal: Administration of the undiluted injectable solution of MONISTAT i.v. by the various intrathecal routes (20 mg per dose) is indicated as an adjunct to intravenous treatment in fungal meningitis. Succeeding intrathecal injections may be alternated between lumbar, cervical, and cisternal punctures every 3 to 7 days. *Bladder instillation:* 200 mg of miconazole in a diluted solution is indicated in the treatment of mycoses of the urinary bladder.

HOW SUPPLIED

MONISTAT i.v. is supplied in 20 ml ampoules.

Store at controlled room temperatures. (15° to 30°C/59° to 86°F)

NDC 50458-200-20

U.S. Patent No. 3,717,655; 3,839,574

Manufactured by TAYLOR PHARMACAL CO for
JANSSEN PHARMACEUTICA Inc.
Piscataway, NJ 08854
Rev. Jan. 1982, Oct. 1984

MONISTAT i.v.™

Organism	Dosage Range*	Duration of Successful Therapy (weeks)
Candidiasis	600 to 1800 mg per day	1 to > 20
Cryptococcosis	1200 to 2400 mg per day	3 to > 12
Coccidioidomycosis	1800 to 3600 mg per day	3 to > 20
Petriellidiosis (Allescheriosis)	600 to 3000 mg per day	5 to > 20
Paracoccidioidomycosis	200 to 1200 mg per day	2 to > 16

*May be divided over 3 infusions.

NIZORAL®
[nī'zōr-ăl]
(ketoconazole) 2% Cream

DESCRIPTION

NIZORAL® (ketoconazole) 2% Cream contains the broad spectrum synthetic antifungal agent, ketoconazole 2%, formulated in an aqueous cream vehicle consisting of propylene glycol, stearyl and cetyl alcohols, sorbitan monostearate, polysorbate 60, isopropyl myristate, sodium sulfite anhydrous, polysorbate 80 and purified water.

Ketoconazole is *cis*-1-acetyl-4-[4-[[2-(2,4-dichlorophenyl)-2-(1*H*-imidazol-1-ylmethyl)-1, 3-dioxolan-4-yl] methoxy] phenyl]piperazine.

CLINICAL PHARMACOLOGY

When NIZORAL® (ketoconazole) 2% Cream was applied dermally to intact or abraded skin of Beagle dogs for 28 consecutive days at a dose of 80 mg, plasma concentrations did not significantly differ from the lower detection limit (2 ng/ml) of the method employed.

After a single topical application to the chest, back and arms of normal volunteers, systemic absorption of ketoconazole was not detected at the 5 ng/ml level in blood over a 72-hour period.

Two dermal irritancy studies, a human sensitization test, a phototoxicity study and a photoallergy study conducted in 38 male and 62 female volunteers showed no contact sensitization of the delayed hypersensitivity type, no irritation, no phototoxicity and no photoallergenic potential due to NIZORAL® (ketoconazole) 2% Cream.

Microbiology: Ketoconazole is a broad spectrum synthetic antifungal agent which inhibits the growth of the following common dermatophytes and yeasts by altering the permeability of the cell membrane: dermatophytes; *Trichophyton rubrum, T. mentagrophytes, T. tonsurans, Microsporum canis, M. audouini, M. gypseum* and *Epidermophyton floccosum;* yeasts; *Candida albicans* and *C. tropicalis;* and the organism responsible for tinea versicolor, *Malassezia furfur (Pityrosporum orbiculare).* Development of resistance to ketoconazole has not been reported.

Mode of Action: *In vitro* studies suggest that ketoconazole impairs the synthesis of ergosterol, which is a vital component of fungal cell membranes.

INDICATIONS AND USAGE

NIZORAL® (ketoconazole) 2% Cream is indicated for the topical treatment of tinea corporis and tinea cruris caused by *Trichophyton rubrum, T. mentagrophytes** and *Epidermophyton floccosum;* and in the treatment of tinea (pityriasis) versicolor caused by *Malassezia furfur (Pityrosporum orbiculare).*

*Efficacy for this organism in this organ system was studied in fewer than ten infections.

CONTRAINDICATIONS

NIZORAL® (ketoconazole) 2% Cream is contraindicated in persons who have shown hypersensitivity to the active or excipient ingredients of this formulation.

WARNINGS

NIZORAL® (ketoconazole) 2% Cream is not for ophthalmic use.

PRECAUTIONS

General: If a reaction suggesting sensitivity or chemical irritation should occur, use of the medication should be discontinued.

Carcinogenesis, Mutagenesis, Impairment of Fertility: A long-term feeding study in Swiss Albino mice and in Wistar rats showed no evidence of oncogenic activity. The dominant lethal mutation test in male and female mice revealed that single oral doses of ketoconazole as high as 80 mg/kg produced no mutation in any stage of germ cell development. The Ames' *Salmonella* microsomal activator assay was also negative.

Pregnancy: Teratogenic effects: Pregnancy Category C: Ketoconazole has been shown to be teratogenic (syndactylia and oligodactylia) in the rat when given orally in the diet at 80 mg/kg/day, (10 times the maximum recommended human dose). However, these effects may be related to maternal toxicity, which was seen at this and higher dose levels. There are no adequate and well-controlled studies in pregnant women. Ketoconazole should be used during pregnancy only if the potential benefit justifies the potential risk to the fetus.

Nursing Mothers: It is not known whether NIZORAL® (ketoconazole) 2% Cream administered topically could result in sufficient systemic absorption to produce detectable quantities in breast milk. Nevertheless, caution should be exercised when NIZORAL® (ketoconazole) 2% Cream is administered to a nursing woman.

Pediatric Use: Safety and effectiveness in children have not been established.

ADVERSE REACTIONS

During clinical trials 43 (5.0%) of 867 patients treated with NIZORAL® (ketoconazole) 2% Cream and 3 (1.8%) of 167 patients treated with placebo reported side effects consisting mainly of severe irritation, pruritus and stinging. One of the patients treated with active cream developed a painful allergic reaction.

DOSAGE AND ADMINISTRATION

It is recommended that NIZORAL® (ketoconazole) 2% Cream be applied once daily to cover the affected and immediate surrounding area in patients with tinea corporis, tinea cruris and tinea (pityriasis) versicolor. Early relief of symptoms is experienced by the majority of patients and clinical improvement may be seen fairly soon after treatment is begun; however, tinea cruris and corporis should be treated for two weeks in order to reduce the possibility of recurrence. Patients with tinea versicolor usually exhibit clinical and mycological clearing after two weeks of treatment. If a patient shows no clinical improvement after the treatment period, the diagnosis should be redetermined.

HOW SUPPLIED

NIZORAL® (ketoconazole) 2% Cream is supplied in 15 (NDC 50458-221-15) and 30 (NDC 50458-221-30) gm tubes.

Rev. Jan. 1986, May 1986

U.S. Patent No. 4,335,125

Manufactured by:
ALTANA, INC.
Melville, N.Y. 11747
Distributed by:
JANSSEN PHARMACEUTICA Inc.
Piscataway, N.J. 08854

NIZORAL® ℞
[nī'zōr-ăl]
(ketoconazole)
Tablets

> **WARNING:** Ketoconazole has been associated with hepatic toxicity, including some fatalities. Patients receiving this drug should be informed by the physician of the risk and should be closely monitored. See WARNINGS and PRECAUTIONS sections.

DESCRIPTION

NIZORAL® (ketoconazole) is a synthetic broad-spectrum antifungal agent available in scored white tablets, each containing 200 mg ketoconazole base for oral administration. Inactive ingredients are colloidal silicon dioxide, corn starch, lactose, magnesium stearate, microcrystalline cellulose, and povidone. Ketoconazole is cis-1-acetyl-4-[4-[[2-(2, 4-dichlorophenyl) -2- (1H-imidazol-1-ylmethyl)-1,3-dioxolan-4-yl] methoxyl]phenyl]piperazine.

Ketoconazole is a white to slightly beige, odorless powder, soluble in acids, with a molecular weight of 531.44.

CLINICAL PHARMACOLOGY

Mean peak plasma levels of approximately 3.5μg/ml are reached within 1 to 2 hours, following oral administration of a single 200 mg dose taken with a meal. Subsequent plasma elimination is biphasic with a half life of 2 hours during the first 10 hours and 8 hours thereafter. Following absorption from the gastrointestinal tract, NIZORAL (ketoconazole) is converted into several inactive metabolites. The major identified metabolic pathways are oxidation and degradation of the imidazole and piperazine rings, oxidative O-dealkylation and aromatic hydroxylation. About 13% of the dose is excreted in the urine, of which 2 to 4% is unchanged drug. The major route of excretion is through the bile into the intestinal tract. *In vitro*, the plasma protein binding is about 99%, mainly to the albumin fraction. Only a negligible proportion of NIZORAL reaches the cerebral-spinal fluid. NIZORAL is a weak dibasic agent and thus requires acidity for dissolution and absorption.

NIZORAL is active against clinical infections with *Blastomyces dermatitidis, Candida spp., Coccidioides immitis, Histoplasma capsulatum, Paracoccidioides brasiliensis,* and *Phialophora spp.* It is also active against *Trichophyton spp., Epidermophyton spp.,* and *Microsporum spp.* NIZORAL is active *in vitro* against a variety of fungi and yeast. In animal models, activity has been demonstrated against *Candida spp., Blastomyces dermatitidis, Histoplasma capsulatum, Malassezia furfur, Coccidioides immitis,* and *Cryptococcus neoformans.*

Mode of Action: *In vitro* studies suggest that NIZORAL impairs the synthesis of ergosterol, which is a vital component of fungal cell membranes.

INDICATIONS AND USAGE

NIZORAL (ketoconazole) is indicated for the treatment of the following systemic fungal infections: candidiasis, chronic mucocutaneous candidiasis, oral thrush, candiduria, blastomycosis, coccidioidomycosis, histoplasmosis, chromomycosis, and paracoccidioidomycosis. NIZORAL should not be used for fungal meningitis because it penetrates poorly into the cerebral-spinal fluid.

NIZORAL is also indicated for the treatment of patients with severe recalcitrant cutaneous dermatophyte infections who have not responded to topical therapy or oral griseofulvin, or who are unable to take griseofulvin.

CONTRAINDICATIONS

NIZORAL is contraindicated in patients who have shown hypersensitivity to the drug.

WARNINGS

Hepatotoxicity, primarily of the hepatocellular type, has been associated with the use of NIZORAL (ketoconazole), including rare fatalities. The reported incidence of hepatotoxicity has been about 1:10,000 exposed patients, but this probably represents some degree of under-reporting, as is the case for most reported adverse reactions to drugs. The median duration of ketoconazole therapy in patients who developed symptomatic hepatotoxicity was about 28 days, although the range extended to as low as 3 days. The hepatic injury has usually, but not always, been reversible upon discontinuation of NIZORAL (ketoconazole) treatment. Several cases of hepatitis have been reported in children.

Prompt recognition of liver injury is essential. Liver function tests (such as SGGT, alkaline phosphatase, SGPT, SGOT and bilirubin) should be measured before starting treatment and at frequent intervals during treatment. Patients receiving ketoconazole concurrently with other potentially hepatotoxic drugs should be carefully monitored, particularly those patients requiring prolonged therapy or those who have had a history of liver disease.

Most of the reported cases of hepatic toxicity have to date been in patients treated for onychomycosis. Of 180 patients worldwide developing idiosyncratic liver dysfunction during ketoconazole therapy, 61.3% had onychomycosis and 16.8% had chronic recalcitrant dermatophytoses.

Transient minor elevations in liver enzymes have occurred during ketoconazole treatment. The drug should be discontinued if these persist, if the abnormalities worsen, or if the abnormalities become accompanied by symptoms of possible liver injury.

In rare cases anaphylaxis has been reported after the first dose. Several cases of hypersensitivity reactions including urticaria have also been reported.

In European clinical trials involving 350 patients with metastatic prostatic cancer, eleven deaths were reported within two weeks of starting treatment with high doses of ketoconazole (1200 mg/day). It is not possible to ascertain from the information available whether death was related to ketoconazole therapy in these patients with serious underlying disease. However, high doses of ketoconazole are known to suppress adrenal corticosteroid secretion.

In female rats treated three to six months with ketoconazole at dose levels of 80 mg/kg and higher, increased fragility of long bones, in some cases leading to fracture, was seen. The maximum "no-effect" dose level in these studies was 20 mg/kg (2.5 times the maximum recommended human dose). The mechanism responsible for this phenomenon is obscure. Limited studies in dogs failed to demonstrate such an effect on the metacarpals and ribs.

PRECAUTIONS

General: NIZORAL (ketoconazole) has been demonstrated to lower serum testosterone. Once therapy with NIZORAL has been discontinued, serum testosterone levels return to baseline values. Testosterone levels are impaired with doses of 800 mg per day and abolished by 1600 mg per day. NIZORAL also decreases ACTH induced corticosteroid serum levels at similar high doses. The recommended dose of 200 mg–400 mg daily should be followed closely.

In four subjects with drug-induced achlorhydria, a marked reduction in NIZORAL (ketoconazole) absorption was observed. NIZORAL requires acidity for dissolution. If concomitant antacids, anticholinergics, and H_2-blockers are needed, they should be given at least two hours after NIZORAL administration. In cases of achlorhydria, the patients should be instructed to dissolve each tablet in 4 ml aqueous solution of 0.2 N HCl. For ingesting the resulting mixture, they should use a drinking straw so as to avoid contact with the teeth. This administration should be followed with a cup of tap water.

Information for patients: Patients should be instructed to report any signs and symptoms which may suggest liver dysfunction so that appropriate biochemical testing can be done. Such signs and symptoms may include unusual fatigue, anorexia, nausea and/or vomiting, jaundice, dark urine or pale stools (see WARNINGS).

Drug Interactions: Imidazole compounds like ketoconazole may enhance the anticoagulant effect of coumarin-like drugs. In simultaneous treatment with imidazole drugs and coumarin drugs, the anticoagulant effect should be carefully titrated and monitored.

Concomitant administration of rifampin with ketoconazole reduces the blood levels of the latter. INH (Isoniazid) is also reported to affect ketoconazole concentrations adversely. These drugs should not be given concomitantly.

Ketoconazole increases the blood level of cyclosporin A. Blood levels of cyclosporin A should be monitored if the two drugs are given concomitantly.

Concomitant administration of ketoconazole with phenytoin may alter the metabolism of one or both of the drugs. It is suggested to monitor both ketoconazole and phenytoin.

Because severe hypoglycemia has been reported in patients concomitantly receiving oral miconazole (an imidazole) and oral hypoglycemic agents, such a potential interaction involving the latter agents when used concomitantly with ketoconazole (an imidazole) can not be ruled out.

Carcinogenesis, Mutagenesis, Impairment of Fertility: The dominant lethal mutation test in male and female mice revealed that single oral doses of NIZORAL (ketoconazole) as high as 80 mg/kg produced no mutation in any stage of germ cell development. The *Ames Salmonella* microsomal activator assay was also negative. A long term feeding study in Swiss Albino mice and in Wistar rats showed no evidence of oncogenic activity.

Pregnancy: Teratogenic effects: *Pregnancy Category C.* NIZORAL (ketoconazole) has been shown to be teratogenic (syndactylia and oligodactylia) in the rat when given in the diet at 80 mg/kg/day, (10 times the maximum recommended human dose). However, these effects may be related to maternal toxicity, evidence of which also was seen at this and higher dose levels.

There are no adequate and well controlled studies in pregnant women, NIZORAL should be used during pregnancy only if the potential benefit justifies the potential risk to the fetus.

Nonteratogenic effects: NIZORAL has also been found to be embryotoxic in the rat when given in the diet at doses higher than 80 mg/kg during the first trimester of gestation.

In addition, dystocia (difficult labor) was noted in rats administered NIZORAL during the third trimester of gestation. This occurred when NIZORAL was administered at doses higher than 10 mg/kg (higher than 1.25 times the maximum human dose).

It is likely that both the malformations and the embryotoxicity resulting from the administration of NIZORAL (ketoconazole) during gestation are a reflection of the particular sensitivity of the female rat to this drug. For example, the oral LD_{50} of NIZORAL given by gavage to the female rat is 166mg/kg whereas in the male rat the oral LD_{50} is 287 mg/kg.

Nursing Mothers: Since NIZORAL is probably excreted in the milk, mothers who are under treatment should not breast feed.

Pediatric Use: NIZORAL has not been systematically studied in children of any age, and essentially no information is available on children under 2 years. NIZORAL should not be used in pediatric patients unless the potential benefit outweighs the risks.

ADVERSE REACTIONS

In rare cases anaphylaxis has been reported after the first dose. Several cases of hypersensitivity reactions including urticaria have also been reported. However, the most frequent adverse reactions were nausea and/or vomiting in approximately 3%, abdominal pain in 1.2%, pruritus in 1.5%, and the following in less than 1% of the patients: headache, dizziness, somnolence, fever and chills, photophobia, diarrhea, gynecomastia, impotence, thrombocytopenia, leukopenia, hemolytic anemia, and bulging fontanelles. Oligospermia has been reported in investigational studies with the drug at dosages above those currently approved. Although oligospermia has not been reported at dosages up to 400 mg daily, sperm counts have been obtained infrequently in patients treated with these dosages. Most of these reactions were mild and transient and rarely required discontinuation of NIZORAL (ketoconazole). In contrast, the rare occurrences of hepatic dysfunction require special attention (see WARNINGS).

OVERDOSAGE

In the event of accidental overdosage, supportive measures, including gastric lavage with sodium bicarbonate, should be employed.

DOSAGE AND ADMINISTRATION

Adults: The recommended starting dose of NIZORAL is a single daily administration of 200 mg (one tablet). In very serious infections or if clinical responsiveness is insufficient within the expected time, the dose of NIZORAL may be increased to 400 mg (two tablets) once daily.

Children: In small numbers of children over 2 years of age, a single daily dose of 3.3 to 6.6 mg/kg has been used. NIZORAL (ketoconazole) has not been studied in children under 2 years of age.

There should be laboratory as well as clinical documentation of infection prior to starting ketoconazole therapy. Treatment should be continued until tests indicate that active fungal infection has subsided. Inadequate periods of treatment may yield poor response and lead to early recurrence of clinical symptoms. Minimum treatment for candidiasis is one or two weeks. Patients with chronic mucocutaneous candidiasis usually require maintenance therapy. Minimum treatment for the other indicated systemic mycoses is six months.

Minimum treatment for recalcitrant dermatophyte infections is four weeks in cases involving glabrous skin. Palmar and plantar infections may respond more slowly. Apparent cures may subsequently recur after discontinuation of therapy in some cases.

HOW SUPPLIED

NIZORAL (ketoconazole) is available as white, scored tablets containing 200 mg of ketoconazole debossed "JANSSEN" and on the reverse side debossed "NIZORAL". They are supplied in bottles of 100 tablets and in blister packs of 10 × 10 tablets.

U.S. Patent 4,335,125
NDC 50458-220-01
(10 ×10 tablets—blister)
NDC 50458-220-10
(100 tablets)
Rev. Sept. 1984, July 1986
Janssen Pharmaceutica Inc.
Piscataway
New Jersey 08854
USA

Shown in Product Identification Section, page 411

SUBLIMAZE® Ⓒ℞

[sa ′blĭ-māz]
(fentanyl citrate) Injection
CAUTION: Federal Law Prohibits Dispensing Without Prescription

DESCRIPTION

SUBLIMAZE (fentanyl citrate) is a potent narcotic analgesic. Each milliliter of solution contains fentanyl citrate equivalent to 50 ug of fentanyl base, adjusted to pH 4.0 –7.5 with sodium hydroxide. SUBLIMAZE is chemically identified as N-(1-phenethyl-4-piperidyl) propionanilide citrate (1:1) with a molecular weight of 528.61.

SUBLIMAZE is a sterile, non-pyrogenic, preservative free aqueous solution for intravenous or intramuscular injection.

CLINICAL PHARMACOLOGY

SUBLIMAZE (fentanyl citrate) is a narcotic analgesic. A dose of 100 ug (0.1 mg) (2.0 ml) is approximately equivalent in analgesic activity to 10 mg of morphine or 75 mg of meperidine. The principal actions of therapeutic value are analgesia and sedation. Alterations in respiratory rate and alveolar ventilation, associated with narcotic analgesics, may last longer than the analgesic effect. As the dose of narcotic is increased, the decrease in pulmonary exchange becomes greater. Large doses may produce apnea. SUBLIMAZE appears to have less emetic activity than either morphine or meperidine. Histamine assays and skin wheal testing in man indicate that clinically significant histamine release rarely occurs with SUBLIMAZE. Recent assays in man show no clinically significant histamine release in dosages up to 50 ug/kg (0.05 mg/kg) (1 ml/kg). SUBLIMAZE preserves cardiac stability, and blunts stress-related hormonal changes at higher doses.

Continued on next page

Janssen—Cont.

The pharmacokinetics of SUBLIMAZE can be described as a three-compartment model, with a distribution time of 1.7 minutes, redistribution of 13 minutes and a terminal elimination half life of 219 minutes. The volume of distribution for SUBLIMAZE is 4 L/kg.
SUBLIMAZE plasma protein binding capacity increases with increasing ionization of the drug. Alterations in pH may affect its distribution between plasma and the central nervous system. It accumulates in skeletal muscle and fat, and is released slowly into the blood. SUBLIMAZE, which is primarily transformed in the liver, demonstrates a high first pass clearance and releases approximately 75% of an intravenous dose in urine, mostly as metabolites with less than 10% representing the unchanged drug. Approximately 9% of the dose is recovered in the feces, primarily as metabolites.
The onset of action of SUBLIMAZE is almost immediate when the drug is given intravenously; however, the maximal analgesic and respiratory depressant effect may not be noted for several minutes. The usual duration of action of the analgesic effect is 30 to 60 minutes after a single intravenous dose of up to 100 ug (0.1 mg) (2.0 ml). Following intramuscular administration, the onset of action is from seven to eight minutes, and the duration of action is one to two hours. As with longer acting narcotic analgesics, the duration of the respiratory depressant effect of SUBLIMAZE may be longer than the analgesic effect. The following observations have been reported concerning altered respiratory response to CO_2 stimulation following administration of SUBLIMAZE to man.

1. DIMINISHED SENSITIVITY TO CO_2 STIMULATION MAY PERSIST LONGER THAN DEPRESSION OF RESPIRATORY RATE. (Altered sensitivity to CO_2 stimulation has been demonstrated for up to four hours following a single dose of 600 ug (0.6 mg) (12 ml) SUBLIMAZE to healthy volunteers.) SUBLIMAZE frequently slows the respiratory rate, duration and degree of respiratory depression being dose related.
2. The peak respiratory depressant effect of a single intravenous dose of SUBLIMAZE is noted 5 to 15 minutes following injection. See also WARNINGS and PRECAUTIONS concerning respiratory depression.

INDICATIONS AND USAGE

SUBLIMAZE (fentanyl citrate) is indicated:
—for analgesic action of short duration during the anesthetic periods, premedication, induction and maintenance, and in the immediate postoperative period (recovery room) as the need arises.
—for use as a narcotic analgesic supplement in general or regional anesthesia.
—for administration with a neuroleptic such as INAPSINE® (droperidol) Injection as an anesthetic premedication, for the induction of anesthesia and as an adjunct in the maintenance of general and regional anesthesia.
—for use as an anesthetic agent with oxygen in selected high risk patients, such as those undergoing open heart surgery or certain complicated neurological or orthopedic procedures.

CONTRAINDICATIONS

SUBLIMAZE (fentanyl citrate) is contraindicated in patients with known intolerance to the drug.

WARNINGS

SUBLIMAZE (fentanyl citrate) SHOULD BE ADMINISTERED ONLY BY PERSONS SPECIFICALLY TRAINED IN THE USE OF INTRAVENOUS ANESTHETICS AND MANAGEMENT OF THE RESPIRATORY EFFECTS OF POTENT OPIOIDS.
AN OPIOID ANTAGONIST, RESUSCITATIVE AND INTUBATION EQUIPMENT AND OXYGEN SHOULD BE READILY AVAILABLE.
See also discussion of narcotic antagonists in PRECAUTIONS and OVERDOSAGE.
If SUBLIMAZE is administered with a tranquilizer such as INAPSINE (droperidol), the user should become familiar with the special properties of each drug, particularly the widely differing duration of action. In addition, when such a combination is used, fluids and other countermeasures to manage hypotension should be available.
As with other potent narcotics, the respiratory depressant effect of SUBLIMAZE may persist longer than the measured analgesic effect. The total dose of all narcotic analgesics administered should be considered by the practitioner before ordering narcotic analgesics during recovery from anesthesia. It is recommended that narcotics, when required, should be used in reduced doses initially, as low as ¼ to ⅓ those usually recommended.
SUBLIMAZE may cause muscle rigidity, particularly involving the muscles of respiration. In addition, skeletal muscle movements of various groups in the extremities, neck and external eye have been reported during induction of anesthesia with fentanyl; these reported movements have, on rare occasions, been strong enough to pose patient management problems. This effect is related to the dose and speed of injection and its incidence can be reduced by: 1) administration of up to ¼ of the full paralyzing dose of a non-depolarizing neuromuscular blocking agent just prior to administration of SUBLIMAZE; 2) administration of a full paralyzing dose of a neuromuscular blocking agent following loss of eyelash reflex when SUBLIMAZE is used in anesthetic doses titrated by slow intravenous infusion; or, 3) simultaneous administration of SUBLIMAZE and a full paralyzing dose of a neuromuscular blocking agent when SUBLIMAZE is used in rapidly administered anesthetic dosages. The neuromuscular blocking agent used should be compatible with the patient's cardiovascular status.
Adequate facilities should be available for postoperative monitoring and ventilation of patients administered anesthetic doses of SUBLIMAZE. Where moderate or high doses are used (above 10 ug/kg), there must be adequate facilities for postoperative observation, and ventilation if necessary, of patients who have received SUBLIMAZE. It is essential that these facilities be fully equipped to handle all degrees of respiratory depression.
SUBLIMAZE may also produce other signs and symptoms characteristic of narcotic analgesics including euphoria, miosis, bradycardia and bronchoconstriction.
Severe and unpredictable potentiation by MAO inhibitors has been reported for other narcotic analgesics. Although this has not been reported for fentanyl, there are insufficient data to establish that this does not occur with fentanyl. Therefore, when fentanyl is administered to patients who have received MAO inhibitors within 14 days, appropriate monitoring and ready availability of vasodilators and beta-blockers for the treatment of hypertension is indicated.
Head Injuries and Increased Intracranial Pressure—SUBLIMAZE should be used with caution in patients who may be particularly susceptible to respiratory depression, such as comatose patients who may have a head injury or brain tumor. In addition, SUBLIMAZE may obscure the clinical course of patients with head injury.

PRECAUTIONS

General: The initial dose of SUBLIMAZE (fentanyl citrate) should be appropriately reduced in elderly and debilitated patients. The effect of the initial dose should be considered in determining incremental doses.
Nitrous oxide has been reported to produce cardiovascular depression when given with higher doses of SUBLIMAZE.
Certain forms of conduction anesthesia, such as spinal anesthesia and some peridural anesthetics, can alter respiration by blocking intercostal nerves. Through other mechanisms (see CLINICAL PHARMACOLOGY) SUBLIMAZE can also alter respiration. Therefore, when SUBLIMAZE is used to supplement these forms of anesthesia, the anesthetist should be familiar with the physiological alterations involved, and be prepared to manage them in the patients selected for these forms of anesthesia.
When a tranquilizer such as INAPSINE (droperidol) is used with SUBLIMAZE, pulmonary arterial pressure may be decreased. This fact should be considered by those who conduct diagnostic and surgical procedures where interpretation of pulmonary arterial pressure measurements might determine final management of the patient. When high dose or anesthetic dosages of SUBLIMAZE are employed, even relatively small dosages of diazepam may cause cardiovascular depression.
When SUBLIMAZE is used with a tranquilizer such as INAPSINE (droperidol), hypotension can occur. If it occurs, the possibility of hypovolemia should also be considered and managed with appropriate parenteral fluid therapy. Repositioning the patient to improve venous return to the heart should be considered when operative conditions permit. Care should be exercised in moving and positioning of patients because of the possibility of orthostatic hypotension. If volume expansion with fluids plus other countermeasures do not correct hypotension, the administration of pressor agents other than epinephrine should be considered. Because of the alpha-adrenergic blocking action of INAPSINE (droperidol), epinephrine may paradoxically decrease the blood pressure in patients treated with INAPSINE (droperidol).
Elevated blood pressure, with and without pre-existing hypertension, has been reported following administration of SUBLIMAZE combined with INAPSINE (droperidol). This might be due to unexplained alterations in sympathetic activity following large doses; however, it is also frequently attributed to anesthetic and surgical stimulation during light anesthesia.
When INAPSINE (droperidol) is used with SUBLIMAZE and the EEG is used for postoperative monitoring, it may be found that the EEG pattern returns to normal slowly.
Vital signs should be monitored routinely.
Respiratory depression caused by opioid analgesics can be reversed by opioid antagonists such as naloxone. Because the duration of respiratory depression produced by SUBLIMAZE may last longer than the duration of the opioid antagonist action, appropriate surveillance should be maintained. As with all potent opioids, profound analgesia is accompanied by respiratory depression and diminished sensitivity to CO_2 stimulation which may persist into or recur in the postoperative period. Intraoperative hyperventilation may further alter postoperative response to CO_2. Appropriate postoperative monitoring should be employed to ensure that adequate spontaneous breathing is established and maintained in the absence of stimulation prior to discharging the patient from the recovery area.
Impaired Respiration: SUBLIMAZE should be used with caution in patients with chronic obstructive pulmonary disease, patients with decreased respiratory reserve, and others with potentially compromised respiration. In such patients, narcotics may additionally decrease respiratory drive and increase airway resistance. During anesthesia, this can be managed by assisted or controlled respiration.
Impaired Hepatic or Renal Function: SUBLIMAZE should be administered with caution to patients with liver and kidney dysfunction because of the importance of these organs in the metabolism and excretion of drugs.
Cardiovascular Effects: SUBLIMAZE may produce bradycardia, which may be treated with atropine. SUBLIMAZE should be used with caution in patients with cardiac bradyarrhythmias.
Drug Interactions: Other CNS depressant drugs (e.g. barbiturates, tranquilizers, narcotics and general anesthetics) will have additive or potentiating effects with SUBLIMAZE. When patients have received such drugs, the dose of SUBLIMAZE required will be less than usual. Following the administration of SUBLIMAZE, the dose of other CNS depressant drugs should be reduced.
Carcinogenesis, Mutagenesis, Impairment of Fertility: No carcinogenicity or mutagenicity studies have been conducted with SUBLIMAZE. Reproduction studies in rats revealed a significant decrease in the pregnancy rate of all experimental groups. This decrease was most pronounced in the high dosed group (1.25 mg/kg—12.5X human dose) in which one of twenty animals became pregnant.
Pregnancy—Category C: SUBLIMAZE has been shown to impair fertility and to have an embryocidal effect in rats when given in doses 0.3 times the upper human dose for a period of 12 days. No evidence of teratogenic effects have been observed after administration of SUBLIMAZE to rats. There are no adequate and well-controlled studies in pregnant women. SUBLIMAZE should be used during pregnancy only if the potential benefit justifies the potential risk to the fetus.
Labor and Delivery: There are insufficient data to support the use of SUBLIMAZE in labor and delivery. Therefore, such use is not recommended.
Nursing Mothers: It is not known whether this drug is excreted in human milk. Because many drugs are excreted in human milk, caution should be exercised when SUBLIMAZE is administered to a nursing woman.
Pediatric Use: The safety and efficacy of SUBLIMAZE in children under two years of age has not been established.
Rare cases of unexplained clinically significant methemoglobinemia have been reported in premature neonates undergoing emergency anesthesia and surgery which included combined use of fentanyl, pancuronium and atropine. A direct cause and effect relationship between the combined use of these drugs and the reported cases of methemoglobinemia has not been established.

ADVERSE REACTIONS

As with other narcotic analgesics, the most common serious adverse reactions reported to occur with SUBLIMAZE (fentanyl citrate) are respiratory depression, apnea, rigidity, and bradycardia; if these remain untreated, respiratory arrest, circulatory depression or cardiac arrest could occur. Other adverse reactions that have been reported are hypertension, hypotension, dizziness, blurred vision, nausea, emesis, laryngospasm, and diaphoresis.
It has been reported that secondary rebound respiratory depression may occasionally occur postoperatively. Patients should be monitored for this possibility and appropriate countermeasures taken as necessary.
When a tranquilizer such as INAPSINE (droperidol) is used with SUBLIMAZE, the following adverse reactions can occur: chills and/or shivering, restlessness, and postoperative hallucinatory episodes (sometimes associated with transient periods of mental depression); extrapyramidal symptoms (dystonia, akathisia, and oculogyric crisis) have been observed up to 24 hours postoperatively. When they occur, extrapyramidal symptoms can usually be controlled with anti-parkinson agents. Postoperative drowsiness is also frequently reported following the use of INAPSINE (droperidol).

DRUG ABUSE AND DEPENDENCE

SUBLIMAZE (fentanyl citrate) is a Schedule II controlled drug substance that can produce drug dependence of the morphine type and therefore has the potential for being abused.

OVERDOSAGE

Manifestations: The manifestations of SUBLIMAZE (fentanyl citrate) overdosage are an extension of its pharmaco-

SUBLIMAZE®

DOSAGE RANGE CHART

TOTAL DOSAGE

Low Dose—2 ug/kg (0.002 mg/kg) (0.04 ml/kg) SUBLIMAZE. SUBLIMAZE in small doses is most useful for minor, but painful, surgical procedures. In addition to the analgesia during surgery, SUBLIMAZE may also provide some pain relief in the immediate postoperative period.	**Moderate Dose**—2–20 ug/kg (0.002–0.02 mg/kg) (0.04–0.4 ml/kg) SUBLIMAZE. Where surgery becomes more major, a larger dose is required. With this dose, in addition to adequate analgesia, one would expect to see some abolition of the stress response. However, respiratory depression will be such that artificial ventilation during anesthesia is necessary and careful observation of ventilation postoperatively is essential.	**High Dose**—20–50 ug/kg (0.02–0.05 mg/kg) (0.4–1 ml/kg) SUBLIMAZE. During open heart surgery and certain more complicated neurosurgical and orthopedic procedures where surgery is more prolonged, and in the opinion of the anesthesiologist, the stress response to surgery would be detrimental to the well being of the patient, dosages of 20–50 ug/kg (0.02–0.05 mg) (0.4–1 ml) of SUBLIMAZE with nitrous oxide/oxygen have been shown to attenuate the	stress response as defined by increased levels of circulating growth hormone, catecholamine, ADH and prolactin. When dosages in this range have been used during surgery, postoperative ventilation and observation are essential due to extended post operative respiratory depression The main objective of this technique would be to produce "stress free" anesthesia.

logic actions (see CLINICAL PHARMACOLOGY) as with other opioid analgesics. The intravenous LD_{50} of SUBLIMAZE is 3 mg/kg in rats, 1 mg/kg in cats, 14 mg/kg in dogs and 0.03 mg/kg in monkeys.

Treatment: In the presence of hypoventilation or apnea, oxygen should be administered and respiration should be assisted or controlled as indicated. A patent airway must be maintained; an oropharyngeal airway or endotracheal tube might be indicated. If depressed respiration is associated with muscular rigidity, an intravenous neuromuscular blocking agent might be required to facilitate assisted or controlled respiration. The patient should be carefully observed for 24 hours; body warmth and adequate fluid intake should be maintained. If hypotension occurs and is severe or persists, the possibility of hypovolemia should be considered and managed with appropriate parenteral fluid therapy. A specific narcotic antagonist such as nalorphine, levallorphan or naloxone should be available for use as indicated to manage respiratory depression. This does not preclude the use of more immediate countermeasures. The duration of respiratory depression following overdosage of SUBLIMAZE may be longer than the duration of narcotic antagonist action. Consult the package insert of the individual narcotic antagonists for details about use.

DOSAGE AND ADMINISTRATION

50 ug = 0.05 mg = 1 ml

Dosage should be individualized. Some of the factors to be considered in determining the dose are age, body weight, physical status, underlying pathological condition, use of other drugs, type of anesthesia to be used and the surgical procedure involved. Dosage should be reduced in elderly or debilitated patients (see PRECAUTIONS).

Vital signs should be monitored routinely.

I. Premedication—Premedication (to be appropriately modified in the elderly, debilitated and those who have received other depressant drugs)—50 to 100 ug (0.05 to 0.1 mg) (1 to 2 ml) may be administered intramuscularly 30 to 60 minutes prior to surgery.
II. Adjunct to General Anesthesia—See Dosage Range Chart
III. Adjunct to Regional Anesthesia—50 to 100 ug (0.05 to 0.1 mg) (1 to 2 ml) may be administered intramuscularly or slowly intravenously, over one to two minutes, when additional analgesia is required.
IV. Postoperatively (recovery room)—50 to 100 ug (0.05 to 0.1 mg) (1 to 2 ml) may be administered intramuscularly for the control of pain, tachypnea and emergence delirium. The dose may be repeated in one to two hours as needed.

Usage in Children: For induction and maintenance in children 2 to 12 years of age, a reduced dose as low as 2 to 3 ug/kg is recommended.

[See table above].

[See table below].

As a General Anesthetic

When attenuation of the responses to surgical stress is especially important, doses of 50 to 100 ug/kg (0.05 to 0.1 mg/kg) (1 to 2 ml/kg) may be administered with oxygen and a muscle relaxant. This technique has been reported to provide anesthesia without the use of additional anesthetic agents. In certain cases, doses up to 150 ug/kg (0.15 mg/kg) (3 ml/kg) may be necessary to produce this anesthetic effect. It has been used for open heart surgery and certain other major surgical procedures in patients for whom protection of the myocardium from excess oxygen demand is particularly indicated, and for certain complicated neurological and orthopedic procedures.

As noted above, it is essential that qualified pesonnel and adequate facilities be available for the management of respiratory depression.

See WARNINGS and PRECAUTIONS for use of SUBLIMAZE (fentanyl citrate) with other CNS depressants, and in patients with altered response.

Parenteral drug products should be inspected visually for particulate matter and discoloration prior to administration, whenever solution and container permit.

HOW SUPPLIED

SUBLIMAZE (fentanyl citrate) Injection is available as:

NDC 50458-030-02 50 ug/ml, 2 ml ampoules in packages of 10
NDC 50458-030-05 50 ug/ml, 5 ml ampoules in packages of 10
NDC 50458-030-10 50 ug/ml, 10 ml ampoules in packages of 5
NDC 50458-030-20 50 ug/ml, 20 ml ampoules in packages of 5

PROTECT FROM LIGHT. STORE AT ROOM TEMPERATURE 15°C–30°C (59°F–86°F).

JANSSEN PHARMACEUTICA INC.
Piscataway, NJ 08854
U.S. Patent No. 3,164,600
Revised January 1981, December 1985

SUBLIMAZE®

DOSAGE RANGE CHART

MAINTENANCE DOSE

Low Dose—2 ug/kg (0.002 mg/kg) (0.04 ml/kg) SUBLIMAZE. Additional dosages of SUBLIMAZE are infrequently needed in these minor procedures.	**Moderate Dose**—2–20 ug/kg (0.002–0.02 mg/kg) (0.04–0.4 ml/kg) SUBLIMAZE. 25 to 100 ug (0.025 to 0.1 mg) (0.5 to 2.0 ml) may be administered intravenously or intramuscularly when movement and/or changes in vital signs indicate surgical stress or lightening of analgesia.	**High Dose**—20–50 ug/kg (0.02–0.05 mg/kg) (0.4–1.0 ml/kg) SUBLIMAZE. Maintenance dosage (ranging from 25 ug (0.025 mg) (0.5 ml) to one half the initial loading dose) will be dictated by the changes in vital signs which indicate stress and lightening of analgesia. However, the additional dosage selected must be individualized especially if the anticipated remaining operative time is short.

SUFENTA® Ⓒ℞

[su-fen'ta]
(sufentanil citrate)
Injection

CAUTION

Federal Law Prohibits Dispensing Without Prescription

DESCRIPTION

SUFENTA® (sufentanil citrate) is a potent opioid analgesic chemically designated as N-[4-(methoxymethyl)-1-[2-(2-thienyl) ethyl]-4-piperidinyl]-N- phenylpropanamide 2-hydroxy-1,2,3-propanetricarboxylate (1:1) with a molecular weight of 578.68.

SUFENTA is a sterile, preservative free, aqueous solution containing sufentanil citrate equivalent to 50 ug per ml of sufentanil base for intravenous injection. The solution has a pH range of 3.5–6.0.

CLINICAL PHARMACOLOGY

SUFENTA is an opioid analgesic. When used in balanced general anesthesia, SUFENTA has been reported to be as much as 10 times as potent as fentanyl. When administered as a primary anesthetic agent with 100% oxygen, SUFENTA is approximately 5 to 7 times as potent as fentanyl. (See dosage chart for more complete information on the use of SUFENTA.) At doses of up to 8 ug/kg, SUFENTA provides profound analgesia; at doses ≥ 8 ug/kg, SUFENTA produces a deep level of anesthesia. SUFENTA produces a dose related attenuation of catecholamine release, particularly norepinephrine.

The pharmacokinetics of SUFENTA can be described as a three-compartment model, with a distribution time of 1.4 minutes, redistribution of 17.1 minutes and an elimination half-life of 164 minutes. The liver and small intestine are the major sites of biotransformation. Approximately 80% of the administered dose is excreted within 24 hours and only 2% of the dose is eliminated as unchanged drug. Plasma protein binding of SUFENTA is approximately 92.5%.

SUFENTA has an immediate onset of action, with relatively limited accumulation. Rapid elimination from tissue storage sites allows for relatively more rapid recovery as compared with equipotent dosages of fentanyl. At dosages of SUFENTA of 1–2 ug/kg, recovery times are comparable to those observed with fentanyl; at dosages of > 2–6 ug/kg, recovery times are comparable to enflurane, isoflurane and fentanyl. Within the anesthetic dosage range of 8–30 ug/kg of SUFENTA, recovery times are more rapid compared to equipotent fentanyl dosages.

At dosages of ≥ 8 ug/kg, SUFENTA produces hypnosis and anesthesia without the use of additional anesthetic agents. A deep level of anesthesia is maintained at these dosages, as demonstrated by EEG patterns. Dosages of up to 25 ug/kg attenuate the sympathetic response to surgical stress. The catecholamine response, particularly norepinephrine, is further attenuated at doses of SUFENTA of 25–30 ug/kg, with hemodynamic stability and preservation of favorable myocardial oxygen balance.

The vagolytic effects of pancuronium may produce a dose dependent elevation in heart rate during SUFENTA-oxygen anesthesia. The vagolytic effect of pancuronium may be reduced in patients administered nitrous oxide with SUFENTA. The use of moderate doses of pancuronium or of

Continued on next page

Janssen—Cont.

a less vagolytic neuromuscular blocking agent may be used to maintain a stable lower heart rate and blood pressure during SUFENTA-oxygen anesthesia.
Preliminary data suggest that in patients administered high doses of SUFENTA, initial dosage requirements for nueromuscular blocking agents are generally lower as compared to patients given fentanyl or halothane, and comparable to patients given enflurane.
Bradycardia is infrequently seen in patients administered SUFENTA-oxygen anesthesia. The use of nitrous oxide with high doses of SUFENTA may decrease mean arterial pressure, heart rate and cardiac output.
Assays of histamine in patients administered SUFENTA have shown no elevation in plasma histamine levels and no indication of histamine release.
SUFENTA at 20 ug/kg has been shown to provide more adequate reduction in intracranial volume than equivalent doses of fentanyl, based upon requirements for furosemide and anesthesia supplementation in one study of patients undergoing craniotomy. During carotid endarterectomy, SUFENTA-nitrous oxide/oxygen produced reductions in cerebral blood flow comparable to those of enflurane-nitrous oxide/oxygen. During cardiovascular surgery, SUFENTA-oxygen produced EEG patterns similar to fentanyl-oxygen; these EEG changes were judged to be compatible with adequate general anesthesia.
The intraoperative use of SUFENTA at anesthetic dosages maintains cardiac output, with a slight reduction in systemic vascular resistance during the initial postoperative period. The incidence of postoperative hypertension, need for vasoactive agents and requirements for postoperative analgesics are generally reduced in patients administered moderate or high doses of SUFENTA as compared to patients given inhalation agents.
Skeletal muscle rigidity is related to the dose and speed of administration of SUFENTA. This muscular rigidity may occur unless preventative measures are taken (see WARNINGS).
Decreased respiratory drive and increased airway resistance occur with SUFENTA. The duration and degree of respiratory depression are dose related when SUFENTA is used at sub-anesthetic dosages. At high doses, a pronounced decrease in pulmonary exchange and apnea may be produced.

SUFENTA® **ADULT DOSAGE RANGE CHART**

TOTAL DOSAGE	MAINTENANCE DOSAGE
ADMINISTRATION WITH NITROUS OXIDE/OXYGEN FOR SURGICAL PROCEDURES LASTING UP TO EIGHT HOURS: **•TOTAL DOSAGE REQUIREMENTS OF 1 UG/KG/HR OR LESS ARE RECOMMENDED**	
1–2 ug/kg: Expected duration of anesthesia 1–2 hours. Approximately 75% or more of total SUFENTA dosage may be administered prior to intubation. Administered with nitrous oxide/oxygen in patients undergoing general surgery in which endotracheal intubation and mechanical ventilation are required.	**10–25 ug (0.2–0.5 ml):** as needed when movement and/or changes in vital signs indicate surgical stress or lightening of analgesia. Supplemental dosages should be individualized and adjusted to the remaining operative time anticipated.
2–8 ug/kg: Expected duration of anesthesia 2–8 hours. Approximately 50 to 75% of total SUFENTA dosage may be administered prior to intubation. Administered with nitrous oxide/oxygen in patients undergoing more complicated major surgical procedures. At dosages in this range, SUFENTA has been shown to provide some attenuation of sympathetic reflex activity in response to surgical stimuli, provide hemodynamic stability, and provide relatively rapid recovery.	**10–50 ug (0.2–1 ml):** as determined by changes in vital signs that indicate stress or lightening of analgesia. Supplemental dosages should be individualized, and adjusted to the remaining operative time anticipated.
ADMINISTRATION WITH 100% OXYGEN	
8–30 ug/kg: (anesthetic doses) administered with 100% oxygen and a muscle relaxant. SUFENTA has been found to produce sleep at dosages ≥ 8 ug/kg and to maintain a deep level of anesthesia without the use of additional anesthetic agents. At dosages in this range of up to 25 ug/kg, catecholamine release is attentuated. Dosages of 25–30 ug/kg have been shown to block sympathetic responses including catecholamine release. High doses are indicated in patients undergoing major surgical procedures, such as cardiovascular surgery and neurosurgery in the sitting position with maintenance of favorable myocardial and cerebral oxygen balance. Postoperative mechanical ventilation and observation are essential at these dosages due to extended postoperative respiratory depression.	**25–50 ug (0.5–1 ml):** as determined by changes in vital signs that indicate stress and lightening of anesthesia.

INDICATIONS AND USAGE

SUFENTA (sufentanil citrate) is indicated:
as an analgesic adjunct in the maintenance of balanced general anesthesia.
as a primary anesthetic agent for the induction and maintenance of anesthesia with 100% oxygen in patients undergoing major surgical procedures, such as cardiovascular surgery or neurosurgical procedures in the sitting position, to provide favorable myocardial and cerebral oxygen balance or when extended postoperative ventilation is anticipated.
SEE DOSAGE CHART FOR MORE COMPLETE INFORMATION ON THE USE OF SUFENTA.

CONTRAINDICATIONS

SUFENTA is contraindicated in patients with known hypersensitivity to the drug.

WARNINGS

SUFENTA should be administered only by persons specifically trained in the use of intravenous anesthetics and management of the respiratory effects of potent opioids.
An opioid antagonist, resuscitative and intubation equipment and oxygen should be readily available.
SUFENTA may cause skeletal muscle rigidity, particularly of the truncal muscles. The incidence and severity of muscle rigidity is dose related. Administration of SUFENTA may produce muscular rigidity with a more rapid onset than that seen with fentanyl. SUFENTA may produce muscular rigidity that involves the skeletal muscles of the neck and extremities. The incidence can be reduced by: 1) administration of up to ¼ of the full paralyzing dose of a non-depolarizing neuromuscular blocking agent just prior to administration of SUFENTA at dosages of up to 8 ug/kg, 2) administration of a full paralyzing dose of a neuromuscular blocking agent following loss of consciousness when SUFENTA is used in anesthetic dosages (above 8 ug/kg) titrated by slow intravenous infusion, or, 3) simultaneous administration of SUFENTA and a full paralyzing dose of a neuromuscular blocking agent when SUFENTA is used in rapidly administered anesthetic dosages (above 8 ug/kg).
The neuromuscular blocking agent used should be compatible with the patient's cardiovascular status. Adequate facilities should be available for postoperative monitoring and ventilation of patients administered SUFENTA. It is essential that these facilities be fully equipped to handle all degrees of respiratory depression.

PRECAUTIONS

General: The initial dose of SUFENTA should be appropriately reduced in elderly and debilitated patients. The effect of the initial dose should be considered in determining supplemental doses.
Vital signs should be monitored routinely.
Nitrous oxide may produce cardiovascular depression when given with high doses of SUFENTA (see CLINICAL PHARMACOLOGY).
The hemodynamic effects of a particular muscle relaxant and the degree of skeletal muscle relaxation required should be considered in the selection of a neuromuscular blocking agent.
High doses of pancuronium may produce increases in heart rate during SUFENTA-oxygen anesthesia. Bradycardia has been reported infrequently with SUFENTA-oxygen anesthesia and has been responsive to atropine.
Respiratory depression caused by opioid analgesics can be reversed by opioid antagonists such as naloxone. Because the duration of respiratory depression produced by SUFENTA may last longer than the duration of the opioid antagonist action, appropriate surveillance should be maintained. As with all potent opioids, profound analgesia is accompanied by respiratory depression and diminished sensitivity to CO_2 stimulation which may persist into or recur in the postoperative period. Appropriate postoperative monitoring should be employed to ensure that adequate spontaneous breathing is established and maintained prior to discharging the patient from the recovery area.
Interaction with Other Central Nervous System Depressants: Both the magnitude and duration of central nervous system and cardiovascular effects may be enhanced when SUFENTA is administered to patients receiving barbiturates, tranquilizers, other opioids, general anesthetics or other CNS depressants. In such cases of combined treatment, the dose of one or both agents should be reduced.
Head Injuries: SUFENTA may obscure the clinical course of patients with head injuries.
Impaired Respiration: SUFENTA should be used with caution in patients with pulmonary disease, decreased respiratory reserve or potentially compromised respiration. In such patients, opioids may additionally decrease respiratory drive and increase airway resistance. During anesthesia, this can be managed by assisted or controlled respiration.
Impaired Hepatic or Renal Function: In patients with liver or kidney dysfunction, SUFENTA should be administered with caution due to the importance of these organs in the metabolism and excretion of SUFENTA.
Carcinogenesis, Mutagenesis and Impairment of Fertility: No long-term animal studies of SUFENTA have been performed to evaluate carcinogenic potential. The micronucleus test in female rats revealed that single intravenous doses of SUFENTA as high as 80 ug/kg (approximately 2.5 times the upper human dose) produced no structural chromosome mutations. The Ames *Salmonella typhimurium* metabolic activating test also revealed no mutagenic activity. See ANIMAL TOXICOLOGY for reproduction studies in rats and rabbits.
Pregnancy Category C: SUFENTA has been shown to have an embryocidal effect in rats and rabbits when given in doses 2.5 times the upper human dose for a period of 10 days to over 30 days. These effects were most probably due to maternal toxicity (decreased food consumption with increased mortality) following prolonged administration of the drug.
No evidence of teratogenic effects have been observed after administration of SUFENTA in rats and rabbits.
There are no adequate and well-controlled studies in pregnant women. SUFENTA should be used during pregnancy only if the potential benefit justifies the potential risk to the fetus.
Labor and Delivery: There are insufficient data to support the use of SUFENTA in labor and delivery. Therefore, such use is not recommended.
Nursing Mothers: It is not known whether this drug is excreted in human milk. Because many drugs are excreted in human milk, caution should be exercised when SUFENTA is administered to a nursing woman.
Pediatric Use: The safety and effficacy of SUFENTA in children under two years of age undergoing cardiovascular surgery has been documented in a limited number of cases.
Animal Toxicology: The intravenous LD_{50} of SUFENTA is 16.8 to 18.0 mg/kg in mice, 11.8 to 13.0 mg/kg in guinea pigs and 10.1 to 19.5 mg/kg in dogs. Reproduction studies performed in rats and rabbits given doses of up to 2.5 times the upper human dose for a period of 10 to over 30 days revealed high maternal mortality rates due to decreased food consumption and anoxia, which preclude any meaningful interpretation of the results.

ADVERSE REACTIONS

The most common adverse reactions of opioids are respiratory depression and skeletal muscle rigidity. See CLINICAL PHARMACOLOGY, WARNINGS and PRECAUTIONS on the management of respiratory depression and skeletal muscle rigidity.
The most frequent adverse reactions in clinical trials involving 320 patients administered SUFENTA were: hypotension (7%), hypertension (3%), chest wall rigidity (3%) and bradycardia (3%).

Other adverse reactions with a reported incidence of less than 1% were:
Cardiovascular: tachycardia, arrhythmia
Gastrointestinal: nausea, vomiting
Respiratory: apnea, postoperative respiratory depression, bronchospasm
Dermatological: itching, erythema
Central Nervous System: chills
Miscellaneous: intraoperative muscle movement

DRUG ABUSE AND DEPENDENCE
SUFENTA (sufentanil citrate) is a Schedule II controlled drug substance that can produce drug dependence of the morphine type and therefore has the potential for being abused.

OVERDOSAGE
Overdosage would be manifested by an extension of the pharmacological actions of SUFENTA (see CLINICAL PHARMACOLOGY) as with other potent opioid analgesics. However, no experiences of overdosage with SUFENTA have been established during clinical trials. The intravenous LD_{50} of SUFENTA in male rats is 9.34 to 12.5 mg/kg (see ANIMAL TOXICOLOGY for LD_{50}s in other species). Intravenous administration of an opioid antagonist such as naloxone should be employed as a specific antidote to manage respiratory depression. The duration of respiratory depression following overdosage with SUFENTA may be longer than the duration of action of the opioid antagonist. Administration of an opioid antagonist should not preclude more immediate countermeasures. In the event of overdosage, oxygen should be administered and ventilation assisted or controlled as indicated for hypoventilation or apnea. A patent airway must be maintained, and a nasopharyngeal airway or endotracheal tube may be indicated. If depressed respiration is associated with muscular rigidity, a neuromuscular blocking agent may be required to facilitate assisted or controlled respiration. Intravenous fluids and vasopressors for the treatment of hypotension and other supportive measures may be employed.

DOSAGE AND ADMINISTRATION
The dosage of SUFENTA should be individualized in each case according to body weight, physical status, underlying pathological condition, use of other drugs, and type of surgical procedure and anesthesia. In obese patients (more than 20% above ideal total body weight), the dosage of SUFENTA should be determined on the basis of lean body weight. Dosage should be reduced in elderly and debilitated patients (see PRECAUTIONS).
Vital signs should be monitored routinely.
See dosage range chart for the use of SUFENTA by intravenous injection 1) in doses of up to 8 ug/kg as an analgesic adjunct to general anesthesia, and 2) in doses ≥ 8 ug/kg as a primary anesthetic agent for induction and maintenance of anesthesia with 100% oxygen.
Usage in Children: For induction and maintenance of anesthesia in children less than 12 years of age undergoing cardiovascular surgery, an anesthetic dose of 10–25 ug/kg administered with 100% oxygen is generally recommended. Supplemental dosages of up to 25–50 ug are recommended for maintenance, based on response to initial dose and as determined by changes in vital signs indicating surgical stress or lightening of anesthesia.
Premedication: The selection of preanesthetic medications should be based upon the needs of the individual patient.
Neuromuscular Blocking Agents: The neuromuscular blocking agent selected should be compatible with the patient's condition, taking into account the hemodynamic effects of a particular muscle relaxant and the degree of skeletal muscle relaxation required (see CLINICAL PHARMACOLOGY, WARNINGS and PRECAUTIONS).
[See table on preceding page].
In patients administered high (anesthetic) doses of SUFENTA, it is essential that qualified personnel and adequate facilities are available for the management of postoperative respiratory depression.
Also see WARNINGS and PRECAUTIONS sections.
For purposes of administering small volumes of SUFENTA accurately, the use of a tuberculin syringe or equivalent is recommended.
Parenteral drug products should be inspected visually for particulate matter and discoloration prior to administration, whenever solution and container permit.

HOW SUPPLIED
SUFENTA (sufentanil citrate) Injection for intravenous use is available as:
NDC 50458-050-01 50 ug/ml, 1 ml ampoules in packages of 10
NDC 50458-050-02 50 ug/ml, 2 ml ampoules in packages of 10
NDC 50458-050-05 50 ug/ml, 5 ml ampoules in packages of 10
Protect from light. Store at room temperature 15°–30°C (59°–86°F).
U.S. Patent No. 3,998,834
January 1986, March 1986

Vermox®	Pinworm (enterobiasis)	Whipworm (trichuriasis)	Common Roundworm (ascariasis)	Hookworm
Cure rates mean	95%	68%	98%	96%
Egg reduction mean	—	93%	99%	99%

VERMOX® ℞
[vĕr'mŏx]
(mebendazole)
Chewable Tablets

DESCRIPTION
VERMOX® (mebendazole) is a (synthetic) broad-spectrum anthelmintic available as chewable tablets, each containing 100 mg of mebendazole. Inactive ingredients are: colloidal silicon dioxide, corn starch, hydrogenated vegetable oil, magnesium stearate, microcrystalline cellulose, sodium lauryl sulfate, sodium saccharin, sodium starch glycolate, talc, tetrarome orange, and FD&C yellow No. 6.
Mebendazole is methyl 5-benzoylbenzimidazole-2-carbamate.
Mebendazole is a white to slightly yellow powder with a molecular weight of 295.29. It is less than 0.05% soluble in water, dilute mineral acid solutions, alcohol, ether and chloroform, but is soluble in formic acid.

CLINICAL PHARMACOLOGY
Following administration of 100 mg twice daily for three consecutive days, plasma levels of VERMOX® and its primary metabolite, the 2-amine, do not exceed 0.03 μg/ml and 0.09 μg/ml, respectively. All metabolites are devoid of anthelmintic activity. In man, approximately 2% of administered VERMOX® is excreted in urine and the remainder in the feces as unchanged drug or a primary metabolite.
Mode of Action: VERMOX® inhibits the formation of the worms' microtubules and causes the worms' glucose depletion.

INDICATIONS AND USAGE
VERMOX® is indicated for the treatment of *Enterobius vermicularis* (pinworm), *Trichuris trichiura* (whipworm), *Ascaris lumbricoides* (common roundworm), *Ancylostoma duodenale* (common hookworm), *Necator americanus* (American hookworm) in single or mixed infections.
Efficacy varies as a function of such factors as pre-existing diarrhea and gastrointestinal transit time, degree of infection, and helminth strains. Efficacy rates derived from various studies are shown in the table above:
[See table above].

CONTRAINDICATIONS
VERMOX® is contraindicated in persons who have shown hypersensitivity to the drug.

WARNINGS
There is no evidence that VERMOX®, even at high doses, is effective for hydatid disease.

PRECAUTIONS
Information for Patients: Patients should be informed of the potential risk to the fetus in women taking VERMOX® during pregnancy, especially during the first trimester (see Use in Pregnancy).
Patients should also be informed that cleanliness is important to prevent reinfection and transmission of the infection.
Carcinogenesis, Mutagenesis: In carcinogenicity tests of VERMOX® in mice and rats, no carcinogenic effects were seen at doses as high as 40 mg/kg given daily over two years. Dominant lethal mutation tests in mice showed no mutagenicity at single doses as high as 640 mg/kg. Neither the spermatocyte test, the F_1 translocation test, nor the Ames test indicated mutagenic properties.
Impairment of Fertility: Doses up to 40 mg/kg in mice, given to males for 60 days and to females for 14 days prior to gestation, had no effect upon fetuses and offspring, though there was slight maternal toxicity.
Use in Pregnancy: Pregnancy Category C. VERMOX® has shown embryotoxic and teratogenic activity in pregnant rats at single oral doses as low as 10 mg/kg. In view of these findings the use of VERMOX® is not recommended in pregnant women. In humans, a post-marketing survey has been done of a limited number of women who inadvertently had consumed VERMOX® during the first trimester of pregnancy. The incidence of spontaneous abortion and malformation did not exceed that in the general population. In 170 deliveries on term, no teratogenic risk of VERMOX® was identified. During pregnancy, especially during the first trimester, VERMOX® should be used only if the potential benefit justifies the potential risk to the fetus.
Nursing Mothers: It is not known whether VERMOX® is excreted in human milk. Because many drugs are excreted in human milk, caution should be exercised when VERMOX® is administered to a nursing woman.
Pediatric Use: The drug has not been extensively studied in children under two years; therefore, in the treatment of children under two years the relative benefit/risk should be considered.

ADVERSE REACTIONS
Transient symptoms of abdominal pain and diarrhea have occurred in cases of massive infection and expulsion of worms.

OVERDOSAGE
In the event of accidental overdosage gastrointestinal complaints lasting up to a few hours may occur. Vomiting and purging should be induced.

DOSAGE AND ADMINISTRATION
The same dosage schedule applies to children and adults. The tablet may be chewed, swallowed, or crushed and mixed with food.
[See table below].
If the patient is not cured three weeks after treatment, a second course of treatment is advised. No special procedures, such as fasting or purging, are required.

HOW SUPPLIED
VERMOX® is available as chewable tablets, each containing 100 mg of mebendazole, and is supplied in boxes of thirty-six tablets.
NDC 50458-110-30 (36 tablets-blister)
VERMOX® (mebendazole) is an original product of Janssen Pharmaceutica n.v. B-2340 Beerse, Belgium.
JANSSEN PHARMACEUTICA INC.
Piscataway, NJ 08854
Rev. August 1984, Sept 1986
U.S. Patent 3,657,267
Shown in Product Identification Section, page 411

Johnson & Johnson Products Inc.
A Johnson & Johnson Company
PATIENT CARE DIVISION
501 GEORGE STREET
NEW BRUNSWICK, NJ 08903

DEBRISAN®
[deb'ri-san]
wound cleaning beads and paste.
Draws Exudate from Wet Ulcers and Wounds

DESCRIPTION
DEBRISAN® consists of spherical hydrophilic beads of dex-
Continued on next page

Vermox®

	Pinworm (enterobiasis)	Whipworm (trichuriasis)	Common Roundworm (ascariasis)	Hookworm
Dose	1 tablet, once	1 tablet morning and evening for 3 consecutive days.	1 tablet morning and evening for 3 consecutive days.	1 tablet morning and evening for 3 consecutive days.

Johnson & Johnson—Cont.

tranomer, 0.1–0.3mm in diameter; the paste is a mixture of the beads and polyethylene glycol. The beads are composed of a three dimensional network of macromolecular chains of cross-linked dextran which is large enough to allow substances with a molecular weight of less than 1000 to enter freely. Substances with a molecular weight of 1000–5000 enter the beads less freely, while those with a molecular weight greater than 5000 remain in the interspaces between the beads.

Characteristics: Because of its hydrophilic properties, each gram of DEBRISAN® beads absorbs approximately 4 ml. of fluid. The beads swell to approximately four times their original size. This swelling causes significant suction forces and capillary action in the spaces between the beads. This action is continuous as long as unsaturated beads or paste is in proximity to the ulcer or wound.

When DEBRISAN® beads or paste are applied to the surface of wet ulcers or wounds suction forces begin removing various exudates and particles that tend to impede tissue repair. For example, low molecular weight components of wound exudates are drawn up within the DEBRISAN® beads while higher molecular weight components, such as plasma proteins, and fibrinogen are found between the swollen beads. Removal of these latter components, particularly fibrin and fibrinogen, retards eschar formation. Additionally, there is *in vitro* evidence that the suction forces created by the beads remove bacteria and inflammatory exudates from the surface of the wound.

The use of DEBRISAN® beads or paste to remove exudates continuously from the surface of the wound results in a concomitant reduction of inflammation and edema.

INDICATIONS

DEBRISAN® beads and paste are indicated for use in cleaning wet ulcers and wounds such as venous stasis ulcers, decubitus ulcers, and infected traumatic and surgical wounds. DEBRISAN® beads are also indicated for use in cleaning infected burns.

PRECAUTIONS

To minimize the possibility of cross-contamination, contents of a DEBRISAN® bead container should be limited to use in one patient.

When treating cratered decubitus ulcers, do not pack the wounds tightly. Allow for expansion of the beads. Do not use DEBRISAN® beads or paste in deep fistulas, sinus tracts, or any body cavity where complete removal is not assured.

Once the DEBRISAN® is saturated it should be removed. This avoids encrustation which makes removal more difficult. All DEBRISAN® must be removed before any surgical procedure to close the wound (*ie* graft or flap).

Wounds may appear larger during the first few days of treatment due to the reduction of edema.

DEBRISAN® beads and paste are not effective in cleaning dry wounds.

Not all wounds require treatment with DEBRISAN® to complete healing. When the wound is no longer wet and a healthy granulation base has been established, the application of DEBRISAN® beads or paste should be discontinued.

Treatment of the underlying condition (venous or arterial flow, pressure, etc.) should be addressed, in addition to using DEBRISAN® beads or paste.

ADVERSE REACTIONS

Upon application and/or removal of DEBRISAN® beads, transitory pain, bleeding, blistering and erythema have been reported in isolated cases.

DIRECTIONS FOR USE

Applying DEBRISAN®

Debride and wash the area in the usual manner. **DEBRISAN® beads and paste are not enzymes and will not debride.** Leave the area moist since this facilitates the action of DEBRISAN®

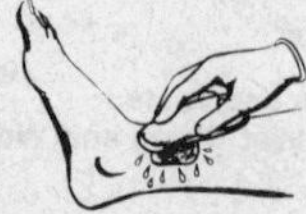

Apply DEBRISAN® beads or paste to at least 1/4 inch (6mm) thickness. At least 1/4 inch thickness is required to achieve desired suction effects.

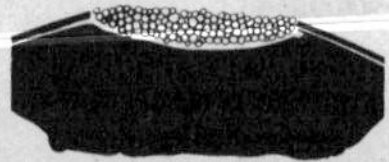

Apply a dressing. Close all four sides.

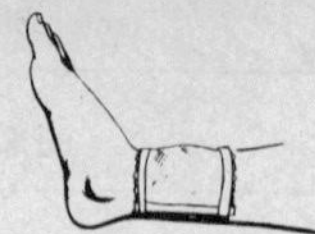

Use of paste

A paste mixture of DEBRISAN® beads may be used for application on irregular body surfaces or hard to reach areas. Three methods of application are possible:

1. DEBRISAN® may be purchased in a convenient, premixed paste form.
2. A paste mixture may be prepared by carefully pouring a small amount of glycerin on a dry dressing large enough to cover the wound and adding a sufficient amount of DEBRISAN® beads to make a layer at least 1/4 inch thick.

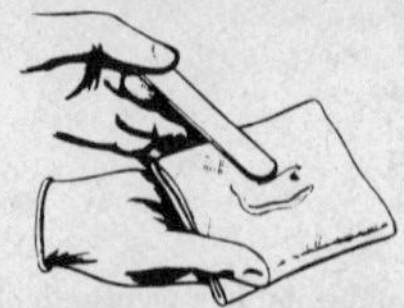

3. Or, DEBRISAN® beads (3 parts) may be mixed with glycerin (1 part) in a receptacle and applied directly to the wound with a spatula. Do not mix with any substance other than glycerin.

In any case, dress the wound in the usual manner. Use fresh paste for each application. Do not reuse. **Removing DEBRISAN®**

When DEBRISAN® beads or paste become saturated, a color change will be noted indicating that they should be removed. Removal should be as complete as possible and is best achieved by irrigation. Occasionally vigorous irrigation, soaking, or whirlpool may be required to remove patches of DEBRISAN® that adhere to the wound.

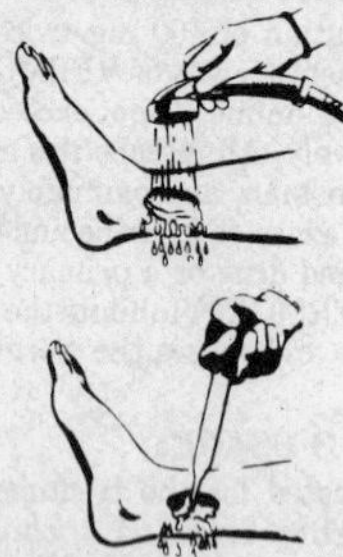

Reapply DEBRISAN® beads or paste every 12 hours, or more frequently if necessary. Reduce the number of applications as the exudate diminishes.

When to Discontinue:

When the area is free of exudate and edema.

When a healthy granulation base is present.

The patient should consult the physician if the condition worsens or persists beyond the expected length of treatment (normally 14–21 days).

HOW SUPPLIED

DEBRISAN® beads are supplied sterile, in containers of 25, 60, 120 grams each and 4 gram packets in boxes of 7 or 14.

DEBRISAN® paste is also available in a pre-mixed sterile form, in 10 gram foil packets, six per box.

Store in a dry place below 85°F.

Avoid contact with eyes.

For external use only.

Spilling beads or paste onto the floor will result in a slippery surface.

Materials Available: Free samples and clinical literature available to physicians. Call 800-526-2459.

MANUFACTURED IN SWEDEN FOR
JOHNSON & JOHNSON PRODUCTS INC.
A Johnson & Johnson company
NEW BRUNSWICK, NEW JERSEY 08903
©J&JPI83

INSTAT™ ℞

[*in 'stat*]
collagen absorbable hemostat

DESCRIPTION

INSTAT Collagen Absorbable Hemostat is a purified and lyophilized bovine dermal collagen. The material, prepared as a sponge-like pad, is lightly crosslinked, sterile, non-pyrogenic, and absorbable. Hemostatic activity, which is an inherent property of collagen, is largely dependent on the basic helical structure of this protein. The helical structure of native collagen is preserved during the manufacture of INSTAT. When collagen comes into contact with blood, platelets aggregate on the collagen and release coagulation factors which, together with plasma factors result in the formation of fibrin, and finally in the formation of a clot.

INDICATIONS

INSTAT Collagen Absorbable Hemostat is indicated in surgical procedures (other than in neurosurgical, unrological and ophthalmological surgery) for use as an adjunct to hemostasis when control of bleeding by ligature or other conventional methods is ineffective or impractical.

CONTRAINDICATIONS

INSTAT Collagen Absorbable Hemostat should not be used in the closure of skin incisions as it may interfere with the healing of skin edges. This interference is due to simple mechanical interposition of dry collagen and not due to any intrinsic interference with wound healing. It has been reported with another absorbable collagen hemostat that, in filling porosities of cancellous bone, collagen may reduce the bonding strength of methylmethacrylate. Therefore, INSTAT should not be applied on bone surfaces to which prosthetic materials are to be attached with methylmethacrylate adhesives.

WARNINGS

INSTAT Collagen Absorbable Hemostat is inactivated by autoclaving. It should not be resterilized. As with any foreign substance, use in contaminated wounds may enhance infection.

INSTAT should not be used in instances of pumping arterial hemorrhage.

INSTAT should not be used where blood or other fluids have pooled or in cases where the point of hemorrhage is submerged. INSTAT will not act as a tampon or plug in a bleeding site nor will it close off an area of blood collecting behind a tampon.

Only the amount of INSTAT necessary to provide hemostasis should be used. The long-term effects of leaving **in situ** are unknown. Opened, unused INSTAT should be discarded because it cannot be resterilized.

PRECAUTIONS

As with other hemostatic agents, it is not recommended that INSTAT Collagen Absorbable Hemostat be left in an infected or contaminated space, nor is it recommended for use in persons known to be sensitive to materials of bovine origin. When placed into cavities or closed spaces, care should be exercised to avoid overpacking INSTAT as it may absorb fluid and expand and press against neighboring structures.

Safety of this product has not been established in children and pregnant women; therefore, INSTAT should only be used when benefit to risk clearly warrants its use.

INSTAT is not intended to be used to treat systemic coagulation disorders.

ADVERSE REACTIONS

INSTAT Collagen Absorbable Hemostat is a collagen product. Although several types of post-operative complications were observed in INSTAT treated patients, none were attributed to INSTAT except one case of fibrotic reaction where INSTAT involvement could not be ruled out. Adverse reactions reported for other collagen hemostats include hematoma, potentiation of infection, wound dehiscence, inflammation and edema. Other reported adverse reactions that may be related to the use of collagen hemostats include adhesion formation, allergic reaction, foreign body reaction and subgaleal seroma (in a single case). The use of microfibrillar collagen in dental extraction sockets has been reported to increase the incidence of alveolalgia. The possibility that all of the above reactions may occur with INSTAT cannot be excluded.

ADMINISTRATION

INSTAT Collagen Absorbable Hemostat is applied directly to the bleeding surface with pressure. INSTAT can be cut to size. The amount needed and the period of time necessary to apply pressure will vary with the type and amount of bleeding to be controlled. Hemostasis time depends upon the type of surgery and degree of pretreatment bleeding. It usually occurred between 2 to 5 minutes with INSTAT.

INSTAT maintains its integrity in the presence of blood and is not dispersed when wet. It is easily removed from the site following hemostasis. It is most effective when used dry.

INSTAT may be left **in situ** whenever necessary. However, the surgeon, at his discretion, should remove any excess of INSTAT prior to wound closure. Animal implant studies have demonstrated that absorption and tissue reaction to INSTAT are similar to those observed with another absorbable collagen hemostatic agent. In these studies, on visual examination, most of INSTAT was found to be absorbed in 8 to 10 weeks after implantation.

CLINICAL STUDIES

The safety, effectiveness and handling characteristics of INSTAT Collagen Absorbable Hemostat were evaluated in a variety of surgical procedures. The median time to hemostasis for INSTAT was 3 minutes. Passive Hemagglutination Assay (PHA) and Enzyme- Linked Immunoabsorbent Assay

(ELISA) methods have been used to evaluate the immunologic potential for INSTAT to produce antibodies in patients. These assays revealed mild elevation of antibody titers in both INSTAT treated patients and patients treated with a collagen control hemostat, confirming that INSTAT, like other collagen hemostats, is a weak antigen.

HOW SUPPLIED

INSTAT Collagen Absorbable Hemostat is supplied in a sponge-like form in peelable plastic envelopes in the following sizes:
1 in. × 2 in. (2.5 cm × 5.1 cm)
3 in. × 4 in. (7.6 cm × 10.2 cm)
The sterility of the product is guaranteed unless the individual envelope is damaged or opened.
Caution: Federal law restricts this device to sale, distribution, and use by or on the order of a physician.

MATERIALS AVAILABLE

Free samples and clinical literature available to physicians, Call 800-526-2459.

SURGICEL® and SURGICEL® NU-KNIT Absorbable Hemostat ℞

[ser'ji-sel]
(oxidized regenerated cellulose)

For surgical use
(For dental application of this product, reference should be made to the package insert for dental use.)

DESCRIPTION

SURGICEL Absorbable Hemostat is a chemically-sterilized, absorbable knitted fabric prepared by the controlled oxidation of regenerated cellulose. The fabric is white with a pale yellow cast and has a faint, caramel-like aroma. It is strong and can be sutured or cut without fraying. It is stable and can be stored at controlled room temperature. A slight discoloration may occur with age, but this does not affect performance.

ACTIONS

The mechanism of action whereby SURGICEL Absorbable Hemostat accelerates clotting is not completely understood, but it appears to be a physical effect rather than any alteration of the normal physiologic clotting mechanism. After SURGICEL has been saturated with blood, it swells into a brownish or black gelatinous mass which aids in the formation of a clot, thereby serving as a hemostatic adjunct in the control of local hemorrhage. When used properly in minimal amounts, SURGICEL is absorbed from the sites of implantation with practically no tissue reaction. Absorption depends upon several factors including the amount used, degree of saturation with blood, and the tissue bed.
In addition to its local hemostatic properties, SURGICEL Absorbable Hemostat is bactericidal **in vitro** against a wide range of gram positive and gram negative organisms including aerobes and anaerobes. SURGICEL is bactericidal **in vitro** against strains of species including those of:
Staphylococcus aureus
Staphylococcus epidermidis
Micrococcus luteus
Streptococcus pyogenes Group A
Streptococcus pyogenes Group B
Bacillus subtilis
Proteus vulgaris
Corynebacterium serosis
Mycobacterium phlei
Clostridium tetani
Streptococcus salivarius
Branhamella catarrhalis
Escherichia coli
Klebsiella aerogenes
Lactobacillus sp.
Salmonella enteritidis
Shigella dysenteriae
Serratia marscescens
Clostridium perfringens
Bacteroides fragilis
Enterococcus
Enterbacter cloacae
Pseudomonas aeruginosa
Pseudomonas stutzeri
Proteus mirabilis
Studies conducted in animals show that SURGICEL in contrast to other hemostatic agents does not tend to enhance experimental infection.

INDICATIONS

SURGICEL Absorbable Hemostat (oxidized regenerated cellulose) is used adjunctively in surgical procedures to assist in the control of capillary, venous, and small arterial hemorrhage when ligation or other conventional methods of control are impractical or ineffective.

CONTRAINDICATIONS

Although packing or wadding sometimes is medically necessary, SURGICEL Absorbable Hemostat should not be used in this manner unlss it is to be removed after hemostasis is achieved.
SURGICEL should not be used for implantation in bone defects, such as fractures, since there is a possibility of interference with callus formation and a theoretical chance of cyst formation.
When SURGICEL is used to help achieve hemostasis around the spinal cord in laminectomies, or around the optic nerve and chiasm, it must always be removed after hemostasis is achieved since it will swell and could exert unwanted pressure.
SURGICEL should not be used to control hemorrhage from large arteries.
SURGICEL should not be used on non-hemorrhagic serous oozing surfaces, since body fluids other than whole blood, such as serum, do not react with SURGICEL to produce satisfactory hemostatic effect.

WARNINGS

SURGICEL Absorbable Hemostat is supplied sterile and should not be autoclaved because autoclaving causes physical breakdown of the product.
SURGICEL is not intended as a substitute for careful surgery and the proper use of sutures and ligatures.
Closing SURGICEL in a contaminated wound without drainage may lead to complications and should be avoided.
The hemostatic effect of SURGICEL is greater when it is applied dry; therefore it should not be moistened with water or saline.
SURGICEL should not be impregnated with anti-infective agents or with other materials such as buffering or hemostatic substances. Its hemostatic effect is not enhanced by the addition of thrombin, the activity of which is destroyed by the low pH of the product.
Although SURGICEL Absorbable Hemostat may be left in situ when necessary, it is advisable to remove it once hemostasis is achieved. It must always be removed from the site of application after use in laminectomy procedures and from foramina in bone when hemostasis is obtained. This is because SURGICEL, by swelling, may cause nerve damage by pressure in a bony confine. Paralysis has been reported when used around the spinal cord, particularly in surgery for herniated intervertebral disc.
Although SURGICEL is bactericidal against a wide range of pathogenic microorganisms, it is not intended as a substitute for systemically administered therapeutic or prophylactic antimicrobial agents to control or prevent post-operative infections.

PRECAUTIONS

Use only as much SURGICEL Absorbable Hemostat as is necessary for hemostasis, holding it in place until bleeding stops. Remove any excess before surgical closure in order to facilitate absorption and minimize the possibility of foreign body reaction.
SURGICEL should be applied loosely against the bleeding surface. Wadding or packing should be avoided, especially within rigid cavities where swelling may intefere with normal function or possibly cause necrosis.
In urological procedures, minimal amounts of SURGICEL should be used and care must be exercised to prevent plugging of the urethra, ureter, or a catheter by dislodged portions of the product.
Since absorption of SURGICEL could be prevented in chemically cauterized areas, its use should not be preceded by application of silver nitrate or any other escharotic chemicals.
If SURGICEL is used temporarily to line the cavity of large open wounds, it should be placed so as not to overlap the skin edges. It should also be removed from open wounds by forceps or by irrigation with sterile water or saline solution after bleeding has stopped.
Precautions should be taken in otorhinolaryngologic surgery to assure that none of the material is aspirated by the patient. (Examples: controlling hemorrhage after tonsillectomy and controlling epistaxis.)
Care should be taken not to apply SURGICEL too tightly when it is used as a wrap during vascular surgery (See "ADVERSE REACTIONS" section).

ADVERSE REACTIONS

"Encapsulation" of fluid and foreign body reactions have been reported.
There have been two reports of stenotic effect when SURGICEL Absorbable Hemostat has been applied as a wrap during vascular surgery. Although it has not been established that the stenosis was directly related to the use of SURGICEL, it is important to be cautious and avoid applying the material tightly as a wrapping.
Possible prolongation of drainage in cholecystectomies and difficulty passing urine per urethra after prostatectomy have been reported. There has been one report of a blocked ureter after kidney resection, in which postoperative catheterization was required.
Occasional reports of "burning" and "stinging" sensations and sneezing when SURGICEL has been used as packing in epistaxis, are believed due to the low pH of the product.
Burning has been reported when SURGICEL was applied after nasal polyp removal and after hemorrhoidectomy. Headache, burning, stinging, and sneezing in epistaxis and other rhinological procedures, and stinging when SURGICEL was applied on surface wounds (varicose ulcerations, dermabrasions, and donor sites) also have been reported.

DOSAGE AND ADMINISTRATION

Sterile technique should be observed in removing SURGICEL Absorbable Hemostat from its envelope. Minimal amounts of SURGICEL in appropriate size are laid on the bleeding site or held firmly against the tissues until hemostasis is obtained.
Opened, unused SURGICEL should be discarded, because it cannot be resterilized.

HOW SUPPLIED

Sterile SURGICEL Absorbable Hemostat (oxidized regenerated cellulose) is supplied as knitted fabric strips in envelopes in the following sizes.
2 in. × 14 in. (28 sq. in.) (5.1 × 35.6 cm. (180.6 sq. cm.))
4 in. × 8 in. (32 sq. in.) (10.2 × 20.3 cm. (206.5 sq. cm.))
2 in. × 3 in. (6 sq. in.) (5.1 × 7.6 cm. (38.7 sq. cm.))
½ in. × 2 in. (1 sq. in.) (1.3 × 5.1 cm. (6.5 sq. cm.))
SURGICEL NU-KNIT
3 in. ×4 in. (12 sq. in.) (7.6 × 10.2 cm. (30.5 sq. cm.))
1 in. × 1 in (1 sq. in.) (2.5 × 2.5 cm. (6.5 sq. cm.))

CLINICAL STUDIES

SURGICEL® Absorbable Hemostat (oxidized regenerated cellulose) has been found useful in helping to control capillary or venous bleeding in a variety of surgical applications, including abdominal, thoracic, neurosurgical, and orthopedic, as well as in otorhinolaryngologic procedures. Examples include gallbladder surgery, partial hepatectomy, hemorrhoidectomy, resections or injuries of the pancreas, spleen, kidney, prostate, bowel, breast or thyroid, and in amputations. (1,3)
SURGICEL has been applied as a surface dressing on donor sites and superficial open wounds, controlling bleeding adequately, and causing no delay in healing or interference with epithelization (4,6). It also has been applied after dermabrasion, punch biopsy, excision biopsy, curettage, finger and toenail removal, and to traumatic wounds. In the foregoing applications, bleeding was controlled and the SURGICEL was absorbed from the sites where it was applied. (5)
In cardiovascular surgery, investigators have found SURGICEL useful in helping to control bleeding from implanted textile grafts, including those of the abdominal aorta. (2,7) Such grafts may leak or weep considerably, even when preclotted, but this seepage can be controlled by covering the graft with a layer or two of SURGICEL after the graft is in place and before releasing the proximal and distal clamps. When the flow has been reestablished and all the bleeding controlled, the fabric either can be removed or left in situ, since absorption of SURGICEL has been shown to occur without constriction of the graft or other untoward incident when proper wrapping technique is employed.
Otorhinolaryngologic experience with SURGICEL includes adjunctive use in controlling bleeding resulting from epistaxis, tonsillectomy, adenoidectomy, removal of nasal polyps, repair of deviated septum, tympanoplasty, stapes surgery, surgery for sinusitis, and removal of tumors. (8,9)
SURGICEL has been reported useful as a hemostatic adjunct in such gynecologic procedures as oophorectomy, hysterectomy, conization of the cervix, and repair of cystorectocele. (1,10)

ANIMAL PHARMACOLOGY

The effects of SURGICEL Absorbable Hemostat, absorbable gelatin sponge, and microfibrillar collagen hemostat were compared in a standardized infection model consisting of intra-abdominal and intrahepatic abscesses in mice. This infection mimics the common characteristics of human infection with nonspore-forming anaerobic bacteria, including a chronic and progressive course. SURGICEL did not increase the infectivity of normally subinfectious inocula of mixed anaerobic species in mice. With the other hemostatic agents, microfibrillar collagen hemostat and absorbable gelatin sponge, an enhancement of infectivity of anaerobic mixtures has been shown. SURGICEL Absorbable Hemostat, in contrast to these hemostatic agents, did not enhance or provide a site for bacterial growth.
It was also found that aerobic pathogens did not grow in the presence of SURGICEL Absorbable Hemostat. In these studies (11), SURGICEL® Absorbable Hemostat was placed in contaminated incisions of guinea pigs and markedly reduced bacterial growth of three different strains of common pathogens.
In a dog model (12), it was shown that bacterial contamination of implanted teflon patches in the aorta could be reduced by wrapping the area of the patch with SURGICEL

Continued on next page

Johnson & Johnson—Cont.

prior to pathogen challenge. Also, in another study (13), SURGICEL Absorbable Hemostat and an absorbable gelatin sponge were placed in two splenotomy sites in large mongrel dogs and the animals were then challenged intravenously and the number of organisms from the splenotomy sites were measured over a period of time. The number of organisms at the site of SURGICEL Absorbable Hemostat was significantly lower than that in the control, or the absorbable gelatin sponge site.

REFERENCES

1. Degenshein, G., Hurwitz, A., and S. Ribacoff: Experience with regenerated oxidized celluose. ***New York State Journal of Medicine 63*** (18):2639–2643, 1963.
2. Hurwitt, E.: A new absorbable hemostatic packing. ***Bulletin de la Societe Internationale de Chirurgle XXI*** (3):237–242, 1962.
3. Venn, R.: Reduction of postsurgical blood-replacement needs with SURGICEL hemostasis. ***Medical Times 93*** (10):1113–1116, 1965.
4. Miller, J., Ginsberg, M., McElfatrick, G., and H. Johnson: Clinical experience with oxidized regenerated cellulose. ***Experimental Medicine and Surgery 19*** (2–3):202–206, (June-Sept.) 1961.
5. Blau, S., Kanof, N., and L. Simonson: Absorbable hemostatic gauze SURGICEL in dermabrasions and dermatologic surgery. ***Acta Dermato-Venerelogica 40***:358–361, 1960.
6. Shea, P., Jr.: Management of the donor site: a new dressing technic ***Journal of the Medical Associaion of Georgia 51*** (9):437–440, 1962.
7. Denck, H.: Use of resorbable oxycellulose in surgery. ***Chirurg 33*** (11):486–488, 1962.
8. Tibbels, E., Jr.: Evaluation of a new method of epistaxis management ***Laryngoscope LXXIII*** (3):306–314, 1963.
9. Huggins, S.: Control of hemorrhage in otorhinolaryngologic surgery with oxidized regenerated cellulose. ***Eye, Ear, Nose and Throat Monthly 48*** (7): (July) 1969.
10. Crisp, W.E., Shalauta, H., and W.A. Bennett: Shallow conization of the cervix. ***Obstetrics and Gynecology 31*** (6):755–758, 1968.
11. Dineen, P.: Antibacterial activity of oxidized regenerated cellulose. ***Surgery, Gynecology and Obstetrics 142***:481–486, 1976.
12. Dineen, P.: The effect of oxidized regenerated cellulose on experimental intravascular infection. ***Surgery 82***:576–579, 1977.
13. Dineen, P.: The effect of oxidized regenerated cellulose on experimental infected splenotomies. ***Journal of Surgical Research 23***:114–116, 1977.

Materials Available: Free samples and clinical literature available to physicians. Call 800-526-2459.

KabiVitrum, Inc.
1311 HARBOR BAY PARKWAY
ALAMEDA, CA 94501

KABIKINASE® ℞
[*kă ′be-ki ″nās*]
(Streptokinase)

DESCRIPTION

KABIKINASE® (streptokinase) is a purified preparation of a bacterial protein elaborated by group C β-hemolytic streptococci. It is supplied as a water soluble white lyophilized powder for intravenous infusion following reconstitution and dilution. KABIKINASE® (streptokinase) contains 11.0 mg Sodium L-Glutamate and 14.5 mg Albumin Human per 100,000 IU of streptokinase as stabilizers.

HOW SUPPLIED

KABIKINASE® (streptokinase) is supplied as a lyophilized powder in 5 ml vials containing 250,000, 600,000 or 750,000 IU per vial of purified streptokinase, and shipped in cartons containing 10 vials.
In each vial there is a 10% overfill above that stated on the label. Each vial also contains 11.0 mg of Sodium L-Glutamate per 100,000 IU of streptokinase and 14.5 mg of Albumin Human per 100,000 IU of streptokinase as stabilizers.
250,000 IU NDC 0601-0110-59
600,000 IU NDC 0601-0110-67
750,000 IU NDC 0601-0119-35

RHESONATIV® ℞
[*rēson ′i-tiv*]
Rh_o(D) Immune Globulin (Human)

DESCRIPTION

Rhesonativ, Rh_o(D) Immune Globulin (Human) is a sterile lyophilized water soluble powder containing anti-Rh_o(D) for intramuscular injection following reconstitution.
It contains Human Immunoglobulin anti-Rh_o(D) 0.2 g, Glycine 70 mg and Sterile Water for Injection, USP 2 ml.
The immune globulin is prepared by a cold ethanol fractionation method from human venous plasma with a high anti-Rh_o(D) titre.
All plasma used in the manufacture of this product was tested for hepatitis B surface antigen (HBsAg) by a licensed third generation test and found to be nonreactive.
The content of IgA in Rhesonativ does not exceed 0.05% of the total protein content.
Rhesonativ contains no preservative and is thus free of mercury.

HOW SUPPLIED

Rhesonativ® is supplied in a package containing:
—Rhesonativ, 1 vial of sterile powder
—Sterile Water for Injection, USP 2 ml
—Package circular
NDC 0601-0107-05

EDUCATIONAL MATERIAL

Videocassettes
Streptokinase Therapy
An Interdisciplinary Approach
Intracoronary Administration Acute Myocardial Infarction
20 minute videocassette
Treatment of Deep Vein Thrombosis
20 minute videocassette

Kenwood Laboratories
a division of
BRADLEY PHARMACEUTICALS, INC.
383 ROUTE 46 WEST
FAIRFIELD, NJ 07006-2402

GLUTOFAC® Tablets

COMPOSITION

Each tablet contains: Saccharomyces Siccum (a selected Brewer's Yeast)—390 mg. (Contains Glucose Tolerance Factor—Chromium Complex)

		% U.S. RDA
Vitamin C (Ascorbic Acid)	250 mg.	416
Thiamine Hydrochloride (Vitamin B1)	15 mg.	1000
Riboflavin (Vitamin B2)	10 mg.	588
Niacinamide	50 mg.	250
Vitamin B6 (Pyridoxine Hydrochloride)	50 mg.	2500
Calcium Pantothenate	20 mg.	200
Magnesium Sulfate*	70 mg.	17
Zinc Sulfate+	80 mg.	533

*As 50 mg. Dried Magnesium Sulfate
+As 50 mg. Dried Zinc Sulfate

INDICATION

For patients with nutritional deficiencies resulting from diabetes mellitus, physiologic stress, alcoholism and for other acute and chronic depletional states.

DOSAGE

Adults: One (1) tablet three (3) times daily or as directed by a physician.

SUPPLIED

Bottles of 90 and 500.

I•L•X® B_{12} Elixir
Crystalline

COMPOSITION

Each three (3) teaspoonfuls (15cc) contains:

		% U.S. RDA
Elemental Iron (from Iron Ammonium Citrate, Brown)	102 mg.	566
Liver Fraction 1	98 mg.	
Thiamine Hydrochloride (Vitamin B1)	5 mg.	333
Riboflavin (Vitamin B2)	2 mg.	117
Nicotinamide	10 mg.	50
Vitamin B12 Crystalline (Cyanocobalamin)	10 mcg.	166

Alcohol 8% by Volume

ACTION AND USES

A readily assimilated hematinic elixir for oral therapy in the treatment or prevention of nutritional and iron deficiency anemias (hypochromic anemia).

ADMINISTRATION AND DOSAGE

As a hematinic. One (1) teaspoonful three (3) times daily or as directed by physician.

HOW SUPPLIED

12 ounce bottles.

I•L•X® B_{12} Tablets
Crystalline

COMPOSITION

Each tablet contains:

		% U.S. RDA
Elemental Iron (from Ferrous Gluconate 5 gr.)	38 mg.	211
Vitamin C	60 mg.	100
Cyanocobalamin (Vit. B12 Crystalline)	10 mcg.	166
Liver (Desiccated)	2 gr.	
Thiamine Hydrochloride (Vitamin B1)	2 mg.	133
Riboflavin (Vitamin B2)	2 mg.	118
Niacinamide	20 mg.	100

INDICATIONS

A readily assimilated oral hematinic for the treatment or prevention of nutritional and iron deficiency anemias (hypochromic anemia) such as those commonly seen in older patients, in convalescence from surgical procedures or medical diseases, and anemias of pregnancy.

ADMINISTRATION AND DOSAGE

Adults: One (1) tablet three (3) times a day after meals or as directed by physician.

HOW SUPPLIED

Bottles of 100.

The following are additional KENWOOD LABORATORIES products for which literature is available upon request:

Product Name	How Supplied
APATATE® Liquid (Therapeutic combination of B_1 and B_{12} with B_6 for nutritional supplementation)	4 oz. and 8 oz. bottles
BONACAL® PLUS Tablets (Prenatal formulation containing fat- and water-soluble vitamins, iron and minerals)	Bottles of 100
I•L•X® Elixir (High-potency hematinic; formulated with iron, liver and vitamins)	12 oz. bottles
KENWOOD THERAPEUTIC LIQUID (Non-alcoholic nutritional formulation of eight fat- and water-soluble vitamins and five minerals)	12 oz. bottles
POSTERISAN® Hemorrhoidal Ointment	25 gm. tubes
Hemorrhoidal Suppositories	Boxes of 10 and 20

Key Pharmaceuticals
GALLOPING HILL ROAD
KENILWORTH, NJ 07033

GENAPAX® ℞
(gentian violet) tampons

DESCRIPTION

Each **GENAPAX®** (gentian violet) tampon contains 5 mg of gentian violet, a topical antifungal, on the anterior portion of a conventional vaginal tampon. The structural formula of gentian violet ($C_{25}H_{30}ClN_3$); n-(4-bis(4-(dimethylamino)-phenyl)methylene-2, 5-cyclohexadien-1-ylidene)-N-methylmethanaminium chloride is as follows:
[See Chemical Formula at top of next column].

CLINICAL PHARMACOLOGY

GENAPAX provides a simple and effective mode of administration of gentian violet in the treatment of monilial vaginitis and eliminates the messiness associated with gentian violet solutions. **GENAPAX** tampons: 1) separate the walls of the vagina; 2) convey soluble medication to the cervix and to the surface of the vaginal vault; 3) keep medication in prolonged contact with vaginal mucosa; 4) provide for the absorption of exudates; and 5) serve as a mechanical barrier to prevent leakage. The mechanism of antifungal action of gentian violet is not known. No information is available on the systemic absorption of gentian violet following topical application.

INDICATIONS AND USAGE

GENEPAX is indicated in the treatment of vaginal infections caused by *Candida albicans*. The diagnosis should be confirmed by KOH smears and/or cultures. Other pathogens associated with vaginitis (*Trichomonis* and *Haemophilus vaginalis* [Gardnerella]) should be ruled out by appropriate methods.

CONTRAINDICATIONS

Patients known to be hypersensitive to gentian violet.

WARNINGS

Although topical gentian violet is usually well tolerated, the drug may cause irritation or sensitivity reactions. Discoloration of the skin may occur when gentian violet is applied to granulation tissue; therefore, the drug should not be used on ulcerative lesions.

Tampons are associated with Toxic Shock Syndrome (TSS). TSS is a rare but serious disease that may cause death. Please refer to Patient Package Insert for more information concerning TSS.

PRECAUTIONS

Do not use in the presence of extensive excoriation or ulceration. Patients should be advised to refrain from coitus during treatment.

Carcinogenesis, mutagenesis, and impairment of fertility: Long-term animal studies have not been performed to evaluate the carcinogenic potential, mutagenic potential, or the effect of gentian violet on fertility.

Pregnancy

Category C—Animal reproduction studies have not been conducted with gentian violet. It is not known whether gentian violet can cause fetal harm when administered to a pregnant woman or can affect reproductive capacity. Therefore, gentian violet is not recommended for use in pregnant women.

Nursing Mothers

Studies have not been performed to evaluate breast milk excretion, so caution should be exercised when **GENAPAX** is administered to a nursing woman.

DOSAGE AND ADMINISTRATION

Patients should be instructed to insert a **GENAPAX** tampon intravaginally for 3 to 4 hours, once or twice daily, for a period of 12 days. In resistant cases, use an additional **GENAPAX** overnight. **GENAPAX** tampons should be inserted in the same manner as the usual tampons utilized for menstrual hygiene. Treatment should be continued through menstruation. If infection persists, a second course of treatment may be required.

HOW SUPPLIED

GENAPAX (gentian violet) tampons are available in boxes of 12 tampons, each individually sealed. Store at 15–30°C (59–86°F).

NDC 0369-0046-12 0686
I004613

Key Pharmaceuticals, Inc.
Kenilworth, New Jersey 07033

INHAL-AID®

Drug Delivery System for Metered Dose Inhalers.

PRESCRIBING INFORMATION:

Inhal-Aid is a drug delivery system that helps deliver oral aerosolized medication from metered dose inhalers (MDIs) to the lungs. It can improve the delivery of these medications by making it simpler for patients to use them. Studies document that almost half of the patients who use MDIs use them incorrectly because they have difficulty coordinating inhalation with the fast release of medication from the MDI. This is a major factor limiting aerosol delivery to the airways. Inhal-Aid's collecting chamber holds the medication and allows patients to breathe medication through the mouthpiece without having to carefully time inhalation with activation of the MDI.

The incentive flow indicator provides a visual means of identifying inspiratory effort and sustained breathing via a sensitive float mechanism activated by the patient's negative inspiratory effort. The design is such that children can adequately perform the maneuver.

CAUTION

The usual caution should be exercised in dosing medications and evaluating patient response. The prescribing information for the marketed MDIs varies with respect to dosing, administration, etc. We recommend that these be followed when using Inhal-Aid.

INHAL-AID contains a clear plastic **collecting chamber** and can be utilized with any of the currently marketed metered-dose inhalers via a **universal adapter.** Connected at the end opposite the universal adapter is a T-tube with a **mouthpiece** on one end, a one-way valve on the other and a vertical **incentive indicator** (incentive spirometer device). The junction between the collecting chamber and the mouthpiece-containing T-tube also contains a **one-way valve.** Inhaling through the mouthpiece draws air through four small holes in the collecting chamber. The contents of the 700-ml collecting chamber are thus progressively inhaled with each successive inspiration by passing through the one-way valve in the collecting chamber through the mouthpiece and into the lungs. Exhaled air passes straight through the T-tube and out the one-way valve opposite the mouthpiece. The aerosol in the collecting chamber therefore leaves only during inhalation and cannot be blown out through the venting holes during exhalation.

NOTE: INHAL-AID should be replaced every 9–12 months or as needed. A prescription will be needed to obtain a new one.

Assembly Instructions

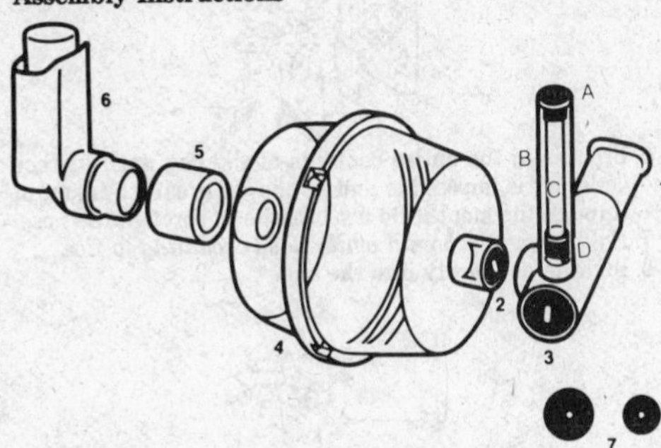

1. Mouthpiece and incentive indicator assembled.
   The incentive indicator has 4 parts:
   A. Orange cap
   B. Outer flow-tube
   C. Inner flow-tube
   D. Orange float
2. Small rubber valve.
3. Large rubber valve.
4. Collecting chamber (700 ml reservoir); the 2 parts are held together by prongs fitting into the 4 small openings.
5. Blue rubber "spray inhaler" adapter.
6. Typical "spray inhaler" and mouthpiece (not included).
7. Extra set of rubber valves. 8
8. Nose clips.

INHAL-AID is supplied partly assembled. The parts include:

— collecting chamber (4) with blue rubber "spray inhaler" (metered dose inhaler-MDI) adapter (5) attached
— mouthpiece with incentive indicator attached (1)
— package of extra rubber valves (7)
— nose clips (8)

Your patient should:

1. Remove the parts. Place the collecting chamber on a flat surface. Check to see that the small rubber valve (2) is firmly in place.

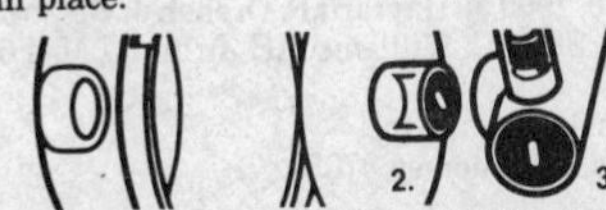

2. Connect the mouthpiece (with incentive indicator attached) to the opening that has the small rubber valve. Check to see that the large rubber valve (3) at the back of the mouthpiece is firmly in place.
3. Check the INHAL-AID. If it is assembled correctly, patients should be able to breathe freely and see the orange float go up to the top of the incentive indicator as they breathe in.
4. To administer the medication, connect the MDI with mouthpiece to the blue rubber adapter. The incentive indicator and MDI container must point upward. This is necessary for INHAL-AID to work properly.
5. INHAL-AID comes with nose clips for patients who may have trouble breathing **only** through their mouth.
6. The small and large rubber valves are needed for INHAL-AID to function properly. A package of extra valves is included in case the original set is damaged or lost.

DIRECTIONS FOR USE:

Your patient should:

1. Shake MDI and its mouthpiece before placing it straight into the blue rubber adapter as far as it will go. The incentive indicator and "spray inhaler" container should both point upward. The blue adapter has one side with a smaller opening and one side with a larger opening. The mouthpiece of the MDI should fit snugly.

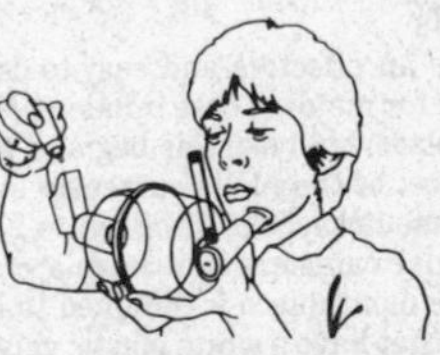

2. Place mouthpiece in mouth and close lips tightly around it.
3. Push the top of the MDI down with a finger while supporting the bottom with the thumb to release medication into the collecting chamber.

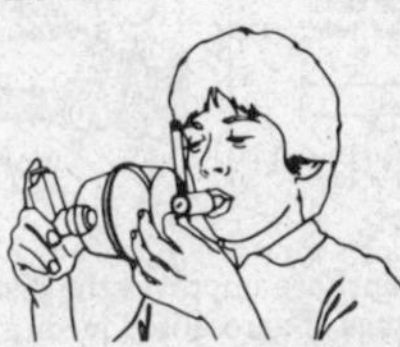

NOTE: Patients should be reminded of the correct dosage schedule.

4. **Breathe in slowly** through the mouthpiece. By teaching patients to **slowly raise** the orange float to the top of the incentive indicator and to keep it at the top as long as possible, they can improve the delivery of medication to their lungs.
5. **Once a breath is taken, hold while slowly counting to five,** when possible. This can help to increse the amount of medication that stays in the lungs.
6. Breathe out slowly **through** the mouthpiece. Do not remove the mouthpiece from the mouth.

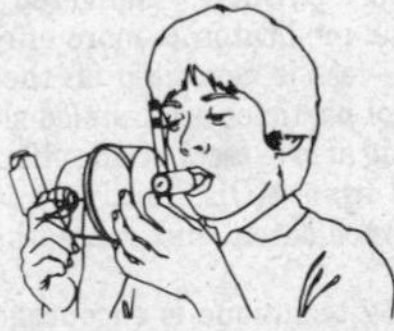

7. Repeat the breathing in and out steps (numbers 4, 5, 6) four more times keeping the lips closed tightly around the mouthpiece. This will help to get the medication from the collecting chamber.

IMPORTANT CLEANING INSTRUCTIONS

Your patient should:

1. Remove the incentive indicator unit from the mouthpiece. The incentive indicator should not be taken apart or washed.
2. Remove mouthpiece (with incentive indicator attached) from the collecting chamber.
3. Take the collecting chamber apart by holding each of the two halves and twisting to release the prongs while pulling apart. (To put the chamber back together, place the prongs into the small openings and snap closed.)
4. Rinse the INHAL-AID parts with **warm, not hot, water.** After rinsing, shake parts to remove most of the water and let air-dry in a clean dust-free area before reassembling. **Do not dry** near artificial heat source such as a dishwasher or oven.

NOTE: Inhal-Aid is designed for single-patient use and single-drug use. Even if the patient cannot exactly follow each step, the rising orange float (slowly moving it off the bottom of the incentive indicator) shows that medication is being delivered. Replace the Inhal-Aid every 9–12 months or as needed.

Children and other first time users should practice the breathing in and out steps before using the medication.

CAUTION: Federal law restricts this device to sale by or on the order of a physician.

Continued on next page

Key—Cont.

References

1. Sackner MA, Brown LK, Kim CS: *Chest 80* (suppl): 915–918, 1981. 2. Tobin MJ, Jenouri G, Danta I, et al; *Am Rev Respir Dis* 126:670–675, 1982. 3. Saunders KB: *Br. Med J* 1:1037–1038, 1965. 4. Gayrard P, Orehek J: *Respiration* 40:47–52, 1980. 5. Shim C, Williams MH Jr: *Am J. Med* 69:891–894, 1980

Revised 01/85

Key Pharmaceuticals, Inc.
Kenilworth, New Jersey 07033

INSPIREASE®
Drug delivery system for metered dose inhalers

Prescribing Information

DESCRIPTION

InspirEase™ is an effective and easy-to-use portable drug delivery system for metered dose inhalers (MDIs). Its components are a replaceable reservoir bag and two mouthpieces adaptable to most of the MDIs currently available.
The *light blue* mouthpiece is designed to be used with metered dose inhaler canisters that have a metal valve stem. The *darker blue* mouthpiece is designed to be used with inhaler canisters that have a white plastic valve stem. A carrying case is supplied for transporting and storing InspirEase and the MDI container.

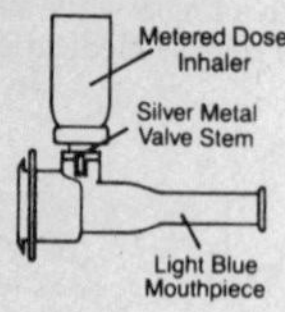

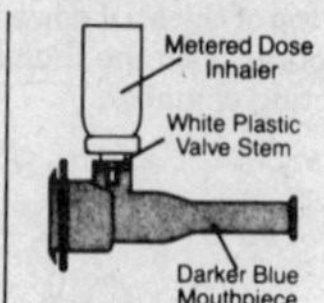

Indicatons: InspirEase improves the distribution and deposition in the lungs of aerosolized medication from MDIs.

1. Minimal patient skill is required for use.
A significant number of patients fail to derive full benefit from their MDIs. This is sometimes due to inadequate instruction or to misuse of the device by anxious, breathless patients. The correct use of an MDI requires greater skill than is immediately apparent.[1–5]
Studies have demonstrated that nearly 50% of patients had difficulty coordinating MDI activation with inspiration.[3–5] This is a major factor limiting aerosol delivery to the airways.[2] With MDIs alone, the patient has to carefully time each inspiraton with activation of the inhaler. InspirEase eliminates the need for the patient to coordinate inspiration with activation of the MDI.
2. Medicaton is more effectively delivered to the airways.
With InspirEase, medicaton is more effectively delivered to the airways—less is deposited on the oropharynx, because the aerosol particles are inhaled slowly and evenly. The reservoir bag acts as a collecting chamber for the medication emitted from MDIs. This permits the patient to calmly inhale medicaton and rebreathe with a second breath.
3. Proper breathing technique is encouraged.
InspirEase has visual and auditory signals to help patients assess the rate and depth of each inhalation. Slow, deep inspiration results in deflaton of the reservoir bag and *no* whistling sound. Rapid inspiration (greater than 0.3 L/s) produces a whistling sound from the flow rate monitor. This signals the patients to inhale more slowly. Patients can see and feel the bag collapsing.
The volume of the fully extended reservoir bag is approximately 700 ml, which is approximately 1½ to 2 times the average adult tidal volume.

CAUTION: The usual caution should be exercised in dosing medications and evaluating patient response. The prescribing information for the marketed MDIs varies with respect to dosing, administration, etc. We recommend that these be followed when using InspirEase.

Directions for Use:

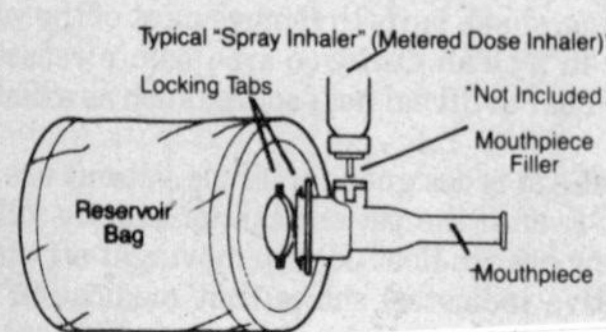

Your patient should:

1. Select the appropriate mouthpiece that fits his or her inhaler. Connect it to the reservoir bag by lining up *locking tabs*, pushing them into the bag and twisting clockwise to lock.

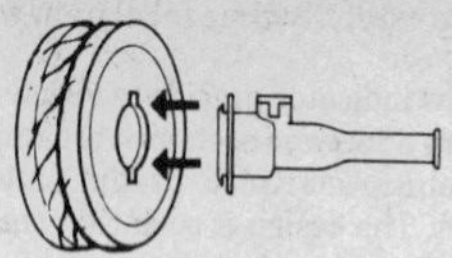

2. Untwist the reservoir bag gently to open it to its full size. Shake drug canister well before placing its stem into the *mouthpiece filler.* Make sure it fits snugly.

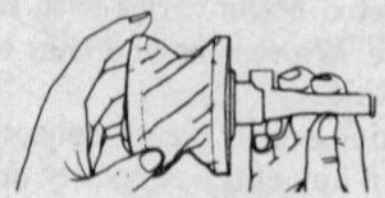

3. Place mouthpiece in mouth and close lips tightly around it.
4. Press down on drug canister to release one dose into the bag.
NOTE: Patients should be remined of the correct dosage schedule.

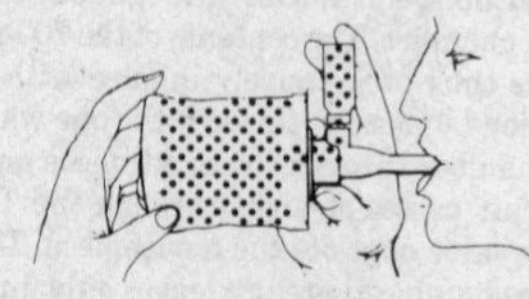

5. Breathe in slowly through the mouthpiece. If a whistling sound is produced, inhalation should be slowed until the sound stop.

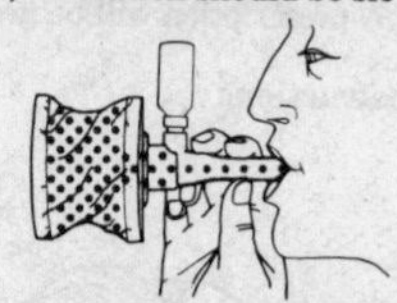

6. Breathe in the entire contents of the bag until further deflation is impossible and no more air can be taken in through the mouth. Do not breathe in through the nose.
7. *Hold his or her breath while slowly counting to five.*
8. Breathe out slowly into the bag.

9. Repeat the inhale/exhale cycle (steps 5 through 8) a second time, keeping lips tightly closed around the mouthpiece.
10. Remove the mouthpiece from mouth. Take drug canister off the reservoir bag. Unlock mouthpiece from the bag and store all components in carrying case.

IMPORTANT CLEANING INSTRUCTIONS

Your patients should:

1. Clean only the mouthpiece thoroughly, with warm (not hot) running water *at least* once a day. *InspirEase is not dishwasher safe. Always clean by hand.*
2. Wait until mouthpiece is *completely dry* before placing in carrying case.
3. Replace reservoir bags every two to three weeks, or as needed, depending on the rate of use. *However, if there is a hole or tear in it, replace immediately.*
4. Replace mouthpiece as needed or immediately if any part of the mouthpiece breaks.

NOTE: *InspirEase is designed for single-patient use and single-drug use.* Effectiveness in children below the age of 6 has not been established.

CAUTION: Federal law restricts this device to sale by or on the order of a physician.

Revised 01/85

REFERENCES

1. Sackner MA, Brown LK, Kim CS: *Chest* 80 (suppl): 915-918, 1981. **2.** Tobin MJ, Jenouri G, Danta I, et al: *Am Rev Respir Dis* 126:670-675, 1982. **3.** Saunders KB:*Br Med J* 1:1037-1038, 1965. **4.** Gayrard P, Orehek J: *Respiration* 40:47-52, 1980. **5.** Shim C, Williams MH Jr: *Am J Med* 69:891-894, 1980.

Key Pharmaceuticals, Inc.
Kenilworth, New Jersey 07033

IRCON®-FA ℞
[*ir ′kon*]

DESCRIPTION

IRCON-FA contains 1.0 mg of folic acid, and 250 mg of ferrous fumarate equivalent to 82 mg of elemental iron.

ACTIONS

IRCON-FA is a prenatal supplemental hematinic agent specifically intended for prophylaxis against two common types of anemia developing as a result of pregnancy. The use of prophylactic iron and prophylactic folic acid during pregnancy is well accepted. Child bearing (per pregnancy) has an iron "cost" of about 725 mg. It has been shown that 78 mg of elemental iron, taken orally each day during the last half of pregnancy, will protect against iron deficiency anemia; half this dose is insufficient to maintain iron stores. Two hundred fifty mg of ferrous fumarate contain approximately 82 mg of iron. Absorption characteristics of ferrous fumarate are identical to those of ferrous sulfate.
A deficiency of folic acid, typically during pregnancy, has long been known to cause a megaloblastic anemia, similar in some respects to Addisonian pernicious anemia. The vitamin is not storable in the body and the combination of fetal demand during pregnancy and misnourishment can lead to a deficiency, hence anemia. The average daily requirement of folic acid during pregnancy is unknown. It has been found that a dosage of 20 mcg/day is inadequate. In other instances doses of 1000 mcg/day orally have been found to produce a prompt hematological response in megaloblastic anemia of pregnancy.
Daily doses of folic acid greater than 1.0 mg/day have not been shown to be necessary, even in cases of overt folate deficiency anemia. The estimated minimum daily requirement for folic acid in late pregnancy when folate depletion is present is said to be greater than 200 mcg and possibly 400 mcg or more. IRCON-FA contains 1000 mcg. Folic acid is nontoxic and has commonly been given in several times this daily dose. Though folic acid dietary deficiency in the United States is rare, prophylaxis during pregnancy is considered to be justified in view of the possible serious consequences of its depletion, both for the mother (megaloblastic anemia) and the fetus.
Finally it has been observed that the rapid production of red blood cells following treatment with iron alone may deplete the body of folate if there is inadequate intake; combining the two substances avoids this complication.

INDICATIONS

For maintenance of maternal hematopoiesis during pregnancy, particularly when diet is abnormal or substandard.

CONTRAINDICATIONS

1) Pernicious anemia. Although rare in the population likely to receive IRCON-FA this megaloblastic anemia must be borne in mind. It is due to faulty or blocked absorption of vitamin B12, or extrinsic factor, on either a genetic, immunologic or surgical basis. The particular danger of missing a diagnosis of pernicious anemia–in relation to folic acid therapy–is that folic acid can mask PA by causing a hematologic remission while allowing the neurological complications of the disease to proceed apace. Thus, before IRCON-FA is prescribed for megaloblastic anemia in pregnancy, appropriate diagnostic exclusion of Addisonian pernicious anemia should be carried out.

2) Anemias other than those due to iron deficiency.

WARNING

Folic acid alone is improper therapy in the treatment of pernicious anemia and other megaloblastic anemias where vitamin B_{12} is deficient.

PRECAUTIONS

1) If, at the time of initial examination, definite anemia is found, a diagnosis of its cause should be made.

2) IRCON-FA is primarily intended to prevent the development of anemia due to a deficiency of either iron or folic acid by reason of the demands of pregnancy. It is not intended for the treatment of these disorders in fully developed form.

3) Blood examinations including hemoglobin and hematocrit should be done at the usual intervals to make certain that therapy is adequate.

4) Use with care in the presence of peptic ulcer, regional enteritis and ulcerative colitis.

5) Folic acid especially in doses above 1.0 mg daily may obscure pernicious anemia, in that hematologic remission may occur while neurological manifestations remain progressive.

ADVERSE REACTIONS

1) Ferrous fumarate gastric distress, abdominal cramps, diarrhea.

2) Folic acid allergic sensitization has been reported following both oral and parenteral administration of folic acid.

ADMINISTRATION AND DOSAGE

The usual dose in the second and third trimester of pregnancy is one tablet daily, taken in the morning between breakfast and lunch with a glass of water or milk. If hyperemesis gravidarum is a problem, the dose may be taken in mid-afternoon.

HOW SUPPLIED

IRCON-FA tablets are available in bottles of 100.

CAUTION

FEDERAL LAW PROHIBITS DISPENSING WITHOUT A PRESCRIPTION.

Revised 0286 I005604

Manufactured for
Key Pharmaceuticals, Inc.
Kenilworth, New Jersey 07033

K-DUR™ ℞

[*kay-dur*]
Microburst Release System™
(Potassium Chloride)
Sustained Release Tablets

DESCRIPTION

Each K-DUR™ 10 tablet contains 750 mg of potassium chloride (equivalent to 10 mEq).

Each K-DUR 20 tablet contains 1500 mg of potassium chloride (equivalent to 20 mEq).

K-DUR is an electrolyte replenisher. Its chemical name is potassium chloride, and its structural formula is KCl. Potassium chloride USP is a white, granular powder of colorless crystals. It is odorless and has a saline taste. Its solutions are neutral to litmus. It is freely soluble in water and insoluble in alcohol.

K-DUR is a tablet formulation (not enteric coated or wax matrix) containing individually coated potassium chloride crystals (micro-crystalloids) which disperse upon tablet disintegration. In simulated gastric fluid at 37°C and in the absence of outside agitation, K-DUR begins disintegrating into the micro-crystalloids within seconds and completely disintegrates within one minute. The micro-crystalloids are formulated to provide a controlled release of potassium chloride. The dispersibility of the micro-crystalloids is intended to minimize the possibility of a high local concentration near the gastrointestinal mucosa and the ability of the KCl to cause stenosis or ulceration.

Inactive Ingredients: Crospovidone, Ethylcellulose, Hydroxypropyl Cellulose, Magnesium Stearate, and Microcrystalline Cellulose.

CLINICAL PHARMACOLOGY

Potassium ion is the principal intracellular cation of most body tissues. Potassium ions participate in a number of essential physiological processes including the maintenance of intracellular tonicity, the transmission of nerve impulses, the contraction of cardiac, skeletal and smooth muscle and the maintenance of normal renal function. Potassium depletion may occur whenever the rate of potassium loss through renal excretion and/or loss from the gastrointestinal tract exceeds the rate of potassium intake. Such depletion usually develops slowly as a consequence of prolonged therapy with oral diuretics, primary or secondary hyperaldosteronism, diabetic ketoacidosis, severe diarrhea, or inadequate replacement of potassium in patients on prolonged parenteral nutrition.

Potassium depletion due to these causes is usually accompanied by a concomitant deficiency of chloride and is manifested by hypokalemia and metabolic alkalosis. Potassium depletion may produce weakness, fatigue, disturbances of cardiac rhythm (primarily ectopic beats), prominent U-waves in the electrocardiogram, and in advanced cases, flaccid paralysis and/or impaired ability to concentrate urine.

Potassium depletion associated with metabolic alkalosis is managed by correcting the fundamental cause of the deficiency whenever possible and administering supplemental potassium chloride, in the form of high potassium food or potassium chloride solution or tablets. In rare circumstances (e.g., patients with renal tubular acidosis) potassium depletion may be associated with metabolic acidosis and hyperchloremia. In such patients potassium replacement should be accomplished with potassium salts other than the chloride, such as potassium bicarbonate, potassium citrate, potassium acetate, or potassium gluconate.

INDICATIONS AND USAGE

BECAUSE OF REPORTS OF INTESTINAL AND GASTRIC ULCERATION AND BLEEDING WITH SLOW-RELEASE POTASSIUM CHLORIDE PREPARATIONS, THESE DRUGS SHOULD BE RESERVED FOR THOSE PATIENTS WHO CANNOT TOLERATE OR REFUSE TO TAKE LIQUID OR EFFERVESCENT POTASSIUM PREPARATIONS OR FOR PATIENTS IN WHOM THERE IS A PROBLEM OF COMPLIANCE WITH THESE PREPARATIONS.

1. For therapeutic use in patients with hypokalemia with or without metabolic alkalosis, in digitalis intoxication and in patients with hypokalemic familial periodic paralysis.
2. For the prevention of potassium depletion when the dietary intake is inadequate in the following conditions: Patients receiving digitalis and diuretics for congestive heart failure, hepatic cirrhosis with ascites, states of aldosterone excess with normal renal function, potassium-losing nephropathy, and with certain diarrheal states.
3. The use of potassium salts in patients receiving diuretics for uncomplicated essential hypertension is often unnecessary when such patients have a normal dietary pattern. Serum potassium should be checked periodically, however, and if hypokalemia occurs, dietary supplementation with potassium-containing foods may be adequate to control milder cases. In more severe cases supplementation with potassium salts may be indicated.

CONTRAINDICATIONS

Potassium supplements are contraindicated in patients with hyperkalemia since a further increase in serum potassium concentration in such patients can produce cardiac arrest. Hyperkalemia may complicate any of the following conditions: Chronic renal failure, systemic acidosis such as diabetic acidosis, acute dehydration, extensive tissue breakdown as in severe burns, adrenal insufficiency, or the administration of a potassium-sparing diuretic (e.g., spironolactone, triamterene).

Wax-matrix potassium chloride preparations have produced esophageal ulceration in certain cardiac patients with esophageal compression due to enlarged left atrium.

All solid dosage forms of potassium chloride supplements are contraindicated in any patient in whom there is cause for arrest or delay in tablet passage through the gastrointestinal tract. In these instances, potassium supplementation should be with a liquid preparation.

WARNINGS

Hyperkalemia—In patients with impaired mechanisms for excreting potassium, the administration of potassium salts can produce hyperkalemia and cardiac arrest. This occurs most commonly in patients given potassium by the intravenous route but may also occur in patients given potassium orally. Potentially fatal hyperkalemia can develop rapidly and be asymptomatic. The use of potassium salts in patients with chronic renal disease, or any other condition which impairs potassium excretion, requires particularly careful monitoring of the serum potassium concentration and appropriate dosage adjustment.

Interaction with Potassium Sparing Diuretics—Hypokalemia should not be treated by the concomitant administration of potassium salts and a potassium-sparing diuretic (e.g., spironolactone or triamterene) since the simultaneous administration of these agents can produce severe hyperkalemia.

Gastrointestinal Lesions—Potassium chloride tablets have produced stenotic and/or ulcerative lesions of the small bowel and deaths. These lesions are caused by a high localized concentration of potassium ion in the region of a rapidly dissolving tablet, which injures the bowel wall and thereby produces obstruction hemorrhage or perforation.

K-DUR tablets contain micro-crystalloids which disperse upon disintegration of the tablet. These micro-crystalloids are formulated to provide a controlled release of potassium chloride. The dispersibility of the micro-crystalloids and the controlled release of ions from them are intended to minimize the possibility of a high local concentration near the gastrointestinal mucosa and the ability of the KCl to cause stenosis or ulceration. Other means of accomplishing this (e.g., incorporation of potassium chloride into a wax matrix) have reduced the frequency of such lesions to less than one per 100,000 patient years (compared to 40–50 per 100,000 patient years with enteric-coated potassium chloride) but have not eliminated them. The frequency of GI lesions with K-DUR tablets is, at present, unknown. K-DUR tablets should be discontinued immediately and the possibility of bowel obstruction or perforation considered if severe vomiting, abdominal pain, distention, or gastrointestinal bleeding occurs.

Metabolic Acidosis—Hypokalemia in patients with metabolic acidosis should be treated with an alkalinizing potassium salt such as potassium bicarbonate, potassium citrate, potassium acetate, or potassium gluconate.

PRECAUTIONS

The diagnosis of potassium depletion is ordinarily made by demonstrating hypokalemia in a patient with a clinical history suggesting some cause for potassium depletion. In interpreting the serum potassium level, the physician should bear in mind that acute alkalosis per se can produce hypokalemia in the absence of a deficit in total body potassium while acute acidosis per se can increase the serum potassium concentration into the normal range even in the presence of a reduced total body potassium. The treatment of potassium depletion, particularly in the presence of cardiac disease, renal disease, or acidosis requires careful attention to acid-base balance and appropriate monitoring of serum electrolytes, the electrocardiogram, and the clinical status of the patient.

Information for Pateints: Physicians should consider reminding the patient of the following:

To take each dose without crushing, chewing, or sucking the tablets.

To take this medicine only as directed. This is especially important if the patient is also taking both diuretics and digitalis preparations.

To check with the physician if there is trouble swallowing tablets or if the tablets seem to stick in the throat.

To check with the doctor at once if tarry stools or other evidence of gastrointestinal bleeding is noticed.

Laboratory Tests: Regular serum potassium determinations are recommended. In addition, during the treatment of potassium depletion, careful attention should be paid to acid-base balance, other serum electrolyte levels, the electrocardiogram, and the clinical status of the patient, particularly in the presence of cardiac disease, renal disease, or acidosis.

Drug Interactions: Potassium-sparing diuretics; see WARNINGS.

Carcinogenesis, Mutagenesis, Impairment of Fertility: Long-term carcinogenicity studies in animals have not been performed.

Pregnancy Category C: Animal reproduction studies have not been conducted with K-DUR. It is also not known whether K-DUR can cause fetal harm when administered to a pregnant woman or can affect reproduction capacity. K-DUR should be given to a pregnant woman only if clearly needed.

Nursing Mothers: The normal potassium ion content of human milk is about 13 mEq per liter. Since oral potassium becomes part of the body potassium pool, so long as body potassium is not excessive, the contribution of potassium chloride supplementation should have little or no effect on the level in human milk.

Pediatric Use: Safety and effectiveness in children have not been established.

ADVERSE REACTIONS

One of the most severe adverse effects is hyperkalemia (see CONTRAINDICATIONS, WARNINGS, and OVERDOSAGE). There have also been reports of upper and lower gastrointestinal conditions including obstruction, bleeding, ulceration, and perforation (see CONTRAINDICATIONS and WARNINGS): other factors known to be associated with such conditions were present in many of these patients.

The most common adverse reactions to oral potassium salts are nausea, vomiting, abdominal discomfort, and diarrhea. These symptoms are due to irritation of the gastrointestinal tract and are best managed by taking the dose with meals or reducing the dose.

Skin rash has been reported rarely.

OVERDOSAGE

The administration of oral potassium salts to persons with normal excretory mechanisms for potassium rarely causes serious hyperkalemia. However, if excretory mechanisms are impaired or if potassium is administered too rapidly intravenously, potentially fatal hyperkalemia can result (see CONTRAINDICATIONS and WARNINGS). It is important to recognize that hyperkalemia is usually asymptomatic and may be manifested only by an increased serum potassium concentration and characteristic electrocardiographic changes (peaking of T-waves, loss of P-waves, depression of S-T segment, and prolongation of the QT-interval). Late manifestations include muscle-paralysis and cardiovascular collapse from cardiac arrest.

Treatment measures for hyperkalemia include the following:

1. Elimination of foods and medications containing potassium and of potassium-sparing diuretics.
2. Intravenous administration of 300 to 500 ml/hr of 10% dextrose solution containing 10–20 units of insulin per 1,000 ml.
3. Correction of acidosis, if present, with intravenous sodium bicarbonate.
4. Use of exchange resins, hemodialysis, or peritoneal dialysis.

In treating hyperkalemia, it should be recalled that in patients who have been stabilized on digitalis, too rapid a lowering of the serum potassium concentration can produce digitalis toxicity.

DOSAGE AND ADMINISTRATION

The usual dietary intake of potassium by the average adult is 40 to 80 mEq per day. Potassium depletion sufficient to cause hypokalemia usually requires the loss of 200 or more mEq of potassium from the total body store.

Dosage must be adjusted to the individual needs of each patient but is typically in the range of 20 mEq per day for the prevention of hypokalemia to 40–100 mEq per day or more for the treatment of potassium depletion.

If more than 2 K-DUR 10 mEq tablets or 1 K-DUR 20 mEq tablet is prescribed per day, the total daily dosage should be divided into two or more separate doses and any single dose should not exceed 20 mEq.

Tablets should be taken with a glass of water or other liquid.

Continued on next page

Key—Cont.

	FOR PREVENTION	FOR TREATMENT
K-DUR™ Tablets (10 mEq)	2 tablets per day (20 mEq)	4–10 tablets per day (40–100 mEq)
K-DUR™ Tablets (20 mEq)	1 tablet per day (20 mEq)	2–5 tablets per day (40–100 mEq)

CAUTION

Federal law prohibits dispensing without prescription.

HOW SUPPLIED

K-DUR 10 mEq
(NDC 0369-0010-01) Sustained Release Tablets are available in bottles of 100. K-DUR 10 mEq tablets are white, oblong, imprinted Key 10.
K-DUR 20 mEq
(NDC 0369-0020-01) Sustained Release Tablets are available in bottles of 100. K-DUR 20 mEq tablets are white, oblong, imprinted Key 20 and scored for flexibility of dosing.

STORAGE CONDITIONS

Keep tightly closed. Store at controlled room temperature 15–30°C (59–86°F).
I002000 06/86

Shown in Product Identification Section, page 411

NITRO–DUR® ℞

[*nī'tra-dur*]
(nitroglycerin)
Transdermal Infusion System

DESCRIPTION

The Nitro-Dur Transdermal Infusion System contains nitroglycerin in a gel-like matrix composed of glycerin, water (purified), lactose, polyvinyl alcohol, povidone and sodium citrate to provide a continuous source of the active ingredient. Nitro-Dur is available in dosage strengths which deliver 5mg /24 hrs (10cm^2), and 10 mg/24 hrs (20cm^2), containing 51 mg, and 104 mg of nitroglycerin, respectively, thereby providing a range of dosing levels of nitroglycerin. The excess nitroglycerin remains in the system and serves as the reservoir to facilitate release of the drug. The rated release of the drug is dependent upon the area of the system; approximately 0.5 mg nitroglycerin is released for every cm^2 of system size per 24 hours. Each unit is sealed in polyester-foil-polyethylene laminate. The bandage portion consists of a medical grade non-woven, heat sealable, microporous tape.

CLINICAL PHARMACOLOGY

When the Nitro-Dur system is applied to the skin, nitroglycerin is absorbed continuously through the skin into the systemic circulation. This results in active drug reaching the target organs (heart, extremities) before deactivation by the liver. Nitroglycerin is a smooth muscle relaxant with vascular effects manifested predominantly by venous dilation and pooling. The major beneficial effect of nitroglycerin in angina pectoris is a reduction in myocardial oxygen consumption secondary to vascular smooth muscle relaxation with resultant reduction in cardiac preload and afterload. In recent years there has been an increasing recognition of a direct vasodilator effect of nitroglycerin on the coronary vessels.

In a bioavailability study using healthy volunteers[1], transdermal absorption of nitroglycerin from Nitro-Dur achieved steady state venous plasma levels, and maintained these levels for 24 hours. Detectable plasma levels were attained within 30 minutes after application of the system, and were still detectable 30 minutes after removal of the system. Precise definition of "therapeutic plasma level" is not known at this time. The amount of nitroglycerin released (5 mg, or 10 mg per 24 hours) represents the mean release rate of nitroglycerin from the system as determined from healthy volunteers, and hence, the amount potentially available for absorption through the skin. Absorption will vary among individuals.

INDICATIONS AND USAGE

This drug product has been conditionally approved by the FDA for the prevention and treatment of angina pectoris due to coronary artery disease. The conditional approval reflects a determination that the drug may be marketed while further investigation of its effectiveness is undertaken. A final evaluation of the effectiveness of the product will be announced by the FDA.

CONTRAINDICATIONS

Intolerance of organic nitrate drugs, marked anemia.

WARNINGS

The Nitro-Dur system should be used under careful clinical and/or hemodynamic monitoring in patients with acute myocardial infarction or congestive heart failure.
In terminating treatment of anginal patients, both the dosage and frequency of application must be gradually reduced over a period of 4 to 6 weeks in order to prevent sudden withdrawal reactions, which are characteristic of all vasodilators in the nitroglycerin class.

PRECAUTIONS

Symptoms of hypotension, such as faintness, weakness or dizziness, particularly orthostatic hypotension, may be due to overdosage. If during the course of treatment these symptoms occur, the dosage should be reduced or use of the product discontinued.
Nitro-Dur is not intended for use in the treatment of acute anginal attacks. For this purpose, occasional use of sublingual nitroglycerin may be necessary.
Pregnancy: Pregnancy Category C. Animal reproduction studies have not been conducted with Nitro-Dur. It is also not known whether nitroglycerin can cause fetal harm when administered to a pregnant woman or can affect reproduction capacity. Nitroglycerin should be given to a pregnant woman only if clearly needed.
Nursing Mothers: It is not known whether nitroglycerin is excreted in human milk. Because many drugs are excreted in human milk, caution should be exercised when Nitro-Dur is administered to a nursing woman.

ADVERSE REACTIONS

Transient headache is the most common side effect, especially when higher doses of the drug are administered. Headaches should be treated with mild analgesics while continuing Nitro-Dur therapy. If headache persists, the Nitro-Dur dosage should be reduced or use of the product discontinued.
Adverse reactions reported less frequently include hypotension, increased heart rate, faintness, flushing, dizziness, nausea, vomiting, and dermatitis. Except for dermatitis, these symptoms are attributed to the pharmacologic effects of nitroglycerin. However, they may be symptoms of overdosage. When they persist, the Nitro-Dur dosage should be reduced or use of the product discontinued.

DOSAGE AND ADMINISTRATION

To apply the Nitro-Dur system, tear away the printed foil surface, then peel away the sectioned release liner as you would an adhesive bandage. Apply the Nitro-Dur system firmly to the skin surface. The initial starting dose is usually 5.0 mg/24 hrs (10cm^2 system). To achieve optimum therapeutic effect in some patients, it may be necessary to titrate to a higher dosing strength.
Dosage should be titrated while monitoring clinical response, i.e., blood pressure, episodes of angina and subsequent use of sublingual nitroglycerin. The Nitro-Dur system may remain in place for periods up to 24 hours as required to provide continuous levels of nitroglycerin.
The Nitro-Dur system may be applied to any convenient skin area; a recommended site of application is the arm or chest. A suitable area may be shaved if necessary. Do not apply the Nitro-Dur system to the distal part of the extremities.

STORAGE CONDITIONS

Store at controlled room temperature 15–30°C (59–86°F). Do not refrigerate.

HOW SUPPLIED

Nitro-Dur Transdermal Infusion System, 5mg/24 hrs (10cm^2), and 10 mg/24 hrs (20cm^2) is available in unit dose packages of 28.

CAUTION

Federal law prohibits dispensing without prescription.

PATIENT INSTRUCTIONS FOR APPLICATION

Patient Instructions are furnished with each unit dose package.

Revised 0886

[1]Data on file: Key Pharmaceuticals
Kenilworth, New Jersey 07033

NITRO–DUR® II ℞

[*nī'tra-dur*]
(nitroglycerin)
Transdermal Infusion System

DESCRIPTION

The NITRO-DUR® II Transdermal Infusion System contains nitroglycerin in acrylic-based polymer adhesives with a resinous cross-linking agent to provide a continuous source of the active ingredient. NITRO-DUR II is available in dosage strengths which deliver 2.5mg/24 hrs (5cm^2), 5mg/24 hrs (10cm^2), 7.5mg/24 hrs (15cm^2), 10mg/24 hrs (20cm^2) and 15mg/24 hrs (30cm^2), containing 20mg, 40mg, 60mg, 80mg, and 120mg of nitroglycerin, respectively, thereby providing a range of dosing levels of nitroglycerin. The excess nitroglycerin remains in the system and serves as the reservoir to facilitate release of the drug. The rated release of the drug is dependent upon the area of the system, approximately 0.5mg nitroglycerin is released for every cm^2 of system size per 24 hours.
Each unit is sealed in a paper-polyethylene-foil pouch.

CLINICAL PHARMACOLOGY

When the NITRO-DUR II system is applied to the skin, nitroglycerin is absorbed continuously through the skin into the systemic circulation. This results in active drug reaching the target organs (heart, extremities) before deactivation by the liver. Nitroglycerin is a smooth muscle relaxant with vascular effects manifested predominantly by venous dilation and pooling. The major beneficial effect of nitroglycerin in angina pectoris is a reduction in myocardial oxygen consumption secondary to vascular smooth muscle relaxation with resultant reduction in cardiac preload and afterload.
In recent years there has been an increasing recognition of a direct vasodilator effect of nitroglycerin on the coronary vessels.
In a bioavailability study using healthy volunteers[1], transdermal absorption of nitroglycerin from NITRO-DUR II achieved steady state venous plasma levels, and maintained these levels for 24 hours. Detectable plasma levels were attained within 30 minutes after application of the system, and were still detectable 30 minutes after removal of the system. Precise definition of "therapeutic plasma level" is not known at this time. The amount of nitroglycerin released (2.5mg, 5mg, 7.5mg, 10mg or 15mg per 24 hours) represents the mean release rate of nitroglycerin from the system as determined from healthy volunteers, and hence, the amount potentially available for absorption through the skin. Absorption will vary among individuals.

INDICATIONS AND USAGE

This drug product has been conditionally approved by the FDA for the prevention and treatment of angina pectoris due to coronary artery disease. The conditional approval reflects a determination that the drug may be marketed while further investigation of its effectiveness is undertaken. A final evaluation of the effectiveness of the product will be announced by the FDA.

CONTRAINDICATIONS

Intolerance of organic nitrate drugs, marked anemia.

WARNINGS

The NITRO-DUR II system should be used under careful clinical and/or hemodynamic monitoring in patients with acute myocardial infarction or congestive heart failure.
In terminating treatment of anginal patients, both the dosage and frequency of application must be gradually reduced over a period of 4 to 6 weeks in order to prevent sudden withdrawal reactions, which are characteristic of all vasodilators in the nitroglycerin class.

PRECAUTIONS

Symptoms of hypotension, such as faintness, weakness or dizziness, particularly orthostatic hypotension, may be due to overdosage. If during the course of treatment these symptoms occur, the dosage should be reduced or use of the product discontinued.
NITRO-DUR II is not intended for use in the treatment of acute anginal attacks. For this purpose, occasional use of sublingual nitroglycerin may be necessary.
Pregnancy:
Pregnancy Category C. Animal reproduction studies have not been conducted with NITRO-DUR II. It is also not known whether nitroglycerin can cause fetal harm when administered to a pregnant woman or can affect reproduction capacity. Nitroglycerin should be given to a pregnant woman only if clearly needed.
Nursing Mothers:
It is not known whether nitroglycerin is excreted in human milk. Because many drugs are excreted in human milk, caution should be exercised when NITRO-DUR II is administered to a nursing woman.

ADVERSE REACTIONS

Transient headache is the most common side effect, especially when higher doses of the drug are administered. Headaches should be treated with mild analgesics while continuing NITRO-DUR II therapy. If headache persists, the NITRO-DUR II dosage should be reduced or use of the product discontinued.
Adverse reactions reported less frequently include hypotension, increased heart rate, faintness, flushing, dizziness, nausea, vomiting, and dermatitits. Except for dermatitis, these symptoms are attributed to the pharmacologic effects of nitroglycerin. However, they may be symptoms of overdosage. When they persist, the NITRO-DUR II dosage should be reduced or use of the product discontinued.

DOSAGE AND ADMINISTRATION

To apply the NITRO-DUR II system, tear open the printed pouch and remove the unit. With the clear side and brown lines facing you, bend the unit away from you to break open the plastic along the brown line. Peel away both halves of the plastic starting at the brown line. Apply the NITRO-DUR II system firmly to the skin surface. The initial starting dose is usually 5mg/24 hrs (10cm^2 system). To achieve optimum therapeutic effect in some patients, it may be necessary to titrate to a higher dosing strength.

Dosage should be titrated while monitoring clinical response, i.e., blood pressure, episodes of angina and subsequent use of sublingual nitroglycerin. A 2.5 mg/24 hrs (5cm^2 system) dose is useful principally for decreasing the dosage gradually, though it may provide adequate therapy for some patients when used alone. The NITRO-DUR II system may remain in place for periods up to 24 hours as required to provide continuous levels of nitroglycerin.

The NITRO-DUR II system may be applied to any convenient skin area; a recommended site of application is the arm or chest. A suitable area may be shaved if necessary. Do not apply the NITRO-DUR II system to the distal part of the extremities.

STORAGE CONDITIONS

Store at controlled room temperature 15°-30°C (59°-86°F). Do not refrigerate.

HOW SUPPLIED

NITRO-DUR II Transdermal Infusion System, 2.5mg/24 hrs (5cm^2), 5mg/24 hrs (10cm^2), 7.5mg/24 hrs (15cm^2), 10mg/24 hrs (20cm^2) and 15mg/24 hrs (30cm^2), is avaiable in unit dose packages of 30, and hospital unit dose packages of 100.

CAUTION

Federal law prohibits dispensing without prescription.

PATIENT INSTRUCTIONS FOR APPLICATION

Patient instructions are furnished with each unit dose package.

[1]Data on file: Key Pharmaceuticals, Inc.
Miami, Florida (U.S.A.) 33137

Revised 0585 EDP# 1030150

Shown in Product Identification Section, page 411

NITROGLYN® ℞

[nī'tra-glin]
(nitroglycerin)
sustained release capsules

DESCRIPTION

Nitroglycerin, an organic nitrate, is a vasodilator which has effects on both arteries and veins. The chemical name for nitroglycerin is 1,2,3 propanetriol trinitrate ($C_3H_5N_3O_9$). The compound has a molecular weight of 227.09. The chemical structure is:

$$\begin{array}{l} CH_2—ONO_2 \\ | \\ CH\ —ONO_2 \\ | \\ CH_2—ONO_2 \end{array}$$

M.W. 227.09

Each Nitroglyn® controlled-release (capsule) contains:
2.5 mg nitroglycerin in a special base for prolonged therapeutic effect.
6.5 mg nitroglycerin in a special base for prolonged therapeutic effect.
9 mg nitroglycerin in a special base for prolonged therapeutic effect.

CLINICAL PHARMACOLOGY

The principal pharmacological action of nitroglycerin is relaxation of vascular smooth muscle, producing a vasodilator effect on both peripheral arteries and veins with more predominant effects on the latter. Dilation of the post-capillary vessels, including large veins, promotes peripheral pooling of blood and decreases venuous return to the heart, thereby reducing left ventricular end-diastolic pressure (preload). Arteriolar relaxation reduces systemic vascular resistance and arterial pressure (after-load).

The mechanism by which nitroglycerin relieves angina pectoris is not fully understood. Myocardial oxygen consumption or demand (as measured by the pressure-rate product, tension time index, and stroke work index) is decreased by both the arterial and venuous effects of nitroglycerin and, presumably, a more favorable supply-demand ratio is achieved. While the large epicardial coronary arteries are also dilated by nitroglycerin, the extent to which this action contributes to relief of exertional angina is unclear.

Nitroglycerin is rapidly metabolized in vivo , with a liver reductase enzyme having primary importance in the formation of glycerol nitrate metabolites and inorganic nitrate. Two active major metabolites, 1-2 and 1-3 dinitroglycerols, the products of hydrolysis, although less potent as vasodilators, have longer plasma half-lives than the parent compound, and appear in substantial concentration. The dinitrates are further metabolized to mononitrates (considered biologically inactive with respect to cardiovascular effects) and ultimately glycerol and carbon dioxide. There is extensive first-pass deactivation by the liver of nitroglycerin following gastrointestinal absorption, but the hepatic reductase activity may be saturated by some doses of oral nitroglycerin, resulting in prolonged pharmacologic effects. Hemodynamic studies employing plethysmographic methods in human volunteers have demonstrated that oral nitroglycerin (single dose 6.5 mg) has biologic effects significantly different from placebo for up to 8 hours.

Adequate studies defining the pharmacokinetics of Nitroglyn® Sustained Release Capsules have not been reported. The clinical relevance of nitroglycerin blood levels has not been established, since therapeutic levels of the drug and metabolites have not been defined. Therapeutic doses of nitroglycerin reduce systolic and mean arterial blood pressures, especially when the patient assumes upright posture. Systolic blood pressure is decreased for up to 4 hours after a single dose of 6.5 mg of swallowed controlled release nitroglycerin.

Clinical studies indicate that oral controlled-release nitroglycerin may reduce abnormally elevated left ventricular end-diastolic pressure (LVEDP), a hemodynamic occurrence during acute episodes of angina pectoris. Although there have been no reported, invasively measured, hemodynamic studies of (Nitroglycerin S.R. Capsule) in patients with angina pectoris, controlled clinical trials in patients with congestive heart failure have shown significant decreases in mean LVEDP for as long as 4 hours after a single dose (6.5–19.5 mg) of oral nitroglycerin. The onset of hemodynamic effect from the swallowed form of nitroglycerin is not sufficiently rapid to be of use in aborting an acute episode of angina pectoris.

INDICATIONS AND USAGE

Nitroglyn® Sustained Release Capsules are indicated for the prevention of angina pectoris due to coronary artery disease. Controlled clinical trials have demonstrated that this form of nitroglycerin is effective in improving exercise tolerance in patients with exertional angina pectoris. Controlled clinical studies of 2.6 mg and larger (6.5–26 mg) doses in patients with angina pectoris have shown improvement in treadmill exercise time for at least 4 hours after dosing.

CONTRAINDICATIONS

Nitroglyn® is contraindicated in patients who have shown purported hypersensitivity or idiosyncrasy to it or other nitrates or nitrites.

WARNINGS

The use of any form of nitroglycerin during the early days of acute myocardial infarction requires particular attention to hemodynamic monitoring and clinical status. In general, a long-acting dosage form such as Nitroglyn® Sustained Release Capsules should not be used because its effects are difficult to terminate rapidly should excessive hypotension or tachycardia develop.

PRECAUTIONS

General: Severe hypotension, particularly with upright posture, may occur even with small doses of nitroglycerin. The drug therefore should be used with caution in subjects who may have volume depletion from diuretic therapy or in patients who have low systolic blood pressure (e.g, below 90 mm Hg). Paradoxical bradycardia and increased angina pectoris may accompany nitroglycerin-induced hypotension. Nitrate therapy may aggravate the angina caused by hypertrophic cardiomyopathy.

Tolerance to this drug and cross-tolerance to other nitrates and nitrites may occur. Tolerance to the vascular and antianginal efects of nitrates has been demonstrated in clinical trials, experience through occupational exposure, and in isolated tissue experiments in the laboratory.

The importance of tolerance to the use of nitroglycerin in the management of patients with angina pectoris has not been determined. In controlled clinical trials in patients with angina pectoris, sustained therapy with some nitrate preparations resulted in significantly less and shorter duration of improvement in exercise time on stress testing than did acute therapy. However, a controlled study of repetitive doses of oral nitroglycerin showed treadmill performance to be significantly better with drug than with placebo in 18 patients with angina pectoris after 2 weeks of therapy.

In industrial workers continuously exposed to nitroglycerin, tolerance clearly occurs. Moreover, physical dependence also occurs since chest pain, acute myocardial infarction, and even sudden death have occured during temporary withdrawal of nitroglycerin from the workers. In various clinical trials in angina patients, there are reports of anginal attacks being more easily provoked and of rebound in the hemodynamic effects soon after nitrate withdrawal. The relative importance of these observations to the routine, clinical use of nitroglycerin is not known. However, it seems prudent to gradually withdraw patients from nitroglycerin when the therapy is being terminated, rather than stopping the drug abruptly.

Drug Interactions: Alcohol may enhance sensitivity to the hypotensive effects of nitrates.

Nitroglyn® acts directly on vascular muscle. Therefore, any other agents that depend on vascular smooth muscle as the final common path can be expected to have decreased or increased effect depending upon the agent.

Marked symptomatic orthostatic hypotension has been reported when calcium channel blockers and oral controlled-release nitroglycerin were used in combination. Dose adjustments of either class of agents may be necessary.

Carcinogenesis, Mutagenesis, Impairment of Fertility: No long-term studies in animals have been performed to evaluate carcinogenic potential of Nitroglyn® Sustained Release Capsules.

Pregnancy: Pregnancy Category C. Animal reproduction studies have not been conducted with Nitroglyn® Sustained Release Capsules. It is also not known whether nitroglycerin can cause fetal harm when administered to a pregnant woman or can affect reproduction capacity. Nitroglyn® should be given to a pregnant woman only if clearly needed.

Nursing Mothers: It is not known whether nitroglycerin is excreted in human milk. Because many drugs are excreted in human milk, caution should be exercised when (Nitroglyn® Sustained Release Capsule) is administered to a nursing woman.

Pediatric Use: Safety and effectiveness in children have not been established.

ADVERSE REACTIONS

Adverse reactions to Nitroglyn® Sustained Release Capsules, particularly headache and hypotension, are generally dose-related. In clinical trials at various doses of nitroglycerin, the following adverse effects have been observed:

Headache, which may be severe and persistent, is the most commonly reported side effect of nitroglycerin, with an incidence in the order of about 50% in some studies. Cutaneous vasodilation with flushing may occur. Transient episodes of dizziness and weakness, as well as other signs of cerebral ischemia associated with postural hypotension, may occasionally develop. An occasional individual may exhibit marked sensitivity to the hypotensive effects of nitrates and severe responses (nausea, vomiting, weakness, restlessness, pallor, perspiration, and collapse) may occur even with therapeutic doses of nitrates. Drug rash and/or exfoliative dermatitis have been reported in patients receiving nitrate therapy. Nausea and vomiting appear to be uncommon.

OVERDOSAGE

Signs and Symptoms: Nitrate overdosage may result in: severe hypotension, persistant throbbing headache, vertigo, palpitation, visual disturbance, flushing and perspiring skin (later becoming cold and cyanotic), nausea and vomiting (possibly with colic and even bloody diarrhea), syncope (especially in the upright posture), methemoglobinemia with cyanosis and anorexia, initial hyperpnea, dyspnea and slow breathing, slow pulse (dicrotic and intermittent), heart block, increased intracranial pressure with cerebral syptoms of confusion and moderate fever, paralysis and coma followed by chronic convulsions, and possibly death due to circulatory collapse.

Treatment of Overdosage: Keep the patient recumbent in a shock position and confortably warm. Gastric lavage may be of use if the medication has only recently been swallowed. Passive movement of the extremities may aid venuous return. Administer oxygen and artificial ventilation if necessary. If methemoglobinemia is present, administration of methylene blue (1% solution), 1–2 mg/kg intravenously, may be required.

Methemoglobin: Case reports of clinically significant methemoglobinemia are rare at conventional doses of organic nitrates. The formation of methemoglobin is dose-related and in the case of genetic abnormalities of hemoglobin that favor methemoglobin formation, even conventional doses of organic nitrates could produce harmful concentrations of methemoglobin.

WARNING

Epinephrine is ineffective in reversing the severe hypotensive events associated with overdose. It and related compounds are contraindicated in this situation.

DOSAGE AND ADMINISTRATION

The usual starting dose for Nitroglyn® Sustained Release Capsules is (2.5 mg or 2.6 mg) taken 3 or 4 times daily.

Controlled trials have been carried out to 5 hours after dosing; therefore, it is not known whether the drug is effective in prevention of exertional angina beyond 5 hours after dosing.

Nitroglyn® Sustained Release Capsules should be TITRATED upward until a dose effective in controlling angina is determined or until side effects limit the dose. The dose generally may be increased by (2.5 or 2.6) mg increments 2 to 4 times daily over a period of days or weeks. Doses as high as 26 mg given 4 times daily have been reported effective in angina pectoris patients.

Continued on next page

Key—Cont.

Administer the smallest effective dose 3 to 4 times daily unless clinical response suggests a different regimen. At initiation of therapy or change in dosage, the blood pressure (patient standing) should be monitored.
Nitroglyn® Sustained Release Capsules must be swallowed. They are NOT FOR CHEWING OR FOR SUBLINGUAL USE. Nitroglyn® Sustained Release Capsules are not intended for immediate relief of anginal attacks.

HOW SUPPLIED

Nitroglyn® Sustained Release Capsules 2.5 mg are available in bottles of 100 capsules.
Nitroglyn® Sustained Release Capsules 6.5 mg are available in bottles of 100 capsules.
Nitroglyn® Sustained Release Capsules 9 mg are available in bottles of 100 capsules.

CAUTION

Federal law prohibits dispensing without prescription.

STORAGE

Store at a controlled room temperature—15–30°C (59°–86°F). Dispense only in the original unopened container.

Revised: 4/85
Distributed By:
KEY PHARMACEUTICALS, INC.
Kenilworth, New Jersey 07033
Manufactured By:
KV PHARMACEUTICAL COMPANY
St. Louis, Missouri 63144

QUINORA® ℞

[*kwin-ō-ra*]
(quinidine sulfate tablets, USP)

DESCRIPTION

Quinora contains quinidine sulfate with no color additives in the base. Quinidine sulfate occurs as minute needle-like white crystals (frequently cohering in masses) or fine white powder. It is odorless, has a very bitter taste, and darkens on exposure to light. It is slightly soluble in water, soluble in alcohol and in chloroform, and insoluble in ether.
Quinidine sulfate is the sulfate salt of quinidine (6-methoxy-(5-vinyl-2 quinuclidinyl)-4-quinoline-methanol), a dextrorotatory isomer of quinine.
M.W. = 799.95
Each **Quinora** 300 mg tablet contains 300 mg quinidine sulfate (equivalent to 264 mg of quinidine base).

CLINICAL PHARMACOLOGY

Quinidine is generally regarded as a myocardial depressant because it decreases myocardial excitability, conduction velocity and contractility of the myocardium. Besides these direct effects, quinidine exerts some indirect activity on the heart through an anticholinergic action. Large oral doses may reduce the arterial pressure by means of peripheral vasodilation. Hypotension of a serious degree is more likely with the parenteral use of the drug.
Quinidine is rapidly absorbed from the gastrointestinal tract. The peak concentrations in plasma are attained in 60 to 90 minutes and activity persists 6 to 8 hours or more. Quinidine is metabolized in the liver and excreted by the kidney. Ten to 50% of quinidine is excreted in the urine as unchanged drug within 24 hours.
Plasma levels of quinidine can be measured. Values vary according to the assay employed. Traditionally, plasma concentrations for effective use of quinidine have been reported to range from 2–7 mcg/ml, and levels of 8 mcg/ml or greater are associated with toxicity. The information is based upon less specific analytic methods which quantitate metabolites as well as intact quinidine. However, plasma quinidine concentrations will be lower using more specific assays. Therefore, clinicians requesting serum quinidine determinations should be aware of the method of analysis. There is a wide individual variation in response to quinidine therapy. In all cases, the physician should carefully consider patient response and evidence of toxicity along with blood levels in determining optimal quinidine therapy.

INDICATIONS AND USAGE

Quinidine sulfate is indicated in the treatment of:
1. Premature atrial and ventricular contractions
2. Paroxysmal atrial tachycardia
3. Paroxysmal atrioventricular (AV) junctional rhythm
4. Atrial flutter
5. Paroxysmal atrial fibrillation
6. Established atrial fibrillation when therapy is appropriate
7. Paroxysmal ventricular tachycardia when not associated with complete heart block
8. Maintenance therapy after electrical conversion of atrial fibrillation and/or flutter.

CONTRAINDICATIONS

Hypersensitivity or idiosyncrasy to the drug, history of thrombocytopenic purpura associated with previous quinidine administration, digitalis intoxication manifested by AV conduction disorders, complete AV block with an AV nodal or idioventricular pacemaker, left bundle branch block or other severe intraventricular conduction defects with marked QRS widening. Ectopic impulses and abnormal rhythms due to escape mechanisms. Also, myasthenia gravis.

WARNINGS

In the treatment of atrial flutter, reversion to sinus rhythm may be preceded by a progressive reduction in the degree of AV block to a 1:1 ratio, which results in extremely rapid ventricular rate. This possible hazard may be decreased by digitalization prior to administration of quinidine.
In susceptible individuals, such as those with marginally compensated cardiovascular disease, quinidine may produce clinically important depression of cardiac function such as hypotension, bradycardia, or heartblock. Quinidine therapy should be carefully monitored in such individuals.
Evidence of quinidine cardiotoxicity (excessive prolongation of Q-T interval, 50% widening of QRS complex, frequent ventricular ectopic beats) mandates immediate discontinuation of the drug and subsequent close observation (electrocardiographic monitoring) of the patient.
Quinidine should be used with extreme caution when there is incomplete AV block, since complete block and asystole may result. The drug may cause unpredictable abnormalities of rhythm in digitalized hearts, and it should be used with special caution in the presence of digitalis intoxication.
The effect of quinidine is enhanced by potassium and reduced if hypokalemia is present.
The depressant actions of quinidine on cardiac contractility and arterial blood pressure limit its use in congestive heart failure and in hypotensive states unless these conditions are due to or aggravated by the arrhythmia. The potential disadvantages and benefits must be weighed.
Patients taking quinidine occasionally have syncopal episodes which usually result from ventricular tachycardia or fibrillation. This syndrome has not been shown to be related to dose or plasma levels. Syncopal episodes frequently terminate spontaneously or in response to treatment, but sometimes are fatal.
Recent reports have described increased, potentially toxic, digoxin plasma levels when quinidine is administered concurrently. When concurrent use is necessary, digoxin dosage should be reduced, its plasma concentration should be monitored and the patient observed closely for digitalis intoxication.
Caution should be used when quinidine is administered concurrently with coumarin anticoagulants. This combination may reduce prothrombin levels and cause bleeding.

PRECAUTIONS

General:
A preliminary test dose of a single tablet of quinidine sulfate may be administered to determine if the patient has an idiosyncrasy to quinidine. Hypersensitivity to quinidine, although rare, should constantly be considered, especially during the first weeks of therapy. Hospitalization for close clinical observation, electrocardiographic monitoring, and possible determination of plasma quinidine levels is indicated when large doses are used, or with patients who present an increased risk.
Quinidine should be used with caution in patients exhibiting renal, cardiac or hepatic insufficiency because of potential accumulation of quinidine in plasma leading to toxicity.
A few cases of hepatotoxicity, including granulomatous hepatitis, due to quinidine hypersensitivity have been reported in patients taking quinidine. Unexplained fever and/or elevation of hepatic enzymes, particularly in the early stages of therapy, warrant consideration of possible hepatotoxicity. Monitoring liver function during the first 4–8 weeks should be considered. Cessation of quinidine in these cases usually results in the disappearance of toxicity.

Drug Interactions

Drug	Effect
Quinidine with anticholinergic drugs	Additive vagolytic effect
Quinidine with cholinergic drugs	Antagonism of cholinergic effects
Quinidine with carbonic anhydrase inhibitors, sodium bicarbonate, thiazide diuretics	Alkalinization of urine resulting in decreased excretion of quinidine
Quinidine with courmarin anticoagulants	Reduction of clotting factor concentrations (see WARNINGS)
Quinidine with tubocurarine, succinylcholine, decamethonium and pancuronium	Potentiation of neuromuscular blockade
Quinidine with phenothiazines and reserpine	Additive cardiac depressive effects
Quinidine with hepatic enzyme-inducing drugs (phenobarbital, phenytoin, rifampin)	Decreased plasma half-life of quinidine
Quinidine with digoxin	Increased plasma concentrations of digoxin (see WARNINGS)

Laboratory Tests:
Continuous electrocardiographic monitoring and determination of plasma quinidine levels are indicated when large doses (more than 2 g/day) are used.
Carcinogenesis, Mutagenesis and Impairment of Fertility:
Long term studies in animals have not been performed to evaluate the carcinogenic potential of quinidine. There is currently no evidence of quinidine-induced mutagenesis or impairment of fertility.
Usage in Pregnancy:
Teratogenic Effects: Pregnancy Category C. Animal reproduction studies have not been conducted with quinidine. There are no adequate and well-controlled studies in pregnant women. Quinidine should be given to a pregnant woman only if clearly needed.
Nonteratogenic Effects: Like quinine, quinidine has been reported to have oxytocic properties. The significance of this property in the clinical setting has not been established.
Nursing Mothers:
Caution should be exercised when quinidine is administered to a nursing mother due to passage of the drug into breast milk.
Usage in Children:
There are no adequate and well-controlled studies establishing the safety and effectiveness of quinidine sulfate in children.

ADVERSE REACTIONS

Symptoms of cinchonism, ringing in the ears, headache, nausea, and/or disturbed vision may appear in sensitive patients after a single dose of the drug. The most frequently encountered side effects to quinidine are gastrointestinal in nature. These gastrointestinal effects include nausea, vomiting, abdominal pain and diarrhea. Less frequently encountered adverse reaitons:
Cardiovascular: Widening of QRS complex, cardiac asystole, ventricular ectopic beats, idioventricular rhythms (including ventricular tachycardia and fibrillation), paradoxical tachycardia, arterial embolism, hypotension.
Hematologic: Acute hemolytic anemia, hypoprothrombinemia, thrombocytopenia (purpura), agranulocytosis.
Central Nervous System: Headache, fever, vertigo, apprehension, excitement, confusion, delirium and syncope, distubed hearing (tinnitus, decreased auditory acuity), disturbed vision (mydriasis, blurred vision, disturbed color perception, reduced vision field, photophobia, diplopia, night blindness, scotomata), optic neuritis.
Dermatologic: Rash, cutaneous flushing with intense pruritus, urticaria. Photosensitivity has also been reported.
Hypersensitivity Reactions: Angioedema, acute asthmatic episode, vascular collapse, respiratory arrest, hepatic toxicity, including granulomatous hepatitis (see PRECAUTIONS). Although extremely rare, there have also been reports of lupus erythematosus in patients taking quinidine. A positive association with quinidine therapy has not been established.

OVERDOSAGE

Respiration must be maintained. Emesis can be undertaken to remove ingested drug followed by activated charcoal. Hypotension should be treated with fluids and in the absence of arrhythmias, norepinephrine with electrocardiographic control can be used. $\frac{1}{6}$ molar sodium lactate injection increases serum binding of quinidine and lowers serum potassium. Forced diuresis will increase the rate of quinidine excretion.

DOSAGE AND ADMINISTRATION

A preliminary test dose of a single tablet of quinidine sulfate should be administered to determine whether the patient has an idiosyncrasy to it. Continuous electrocardiographic monitoring is recommended in all cases in which quinidine is used in large doses.
Usual Adult Dose:
Premature Atrial and Ventricular Contractions:—200 to 300 mg, 3 or 4 times daily.
Paroxysmal Supraventricular Tachycardias:—400 to 600 mg, every 2 or 3 hours until the paroxysm is terminated.
Atrial Flutter:—Quinidine should be administered after digitalization for this indication. Dosage is to be individualized.
Conversion of Atrial Fibrillation:—Various schedules of quinidine administration have been in clinical use. A widely used technique is the administration of 200 mg of quinidine sulfate orally every 2 or 3 hours for 5 to 8 doses, with subsequent daily increase of the individual dose until sinus

rhythm is restored or toxic effects occur. The total daily dose should not exceed 3 to 4 grams in any regimen. Prior to quinidine administration, the ventricular rate and congestive failure (if present) should be brought under control by digitalis therapy.

Usual Maintenance Therapy:—200 to 300 mg, three or four times daily. Athough most patients may be maintained in normal rhythm on a dosage of 200 to 300 mg of quinidine sulfate every 6 to 8 hours, other patients may require larger doses or more frequent administration than the usually recommended schedule. Such increased dosage should be instituted only after careful clinical and laboratory evaluation of the patient, including monitoring of plasma quinidine levels and, if possible, serial electrocardiograms.

Gastrointestinal disturbances, if they occur, may be minimized by administering the drug with food.

HOW SUPPLIED

Quinora 300 mg tablets are available in bottles of 100 and 1000 tablets and unit dose packages of 100 tablets.

300 mg Tablet: NDC 0369-0073-01: round, flat, beveled, white to off-white, unscored, tablet debossed QUINORA 300 on one side.

STORAGE CONDITIONS

Tablets must be dispensed in tight, light resistant containers as defined in the U.S.P.

Tablets must be stored at controlled room temperature 15–30°C (59°–86°F).

Caution

FEDERAL LAW PROHIBITS DISPENSING WITHOUT PRESCRIPTION.

Key Pharmaceuticals
Kenilworth, New Jersey 07033

Revised 0286 I007206

THEO-DUR® ℞

[thē-a-dur]
(theophylline anhydrous sustained action tablets)

DESCRIPTION

THEO-DUR sustained action tablets contain anhydrous theophylline, a bronchodilator, in a sustained release formulation which allows a 12-hour dosing interval for a majority of patients and a 24-hour dosing interval for selected patients (see DOSAGE AND ADMINISTRATION section for description of appropriate patient populations). THEO-DUR contains no color additives and is available in three strengths: 100 mg, 200 mg and 300 mg.

The structural formula of theophylline, 1,3-dimethylxanthine is:

Anhydrous theophylline is a white, odorless, crystalline powder having a bitter taste.

CLINICAL PHARMACOLOGY

Theophylline directly relaxes the smooth muscle of the bronchial airways and pulmonary blood vessels, thus acting mainly as a bronchodilator and smooth muscle relaxant. The drug also produces other actions typical of the xanthine derivatives: coronary vasodilator, cardiac stimulant, diuretic, cerebral stimulant, and skeletal muscle stimulant. The actions of theophylline may be mediated through inhibition of phosphodiesterase and a resultant increase in intracellular cyclic AMP.

In vitro theophylline has been shown to act synergistically with beta agonists that increase intracellular cyclic AMP through the stimulation of adenyl cyclase, but synergism has not been demonstrated in patient studies. More data are needed to determine if theophylline and beta agonists have a clinically important additive effect *invivo.* Apparently, no development of tolerance occurs with chronic use of theophylline.

PHARMACOKINETICS

The half-life of theophylline is influenced by a number of known variables. It is prolonged in patients suffering from chronic alcoholism, impaired hepatic or renal function, congestive heart failure, and in patients receiving macrolide antibiotics and cimetidine. Older adults (over age 55) and patients with chronic obstructive pulmonary disease, with or without cor pulmonale, may also have much slower clearance rates. For such patients, the theophylline half-life may exceed 24 hours.

Newborns and neonates have extremely slow clearance rates compared to older infants (over 6 months) and children, and may also have a theophylline half-life of over 24 hours. High fever for prolonged periods may also reduce the rate of theophylline elimination.

THEOPHYLLINE ELIMINATION CHARACTERISTICS

Theophylline Clearance Rates (mean ± S.D.)	Half-life Average (mean ± S.D.)
Children (over 6 months of age)	
1.45 ± 0.58 ml/kg/min	3.7 ± 1.1 hrs.
Adult non-smokers uncomplicated asthma	
0.65 ± 0.19 ml/kg/min	8.7 ± 2.2 hrs.

The half-life of theophylline in smokers (1 to 2 packs/day) averages 4–5 hours, much shorter than the half-life in nonsmokers which averages 7–9 hours. The increase in theophylline clearance caused by smoking is probably the result of induction of drug-metabolizing enzymes that do not readily normalize after cessation of smoking. It appears that between 3 months and 2 years may be necessary for normalization of the effect of smoking on theophylline pharmacokinetics.

In single dose studies with 18 subjects, THEO-DUR, at 8 mg/kg body weight, produced mean peak theophylline blood levels of 7.5 ± 1.9 mcg/ml at 9.2 ± 1.9 hours following administration. In multiple dose, steady-state, 3 and 5 day studies with 12 subjects, THEO-DUR administered at 8mg/kg twice daily, achieved an average peak-trough difference of 4 mcg/ml. The Cmax and Cmin were 13.9 ± 6.9 and 9.9 ± 6.0, respectively. In a multiple dose (300–500 mg BID), steady-state, 5 day study involving 14 normal, nonfasting, subjects with theophylline half-lives between 5.8 and 12.3 hours (mean 8.0 ± 1.8 hours), THEO-DUR, dosed twice daily, produced mean Cmax and Cmin levels of 12.2 ± 2.0 and 10.2 ± 1.6 mcg/ml, respectively, over the a.m. dosing interval and Cmax and Cmin of 11.6 ± 1.6 and 8.7 ± 1.8 mcg/ml, respectively, over the p.m. dosing interval. In the same subjects, THEO-DUR given once daily, in the morning, in doses ranging from 600–1000 mg (same daily dose as for BID, above) produced a mean Cmax and Cmin of 14.4 ± 2.2 and 5.5 ± 2.0, respectively and a mean fraction of fluctuation of 0.63 ± 0.11 [Cmax -Cmin/ Cmax]. Average peak-trough differences over 24 hours were 8.9 ± 1.3 and 3.7 ± 1.2 mcg/ml when THEO-DUR was given once or twice daily, respectively. In both the twice daily and once daily dosing regimens, THEO-DUR exhibited complete bioavailability when compared to an immediate release product.

INDICATIONS

THEO-DUR is indicated for relief and/or prevention of symptoms of bronchial asthma and for reversible bronchospasm associated with chronic bronchitis and emphysema.

CONTRAINDICATIONS

THEO-DUR is contraindicated in individuals who have shown hypersensitivity to theophylline or any of the tablet components.

WARNINGS

Status asthmaticus should be considered a medical emergency and is defined as that degree of bronchospasm which is not rapidly responsive to usual doses of conventional bronchodilators. Optimal therapy for such patients frequently requires both *additional medication,* parenterally administered, and *close monitoring,* preferably in an intensive care setting.

Although increasing the dose of theophylline may bring about relief, such treatment may be associated with toxicity. The likelihood of such toxicity developing increases significantly when the serum theophylline concentration exceeds 20 mcg/ml. Therefore, determination of serum theophylline levels is recommended to assure maximal benefit without excessive risk.

Serum levels above 20 mcg/ml are rarely found after appropriate administration of the recommended doses. However, in individuals in whom theophylline plasma clearance is reduced *for any reason,* even conventional doses may result in increased serum levels and potential toxicity. Reduced theophylline clearance has been documented in the following readily identifiable groups: 1) patients with impaired renal or liver function; 2) patients over 55 years of age, particularly males and those with chronic lung disease; 3) those with cardiac failure from any cause; 4) neonates; and 5) those patients taking certain drugs (macrolide antibiotics and cimetidine). Decreased clearance of theophylline may be associated with either influenza immunization or active infection with influenza.

Reduction of dosage and laboratory monitoring is especially appropriate in the above individuals.

Less serious signs of theophylline toxicity, i.e. nausea and restlessness, may appear in up to 50% of patients. Unfortunately, however, serious side effects such as ventricular arrhythmias, convulsions or even death may appear as the first sign of toxicity without any previous warning. Stated differently; *serious toxicity is not reliably preceded by less severe side effects.*

Many patients who require theophylline may exhibit tachycardia due to their underlying disease process so that the cause/effect relationship to elevated serum theophylline concentrations may not be appreciated.

Theophylline products may cause dysrhythmia and/or worsen pre-existing arrhythmias and any significant change in rate and/or rhythm warrants monitoring and further investigation.

The occurrence of arrhythmias and sudden death (with histological evidence of necrosis of the myocardium) has been recorded in laboratory animals (minipigs, rodents and dogs) when theophylline and beta agonists were administered concomitantly, although not when either was administered alone. The significance of these findings when applied to human usage is currently unknown.

PRECAUTIONS

THEO-DUR TABLETS SHOULD NOT BE CHEWED OR CRUSHED.

General: Theophylline half-life is shorter in smokers than in non-smokers. Therefore, smokers may require larger or more frequent doses. Morphine and curare should be used with caution in patients with airway obstruction as they may suppress respiration and stimulate histamine release. Alternative drugs should be used when possible. Theophylline should not be administered concurrently with other xanthine medications. Use with caution in patients with severe cardiac disease, severe hypoxemia, hypertension, hyperthyroidism, acute myocardial injury, cor pulmonale, congestive heart failure, liver disease, in the elderly (especially males) and in neonates. In particular, great caution should be used in giving theophylline to patients with congestive heart failure. Frequently, such patients have markedly prolonged theophylline serum levels with theophylline persisting in serum for long periods following discontinuation of the drug. Individuals who are rapid metabolizers of theophylline, such as the young, smokers, and some non-smoking adults, may not be suitable candidates for once-daily dosing. These individuals will generally need to be dosed at 12 hourly or sometimes 8 hourly intervals. Such patients may exhibit symptoms of bronchospasm near the end of a dosing interval, or may have wider peak-to-trough differences than desired.

Use theophylline cautiously in patients with history of peptic ulcer. Theophylline may occasionally act as a local irritant to the G.I. tract although gastrointestinal symptoms are more commonly centrally mediated and associated with serum drug concentrations over 20 mcg/ml.

Information for Patients: The physician should reinforce the importance of taking only the prescribed dose and time interval between doses. THEO-DUR tablets should not be chewed or crushed. When dosing THEO-DUR on a once daily (q24h) basis, tablets should be taken whole and not split. As with any controlled-release theophylline product, the patient should alert the physician if symptoms occur repeatedly, especially near the end of the dosing interval.

Drug Interactions: Toxic synergism with ephedrine has been documented and may occur with some other sympathomimetic bronchodilators. In addition, the following drug interactions have been demonstrated:

Drug	Effect
Aminophylline with Lithium Carbonate	Increased excretion of Lithium Carbonate
Aminophylline with Propranolol	Antagonism of Propranolol effect
Theophylline with Cimetidine	Increased theophylline blood levels
Theophylline with troleandomycin, erythromycin	Increased theophylline blood levels

Drug-Laboratory Test Interactions: When plasma levels of theophylline are measured by spectrophotometric methods, coffee, tea, cola beverages, chocolate, and acetaminophen contribute falsely high values.

Carcinogenesis, Mutagenesis, and Impairment of Fertility: Long-term animal studies have not been performed to evaluate the carcinogenic potential, mutagenic potential, or the effect on fertility of xanthine compounds.

Pregnancy: Category C-Animal reproduction studies have not been conducted with theophylline. It is not known whether theophylline can cause fetal harm when administered to a pregnant woman or can affect reproduction capacity. Xanthines should be given to a pregnant woman only if clearly needed.

Nursing Mothers: It has been reported that theophylline distributes readily into breast milk and may cause adverse effects in the infant. Caution must be used if prescribing xanthine to a mother who is nursing, taking into account the risk-benefit of this therapy.

Pediatric Use: Safety and effectiveness of THEO-DUR administered:

1. Every 24 hours in children under 12 years of age, have not been established.

Continued on next page

Key—Cont.

2. Every 12 hours in children under 6 years of age, have not been established.

ADVERSE REACTIONS

The most consistent adverse reactions are usually due to overdose and are:

1. *Gastrointestinal:* nausea, vomiting, epigastric pain, hematemesis, diarrhea.
2. *Central nervous system:* headaches, irritability, restlessness, insomnia, reflex hyperexcitability, muscle twitching, clonic and tonic generalized convulsions.
3. *Cardiovascular:* palpitation, tachycardia, extrasystoles, flushing, hypotension, circulatory failure, ventricular arrhythmias.
4. *Respiratory:* tachypnea.
5. *Renal:* albuminuria, increased excretion of renal tubular and red blood cells, potentiation of diuresis.
6. *Others:* rash, hyperglycemia and inappropriate ADH syndrome.

OVERDOSAGE

Management:

If potential oral overdose is established and seizure has not occurred:

A. Induce vomiting.
B. Administer a cathartic (this is particularly important if sustained-release preparations have been taken).
C. Administer activated charcoal.

If patient is having a seizure:

A. Establish an airway.
B. Administer oxygen.
C. Treat the seizure with intravenous diazepam, 0.1 to 0.3 mg/kg up to 10 mg.
D. Monitor vital signs, maintain blood pressure and provide adequate hydration.

Post Seizure Coma:

A. Maintain airway and oxygenation.
B. If a result of oral medication, follow above recommendations to prevent absorption of the drug, but intubation and lavage will have to be performed instead of inducing emesis, and the cathartic and charcoal will need to be introduced via a large bore gastric lavage tube.
C. Continue to provide full supportive care and adequate hydration while waiting for drug to be metabolized. In general, the drug is metabolized sufficiently rapid so as not to warrant consideration of dialysis; however, if serum levels exceed 50 mcg/ml, charcoal hemoperfusion may be indicated.

DOSAGE AND ADMINISTRATION

For most patients, *effective use* of theophylline, i.e. associated with optimal likelihood of benefit combined with minimal risk of toxicity, is considered to occur when serum levels are maintained between 10 and 20 mcg/ml. Levels above 20 mcg/ml may produce toxicity, and in a small number of patients, toxicity may even be seen with serum levels between 15–20 mcg/ml, particularly during initiation of therapy.

There is considerable variation from patient to patient in the dosage required to achieve and maintain therapeutic and safe levels, primarily due to variable rates of elimination. Therefore, it is essential that not only must dosage be individualized, but titration and monitoring of serum levels be utilized where available. When serum concentration cannot be obtained, restriction of dosage to the amounts and intervals recommended in the guidelines listed below becomes essential. Dosage should be calculated on the basis of lean (ideal) body weight where mg/kg doses are presented. Theophylline does not distribute into fatty tissue. Giving theophylline with food may prevent some local gastric irritation and though absorption is slower, it is still complete.

As a practical consideration, it is not always possible to obtain serum level determinations. Under such conditions, restriction of the daily dose (in otherwise healthy adults) to not greater than 16 mg/kg/day or up to 900 mg (of anhydrous theophylline) will result in relatively few patients exceeding serum levels of 20 mcg/ml and the resultant risk of toxicity. THEO-DUR is not intended for patients experiencing an acute episode of bronchospasm (associated with asthma, chronic bronchitis, or emphysema). Such patients require *rapid* relief of symptoms and should be treated with an immediate-release or intravenous theophylline preparation (or other bronchodilators) and not with controlled release products.

Dosage Guidelines:

WARNING: DO NOT ATTEMPT TO MAINTAIN ANY DOSE THAT IS NOT TOLERATED.

Dosage guidelines are approximations only, and the wide range of clearance of theophylline among individuals (particularly those with concomitant disease) makes indiscriminate usage hazardous. It is recommended that dosing be considered in two stages: initiation of therapy with THEO-DUR, and titration, adjustment, and chronic maintenance.

Initiation of therapy:

It is recommended that the appropriate dosage be established using an immediate-release preparation. Slow clinical titration is generally preferred to help assure acceptance and safety of the medication. Then, if the total 24 hour dose can be given by use of the available strengths of this product, the patient can usually be switched to THEO-DUR giving one-half of the daily dose at 12 hour intervals. However, certain patients, such as the young, smokers and some nonsmoking adults are likely to metabolize theophylline rapidly and require dosing at 8 hour intervals. Such patients can generally be identified as having trough serum concentrations lower than desired or repeatedly exhibiting symptoms near the end of a dosing interval.

Alternatively, therapy can be initiated with THEO-DUR since it is available in dosage forms/strengths which permit titration and adjustment of dosage as outlined in the following dosing guidelines. It is recommended that for children under 25 kg, proper dosage be established with a liquid preparation to permit titration in small increments.

THE AVERAGE INITIAL ADULT AND CHILDREN'S (over 25 kg) DOSE IS ONE THEO-DUR 200 mg TABLET q12h.

Titration, Adjustment and Chronic Maintenance:

If the desired response is not achieved with the above AVERAGE INITIAL DOSE recommendations, there are no adverse reactions and the serum theophylline level cannot be measured, dosage adjustment should proceed by increasing the dose in approximately 25% increments at three day intervals. Following each adjustment, if the clinical reponse is satisfactory, then that dosage level should be maintained. Dosage increases may be made in this manner up to the following:

MAXIMUM DOSE WITHOUT MEASUREMENT OF SERUM CONCENTRATION

	Dose Per Interval
Children (25–35 kg)	250 mg q12h
Adults and Children (35–70 kg)	300 mg q12h
Adults (over 70 kg)	450 mg q12h

If an increased dose is not tolerated because of headaches or stomach upset (nausea, vomiting, diarrhea, etc.), decrease dose to previous tolerated level. Do not exceed the above recommended doses unless serum theophylline levels can be measured.

If serum theophylline levels can be measured and the concentration is between 10 and 20 mcg/ml, maintain dose if tolerated. CHECK SERUM CONCENTRATION AT APPROXIMATELY 8 HOURS AFTER A DOSE WHEN NONE HAVE BEEN MISSED OR ADDED FOR AT LEAST 3 DAYS. RECHECK SERUM THEOPHYLLINE CONCENTRATION AT 6 TO 12 MONTH INTERVALS. THIS INTERVAL MAY NEED TO BE MORE FREQUENT IN SOME INDIVIDUALS.

Take the following action if the measured serum theophylline concentration is too high.

20 to 25 mcg/ml—Decrease dose by about 10% and serum theophylline levels should be rechecked after 3 days.*

25 to 30 mcg/ml—Skip next dose and decrease subsequent doses by 25% and serum theophylline levels should be rechecked after 3 days.

Over 30 mcg/ml—Skip next 2 doses and decrease subsequent doses by 50% and serum theophylline levels should be rechecked after 3 days.

Take the following action if the measured serum theophylline concentration is too low. 7.5 to 10 mcg/ml—Increase dose by 25%.**

5 to 7.5 mcg/ml—Increase dose by 25% RECHECK SERUM THEOPHYLLINE FOR GUIDANCE IN FURTHER DOSAGE ADJUSTMENT.

*Finer adjustments in dosage may be needed for some patients.

** Dividing the daily dosage into 3 doses administered at 8 hour intervals may be indicated if symptoms occur repeatedly at the end of a dosing interval.

Once-Daily Dosing:

The slow absorption rate of this preparation may allow once-daily administration in adult non-smokers with appropriate total body clearance and other patients with low dosage requirements. Once-daily dosing should be considered only after the patient has been gradually and satisfactorily titrated to therapeutic levels with q12h dosing. Once-daily dosing should be based on twice the q12h dose and should be initiated at the end of the last q12h dosing interval. The trough concentration (Cmin) obtained following conversion to once-daily dosing may be lower (especially in high clearance patients) and the peak concentration (Cmax) may be higher (especially in low clearance patients) than that obtained with q12h dosing. If symptoms recur, or signs of toxicity appear during the once-daily dosing interval, dosing on the q12h basis should be reinstituted.

It is essential that serum theophylline concentrations be monitored before and after transfer to once-daily dosing.

Food and posture, along with changes associated with circadian rhythm, may influence the rate of absorption and/or clearance rates of theophylline from controlled-release dosage forms administered at night. The exact relationship of these and other factors to nighttime serum concentrations and the clinical significance of such findings require additional study. Therefore, it is not recommended that THEO-DUR, when used as a once-a-day product, be administered at night.

THEO-DUR, when used as a once-a-day product, must be taken whole and not broken. DOSAGE ADJUSTMENT BASED ON SERUM THEOPHYLLINE CONCENTRATION MEASUREMENTS WHEN THESE INSTRUCTIONS HAVE NOT BEEN FOLLOWED MAY RESULT IN RECOMMENDATIONS THAT PRESENT RISK OF TOXICITY TO THE PATIENT. Caution should be exercised for younger children who cannot complain of minor side effects. Older adults, those with cor pulmonale, congestive heart failure, and/or liver disease may have unusually low dosage requirements and thus may experience toxicity at the maximal dosage recommended above.

It is important that no patient be maintained on any dosage that is not tolerated. In instructing patients to increase dosage according to the schedule above, they should be instructed not to take a subsequent dose if apparent side effects occur and to resume therapy at a lower dose once adverse effects have disappeared.

HOW SUPPLIED

THEO-DUR 100 mg, 200 mg and 300 mg sustained action tablets are available in bottles of 100, 500, 1000 and 5000, and in unit dose packages of 100.

100 mg tablet: NDC 0369-0804: round, white to off-white, debossed THEO-DUR 100 on one side and scored on the other side.

200 mg tablet: NDC 0369-0805: oval, white to off-white, debossed THEO-DUR 200 on one side and scored on the other side.

300 mg tablet: NDC 0369-0803: capsule shaped, white to off-white debossed THEO-DUR 300 on one side and scored on the other side.

STORAGE CONDITIONS

Keep tightly closed. Store at controlled room temperature 15–30°C (59–86°F).

CAUTION

Federal Law Prohibits Dispensing Without Prescription.

Revised 12/83

KEY PHARMACEUTICALS, INC.
Kenilworth, New Jersey 07033

Shown in Product Identification Section, page 411

THEO-DUR® SPRINKLE ℞

[*thē-a-dur*]

(theophylline anhydrous sustained action capsules)

DESCRIPTION

THEO-DUR SPRINKLE Sustained Action Capsules contain 50 mg, 75 mg, 125 mg or 200 mg theophylline anhydrous in the form of long acting, microencapsulated beads within a hard gelatin capsule and are intended for oral administration.

The theophylline has been microencapsulated in a proprietary coating of polymers to mask the bitter taste associated with the drug, while providing a prolonged effect. The entire contents of a THEO-DUR SPRINKLE capsule is intended to be sprinkled on a small amount of soft food immediately prior to ingestion, or may be swallowed whole. SUBDIVIDING THE CONTENTS OF A CAPSULE IS NOT RECOMMENDED. Each capsule is oversized to allow ease of opening.

Theophylline is a bronchodilator and is a member of the xanthine class of chemical compounds related to both theobromine and caffeine. Theophylline is a white, odorless, crystalline powder having a bitter taste. Theophylline is 3.7-dihydro-1,3-dimethyl-1*h*-purine-2,6-dione represented by the following structural formula:

CLINICAL PHARMACOLOGY

Theophylline directly relaxes the smooth muscle of the bronchial airways and pulmonary blood vessels, thus acting mainly as a bronchodilator and smooth muscle relaxant. The drug also produces other actions typical of the xanthine derivatives: cardiac stimulation, coronary vasodilation, stimulation of skeletal muscles, cerebral stimulation, and diuresis. The actions of theophylline may be mediated through inhibition of phosphodiesterase and a resultant increase in intracellular cyclic AMP.

In vitro theophylline has been shown to act synergistically with beta agonists that increase intracellular cyclic AMP through the stimulation of adenyl cyclase, but synergism has not been demonstrated in patient studies. More data are needed to determine if theophylline and beta agonists have a clinically important additive effect *in vivo* . Apparently, no development of tolerance occurs with chronic use of theophylline.

Pharmacokinetics: The half-life of theophylline is influenced by a number of known variables. It is prolonged in patients suffering from chronic alcoholism, impaired hepatic or renal function, congestive heart failure, and in patients receiving macrolide antibiotics and cimetidine. Older adults (over age 55) and patients with chronic obstructive pulmonary disease, with or without cor pulmonale, may also have much slower clearance rates. For such patients, the theophylline half-life may exceed 24 hours.

Newborns and neonates have extremely slow clearance rates compared to older infants (over 6 months) and children, and may also have a theophylline half-life of over 24 hours. High fever for prolonged periods may also reduce the rate of theophylline elimination.

THEOPHYLLINE ELIMINATION CHARACTERISTICS

Theophylline Clearance Rates (mean±S.D.)	Half-Life Average (mean±S.D.)
Children (over 6 months of age)	
1.45±0.58 ml/kg/min	3.7±1.1 hrs
Adult non-smokers uncomplicated asthma	
0.65±0.19 ml/kg/min	8.7±2.2 hrs

The half-life of theophylline in smokers (1 to 2 packs/day) averages 4–5 hours, much shorter than the half-life in nonsmokers which averages 7–9 hours. The increase in theophylline clearance caused by smoking is probably the result of induction of drug-metabolizing enzymes that do not readily normalize after cessation of smoking. It appears that between 3 months and 2 years may be necessary for normalization of the effect of smoking on theophylline pharmacokinetics.

In two separate single dose studies utilizing different subjects, the following bioavailability parameters were observed. THEO-DUR SPRINKLE administered in a 500 mg dose as pellets on applesauce to 6 healthy adults produced mean peak theophylline serum levels of 9.03 ±2.59 mcg/ml at 8.67 ±1.03 hours following administration. Administration of two lots of THEO-DUR SPRINKLE as intact capsules in a 600 mg dose to 6 healthy adults produced mean peak theophylline serum levels of 9.08 ±1.30 mcg/ml and 7.60 ±0.95 mcg/ml at 8.33 ±1.50 and 8.67 ±3.01 hours after administration respectively. In these studies THEO-DUR SPRINKLE exhibited complete bioavailability when compared to an immediate release product. In both of these studies, the subjects fasted for 10 hours prior to dosing and for 4 hours after dosing.

In a multiple dose, two-way, crossover study with 18 healthy, normal adults, the bioavailability from THEO-DUR SPRINKLE administered as intact capsules was evaluated using THEO-DUR Sustained Action Tablets as the reference product. Fifteen subjects received 400 mg at 7:00 AM and 7:00 PM while three subjects received 200 mg because of low theophylline clearance. All meals and snacks were provided to the subjects during the course of this study, with breakfast at 9:00 AM, lunch at 12:30 PM a snack at 3:00 PM, and dinner at 9:00 PM. THEO-DUR SPRINKLE produced mean Cmax and Cmin levels of 10.4 ±2.6 and 6.9 ±1.8 mcg/ml as compared to a Cmax and Cmin of 10.5 ±2.8 and 7.5 ±2.7 mcg/ml for THEO-DUR tablets. The mean percent fluctuation normalized to Css was 38.8 ±8.5% for THEO-DUR SPRINKLE and 33.4 ±9.7% for THEO-DUR tablets [100(Cmax-Cmin)/Css where Css = AUC_{0-12}/dosing interval]. The mean percent fluctuation when normalized to Cmin was 51.9 ±15.4% for THEO-DUR SPRINKLE and 43.9 ±17.4% for THEO-DUR tablets [% fluctuation = 100 (Cmax-Cmin)/Cmin]. The average peak-trough differences over 12 hours for THEO-DUR SPRINKLE and THEO-DUR tablets were 3.5 ±1.2 and 3.0 ±0.7 mcg/ml respectively. The AUC for THEO-DUR SPRINKLE was 108.4 ±26.0 while that for THEO-DUR tablets was 112.1 ±32.5 mcg-hr/ml. In a separate study, THEO-DUR exhibited complete bioavailability when compared to an immediate release product. This would suggest that bioavailability from THEO-DUR SPRINKLE was complete and not statistically different from that of the THEO-DUR tablets.

INDICATIONS AND USE

For relief and/or prevention of symptoms of asthma and for reversible bronchospasm associated with chronic bronchitis and emphysema.

CONTRAINDICATIONS

THEO-DUR SPRINKLE is contraindicated in individuals who have shown hypersensitivity to theophylline or any of the capsule components.

WARNINGS

Status asthmaticus should be considered a medical emergency and is defined as that degree of bronchospasm which is not rapidly responsive to usual doses of conventional bronchodilators. Optimal therapy for such patients frequently requires both *additional medication*, parenterally administered, and *close monitoring*, preferably in an intensive care setting. Although increasing the dose of theophylline may bring about relief, such treatment may be associated with toxicity. The likelihood of such toxicity developing increases significantly when the serum theophylline concentration exceeds 20 mcg/ml. Therefore, determination of serum theophylline levels is recommended to assure maximal benefit without excessive risk.

Serum levels above 20 mcg/ml are rarely found after appropriate administration of the recommended doses. However, in individuals in whom theophylline plasma clearance is reduced for any reason, even conventional doses may result in increased serum levels and potential toxicity. Reduced theophylline clearance has been documented in the following readily identifiable groups: 1) patients with impaired renal or liver function; 2) patients over 55 years of age, particularly males and those with chronic lung disease; 3) those with cardiac failure from any cause; 4) neonates; and 5) those patients taking certain drugs (macrolide antibiotics and cimetidine). Decreased clearance of theophylline may be associated with either influenza immunization or active infection with influenza.

Reduction of dosage and laboratory monitoring is especially appropriate in the above individuals.

Less serious signs of theophylline toxicity (i.e., nausea and restlessness) may occur frequently when initiating therapy, but are usually transient; when such signs are persistent during maintenance therapy, they are often associated with serum concentrations above 20 mcg/ml.

Unfortunately, however, serious side effects such as ventricular arrhythmias, convulsions or even death may appear as the first sign of toxicity without any previous warning. *Stated differently; serious toxicity is not reliably preceded by less severe side effects.*

Many patients who require theophylline may exhibit tachycardia due to their underlying disease process so that the cause/effect relationship to elevated serum theophylline concentrations may not be appreciated.

Theophylline products may cause dysrhythmia and/or worsen pre-existing arrhythmias and any significant change in rate and/or rhythm warrants monitoring and futher investigation.

The occurrence of arrhythmias and sudden death (with histological evidence of necrosis of the myocardium) has been recorded in laboratory animals (minipigs, rodents and dogs) when theophylline and beta agonists were administered concomitantly, although not when either was administered alone. The significance of these findings when applied to human usage is currently unknown.

PRECAUTIONS

THE CONTENTS OF THE THEO-DUR SPRINKLE CAPSULE SHOULD NOT BE CHEWED OR CRUSHED.

General: Mean half-life in smokers is shorter than nonsmokers. Therefore, smokers may require larger or more frequent doses of theophylline. Morphine and curare should be used with caution in patients with airway obstruction as they may suppress respiration and stimulate histamine release. Alternative drugs should be used when possible.

Theophylline should not be administered concurrently with other xanthine preparations. Use with caution in patients with severe cardiac disease, severe hypoxemia, hypertension, hyperthyroidism, acute myocardial injury, cor pulmonale, congestive heart failure, alcoholism, liver disease and in the elderly, especially males, and in neonates. Great caution should be used in giving theophylline to patients with congestive heart failure. Frequently, such patients have shown markedly prolonged theophylline blood levels with theophylline persisting in serum for long periods following discontinuation of the drug. Use theophylline cautiously in patients with a history of peptic ulcer. Theophylline may occasionally act as a local gastrointestinal irritant although G.I. symptoms are more commonly centrally mediated and associated with serum drug concentrations over 20 mcg/ml.

Information for Patients: The physician should reinforce the importance of taking only the prescribed dose at the prescribed time intervals. The patient should alert the physician if symptoms occur repeatedly, especially near the end of a dosing interval.

When prescribing administration by the sprinkle method, details of the proper technique should be explained to the patient (see DOSAGE AND ADMINISTRATION Sprinkling Contents on Food).

Patients should be informed of the need to take this drug in the fasting state, and that drug administration should be one hour before, or two hours after meals (see PRECAUTIONS, Drug-Food Interactions and DOSAGE AND ADMINISTRATION).

Drug Interactions:

Drug-Drug: Toxic synergism with ephedrine has been documented and may occur with some other sympathomimetic bronchodilators. In addition, the following drug interactions have been demonstrated.

Drug	Effect
Theophylline with Lithium Carbonate	Increased excretion of Lithium Carbonate
Theophylline with Propranolol	Increased theophylline serum concentrations Antagonism of Propranolol effect
Theophylline with troleandomycin or erythromycin	Increased theophylline serum concentrations
Theophylline with Cimetidine	Increased theophylline serum concentrations

Drug-Food: THEO-DUR SPRINKLE has not been adequately studied to determine the extent of alteration of bioavailability when it is given with food as compared to the fasting state.

However, there is data to indicate that drug administration at the time of food ingestion will result in significantly lower peak serum concentrations and reduced extent of absorption (bioavailability).

The influence of the type and amount of food as well as the time interval between drug and food, on performance of THEO-DUR SPRINKLE is under study.

Drug/Laboratory Test Interactions: When plasma levels of theophylline are measured by spectrophotometric methods, coffee, tea, cola beverages, chocolate, and acetaminophen contribute falsely high values.

Carcinogenesis, Mutagenesis, and Impairment of Fertility: Long-term animal studies have not been performed to evaluate the carcinogenic potential, mutagenic potential, or the effect on fertility of xanthine compounds.

Pregnancy: Pregnancy Category C: Animal reproduction studies have not been conducted with theophylline. It is not known whether theophylline can cause fetal harm when administered to a pregnant woman or can affect reproduction capacity. Theophylline should be give to a preganant woman only if clearly needed.

Nursing Mothers: It has been reported that theophylline distributes readily into breast milk and may cause adverse effects in the infant. Caution must be used if prescribing xanthines to a mother who is nursing, taking into account the risk-benefit of this therapy.

Pediatric Use: Safety and effectiveness in children under 6 years of age have not been established with this product.

ADVERSE REACTIONS

The most consistent adverse reactions are usually due to overdose and are:

Gastrointestinal: nausea, vomiting, epigastric pain, hematemesis, diarrhea.

Central nervous system: headaches, irritability, restlessness, insomnia, reflex hyperexcitability, muscle twitching, clonic and tonic generalized convulsions.

Cardiovascular: palpitation, tachycardia, extrasystoles, flushing, hypotension, circulatory failure, ventricular arrhythmias.

Respiratory: tachypnea.

Renal: albuminuria, increased excretion of renal tubular cells and red blood cells, potentiation of diuresis.

Other: hyperglycemia and inappropriate ADH syndrome and rash.

OVERDOSAGE

Management:

A. If potential oral overdose is established and seizure has not occurred:
   1. Induce vomiting.
   2. Administer a cathartic (this is particulary important if sustained-released preparations have been taken).
   3. Administer activated charcoal.
   4. Monitor vital signs, maintain blood pressure and provide adequate hydration.

B. If patient is having a seizure:
   1. Establish an airway.
   2. Administer oxygen.
   3. Treat the seiure with intravenous diazepam, 0.1 to 0.3 mg/kg up to a total dose of 10 mg.
   4. Monitor vital signs, maintain blood pressure and provide adequate hydration.

Continued on next page

Key—Cont.

C. Post Seizure Coma:
1. Maintain airway and oxygenation.
2. If a result of oral medication, follow above recommendations to prevent absorption of the drug, but intubation and lavage will have to be performed instead of inducing emesis, and the cathartic and charcoal will need to be introduced via a large bore gastric lavage tube.
3. Continue to provide full supportive care and adequate hydration while waiting for drug to be metabolized. In general, the drug is metabolized sufficiently rapidly so as to not warrant consideration of dialysis. However, if serum levels exceed 50 mcg/ml, charcoal hemoperfusion may be indicated.

DOSAGE AND ADMINISTRATION

There is data to indicate that administration of THEO-DUR SPRINKLE at the time of food ingestion will result in significantly lower peak serum concentrations and reduced extent of absorption (bioavailability).
Therefore, the patient should be instructed to take this medication at least one hour before or two hours after a meal (See PRECAUTIONS, Drug-Food Interactions).
For most patients, effective use of theophylline, i.e. associated with optimal likelihood of benefit combined with minimal risk of toxicity, is considered to occur when serum levels are maintained between 10 and 20 mcg/ml. Levels above 20 mcg/ml may produce toxicity and in a small number of patients, toxicity may even be seen with serum levels between 15–20 mcg/ml, particularly during initation of therapy.
There is considerable variation from patient to patient in the dosage required to achieve and maintain therapeutic and safe levels, primarily due to variable rates of elimination. Therefore, it is essential that not only must dosage be individualized but titration and monitoring of serum levels be utilized where available. When serum concentrations cannot be obtained, restriction of dosage to the amounts and intervals recommended in the guidelines listed below becomes essential. Dosage should be calculated on the basis of lean (ideal) body weight where mg/kg doses are presented. Theophylline does not distribute into fatty tissue.
As a practical consideration, it is not always possible to obtain serum level determinations. Under such conditions, restriction of the daily dose (in otherwise healthy adults) to not greater than 13 mg/kg/day of anhydrous theophylline in divided doses will result in relatively few patients exceeding serum levels of 20 mcg/ml and the resultant risk of toxicity.
Sprinkling Contents on Food: *THEO-DUR SPRINKLE may be administered by carefully opening the capsule and sprinkling the beaded contents on a spoonful of soft food such as applesauce or pudding. The soft food should be swallowed immediately without chewing and followed with a glass of cool water or juice to ensure complete swallowing of the beads. It is recommended that the food used should not be hot and should be soft enough to be swallowed without chewing. Any bead/food mixture should be used immediately and not stored for future use. The small amount of food (one spoonful) used to administer the dose will not alter the bioavailablity of THEO-DUR SPRINKLE, however, the dosing should be at least one hour before or two hours after a meal. SUBDIVIDING THE CONTENTS OF A CAPSULE IS NOT RECOMMENDED.*
Dosage Guidelines: Because administration of Theo-Dur Sprinkle at the time of food ingestion has been shown to result in significantly lower peak serum concentrations and reduced extent of absorption (bioavailability), patients should be instructed to take this medication at least one hour before or two hours after a meal (See PRECAUTIONS, Drug-Food Interactions).
Taking THEO-DUR SPRINKLE at 12 hour intervals under the above restrictive recommendations in regard to food ingestion may be difficult for the patient to follow. Under such circumstances, consideration should be given to prescribing this drug every 8 hours (giving one third of the 24 hour dosage requirement with each dose), if this regimen would more easily permit dosing under fasting conditions.
I. Acute Symptoms: THEO-DUR SPRINKLE is not intended for patients experiencing an acute episode of bronchospasm (associated with asthma, chronic bronchitis, or emphysema). Such patients require rapid relief of symptoms and should be treated with an immediate-release or intravenous theophylline preparation (or other bronchodilators) and not with controlled release products.
II. Chronic Therapy:
A. Initating Therapy with an Immediate-Release Product: It is recommended that the appropriate dosage be established using an immediate-release preparation. Children weighing less than 25 kg should have their daily dosage requirements established with a liquid preparation to permit small dosage increments. Slow clinical titration is generally preferred to help assure acceptance and safety of the medication, and to allow the patient to develop tolerance to transient caffeine-like side effects. Then, if the total 24 hour dose can be given by use of the sustained release product, the patient can usually be switched to THEO-DUR SPRINKLE giving one-half of the daily dose at 12 hour intervals. Patients who metabolize theophylline rapidly such as the young, smokers, and some non-smoking adults are the most likely candidates for dosing at 8-hour intervals. Such patients can generally be identified as having trough serum concentrations lower than desired or repeatedly exhibiting symptoms near the end of a dosing interval.
B. Initating Therapy with THEO-DUR SPRINKLE: Alternatively, therapy can be initiated with THEO-DUR SPRINKLE since they are available in dosage strengths which permit titration and adjustments of dosage in adults and older children:

Initial Dose	16 mg/kg/24 hours or 400 mg/24 hours (whichever is less) of anhydrous theophylline in 2 divided doses 12-hour intervals.
Increasing Dose	The above dosage may be increased in approximately 25 percent increments at 3-day intervals so long as the drug is tolerated; until clinical reponse is satisfactory or the maximum dose as indicated in section III (below) is reached. The serum concentration may be checked at these intervals, but at a minimum, should be determined at the end of this adjustment period.

III. Maintenance Dose of Theophylline where the Serum Concentration is not Measured:
WARNING: DO NOT ATTEMPT TO MAINTAIN ANY DOSE THAT IS NOT TOLERATED.
Not to exceed the following:

			Dose per 12 hours
Age	6–9 years	24mg/kg/day	12.0 mg/kg
Age	9–12 years	20mg/kg/day	10.0 mg/kg
Age	12–16 years	18 mg/kg/day	9.0 mg/kg
Age	Over 16 years	13 mg/kg/day or 900 mg	6.5 mg/kg

(WHICHEVER IS LESS)

IV. Measurement of Serum Theophylline Concentrations During Chronic Therapy: If the above maximum doses are to be maintained or exceeded, serum theophylline measurement is recommended. The serum sample should be obtained at the time of peak absorption: 1 to 2 hours after administration for immediate-release products and 5 to 10 hours after dosing for THEO-DUR SPRINKLE. It is important that the patient will have missed no doses during the previous 48 hours and that the dosing intervals will have been reasonably typical with no added doses during that period of time. DOSAGE ADJUSTMENT BASED ON SERUM THEOPHYLLINE CONCENTRATION MEASUREMENTS WHEN THESE INSTRUCTIONS HAVE NOT BEEN FOLLOWED MAY RESULT IN RECOMMENDATIONS THAT PRESENT RISK OF TOXICITY TO THE PATIENT.
V. Final Adjustment of Dosage (see Table 1)
Table 1—Dosage adjustment after serum theophylline measurement

If serum theophylline is:		Directions:
Within normal Limits	10 to 20 mcg/ml	Maintain dosage if tolerated. Recheck serum theophylline concentration at 6- to 12-month intervals*
Too high	20 to 25 mcg/ml	Decrease doses by about 10%. Recheck serum theophylline concentration at 6- to 12-month intervals*
	25 to 30 mcg/ml	Skip next dose and decrease subsequent doses by about 25%.
	over 30 mcg/ml	Skip next 2 doses and decrease subsequent doses by 50%. Recheck serum theophylline.
Too low	7.5 to 10 mcg/ml	Increase dose by about 25%.** Recheck serum theophylline concentration at 6- to 12-month intervals.*
	5 to 7.5 mcg/ml	Increase dose by about 25% to the nearest dose increment and recheck serum theophylline for guidance in further dosage adjustment (another increase will probably be needed, but this provides a safety check).

*Finer adjustments in dosage may be needed for some patients.
**The total daily dose may need to be administered at more frequent intervals if symptoms occur repeatedly at the end of a dosing interval.

From the Journal of Respiratory Diseases 2(7):16.1981.
Caution should be exercised for younger children who cannot complain of minor side effects. Those with cor pulmonale, congestive heart failure, and/or liver disease may have unusually low dosage requirements and thus may experience toxicity at the maximal dosage recommended above. It is important that no patient be maintained on any dosage that is not tolerated. In instructing patients to increase dosage according to the schedule above, they should be instructed not to take a subsequent dose if apparent side effects occur and to resume therapy at a lower dose once adverse effects have disappeared.

HOW SUPPLIED

THEO-DUR SPRINKLE 50, 75, 125 and 200 mg Sustained Action Capsules are available in bottles of 100.
50 mg capsule: NDC 0369-0850: white opaque capsule body with clear cap embossed in black, THIS END UP THEO-DUR® SPRINKLE 50 mg
75 mg capsule: NDC 0369-0875: white opaque capsule body with clear cap embossed in green, THIS END UP THEO-DUR® SPRINKLE 75 mg
125 mg capsule: NDC 0369-0812: white opaque capsule body with clear cap embossed in red, THIS END UP THEO-DUR® SPRINKLE 125 mg
200 mg capsule: NDC 0369-0820: white opaque capsule body with clear cap embossed in blue, THIS END UP THEO-DUR® SPRINKLE 200 mg

STORAGE CONDITIONS

Keep tightly closed. Store at controlled room temperature 15–30°C (59–86°F).

CAUTION

Federal law prohibits dispensing without prescription.
Keep this and all medications out of the reach of children.
Revised 0585
EDP#1-085006
KEY PHARMACEUTICALS, INC.
Kenilworth, New Jersey 07033
Shown in Product Identification Section, page 411

TYZINE®
(tetrahydrozoline HCl)
NASAL SOLUTION

DESCRIPTION

Tyzine® Nasal Solution contains tetrahydrozoline hydrochloride, 2-(1,2,3,4-Tetrahydro-1-naphthyl)-2-imidazoline monohydrochloride, as a nasal decongestant.
Tyzine Nasal Solution is available for topical nasal application as 0.1% nasal solution and as 0.05% pediatric nasal drops. The nasal solution is a solution of tetrahydrozoline hydrochloride in water, with sodium chloride, sodium citrate, edetate disodium, and benzalkonium chloride, with hydrochloric acid to adjust the pH.

CLINICAL PHARMACOLOGY

Tyzine Nasal Solution (tetrahydrozoline hydrochloride), a sympathomimetic amine, possesses vasoconstrictor and decongestant actions when applied to the nasal mucosa, resulting in vasoconstriction of the smaller arterioles of the nasal passages. Information on the absorption, distribution and elimination of the drug is not available.

INDICATIONS AND USAGE

Tyzine Nasal Solution is indicated for decongestion of nasal and nasopharyngeal mucosa.

CONTRAINDICATIONS

Tyzine Nasal Solution is contraindicated for patients who have shown previous hypersensitivity to its components. The 0.1% solution is contraindicated in children under six years of age. **Tyzine** Nasal Solution is not to be used for infants under two years of age. **Tyzine** Pediatric Nasal Solution should be used for children between the ages of 2 and 6 years (See "Dosage and Administration"). **Tyzine** Nasal Solution should not be used by patients under treatment with Monoamine Oxidase (MAO) Inhibitors.

WARNINGS

Overdosage in children may produce profound sedation. This may be accompanied by profuse sweating, hypotension or even shock (See "Overdosage").
General:
Avoid doses greater or more frequent than those recommended below. Excessive dosage in children may, on rare occasions, cause severe drowsiness. Profuse sweating may accompany this effect. Overdosage may also cause marked hypotension or even shock. Use cautiously in patients with cardiovascular disease (e.g., coronary artery disease, hypertension), and metabolic-endocrine diseases (e.g., hyperthyroidism, diabetes).
Information for Patients:
Patients should be advised to follow the prescribed dosage regimen. The spray should be administered with the head held upright. To spray, squeeze bottle quickly and firmly and sniff briskly. Instillation of the nose drops can be most conveniently accomplished with the patient in the lateral head-low position.

Drug Interactions:

DRUG	EFFECT
Monoamine Oxidase (MAO) Inhibitors	Hypertension

Pregnancy:

Pregnancy Category C. Animal reproduction studies have not been conducted with **Tyzine**. It is also not known whether **Tyzine** Nasal Solution can cause fetal harm when administered to a pregnant woman or can affect reproduction capacity. **Tyzine** Nasal Solution should be given to a pregnant woman only if clearly needed.

Nursing Mothers:

It is not known whether this drug is secreted in human milk. Because many drugs are secreted in human milk, caution should be exercised when **Tyzine** Nasal Solution is administered to a nursing woman.

ADVERSE REACTIONS

Local application of **Tyzine** Nasal Solution can be associated with burning, stinging, sneezing, or dryness of the mucosa. Occasionally, systemic sympathomimetic effects can occur, including headaches, drowsiness, weakness, tremors, lightheadedness, insomnia, and palpitations. Rebound congestion can also occur, and is characterized by chronic swelling of the nasal mucosa resulting in chronic redness, swelling and rhinitis. If adverse reactions occur, discontinue use.

OVERDOSAGE

The administration or ingestion of overdoses of **Tyzine** (tetrahydrozoline hydrochloride) Nasal Solution may result in oversedation in young children. Overdoses have caused hypertension, bradycardia, drowsiness and rebound hypotension in adults; a shock-like syndrome with hypotension and bradycardia may also occur. In either case, the treatment of overdosage is usually that of watchful expectancy and general supportive measures. The patient should be kept warm, fluid balance should be maintained orally, if possible, and parenterally, if necessary.

If the respiratory rate drops to 10 or below, the patient should be given oxygen, and respiration assisted. Blood pressure should be watched carefully to prevent a hypotensive crisis.

There is no known antidote for **Tyzine** Nasal Solution. The use of stimulants is contraindicated. To date, we have had no report of fatalities resulting from overdosages of **Tyzine** Nasal Solution and while the symptoms resulting from **Tyzine** Nasal Solution overdosage may be alarming, they are self-limiting and the patient recovers with no sequelae.

DOSAGE AND ADMINISTRATION

Adults and Children 6 years and over:

It is recommended that 2 to 4 drops of **Tyzine** 0.1% Nasal Solution be instilled in each nostril as needed, never more often than every three hours. Less frequent administration is usually sufficient since relief is maintained for four hours or longer in most cases, and often for as long as eight hours. Bedtime instillation usually assures sleep undisturbed by the need for remedication before morning, or by insomnia from central stimulation.

Children 2 to 6 years of age:

It is recommended that 2 to 3 drops of **Tyzine** 0.05% Pediatric Nasal Drops be instilled in each nostril as needed and never more often than every three hours. Relief usually lasts for several hours so that instillations are usually needed only every four to six hours.

Instillation of nose drops can be most conveniently accomplished with the patient in the lateral head-low position.

HOW SUPPLIED

Tyzine Nasal Solution (0.1%) is available in:

—1 fl. oz. (30 cc) bottles—NDC 0369-4760-30

—1 pint (473 cc) bottles—NDC 0369-4760-16

—½ fl. oz. (15 cc) nasal spray bottles—NDC 0369-4760-15

Tyzine Pediatric Nasal Drops (0.05%) is available in:

—½ fl. oz. (15 cc) bottles—NDC 0369-4770-15

Recommended Storage: Store below 86° F (30°C).

CAUTION

FEDERAL LAW PROHIBITS DISPENSING WITHOUT PRESCRIPTION.

I476005

Key Pharmaceuticals

Kenilworth, NJ 07033

Revised 0286

Knoll Pharmaceuticals

A Unit of BASF K&F Corporation

WHIPPANY, NJ 07981

BASF Group

AKINETON® TABLETS AND AMPULES ℞

[ā-kĭn 'ĕ-ton]

biperiden hydrochloride and biperiden lactate

DESCRIPTION

Each AKINETON® Tablet for oral administration contains 2 mg biperiden hydrochloride. Other ingredients include corn syrup, lactose, magnesium stearate, potato starch, and talc. Each 1 mL AKINETON Ampule for intramuscular or intravenous administration contains 5 mg biperiden lactate in an aqueous 1.4 percent sodium lactate solution. No added preservative. AKINETON is an anticholinergic agent. Biperiden is α-5-Norbornen-2-yl-α-phenyl-1-piperidine-propanol. It is a white, crystalline, odorless powder, slightly soluble in water and alcohol. It is stable in air at normal temperatures. Biperiden may be represented by the following structural formula:

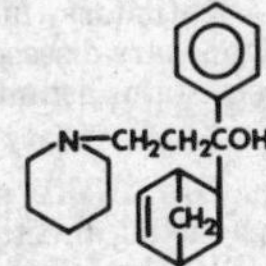

CLINICAL PHARMACOLOGY

AKINETON is a weak peripheral anticholinergic agent. It has, therefore, some antisecretory, antispasmodic and mydriatic effects. In addition, AKINETON possesses nicotinolytic activity. Parkinsonism is thought to result from an imbalance between the excitatory (cholinergic) and inhibitory (dopaminergic) systems in the corpus striatum. The mechanism of action of centrally active anticholinergic drugs such as AKINETON is considered to relate to competitive antagonism of acetylcholine at cholinergic receptors in the corpus striatum, which then restores the balance.

The parenteral form of AKINETON is an effective and reliable agent for the treatment of acute episodes of extrapyramidal disturbances sometimes seen during treatment with neuroleptic agents. Akathisia, akinesia, dyskinetic tremors, rigor, oculogyric crisis, spasmodic torticollis, and profuse sweating are markedly reduced or eliminated. With parenteral AKINETON, these drug-induced disturbances are rapidly brought under control. Subsequently, this can usually be maintained with oral doses which may be given with tranquilizer therapy in psychotic and other conditions requiring an uninterrupted therapeutic program.

Pharmacokinetics and Metabolism: Only limited pharmacokinetic studies of biperiden in humans are available. The serum concentration at 1 to 1.5 hours following a single, 4 mg oral dose was 4–5 ng/mL. Plasma levels (0.1–0.2 ng/mL) could be determined up to 48 hours after dosing. Six hours after an oral dose of 250 mg/kg in rats, 87% of the drug had been absorbed. The metabolism of AKINETON is also incompletely understood, but does involve hydroxylation. In normal volunteers a single 10 mg intravenous dose of biperiden seemed to cause a transient rise in plasma cortisol and prolactin. No change in GH, LH, FSH, or TSH levels were seen. Biperiden lactate (10 mg/mL) was not irritating to the tissue of rabbits when injected intramuscularly (1.0 mL) into the sacrospinalis muscles and intradermally (0.25 mL) and subcutaneously (0.5 mL) into the shaved abdominal skin.

INDICATIONS AND USAGE

- As an adjunct in the therapy of all forms of parkinsonism (idiopathic, post-encephalitic, arteriosclerotic)
- Control of extrapyramidal disorders secondary to neuroleptic drug therapy (e.g., phenothiazines)

CONTRAINDICATIONS

1) Hypersensitivity to biperiden 2) Narrow angle glaucoma 3) Bowel obstruction 4) Megacolon

WARNINGS

Isolated instances of mental confusion, euphoria, agitation and disturbed behavior have been reported in susceptible patients. Also, the central anticholinergic syndrome can occur as an adverse reaction to properly prescribed anticholinergic medication, although it is more frequently due to overdosage. It may also result from concomitant administration of an anticholinergic agent and a drug that has secondary anticholinergic actions (see Drug Interactions and Overdosage sections). Caution should be observed in patients with manifest glaucoma, though no prohibitive rise in intraocular pressure has been noted following either oral or parenteral administration. Patients with prostatism, epilepsy or cardiac arrhythmia should be given this drug with caution. Occasionally, drowsiness may occur, and patients who drive a car or operate any other potentially dangerous machinery should be warned of this possibility. As with other drugs acting on the central nervous system, the consumption of alcohol should be avoided during AKINETON therapy.

PRECAUTIONS

Drug Interactions: The central anticholinergic syndrome can occur when anticholinergic agents such as AKINETON are administered concomitantly with drugs that have secondary anticholinergic actions, e.g., certain narcotic analgesics such as meperidine, the phenothiazines and other antipsychotics, tricyclic antidepressants, certain antiarrhythmics such as the quinidine salts, and antihistamines. See Overdosage section for signs and symptoms of the central anticholinergic syndrome, and for treatment.

Pregnancy: Pregnancy Category C. Animal reproduction studies have not been conducted with AKINETON. It is also not known whether AKINETON can cause fetal harm when administered to a pregnant woman or can affect reproduction capacity. AKINETON should be given to a pregnant woman only if clearly needed.

Nursing Mothers: It is not known whether this drug is excreted in human milk. Because many drugs are excreted in human milk, caution should be exercised when AKINETON is administered to a nursing woman.

Pediatric Use: Safety and effectiveness in children have not been established.

ADVERSE REACTIONS

Atropine-like side effects such as dry mouth; blurred vision; drowsiness; euphoria or disorientation; urinary retention; postural hypotension; constipation; agitation; disturbed behavior may be seen. There usually are no significant changes in blood pressure or heart rate in patients who have been given the parenteral form of AKINETON. Mild transient postural hypotension and bradycardia may occur. These side effects can be minimized or avoided by slow intravenous administration. No local tissue reactions have been reported following intramuscular injection. If gastric irritation occurs following oral administration, it can be avoided by administering the drug during or after meals.

The central anticholinergic syndrome can occur as an adverse reaction to properly prescribed anticholinergic medication. See Overdosage section for signs and symptoms of the central anticholinergic syndrome, and for treatment.

OVERDOSAGE

Signs and Symptoms: Overdosage with AKINETON produces typical central symptoms of atropine intoxication (the central anticholinergic syndrome). Correct diagnosis depends upon recognition of the peripheral signs of parasympathetic blockade including dilated and sluggish pupils; warm, dry skin; facial flushing; decreased secretions of the mouth, pharynx, nose, and bronchi; foul-smelling breath; elevated temperature, tachycardia, cardiac arrhythmias, decreased bowel sounds, and urinary retention. Neuropsychiatric signs such as delirium, disorientation, anxiety, hallucinations, illusions, confusion, incoherence, agitation, hyperactivity, ataxia, loss of memory, paranoia, combativeness, and seizures may be present. The condition can progress to stupor, coma, paralysis, and cardiac and respiratory arrest, and death.

Treatment: Treatment of acute overdose revolves around symptomatic and supportive therapy. If AKINETON was administered orally, gastric lavage or other measures to limit absorption should be instituted. A small dose of diazepam or a short acting barbiturate may be administered if CNS excitation is observed. Phenothiazines are contraindicated because the toxicity may be intensified due to their antimuscarinic action, causing coma. Respiratory support, artificial respiration or vasopressor agents may be necessary. Hyperpyrexia must be reversed, fluid volume replaced and acid-base balance maintained. Urinary catheterization may be necessary.

Routine use of physostigmine for overdose is controversial. Delirium, hallucinations, coma, and supraventricular tachycardia (not ventricular tachycardias or conduction defects) seem to respond. If indicated, 1 mg (half this amount for children or the elderly) may be given intramuscularly or by slow intravenous infusion. If there is no response within 20 minutes, an additional 1 mg dose may be given; this may be repeated until a total of 4 mg has been administered, a reversal of the toxic effects occur or excessive cholinergic signs are seen. Frequent monitoring of clinical signs should be done. Since physostigmine is rapidly destroyed, additional injections may be required every one or two hours to maintain control. The relapse intervals tend to lengthen as the toxic anticholinergic agent is metabolized, so the patient should be carefully observed for 8 to 12 hours following the last relapse.

Toxicity in Animals: The LD_{50} of biperiden in the white mouse is 545 mg/kg orally, 195 mg/kg subcutaneously, and 56 mg/kg intravenously. The acute oral toxicity (LD_{50}) in rats is 750 mg/kg. The intraperitoneal toxicity (LD_{50}) of biperiden lactate in rats was 270 mg/kg and the intravenous

Continued on next page

Knoll—Cont.

toxicity (LD_{50}) in dogs is 222 mg/kg. In dogs under general anesthesia, respiratory arrest occurred at 33 mg/kg (intravenous) and circulatory standstill at 45 mg/kg (intravenous). The oral LD_{50} in dogs was 340 mg/kg. Chronic toxicity studies in both rat and dog have been reported.

DOSAGE AND ADMINISTRATION

Drug-Induced Extrapyramidal Symptoms:
Parenteral: The average adult dose is 2 mg intramuscularly or intravenously. May be repeated every half-hour until there is resolution of symptoms, but not more than four consecutive doses should be given in a 24-hour period.
Note: Parenteral drug products should be inspected visually for particulate matter and discoloration prior to administration, whenever solution and container permit.
Oral: One tablet one to three times daily.
Parkinson's Disease: Oral: The usual beginning dose is one tablet three or four times daily. The dosage should be individualized with the dose titrated upward to a maximum of 8 tablets (16 mg) per 24 hours.

HOW SUPPLIED

AKINETON Tablets, 2 mg each, white, embossed on one face with a triangle, bisected on the reverse and imprinted with the number "11".
Bottles of 100—NDC #0044-0120-02.
Bottles of 1000—NDC #0044-0120-04.
Shown in Product Identification Section, page 411
AKINETON Ampules, 1 mL each containing 5 mg biperiden lactate per mL.
Boxes of 10—NDC #0044-0110-01.
Storage: All dosage forms of AKINETON should be stored at 59°-86°F, (15°-30°C.).
Revised Oct 1985 5422A

DILAUDID® Ⓒ ℞

[dī″law′did]
(hydromorphone hydrochloride)

DESCRIPTION

DILAUDID (hydromorphone hydrochloride) (**WARNING:** May be habit forming), a hydrogenated ketone of morphine, is a narcotic analgesic. It is available in:
Ampules (for parenteral administration) containing 1 mg, 2 mg, and 4 mg hydromorphone hydrochloride per mL with 0.2% sodium citrate, 0.2% citric acid solution. DILAUDID ampules are sterile.
Multiple Dose Vials (for parenteral administration) containing 20 mL of solution. Each mL contains 2 mg hydromorphone hydrochloride and 0.5 mg edetate disodium with 1.8 mg methylparaben and 0.2 mg propylparaben as preservatives. Sodium hydroxide or hydrochloric acid is used for pH adjustment. DILAUDID multiple dose vials are sterile.
Color Coded Tablets (for oral administration) containing 1 mg, 2 mg, 3 mg and 4 mg hydromorphone hydrochloride.
Suppositories (for rectal administration) containing 3 mg hydromorphone hydrochloride in a cocoa butter base with silicon dioxide.
Powder (for prescription compounding) containing hydromorphone hydrochloride.
The structural formula of DILAUDID (hydromorphone hydrochloride) is:

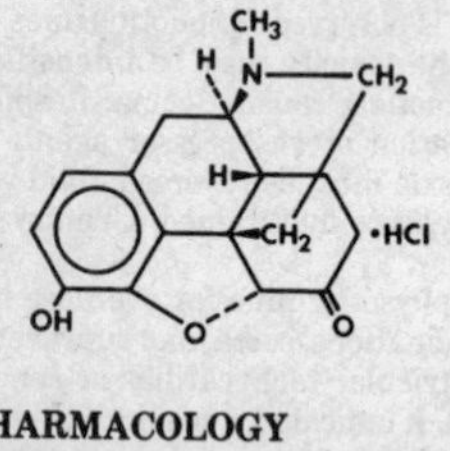

CLINICAL PHARMACOLOGY

DILAUDID is a narcotic analgesic; its principal therapeutic effect is relief of pain. The precise mechanism of action of DILAUDID and other opiates is not known, although it is believed to relate to the existence of opiate receptors in the central nervous system. There is no intrinsic limit to the analgesic effect of DILAUDID; like morphine, adequate doses will relieve even the most severe pain. Clinically, however, dosage limitations are imposed by the adverse effects, primarily respiratory depression, nausea, and vomiting, which can result from high doses.
DILAUDID has diverse additional actions. It produces drowsiness, changes in mood and mental clouding; depresses the respiratory center and the cough center, stimulates the vomiting center, produces pinpoint constriction of the pupil, enhances parasympathetic activitiy, elevates cerebrospinal fluid pressure, increases biliary pressure, produces transient hyperglycemia.
Generally, the analgesic action of parenterally administered DILAUDID is apparent within 15 minutes and usually remains in effect for more than five hours. The onset of action of oral DILAUDID is somewhat slower, with measurable analgesia occurring within 30 minutes.
Radioimmunoassay techniques have recently been developed for the analysis of DILAUDID in human plasma. In humans the half-life of a DILAUDID 4 mg tablet is 2.6 hours. In a random crossover study in six subjects, 4mg of *oral* DILAUDID produced a mean concentration/time curve similar to that of 2mg DILAUDID I.V., after the first hour.

INDICATIONS AND USAGE

DILAUDID is indicated for the relief of moderate to severe pain such as that due to:
Surgery
Cancer
Trauma (soft tissue & bone)
Biliary Colic
Myocardial Infarction
Burns
Renal Colic

CONTRAINDICATIONS

DILAUDID is contraindicated in patients with a known hypersensitivity to hydromorphone; in the presence of an intracranial lesion associated with increased intracranial pressure; and whenever ventilatory function is depressed (chronic obstructive pulmonary disease, cor pulmonale, emphysema, kyphoscoliosis, status asthmaticus).

WARNINGS

Respiratory Depression: DILAUDID produces dose-related respiratory depression by acting directly on brain stem respiratory centers. DILAUDID also affects centers that control respiratory rhythm, and may produce irregular and periodic breathing.
Head Injury and Increased Intracranial Pressure: The respiratory depressant effects of narcotics and their capacity to elevate cerebrospinal fluid pressure may be markedly exaggerated in the presence of head injury, other intracranial lesions or a pre-existing increase in intracranial pressure. Furthermore, narcotics produce adverse reactions which may obscure the clinical course of patients with head injuries.
Acute Abdominal Conditions: The administration of narcotics may obscure the diagnosis or clinical course of patients with acute abdominal conditions.

PRECAUTIONS

Special Risk Patients: DILAUDID should be used with caution in elderly or debilitated patients and those with impaired renal or hepatic function, hypothyroidism, Addison's disease, prostatic hypertrophy or urethral stricture. As with any narcotic analgesic agent, the usual precautions should be observed and the possibility of respiratory depression should be kept in mind.
Cough Reflex: DILAUDID suppresses the cough reflex; as with all narcotics, caution should be exercised when DILAUDID is used postoperatively and in patients with pulmonary disease.
Usage in Ambulatory Patients: Narcotics may impair the mental and/or physical abilities required for the performance of potentially hazardous tasks such as driving a car or operating machinery; patients should be cautioned accordingly.
Drug Interactions: Patients receiving other narcotic analgesics, general anesthetics, phenothiazines, tranquilizers, sedative-hypnotics, tricyclic antidepressants or other CNS depressants (including alcohol) concomitantly with DILAUDID may exhibit an additive CNS depression. When such combined therapy is contemplated, the dose of one or both agents should be reduced.
Parenteral Administration: The parenteral form of DILAUDID may be given intravenously, but the injection should be given very slowly. Rapid intravenous injection of narcotic analgesics increases the possibility of side effects such as hypotension and respiratory depression.
Pregnancy: Pregnancy Category C. DILAUDID has been shown to be teratogenic in hamsters when given in doses 600 times the human dose. There are no adequate and well-controlled studies in pregnant women. DILAUDID should be used during pregnancy only if the potential benefit justifies the potential risk to the fetus.
Nonteratogenic effects: Babies born to mothers who have been taking opioids regularly prior to delivery will be physically dependent. The withdrawal signs include irritability and excessive crying, tremors, hyperactive reflexes, increased respiratory rate, increased stools, sneezing, yawning, vomiting, and fever. The intensity of the syndrome does not always correlate with the duration of maternal opioid use or dose. There is no consensus on the best method of managing withdrawal. Chlorpromazine 0.7 to 1.0 mg/kg q6h, phenobarbital 2 mg/kg q6h, and paregoric 2 to 4 drops/kg q4h, have been used to treat withdrawal symptoms in infants. The duration of therapy is 4 to 28 days, with the dosages decreased as tolerated.
Labor and Delivery: As with all narcotics, administration of DILAUDID to the mother shortly before delivery may result in some degree of respiratory depression in the newborn, especially if higher doses are used.
Nursing Mothers: It is not known whether this drug is excreted in human milk. Because many drugs are excreted in human milk and because of the potential for serious adverse reactions in nursing infants from DILAUDID, a decision should be made whether to discontinue nursing or to discontinue the drug, taking into account the importance of the drug to the mother.
Pediatric Use: Safety and effectiveness in children have not been established.
FD&C Yellow No. 5: DILAUDID 1 mg, 2 mg and 4 mg color coded tablets contain FD&C Yellow No. 5 (tartrazine) dye which may cause allergic-type reactions (including bronchial asthma) in certain susceptible individuals. Although the overall incidence of FD&C Yellow No. 5 (tartrazine) dye sensitivity in the general population is low, it is frequently seen in patients who also have aspirin hypersensitivity.

ADVERSE REACTIONS

Central Nervous System: Sedation, drowsiness, mental clouding, lethargy, impairment of mental and physical performance, anxiety, fear, dysphoria, dizziness, psychic dependence, mood changes.
Gastrointestinal System: Nausea and vomiting occur more frequently in ambulatory than in recumbent patients. The antiemetic phenothiazines are useful in suppressing these effects; however, some phenothiazine derivatives seem to be antianalgesic and increase the amount of narcotic required to produce pain relief, while other phenothiazines reduce the amount of narcotic required to produce a given level of analgesia. Prolonged administration of DILAUDID may produce constipation. Opiate agonist-induced increase in intraluminal pressure may endanger surgical anastomosis.
Cardiovascular System: Circulatory depression, peripheral circulatory collapse and cardiac arrest have occurred after rapid intravenous injection. Orthostatic hypotension and fainting may occur if a patient stands up suddenly after receiving an injection of DILAUDID.
Genitourinary System: Ureteral spasm, spasm of vesical sphincters and urinary retention have been reported.
Respiratory Depression: DILAUDID produces dose-related respiratory depression by acting directly on brain stem respiratory centers. DILAUDID also affects centers that control respiratory rhythm, and may produce irregular and periodic breathing. If significant respiratory depression occurs, it may be antagonized by the use of naloxone hydrochloride. The usual adult dose of 0.4 to 0.8 mg given *intramuscularly* or *intravenously*, promptly reverses the effects of morphine-like opioid agonists such as DILAUDID. In patients who are physically dependent, small doses of naloxone may be sufficient not only to antagonize respiratory depression, but also to precipitate withdrawal phenomena. The dose of naloxone should therefore be adjusted accordingly in such patients. Since the duration of action of DILAUDID may exceed that of the antagonist, the patient should be kept under continued surveillance; repeated doses of the antagonist may be required to maintain adequate respiration. Apply other supportive measures when indicated.

DRUG ABUSE AND DEPENDENCE

DILAUDID is a Schedule Ⓒ narcotic. Psychic dependence, physical dependence, and tolerance may develop upon repeated administration of narcotics; therefore, DILAUDID should be prescribed and administered with caution. However, psychic dependence is unlikely to develop when DILAUDID is used for a short time for the treatment of pain. Physical dependence, the condition in which continued administration of the drug is required to prevent the appearance of a withdrawal syndrome, usually assumes clinically significant proportions only after several weeks of continued narcotic use, although some mild degree of physical dependence may develop after a few days of narcotic therapy. Tolerance, in which increasingly large doses are required in order to produce the same degree of analgesia, is manifested initially by a shortened duration of analgesic effect, and subsequently by decreases in the intensity of analgesia. The rate of development of tolerance varies among patients.

OVERDOSAGE

Signs and Symptoms: Serious overdosage with DILAUDID is characterized by respiratory depression (a decrease in respiratory rate and/or tidal volume, Cheyne-Stokes respiration, cyanosis), extreme somnolence progressing to stupor or coma, skeletal muscle flaccidity, cold and clammy skin, and sometimes bradycardia and hypotension. In severe overdosage, particularly by the intravenous route, apnea, circulatory collapse, cardiac arrest, and death may occur.
Treatment: Primary attention should be given to the reestablishment of adequate respiratory exchange through provision of a patent airway and institution of assisted or controlled ventilation. The narcotic antagonist naloxone hydrochloride is a specific antidote against respiratory depression which may result from overdosage or unusual sensitivity to narcotics, including DILAUDID. Therefore, naloxone hydrochloride should be administered as described under **Adverse**

Reactions (see *Respiratory Depression*) in conjunction with ventilatory assistance.

Since the duration of action of DILAUDID may exceed that of the antagonist, the patient should be kept under continued surveillance; repeated doses of the antagonist may be required to maintain adequate respiration. An antagonist should not be administered in the absence of clinically significant respiratory or cardiovascular depression. Oxygen, intravenous fluids, vasopressors, and other supportive measures should be employed as indicated.

In cases of overdosage with oral DILAUDID, gastric lavage or induced emesis may be useful in removing unabsorbed drug from conscious patients.

DOSAGE AND ADMINISTRATION

Parenteral The usual starting dose is 1–2 mg *subcutaneously* or *intramuscularly* every 4 to 6 hours as necessary for pain control. The dose should be adjusted according to the severity of pain, as well as the patient's underlying disease, age, and size. Patients with terminal cancer may be tolerant to narcotic analgesics and may, therefore, require higher doses for adequate pain relief. Intravenous or subcutaneous administration is usually not painful. Should intravenous administration be necessary, the injection should be given *slowly*, over at least 2 to 3 minutes, depending on the dose. A gradual increase in dose may be required if analgesia is inadequate, tolerance occurs, or if pain severity increases. The first sign of tolerance is usually a reduced duration of effect.

NOTE: Parenteral drug products should be inspected visually for particulate matter and discoloration prior to administration, whenever solution and container permit. A slight yellowish discoloration may develop in DILAUDID ampules and multiple dose vials. No loss of potency has been demonstrated.

Oral: The usual oral dose is 2 mg every 4 to 6 hours as necessary. The dose must be individually adjusted according to severity of pain, patient response and patient size. More severe pain may require 4 mg or more every 4 to 6 hours. If the pain increases in severity, analgesia is not adequate or tolerance occurs, a gradual increase in dosage may be required. If pain is exceedingly severe, or if prompt response is desired, parenteral DILAUDID should be used initially in adequate amounts to control the pain.

Rectal: DILAUDID suppositories (3 mg) may provide longer duration of relief which could obviate additional medication during the sleeping hours. The usual adult dose is one (1) suppository inserted rectally every 6 to 8 hours or as directed by physician.

HOW SUPPLIED

Ampules: 1 mg, 2 mg and 4 mg hydromorphone hydrochloride per mL with 0.2% sodium citrate, 0.2% citric acid solution. No added preservative.

1 mg/mL ampules—Boxes of 10—
NDC# 0044-1011-01.
2 mg/mL ampules—Boxes of 10—
NDC# 0044-1012-01.
Boxes of 25—NDC# 0044-1012-09.
4 mg/mL ampules—Boxes of 10—
NDC# 0044-1014-01.

Multiple Dose Vials: 20 mL sterile solution, each mL contains 2 mg hydromorphone hydrochloride and 0.5 mg edetate disodium with 1.8 mg methylparaben and 0.2 mg propylparaben as preservatives. pH adjusted with sodium hydroxide or hydrochloric acid.

2 mg/mL—20 mL multiple dose vials
NDC# 0044-1062-05.

Oral Color Coded Tablets: (NOT FOR INJECTION)

1 mg tablet (green)—Bottles of 100—
NDC# 0044-1021-02.
2 mg tablet (orange)—Bottles of 100—
NDC# 0044-1022-02.
Strip Pack of 100 (4 × 25)—
NDC# 0044-1022-45
Bottles of 500—NDC# 0044-1022-03.
3 mg tablet (pink)—Bottles of 100—
NDC# 0044-1023-02.
4 mg tablet (yellow)—Bottles of 100—
NDC# 0044-1024-02.
Strip Pack of 100 (4 × 25)—
NDC# 0044-1024-45
Bottles of 500—NDC# 0044-1024-03.

Rectal Suppositories: 3 mg hydromorphone hydrochloride in cocoa butter base with 1% colloidal silica as an inactive ingredient.

Boxes of 6—NDC# 0044-1053-01.

Powder: For prescription compounding.

15 grain vial—NDC# 0044-1040-01.

Storage: Parenteral and oral dosage forms of DILAUDID should be stored at 59°–86°F. (15°–30°C.).

Protect from light.

DILAUDID suppositories should be stored in a refrigerator.

DEA order form required.

A Schedule Ⓒ II Narcotic. 6663C

Revised Oct 1985

Shown in Product Identification Section, page 411

DILAUDID® COUGH SYRUP Ⓒ II ℞

[*dī″law′dĭd*]

(hydromorphone hydrochloride)

DESCRIPTION

Each 5 mL (1 teaspoonful) contains 1 mg DILAUDID (hydromorphone hydrochloride) (**WARNING:** May be habit forming) and 100 mg guaifenesin in a peach-flavored syrup containing 5% alcohol. DILAUDID is a hydrogenated ketone of morphine; it is a narcotic analgesic and antitussive.

CLINICAL PHARMACOLOGY

DILAUDID (hydromorphone hydrochloride) is a centrally acting narcotic antitussive which acts directly on the cough reflex center.

DILAUDID is also a narcotic analgesic; its principal therapeutic effect is relief of pain. The precise mechanism of action of DILAUDID and other opiates is not known, although it is believed to relate to the existence of opiate receptors in the central nervous system. There is no intrinsic limit to the analgesic effect of DILAUDID; like morphine, adequate doses will relieve even the most severe pain. Clinically, however, dosage limitations are imposed by the adverse effects, primarily respiratory depression, nausea, and vomiting, which can result from high doses.

DILAUDID has diverse additional actions. It produces drowsiness, changes in mood and mental clouding, depresses the respiratory center and the cough center, stimulates the vomiting center, produces pinpoint constriction of the pupil, enhances parasympathetic activity, elevates cerebrospinal fluid pressure, increases biliary pressure, produces transient hyperglycemia.

Generally, the analgesic action of parenterally administered DILAUDID is apparent within 15 minutes and usually remains in effect for more than five hours. The onset of action of oral DILAUDID is somewhat slower, with measurable analgesia occurring within 30 minutes.

Radioimmunoassay techniques have recently been developed for the analysis of DILAUDID in human plasma. In humans the half-life of a DILAUDID 4 mg tablet is 2.6 hours. In a random crossover study in six subjects, 4 mg of *oral* DILAUDID produced a mean concentration/time curve similar to that of 2 mg DILAUDID I.V., after the first hour.

Guaifenesin (glyceryl guaiacolate) reduces the viscosity of secretions, thereby increasing the efficiency of the cough reflex and of ciliary action in removing accumulated secretions from the trachea and bronchi. Unlike many other expectorants, guaifenesin rarely causes gastric irritation.

INDICATIONS AND USAGE

DILAUDID Cough Syrup is indicated for the control of persistent, exhausting cough or dry, non-productive cough.

CONTRAINDICATIONS

DILAUDID Cough Syrup is contraindicated in patients known to have a hypersensitivity to hydromorphone; in the presence of an intracranial lesion associated with increased intracranial pressure; and whenever ventilatory function is depressed (chronic obstructive pulmonary disease, cor pulmonale, emphysema, kyphoscoliosis, status asthmaticus).

WARNINGS

Respiratory Depression: DILAUDID may produce dose-related respiratory depression by acting directly on brain stem respiratory centers. DILAUDID also affects centers that control respiratory rhythm and may produce irregular and periodic breathing.

Head Injury and Increased Intracranial Pressure: The respiratory depressant effects of narcotics and their capacity to elevate cerebrospinal fluid pressure may be markedly exaggerated in the presence of head injury, other intracranial lesions or a preexisting increase in intracranial pressure. Furthermore, narcotics produce effects which may obscure the clinical course of patients with head injuries.

Acute Abdominal Conditions: The administration of narcotics may obscure the diagnosis or clinical course of patients with acute abdominal conditions.

PRECAUTIONS

Special Risk Patients: DILAUDID Cough Syrup should be used with caution in elderly or debilitated patients and those with impaired renal or hepatic function, hypothyroidism, Addison's disease, prostatic hypertrophy or urethral stricture. As with any narcotic analgesic agent, the usual precautions should be observed and the possibility of respiratory depression should be kept in mind.

Cough Reflex: DILAUDID Cough Syrup suppresses the cough reflex; as with all narcotics, caution should be exercised when DILAUDID Cough Syrup is used postoperatively and in patients with pulmonary disease.

Usage in Ambulatory Patients: Narcotics may impair the mental and/or physical abilities required for the performance of potentially hazardous tasks such as driving a car or operating machinery; patients should be cautioned accordingly.

Drug Interactions: Patients receiving other narcotic analgesics, general anesthetics, phenothiazines, tranquilizers, sedative-hypnotics, tricyclic antidepressants or other CNS depressants (including alcohol) concomitantly with DILAUDID Cough Syrup may exhibit an additive CNS depression. When such combined therapy is contemplated, the dose of one or both agents should be reduced.

Usage in Pregnancy: Pregnancy Category C. DILAUDID has been shown to be teratogenic in hamsters when given in doses 600 times the human dose. There are no adequate and well-controlled studies in pregnant women. DILAUDID Cough Syrup should be used during pregnancy only if the potential benefit justifies the potential risk to the fetus.

Nonteratogenic effects: Babies born to mothers who have been taking opioids regularly prior to delivery will be physically dependent. The withdrawal signs include irritability and excessive crying, tremors, hyperactive reflexes, increased respiratory rate, increased stools, sneezing, yawning, vomiting, and fever. The intensity of the syndrome does not always correlate with the duration of maternal opioid use or dose. There is no consensus on the best method of managing withdrawal. Chlorpromazine 0.7 to 1.0 mg/kg q6h, phenobarbital 2 mg/kg q6h, and paregoric 2 to 4 drops/kg q4h, have been used to treat withdrawal symptoms in infants. The duration of therapy is 4 to 28 days, with the dosage decreased as tolerated.

Labor and Delivery: As with all narcotics, administration of DILAUDID Cough Syrup to the mother shortly before delivery may result in some degree of respiratory depression in the newborn, especially if higher doses are used.

Nursing Mothers: It is not known whether this drug is excreted in human milk. Because many drugs are excreted in human milk and because of the potential for serious adverse reactions in nursing infants from DILAUDID Cough Syrup, a decision should be made whether to discontinue nursing or to discontinue the drug, taking into account the importance of the drug to the mother.

Pediatric Use: Safety and effectiveness in children have not been established.

FD&C Yellow No. 5: DILAUDID Cough Syrup contains FD&C Yellow No. 5 (tartrazine) dye which may cause allergic-type reactions (including bronchial asthma) in certain susceptible individuals. Although the overall incidence of FD&C Yellow No. 5 (tartrazine) dye sensitivity in the general population is low, it is frequently seen in patients who also have aspirin hypersensitivity.

ADVERSE REACTIONS

Central Nervous System: Sedation, drowsiness, mental clouding, lethargy, impairment of mental and physical performance, anxiety, fear, dysphoria, dizziness, psychic dependence, mood changes.

Gastrointestinal System: Nausea and vomiting occur more frequently in ambulatory than in recumbent patients. Some of the antiemetic phenothiazines are useful in suppressing these effects. Prolonged administration of DILAUDID Cough Syrup may produce constipation. Opiate agonist-induced increase in intraluminal pressure may endanger surgical anastomosis.

Genitourinary System: Ureteral spasm, spasm of vesical sphincters and urinary retention have been reported.

Respiratory Depression: DILAUDID may produce dose-related respiratory depression by acting directly on brain stem respiratory centers. DILAUDID also affects centers that control respiratory rhythm, and may produce irregular and periodic breathing. If significant respiratory depression occurs, it can be antagonized by the use of naloxone hydrochloride. The usual adult dose of 0.4 to 0.8 mg given intramuscularly or intravenously, promptly reverses the effects of morphine-like opioid agonists such as DILAUDID. In patients who are physically dependent, small doses of naloxone may be sufficient not only to antagonize respiratory depression, but also to precipitate withdrawal phenomena. The dose of naloxone should therefore be adjusted accordingly in such patients. Sine the duration of action of DILAUDID may exceed that of the antagonist, the patient should be kept under continued surveillance; repeated doses of the antagonist may be required to maintain adequate respiration. Apply other supportive measures when indicated.

DRUG ABUSE AND DEPENDENCE

DILAUDID is a Schedule Ⓒ II narcotic. Psychic dependence, physical dependence, and tolerance may develop upon repeated administration of narcotics; therefore, DILAUDID Cough Syrup should be prescribed and administered with caution. However, psychic dependence is unlikely to develop when DILAUDID Cough Syrup is used for a short time as indicated. Physical dependence, the condition in which continued administration of the drug is required to prevent the appearance of a withdrawal syndrome, usually assumes clinically significant proportions only after several weeks of continued narcotic use, although some mild degree of physical dependence may develop after few days of narcotic therapy.

Continued on next page

Knoll—Cont.

OVERDOSAGE

Signs and Symptoms: Serious overdosage with DILAUDID Cough Syrup is characterized by respiratory depression (a decrease in respiratory rate and/or tidal volume, Cheyne-Stokes respiration, cyanosis), extreme somnolence progressing to stupor or coma, skeletal muscle flaccidity, cold and clammy skin, and sometimes bradycardia and hypotension. In severe overdosage particularly by the intravenous route, apnea, circulatory collapse, cardiac arrest and death may occur.
Treatment: Primary attention should be given to the reestablishment of adequate respiratory exchange through provision of a patent airway and the institution of assisted or controlled ventilation. The narcotic antagonist naloxone hydrochloride is a specific antidote against respiratory depression which may result from overdosage or unusual sensitivity to narcotics, including DILAUDID. Therefore, naloxone hydrochloride should be administered as described under ADVERSE REACTIONS (see Respiratory Depression) in conjunction with ventilatory assistance.
Since the duration of action of Dilaudid may exceed that of the antagonist, the patient should be kept under continued surveillance; repeated doses of the antagonist may be required to maintain adequate respiration. An antagonist should not be administered in the absence of clinically significant respiratory or cardiovascular depression. Oxygen, intravenous fluids, vasopressors and other supportive measures should be employed as indicated.
In cases of overdosage with oral DILAUDID, gastric lavage or induced emesis may be useful in removing unabsorbed drug from conscious patients.

DOSAGE AND ADMINISTRATION

The usual adult dose of DILAUDID Cough Syrup is one teaspoonful (5 mL) every 3 to 4 hours.

HOW SUPPLIED

Bottles of 1 pint (473 mL)—NDC #0044-1080-01.
Storage: Store at 59°–86°F. (15°–30°C.).
A Schedule Ⓒ Narcotic.
DEA order form required.
Revised Oct 1985 8073

DILAUDID–HP® INJECTION Ⓒ ℞

[*dī″law′did*]
10 mg/mL
(hydromorphone hydrochloride)

WARNING

DILAUDID-HP® (HIGH POTENCY) IS A HIGHLY CONCENTRATED SOLUTION OF HYDROMORPHONE INTENDED FOR USE IN NARCOTIC-TOLERANT PATIENTS. DO NOT CONFUSE DILAUDID-HP WITH STANDARD PARENTERAL FORMULATIONS OF DILAUDID OR OTHER NARCOTICS. OVERDOSE AND DEATH COULD RESULT.

DESCRIPTION

DILAUDID (hydromorphone hydrochloride) (WARNING: May be habit forming), a hydrogenated ketone of morphine, is a narcotic analgesic, HIGH POTENCY DILAUDID is available in AMBER ampules for subcutaneous (SC) or intramuscular (IM) administration. Each 1 mL of sterile solution contains 10 mg hydromorphone hydrochloride with 0.2% sodium citrate, 0.2% citric acid solution.
The structural formula of DILAUDID (hydromorphone hydrochloride) is:

CH_3 H N CH_2 H CH_2 • HCl OH O O

CLINICAL PHARMACOLOGY

Many of the effects described below are common to the class of narcotic analgesics. In some instances, data may not exist to demonstrate that DILAUDID-HP possesses similar or different effects than those observed with other narcotic analgesics. However, in the absence of data to the contrary, it is assumed that DILAUDID-HP would possess these effects.
Central Nervous System: Narcotic analgesics have multiple actions but exert their primary effects on the central nervous system and organs containing smooth muscle. The principal actions of therapeutic value are analgesia and sedation. A significant feature of the analgesia is that it occurs without loss of consciousness. Narcotic analgesics also suppress the cough reflex and cause respiratory depression, mood changes, mental clouding, euphoria, dysphoria, nausea, vomiting and electroencephalographic changes. The precise mode of analgesic action of narcotic analgesics is unknown. However, specific CNS opiate receptors have been identified. Narcotics are believed to express their pharmacological effects by combining with these receptors.
Narcotics depress the cough reflex by direct effect on the cough center in the medulla.
Narcotics produce respiratory depression by direct effect on brain stem respiratory centers. The mechanism of respiratory depression also involves a reduction in the responsiveness of the brain stem respiratory centers to increases in carbon dioxide tension.
Narcotics cause miosis. Pinpoint pupils are a common sign of narcotic overdose but are not pathognomonic (e.g., pontine lesions of hemorrhagic or ischemic origin may produce similar findings) and marked mydriasis occurs when asphyxia intervenes.
Gastrointestinal Tract and Other Smooth Muscle: Gastric, biliary and pancreatic secretions are decreased by narcotics. Narcotics cause a reduction in motility associated with an increase in tone in the antrum portion of the stomach and duodenum. Digestion of food in the small intestine is delayed and propulsive contractions are decreased. Propulsive peristaltic waves in the colon are decreased, and tone may be increased to the point of spasm. The end result is constipation. Narcotics can cause a marked increase in biliary tract pressure as a result of spasm of the sphincter of Oddi.
Cardiovascular System: Certain narcotics produce peripheral vasodilation which may result in orthostatic hypotension. Release of histamine may occur with narcotics and may contribute to narcotic-induced hypotension. Other manifestations of histamine release and/or peripheral vasodilation may include pruritis, flushing, and red eyes.
Effects on the myocardium after i.v. administration of narcotics are not significant in normal persons, vary with different narcotic analgesic agents and vary with the hemodynamic state of the patient, state of hydration and sympathetic drive.
Pharmacokinetics: In normal human volunteers hydromorphone is metabolized primarily in the liver. It is excreted primarily as the glucuronidated conjugate, with small amounts of parent drug and minor amounts of 6-hydroxy reduction metabolites.
Following intravenous administration of DILAUDID to normal volunteers, the mean half-life of elimination was 2.64 +/− 0.88 hours. The mean volume of distribution was 91.5 liters, suggesting extensive tissue uptake. DILAUDID is rapidly removed from the blood stream and distributed to skeletal muscle, kidneys, liver, intestinal tract, lungs, spleen and brain. DILAUDID also crosses the placental membranes.
In terms of area under the analgesic time-effect curve, hydromorphone is approximately 8 times more potent than morphine (i.e., 1.3 mg of hydromorphone produces analgesia equal to that produced by 10 mg of morphine). After intramuscular administration, hydromorphone has a slightly more rapid onset and slightly shorter duration of action than morphine. The duration of DILAUDID analgesia in the nontolerant patient with usual doses may be up to 4–5 hours. However, in tolerant subjects, duration will vary substantially depending on tolerance and dose. Dose should be adjusted so that 3–4 hours of pain relief may be achieved.

INDICATIONS AND USAGE

DILAUDID-HP (hydromorphone hydrochloride) is indicated for the relief of moderate to severe pain in narcotic tolerant patients who require larger than usual doses of narcotics to provide adequate pain relief. Because DILAUDID-HP contains 10 mg of hydromorphone per mL, a smaller injection volume can be used than with other parenteral narcotic formulations. Discomfort associated with the intramuscular or subcutaneous injection of an unusually large volume of solution can therefore be avoided.
Contraindications: DILAUDID-HP is contraindicated in: patients who are not already receiving large amounts of parenteral narcotics, patients with known hypersensitivity to the drug, patients with respiratory depression in the absence of resuscitative equipment, and in patients with status asthmaticus. DILAUDID-HP is also contraindicated for use in obstetrical analgesia.
Warnings—Drug Dependence: DILAUDID-HP can produce drug dependence of the morphine type and therefore has the potential for being abused. Psychic dependence, physical dependence and tolerance may develop upon repeated administration of DILAUDID-HP, and it should be prescribed and administered with the same degree of caution appropriate for the use of morphine. Since DILAUDID-HP is indicated for use in patients who are already tolerant to and hence physically dependent on narcotics, abrupt discontinuance in the administration of DILAUDID-HP is likely to result in a withdrawal syndrome. (See ***Drug Abuse and Dependence***).
Infants born to mothers physically dependent on DILAUDID-HP will also be physically dependent and may exhibit respiratory difficulties and withdrawal symptoms (see ***Drug Abuse and Dependence***).
Impaired Respiration: Respiratory depression is the chief hazard of DILAUDID-HP. Respiratory depression occurs most frequently in the elderly, in the debilitated, and in those suffering from conditions accompanied by hypoxia or hypercapnia when even moderate therapeutic doses may dangerously decrease pulmonary ventilation.
DILAUDID-HP should be used with extreme caution in patients with chronic obstructive pulmonary disease or cor pulmonale, patients having a substantially decreased respiratory reserve, hypoxia, hypercapnia, or preexisting respiratory depression. In such patients even usual therapeutic doses of narcotic analgesics may decrease respiratory drive while simultaneously increasing airway resistance to the point of apnea.
Head Injury and Increased Intracranial Pressure: The respiratory depressant effects of DILAUDID-HP with carbon dioxide retention and secondary elevation of cerebrospinal fluid pressure may be markedly exaggerated in the presence of head injury, other intracranial lesions, or preexisting increase in intracranial pressure. Narcotic analgesics including DILAUDID-HP (hydromorphone hydrochloride) may produce effects which can obscure the clinical course and neurologic signs of further increase in pressure in patients with head injuries.
Hypotensive Effect: Narcotic analgesics, including DILAUDID-HP, may cause severe hypotension in an individual whose ability to maintain his blood pressure has already been compromised by a depleted blood volume, or a concurrent administration of drugs such as phenothiazines or general anesthetics (see also ***Precautions—Drug Interactions***).
DILAUDID-HP may produce orthostatic hypotension in ambulatory patients.
DILAUDID-HP should be administered with caution to patients in circulatory shock, since vasodilation produced by the drug may further reduce cardiac output and blood pressure.

PRECAUTIONS

General: Because of its high concentration, the delivery of precise doses of DILAUDID-HP may be difficult if low doses of hydromorphone are required. Therefore, DILAUDID-HP should be used only if the amount of hydromorphone required can be delivered accurately with this formulation.
In general, narcotics should be given with caution and the initial dose should be reduced in the elderly or debilitated and those with severe impairment of hepatic, pulmonary or renal function; myxedema or hypothyroidism; adrenocortical insufficiency (e.g., Addison's Disease); CNS depression or coma; toxic psychoses; prostatic hypertrophy or urethral stricture; gallbladder disease; acute alcoholism; delirium tremens; or kyphoscoliosis.
In the case of DILAUDID-HP, however, the patient is presumed to be receiving a narcotic to which he or she exhibits tolerance and the initial dose of DILAUDID-HP selected should be estimated based on the relative potency of hydromorphone and the narcotic previously used by the patient. See ***Dosage and Administration*** section.
The administration of narcotic analgesics including DILAUDID-HP may obscure the diagnosis or clinical course in patients with acute abdominal conditions and may aggravate preexisting convulsions in patients with convulsive disorders.
Narcotic analgesics including DILAUDID-HP (hydromorphone hydrochloride) should also be used with caution in patients about to undergo surgery of the biliary tract since it may cause spasm of the sphincter of Oddi.
Drug Interactions: The concomitant use of other central nervous system depressants including sedatives or hypnotics, general anesthetics, phenothiazines, tranquilizers and alcohol may produce additive depressant effects. Respiratory depression, hypotension and profound sedation or coma may occur. When such combined therapy is contemplated, the dose of one or both agents should be reduced. Narcotic analgesics, including DILAUDID-HP, may enhance the action of neuromuscular blocking agents and produce an increased degree of respiratory depression.
Pregnancy—Category C:
Human: Adequate animal studies on reproduction have not been performed to determine whether hydromorphone affects fertility in males or females. There are no well-controlled studies in women. Reports based on marketing experience do not identify any specific teratogenic risks following routine (short-term) clinical use. Although there is no clearly defined risk, such reports do not exclude the possibility of infrequent or subtle damage to the human fetus. DILAUDID-HP should be used in pregnant women only when clearly needed (see ***Labor and Delivery*** and ***Drug Abuse and Dependence***).
Animal: Literature reports of hydromorphone hydrochloride administration to pregnant Syrian hamsters show that DILAUDID is teratogenic at a dose of 20 mg/kg which is 600 times the human dose. A maximal teratogenic effect (50% of fetuses affected) in the Syrian hamster was observed at a dose of 125 mg/kg.

Labor and Delivery: DILAUDID-HP is contraindicated in Labor and Delivery (see ***Contraindications*** section).
Nursing Mothers: Low levels of narcotic analgesics have been detected in human milk. As a general rule, nursing should not be undertaken while a patient is receiving DILAUDID-HP since it, and other drugs in this class, may be excreted in the milk.
Pediatric Use: Safety and effectiveness in children have not been established.

ADVERSE REACTIONS

The adverse effects of DILAUDID-HP are similar to those of other narcotic analgesics, and represent established pharmacological effects of the drug class. The major hazards include respiratory depression and apnea. To a lesser degree, circulatory depression, respiratory arrest, shock and cardiac arrest have occurred.
The most frequently observed adverse effects are lightheadedness, dizziness, sedation, nausea, vomiting, and sweating. These effects seem to be more prominent in ambulatory patients and in those not experiencing severe pain. Some adverse reactions in ambulatory patients may be alleviated if the patient lies down.

Less Frequently Observed With Narcotic Analgesics:
General and CNS: Dysphoria, euphoria, weakness, headache, agitation, tremor, uncoordinated muscle movements, alterations of mood (nervousness, apprehension, depression, floating feelings, dreams), muscle rigidity, paresthesia, muscle tremor, blurred vision, nystagmus, diplopia and miosis, transient hallucinations* and disorientation, visual disturbances, insomnia and increased intracranial pressure may occur.
* Hallucinations, although unusual with pure agonist narcotics, have been observed in one patient following both a 6 mg and a 4 mg DILAUDID-HP dose. However, the patient was receiving several concomitant medications during the second episode and a causal relationship cannot be established.
Cardiovascular: Flushing of the face, chills, tachycardia, bradycardia, palpitation, faintness, syncope, hypotension and hypertension have been reported.
Respiratory: Bronchospasm and laryngospasm have been known to occur.
Gastrointestinal: Dry mouth, constipation, biliary tract spasm, anorexia, diarrhea, cramps and taste alterations have been reported.
Genitourinary: Urinary retention or hesitancy, and antidiuretic effects have been reported.
Dermatologic: Pruritis, urticaria, other skin rashes, wheal and flare over the vein with intravenous injection, and diaphoresis have been reported with narcotic analgesics.
Other: In clinical trials, neither local tissue irritation nor induration was observed at the site of subcutaneous injection of DILAUDID-HP; pain at the injection site was rarely observed. However, local irritation and induration have been seen following parenteral injection of other narcotic drug products.

DRUG ABUSE AND DEPENDENCE

Narcotic analgesics may cause psychological and physical dependence (see ***Warnings***). Physical dependence results in withdrawal symptoms in patients who abruptly discontinue the drug. Withdrawal symptoms also may be precipitated in the patient with physical dependence by the administration of a drug with narcotic antagonist activity, e.g., naloxone (see also ***Overdosage***). Physical dependence usually does not occur to a clinically significant degree until after several weeks of continued narcotic usage. Tolerance, in which increasingly large doses are required in order to produce the same degree of analgesia, is initially manifested by a shortened duration of analgesic effect, and subsequently, by decreases in the intensity of analgesia. In chronic pain patients, and in narcotic-tolerant cancer patients, the dose of DILAUDID-HP (hydromorphone hydrochloride) should be guided by the degree of tolerance manifested.
In chronic pain patients in whom narcotic analgesics including DILAUDID-HP are abruptly discontinued, a severe abstinence syndrome should be anticipated. This may be similar to the abstinence syndrome noted in patients who withdraw from heroin. The latter abstinence syndrome may be characterized by restlessness, lacrimation, rhinorrhea, yawning, perspiration, gooseflesh, restless sleep or "yen" and mydriasis during the first 24 hours. These symptoms may increase in severity and over the next 72 hours may be accompanied by increasing irritability, anxiety, weakness, twitching and spasms of muscles, kicking movements, severe backache, abdominal and leg pains, abdominal and muscle cramps, hot and cold flashes, insomnia, nausea, anorexia, vomiting, intestinal spasm, diarrhea, coryza and repetitive sneezing, increase in body temperature, blood pressure, respiratory rate and heart rate.
Because of excessive loss of fluids through sweating, or vomiting and diarrhea, there is usually marked weight loss, dehydration, ketosis, and disturbances in acid-base balance. Cardiovascular collapse can occur. Without treatment most observable symptoms disappear in 5–14 days; however, there appears to be a phase of secondary or chronic abstinence which may last for 2–6 months characterized by insomnia, irritability, muscular aches, and autonomic instability.
In the treatment of physical dependence on DILAUDID-HP, the patient may be detoxified by gradual reduction of the dosage, although this is unlikely to be necessary in the terminal cancer patient. If abstinence symptoms become severe, the patient may be given methadone. Temporary administration of tranquilizers and sedatives may aid in reducing patient anxiety. Gastrointestinal disturbances or dehydration should be treated accordingly.

OVERDOSAGE

Serious overdosage with DILAUDID-HP is characterized by respiratory depression, somnolence progressing to stupor or coma, skeletal muscle flaccidity, cold and clammy skin, constricted pupils, and sometimes bradycardia and hypotension. In serious overdosage, particularly following intravenous injection, apnea, circulatory collapse, cardiac arrest and death may occur.
In the treatment of overdosage primary attention should be given to the reestablishment of adequate respiratory exchange through provision of a patent airway and institution of assisted or controlled ventilation.
Narcotic-Tolerant Patient: Since tolerance to the respiratory and CNS depressant effects of narcotics develops concomitantly with tolerance to their analgesic effects, serious respiratory depression due to an acute overdose is unlikely to be seen in narcotic-tolerant patients receiving DILAUDID-HP for chronic pain.
NOTE: In such an individual who is physically dependent on narcotics, administration of the usual dose of the antagonist will precipitate an acute withdrawal syndrome. The severity will depend on the degree of physical dependence and the dose of the antagonist administered. Use of a narcotic antagonist in such a person should be avoided. If necessary to treat serious respiratory depression in the physically-dependent patient, the antagonist should be administered with extreme care and by titration with smaller than usual doses of the antagonist.
Non-Tolerant Patient: The narcotic antagonist, naloxone, is a specific antidote against respiratory depression which may result from overdosage, or unusual sensitivity to DILAUDID-HP. A dose of naloxone (usually 0.4 to 2.0 mg) should be administered intravenously, if possible, simultaneously with respiratory resuscitation. The dose can be repeated in 3 minutes. Naloxone should not be administered in the absence of clinically significant respiratory or circulatory depression. Naloxone should be administered cautiously to persons who are known, or suspected to be physically dependent on DILAUDID-HP. In such cases, an abrupt or complete reversal of narcotic effects may precipitate an acute abstinence syndrome.
Since the duration of action of DILAUDID may exceed that of the antagonist, the patient should be kept under continued surveillance; repeated doses of the antagonist may be required to maintain adequate respiration. Apply other supportive measures when indicated.
Supportive measures (including oxygen, vasopressors) should be employed in the management of circulatory shock and pulmonary edema accompanying overdose as indicated. Cardiac arrest or arrhythmias may require cardiac massage or defibrillation.

STRONG ANALGESICS AND STRUCTURALLY RELATED DRUGS USED IN THE TREATMENT OF CANCER PAIN*

	IM or SC Administration	
Nonproprietary (Trade) Names	Dose, mg Equianalgesic to 10 mg of IM Morphine†	Duration Compared With Morphine
Morphine sulfate	10	Same
Papaveretum (Pantopon)	20	Same
Hydromorphone hydrochloride (DILAUDID)	1.3	Slightly shorter
Oxymorphone hydrochloride (Numorphan)	1.1	Slightly shorter
Nalbuphine hydrochloride (Nubain)	12	Same
Heroin, diamorphine hydrochloride (NA in U.S.)	4–5	Slightly shorter
Levorphanol tartrate (Levo-Dromoran)	2.3	Same
Butorphanol tartrate (Stadol)	1.5–2.5	Same
Pentazocine lactate or hydrochloride (Talwin)	60	Shorter
Meperidine, pethidine hydrochloride (Demerol)	80	Shorter
Methadone hydrochloride (Dolophine)	10	Same

DOSAGE AND ADMINISTRATION

Parenteral: **DILAUDID-HP SHOULD BE GIVEN ONLY TO PATIENTS WHO ARE ALREADY RECEIVING LARGE DOSES OF NARCOTICS.** DILAUDID-HP is indicated for relief of moderate to severe pain in narcotic tolerant patients. Thus, these patients will already have been treated with other narcotic analgesics. If the patient is being changed from regular DILAUDID to DILAUDID-HP, similar doses should be used, depending on the patient's clinical response to the drug. If DILAUDID-HP is substituted for a different narcotic analgesic, the following equivalency table should be used as a guide to determine the appropriate starting dose of DILAUDID-HP (hydromorphone hydrochloride). [See table above].
* from Beaver WT
Management of cancer pain with parenteral medication J. Am. Med. Assoc. 244:2653–2657 (1980)
† (in terms of the area under the analgesic time-effect curve.)

In open clinical trials with DILAUDID-HP in patients with terminal cancer, doses ranged from 1–14 mg subcutaneously or intramuscularly; one patient received 30 mg subcutaneously on two occasions. In these trials, both subcutaneous and intramuscular injections of DILAUDID-HP were well-tolerated, with minimal pain and/or burning at the injection site. Mild erythema was rarely noted after intramuscular injection. There was no induration after either intramuscular or subcutaneous administration of DILAUDID-HP. Subcutaneous injections of DILAUDID-HP were particularly well accepted when administered with a short, 30-gauge needle.
Experience with administration of DILAUDID-HP by the intravenous route is limited. Should intravenous administration be necessary, the injection should be given slowly, over at least 2 to 3 minutes. The intravenous route is usually painless.
A gradual increase in dose may be required if analgesia is inadequate, tolerance occurs, or if pain severity increases. The first sign of tolerance is usually a reduced duration of effect.
NOTE: Parenteral drug products should be inspected visually for particulate matter and discoloration prior to administration, whenever solution and container permit. A slight yellowish discoloration may develop in DILAUDID-HP ampules. No loss of potency has been demonstrated.

HOW SUPPLIED

DILAUDID-HP *amber* ampules contain 10 mg hydromorphone hydrochloride per mL with 0.2% sodium citrate and 0.2% citric acid solution. No added preservative.
NOTE: DILAUDID-HP ampules are *amber* in color and marked with a distinctive violet-colored identification band.
HIGH POTENCY 10 mg/mL—Box of 10 ampules NDC 0044-1017-10

STORAGE

Parenteral forms of DILAUDID should be stored at 59°–86°F. (15–30°C). Protect from light.
DEA Order Form Required
A Schedule ⓒII Narcotic.
January, 1984 6642
Shown in Product Identification Section, page 411

Continued on next page

Knoll—Cont.

ISOPTIN® ℞
[*ī-sŏp″tĭn*]
(verapamil hydrochloride)
Intravenous Injection

DESCRIPTION

ISOPTIN® (verapamil hydrochloride) is a calcium antagonist or slow channel inhibitor. ISOPTIN is available in 5 mg per 2 mL and 10 mg per 4 mL ampules, 5 mg per 2 mL and 10 mg per 4 mL syringes, 5 mg/2 mL and 10 mg/4 mL single dose vials (for intravenous administration). Each 1 mL of solution contains 2.5 mg verapamil HCl and 8.5 mg sodium chloride in water for injection. Hydrochloric acid is used for pH adjustment. The pH of the solution is between 4.1 and 6.0. Protect contents from light. ISOPTIN ampules, syringes and vials are sterile.
The structural formula of verapamil HCl is given below:

$C_{27}H_{38}N_2O_4 \cdot HCl$ M.W. = 491.08
Benzeneacetonitrile, α-[3-[[2-(3,4-dimethoxyphenyl) ethyl] methylamino] propyl] - 3,4-dimethoxy-α-(1-methylethyl) hydrochloride
Verapamil HCl is an almost white, crystalline powder, practically free of odor, with a bitter taste. It is soluble in water, chloroform and methanol. Verapamil HCl is not chemically related to other antiarrhythmic drugs.

CLINICAL PHARMACOLOGY

Mechanism of Action: ISOPTIN (verapamil HCl) inhibits the calcium ion (and possibly sodium ion) influx through slow channels into conductile and contractile myocardial cells and vascular smooth muscle cells. The antiarrhythmic effect of ISOPTIN appears to be due to its effect on the slow channel in cells of the cardiac conduction system. The vasodilatory effect of ISOPTIN appears to be due to its effect on blockade of calcium channels as well as α-receptors.
In the isolated rabbit heart, concentrations of ISOPTIN that markedly affect SA nodal fibers or fibers in the upper and middle regions of the AV node, have very little effect on fibers in the lower AV node (NH region) and no effect on atrial action potentials or His bundle fibers.
Electrical activity in the SA and AV nodes depends, to a large degree, upon calcium influx through the slow channel. By inhibiting this influx, ISOPTIN slows AV conduction and prolongs the effective refractory period within the AV node in a rate-related manner. This effect results in a reduction of the ventricular rate in patients with atrial flutter and/or atrial fibrillation and a rapid ventricular response.
By interrupting reentry at the AV node, ISOPTIN can restore normal sinus rhythm in patients with paroxysmal supraventricular tachycardias (PSVT), including PSVT associated with Wolff-Parkinson-White syndrome.
ISOPTIN does not induce peripheral arterial spasm.
ISOPTIN has a local anesthetic action that is 1.6 times that of procaine on an equimolar basis. It is not known whether this action is important at the doses used in man.
ISOPTIN does not alter total serum calcium levels.
Hemodynamics: ISOPTIN (verapamil HCl) reduces afterload and myocardial contractility. The commonly used intravenous doses of 5–10 mg ISOPTIN produce transient, usually asymptomatic, reduction in normal systemic arterial pressure, systemic vascular resistance and contractility; left ventricular filling pressure is slightly increased. In most patients, including those with organic cardiac disease, the negative inotropic action of ISOPTIN is countered by reduction of afterload, and cardiac index is usually not reduced. However, in patients with moderately severe to severe cardiac dysfunction (pulmonary wedge pressure above 20 mm Hg, ejection fraction less than 30%), acute worsening of heart failure may be seen. Peak therapeutic effects occur within 3 to 5 minutes after a bolus injection.
Pharmacokinetics: Intravenously administered ISOPTIN (verapamil HCl) has been shown to be rapidly metabolized. Following intravenous infusion in man, verapamil is eliminated bi-exponentially, with a rapid early distribution phase (half-life about 4 minutes) and a slower terminal elimination phase (half-life 2–5 hours). In healthy men, orally administered ISOPTIN undergoes extensive metabolism in the liver; 12 metabolites having been identified, most in only trace amounts. The major metabolites have been identified as various N- and O-dealkylated products of ISOPTIN. Approximately 70% of an administered dose is excreted in the urine and 16% or more in the feces within 5 days. About 3–4% is excreted as unchanged drug.

INDICATIONS AND USAGE

Intravenous ISOPTIN (verapamil HCl) is indicated for the following:

- Rapid conversion to sinus rhythm of paroxysmal supraventricular tachycardias, including those associated with accessory bypass tracts (Wolff-Parkinson-White [W-P-W] and Lown-Ganong-Levine [L-G-L] syndromes). When clinically advisable, appropriate vagal maneuvers (e.g. Valsalva maneuver) should be attempted prior to ISOPTIN administration.
- Temporary control of rapid ventricular rate in atrial flutter or atrial fibrillation **except** when the atrial flutter and/or atrial fibrillation are associated with accessory bypass tracts (Wolff-Parkinson-White [W-P-W] and Lown-Ganong-Levine [L-G-L] syndromes).

In controlled studies in the United States, about 60% of patients with supraventricular tachycardia converted to normal sinus rhythm within 10 minutes after intravenous ISOPTIN. Uncontrolled studies reported in the world literature describe a conversion rate of about 80%. About 70% of patients with atrial flutter and/or fibrillation with a fast ventricular rate respond with a decrease in ventricular rate of at least 20%. Conversion of atrial flutter or fibrillation to sinus rhythm is uncommon (about 10%) after ISOPTIN and may reflect the spontaneous conversion rate, since the conversion rate after placebo was similar. Slowing of the ventricular rate in patients with atrial fibrillation/flutter lasts 30–60 minutes after a single injection.
Because a small fraction (< 1.0%) of patients treated with ISOPTIN respond with life-threatening adverse responses (rapid ventricular rate in atrial flutter/fibrillation and an accessory bypass tract, marked hypotension, or extreme bradycardia/asystole—see Contraindications and Warnings), the initial use of intravenous ISOPTIN should, if possible, be in a treatment setting with monitoring and resuscitation facilities, including DC-cardioversion capability (see Suggested Treatment of Acute Cardiovascular Adverse Reactions). As familiarity with the patient's response is gained, use in an office setting may be acceptable.
Cardioversion has been used safely and effectively after intravenous ISOPTIN.

CONTRAINDICATIONS

Intravenous ISOPTIN (verapamil HCl) is contraindicated in:

1. Severe hypotension or cardiogenic shock
2. Second- or third-degree AV block (except in patients with a functioning artificial ventricular pacemaker)
3. Sick sinus syndrome (except in patients with a functioning artificial ventricular pacemaker)
4. Severe congestive heart failure (unless secondary to a supraventricular tachycardia amenable to verapamil therapy)
5. Patients receiving **intravenous** beta adrenergic blocking drugs (e.g., propranolol). **Intravenous** verapamil and **intravenous** beta adrenergic blocking drugs should not be administered in close proximity to each other (within a few hours), since both may have a depressant effect on myocardial contractility and AV conduction.
6. Patients with atrial flutter or atrial fibrillation and an accessory bypass tract (e.g. Wolff-Parkinson-White, Lown-Ganong-Levine syndromes) are at risk to develop ventricular tachyarrhythmia including ventricular fibrillation if verapamil is administered. Therefore the use of verapamil in these patients is contraindicated.
7. Ventricular Tachycardia. Administration of intravenous verapamil to patients with wide-complex ventricular tachycardia (QRS ≥0.12 sec) can result in marked hemodynamic deterioration and ventricular fibrillation. Proper pre-therapy diagnosis and differentiation from wide complex supraventricular tachycardia is imperative in the emergency room setting.
8. Known hypersensitivity to verapamil hydrochloride.

WARNINGS

ISOPTIN SHOULD BE GIVEN AS A SLOW INTRAVENOUS INJECTION OVER AT LEAST A TWO MINUTE PERIOD OF TIME. (See Dosage and Administration)
Hypotension: Intravenous ISOPTIN (verapamil HCl) often produces a decrease in blood pressure below baseline levels that is usually transient and asymptomatic but may result in dizziness. Systolic pressure less than 90 mm Hg and/or diastolic pressure less than 60 mm Hg was seen in 5–10% of patients in controlled U.S. trials in supraventricular tachycardia and in about 10% of the patients with atrial flutter/fibrillation. The incidence of symptomatic hypotension observed in studies conducted in the U.S. was approximately 1.5%. Three of the five symptomatic patients required intravenous pharmacologic treatment (levarterenol bitartrate, metaraminol bitartrate, or 10% calcium gluconate). All recovered without sequelae.
Extreme Bradycardia/Asystole: ISOPTIN (verapamil HCl) affects the AV and SA nodes and rarely may produce second- or third-degree AV block, bradycardia and, in extreme cases, asystole. This is more likely to occur in patients with a sick sinus syndrome (SA nodal disease), which is more common in older patients. Bradycardia associated with sick sinus syndrome was reported in 0.3% of the patients treated in controlled double-blind trials in the United States. The total incidence of bradycardia (ventricular rate less than 60 beats/min) was 1.2% in these studies. Asystole in patients other than those with sick sinus syndrome is usually of short duration (few seconds or less), with spontaneous return to AV nodal or normal sinus rhythm. If this does not occur promptly, appropriate treatment should be initiated immediately. (See Adverse Reactions and Treatment of Adverse Reactions.)
Heart Failure: When heart failure is not severe or rate related, it should be controlled with digitalis glycosides and diuretics, as appropriate, before ISOPTIN is used. In patients with moderately severe to severe cardiac dysfunction (pulmonary wedge pressure above 20 mm Hg, ejection fraction less than 30%), acute worsening of heart failure may be seen.
Concomitant Antiarrhythmic Therapy:
Digitalis: Intravenous verapamil has been used concomitantly with digitalis preparations without the occurrence of serious adverse effects. However, since both drugs slow AV conduction, patients should be monitored for AV block or excessive bradycardia.
Procainamide: Intravenous verapamil has been administered to a small number of patients receiving oral procainamide without the occurrence of serious adverse effects.
Quinidine: Intravenous verapamil has been administered to a small number of patients receiving oral Quinidine without the occurrence of serious adverse effects. However, three patients have been described in whom the combination resulted in an exaggerated hypotensive response presumably from the combined ability of both drugs to antagonize the effects of catecholamines on α-adrenergic receptors. Caution should therefore be used when employing this combination of drugs.
Beta Adrenergic Blocking Drugs: Intravenous verapamil has been administered to patients receiving oral beta blockers without the development of serious adverse effects. However, since both drugs may depress myocardial contractility or AV conduction, the possibility of detrimental interactions should be considered. The concomitant administration of **intravenous** beta blockers and **intravenous** verapamil has resulted in serious adverse reactions (see Contraindications), especially in patients with severe cardiomyopathy, congestive heart failure or recent myocardial infarction.
Disopyramide: Until data on possible interactions between verapamil and all forms of disopyramide phosphate are obtained, disopyramide should not be administered within 48 hours before or 24 hours after verapamil administration.
Heart Block: ISOPTIN (verapamil HCl) prolongs AV conduction time. While high degree AV block has not been observed in controlled clinical trials in the U.S., a low percentage (less than 0.5%) has been reported in the world literature. Development of second- or third-degree AV block or unifascicular, bifascicular or trifascicular bundle branch block requires reduction in subsequent doses or discontinuation of verapamil and institution of appropriate therapy, if needed. (See Treatment of Acute Cardiovascular Adverse Reactions.)
Hepatic and Renal Failure: Significant hepatic and renal failure should not increase the effects of a single intravenous dose of ISOPTIN (verapamil HCl) but may prolong its duration. Repeated injections of intravenous ISOPTIN in such patients may lead to accumulation and an excessive pharmacologic effect of the drug. There is no experience to guide use of multiple doses in such patients and this generally should be avoided. If repeated injections are essential, blood pressure and PR interval should be closely monitored and smaller repeat doses should be utilized. Data on the clearance of verapamil by dialysis are not yet available.
Premature Ventricular Contractions: During conversion to normal sinus rhythm, or marked reduction in ventricular rate, a few benign complexes of unusual appearance (sometimes resembling premature ventricular contractions) may be seen after treatment with ISOPTIN (verapamil HCl). Similar complexes are seen during spontaneous conversion of supraventricular tachycardias, after D.C.-cardioversion and other pharmacologic therapy. These complexes appear to have no clinical significance.
Duchenne's Muscular Dystrophy: Intravenous ISOPTIN (verapamil HCl) can precipitate respiratory muscle failure in these patients and should, therefore, be used with caution.
Increased Intracranial Pressure: Intravenous ISOPTIN (verapamil HCl) has been seen to increase intracranial pressure in patients with supratentorial tumors at the time of anesthesia induction. Caution should be taken and appropriate monitoring performed.

PRECAUTIONS

Drug Interactions: (See Warnings: Concomitant Antiarrhythmic Therapy) Intravenous ISOPTIN (verapamil HCl) has been used concomitantly with other cardioactive drugs (especially digitalis) without evidence of serious negative drug interactions. In rare instances, including when patients with severe cardiomyopathy, congestive heart failure or recent myocardial infarction were given **intravenous** beta-adrenergic blocking agents or disopyramide concomitantly with intravenous verapamil, serious adverse effects have occurred. Concomitant use of ISOPTIN with α-adrenergic blockers may result in an exaggerated hypotensive response. Two animal studies suggest concomitant use of intravenous verapamil and intravenous dantrolene sodium may result in cardiovascular collapse. The clinical relevance of these findings is unknown. Animal studies and a clinical report suggest that concomitant use of inhalation anesthetics and calcium antagonists may result in excessive cardiovascular depression. Careful titration of dose is warranted. Clinical data and animal studies suggest that verapamil may potentiate the activity of neuromuscular blocking agents (curare-like and depolarizing). It may be necessary to decrease the dose of verapamil and/or dose of the neuromuscular blocking agent when the drugs are used concomitantly. Cimetidine has no effect on intravenous ISOPTIN kinetics. As verapamil is highly bound to plasma proteins, it should be administered with caution to patients receiving other highly protein bound drugs.

Pregnancy: Pregnancy Category C. Reproduction studies have been performed in rabbits and rats at oral verapamil doses up to 1.5 (15 mg/kg/day) and 6 (60 mg/kg/day) times the human oral daily dose, respectively, and have revealed no evidence of teratogenicity. In the rat, however, this multiple of the human dose was embryocidal and retarded fetal growth and development, probably because of adverse maternal effects reflected in reduced weight gains of the dams. This oral dose has also been shown to cause hypotension in rats. There are no adequate and well-controlled studies in pregnant women. Because animal reproduction studies are not always predictive of human response, this drug should be used during pregnancy only if clearly needed.

Labor and Delivery: There have been few controlled studies to determine whether the use of verapamil during labor or delivery has immediate or delayed adverse effects on the fetus, or whether it prolongs the duration of labor or increases the need for forceps delivery or other obstetric intervention. Such adverse experiences have not been reported in the literature, despite a long history of use of intravenous ISOPTIN in Europe in the treatment of cardiac side effects of beta-adrenergic agonist agents used to treat premature labor.

Nursing Mothers: ISOPTIN crosses the placental barrier and can be detected in umbilical vein blood at delivery. Also, ISOPTIN is excreted in human milk. Because of the potential for adverse reactions in nursing infants from verapamil, nursing should be discontinued while verapamil is administered.

Pediatrics: Controlled studies with verapamil have not been conducted in pediatric patients, but uncontrolled experience with intravenous administration in more than 250 patients, about half under 12 months of age and about 25% newborn, indicates that results of treatment are similar to those in adults. **However, in rare instances, severe hemodynamic side effects have occurred following the intravenous administration of verapamil in neonates and infants. Caution should therefore be used when administering verapamil to this group of pediatric patients.**

The most commonly used single doses in patients up to 12 months of age have ranged from 0.1 to 0.2 mg/kg of body weight, while in patients aged 1 to 15 years, the most commonly used single doses ranged from 0.1 to 0.3 mg/kg of body weight. Most of the patients received the lower dose of 0.1 mg/kg once but, in some cases, the dose was repeated once or twice every 10 to 30 minutes.

ADVERSE REACTIONS

The following reactions were reported with intravenous ISOPTIN (verapamil HCl) use in controlled U.S. clinical trials involving 324 patients:

Cardiovascular: Symptomatic hypotension (1.5%); bradycardia (1.2%); severe tachycardia (1.0%). The worldwide experience in open clinical trials in more than 7,900 patients was similar.

Central Nervous System Effects: Dizziness (1.2%); headache (1.2%). Occasional cases of seizures during verapamil injection have been reported.

Gastrointestinal: Nausea (0.9%); abdominal discomfort (0.6%).

In rare cases of hypersensitive patients, broncho/laryngeal spasm accompanied by itch and urticaria have been reported.

The following reactions were reported in single patients: emotional depression, rotary nystagmus, sleepiness, vertigo, muscle fatigue or diaphoresis.

[See table above].

OVERDOSAGE

Treatment of overdosage should be supportive and individualized. Beta-adrenergic stimulation and/or parenteral administration of calcium solutions (calcium chloride) have been effectively used in treatment of deliberate overdosage with oral ISOPTIN (verapamil HCl). Clinically significant hypotensive reactions or high degree AV block should be treated with vasopresssor agents or cardiac pacing, respectively. Asystole should be handled by the usual measures including isoproterenol hydrochloride, other vasopressor

Suggested Treatment of Acute Cardiovascular Adverse Reactions*

The frequency of these adverse reactions was quite low and experience with their treatment has been limited.

Adverse Reaction	Proven Effective Treatment	Supportive Treatment
1. Symptomatic hypotension requiring treatment	Calcium chloride (IV) Levarterenol bitartrate (IV) Metaraminol bitartrate (IV) Isoproterenol HCl (IV) Dopamine (IV)	Intravenous fluids Trendelenburg position
2. Bradycardia, AV block, Asystole	Isoproterenol HCl (IV) Calcium chloride (IV) Cardiac pacing Levarterenol bitartrate (IV) Atropine (IV)	Intravenous fluids (slow drip)
3. Rapid ventricular rate (due to antegrade conduction in flutter/fibrillation with W-P-W or L-G-L syndromes)	D.C.-cardioversion (high energy may be required) Procainamide (IV) Lidocaine (IV)	Intravenous fluids (slow drip)

* Actual treatment and dosage should depend on the severity of the clinical situation and the judgment and experience of the treating physician.

agents or cardiopulmonary resuscitation. (See Treatment of Cardiovascular Adverse Reactions.)

DOSAGE AND ADMINISTRATION

(For Intravenous Use Only): ISOPTIN SHOULD BE GIVEN AS A SLOW INTRAVENOUS INJECTION OVER AT LEAST A TWO MINUTE PERIOD OF TIME.

The recommended intravenous doses of ISOPTIN are as follows:

ADULT: Initial dose: 5–10 mg (0.075–0.15 mg/kg body weight) given as an intravenous bolus over at least 2 minutes.

Repeat dose: 10 mg (0.15 mg/kg body weight) 30 minutes after the first dose if the initial response is not adequate. An optimal interval for subsequent I.V. doses has not been determined, and should be individualized for each patient.

Older Patients: The dose should be administered over at least 3 minutes to minimize the risk of untoward drug effects.

PEDIATRIC: Initial dose:

0–1 year: 0.1–0.2 mg/kg body weight (usual single dose range 0.75–2 mg) should be administered as an intravenous bolus over at least 2 minutes **under continuous ECG monitoring.**

1–15 years: 0.1–0.3 mg/kg body weight (usual single dose range 2–5 mg) should be administered as an intravenous bolus over at least 2 minutes. **Do not exceed 5 mg.**

Repeat dose:

0–1 year: 0.1–0.2 mg/kg body weight (usual single dose range 0.75–2 mg) 30 minutes after the first dose if the initial response is not adequate **(under continuous ECG monitoring).** An optimal interval for subsequent I.V. doses has not been determined, and should be individualized for each patient.

1–15 years: 0.1–0.3 mg/kg body weight (usual single dose range 2–5 mg) 30 minutes after the first dose if the initial response is not adequate. **Do not exceed 10 mg as a single dose.** An optimal interval for subsequent I.V. doses has not been determined, and should be individualized for each patient.

NOTE

Parenteral drug products should be inspected visually for particulate matter and discoloration prior to administration, whenever solution and container permit. ISOPTIN is physically compatible and chemically stable for at least 24 hours at 25°C protected from light in most common large volume parenteral solutions. Admixing ISOPTIN with albumin, amphotericin B, hydralazine HCl and trimethoprim with sulfamethoxazole should be avoided. ISOPTIN will precipitate in any solution with a pH above 6.0.

HOW SUPPLIED

Each 1 mL of sterile solution contains 2.5 mg verapamil HCl and 8.5 mg sodium chloride. pH adjusted with hydrochloric acid.

5 mg/2 mL ampule—Individual unit carton—NDC 0044-1815-01

Space saver pack of 10 ampules—NDC 0044-1815-07

*5 mg/2 mL syringe—Carton of 5 syringes—NDC 0044-1815-25

5 mg/2 mL vial—Single dose. No preservative. Individual unit carton—NDC 0044-1816-21

10 mg/4 mL ampule—Individual unit carton—NDC 0044-1815-11

Space saver pack of 10 ampules—NDC 0044-1815-17

*10 mg/4 mL syringe—Carton of 5 syringes—NDC 0044-1815-45

10 mg/4 mL vial—Single dose. No preservative. Individual unit carton—NDC 0044-1816-41

*Syringes manufactured for Knoll Pharmaceuticals, Whippany, New Jersey 07981 by Taylor Pharmacal Company. Decatur, Illinois 62525

Storage: 59°–86°F, (15°–30°C). Protect from light.

Revised Feb 1986 Print No. 1189B

Shown in Product Identification Section, page 411

ISOPTIN® ℞

[ī-sŏp″tĭn]

(verapamil hydrochloride)
Oral Tablets

DESCRIPTION

ISOPTIN (verapamil hydrochloride) is a calcium ion influx inhibitor (slow channel blocker or calcium ion antagonist). ISOPTIN is available for oral administration as round, scored, film-coated tablets containing 80 mg or 120 mg verapamil hydrochloride.

The structural formula of verapamil HCl is given below:

$$(CH_3O)_2C_6H_3-C(CN)(CH(CH_3)_2)-(CH_2)_3N(CH_3)CH_2CH_2-C_6H_3(OCH_3)_2 \cdot HCl$$

$C_{27}H_{38}N_2O_4 \cdot HCl$ M.W. = 491.08

Benzeneacetonitrile,
α-[3-[[2-(3,4-dimethoxyphenyl) ethyl] methylamino] propyl]-3,4-dimethoxy-α-(1-methylethyl) hydrochloride

Verapamil HCl is an almost white, crystalline powder, practically free of odor, with a bitter taste. It is soluble in water, chloroform and methanol. Verapamil HCl is not chemically related to other cardioactive drugs.

CLINICAL PHARMACOLOGY

ISOPTIN is a calcium ion influx inhibitor (slow channel blocker or calcium ion antagonist) which exerts its pharmacologic effects by modulating the influx of ionic calcium across the cell membrane of the arterial smooth muscle as well as in conductile and contractile myocardial cells.

Mechanism of Action: The precise mechanism of action of ISOPTIN as an antianginal agent remains to be fully determined but includes the following mechanisms:

1. **Relaxation and prevention of coronary artery spasm**
ISOPTIN dilates the main coronary arteries and coronary arterioles, both in normal and ischemic regions, and is a potent inhibitor of coronary artery spasm, whether spontaneous or ergonovine-induced. This property increases myocardial oxygen delivery in patients with coronary artery spasm, and is responsible for the effectiveness of ISOPTIN in vasospastic (Prinzmetal's or variant) as well as unstable angina at rest. Whether this effect plays any role in classical effort angina is not clear, but studies of exercise tolerance have not shown an increase in the maximum exercise rate-pressure product, a widely accepted measure of oxygen utilization. This suggests that, in general, relief of spasm or dilation of coronary arteries is not an important factor in classical angina.
2. **Reduction of oxygen utilization**
ISOPTIN regularly reduces arterial pressure at rest and at a given level of exercise by dilating peripheral arterioles and reducing the total peripheral resistance (afterload) against which the heart works. This unloading of the heart reduces myocardial energy consump-

Continued on next page

Knoll—Cont.

tion and oxygen requirements and probably accounts for the effectiveness of ISOPTIN in chronic stable effort angina.

Electrical activity through the SA and AV nodes depends, to a significant degree, upon calcium influx through the slow channel. By inhibiting this influx, ISOPTIN slows AV conduction and prolongs the effective refractory period within the AV node in a rate-related manner. It can interfere with sinus node impulse generation and induce sinus arrest in patients with sick sinus syndrome and also can induce atrioventricular block, although this has been seen rarely in clinical use.

ISOPTIN may shorten the antegrade effective refractory period of accessory bypass tracts. ISOPTIN does not alter the normal atrial action potential or intraventricular conduction time, but depresses amplitude, velocity of depolarization and conduction in depressed atrial fibers.

ISOPTIN has a local anesthetic action that is 1.6 times that of procaine on an equimolar basis. It is not known whether this action is important at the doses used in man.

ISOPTIN does not alter total serum calcium levels.

Pharmacokinetics and Metabolism: More than 90% of the orally administered dose of ISOPTIN is absorbed. Because of rapid biotransformation of verapamil during its first pass through the portal circulation, absolute bioavailability ranges from 20% to 35%. Peak plasma concentrations are reached between 1 and 2 hours after oral administration. Chronic oral administration of 120 mg of ISOPTIN every 6 hours resulted in plasma levels of verapamil ranging from 125 to 400 ng/mL with higher values reported occasionally. A close relationship exists between verapamil plasma concentration and prolongation of the PR interval. The mean elimination half-life in single dose studies ranged from 2.8 to 7.4 hours. In these same studies, after repetitive dosing, the half-life increased to a range from 4.5 to 12.0 hours (after less than 10 consecutive doses given 6 hours apart). Half-life may increase during titration due to saturation of hepatic enzyme systems as plasma verapamil levels rise.

In healthy men, orally administered ISOPTIN undergoes extensive metabolism in the liver. Twelve metabolites have been identified in plasma; all except norverapamil are present in trace amounts only. Norverapamil can reach steady-state plasma concentrations approximately equal to those of verapamil itself. The major metabolites of verapamil have been identified as various N- and O-dealkylated products of ISOPTIN. Approximately 70% of an administered dose is excreted as metabolites in the urine and 16% or more in the feces within 5 days. About 3% to 4% is excreted in the urine as unchanged drug. Approximately 90% is bound to plasma proteins. In patients with hepatic insufficiency, metabolism is delayed and elimination half-life prolonged up to 14 to 16 hours (see Precautions); the volume of distribution is increased and plasma clearance reduced to about 30% of normal. Verapamil clearance values suggest that patients with liver dysfunction may attain therapeutic verapamil plasma concentrations with one-third of the oral daily dose required for patients with normal liver function.

Hemodynamics and Myocardial Metabolism: In animals and man, ISOPTIN reduces afterload and myocardial contractility. In most patients, including those with organic cardiac disease, the negative inotropic action of ISOPTIN is countered by reduction of afterload and cardiac index is usually not reduced. In patients with severe left ventricular dysfunction however, (e.g., pulmonary wedge pressure above 20 mm Hg or ejection fraction lower than 30%), or in patients on beta-adrenergic blocking agents or other cardiodepressant drugs, deterioration of ventricular function may occur (see Drug Interactions).

Pulmonary Function: ISOPTIN does not induce bronchoconstriction and hence, does not impair ventilatory function.

INDICATIONS AND USAGE

ISOPTIN is indicated for the treatment of angina pectoris including:

1. Angina at rest including:
   - Vasospastic (Prinzmetal's variant) angina
   - Unstable (crescendo, pre-infarction) angina
2. Chronic stable angina (classic effort-associated angina)

CONTRAINDICATIONS

Verapamil HCl is contraindicated in:

1. Severe left ventricular dysfunction (see Warnings)
2. Hypotension (less than 90 mm Hg systolic pressure) or cardiogenic shock
3. Sick sinus syndrome (except in patients with a functioning artificial ventricular pacemaker)
4. Second- or third-degree AV block

WARNINGS

Heart Failure: Verapamil has a negative inotropic effect which, in most patients, is compensated by its afterload reduction (decreased peripheral vascular resistance) properties without a net impairment of ventricular performance. In clinical experience with 1166 patients, 11 (0.9%) developed congestive heart failure or pulmonary edema. Congestive heart failure/pulmonary edema led to discontinuation or reduction in dosage of verapamil in 6 (0.5%) patients. Verapamil should be avoided in patients with severe left ventricular dysfunction (e.g., ejection fraction less than 30% or moderate to severe symptoms of cardiac failure) and in patients with any degree of ventricular dysfunction if they are receiving a beta blocker (see Drug Interactions). Patients with milder ventricular dysfunction should, if possible, be controlled with optimum doses of digitalis and/or diuretics before verapamil treatment (**Note interactions with digoxin under: Precautions).**

Hypotension: Occasionally, the pharmacologic action of verapamil may produce a decrease in blood pressure below normal levels which may result in dizziness or symptomatic hypotension. Hypotension is usually asymptomatic, orthostatic, mild and can be controlled by a decrease in the ISOPTIN dose. The incidence of hypotension observed in 1166 patients enrolled in clinical trials was 2.9%.

Elevated Liver Enzymes: Elevations of transaminases with and without concomitant elevations in alkaline phosphatase and bilirubin have been reported. Such elevations have sometimes been transient and may disappear even in the face of continued verapamil treatment; however, four cases of hepatocellular injury produced by verapamil have been proven by rechallenge. Two of these four cases had clinical symptoms of malaise, fever, and/or right upper quadrant pain in addition to elevations of SGOT, SGPT and alkaline phosphatase. Periodic monitoring of liver function in patients receiving verapamil is therefore prudent.

Atrial Flutter/Fibrillation with Accessory Bypass Tract: Patients with atrial flutter or fibrillation and an accessory AV pathway (e.g., Wolff-Parkinson-White or Lown-Ganong-Levine syndromes) may develop increased antegrade conduction across the aberrant pathway bypassing the AV node, producing a very rapid ventricular response after receiving verapamil (or digitalis). Treatment is usually D.C.-cardioversion. Cardioversion has been used safely and effectively after oral ISOPTIN.

Atrioventricular Block: The effect of verapamil on AV conduction and the SA node leads to first-degree AV block and transient bradycardia, sometimes accompanied by nodal escape rhythms, fairly commonly during the peaks of serum concentration. Higher degrees of AV block, however, were infrequently (0.8%) observed. Marked first-degree block or progressive development to second- or third-degree AV block requires a reduction in dosage or, in rare instances, discontinuation of verapamil HCl and institution of appropriate therapy depending upon the clinical situation.

Patients with Hypertrophic Cardiomyopathy (IHSS): In 120 patients with hypertrophic cardiomyopathy (most of them refractory or intolerant to propranolol) who received therapy with verapamil at doses up to 720 mg/day, a variety of serious adverse effects were seen. Three patients died in pulmonary edema; all had severe left ventricular outflow obstruction and a past history of left ventricular dysfunction. Eight other patients had pulmonary edema and/or severe hypotension; abnormally high (over 20 mm Hg) capillary wedge pressure and a marked left ventricular outflow obstruction were present in most of these patients. Concomitant administration of quinidine preceded the severe hypotension in 3 of the 8 patients (2 of whom developed pulmonary edema). Sinus bradycardia occurred in 11% of the patients, second-degree AV block in 4% and sinus arrest in 2%. It must be appreciated that this group of patients had a serious disease with a high mortality rate. Most adverse effects responded well to dose reduction and only rarely did verapamil have to be discontinued.

PRECAUTIONS

General

Use in Patients with Impaired Hepatic Function: Since verapamil is highly metabolized by the liver, it should be administered cautiously to patients with impaired hepatic function. Severe liver dysfunction prolongs the elimination half-life of verapamil to about 14 to 16 hours; hence, approximately 30% of the dose given to patients with normal liver function should be administered to these patients. Careful monitoring for abnormal prolongation of the PR interval or other signs of excessive pharmacologic effects (See Overdosage) should be carried out.

Use in Patients with Impaired Renal Function: About 70% of an administered dose of verapamil is excreted as metabolites in the urine. Until further data are available, verapamil should be administered cautiously to patients with impaired renal function. These patients should be carefully monitored for abnormal prolongation of the PR interval or other signs of overdosage (see Overdosage).

Drug Interactions

Beta Blockers: Controlled studies in small numbers of patients suggest that the concomitant use of ISOPTIN and beta-blocking agents may be beneficial in patients with chronic stable angina but available information is not sufficient to predict with confidence the effects of concurrent treatment, especially in patients with left ventricular dysfunction or cardiac conduction abnormalities.

The combination can have adverse effects on cardiac function. In one study of 15 patients treated with high doses of propranolol (median dose: 480 mg/day, range 160 to 1280 mg/day) for severe angina, with preserved left ventricular function (ejection fraction greater than 35%), the hemodynamic effects of additional therapy with ISOPTIN (verapamil HCl) were assessed using invasive methods. The addition of verapamil to high dose beta blockers induced modest negative inotropic and chronotropic effects which were not severe enough to limit short-term (48 hours) combination therapy in this study. These modest cardiodepressant effects persist for greater than 6, but less than 30 hours after abrupt withdrawal of beta blockers and were closely related to plasma levels of propranolol. The primary verapamil/beta-blocker interaction in this study appeared to be hemodynamic rather than electrophysiologic.

In three other studies involving 51 patients, verapamil did not induce negative inotropic or chronotropic effects in patients with preserved left ventricular function receiving low or moderate doses of propranolol (less than or equal to 320 mg/day). Because of the still limited experience with combination therapy verapamil should be used alone, if possible. If combined therapy is used, close surveillance of vital signs and clinical status should be carried out and the need for concomitant treatment with propranolol reassessed periodically. Combined therapy should usually be avoided in patients with atrioventricular conduction abnormalities and those with depressed left ventricular function.

Digitalis: Chronic verapamil treatment increases serum digoxin levels by 50% to 70% during the first week of therapy and this can result in digitalis toxicity. Maintenance digitalization doses should be reduced when verapamil is administered and the patient should be carefully monitored to avoid over- or underdigitalization. Whenever overdigitalization is suspected, the daily dose of digoxin should be reduced or temporarily discontinued. Upon discontinuation of ISOPTIN (verapamil HCl), the patient should be monitored to avoid underdigitalization.

Antihypertensive Agents: Verapamil administered concomitantly with oral antihypertensive agents (e.g., vasodilators, diuretics) may have an additive effect on lowering blood pressure. Patients receiving these combinations should be appropriately monitored. In patients who have recently received drugs such as methyldopa, which attenuate alpha-adrenergic response, combined therapy of verapamil and propranolol should probably be avoided (severe hypotension may occur).

Disopyramide: Until data on possible interactions between verapamil and disopyramide phosphate are obtained, disopyramide should not be administered within 48 hours before or 24 hours after verapamil administration.

Quinidine: In a small number of patients with hypertrophic cardiomyopathy (IHSS), concomitant use of verapamil and quinidine resulted in significant hypotension. Until further data are obtained, combined therapy of verapamil and quinidine in patients with hypertrophic cardiomyopathy should probably be avoided.

Nitrates: Verapamil has been given concomitantly with short- and long-acting nitrates without any undesirable drug interactions. The pharmacologic profile of both drugs and the clinical experience suggest beneficial interactions.

Carcinogenesis, Mutagenesis, Impairment of Fertility: Adequate animal carcinogenicity studies have not been performed with verapamil. An 18 month toxicity study in rats, at a low multiple (6 fold) of the maximum recommended human dose, and not the maximum tolerated dose, did not suggest a tumorigenic potential. A two year carcinogenicity study will be carried out in rats.

Verapamil was not mutagenic in the Ames test in 5 test strains at 3 mg per plate, with or without metabolic activation.

Studies in female rats at daily dietary doses up to 5.5 times (55 mg/kg/day) the maximum recommended human dose did not show impaired fertility. Effects on male fertility have not been determined.

Pregnancy: Pregnancy Category C. Reproduction studies have been performed in rabbits and rats at oral doses up to 1.5 (15 mg/kg/day) and 6 (60 mg/kg/day) times the human oral daily dose, respectively, and have revealed no evidence of teratogenicity. In the rat, however, this multiple of the human dose was embryocidal and retarded fetal growth and development, probably because of adverse maternal effects reflected in reduced weight gains of the dams. This oral dose has also been shown to cause hypotension in rats. There are no adequate and well-controlled studies in pregnant women. Because animal reproduction studies are not always predictive of human response, this drug should be used during pregnancy only if clearly needed.

Labor and Delivery: It is not known whether the use of verapamil during labor or delivery has immediate or delayed adverse effects on the fetus, or whether it prolongs the duration of labor or increases the need for forceps delivery or other obstetric intervention. Such adverse experiences have not been reported in the literature, despite a long history of use of ISOPTIN in Europe in the treatment of cardiac side effects of beta-adrenergic agonist agents used to treat premature labor.

Nursing Mothers: It is not known whether this drug is excreted in human milk. Because many drugs are excreted in human milk and because of the potential for adverse reactions in nursing infants from verapamil, nursing should be discontinued while verapamil is administered. Studies in rats at 2.5 times the maximum recommended human dose revealed no evidence of an effect of verapamil on lactation or weaning.

Animal Pharmacology and/or Animal Toxicology: Chronic animal toxicology studies indicate that verapamil causes lenticular and/or suture line changes at 30 mg/kg/day or greater and frank cataracts at 62.5 mg/kg/day or greater in the beagle dog but not the rat. These effects are thought to be species-specific. Development of cataracts due to verapamil has not been reported in man.

ADVERSE REACTIONS

Serious adverse reactions are rare when ISOPTIN therapy is initiated with upward dose titration within the recommended single and total daily dose. The following reactions to orally administered ISOPTIN were reported from clinical experience in 1166 patients with angina or arrhythmia. Adverse reactions occurred at a similar rate in controlled clinical trials and uncontrolled clinical experience.

Cardiovascular: Hypotension (2.9%), peripheral edema (1.7%), AV block (third-degree)(0.8%), bradycardia (HR <50/min, 1.1%), congestive heart failure or pulmonary edema (0.9%).

Central Nervous System: Dizziness (3.6%), headache (1.8%), fatigue (1.1%).

Gastrointestinal: Constipation (6.3%), nausea (1.6%). Elevations of liver enzymes have been reported (see **Warnings**).

The following reactions, reported in less than 0.5%, occurred under circumstances where a causal relationship is uncertain and are therefore mentioned to alert the physician to a possible relationship: ecchymosis, bruising, gynecomastia, psychotic symptoms, confusion, paresthesia, insomnia, somnolence, equilibrium disorder, blurred vision, syncope, muscle cramp, shakiness, claudication, hair loss, macules, spotty menstruation. In addition, more serious adverse events were observed, not readily distinguishable from the natural history of the disease in these patients. Of the 1166 patients evaluated 16 (1.4%) had myocardial infarctions. Nine of these 16 patients had myocardial infarctions while being treated for unstable angina, 4 of these were receiving placebo, the remaining 5 received verapamil.

The daily dose of verapamil was reduced in 6.3% and discontinued in 5.5% of the 1166 patients. In general, the highest incidence of adverse reactions was seen in the dose titration periods in all the studies.

Treatment of Acute Cardiovascular Adverse Reactions: The frequency of cardiovascular adverse reactions which require therapy is rare; hence, experience with their treatment is limited. Whenever severe hypotension or complete AV block occur following oral administration of verapamil, the appropriate emergency measures should be applied immediately, e.g., intravenously administered isoproterenol HCl, levarterenol bitartrate, atropine (all in the usual doses), or calcium gluconate (10% solution). In patients with hypertrophic cardiomyopathy (IHSS), alpha-adrenergic agents (phenylephrine, metaraminol bitartrate or methoxamine) should be used to maintain blood pressure and isoproterenol and levarterenol should be avoided. If further support is necessary, inotropic agents (dopamine or dobutamine) may be administered. Actual treatment and dosage should depend on the severity of the clinical situation and the judgment and experience of the treating physician.

OVERDOSAGE

Treatment of overdosage should be supportive. Beta-adrenergic stimulation or parenteral administration of calcium solutions may increase calcium ion flux across the slow channel, and have been used effectively in treatment of deliberate overdosage with verapamil. Clinically significant hypotensive reactions or fixed high degree AV block should be treated with vasopressor agents or cardiac pacing, respectively. Asystole should be handled by the usual measures including cardiopulmonary resuscitation.

DOSAGE AND ADMINISTRATION

The dose of verapamil must be individualized by titration. ISOPTIN is available in 80 mg and 120 mg scored tablets. The usual initial dose is 80 mg three or four times a day. Dosage may be increased at daily (e.g., patients with unstable angina) or weekly intervals until optimum clinical response is obtained. In general, maximum effects of any given dosage would be apparent during the first 24 to 48 hours of therapy, but note that between 24 to 48 hours the half-life of verapamil increases, hence maximum response may be delayed. The total daily dose for most patients ranges from 320 to 480 mg. The usefulness and safety of dosages exceeding 480 mg per day in angina pectoris have not been established.

HOW SUPPLIED

ISOPTIN tablets are supplied as round, scored, film-coated tablets containing either 80 mg or 120 mg of verapamil hydrochloride and embossed with "ISOPTIN 80" or "ISOPTIN 120" on one side and with "Knoll" on the reverse side.

80 mg (yellow)—
- Bottle of 100—NDC #0044-1822-02
- Bottle of 500—NDC #0044-1822-05
- Bottle of 1000—NDC #0044-1822-04
- Hospital Unit Dose (100 tablets—Strips of 10)—NDC #0044-1822-10

120 mg (white)—
- Bottle of 100—NDC #0044-1823-02
- Bottle of 500—NDC #0044-1823-05
- Bottle of 1000—NDC #0044-1823-04
- Hospital Unit Dose (100 tablets—Strips of 10)—NDC #0044-1823-10

Storage: 15° to 30°C, 59° to 86°F.

Revised August 1984 Print #2425

Shown in Product Identification Section, page 412

QUADRINAL® Tablets ℞

[kwă 'drĭ-nawl]

DESCRIPTION

Each QUADRINAL™ Tablet contains ephedrine hydrochloride 24 mg; phenobarbital 24 mg [**Warning:** May be habit forming]; theophylline calcium salicylate 130 mg (equivalent to 65 mg anhydrous theophylline); potassium iodide 320 mg. Other ingredients include magnesium stearate, potato starch, sodium thiosulfate and talc.

QUADRINAL contains two bronchodilators, theophylline and ephedrine. Phenobarbital serves as a mild sedative to help counteract central nervous system stimulation which may be caused by ephedrine. Wheezing and coughing are relieved by improved bronchodilation while the expectorant action of potassium iodide helps to remove secretions from the bronchial tree. Dyspnea is thus relieved or prevented and acute episodes of bronchospasm are often eliminated with consequent lessening of apprehension and distress.

CLINICAL PHARMACOLOGY

Theophylline directly relaxes the smooth muscle of the bronchial airways and pulmonary blood vessels, thus acting mainly as a bronchodilator, pulmonary vasodilator and smooth muscle relaxant. It also possesses other actions typical of the xanthine derivatives: coronary vasodilator, diuretic, and cardiac, cerebral, and skeletal muscle stimulant. The actions of theophylline may be mediated through inhibition of phosphodiesterase and a resultant increase in intracellular cyclic AMP which could mediate smooth muscle relaxation.

In vitro, theophylline has been shown to react synergistically with beta agonists (such as isoproterenol) that increase intracellular cyclic AMP through the stimulation of adenyl cyclase, but synergism has not been demonstrated in clinical studies and more data are needed to determine if theophylline and beta agonists have clinically important additive effects **in vivo**.

Apparently, tolerance does not develop with chronic use of theophylline.

The half-life is shortened with cigarette smoking. The half-life is prolonged in alcoholism, reduced hepatic or renal function, congestive heart failure, and in patients receiving cimetidine or antibiotics such as troleandomycin (TAO, Cyclamycin), erythromycin, lincomycin and clindamycin. High fever for prolonged periods may decrease theophylline elimination.

Theophylline Elimination Characteristics

	Theophylline Clearance Rates (mean ± S.D.)	Half-life Average (mean ± S.D.)
Children (over 6 months of age)	1.45 ± 0.58 mL/kg/min	3.7 ± 1.1 hrs.
Adult non-smokers with uncomplicated asthma	0.65 ± 0.19 mL/kg/min	8.7 ± 2.2 hrs.

Newborn infants have extremely slow clearances with half-lives exceeding 24 hours. These approach those seen for older children after about 3–6 months.

Older adults with chronic obstructive pulmonary disease, patients with cor pulmonale or other causes of heart failure, and patients with liver pathology may have much lower clearances with half-lives that may exceed 24 hours. The half-life is prolonged in alcoholism, reduced hepatic or renal function, congestive heart failure, and in patients receiving cimetidine or antibiotics such as troleandomycin (TAO, Cyclamycin), erythromycin, lincomycin and clindamycin. High fever for prolonged periods may decrease theophylline elimination.

The half-life of theophylline in smokers (1 to 2 packs/day) averaged 4 to 5 hours in various studies, much shorter than the 7 to 9 hour half-life in nonsmokers. The increase in theophylline clearance caused by smoking is probably the result of induction of drug-metabolizing enzymes that do not readily normalize after cessation of smoking. It appears that between 3 months and 2 years may be necessary for normalization of the effect of smoking on theophylline pharmacokinetics.

INDICATIONS

For chronic respiratory disease in which tenacious mucus and bronchospasm are dominant symptoms, such as bronchial asthma, chronic bronchitis and pulmonary emphysema.

CONTRAINDICATIONS

Use of QUADRINAL is contraindicated in patients with enlarged thyroid or goiter or with known sensitivity to theophylline, potassium iodide, ephedrine or sympathomimetics, or barbiturates.

The iodide in QUADRINAL can cause fetal harm when administered to a pregnant woman. Development of goiter has been reported in infants whose mothers received iodide-containing medications during pregnancy. A few neonatal deaths resulting from tracheal obstruction due to congenital goiters have been reported. Use of barbiturates during pregnancy may cause physical dependence with resulting withdrawal symptoms in the neonate; may cause birth defects; may be associated with neonatal hemorrhage due to reduction in levels of vitamin K-dependent clotting factors in the neonate; may cause respiratory depression in the neonate. QUADRINAL is contraindicated in women who are or may become pregnant. If this drug is used during pregnancy, or if the patient becomes pregnant while taking this drug, the patient should be apprised of the potential hazard to the fetus.

WARNINGS

QUADRINAL contains theophylline calcium salicylate. Salicylates have been reported to be associated with the development of Reyes syndrome in children and teenagers with chicken pox or flu.

Excessive theophylline doses may be associated with toxicity; determination of serum theophylline levels is recommended to assure maximal benefit without excessive risk. Incidence of toxicity increases at serum levels greater than 20 mcg/mL. Because of the theophylline content of QUADRINAL, it is unlikely that toxic levels of theophylline would be reached unless a serious overdosage occurs.

Morphine, curare, and stilbamidine should be used with caution in patients with airflow obstruction since they stimulate histamine release and can induce asthmatic attacks. They may also suppress respiration leading to respiratory failure. Alternative drugs should be chosen whenever possible.

There is an excellent correlation between clinical manifestations of toxicity and high blood levels of theophylline resulting from conventional doses in patients with lowered body plasma clearances (due to transient cardiac decompensation), patients with liver dysfunction or chronic obstructive lung disease, and patients who are older than 55 years of age, particularly males. In about 50% of patients, nausea and restlessness precede more severe manifestations of toxicity. In other patients, ventricular arrhythmias or seizures may be the first signs of toxicity. These more serious side effects are more likely to occur after intravenous administration of theophylline. Many patients who have high theophylline serum levels exhibit a tachycardia, and theophylline may worsen preexisting arrhythmias.

PRECAUTIONS

Mean half-life in smokers is shorter than in nonsmokers; therefore, smokers may require larger doses of theophylline. QUADRINAL, like all theophylline products, should not be administered concurrently with other xanthine medications. Use with caution in patients with severe cardiac disease, severe hypoxemia, hypertension, hyperthyroidism, acute myocardial injury, cor pulmonale, congestive heart failure, liver disease, peptic ulcer and in the elderly (especially males) and in neonates. Great caution should be used especially in giving theophylline to patients in congestive heart failure; such patients have shown markedly prolonged theophylline blood level curves with theophylline persisting in serum for long periods following discontinuation of the drug. Theophylline may occasionally act as a local irritant to the G.I. tract although gastrointestinal symptoms are more commonly central in origin and associated with serum concentrations over 20 mcg/mL.

Ephedrine-containing medications should be used with caution in patients with cardiovascular disease, diabetes mellitus, predisposition to glaucoma, hypertension, hyperthyroidism, or prostatic hypertrophy.

Potassium iodide may aggravate acne in adolescents and adults.

Continued on next page

Knoll—Cont.

Phenobarbital should be used with caution in patients with a history of drug abuse or dependence, impaired renal or hepatic function, hyperkinesis, uncontrolled pain, or history of porphyria.

Usage in Pregnancy: Pregnancy Category X. See "Contraindications" section.

Nursing Mothers: Because of the potential for serious adverse reactions in nursing infants from the potassium iodide, ephedrine and phenobarbital in QUADRINAL, a decision should be made whether to discontinue nursing or to discontinue the drug, taking into account the importance of the drug to the mother.

Pediatric Use: QUADRINAL is indicated for use in children on a short term basis. Chronic use should be reserved for patients in whom other expectorants have not been effective. If QUADRINAL is used chronically in children, the patient should be observed for signs of thyroid enlargement and worsening of acne.

Geriatric Patients: Geriatric patients may be more sensitive to the effects of ephedrine.

ADVERSE REACTIONS

The most frequent adverse reactions to theophylline are usually due to overdose (serum levels in excess of 20 mcg/mL) and are: nausea, vomiting, epigastric pain, hematemesis, diarrhea, headaches, irritability, restlessness, insomnia, reflex hyperexcitability, muscle twitching, clonic and tonic generalized convulsions, palpitations, tachycardia, extra systoles, flushing, hypotension, circulatory failure, ventricular arrhythmias, tachypnea, albuminuria, increased excretion of renal tubular cells and red blood cells, potentiation of diuresis, hyperglycemia and inappropriate ADH syndrome.

Thyroid adenoma, goiter and myxedema are possible side effects of potassium iodide.

Hypersensitivity to iodides may be manifested by angioneurotic edema, cutaneous and mucosal hemorrhages, and symptoms resembling serum sickness, such as fever, arthralgia, lymph node enlargement and eosinophilia.

Chronic ingestion of iodides may result in chronic iodide poisoning, or iodism. Initial symptoms include an unpleasant brassy taste, burning in the mouth and throat, soreness of the teeth and gums, increased salivation, coryza, sneezing, irritation of the eyes with swelling of the eyelids, headache, cough, skin lesions, diarrhea, gastric irritation, anorexia, fever and depression. The symptoms of iodism disappear spontaneously within a few days after stopping the administration of iodide. Therefore, treatment consists of stopping QUADRINAL therapy and providing supportive measures as indicated by the symptoms. Abundant fluid and sodium chloride intake may hasten iodide elimination. In severe cases, the use of mannitol to establish an osmotic diuresis may be appropriate. Potassium iodide may produce hyperkalemia and, if ingested chronically, may lead to goiter.

Adverse reactions to ephedrine include nervousness, restlessness, trouble in sleeping, irregular heartbeat, difficult or painful urination, dizziness or light-headedness, headache, loss of appetite, nausea or vomiting, trembling, troubled breathing, unusual increase in sweating, unusual paleness, feeling of warmth, and weakness. Tolerance to ephedrine may develop with prolonged or excessive use.

Adverse reactions to phenobarbital include mental confusion or depression, shortness of breath or troubled breathing, skin rash, hives, swelling of eyelids, face or lips, wheezing or tightness in chest, sore throat and fever, unusual bleeding or bruising, unusual excitement, tiredness or weakness, unusually slow heartbeat, yellowing of eyes or skin.

DRUG INTERACTIONS

Toxic synergism of theophylline with ephedrine has been documented and may occur with some other sympathomimetic bronchodilators.

[See table below].

OVERDOSAGE

A. If potential overdose is established and seizure has not occurred and patient is conscious:
   1) Induce vomiting.
   2) Administer a cathartic.
   3) Administer activated charcoal.
B. If patient is having a seizure:
   1) Establish an airway.
   2) Administer O_2.
   3) Treat the seizure with intravenous diazepam, 0.1 to 0.3 mg/kg up to 10 mg.
   4) Monitor vital signs, maintain blood pressure and provide adequate hydration.
C. Post-seizure coma:
   1) Maintain airway and oxygenation.
   2) Following above recommendations to prevent absorption of drug, but intubation and lavage will have to be performed instead of inducing emesis, and introduce the cathartic and charcoal via a large bore gastric lavage tube.
   3) Continue to provide full supportive care and adequate hydration while waiting for drug to be metabolized. In general, the drug is metabolized sufficiently rapidly so as not to require dialysis.

DOSAGE AND ADMINISTRATION

When rapidly absorbed products such as uncoated tablets with rapid dissolution are used, dosing to maintain "around the clock" blood levels generally requires administration every 6 hours in children; dosing intervals up to 8 hours may be satisfactory for adults because of their slower elimination rate.

Drug	Effect
Aminophylline with lithium carbonate	Increased excretion of lithium carbonate
Potassium iodide with lithium	Increased hypothyroid and goiterogenic effects
Aminophylline with propranolol	Antagonism of propranolol effect
Theophylline with furosemide	Increased diuresis
Theophylline with hexamethonium	Decreased hexamethonium induced chronotropic effect
Theophylline with reserpine	Reserpine-induced tachycardia
Theophylline with chlordiazepoxide	Chlordiazepoxide-induced fatty acid mobilization
Theophylline with troleandomycin (TAO, Cyclamycin), erythromycin, lincomycin, clindamycin	Increased theophylline plasma levels
Theophylline with phenytoin	Decreased phenytoin levels
Theophylline with cimetidine	Increased theophylline blood levels
Ephedrine with digitalis glycosides or anesthetics	May cause cardiac arrhythmias
Ephedrine with ergonovine, methylergonovine or oxytocin	Hypertension
Ephedrine with guanethidine	Decreased hypotensive effect
Ephedrine with MAO inhibitors	Potentiation of pressor effect of ephedrine
Ephedrine with reserpine	Decreased pressor effect of ephedrine
Ephedrine with other sympathomimetics	Increased effects of either medication
Ephedrine with tricyclic antidepressants	May antagonize the pressor action of ephedrine
Phenobarbital with alcohol, general anesthetics, other CNS depressants, or MAO inhibitors	Increased effects of either medication
Phenobarbital with oral anticoagulants	Decreased anticoagulant effects
Phenobarbital with corticosteroids, digitalis, digitoxin, doxycycline, tricyclic antidepressants, griseofulvin or phenytoin	Decreased effects of these drugs

Pulmonary function measurements before and after a period of treatment permit an objective assessment of response to QUADRINAL.

Usual dose:

Adults—One tablet 3 or 4 times daily; if needed, an additional one tablet upon retiring for nighttime relief. In severe attacks, the usual dose may be increased by one half.

Children 6 to 12 years—one half tablet three times daily.

Children under 6 years—dose is proportionately less.

HOW SUPPLIED

QUADRINAL Tablets— white, round, bi-convex tablets, engraved with a triangle on one side, bisected on the other side and imprinted with the number "14".

Bottles of 100—NDC #0044-4520-02.

Bottles of 1000—NDC #0044-4520-04.

STORAGE

59°-86°F, (15°-30°C).

Revised April 1985 8442

Shown in Product Identification Section, page 412

SANTYL® Ointment ℞

[*săn 'tĭl*]

(collagenase)

DESCRIPTION

SANTYL® OINTMENT is a sterile enzymatic debriding ointment which contains 250 collagenase units per gram of white petrolatum USP. The enzyme collagenase is derived from the fermentation by *Clostridium histolyticum.* It possesses the unique ability to digest native and denatured collagen in necrotic tissue.

CLINICAL PHARMACOLOGY

Since collagen accounts for 75% of the dry weight of skin tissue, the ability of collagenase to digest collagen in the physiological pH range and temperature makes it particularly effective in the removal of detritus.[1] Collagenase thus contributes towards the formation of granulation tissue and subsequent epithelization of dermal ulcers and severely burned areas.[2,3,4,5,6] Collagen in healthy tissue or in newly formed granulation tissue is not attacked.[2,3,4,5,6,7,8]

INDICATIONS

Santyl Ointment is indicated for debriding chronic dermal ulcers[2,3,4,5,6,8,9,10,11,12,13,14,15,16,17,18] and severely burned areas.[3,4,5,7,16,19,20,21]

CONTRAINDICATIONS

Santyl Ointment is contraindicated in patients who have shown local or systemic hypersensitivity to collagenase.

PRECAUTIONS

The optimal pH range of collagenase is 6 to 8. Higher or lower pH conditions will decrease the enzyme's activity and appropriate precautions should be taken. The enzymatic activity is also adversely affected by detergents, hexachlorophene and heavy metal ions such as mercury and silver which are used in some antiseptics. When it is suspected such materials have been used, the site should be carefully cleansed by repeated washings with normal saline before Santyl Ointment is applied. Soaks containing metal ions or acidic solutions such as Burow's solution should be avoided because of the metal ion and low pH. Cleansing materials such as hydrogen peroxide, Dakin's solution, and sterile saline are compatible with Santyl Ointment.

Debilitated patients should be closely monitored for systemic bacterial infections because of the theoretical possibility that debriding enzymes may increase the risk of bacteremia.

A slight transient erythema has been noted occasionally in the surrounding tissue, particularly when Santyl Ointment was not confined to the lesion. Therefore, the ointment should be applied carefully within the area of the lesion.

ADVERSE REACTIONS

No allergic sensitivity or toxic reactions have been noted in the recorded clinical investigations. However, one case of systemic manifestations of hypersensitivity to collagenase in a patient treated for more than one year with a combination of collagenase and cortisone has been reported to us.

OVERDOSAGE

Action of the enzyme may be stopped, should this be desired, by the application of Burow's solution USP (pH 3.6–4.4) to the lesion.

DOSAGE AND ADMINISTRATION

Santyl Ointment should be applied once daily (or more frequently if the dressing becomes soiled, as from incontinence) in the following manner:

(1) Prior to application the lesion should be cleansed of debris and digested material by gently rubbing with a gauze pad saturated with hydrogen peroxide or Dakin's solution followed by sterile normal saline.

(2) Whenever infection is present it is desirable to use an appropriate topical antibacterial agent. Neomycin-

Bacitracin-Polymyxin B (Neosporin) powder has been found to be compatible with Santyl Ointment. The antibiotic should be applied to the lesion prior to the application of Santyl Ointment. Should the infection not respond, therapy with Santyl Ointment should be discontinued until remission of the infection.

(3) Santyl Ointment should be applied directly to deep lesions with a wooden tongue depressor or spatula. For shallow lesions, Santyl Ointment may be applied to a sterile gauze pad which is then applied to the wound and properly secured.

(4) Crosshatching thick eschar with a #10 blade allows collagenase more surface contact with necrotic debris. It is also desirable to remove, with forceps and scissors, as much loosened detritus as can be done readily.

(5) All excess ointment should be removed each time dressing is changed.

(6) Use of Santyl Ointment should be terminated when debridement of necrotic tissue is complete and granulation tissue is well established.

HOW SUPPLIED

Santyl Ointment contains 250 units of collagenase enzyme per gram of white petrolatum USP. The potency assay of collagenase is based on the digestion of undenatured collagen (from bovine Achilles tendon) at pH 7.2 and 37°C for 24 hours. The number of peptide bonds cleaved are measured by reaction with ninhydrin. Amino groups released by a trypsin digestion control are subtracted. One net collagenase unit will solubilize ninhydrin reactive material equivalent to 4 micromoles of leucine.

REFERENCES

1— Mandl, I., Adv. Enzymol. 23:163, 1961.
2— Boxer, A.M., Gottesman, N., Bernstein, H., & Mandl, I., Geriatrics 24:75, 1969.
3— Mazurek, I., Med. Welt 22:150, 1971.
4— Zimmerman, W.E., in "Collagenase," I. Mandl, ed., Gordon & Breach, Science Publishers, New York, 1971, p. 131, p. 185.
5— Vetra, H., & Whittaker, D., Geriatrics 30:53, 1975.
6— Rao, D.B., Sane, P.G., & Georgiev, E.L., J. Am. Geriatrics Soc. 23:22, 1975.
7— Vrabec, R., Moserova, J., Konickova, Z., Behounkova, E., & Blaha, J., J. Hyg. Epidemiol. Microbiol. Immunol. 18:496, 1974.
8— Lippmann, H.I., Arch. Phys. Med. Rehabil. 54:588, 1973.
9— German, F.M., in "Collagenase," I. Mandl, ed. Gordon & Breach, Science Publishers, New York, 1971, p. 165.
10— Haimovici, H. & Strauch, B., in "Collagenase," I. Mandl, ed., Gordon & Breach, Science Publishers, New York, 1971, p. 177.
11— Lee, L.K., & Ambrus, J.L., Geriatrics 30:91, 1975.
12— Locke, R.K., & Heifitz, N.M., J. Am. Pod. Assoc. 65:242, 1975.
13— Varma, A.O., Bugatch, E., & German, F.M., Surg. Gynecol. Obstet. 136:281, 1973.
14— Barrett, D., Jr., & Klibanski, A., Am. J. Nurs. 73:849, 1973.
15— Bardfeld, L.A., J. Pod. Ed. 1:41, 1970.
16— Blum, G., Schweiz. Rundschau Med. Praxis 62:820, 1973. Abstr. in Dermatology Digest, Feb. 1974, p. 36.
17— Zaruba, F., Lettl, A., Brozkova, L., Skrdlantova, H., & Krs, V., J. Hyg. Epidemiol. Microbiol. Immunol. 18:499, 1974.
18— Altman, M.I., Goldstein, L., Horowitz, S., J. Am. Pod. Assoc. 68:11, 1978.
19— Rehn, V.J., Med. Klin. 58:799, 1963.
20— Krauss, H., Koslowski, L., & Zimmermann, W.E., Langenbecks Arch. Klin. Chir. 303:23, 1963.
21— Gruenagel, H.H., Med. Klin. 58:442, 1963.

Manufactured for:
Knoll Pharmaceuticals, distributor
30 N. Jefferson Road
Whippany, NJ 07981
Tel. No. 201-887-8300
by **Advance Biofactures Corp.**
35 Wilbur Street
Lynbrook, NY 11563
Revised March 1981 6090

VICODIN® TABLETS Ⓒ℞

[vī'kō-dĭn]

DESCRIPTION

Each VICODIN® tablet contains:

hydrocodone bitartrate .... 5 mg
(**WARNING:** May be habit forming.)
acetaminophen .... 500 mg

Other ingredients include colloidal silicon dioxide, corn starch, croscarmellose sodium, dibasic calcium phosphate, magnesium stearate, microcrystalline cellulose, povidone, stearic acid and sulfites.

Hydrocodone bitartrate is an opioid analgesic and antitussive and occurs as fine, white crystals or as a crystalline powder. It is affected by light. The structural formula of hydrocodone bitartrate is:

Acetaminophen is a nonopiate, nonsalicylate analgesic and antipyretic which occurs as a white, odorless, crystalline powder possessing a slightly bitter taste. It may be represented by the following structural formula:

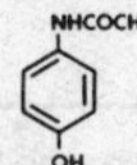

CLINICAL PHARMACOLOGY

Hydrocodone is a semisynthetic narcotic analgesic and antitussive with multiple actions qualitatively similar to those of codeine. Most of these involve the central nervous system and smooth muscle. The precise mechanism of action of hydrocodone and other opiates is not known, although it is believed to relate to the existence of opiate receptors in the central nervous system. In addition to analgesia, narcotics may produce drowsiness, changes in mood and mental clouding.

Radioimmunoassay techniques have recently been developed for the analysis of hydrocodone in human plasma. After a 10 mg oral dose of hydrocodone bitartrate, a mean peak serum drug level of 23.6 ng/mL and an elimination half-life of 3.8 hours were found.

The analgesic action of acetaminophen involves peripheral and central influences, but the specific mechanism is as yet undetermined. Antipyretic activity is mediated through hypothalamic heat regulating centers. Acetaminophen inhibits prostaglandin synthetase. Therapeutic doses of acetaminophen have negligible effects on the cardiovascular or respiratory systems; however, toxic doses may cause circulatory failure and rapid, shallow breathing. Acetaminophen is rapidly and almost completely absorbed from the gastrointestinal tract, producing maximum serum concentrations within 30 minutes to one hour. The plasma half-life in adults and children ranges from 0.90 hours to 3.25 hours with an average of approximately 2 hours. The drug distributes uniformly in most body fluids and is approximately 25% protein bound. Acetaminophen is conjugated in the liver, with less than 3% of the dose excreted unchanged in 24 hours. The primary metabolic pathway is conjugation to sulfate and glucuronide byproducts. A minor oxidative pathway forms cysteine and mercapturic acid. These compounds are subsequently excreted by the kidneys into the urine.

INDICATIONS AND USAGE

For the relief of moderate to moderately severe pain.

CONTRAINDICATIONS

Hypersensitivity to acetaminophen or hydrocodone.

WARNINGS

Respiratory Depression: At high doses or in sensitive patients, hydrocodone may produce dose-related respiratory depression by acting directly on brain stem respiratory centers. Hydrocodone also affects centers that control respiratory rhythm, and may produce irregular and periodic breathing. If significant respiratory depression occurs, it may be antagonized by the use of naloxone hydrochloride, 0.005 mg/kg intravenously. Since the duration of action of hydrocodone may exceed that of the antagonist, the patient should be kept under continued surveillance and repeated doses of the antagonist should be administered as needed to maintain adequate respiration. Apply other supportive measures when indicated.

Head Injury and Increased Intracranial Pressure: The respiratory depressant effects of narcotics and their capacity to elevate cerebrospinal fluid pressure may be markedly exaggerated in the presence of head injury, other intracranial lesions or a preexisting increase in intracranial pressure. Furthermore, narcotics produce adverse reactions which may obscure the clinical course of patients with head injuries.

Acute Abdominal Conditions: The administration of narcotics may obscure the diagnosis or clinical course of patients with acute abdominal conditions.

PRECAUTIONS

Special Risk Patients: As with any narcotic analgesic agent, VICODIN should be used with caution in elderly or debilitated patients and those with severe impairment of hepatic or renal function, hypothyroidism, Addison's disease, prostatic hypertrophy or urethral stricture. The usual precautions should be observed and the possibility of respiratory depression should be kept in mind.

Information for Patients: VICODIN, like all narcotics, may impair the mental and/or physical abilities required for the performance of potentially hazardous tasks such as driving a car or operating machinery; patients should be cautioned accordingly.

Cough Reflex: Hydrocodone suppresses the cough reflex; as with all narcotics, caution should be exercised when VICODIN is used postoperatively and in patients with pulmonary disease.

Drug Interactions: Patients receiving other narcotic analgesics, antipsychotics, antianxiety agents, or other CNS depressants (including alcohol) concomitantly with VICODIN may exhibit an additive CNS depression. When combined therapy is contemplated, the dose of one or both agents should be reduced.

The use of MAO inhibitors or tricyclic antidepressants with hydrocodone preparations may increase the effect of either the antidepressant or hydrocodone.

The concurrent use of anticholinergics with hydrocodone may produce paralytic ileus.

Usage in Pregnancy: Pregnancy Category C. Hydrocodone has been shown to be teratogenic in hamsters when given in doses 700 times the human dose. There are no adequate and well-controlled studies in pregnant women. VICODIN should be used during pregnancy only if the potential benefit justifies the potential risk to the fetus.

Nonteratogenic effects: Babies born to mothers who have been taking opioids regularly prior to delivery will be physically dependent. The withdrawal signs include irritability and excessive crying, tremors, hyperactive reflexes, increased respiratory rate, increased stools, sneezing, yawning, vomiting, and fever. The intensity of the syndrome does not always correlate with the duration of maternal opioid use or dose. There is no consensus on the best method of managing withdrawal. Chlorpromazine 0.7 to 1.0 mg/kg q6h, and paregoric 2 to 4 drops/kg q4h, have been used to treat withdrawal symptoms in infants. The duration of therapy is 4 to 28 days, with the dosage decreased as tolerated.

Labor and Delivery: As with all narcotics, administration of VICODIN to the mother shortly before delivery may result in some degree of respiratory depression in the newborn, especially if higher doses are used.

Nursing Mothers: It is not known whether this drug is excreted in human milk. Because many drugs are excreted in human milk and because of the potential for serious adverse reactions in nursing infants from VICODIN, a decision should be made whether to discontinue nursing or to discontinue the drug, taking into account the importance of the drug to the mother.

Pediatric Use: Safety and effectiveness in children have not been established.

ADVERSE REACTIONS

Central Nervous System: Sedation, drowsiness, mental clouding, lethargy, impairment of mental and physical performance, anxiety, fear, dysphoria, dizziness, psychic dependence, mood changes.

Gastrointestinal System: Nausea and vomiting may occur; they are more frequent in ambulatory than in recumbent patients. The antiemetic phenothiazines are useful in suppressing these effects; however, some phenothiazine derivatives seem to be antianalgesic and to increase the amount of narcotic required to produce pain relief, while other phenothiazines reduce the amount of narcotic required to produce a given level of analgesia. Prolonged administration of VICODIN may produce constipation.

Genitourinary System: Ureteral spasm, spasm of vesical sphincters and urinary retention have been reported.

Respiratory Depression: VICODIN may produce dose-related respiratory depression by acting directly on brain stem respiratory centers. Hydrocodone also affects centers that control respiratory rhythm, and may produce irregular and periodic breathing. If significant respiratory depression occurs, it may be antagonized by the use of naloxone hydrochloride, 0.005 mg/kg intravenously. Since the duration of action of hydrocodone may exceed that of the antagonist, the patient should be kept under continued surveillance and repeated doses of the antagonist should be administered as needed to maintain adequate respiration. Apply other supportive measures when indicated.

DRUG ABUSE AND DEPENDENCE

VICODIN is subject to the Federal Controlled Substances Act (Schedule Ⓒ).

Psychic dependence, physical dependence, and tolerance may develop upon repeated administration of narcotics; therefore, VICODIN should be prescribed and administered with caution. However, psychic dependence is unlikely to develop when VICODIN is used for a short time for the treatment of pain. Physical dependence, the condition in which continued administration of the drug is required to prevent the appearance of a withdrawal syndrome, assumes clini-

Continued on next page

Knoll—Cont.

cally significant proportions only after several weeks of continued narcotic use, although some mild degree of physical dependence may develop after a few days of narcotic therapy. Tolerance, in which increasingly large doses are required in order to produce the same degree of analgesia, is manifested initially by a shortened duration of analgesic effect, and subsequently by decreases in the intensity of analgesia. The rate of development of tolerance varies among patients.

OVERDOSAGE

Hydrocodone

Signs and Symptoms: Serious overdose with hydrocodone is characterized by respiratory depression (a decrease in respiratory rate and/or tidal volume, Cheyne-Stokes respiration, cyanosis), extreme somnolence progressing to stupor or coma, skeletal muscle flaccidity, cold and clammy skin, and sometimes bradycardia and hypotension. In severe overdosage, apnea, circulatory collapse, cardiac arrest and death may occur.

Treatment: Primary attention should be given to the reestablishment of adequate respiratory exchange through provision of a patent airway and the institution of assisted or controlled ventilation. The narcotic antagonist naloxone is a specific antidote against respiratory depression which may result from overdosage or unusual sensitivity to narcotics, including hydrocodone. Therefore, 0.005 mg/kg of naloxone should be administered, preferably by the intravenous route, and simultaneously with efforts at respiratory resuscitation. Since the duration of action of hydrocodone may exceed that of the antagonist, the patient should be kept under continued surveillance and repeated doses of the antagonist should be administered as needed to maintain adequate respiration. An antagonist should not be administered in the absence of clinically significant respiratory or cardiovascular depression. Oxygen, intravenous fluids, vasopressors and other supportive measures should be employed as indicated.

Gastric emptying may be useful in removing unabsorbed drug.

Acetaminophen

Signs and Symptoms: Acetaminophen in massive overdosage may cause hepatic toxicity in some patients. In all cases of suspected overdose, immediately call your Regional Poison Center or the Rocky Mountain Poison Center's toll free number (800/525-6115) for assistance in diagnosis and for directions in the use of N-acetylcysteine as an antidote.

In adults, hepatic toxicity has rarely been reported with acute overdoses of less than 10 grams and fatalities with less than 15 grams. Importantly, young children seem to be more resistant than adults to the hepatotoxic effect of an acetaminophen overdose. Despite this, the measures outlined below should be initiated in any adult or child suspected of having ingested an acetaminophen overdose.

Early symptoms following a potentially hepatotoxic overdose may include: nausea, vomiting, diaphoresis and general malaise. Clinical and laboratory evidence of hepatic toxicity may not be apparent until 48 to 72 hours post-ingestion.

Treatment: The stomach should be emptied promptly by lavage or by induction of emesis with syrup of ipecac. Patients' estimates of the quantity of a drug ingested are notoriously unreliable. Therefore, if an acetaminophen overdose is suspected, a serum acetaminophen assay should be obtained as early as possible, but no sooner than four hours following ingestion. Liver function studies should be obtained initially and repeated at 24-hour intervals.

The antidote, N-acetylcysteine, should be administered as early as possible, and within 16 hours of the overdose ingestion for optimal results. Following recovery, there are no residual, structural or functional hepatic abnormalities.

DOSAGE AND ADMINISTRATION

Dosage should be adjusted according to the severity of the pain and the response of the patient. However, tolerance to hydrocodone can develop with continued use and the incidence of untoward effects is dose related.

The usual dose is one tablet every six hours as needed for pain. If necessary, this dose may be repeated at four hour intervals. In cases of more severe pain, two tablets every six hours (up to 8 tablets in 24 hours) may be required.

HOW SUPPLIED

White, capsule shaped tablet bisected on one side and imprinted with "VICODIN" on the other side.

Bottles of 100—NDC #0044-0727-02.

Hospital Unit Dose Package—100 tablets (4×25 tablets)—NDC #0044-0727-41.

Bottles of 500—NDC #0044-0727-03

Storage: VICODIN should be stored at 59°- 86°F. (15°-30°C.).

A Schedule Ⓒ Narcotic.

Revised June, 1985 5750

Shown in Product Identification Section, page 412

EDUCATIONAL MATERIAL

Continuing Education Booklets

"Calcium in Cardiac Metabolism" (3 credits)
Home Study Module - Pharmacists
"Cardiac Arrhythmias" (2 credits)
Home Study Module - Pharmacists
"Treatment of Cardiac Arrhythmias" (3 credits)
Home Study Module - Pharmacists
"Angina Pectoris" (2 credits)
Home Study Module - Pharmacists
"Management of Angina Pectoris" (3 credits)
Home Study Module - Pharmacists
"Management of Essential Hypertension" (3 credits)
Home Study Module - Pharmacists

Kramer Pharmacal, Inc.
8778 S.W. 8TH STREET
MIAMI, FL 33174

EPATROL OTC
[*e-pa'-trōl*]
Capsules

DESCRIPTION

Each Epatrol capsule provides:

Eicosapentaenoic acid (EPA)	300mg
Docosahexaenoic acid (DHA)	200mg
Total Omega 3 fatty acids	500mg
Vitamin E	1 I.U.

Contains no added chemicals, preservatives, sugar, starches, flavoring or colors. EPATROL provides 500mg, the highest content available of the Omega 3 fatty acids.

INDICATIONS

Recent medical studies have shown that there are health benefits to be obtained from increased consumption of fish, particularly deep sea cold water fish such as salmon, mackerel and sardines which are high in Omega 3 fatty acids. Americans who cannot eat a diet rich in fish may wish to supplement their dietary intake of these essential omega 3 fatty acids with the fish oil concentrate provided in EPATROL capsules.

SUGGESTED DOSAGE

One to three capsules of EPATROL with each meal as a dietary supplement.

HOW SUPPLIED

EPATROL is available in bottles containing 60 soft gelatin capsules. (NDC 52083-399-60)

FUNGI-NAIL®
[*fun'gi-nāl*]
Tincture

COMPOSITION

Resorcinol 1%; Salicylic Acid 2%; Parachlorometaxylenol 2%; Benzocaine 0.5%; Acetic Acid 2.5%; Propylene glycol, Hydroxypropylmethyl Cellulose, Alcohol 50%.

INDICATIONS

For topical treatment of ringworm infections of the nails tinea unguium (onychomycosis), and other fungus and bacterial infections of the skin.

PRECAUTIONS

Avoid contact with eyes and mucous membranes. Do not use on broken skin or irritated areas.

DOSAGE AND ADMINISTRATION

Apply to affected nails and other affected areas of the skin twice daily.

HOW SUPPLIED

1 oz. bottle with brush applicator. (NDC 52083-629-26)

YOHIMEX™ Tablets ℞
[*yō-him'eks*]

DESCRIPTION

Yohimbine is an indoalkylamine alkaloid with chemical similarity to reserpine. It is a 3α-15α-20β-17α hydroxy Yohimbine-16α- carboxylic acid methylester. The alkaloid is found in Rubaceae and related trees and in Rauwolfia Serpentina(L) Benth.

Each pink tablet contains: Yohimbine Hydrochloride 5 mg ($^1/_{12}$ grain).

ACTIONS

Yohimbine blocks presynaptic alpha-2 adrenergic receptors. Its action on peripheral blood vessels is similar to that of reserpine, though its of short duration and weaker. Yohimbine's peripheral autonomic nervous system effect is to increase parasympathetic (cholinergic) and decrease sympathetic (adrenergic) activity. It is to be noted that in males sexual performance, erection is linked to cholinergic activity and to alpha-2—adrenergic blockade which may theoretically result in increased penile inflow, decreased penile outflow, or both. Yohimbine exerts a stimulating action on mood and can increase anxiety. These actions have not been adequately studied or related to dosage although it appears to require high doses of Yohimbine. Yohimbine has a mild antidiuretic action, probably via hypothalamus stimulation and release of posterior pituitary hormone. As reported, Yohimbine exerts no significant influence on cardiac stimulation and other effects mediated by β-adrenergic receptors. Its effect on blood pressure, if any, would be to lower it; however, no adequate studies are at hand to quantitate this terms of Yohimbine dosage.

INDICATIONS

Yohimex is indicated as a sympathicolytic and mydriatic. At present time, there is growing interest among urologists to use Yohimbine experimentally for the treatment and the diagnostic classification of certain types of male erectile impotence.

CONTRAINDICATIONS

Sensitivity to the drug and renal diseases. No additional contraindications can be offered due to the limited and inadequate information available.

WARNING

Generally, Yohimex is not proposed for use in females and certainly must not be used during pregnancy. This drug is not proposed for use in pediatric, cardio-renal patients with gastric or duodenal history, nor geriatric patients. It should not be used in conjunction with mood modifying agents such as antidepressants, nor in psychiatric patients.

ADVERSE REACTIONS

Yohimbine HCl readily penetrates the CNS and produces a complex patterns of responses in lower doses than required to produce peripheral adrenergic blockade. These includes: antidiuresis, a general picture of central excitation including elevation of blood pressure and heart rate increased motor activity, tremor and irritability. Dizziness, headache, and skin flushing reactions have been reported following oral administration of Yohimbine HCl.

DOSAGE

Experimental dosage reported in the treatment of erectile impotence is of 1 tablet (5 mg of Yohimbine HCl) three times a day, to adult males taken orally. The occasional side effects reported with this dosage are nausea, dizziness, or nervousness. If side effects occurs, the dosage is to be reduced to ½ tablet 3 times a day followed by gradual increases to 1 tablet 3 times a day. The therapy reported is not more than 10 weeks.

HOW SUPPLIED

Yohimex Tablets in bottles of 100's (NDC 52083-842-10).
Revised: 7/84

Kremers Urban Company
P.O. BOX 2038
5600 W. COUNTY LINE ROAD
MILWAUKEE, WI 53201

CALCIFEROL™
[*kal-si'fur-ol*]
(Ergocalciferol USP, Vitamin D_2)
50,000 USP Unit Tablets ℞
500,000 USP Units/mL in Oil for Injection ℞
8,000 USP Units/mL Drops (Oral Solution) OTC

DESCRIPTION

CALCIFEROL™, also known as ergocalciferol or Vitamin D_2 is a Vitamin D analog. It occurs as white crystals and is insoluble in water and soluble in alcohol and in fatty oils. CALCIFEROL Tablets contain 1.25 mg (50,000 USP units) of Ergocalciferol (Vitamin D_2). CALCIFEROL in Oil for Injection is a sterile solution of Vitamin D_2 in sesame oil for intramuscular use only. Each mL of CALCIFEROL in Oil for Injection contains 500,000 USP units of Ergocalciferol. CALCIFEROL Drops, oral solution, contains 8,000 USP units of Vitamin D_2 in Propylene Glycol per mL (200 USP units per drop).

INACTIVE INGREDIENTS

CALCIFEROL Tablets: Colloidal Silicon Dioxide, Dibasic Calcium Phosphate, Diethylphthalate, Ethylcellulose, Hydrogenated Vegetable Oil, Hydroxypropyl Methylcellulose,

Microcrystalline Cellulose, Pharmaceutical Glaze, Silicon Dioxide, Sodium Starch Glycolate, Talc, Titanium Dioxide, plus colors.
CALCIFEROL in Oil for Injection: Sesame oil.
CALCIFEROL Drops: Propylene Glycol.

PHARMACOLOGY

CALCIFEROL in its activated form (1,25-dihydroxy ergocalciferol) along with parathyroid hormone and calcitonin, regulates calcium metabolism. Vitamin D deficiency leads to rickets in children and osteomalacia in adults. The administration of Vitamin D completely reverses the symptoms of nutritional rickets or osteomalacia unless permanent deformities have already occurred. In humans, activated CALCIFEROL functions primarily to increase intestinal absorption of calcium and phosphorus. It is also required for normal mineralization of bone and stimulates resorption of bone matrix.
After intramuscular injection, ergocalciferol appears in chylomicrons of lymph and then associates primarily with a specific alpha-globulin and with albumin. The plasma half-life of ergocalciferol is approximately 24 hours. Ergocalciferol is stored in the liver, fat, and muscle for prolonged periods.
CALCIFEROL taken orally is readily absorbed from the gastrointestinal tract if fat absorption is normal. The presence of bile is necessary for absorption of Vitamin D and its analogs. In patients with hepatic, biliary, or GI disease, the absorption of Vitamin D may decrease. Once absorbed, ergocalciferol appears in chylomicrons of lymph and then associates primarily with a specific alpha-globulin and with albumin.

INDICATIONS AND USES

CALCIFEROL is indicated for use in the treatment of hypoparathyroidism and refractory rickets. CALCIFEROL is used to increase serum calcium concentration to prevent or treat rickets or osteomalacia. Patients with gastrointestinal, liver or biliary disease associated with malabsorption of Vitamin D require intramuscular administration of Vitamin D.

CONTRAINDICATIONS

CALCIFEROL should not be given to patients with hypercalcemia or evidence of Vitamin D toxicity.

WARNING

Overdosage of any form of Vitamin D is dangerous. Progressive hypercalcemia due to overdosage of Vitamin D and its metabolites may be so severe as to require emergency attention. Chronic hypercalcemia can lead to generalized vascular calcification, nephrocalcinosis and other soft tissue calcification. Radiographic evaluation of suspect anatomical regions may be useful in the early detection of this condition.

PRECAUTIONS

Treatment of patients with coronary disease, impaired renal function, and arteriosclerosis, especially in the elderly, should be cautious.
Large doses of Vitamin D are potentially dangerous; therefore, early in treatment or during dosage adjustment, serum calcium should be determined twice weekly. Similarly, phosphate, magnesium, and alkaline phosphatase and 24 hour urinary calcium and phosphate should be determined periodically. A fall in serum alkaline phosphatase levels usually precedes the appearance of hypercalcemia and may be an indication of impending hypercalcemia. Should hypercalcemia develop, the drug should be discontinued immediately.

ADVERSE REACTIONS

Excessive Vitamin D intake can produce vitamin toxicity. The early and late signs and symptoms of Vitamin D intoxication associated with hypercalcemia may include weakness and headache, vomiting, muscle pain, bone pain, anorexia, weight loss, hypertension, and cardiac arrhythmias.

DRUG ABUSE AND DEPENDENCE

The information on drug abuse and dependence is limited to an existent literature survey and marketing experience. Such experience has revealed no evidence of drug abuse and dependence associated with use of CALCIFEROL.

OVERDOSAGE

Use of CALCIFEROL in excessive quantities in patients can cause hypercalcemia, hypercalciuria and hyperphosphatemia. High intake of calcium and phosphate concomitant with CALCIFEROL can lead to similar abnormalities.
Treatment of Vitamin D intoxication consists of withdrawal of the drug and calcium supplements, administration of low-calcium diet, oral or parenteral fluids, and if needed, glucocorticoids or other drugs to decrease serum calcium levels. When serum calcium levels have returned to within normal limits, CALCIFEROL therapy may be reinstituted at a dose lower than prior therapy. Serum calcium levels should be determined at least twice weekly after all dosage changes and subsequent dosage titration. Persistent or markedly elevated serum calcium levels may be corrected by dialysis against a calcium free dialysate.

DOSAGE AND ADMINISTRATION

The optimal daily dose of CALCIFEROL must be carefully determined for each patient. Patients with refractory rickets may need 50,000 to 500,000 units per day. After oral therapy with CALCIFEROL is instituted, normal serum calcium and phosphate levels may be observed within 2 weeks. Roentgenographic evidence of healing of bone may be seen within 4 weeks after administration of a fixed maintenance dose. During therapy with CALCIFEROL, the dosage must be individualized and carefully adjusted to avoid hypercalcemia. Determinations of serum calcium, phosphate, alkaline phosphatase, total protein, creatine and BUN should be made every two weeks or more frequently as needed. Until the condition stabilizes, monthly radiographic evaluation is helpful. In treatment of hypoparathyroidism, 50,000 to 400,000 units per day are recommended. In recommending CALCIFEROL, it is assumed that each patient is receiving an adequate daily intake of calcium. The recommended daily allowance for calcium in adults is 1 gram.

HOW SUPPLIED

CALCIFEROL Tablets are yellow with a "KU1" imprint, bottles of 100 (NDC 0091-3150-01).
CALCIFEROL in Oil for Injection is supplied in 1 mL ampules and packaged in boxes of 5 (NDC 0091-1150-05).
CALCIFEROL Drops, oral solution, is supplied in 60 mL bottle with dropper (NDC 0091-4150-60).

Store at controlled room temperature 59–86°F (15–30°C).

Shown in Product Identification Section, page 412

FEDAHIST® Products
[fed 'a-hist"]

FEDAHIST® Expectorant OTC
FEDAHIST® Syrup OTC
FEDAHIST® Tablets OTC
FEDAHIST® Gyrocaps® ℞

DESCRIPTION

FEDAHIST® is a combination of pseudoephedrine hydrochloride (1-phenyl-2 methylaminopropan-1-ol hydrochloride) and chlorpheniramine maleate (2-[p-chloro-α(2-dimethylaminoethyl) benzyl] pyridine maleate 1:1) as an oral antihistamine decongestant.

FEDAHIST Expectorant, nonalcoholic, contains in each 5 mL (teaspoonful):

Guaifenesin	100 mg
Pseudoephedrine Hydrochloride	30 mg
Chlorpheniramine Maleate	2 mg

FEDAHIST Syrup, nonalcoholic, contains in each 5 mL (teaspoonful):

Pseudoephedrine Hydrochloride	30 mg
Chlorpheniramine Maleate	2 mg

FEDAHIST Tablets contain:

Pseudoephedrine Hydrochloride	60 mg
Chlorpheniramine Maleate	4 mg

FEDAHIST Gyrocaps, timed release capsules formulated in a special base that provides for a prolonged, therapeutic effect contain:

Pseudoephedrine Hydrochloride	65 mg
Chlorpheniramine Maleate	10 mg

INACTIVE INGREDIENTS

FEDAHIST Expectorant: Citric Acid, FD&C Red No. 40, Flavors, Glycerin, Methylparaben, Saccharin Sodium, Sodium Benzoate, Sorbitol Solution, Sucrose, and Purified Water.
FEDAHIST Syrup: Citric Acid, FD&C Blue No. 1, FD&C Red No. 40, Flavors, Glycerin, Methylparaben, Saccharin Sodium, Sodium Benzoate, Sorbitol Solution, Sucrose, and Purified Water.
FEDAHIST Tablets: Colloidal Silicon Dioxide, Lactose, Magnesium Stearate, Microcrystalline Cellulose, Stearic Acid, and Talc.
FEDAHIST Gyrocaps: Carnauba wax, Lactose, Pharmaceutical Glaze, Starch, Stearic Acid, Sucrose, Talc, plus color.

CLINICAL PHARMACOLOGY

FEDAHIST provides the antihistaminic activity of chlorpheniramine maleate with the vasoconstrictive actions of pseudoephedrine hydrochloride.
At the recommended oral dosage, pseudoephedrine has little or no pressor effects in normotensive adults, and is not known to produce drowsiness.
Chlorpheniramine is an antihistamine which acts on H_1 receptors as an antagonist. It is well absorbed and has a duration of 4 to 6 hours. (The Timecaps formulation provides a longer therapeutic effect up to 12 hours.) Plasma half-life is approximately 22 hours. Degradation products of chlorpheniramine's metabolic transformation by the liver are almost completely excreted in 24 hours via the kidney. The alkylamines, of which chlorpheniramine is the prototype, are among the most potent H_1 blockers. Although not so prone as others to cause drowsiness, a significant proportion of patients do experience this effect. CNS stimulation is more common in chlorpheniramine than in other groups of H_1 blockers.
Pseudoephedrine is a sympathomimetic amine with peripheral effects similar to epinephrine and central effects similar to, but less intense than, amphetamines. Therefore, it has the potential for excitatory side effects. Pseudoephedrine at the recommended oral dosage has little or no pressor effect in normotensive adults.
Pseudoephedrine is an orally effective nasal decongestant. Patients taking pseudoephedrine orally have not been reported to experience the rebound congestion sometimes experienced with frequent repeated use of topical decongestants.

INDICATIONS AND USAGE

FEDAHIST® is indicated for the symptomatic relief of seasonal and perennial allergic rhinitis, and eustachian tube congestion.

CONTRAINDICATIONS

Use in Newborn or Premature Infants: This drug should not be used in newborn or premature infants.
Antihistamines are contraindicated in the following conditions: Hypersensitivity to chlorpheniramine maleate and other antihistamines of similar chemical structure; monoamine oxidase inhibitor therapy (see Drug Interactions Section).
FEDAHIST is also contraindicated in patients with hypersensitivity or idiosyncrasy to sympathomimetic amines. Sympathomimetic amines are contraindicated in patients with severe hypertension, severe coronary artery disease, and in patients on MAO inhibitor therapy. Patient idiosyncrasy to adrenergic agents may be manifested by insomnia, dizziness, weakness, tremor or arrhythmias.

WARNINGS

Antihistamines should be used with considerable caution in patients with: narrow angle glaucoma; stenosing peptic ulcer; pyloroduodenal obstruction; symptomatic prostatic hypertrophy; bladder neck obstruction.
Use in Children: In infants and children especially, antihistamines in **overdosage** may cause hallucinations, convulsions or death.
As in adults, antihistamines may diminish mental alertness in children. In the young child particularly, they may produce excitation.
Use with CNS Depressants: Chlorpheniramine maleate has additive effects with alcohol and other CNS depressants (hypnotics, sedatives, tranquilizers, etc.)
Use in Activities Requiring Mental Alertness: Patients should be warned about engaging in activities requiring mental alertness, such as driving a car or operating appliances, machinery, etc.
Use in the Elderly (approximately 60 years or older): Antihistamines are more likely to cause dizziness, sedation, hypotension in elderly patients.
The elderly are more likely to have adverse reactions to sympathomimetics. Overdosage of sympathomimetics in this age group may cause hallucinations, convulsions, CNS depression, and death. Therefore, safe use of a short-acting sympathomimetic should be demonstrated in the individual elderly patient before considering the use of a sustained-action formulation.
Sympathomimetic amines should be used judiciously and sparingly in patients with hypertension, diabetes mellitus, ischemic heart disease, increased intraocular pressure, hyperthyroidism, and prostatic hypertrophy. Sympathomimetics may produce central nervous system stimulation with convulsions or cardiovascular collapse with accompanying hypotension.
Do not exceed recommended dosage.

PRECAUTIONS

General: Chlorpheniramine maleate has an atropine-like action and therefore should be used with caution in patients with: a history of bronchial asthma, increased intraocular pressure, hyperthyroidism, cardiovascular disease and hypertension.
Pseudoephedrine should be used with caution in patients with diabetes, hypertension, cardiovascular disease and hyper-reactivity to ephedrine.
Drug Interactions: MAO inhibitors prolong and intensify the anticholinergic (drying) effects of antihistamines. MAO inhibitors and beta adrenergic blockers increase the effects of pseudoephedrine (sympathomimetics).
Sympathomimetics may reduce the antihypertensive effects of methyldopa, mecamylamine, reserpine and veratrum alkaloids.
Carcinogenicity: Studies show that the ingredients in FEDAHIST have no carcinogenic effects on animals or humans.
Use in Pregnancy: The safety of the ingredients in FEDAHIST for use during pregnancy has not been established.
Pregnancy Category C: Animal reproduction studies have not been conducted with FEDAHIST. It is also not known

Continued on next page

Kremers Urban—Cont.

whether FEDAHIST can cause fetal harm when administered to a pregnant woman or can affect reproduction capacity.
There have been no reports that pseudoephedrine increases the risk of fetal abnormalities if administered during pregnancy. If this drug is used during pregnancy, the possibility of fetal harm appears remote. Because studies cannot rule out the possibility of harm, however, FEDAHIST should be used during pregnancy only if clearly needed.

Nonteratogenic Effects

Nursing Mothers: Because of the potential for serious adverse reactions in nursing infants from FEDAHIST a decision should be made whether to discontinue nursing or to discontinue the drug, taking into account the importance of the drug to the mother.

ADVERSE REACTIONS

Slight to moderate drowsiness occurs relatively infrequently with chlorpheniramine maleate. Other possible side effects common to antihistamines in general include:
General: Urticaria, drug rash, anaphylactic shock, photosensitivity, excessive perspiration, chills, dryness of mouth, nose, and throat.
Cardiovascular System: Hypotension, headache, palpitations, tachycardia, extrasystoles.
Hematologic System: Hemolytic anemia, thrombocytopenia, agranulocytosis.
Nervous System: Sedation, dizziness, disturbed coordination, fatigue, confusion, restlessness, excitation, nervousness, tremor, irritability, insomnia, euphoria, paresthesias, blurred vision, diplopia, vertigo, tinnitus, acute labryinthitis, hysteria, neuritis, convulsions.
Gastrointestinal System: Epigastric distress, anorexia, nausea, vomiting, diarrhea, constipation.
Genitourinary System: Urinary frequency, difficult urination, urinary retention, early menses.
Respiratory System: Thickening of bronchial secretions, tightness of chest and wheezing, nasal stuffiness.
Individuals hyper-reactive to pseudoephedrine may display reactions such as tachycardia, palpitations, headache, dizziness or nausea. Sympathomimetic drugs have been associated with certain untoward reactions including fear, anxiety, tenseness, restlessness, tremor, weakness, pallor, respiratory difficulty, dysuria, insomnia, hallucinations, convulsions, CNS depression, arrhythmias, and cardiovascular collapse with hypotension.

OVERDOSAGE

In the event of overdosage, emergency treatment should be started immediately. Manifestations of antihistamine overdosage may vary from central nervous system depression (sedation, apnea, cardiovascular collapse) to stimulation (insomnia, hallucinations, tremors or convulsions). Other signs and symptoms may be dizziness, tinnitus, ataxia, blurred vision and hypotension. Stimulation is particularly likely in children, as are atropine-like signs and symptoms (dry mouth; fixed, dilated pupils; flushing, hyperthermia and gastrointestinal symptoms).
Treatment: The patient should be induced to vomit, even if emesis has occurred spontaneously. Pharmacologic vomiting by the administration of ipecac syrup is a preferred method. However, vomiting should not be induced in patients with impaired consciousness. The action of ipecac is facilitated by physical activity and by the administration of eight to twelve fluid ounces of water. If emesis does not occur within fifteen minutes, the dose of ipecac should be repeated. Precautions against aspiration must be taken, especially in infants and children. Following emesis, any drug remaining in the stomach may be absorbed by activated charcoal administered as a slurry with water. If vomiting is unsuccessful, or contraindicated, gastric lavage should be performed. Isotonic and one-half isotonic saline are the lavage solutions of choice. Saline cathartics, such as milk of magnesia, draw water into the bowel by osmosis and, therefore, may be valuable for their action in rapid dilution of bowel content. After emergency treatment the patient should continue to be medically monitored. Treatment of the signs and symptoms of overdosage is symptomatic and supportive.
Stimulants (analeptic agents) should not be used. Vasopressors may be used to treat hypotension. Short-acting barbiturates, diazepam or paraldehyde may be administered to control seizures. Hyperpyrexia, especially in children, may require treatment with tepid water sponge baths or a hypothermic blanket. Apnea is treated with ventilatory support.

DOSAGE AND ADMINISTRATION

FEDAHIST Gyrocaps: Adults and children 12 years and older: one capsule twice a day. Not recommended for children under 12 years.
FEDAHIST Expectorant: Adults and children 12 years and over: two teaspoonfuls every 6 hours not to exceed 8 teaspoonfuls in 24 hours.
Children 6 to 12 years: one teaspoonful every 6 hours not to exceed 4 teaspoonfuls in 24 hours.
Children 2 to under 6 years; one-half teaspoonful every 6 hours not to exceed 2 teaspoonfuls in 24 hours.
Do not give to children under 6 years except under the advice and supervision of a physician.
FEDAHIST Tablets: Adults and children 12 and over: one tablet every 6 hours not to exceed 4 tablets in 24 hours.
Children 6 to under 12 years: one-half tablet every 6 hours not to exceed 2 tablets in 24 hours.
Do not give to children under 6 years except under the advice and supervision of a physician.
FEDAHIST Syrup: Adults and children 12 years and over: two teaspoonfuls every 6 hours not to exceed 8 teaspoonfuls in 24 hours.
Children 6 to under 12 years: one teaspoonful every 6 hours not to exceed 4 teaspoonfuls in 24 hours.
Children 2 to under 6 years: one-half teaspoonful every 6 hours not to exceed 2 teaspoonfuls in 24 hours.
Do not give to children under 6 years except under the advice and supervision of a physician.

SUPPLIED

FEDAHIST Expectorant is a red colored and cherry flavored syrup, 4 oz. bottles, (NDC 0091-0054-04).
FEDAHIST Syrup is a grape colored and flavored syrup, 4 oz. bottles, (NDC 0091-0052-04).
FEDAHIST Tablets are white, oval, scored and embossed, bottles of 100, (NDC 0091-0050-01).
FEDAHIST Gyrocaps are two colored, embossed capsules, bottles of 100, (NDC 0091-1053-01).
Store at controlled room temperature 59–86°F (15–30°C).
Fedahist ® Gyrocaps ® and Tablets Shown in Product Identification Section, page 412

GEMNISYN™ Tablets

(See PDR For Nonprescription Drugs)

KUDROX® Suspension

(See PDR For Nonprescription Drugs)

KUTRASE® Capsules ℞

[qū 'trās]

DESCRIPTION

KUTRASE® is a unique formulation containing 4 standardized digestive enzymes, an antispasmodic-anticholinergic agent and a non-barbiturate sedative.
Each green and white capsule contains:

Amylase	30 mg
Protease	6 mg
Lipase	75 mg
Cellulase	2 mg
Phenyltoloxamine citrate	15 mg
LEVSIN® (Hyoscyamine Sulfate)	0.0625 mg

INACTIVE INGREDIENTS

Ethylcellulose, Gelatin, Lactose, Magnesium Stearate, Pharmaceutical Glaze, Iron Oxide, Titanium Dioxide, Vanillin, plus colors.

CLINICAL PHARMACOLOGY

Diminution of secretions from exocrine glands is often a result of normal aging process. KUTRASE provides a balanced combination of natural proteolytic, amylolytic, cellulolytic and lipolytic enzymes to enhance digestion of proteins, starch and fat in the gastrointestinal tract. These enzymes do not exert any systemic pharmacologic effects. KUTRASE should be considered an enzyme supplement and not an enzyme replacement therapy. Enzymes in KUTRASE are basically derived from vegetable sources and possess a broad spectrum of pH activity. Enzymes are promptly released from the capsule and are bioavailable for digestion of food in the stomach and intestines. LEVSIN (Hyoscyamine Sulfate) provides a potent spasmolytic effect in reducing gastrointestinal hypermotility and intestinal spasm. A mild sedative effect is provided by Phenyltoloxamine Citrate.

INDICATIONS AND USAGE

KUTRASE is indicated for the relief of the symptoms of functional indigestion devoid of organic pathology commonly referred to as nervous indigestion and colloquially as "butterflies". The symptoms are bloating, gas, and fullness.

CONTRAINDICATIONS

Glaucoma, obstructive uropathy, obstructive disease of the gastrointestinal tract (as in achalasia, pyloroduodenal stenosis); paralytic ileus, intestinal atony of the elderly or debilitated patients; unstable cardiovascular status in acute hemorrhage; severe ulcerative colitis; toxic megacolon, complicating ulcerative colitis; myasthenia gravis, or a hypersensitivity to any of the ingredients.

WARNINGS

In the presence of high environmental temperature, heat prostration can occur with drug use (fever and heat stroke due to decreased sweating). Diarrhea may be an early symptom of incomplete intestinal obstruction, especially in patients with ileostomy or colostomy. In this instance, treatment with this drug would be inappropriate. KUTRASE may produce drowsiness or blurred vision. In this event, the patient should be warned not to engage in activities requiring mental alertness such as operating a motor vehicle or other machinery or to perform hazardous work while taking this drug.

PRECAUTIONS

Use with caution in patients with autonomic neuropathy, hyperthyroidism, coronary heart disease, congestive heart failure, cardiac arrhythmias, and hypertension. Investigate any tachycardia before giving any anticholinergic drugs since they may increase the heart rate. Use with caution in patients with hiatal hernia associated with reflux esophagitis.
Carcinogenesis, mutagenesis — Long-term studies in animals have not been performed to evaluate carcinogenic potential.
Pregnancy Category C—Animal reproduction studies have not been conducted with KUTRASE. It is not known whether KUTRASE can cause fetal harm when administered to a pregnant woman or can affect reproduction capacity. KUTRASE should be given to a pregnant woman only if clearly needed.

ADVERSE REACTIONS

Occasionally a slight looseness of the stools may be noticed. Other adverse reactions may include dryness of the mouth; urinary hesitancy and retention; blurred vision and tachycardia; palpitations; mydriasis; cycloplegia; increased ocular tension; headache; nervousness; drowsiness; weakness; suppression of lactation, and allergic reactions or drug idiosyncrasies, urticaria and other dermal manifestations and decreased sweating.

DRUG ABUSE AND DEPENDENCE

The information on drug abuse and dependence is limited to uncontrolled data derived from marketing experience. Such experience has revealed no evidence of drug abuse and dependence associated with KUTRASE.

OVERDOSAGE

The signs and symptoms of overdose are headache, nausea, vomiting, blurred vision, dilated pupils, hot dry skin, dizziness, dryness of the mouth, difficulty in swallowing. Measures to be taken are immediate lavage of the stomach and injection of physostigmine 0.5 to 2 mg intravenously and repeated as necessary up to a total of 5 mg. Fever may be treated symptomatically. Excitement to a degree which demands attention may be managed with sodium thiopental 2% solution given slowly intravenously. In the event of paralysis of the respiratory muscles, artificial respiration should be instituted.

ADMINISTRATION AND DOSAGE

The dosage of KUTRASE should be adjusted to the needs of the individual patient to assure symptomatic control with a minimum of adverse effects. The usual dose is one or two capsules at meal times, preferably taken during the course of the meal.

SUPPLIED

KUTRASE capsules are green and white with a "Kremers-Urban 475" imprint.

Bottles of 100 capsules	NDC 0091-3475-01
Bottles of 500 capsules	NDC 0091-3475-05

Store at controlled room temperature 59–86°F (15–30°C).
Shown in Product Identification Section, page 412

KU-ZYME® Capsules ℞

[qū ' zīm]

DESCRIPTION

KU-ZYME® is a digestive aid containing 4 digestive enzymes which are highly purified, accurately standardized and potent.
Each yellow and white capsule contains:

Amylase	30 mg
Protease	6 mg
Lipase	75 mg
Cellulase	2 mg

INACTIVE INGREDIENTS

Gelatin, Lactose, Magnesium Stearate, Pharmaceutical Glaze, Titanium Dioxide, Iron Oxide, Vanillin, plus colors.

CLINICAL PHARMACOLOGY

Diminution of secretions from exocrine glands is often a result of normal aging process. KU-ZYME provides a balanced combination of natural proteolytic, amylolytic, cellulolytic and lipolytic enzymes to enhance digestion of proteins, starch and fat in the gastrointestinal tract. These enzymes do not exert any systemic pharmacologic effects. KU-ZYME should be considered an enzyme supplement and not an enzyme replacement therapy. Enzymes in KU-ZYME are basically derived from vegetable sources and possess a broad spectrum of pH activity. Enzymes are promptly released from the capsule and are bioavailable for digestion of food in the stomach and intestines.

INDICATIONS AND USAGE
For the relief of functional indigestion when due to enzyme deficiency or imbalance. KU-ZYME relieves symptoms due to faulty digestion including the sensation of fullness after meals, dyspepsia, flatulence, abdominal distention and intolerance to certain foods.

CONTRAINDICATIONS
There are no known contraindications to the administration of digestive enzymes. These enzymes do not attack living tissues and do not present any danger to the patient with ulceration or inflammation in the digestive tract.

WARNINGS
Do not administer to patients who are allergic to pork products.

PRECAUTIONS
Long-term studies in animals have not been performed to evaluate carcinogenic potential.
Pregnancy Category C—Animal reproduction studies have not been conducted with KU-ZYME. It is not known whether KU-ZYME can cause fetal harm when administered to a pregnant woman or can affect reproduction capacity. KU-ZYME should be given to a pregnant woman only if clearly needed.

ADVERSE REACTIONS
Virtually unknown. Occasionally a slight looseness of stools may be noticed. If so, dosage should be reduced.

OVERDOSAGE
No systemic toxicity occurs. Excessive dosage may, however produce a laxative effect.

DOSAGE AND ADMINISTRATION
For most patients, one capsule of KU-ZYME taken during the course of a meal will relieve symptoms due to a digestive deficiency. In patients (especially children) who experience difficulty in swallowing the capsule, it may be opened and the contents sprinkled on the food. In a few cases, where enzyme deficiency is marked (e.g. following gastrectomy, pancreatitis) the dosage may be doubled.

SUPPLIED
KU-ZYME capsules are yellow and white with a "Kremers-Urban 522" imprint.

Bottles of 100 capsules	(NDC 0091-3522-01)
Bottles of 500 capsules	(NDC 0091-3522-05)

Store at controlled room temperature 59–86°F (15–30°C).
Shown in Product Identification Section, page 412

KU-ZYME® HP Capsules ℞
[qū' zīm]
(Pancrelipase Capsules USP)

DESCRIPTION
KU-ZYME® HP (Pancrelipase USP) is a standardized concentrate of pancreatic enzymes. Each white capsule contains:

Lipase	8,000 USP units
Protease	30,000 USP units
Amylase	30,000 USP units

INACTIVE INGREDIENTS
Gelatin, Iron Oxide, Lactose, Magnesium Stearate, Pharmaceutical Glaze, and Titanium Dioxide.

CLINICAL PHARMACOLOGY
Pancrelipase USP is a pancreatic enzyme concentrate which hydrolyzes fats to glycerol and fatty acids, changes protein into proteoses and derived substances, and converts starch into dextrins and sugars. The administration of Pancrelipase reduces the fat and nitrogen content in the stool. Pancreatic enzymes are normally secreted in great excess. Generally, steatorrhea and malabsorption occur only after a 90 percent or greater reduction in secretion of lipase and proteolytic enzymes. It has been estimated that approximately 8,000 units of lipase per hour should be delivered into the duodenum postprandially. Even if all the enzymes taken orally reached the proximal intestine in active form, ingestion of 24,000 units of lipase (8,000 units per hour) for 3 postprandial hours would be required. If one could deliver sufficient pancreatic enzymes to the small intestine, malabsorption could be corrected. It is rarely possible to achieve complete relief of steatorrhea although major improvement in fat absorption can be achieved in most patients.

INDICATIONS
KU-ZYME HP is effective in patients with deficient exocrine pancreatic secretions. Thus, KU-ZYME HP may be used as enzyme replacement therapy in cystic fibrosis, chronic pancreatitis, post pancreatectomy, in ductal obstructions caused by cancer of the pancreas, pancreatic insufficiency and for steatorrhea of malabsorption syndrome and post gastrectomy (Billroth II and Total). May also be used as a presumptive test for pancreatic function, especially in pancreatic insufficiency due to chronic pancreatitis.

CONTRAINDICATIONS
There are no known contraindications for the use of pancrelipase although sensitivity to pork protein may preclude its use.

WARNINGS
Pancreatic exocrine replacement therapy should not delay or supplant treatment of the primary disorder. Use with caution in patients known to be hypersensitive to pork or enzymes.

PRECAUTIONS
Drug interactions—The serum iron response to oral iron may be decreased by concomitant administration of pancreatic extracts.
Carcinogenicity, Mutagenicity, and Impairment of Fertility—There have been no studies in animals to evaluate the carcinogenic, mutagenic or impairment of fertility potential of pancrelipase.

ADVERSE REACTIONS
High doses may cause nausea, abdominal cramps and/or diarrhea in certain patients.

DOSAGE AND ADMINISTRATION
Dosage should be adjusted to individual patient needs. Suggested dosage is 1 to 3 capsules with meals and 1 capsule with any food between meals. In severe deficiencies, the dose may be increased to 8 capsules with meals or the frequency of administration may increase to hourly intervals if nausea, cramps and/or diarrhea do not occur.
Caution: Federal law prohibits dispensing without prescription.

SUPPLIED
White capsules with a "Kremers-Urban 525" imprint, bottles of 100. (NDC 0091-3525-01)
Store at a temperature not exceeding 25°C (77°F).
Shown in Product Identification Section, page 412

LACTRASE® Capsules OTC
[lăk'trās]
(Lactase Enzyme)

DESCRIPTION
LACTRASE®, also known as lactase, is a natural enzyme produced by a unique fermentation process. LACTRASE is a biochemically beta-D-galactosidase. Each light brown and white capsule contains 125 mg of standardized enzyme dispersed in a lactose free base.

ACTION
Lactose is a non-absorbable disaccharide found as a common constituent in most dairy products. Under normal conditions, dietary lactose is hydrolyzed in the jejunum and proximal ileum by beta-D-galactosidase or lactase. Lactase is produced in the brush border of the columnar epithelial cells of the intestinal villi. Lactase hydrolyzes lactose into two monosaccharides, glucose and galactose, that are readily absorbed by the intestine.

LACTOSE INTOLERANCE
Though lactase is normally present in adequate quantities in infants, in many populations its concentration naturally declines starting at about 4–5 years of age and is low in a substantial number of individuals by their teens or early 20's. Within certain geographic and ethnic groups, especially in adult Blacks, Orientals, American Indians, and eastern European Jews, the lactase activity may be low even earlier. Although many of them can easily digest smaller quantities of lactose in milk, after consumption of an excessive volume of milk or dairy products, they may exhibit symptoms of lactose intolerance.
When available lactase is insufficient to split the lactose, the unabsorbable sugar remains in the small intestine for an extended period, presenting an osmotic load that increases and retains intraluminal fluid and intensifies intestinal motility; thus the individual reports a bloated feeling and cramps. The undigested lactose is decomposed by the intestinal flora in the lower intestine and excessive carbon dioxide and hydrogen is produced. These gases contribute to flatulence and increased abdominal discomfort. The lactic acid and other short chain acids raise the osmolality, hinder fluid reabsorption and decrease transit time of the contents of the colon, leading to diarrhea. Often hydrogen is noticed in the expired breath of a lactase deficient patient.

INDICATIONS
LACTRASE is indicated for individuals exhibiting symptoms of lactose intolerance or lactase insufficiency as identified by a lactose tolerance test or by symptoms of gastrointestinal disturbances after consumption of milk or dairy products.

PRECAUTIONS
It should be noted that in diabetic persons who use LACTRASE, the milk sugar will be metabolically available and must be taken into account (approximately 25 g of glucose and 25 g of galactose per quart of milk). Individuals with galactosemia may not have milk in any form, lactose enzyme modified or not.

DIRECTIONS FOR USE
Generally, one or two LACTRASE Capsules swallowed with milk or dairy products is all that is necessary to digest the milk sugar contained in a normal serving. If the individual is severely intolerant to lactose, additional capsules may be taken until a satisfactory response is achieved as recognized by resolution of the symptoms. LACTRASE Capsules are safe to take and higher quantities in severe cases will be well-tolerated.
If the individual cannot swallow capsules, the contents of the capsules may be sprinkled onto dairy products before consuming. LACTRASE will not alter the taste of the dairy product when used in this manner.
Milk may also be pre-treated with LACTRASE; simply add the contents from one or two capsules to each quart of milk, shake gently, and store the milk in the refrigerator for 24 hours. The LACTRASE will break down milk sugars to digestible simple sugars. LACTRASE powder will not alter the appearance of milk, however the taste may be slightly sweeter than untreated milk.

HOW SUPPLIED
LACTRASE Capsules are brown and white and are imprinted, "KREMERS-URBAN 500". They are supplied in bottles of 100 capsules (NDC 0091-3500-01), and in bottles of 20 capsules (NDC 0091-3500-20).

Store at controlled room temperature 59–86°F (15–30°C).
Shown in Product Identification Section, page 412

LEVSIN® Products ℞
[lev'sin]
(Hyoscyamine Sulfate USP)

LEVSIN® Tablets
LEVSIN® Injection
LEVSIN® Elixir
LEVSIN® Drops (Oral Solution)
LEVSINEX™ TIMECAPS™

DESCRIPTION
LEVSIN Tablets contain 0.125 mg Hyoscyamine Sulfate.
LEVSIN Injection contains 0.5 mg/mL of Hyoscyamine Sulfate.
LEVSIN Elixir contains Hyoscyamine Sulfate 0.125 mg/5 mL (Teaspoonful and contains 20% alcohol).
LEVSIN Drops, oral solution, contain Hyoscyamine Sulfate 0.125 mg/mL and contains 5% alcohol.
LEVSINEX TIMECAPS contain Hyoscyamine Sulfate 0.375 mg in a sustained release formulation designed for b.i.d. dosage.

INACTIVE INGREDIENTS
LEVSIN Tablets: Acacia, Confectioner's Sugar, Lactose, Powdered Cellulose, Starch, and Stearic Acid.
LEVSIN Injection: 1 mL—Water For Injection, Hydrochloric Acid. 10 mL—Benzyl Alcohol, Sodium Metabisulfite, Isotonic Sodium Chloride, Water For Injection.
LEVSIN Elixir: Alcohol, Flavor, Glycerin, Sorbitol Solution, Sucrose, Purified Water, plus colors.
LEVSIN Drops: Alcohol, Flavor, Glycerin, Sodium Citrate, Sorbitol Solution, Sucrose, Purified Water, plus colors.
LEVSINEX TIMECAPS: Calcium Stearate, Gelatin, Iron Oxide, Pharmaceutical Glaze, Povidone, Starch, Sucrose, Talc, Titanium Dioxide, plus colors.

CLINICAL PHARMACOLOGY
LEVSIN is chemically pure Hyoscyamine Sulfate, one of the principal anticholinergic/ antispasmodic components of Belladonna alkaloids. LEVSIN inhibits specifically the actions of acetylcholine on structures innervated by postganglionic cholinergic nerves and on smooth muscles that respond to acetylcholine but lack cholinergic innervation. These peripheral cholinergic receptors are present in the autonomic effector cells of the smooth muscle, cardiac muscle, the sinoatrial node, the atrioventricular node and the exocrine glands. It is completely devoid of any action in the autonomic ganglia. LEVSIN inhibits gastrointestinal propulsive motility and decreases gastric acid secretion. LEVSIN also controls excessive pharyngeal, tracheal, and bronchial secretions. LEVSIN is absorbed totally and completely by sublingual administration as well as oral administration. Once absorbed, LEVSIN disappears rapidly from the blood and is distributed throughout the entire body. The half-life of LEVSIN is $3\frac{1}{2}$ hours and the majority of drug is excreted in the urine unchanged within the first 12 hours. Only traces of this drug are found in breast milk.

Continued on next page

Kremers Urban—Cont.

INDICATIONS AND USAGE

LEVSIN is effective as adjunctive therapy in the treatment of peptic ulcer. It can also be used to control gastric secretion, visceral spasm, and hypermotility in spastic colitis, spastic bladder, cystitis, pylorospasm, and associated abdominal cramps. May be used in functional intestinal disorders to reduce symptoms such as those seen in mild dysenteries and diverticulitis. For use as adjunctive therapy in the treatment of irritable bowel syndrome (irritable colon, spastic colon, mucous colitis, and functional gastrointestinal disorders) and acute enterocolitis. Also as adjunctive therapy in the treatment of neurogenic bowel disturbances (including the splenic flexure syndrome and neurogenic colon). Also used in the treatment of infant colic (elixir and drops). LEVSIN is indicated along with morphine and other narcotics in symptomatic relief of biliary and renal colic; as a "drying agent" in the relief of symptoms of acute rhinitis; in the therapy of parkinsonism to reduce rigidity and tremors and to control associated sialorrhea, and hyperhidrosis. May be used in the therapy of poisoning by anticholinesterase agents.

CONTRAINDICATIONS

Glaucoma; obstructive uropathy (for example, bladder neck obstruction due to prostatic hypertrophy); obstructive disease of the gastrointestinal tract (as in achalasia, pyloroduodenal stenosis); paralytic ileus; intestinal atony of the elderly or debilitated patients; unstable cardiovascular status in acute hemorrhage; severe ulcerative colitis; toxic megacolon complicating ulcerative colitis; myasthenia gravis.

WARNINGS

In the presence of high environmental temperature, heat prostration can occur with drug use (fever and heat stroke due to decreased sweating). Diarrhea may be an early symptom of incomplete intestinal obstruction, especially in patients with ileostomy or colostomy. In this instance, treatment with this drug would be inappropriate and possibly harmful. Like other anticholinergic agents, LEVSIN may produce drowsiness or blurred vision. In this event, the patient should be warned not to engage in activities requiring mental alertness such as operating a motor vehicle or other machinery or to perform hazardous work while taking this drug.

PRECAUTIONS

Use with caution in patients with autonomic neuropathy, hyperthyroidism, coronary heart disease, congestive heart failure, cardiac arrhythmias, and hypertension. Investigate any tachycardia before giving any anticholinergic drugs since they may increase the heart rate. Use with caution in patients with hiatal hernia associated with reflux esophagitis.

ADVERSE REACTIONS

Adverse reactions may include dryness of the mouth; urinary hesitancy and retention; blurred vision and tachycardia; palpitations; mydriasis; cycloplegia; increased ocular tension; headache; nervousness; drowsiness; weakness; suppression of lactation; allergic reactions or drug idiosyncrasies; urticaria and other dermal manifestations; and decreased sweating.

DRUG ABUSE AND DEPENDENCE

The information on drug abuse and dependence is limited to uncontrolled data derived from marketing experience. Such experience has revealed no evidence of drug abuse and dependence associated with LEVSIN.

OVERDOSAGE

The signs and symptoms of overdose are headache, nausea, vomiting, blurred vision, dilated pupils, hot/dry skin, dizziness, dryness of the mouth, difficulty in swallowing. Overdosage may be treated with immediate lavage of the stomach and injection of physostigmine 0.5 to 2 mg intravenously and repeated as necessary up to a total of 5 mg. Fever may be treated symptomatically (alcohol sponging, ice packs). Excitement to a degree which demands attention may be managed with sodium thiopental 2% solution given slowly intravenously or chloral hydrate (100/200 mL of a 2% solution) by rectal infusion. In the event of progression of the curare-like effect to paralysis of the respiratory muscles, artificial respiration should be instituted and maintained until effective respiratory action returns.

DOSAGE AND ADMINISTRATION

The dosage of LEVSIN products should be adjusted to the needs of the individual patient to assure symptomatic control with a minimum of adverse effects.

LEVSIN Tablets: One or two tablets three to four times a day according to condition and severity of symptoms. May be taken orally or sublingually.

LEVSIN Elixir: Adults, one or two teaspoonfuls of elixir three to four times a day according to conditions and severity of symptoms.

Children (Elixir)

Body Weight	Starting Dosage
10 lb	0.5 mL to 0.75 mL
20 lb	1.25 mL (1/4 tsp) to 2.0 mL
30 lb	2.5 mL (1/2 tsp)
50 lb	3/4 tsp to 1 tsp
75–80 lb	1 tsp to 1 1/2 tsp

Doses may be repeated every 4 hours as needed; dosage adjustment may be necessary.

LEVSIN Drops:

Infants

Body Weight	Starting Dosage (in drops)
5 lb	3
7.5 lb	4
10 lb	6
15 lb	7
20 lb	9

Children 1–10 years: 1/2–1 mL

Adults: 1–2 mL

Doses may be repeated every 4 hours as needed; dosage adjustment may be necessary according to conditions and severity of symptoms.

LEVSIN Injection may be administered subcutaneously, intramuscularly, or intravenously without dilution. The usual recommended dose of LEVSIN in the treatment of gastrointestinal disorders is 0.5 to 1.0 mL (0.25 to 0.5 mg) administered at four-hour intervals three to four times daily. Some patients may need only a single dose, others may require administration 2, 3, or 4 times a day. For hypotonic duodenography, LEVSIN Injection may be used five to ten minutes prior to the diagnostic procedure. The usual dose is 0.5 to 1.0 mL (0.25 mg to 0.5 mg).

IN ANESTHESIA: As pre-anesthetic medication, the recommended dose of LEVSIN Injection is 5 μg/kg of body weight, given thirty to sixty minutes prior to the anticipated time of induction of anesthesia, or at the time the pre-anesthetic narcotic or sedatives are administered. In intraoperative medication, LEVSIN Injectable may be used during surgery to counteract drug induced bradycardia. It should be administered intravenously in increments of 0.25 mL and repeated as needed. To achieve reversal of neuromuscular blockage, the recommended dose of LEVSIN Injectable is 0.2 mg for each 1 mg of neostigmine or the equivalent dose of physostigmine and pyridostigmine.

LEVSINEX TIMECAPS: Adults: The usual dose is one TIMECAP every 12 hours. For patients requiring higher anticholinergic therapy, the dosage may be increased to two TIMECAPS every 12 hours or one Timecap every 8 hours.

Children over 2 years: One capsule every 12 hours. Dosage may be increased to one capsule every 8 hours if needed.

Caution: Federal law prohibits dispensing without prescription.

HOW SUPPLIED

LEVSIN Tablets are white and scored with "K-U" imprint on one side and "531" imprinted on the other.

Bottles of 100 tablets	(NDC 0091-3531-01)
Bottles of 500 tablets	(NDC 0091-3531-05)

LEVSIN Elixir is orange colored and flavored and contains 20% alcohol, pints (473 mL), (NDC 0091-4532-16).

LEVSIN Drops, oral solution, is orange colored and flavored, contains 5% alcohol, supplied in a 15 mL dropper bottle, (NDC 0091-4538-15).

LEVSIN Injection is supplied in 1 mL ampules and packaged in boxes of 5, (NDC 0091-1536-05), and 10 mL vials, (NDC 0091-1536-10).

LEVSINEX TIMECAPS are brown and clear capsules containing brown and white beadlets, they are imprinted with "KREMERS URBAN 537", bottles of 100, (NDC 0091-3537-01).

LEVSIN with Phenobarbitol Products, call K-U (1-800-558-5114) for complete prescribing information.

LEVSIN with Phenobarbital Tablets are pink and scored with "K-U" imprint on one side and "534" imprinted on the other.

Bottles of 100 tablets	(NDC 0091-3534-01)
Bottles of 500 tablets	(NDC 0091-3534-05)

LEVSIN with Phenobarbital Elixer is red colored and raspberry flavored and contains 20% alcohol, pints (473 mL), (NDC 0091-4530-16).

LEVSIN with Phenobarbital Drops, oral solution, is red colored and cherry flavored, contains 5% alcohol, supplied in a 15 mL dropper bottle, (NDC 0091-4536-15).

LEVSINEX with Phenobarbital TIMECAPS are pink and clear capsules containing pink and white beadlets, they are imprinted with "KREMERS URBAN 539", bottles of 100, (NDC 0091-3539-01).

Store at controlled room temperatue 59–86°F (15–30°C).

Shown in Product Identification Section, page 412

MILKINOL®

(See PDR For Nonprescription Drugs)

PRE-PEN® ℞

[prē 'pen]

(Benzylpenicilloyl-polylysine USP)

Skin Test Antigen

DESCRIPTION

PRE-PEN® is a sterile solution of benzylpenicilloyl-polylysine in a concentration of 6.0×10^{-5}M (penicilloyl) in 0.01 M phosphate buffer and 0.15 M sodium chloride. The benzylpenicilloyl-polylysine in PRE-PEN is a derivative of poly-l-lysine, where the epsilon amino groups are substituted with benzylpenicilloyl groups (50-70%) forming benzylpenicilloyl alpha amide. Each single dose ampule contains 0.25 mL of PRE-PEN.

INACTIVE INGREDIENTS

Sodium Chloride, and Sodium Phosphate.

ACTION

PRE-PEN (benzylpenicilloyl-polylysine) reacts specifically with benzylpenicilloyl skin sensitizing antibodies (reagins: IgE class) to initiate release of chemical mediators which produce an immediate wheal and flare reaction at a skin test site. All individuals exhibiting a positive skin test to PRE-PEN possess reagins against the benzylpenicilloyl group which is a haptene. A haptene is a low molecular weight chemical which, when conjugated to a carrier, e.g., poly-l-lysine, has the properties under appropriate conditions of an antigen with the haptene's specificity.

It is to be noted that individuals who have previously received therapeutic penicillin may have positive skin test reactions to PRE-PEN as well as to a number of other non-benzylpenicilloyl haptenes. The latter are designated as minor determinants, in that they are present in lesser amounts than the major determinant, benzylpenicilloyl. The minor determinants may nevertheless be associated with examples of significant clinical hypersensitivity.

Virtually everyone who receives penicillin develops specific antibodies to the drug as measured by hemagglutination studies, but (a) positive skin tests to various penicillin and penicillin-derived reagents become positive in less than 10% of patients who have tolerated penicillin in the past and (b) allergic responses are infrequent (less than 1%).

Many individuals reacting positively to PRE-PEN will not develop a systemic allergic reaction on subsequent exposure to therapeutic penicillin. Thus, the PRE-PEN skin test facilitates assessing the local allergic skin reactivity of a patient to benzylpenicilloyl.

INDICATIONS

PRE-PEN is useful as an adjunct in assessing the risk of administering penicillin (benzylpenicillin or penicillin G) when it is the preferred drug of choice in adult patients who have previously received penicillin and have a history of clinical penicillin hypersensitivity. In this situation, a negative skin test to PRE-PEN is associated with an incidence of allergic reactions of less than 5% after the administration of therapeutic penicillin, whereas the incidence may be more than 20% in the presence of a positive skin test to PRE-PEN.

These allergic reactions are predominantly dermatologic. Because of the extremely low incidence of anaphylactic reactions, there are insufficient data at present to document that a decreased incidence of anaphylactic reactions following the administration of penicillin will occur in patients with a negative skin test to PRE-PEN. Similarly, when deciding the risk of proposed penicillin treatment, there are not enough data at present to permit relative weighting in individual cases of a history of clinical penicillin hypersensitivity as compared to positive skin tests to PRE-PEN and/or minor penicillin determinants.

It should be borne in mind that no reagent, test, or combination of tests will completely assure that a reaction to penicillin therapy will not occur.

CONTRAINDICATIONS

PRE-PEN is contraindicated in those patients who have exhibited either a systemic or marked local reaction to its previous administration. Patients known to be extremely hypersensitive to penicillin should not be skin tested.

WARNINGS

There is insufficient data to assess the potential danger of sensitization to penicillin from repeated skin testing with PRE-PEN.

Rarely, a systemic allergic reaction (see below) may follow a skin test with PRE-PEN. This can be avoided by making the first application by scratch test and very carefully following the instructions below in administering the intradermal test, using the intradermal route only if the scratch test has been entirely negative.

Skin testing with penicillin and/or other penicillin-derived reagents should not be performed simultaneously.

No controlled studies have been made of the safety of PRE-PEN skin testing in pregnant women and therefore, the hazard of skin testing of such patients should be weighed against the hazards of penicillin therapy without skin testing.

PRECAUTIONS

There is insufficient data derived from well-controlled studies to determine the value of the PRE-PEN skin test as a means of assessing the risk of administering therapeutic penicillin (when penicillin is the preferred drug of choice) in the following situations:

(1) Adult patients who give no history of clinical penicillin hypersensitivity.
(2) Pediatric patients.

In addition, there are no data at present to assess the clinical value of PRE-PEN where exposure to penicillin is suspected as a cause of a drug reaction and in patients who are undergoing routine allergy evaluation.

Furthermore, there are no data relating the clinical value of PRE-PEN skin tests to the risk of administering semi-synthetic penicillins (phenoxymethyl penicillin, ampicillin, carbenicillin, dicloxacillin, methicillin, nafcillin, oxacillin, phenethicillin) and cephalosporin-derived antibiotics.

Recognition that the following clinical outcomes are possible makes it imperative for the physician to weigh risk to benefit in every instance where the decision to administer or not to administer penicillin is based in part on a PRE-PEN skin test.

(1) An allergic reaction to therapeutic penicillin may occur in a patient with a negative skin test to PRE-PEN.
(2) It is possible for a patient to have an anaphylactic reaction to therapeutic penicillin in the presence of a negative PRE-PEN skin test and a negative history of clinical penicillin hypersensitivity.
(3) If penicillin is the absolute drug of choice in a life-threatening situation, successful desensitization with therapeutic penicillin may be possible irrespective of a positive skin test and/or a positive history of clinical penicillin hypersensitivity.

ADVERSE REACTIONS

Occasionally, patients may develop an intense local inflammatory response at the skin test site. Rarely, patients will develop a systemic allergic reaction, manifested by generalized erythema, pruritus, angioneurotic edema, urticaria, dyspnea, and/or hypotension. The usual methods of treating a skin test antigen induced reaction—the application of a venous occlusion tourniquet proximal to the skin test site and administration of epinephrine (and, at times, an injection of an antihistamine) — are recommended and will usually control the reaction. As a rule, systemic allergic reactions following skin test procedures are of short duration and controllable, but the patient should be kept under observation for several hours.

Skin Testing Dosage and Technique:

SCRATCH TESTING

Skin testing is usually performed on the inner volar aspect of the forearm. The skin test material should **always** be applied first by the scratch technique. After preparing the skin surface, a sterile 20 gauge needle should be used to make a 3–5 mm scratch of the epidermis. Very little pressure is required to break the epidermal continuity. If bleeding occurs, prepare a second site and scratch more lightly with the needle—sufficient to produce a non-bleeding scratched surface. Apply a small drop of PRE-PEN solution to the scratch and rub gently with an applicator, toothpick, or the side of the needle. Observe for the appearance of a wheal, erythema, and the occurrence of itching at the test site during the succeeding 15 minutes at which time the solution over the scratch is wiped off. A positive reaction is unmistakable and consists of the development within 10 minutes of a pale wheal, usually with pseudopods, surrounding the scratch site and varying in diameter from 5 to 15 mm (or more). This wheal may be surrounded by a variable diameter of erythema, and accompanied by a variable degree of itching. The most sensitive individuals develop itching almost instantly, and the wheal and erythema are prompt in their appearance.

As soon as a positive response as defined above is clearly evident, the solution over the scratch should be immediately wiped off. If the scratch test is either negative or equivocally positive (less than 5 mm wheal and little or no erythema, and no itching), an intradermal test may be performed.

THE INTRADERMAL TEST

Using a tuberculin syringe with a 3/8" to 5/8" long, 26 to 30 gauge, short bevel needle, withdraw the contents of the ampule. Prepare a sterile skin test area on the upper, outer arm, sufficiently below the deltoid muscle to permit proximal application of a tourniquet later, if necessary. Be sure to eject all air from the syringe through the needle, then insert the needle, bevel up immediately below the skin surface. Inject an amount of PRE-PEN sufficient to raise the smallest possible perceptible bleb. This volume will be between 0.01 and 0.02 mL. Using a separate syringe and needle, inject a like amount of saline as a control at least 1½ inches removed from the test site. Most skin reactions will develop within 5–15 minutes and response to the skin test is read as follows:

(—) Negative response—no increase in size of original bleb and/or no greater reaction than the control site.
(±) Ambiguous response—wheal being only slightly larger than initial injection bleb, with or without accompanying erythematous flare and larger than the control site.
(+) Positive response—itching and marked increase in size of original bleb. Wheal may exceed 20 mm in diameter and exhibit pseudopods.

The control site should be completely reactionless. If it exhibits a wheal greater than 2–3 mm, repeat the test, and if the same reaction is observed, a physician experienced with allergy skin testing should be consulted.

HOW SUPPLIED

PRE-PEN is supplied in ampules containing 0.25 mL and packaged in boxes of 5 (NDC 0091-1640-05).

PRE-PEN is stable only when kept under refrigeration. It is, therefore, recommended that test materials subjected to ambient temperatures for over a day be discarded.

EDUCATIONAL MATERIAL

Booklet

"Lactose Intolerance: The Villain Wears a Masque of White"

For people who cannot digest dairy products because they lack the enzymes necessary for the digestion of milk sugar, this pamphlet explains how the problem comes about, its symptoms and how it can be treated with LACTRASE®, an enzyme supplement. A table addressing the lactose content of food is included.

FREE TO HEALTH PROFESSIONALS AND CONSUMERS

Lactaid Inc.
P.O. BOX 111
PLEASANTVILLE, NJ 08232-0111

LACTAID®
Lactaid liquid drops
and
Lactaid Tablets
(lactase enzyme)

DESCRIPTION

LIQUID: Each 5 drop dosage contains not less than 1000 NLU (Neutral Lactase Units) of Beta-D-galactosidase derived from Kluyveromyces lactis yeast. The enzyme is in a liquid carrier of glycerol (50%), water (30%), and inert yeast dry matter (20%). 4–5 drops hydrolyzes approximately 70% of the lactose in 1 quart of milk at refrigerator temperature, @ 42°F–6°C in 24 hours, or will do the same in 2 hours @ 85°F–30°C. Additional time and/or enzyme required for 100% lactose conversion. 1 U.S. quart of milk will contain approximately 50 gm lactose prior to lactose hydrolysis and will contain 15 gm or less, after 70% conversion.

ACTION

Hydrolysis converts the lactose into its simple sugar components: glucose and galactose.

INDICATIONS

Lactase insufficiency in the patient, suspected from g.i. disturbances after consumption of milk or milk content products: e.g., bloat, distension, flatulence, diarrhea; or identified by a lactose tolerance test.

USAGE

Added to milk. 4–10 drops per quart of milk depending on level of lactose conversion desired.

OTHER USES

In vivo activity has been demonstrated, indicating usage in tube feedings and other lactose-content solid and liquid foods, with addition at time of consumption.

HOW SUPPLIED

Lactase enzyme in a stable liquid form, in sales units of 4, 12, 30 and 75 one-quart dosages at 5 drops per dose.

TABLETS: Each tablet contains not less than 3300 FCC lactase units of Beta-D-Galactosidase from Aspergillis oryzae. 1 to 2 tablets taken with a meal will normally handle a lactose challenge equal to 1 glass of milk. In severe cases, 3 tablets may be required.

HOW SUPPLIED

In bottles of 100 and boxes of 12.

TOXICITY

None.

DRUG INTERACTIONS

None. Both liquid and tablets are classified as food, not drugs.

PRECAUTIONS

Diabetics should be aware that the milk sugar will now be metabolically available and must be taken into account (25 gm glucose and 25 gm galactose per quart @ 100% hydrolysis). No reports received of any diabetics' reactions. Galactosemics may not have milk in any form, lactase enzyme modified or not.

Also in most areas of the U.S.: Fresh hydrolyzed lowfat milk from dairies, ready to drink, sold in food markets. Lactose hydrolysis level: 70%. If desired, further conversion of the dairy-treated milk can be done at home or institution with the Lactaid liquid enzyme. Also in some areas: Lactaid lactose reduced cottage cheese, American process cheese, ice cream.

Any person or institution unable to locate Lactaid enzyme locally can order direct from Lactaid Inc. retail or wholesale. Samples and full product information to doctors, institutions and nutritionists on request. Call toll-free 800-257-8650.

Shown in Product Identification Section, page 412

EDUCATIONAL MATERIAL

Samples and literature available to physicians and dietitians upon request.

Lafayette Pharmacal, Inc.
4200 SOUTH HULEN STREET
FORT WORTH, TX 76109

SUGAR-FREE
KONSYL®
[kon-sil']
Refined Psyllium Hydrophilic Mucilloid

(See PDR For Nonprescription Drugs)

KONSYL®-D
[kon-sil'-d]
(FORMERLY L.A. FORMULA)
Refined Psyllium Hydrophilic Mucilloid With Dextrose Added

(See PDR For Nonprescription Drugs)

Lakeside Pharmaceuticals
Division of Merrell Dow Pharmaceuticals Inc.
CINCINNATI, OH 45242-9553

BENTYL® ℞
[bĕn'tĭl]
(dicyclomine hydrochloride USP)
Tablets, Capsules, Syrup, Injection

CAUTION: Federal law prohibits dispensing without prescription.

DESCRIPTION

1. Bentyl capsules contain 10 mg dicyclomine hydrochloride USP. Bentyl 10 mg capsules also contain calcium sulfate, corn starch, FD&C Blue No. 1, FD&C Red No. 3, gelatin, lactose, magnesium stearate, pregelatinized corn starch, and titanium dioxide.
2. Bentyl tablets contain 20 mg dicyclomine hydrochloride USP. Bentyl 20 mg tablets also contain acacia, dibasic calcium phosphate, corn starch, FD&C Blue No. 1, lactose, magnesium stearate, pregelatinized corn starch, and sucrose.
3. Bentyl syrup contains 10 mg dicyclomine hydrochloride USP in each 5 ml (1 teaspoonful). Bentyl syrup also contains citric acid, D&C Red No. 33, FD&C Blue No. 1, FD&C Red No. 40, FD&C Yellow No. 6, flavors, glucose, methylparaben, propylene glycol, propylparaben, saccharin sodium, and water.
4. Bentyl Injection
   Ampul—2 ml—Each ml contains 10 mg dicyclomine hydrochloride USP, in water for injection, made isotonic with sodium chloride.
   Vial—10 ml—Each ml contains 10 mg dicyclomine hydrochloride USP, in water for injection, made isotonic with sodium chloride. 0.5% chlorobutanol hydrous (chloral derivative) added as a preservative.

Continued on next page

Information on Lakeside Pharmaceuticals products is based on labeling in effect in May, 1986.

Lakeside—Cont.

Prefilled Syringe—2 ml—Each ml contains 10 mg dicyclomine hydrochloride USP, in water for injection, made isotonic with sodium chloride.

INDICATIONS

For the treatment of Functional Bowel/Irritable Bowel Syndrome (irritable colon, spastic colon, and mucous colitis).

CLINICAL PHARMACOLOGY

Bentyl relieves smooth muscle spasm of the gastrointestinal tract.

In two controlled clinical trials, 82 percent of the patients treated with initial doses of 160 mg daily demonstrated a favorable clinical response. In these trials, however, 61 percent of the patients on the drug experienced one or more of the following typical anticholinergic side effects: (See "Adverse Reactions" for full information).

Side effect	Dicyclomine hydrochloride (40 mg q.i.d.) %	Placebo %
Dry Mouth	33	5
Dizziness	29	2
Blurred Vision	27	2
Nausea	14	6
Light-headedness	11	3
Drowsiness	9	1
Weakness	7	1
Nervousness	6	2

In these trials, approximately 9 percent of the dicyclomine (and 2 percent of the placebo) patients discontinued therapy because of one or more of these side effects. For the most part, however, these side effects were neither severe nor intolerable, and generally did not interfere with successful treatment of the patient. In 25 percent of the patients who had these side effects, the side effects disappeared or were tolerated with no dose reduction. A total of 28 percent of the patients in these trials had their dose reduced (to an average dose of 90 mg daily) because of side effects. These patients generally continued to experience a favorable clinical response and their side effects either disappeared or were tolerated.

CONTRAINDICATIONS

Obstructive uropathy (for example, bladder neck obstruction due to prostatic hypertrophy); obstructive disease of the gastrointestinal tract (as in achalasia, pyloroduodenal stenosis); paralytic ileus, intestinal atony of the elderly or debilitated patient; unstable cardiovascular status in acute hemorrhage; severe ulcerative colitis; toxic megacolon complicating ulcerative colitis; myasthenia gravis; and glaucoma.

Infants less than 6 months of age. (See PRECAUTIONS and WARNINGS.)

WARNINGS

In the presence of a high environmental temperature, heat prostration can occur with drug use (fever and heat stroke due to decreased sweating).

Diarrhea may be an early symptom of incomplete intestinal obstruction, especially in patients with ileostomy or colostomy. In this instance, treatment with this drug would be inappropriate and possibly harmful.

Bentyl may produce drowsiness or blurred vision. In this event, the patient should be warned not to engage in activities requiring mental alertness such as operating a motor vehicle or other machinery or perform hazardous work while taking this drug.

Anticholinergic psychosis has been reported in sensitive individuals given anticholinergic drugs. CNS signs and symptoms include confusion, disorientation, short-term memory loss, hallucinations, dysarthria, ataxia, coma, euphoria, decreased anxiety, fatigue, insomnia, agitation and mannerisms, and inappropriate affect. These CNS signs and symptoms usually resolve within 12 to 24 hours after discontinuation of the drug.

There are reports of infants who, in their first 3 months of life, were given dicyclomine hydrochloride syrup and evidenced respiratory symptoms (breathing difficulty, shortness of breath, breathlessness, respiratory collapse, apnea), as well as seizures, syncope, asphyxia, pulse rate fluctuations, muscular hypotonia, and coma. In some instances, these symptoms occurred within minutes of ingestion and lasted up to 20 to 30 minutes. The symptoms were reported in association with dicyclomine hydrochloride syrup therapy but the cause and effect relationship has neither been disproved nor proved. The timing and nature of the reactions suggest that they may have been a consequence of local irritation, aspiration and/or sensitization.

Worldwide, a few deaths have been reported in infants three months of age or less who had been given dicyclomine hydrochloride syrup. Two of these were reported to have been associated with excessively high dicyclomine blood levels.

Although no causal relationship between these effects, observed in infants, and dicyclomine administration has been established, Bentyl is contraindicated in infants less than 6 months of age. (See CONTRAINDICATIONS.)

PRECAUTIONS

Although studies have failed to demonstrate adverse effects of dicyclomine hydrochloride in patients with prostatic hypertrophy, it should be prescribed with caution in patients known to have or suspected of having prostatic hypertrophy.

Use with caution in patients with:

- Autonomic neuropathy.
- Hepatic or renal disease.
- Ulcerative colitis. Large doses may suppress intestinal motility to the point of producing a paralytic ileus and the use of this drug may precipitate or aggravate the serious complication of toxic megacolon.
- Hyperthyroidism, coronary heart disease, congestive heart failure, cardiac arrhythmias, and hypertension.
- Hiatal hernia associated with reflux esophagitis since anticholinergic drugs may aggravate this condition.

Do not rely on the use of the drug in the presence of complication of biliary tract disease.

Investigate any tachycardia before giving anticholinergic (atropine-like) drugs since they may increase the heart rate.

With overdosage, a curare-like action may occur.

Pediatric Use (See CONTRAINDICATIONS and WARNINGS.)

Safety and effectiveness in children have not been adequately established.

ADVERSE REACTIONS

Anticholinergics/antispasmodics produce certain effects which may be physiologic or toxic depending upon the individual patient's response. The physician must delineate these.

Adverse reactions may include xerostomia; urinary hesitancy and retention; blurred vision and tachycardia; palpitations; mydriasis; cycloplegia; increased ocular tension; loss of taste; headache; nervousness; drowsiness; weakness; dizziness; insomnia; nausea; vomiting; impotence; suppression of lactation; constipation; bloated feeling; severe allergic reaction or drug idiosyncrasies including anaphylaxis; urticaria and other dermal manifestations; some degree of mental confusion and/or excitement, especially in elderly persons; and decreased sweating.

With the injectable form there may be a temporary sensation of light-headedness and occasionally local irritation.

DOSAGE AND ADMINISTRATION

DOSAGE MUST BE ADJUSTED TO INDIVIDUAL PATIENT NEEDS. (See CLINICAL PHARMACOLOGY.)

Adults—oral

The only oral dose clearly shown to be effective is 160 mg per day (in four equally divided doses). Since this dose is associated with a significant incidence of side effects, it is prudent to begin with 80 mg per day (in four equally divided doses). Depending upon the patient's response, during the first week of therapy the dose should be increased to 160 mg per day unless side effects limit dosage escalation.

If efficacy is not achieved within two weeks or side effects require doses below 80 mg per day, the drug should be discontinued. Documented safety data are not available for doses of 80 to 160 mg daily for periods longer than two weeks.

Adults—intramuscular injection

The intramuscular dosage form is to be used temporarily when the patient cannot take oral medication. Intramuscular injection is about twice as bioavailable as oral dosage forms; consequently the recommended intramuscular dose is 80 mg daily (in four divided doses). Oral dicyclomine should be started as soon as possible and the intramuscular form should not be used for periods longer than one or two days.

NOT FOR INTRAVENOUS USE.

MANAGEMENT OF OVERDOSE

The signs and symptoms of overdose are headache, nausea, vomiting, blurred vision, dilated pupils, hot, dry skin, dizziness, dryness of the mouth, difficulty in swallowing, CNS stimulation.

Treatment should consist of gastric lavage, emetics, and activated charcoal. Barbiturates may be used either orally or intramuscularly for sedation but they should not be used if Bentyl with Phenobarbital has been ingested. If indicated, parenteral cholinergic agents such as Urecholine® (bethanecol chloride USP) should be used.

HOW SUPPLIED

20 mg Tablets debossed MERRELL 123 or BENTYL 20

Bottles of 100, 500, and 1,000 and unit dose dispenser of 100

To prevent fading, avoid exposure to direct sunlight. Store at room temperature, preferably below 86°F (30°C).

Syrup

16-ounce bottles

Store at room temperature, preferably below 86°F (30°C). Protect from excessive heat.

10 mg Capsules imprinted MERRELL 120/BENTYL® or BENTYL 10

Bottles of 100, 500, and unit dose dispenser of 100

Store at room temperature, preferably below 86°F (30°C).

Injection

10 ml multiple dose vials

Boxes of five 2 ml ampuls

Cartons of five 2 ml prefilled syringes

Store at room temperature, preferably below 86°F (30°C). Protect from freezing.

Product Information as of February, 1985

Injectable dosage forms manufactured by
CONNAUGHT LABORATORIES, INC.
Swiftwater, Pennsylvania 18370 or
TAYLOR PHARMACAL COMPANY
Decatur, Illinois 62525 for
LAKESIDE PHARMACEUTICALS
Division of Merrell Dow Pharmaceuticals Inc.
Cincinnati, Ohio 45215, U.S.A.

Shown in Product Identification Section, page 412

BRICANYL® ℞

[brĭk 'ă-nĭl]
(terbutaline sulfate USP)
Subcutaneous Injection

CAUTION: Federal law prohibits dispensing without prescription.

DESCRIPTION

Bricanyl (terbutaline sulfate USP) Subcutaneous Injection is a sterile isotonic solution containing, per ml, 1.0 mg terbutaline sulfate (equivalent to 0.82 mg free base) and 8.9 mg sodium chloride in water for injection. Hydrochloric acid is used to adjust pH to 3.0–5.0.

Terbutaline sulfate (5-[2-[(1,1-dimethylethyl)amino]-1-hydroxyethyl]-1,3-benzenediol sulfate) is a beta-adrenergic agonist bronchodilator having the chemical structure:

$$[(HO)_2C_6H_3\text{-}CH(OH)CH_2NHC(CH_3)_3]_2 \cdot H_2SO_4$$

CLINICAL PHARMACOLOGY

Bricanyl is a beta-adrenergic receptor agonist which has been shown by *in vitro* and *in vivo* pharmacological studies in animals to exert a preferential effect on $beta_2$-adrenergic receptors such as those located in bronchial smooth muscle. However, controlled clinical studies on patients who were administered the drug have not revealed a preferential $beta_2$-adrenergic effect.

It has been postulated that beta-adrenergic agonists produce many of their pharmacologic effects by activation of adenyl cyclase, the enzyme which catalyzes the conversion of adenosine triphosphate to cyclic adenosine monophosphate.

Bricanyl Injection has been shown in controlled clinical studies to relieve acute bronchospasm in acute and chronic obstructive pulmonary disease, resulting in a clinically significant increase in pulmonary flow rates, e.g., an increase of 15% or greater in FEV_1 in some patients. Following administration of 0.25 mg by subcutaneous injection, a measurable change in flow rate is usually observed within five minutes, and a clinically significant increase in FEV_1 occurs by 15 minutes following the injection. The maximum effect usually occurs within 30–60 minutes and clinically significant bronchodilator activity has been observed to persist for 90 minutes to four hours in most patients. The duration of clinically significant improvement is comparable to that found with equimilligram doses of epinephrine.

Subcutaneously administered Bricanyl shows peak plasma concentrations 15–30 minutes after injection (0.5 mg dose, mean peak plasma level 7.6 μg/L). Approximately $\frac{1}{3}$ is metabolized (inactive), the majority of the dose being excreted in urine unchanged. A half-life of 3–4 hours has been reported.

Terbutaline crosses the placenta. After single dose IV administration of terbutaline to 22 women in late pregnancy who were delivered by elective Caesarean section due to clinical reasons, umbilical blood levels of terbutaline were found to range from 11 to 48% of the maternal blood levels.

INDICATIONS AND USAGE

Bricanyl is indicated as a bronchodilator for the relief of reversible bronchospasm in patients with obstructive airway diseases such as asthma, bronchitis and emphysema.

CONTRAINDICATIONS

Bricanyl is contraindicated in patients with a history of hypersensitivity to any of its components or sympathomimetic amines.

WARNINGS

Usage in Labor and Delivery: Bricanyl is not indicated for the management of preterm labor. Serious adverse reactions have been reported following administration of terbutaline sulfate to women in labor. These reports have included transient hypokalemia, pulmonary edema (sometimes after delivery) and hypoglycemia in the mother and hypoglycemia in the neonatal child. Maternal death has been reported with terbutaline sulfate and other drugs of this class.

PRECAUTIONS

General

Terbutaline sulfate is a sympathomimetic amine and as such should be used with caution in patients with cardiovascular disorders (including arrhythmias, coronary insufficiency and hypertension), in patients with hyperthyroidism or diabetes mellitus, history of seizures, or in patients who are unusually responsive to sympathomimetic amines. Age-related differences in the hemodynamic response to beta-adrenergic receptor stimulation have been reported.

Patients susceptible to hypokalemia should be monitored because transient early falls in serum potassium levels have been reported with beta agonists.

Large doses of intravenous terbutaline sulfate have been reported to aggravate pre-existing diabetes and ketoacidosis. Immediate hypersensitivity reactions and exacerbation of bronchospasm have been reported after terbutaline administration.

Preparation of Other Dosage Forms: Use of the subcutaneous injection for preparation of other dosage forms, e.g., IV infusion, is not appropriate. Sterility, stability, and accurate dosing cannot be assured if the ampuls are not used in accordance with DOSAGE AND ADMINISTRATION.

Information for Patients

Patients should be advised regarding the potential adverse reactions associated with Bricanyl.

Drug Interactions

Other sympathomimetic bronchodilators or epinephrine should not be used concomitantly with terbutaline sulfate since their combined effect on the cardiovascular system may be deleterious to the patient. Terbutaline sulfate should be administered with caution in patients being treated with monoamine oxidase (MAO) inhibitors or tricyclic antidepressants, since the action of terbutaline sulfate on the vascular system may be potentiated.

Beta-adrenergic receptor blocking agents not only block the pulmonary effect of terbutaline but may produce severe asthmatic attacks in asthmatic patients. Therefore, patients requiring treatment for both bronchospastic disease and hypertension should be treated with medication other than beta-adrenergic blocking agents for their hypertension.

Carcinogenesis, Mutagenesis, Impairment of Fertility

A two year oral carcinogenesis bioassay of terbutaline sulfate (50, 500, 1000 and 2000 mg/kg, corresponding to 5,000, 50,000, 100,000, and 200,000 times the recommended daily adult subcutaneous dose, respectively) in the Sprague-Dawley rat revealed drug-related changes in the female genital system. Females showed dose-related increases in leiomyomas of the mesovarium: 3 (5%) at 50 mg/kg, 17 (28%) at 500 mg/kg, 21 (35%) at 1000 mg/kg, and 23 (38%) at 2000 mg/kg, which were significant at the three highest levels. None occurred in female controls. The incidence of ovarian cysts was significantly elevated at all dose levels except at 2000 mg/kg and hyperplasia of the mesovarium was increased significantly at 500 and 2000 mg/kg. A 21-month oral study of terbutaline sulfate (5, 50 and 200 mg/kg, corresponding to 500, 5,000 and 20,000 times the recommended daily adult subcutaneous dose, respectively) in the mouse revealed no evidence of carcinogenicity.

Studies of terbutaline sulfate have not been conducted to determine mutagenic potential.

An oral reproduction study of terbutaline sulfate (up to 50 mg/kg, corresponding to 5,000 times the human subcutaneous dose) in the rat revealed no adverse effects on fertility.

Pregnancy

Teratogenic Effects

Pregnancy Category B: Reproduction studies in mice (up to 1.1 mg/kg subcutaneously, corresponding to 110 times the human subcutaneous dose) and in rats and rabbits (up to 50 mg/kg orally, corresponding to 5000 times the human subcutaneous dose) have revealed no evidence of impaired fertility or harm to the fetus due to terbutaline. There are, however, no adequate and well-controlled studies in pregnant women. Because animal reproduction studies are not always predictive of human response, this drug should be used during pregnancy only if clearly needed.

Labor and Delivery

Usage in Labor and Delivery: The safe use of Bricanyl Subcutaneous Injection for mangement of preterm labor or for other uses during labor and delivery has not been established. (See WARNINGS.)

Nursing Mothers

Terbutaline is excreted in breast milk. Caution should be exercised when Bricanyl is administered to a nursing woman.

Pediatric Use

Safety and effectiveness in children below the age of 12 have not been established.

ADVERSE REACTIONS

The adverse reactions of terbutaline sulfate are similar in nature to those of other sympathomimetic agents.

The most commonly observed side effects are tremor and nervousness. These occur more frequently at doses in excess of 0.25 mg. Other commonly reported reactions include increased heart rate, palpitations and dizziness. Other reported reactions include headache, drowsiness, vomiting, nausea, sweating, and muscle cramps. These reactions are generally transient and usually do not require treatment.

OVERDOSAGE

Overdosage information is limited. Excessive adrenergic receptor stimulation may augment the signs and symptoms listed under ADVERSE REACTIONS and may be accompanied by other adrenergic effects.

Signs and symptoms of overdosage may include the following—*CARDIOVASCULAR:* tachycardia of varying degrees, transient arrhythmias and extrasystoles. A significant drop in blood pressure may occur due to peripheral vasodilation. *NEUROMUSCULAR:* tremors of varying degrees, nervousness, drowsiness, muscle cramps, headache, and sweating. *GASTROINTESTINAL:* nausea and vomiting. *ENDOCRINE:* varying degrees of hyperglycemia and rise in insulin levels which could be followed by rebound hypoglycemia. Hypokalemia in the early stages may occur. The duration of these signs and symptoms will be dependent on the degree of overdosage.

In the case of terbutaline overdosage, the patient should be treated symptomatically for sympathomimetic overdosage with careful consideration to the appropriateness of any chosen therapy and possible effect on the patient's underlying disease state. (See also WARNINGS.)

Studies in mice, rats, rabbits and dogs have established the LD_{50} of terbutaline to be 1–9 g/kg orally and 0.3–1.6 g/kg subcutaneously.

It is not known whether terbutaline is dialyzable.

DOSAGE AND ADMINISTRATION

Parenteral drug products should be inspected visually for particulate matter and discoloration prior to administration, whenever solution and container permit.

The usual subcutaneous dose of Bricanyl is 0.25 mg (0.25 ml, ¼ ampul contents) injected into the lateral deltoid area. If significant clinical improvement does not occur by 15–30 minutes, a second dose of 0.25 mg may be administered. A total dose of 0.5 mg should not be exceeded within a four hour period. If a patient fails to respond to a second 0.25 mg (0.25 ml) dose within 15–30 minutes, other therapeutic measures should be considered.

HOW SUPPLIED

Each 2 ml size ampul contains 1.0 ml of solution (1.0 mg terbutaline sulfate).

Note: 0.25 ml of solution will provide the usual clinical dose 0.25 mg.

NDC 0068-0702-20: package of 10 Ampuls

Solutions of terbutaline sulfate are sensitive to excessive heat and light. Ampuls should therefore be stored at controlled room temperature in their original carton to provide protection from light until dispensed. Solutions should not be used if discolored.

Product Information as of April, 1986

Manufactured by
Astra Pharmaceutical Products, Inc.
Westboro, Mass. 01581, U.S.A. for
LAKESIDE PHARMACEUTICALS
Division of Merrell Dow Pharmaceuticals Inc.
Cincinnati, Ohio 45215, U.S.A.
U.S. Patent No. 3,937,838

Shown in Product Identification Section, page 412

BRICANYL® ℞

[brĭk′ă-nĭl]
(terbutaline sulfate)
Tablets

CAUTION: Federal law prohibits dispensing without prescription.

DESCRIPTION

Bricanyl (terbutaline sulfate USP) Tablets, for oral administration, contain 2.5 mg or 5.0 mg of terbutaline sulfate (equivalent to 2.05 mg and 4.1 mg free base, respectively). Both the 2.5 and 5.0 mg tablets contain the following inactive ingredients: corn starch (or pregelatinized corn starch), lactose, magnesium stearate, microcrystalline cellulose, and povidone.

Terbutaline sulfate (5-[2-[(1,1-dimethylethyl)amino]-1-hydroxyethyl]-1,3-benzenediol sulfate) is a beta-adrenergic agonist bronchodilator having the chemical structure:

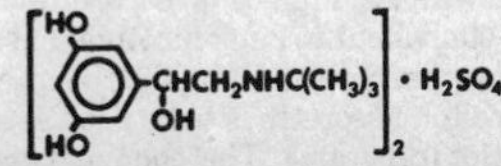

CLINICAL PHARMACOLOGY

Bricanyl is a beta-adrenergic receptor agonist which has been shown by *in vitro* and *in vivo* pharmacological studies in animals to exert a preferential effect on $beta_2$-adrenergic receptors such as those located in bronchial smooth muscle. However, controlled clinical studies on patients who were administered the drug have not revealed a preferential $beta_2$-adrenergic effect.

It has been postulated that beta-adrenergic agonists produce many of their pharmacologic effects by activation of adenyl cyclase, the enzyme which catalyzes the conversion of adenosine triphosphate to cyclic adenosine monophosphate.

Bricanyl Tablets have been shown in controlled clinical studies to relieve bronchospasm in chronic obstructive pulmonary disease such as asthma, chronic bronchitis and emphysema. This action was manifested by a clinically significant increase in pulmonary function as demonstrated by an increase of 15% or more in some patients. A measurable change in pulmonary function usually occurs within 30 minutes following administration. The maximum effect usually occurs within 120–180 minutes. There is a clinically significant decrease in airway and pulmonary resistance which persists for at least 4 hours or longer in most patients. Significant bronchodilator action as measured by various pulmonary function determinations (airway resistance, MMEFR, PEFR) has been demonstrated in studies for periods up to 8 hours in many patients.

Clinical studies have evaluated the effectiveness of oral Bricanyl for periods up to 12 months and the drug continued to produce significant improvement of pulmonary function throughout the period of treatment.

Orally administered terbutaline sulfate is 30–70% absorbed in the GI tract (food reduces bioavailability by one third). Sixty percent of the absorbed oral dose is metabolized via first pass conjugation in the gut wall and liver. There are no known active metabolites. After single oral doses, peak concentrations are found ½ to 5 hours after administration. As a rough guideline, each mg of orally administered terbutaline sulfate (in fasting adults) produces an average peak serum concentration of 1 μg/L. It has a half-life of 3–4 hours. It is excreted in the urine.

Terbutaline crosses the placenta. After single dose IV administration of terbutaline to 22 women in late pregnancy who were delivered by elective Caesarean section due to clinical reasons, umbilical blood levels of terbutaline were found to range from 11 to 48% of the maternal blood levels.

INDICATIONS AND USAGE

Bricanyl is indicated as a bronchodilator for the relief of reversible bronchospasm in patients with obstructive airway diseases such as asthma, bronchitis and emphysema.

CONTRAINDICATIONS

Bricanyl is contraindicated in patients with a history of hypersensitivity to any of its components or sympathomimetic amines.

WARNINGS

Usage in Labor and Delivery: Bricanyl is not indicated for the management of preterm labor. Serious adverse reactions have been reported following administration of terbutaline sulfate to women in labor. These reports have included transient hypokalemia, pulmonary edema (sometimes after delivery) and hypoglycemia in the mother and hypoglycemia in the neonatal child. Maternal death has been reported with terbutaline sulfate and other drugs of this class.

PRECAUTIONS

General

Terbutaline sulfate is a sympathomimetic amine and as such should be used with caution in patients with cardiovascular disorders (including arrhythmias, coronary insufficiency and hypertension), in patients with hyperthyroidism or diabetes mellitus, history of seizures, or in patients who are unusually responsive to sympathomimetic amines. Age-related differences in the hemodynamic response to beta-adrenergic receptor stimulation have been reported.

Patients susceptible to hypokalemia should be monitored because transient early falls in serum potassium levels have been reported with beta agonists.

Large doses of intravenous terbutaline sulfate have been reported to aggravate pre-existing diabetes and ketoacidosis. The relevance of this observation to the use of Bricanyl Tablets is unknown.

Immediate hypersensitivity reactions and exacerbation of bronchospasm have been reported after terbutaline administration.

Information for Patients

The patient should be advised regarding the potential adverse reactions associated with Bricanyl and that: (1) the action of Bricanyl Tablets may last up to 8 hours and there-

Continued on next page

Information on Lakeside Pharmaceuticals products is based on labeling in effect in May, 1986.

Lakeside—Cont.

fore should not be used more frequently than recommended. (2) the number or frequency of doses should not be increased without medical consultation, (3) medical consultation should be sought promptly if symptoms get worse, and (4) other medicines should not be used while taking Bricanyl without consulting the physician.

Drug Interactions

Other sympathomimetic bronchodilators or epinephrine should not be used concomitantly with terbutaline sulfate since their combined effect on the cardiovascular system may be deleterious to the patient. This recommendation does not preclude the judicious use of an aerosol bronchodilator of the adrenergic stimulant type in patients receiving Bricanyl Tablets. Such concomitant use, however, should be individualized and not given on a routine basis. If regular coadministration is required, alternative therapy should be considered.

Terbutaline sulfate should be administered with caution in patients being treated with monoamine oxidase (MAO) inhibitors or tricyclic antidepressants, since the action of terbutaline sulfate on the vascular system may be potentiated.

Beta-adrenergic receptor blocking agents not only block the pulmonary effect of terbutaline but may produce severe asthmatic attacks in asthmatic patients. Therefore, patients requiring treatment for both bronchospastic disease and hypertension should be treated with medication other than beta-adrenergic blocking agents for their hypertension.

Carcinogenesis, Mutagenesis, Impairment of Fertility

A two year oral carcinogenesis bioassay of terbutaline sulfate (50, 500, 1000 and 2000 mg/kg, corresponding to 167, 1667, 3333, and 6667 times the recommended daily adult oral dose, respectively) in the Sprague-Dawley rat revealed drug-related changes in the female genital system. Females showed dose-related increases in leiomyomas of the mesovarium: 3 (5%) at 50 mg/kg, 17 (28%) at 500 mg/kg, 21 (35%) at 1000 mg/kg, and 23 (38%) at 2000 mg/kg, which were significant at the three highest levels. None occurred in female controls. The incidence of ovarian cysts was significantly elevated at all dose levels except at 2000 mg/kg and hyperplasia of the mesovarium was increased significantly at 500 and 2000 mg/kg. A 21-month oral study of terbutaline sulfate (5, 50 and 200 mg/kg, corresponding to 17, 167 and 667 times the recommended daily adult oral dose, respectively) in the mouse revealed no evidence of carcinogenicity.

Studies of terbutaline sulfate have not been conducted to determine mutagenic potential.

An oral reproduction study of terbutaline sulfate up to 50 mg/kg (corresponding to 167 times the human oral dose) in the rat revealed no adverse effects on fertility.

Pregnancy

Teratogenic Effects

Pregnancy Category B: Reproduction studies in mice (up to 1.1 mg/kg subcutaneously, corresponding to 4 times the human oral dose) and in rats and rabbits (up to 50 mg/kg orally, corresponding to 167 times the human oral dose) have revealed no evidence of impaired fertility or harm to the fetus due to terbutaline. There are, however, no adequate and well-controlled studies in pregnant women. Because animal reproduction studies are not always predictive of human response, this drug should be used during pregnancy only if clearly needed.

Labor and Delivery

Usage in Labor and Delivery: The safe use of Bricanyl Tablets for mangement of preterm labor or for other uses during labor and delivery has not been established. (See WARNINGS.)

Nursing Mothers

Terbutaline is excreted in breast milk. Caution should be exercised when Bricanyl is administered to a nursing woman.

Pediatric Use

Safety and effectiveness in children below the age of 12 have not been established.

ADVERSE REACTIONS

The adverse reactions of terbutaline sulfate are similar in nature to those of other sympathomimetic agents.

The most commonly observed side effects are tremor and nervousness. The frequency of these side effects appear to diminish with continued therapy. Other commonly reported reactions include increased heart rate, palpitations and dizziness. Other reported reactions include headache, drowsiness, vomiting, nausea, sweating, and muscle cramps. These reactions are generally transient and usually do not require treatment.

OVERDOSAGE

Overdosage information is limited. Excessive adrenergic receptor stimulation may augment the signs and symptoms listed under ADVERSE REACTIONS and may be accompanied by other adrenergic effects.

Signs and symptoms of overdosage may include the following—*CARDIOVASCULAR:* tachycardia of varying degrees, transient arrhythmias and extrasystoles. A significant drop in blood pressure may occur due to peripheral vasodilation. *NEUROMUSCULAR:* tremors of varying degrees, nervousness, drowsiness, muscle cramps, headache, and sweating. *GASTROINTESTINAL:* nausea and vomiting. *ENDOCRINE:* varying degrees of hyperglycemia and rise in insulin levels which could be followed by rebound hypoglycemia. Hypokalemia in the early stages may occur. The duration of these signs and symptoms will be dependent on the degree of overdosage.

Treat the alert patient who has taken excessive oral medication by emptying the stomach by means of induced emesis, followed by gastric lavage. In the unconscious patient, secure the airway with a cuffed endotracheal tube before beginning lavage (do not induce emesis). Instillation of activated charcoal slurry may help reduce absorption of terbutaline sulfate. Maintain adequate respiratory exchange. Provide cardiac and respiratory support as needed. Continue observation until symptom-free. Careful consideration should be given to the appropriateness of any chosen therapy and possible effect on the patient's underlying disease state. (See also WARNINGS.)

Studies in mice, rats, rabbits and dogs have established the LD_{50} of terbutaline to be 1–9 g/kg orally and 0.3–1.6 g/kg subcutaneously.

It is not known whether terbutaline is dialyzable.

DOSAGE AND ADMINISTRATION

ADULTS: Usual dose is 5 mg three times daily. Dosing may be initiated at 2.5 mg three or four times daily and titrated upward depending on clinical response. A total dose of 15 mg in a 24 hour period should not be exceeded.

CHILDREN (12–15 yrs): 2.5 mg three times daily.

If a previously effective dosage regimen fails to provide the usual relief, medical advice should be sought immediately as this is often a sign of seriously worsening asthma which would require reassessment of therapy.

HOW SUPPLIED

2.5 mg Tablets (*round,* white, debossed "BRICANYL 2½"):
NDC 0068-0725-61: Bottle of 100
NDC 0068-0725-71: Bottle of 1000

5.0 mg Tablets (*square,* white, scored, debossed "BRICANYL 5"):
NDC 0068-0750-61: Bottle of 100
NDC 0068-0750-71: Bottle of 1000

Store at controlled room temperature (59°–86°F) (15°–30°C).

Product Information as of March, 1986

Shown in Product Identification Section, page 412

CĒPACOL® Mouthwash/Gargle
[*sēp 'ă-cōl*]

(See PDR For Nonprescription Drugs)

CĒPACOL® Throat Lozenges
[*sēp 'ă-cōl*]

(See PDR For Nonprescription Drugs)

CĒPACOL® Anesthetic Lozenges (Troches)
[*sēp 'ă-cōl*]

(See PDR For Nonprescription Drugs)

CĒPASTAT® Lozenges
[*sēp 'ă-stăt*]

(See PDR For Nonprescription Drugs)

Cherry Flavor
CĒPASTAT® Sore Throat Lozenges
[*sēp 'ă-stăt*]

(See PDR For Nonprescription Drugs)

NICORETTE® ℞
[*nĭk 'ō-rĕt* "]
(nicotine polacrilex)

Caution: Federal law prohibits dispensing without prescription.

DESCRIPTION

Nicorette (nicotine polacrilex) contains nicotine bound to an ion exchange resin in a sugar-free flavored chewing gum base. Nicotine is absorbed through the buccal mucosa when Nicorette is chewed. Each piece of Nicorette contains nicotine polacrilex equivalent to 2 mg nicotine and also contains flavors, glycerin, gum base, sodium bicarbonate, sodium carbonate, and sorbitol. Nicorette is to be used as an adjunct to smoking cessation programs. The chemical name for nicotine is (*S*)-3-(1-methyl-2-pyrrolidinyl)pyridine.

CLINICAL PHARMACOLOGY

Nicotine is an agonist at nicotinic receptors in the peripheral and central nervous systems. In man, as in animals, nicotine has been shown to produce both behavioral stimulation and depression.

Nicotine's effects are generally dose-dependent, and extremely high doses (achievable through parenteral, rectal, and perhaps percutaneous routes), can produce toxic symptoms, i.e., delirium. These effects can occur in nicotine-tolerant individuals. In nonsmokers, CNS mediated symptoms of hiccups, nausea, and emesis are commonly associated with the use of even small doses of inhaled smoke or chewed Nicorette gum. However, in smokers, these symptoms occur only with much larger doses.

Nicotine has actions at the sympathetic ganglia and on the chemoreceptors of the aorta and carotid bodies. Nicotine also affects the adrenal medulla, with the attendant release of catecholamines. The overall effect on the cardiovascular system leads to acceleration of the heart, peripheral vasoconstriction, and elevation of blood pressure with an attendant increase in the work of the heart. Nicotine may induce vasospasm and cardiac arrhythmias. Tolerance does not develop to the catecholamine-releasing effects of nicotine.

Results of cardiovascular studies comparing Nicorette with cigarettes document that each source of nicotine produces similar dose-dependent effects on cardiovascular performance (see *Biopharmaceutics and Pharmacokinetics* section). However, if Nicorette gum (2 mg/piece) is used by smokers at a rate not exceeding one piece per hour, the cardiovascular effects produced do not differ from those seen with placebo.

Reinforcement of cigarette smoking behavior is considered to have both psychological (or learned) and pharmacological components. Buffered nicotine-containing gum is designed to provide an alternative source of nicotine for nicotine-dependent individuals acutely withdrawing from tobacco smoking.

Biopharmaceutics and Pharmacokinetics

The nicotine in Nicorette is bound to an ion exchange resin and is released only during chewing; nicotine will not be released in significant amounts if the gum is swallowed. The blood level of nicotine obtained with Nicorette will depend upon the vigor and duration of chewing.

In studies comparing the nicotine blood level achieved with Nicorette to that achieved with smoking, it was found that the trough level of nicotine obtained by smoking one cigarette per hour is approximately twice that of chewing one 2 mg Nicorette.

The pronounced early peak in nicotine blood levels seen with the inhalation of cigarette smoke is not observed with the chewing of Nicorette. Swallowing Nicorette does not produce clinically significant blood levels of nicotine. Nicotine is metabolized mainly by the liver, but may also be metabolized to a lesser extent by the kidney and the lung. The principal metabolites are cotinine and nicotine-1'-N-oxide. Both nicotine and its metabolites are excreted through the kidneys with about 10 to 20% of absorbed nicotine excreted unchanged in the urine. Excretion of nicotine is increased in acid urine and by high urine output. The metabolism of nicotine absorbed buccally from Nicorette is qualitatively similar to the metabolism observed when nicotine is absorbed through inhalation of cigarette smoke.

INDICATION AND USAGE

Nicorette is indicated as a temporary aid to the cigarette smoker seeking to give up his or her smoking habit while participating in a behavioral modification program under medical supervision.

The efficacy of Nicorette as an aid to smoking cessation was demonstrated in clinical studies which showed that Nicorette gum, in comparison to control chewing gums, increased the likelihood of smoking cessation among participants in behavior modification programs. As used in the context of this labeling, behavioral modification refers to supervised programs of education, counselling and psychological support. The efficacy of Nicorette use without concomitant participation in a behavioral modification program has not been established.

In general, smokers who have a high 'physical' type of nicotine dependence are most likely to benefit from the use of Nicorette. The following subject characteristics are correlated with a 'physical' type of nicotine dependence: (1) smoke more than 15 cigarettes per day, (2) prefer brands of cigarettes with nicotine levels of greater than 0.9 mg, (3) usually inhale the smoke, (4) smoke the first cigarette within 30 minutes of arising, (5) find the first cigarette in the morning the hardest to give up, (6) smoke more frequently during the morning than the rest of the day, (7) find it difficult to refrain from smoking in places where it is forbidden, or (8) smoke even when they are so ill they are confined to bed most of the day.

The benefits of Nicorette use beyond three months has not been demonstrated.

CONTRAINDICATIONS

Nicorette is contraindicated in non-smokers.

Nicorette is contraindicated in patients during the immediate post-myocardial infarction period, patients with life-threatening arrhythmias, and patients with severe or worsening angina pectoris (see WARNINGS). Also, Nicorette is contraindicated in patients with active temporomandibular joint disease.

Current medical opinion indicates that nicotine in any form may be harmful to an unborn child. Nicorette and cigarettes both contain nicotine.

Nicorette may cause fetal harm when administered to a pregnant woman.

Use of cigarettes or Nicorette during the last trimester has been associated with a decrease in fetal breathing movements. These effects may be the result of decreased placental perfusion caused by nicotine. One miscarriage during Nicorette therapy has been reported, and the relation to drug therapy as a contributing factor cannot be excluded. Studies in pregnant rhesus monkeys have shown that maternal nicotine administration produced acidosis, hypoxia and hypercarbia in the fetus.

Nicotine has been shown to be teratogenic in mice treated subcutaneously with 25 mg/kg, which is approximately 300 times the human buccal dose. Studies in rats and monkeys have not demonstrated a teratogenic effect of nicotine in doses which would occur during cigarette smoking.

Nicorette is therefore contraindicated in women who are or may become pregnant, and female patients should be advised to take adequate precautions to avoid becoming pregnant. The physician may wish to consider a pregnancy test before instituting therapy with Nicorette. If this drug is used during pregnancy, or if the patient becomes pregnant while taking this drug, the patient should be apprised of the potential hazard to the fetus.

WARNINGS

The risks of nicotine in patients with certain cardiovascular and endocrine diseases should be carefully weighed against the benefits of including Nicorette in a smoking cessation program in these patients. Specifically, patients with coronary heart disease (history of myocardial infarction and/or angina pectoris), serious cardiac arrhythmias, or vasospastic diseases (Buerger's disease, Prinzmetal variant angina) should be carefully screened and evaluated before Nicorette is prescribed.

As the action of nicotine on the adrenal medulla (release of catecholamines) does not appear to be affected by tolerance, Nicorette should be used with caution in patients with hyperthyroidism, pheochromocytoma or insulin-dependent diabetes. Cigarette smoking is felt to play a perpetuating role in hypertension and peptic ulcer disease. Therefore, Nicorette should be used in patients with systemic hypertension or inactive peptic ulcer only when the benefits of including Nicorette in a smoking cessation program outweigh the risks.

PRECAUTIONS

Nicorette should be used with caution in patients with oral or pharyngeal inflammation and in patients with a history of esophagitis or peptic ulcer.

The dosage form of Nicorette dictates that it be used with caution in patients whose dental problems might be exacerbated by chewing gum.

Nicorette is sugar-free and has been formulated to minimize stickiness. As with other gums, however, the degree to which Nicorette may stick to dentures, dental caps or partial bridges may depend on the materials from which they are made and other factors such as amount of saliva produced, possible interaction with denture adhesives, denture cleaning compounds, dryness of mouth due to other causes and salivary constituents. Should an excessive degree of stickiness to dental work occur, there is the possibility that as with other gums, Nicorette may damage dental work; if this should occur, the patient should discontinue its use and consult a physician or dentist.

The sustained use of Nicorette by ex-smokers is not to be encouraged because the chronic consumption of nicotine is toxic and addicting. The physician must, however, weigh the relative risks of a possible return to smoking and continued, long-term use of the gum.

Information for Patients: The patient instruction sheet is attached at the end of the professional labeling text. It is intended for detachment by the pharmacist and inclusion in the package of Nicorette dispensed to the patient. It contains important selected information on patient selection, risks, adverse effects and instructions on how to use Nicorette properly.

Drug Interactions: Smoking cessation, with or without nicotine substitutes, may alter response to concomitant medication in ex-smokers. Smoking is considered to increase metabolism and thus lower blood levels of drugs such as phenacetin, caffeine, theophylline, imipramine and pentazocine, through enzyme induction. Cessation of smoking may result in increased levels of these drugs. Absorption of glutethimide may be decreased, and the "first pass" metabolism of propoxyphene decreased by smoking cessation. Other reported effects of smoking, which do not involve enzyme induction, include reduced diuretic effects of furosemide and decreased cardiac output, and increased blood pressure with propranolol, which may also relate to the hormonal effects of nicotine. Smoking cessation may reverse these actions.

Treatment Emergent
Symptom Incidence for the 2 mg Gum

	U.S.		British	
	Drug	Placebo	Drug	Placebo
Number of Subjects Reporting	94	95	58	58
Percent of Subjects Reporting				
Autonomic				
Excess Salivation	2.1	0.0		
CNS				
Insomnia	1.1	1.1		
Dizziness/Light-headedness	2.1	2.1	19.0	13.8
Irritable/Fussy	1.1	1.1		
Headache	1.1	5.3	24.1	29.3
Gastrointestinal				
Nonspecific GI Distress	9.6	6.3		
Eructation	6.4	1.1		
Indigestion			41.4	20.7
Nausea/Vomiting	18.1	4.2	31.0	15.5
Reactions Referable to Mouth, Throat, Jaw, or Teeth				
Mouth or Throat Soreness	37.2	31.6	56.9	53.4
Jaw Muscle Ache	18.1	9.5	44.8	44.8
Others				
Anorexia	1.1	1.1		
Hiccups	14.9	0.0	22.4	3.4

Both smoking and nicotine can increase circulating cortisol and catecholamines. Therapy with adrenergic agonists or with adrenergic blockers may need to be adjusted according to changes in nicotine therapy or smoking status.

Carcinogenesis, Mutagenesis, Impairment of Fertility
Nicotine was not mutagenic in the Ames *Salmonella* test. Literature reports indicate that nicotine is neither an initiator nor a tumor-promoter in mice. There is inconclusive evidence to suggest that cotinine, an oxidized metabolite of nicotine, may be carcinogenic in rats. Cotinine was not mutagenic in the Ames *Salmonella* test.

Studies have shown a decrease of litter size in rats treated with nicotine during the time of fertilization.

Pregnancy: Pregnancy Category X. See "Contraindications" section.

Nursing Mothers: Nicotine passes freely into the breast milk. Because of the potential for serious adverse reactions in nursing infants from nicotine, a decision should be made whether to discontinue nursing or to discontinue the drug, taking into account the importance of the drug to the mother.

Pediatric Use: Safety and effectiveness in children and adolescents who smoke has not been evaluated.

ADVERSE REACTIONS

Adverse reactions reported in association with the use of Nicorette include both local effects and systemic effects representing the pharmacologic action of nicotine.

Local side effects: Mechanical effects of gum chewing include traumatic injury to oral mucosa or teeth, jaw ache, and eructation secondary to air swallowing. These side effects may be minimized by modifying chewing technique.

Systemic side effects: Although the systemic effects seen in trials were generally similar, the reported frequency of adverse drug effects was highly variable, as illustrated by the variation observed in adverse event incidence estimated from the results of two well-controlled studies (one performed in the United States, and the other in England) designed to evaluate the safety and efficacy of Nicorette. (See table, below.) Given this variability, the table can be used only as an indication of the relative frequency of adverse events reported in representative clinical trials. It can not predict expected incidences of these effects during the course of usual medical practice.

[See table above].

In addition to the more frequently reported effects listed in the table above, the following events were reported at a rate of less than one percent in clinical trials with Nicorette: systemic nicotine intoxication (see below), laxative effect, constipation, vomiting, hoarseness, dry mouth, flushing, sneezing, cough, euphoria, insomnia and gas pains. One miscarriage during Nicorette therapy has been reported, and a relation to drug therapy as a contributing factor cannot be excluded.

The only potentially serious systemic adverse effect observed among the 152 patients evaluated in the controlled clinical trials used to support the efficacy of Nicorette was cardiac irritability; a patient displayed what may have been nicotine-induced, but reversible, atrial fibrillation. Cardiac irritability is a well known consequence of cigarette smoking.

Adverse reactions reported in settings other than controlled clinical trials are similar to those reported in the trials. A 46-year-old male patient participating in a clinical trial of Nicorette was reported to have developed nicotine intoxication requiring hospitalization. After 4 days, he was discharged, fully recovered. He died suddenly one month later. Nicorette was not used during this one-month interval. The relationship of the patient's death to his prior treatment is undetermined.

DRUG ABUSE AND DEPENDENCE

While nicotine dependence from the use of substances other than tobacco products has not been reported, the possibility of transference of nicotine dependence to Nicorette exists. The use of the Nicorette gum beyond three months has not been demonstrated to increase the smoking cessation rate. To minimize the risk of dependence, patients should be encouraged to gradually withdraw or stop gum usage altogether at 3 months. Usage beyond three months should be discouraged. In patients who have used the gum for longer periods, gradual withdrawal should be instituted.

OVERDOSAGE

Overdosage could occur if many pieces were chewed simultaneously or in rapid succession. Risk of poisoning by swallowing the gum is small because absorption in the absence of chewing is slow and incomplete. The consequences of overdose will most likely be minimized by the early nausea and vomiting known to occur with excessive nicotine intake. However, toxic systemic effects may occur. Should an overdose occur, the symptoms would be those of acute nicotine poisoning. Symptoms and signs include nausea, salivation, abdominal pain, vomiting, diarrhea, cold sweat, headache, dizziness, disturbed hearing and vision, mental confusion and marked weakness. Faintness and prostration will likely ensue and hypotension may occur; breathing is difficult; the pulse may be rapid, weak and irregular; collapse may follow by terminal convulsions. Death may result within a few minutes from respiratory failure caused by paralysis of the muscles of respiration.

The oral LD_{50} for nicotine in rodents varies with species but is in excess of 24 mg/kg. Death in rodents was due to respiratory paralysis. The oral minimum lethal dose of nicotine in dogs is greater than 5 mg/kg. The oral minimum lethal dose for nicotine in human adults is 40–60 mg.

TREATMENT OF OVERDOSAGE

In view of the lack of actual experience in the treatment of Nicorette overdose, the procedures recommended are those that have been suggested for the treatment of acute nicotine poisoning.

If emesis has not occurred, it should be induced with ipecac syrup in conscious patients. A saline cathartic will speed gastrointestinal passage of the gum. In unconscious patients with a secure airway, gastric lavage with a wide-bore tube followed by suspension of activated charcoal will aid in nicotine removal. Mechanical ventilation for respiratory paralysis may be necessary in severe nicotine poisoning. Hypotension and/or cardiovascular collapse may occur and should be treated vigorously.

DOSAGE AND ADMINISTRATION

Nicorette is an adjunct to smoking cessation programs (see *Indication and Usage* section), and dosage should be individualized. A patient who is a candidate for Nicorette therapy must desire to stop smoking and should be instructed to *stop smoking immediately*. The patient should be given an in-

Continued on next page

Information on Lakeside Pharmaceuticals products is based on labeling in effect in May, 1986.

Lakeside—Cont.

struction sheet on Nicorette gum chewing, and be allowed to read the instruction sheet and ask any questions. The patient should arrange for followup visits at intervals not greater than one month. At followup visits the patient's progress in smoking cessation should be evaluated and the continued usage of Nicorette reassessed. It is recommended that patients be evaluated at not greater than monthly intervals and that those successful abstainers at three months should stop using gum or gradually withdraw from gum usage. Patients who chew gum beyond a three-month period should be considered as possibly using Nicorette as a substitute source of nicotine for their nicotine dependence. (See *Drug Abuse and Dependence* section.)

At the initial office or group visit, patients should be instructed to chew one piece of gum whenever they have the urge to smoke. Each piece should be chewed slowly and intermittently for about 30 minutes. The aim of this chewing is to promote even, slow, buccal absorption of the nicotine released from the buffered gum. Chewing quickly can release the nicotine too rapidly, leading to effects similar to oversmoking, e.g., nausea, hiccups or irritation of the throat.

As the nature of adverse effects experienced by an individual patient will be primarily related to the balance between the degree of nicotine tolerance and the rate and degree of absorption of nicotine from the gum, it is important for the patient to learn to chew the gum slowly and to self-titrate the nicotine dose, in order to minimize side effects. (SEE PATIENT INSTRUCTION SHEET AT END OF PRODUCT LABELING.)

Most patients require approximately 10 pieces of gum per day during the first month of treatment. Patients should be instructed not to exceed 30 pieces of the Nicorette per day.

Patients should be assessed after one month of treatment to determine smoking status, and the use of Nicorette as an adjunct should be reevaluated.

Most patients who have returned to smoking in Nicorette assisted programs did so within six months of treatment. Therefore, a gradual withdrawal from Nicorette should be instituted if gum consumption has not been spontaneously reduced by the patient by six months. The use of Nicorette beyond six months is not recommended.

HOW SUPPLIED

Nicorette is available in 2 mg (beige) square chewing pieces, packaged in child-resistant blister strips of 12 chewing pieces per strip with 8 strips per box.

Boxes of 96 chewing pieces, 2 mg (NDC 0068-0045-55). Store at room temperature, below 86°F (30°C). Protect from light.

Product Information as of May, 1985

Manufactured by AKTIEBOLAGET LEO, Helsingborg, Sweden for

LAKESIDE PHARMACEUTICALS
Division of Merrell Dow Pharmaceuticals Inc.
Cincinnati, Ohio 45215, U.S.A.

NICORETTE®

(nicotine polacrilex)

INSTRUCTIONS FOR USE

You must read these instructions carefully before using Nicorette. While this pamphlet contains important information about Nicorette, it does not contain all information about the drug. If you have questions on the use of Nicorette, you should consult your physician.

WARNING TO FEMALE PATIENTS: NICORETTE CONTAINS NICOTINE WHICH MAY CAUSE FETAL HARM WHEN ADMINISTERED TO A PREGNANT WOMAN. DO NOT TAKE NICORETTE IF YOU ARE PREGNANT OR NURSING. TAKE PRECAUTIONS TO AVOID PREGNANCY WHILE USING NICORETTE, BUT IF YOU SUSPECT YOU ARE PREGNANT, STOP MEDICATION AND TELL YOUR DOCTOR AT ONCE.

THIS DRUG HAS BEEN PRESCRIBED FOR YOU BY YOUR PHYSICIAN. DO NOT LET ANYONE ELSE USE IT. KEEP THIS AND ALL OTHER DRUGS OUT OF THE REACH OF CHILDREN.

1. Starting now you must give up smoking completely. Gradually cutting down your tobacco consumption will not work.
2. Your physician has prescribed Nicorette as part of a program to help you stop smoking.
3. Whenever you feel that you want to smoke, put *one* piece of gum into your mouth.
4. When you chew the gum, nicotine is slowly released and is absorbed through the lining of your mouth.
5. Chew the gum *very slowly* until you taste it or feel a slight tingling in your mouth. (This is *usually* after about 15 chews—the number of chews is not the same for all people.) Because of its nicotine content, the gum does not taste like ordinary chewing gum.
6. As soon as you get the taste of the gum, stop chewing.
7. After the taste or tingling is almost gone (about one minute), chew *slowly* again until you taste the gum. Then stop chewing again.
8. The gum should be chewed slowly and intermittently for about 30 minutes to release most of the nicotine.
9. Most people find that 10 to 12 pieces per day of 2 mg Nicorette are enough to control their urge to smoke. Depending on your needs, you can adjust the rate of chewing and the time between pieces.
10. WARNING: If you chew the gum too fast, you may get effects like people get when they inhale a cigarette for the first time, or when they smoke too fast. These effects include light-headedness, nausea and vomiting, throat and mouth irritation, hiccups, and stomach upset. Most of these side effects are controlled by chewing more slowly. See instructions above. Some other effects sometimes seen—particularly during the first few days of using the gum —include mouth ulcers, jaw muscle ache, headaches, heart palpitations, and more than the usual amount of saliva in the mouth. In addition, the mechanical effects of gum chewing (any gum) include traumatic injury to oral mucosa or teeth, jaw ache and belching from swallowing air. These side effects may be minimized by proper chewing technique (see steps 5 through 8 above). *There are other side effects which have been infrequently reported with the use of Nicorette. Your physician can answer any questions you may have as to possible side effects. Report any disturbing symptoms to your doctor.*
11. *Not more than 30 pieces of 2 mg gum should be chewed in any one day.*
12. If you accidentally swallow a piece of gum, you should not experience adverse effects. If you do experience adverse effects, call your doctor. Overdosage could occur if many pieces are chewed simultaneously or in rapid succession. IN CASE OF ACCIDENTAL OVERDOSE OR IF A CHILD CHEWS OR SWALLOWS ONE OR MORE PIECES OF THE GUM, YOU SHOULD CONTACT YOUR PHYSICIAN OR LOCAL POISON CONTROL CENTER IMMEDIATELY.
13. As your urge to smoke fades, gradually reduce the number of pieces of gum you chew each day. This may be possible within two to three months. Unless your physician tells you otherwise, do not attempt to stop using the gum until your craving is satisfied with one or two pieces a day, but do not use the gum for more than 6 months.
14. Remember to carry the gum with you at all times in case you feel the sudden urge to smoke again. DO NOT FORGET THAT ONE CIGARETTE IS ENOUGH TO START YOU ON THE SMOKING HABIT AGAIN.

PLEASE NOTE: Nicorette is sugar-free and has been formulated to minimize stickiness. As with other gums, however, the degree to which Nicorette may stick to your dentures, dental caps or partial bridges may depend on the materials from which they are made and other factors. Should an excessive degree of stickiness to your dental work occur, there is the possibility that as with other gums, Nicorette may damage dental work, and you should discontinue its use and consult your physician or dentist.

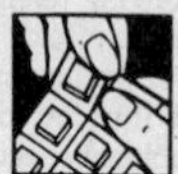

To remove the gum, tear off single unit

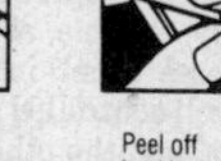

Peel off backing starting at corner with loose edge

Push gum through foil

Shown in Product Identification Section, page 412

NOVAHISTINE® COUGH & COLD FORMULA

[*nō″vă-his′tēn*]

(See PDR For Nonprescription Drugs)

NOVAHISTINE® DH Ⓒ

[*nō″vă-his′tēn*]

Antitussive-Decongestant-Antihistamine

DESCRIPTION

Each 5 ml teaspoonful contains Codeine Phosphate, 10 mg (Warning: may be habit forming), Pseudoephedrine Hydrochloride, 30 mg, Chlorpheniramine Maleate, 2 mg. Also contains: Alcohol, 5%, FD&C Blue No. 1, FD&C Red No. 40, Flavors, Glycerin, Hydrochloric Acid, Invert Sugar, Saccharin Sodium, Sodium Chloride, Sorbitol, and Water.

ACTIONS

Antitussive, decongestant and antihistaminic actions. Codeine, at the recommended dose, causes suppression of the cough reflex by a direct effect on the cough center in the medulla of the brain. Codeine has antitussive, mild analgesic and sedative effects.

Pseudoephedrine hydrochloride, an orally effective nasal decongestant, is a sympathomimetic amine with peripheral effects similar to epinephrine and central effects similar to, but less intense than, amphetamines. Therefore, it has the potential for excitatory side effects. Pseudoephedrine at the recommended oral dosage has little or no pressor effect in normotensive adults. Patients taking pseudoephedrine orally have not been reported to experience the rebound congestion sometimes experienced with frequent, repeated use of topical decongestants. Pseudoephedrine is not known to produce drowsiness.

Chlorpheniramine possesses antihistaminic, mild anticholinergic and sedative effects. It antagonizes many of the pharmacologic actions of histamine. It prevents released histamine from dilating capillaries and causing edema of the respiratory mucosa.

INDICATIONS

For the temporary relief of cough associated with minor throat and bronchial irritation or nasal congestion due to the common cold, sinusitis, and hay fever (allergic rhinitis).

A minimum dosage of codeine is provided for the symptomatic relief of nonproductive cough. Decongestants have been used to relieve eustachian salpingitis, aerotitis, otitis, and serous otitis media. Chlorpheniramine maleate provides temporary relief from runny nose, sneezing, itching of nose or throat, and itchy and watery eyes as may occur in hay fever (allergic rhinitis).

May be used as supportive therapy for acute otitis media and relief of mild otalgia.

May be given concomitantly, when indicated, with analgesics and antibiotics.

CONTRAINDICATIONS

Patients with severe hypertension, severe coronary artery disease, and in patients on MAO inhibitor therapy.

Nursing Mothers: Pseudoephedrine is contraindicated in nursing mothers because of the higher than usual risk for infants from sympathomimetic amines.

Hypersensitivity: This drug is contraindicated in patients with hypersensitivity or idiosyncrasy to its ingredients. Patient idiosyncrasy to adrenergic agents may be manifested by insomnia, dizziness, weakness, tremor or arrhythmias.

WARNINGS

Codeine should be prescribed and administered with the same degree of caution as all oral medications containing a narcotic analgesic. Codeine appears in the milk of nursing mothers.

If sympathomimetic amines are used in patients with hypertension, diabetes mellitus, ischemic heart disease, hyperthyroidism, increased intraocular pressure or prostatic hypertrophy, judicious caution should be exercised. See, however, Contraindications. Sympathomimetics may produce CNS stimulation with convulsions or cardiovascular collapse with accompanying hypotension. Do not exceed recommended dosage.

The elderly (60 years and older) are more likely to have adverse reactions to sympathomimetics. Safety for use during pregnancy has not been established.

Antihistamines may cause excitability, especially in children.

PRECAUTIONS

If cough persists for more than one week, tends to recur or is accompanied by fever, rash or headache, discontinue treatment. Other medications containing a narcotic analgesic, phenothiazines, tranquilizers, sedatives, hypnotics and other CNS depressants, including alcohol, may have an additive CNS depressant effect when used concomitantly. The dose should be reduced when such combined therapy is contemplated.

Caution should be exercised if used in patients with high blood pressure, heart disease, asthma, emphysema, diabetes, thyroid disease and hyperreactivity to ephedrine.

The antihistamine may cause drowsiness, and ambulatory patients who operate machinery or motor vehicles should be cautioned accordingly.

ADVERSE REACTIONS

Nausea, vomiting, constipation, dizziness, sedation, palpitations or pruritus may occur. More frequent or higher than recommended dosage may cause respiratory depression, especially in patients with respiratory disease associated with carbon dioxide retention.

Drugs containing sympathomimetic amines have been associated with certain untoward reactions including fear, anxiety, tenseness, restlessness, tremor, weakness, pallor, respiratory difficulty, dysuria, insomnia, hallucinations, convulsions, CNS depression, arrhythmias and cardiovascular collapse with hypotension.

Patients sensitive to antihistamine drugs may experience mild sedation. Other side effects from antihistamines may include dry mouth, dizziness, weakness, anorexia, nausea, vomiting, headache, nervousness, polyuria, heartburn, diplopia, dysuria, and very rarely, dermatitis.

DRUG INTERACTIONS

Codeine may potentiate the effects of other narcotics, general anesthetics, tranquilizers, sedatives and hypnotics, tricyclic antidepressants, MAO inhibitors, alcohol and other CNS depressants.

Beta adrenergic blockers and MAO inhibitors potentiate the sympathomimetic effects of pseudoephedrine. Sympathomimetics may reduce the antihypertensive effects of methyldopa, mecamylamine, reserpine and veratrum alkaloids.

Antihistamines have been shown to enhance one or more of the effects of alcohol, tricyclic antidepressants, barbiturates and other CNS depressants.

DOSAGE

Adults, 2 teaspoonfuls; children 50–90 lbs, ½ to 1 teaspoonful; 25–50 lbs, ¼ to ½ teaspoonful. Repeat every 4 to 6 hours. May be given to children under 2 at the discretion of the physician. *Do not exceed 4 doses in a 24-hour period.*

Product label dosage is as follows: Adults, 2 teaspoonfuls; children 6 to 12 years, 1 teaspoonful. May be given every 4 to 6 hours, *but do not exceed 4 doses in 24 hours.* For children under 6 years, consult a physician.

HOW SUPPLIED

In 4 fluid ounce bottles (NDC 0068-1027-04), and pints (NDC 0068-1027-16).

Product Information as of May, 1986

Shown in Product Identification Section, page 412

NOVAHISTINE® DMX

[*nō″vă-hĭs′tēn*]

Antitussive-Decongestant-Expectorant Liquid

(See PDR For Nonprescription Drugs)

NOVAHISTINE® ELIXIR

[*nō″vă-hĭs′tēn*]

Decongestant—Antihistaminic

(See PDR For Nonprescription Drugs)

NOVAHISTINE® EXPECTORANT Ⓒ

[*nō″vă-hĭs′tēn*]

Antitussive-Decongestant-Expectorant

DESCRIPTION

Each 5 ml teaspoonful contains Codeine Phosphate, 10 mg (Warning: may be habit forming), Pseudoephedrine Hydrochloride, 30 mg, Guaifenesin (glyceryl guaiacolate), 100 mg. Also contains: Alcohol, 7.5%, D&C Yellow No. 10, FD&C Blue No. 1, FD&C Red No. 40, Flavors, Glycerin, Hydrochloric Acid, Invert Sugar, Saccharin Sodium, Sodium Chloride, Sodium Gluconate, Sorbitol, and Water.

ACTIONS

Expectorant, antitussive and decongestant actions. Codeine, at the recommended dose, causes suppression of the cough reflex by a direct effect on the cough center in the medulla of the brain. Codeine has antitussive and mild analgesic and sedative effects.

Pseudoephedrine hydrochloride, an orally effective nasal decongestant, is a sympathomimetic amine with peripheral effects similar to epinephrine and central effects similar to, but less intense than, amphetamines. Therefore, it has the potential for excitatory side effects. Pseudoephedrine at the recommended oral dosage has little or no pressor effect in normotensive adults. Patients taking pseudoephedrine orally have not been reported to experience the rebound congestion sometimes experienced with frequent, repeated use of topical decongestants. Pseudoephedrine is not known to produce drowsiness.

Guaifenesin helps drainage of bronchial tubes by thinning the mucus, and facilitates expectoration by loosening phlegm and bronchial secretions.

INDICATIONS

For loosening tenacious pulmonary secretions associated with cough and respiratory congestion.

A minimum dosage of codeine phosphate is provided for the symptomatic relief of nonproductive cough. Decongestants have been used to relieve eustachian tube congestion associated with acute eustachian salpingitis, aerotitis, otitis and serous otitis media. Guaifenesin helps loosen phlegm (sputum) and bronchial secretions.

May be used as supportive therapy for acute otitis media and relief of mild otalgia.

May be given concomitantly, when indicated, with analgesics and antibiotics.

CONTRAINDICATIONS

Patients with severe hypertension, severe coronary artery disease, and in patients on MAO inhibitor therapy.

Nursing Mothers: Pseudoephedrine is contraindicated in nursing mothers because of the higher than usual risk for infants from sympathomimetic amines.

Hypersensitivity: This drug is contraindicated in patients with hypersensitivity or idiosyncrasy to its ingredients. Patient idiosyncrasy to adrenergic agents may be manifested by insomnia, dizziness, weakness, tremor or arrhythmias.

WARNINGS

Codeine should be prescribed and administered with the same degree of caution as all oral medications containing a narcotic analgesic. Codeine appears in the milk of nursing mothers.

If sympathomimetic amines are used in patients with hypertension, diabetes mellitus, ischemic heart disease, hyperthyroidism, increased intraocular pressure and prostatic hypertrophy, judicious caution should be exercised. See, however, Contraindications. Sympathomimetics may produce CNS stimulation with convulsions or cardiovascular collapse with accompanying hypotension. Do not exceed recommended dosage.

The elderly (60 years and older) are more likely to have adverse reactions to sympathomimetics. Safety for use during pregnancy has not been established.

PRECAUTIONS

If cough persists for more than one week, tends to recur or is accompanied by fever, rash or headache, discontinue treatment.

Other medications containing a narcotic analgesic, phenothiazines, tranquilizers, sedatives, hypnotics, and other CNS depressants, including alcohol, may have an additive CNS depressant effect when used concomitantly. The dose should be reduced when such combined therapy is contemplated.

Caution should be exercised if used in patients with high blood pressure, heart disease, asthma, emphysema, diabetes, thyroid disease and hyperreactivity to ephedrine.

ADVERSE REACTIONS

Nausea, vomiting, constipation, dizziness, sedation, palpitations, or pruritus may occur. More frequent or higher than recommended dosage may cause respiratory depression, especially in patients with respiratory disease associated with carbon dioxide retention.

Drugs containing sympathomimetic amines have been associated with certain untoward reactions including fear, anxiety, tenseness, restlessness, tremor, weakness, pallor, respiratory difficulty, dysuria, insomnia, hallucinations, convulsions, CNS depression, arrhythmias and cardiovascular collapse with hypotension.

Note: Guaifenesin interferes with the colorimetric determination of 5-hydroxyindoleacetic acid (5-HIAA) and vanillylmandelic acid (VMA).

DRUG INTERACTIONS

Codeine may potentiate the effects of other narcotics, general anesthetics, tranquilizers, sedatives and hypnotics, tricyclic antidepressants, MAO inhibitors, alcohol and other CNS depressants.

Beta adrenergic blockers and MAO inhibitors potentiate the sympathomimetic effects of pseudoephedrine. Sympathomimetics may reduce the antihypertensive effects of methyldopa, mecamylamine, reserpine and veratrum alkaloids.

DOSAGE

Adults, 2 teaspoonfuls; children 50–90 lbs, ½ to 1 teaspoonful; 25–50 lbs, ¼ to ½ teaspoonful. Repeat every 4 to 6 hours. May be given to children under 2 at the discretion of the physician. *Do not exceed 4 doses in a 24-hour period.*

Product label dosage is as follows: Adults, 2 teaspoonfuls; children 6 to 12 years, 1 teaspoonful; children 2 to 5 years, ½ teaspoonful. May be given every 4 to 6 hours but *do not exceed 4 doses in 24 hours.* For children under 2 years, consult a physician.

HOW SUPPLIED

As a liquid in 4 fluid ounce bottles (NDC 0068-1028-04) and pints (NDC 0068-1028-16).

Product Information as of May, 1986

Shown in Product Identification Section, page 412

SINGLET®

[*sĭn′glĕt*]

Long-Acting Tablets

Decongestant-Antihistamine-Analgesic

(See PDR For Nonprescription Drugs)

TENUATE® Ⓒ ℞

[*tĕn′ū-āt*]

(diethylpropion hydrochloride USP)

TENUATE DOSPAN®

(diethylpropion hydrochloride USP)

controlled-release tablets

CAUTION: Federal law prohibits dispensing without prescription.

DESCRIPTION

Tenuate is available for oral administration in immediate-release tablets containing 25 mg diethylpropion hydrochloride and in controlled-release tablets containing 75 mg diethylpropion hydrochloride. The inactive ingredients in each immediate-release tablet are: corn starch, lactose, magnesium stearate, pregelatinized corn starch, talc, and tartaric acid. The inactive ingredients in each controlled-release tablet are: carbomer 934P, mannitol, povidone, tartaric acid, zinc stearate.

Diethylpropion hydrochloride, a sympathomimetic agent, is 1-phenyl-2-diethylamino-1-propanone hydrochloride.

In Tenuate Dospan tablets, diethylpropion hydrochloride is dispersed in a hydrophilic matrix. On exposure to water the diethylpropion hydrochloride is released at a relatively uniform rate as a result of slow hydration of the matrix. The result is controlled-release of the anorexic agent.

ACTIONS

Tenuate is a sympathomimetic amine with some pharmacologic activity similar to that of the prototype drugs in this class used in obesity, the amphetamines. Actions include some central nervous system stimulation and elevation of blood pressure. Tolerance has been demonstrated with all drugs of this class in which these phenomena have been looked for.

Drugs of this class used in obesity are commonly known as "anorectics" or "anorexigenics." It has not been established, however, that the action of such drugs in treating obesity is primarily one of appetite suppression. Other central nervous system actions, or metabolic effects may be involved, for example.

Adult obese subjects instructed in dietary management and treated with "anorectic" drugs lose more weight on the average than those treated with placebo and diet, as determined in relatively short-term clinical trials.

The magnitude of increased weight loss of drug-treated patients over placebo-treated patients is some fraction of a pound a week. However, some patients lose more weight than this and some lose less. The rate of weight loss is greatest in the first weeks of therapy for both drug and placebo subjects and tends to decrease in succeeding weeks. The possible origins of the increased weight loss due to the various drug effects are not established. The amount of weight loss associated with the use of an "anorectic" drug varies from trial to trial, and the increased weight loss appears to be related in part to variables other than the drug prescribed, such as the physician/investigator relationship, the population treated, and the diet prescribed. Studies do not permit conclusions as to the relative importance of the drug and non-drug factors on weight loss.

The natural history of obesity is measured in years, whereas most studies cited are restricted to a few weeks duration; thus, the total impact of drug-induced weight loss over that of diet alone must be considered clinically limited.

The controlled-release characteristics of Tenuate Dospan have been demonstrated by studies in humans in which plasma levels of diethylpropion-related material were measured by phosphorescence analysis. Plasma levels obtained with the 75 mg Dospan formulation administered once daily indicated a more gradual release than the standard formulation. The formulation has not been shown superior in effectiveness to the same dosage of the standard, noncontrolled-release formulation.

INDICATION

Tenuate and Tenuate Dospan are indicated in the management of exogenous obesity as a short-term adjunct (a few weeks) in a regimen of weight reduction based on caloric restriction. The limited usefulness of agents of this class (see ACTIONS) should be measured against possible risk factors inherent in their use such as those described below.

CONTRAINDICATIONS

Advanced arteriosclerosis, hyperthyroidism, known hypersensitivity, or idiosyncrasy to the sympathomimetic amines, glaucoma.

Continued on next page

Information on Lakeside Pharmaceuticals products is based on labeling in effect in May, 1986.

Lakeside—Cont.

Agitated states.
Patients with a history of drug abuse.
During or within 14 days following the administration of monoamine oxidase inhibitors, (hypertensive crises may result).

WARNINGS

If tolerance develops, the recommended dose should not be exceeded in an attempt to increase the effect; rather, the drug should be discontinued. Tenuate may impair the ability of the patient to engage in potentially hazardous activities such as operating machinery or driving a motor vehicle; the patient should therefore be cautioned accordingly.
When central nervous system active agents are used, consideration must always be given to the possibility of adverse interactions with alcohol.

Drug Dependence
Tenuate has some chemical and pharmacologic similarities to the amphetamines and other related stimulant drugs that have been extensively abused. There have been reports of subjects becoming psychologically dependent on diethylpropion. The possibility of abuse should be kept in mind when evaluating the desirability of including a drug as part of a weight reduction program. Abuse of amphetamines and related drugs may be associated with varying degrees of psychologic dependence and social dysfunction which, in the case of certain drugs, may be severe. There are reports of patients who have increased the dosage to many times that recommended. Abrupt cessation following prolonged high dosage administration results in extreme fatigue and mental depression; changes are also noted on the sleep EEG. Manifestations of chronic intoxication with anorectic drugs include severe dermatoses, marked insomnia, irritability, hyperactivity, and personality changes. The most severe manifestation of chronic intoxication is psychosis, often clinically indistinguishable from schizophrenia.

Use in Pregnancy
Although rat and human reproductive studies have not indicated adverse effects, the use of Tenuate by women who are pregnant or may become pregnant requires that the potential benefits be weighed against the potential risks.

Use in Nursing Mothers
Since diethylpropion hydrochloride and/or its metabolites have been shown to be excreted in human milk, caution should be exercised when Tenuate or Tenuate Dospan is administered to a nursing woman.

Use in Children
Tenuate is not recommended for use in children under 12 years of age.

PRECAUTIONS

Caution is to be exercised in prescribing Tenuate for patients with hypertension or with symptomatic cardiovascular disease, including arrhythmias. Tenuate should not be administered to patients with severe hypertension.
Insulin requirements in diabetes mellitus may be altered in association with the use of Tenuate and the concomitant dietary regimen.
Tenuate may decrease the hypotensive effect of guanethidine.
The least amount feasible should be prescribed or dispensed at one time in order to minimize the possibility of overdosage.
Reports suggest that Tenuate may increase convulsions in some epileptics. Therefore, epileptics receiving Tenuate should be carefully monitored. Titration of dose or discontinuance of Tenuate may be necessary.

ADVERSE REACTIONS

Cardiovascular: Palpitation, tachycardia, elevation of blood pressure, precordial pain, arrhythmia. One published report described T-wave changes in the ECG of a healthy young male after ingestion of diethylpropion hydrochloride.
Central Nervous System: Overstimulation, nervousness, restlessness, dizziness, jitteriness, insomnia, anxiety, euphoria, depression, dysphoria, tremor, dyskinesia, mydriasis, drowsiness, malaise, headache; rarely psychotic episodes at recommended doses. In a few epileptics an increase in convulsive episodes has been reported.
Gastrointestinal: Dryness of the mouth, unpleasant taste, nausea, vomiting, abdominal discomfort, diarrhea, constipation, other gastrointestinal disturbances.
Allergic: Urticaria, rash, ecchymosis, erythema.
Endocrine: Impotence, changes in libido, gynecomastia, menstrual upset.
Hematopoietic System: Bone marrow depression, agranulocytosis, leukopenia.
Miscellaneous: A variety of miscellaneous adverse reactions has been reported by physicians. These include complaints such as dyspnea, hair loss, muscle pain, dysuria, increased sweating, and polyuria.

DOSAGE AND ADMINISTRATION

Tenuate (diethylpropion hydrochloride) immediate-release:
One 25 mg tablet three times daily, one hour before meals, and in midevening if desired to overcome night hunger.
Tenuate Dospan (diethylpropion hydrochloride) controlled-release:
One 75 mg tablet daily, swallowed whole, in midmorning.
Tenuate is not recommended for use in children under 12 years of age.

OVERDOSAGE

Manifestations of acute overdosage include restlessness, tremor, hyperreflexia, rapid respiration, confusion, assaultiveness, hallucinations, panic states.
Fatigue and depression usually follow the central stimulation.
Cardiovascular effects include arrhythmias, hypertension or hypotension and circulatory collapse. Gastrointestinal symptoms include nausea, vomiting, diarrhea, and abdominal cramps. Overdose of pharmacologically similar compounds has resulted in fatal poisoning, usually terminating in convulsions and coma.
Management of acute Tenuate intoxication is largely symptomatic and includes lavage and sedation with a barbiturate. Experience with hemodialysis or peritoneal dialysis is inadequate to permit recommendation in this regard. Intravenous phentolamine (Regitine®) has been suggested on pharmacologic grounds for possible acute, severe hypertension, if this complicates Tenuate overdosage.

HOW SUPPLIED

NDC 0068-0697-61
25 mg immediate-release tablets in bottles of 100
Each white, round, tablet is debossed TENUATE 25 or MERRELL 697
Keep tightly closed. Store at room temperature, preferably below 86°F.
Protect from excessive heat.
NDC 0068-0698-61
75 mg controlled-release tablets in bottles of 100
NDC 0068-0698-62
75 mg controlled-release tablets in bottles of 250
Each white, capsule-shaped, tablet is debossed TENUATE 75 or MERRELL 698
Keep tightly closed. Store at room temperature, below 86°F.

Product Information as of January, 1985
Shown in Product Identification Section, page 412

Information on Lakeside Pharmaceuticals products is based on labeling in effect in May, 1986.

The Lannett Company, Inc.
9000 STATE ROAD
PHILADELPHIA, PA 19136

ACNEDERM™ LOTION

(See PDR For Nonprescription Drugs)

CODALAN™ Ⓒ℞

COMPOSITION

Each tablet contains: Codeine Phosphate* 8 mg. in No. 1; 15 mg. in No. 2; 30 mg. in No. 3; Acetaminophen 150 mg., Salicylamide 230 mg.; and caffeine 30 mg.
*Warning: May be habit-forming.

ACTION AND USES

Analgesic, antitussive. Indicated for the relief of pain of all degrees of severity up to that which requires morphine.

ADMINISTRATION AND DOSAGE

One (No. 1, No. 2 or No. 3) as required to relieve pain.

HOW SUPPLIED

No. 1 orange color, No. 2 white color, No. 3 green color; all strengths in bottles of 100, 500 and 1000.

LITERATURE AVAILABLE

Complete Data Card.

DISONATE™ Capsules, Liquid and Syrup
(dioctyl sodium sulfosuccinate)

COMPOSITION

Docusate Sodium, U.S.P. (Dioctyl sodium sulfosuccinate), an effective stool-softener.

ACTION AND USES

Disonate keeps stools soft for easy passage. It is not a laxative and does not irritate the intestinal tract. Useful in treating constipation due to hard stools; in painful anorectal conditions, in cardiac and other patients who must avoid straining at stool.

DOSAGE

Adults and older children 60 to 240 mg. daily. Children 6 to 12 years of age 40 to 120 mg. daily. Higher doses are recommended for initial therapy and the effect on stools is usually apparent one to three days after the initial dose. Divided dosage may be used and dosage should be adjusted to individual response.

HOW SUPPLIED

Capsules of 100 mg., and 240 mg. Bottles of 100, 500 and 1000 capsules. Solution, 10 mg/cc Pint Bottle. Syrup, 20 mg/5 cc Pint and Gallon Bottle.

LITERATURE AVAILABLE

Yes.

LANIAZID SYRUP™ ℞
(Isoniazid Syrup, USP)

Each 5 mL (teaspoonful) contains:
Isoniazid, USP, 50 mg in a raspberry flavored Sorbitol Solution base.

HOW SUPPLIED

16 FL OZ bottles
LITERATURE AVAILABLE

MAGNATRIL™ SUSPENSION AND TABLETS

(See PDR For Nonprescription Drugs)

QUINALAN™
(Sustained release tablets of Quinidine Gluconate)

Each tablet contains:
324 mgs. of Quinidine Gluconate in a specifically designed base for sustained release of the drug in the gastrointestinal tract.

HOW SUPPLIED

In white to yellowish white convex tablets, each containing 324 mg. of Quinidine Gluconate, and with a single score on one side and the letter "Q" on the other.
In bottles of 100, 250, and 500 tablets.
LITERATURE AVAILABLE

LaSalle Laboratories, Inc.
Subsidiary of Mallard, Inc.
3021 WABASH AVENUE
DETROIT, MI 48216

FETRIN ℞
Hematinic with Vitamins B-12 & C

DESCRIPTION

Each sustained release capsule contains:
Ferrous Fumarate (equivalent to 66 mg. elemental Iron) .... 200 mg.
Ascorbic Acid .... 60 mg.
Cyanocobalamin .... 5 mcg.
With Intrinsic Factor

HOW SUPPLIED

Bottles of 100 capsules.

LITERATURE

Available on request.

PACAPS ℞

DESCRIPTION

Each capsule contains:
Butalbital .... 50 mg.
(May be habit forming)
Caffeine .... 40 mg.
Acetaminophen .... 325 mg.

HOW SUPPLIED

Available in bottles of 100 capsules.

LITERATURE

Available on request.

PROTID, Improved Formula ℞

DESCRIPTION

Each timed release tablet contains:
Acetaminophen .... 500 mg.
Chlorpheniramine Maleate .... 8 mg.
Phenylephrine HCl .... 40 mg.

HOW SUPPLIED
Bottles of 100 tablets.

LITERATURE
Available on request.

Laser, Inc.
2000 N. MAIN ST.
P.O. BOX 905
CROWN POINT, IN 46307

DALLERGY® SYRUP, TABLETS, CAPSULES ℞

Each 5 ml. of syrup contains: chlorpheniramine maleate 2 mg., phenylephrine hydrochloride 10 mg., methscopolamine nitrate 0.625 mg. Each tablet contains: chlorpheniramine maleate 4 mg., phenylephrine hydrochloride 10 mg., methscopolamine nitrate 1.25 mg. Each sustained-release capsule contains: chlorpheniramine maleate 8 mg., phenylephrine hydrochloride 20 mg., methscopolamine nitrate 2.5 mg.

DALLERGY® -JR. CAPSULES ℞

Each Sustained-Release Capsule contains: Brompheniramine Maleate, 6 mg., Pseudoephedrine Hydrochloride 60 mg.

DONATUSSIN DC SYRUP C-III ℞

Each 5 ml. contains: hydrocodone bitartrate 2.5 mg. (WARNING: May be habit forming), phenylephrine hydrochloride 7.5 mg., guaifenesin 50 mg. Red syrup.

DONATUSSIN DROPS ℞

Each ml. contains: chlorpheniramine maleate 1 mg., phenylephrine hydrochloride 2 mg., guaifenesin 20 mg.

LACTOCAL-F TABLETS ℞

Multivitamin, Multimineral supplement for pregnant or lactating women. Orange, film-coated tablet.

RESPAIRE®-SR CAPSULES 60 & 120 ℞

Each Sustained-Release RESPAIRE-60 SR Capsule contains pseudoephedrine hydrochloride 60 mg. and guaifenesin 200 mg. Each Sustained-Release RESPAIRE-120 SR Capsule contains pseudoephrine hydrochloride 120 mg. and guaifenesin 250 mg.

THEOSPAN® -SR CAPSULES ℞
(theophylline anhydrous, 130 mg. & 260 mg.)

Each sustained-release THEOSPAN-SR Capsule 130 mg. contains theophylline anhydrous 130 mg. Each sustained-release THEOSPAN-SR Capsule 260 mg. contains theophylline anhydrous 260 mg.

THEOSTAT® 80 SYRUP ℞
(theophylline anhydrous)

Each 15 ml. contains theophylline anhydrous 80 mg., alcohol 1%. Dye-free cherry-vanilla flavor.

TRIMSTAT® TABLETS C-III ℞
(phendimetrazine tartrate)

Each tan tablet contains: phendimetrazine tartrate 35 mg., embossed Laser, 35 .

Products are cross-indexed by generic and chemical names in the
YELLOW SECTION

Lederle Laboratories
A Division of American Cyanamid Co.
ONE CYANAMID PLAZA
WAYNE, NJ 07470

Lederle Parenterals, Inc.
CAROLINA, PUERTO RICO 00630

Lederle Piperacillin, Inc.
CAROLINA, PUERTO RICO 00630

LEDERMARK® Product Identification Code

To provide quick and positive identification of Lederle products, we have imprinted an alphanumeric code on the tablet and capsule products. In order that you may quickly identify a product by its code, following is an alphanumeric list of LEDERMARK codes with their corresponding product names.

A1	ARISTOCORT® Tabs., 1 mg.
A2	ARISTOCORT® Tabs., 2 mg.
A3	ACHROMYCIN® V Caps., 250 mg.
A4	ARISTOCORT® Tabs., 4 mg.
A4	ARISTO-PAK® Tabs., 4 mg.
A5	ACHROMYCIN® V Caps., 500 mg.
A8	ARISTOCORT® Tabs., 8 mg.
A9	ARTANE® SEQUELS®, 5 mg.
A10	AMICAR® Tabs., 500 mg.
A11	ARTANE® Tabs., 2 mg.
A12	ARTANE® Tabs., 5 mg.
A13	ASENDIN® Tabs., 25 mg.
A15	ASENDIN® Tabs., 50 mg.
A17	ASENDIN® Tabs., 100 mg.
A18	ASENDIN® Tabs., 150 mg.
A19	Acetaminophen Tabs., 500 mg.
A20	Acetaminophen Caps., 500 mg.
A21	Acetaminophen Tabs., USP, 325 mg.
A23	Acetaminophen w/Codeine Tabs., 30 mg.
A24	Amitriptyline HCl Tabs., USP, 10 mg.
A25	Amitriptyline HCl Tabs., USP, 25 mg.
A26	Amitriptyline HCl Tabs., USP, 50 mg.
A27	Amitriptyline HCl Tabs., USP, 75 mg.
A28	Amitriptyline HCl Tabs., USP, 100 mg.
A31	Ampicillin Trihydrate Caps., USP, 250 mg.
A32	Ampicillin Trihydrate Caps., USP, 500 mg.
A33	Amoxicillin Capsules, USP, 250 mg.
A34	Amoxicillin Capsules, USP, 500 mg.
A36	Ascorbic Acid Tabs., USP, 250 mg.
A37	Ascorbic Acid Tabs., USP, 500 mg.
A39	Acetaminophen w/Codeine Tablets, 60 mg.
A43	Allopurinol Tablets, 100 mg.
A44	Allopurinol Tablets, 300 mg.
B10	Benztropine Mesylate Tabs., USP, 1 mg.
B11	Benztropine Mesylate Tabs., USP, 2 mg.
C600	CALTRATE® 600 Tabs.
C40	CALTRATE® 600 + D Tabs.
C45	CALTRATE® 600 + Iron Tabs.
C1	CENTRUM® Tabs.
C2	CENTRUM, JR.® Tabs.
C39	CENTRUM, JR® Extra C Tabs.
C7	Chlorthalidone Tabs., USP, 25 mg.
C9	Chlordiazepoxide HCl Caps., USP, 5 mg.
C10	Chlordiazepoxide HCl Caps., USP, 10 mg.
C11	Chlordiazepoxide HCl Caps., USP, 25 mg.
C13	Chlorothiazide Tabs., USP, 250 mg.
C14	Chlorothiazide Tabs., USP, 500 mg.
C15	Chlorthalidone Tabs., USP, 50 mg.
C16	Chlorpheniramine Maleate Tabs., USP, 4 mg.
C17	Chlorpheniramine Maleate T.D. Caps., 8 mg.
C18	Chlorpheniramine Maleate T.D. Caps., 12 mg.
C19	Chlorzoxazone w/Acetaminophen Tabs., 250 mg/300 mg.
C22	Chlorpromazine HCl Tabs., USP, 25 mg.
C23	Chlorpromazine HCl Tabs., USP, 50 mg.
C24	Chlorpromazine HCl Tabs., USP, 100 mg.
C25	Chlorpromazine HCl Tabs., USP, 200 mg.
C30	Cloxacillin Sodium Caps., USP, 250 mg.
C31	Cloxacillin Sodium Caps., USP, 500 mg.
C33	Leucovorin Calcium Tabs., 5 mg.
C37	Chlorpropamide Tablets, USP, 100 mg.
C38	Chlorpropamide Tablets, USP, 250 mg.
C42	Clonidine HCL Tabs., USP, 0.1 mg.
C43	Clonidine HCL Tabs., USP, 0.2 mg.
C44	Clonidine HCL Tabs., USP, 0.3 mg.
D1	DIAMOX® Tabs., 125 mg.
D2	DIAMOX® Tabs., 250 mg.
D3	DIAMOX® SEQUELS® 500 mg.
D9	DECLOMYCIN® Caps., 150 mg.
D11	DECLOMYCIN® Tabs., 150 mg.
D12	DECLOMYCIN® Tabs., 300 mg.
D16	Dicloxacillin Sodium Capsules, USP, 250 mg.
D17	Dicloxacillin Sodium Capsules, USP, 500 mg.
D22	Doxycycline Hyclate Caps., USP, 50 mg.
D23	Dicyclomine HCl Caps, USP, 10 mg.
D24	Dicyclomine HCl Tabs., USP, 20 mg.
D25	Doxycycline Hyclate Caps., USP, 100 mg.
D27	Ergoloid Mesylates Sublingual Tabs., 0.5 mg.
D28	Ergoloid Mesylates Sublingual Tabs., 1.0 mg.
D31	Diphenoxylate HCl 2.5 mg. and Atropine Sulfate 0.025 mg. Tabs., USP
D32	Docusate Sodium (DSS), USP, Caps., 100 mg.
D33	Docusate Sodium (DSS), USP, Caps., 250 mg.
D34	Docusate Sodium (DSS), 100 mg., USP, w/Casanthranol 30 mg., Caps.
D35	DOLENE® AP-65 Tabs.
D36	DOLENE® Caps., USP, 65 mg.
D41	Doxycycline Hyclate Tabs., 100 mg.
D42	DOLENE COMPOUND-65 Caps.
D43	Disopyramide Phosphate Capsules, 150 mg.
D44	Dipyridamole Tabs., 25 mg.
D45	Dipyridamole Tabs., 50 mg.
D46	Dipyridamole Tabs., 75 mg.
D51	Diazepam Tabs., USP, 2 mg.
D52	Diazepam Tabs., USP, 5 mg.
D53	Diazepam Tabs., USP, 10 mg.
D62	Disopyramide Phosphate Capsules, USP, 100 mg.
E2	Erythromycin Stearate Tabs., USP, 250 mg.
E3	Ergoloid Mesylates Tabs., oral, 1 mg.
E5	Erythromycin Stearate Tabs., USP, 500 mg.
E10	Erythromycin Ethylsuccinate Tabs., 400 mg.
F1	FOLVITE® Tabs., 1 mg.
F2	FERRO-SEQUELS®
F4	FILIBON® Tabs.
F5	FILIBON® F.A. Tabs.
F6	FILIBON® FORTE Tabs.
F11	Furosemide Tabs., USP, 20 mg.
F12	Furosemide Tabs., USP, 40 mg.
F13	Furosemide Tablets, USP, 80 mg.
F15	Flurazepam Caps., USP, 15 mg.
F20	Ferrous Sulfate Tabs., USP, 300 mg.
F21	Ferrous Gluconate Tabs., USP, 300 mg.
F30	Flurazepam Caps., USP, 30 mg.
G1	GEVRAL® Tabs.
G2	GEVRAL® T Tabs.
H1	HYDROMOX® Tabs., 50 mg.
H2	HYDROMOX® R Tabs.
H11	Hydralazine HCl Tabs., USP, 25 mg.
H12	Hydralazine HCl Tabs., USP, 50 mg.
H14	Hydrochlorothiazide Tabs., USP, 25 mg.
H15	Hydrochlorothiazide Tabs., USP, 50 mg.
H17	Hydroxyzine HCl Tabs., 10 mg.
H18	Hydroxyzine HCl Tabs., 25 mg.
H22	Reserpine, Hydralazine HCl and Hydrochlorothiazide Tabs., USP
I11	Imipramine HCl Tabs., USP, 10 mg.
I12	Imipramine HCl Tabs., USP, 25 mg.
I13	Imipramine HCl Tabs., USP, 50 mg.
I15	Isosorbide Dinitrate Tabs., 5 mg.
I16	Isosorbide Dinitrate Tabs., 10 mg.
I17	Isosorbide Dinitrate Tab., USP, 2.5 mg. Sublingual
I18	Isosorbide Dinitrate Tabs., USP, 5 mg. Sublingual
I19	Indomethacin Capsules, USP, 25 mg.
I20	Indomethacin Capsules, USP, 50 mg.
I21	Isoxsuprine HCl Tabs., USP, 10 mg.
I22	Isoxsuprine HCl Tabs., USP, 20 mg.
I23	Isosorbide Dinitrate S.A. Tablets, 40 mg.
I24	Isosorbide Dinitrate Tabs., 20 mg.
I28	Ibuprofen Tabs., USP, 400 mg.
I29	Ibuprofen Tabs., USP, 600 mg.
L1	LOXITANE® Caps., 5 mg.
L2	LOXITANE® Caps., 10 mg.
L3	LOXITANE® Caps., 25 mg.
L4	LOXITANE® Caps., 50 mg.
L6	LEDERPLEX® Caps.
L9	LEDERCILLIN® VK Tabs., USP, 500 mg.
L10	LEDERCILLIN® VK Tabs., USP, 250 mg.
L11	Levothyroxine Sodium Tabs., USP, 0.1 mg.
L12	Levothyroxine Sodium Tabs., USP, 0.2 mg.
L13	Levothyroxine Sodium Tabs., USP, 0.3 mg.
L15	Brompheniramine maleate 12 mg., phenylephrine HCl 15 mg., and phenylpropanolamine HCl 15 mg. Sustained Release Tablets
L17	Levothyroxine Sodium Tabs., USP, 0.15 mg.
L30	Lorazepam Tabs., 0.5 mg.
L31	Lorazepam Tabs., 1 mg.

Continued on next page

The information on each product appearing here is based on labelling effective in August, 1986 and is either the entire official brochure or an accurate condensation therefrom. Information concerning all Lederle products may be obtained from the Professional Services Department, Lederle Laboratories, Pearl River, New York, 10965.

Lederle—Cont.

L32	Lorazepam Tabs., 2 mg.
M1	Methotrexate Tabs., 2.5 mg.
M2	MINOCIN® Caps, 50 mg.
M3	MINOCIN® Tabs., 50 mg.
M4	MINOCIN® Caps, 100 mg.
M5	MINOCIN® Tabs., 100 mg.
M6	MYAMBUTOL® Tabs., 100 mg.
M7	MYAMBUTOL® Tabs., 400 mg.
M8	MAXZIDE® Tabs., 75 mg./50 mg.
M10	MATERNA® 1.60 Tabs.
M12	Meclizine HCl Tabs., USP, 12.5 mg.
M13	Meclizine HCl Tabs., USP, 25 mg.
M19	Methocarbamol Tabs., USP, 500 mg.
M20	Methocarbamol Tabs., USP, 750 mg.
M21	Methyldopa Tablets, USP, 125 mg.
M22	Methyldopa Tablets, USP, 250 mg.
M23	Methyldopa Tablets, USP, 500 mg.
M25	Methyclothiazide Tabs., 5 mg.
M26	Metronidazole Tabs., 250 mg.
M27	Metronidazole Tabs., USP, 500 mg.
M28	Metoclopromide Tabs., 10 mg.
M35	Medroxyprogesterone Acetate Tabs., 10 mg.
N1	NEPTAZANE® Tabs., 50 mg.
N5	NILSTAT® Oral Tabs.
N6	NILSTAT® Vaginal Tabs.
N10	Neomycin Sulfate Tabs., USP, 500 mg.
N20	Nitroglycerin SR Caps., 2.5 mg.
N21	Nitroglycerin SR Caps., 6.5 mg.
N22	Nitroglycerin SR Caps., 9 mg.
N23	Nylidrin HCl Tabs., USP, 6 mg.
N24	Nylidrin HCl Tabs., USP, 12 mg.
P1	PATHIBAMATE® 200 Tabs.
P2	PATHIBAMATE® 400 Tabs.
P4	PATHILON® Tabs., 25 mg.
P7	PERIHEMIN® Caps.
P8	PERITINIC® Tabs.
P9	PRONEMIA® Caps.
P11	Papaverine HCl Time Release Caps., 150 mg.
P13	Papaverine HCl Tabs., USP, 100 mg.
P17	Penicillin G Potassium Tabs., USP, 400,000 Units
P21	Phenobarbital Tabs., USP, 30 mg.
P24	Prednisone Tabs., USP, 5 mg.
P25	Probenecid Tabs., USP, 500 mg.
P26	Probenecid with Colchicine Tabs., 500 mg/0.5 mg.
P29	Procainamide HCl Caps., USP, 250 mg.
P30	Procainamide HCl Caps., USP, 375 mg.
P31	Procainamide HCl Caps., USP, 500 mg.
P33	Propylthiouracil Tabs., USP, 50 mg.
P34	Pseudoephedrine HCl Tabs., USP, 60 mg.
P35	Pseudoephedrine HCl Tabs., USP, 30 mg.
P36	Pyrazinamide Tabs., 500 mg.
P37	Pyridoxine HCl (Vitamin B-6) Tabs., USP, 25 mg.
P38	Pyridoxine HCl (Vitamin B-6) Tabs., USP, 50 mg.
P39	Propoxyphene Napsylate w/Acetaminophen Tabs., 100 mg/650 mg.
P44	Propranolol HCl Tabs., USP, 10 mg.
P45	Propranolol HCl Tabs., USP, 20 mg.
P46	Propranolol HCl Tabs., USP, 40 mg.
P47	Propranolol HCl Tabs., USP, 80 mg.
P48	Procainamide S.R. Tabs., 250 mg.
P49	Procainamide S.R. Tabs., 500 mg.
P50	Procainamide S.R. Tabs., 750 mg.
Q11	Quinidine Sulfate Tabs., USP, 200 mg.
Q13	Quinidine Gluconate S.R.Tabs., 324 mg.
Q15	Quinine Sulfate Caps., USP, 325 mg.
S1	STRESSTABS® 600
S2	STRESSTABS® 600 w/Iron
S3	STRESSTABS® 600 w/Zinc
S5	STRESSCAPS®
S12	Spironolactone with Hydrochlorothiazide Tabs., 25 mg/25 mg.
S13	Spironolactone Tabs., USP, 25 mg.
S14	Sulfasalazine Tabs., 0.5 Gram
S22	SPARTUS® Tablets
S23	SPARTUS® +Iron Tablets
T1	TriHEMIC® 600 Tabs.
T10	Thioridazine HCl USP, 10 mg.
T11	Thiamine HCl (Vitamin B-1) Tabs., 50 mg.
T12	Thiamine HCl (Vitamin B-1) Tabs., 100 mg.
T13	Sulfamethoxazole & Trimethoprim Tablets, 400 mg/80 mg.
T14	Thyroid Tabs., USP, 60 mg.
T16	Sulfamethoxazole & Trimethoprim Tablets, 800 mg/160 mg.
T17	Tolbutamide Tabs., USP, 500 mg.
T19	Tolazamide Tabs., USP, 100 mg.
T20	Tolazamide Tabs., USP, 100 mg.
T22	Tolazamide Tabs., USP, 500 mg.
T23	Triprolidine HCl and Pseudoephedrine HCl Tabs., 2.5 mg/60 mg.
T25	Thioridazine HCl Tabs., USP, 25 mg.
T27	Thioridazine HCl Tabs., USP, 50 mg.
T28	Thioridazine HCl Tabs., USP, 100 mg.
V11	Vitamin A Caps., Natural USP, 25,000 I.U.
V14	Vitamin C Chewable Tabs., 250 mg.
V15	Vitamin C Chewable Tabs., 500 mg.
V19	Vitamin E Caps., Natural, USP, 400 I.U.
V21	Vitamin E Caps., USP., 200 I.U.
V22	Vitamin E Caps., USP., 400 I.U.
V23	Vitamin E Caps., USP, 600 I.U.
V24	Vitamin E Caps., USP, 1,000 I.U.

LEDERLE STANDARD PRODUCTS

PRODUCT IDENTITY CODE NO.	PRODUCT
—	Acetaminophen Liquid, USP, 160mg/5ml
A19	Acetaminophen Tablets, 500mg
A20	Acetaminophen Capsules, USP, 500mg
A21	Acetaminophen Tablets, USP, 325mg
A23	Acetaminophen w/Codeine Tablets, 30mg
A39	Acetaminophen w/Codeine Tablets, 60 mg
A43	Allopurinol Tablets, USP, 100 mg
A44	Allopurinol Tablets, USP, 300 mg
A24	Amitriptyline HCl Tablets, USP, 10mg
A25	Amitriptyline HCl Tablets, USP, 25mg
A26	Amitriptyline HCl Tablets, USP, 50mg
A27	Amitriptyline HCl Tablets, USP, 75mg
A28	Amitriptyline HCl Tablets, USP, 100mg
A31	Ampicillin Trihydrate Capsules, USP, 250mg
A32	Ampicillin Trihydrate Capsules, USP, 500mg
—	Ampicillin Trihydrate for Oral Suspension, USP, 125mg/5ml
—	Ampicillin Trihydrate for Oral Suspension, USP, 250mg/5ml
A33	Amoxicillin Capsules, USP, 250 mg
A34	Amoxicillin Capsules, USP, 500 mg
—	Amoxicillin Suspension 125 mg/5 ml
—	Amoxicillin Suspension 250 mg/5 ml
A36	Ascorbic Acid Tablets, USP, 250mg
A37	Ascorbic Acid Tablets, USP, 500mg
B10	Benztropine Mesylate Tablets, USP, 1 mg
B11	Benztropine Mesylate Tablets, USP, 2 mg
—	Brompheniramine Compound Elixir
L15	Brompheniramine Maleate, N.F., 12mg, Phenylephrine HCl 15mg, and Phenylpropanolamine HCl 15mg Sustained Release Tablets (Formerly LEDER-BP™ SEQUELS®)
—	Brompheniramine Maleate With Codeine, D.C., Cough Syrup
C 9	Chlordiazepoxide HCl Capsules, USP, 5mg
C10	Chlordiazepoxide HCl Capsules, USP, 10mg
C11	Chlordiazepoxide HCl Capsules, USP, 25mg
C13	Chlorothiazide Tablets, USP, 250mg
C14	Chlorothiazide Tablets, USP, 500mg
C16	Chlorpheniramine Maleate Tablets, USP, 4mg
C17	Chlorpheniramine Maleate T.D. Capsules, 8mg
C18	Chlorpheniramine Maleate T.D. Capsules, 12mg
C22	Chlorpromazine HCl Tablets, USP, 25mg
C23	Chlorpromazine HCl Tablets, USP, 50mg
C24	Chlorpromazine HCl Tablets, USP, 100mg
C25	Chlorpromazine HCl Tablets, USP, 200mg
—	Chlorpromazine HCl Liquid Concentrate 100mg/ml
C37	Chlorpropamide Tablets, USP, 100 mg
C38	Chlorpropamide Tablets, USP, 250 mg
C 7	Chlorthalidone Tablets, USP, 25mg
C15	Chlorthalidone Tablets, USP, 50mg
C19	Chlorzoxazone w/Acetaminophen Tablets 250mg/300mg
C42	Clonidine HCl Tablets, USP, 0.1 mg
C43	Clonidine HCl Tablets, USP, 0.2 mg
C44	Clonidine HCl Tablets, USP, 0.3 mg
C30	Cloxacillin Sodium Capsules, USP, 250mg
C31	Cloxacillin Sodium Capsules, USP, 500mg
D51	Diazepam Tablets, USP, 2 mg
D52	Diazepam Tablets, USP, 5 mg
D53	Diazepam Tablets, USP, 10 mg
D16	Dicloxacillin Sodium Capsules, USP, 250 mg
D17	Dicloxacillin Sodium Capsules, USP, 500 mg
D23	Dicyclomine HCl Capsules, USP, 10mg
D24	Dicyclomine HCl Tablets, USP, 20mg
—	Diphenhydramine HCl Elixir, USP, 12.5mg/5ml
—	Diphenhydramine HCl Cough Syrup, 12.5mg/5ml
D31	Diphenoxylate HCl 2.5mg + Atropine Sulfate 0.025mg Tablets, USP
D44	Dipyridamole Tablets, 25mg
D45	Dipyridamole Tablets, 50mg
D46	Dipyridamole Tablets, 75mg
D62	Disopyramide Phosphate Capsules, USP, 100 mg
D43	Disopyramide Phosphate Capsules, USP, 150 mg
D32	Docusate Sodium, (DSS) USP, Capsules, 100mg
D33	Docusate Sodium, (DSS) USP, Capsules, 250mg
D34	Docusate Sodium, (DSS) USP, 100mg, w/Casanthranol, 30mg, Capsules
—	Docusate Sodium (DSS) Syrup, USP, 20mg/5ml
—	Docusate Sodium (DSS) 60 mg/15 ml, w/Casanthranol, 30 mg/15 ml syrup
D36	DOLENE® Capsules, Propoxyphene HCl, Plain, 65mg
D35	DOLENE® AP-65 Tablets, Propoxyphene HCl, Acetaminophen
D42	DOLENE® Compound-65 Capsules, Propoxyphene HCl, Aspirin, and Caffeine
D22	Doxycycline Hyclate Capsules, USP, 50mg
D25	Doxycycline Hyclate Capsules, USP, 100mg
D41	Doxycycline Hyclate Tablets, USP, 100mg
E 3	Ergoloid Mesylates Tablets, Oral 1mg
D27	Ergoloid Mesylates Tablets, Sublingual, 0.5mg
D28	Ergoloid Mesylates Tablets, Sublingual, 1.0mg
—	Erythromycin Estolate Oral Suspension, 125mg/5ml
—	Erythromycin Estolate Oral Suspension, 250mg/5ml
E10	Erythromycin Ethylsuccinate Tablets, USP, 400mg
—	Erythromycin Ethylsuccinate Oral Suspension, 200mg/5ml
—	Erythromycin Ethylsuccinate Oral Suspension, 400mg/5ml
E 2	Erythromycin Stearate Tablets, USP, 250mg
E 5	Erythromycin Stearate Tablets, USP, 500mg
F21	Ferrous Gluconate Iron Supplement Tablets, USP, 300mg
—	Ferrous Sulfate Elixir, 220mg/5ml
F20	Ferrous Sulfate Tablets, USP, 300mg
F15	Flurazepam Capsules, USP, 15 mg
F30	Flurazepam Capsules, USP, 30 mg
F11	Furosemide Tablets, USP, 20mg
F12	Furosemide Tablets, USP, 40mg
F13	Furosemide Tablets, USP, 80mg
—	Guaifenesin Syrup, USP, 100mg/5ml
—	Guaifenesin, 100mg, w/D-Methorphan Hydrobromide Syrup, 15mg/5ml
H11	Hydralazine HCl Tablets, USP, 25mg
H12	Hydralazine HCl Tablets, USP, 50mg
H14	Hydrochlorothiazide Tablets, USP, 25mg
H15	Hydrochlorothiazide Tablets, USP, 50mg
H17	Hydroxyzine HCl Tablets, 10mg
H18	Hydroxyzine HCl Tablets, 25mg
I28	Ibuprofen Tablets, USP, 400 mg
I29	Ibuprofen Tablets, USP, 600 mg
I11	Imipramine HCl Tablets, USP, 10mg
I12	Imipramine HCl Tablets, USP, 25mg
I13	Imipramine HCl Tablets, USP, 50mg
I19	Indomethacin Capsules, USP, 25 mg
I20	Indomethacin Capsules, USP, 50 mg
I15	Isosorbide Dinitrate Tablets, oral, 5mg
I16	Isosorbide Dinitrate Tablets, oral, 10mg
I24	Isosorbide Tablets, 20 mg
I17	Isosorbide Dinitrate Tablets, Sublingual, 2.5mg
I18	Isosorbide Dinitrate Tablets, USP, Sublingual, 5.0mg
I23	Isosorbide Dinitrate S.A. Tablets, USP, 40 mg
I21	Isoxsuprine HCl Tablets, USP, 10mg
I22	Isoxsuprine HCl Tablets, USP, 20mg
—	LEDERCILLIN® VK, for Oral Solution, 125mg/5ml
—	LEDERCILLIN® VK, for Oral Solution, 250mg/5ml
L10	LEDERCILLIN® VK, USP, Tablets, 250mg
L 9	LEDERCILLIN® VK, USP, Tablets, 500mg
L11	Levothyroxine Sodium Tabs., USP, 0.1mg
L17	Levothyroxine Sodium Tabs., USP, 0.15 mg
L12	Levothyroxine Sodium Tabs., USP, 0.2mg
L13	Levothyroxine Sodium Tabs., USP, 0.3mg
L30	Lorazepam Tablets, 0.5 mg
L31	Lorazepam Tablets, 1.0 mg
L32	Lorazepam Tablets, 2.0 mg
M12	Meclizine HCl Tablets, USP, 12.5mg
M13	Meclizine HCl Tablets, USP, 25mg
M35	Medroxyprogesterone Acetate Tablets, 10 mg
—	Methenamine Mandelate Suspension, 500mg/5ml

M19	Methocarbamol Tablets, USP, 500mg
M20	Methocarbamol Tablets, USP, 750mg
M25	Methyclothiazide Tablets, 5mg
M21	Methyldopa Tablets, USP, 125 mg
M22	Methyldopa Tablets, USP, 250 mg
M23	Methyldopa Tablets, USP, 500 mg
M28	Metoclopramide Tablets, 10mg
M26	Metronidazole Tablets, USP, 250mg
M27	Metronidazole Tablets, USP, 500mg
N10	Neomycin Sulfate Tablets, USP, 500mg
N20	Nitroglycerin S.R. Capsules, 2.5mg
N21	Nitroglycerin S.R. Capsules, 6.5mg
N22	Nitroglycerin S.R. Capsules, 9 mg
N23	Nylidrin HCl Tablets, USP, 6mg
N24	Nylidrin HCl Tablets, USP, 12mg
P11	Papaverine HCl T.R. Capsules, 150mg
P13	Papaverine HCl Tablets, USP, 100mg
P17	Penicillin G Potassium Tablets, USP, 400,000 Units
P21	Phenobarbital Tablets, USP, 30mg (1/2 gr)
—	Potassium Chloride Liquid 10%
—	Potassium Chloride Liquid 20%
—	Potassium Gluconate Elixir, USP, 4.68gm/15ml
P24	Prednisone Tablets, USP, 5mg
P25	Probenecid Tablets, USP, 500mg
P26	Probenecid w/Colchicine Tablets, 500mg/0.5mg
P29	Procainamide HCl Capsules, USP, 250mg
P30	Procainamide HCl Capsules, USP, 375mg
P31	Procainamide HCl Capsules, USP, 500mg
P48	Procainamide HCl S.R. Tablets, 250 mg
P49	Procainamide HCl S.R. Tablets, 500 mg
P50	Procainamide HCl S.R. Tablets, 750 mg
—	Promethazine HCl Syrup, Plain, 6.25mg/5ml
—	Promethazine HCl Syrup w/Codeine, 10mg/5ml
—	Promethazine HCl Syrup VC w/Codeine, 10mg/5ml
—	Promethazine HCl Syrup VC, Plain
P39	Propoxyphene Napsylate with Acetaminophen Tablets, USP, 100mg/650mg
P44	Propranolol HCl Tablets, USP, 10 mg
P45	Propranolol HCl Tablets, USP, 20 mg
P46	Propranolol HCl Tablets, USP, 40 mg
P47	Propranolol HCl Tablets, USP, 80 mg
P33	Propylthiouracil Tablets, USP, 50mg
—	Pseudoephedrine HCl USP, Syrup, 30mg/5ml
P35	Pseudoephedrine HCl Tablets, USP, 30mg
P34	Pseudoephedrine HCl Tablets, USP, 60mg
P36	Pyrazinamide Tablets, 500mg
P37	Pyridoxine HCl (Vitamin B-6) Tablets, USP, 25mg
P38	Pyridoxine HCl (Vitamin B-6) Tablets, USP, 50mg
Q13	Quinidine Gluconate Sustained Release Tablets, 324mg
Q11	Quinidine Sulfate Tablets, USP, 200mg
Q15	Quinine Sulfate Capsules, USP, 325mg
H22	Reserpine 0.1mg, Hydrochlorothiazide 15mg and Hydralazine HCl 25mg Combination Tablets
S13	Spironolactone Tablets, USP, 25mg
S12	Spironolactone w/Hydrochlorothiazide Tablets, 25mg/25mg
	Sulfamethoxazole and Trimethoprim Pediatric Suspension, 200 mg/40 mg per 5 ml
T13	Sulfamethoxazole and Trimethoprim Tablets 400 mg/80 mg
T16	Sulfamethoxazole and Trimethoprim Tablets, 800 mg/160 mg
S14	Sulfasalazine Tablets, 0.5mg
T11	Thiamine HCl (Vitamin B-1) Tablets, 50mg
T12	Thiamine HCl (Vitamin B-1) Tablets, 100mg
T10	Thioridazine HCl Tablets, USP, 10mg
T25	Thioridazine HCl Tablets, USP, 25mg
T27	Thioridazine HCl Tablets, USP, 50mg
T28	Thioridazine HCl Tablets, USP, 100mg
T14	Thyroid Tablets, USP, 60mg
T19	Tolazamide Tablets, USP, 100 mg
T20	Tolazamide Tablets, USP, 250 mg
T22	Tolazamide Tablets, USP, 500 mg
T17	Tolbutamide Tablets, USP, 500mg
—	Triprolidine HCl with Pseudoephedrine HCl Syrup 1.25mg/30mg per 5ml
T23	Triprolidine HCl with Pseudoephedrine HCl Tablets 2.5mg/60mg
V11	Vitamin A Capsules, Natural, USP, 25,000 I.U.
V14	Vitamin C Chewable Tablets, 250mg
V15	Vitamin C Chewable Tablets, 500mg
V19	Vitamin E Capsules, Natural, USP, 400 I.U.
V21	Vitamin E Capsules, USP, 200 I.U.
V22	Vitamin E Capsules, USP, 400 I.U.
V23	Vitamin E Capsules, USP, 600 I.U.
V24	Vitamin E Capsules, USP, 1000 I.U.

ACHROMYCIN® ℞

[a-krō-mī-cin]

Sterile Tetracycline Hydrochloride
Intramuscular/Intravenous

ACHROMYCIN® *tetracycline hydrochloride* is an antibiotic isolated from *Streptomyces aureofaciens.* Chemically it is the hydrochloride of 4-dimethylamino-1,4,4a,5,5a,6,11,12a-octahydro-3, 6, 10, 12, 12a-pentahydroxy-6-methyl-1,11-dioxo-2-naphthacenecarboxamide.

ACTIONS

The tetracyclines are primarily bacteriostatic and are thought to exert their antimicrobial effect by the inhibition of protein synthesis. Tetracyclines are active against a wide range of Gram-negative and Gram-positive organisms. The drugs in the tetracycline class have closely similar antimicrobial spectra, and cross-resistance among them is common. Microorganisms may be considered susceptible if the MIC (minimum inhibitory concentration) is not more than 4.0 mcg/ml and intermediate if the MIC is 4.0 to 12.5 mcg/ml. Susceptibility plate testing: A tetracycline disc may be used to determine microbial susceptibility to drugs in the tetracycline class. If the Kirby-Bauer method of disc susceptibility testing is used, a 30 mcg tetracycline disc should give a zone of at least 19 mm, when tested against a tetracycline-susceptible bacterial strain.

Tetracyclines are readily absorbed and are bound to plasma proteins in varying degree. They are concentrated by the liver in the bile and excreted in the urine and feces at high concentrations and in a biologically active form.

INDICATIONS

ACHROMYCIN® *tetracycline HCl* is indicated for treatment of infections caused by the following microorganisms:

Rickettsiae: (Rocky Mountain spotted fever, typhus fever and the typhus group, Q fever, rickettsialpox and tick fevers).
Mycoplasma pneumoniae (PPLO, Eaton Agent)
Agents of psittacosis and ornithosis,
Agents of lymphogranuloma venereum and granuloma inguinale,
The spirochetal agent of relapsing fever (*Borrelia recurrentis*).
The following Gram-negative microorganisms:
Haemophilus ducreyi (chancroid),
Pasteurella pestis and *Pasteurella tularensis,*
Bartonella bacilliformis,
Bacteroides species,
Vibrio comma and Vibrio fetus,
Brucella species (in conjunction with streptomycin).

Because many strains of the following groups of microorganisms have been shown to be resistant to tetracyclines, culture and susceptibility testing are recommended.

Tetracycline is indicated for treatment of infections caused by the following Gram-negative microorganisms, when bacteriologic testing indicates appropriate susceptibility to the drug:

Escherichia coli,
Enterobacter aerogenes (formerly *Aerobacter aerogenes*),
Shigella species,
Mima species and *Herellea* species,
Haemophilus influenzae (respiratory infections),
Klebsiella species (respiratory and urinary infections).

Tetracycline is indicated for treatment of infections caused by the following Gram-positive microorganisms when bacteriologic testing indicates appropriate susceptibility to the drug:

Streptococcus species:
Up to 44% of strains of *Streptococcus pyogenes* and 74% of *Streptococcus faecalis* have been found to be resistant to tetracycline drugs. Therefore, tetracyclines should not be used for streptococcal disease unless the organism has been demonstrated to be sensitive.

For upper respiratory infections due to Group A beta-hemolytic streptococci, penicillin is the usual drug of choice, including prophylaxis of rheumatic fever.

Diplococcus pneumoniae,
Staphylococcus aureus, skin and soft tissue infections.

Tetracyclines are not the drug of choice in the treatment of any type of staphylococcal infection.

When penicillin is contraindicated, tetracyclines are alternative drugs in the treatment of infections due to:

Neisseria gonorrhoeae and (Neisseria meningitidis)
Treponema pallidum and *Treponema pertenue* (syphillis and yaws),
Listeria monocytogenes,
Clostridium species,
Bacillus anthracis,
Fusobacterium fusiforme (Vincent's infection),
Actinomyces species.

In acute intestinal amebiasis, the tetracyclines may be a useful adjunct to amebicides. ACHROMYCIN® *tetracycline HCl* is indicated in the treatment of trachoma, although the infectious agent is not always eliminated, as judged by immunofluorescence.

Inclusion conjunctivitis may be treated with oral tetracyclines or with a combination of oral and topical agents.

CONTRAINDICATIONS

This drug is contraindicated in persons who have shown hypersensitivity to any of the tetracyclines.

WARNINGS

THE USE OF DRUGS OF THE TETRACYCINE CLASS DURING TOOTH DEVELOPMENT (LAST HALF OF PREGNANCY, INFANCY AND CHILDHOOD TO THE AGE OF 8 YEARS) MAY CAUSE PERMANENT DISCOLORATION OF THE TEETH (YELLOW-GRAY-BROWN). This adverse reaction is more common during long-term use of the drugs but has been observed following repeated short-term courses. Enamel hypoplasia has also been reported. TETRACYCLINES, THEREFORE, SHOULD NOT BE USED IN THIS AGE GROUP UNLESS OTHER DRUGS ARE NOT LIKELY TO BE EFFECTIVE OR ARE CONTRA-INDICATED.

If renal impairment exists, even usual oral or parenteral doses may lead to excessive systemic accumulation of the drug and possible liver toxicity. Under such conditions, lower than usual total doses are indicated and, if therapy is prolonged, serum level determinations of the drug may be advisable. This hazard is of particular importance in the parenteral administration of tetracyclines to pregnant or postpartum patients with pyelonephritis. When used under these circumstances, the blood level should not exceed 15 micrograms/ml and liver function tests should be made at frequent intervals. Other potentially hepatotoxic drugs should not be prescribed concomitantly.

(In the presence of renal dysfunction, particularly in pregnancy, intravenous tetracycline therapy in daily doses exceeding 2 grams has been associated with deaths due to liver failure.)

Photosensitivity manifested by an exaggerated sunburn reaction has been observed in some individuals taking tetracyclines. Patients apt to be exposed to direct sunlight or ultraviolet light should be advised that this reaction can occur with tetracycline drugs, and treatment should be discontinued at the first evidence of skin erythema.

The antianabolic action of the tetracyclines may cause an increase in BUN. While this is not a problem in those with normal renal function, in patients with significantly impaired function, higher serum levels of tetracycline may lead to azotemia, hyperphosphatemia, and acidosis.

Usage In Pregnancy

(See above "Warnings" about use during tooth development). Results of animal studies indicate that tetracyclines cross the placenta, are found in fetal tissues and can have toxic effects on the developing fetus (often related to retardation of skeletal development). Evidence of embryotoxicity has also been noted in animals treated early in pregnancy.

Usage in newborns, infants, and children (See above "Warnings" about use during tooth development.)

All tetracyclines form a stable calcium complex in any bone-forming tissue. A decrease in the fibula growth rate has been observed in prematures given oral tetracycline in doses of 25 mg/kg every 6 hours. This reaction was shown to be reversible when the drug was discontinued.

Tetracyclines are present in the milk of lactating women who are taking a drug in this class.

PRECAUTIONS

As with other antibiotic preparations, use of this drug may result in overgrowth of nonsusceptible organisms, including fungi. If superinfection occurs, the antibiotic should be discontinued and appropriate therapy should be instituted.

In venereal diseases when coexistent syphilis is suspected, darkfield examination should be done before treatment is started and the blood serology repeated monthly for at least 4 months.

Because tetracyclines have shown to depress plasma prothrombin activity, patients who are on anticoagulant therapy may require downward adjustment of their anticoagulant dosage.

In long-term therapy, periodic laboratory evaluation of organ systems, including hematopoietic, renal and hepatic studies should be performed.

All infections due to Group A beta-hemolytic streptococci should be treated for at least ten days.

Since bacteriostatic drugs may interfere with the bactericidal action of penicillin, it is advisable to avoid giving tetracycline in conjunction with penicillin.

Continued on next page

The information on each product appearing here is based on labelling effective in August, 1986 and is either the entire official brochure or an accurate condensation therefrom. Information concerning all Lederle products may be obtained from the Professional Services Department, Lederle Laboratories, Pearl River, New York, 10965.

Lederle—Cont.

ADVERSE REACTIONS

Local irritation may be present after intramuscular injection. The injection should be deep, with care taken not to injure the sciatic nerve nor inject intravascularly.

Gastrointestinal: Anorexia, nausea, vomiting, diarrhea, glossitis, dysphagia, enterocolitis, and inflammatory lesions (with monilial overgrowth) in the anogenital region. Hepatic toxicity has been reported rarely. These reactions have been caused by both the oral and parenteral administration of tetracyclines.

Skin: Maculopapular and erythematous rashes. Exfoliative dermatitis has been reported but is uncommon. Photosensitivity is discussed above. (See "Warnings")

Renal toxicity: Rise in BUN has been reported and is apparently dose related. (See "Warnings")

Hypersensitivity reactions: Urticaria, angioneurotic edema, anaphylaxis, anaphylactoid purpura, pericarditis and exacerbation of systemic lupus erythematosus.

Bulging fontanels have been reported in young infants following full therapeutic dosage. This sign disappeared rapidly when the drug was discontinued.

Blood: Hemolytic anemia, thrombocytopenia, neutropenia, and eosinophilia have been reported.

When given over prolonged periods, tetracyclines have been reported to produced brown-black microscopic discoloration of thyroid glands. No abnormalities of thyroid function studies are known to occur.

PREPARATION OF SOLUTION

Intravenous

Vials of ACHROMYCIN® *sterile tetracycline hydrochloride,* intravenous should be initially reconstituted by adding 5 ml of Sterile Water for Injection to 250 mg vial and 10 ml of Sterile Water for Injection to the 500 mg vial, and then further diluted prior to administration to at least 100 ml (up to 1000 ml) with any of the following diluents:

Ringer's Injection, USP
Sodium Chloride Injection, USP
Dextrose Injection, USP
(5% Dextrose in Sterile Water for Injection, USP)
Dextrose and Sodium Chloride Injection, USP (5% in Sodium Chloride Injection, USP)
Lactated Ringer's Injection, USP
Protein Hydrolysate Injection, Low Sodium, USP 5%
5% with Dextrose 5%
5% with Invert Sugar 10%

The initial reconstituted solutions are stable at room temperature for 12 hours without significant loss of potency. The final dilution for administration should be administered immediately.

Note: The use of solutions containing calcium should be avoided as these tend to form precipitates (especially in neutral to alkaline solution) and, therefore, should not be used unless necessary. However, Ringer's Injection, USP and Lactated Ringer's Injection, USP can be used with caution since the calcium ion content in these diluents does not normally precipitate tetracycline in an acid media.

Intramuscular

Add 2 ml of Sterile Water for Injection USP (or Sodium Chloride Injection USP) to the 100 mg or 250 mg vial. The resulting solution may be stored at room temperature and should not be used after 24 hours.

DOSAGE AND ADMINISTRATION

Intravenous administration: **Note:** Rapid administration is to be avoided. Parenteral therapy is indicated only when oral therapy is not adequate or tolerated. Oral therapy should be instituted as soon as possible. If intravenous therapy is given over prolonged periods of time, thrombophlebitis may result.

Adults: The usual adult dose: 250 to 500 mg every 12 hours and should not exceed 500 mg every six hours. The drug may be dissolved and then diluted in 100–1,000 ml of Dextrose 5% in water, Isotonic Sodium Chloride Solution or Ringer's Solution, but not in other solutions containing calcium (a precipitate may form).

For children above 8 years of age: The usual dosage: 12mg/kg/day, divided into 2 doses, but from 10 to 20 mg/kg/day may be given, depending on the severity of the infection.

Gonorrhea patients sensitive to penicillin may be treated with tetracycline administered as an initial oral dose of 1.5 grams followed by 0.5 grams every six hours for four days, a total dosage of 9 grams. Intravenous therapy should be reserved for situations in which oral therapy is not feasible.

In patients with renal impairment: (See "Warnings").

Total dosage should be decreased by reduction of recommended individual doses and/or by extending time intervals between doses.

Intramuscular administration, Adults: The usual daily dose is 250 mg administered once every 24 hours or 300 mg given in divided doses at 8- to 12-hour intervals.

For children above 8 years of age: 15–25 mg/kg body weight up to a maximum of 250 mg per single daily injection. Dosage may be divided and given at 8- to 12-hour intervals.

Gonorrhea patients sensitive to penicillin may be treated with tetracycline administered as an initial oral dose of 1.5 grams followed by 0.5 grams every six hours for four days, a total dosage of 9 grams. Intramuscular therapy should be reserved for situations in which oral therapy is not feasible.

In patients with renal impairment: (See "Warnings").

Total dosage should be decreased by reduction of recommended individual doses and/or by extending time intervals between doses.

The intramuscular administration of ACHROMYCIN® *sterile tetracycline hydrochloride* produces lower blood levels than oral administration in the recommended dosages. Patients placed on intramuscular tetracyclines should be changed to the oral dosage form as soon as possible. If rapid, high blood levels are needed, ACHROMYCIN should be administered intravenously.

ACHROMYCIN intramuscular should be injected deeply into a large muscle mass such as the gluteal region. Inadvertent injection into the subcutaneous or fat layers may cause pain and induration, which can be relieved by applying an ice pack.

HOW SUPPLIED

Intramuscular:

Sterile Tetracycline Hydrochloride

100 mg/vial NDC 0005-4772-94	250 mg/vial NDC 0005-5357-95

Procaine HCl

40 mg/vial	40 mg/vial

Magnesium Chloride

46.84 mg/vial	46.84 mg/vial

Ascorbic Acid

250 mg/vial packages of 1 and 100 vials	275 mg/vial packages of 1 and 100 vials

Intravenous:

Sterile Tetracycline Hydrochloride 250 mg with 625 mg ascorbic acid/vial NDC 0005-5352-95

Sterile Tetracycline Hydrochloride 500 mg with 1250 mg ascorbic acid/vial NDC 0005-4771-96

Store at Controlled Room Temperature 15°-30°C (59°-86°F).

ACHROMYCIN® ℞

[*a-krō-mī-cin*]
tetracycline hydrochloride
Ophthalmic Suspension 1.0%
Sterile

DESCRIPTION

ACHROMYCIN® *tetracycline hydrochloride* Ophthalmic Suspension, Sterile contains 10 mg of tetracycline hydrochloride per ml with Plastibase 50W and Light Mineral Oil as inactive ingredients.

Chemically, ACHROMYCIN is: [4S-(4α,4aα,5aα,6β,12aα)]-4-(dimethylamino)-1,4,4a,5,5a,6,11,12a-octahydro-3,6, 10,12, 12a,pentahydroxy-6-methyl -1,11- dioxo-2-naphthacenecarboxamide monohydrochloride.

INDICATIONS

For the treatment of superficial ocular infections susceptible to ACHROMYCIN® *tetracycline hydrochloride.*

For prophylaxis of ophthalmia neonatorum due to *Neisseria gonorrhoeae* or *Chlamydia trachomatis.* The Centers for Disease Control (USPHS) and the Committee on Drugs, the Committee on Fetus and Newborn, and the Committee on Infectious Diseases of the American Academy of Pediatrics recommend 1% silver nitrate solution in single-dose ampoules or single-use tubes of an ophthalmic ointment containing 0.5% erythromycin or 1% tetracycline as "effective and acceptable regimens for prophylaxis of gonococcal ophthalmia neonatorum."[1] (For infants born to mothers with clinically apparent gonorrhea, intravenous or intramuscular injections of aqueous crystalline penicillin G should be given: a single dose of 50,000 units for term infants or 20,000 units for infants of low birth weight. Topical prophylaxis alone is inadequate for these infants.[1])

The following organisms have demonstrated susceptibility to ACHROMYCIN:

Staphylococcus aureus,
Streptococci including *Streptococcus pneumoniae,*
E. coli,
Neisseria species,
Chlamydia trachomatis.

When treating trachoma a concomitant oral tetracycline is helpful.

Other organisms, not known to cause superficial eye infections, but with demonstrated susceptibility to ACHROMYCIN, have been omitted from the above list.

ACHROMYCIN does not provide adequate coverage against:

Haemophilus influenzae
Klebsiella/Enterobacter species
Pseudomonas aeruginosa
Serratia marcescens.

CONTRAINDICATIONS

This product is contraindicated in persons who have shown hypersensitivity to any of the tetracyclines.

PRECAUTIONS

The use of antibiotics occasionally may result in overgrowth of nonsusceptible organisms. Constant observation of the patient is essential. If new infections appear during therapy, appropriate measures should be taken.

ADVERSE REACTIONS

Dermatitis and allied symptomatology have been reported. If adverse reaction or idiosyncrasy occurs, discontinue medication and institute appropriate therapy.

DOSAGE AND ADMINISTRATION

For most susceptible bacterial infections shake well, then gently squeeze the plastic dropper bottle to instill two drops in the affected eye, or, if necessary, in both eyes, two or four times daily, or more frequently, depending upon the severity of the infection. Very severe infections may require days of treatment, whereas other cases may be cured by instillation with much less frequency for 48 hours.

In acute and chronic trachoma instill two drops in each eye two to four times daily. This treatment should be continued for one to two months, except that certain individual or complicated cases may require a longer duration. A concomitant oral tetracycline is helpful.

For unit dose administration and convenience, the dispenser may be used. Immediately prior to use, simultaneously roll, invert, and squeeze dispenser between thumb and fingers. Repeat several times to mix contents well. Use aseptic technique to cut the tip of the dispenser, thereby maintaining sterility. Discard first two drops before instilling drops in eye(s). Instill two drops in eye(s), then discard dispenser.

HOW SUPPLIED

ACHROMYCIN® *tetracycline hydrochloride* Ophthalmic Suspension, 1.0% Sterile is supplied as follows:

NDC 0005-3505-12 - 50 × 0.5 ml Unit Dose Dispenser
NDC 0005-3505-18 - 4 ml plastic dropper-type bottle

Store at Controlled Room Temperature 15°-30° C (59°-86° F).

REFERENCE

1. American Academy of Pediatrics: Prophylaxis and treatment of neonatal gonococcal infections, Pediatr, 65:1047, 1980.

A.H.F.S. 52:04:04

Shown in Product Identification Section, page 412

ACHROMYCIN® V ℞

[*a-krō-mī-cin*]
tetracycline HCl
for ORAL USE

DESCRIPTION

ACHROMYCIN V *tetracycline HCl* is an antibiotic isolated from *Streptomyces aureofaciens.* Chemically it is the monohydrochloride of [4S-(4α,4aα,5aα,6β,12aα,)]-4-(Dimethylamino)-1, 4,4a,5,5a, 6,11,12a-octahydro-3,6,10,12,12a-pentahydroxy-6-methyl-1,11-dioxo-2-naphthacenecarboxamide.

ACHROMYCIN V oral dosage forms contain the following inactive ingredients:

Capsules: Blue 1, Gelatin, Lactose, Magnesium Stearate, Red 28, Titanium Dioxide, Yellow 6, Yellow 10 and other ingredients.

Oral Suspension: Blue 1, Citric Acid, Edetate Calcium Disodium, Flavoring, Magnesium Aluminum Silicate, Methylparaben, Polysorbate 80, Propylparaben, Red 40, Sodium Citrate, Sucrose.

ACTIONS

The tetracyclines are primarily bacteriostatic and are thought to exert their antimicrobial effect by the inhibition of protein synthesis. Tetracyclines are active against a wide range of Gram-negative and Gram-positive organisms.

The drugs in the tetracycline class have closely similar antimicrobial spectra, and cross-resistance among them is common. Microorganisms may be considered susceptible if the MIC (minimum inhibitory concentration) is not more than 4.0 mcg/ml and intermediate if the MIC is 4.0 to 12.5 mcg/ml.

Susceptibility plate testing: A tetracycline disc may be used to determine microbial susceptibility to drugs in the tetracycline class. If the Kirby-Bauer method of disc susceptibility testing is used, a 30 mcg tetracycline HCl disc should give a zone of at least 19 mm. when tested against a tetracycline-susceptible bacterial strain.

Tetracyclines are readily absorbed and are bound to plasma proteins in varying degree. They are concentrated by the liver in the bile and excreted in the urine and feces at high concentrations and in a biologically active form.

INDICATIONS

ACHROMYCIN V is indicated in infections caused by the following microorganisms.

Rickettsiae: (Rocky Mountain spotted fever, typhus fever, and the typhus group, Q fever, rickettsialpox, tick fevers).

Mycoplasma pneumoniae (PPLO, Eaton agent).

Agents of psittacosis and ornithosis.

Agents of lymphogranuloma venereum and granuloma inguinale.

The spirochetal agent of relapsing fever (*Borrelia recurrentis*).

The following Gram-negative microorganisms:
Haemophilus ducreyi (chancroid),
Pasteurella pestis and *Pasteurella tularensis*,
Bartonella bacilliformis,
Bacteroides species,
Vibrio comma and *Vibrio fetus*,
Brucella species (in conjunction with streptomycin).

Because many strains of the following groups of microorganisms have been shown to be resistant to tetracyclines, culture and susceptibility testing are recommended.

ACHROMYCIN is indicated for treatment of infections caused by the following Gram-negative microorganisms, when bacteriologic testing indicates appropriate susceptibility to the drug:
Escherichia coli,
Enterobacter aerogenes (formerly *Aerobacter aerogenes*),
Shigella species,
Mima species and *Herellea* species,
Haemophilus influenzae (respiratory infections),
Klebsiella species (respiratory and urinary infections).

ACHROMYCIN® *tetracycline HCl* is indicated for treatment of infections caused by the following Gram-positive microorganisms when bacteriologic testing indicates appropriate susceptibility to the drug:

Streptococcus species:
Up to 44% of strains of *Streptococcus pyogenes* and 74% of *Streptococcus faecalis* have been found to be resistant to tetracycline drugs. Therefore, tetracyclines should not be used for streptococcal disease unless the organism has been demonstrated to be sensitive.

For upper respiratory infections due to Group A beta-hemolytic streptococci, penicillin is the usual drug of choice, including prophylaxis of rheumatic fever.

Diplococcus pneumoniae,
Staphylococcus aureus, skin and soft tissue infections. Tetracyclines are not the drugs of choice in the treatment of any type of staphylococcal infection.

When penicillin is contraindicated, tetracyclines are alternative drugs in the treatment of infections due to:
Neisseria gonorrhoeae,
Treponema pallidum and *Treponema pertenue* (syphilis and yaws),
Listeria monocytogenes,
Clostridium species,
Bacillus anthracis,
Fusobacterium fusiforme (Vincent's infection)
Actinomyces species.

In acute intestinal amebiasis, the tetracyclines may be a useful adjunct to amebicides.

In severe acne, the tetracyclines may be useful adjunctive therapy.

ACHROMYCIN V is indicated in the treatment of trachoma, although the infectious agent is not always eliminated, as judged by immunofluorescence.

Inclusion conjunctivitis may be treated with oral tetracyclines or with a combination of oral and topical agents.

ACHROMYCIN is indicated for the treatment of uncomplicated urethral, endocervical or rectal infections in adults caused by *Chlamydia trachomatis*.[1]

CONTRAINDICATIONS

This drug is contraindicated in persons who have shown hypersensitivity to any of the tetracyclines.

WARNINGS

THE USE OF DRUGS OF THE TETRACYCLINE CLASS DURING TOOTH DEVELOPMENT (LAST HALF OF PREGNANCY, INFANCY AND CHILDHOOD TO THE AGE OF 8 YEARS) MAY CAUSE PERMANENT DISCOLORATION OF THE TEETH (YELLOW-GRAY-BROWN). This adverse reaction is more common during long-term use of the drugs but has been observed following repeated short-term courses. Enamel hypoplasia has also been reported. TETRACYCLINE DRUGS, THEREFORE, SHOULD NOT BE USED IN THIS AGE GROUP UNLESS OTHER DRUGS ARE NOT LIKELY TO BE EFFECTIVE OR ARE CONTRAINDICATED.

If renal impairment exists, even usual oral or parental doses may lead to excessive systemic accumulation of the drug and possible liver toxicity. Under such conditions, lower than usual total doses are indicated and, if therapy is prolonged, serum level determinations of the drug may be advisable.

Photosensitivity manifested by an exaggerated sunburn reaction has been observed in some individuals taking tetracyclines. Patients apt to be exposed to direct sunlight or ultraviolet light should be advised that this reaction can occur with tetracycline drugs, and treatment should be discontinued at the first evidence of skin erythema.

The anti-anabolic action of the tetracyclines may cause an increase in BUN. While this is not a problem in those with normal renal function, in patients with significantly impaired function, higher serum levels of tetracycline may lead to azotemia, hyperphosphatemia, and acidosis.

Usage in pregnancy (See above "Warnings" about use during tooth development). Results of animal studies indicate that tetracyclines cross the placenta, are found in fetal tissues and can have toxic effects on the developing fetus (often related to retardation of skeletal development). Evidence of embryotoxicity has also been noted in animals treated early in pregnancy.

Usage in newborns, infants, and children (See above "Warnings" about use during tooth development).

All tetracyclines form a stable calcium complex in any bone-forming tissue. A decrease in the fibula growth rate has been observed in prematures given oral tetracycline in doses of 25 mg/kg every six hours. This reaction was shown to be reversible when the drug was discontinued.

Tetracyclines are present in the milk of lactating women who are taking a drug in this class.

PRECAUTIONS

As with other antibiotic preparations, use of this drug may result in over-growth of nonsusceptible organisms, including fungi. If superinfection occurs, the antibiotic should be discontinued and appropriate therapy should be instituted.

In veneral diseases when coexistent syphilis is suspected, darkfield examination should be done before treatment is started and the blood serology repeated monthly for at least 4 months.

Because tetracyclines have been shown to depress plasma prothrombin activity, patients who are on anticoagulant therapy may require downward adjustment of their anticoagulant dosage.

In long-term therapy, periodic laboratory evaluation of organ systems, including hematopoietic, renal and hepatic studies should be performed.

All infections due to Group A beta-hemolytic streptococci should be treated for at least ten days.

Since bacteriostatic drugs may interfere with the bactericidal action of penicillin, it is advisable to avoid giving tetracycline in conjunction with penicillin.

ADVERSE REACTIONS

Gastrointestinal: Anorexia, nausea, vomiting, diarrhea, glossitis, dysphagia, enterocolitis, and inflammatory lesions (with monilial overgrowth) in the anogenital region. Hepatic toxicity has been reported rarely. These reactions have been caused by both the oral and parenteral administration of tetracyclines.

Skin: Maculopapular and erythematous rashes. Exfoliative dermatitis has been reported but is uncommon. Photosensitivity is discussed above. (See "Warnings").

Renal toxicity: Rise in BUN has been reported and is apparently dose related (See "Warnings").

Hypersensitivity reactions: Urticaria, angioneurotic edema, anaphylaxis, anaphylactoid purpura, pericarditis and exacerbation of systemic lupus erythematosus.

Bulging fontanels have been reported in young infants following full therapeutic dosage. This sign disappeared rapidly when the drug was discontinued.

Blood: Hemolytic anemia, thrombocytopenia, neutropenia and eosinophilia have been reported.

When given over prolonged periods, tetracyclines have been reported to produce brown-black microscopic discoloration of thyroid glands. No abnormalities of thyroid function studies are known to occur.

DOSAGE AND ADMINISTRATION

Therapy should be continued for at least 24–48 hours after symptoms and fever have subsided.

Concomitant therapy: Antacids containing aluminum, calcium, or magnesium impair absorption and should not be given to patients taking oral tetracycline.

Foods and some dairy products also interfere with absorption. Oral forms of tetracycline should be given one hour before or two hours after meals.

In patients with renal impairment: (See "Warnings"). Total dosage should be decreased by reduction of recommended individual doses and/or by extending time intervals between doses.

In the treatment of streptococcal infections, a therapeutic dose of tetracycline should be administered for at least ten days.

Adults: Usual daily dose, 1–2 grams divided in two or four equal doses, depending on the severity of the infection.

For children above eight years of age: usual daily dose, 10–20 mg (25–50 mg/kg) per pound of body weight divided in two or four equal doses.

For treatment of brucellosis, 500 mg tetracycline four times daily for three weeks should be accompanied by streptomycin, 1 gram intramuscularly twice daily the first week and once daily the second week.

For treatment of syphilis, a total of 30–40 grams in equally divided doses over a period of 10–15 days should be given. Close followup, including laboratory tests, is recommended.

Gonorrhea patients sensitive to pencillin may be treated with tetracycline, administered as an initial oral dose of 1.5 grams followed by 0.5 grams every six hours for four days to a total dosage of 9 grams.

Uncomplicated urethral, endocervical, or rectal infection in adults caused by *Chlamydia trachomatis:* 500 mg, by mouth, four times a day for at least seven days.[1]

HOW SUPPLIED

ACHROMYCIN® V *Tetracycline HCl* oral dosage forms are available as follows:

CAPSULES

500 mg - Two-piece, hard shell, elongated, opaque capsules with a blue cap and a yellow body, printed with Lederle over A5 on one half and Lederle over 500 mg on the other in gray ink, supplied as follows:
NDC 0005-4875-23—Bottles of 100
NDC 0005-4875-34—Bottles of 1,000
NDC 0005-4875-59—Unit of Issue 12 × 20's
NDC 0005-4875-60—Unit Dose 10 × 10's

250 mg - Two-piece, hard shell, opaque capsules with a blue cap and yellow body, printed with Lederle over A3 on one half and Lederle over 250 mg on the other in gray ink, are supplied as follows:
NDC 0005-4880-23—Bottles of 100
NDC 0005-4880-34—Bottles of 1,000
NDC 0005-4880-59—Unit of Issue 12 × 20's
NDC 0005-4880-60—Unit Dose 10 × 10's
NDC 0005-4880-61—Unit of Issue 12 × 40's
NDC 0005-4880-63—Unit of Issue 12 × 28's
NDC 0005-4880-65—Unit of Issue 12 × 100's

Store at Controlled Room Temperature 15°-30°C (59°-86°F)

ORAL SUSPENSION

Tetracycline equivalent to 125 mg Tetracycline HCl per teaspoonful (5 ml). Preserved with Methylparaben 0.12% and Propylparaben 0.03%, cherry-flavored, is supplied as follows:
NDC 0005-5410-56—Bottles of 2 Fl. Oz. (60 ml)
NDC 0005-5410-65—Bottles of 16 Fl. Oz. (473 ml)

Store at Controlled Room Temperature 15°-30°C (59°-86°F)

DO NOT FREEZE

Reference: 1. CDC Sexually Transmitted Diseases Treatment Guidelines 1982.

Military Depots:
NSN 6505-01-059-8997-250 mg.—40's
NSN 6505-00-655-8355-250 mg.—100's
NSN 6505-00-963-4924-250 mg.—1000's

Shown in Product Identification Section, page 412

ACHROMYCIN
tetracycline HCl
3% Ointment
(For topical use)—

½ oz. tube—NDC 0005-4796-56
1 oz. tube—NDC 0005-4796-55
℞ not required

AMICAR® ℞
[*ă-mĭ-car*]
Aminocaproic Acid
Intravenous, Syrup, and Tablets USP

DESCRIPTION

AMICAR® *aminocaproic acid* is 6-amino-hexanoic acid which acts as an effective inhibitor of fibrinolysis.

AMICAR Intravenous contains 250 mg/ml Aminocaproic Acid, Benzyl Alcohol, 0.9% and Water for Injection, qs 100%. Hydrochloric acid may be added during manufacture to adjust pH to approximately 6.8.

AMICAR Syrup, 25%, contains 250 mg/ml of Aminocaproic Acid and the following inactive ingredients: Citric Acid, Flavorings, Potassium Sorbate, Preservatives, Sodium Saccharin and Sorbitol.

Each AMICAR Tablet contains 500 mg of Aminocaproic Acid and the following inactive ingredients: Magnesium Stearate, Stearic Acid and Povidone.

ACTIONS

The beneficial fibrinolysis-inhibitory effects of AMICAR appear to be principally via inhibition of plasminogen activa-

Continued on next page

The information on each product appearing here is based on labelling effective in August, 1986 and is either the entire official brochure or an accurate condensation therefrom. Information concerning all Lederle products may be obtained from the Professional Services Department, Lederle Laboratories, Pearl River, New York, 10965.

Lederle—Cont.

tor substances and, to a lesser degree, through antiplasmin activity. The drug is absorbed rapidly following oral administration. Whether administered by the oral or intravenous route, a major portion of the compound is recovered unmetabolized in the urine. The renal clearance of AMICAR is high (about 75% of the creatinine clearance). Thus the drug is excreted rapidly. After prolonged administration, AMICAR distributes throughout both the extravascular and intravascular compartments of the body and readily penetrates human red blood and other tissue cells.

INDICATIONS

AMICAR is useful in enhancing hemostasis when fibrinolysis contributes to bleeding. In life-threatening situations, fresh whole blood transfusions, fibrinogen infusions, and other emergency measures may be required.

Fibrinolytic bleeding may frequently be associated with *surgical complications* following heart surgery (with or without cardiac bypass procedures) and portacaval shunt; *hematological disorders* such as aplastic anemia, *abruptio placentae, hepatic cirrhosis, neoplastic disease* such as carcinoma of the prostate, lung, stomach, and cervix.

Urinary fibrinolysis, usually a normal physiological phenomenon, may frequently be associated with life-threatening complications following severe trauma, anoxia and shock. Symptomatic of such complications is *surgical hematuria* (following prostatectomy and nephrectomy) or *nonsurgical hematuria* (accompanying polycystic or neoplastic diseases of the genitourinary system). (See WARNINGS)

CONTRAINDICATIONS

AMICAR should not be used when there is evidence of an active intravascular clotting process.

When there is uncertainty as to whether the cause of bleeding is primary fibrinolysis or disseminated intravascular coagulation (DIC), this distinction must be made before administering AMICAR. The following tests can be applied to differentiate the two conditions:

- Platelet count is usually decreased in DIC but normal in primary fibrinolysis.
- Protamine Paracoagulation test is positive in DIC; a precipitate forms when protamine sulphate is dropped into citrated plasma. The test is negative in the presence of primary fibrinolysis.
- The euglobulin clot lysis test is abnormal in primary fibrinolysis, but normal in DIC.

AMICAR must not be used in the presence of DIC without concomitant heparin.

WARNINGS

Safe use of AMICAR® *aminocaproic acid* has not been established with respect to adverse effects upon fetal development. Therefore, it should not be used in women of childbearing potential and particularly during early pregnancy, unless in the judgement of the physician the potential benefits outweigh the possible hazards. Antifertility effects, consistent with the drug's antifibrinolytic activity, have been suggested in some rodent studies.

In patients with upper urinary tract bleeding, AMICAR administration has been known to cause intrarenal obstruction in the form of glomerular capillary thrombosis, or clots in the renal pelvis and ureters. For this reason, AMICAR should not be used in hematuria of upper urinary tract origin, unless the possible benefits outweigh the risk.

PRECAUTIONS

AMICAR has a very specific action in that it inhibits both plasminogen activator substances and, to a lesser degree, plasmin activity. The drug should NOT be administered without a definite diagnosis, and/or laboratory findings indicative of hyperfibrinolysis (hyperplasminemia).*

*Stefanini, M. and Dameshek, W.: The Hemorrhagic Disorders, Ed. 2, New York, Grune and Stratton, pp. 510–514, 1962.

The use of AMICAR should be accompanied by tests designed to determine the amount of fibrinolysis present. There are presently available (a) general tests, such as those for the determination of the lysis of a clot of blood or plasma and (b) more specific tests for the study of various phases of fibrinolytic mechanisms. These latter tests include both semiquantitative and quantitative techniques for the determination of profibrinolysin, fibrinolysin, and antifibrinolysin.

Animal experiments indicate particular caution should be taken in administering AMICAR to patients with cardiac, hepatic or renal diseases.

Demonstrable animal pathology in some cases has shown endocardial hemorrhages and myocardial fat degeneration. Rarely, skeletal muscle weakness with necrosis of muscle fibers has been reported clinically. The possibility of cardiac muscle damage should be considered also when skeletal myopathy occurs. CPK levels should be monitored in patients on long-term therapy. AMICAR administration should be stopped if a rise in CPK is noted.

The use of this drug should thus be restricted to patients in whom the benefit expected would outweigh the potential hazard. Physicians are cautioned in the use of this product because of animal data showing rat teratogenicity and kidney concretions.

Rapid intravenous administration of the drug should be avoided since this may induce hypotension, bradycardia, and /or arrhythmia.

One case of *cardiac* and *hepatic lesions* observed in man has been reported. The patient received 2 grams of aminocaproic acid every six hours for a total dose of 26 grams. Death was due to continued cerebrovascular hemorrhage. Necrotic changes in the heart and liver were noted at autopsy.

Fibrinolysis is a normal process, presumably active at all times to ensure the fluidity of blood. Inhibition of fibrinolysis by aminocaproic acid *may* theoretically result in clotting or thrombosis. However, there is no definite evidence that administration of aminocaproic acid has been responsible for the few reported cases of *intravascular clotting* which followed this treatment. Rather, it appears that such intravascular clotting was most likely due to the patient's preexisting clinical condition, eg, the presence of DIC.

It has been postulated that *extravascular clots* formed *in vivo* may not undergo spontaneous lysis as do normal clots.

Reports have appeared in the literature of an increased incidence of certain neurological deficits, such as hydrocephalus, cerebral ischemia, or cerebral vasospasm, associated with the use of fibrinolytic agents in the treatment of subarachnoid hemorrhage. All of these events have also been described as part of the natural course of SAH, or as a consequence of diagnostic procedures such as angiography. Drug relatedness remains unclear.

ADVERSE REACTIONS

Occasionally nausea, cramps, diarrhea, hypotension, dizziness, tinnitus, malaise, conjunctival suffusion, nasal stuffiness, headache, myopathy, and skin rash have been reported as results of the administration of aminocaproic acid. The myopathy may be accompanied with general weakness, fatigue, and elevated serum enzymes. Rarely, rhabdomyolysis with myoglobinuria and renal failure may occur. Only rarely has it been necessary to discontinue or reduce medication because of one or more of these effects.

There have also been some reports of dry ejaculation during the period of AMICAR® *aminocaproic acid* treatment. These have been reported to date only in hemophilia patients who received the drug after undergoing dental surgical procedures. However, this symptom resolved in all patients within 24 to 48 hours of completion of therapy.

Two cases of convulsions occurring following intravenous administration of AMICAR have been reported. However, definite associations between the seizures and the drug have not been established.

Thrombophlebitis, a possibility with all intravenous therapy, should be guarded against by strict attention to the proper insertion of the needle and the fixing of its position.

DOSAGE AND ADMINISTRATION

Initial Therapy: An initial priming dose of 5 grams of AMICAR administered either orally or intravenously followed by 1.0 to 1.25 gram doses at hourly intervals thereafter should achieve and sustain plasma levels of 0.130 mg/ml of the drug. This is the concentration apparently necessary for the inhibition of fibrinolysis. Administration of more than 30 grams in any 24-hour period is not recommended.

Intravenous: AMICAR Intravenous is administered by infusion, utilizing the usual compatible intravenous vehicles (eg, Sterile Water for Injection, physiologic saline, 5% dextrose or Ringer's Solution). RAPID INJECTION OF AMICAR INTRAVENOUS UNDILUTED INTO A VEIN IS NOT RECOMMENDED.

For the treatment of *acute* bleeding syndromes due to elevated fibrinolytic activity, it is suggested that 16 to 20 ml (4.0 to 5.0 grams) of AMICAR® *aminocaproic acid* Intravenous in 250 ml of diluent be administered by infusion during the first hour of treatment, followed by a continuing infusion at the rate of 4 ml (1.0 gram) per hour in 50 ml of diluent. This method of treatment would ordinarily be continued for about eight hours or until the bleeding situation has been controlled.

Oral Therapy: If the patient is able to take medication by mouth, an identical dosage regimen may be followed by administering AMICAR Tablets or 25% Syrup as follows: For the treatment of *acute* bleeding syndromes due to elevated fibrinolytic activity, it is suggested that 10 tablets (5.0 grams) or 4 teaspoonfuls of syrup (5.0 grams) of AMICAR be administered during the first hour of treatment, followed by a continuing rate of 2 tablets (1.0 gram) or 1 teaspoonful of syrup (1.25 grams) per hour. This method of treatment would ordinarily be continued for about eight hours or until the bleeding situation has been controlled.

HOW SUPPLIED

*AMICAR *Intravenous:* Each 20 ml vial contains 5.0 grams of aminocaproic acid (250 mg per ml) as an aqueous solution, with 0.9% benzyl alcohol as a preservative. The pH is adjusted to approx. 6.8 with hydrochloric acid. 20 ml vials, Product No. NDC 0205-4668-37.

Each 96 ml vial contains 24 grams of aminocaproic acid (250 mg per ml) as an aqueous solution, with 0.9% benzyl alcohol as a preservative. The pH is adjusted to approx. 6.8 with hydrochloric acid. 96 ml vials, Product No. NDC 0205-4668-73.

Store at Controlled Room Temperature 15°–30°C (59°–86°F)

Lederle Parenterals, Inc.
Carolina, Puerto Rico 00630

AMICAR *Lederle 25% Syrup:* Each ml of raspberry flavored syrup contains 250 mg of aminocaproic acid. 16 fl oz bottles, Product No. NDC 0005-4667-65.

AMICAR *Lederle Tablets:* Each round, white tablet, engraved with LL on one side and scored on the other with A to the left of the score and 10 on the right, contains 500 mg of aminocaproic acid. Bottles of 100, Product No. NDC 0005-4665-23.

Store at Controlled Room Temperature 15°–30°C (59°–86°F).

* Manufactured for
LEDERLE LABORATORIES DIVISION
American Cyanamid Company
Pearl River, NY 10965

Shown in Product Identification Section, page 412

ARISTOCORT® ℞

[*a-ris-tō-cort*]
triamcinolone
TABLETS
ARISTOCORT®
triamcinolone diacetate
SYRUP

DESCRIPTION

ARISTOCORT® *triamcinolone* is a synthetic adrenocorticosteroid. The tablets contain triamcinolone, 9-Fluoro-11β,16α,17,21-tetrahydroxypregna-1,4-diene-3,20-dione.

Syrup contains triamcinolone diacetate which is 9-Fluoro-11β,16α,17,21-tetrahydroxypregna-1,4-diene-3,20-dione 16,21-diacetate. It is readily absorbed from the gastrointestinal tract.

INACTIVE INGREDIENTS

ARISTOCORT *triamcinolone* Tablets contain 1, 2, 4, or 8 mg triamcinolone and the following inactive ingredients: Cornstarch, Dibasic Calcium Phosphate, Docusate Sodium, Lactose, Magnesium Stearate, Microcrystalline Cellulose, Red 30, Sodium Benzoate, Sodium Starch Glycolate and Yellow 10.

INACTIVE INGREDIENTS

Syrup contains Flavorings, Kaolin, Magnesium Aluminum Silicate, Methylparaben, Monobasic Sodium Phosphate, Propylparaben, Red 33, Red 40, Sodium Phosphate, Sucrose.

ACTION

ARISTOCORT is primarily glucocorticoid in action and has potent anti-inflammatory, hormonal, and metabolic effects common to cortisone-like drugs. It is essentially devoid of mineralocorticoid activity when administered in therapeutic doses, causing little or no sodium retention, with potassium excretion minimal or absent. The body's immune responses to diverse stimuli are also modified by its action.

INDICATIONS

1. Endocrine Disorders:

Primary or secondary adrenocortical insufficiency (hydrocortisone or cortisone is the first choice; synthetic analogs may be used in conjunction with mineralocorticoids where applicable. In infancy mineralocorticoid supplementation is of particular importance).

Congenital adrenal hyperplasia.
Nonsuppurative thyroiditis.
Hypercalcemia associated with cancer.

2. Rheumatic Disorders:

As adjunctive therapy for short-term administration (to tide the patient over an acute episode or exacerbation) in:

Psoriatic arthritis.
Rheumatoid arthritis including juvenile rheumatoid arthritis (selected cases may require low-dose maintenance therapy).
Ankylosing spondylitis.
Acute and subacute bursitis.
Acute nonspecific tenosynovitis.
Acute gouty arthritis.
Posttraumatic osteoarthritis.
Synovitis of osteoarthritis.
Epicondylitis.

3. Collagen Diseases:

During an exacerbation or as maintenance therapy in selected cases of—

Systemic lupus erythematosus.
Acute rheumatic carditis.

4. Dermatologic Diseases:
Pemphigus.
Bullous dermatitis herpetiformis.
Severe erythema multiforme (Stevens-Johnson syndrome).
Exfoliative dermatitis.
Mycosis fungoides.
Severe psoriasis.
Severe seborrheic dermatitis.
5. Allergic States:
Control of severe or incapacitating allergic conditions intractable to adequate trials of conventional treatment:
Seasonal or perennial allergic rhinitis.
Bronchial asthma.
Contact dermatitis.
Atopic dermatitis.
Serum sickness.
Drug hypersensitivity reactions.
6. Ophthalmic Diseases:
Severe acute and chronic allergic and inflammatory processes involving the eye and its adnexa such as—
Allergic conjunctivitis.
Keratitis.
Allergic corneal marginal ulcers.
Herpes zoster ophthalmicus.
Iritis and iridocyclitis.
Chorioretinitis.
Anterior segment inflammation.
Diffuse posterior uveitis and choroiditis.
Optic neuritis.
Sympathetic ophthalmia.
7. Respiratory Diseases:
Symptomatic sarcoidosis.
Loeffler's syndrome not manageable by other means.
Berylliosis.
Fulminating or disseminated pulmonary tuberculosis when used concurrently with appropriate antituberculous chemotherapy.
Aspiration pneumonitis.
8. Hematologic Disorders:
Idiopathic thrombocytopenic purpura in adults.
Secondary thrombocytopenia in adults.
Acquired (autoimmune) hemolytic anemia.
Erythroblastopenia (RBC anemia).
Congenital (erythroid) hypoplastic anemia.
9. Neoplastic Diseases:
For palliative management of:
Leukemias and lymphomas in adults.
Acute leukemia of childhood.
10. Edematous States:
To induce a diuresis or remission of proteinuria in the nephrotic syndrome, without uremia, of the idiopathic type or that due to lupus erythematosus.
11. Gastrointestinal Diseases:
To tide the patient over a critical period of the disease in:
Ulcerative colitis.
Regional enteritis.
12. Nervous System:
Acute exacerbations of multiple sclerosis.
13. Miscellaneous:
Tuberculous meningitis with subarachnoid block or impending block when used concurrently with appropriate antituberculous chemotherapy.
Trichinosis with neurologic or myocardial involvement.

CONTRAINDICATIONS

Systemic fungal infections.
Sensitivity to the drug or any of its components.

WARNINGS

In patients on corticosteroid therapy subjected to unusual stress, increased dosage of rapidly acting corticosteroids before, during, and after the stressful situation is indicated.
Corticosteroids may mask some signs of infection, and new infections may appear during their use. There may be decreased resistance and inability to localize infection when corticosteroids are used.
Prolonged use of corticosteroids may produce posterior subcapsular cataracts, glaucoma with possible damage to the optic nerves, and may enhance the establishment of secondary ocular infections due to fungi or viruses.
Usage in pregnancy: Since adequate human reproduction studies have not been done with corticosteroids, the use of these drugs in pregnancy, nursing mothers or women of childbearing potential requires that the possible benefits of the drug be weighed against the potential hazards to the mother and embryo or fetus. Infants born of mothers who have received substantial doses of corticosteroids during pregnancy should be carefully observed for signs of hypoadrenalism.
Average and large doses of hydrocortisone or cortisone can cause elevation of blood pressure, salt and water retention, and increased excretion of potassium. These effects are less likely to occur with ARISTOCORT® *triamcinolone* except when used in large doses. Dietary salt restriction and potassium supplementation may be necessary. All corticosteroids increase calcium excretion.
While on Corticosteroid Therapy Patients Should Not Be Vaccinated Against Smallpox. Other Immunization Procedures Should Not Be Undertaken in Patients Who Are on Corticosteroids, Especially on High Doses, Because of Possible Hazards of Neurological Complications and a Lack of Antibody Response.
The use of triamcinolone in active tuberculosis should be restricted to those cases of fulminating or disseminated tuberculosis in which the corticosteroid is used for the management of the disease in conjunction with appropriate antituberculous regimen.
If corticosteroids are indicated in patients with latent tuberculosis or tuberculin reactivity, close observation is necessary as reactivation of the disease may occur. During prolonged corticosteroid therapy, these patients should receive chemoprophylaxis.

PRECAUTIONS

Drug-induced secondary adrenocortical insufficiency may be minimized by gradual reduction of dosage. This type of relative insufficiency may persist for months after discontinuation of therapy; therefore, in any situation of stress occurring during that period, hormone therapy should be reinstituted. Since mineralocorticoid secretion may be impaired, salt and/or a mineralocorticoid should be administered concurrently.
There is an enhanced effect of corticosteroids on patients with hypothyroidism and in those with cirrhosis.
Corticosteroids should be used cautiously in patients with ocular herpes simplex because of possible corneal perforation.
The lowest possible dose of corticosteroid should be used to control the condition under treatment, and when reduction in dosage is possible, the reduction should be gradual.
Psychic derangements may appear when corticosteroids are used, ranging from euphoria, insomnia, mood swings, personality changes, and severe depression to frank psychotic manifestations. Also, existing emotional instability or psychotic tendencies may be aggravated by corticosteroids.
Aspirin should be used cautiously in conjunction with corticosteroids in hypoprothrombinemia.
Steroids should be used with caution in nonspecific ulcerative colitis if there is a probability of impending perforation, abscess or other pyogenic infection, diverticulitis, fresh intestinal anastomoses, active or latent peptic ulcer, renal insufficiency, hypertension, osteoporosis, and myasthenia gravis.
Growth and development of infants and children on prolonged corticosteroid therapy should be carefully observed.
Although controlled clinical trials have shown corticosteroids to be effective in speeding the resolution of acute exacerbations of multiple sclerosis, they do not show that they affect the ultimate outcome or natural history of the disease. The studies do show that relatively high doses of corticosteroids are necessary to demonstrate a significant effect. (See DOSAGE AND ADMINISTRATION).
Since complications of treatment with glucocorticoid are dependent on the size of the dose and the duration of treatment, a risk/benefit decision must be made in each individual case as to dose and duration of treatment and as to whether daily or intermittent therapy should be used.

ADVERSE REACTIONS

Fluid and Electrolyte Disturbances.
Sodium retention.
Fluid retention.
Congestive heart failure in susceptible patients.
Potassium loss.
Hypokalemic alkalosis.
Hypertension.
Musculoskeletal.
Muscle weakness.
Steroid myopathy.
Loss of muscle mass.
Osteoporosis.
Vertebral compression fractures.
Aseptic necrosis of femoral and humeral heads.
Pathologic fracture of long bones.
Gastrointestinal.
Peptic ulcer with possible subsequent perforation and hemorrhage.
Pancreatitis.
Abdominal distention.
Ulcerative esophagitis.
Dermatologic.
Impaired wound healing.
Thin fragile skin.
Petechiae and ecchymoses.
Facial erythema.
Increased sweating.
May suppress reactions to skin tests.
Neurological.
Convulsions.
Increased intracranial pressure with papilledema (pseudotumor cerebri) usually after treatment.
Vertigo.
Headache.
Endocrine.
Menstrual irregularities.
Development of cushingoid state.
Suppression of growth in children.
Secondary adrenocortical and pituitary unresponsiveness, particularly in times of stress, as in trauma, surgery or illness.
Decreased carbohydrate tolerance.
Manifestations of latent diabetes mellitus.
Increased requirements for insulin or oral hypoglycemic agents in diabetics.
Ophthalmic.
Posterior subcapsular cataracts.
Increased intraocular pressure.
Glaucoma.
Exophthalmos.
Metabolic.
Negative nitrogen balance due to protein catabolism.
Hypersensitivity Reactions:
Anaphylactoid reactions have been reported, rarely, with products of this class.

DOSAGE AND ADMINISTRATION

General Principles:

1. The initial dosage of ARISTOCORT® *triamcinolone* may vary from 4 mg to 48 mg per day depending on the specific disease entity being treated. In situations of less severity lower doses will generally suffice while in selected patients higher initial doses may be required. The initial dosage should be maintained or adjusted until a satisfactory response is noted. If after a reasonable period of time there is a lack of satisfactory clinical response, the drug should be discontinued and the patient transferred to other appropriate therapy. *IT SHOULD BE EMPHASIZED THAT DOSAGE REQUIREMENTS ARE VARIABLE AND MUST BE INDIVIDUALIZED ON THE BASIS OF THE DISEASE UNDER TREATMENT AND THE RESPONSE OF THE PATIENT.* After a favorable response is noted, the proper maintenance dosage should be determined by decreasing the initial drug dosage in small increments at appropriate time intervals until the lowest dosage is reached which will maintain an adequate clinical response. It should be kept in mind that constant monitoring is needed in regard to drug dosage. Included in the situations which may make dosage adjustments necessary are changes in clinical status secondary to remissions or exacerbations in the disease process, the patient's individual drug responsiveness, and the effect of patient exposure to stressful situations not directly related to the disease entity under treatment; in this latter situation it may be necessary to increase the dosage of ARISTOCORT® *triamcinolone* for a period of time consistent with the patient's condition. If after long-term therapy the drug is to be stopped, it is recommended that it be withdrawn gradually rather than abruptly.

2. Dosage should be individualized according to the severity of the disease and the response of the patient. For infants and children, the recommended dosage should be governed by the same considerations rather than by strict adherence to the ratio indicated by age or body weight.

3. Hormone therapy is an adjunct to, and not a replacement for, conventional therapy.

4. The severity, prognosis and expected duration of the disease, and the reaction of the patient to medication are primary factors in determining dosage.

5. If a period of spontaneous remission occurs in a chronic condition, treatment should be discontinued.

6. Blood pressure, body weight, routine laboratory studies, including two-hour postprandial blood glucose and serum potassium, and a chest x-ray should be obtained at regular intervals during prolonged therapy. Upper GI x-rays are desirable in patients with known or suspected peptic ulcer disease.

7. Suppression of autogenous pituitary function, a common effect of exogenous corticosteroid administration, may be reduced, modified or minimized by revision of dose schedules. The time of maximum corticoid effect is from midnight to 8 am and minimal during the intervening hours. Use of a single daily dose at or about 8 am will be effective in most conditions, will lower corticoid overload and will cause the least interference with the diurnal system of endogenous secretion and hypothalamopituitary-adrenal function; alternate-day dosage in some conditions in certain severe disorders requiring long-term and/or high dose maintenance levels have proven both clinically effective and less likely to

Continued on next page

The information on each product appearing here is based on labelling effective in August, 1986 and is either the entire official brochure or an accurate condensation therefrom. Information concerning all Lederle products may be obtained from the Professional Services Department, Lederle Laboratories, Pearl River, New York, 10965.

Lederle—Cont.

produce adverse reactions. The maximum daily morning dose not associated with lasting adrenocorticoid suppression is 8 mg.

8. *Alternate-Day Therapy.* After the conventional dose has been established, some patients may be maintained on alternate-day therapy. It has been shown that the activity of the adrenal cortex varies throughout the day, being greatest from about midnight to 8 am. Exogenous corticoid suppresses this activity least when given at the time of maximum activity. A 48-hour interval appears to be necessary since shorter intervals are accompanied by adrenal suppression similar to that of conventional daily divided doses. Therefore, with the alternate-day dose plan, a total 48-hour requirement is given every other day at 8 am. As with other regimens, the minimum effective dose level should be sought.

9.* *Intermittent-Type Therapy.* An additional modification of corticosteroid usage has been recommended and used for treatment of disorders often requiring long-term administration of medium or high dose range. It is generally recommended that treatment be initiated with a single calculated dose of ARISTOCORT given once daily and continued daily until clinical response is adequate or appropriate. The time of maximum corticoid effect is from midnight to 8 am and minimal during the intervening hours. Therefore, dosage beginning at or after 8 am will offer good effect and lower corticoid overload. Thereafter, the patient is maintained on a calculated single daily dose given each morning for three to four consecutive days, followed by a "rest period" of three days, during which no corticosteroid is administered. This schedule is continued for as long as therapeutically indicated.

*For syrup only.

Specific Dosage Recommendations:

1. *Endocrine Disorders:* Wide variation in dosage requirements for the endocrine disorders such as *congenital adrenal hyperplasia, nonsuppurative thyroiditis,* and *hypercalcemia* associated with *cancer* precludes specific recommendation except for *adrenocortical insufficiency* where the dose is usually 4 mg to 12 mg daily in addition to mineralocorticoid therapy.

2. *Rheumatic Disorders: Rheumatoid arthritis; acute gouty arthritis; ankylosing spondylitis;* and *selected cases of psoriatic arthritis;* in *acute* and *subacute bursitis;* and in *acute nonspecific tenosynovitis.* The initial suppressive dose of ARISTOCORT in these conditions ranges from 8 mg to 16 mg per day, although the occasional patient may require higher doses. Patients may show an early or a delayed effect, characterized by a reduction in the inflammatory reaction and in joint swelling, together with alleviation of pain and stiffness, resulting in an increased range of motion of the affected joints or tissues. Maintenance doses are adjusted to keep symptoms at a level tolerable to the patient. Rapid reduction of the steroid or its abrupt discontinuance may result in recurrence or even exacerbation of signs and symptoms. Short-term administration is desirable as a rule. ARISTOCORT® *triamcinolone* is ordinarily administered as a single morning dose, daily or on alternate days, depending on the need of the patient. Occasional patients may secure more effective relief on divided daily doses, either two to four times daily.

3. *Collagen Diseases: Systemic Lupus Erythematosus.* The initial dose is usually 20 mg to 32 mg daily continued until the desired response is obtained, when reduced maintenance levels are sought. Patients with more severe symptoms may require higher initial doses, 48 mg or more daily, and higher maintenance doses. Although some patients with systemic lupus erythematosus appear to have spontaneous remissions or to tolerate the disorder in its milder forms for prolonged periods of time, adjustment of dosage scheduling to reduce adverse suppression of the pituitary-adrenal axis may be useful. Intermittent higher doses may be given daily for three or four successive days followed by a rest period of several days; this regimen being repeated each week.

Acute Rheumatic Carditis. In severely ill patients with carditis, pericardial effusion and/or congestive heart failure, corticosteroid therapy is effective in the control of the acute and severe inflammatory changes and may be lifesaving. Initial doses of ARISTOCORT may be from 20 mg to 60 mg daily, and clinical response is usually rapid and the drug can then be reduced. Maintenance therapy should be continued for at least 6 to 8 weeks and is seldom required beyond a period of 3 months. Corticosteroid therapy does not preclude conventional treatment, including antibiotics and salicylization.

4. *Dermatological Disorders: Pemphigus; bullous dermatitis herpetiformis, severe erythema multiforme* (Stevens-Johnson syndrome); *exfoliative dermatitis;* and *mycosis fungoides.* The initial dose is 8 mg to 16 mg daily. In these conditions, as well as in certain allergic dermatoses, *alternate-day* administration has been found effective and apparently less likely to produce adverse side effects.

Severe psoriasis: ARISTOCORT may produce reduction or remission of the disabling skin manifestations following initial doses of 8 mg to 16 mg daily. The period of maintenance is dependent on the clinical response. Corticosteroid reduction or discontinuation of therapy should be attempted with caution since relapse may occur and may appear in a more aggravated form, the so-called "rebound phenomenon."

5. *Allergic States:* ARISTOCORT® *triamcinolone* is administered in doses of 8 mg to 12 mg daily in acute seasonal or perennial *allergic rhinitis.* Intractable cases may require high initial and maintenance doses. In *bronchial asthma,* 8 mg to 16 mg daily are usually effective. The usual therapeutic measures for control of bronchial asthma should be carried out in addition to ARISTOCORT therapy. In both allergic rhinitis and bronchial asthma, therapy is directed at alleviation of acute distress and chronic long-term use of corticosteroids is neither desirable nor often essential. Some patients may be maintained on alternate-day therapy. In such conditions as *contact dermatitis* and *atopic dermatitis,* topical therapy may be supplemented with short courses of ARISTOCORT by mouth in doses of 8 mg to 16 mg daily. In severely ill patients with *serum sickness,* epinephrine may be the drug of choice for immediate therapy, often supplemented by antihistamines. ARISTOCORT is frequently useful as adjunctive treatment in such cases, with the dosage determined by the severity of the disorder, the speed with which therapeutic response is desired and the response of the patient to initial therapy.

6. *Ophthalmological Diseases: Allergic conjunctivitis; keratitis; allergic corneal marginal ulcers, iritis* and *iridocyclitis; chorioretinitis; anterior segment inflammation; diffuse posterior uveitis* and *choroiditis; optic neuritis* and *sympathetic ophthalmia.* Initial doses range from 12 mg to 40 mg daily depending on the severity of the condition, the nature and degree of involvement of ocular structure, but response is usually rapid and therapy of short-term duration.

7. *Respiratory Diseases: Symptomatic sarcoidosis; Loeffler's Syndrome; berylliosis;* and in certain cases of *fulminating* or *disseminated pulmonary tuberculosis* when concurrently accompanied by appropriate antituberculous chemotherapy. Initial doses are usually in the range of 16 mg to 48 mg daily.

8. *Hematologic Disorders: Idiopathic* and *secondary thrombocytopenia in adults, acquired (autoimmune) hemolytic anemia; erythroblastopenia (RBC anemia); congenital (erythroid) hypoplastic anemia.* ARISTOCORT is used to produce a remission of symptoms and may, in some instances, produce an apparent regression of abnormal cellular blood elements to normal states, temporary or permanent. The recommended dose varies between 16 mg and 60 mg daily, with reduction after adequate clinical response.

9. *Neoplastic Diseases: Acute leukemia in childhood.* The usual dose of ARISTOCORT is 1 mg per kilogram of body weight daily, although as much as 2 mg per kilogram may be necessary. Initial response is usually seen within 6 to 21 days and therapy continued from 4 to 6 weeks.

Acute leukemia and *lymphoma in adults.* The usual dose of ARISTOCORT® *triamcinolone* is 16 mg to 40 mg daily, although it may be necessary to give as much as 100 mg daily in leukemia. ARISTOCORT therapy in these neoplasias is only palliative and not curative. Other therapeutic and supportive measures must be used when appropriate.

10. *Edematous States: Nephrotic syndrome:* ARISTOCORT may be used to induce a diuresis or remission of proteinuria in the *nephrotic syndrome,* without uremia, of the idiopathic type or that due to *lupus erythematosus.* The average dose is 16 mg to 20 mg (up to 48 mg) daily until diuresis occurs. The diuresis may be massive and usually occurs by the 14th day, but occasionally may be delayed. After diuresis begins it is advisable to continue treatment until maximal or complete chemical and clinical remission occurs, at which time the dosage should be reduced gradually and then discontinued. In less severe cases maintenance dosages of as little as 4 mg daily may be adequate. Alternatively and when maintenance therapy may be prolonged, ARISTOCORT may be administered on alternate-day dose schedules.

11. *Miscellaneous: Tuberculous meningitis:* ARISTOCORT may be useful when accompanied by appropriate antituberculous therapy when there is subarachnoid block or impending block. The average dosage is 32 mg to 48 mg daily in either single or divided doses.

[See table below].

	Anti-inflammatory Relative Potency		Frequently Used Tablet Strength (mg)		Tablet × Potency Equivalent Value
Hydrocortisone	1	×	20	=	20
Prednisolone	4	×	5	=	20
ARISTOCORT® *triamcinolone*	5	×	4	=	20
Dexamethasone	25	×	0.75	=	18.75

HOW SUPPLIED

1 mg Tablets—oblong, flat, scored, yellow; Engraved LL A1 Bottles of 50 NDC 0005-4409-18.

2 mg Tablets—oblong, flat, scored, pink; Engraved LL A2 Bottles of 100 NDC 0005-4405-23.

4 mg Tablets—oblong, flat, scored, white; Engraved LL A4 Bottles of 30 NDC 0005-4406-13; Bottles of 100 NDC-0005-4406-23; ARISTO-PAK® 16s Engraved LL 4 (for 6 days' therapy) NDC 0005-4406-07.

8 mg Tablets—oblong, flat, scored, yellow; Engraved LL A8 Bottles of 50 NDC 005-4444-18.

Syrup 2 mg/5 ml triamcinolone diacetate; cherry flavored; Bottles of 4 fl oz NDC 0005-4421-58.

Store at Controlled Room Temperature 15°-30°C (59°-86°F).

A.H.F.S. 68:04

Tablets, and ARISTO-PAK 4 mg Shown in Product Identification Section, page 412

ARISTOCORT® ℞

[*a-ris-tō-cort*]

triamcinolone acetonide

Topical Products

[See table above].

ARISTOCORT® Triamcinolone Acetonide TOPICAL PRODUCTS

	Cream 0.025%	Cream 0.1%	Cream 0.5%	Ointment 0.1%	Ointment 0.5%
Each gram contains Triamcinolone Acetonide	0.25 mg.	1 mg.	5 mg.	1 mg.	5 mg.
Preservatives:					
Sorbic Acid	0.1%	0.1%	0.1%		
Potassium Sorbate	0.1%	0.1%	0.1%		
Inactive Ingredients:	In a water base: Mono and Diglycerides, Squalane NF, Polysorbate 80 Cetyl Esters Wax, Polysorbate 60, Stearyl Alcohol, Tenox II, and Sorbitol Solution, USP			White Petrolatum	
Dosage and Administration	Apply to the affected areas as a thin film three to four times daily. The cream should be rubbed in gently and thoroughly until it disappears. Occlusive dressings may be used for the management of psoriasis or recalcitrant conditions. If an infection develops, the use of occlusive dressings should be discontinued and appropriate antimicrobial therapy instituted.			Apply to the affected areas three to four times daily.	

The topical corticosteroids constitute a class of primarily synthetic steroids used as antiinflammatory and anti-pruritic agents.

CLINICAL PHARMACOLOGY

Topical corticosteroids share anti-inflammatory, antipruritic, and vasoconstrictive actions.

The mechanism of anti-inflammatory activity of the topical corticosteroids is unclear. Various laboratory methods, including vasoconstrictor assays, are used to compare and predict potencies and/or clinical efficacies of the topical corticosteroids. There is some evidence to suggest that a recognizable correlation exists between vasoconstrictor potency and therapeutic efficacy in man.

PHARMACOKINETICS

The extent of percutaneous absorption of topical corticosteroids is determined by many factors including the vehicle, the integrity of the epidermal barrier, and the use of occlusive dressings.

Topical corticosteroids can be absorbed from normal intact skin. Inflammation and/or other disease processes in the skin increase percutaneous absorption. Occlusive dressings substantially increase the percutaneous absorption of topical corticosteroids. Thus, occlusive dressings may be a valuable therapeutic adjunct for treatment of resistant dermatoses. (See **DOSAGE AND ADMINISTRATION**). Once absorbed through the skin, topical corticosteroids are handled through pharmacokinetic pathways similar to systemically administered corticosteroids. Corticosteroids are bound to plasma proteins in varying degrees. Corticosteroids are metabolized primarily in the liver and are then excreted by the kidneys. Some of the topical corticosteroids and their metabolites are also excreted into the bile.

INDICATIONS AND USAGE

Topical corticosteroids are indicated for the relief of the inflammatory and pruritic manifestations of corticosteroid-responsive dermatoses.

CONTRAINDICATIONS

Topical corticosteroids are contraindicated in those patients with a history of hypersensitivity to any of the components of the preparation.

PRECAUTIONS

General

Systemic absorption of topical corticosteroids has produced reversible hypothalamic-pituitary-adrenal (HPA) axis suppression, manifestations of Cushing's syndrome, hyperglycemia, and glucosuria in some patients.

Conditions which augment systemic absorption include the application of the more potent steroids, use over large surface areas, prolonged use, and the addition of occlusive dressings.

Therefore, patients receiving a large dose of a potent topical steroid applied to a large surface area or under an occlusive dressing should be evaluated periodically for evidence of HPA axis suppression by using the urinary free cortisol and ACTH stimulation tests. If HPA axis suppression is noted, an attempt should be made to withdraw the drug, to reduce the frequency of application, or to substitute a less potent steroid.

Recovery of HPA axis function is generally prompt and complete upon discontinuation of the drug. Infrequently, signs and symptoms of steroid withdrawal may occur, requiring supplemental systemic corticosteroids.

Children may absorb proportionally larger amounts of topical corticosteroids and thus be more susceptible to systemic toxicity. (See **PRECAUTIONS-Pediatric Use**).

If irritation develops, topical corticosteroids should be discontinued and appropriate therapy instituted.

In the presence of dermatological infections, the use of an appropriate antifungal or antibacterial agent should be instituted. If a favorable response does not occur promptly, the corticosteroid should be discontinued until the infection has been adequately controlled.

Information for the Patient

Patients using topical corticosteroids should receive the following information and instructions:

1. This medication is to be used as directed by the physician. It is for external use only. Avoid contact with the eyes.
2. Patients should be advised not to use this medication for any disorder other than for which it was prescribed.
3. The treated skin area should not be bandaged or otherwise covered or wrapped as to be occlusive unless directed by the physician.
4. Patients should report any signs of local adverse reactions especially under occlusive dressing.
5. Parents of pediatric patients should be advised not to use tight-fitting diapers or plastic pants on a child being treated in the diaper area, since these garments may constitute occlusive dressings.

Laboratory Tests

The following tests may be helpful in evaluating the HPA axis suppression:

Urinary free cortisol test
ACTH stimulation test

Carcinogenesis, Mutagenesis, and Impairment of Fertility

Long-term animal studies have not been performed to evaluate the carcinogenic potential or the effect on fertility of topical corticosteroids.

Studies to determine mutagenicity with prednisolone and hydrocortisone have revealed negative results.

Pregnancy Category C

Corticosteroids are generally teratogenic in laboratory animals when administered systemically at relatively low dosage levels. The more potent corticosteroids have been shown to be teratogenic after dermal application in laboratory animals. There are no adequate and well-controlled studies in pregnant women on teratogenic effects from topically applied corticosteroids. Therefore, topical corticosteroids should be used during pregnancy only if the potential benefit justifies the potential risk to the fetus. Drugs of this class should not be used extensively on pregnant patients, in large amounts, or for prolonged periods of time.

Nursing Mothers

It is not known whether topical administration of corticosteroids could result in sufficient systemic absorption to produce detectable quantities in breast milk. Systemically administered corticosteroids are secreted into breast milk in quantities *not* likely to have a deleterious effect on the infant. Nevertheless, caution should be exercised when topical corticosteroids are administered to a nursing woman.

Pediatric Use

Pediatric patients may demonstrate greater susceptibility to topical corticosteroid-induced HPA axis suppression and Cushing's syndrome than mature patients because of a larger skin surface area to body weight ratio. Hypothalamic-pituitary-adrenal (HPA) axis suppression, Cushing's syndrome, and intracranial hypertension have been reported in children receiving topical corticosteroids. Manifestations of adrenal suppression in children include linear growth retardation, delayed weight gain, low plasma cortisol levels, and absence of response to ACTH stimulation. Manifestations of intracranial hypertension include bulging fontanels, headaches, and bilateral papilledema.

Administration of topical corticosteroids to children should be limited to the least amount compatible with an effective therapeutic regimen. Chronic corticosteroid therapy may interfere with the growth and development of children.

ADVERSE REACTIONS

The following local adverse reactions are reported infrequently with topical corticosteroids, but may occur more frequently with the use of occlusive dressings. These reactions are listed in an approximate decreasing order of occurrence:

Burning	Perioral dermatitis
Itching	Allergic contact dermatitis
Irritation	Maceration of the skin
Dryness	Secondary infection
Folliculitis	Skin Atrophy
Hypertrichosis	Striae
Acneiform eruptions	Miliaria
Hypopigmentation	

OVERDOSAGE

Topically applied corticosteroids can be absorbed in sufficient amounts to produce systemic effects (See **PRECAUTIONS**).

HOW SUPPLIED

Cream 0.025%
15 gram tubes— NDC 0005-5130-09
60 gram tubes— NDC 0005-5130-40
240 gram jars— NDC 0005-5130-57
5.25 lb. jars— NDC 0005-5130-54

Cream 0.1%
15 gram tubes— NDC 0005-5131-09
60 gram tubes— NDC 0005-5131-40
240 gram jars— NDC 0005-5131-57
5.25 lb. jars— NDC 0005-5131-54

Cream 0.5%
15 gram tubes— NDC 0005-5132-09
240 gram jars— NDC 0005-5132-57

Ointment 0.1%
15 gram tubes— NDC 0005-5175-09
60 gram tubes— NDC 0005-5175-40
240 gram jars— NDC 0005-5175-57
5 lb. jars— NDC 0005-5175-70

Ointment 0.5%
15 gram tubes— NDC 0005-5178-09
240 gram jars— NDC 00055-5178-57

Store at Controlled Room Temperature 15°–30° C (59°–86°F)
Do Not Freeze.

Shown in Product Identification Section, page 412

Suspensions
ARISTOCORT® ℞
[*a-ris-tō-cort*]
Sterile triamcinolone diacetate
Forte parenteral 40 mg/ml
Intralesional 25 mg/ml

NOT FOR INTRAVENOUS USE

FORTE PARENTERAL:

DESCRIPTION

A sterile suspension of 40 mg/ml. of *triamcinolone diacetate* (micronized) suspended in a vehicle consisting of:

Polysorbate 80 NF	0.20%
Polyethylene Glycol 4000 NF	3%
Sodium Chloride	0.85%
Benzyl Alcohol	0.90%
Water for Injection q.s.	100%

Hydrochloric Acid and/or sodium hydroxide may be used during manufacture to adjust pH of suspension to 6.0.

This preparation is a slightly soluble suspension suitable for parenteral administration through a 24-gauge needle (or larger), but NOT suitable for intravenous use. It may be administered by the intramuscular, intra-articular, or intrasynovial routes, depending upon the situation. The response to each glucocorticoid varies considerably with each type of disease indication and each corticosteroid prescribed. Irreversible clumping occurs when product is frozen.

The chemical name for triamcinolone diacetate is (11β, 16α)-16,21-bis(acetyloxy)-9-fluoro-11,17-dihydroxy-pregna-1,4-diene-3,20-dione.Its molecular weight is 478.51.

ACTION

ARISTOCORT is primarily glucocorticoid in action and has potent anti-inflammatory, hormonal and metabolic effects common to cortisone-like drugs. It is essentially devoid of mineralocorticoid activity when administered in therapeutic doses, causing little or no sodium retention, with potassium excretion minimal or absent. The body's immune responses to diverse stimuli are also modified by its action.

INDICATIONS

Where oral therapy is not feasible or temporarily desirable in the judgment of the physician, sterile *triamcinolone diacetate* suspension, 40 mg/ml, is indicated for intramuscular use as follows:

1. Endocrine disorders.
   Primary or secondary adrenocortical insufficiency (hydrocortisone or cortisone is the drug of choice; synthetic analogs may be used in conjunction with mineralocorticoids where applicable; in infancy, mineralocorticoid supplementation is of particular importance).
   Preoperatively and in the event of serious trauma or illness, in patients with known adrenal insufficiency or when adrenocortical reserve is doubtful.
   Congenital adrenal hyperplasia.
   Nonsuppurative thyroiditis.
   Hypercalcemia associated with cancer.
2. Rheumatic disorders. As adjunctive therapy for short-term administration to tide the patient over an acute episode or exacerbation) in:
   Post-traumatic osteoarthritis.
   Synovitis of osteoarthritis.
   Rheumatoid arthritis, including juvenile rheumatoid arthritis (selected cases may require low-dose maintenance therapy).
   Acute and subacute bursitis.
   Epicondylitis.
   Acute nonspecific tenosynovitis.
   Acute gouty arthritis.
   Psoriatic arthritis.
   Ankylosing spondylitis.
3. Collagen diseases. During an exacerbation or as maintenance therapy in selected cases of:
   Systemic lupus erythematosus.
   Acute rheumatic carditis.
4. Dermatologic diseases. Pemphigus.
   Severe erythema multiforme (Stevens-Johnson syndrome).
   Exfoliative dermatitis.
   Bullous dermatitis herpetiformis.
   Severe seborrheic dermatitis.
   Severe psoriasis.
   Mycosis fungoides.

Continued on next page

The information on each product appearing here is based on labelling effective in August, 1986 and is either the entire official brochure or an accurate condensation therefrom. Information concerning all Lederle products may be obtained from the Professional Services Department, Lederle Laboratories, Pearl River, New York, 10965.

Lederle—Cont.

5. Allergic states. Control of severe or incapacitating allergic conditions intractable to adequate trials of conventional treatment in:
   Bronchial asthma.
   Contact dermatitis.
   Seasonal or perennial allergic rhinitis.
   Drug hypersensitivity reactions.
   Urticarial transfusion reactions.
   Atopic dermatitis.
   Serum sickness.
   Acute noninfectious laryngeal edema (epinephrine is the drug of first choice).
6. Ophthalmic diseases. Severe acute and chronic allergic and inflammatory processes involving the eye, such as:
   Herpes zoster ophthalmicus.
   Iritis, iridocyclitis.
   Chorioretinitis.
   Sympathetic ophthalmia.
   Diffuse posterior uveitis and choroiditis.
   Optic neuritis.
   Keratitis.
   Allergic conjunctivitis.
   Allergic corneal marginal ulcers.
7. Gastrointestinal diseases. To tide the patient over a critical period of disease in:
   Ulcerative colitis - (Systemic therapy).
   Regional enteritis - (Systemic therapy).
8. Respiratory diseases.
   Symptomatic sarcoidosis.
   Berylliosis.
   Fulminating or disseminated pulmonary tuberculosis when used concurrently with appropriate antituberculous chemotherapy.
   Aspiration pneumonitis.
   Loeffler's syndrome not manageable by other means.
9. Hematologic disorders.
   Acquired (autoimmune) hemolytic anemia.
   Secondary thrombocytopenia in adults.
   Erythroblastopenia (RBC anemia).
   Congenital (erythroid) hypoplastic anemia.
10. Neoplastic diseases. For palliative management of:
    Leukemias and lymphomas in adults.
    Acute leukemia of childhood.
11. Edematous state. To induce diuresis or remission of proteinuria in the nephrotic syndrome, without uremia, of the idiopathic type or that due to lupus erythematosus.
12. Nervous System.
    Acute exacerbations of multiple sclerosis.
13. Miscellaneous. Tuberculous meningitis with subarachnoid block or impending block when used concurrently with appropriate antituberculous chemotherapy.
    Trichinosis with neurologic or myocardial involvement.

ARISTOCORT® *triamcinolone diacetate* FORTE 40 mg/ml. is indicated for intra-articular or soft tissue use as follows:
As adjunctive therapy for short-term administration (to tide the patient over an acute episode or exacerbation) in:
Synovitis of osteoarthritis.
Rheumatoid arthritis.
Acute and subacute bursitis.
Acute gouty arthritis.
Epicondylitis.
Acute nonspecific tenosynovitis.
Post-traumatic osteoarthritis.

ARISTOCORT FORTE is indicated for intralesional use as follows:
Keloids
Localized hypertrophic, infiltrated, inflammatory lesions of: lichen planus, psoriatic plaques, granuloma annulare and lichen simplex chronicus (neurodermatitis).
Discoid lupus erythematosus.
Necrobiosis lipoidica diabeticorum.
Alopecia areata.
It may also be useful in cystic tumors of an aponeurosis or tendon (ganglia).

INTRALESIONAL:

DESCRIPTION

ARISTOCORT *triamcinolone diacetate,* possesses glucocorticoid properties while being essentially devoid of mineralocorticoid activity thus causing little or no sodium retention.
Supplied as a sterile suspension of 25 mg/ml micronized triamcinolone diacetate in the following vehicle:

Polysorbate 80 NF	0.20%
Polyethylene Glycol 3350 NF	3%
Sodium Chloride	0.85%
Benzyl Alcohol	0.90%
Water for Injection q.s.	100%

Hydrochloric Acid to approx. pH 6

Chemically triamcinolone diacetate is Pregna - 1, 4 - diene - 3, 20 - dione, 16, 21 - bis(acetyloxy) - 9 - fluoro - 11, 17-dihydroxy-,(11β, 16α)- or 9-Fluoro-11β, 16α, 17, 21-tetrahydroxypregna-1, 4-diene-3,20-dione 16,21-diacetate. Molecular weight is 478.51.

ACTIONS

Naturally occurring glucocorticoids (hydrocortisone), which also have salt-retaining properties, are used as replacement therapy in adrenocortical deficiency states. Their synthetic analogs are primarily used for their potent anti-inflammatory effects in disorders of many organ systems.
Glucocorticoids cause profound and varied metabolic effects. In addition, they modify the body's immune responses to diverse stimuli.

INDICATIONS

ARISTOCORT® *triamcinolone diacetate* INTRALESIONAL is indicated by the intralesional route for:
Keloids
Localized hypertrophic, infiltrated, inflammatory lesions of:
lichen planus, psoriatic plaques, granuloma annulare and lichen simplex chronicus (neurodermatitis).
Discoid lupus erythematosus.
Necrobiosis lipoidica diabeticorum.
Alopecia areata.
It may also be useful in cystic tumors of an aponeurosis or tendon (ganglia).
When used intra-articularly it is also indicated for:
Adjunctive therapy for short-term administration (to tide the patient over an acute episode or exacerbation) in:
Synovitis of osteoarthritis.
Rheumatoid arthritis.
Acute and subacute bursitis.
Acute gouty arthritis.
Epicondylitis.
Acute nonspecific tenosynovitis.
Post-traumatic osteoarthritis.

FORTE AND INTRALESIONAL:

CONTRAINDICATIONS

Systemic fungal infections.

WARNINGS

In patients on corticosteroid therapy subjected to any unusual stress, increased dosage of rapidly acting corticosteroids before, during, and after the stressful situation is indicated.
Corticosteroids may mask some signs of infection, and new infections may appear during their use. There may be decreased resistance and inability to localize infection when corticosteroids are used.
Prolonged use of corticosteroids may produce posterior subcapsular cataracts, glaucoma with possible damage to the optic nerves, and may enhance the establishment of secondary ocular infections due to fungi or viruses.
Usage in pregnancy
Since adequate human reproduction studies have not been done with corticosteroids, the use of these drugs in pregnancy, nursing mothers, or women of childbearing potential requires that the possible benefits of the drug be weighed against the potential hazards to the mother and embryo or fetus. Infants born of mothers who have received substantial doses of corticosteroids during pregnancy should be carefully observed for signs of hypoadrenalism.
Average and large doses of cortisone or hydrocortisone can cause elevation of blood pressure, salt and water retention, and increased excretion of potassium. These effects are less likely to occur with the synthetic derivatives except when used in large doses. Dietary salt restriction and potassium supplementation may be necessary. All corticosteroids increase calcium excretion.
While on Corticosteroid Therapy Patients Should Not Be Vaccinated Against Smallpox. Other Immunization Procedures Should Not Be Undertaken in Patients Who Are on Corticosteroids, Especially in High Doses, Because of Possible Hazards of Neurological Complications and Lack of Antibody Response.
The use of ARISTOCORT® *triamcinolone diacetate* in active tuberculosis should be restricted to those cases of fulminating or disseminated tuberculosis in which the corticosteroid is used for the management of the disease in conjunction with appropriate antituberculous regimen.
If corticosteroids are indicated in patients with latent tuberculosis or tuberculin reactivity, close observation is necessary as reactivation of the disease may occur. During prolonged corticosteroid therapy, these patients should receive chemoprophylaxis.
Because rare instances of anaphylactoid reactions have occurred in patients receiving parenteral corticosteroid therapy, appropriate precautionary measures should be taken prior to administration, especially when the patient has a history of allergy to any drug.
Postinjection flare (following intra-articular use) and Charcot-like arthropathy have been associated with parenteral corticosteroid therapy.
Intralesional or sublesional injection of excessive dosage whether by single or multiple injection into any given area may cause cutaneous or subcutaneous atrophy.

PRECAUTIONS

Drug-induced secondary adrenocortical insufficiency may be minimized by gradual reduction of dosage. This type of relative insufficiency may persist for months after discontinuation of therapy; therefore, in any situation of stress occurring during that period, hormone therapy should be reinstituted.
Since mineralocorticoid secretion may be impaired, salt and/or a mineralocorticoid should be administered concurrently.
There is an enhanced effect of corticosteroids in patients with hypothyroidism and in those with cirrhosis.
Corticosteroids should be used cautiously in patients with ocular herpes simplex for fear of corneal perforation.
The lowest possible dose of corticosteroid should be used to control the condition under treatment, and when reduction in dosage is possible, the reduction must be gradual.
Psychic derangements may appear when corticosteroids are used, ranging from euphoria, insomnia, mood swings, personality changes, and severe depression to frank psychotic manifestations. Also, existing emotional instability or psychotic tendencies may be aggravated by corticosteroids.
Aspirin should be used cautiously in conjunction with corticosteroids in hypoprothrombinemia.
Steroids should be used with caution in nonspecific ulcerative colitis, if there is a probability of impending perforation, abscess or other pyogenic infection, also in diverticulitis, fresh intestinal anastomoses, active or latent peptic ulcer, renal insufficiency, hypertension, osteoporosis, and myasthenia gravis.
Growth and development of infants and children on prolonged corticosteroid therapy should be carefully followed.
The following additional precautions apply for parenteral corticosteroids. Intra-articular injection of a corticosteroid may produce systemic as well as local effects.
Appropriate examination of any joint fluid present is necessary to exclude a septic process.
A marked increase in pain accompanied by local swelling, further restriction of joint motion, fever, and malaise are suggestive of septic arthritis. If this complication occurs and the diagnosis of sepsis is confirmed, appropriate antimicrobial therapy should be instituted.
Local injection of a steroid into a previously infected joint is to be avoided.
Corticosteroids should not be injected into unstable joints.
The slower rate of absorption by intramuscular administration should be recognized.
Atrophy at the site of injection has been reported.
Routine laboratory studies, such as urinalysis, two-hour postprandial blood sugar, determination of blood pressure and body weight, and a chest x-ray should be made at regular intervals during prolonged therapy. Upper GI x-rays are desirable in patients with an ulcer history or significant dyspepsia.
Accidental injection into soft tissue during intra-articular administration decreases local effectiveness in the joint and, by increasing rate of absorption, may produce systemic effects.
Although controlled clinical trials have shown corticosteroids to be effective in speeding the resolution of acute exacerbations of multiple sclerosis they do not show that they affect the ultimate outcome or natural history of the disease. The studies do show that relatively high doses of corticosteroids are necessary to demonstrate a significant effect. (See Dosage and Administration).
Since complications of treatment with glucocorticoid are dependent on the size of the dose and the duration of treatment a risk/benefit decision must be made in each individual case as to dose and duration of treatment and as to whether daily or intermittent therapy should be used.

ADVERSE REACTIONS

Fluid and electrolyte disturbances:
  Sodium retention.
  Fluid retention.
  Congestive heart failure in susceptible patients.
  Potassium loss.
  Hypokalemic alkalosis.
  Hypertension.
Musculoskeletal:
  Muscle weakness.
  Steroid myopathy.
  Loss of muscle mass.
  Osteoporosis.
  Vertebral compression fractures.
  Aseptic necrosis of femoral and humeral heads.
  Pathologic fracture of long bones.
Gastrointestinal:
  Peptic ulcer with possible subsequent perforation and hemorrhage.

Pancreatitis.
Abdominal distention.
Ulcerative esophagitis.

Dermatologic:
Impaired wound healing.
Thin fragile skin.
Petechiae and ecchymoses.
Facial erythema.
Increased sweating.
May suppress reactions to skin tests.

Neurological:
Increased intracranial pressure with papilledema (pseudotumor cerebri) usually after treatment.
Convulsions.
Vertigo.
Headache.

Endocrine:
Menstrual irregularities.
Development of cushingoid state.
Suppression of growth in children.
Secondary adrenocortical and pituitary unresponsiveness, particularly in times of stress, as in trauma, surgery, or illness.
Decreased carbohydrate tolerance.
Manifestations of latent diabetes mellitus.
Increased requirements for insulin or oral hypoglycemic agents in diabetics.

Ophthalmic:
Posterior subcapsular cataracts.
Increased intraocular pressure.
Glaucoma.
Exophthalmos.

Metabolic:
Negative nitrogen balance due to protein catabolism.

The following additional adverse reactions are related to parenteral and intralesional corticosteroid therapy:
Rare instances of blindness associated with intralesional therapy around the orbit or intranasally.
Hyperpigmentation or hypopigmentation.
Subcutaneous and cutaneous atrophy.
Sterile abscess.

Anaphylactoid reactions have been reported rarely with products of this class.

DOSAGE AND ADMINISTRATION

General

The initial dosage of ARISTOCORT® *triamcinolone diacetate* may vary from 3 to 48 mg per day depending on the specific disease entity being treated. In situations of less severity, lower doses will generally suffice while in selected patients higher initial doses may be required. Usually the parenteral dosage ranges are one-third to one-half the oral dose given every 12 hours. However, in certain overwhelming, acute, life-threatening situations, administration in dosages exceeding the usual dosages may be justified and may be in multiples of the oral dosages.

The initial dosage should be maintained or adjusted until a satisfactory response is noted. If after a reasonable period of time there is a lack of satisfactory clinical response, ARISTOCORT should be discontinued and the patient transferred to other appropriate therapy. It Should Be Emphasized That Dosage Requirements Are Variable and Must Be Individualized on the Basis of the Disease Under Treatment and the Response of the Patient. After a favorable response is noted, the proper maintenance dosage should be determined by decreasing the initial drug dosage in small increments at appropriate time intervals until the lowest dosage which will maintain an adequate clinical response is reached. It should be kept in mind that constant monitoring is needed in regard to drug dosage. Included in the situations which may make dosage adjustments necessary are changes in clinical status secondary to remissions or exacerbations in the disease process, the patient's individual drug responsiveness, and the effect of patient exposure to stressful situations not directly related to the disease entity under treatment; in this latter situation, it may be necessary to increase the dosage of ARISTOCORT® *triamcinolone diacetate* for a period of time consistent with the patient's condition. If after long-term therapy the drug is to be stopped, it is recommended that it be withdrawn gradually rather than abruptly.

For intra-articular, intralesional and soft tissue use, a lesser initial dosage range of triamcinolone diacetate may produce the desired effect when the drug is administered to provide a localized concentration. The site of the injection and the volume of the injection should be carefully considered when triamcinolone diacetate is administered for this purpose.

Specific

Forte:

ARISTOCORT FORTE Parenteral is sterile *triamcinolone diacetate* (40 mg/ml) suspended in a suitable vehicle. The full-strength suspension may be employed. If preferred, the suspension may be diluted with normal saline or water. The diluent may also be prepared by mixing equal parts of normal saline and 1% procaine hydrochloride or other similar local anesthetics. The use of diluents containing preservatives such as methylparaben, propylparaben, phenol, etc., must be avoided as these preparations tend to cause flocculation of the steroid. These dilutions retain full potency for at least one week. Topical ethyl chloride spray may be used locally prior to injection. Since this product has been designed for ease of administration, a small bore needle (not smaller than 24 gauge) may be used.

Equivalence Table

	Anti-inflammatory Relative Potency		Frequently Used Tablet Strength (mg)		Tablet × Potency Equivalent Value
Hydrocortisone	1	×	20	=	20
Prednisolone	4	×	5	=	20
ARISTOCORT® triamcinolone	5	×	4	=	20
Dexamethasone	25	×	0.75	=	18.75

Intramuscular: Although ARISTOCORT FORTE Parenteral may be administered intramuscularly for initial therapy, most physicians prefer to adjust the dose orally until adequate control is attained. Intramuscular administration provides a sustained or depot action which can be used to supplement or replace initial oral therapy. With intramuscular therapy, greater supervision of the amount of steroid used is made possible in the patient who is inconsistent in following an oral dosage schedule. In maintenance therapy, the patient-to-patient response is not uniform and, therefore, the dose must be individualized for optimal control.

Although triamcinolone diacetate may possess greater anti-inflammatory potency than many glucocorticoids, this is only dose-related since side effects, such as osteoporosis, peptic ulcer, etc., related to glucocorticoid activity, have not been diminished.

The average dose is 40 mg (1 ml) administered intramuscularly once a week for conditions in which anti-inflammatory action is desired.

In general, a single parenteral dose 4 to 7 times the oral daily dose may be expected to control the patient from 4 to 7 days up to 3 to 4 weeks. Dosage should be adjusted to the point where adequate but not necessarily complete relief of symptoms is obtained.

Intra-Articular and Intrasynovial: The usual dose varies from 5 to 40 mg. The average for the knee, for example, is 25 mg. The duration of effect varies from one week to 2 months. However, acutely inflamed joints may require more frequent injections.

A lesser initial dosage range of triamcinolone diacetate may produce the desired effect when the drug is administered to provide a localized concentration. The site of the injection and the volume of the injection should be carefully considered when triamcinolone diacetate is administered for this purpose.

A specific dose depends largely on the size of the joint. Strict surgical asepsis is mandatory. The physician should be familiar with anatomical relationships as described in standard text books. ARISTOCORT FORTE Parenteral may be used in any accessible joint except the intervertebrals. In general, intrasynovial therapy is suggested under the following circumstances:

1. When systemic steroid therapy is contraindicated because of side effects such as peptic ulcer.
2. When it is desirable to secure relief in one or two specific joints.
3. When good systemic maintenance fails to control flare-ups in a few joints and it is desirable to secure relief without increasing oral therapy.

Such treatment should not be considered to constitute a cure; for although this method will ameliorate the joint symptoms, it does not preclude the need for the conventional measures usually employed.

It is suggested that infiltration of the soft tissue by local anesthetic precede intra-articular injection. A 24-gauge or larger needle on a dry syringe may be inserted into the joint and excess fluid aspirated. For the first few hours following injection, there may be local discomfort in the joint but this is usually followed rapidly by effective relief of pain and improvement in local function.

[See table above].

Intralesional

When ARISTOCORT INTRALESIONAL is administered by injection strict aseptic technique is mandatory. Full strength suspensions may be employed, or if preferred, the suspension may be diluted, either to a 1:1 or 1:10 concentration, thus obtaining a working concentration of 12.5 mg/ml or approximately 2.5 mg/ml respectively. Normal (isotonic) saline solution alone or equal parts of normal (isotonic) saline solution and 1% procaine or other local anesthetics, may be used as diluents. These dilutions usually retain full potency for at least one week. Topical ethyl chloride spray may be used as a local anesthetic. The use of diluents containing preservatives such as methylparaben, propylparaben, phenol, etc must be avoided as these preparations tend to cause flocculations of the steroid. Since this product has been designed for ease of administration, a small bore needle (not smaller than 24 gauge) may be used.

Intralesional or Sublesional: For small lesions, injection is usually well tolerated and a local anesthetic is not necessary. The location and type of lesion will determine the route of injection: intralesional, sublesional, intradermal, subdermal, intracutaneous, or subcutaneous. The size of the lesion will determine: the total amount of drug needed, the concentration used, and the number and pattern of injection sites utilized (eg from a total of 5 mg ARISTOCORT INTRALESIONAL in a 2 ml volume divided over several locations in small lesions, ranging up to 48 mg total ARISTOCORT INTRALESIONAL for large psoriatic plaques). Avoid injecting too superficially. In general, no more than 12.5 mg per injection site should be used. An average of 25 mg is the usual limit for any one lesion. Large areas require multiple injections with smaller doses per injection.

For a majority of conditions, sublesional injection directly through the lesion into the deep dermal tissue is suggested. In cases where it is difficult to inject intradermally, the suspension may be introduced subcutaneously, as superficially as possible.

Two or three injections at one to two week intervals may suffice as an average course of treatment for many conditions. Within 5-7 days after initial injection involution of the lesion can usually be seen, with pronounced clearing towards normal tissue after 12-14 days. Multiple injections of small amounts of equal strength may be convenient in alopecia areata and in psoriasis where there are large or confluent lesions. This is best accomplished by a series of fan-like injections ½ to 1 inch apart.

Alopecia areata and totalis require an average dose of 25 mg to 30 mg in a concentration of 10 mg/ml. subcutaneously 1 to 2 times a week, to stimulate hair regrowth. Results may be expected in 3 to 6 weeks on this dosage, and hair growth may last 3-6 months after initial injection. No more than 0.5 ml should be given in any one site, because excessive deposition may produce local skin atrophy. Continued periodic local injections may be necessary to maintain response and continued hair growth. Use of more dilute solutions diminishes the incidence and degree of local atrophy in the injection site.

In keloids and similar dense scars, injections are usually made directly into the lesion.

Injections may be repeated as required, but probably a total of no more than 75 mg of ARISTOCORT® *triamcinolone diacetate* a week should be given to any one patient. The need for repeated injections is best determined by clinical response. Remissions may be expected to last from a few weeks up to eleven months.

Intra-articular or Intrasynovial: Strict surgical asepsis is mandatory. The physician should be familiar with anatomical relationships as described in standard text books. A recent paper details the anatomy and the technical approach in arthrocentesis.

It is usually recommended that infiltration by local anesthetic of the soft tissue precede intra-articular injection. A 22-gauge or larger needle on a dry syringe should be inserted into the joint and excess fluid if present should be aspirated. The specific dose depends primarily on the size of the joint. The usual dose varies from 5 mg to 40 mg with the average for the knee being 25 mg. Smaller joints as in the fingers require 2 mg to 5 mg The duration of effect varies from one week to two months. However, acutely inflamed joints may require more frequent injections. Accidental injection into soft tissue is usually not harmful but decreases the local effectiveness. Injection into subcutaneous lipoid tissue may produce "pseudo-atrophy" with a persistent depression of the overlying dermis, lasting several weeks or months.

Administration and dosage of ARISTOCORT INTRALESIONAL must be individualized according to the nature, severity and chronicity of the disease or disorder treated, and should be undertaken with a view of the patient's entire clinical condition. Corticosteroid therapy is considered an adjunct to and not usually a replacement for conventional therapy. Therapy with ARISTOCORT INTRALESIONAL,

Continued on next page

The information on each product appearing here is based on labelling effective in August, 1986 and is either the entire official brochure or an accurate condensation therefrom. Information concerning all Lederle products may be obtained from the Professional Services Department, Lederle Laboratories, Pearl River, New York, 10965.

Lederle—Cont.

as with all steroids, is of the suppressive type, related to its anti-inflammatory effect. The dose should be regulated during therapy according to the degree of therapeutic response, and should be reduced gradually to maintenance levels, whereby the patient obtains adequate or acceptable control of symptoms. When such control occurs, consideration should be given to gradual decrease in dosage and eventual cessation of therapy. Remission of symptoms may be due to therapy or may be spontaneous and a therapeutic test of gradual withdrawal of steroid treatment is usually indicated.

HOW SUPPLIED

***Intralesional:** (25 mg/ml); 5 ml. Vials NDC 0205-4422-31.
***Forte:** (40 mg/ml); 1 ml and 5 ml Vials NDC 0205-4450-24, NDC 0205-4450-31.
Store at Controlled Room Temperature 15°-30°C (59°-86°F).
*Manufactured for
LEDERLE LABORATORIES DIVISION
American Cyanamid Company
Pearl River, NY 10965
by
LEDERLE PARENTERALS INC.
Carolina, Puerto Rico 00630

ARISTOCORT A® ℞

[a-ris-tō-cort]
Triamcinolone Acetonide Cream
ARISTOCORT A® ℞
Triamcinolone Acetonide Ointment

DESCRIPTION

Each gram of 0.025% Cream contains 0.25 mg of the highly active steroid, Triamcinolone Acetonide (a derivative of triamcinolone); each gram of 0.1% Cream contains 1 mg Triamcinolone Acetonide; each gram of 0.5% Cream contains 5 mg of Triamcinolone Acetonide; all in AQUATAIN™, a specially formulated cream base composed of emulsifying wax NF, isopropyl palmitate, glycerin USP, sorbitol solution USP, lactic acid, 2% benzyl alcohol, and purified water. AQUATAIN is non-staining, water-washable, paraben-free, spermaceti-free, and has a light texture and consistency.
Each gram of 0.1% Ointment contains 1 mg Triamcinolone Acetonide in a specially formulated ointment base composed of emulsifying wax NF, white petrolatum, and propylene glycol, Tenox II (butylated hydroxyanisole, propyl gallate, citric acid, propylene glycol) and lactic acid.
The topical corticosteroids constitute a class of primarily synthetic steroids used as anti-inflammatory and antipruritic agents.

CLINICAL PHARMACOLOGY

Topical corticosteroids share anti-inflammatory, anti-pruritic and vasoconstrictive actions.
The mechanism of anti-inflammatory activity of the topical corticosteroids is unclear. Various laboratory methods, including vasoconstrictor assays, are used to compare and predict potencies and/or clinical efficacies of the topical corticosteroids. There is some evidence to suggest that a recognizable correlation exists between vasoconstrictor potency and therapeutic efficacy in man.
Pharmacokinetics: The extent of percutaneous absorption of topical corticosteroids is determined by many factors including the vehicle, the integrity of the epidermal barrier, and the use of occlusive dressings.
Topical corticosteroids can be absorbed from normal intact skin. Inflammation and/or other disease processes in the skin increase percutaneous absorption. Occlusive dressings substantially increase the percutaneous absorption of topical corticosteroids. Thus, occlusive dressings may be a valuable therapeutic adjunct for treatment of resistant dermatoses. (See *DOSAGE AND ADMINISTRATION*).
Once absorbed through the skin, topical corticosteroids are handled through pharmacokinetic pathways similar to systemically administered corticosteroids. Corticosteroids are bound to plasma proteins in varying degrees.
Corticosteroids are metabolized primarily in the liver and are then excreted by the kidneys. Some of the topical corticosteroids and their metabolites are also excreted into the bile.

INDICATIONS AND USAGE

Topical corticosteroids are indicated for the relief of the inflammatory and pruritic manifestations of corticosteroid-responsive dermatoses.

CONTRAINDICATIONS

Topical corticosteroids are contraindicated in those patients with a history of hypersensitivity to any of the components of the preparation.

PRECAUTIONS

General: Systemic absorption of topical corticosteroids has produced reversible hypothalamic-pituitary-adrenal (HPA) axis suppression, manifestations of Cushing's syndrome, hyperglycemia, and glucosuria in some patients.
Conditions which augment systemic absorption include the application of the more potent steroids, use over large surface areas, prolonged use, and the addition of occlusive dressings.
Therefore, patients receiving a large dose of a potent topical steroid applied to a large surface area or under an occlusive dressing should be evaluated periodically for evidence of HPA axis suppression by using the urinary free cortisol and ACTH stimulation tests. If HPA axis suppression is noted, an attempt should be made to withdraw the drug, to reduce the frequency of application, or to substitute a less potent steroid.
Recovery of HPA axis function is generally prompt and complete upon discontinuation of the drug. Infrequently, signs and symptoms of steroid withdrawal may occur, requiring supplemental systemic corticosteroids.
Children may absorb proportionally larger amounts of topical corticosteroids and thus be more susceptible to systemic toxicity. (See *PRECAUTIONS—Pediatric Use*).
If irritation develops, topical corticosteroids should be discontinued and appropriate therapy instituted.
In the presence of dermatological infections, the use of an appropriate antifungal or antibacterial agent should be instituted. If a favorable response does not occur promptly, the corticosteroid should be discontinued until the infection has been adequately controlled.
Information for the Patient: Patients using topical corticosteroids should receive the following information and instructions:
1. This medication is to be used as directed by the physician. It is for external use only. Avoid contact with the eyes.
2. Patients should be advised not to use this medication for any disorder other than for which it was prescribed.
3. The treated skin area should not be bandaged or otherwise covered or wrapped as to be occlusive unless directed by the physician.
4. Patients should report any signs of local adverse reactions especially under occlusive dressing.
5. Parents of pediatric patients should be advised not to use tight-fitting diapers or plastic pants on a child being treated in the diaper area, as these garments may constitute occlusive dressings.

Laboratory Tests: The following tests may be helpful in evaluating the HPA axis suppression:
Urinary free cortisol test
ACTH stimulation test
Carcinogenesis, Mutagenesis, and Impairment of Fertility: Long-term animal studies have not been performed to evaluate the carcinogenic potential or the effect on fertility of topical corticosteroids.
Studies to determine mutagenicity with prednisolone and hydrocortisone have revealed negative results.
Pregnancy Category C: Corticosteroids are generally teratogenic in laboratory animals when administered systemically at relatively low dosage levels. The more potent corticosteroids have been shown to be teratogenic after dermal application in laboratory animals. There are no adequate and well-controlled studies in pregnant women on teratogenic effects from topically applied corticosteroids. Therefore, topical corticosteroids should be used during pregnancy only if the potential benefit justifies the potential risk to the fetus. Drugs of this class should not be used extensively on pregnant patients, in large amounts, or for prolonged periods of time.
Nursing Mothers: It is not known whether topical administration of corticosteroids could result in sufficient systemic absorption to produce detectable quantities in breast milk. Systemically administered corticosteroids are secreted into breast milk in quantities *not* likely to have a deleterious effect on the infant. Nevertheless, caution should be exercised when topical corticosteroids are administered to a nursing woman.
Pediatric Use: Pediatric patients may demonstrate greater susceptibility to topical corticosteroid-induced HPA axis suppression and Cushing's syndrome than mature patients because of a larger skin surface area to body weight ratio.
Hypothalamic-pituitary-adrenal (HPA) axis suppression, Cushing's syndrome, and intracranial hypertension have been reported in children receiving topical corticosteroids. Manifestations of adrenal suppression in children include linear growth retardation, delayed weight gain, low plasma cortisol levels, and absence of response to ACTH stimulation. Manifestations of intracranial hypertension include bulging fontanels, headaches, and bilateral papilledema.
Administration of topical corticosteroids to children should be limited to the least amount compatible with an effective therapeutic regimen. Chronic corticosteroid therapy may interfere with the growth and development of children.

ADVERSE REACTIONS

The following local adverse reactions are reported infrequently with topical corticosteroids, but may occur more frequently with the use of occlusive dressings. These reactions are listed in an approximate decreasing order of occurrence:
Burning
Itching
Irritation
Dryness
Folliculitis
Hypertrichosis
Acneform eruptions
Hypopigmentation
Perioral dermatitis
Allergic contact dermatitis
Maceration of the skin
Secondary infection
Skin Atrophy
Striae
Miliaria

OVERDOSAGE

Topically applied corticosteroids can be absorbed in sufficient amounts to produce systemic effects (See *PRECAUTIONS*).

DOSAGE AND ADMINISTRATION

Topical corticosteroids are generally applied to the affected area as a thin film from three to four times daily depending on the severity of the condition.
Occlusive dressings may be used for the management of psoriasis or recalcitrant conditions.
If an infection develops, the use of occlusive dressings should be discontinued and appropriate antimicrobial therapy instituted.

HOW SUPPLIED

0.025% Cream:
15 gram tubes—NDC 0005-5169-09
60 gram tubes—NDC 0005-5169-40
0.1% Cream:
15 gram tubes—NDC 0005-5191-09
60 gram tubes—NDC 0005-5191-40
240 gram jars—NDC 0005-5191-57
0.5% Cream:
15 gram tubes—NDC 0005-5192-09
0.1% Ointment:
15 gram tubes—NDC 0005-5468-09
60 gram tubes—NDC 0005-5468-40
Store at Controlled Room Temperature 15°-30°C (59°-86°F)
Do Not Freeze
60 gm tube VA: NSN 6505-01-107-1731
60 gm tube Military: NSN 6505-01-107-1731
Shown in Product Identification Section, page 413

ARISTOSPAN® ℞

[a-ris-tō-span]
Sterile Triamcinolone Hexacetonide Suspension, USP
For Intralesional Administration
5 mg/ml—Parenteral
For Intra-articular Administration
20 mg/ml—Parenteral
NOT FOR INTRAVENOUS USE

DESCRIPTION

Intralesional:
A sterile suspension containing 5 mg/ml of micronized triamcinolone hexacetonide in the following inactive ingredients:
Polysorbate 80 NF .... 0.20% w/v
Sorbitol Solution USP .... 50.00% v/v
Water for Injection qs ad .... 100.00% V
Hydrochloric Acid and Sodium Hydroxide, if required, to adjust pH to 4.5–6.5.
Preservative:
Benzyl Alcohol .... 0.90% w/v
Intra-articular:
A sterile suspension containing 20 mg/ml of micronized triamcinolone hexacetonide in the following inactive ingredients:
Polysorbate 80 NF .... 0.40% w/v
Sorbitol Solution USP .... 50.00% v/v
Water for Injection qs ad .... 100.00% V
Hydrochloric Acid and Sodium Hydroxide, if required, to adjust pH to 4.5–6.5.
Preservative:
Benzyl Alcohol .... 0.90% w/v
The hexacetonide ester of the potent glucocorticoid triamcinolone is relatively insoluble (0.0002% at 25° C. in water). When injected intralesionally, sublesionally, or intra-articularly, it can be expected to be absorbed slowly from the injection site.
Chemically triamcinolone hexacetonide USP is 9-Fluoro-11β, 16α, 17,21-tetrahydroxypregna-1,4-diene-3,20-dione cyclic 16,17-acetal with acetone 21-(3,3-dimethylbutyrate). Molecular weight 532.65.

ACTIONS

Naturally occurring glucocorticoids (hydrocortisone), which also have salt-retaining properties, are used as replacement therapy in adrenocortical deficiency states. Their synthetic analogs are primarily used for their potent anti-inflammatory effects in disorders of many organ systems.

Glucocorticoids cause profound and varied metabolic effects. In addition, they modify the body's immune responses to diverse stimuli.

INDICATIONS

Intralesional or sublesional ARISTOSPAN® *sterile triamcinolone hexacetonide suspension* is indicated for the following:

Keloids.

Localized hypertrophic, infiltrated, inflammatory lesions of: lichen planus, psoriatic plaques, granuloma annulare and lichen simplex chronicus (neurodermatitis).

Discoid lupus erythematosus.

Necrobiosis lipoidica diabeticorum.

Alopecia areata.

They may also be useful in cystic tumors of an aponeurosis or tendon (ganglia).

Intra-articular:

As adjunctive therapy for short-term administration (to tide the patient over an acute episode or exacerbation) in:

Synovitis of osteoarthritis

Acute and subacute bursitis

Epicondylitis

Posttraumatic osteoarthritis

Rheumatoid arthritis

Acute gouty arthritis

Acute nonspecific tenosynovitis

CONTRAINDICATIONS

Systemic fungal infections.

WARNINGS

In patients on corticosteroid therapy subjected to any unusual stress, increased dosage of rapidly acting corticosteroids before, during, and after the stressful situation is indicated.

Corticosteroids may mask some signs of infection, and new infections may appear during their use. There may be decreased resistance and inability to localize infection when corticosteroids are used.

Prolonged use of corticosteroids may produce posterior subcapsular cataracts, glaucoma with possible damage to the optic nerves and may enhance the establishment of secondary ocular infections due to fungi or viruses.

Usage in pregnancy

Since adequate human reproduction studies have not been done with corticosteroids, the use of these drugs in pregnancy, nursing mothers, or women of childbearing potential requires that the possible benefits of the drug be weighed against the potential hazards to the mother and embryo or fetus.

Infants born of mothers who have received substantial doses of corticosteroids during pregnancy should be carefully observed for signs of hypoadrenalism.

Average and large doses of cortisone or hydrocortisone can cause elevation of blood pressure, salt and water retention, and increased excretion of potassium. These effects are less likely to occur with the synthetic derivatives except when used in large doses. Dietary salt restriction and potassium supplementation may be necessary. All corticosteroids increase calcium excretion.

While on Corticosteroid Therapy Patients Should Not Be Vaccinated Against Smallpox. Other Immunization Procedures Should Not Be Undertaken in Patients Who Are on Corticosteroids, Especially in High Doses, Because of Possible Hazards of Neurological Complications and Lack of Antibody Response.

The use of ARISTOSPAN® *sterile triamcinolone hexacetonide suspension* in active tuberculosis should be restricted to those cases of fulminating or disseminated tuberculosis in which the corticosteroid is used for the management of the disease in conjunction with appropriate antituberculous regimen.

If corticosteroids are indicated in patients with latent tuberculosis or tuberculin reactivity, close observation is necessary as reactivation of the disease may occur. During prolonged corticosteroid therapy, these patients should receive chemoprophylaxis.

Because rare instances of anaphylactoid reactions have occurred in patients receiving parenteral corticosteroid therapy, appropriate precautionary measures should be taken prior to administration, especially when the patient has a history of allergy to any drug.

Intralesional or sublesional injection of excessive dosage whether by single or multiple injection into any given area may cause cutaneous or subcutaneous atrophy.

Post injection flare (following intra-articular use) and Charcot-like arthropathy have been associated with parenteral corticosteroid therapy.

PRECAUTIONS

Drug-induced secondary adrenocortical insufficiency may be minimized by gradual reduction of dosage. This type of relative insufficiency may persist for months after discontinuation of therapy; therefore, in any situation of stress occurring during that period, hormone therapy should be reinstituted. Since mineralocorticoid secretion may be impaired, salt and/or a mineralocorticoid should be administered concurrently.

There is an enhanced effect of corticosteroids in patients with hypothyroidism and in those with cirrhosis.

Corticosteroids should be used cautiously in patients with ocular herpes simplex for fear of corneal perforation.

The lowest possible dose of corticosteroid should be used to control the condition under treatment, and when reduction in dosage is possible, the reduction must be gradual.

Psychic derangements may appear when corticosteroids are used, ranging from euphoria, insomnia, mood swings, personality changes, and severe depression to frank psychotic manifestations. Also, existing emotional instability or psychotic tendencies may be aggravated by corticosteroids.

Aspirin should be used cautiously in conjunction with corticosteroids in hypoprothrombinemia.

Steroids should be used with caution in nonspecific ulcerative colitis, if there is a probability of impending perforation, abscess or other pyogenic infection, also in diverticulitis, fresh intestinal anastomoses, active or latent peptic ulcer, renal insufficiency, hypertension, osteoporosis, and myasthenia gravis.

Growth and development of infants and children on prolonged corticosteroid therapy should be carefully followed.

The following additional precautions apply for parenteral corticosteroids.

Intra-articular injection of a corticosteroid may produce systemic as well as local effects.

Appropriate examination of any joint fluid present is necessary to exclude a septic process..

A marked increase in pain accompanied by local swelling, further restriction of joint motion, fever, and malaise are suggestive of septic arthritis. If this complication occurs and the diagnosis of sepsis is confirmed, appropriate antimicrobial therapy should be instituted.

Local injection of a steroid into a previously infected joint is to be avoided.

Corticosteroids should not be injected into unstable joints.

The slower rate of absorption by intramuscular administration should be recognized.

Atrophy at the site of injection has been reported.

Routine laboratory studies, such as urinalysis, two-hour postprandial blood sugar, determination of blood pressure and body weight, and a chest x-ray should be made at regular intervals during prolonged therapy. Upper GI x-rays are desirable in patients with an ulcer history or significant dyspepsia.

ADVERSE REACTIONS

Fluid and electrolyte disturbances:

Sodium retention.

Fluid retention.

Congestive heart failure in susceptible patients.

Potassium loss.

Hypokalemic alkalosis.

Hypertension.

Musculoskeletal:

Muscle weakness.

Steroid myopathy.

Loss of muscle mass.

Osteoporosis.

Vertebral compression fractures.

Aseptic necrosis of femoral and humeral heads.

Pathologic fracture of long bones.

Gastrointestinal:

Peptic ulcer with possible subsequent perforation and hemorrhage.

Pancreatitis.

Abdominal distention.

Ulcerative esophagitis.

Dermatologic:

Impaired wound healing.

Thin fragile skin.

Petechiae and ecchymoses.

Facial erythema.

Increased sweating.

May suppress reactions to skin tests.

Neurological:

Convulsions.

Increased intracranial pressure with papilledema (pseudotumor cerebri) usually after treatment.

Vertigo.

Headache.

Endocrine:

Menstrual irregularities.

Development of cushingoid state.

Suppression of growth in children.

Secondary adrenocortical and pituitary unresponsiveness, particularly in times of stress, as in trauma, surgery, or illness.

Decreased carbohydrate tolerance.

Manifestations of latent diabetes mellitus.

Increased requirements for insulin or oral hypoglycemic agents in diabetics.

Ophthalmic:

Posterior subcapsular cataracts.

Increased intraocular pressure.

Glaucoma.

Exophthalmos.

Metabolic:

Negative nitrogen balance due to protein catabolism.

The following additional adverse reactions are related to parenteral and intralesional corticosteroid therapy:

Rare instances of blindness associated with intralesional therapy around the orbit or intranasally.

Hyperpigmentation or hypopigmentation.

Subcutaneous and cutaneous atrophy.

Sterile abscess.

Anaphylactoid reactions have been reported rarely with products of this class.

DOSAGE AND ADMINISTRATION

General

The initial dosage of ARISTOSPAN® *sterile triamcinolone hexacetonide suspension* may vary from 2 to 48 mg per day depending on the specific disease entity being treated. In situations of less severity, lower doses will generally suffice while in selected patients higher initial doses may be required. Usually the parenteral dosage ranges are one-third to one-half the oral dose given every 12 hours. However, in certain overwhelming, acute, life-threatening situations, administration in dosages exceeding the usual dosages may be justified and may be in multiples of the oral dosages.

The initial dosage should be maintained or adjusted until a satisfactory response is noted. If after a reasonable period of time there is a lack of satisfactory clinical response, ARISTOSPAN should be discontinued and the patient transferred to other appropriate therapy. It Should Be Emphasized That Dosage Requirements Are Variable and Must Be Individualized on the Basis of the Disease Under Treatment and the Response of the Patient. After a favorable response is noted, the proper maintenance dosage should be determined by decreasing the initial drug dosage in small increments at appropriate time intervals until the lowest dosage which will maintain an adequate clinical response is reached. It should be kept in mind that constant monitoring is needed in regard to drug dosage. Included in the situations which may make dosage adjustments necessary are changes in clinical status secondary to remissions or exacerbations in the disease process, the patient's individual drug responsiveness, and the effect of patient exposure to stressful situations not directly related to the disease entity under treatment; in this latter situation it may be necessary to increase the dosage of ARISTOSPAN for a period of time consistent with the patient's condition. If after long-term therapy the drug is to be stopped, it is recommended that it be withdrawn gradually rather than abruptly.

Directions for Use

Strict aseptic administration technique is mandatory. Topical ethylchloride spray may be used locally before injection. The syringe should be gently agitated to achieve uniform suspension before use. Since this product has been designed for ease of administration, a small bore needle (not smaller than 24 gauge) may be used.

Dilution—Intralesional 5 mg/ml

ARISTOSPAN suspension may be diluted, if desired, with Dextrose and Sodium Chloride Injection USP, (5% and 10% Dextrose), Sodium Chloride Injection USP, or Sterile Water for Injection USP.

The optimum dilution, ie, 1:1, 1:2, 1:4, should be determined by the nature of the lesion, its size, the depth of injection, the volume needed, and location of the lesion. In general, more superficial injections should be performed with greater dilution. Certain conditions, such as keloids, require a less dilute suspension such as 5 mg/ml, with variation in dose and dilution as dictated by the condition of the individual patient. Subsequent dosage, dilution, and frequency of injections are best judged by the clinical response.

The suspension may also be mixed with 1% or 2% Lidocaine Hydrochloride, using the formulations which do not contain parabens. Similar local anesthetics may also be used. Dilu-

Continued on next page

The information on each product appearing here is based on labelling effective in August, 1986 and is either the entire official brochure or an accurate condensation therefrom. Information concerning all Lederle products may be obtained from the Professional Services Department, Lederle Laboratories, Pearl River, New York, 10965.

Lederle—Cont.

ents containing methylparaben, propylparaben, phenol, etc, should be avoided since these compounds may cause flocculation of the steroid. These dilutions will retain full potency for one week, but care should be exercised to avoid contamination of the vial's contents and the dilutions should be discarded after seven days.

Intralesional or Sublesional

Average Dose—up to 0.5 mg per square inch of affected skin injected intralesionally or sublesionally. The frequency of subsequent injections is best determined by the clinical response. If desired, the vial may be diluted as indicated under DIRECTIONS FOR USE.

A lesser initial dosage range of ARISTOSPAN® *triamcinolone hexacetonide* may produce the desired effect when the drug is administered to provide a localized concentration. The site of the injection and the volume of the injection should be carefully considered when ARISTOSPAN is administered for this purpose.

Dilution—Intra-articular 20 mg/ml

ARISTOSPAN suspension may be mixed with 1% or 2% Lidocaine Hydrochloride, using the formulations which do not contain parabens. Similar local anesthetics may also be used. Diluents containing methylparaben, propylparaben, phenol, etc, should be avoided since these compounds may cause flocculation of the steroid. These dilutions will retain full potency for one week, but care should be exercised to avoid contamination.

Intra-articular

Average dose—2 to 20 mg (0.1 ml to 1.0 ml)

The dose depends on the size of the joint to be injected, the degree of inflammation, and the amount of fluid present. In general, large joints (such as knee, hip, shoulder) require 10 to 20 mg. For small joints (such as interphalangeal, metacarpophalangeal), 2 to 6 mg may be employed. When the amount of synovial fluid is increased, aspiration may be performed before administering ARISTOSPAN. Subsequent dosage and frequency of injections can best be judged by clinical response.

The usual frequency of injection into a single joint is every three or four weeks, and injection more frequently than that is generally not advisable. To avoid possible joint destruction from repeated use of intra-articular corticosteroids, injection should be as infrequent as possible, consistent with adequate patient care. Attention should be paid to avoiding deposition of drug along the needle path which might produce atrophy.

HOW SUPPLIED

*Intralesional, 5 ml (in a 12.5 ml vial) NDC 0205-4502-31 Color Code Violet Cap.

*Intra-articular, 1 ml vial and 5 ml vial NDC 0205-4505-24, NDC 0205-4505-31.

A.H.F.S. 68:04

Military Depots: NSN-6505-00-148-6985, 5 ml vial

Store at Controlled Room Temperature 15°–30°C (59°–86°F).

DO NOT FREEZE

*Manufactured for
LEDERLE LABORATORIES DIVISION
American Cyanamid Company
Pearl River, NY 10965
by
LEDERLE PARENTERALS INC.
Carolina, Puerto Rico 00630

ARTANE® ℞

[*ar-tāne*]

trihexyphenidyl HCl

Tablets, Elixir, and SEQUELS—
Sustained Release Capsules

DESCRIPTION

ARTANE® *trihexyphenidyl HCl* is a synthetic antispasmodic drug available in the following forms:

TABLETS: Containing 2 mg and 5 mg ARTANE® *trihexyphenidyl HCl;* each strength also containing as inactive ingredients: Cornstarch, Dibasic Calcium Phosphate, Magnesium Stearate and Modified Starch.

ELIXIR: Containing 2 mg/5 ml ARTANE® *trihexyphenidyl HCl* in a clear, colorless, lime-mint flavored preparation; also containing as inactive ingredients: Alcohol, Citric Acid, Flavorings, Methylparaben, Propylparaben, Sodium Chloride and Sorbitol.

SEQUELS: Containing 5 mg ARTANE® *trihexyphenidyl HCl* as sustained release soft shell capsules; also containing as inactive ingredients: Beeswax, Benzoin Gum, Blue 1, Dibasic Calcium Phosphate, Ethylcellulose, Ethyl Vanillin, Gelatin, Glycerin, Glyceryl Stearate, Magnesium Stearate, Methylparaben, Mineral Oil, Non-pareil Seeds, Propylene Glycol, Propylparaben, Silica Gel, Sucrose, Talc, and Terpene Resin.

ACTIONS

ARTANE is the substituted piperidine salt, 3-(1-piperidyl)-1-phenyl-cyclohexyl-1-propanol hydrochloride, which exerts a direct inhibitory effect upon the parasympathetic nervous system. It also has a relaxing effect on smooth musculature; exerted both directly upon the muscle tissue itself and indirectly through an inhibitory effect upon the parasympathetic nervous system. Its therapeutic properties are similar to those of atropine, although undesirable side effects are ordinarily less frequent and severe than with the latter.

INDICATIONS

This drug is indicated as an adjunct in the treatment of all forms of parkinsonism (postencephalitic, arteriosclerotic, and idiopathic). It is often useful as adjuvant therapy when treating these forms of parkinsonism with levodopa. Additionally, it is indicated for the control of extrapyramidal disorders caused by central nervous system drugs such as the dibenoxazepines, phenothiazines, thioxanthenes, and butyrophenones.

SEQUELS—For maintenance therapy after patients have been stabilized on trihexyphenidyl hydrochloride in conventional dosage forms (tablets or elixir).

WARNING

Patients to be treated with ARTANE should have a gonioscope evaluation and close monitoring of intraocular pressures at regular periodic intervals.

PRECAUTIONS

Although trihexyphenidyl HCl is *not* contraindicated for patients with cardiac, liver, or kidney disorders, or with hypertension, such patients should be maintained under close observation.

Since the use of trihexyphenidyl HCl may, in some cases, continue indefinitely and since it has atropine-like properties, patients should be subjected to constant and careful long-term observation to avoid allergic and other untoward reactions. Inasmuch as trihexyphenidyl HCl possesses some parasympatholytic activity, it should be used with caution in patients with glaucoma, obstructive disease of the gastrointestinal or genitourinary tracts, and in elderly males with possible prostatic hypertrophy. Geriatric patients, particularly over the age of 60, frequently develop increased sensitivity to the actions of drugs of this type, and hence, require strict dosage regulation. Incipient glaucoma may be precipitated by parasympatholytic drugs such as trihexyphenidyl HCl.

Tardive dyskinesia may appear in some patients on long-term therapy with antipsychotic drugs or may occur after therapy with these drugs has been discontinued. Antiparkinsonism agents do not alleviate the symptoms of tardive dyskinesia, and in some instances may aggravate them. ARTANE® *trihexyphenidyl HCl* is not recommended for use in patients with tardive dyskinesia.

ADVERSE REACTIONS

Minor side effects, such as dryness of the mouth, blurring of vision, dizziness, mild nausea or nervousness, will be experienced by 30% to 50% of all patients. These sensations, however, are much less troublesome with ARTANE than with belladonna alkaloids and are usually less disturbing than unalleviated parkinsonism. Such reactions tend to become less pronounced, and even to disappear, as treatment continues. Even before these reactions have remitted spontaneously, they may often be controlled by careful adjustment of dosage form, amount of drug, or interval between doses.

Isolated instances of suppurative parotitis secondary to excessive dryness of the mouth, skin rashes, dilatation of the colon, paralytic ileus, and certain psychiatric manifestations such as delusions and hallucinations, plus one doubtful case of paranoia all of which may occur with any of the atropine-like drugs, have been rarely reported with ARTANE.

Patients with arteriosclerosis or with a history of idiosyncrasy to other drugs may exhibit reactions of mental confusion, agitation, disturbed behavior, or nausea and vomiting. Such patients should be allowed to develop a tolerance through the initial administration of a small dose and gradual increase in dose until an effective level is reached. If a severe reaction should occur, administration of the drug should be discontinued for a few days and then resumed at a lower dosage. Psychiatric disturbances can result from indiscriminate use (leading to overdosage) to sustain continued euphoria.

Potential side effects associated with the use of any atropine-like drugs include constipation, drowsiness, urinary hesitancy or retention, tachycardia, dilation of the pupil, increased intraocular tension, weakness, vomiting, and headache.

The occurrence of angle-closure glaucoma due to long-term treatment with trihexyphenidyl hydrochloride has been reported.

DOSAGE AND ADMINISTRATION

Dosage should be individualized. The initial dose should be low and then increased gradually, especially in patients over 60 years of age. Whether ARTANE may best be given before or after meals should be determined by the way the patient reacts. Postencephalitic patients, who are usually more prone to excessive salivation, may prefer to take it after meals and may, in addition, require small amounts of atropine which, under such circumstances, is sometimes an effective adjuvant. If ARTANE® *trihexyphenidyl HCl* tends to dry the mouth excessively, it may be better to take it before meals, unless it causes nausea. If taken after meals, the thirst sometimes induced can be allayed by mint candies, chewing gum or water.

ARTANE ® trihexyphenidyl HCl in Idiopathic parkinsonism

As initial therapy for parkinsonism, 1 mg of ARTANE in tablet or elixir form may be administered the first day. The dose may then be increased by 2 mg increments at intervals of three to five days, until a total of 6 to 10 mg is given daily. The total daily dose will depend upon what is found to be the optimal level. Many patients derive maximum benefit from this daily total of 6 to 10 mg, but some patients, chiefly those in the postencephalitic group, may require a total daily dose of 12 to 15 mg.

ARTANE in Drug-Induced parkinsonism

The size and frequency of dose of ARTANE needed to control extrapyramidal reactions to commonly employed tranquilizers, notably the phenothiazines, thioxanthenes, and butyrophenones, must be determined empirically. The total daily dosage usually ranges between 5 and 15 mg although, in some cases, these reactions have been satisfactorily controlled on as little as 1 mg daily. It may be advisable to commence therapy with a single 1 mg dose. If the extrapyramidal manifestations are not controlled in a few hours, the subsequent doses may be progressively increased until satisfactory control is achieved. Satisfactory control may sometimes be more rapidly achieved by temporarily reducing the dosage of the tranquilizer on instituting ARTANE therapy and then adjusting dosage of both drugs until the desired ataractic effect is retained without onset of extrapyramidal reactions.

It is sometimes possible to maintain the patient on a reduced ARTANE dosage after the reactions have remained under control for several days. Instances have been reported in which these reactions have remained in remission for long periods after ARTANE therapy was discontinued.

Concomitant Use of ARTANE with Levodopa

When ARTANE is used concomitantly with levodopa, the usual dose of each may need to be reduced. Careful adjustment is necessary, depending on side effects and degree of symptom control. ARTANE dosage of 3 to 6 mg daily, in divided doses, is usually adequate.

Concomitant Use of ARTANE with Other Parasympathetic Inhibitors

ARTANE may be substituted, in whole or in part, for other parasympathetic inhibitors. The usual technique is partial substitution initially, with progressive reduction in the other medication as the dose of trihexyphenidyl HCl is increased.

ARTANE TABLETS and ELIXIR—The total daily intake of ARTANE tablets or elixir is tolerated best if divided into 3 doses and taken at mealtimes. High doses (> 10 mg daily) may be divided into 4 parts, with 3 doses administered at mealtimes and the fourth at bedtime.

ARTANE SEQUELS—Because of the relatively high dosage in each controlled release capsule, this dosage form should not be used for initial therapy. After patients are stabilized on trihexyphenidyl HCl in conventional dosage forms (tablet or elixir), for convenience of administration they may be switched to the controlled release capsules on a milligram per milligram total daily dose basis, as a single dose after breakfast or in two divided doses 12 hours apart. Most patients will be adequately maintained on the controlled release form, but some may develop an exacerbation of parkinsonism and have to be returned to the conventional form.

HOW SUPPLIED

ARTANE® *trihexyphenidyl HCl* is available as follows:

TABLETS: 2 mg—round, flat, scored, white tablets, engraved ARTANE above 2 on one side and LL above A11 below the score on the other side, are supplied as follows:

NDC 0005-4434-23—Bottles of 100
NDC 0005-4434-34—Bottles of 1000
NDC 0005-4434-60—Unit Dose 10 × 10s

5 mg—round, flat, scored, white tablets; engraved ARTANE above 5 on one side and LL above A12 below the score on the other side, are supplied as follows:

NDC 0005-4436-23—Bottles of 100
NDC 0005-4436-34—Bottles of 1000
NDC 0005-4436-60—Unit Dose 10 × 10s

Store at Controlled Room Temperature 15°–30°C (59°–86°F).

ELIXIR: 2 mg/5ml—NDC 0005-4440-65—Bottles of 16 fl. oz.

Store at Controlled Room Temperature 15°–30°C (59°–86°F).

DO NOT FREEZE

SEQUELS SUSTAINED RELEASE CAPSULES: 5 mg—soft shell, oval shaped, clear blue, printed A9L, are supplied as follows:

NDC 0005-4438-32—Unit-of-Issue 60s with CRC
NDC 0005-4438-31—Bottles of 500

VA depot NSN 6505-00-890-1378—16 oz.

Store at Controlled Room Temperature 15°–30° C (59°–86° F).

Shown in Product Identification Section, page 413

ASENDIN® ℞
[*a-sen-din*]
amoxapine

DESCRIPTION

ASENDIN® *amoxapine* is an antidepressant of the dibenzoxazepine class, chemically distinct from the dibenzazepines, dibenzocycloheptenes, and dibenzoxepines.
It is designated chemically as 2-chloro-11-(1-piperazinyl) dibenz-[b,f][1,4]oxazepine. The molecular weight is 313.8. The empirical formula is $C_{17}H_{16}ClN_3O$.
ASENDIN is supplied for oral administration as 25 mg, 50 mg, 100 mg, and 150 mg tablets.
Inactive Ingredients
All tablets contain Cornstarch, Dibasic Calcium Phosphate, Modified Food Starch, Magnesium Stearate and Stearic Acid. Additionally, the 50 mg and 150 mg tablets contain Yellow 6 and the 100 mg tablet contains Blue 2.

CLINICAL PHARMACOLOGY

ASENDIN is an antidepressant with a mild sedative component to its action. The mechanism of its clinical action in man is not well understood. In animals, amoxapine reduced the uptake of norepinephrine and serotonin and blocked the response of dopamine receptors to dopamine. Amoxapine is not a monoamine oxidase inhibitor.
ASENDIN is absorbed rapidly and reaches peak blood levels approximately 90 minutes after ingestion. It is almost completely metabolized. The main route of excretion is the kidney. *In vitro* tests show that amoxapine binding to human serum is approximately 90%.
In man, amoxapine serum concentration declines with a half-life of eight hours. However, the major metabolite, 8-hydroxyamoxapine, has a biologic half-life of 30 hours. Metabolites are excreted in the urine in conjugated form as glucuronides.
Clinical studies have demonstrated that ASENDIN has a more rapid onset of action than either amitriptyline or imipramine. The initial clinical effect may occur within four to seven days and occurs within 2 weeks in over 80% of responders.

INDICATIONS AND USAGE

ASENDIN is indicated for the relief of symptoms of depression in patients with neurotic or reactive depressive disorders as well as endogenous and psychotic depressions. It is indicated for depression accompanied by anxiety or agitation.

CONTRAINDICATIONS

ASENDIN is contraindicated in patients who have shown prior hypersensitivity to dibenzoxazepine compounds. It should not be given concomitantly with monoamine oxidase inhibitors. Hyperpyretic crises, severe convulsions, and deaths have occurred in patients receiving tricyclic antidepressants and monoamine oxidase inhibitors simultaneously. When it is desired to replace a monoamine oxidase inhibitor with ASENDIN, a minimum of 14 days should be allowed to elapse after the former is discontinued. ASENDIN should then be initiated cautiously with gradual increase in dosage until optimum response is achieved. The drug is not recommended for use during the acute recovery phase following myocardial infarction.

WARNINGS

Tardive Dyskinesia:
Tardive dyskinesia, a syndrome consisting of potentially irreversible, involuntary, dyskinetic movements may develop in patients treated with neuroleptic (ie, antipsychotics) drugs. (Amoxapine is not an antipsychotic, but it has substantive neuroleptic activity). Although the prevalence of the syndrome appears to be highest among the elderly, especially elderly women, it is impossible to rely upon prevalence estimates to predict, at the inception of neuroleptic treatment, which patients are likely to develop the syndrome. Whether neuroleptic drug products differ in their potential to cause tardive dyskinesia is unknown.
Both the risk of developing the syndrome and the likelihood that it will become irreversible are believed to increase as the duration of treatment and the total cumulative dose of neuroleptic drugs administered to the patient increase. However, the syndrome can develop, although much less commonly, after relatively brief treatment periods at low doses.
There is no known treatment for established cases of tardive dyskinesia, although the syndrome may remit, partially or completely, if neuroleptic treatment is withdrawn. Neuroleptic treatment itself, however, may suppress (or partially suppress) the signs and symptoms of the syndrome and thereby may possibly mask the underlying disease process. The effect that symptomatic suppression has upon the long-term course of the syndrome is unknown.
Given these considerations, neuroleptics should be prescribed in a manner that is most likely to minimize the occurrence of tardive dyskinesia. Chronic neuroleptic treatment should generally be reserved for patients who suffer from a chronic illness that, 1) is known to respond to neuroleptic drugs, and, 2) for whom alternative, equally effective, but potentially less harmful treatments are not available or appropriate. In patients who do require chronic treatment, the smallest dose and the shortest duration of treatment producing a satisfactory clinical response should be sought. The need for continued treatment should be reassessed periodically.
If signs and symptoms of tardive dyskinesia appear in a patient on neuroleptics, drug discontinuation should be considered. However, some patients may require treatment despite the presence of the syndrome.
(For further information about the description of tardive dyskinesia and its clinical detection, please refer to the sections on Information for Patients and Adverse Reactions.)
ASENDIN® *amoxapine* should be used with caution in patients with a history of urinary retention, angle-closure glaucoma, or increased intraocular pressure. Patients with cardiovascular disorders should be watched closely. Tricyclic antidepressant drugs, particularly when given in high doses, can induce sinus tachycardia, changes in conduction time, and arrhythmias. Myocardial infarction and stroke have been reported with drugs of this class.
Extreme caution should be used in treating patients with a history of convulsive disorder or those with overt or latent seizure disorders.

PRECAUTIONS

General:
In prescribing the drug, it should be borne in mind that the possibility of suicide is inherent in any severe depression, and persists until a significant remission occurs; the drug should be dispensed in the smallest suitable amount. Manic depressive patients may experience a shift to the manic phase. Schizophrenic patients may develop increased symptoms of psychosis; patients with paranoid symptomatology may have an exaggeration of such symptoms. This may require reduction of dosage or the addition of a major tranquilizer to the therapeutic regimen. Antidepressant drugs can cause skin rashes and/or "drug fever" in susceptible individuals. These allergic reactions may, in rare cases, be severe. They are more likely to occur during the first few days of treatment, but may also occur later. ASENDIN® *amoxapine* should be discontinued if rash and/or fever develop. Amoxapine possesses a degree of dopamine-blocking activity which may cause extrapyramidal symptoms in <1% of patients. Rarely, symptoms indicative of tardive dyskinesia have been reported.
Information for the patient:
Given the likelihood that some patients exposed chronically to neuroleptics will develop tardive dyskinesia, it is advised that all patients in whom chronic use is contemplated be given, if possible, full information about this risk. The decision to inform patients and/or their guardians must obviously take into account the clinical circumstances and the competency of the patient to understand the information provided.
Patients should be warned of the possibility of drowsiness that may impair performance of potentially hazardous tasks such as driving an automobile or operating machinery.
Drug interactions:
See "Contraindications" about concurrent usage of tricyclic antidepressants and monoamine oxidase inhibitors. Paralytic ileus may occur in patients taking tricyclic antidepressants in combination with anticholinergic drugs. ASENDIN may enhance the response to alcohol and the effects of barbiturates and other CNS depressants. Serum levels of several tricyclic antidepressants have been reported to be significantly increased when cimetidine is administered concurrently. Although such an interaction has not been reported to date with ASENDIN, specific interaction studies have not been done, and the possibility should be considered.
Therapeutic interactions:
Concurrent administration with electroshock therapy may increase the hazards associated with such therapy.
Carcinogenesis, impairment of fertility:
In a 21-month toxicity study at three dose levels in rats, pancreatic islet cell hyperplasia occurred with slightly increased incidence at doses 5–10 times the human dose. Pancreatic adenocarcinoma was detected in low incidence in the mid-dose group only, and may possibly have resulted from endocrine-mediated organ hyperfunction. The significance of these findings to man is not known.
Treatment of male rats with 5 to 10 times the human dose resulted in a slight decrease in the number of fertile matings. Female rats receiving oral doses within the therapeutic range displayed a reversible increase in estrous cycle length.
Pregnancy. Pregnancy category C:
Studies performed in mice, rats, and rabbits have demonstrated no evidence of teratogenic effect due to ASENDIN. Embryotoxicity was seen in rats and rabbits given oral doses approximating the human dose. Fetotoxic effects (intrauterine death, stillbirth, decreased birth weight) were seen in animals studied at oral doses 3 to 10 times the human dose. Decreased postnatal survival (between days 0–4) was demonstrated in the offspring of rats at 5 to 10 times the human dose. There are no adequate and well-controlled studies in pregnant women. ASENDIN® *amoxapine* should be used during pregnancy only if the potential benefit justifies the potential risk to the fetus.
Nursing mothers:
ASENDIN, like many other systemic drugs, is excreted in human milk. Because effects of the drug on infants are unknown, caution should be exercised when ASENDIN is administered to nursing women.
Pediatric use:
Safety and effectiveness in children below the age of 16 have not been established.

ADVERSE REACTIONS

Adverse reactions reported in controlled studies in the United States are categorized with respect to incidence below. Following this is a listing of reactions known to occur with other antidepressant drugs of this class but not reported to date with ASENDIN.
Incidence Greater Than 1%
The most frequent types of adverse reactions occurring with ASENDIN® *amoxapine* in controlled clinical trials were sedative and anticholinergic: these included drowsiness (14%), dry mouth (14%), constipation (12%), and blurred vision (7%).
Less frequently reported reactions are:
CNS and Neuromuscular—anxiety, insomnia, restlessness, nervousness, palpitations, tremors, confusion, excitement, nightmares, ataxia, alterations in EEG patterns.
Allergic—edema, skin rash.
Endocrine—elevation of prolactin levels.
Gastrointestinal—nausea.
Other—dizziness, headache, fatigue, weakness, excessive appetite, increased perspiration.
Incidence Less Than 1%
Anticholinergic—disturbances of accommodation, mydriasis, delayed micturition, urinary retention, nasal stuffiness.
Cardiovascular—hypotension, hypertension, syncope, tachycardia.
Allergic—drug fever, urticaria, photosensitization, pruritus, rarely, vasculitis, hepatitis.
CNS and Neuromuscular—tingling, paresthesias of the extremities, tinnitus, disorientation, seizures, hypomania, numbness, incoordination, disturbed concentration, hyperthermia, extrapyramidal symptoms, including, rarely, tardive dyskinesia. Neuroleptic malignant syndrome has been reported.
Hematologic—leukopenia, agranulocytosis.
Gastrointestinal—epigastric distress, vomiting, flatulence, abdominal pain, peculiar taste, diarrhea.
Endocrine—increased or decreased libido, impotence, menstrual irregularity, breast enlargement and galactorrhea in the female, syndrome of inappropriate antidiuretic hormone secretion.
Other—lacrimation, weight gain or loss, altered liver function.
Drug Relationship Unknown: The following reactions have been reported very rarely, and occurred under uncontrolled circumstances where a drug relationship was difficult to assess. These observations are listed to serve as alerting information to physicians.
Anticholinergic—paralytic ileus.
Cardiovascular—atrial arrhythmias (including atrial fibrillation), myocardial infarction, stroke, heart block.
CNS and Neuromuscular—hallucinations.
Hematologic—thrombocytopenia, eosinophilia, purpura, petechiae.
Gastrointestinal—parotid swelling.
Endocrine—change in blood glucose levels.
Other—pancreatitis, hepatitis, jaundice, urinary frequency, testicular swelling, anorexia, alopecia.
Additional Adverse Reactions: The following reactions have been reported with other antidepressant drugs, but not with ASENDIN® *amoxapine*.
Anticholinergic—sublingual adenitis, dilation of the urinary tract.
CNS and Neuromuscular—delusions.
Gastrointestinal—stomatitis, black tongue.
Endocrine—gynecomastia.

OVERDOSAGE

Signs and Symptoms
Toxic manifestations of ASENDIN overdosage differ significantly from those of other tricyclic antidepressants. Serious

Continued on next page

The information on each product appearing here is based on labelling effective in August, 1986 and is either the entire official brochure or an accurate condensation therefrom. Information concerning all Lederle products may be obtained from the Professional Services Department, Lederle Laboratories, Pearl River, New York, 10965.

Lederle—Cont.

cardiovascular effects are seldom if ever observed. However, CNS effects—particularly grand mal convulsions—occur frequently, and treatment should be directed primarily toward prevention or control of seizures. Status epilepticus may develop and constitutes a neurologic emergency. Coma and acidosis are other serious complications of substantial ASENDIN overdosage in some cases.
Renal failure may develop two to five days after toxic overdosage in patients who may appear otherwise recovered. Acute tubular necrosis with rhabdomyolysis and myoglobinuria is the most common renal complication in such cases. This reaction probably occurs in less than 5% of overdose cases, and typically in those who have experienced multiple seizures.

Treatment

Treatment of ASENDIN overdosage should be symptomatic and supportive, but with special attention to prevention or control of seizures. If the patient is conscious, induced emesis followed by gastric lavage with appropriate precautions to prevent pulmonary aspiration should be accomplished as soon as possible. Following lavage, activated charcoal may be administered to reduce absorption, and repeated administrations may facilitate drug elimination. An adequate airway should be established in comatose patients and assisted ventilation instituted if necessary. Seizures may respond to standard anticonvulsant therapy such as intravenous diazepam and/or phenytoin. The value of physostigmine appears less certain. Status epilepticus, should it develop, requires vigorous treatment such as that described by Delgado-Escueta et al (*N Engl J Med* 1982; 306:1337-1340).
Convulsions, when they occur, typically begin within 12 hours after ingestion. Because seizures may occur precipitously in some overdosage patients who appear otherwise relatively asymptomatic, the treating physician may wish to consider prophylactic administration of anticonvulsant medication during this period.
Treatment of renal impairment, should it occur, is the same as that for non-drug-induced renal dysfunction.
Serious cardiovascular effects are remarkably rare following ASENDIN® *amoxapine* overdosage, and the ECG typically remains within normal limits except for sinus tachycardia. Hence, prolongation of the QRS interval beyond 100 milliseconds within the first 24 hours is *not* a useful guide to the severity of overdosage with this drug.
Fatalities and, rarely, neurologic sequelae have resulted from prolonged status epilepticus in ASENDIN overdosage patients. While the lethal dose appears higher than that of other tricyclic antidepressants (80% of lethal ASENDIN overdosages have involved ingestion of 3 grams or more), many factors other than amount ingested are important in assessing probability of survival. These include age and physical condition of the patient, concomitant ingestion of other drugs, and especially the interval between drug ingestion and initiation of emergency treatment.

DOSAGE AND ADMINISTRATION

Effective dosage of ASENDIN may vary from one patient to another. Usual effective dosage is 200 mg to 300 mg daily. Three weeks constitute an adequate period of trial, providing dosage has reached 300 mg daily (or lower level of tolerance) for at least 2 weeks. If no response is seen at 300 mg, dosage may be increased, depending upon tolerance, up to 400 mg daily. Hospitalized patients who have been refractory to antidepressant therapy and who have no history of convulsive seizures may have dosage raised cautiously up to 600 mg daily in divided doses.
ASENDIN may be given in a single daily dose, not to exceed 300 mg, preferably at bedtime. If the total daily dosage exceeds 300 mg, it should be given in divided doses.

Initial Dosage for Adults:

Usual starting dosage is 50 mg two or three times daily. Depending upon tolerance, dosage may be increased to 100 mg two or three times daily by the end of the first week. (Initial dosage of 300 mg daily may be given, but notable sedation may occur in some patients during the first few days of therapy at this level.) Increases above 300 mg daily should be made only if 300 mg daily has been ineffective during a trial period of at least 2 weeks. When effective dosage is established, the drug may be given in a single dose (not to exceed 300 mg) at bedtime.

Elderly Patients:

In general, lower dosages are recommended for these patients. Recommended starting dosage of ASENDIN is 25 mg two or three times daily. If no intolerance is observed, dosage may be increased by the end of the first week to 50 mg two or three times daily. Although 100 mg to 150 mg daily may be adequate for many elderly patients, some may require higher dosage. Careful increases up to 300 mg daily are indicated in such cases.
Once an effective dosage is established, ASENDIN may conveniently be given in a single bedtime dose, not to exceed 300 mg.

Maintenance:

Recommended maintenance dosage of ASENDIN is the lowest dose that will maintain remission. If symptoms reappear, dosage should be increased to the earlier level until they are controlled.
For maintenance therapy at dosages of 300 mg or less, a single dose at bedtime is recommended.

HOW SUPPLIED

ASENDIN® *amoxapine* Tablets are supplied as follows:
25 mg—White, heptagon-shaped tablets, engraved on one side with LL above 25 and with A13 on the other scored side. (Product No. NDC 0005-5389-23)—Bottles of 100
50 mg—Orange, heptagon-shaped tablets, engraved on one side with LL above 50 and with A15 on the other scored side. (Product No. NDC 0005-5390-23)—Bottles of 100 (Product No. NDC 0005-5390-31)—Bottles of 500 (Product No. NDC 0005-5390-60)—10 ×10 Unit Dose
100 mg—Blue, heptagon-shaped tablets, engraved on one side with LL above 100 and with A17 on the other scored side. (Product No. NDC 0005-5391-23)—Bottles of 100 (Product No. NDC 0005-5391-60)—10×10 Unit Dose
150 mg—Peach, heptagon-shaped tablets, engraved on one side with LL above 150 and with A18 on the other scored side. (Product No. NDC 0005-5392-38)—Bottles of 30 with CRC

VA and Military Depots: Tablets 50 mg, 100s NSN 6505-01-111-3195 100 mg 100s NSN 6505-01-111-3194

Store at Controlled Room Temperature 15°–30° C (59°–86° F).
LEDERLE LABORATORIES DIVISION
American Cyanamid Company, Pearl River, NY 10965

Shown in Product Identification Section, page 413

AUREOMYCIN®

[or-ĕō-mī-cin]
chlortetracycline HCl 3%
OINTMENT

HOW SUPPLIED

½ and 1 oz tubes. Rx not required NDC 0005-4442-56, NDC 0005-4442-55.

CALTRATE® 600

High Potency Calcium Supplement

(See PDR For Nonprescription Drugs)

CALTRATE® 600 +D

High Potency Calcium Supplement

(See PDR For Nonprescription Drugs)

CALTRATE® 600 + Iron and Vitamin D

(See PDR For Nonprescription Drugs)

Advanced Formula

CENTRUM®

[sĕn-trŭm]
High Potency
Multivitamin-Multimineral Formula

(See PDR For Nonprescription Drugs)

Children's Chewable

CENTRUM, Jr.®

[sĕn-trŭm]
Vitamin/Mineral Formula + Iron

(See PDR For Nonprescription Drugs)

Advanced Formula
Children's Chewable

CENTRUM, Jr.®

[sĕn-trŭm]
Vitamin/Mineral Formula + Extra C

(See PDR For Nonprescription Drugs)

CHOLERA VACCINE ℞

[kŏl-ĕra]
(India Strains)

HOW SUPPLIED

1 ml vial (1 immunization) NDC 0005-1976-24
COMPLETE INFORMATION FURNISHED IN THE PACKAGE.

CYCLOCORT® ℞

[sī-clō-cŏrt]
Amcinonide Topical Cream 0.1%
with AQUATAIN™ hydrophilic base

CYCLOCORT® ℞

Amcinonide Ointment 0.1%

DESCRIPTION

0.1% topical cream.

Each gram of CYCLOCORT Topical Cream contains 1 mg of the active steroid Amcinonide in AQUATAIN, a specially formulated cream base composed of emulsifying wax NF, isopropyl palmitate, glycerin USP, sorbitol solution USP, lactic acid, 2% benzyl alcohol and purified water. AQUATAIN is non-staining, water-washable, paraben-free, spermaceti-free and has a light texture and consistency. Amcinonide is (11β, 16α) - 21-(acetyloxy)-16, 17-[cyclopentylidenebis(oxy)]-9-fluoro-11-hydroxypregna-1,4-diene-3,20-dione.

0.1% topical ointment.

Each gram of CYCLOCORT Ointment contains 1 mg of the active steroid amcinonide in a specially formulated base composed of petrolatum, white USP; benzyl alcohol NF, emulsifying wax NF; and Tenox II (butylated hydroxyanisole, propyl gallate, citric acid, propylene glycol).
The topical corticosteroids constitute a class of primarily synthetic steroids used as anti-inflammatory and antipruritic agents.

CLINICAL PHARMACOLOGY

Topical corticosteroids share anti-inflammatory, antipruritic and vasoconstrictive actions.
The mechanism of anti-inflammatory activity of the topical corticosteroids is unclear. Various laboratory methods, including vasoconstrictor assays, are used to compare and predict potencies and/or clinical efficacies of the topical corticosteroids. There is some evidence to suggest that a recognizable correlation exists between vasoconstrictor potency and therapeutic efficacy in man.
Pharmacokinetics: The extent of percutaneous absorption of topical corticosteroids is determined by many factors including the vehicle, the integrity of the epidermal barrier, and the use of occlusive dressings.
Topical corticosteroids can be absorbed from normal intact skin. Inflammation and/or other disease processes in the skin increase percutaneous absorption. Occlusive dressings substantially increase the percutaneous absorption of topical corticosteroids. Thus, occlusive dressings may be a valuable therapeutic adjunct for treatment of resistant dermatoses. (See *DOSAGE AND ADMINISTRATION*).
Once absorbed through the skin, topical corticosteroids are handled through pharmacokinetic pathways similar to systemically administered corticosteroids. Corticosteroids are bound to plasma proteins in varying degrees. Corticosteroids are metabolized primarily in the liver and are then excreted by the kidneys. Some of the topical corticosteroids and their metabolities are also excreted into the bile.

INDICATIONS AND USAGE

Topical corticosteroids are indicated for the relief of the inflammatory and pruritic manifestations of corticosteroid-responsive dermatoses.

CONTRAINDICATIONS

Topical corticosteroids are contraindicated in those patients with a history of hypersensitivity to any of the components of the preparation.

PRECAUTIONS

General: Systemic absorption of topical corticosteroids has produced reversible hypothalamic-pituitary-adrenal (HPA) axis suppression, manifestations of Cushing's syndrome, hyperglycemia, and glucosuria in some patients.
Conditions which augment systemic absorption include the application of the more potent steroids, use over large surface areas, prolonged use, and the addition of occlusive dressings.
Therefore, patients receiving a large dose of a potent topical steroid applied to a large surface area or under an occlusive dressing should be evaluated periodically for evidence of HPA axis suppression by using the urinary free cortisol and ACTH stimulation tests. If HPA axis suppression is noted, an attempt should be made to withdraw the drug, to reduce the frequency of application, or to substitute a less potent steroid.
Recovery of HPA axis function is generally prompt and complete upon discontinuation of the drug. Infrequently, signs and symptoms of steroid withdrawal may occur, requiring supplemental systemic corticosteroids.
Children may absorb proportionally larger amounts of topical corticosteroids and thus be more susceptible to system toxicity. (See *PRECAUTIONS—Pediatric Use*). If irritation develops, topical corticosteroids should be discontinued and appropriate therapy instituted.
In the presence of dermatological infections, the use of an appropriate antifungal or antibacterial agent should be instituted. If a favorable response does not occur promptly, the

corticosteroid should be discontinued until the infection has been adequately controlled.
The product is not for ophthalmic use.
Information for the Patient: Patients using topical corticosteroids should receive the following information and instructions:
1. This medication is to be used as directed by the physician. It is for external use only. Avoid contact with the eyes.
2. Patients should be advised not to use this medication for any disorder other than for which it was prescribed.
3. The treated skin area should not be bandaged or otherwise covered or wrapped as to be occlusive unless directed by the physician.
4. Patients should report any signs of local adverse reactions especially under occlusive dressing.
5. Parents of pediatric patients should be advised not to use tight-fitting diapers or plastic pants on a child being treated in the diaper area, as these garments may constitute occlusive dressings.

Laboratory Tests: The following tests may be helpful in evaluating the HPA axis suppression:
Urinary free cortisol test.
ACTH stimulation test.
Carcinogenesis, Mutagenesis, and Impairment of Fertility: Long-term animal studies have not been performed to evaluate the carcinogenic potential or the effect on fertility of topical corticosteroids.
Studies to determine mutagenicity with prednisolone and hydrocortisone have revealed negative results.
Pregnancy Category C: Corticosteroids are generally teratogenic in laboratory animals when administered systemically at relatively low dosage levels. The more potent corticosteroids have been shown to be teratogenic after dermal application in laboratory animals. There are no adequate and well-controlled studies in pregnant women on teratogenic effects from topically applied corticosteroids. Therefore, topical corticosteroids should be used during pregnancy only if the potential benefit justifies the potential risk to the fetus. Drugs of this class should not be used extensively on pregnant patients, in large amounts, or for prolonged periods of time.
Nursing Mothers: It is not known whether topical administration of corticosteroids could result in sufficient systemic absorption to produce detectable quantities in breast milk. Systemically administered corticosteroids are secreted into breast milk in quantities *not* likely to have a deleterious effect on the infant. Nevertheless, caution should be exercised when topical corticosteroids are administered to a nursing woman.
Pediatric Use: Pediatric patients may demonstrate greater susceptibility to topical corticosteroid-induced HPA axis suppression and Cushing's syndrome than mature patients because of a larger skin surface area to body weight ratio.
Hypothalamic-pituitary-adrenal (HPA) axis suppression, Cushing's syndrome, and intracranial hypertension have been reported in children receiving topical corticosteroids. Manifestations of adrenal suppression in children include linear growth retardation, delayed weight gain, low plasma cortisol levels, and absence of response to ACTH stimulation. Manifestations of intracranial hypertension include bulging fontanelles, headaches, and bilateral papilledema.
Administration of topical corticosteroids to children should be limited to the least amount compatible with an effective therapeutic regimen. Chronic corticosteroid therapy may interfere with the growth and development of children.

ADVERSE REACTIONS

The following local adverse reactions are reported infrequently with topical corticosteroids, but may occur more frequently with the use of occlusive dressings. These reactions are listed in an approximate decreasing order of occurrence: burning, itching, irritation, dryness, folliculitis, hypertrichosis, acneiform eruptions, hypopigmentation, perioral dermatitis, allergic contact dermatitis, maceration of the skin, secondary infection, skin atrophy, striae, miliaria.

OVERDOSAGE

Topically applied corticosteroids can be absorbed in sufficient amounts to produce systemic effects (See *PRECAUTIONS*).

DOSAGE AND ADMINISTRATION

CYCLOCORT Cream 0.1% should be applied to the affected area as a thin film from two to three times daily, depending on the severity of the condition. CYCLOCORT Ointment 0.1% should be applied to the affected area as a thin film twice daily, depending on the severity of the condition.
Occlusive dressings may be used for the management of psoriasis or recalcitrant conditions.
If an infection develops, the use of occlusive dressings should be discontinued and appropriate antimicrobial therapy instituted.

HOW SUPPLIED

CYCLOCORT® Amcinonide Cream 0.1% (1 mg/gm) with AQUATAIN hydrophilic base is available as follows:
15 gram tubes—NDC 0005-9183-09
30 gram tubes—NDC 0005-9183-32
60 gram tubes—NDC 0005-9183-40
CYCLOCORT® Amcinonide Topical Ointment 0.1% (1 mg/gm) is available as follows:
15 gram tubes—NDC 0005-9345-09
30 gram tubes—NDC 0005-9345-32
60 gram tubes—NDC 0005-9345-40
Store at Controlled Room Temperature 15°–30°C (59–86°F)
60 gram tube VA NSN 6505-01-093-7968
Military Depot: Cyclocort Cream 0.1% NSN 6505-01-139-5001, 15 gm tube NSN 6505-01-093-7968, 60 gm tube; Cyclocort Ointment 0.1% NSN 6505-01-150-3824
Shown in Product Identification Section, page 413

DECLOMYCIN® ℞

[*dĕk-lō-mī-sĭn*]
Demeclocycline Hydrochloride
For Oral Use

DESCRIPTION

DECLOMYCIN® *demeclocycline hydrochloride* is an antibiotic isolated from a mutant strain of *Streptomyces aureofaciens*. Chemically it is [4S-(4α,4aα,5aα,6β,12aα)]-7-Chloro-4-dimethylamino)-1,4,4a,5,5a,6,11,12a-octahydro- 3,6,10,12, 12a-pentahydroxy-1,11-dioxo -2- naphthacenecarboxamide monohydrochloride.

Inactive Ingredients

DECLOMYCIN® *demeclocycline hydrochloride* contains the following inactive ingredients:
Capsules: Benzoin Gum, Blue 1, Cornstarch, Ethyl Vanillin, Gelatin, Glycerin, Methylparaben, Mineral Oil, Propylene Glycol, Propylparaben, Red 33, Red 40, Silica Aerogel, Terpene Resin, Titanium Dioxide, Yellow 6.
Tablets: Alginic Acid, Cornstarch, Ethylcellulose, Hydroxypropyl Methylcellulose, Magnesium Stearate, Red 7, Sorbitol, Titanium Dioxide, and other ingredients.

ACTIONS

The tetracyclines are primarily bacteriostatic and are thought to exert their antimicrobial effect by the inhibition of protein synthesis. Tetracyclines are active against a wide range of Gram-negative and Gram-positive organisms.
The drugs in the tetracycline class have closely similar antimicrobial spectra, and cross-resistance among them is common. Microorganisms may be considered susceptible if the MIC (minimum inhibitory concentration) is not more than 4.0 mcg/ml and intermediate if the MIC is 4.0 to 12.5 mcg/ml.
Susceptibility plate testing: A tetracycline disc may be used to determine microbial susceptibility to drugs in the tetracycline class. If the Kirby-Bauer method of disc susceptibility testing is used, a 30 mcg tetracycline disc should give a zone of at least 19 mm when tested against a tetracycline-susceptible bacterial strain.
Tetracyclines are readily absorbed and are bound to plasma proteins in varying degree. They are concentrated by the liver in the bile and excreted in the urine and feces at high concentrations and in a biologically active form.

INDICATIONS

DECLOMYCIN is indicated in infections caused by the following microorganisms:
Rickettsiae: (Rocky Mountain spotted fever, typhus fever and the typhus group, Q fever, rickettsialpox, tick fevers.)
Mycoplasma pneumoniae (PPLO, Eaton agent).
Agents of psittacosis and ornithosis.
Agents of lymphogranuloma venereum and granuloma inguinale.
The spirochetal agent of relapsing fever (*Borrelia recurrentis*).
The following Gram-negative microorganisms:
Haemophilus ducreyi (chancroid),
Pasteurella pestis and *Pasteurella tularensis,*
Bartonella bacilliformis,
Bacteroides species,
Vibrio comma and *Vibrio fetus.*
Brucella species (in conjunction with streptomycin).
Because many strains of the following groups of microorganisms have been shown to be resistant to tetracyclines, culture and susceptibility testing are recommended.
Demeclocycline is indicated for treatment of infections caused by the following Gram-negative microorganisms, when bacteriologic testing indicates appropriate susceptibility to the drug:
Escherichia coli,
Enterobacter aerogenes (formerly *Aerobacter aerogenes*),
Shigella species,
Mima species and *Herellea* species,
Haemophilus influenzae (respiratory infections),
Klebsiella species (respiratory and urinary infections).
DECLOMYCIN is indicated for treatment of infections caused by the following Gram-positive microorganisms when bacteriologic testing indicates appropriate susceptibility to the drug:
Streptococcus species:
Up to 44% of strains of *Streptococcus pyogenes* and 74% of *Streptococcus faecalis* have been found to be resistant to tetracycline drugs. Therefore, tetracyclines should not be used for streptococcal disease unless the organism has been demonstrated to be sensitive.
For upper respiratory infections due to Group A beta-hemolytic streptococci, penicillin is the usual drug of choice, including prophylaxis of rheumatic fever.
Diplococcus pneumoniae,
Staphylococcus aureus, skin and soft tissue infections. Tetracyclines are not the drugs of choice in the treatment of any type of staphylococcal infection.
When penicillin is contraindicated, tetracyclines are alternative drugs in the treatment of infections due to:
Neisseria gonorrhoeae,
Treponema pallidum and *Treponema pertenue* (syphilis and yaws),
Listeria monocytogenes,
Clostridium species,
Bacillus anthracis,
Fusobacterium fusiforme (Vincent's infection),
Actinomyces species.
In acute intestinal amebiasis, the tetracyclines may be a useful adjunct to amebicides.
DECLOMYCIN® *demeclocycline hydrochloride* is indicated in the treatment of trachoma, although the infectious agent is not always eliminated, as judged by immunofluorescence.
Inclusion conjunctivitis may be treated with oral tetracyclines or with a combination of oral and topical agents.

CONTRAINDICATIONS

This drug is contraindicated in persons who have shown hypersensitivity to any of the tetracyclines.

WARNINGS

THE USE OF DRUGS OF THE TETRACYCLINE CLASS DURING TOOTH DEVELOPMENT (LAST HALF OF PREGNANCY, INFANCY, AND CHILDHOOD TO THE AGE OF 8 YEARS) MAY CAUSE PERMANENT DISCOLORATION OF THE TEETH (YELLOW-GRAY-BROWN). This adverse reaction is more common during long-term use of the drugs but has been observed following repeated short-term courses. Enamel hypoplasia has also been reported. TETRACYCLINE DRUGS, THEREFORE, SHOULD NOT BE USED IN THIS AGE GROUP UNLESS OTHER DRUGS ARE NOT LIKELY TO BE EFFECTIVE OR ARE CONTRAINDICATED.
If renal impairment exists, even usual oral or parenteral doses may lead to excessive systemic accumulation of the drug and possible liver toxicity. Under such conditions, lower-than-usual total doses are indicated and, if therapy is prolonged, serum level determinations of the drug may be advisable.
Phototoxic reactions can occur in individuals taking demeclocycline, and are characterized by severe burns of exposed surfaces resulting from direct exposure of patients to sunlight during therapy with moderate or large doses of demeclocycline. Patients apt to be exposed to direct sunlight or ultraviolet light should be advised that this reaction can occur, and treatment should be discontinued at the first evidence of skin erythema.
The antianabolic action of the tetracyclines may cause an increase in BUN. While this is not a problem in those with normal renal function, in patients with significantly impaired function, higher serum levels of tetracycline may lead to azotemia, hyperphosphatemia, and acidosis.
Administration of DECLOMYCIN® *demeclocycline* has resulted in appearance of the diabetes insipidus syndrome (polyuria, polydipsia, and weakness) in some patients on long-term therapy. The syndrome has been shown to be nephrogenic, dose-dependent, and reversible on discontinuance of therapy.
Usage in pregnancy (See above "Warnings" about use during tooth development).
Results of animal studies indicate that tetracyclines cross the placenta, are found in fetal tissues, and can have toxic effects on the developing fetus (often related to retardation of skeletal development). Evidence of embryotoxicity has also been noted in animals treated early in pregnancy.
Usage in newborns, infants, and children (See above "Warnings" about use during tooth development).
All tetracyclines form a stable calcium complex in any bone-forming tissue. A decrease in the fibula growth rate has been

Continued on next page

The information on each product appearing here is based on labelling effective in August, 1986 and is either the entire official brochure or an accurate condensation therefrom. Information concerning all Lederle products may be obtained from the Professional Services Department, Lederle Laboratories, Pearl River, New York, 10965.

Lederle—Cont.

observed in prematures given oral tetracycline in doses of 25 mg/kg every six hours. This reaction was shown to be reversible when the drug was discontinued.

Tetracyclines are present in the milk of lactating women who are taking a drug in this class.

PRECAUTIONS

As with other antibiotic preparations, use of this drug may result in overgrowth of nonsusceptible organisms, including fungi. If superinfection occurs, the antibiotic should be discontinued and appropriate therapy should be instituted.

In venereal diseases when coexistent syphilis is suspected, darkfield examination should be done before treatment is started and the blood serology repeated monthly for at least four months.

Because the tetracyclines have been shown to depress plasma prothrombin activity, patients who are on anticoagulant therapy may require downward adjustment of their anticoagulant dosage.

In long-term therapy, periodic laboratory evaluation of organ systems, including hematopoietic, renal, and hepatic, studies should be performed.

All infections due to Group A beta-hemolytic streptococci should be treated for at least ten days.

Since bacteriostatic drugs may interfere with the bactericidal action of penicillin, it is advisable to avoid giving demeclocycline in conjunction with penicillin.

Interpretation of Bacteriologic Studies: Following a course of therapy, persistence for several days in both urine and blood of bacteriosuppressive levels of demeclocycline may interfere with culture studies. These levels should not be considered therapeutic.

ADVERSE REACTIONS

Gastrointestinal: Anorexia, nausea, vomiting, diarrhea, glossitis, dysphagia, enterocolitis, and inflammatory lesions (with monilial overgrowth) in the anogenital region. Hepatic toxicity has been reported rarely. These reactions have been caused by both the oral and parenteral administration of tetracyclines.

Skin: Maculopapular and erythematous rashes. Exfoliative dermatitis has been reported but is uncommon. Photosensitivity is discussed above. (See "Warnings").

Renal toxicity: Rise in BUN has been reported and is apparently dose related. Nephrogenic diabetes insipidus. (See "Warnings").

Hypersensitivity reactions: Urticaria, angioneurotic edema, anaphylaxis, anaphylactoid purpura, pericarditis, and exacerbation of systemic lupus erythematosus.

Bulging fontanels have been reported in young infants following full therapeutic dosage. This sign disappeared rapidly when the drug was discontinued.

Blood: Hemolytic anemia, thrombocytopenia, neutropenia, and eosinophilia have been reported.

When given over prolonged periods, tetracyclines have been reported to produce brown-black microscopic discoloration of thyroid glands. No abnormalities of thyroid function studies are known to occur.

DOSAGE AND ADMINISTRATION

Therapy should be continued for at least 24 to 48 hours after symptoms and fever have subsided.

Concomitant therapy: Antacids containing aluminum, calcium, or magnesium impair absorption and should not be given to patients taking oral tetracycline.

Foods and some dairy products also interfere with absorption. Oral forms of tetracycline should be given one hour before or two hours after meals.

In patients with renal impairment: (See "Warnings"). Total dosage should be decreased by reduction of recommended individual doses and/or by extending time intervals between doses.

In the treatment of streptococcal infections, a therapeutic dose of demeclocycline should be administered for at least ten days.

Adults: Usual daily dose—Four divided doses of 150 mg each or two divided doses of 300 mg each.

For children above eight years of age: Usual daily dose, 3 mg to 6 mg per pound body weight per day, depending upon the severity of the disease, divided into 2 to 4 doses.

Gonorrhea patients sensitive to penicillin may be treated with demeclocycline administered as an initial oral dose of 600 mg followed by 300 mg every 12 hours for four days to a total of 3 grams.

HOW SUPPLIED

DECLOMYCIN Capsules: 150 mg *demeclocycline hydrochloride* two-tone, coral colored, soft gelatin capsules, printed with LL followed by D9 on the light side in blue ink, are supplied as follows: NDC 0005-9208-23—Bottles of 100

Tablets: 150 mg *demeclocycline hydrochloride* round, convex, red, film-coated tablets, engraved with LL on one side and D11 on the other, are supplied as follows:

NDC 0005-9218-23—Bottles of 100

300 mg *demeclocycline hydrochloride* round, convex, red, film-coated tablets, engraved with LL on one side and D12 on the other, are supplied as follows:

NDC 0005-9270-29—Bottles of 48

Store at Controlled Room Temperature 15°–30°C (59°–86°F).

Oral Suspension: Tetracycline HCl equivalent to 125 mg tetracycline per teaspoonful (5 ml), preserved with Methylparaben 0.12% and Propylparaben 0.03%, cherry-flavored, is supplied as follows:

NDC 0005-5410-56 – Bottles of 2 fl oz (60 ml)

NDC 0005-5410-65 – Bottles of 16 fl oz (473 ml)

Store at Controlled Room Temperature 15°–30°C (59°–86°F). DO NOT FREEZE.

Reference: 1. CDC Sexually Transmitted Diseases Treatment Guidelines 1982.

Shown in Product Identification Section, page 413

DIAMOX® ℞

[*dīa-mŏx*]

Acetazolamide

SEQUELS® Sustained Release Capsules 500 mg

DESCRIPTION

DIAMOX® *acetazolamide* SEQUELS Lederle are sustained-release capsules each containing 500 mg of acetazolamide.

Inactive Ingredients: Bees Wax, Benzoin Gum, Blue 1, Cornstarch, Ethylcellulose, Gelatin, Glycerin, Magnesium Stearate, Methylparaben, Mineral Oil, Mono and Diglycerides, Propylene Glycol, Propylparaben, Silica, Sucrose, Talc, Terpene Resin, Vanillin, Yellow 6.

ACTIONS

DIAMOX is a potent carbonic anhydrase inhibitor, effective in the control of fluid secretion (eg, some types of glaucoma), in the treatment of certain convulsive disorders (eg, epilepsy), and in the promotion of diuresis in instances of abnormal fluid retention (eg, cardiac edema).

DIAMOX is not a mercurial diuretic. Rather it is a nonbacteriostatic sulfonamide possessing a chemical structure and pharmacological activity distinctly different from the bacteriostatic sulfonamides.

DIAMOX is an enzyme inhibitor which acts specifically on carbonic anhydrase, the enzyme which catalyzes the reversible reaction involving the hydration of carbon dioxide and the dehydration of carbonic acid. In the eye, this inhibitory action of acetazolamide decreases the secretion of aqueous humor and results in a drop in intraocular pressure, a reaction considered desirable in cases of glaucoma and even in certain nonglaucomatous conditions. Evidence seems to indicate that DIAMOX has utility as an adjuvant in the treatment of certain dysfunctions of the central nervous system (eg, epilepsy). Inhibition of carbonic anhydrase in this area appears to retard abnormal, paroxysmal, excessive discharge from central nervous system neurons. The diuretic effect of DIAMOX is due to its action in the kidney on the reversible reaction involving hydration of carbon dioxide and dehydration of carbonic acid. The result is renal loss of HCO_3 ion, which carries out sodium, water, and potassium. Alkalinization of the urine and promotion of diuresis are thus effected.

DIAMOX® *acetazolamide* SEQUELS Sustained Release Capsules provide prolonged action to inhibit aqueous humor secretion for 18 to 24 hours after each dose, whereas tablets act for only 8 to 12 hours. The prolonged/continuous effect of SEQUELS permits a reduction in dosage frequency.

Blood level concentrations of acetazolamide peak between 8 to 12 hours after administration of DIAMOX SEQUELS, compared to two to four hours with tablets.

Placebo-controlled clinical trials have shown that prophylactic administration of DIAMOX at a dose of 250 mg every 8 to 12 hours (or a 500 mg controlled release capsule once daily) before and during rapid ascent to altitude results in fewer and/or less severe symptoms (such as headache, nausea, shortness of breath, dizziness, drowsiness, and fatigue) of acute mountain sickness (AMS). Pulmonary function (eg, minute ventilation, expired vital capacity, and peak flow) is greater in the DIAMOX treated group, both in subjects with AMS and asymptomatic subjects. The DIAMOX treated climbers also had less difficulty in sleeping.

INDICATIONS

For adjunctive treatment of: chronic simple (open-angle) glaucoma, secondary glaucoma, and preoperatively in acute angle-closure glaucoma where delay of surgery is desired in order to lower intraocular pressure. DIAMOX is also indicated for the prevention or amelioration of symptoms associated with acute mountain sickness in climbers attempting rapid ascent and in those who are very susceptible to acute mountain sickness despite gradual ascent.

CONTRAINDICATIONS

Acetazolamide therapy is contraindicated in situations in which sodium and/or potassium blood serum levels are depressed, in cases of marked kidney and liver disease or dysfunction, suprarenal gland failure, and hyperchloremic acidosis.

Long-term administration of DIAMOX® *acetazolamide* is contraindicated in patients with chronic noncongestive angle-closure glaucoma since it may permit organic closure of the angle to occur while the worsening glaucoma is masked by lowered intraocular pressure.

WARNING

Studies of acetazolamide in rats and mice have demonstrated teratogenic and embryocidal effects at doses in excess of ten times those recommended in human beings. There is no evidence of these effects in human beings. However, acetazolamide should not be used in pregnancy, especially during the first trimester, unless the benefits to be expected outweigh these potential adverse effects.

PRECAUTIONS

Increasing the dose does not increase the diuresis and may increase the incidence of drowsiness and/or paresthesia. Increasing the dose often results in a decrease in diuresis. Under certain circumstances, however, very large doses have been given in conjunction with other diuretics in order to secure diuresis in complete refractory failure.

Adverse reactions common to all sulfonamide derivatives may occur: anaphylaxis, fever, rash (including erythema multiforme, Stevens-Johnson syndrome, toxic epidermal necrolysis), crystalluria, renal calculus, bone marrow depression, thrombocytopenia purpura, hemolytic anemia, leukopenia, pancytopenia, and agranulocytosis. Precaution is advised for early detection of such reactions and the drug should be discontinued and appropriate therapy instituted.

To monitor for hematologic reactions, common to all sulfonamides, it is recommended that a baseline CBC and platelet count be obtained on patients prior to initiating DIAMOX therapy and at regular intervals during therapy. If significant changes occur, early discontinuance and institution of appropriate therapy are important.

In patients with pulmonary obstruction or emphysema where alveolar ventilation may be impaired, DIAMOX® *acetazolamide*, which may aggravate acidosis, should be used with caution.

Precaution is advised for patients receiving concomitant high-dose aspirin and DIAMOX, as anorexia, tachypnea, lethargy, and coma have been rarely reported due to a possible drug interaction.

Gradual ascent is desirable to try to avoid acute mountain sickness. If rapid ascent is undertaken and DIAMOX is used, it should be noted that such use does not obviate the need for prompt descent if severe forms of high altitude sickness occur, ie, high altitude pulmonary edema (HAPE) or high altitude cerebral edema.

ADVERSE REACTIONS

Adverse reactions during short-term therapy are minimal. Those effects which have been noted include: paresthesias, particularly a "tingling" feeling in the extremities, some loss of appetite, polyuria, and occasional instances of drowsiness and confusion. Rarely, photosensitivity has been reported.

During long-term therapy, an acidotic state may occasionally supervene. This can usually be corrected by the administration of bicarbonate.

Transient myopia has been reported. This condition invariably subsides upon diminution or discontinuance of the medication.

Other occasional adverse reactions include: urticaria, melena, hematuria, glycosuria, hepatic insufficiency, flaccid paralysis, and convulsions.

DOSAGE AND ADMINISTRATION

Glaucoma: The recommended dose is 1 capsule (500 mg) two times a day. Usually 1 capsule is administered in the morning and 1 capsule in the evening. It may be necessary to adjust the dose but it has usually been found that dosage in excess of 2 capsules (1 gram) does not produce an increased effect. The dosage should be adjusted with careful individual attention both to symptomatology and intraocular tension. In all cases, continuous supervision by a physician is advisable.

In those unusual instances where adequate control is not obtained by the twice-a-day administration of DIAMOX® *acetazolamide* SEQUELS Sustained Release Capsules, the desired control may be established by means of DIAMOX (Tablets or Parenteral). Use tablets or parenteral in accordance with the more frequent dosage schedules recommended for these dosage forms, such as 250 mg every four hours, or an initial dose of 500 mg followed by 250 mg or 125 mg every four hours, depending on the case in question.

Acute Mountain Sickness: Dosage is 500 mg to 1000 mg daily, in divided doses using tablets or sustained release capsules as appropriate. In circumstances of rapid ascent, such as in rescue or military operations, the higher dose level of 1000 mg is recommended. It is preferable to initiate dosing 24 to 48 hours before ascent and to continue for 48 hours while at high altitude, or longer, as necessary to control symptoms.

HOW SUPPLIED

DIAMOX® *acetazolamide* SEQUELS®, orange capsules printed with "Diamox" over D3 are supplied as follows:
NDC 0005-4465-13—Bottles of 30
NDC 0005-4465-23—Bottles of 100
Store at Controlled Room Temperature 15°-30°C (59°-86°F).
LEDERLE LABORATORIES DIVISION
American Cyanamid Company
Pearl River, NY 10965
MILITARY: NSN 6505-00-880-4949 (100s)
VA: NSN 6505-00-880-4949A (100s)
Shown in Product Identification Section, page 413

DIAMOX® ℞

[*dīa-mŏx*]
Acetazolamide Tablets and
DIAMOX
Sterile Acetazolamide Sodium Parenteral
Tablets 250 mg:

DESCRIPTION

Tablets: 125 mg of acetazolamide, round, flat-faced, beveled, white tablets engraved with DIAMOX and 125 on one side and scored in half on the other side. Engraved with LL on the right of the score and D1 on the left.
250 mg of acetazolamide, round, convex, white tablets engraved with DIAMOX and 250 on one side and scored in quarters on the other side. Engraved with LL in the upper right quadrant and D2 in the lower left quadrant.
Inactive Ingredients: Calcium Phosphate Dibasic, Cornstarch, Magnesium Stearate, Povidone, Sodium Starch Glycolate.
Parenteral: Each vial contains acetazolamide 500 mg (as sodium salt) and pH adjusted to approximately 9.2 with sodium hydroxide and, if necessary, hydrochloric acid.

ACTIONS

DIAMOX® *acetazolamide* is a potent carbonic anhydrase inhibitor, effective in the control of fluid secretion (eg, some types of glaucoma), in the treatment of certain convulsive disorders (eg, epilepsy), and in the promotion of diuresis in instances of abnormal fluid retention (eg, cardiac edema).
DIAMOX is not a mercurial diuretic. Rather it is a nonbacteriostatic sulfonamide possessing a chemical structure and pharmacological activity distinctly different from the bacteriostatic sulfonamides.
DIAMOX is an enzyme inhibitor which acts specifically on carbonic anhydrase, the enzyme which catalyzes the reversible reaction involving the hydration of carbon dioxide and the dehydration of carbonic acid. In the eye, this inhibitory action of acetazolamide decreases the secretion of aqueous humor and results in a drop in intraocular pressure, a reaction considered desirable in cases of glaucoma and even in certain nonglaucomatous conditions. Evidence seems to indicate that DIAMOX has utility as an adjuvant in the treatment of certain dysfunctions of the central nervous system (eg, epilepsy). Inhibition of carbonic anhydrase in this area appears to retard abnormal, paroxysmal, excessive discharge from central nervous system neurons. The diuretic effect of DIAMOX is due to its action in the kidney on the reversible reaction involving hydration of carbon dioxide and dehydration of carbonic acid. The result is renal loss of HCO_3 ion, which carries out sodium, water, and potassium. Alkalinization of the urine and promotion of diuresis are thus effected.
Placebo-controlled clinical trials have shown that prophylactic administration of DIAMOX at a dose of 250 mg every 8 to 12 hours (or a 500 mg controlled release capsule once daily) before and during rapid ascent to altitude results in fewer and/or less severe symptoms (such as headache, nausea, shortness of breath, dizziness, drowsiness, and fatigue) of acute mountain sickness (AMS). Pulmonary function (eg, minute ventilation, expired vital capacity, and peak flow) is greater in the DIAMOX treated group, both in subjects with AMS and asymptomatic subjects. The DIAMOX treated climbers also had less difficulty in sleeping.

INDICATIONS

For adjunctive treatment of: edema due to congestive heart failure; drug-induced edema; centrencephalic epilepsies (petit mal, unlocalized seizures); chronic simple (open-angle) glaucoma, secondary glaucoma, and preoperatively in acute angle-closure glaucoma where delay of surgery is desired in order to lower intraocular pressure. DIAMOX is also indicated for the prevention or amelioration of symptoms associated with acute mountain sickness in climbers attempting rapid ascent and in those who are very susceptible to acute mountain sickness despite gradual ascent.

CONTRAINDICATIONS

DIAMOX® *acetazolamide* therapy is contraindicated in situations in which sodium and/or potassium blood serum levels are depressed, in cases of marked kidney and liver disease or dysfunction, suprarenal gland failure, and hyperchloremic acidosis.
Long-term administration of DIAMOX® *acetazolamide* is contraindicated in patients with chronic noncongestive angle-closure glaucoma since it may permit organic closure of the angle to occur while the worsening glaucoma is masked by lowered intraocular pressure.

WARNING

Studies of acetazolamide in rats and mice have demonstrated teratogenic and embryocidal effects at doses in excess of ten times those recommended in human beings. There is no evidence of these effects in human beings. However, DIAMOX should not be used in pregnancy, especially during the first trimester, unless the benefits to be expected outweigh these potential adverse effects.

PRECAUTIONS

Increasing the dose does not increase the diuresis and may increase the incidence of drowsiness and/or paresthesia. Increasing the dose often results in a decrease in diuresis. Under certain circumstances, however, very large doses have been given in conjunction with other diuretics in order to secure diuresis in complete refractory failure.
Adverse reactions common to all sulfonamide derivatives may occur: anaphylaxis, fever, rash (including erythema multiforme, Stevens-Johnson syndrome, toxic epidermal necrolysis), crystalluria, renal calculus, bone marrow depression, thrombocytopenic purpura, hemolytic anemia, leukopenia, pancytopenia, and agranulocytosis. Precaution is advised for early detection of such reactions and the drug should be discontinued and appropriate therapy instituted. To monitor for hematologic reactions, common to all sulfonamides, it is recommended that a baseline CBC and platelet count be obtained on patients prior to initiating DIAMOX therapy and at regular intervals during therapy. If significant changes occur, early discontinuance and institution of appropriate therapy are important.
In patients with pulmonary obstruction or emphysema where alveolar ventilation may be impaired, DIAMOX® *acetazolamide,* which may precipitate or aggravate acidosis, should be used with caution.
Precaution is advised for patients receiving concomitant high-dose aspirin and DIAMOX® *acetazolamide,* as anorexia, tachypnea, lethargy, and coma have been rarely reported due to a possible drug interaction.
Gradual ascent is desirable to try to avoid acute mountain sickness. If rapid ascent is undertaken and DIAMOX is used, it should be noted that such use does not obviate the need for prompt descent if severe forms of high altitude sickness occur, ie, high altitude pulmonary edema (HAPE) or high altitude cerebral edema.

ADVERSE REACTIONS

Adverse reactions during short-term therapy are minimal. Those effects which have been noted include: paresthesias, particularly a "tingling" feeling in the extremities, some loss of appetite, polyuria, and occasional instances of drowsiness and confusion. Rarely, photosensitivity has been reported.
During long-term therapy, an acidotic state may occasionally supervene. This can usually be corrected by the administration of bicarbonate.
Transient myopia has been reported. This condition invariably subsides upon diminution or discontinuance of the medication.
Other occasional adverse reactions include: urticaria, melena, hematuria, glycosuria, hepatic insufficiency, flaccid paralysis, and convulsions.

DOSAGE AND ADMINISTRATION

Preparation and Storage of Parenteral Solution: Each 500 mg vial containing DIAMOX *sterile acetazolamide sodium* Parenteral should be reconstituted with at least 5 ml of Sterile Water for Injection prior to use. Reconstituted solutions retain potency for one week if refrigerated. Since this product contains no preservative, use within 24 hours of reconstitution is strongly recommended. The direct intravenous route of administration is preferred.
Intramuscular administration may be employed but is painful, due to the alkaline pH of the solution.
Glaucoma: DIAMOX® *acetazolamide* should be used as an adjunct to the usual therapy. The dosage employed in the treatment of *chronic simple (open-angle) glaucoma* ranges from 250 mg to 1 gram of DIAMOX per 24 hours, usually in divided doses for amounts over 250 mg. It has usually been found that a dosage in excess of 1 gram per 24 hours does not produce an increased effect. In all cases, the dosage should be adjusted with careful individual attention both to symptomatology and ocular tension. Continuous supervision by a physician is advisable.
In the treatment of secondary glaucoma and in the preoperative treatment of some cases of *acute congestive (closed-angle) glaucoma,* the preferred dosage is 250 mg every four hours, although some cases have responded to 250 mg twice daily on short-term therapy. In some acute cases, it may be more satisfactory to administer an initial dose of 500 mg followed by 125 mg or 250 mg every four hours depending on the individual case. Intravenous therapy may be used for rapid relief of ocular tension in acute cases. A complementary effect has been noted when DIAMOX has been used in conjunction with miotics or mydriatics as the case demanded.
Epilepsy: It is not clearly known whether the beneficial effects observed in epilepsy are due to direct inhibition of carbonic anhydrase in the central nervous system or whether they are due to the slight degree of acidosis produced by the divided dosage. The best results to date have been seen in petit mal in children. Good results, however, have been seen in patients, both children and adult, in other types of seizures such as grand mal, mixed seizure patterns, myoclonic jerk patterns, etc. The suggested total daily dose is 8 mg to 30 mg per kg in divided doses. Although some patients respond to a low dose, the optimum range appears to be from 375 mg to 1000 mg daily. However, some investigators feel that daily doses in excess of 1 gram do not produce any better results than a 1 gram dose. When DIAMOX is given in combination with other anticonvulsants, it is suggested that the starting dose should be 250 mg once daily in addition to the existing medications. This can be increased to levels as indicated above.
The change from other medication to DIAMOX should be gradual in accordance with usual practice in epilepsy therapy.
Congestive Heart Failure: For diuresis in congestive heart failure, the starting dose is usually 250 mg to 375 mg once daily in the morning (5 mg/kg). If after an initial response, the patient fails to continue to lose edema fluid, do not increase the dose but allow for kidney recovery by skipping medication for a day. DIAMOX® *acetazolamide* yields best diuretic results when given on alternate days, or for two days alternating with a day of rest.
Failure in therapy may be due to overdosage or too frequent dosage. The use of DIAMOX does not eliminate the need for other therapy such as digitalis, bed rest, and salt restriction.
Drug-Induced Edema: Recommended dosage is 250 mg to 375 mg of DIAMOX once a day for one or two days, alternating with a day of rest.
Acute Mountain Sickness: Dosage is 500 mg to 1000 mg daily in divided doses, using tablets or sustained release capsules as appropriate. In circumstances of rapid ascent, such as in rescue or military operations, the higher dose level of 1000 mg is recommended. It is preferable to initiate dosing 24 to 48 hours before ascent and to continue for 48 hours while at high altitude, or longer, as necessary to control symptoms.
Note: The dosage recommendations for glaucoma and epilepsy differ considerably from those for congestive heart failure, since the first two conditions are not dependent upon carbonic anhydrase inhibition in the kidney which requires intermittent dosage if it is to recover from the inhibitory effect of the therapeutic agent.

HOW SUPPLIED

Tablets—125 mg—Round, flat-faced, beveled, white tablets engraved with Diamox and 125 on one side and scored in half on the other side. Engraved with LL on the right of the score and D1 on the left, are supplied as follows:
NDC 0005-4398-23—Bottles of 100
250 mg—Round, convex, white tablets engraved with Diamox and 250 on one side and scored in quarters on the other side. Engraved with LL in the upper right quadrant and D2 in the lower left quadrant, are supplied as follows:
NDC 0005-4469-23—bottles of 100
NDC 0005-4469-34—bottles of 1000
NDC 0005-4469-60—Unit Dose 10 x 10
Store at Controlled Room Temperature 15°-30°C (59°-86°F).
LEDERLE LABORATORIES DIVISION
American Cyanamid Company, Pearl River, NY 10965
Parenteral—500 mg vial of cryodesiccated powder—
Product Number NDC 0205-4466-96
Store at Controlled Room Temperature 15°-30°C (59°-86°F).
LEDERLE PARENTERALS, INC.
Carolina, Puerto Rico 00630
Shown in Product Identification Section, page 413

DIPHTHERIA AND TETANUS TOXOIDS ADSORBED PUROGENATED® ℞

For Pediatric Use
NDC 0005-1858-31

HOW SUPPLIED

5 ml vials (5 immunizations).
COMPLETE INFORMATION FURNISHED IN THE PACKAGE.

Continued on next page

The information on each product appearing here is based on labelling effective in August, 1986 and is either the entire official brochure or an accurate condensation therefrom. Information concerning all Lederle products may be obtained from the Professional Services Department, Lederle Laboratories, Pearl River, New York, 10965.

Lederle—Cont.

FERRO-SEQUELS®
[*fĕrrō sē-quls*]
Sustained Release
Iron Capsules

COMPOSITION

Each capsule contains 150 mg of ferrous fumarate, equivalent to approximately 50 mg of elemental iron, and 100 mg of docusate sodium (DSS).
Inactive Ingredients: Acacia, Beeswax, Blue 1, Cornstarch with Magnesium Oxide, Gelatin, Glyceryl Stearate, Magnesium Stearate, Mono- and Di-Glycerides, Mineral Oil, Silica Gel, Sucrose, Titanium Dioxide, Yellow 6, Yellow 10.

INDICATIONS

For the treatment of iron-deficiency anemias.

WARNING

As with any drug, if you are pregnant or nursing a baby, seek the advice of a health professional before using this product. Keep this and all medications out of the reach of children. In case of accidental overdose, seek professional assistance or contact a Poison Control Center immediately.

DOSAGE

1 capsule, once or twice daily or as prescribed by the physician.

HOW SUPPLIED

Bottles of 30 capsules, NDC 0005-4612-13
Bottles of 100 capsules, NDC 0005-4612-23 Unit Dose Pkg., 10-10s, NDC 0005-4612-60
Bottles of 1,000 capsules, NDC 0005-4612-34
Store at Controlled Room Temperature 15°-30° C (59°-86° F).
Capsules (light green) Printed Lederle FERRO-SEQUELS F2
Military Depots
30s....................NSN 6505-00-149-0103
Individually sealed 100s (Unit Dose) NSN 6505-00-131-8870
1000s....................NSN 6505-00-074-2981

Shown in Product Identification Section, page 413

FILIBON®
[*fĭl-ă-bŏn*]
prenatal tablets

Each tablet contains:

	For Pregnant or Lactating Women Percentage of U.S. Recommended Daily Allowance (U.S. RDA)
Vitamin A (as Acetate)	5000 I.U. (63%)
Vitamin D_2	400 I.U. (100%)
Vitamin E (as *dl*-Alpha Tocopheryl Acetate)	30 I.U. (100%)
Vitamin C (as Ascorbic Acid)	60 mg (100%)
Folic Acid	0.4 mg (50%)
Vitamin B_1 (as Thiamine Mononitrate)	1.5 mg (88%)
Vitamin B_2 (as Riboflavin)	1.7 mg (85%)
Niacinamide	20 mg (100%)
Vitamin B_6 (as Pyridoxine Hydrochloride)	2 mg (80%)
Vitamin B_{12} (as Cyanocobalamin)	6 mcg (75%)
Calcium (as Calcium Carbonate)	125 mg (10%)
Iodine (as Potassium Iodide)	150 mcg (100%)
Iron (as Ferrous Fumarate)	18 mg (100%)
Magnesium (as Magnesium Oxide)	100 mg (22%)

Inactive Ingredients:
BHA, BHT, Dextrose, Ethylcellulose, Gelatin, Hydrolyzed Protein, Hydroxypropyl Methylcellulose, Lactose, Magnesium Stearate, Methylparaben, Modified Food Starch, Mono- and Di-glycerides, Polacrilin, Polysorbate 60, Povidone, Propylparaben, Red 30, Silica Gel, Sodium Benzoate, Sodium Bisulfite, Sodium Lauryl Sulfate, Sorbic Acid, Stearic Acid, Sucrose, Titanium Dioxide, Tricalcium Phosphate and other ingredients.

RECOMMENDED INTAKE

1 daily, or as prescribed by the physician.

HOW SUPPLIED

Bottles of 100 NDC 0005-4294-23

Shown in Product Identification Section, page 413

FILIBON® F.A. ℞
[*fĭl-ă-bŏn*]
prenatal tablets

Each tablet contains:

	Percentage of U.S. Recommended Daily Allowance (U.S. RDA)
Vitamin A (as Acetate)	8000 I.U. (100%)
Vitamin D	400 I.U. (100%)
Vitamin E (as *dl*-Alpha Tocopheryl Acetate)	30 I.U. (100%)
Vitamin C (as Ascorbic Acid)	60 mg (100%)
Folic Acid	1 mg (125%)
Vitamin B_1 (as Thiamine Mononitrate)	1.7 mg (100%)
Vitamin B_2 (as Riboflavin)	2 mg (100%)
Niacinamide	20 mg (100%)
Vitamin B_6 (as Pyridoxine Hydrochloride)	4.0 mg (160%)
Vitamin B_{12} (as Cyanocobalamin)	8 mcg (100%)
Calcium (as Calcium Carbonate)	250 mg (19%)
Iodine (as Potassium Iodide)	150 mcg (100%)
Iron (as Ferrous Fumarate)	45 mg (250%)
Magnesium (as Magnesium Oxide)	100 mg (22%)

DESCRIPTION

Multivitamin-Multimineral Supplement for pregnant or lactating women. A Phosphorus-Free Vitamin and Mineral Dietary Supplement for use in prenatal care and lactation.

RECOMMENDED INTAKE

1 tablet daily.

CAUTION

Federal law prohibits dispensing without prescription.

PRECAUTION

Folic acid may obscure pernicious anemia in that the peripheral blood picture may revert to normal while neurological manifestations remain progressive.
Inactive Ingredients:
BHA, BHT, Blue 2, Dextrose, Ethylcellulose, Gelatin, Hydrolyzed Protein, Hydroxypropyl Methylcellulose, Lactose, Magnesium Stearate, Methylparaben, Modified Food Starch, Mono- and Di-glycerides, Polacrilin, Polysorbate 60, Povidone, Propylparaben, Red 30, Silica Gel, Sodium Benzoate, Sodium Lauryl Sulfate, Sodium Starch Glycolate, Sorbic Acid, Stearic Acid, Sucrose, Titanium Dioxide.
Professional literature available on request.

HOW SUPPLIED

Capsule-shaped tablets (film-coated, pink) engraved LL-F5—bottles of 100 NDC 0005-4225-23.

Shown in Product Identification Section, page 413

FILIBON® FORTE ℞
[*fĭl-ă-bŏn for-tā*]
prenatal tablets

Each tablet contains:

	Percentage of U.S. Recommended Daily Allowance (U.S. RDA)
Vitamin A (as Acetate)	8000 I.U. (100%)
Vitamin D_2	400 I.U. (100%)
Vitamin E (as *dl*-Alpha Tocopheryl Acetate)	45 I.U. (150%)
Vitamin C (Ascorbic Acid)	90 mg (150%)
Folic Acid	1 mg (125%)
Vitamin B_1 (as Thiamine Mononitrate)	2 mg (118%)
Vitamin B_2 (as Riboflavin)	2.5 mg (125%)
Niacinamide	30 mg (150%)
Vitamin B_6 (as Pyridoxine Hydrochloride)	3 mg (120%)
Vitamin B_{12} (as Cyanocobalamin)	12 mcg (150%)
Calcium (as Calcium Carbonate)	300 mg (23%)
Iodine (as Potassium Iodide)	200 mg (133%)
Iron (as Ferrous Fumarate)	45 mg (250%)
Magnesium (as Magnesium Oxide)	100 mg (22%)

RECOMMENDED INTAKE

1 tablet daily. This dosage provides 23% and 22% the Recommended Daily Allowance of calcium and magnesium respectively, therefore, supplementation of the diet by milk or other sources of calcium may be advisable.

CAUTION: Federal law prohibits dispensing without prescription.

PRECAUTION

Folic Acid may obscure pernicious anemia in that the peripheral blood picture may revert to normal while neurological manifestations remain progressive.
Inactive Ingredients
Amberlite® Resin, BHA, BHT, Dextrose, Ethylcellulose, Gelatin, Hydroxypropyl Methylcellulose, Lactose, Magnesium Stearate, Methylparaben, Modified Food Starch, Mono- and Di-glycerides, Polysorbate 60, Potassium Sorbate, Povidone, Propylparaben, Red 30, Silica Gel, Sodium Benzoate, Sodium Lauryl Sulfate, Sodium Starch, Glycolate, Sorbic Acid, Stearic Acid, Sucrose.

HOW SUPPLIED

Tablets—bottles of 100 NDC 0005-4226-23.

Shown in Product Identification Section, page 413

FOLVITE® ℞
[*fōl-vīt*]
folic acid
Tablets—Parenteral Solution

DESCRIPTION

Folic acid, *N*-[4[[(2-Amino-1,4-dihydro-4-oxo-6-ptendinyl) methyl]-amino]benzoyl]-L-glutamic acid, is a complex organic compound present in liver, yeast, and natural sources; it also may be prepared synthetically.
Tablets
1 mg Folic Acid
Inactive Ingredients: Alginic Acid, Dibasic Calcium Phosphate, Magnesium Stearate, Yellow 6.
Parenteral
Each ml of FOLVITE *folic acid* -Solution contains sodium folate equivalent to 5 mg of FOLIC ACID.
Inactive Ingredients: Sequestrene Sodium 0.2% and Water for Injection q.s. 100%, Sodium Hydroxide to approx. pH 9, Preservative: Benzyl Alcohol 1.5%
Inactive Ingredients: Sequestrene Sodium 0.2% and Water for Injection q.s. 100%. Sodium Hydroxide to approx. pH 9. Preservative: Benzyl Alcohol 1.5%.

ACTIONS

In man, an exogenous source of folate is required for nucleoprotein synthesis and maintenance of normal erythropoiesis. Folic Acid, whether given by mouth or parenterally, stimulates specifically the production of red blood cells, white blood cells, and platelets in persons suffering from certain megaloblastic anemias.

INDICATIONS

Folic Acid is effective in the treatment of megaloblastic anemias due to a deficiency of Folic Acid as may be seen in tropical or nontropical sprue, in anemias of nutritional origin, pregnancy, infancy, or childhood.

WARNINGS

Folic Acid alone is improper therapy in the treatment of pernicious anemia and other megaloblastic anemias where Vitamin B_{12} is deficient.

PRECAUTIONS

Folic acid in doses above 0.1 mg daily may obscure pernicious anemia in that hematologic remission can occur while neurological manifestations remain progressive.

ADVERSE REACTIONS

Allergic sensitization has been reported following both oral and parenteral administration of Folic Acid.

DOSAGE AND ADMINISTRATION

Oral administration: Folic Acid is well absorbed and may be administered orally with satisfactory results except in severe instances of intestinal malabsorption.
Parenteral administration: Intramuscular, intravenous, and subcutaneous routes may be used if the disease is exceptionally severe or if gastrointestinal absorption may be, or is known to be, impaired.
Usual therapeutic dosage—In adults and children (regardless of age): up to 1.0 mg daily. Resistant cases may require larger doses.
Maintenance level: When clinical symptoms have subsided and the blood picture has become normal, a maintenance level should be used, ie, 0.1 mg for infants and up to 0.3 mg for children under 4 years of age, 0.4 mg for adults and children 4 or more years of age, and 0.8 mg for pregnant and lactating women, per day, but never less than 0.1 mg per day. Patients should be kept under close supervision and adjustment of the maintenance level made if relapse appears imminent. In the presence of alcoholism, hemolytic anemia, anticonvulsant therapy, or chronic infection, the maintenance level may need to be increased.

HOW SUPPLIED

Tablets Round, flat-faced, beveled, scored, yellow-orange tablets engraved with LL on one side and F above and 1 below the score on the other side, are supplied as follows:

NDC 0005-4165-23—Bottles of 100
NDC 0005-4165-34—Bottles of 1000
NDC 0005-4165-60—Unit Dose 10 x 10's
***Parenteral Solution**, 5 mg/ml—10 ml vials NDC 0205-4154-34.
Military Depots:
Folvite Solution, 5 mg/ml................ NSN 6505-00-150-7552
Store at Controlled Room Temperature 15°-30°C (59°-86°F).
A.H.F.S. 88:08
*Manufactured for
LEDERLE LABORATORIES DIVISION
American Cyanamid Company
Pearl River, NY 10965
by
LEDERLE PARENTERALS INC.
Carolina, Puerto Rico 00630

FOOTWORK™
Athlete's Foot Remedy

(See PDR For Nonprescription Drugs)

GEVRABON®
[jĕv-ra-bŏn]
(vitamin-mineral supplement)

(See PDR For Nonprescription Drugs)

GEVRAL®
[jĕv-ral]
Multivitamin and Multimineral Supplement for Adults and Children 4 or More Years of Age
TABLETS

(See PDR For Nonprescription Drugs)

GEVRAL® T
[jĕv-ral]
High Potency Multivitamin and Multimineral Supplement for Adults and Children 4 or More Years of Age
TABLETS

(See PDR For Nonprescription Drugs)

HIB-IMUNE® ℞
Haemophilus b Polysaccharide Vaccine

DESCRIPTION

Haemophilus b polysaccharide vaccine, HIB-IMUNE®, is a highly purified capsular polysaccharide, polyribosylribitol phosphate isolated from *Haemophilus influenzae* type b. It is intended for intramuscular or subcutaneous use.
HIB-IMUNE® is indicated for immunization against the various invasive diseases caused by *H influenzae* type b (Hib).
HIB-IMUNE is a lyophilized preparation of Hib polysaccharide with sucrose NF as a stabilizer. The Hib polysaccharide and sucrose are mixed before lyophilization. When reconstituted as directed, each 0.5 ml dose contains 25 micrograms (mcg) of Hib polysaccharide and 4 milligrams (mg) of sucrose. Thimerosal (a mercury derivative) which is used as a preservative, is present in the diluent at a concentration of 1:10,000.

CLINICAL PHARMACOLOGY

H influenzae is a Gram-negative coccobacillus which causes a wide variety of clinical diseases in a significant number of persons.[1] Of the typeable and nontypeable strains, Hib is the most virulent and accounts for approximately 95% of serious systemic infections due to *H influenzae* in children.[1] Nontypeable (noncapsulated) strains of *H influenzae* commonly colonize the human respiratory tract and are a major cause of respiratory mucosal infection and otitis media, but rarely result in bacteremic disease. Hib strains account for 5% to 10% of *H influenzae* causing otitis media.[2]
An estimated 15,000 to 20,000 cases of invasive disease caused by Hib, including meningitis, epiglottitis, sepsis, cellulitis, septic arthritis, pneumonia, and osteomyelitis, occur annually in the United States[3]. Children under 5 years of age are the major group at risk for Hib disease, although invasive disease has been reported in all age groups. Several population-based studies conducted in the US over the past ten years indicate that a child's cumulative risk of developing Hib disease at some time during the first 5 years of life is about 1:200. Thirty-five to 40% of Hib disease occurs in children 18 months of age or older, with 25% occurring in children 2 years old or more.[2,4]
The incidence of systemic Hib disease is increased in certain children. Recent studies indicate that Hib can cause systemic disease among previously healthy children attending nursery school or day care centers, and that attendance at these facilities significantly increases the risk of developing systemic Hib disease.[5–7] There have also been reports of the spread of Hib disease among institutionalized children.[8] Furthermore, the risk of acquiring systemic Hib disease for a child in intimate contact with one who has developed Hib disease is up to 400 times that of a child in the general populatin.[5] The incidence of systemic Hib disease is also increased in children with conditions such as asplenia, sickle cell disease[9] malignancies associated with immunosuppression[10], and antibody deficiency syndromes.[11]
Hib is the leading cause of meningitis in children in the US. Approximately 8,000 to 12,000 cases of meningitis due to Hib occur annually in the US.[2,12] Although mortality has been reduced by antibiotic therapy to between 5% and 10%, significant, long-term neurologic sequelae, such as mental retardation, deafness, blindness, and seizure disorders occur in up to a third of survivors.[13–15] When parameters such as behavior disorders and decreased school performance are included, only about 50% of survivors remain free of detectable defects.[16] Hib meningitis is regarded as the leading cause of acquired mental retardation in the US.[17] Hib is also the major cause of epiglottitis, an infection which can lead to life-threatening airway obstruction and usually occurs between the ages of 2 and 7 years.[18]
Antibiotics have been only partially effective in reducing the morbidity and mortality of disease due to *H influenzae* type b. Control of disease due to Hib is becoming more difficult because of plasmid-borne resistance to ampicillin and chloramphenicol.[3,13] A survey by the Centers for Disease Control in 1975–1976 showed the prevalence of ampicillin-resistant Hib isolates from cultures of blood and cerebrospinal fluid to 4.5%. By 1980–1981, ampicillin-resistant rates of up to 28% were reported.[3]
The incidence, morbidity and mortality associated with invasive disease due to Hib, the recognition of its transmissibility, and the emergence of strains of Hib with increased resistance to one or more commonly used antibiotics emphasize the importance of vaccine prophylaxis against this disease in children.
The ability of polysaccharide vaccines to induce an immune response has been well demonstrated by clinical trials with meningococcal A and C vaccines as well as the pneumococcal vaccines. Human protection against disease due to *H influenzae* type b is associated with the presence of antibody to Hib polysaccharide.[17,19–24]
Physicochemical properties of polysaccharide vaccines have been related to their ability to induce protective immunity, and a direct relationship has been shown between molecular size and protective immunity.[25–27] In comparison with the *Haemophilus* b polysaccharide vaccine shown to be efficacious in Finland, the present vaccine, HIB-IMUNE® *Haemophilus b polysaccharide vaccine,* is of comparable molecular size and has a lower endotoxin content.[22,28]
The precise protective level of *Haemophilus* b polysaccharide antibody has not been established. However, based on evidence from passive protection in the infant rat model and from experience with agammaglobulinemic children, a serum antibody concentration of 0.15 mcg/ml correlates with protection.[2,19,20] In the Finnish trial, levels of antibody greater than 1 mcg/ml as determined by the Finnish assay, in three-week post immunization sera, correlated with clinical protection.[2,22,29]
Variability has been observed in results obtained by various laboratories using different radioimmunoassays for the measurement of *Haemophilus* b polysaccharide antibody. For this reason, 74 pairs of sera from 24 to 26-month old children were randomly selected from *Haemophilus* b polysaccharide immunization studies conducted in several centers. When these sera were analyzed by a single radioimmunoassay, antibody responses of the children from the different studies were not significantly different.[30]
The efficacy of *Haemophilus* b polysaccharide vaccine has been demonstrated in human populations. In a large-scale efficacy trial conducted in Finland, approximately 50,000 children 3 months through 5 years of age were immunized with a *Haemophilus* b polysaccharide vaccine. Among children 18 months through 5 years of age, 90% protective efficacy (95% confidence limits, 55% to 98%) was demonstrated against all forms of invasive Hib disease for the four-year follow-up period. A significant difference in incidence of Hib disease was demonstrated between immunized and nonimmunized children over 2 years of age. None of more than 4,000 children vaccinated at 18 through 23 months of age developed bacteremic Hib disease during the four-years of follow-up. However, the number of cases of bacteremic Hib disease in the control group was too small to permit a statistically valid assessment of *Haemophilus* b polysaccharide vaccine efficacy in that age group. Children younger than 18 months of age had little immunologic response to the vaccine and were not protected.[17,22]
Follow-up antibody data from the Finnish trial demonstrated that the persistence of elevated serum antibody levels after immunization with *Haemophilus* b polysaccharide vaccine was age dependent. Elevated serum antibody levels were detectable for longer than one and one-half years but fewer than three and one-half years in children who were vaccinated at 18 through 35 months of age, and for at least three and one-half years in children who were 3 through 5 years of age, when first vaccinated.[23] Therefore, a second dose of vaccine may be needed to maintain immunity throughout the period of risk, particularly for those in the youngest age group considered for vaccination, those 18 to 23 months of age.[2] Studies in children are ongoing to determine the need and timing for revaccination.

INDICATIONS AND USAGE

Haemophilus b polysaccharide vaccine is recommended for routine use by the Committee on Infectious Diseases of the American Academy of Pediatrics and the Immunization Practices Advisory Committee of the US Public Health Services.[2,31]
HIB-IMUNE® *Haemophilus b polysaccharide vaccine* is indicated for immunization against the invasive disease caused by *H influenzae* type b in children from 24 months through 5 years of age. Routine revaccination of these children is not recommended at this time.[2]
Immunization of children 18 through 23 months of age, particularly those in known high-risk groups, may be considered. Initial vaccination at 18 months may be recommended for the following groups:[2]
(1) Children attending day care facilities.
(2) Children with chronic illnesses known to be associated with an increased risk of Hib disease, eg, anatomic or functional asplenia such as sickle cell anemia or splenectomy, and malignancies associated with immunosuppression. Limited data are available on the immune response to the Hib vaccine in these risk groups.

The precise efficacy of the vaccine among children 18 through 23 months of age is not known; however, this age group accounts for approximately 12% of all invasive Hib disease among children under 5 years of age, and Hib vaccine has been shown by serologic methods to be immunogenic in most children of this age group. Physicians and parents should be informed that the vaccine is not likely to be as effective in this age group as in older children. These younger children may need a second dose of vaccine within 18 months following the initial dose to ensure prtoection.[2]
HIB-IMUNE will not protect children younger than 18 months of age and will not protect against *H influenzae* other than type b or other microorganisms that cause meningitis or septic disease.
HIB-IMUNE® *Haemophilus b polysaccharide vaccine* should be reconstituted with the diluent provided (phosphate buffered saline).
Simultaneous administration of *Haemophilus* b polysaccharide and DTP vaccines at separate sites can be performed, because no impairment of the immune response to the individual antigens occurs under these circumstances. Simultaneous administration with DTP does not result in reaction rates above those expected with separate administration.[2,32]

CONTRAINDICATIONS

Hypersensitivity to any component of the vaccine, including thimerosal, a mercury derivative.

WARNINGS

HIB-IMUNE will not protect children younger than 18 months of age and will not protect against *Haemophilus influenzae* other than type b or other microorganisms that cause meningitis or septic disease.
The expected antibody response may not be obtained in patients with impaired immune responsiveness, which may be due to a genetic defect or use of immunosuppressive agents.
A temporal association of neurologic disorders has been reported following the parenteral injection of many biological products and should always be carefully considered when an immunization is indicated.

PRECAUTIONS

General: As with any parenteral vaccine, epinephrine (1:1000) should be available for immediate use should an anaphylactoid reaction occur.
HIB-IMUNE® should be injected intramuscularly or subcutaneously. Do not inject intravenously.
Any febrile illness or acute infection is reason for delaying use of HIB-IMUNE.
When administering HIB-IMUNE, a separate sterile syringe and needle should be used for each patient to prevent transmission of hepatitis B (homologous serum hepatitis) or other infectious agents.
Pregnancy: Pregnancy Category C: Animal reproduction studies have not been conducted with HIB-IMUNE. It is not

Continued on next page

The information on each product appearing here is based on labelling effective in August, 1986 and is either the entire official brochure or an accurate condensation therefrom. Information concerning all Lederle products may be obtained from the Professional Services Department, Lederle Laboratories, Pearl River, New York, 10965.

Lederle—Cont.

known whether HIB-IMUNE can cause fetal harm when administered to a pregnant woman or can affect reproductive capacity. HIB-IMUNE is not recommended for use in a pregnant woman.

Nursing Mothers: It is not known whether this vaccine is secreted in human milk. HIB-IMUNE is not recommended for use in a nursing mother.

Infants: The use of HIB-IMUNE in children younger than 18 months of age is not recommended. Please see Indications and Usage Section.

ADVERSE REACTIONS

Different preparations of *Haemophilus* b polysaccharide vaccine produced by different procedures and administered at different doses have been evaluated in several field studies in a total of over 60,000 children.[2,17,24] Objectively observed side effects, eg, erythema and induration at the injection site and fever, have generally been minor and lasted 24 hours or less. In the Finnish field trial, one child had a possible anaphylactoid reaction; following an injection of epinephrine, the child recovered rapidly and without complications.[2]

In clinical trials involving the administration of HIB-IMUNE, reconstituted with phosphate buffered saline, to over 600 children (18 months of age and older), local adverse reactions such as erythema, warmth, swelling and tenderness at the site of injection were observed. Erythema or swelling that was considered to be significant occurred in approximately 1% of subjects. In general, local reactions have been mild with a peak occurrence at approximately six hours and resolution within 24 hours.[33]

Systemic reactions observed included fever, irritability, anorexia, and sleep disturbance. Fever exceeding 38.5°C (101.3°F) was observed in approximately 2% of subjects within 24 hours after immunization.[33]

As with any vaccine, there is the possiblity that broad use of the vaccine could reveal rare adverse events not observed in the clinical trials. Since the introduction of *Haemophilus* b polysaccharide vaccine in the U.S. for routine use, a number of infrequent adverse reactions have been reported temporarily associated with administration of the vaccine including seizures, rashes, and sleep disturbance.[30] A cause and effect relationship has not been established.

A temporal association of neurologic disorders has been reported following the parenteral injection of many biological products and should always be carefully considered when an immunization is indicated.

Simultaneous administration of *Haemophilus* b polysaccharide and DTP vaccines at separate sites does not result in reaction rates above those expected with separate administration.[2,32]

DOSAGE AND ADMINISTRATION

FOR INTRAMUSCULAR OR SUBCUTANEOUS ADMINISTRATION. DO NOT INJECT INTRAVENOUSLY. The immunization schedule for HIB-IMUNE® *Haemophilus b Polysaccharide Vaccine* consists of a single 0.5 ml dose.

Each 0.5 ml dose of reconstituted HIB-IMUNE contains 25 mcg of Hib polysaccharide and 4 mg sucrose.

Reconstitute contents of each vial with 0.6 ml of the phosphate buffered saline diluent. When reconstituted, HIB-IMUNE is a clear, colorless liquid. After reconstitution, shake the vial gently before drawing a 0.5 ml dose of vaccine into a syringe. Reconstituted vials should be used as soon as possible. Discard unused reconstituted vials after eight hours. Discard unused and unreconstituted vials beyond expiration date.

The duration of the protective effect of HIB-IMUNE is unknown at present. The longevity of immunity and the suggested time for reimmunization, if needed, remain to be determined. Studies to determine the need, timing and safety of revaccination are being conducted.

HOW SUPPLIED

HIB-IMUNE is supplied as a box of 5 single-dose vials of lyophilized vaccine and 5 single-dose vials of diluent (phosphate buffered saline), which contains thimerosal (mercury derivative) 1:10,000 as preservative.

Product No. NDC 0005-1984-46.

STORAGE

Store vials in a refrigerator at temperatures of 2°C–8°C (36°–46°F.) DO NOT FREEZE.

MILITARY AND VA DEPOTS:

NSN 6505-01-230-8713

5 single-dose vials of lyophilized vaccine and 5 single-dose vials of diluent (phosphate buffered saline)

REFERENCES

1. Kaplan SL and Feigin RD; Infections due to *Haemophilus Influenzae*, in Nelson WE, Behrman RE, Vaughan VC III (eds): *Textbook of Pediatrics*, 12, Philadelphia, WB Saunders Co, 1983, pp 655-658.
2. Recommendation of the Immunization Practices Advisory Committee (ACIP): Polysaccharide vaccine for prevention of *Haemophilus influenzae* type b disease. *MMWR* 1985; 34(15):201–205.
3. Ampicillin and chloramphenicol resistance in systemic *Haemophilus influenzae* disease. *MMWR* 1984; 33:35–37.
4. Cochi SL, Broome CV, Hightower AW: Assessment of strategies for immunization of US children with *Haemophilus influenzae* type b polysaccharide vaccine: A cost-effectiveness model. *JAMA* 1985; 253:521–529.
5. Granoff D, Daum RS: Spread of *Haemophilus influenzae* type b: Recent epidemiologic and therapeutic considerations. *J Pediatr* 1980; 97:854–860.
6. Redmond SR, Pichichero ME: *Haemophilus influenzae* type b disease: An epidemiologic study with special reference to day care centers. *JAMA* 1984; 252:2581–2584.
7. Istre GR, Conner JS, Broome CV, et al: Risk factors for primary invasive *Haemophilus influenzae* disease: Increased risk from day care attendance and school-aged household members. *J Pediatr* 1985; 106:190–195.
8. Band JD: Chemoprophylaxis of *Haemophilus influenzae* Type b Disease: A strategy for preventing secondary cases, in Sell SH, Wright PF, (eds): *Haemophilus influenzae. Epidemiology, Immunology, and Prevention of Diseases.* New York, : Elsevier Biomedical, 1982, pp 309–315.
9. Ward J, Smith AL: *Haemophilus influenzae* bacteremia in children with sickle cell disease. *J Pediatr* 1976; 88:261–263.
10. Siber GR: Bacteremias due to *Haemophilus influenzae* and *Streptococcus pneumoniae:* their occurrence and course in children with cancer. *Am J Dis Child* 1980; 134:668–672.
11. Cherry JD, Feigin RD: Infections in the Compromised Host, in Stiehm ER, Fulginitti VA (eds): *Immunologic Disorders of Infants and Children.* Philadelphia, WB Saunders Co, 1980; 715 –744.
12. Prevention of Secondary Cases of *Haemophilus influenzae* type b disease. *MMWR* 1982; 31:672–680.
13. Hill JC: Summary of a Workshop on *Haemophilus influenzae* type b vaccines, from the National Institute of Allergy and Infectious Diseases. *J Inf Dis* 1983; 148(1):167–175.
14. Sell S: The clinical importance of *Haemophilus influenzae* infections in children. *Ped Clin North Am* 1970; 17:415–426.
15. Lindberg J, Rosenhall U, Nylen O, et al: Long-term outcome of *Haemophilus influenzae* type b meningitis related to antibiotic treatment. *Pediatr* 1977; 60:1–6.
16. Sell SH: Long-term sequelae of bacterial meningitis in children. *Pediatr Infect Dis* 1983; 2:90–93.
17. Peltola H, Kayhty H, Sironen A, et al: *Haemophilus influenzae* type b capsular polysaccharide vaccine in children: A double-blind field study of 100,000 vaccinees 3 months to 5 years of age in Finland. *Pediatr* 1977: 60:730–737.
18. Fraser DW: *Haemophilus influenzae* in the Pediatr community and the home, in Sell SH, Wright PF (eds): *Haemophilus influenzae, Epidemiology, Immunology, and Prevention of Diseases.* 1982, pp 11–22.
19. Smith DH, Peter G, Ingram DL, et al: Responses of children immunized with the capsular polysaccharide of *Haemophilus influenzae* type b. *Pediatr* 1973; 52:637–644.
20. Robbins JB, Parke JC Jr, Schneerson R, et al: Quantitative measurement of "natural" and immunization induced *Haemophilus influenzae* type b capsular polysaccharide antibodies. *Pediatr Res* 1973; 7:103–110.
21. Peltola H, Virtanen M, Makela PH: Efficacy of *Haemophilus influenzae* type b capsular polysaccharide vaccine on the incidence of epiglottis and meningitis. *Pathol Biol* (Paris) 1983; 31:141–143.
22. Peltola H, Kayhty H, Virtanen M, et al: Prevention of *Haemophilus influenzae* type b bacteremic infections with the capsular polysaccharide vaccine. *N Engl J Med* 1984; 310:1561–1566.
23. Kayhty H, Karanko V, Peltola H, et al: Serum antibodies after vaccination with *Haemophilus influenzae* type b capsular polysaccharide and responses to reimmunization: No evidence of immunologic tolerance or memory. *Pediatr* 1984; 74:857–865.
24. Parke JC, Schneerson R, Robbins JB, et al: Interim report of a controlled field trial of immunization with capsular polysaccharides of *Haemophilus influenzae* type b and Group C *Neisseria meningitis* in Mecklenburg County, North Carolina, (March 1974–March 1976) *J Infect Dis* 1977; 136(Suppl.):S51–S56.
25. Kabat EA, Bezer AE: The effect of variation in molecular weight on the antigenicity of dextran in man. *Arch Biochem Biophys* 1958; 78:306–318.
26. Gotschlich EC, Rey M, Triau R, et al: Quantitative determination of the human immune response to immunization with meningococcal vaccines. *J Clin Invest* 1972; 51:89–96.
27. Gold R: Immunogenicity of meningococcal polysaccharides, in man, in Rudbach B, Baker R (eds): *Immunology of Bacterial Polysaccharides.* New York, Elsevier 1979, pp 121–151.
28. Kuronen T, Peltola H, Nors T, et al: Adverse reactions and endotoxin content of polysaccharide vaccines. *Develop Biol Standard* 1977; 34:117–125.
29. Kayhty H, Peltola H, Karanko V, et al: The protective level of serum antibodies to the capsular polysaccharide of *Haemophilus influenzae* type b. *J Infect Dis* 1983; 147:1100.
30. Data on file at Office of Biologics Research and Review (OBRR).
31. Committee on Infections Diseases. Haemophilus type b Polysaccharide vaccine. *Pediatr* 1985; 76:322–324.
32. Lepow ML, Peter G, Glode MP, et al: Response of infants to *Haemophilus influenzae* type b polysaccharide and diptheria-tetanus-pertussis vaccine in combination. *J Infect Dis* 1984; 149:950–955.
33. Data on file at Lederle Laboratories.

HYDROMOX® ℞

[*hū-drō-mŏx*]
quinethazone
Tablets

DESCRIPTION

Chemistry: HYDROMOX is a quinazoline derivative, in which a cyclic carbamyl group replaces the cyclic sulfamyl group present in the thiazide derivatives.

Chemical name: 7 - Chloro - 2 - ethyl - 1, 2, 3, 4-tetrahydro-4-oxo-6-quinazolinesulfonamide.

HYDROMOX tablets contain the following inactive ingredients: Cornstarch, Dibasic Calcium Phosphate, Magnesium Stearate, Modified Food Starch.

ACTIONS

HYDROMOX produces urinary excretion of sodium and chloride in approximately equivalent amounts (saluresis), while potassium is excreted to a much lesser degree. The saluretic effect of HYDROMOX is rapid and relatively prolonged, beginning within two hours after administration, reaching a peak at six hours, and lasting for 18 to 24 hours. While HYDROMOX is chemically different, it is pharmacologically genetic to the benzothiadiazine group of drugs.

The dominant action of quinethazone is to increase the renal excretion of sodium and chloride and an accompanying volume of water. This results from inhibition of the tubular mechanism of electrolyte reabsorption. The renal effect is virtually independent of alterations in acid-base balance.

HYDROMOX, like other drugs in this class, inhibits the proximal reabsorption of sodium and chloride. The excretion of potassium results from increased potassium secretion by the distal tubule where potassium is exchanged for sodium.

HYDROMOX may exert its antihypertensive effect by diuresis and sodium loss and/or on vascular function to reduce peripheral resistance.

INDICATIONS

HYDROMOX Lederle, a nonmercurial oral diuretic agent, is indicated as adjunctive therapy in edema associated with congestive heart failure, hepatic cirrhosis, and corticosteroid and estrogen therapy.

HYDROMOX has also been found useful in edema due to various forms of renal dysfunction such as: nephrotic syndrome, acute glomerulonephritis, and chronic renal failure.

HYDROMOX® *quinethazone* is indicated in the management of hypertension either as the sole therapeutic agent or to enhance the effectiveness of other antihypertensive drugs in the more severe forms of hypertension.

Usage in Pregnancy: The routine use of diuretics in an otherwise healthy woman is inappropriate and exposes mother and fetus to unnecessary hazard. Diuretics do not prevent development of toxemia of pregnancy, and there is no satisfactory evidence that they are useful in the treatment of developed toxemia.

Edema during pregnancy may arise from pathological causes or from the physiologic and mechanical consequences of pregnancy. Diuretics are indicated in pregnancy when edema is due to pathologic causes, just as they are in the absence of pregnancy (however, see Warnings, below). Dependent edema in pregnancy, resulting from restriction of venous return by the expanded uterus, is properly treated through elevation of the lower extremities and use of support hose; use of diuretics to lower intravascular volume in this case is illogical and unnecessary. There is hypervolemia during normal pregnancy which is harmful to neither the fetus nor the mother (in the absence of cardiovascular disease), but which is associated with edema, including generalized edema, in the majority of pregnant women. If this edema produces discomfort, increased recumbency will often provide relief. In rare instances, this edema may cause extreme discomfort which is not relieved by rest. In these cases, a short course of diuretics may provide relief and may be appropriate.

CONTRAINDICATIONS

A. Anuria.

B. Hypersensitivity to this or other sulfonamide-derived drugs.

WARNINGS

Diuretics should be used with caution in severe renal disease. In patients with renal disease, diuretics may precipitate azotemia. Cumulative effects of the drug may develop in patients with impaired renal function.

Diuretics should be used with caution in patients with impaired hepatic function or progressive liver disease, since minor alterations of fluid and electrolyte balance may precipitate hepatic coma.

Quinethazone may add to or potentiate the action of other antihypertensive drugs. Potentiation occurs with ganglionic or peripheral adrenergic-blocking drugs.

Sensitivity reactions may occur in patients with a history of allergy or bronchial asthma.

The possibility of exacerbation or activation of systemic lupus erythematosus has been reported.

Usage in Pregnancy: HYDROMOX crosses the placental barrier and appears in cord blood. The use of quinethazone in pregnant women requires that the anticipated benefit be weighed against possible hazards to the fetus. These hazards include fetal or neonatal jaundice, thrombocytopenia, and possible other adverse reactions which have occurred in the adult.

Nursing Mothers: HYDROMOX appears in breast milk. If use of the drug is deemed essential, the patient should stop nursing.

PRECAUTIONS

(1) HYDROMOX should be used with caution in patients with impaired hepatic function or progressive liver disease, since minor alterations of fluid and electrolyte balance may precipitate hepatic coma. (2) Whereas electrolyte abnormalities are often present in such conditions as heart failure and cirrhosis as a result of underlying disease process, they may also be aggravated or may be produced independently by any potent diuretic affecting electrolyte excretion. Caution is especially important during prolonged or intensive therapy and when salt intake is restricted or during concomitant use of steroids or ACTH. Hypokalemia attributable to HYDROMOX® *quinethazone* therapy has been mild and infrequent, and other electrolyte abnormalities have been rare.

The possibility of potassium depletion and its toxic sequelae must be kept in mind, particularly in cirrhotics and patients receiving digitalis. As a preventive measure the use of foods rich in potassium, such as orange juice, or supplements of potassium chloride may be desirable. (3) In patients with impaired renal function, azotemia and/or excessive drug accumulation may develop. (4) As with other potent diuretics, when HYDROMOX is added to a regimen that includes ganglionic-blocking agents, the dosage of these latter preparations should be reduced to avoid a sudden drop in blood pressure. Reduction of dosage is also necessary when one or more of these antihypertensive agents is added to an established HYDROMOX regimen. (5) As with the thiazide diuretics, increases of serum uric acid may occur but precipitation of gout has been rare. (6) A decreased glucose tolerance as evidenced by hyperglycemia and glycosuria, thus aggravating or provoking diabetes mellitus, has occurred. (7) HYDROMOX may decrease arterial responsiveness to norepinephrine and therefore should be withdrawn 48 hours before elective surgery. If emergency surgery is indicated, preanesthetic and anesthetic agents should be administered in reduced dosage. Quinethazone may also increase the responsiveness to tubocurarine. The antihypertensive effects of the drug may be enhanced in the post-sympathectomy patient. (8) Sensitivity reactions may be more likely to occur in patients with a history of allergy or bronchial asthma. (9) The possibility of exacerbation or activation of systemic lupus erythematosus has been suggested for sulfonamide-derived drugs.

ADVERSE REACTIONS

The following adverse reactions have been reported with the diuretic drugs, some of which may be expected to occur with quinethazone:

A. *Gastrointestinal System Reactions:* 1. anorexia, 2. gastric irritation, 3. nausea, 4. vomiting, 5. cramping, 6. diarrhea, 7. constipation, 8. jaundice (intrahepatic cholestatic jaundice), 9. pancreatitis, 10. hyperglycemia, 11. glycosuria.

B. *Central Nervous System Reactions:* 1. dizziness, 2. vertigo, 3. paresthesias, 4. headache, 5. xanthopsia.

C. *Hematologic Reactions:* 1. leukopenia, 2. thrombocytopenia, 3. agranulocytosis, 4. aplastic anemia.

D. *Dermatologic—Hypersensitivity Reactions:* 1. purpura, 2. photosensitivity, 3. rash, 4. urticaria, 5. necrotizing angiitis (vasculitis) (cutaneous vasculitis).

E. *Cardiovascular Reactions:* 1. orthostatic hypotension may occur and may be potentiated by alcohol, barbiturates, or narcotics.

F. *Miscellaneous:* 1. muscle spasm, 2. weakness, 3. restlessness.

Whenever adverse reactions are moderate or severe, thiazide dosage should be reduced or therapy withdrawn.

Dosage: Average Adult Dosage: One or two 50 mg tablets, orally, once a day. Because of its relatively prolonged duration of activity, a single daily dose is generally sufficient. Occasionally, 1 tablet (50 mg) is administered twice a day. Infrequently, a total daily dose of 3 to 4 tablets (150 to 200 mg) may be necessary. The dosage employed depends upon the severity of the condition being treated and the responsiveness of the patient, and often must be adjusted at the beginning or during the course of therapy. When HYDROMOX® *quinethazone* is used in combination with other antihypertensive agents, the dosage of each drug may often be reduced because of potentiation. (See under PRECAUTIONS concerning the necessity for dosage adjustment when one or more of these drugs is added to an already established therapeutic regime.)

HOW SUPPLIED

HYDROMOX® *quinethazone* tablets, are round, white, flat-faced, scored, beveled, engraved with H above and 1 below the score on one side and LL on the other side, supplied as follows:

NDC 0005-4458-23—Bottles of 100

Store at Controlled Room Temperature 15°-30° C (59°-86° F).

Shown in Product Identification Section, page 413

HYDROMOX® R ℞

[hī-drō-mŏx]

Quinethazone-Reserpine
TABLETS

WARNINGS

This fixed combination drug is not indicated for initial therapy of hypertension. Hypertension requires therapy titrated to the individual patient. If the fixed combination represents the dosage so determined, its use may be more convenient in patient management. The treatment of hypertension is not static, but must be reevaluated as conditions in each patient warrant.

DESCRIPTION

HYDROMOX® R *quinethazone-reserpine* tablets each contain 50 mg quinethazone and 0.125 mg reserpine. Quinethazone is a nonmercurial oral diuretic agent, effective in the treatment of edema and hypertension. It is chemically distinct from the benzothiadiazine series of compounds. Reserpine, an antihypertensive agent, has been combined with quinethazone in a dosage form designed to be useful in the treatment of hypertension with or without edema.

Chemistry: Quinethazone is a quinazoline derivative, in which a carbamyl group replaces the cyclic sulfamyl group present in the thiazide derivatives.

Quinethazone is 7-Chloro-2-ethyl-1,2,3,4-tetrahydro-4-oxo-6-quinazoline-sulfonamide.

Reserpine is 3β,16β,17α,18β,20α)-11,17-Dimethoxy-18-[(3,4,5-trimethoxybenzoyl)oxy]-yohimban-16-carboxylic acid methyl ester.

HYDROMOX R also contains the following inactive ingredients: Cornstarch, Dibasic Calcium Phosphate, Magnesium Stearate, Methylcellulose, Yellow 10.

ACTIONS

HYDROMOX produces urinary excretion of sodium and chloride in approximately equivalent amounts (saluresis), while potassium is excreted to a much lesser degree. The saluretic effect of HYDROMOX is rapid and relatively prolonged, beginning within two hours after administration, reaching a peak at six hours, and lasting for 18 to 24 hours. While quinethazone is chemically different from the benzothiadiazine group of drugs, its pharmacologic effects are similar to those elicited by benzothiadiazine derivatives.

The dominant action of quinethazone is to increase the renal excretion of sodium and chloride and an accompanying volume of water. This results from inhibition of the tubular mechanism of electrolyte reabsorption. The renal effect is virtually independent of alterations in acid-base balance.

Quinethazone, like other drugs in its class, inhibits the proximal reabsorption of sodium and chloride. The excretion of potassium results from increased potassium secretion by the distal tubule where potassium is exchanged for sodium.

Quinethazone may exert its antihypertensive effect by diuresis and sodium loss and/or on vascular function to reduce peripheral resistance.

Reserpine is an antihypertensive agent which produces a mild type of sedation that is tranquilizing rather than hypnotic. The most prominent actions of reserpine are upon the cardiovascular and central nervous systems. In clinical hypertension, reserpine produces a gradual and moderate fall in both systolic and diastolic blood pressures after oral administration for several days to two to three weeks. Its effects persist about three to four weeks after medication is withdrawn. With an increase in dose, a prolongation of hypotensive effect, rather than an intensification of blood pressure fall, tends to occur. The doses employed in the therapy of hypertension are smaller than those used in psychiatric disorders.

The dosage form combining quinethazone with reserpine is designed to provide effective antihypertensive action in patients who have failed to show satisfactory response to the use of quinethazone or reserpine alone. This combination of quinethazone and reserpine frequently permits use of a lower dosage of each agent and hence tends to produce the desired antihypertensive effect while eliminating, or at least minimizing, adverse reactions. Blood pressure reductions averaging about -30/-15 have been demonstrated within the first two weeks of treatment. Continuation of therapy beyond two weeks may be expected to produce further *small* drops in blood pressure. The enhanced reduction in blood pressure produced by quinethazone with reserpine appears to be an additive rather than a potentiating effect.

INDICATIONS

HYDROMOX® R *quinethazone-reserpine* tablets are indicated in the management of hypertension (see box WARNINGS) either as the sole therapeutic agent or to enhance the effectiveness of other antihypertensive drugs in the more severe forms of hypertension.

Usage in Pregnancy

The routine use of diuretics in an otherwise healthy woman is inappropriate and exposes mother and fetus to unnecessary hazard. Diuretics do not prevent development of toxemia of pregnancy, and there is no satisfactory evidence that they are useful in the treatment of developed toxemia.

Edema during pregnancy may arise from pathological causes or from the physiologic and mechanical consequences of pregnancy. Diuretics are indicated in pregnancy when edema is due to pathologic causes, just as they are in the absence of pregnancy (however, see WARNINGS, below). Dependent edema in pregnancy, resulting from restriction of venous return by the expanded uterus, is properly treated through elevation of the lower extremities and use of support hose; use of diuretics to lower intravascular volume in this case is illogical and unnecessary. There is hypervolemia during normal pregnancy which is harmful to neither the fetus nor the mother (in the absence of cardiovascular disease), but which is associated with edema, including generalized edema, in the majority of pregnant women. If this edema produces discomfort, increased recumbency will often provide relief. In rare instances, this edema may cause extreme discomfort which is not relieved by rest. In these cases, a short course of diuretics may provide relief and may be appropriate.

CONTRAINDICATIONS

A. Anuria.

B. Hypersensitivity to this or other sulfonamide-derived drugs.

C. Progressively impaired renal function. Since reserpine may increase gastric secretion and motility, its use alone or in combination requires caution and is sometimes contraindicated in patients with a history of peptic or duodenal ulcer or other gastrointestinal disorders.

D. HYDROMOX® R *quinethazone-reserpine* tablets should not be administered to patients with severe hepatic dysfunction. The use of the drug should be avoided in patients with a history of mental depression or psychosis. HYDROMOX R should not be used by patients who are known to be hypersensitive to either agent.

E. History of mental depression.

WARNINGS

Diuretics should be used with caution in severe renal disease. In patients with renal disease, diuretics may precipitate azotemia.

Cumulative effects of the drug may develop in patients with impaired renal function.

Diuretics should be used with caution in patients with impaired hepatic function or progressive liver disease, since minor alterations of fluid and electrolyte balance may precipitate hepatic coma.

HYDROMOX R may add to or potentiate the action of other antihypertensive drugs. Potentiation occurs with ganglionic or peripheral adrenergic blocking drugs.

Sensitivity reactions may occur in patients with a history of allergy or bronchial asthma.

The possibility of exacerbation or activation of systemic lupus erythematosus has been reported with sulfonamide-derived drugs.

Reserpine may cause mental depression. Recognition of depression may be difficult because this condition may often be disguised by somatic complaints (Masked Depression). The

Continued on next page

The information on each product appearing here is based on labelling effective in August, 1986 and is either the entire official brochure or an accurate condensation therefrom. Information concerning all Lederle products may be obtained from the Professional Services Department, Lederle Laboratories, Pearl River, New York, 10965.

Lederle—Cont.

drug should be discontinued at first signs of depression such as despondency, early morning insomnia, loss of appetite, impotence, or self-deprecation. Drug-induced depression may persist for several months after drug withdrawal and may be severe enough to result in suicide.

Usage in Pregnancy

HYDROMOX R crosses the placental barrier and appears in cord blood. The use of HYDROMOX R in pregnant women requires that the anticipated benefit be weighed against possible hazards to the fetus. These hazards include fetal or neonatal jaundice, thrombocytopenia, and possibly other adverse reactions which have occurred in the adult.

Nursing Mothers

HYDROMOX R appears in breast milk. If use of the drug is deemed essential, the patient should stop nursing.

Reserpine has been reported to cause central nervous system depression of the newborn infant when given to the mother in the immediate antepartum period.

HYDROMOX R should be discontinued promptly if any symptoms of mental depression occur with the use of the drug.

PRECAUTIONS

Quinethazone:

(1) Quinethazone should be used with caution in patients with impaired hepatic function or progressive liver disease, since minor alterations of fluid and electrolyte balance may precipitate hepatic coma.

(2) Whereas electrolyte abnormalities are often present in such conditions as heart failure and cirrhosis as a result of underlying disease process, they may also be aggravated or may be produced independently by any potent diuretic affecting electrolyte excretion. Caution is especially important during prolonged or intensive therapy and when salt intake is restricted or during concomitant use of steroids or ACTH. Hypokalemia attributable to HYDROMOX® *quinethazone* therapy has been mild and infrequent, and other electrolyte abnormalities have been rare.
The possibility of potassium depletion and its toxic sequelae must be kept in mind, particularly in cirrhotics and patients receiving digitalis. As a preventive measure the use of foods rich in potassium, such as orange juice, or supplements of potassium chloride may be desirable.

(3) In patients with impaired renal function, azotemia and/or excessive drug accumulation may develop.

(4) As with other potent diuretics, when HYDROMOX® *quinethazone* is added to a regimen that includes ganglionic-blocking agents, the dosage of these latter preparations should be reduced to avoid a sudden drop in blood pressure. Reduction of dosage is also necessary when one or more of these antihypertensive agents is added to an established HYDROMOX® regimen.

(5) As with the thiazide diuretics, increases of serum uric acid may occur but precipitation of gout has been rare.

(6) A decreased glucose tolerance as evidenced by hyperglycemia and glycosuria, thus aggravating or provoking diabetes mellitus, has occurred.

(7) Quinethazone may decrease arterial responsiveness to norepinephrine and therefore should be withdrawn 48 hours before elective surgery. If emergency surgery is indicated, preanesthetic and anesthetic agents should be administered in reduced dosage. Quinethazone may also increase the responsiveness to tubocurarine. The antihypertensive effects of the drug may be enhanced in the post-sympathectomy patient.

(8) Sensitivity reactions may be more likely to occur in patients with a history of allergy or bronchial asthma.

(9) The possibility of exacerbation or activation of systemic lupus erythematosus has been suggested for sulfonamide-derived drugs.

Reserpine:

Reserpine may precipitate biliary colic in patients with gallstones, or bronchial asthma in susceptible patients. Reserpine preparations should be used with caution in patients with a history of peptic ulcer, ulcerative colitis, and other gastrointestinal disorders. It may cause severe depression and suicidal risk and may produce pseudoparkinsonism (a paralysis agitans-like syndrome).

Administration of reserpine should be discontinued two weeks or more before electroconvulsant therapy if possible to preclude severe, even fatal, reactions.

Reserpine may cause cardiotoxic effects, eg, premature ventricular contractions and other arrhythmias, possible sensitization to digitalis (which might be further complicated by any hypokalemic effects of quinethazone), fluid retention, and congestive failure.

Animal tumorigenicity: Rodent studies have shown that reserpine is an animal tumorigen, causing an increased incidence of mammary fibroadenomas in female mice, malignant tumors of the seminal vesicles in male mice, and malignant adrenal medullary tumors in male rats. These findings arose in two-year studies in which the drug was administered in the feed at concentrations of 5 and 10 ppm—about 100 to 300 times the usual human dose. The breast neoplasms are thought to be related to reserpine's prolactin-elevating effect. Several other prolactin-elevating drugs have also been associated with an increased incidence of mammary neoplasia in rodents.

The extent to which these findings indicate a risk to humans is uncertain. Tissue culture experiments show that about one-third of human breast tumors are prolactin-dependent *in vitro*, a factor of considerable importance if the use of the drug is contemplated in a patient with previously detected breast cancer. The possibility of an increased risk of breast cancer in reserpine users has been studied extensively; however, no firm conclusion has emerged. Although a few epidemiologic studies have suggested a slightly increased risk (less than twofold in all studies except one) in women who have used reserpine, other studies of generally similar design have not confirmed this. Epidemiologic studies conducted using other drugs (neuroleptic agents) that, like reserpine, increase prolactin levels, and therefore would be considered rodent mammary carcinogens, have not shown an association between chronic administration of the drug and human mammary tumorigenesis. While long-term clinical observation has not suggested such an association, the available evidence is considered too limited to be conclusive at this time. An association of reserpine intake with pheochromocytoma or tumors of the seminal vesicles has not been explored.

ADVERSE REACTIONS

The following adverse reactions have been reported with the diuretic drugs, some of which may be expected to occur with quinethazone:

A. Gastrointestinal System Reactions
   1. anorexia
   2. gastric irritation
   3. nausea
   4. vomiting
   5. cramping
   6. diarrhea
   7. constipation
   8. jaundice (intrahepatic cholestatic jaundice)
   9. pancreatitis
   10. hyperglycemia
   11. glycosuria

B. Central Nervous System Reactions
   1. dizziness
   2. vertigo
   3. paresthesias
   4. headache
   5. xanthopsia

C. Hematologic Reactions
   1. leukopenia
   2. thrombocytopenia
   3. agranulocytosis
   4. aplastic anemia

D. Dermatologic—Hypersensitivity Reactions
   1. purpura
   2. photosensitivity
   3. rash
   4. urticaria
   5. necrotizing angiitis (vasculitis) (cutaneous vasculitis)

E. Cardiovascular Reactions
   1. orthostatic hypotension may occur and may be potentiated by alcohol, barbiturates, or narcotics

F. Miscellaneous
   1. muscle spasm
   2. weakness
   3. restlessness

Reserpine:

With reserpine, nasal congestion, weight gain, and diarrhea are the most frequently noted side effects. The drug may reactivate old peptic ulcers because it increases hydrochloric acid secretion by the stomach. More serious reactions are excessive drowsiness, fatigue, weakness, insomnia, nightmares, excitement, irrational behavior, and incipient parkinsonism. Sodium retention edema may occur when reserpine is used.

Whenever adverse reactions are moderate or severe, thiazide dosage should be reduced or therapy withdrawn.

DOSAGE AND ADMINISTRATION

Dosage: As determined by individual titration (see box WARNINGS).

Usual Initial Adult Loading Dosage: If considered necessary, 3 to 4 HYDROMOX R tablets (150 mg quinethazone with 0.375 mg reserpine to 200 mg quinethazone with 0.5 mg reserpine) may be administered orally, once a day, for not more than two weeks.

Average (or Maintenance) Adult Dosage: 1 to 2 HYDROMOX R tablets (50 mg quinethazone with 0.125 mg reserpine to 100 mg quinethazone with 0.25 mg reserpine) administered orally, once a day.

Because of the relatively prolonged effect of HYDROMOX R, a single daily dose is usually sufficient. Occasionally 1 tablet is administered twice a day, but ordinarily medication is administered only in the morning to avoid the inconvenience of nocturia.

With the exception of the initial loading phase, a total dose of 3 to 4 tablets of HYDROMOX R *quinethazone-reserpine* is not recommended since the 0.375 mg to 0.5 mg of reserpine thus provided is more than is routinely necessary for a hypotensive effect and serves to increase the risk of adverse reactions. If more than 100 mg of quinethazone per day is desired, it is recommended that HYDROMOX quinethazone tablets be used to supplement HYDROMOX R tablets.

The dosage of HYDROMOX R to be employed depends upon the severity of the condition being treated and the responsiveness of the individual patient and often must be adjusted at the beginning of, or during the course of, therapy. Reduction of dosage is often possible after two weeks, when as little as 1 tablet a day may be sufficient for maintenance.

When HYDROMOX R tablets are used in combination with other antihypertensive drugs, the dosage of each drug may often be reduced because of potentiation. (See under PRECAUTIONS concerning the necessity for dosage adjustment when one or more of these drugs is added to an already established therapeutic regimen.)

HOW SUPPLIED

HYDROMOX® R quinethazone-reserpine tablets, each containing 50 mg quinethazone and 0.125 mg reserpine, are round, yellow, scored tablets, engraved with LL on one side and H above and 2 below the score on the other side, supplied as follows:

NDC 0005-4457-23—bottles of 100
NDC 0005-4457-31—bottles of 500

Store at Controlled Room Temperature 15°–30° C (59°–86° F).

Shown in Product Identification Section, page 413

INCREMIN®

[*in-cre-min*]

WITH IRON • SYRUP

(vitamins B_1, B_6, B_{12}-lysine-iron)

Dietary Supplement

(See PDR For Nonprescription Drugs)

LEDERPLEX®

[*lěder-plěx*]

Dietary Supplement of B-Complex Vitamins for Adults and Children 4 or More Years of Age

Capsules—Liquid

(See PDR For Nonprescription Drugs)

LEUCOVORIN CALCIUM INJECTION ℞

[*lu-cō-vor-in*]

DESCRIPTION

Each 1 ml ampul of Leucovorin Calcium *Lederle* contains Leucovorin 3 mg as the calcium salt which is the form preferred for intramuscular injection. Preservative: Benzyl Alcohol 0.9% w/v. The inactive ingredients are Sodium Chloride 0.56% w/v, Water for Injection qs 100% and sodium hydroxide or hydrochloric acid is used to adjust the pH to approximately 7.7.

Each 50 mg vial of Leucovorin Calcium cryodesiccated powder when reconstituted with 5 ml of sterile diluent contains Leucovorin 10 mg per ml as the calcium salt, which is the form preferred for intramuscular injection; contains no preservative. Dilute only with Bacteriostatic Water for Injection USP which contains benzyl alcohol. The inactive ingredients are sodium chloride 40 mg/vial, and sodium hydroxide or hydrochloric acid qs to pH approximately 8.1. When reconstituted as directed, the resulting solution must be used within seven days. If the product is reconstituted with Water for Injection USP, use immediately.

ACTIONS

Leucovorin (folinic acid) is the formyl derivative and active form of folic acid.

Leucovorin Calcium is useful clinically in circumventing the action of folate reductase. There is no evidence that intramuscular doses of greater than 1 mg have greater efficacy than those of 1 mg.

INDICATIONS

Indicated (a) to diminish the toxicity and counteract the effect of inadvertently administered overdosages of folic acid antagonists (See Warnings); (b) in the treatment of the megaloblastic anemias due to sprue, nutritional deficiency, pregnancy, and infancy when oral therapy is not feasible.

CONTRAINDICATIONS

Not to be administered for the treatment of pernicious anemia or other megaloblastic anemias where Vitamin B_{12} is deficient.

WARNINGS
Leucovorin is improper therapy for pernicious anemia and other megaloblastic anemias secondary to lack of Vitamin B_{12}. A hematologic remission may occur while neurologic manifestations remain progressive.
In the treatment of overdosage of folic acid antagonists, Leucovorin must be administered within one hour, if possible, and is usually ineffective if administered after a delay of four hours.

PRECAUTIONS
In the presence of pernicious anemia a hematologic remission may occur while neurologic manifestations remain progressive.

ADVERSE REACTIONS
Allergic sensitization has been reported following both oral and parenteral administration of folic acid.

DOSAGE
Megaloblastic anemia: No more than or up to 1 mg daily. There is no evidence that intramuscular doses greater than 1 mg daily have greater efficacy than those of 1 mg; additionally, loss of folate in the urine becomes roughly logarithmic as the amount administered exceeds 1 mg.
For the treatment of overdosage of folic acid antagonists: To be given in amounts equal to the weight of the antagonist given.

HOW SUPPLIED
6 — 1 ml ampuls NDC 0205-4004-51.
50 mg vials of cryodesiccated powder NDC 0205-5330-92.
Military Depot
NSN 6505-01-054-7008, 50 mg/vial
VA Depots
NSN 6505-01-054-7008, 50 mg/vial for IM use
Manufactured for
LEDERLE LABORATORIES DIVISION
American Cyanamid Company
Pearl River, NY 10965
by
LEDERLE PARENTERALS INC.
Carolina, Puerto Rico 00630
Shown in Product Identification Section, page 413

LEUCOVORIN CALCIUM TABLETS ℞

DESCRIPTION
Leucovorin Calcium Tablets contain 5 mg leucovorin as the calcium salt of N-[p-[[(2-amino-5-formyl-1,4,5,6,7,8-hexahydro-4-oxo-6-pteridinyl)-methyl]amino]benzoyl]-L-glutamic acid. This is equivalent to 5.40 mg of anhydrous Leucovorin Calcium.
Leucovorin Calcium Tablets also contain the following inactive ingredients: Corn Starch, Dibasic Calcium Phosphate, Magnesium Stearate, Modified Food Starch.
Leucovorin is a water soluble vitamin in the folate group; it is useful as an antidote to drugs which act as folic acid antagonists. These tablets are intended for oral administration only.

CLINICAL PHARMACOLOGY
Leucovorin is a mixture of the diastereoisomers of the 5-formyl derivative of tetrahydrofolic acid. The biologically active component of the mixture is the (-)-L-isomer, known as *Citrovorum factor*, or (-)-folinic acid. Leucovorin does *not* require reduction by the enzyme dihydrofolate reductase in order to participate in reactions utilizing folates as a source of "one-carbon" moieties. Following oral administration, leucovorin is rapidly absorbed and enters the general body pool of reduced folates.[1] The increase in plasma and serum folate activity (determined microbiologically with *Lactobacillus casei*) seen after oral administration of leucovorin is predominantly due to 5-methyltetrahydrofolate.[1,2,3,4,5,6]
Following a 20 mg dose of Leucovorin Calcium, the mean maximum serum total reduced folate concentrations were:[4]
Tablet—364 ± 12.1 ng/ml at 2.0 ± 0.07 hours
Solution—375 ± 12.8 ng/ml at 2.1 ± 0.11 hours
Parenteral—355 ± 17.2 ng/ml at 0.96 ± 0.10 hours
The half-life of plasma 5-formyl tetrahydrofolate as 1.5 ± 0.08 hours and that of the 5-methyltetrahydrofolate was 3.0 ± 0.09 hours.
Oral tablets produced equivalent bioavailability (8% difference) when compared to the parenteral administration. The parenteral solution also provided equal bioavailability to the tablets when administered orally (2% difference).[4]

INDICATIONS AND USAGE
Leucovorin Calcium is indicated for the prophylaxis and treatment of undesired hematopoietic effects of folic acid antagonists (see WARNINGS).

CONTRAINDICATIONS
Leucovorin is improper therapy for pernicious anemia and other megaloblastic anemias secondary to the lack of vitamin B_{12}. A hematologic remission may occur while neurologic manifestations remain progressive.

WARNINGS
In the treatment of accidental overdosage of folic acid antagonists, leucovorin should be administered as promptly as possible. As the time interval between antifolate administration (eg, methotrexate) and leucovorin rescue increases, leucovorin's effectiveness in counteracting hematologic toxicity diminishes.

PRECAUTIONS
General: Following chemotherapy with folic acid antagonists, parenteral administration of leucovorin is preferable to oral dosing if there is a possibility that the patient may vomit and not absorb the leucovorin. In the presence of pernicious anemia, a hematologic remission may occur while neurologic manifestations remain progressive. Leucovorin has no effect on other toxicities of methotrexate, such as the nephrotoxicity resulting from drug precipitation in the kidney.
Drug Interactions: Folic acid in large amounts may counteract the antiepileptic effect of phenobarbital, phenytoin, and primidone, and increase the frequency of seizures in susceptible children.
Pregnancy: Teratogenic Effects: Pregnancy Category C. Animal reproduction studies have not been conducted with leucovorin. It is also not known whether leucovorin can cause fetal harm when administered to a pregnant woman or can affect reproduction capacity. Leucovorin should be given to a pregnant woman only if clearly needed.
Nursing Mothers: It is not known whether this drug is excreted in human milk. Because many drugs are excreted in human milk, caution should be exercised when leucovorin is administered to a nursing mother.
Pediatric Use: (See—Drug Interactions)

ADVERSE REACTIONS
Allergic sensitization has been reported following both oral and parenteral administration of folic acid.

OVERDOSAGE
Excessive amounts of leucovorin may nullify the chemotherapeutic effect of folic acid antagonists.

DOSAGE AND ADMINISTRATION
Leucovorin is a specific antidote for the hematopoietic toxicity of methotrexate and other strong inhibitors of the enzyme dihydrofolate reductase. Leucovorin rescue must begin within 24 hours of antifolate administration. A conventional leucovorin rescue dosage schedule is 10 mg/m^2 orally or parenterally followed by 10 mg/m^2 orally every six hours for 72 hours. If, however, at 24 hours following methotrexate administration the serum creatinine is 50% or greater than the premethotrexate serum creatinine, the leucovorin dosage should be immediately increased to 100 mg/m^2 every three hours until the serum methotrexate level is below 5×10^{-8}M.[7,8]
The recommended dose of leucovorin to counteract hematologic toxicity from folic acid antagonists with less affinity for mammalian dihydrofolate reductase than methotrexate (ie, trimethoprim, pyrimethamine) is substantially less and 5 to 15 mg of leucovorin per day has been recommended by some investigators.[9,10,11]

HOW SUPPLIED
Leucovorin Calcium Tablets are round, unscored, yellowish white, engraved 5 on one side and C33 on the other each containing 5 mg of leucovorin as the calcium salt, supplied as follows:
NDC 0005-4536-38—Bottles of 30 with CRC.
Store at Controlled Room Temperature 15°-30°C (59°-86°F.)

REFERENCES

1. Nixon PF and Bertino JR: Effective Absorption and Utilization of Oral Formyltetrahydrofolate in Man. *N Engl J Med 286* (4):175–179, Jan 27, 1972.
2. Ratanasthien K, Blair JA, Leeming RJ, Cooke WT and Melikian V: Folates in Human Serum. *J Clin Pathol 27:* 875–879, 1974.
3. Mehta BM, Gisolfi AL, Hutchison DJ, Nirenberg A, Kellick MG and Rosen G: Serum Distribution of Citrovorum Factor and 5-methyltetrahydrofolate Following Oral and I.M. Administration of Calcium Leucovorin in Normal Adults. *Cancer Treat Rep 62* (3):345–350, Mar 1978.
4. Data on file, Clinical Research, Lederle Laboratories, Pearl River, NY 10965.
5. Whitehead VM, Pratt R, Viallet A and Cooper BA: Intestinal Conversion of Folinic Acid to 5-methyltetrahydrofolate in Man. *Br J Haematol 22*:63–72, 1972.
6. Herbert V: Aseptic Addition for *Lactobacillus casei* Assay of Folate Activity in Human Serum. *J Clin Path 19*:12–16, 1966.
7. Bleyer WA: The Clinical Pharmacology of Methotrexate. *Cancer: 41* (1):36–51, 1978.
8. Frei, E, Blum RH, Pitman SW, *et al:* High Dose Methotrexate with Leucovorin Rescue: Rationale and Spectrum of Antitumor Activity *Am J Med 68*:370–376, 1980.
9. Golde DW, Bersch N, Quan SG: Trimethoprim and Sulphamethoxazole Inhibition of Haematopoiesis *in Vitro, Br J Haematol, 40* (3):363–367, 1978.
10. Stein berg SE, Campbell CL, Rabinovitch PS, *et al:* The Effect of Trimethoprim/Sulfamethoxazole on Friend Erythroleukemia Cells. *Blood, 55* (3):501–504, 1980.
11. Mahmound AAF and Warren KS: Algorithms in the Diagnosis and Management of Exotic Disease. XX. Toxoplasmosis. *J Infect Dis 135* (3):493–496, 1977.

Shown in Product Identification Section, page 413

LOXITANE® ℞
[*lŏks-ĭ-tāne*]
Loxapine Succinate
Capsules

LOXITANE® C ℞
Loxapine Hydrochloride
Oral Concentrate

LOXITANE® IM ℞
Loxapine Hydrochloride
For Intramuscular Use Only

DESCRIPTION
LOXITANE® *loxapine*, a dibenzoxazepine compound, represents a new subclass of tricyclic antipsychotic agent, chemically distinct from the thioxanthenes, butyrophenones, and phenothiazines. Chemically, it is 2-chloro-11-(4-methyl-1-piperazinyl)-dibenz[*b,f*][1,4]oxazepine. It is present in capsules as the succinate salt, and in the concentrate and parenteral primarily as the hydrochloride salt.
CAPSULES—Each capsule contains loxapine succinate equivalent to 5, 10, 25, or 50 mg of loxapine base and the following inactive ingredients: Blue 1, Gelatin, Lactose, Magnesium Stearate, Titanium Dioxide, and Yellow 10. Additionally, the 5 mg capsule contains Red 33, the 10 mg capsule contains Red 28 and Red 33, and the 25 mg capsule contains Yellow 6 as inactive ingredients.
ORAL CONCENTRATE—Each ml contains loxapine hydrochloride equivalent to 25 mg of loxapine base and propylene glycol as an inactive ingredient.
INTRAMUSCULAR—(Sterile)—Not for Intravenous Use —Each ml contains loxapine hydrochloride equivalent to 50 mg of loxapine base.
Inactive Ingredients: Polysorbate 80 NF 5% w/v; Propylene Glycol 70% v/v; and Water for Injection qs ad 100% v.
Sodium hydroxide and hydrochloric acid are used to adjust pH to approx. 5.8 during manufacture.

ACTIONS
Pharmacologically, loxapine is a tranquilizer for which the exact mode of action has not been established. However, changes in the level of excitability of subcortical inhibitory areas have been observed in several animal species in association with such manifestations of tranquilization as calming effects and suppression of aggressive behavior.
In normal human volunteers, signs of sedation were seen within 20 to 30 minutes after administration, were most pronounced within one and one-half to three hours, and lasted through 12 hours. Similar timing of primary pharmacologic effects was seen in animals.
Absorption of LOXITANE following oral or parenteral administration is virtually complete. The drug is removed rapidly from the plasma and distributed in tissues. Animal studies suggest an initial preferential distribution in lungs, brain, spleen, heart, and kidney. Loxapine is metabolized extensively and is excreted mainly in the first 24 hours. Metabolites are excreted in the urine in the form of conjugates and in the feces unconjugated.

INDICATIONS
LOXITANE is indicated for the management of the manifestations of psychotic disorders. The antipsychotic efficacy of LOXITANE® *loxapine* was established in clinical studies which enrolled newly hospitalized and chronically hospitalized acutely ill schizophrenic patients as subjects.

CONTRAINDICATIONS
LOXITANE is contraindicated in comatose or severe drug-induced depressed states (alcohol, barbiturates, narcotics, etc).
LOXITANE is contraindicated in individuals with known hypersensitivity to dibenzoxazepines.

WARNINGS
Tardive Dyskinesia: Tardive dyskinesia, a syndrome consisting of potentially irreversible, involuntary, dyskinetic movements, may develop in patients treated with neuroleptic (antipsychotic) drugs. Although the prevalence of the

Continued on next page

The information on each product appearing here is based on labelling effective in August, 1986 and is either the entire official brochure or an accurate condensation therefrom. Information concerning all Lederle products may be obtained from the Professional Services Department, Lederle Laboratories, Pearl River, New York, 10965.

Lederle—Cont.

syndrome appears to be highest among the elderly, especially elderly women, it is impossible to rely upon prevalence estimates to predict, at the inception of neuroleptic treatment, which patients are likely to develop the syndrome. Whether neuroleptic drug products differ in their potential to cause tardive dyskinesia is unknown.

Both the risk of developing the syndrome and the likelihood that it will become irreversible are believed to increase as the duration of treatment and the total cumulative dosage of neuroleptic drugs administered to the patient increases. However, the syndrome can develop, although much less commonly, after relatively brief treatment periods at low dosages.

There is no known treatment for established cases of tardive dyskinesia, although the syndrome may remit, partially or completely, if neuroleptic treatment is withdrawn. Neuroleptic treatment, itself, however, may suppress (or partially suppress) the signs and symptoms of the syndrome, and thereby may possibly mask the underlying disease process. The effect that symptomatic suppression has upon the long-term course of the syndrome is unknown.

Given these considerations, neuroleptics should be prescribed in a manner that is most likely to minimize the occurrence of tardive dyskinesia. Chronic neuroleptic treatment should generally be reserved for patients who suffer from a chronic illness that 1) is known to respond to neuroleptic drugs, and, 2) for whom alternative, equally effective, but potentially less harmful treatments are *not* available or appropriate. In patients who do require chronic treatment, the smallest dose and the shortest duration of treatment producing a satisfactory clinical response should be sought. The need for continued treatment should be reassessed periodically.

If signs and symptoms of tardive dyskinesia appear in a patient on neuroleptics, drug discontinuation should be considered. However, some patients may require treatment despite the presence of the syndrome. (See ADVERSE REACTIONS and Information for Patients sections.)

LOXITANE, like other tranquilizers, may impair mental and/or physical abilities, especially during the first few days of therapy. Therefore, ambulatory patients should be warned about activities requiring alertness (eg, operating vehicles or machinery) and about concomitant use of alcohol and other CNS depressants.

LOXITANE has not been evaluated for the management of behavioral complications in patients with mental retardation, and, therefore, it cannot be recommended.

PRECAUTIONS

General:

LOXITANE® *loxapine* should be used with extreme caution in patients with a history of convulsive disorders since it lowers the convulsive threshold. Seizures have been reported in patients receiving LOXITANE at antipsychotic dosage levels, and may occur in epileptic patients even with maintenance of routine anticonvulsant drug therapy.

LOXITANE has an antiemetic effect in animals. Since this effect may also occur in man, LOXITANE may mask signs of overdosage of toxic drugs and may obscure conditions such as intestinal obstruction and brain tumor.

LOXITANE should be used with caution in patients with cardiovascular disease. Increased pulse rates have been reported in the majority of patients receiving antipsychotic doses; transient hypotension has been reported. In the presence of severe hypotension requiring vasopressor therapy, the preferred drugs may be norepinephrine and angiotensin. Usual doses of epinephrine may be ineffective because of inhibition of its vasopressor effect by LOXITANE.

The possiblity of ocular toxicity from loxapine cannot be excluded at this time. Therefore, careful observation should be made for pigmentary retinopathy and lenticular pigmentation, since these have been observed in some patients receiving certain other antipsychotic drugs for prolonged periods.

Because of possible anticholinergic action, the drug should be used cautiously in patients with glaucoma or a tendency to urinary retention, particularly with concomitant administration of anticholinergic-type antiparkinson medication.

Experience to date indicates the possibility of a slightly higher incidence of extrapyramidal effects following intramuscular administration than normally anticipated with oral formulations. The increase may be attributable to higher plasma levels following intramuscular injection.

Neuroleptic drugs elevate prolactin levels; the elevation persists during chronic administration. Tissue culture experiments indicate that approximately one third of human breast cancers are prolactin-dependent *in vitro*, a factor of potential importance if the prescription of these drugs is contemplated in a patient with a previously detected breast cancer. Although disturbances such as galactorrhea, amenorrhea, gynecomastia, and impotence have been reported, the clinical significance of elevated serum prolactin levels is unknown for most patients. An increase in mammary neoplasms has been found in rodents after chronic administration of neuroleptic drugs. Neither clinical studies nor epidemiologic studies conducted to date, however, have shown an association between chronic administration of these drugs and mammary tumorigenesis; the available evidence is considered too limited to be conclusive at this time.

Information for Patients

Given the likelihood that some patients exposed chronically to neuroleptics will develop tardive dyskinesia, it is advised that all patients in whom chronic use is contemplated be given, if possible, full information about this risk. The decision to inform patients and/or their guardians must obviously take into account the clinical circumstances and the competency of the patient to understand the information provided.

Usage in Pregnancy: Safe use of LOXITANE® loxapine during pregnancy or lactation has not been established; therefore, its use in pregnancy, in nursing mothers, or in women of childbearing potential requires that the benefits of treatment be weighed against the possible risks to mother and child. No embryotoxicity or teratogenicity was observed in studies in rats, rabbits, or dogs although, with the exception of one rabbit study, the highest dosage was only two times the maximum recommended human dosage, and in some studies it was below this dosage. Perinatal studies have shown renal papillary abnormalities in offspring of rats treated from midpregnancy with doses of 0.6 and 1.8 mg/kg, doses which approximate the usual human dose but which are considerably below the maximum recommended human dose.

Nursing Mothers: The extent of the excretion of LOXITANE or its metabolites in human milk is not known. However, LOXITANE and its metabolites have been shown to be transported into the milk of lactating dogs. LOXITANE administration to nursing women should be avoided if clinically possible.

Usage in Children: Studies have not been performed in children; therefore, this drug is not recommended for use in children below the age of 16.

ADVERSE REACTIONS

CNS Effects: Manifestations of adverse effects on the central nervous system, other than extrapyramidal effects, have been seen infrequently. Drowsiness, usually mild, may occur at the beginning of therapy or when dosage is increased. It usually subsides with continued LOXITANE therapy. The incidence of sedation has been less than that of certain aliphatic phenothiazines and slightly more than the piperazine phenothiazines. Dizziness, faintness, staggering gait, shuffling gait, muscle twitching, weakness, insomnia, agitation, tension, seizures, akinesia, slurred speech, numbness, and confusional states have been reported. Neuroleptic malignant syndrome (NMS) has been reported.

Extrapyramidal Reactions—Neuromuscular (extrapyramidal) reactions during the administration of LOXITANE® *loxapine* have been reported frequently, often during the first few days of treatment. In most patients, these reactions involved parkinsonian-like symptoms such as tremor, rigidity, excessive salivation, and masked facies. Akathisia (motor restlessness) also has been reported relatively frequently. These symptoms are usually not severe and can be controlled by reduction of LOXITANE dosage or by administration of antiparkinson drugs in usual dosage. Dystonic and dyskinetic reactions have occurred less frequently, but may be more severe. Dystonias include spasms of muscles of the neck and face, tongue protrusion, and oculogyric movement. Dyskinetic reactions have been described in the form of choreoathetoid movements. These reactions sometimes require reduction or temporary withdrawal of loxapine dosage in addition to appropriate counteractive drugs.

Persistent Tardive Dyskinesia—As with all antipsychotic agents, tardive dyskinesia may appear in some patients on long-term therapy or may appear after drug therapy has been discontinued. The risk appears to be greater in elderly patients on high-dose therapy, especially females. The symptoms are persistent and in some patients appear to be irreversible. The syndrome is characterized by rhythmical involuntary movement of the tongue, face, mouth, or jaw (eg, protrusion of tongue, puffing of cheeks, puckering of mouth, chewing movements). Sometimes these may be accompanied by involuntary movements of extremities.

There is no known effective treatment for tardive dyskinesia; antiparkinson agents usually do not alleviate the symptoms of this syndrome. It is suggested that all antipsychotic agents be discontinued if these symptoms appear. Should it be necessary to reinstitute treatment, or increase the dosage of the agent, or switch to a different antipsychotic agent, the syndrome may be masked. It has been suggested that fine vermicular movements of the tongue may be an early sign of the syndrome, and if the medication is stopped at that time the syndrome may not develop.

Cardiovascular Effects: Tachycardia, hypotension, hypertension, orthostatic hypotension, lightheadedness, and syncope have been reported.

A few cases of ECG changes similar to those seen with phenothiazines have been reported. It is not known whether these were related to LOXITANE® *loxapine* administration.

Hematologic: Rarely, agranulocytosis, thrombocytopenia, leukopenia.

Skin: Dermatitis, edema (puffiness of face), pruritus, rash, alopecia, and seborrhea have been reported with loxapine.

Anticholinergic Effects: Dry mouth, nasal congestion, constipation, blurred vision, urinary retention, and paralytic ileus have occurred.

Gastrointestinal: Nausea and vomiting have been reported in some patients. Hepatocellular injury (ie, SGOT/SGPT elevation) has been reported in association with loxapine administration and rarely, jaundice and/or hepatitis questionably related to LOXITANE treatment.

Other Adverse Reactions: Weight gain, weight loss, dyspnea, ptosis, hyperpyrexia, flushed facies, headache, paresthesia, and polydipsia have been reported in some patients. Rarely, galactorrhea, amenorrhea, gynecomastia, and menstrual irregularity of uncertain etiology have been reported.

DOSAGE AND ADMINISTRATION

LOXITANE is administered, usually in divided doses, two to four times a day. Daily dosage (in terms of base equivalents) should be adjusted to the individual patient's needs as assessed by the severity of symptoms and previous history of response to antipsychotic drugs.

Oral Administration

Initial dosage of 10 mg twice daily is recommended, although in severely disturbed patients, initial dosage up to a total of 50 mg daily may be desirable. Dosage should then be increased fairly rapidly over the first seven to ten days until there is effective control of psychotic symptoms. The usual therapeutic and maintenance range is 60 mg to 100 mg daily. However, as with other antipsychotic drugs, some patients respond to lower dosage and others require higher dosage for optimal benefit. Daily dosage higher than 250 mg is not recommended.

LOXITANE C Oral Concentrate should be mixed with orange or grapefruit juice shortly before administration. Use only the enclosed calibrated (10 mg, 15 mg, 25 mg, 50 mg) dropper for dosage.

Maintenance Therapy

For maintenance therapy, dosage should be reduced to the lowest level compatible with symptom control; many patients have been maintained satisfactorily at dosages in the range of 20 mg to 60 mg daily.

Intramuscular Administration

LOXITANE IM is used for prompt symptomatic control in the acutely agitated patient and in patients whose symptoms render oral medication temporarily impractical. During clinical trial there were only rare reports of significant local tissue reaction.

LOXITANE IM is administered by intramuscular (not intravenous) injection in doses of 12.5 mg (1/4 ml) to 50 mg (1 ml) at intervals of four to six hours or longer, both dose and interval depending on patient response. Many patients have responded satisfactorily to twice-daily dosage. As described above for oral administration, attention is directed to the necessity for dosage adjustment on an individual basis over the early days of loxapine administration.

Once the desired symptomatic control is achieved and the patient is able to take medication orally, loxapine should be administered in capsule or oral concentrate form. Usually this should occur within five days.

OVERDOSAGE

Signs and symptoms of overdosage will depend on the amount ingested and individual patient tolerance. As would be expected from the pharmacologic actions of the drug, the clinical findings may range from mild depression of the CNS and cardiovascular systems to profound hypotension, respiratory depression, and unconsciousness. The possibility of occurrence of extrapyramidal symptoms and/or convulsive seizures should be kept in mind. Renal failure following loxapine overdosage has also been reported.

The treatment of overdosage is essentially symptomatic and supportive. Early gastric lavage and extended dialysis might be expected to be beneficial. Centrally acting emetics may have little effect because of the antiemetic action of loxapine. In addition, emesis should be avoided because of the possibility of aspiration of vomitus. Avoid analeptics, such as pentylenetetrazol, which may cause convulsions. Severe hypotension might be expected to respond to the administration of levarterenol or phenylephrine. EPINEPHRINE SHOULD NOT BE USED SINCE ITS USE IN A PATIENT WITH PARTIAL ADRENERGIC BLOCKADE MAY FURTHER LOWER THE BLOOD PRESSURE. Severe extrapyramidal reactions should be treated with anticholinergic antiparkinson agents or diphenhydramine hydrochloride, and anticonvulsant therapy should be initiated as indicated. Additional measures include oxygen and intravenous fluids.

HOW SUPPLIED

LOXITANE® *loxapine succinate* Capsules are available in the following base equivalent strengths:

5 mg—Hard shell, opaque, dark green capsules printed with Lederle over L1 on one half and 5 mg on the other, are supplied as follows:
NDC 0005-5359-23—Bottles of 100
NDC 0005-5359-60—Unit Dose 10 × 10
10 mg—Hard shell, opaque, with yellow body and a dark green cap, printed with Lederle over L2 on one half and 10 mg on the other, are supplied as follows:
NDC 0005-5360-23—Bottles of 100
NDC 0005-5360-34—Bottles of 1000
NDC 0005-5360-60—Unit Dose 10 × 10
25 mg—Hard shell, opaque, with a light green body and a dark green cap, printed with Lederle over L3 on one half and 25 mg on the other, are supplied as follows:
NDC 0005-5361-23—Bottles of 100
NDC 0005-5361-34—Bottles of 1000
NDC 0005-5361-60—Unit Dose 10 × 10
50 mg—Hard shell, opaque, with a blue body and a dark green cap, printed with Lederle over L4 on one half and 50 mg on the other, are supplied as follows:
NDC 0005-5362-23—Bottles of 100
NDC 0005-5362-34—Bottles of 1000
NDC 0005-5362-60—Unit Dose 10 × 10
Store at Controlled Room Temperature 15°-30° C (59°-86° F).
LOXITANE® C *loxapine hydrochloride* Oral Concentrate is supplied as follows:
NDC 0005-5387-58—4 fl oz (120 ml) with calibrated dropper.
Each ml contains loxapine HC1 equivalent to 25 mg of loxapine base.
Store at Controlled Room Temperature 15°-30° C (59°-86° F).
DO NOT FREEZE.
LEDERLE LABORATORIES DIVISION
American Cyanamid Company, Pearl River, NY 10965
LOXITANE® IM *loxapine hydrochloride* for Intramuscular Use Only is supplied as follows:
NDC 0205-5385-55—sterile 10—1 ml ampuls
NDC 0205-5385-34—10 ml multidose vials
Each ml contains loxapine HC1 equivalent to 50 mg of loxapine base.
Keep package closed to protect from light. Intensification of the straw color to a light amber will not alter potency or therapeutic efficacy; if noticeably discolored, ampul or vial should not be used.
Store at Controlled Room Temperature 15°-30° C (59°-86° F).
DO NOT FREEZE.

LOXITANE®
loxapine succinate
Capsules
VA Depot:
NSN 6505-01-048-3179A, 25 mg (1000s)
NSN 6505-01-048-3718A, 50 mg (1000s)
LOXITANE® C
loxapine hydrochloride
Oral Concentrate
For Oral Use
VA Depot: NSN 6505-01-026-0101A
4 oz
LOXITANE® IM
loxapine hydrochloride
For Intramuscular Use Only
LEDERLE PARENTERALS, INC.
Carolina, Puerto Rico 00630
Shown in Product Identification Section, page 413

MATERNA® 1•60 ℞

[ma-ter-na]
Prenatal Vitamin and Mineral Tablets
For the woman full of life®

DESCRIPTION

Each tablet contains:

		For Pregnant or Lactating Women % of U.S. RDA
Vitamin A Acetate	8,000 I.U.	(100%)
Vitamin D	400 I.U.	(100%)
Vitamin E (as *dl*-Alpha Tocopheryl Acetate)	30 I.U.	(100%)
Vitamin C (Ascorbic Acid)	100 mg	(167%)
Folic Acid	1 mg	(125%)
Thiamine (as Thiamine Mononitrate Vitamin B_1)	3 mg	(224%)
Riboflavin (Vitamin B_2)	3.4 mg	(170%)
Vitamin B_6 (as Pyridoxine Hydrochloride)	4 mg	(160%)
Niacinamide	20 mg	(100%)
Vitamin B_{12} (Cyanocobalamin)	12 mcg	(150%)
Calcium (as Calcium Carbonate)	250 mg	(19%)
Iodine (as Potassium Iodide)	0.3 mg	(200%)
Iron (as Ferrous Fumarate)	60 mg	(333%)
Magnesium (as Magnesium Oxide)	25 mg	(6%)
Copper (as Cupric Oxide)	2 mg	(100%)
Zinc (as Zinc Sulfate)	25 mg	(167%)

Inactive Ingredients: BHA, BHT, Ethylcellulose, Gelatin, Hydrolyzed Protein, Hydroxypropyl Methylcellulose, Lactose, Magnesium Stearate, Methylparaben, Modified Food Starch, Mono- and Di-glycerides, Polacrilin, Potassium Sorbate, Povidone, Propylparaben, Red 30, Silica Gell, Sodium Benzoate, Sodium Starch Glycolate, Sorbic Acid, Stearic Acid, Sucrose, Titanium Dioxide, and other ingredients.
Caution: Federal law prohibits dispensing without prescription.
A PHOSPHORUS-FREE VITAMIN AND MINERAL DIETARY SUPPLEMENT, FOR USE DURING PREGNANCY AND LACTATION.

RECOMMENDED INTAKE

1 daily with or without food or as prescribed by physician.

WARNING

Keep out of the reach of children.
Notice: Contact with moisture may produce surface discoloration or erosion of the tablet.

PRECAUTION

Folic acid may obscure pernicious anemia in that the peripheral blood picture may revert to normal while neurological manifestations remain progressive.
Allergic sensitization has been reported following both oral and parenteral administraion of Folic Acid.
Store at Controlled Room Temperature 15-30°C (59-86°F).

HOW SUPPLIED

Bottles of 100.
NDC 0005-5536-23
Control No.
PATENTED
U.S. Pat. No. 4,431,634
© 1984
LEDERLE LABORATORIES DIVISION
American Cyanamid Company, Pearl River, N.Y. 10965
Shown in Product Identification Section, page 413

MAXZIDE™ TABLETS

triamterene 75 mg
hydrochlorothiazide 50 mg

DESCRIPTION

Each yellow, scored MAXZIDE tablet for oral use contains 75 mg of triamterene, a potassium-conserving diuretic and 50 mg of hydrochlorothiazide, a natriuretic agent.

Inactive Ingredients
Colloidal Silicon Dioxide, Croscarmellose Sodium, Magnesium Stearate, Microcrystalline Cellulose, Powdered Cellulose, Sodium Lauryl Sulfate, Yellow 10.
Triamterene is 2,4,7-triamino-6-phenylpteridine. Triamterene is practically insoluble in water, benzene, chloroform, ether and dilute alkali hydroxides. It is soluble in formic acid and sparingly soluble in methoxyethanol. Triamterene is very slightly soluble in acetic acid, alcohol and dilute mineral acids. Its molecular weight is 253.27.
Hydrochlorothiazide is 6-chloro-3,4-dihydro-2H-1,2,4, benzothiadiazine-7-sulfonamide 1, 1-dioxide. Hydrochlorothiazide is slightly soluble in water and freely soluble in sodium hydroxide solution, n-butylamine and dimethylformamide. It is sparingly soluble in methanol and insoluble in ether, chloroform, and dilute mineral acids. Its molecular weight is 297.73.

CLINICAL PHARMACOLOGY

MAXZIDE is a diuretic antihypertensive drug product, principally due to its hydrochlorothiazide component; the triamterene component of MAXZIDE reduces the excessive potassium loss which may occur with hydrochlorothiazide use.

Hydrochlorothiazide
Hydrochlorothiazide is a diuretic and antihypertensive agent. It blocks the renal tubular absorption of sodium and chloride ions. This natriuresis and diuresis is accompanied by a secondary loss of potassium and bicarbonate. Onset of hydrochlorothiazide's diuretic effect occurs within two hours and the peak action takes place in four hours. Diuretic activity persists for approximately six to twelve hours.
The exact mechanism of hydrochlorothiazide's antihypertensive action is not known although it may relate to the excretion and redistribution of body sodium. Hydrochlorothiazide does not affect normal blood pressure.
Following oral administration, peak hydrochlorothiazide plasma levels are attained in approximately two hours. It is excreted rapidly and unchanged in the urine.

Triamterene
Triamterene is a potassium-conserving (antikaliuretic) diuretic with relatively weak natriuretic properties. It exerts its diuretic effect on the distal renal tubule to inhibit the reabsorption of sodium in exchange for potassium and hydrogen. With this action, triamterene increases sodium excretion and reduces the excessive loss of potassium and hydrogen associated with hydrochlorothiazide. Triamterene is not a competitive antagonist of the mineralocorticoids and its potassium-conserving effect is observed in patients with Addison's disease, ie, without aldosterone. Triamterene's onset and duration of activity is similar to hydrochlorothiazide. No predictable antihypertensive effect has been demonstrated with triamterene.
Triamterene is rapidly absorbed following oral administration. Peak plasma levels are achieved within one hour after dosing. Triamterene is primarily metabolized to the sulfate conjugate of hydroxytriamterene. Both the plasma and urine levels of this metabolite greatly exceed triamterene levels.
The amount of triamterene added to 50 mg of hydrochlorothiazide in MAXZIDE tablets was determined from steady-state dose response evaluations in which various doses of liquid preparations of triamterene were administered to hypertensive persons who developed hypokalemia with hydrochlorothiazide (50 mg/day). Daily doses of 75 mg triamterene produced maximal increases in serum potassium levels. Doses exceeding 75 mg daily provided no additional elevations in serum potassium levels. Ordinarily, triamterene does not entirely reverse the kaliuretic effect of hydrochlorothiazide. In some individuals, however, it may induce hyperkalemia (see WARNINGS).
The triamterene and hydrochlorothiazide components of MAXZIDE™ *triamterene 75 mg/hydrochlorothiazide 50 mg* are well absorbed and are bioequivalent to liquid preparations of the individual components administered orally. The hydrochlorothiazide component of MAXZIDE is bioequivalent to single-entity hydrochlorothiazide tablet formulations.

INDICATIONS AND USAGE

1. MAXZIDE is indicated for the treatment of hypertension or edema in patients who develop hypokalemia on hydrochlorothiazide alone.
2. MAXZIDE (triamterene and hydrochlorothiazide) is also indicated for those patients who require a thiazide diuretic and in whom the development of hypokalemia cannot be risked (eg, patients on concomitant digitalis preparations, or with a history of cardiac arrhythmias, etc).

This fixed combination drug is not indicated for the initial therapy of edema or hypertension except in individuals in whom the development of hypokalemia cannot be risked.
MAXZIDE may be used alone or in combination with other antihypertensive drugs such as beta-blockers. Since MAXZIDE may enhance the actions of these drugs, dosage adjustments may be necessary.

Usage in Pregnancy
The routine use of diuretics in an otherwise healthy woman is inappropriate and exposes mother and fetus to unnecessary hazard. Diuretics do not prevent development of toxemia in pregnancy, and there is no satisfactory evidence that they are useful in the treatment of developed toxemia.
Edema during pregnancy may arise from pathological causes or from the physiologic and mechanical consequences of pregnancy. Thiazides are indicated in pregnancy when edema is due to pathologic causes, just as they are in absence of pregnancy. Dependent edema in pregnancy, resulting from restriction of venous return by the expanded uterus, is properly treated through elevation of the lower extremities and use of support hose; use of diuretics to lower intravascular volume in this case is illogical and unnecessary. There is hypervolemia during normal pregnancy which is harmful to neither the fetus nor the mother (in the absence of cardiovascular disease), but which is associated with edema, including generalized edema, in the majority of pregnant women. If this edema produces discomfort, increased recumbency will often provide relief. In rare instances, this edema may cause extreme discomfort which is not relieved by rest. In these cases, a short course of diuretics may provide relief and may be appropriate.

CONTRAINDICATIONS

Hyperkalemia
MAXZIDE should not be used in the presence of elevated serum potassium levels (greater than 5.5 mEq/liter). If hyperkalemia develops, this drug should be discontinued and a thiazide alone should be substituted.

Antikaliuretic Therapy or Potassium Supplementation
MAXZIDE should not be given to patients receiving other potassium conserving agents such as spironolactone, amiloride HCl, or other formulations containing triamterene. Concomitant potassium supplementation in the form of medication, potassium-containing salt substitute, or potassium-enriched diets should also not be used.

Continued on next page

The information on each product appearing here is based on labelling effective in August, 1986 and is either the entire official brochure or an accurate condensation therefrom. Information concerning all Lederle products may be obtained from the Professional Services Department, Lederle Laboratories, Pearl River, New York, 10965.

Lederle—Cont.

Impaired Renal Function
MAXZIDE is contraindicated in patients with anuria, acute and chronic renal insufficiency or significant renal impairment.

Hypersensitivity
MAXZIDE should not be used in patients who are hypersensitive to triamterene or hydrochlorothiazide or other sulfonamide-derived drugs.

WARNINGS

Hyperkalemia

Abnormal elevation of serum potassium levels (greater than or equal to 5.5 mEq/liter) can occur with all potassium-conserving diuretic combinations, including MAXZIDE. Hyperkalemia is more likely to occur in patients with renal impairment, diabetes (even without evidence of renal impairment), or elderly or severely ill patients. Since uncorrected hyperkalemia may be fatal, serum potassium levels must be monitored at frequent intervals especially in patients first receiving MAXZIDE, when dosages are changed, or with any illness that may influence renal function.

If hyperkalemia is suspected (warning signs include paresthesias, muscular weakness, fatigue, flaccid paralysis of the extremities, bradycardia, and shock), an electrocardiogram (ECG) should be obtained. However, it is important to monitor serum potassium levels because mild hyperkalemia may not be associated with ECG changes.
If hyperkalemia is present, MAXZIDE™ *triamterene 75 mg/hydrochlorothiazide 50 mg* should be discontinued immediately and a thiazide only should be substituted. If the serum potassium exceed 6.5 mEq/liter, more vigorous therapy is required. The clinical situation dictates the procedures to be employed. These include the intravenous administration of calcium chloride solution, sodium bicarbonate solution, and/or the oral or parenteral administration of glucose with a rapid-acting insulin preparation. Cationic exchange resins such as sodium polystyrene sulfonate may be orally or rectally administered. Persistent hyperkalemia may require dialysis.
The development of hyperkalemia associated with potassium-sparing diuretics is accentuated in the presence of renal impairment (see CONTRAINDICATIONS). Patients with mild renal functional impairment should not receive this drug without frequent and continuing monitoring of serum electrolytes. Cumulative drug effects may be observed in patients with impaired renal function. The renal clearances of hydrochlorothiazide and the pharmacologically active metabolite of triamterene, the sulfate ester of hydroxytriamterene, have been shown to be reduced and the plasma levels increased following MAXZIDE administration to elderly patients and patients with impaired renal function.
Hyperkalemia has been reported in diabetic patients with the use of potassium-conserving agents even in the absence of apparent renal impairment. Accordingly, MAXZIDE should be avoided in diabetic patients. If it is employed, serum electrolytes must be frequently monitored.

Metabolic or Respiratory Acidosis
Potassium-conserving therapy should also be avoided in severely ill patients in whom respiratory or metabolic acidosis may occur. Acidosis may be associated with rapid elevations in serum potassium levels. If MAXZIDE is employed, frequent evaluations of acid/base balance and serum electrolytes are necessary.

PRECAUTIONS

General

Electrolyte Imbalance and BUN Increases
Patients receiving MAXZIDE should be carefully monitored for fluid or electrolyte imbalances, ie, hyponatremia, hypochloremic alkalosis, hypokalemia, and hypomagnesemia. Determination of serum electrolytes to detect possible electrolyte imbalance should be performed at appropriate intervals. Serum and urine electrolyte determinations are especially important and should be frequently performed when the patient is vomiting or receiving parenteral fluids. Warning signs or symptoms of fluid and electrolyte imbalance include: dryness of mouth, thirst, weakness, lethargy, drowsiness, restlessness, muscle pains or cramps, muscular fatigue, hypotension, oliguria, tachycardia and gastrointestinal disburbances such as nausea and vomiting.
Any chloride deficit thiazide therapy is generally mild and usually does not require any specific treatment except under extraordinary circumstances (as in liver disease or renal disease). Dilutional hyponatremia may occur in edematous patients in hot weather; appropriate therapy is water restriction, rather than administration of salt, except in rare instances when the hyponatremia is life threatening. In actual salt depletion, appropriate replacement is the therapy of choice.
Hypokalemia may develop with thiazide therapy, especially with brisk diuresis, when severe cirrhosis is present, or during concomitant use of corticosteroids, ACTH, amphotericin B, or after prolonged thiazide therapy. However, hypokalemia of this type is usually prevented by the triamterene component of MAXZIDE™ *triamterene 75 mg/hydrochlorothiazide 50 mg.*
Interference with adequate oral electrolyte intake will also contribute to hypokalemia. Hypokalemia can sensitize or exaggerate the response of the heart to the toxic effects of digitalis (eg, increased ventricular irritability).
MAXZIDE may produce an elevated blood urea nitrogen level (BUN), creatinine level or both. This is probably not the result of renal toxicity but is secondary to a reversible reduction of the glomerular filtration rate or a depletion of the intravascular fluid volume. Periodic BUN and creatinine determinations should be made especially in elderly patients, patients with suspected or confirmed hepatic disease, or renal insufficiencies. If azotemia increases, MAXZIDE should be discontinued.

Hepatic Coma
MAXZIDE should be used with caution in patients with impaired hepatic function or progressive liver disease, since minor alterations of fluid and electrolyte balance may precipitate hepatic coma.

Renal Stones
Triamterene has been reported in renal stones in association with other calculus components. MAXZIDE should be used with caution in patients with histories of renal lithiasis.

Folic Acid Deficiency
Triamterene is a weak folic acid antagonist and may contribute to the appearance of megaloblastosis in instances where folic acid stores are decreased. In such patients, periodic blood evaluations are recommended.

Hyperuricemia
Hyperuricemia may occur or acute gout may be precipitated in certain patients receiving thiazide therapy.

Metabolic and Endocrine Effects
The thiazides may decrease serum PBI levels without signs of thyroid disturbance.
Calcium excretion is decreased by thiazides. Pathological changes in the parathyroid gland with hypercalcemia and hypophosphatemia have been observed in a few patients on prolonged thiazide therapy. The common complications of hyperparathyroidism such as renal lithiasis, bone resorption, and peptic ulceration have not been seen. Thiazides should be discontinued before carrying out tests for parathyroid function.
Insulin requirements in diabetic patients may be increased, decreased, or unchanged. Diabetes mellitus which has been latent may become manifest during thiazide administration.

Hypersensitivity
Sensitivity reactions to thiazides may occur in patients with or without a history of allergy or bronchial asthma.
Possible exacerbation or activation of systemic lupus erythematosus by thiazides has been reported.

Drug Interactions
Thiazides may add to or potentiate the action of other antihypertensive drugs.
The thiazides may decrease arterial responsiveness to norepinephrine. This diminution is not sufficient to preclude effectiveness of the pressor agent for therapeutic use. Thiazides have also been shown to increase responsiveness to tubocurarine.
Lithium generally should not be given with diuretics because they reduce its renal clearance and add a high risk of lithium toxicity. Refer to the package insert on lithium before use of such concomitant therapy.
Acute renal failure has been reported in a few patients receiving indomethacin and other formulations containing triamterene and hydrochlorothiazide. Caution is therefore advised when administering nonsteroidal anti-inflammatory agents with MAXZIDE™ *triamterene 75 mg/hydrochlorothiazide 50 mg.*

Drug/Laboratory Test Interactions
Triamterene and quinidine have similar fluorescence spectra; thus, MAXZIDE may interfere with the measurement of quinidine.

Pregnancy Category C
The safe use of MAXZIDE in pregnancy has not been established. Animal reproduction studies have not been conducted with MAXZIDE. It is also not known if MAXZIDE can cause fetal harm when administered to a pregnant woman or can affect reproductive capacity. Thiazides cross the placental barrier and appear in cord blood. The use of thiazides in pregnant women requires that the anticipated benefit be weighed against possible hazards to the fetus. These hazards include fetal or neonatal jaundice, thrombocytopenia, pancreatitis and possibly other adverse reactions which have occurred in the adult. MAXZIDE should be given to a pregnant woman only if clearly needed.

Nursing Mothers
Thiazides appear in breast milk. If the use of MAXZIDE is deemed essential, the patient should stop nursing.

Pediatric Use
The safety and effectiveness of MAXZIDE in children has not been established.

ADVERSE REACTIONS

Side effects observed in association with the use of MAXZIDE include drowsiness and fatigue, insomnia, muscle cramps and weakness, headache, nausea, appetite disturbance, vomiting, diarrhea, constipation, urine discoloration, dizziness, decreased sexual performance, shortness of breath and chest pain, dry mouth, depression and anxiety. Rare incidents of acute interstitial nephritis and acute renal failure have been reported with the use of MAXZIDE. These adverse reactions are common to other triamterene and hydrochlorothiazide-containing products. Other adverse reactions which have been reported with the individual active drugs include:

Hydrochlorothiazide
Gastrointestinal: anorexia, gastric irritation, cramping, jaundice (intrahepatic cholestatic jaundice), pancreatitis, sialadenitis.
Central Nervous System: vertigo, paresthesias, xanthopsia.
Hematologic: leukopenia, agranulocytosis, thrombocytopenia, aplastic anemia, hemolytic anemia, megaloblastosis.
Cardiovascular: orthostatic hypotension (may be aggravated by alcohol, barbiturates, or narcotics).
Hypersensitivity: anaphylaxis, purpura, photosensitivity, rash, urticaria, necrotizing angiitis (vasculitis, cutaneous vasculitis), fever, respiratory distress including pneumonitis.
Other: hyperglycemia, glycosuria, hyperuricemia, restlessness, transient blurred vision.

Triamterene
Hypersensitivity: anaphylaxis, photosensitivity, and rash.
Other: Triamterene has been reported in renal stones in association with other calculus materials. Triamterene has been associated with blood dyscrasias.
Whenever adverse reactions are moderate to severe, therapy should be reduced or withdrawn.

OVERDOSAGE

No specific data are available regarding MAXZIDE™ *triamterene 75 mg/hydrochlorothiazide 50 mg* overdosage in humans and no specific antidote is available.
Fluid and electrolyte imbalances are the most important concerns. Excessive doses of the triamterene component may elicit hyperkalemia, dehydration, nausea, vomiting and weakness and possibly hypotension. Overdosing with hydrochlorothiazide has been associated with hypokalemia, hypochloremia, hyponatremia, dehydration, lethargy (may progress to coma), and gastrointestinal irritation. Treatment is symptomatic and supportive. Therapy with MAXZIDE should be discontinued. Induce emesis or institute gastric lavage. Monitor serum electrolyte levels and fluid balance. Institute supportive measures as required to maintain hydration, electrolyte balance, respiratory, cardiovascular, and renal function.

DOSAGE AND ADMINISTRATION

The recommended dosage of MAXZIDE is one tablet daily with appropriate monitoring of serum potassium levels (see WARNINGS). Patients receiving 50 mg of hydrochlorothiazide who become hypokalemic may be transferred to MAXZIDE directly. In patients requiring 50 mg of hydrochlorothiazide in whom hypokalemia cannot be risked, therapy may be initiated with MAXZIDE. There is no clinical experience with doses exceeding one tablet daily.
Clinical studies have shown that patients already taking less bioavailable formulations of triamterene and hydrochlorothiazide, (totaling 50–100 mg of hydrochlorothiazide and 100–200 mg of triamterene) may be safely changed to one MAXZIDE tablet per day.
Clinical studies have not been completed with one-half MAXZIDE tablet (25 mg hydrochlorothiazide and 37.5 mg triamterene) given once daily. Patients changed from the less bioavailable formulations in daily doses of 25 mg hydrochlorothiazide and 50 mg triamterene to one-half MAXZIDE tablet, will absorb approximately two times more hydrochlorothiazide and triamterene. All patients changed from less bioavailable formulations to MAXZIDE should be monitored clinically and for serum potassium after the transfer.

HOW SUPPLIED

MAXZIDE tablets are bow-tie shaped, flat-faced beveled, light yellow tablets, engraved with MAXZIDE on one side and scored on the other with LL on left and M8 on right of the score. Each tablet contains 75 mg of triamterene, USP and 50 mg of hydrochlorothiazide, USP.
They are supplied as follows:
NDC 0005-4460-43—Bottles of 100 with CRC
NDC 0005-4460-31—Bottles of 500
NDC 0005-4460-60—Unit Dose 10 × 10s
Store at Controlled Room Temperature 15°-30° C (59°-86° F).
Protected from light.
Dispense in a tight, light-resistant, child-resistant container.

Military and VA Numbers:
100s NSN 6505-01-196-5402
Unit Dose NSN 6501-01-196-5403
500s NSN 6501-01-206-5068
30s NSN 6505-01-223-8008
Manufactured for
LEDERLE LABORATORIES DIVISION
American Cyanamid Company, Pearl River, NY 10965
by
MYLAN PHARMACEUTICALS, INC.
Morgantown, West Virginia 26505
Shown in Product Identification Section, page 413

METHOTREXATE ℞

[*meth-ō-trĕx-āte*]
Tablets and Parenteral

WARNING
METHOTREXATE MUST BE USED ONLY BY PHYSICIANS EXPERIENCED IN ANTIMETABOLITE CHEMOTHERAPY.
BECAUSE OF THE POSSIBILITY OF FATAL OR SEVERE TOXIC REACTIONS, THE PATIENT SHOULD BE FULLY INFORMED BY THE PHYSICIAN OF THE RISKS INVOLVED AND SHOULD BE UNDER HIS CONSTANT SUPERVISION.
DEATHS HAVE BEEN REPORTED WITH THE USE OF METHOTREXATE IN THE TREATMENT OF PSORIASIS.
IN THE TREATMENT OF PSORIASIS, METHOTREXATE SHOULD BE RESTRICTED TO SEVERE, RECALCITRANT, DISABLING PSORIASIS WHICH IS NOT ADEQUATELY RESPONSIVE TO OTHER FORMS OF THERAPY, BUT ONLY WHEN THE DIAGNOSIS HAS BEEN ESTABLISHED, AS BY BIOPSY AND/OR AFTER DERMATOLOGIC CONSULTATION.

1. Methotrexate may produce marked depression of bone marrow, anemia, leukopenia, thrombocytopenia and bleeding.
2. Methotrexate may be hepatotoxic, particularly at high dosage or with prolonged therapy. Liver atrophy, necrosis, cirrhosis, fatty changes, and periportal fibrosis have been reported. Since changes may occur without previous signs of gastrointestinal or hematologic toxicity, it is imperative that hepatic function be determined prior to initiation of treatment and monitored regularly throughout therapy. Special caution is indicated in the presence of preexisting liver damage or impaired hepatic function. Concomitant use of other drugs with hepatotoxic potential (including alcohol) should be avoided.
3. Methotrexate has caused fetal death and/or congenital anomalies. Therefore, it is not recommended in women of childbearing potential unless there is appropriate medical evidence that the benefits can be expected to outweigh the considered risks. Pregnant psoriatic patients should not receive Methotrexate.
4. Impaired renal function is usually a contraindication.
5. Diarrhea and ulcerative stomatitis are frequent toxic effects and require interruption of therapy; otherwise hemorrhagic enteritis and death from intestinal perforation may occur.

METHOTREXATE HAS BEEN ADMINISTERED IN VERY HIGH DOSAGE FOLLOWED BY LEUCOVORIN RESCUE IN EXPERIMENTAL TREATMENT OF CERTAIN NEOPLASTIC DISEASES. THIS PROCEDURE IS INVESTIGATIONAL AND HAZARDOUS.

DESCRIPTION

Methotrexate Lederle (formerly A-methopterin) is an antimetabolite used in the treatment of certain neoplastic diseases. Chemically Methotrexate is N-[4-[[(2,4-Diamino-6-pteridinyl) methyl]methylamino]benzoyl]-L-glutamic acid.
Methotrexate Tablets contain an amount of Methotrexate Sodium equivalent to 2.5 mg of Methotrexate and the following inactive ingredients: Cornstarch, Lactose, Magnesium Stearate and Modified Food Starch.
Methotrexate Sodium Parenteral, preserved, is available both in 2.5 mg/ml and 25 mg/ml strengths each available in 2 ml vials.
Each 2.5 mg/ml (5.0 mg) vial contains per 2 ml: Methotrexate Sodium equivalent to 5 mg Methotrexate, 0.90% w/v of benzyl alcohol as a preservative, and the following inactive ingredients: sodium chloride 0.630% w/v and Water for Injection qs ad 100% V. sodium hydroxide and, if necessary, hydrochloric acid to adjust pH to approx. 8.5.
Each 25 mg/ml (50 mg) vial contains per 2 ml: Methotrexate Sodium equivalent to 50 mg Methotrexate, 0.90% w/v of benzyl alcohol as a preservative, and the following inactive ingredients: sodium chloride 0.260% w/v and Water for Injection qs ad 100% V. sodium hydroxide and, if necessary, hydrochloric acid to adjust pH to approx. 8.5.
If desired, the solution may be further diluted with a compatible medium such as Sodium Chloride Injection, USP. Storage for 24 hours at a temperature of 21° to 25° C results in a product which is within 90% of label potency.
Methotrexate LPF® Sodium Parenteral, Isotonic, preservative-free, single use only, is available in 2 ml (50 mg), 4 ml (100 mg), and 8 ml (200 mg) vials.
Each 25 mg/ml, 2 ml (50 mg) vial contains: Methotrexate Sodium equivalent to 50 mg Methotrexate, and the following inactive ingredients: sodium chloride 0.490% w/v and Water for Injection qs ad 100% V. sodium hydroxide and, if necessary, hydrochloric acid to adjust pH to approx. 8.5. Contains approximately 0.43 milliequivalents of sodium per vial and is an isotonic solution.
Each 25 mg/ml, 4 ml (100 mg) vial contains: Methotrexate Sodium equivalent to 100 mg Methotrexate, and the following inactive ingredients: sodium chloride 0.490% w/v and Water for Injection qs ad 100% V. sodium hydroxide and, if necessary, hydrochloric acid to adjust pH to approx. 8.5. Contains approximately 0.86 milliequivalents of sodium per vial and is an isotonic solution.
Each 25 mg/ml, 8 ml (200 mg) vial contains: Methotrexate Sodium equivalent to 200 mg Methotrexate, and the following inactive ingredients: sodium chloride 0.490% w/v and Water for Injection qs ad 100% V. sodium hydroxide and, if necessary, hydrochloric acid to adjust pH to approx. 8.5. Contains approximately 1.72 milliequivalents of sodium per vial and is an isotonic solution.
If desired, the solution may be further diluted immediately prior to use with an appropriate sterile, preservative-free medium such as 5% Dextrose Solution, USP, or Sodium Chloride Injection, USP.
Each Low Sodium 20 mg vial of sterile cryodesiccated powder, for single use only, contains: Methotrexate Sodium equivalent to 20 mg Methotrexate. Contains no preservative. Sodium hydroxide and, if necessary, hydrochloric acid added during manufacture to adjust pH. Contains approximately 0.14 milliequivalents of sodium per vial.
Each Low Sodium 50 mg vial of sterile cryodesiccated powder, for single use only, contains: Methotrexate Sodium equivalent to 50 mg Methotrexate. Contains no preservative. Sodium hydroxide and, if necessary, hydrochloric acid added during manufacture to adjust pH. Contains approximately 0.33 milliequivalents of sodium per vial.
Each Low Sodium 100 mg vial of sterile cryodesiccated powder, for single use only, contains: Methotrexate Sodium equivalent to 100 mg Methotrexate. Contains no preservative. Sodium hydroxide and, if necessary, hydrochloric acid added during manufacture to adjust pH. Contains approximately 0.65 milliequivalents of sodium per vial.

ACTION

Methotrexate has as its principal mechanism of action the competitive inhibition of the enzyme folic acid reductase. Folic acid must be reduced to tetrahydrofolic acid by this enzyme in the process of DNA synthesis and cellular replication. Methotrexate inhibits the reduction of folic acid and interferes with tissue-cell reproduction.
Actively proliferating tissues such as malignant cells, bone marrow, fetal cells, dermal epithelium, buccal and intestinal mucosa, and cells of the urinary bladder are, in general, more sensitive to this effect of Methotrexate. Cellular proliferation in malignant tissue is greater than in most normal tissue and thus Methotrexate may impair malignant growth without irreversible damage to normal tissues.
Orally administered Methotrexate is absorbed rapidly in most, but not all patients, and reaches peak serum levels in one to two hours. After parenteral injection, peak serum levels are seen in about one-half this period. Approximately one-half the absorbed Methotrexate is reversibly bound to serum protein, but exchanges with body fluids easily and diffuses into the body tissue cells.
Excretion of single daily doses occurs through the kidneys in amounts from 55% to 88% or higher within 24 hours. Repeated doses daily result in more sustained serum levels and some retention of Methotrexate over each 24-hour period which may result in accumulation of the drug within the tissues. The liver cells appear to retain certain amounts of the drug for prolonged periods even after a single therapeutic dose. Methotrexate is retained in the presence of impaired renal function and may increase rapidly in the serum and in the tissue cells under such conditions. Methotrexate does not penetrate the blood cerebrospinal fluid barrier in therapeutic amounts when given orally or parenterally. High concentrations of the drug when needed may be attained by direct intrathecal administration.
In psoriasis, the rate of production of epithelial cells in the skin is greatly increased over normal skin. This differential in reproductive rates is the basis for the use of Methotrexate to control the psoriatic process.

INDICATIONS

Antineoplastic Chemotherapy
Methotrexate is indicated for the treatment of gestational choriocarcinoma, and in patients with chorioadenoma destruens and hydatidiform mole.
Methotrexate is indicated for the palliation of acute lymphocytic leukemia. It is also indicated in the treatment and prophylaxis of meningeal leukemia. Greatest effect has been observed in palliation of acute lymphoblastic (stem-cell) leukemias in children. In combination with other anticancer drugs or suitable agents Methotrexate may be used for induction of remission, but it is most commonly used, as described in the literature, in the maintenance of induced remissions.
Methotrexate may be used alone or in combination with other anticancer agents in the management of breast cancer, epidermoid cancers of the head and neck, and lung cancer, particularly squamous cell and small cell types.
Methotrexate is also effective in the treatment of the advanced stages (III and IV, Peters Staging Systems) of lymphosarcoma, particularly in those cases in children and in advanced cases of mycosis fungoides.
Psoriasis Chemotherapy **[See Box Warnings at top of Insert]**
Because of high risk attending its use, Methotrexate is only indicated in the symptomatic control of severe, recalcitrant, disabling psoriasis which is not adequately responsive to other forms of therapy, *but only when the diagnosis has been established, as by biopsy and/or after dermatologic consultation.*

CONTRAINDICATIONS

Pregnant psoriatic patients should not receive Methotrexate.
Psoriatic patients with severe renal or hepatic disorders should not receive Methotrexate.
Psoriatic patients with preexisting blood dyscrasias, such as bone marrow hypoplasia, leukopenia, thrombocytopenia or anemia, should not receive Methotrexate.

WARNINGS

See Box Warnings

PRECAUTIONS

Methotrexate has a high potential toxicity, usually dose-related. The physician should be familiar with the various characteristics of the drug and its established clinical usage. Patients undergoing therapy should be subject to appropriate supervision so that signs or symptoms of possible toxic effects or adverse reactions may be detected and evaluated with minimal delay. Pretreatment and periodic hematologic studies are essential to the use of Methotrexate in chemotherapy because of its common effect of hematopoietic suppression. This may occur abruptly and on apparent safe dosage, and any profound drop in blood-cell count indicates immediate stopping of the drug and appropriate therapy. In patients with malignant disease who have preexisting bone marrow aplasia, leukopenia, thrombocytopenia or anemia, the drug should be used with caution, if at all.
Methotrexate is excreted principally by the kidneys. Its use in the presence of impaired renal function may result in accumulation of toxic amounts or even additional renal damage. The patient's renal status should be determined prior to and during Methotrexate therapy and proper caution exercised should significant renal impairment be disclosed. Drug dosage should be reduced or discontinued until renal function is improved or restored.
In general, the following laboratory tests are recommended as part of essential clinical evaluation and appropriate monitoring of patients chosen for or receiving Methotrexate therapy: complete hemogram; hematocrit; urinalysis; renal function tests; and liver function tests. A chest x-ray is also recommended. The purpose is to determine any existing organ dysfunction or system impairment. The tests should be performed prior to therapy, at appropriate periods during therapy and after termination of therapy. It may be useful or important to perform liver biopsy or bone marrow aspiration studies where high dose or long-term therapy is being followed.
Methotrexate is bound in part to serum albumin after absorption and toxicity may be increased because of displacement by certain drugs such as salicylates, sulfonamides, phenytoin, phenylbutazone, and some antibacterials as tetracycline, chloramphenicol and para-amino-benzoic acid. These drugs, especially salicylates, phenylbutazone, and sulfonamides, whether antibacterial, hypoglycemic or di-

Continued on next page

The information on each product appearing here is based on labelling effective in August, 1986 and is either the entire official brochure or an accurate condensation therefrom. Information concerning all Lederle products may be obtained from the Professional Services Department, Lederle Laboratories, Pearl River, New York, 10965.

Lederle—Cont.

uretic, should not be given concurrently until the significance of these findings is established.

Vitamin preparations containing folic acid or its derivatives may alter responses to Methotrexate.

Methotrexate should be used with extreme caution in the presence of infection, peptic ulcer, ulcerative colitis, debility, and in extreme youth and old age.

If profound leukopenia occurs during therapy, bacterial infection may occur or become a threat. Cessation of the drug and appropriate antibiotic therapy is usually indicated. In severe bone marrow depression, blood or platelet transfusions may be necessary.

Since it is reported that Methotrexate may have an immunosuppressive action, this factor must be taken into consideration in evaluating the use of the drug where immune responses in a patient may be important or essential.

In all instances where the use of Methotrexate is considered for chemotherapy, the physician must evaluate the need and usefulness of the drug against the risks of toxic effects or adverse reaction. Most such adverse reactions are reversible if detected early. When such effects or reactions do occur, the drug should be reduced in dosage or discontinued and appropriate corrective measures should be taken, according to the clinical judgment of the physician. Reinstitution of Methotrexate therapy should be carried out with caution, with adequate consideration of further need for the drug and alertness as to possible recurrence of toxicity.

ADVERSE REACTIONS

The most common adverse reactions include ulcerative stomatitis, leukopenia, nausea and abdominal distress. Others reported are malaise, undue fatigue, chills and fever, dizziness and decreased resistance to infection. In general, the incidence and severity of side effects are considered to be dose-related. Adverse reactions as reported for the various systems are as follows:

Skin: erythematous rashes, pruritus, urticaria, photosensitivity, depigmentation, alopecia, ecchymosis, telangiectasia, acne, furunculosis. Lesions of psoriasis may be aggravated by concomitant exposure to ultraviolet radiation.

Blood: bone marrow depression, leukopenia, thrombocytopenia, anemia, hypogammaglobulinemia, hemorrhage from various sites, septicemia.

Alimentary System: gingivitis, pharyngitis, stomatitis, anorexia, vomiting, diarrhea, hematemesis, melena, gastrointestinal ulceration and bleeding, enteritis, hepatic toxicity resulting in acute liver atrophy, necrosis, fatty metamorphosis, periportal fibrosis, or hepatic cirrhosis.

Urogenital System: renal failure, azotemia, cystitis, hematuria; defective oogenesis or spermatogenesis, transient oligospermia, menstrual dysfunction; infertility, abortion, fetal defects, severe nephropathy.

Pulmonary System: Interstitial Pneumonitis. Deaths have been reported and chronic interstitial obstructive pulmonary disease has occasionally occurred.

Central Nervous System: headaches, drowsiness, blurred vision. Aphasia, hemiparesis, paresis and convulsions have also occurred following administration of Methotrexate.

There have been reports of leucoencephalopathy following intravenous administration of Methotrexate to patients who have had craniospinal irradiation.

After the intrathecal use of Methotrexate, the central nervous system toxicity which may occur can be classified as follows: (1) chemical arachnoiditis manifested by such symptoms as headache, back pain, nuchal rigidity, and fever; (2) paresis, usually transient, manifested by paraplegia associated with involvement with one or more spinal nerve roots; (3) leucoencephalopathy manifested by confusion, irritability, somnolence, ataxia, dementia, and occasionally major convulsions.

Other reactions related to or attributed to the use of Methotrexate such as metabolic changes, precipitating diabetes, osteoporotic effects, abnormal tissue cell changes, and even sudden death have been reported.

DOSAGE AND ADMINISTRATION

Antineoplastic chemotherapy

Oral administration in tablet form is often preferred since absorption is rapid and effective serum levels are obtained. Methotrexate sodium parenteral may be given by intramuscular, intravenous, intraarterial or intrathecal route. Initial treatment is usually undertaken with the patient under hospital care.

For conversion of mg/kg b.w. to mg/M^2 of body surface or the reverse, a ratio of 1:30 is given as a guideline. The conversion factor varies between 1:20 and 1:40 depending on age and body build.

Choriocarcinoma and similar trophoblastic diseases: Methotrexate is administered orally or intramuscularly in doses of 15 mg to 30 mg daily for a five day course. Such courses are usually repeated for three to five times as required, with rest periods of one or more weeks interposed between courses, until any manifesting toxic symptoms subside. The effectiveness of therapy is ordinarily evaluated by 24 hour quantitative analysis of urinary chorionic gonadotropin hormone (CGH), which should return to normal or less than 50 IU/24 hr. usually after the third or fourth course and usually be followed by a complete resolution of measurable lesions in four to six weeks. One to two courses of Methotrexate after normalization of CGH is usually recommended. Before each course of the drug careful clinical assessment is essential. Cyclic combination therapy of Methotrexate with other antitumor drugs has been reported as being useful. Since hydatidiform mole may precede or be followed by choriocarcinoma, prophylactic chemotherapy with Methotrexate has been recommended. Chorioadenoma destruens is considered to be an invasive form of hydatidiform mole. Methotrexate is administered in these disease states in doses similar to those recommended for choriocarcinoma.

Leukemia: acute lymphatic (lymphoblastic) leukemia in children and young adolescents is the most responsive to present day chemotherapy. In young adults and older patients, clinical remission is more difficult to obtain and early relapse is more common. In chronic lymphatic leukemia, the prognosis for adequate response is less encouraging.

Methotrexate alone or in combination with steroids was used initially for induction of remission of lymphoblastic leukemias. More recently corticosteroid therapy in combination with other antileukemic drugs or in cyclic combinations with Methotrexate included appear to produce rapid and effective remissions. When used for induction, Methotrexate in doses of 3.3 mg/M^2 in combination with prednisone 60 mg/M^2, given daily, produced remission in 50% of patients treated, usually within a period of four to six weeks. Methotrexate alone or in combination with other agents appears to be the drug of choice for securing maintenance of drug-induced remissions. When remission is achieved and supportive care has produced general clinical improvement, maintenance therapy is initiated, as follows: Methotrexate is administered two times weekly either by mouth or intramuscularly in doses of 30 mg/M^2. It has also been given in doses of 2.5 mg/kg intravenously every 14 days. If and when relapse does occur, reinduction of remission can again usually be obtained by repeating the initial induction regimen. Various experts have recently introduced a variety of dosage schedules for both induction and maintenance of remission with various combinations of alkylating and antifolic agents. Multiple drug therapy with several agents, including Methotrexate given concomitantly is gaining increasing support in both the acute and chronic forms of leukemia. The physician should familiarize himself with the new advances in antileukemic therapy.

Acute granulocytic leukemia is rare in children but common in adults. This form of leukemia responds poorly to chemotherapy and remissions are short with relapses common, and resistance to therapy develops rapidly.

Meningeal leukemia: Patients with leukemia are subject to leukemic invasion of the central nervous system. This may manifest characteristic signs or symptoms or may remain silent and be diagnosed only by examination of the cerebrospinal fluid which contains leukemic cells in such cases. Therefore, the CSF should be examined in all leukemic patients. Since passage of Methotrexate from blood serum to the cerebrospinal fluid is minimal, for adequate therapy the drug is administered intrathecally. It is now common practice because of the noted increased frequency of meningeal leukemia to administer Methotrexate intrathecally as prophylaxis in all cases of lymphocytic leukemia.

By intrathecal injection, the sodium salt of Methotrexate is administered in solution in doses of 12 mg per square meter of body surface or in an empirical dose of 15 mg. The solution is made in a strength of 1 mg per ml with an appropriate, sterile, preservative-free medium such as Sodium Chloride Injection, USP.

For the treatment of meningeal leukemia, Methotrexate is given at intervals of two to five days. Methotrexate is administered until the cell count of the cerebrospinal fluid returns to normal. At this point one additional dose is advisable.

For prophylaxis against meningeal leukemia, the dosage is the same as for treatment except for the intervals of administration. On this subject, it is advisable for the physician to consult the medical literature.

Large doses may cause convulsions. Untoward side effects may occur with any given intrathecal injection and are commonly neurological in character. Methotrexate given by intrathecal route appears significantly in the systemic circulation and may cause systemic Methotrexate toxicity. Therefore, systemic antileukemic therapy with the drug should be appropriately adjusted, reduced or discontinued. Focal leukemic involvement of the central nervous system may not respond to intrathecal chemotherapy and is best treated with radiotherapy.

Lymphomas: In Burkitt's Tumor, Stages I-II, Methotrexate has produced prolonged remissions in some cases. Recommended dosage is 10 mg to 25 mg per day orally for four to eight days. In Stage III, Methotrexate is commonly given concomitantly with other antitumor agents. Treatment in all stages usually consists of several courses of the drug interposed with seven to ten day rest periods. Lymphosarcomas in Stage III may respond to combined drug therapy with Methotrexate given in doses of 0.625 mg to 2.5 mg/kg daily. Hodgkin's disease responds poorly to Methotrexate and to most types of chemotherapy.

Mycosis fungoides: Therapy with Methotrexate appears to produce clinical remissions in one half of the cases treated. Dosage is usually 2.5 mg to 10 mg daily by mouth for weeks or months. Dose levels of drug and adjustment of dose regimen by reduction or cessation of drug are guided by patient response and hematologic monitoring. Methotrexate has also been given intramuscularly in doses of 50 mg once weekly or 25 mg two times weekly.

Psoriasis Chemotherapy

The patient should be fully informed of the risks involved and should be under constant supervision of the physician.

Assessment of renal function, liver function, and blood elements should be made by history, physical examination, and laboratory tests (such as CBC, urinalysis, serum creatinine, liver function studies, and liver biopsy if indicated) before beginning Methotrexate, periodically during Methotrexate therapy, and before reinstituting Methotrexate therapy after a rest period. Appropriate steps should be taken to avoid conception during and for at least eight weeks following Methotrexate therapy.

There are three commonly used general types of dosage schedules:

1) weekly oral or parenteral intermittent large doses
2) divided dose intermittent oral schedule over a 36-hour period
3) daily oral with a rest period

All schedules should be continually tailored to the individual patient. Dose schedules cited below pertain to an average 70 kg adult. An initial test dose one week prior to initiation of therapy is recommended to detect any idiosyncrasy. A suggested dose range is 5 mg to 10 mg parenterally.

Recommended starting dose schedules:

1. Weekly single oral, IM or IV dose schedule: 10 mg to 25 mg per week until adequate response is achieved. With this dosage schedule, 50 mg per week should ordinarily not be exceeded.
2. Divided oral dose schedule: 2.5 mg at 12 hour intervals for three doses or at eight hour intervals for four doses each week. With this dosage schedule, 30 mg per week should not be exceeded.
3. Daily oral dose schedule: 2.5 mg daily for five days followed by at least a two day rest period. With this dosage schedule, 6.25 mg per day should not be exceeded.

SPECIAL NOTE: Available data suggest that schedule 3 may carry an increased risk of serious liver pathology.

Dosages in each schedule may be gradually adjusted to achieve optimal clinical response, but not to exceed the maximum stated for each schedule.

Once optimal clinical response has been achieved, each dosage schedule should be reduced to the lowest possible amount of drug and to the longest possible rest period. The use of Methotrexate may permit the return to conventional topical therapy, which should be encouraged.

Procedures for proper handling and disposal of anticancer drugs should be considered. Several guidelines on this subject have been published.[1–6] There is no general agreement that all of the procedures recommended in the guidelines are necessary or appropriate.

ANTIDOTE FOR OVERDOSAGE

Leucovorin (citrovorum factor) is a potent agent for neutralizing the immediate toxic effects of Methotrexate on the hematopoietic system. Where large doses or overdoses are given, Calcium Leucovorin may be administered by intravenous infusion in doses up to 75 mg within 12 hours, followed by 12 mg intramuscularly every six hours for four doses. Where average doses of Methotrexate appear to have an adverse effect, 2 ml to 4 ml (6 mg to 12 mg) of Calcium Leucovorin may be given intramuscularly every six hours for four doses. In general, where overdosage is suspected, the dose of Leucovorin should be equal to or higher than the offending dose of Methotrexate and should best be administered within the first hour. Use of Calcium Leucovorin after an hour delay is much less effective.

CAUTION. Pharmacist: Because of its potential to cause severe toxicity, Methotrexate therapy requires close supervision of the patient by the physician. Pharmacists should dispense no more than a seven (7) day supply of the drug at one time. Refill of such prescriptions should be by direct order (written or oral) of the physician only.

Reconstitution of Low Sodium Cryodesiccated Powders

Dilute immediately prior to use.

For IV or IM administration, reconstitute to a concentration of no greater than 25 mg/ml with an appropriate sterile, preservative-free medium such as Sodium Chloride Injection, USP (IM) or 5% Dextrose Solution, USP (IV).

For intrathecal injection, reconstitute to a concentration of 1 mg/ml with an appropriate sterile, preservative-free medium such as Sodium Chloride Injection, USP.

HOW SUPPLIED

Parenterals:

Low Sodium Cryodesiccated Powders—Preservative Free, Single Use Only

20 mg vial—Product No. NDC 0205-4654-90 (Dark Blue Cap)
50 mg vial—Product No. NDC 0205-9337-92 (Violet Cap)
100 mg vial—Product No. NDC 0205-9338-94 (Green Cap)
Store at Controlled Room Temperature 15°-30° C (59°-86°F)
Protect from light.

Isotonic Liquids—Preservative Free, Single Use Only
Methotrexate LPF® Sodium

25 mg/ml—2 ml (50 mg) vials—Product No. NDC 0205-5325-26 (Brown Cap)
25 mg/ml—4 ml (100 mg) vials—Product No. NDC 0205-5326-18 (Light Blue Cap)
25 mg/ml—8 ml (200 mg) vials—Product No. NDC 0205-5327-30
25 mg/ml—8 ml (200 mg) vials—25 per box, Product No. NDC-0205-5327-19 (Orange Cap)
Store at Controlled Room Temperature 15°-30° C (59°-86°F)
Protect from light.

Isotonic Liquids—Preserved

2.5 mg per ml—2 ml vials—Product No. NDC 0205-4554-26 (White Cap)
25 mg per ml—2 ml vials—Product NDC 0205-4556-26 (Red Cap)
Store at Controlled Room Temperature 15°-30° C (59°-86°F)
Protect from light.
*LEDERLE PARENTERALS, INC.
Carolina, Puerto Rico 00630

Oral:

Description

Methotrexate Tablets contain an amount of Methotrexate Sodium equivalent to 2.5 mg of Methotrexate and are round, convex, yellow tablets, engraved with LL on one side, scored in half on the other side, and engraved with M above the score, and 1 below.

2.5 mg Tablets—Bottles of 100—Product No. NDC 0005-4507-23
Store at Controlled Room Temperature 15°-30°C (59°-86°F)
Protect from light.

REFERENCES

1. Recommendations for the Safe Handling of Parenteral Antineoplastic Drugs. NIH Publication No. 83-2621. For sale by the Superintendent of Documents, US Government Printing Office, Washington, DC 20402.
2. AMA Council Report. Guidelines for Handling Parenteral Antineoplastics. *JAMA*, March 15, 1985.
3. National Study Commission on Cytotoxic Exposure—Recommendations for Handling Cytotoxic Agents. Available from Louis P. Jeffrey, Sc. D., Director of Pharmacy Services, Rhode Island Hospital, 593 Eddy Street, Providence, Rhode Island 02902.
4. Clinical Oconological Society of Australia: Guidelines and recommendations for safe handling of antineoplastic agents. *Med J Australia* 1:426-428 1983.
5. Jones R. B., et al. Safe handling of chemotherapeutic agents: A report from the Mount Sinai Medical Center, Ca. *A Cancer Journal for Clinicians* Sept/Oct, 258-263 1983.
6. American Society of Hospital Pharmacists technical assistance bulletin on handling cytotoxic drugs in hospitals. *Am J Hosp Pharm* 42:131-137 1985.

LEDERLE LABORATORIES DIVISION
American Cyanamid Company
Pearl River, NY 10965

Military Depot:
Sodium Parenteral
50 mg vial NSN 6505-01-020-2367
NSN 6505-01-125-6505

VA Depots:
Methotrexate LPF®
Sodium Parenteral
50 mg/ml 2 ml, NSN 6505-01-125-6503
100 mg/ml 4 ml, NSN 6505-01-125-6504
200 mg/ml 8 ml, NSN 6505-01-125-6505

Shown in Product Identification Section, page 413

MINOCIN® ℞

[*mī-nō-sĭn*]
Sterile
minocycline hydrochloride
Intravenous
100 mg/Vial

DESCRIPTION

MINOCIN® *minocycline hydrochloride*, a semisynthetic derivative of tetracycline, is named [4S-(4α, 4aα, 5aα, 12aα)]-4,7-bis(dimethylamino) -1,4,4a,5,5a,6,11,12a-octahydro-3,10, 12,12a-tetrahydroxy-1,11-dioxo-2-naphthacenecarboxamide monohydrochloride.

Each vial, dried by cryodesiccation, contains sterile minocycline hydrochloride equivalent to 100 mg minocycline. When reconstituted with 5 ml of Sterile Water For Injection the pH ranges from 2.0 to 2.8.

ACTIONS

Microbiology—The tetracyclines are primarily bacteriostatic and are thought to exert their antimicrobial effect by the inhibition of protein synthesis. Minocycline HCl is a tetracycline with antibacterial activity comparable to other tetracyclines with activity against a wide range of Gram-negative and Gram-positive organisms.

Tube dilution testing: Microorganisms may be considered susceptible (likely to respond to minocycline therapy) if the minimum inhibitory concentration (MIC) is not more than 4.0 mcg/ml. Microorganisms may be considered intermediate (harboring partial resistance) if the MIC is 4.0 mcg/ml to 12.5 mcg/ml and resistant (not likely to respond to minocycline therapy) if the MIC is greater than 12.5 mcg/ml.

Susceptibility plate testing: If the Kirby-Bauer method of susceptibility testing (using a 30 mcg tetracycline disc) gives a zone of 18 mm or greater, the bacterial strain is considered to be susceptible to any tetracycline. Minocycline shows moderate *in vitro* activity against certain strains of staphylococci which have been found resistant to other tetracyclines. For such strains, minocycline susceptibility powder may be used for additional susceptibility testing.

Human Pharmacology—Following a single dose of 200 mg administered to ten healthy male volunteers, serum levels ranged from 2.52 to 6.63 mcg/ml (average 4.18); after 12 hours they ranged from 0.82 to 2.64 mcg/ml (average 1.38). In a group of five healthy male volunteers serum levels of 1.4–1.8 mcg/ml were maintained at 12 and 24 hours with doses of 100 mg every 12 hours for three days. When given 200 mg once daily for three days the serum levels had fallen to approximately 1 mcg/ml at 24 hours. The serum half-life following I.V. doses of 100 mg every 12 hours or 200 mg once daily did not differ significantly and ranged from 15 to 23 hours. The serum half-life following a single 200 mg oral dose in 12 essentially normal volunteers ranged from 11 to 17 hours, in seven patients with hepatic dysfunction ranged from 11 to 16 hours, and in five patients with renal dysfunction from 18 to 69 hours.

Intravenously administered minocycline appears similar to oral doses in excretion. The urinary and fecal recovery of oral minocycline when administered to 12 normal volunteers is one half to one third that of other tetracyclines.

INDICATIONS

MINOCIN® *minocycline HCl* is indicated in infections caused by the following microorganisms:

Rickettsiae: (Rocky Mountain spotted fever, typhus fever and the typhus group, Q fever, rickettsialpox, tick fevers).
Mycoplasma pneumoniae (PPLO, Eaton agent).
Agents of psittacosis and ornithosis.
Agents of lymphogranuloma venereum and granuloma inguinale.
The spirochetal agent of relapsing fever (*Borrelia recurrentis*).

The following Gram-negative microorganisms:

Haemophilus ducreyi (chancroid),
Pasteurella pestis and *Pasteurella tularensis*,
Bartonella bacilliformis,
Bacteroides species,
Vibrio comma and *Vibrio fetus*,
Brucella species (in conjunction with streptomycin).

Because many strains of the following groups of microorganisms have been shown to be resistant to tetracyclines, culture and susceptibility testing are recommended.

MINOCIN is indicated for treatment of infections caused by the following Gram-negative microorganisms, when bacteriologic testing indicates appropriate susceptibility to the drug:

Escherichia coli,
Enterobacter aerogenes (formerly *Aerobacter aerogenes*),
Shigella species,
Mima species and *Herellea* species,
Haemophilus influenzae (respiratory infections),
Klebsiella species (respiratory and urinary infections).

MINOCIN is indicated for treatment of infections caused by the following Gram-positive microorganisms when bacteriologic testing indicates appropriate susceptibility to the drug:

Streptococcus species:

Up to 44% of strains of *Streptococcus pyogenes* and 74% of *Streptococcus faecalis* have been found to be resistant to tetracycline drugs. Therefore, tetracyclines should not be used for streptococcal disease unless the organism has been demonstrated to be sensitive.

For upper respiratory infections due to Group A beta-hemolytic streptococci, penicillin is the usual drug of choice, including prophylaxis of rheumatic fever.

Diplococcus pneumoniae,
Staphylococcus aureus, skin and soft tissue infections.

Tetracyclines are not the drug of choice in the treatment of any type of staphylococcal infection.

When penicillin is contraindicated, tetracyclines are alternative drugs in the treatment of infections due to:

Neisseria gonorrhoeae, and *Neisseria meningitidis*,
Treponema pallidum and *Treponema pertenue* (syphilis and yaws),
Listeria monocytogenes,
Clostridium species,
Bacillus anthracis,
Fusobacterium fusiforme (Vincent's infection),
Actinomyces species.

In acute intestinal amebiasis, the tetracyclines may be a useful adjunct to amebicides.

MINOCIN is indicated in the treatment of trachoma, although the infectious agent is not always eliminated as judged by immunofluorescence.

Inclusion conjunctivitis may be treated with oral tetracyclines or with a combination of oral and topical agents.

CONTRAINDICATIONS

This drug is contraindicated in persons who have shown hypersensitivity to any of the tetracyclines.

WARNINGS

In the presence of renal dysfunction, particularly in pregnancy, intravenous tetracycline therapy in daily doses exceeding 2 grams has been associated with deaths through liver failure.

When the need for intensive treatment outweighs its potential dangers (mostly during pregnancy or in individuals with known or suspected renal or liver impairment), it is advisable to perform renal and liver function tests before and during therapy. Also tetracycline serum concentrations should be followed.

If renal impairment exists, even usual oral or parenteral doses may lead to excessive systemic accumulation of the drug and possible liver toxicity. Under such conditions, lower-than-usual total doses are indicated, and, if therapy is prolonged, serum level determinations of the drug may be advisable. This hazard is of particular importance in the parenteral administration of tetracyclines to pregnant or postpartum patients with pyelonephritis. When used under these circumstances, the blood level should not exceed 15 micrograms/ml and liver function tests should be made at frequent intervals. Other potentially hepatotoxic drugs should not be prescribed concomitantly.

THE USE OF TETRACYCLINES DURING TOOTH DEVELOPMENT (LAST HALF OF PREGNANCY, INFANCY AND CHILDHOOD TO THE AGE OF 8 YEARS) MAY CAUSE PERMANENT DISCOLORATION OF THE TEETH (YELLOW-GRAY-BROWN). This adverse reaction is more common during long-term use of the drugs but has been observed following repeated short-term courses. Enamel hypoplasia has also been reported. TETRACYCLINES, THEREFORE, SHOULD NOT BE USED IN THIS AGE GROUP UNLESS OTHER DRUGS ARE NOT LIKELY TO BE EFFECTIVE OR ARE CONTRAINDICATED.

Photosensitivity manifested by an exaggerated sunburn reaction has been observed in some individuals taking tetracyclines. Patients apt to be exposed to direct sunlight or ultraviolet light should be advised that this reaction can occur with tetracycline drugs, and treatment should be discontinued at the first evidence of skin erythema. Studies to date indicate that photosensitivity is rarely reported with MINOCIN® *minocycline HCl*.

The antianabolic action of the tetracyclines may cause an increase in BUN. While this is not a problem in those with normal renal function, in patients with significantly impaired function, higher serum levels of tetracycline may lead to azotemia, hyperphosphatemia, and acidosis.

CNS side effects including lightheadedness, dizziness or vertigo have been reported. Patients who experience these symptoms should be cautioned about driving vehicles or using hazardous machinery while on minocycline therapy. These symptoms may disappear during therapy and usually disappear rapidly when the drug is discontinued.

Usage in Pregnancy—(See above "Warnings" about use during tooth development).

Results of animal studies indicate that tetracyclines cross the placenta, are found in fetal tissues and can have toxic effects on the developing fetus (often related to retardation of skeletal development). Evidence of embryotoxicity has also been noted in animals treated early in pregnancy.

The safety of minocycline HCl for use during pregnancy has not been established.

Usage in newborns, infants, and children—(See above "Warnings" about use during tooth development).

All tetracyclines form a stable calcium complex in any bone forming tissue. A decrease in the fibula growth rate has been

Continued on next page

The information on each product appearing here is based on labelling effective in August, 1986 and is either the entire official brochure or an accurate condensation therefrom. Information concerning all Lederle products may be obtained from the Professional Services Department, Lederle Laboratories, Pearl River, New York, 10965.

Lederle—Cont.

observed in prematures given oral tetracycline in doses of 25 mg/kg every six hours. This reaction was shown to be reversible when the drug was discontinued.
Tetracyclines are present in the milk of lactating women who are taking a drug in this class.

PRECAUTIONS

As with other antibiotic preparations, use of this drug may result in overgrowth of nonsusceptible organisms, including fungi. If superinfection occurs, the antibiotic should be discontinued and appropriate therapy should be instituted.
In venereal diseases when coexistent syphilis is suspected, darkfield examination should be done before treatment is started and the blood serology repeated monthly for at least four months.
Because tetracyclines have been shown to depress plasma prothrombin activity, patients who are on anticoagulant therapy may require downward adjustment of their anticoagulant dosage.
In long-term therapy, periodic laboratory evaluation of organ systems, including hematopoietic, renal, and hepatic studies should be performed.
All infections due to Group A beta-hemolytic streptococci should be treated for at least ten days.
Since bacteriostatic drugs may interfere with the bactericidal action of penicillin, it is advisable to avoid giving tetracycline in conjunction with penicillin.

ADVERSE REACTIONS

Gastrointestinal: Anorexia, nausea, vomiting, diarrhea, glossitis, dysphagia, enterocolitis, inflammatory lesions (with monilial overgrowth) in the anogenital region and increases in liver enzymes; rarely hepatitis.
These reactions have been caused by both the oral and parenteral administration of tetracyclines.
Skin: Maculopapular and erythematous rashes. Exfoliative dermatitis has been reported but is uncommon. Photosensitivity is discussed above. (See "Warnings").
Tooth discoloration has been reported rarely in adults.
Renal toxicity: Rise in BUN has been reported and is apparently dose related (See "Warnings").
Hypersensitivity reactions: Urticaria, angioneurotic edema, anaphylaxis, anaphylactoid purpura, pericarditis, exacerbation of systemic lupus erythematosus and, rarely, pulmonary infiltrates with eosinophilia.
Bulging fontanels have been reported in young infants following full therapeutic dosage. Pseudotumor Cerebri has very rarely been reported in adults. These signs disappeared rapidly when the drug was discontinued.
Blood: Hemolytic anemia, thrombocytopenia, neutropenia and eosinophilia have been reported.
CNS: (See "Warnings").
When given over prolonged periods, tetracyclines have been reported to produce brown-black microscopic discoloration of thyroid glands. No abnormalities of thyroid function studies are known to occur.

DOSAGE AND ADMINISTRATION

Note: Rapid administration is to be avoided. Parenteral therapy is indicated only when oral therapy is not adequate or tolerated. Oral therapy should be instituted as soon as possible. If intravenous therapy is given over prolonged periods of time, thrombophlebitis may result.
Adults: Usual adult dose: 200 mg followed by 100 mg every 12 hours and should not exceed 400 mg in 24 hours. The drug should be initially dissolved and then further diluted to 500 to 1,000 ml with either Sodium Chloride Injection USP, Dextrose Injection USP, Dextrose and Sodium Chloride Injection USP, Ringer's Injection USP, or Lactated Ringer's Injection USP but not in other solutions containing calcium (a precipitate may form).
The reconstituted solutions are stable at room temperature for 24 hours without significant loss of potency. Any unused portions must be discarded after that period. The final dilution for administration should be administered immediately.
For children above eight years of age: Usual pediatric dose: 4 mg/kg followed by 2 mg/kg every 12 hours.
In patients with renal impairment: (See "Warnings").
Total dosage should be decreased by reduction of recommended individual doses and/or by extending time intervals between doses.

HOW SUPPLIED

100 mg vials of sterile cryodesiccated powder
Product No. NDC 0205-5305-94
Store at Controlled Room Temperature 15°-30°C (59°-86°F).
Military Depot: Intravenous—100 mg vial—NSN 6505-00-149-0574
*Manufactured for
LEDERLE LABORATORIES DIVISION
American Cyanamid Company
Pearl River, NY 10965
by
LEDERLE PARENTERALS, INC.
Carolina, Puerto Rico 00630

Shown in Product Identification Section, page 413

MINOCIN® ℞

[*mī-nō-sĭn*]
Minocycline Hydrochloride Tablets for Oral Use

DESCRIPTION

MINOCIN® *minocycline hydrochloride*, a semisynthetic derivative of tetracycline, is named [4*S*-(4α,4aα,5aα,12aα)]-4,7-bis(dimethylamino)- 1,4,4a,5,5a,6,11,12a-octahydro-3,10, 12, 12a-tetrahydroxy-1,11-dioxo-2-naphthacenecarboxamide monohydrochloride.
MINOCIN Capsules contain minocycline HCl equivalent to 50 or 100 mg minocycline and the following inactive ingredients: Cornstarch, Magnesium Stearate, Titanium Dioxide and Yellow 6. Additionally, the 100 mg capsules contain Blue 1 and Red 28 as inactive ingredients.
MINOCIN Oral Suspension contains minocycline HCl equivalent to 50 mg of minocycline per 5 ml (10 mg/ml) and the following inactive ingredients: Alcohol, Butylparaben, Calcium Hydroxide, Cellulose, Decaglyceryl Tetraoleate, Edetate Calcium Disodium, Glycol, Guar Gum, Polysorbate 80, Propylparaben, Propylene Glycol, Sodium Saccharin, Sodium Sulfite and Sorbitol.
MINOCIN Tablets contain minocycline HCl equivalent to 50 or 100 mg minocycline and the following inactive ingredients: Lactose, Microcrystalline Cellulose, Magnesium Stearate, Povidone, Sodium Lauryl Sulfate, Sodium Starch Glycolate, Sorbitol, Stearic Acid, Titanium Dioxide, Yellow 6, Yellow 10 and other ingredients.

ACTIONS

Microbiology—The tetracyclines are primarily bacteriostatic and are thought to exert their antimicrobial effect by the inhibition of protein synthesis. Minocycline HCl is a tetracycline with antibacterial activity comparable to other tetracyclines with activity against a wide range of Gram-negative and Gram-positive organisms.
Tube dilution testing: Microorganisms may be considered susceptible (likely to respond to minocycline therapy) if the minimum inhibitory concentration (MIC) is not more than 4.0 mcg/ml. Microorganisms may be considered intermediate (harboring partial resistance) if the MIC is 4.0 to 12.5 mcg/ml and resistant (not likely to respond to minocycline therapy) if the MIC is greater than 12.5 mcg/ml.
Susceptibility plate testing: If the Kirby-Bauer method of susceptibility testing (using a 30 mcg tetracycline disc) gives a zone of 18 mm or greater, the bacterial strain is considered to be susceptible to any tetracycline. Minocycline shows moderate *in vitro* activity against certain strains of staphylococci which have been found resistant to other tetracyclines. For such strains minocycline susceptibility powder may be used for additional susceptibility testing.
Human Pharmacology—Following a single dose of two 100 mg of minocycline HCl capsules administered to ten normal adult volunteers, serum levels ranged from 0.74 to 4.45 mcg/ml in one hour (average 2.24); after 12 hours, they ranged from 0.34 to 2.36 mcg/ml (average 1.25). The serum half-life following a single 200 mg dose in 12 essentially normal volunteers ranged from 11 to 17 hours; in seven patients with hepatic dysfunction, ranged from 11 to 16 hours; and in five patients with renal dysfunction, from 18 to 69 hours. The urinary and fecal recovery of minocycline when administered to 12 normal volunteers is one half to one third that of other tetracyclines.

INDICATIONS

MINOCIN® *minocycline HCl* is indicated in infections caused by the following microorganisms:

Rickettsiae: (Rocky Mountain spotted fever, typhus fever and the typhus group, Q fever, rickettsialpox, tick fevers).
Mycoplasma pneumoniae (PPLO, Eaton agent).
Agents of psittacosis and ornithosis.
Agents of lymphogranuloma venereum and granuloma inguinale.
The spirochetal agent of relapsing fever (*Borrelia recurrentis*).

The following Gram-negative microorganisms:

Haemophilus ducreyi (chancroid),
Pasteurella pestis and *Pasteurella tularensis,*
Bartonella bacilliformis,
Bacteroides species,
Vibrio comma and *Vibrio fetus,*
Brucella species (in conjunction with streptomycin).

Because many strains of the following groups of microorganisms have been shown to be resistant to tetracyclines, culture and susceptibility testing are recommended.
MINOCIN is indicated for treatment of infections caused by the following Gram-negative microorganisms when bacteriologic testing indicates appropriate susceptibility to the drug:

Escherichia coli,
Enterobacter aerogenes (formerly *Aerobacter aerogenes*),
Shigella species,
Acinetobacter calcoaceticus (syn. *Herellea*, Mima),
Haemophilus influenzae (respiratory infections),
Klebsiella species (respiratory and urinary infections).

MINOCIN is indicated for treatment of infections caused by the following Gram-positive microorganisms when bacteriologic testing indicates appropriate susceptibility to the drug:
Streptococcus species:
Up to 44% of strains of *Streptococcus pyogenes* and 74% of *Streptococcus faecalis* have been found to be resistant to tetracycline drugs. Therefore, tetracyclines should not be used for streptococcal disease unless the organism has been demonstrated to be sensitive.
For upper respiratory infections due to Group A beta-hemolytic streptococci, penicillin is the usual drug of choice, including prophylaxis of rheumatic fever.

Diplococcus pneumoniae,
Staphylococcus aureus, skin and soft tissue infections.

Tetracyclines are not the drugs of choice in the treatment of any type of staphylococcal infection.
MINOCIN is indicated for the treatment of uncomplicated gonococcal urethritis in men due to *Neisseria gonorrhoeae.*
When penicillin is contraindicated, tetracyclines are alternative drugs in the treatment of infections due to:

Neisseria gonorrhoeae (in women),
Treponema pallidum and *Treponema pertenue* (syphilis and yaws),
Listeria monocytogenes,
Clostridium species,
Bacillus anthracis,
Fusobacterium fusiforme (Vincent's infection),
Actinomyces species.
In acute intestinal amebiasis, the tetracyclines may be a useful adjunct to amebicides.

In severe acne, the tetracyclines may be useful adjunctive therapy.
MINOCIN® *minocycline HCl* is indicated in the treatment of trachoma, although the infectious agent is not always eliminated, as judged by immunofluorescence.
Minocycline hydrochloride is indicated for the treatment of uncomplicated urethral, endocervical or rectal infections in adults caused by *Chlamydia trachomatis* or *Ureaplasma urealyticum.*[1]
Inclusion conjunctivitis may be treated with oral tetracyclines or with a combination of oral and topical agents.
Minocycline is indicated in the treatment of asymptomatic carriers of *N meningitidis* to eliminate meningococci from the nasopharynx.
In order to preserve the usefulness of MINOCIN in the treatment of asymtomatic meningococcal carriers, diagnostic laboratory procedures, including serotyping and susceptibility testing, should be performed to establish the carrier state and the correct treatment. It is recommended that the drug be reserved for situations in which the risk of meningococcal meningitis is high.
Minocycline by oral administration is not indicated for the treatment of meningococcal infection.
Although no controlled clinical efficacy studies have been conducted, limited clinical data show that oral minocycline hydrochloride has been used successfully in the treatment of infections caused by Mycobacterium marinum.

CONTRAINDICATIONS

This drug is contraindicated in persons who have shown hypersensitivity to any of the tetracyclines.

WARNINGS

THE USE OF DRUGS OF THE TETRACYCLINE CLASS DURING TOOTH DEVELOPMENT (LAST HALF OF PREGNANCY, INFANCY, AND CHILDHOOD TO THE AGE OF 8 YEARS) MAY CAUSE PERMANENT DISCOLORATION OF THE TEETH (YELLOW-GRAY-BROWN). This adverse reaction is more common during long-term use of the drugs but has been observed following repeated short-term courses. Enamel hypoplasia has also been reported. TETRACYCLINE DRUGS, THEREFORE, SHOULD NOT BE USED IN THIS AGE GROUP UNLESS OTHER DRUGS ARE NOT LIKELY TO BE EFFECTIVE OR ARE CONTRAINDICATED.
If renal impairment exists, even usual oral or parenteral doses may lead to excessive systemic accumulation of the drug and possible liver toxicity. Under such conditions, lower-than-usual total doses are indicated, and if therapy is prolonged, serum level determinations of the drug may be advisable.
Photosensitivity manifested by an exaggerated sunburn reaction has been observed in some individuals taking tetracyclines. Patients apt to be exposed to direct sunlight or ultraviolet light should be advised that this reaction can occur with tetracycline drugs, and treatment should be discontinued at the first evidence of skin erythema. Studies to date indicate that photosensitivity is rarely reported with MINOCIN® *minocycline HCl.*

The anti-anabolic action of the tetracyclines may cause an increase in BUN. While this is not a problem in those with normal renal function, in patients with significantly impaired function, higher serum levels of tetracycline may lead to azotemia, hyperphosphatemia, and acidosis.
CNS side effects including lightheadedness, dizziness, or vertigo have been reported. Patients who experience these symptoms should be cautioned about driving vehicles or using hazardous machinery while on minocycline therapy. These symptoms may disappear during therapy and usually disappear rapidly when the drug is discontinued.
Usage in pregnancy (See above "Warnings" about use during tooth development). Results of animal studies indicate that tetracyclines cross the placenta, are found in fetal tissues and can have toxic effects on the developing fetus (often related to retardation of skeletal development). Evidence of embryotoxicity has also been noted in animals treated early in pregnancy.
The safety of minocycline HCl for use during pregnancy has not been established.
Usage in newborns, infants, and children (See above "Warnings" about use during tooth development).
All tetracyclines form a stable calcium complex in any bone-forming tissue. A decrease in the fibula growth rate has been observed in prematures given oral tetracycline in doses of 25 mg/kg every six hours. This reaction was shown to be reversible when the drug was discontinued.
Tetracyclines are present in the milk of lactating women who are taking a drug in this class.

PRECAUTIONS

As with other antibiotic preparations, use of this drug may result in overgrowth of nonsusceptible organisms, including fungi. If superinfection occurs, the antibiotic should be discontinued and appropriate therapy should be instituted.
In venereal diseases when coexistent syphilis is suspected, darkfield examination should be done before treatment is started and the blood serology repeated monthly for at least four months.
Because tetracyclines have been shown to depress plasma prothrombin activity, patients who are on anticoagulant therapy may require downward adjustment of their anticoagulant dosage.
In long-term therapy, periodic laboratory evaluation of organ systems, including hematopoietic, renal and hepatic studies should be performed.
All infections due to Group A beta-hemolytic streptococci should be treated for at least ten days.
Since bacteriostatic drugs may interfere with the bactericidal action of penicillin, it is advisable to avoid giving tetracycline in conjunction with penicillin.

ADVERSE REACTIONS

Gastrointestinal: Anorexia, nausea, vomiting, diarrhea, glossitis, dysphagia, enterocolitis, inflammatory lesions (with monilial overgrowth) in the anogenital region, and increases in liver enzymes; rarely, hepatitis.
These reactions have been caused by both the oral and parenteral administration of tetracyclines.
Skin: Maculopapular and erythematous rashes. Exfoliative dermatitis has been reported but is uncommon. Photosensitivity is discussed above. (See "Warnings").
Pigmentation of the skin and mucous membranes has been reported.
Tooth discoloration has been reported rarely in adults.
Renal toxicity: Rise in BUN has been reported and is apparently dose-related (See "Warnings").
Hypersensitivity reactions: Urticaria, angioneurotic edema, anaphylaxis, anaphylactoid purpura, pericarditis, exacerbation of systemic lupus erythematosus and, rarely, pulmonary infiltrates with eosinophilia. Bulging fontanels have been reported in young infants following full therapeutic dosage. Pseudotumor Cerebri has very rarely been reported in adults. These signs disappeared rapidly when the drug was discontinued.
Blood: Hemolytic anemia, thrombocytopenia, neutropenia and eosinophilia have been reported.
CNS: (See "Warnings.")
When given over prolonged periods, tetracyclines have been reported to produce brown-black microscopic discoloration of thyroid glands. No abnormalities of thyroid function studies are known to occur.

DOSAGE AND ADMINISTRATION

Therapy should be continued for at least 24–48 hours after symptoms and fever have subsided.
Concomitant therapy: Antacids containing aluminum, calcium, or magnesium impair absorption and should not be given to patients taking oral tetracycline.
Studies to date have indicated that the absorption of MINOCIN is not notably influenced by foods and dairy products.
In patients with renal impairment: (See "Warnings.") Total dosage should be decreased by reduction of recommended individual doses and/or extending time intervals between doses.
In the treatment of streptococcal infections, a therapeutic dosage of tetracycline should be administered for at least ten days.
ADULTS: The usual dosage of MINOCIN® *minocycline HCl* is 200 mg initially followed by 100 mg every 12 hours. Alternatively, if more frequent doses are preferred, two or four 50 mg capsules or tablets may be given initially, followed by one 50 mg capsule or tablet four times daily.
For children above 8 years of age: The usual dosage of MINOCIN is 4 mg/kg initially followed by two mg/kg every 12 hours.
For treatment of syphilis, the usual dosage of MINOCIN should be administered over a period of 10 to 15 days. Close followup, including laboratory tests, is recommended.
Gonorrhea patients sensitive to penicillin may be treated with MINOCIN, administered as 200 mg initially, followed by 100 mg every 12 hours for a minimum of four days, with post-therapy cultures within two to three days.
In the treatment of meningococcal carrier state recommended dosage is 100 mg every 12 hours for five days.
Mycobacterium marinum infections: Although optimal doses have not been established, 100 mg twice a day for 6 to 8 weeks have been used successfully in a limited number of cases.
Uncomplicated urethral, endocervical, or rectal infection in adults caused by *Chlamydia trachomatis* or *Ureaplasma urealyticum:* 100 mg, by mouth, 2 times a day for at least seven days.[1]
In the treatment of uncomplicated gonococcal urethritis in men, 100 mg twice a day orally for 5 days is recommended.

HOW SUPPLIED

CAPSULES
Minocycline hydrochloride equivalent to 100 mg minocycline.
Hardshell orange and purple with Lederle over M4 printed on one half and MINOCIN over 100 mg on the other.
NDC 0005-5301-18 Bottle of 50s
NDC 0005-5301-23 Bottle of 100s
NDC 0005-5301-60 Unit Dose (strips) 10×10s
Store at Controlled Room Temperature 15°–30° C (59°–86° F)
Minocycline hydrochloride equivalent to 50 mg minocycline.
Hardshell orange with Lederle over M2 printed on one half and MINOCIN over 50 mg on the other.
NDC 0005-5300-23 Bottle of 100s
NDC 0005-5300-60 Unit Dose (strips) 10×10s
Store at Controlled Room Temperature 15°–30° C (59°–86° F)
ORAL SUSPENSION
Minocycline hydrochloride equivalent to 50 mg minocycline per teaspoonful (5 ml). Preserved with propylparaben 0.10% and butylparaben 0.06% with Alcohol USP 5% v/v, custard-flavored.
NDC 0005-5313-56 Bottle 2 fl. oz. (60 ml)
Store at Controlled Room Temperature 15°–30° C (59°–86° F)
DO NOT FREEZE
TABLETS
Minocycline hydrochloride equivalent to 100 mg minocycline. Round, convex, orange film-coated tablet engraved with M over bisect and 5 under bisect on one side of the tablet and LL on the other.
NDC 0005-9376-18 Bottle of 50s
Store at Controlled Room Temperature 15°–30° C (59°–86° F)
Minocycline hydrochloride equivalent to 50 mg minocycline. Round, convex, orange film-coated tablet engraved with M3 on one side and LL on the other.
NDC 0005-9375-23 Bottle of 100s
Store at Controlled Room Temperature 15°–30° C (59°–86° F)
Animal Pharmacology and Toxicology: MINOCIN minocycline HCl has been found to produce high blood concentrations following oral dosage to various animal species and to be extensively distributed to all tissues examined in ^{14}C-labeled drug studies in dogs. MINOCIN has been found experimentally to produce discoloration of the thyroid glands. This finding has been observed in rats and dogs. Changes in thyroid function have also been found in these animal species. However, no change in thyroid function has been observed in humans.
Reference: 1. CDC Sexually Transmitted Diseases Treatment Guidelines 1982.
LEDERLE LABORATORIES DIVISION
American Cyanamid Company, Pearl River, NY 10965
Shown in Product Identification Section, page 413

MYAMBUTOL® ℞

[*mī-am-bū-tōl*]
ethambutol hydrochloride
Tablets

DESCRIPTION

MYAMBUTOL® *ethambutol hydrochloride Lederle* is an oral chemotherapeutic agent which is specifically effective against actively growing microorganisms of the genus *Mycobacterium,* including *M tuberculosis.*
MYAMBUTOL tablets contain the following inactive ingredients: 100 mg—Blue 2, Ethylcellulose, Gelatin, Hydroxypropyl Methylcellulose, Magnesium Stearate, Sorbitol, Stearic Acid, Sucrose, Titanium Dioxide and other ingredients. 400 mg—Gelatin, Hydroxypropyl Methylcellulose, Magnesium Stearate, Sodium Lauryl Sulfate, Sorbitol, Stearic Acid, Sucrose, Titanium Dioxide and other ingredients.

ACTION

MYAMBUTOL, following a single oral dose of 25 mg/kg of body weight, attains a peak of 2 to 5 micrograms/ml in serum two to four hours after administration. When the drug is administered daily for longer periods of time at this dose, serum levels are similar. The serum level of MYAMBUTOL falls to undetectable levels by 24 hours after the last dose except in some patients with abnormal renal function. The intracellular concentrations of erythrocytes reach peak values approximately twice those of plasma and maintain this ratio throughout the 24 hours.
During the 24-hour period following oral administration of MYAMBUTOL, approximately 50% of the initial dose is excreted unchanged in the urine, while an additional 8% to 15% appears in the form of metabolites. The main path of metabolism appears to be an initial oxidation of the alcohol to an aldehydic intermediate, followed by conversion to a dicarboxylic acid. From 20% to 22% of the initial dose is excreted in the feces as unchanged drug. No drug accumulation has been observed with consecutive single daily doses of 25 mg/kg in patients with normal kidney function, although marked accumulation has been demonstrated in patients with renal insufficiency.
MYAMBUTOL diffuses into actively growing *mycobacterium* cells such as tubercle bacilli. MYAMBUTOL appears to inhibit the synthesis of one or more metabolites, thus causing impairment of cell metabolism, arrest of multiplication, and cell death. No cross resistance with other available antimycobacterial agents has been demonstrated.
MYAMBUTOL has been shown to be effective against strains of *Mycobacterium tuberculosis* but does not seem to be active against fungi, viruses, or other bacteria.
Mycobacterium tuberculosis strains previously unexposed to MYAMBUTOL have been uniformly sensitive to concentrations of 8 or less μg/ml, depending on the nature of the culture media. When MYAMBUTOL has been used alone for treatment of tuberculosis, tubercle bacilli from these patients have developed resistance to MYAMBUTOL by *in vitro* susceptibility tests; the development of resistance has been unpredictable and appears to occur in a step-like manner. No cross resistance between MYAMBUTOL and other antituberculous drugs has been reported. MYAMBUTOL has reduced the incidence of the emergence of mycobacterial resistance to isoniazid when both drugs have been used concurrently.
An agar diffusion microbiologic assay, based upon inhibition of *Mycobacterium smegmatis* (ATCC 607) may be used to determine concentrations of MYAMBUTOL® *ethambutol hydrochloride* in serum and urine. This technique has not been published, but further information can be obtained upon inquiry to Lederle Laboratories.

ANIMAL PHARMACOLOGY

Toxicological studies in dogs on high prolonged doses produced evidence of myocardial damage and failure, and depigmentation of the tapetum lucidum of the eyes, the significance of which is not known. Degenerative changes in the central nervous system, apparently not dose-related, have also been noted in dogs receiving ethambutol hydrochloride over a prolonged period.
In the rhesus monkey, neurological signs appeared after treatment with high doses given daily over a period of several months. These were correlated with specific serum levels of ethambutol hydrochloride and with definite neuroanatomical changes in the central nervous system. Focal interstitial carditis was also noted in monkeys which received ethambutol hydrochloride in high doses for a prolonged period.
When pregnant mice or rabbits were treated with high doses of ethambutol hydrochloride, fetal mortality was slightly but not significantly ($P > 0.05$) increased. Female rats treated with ethambutol hydrochloride displayed slight but insignificant ($P > 0.05$) decreases in fertility and litter size.
In fetuses born of mice treated with high doses of MYAMBUTOL during pregnancy, a low incidence of cleft palate, exencephaly and abnormality of the vertebral column were observed. Minor abnormalities of the cervical vertebra were seen in the newborn of rats treated with high doses of MYAMBUTOL during pregnancy. Rabbits receiving high doses of MYAMBUTOL during pregnancy gave birth to

Continued on next page

The information on each product appearing here is based on labelling effective in August, 1986 and is either the entire official brochure or an accurate condensation therefrom. Information concerning all Lederle products may be obtained from the Professional Services Department, Lederle Laboratories, Pearl River, New York, 10965.

two fetuses with monophthalmia, one with a shortened right forearm accompanied by bilateral wrist-joint contracture and one with harelip and cleft palate.

INDICATIONS

MYAMBUTOL is indicated for the treatment of pulmonary tuberculosis. It should not be used as the sole antituberculous drug, but should be used in conjunction with at least one other antituberculous drug. Selection of the companion drug should be based on clinical experience, considerations of comparative safety and appropriate *in vitro* susceptibility studies.

In patients who have not received previous antituberculous therapy, ie initial treatment, the most frequently used regimens have been the following:

MYAMBUTOL plus isoniazid

MYAMBUTOL plus isoniazid plus streptomycin.

In patients who have received previous antituberculous therapy, mycobacterial resistance to other drugs used in initial therapy is frequent. Consequently, in such retreatment patients, MYAMBUTOL should be combined with at least one of the second line drugs not previously administered to the patient and to which bacterial susceptibility has been indicated by appropriate *in vitro* studies. Antituberculous drugs used with MYAMBUTOL have included cycloserine, ethionamide, pyrazinamide, viomycin and other drugs. Isoniazid, aminosalicylic acid, and streptomycin have also been used in multiple drug regimens. Alternating drug regimens have also been utilized.

CONTRAINDICATIONS:

MYAMBUTOL® *ethambutol hydrochloride* is contraindicated in patients who are known to be hypersensitive to this drug. It is also contraindicated in patients with known optic neuritis unless clinical judgment determines that it may be used.

PRECAUTIONS

The effects of combinations of MYAMBUTOL with other antituberculous drugs on the fetus is not known. While administration of this drug to pregnant human patients has produced no detectable effect upon the fetus, the possible teratogenic potential in women capable of bearing children should be weighed carefully against the benefits of therapy.

There are published reports of five women who received the drug during pregnancy without apparent adverse effect upon the fetus.

MYAMBUTOL is not recommended for use in children under thirteen years of age since safe conditions for use have not been established.

Patients with decreased renal function need the dosage reduced as determined by serum levels of MYAMBUTOL, since the main path of excretion of this drug is by the kidneys.

Because this drug may have adverse effects on vision, physical examination should include ophthalmoscopy, finger perimetry and testing of color discrimination. In patients with visual defects such as cataracts, recurrent inflammatory conditions of the eye, optic neuritis, and diabetic retinopathy, the evaluation of changes in visual acuity is more difficult, and care should be taken to be sure the variations in vision are not due to the underlying disease conditions. In such patients, consideration should be given to relationship between benefits expected and possible visual deterioration since evaluation of visual changes is difficult. (For recommended procedures, see next paragraphs under ADVERSE REACTIONS).

As with any potent drug, periodic assessment of organ system functions, including renal, hepatic, and hematopoietic, should be made during long-term therapy.

ADVERSE REACTIONS

MYAMBUTOL may produce decreases in visual acuity which appear to be due to optic neuritis and to be related to dose and duration of treatment. The effects are generally reversible when administration of the drug is discontinued promptly.

In rare cases recovery may be delayed for up to one year or more and the effect may possibly be irreversible in these cases.

Patients should be advised to report promptly to their physician any change of visual acuity. The change in visual acuity may be unilateral or bilateral and hence *each eye must be tested separately and both eyes tested together.* Testing of visual acuity should be performed before beginning MYAMBUTOL therapy and periodically during drug administration, except that it should be done monthly when a patient is on a dosage of more than 15 mg per kg per day. Snellen eye charts are recommended for testing of visual acuity. Studies have shown that there are definite fluctuations of one or two lines of the Snellen chart in the visual acuity of many tuberculous patients *not* receiving MYAMBUTOL® *ethambutol hydrochloride.*

The following table may be useful in interpreting possible changes in visual acuity attributable to MYAMBUTOL. [See table below].

In general, changes in visual acuity less than those indicated under "Significant Number of Lines" and "Decreases-Number of Points", may be due to chance variation, limitations of the testing method or physiologic variability. Conversely, changes in visual acuity equaling or exceeding those under "Significant Number of Lines" and "Decreases-Number of Points" indicate need for retesting and careful evaluation of the patient's visual status. If careful evaluation confirms the magnitude of visual change and fails to reveal another cause, MYAMBUTOL should be discontinued and the patient reevaluated at frequent intervals. Progressive decreases in visual acuity during therapy must be considered to be due to MYAMBUTOL.

If corrective glasses are used prior to treatment, these must be worn during visual acuity testing. During one to two years of therapy, a refractive error may develop which must be corrected in order to obtain accurate test results. Testing the visual acuity through a pinhole eliminates refractive error.

Patients developing visual abnormality during MYAMBUTOL treatment may show subjective visual symptoms before, or simultaneously with, the demonstration of decreases in visual acuity, and all patients receiving MYAMBUTOL should be questioned periodically about blurred vision and other subjective eye symptoms.

Recovery of visual acuity generally occurs over a period of weeks to months after the drug has been discontinued. Patients have then received MYAMBUTOL again without recurrence of loss of visual acuity.

Other adverse reactions reported include: anaphylactoid reactions, dermatitis pruritus and joint pain; anorexia, nausea, vomiting, gastrointestinal upset, abdominal pain; fever, malaise, headache, and dizziness; mental confusion, disorientation and possible hallucinations. Numbness and tingling of the extremities due to peripheral neuritis have been reported infrequently.

Elevated serum uric acid levels occur and precipitation of acute gout has been reported. Transient impairment of liver function as indicated by abnormal liver function tests is not an unusual finding. Since MYAMBUTOL is recommended for therapy in conjunction with one or more other antituberculous drugs, these changes may be related to the concurrent therapy.

DOSAGE AND ADMINISTRATION

MYAMBUTOL® *ethambutol hydrochloride* should not be used alone, in initial treatment or in retreatment. MYAMBUTOL should be administered on a once every 24-hour basis only. Absorption is not significantly altered by administration with food. Therapy, in general, should be continued until bacteriological conversion has become permanent and maximal clinical improvement has occurred.

MYAMBUTOL is not recommended for use in children under thirteen years of age since safe conditions for use have not been established.

Initial Treatment: In patients who have not received previous antituberculous therapy, administer MYAMBUTOL 15 mg per kg (7 mg per pound) of body weight, as a single oral dose once every 24 hours. In the more recent studies, isoniazid has been administered concurrently in a single, daily, oral dose.

Retreatment: In patients who have received previous antituberculous therapy, administer MYAMBUTOL 25 mg per kg (11 mg per pound) of body weight, as a single oral dose once every 24 hours. Concurrently administer at least one other antituberculous drug to which the organisms have been demonstrated to be susceptible by appropriate *in vitro* tests. Suitable drugs usually consist of those not previously used in the treatment of the patient. After 60 days of MYAMBUTOL administration, decrease the dose to 15 mg per kg (7 mg per pound) of body weight, and administer as a single oral dose once every 24 hours.

During the period when a patient is on a daily dose of 25 mg/kg, monthly eye examinations are advised.

See Table for easy selection of proper weight-dose tablet(s).

Weight-Dose Table

15 mg/kg (7 mg/lb) Schedule

Weight Range Pounds	Kilograms	Daily Dose In mg
Under 85 lbs	Under 37 kg	500
85–94.5	37–43	600
95–109.5	43–50	700
110–124.5	50–57	800
125–139.5	57–64	900
140–154.5	64–71	1000
155–169.5	71–79	1100
170–184.5	79–84	1200
185–199.5	84–90	1300
200–214.5	90–97	1400
215 and Over	Over 97	1500
25 mg/kg (11 mg/lb) Schedule		
Under 85 lbs	Under 38 kg	900
85–92.5	38–42	1000
93–101.5	42–45.5	1100
102–109.5	45.5–50	1200
110–118.5	50–54	1300
119–128.5	54–58	1400
129–136.5	58–62	1500
137–146.5	62–67	1600
147–155.5	67–71	1700
156–164.5	71–75	1800
165–173.5	75–79	1900
174–182.5	79–83	2000
183–191.5	83–87	2100
192–199.5	87–91	2200
200–209.5	91–95	2300
210–218.5	95–99	2400
219 and Over	Over 99	2500

HOW SUPPLIED

MYAMBUTOL Tablets 100 mg round, convex, white, coated tablets engraved M6 on one side and LL on the other, are supplied as follows:

NDC 0005-5015-23 - Bottles of 100

NDC 0005-5015-34 Bottles of 1000

400 mg - round, convex, white, scored, film-coated tablets engraved with LL on one side and M to the left and 7 to the right of the score on the other side, are supplied as follows:

NDC 0005-5084-62 Unit-of-Issue 100s with CRC

NDC 0005-5084-34 Bottles of 1000

NDC 0005-5084-60 - Unit Dose 10 × 10s

Store at Controlled Room Temperature 15°–30°C (59°–86°F).

AHFS 8:16

Tablets, 100 mg

Military Depot NSN 6505-00-403-7645, 100s

Tablets 400 mg

Military Depot NSN 6505-00-812-2579, 100s

VA Depot NSN 6505-00-812-2543, 1000s

Shown in Product Identification Section, page 413

MYAMBUTOL

VISUAL ACUITY TABLE

Initial Snellen Reading	Reading Indicating Significant Decrease	Significant Number of Lines	Decreases Number of Points
20/13	20/25	3	12
20/15	20/25	2	10
20/20	20/30	2	10
20/25	20/40	2	15
20/30	20/50	2	20
20/40	20/70	2	30
20/50	20/70	1	20

NEOLOID®

[*nēo-loid*]

EMULSIFIED CASTOR OIL

For the treatment of isolated bouts of constipation

PEPPERMINT FLAVORED - SHAKE WELL

CONTAINS

Castor Oil USP 36.4% (w/w) with 0.1% (w/w) Sodium Benzoate and 0.2% (w/w) Potassium Sorbate added as preservatives, emulsifying and flavoring agents in water. Also contains the following inactive ingredients: Citric Acid, Glyceryl Monostearate, Polysorbate 80, Propylene Glycol, Sodium Alginate, Sodium Saccharin, Stearic Acid, Tenox II. NEOLOID is an emulsion with an exceptionally bland, pleasant taste.

DOSAGE

Infants ½ to 1½ teaspoonfuls; children, adjust between infant and adult dose. Average adult dose, 2 to 4 tablespoonfuls, or as prescribed by the physician. Not to be used when abdominal pain, nausea, vomiting, or other symptoms of appendicitis are present. Frequent or continued use of this preparation may result in dependence on laxatives. Do not use during pregnancy except on a physician's advice. Keep this and all drugs out of the reach of children.

WARNING

As with any drug, if you are pregnant or nursing a baby, seek the advice of a health professional before using this product. In case of accidental overdose, seek professional assistance or contact a Poison Control Center immediately.

Store at Room Temperature.

DO NOT FREEZE

NET 4 Fl. Oz. (118 ml) NDC 0005-5442-58.

NEPTAZANE® ℞

[*nĕp-ta-zāne*]
methazolamide

DESCRIPTION

NEPTAZANE® *methazolamide*, a sulfonamide derivative, is a white crystalline powder, weakly acid, and slightly soluble in water. It is available as a 50 mg white convex scored tablet. The chemical name for methazolamide is: *N*-[5-(aminosulfonyl)-3-methyl-1,3,4-thiadiazol-2(3*H*)-ylidene]-acetamide.
NEPTAZANE 50 mg tablets contain the following inactive ingredients: Acacia, Alginic Acid, Cornstarch, Calcium Phosphate Dibasic, Gelatin, and Magnesium Stearate.

ACTION

NEPTAZANE is a potent inhibitor of the enzyme carbonic anhydrase. It is absorbed somewhat slowly from the gastrointestinal tract and disappears more slowly from the plasma than does acetazolamide, which may account for the delay in onset and duration of its activity. It is distributed throughout the body and can be assayed in the blood plasma, the cerebrospinal fluid, the aqueous humor of the eye, the red blood cell, in the bile, and the extracellular fluid. Urinary excretion accounts for only 15% of NEPTAZANE in man. It is not cumulative in its concentration. The drug is considered nonbactericidal. Although concentration in the cerebrospinal fluid is high, it is not considered an effective anticonvulsant.
NEPTAZANE does have a diuretic effect, resulting in increase in urinary volume, with excretion of sodium and potassium and chloride, but it is less active than acetazolamide. This effect is transient and of low degree and the drug is not used as a diuretic. Serum electrolyte changes in sodium, potassium and chloride are minimal and return to pretreatment levels after daily administration for three to four days. Inhibition of renal bicarbonate reabsorption produces an alkaline urine. Plasma bicarbonate decreases temporarily, and a relative and transient metabolic acidosis may occur due to a disequilibrium in CO_2 transport in the red cell. This is quickly restored to balance by the initiation of compensatory mechanisms. Urinary citrate excretion is decreased by 40% on doses of 100 mg every eight hours with variations in urinary volume output. Uric acid output was decreased 36% in the first 24-hour period and varied thereafter. The oral administration of the drug by inhibition of carbonic anhydrase in the various tissues of the eye causes a decrease in the rate of aqueous humor formation. Various authors differ somewhat as to the time of onset of intraocular pressure fall, of the peak of activity, and the duration of the effect on the pressure, of a 24-hour period of ingestion, but on the average, the onset of fall in intraocular pressure occurs within two to four hours, with peak of fall in six to eight hours, the effect lasting from 10 to 18 hours.

INDICATIONS

For adjunctive treatment of: chronic simple (open angle) glaucoma, secondary glaucoma, and preoperatively in acute angle-closure glaucoma where delay of surgery is desired in order to lower intraocular pressure.

CONTRAINDICATIONS

Severe or absolute glaucoma and chronic noncongestive angle-closure glaucoma. It is of doubtful use in glaucoma due to severe peripheral anterior synechiae or hemorrhagic glaucoma.
NEPTAZANE® *methazolamide* is contraindicated in patients with adrenocortical insufficiency, hepatic insufficiency, renal insufficiency, or an electrolyte imbalance state such as hyperchloremic acidosis, and sodium and potassium depletion states.

WARNING

Studies in rats have demonstrated teratogenic effects (skeletal anomalies) at high doses. There is no evidence of these effects in human beings and no fetal defects have been reported. However, NEPTAZANE should not be used in women of childbearing potential or in pregnancy, especially in the first trimester, unless the benefits to be gained in the control of glaucoma outweigh potential adverse effects.

PRECAUTIONS

Potassium excretion is increased initially, upon administration of NEPTAZANE, and in patients with cirrhosis or hepatic insufficiency could precipitate a hepatic coma. It should be used with caution in patients on steroid therapy because of the potentiality of hypokalemic state.
Adequate and balanced electrolyte intake is essential in all patients whose concomitant clinical condition may occasion electrolyte imbalance.
In patients with pulmonary obstruction or emphysema where alveolar ventilation may be impaired, NEPTAZANE, which may precipitate or aggravate acidosis, should be used with caution.
Adverse reactions common to all sulfonamide derivatives may occur: fever, rash (including erythema multiforme, Stevens-Johnson syndrome, toxic epidermal necrolysis), crystalluria, renal calculus, bone marrow depression, thrombocytopenic purpura, hemolytic anemia, leukopenia, pancytopenia, and agranulocytosis. Precaution is advised for early detection of such reactions, and the drug should be discontinued and appropriate therapy instituted.
Precaution is advised for patients receiving concomitant high-dose aspirin and NEPTAZANE, as anorexia, tachypnea, lethargy, and coma have been rarely reported due to possible drug interactions of drugs of this class.

ADVERSE REACTIONS

Most adverse reactions to NEPTAZANE have been relatively mild in character and disappear upon withdrawal of the drug or adjustment of dosage. They are as follows: anorexia, nausea, vomiting, malaise, fatigue or drowsiness, headache, vertigo, mental confusion, depression, and paresthesias of fingers, toes, hands or feet and occasionally at the mucocutaneous junction of the lips, mouth, and anus. Rarely, photosensitivity has been reported.
Urinary citrate excretion is decreased during the administration of NEPTAZANE as is uric acid output, but urinary calculi have been reported only rarely. The effect on citrate excretion is less than that reported from the administration of acetazolamide.
In order to monitor for hematologic reactions common to all sulfonamides, it is recommended that a baseline CBC and platelet count be obtained on all patients prior to initiating NEPTAZANE therapy and at regular intervals during therapy. Early detection of such reactions is important, and the drug should be discontinued, and appropriate therapy instituted if significant changes occur in these laboratory parameters.

DOSAGE AND ADMINISTRATION

The effective therapeutic dose administered in tablet form varies from 50 mg to 100 mg two to three times daily. The drug may be used concomitantly with miotic and osmotic agents. It is not available for parenteral use.

HOW SUPPLIED

NEPTAZANE® *methazolamide* Tablets, 50 mg, round, scored, white tablets engraved with LL on one side and N above and 1 below the score on the other side, are supplied as follows: NDC 0005-4570-23—Bottles of 100
Military Depots:
Tablets, 50 mg—100s
NSN 6505-00-065-4205
Store at Controlled Room Temperature 15°–30°C (59°–86°F).
Shown in Product Identification Section, page 413

NILSTAT® ℞

[*nĭl-stăt*]
Nystatin Oral Suspension

DESCRIPTION

This antifungal agent is obtained from *Streptomyces noursei*. It is now known to be a mixture, but the composition has not been completely elucidated. Nystatin A is closely related to amphotericin B. Each is a macrocyclic lactone containing a ketal ring, an *all-trans* polyene system, and a mycosamine (3-amino-3-deoxyrhamose) moiety.
NILSTAT® *nystatin* Oral Suspension is a cherry-flavored, ready-to-use suspension containing 100,000 units of nystatin per ml. NILSTAT contains the following inactive ingredients: Edetate Calcium Disodium, Flavor, Magnesium Aluminum Silicate, Methylparaben, Polysorbate 80, Propylparaben, Sucrose, Yellow 10.

ACTIONS

Nystatin probably acts by binding to sterols in the cell membrane of the fungus with a resultant change in membrane permeability allowing leakage of intracellular components. It is absorbed very sparingly following oral administration, with no detectable blood levels when given in the recommended doses.

INDICATIONS

For the treatment of infections of the oral cavity caused by *Candida* (Monilia) *albicans*.

CONTRAINDICATIONS

Hypersensitivity to the drug.

ADVERSE REACTIONS

Nausea and vomiting, Gastrointestinal distress, Diarrhea.

DOSAGE AND ADMINISTRATION

Infants: 2 ml (200,000 units) four times daily (1 ml in each side of mouth).
Children and adults: 4-6 ml (400,000 to 600,000 units) four times daily (one-half of dose in each side of mouth).
Note: Limited clinical studies in premature and low birth weight infants indicate that 1 ml four times daily is effective. Local treatment should be continued at least 48 hours after perioral symptoms have disappeared and cultures returned to normal.
It is recommended that the drug be retained in the mouth as long as possible before swallowing.

HOW SUPPLIED

NILSTAT® *nystatin* Oral Suspension, is a cherry flavored, ready-to-use suspension containing 100,000 units of nystatin per ml, supplied as follows:
60 ml bottle with dropper NDC 0005-5429-18 and 16 fl oz bottle NDC 0005-5429-65.
Store at Controlled Room Temperature 15°–30°C (59°–86°F).
DO NOT FREEZE.

NILSTAT® ℞

[*nĭl-stăt*]
Nystatin, USP
For Extemporaneous Preparation of Oral Suspension

DESCRIPTION

Nystatin, USP is an antifungal antibiotic which is both fungistatic and fungicidal *in vitro* against a wide variety of yeasts and yeast-like fungi. It is a polyene antibiotic of undetermined structural formula that is obtained from *Streptomyces noursei*. Nystatin, USP, which contains no excipients or preservatives, is a ready-to-use non-sterile powder for oral administration available in bottles of 150 million, 1 billion and 2 billion units.

CLINICAL PHARMACOLOGY

Nystatin probably acts by binding to sterols in the cell membrane of the fungus with a resultant change in membrane permeability allowing leakage of intracellular components. It is absorbed very sparingly following oral administration, with no detectable blood levels when given in the recommended doses. Most of the orally administered nystatin is passed unchanged in the stool.

INDICATIONS AND USAGE

For treatment of infections of the oral cavity caused by *Candida albicans* (monilia).

CONTRAINDICATIONS

Hypersensitivity to the drug.

ADVERSE REACTIONS

Large oral doses of nystatin have occasionally produced diarrhea, gastrointestinal distress, nausea and vomiting.

DOSAGE AND ADMINISTRATION

Adults and older children: add ⅛ tsp (500,000 units) of nystatin, USP to approximately ½ to 1 cup (120 to 240 ml, or 4 to 8 oz.) of water and stir well. The entire dose should then be used to thoroughly rinse the mouth and the dose should be retained in the mouth as long as possible before swallowing. This dose should be given orally four times daily, and should be continued for at least 48 hours after perioral symptoms have disappeared and cultures have returned to normal.
One-eighth tsp. of nystatin, USP is equivalent to the recommended dose for adults and children of NILSTAT® Oral Suspension (4 to 6 ml, or 400,000 to 600,000 units). This product contains no preservative and therefore should be used immediately after mixing and should not be stored.

HOW SUPPLIED

Bottles containing 150 million units, 1 billion units and bottles containing 2 billion units—(1 billion units is approximately 170–200 grams, depending on potency of powder).
NDC 0005-5421-12—150 Million Units
NDC 0005-5421-10—One Billion Units
NDC 0005-5421-11—Two Billion Units
Store under refrigeration 2°–8° C (36°–46° F) in tight, light resistant containers.
Note: The potency of this product cannot be assured for longer than 90 days after the container is first opened.

NILSTAT® ℞

[*nĭl-stăt*]
Nystatin Vaginal Tablets USP

DESCRIPTION

NILSTAT® *nystatin* Vaginal Tablets, USP are oblong shaped vaginal tablets, each containing 100,000 units nystatin, USP and the following inactive ingredients: Cornstarch, Lactose, Magnesium Stearate, Povidone and Sorbitol. Nystatin is a polyene antibiotic of undetermined structural formula that is obtained from *Streptomyces noursei*.

Continued on next page

The information on each product appearing here is based on labelling effective in August, 1986 and is either the entire official brochure or an accurate condensation therefrom. Information concerning all Lederle products may be obtained from the Professional Services Department, Lederle Laboratories, Pearl River, New York, 10965.

Lederle—Cont.

CLINICAL PHARMACOLOGY

Nystatin is an antifungal antibiotic which is both fungistatic and fungicidal *in vitro* against a wide variety of yeasts and yeast-like fungi. It probably acts by binding to sterols in the cell membrane of the fungus with a resultant change in membrane permeability allowing leakage of intracellular components. It exhibits no appreciable activity against bacteria or trichomonads.

INDICATIONS AND USAGE

NILSTAT® *nystatin* Vaginal Tablets, USP are effective for the local treatment of vulvovaginal candidiasis (moniliasis). The diagnosis should be confirmed, prior to therapy, by KOH smears and/or cultures. Other pathogens commonly associated with vulvovaginitis (Trichomonas and *Haemophilus vaginalis)* do not respond to nystatin and should be ruled out by appropriate laboratory methods.

CONTRAINDICATIONS

This preparation is contraindicated in patients with a history of hypersensitivity to any of its components.

PRECAUTIONS

General:
Discontinue treatment if sensitization or irritation is reported during use.
Laboratory Tests:
If there is a lack of response to NILSTAT® *nystatin* Vaginal Tablets, USP, appropriate microbiological studies should be repeated to confirm the diagnosis and rule out other pathogens, before instituting another course of antimycotic therapy.
Usage in Pregnancy:
No adverse effects or complications have been attributed to nystatin in infants born to women treated with nystatin vaginal tablets.

ADVERSE REACTIONS

Nystatin is virtually nontoxic and nonsensitizing and is well tolerated by all age groups, even on prolonged administration. Rarely, irritation or sensitization may occur (see PRECAUTIONS).

DOSAGE AND ADMINISTRATION

The usual dosage is one tablet (100,000 units nystatin) daily for two weeks. The tablets should be deposited high in the vagina by means of the applicator. "Instructions for the Patient" are enclosed in each package.
Even though symptomatic relief may occur within a few days, treatment should be continued for the full course.
It is important that therapy be continued during menstruation. Adjunctive measures such as therapeutic douches are unnecessary and sometimes inadvisable. Cleansing douches may be used by nonpregnant women, if desired, for esthetic purposes.

HOW SUPPLIED

NILSTAT *nystatin* Vaginal Tablets, USP, 100,000 units per tablet are oval-shaped, pale yellow, uncoated, engraved with LL on one side and N6 on the other, supplied as follows:
Packages of 15 and 30 Vaginal Tablets with Applicator. 15 tablets: NDC 0005-5428-06; 30 tablets: NDC 0005-5428-08.
Shown in Product Identification Section, page 413

NILSTAT® ℞

[*nĭl-stăt*]
NYSTATIN ORAL TABLETS, USP
(Film-Coated)
500,000 Units/Tablet

DESCRIPTION

This antifungal agent is obtained from *Streptomyces noursei.* It is now known to be a mixture, but the composition has not been completely elucidated. Nystatin A is closely related to amphotericin B. Each is a macrocylic lactone containing a ketal ring, an *all-trans* polyene system, and a mycosamine (3-amino-3-deoxyrhamose) moiety.
NILSTAT® *nystatin* Oral Tablets, USP—*Lederle* are available as coated tablets. Each nystatin Oral Tablet, USP *Lederle* provides 500,000 units nystatin. NILSTAT tablets also contain the following inactive ingredients: Cornstarch, Ethylcellulose, Magnesium Stearate, Methylcellulose, Red 30, Stearic Acid, Titanium Dioxide, and other ingredients.

ACTIONS

Nystatin probably acts by binding to sterols in the cell membrane of the fungus with a resultant change in membrane permeability allowing leakage of intracellular components. It is absorbed very sparingly following oral administration, with no detectable blood levels when given in the recommended doses.

INDICATIONS

For the treatment of intestinal moniliasis.

CONTRAINDICATIONS

Hypersensitivity to the drug.

ADVERSE REACTIONS

Nausea and vomiting. Gastrointestinal distress. Diarrhea.

DOSAGE AND ADMINISTRATION

Usual dosage: 500,000 to 1 million units tid. Treatment should generally be continued for at least 48 hours after clinical cure to prevent relapse.

HOW SUPPLIED

NILSTAT® *nystatin* Oral Tablets, USP (500,000 units per tablet), round, convex, pink film-coated tablets, engraved with LL on one side and N5 on the other, are supplied as follows:
NDC 0005-5426-23—Bottles of 100
NDC 0005-5426-60—Unit Dose 10 × 10s
Store at Controlled Room Temperature 15°–30° C (59°–86° F).
Shown in Product Identification Section, page 413

NILSTAT®

[*nĭl-stăt*]
NYSTATIN
TOPICAL CREAM USP
100,000 U. per Gram

DESCRIPTION

NILSTAT® *nystatin* Topical Cream, contains 100,000 units Nystatin per gram and the following inactive ingredients in a vanishing cream water base: Emulsifying Wax NF, Isopropyl Myristate, Glycerin, Lactic Acid and Sodium Hydroxide. It is preserved with 0.2% Sorbic Acid.

ACTIONS

Microbiology: Nystatin is an antifungal antibiotic produced by a strain of*Streptomyces noursei.* Nystatin is useful in the treatment of infections caused by *Candida (Monilia) albicans.* Nystatin has no appreciable activity against bacteria.
Human Pharmacology: No detectable blood levels are obtained following topical or vaginal application.

INDICATIONS

For the treatment of cutaneous or mucocutaneous mycotic infections caused by *Candida* species (*Monilia*).

CONTRAINDICATIONS

All nystatin preparations are contraindicated in patients with a history of hypersensitivity to nystatin.

ADVERSE REACTIONS

Nystatin USP is virtually nontoxic and nonsensitizing and is well tolerated by all age groups, even on prolonged administration.

DOSAGE AND ADMINISTRATION

Apply liberally to affected areas twice daily or as indicated until healing is complete.

HOW SUPPLIED

15 gram tubes and 240 gram jars. Product No. 5433
Shown in Product Identification Section, page 413

NILSTAT®

[*nĭl-stăt*]
NYSTATIN
TOPICAL OINTMENT
100,000 U. per Gram

DESCRIPTION

NILSTAT® *nystatin* Topical Ointment, contains 100,000 units Nystatin, per gram and the following inactive ingredients: Light Mineral Oil and Plastibase 50 W.

ACTIONS

Microbiology: Nystatin is an antifungal antibiotic produced by a strain of *Streptomyces noursei.* Nystatin is useful in the treatment of infections caused by *Candida (Monilia) albicans.* Nystatin has no appreciable activity against bacteria.
Human Pharmacology: No detectable blood levels are obtained following topical or vaginal application.

INDICATIONS

For the treatment of cutaneous or mucocutaneous mycotic infections caused by *Candida* species (*Monilia*).

CONTRAINDICATIONS

All nystatin preparations are contraindicated in patients with a history of hypersensitivity to nystatin.

ADVERSE REACTIONS

Nystatin USP is virtually nontoxic and nonsensitizing and is well tolerated by all age groups, even on prolonged administration.

DOSAGE AND ADMINISTRATION

Apply liberally to affected areas twice daily or as indicated until healing is complete.
Military Depot: 240 gm jar, NSN 6505-01-063- 1141

HOW SUPPLIED

15 gram tubes
Product No. NDC 0005-5432-09
Shown in Product Identification Section, page 413

ORIMUNE® ℞

[*or-ĭ-mune*]
POLIOVIRUS VACCINE
LIVE ORAL TRIVALENT
0.5 ml Dose Contains Sorbitol
SABIN STRAINS TYPES 1, 2 and 3
FOR ORAL ADMINISTRATION—NOT FOR INJECTION

DESCRIPTION

Manufacture and Composition: Poliovirus vaccine live oral trivalent ORIMUNE® is a mixture of three types of attenuated polioviruses which have been propagated in monkey kidney cell culture. The cells are grown in the presence of Eagle's Basal Medium consisting of Earle's Balanced Salt Solution containing amino acids, antibiotics and calf serum. After cell growth, the medium is removed and replaced with fresh medium containing the inoculating virus but no calf serum. The final vaccine is diluted with a modified cell culture maintenance medium containing sorbitol. Each dose (0.5 ml) contains less than 25 micrograms of each of the antibiotics, streptomycin and neomycin.
The potency is expressed in terms of the amount of virus contained in the recommended dose as tissue culture infective doses ($TCID_{50}$). The human dose of vaccine containing all three virus types shall be constituted to have infectivity titers in the final container material of $10^{5.4}$ to $10^{6.4}$ for Type 1, $10^{4.5}$ to $10^{5.5}$ for Type 2, and $10^{5.2}$ to $10^{6.2}$ for Type 3.[1]

CLINICAL PHARMACOLOGY

Administration of attenuated, live oral poliovirus vaccine (OPV) simulates natural infection, inducing active mucosal and systemic immunity without producting untoward symptoms of disease. For optimal mucosal immunity to occur, it is necessary for the virus to multiply in the intestinal tract. A primary series of trivalent vaccine is designed to produce an antibody response to poliovirus Types 1, 2, and 3. This response is comparable to the immunity induced by the natural disease. The antibodies thus formed help protect the individual against clinical poliomyelitis infection by any of the three types of poliovirus. Multiple doses of OPV in the primary series are not administered as boosters, but to insure that immunity to all three types of poliovirus has been achieved.[2] When used in the prescribed manner for immunization, type specific neutralizing antibodies will be induced in 90% or more of susceptibles.

INDICATIONS AND USAGE

This vaccine is indicated for use in the prevention of poliomyelitis caused by poliovirus Types 1, 2, and 3.
Infants starting at 6 to 12 weeks of age, *all unimmunized children* and *adolescents* up to age 18 are the usual candidates for routine prophylaxis.
The Immunization Practices Advisory Committee (ACIP) of the Public Health Service states that trivalent oral poliovirus vaccine (OPV) and inactivated poliovirus vaccine (IPV) are both effective in preventing poliomyelitis.
The choice of OPV as the preferred poliovirus vaccine for primary administration to children in the United States has been made by the ACIP, the Committee on Infectious Diseases of the American Academy of Pediatrics, and a special expert committee of the Institute of Medicine, National Academy of Science.[2,3,4] OPV is preferred because it induces intestinal immunity, is simple to administer, is well accepted by patients, results in immunization of some contacts of vaccinated persons, and has a record of having essentially eliminated disease associated with wild poliovirus in this country.[3] OPV is also recommended for control of epidemic poliomyelitis.[2,3]
Past history of clinical poliomyelitis or prior vaccination with IPV in otherwise healthy individuals does not preclude the administration of OPV when otherwise indicated.
Serologic evidence indicates that measles and rubella vaccines or combinations (measles-mumps-rubella vaccine) given simultaneously with trivalent oral poliovirus vaccine can be expected to give adequate antibody response.[5]
Routine poliomyelitis immunization for adults residing in the continental United States is not necessary because of extreme unlikelihood of exposure. However, primary immunization with IPV is recommended whenever feasible for those unimmunized adults subject to *increased risk* of exposure, as by travel to or contact with epidemic or endemic areas and for those employed in hospitals, medical laboratories, clinics, or sanitation facilities. If less than 4 weeks are available before protection is needed, a single dose of TOPV

is recommended, with the remaining doses of vaccine given later if the person remains at increased risk. Immunization with IPV may be indicated for unimmunized parents and those in other special situations where, in the judgment of the attending physician, protection may be needed.[3] (See CONTRAINDICATIONS and ADVERSE REACTIONS.)

Community Programs: Poliovirus Vaccine Live Oral Trivalent ORIMUNE® has been recommended for epidemic control. Within an epidemic area, OPV should be provided for all persons over 6 weeks of age who have not been completely immunized or whose immunization status is unknown, with the exceptions noted under immunodeficiency.[2,3] (See CONTRAINDICATIONS.)

In certain tropical endemic areas, where poliomyelitis has been increasing in recent years, the physician may wish to administer OPV to the infant at birth. Because successful immunization is less likely in newborn infants, a complete series of OPV should follow the neonatal dose beginning when the infants are 2 months old.[2] If the physician chooses to immunize the infant at birth, it may be wise to wait until the child is three days old, and it may be prudent to recommend abstention from breastfeeding for two to three hours before and after oral vaccination to permit the establishment of the vaccine viruses in the gut.[6]

CONTRAINDICATIONS

Under no circumstances should this vaccine be administered parenterally.

Administration of the vaccine should be postponed or avoided in those experiencing any acute illness and in those with any advanced debilitated condition or persistent vomiting or diarrhea.

Other viruses (including poliovirus and other enterovirus) may interfere with the desired response to this vaccine, since their presence in the intestinal tract may intefere with the replication of the attenuated strains of poliovirus in the vaccine.

ORIMUNE *must not* be administered to patients with immune deficiency diseases such as combined immunodeficiency, hypogammaglobulinemia and agammaglobulinemia. Further, *Poliovirus vaccine live oral trivalent* ORIMUNE® *must not* be administered to patients with altered immune states, such as those occurring in thymic abnormalities, leukemia, lymphoma, or generalized malignancy or by lowered resistance from therapy with corticosteroids, alkylating drugs, antimetabolites, or radiation. Because vaccine viruses are excreted by the vaccinee, and may spread to contacts, ORIMUNE should not be used in families with immunodeficient members.[2]

Recipients of the vaccine should avoid close household-type contact with all persons with altered immune status for at least 6 to 8 weeks.

Because of the possibility of immunodeficiency in other children born to a family in which there has been one such case, OPV should not be given to a member of a household in which there is a family history of immunodeficiency until the immune status of the intended recipient and other children in the family is determined to be normal.

IPV is preferred for immunizing all persons in the above described circumstances regarding immunodeficiency.

WARNINGS

Under no circumstances should this vaccine be administered parenterally.

Administration of the vaccine should be postponed or avoided in those experiencing any acute illness and in those with any advanced debilitated condition or persistent vomiting or diarrhea.

Other viruses (including poliovirus and other enterovirus) may interfere with the desired response to this vaccine, since their presence in the intestinal tract may interfere with the replication of the attenuated strains of poliovirus in the vaccine.

PRECAUTIONS

Preliminary data indicate that Immune Globulin (Human) (IG) does not appear to interfere with immunization with OPV.[7] However, until more data are available, it would seem prudent not to administer OPV shortly after Immune Globulin (IG) unless such a procedure is unavoidable, for example, with unexpected travel to or contact with epidemic or endemic areas. If OPV is given with or shortly after IG, the dose probably should be repeated after three months if immunization is still indicated.[8]

The vaccine is not effective in modifying or preventing cases of existing and/or incubating poliomyelitis.

Use in Pregnancy: Pregnancy Category C: Animal reproduction studies have not been conducted with Poliovirus Vaccine Oral Trivalent. It is also not known whether OPV can cause fetal harm when administered to a pregnant woman or can affect reproduction capacity.

Although there is no convincing evidence documenting adverse effects of either OPV or IPV on the developing fetus or pregnant women, it is prudent on theoretical grounds to avoid vaccinating pregnant women. However, if immediate protection against poliomyelitis is needed, OPV is recommended.[3] (See CONTRAINDICATIONS and ADVERSE REACTIONS.)

ADVERSE REACTIONS

Paralytic disease following the ingestion of live poliovirus vaccines has been, on rare occasion, reported in individuals receiving the vaccine, and in persons who were in close contact with vaccinees.[2,3,4,9,10,11,12] The vaccine viruses are shed in the vaccinee's stools for at least six to eight weeks as well as via the pharyngeal route. Most reports of paralytic disease following ingestion of the vaccine or contact with a recent vaccinee are based on epidemiological analysis and temporal association between vaccination or contact and the onset of symptoms. Most authorities believe that a causal relationship exists.[2,10,13,14]

Prior to administration of the vaccine, the attending physician should warn or specifically direct personnel acting under his authority to convey the warnings to the vaccinee, parent, guardian, or other responsible person of the possibility of vaccine-associated paralysis, particularly to susceptible family members and other close personal contacts.[3] The Centers for Disease Control report that during 1972 to 1983, 278.8 million OPV doses were distributed in the United States. During this same period, 87 vaccine-associated cases in apparently immunologically normal individuals were reported. Thirty-two occurred among vaccine recipients (one case per 8.7 million OPV doses distributed), and 55 cases occurred among household and nonhousehold contacts of vaccinees (1 case per 5.1 million doses distributed). Sixteen other vaccine-associated cases have been reported in persons (recipients or contacts) with immune deficiency conditions.[15,16] Because the number of susceptible vaccine recipients or contacts of recipients is not known, the true risk of vaccine-associated poliomyelitis is impossible to determine precisely.[15,16]

When the attenuated vaccine strains are to be introduced into a household with adults who have not been adequately vaccinated or whose immune status cannot be determined, the risk of vaccine-associated paralysis can be reduced by giving these adults three doses of IPV a month apart before the children receive *Poliovirus vaccine live oral trivalent* ORIMUNE®.[3] The children may receive the first dose of ORIMUNE at the same visit that the adult receives the third dose of IPV. The CDC reports that no paralytic reactions to IPV are known to have occurred since the 1955 cluster of poliomyelitis cases caused by vaccine that contained live polioviruses that had escaped inactivation.[3]

The ACIP states: "Because of the overriding importance of ensuring prompt and complete immunization of the child and the extreme rarity of OPV-associated disease in contacts, the Committee recommends the administration of OPV to a child regardless of the poliovirus-vaccine status of adult household contacts. This is the usual practice in the United States. The responsible adult should be informed of the small risk involved. An acceptable alternative, if there is a strong assurance that ultimate, full immunization of the child will not be jeopardized or unduly delayed, is to immunize adults according to the schedule outlined above before giving OPV to the child."[3]

The ACIP has concluded that "Oral polio vaccine remains the vaccine of choice for primary immunization of children."[3]

DOSAGE AND ADMINISTRATION

ORIMUNE is to be administered *orally, under the supervision of a physician. Under no circumstances should this vaccine be administered parenterally.* For convenience, the vaccine is supplied in a disposable pipette containing a single dose of 0.5 ml. The vaccine can be administered directly or mixed with distilled water, tap water free of chlorine, simple syrup NF, or milk. Alternatively, it may be adsorbed on any one of a number of foods such as bread, cake, or cube sugar. Breast feeding does not interfere with successful immunization.[3]

Initial Administration (Primary Series)

Infants: The primary series is three doses. The ACIP and the American Academy of Pediatrics recommends that the three-dose immunization series be started at 6 to 12 weeks of age, commonly with the first DTP inoculation at 2 months of age. The second dose should be given not less than 6 and preferably 8 weeks later, commonly at 4 months of age. The third dose is an integral part of the primary immunization and should be administered 8 to 12 months after the second dose, commonly at 18 months of age. An optional dose of OPV may be given at 6 months of age in areas where poliomyelitis is endemic.[2,3]

Older Children and Adolescents (up to age 18): Two doses, given not less than 6 and preferably 8 weeks apart and the third dose 6 to 12 months after the second dose.[2,3]

Adults: See INDICATIONS and ADVERSE REACTIONS. Where *Poliovirus vaccine live oral trivalent* ORIMUNE® is given to unimmunized adults, the dosage is as indicated for children and adolescents.

Booster Doses—School Entrance: On entering elementary school, all children who have completed the primary series should be given a single follow-up dose of trivalent oral poliovirus vaccine.[2,3] All others should complete the primary series. The fourth supplemental dose is not required in those who received the third primary dose on or after their fourth birthday.[3] The ACIP does not recommend routine booster doses of vaccine on the basis of current information, beyond that given at the time of entering school.[3] It has been shown that over 95% of children studied five years after full immunization with oral poliovirus vaccine had protective antibodies to all three types of poliovirus.[17]

Increased Risk: If an individual who has completed a primary series is subjected to a substantially increased risk by virtue of contact, travel, or occupation, a single dose of OPV has been suggested.[3]

STORAGE

To maintain potency, it is necessary to store this vaccine at a temperature which will maintain ice continuously in a solid state. This vaccine may remain fluid at temperatures above −14°C (+7°F) because of its sorbitol content. If frozen, the vaccine must be completely thawed prior to use. A container of vaccine that has been frozen and then is thawed may be carried through a maximum of 10 freeze-thaw cycles, provided the temperature does not exceed 8°C (46°F) during the periods of thaw, and provided the total cumulative duration of thaw does not exceed 24 hours. If the 24-hour period is exceeded, the vaccine then must be used within 30 days, during which time it must be stored at a temperature between 2°–8°C (36°–46°F).

Color Change: This vaccine contains phenol red as a pH indicator. The usual color of the vaccine is pink, although some containers of vaccine, shipped or stored in dry ice, may exhibit a yellow coloration due to the very low temperature or possible absorption of carbon dioxide. The color of the vaccine prior to use (red-pink-yellow) has no effect on the virus or efficacy of the vaccine.

DISCLAIMER OF REPRESENTATIONS AND WARRANTIES

This vaccine has been produced and tested in accordance with the regulations of the United States Food and Drug Administration for the production of Poliovirus Vaccine, Live, Oral, Trivalent ORIMUNE®. The manufacturer makes no representation or warranty, expressed or implied, with respect to the merchantability or fitness for use of this vaccine other than that the vaccine has been produced in accordance with the standards for its production prescribed by the United States Food and Drug Administration and applicable thereto at the time of its release by the manufacturer. While the use of this preparation and other measures described herein are consistent with accepted standards of medical practice, their use as described cannot be expected necessarily to assure a specific result.

DIRECTIONS FOR USE: Pull off the protective caps and squeeze to expel contents.

HOW SUPPLIED

2084-08-10 (0.5 ml) DISPETTES®
2084-12-50 (0.5 ml) DISPETTES

REFERENCES

1. *Code of Federal Regulations.* 21 CFR §630.17; p 97 (revised Apr 1985).
2. Report of the Committee on the Control of Infectious Diseases. *Amer Acad of Pediatr* 1982; 19:207–211.
3. Recommendations of the Public Health Service Immunization Practices Advisory Committee [ACIP]. *MMWR* 1982; 31:22–34.
4. Nightingale EO: Recommendations for a national policy on poliomyelitis vaccination. *N Engl J Med* 1977; 297:249–253.
5. Recommendations of ACIP Simultaneous Administration of Certain Live Virus Vaccines. *MMWR* 1972; 21:403.
6. Welsh JH, et al: Anti-infective properties of breast milk. *J Pediatr* 1979; 94:1–9.
7. Melnick, JL: Advantages and disadvantages of killed and live poliomyelitis vaccines. *Bull WHO* 1978; 56:21–38.
8. Immunization Practices Advisory Committee [ACIP], general recommendations on immunization. *MMWR* 1980; 29:75–83.
9. Henderson, DA, et al. Paralytic disease associated with oral polio vaccines. *JAMA* 1964; 190:41–48.
10. Morse, LJ, et al. Vaccine-acquired paralytic poliomyelitis in an unvaccinated mother. *JAMA* 1966; 197:1034–1035.
11. Swanson, PD, et al. Poliomyelitis associated with type 2 virus. *JAMA* 1967; 201:771–773.

Continued on next page

The information on each product appearing here is based on labelling effective in August, 1986 and is either the entire official brochure or an accurate condensation therefrom. Information concerning all Lederle products may be obtained from the Professional Services Department, Lederle Laboratories, Pearl River, New York, 10965.

Lederle—Cont.

12. Balduzzi, P, et al. Paralytic poliomyelitis in a contact of a vaccinated child. *New Engl J Med* 1967; 276:796–797.
13. *Neurotropic Diseases Surveillance Annual Poliomyelitis Summary 1971.* Atlanta, Centers for Disease Control, March 1973.
14. Evidence on the safety and efficacy of live poliomyelitis vaccines currently in use, with special reference to type 3 poliovirus, *Bull WHO* 1969; 40:925–945.
15. Paralytic Poliomyelitis—United States 1982 and 1983 *MMWR* 1984; 33:637.
16. Nkowane B: Update on paralytic poliomyelitis. Immunization Practices Advisory Committee Meeting, September 1984.
17. Krugman, RD, et al. Antibody persistence after primary immunization with trivalent oral poliovirus vaccine. *Pediatrics* 1977; 60:80–82.

PATHIBAMATE®-200 ℞

[*path-ĭ-bă-māte*]
tridihexethyl chloride-meprobamate

PATHIBAMATE®-400 ℞

tridihexethyl chloride-meprobamate
Tablets

DESCRIPTION

PATHILON® *tridihexethyl chloride* is a synthetic quaternary ammonium compound. Meprobamate is 2-methyl-2-propyltrimethylene dicarbamate.

Each PATHIBAMATE, 200 mg Tablet contains 200 mg of meprobamate and 25 mg of trihexethyl chloride and the following inactive ingredients: Acacia, Alginic Acid, Carnauba Wax, Cornstarch, Dibasic Calcium Phosphate, Ethyl Cellulose, Gelatin, Kaolin, Magnesium Stearate, Shellac, Stearic Acid, Sucrose, Talc, Yellow 6 and Yellow 10.

Each PATHIBAMATE, 400 mg Tablet contains 400 mg of meprobamate and 25 mg of trihexethyl chloride and the following inactive ingredients: Alginic Acid, Blue 1, Cornstarch, Ethyl Cellulose, Magnesium Stearate, Stearic Acid and Yellow 10.

ACTIONS

PATHIBAMATE tridihexethyl chloride-meprobamate combines tridihexethyl chloride, an anticholinergic agent with meprobamate, a tranquilizing agent.

Tridihexethyl chloride

Tridihexethyl chloride possesses antimuscarinic actions. Gastrointestinal actions include reduction in both gastric secretion and gastrointestinal motility.

Meprobamate

Meprobamate is a carbamate derivative which has been shown in animal studies to have effects at multiple sites in the central nervous system, including the thalamus and limbic system.

INDICATIONS

Based on a review of this drug by the National Academy of Sciences-National Research Council and/or other information, FDA has classified the indications as follows:

Possibly Effective: as adjunctive therapy in peptic ulcer and in the irritable bowel syndrome (irritable colon, spastic colon, mucous colitis, and functional gastrointestinal disorders), especially when accompanied by anxiety or tension. It should be used as an adjunct to other appropriate measures such as proper diet and antacids.

CONTRAINDICATIONS

Tridihexethyl chloride

Allergic or idiosyncratic reactions to tridihexethyl chloride or related compounds; glaucoma; obstructive uropathy (eg, bladder neck obstruction due to prostatic hypertrophy); obstructive disease of the gastrointestinal tract (as in achalasia, paralytic ileus, pyloroduodenal stenosis, etc.); intestinal atony of the elderly or debilitated patient; unstable cardiovascular status in acute hemorrhage; severe ulcerative colitis; toxic megacolon complicating ulcerative colitis; myasthenia gravis.

Meprobamate

Acute intermittent porphyria as well as allergic or idiosyncratic reactions to meprobamate or related compounds such as carisoprodol, mebutamate, tybamate, or carbromal.

WARNINGS

Tridihexethyl chloride

In the presence of a high environment temperature, heat prostration can occur with drug use (fever and heat stroke due to decreased sweating).

Diarrhea may be an early symptom of incomplete intestinal obstruction, especially in patients with ileostomy or colostomy. In this instance treatment with this drug would be inappropriate and possibly harmful.

This drug may produce drowsiness or blurred vision. In this event, the patient should be warned not to engage in activities requiring mental alertness such as operating a motor vehicle or other machinery or perform hazardous work while taking this drug.

Meprobamate

Drug Dependence—Physical dependence, psychological dependence, and abuse have occurred. When chronic intoxication from prolonged use occurs, it usually involves ingestion of greater than recommended doses and is manifested by ataxia, slurred speech, and vertigo. Therefore, careful supervision of dose and amounts prescribed is advised, as well as avoidance of prolonged administration, especially for alcoholics and other patients with a known propensity for taking excessive quantities of drugs. Sudden withdrawal of the drug after prolonged and excessive use may precipitate recurrence of pre-existing symptoms, such as anxiety, anorexia, or insomnia, or withdrawal reactions, such as vomiting, ataxia, tremors, muscle twitching, confusional states, hallucinosis, and, rarely, convulsive seizures. Such seizures are more likely to occur in persons with central nervous system damage or pre-existent or latent convulsive disorders. Onset of withdrawal symptoms occurs usually within 12 to 48 hours after discontinuation of meprobamate; symptoms usually cease within the next 12 to 48 hours.

When excessive dosage has continued for weeks or months, dosage should be reduced gradually over a period of one or two weeks rather than abruptly stopped. Alternatively, a short-acting barbiturate may be substituted, then gradually withdrawn.

Potentially Hazardous Tasks—Patients should be warned that this drug may impair the mental and/ or physical abilities required for the performance of potentially hazardous tasks such as driving a motor vehicle or operating machinery.

Additive Effects—Since the effects of meprobamate and alcohol or meprobamate and other CNS depressants or psychotropic drugs may be additive, appropriate caution should be exercised with patients who take more than one of these agents simultaneously.

***Usage in Pregnancy and Lactation*—An increased risk of congenital malformations associated with the use of minor tranquilizers (meprobamate, chlordiazepoxide, and diazepam) during the first trimester of pregnancy has been suggested in several studies. Because use of these drugs is rarely a matter of urgency, their use during this period should also always be avoided. The possibility that a woman of childbearing potential may be pregnant at the time of institution of therapy should be considered. Patients should be advised that if they become pregnant during therapy or intend to become pregnant, they should communicate with their physicians about the desirability of discontinuing the drug.**

Meprobamate passes the placental barrier. It is present both in umbilical cord blood at or near maternal plasma levels and in breast milk of lactating mothers at concentrations two to four times that of maternal plasma. When use of meprobamate is contemplated in breast-feeding patients, the drug's higher concentrations in breast milk as compared to maternal plasma levels should be considered.

PRECAUTIONS

Tridihexethyl chloride

Use with caution in patients with:

- Autonomic neuropathy.
- Hepatic or renal disease.
- Early evidence of ileus as in peritonitis.
- Ulcerative colitis-large doses may suppress intestinal motility to the point of producing a paralytic ileus and the use of this drug may precipitate or aggravate the serious complication of toxic megacolon.
- Hyperthyroidism, coronary heart disease, congestive heart failure, cardiac arrhythmias, hypertension and non-obstructing prostatic hypertrophy.
- Hiatal hernia associated with reflux esophagitis since anticholinergic drugs may aggravate this condition.
- It should be noted that the use of anticholinergic drugs in the treatment of gastric ulcer may produce a delay in gastric emptying time and may complicate such therapy (antral stasis).
- Do not rely on the use of the drug in the presence of complication of biliary tract disease.
- Investigate any tachycardia before giving anticholinergic (atropine-like) drugs since they may increase the heart rate.
- With overdosage, a curare-like action may occur.

Meprobamate

The lowest effective dose should be administered, particularly to elderly and/or debilitated patients, in order to preclude oversedation.

The possibility of suicide attempts should be considered and the least amount of drug feasible should be dispensed at any one time.

Meprobamate is metabolized in the liver and excreted by the kidney; to avoid its excess accumulation, caution should be exercised in administration to patients with compromised liver or kidney function.

Meprobamate occasionally may precipitate seizures in epileptic patients.

ADVERSE REACTIONS

In evaluating adverse reactions to this combination, consider the possibility of adverse reactions that can occur with either component, as listed below:

Tridihexethyl chloride

Adverse reactions may be physiologic or toxic, depending upon the individual patient's response, and may include xerostomia; urinary hesitancy and retention; tachycardia; palpitations; blurred vision; mydriasis; cycloplegia; increased ocular tension; loss of taste; headaches; nervousness; drowsiness; weakness; dizziness; insomnia; nausea; vomiting; impotence; suppression of lactation; constipation; bloated feeling; severe allergic reaction or drug idiosyncrasies including anaphylaxis; urticaria and other dermal manifestations; decreased sweating; some degree of mental confusion and/or excitement especially in elderly persons.

Meprobamate

Central Nervous System—Drowsiness, ataxia, dizziness, slurred speech, headache, vertigo, weakness, paresthesias, impairment of visual accommodation, euphoria, overstimulation, paradoxical excitement, fast EEG activity.

Gastrointestinal—Nausea, vomiting, diarrhea.

Cardiovascular—Palpitations, tachycardia, various forms of arrhythmia, transient ECG changes, syncope; also, hypotensive crises (including one fatal case).

Allergic or Idiosyncratic—Allergic or idiosyncratic reactions are usually seen within the period of the first to fourth dose in patients having had no previous contact with the drug. Milder reactions are characterized by an itchy, urticarial, or erythematous maculopapular rash which may be generalized or confined to the groin. Other reactions have included leukopenia, acute nonthrombocytopenic purpura, petechiae, ecchymoses, eosinophilia, peripheral edema, adenopathy, fever, fixed drug eruption with cross reaction to carisoprodol, and cross sensitivity between meprobamate/mebutamate and meprobamate/carbromal.

More severe hypersensitivity reactions, rarely reported, include hyperpyrexia, chills, angioneurotic edema, bronchospasm, oliguria, and anuria. Also, anaphylaxis, erythema multiforme, exfoliative dermatitis, stomatitis, proctitis, Stevens-Johnson syndrome, and bullous dermatitis, including one fatal case of the latter following administration of meprobamate in combination with prednisolone.

In case of allergic or idiosyncratic reactions to meprobamate, discontinue the drug and initiate appropriate symptomatic therapy, which may include epinephrine, antihistamines, and in severe cases, corticosteroids. In evaluating possible allergic reactions, also consider allergy to excipients (information on excipients is available to physicians on request).

Hematologic (See also *Allergic or Idiosyncratic.*) —Agranulocytosis and aplastic anemia have been reported, although no causal relationship has been established. These cases rarely were fatal. Rare cases of thrombocytopenic purpura have been reported.

Other—Exacerbation of porphyric symptoms.

DOSAGE AND ADMINISTRATION

The usual adult dose of PATHIBAMATE *tridihexethyl chloride-meprobamate*-400 (meprobamate 400 mg. + tridihexethyl chloride 25 mg.) is one tablet three times a day at mealtimes, and two tablets at bedtime. If a greater anticholinergic effect is desired, the usual adult dose is two PATHIBAMATE *tridihexethyl chloride-meprobamate*-200 (meprobamate 200 mg. + tridihexethyl chloride 25 mg.) tablets three times a day at mealtimes, and two tablets at bedtime. Doses of meprobamate above 2400 mg. daily are not recommended. Not for use in children under age 12.

OVERDOSAGE

Overdosage information on this combination is lacking. However, consider the possibility of signs and symptoms that can occur with either component, as listed below:

Tridihexethyl chloride

Acute overdosage of anticholinergic agents can produce dry mouth, difficulty swallowing, marked thirst; blurred vision, photophobia; flushed, hot, dry skin; rash; hyperthermia; palpitations, tachycardia with weak pulse, elevated blood pressure; urinary urgency with difficulty in micturition; abdominal distention; restlessness, confusion, delirium and other signs suggestive of an acute organic psychosis. Treatment should include removal of remaining drug from stomach after administration of Universal Antidote, and supportive and symptomatic therapy as indicated. Universal Antidote is a mixture of 2 parts activated charcoal, 1 part magnesium oxide, and 1 part tannic acid, given as ½ ounce in a half glass of warm water.

Meprobamate

Suicidal attempts with meprobamate have resulted in drowsiness, lethargy, stupor, ataxia, coma, shock, vasomotor and respiratory collapse. Some suicidal attempts have been fatal.

The following data on meprobamate tablets have been reported in the literature and from other sources. These data are not expected to correlate with each case (considering factors such as individual susceptibility and length of time from ingestion to treatment), but represent the *usual ranges* reported.

Acute simple overdose (meprobamate alone): Death has been reported with ingestion of as little as 12 grams meprobamate and survival with as much as 40 grams.

Blood Levels:

0.5-2.0 mg.% represents the usual blood level range of meprobamate after therapeutic doses. The level may occasionally be as high as 3.0 mg.%.

3-10 mg.% usually corresponds to findings of mild to moderate symptoms of overdosage, such as stupor or light coma.

10-20 mg.% usually corresponds to deeper coma, requiring more intensive treatment. Some fatalities occur.

At levels greater than 20 mg.%, more fatalities than survivals can be expected.

Acute combined overdose (meprobamate with alcohol or other CNS depressants or psychotropic drugs): Since effects can be additive, a history of ingestion of a low dose of meprobamate plus any of these compounds (or of a relatively low blood or tissue level) cannot be used as a prognostic indicator.

In cases where excessive doses have been taken, sleep ensues rapidly; and blood pressure, pulse, and respiratory rates are reduced to basal levels. Any drug remaining in the stomach should be removed and symptomatic therapy given. Should respiration or blood pressure become compromised, respiratory assistance, central nervous system stimulants, and pressor agents should be administered cautiously as indicated. Meprobamate is metabolized in the liver and excreted by the kidney. Diuresis, osmotic (mannitol) diuresis, peritoneal dialysis, and hemodialysis have been used successfully. Careful monitoring of urinary output is necessary and caution should be taken to avoid overhydration. Relapse and death, after initial recovery, have been attributed to incomplete gastric emptying and delayed absorption. Meprobamate can be measured in biological fluids by two methods: colorimetric (Hoffman, A.J. and Ludwig, B.J.: *J Amer Pharm Assn 48:* 740,1959) and gas chromatographic (Douglas, J.F. et al: *Anal Chem 39:* 956, 1967).

HOW SUPPLIED

PATHIBAMATE-400 tablets containing 400 mg meprobamate and 25 mg tridihexethyl chloride are round and pale greenish yellow, engraved with Lederle on one side and P2 on the other, supplied as follows:

NDC 0005-5071-23—bottles of 100
NDC 0005-5071-34—bottles of 1000

PATHIBAMATE-200 tablets containing 200 mg meprobamate and 25 mg tridihexethyl chloride are round, yellow, coated, printed with LL above P1 in red ink on one side, supplied as follows:

NDC 0005-5070-23—bottles of 100
NDC 0005-5070-34—bottles of 1000

Store at Controlled Room Temperature 15°-30°C (59°-86°F).

Shown in Product Identification Section, page 413

PATHILON® ℞

[păth-ĭ-lon]
Tridihexethyl Chloride Tablets

DESCRIPTION

PATHILON® *tridihexethyl chloride* is a synthetic anticholinergic quaternary ammonium compound.

Pathilon tablets contain 25 mg of tridihexethyl chloride and the following inactive ingredients: Cornstarch, Dibasic Calcium Phosphate, Ethylcellulose, Hydroxypropyl Methylcellulose, Magnesium Stearate, Red 7, Sodium Starch Glycolate, Stearic Acid, Titanium Dioxide, and other ingredients.

ACTIONS

PATHILON relieves pain by reducing spasm of the gastrointestinal tract.

INDICATIONS

Effective for use as adjunctive therapy in the treatment of peptic ulcer.

CONTRAINDICATIONS

Glaucoma; obstructive uropathy (for example, bladder neck obstruction due to prostatic hypertrophy); obstructive disease of the gastrointestinal tract (as in achalasia, paralytic ileus, pyloroduodenal stenosis, etc.); intestinal atony of the elderly or debilitated patient; unstable cardiovascular status in acute hemorrhage; severe ulcerative colitis; toxic megacolon complicating ulcerative colitis; myasthenia gravis.

WARNINGS

USE IN PREGNANCY—The use of any drug in pregnancy, lactation, or in women of child-bearing potential requires that the potential benefit of the drug be weighed against its possible hazards to the mother and child. As with all anticholinergic drugs, an inhibiting effect on lactation may occur.

In the presence of a high environmental temperature, heat prostration can occur with drug use (fever and heat stroke due to decreased sweating).

Diarrhea may be an early symptom of incomplete intestinal obstruction, especially in patients with ileostomy or colostomy. In this instance, treatment with this drug would be inappropriate and possibly harmful.

PATHILON may produce drowsiness or blurred vision. In this event, the patient should be warned not to engage in activities requiring mental alertness such as operating a motor vehicle or other machinery or perform hazardous work while taking this drug.

PRECAUTIONS

Use with caution in patients with:

Autonomic neuropathy.
Hepatic or renal disease.
Early evidence of ileus as in peritonitis.
Ulcerative colitis—large doses may suppress intestinal motility to the point of producing a paralytic ileus and the use of this drug may precipitate or aggravate the serious complication of toxic megacolon.
Hyperthyroidism, coronary heart disease, congestive heart failure, cardiac arrhythmias, hypertension and non-obstructing prostatic hypertrophy.
Hiatal hernia associated with reflux esophagitis since anticholinergic drugs may aggravate this condition.

It should be noted that the use of anticholinergic drugs in the treatment of gastric ulcer may produce a delay in gastric emptying time and may complicate such therapy (antral stasis).

Do not rely on the use of the drug in the presence of complication of biliary tract disease.

Investigate any tachycardia before giving anticholinergic (atropine-like) drugs since they may increase the heart rate.

With overdosage, a curare-like action may occur.

ADVERSE REACTIONS

Anticholinergics produce certain effects which may be physiologic or toxic, depending upon the individual patient's response. The physician must delineate these.

Adverse reactions may include: xerostomia; urinary hesitancy and retention; blurred vision and tachycardia; palpitations; mydriasis; dilatation of the pupil; cycloplegia; increased ocular tension; loss of taste; headaches; nervousness; drowsiness; weakness; dizziness; insomnia; nausea; vomiting; impotence; suppression of lactation; constipation; bloated feeling; severe allergic reaction or drug idiosyncrasies including anaphylaxis; urticaria and other dermal manifestation; some degree of mental confusion and/or excitement, especially in elderly persons.

Decreased sweating is another adverse reaction that may occur. It should be noted that adrenergic innervation of the eccrine sweat glands on the palms and soles make complete control of sweating impossible. An end point of complete anhidrosis cannot occur because large doses of drug would be required, and this would produce severe side effects from parasympathetic paralysis.

DOSAGE AND ADMINISTRATION

For effective therapeutic results, in particular with anticholinergic drugs, it is absolutely necessary to titrate dosage against the patient's individual needs and response.

The average oral adult dose is 25 mg to 50 mg of PATHILON® *tridihexethyl chloride,* three to four times per day. The usual bedtime dose has been 50 mg. A few patients are well-controlled on as little as 10 mg three times per day, while some require as much as 75 mg four times per day. The suggested initial dose is 25 mg three times per day before meals and 50 mg at bedtime.

OVERDOSAGE

Tridihexethyl chloride

Acute overdosage of anticholinergic agents can produce dry mouth, difficulty swallowing, marked thirst; blurred vision, photophobia; flushed, hot, dry skin; rash; hyperthermia; palpitations, tachycardia with weak pulse, elevated blood pressure; urinary urgency with difficulty in micturition; abdominal distention; restlessness, confusion, delirium and other signs suggestive of an acute organic psychosis. Treatment should include removal of remaining drug from stomach after administration of Universal Antidote, and supportive and symptomatic therapy as indicated. Universal Antidote is a mixture of 2 parts activated charcoal, 1 part magnesium oxide, and 1 part tannic acid, given as ½ ounce in a half glass of warm water.

HOW SUPPLIED

PATHILON® *tridihexethyl chloride* Tablets, 25 mg—round, convex, pink, film-coated tablets printed P4 one side and LL on the other. NDC-0005-5079-23—Bottles of 100

Store at Controlled Room Temperature 15°-30°C (59°-86°F).

Shown in Product Identification Section, page 413

PERIHEMIN® ℞

[perĭ-hĭm-ĭn]
hematinic Capsules

DESCRIPTION

PERIHEMIN® *hematinic* Capsules for children over 12 and adults.

Each capsule contains: Vitamin B_{12} (as Cyanocobalamin U.S.P.) 5 mcg.; Intrinsic Factor Concentrate 25 mg.; Ferrous Fumarate 168 mg., (Elemental Iron 55 mg.); Folic Acid 0.33 mg.; Ascorbic Acid (C) 50 mg.

Inactive Ingredients:

Benzoin Gum, Blue 1, Cornstarch, Ethyl Cellulose, Ethyl Vanillin, Gelatin, Glycerin, Methylparaben, Mineral Oil, Propylparaben, Red 40, Silica Aerogel, Sucrose, Terpene Resin, Titanium Dioxide, Yellow 6.

ACTIONS

PERIHEMIN *Lederle* is a general hematinic for the oral treatment of the common anemias. It contains the common substances used in the prevention and treatment of anemic conditions produced or aggravated by insufficient food intake.

INDICATIONS

PERIHEMIN is primarily indicated in the hypochromic, microcytic anemias due to insufficient iron intake or absorption. It is also useful in the treatment of macrocytic hyperchromic anemias where an increased intake of oral B_{12} or folic acid is desirable.

WARNINGS

Folic acid alone is improper therapy in the treatment of pernicious anemia and other megaloblastic anemias where vitamin B_{12} is deficient.

PRECAUTIONS

Some patients affected with pernicious anemia may not respond to orally administered Vitamin B_{12} with intrinsic factor concentrate and there is no known way to predict which patients will respond or which patients may cease to respond. Periodic examinations and laboratory studies of pernicious anemia patients are essential and recommended.

Folic acid especially in doses above 0.1 mg. daily may obscure pernicious anemia, in that hematologic remission can occur while neurological manifestations remain progressive.

Overdosage or accidental overingestion of iron-containing compounds may lead to gastrointestinal hemorrhage in children. If symptoms of intolerance develop, the drug should be temporarily or permanently discontinued.

PERIHEMIN *hematinic* preparations should not be relied on to correct the serious folic acid deficiency characterizing sprue or the malabsorption syndromes. In these conditions therapeutic amounts of folic acid should be administered.

ADVERSE REACTIONS

Allergic sensitization has been reported following both oral and parenteral administration of Folic acid.

DOSAGE

PERIHEMIN Capsules for children over 12 and adults.
1 capsule 3 times daily with or after meals.

HOW SUPPLIED

Capsules—Oval shaped, red soft gelatin printed with LL and P7 in blue ink, are supplied as follows: Bottles of 100 NDC 0005-5121-23

Store at Controlled Room Temperature 15°-30°C (59°-86°F).

PERITINIC

[perĭ-tĭn-ik]
Hematinic with Vitamins and Fecal Softener Tablets (Film Coated)

In the prevention of nutritional anemias, certain vitamin deficiencies and iron-deficiency anemias.

RECOMMENDED INTAKE

Adults, 1 or 2 tablets daily.

WARNING

As with any drug, if you are pregnant or nursing a baby, seek the advice of a health professional before using this product.

Keep out of the reach of children.

In case of accidental overdose, seek professional assistance or contact a Poison Control Center immediately.

Continued on next page

The information on each product appearing here is based on labelling effective in August, 1986 and is either the entire official brochure or an accurate condensation therefrom. Information concerning all Lederle products may be obtained from the Professional Services Department, Lederle Laboratories, Pearl River, New York, 10965.

Lederle—Cont.

60 TABLETS
Each tablet contains:

Elemental Iron (as Ferrous Fumarate)	100 mg	
Docusate Sodium USP (DSS) (to counteract the constipating effect of iron)	100 mg	
Vitamin B_1 (as Thiamine Mononitrate)	7.5 mg	(7½ MDR)
Vitamin B_2 (Riboflavin)	7.5 mg	(6¼ MDR)
Vitamin B_6 (Pyridoxine Hydrochloride)	7.5 mg	
Vitamin B_{12} (Cyanocobalamin)	50 mcg	
Vitamin C (Ascorbic Acid)	200 mg	(6⅔ MDR)
Niacinamide	30 mg	(3 MDR)
Folic Acid	0.05 mg	
Pantothenic Acid (as D-Pantothenyl Alcohol)	15 mg	

MDR—Adult Minimum Daily Requirement
Inactive Ingredients: Alginic Acid, Amberlite Resin, Blue 2, Ethyl Cellulose, Hydroxypropyl Methylcellulose, Lactose, Magnesium Stearate, Modified Food Starch, Povidone, Red 40, Silica Gel, Titanium Dioxide, Yellow 6, and other ingredients.
Embossed LL and P8
NDC 0005-5124-19

PIPRACIL® ℞
[*pĭp-ra-sĭl*]
sterile piperacillin sodium
For Intravenous and Intramuscular Use

DESCRIPTION

PIPRACIL® *sterile piperacillin sodium* is a semisynthetic broad spectrum penicillin for parenteral use derived from *d* (-) α-aminobenzylpenicillin. The chemical name of piperacillin sodium is [2*S*-[2α,5α,6β(*S* *)]]-6-[[[[(4-ethyl-2,3-dioxo-1-piperazinyl) carbonyl]amino]phenylacetyl]amino] -3,3-dimethyl-7-oxo-4-thia-1-azabicyclo[3.2.0]heptane-2-carboxylic acid, monosodium salt.

PIPRACIL is a white to off-white hygroscopic cryodesiccated crystalline powder which is readily soluble in water and gives a colorless to pale yellow solution. The pH of the aqueous solution is 5.5 to 7.5. One gram contains 1.85 mEq (42.5 mg) of sodium (Na^+).

CLINICAL PHARMACOLOGY

Intravenous Administration. In healthy adult volunteers, mean serum levels immediately after a two- to three-minute intravenous injection of 2, 4, or 6 grams were 305, 412, and 775 mcg/ml. Serum levels lack dose proportionality. [See table below].

A 30-minute infusion of 6 grams every six hours gave, on the fourth day, a mean peak serum concentration of 420 mcg/ml.

Intramuscular Administration. PIPRACIL is rapidly absorbed after intramuscular injection. In healthy volunteers, the mean peak serum concentration occurs approximately 30 minutes after a single dose of 2 g and is about 36 mcg/ml. The oral administration of 1 g probenecid before injection produces an increase in piperacillin peak serum level of about 30%. The area under the curve (AUC) is increased by approximately 60%.

General. PIPRACIL is not absorbed when given orally. Peak serum concentrations are attained approximately 30 minutes after intramuscular injections and immediately after completion of intravenous injection or infusion. The serum half-life in healthy volunteers ranges from 36 minutes to one hour and 12 minutes. The mean elimination half-life of PIPRACIL in healthy adult volunteers is 54 minutes following administration of 2 grams and 63 minutes following 6 grams. As with other penicillins, PIPRACIL is eliminated primarily by glomerular filtration and tubular secretion; it is excreted rapidly as unchanged drug in high concentrations in the urine. Approximately 60% to 80% of the administered dose is excreted in the urine in the first 24 hours. Piperacillin urine concentrations, determined by microbioassay, were as high as 14,100 mcg/ml following a 6 g intravenous dose and 8,500 mcg/ml following a 4 g intravenous dose. These urine drug concentrations remained well above 1,000 mcg/ml throughout the dosing interval. The elimination half-life is increased two-fold in mild to moderate renal impairment and five- to six-fold in severe impairment.

PIPRACIL binding to human serum proteins is 16%. The drug is widely distributed in human tissues and body fluids, including bone, prostate, and heart, and reaches high concentrations in bile. After a 4 gram bolus, maximum biliary concentrations averaged 3205 mcg/ml. It penetrates into the cerebral spinal fluid in the presence of inflamed meninges. Because PIPRACIL is excreted by the biliary route as well as by the renal route, it can be used safely in appropriate dosage (see DOSAGE AND ADMINISTRATION) in patients with severely restricted kidney function, and can be used effectively in treatment of hepatobiliary infections.

Microbiology:
PIPRACIL is an antibiotic which exerts its bactericidal activity by inhibiting both septum and cell wall synthesis. It is active against a variety of Gram-positive and Gram-negative aerobic and anaerobic bacteria. *In vitro,* piperacillin is active against most strains of clinical isolates of the following microorganisms:

Aerobic and facultatively anaerobic organisms
Gram-negative bacteria
Escherichia coli
Proteus mirabilis
Proteus vulgaris
Morganella morganii (formerly *Proteus morganii)*
Providencia rettgeri (formerly *Proteus rettgeri)*
Serratia species including *S marcescens* and *S liquefaciens*
Klebsiella pneumoniae
Klebsiella species
Enterobacter species including *E aerogenes* and *E cloacae*
Citrobacter species including *C freundii* and *C diversus*
Salmonella species*
Shigella species*
Pseudomonas aeruginosa
Pseudomonas species including *P cepacia,* * *P maltophilia,** and *P fluorescens*
Acinetobacter species (formerly *Mima-Herellea*)
Haemophilus influenzae (non-β-lactamase-producing strains)
Neisseria gonorrhoeae
*Neisseria meningitidis**
Moraxella species*
Yersinia species* (formerly *Pasteurella)*
Gram-positive bacteria
Group D streptococci including
  Enterococci *(Streptococcus faecalis, S faecium)*
  Non-enterococci*
Beta-hemolytic streptococci including
  Group A *Streptococcus (S pyogenes)*
  Group B *Streptococcus (S agalactiae)*
Streptococcus pneumoniae
Streptococcus viridans
Staphylococcus aureus (non-penicillinase-producing)*
Staphylococcus epidermidis (non-penicillinase-producing)*
Anaerobic bacteria
Actinomyces species*
Bacteroides species including
  B fragilis group *(B fragilis, B vulgatus)*
  Non-*B fragilis (B melaninogenicus)*
  *B asaccharolyticus**
Clostridium species including
  C perfringens and *C difficile**
Eubacterium species
Fusobacterium species including
  F nucleatum and *F necrophorum*
Peptococcus species
Peptostreptococcus species
Veillonella species

*Piperacillin has been shown to be active *in vitro* against these organisms; however, clinical efficacy has not yet been established.

In vitro, PIPRACIL® *sterile piperacillin sodium* is inactivated by staphylococcal β-lactamases, and β-lactamases produced by Gram-negative bacteria. However, it is active against β-lactamase-producing gonococci.

Many strains of Gram-negative organisms resistant to certain antibiotics have been found to be susceptible to PIPRACIL.

PIPRACIL has excellent activity against Gram-positive organisms, including enterococci *(S faecalis).* It is active against obligate anaerobes such as *Bacteroides* species and also against *C difficile* (which has been associated with pseudomembranous colitis).

Piperacillin is active against many Gram-negative bacteria including *Enterobacteriaceae, Klebsiella, Serratia, Pseudomonas, E coli, Proteus,* and *Citrobacter,* and in addition it is active against anaerobes and enterococci. *In vitro* tests show PIPRACIL to act synergistically with aminoglycoside antibiotics against most isolates of *P aeruginosa.*

Susceptibility Testing:
The use of 100 mcg piperacillin antibiotic disk with susceptibility test methods which measure zone diameter gives an accurate estimation of susceptibility of organisms to PIPRACIL. The following standard procedure† has been recommended for use with disks for testing antimicrobials.

† NCCLS Approved Standard; M2-A2 (Formerly ASM-2) Performance Standards for Antimicrobic Disk Susceptibility Tests, Second Edition, available from the National Committee of Clinical Laboratory Standards.

With this type of procedure, a report of "susceptible" from the laboratory indicates that the infecting organism is likely to respond to therapy. A report of "intermediate susceptibility" suggests that the organism would be susceptible if high dosage is used or if the infection is confined to tissue and fluids (eg, urine) in which high antibiotic levels are obtained. A report of "resistant" indicates that the infecting organism is not likely to respond to therapy. With the piperacillin disk, a zone of 18 mm or greater indicates susceptibility, zone sizes of 14 mm or less indicate resistance, and zone sizes of 15 to 17 mm indicate intermediate susceptibility.

Haemophilus and *Neisseria* species which give zones of ≥ 29 mm are susceptible; resistant strains give zones of ≤ 28 mm. The above interpretive criteria are based on the use of the standardized procedure. Antibiotic susceptibility testing requires carefully prescribed procedures. Susceptibility tests are biased to a considerable degree when different methods are used.

The standardized procedure requires the use of control organisms. The 100 mcg piperacillin disk should give zone diameters between 24 and 30 mm for *E coli* ATCC No. 25922 and between 25 and 33 mm for *P aeruginosa* ATCC No. 27853.

Dilution methods such as those described in the International Collaborative Study‡ have been used to determine susceptibility of the following organisms to PIPRACIL.

‡*Acta Pathol Microbiol Scand* 1971; (B) Suppl. 217.

Enterobacteriaceae, Pseudomonas species and *Acinetobacter* sp are considered susceptible if the minimal inhibitory concentration (MIC) of piperacillin is no greater than 64 mcg/ml and are considered resistant if the MIC is greater than 128 mcg/ml.

PIPERACILLIN SERUM LEVELS IN ADULTS (mcg/ml) after a two- to three-minute IV INJECTION

DOSE	0	10 min	20 min	30 min	1 hr	1.5 hr	2 hr	3 hr	4 hr	6 hr	8 hr
2	**305** (159–615)	**202** (164–225)	**156** (52–165)	**67** (41–88)	**40** (25–57)	**24** (18–31)	**20** (14–24)	**8** (3–11)	**3** (2–4)	**2** (<0.6–3)	—
4	**412** (389–484)	**344** (315–379)	**295** (269–330)	**117** (98–138)	**93** (78–110)	**60** (50–67)	**36** (26–51)	**20** (17–24)	**8** (7–11)	**4** (3.7–4.1)	**0.9** (0.7–1)
6	**775** (695–849)	**609** (530–670)	**563** (492–630)	**325** (292–363)	**208** (180–239)	**138** (115–175)	**90** (71–113)	**38** (29–53)	**33** (25–44)	**8** (3–19)	**3.2** (<2–6)

PIPERACILLIN SERUM LEVELS IN ADULTS (mcg/ml) after a 30-minute IV INFUSION

DOSE	0	5 min	10 min	15 min	30 min	45 min	1 hr	1.5 hr	2 hr	4 hr	6 hr	7.5 hr
4	**244** (155–298)	**215** (169–247)	**186** (140–209)	**177** (142–213)	**141** (122–156)	**146** (110–265)	**105** (85–133)	**72** (53–105)	**53** (36–69)	**15** (6–24)	**4** (1–9)	**2** (0.5–3)
6	**353** (324–371)	**298** (242–339)	**298** (232–331)	**272** (219–314)	**229** (185–249)	**180** (144–209)	**149** (117–171)	**104** (89–113)	**73** (66–94)	**22** (12–39)	**16** (5–49)	— —

Haemophilus and *Neisseria* species are considered susceptible if the MIC of PIPRACIL is less than or equal to 1 mcg/ml. When anaerobic organisms are isolated from infection sites, it is recommended that other tests such as the modified Broth-Disk Method§ be used to determine the antibiotic susceptibility of these slow-growing organisms.

§ Wilkins TD, Thiel T: *Antimicrob Agents Chemother* 1973; 3:350–356.

INDICATIONS AND USAGE

Therapeutic: PIPRACIL is indicated for the treatment of serious infections caused by susceptible strains of the designated organisms in the conditions as listed below.

Intra-abdominal Infections including hepatobiliary and surgical infections caused by *E coli, P aeruginosa,* enterococci, *Clostridium* sp, anaerobic cocci, and *Bacteroides* sp, including *B fragilis.*

Urinary Tract Infections caused by *E coli, Klebsiella* sp, *P aeruginosa, Proteus* sp, including *P mirabilis* and enterococci.

Gynecologic Infections including endometritis, pelvic inflammatory disease, pelvic cellulitis caused by *Bacteroides* sp, including *B fragilis,* anaerobic cocci, *Neisseria gonorrhoeae,* and enterococci *(Streptococcus faecalis).*

Septicemia including bacteremia caused by *E coli, Klebsiella* sp, *Enterobacter* sp, *Serratia* sp, *P mirabilis, S pneumoniae,* enterococci, *P aeruginosa, Bacteroides* sp, and anaerobic cocci.

Lower Respiratory Tract Infections caused by *E coli, Klebsiella* sp, *Enterobacter* sp, *P aeruginosa, Serratia* sp, *H influenzae, Bacteroides* species, and anaerobic cocci. Although improvement has been noted in patients with cystic fibrosis, lasting bacterial eradication may not necessarily be achieved.

Skin and Skin Structure Infections caused by *E coli, Klebsiella* sp, *Serratia* sp, *Acinetobacter* sp, *Enterobacter* sp, *P aeruginosa,* indole-positive *Proteus* sp, *P mirabilis, Bacteroides* sp, including *B fragilis,* anaerobic cocci, and enterococci.

Bone and Joint Infections caused by *P aeruginosa,* enterococci, *Bacteroides* sp, and anaerobic cocci.

Gonococcal Infections. PIPRACIL has been effective in the treatment of uncomplicated gonococcal urethritis.

PIPRACIL® *sterile piperacillin sodium* has also been shown to be clinically effective for the treatment of infections at various sites caused by *Streptococcus* species including Group A β-hemolytic *Streptococcus* and *S pneumoniae;* however, infections caused by these organisms are ordinarily treated with more narrow spectrum penicillins. Because of its broad spectrum of bactericidal activity against Gram-positive and Gram-negative aerobic and anaerobic bacteria, PIPRACIL is particularly useful for the treatment of mixed infections and presumptive therapy prior to the identification of the causative organisms.

Also, PIPRACIL may be administered as single drug therapy in some situations where normally two antibiotics might be employed.

PIPRACIL has been successfully used with aminoglycosides, especially in patients with impaired host defenses. Both drugs should be used in full therapeutic doses.

Appropriate cultures should be made for susceptibility testing before initiating therapy and therapy adjusted, if appropriate, once the results are known.

Prophylaxis: PIPRACIL is indicated for prophylactic use in surgery including intra-abdominal (gastrointestinal and biliary) procedures, vaginal hysterectomy, abdominal hysterectomy, and cesarean section. Effective prophylactic use depends on the time of administration and PIPRACIL should be given one-half to one hour before the operation so that effective levels can be achieved in the wound prior to the procedure.

The prophylactic use of piperacillin should be stopped within 24 hours, since continuing administration of any antibiotic increases the possibility of adverse reactions, but in the majority of surgical procedures, does not reduce the incidence of subsequent infections. If there are signs of infection, specimens for culture should be obtained for identification of the causative organism so that appropriate therapy can be instituted.

CONTRAINDICATIONS

A history of allergic reactions to any of the penicillins and/or cephalosporins.

WARNINGS

Serious and occasionally fatal hypersensitivity (anaphylactic) reactions have been reported in patients receiving therapy with penicillins. These reactions are more apt to occur in persons with a history of sensitivity to multiple allergens. There have been reports of patients with a history of penicillin hypersensitivity who have experienced severe hypersensitivity reactions when treated with a cephalosporin. Before initiating therapy with PIPRACIL, careful inquiry should be made concerning previous hypersensitivity reactions to penicillins, cephalosporins, and other allergens. If an allergic reaction occurs during therapy with PIPRACIL, the antibiotic should be discontinued. The usual agents (antihistamines, pressor amines, and corticosteroids) should be readily available. SERIOUS ANAPHYLACTOID REACTIONS REQUIRE IMMEDIATE EMERGENCY TREATMENT WITH EPINEPHRINE. OXYGEN AND INTRAVENOUS CORTICOSTEROIDS AND AIRWAY MANAGEMENT INCLUDING INTUBATION SHOULD ALSO BE ADMINISTERED AS NECESSARY.

PRECAUTIONS

General. While piperacillin possesses the characteristic low toxicity of the penicillin group of antibiotics, periodic assessment of organ system functions, including renal, hepatic, and hematopoietic, during prolonged therapy is advisable.

Bleeding manifestations have occurred in some patients receiving β-lactam antibiotics, including piperacillin. These reactions have sometimes been associated with abnormalities of coagulation tests such as clotting time, platelet aggregation and prothrombin time and are more likely to occur in patients with renal failure.

If bleeding manifestations occur, the antibiotic should be discontinued and appropriate therapy instituted.

The possibility of the emergence of resistant organisms which might cause superinfections should be kept in mind, particularly during prolonged treatment. If this occurs, appropriate measures should be taken.

As with other penicillins, patients may experience neuromuscular excitability or convulsions if higher than recommended doses are given intravenously.

PIPRACIL® *sterile piperacillin sodium* is a monosodium salt containing 1.85 milliequivalents of Na^+ per gram. This should be considered when treating patients requiring restricted salt intake. Periodic electrolyte determinations should be made in patients with low potassium reserves, and the possibility of hypokalemia should be kept in mind with patients who have potentially low potassium reserves and who are receiving cytotoxic therapy or diuretics. Antimicrobials used in high doses for short periods to treat gonorrhea may mask or delay the symptoms of incubating syphilis. Therefore, prior to treatment, patients with gonorrhea should also be evaluated for syphilis. Specimens for darkfield examination should be obtained from patients with any suspected primary lesion, and serologic tests should be performed. In all cases where concomitant syphilis is suspected, monthly serological tests should be made for a minimum of four months.

As with other semisynthetic penicillins, PIPRACIL therapy has been associated with an increased incidence of fever and rash in cystic fibrosis patients.

Drug Interactions. The mixing of PIPRACIL with an aminoglycoside *in vitro* can result in substantial inactivation of the aminoglycosides.

Pregnancy—Pregnancy Category B. Although reproduction studies in mice and rats performed at doses up to four times the human dose have shown no evidence of impaired fertility or harm to the fetus, safety of PIPRACIL use in pregnant women has not been determined by adequate and well-controlled studies. Because animal reproduction studies are not always predictive of human response, this drug should be used during pregnancy only if clearly needed. It has been found to cross the placenta in rats.

Nursing Mothers. Caution should be exercised when PIPRACIL is administered to nursing mothers. It is excreted in low concentrations in milk.

Pediatric Use. Dosages for children under the age of 12 have not been established. The safety of PIPRACIL in neonates is not known. In dog neonates dilated renal tubules and peritubular hyalinization occurred following administration of PIPRACIL.

ADVERSE EFFECTS

PIPRACIL is generally well tolerated. The most common adverse reactions have been local in nature, following intravenous or intramuscular injection. The following adverse reactions may occur.

Local Reactions. In clinical trials thrombophlebitis was noted in 4% of patients. Pain, erythema, and/or induration at the injection site occurred in 2% of patients. Less frequent reactions including ecchymosis, deep vein thrombosis and hematomas have also occurred.

Gastrointestinal. Diarrhea and loose stools were noted in 2% of patients. Other less frequent reactions included vomiting, nausea, increases in liver enzymes (LDH, SGOT, SGPT), hyperbilirubinemia, cholestatic hepatitis, bloody diarrhea and, rarely, pseudomembranous colitis.

Hypersensitivity Reactions. Anaphylactoid Reactions (see WARNINGS). Rash was noted in 1% of patients. Other less frequent findings included pruritus, vesicular eruptions, positive Coombs tests.

Renal. Elevations of creatinine or BUN and, rarely, interstitial nephritis.

Central Nervous System. Headache, dizziness, fatigue.

Hemic and Lymphatic. Reversible leukopenia, neutropenia, thrombocytopenia and/or eosinophilia have been reported. As with other β-lactam antibiotics, reversible leukopenia (neutropenia) is more apt to occur in patients receiving prolonged therapy at high dosages or in association with drugs known to cause this reaction.

Serum Electrolytes. Individuals with liver disease, or individuals receiving cytotoxic therapy or diuretics, were reported rarely to demonstrate a decrease in serum potassium concentrations with high doses of piperacillin.

Skeletal. Rarely, prolonged muscle relaxation.

Other. Superinfection, including candidiasis. Hemorrhagic manifestations.

DOSAGE AND ADMINISTRATION

PIPRACIL ® *sterile piperacillin sodium* may be administered by the intramuscular route or intravenously or given in a three-to five-minute intravenous injection. The usual dosage of PIPRACIL for serious infections is 3 to 4 grams given every four to six hours as a 20-to 30-minute infusion. For serious infections, the intravenous route of administration should be used.

PIPRACIL should not be mixed with an aminoglycoside in a syringe or infusion bottle since this can result in inactivation of the aminoglycoside.

The maximum daily dose for adults is usually 24 g/day, although higher doses have been used.

Intramuscular injections should be limited to 2 g per injection site. This route of administration has been used primarily in the treatment of patients with uncomplicated gonorrhea and urinary tract infections.

[See tables on next page].

Infants and Children. Dosages in infants and children under 12 years of age have not been established.

PRODUCT RECONSTITUTION/DOSAGE PREPARATION

Diluents for Reconstitution

Sterile Water for Injection
†Bacteriostatic Water for Injection
Sodium Chloride Injection
†Bacteriostatic Sodium Chloride Injection
Dextrose 5% in Water
Dextrose 5% and 0.9% Sodium Chloride
‡Lidocaine HCl 0.5–1% (without epinephrine)

†Either Parabens or Benzyl Alcohol
‡For Intramuscular Use Only. Lidocaine is contraindicated in patients with a known history of hypersensitivity to local anesthetics of the amide type.

Intravenous Solutions

Dextrose 5% in Water
0.9% Sodium Chloride
Dextrose 5% and 0.9% Sodium Chloride
Lactated Ringer's Injection
Dextran 6% in 0.9% Sodium Chloride

Intravenous Admixtures

Normal Saline [+ KCl 40 mEq]
5% Dextrose in Water/ [+ KCl 40 mEq]
5% Dextrose/Normal Saline [+ KCl 40 mEq]
Ringer's Injection [+ KCl 40 mEq]
Lactated Ringer's Injection, [+ KCl 40 mEq]

Intravenous Administration

Reconstitution Directions. Reconstitute each gram of PIPRACIL with at least 5 ml of a suitable diluent (except Lidocaine HCl 0.5–1% without epinephrine) listed above. Shake well until dissolved. Reconstituted solution may be further diluted to the desired volume (eg, 50 or 100 ml) in the above listed intravenous solutions and admixtures.

Reconstitution Directions for PHARMACY BULK VIAL. Reconstitute the 40 gram vial with 172 ml of a suitable diluent (except Lidocaine HCl 0.5–1% without epinephrine) listed above to achieve a concentration of 1 gram per 5 ml.

Directions for Administration

Intermittent IV Infusion —Infuse diluted solution over period of about 30 minutes. During infusion it is desirable to discontinue the primary intravenous solution.

Intravenous Injection (Bolus) — Reconstituted solution should be injected slowly over a three-to five-minute period to help avoid vein irritation.

Intramuscular Administration

Reconstitution Directions. Reconstitute each gram of PIPRACIL with 2 ml of a suitable diluent listed above to achieve a concentration of 1 g per 2.5 ml. Shake well until dissolved.

Directions for Administration

When indicated by clinical and bacteriological findings, intramuscular administration of 6 to 8 grams daily of PIPRACIL, in divided doses, may be utilized for initiation of

Continued on next page

The information on each product appearing here is based on labelling effective in August, 1986 and is either the entire official brochure or an accurate condensation therefrom. Information concerning all Lederle products may be obtained from the Professional Services Department, Lederle Laboratories, Pearl River, New York, 10965.

Lederle—Cont.

therapy. In addition, intramuscular administration of the drug may be considered for maintenance therapy after clinical and bacteriologic improvement has been obtained with intravenous piperacillin sodium treatment.
Intramuscular administration should not exceed 2 grams per injection at any one site.
The preferred site is the upper outer quadrant of the buttock (ie, gluteus maximus).
The deltoid area should be used only if well-developed, and then only with caution to avoid radial nerve injury. Intramuscular injections should not be made into the lower or mid-third of the upper arm.

Stability of PIPRACIL Following Reconstitution
PIPRACIL is stable in both glass and plastic containers when reconstituted with recommended diluents and when diluted with the intravenous solutions and intravenous admixtures indicated above.
Extensive stability studies have demonstrated chemical stability (potency, pH, and clarity) through 24 hours at room temperature, up to one week refrigerated, and up to one month frozen (−10° to −20°C). (Note: The 40 g Pharmacy Bulk Vial should not be frozen after reconstitution.) Appropriate consideration of aseptic technique and individual hospital policy, however, may recommend discarding unused portions after storage for 48 hours under refrigeration and recommend discarding after 24 hours storage at room temperature.
Additional stability data available upon request.

HOW SUPPLIED

PIPRACIL® *sterile cryodesiccated piperacillin sodium* is available in vials containing sterile freeze-dried piperacillin sodium powder equivalent to 2, 3, 4, and 40 grams of piperacillin. One gram of piperacillin (as a monosodium salt) contains 1.85 mEq (42.5 mg) of sodium.

Product Numbers:
2 gram/vial—NDC 0206-3879-14
2 gram/vial—10 per box—NDC 0206-3879-16
3 gram/vial—NDC 0206-3882-06
3 gram/vial—25 per box—NDC 0206-3882-21
4 gram/vial—NDC 0206-3880-18
4 gram/vial—25 per box—NDC 0206-3880-22
2 gram infusion bottle—10 per box—NDC 0206-3879-47
3 gram infusion bottle—10 per box—NDC 0206-3882-65
4 gram infusion bottle—10 per box—NDC 0206-3880-66
40 gram Pharmacy Bulk Vial—NDC 0206-3877-60
This product should be stored at controlled room temperature 15°-30°C (59°-86°F).
3 gm vial (25s)
MILITARY NSN 6505-01-130-4451
3 gm infusion bottle (10s)
MILITARY NSN 6505-01-137-0039
4 gm vial (25s)
MILITARY NSN 6505-01-130-4452
2 gm (10s)
VA NSN 6505-01-148-5040
3 gm vial (25s)
VA NSN 6505-01-130-4451
3 gm infusion bottle (10s)
VA NSN 6505-01-137-0039
4 gm vial (25s)
VA NSN 6505-01-130-4452
LEDERLE PIPERACILLIN, INC.

Carolina, Puerto Rico 00630
Shown in Product Identification Section, page 413

PIPRACIL DOSAGE RECOMMENDATIONS

Type of Infections	Usual Total Daily Dosage	Frequency of Administration
Serious infections such as septicemia, nosocomial pneumonia, intra-abdominal infections, aerobic and anaerobic gynecologic infections, and skin and soft-tissue infections	12–18 g IV (200–300 mg/kg)	Every four to six hours
Complicated urinary tract infections	8–16 g IV (125–200 mg/kg)	Every six to eight hours
Uncomplicated urinary tract infections and most community-acquired pneumonia	6–8 g IM or IV (100–125 mg/kg)	Every six to 12 hours
Uncomplicated gonorrhea infections	2 g IM*	Single dose

*One gram of probenecid given orally one-half hour prior to injection.

The average duration of PIPRACIL treatment is from seven to ten days, except in the treatment of gynecologic infections, in which it is from three to ten days; the duration should be guided by the patient's clinical and bacteriological progress. For most acute infections, treatment should be continued for at least 48 to 72 hours after the patient becomes asymptomatic. Antibiotic therapy for Group A β-hemolytic streptococcal infections should be maintained for at least ten days to reduce the risk of rheumatic fever or glomerulonephritis.
When PIPRACIL is given concurrently with aminoglycosides, both drugs should be used in full therapeutic doses.

Renal Impairment — Dosage in Renal Impairment

Creatinine Clearance ml/min	Urinary Tract Infection (uncomplicated)	Urinary Tract Infection (complicated)	Serious Systemic Infection
>40	No dosage adjustment necessary		
20–40	No dosage adjustment necessary	9 g/day (3 g every 8 h)	12 g/day (4 g every 8 h)
<20	6 g/day (3 g every 12 h)	6 g/day (3 g every 12 h)	8 g/day (4 g every 12 h)

For patients on hemodialysis the maximum daily dose is 6 g/day (2 g every 8 h). In addition, because hemodialysis removes 30%–50% of piperacillin in four hours, 1g additional dose should be administered following each dialysis period.
For patients with renal failure and hepatic insufficiency, measurement of serum levels of PIPRACIL® *sterile piperacillin sodium* will provide additional guidance for adjusting dosage.

Prophylaxis

INDICATION	1st Dose	2nd Dose	3rd Dose
Intra-abdominal Surgery	2 g IV just prior to surgery	2 g during surgery	2 g every 6 h postop for no more than 24 h
Vaginal Hysterectomy	2 g IV just prior to surgery	2 g 6 h after 1st dose	2 g 12 h after 1st dose
Cesarean Section	2 g IV after cord is clamped	2 g 4 h after 1st dose	2 g 8 h after 1st dose
Abdominal Hysterectomy	2 g IV just prior to surgery	2 g on return to recovery room	2 g after 6 h

PNU-IMUNE® 23 ℞

[*new-ĭ-mune*]
Pneumococcal Vaccine, Polyvalent

DESCRIPTION

Pneumococcal Vaccine Polyvalent, PNU-IMUNE® 23 is a sterile liquid vaccine for intramuscular or subcutaneous use, consisting of a mixture of purified capsular polysaccharides from 23 pneumococcal types:
[See table on next page].
It is indicated for immunization against infections caused by the 23 most prevalent types of pneumococci responsible for approximately 90% of serious pneumococcal disease in the United States and the rest of the world.[1-5] Each of the pneumococcal polysaccharide types is produced separately by Lederle Laboratories to give a high degree of purity. After an individual pneumococcal type is grown, the polysaccharide is separated from the cell and purified by a series of steps including ethanol fractionation. The resultant 23 purified polysaccharides are combined in amounts to give 25 micrograms of each type per dose (0.5 ml) in the final vaccine. Thimerosal (a mercury derivative) at a final concentration of 0.01% is added as a preservative.

CLINICAL PHARMACOLOGY

Pneumococci are the etiologic agents for a significant number of the pneumonias occurring throughout the world. The emergence of strains of pneumococci with increased resistance to one or more of the common antibiotics[4] and recent isolations of pneumococci with multiple-antibiotic resistance[6] emphasize the importance of vaccine prophylaxis against pneumococcal disease.
Based on projections from limited observations in the United States, it has been estimated that 150,000 to 570,000 cases of pneumococcal pneumonia may occur annually. The overall case fatality rate ranges from 5% to 7%.[2] As many as 60% of all deaths among patients with pneumococcal bacteremia treated with penicillin or tetracycline occur within five days of onset of the illness.[6] Thus vaccination offers an effective means for further reducing the mortality and morbidity of this disease. Populations at high risk are the elderly,[7-8] individuals with immune deficiencies, asplenics and patients with splenic deficiencies including sickle cell anemia and other severe hemoglobinopathies, alcoholics and patients with the following diseases: chronic respiratory illness, the nephrotic syndrome, multiple myeloma, Hodgkin's disease and cirrhosis.[2] Antibiotics have only been partially effective in reducing the mortality of pneumococcal pneumonia. The pneumococcus is also a major infectious agent in meningitis[9] and otitis media. Other illnesses caused by pneumococci include sinus infection, arthritis and conjunctivitis. The annual incidence of pneumococcal meningitis is approximately 1.5 to 2.5 per 100,000 population. One-half of the cases occur in children in whom the fatality rate is about 40%.[1,8]
The polysaccharide capsules of pneumococci endow these organisms with resistance to the phagocytic action of polymorphonuclear leukocytes and monocytes. The opsonin activity of type-specific antibody facilitates their destruction in the body by complement-mediated activities.
The protection induced by the vaccine is of long duration but its extent is not yet known. Elevated antibody levels have been shown to persist for at least 5 years after immunization with other pneumococcal vaccines.[10]
Children under 2 years of age do not respond adequately to some of the important polysaccharide types.[12]
PNU-IMUNE® 23 *pneumococcal vaccine, polyvalent* has not been studied in children under 2 years of age. Recipients of polyvalent vaccines acquired less nasopharyngeal carriage of pneumococcal types included in the vaccine.[2,11]
A repeat (booster) injection of pneumococcal vaccine *should not be given* to previously vaccinated subjects regardless of the time interval from the previous injection. Available data indicate that revaccination may result in more frequent and severe local reactions at the site of injection, especially in persons who have retained high antibody titers. Such adverse reactions have occurred with booster doses given after long intervals from the initial vaccination. There is also evidence that booster doses do not result in increased antibody titers.[2]
In clinical studies with PNU-IMUNE 23, more than 90% of all adults showed a twofold or greater increase in geometric

mean antibody titer for each vaccine capsular type.[13]
Patients over the age of 2 years with anatomical or functional asplenia and otherwise intact lymphoid function responded to PNU-IMUNE 23 and other comparable pneumococcal vaccines with a serological conversion comparable to that observed in healthy individuals of the same age.[14]
Polyvalent pneumococcal vaccines, from other sources, were shown to be effective in preventing pneumococcal disease. Controlled field trials in South Africa involving 12,000 gold miners have shown a 6-valent and a 13-valent pneumococcal vaccine to be 78.5% effective in preventing type-specific pneumococcal pneumonia and 82.3% effective in preventing pneumococcal bacteremia with the types in the vaccine.[15] In a preliminary study of an 8-valent polysaccharide vaccine in a group consisting of 77 patients with sickle cell disease and 19 asplenic persons, there were no pneumococcal infections in the immunized patients within two years of immunization. There were eight cases of pneumococcal infection in 106 unimmunized, age-matched patients with sickle cell disease. Antibody response of the asplenic patients was comparable to normal controls.[16]
In a study carried out by Austrian, et al,[15] with 13-valent pneumococcal vaccines prepared for the National Institute of Allergy and Infectious Disease, the reduction in pneumonias caused by the capsular types in the vaccines was 79%. Reduction in type-specific pneumococcal bacteremia was 82%.
In a double-blind study of a 14-valent pneumococcal vaccine carried out in Papua, New Guinea, pneumococcal infection was less in the vaccinated group by 84%. Mortality from pneumonia was less by 44%.[17]
Pneumococcal polysaccharide vaccine was found to significantly reduce clinical cases of pneumococcal otitis media in a six-month post-vaccination period of observation. In a controlled study there were 455 children ages two to six years with a history of prior episodes of otitis media. Two hundred seventy-four of these patients received 14-valent pneumococcal vaccine. Overall, there was a 73% reduction in frequency of cases caused by serotypes in the pneumococcal vaccine, other than type 6 for which no protection was found. These Finnish otitis studies revealed a marked fall-off protective efficacy later than six months after immunization.[18]

INDICATIONS AND USAGE

PNU-IMUNE® 23 *pneumococcal vaccine, polyvalent* is indicated for immunization against pneumococcal disease caused by those pneumococcal types included in the vaccine.
Use in preventing pneumococcal otitis media. Children 2 years or older who, in the judgment of the physician, are clearly in need of protection due to a risk of developing otitis media. (See CLINICAL PHARMACOLOGY for clinical data.)
Use in Selected Individuals. Persons over 2 years of age as follows: (1) who have anatomical asplenia or who have splenic dysfunction due to sickle cell disease or other causes; (2) persons with chronic illnesses in which there is an increased risk of pneumococcal disease, such as diabetes mellitus, functional impairment of cardiorespiratory, hepatic and renal systems; (3) persons 50 years of age or older, and (4) patients about to undergo immunosuppressive therapy.[2] It is reasonable to assume that patients on immunosuppressive therapy are at increased risk of pneumococcal disease. When possible, vaccination should be given at least ten days and preferably more than 14 days prior to initiation of such immunosuppressive therapy. Impairment of antibody response in Hodgkin's disease patients receiving radiotherapy, chemotherapy or both, was demonstrated.[20]
Use in Communities. Persons over 2 years of age as follows: (1) closed groups such as those in residential schools, nursing homes and other institutions; (2) groups epidemiologically at risk in the community when there is a generalized outbreak in the population due to a single pneumococcal type included in the vaccine, and (3) patients at high risk of influenza complications, particularly pneumonia.[11]
Simultaneous administration of pneumococcal polysaccharide vaccine and whole-virus influenza vaccine has been found to give satisfactory antibody response without increasing the incidence of side effects. Although not yet studied, simultaneous administration of the pneumococcal vaccine and split-virus influenza vaccine may also be expected to yield satisfactory results.[2,19]

CONTRAINDICATIONS

Children below 2 years of age. While pneumococcal polysaccharide vaccines have been shown to be highly immunogenic and effective in adults, their usefulness in children is still being evaluated. Although some pneumococcal polysaccharides have been reported to be immunogenic from the age of 3 months (particularly serotype 3), serum antibody responses to most of the polysaccharides present in the 14-valent vaccine have been shown to be poor in children under 2 years of age.[22]
Hypersensitivity. Known hypersensitivity to any component of the vaccine including hypersensitivity to thimerosal. Remedial measures for anaphylactoid reactions, including epinephrine injection (1:1000), must be available for immediate use.

Nomenclature	Pneumococcal Types																						
Danish	1	2	3	4	5	6B	7F	8	9N	9V	10A	11A	12F	14	15B	17F	18C	19A	19F	20	22F	23F	33F
U.S.	1	2	3	4	5	26	51	8	9	68	34	43	12	14	54	17	56	57	19	20	22	23	70

Patients on Immunosuppressive Therapy. Immunization of patients should not be attempted less than ten days prior to or during treatment with immunosuppressive drugs or irradiation. Administration of vaccine to patients on such therapy for Hodgkin's disease resulted in reduction of preexisting antibody levels.[20]
Previously vaccinated subjects. The use of PNU-IMUNE® 23 *pneumococcal vaccine, polyvalent* is contraindicated in persons who have been immunized with any polyvalent pneumococcal vaccine.

WARNINGS

PNU-IMUNE 23 is not an effective agent for prophylaxis against pneumococcal disease caused by types not present in the vaccine. The vaccine may not be effective in patients undergoing treatment causing therapeutic suppression of the immune-response system.
Patients who have received extensive chemotherapy and/or splenectomy for the treatment of Hodgkin's disease have been shown to have an impaired serum antibody response to pneumococcal vaccine.[20]
A repeat (booster) injection of pneumococcal vaccine *should not be given* to previously vaccinated subjects regardless of the time interval from the previous injection. Available data indicate that revaccination may result in more frequent and severe local reactions at the site of injection, especially in persons who have retained high antibody titers. Such adverse reactions have occurred with booster doses given after long intervals from the initial vaccination. There is also evidence that booster doses do not result in increased antibody titers.[2]
Intradermal administration may cause severe local reactions.

PRECAUTIONS

General. The vaccine should be injected subcutaneously or intramuscularly. *Do not inject intravenously.*
In the presence of any febrile respiratory illness or other active infection, the vaccine should not be used.
The parenteral administration of any biological product should be surrounded by every known precaution for the prevention and arrest of allergic and other untoward reactions. (See CONTRAINDICATIONS.)
When administering this vaccine, a separate heat-sterilized syringe and needle or a new disposable equivalent should be used for each patient to prevent transmission of hepatitis B (homologous serum hepatitis) or other infectious agents.
Patients who have had episodes of pneumococcal pneumonia or other pneumococcal infection may have high levels of preexisting pneumococcal antibodies which may result in increased reactions to PNU-IMUNE 23, mostly local, but occasionally systemic.[21] Caution should be exercised if such patients are considered for vaccination with PNU-IMUNE 23.
Pregnancy Category C: Animal reproduction studies have not been conducted with PNU-IMUNE 23. It is also not known whether PNU-IMUNE 23 can cause fetal harm when administered to a pregnant woman or can affect reproduction capacity. PNU-IMUNE 23 is not recommended for use in pregnant women.
It is not known whether the drug is excreted in human milk. Because many drugs are excreted in human milk, caution should be exercised when PNU-IMUNE® 23 *pneumococcal vaccine, polyvalent* is administered to a nursing woman.
Pediatric Use. PNU-IMUNE 23 has not been studied in children under 2 years of age. While pneumococcal polysaccharide vaccines have been shown to be highly immunogenic and effective in adults, their usefulness in children is still being evaluated. Although some pneumococcal polysaccharides have been reported to be immunogenic from the age of 3 months (particularly serotype 3), serum antibody responses to most of the polysaccharides present in the 14-valent vaccine have been shown to be poor in children under two years of age.[22]

ADVERSE REACTIONS

PNU-IMUNE 23 is associated with a relatively low incidence of adverse reactions. The adverse reactivity observed in clinical studies was not serious and of short duration.
In a study of 32 individuals who received PNU-IMUNE 23, 23 (72%) experienced a local reaction characterized by local soreness at the injection site within three days after vaccination.
Low grade fever (less than 100°F) and mild myalgia occur occasionally with PNU-IMUNE 23 and are usually confined to the 24-hour period following vaccination. Rash and arthralgia have been reported rarely.
Although rare, fever over 102° and marked local swelling has been reported with pneumococcal polysaccharide vaccine.
Patients with otherwise stabilized idiopathic thrombocytopenic purpura have, on rare occasions, experienced a relapse in their thrombocytopenia, occurring two to 14 days after vaccination, and lasting up to 2 weeks.[23]
Reactions of greater severity, or extent are unusual. Rarely, anaphylactoid reactions have been reported.
A repeat (booster) injection of pneumococcal vaccine *should not be given* to previously vaccinated subjects regardless of the time interval from the previous injection. Available data indicate that revaccination may result in more frequent and severe local reactions at the site of injection, especially in persons who have retained high antibody titers. Such adverse reactions have occurred with booster doses given after long intervals from the initial vaccination. There is also evidence that booster doses do not result in increased antibody titers.[2]
Temporal association of neurological disorders have been reported following parenteral injections of biological products.

DOSAGE AND ADMINISTRATION

Do not inject intravenously. The immunization schedule consists of a single 0.5 ml dose given subcutaneously or intramuscularly.
Parenteral drug products should be inspected visually for particulate matter and discoloration prior to administration, whenever solution and container permit.
PNU-IMUNE 23 *must not* be administered to persons who have been immunized previously with any polyvalent pneumococcal vaccine.
A repeat (booster) injection of pneumococcal vaccine *should not be given* to previously vaccinated subjects regardless of the time interval from the previous injection. Available data indicate that revaccination may result in more frequent and severe local reactions at the site of injection, especially in persons who have retained high antibody titers. Such adverse reactions have occurred with booster doses given after long intervals from the initial vaccination. There is also evidence that booster doses do not result in increased antibody titers.[2]

Directions for Use of the LEDERJECT® Disposable Syringe.

1. Twist the plunger rod clockwise to be sure that rod is secure to rubber plunger base.
2. Hold needle shield in place with index finger and thumb of one hand while with the other thumb exert light pressure on plunger rod until the plunger base has been freed and demonstrates slight movement when pressure is applied.
3. Grasp the rubber needle shield at its base; twist and pull to remove.
4. Pull back plunger rod slowly and carefully to insure smooth plunger operation.
5. Expel the air bubble.

Storage and Use: Store syringes and unopened or opened vials at 2°–8°C (35°–46°F).
The vaccine is used directly as supplied. No dilution or reconstitution is necessary. Thimerosal (a mercury derivative) is present in the vaccine as a preservative at a final concentration of 0.01%. Discard unused vials beyond expiration date.

HOW SUPPLIED

PNU-IMUNE® 23 *pneumococcal vaccine, polyvalent* is supplied as follows:
NDC 0005-2309-31 5 dose vial, for use with syringe only.
NDC 0005-2309-33 5 × One dose LEDERJECT® Disposable Syringes.

References:

1. Austrian, R "Surveillance of Pneumococcal Infection for Field Trials of Polyvalent Vaccines." Annual Contract Prog. Report to the Nat. Inst. of Allerg. and Inf. Dis. (1975) Updated to Dec. 1977, personal communication.
2. Recommendation of the Immunization Practices Advisory Committee, Morb. Mort. Weekly Report 30 (33):410–419 August 28, 1981.
3. Lund, E "Distribution of Pneumococcal Types at Different Times and Different Areas" in *Bayer Symposium III. Bacterial Infections.* "Changes in Their Causative Agents, Trends and Possible Basis." M Finland, W Marget and K Bartman (eds.) Berlin, Springer-Verlag:49, (1971).
4. Mufson, MA, Kruss, DM, Wasil, RE and Metzger, WI "Capsular Types and Outcome of Bacteremic Pneumococcal Disease in the Antibiotic Era." Arch. Int. Med., 134:505, (1974).

Continued on next page

The information on each product appearing here is based on labelling effective in August, 1986 and is either the entire official brochure or an accurate condensation therefrom. Information concerning all Lederle products may be obtained from the Professional Services Department, Lederle Laboratories, Pearl River, New York, 10965.

Lederle—Cont.

5. Robbins, JB, Austrian, R, Lee, CJ, Rastogi, SC, Schiffman, G, Henrichsen, J, Mäkelä, PH, Broome, CV, Facklam, RR, Tiesjema, RH, and Parke, JC, Jr. "Consideration for Formulating the Second Generation Pneumococcal Capsule Polysaccharide Vaccine with Emphasis on the Cross-Reactive Types Within Groups." J. Infec. Dis. 148(6):1136–1159, 1983.
6. Epidemiologic Notes and Reports, Multiple-Antibiotic Resistance of Pneumococci—South Africa Morb. Mort. Weekly Report 26 (35):285–286 September 2, 1977.
7. Austrian, R, and Gold, J "Pneumococcal Bacteremia with Especial Reference to Bacteremic Pneumococcal Pneumonia." Ann. Int. Med., 60:759, (1964).
8. Valenti, WM, Jenzer, M and Bently, W "Type-Specific Pneumococcal Respiratory Disease in the Elderly and Chronically Ill." Am. Rev. Resp. Dis., 117:233, (1978).
9. Fraser, DW, Geil, CC, and Feldman, RA "Meningitis in Bernalillo County, New Mexico. A Comparison with Three Other American Populations." Am. J. Epidemiol., 100:29, (1974).
10. Mufson, MA, Krause, HE and Schiffman, G "Long Term Persistence of Antibody Following Immunization with Pneumococcal Polysaccharide Vaccine" Proc. Soc. Exptl. Biol. & Med. 173(2):270–275, 1983.
11. Mufson, MA and Krause, HE "Role of Antibody in Prevention of Acquisition of Pneumococcal Carriage Among Vaccinees." Clin. Res., 24:577A, (1976).
12. Report of the Committee on Infectious Diseases. Pneumococcal Infections. Amer. Acad. of Ped. 19th Edition: 205–206, 1982.
13. Data on File, Lederle Laboratories.
14. Sullivan, JL, Ochs, HD, Schiffman, G, Hammerschlag, MR, Miser, J, Vichinsky, E, and Wedgwood, RJ "Immune Response After Splenectomy." Lancet, 178, (1978).
15. Austrian, R, Douglas, RM, Schiffman, G, Coetzee, AM, Koornhof, HJ, Hayden-Smith, S and Reid, RDW "Prevention of Pneumococcal Pneumonia by Vaccination." Trans. Asc. Am. Physicians, 89:184, (1976).
16. Amman, AJ, Addiego, K, Wara, DW, Lubin, B, Smith, WB and Mentzer, WC "Polyvalent Pneumococcal-Polysaccharide Immunization of Patients with Sickle-Cell Anemia and Patients with Splenectomy." New Eng. J. Med., 297:897, (1977).
17. Riley, ID, Andrews, M, Howard, R, Tarr, PI, Pfeiffer, M, Challands, P and Jennison, G "Immunization with Polyvalent Pneumococcal Vaccine." Lancet, 1338, (1977).
18. Makela, PH, Sibakov, M, Herva, E, Henrichsen, J, Luotonen, J, Timonen, M, Lienonen, M, Koskela, M, Pukander, J, Pontynen, S, Gronroos, P, Karma, P Pneumococcal Vaccine and Otitis Media. Lancet 547-551, 1980.
19. DeStefano, F, Goodman, RA, Noble, GR, McClary, GD, Smith, SJ and Broome, CV "Simultaneous Administration of Influenza and Pneumococcal Vaccines" JAMA 247:2551–2554, (1982).
20. Siber, GR, Weitzman, SA, Aisenberg, AC, Weinstein, HJ, and Schiffman, G "Impaired Antibody Response to Pneumococcal Vaccine After Treatment for Hodgkin's Disease." New Eng. J. Med., 299:442, (1978).
21. Pönkä, A and Leinonen, M "Adverse Reactions to Polyvalent Pneumococcal Vaccine." Scand. J. Infect. Dis., 14:67–71, (1982).
22. Douglas, RM, Paton, JC, Duncan, SJ, and Hansman, DJ "Antibody Response to Pneumococcal Vaccination in Children Younger than Five Years of Age." J. Infec. Dis., (1):13-137, (1983).
23. Kelton, JG "Vaccination-Associated Relapse of Immune Thrombocytopenia." J. Am. Med. Assoc., 245(4):369-371, 1981).

LEDERLE LABORATORIES DIVISION
American Cyanamid Company, Pearl River, NY 10965

PRONEMIA® ℞
[*prō-nēēm-ēa*]
hematinic
Capsules

COMPOSITION
Each capsule contains: Vitamin B_{12} (as Cobalamin Concentrate) 15 mcg, Intrinsic Factor Concentrate 75 mg, Ferrous Fumarate 350 mg (Elemental Iron 115 mg), Ascorbic Acid (Vitamin C) 150 mg, and Folic Acid 1 mg and the following inactive ingredients: Acacia, Benzoin Gum, Blue 1, Cornstarch, Dibasic Calcium Phosphate, Ethylcellulose, Ethyl Vanillin, Gelatin, Glycerin, Methylparaben, Mineral Oil, Propylene Glycol, Propylparaben, Red 40, Silica Aerogel, Sucrose, Terpene Resin, Titanium Dioxide, Yellow 6.

INDICATIONS
Indicated for treatment and maintenance in common anemias, including iron-deficiency anemia, megaloblastic anemias of pregnancy, and those of nutritional origin. All of the other means that are recognized as suited to the treatment of these anemias should also be employed. If cases prove resistant to this form of therapy, further exploration of the etiology and additional therapeutic measures should be instituted.

WARNINGS
Folic Acid alone is improper therapy in the treatment of pernicious anemia and other megaloblastic anemias where vitamin B_{12} is deficient.

PRECAUTIONS
Some patients affected with pernicious anemia may not respond to orally administered Vitamin B_{12} with intrinsic factor concentrate and there is no known way to predict which patients will respond or which patients may cease to respond. Periodic examinations and laboratory studies of pernicious anemia patients are essential and recommended.
If any symptoms of intolerance occur, the drug should be temporarily or permanently discontinued.
Folic Acid in doses above 0.1 mg daily may obscure pernicious anemia, in that hematologic remission can occur while neurological manifestations remain progressive.

ADVERSE REACTIONS
Allergic sensitization has been reported following both oral and parenteral administration of Folic Acid.

ADMINISTRATION AND DOSAGE
One capsule daily with or after meals to treat and maintain the average uncomplicated case of anemia.

HOW SUPPLIED
Capsules—maroon, soft gelatin capsules printed with LL and P9 in blue ink are supplied as follows:
NDC 0005-5150-23—bottles of 100
Store at Controlled Room Temperature 15°-30°C (59°-86°F).

SPARTUS®
[*spar-tus*]
High Potency Vitamins & Minerals plus Electrolytes

(See PDR For Nonprescription Drugs)

SPARTUS® + Iron
[*spar-tus*]
High Potency Vitamins & Minerals plus Electrolytes

(See PDR For Nonprescription Drugs)

STRESSCAPS®
[*strĕs-caps*]
Stress Formula B+C Vitamins

(See PDR For Nonprescription Drugs)

STRESSTABS® 600, Advanced Formula
[*strĕs-tabs*]
High Potency
Stress Formula Vitamins

(See PDR For Nonprescription Drugs)

STRESSTABS® 600 with IRON,
[*strĕs-tabs*]
Advanced Formula
High Potency
Stress Formula Vitamins

(See PDR For Nonprescription Drugs)

STRESSTABS® 600 with ZINC,
[*strĕs-tabs*]
Advanced Formula
High Potency
Stress Formula Vitamins

(See PDR For Nonprescription Drugs)

TETANUS AND DIPHTHERIA TOXOIDS, ADSORBED PUROGENATED® ℞

HOW SUPPLIED
5 ml vial (10 immunizations): NDC 0005-1875-31
10 × 0.5 ml LEDERJECT® Disposable Syringe NDC 0005-1875-47
COMPLETE INFORMATION FURNISHED IN THE PACKAGE.

TETANUS TOXOID, ADSORBED PUROGENATED® ℞

HOW SUPPLIED
5 ml vial (10 immunizations);
10 x 5 ml NDC 0005-1938-31 and 10 x 0.5 ml LEDERJECT® Disposable Syringe. NDC 0005-1938-47
COMPLETE INFORMATION FURNISHED IN THE PACKAGE.

TETANUS TOXOID PUROGENATED® ℞
(Tetanus Toxoid fluid)

HOW SUPPLIED
7.5 ml. vial (15 immunizations);
10 x 0.5 ml. NDC 0005-1942-33 and 10 x 0.5 ml. LEDERJECT® Disposable Syringe. NDC 0005-1942-47
COMPLETE INFORMATION FURNISHED IN THE PACKAGE.

THIOTEPA ℞
[*thīō-tĕpa*]
N,N',N''-triethylenethiophosphoramide parenteral
Sterile

THIOTEPA Lederle is a polyfunctional alkylating agent used in the chemotherapy of certain neoplastic diseases.

DESCRIPTION
Thiotepa is the ethylenimine-type compound N, N', N''-Triethylenethiophosphoramide and is available in powder form in vials which contain a sterile mixture of 15 mg Thiotepa, 80 mg NaCl, and 50 mg $NaHCO_3$. Thiotepa has also been known as TESPA and TSPA and is not the same as TEPA. Thiotepa is stable in alkaline medium and unstable in acid medium. When reconstituted with Sterile Water for Injection, the resulting solution has a pH of approximately 7.6.

ACTION
Thiotepa is a cytotoxic agent of the polyfunctional alkylating type (more than one reactive ethylenimine group) related chemically and pharmacologically to nitrogen mustard. Its radiomimetic action is believed to occur through the release of ethylenimine radicals which, like irradiation, disrupt the bonds of DNA. One of the principal bond disruptions is initiated by alkylation of guanine at the N-7 position, which severs the linkage between the purine base and the sugar and liberates alkylated guanines. On the basis of tissue concentration studies, it is reported that Thiotepa has no differential affinity for neoplasms. Most of the drug appears to be excreted unchanged in the urine.

INDICATIONS
Thiotepa has been tried with varying results in the palliation of a wide variety of neoplastic diseases. However, the most consistent results have been seen in the following tumors:

1. Adenocarcinoma of the breast.
2. Adenocarcinoma of the ovary.
3. For controlling intracavitary effusions secondary to diffuse or localized neoplastic disease of various serosal cavities.
4. For the treatment of superficial papillary carcinoma of the urinary bladder.

While now largely superseded by other treatments, Thiotepa has been effective against other lymphomas, such as lymphosarcoma and Hodgkin's disease.

CONTRAINDICATIONS
Therapy is probably contraindicated in cases of existing hepatic, renal, or bone-marrow damage. However, if the need overweighs the risk in such patients, Thiotepa may be used in low dosage, and accompanied by hepatic, renal, and hemopoietic function tests.
Thiotepa is contraindicated in patients with a known hypersensitivity (allergy) to this preparation.

WARNINGS
The administration of Thiotepa to pregnant women is not recommended except in cases where the benefit to be gained outweighs the risk of teratogenicity involved.
Thiotepa is highly toxic to the hematopoietic system. A rapidly falling white blood cell or platelet count indicates the necessity for discontinuing or reducing the dosage of Thiotepa. Weekly blood and platelet counts are recommended during therapy and for at least three weeks after therapy has been discontinued.
Thiotepa is a polyfunctional alkylating agent, capable of cross-linking the DNA within a cell and changing its nature. The replication of the cell is, therefore, altered, and Thiotepa may be described as mutagenic. An *in vitro* study has shown that it causes chromosomal aberrations of the chromatid type and that the frequency of induced aberrations increases with the age of the subject.

Like all alkylating agents, Thiotepa is carcinogenic. Carcinogenicity is shown most clearly in mouse studies, but there is strong circumstantial evidence of carcinogenicity in man.

PRECAUTIONS

The serious complication of excessive Thiotepa therapy, or sensitivity to the effects of Thiotepa, is bone-marrow depression. If proper precautions are not observed, Thiotepa may cause leukopenia, thrombocytopenia, and anemia. Death from septicemia and hemorrhage has occurred as a direct result of hematopoietic depression by Thiotepa.

It is not advisable to combine, simultaneously or sequentially, cancer chemotherapeutic agents or a cancer chemotherapeutic agent and a therapeutic modality having the same mechanism of action. Therefore, Thiotepa combined with other alkylating agents such as nitrogen mustard or cyclophosphamide or Thiotepa combined with irradiation would serve to intensify toxicity rather than to enhance therapeutic response. If these agents must follow each other, it is important that recovery from the first agent, as indicated by white blood cell count, be complete before therapy with the second agent is instituted.

The most reliable guide to Thiotepa toxicity is the white blood cell count. If this falls to 3000 or less, the dose should be discontinued. Another good index of Thiotepa toxicity is the platelet count; if this falls to 150,000, therapy should be discontinued. Red blood cell count is a less accurate indicator of Thiotepa toxicity.

Other drugs which are known to produce bone-marrow depression should be avoided.

There is no known antidote for overdosage with Thiotepa. Transfusions of whole blood or platelets or leukocytes have proved beneficial to the patient in combating hematopoietic toxicity.

ADVERSE REACTIONS

Apart from its effect on the blood-forming elements, Thiotepa may cause other adverse reactions. These include pain at the site of injection, nausea, vomiting, anorexia, dizziness, headache, amenorrhea, and interference with spermatogenesis.

Febrile reaction and weeping from a subcutaneous lesion may occur as the result of breakdown of tumor tissue.

Allergic reactions are rare, but hives and skin rash have been noted occasionally. One case of alopecia has been reported. In addition, a patient who had received Thiotepa and other anticancer agents experienced prolonged apnea after succinylcholine was administered prior to surgery. It was theorized that this was caused by decrease of pseudocholinesterase activity caused by the anticancer drugs.

DOSAGE

Parenteral routes of administration are most reliable since absorption of Thiotepa from the gastrointestinal tract is variable.

Since Thiotepa is nonvesicant, intravenous doses may be given directly and rapidly without need for slow drip or large volumes of diluent. Some physicians prefer to give Thiotepa directly into the tumor mass. This may be effected transrectally, transvaginally, or intracerebrally. The technique is discussed in the appropriate section which follows. For the control of malignant effusions, Thiotepa is instilled directly into the cavity involved.

Dosage must be carefully individualized. A slow response to Thiotepa may be deceptive and may occasion unwarranted frequency of administration with subsequent signs of toxicity. After maximum benefit is obtained by initial therapy, it is necessary to continue patient on maintenance therapy (one to four week intervals). In order to continue optimal effect, maintenance doses should be no more frequent than weekly in order to preserve correlation between dose and blood counts.

Initial and Maintenance Doses: Initially the higher dose in the given range is commonly administered. The maintenance dose should be adjusted weekly on the basis of pretreatment control blood counts and subsequent blood counts.

Intravenous Administration: Thiotepa may be given by rapid intravenous administration in doses of 0.3–0.4 mg/kg. Doses should be given at one to four week intervals.

For conversion of mg/kg of body weight to mg/M^2 of body surface or the reverse, a ratio of 1:30 is given as a guideline. The conversion factor varies between 1:20 and 1:40 depending on age and body build.

Intratumor Administration: Thiotepa in initial doses of 0.6–0.8 mg/kg may be injected directly into a tumor by means of a 22-gauge needle. A small amount of local anesthetic is injected first; then the syringe is removed and the Thiotepa solution is injected through the same needle. The drug is diluted in Sterile Water for Injection, 10 mg per 1 ml. Maintenance doses at one to four week intervals range from 0.07 mg/kg to 0.8 mg/kg depending on the condition of the patient.

Intracavitary Administration: The dosage recommended is 0.6–0.8 mg/kg. Administration is usually effected through the same tubing which is used to remove the fluid from the cavity involved.

Intravesical Administration: Patients with papillary carcinoma of the bladder are dehydrated for 8 to 12 hours prior to treatment. Then 60 mg of Thiotepa in 30–60 ml of Sterile Water for Injection is instilled into the bladder by catheter. For maximum effect, the solution should be retained for two hours. If the patient finds it impossible to retain 60 ml for two hours, the dose may be given in a volume of 30 ml. If desired, the patient may be positioned every 15 minutes for maximum area contact. The usual course of treatment is once a week for 4 weeks. The course may be repeated if necessary, but second and third courses must be given with caution since bone-marrow depression may be increased. Deaths have occurred after intravesical administration, caused by bone-marrow depression from systemically absorbed drug.

Preparation of Solution: The powder should be reconstituted preferably in Sterile Water for Injection. The amount of diluent most often used is 1.5 ml. resulting in a drug concentration of 5 mg in each 0.5 ml of solution. Larger volumes are usually employed for intracavity use, intravenous drip, or perfusion therapy. The 1.5 ml reconstituted preparation may be added to larger volumes of other diluents: Sodium Chloride Injection USP, Dextrose Injection USP, Dextrose and Sodium Chloride Injection USP, Ringer's Injection USP, or Lactated Ringer's Injection USP. Reconstituted solutions should be clear to slightly opaque but solutions that are grossly opaque or precipitated should not be used.

Since the original powder form contains 15 mg Thiotepa, 80 mg NaCl, 50 mg $NaHCO_3$, the addition of Sterile Water for Injection produces an isotonic solution. The addition of other diluents may result in hypertonic solutions, which may cause mild to moderate discomfort on injection.

For local use into single or multiple sites, Thiotepa may be mixed with procaine HCl 2%, epinephrine HCl 1:1000, or both.

Procedures for proper handling and disposal of anti-cancer drugs should be considered. Several guidelines on this subject have been published.[1–6] There is no general agreement that all of the procedures recommended in the guidelines are necessary or appropriate.

Whether in its original powder form or in reconstituted solution, Thiotepa must be stored in the refrigerator at 2°–8° C. (35°–46° F.).

Reconstituted solutions may be kept for five days in a refrigerator without substantial loss of potency.

HOW SUPPLIED

15 mg vials, sterile, for parenteral use—NDC 0005-4650-91.
Military Depot:
15 mg vial
NSN 6505-01-047-3872

Shown in Product Identification Section, page 413

REFERENCES

1. Recommendations for the Safe Handling of Parenteral Antineoplastic Drugs. NIH Publication No. 83-2621. For sale by the Superintendent of Documents, U.S. Government Printing Office, Washington, D.C. 20402.
2. AMA Council Report. Guidelines for Handling Parenteral Antineoplastics. JAMA, March 15, 1985.
3. National Study Commission on Cytotoxic Exposure—Recommendations for Handling Cytotoxic Agents. Available from Louis P. Jeffrey, Sc. D., Director of Pharmacy Services, Rhode Island Hospital, 593 Eddy Street, Providence, Rhode Island 02902.
4. Clinical Oncological Society of Australia: Guidelines and recommendations for safe handling of antineoplastic agents. Med J Australia 1983, 1:426–428.
5. Jones, R.B., et al. Safe handling of chemotherapeutic agents: A report from the Mount Sinai Medical Center. Ca—A Cancer Journal for Clinicians Sept/Oct 1983, 258–263.
6. American Society of Hospital Pharmacists technical assistance bulletin on handling cytotoxic drugs in hospitals. Am J Hosp Pharm 1985, 42:131–137.

Lederle Laboratories Division
American Cyanamid Company
Pearl River, N.Y. 10965

TriHEMIC® 600 ℞

[*trī-hĕm-ĭk*]
hematinic
Tablets

DESCRIPTION

Each tablet contains:

Vitamin C (Ascorbic Acid)	600 mg
Vitamin B_{12} (Cyanocobalamin)	25 mcg
Intrinsic Factor Concentrate	75 mg
Folic Acid	1 mg
Vitamin E (*dl*-Alpha Tocopheryl Acetate)	30 Int. Units
Elemental Iron (as 350 mg of Ferrous Fumarate)	115 mg
Docusate Sodium USP (DSS)	50 mg

Inactive Ingredients
Blue 2, Cornstarch, Ethylcellulose, Ethyl Vanillin, Hydrolyzed Protein, Hydroxypropyl Methylcellulose, Lactose, Magnesium Stearate, Polacrilin, Povidone, Red 3, Silica Gel, Sodium Benzoate, Sorbic Acid, Titanium Dioxide, Yellow 6, and other ingredients.

ACTIONS

TriHEMIC® 600 *hematinic* is a preparation containing those ingredients essential to normal erythropoiesis, plus a stool softener to counteract the constipating effects of iron.

INDICATIONS

TriHEMIC 600 is a multiphasic preparation for use in the treatment of most megaloblastic, macrocytic and iron-deficiency anemias, in the anemias of pregnancy, in those anemias occurring in a variety of malabsorption syndromes, and those of nutritional origin. It is a useful adjuvant in patients in whom erythropoiesis is suppressed due to severe infections, malignancies or to the toxic effects of certain chemotherapeutic agents. A deficiency of Vitamin E may increase the fragility of red blood cells, with resultant enhanced hemolysis. Vitamin C is present to aid in the absorption of iron.

WARNINGS

Folic Acid alone is improper therapy in the treatment of pernicious anemia and other megaloblastic anemias where Vitamin B_{12} is deficient.

PRECAUTIONS

Some patients affected with pernicious anemia may not respond to orally administered Vitamin B_{12} with intrinsic factor concentrate and there is no known way to predict which patients will respond or which patients may cease to respond. Periodic examinations and laboratory studies of pernicious anemia patients are essential and recommended.

If any symptoms of intolerance occur, the drug should be temporarily or permanently discontinued.

Folic Acid in doses above 0.1 mg daily may obscure pernicious anemia, in that hematologic remission can occur while neurological manifestations remain progressive.

ADVERSE REACTIONS

Gastrointestinal intolerance may develop and be manifest by nausea, vomiting, diarrhea, or abdominal pain. Skin rashes of various types may occur. Such reactions can necessitate temporary or permanent changes in dosage or usage.

Allergic sensitization has been reported following both oral and parenteral administration of Folic Acid.

DOSAGE AND ADMINISTRATION

One tablet daily. Adjustment of dosage is dependent on patient response and the physician's clinical judgment.

HOW SUPPLIED

TriHEMIC® 600 *hematinic* Tablets are capsule-shaped, red, film coated, engraved T1 on one side and LL on the other, are supplied as follows:

NDC 0005-4590-13—Bottles of 30
NDC 0005-4590-31—Bottles of 500

Store at Controlled Room Temperature 15°–30° C (59°–86° F).

Shown in Product Identification Section, page 414

TRI-IMMUNOL® ℞

[*trī-ĭm-u-nōl*]
diphtheria and tetanus toxoids and pertussis vaccine adsorbed

DESCRIPTION

Diphtheria and Tetanus Toxoids and Pertussis Vaccine Adsorbed, TRI-IMMUNOL®, Lederle, is a combination of *Purogenated* Diphtheria Toxoid Aluminum Phosphate-Adsorbed, *Purogenated* Tetanus Toxoid Aluminum Phosphate-Adsorbed, and Pertussis Vaccine.

The diphtheria toxin is produced according to the method of Mueller and Miller and is detoxified by use of formaldehyde. The tetanus toxin is produced by the method of Mueller and Miller and is detoxified by the use of formaldehyde. The toxoids are refined by the Pillemer alcohol fractionation method and are diluted with a solution containing potassium phosphate monobasic, sodium phosphate dibasic, glycine, and thimerosal (mercury derivative) as a preservative. Pertussis Vaccine is prepared by growing Phase 1 *B pertussis* in a modified Cohen-Wheeler broth containing acid hydrolysate of casein. The *B pertussis* culture is harvested, inactivated, and then suspended in a solution containing potas-

Continued on next page

The information on each product appearing here is based on labelling effective in August, 1986 and is either the entire official brochure or an accurate condensation therefrom. Information concerning all Lederle products may be obtained from the Professional Services Department, Lederle Laboratories, Pearl River, New York, 10965.

Lederle—Cont.

sium phosphate monobasic, sodium phosphate dibasic, sodium chloride, and thimerosal (mercury derivative) as a preservative and is then combined with the refined Diphtheria and Tetanus Toxoids in physiological saline (NaCl) diluent containing thimerosal (mercury derivative) as a preservative. The final concentration of thimerosal (mercury derivative) in the combined vaccine is 1:10,000. The aluminum content of the final product does not exceed 0.80 mg per 0.5 ml dose.

The total immunizing dose contains 12 units of pertussis vaccine.

The primary immunization against diphtheria, tetanus, and pertussis consists of four 0.5 ml doses when administered as recommended.[1,2]

CLINICAL PHARMACOLOGY

Simultaneous immunization against diphtheria, tetanus, and pertussis during infancy and childhood has been a routine practice in the United States since the late 1940s. It has played a major role in markedly reducing the incidence of cases and deaths from each of these diseases.

Diphtheria is primarily a localized and generalized intoxication caused by diphtherial toxin, an extracellular protein metabolite of toxinogenic strains of *Corynebacterium diphtheriae.* While the incidence of diphtheria has decreased from about 20 cases per 100,000 population before the general use of diphtheria toxoid[1,3] to about 56 cases reported between 1976 and 1981, the ratio of fatalities to attack rate has remained constant at about 5% to 10%. The highest case fatality rates are in the very young and the elderly. Diphtheria toxoid induces antitoxin. Following adequate immunization with diphtheria toxoid, it is thought that protection lasts at least ten years.[1] It significantly reduces both the risk of developing diphtheria and the severity of clinical illness. It does not, however, eliminate carriage of *C diphtheria* in the pharynx or on the skin.[1] A serum level ≥0.01 toxin neutralization units/ml is generally considered protective.[4]

Tetanus is an intoxication manifested primarily by neuromuscular dysfunction, caused by a potent exotoxin elaborated by *Clostridium tetani.* The incidence of tetanus has dropped dramatically with the routine use of tetanus toxoid, remaining relatively constant over the last decade at about 100 cases reported annually. Spores of *C tetani* are ubiquitous, and there is essentially no natural immunity to tetanus toxin. Thus, universal primary immunization with tetanus toxoid with subsequent maintenance of adequate antitoxin levels by means of timed boosters is necessary to protect all age groups.[1] Tetanus toxoid is highly effective, with a failure rate in fully immunized persons of less than 4 per 100 million.[5] Protective levels of serum antitoxin (≥0.01 toxin neutralization units/ml)[4] are achieved and persist for at least 10 years after full immunization.[1]

Pertussis is a disease of the respiratory tract caused by *Bordetella pertussis.* This Gram-negative coccobacillus produces an array of biologically active components that escape from the site of infection and produce systemic effects, including an endotoxin-related febrile response, attenuation of the host's febrile and inflammatory responses, lymphocytosis, leukocytosis, effects on glucose homeostasis, and possible neurotoxicity. The role of each of the different components in the pathogenesis of and immunity to pertussis is not well understood.

Pertussis is a highly communicable disease, which, unique for a bacterial disease, has an attack rate in unimmunized populations of over 90%.[3] As a result of immunization with pertussis vaccine, the number of reported cases and associated mortality has declined from about 120,000 cases and 1,100 deaths in 1950[6] to an annual average of about 2,300 cases and 10 fatalities over the last 10 years.[7] Accurate data do not exist, as bacteriological confirmation of pertussis can be obtained in less than half of the cases. Most reported illnesses from *B pertussis* occur in infants and young children; two thirds of reported deaths occur in children less than one year old. Older children and adults, in whom classic signs are often absent, may go undiagnosed and serve as reservoirs of disease.[1]

Evidence of the efficacy of pertussis vaccine can be provided by the recent British experience, where a reduction in the number of immunized individuals from 79% in 1973, to 31% in 1978 resulted in an epidemic of 102,500 pertussis cases and 36 deaths between late 1977 and 1980, and 1,440 cases per week reported during the winter of 1981–82. A similar situation occurred in Japan.[8]

Because the incidence and severity of pertussis decrease with age, routine pertussis immunization is not recommended for persons 7 years of age or older.[1]

INDICATION AND USAGE

Diphtheria and Tetanus Toxoids and Pertussis Vaccine Adsorbed is indicated for active immunization of infants and children through 6 years of age against diphtheria, tetanus, and pertussis.[1,2]

CONTRAINDICATIONS

IMMUNIZATION SHOULD BE DEFERRED DURING THE COURSE OF ANY ACUTE ILLNESS. THE OCCURRENCE OF ANY TYPE OF NEUROLOGICAL SYMPTOMS OR SIGNS, INCLUDING ONE OR MORE CONVULSIONS (SEIZURES) FOLLOWING ADMINISTRATION OF THIS PRODUCT IS A CONTRAINDICATION TO FURTHER USE. USE OF THIS PRODUCT IS ALSO CONTRAINDICATED IF THE CHILD HAS A PERSONAL OR FAMILY HISTORY OF CENTRAL NERVOUS SYSTEM DISORDERS.

THE PRESENCE OF ANY EVOLVING OR CHANGING DISORDER AFFECTING THE CENTRAL NERVOUS SYSTEM IS A CONTRAINDICATION TO ADMINISTRATION OF DTP REGARDLESS OF WHETHER THE SUSPECTED NEUROLOGICAL DISORDER IS ASSOCIATED WITH OCCURRENCE OF SEIZURE ACTIVITY OF ANY TYPE.

The Committee on Infectious Diseases of the American Academy of Pediatrics recommends that pertussis vaccine should be withheld when a previous dose has been followed by convulsion, encephalitis, focal neurological signs or collapse. Moreover, infants who experience excessive somnolence, excessive screaming (persistent crying or screaming for three or more hours' duration), or temperature more than 105°F (40.5°C), should not resume additional doses of the vaccine.[2]

The Immunization Practices Advisory Committee (ACIP) of the U.S. Public Health Service recommends that hypersensitivity to vaccine components, presence of an evolving neurologic disorder, or a history of a severe reaction (usually within 48 hours) following a previous dose all remain definitive contraindications to the receipt of pertussis vaccine. Severe reactions include collapse or shock, persistent screaming episode, temperature 40.5° C (105° F) or greater, convulsion(s) with or without accompanying fever, severe alterations of consciousness, generalized and/or local neurologic signs, or systemic allergic reactions.[9]

Immunosuppressive therapy, including irradiation, corticosteroids, antimetabolites, alkylating agents, and cytotoxic agents may result in aberrant responses to active immunization procedures. Administration should be deferred in individuals receiving such therapy.

The clinical judgement of the attending physician should prevail at all times.

Elective immunization of patients over the age of 6 months should be deferred during an outbreak of poliomyelitis.

WARNING

THIS PRODUCT IS NOT RECOMMENDED FOR IMMUNIZING PERSONS AFTER THEIR SEVENTH BIRTHDAY. DO NOT ATTEMPT ROUTINE IMMUNIZATION IF THE CHILD HAS A PERSONAL OR FAMILY HISTORY OF CENTRAL NERVOUS SYSTEM DISORDERS. SHOULD ANY SYMPTOMATOLOGY RELATED TO NEUROLOGICAL DISORDERS DEVELOP FOLLOWING ADMINISTRATION, DO NOT ATTEMPT FURTHER ADMINISTRATION OF PERTUSSIS VACCINE. CONVULSION, ENCEPHALITIS, FOCAL NEUROLOGIC SIGNS, COLLAPSE, SHOCK, EXCESSIVE SCREAMING (PERSISTENT CRYING OR SCREAMING FOR THREE OR MORE HOURS DURATION), EXCESSIVE SOMNOLENCE, SEVERE ALTERATION OF CONSCIOUSNESS, SYSTEMIC ALLERGIC REACTIONS OR TEMPERATURE MORE THAN 105° F (40.5° C) ARE CONTRAINDICATIONS FOR ANY FURTHER USE OF PERTUSSIS VACCINE.

If such disorders are found, the infants or children should be given diphtheria and tetanus toxoids (DT) instead of DTP. If DT is used, three doses at least 4 weeks apart, followed by a fourth dose 6 to 12 months later, are recommended for infants. For children 1 year of age or older, two doses of DT at least 4 weeks apart followed by a third dose 6 to 12 months later, are recommended.[9]

The occurrence of sudden-infant-death syndrome (SIDS) has been reported following administration of DTP.[10,11,12] A causal relationship between DTP immunization and the syndrome has not been established.[13,14]

Prior to administration of this vaccine, health care personnel should inform the parent, guardian, or other responsible adult of the benefits and risks to the child of DTP vaccine. For recent information about the estimated range of risks of severe reactions following DTP administration, consult references 1, 15, 16, 17, 18, and 21.

DTP should not be given to infants or children with thrombocytopenia or any coagulation disorder that would contraindicate intramuscular injection unless the potential benefit clearly outweighs the risk of administration.

If the vaccine is used in persons receiving immunosuppressive therapy, the expected antigenic response may not be obtained.

Special care should be taken so the injection is not made into a blood vessel.

PRECAUTIONS

A. **General:**

1. This product should be used for the age group between 2 months and the 7th birthday.
2. A separate sterile syringe and needle or a sterile disposable unit should be used for each individual patient to prevent transmission of hepatitis or other infectious agents from one person to another.
3. *Since this product contains both a bacterial suspension and an adjuvant, shake vigorously before withdrawing each dose from multiple dose vials.*
4. Before the injection of any biological, the physician should take all precautions known for prevention of allergic or any other side reactions. This should include: A review of the patient's history regarding possible sensitivity; the ready availability of epinephrine 1:1000 and other appropriate agents used for control of immediate allergic reactions; and a knowledge of the recent literature pertaining to use of the biological concerned, including the nature of side effects and adverse reactions that may follow its use.

B. **Information for Patient:**

1. Prior to administration of any dose of DTP, the parent or guardian should be asked about the recent health status of the infant or child to be injected.
2. WHEN AN INFANT OR CHILD IS RETURNED FOR THE NEXT DOSE IN THE SERIES, THE PARENT SHOULD BE QUESTIONED CONCERNING OCCURRENCE OF ANY SYMPTOM AND/OR SIGNS OF AN ADVERSE REACTION AFTER THE PREVIOUS DOSE (SEE CONTRAINDICATIONS; ADVERSE REACTIONS).

ADVERSE REACTIONS

Local reactions, manifested by erythema and induration with or without tenderness, are common after administration of DTP. Such local reactions are usually self-limited and require no therapy. A nodule may be palpable at the injection site for a few weeks.

Abscess formation at the site of injection has been reported.[15,16,17] Cervical lymphadenopathy has been reported following DTP injections into the arm.[18]

Mild to moderate temperature elevations frequently follow DTP administration and are often accompanied by fretfulness, drowsiness, vomiting, and anorexia.[15,16,19] Approximately 50% of DTP recipients will develop temperature elevations > 38° C (100.4° F) after one or more doses of the series; approximately 6% > 39° C (102.2° F); and approximately 1.5% > 40° C (104° F). Some data suggest that febrile reactions are more likely to occur in those who have experienced such responses after prior doses.[16]

SIGNIFICANT REACTIONS ATTRIBUTED TO THE PERTUSSIS VACCINE COMPONENT HAVE BEEN: HIGH FEVER OF 40.5° C (105° F), A TRANSIENT SHOCK-LIKE EPISODE, EXCESSIVE SCREAMING (PERSISTENT CRYING OR SCREAMING FOR THREE OR MORE HOURS DURATION), SOMNOLENCE, CONVULSIONS, AND ENCEPHALOPATHY. THESE REACTIONS HAVE BEEN REPORTED TO OCCUR RARELY FOLLOWING THE INJECTION OF THIS PRODUCT AND THEY MAY BE FATAL OR RESULT IN PERMANENT DAMAGE TO THE CENTRAL NERVOUS SYSTEM. PERTUSSIS VACCINE HAS BEEN ASSOCIATED WITH A GREATER PROPORTION OF ADVERSE REACTIONS THAN MANY OTHER CHILDHOOD IMMUNIZATIONS.[13,21] SHOULD SYMPTOMATOLOGY REFERABLE TO THE CENTRAL NERVOUS SYSTEM DEVELOP FOLLOWING ADMINISTRATION, FURTHER IMMUNIZATION WITH THIS PRODUCT IS CONTRAINDICATED (SEE CONTRAINDICATIONS). SUCH REACTIONS ALMOST ALWAYS APPEAR WITHIN 24 TO 48 HOURS AFTER INJECTION, BUT HAVE BEEN THOUGHT TO OCCUR AFTER AN INTERVAL AS LONG AS SEVEN DAYS.

NEUROLOGICAL COMPLICATIONS FOLLOWING TETANUS TOXOID ADMINISTRATION, SUCH AS PARALYSIS OF THE RADIAL NERVE,[22] RECURRENT PHARYNGEAL NERVE,[23] COCHLEAR LESION,[24] BRACHIAL PLEXUS NEUROPATHY[25,26,] AND A CASE OF DIFFICULTY IN SWALLOWING, ACCOMMODATION PARESIS, AND EEG DISTURBANCES[27] HAVE BEEN REPORTED. IN THE DIFFERENTIAL DIAGNOSIS OF POLYRADICULONEUROPATHIES FOLLOWING ADMINISTRATION OF TETANUS TOXOID, TETANUS TOXOID SHOULD BE CONSIDERED AS A POSSIBLE ETIOLOGY.[28]

DOSAGE AND ADMINISTRATION

Shake vigorously before withdrawing each dose from the multiple dose vials.

Before injection, the skin over the site to be injected should be cleansed and prepared with a suitable germicide. After insertion of the needle, aspirate to help avoid inadvertent injection into a blood vessel. Expel the dose slowly and terminate the dose with a small bubble of air (0.1 to 0.2 ml).

The basic immunizing course for infants and children through 6 years of age consists of three doses of 0.5 ml each at 4- to 8-week intervals, followed by a fourth dose of 0.5 ml approximately one year after the third dose.

It is recommended that active immunization against diphtheria, tetanus, and pertussis be started at 2 months of

age.[1,2] All doses should be injected intramuscularly, preferably into the midlateral muscles of the thigh or deltoid, with care to avoid major peripheral nerve trunks.
Interruption of the recommended schedule with a delay between doses does not interfere with the final immunity achieved; nor does it necessitate starting the series over again, regardless of the length of time elapsed between doses.[1]
A recall (booster) dose of 0.5 ml is indicated at age 4–6 years, preferably prior to entrance into kindergarten or elementary school. However, if the fourth dose of the basic immunizing series was administered after the fourth birthday, a recall (booster) of DTP prior to school entry is not considered necessary.[1]
For either basic or recall (booster) immunization against tetanus and diphtheria of individuals 7 years of age and older, the use of Tetanus and Diphtheria Toxoids Adsorbed (*For Adult Use*) is recommended.[1,2]
Parenteral drug products should be inspected visually for particulate matter and discoloration prior to administration whenever solution and container permit.

HOW SUPPLIED

Diphtheria and Tetanus Toxoids and Pertussis Vaccine Adsorbed, Aluminum Phosphate Adsorbed, is available in vials of 7.5 ml. Product 1948-33

STORAGE

Keep between 2° and 8° C (35°–46° F). DO NOT FREEZE.

REFERENCES

1. Recommendation of the Immunization Practices Advisory Committee (ACIP): Diphtheria, tetanus and pertussis: Guidelines for vaccine prophylaxis and other preventive measures. MMWR 30:392–407, 1981.
2. American Academy of Pediatrics, Report of the Committee on Infectious Diseases. Pertussis Vaccine Pediatrics. 74(2) 303, August 1984.
3. Centers for Disease Control. Diphtheria Surveillance Report #12, 1971–1975 Summary, July 1978.
4. Barkin, R.M. et al. DTP reaction and serologic response with a reduced dose schedule. J. Pediatrics 105:189, 1984.
5. Bennett, John V., "Tetanus" in Infectious Diseases, Hoeprich, P.D. (ed), Harper & Row, Inc., pp. 303–307, 1972.
6. Annual Supplement: Reported incidence of notifiable diseases in the United States. MMWR, 1970.
7. Diphtheria, Tetanus and Pertussis: Guideline for vaccine prophylaxis and other preventive measures. MMWR 30(32):392–396, 1981.
8. Manclark, C.R. and Cowell, J.L. Pertussis Vaccine. In R. Germanier (ed), Bacterial Vaccines Academic Press, Inc., NY pp. 60–106, 1984.
9. Recommendation of the Immunization Practices Advisory Committee (ACIP): Supplementary statement of contraindications to receipt of pertussis vaccine. MMWR 33:169, 1984.
10. Bernier, R., et al.: Diphtheria-tetanus toxoids-pertussis vaccination and sudden infant deaths in Tennessee. J. Pediatrics, 101:149, 1982.
11. Baraff, L. et al.: Possible temporal association between diphtheria-tetanus toxoid-pertussis vaccination and sudden infant death syndrome. Ped. Inf. Dis. 2:7, 1983.
12. Fulginiti, V.: Sudden infant death syndrome, diphtheria-tetanus toxoid-pertussis vaccination and visits to the doctor: Chance association or cause and effect. Ped. Inf. Dis. 2:5, 1983.
13. Hinman, A.R.: The Pertussis Controversy. Public Health Reports. 99(3) 255, 1984.
14. Hoffman, H. et al.: SIDS and DTP Proceedings of the 17th Immunization Conference. Pub. No. 546-007-8224, Centers for Disease Control, pp. 79–88. May 18–19, 1982.
15. Cody, C. et al.: Nature and rates of adverse reactions associated with DTP and DT immunizations in infants and children. Pediatrics 68:650, 1981.
16. Baraff, L. et al.: DTP-associated reactions: An analysis by injection site, manufacturer, prior reactions and dose. Pediatrics 73:31, 1984.
17. Bernier, R. et al.: Abscesses complicating DTP vaccination. Am. J. Dis. Child. 135, 826, 1981.
18. Omokoku, B., Castells, S.: Post-DPT inoculation caused lymphadenitis in children. NY State J. Med. 81:1667, 1981.
19. Barkin, R., Pichichero, M.: Diphtheria-pertussis-tetanus vaccine: Reactogenicity of commercial products. Pediatrics 63:256, 1979.
20. Hopkins, R.: Reactions to DTP vaccine, by lot and manufacturer: Results of a survey in Montana. International Symposium on Pertussis, Bethesda, Maryland, 1979, DHEW Pub. No. (NIH) 79–1820, p. 300.
21. Miller, D.L. et al.: Pertussis Immunization and Serious Acute Neurological Illness in Children. Brit. Med. J. 282, 1595–1599, 1981.
22. Blumstein, G.I., Kreithen, H.: Peripheral neuropathy following tetanus toxoid administration, J.A.M.A. 198:1030–1031, 1966.
23. Eicher, W., Neundorfer, B.: Recurrenslahmung nach Tetanustoxoid-Auffrischimpfung. Munch. med. Wschr. 34:1692–1695, 1969.
24. Wirth, G., Reversible Kochlearisschadigung nach Tetanol-Injektion. Munch. med. Wschr. 107: 379–381, 1965.
25. Gersbach, P., Waridel, D.: Paralysis apres prevention antitetanique. Schweiz. med. Wschr. 106: 150–153, 1976.
26. Tsairis, P., Duck, P.J., Mulder, D.W.: Natural history of brachial plexus neuropathy. Arch. Neurol. 27: 109–117, 1972.
27. Harrer, G., Melnizky, U., Wendt, H.: Akkomodation-sparese und Schlucklahmung nach Tetanus-Toxoid-Auffrischimpfung. Wien. med. Wschr. 15: 296–297, 1971.
28. Schlenska, G.K.: Unusual neurological complications following tetanus toxoid administration. J. Neurol. 215: 209–302, 1977.

LEDERLE LABORATORIES DIVISION
American Cyanamid Company, Pearl River, NY 10965

ZINCON® Pyrithione Zinc 1%
[*zink 'on*]
Formula Dandruff Shampoo

(See PDR For Nonprescription Drugs)

EDUCATIONAL MATERIAL

Films
Product: ASENDIN® *amoxapine*
Film Titles
Antidepressant Therapy—Why Aren't We Content?
Lionel Corbett, M.D. At My Age What Does It Matter?
Lionel Corbett, M.D. The Missing Twenty
Product: LOXITANE® *loxapine*
Film Titles
New Techniques in the Diagnosis and Treatment Evaluation of Schizophrenia
Neuroleptic Side Effects: Medicolegal Aspects
Today's Clinical Perceptions of a Chemically Distinct Neuroleptic Rapid Rehabilitation of the Schizophrenic Patient
LOXITANE IM and the Psychiatric Emergency
Free Samples available for ASENDIN, LOXITANE and PATHIBAMATE.
Product: PIPRACIL® *piperacillin sodium*
Film Titles
Considerations in Cost Effective Antimicrobial Therapy
Mechanisms of Bacterial Resistance
Aspiration Pneumonia in the Surgery Patient
Aspiration Pneumonia in the Medical Patient
Call: 800-L-E-D-E-R-L-E—between the hours of 8:30 am and 4:30 pm
Product: MAXZIDE™ *75 triamterene/50 mg hydrochlorothiazide*

Brochures
Patient Information Brochure

Slide Lecture Kits
The Role of Diuretics, Potassium, Magnesium, and Calcium in Hypertension
MAXZIDE: A New Formulation of Triamterene/Hydrochlorothiazide
Free Samples available for MAXZIDE
Call: 800-L-E-D-E-R-L-E—between the hours of 8:30 am and 4:30 pm

Leeming Division
Pfizer, Inc. 100 JEFFERSON ROAD PARSIPPANY, NJ 07054

BEN-GAY® EXTERNAL
[*ben-gā '*]
ANALGESIC PRODUCTS

(See PDR For Nonprescription Drugs)

BONINE®
(meclizine hydrochloride)
Chewable Tablets

ACTIONS

BONINE is an antihistamine which shows marked protective activity against nebulized histamine and lethal doses of intravenously injected histamine in guinea pigs. It has a marked effect in blocking the vasodepressor response to histamine, but only a slight blocking action against acetylcholine. Its activity is relatively weak in inhibiting the spasmogenic action of histamine on isolated guinea pig ileum.

INDICATIONS

BONINE is effective in the management of nausea, vomiting and dizziness associated with motion sickness.

CONTRAINDICATIONS

Meclizine HCl is contraindicated in individuals who have shown a previous hypersensitivity to it.

WARNINGS

Since drowsiness may, on occasion, occur with the use of this drug, patients should be warned of this possibility and cautioned against driving a car or operating dangerous machinery.
Patients should avoid alcoholic beverages while taking this drug. Due to its potential anticholinergic action, this drug should be used with caution in patients with asthma, glaucoma, or enlargement of the prostate gland.
Usage in Children:
Clinical studies establishing safety and effectiveness in children have not been done; therefore, usage is not recommended in children under 12 years of age.
Usage in Pregnancy:
As with any drug, if you are pregnant or nursing a baby, seek advice of a health care professional before taking this product.

ADVERSE REACTIONS

Drowsiness, dry mouth, and on rare occasions, blurred vision have been reported.

DOSAGE AND ADMINISTRATION

For motion sickness 1 or 2 tablets of BONINE should be taken one hour prior to embarkation. Thereafter, the dose may be repeated every 24 hours for the duration of the journey.

HOW SUPPLIED

BONINE (meclizine HCl) is available in convenient packets of 8 chewable tablets of 25 mg. meclizine HCl.

CORYBAN®-D CAPSULES
Decongestant Cold Capsules

(See 1987 PDR For Nonprescription Drugs)

CORYBAN®-D COUGH SYRUP
With Decongestant
(Sugar and Saccharin Free Formula)

(See 1987 PDR For Nonprescription Drugs)

DESITIN® OINTMENT
[*des "i-tin '*]

(See PDR For Nonprescription Drugs)

LI-BAN® Spray
Lice Control Spray

THIS PRODUCT IS NOT FOR USE ON HUMANS OR ANIMALS

ACTIVE INGREDIENT

(5-Benzyl-3-Furyl) methyl 2, 2-dimethyl-3-(2-methylpropenyl) cyclopropanecarboxylate	0.500%
Related Compounds	0.068%
Aromatic petroleum hydrocarbons	0.664%
Inert Ingredients	98.768%
	100.000%

ACTIONS

A highly active synthetic pyrethroid for the control of lice and louse eggs on garments, bedding, furniture and other inanimate objects.

WARNINGS

Avoid contamination of feed and foodstuffs. Cover or remove fishbowls. HARMFUL IF SWALLOWED. This product is not for use on humans or animals. If lice infestations should occur on humans, consult either your physician or pharmacist for a product for use on humans.

PHYSICAL AND CHEMICAL HAZARDS

Contents under pressure. Do not use or store near heat or open flame. Do not puncture or incinerate container. Exposure to temperatures above 130° F may cause bursting.
CAUTION: Avoid spraying in eyes. Avoid breathing spray mist. Use only in well ventilated areas. Avoid contact with skin. In case of contact wash immediately with soap and water. Vacate room after treatment and ventilate before reoccupying.

Continued on next page

Leeming—Cont.

Statement of Practical Treatment:
If inhaled: Remove affected person to fresh air. Apply artifical respiration if indicated.
In in eyes: Flush with plenty of water. Contact physician if irritation persists.
If on skin: Wash affected areas immediately with soap and water.

DIRECTION FOR USE

It is a violation of Federal law to use this product in a manner inconsistent with its labeling.
Shake well before each use. Remove protective cap. Aim spray opening away from person. Push button to spray.
To kill lice and louse eggs: Spray in an inconspicuous area to test for possible staining or discoloration. Inspect again after drying, then proceed to spray entire area to be treated. Hold container upright with nozzle away from you. Depress valve and spray from a distance of 8 to 10 inches.
Spray each square foot for 3 seconds. Spray only those garments, parts of bedding, including mattresses and furniture that cannot be either laundered or dry cleaned.
Allow all sprayed articles to dry thoroughly before use. Repeat treatment as necessary.
Buyer assumes all risks of use, storage or handling of this material not in strict accordance with direction given herewith.
DISPOSAL OF CONTAINER
Wrap container and dispose of in trash. Do not incinerate.

HOW SUPPLIED

5 ounce aerosol can.

RID®
Lice Treatment Kit

DESCRIPTION

Rid contains a liquid pediculicide whose active ingredients are: pyrethrins 0.3% and piperonyl butoxide, technical 3.00%, equivalent to 2.4% (butylcarbityl) (6-propylpiperonyl) ether and to 0.6% related compounds. Also contains petroleum distillate 1.20% and benzyl alcohol 2.4%. Inert ingredients 93.1%.

ACTIONS

RID kills head lice (Pediculus humanus capitis), body lice (Pediculus humanus humanus), and pubic or crab lice (Phthirus pubis), and their eggs.
The pyrethrins act as a contact poison and affect the parasite's nervous system, resulting in paralysis and death. The efficacy of the pyrethrins is enhanced by the synergist, piperonyl butoxide.

INDICATIONS

RID is indicated for the treatment of infestations of head lice, body lice and pubic (crab) lice and their eggs.

WARNING

RID should be used with caution by ragweed sensitized persons.

PRECAUTIONS

This product is for external use only. It is harmful if swallowed. It should not be inhaled. It should be kept out of the eyes and contact with mucous membranes should be avoided. If accidental contact with eyes occurs, flush immediately with water. In case of infection or skin irritation, discontinue use and consult a physician. Consult a physician if infestation of eyebrows or eyelashes occurs. Avoid contamination of feed or foodstuffs.

STORAGE AND DISPOSAL

Do not store below 32°F (0°C). Do not reuse empty container. Wrap in several layers of newspaper and discard in trash.

DOSAGE AND ADMINISTRATION

(1) Shake well. Apply undiluted RID to dry hair and scalp or to any other infested area until entirely wet. Do not use on eyelashes or eyebrows. (2) Allow RID to remain on area for 10 minutes but no longer. (3) Wash thoroughly with warm water and soap or shampoo. (4) Dead lice and eggs should be removed with special nit comb provided. (5) Repeat treatment in 7 to 10 days to kill any newly hatched lice. Do not exceed two consecutive applications within 24 hours.
Since lice infestations are spread by contact, each family member should be examined carefully. If infested, he or she should be treated promptly to avoid spread or reinfestation of previously treated individuals. Contaminated clothing and other articles, such as hats, etc., should be dry cleaned, boiled or otherwise treated until decontaminated to prevent reinfestation or spread.

HOW SUPPLIED

In 2 and 4 fl. oz. plastic bottles. Exclusive nit removal comb that removes all the nits and patient instruction booklet (English and Spanish) are included in each package of RID.

TERRAMYCIN® OINTMENT
(oxytetracycline hydrochloride topical ointment with polymyxin B sulfate)

(See 1987 PDR For Nonprescription Drugs)

UNISOM® NIGHTTIME OTC
[yu 'na-som]
SLEEP-AID
(doxylamine succinate)

DESCRIPTION

Pale blue oval scored tablets containing 25 mg. of doxylamine succinate, 2-(α-(2-dimethylaminoethoxy)α-methylbenzyl) pyridine succinate.

ACTION AND USES

Doxylamine succinate is an antihistamine of the ethanolamine class, which characteristically shows a high incidence of sedation. In a comparative clinical study of over 20 antihistamines on more than 3000 subjects, doxylamine succinate 25 mg. was one of the three most sedating antihistamines, producing a significantly reduced latency to end of wakefulness and comparing favorably with established hypnotic drugs such as secobarbital and pentobarbital in sedation activity. It was chosen as the antihistamine, based on dosage, causing the earliest onset of sleep. In another clinical study, doxylamine succinate 25 mg. scored better than secobarbital 100 mg. as a nighttime hypnotic. Two additional, identical clinical studies, involving a total of 121 subjects demonstrated that doxylamine succinate 25 mg. reduced the sleep latency period by a third, compared to placebo. Duration of sleep was 26.6% longer with doxylamine succinate, and the quality of sleep was rated higher with the drug than with placebo. An EEG study on 6 subjects confirmed the results of these studies. In yet another study, no statistically significant difference was found between doxylamine succinate and flurazepam in the average time required for 200 patients with mild to moderate insomnia to fall asleep over 5 nights following a nightly dose of doxylamine succinate 25 mg. or flurazepam 30 mg., nor was any statistically significant difference found in the total time the 200 patients slept. Patients on doxylamine succinate awoke an average of 1.2 times per night while those on flurazepam awoke an average of 0.9 times per night. In either case the patients awoke rested the following morning. On a rating scale of 1 to 5, doxylamine succinate was given a 3.0, flurazepam a 3.4 by patients rating the degree of restfulness provided by their medication (5 represents "very well rested"). Although statistically significant, the difference between doxylamine succinate 25 mg. and flurazepam 30 mg. in the number of awakenings and degree of restfulness are clinically insignificant.

ADMINISTRATION AND DOSAGE

One tablet 30 minutes before retiring. Not for children under 12 years of age.

SIDE EFFECTS

Occasional anticholinergic effects may be seen.

PRECAUTIONS

Unisom® should be taken only at bedtime.

CONTRAINDICATIONS

Asthma, glaucoma, enlargement of the prostate gland. This product should not be taken by pregnant women or those who are nursing a baby.

WARNINGS

Should be taken with caution if alcohol is being consumed. Product should not be taken if patient is concurrently on any other drug, without prior consultation with physician. Should not be taken for longer than two weeks unless approved by physician.

HOW SUPPLIED

Boxes of 8, 16, 32 or 48 tablets.

WART-OFF™
Liquid

ACTIVE INGREDIENT

Salicylic Acid, U.S.P., 17%, in Flexible Collodion, U.S.P. Wart-Off™ Solution contains approx. 20.5% Alcohol and 54.2% Ether—small losses are unavoidable.

INDICATIONS

Removal of Warts

WARNINGS

Keep this and all medications out of reach of children to avoid accidental poisoning.
Flammable—Do not use near fire or flame. For external use only. In case of accidental ingestion, contact a physician or a Poison Control Center immediately. Do not use near eyes or on mucous membranes. Diabetics or other people with impaired circulation should not use Wart-Off™. Do not use on moles, birthmarks or unusual warts with hair growing from them. If wart persists, see your physician. If pain should develop, consult your physician. **Do not apply to surrounding skin.**

DOSAGE AND ADMINISTRATION

Instructions For Use: Read warning and enclosed instructional brochure. Do not apply to surrounding skin. Make sure that surrounding skin is protected from accidental application. Apply Wart-Off™ to warts only. Before applying, soak affected area in hot water for several minutes. If any tissue has loosened, remove by rubbing surface of wart gently with cleaning brush enclosed in Wart-Off™ package. Dry thoroughly. Warts are contagious, so dont'share your towel. Apply once or twice daily. Using pinpoint applicator attached to cap, apply one drop at a time until entire wart is covered. Lightly cover with small adhesive bandage. Replace cap tightly. This treatment may be used daily for three to four weeks if necessary.

HOW SUPPLIED

0.5 fluid ounce bottle with special pinpoint plastic applicator, cleaning brush and instructional brochure.

Legere Pharmaceuticals
7326 E. EVANS ROAD
SCOTTSDALE, AZ 85260

Product Number	Product Name	
1038	ACE + Z Tablets	OTC
	Vitamin A	5000 I.U.
	Vitamin C	1000 mg.
	Vitamin E (Succinate)	50 I.U.
	Magnesium (oxide)	100 mg.
	Zinc Sulfate	100 mg.
1066	ACETACO Tablets	℞ Ⓒ III
	Acetaminophen	300 mg.
	Codeine Phosphate	30 mg.
046	ALLERDRYL 50 10 ml.	℞
	Diphenhydramine HCL.	50 mg.
095	B-S-P 5 ml.	℞
	Betamethasone Sodium	
	Phosphate	4 mg.
	B-S-P LA	℞
	Betamethasone Sodium	
	Phosphate	3 mg.
	Betamethasone Acetate	
	Suspension	3 mg.
086	CEE-500 5 ml.	℞
	Ascorbic Acid	500 mg.
1073	CEE-1000 T.D. Tablets	OTC
	Ascorbic Acid	1000 mg.
055	CINALONE 40 5 ml.	℞
	Triamcinolone Diacetate	40 mg.
101	CINONIDE 40 5 ml.	℞
	Triamcinolone Acetonide	40 mg.
004	COBOLIN-M 30 ml.	℞
	Cyanocobalamin	1000 mcg.
062	DEPO-PREDATE 80 10 ml.	℞
	Methylprednisolone Acetate	80 mg.
121	DEPO-PREDATE 40 10 ml.	℞
	Methylprednisolone Acetate	40 mg.
010	DEXASONE 4 5 ml.	℞
	Dexamethasone Phosphate	4 mg.
011	DEXASONE LA 5 ml.	℞
	Dexamethasone Acetate	8 mg.
113	DEXASONE 10 5 ml.	℞
	Dexamethasone Sodium	
	Phosphate	10 mg.
1058	DEXOL T.D. Tablets	OTC
	Pantothenic Acid	1000 mg.
074	DEXOL 300 30 ml.	℞
	Dexpanthanol	300 mg.
065	DEXTRARON-50 10 ml.	℞
	Iron Dextran	50 mg.
1111	DI-ATRO Tablets	℞ Ⓒ
	Diphenoxylate HCl	2.5 mg.
	Atropine Sulfate	0.025 mg.
1130	DIEUTRIM Capsules	℞
	Phenylpropanolamine HCl	75 mg.
	Benzocaine	9 mg.
	Carboxymethylcellulose	75 mg.
0122	DI-HYDROTIC 10 ml.	℞
	Polymixin B Sulfate	10,000 units
	Neomycin Sulfate (Equiv.	
	to Neomycin base)	3.5 mg.
	Hydrocortisone 1%	10 mg.
015	E-CYPIONATE 10 ml.	℞
	Estradiol Cypionate	5 mg.
019	ESTRONE 10 ml.	℞
	Estrone	2 mg.
114	KABOLIN 2 ml.	℞
	Nandrolone Decanoate	50 mg.

026	LIDOCAINE 1% 50 ml.	℞
	Lidocaine Hydrochloride	10 mg.
027	LIDOCAINE 2%	℞
	Lidocaine Hydrochloride	20 mg.
1129	LIPO-B-C	OTC
	Vitamin C	500 mg.
	Vitamin B-1	50 mg.
	Vitamin B-2	50 mg.
	Vitamin B-6	50 mg.
	Vitamin B-12	50 mcg.
	Niacinamide	50 mg.
	Folic Acid	100 mcg.
	Calcium Pantothenate	50 mg.
	Biotin	50 mcg.
	Choline	50 mg.
	Inositol	50 mg.
	Paba	30 mg.
059	LIVOLEX 30 ml.	℞
	Liver Vitamins and Iron	
117	MENAVAL 20 10 ml.	℞
	Estradiol Valerate	20 mg.
023	MENAVAL 40 10 ml.	℞
	Estradiol Valerate	40 mg.
028	MERSALYL-THEOPHYL-LINE 30 ml.	℞
	Sodium Mersalyl	100 mg.
	Theophylline	50 mg.
064	MYOTROL 10 ml.	℞
	Orphenadrine Citrate	300 mg.
018	NATURAL ESTROGENIC SUBSTANCE	℞
	Each ml.—2 ml. Estrone Suspension	2 mg.
049	NEUCALM 50 10 ml.	℞
	Hydroxyzine HCl	50 mg.
1063	O. B. THERA Tablets	OTC
	Pre-natal Vitamins	
1022	PHENAZINE Tablets and Capsules	℞ C-III
	Phendimetrazine Tartrate	35 mg.
031	PREDATE 50 10 ml.	℞
	Prednisolone Acetate Suspension	50 mg.
032	PREDATE S 10 ml.	℞
	Prednisolone Sodium Phosphate	20 mg.
033	PREDATE TBA 10 ml.	℞
	Prednisolone Tebutate Suspension	20 mg.
1064	PREVENZYME Tablets	OTC
	Pancreatin	600 mg.
	Pepsin	225 mg.
	Amylase	15 mg.
	Diastase	150 mg.
	Papain	150 mg.
	Glutamic Acid HCL	30 mg.
	Betaine HCL	30 mg.
602	PROBAHIST	℞
	Brompheniramine maleate	10 mg.
1132	PROBAHIST Capsules	℞
	Pseudoephedrine	120 mg.
	Chlorpheniramine	8 mg.
088	PRODROX 250 5 ml.	℞
	Hydroxyprogesterone Caproate	250 mg.
081	PROGESTERONE 50 10 ml.	℞
	Progesterone	50 mg.
034	PROMET 50 10 ml.	℞
	Promethazine Hydrochloride	50 mg.
1133	PT 105 Capsules	℞ C-III
	Phendimetrazine	105 mg.
	Phendimetrazine Tartrate	35 mg.
073	RODEX 30 ml.	℞
	Pyridoxine HCl	100 mg.
1037	RODEX T.D. Capsules	OTC
	Pyridoxine	150 mg.
054	STEMETIC 20 ml.	℞
	Trimethobenzamide HCl	100 mg.
039	T-CYPIONATE 10 ml.	℞
	Testosterone Cypionate	200 mg.
051	T-E CYPIONATE 10 ml.	℞
	Testosterone Cypionate	50 mg.
	Estradiol Cypionate	2 mg.
1025	TERAMINE Capsules	℞ C-IV
	Phentermine HCl	30 mg.
050	TESTAVAL 90/4 10 ml.	℞
	Testosterone Enanthate	90 mg.
	Estradiol Valerate	4 mg.
030	TESTOSTERONE SUS-PENSION 10 ml.	℞
	Testosterone 100 Aqueous	100 mg.
1120	THERA-RON Tablets	OTC
	Multi-Vitamins	
445	T-QUIL	C-IV
	Diazepam	5 mg.
1013	TRIAZIDE Tablets	℞
	Trichlormethiazide	4 mg.
2001	VAGIMIDE CREAM 4 oz.	℞
	Sulfanilamide	15%
	Allantoin	2.0%
	Aminacrine HCl	0.2%
1044	VITABESE Capsules	OTC
	Multi-Vitamins	

Lemmon Ethical Division
Lemmon Company
SELLERSVILLE, PA 18960

ADIPEX-P® C-IV ℞
[*ă'dĭ-pĕx*]
(phentermine hydrochloride 37.5 mg)

DESCRIPTION

Each blue and white capsule or tablet contains:
Phentermine Hydrochloride, 37.5 mg. (equivalent to 30 mg. of Phentermine base)
Phentermine hydrochloride is designated chemically as phenyl-tert-butylamine hydrochloride. It is a white crystalline powder, very soluble in water and alcohol.
Adipex-P capsules contain the inactive ingredients Corn Starch, Gelatin, Lactose, Magnesium Stearate, and Coloring.
Adipex-P Tablets contain the inactive ingredients Acacia, Confectioner's Sugar, Corn Starch, Lactose, Magnesium Stearate, Stearic Acid, and Coloring.

ACTIONS

Phentermine hydrochloride is a sympathomimetic amine with pharmacologic activity similar to the prototype drugs of this class used in obesity, the amphetamines. Actions include central nervous system stimulation and elevation of blood pressure. Tachyphylaxis and tolerance have been demonstrated with all drugs of this class in which these phenomena have been looked for.
Drugs of this class used in obesity are commonly known as "anorectics" or "anorexigenics". It has not been established, however, that the action of such drugs in treating obesity is primarily one of appetite suppression. Other central nervous system actions, or metabolic effects, may be involved, for example.
Adult obese subjects instructed in dietary management and treated with "anorectic" drugs, lose more weight on the average than those treated with placebo and diet, as determined in relatively short-term clinical trials. The magnitude of increased weight loss of drug-treated patients over placebo-treated patients is only a fraction of a pound a week. The rate of weight loss is greatest in the first weeks of therapy for both drug and placebo subjects and tends to decrease in succeeding weeks. The possible origins of the increased weight loss due to the various drug effects are not established. The amount of weight loss associated with the use of an "anorectic" drug varies from trial to trial, and the increased weight loss appears to be related in part to variables other than the drug prescribed, such as the physician-investigator, the population treated, and the diet prescribed. Studies do not permit conclusions as to the relative importance of the drug and non-drug factors on weight loss.
The natural history of obesity is measured in years, whereas, the studies cited are restricted to a few weeks duration; thus, the total impact of drug-induced weight loss over that of diet alone must be considered clinically limited.

INDICATIONS

Adipex-P (phentermine hydrochloride) is indicated in the management of exogenous obesity as a short term adjunct (a few weeks) in a regimen of weight reduction based on caloric restriction.
The limited usefulness of agents of this class (see ACTIONS) should be measured against possible risk factors inherent in their use such as those described below.

CONTRAINDICATIONS

Advanced arteriosclerosis, symptomatic cardiovascular disease, moderate to severe hypertension, hyperthyroidism, known hypersensitivity or idiosyncrasy to the sympathomimetic amines, glaucoma.
Agitated states.
Patients with a history of drug abuse.
During or within 14 days following the administration of monoamine oxidase inhibitors (hypertensive crisis may result).

WARNINGS

Tolerance to the anorectic effect usually develops within a few weeks. When this occurs, the recommended dose should not be exceeded in an attempt to increase the effect; rather, the drug should be discontinued. Phentermine hydrochloride may impair the ability of the patient to engage in potentially hazardous activities such as operating machinery or driving a motor vehicle; the patient should therefore be cautioned accordingly.

DRUG DEPENDENCE

Phentermine hydrochloride is related chemically and pharmacologically to the amphetamines. Amphetamines and related stimulant drugs have been extensively abused, and the possibility of abuse of phentermine hydrochloride should be kept in mind when evaluating the desirability of including a drug as part of a weight reduction program. Abuse of amphetamines and related drugs may be associated with intense psychological dependence and severe social dysfunction. There are reports of patients who have increased the dosage to many times that recommended. Abrupt cessation following prolonged high dosage administration results in extreme fatigue and mental depression; changes are also noted in the sleep EEG. Manifestations of chronic intoxication with anorectic drugs include severe dermatoses, marked insomnia, irritability, hyperactivity, and personality changes. The most severe manifestation of chronic intoxications is psychosis, often clinically indistinguishable from schizophrenia.

USAGE IN PREGNANCY

No reproduction studies or teratology studies of phentermine hydrochloride, in animals or humans, have been published. Therefore, use of phentermine hydrochloride by women who are or may become pregnant, requires that the potential benefit be weighed against the possible hazard to mother and infant.

USAGE IN CHILDREN

Phentermine hydrochloride is not recommended for use in children under 12 years of age.

PRECAUTIONS

Caution is to be exercised in prescribing phentermine hydrochloride for patients with even mild hypertension.
Insulin requirements in diabetes mellitus may be altered in association with the use of phentermine hydrochloride and the concomitant dietary regimen.
Phentermine hydrochloride may decrease the hypotensive effect of guanethidine.
The least amount feasible should be prescribed or dispensed at one time in order to minimize the possibility of overdosage.

ADVERSE REACTIONS

Cardiovascular: Palpitation, tachycardia, elevation of blood pressure.
Central Nervous System: Overstimulation, restlessness, dizziness, insomnia, euphoria, dysphoria, tremor, headache; rarely psychotic episodes at recommended doses.
Gastrointestinal: Dryness of the mouth, unpleasant taste, diarrhea, constipation, other gastrointestinal disturbances.
Allergic: Urticaria.
Endocrine: Impotence, changes in libido.

DOSAGE AND ADMINISTRATION

The usual adult dose is one capsule or tablet (37.5 mg) daily, administered before breakfast or 1-2 hours after breakfast. For tablets, dosage may be adjusted to the patient's need. For some patients ½ tablet (18.75 mg) daily may be adequate, while in some cases it may be desirable to give ½ tablet (18.75 mg) two times a day.
Phentermine hydrochloride is not recommended for use in children under 12 years of age.

OVERDOSAGE

Manifestations of acute overdosage with phentermine hydrochloride include restlessness, tremor, hyperreflexia, rapid respiration, confusion, assaultive behavior hallucinations, panic states.
Fatigue and depression usually follow the central stimulation.
Cardiovascular effects include arrhythmias, hypertension or hypotension and circulatory collapse. Gastrointestinal symptoms include nausea, vomiting, diarrhea, and abdominal cramps. In fatal poisoning, death is usually preceded by convulsions and coma.
Management of acute phentermine hydrochloride intoxication is largely symptomatic and includes lavage and sedation with a barbiturate. Experience with hemodialysis or peritoneal dialysis is inadequate to permit recommendation in this regard. Acidification of the urine increases phentermine hydrochloride excretion. Intravenous phentolamine (Regitine) has been suggested for possible acute, severe hypertension, if this complicates phentermine hydrochloride overdosage.

HOW SUPPLIED

Available in tablets and capsules containing 37.5 mg phentermine hydrochloride (equivalent to 30 mg phentermine base). Each blue and white, oblong, scored tablet is imprinted with "LEMMON"/"9"—"9". The #3 capsule has an opaque white body and an opaque light blue cap. Each capsule is

Continued on next page

Lemmon—Cont.

imprinted with "Adipex-P"-"37.5" on the cap and two blue stripes on the body.
Tablets are packaged in bottles of 100 (NDC 0093-0009-01); 400 (NDC 0093-0009-26); and 1000 (NDC 0093-0009-10).
Capsules are packaged in bottles of 100 (NDC 0093-0019-01); and 400 (NDC 0093-0019-26).

Shown in Product Identification Section, page 415

PROPACET™ 100 Ⓒ℞

[*prō´pă-cĕt*]
(propoxyphene napsylate w/acetaminophen tablets USP)

DESCRIPTION
Each tablet contains Propoxyphene Napsylate 100 mg and Acetaminophen 650 mg.
Propoxyphene Napsylate differs from propoxyphene hydrochloride in that it allows more stable liquid dosage forms and tablet formulations. A dose of 100 mg of propoxyphene napsylate is required to supply an amount of propoxyphene equivalent to 65 mg of propoxyphene hydrochloride due to differences in molecular weight.

HOW SUPPLIED
Tablets, oblong, film coated, white, imprinted "Propacet 100" "LEMMON". Available in bottles of 100 tablets (NDC 0093-0590-01) and 500 tablets (NDC 0093-0590-05) and 4×25—tablet unit dose dispensits (NDC 0093-0590-45).

Shown in Product Identification Section, page 415

RHUS TOX ANTIGEN™ ℞

[*rŭs tŏx ant-ĭ-jen*]
(poison ivy extract)

COMPOSITION
Each ml. of sterile solution contains 40 mg. poison ivy extract in a 35 per cent aqueous-alcoholic menstruum, with 4 per cent benzyl alcohol to reduce pain of injection; pH adjusted with lactic acid.

INDICATIONS
For prophylaxis and treatment of rhus dermatitis.

PRECAUTIONS
Attention is directed to reports that renal complications may follow extensive dermatitis of various types, and that with severe rhus dermatitis there may be an aggravation of symptoms following administration of poison ivy extract.

DOSAGE AND ADMINISTRATION
Specific Treatment of Rhus Dermatitis—1 ml. intramuscularly every 12 to 24 hours until symptoms are controlled. A minimum of four injections is recommended even if symptoms are alleviated within a few hours; the tendency to future attacks will be lessened. Children usually tolerate the same dose as adults.
Prophylactic Treatment—Susceptible persons can usually be protected against attacks of rhus dermatitis for a season or longer by preseasonal injections of RHUS TOX ANTIGEN. Dose: 1 ml. intramuscularly every 4 to 7 days for four or more injections. In very sensitive individuals it may be advisable to start with a smaller dose—0.25 to 0.5 ml.—and increase the dose gradually to 1 ml., giving a total of 4 ml. or more.

NOTE
The patient usually complains of a burning sensation at site of the injection. This is due to the alcohol and disappears in a few seconds. In some individuals, localized soreness or a dull ache may be noted for 24 to 48 hours.

HOW SUPPLIED
Boxes of four 1 ml. vials. Refrigeration not required. Full prescribing information is available on request (NDC 0093-0401).

SOFARIN™ ℞

[*sōfăr´in*]
(warfarin sodium tablets USP)

DESCRIPTION
Each crystalline warfarin sodium tablet for oral administration contains 2 mg, 2.5 mg, or 5 mg of warfarin sodium, USP. Crystalline warfarin sodium, a prothrombinopenic anticoagulant, is chemically crystalline warfarin sodium isopropanol clathrate. On a dose-for-dose basis, crystalline warfarin sodium is therapeutically equivalent to amorphous warfarin sodium.

HOW SUPPLIED
As 2 mg—round, lavender, single-scored tablets embossed with "SOFARIN" "93" on the plain side and "2" on the scored side. NDC 0093-0143-01 (100's). As 2.5 mg—round, orange, single-scored tablets embossed with "SOFARIN" "93" on the plain side and "2½" on the scored side. NDC 0093-0144-01 (100's). As 5 mg—round, pink, single-scored tablets embossed with "SOFARIN" "93" on the plain side and "5" on the scored side. NDC 0093-0145-01 (100's), NDC 0093-0145-10 (1000's)

Shown in Product Identification Section, page 415

These fine products are also available:

Acetaminophen and Codeine Ⓒ℞

Tablets #2	100	NDC 0093-0050-01
	500	NDC 0093-0050-05
	1000	NDC 0093-0050-10
Tablets #3	100	NDC 0093-0150-01
	500	NDC 0093-0150-05
	1000	NDC 0093-0150-10
Tablets #4	100	NDC 0093-0350-01
	500	NDC 0093-0350-05
	1000	NDC 0093-0350-10

Beta-Val™ ℞
(betamethasone valerate)

Cream 0.1%	15 gm‡	NDC 0093-0673-15
	45 gm‡	NDC 0093-0673-95

***Cotrim™** ℞
(sulfamethoxazole with trimethoprim)

Tablets	100	NDC 0093-0188-01
	500	NDC 0093-0188-05
Double Strength Tablets	100	NDC 0093-0189-01
	500	NDC 0093-0189-05
Pediatric Suspension	16 oz	NDC 0093-0190-16

***Doxy-Lemmon™** ℞
(doxycycline hyclate)

100 mg Capsules	50	NDC 0093-0743-53
	unit dose	NDC 0093-0743-93,
	10 capsules per strip, 10 strips per pack	
	500	NDC 0093-0743-05
50 mg Capsules	50	NDC 0093-0742-53
100 mg Tablets	50	NDC 0093-0484-53
	500	NDC 0093-0484-05
	unit dose	NDC 0093-0484-93,
	10 tablets per strip, 10 strips per pack	

Glucamide™ ℞
(chlorpropamide)

100 mg Tablets	100	NDC 0093-0010-01
	250	NDC 0093-0010-52
	500	NDC 0093-0010-05
	1000	NDC 0093-0010-10
250 mg Tablets	100	NDC 0093-0007-01
	250	NDC 0093-0007-52
	500	NDC 0093-0007-05
	1000	NDC 0093-0007-10
	unit dose	NDC 0093-0007-93,
	10 tablets per strip, 10 strips per pack	

Indo-Lemmon™ ℞
(indomethacin)

25 mg Capsules	100	NDC 0093-0585-01
	500	NDC 0093-0585-05
	1000	NDC 0093-0585-10
50 mg Capsules	100	NDC 0093-0587-01
	500	NDC 0093-0587-05
	1000	NDC 0093-0587-10

***Metryl™** ℞
(metronidazole)

250 mg Tablets	100	NDC 0093-0551-01
	250	NDC 0093-0551-52
	500	NDC 0093-0551-05
	unit dose	NDC 0093-0551-93,
	10 tablets per strip, 10 strips per pack	
500 mg Tablets	50	NDC 0093-0500-53
	100	NDC 0093-0500-01
	500	NDC 0093-0500-05

Myco-Triacet™ II ℞
(nystatin, triamcinolone acetonide)

Cream	15 gm‡	NDC 0093-0232-15
	30 gm‡	NDC 0093-0232-30
	60 gm‡	NDC 0093-0232-92
Ointment	15 gm‡	NDC 0093-0701-15
	30 gm	NDC 0093-0701-30

Nystatin ℞

Oral Tablets (500,000 units)	100	NDC 0093-0983-01
	unit dose	NDC 0093-0983-93,
	10 tablets per strip. 10 strips per pack	
Vaginal Tablets (100,000 units)	15	NDC 0093-0943-51
	30	NDC 0093-0943-56
Cream (100,000 units)	15 gm‡	NDC 0093-0955-15

Otocort® Sterile Ear Drops ℞
(neomycin sulfate, polymyxin B sulfate, hydrocortisone)

Solution	10 ml‡	NDC 0093-0047-43
Suspension	10 ml‡	NDC 0093-0363-43

* Literature available
‡ Minimum quantity shipped in shelf cartons of 12

Eli Lilly and Company
**LILLY CORPORATE CENTER
INDIANAPOLIS, IN 46285**

LEGEND

Aspirol®—*Inhalant in an Ampoule, Lilly*
Disket®—*Dispersible Tablet, Lilly*
Enseal®—*Enteric-Release Tablet, Lilly*
Faspak®—*Flexible Plastic Bag, Lilly*
Gelseal®—*Filled Elastic Capsule, Lilly*
Identi-Code®—*Formula Identification Code, Lilly*
Identi-Dose®—*Unit Dose Medication, Lilly*
Pulvule®—*Filled Gelatin Capsule, Lilly*
Redi Vial®—*Dual Compartment Vial, Lilly*
℞Pak—*Prescription Package, Lilly*
Solvet®—*Soluble Tablet, Lilly*
Traypak™—*Multivial Carton, Lilly*

IDENTI-CODE® Index

Illustrations of examples of products bearing Identi-Code® appear in Product Identification Section.

Identi-Code®	Product Name
A01-A36 (Enseals®)	
A01	**Ammonium Chloride** Composition (Each Enseal®): Ammonium Chloride, USP, 7½ grs (486 mg)
A02	**Ferrous Sulfate** Composition (Each Enseal®): Ferrous Sulfate, USP, 5 grs (324 mg) (equiv. to 65 mg elemental iron), Red
A04	**Pancreatin** Composition (Each Enseal®): Pancreatin, Triple Strength, equivalent to 1 g Pancreatin, USP
A05	**Potassium Chloride** Composition (Each Enseal®): Potassium chloride, 300 mg
A06	**Potassium Iodide** Composition (Each Enseal®): Potassium Iodide, USP, 300 mg
A09	**Sodium Chloride** Composition (Each Enseal®): Sodium Chloride, USP, 15½ grs (1.004 g)
A10	**Sodium Salicylate** Composition (Each Enseal®): Sodium Salicylate, USP, 5 grs (324 mg)
A11	**Sodium Salicylate** Composition (Each Enseal®): Sodium Salicylate, USP, 10 grs (648 mg)
A12	**Ammonium Chloride** Composition (Each Enseal®): Ammonium Chloride, USP, 15 grs (972 mg)
A14	**Thyroid** Composition (Each Enseal®): Thyroid, USP, 30 mg
A15	**Thyroid** Composition (Each Enseal®): Thyroid, USP, 60 mg
A16	**Thyroid** Composition (Each Enseal®): Thyroid, USP, 120 mg
A17	**Thyroid** Composition (Each Enseal®): Thyroid, USP, 200 mg
A19	**Diethylstilbestrol** Composition (Each Enseal®): Diethylstilbestrol, USP, 0.1 mg
A20	**Diethylstilbestrol** Composition (Each Enseal®): Diethylstilbestrol, USP, 0.25 mg
A21	**Diethylstilbestrol** Composition (Each Enseal®): Diethylstilbestrol, USP, 0.5 mg
A22	**Diethylstilbestrol** Composition (Each Enseal®): Diethylstilbestrol, USP, 1 mg
A24	**Seconal® Sodium** Composition (Each Enseal®): Secobarbital sodium, 100 mg

A25 **A.S.A.®**
Composition (Each Enseal®): Aspirin, USP, 5 grs (324 mg)

A26 **Ox Bile Extract**
Composition (Each Enseal®): Ox bile extract, 5 grs (324 mg)

A30 **Aminosalicylic Acid**
Composition (Each Enseal®): Aminosalicylic Acid, USP, 500 mg

A31 **Potassium Chloride**
Composition (Each Enseal®): Potassium chloride, 1 g

A32 **A.S.A.®**
Composition (Each Enseal®): Aspirin, USP, 10 grs (648 mg)

A33 **Diethylstilbestrol**
Composition (Each Enseal®): Diethylstilbestrol, USP, 5 mg

A36 **Ferrous Sulfate**
Composition (Each Enseal®): Ferrous Sulfate, USP, 5 grs (324 mg) (equiv. to 65 mg elemental iron), Green

C06-C71 (Coated Tablets)

C06 **Cascara**
Composition (Each Coated Tablet): Cascara, USP, 5 grs (324 mg)

C07 **Cascara Compound**
Composition (Each Coated Tablet): Ext. cascara, 16 mg; aloin, 16 mg; podophyllum resin, 10 mg; ext. belladonna, 8 mg (total alkaloids, 0.1 mg); oleoresin ginger, 4 mg

C09 **Digiglusin®**
Composition (Each Coated Tablet): Digitalis glucosides, 1 USP digitalis unit

C11 **Rhinitis, Full Strength**
Composition (Each Coated Tablet): Camphor, 32.5 mg; quinine sulfate, 32.5 mg; ext. belladonna leaf, 5.8 mg (total alkaloids, $\frac{1}{960}$ gr)

C13 **Ferrous Sulfate**
Composition (Each Coated Tablet): Ferrous Sulfate, USP, 5 grs (324 mg) (equiv. to 65 mg elemental iron)

C16 **Pagitane® Hydrochloride**
Composition (Each Coated Tablet): Cycrimine Hydrochloride, USP, 1.25 mg

C17 **Pagitane® Hydrochloride**
Composition (Each Coated Tablet): Cycrimine Hydrochloride, USP, 2.5 mg

C27 **V-Cillin K®**
Composition (Each Coated Tablet): Penicillin V Potassium, USP, 125 mg

C29 **V-Cillin K®**
Composition (Each Coated Tablet): Penicillin V Potassium, USP, 250 mg

C36 **Quinine Sulfate**
Composition (Each Coated Tablet): Quinine Sulfate, USP, 5 grs (324 mg)

C46 **V-Cillin K®**
Composition (Each Coated Tablet): Penicillin V Potassium, USP, 500 mg

C47 **Hepicebrin®**
Composition (Each Coated Tablet): Vitamin A acetate, 5000 IU (1.5 mg); vitamin D (as ergocalciferol), 400 IU (10 mcg); ascorbic acid (vitamin C), 75 mg; thiamine mononitrate (vitamin B_1), 2 mg; riboflavin (vitamin B_2), 3 mg; niacinamide, 20 mg (USP)

C51 **Darvocet-N® 50**
Composition (Each Coated Tablet): Propoxyphene napsylate, 50 mg; acetaminophen, 325 mg (USP)

C53 **Darvon-N®**
Composition (Each Coated Tablet): Propoxyphene Napsylate, USP, 100 mg

C54 **Darvon-N® with A.S.A.®**
Composition (Each Coated Tablet): Propoxyphene napsylate, 100 mg; aspirin, 325 mg (USP)

C63 **Darvocet-N® 100**
Composition (Each Coated Tablet): Propoxyphene napsylate, 100 mg; acetaminophen, 650 mg (USP)

C71 **Multicebrin®**
Composition (Each Coated Tablet): Thiamine (vitamin B_1), 3 mg; riboflavin (vitamin B_2), 3 mg; pyridoxine (vitamin B_6), 1.2 mg; pantothenic acid, 5 mg; niacinamide, 25 mg; vitamin B_{12} (activity equivalent), 3 mcg; ascorbic acid (vitamin C), 75 mg; *dl*-alpha tocopheryl acetate (vitamin E), 6.6 IU (6.6 mg); vitamin A, 10,000 IU (3 mg); vitamin D, 400 IU (10 mcg)

F03-H72 (Pulvules®)

F03 **Zentinic®**
Composition (Each Pulvule®): Iron, elemental (as ferrous fumarate), 100 mg; folic acid, 0.05 mg; thiamine mononitrate (vitamin B_1), 7.5 mg; riboflavin (vitamin B_2), 7.5 mg; pyridoxine hydrochloride (vitamin B_6), 7.5 mg; vitamin B_{12} (activity equivalent), 50 mcg; pantothenic acid (as calcium pantothenate), 15 mg; niacinamide, 30 mg; ascorbic acid (vitamin C), 200 mg

F04 **Seromycin®**
Composition (Each Pulvule®): Cycloserine, USP, 250 mg

F11 **A.S.A.®**
Composition (Each Pulvule®): Aspirin, USP, 5 grs (324 mg), Clear

F12 **A.S.A.®**
Composition (Each Pulvule®): Aspirin, USP, 5 grs (324 mg), Pink

F14 **Ephedrine and Amytal®**
Composition (Each Pulvule®): Ephedrine sulfate, 25 mg; amobarbital, 50 mg

F15 **Lextron®**
Composition (Each Pulvule®): Liver-stomach concentrate (as intrinsic powder), 50 mg; iron, elemental (as iron and ammonium citrates green), 30 mg; vitamin B_{12} (activity equivalent), 2 mcg; thiamine hydrochloride (vitamin B_1), 1 mg; riboflavin (vitamin B_2), 0.25 mg; with other factors of vitamin B complex present in the liver-stomach concentrate

F16 **Lextron® Ferrous**
Composition (Each Pulvule®): Liver-stomach concentrate (as intrinsic powder), 50 mg; iron, elemental (as ferrous sulfate), 35 mg; vitamin B_{12} (activity equivalent), 2 mcg; thiamine hydrochloride (vitamin B_1), 1 mg; riboflavin (vitamin B_2), 0.25 mg; with other factors of vitamin B complex present in the liver-stomach concentrate

F19 **Extralin®**
Composition (Each Pulvule®): Liver-stomach concentrate (as intrinsic powder), 50 mg

F21 **Extralin® B**
Composition (Each Pulvule®): Liver-stomach concentrate (as intrinsic powder), 67 mg; vitamin B_{12} (activity equivalent), 3 mcg; thiamine hydrochloride (vitamin B_1), 1 mg; riboflavin (vitamin B_2), 0.25 mg; with other factors of vitamin B complex present in the liver-stomach concentrate

F22 **Lextron® F. G.**
Composition (Each Pulvule®): Liver-stomach concentrate (as intrinsic powder), 50 mg; iron, elemental (as ferrous gluconate), 20 mg; vitamin B_{12} (activity equivalent), 2 mcg; thiamine hydrochloride (vitamin B_1), 1 mg; riboflavin (vitamin B_2), 0.25 mg; with other factors of vitamin B complex present in the liver-stomach concentrate

F23 **Amytal® Sodium**
Composition (Each Pulvule®): Amobarbital Sodium, USP, 65 mg

F24 **Ephedrine Sulfate**
Composition (Each Pulvule®): Ephedrine Sulfate, USP, 25 mg

F25 **Ephedrine Sulfate**
Composition (Each Pulvule®): Ephedrine Sulfate, USP, 50 mg

F26 **Quinine Sulfate**
Composition (Each Pulvule®): Quinine Sulfate, USP, 2 grs (130 mg)

F27 **Quinine Sulfate**
Composition (Each Pulvule®): Quinine Sulfate, USP, 3 grs (194 mg)

F29 **Quinine Sulfate**
Composition (Each Pulvule®): Quinine Sulfate, USP, 5 grs (324 mg)

F31 **Acidulin®**
Composition (Each Pulvule®): Glutamic acid hydrochloride, 340 mg

F32 **Digitalis**
Composition (Each Pulvule®): Digitalis, USP, 100 mg

F33 **Amytal® Sodium**
Composition (Each Pulvule®): Amobarbital Sodium, USP, 200 mg

F34 **Carbarsone**
Composition (Each Pulvule®): Carbarsone, USP, 250 mg

F36 **Copavin®**
Composition (Each Pulvule®): Codeine sulfate, 15 mg; papaverine hydrochloride, 15 mg

F39 **Quinidine Sulfate**
Composition (Each Pulvule®): Quinidine Sulfate, USP, 200 mg

F40 **Seconal® Sodium**
Composition (Each Pulvule®): Secobarbital Sodium, USP, 100 mg

F41 **Bilron®**
Composition (Each Pulvule®): Iron bile salts, 300 mg

F42 **Seconal® Sodium**
Composition (Each Pulvule®): Secobarbital Sodium, USP, 50 mg

F43 **Vitamin B Complex (Betalin® Compound)**
Composition (Each Pulvule®): Thiamine (vitamin B_1), 1 mg; riboflavin (vitamin B_2), 2 mg; pyridoxine (vitamin B_6), 0.4 mg; pantothenic acid, 3.333 mg; niacinamide, 10 mg; vitamin B_{12} (activity equivalent), 1 mcg

F44 **Ferrous Gluconate**
Composition (Each Pulvule®): Ferrous Gluconate, USP, 5 grs (324 mg)

F52 **Dibasic Calcium Phosphate with Vitamin D**
Composition (Each Pulvule®): Dibasic calcium phosphate, anhydrous, equivalent to 500 mg of dibasic calcium phosphate dihydrate; vitamin D synthetic, 33 IU (0.825 mcg)

F54 **Dicumarol**
Composition (Each Pulvule®): Dicumarol, USP, 50 mg

F56 **Calcium Gluconate with Vitamin D**
Composition (Each Pulvule®): Calcium gluconate, 325 mg; vitamin D synthetic, 0.825 mcg

F61 **Bilron®**
Composition (Each Pulvule®): Iron bile salts, 150 mg

F63 **Dibasic Calcium Phosphate with Vitamin D and Iron**
Composition (Each Pulvule®): Dibasic calcium phosphate, anhydrous, equivalent to 500 mg of dibasic calcium phosphate dihydrate; vitamin D, 33 IU (0.825 mcg); iron (as iron pyrophosphate), 10 mg

F64 **Tuinal®**
Composition (Each Pulvule®): Secobarbital sodium, 25 mg; amobarbital sodium, 25 mg (USP)

F65 **Tuinal®**
Composition (Each Pulvule®): Secobarbital sodium, 50 mg; amobarbital sodium, 50 mg (USP)

F66 **Tuinal®**
Composition (Each Pulvule®): Secobarbital sodium, 100 mg; amobarbital sodium, 100 mg (USP)

F71 **Dicumarol**
Composition (Each Pulvule®): Dicumarol, USP, 25 mg

F72 **Seconal® Sodium**
Composition (Each Pulvule®): Secobarbital Sodium, USP, 30 mg

F74 **Tycopan®**
Composition: Three Pulvules® contain thiamine mononitrate (vitamin B_1), 10 mg; riboflavin (vitamin B_2), 8 mg; pyridoxine hydrochloride (vitamin B_6), 10 mg; pantothenic acid (as calcium pantothenate), 60 mg; niacinamide, 60 mg; vitamin B_{12} (activity equivalent), 15 mcg; ascorbic acid (vitamin C), 200 mg; *dl*-alpha tocopheryl acetate (vitamin E), 22 IU (22 mg); biotin, 0.16 mg; folic acid, 0.45 mg; aminobenzoic acid, 33 mg; inositol, 160 mg; choline (as choline bitartrate), 160 mg; lipoic acid, 0.3 mg; vitamin A synthetic, 20,000 IU (6 mg); vitamin D synthetic, 1000 IU (25 mcg)

F92 **Extralin® F**
Composition (Each Pulvule®): Special Liver-Stomach Concentrate, Lilly (containing intrinsic factor), 390 mg; Cobalamin Concentrate, USP, equivalent to cobalamin, 15 mcg (the total vitamin B_{12} activity in the Special Liver-Stomach Concentrate, Lilly, and the Cobalamin Concentrate, USP, is 30 mcg); folic acid, 1 mg

F96 **Reticulex®**
Composition (Each Pulvule®): Liver-stomach concentrate (as intrinsic powder), 222 mg; vitamin B_{12} (activity equivalent), 10 mcg; iron, elemental (as ferrous sulfate), 75 mg; ascorbic acid (vitamin C), 50 mg; folic acid, 0.3 mg

H02 **Darvon®**
Composition (Each Pulvule®): Propoxyphene Hydrochloride, USP, 32 mg

H03 **Darvon®**
Composition (Each Pulvule®): Propoxyphene Hydrochloride, USP, 65 mg

H04 **Darvon® with A.S.A.®**
Composition (Each Pulvule®): Propoxyphene hydrochloride, 65 mg; aspirin, 325 mg

Continued on next page

* **Identi-Code® symbol.**

Lilly—Cont.

H10 **En-Cebrin® F**
Composition (Each Pulvule®): Vitamin A synthetic, 4000 IU (1.2 mg); thiamine mononitrate (vitamin B_1), 3 mg; riboflavin (vitamin B_2), 2 mg; niacinamide, 10 mg; pyridoxine hydrochloride (vitamin B_6), 2 mg; folic acid, 1 mg; vitamin B_{12} (activity equivalent), 5 mcg; pantothenic acid (as calcium pantothenate), 5 mg; ascorbic acid (vitamin C), 50 mg; vitamin D synthetic, 400 IU (10 mcg); calcium (as the carbonate), 250 mg; iron (as ferrous fumarate), 30 mg; iodine (as potassium iodide), 0.15 mg; copper (as the sulfate), 1 mg; magnesium (as the hydroxide), 5 mg; manganese (as the glycerophosphate), 1 mg; zinc (as the chloride), 1.5 mg

H12 **En-Cebrin®**
Composition (Each Pulvule®): Vitamin A, 4000 IU (1.2 mg); thiamine mononitrate (vitamin B_1), 3 mg; riboflavin (vitamin B_2), 2 mg; niacinamide, 10 mg; pyridoxine (vitamin B_6), 1.7 mg; vitamin B_{12} (activity equivalent), 5 mcg; pantothenic acid, 5 mg; ascorbic acid (vitamin C), 50 mg; vitamin D, 400 IU (10 mcg); calcium (as the carbonate), 250 mg; iron (as ferrous fumarate), 30 mg; iodine (as potassium iodide), 0.15 mg; copper (as the sulfate), 1 mg; magnesium (as the hydroxide), 5 mg; manganese (as the glycerophosphate), 1 mg; zinc (as the chloride), 1.5 mg

H17 **Aventyl® HCl**
Composition (Each Pulvule®): Nortriptyline Hydrochloride, USP, 10 mg (equiv. to base)

H19 **Aventyl® HCl**
Composition (Each Pulvule®): Nortriptyline Hydrochloride, USP, 25 mg (equiv. to base)

H72 **Theracebrin®**
Composition (Each Pulvule®): Thiamine (as the mononitrate) (vitamin B_1), 15 mg; riboflavin (vitamin B_2), 10 mg; pyridoxine (as the hydrochloride) (vitamin B_6), 2.5 mg; pantothenic acid (as *d*-calcium pantothenate), 20 mg; niacinamide, 150 mg; vitamin B_{12} (activity equivalent), 10 mcg; ascorbic acid (vitamin C), 150 mg; *dl*-alpha tocopheryl acetate (vitamin E), 18.5 IU (18.5 mg); vitamin A synthetic, 25,000 IU (7.5 mg); vitamin D synthetic, 1500 IU (37.5 mcg)

3061 **Ceclor®**
Composition (Each Pulvule®): Cefaclor, USP, 250 mg

3062 **Ceclor®**
Composition (Each Pulvule®): Cefaclor, USP, 500 mg

3075 **Histadyl® and A.S.A.®**
Composition (Each Pulvule®): Chlorpheniramine maleate, 4 mg; aspirin, 325 mg

3110 **Darvon® Compound**
Composition (Each Pulvule®): Propoxyphene hydrochloride, 32 mg; aspirin, 389 mg; caffeine, 32.4 mg

3111 **Darvon® Compound-65**
Composition (Each Pulvule®): Propoxyphene hydrochloride, 65 mg; aspirin, 389 mg; caffeine, 32.4 mg

3113 **A.S.A.® and Codeine Compound, No. 3**
Composition (Each Pulvule®): Codeine phosphate, 30 mg; aspirin, 380 mg; caffeine, 30 mg

---

J02-J99 (Compressed Tablets)

J02 **Atropine Sulfate**
Composition (Each Compressed Tablet): Atropine Sulfate, USP, 0.4 mg

J03 **Belladonna Extract**
Composition (Each Compressed Tablet): Belladonna Extract, USP, 15 mg (1/4 gr) (total alkaloids, 0.187 mg)

J04 **Bismuth Subcarbonate**
Composition (Each Compressed Tablet): Bismuth subcarbonate, 5 grs (324 mg)

J05 **Citrated Caffeine**
Composition (Each Compressed Tablet): Citrated caffeine, 1 gr (64.8 mg)

J09 **Codeine Sulfate**
Composition (Each Compressed Tablet): Codeine Sulfate, USP, 15 mg

J10 **Codeine Sulfate**
Composition (Each Compressed Tablet): Codeine Sulfate, USP, 30 mg

J11 **Codeine Sulfate**
Composition (Each Compressed Tablet): Codeine Sulfate, USP, 60 mg

J13 **Colchicine**
Composition (Each Compressed Tablet): Colchicine, USP, 0.6 mg

J20 **Quinidine Sulfate**
Composition (Each Compressed Tablet): Quinidine Sulfate, USP, 200 mg

J23 **Soda Mint**
Composition (Each Compressed Tablet): Sodium bicarbonate, 5 grs; oil peppermint

J24 **Sodium Bicarbonate**
Composition (Each Compressed Tablet): Sodium Bicarbonate, USP, 5 grs (324 mg)

J25 **Thyroid**
Composition (Each Compressed Tablet): Thyroid, USP, 60 mg

J26 **Thyroid**
Composition (Each Compressed Tablet): Thyroid, USP, 120 mg

J29 **Thyroid**
Composition (Each Compressed Tablet): Thyroid, USP, 30 mg

J30 **Thyroid**
Composition (Each Compressed Tablet): Thyroid, USP, 15 mg

J31 **Phenobarbital**
Composition (Each Compressed Tablet): Phenobarbital, USP, 15 mg

J32 **Phenobarbital**
Composition (Each Compressed Tablet): Phenobarbital, USP, 30 mg

J33 **Phenobarbital**
Composition (Each Compressed Tablet): Phenobarbital, USP, 100 mg

J36 **Ergotrate® Maleate**
Composition (Each Compressed Tablet): Ergonovine Maleate, USP, 0.2 mg

J37 **Phenobarbital**
Composition (Each Compressed Tablet): Phenobarbital, USP, 60 mg

J41 **Niacin**
Composition (Each Compressed Tablet): Niacin, USP, 20 mg

J42 **Niacin**
Composition (Each Compressed Tablet): Niacin, USP, 100 mg

J43 **Niacin**
Composition (Each Compressed Tablet): Niacin, USP, 50 mg

J45 **Pyridoxine Hydrochloride (Hexa-Betalin®)**
Composition (Each Compressed Tablet): Pyridoxine Hydrochloride, USP, 25 mg

J46 **Niacinamide**
Composition (Each Compressed Tablet): Niacinamide, USP, 50 mg

J47 **Riboflavin**
Composition (Each Compressed Tablet): Riboflavin, USP, 5 mg

J49 **Diethylstilbestrol**
Composition (Each Compressed Tablet): Diethylstilbestrol, USP, 0.1 mg

J50 **Diethylstilbestrol**
Composition (Each Compressed Tablet): Diethylstilbestrol, USP, 0.25 mg

J51 **Diethylstilbestrol**
Composition (Each Compressed Tablet): Diethylstilbestrol, USP, 0.5 mg

J52 **Diethylstilbestrol**
Composition (Each Compressed Tablet): Diethylstilbestrol, USP, 1 mg

J53 **Pantholin®**
Composition (Each Compressed Tablet): Calcium Pantothenate, USP, 10 mg

J54 **Diethylstilbestrol**
Composition (Each Compressed Tablet): Diethylstilbestrol, USP, 5 mg

J56 **Pyridoxine Hydrochloride (Hexa-Betalin®)**
Composition (Each Compressed Tablet): Pyridoxine Hydrochloride, USP, 10 mg

J57 **Crystodigin®**
Composition (Each Compressed Tablet): Digitoxin, USP, 0.2 mg

J60 **Crystodigin®**
Composition (Each Compressed Tablet): Digitoxin, USP, 0.1 mg

J61 **Papaverine Hydrochloride**
Composition (Each Compressed Tablet): Papaverine Hydrochloride, USP, 30 mg

J62 **Papaverine Hydrochloride**
Composition (Each Compressed Tablet): Papaverine Hydrochloride, USP, 60 mg

J63 **Riboflavin**
Composition (Each Compressed Tablet): Riboflavin, USP, 10 mg

J64 **Dolophine® Hydrochloride**
Composition (Each Compressed Tablet): Methadone Hydrochloride, USP, 5 mg

J69 **Propylthiouracil**
Composition (Each Compressed Tablet): Propylthiouracil, USP, 50 mg

J72 **Dolophine® Hydrochloride**
Composition (Each Compressed Tablet): Methadone Hydrochloride, USP, 10 mg

J73 **Methyltestosterone**
Composition (Each Compressed Tablet): Methyltestosterone, USP, 10 mg

J74 **Methyltestosterone**
Composition (Each Compressed Tablet): Methyltestosterone, USP, 25 mg

J75 **Crystodigin®**
Composition (Each Compressed Tablet): Digitoxin, USP, 0.05 mg

J76 **Crystodigin®**
Composition (Each Compressed Tablet): Digitoxin, USP, 0.15 mg

J94 **Tapazole®**
Composition (Each Compressed Tablet): Methimazole, USP, 5 mg

J95 **Tapazole®**
Composition (Each Compressed Tablet): Methimazole, USP, 10 mg

J96 **Tylosterone®**
Composition (Each Compressed Tablet): Diethylstilbestrol, 0.25 mg; methyltestosterone, 5 mg

J97 **Paveril® Phosphate**
Composition (Each Compressed Tablet): Dioxyline phosphate, 100 mg

J99 **Sandril®**
Composition (Each Compressed Tablet): Reserpine, USP, 0.1 mg

S05-S17 (Suppositories)

S05 **Seconal® Sodium**
Composition (Each Suppository): Secobarbital sodium, 120 mg

S07 **Diethylstilbestrol**
Composition (Each Suppository): Diethylstilbestrol, USP, 0.1 mg

S09 **Diethylstilbestrol**
Composition (Each Suppository): Diethylstilbestrol, USP, 0.5 mg

S11 **Seconal® Sodium**
Composition (Each Suppository): Secobarbital sodium, 200 mg

S14 **Seconal® Sodium**
Composition (Each Suppository): Secobarbital sodium, 60 mg

S15 **A.S.A.®**
Composition (Each Suppository): Aspirin, USP, 5 grs (324 mg)

S16 **A.S.A.®**
Composition (Each Suppository): Aspirin, USP, 10 grs (648 mg)

S17 **Seconal® Sodium**
Composition (Each Suppository): Secobarbital sodium, 30 mg

T01-U56 (Compressed Tablets)

T01 **Zentron® Chewable**
Composition (Each Compressed Tablet): Iron, elemental (as ferrous fumarate), 20 mg; thiamine mononitrate (vitamin B_1), 1 mg; riboflavin (vitamin B_2), 1 mg; pyridoxine hydrochloride (vitamin B_6), 1 mg; cyanocobalamin (vitamin B_{12} crystalline), 5 mcg; pantothenic acid (as panthenol), 1 mg; niacinamide, 5 mg; ascorbic acid (vitamin C), 100 mg

T05 **A.S.A.®**
Composition (Each Compressed Tablet): Aspirin, USP, 5 grs (324 mg)

T06 **A.S.A.®**
Composition (Each Compressed Tablet): Aspirin, USP, 5 grs (324 mg), Pink

T13 **Calcium Lactate**
Composition (Each Compressed Tablet): Calcium Lactate, USP, 5 grs (324 mg)

T14 **Calcium Lactate**
Composition (Each Compressed Tablet): Calcium Lactate, USP, 10 grs (648 mg)

T20 **Methenamine**
Composition (Each Compressed Tablet): Methenamine, USP, 7 1/2 grs (500 mg)

T21 **Methenamine and Sodium Biphosphate**
Composition (Each Compressed Tablet): Methenamine, 325 mg; sodium biphosphate, 325 mg (USP)

T23 **Sodium Chloride**
Composition (Each Compressed Tablet): Sodium Chloride, USP, 2.25 g

T24 **Sodium Chloride**
Composition (Each Compressed Tablet): Sodium Chloride, USP, 1 g

T26 **Pancreatin**
Composition (Each Compressed Tablet): Pancreatin, Single Strength, equivalent to 325 mg Pancreatin, USP

T29 **Sodium Bicarbonate**
Composition (Each Compressed Tablet): Sodium Bicarbonate, USP, 10 grs (648 mg)

T32 **Amytal®**
Composition (Each Compressed Tablet): Amobarbital, USP, 100 mg

T35 **Calcium Carbonate**
Composition (Each Compressed Tablet): Calcium Carbonate, USP, Aromatic, 10 grs (648 mg)

T36 **Calcium Gluconate**
Composition (Each Compressed Tablet): Calcium Gluconate, USP, 1 g

T37 **Amytal®**
Composition (Each Compressed Tablet): Amobarbital, USP, 50 mg

T39 **Calcium Gluconate**
Composition (Each Compressed Tablet): Calcium Gluconate, USP, 7½ grs (486 mg)

T40 **Amytal®**
Composition (Each Compressed Tablet): Amobarbital, USP, 15 mg

T44 **Calcium Gluconate with Vitamin D**
Composition (Each Compressed Tablet): Calcium gluconate, 1 g; vitamin D synthetic, 1.65 mcg

T45 **Vitamin C (Cevalin®)**
Composition (Each Compressed Tablet): Ascorbic Acid, USP, 100 mg

T46 **Sulfapyridine**
Composition (Each Compressed Tablet): Sulfapyridine, USP, 0.5 g

T52 **Thiamine Hydrochloride (Betalin® S)**
Composition (Each Compressed Tablet): Thiamine Hydrochloride, USP, 10 mg

T53 **Niacinamide**
Composition (Each Compressed Tablet): Niacinamide, USP, 100 mg

T54 **Sulfadiazine**
Composition (Each Compressed Tablet): Sulfadiazine, USP, 0.5 g

T55 **Papaverine Hydrochloride**
Composition (Each Compressed Tablet): Papaverine Hydrochloride, USP, 100 mg

T56 **Amytal®**
Composition (Each Compressed Tablet): Amobarbital, USP, 30 mg

T59 **Thiamine Hydrochloride (Betalin® S)**
Composition (Each Compressed Tablet): Thiamine Hydrochloride, USP, 25 mg

T60 **Vitamin C (Cevalin®)**
Composition (Each Compressed Tablet): Ascorbic Acid, USP, 250 mg

T61 **Dibasic Calcium Phosphate**
Composition (Each Compressed Tablet): Dibasic calcium phosphate, anhydrous, equivalent to 7½ grs (486 mg) of dibasic calcium phosphate dihydrate (USP)

T62 **Thiamine Hydrochloride (Betalin® S)**
Composition (Each Compressed Tablet): Thiamine Hydrochloride, USP, 50 mg

T63 **Thiamine Hydrochloride (Betalin® S)**
Composition (Each Compressed Tablet): Thiamine Hydrochloride, USP, 100 mg

T67 **Vitamin C (Cevalin®)**
Composition (Each Compressed Tablet): Ascorbic Acid, USP, 500 mg

T72 **Pyridoxine Hydrochloride (Hexa-Betalin®)**
Composition (Each Compressed Tablet): Pyridoxine Hydrochloride, USP, 50 mg

T73 **Papaverine Hydrochloride**
Composition (Each Compressed Tablet): Papaverine Hydrochloride, USP, 200 mg

T75 **Neotrizine®**
Composition (Each Compressed Tablet): Sulfadiazine, 167 mg; sulfamerazine, 167 mg sulfamethazine, 167 mg (USP)

T91 **Paveril® Phosphate**
Composition (Each Compressed Tablet): Dioxyline phosphate, 200 mg

T93 **Isoniazid**
Composition (Each Compressed Tablet): Isoniazid, USP, 100 mg

T96 **Neomycin Sulfate**
Composition (Each Compressed Tablet): Neomycin Sulfate, USP, 500 mg (equiv. to 350 mg base)

T99 **Haldrone®**
Composition (Each Compressed Tablet): Paramethasone Acetate, USP, 1 mg

---

U01 **Haldrone®**
Composition (Each Compressed Tablet): Paramethasone Acetate, USP, 2 mg

U03 **Dymelor®**
Composition (Each Compressed Tablet): Acetohexamide, USP, 250 mg

U07 **Dymelor®**
Composition (Each Compressed Tablet): Acetohexamide, USP, 500 mg

U09 **Anhydron®**
Composition (Each Compressed Tablet): Cyclothiazide, USP, 2 mg

U23 **Isoniazid**
Composition (Each Compressed Tablet): Isoniazid, USP, 300 mg

U29 **Reserpine (Sandril®)**
Composition (Each Compressed Tablet): Reserpine, USP, 0.25 mg

U53 **Methadone Hydrochloride**
Composition (Each Disket®): Methadone Hydrochloride, USP, 40 mg

U56 **Folic Acid**
Composition (Each Compressed Tablet): Folic Acid, USP, 1 mg

4067 **A.S.A.® and Codeine Compound, No. 3**
Composition (Each Compressed Tablet): Codeine phosphate, 30 mg; aspirin, 80 mg; caffeine, 30 mg

W07-W16 (Miscellaneous)

W07 **V-Cillin K®, for Oral Solution**
Composition (When Mixed as Directed): Each 5 ml contain penicillin V potassium equivalent to penicillin V, 125 mg (USP).

W16 **V-Cillin K®, for Oral Solution**
Composition (When Mixed as Directed): Each 5 ml contain penicillin V potassium equivalent to penicillin V, 250 mg (USP).

5057 **Ceclor®, for Oral Suspension**
Composition (When Mixed as Directed): Each 5 ml contain cefaclor, 125 mg (USP).

5058 **Ceclor®, for Oral Suspension**
Composition (When Mixed as Directed): Each 5 ml contain cefaclor, 250 mg (USP).

UNIT-DOSE PACKAGING

Dispenser Strip
Identi-Dose® (unit dose medication, Lilly)
Reverse-Numbered Package
Closed-circuit control of medication from pharmacy to nurse to patient and return. Simplifies counting and dispensing whether in single-unit or prescription-size quantities. Fits into any dispensing system for ready identification and legibility, better inventory control, protection from contamination, easier handling and recording under Medicare, prevention of drug loss through pilferage or spilling, better control of Federal Controlled Substances, and less chance of medication errors.
The following products are available through normal channels of supply:

Dispenser Strip
Pulvules®
No.
C-II 303 Tuinal®, 100 mg

Identi-Dose® (ID100)
Pulvules®
No.
C-II 240 Seconal® Sodium, 100 mg
C-II 303 Tuinal®, 100 mg
C-II 304 Tuinal®, 200 mg
C-IV 364 Darvon®, 32 mg
C-IV 365 Darvon®, 65 mg
C-IV 369 Darvon® Compound-65
387 Aventyl® HCl, 10 mg
389 Aventyl® HCl, 25 mg
3061 Ceclor®, 250 mg
3062 Ceclor®, 500 mg
Tablets
No.
100 Multicebrin®
186 A.S.A.®, 5 grs
C-II 558 Codeine Sulfate, USP, 30 mg
1125 Quinidine Sulfate, USP, 200 mg
C-IV 1544 Phenobarbital, USP, 15 mg
C-IV 1545 Phenobarbital, USP, 30 mg
C-IV 1546 Phenobarbital, USP, 100 mg
1572 Ergotrate® Maleate, 0.2 mg
C-IV 1574 Phenobarbital, USP, 60 mg
1671 Papaverine Hydrochloride, USP, 100 mg
1703 Crystodigin®, 0.1 mg
1803 Neomycin Sulfate, USP, 500 mg
1842 Dymelor®, 250 mg
1843 Dymelor®, 500 mg, Yellow
C-IV 1883 Darvon-N®, 100 mg
C-IV 1890 Darvocet-N® 50
C-IV 1893 Darvocet-N® 100
Miscellaneous
M-126 V-Cillin K®, for Oral Solution, 125 mg
M-142 V-Cillin K®, for Oral Solution, 250 mg

Reverse-Numbered Package (RN500)
Pulvules®
No.
C-IV 365 Darvon®, 65 mg
Tablets
No.
C-IV 1893 Darvocet-N® 100

Single-Cut Identi-Dose® (ID500)
Tablets
No.
C-IV 1893 Darvocet-N® 100

C-II, C-III, C-IV Federal Controlled Substances.

FASPAK® ℞
AMPICILLIN SODIUM
Sterile USP
[ăm′-pĭ-sĭl″-lĭn]
For Intravenous Injection

DESCRIPTION

Ampicillin is a synthetic penicillin with a broad spectrum of bactericidal activity against penicillin-susceptible gram-positive organisms and many common gram-negative pathogens.
Sterile Ampicillin Sodium, USP, is supplied in Faspak® (flexible plastic bag, Lilly) containing 500 mg ampicillin activity (No. 7204) and 1 g ampicillin activity (No. 7205). The total sodium content is approximately 65 mg (2.84 mEq sodium ion) per g of ampicillin activity. These Faspaks are for intravenous administration only (see Dosage and Administration for directions for use).

CLINICAL PHARMACOLOGY

Ampicillin diffuses readily into most body tissues and fluids. However, substantial penetration into the cerebrospinal fluid and brain occurs only when the meninges are inflamed. Ampicillin is excreted largely unchanged in the urine, and its excretion can be delayed by concurrent administration of probenecid. The active form appears in the bile in higher concentrations than those found in serum. Ampicillin is the least serum-bound of all the penicillins, averaging about 20% compared to approximately 60 to 90% for other penicillins.
Microbiology—The following bacteria have been shown in in vitro studies to be susceptible to ampicillin.
Gram-positive organisms: Hemolytic and nonhemolytic streptococci. *Streptococcus (Diplococcus) pneumoniae*, non-penicillinase-producing staphylococci, *Clostridia* spp., *Bacillus anthracis*, *Listeria monocytogenes*, and most strains of enterococci.
Gram-positive organisms: *Haemophilis influenzae* (non-beta-lactamase-producing), *Neisseria gonorrhoeae*, *N. meningitidis*, *Proteus mirabilis*, and many strains of *Salmonella*, *Shigella*, and *Escherichia coli*.
Ampicillin does not resist destruction by penicillinase. Ampicillin Susceptibility Test Discs, 10 mcg, should be used to estimate the in vitro susceptibility of bacteria to ampicillin.

INDICATIONS AND USAGE

Ampicillin is inidcated for the treatment of infections due to susceptible gram-positive organisms including streptococci, pneumococci, penicillin G-susceptible staphylococci, and enterococci, and susceptible strains of gram-negative bacteria including non-beta-lactamase-producing *H. influenzae*, *E. coli*, *P. mirabilis*, *N. gonorrhoeae*, *N. meningitidis*, *Shigella*, *H., typhosa*, and other *Salmonella*.
Bacteriology studies to determine the causative organisms and their susceptibility to ampicillin should be peformed. Therapy may be instituted prior to obtaining results of susceptibility testing. Parenteral ampicillin should be reserved for moderately severe and severe infections and for patients who are unable to take the oral forms. A change to oral ampicillin may be made as soon as appropriate. Indicated surgical procedures should be performed.

Continued on next page

• **Identi-Code® symbol.**

Lilly—Cont.

CONTRAINDICATIONS
A history of a previous hypersensitivity reaction to any of the penicillins is a contraindication.

WARNINGS
Serious and occasionally fatal hypersensitivity (anaphylactoid) reactions have been reported in patients on penicillin therapy. Anaphylaxis is more frequent following parenteral therapy. These reactions are more apt to occur in individuals with a history of sensitivity to multiple allergens.
There have been well-documented reports of individuals with a history of cephalophorin hypersensitivity reactions who have experienced severe hypersensitivity reactions when treated with a penicillin. Before instituting therapy with a penicillin, careful inquiry should be made concerning previous hypersensitivity reactions to penicillins, cephalosporins, and other allergens.
Serious anaphylactoid reactions require immediate emergency treatment with epinephrine. Oxygen, intravenous steroids, and airway management, including intubation, should also be administered as indicated.
Usage in Pregnancy—Safety for use in pregnancy has not been established.

PRECAUTIONS
The possibility of superinfections with mycotic organisms or bacterial pathogens should be kept in mind during therapy. In such cases, discontinue the drug and substitute appropriate treatment.
As with any potent drug, periodic assessment of organ system function, including renal, hepatic, and hematopoietic, should be made during prolonged therapy.
With high urine concentrations of ampicillin, false-positive glucose reactions may occur in Clinitest® tablets or Benedict's or Fehling's solutions are used. Therefore, it is recommended that glucose tests based on enzymatic glucose oxidase reactions (such as Tes-Tape [Glucose Enzymatic Test Strip, USP, Lilly] or Clinistix®) be used.

ADVERSE REACTIONS
As with other penicillins, it may be expected that untoward reactions will be essentially limited to sensitivity phenomenona. They are more likely to occur in individuals who have previously demonstrated hypersensitivity to penicillins and in those with a history of allergy, asthma, hay fever, or urticaria.
The following adverse reactions have been reported as associated with the use of ampicillin:
Gastrointestinal—Glossitis, stomatitis, black "hairy" tongue, nausea, vomiting, enterocolitis, pseudomembranous colitis, and diarrhea. (These reactions are usually associated with oral dosage forms.)
Hypersensitivity Reactions—Skin rashes and urticaria have been reported frequently. Cases of exfoliative dermatitis and erythema multiforme have been reported. Anaphylaxis is the most serious reaction experienced and has usually been associated with the parenteral dosage form.
Note: Urticaria, other skin rashes, and serum sickness-like reactions may be controlled with antihistamines and, if necessary, systemic corticosteroids. Whenever such reactions occur, ampicillin should be discontinued, unless, in the opinion of the physician, the condition being treated is life-threatening and amenable only to ampicillin therapy. Serious anaphylactic reactions require the immediate use of epinephrine, oxygen, and intravenous steroids.
Liver—A moderate rise in serum glutamic oxaloacetic transaminases (SGOT) has been noted, particularly in infants, but the significance of this finding is unknown. Mild transitory SGOT elevations have been observed in individuals receiving larger (2 to 4 times) than usual and often-repeated intramuscular injections. Evidence indicates that glutamic oxaloacetic transaminase is released at the site of intramuscular injection of ampicillin sodium and that the presence of increased amount of this enzyme in the blood does not necessarily indicate liver involvement.
Hemic and Lymphatic Systems—Anemia, thrombocytopenia, thrombocytopenic purpura, eosinophilia, leukopenia, and agranulocytosis have been reported during therapy with the penicillins. These reactions are usually reversible on discontinuation of therapy and are believed to be hypersensitivity phenomena.
Other—Since infectious mononucleosis is viral in origin, ampicillin should not be used in the treatment. A high percentage of patients with mononucleosis who received ampicillin developed a skin rash.

DOSAGE AND ADMINISTRATION
Directions for use: Faspak units (for intravenous use) use Sterile Water for Injection or Sodium Chloride Injection for reconstitution.
Add 50 or 100 ml of water or saline to the contents of Faspaks Ampicillin Sodium, and shake to dissolve. Use only freshly prepared solutions. See stability section and label instructions for storage conditions.

CAUTION: Administer slowly by intravenous route over a period of at least 10–15 minutes. More rapid administration may result in major motor seizures.
The use of water for injection as the diluent for reconstitution of Faspak Ampicillin Sodium results in hypotonic solutions having the following osmolalities:

0.5 g ampicillin sodium plus 100 ml water for injection—	29 milliosmols
0.5 g ampicillin sodium plus 50 ml water for injection—	60 milliosmols
1 g ampicillin sodium plus 100 ml water for injection—	60 milliosmols
1 g ampicillin sodium plus 50 ml water for injection—	120 milliosmols

Slow intravenous administration is therefore advisable.
Faspak units of Sterile Ampicillin Sodium are provided for intravenous use. The following intravenous dosages are recommended.
Infections of the respiratory tract and soft tissues:
Patients weighing 40 kg (88 lb) or more: 250 to 500 mg every 6 hours.
Patients weighing less than 40 kg (88 lb): 25 to 50 mg/kg/day in equally divided doses at 6- to 8-hour intervals.
Infections of the gastrointestinal and genitourinary tracts (including those caused by N. gonorrhoeae *in females).*
Patient weighing 40 kg (88 lb) or more: 500 mg every 6 hours.
Patients weighing less than 40 kg (88 lb): 50 mg/kg/day in equally divided doses at 6- to 8-hour intervals.
In the treatment of chronic urinary tract and intestinal infections, frequent bacteriologic and clinical appraisal is necessary. Smaller doses than those recommended above should not be used. Higher doses should be used for stubborn or severe infections. In stubborn infections, therapy may be required for several weeks. It may be necessary to continue clinical and/or bacteriologic follow-up for several months after cessation of therapy.
Urethritis in males due to N. gonorrhoeae:
Adults: Two doses of 500 mg each at an interval of 8 to 12 hours. Treatment may be repeated if necessary or extended if required.
In the treatment of complications of gonorrheal urethritis, such as prostatitis and epididymitis, prolonged and intensive therapy is recommended. Cases of gonorrhea with a suspected primary lesion of syphilis should have darkfield examinations before receiving treatment. In all other cases where concomitant syphilis is suspected, monthly serologic tests should be made for a minimum of 4 months. A change to oral ampicillin may be made when appropriate.
Bacterial Meningitis
Adults and Children: 150 to 200 mg/kg/day in equally divided doses every 3 to 4 hours.
Septicemia
Adults and Children: 150 to 200 mg/kg/day.
Treatment of all infections should be continued for a minimum of 48 to 72 hours beyond the time that the patient becomes asymptomatic or evidence of bacterial eradication has been obtained. A minimum 10-day treatment is recommended for any infection caused by Group A beta-hemolytic streptococci to help prevent the occurrence of acute rheumatic fever or acute glomerulonephritis.

STABILITY
Reconstituted solutions of ampicillin sodium are stable for the time periods and with the concentrations and diluents stated in the following table:

Room Temperature (25°C)		
Diluent	*Concentrations*	*Stability Period*
Sterile Water for Injection	5 to 20 mg/ml	8 hrs
Isotonic Sodium Chloride Injection	5 to 20 mg/ml	8 hrs
Refrigerated (5°C)		
Diluent	*Concentrations*	*Stability Period*
Sterile Water for Injection	5 to 20 mg/ml	72 hrs
Isotonic Sodium Chloride Injection	5 to 20 mg/ml	72 hrs

Only the solutions listed above should be used for the intravenous infusion of Faspak Ampicillin Sodium. The concentrations should fall within the range specified. The drug concentration and the rate and volume of the infusion should be adjusted so that the total dose of ampicillin is admininistered during the stated time period.

HOW SUPPLIED
℞ **Sterile Ampicillin Sodium, USP,** Faspak® *(flexible plastic bag, Lilly)* of 96: *No. 7204,* 500 mg (equivalent to ampicillin) (NDC 0002-7204-74) and *No. 7205,* 1 g (equivalent to ampicillin) (NDC 0002-7205-74).

[082384]

BREVITAL® SODIUM Ⓒ
[*brĕv ′ĭ-tăl sō ′dĭ-ŭm*]
(methohexital sodium)
For Injection, USP
For Intravenous Use

WARNING
This drug should be administered by persons qualified in the use of intravenous anesthetics and with the ready availability of appropriate resuscitative equipment for prevention and treatment of anesthetic emergencies.

DESCRIPTION
Brevital® Sodium (Methohexital Sodium for Injection, USP, Lilly) is sodium *α-dl*-1 - methyl - 5 - allyl - 5 - (1-methyl - 2 - pentynyl) barbiturate. It differs chemically from the established barbiturate anesthetics in that it contains no sulfur.

ACTION
Methohexital sodium is a rapid, ultrashort-acting barbiturate anesthetic agent.

INDICATIONS
For induction of anesthesia, for supplementing other anesthetic agents, as intravenous anesthesia for short surgical procedures with minimum painful stimuli, or as an agent for inducing a hypnotic state.

CONTRAINDICATIONS
Methohexital sodium is contraindicated when general anesthesia is contraindicated, in patients with latent or manifest porphyria, or in patients with a known hypersensitivity to barbiturates.

WARNINGS
May be habit-forming.
Repeated or continuous infusion may cause cumulative effects resulting in prolonged somnolence and respiratory and circulatory depression.
Usage in Pregnancy—Safe use of methohexital sodium has not been established with respect to possible adverse effects on human fetal development. Therefore, if methohexital sodium is to be given to women who are pregnant, the benefits to the mother should be weighed against possible risks to the fetus. When administered to pregnant rabbits and rats at four and seven times the human dose respectively, methohexital sodium produced no evidence of teratogenicity and no fetal abnormalities.

PRECAUTIONS
Respiratory depression, apnea, or hypotension may occur owing to variations in tolerance from individual to individual or to the physical status of the patient. Caution should be exercised in debilitated patients or in those with impaired function of respiratory, circulatory, renal, hepatic, or endocrine systems.
Methohexital sodium should be used with extreme caution in patients in status asthmaticus.
Extravascular injection may cause pain, swelling, ulceration, and necrosis. Intra-arterial injection is dangerous and may produce gangrene of an extremity. The central-nervous-system (CNS) depressant effect of methohexital sodium may be additive with that of other CNS depressants, including alcohol.

ADVERSE REACTIONS
The following reactions have been reported:
- Circulatory depression
- Thrombophlebitis
- Pain at injection site
- Respiratory depression, including apnea
- Laryngospasm
- Bronchospasm
- Salivation
- Hiccups
- Skeletal-muscle hyperactivity (twitching to convulsive-like movements)
- Emergence delirium
- Headache
- Injury to nerves adjacent to injection site
- Nausea
- Emesis

Acute allergic reactions, such as erythema, pruritus, urticaria, rhinitis, dyspnea, hypotension, restlessness, anxiety, abdominal pain, and peripheral vascular collapse, have been reported with the use of Brevital® Sodium (methohexital sodium, Lilly).

DOSAGE AND ADMINISTRATION
Preanesthetic medication is generally advisable. Brevital® Sodium (methohexital sodium, Lilly) may be used with any of the recognized preanesthetic medications, but the phenothiazines are less satisfactory than the combination of an opiate and a belladonna derivative.

Facilities for assisting respirations and administering oxygen are necessary adjuncts for intravenous anesthesia.
[See table to right].
For continuous drip anesthesia, prepare a 0.2% solution by adding 500 mg of Brevital Sodium to 250 ml of diluent. For this dilution, we recommend as solvents either 5% glucose solution or isotonic (0.9%) sodium chloride solution instead of distilled water in order to avoid extreme hypotonicity.
Administration —A 1% solution is recommended for induction of anesthesia and for maintenance by intermittent injection. Dosage of all intravenous barbiturates must be individualized according to the patient's response. The usual range for Brevital® Sodium (methohexital sodium, Lilly) is 5 to 12 ml of a 1% solution (50 to 120 mg). This induction dose will provide anesthesia for five to seven minutes. The rate of injection is not fixed, but it is usually found to be about 1 ml of the 1% solution (10 mg) in five seconds. If intermittent injection of a 1% solution is used for maintenance, additional amounts of about 2 to 4 ml (20 to 40 mg) will be required every four to seven minutes.
Some anesthesiologists have preferred the continuous drip method of maintenance with a 0.2% solution. The rate of flow must be individualized for each patient. As a guide, 1 drop per second may be used.
Storage —Brevital Sodium is stable in Sterile Water for Injection at room temperature (25°C or below) for at least *six weeks.* Dextrose Injection (5%) or isotonic (0.9%) sodium chloride injection may be used as diluents, but these solutions are not stable for much more than *24 hours.* Solutions may be stored and used as long as they remain clear and colorless.

COMPATIBILITY INFORMATION

Solutions of Brevital® Sodium (methohexital sodium, Lilly) should not be mixed with acid solutions such as atropine sulfate, Metubine® Iodide (Metocurine Iodide Injection, USP, Lilly), and succinylcholine chloride. However, because of numerous requests from anesthesiologists for information regarding the chemical compatibility of these mixtures, the following is provided.
The soluble sodium salts of barbiturates are the forms used for intravenous administration. Solubility is maintained only at a relatively high (basic) *p*H. The accompanying chart contains information obtained from compatibility studies in which a 1% solution of Brevital Sodium was mixed with therapeutic amounts of agents whose solutions have a low (acid) *p*H.
Solutions of Brevital Sodium are incompatible with silicone and should not be allowed to come in contact with rubber stoppers or parts of disposable syringes that have been treated with silicone.
[See table below].

Preparation of Solutions of Brevital® Sodium (methohexital sodium)

Preparation of Solution —FOLLOW DILUTING INSTRUCTIONS EXACTLY.
Diluents —DO NOT USE DILUENTS CONTAINING BACTERIOSTATS.
Sterile Water for Injection is the preferred diluent.
Dextrose Injection (5%) or Sodium Chloride Injection (0.9%) may be used.
(Brevital Sodium is not compatible with Lactated Ringer's Injection.)
Dilution Instructions —For a 1% solution (10 mg/ml), contents of vials should be diluted as follows:
Vials No. 660 (500 mg)—add 50 ml of diluent
Vials No. 760 (500 mg)—add 50 ml of accompanying diluent
Vials No. 664 (2.5 g)—add 250 ml of diluent
Vials No. 662 (5 g)—add 500 ml of diluent

Vial No.	Amount of Diluent to Be Added to the Vial	For 1% Solution Dilute to
663 (2.5 g)	15 ml	250 ml
659 (5 g)	30 ml	500 ml

When the first dilution is made with Vials No. 663 or No. 659, the solution in the vial will be yellow. When further diluted to make a 1% solution, it must be *clear and colorless* or should not be used.

HOW SUPPLIED

Vials Brevital® Sodium (Methohexital Sodium for Injection, USP) are supplied as follows:
(Ⓒ) *No. 660,* 500 mg, 50-ml size, multiple dose, rubber-stoppered (Dry Powder), in singles (10 per carton) (NDC 0002-1446-01) and in packages of 25 (NDC 0002-1446-25).
Each vial contains—
Brevital® Sodium (methohexital sodium, Lilly) ....500 mg
Anhydrous Sodium Carbonate.... 30 mg
Contains no preservative.
(Ⓒ) *No. 760,* 500 mg, 50-ml size, multiple dose, rubber-stoppered (Dry Powder), in singles (10 per carton) (NDC 0002-1465-01). Each package contains one 50-ml vial of Sterile Water for Injection.
Each vial contains—
Brevital® Sodium (methohexital sodium, Lilly) ....500 mg
Anhydrous Sodium Carbonate.... 30 mg
Contains no preservative.
(Ⓒ) *No. 663,* 2.5 g, rubber-stoppered (Dry Powder), in singles (10 per carton) (NDC 0002-1448-01) and in packages of 25 (NDC 0002-1448-25).
Each vial contains—
Brevital® Sodium (methohexital sodium, Lilly) ....2.5 g
Anhydrous Sodium Carbonate ....150 mg
Contains no preservative.
(Ⓒ) *No. 664,* 2.5 g, 250-ml size, multiple dose, rubber-stoppered (Dry Powder), in singles (NDC 0002-1449-01) and in packages of 25 (NDC 0002-1449-25).
Each vial contains—
Brevital® Sodium (methohexital sodium, Lilly) ....2.5 g
Anhydrous Sodium Carbonate ....150 mg
Contains no preservative.
(Ⓒ) *No. 659,* 5 g, rubber-stoppered (Dry Powder), in singles (10 per carton) (NDC 0002-1445-01).
Each vial contains—
Brevital® Sodium (methohexital sodium, Lilly) ....5 g
Anhydrous Sodium Carbonate ....300 mg
Contains no preservative.
(Ⓒ) *No. 662,* 5 g, 500-ml size, multiple dose, rubber-stoppered (Dry Powder), in singles (NDC 0002-1447-01) and in packages of 25 (NDC 0002-1447-25).
Each vial contains—
Brevital® Sodium (methohexital sodium, Lilly) ....5 g
Anhydrous Sodium Carbonate ....300 mg
Contains no preservative. [101784]

Compatibility of Brevital® Sodium (methohexital sodium) with Solutions Having a Low *p*H

Active Ingredient	Potency per ml	Volume Used	Physical Change: Immediate	Physical Change: 15 min	Physical Change: 30 min	Physical Change: 1 hr
BREVITAL SODIUM	10 mg	10 ml	CONTROL			
Atropine sulfate	1/150 gr	1 ml	None	Haze		
Atropine sulfate	1/100 gr	1 ml	None	Ppt.	Ppt.	
Succinylcholine chloride	0.5 mg	4 ml	None	None	Haze	
Succinylcholine chloride	1 mg	4 ml	None	None	Haze	
Metocurine iodide	0.5 mg	4 ml	None	None	Ppt.	
Metocurine iodide	1 mg	4 ml	None	None	Ppt.	
Scopolamine hydrobromide	1/120 gr	1 ml	None	None	None	Haze
Tubocurarine chloride	3 mg	4 ml	None	Haze		

CAPASTAT® SULFATE ℞

[kăp 'a-stăt sŭl 'fāt]
(capreomycin sulfate)
Sterile, USP
Not for Pediatric Use

Warnings

The use of capreomycin in patients with renal insufficiency or preexisting auditory impairment must be undertaken with great caution, and the risk of additional eighth-nerve impairment or renal injury should be weighed against the benefits to be derived from therapy.
Refer to animal pharmacology section for additional information.
Since other parenteral antituberculosis agents (streptomycin, viomycin) also have similar and sometimes irreversible toxic effects, particularly on eighth-cranial-nerve and renal function, simultaneous administration of these agents with capreomycin is not recommended. Use with nonantituberculosis drugs (polymyxin, colistin sulfate, gentamicin, tobramycin, vancomycin, kanamycin, and neomycin) having ototoxic or nephrotoxic potential should be undertaken only with great caution.
Usage in Pregnancy—The safety of the use of capreomycin in *pregnancy* has not been determined.
Pediatric Usage—Safety of the use of capreomycin in infants and children has not been established.

DESCRIPTION

Capastat® Sulfate (capreomycin sulfate, Lilly) is a polypeptide antibiotic isolated from *Streptomyces capreolus.* It is a complex of four microbiologically active components which have been characterized in part; however, complete structural determination of all the components has not been established.
Capreomycin is supplied as the disulfate salt and is soluble in water. In complete solution, it is almost colorless.

ACTIONS

Human Pharmacology —Capastat® Sulfate (capreomycin sulfate, Lilly) is not absorbed in significant quantities from the gastrointestinal tract and must be administered parenterally. In two studies of ten patients each, peak serum concentrations following 1 g of capreomycin given intramuscularly were achieved one to two hours after administration, and average peak levels reached were 28 and 32 mcg/ml respectively (range, 20 to 47 mcg/ml). Low serum concentrations were present at 24 hours. However, 1 g of capreomycin daily for 30 days or more produced no significant accumulation in subjects with normal renal function. Two patients with marked reduction of renal function had high serum concentrations 24 hours after administration of the drug. When a 1-g dose of capreomycin was given intramuscularly to normal volunteers, 52 percent was excreted in the urine within 12 hours.
Paper chromatographic studies indicated that capreomycin is excreted essentially unaltered. Urine concentrations averaged 1.68 mg/ml (average urine volume, 228 ml) during the six hours following a 1-g dose.
Microbiology—Capreomycin is active against human strains of *Mycobacterium tuberculosis.*
The susceptibility of strains of *M. tuberculosis* in vitro varies with the media and techniques employed. In general, the minimum inhibitory concentrations for *M. tuberculosis* are lowest in liquid media that are free of egg protein (7H10 or Dubos) and range from 1 to 5 mcg/ml when the indirect method is used. Comparable inhibitory concentrations are obtained when 7H10 agar is used for direct susceptibility testing. When indirect susceptibility tests are performed on standard tube slants with 7H10 media, susceptible strains are inhibited by 10 to 25 mcg/ml. Egg-containing media, such as Löwenstein-Jensen or ATS, require concentrations of 25 to 50 mcg/ml to inhibit susceptible strains.
Cross-Resistance—Frequent cross-resistance occurs between capreomycin and viomycin. Varying degrees of cross-resistance between capreomycin and kanamycin and neomycin have been reported. No cross-resistance has been observed between capreomycin and isoniazid, aminosalicylic acid, cycloserine, streptomycin, ethionamide, or ethambutol.

INDICATIONS

Capreomycin, which is to be used concomitantly with other appropriate antituberculosis agents, is indicated in pulmonary infections caused by capreomycin-susceptible strains of *M. tuberculosis* when the primary agents (isoniazid, aminosalicylic acid, and streptomycin) have been ineffective or cannot be used because of toxicity or the presence of resistant tubercle bacilli.
Susceptibility studies should be performed to determine the presence of a capreomycin-susceptible strain of *M. tuberculosis.*

CONTRAINDICATION

Capreomycin is contraindicated in those patients who are hypersensitive to it.

Continued on next page

• **Identi-Code® symbol.**

Lilly—Cont.

PRECAUTIONS

Audiometric measurements and assessment of vestibular function should be performed prior to initiation of therapy with capreomycin and at regular intervals during treatment.

Regular tests of renal function should be made throughout the period of treatment, and reduced dosage should be employed in patients with known or suspected renal impairment.

Renal injury, with tubular necrosis, elevation of the blood urea nitrogen (BUN) or nonprotein nitrogen (NPN), and abnormal urinary sediment, has been noted. Renal function studies should be made both before capreomycin therapy is started and on a weekly basis during treatment. Slight elevation of the BUN or NPN has been observed in a significant number of patients receiving prolonged therapy. The appearance of casts, red cells, and white cells in the urine has been noted in a high percentage of these cases. Elevation of the BUN above 30 mg/100 ml or any other evidence of decreasing renal function with or without a rise in BUN levels calls for careful evaluation of the patient, and the dosage should be reduced or the drug completely withdrawn. The clinical significance of abnormal urine sediment and slight elevation in the BUN (or total NPN) observed during long-term capreomycin therapy has not been established.

Since hypokalemia may occur during capreomycin therapy, serum potassium levels should be determined frequently.

The peripheral neuromuscular blocking action that has been attributed to other polypeptide antibiotics (colistin sulfate, polymyxin A sulfate, paromomycin, and viomycin) and aminoglycoside antibiotics (streptomycin, dihydrostreptomycin, neomycin, and kanamycin) has been studied with capreomycin. A partial neuromuscular block was demonstrated after large intravenous doses of capreomycin. This action was enhanced by ether anesthesia (as has been reported for neomycin) and was antagonized by neostigmine.

Caution should be exercised in the administration of antibiotics, including capreomycin, to any patient who has demonstrated some form of allergy, particularly to drugs.

ADVERSE REACTIONS

Nephrotoxicity—In 36 percent of 722 patients treated with capreomycin, elevation of the BUN above 20 mg/100 ml and of the NPN above 35 mg/100 ml has been observed. In many instances, there was also depression of PSP excretion and abnormal urine sediment. In 10 percent of this series, the BUN elevation exceeded 30 mg/100 ml or the NPN exceeded 50 mg/100 ml.

Toxic nephritis was reported in one patient with tuberculosis and portal cirrhosis who was treated with capreomycin (1 g) and aminosalicylic acid daily for one month. This patient developed renal insufficiency and oliguria and died. Autopsy showed subsiding acute tubular necrosis.

Ototoxicity—Subclinical auditory loss was noted in approximately 11 percent of patients undergoing treatment with capreomycin. This has been a 5 to 10-decibel loss in the 4000 to 8000-CPS range. Clinically apparent hearing loss occurred in 3 percent of 722 subjects. Some audiometric changes were reversible. Other cases with permanent loss were not progressive following withdrawal of capreomycin.

Tinnitus and vertigo have occurred.

Liver—Serial tests of liver function have demonstrated a decrease in BSP excretion without change in SGOT or SGPT in the presence of preexisting liver disease. Abnormal results in liver function tests have occurred in many persons receiving capreomycin in combination with other antituberculosis agents which also are known to cause changes in hepatic function. The role of capreomycin in producing these abnormalities is not clear; however, periodic determinations of liver function are recommended.

Blood—Leukocytosis and leukopenia have been observed. The majority of patients treated have had eosinophilia exceeding 5 percent while receiving daily injections of capreomycin. This has subsided with reduction of the capreomycin dosage to 2 or 3 g weekly. Rare cases of thrombocytopenia have been reported.

Pain and induration at the injection sites have been observed. Excessive bleeding at the injection site has been reported. Sterile abscesses have been noted.

Hypersensitivity—Urticaria and maculopapular skin rashes associated in some cases with febrile reactions have been reported when capreomycin and other antituberculosis drugs were given concomitantly.

DOSAGE AND ADMINISTRATION

Capastat® Sulfate (capreomycin sulfate, Lilly) should be dissolved in 2 ml of 0.9% Sodium Chloride Injection or Sterile Water for Injection. Two to three minutes should be allowed for complete solution. For administration of a 1-g dose, the entire contents of the vial should be given. For dosages less than 1 g, the accompanying dilution table may be used. [See table below].

The solution may acquire a pale straw color and darken with time, but this is not associated with loss of potency or the development of toxicity. After reconstitution, solutions of Capastat Sulfate may be stored for 48 hours at room temperature and up to 14 days under refrigeration.

Capastat Sulfate should be given by deep intramuscular injection into a large muscle mass, since superficial injections may be associated with increased pain and the development of sterile abscesses.

Capreomycin is always administered in combination with at least one other antituberculosis agent to which the patient's strain of tubercle bacilli is susceptible. The usual dose is 1 g daily (not to exceed 20 mg/kg/day) given intramuscularly for 60 to 120 days, followed by 1 g intramuscularly two or three times weekly. (*Note*—Therapy for tuberculosis should be maintained for 18 to 24 months. If facilities for administering injectable medication are not available, a change to appropriate oral therapy is indicated on the patient's release from the hospital.)

ANIMAL PHARMACOLOGY

In addition to renal and eighth-cranial-nerve toxicity demonstrated in animal toxicology studies, two dogs have developed cataracts while on doses of 62 mg/kg and 100 mg/kg for prolonged periods.

In teratology studies, a low incidence of "wavy ribs" was noted in litters of female rats treated with daily doses of 50 mg/kg or more of capreomycin.

HOW SUPPLIED

(℞) *Vials No. 718, Capastat® Sulfate (Sterile Capreomycin Sulfate, USP),* equivalent to 1 g capreomycin activity, 10-ml size, rubber-stoppered (Dry Powder), in singles (NDC 0002-1485-01) (10 per carton).

[110585]

DILUTION TABLE FOR CAPASTAT® SULFATE (capreomycin sulfate)

Diluent Added to 1-g Vial	Volume of Capastat Sulfate Solution	Concentration* (Approx.)
2.15 ml	2.85 ml	350 mg/ml
2.63 ml	3.33 ml	300 mg/ml
3.3 ml	4 ml	250 mg/ml
4.3 ml	5 ml	200 mg/ml

*Stated in terms of mg of capreomycin activity.

CECLOR® ℞

[sē'klôr]

(cefaclor)

DESCRIPTION

Ceclor® (cefaclor, Lilly) is a semisynthetic cephalosporin antibiotic for oral administration. It is chemically designated as 3-chloro-7-D-(2-phenylglycinamido)-3-cephem-4-carboxylic acid. Ceclor is available in 250-mg and 500-mg Pulvules® and in a powder for oral suspension containing 125 or 250 mg/5 ml.

CLINICAL PHARMACOLOGY

Cefaclor is well absorbed after oral administration to fasting subjects. Total absorption is the same whether the drug is given with or without food; however, when it is taken with food, the peak concentration achieved is 50 to 75 percent of that observed when the drug is administered to fasting subjects and generally appears from three-fourths to one hour later. Following administration of 250-mg, 500-mg, and 1-g doses to fasting subjects, average peak serum levels of approximately 7, 13, and 23 mcg/ml respectively were obtained within 30 to 60 minutes. Approximately 60 to 85 percent of the drug is excreted unchanged in the urine within eight hours, the greater portion being excreted within the first two hours. During this eight-hour period, peak urine concentrations following the 250-mg, 500-mg, and 1-g doses were approximately 600, 900, and 1900 mcg/ml respectively. The serum half-life in normal subjects is 0.6 to 0.9 hour. In patients with reduced renal function, the serum half-life of cefaclor is slightly prolonged. In those with complete absence of renal function, the biologic half-life of the intact molecule is 2.3 to 2.8 hours. Excretion pathways in patients with markedly impaired renal function have not been determined. Hemodialysis shortens the half-life by 25 to 30 percent.

Microbiology—In vitro tests demonstrate that the bactericidal action of the cephalosporins results from inhibition of cell-wall synthesis. Cefaclor is usually active against the following organisms in vitro and in clinical infections:

- Staphylococci, including coagulase-positive, coagulase-negative, and penicillinase-producing strains
- *Streptococcus pyogenes* (group A beta-hemolytic streptococci)
- *S. pneumoniae* (formerly *Diplococcus pneumoniae*)
- *Escherichia coli*
- *Proteus mirabilis*
- *Klebsiella* species
- *Haemophilus influenzae,* including some beta-lactamase-producing ampicillin-resistant strains

Note: Pseudomonas species, *Acinetobacter calcoaceticus* (formerly *Mima* and *Herellea* species), and most strains of enterococci (*S. faecalis,* group D streptococci), *Enterobacter* species, indole-positive *Proteus,* and *Serratia* species are resistant to cefaclor. When tested by in vitro methods, staphylococci exhibit cross-resistance between cefaclor and methicillin-type antibiotics.

Disc Susceptibility Tests—Quantitative methods that require measurement of zone diameters give the most precise estimates of antibiotic susceptibility. One such procedure* has been recommended for use with discs for testing susceptibility to cephalothin. The currently accepted zone diameter interpretative criteria for the cephalothin disc are appropriate for determining bacterial susceptibility to cefaclor. With this procedure, a report from the laboratory of "resistant" indicates that the infecting organism is not likely to respond to therapy. A report of "intermediate susceptibility" suggests that the organism would be susceptible if the infection is confined to tissues and fluids (e.g., urine) in which high antibiotic levels can be obtained or if high dosage is used.

INDICATIONS AND USAGE

Ceclor® (cefaclor, Lilly) is indicated in the treatment of the following infections when caused by susceptible strains of the designated microorganisms:

Otitis media caused by *S. pneumoniae (D. pneumoniae), H. influenzae,* staphylococci, and *S. pyogenes* (group A beta-hemolytic streptococci)

Lower respiratory infections, including pneumonia caused by *S. pneumoniae (D. pneumoniae), H. influenzae,* and *S. pyogenes* (group A beta-hemolytic streptococci)

Upper respiratory infections, including pharyngitis and tonsillitis caused by *S. pyogenes* (group A beta-hemolytic streptococci)

Note: Penicillin is the usual drug of choice in the treatment and prevention of streptococcal infections, including the prophylaxis of rheumatic fever. Ceclor is generally effective in the eradication of streptococci from the nasopharynx; however, substantial data establishing the efficacy of Ceclor in the subsequent prevention of rheumatic fever are not available at present.

Urinary tract infections, including pyelonephritis and cystitis caused by *E. coli, P. mirabilis, Klebsiella* species, and coagulase-negative staphylococci

Skin and skin-structure infections caused by *Staphylococcus aureus* and *S. pyogenes* (group A beta-hemolytic streptococci)

Appropriate culture and susceptibility studies should be performed to determine susceptibility of the causative organism to Ceclor.

CONTRAINDICATION

Ceclor® (cefaclor, Lilly) is contraindicated in patients with known allergy to the cephalosporin group of antibiotics.

WARNINGS

IN PENICILLIN-SENSITIVE PATIENTS, CEPHALOSPORIN ANTIBIOTICS SHOULD BE ADMINISTERED CAUTIOUSLY. THERE IS CLINICAL AND LABORATORY EVIDENCE OF PARTIAL CROSS-ALLERGENICITY OF THE PENICILLINS AND THE CEPHALOSPORINS, AND THERE ARE INSTANCES IN WHICH PATIENTS HAVE HAD REACTIONS, INCLUDING ANAPHYLAXIS, TO BOTH DRUG CLASSES.

Antibiotics, including Ceclor® (cefaclor, Lilly), should be administered cautiously to any patient who has demonstrated some form of allergy, particularly to drugs.

Pseudomembranous colitis has been reported with virtually all broad-spectrum antibiotics (including macrolides, semisynthetic penicillins, and cephalosporins); therefore, it is important to consider its diagnosis in patients who develop diarrhea in association with the use of antibiotics. Such colitis may range in severity from mild to life-threatening.

Treatment with broad-spectrum antibiotics alters the normal flora of the colon and may permit overgrowth of clostridia. Studies indicate that a toxin produced by *Clostridium difficile* is one primary cause of antibiotic-associated colitis.

Mild cases of pseudomembranous colitis usually respond to drug discontinuance alone. In moderate to severe cases, management should include sigmoidoscopy, appropriate bacteriologic studies, and fluid, electrolyte, and protein supplementation. When the colitis does not improve after the drug has been discontinued, or when it is severe, oral vancomycin is the drug of choice for antibiotic-associated pseudomembranous colitis produced by *C. difficile*. Other causes of colitis should be ruled out.

PRECAUTIONS

General Precautions—If an allergic reaction to cefaclor occurs, the drug should be discontinued, and, if necessary, the patient should be treated with appropriate agents, e.g., pressor amines, antihistamines, or corticosteroids.

Prolonged use of Ceclor® (cefaclor, Lilly) may result in the overgrowth of nonsusceptible organisms. Careful observation of the patient is essential. If superinfection occurs during therapy, appropriate measures should be taken.

Positive direct Coombs' tests have been reported during treatment with the cephalosporin antibiotics. In hematologic studies or in transfusion cross-matching procedures when antiglobulin tests are performed on the minor side or in Coombs' testing of newborns whose mothers have received cephalosporin antibiotics before parturition, it should be recognized that a positive Coombs' test may be due to the drug.

Ceclor should be administered with caution in the presence of markedly impaired renal function. Under such conditions, careful clinical observation and laboratory studies should be made because safe dosage may be lower than that usually recommended.

As a result of administration of Ceclor, a false-positive reaction for glucose in the urine may occur. This has been observed with Benedict's and Fehling's solutions and also with Clinitest® tablets but not with Tes-Tape® (Glucose Enzymatic Test Strip, USP, Lilly).

Broad-spectrum antibiotics should be prescribed with caution in individuals with a history of gastrointestinal disease, particularly colitis.

Usage in Pregnancy—Pregnancy Category B—Reproduction studies have been performed in mice and rats at doses up to 12 times the human dose and in ferrets given three times the maximum human dose and have revealed no evidence of impaired fertility or harm to the fetus due to Ceclor. There are, however, no adequate and well-controlled studies in pregnant women. Because animal reproduction studies are not always predictive of human response, this drug should be used during pregnancy only if clearly needed.

Nursing Mothers—Small amounts of Ceclor have been detected in mother's milk following administration of single 500-mg doses. Average levels were 0.18, 0.20, 0.21, and 0.16 mcg/ml at two, three, four, and five hours respectively. Trace amounts were detected at one hour. The effect on nursing infants is not known. Caution should be exercised when Ceclor is administered to a nursing woman.

Usage in Children—Safety and effectiveness of this product for use in infants less than one month of age have not been established.

ADVERSE REACTIONS

Adverse effects considered related to therapy with Ceclor® (cefaclor, Lilly) are listed below:

Gastrointestinal symptoms occur in about 2.5 percent of patients and include diarrhea (1 in 70).

Symptoms of pseudomembranous colitis may appear either during or after antibiotic treatment. Nausea and vomiting have been reported rarely. As with some penicillins and some other cephalosporins, transient hepatitis and cholestatic jaundice have been reported rarely.

Hypersensitivity reactions have been reported in about 1.5 percent of patients and include morbilliform eruptions (1 in 100). Pruritus, urticaria, and positive Coombs' tests each occur in less than 1 in 200 patients. Cases of serum-sickness-like reactions (erythema multiforme or the above skin manifestations accompanied by arthritis/arthralgia and, frequently, fever) have been reported. These reactions are apparently due to hypersensitivity and have usually occurred during or following a second course of therapy with Ceclor. Such reactions have been reported more frequently in children than in adults. Signs and symptoms usually occur a few days after initiation of therapy and subside within a few days after cessation of therapy. No serious sequelae have been reported. Antihistamines and corticosteroids appear to enhance resolution of the syndrome.

Cases of anaphylaxis have been reported, half of which have occurred in patients with a history of penicillin allergy.

Other effects considered related to therapy include eosinophilia (1 in 50 patients) and genital pruritus or vaginitis (less than 1 in 100 patients).

Causal Relationship Uncertain—CNS—Rarely, reversible hyperactivity, nervousness, insomnia, confusion, hypertonia, dizziness, and somnolence have been reported.

Transitory abnormalities in clinical laboratory test results have been reported. Although they were of uncertain etiology, they are listed below to serve as alerting information for the physician.

Hepatic—Slight elevations in SGOT, SGPT, or alkaline phosphatase values (1 in 40).

Hematopoietic—Transient fluctuations in leukocyte count, predominantly lymphocytosis occurring in infants and young children (1 in 40).

Renal—Slight elevations in BUN or serum creatinine (less than 1 in 500) or abnormal urinalysis (less than 1 in 200).

DOSAGE AND ADMINISTRATION

Ceclor® (cefaclor, Lilly) is administered orally.

Adults—The usual adult dosage is 250 mg every eight hours. For more severe infections (such as pneumonia) or those caused by less susceptible organisms, doses may be doubled. Doses of 4 g/day have been administered safely to normal subjects for 28 days, but the total daily dosage should not exceed this amount.

Children—The usual recommended daily dosage for children is 20 mg/kg/day in divided doses every eight hours, as indicated:

	Ceclor Suspension	
Child's Weight	125 mg/5 ml	250 mg/5 ml
9 kg	½ tsp t.i.d.	
18 kg	1 tsp t.i.d.	½ tsp t.i.d.

In more serious infections, otitis media, and infections caused by less susceptible organisms, 40 mg/kg/day are recommended, with a maximum dosage of 1 g/day.

Ceclor may be administered in the presence of impaired renal function. Under such a condition, the dosage usually is unchanged (*see* PRECAUTIONS).

In the treatment of beta-hemolytic streptococcal infections, a therapeutic dosage of Ceclor should be administered for at least ten days.

HOW SUPPLIED

(℞) *Ceclor® (Cefaclor, USP), for Oral Suspension, M-5057*, 125 mg/5 ml (strawberry flavor) and *M-5058*, 250 mg/5 ml (strawberry flavor), in 75 (NDC 0002-5057-18 and NDC 0002-5058-18) and 150-ml-size (NDC 0002-5057-68 and NDC 0002-5058-68) packages.

Directions for mixing are included on the label. After mixing, store in a refrigerator. Shake well before using. Keep tightly closed. The mixture may be kept for 14 days without significant loss of potency. Discard unused portion after 14 days.

(℞) *Pulvules® Ceclor® (Cefaclor, USP): No. 3061*, 250 mg (White Opaque Body, Purple Opaque Cap), and *No. 3062*, 500 mg (Gray Opaque Body, Purple Opaque Cap), in bottles of 15 (NDC 0002-3061-15 and NDC 0002-3062-15) and 100 (NDC 0002-3061-02 and NDC 0002-3062-02) and in 10 strips of 10 individually labeled blisters each containing one Pulvule (ID100) (NDC 0002-3061-33 and NDC 0002-3062-33).

M-5057—150 ml—6505-01-141-9488
M-5058—75 ml—6505-01-152-3607
M-5058—150 ml—6505-01-141-9489
Pulvules® No. 3061—100's—6505-01-150-2101

Shown in Product Identification Section, page 415

* Bauer, A. W., Kirby, W. M. M., Sherris, J. C., and Turck, M.: Antibiotic Susceptibility Testing by a Standardized Single Disk Method, Am. J. Clin. Pathol, *45*: 493, 1966; Standardized Disc Susceptibility Test, Federal Register, *39*: 19182–19184, 1974.

[030486]

CEFACLOR, *see* Ceclor® (cefaclor, Lilly).

CEFAMANDOLE NAFATE, *see* Mandol® (cefamandole nafate, Lilly).

CEFAZOLIN SODIUM, *see* Kefzol® (cefazolin sodium, Lilly).

CEFTAZIDIME, *see* Tazidime™ (ceftazidime, Lilly).

CEFUROXIME SODIUM, *see* Kefurox™ (cefuroxime sodium, Lilly).

CEPHALOTHIN SODIUM, *see* Keflin® (cephalothin sodium, Lilly).

CRYSTODIGIN® ℞

[*krĭs-tō-dĭj ′ĭn*]
(digitoxin)
Tablets, USP

DESCRIPTION

Crystodigin® (digitoxin, Lilly) is a crystalline-pure single cardiac glycoside obtained from *Digitalis purpurea* and is identical in pharmacologic action with whole-leaf digitalis. Digitoxin is the most slowly excreted of all digitalis compounds (excretion time is 14 to 21 days). It is most useful in patients with impaired renal function, since excretion and metabolism are independent of renal function.

Crystodigin is noted for its uniform potency, complete absorption, and lack of gastrointestinal irritation. It permits accurate dosage adjustments to produce maximum therapeutic effect smoothly and dependably.

Crystodigin, for oral administration, is available in tablets containing 0.05, 0.1, or 0.15 mg crystalline digitoxin.

The tablets may contain any or all of the following: D & C Yellow No. 10, F D & C Red No. 40, F D & C Yellow No. 6, lactose, magnesium stearate, povidone, and starch.

Digitoxin is a cardiotonic glycoside. The chemical name is card-20 (22) - enolide,3-[(*O*-2,6-dideoxy-β- D -*ribo* -hexopyranosyl-(1→4)-*O*-2,6 - dideoxy-β- D - *ribo* -hexopyranosyl-(1→4) -2,6- dideoxy- β-D- *ribo*- hexopyranosyl) oxy]-14-hydroxy,(3β,5β) -. The empirical formula of digitoxin is $C_{41}H_{64}O_{13}$.

CLINICAL PHARMACOLOGY

The cellular basis for the inotropic effects of digitalis is probably enhancement of excitation-contraction coupling, that process by which chemical energy is converted into mechanical energy when triggered by membrane depolarization. Most evidence relates this process to the entry of calcium ions into the cell during depolarization of the membrane and / or to the release of calcium from intracellular binding sites on the sarcoplasmic reticulum. The free calcium ion mediates the interaction of actin and myosin, resulting in contraction.

The amount of glycoside absorbed depends largely on its polarity, which is a function of the net electronic charge on the molecule. The more nonpolar or lipid soluble, the better is the absorption, because of the greater permeability of lipid membrane of the intestinal mucosa for lipid-soluble substances. The nonpolar, lipophilic digitoxin is completely absorbed; the oral dose, therefore, is the same as the intravenous dose. Other glycosides are not as well absorbed.

Nonpolar digitoxin is over 90 percent bound to tissue proteins. The firm binding of digitoxin to protein is responsible for its long half-life (seven to nine days).

Digitoxin differs from other commonly used glycosides not only in its firm binding to protein but also because it is metabolized in the liver, with the only active metabolite being digoxin, which represents only a small fraction of the total metabolites. All other metabolites are inert and are probably excreted as such in the urine. The portion of digitoxin that is not metabolized is excreted in the bile to the intestines and recycled to the liver until it is completely metabolized. The portion of digitoxin that is bound to protein is in equilibrium with free digitoxin in the serum. Thus, as more and more of the free digitoxin is metabolized after a single dose, there is proportionately less bound digitoxin.

INDICATIONS AND USAGE

Crystodigin® (digitoxin, Lilly) is indicated in the treatment of heart failure, atrial flutter, atrial fibrillation, and supraventricular tachycardia. Parenteral administration of Crystodigin is indicated for neonates and immature infants.

CONTRAINDICATIONS

If the indications are carefully observed, there are few contraindications to digitalis therapy except toxic response to digitalis or idiosyncrasy, ventricular tachycardia, beriberi heart disease, and some instances of the hypersensitive carotid sinus syndrome.

Patients already taking digitalis preparations must not be given the rapid digitalizing dose of Crystodigin® (digitoxin, Lilly) or parenteral calcium.

WARNINGS

Many of the arrhythmias for which digitalis is advised are identical with those reflecting digitalis intoxication. When the possibility of digitalis intoxication cannot be excluded, cardiac glycosides should be withheld temporarily if the clinical situation permits.

The patient with congestive heart failure may complain of nausea and vomiting. Since these symptoms may also be associated with digitalis intoxication, a clinical determination of their cause must be attempted before further administration of the drug.

Cases of idiopathic hypertrophic subaortic stenosis must be managed with extreme care. Unless cardiac failure is severe, it is doubtful whether digitalis should be employed.

Children—During the first month of life, infants have a sharply defined tolerance to digitalis. Impaired renal function must also be considered. Premature and immature infants are particularly sensitive, and reduction in dosage may be necessary.

The presence of acute glomerulonephritis accompanied by congestive failure requires extreme care in digitalization. A relatively low total dose, administered in divided doses, and concomitant use of reserpine or other antihypertensive agents have been recommended. Constant ECG monitoring

Continued on next page

• **Identi-Code® symbol.**

Lilly—Cont.

is essential. Digitalis should be discontinued as soon as possible.

Patients with rheumatic carditis, especially when severe, are unusually sensitive to digitalis and prone to disturbances of rhythm. If heart failure develops, digitalization may be tried with relatively low doses; these must be cautiously increased until a beneficial effect is obtained. If a therapeutic trial does not result in improvement, the drug should be discontinued.

NOTE: Digitalis glycosides are an important cause of accidental poisoning in children.

PRECAUTIONS

General Precautions—When the risk of digitalis intoxication is great, the use of a short-acting, rapidly eliminated glycoside, such as digoxin, is advisable. Although intoxication cannot always be prevented by the selection of one glycoside over another, certain glycosides may be preferred in patients who have fixed disabilities (e.g., liver impairment, drug intolerance). However, digitoxin can be used in patients with impaired renal function.

Newborn infants with heart disease, especially prematures, are particularly susceptible to digitalis intoxication, and frequent electrocardiographic monitoring is essential in these patients. Special care must likewise be exercised in elderly patients receiving digitalis because their body mass tends to be small and renal clearance is likely to be reduced. In addition, digitalis must be used cautiously in the presence of active heart disease, such as acute myocardial infarction or acute myocarditis. In patients with acute or unstable chronic atrial fibrillation, digitalis may not normalize the ventricular rate even when the serum concentration exceeds the usual therapeutic level. Although these patients may be less sensitive to the toxic effects of digitalis than are patients with normal sinus rhythm, dosage should not be increased to potentially toxic levels.

Hypokalemia predisposes to digitalis toxicity, and even a moderate decrease in the concentration of serum potassium can precipitate serious arrhythmias.

Impaired liver function may necessitate reduction in dosage of any digitalis preparation, including digitoxin.

Sensitive radioimmunoassay techniques have been developed for measuring serum levels of digitoxin, and these procedures can be instituted in almost any hospital. Serum levels must, however, be evaluated in conjunction with clinical history and the results of the electrocardiogram and other laboratory tests. A therapeutic serum level for one patient may be excessive or inadequate for another patient.

Drug Interactions—The synthesis of microsomal enzymes that metabolize digitoxin in the liver is subject to stimulation by a number of drugs, such as antihistamines, anticonvulsants, barbiturates, oral hypoglycemic agents, and others.

When digitoxin is the glycoside used for digitalis maintenance, drugs that are liver-microsomal-enzyme inducers should not be used at the same time. Phenobarbital, phenylbutazone, and diphenylhydantoin will increase the rate of metabolism of digitoxin. In patients receiving 60 mg of phenobarbital three times a day for 12 weeks, the steady-state concentration of digitoxin in plasma fell approximately 50 percent when the drugs were administered concurrently and returned to previous levels when phenobarbital was discontinued.

When drugs that increase the rate of metabolism of digitoxin in the liver are discontinued, toxicity may occur.

Hypokalemia is most frequently encountered in patients receiving concomitant diuretic therapy, because the most widely used and most effective diuretics (i.e., thiazides and furosemide) increase the urinary loss of potassium. Prescribing a potassium-sparing agent (spironolactone or triamterene) together with the potassium-wasting diuretic is a reliable means for maintaining the serum potassium level. Alternatively, potassium chloride supplements may be prescribed.

Mineralocorticoids (e.g., prednisone) and, rarely, certain antibiotics (e.g., amphotericin B) may also cause increased excretion of potassium.

Usage in Pregnancy—Pregnancy Category C—Animal reproduction studies have not been conducted with Crystodigin. It is also not known whether this drug can cause fetal harm when administered to a pregnant woman or can affect reproduction capacity. Crystodigin should be given to a pregnant woman only if clearly needed.

Labor and Delivery—No information is available concerning the use of Crystodigin in labor and delivery.

Nursing Mothers—It is not known whether this drug is excreted in human milk. Because many drugs are excreted in human milk, caution should be exercised when Crystodigin is administered to a nursing woman.

ADVERSE REACTIONS

Anorexia, nausea, and vomiting have been reported. These effects are central in origin, but following large oral doses, there is also a local emetic action. Abdominal discomfort or pain and diarrhea may also occur.

OVERDOSAGE

Overdosage causes side effects, such as mental depression, anorexia, nausea, vomiting, premature beats, complete heart block, AV dissociation, ventricular tachycardia, ventricular fibrillation, restlessness, yellow vision, mental confusion, disorientation, and delirium.

Alterations in cardiac rate and rhythm occurring in digitalis poisoning may simulate almost any known type of arrhythmia seen clinically. Extrasystoles are probably the most frequent effect. An electrocardiogram is necessary in the clinical management of the patient to aid in the differentiation of arrhythmia due to digitalis poisoning from that due to heart disease. Older patients and particularly those with disease of the coronary arteries and impaired myocardial blood supply are more susceptible to these untoward effects. Sinus arrhythmia may occur early as a minor toxic effect. Paroxysmal atrial and ventricular tachycardia call for immediate cessation of the drug. Atrial fibrillation can occur following large doses of digitalis. Ventricular fibrillation is the most common cause of death from digitalis poisoning.

Potassium ion is probably the best agent for prompt suppression of digitalis arrhythmias. It can be administered intravenously in the form of potassium chloride at a rate of 0.5 mEq/minute in sodium chloride (isotonic) or dextrose (5 percent) solution containing 50 to 100 mEq of potassium per liter. Administration of the potassium salt in normal saline is preferred. Constant electrocardiographic monitoring is essential during injection of the solution. Since the action of potassium ion lasts only minutes after infusion is discontinued, oral therapy with potassium chloride may be given for prolonged suppression of arrhythmias. Potassium is contraindicated in the presence of renal failure. Diphenylhydantoin may be used if potassium fails or is contraindicated. If both potassium and diphenylhydantoin fail, procainamide and quinidine can be used. Disodium edetate has been used for terminating digitalis-induced ventricular arrhythmias and abnormalities of atrioventricular conduction.

DOSAGE AND ADMINISTRATION

Adults: Slow Digitalization—0.2 mg twice daily for a period of four days, followed by maintenance dosage. *Rapid Digitalization*—Preferably 0.6 mg initially, followed by 0.4 mg and then 0.2 mg at intervals of four to six hours. *Maintenance Dosage*—Ranges from 0.05 to 0.3 mg daily, the most common dose being 0.15 mg daily.

Children: Digitalization must be individualized. Generally, premature and immature infants are particularly sensitive and require reduced parenteral dosage of Crystodigin that must be determined by careful titration.

After the neonatal period, the dose is as follows:

Under one year of age—0.045 mg/kg
One to two years of age—0.04 mg/kg
Over two years of age—0.03 mg/kg (0.75 mg/m^2)

The total dose should be divided into three, four, or more portions, with six hours or more between doses.

For a maintenance dose, the patient should be given one-tenth of the digitalizing dose.

HOW SUPPLIED

(℞) *Tablets Crystodigin® (Digitoxin Tablets, USP)* (scored): *No. 1736, J75,** 0.05 mg, Orange, in bottles of 100 (NDC 0002-1075-02); *No. 1703, J60,** 0.1 mg, Pink, in bottles of 100 (NDC 0002-1060-02) and 500 (NDC 0002-1060-03); *No. 1737, J76,** 0.15 mg, Yellow, in bottles of 100 (NDC 0002-1076-02).

[011786]

Shown in Product Identification Section, page 415

CYCLOSERINE, *see* Seromycin® (cycloserine, Lilly).

DARVOCET-N® 50 Ⓒ

[där'vō-sĕt ĕn]

and

DARVOCET-N® 100

(propoxyphene napsylate and acetaminophen)

USP

DARVON-N®

[där'vŏn ĕn]

(propoxyphene napsylate)

USP

DARVON-N® WITH A.S.A.®

[där'vŏn ĕn wĭth ā'ĕs-ā]

(propoxyphene napsylate and aspirin)

USP

DESCRIPTION

Propoxyphene napsylate (Darvon-N®) is an odorless white crystalline solid with a bitter taste. It is very slightly soluble in water and soluble in methanol, ethanol, chloroform, and acetone. Chemically, it is α-(+)- 4-(Dimethylamino) -3 - methyl - 1, 2 - diphenyl - 2 - butanol Propionate (ester) 2-Naphthalene-sulfonate (salt) Hydrate.

Propoxyphene napsylate differs from propoxyphene hydrochloride in that it allows more stable liquid dosage forms and tablet formulations. Because of differences in molecular weight, a dose of 100 mg of propoxyphene napsylate is required to supply an amount of propoxyphene equivalent to that present in 65 mg of propoxyphene hydrochloride.

Each tablet of Darvocet-N 50 contains 50 mg propoxyphene napsylate and 325 mg acetaminophen.

Each tablet of Darvocet-N 100 contains 100 mg propoxyphene napsylate and 650 mg acetaminophen.

Tablets Darvocet-N 50 and Darvocet-N 100 also contain amberlite, cellulose, F D & C Yellow No. 6, magnesium stearate, stearic acid, titanium dioxide, and other inactive ingredients.

Each 5 ml of Suspension Darvon-N contain 50 mg propoxyphene napsylate.

Each tablet of Darvon-N contains 100 mg propoxyphene napsylate.

Each tablet and suspension of Darvon-N may also contain any or all of the following: butylparaben, cellulose, D & C Yellow No. 10, F D & C Yellow No. 6, flavors, glucose, hydroxypropyl methylcellulose, iron oxide, lactose, magnesium stearate, methylparaben, propylparaben, saccharin, silicon dioxide, silicone, sodium-2-naphthalene sulfonate, starch, stearic acid, sucrose, titanium dioxide, and other inactive ingredients.

Each tablet of Darvon-N with A.S.A. contains 100 mg propoxyphene napsylate and 325 mg aspirin.

Each tablet Darvon-N with A.S.A. also contains cellulose, F D & C Yellow No. 6, silicon dioxide, starch, stearic acid, titanium dioxide, yellow iron oxide, and other inactive ingredients.

CLINICAL PHARMACOLOGY

Propoxyphene is a centrally acting narcotic analgesic agent. Equimolar doses of propoxyphene hydrochloride or napsylate provide similar plasma concentrations. Following administration of 65, 130, or 195 mg of propoxyphene hydrochloride, the bioavailability of propoxyphene is equivalent to that of 100, 200, or 300 mg respectively of propoxyphene napsylate. Peak plasma concentrations of propoxyphene are reached in two to two and one-half hours. After a 100-mg oral dose of propoxyphene napsylate, peak plasma levels of 0.05 to 0.1 mcg/ml are achieved. As shown in Figure 1, the napsylate salt tends to be absorbed more slowly than the hydrochloride. At or near therapeutic doses, this difference is small when compared with that among subjects and among doses. (See Figure 1)

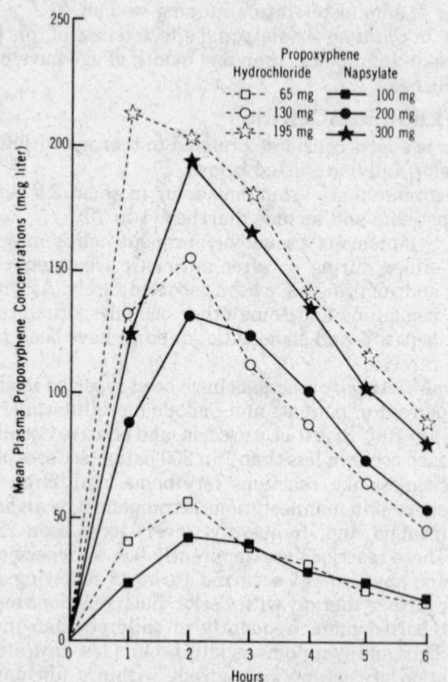

Figure 1. Mean plasma concentrations of propoxyphene in eight human subjects following oral administration of 65 and 130 mg of the hydrochloride salt and 100 and 200 mg of the napsylate salt and in seven given 195 mg of the hydrochloride and 300 mg of the napsylate salt

Because of this several hundredfold difference in solubility, the absorption rate of very large doses of the napsylate salt is significantly lower than that of equimolar doses of the hydrochloride.

Repeated doses of propoxyphene at six-hour intervals lead to increasing plasma concentrations, with a plateau after the ninth dose at 48 hours.

Propoxyphene is metabolized in the liver to yield norpropoxyphene. Propoxyphene has a half-life of six to 12 hours, whereas that of norpropoxyphene is 30 to 36 hours.

Norpropoxyphene has substantially less central-nervous-system-depressant effect than propoxyphene but a greater local anesthetic effect, which is similar to that of amitriptyline and antiarrhythmic agents, such as lidocaine and quinidine.
In animal studies in which propoxyphene and norpropoxyphene were continuously infused in large amounts, intracardiac conduction time (PR and QRS intervals) was prolonged. Any intracardiac conduction delay attributable to high concentrations of norpropoxyphene may be of relatively long duration.

ACTIONS

Propoxyphene is a mild narcotic analgesic structurally related to methadone. The potency of propoxyphene napsylate is from two-thirds to equal that of codeine.
Darvocet-N 50 and Darvocet-N 100 provide the analgesic activity of propoxyphene napsylate and the antipyretic-analgesic activity of acetaminophen.
The combination of propoxyphene and acetaminophen produces greater analgesia than that produced by either propoxyphene or acetaminophen administered alone.
The combination of propoxyphene with aspirin produces greater analgesia than that produced by either drug administered alone.

INDICATIONS

Darvocet-N 50, Darvocet-N 100, and Darvon-N with A.S.A. are indicated for the relief of mild to moderate pain, either when pain is present alone or when it is accompanied by fever.
Darvon-N® (propoxyphene napsylate, Lilly) is indicated for the relief of mild to moderate pain.

CONTRAINDICATIONS

Hypersensitivity to propoxyphene, acetaminophen, or aspirin.

WARNINGS

- **Do not prescribe propoxyphene for patients who are suicidal or addiction-prone.**
- **Prescribe propoxyphene with caution for patients taking tranquilizers or antidepressant drugs and patients who use alcohol in excess.**
- **Tell your patients not to exceed the recommended dose and to limit their intake of alcohol.**

Propoxyphene products in excessive doses, either alone or in combination with other CNS depressants, including alcohol, are a major cause of drug-related deaths. Fatalities within the first hour of overdosage are not uncommon. In a survey of deaths due to overdosage conducted in 1975, in approximately 20 percent of the fatal cases, death occurred within the first hour (5 percent occurred within 15 minutes). Propoxyphene should not be taken in doses higher than those recommended by the physician. The judicious prescribing of propoxyphene is essential to the safe use of this drug. With patients who are depressed or suicidal, consideration should be given to the use of non-narcotic analgesics. Patients should be cautioned about the concomitant use of propoxyphene products and alcohol because of potentially serious CNS-additive effects of these agents. Because of its added depressant effects, propoxyphene should be prescribed with caution for those patients whose medical condition requires the concomitant administration of sedatives, tranquilizers, muscle relaxants, antidepressants, or other CNS-depressant drugs. Patients should be advised of the additive depressant effects of these combinations.
Many of the propoxyphene-related deaths have occurred in patients with previous histories of emotional disturbances or suicidal ideation or attempts as well as histories of misuse of tranquilizers, alcohol, and other CNS-active drugs. Some deaths have occurred as a consequence of the accidental ingestion of excessive quantities of propoxyphene alone or in combination with other drugs. Patients taking propoxyphene should be warned not to exceed the dosage recommended by the physician.

Drug Dependence—Propoxyphene, when taken in higher-than-recommended doses over long periods of time, can produce drug dependence characterized by psychic dependence and, less frequently, physical dependence and tolerance. Propoxyphene will only partially suppress the withdrawal syndrome in individuals physically dependent on morphine or other narcotics. The abuse liability of propoxyphene is qualitatively similar to that of codeine although quantitatively less, and propoxyphene should be prescribed with the same degree of caution appropriate to the use of codeine.
Usage in Ambulatory Patients—Propoxyphene may impair the mental and/or physical abilities required for the performance of potentially hazardous tasks, such as driving a car or operating machinery. The patient should be cautioned accordingly.
Warning—Reyes syndrome is a rare but serious disease which can follow flu or chickenpox in children and teenagers. While the cause of Reyes syndrome is unknown, some reports claim aspirin (or salicylates) may increase the risk of developing this disease.

PRECAUTIONS

General—Propoxyphene should be administered with caution to patients with hepatic or renal impairment, since higher serum concentrations or delayed elimination may occur.
Salicylates should be used with extreme caution in the presence of peptic ulcer or coagulation abnormalities.
Drug Interactions—The CNS-depressant effect of propoxyphene is additive with that of other CNS depressants, including alcohol.
As is the case with many medicinal agents, propoxyphene may slow the metabolism of a concomitantly administered drug. Should this occur, the higher serum concentrations of that drug may result in increased phamacologic or adverse effects of that drug. Such occurrences have been reported when propoxyphene was administered to patients on antidepressants, anticonvulsants, or warfarinlike drugs.
Salicylates may enhance the effect of anticoagulants and inhibit the uricosuric effect of uricosuric agents.
Usage in Pregnancy—Safe use in pregnancy has not been established relative to possible adverse effects on fetal development. Instances of withdrawal symptoms in the neonate have been reported following usage during pregnancy. Therefore, propoxyphene should not be used in pregnant women unless, in the judgment of the physician, the potential benefits outweigh the possible hazards.
Usage in Nursing Mothers—Low levels of propoxyphene have been detected in human milk. In postpartum studies involving nursing mothers who were given propoxyphene, no adverse effects were noted in infants receiving mother's milk.
Usage in Children—Propoxyphene is not recommended for use in children, because documented clinical experience has been insufficient to establish safety and a suitable dosage regimen in the pediatric age group.
A Patient Information Sheet is available for these products. See text following "HOW SUPPLIED" section below.

ADVERSE REACTIONS

In a survey conducted in hospitalized patients, less than 1 percent of patients taking propoxyphene hydrochloride at recommended doses experienced side effects. The most frequently reported have been dizziness, sedation, nausea, and vomiting. Some of these adverse reactions may be alleviated if the patient lies down.
Other adverse reactions include constipation, abdominal pain, skin rashes, lightheadedness, headache, weakness, euphoria, dysphoria, and minor visual disturbances.
Cases of liver dysfunction have been reported.

DOSAGE AND ADMINISTRATION

These products are given orally. The usual dose of Darvocet-N 50 or Darvocet-N 100 is 100 mg propoxyphene napsylate and 650 mg acetaminophen every four hours as needed for pain.
The usual dose of Darvon-N® (propoxyphene napsylate, Lilly) is 100 mg every four hours as needed for pain.
The usual dose of Darvon-N with A.S.A. is 100 mg propoxyphene napsylate and 325 mg aspirin every four hours as needed for pain.
The maximum recommended dose of propoxyphene napsylate is 600 mg per day.
Consideration should be given to a reduced total daily dosage in patients with hepatic or renal impairment.

MANAGEMENT OF OVERDOSAGE

In all cases of suspected overdosage, call your regional Poison Control Center to obtain the most up-to-date information about the treatment of overdosage. This recommendation is made because, in general, information regarding the treatment of overdosage may change more rapidly than do package inserts.
Initial consideration should be given to the management of the CNS effects of propoxyphene overdosage. Resuscitative measures should be initiated promptly.
Symptoms of Propoxyphene Overdosage—The manifestations of acute overdosage with propoxyphene are those of narcotic overdosage. The patient is usually somnolent but may be stuporous or comatose and convulsing. Respiratory depression is characteristic. The ventilatory rate and/or tidal volume is decreased, which results in cyanosis and hypoxia. Pupils, initially pinpoint, may become dilated as hypoxia increases. Cheyne-Stokes respiration and apnea may occur. Blood pressure and heart rate are usually normal initially, but blood pressure falls and cardiac performance deteriorates, which ultimately results in pulmonary edema and circulatory collapse, unless the respiratory depression is corrected and adequate ventilation is restored promptly. Cardiac arrhythmias and conduction delay may be present. A combined respiratory-metabolic acidosis occurs owing to retained CO_2 (hypercapnea) and to lactic acid formed during anaerobic glycolysis. Acidosis may be severe if large amounts of salicylates have also been ingested. Death may occur.
Treatment of Propoxyphene Overdosage—Attention should be directed first to establishing a patent airway and to restoring ventilation. Mechanically assisted ventilation, with or without oxygen, may be required, and positive pressure respiration may be desirable if pulmonary edema is present. The narcotic antagonist naloxone will markedly reduce the degree of respiratory depression, and 0.4 to 2 mg should be administered promptly, preferably intravenously. If the desired degree of counteraction with improvement in respiratory functions is not obtained, naloxone should be repeated at two to three-minute intervals. The duration of action of the antagonist may be brief. If no response is observed after 10 mg of naloxone have been administered, the diagnosis of propoxyphene toxicity should be questioned. Naloxone may also be administered by continuous intravenous infusion.
Treatment of Propoxyphene Overdosage in Children—The usual inital dose of naloxone in children is 0.01 mg/kg body weight given intravenously. If this dose does not result in the desired degree of clinical improvement, a subsequent increased dose of 0.1 mg/kg body weight may be administered. If an IV route of administration is not available, naloxone may be administered IM or subcutaneously in divided doses. If necessary, naloxone can be diluted with sterile water for injection.
Blood gases, pH, and electrolytes should be monitored in order that acidosis and any electrolyte disturbance present may be corrected promptly. Acidosis, hypoxia, and generalized CNS depression predispose to the development of cardiac arrhythmias. Ventricular fibrillation or cardiac arrest may occur and necessitate the full complement of cardiopulmonary resuscitation (CPR) measures. Respiratory acidosis rapidly subsides as ventilation is restored and hypercapnea eliminated, but lactic acidosis may require intravenous bicarbonate for prompt correction.
Electrocardiographic monitoring is essential. Prompt correction of hypoxia, acidosis, and electrolyte disturbance (when present) will help prevent these cardiac complications and will increase the effectiveness of agents administered to restore normal cardiac function.
In addition to the use of a narcotic antagonist, the patient may require careful titration with an anticonvulsant to control convulsions. Analeptic drugs (for example, caffeine or amphetamine) should not be used because of their tendency to precipitate convulsions.
General supportive measures, in addition to oxygen, include, when necessary, intravenous fluids, vasopressor-inotropic compounds, and, when infection is likely, anti-infective agents. Gastric lavage may be useful, and activated charcoal can adsorb a significant amount of ingested propoxyphene. Dialysis is of little value in poisoning due to propoxyphene. Efforts should be made to determine whether other agents, such as alcohol, barbiturates, tranquilizers, or other CNS depressants, were also ingested, since these increase CNS depression as well as cause specific toxic effects.
Symptoms of Acetaminophen Overdosage—Shortly after oral ingestion of an overdose of acetaminophen and for the next 24 hours, anorexia, nausea, vomiting, and abdominal pain have been noted. The patient may then present no symptoms, but evidence of liver dysfunction may be apparent during the next 24 to 48 hours, with elevated serum transaminase and lactic dehydrogenase levels, an increase in serum bilirubin concentrations, and a prolonged prothrombin time. Death from hepatic failure may result three to seven days after overdosage.
Treatment of Acetaminophen Overdosage—Acetaminophen in massive overdosage may cause hepatic toxicity in some patients. *In all cases of suspected overdose, immediately call your regional poison center or the Rocky Mountain Poison Center's toll-free number* (800-525-6115) for assistance in diagnosis and for directions in the use of N-acetylcysteine as an antidote, a use currently restricted to investigational status. In adults, hepatic toxicity has rarely been reported with acute overdoses of less than 10 g and fatalities with less than 15 g. Importantly, young children seem to be more resistant than adults to the hepatotoxic effect of an acetaminophen overdose. Despite this, the measures outlined below should be initiated in any adult or child suspected of having ingested an acetaminophen overdose.
Clinical and laboratory evidence of hepatic toxicity may not be apparent until 48 to 72 hours postingestion. Early symptoms following a potentially hepatotoxic overdose may include: nausea, vomiting, diaphoresis, and general malaise. The stomach should be emptied promptly by lavage or by induction of emesis with syrup of ipecac. Patients' estimates of the quantity of a drug ingested are notoriously unreliable. Therefore, if an acetaminophen overdose is suspected, a serum acetaminophen assay should be obtained as early as possible, but no sooner than four hours following ingestion. Liver function studies should be obtained initially and re-

Continued on next page

• **Identi-Code® symbol.**

Lilly—Cont.

peated at 24-hour intervals. The antidote, N-acetylcysteine, should be administered as early as possible, and within 16 hours of the overdose ingestion for optimal results. Following recovery, there are no residual, structural, or functional hepatic abnormalities.

Symptoms of Salicylate Overdosage—Such symptoms include central nausea and vomiting, tinnitus and deafness, vertigo and headaches, mental dullness and confusion, diaphoresis, rapid pulse, and increased respiration and respiratory alkalosis.

Treatment of Salicylate Overdosage—When Darvon-N with A.S.A. has been ingested, the clinical picture may be complicated by salicylism.

The treatment of acute salicylate intoxication includes minimizing drug absorption, promoting elimination through the kidneys, and correcting metabolic derangements affecting body temperature, hydration, acid-base balance, and electrolyte balance. The technique to be employed for eliminating salicylate from the bloodstream depends on the degree of drug intoxication.

If the patient is seen within four hours of ingestion, the stomach should be emptied by inducing vomiting or by gastric lavage as soon as possible.

The nomogram of Done is a useful prognostic guide in which the expected severity of salicylate intoxication is based on serum salicylate levels and the time interval between ingestion and taking the blood sample.

Exchange transfusion is most feasible for a small infant. Intermittent peritoneal dialysis is useful for cases of moderate severity in adults. Intravenous fluids alkalinized by the addition of sodium bicarbonate or potassium citrate are helpful. Hemodialysis with the artificial kidney is the most effective means of removing salicylate and is indicated for the very severe cases of salicylate intoxication.

ANIMAL TOXICOLOGY

The acute lethal doses of the hydrochloride and napsylate salts of propoxyphene were determined in four species. The results shown in Figure 2 indicate that, on a molar basis, the napsylate salt is less toxic than the hydrochloride. This may be due to the relative insolubility and retarded absorption of propoxyphene napsylate.

Figure 2. Acute oral toxicity of propoxyphene

	LD_{50} (mg/kg) $\pm$ SE / LD_{50} (mmole/kg)	
Species	Propoxyphene Hydrochloride	Propoxyphene Napsylate
Mouse	282 $\pm$ 39 / 0.75	915 $\pm$ 163 / 1.62
Rat	230 $\pm$ 44 / 0.61	647 $\pm$ 95 / 1.14
Rabbit	*ca.* 82 / 0.22	>183 / >0.32
Dog	*ca.* 100 / 0.27	>183 / >0.32

Some indication of the relative insolubility and retarded absorption of propoxyphene napsylate was obtained by measuring plasma propoxyphene levels in two groups of four dogs following oral administration of equimolar doses of the two salts. As shown in Figure 3, the peak plasma concentration observed with propoxyphene hydrochloride was much higher than that obtained after administration of the napsylate salt.

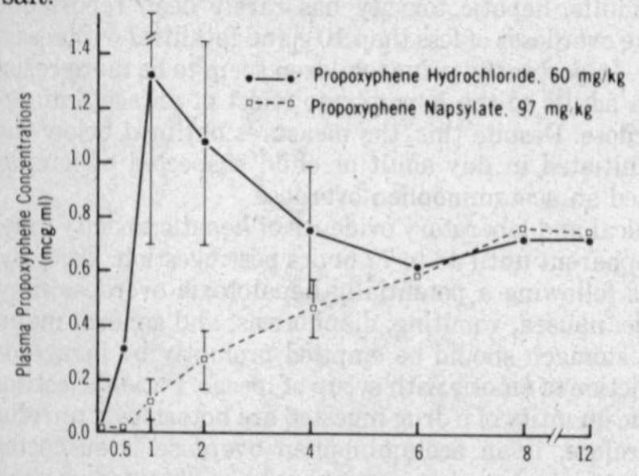

Figure 3. Plasma propoxyphene concentrations in dogs following large doses of the hydrochloride and napsylate salts

Although none of the animals in this experiment died, three of the four dogs given propoxyphene hydrochloride exhibited convulsive seizures during the time interval corresponding to the peak plasma levels. The four animals receiving the napsylate salt were mildly ataxic but not acutely ill.

HOW SUPPLIED

Ⓒ *Darvocet-N* ® *50 (Propoxyphene Napsylate and Acetaminophen, USP), Tablets No. 1890, C51,** Specially Coated, Dark-Orange, in bottles of 500 (NDC 0002-0351-03), in 10 strips of 10 individually labeled blisters each containing 1 tablet (ID100) (NDC 0002-0351-33), and in ℞Paks (prescription packages, Lilly) in bottles of 100 (NDC 0002-0351-02). All ℞Paks have safety closures.

500's—6505-00-279-7469.

Ⓒ *Darvocet-N* ® *100 (Propoxyphene Napsylate and Acetaminophen, USP), Tablets No. 1893, C63,** Specially Coated, Dark-Orange, in bottles of 500 (NDC 0002-0363-03), in 10 strips of 10 individually labeled blisters each containing 1 tablet (ID100) (NDC 0002-0363-33), in 500 single-cut individually labeled blisters each containing 1 tablet (ID500) (NDC 0002-0363-43), in 20 rolls, each consisting of 25 tablets in individual unit-dose packets, reverse-numbered (RN500) (NDC 0002-0363-46), and in ℞Paks in bottles of 100 (NDC 0002-0363-02). All ℞Paks have safety closures.

ID100—6505-00-111-8373

Ⓒ *Darvon-N* ® *(Propoxyphene Napsylate Oral Suspension, USP), Suspension No. M-135,* 50 mg per 5 ml, in 16-fl-oz (473-ml) bottles (NDC 0002-2371-05). *Avoid freezing.*

Ⓒ *Darvon-N* ® *(Propoxyphene Napsylate Tablets, USP), Tablets No. 1883, C53,** 100 mg, Specially Coated, Buff, in bottles of 100 (℞Pak) (NDC 0002-0353-02) and 500 (NDC 0002-0353-03), in 10 strips of 10 individually labeled blisters each containing 1 tablet (ID100) (NDC 0002-0353-33), and in ℞Paks in 20 packages of 50 (NDC 0002-0353-51). All ℞Paks have safety closures.

ID100—6505-00-197-9201; 500's—6505-00-111-8383

Ⓒ *Darvon-N* ® *with A.S.A.* ® *(Propoxyphene Napsylate and Aspirin, USP), Tablets No. 1884, C54,** Specially Coated, Orange, in bottles of 100 (℞Pak) (NDC 0002-0354-02) and 500 (NDC 0002-0354-03). All ℞Paks have safety closures.

500's—6505-00-212-6109

Shown in Product Identification Section, page 415

The following information, including illustrations of dosage forms and the maximum daily dosage of each, is available to patients receiving Darvon products.

Patient Information Sheet

YOUR PRESCRIPTION FOR A DARVON® (PROPOXYPHENE) PRODUCT Ⓒ

Summary: Products containing Darvon are used to relieve pain.

LIMIT YOUR INTAKE OF ALCOHOL WHILE TAKING THIS DRUG. Make sure your doctor knows that you are taking tranquilizers, sleep aids, antidepressants, antihistamines, or any other drugs that make you sleepy. Combining propoxyphene with alcohol or these drugs in excessive doses is dangerous.

Use care while driving a car or using machines until you see how the drug affects you because propoxyphene can make you sleepy. Do not take more of the drug than your doctor prescribed. Dependence has occurred when patients have taken propoxyphene for a long period of time at doses greater than recommended.

The rest of this leaflet gives you more information about propoxyphene. Please read it and keep it for future use.

Uses of Darvon: Products containing Darvon are used for the relief of mild to moderate pain. Products which contain Darvon plus aspirin or acetaminophen are prescribed for the relief of pain or pain associated with fever.

Before Taking Darvon: Make sure your doctor knows if you have ever had an allergic reaction to propoxyphene, aspirin, or acetaminophen. Some forms of propoxyphene products contain aspirin to help relieve the pain. Your doctor should be advised if you have a history of ulcers or if you are taking an anticoagulant ("blood thinner"). The aspirin may irritate the stomach lining and may cause bleeding, particularly if an ulcer is present. Also, bleeding may occur if you are taking an anticoagulant. In a small group of people, aspirin may cause an asthma attack. If you are one of these people, be sure your drug does not contain aspirin.

The effect of propoxyphene in children under 12 has not been studied. Therefore, use of the drug in this age group is not recommended.

Also, due to the possible association betwen aspirin and Reyes syndrome, those propoxyphene products containing aspirin should not be given to children, including teenagers, with chickenpox or flu unless prescribed by a physician. The following propoxyphene products contain aspirin:

Darvon® with A.S.A.® (propoxyphene hydrochloride and aspirin, Lilly)

Darvon® Compound and Darvon® Compound-65 (propoxyphene hydrochloride, aspirin, and caffeine, Lilly)

Darvon-N® with A.S.A.® (propoxyphene napsylate and aspirin, Lilly)

How to Take Darvon: Follow your doctor's directions exactly. Do not increase the amount you take without your doctor's approval. If you miss a dose of the drug, do not take twice as much the next time.

Pregnancy: Do not take propoxyphene during pregnancy unless your doctor knows you are pregnant and specifically recommends its use. Cases of temporary dependence in the newborn have occurred when the mother has taken propoxyphene consistently in the weeks before delivery. As a general principle, no drug should be taken during pregnancy unless it is clearly necessary.

General Cautions: Heavy use of alcohol with propoxyphene is hazardous and may lead to overdosage symptoms (see "Overdose" below). THEREFORE, LIMIT YOUR INTAKE OF ALCOHOL WHILE TAKING PROPOXYPHENE.

Combinations of excessive doses of propoxyphene, alcohol, and tranquilizers are dangerous. Make sure your doctor knows you are taking tranquilizers, sleep aids, antidepressant drugs, antihistamines, or any other drugs that make you sleepy. The use of these drugs with propoxyphene increases their sedative effects and may lead to overdosage symptoms, including death (see "Overdose" below).

Propoxyphene may cause drowsiness or impair your mental and/or physical abilities; therefore, use caution when driving a vehicle or operating dangerous machinery. DO NOT perform any hazardous task until you have seen your response to this drug.

Propoxyphene may increase the concentration in the body of medications such as anticoagulants ("blood thinners"), antidepressants, or drugs used for epilepsy. The result may be excessive or adverse effects of these medications. Make sure your doctor knows if you are taking any of these medications.

Dependence: You can become dependent on propoxyphene if you take it in higher than recommended doses over a long period of time. Dependence is a feeling of need for the drug and a feeling that you cannot perform normally without it.

Overdose: An overdose of Darvon, alone or in combination with other drugs, including alcohol, may cause weakness, difficulty in breathing, confusion, anxiety, and more severe drowsiness and dizziness. Extreme overdosage may lead to unconsciousness and death.

If the propoxyphene product contains acetaminophen, the overdosage symptoms include nausea, vomiting, lack of appetite, and abdominal pain. Liver damage may occur.

When the propoxyphene product contains aspirin, symptoms of taking too much of the drug are headache, dizziness, ringing in the ears, difficulty in hearing, dim vision, confusion, drowsiness, sweating, thirst, rapid breathing, nausea, vomiting, and, occasionally, diarrhea.

In any suspected overdosage situation, contact your doctor or nearest hospital emergency room. GET EMERGENCY HELP IMMEDIATELY.

KEEP THIS DRUG AND ALL DRUGS OUT OF THE REACH OF CHILDREN.

Possible Side Effects: When propoxyphene is taken as directed, side effects are infrequent. Among those reported are drowsiness, dizziness, nausea, and vomiting. If these effects occur, it may help if you lie down and rest.

Less frequently reported side effects are constipation, abdominal pain, skin rashes, lightheadedness, headache, weakness, minor visual disturbances, and feelings of elation or discomfort.

If side effects occur and concern you, contact your doctor.

Other Information: The safe and effective use of propoxyphene depends on your taking it exactly as directed. This drug has been prescribed specifically for you and your present condition. Do not give this drug to others who may have similar symptoms. Do not use it for any other reason.

If you would like more information about propoxyphene, ask your doctor or pharmacist. They have a more technical leaflet (professional labeling) you may read.

Prescription Vial Sticker

Tell your doctor if you are taking tranquilizers, antidepressant drugs, or sleep aids. LIMIT alcohol use with Darvon-N® (propoxyphene napsylate) and Darvon® (propoxyphene hydrochloride) products.

[103085]

DARVON® Ⓒ

[där'von]

(propoxyphene hydrochloride)

Capsules, USP

DARVON® COMPOUND and

[där'vŏn kŏm'pound]

DARVON® COMPOUND-65

(propoxyphene hydrochloride, aspirin, and caffeine)

DARVON® WITH A.S.A®

[där'vŏn with ā'ĕs-ā]

(propoxyphene hydrochloride and aspirin)

DESCRIPTION

Darvon® (propoxyphene hydrochloride, Lilly) is an odorless white crystalline powder with a bitter taste. It is freely soluble in water. Chemically, it is alpha-(+)-4-(Dimethylamino)-3-methyl-1,2-diphenyl-2-butanol Propionate Hydrochloride. Each Pulvule® Darvon contains 32 or 65 mg propoxyphene hydrochloride. Each Pulvule also contains D & C Red No. 33, F D & C Yellow No. 6, gelatin, magnesium stearate, silicone, starch, titanium dioxide, and other inactive ingredients.

Pulvules No. 368 Darvon® Compound		Pulvules No. 369 Darvon® Compound-65
32 mg	Darvon® (propoxyphene hydrochloride, Lilly)	65 mg
389 mg	A.S.A.® (aspirin, Lilly)	389 mg
32.4 mg	Caffeine	32.4 mg

Pulvules Darvon Compound and Darvon Compound-65 may contain any or all of the following: D & C Red No. 33, F D & C Red No. 3, F D & C Yellow No. 6, gelatin, glutamic acid hydrochloride, iron oxide, kaolin, silicone, titanium dioxide, and other inactive ingredients.

Each Pulvule Darvon with A.S.A. contains 65 mg propoxyphene hydrochloride and 325 mg aspirin. Each Pulvule also contains D & C Red No. 33, F D & C Red No. 3, F D & C Yellow No. 6, gelatin, glutamic acid hydrochloride, silicone, starch, titanium dioxide, and other inactive ingredients.

CLINICAL PHARMACOLOGY

Propoxyphene is a centrally acting narcotic analgesic agent. Equimolar doses of propoxyphene hydrochloride or napsylate provide similar plasma concentrations. Following administration of 65, 130, or 195 mg of propoxyphene hydrochloride, the bioavailability of propoxyphene is equivalent to that of 100, 200, or 300 mg respectively of propoxyphene napsylate. Peak plasma concentrations of propoxyphene are reached in two to two and one-half hours. After a 65-mg oral dose of propoxyphene hydrochloride, peak plasma levels of 0.05 to 0.1 mcg/ml are achieved.

Repeated doses of propoxyphene at six-hour intervals lead to increasing plasma concentrations, with a plateau after the ninth dose at 48 hours.

Propoxyphene is metabolized in the liver to yield norpropoxyphene. Propoxyphene has a half-life of six to 12 hours, whereas that of norpropoxyphene is 30 to 36 hours.

Norpropoxyphene has substantially less central-nervous-system-depressant effect than propoxyphene but a greater local anesthetic effect, which is similar to that of amitriptyline and antiarrhythmic agents, such as lidocaine and quinidine.

In animal studies in which propoxyphene and norpropoxyphene were continuously infused in large amounts, intracardiac conduction time (PR and QRS intervals) was prolonged. Any intracardiac conduction delay attributable to high concentrations of norpropoxyphene may be of relatively long duration.

ACTIONS

Propoxyphene is a mild narcotic analgesic structurally related to methadone. The potency of propoxyphene hydrochloride is from two-thirds to equal that of codeine.

The combination of propoxyphene with a mixture of aspirin and caffeine produces greater analgesia than that produced by either propoxyphene or aspirin and caffeine administered alone.

INDICATIONS

Darvon® (propoxyphene hydrochloride, Lilly) is indicated for the relief of mild to moderate pain.

Darvon Compound, Darvon Compound-65, and Darvon with A.S.A. are indicated for the relief of mild to moderate pain, either when pain is present alone or when it is accompanied by fever.

CONTRAINDICATION

Hypersensitivity to propoxyphene, aspirin, or caffeine.

WARNINGS

- **Do not prescribe propoxyphene for patients who are suicidal or addiction-prone.**
- **Prescribe propoxyphene with caution for patients taking tranquilizers or antidepressant drugs and patients who use alcohol in excess.**
- **Tell your patients not to exceed the recommended dose and to limit their intake of alcohol.**

Propoxyphene products in excessive doses, either alone or in combination with other CNS depressants, including alcohol, are a major cause of drug-related deaths. Fatalities within the first hour of overdosage are not uncommon. In a survey of deaths due to overdosage conducted in 1975, in approximately 20 percent of the fatal cases, death occurred within the first hour (5 percent occurred within 15 minutes). Propoxyphene should not be taken in doses higher than those recommended by the physician. The judicious prescribing of propoxyphene is essential to the safe use of this drug. With patients who are depressed or suicidal, consideration should be given to the use of non-narcotic analgesics.

Patients should be cautioned about the concomitant use of propoxyphene products and alcohol because of potentially serious CNS-additive effects of these agents. Because of its added depressant effects, propoxyphene should be prescribed with caution for those patients whose medical condition requires the concomitant administration of sedatives, tranquilizers, muscle relaxants, antidepressants, or other CNS-depressant drugs. Patients should be advised of the additive depressant effects of these combinations.

Many of the propoxyphene-related deaths have occurred in patients with previous histories of emotional disturbances or suicidal ideation or attempts as well as histories of misuse of tranquilizers, alcohol, and other CNS-active drugs. Some deaths have occurred as a consequence of the accidental ingestion of excessive quantities of propoxyphene alone or in combination with other drugs. Patients taking propoxyphene should be warned not to exceed the dosage recommended by the physician.

Drug Dependence—Propoxyphene, when taken in higher-than-recommended doses over long periods of time, can produce drug dependence characterized by psychic dependence and, less frequently, physical dependence and tolerance. Propoxyphene will only partially suppress the withdrawal syndrome in individuals physically dependent on morphine or other narcotics. The abuse liability of propoxyphene is qualitatively similar to that of codeine although quantitatively less, and propoxyphene should be prescribed with the same degree of caution appropriate to the use of codeine.

Usage in Ambulatory Patients—Propoxyphene may impair the mental and/or physical abilities required for the performance of potentially hazardous tasks, such as driving a car or operating machinery. The patient should be cautioned accordingly.

Warning—Reyes syndrome is a rare but serious disease which can follow flu or chickenpox in children and teenagers. While the cause of Reyes syndrome is unknown, some reports claim aspirin (or salicylates) may increase the risk of developing this disease.

PRECAUTIONS

General—Propoxyphene should be administered with caution to patients with hepatic or renal impairment, since higher serum concentrations or delayed elimination may occur.

Salicylates should be used with extreme caution in the presence of peptic ulcer or coagulation abnormalities.

Drug Interactions—The CNS-depressant effect of propoxyphene is additive with that of other CNS depressants, including alcohol.

Salicylates may enhance the effect of anticoagulants and inhibit the uricosuric effect of uricosuric agents.

As is the case with many medicinal agents, propoxyphene may slow the metabolism of a concomitantly administered drug. Should this occur, the higher serum concentrations of that drug may result in increased pharmacologic or adverse effects of that drug. Such occurrences have been reported when propoxyphene was administered to patients on antidepressants, anticonvulsants, or warfarinlike drugs.

Usage in Pregnancy—Safe use in pregnancy has not been established relative to possible adverse effects on fetal development. Instances of withdrawal symptoms in the neonate have been reported following usage during pregnancy. Therefore, propoxyphene should not be used in pregnant women unless, in the judgment of the physician, the potential benefits outweigh the possible hazards.

Usage in Nursing Mothers—Low levels of propoxyphene have been detected in human milk. In postpartum studies involving nursing mothers who were given propoxyphene, no adverse effects were noted in infants receiving mother's milk.

Usage in Children—Propoxyphene is not recommended for use in children, because documented clinical experience has been insufficient to establish safety and a suitable dosage regimen in the pediatric age group.

A Patient Information Sheet is available for these products. See text following "HOW SUPPLIED" section below.

ADVERSE REACTIONS

In a survey conducted in hospitalized patients, less than 1 percent of patients taking propoxyphene hydrochloride at recommended doses experienced side effects. The most frequently reported have been dizziness, sedation, nausea, and vomiting. Some of these adverse reactions may be alleviated if the patient lies down.

Other adverse reactions include constipation, abdominal pain, skin rashes, lightheadedness, headache, weakness, euphoria, dysphoria, and minor visual disturbances.

Cases of liver dysfunction have been reported.

DOSAGE AND ADMINISTRATION

These products are given orally. The usual dosage of Darvon® (propoxyphene hydrochloride, Lilly) is 65 mg every four hours as needed for pain.

The usual dosage of Darvon Compound and Darvon Compound-65 is 32 or 65 mg propoxyphene hydrochloride, 389 mg aspirin, and 32.4 mg caffeine every four hours as needed for pain.

The usual dosage of Darvon with A.S.A. is 65 mg propoxyphene hydrochloride and 325 mg aspirin every four hours as needed for pain.

The maximum recommended dose of propoxyphene hydrochloride is 390 mg per day.

Consideration should be given to a reduced total daily dosage in patients with hepatic or renal impairment.

MANAGEMENT OF OVERDOSAGE

In all cases of suspected overdosage, call your regional Poison Control Center to obtain the most up-to-date information about the treatment of overdose. This recommendation is made because, in general, information regarding the treatment of overdosage may change more rapidly than do package inserts.

Initial consideration should be given to the management of the CNS effects of propoxyphene overdosage. Resuscitative measures should be initiated promptly.

Symptoms of Propoxyphene Overdosage—The manifestations of acute overdosage with propoxyphene are those of narcotic overdosage. The patient is usually somnolent but may be stuporous or comatose and convulsing. Respiratory depression is characteristic. The ventilatory rate and/or tidal volume is decreased, which results in cyanosis and hypoxia. Pupils, initially pinpoint, may become dilated as hypoxia increases. Cheyne-Stokes respiration and apnea may occur. Blood pressure and heart rate are usually normal initially, but blood pressure falls and cardiac performance deteriorates, which ultimately results in pulmonary edema and circulatory collapse, unless the respiratory depression is corrected and adequate ventilation is restored promptly. Cardiac arrhythmias and conduction delay may be present. A combined respiratory-metabolic acidosis occurs owing to retained CO_2 (hypercapnea) and to lactic acid formed during anaerobic glycolysis. Acidosis may be severe if large amounts of salicylates have also been ingested. Death may occur.

Treatment of Propoxyphene Overdosage — Attention should be directed first to establishing a patent airway and to restoring ventilation. Mechanically assisted ventilation, with or without oxygen, may be required, and positive pressure respiration may be desirable if pulmonary edema is present. The narcotic antagonist naloxone will markedly reduce the degree of respiratory depression, and 0.4 to 2 mg should be administered promptly, preferably intravenously. If the desired degree of counteraction with improvement in respiratory functions is not obtained, naloxone should be repeated at two to three-minute intervals. The duration of action of the antagonist may be brief. If no response is observed after 10 mg of naloxone have been administered, the diagnosis of propoxyphene toxicity should be questioned. Naloxone may also be administered by continuous intravenous infusion.

Treatment of Propoxyphene Overdosage in Children—The usual initial dose of naloxone in children is 0.01 mg/kg body weight given intravenously. If this dose does not result in the desired degree of clinical improvement, a subsequent increased dose of 0.1 mg/kg body weight may be administered. If an IV route of administration is not available, naloxone may be administered IM or subcutaneously in divided doses. If necessary, naloxone can be diluted with sterile water for injection.

Blood gases, pH, and electrolytes should be monitored in order that acidosis and any electrolyte disturbance present may be corrected promptly. Acidosis, hypoxia, and generalized CNS depression predispose to the development of cardiac arrhythmias. Ventricular fibrillation or cardiac arrest may occur and necessitate the full complement of cardiopulmonary resuscitation (CPR) measures. Respiratory acidosis rapidly subsides as ventilation is restored and hypercapnea eliminated, but lactic acidosis may require intravenous bicarbonate for prompt correction.

Electrocardiographic monitoring is essential. Prompt correction of hypoxia, acidosis, and electrolyte disturbance (when present) will help prevent these cardiac complications and will increase the effectiveness of agents administered to restore normal cardiac function.

In addition to the use of a narcotic antagonist, the patient may require careful titration with an anticonvulsant to control convulsions. Analeptic drugs (for example, caffeine or amphetamine) should not be used because of their tendency to precipitate convulsions.

Continued on next page

• Identi-Code® symbol.

Lilly—Cont.

General supportive measures, in addition to oxygen, include, when necessary, intravenous fluids, vasopressor-inotropic compounds, and, when infection is likely, anti-infective agents. Gastric lavage may be useful, and activated charcoal can adsorb a significant amount of ingested propoxyphene. Dialysis is of little value in poisoning due to propoxyphene. Efforts should be made to determine whether other agents, such as alcohol, barbiturates, tranquilizers, or other CNS depressants, were also ingested, since these increase CNS depression as well as cause specific toxic effects.

Symptoms of Salicylate Overdosage—Such symptoms include central nausea and vomiting, tinnitus and deafness, vertigo and headaches, mental dullness and confusion, diaphoresis, rapid pulse, and increased respiration and respiratory alkalosis.

Treatment of Salicylate Overdosage—When Darvon Compound, Darvon Compound-65, or Darvon with A.S.A. has been ingested, the clinical picture may be complicated by salicylism.

The treatment of acute salicylate intoxication includes minimizing drug absorption, promoting elimination through the kidneys, and correcting metabolic derangements affecting body temperature, hydration, acid-base balance, and electrolyte balance. The technique to be employed for eliminating salicylate from the bloodstream depends on the degree of drug intoxication.

If the patient is seen within four hours of ingestion, the stomach should be emptied by inducing vomiting or by gastric lavage as soon as possible.

The nomogram of Done is a useful prognostic guide in which the expected severity of salicylate intoxication is based on serum salicylate levels and the time interval between ingestion and taking the blood sample.

Exchange transfusion is most feasible for a small infant. Intermittent peritoneal dialysis is useful for cases of moderate severity in adults. Intravenous fluids alkalinized by the addition of sodium bicarbonate or potassium citrate are helpful. Hemodialysis with the artificial kidney is the most effective means of removing salicylate and is indicated for the very severe cases of salicylate intoxication.

HOW SUPPLIED

Ⓒ *Pulvules Darvon ® (Propoxyphene Hydrochloride Capsules, USP): No. 364, HO2,** 32 mg (No. 4, Light-Pink Opaque), in bottles of 100 (℞Pak) (NDC 0002-0802-02) and 500 (NDC 0002-0802-03) and in 10 strips of 10 individually labeled blisters each containing 1 Pulvule (ID100) (NDC 0002-0802-33); *No. 365, HO3,** 65 mg (No. 3, Light-Pink Opaque), in bottles of 100 (℞Pak) (NDC 0002-0803-02) and 500 (NDC 0002-0803-03), in 10 strips of 10 individually labeled blisters each containing 1 Pulvule (ID100) (NDC 0002-0803-33), and in 20 rolls, each consisting of 25 Pulvules in individual unit-dose packets, reverse-numbered (RN500) (NDC 0002-0803-46). All ℞Paks have safety closures.

Ⓒ *Darvon Compound, Pulvules No. 368, USP, HO5** (No. 0, Light-Pink Opaque Body, Light-Gray Opaque Cap), in bottles of 100 (℞Pak) (NDC 0002-3110-02) and 500 (NDC 0002-3110-03). All ℞Paks have safety closures.

Ⓒ *Darvon Compound-65, Pulvules No. 369, USP, HO6** (No. 0, Red Opaque Body, Light-Gray Opaque Cap), in bottles of 100 (℞Pak) (NDC 0002-3111-02) and 500 (NDC 0002-3111-03) and in 10 strips of 10 individually labeled blisters each containing 1 Pulvule (ID100) (NDC 0002-3111-33). All ℞Paks have safety closures.

Ⓒ *Darvon with A.S.A., Pulvules No. 366, HO4** (No. 0, Red Opaque Body, Light-Pink Opaque Cap), in bottles of 100 (℞Pak) (NDC 0002-0804-02) and 500 (NDC 0002-0804-03). All ℞Paks have safety closures.

Shown in Product Identification Section, page 415

The following information, including illustrations of dosage forms and the maximum daily dosage of each, is available to patients receiving Darvon products.

Patient Information Sheet

YOUR PRESCRIPTION FOR A DARVON®
(PROPOXYPHENE) PRODUCT Ⓒ

Summary: Products containing Darvon are used to relieve pain.

LIMIT YOUR INTAKE OF ALCOHOL WHILE TAKING THIS DRUG. Make sure your doctor knows that you are taking tranquilizers, sleep aids, antidepressants, antihistamines, or any other drugs that make you sleepy. Combining propoxyphene with alcohol or these drugs in excessive doses is dangerous.

Use care while driving a car or using machines until you see how the drug affects you because propoxyphene can make you sleepy. Do not take more of the drug than your doctor prescribed. Dependence has occurred when patients have taken propoxyphene for a long period of time at doses greater than recommended.

The rest of this leaflet gives you more information about propoxyphene. Please read it and keep it for future use.

Uses of Darvon: Products containing Darvon are used for the relief of mild to moderate pain. Products which contain Darvon plus aspirin or acetaminophen are prescribed for the relief of pain or pain associated with fever.

Before Taking Darvon: Make sure your doctor knows if you have ever had an allergic reaction to propoxyphene, aspirin, or acetaminophen. Some forms of propoxyphene products contain aspirin to help relieve the pain. Your doctor should be advised if you have a history of ulcers or if you are taking an anticoagulant ("blood thinner"). The aspirin may irritate the stomach lining and may cause bleeding, particularly if an ulcer is present. Also, bleeding may occur if you are taking an anticoagulant. In a small group of people, aspirin may cause an asthma attack. If you are one of these people, be sure your drug does not contain aspirin.

The effect of propoxyphene in children under 12 has not been studied. Therefore, use of the drug in this age group is not recommended.

Also, due to the possible association between aspirin and Reyes syndrome, those propoxyphene products containing aspirin should not be given to children, including teenagers, with chickenpox or flu unless prescribed by a physician. The following propoxyphene products contain aspirin:

Darvon® with A.S.A.® (propoxyphene hydrochloride and aspirin, Lilly)

Darvon® Compound and Darvon® Compound-65 (propoxyphene hydrochloride, aspirin, and caffeine, Lilly)

Darvon-N® with A.S.A.® (propoxyphene napsylate and aspirin, Lilly)

How to Take Darvon: Follow your doctor's directions exactly. Do not increase the amount you take without your doctor's approval. If you miss a dose of the drug, do not take twice as much the next time.

Pregnancy: Do not take propoxyphene during pregnancy unless your doctor knows you are pregnant and specifically recommends its use. Cases of temporary dependence in the newborn have occurred when the mother has taken propoxyphene consistently in the weeks before delivery. As a general principle, no drug should be taken during pregnancy unless it is clearly necessary.

General Cautions: Heavy use of alcohol with propoxyphene is hazardous and may lead to overdosage symptoms (see "Overdose" below). THEREFORE, LIMIT YOUR INTAKE OF ALCOHOL WHILE TAKING PROPOXYPHENE.

Combinations of excessive doses of propoxyphene, alcohol, and tranquilizers are dangerous. Make sure your doctor knows you are taking tranquilizers, sleep aids, antidepressant drugs, antihistamines, or any other drugs that make you sleepy. The use of these drugs with propoxyphene increases their sedative effects and may lead to overdosage symptoms, including death (see "Overdose" below).

Propoxyphene may cause drowsiness or impair your mental and/or physical abilities: therefore, use caution when driving a vehicle or operating dangerous machinery. DO NOT perform any hazardous task until you have seen your response to this drug.

Propoxyphene may increase the concentration in the body of medications such as anticoagulants ("blood thinners"), antidepressants, or drugs used for epilepsy. The result may be excessive or adverse effects of these medications. Make sure your doctor knows if you are taking any of these medications.

Dependence: You can become dependent on propoxyphene if you take it in higher than recommended doses over a long period of time. Dependence is a feeling of need for the drug and a feeling that you cannot perform normally without it.

Overdose: An overdose of Darvon, alone or in combination with other drugs, including alcohol, may cause weakness, difficulty in breathing, confusion, anxiety, and more severe drowsiness and dizziness. Extreme overdosage may lead to unconsciousness and death.

If the propoxyphene product contains acetaminophen, the overdosage symptoms include nausea, vomiting, lack of appetite, and abdominal pain. Liver damage may occur.

When the propoxyphene product contains aspirin, symptoms of taking too much of the drug are headache, dizziness, ringing in the ears, difficulty in hearing, dim vision, confusion, drowsiness, sweating, thirst, rapid breathing, nausea, vomiting, and, occasionally, diarrhea.

In any suspected overdosage situation, contact your doctor or nearest hospital emergency room. GET EMERGENCY HELP IMMEDIATELY.

KEEP THIS DRUG AND ALL DRUGS OUT OF THE REACH OF CHILDREN.

Possible Side Effects: When propoxyphene is taken as directed, side effects are infrequent. Among those reported are drowsiness, dizziness, nausea, and vomiting. If these effects occur, it may help if you lie down and rest.

Less frequently reported side effects are constipation, abdominal pain, skin rashes, lightheadedness, headache, weakness, minor visual disturbances, and feelings of elation or discomfort.

If side effects occur and concern you, contact your doctor.

Other Information: The safe and effective use of propoxyphene depends on your taking it exactly as directed. This drug has been prescribed specifically for you and your present condition. Do not give this drug to others who may have similar symptoms. Do not use it for any other reason.

If you would like more information about propoxyphene, ask your doctor or pharmacist. They have a more technical leaflet (professional labeling) you may read.

Prescription Vial Sticker

Tell your doctor if you are taking tranquilizers, antidepressant drugs, or sleep aids. LIMIT alcohol use with Darvon-N® (propoxyphene napsylate) and Darvon® (propoxyphene hydrochloride) products.

[110485]

DIETHYLSTILBESTROL ℞

[dī-eth ′ĭl-stĭl-bĕs ′trōl]
USP

1. USE OF ESTROGENS HAS BEEN REPORTED TO INCREASE THE RISK OF ENDOMETRIAL CARCINOMA

Three independent case-control studies have reported an increased risk of endometrial cancer in postmenopausal women exposed to exogenous estrogens for more than one year. This risk was independent of other known risk factors for endometrial cancer. These studies are further supported by the finding that, since 1969, the incidence rate of endometrial cancer has increased sharply in eight different areas of the United States which have population-based cancer reporting systems. The three case-control studies reported that the risk of endometrial cancer in estrogen users was about 4.5 to 13.9 times greater than in nonusers. The risk appears to depend on both the duration of treatment and the dose of estrogen. In view of these findings, the lowest dose that will control symptoms should be utilized when estrogens are used for the treatment of menopausal symptoms, and medication should be discontinued as soon as possible. When prolonged treatment is medically indicated, a reassessment should be made on at least a semiannual basis to determine the need for continued therapy. Although the evidence must be considered preliminary, one study suggests that cyclic administration of low doses of estrogen may carry less risk than does continuous administration; it therefore appears prudent to utilize such a regimen.

Close clinical surveillance of all women taking estrogens is important. In all cases of undiagnosed persistent or recurring abnormal vaginal bleeding, adequate diagnostic measures should be undertaken to rule out malignancy.

At present, there is no evidence that "natural" estrogens are more or less hazardous than "synthetic" estrogens at equivalent estrogenic doses.

2. ESTROGENS SHOULD NOT BE USED DURING PREGNANCY

The use of female sex hormones, both estrogens and progestogens, during early pregnancy may affect the offspring. It has been reported that females exposed *in utero* to diethylstilbestrol, a nonsteroidal estrogen, may have an increased risk of developing later in life a rare form of vaginal or cervical cancer. This risk has been estimated to be 0.14 to 1.4 per 1000 exposures. Furthermore, from 30 to 90 percent of such exposed women have been found to have vaginal adenosis and epithelial changes of the vagina and cervix. Although these changes are histologically benign, it is not known whether they are precursors of malignancy. Even though similar data are not available with the use of other estrogens, it cannot be presumed that they would not induce similar changes.

Several reports suggest that there is an association between intrauterine exposure to female sex hormones and congenital anomalies, including congenital heart defects and limb-reduction defects. One case-control study estimated a 4.7-fold increased risk of limb-reduction defects in infants exposed *in utero* to sex hormones (oral contraceptives, hormone withdrawal tests for pregnancy, or attempted treatment for threatened abortion). Some of these exposures were very short and involved only a few days of treatment. The data suggest that the risk of limb-reduction defects in exposed fetuses is somewhat less than 1 per 1000.

In the past, female sex hormones have been used during pregnancy in an attempt to treat threatened or habitual abortion; however, their efficacy was never conclusively proved or disproved.

If diethylstilbestrol is administered during pregnancy, or if the patient becomes pregnant while taking this drug, she should be apprised of the potential risks to the fetus and of the advisability of pregnancy continuation.

THIS DRUG PRODUCT SHOULD NOT BE USED AS A POSTCOITAL CONTRACEPTIVE

DESCRIPTION

Diethylstilbestrol is a crystalline synthetic estrogenic substance capable of producing all the pharmacologic and therapeutic responses attributed to natural estrogens. Diethylstilbestrol may be administered orally (in the form of Enseals® [enteric-release tablets, Lilly] and tablets). Chemically, diethylstilbestrol is α,α'-diethyl-4,4'-stilbenediol.

INDICATIONS

Diethylstilbestrol is indicated in the treatment of:

1. Moderate to severe *vasomotor* symptoms associated with the menopause (There is no evidence that estrogens are effective for nervous symptoms or depression which might occur during menopause, and they should not be used to treat these conditions.)
2. Atrophic vaginitis
3. Kraurosis vulvae
4. Female hypogonadism
5. Female castration
6. Primary ovarian failure
7. Breast cancer (for palliation only) in appropriately selected women and men with metastatic disease
8. Prostatic carcinoma—palliative therapy of advanced disease

DIETHYLSTILBESTROL SHOULD NOT BE USED FOR ANY PURPOSE DURING PREGNANCY. ITS USE MAY CAUSE SEVERE HARM TO THE FETUS (SEE BOXED WARNING).

CONTRAINDICATIONS

Estrogens should not be used in women (or men) with any of the following conditions:

1. Known or suspected cancer of the breast, except in appropriately selected patients being treated for metastatic disease
2. Known or suspected estrogen-dependent neoplasia
3. Known or suspected pregnancy (see boxed warning)
4. Undiagnosed abnormal genital bleeding
5. Active thrombophlebitis or thromboembolic disorders
6. A past history of thrombophlebitis, thrombosis, or thromboembolic disorders associated with previous use of estrogen (except when used in treatment of breast or prostatic malignancy)

WARNINGS

1. *Induction of Malignant Neoplasms*—In certain animal species, long-term continuous administration of natural and synthetic estrogens increases the frequency of carcinomas of the breast, cervix, vagina, kidney, and liver. There are now reports that prolonged use of estrogens increases the risk of carcinoma of the endometrium in humans (see boxed warning).

At the present time, there is no satisfactory evidence that administration of estrogens to postmenopausal women increases the risk of cancer of the breast. This possibility, however, has been raised by a recent long-term follow-up of one physician's practice. Because of the animal data, there is a need for caution in prescribing estrogens for women with a family history of breast cancer or for women who have breast nodules, fibrocystic disease, or abnormal mammograms.

2. *Gallbladder Disease*—A recent study reported a two-to-threefold increase in the risk of gallbladder disease occurring in women receiving postmenopausal estrogen therapy, similar to the twofold increased risk previously noted in women using oral contraceptives. In the case of oral contraceptives, this increased risk appeared after two years of use.

3. *Effects Similar to Those Caused by Estrogen-Progestogen Oral Contraceptives*—There are several serious adverse effects associated with the use of oral contraceptives; however, most of these adverse effects have not as yet been documented as consequences of postmenopausal estrogen therapy. This may reflect the comparatively low doses of estrogen used in postmenopausal women. It would be expected that these adverse effects are more likely to occur following administration of the larger doses of estrogen used for treating prostatic or breast cancer. It has, in fact, been shown that there is an increased risk of thrombosis with the administration of estrogens for prostatic cancer in men and for postpartum breast engorgement in women.

a. *Thromboembolic Disease*—It is now well established that women taking oral contraceptives run an increased risk of various thromboembolic and thrombotic vascular diseases, such as thrombophlebitis, pulmonary embolism, stroke, and myocardial infarction. Cases of retinal thrombosis, mesenteric thrombosis, and optic neuritis have been reported in users of oral contraceptives. There is evidence that the risk of several of these adverse reactions is related to the dose of the drug. An increased risk of postsurgical thromboembolic complications has also been reported in users of oral contraceptives. If feasible, estrogen therapy should be discontinued at least four weeks before any surgery that may be associated with an increased risk of thromboembolism or that may require periods of prolonged immobilization.

Although an increased rate of thromboembolic and thrombotic disease has not been noted in postmenopausal users of estrogen, this does not rule out the possiblity that such an increase may be present or that it exists in subgroups of women who have underlying risk factors or who are receiving relatively large doses of estrogens. Therefore, estrogens should not be used in persons with active thrombophlebitis or thromboembolic disorders, nor should they be used (except in treatment of malignancy) in persons with a history of such disorders associated with estrogen therapy. Estrogens should be administered cautiously to patients with cerebral vascular or coronary artery disease and only when such therapy is clearly needed.

In a large prospective clinical trial in men, large doses of estrogen (5 mg of conjugated estrogens per day), comparable to those used to treat cancer of the prostate and breast, have been shown to increase the risk of nonfatal myocardial infarction, pulmonary embolism, and thrombophlebitis. When such large doses of estrogen are used, any of the thromboembolic and thrombotic adverse effects associated with the use of oral contraceptives should be considered a clear risk.

b. *Hepatic Adenoma*—Benign hepatic adenomas appear to be associated with the use of oral contraceptives. Although these adenomas are benign and rare, they may rupture and may cause death by intra-abdominal hemorrhage. Such lesions have not yet been reported in association with the administration of other estrogen or progestogen preparations, but they should be considered when abdominal pain and tenderness, abdominal mass, or hypovolemic shock occurs in persons receiving estrogen therapy. Hepatocellular carcinoma has also been reported in women taking estrogen-containing oral contraceptives. The relationship of this malignancy to such drugs is not known at this time.

c. *Elevated Blood Pressure*—Increased blood pressure is not uncommon in women taking oral contraceptives. There is now one report that this may occur with use of estrogens in the menopause, and blood pressure should be monitored during estrogen therapy, especially if high doses are used.

d. *Glucose Tolerance*—A decrease in glucose tolerance has been observed in a significant percentage of patients on estrogen-containing oral contraceptives. For this reason, diabetic patients should be carefully observed while receiving estrogen.

4. *Hypercalcemia*—Administration of estrogens may lead to severe hypercalcemia in patients with breast cancer and bone metastases. If this occurs, the drug should be stopped and appropriate measures taken to reduce the serum calcium level.

PRECAUTIONS

A. General Precautions.

1. A complete medical and family history should be taken prior to initiation of any estrogen therapy. In the pretreatment and periodic physical examinations, special consideration should be given to blood pressure, breasts, abdomen, and pelvic organs, and a Papanicolaou smear should be performed. As a general rule, estrogen should not be prescribed for over a year without another physical examination.

2. Fluid retention—Because estrogens may cause some degree of fluid retention, conditions which might be influenced by this factor, such as epilepsy, migraine, and cardiac or renal dysfunction, require careful observation.

3. Certain patients may develop undesirable manifestations of excessive estrogenic stimulation, such as abnormal or excessive uterine bleeding, mastodynia, etc.

4. Oral contraceptives appear to be associated with an increased incidence of mental depression. Although it is not clear whether this is due to the estrogenic or progestogenic component of the contraceptive agent, patients with a history of depression should be carefully observed.

5. Preexisting uterine leiomyomata may increase in size with administration of estrogens.

6. The pathologist should be advised of estrogen therapy when relevant specimens are submitted.

7. Patients with a past history of jaundice during pregnancy run an increased risk of recurrence of jaundice while receiving estrogen-containing oral contraceptive therapy. If jaundice develops in any patient receiving estrogen, the medication should be discontinued while the cause is investigated.

8. Estrogens may be poorly metabolized in patients with impaired liver function, and they should therefore be administered with caution in such patients.

9. Because estrogens influence the metabolism of calcium and phosphorus, they should be used with caution in patients with metabolic bone diseases associated with hypercalcemia or in patients with renal insufficiency.

10. Because of the effects of estrogens on epiphyseal closure, they should be used judiciously in young patients in whom bone growth is not complete.

11. Certain endocrine and liver function tests may be affected by estrogen-containing oral contraceptives. The following similar changes may be expected with larger doses of estrogen:

a. Increased sulfobromophthalein retention

b. Increased prothrombin and factors VII, VIII, IX, and X; decreased antithrombin 3; increased norepinephrine-induced platelet aggregability

c. Increased thyroid-binding globulin (TBG) leading to increased circulating total thyroid hormone, as measured by PBI, T^4 by column, or T^4 by radioimmunoassay. Free T^3 resin uptake is decreased, reflecting the elevated TBG; free T^4 concentration is unaltered

d. Impaired glucose tolerance

e. Decreased pregnanediol excretion

f. Reduced response to metyrapone test

g. Reduced serum folate concentration

h. Increased serum triglyceride and phospholipid concentration

B. Information for the Patient. *See* text of Patient Package Insert.

C. Pregnancy Category X. *See* Contraindications and boxed warning.

D. Nursing Mothers. As a general principle, any drug should be administered to nursing mothers only when clearly necessary, since many drugs are excreted in human milk.

ADVERSE REACTIONS

(*See* Warnings regarding induction of neoplasia, adverse effects on the fetus, increased incidence of gallbladder disease, and adverse effects similar to those of oral contraceptives, including thromboembolism.) The following additional adverse reactions have been reported with estrogenic therapy, including oral contraceptives:

1. *Genitourinary System*
   - Breakthrough bleeding, spotting, change in menstrual flow
   - Dysmenorrhea
   - Premenstrual-like syndrome
   - Amenorrhea during and after treatment
   - Increase in size of uterine fibromyomata
   - Vaginal candidiasis
   - Change in cervical eversion and in degree of cervical secretion
   - Cystitis-like syndrome
2. *Breasts*
   - Tenderness, enlargement, secretion
3. *Gastrointestinal*
   - Nausea, vomiting
   - Abdominal cramps, bloating
   - Cholestatic jaundice
4. *Skin*
   - Chloasma or melasma which may persist when drug is discontinued
   - Erythema multiforme
   - Erythema nodosum
   - Hemorrhagic eruption
   - Loss of scalp hair
   - Hirsutism
5. *Eyes*
   - Steepening of corneal curvature
   - Intolerance to contact lenses
6. *CNS*
   - Headache, migraine, dizziness
   - Mental depression
   - Chorea
7. *Miscellaneous*
   - Increase or decrease in weight
   - Reduced carbohydrate tolerance
   - Aggravation of porphyria
   - Edema
   - Changes in libido

ACUTE OVERDOSAGE

Numerous reports indicate that serious ill effects do not occur when large doses of estrogen-containing oral contraceptives are ingested by young children. Overdosage of estrogen may cause nausea, and withdrawal bleeding may occur in females.

DOSAGE AND ADMINISTRATION

1. *Given Cyclically for Short-Term Use Only:*

For treatment of moderate to severe *vasomotor* symptoms, atrophic vaginitis, or kraurosis vulvae associated with the menopause.

The lowest dose that will control symptoms should be chosen, and medication should be discontinued as promptly as possible.

Administration should be cyclic (e.g., three weeks on and one week off).

Attempts to discontinue or taper medication should be made at three to six-month intervals.

The usual dosage range is 0.2 to 0.5 mg daily. Patients with atrophic vaginitis may require up to 2 mg daily, and cyclic administration may be necessary for several years.

Continued on next page

• Identi-Code® symbol.

Lilly—Cont.

2. *Given Cyclically:*
   Female hypogonadism
   Female castration
   Primary ovarian failure
   0.2 to 0.5 mg daily
3. *Given Chronically:*
   Inoperable progressing prostatic cancer
   1 to 3 mg daily initially, increased in advanced cases; the dosage may later be reduced to an average of 1 mg daily.
   Inoperable progressing breast cancer in appropriately selected men and postmenopausal women (*see* INDICATIONS)
   15 mg daily

Patients with an intact uterus should be closely monitored for signs of endometrial cancer, and appropriate diagnostic measures should be taken to rule out malignancy in the event of persistent or recurring abnormal vaginal bleeding.

HOW SUPPLIED

(℞) *Enseals—Diethylstilbestrol Tablets, USP (Enteric): No. 46, A19,** 0.1 mg, in bottles of 100 (NDC 0002-0119-02); *No. 49, A22,** 1 mg, in bottles of 100 (NDC 0002-0122-02) and 1000 (NDC 0002-0122-04); and *No. 85, A33,** 5 mg, in bottles of 100 (NDC 0002-0133-02).

(℞) *Tablets—Diethylstilbestrol Tablets, USP: No. 1649, J52,** 1 mg, in bottles of 100 (NDC 0002-1052-02) and 1000 (NDC 0002-1052-04); *No. 1685, J54,** 5 mg, in bottles of 100) (NDC 0002-1054-02). [061384]

DOBUTREX® SOLUTION ℞

[dō ′bū-trĕks]

(dobutamine hydrochloride)
Injection

DESCRIPTION

Dobutrex® Solution (dobutamine hydrochloride injection, Lilly) is (±)-4-[2-[[3-(*p*-hydroxyphenyl)-1-methylpropyl]amino]-ethyl] -pyro- catechol hydrochloride. It is a synthetic catecholamine.

The clinical formulation is supplied in a sterile form for intravenous use only. Each ml contains 12.5 mg dobutamine, 0.24 mg sodium bisulfite (added during manufacture), and water for injection, q.s. Hydrochloric acid and/or sodium hydroxide may have been added during manufacture to adjust the *p*H.

CLINICAL PHARMACOLOGY

Dobutrex® (dobutamine hydrochloride, Lilly) is a direct-acting inotropic agent whose primary activity results from stimulation of the beta receptors of the heart while producing comparatively mild chronotropic, hypertensive, arrhythmogenic, and vasodilative effects. It does not cause the release of endogenous norepinephrine, as does dopamine. In animal studies, dobutamine produces less increase in heart rate and less decrease in peripheral vascular resistance for a given inotropic effect than does isoproterenol.

In patients with depressed cardiac function, both dobutamine and isoproterenol increase the cardiac output to a similar degree. In the case of dobutamine, this increase is usually not accompanied by marked increases in heart rate (although tachycardia is occasionally observed), and the cardiac stroke volume is usually increased. In contrast, isoproterenol increases the cardiac index primarily by increasing the heart rate while stroke volume changes little or declines.

Facilitation of atrioventricular conduction has been observed in human electrophysiologic studies and in patients with atrial fibrillation.

Systemic vascular resistance is usually decreased with administration of dobutamine. Occasionally, minimum vasoconstriction has been observed.

Most clinical experience with dobutamine is short-term—up to several hours in duration. In the limited number of patients who were studied for 24, 48, and 72 hours, a persistent increase in cardiac output occurred in some, whereas the output of others returned toward base-line values.

The onset of action of Dobutrex is within one to two minutes; however, as much as ten minutes may be required to obtain the peak effect of a particular infusion rate.

The plasma half-life of dobutamine in humans is two minutes. The principal routes of metabolism are methylation of the catechol and conjugation. In human urine, the major excretion products are the conjugates of dobutamine and 3-O-methyl dobutamine. The 3-O-methyl derivative of dobutamine is inactive.

Alteration of synaptic concentrations of catecholamines with either reserpine or tricyclic antidepressants does not alter the actions of dobutamine in animals, which indicates that the actions of dobutamine are not dependent on presynaptic mechanisms.

INDICATIONS AND USAGE

Dobutrex® (dobutamine hydrochloride, Lilly) is indicated when parenteral therapy is necessary for inotropic support in the short-term treatment of adults with cardiac decompensation due to depressed contractility resulting either from organic heart disease or from cardiac surgical procedures.

In patients who have atrial fibrillation with rapid ventricular response, a digitalis preparation should be used prior to institution of therapy with Dobutrex.

CONTRAINDICATION

Dobutrex® (dobutamine hydrochloride, Lilly) is contraindicated in patients with idiopathic hypertrophic subaortic stenosis and in patients who have shown previous manifestations of hypersensitivity to Dobutrex.

WARNINGS

1. *Increase in Heart Rate or Blood Pressure*—Dobutrex® (dobutamine hydrochloride, Lilly) may cause a marked increase in heart rate or blood pressure, especially systolic pressure. Approximately 10 percent of patients in clinical studies have had rate increases of 30 beats/minute or more, and about 7.5 percent have had a 50-mm Hg or greater increase in systolic pressure. Reduction of dosage usually reverses these effects promptly. Because dobutamine facilitates atrioventricular conduction, patients with atrial fibrillation are at risk of developing rapid ventricular response. Patients with preexisting hypertension appear to face an increased risk of developing an exaggerated pressor response.
2. *Ectopic Activity*—Dobutrex may precipitate or exacerbate ventricular ectopic activity, but it rarely has caused ventricular tachycardia.
3. *Hypersensitivity*—Reactions suggestive of hypersensitivity associated with administration of Dobutrex, including skin rash, fever, eosinophilia, and bronchospasm, have been reported occasionally.

PRECAUTIONS

1. **During the administration of Dobutrex® (dobutamine hydrochloride, Lilly), as with any adrenergic agent, ECG and blood pressure should be continuously monitored. In addition, pulmonary wedge pressure and cardiac output should be monitored whenever possible to aid in the safe and effective infusion of Dobutrex.**
2. Hypovolemia should be corrected with suitable volume expanders before treatment with Dobutrex is instituted.
3. Animal studies indicate that Dobutrex may be ineffective if the patient has recently received a beta-blocking drug. In such a case, the peripheral vascular resistance may increase.
4. No improvement may be observed in the presence of marked mechanical obstruction, such as severe valvular aortic stenosis.

Usage Following Acute Myocardial Infarction—Clinical experience with Dobutrex following myocardial infarction has been insufficient to establish the safety of the drug for this use. There is concern that any agent which increases contractile force and heart rate may increase the size of an infarction by intensifying ischemia, but it is not known whether dobutamine does so.

Usage in Pregnancy—Reproduction studies performed in rats and rabbits have revealed no evidence of impaired fertility, harm to the fetus, or teratogenic effects due to dobutamine. However, the drug has not been administered to pregnant women and should be used only when the expected benefits clearly outweigh the potential risks to the fetus.

Pediatric Use—The safety and effectiveness of Dobutrex for use in children have not been studied.

Drug Interactions—There was no evidence of drug interactions in clinical studies in which Dobutrex was administered concurrently with other drugs, including digitalis preparations, furosemide, spironolactone, lidocaine, glyceryl trinitrate, isosorbide dinitrate, morphine, atropine, heparin, protamine, potassium chloride, folic acid, and acetaminophen. Preliminary studies indicate that the concomitant use of dobutamine and nitroprusside results in a higher cardiac output and, usually, a lower pulmonary wedge pressure than when either drug is used alone.

ADVERSE REACTIONS

Increased Heart Rate, Blood Pressure, and Ventricular Ectopic Activity—A 10 to 20-mm increase in systolic blood pressure and an increase in heart rate of five to 15 beats/minute have been noted in most patients. (*See* WARNINGS regarding exaggerated chronotropic and pressor effects.) Approximately 5 percent of patients have had increased premature ventricular beats during infusions. These effects are dose related.

Miscellaneous Uncommon Effects—The following adverse effects have been reported in 1 to 3 percent of patients: nausea, headache, anginal pain, nonspecific chest pain, palpitations, and shortness of breath.

No abnormal laboratory values attributable to Dobutrex® (dobutamine hydrochloride, Lilly) have been observed.

Longer-Term Safety—Infusions of up to 72 hours have revealed no adverse effects other than those seen with shorter infusions.

OVERDOSAGE

In case of overdosage, as evidenced by excessive alteration of blood pressure or by tachycardia, reduce the rate of administration or temporarily discontinue Dobutrex® (dobutamine hydrochloride, Lilly) until the patient's condition stabilizes. Because the duration of action of Dobutrex is short, usually no additional remedial measures are necessary.

DOSAGE AND ADMINISTRATION

Note—Do not add Dobutrex® (dobutamine hydrochloride, Lilly) to 5% Sodium Bicarbonate Injection or to any other strongly alkaline solutions. Dobutrex should not be used in conjunction with other agents or diluents containing both sodium bisulfite and ethanol.

Reconstitution and Stability—Dobutrex must be further diluted at the time of administration to at least 50 ml prior to administration in an IV container with one of the following intravenous solutions: 5% Dextrose Injection, 5% Dextrose and 0.45% Sodium Chloride Injection, 5% Dextrose and 0.9% Sodium Chloride Injection, 10% Dextrose Injection, Isolyte® M with 5% Dextrose Injection, Lactated Ringer's Injection, 5% Dextrose in Lactated Ringer's Injection, Normosol®-M in D5-W, 20% Osmitrol® in Water for Injection, 0.9% Sodium Chloride Injection, or Sodium Lactate Injection. Intravenous solutions should be used within 24 hours. Solutions containing Dobutrex may exhibit a pink color that, if present, will increase with time. This color change is due to slight oxidation of the drug, but there is no significant loss of potency during the reconstituted time periods stated above.

Recommended Dosage—The rate of infusion needed to increase cardiac output usually ranges from 2.5 to 10 mcg/kg/min. (see table). On rare occasions, infusion rates up to 40 mcg/kg/min. have been required to obtain the desired effect.

[See table at left].

The rate of administration and the duration of therapy should be adjusted according to the patient's response, as determined by heart rate, presence of ectopic activity, blood pressure, urine flow, and, whenever possible, measurement of central venous or pulmonary wedge pressure and cardiac output.

Concentrations up to 5000 mcg/ml have been administered to humans (250 mg/50 ml). The final volume administered should be determined by the fluid requirements of the patient.

HOW SUPPLIED

(℞) *Vials No. 7175, Dobutrex® Solution (dobutamine hydrochloride injection, Lilly)*, equivalent to 250 mg dobutamine, 20-ml size, rubber-stoppered, in singles (10/carton) (NDC 0002-7175-01). Store at controlled room temperature, 59° to 86°F (15° to 30°C).

[032686]

FSN 6505-01-085-1833

Dobutrex® (dobutamine hydrochloride)—Rates of Infusion for Concentrations of 250, 500, and 1000 mcg/ml

Drug Delivery Rate (mcg/kg/min.)	Infusion Delivery Rate 250 mcg/ml* (ml/kg/min.)	500 mcg/ml† (ml/kg/min.)	1000 mcg/ml‡ (ml/kg/min.)
2.5	0.01	0.005	0.0025
5	0.02	0.01	0.005
7.5	0.03	0.015	0.0075
10	0.04	0.02	0.01
12.5	0.05	0.025	0.0125
15	0.06	0.03	0.015

*250 mg/liter of diluent
†500 mg/liter or 250 mg/500 ml of diluent
‡1000 mg/liter or 250 mg/250 ml of diluent

DOLOPHINE® HYDROCHLORIDE ⓘ
[dō'lō-fēn hī-drō-klō'rīd]
(methadone hydrochloride)
Injection, USP

AMPOULES AND VIALS

CONDITIONS FOR DISTRIBUTION AND USE OF METHADONE PRODUCTS:
Code of Federal Regulations, Title 21, Sec. 291.505

METHADONE PRODUCTS, WHEN USED FOR THE TREATMENT OF NARCOTIC ADDICTION IN DETOXIFICATION OR MAINTENANCE PROGRAMS, SHALL BE DISPENSED ONLY BY APPROVED HOSPITAL PHARMACIES, APPROVED COMMUNITY PHARMACIES, AND MAINTENANCE PROGRAMS APPROVED BY THE FOOD AND DRUG ADMINISTRATION AND THE DESIGNATED STATE AUTHORITY.
APPROVED MAINTENANCE PROGRAMS SHALL DISPENSE AND USE METHADONE IN ORAL FORM ONLY AND ACCORDING TO THE TREATMENT REQUIREMENTS STIPULATED IN THE FEDERAL METHADONE REGULATIONS (21 CFR 291.505).
FAILURE TO ABIDE BY THE REQUIREMENTS IN THESE REGULATIONS MAY RESULT IN CRIMINAL PROSECUTION, SEIZURE OF THE DRUG SUPPLY, REVOCATION OF THE PROGRAM APPROVAL, AND INJUNCTION PRECLUDING OPERATION OF THE PROGRAM.
A METHADONE PRODUCT, WHEN USED AS AN ANALGESIC, MAY BE DISPENSED IN ANY LICENSED PHARMACY.

DESCRIPTION
Dolophine® Hydrochloride (Methadone Hydrochloride, USP, Lilly) (4,4- diphenyl-6-dimethylamino-heptanone-3 hydrochloride) is a white crystalline material which is water soluble.
Each ml contains methadone hydrochloride, 10 mg, and sodium chloride, 0.9 percent. Sodium hydroxide and/or hydrochloric acid may have been added during manufacture to adjust the pH. The 20-ml vials also contain chlorobutanol (chloroform derivative), 0.5 percent, as a preservative.

ACTIONS
Methadone hydrochloride is a synthetic narcotic analgesic with multiple actions quantitatively similar to those of morphine, the most prominent of which involve the central nervous system and organs composed of smooth muscle. The principal actions of therapeutic value are analgesia and sedation and detoxification or temporary maintenance in narcotic addiction. The methadone abstinence syndrome, although qualitatively similar to that of morphine, differs in that the onset is slower, the course is more prolonged, and the symptoms are less severe.
A parenteral dose of 8 to 10 mg of methadone is approximately equivalent in analgesic effect to 10 mg of morphine. With single-dose administration, the onset and duration of analgesic action of the two drugs are similar.
When administered orally, methadone is approximately one-half as potent as when given parenterally. Oral administration results in a delay of the onset, a lowering of the peak, and an increase in the duration of analgesic effect.

INDICATIONS
(See Note below.)
For relief of severe pain.
For detoxification treatment of narcotic addiction.
For temporary maintenance treatment of narcotic addiction.

NOTE

If methadone is administered for treatment of heroin dependence for more than three weeks, the procedure passes from treatment of the acute withdrawal syndrome (detoxification) to maintenance therapy. Maintenance treatment is permitted to be undertaken only by approved methadone programs. This does not preclude the maintenance treatment of an addict who is hospitalized for medical conditions other than addiction and who requires temporary maintenance during the critical period of his stay or whose enrollment has been verified in a program which has approval for maintenance treatment with methadone.

CONTRAINDICATION
Hypersensitivity to methadone.

WARNINGS
Methadone hydrochloride, a narcotic, is a Schedule II controlled substance under the Federal Controlled Substances Act. Appropriate security measures should be taken to safeguard stocks of methadone against diversion.
DRUG DEPENDENCE—METHADONE CAN PRODUCE DRUG DEPENDENCE OF THE MORPHINE TYPE AND, THEREFORE, HAS THE POTENTIAL FOR BEING ABUSED. PSYCHIC DEPENDENCE, PHYSICAL DEPENDENCE, AND TOLERANCE MAY DEVELOP UPON REPEATED ADMINISTRATION OF METHADONE, AND IT SHOULD BE PRESCRIBED AND ADMINISTERED WITH THE SAME DEGREE OF CAUTION APPROPRIATE TO THE USE OF MORPHINE.
Interaction with Other Central-Nervous-System Depressants—Methadone should be used with caution and in reduced dosage in patients who are concurrently receiving other narcotic analgesics, general anesthetics, phenothiazines, other tranquilizers, sedative-hypnotics, tricyclic antidepressants, and other CNS depressants (including alcohol). Respiratory depression, hypotension, and profound sedation or coma may result.
Anxiety—Since methadone, as used by tolerant subjects at a constant maintenance dosage, is not a tranquilizer, patients who are maintained on this drug will react to life problems and stresses with the same symptoms of anxiety as do other individuals. The physician should not confuse such symptoms with those of narcotic abstinence and should not attempt to treat anxiety by increasing the dosage of methadone. The action of methadone in maintenance treatment is limited to the control of narcotic symptoms and is ineffective for relief of general anxiety.
Head Injury and Increased Intracranial Pressure—The respiratory depressant effects of methadone and its capacity to elevate cerebrospinal-fluid pressure may be markedly exaggerated in the presence of increased intracranial pressure. Furthermore, narcotics produce side effects that may obscure the clinical course of patients with head injuries. In such patients, methadone must be used with caution and only if it is deemed essential.
Asthma and Other Respiratory Conditions— Methadone should be used with caution in patients having an acute asthmatic attack, in those with chronic obstructive pulmonary disease or cor pulmonale, and in individuals with a substantially decreased respiratory reserve, preexisting respiratory depression, hypoxia, or hypercapnia. In such patients, even usual therapeutic doses of narcotics may decrease respiratory drive while simultaneously increasing airway resistance to the point of apnea.
Hypotensive Effect—The administration of methadone may result in severe hypotension in an individual whose ability to maintain his blood pressure has already been compromised by a depleted blood volume or concurrent administration of such drugs as the phenothiazines or certain anesthetics.
Use in Ambulatory Patients—Methadone may impair the mental and/or physical abilities required for the performance of potentially hazardous tasks, such as driving a car or operating machinery. The patient should be cautioned accordingly.
Methadone, like other narcotics, may produce orthostatic hypotension in ambulatory patients.
Use in Pregnancy—Safe use in pregnancy has not been established in relation to possible adverse effects on fetal development. Therefore, methadone should not be used in pregnant women unless, in the judgment of the physician, the potential benefits outweigh the possible hazards.
Methadone is not recommended for obstetric analgesia because its long duration of action increases the probability of respiratory depression in the newborn.
Use in Children—Methadone is not recommended for use as an analgesic in children, since documented clinical experience has been insufficient to establish a suitable dosage regimen for the pediatric age group.

PRECAUTIONS
Interaction with Pentazocine—Patients who are addicted to heroin or who are on the methadone maintenance program may experience withdrawal symptoms when given pentazocine.
Interaction with Rifampin—The concurrent administration of rifampin may possibly reduce the blood concentration of methadone to a degree sufficient to produce withdrawal symptoms. The mechanism by which rifampin may decrease blood concentrations of methadone is not fully understood, although enhanced microsomal drug-metabolized enzymes may influence drug disposition.
Acute Abdominal Conditions—The administration of methadone or other narcotics may obscure the diagnosis or clinical course in patients with acute abdominal conditions.
Interaction with Monoamine Oxidase (MAO) Inhibitors—Therapeutic doses of meperidine have precipitated severe reactions in patients concurrently receiving monoamine oxidase inhibitors or those who have received such agents within 14 days. Similar reactions thus far have not been reported with methadone; but if the use of methadone is necessary in such patients, a sensitivity test should be performed in which repeated small incremental doses are administered over the course of several hours while the patient's condition and vital signs are under careful observation.
Special-Risk Patients—Methadone should be given with caution and the initial dose should be reduced in certain patients, such as the elderly or debilitated and those with severe impairment of hepatic or renal function, hypothyroidism, Addison's disease, prostatic hypertrophy, or urethral stricture.

ADVERSE REACTIONS
THE MAJOR HAZARDS OF METHADONE, AS OF OTHER NARCOTIC ANALGESICS, ARE RESPIRATORY DEPRESSION AND, TO A LESSER DEGREE, CIRCULATORY DEPRESSION. RESPIRATORY ARREST, SHOCK, AND CARDIAC ARREST HAVE OCCURRED.
The most frequently observed adverse reactions include lightheadedness, dizziness, sedation, nausea, vomiting, and sweating. These effects seem to be more prominent in ambulatory patients and in those who are not suffering severe pain. In such individuals, lower doses are advisable. Some adverse reactions may be alleviated in the ambulatory patient if he lies down.
Other adverse reactions include the following:
Central Nervous System—Euphoria, dysphoria, weakness, headache, insomnia, agitation, disorientation, and visual disturbances.
Gastrointestinal—Dry mouth, anorexia, constipation, and biliary tract spasm.
Cardiovascular—Flushing of the face, bradycardia, palpitation, faintness, and syncope.
Genitourinary—Urinary retention or hesitancy, antidiuretic effect, and reduced libido and/or potency.
Allergic—Pruritus, urticaria, other skin rashes, edema, and, rarely, hemorrhagic urticaria.
In addition, pain at injection site; local tissue irritation and induration following subcutaneous injection, particularly when repeated.

DOSAGE AND ADMINISTRATION
For Relief of Pain—Dosage should be adjusted according to the severity of the pain and the response of the patient. Occasionally it may be necessary to exceed the usual dosage recommended in cases of exceptionally severe pain or in those patients who have become tolerant to the analgesic effect of narcotics.
Although subcutaneous administration is suitable for occasional use, intramuscular injection is preferred when repeated doses are required.
The usual adult dosage is 2.5 to 10 mg intramuscularly or subcutaneously every three or four hours as necessary.
For Detoxification Treatment—THE DRUG SHALL BE ADMINISTERED DAILY UNDER CLOSE SUPERVISION AS FOLLOWS:
A detoxification treatment course shall not exceed 21 days and may not be repeated earlier than four weeks after completion of the preceding course.
The oral form of administration is preferred. However, if the patient is unable to ingest oral medication, he may be started on the parenteral form initially.
In detoxification, the patient may receive methadone when there are significant symptoms of withdrawal. The dosage schedules indicated below are recommended but could be varied in accordance with clinical judgment. Initially, a single dose of 15 to 20 mg of methadone will often be sufficient to suppress withdrawal symptoms. Additional methadone may be provided if withdrawal symptoms are not suppressed or if symptoms reappear. When patients are physically dependent on high doses, it may be necessary to exceed these levels. Forty mg/day in single or divided doses will usually constitute an adequate stabilizing dosage level. Stabilization can be continued for two to three days, and then the amount of methadone normally will be gradually decreased. The rate at which methadone is decreased will be determined separately for each patient. The dose of methadone can be decreased on a daily basis or at two-day intervals, but the amount of intake shall always be sufficient to keep withdrawal symptoms at a tolerable level. In hospitalized patients, a daily reduction of 20 percent of the total daily dose may be tolerated and may cause little discomfort. In ambulatory patients, a somewhat slower schedule may be needed. If methadone is administered for more than three weeks, the procedure is considered to have progressed from detoxification or treatment of the acute withdrawal syndrome to maintenance treatment, even though the goal and intent may be eventual total withdrawal.

OVERDOSAGE
Symptoms—Serious overdosage of methadone is characterized by respiratory depression (a decrease in respiratory rate and/or tidal volume, Cheyne-Stokes respiration, cyanosis), extreme somnolence progressing to stupor or coma, maximally constricted pupils, skeletal-muscle flaccidity, cold and clammy skin, and, sometimes, bradycardia and hypotension. In severe overdosage, particularly by the intravenous route,

Continued on next page

• **Identi-Code® symbol.**

Lilly—Cont.

apnea, circulatory collapse, cardiac arrest, and death may occur.

Treatment—Primary attention should be given to the reestablishment of adequate respiratory exchange through provision of a patent airway and institution of assisted or controlled ventilation. If a nontolerant person, especially a child, takes a large dose of methadone, effective narcotic antagonists are available to counteract the potentially lethal respiratory depression. **The physician must remember, however, that methadone is a long-acting depressant (36 to 48 hours), whereas the antagonists act for much shorter periods (one to three hours).** The patient must, therefore, be monitored continuously for recurrence of respiratory depression and treated repeatedly with the narcotic antagonist as needed. If the diagnosis is correct and respiratory depression is due only to overdosage of methadone, the use of respiratory stimulants is not indicated.

An antagonist should not be administered in the absence of clinically significant respiratory or cardiovascular depression. Intravenously administered naloxone is the drug of choice to reverse signs of intoxication. Because of the relatively short half-life of naloxone as compared with methadone, repeated injections may be required until the status of the patient remains satisfactory. Naloxone may also be administered by continuous intravenous infusion.

Oxygen, intravenous fluids, vasopressors, and other supportive measures should be employed as indicated.

NOTE: IN AN INDIVIDUAL PHYSICALLY DEPENDENT ON NARCOTICS, THE ADMINISTRATION OF THE USUAL DOSE OF A NARCOTIC ANTAGONIST WILL PRECIPITATE AN ACUTE WITHDRAWAL SYNDROME. THE SEVERITY OF THIS SYNDROME WILL DEPEND ON THE DEGREE OF PHYSICAL DEPENDENCE AND THE DOSE OF THE ANTAGONIST ADMINISTERED. THE USE OF A NARCOTIC ANTAGONIST IN SUCH A PERSON SHOULD BE AVOIDED IF POSSIBLE. IF IT MUST BE USED TO TREAT SERIOUS RESPIRATORY DEPRESSION IN THE PHYSICALLY DEPENDENT PATIENT, THE ANTAGONIST SHOULD BE ADMINISTERED WITH EXTREME CARE AND BY TITRATION WITH SMALLER THAN USUAL DOSES OF THE ANTAGONIST.

HOW SUPPLIED

(Ⓒ) *Dolophine® Hydrochloride (Methadone Hydrochloride Injection, USP): Ampoules No. 456,* 10 mg, 1 ml, in packages of 12 (NDC 0002-1687-12) and 100 (NDC 0002-1687-02). *Vials No. 435,* 10 mg per ml, 20 ml, multiple dose, rubber-stoppered, in singles (10/carton) (NDC 0002-1682-01) and in packages of 25 (NDC 0002-1682-25).

[011786]

DOLOPHINE® HYDROCHLORIDE Ⓒ

[*dō'lō-fēn hī-drō-klō'rīd*]
(methadone hydrochloride)
Tablets, USP

CONDITIONS FOR DISTRIBUTION AND USE OF METHADONE PRODUCTS: *See under* Ampoules Dolophine Hydrochloride.

DESCRIPTION, ACTIONS, INDICATIONS, and CONTRAINDICATIONS

See under Ampoules Dolophine Hydrochloride.

WARNINGS

Tablets Dolophine® Hydrochloride (methadone hydrochloride, Lilly) are for oral administration only and *must not* be used for injection. It is recommended that Tablets Dolophine Hydrochloride, if dispensed, be packaged in child-resistant containers and kept out of the reach of children to prevent accidental ingestion.

See also under Ampoules Dolophine Hydrochloride.

PRECAUTIONS and ADVERSE REACTIONS

See under Ampoules Dolophine Hydrochloride.

DOSAGE AND ADMINISTRATION

For Relief of Pain—Dosage should be adjusted according to the severity of the pain and the response of the patient. Occasionally it may be necessary to exceed the usual dosage recommended in cases of exceptionally severe pain or in those patients who have become tolerant to the analgesic effect of narcotics.

The usual adult dosage is 2.5 to 10 mg every three or four hours as necessary.

See also under Ampoules Dolophine Hydrochloride.

If the patient cannot ingest methadone orally, parenteral administration may be substituted.

OVERDOSAGE

See under Ampoules Dolophine Hydrochloride.

HOW SUPPLIED

(Ⓒ)*Tablets Dolophine® Hydrochloride (Methadone Hydrochloride Tablets, USP): No. 1712, J64,** 5 mg, in bottles of 100 (NDC 0002-1064-02); *No. 1730, J72,**10 mg, in bottles of 100 (NDC 0002-1072-02).

[031284]

DYMELOR® ℞

[*dī'mĕ-lōr*]
(acetohexamide)
Tablets, USP

DESCRIPTION

Dymelor® (acetohexamide, Lilly) is an oral blood-glucose-lowering drug of the sulfonylurea class. Acetohexamide is a white, crystalline, practically odorless powder. It is practically insoluble in water and ether, soluble in pyridine and dilute solutions of alkali hydroxides, and slightly soluble in alcohol and chloroform. Chemically, it is benzenesulfonamide, 4-acetyl-*N*-[[cyclohexylamino]carbony]- or 1-[(*p*-acetylphenyl) sulfonyl]-3-cyclohexylurea. The empirical formula for acetohexamide is $C_{15}H_{20}N_2O_4S$.

Dymelor is supplied in 250 and 500-mg tablets. These products may also contain any or all of the following: amberlite, D&C Yellow No. 10, FD&C Yellow No. 6, magnesium stearate, starch, and talc.

CLINICAL PHARMACOLOGY

Acetohexamide appears to lower the blood glucose acutely by stimulating the release of insulin from the pancreas, an effect that is dependent on functioning beta cells in the pancreatic islets. The mechanism by which acetohexamide lowers blood glucose during long-term administration has not been clearly established.

Acetohexamide is rapidly absorbed from the gastrointestinal tract, and maximum hypoglycemic activity is observed about three hours after ingestion. The total duration of action is 12 to 24 hours. Much of the activity is ascribable to a metabolite, hydroxyhexamide, which has a plasma half-life of approximately six hours; the parent compound, acetohexamide, has a plasma half-life of 1.3 hours. In persons with normal renal and hepatic function, more than 80 percent is excreted, largely as metabolites, in 24 hours.

INDICATIONS AND USAGE

Dymelor® (acetohexamide Lilly) is indicated as an adjunct to diet for lowering the blood glucose in patients with non-insulin-dependent diabetes mellitus (type II) whose hyperglycemia cannot be controlled by diet alone.

In initiating treatment for non-insulin-dependent diabetes, diet should be emphasized as the primary form of treatment. Caloric restriction and weight loss are essential in the obese diabetic patient. Proper dietary management alone may be effective in controlling the blood glucose and symptoms of hyperglycemia. The importance of regular physical activity should also be stressed, and cardiovascular risk factors should be identified and corrective measures taken when possible.

If this treatment program fails to reduce symptoms and/or blood glucose, the use of oral sulfonylurea or insulin should be considered. The use of Dymelor must be viewed by both the physician and patient as a treatment in addition to diet and not as a substitute for diet or as a convenient mechanism for avoiding dietary restraint. Futhermore, loss of blood glucose control with diet alone may be transient, thus requiring only short-term administration of Dymelor.

During maintenance programs, Dymelor should be discontinued if satisfactory lowering of blood glucose is no longer achieved. Judgments should be based on regular clinical and laboratory evaluations.

In considering the use of Dymelor in asymptomatic patients, it should be recognized that controlling the blood glucose in non-insulin-dependent diabetes has not been definitely established as being effective in preventing the long-term cardiovascular or neural complications of diabetes.

CONTRAINDICATIONS

Dymelor® (acetohexamide Lilly) is contraindicated in patients with: (1) known hypersensitivity to the drug: (2) diabetic ketoacidosis, with or without coma. This condition should be treated with insulin.

WARNING

SPECIAL WARNING ON INCREASED RISK OF CARDIOVASCULAR MORTALITY

The administration of oral hypoglycemic drugs has been reported to be associated with increased cardiovascular mortality as compared to treatment with diet alone or diet plus insulin. This warning is based on the study conducted by the University Group Diabetes Program (UGDP), a long-term prospective clinical trial designed to evaluate the effectiveness of glucose-lowering drugs in preventing or delaying vascular complications in patients with non-insulin-dependent diabetes. The study involved 823 patients who were randomly assigned to one of four treatment groups (*Diabetes, 19* (Supp. 2): 747–830, 1970).

UGDP reported that patients treated for five to eight years with diet plus a fixed dose of tolbutamide (1.5 g/day) had a rate of cardiovascular mortality approximately 2½ times that of patients treated with diet alone. A significant increase in total mortality was not observed, but the use of tolbutamide was discontinued on the basis of the increase in cardiovascular mortality, thus limiting the opportunity for the study to show an increase in overall mortality. Despite controversy regarding the interpretation of these results, the findings of the UGDP study provide an adequate basis for this warning. The patient should be informed of the potential risks and advantages of Dymelor® (acetohexamide, Lilly) and of alternative modes of therapy.

Although only one drug in the sulfonylurea class (tolbutamide) was included in this study, it is prudent from a safety standpoint to consider that this warning may also apply to other oral hypoglycemic drugs in this class, in view of their close similarities in mode of action and chemical structure.

PRECAUTIONS

General —Hypoglycemia —All sulfonylurea drugs are capable of producing severe hypoglycemia. Proper patient selection, dosage, and instructions are important for avoiding hypoglycemia episodes. Renal or hepatic insufficiency may cause elevated blood levels of acetohexamide, and the latter may also diminish gluconeogenic capacity, both of which increase the risk of serious hypoglycemic reactions. Elderly, debilitated, or malnourished patients and those with adrenal or pituitary insufficiency are particularly susceptible to the hypoglycemia action of glucose-lowering drugs. Hypoglycemia may be difficult to recognize in the elderly and in people who are taking beta-adrenergic blocking drugs. Hypoglycemia is more likely to occur when caloric intake is deficient, after severe or prolonged exercise, when alcohol is ingested, or when more than one glucose-lowering drug is used.

Loss of Control of Blood Glucose —When a patient stabilized on any diabetic regimen is exposed to stress such as fever, trauma, infection, or surgery, a loss of control may occur. At such times, if may be necessary to discontinue Dymelor® (acetohexamide, Lilly) and administer insulin.

The effectiveness of any oral hypoglycemia drug, including Dymelor, in lowering blood glucose to a desired level decreases in many patients over a period of time; this decrease in effectiveness may be due to progression of the severity of the diabetes or to diminished responsiveness to the drug. This phenomenon is known as secondary failure, to distinguish it from primary failure, in which the drug is ineffective in an individual patient when first given.

Information for Patients —Patients should be informed of the potential risks and advantages of Dymelor and of alternative modes of therapy. They should also be informed about the importance of adherence to dietary instructions, of a regular exercise program, and of regular testing of urine and/or blood glucose.

The risks of hypoglycemia, its symptoms and treatment, and conditions that predispose to its development should be explained to patients and responsible family members. Primary and secondary failure should also be explained.

Laboratory Tests —Blood and urine glucose should be monitored periodically. Measurement of glycosylated hemoglobin may be useful.

Drug Interactions —The hypoglycemia action of sulfonylurea agents may be potentiated by certain drugs, including nonsteroidal anti-inflammatory agents and other drugs that are highly protein bound, salicylates, sulfonamides, chloramphenicol, probenecid, coumarins, monoamine oxidase inhibitors, and beta-adrenergic blocking agents. When such drugs are administered to a patient receiving Dymelor, the patient should be observed closely for hypoglycemia. When such drugs are withdrawn from a patient receiving Dymelor, the patient should be observed closely for loss of control.

Certain drugs tend to produce hyperglycemia and may lead to loss of control. These drugs include the thiazides and other diuretics, corticosteroids, phenothiazines, thyroid products, estrogens, oral contraceptives, phenytoin, nicotinic acid, sympathomimetics, calcium channel blocking drugs, and isoniazid. When such drugs are administered to a patient receiving Dymelor® (acetohexamide, Lilly), the patient should be closely observed for loss of control. When such drugs are withdrawn from a patient receiving Dymelor, the patient should be observed closely for hypoglycemia.

A potential interaction between oral miconazole and oral hypoglycemic agents leading to severe hypoglycemia has been reported. Whether this interaction also occurs with the intravenous, topical, or vaginal preparations of miconazole is not known.

Carcinogenesis, Mutagenesis, and Impairment of Fertility —Long-term studies in rats and mice revealed no evidence of carcinogenicity of acetohexamide. A sister chromatid exchange study performed with acetohexamide showed no evidence of mutagenicity. No animal studies have been conducted to determine whether acetohexamide has the potential to impair fertility.

Pregnancy

Teratogenic Effects—Pregnancy Category C—Dymelor has been shown to be teratogenic in animals receiving large doses of sulfonylurea agents. There are no adequate and well-controlled studies in pregnant women. Dymelor should be used during pregnancy only if the potential benefit justifies the potential risk to the fetus.

Because recent information suggests that abnormal blood glucose levels during pregnancy are associated with a higher incidence of congenital abnormalities, many experts recommend that insulin be used during pregnancy to maintain blood glucose levels as close to normal as possible.

Nonteratogenic Effects—Prolonged severe hypoglycemia (four to ten days) has been reported in neonates born to mothers who were receiving a sulfonylurea drug at the time of delivery. This has been reported more frequently with the use of agents with prolonged half-lives. The use of Dymelor is not recommended for the management of diabetes when complicated by pregnancy.

Nursing Mothers—It is not known whether this drug is excreted in human milk. Because some sulfonylurea drugs are excreted in human milk, and because of the potential for serious adverse reactions in nursing infants from Dymelor, a decision should be made whether to discontinue nursing or to discontinue the drug, taking into account the importance of the drug to the mother.

ADVERSE REACTIONS

Hypoglycemia—*See* PRECAUTIONS and OVERDOSAGE sections.

Gastrointestinal Reactions—Cholestatic jaundice may occur rarely; Dymelor® (acetohexamide, Lilly) should be discontinued if this occurs. Gastrointestinal disturbances, e.g., nausea, epigastric fullness, and heartburn, are the most common reactions and occur in 1 in 40 patients. These reactions tend to be dose related and may disappear when dosage is reduced.

Dermatologic Reactions—Allergic skin reactions, e.g., pruritus, erythema, urticaria, and morbilliform or maculopapular eruptions, occur in less than 1 in 100 patients. These may be transient and may disappear despite continued use of Dymelor; if skin reactions persist, the drug should be discontinued. Porphyria cutanea tarda and photosensitivity reactions have been reported with sulfonylurea agents.

Hematologic Reactions—Leukopenia, agranulocytosis, thrombocytopenia, hemolytic anemia, aplastic anemia, and pancytopenia have been reported with sulfonylurea agents.

Metabolic Reactions—Hepatic porphyria and disulfiram-like reactions have been reported with sulfonylurea agents.

OVERDOSAGE

Overdosage of sulfonylureas, including Dymelor® (acetohexamide, Lilly), can produce hypoglycemia. Mild hypoglycemic symptoms without loss of consciousness or neurologic findings should be treated aggressively with oral glucose and adjustments in drug dosage and/or meal patterns. Close monitoring should continue until the physician is assured that the patient is out of danger. Severe hypoglycemic reactions, with coma, seizure, or other neurologic impairment, occur infrequently but constitute medical emergencies requiring immediate hospitalization. If hypoglycemic coma is diagnosed or suspected, the patient should be given a rapid intravenous injection of concentrated (50%) glucose solution. This should be followed by a continuous infusion of a more dilute (10%) glucose solution at a rate that will maintain the blood glucose at a level about 100 mg/dl. Patients should be closely monitored for a minimum of 24 to 48 hours since hypoglycemia may recur after apparent clinical recovery.

DOSAGE AND ADMINISTRATION

There is no fixed dosage regimen for the management of diabetes mellitus with Dymelor® (acetohexamide, Lilly) or any other hypoglycemic agent. In addition to the usual monitoring of urinary glucose, the patient's blood glucose must also be monitored periodically to determine the minimum effective dose for a patient; to detect primary failure, i.e., inadequate lowering of blood glucose with the recommended dose of medication; and to detect secondary failure, i.e., loss of an adequate blood-glucose-lowering response after an initial period of effectiveness. Glycosylated hemoglobin levels may also be of value in monitoring the patient's response to therapy.

Short-term administration of Dymelor may be sufficient during periods of transient loss of control in patients usually controlled well on diet.

Daily oral dosage of Dymelor may range between 250 mg and 1.5 g. No loading dose is required. Patients who do not respond to 1.5 g daily usually will not respond to a higher dose. For this reason, doses in excess of 1.5 g daily are not recommended.

The majority of patients receiving 1 g or less/day can be controlled on a convenient once-daily dosage. Patients who need 1.5 g/day usually benefit from twice-daily dosage, given before the morning and evening meals.

Various measures have been employed to establish patients on Dymelor, and the following procedures are suggested.

Patients Not Previously Receiving Insulin or Drug Therapy—In mild, stable diabetes (after dietary regulation), therapy may be initiated with 250 mg daily before breakfast; subsequent adjustment of the dosage may be made by increments of 250 to 500 mg every five to seven days as necessary. The 250-mg or 500-mg tablet (scored and easily broken in half) may be used.

Because of reports of hyperresponsiveness of some elderly diabetics to Dymelor, patients in this group should be started with a single dose of 250 mg before breakfast, and their blood and urine sugars should be checked during the first 24 hours of therapy. If control appears to be satisfactory, this dose may be continued on a daily basis or, if necessary, gradually increased. If, however, there appears to be a tendency toward hypoglycemia, this dose should be reduced or the drug should be discontinued.

Patients Receiving Other Oral Agents—When transfer is made from tolbutamine, the initial dose of Dymelor should be about half the tolbutamide dose (e.g., 250 mg of Dymelor in place of 500 mg of tolbutamide), up to maximum of 1.5 g of Dymelor.

When transfer is made from chlorpropamide, the initial dose of Dymelor should be about double the chlorpropamide dose (e.g., 500 mg of Dymelor in place of 250 mg of chlorpropamide).

A transition period usually is required because of the long half-life of chlorpropamide. Subsequent adjustment of dosage should be made according to clinical response. The maximum recommended dose of Dymelor is 1.5 g.

Clinical reports on the efficacy of once-daily dosage of Dymelor indicate that its effect on the blood sugar is better sustained than that of tolbutamide. However, patients requiring more than 1 g of Dymelor daily should be treated with divided doses.

Patients Receiving Insulin—In general, patients who were previously maintained on insulin in small dosage (e.g., up to 20 units/day) may be placed on Dymelor directly and their insulin administration abruptly discontinued. Patients requiring larger doses of insulin, such as 20 to 40 units or more/day, should have an initial reduction of insulin dosage by 25 to 30 percent daily or every other day and subsequent further reduction depending on the response to Dymelor. An initial dose of 250 mg of Dymelor can be used, with readjustment depending on response to therapy. Because of the potential hazards of hypoglycemia in the elderly, patients in this age group should be carefully observed during the transition from insulin to Dymelor.

During the period of insulin withdrawal, the patient should test his urine for sugar and acetone at least three times a day and report the results frequently to his physician so that appropriate adjustments of therapy may be made. In some cases, it may be advisable to consider hospitalization during the transition period from insulin to Dymelor.

It should be noted that, as with other sulfonylureas, primary and secondary failures may occur with Dymelor.

In elderly, debilitated, or malnourished patients and patients with impaired renal or hepatic function, the initial and maintenance doses should be conservative to avoid hypoglycemic reactions (*see* Precautions section).

HOW SUPPLIED

(℞) *Tablets Dymelor ® (Acetohexamide Tablets, USP)* (capsule-shaped, scored): *No. 1842, U03,** 250 mg, White, and *No. 1843, U07,** 500 mg, Yellow, in bottles of 50 (NDC 0002-2103-50 and 2107-50), 200 (NDC 0002-2103-22 and 2107-22), and 500 (NDC 0002-2103-03 and 2107-03) and in 10 strips of 10 individually labeled blisters each containing 1 tablet (ID100) (NDC 0002-2103-33 and 2107-33). Store at controlled room temperature, 59° to 86°F (15° to 30°C).

[091085]

Shown in Product Identification Section, page 415

Tablets No. 1843, 500 mg—50's—6505-00-765-0589; 500's—6505-00-765-2068.

FOLIC ACID ℞

[fō'lĭk ăs'ĭd]

Tablets, USP

DESCRIPTION

Folic acid is a member of the vitamin B complex. Each tablet contains folic acid, 1 mg; lactose, magnesium stearate, starch, and talc.

ACTION

Folic acid acts on megaloblastic bone marrow to produce a normoblastic marrow.

INDICATIONS

It is effective in the treatment of megaloblastic anemias due to a deficiency of folic acid (as may be seen in tropical or nontropical sprue) and in anemias of nutritional origin, pregnancy, infancy, or childhood.

WARNING

Administration of folic acid alone is improper therapy for pernicious anemia and other megaloblastic anemias in which vitamin B_{12} is deficient.

PRECAUTION

Folic acid in doses above 0.1 mg daily may obscure pernicious anemia in that hematologic remission can occur while neurologic manifestations remain progressive.

ADVERSE REACTION

Allergic sensitization has been reported following both oral and parenteral administration of folic acid.

DOSAGE AND ADMINISTRATION

Folic acid is well absorbed and may be administered orally with satisfactory results except in severe instances of intestinal malabsorption.

The usual therapeutic dosage in adults and children (regardless of age) is up to 1 mg daily. Resistant cases may require larger doses.

When clinical symptoms have subsided and the blood picture has become normal, a daily maintenance level should be used, i.e., 0.1 mg for infants and up to 0.3 mg for children under four years of age, 0.4 mg for adults and children four or more years of age, and 0.8 mg for pregnant and lactating women, but never less than 0.1 mg/day. Patients should be kept under close supervision and adjustment of the maintenance level made if relapse appears imminent.

In the presence of alcoholism, hemolytic anemia, anticonvulsant therapy, or chronic infection, the maintenance level may need to be increased.

HOW SUPPLIED

(℞) *Tablets No. 1897, Folic Acid, USP, U56,** 1 mg, in bottles of 100 (NDC 0002-2156-02). [072985]

GLUCAGON FOR INJECTION ℞

[glōō'ka-gŏn]

USP

DESCRIPTION

Glucagon, manufactured by Eli Lilly and Company, is extracted from beef and pork pancreas.

Chemically unrelated to insulin, glucagon is a single-chain polypeptide containing 29 amino acid residues and having a molecular weight of 3483.

The empirical formula is $C_{153}H_{225}N_{43}O_{49}S$.

Crystalline glucagon is a white powder containing less than 0.01 percent zinc. It is relatively insoluble in water but is soluble at a *p*H of less than 3 or more than 9.5. Glucagon is stable in lyophilized form at room temperatures. Glucagon should be used immediately after reconstitution. It may be kept at 5°C (41°F) for up to 48 hours, if necessary.

Vials No. 666, Glucagon for Injection, USP, contain 1 unit (1 mg) of glucagon as the hydrochloride with 49 mg of lactose. (Vials No. 667, Diluting Solution for Glucagon for Injection, USP, 1 ml, contain glycerin, 1.6%, with 0.2% phenol added as a preservative. Sodium hydroxide and/or hydrochloric acid may have been added during manufacture to adjust the *p*H.)

Vials No. 668, Glucagon for Injection, USP, contain 10 units (10 mg) of glucagon as the hydrochloride with 140 mg of lactose. (Vials No. 669, Diluting Solution for Glucagon for Injection, USP, 10 ml, contain glycerin, 1.6%, with 0.2% phenol added as a preservative. Sodium hydroxide and/or hydrochloric acid may have been added during manufacture to adjust the *p*H.) Glucagon should be used immediately after reconstitution. It may be kept at 5°C (41°F) for up to 48 hours, if necessary.

If glucagon is to be given at doses higher than 2 mg, it should be reconstituted with Sterile Water for Injection instead of the diluting solution supplied and used immediately.

CLINICAL PHARMACOLOGY

Glucagon causes an increase in blood glucose concentration and is used in the treatment of hypoglycemic states. It is effective in small doses, and no evidence of toxicity has been reported with its use. Glucagon acts only on liver glycogen, converting it to glucose.

Parenteral administration of glucagon produces relaxation of the smooth muscle of the stomach, duodenum, small bowel, and colon.

The half-life of glucagon in plasma is approximately three to six minutes, which is similar to that of insulin.

INDICATIONS AND USAGE

For the treatment of hypoglycemia: Glucagon is useful in counteracting severe hypoglycemic reactions in diabetic patients or during insulin shock therapy in psychiatric patients. Glucagon is helpful in hypoglycemia only if liver gly-

Continued on next page

* Identi-Code® symbol.

Lilly—Cont.

cogen is available. It is of little or no help in states of starvation, adrenal insufficiency, or chronic hypoglycemia.
The patient with type I diabetes does not have as great a response in blood glucose levels as does the type II stable diabetic. Therefore, supplementary carbohydrate should be given as soon as possible, to the child or adolescent patient especially.
For use as a diagnostic aid: Glucagon is indicated as a diagnostic aid in the radiologic examination of the stomach, duodenum, small bowel, and colon when a hypotonic state would be advantageous.
Glucagon is as effective for this examination as are the anticholinergic drugs, but it has fewer side effects. When glucagon is administered concomitantly with an anticholinergic agent, the response is not significantly greater than when either drug is used alone. However, the addition of the anticholinergic agent results in increased side effects.

CONTRAINDICATION

Since glucagon is a protein, hypersensitivity is a possibility.

WARNINGS

Glucagon should be administered cautiously to patients with a history of insulinoma and/or pheochromocytoma. In patients with insulinoma, intravenous administration of glucagon will produce an initial increase in blood glucose but, because of its insulin-releasing effect, may cause the insulinoma to release its insulin and thus, may subsequently cause hypoglycemia. A patient developing symptoms of hypoglycemia after a dose of glucagon should be given glucose orally, intravenously, or by gavage, whichever is more appropriate.
Exogenous glucagon also stimulates the release of catecholamines. In the presence of pheochromocytoma, glucagon can cause the tumor to release catecholamines, which results in a sudden and marked increase in blood pressure. If a patient suddenly develops a marked increase in blood pressure, 5 to 10 mg of phentolamine mesylate may be administered intravenously in an attempt to control the blood pressure.
Generalized allergic reactions, including urticaria, respiratory distress, and hypotension, have been reported in patients who received glucagon injection.

PRECAUTIONS

General—In the treatment of hypoglycemic shock with glucagon, liver glycogen must be available. Glucose by the intravenous route or by gavage should be considered in the hypoglycemic patient.
Laboratory Tests—Blood glucose determinations may be obtained to follow the patient in hypoglycemic shock until he or she is asymptomatic.
Carcinogenesis, Mutagenesis, Impairment of Fertility—Glucagon is administered in one or two doses to patients in hypoglycemic shock or for diagnostic radiology. The drug has a half-life of approximately three to six minutes. Because glucagon is usually given in a single dose and has a very short half-life, no studies have been done regarding carcinogenesis.
Reproduction studies have been performed in rats at doses up to 2 mg/kg b.i.d. (or 90 to 120 times the human dose) and have revealed no evidence of impaired fertility.
Usage in Pregnancy—Pregnancy Category B—Reproduction studies have been performed in rats at doses up to 2 mg/kg b.i.d., or 90 to 120 times the human dose, and have revealed no evidence of harm to the fetus due to glucagon. There are, however, no adequate and well-controlled studies in pregnant women. Because animal reproduction studies are not always predictive of human response, this drug should be used during pregnancy only if clearly needed.
Nursing Mothers—It is not known whether this drug is excreted in human milk. Because many drugs are excreted in human milk, caution should be exercised when glucagon is administered to a nursing woman. The plasma half-life of glucagon is approximately three to six minutes. If the drug is excreted in human milk during this short period, it will be handled like any other polypeptide, i.e., it will be hydrolyzed and absorbed. Glucagon is not active when taken orally because it is destroyed in the gastrointestinal tract before it is absorbed.

ADVERSE REACTIONS

Glucagon is relatively free of adverse reactions except for occasional nausea and vomiting, which may also occur with hypoglycemia. Generalized allergic reactions have been reported (*see* WARNINGS).

OVERDOSAGE

Symptoms and Treatment—The LD_{50} for glucagon in rats is approximately 300 mg/kg. To date, there have been no reported cases of human overdosage of glucagon. When glucagon was given in large doses to cardiac patients, investigators reported a positive inotropic effect. These investigators administered glucagon in doses of 0.5 to 16 mg/hour by continuous infusion for periods of five to 166 hours. Total doses ranged from 25 to 996 mg, and a 21-month-old child received approximately 8.25 mg in 165 hours. Side effects included nausea, vomiting, and decreasing serum potassium. The serum potassium could be maintained within normal limits with supplemental potassium.
In view of the extremely short half-life of glucagon and its prompt destruction and excretion, the treatment of overdosage is symptomatic, primarily for nausea, vomiting, and possible hypokalemia.

DOSAGE AND ADMINISTRATION

For the treatment of hypoglycemia: The diluent is provided for use only in the preparation of glucagon for *intermittent* parenteral injection and for no other use.
If glucagon is to be given at doses higher than 2 mg, it should be reconstituted with Sterile Water for Injection instead of the diluting solution supplied and used immediately.
Directions for Use of Glucagon—1. Dissolve the lyophilized glucagon in the accompanying solvent.
2. Glucagon should not be used at concentrations greater than 1 unit/ml.
3. Glucagon solutions should not be used unless they are clear and of a water-like consistency.
4. Give 0.5 to 1 unit of glucagon by subcutaneous, intramuscular, or intravenous injection.
5. The patient will usually awaken in five to 20 minutes. If the response is delayed, there is no contraindication to the administration of one or two additional doses of glucagon; however, in view of the deleterious effects of cerebral hypoglycemia and depending on the duration and depth of coma, the use of parenteral glucose *must* be considered by the physician.
6. Intravenous glucose *must* be given if the patient fails to respond to glucagon.
7. When the patient responds, give supplemental carbohydrate to restore the liver glycogen and prevent secondary hypoglycemia.
General Management of Hypoglycemia—The following are helpful measures in the prevention of hypoglycemic reactions due to insulin:
1. Reasonable uniformity from day to day with regard to diet, insulin, and exercise.
2. Careful adjustment of the insulin program so that the type (or types) of insulin, dose, and time (or times) of administration are suited to the individual patient.
3. Frequent testing of the urine so that a change in insulin requirements can be foreseen.
4. Routine carrying of sugar, candy, or other readily absorbable carbohydrate by the patient so that it may be taken at the first warning of an oncoming reaction.
If the patient is unaware of the symptoms of hypoglycemia, he may lapse into insulin shock; therefore, the physician should instruct the patient in this regard when feasible.
It is important that the patient be aroused as quickly as possible, for prolonged hypoglycemic reactions may result in cortical damage. Glucagon or intravenous glucose will awaken the patient sufficiently so that oral carbohydrates may be taken.
Instructions to the Family—Instructions describing the method of using this preparation are included in the literature which accompanies the patient's package. It is advisable for the patient to become familiar with the technique of preparing glucagon for injection before an emergency arises.
CAUTION—Although glucagon may be used for the treatment of hypoglycemia by the patient during an emergency, the physician must still be notified when hypoglycemic reactions occur so that the dose of insulin may be adjusted more accurately.
Insulin Shock Therapy—Dissolve the lyophilized glucagon in the accompanying diluting solution.
After one hour of coma, inject 0.5 to 1 unit of glucagon by the subcutaneous, intramuscular, or intravenous route. Larger doses may be employed if desired.
Glucagon should not be used at concentrations greater than 1 unit/ml.
The patient will usually awaken in ten to 25 minutes. If no response occurs within the desired interval, the dose may be repeated. Upon awakening, the patient should be fed orally as soon as possible and the usual dietary regimen followed.
In a very deep state of coma, such as Stage IV or Stage V of Himwich, intravenous glucose should be given in addition to glucagon for a more immediate response. Glucagon and glucose may be used together without decreasing the efficacy of glucose administration.
For use as a diagnostic aid: Dissolve the lyophilized glucagon in the accompanying diluting solution.
Glucagon should not be used at concentrations greater than 1 unit/ml.
The doses in the accompanying chart may be administered for relaxation of the stomach, duodenum, and small bowel, depending on the time of onset of action and the duration of effect required for the examination. Since the stomach is less sensitive to the effect of glucagon, ½ unit IV or 2 units IM are recommended.
[See table below].
For examination of the colon, it is recommended that a 2-unit dose (2 mg) be administered intramuscularly approximately ten minutes prior to initiation of the procedure. Relaxation of the colon and reduction of discomfort to the patient will allow the radiologist to perform a more satisfactory examination.

HOW SUPPLIED

℞ *Vials Glucagon for Injection, USP:* are supplied in lyophilized form with accompanying diluting solution: *No. 666,* 1 unit (1 mg), rubber-stoppered (Dry Powder), with 49 mg of lactose, in single packages (10 per carton) (NDC 0002-1450-01); *No. 668,* 10 units (10 mg), rubber-stoppered (Dry Powder), multiple dose, with 140 mg of lactose, in single packages (10 per carton) (NDC 0002-1451-01).
Prior to reconstitution, the vials may be stored at controlled room temperature, 59° to 86°F (15° to 30°C).
Glucagon should be used immediately after reconstitution. It may be kept at 5°C (41°F) for up to 48 hours, if necessary.
Glucagon solutions should not be used unless they are clear and of a water-like consistency.
If glucagon is to be given at doses higher than 2 mg, it should be reconstituted with Sterile Water for Injection instead of the diluting solution supplied and used immediately.
Also available:
Glucagon Emergency Kit for Diabetic Insulin Reaction (M-8030) (1's), NDC 0002-8030-01. This emergency kit contains 1 vial of Glucagon for Injection, USP, 1 unit (1 mg) (No. 7286), NDC 0002-7286-01; and 1 Hyporet® (disposable syringe, Lilly) of Diluting Solution for Glucagon for Injection, USP, 1 ml (No. 7287).

[042386]

HUMULIN® L OTC

[*hū'-mū-lin ĕl*]
(Lente human insulin [recombinant DNA origin])
Insulin Zinc Suspension

INFORMATION FOR THE PATIENT

WARNINGS

THIS LILLY HUMAN INSULIN PRODUCT DIFFERS FROM ANIMAL-SOURCE INSULINS BECAUSE IT IS STRUCTURALLY IDENTICAL TO THE INSULIN PRODUCED BY YOUR BODY'S PANCREAS, AND BECAUSE OF ITS UNIQUE MANUFACTURING PROCESS.
ANY CHANGE OF INSULIN SHOULD BE MADE CAUTIOUSLY AND ONLY UNDER MEDICAL SUPERVISION. CHANGES IN REFINEMENT, PURITY, STRENGTH, BRAND (MANUFACTURER), TYPE (REGULAR, NPH, LENTE®, ETC), AND/OR METHOD OF MANUFACTURE (RECOMBINANT DNA VERSUS ANIMAL-SOURCE INSULIN) MAY RESULT IN THE NEED FOR A CHANGE IN DOSAGE.
SOME PATIENTS TAKING HUMULIN® (HUMAN INSULIN, RECOMBINANT DNA ORIGIN, LILLY) WILL REQUIRE A CHANGE IN DOSAGE FROM THAT USED WITH ANIMAL-SOURCE INSULINS. IF AN ADJUSTMENT IS NEEDED, IT MAY OCCUR WITH THE FIRST DOSE OR OVER A PERIOD OF SEVERAL WEEKS.

INSULIN AND DIABETES

Your doctor has explained that you have diabetes. You have learned that the treatment of your diabetes requires injections of insulin.
Insulin is a hormone produced by the pancreas, a large gland that lies near the stomach. This hormone is necessary for the body's correct use of food, especially sugar. Diabetes occurs when the pancreas does not make enough insulin to meet your body's needs.

Dosage of Glucagon as a Diagnostic Aid

Dose	Route of Administration	Time of Onset of Action	Approximate Duration of Effect
¼–½ unit (0.25–0.5 mg)	IV	1 minute	9–17 minutes
1 unit (1 mg)	IM	8–10 minutes	12–27 minutes
2 units (2 mg)*	IV	1 minute	22–25 minutes
2 units (2 mg)*	IM	4–7 minutes	21–32 minutes

***Administration of 2-unit doses produces a higher incidence of nausea and vomiting than do lower doses.**

To control your diabetes, your doctor has prescribed injections of insulin to keep your blood sugar at a nearly normal level and to keep your urine as free of sugar as possible. Each case of diabetes is different. You doctor has told you which insulin to use, how much, and when and how often to inject it. This schedule has been individualized for you. Proper control of your diabetes requires close and constant cooperation with your doctor.

In spite of diabetes, you can lead an active, healthy, and useful life if you eat a balanced diet daily, exercise regularly, and take your insulin injections exactly as prescribed by your doctor.

You have been instructed to test your urine and/or your blood regularly for sugar. If your urine tests consistently show the presence of sugar or your blood tests consistently show above-normal sugar levels, your diabetes is not properly controlled and you must let your doctor know.

USE THE PROPER TYPE OF INSULIN

This insulin, manufactured by Eli Lilly and Company, has the trademark Humulin and is available in three formulations—Regular, NPH, and Lente®. These products can be identified by a large letter that appears on the carton and vial (bottle) label following the name Humulin: Humulin R (regular), Humulin N (NPH), or Humulin L (Lente).

These types of insulin differ mainly in the time they require to take effect and in the length of time their action lasts. Your doctor has prescribed the type of insulin that he/she believes is best for you. **DO NOT USE ANY OTHER INSULIN EXCEPT ON HIS/HER ADVICE AND DIRECTION.**

If you physician has directed you to take Humulin, when you receive your insulin from the pharmacy, always check to see that:

1. The name Humulin appears on the carton and bottle label and is followed by the proper letter designation and name for the insulin formulation: R-Regular; N-NPH; L-Lente.
2. The carton and bottle label are correct for your type of insulin.
3. The human insulin is of recombinant DNA origin.
4. The insulin strength is U-100.
5. The expiration date on the package will allow you to use the insulin before that date.

LENTE HUMAN INSULIN

Humulin® L (Lente Human Insulin, Recombinant DNA Origin, Lilly) is synthesized in a non-disease-producing special laboratory strain of *E. coli* bacteria which has been genetically altered by the addition of the human gene for insulin production. This product is a suspension of zinc-insulin crystals providing a different duration of action than regular insulin. The result is an intermediate-acting insulin with a slower onset of action than regular insulin and a longer duration of activity (up to 24 hours).

Humulin L should look uniformly cloudy, or milky. If the insulin substance (the cloudy material) settles at the bottom of the bottle, the bottle must be carefully rotated before the injection so that the contents are uniformly mixed (see instructions under PREPARING THE DOSE). Do not use a vial of insulin if you see lumps that float or stick to the sides. Also, the insulin should not be used if it is clear and remains clear after the bottle is rotated.

STORAGE

Insulin should be stored in a cold place, preferably in a refrigerator, but not in the freezing compartment. Do not let it freeze or leave it in direct sunlight. If refrigeration is not possible, the bottle of insulin which you are currently using can be kept unrefrigerated as long as it is kept as cool as possible and away from heat and sunlight. Do not use a bottle of insulin after the expiration date stamped on the label.

USE THE CORRECT SYRINGE

Doses of insulin are measured in **units.** The number of units in each milliliter (ml) is clearly stated on the package. It is important to use a syringe which is marked for an insulin preparation with 100 units per ml. Failure to use the proper syringe can lead to a mistake in dosage, and you may receive too little or too much insulin. This can cause serious problems for you, ranging from a blood sugar level that is too low or too high to coma (unconsciousness) or, rarely, death.

IMPORTANT: TO HELP AVOID CONTAMINATION AND POSSIBLE INFECTION, FOLLOW THESE INSTRUCTIONS EXACTLY.

DISPOSABLE SYRINGES

Disposable syringes and needles require no sterilization; they should be used only once and then discarded.

STERILIZING AND ASSEMBLING REUSABLE SYRINGES

Your reusable syringe and needle must be sterilized before each injection—**follow the package directions supplied with your syringe.** Boiling, as described below, is the best method of sterilizing.

1. Put syringe, plunger, and needle in strainer, place in saucepan, and cover with water. Boil for 5 minutes.
2. Remove articles from water. When they have cooled, insert plunger into barrel, and fasten needle to syringe with a slight twist.
3. Push plunger in and out several times until water is completely removed.
(If the syringe, plunger, and needle cannot be boiled, as when you are traveling, they may be sterilized by immersion for at least 5 minutes in Isopropyl Alcohol, 91%. Do not use bathing, rubbing, or medicated alcohol for this sterilization. If the syringe is sterilized with alcohol, it must be absolutely dry before use.)

PREPARING THE DOSE

1. Wash your hands.
2. Gently roll the insulin bottle several times to mix the insulin. Be sure it is completely mixed. Do not shake bottle. Flip off the colored protective cap on the bottle, but **do not** remove the rubber stopper.

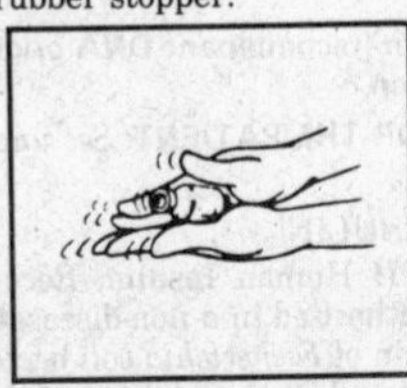

3. Wipe top of bottle with alcohol swab.

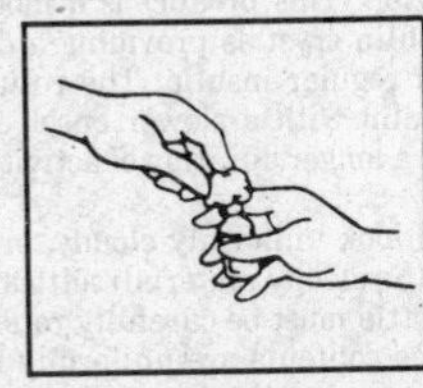

4. Draw air into the syringe by pulling back on the plunger. The amount of air should be equal to your insulin dose.

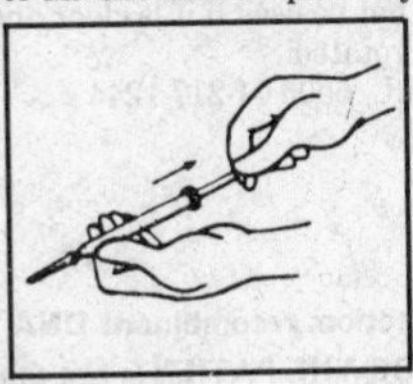

5. Remove the needle cover. Put the needle through rubber top of insulin bottle.

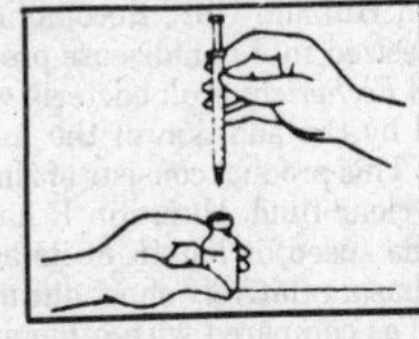

6. Push plunger in. The air injected into the bottle will allow insulin to be easily withdrawn into syringe.

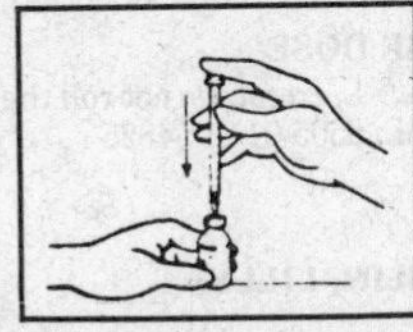

7. Turn bottle and syringe upside down in one hand. Be sure tip of needle is in insulin. Your other hand will be free to move the plunger. Draw back on plunger slowly to draw the correct dose of insulin into syringe.

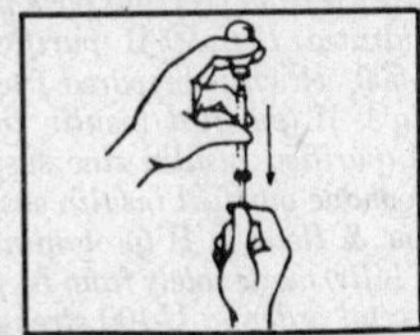

8. Check for air bubbles. The air is harmless. but too large an air bubble will reduce the insulin dose. To remove air bubbles, push insulin back into the bottle and measure your correct dose of insulin.

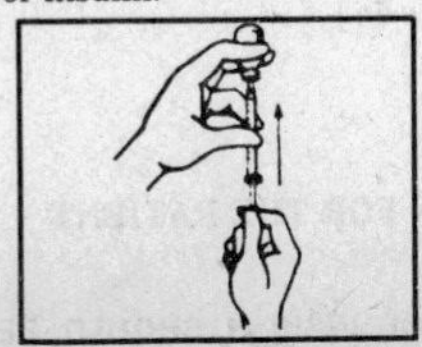

9. Double check your dose. Remove needle from bottle. Cover needle with guard or lay syringe down so that needle does not touch anything.

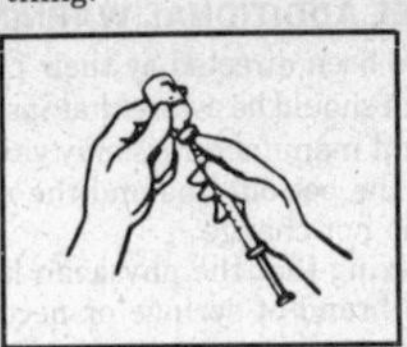

INJECTING THE DOSE

1. Cleanse the skin where the injection is to be made.

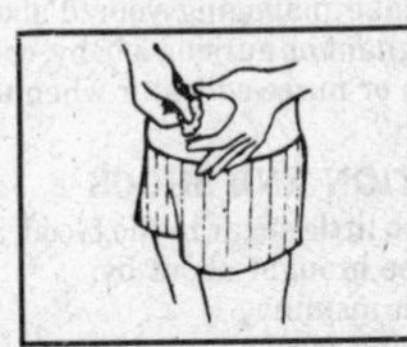

2. With one hand, stabilize the skin by spreading it or pinching up a large area of skin.

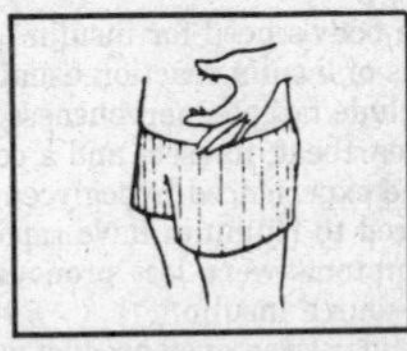

3. Pick up syringe with other hand, and hold it as you would a pencil. Insert needle straight into the skin (90° angle). After the needle is in, pull back the plunger very slightly. If blood comes into the syringe, the needle has entered a blood vessel. Remove the needle and put it at another location. If blood does not appear in the syringe, push the plunger in slowly as far as it will go.

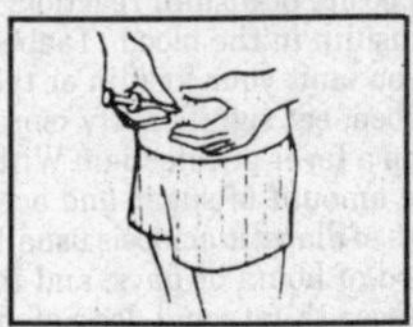

4. To inject the insulin, push plunger all the way down, using less than 5 seconds to inject the dose.

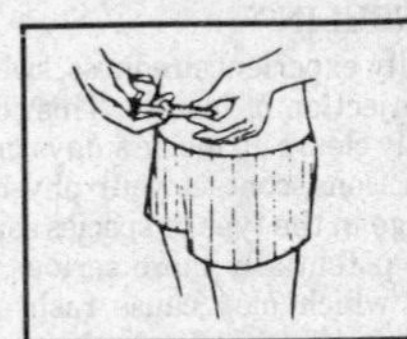

5. Hold alcohol swab near the needle and pull needle straight out of skin. Press alcohol swab over injection site for several seconds.

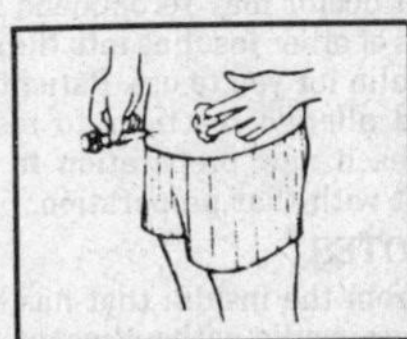

6. Use disposable syringe only once to insure sterility of syringe and needle and accuracy of dose. Destroy syringes as directed.

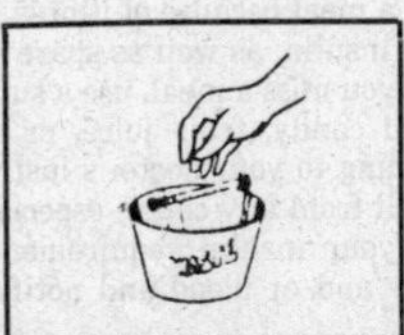

Continued on next page

• **Identi-Code® symbol.**

Lilly—Cont.

7. To avoid tissue damage, always change the site for each injection.

WARNINGS—SEE ADDITIONAL WARNINGS ABOVE

Patients who have been directed by their physicians to mix two types of insulin should be aware that insulin hypodermic syringes of different manufacturers may vary in the amount of space between the bottom line and the needle.
Because of this, do not change:
1. The order of mixing that the physician has prescribed or
2. The model and brand of syringe or needle without first consulting your physician.

The mixing should be done immediately prior to injection. Failure to heed this warning could result in a dosage error.

USAGE IN PREGNANCY

Pregnancy may make managing your diabetes more difficult. If you are pregnant or nursing a baby, consult your physician, pharmacist, or nurse-educator when using this product.

INSULIN REACTION AND SHOCK

Insulin reaction (too little sugar in the blood, also called "hypoglycemia") can be brought about by:
1. Taking too much insulin
2. Missing or delaying meals
3. Exercising or working too hard just before a meal
4. An infection or illness (especially with diarrhea or vomiting)
5. A change in the body's need for insulin

The first symptoms of insulin reaction usually come on suddenly and may include fatigue, nervousness or "shakiness," headache, rapid heartbeat, nausea, and a cold sweat.
A few patients who experienced hypoglycemic reactions after being transferred to Humulin have reported that these early warning symptoms were less pronounced than they were with animal-source insulin.
Eating sugar or a sugar-sweetened product will often correct the condition and prevent more serious symptoms.
If the reaction becomes more severe, breathing will be shallow and the skin pale. Contact a doctor at once if you develop any of these symptoms.

DIABETIC ACIDOSIS AND COMA

Diabetic acidosis may develop if your body has too little insulin. (This is the opposite of insulin reaction, which is the result of too much insulin in the blood.) Diabetic acidosis may be brought on if you omit your insulin or take less than the doctor has prescribed, eat significantly more than your diet calls for, or develop a fever or infection. With acidosis, urine tests show a large amount of sugar and acetone.
The first symptoms of diabetic acidosis usually come on gradually, over a period of hours or days, and include a drowsy feeling, flushed face, thirst, and loss of appetite. Heavy breathing and a rapid pulse are more severe symptoms. It is important that you notify your doctor immediately, because diabetic coma (unconsciousness) can follow.

ALLERGY TO INSULIN

Patients occasionally experience redness, swelling, and itching at the site of injection of insulin. This condition, called local allergy, usually clears up in a few days to a few weeks. If you have local reactions, contact your physician, who may recommend a change in the type or species source of insulin.
Less common, but potentially more serious, is generalized allergy to insulin, which may cause rash over the whole body, shortness of breath, wheezing, reduction in blood pressure, fast pulse, or sweating. Severe cases of generalized allergy may be life-threatening. If you think you are having a generalized allergic reaction to insulin, notify a physician immediately. Your doctor may recommend skin testing, injecting small doses of other insulins into the skin, in order to select the best insulin for you to use. Patients who have had severe generalized allergic reactions to insulin should be skin tested with each new preparation to be used before starting treatment with that preparation.

IMPORTANT NOTES

1. Never change from the insulin that has been prescribed for you to another insulin without instructions from your doctor. Changing the type, strength, species, or manufacturer of insulin can cause problems with your diabetes.
2. Your doctor will tell you what to do if you miss a dose of insulin or miss a meal because of illness. Always keep an extra supply of insulin, as well as spare syringe and needle, on hand. If you miss a meal, use a substitute of sugar, sugar-sweetened candy, fruit juice, or sugar-sweetened beverage according to your doctor's instructions.
3. If you become ill from any cause, especially with nausea and vomiting, your insulin requirements may change. Test your urine and/or blood and notify your doctor at once.
4. Consult your doctor if you notice anything unusual or have doubts about your condition or your use of insulin.
5. Always wear diabetic identification so that appropriate treatment can be given if complications occur away from home.
6. Understand how to manage your diabetes so that your life can be active and healthy.

DIABETES FORECAST is a national magazine designed especially for patients with diabetes and their families and is available on subscription from the American Diabetes Association, National Service Center, 1660 Duke Street, Alexandria, Virginia 22314.
Another publication, **DIABETES COUNTDOWN,** is available from the Juvenile Diabetes Foundation, 60 Madison Avenue, New York, New York 10010.

[101684]

HUMULIN® N — OTC

[*hū 'mŭ-lĭn ĕn*]
(NPH human insulin [recombinant DNA origin])
Isophane Suspension

INFORMATION FOR THE PATIENT: *See under* Humulin® L.

NPH HUMAN INSULIN

Humulin® N (NPH Human Insulin, Recombinant DNA Origin, Lilly) is synthesized in a non-disease-producing special laboratory strain of *Escherichia coli* bacteria which has been genetically altered by the addition of the human gene for insulin production. This product is a modification of a solution of zinc-insulin crystals providing a different duration of action than regular insulin. The result is an intermediate-acting insulin with a slower onset of action than regular insulin and a longer duration of activity (slightly less than 24 hours).
Humulin N should look uniformly cloudy, or milky. If the insulin substance (the cloudy material) settles at the bottom of the bottle, the bottle must be carefully rotated before the injection so that the contents are uniformly mixed (see instructions under Preparing the Dose). Do not use a vial of insulin if you see lumps that float or stick to the sides. Also, the insulin should not be used if it is clear and remains clear after the bottle is rotated.
Humulin N, 100 mL, 6505-01-217-1244

[041086]

HUMULIN® R — OTC

[*hū 'mŭ-lĭn är*]
(insulin human injection, recombinant DNA origin) USP

INFORMATION FOR THE PATIENT: *See under* Humulin® L.

NEUTRAL REGULAR HUMAN INSULIN

Humulin® (Insulin Human, USP, Recombinant DNA Origin, Lilly) is synthesized in a non-disease-producing special laboratory strain of *Escherichia coli* bacteria which has been genetically altered by the addition of the human gene for insulin production. This product consists of zinc-insulin crystals dissolved in a clear fluid. Humulin R has had nothing added to change the speed or length of its action. It takes effect rapidly and has a relatively short duration of activity (six to eight hours) as compared with other insulins.
Humulin R should be clear and colorless. Do not use it if it is cloudy, unusually viscous, precipitated, or even slightly colored.

PREPARING THE DOSE

See under Humulin® L, *except:* Do not roll the insulin bottle.
Humulin R, 100 mL, 6505-01-215-4825

[013085]

ILETIN® (INSULIN, LILLY)—

[*ī 'lĕ-tĭn*]
REGULAR AND MODIFIED INSULIN PRODUCTS

All of the insulins listed below are prepared from a mixture of insulin crystals extracted from beef and pork pancreas, except for Regular (Concentrated) Iletin® II (purified pork insulin injection, Lilly), U-500, which is prepared from pork insulin only. Regular Iletin® II (purified insulin injection, Lilly), Lente® Iletin® II (purified insulin zinc suspension, Lilly), NPH Iletin® II (isophane purified insulin suspension, Lilly), and Protamine, Zinc & Iletin® II (protamine zinc purified insulin suspension, Lilly) made solely from beef or pork source are available on special order in U-100 strength only. When insulin is prepared from a single animal source, the species is indicated on the vial label and on the package.

REGULAR ILETIN® I

[*rĕg 'ū-lĕr ī 'lĕ-tĭn wŭn*]
(Beef-Pork)
(insulin injection)
USP

INFORMATION FOR THE PATIENT

WARNINGS

ANY CHANGE OF INSULIN SHOULD BE MADE CAUTIOUSLY AND ONLY UNDER MEDICAL SUPERVISION. CHANGES IN REFINEMENT, PURITY, STRENGTH (U-40, U-100), BRAND (MANUFACTURER), TYPE (LENTE®, NPH, REGULAR, ETC.), AND SPECIES SOURCE (BEEF, PORK, BEEF-PORK, OR HUMAN) MAY RESULT IN THE NEED FOR A CHANGE IN DOSAGE.
SOME PATIENTS TAKING THIS BEEF-PORK INSULIN WILL REQUIRE SUCH A CHANGE IN DOSAGE. IF AN ADJUSTMENT IS NEEDED, IT MAY OCCUR WITH THE FIRST DOSE OR OVER A PERIOD OF SEVERAL WEEKS.

INSULIN AND DIABETES

Your doctor has explained that you have diabetes. You have learned that the treatment of your diabetes requires injections of insulin.
Insulin is a hormone produced by the pancreas, a large gland that lies near the stomach. This hormone is necessary for the body's correct use of food, especially sugar. Diabetes occurs when the pancreas does not make enough insulin to meet the body's needs.
To control your diabetes, your doctor has prescribed injections of insulin to keep your blood sugar at a nearly normal level and to keep your urine as free of sugar as possible. Each case of diabetes is different. Your doctor has told you which insulin to use, how much, and when and how often to inject it. This schedule has been individualized for you. Proper control of your diabetes requires close and constant cooperation with your doctor.
In spite of diabetes, you can lead an active, healthy, and useful life if you eat a balanced diet daily, exercise regularly, and take your insulin injections exactly as prescribed by your doctor.
You have been instructed to test your urine and/or blood regularly for sugar. If your urine tests consistently show the presence of sugar or your blood tests consistently show above-normal sugar levels, your diabetes is not properly controlled and you must let your doctor know.

USE THE PROPER TYPE OF INSULIN

This insulin, manufactured by Eli Lilly and Company, has the trademark Iletin® I (insulin, Lilly) and is available in various types—Regular, NPH, Protamine Zinc, Lente, Semilente®, and Ultralente®.
These types of insulin differ mainly in the time they require to take effect and in the length of time their action lasts. Your doctor has prescribed the type of insulin that he/she believes is best for you. **Do not use any other type of insulin except on his/her advice and direction.**

REGULAR BEEF-PORK INSULIN

Regular Iletin I, consisting of zinc-insulin crystals dissolved in a clear fluid, is obtained from beef and pork pancreas. Regular beef-pork insulin is "unmodified" (that is, nothing has been added to change the speed or length of its action). It takes effect rapidly and has a relatively short duration of activity (six to eight hours) as compared with other insulins.
Regular beef-pork insulin should be clear and colorless. Do not use it if it is cloudy, unusually viscous, precipitated, or even slightly colored.

STORAGE

Insulin should be stored in a cold place, preferably in a refrigerator, but not in the freezing compartment. Do not let it freeze or leave it in direct sunlight. If refrigeration is not possible, the bottle of insulin which you are currently using can be kept unrefrigerated as long as it is kept as cool as possible and away from heat and sunlight. Do not use a bottle of insulin after the expiration date stamped on the label.

USE THE CORRECT SYRINGE

Doses of insulin are measured in **units.** The number of units in each cubic centimeter (cc) is clearly stated on the package. Two strengths are available for each type of insulin: U-40 (40 units per cc) and U-100 (100 units per cc). It is important that you understand the markings on your syringe, because the volume of insulin you inject depends on the strength, that is, the number of units per cc. For this reason, you should always use a syringe marked for the strength of insulin you are injecting. Failure to use the proper syringe can lead to a mistake in dosage, and you may receive too little or too much insulin. This can cause serious problems for you, ranging from a blood sugar that is too low or too high to coma (unconsciousness) or, rarely, death.
IMPORTANT: TO HELP AVOID CONTAMINATION AND POSSIBLE INFECTION, FOLLOW THESE INSTRUCTIONS EXACTLY.

DISPOSABLE SYRINGES

Disposable syringes and needles require no sterilization; they should be used only once and then discarded.

STERILIZING AND ASSEMBLING REUSABLE SYRINGES

Your reusable syringe and needle must be sterilized before each injection—**follow the package directions supplied with your syringe.** Boiling, as described below, is the best method of sterilizing.

1. Put syringe, plunger, and needle in strainer, place in saucepan, and cover with water. Boil for five minutes.
2. Remove articles from water. When they have cooled, insert plunger into barrel, and fasten needle to syringe with a slight twist.
3. Push plunger in and out several times until water is completely removed. (If the syringe, plunger, and needle cannot be boiled, as when you are traveling, they may be sterilized by immersion for at least five minutes in Isopropyl Alcohol, 91%. Do not use bathing, rubbing, or medicated alcohol for this sterilization. If the syringe is sterilized with alcohol, it must be absolutely dry before use.)

PREPARING THE DOSE

1. Wash your hands.
2. Flip off the colored protective cap on the bottle, but **do not** remove rubber stopper.
3. Wipe top of bottle with alcohol swab.
4. Draw air into the syringe by pulling back on the plunger. The amount of air should be equal to your insulin dose.
5. Remove the needle cover. Put the needle through rubber top of insulin bottle.
6. Push plunger in. The air injected into the bottle will allow insulin to be easily withdrawn into syringe.
7. Turn bottle and syringe upside down in one hand. Be sure tip of needle is in insulin. Your other hand will be free to move the plunger. Draw back on plunger slowly to draw the correct dose of insulin into syringe.
8. Check for air bubbles. The air is harmless, but too large an air bubble will reduce the insulin dose. To remove air bubbles, push insulin back into the bottle and measure your correct dose of insulin.
9. Double check your dose. Remove needle from bottle. Cover needle with guard or lay syringe down so that needle does not touch anything.

INJECTING THE DOSE

1. Clean the skin where the injection is to be made.
2. With one hand, stabilize the skin by spreading it or pinching up a large area of skin.
3. Pick up syringe with other hand, and hold it as you would a pencil. Insert needle straight into the skin (90° angle). After the needle is in, pull back the plunger very slightly. If blood comes into the syringe, the needle has entered a blood vessel. Remove the needle and put it in at another location. If blood does not appear in the syringe, push the plunger in slowly as far as it will go.
4. To inject the insulin, push plunger all the way down, using less than five seconds to inject the dose.
5. Hold alcohol swab near the needle and pull needle straight out of skin. Press alcohol swab over injection site for several seconds.
6. Use disposable syringe only once to insure sterility of syringe and needle and accuracy of dose. Destroy syringes as directed.
7. To avoid tissue damage, always change the site for each injection.

WARNINGS—SEE ADDITIONAL WARNINGS ABOVE

Patients who have been directed by their physicians to mix two types of insulin should be aware that insulin hypodermic syringes of different manufacturers may vary in the amount of space between the bottom line and the needle.

Because of this, do not change:

1. The order of mixing that the physician has prescribed or
2. The model and brand of syringe or needle without first consulting your physician.

The mixing should be done immediately prior to injection. Failure to heed this warning could result in a dosage error.

USAGE IN PREGNANCY

Pregnancy may make managing your diabetes more difficult. If you are pregnant or nursing a baby, consult your physician, pharmacist, or nurse-educator when using this product.

INSULIN REACTION AND SHOCK

Insulin reaction (too little sugar in the blood, also called "hypoglycemia") can be brought about by:

1. Taking too much insulin
2. Missing or delaying meals
3. Exercising or working too hard just before a meal
4. An infection or illness (especially with diarrhea or vomiting)
5. A change in the body's need for insulin

The first symptoms of insulin reaction usually come on suddenly and may include fatigue, nervousness or "shakiness," headache, rapid heartbeat, nausea, and a cold sweat. Eating sugar or a sugar-sweetened product will often correct the condition and prevent more serious symptoms. If the reaction becomes more severe, breathing will be shallow and the skin pale. Contact your doctor at once if you develop any of these symptoms.

DIABETIC ACIDOSIS AND COMA

Diabetic acidosis may develop if your body has too little insulin. (This is the opposite of insulin reaction, which is the result of too much insulin in the blood.) Diabetic acidosis may be brought on if you omit your insulin or take less than the doctor has prescribed, eat significantly more than your diet calls for, or develop a fever or infection. With acidosis, urine tests show a large amount of sugar and acetone.

The first symptoms of diabetic acidosis usually come on gradually, over a period of hours or days, and include a drowsy feeling, flushed face, thirst, and loss of appetite. Heavy breathing and a rapid pulse are more severe symptoms. It is important that you notify your doctor immediately, because diabetic coma (unconsciousness) can follow.

ALLERGY TO INSULIN

Patients occasionally experience redness, swelling, and itching at the site of injection of insulin. This condition, called local allergy, usually clears up in a few days to a few weeks. If you have local reactions, contact your physician, who may recommend a change in the type or species source of insulin. Less common, but potentially more serious, is generalized allergy to insulin, which may cause rash over the whole body, shortness of breath, wheezing, reduction in blood pressure, fast pulse, or sweating. Severe cases of generalized allergy may be life-threatening. If you think you are having a generalized allergic reaction to insulin, notify a physician immediately. Your doctor may recommend skin testing, injecting small doses of other insulins into the skin, in order to select the best insulin for you to use. Patients who have had severe generalized allergic reactions to insulin should be skin tested with each new preparation to be used before starting treatment with that preparation.

IMPORTANT NOTES

1. Never change from the insulin that has been prescribed for you to another insulin without instructions from your doctor. Changing the type, strength, species, or manufacturer of insulin can cause problems with your diabetes.
2. Your doctor will tell you what to do if you miss a dose of insulin or miss a meal because of illness. Always keep an extra supply of insulin, as well as spare syringe and needle, on hand. If you miss a meal, use a substitute of sugar, sugar-sweetened candy, fruit juice, or sugar-sweetened beverage according to your doctor's instructions.
3. If you become ill from any cause, especially with nausea and vomiting, your insulin requirement may change. Test your urine and /or blood and notify your doctor at once.
4. Consult your doctor if you notice anything unusual or have doubts about your condition or your use of insulin.
5. Always wear diabetic identification so that appropriate treatment can be given if complications occur away from home.
6. Understand how to manage your diabetes so that your life can be active and healthy.

HOW SUPPLIED

Regular Iletin ® I (Insulin Injection, USP) (Beef-Pork) is supplied in rubber-stoppered vials as follows:

CP-240, U-40, 40 units/cc, 10 cc (400 units) (NDC 0002-8240-01).

CP-210, U-100, 100 units/cc, 10 cc (1000 units) (NDC 0002-8210-01). The above products are supplied 10 per carton. *Refrigerate. Avoid freezing.*

CP-210—6505-01-141-94964
[031584]

REGULAR (CONCENTRATED) ILETIN® II, U-500 ℞

[*rĕg-ū-lĕr ī'lĕ-tĭn*]
(insulin injection, USP, purified pork)

WARNINGS

ANY CHANGE OF INSULIN SHOULD BE MADE CAUTIOUSLY AND ONLY UNDER MEDICAL SUPERVISION. CHANGES IN PURITY, STRENGTH (U-40, U-100), BRAND (MANUFACTURER), TYPE (LENTE®, NPH, REGULAR, ETC.), AND/OR SPECIES SOURCE (BEEF, PORK, BEEF-PORK, OR HUMAN) MAY RESULT IN THE NEED FOR A CHANGE IN DOSAGE. SEE BELOW.

IT IS NOT POSSIBLE TO IDENTIFY WHICH PATIENTS WILL REQUIRE A REDUCTION IN DOSE TO AVOID HYPOGLYCEMIA WHEN USING THIS INSULIN. HOWEVER, IT IS KNOWN THAT A SMALL NUMBER OF PATIENTS MAY REQUIRE A SIGNIFICANT CHANGE. ADJUSTMENT MAY BE NEEDED WITH THE FIRST DOSE OR OCCUR OVER A PERIOD OF SEVERAL WEEKS. BE AWARE OF THE POSSIBILITY OF SYMPTOMS OF EITHER HYPOGLYCEMIA OR HYPERGLYCEMIA.

This insulin is prepared from pork pancreas only. The dose of pork insulin for patients with insulin resistance due to antibodies to beef insulin may be only a fraction of that of beef insulin.

This insulin preparation contains 500 units of insulin in each milliliter. Extreme caution must be observed in the measurement of dosage because inadvertent overdose may result in irreversible insulin shock. Serious consequences may result if it is used other than under constant medical supervision.

DESCRIPTION

This Lilly pork insulin product differs from previous pork insulin preparations because it has undergone additional steps of chromatographic purification.

Regular (Concentrated) Iletin® II (insulin injection, USP, purified pork, Lilly), U-500, is an aqueous solution made from the antidiabetic principle of pork pancreas as stated on the label. Each milliliter contains 500 units of regular (unmodified) insulin and approximately 1.6 percent glycerin (w/v), with approximately 0.25 percent m-cresol (w/v) as a preservative. Sodium hydroxide and hydrochloric acid are added during manufacture to adjust the pH. All preparations of Iletin® II (insulin, purified pork, Lilly) are made from zinc-insulin crystals.

Adequate insulin dosage permits the diabetic patient to utilize carbohydrates and fats in a comparatively satisfactory manner. Regardless of concentration, the action of insulin is basically the same: to enable carbohydrate metabolism to occur and thus to prevent the production of ketone bodies by the liver. Although, under usual circumstances, diabetes can be controlled with doses in the vicinity of 40 to 60 units or less, an occasional patient develops such resistance or becomes so unresponsive to the effect of insulin that daily doses of several hundred, or even several thousand, units are required. Fortunately, there seems to be no condition of absolute resistance; all resistant patients will apparently respond to some dose, if it is large enough.

Occasionally, a cause of the insulin resistance can be found (such as hemochromatosis, cirrhosis of the liver, some complicating disease of the endocrine glands other than the pancreas, allergy, or infection), but in other cases, no cause of the high insulin requirement can be determined.

Iletin II, U-500, is unmodified by any agent that might prolong its action; however, clinical experience has shown that it frequently has a time action similar to a repository insulin preparation and that a single dose may show activity over a 24-hour period. This effect has been credited to the high concentration of the preparation.

INDICATIONS

Iletin® II (purified pork insulin injection, Lilly), U-500, is especially useful for the treatment of diabetic patients with marked insulin resistance (daily requirements more than 200 units), since a large dose may be administered subcutaneously in a reasonable volume.

PRECAUTIONS

Every patient exhibiting insulin resistance who requires Iletin® II (purified pork insulin injection, Lilly), U-500, for the control of diabetes should be held under close observation until dosage is established. The response will vary among patients. Some can be controlled with a single dose daily; others may require two or three injections per day. Most patients will show a "tolerance" to insulin, so that minor variations in dosage can occur without the development of untoward symptoms of insulin shock.

Insulin resistance is frequently self-limited; after several weeks or months during which high dosage is required, responsiveness to the pharmacologic effect of insulin may be regained and dosage can be reduced.

Insulin should be kept in a cold place, preferably in a refrigerator. Do not inject insulin that is not water-clear. Discoloration, turbidity, or unusual viscosity indicates deterioration or contamination.

Use of a package of insulin should not be started after the expiration date stamped on it.

ADVERSE REACTIONS

As with other insulin preparations, hypoglycemic reactions may be associated with the administration of Iletin® II (purified pork insulin injection, Lilly), U-500. However, deep secondary hypoglycemic reactions may develop 18 to 24 hours after the original injection of Iletin II, U-500. Consequently, patients should be carefully observed, and prompt treatment of such reactions should be initiated with glucagon injections and/or with glucose by intravenous injection or gavage.

Continued on next page

• Identi-Code® symbol.

Lilly—Cont.

ALLERGIC REACTIONS

Erythema, swelling, or pruritus may occur at injection sites. Such localized allergic manifestations usually resolve within a few days to a few weeks.

Less common, but potentially more serious, is systemic allergy to insulin, which may cause generalized urticaria, dyspnea, or wheezing and may, on continued administration of the insulin, progress to anaphylaxis.

If a severe allergic reaction occurs, the drug should be discontinued and the patient treated with the usual agents (e.g., epinephrine, antihistamines, or corticosteroids). Patients who have experienced severe systemic allergic symptoms should be skin tested with another insulin preparation before its initiation. Desensitization procedures may permit resumption of insulin administration.

DOSAGE AND ADMINISTRATION

Iletin® II (purified pork insulin injection, Lilly), U-500, can be administered by both the subcutaneous and the intramuscular routes. It is inadvisable to inject Iletin II, U-500, intravenously because of the possible development of allergic or anaphylactoid reactions.

It is recommended that a tuberculin type of syringe be utilized for the measurement of dosage. Variations in dosage are frequently possible in the insulin-resistant patient, since the individual is unresponsive to the pharmacologic effect of the insulin. Nevertheless, accuracy of measurement is to be encouraged because of the potential danger of the preparation.

HOW SUPPLIED

℞ *CP-2500, Regular (Concentrated) Iletin® II (purified pork insulin injection, Lilly), U-500,* 500 units/cc, 20 cc, rubber-stoppered vials (10,000 units) (10 per carton) (NDC 0002-8500-01). *Refrigerate. Avoid freezing.*

[013185]

LENTE® ILETIN® I
[*lĕn-ta ī-lĕ-tĭn*]
(Beef-Pork)
(insulin zinc suspension)
USP

SEMILENTE® ILETIN® I
[*sĕm 'ī-lĕn 'ta ī 'lĕ-tĭn*]
(Beef-Pork)
(prompt insulin zinc suspension)
USP

ULTRALENTE® ILETIN® I
[*ŭl 'tra-lĕn 'ta ī 'lĕ-tĭn*]
(Beef-Pork)
(extended insulin zinc suspension)
USP

INFORMATION FOR THE PATIENT

WARNINGS, Insulin and Diabetes, and Use of Proper Type of Insulin: *See under* Regular Iletin® I.

LENTE BEEF-PORK INSULIN

Lente beef-pork insulin is obtained from beef and pork pancreas. Insulin has been combined with zinc to form small crystals. Lente beef-pork insulin has an intermediate time of activity. Its action starts more slowly than does that of regular beef-pork insulin and lasts somewhat longer (slightly over 24 hours).

Lente beef-pork insulin should look uniformly cloudy or milky. If the insulin substance (the cloudy material) settles at the bottom of the vial, the vial must be carefully rotated before the injection so that the contents are uniformly mixed (see instructions under Preparing the Dose). Do not use a vial of insulin if you see lumps that float or stick to the sides. Also, the insulin should not be used if it is clear and remains clear after the vial is rotated.

SEMILENTE BEEF-PORK INSULIN

Semilente beef-pork insulin comes from beef and pork pancreas. Insulin has been combined with zinc to form small crystals. Semilente beef-pork insulin has a short period of activity. Its action starts nearly as rapidly as that of regular insulin and lasts slightly longer (approximately 12 to 16 hours). This type of insulin will shorten the action time of Lente insulin (an intermediate-acting form) when they are mixed.

Semilente beef-pork insulin should look uniformly cloudy or milky. If the insulin substance (the cloudy material) settles at the bottom of the vial, the vial must be carefully rotated before the injection so that the contents are uniformly mixed (see instructions under Preparing the Dose). Do not use a vial of insulin if you see lumps that float or stick to the sides. Also, the insulin should not be used if it is clear and remains clear after the vial is rotated.

ULTRALENTE BEEF-PORK INSULIN

Ultralente beef-pork insulin comes from beef and pork pancreas. Insulin has been combined with zinc to form small crystals. Ultralente beef-pork insulin takes effect very gradually and, in comparison with regular insulin, has a long period of activity (more than 36 hours). This type of insulin will lengthen the action time of Lente insulin (an intermediate-acting form) when they are mixed.

Ultralente beef-pork insulin should look uniformly cloudy or milky. If the insulin substance (the cloudy material) settles at the bottom of the vial, the vial must be carefully rotated before the injection so that the contents are uniformly mixed (see instructions under Preparing the Dose). Do not use a vial of insulin if you see lumps that float or stick to the sides. Also, the insulin should not be used if it is clear and remains clear after the vial is rotated.

Storage, Use the Correct Syringe, Disposable Syringes, and Sterilizing and Assembling Reusable Syringes: *See under* Regular Iletin® I.

PREPARING THE DOSE

1. Wash your hands.
2. Gently roll the insulin bottle several times to mix the insulin. Be sure it is completely mixed. Do not shake bottle. Flip off the colored protective cap on the bottle, but **do not** remove the rubber stopper. *See also under* Regular Iletin® I.

Injecting the Dose, Warnings, Usage in Pregnancy, Insulin Reaction and Shock, Diabetic Acidosis and Coma, Allergy to Insulin, and **Important Notes:** *See under* Regular Iletin® I.

HOW SUPPLIED

Lente ® Iletin ® I (Insulin Zinc Suspension, USP) is supplied in rubber-stoppered vials as follows:

CP-440, U-40, 40 units/cc, 10 cc (400 units) (NDC 0002-8440-01).

CP-410, U-100, 100 units/cc, 10 cc (1000 units) (NDC 0002-8410-01).

Semilente ® Iletin ® I (Prompt Insulin Zinc Suspension, USP) is supplied in rubber-stoppered vials as follows:

CP-540, U-40, 40 units/cc, 10 cc (400 units) (NDC 0002-8540-01).

CP-510, U-100, 100 units/cc, 10 cc (1000 units) (NDC 0002-8510-01).

Ultralente ® Iletin ® I (Extended Insulin Zinc Suspension, USP) is supplied in rubber-stoppered vials as follows:

CP-640, U-40, 40 units/cc, 10 cc (400 units) (NDC 0002-8640-01).

CP-610, U-100, 100 units/cc, 10 cc (1000 units) (NDC 0002-8610-01).

The above products are supplied 10/carton. *Refrigerate. Avoid freezing.*

CP-410—6505-01-142-5588
[031484]

NPH ILETIN® I
[*ĕn 'pē-āch ī 'lĕ-tĭn*]
(Beef-Pork)
(isophane insulin suspension)
USP

INFORMATION FOR THE PATIENT

WARNINGS, Insulin and Diabetes, and Use of Proper Type of Insulin: *See under* Regular Iletin® I.

NPH BEEF-PORK INSULIN

NPH beef-pork insulin is obtained from beef and pork pancreas. Insulin has been combined with protamine and zinc so that its action is similar to that of a mixture of Regular and Protamine Zinc insulins. The result is an intermediate-acting insulin with a slower speed of action than Regular insulin and a shorter time of activity than Protamine Zinc insulin. The effect of NPH beef-pork insulin lasts slightly more than 24 hours.

NPH beef-pork insulin should look uniformly cloudy or milky. If the insulin substance (the cloudy material) settles at the bottom of the vial, the vial must be carefully rotated before the injection so that the contents are uniformly mixed (see instructions under Preparing the Dose). Do not use a vial of insulin if you see lumps that float or stick to the sides. Also, the insulin should not be used if it is clear and remains clear after the vial is rotated.

Storage, Use the Correct Syringe, Disposable Syringes, and Sterilizing and Assembling Reusable Syringes: *See under* Regular Iletin® I.

Preparing the Dose: *See under* Lente® Iletin® I and Regular Iletin® I.

Injecting the Dose, Warnings, Usage in Pregnancy, Insulin Reaction and Shock, Diabetic Acidosis and Coma, Allergy to Insulin, and Important Notes: *See under* Regular Iletin® I.

HOW SUPPLIED

NPH Iletin® I (Isophane Insulin Suspension, USP) is supplied in rubber-stoppered vials as follows:

CP-340, U-40, 40 units/cc, 10 cc (400 units) (NDC 0002-8340-01).

CP-310, U-100, 100 units/cc, 10 cc (1000 units) (NDC 0002-8310-01).

The above products are supplied 10/carton. *Refrigerate. Avoid freezing.*

CP-310—6505-01-141-9463
[031484]

PROTAMINE, ZINC & ILETIN® I
[*prō 'ta-mēn zĭngk ănd ī 'lĕ-tĭn*]
(Beef-Pork)
(protamine zinc insulin suspension)
USP

INFORMATION FOR THE PATIENT

WARNINGS, Insulin and Diabetes, and Use of Proper Type of Insulin: *See under* Regular Iletin® I.

PROTAMINE ZINC BEEF-PORK INSULIN

Protamine zinc beef-pork insulin is obtained from beef and pork pancreas. Protamine and zinc have been added to lengthen the time of action. Protamine zinc beef-pork insulin takes effect gradually and, in comparison with regular beef-pork insulin, has a long period of activity (well over 24 hours).

Protamine zinc beef-pork insulin should look uniformly cloudy or milky. If the insulin substance (the cloudy material) settles at the bottom of the vial, the vial must be carefully rotated before the injection so that the contents are uniformly mixed (see instructions under Preparing the Dose). Do not use a vial of insulin if you see lumps that float or stick to the sides. Also, the insulin should not be used if it is clear and remains clear after the vial is rotated.

Storage, Use the Correct Syringe, Disposable Syringes, and Sterilizing and Assembling Reusable Syringes: *See under* Regular Iletin® I.

Preparing the Dose: *See under* Lente® Iletin® I and Regular Iletin® I.

Injecting the Dose, Warnings, Usage in Pregnancy, Insulin Reaction and Shock, Diabetic Acidosis and Coma, Allergy to Insulin, and **Important Notes:** *See under* Regular Iletin® I.

HOW SUPPLIED

Protamine, Zinc & Iletin® I (Protamine Zinc Insulin Suspension, USP) is supplied in rubber-stoppered vials as follows:

CP-140, U-40, 40 units/cc, 10 cc (400 units) (NDC 0002-8140-01).

CP-110, U-100, 100 units/cc, 10 cc (1000 units) (NDC 0002-8110-01).

The above products are supplied 10/carton. *Refrigerate. Avoid freezing.*

[031484]

KEFLIN® ℞
[*kĕf 'lĭn*]
(cephalothin sodium)
For Injection, USP
Neutral

DESCRIPTION

Keflin® (cephalothin sodium, Lilly), Neutral, is a semisynthetic cephalosporin antibiotic for parenteral use. It is the sodium salt of 7-(thiophene-2-acetamido) cephalosporanic acid. Sodium bicarbonate has been added to result in reconstituted solutions having a pH ranging between 6 and 8.5. The total sodium content is approximately 63 mg (2.8 mEq sodium ion) per g of Keflin.

Cephalothin was synthesized in the Lilly Research Laboratories by the reaction of thiophene-2-acetic acid with 7-aminocephalosporanic acid. The cephalosporanic acid nucleus is obtained from cephalosporin C, which is produced by the fungus *Cephalosporium.* Cephalothin is supplied as the sodium salt of 7-(thiophene-2-acetamido) cephalosporanic acid.

Cephalothin is a cream-colored crystalline solid which is stable in the dry state and moderately soluble in distilled water (250 to 300 mg/ml).

Keflin, Neutral, contains 30 mg of sodium bicarbonate/g of cephalothin sodium. Free cephalothin acid does not form within this range, and the solubility and freezability are thereby enhanced.

The molecular weight of cephalothin sodium is 418.4.

CLINICAL PHARMACOLOGY

Human Pharmacology—Keflin® (cephalothin sodium, Lilly) is a broad-spectrum antibiotic for parenteral administration. After administration of a 500-mg dose intramuscularly to normal volunteers, the average peak serum antibiotic level was 10 mcg/ml at one-half hour; with a 1-g dose, the average was about 20 mcg/ml. Following a single 1-g intravenous dose of Keflin, blood levels have been about 30 mcg/ml at 15 minutes, have ranged from 3 to 12 mcg at one hour, and have declined to about 1 mcg at four hours. With continuous infusion, at the rate of 500 mg/hour, levels have been from 14 to 20 mcg/ml of serum. Dosages of 2 g given intravenously over a 30-minute period have produced serum concentrations of 80 to 100 mcg/ml one-half hour after the infusion;

levels ranged from 10 to 40 mcg/ml at one hour and from 3 to 6 mcg/ml at two hours and were not assayable after five hours.

Sixty to 70 percent of an intramuscular dose is excreted by the kidneys in the first six hours; this results in high urine levels, e.g., 800 mcg/ml of urine after a 500-mg dose and 2500 mcg/ml following 1 g. Probenecid slows tubular excretion and almost doubles peak blood levels.

Spinal-fluid levels have ranged from 0.4 to 1.4 mcg/ml in a child and from 0.15 to 5 mcg/ml in adults with meningeal inflammatory states. The antibiotic passes readily into other body fluids, e.g., pleural, joint, and ascitic fluids. Studies of amniotic fluid and cord blood show prompt transfer of Keflin across the placenta.

Following single 1-g intramuscular doses of cephalothin, peak maternal levels were reached between 31 and 45 minutes after injection; the peak levels in the infants occurred about 15 minutes later. All plasma levels in the infants were far below those of the mothers.

Secondary aqueous-humor levels have averaged 0.5 mcg/ml 30 minutes after a single 1-g intravenous dose. The antibiotic has been detected in bile.

Microbiology—The in vitro bactericidal action of cephalothin results from inhibition of cell-wall synthesis.

Keflin is usually active against the following organisms in vitro:

- Beta-hemolytic and other streptococci (many strains of enterococci, e.g., *Streptococcus faecalis,* are relatively resistant)
- Staphylococci, including coagulase-positive, coagulase-negative, and penicillinase-producing strains
- *S. (Diplococcus) pneumoniae*
- *Haemophilus influenzae*
- *Escherichia coli* and other coliform bacteria
- *Klebsiella*
- *Proteus mirabilis*
- *Salmonella* sp.
- *Shigella* sp.

Pseudomonas organisms are resistant to Keflin, as are most indole-producing *Proteus* species and motile *Enterobacter* species.

Susceptibility Plate Tests—If the Bauer-Kirby-Sherris-Turck method of disc susceptibility testing is used (*Am. J. Clin. Pathol., 45:* 493, 1966; *Federal Register, 39:* 19182-19184, 1974), a disc containing 30 mcg cephalothin should give a zone of over 17 mm when tested against a cephalothin-susceptible bacterial strain and a zone of over 14 mm with an organism of intermediate susceptibility.

INDICATIONS AND USAGE

Keflin® (cephalothin sodium, Lilly) is indicated for the treatment of serious infections caused by susceptible strains of the designated microorganisms in the diseases listed below. Culture and susceptibility studies should be performed. Therapy may be instituted before results of susceptibility studies are obtained.

- Respiratory tract infections caused by *S. pneumoniae,* staphylococci (penicillinase and non-penicillinase-producing), group A beta-hemolytic streptococci, *Klebsiella,* and *H. influenzae*
- Skin and soft-tissue infections, including peritonitis, caused by staphylococci (penicillinase and non-penicillinase-producing), group A beta-hemolytic streptococci, *E. coli, P. mirabilis,* and *Klebsiella*
- Genitourinary tract infections caused by *E. coli, P. mirabilis,* and *Klebsiella*
- Septicemia, including endocarditis, caused by *S. pneumoniae,* staphylococci (penicillinase and non-penicillinase-producing), group A beta-hemolytic streptococci, *S. viridans, E. coli, P. mirabilis,* and *Klebsiella*
- Gastrointestinal infections caused by *Salmonella* and *Shigella* species
- Meningitis caused by *S. pneumoniae,* group A beta-hemolytic streptococci, and staphylococci (penicillinase and non-penicillinase-producing)

  NOTE: Inasmuch as only low levels of Keflin are found in the cerebrospinal fluid, the drug is not reliable in the treatment of meningitis and cannot be recommended for that purpose. Keflin has, however, proved to be effective in a number of cases of meningitis and may be considered for unusual circumstances in which other, more reliably effective antibiotics cannot be used.
- Bone and joint infections caused by staphylococci (penicillinase and non-penicillinase-producing)

The prophylactic administration of Keflin preoperatively, intraoperatively, and postoperatively may reduce the incidence of certain postoperative infections in patients undergoing surgical procedures (e.g., vaginal hysterectomy) that are classified as contaminated or potentially contaminated. The perioperative use of Keflin also may be effective in surgical patients in whom infection at the operative site would present a serious risk, e.g., during open-heart surgery and prosthetic arthroplasty.

The prophylactic administration of Keflin should be discontinued within a 24-hour period after the surgical procedure. If there are signs of infection, specimens for culture should be obtained for the identification of the causative organism so that appropriate therapy may be instituted. (*See* DOSAGE AND ADMINISTRATION.)

NOTE: If the susceptibility tests show that the causative organism is resistant to Keflin, other appropriate antibiotic therapy should be instituted.

CONTRAINDICATION

Keflin ® (cephalothin sodium, Lilly) is contraindicated in persons who have shown hypersensitivity to cephalosporin antibiotics.

WARNINGS

BEFORE CEPHALOTHIN THERAPY IS INSTITUTED, CAREFUL INQUIRY SHOULD BE MADE CONCERNING PREVIOUS HYPERSENSITIVITY REACTIONS TO CEPHALOSPORINS AND PENICILLIN. CEPHALOSPORIN C DERIVATIVES SHOULD BE GIVEN CAUTIOUSLY TO PENICILLIN-SENSITIVE PATIENTS.

SERIOUS ACUTE HYPERSENSITIVITY REACTIONS MAY REQUIRE EPINEPHRINE AND OTHER EMERGENCY MEASURES.

There is some clinical and laboratory evidence of partial cross-allergenicity of the penicillins and the cephalosporins. Patients have been reported to have had severe reactions (including anaphylaxis) to both drugs.

Any patient who has demonstrated some form of allergy, particularly to drugs, should receive antibiotics cautiously and then only when absolutely necessary. No exception should be made with regard to Keflin® (cephalothin sodium, Lilly).

Pseudomembranous colitis has been reported with virtually all broad-spectrum antibiotics (including macrolides, semisynthetic penicillins, and cephalosporins); therefore, it is important to consider its diagnosis in patients who develop diarrhea in association with the use of antibiotics. Such colitis may range in severity from mild to life-threatening.

Treatment with broad-spectrum antibiotics alters the normal flora of the colon and may permit overgrowth of clostridia. Studies indicate that a toxin produced by *Clostridium difficile* is one primary cause of antibiotic-associated colitis. Mild cases of pseudomembranous colitis usually respond to drug discontinuance alone. In moderate to severe cases, management should include sigmoidoscopy, appropriate bacteriologic studies, and fluid, electrolyte, and protein supplementation. When the colitis does not improve after the drug has been discontinued, or when it is severe, oral vancomycin is the drug of choice for antibiotic-associated pseudomembranous colitis produced by *C. difficile.* Other causes of colitis should be ruled out.

PRECAUTIONS

General Precautions—Patients should be followed carefully so that any side effects or unusual manifestations of drug idiosyncrasy may be detected. If an allergic reaction to Keflin® (cephalothin sodium, Lilly) occurs, the drug should be discontinued and the patient treated with the usual agents (e.g., epinephrine or other pressor amines, antihistamines, or corticosteroids).

Although Keflin rarely produces alteration in kidney function, evaluation of renal status is recommended, especially in seriously ill patients receiving maximum doses. Patients with impaired renal function should be placed on the dosage schedule recommended under DOSAGE AND ADMINISTRATION. Usual doses in such individuals may result in excessive serum concentrations.

When intravenous doses of cephalothin larger than 6 g daily are given by infusion for periods longer than three days, they may be associated with thrombophlebitis, and the veins may have to be alternated. The addition of 10 to 25 mg of hydrocortisone to intravenous solutions containing 4 to 6 g of cephalothin may reduce the incidence of thrombophlebitis. The use of small IV needles in the larger available veins may be preferred.

Prolonged use of Keflin may result in the overgrowth of nonsusceptible organisms. Constant observation of the patient is essential. If superinfection occurs during therapy, appropriate measures should be taken.

A false-positive reaction for glucose in the urine may occur with Benedict's or Fehling's solution or with Clinitest® tablets but not with Tes-Tape® (Glucose Enzymatic Test Strip, USP, Lilly).

An increased incidence of nephrotoxicity has been reported following concomitant administration of cephalosporins and aminoglycoside antibiotics.

Broad-spectrum antibiotics should be prescribed with caution in individuals with a history of gastrointestinal disease, particularly colitis.

Usage in Pregnancy—Pregnancy Category B—Reproduction studies have been performed in rabbits given doses of 200 mg/kg and have revealed no evidence of impaired fertility or harm to the fetus due to Keflin. There are, however, no adequate and well-controlled studies in pregnant women. Because animal reproduction studies are not always predictive of human response, this drug should be used during pregnancy only if clearly needed.

Nursing Mothers—Caution should be exercised when Keflin is administered to a nursing woman.

ADVERSE REACTIONS

Hypersensitivity—Maculopapular rash, urticaria, reactions resembling serum sickness, and anaphylaxis have been reported. Eosinophilia and drug fever have been observed to be associated with other allergic reactions. These reactions are most likely to occur in patients with a history of allergy, particularly to penicillin.

Blood—Neutropenia, thrombocytopenia, and hemolytic anemia have been reported. Some individuals, particularly those with azotemia, have developed positive direct Coombs' tests during cephalothin therapy.

Liver—Transient rise in SGOT and alkaline phosphatase has been noted.

Kidney—Rise in BUN and decreased creatinine clearance have been reported, particularly in patients with prior renal impairment. The role of Keflin® (cephalothin sodium, Lilly) in renal changes is difficult to assess, because other factors predisposing to prerenal azotemia or to acute renal failure usually have been present.

Local Reactions—Pain, induration, tenderness, and elevation of temperature have been reported following repeated intramuscular injections. Thrombophlebitis has occurred and is usually associated with daily doses of more than 6 g given by infusion for longer than three days.

Gastrointestinal—Symptoms of pseudomembranous colitis may appear either during or after antibiotic treatment. Nausea and vomiting have been reported rarely.

DOSAGE AND ADMINISTRATION

In adults, the usual dosage range is 500 mg to 1 g of cephalothin every four to six hours. A dosage of 500 mg every six hours is adequate in uncomplicated pneumonia, furunculosis with cellulitis, and most urinary tract infections. In severe infections, this may be increased by giving the injections every four hours or, when the desired response is not obtained, by raising the dose to 1 g. In life-threatening infections, doses up to 2 g every four hours may be required.

For perioperative prophylactic use to prevent postoperative infection in contaminated or potentially contaminated surgery in adults, the following doses are recommended:

(a) 1 to 2 g administered IV just prior to surgery (approximately one-half to one hour before the initial incision);

(b) 1 to 2 g during surgery (administration modified according to the duration of the operative procedure); and

(c) 1 to 2 g every six hours postoperatively for 24 hours.

In children, 20 to 30 mg/kg may be given at the times designated above.

Since Keflin has a serum half-life of 30 to 50 minutes, it is important that (1) the preoperative dose be given just prior to the start of surgery so that adequate antibiotic levels are present in the serum and tissues at the time of initial surgical incision; and (2) Keflin be administered, if necessary, at appropriate intervals during surgery to provide sufficient levels of the antibiotic at the anticipated moments of greatest exposure to infective organisms.

When renal function is reduced, an intravenous loading dose of 1 to 2 g may be given. Continued dosage schedule should be determined by degree of renal impairment, severity of infection, and susceptibility of the causative organism. The maximum doses administered should be based on the following recommendations.

DOSAGE OF KEFLIN®
(CEPHALOTHIN SODIUM, LILLY)
WHEN RENAL FUNCTION IS IMPAIRED

STATUS OF RENAL FUNCTION	MAXIMUM ADULT DOSAGE (Maintenance)
Mild Impairment (C_{cr}=80–50 ml/min)	2 g q. 6 h.
Moderate Impairment (C_{cr}=50–25 ml/min)	1.5 g q. 6 h.
Severe Impairment (C_{cr}=25–10 ml/min)	1 g q. 6 h.
Marked Impairment (C_{cr}=10–2 ml/min)	0.5 g q. 6 h.
Essentially No Function (C_{cr}= <2 ml/min)	0.5 g q. 8 h.

In infants and children, the dosage should be proportionately less in accordance with age, weight, and severity of infection. Daily administration of 100 mg/kg (80 to 160 mg/kg or 40 to

Continued on next page

Lilly—Cont.

80 mg/lb) in divided doses has been found effective for most infections susceptible to Keflin® (cephalothin sodium, Lilly).
Antibiotic therapy in beta-hemolytic streptococcal infections should continue for at least ten days. In staphylococcal infections, surgical procedures, such as incision and drainage, should be carried out in all cases when indicated.
Keflin may be given intravenously or by deep intramuscular injection into a large muscle mass, such as the gluteus or lateral aspect of the thigh, to minimize pain and induration.
Intramuscular—Each g of cephalothin should be diluted with 4 ml of Sterile Water for Injection. If the vial contents do not completely dissolve, an additional small amount of diluent (e.g., 0.2 to 0.4 ml) may be added and the contents warmed slightly.
Intravenous—The intravenous route may be preferable for patients with bacteremia, septicemia, or other severe or life-threatening infections who may be poor risks because of lowered resistance resulting from such debilitating conditions as malnutrition, trauma, surgery, diabetes, heart failure, or malignancy, particularly if shock is present or impending.
For these infections in patients with normal renal function, the intravenous dosage is 4 to 12 g of cephalothin daily. In conditions such as septicemia, 6 to 8 g/day may be given intravenously for several days at the beginning of therapy; then, depending on the clinical response and laboratory findings, the dosage may gradually be reduced.
For patients who are to receive cephalothin intravenously, it is convenient to use the 1 or 2-g 100-ml-size vial (*see* PRECAUTIONS).
For intermittent intravenous administration, a solution containing 1 g cephalothin in 10 ml of diluent may be slowly injected directly into the vein over a period of three to five minutes or may be given through the tubing when the patient is receiving parenteral solutions.
Intermittent intravenous infusion with a Y-type administration set can also be accomplished while bulk intravenous solutions are being infused. However, during infusion of the solution containing Keflin® (cephalothin sodium, Lilly), it is desirable to discontinue the other solution. When this technique is employed, careful attention should be paid to the volume of the solution containing Keflin so that the calculated dose will be infused.
For continuous intravenous infusion, 1 or 2 g of cephalothin, diluted and well mixed with at least 10 ml of Sterile Water for Injection, may be added to an IV bottle containing one of the following intravenous solutions: Acetated Ringer's Injection, 5% Dextrose Injection, 5% Dextrose in Lactated Ringer's Injection, Ionosol® B in D5-W, Isolyte® M with 5% Dextrose, Lactated Ringer's Injection, Normosol®-M in D5-W, Plasma-Lyte® Injection, Plasma-Lyte®-M Injection in 5% Dextrose, Ringer's Injection, or 0.9% Sodium Chloride Injection. The choice of solution and the volume to be employed are dictated by fluid and electrolyte management.
Intraperitoneal—In peritoneal dialysis procedures, cephalothin has been added to dialysis fluid in concentrations up to 6 mg/100 ml and instilled into the peritoneal space throughout an entire dialysis (16 to 30 hours). Careful assay procedures have shown that 44 percent of the administered drug was absorbed into the bloodstream. Serum levels of 10 mcg/ml were reported, with no evidence of accumulation and no untoward local or systemic reactions.
The intraperitoneal administration of solutions containing 0.1 to 4 percent Keflin in saline has been used in treating patients with peritonitis or contaminated peritoneal cavities. (The total daily dosage of Keflin should take into account the amount given by the intraperitoneal route.)

STABILITY

While stored under *refrigeration,* the solution has a satisfactory potency for 96 hours after reconstitution. Solutions may precipitate; they can be redissolved by being warmed to room temperature with constant agitation. Kept at *room temperature,* solutions for intramuscular injection should be given within 12 hours after being mixed. Intravenous infusions should be started within 12 hours and completed within 24 hours. For prolonged infusions, replace with a freshly prepared solution at least every 24 hours.
The concentrated solution will darken, especially at room temperature. Slight discoloration of the solution is permissible.
Solutions of Keflin® (cephalothin sodium, Lilly) in Sterile Water for Injection, 5% Dextrose Injection, or 0.9% Sodium Chloride Injection that are frozen immediately after reconstitution in Faspak containers and the conventional vials in which the drugs are supplied are stable for as long as 12 weeks when stored at −20°C. **If the product is warmed, care should be taken to avoid heating it after the thawing is complete. Once thawed, the solution should not be refrozen.**

HOW SUPPLIED

(℞) *Vials Keflin® (Cephalothin Sodium for Injection, USP), Neutral,* rubber-stoppered (Dry Powder): *No. 7001,* 1 g (equivalent to cephalothin), 10-ml size, in singles (NDC 0002-7001-01) (10/carton) and Traypak™ (multivial carton, Lilly) of 25 (NDC 0002-7001-25); *No. 7000,* 1 g (equivalent to cephalothin), 100-ml size (NDC 0002-7000-10), *No. 7003,* 2 g (equivalent to cephalothin), 20-ml size (NDC 0002-7003-10), *No. 7002,* 2 g (equivalent to cephalothin), 100-ml size (NDC 0002-7002-10), and *No. 7004,* 4 g (equivalent to cephalothin), 50-ml size (NDC 0002-7004-10), in Traypak of 10; *No. 7020,* 20 g (equivalent to cephalothin), 200-ml size, in Traypak of 6 (NDC 0002-7020-16).
(℞) *Faspak ® (flexible plastic bag, Lilly): No. 7190,* 1 g (equivalent to cephalothin), in Faspak of 96 (NDC 0002-7190-74); *No. 7191,* 2 g, in Faspak of 96 (NDC 0002-7191-74).
(℞) *ADD-Vantage® (vials and diluent containers, Abbott) Vials: No. 7260,* 1 g (equivalent to cephalothin), in Traypak of 25 (NDC 0002-7260-25); *No. 7261,* 2 g (equivalent to cephalothin), in Traypak of 10 (NDC 0002-7261-10).
The above ADD-Vantage Vials are to be used only with Abbott Laboratories Diluent Containers containing:

0.9% Sodium Chloride Injection, USP, 50 ml, NDC 0074-7101-13; 100 ml, NDC 0074-7101-23, or 5% Dextrose Injection, USP, 50 ml, NDC 0074-7100-13; 100 ml, NDC 0074-7100-23 [031385]

No. 7001, 1 g—1's and 25's—6505-00-000-0072

KEFUROX™ ℞

[*kĕf'ōō-rŏcks*]
(sterile cefuroxime sodium)

DESCRIPTION

Kefurox™ (sterile cefuroxime sodium, Lilly) is a semisynthetic, broad-spectrum cephalosporin antibiotic for parenteral administration. It has the chemical formula (6R,7R)-7-[2-(2-Furyl) glyoxylamido]-3-(hydroxymethyl)-8-oxo-5-thia-1-azabicyclo [4.2.0] oct-2-ene-2-carboxyl-acid (Z)-mono(0-methyloxime) carbamate (ester), monosodium salt (USAN).
Kefurox contains approximately 54.2 mg (2.4 mEq) of sodium per gram of cefuroxime activity. Solutions of Kefurox range from light yellow to amber, depending on the concentration and diluent used. The *p* H of freshly reconstituted solutions usually ranges from 6.0 to 8.5.

CLINICAL PHARMACOLOGY

After intramuscular injection of a 750-mg dose of cefuroxime to normal volunteers, the mean peak serum concentration was 27 mcg/ml. The peak occurred at approximately 45 minutes (range 15–60 minutes). Following intravenous doses of 750 mg and 1.5 g, serum concentrations were approximately 50 mcg/ml and 100 mcg/ml respectively at 15 minutes. Therapeutic serum concentrations of approximately 2 mcg/ml or more were maintained for 5.3 hours and 8 hours or more, respectively. There was no evidence of accumulation of cefuroxime in the serum following intravenous administration of 1.5 g doses every 8 hours to normal volunteers. The serum half-life after either intramuscular or intravenous injections is approximately 80 minutes.
Approximately 89% of a dose of cefuroxime is excreted by the kidneys over an 8 hour period, resulting in high urinary concentrations.
Following the intramuscular administration of a 750 mg single dose, urinary concentrations averaged 1300 mcg/ml during the first 8 hours. Intravenous doses of 750 mg and 1.5 g produced urinary levels averaging 1150 mcg/ml and 2500 mcg/ml, respectively, during the first 8-hour period.
The concomitant oral administration of probenecid with cefuroxime slows tubular secretion, decreases renal clearance by approximately 40%, increases the peak serum level by approximately 30%, and increases the serum half-life by approximately 30%. Kefurox is detectable in therapeutic concentrations in pleural fluid, joint fluid, bile, sputum, bone, cerebrospinal fluid (in patients with meningitis), and aqueous humor.
Cefuroxime is approximately 50% bound to serum protein.
Microbiology—Cefuroxime has in vitro activity against a wide range of Gram-positive and Gram-negative organisms and it is highly stable in the presence of beta-lactamases of certain Gram-negative bacteria. The bactericidal action of cefuroxime results from inhibition of cell-wall synthesis.
Cefuroxime is usually active against the following organisms in vitro.
Gram-Negative—*Haemophilus influenzae* (including ampicillin-resistant strains), *Haemophilus parainfluenzae, Neisseria gonorrhoeae* (including penicillinase and non- penicillinase-producing strains), *Neisseria meningitidis, Escherichia coli, Klebsiella* species (including *K. pneumoniae), Enterobacter* species, *Citrobacter* species, *Salmonella* species, *Shigella* species, *Proteus mirabilis, Proteus inconstans* (formerly *Providencia), Providencia rettgeri* (formerly *Proteus rettgeri), Morganella morganii* (formerly *Proteus morganii).*
Some strains of *M. morganii, E. cloacae,* and *Citrobacter* species have been shown by in vitro tests to be resistant to cefuroxime and other cephalosporins.
Gram-Positive—*Staphylococcus aureus* (including penicillinase and non-penicillinase-producing strains), *Staphylococcus epidermidis, Streptococcus pyogenes* (and other streptococci), *Streptococcus pneumoniae* (formerly *Diplococcis pneumoniae*).
Certain strains of enterococci, e.g. *Streptococcus faecalis,* are resistant.
Anaerobic Organisms—Gram-positive and Gram-negative cocci (including *Peptococcus* and *Peptostreptococcus* species), Gram-positive bacilli (including *Clostridium* species), Gram-negative bacilli (including *Bacteroides* and *Fusobacterium* species). Most strains of *Bacteroides fragilis* are resistant.
Pseudomonas and *Campylobacter* species, *Acinetobacter calcoaceticus* (formerly *Mima* and *Herellea* species), and most strains of *Serratia* and *Proteus vulgaris* are resistant to cephalosporins. Methicillin-resistant staphylococci, *Clostridium difficile,* and *Listeria monocytogenes* are resistant to cefuroxime.
Susceptibility Tests—Diffusion Techniques—Quantitative methods that require measurement of zone diameters give the most precise estimates of antibiotic susceptibility. One such procedure[1] has been recommended for use with discs to test susceptibility to cefuroxime. Interpretation involves correlation of the diameters obtained in the disc test with minimum inhibitory concentration (MIC) values for cefuroxime.
Reports from the laboratory giving results of the standardized single-disc susceptibility test[1] using a 30 mcg cefuroxime disc should be interpreted according to the following criteria:

1. Bauer, A. W., Kirby, W. M. M., Sherris, J. C., and Turck, M.: Antibiotic Susceptibility Testing by a Standardized Single Disc Method, Am. J. Clin. Pathol.,*45*:493,1966. Standardized Disc Susceptibility Test, Federal Register, *39*:19182-19184, 1974. National Committee for Clinical Laboratory Standards, Approved Standard: ASM-2 Performance Standards for Antimicrobial Disc Susceptibility Tests, July, 1975.

Susceptible organisms produce zone sizes of 18 mm or greater, indicating that the tested organism is likely to respond to therapy.
Organisms that produce zones of 15 to 17 mm are expected to be susceptible if high dosage is used or if the infection is confined to tissues and fluids (eg, urine), in which high antibiotic levels are attained.
Resistant organisms produce zones of 14 mm or less, indicating that other therapy should be selected.
For gram-positive isolates, the test may be performed with either the cephalosporin-class disc (30 mcg cephalothin) or the cefuroxime disc (30 mcg cefuroxime) and a zone of 18 mm or greater indicates a cefuroxime-susceptible organism.
Gram-negative organisms should be tested with the cefuroxime disc (using the above criteria), since cefuroxime has been shown by in vitro tests to have activity against certain strains of *Enterobacteriaceae* found resistant when tested with the cephalosporin-class disc. Gram-negative organisms having zones of less than 18 mm around the cephalothin disc are not necessarily of intermediate susceptibility or resistant to cefuroxime. The cefuroxime disc should not be used for testing susceptibility to other cephalosporins.
Standardized procedures require the use of laboratory control organisms. The 30 mcg cefuroxime disc should give zone diameters between 27 and 35 mm for *S. aureus* ATCC 25923. For *E. coli* ATCC 25922, the zone diameters should be between 20 and 26 mm.
Dilution Techniques—A bacteria isolate may be considered susceptible if the MIC value for cefuroxime is not more than 16 mcg/ml. Organisms are considered resistant if the MIC is greater than 32 mcg/ml.
As with standard diffusion methods, dilution procedures require the use of laboratory control organisms. Standard cefuroxime powder should give MIC values in the range of 0.5 mcg/ml and 2 mcg/ml for *S. aureus* ATCC 25923. For *E. coli* ATCC 25922, the MIC range should be between 2 mcg/ml and 8 mcg/ml.

INDICATIONS AND USAGE

Kefurox™ (sterile cefuroxime sodium, Lilly) is indicated for the treatment of infections caused by susceptible strains of the designated microorganisms in the diseases listed below:
Lower Respiratory Infections, including pneumonia caused by *S. pneumoniae* (formerly *Diplococcus pneumoniae), H. influenzae* (including ampicillin-resistant strains), *Klebsiella* species, *S. aureus* (penicillinase and non-penicillinase-producing), *S. pyogenes,* and *E. coli.*
Urinary Tract Infections caused by *E. coli* and *Klebsiella* species.
Skin and Skin Structure Infections caused by *S. aureus* (penicillinase and non-penicillinase-producing), *S. pyogenes, E. coli, Klebsiella* species, and *Enterobacter* species.
Septicemia caused by *S. aureus* (penicillinase and non-penicillinase-producing), *S. pneumoniae, E. coli, H. influenzae* (including ampicillin-resistant strains), and *Klebsiella* species.
Meningitis caused by *S. pneumoniae, H. influenzae* (including ampicillin-resistant strains), *N. meningitidis,* and *S. aureus* (penicillinase and non-penicillinase-producing).

Gonorrhea —Uncomplicated and disseminated gonococcal infections due to *N. gonorrhoeae* (penicillinase and non-penicillinase-producing strains) in both males and females.

Clinical microbiologic studies in skin and skin structure infections frequently reveal the growth of susceptible strains of both aerobic and anaerobic organisms. Kefurox has been used successfully in these mixed infections in which several organisms have been isolated. Appropriate cultures and susceptibility studies should be performed to determine the susceptibility of the causative organisms to Kefurox.

Therapy may be started while awaiting the results of these studies; however, once these results become available, the antibiotic treatment should be adjusted accordingly. In certain cases of confirmed or suspected gram-positive or gram-negative sepsis or in patients with other serious infections in which the causative organism has not been identified, Kefurox may be used concomitantly with an aminoglycoside (*see* PRECAUTIONS). The recommended doses of both antibiotics may be given depending on the severity of the infection and the patient's condition.

Prevention: The preoperative prophylactic administration of Kefurox may prevent the growth of susceptible disease-causing bacteria and, thereby, may reduce the incidence of certain postoperative infections in patients undergoing surgical procedures (eg, vaginal hysterectomy) that are classified as clean-contaminated or potentially contaminated procedures. Effective prophylactic use of antibiotics in surgery depends on the time of administration. Kefurox should usually be given ½ to 1 hour before the operation to allow sufficient time to achieve effective antibiotic concentrations in the wound tissues during the procedure. The dose should be repeated intraoperatively if the surgical procedure is lengthy. Prophylactic administration is usually not required after the surgical procedure ends and should be stopped within 24 hours. In the majority of surgical procedures, continuing prophylactic administration of any antibiotic does not reduce the incidence of subsequent infections but will increase the possibility of adverse reactions and the development of bacterial resistance. The perioperative use of Kefurox has also been effective during open heart surgery for surgical patients in whom infections at the operative site would present a serious risk. For these patients, it is recommended that therapy with Kefurox be continued for at least 48 hours after the surgical procedure ends. If an infection is present, specimens for culture should be obtained for the identification of the causative organism and appropriate antimicrobial therapy should be instituted.

CONTRAINDICATIONS

Kefurox™ (sterile cefuroxime sodium, Lilly) is contraindicated in patients with known allergy to the cephalosporin group of antibiotics.

WARNINGS

BEFORE THERAPY WITH KEFUROX IS INSTITUTED, CAREFUL INQUIRY SHOULD BE MADE TO DETERMINE WHETHER THE PATIENT HAS HAD PREVIOUS HYPERSENSITIVITY REACTIONS TO CEPHALOSPORINS, PENICILLINS, OR OTHER DRUGS. THIS PRODUCT SHOULD BE GIVEN CAUTIOUSLY TO PENICILLIN-SENSITIVE PATIENTS. ANTIBIOTICS SHOULD BE ADMINISTERED WITH CAUTION TO ANY PATIENT WHO HAS DEMONSTRATED SOME FORM OF ALLERGY, PARTICULARLY TO DRUGS. IF AN ALLERGIC REACTION TO KEFUROX™ (STERILE, CEFUROXIME SODIUM, LILLY) OCCURS, DISCONTINUE THE DRUG, SERIOUS ACUTE HYPERSENSITIVITY REACTIONS MAY REQUIRE EPINEPHRINE AND OTHER EMERGENCY MEASURES.

Pseudomembranous colitis has been reported with the use of cephalosporins (and other broad-spectrum antibiotics); therefore, it is important to consider its diagnosis in patients who develop diarrhea in association with antibiotic use.

Treatment with broad-spectrum antibiotics alters normal flora of the colon and may permit overgrowth of Clostridia. Studies indicate a toxin produced by *C. difficile* is one primary cause of antibiotic-associated colitis. Cholestyramine and colestipol resins have been shown to bind the toxin in vitro.

Mild cases of colitis may respond to drug discontinuance alone. Moderate to severe cases should be managed with fluid, electrolyte, and protein supplementation as indicated. When the colitis is not relieved by drug discontinuance or when it is severe, oral vancomycin is the treatment of choice for antibiotic-associated pseudomembranous colitis produced by *C. difficile.* Other causes of colitis should also be considered.

PRECAUTIONS

Although Kefurox™ (sterile cefuroxime sodium, Lilly) rarely produces alterations in kidney function, evaluation of renal status during therapy is recommended, especially in seriously ill patients receiving the maximum doses. Cephalosporins should be given with caution to patients receiving concurrent treatment with potent diuretics, as these regimens are suspected of adversely affecting renal function.

The total daily dose of Kefurox™ (sterile cefuroxime sodium, Lilly) should be reduced in patients with transient or persistent renal insufficiency (*see* DOSAGE), because high and prolonged serum antibiotic concentrations can occur in such individuals from usual doses.

As with other antibiotics, prolonged use of Kefurox may result in overgrowth of nonsusceptible organisms. Careful observation of the patient is essential. If superinfection does occur during therapy, appropriate measures should be taken.

Broad-spectrum antibiotics should be prescribed with caution in individuals with a history of gastrointestinal disease, particularly colitis.

Nephrotoxicity has been reported following concomitant administration of aminoglycoside antibiotics and cephalosporins.

Interference with Laboratory Tests —A false positive reaction for glucose in the urine may occur with copper reduction tests (Benedict's or Fehling's solution or with Clinitest® tablets), but not with enzyme-based tests for glycosuria (eg, Tes-Tape®). A false negative reaction may occur in the ferricyanide test for blood glucose.

Cefuroxime does not interfere with the assay of serum and urine creatinine by the the alkaline picrate method.

Carcinogenesis, Mutagenesis, and Impairment of Fertility —Although no long-term studies in animals have been performed to evaluate carcinogenic potential, no mutagenic potential of cefuroxime was found in standard laboratory tests.

Reproductive studies revealed no impairment of fertility in animals.

Usage in Pregnancy—Pregnancy Category B —Reproduction studies have been performed in mice and rabbits at doses up to 60 times the human dose and have revealed no evidence of impaired fertility or harm to the fetus due to cefuroxime. There are, however, no adequate, well-controlled studies in pregnant women. Because animal reproduction studies are not always predictive of human response, this drug should be used during pregnancy only if clearly needed.

Nursing Mothers —Since Kefurox is excreted in human milk, caution should be exercised when Kefurox is administered to a nursing woman.

Pediatric Use —Safety and effectiveness in children below the age of 3 months have not been established. Accumulation of other members of the cephalosporin class in newborn infants (with resulting prolongation of drug half-life) has been reported.

ADVERSE REACTIONS

Kefurox™ (sterile cefuroxime sodium, Lilly) is generally well tolerated. The most common adverse effects have been local reactions following intravenous administration. Other adverse reactions have been encountered only rarely.

Local Reactions —Thrombophlebitis has occurred with intravenous administration in 1 in 60 patients.

Gastrointestinal —Gastrointestinal symptoms occurred in 1 in 150 patients and included diarrhea (1 in 220 patients) and nausea (1 in 440 patients). Symptoms of pseudomembranous colitis can appear during or after antibiotic treatment.

Hypersensitivity Reactions —Hypersensitivity reactions have been reported in less than 1% of the patients treated with Kefurox and include rash (1 in 125). Pruritus and urticaria and positive Coombs test each occurred in less than 1 in 250 patients.

Blood —A decrease in hemoglobin and hematocrit has been observed in 1 in 10 patients and transient eosinophilia in 1 in 14 patients. Less common reactions seen were transient neutropenia (less than 1 in 100 patients) and leukopenia (1 in 750 patients). A similar pattern and incidence was seen with other cephalosporins used in controlled studies.

Hepatic —Transient rise in SGOT and SGPT (1 in 25 patients), alkaline phosphatase (1 in 50 patients), LDH (1 in 75 patients) and bilirubin (1 in 500 patients) levels has been noted.

Kidney —Elevations in serum creatinine and/or blood urea nitrogen and a decreased creatinine clearance have been observed, but their relationship to cefuroxime is unknown.

DOSAGE AND ADMINISTRATION

Adults—The usual adult dosage range for Kefurox™ (sterile cefuroxime sodium, Lilly) is 750 mg to 1.5 g every 8 hours, usually for 5 to 10 days. In uncomplicated urinary tract infections, skin and skin structure infections, disseminated gonococcal infections and uncomplicated pneumonia, a 750 mg dose every 8 hours is recommended. In severe or complicated infections, a 1.5 g dose every 8 hours is recommended. In life-threatening infections or infections due to less susceptible organisms, 1.5 g every 6 hours may be required. In bacterial meningitis, the dose should not exceed 3.0 g every 8 hours. The recommended dose for uncomplicated gonococcal infection is 1.5 g intramuscularly, given as a single dose at two different sites together with 1.0 g of oral probenecid. For preventive use for clean-contaminated or potentially contaminated surgical procedures, a 1.5 g dose administered intravenously just prior to surgery (approximately ½ to 1 hour before the initial incision) is recommended. Thereafter, give 750 mg intravenously or intramuscularly every 8 hours when the procedure is prolonged.

For preventive use during open heart surgery, a 1.5 g dose administered intravenously at the induction of anesthesia and every 12 hours thereafter for a total of 6.0 g is recommended.

Impaired Renal Function —When renal function is impaired, a reduced dosage must be employed. Dosage should be determined by the degree of renal impairment and the susceptibility of the causative organism (see Table 1).

TABLE 1: Dosage of Kefurox™ (Sterile Cefuroxime Sodium) in Adults With Reduced Renal Function

Creatinine Clearance (ml/min.)	Dose	Frequency
>20	750 mg–1.5 g	Every 8 hours
10–20	750 mg	Every 12 hours
<10	750 mg	Every 24 hours*

*Since Kefurox is dialyzable, patients on hemodialysis should be given a further dose at the end of the dialysis.

When only serum creatinine is available, the following formula (based on sex, weight, and age of the patient) may be used to convert this value into creatinine clearance. The serum creatinine should represent a steady state of renal function.

$$\text{Male: } \frac{\text{Weight (kg)} \times (140-\text{age})}{72 \times \text{serum creatinine (mg/100 ml)}}$$

Females: 0.9 × above value

Note: As with antibiotic therapy in general, administration of Kefurox should be continued for a minimum of 48 to 72 hours after the patient becomes asymptomatic or after evidence of bacterial eradication has been obtained; a minimum of 10 days of treatment is recommended in infections caused by *Streptococcus pyogenes* in order to guard against the risk of rheumatic fever or glomerulonephritis; frequent bacteriologic and clinical appraisal is necessary during therapy of chronic urinary tract infection and may be required for several months after therapy has been completed; persistent infections may require treatment for several weeks; and doses smaller than those indicated above should not be used. In staphylococcal and other infections involving a collection of pus, surgical drainage should be carried out when indicated.

Infants and Children Above 3 Months of Age —Administration of 50 to 100 mg/kg/day in equally divided doses every 6 to 8 hours has been successful for most infections susceptible to cefuroxime. The higher dose of 100 mg/kg/day (not to exceed the maximum adult dose) should be used for the more severe or serious infections.

In cases of bacterial meningitis, larger doses of Kefurox are recommended, initially 200 to 240 mg/kg/day intravenously in divided doses every 6 to 8 hours.

In children with renal insufficiency, the frequency of dosage should be modified consistent with the recommendations for adults.

Preparation of Solution and Suspension —The directions for preparing Kefurox for both intravenous and intramuscular use are summarized in Table 2.

For Intramuscular Use —Each 750 mg vial of Kefurox should be reconstituted with 3.6 ml of Sterile Water for Injection. Shake gently to disperse and withdraw 3.6 ml of the resulting suspension for injection.

For Intravenous Use —Each 750 mg vial should be reconstituted with 9.0 ml of Sterile Water for Injection. Withdraw 8.0 ml of the resulting solution for injection.

Each 1.5 g vial should be reconstituted with 16.0 ml of Sterile Water for Injection and the solution completely withdrawn for injection.

For infusion, each 750 mg or 1.5 g dose should be reconstituted with 50 to 100 ml of Sterile Water for Injection, 5% Dextrose Injection, 0.9% Sodium Chloride Injection, or any of the solutions listed under the Intravenous portion of the Compatibility and Stability section. If Sterile Water for Injection is used as the diluent, reconstitute with approximately 20 ml/g to avoid a hypotonic solution.

[See table on bottom next page].

Administration —After reconstitution, Kefurox™ (sterile cefuroxime sodium, Lilly) may be given intravenously or by deep intramuscular injection into a large muscle mass (such as the gluteus or lateral part of the thigh). Prior to injecting intramuscularly, aspiration is necessary to avoid inadvertent injection into a blood vessel.

Intravenous Administration —The intravenous route may be preferable for patients with bacterial septicemia or other severe or life-threatening infections or for patients who may

Continued on next page

• **Identi-Code® symbol.**

Lilly—Cont.

be poor risks because of lowered resistance, particularly if shock is present or impending.

For Direct Intermittent Intravenous Administration —Slowly inject the solution into a vein over a period of 3–5 minutes or give it through the tubing system by which the patient is also receiving other intravenous solutions.

For Intermittent Intravenous Infusion with a Y-Type Administration Set —Dosing can be accomplished through the tubing system by which the patient may be receiving other intravenous solutions. However, during infusion of the solution containing Kefurox, it is advisable to temporarily discontinue administration of any other solutions at the same site.

For Continuous Intravenous Infusion —A solution of Kefurox may be added to an intravenous bottle containing one of the following fluids:

0.9% Sodium Chloride Injection, 5% Dextrose Injection, 10% Dextrose Injection, 5% Dextrose and 0.9% Sodium Chloride Injection, 5% Dextrose and 0.45% Sodium Chloride Injection, or M/6 Sodium Lactate Injection

Solutions of Kefurox, like those of most beta-lactam antibiotics, should not be added to solutions of aminglycoside antibiotics because of potential interaction.

However, if concurrent therapy with Kefurox and an aminoglycoside is indicated, each of these antibiotics can be administered separately to the same patient.

Compatibility and Stability —Intramuscular—When reconstituted as directed with Sterile Water for Injection, suspensions of Kefurox™ (sterile cefuroxime sodium, Lilly) for intramuscular injection maintain satisfactory potency for 24 hours at room temperature and for 48 hours under refrigeration (5°C).

After the periods mentioned above, any unused suspensions should be discarded.

Intravenous—When the 750 mg and 1.5 g vials are reconstituted as directed with Sterile Water for Injection, the solutions of Kefurox for intravenous administration maintain satisfactory potency for 24 hours at room temperature and for 48 hours under refrigeration (5°C). More dilute solutions, such as 750 mg or 1.5 g plus 50 to 100 ml of Sterile Water for Injection, 5% Dextrose Injection or 0.9% Sodium Chloride Injection, maintain satisfactory potency for 24 hours at room temperature and for 7 days under refrigeration.

These solutions may be further diluted to concentrations of between 1 mg/ml and 30 mg/ml in the following solutions and will lose not more than 10% activity for 24 hour at room temperature or for at least 7 days under refrigeration: 0.9% Sodium Chloride Injection, M/6 Sodium Lactate Injection, Ringer's Injection USP, Lactated Ringer's Injection USP, 5% Dextrose and 0.9% Sodium Chloride Injection, 5% Dextrose Injection, 5% Dextrose and 0.45% Sodium Chloride Injection, 5% Dextrose and 0.225% Sodium Chloride Injection, 10% Dextrose Injection, and 10% Invert Sugar in Water for Injection.

Unused solutions should be discarded after the time periods mentioned above.

Kefurox has also been found compatible for 24 hours at room temperature when admixed in intravenous infusion with: Heparin (10 and 50 units/ml) in 0.9% Sodium Chloride Injection and Potassium Chloride (10 and 40 mEq/L) in 0.9% Sodium Chloride Injection.

Note: Parenteral drug products should be inspected visually for particulate matter and discoloration prior to administration whenever solution and container permit.

As with other cephalosporins, however, cefuroxime powder as well as solutions and suspensions tend to darken, depending on storage conditions, without adversely affecting product potency.

TABLE 2
Preparation of Solution and Suspension
(Glass Vials and ADD-Vantage)

Strength	Amount of Diluent to Be Added (ml)	Volume to Be Withdrawn (ml)	Approximate Concentration (mg/ml)
750 mg/10 ml vial	3.6 (IM)	3.6*	200
750 mg/10 ml vial	9 (IV)	8	100
1.5 g/20 ml vial	16 (IV)	Total	100
750 mg/100 ml bottle	50 (IV)	—	15
750 mg/100 ml bottle	100 (IV)	—	7.5
1.5 g/100 ml bottle	50 (IV)	—	30
1.5 g/100 ml bottle	100 (IV)	—	15
750 mg/ADD-Vantage†	50 (IV)	—	15
750 mg/ADD-Vantage†	100 (IV)	—	7.5
1.5 g/ADD-Vantage†	50 (IV)	—	30
1.5 g/ADD-Vantage†	100 (IV)	—	15

* KEFUROX™ (sterile cefuroxime sodium, Lilly) is a suspension of IM concentrations.
† See ADD-Vantage instructions for use.

HOW SUPPLIED

℞ *Vials Kefurox™ (sterile cefuroxime sodium, Lilly): No. 7271,* 750 mg,* 10-ml size, Traypak™ (multivial carton, Lilly) of 25 (NDC 0002-7271-25); *No. 7272,* 1.5 g,* 20-ml size, Traypak of 10 (NDC 0002-7272-10); *No. 7273,* 750 mg,* 100-ml size, Traypak of 10 (NDC 0002-7273-10); *No. 7274,* 1.5 g,* 150-ml size, Traypak of 10 (NDC 0002-7274-10).

℞ *ADD-Vantage® (vials and diluent containers, Abbott) Vials: No. 7278,* 750 mg,* Traypak of 25 (NDC 0002-7278-25); *No. 7279,* 1.5 g,* Traypak of 10 (NDC 0002-7279-10).

The above ADD-Vantage Vials are to be used with Abbott Laboratories' ADD-Vantage Diluent Container containing:

0.9% Sodium Chloride Injection, USP, 50 ml, NDC 0074-7101-13; 100 ml, NDC 0074-7101-23, or

5% Dextrose Injection, USP, 50 ml, NDC 0074-7100-13; 100 ml, NDC 0074-7100-23

*Equivalent to cefuroxime. [121284]

KEFZOL® ℞

[*kĕf'zōl*]
(cefazolin sodium)
Sterile, USP

DESCRIPTION

Kefzol® (cefazolin sodium, Lilly) is a semisynthetic cephalosporin for parenteral administration. It is the sodium salt of 3- [[(5-methyl-1,3,4-thiadiazol-2-yl)-thio]methyl] -7- [2 - (1H-tetrazol-1-yl)acetamido] -3- cephem-4-carboxylic acid. The sodium content is 48.3 mg/g of cefazolin sodium. In addition to cefazolin sodium, the Faspak® (flexible plastic bag, Lilly) and the ADD-Vantage® System vial also contain 0.04% polysorbate 80.

The molecular formula is $C_{14}H_{14}N_8O_4S_3$ (sodium salt). The molecular weight is 476.5.

The dry crystalline powder is stable for at least two years when stored at room temperature (25°C). After reconstitution, the solution should be stored in a refrigerator and used within 96 hours. If kept at room temperature, the solution should be used within 24 hours.

The *p*H of the reconstituted solution is between 4.5 and 6.

CLINICAL PHARMACOLOGY

Human Pharmacology —Table 1 demonstrates the blood levels and duration of cefazolin following intramuscular administration.

TABLE 1. SERUM CONCENTRATIONS AFTER INTRAMUSCULAR ADMINISTRATION

Dose	Serum Concentrations (mcg/ml) ½ hr	1 hr	2 hr	4 hr	6 hr	8 hr
250 mg	15.5	17	13	5.1	2.5	
500 mg	36.2	36.8	37.9	15.5	6.3	3
1 g*	60.1	63.8	54.3	29.3	13.2	7.1

*Average of two studies

Clinical pharmacology studies in patients hospitalized with infections indicate that cefazolin produces mean peak serum levels approximately equivalent to those seen in normal volunteers.

In a study (using normal volunteers) of constant intravenous infusion with dosages of 3.5 mg/kg for one hour (approximately 250 mg) and 1.5 mg/kg the next two hours (approximately 100 mg), cefazolin produced a steady serum level at the third hour of approximately 28 mcg/ml. Table 2 shows the average serum concentrations after IV injection of a single 1-g dose; average half-life was 1.4 hours.

TABLE 2. SERUM CONCENTRATIONS AFTER 1-G INTRAVENOUS DOSE

Serum Concentrations (mcg/ml) 5 min	15 min	30 min	1 hr	2 hr	4 hr
188.4	135.8	106.8	73.7	45.6	16.5

Controlled studies on adult normal volunteers receiving 1 g four times a day for ten days, monitoring CBC, SGOT, SGPT, bilirubin, alkaline phosphatase, BUN, creatinine, and urinalysis, indicated no clinically significant changes attributed to cefazolin.

Cefazolin is excreted unchanged in the urine primarily by glomerular filtration and, to a lesser degree, by tubular secretion. Following intramuscular injection of 500 mg, 56 to 89 percent of the administered dose is recovered within six hours and 80 to nearly 100 percent in 24 hours. Cefazolin achieves peak urine concentrations greater than 1000 mcg/ml and 4000 mcg/ml respectively following 500-mg and 1-g intramuscular doses.

In patients undergoing peritoneal dialysis (2 L/hr), mean serum levels of cefazolin were approximately 10 and 30 mcg/ml after 24 hours' instillation of a dialyzing solution containing 50 mg/L and 150 mg/L respectively. Mean peak levels were 29 mcg/ml (range 13-44 mcg/ml) with 50 mg/L (three patients), and 72 mcg/ml (range 26-142 mcg/ml) with 150 mg/L (six patients). Intraperitoneal administration of cefazolin is usually well tolerated.

When cefazolin is administered to patients with unobstructed biliary tracts, high concentrations well over serum levels occur in the gallbladder tissue and bile. In the presence of obstruction, however, concentration of the antibiotic is considerably lower in bile than in serum.

Cefazolin readily crosses an inflamed synovial membrane, and the concentration of the antibiotic achieved in the joint space is comparable to levels measured in the serum.

Cefazolin readily crosses the placental barrier into the cord blood and amniotic fluid. It is present in very low concentrations in the milk of nursing mothers.

Microbiology —In vitro tests demonstrate that the bactericidal action of cephalosporins results from inhibition of cell-wall synthesis. Kefzol® (cefazolin sodium, Lilly) is active against the following organisms in vitro and in clinical infections.

- *Staphylococcus aureus* (including penicillinase-producing strains)
- *Staphylococcus epidermidis*
- Group A beta-hemolytic streptococci and other strains of streptococci (many strains of enterococci are resistant)
- *Streptococcus (Diplococcus) pneumoniae*
- *Escherichia coli*
- *Proteus mirabilis*
- *Klebsiella* species
- *Enterobacter aerogenes*
- *Haemophilus influenzae*

Most strains of indole-positive *Proteus* (*P. vulgaris*), *Enterobacter cloncae, Morganella morganii,* and *Providencia rettgeri* are resistant. *Serratia, Pseudomonas, Mima,* and *Herellea* species are almost uniformly resistant to cefazolin.

Disc Susceptibility Tests —Quantitative methods that require measurement of zone diameters give the most precise estimates of antibiotic susceptibility. One such procedure* has been recommended for use with discs for testing susceptibility to cephalosporin-class antibiotics. Interpretations correlate diameters of the disc test with MIC values for Kefzol® (cefazolin sodium, Lilly). With this procedure, a report from the laboratory of "susceptible" indicates that the infecting organism is likely to respond to therapy. A report of "resistant" indicates that the infecting organism is not likely to respond to therapy. A report of "intermediate susceptibility" suggests that the organism would be susceptible if high dosage is used or if the infection is confined to tissues and fluids (e.g., urine) in which high antibiotic levels are attained.

*National Committee for Clinical Laboratory Standards (NCCLS), 1983. Performance Standards for Antimicrobial Disk Susceptibility Tests, Tentative Standard, M2-T3, NCCLS, Villanova, PA 19085.

For gram-positive isolates, a zone of 18 mm is indicative of a cefazolin-susceptible organism when tested with either the cephalosporin-class disc (30 mcg cephalothin) or the cefazolin disc (30 mcg cefazolin).

Gram-negative organisms should be tested with the cefazolin disc (using the above criteria), since cefazolin has been shown by in vitro tests to have activity against certain strains of *Enterobacteriaceae* found resistant when tested with the cephalothin disc. Gram-negative organisms having zones of less than 18 mm around the cephalothin disc may be susceptible to cefazolin.

The cefazolin disc should not be used for testing susceptibility to other cephalosporins.

Dilution Techniques —A bacterial isolate may be considered susceptible if the minimum inhibitory concentration (MIC) for cefazolin is not more than 16 mcg/ml. Organisms are considered resistant if the MIC is equal to or greater than 64 mcg/ml.

INDICATIONS AND USAGE

Kefzol® (cefazolin sodium, Lilly) is indicated in the treatment of the following serious infections due to susceptible organisms:

Respiratory tract infections due to *S. pneumoniae, Klebsiella* species, *H. influenzae, S. aureus* (including penicillinase-producing strains), and group A beta-hemolytic streptococci

Injectable penicillin G benzathine is considered to be the drug of choice in the treatment and prevention of streptococcal infections, including the prophylaxis of rheumatic fever. Kefzol is effective in the eradication of streptococci from the nasopharynx; however, data establishing the efficacy of Kefzol in the subsequent prevention of rheumatic fever are not available at present.

Genitourinary tract infections due to *E. coli, P. mirabilis, Klebsiella* species, and some strains of *Enterobacter* and enterococci

Skin and skin-structure infections due to *S. aureus* (including penicillinase-producing strains) and group A beta-hemolytic streptococci and other strains of streptococci

Biliary tract infections due to *E. coli*, various strains of streptococci, *P. mirabilis, Klebsiella* species, and *S. aureus*

Bone and joint infections due to *S. aureus*

Septicemia due to *S. pneumoniae, S. aureus* (penicillin-sensitive and penicillin-resistant), *P. mirabilis, E. coli,* and *Klebsiella* species

Endocarditis due to *S. aureus* (penicillin-sensitive and penicillin-resistant) and group A beta-hemolytic streptococci

Appropriate culture and susceptibility studies should be performed to determine susceptibility of the causative organism to Kefzol.

Perioperative Prophylaxis—The prophylactic administration of Kefzol preoperatively, intraoperatively, and postoperatively may reduce the incidence of certain postoperative infections in patients undergoing surgical procedures that are classified as contaminated or potentially contaminated (e.g., vaginal hysterectomy or cholecystectomy in high-risk patients such as those over 70 years of age, with acute cholecystitis, obstructive jaundice, or common-bile-duct stones).

The perioperative use of Kefzol also may be effective in surgical patients in whom infection at the operative site would present a serious risk (e.g., during open-heart surgery and prosthetic arthroplasty).

The prophylactic administration of Kefzol should usually be discontinued within a 24-hour period after the surgical procedure. In surgery in which the occurrence of infection may be particularly devastating (e.g., open-heart surgery and prosthetic arthroplasty), the prophylactic administration of Kefzol may be continued for three to five days following the completion of surgery. If there are signs of infection, specimens for culture should be obtained for the identification of the causative organism so that appropriate therapy may be instituted. (*See* DOSAGE AND ADMINISTRATION.)

CONTRAINDICATION

Kefzol® (cefazolin sodium, Lilly) is contraindicated in patients with known allergy to the cephalosporin group of antibiotics.

WARNINGS

BEFORE CEFAZOLIN THERAPY IS INSTITUTED, CAREFUL INQUIRY SHOULD BE MADE CONCERNING PREVIOUS HYPERSENSITIVITY REACTIONS TO CEPHALOSPORINS AND PENICILLIN. CEPHALOSPORIN C DERIVATIVES SHOULD BE GIVEN CAUTIOUSLY TO PENICILLIN-SENSITIVE PATIENTS.

SERIOUS ACUTE HYPERSENSITIVITY REACTIONS MAY REQUIRE EPINEPHRINE AND OTHER EMERGENCY MEASURES.

There is some clinical and laboratory evidence of partial cross-allergenicity of the penicillins and the cephalosporins. Patients have been reported to have had severe reactions (including anaphylaxis) to both drugs.

Antibiotics, including Kefzol® (cefazolin sodium, Lilly), should be administered cautiously to any patient who has demonstrated some form of allergy, particularly to drugs.

Pseudomembranous colitis has been reported with virtually all broad-spectrum antibiotics (including macrolides, semisynthetic penicillins, and cephalosporins); therefore, it is important to consider its diagnosis in patients who develop diarrhea in association with the use of antibiotics. Such colitis may range in severity from mild to life-threatening.

Treatment with broad-spectrum antibiotics alters the normal flora of the colon and may permit overgrowth of clostridia. Studies indicate that a toxin produced by *Clostridium difficile* is one primary cause of antibiotic-associated colitis. Mild cases of pseudomembranous colitis usually respond to drug discontinuance alone. In moderate to severe cases, management should include sigmoidoscopy, appropriate bacteriologic studies, and fluid, electrolyte, and protein supplementation. When the colitis does not improve after the drug has been discontinued, or when it is severe, oral vancomycin is the drug of choice for antibiotic-associated pseudomembranous colitis produced by *C. difficile*. Other causes of colitis should be ruled out.

Usage in Infants—Safety for use in prematures and infants under one month of age has not been established.

PRECAUTIONS

General Precautions—If an allergic reaction to Kefzol® (cefazolin sodium, Lilly) occurs, the drug should be discontinued and the patient treated with the usual agents (e.g., epinephrine or other pressor amines, antihistamines, or corticosteroids).

Prolonged use of Kefzol may result in the overgrowth of nonsusceptible organisms. Careful clinical observation of the patient is essential. If superinfection occurs during therapy, appropriate measures should be taken.

When Kefzol is administered to patients with low urinary output because of impaired renal function, lower daily dosage is required (see dosage instructions).

Drug Interactions—Probenecid may decrease renal tubular secretion of cephalosporins when used concurrently, which results in increased and more prolonged cephalosporin blood levels.

Drug/Laboratory Test Interactions—A false-positive reaction for glucose in the urine may occur with Benedict's solution, Fehling's solution, or Clinitest® tablets but not with enzyme-based tests, such as Clinistix® and Tes-Tape® (Glucose Enzymatic Test Strip, USP, Lilly).

Positive direct and indirect antiglobulin (Coombs') tests have occurred; these may also occur in neonates whose mothers received cephalosporins before delivery.

Broad-spectrum antibiotics should be prescribed with caution in individuals with a history of gastrointestinal disease, particularly colitis.

Carcinogenesis, Mutagenesis—Mutagenicity studies and long-term studies in animals to determine the carcinogenic potential of cefazolin have not been performed.

Usage in Pregnancy—Pregnancy Category B—Reproduction studies have been performed in rats given doses of 500 mg or 1 g of cefazolin/kg and have revealed no evidence of impaired fertility or harm to the fetus due to Kefzol. There are, however, no adequate and well-controlled studies in pregnant women. Because animal reproduction studies are not always predictive of human response, this drug should be used during pregnancy only if clearly needed.

Labor and Delivery—When cefazolin has been administered prior to cesarean section, drug levels in cord blood have been approximately one-quarter to one-third of maternal drug levels. The drug appears to have no adverse effect on the fetus.

Nursing Mothers—Cefazolin is present in very low concentrations in the milk of nursing mothers. Caution should be exercised when cefazolin is administered to a nursing woman.

ADVERSE REACTIONS

The following reactions have been reported:

Hypersensitivity—Drug fever, skin rash, vulvar pruritus, and eosinophilia have occurred.

Blood—Neutropenia, leukopenia, thrombocythemia, and positive direct and indirect Coombs' tests have occurred.

Renal—Transient rise in BUN levels has been observed without clinical evidence of renal impairment.

Hepatic—Transient rise in SGOT, SGPT, and alkaline phosphatase levels has been observed rarely. As with some penicillins and some other cephalosporins, transient hepatitis and cholestatic jaundice have been reported rarely.

Gastrointestinal—Symptoms of pseudomembranous colitis may appear either during or after antibiotic treatment. Nausea and vomiting have been reported rarely. Anorexia, diarrhea, and oral candidiasis (oral thrush) have been reported.

Other—Pain on intramuscular injection, sometimes with induration, has occurred infrequently. Phlebitis at the site of injection has been noted. Other reactions have included genital and anal pruritus, genital moniliasis, and vaginitis.

DOSAGE AND ADMINISTRATION

Kefzol® (cefazolin sodium, Lilly) may be administered intramuscularly or intravenously after reconstitution.

Intramuscular Administration—Reconstitute with 0.9% Sodium Chloride Injection, Sterile Water for Injection, or Bacteriostatic Water for Injection according to Table 3. Shake well until dissolved. Kefzol should be injected into a large muscle mass. Pain on injection is infrequent with Kefzol.

[See table above].

TABLE 3. DILUTION TABLE FOR KEFZOL® (CEFAZOLIN SODIUM)

Vial Size	Diluent to Be Added	Approximate Available Volume	Approximate Average Concentration
250 mg	2 ml	2 ml	125 mg/ml
500 mg	2 ml	2.2 ml	225 mg/ml
1 g*	2.5 ml	3 ml	330 mg/ml

* The 1-g vial should be reconstituted only with Sterile Water for Injection or Bacteriostatic Water for Injection.

Intravenous Administration—Kefzol® (cefazolin sodium, Lilly) may be administered by intravenous injection or by continuous or intermittent infusion. Total daily dosages are the same as with intramuscular injection.

Intermittent intravenous infusion: Kefzol can be administered along with primary intravenous fluid management programs in a volume control set or in a separate, secondary IV bottle. Reconstituted 500 mg or 1 g of Kefzol may be diluted in 50 to 100 ml of one of the following intravenous solutions: 0.9% Sodium Chloride Injection, 5% or 10% Dextrose Injection, 5% Dextrose in Lactated Ringer's Injection, 5% Dextrose and 0.9% Sodium Chloride Injection (also may be used with 5% Dextrose and 0.45% or 0.2% Sodium Chloride Injection), Lactated Ringer's Injection, 5% or 10% Invert Sugar in Sterile Water for Injection, Ringer's Injection, Normosol®-M in D5-W, Ionosol® B with Dextrose 5%, or Plasma-Lyte® with 5% Dextrose.

Direct intravenous injection: Dilute the reconstituted 500 mg or 1 g of Kefzol in a minimum of 10 ml of Sterile Water for Injection. Inject solution slowly over three to five minutes. It may be administered directly into a vein or through the tubing for a patient receiving the above parenteral fluids.

Dosage—The usual adult dosages are given in Table 4.

TABLE 4. USUAL ADULT DOSAGE OF KEFZOL® (CEFAZOLIN SODIUM)

Type of Infection	Dose	Frequency
Pneumococcal pneumonia	500 mg	q. 12 h.
Mild infections caused by susceptible gram-positive cocci	250 to 500 mg	q. 8 h.
Acute uncomplicated urinary tract infections	1 g	q. 12 h.
Moderate to severe infections	500 mg to 1 g	q. 6 to 8 h.
Severe, life-threatening infections (e.g., endocarditis, septicemia)	1 g to 1.5 g	q. 6 h.

* In rare instances, doses up to 12 g of cefazolin per day have been used.

Dosage Adjustment for Patients with Reduced Renal Function—Kefzol may be used in patients with reduced renal function with the following dosage adjustments: Patients with a creatinine clearance of 55 ml/min. or greater or a serum creatinine of 1.5 mg % or less can be given full doses. Patients with creatinine clearance rates of 35 to 54 ml/min. or serum creatinine of 1.6 to 3.0 mg % can also be given full doses, but dosage should be restricted to at least eight-hour intervals. Patients with creatinine clearance rates of 11 to 34 ml/min. or serum creatinine of 3.1 to 4.5 mg % should be given one-half the usual dose every 12 hours. Patients with creatinine clearance rates of 10 ml/min. or less or serum creatinine of 4.6 mg % or greater should be given one-half the usual dose every 18 to 24 hours. All reduced dosage recommendations apply after an initial loading dose appropriate to the severity of the infection. Patients undergoing peritoneal dialysis: See *Human Pharmacology*.

Perioperative Prophylactic Use—To prevent postoperative infection in contaminated or potentially contaminated surgery, the recommended doses are as follows:

a. 1 g IV or IM administered one-half to one hour prior to the start of surgery.

Continued on next page

• **Identi-Code® symbol.**

Lilly—Cont.

b. For lengthy operative procedures (e.g., two hours or more), 0.5 to 1 g IV or IM during surgery (administration modified according to the duration of the operative procedure).

c. 0.5 to 1 g IV or IM every six to eight hours for 24 hours postoperatively.

It is important that (1) the preoperative dose be given just (one-half to one hour) prior to the start of surgery so that adequate antibiotic levels are present in the serum and tissues at the time of the initial surgical incision and (2) Kefzol be administered, if necessary, at appropriate intervals during surgery to provide sufficient levels of the antibiotic at the anticipated moments of greatest exposure to infective organisms.

In surgery in which the occurrence of infection may be particularly devastating (e.g., open-heart surgery and prosthetic arthroplasty), the prophylactic administration of Kefzol may be continued for three to five days following the completion of surgery.

In children, a total daily dosage of 25 to 50 mg/kg (approximately 10 to 20 mg/lb) of body weight, divided into three or four equal doses, is effective for most mild to moderately severe infections (Table 5). Total daily dosage may be increased to 100 mg/kg (45 mg/lb) of body weight for severe infections.

TABLE 5. PEDIATRIC DOSAGE GUIDE FOR KEFZOL® (CEFAZOLIN SODIUM)

Weight		25 mg/kg/Day Divided into 3 Doses		25 mg/kg/Day Divided into 4 Doses	
lb	kg	Approximate Single Dose (mg q. 8 h.)	Vol. (ml) Needed with Dilution of 125 mg/ml	Approximate Single Dose (mg q. 6 h.)	Vol. (ml) Needed with Dilution of 125 mg/ml
10	4.5	40 mg	0.35 ml	30 mg	0.25 ml
20	9	75 mg	0.6 ml	55 mg	0.45 ml
30	13.6	115 mg	0.9 ml	85 mg	0.7 ml
40	18.1	150 mg	1.2 ml	115 mg	0.9 ml
50	22.7	190 mg	1.5 ml	140 mg	1.1 ml

Weight		50 mg/kg/Day Divided into 3 Doses		50 mg/kg/Day Divided into 4 Doses	
lb	kg	Approximate Single Dose (mg q. 8 h.)	Vol. (ml) Needed with Dilution of 225 mg/ml	Approximate Single Dose (mg q. 6 h.)	Vol. (ml) Needed with Dilution of 225 mg/ml
10	4.5	75 mg	0.35 ml	55 mg	0.25 ml
20	9	150 mg	0.7 ml	110 mg	0.5 ml
30	13.6	225 mg	1 ml	170 mg	0.75 ml
40	18.1	300 mg	1.35 ml	225 mg	1 ml
50	22.7	375 mg	1.7 ml	285 mg	1.25 ml

In children with mild to moderate renal impairment (creatinine clearance of 70 to 40 ml/min.), 60 percent of the normal daily dose given in divided doses every 12 hours should be sufficient. In patients with moderate impairment (creatinine clearance of 40 to 20 ml/min.), 25 percent of the normal daily dose given in divided doses every 12 hours should be sufficient. In children with severe impairment (creatinine clearance of 20 to 5 ml/min.), 10 percent of the normal daily dose given every 24 hours should be adequate. All dosage recommendations apply after an initial loading dose.

Since safety for use in premature infants and in infants under one month of age has not been established, the use of Kefzol in these patients is not recommended.

STABILITY

Reconstituted Kefzol® (cefazolin sodium, Lilly) and dilutions of Kefzol in the recommended intravenous fluids are stable for 24 hours at room temperature and for 96 hours if stored under refrigeration (5°C).

Solutions of Kefzol in Sterile Water for Injection, 5% Dextrose Injection, or 0.9% Sodium Chloride Injection that are frozen immediately after reconstitution in the Faspak containers and the conventional vials in which the drugs are supplied are stable for as long as 12 weeks when stored at −20°C. **If the product is warmed, care should be taken to avoid heating it after the thawing is complete. Once thawed, the solution should not be refrozen.**

Parenteral drug products should be inspected visually for particulate matter and discoloration prior to administration, whenever solution and container permit.

HOW SUPPLIED

(℞) *Vials Kefzol® (Sterile Cefazolin Sodium, USP),* rubber-stoppered (Dry Powder): *No. 766,* 250 mg (equivalent to cefazolin), 10-ml size (NDC 0002-1496-01), in singles (10/carton); *No. 767,* 500 mg (equivalent to cefazolin), and *No. 768,* 1 g (equivalent to cefazolin), 10-ml size, in singles (NDC 0002-1497-01 and NDC 0002-1498-01) (10/carton) and in Traypak® (multivial carton, Lilly) of 25 (NDC 0002-1497-25 and NDC 0002-1498-25); *No. 7018,* 500 mg (equivalent to cefazolin) (NDC 0002-7018-10), and *No. 7011,* 1 g (equivalent to cefazolin) (NDC 0002-7011-10), 100-ml size, in Traypak of 10; *No. 7014,* 10 g (equivalent to cefazolin), 100-ml size, in Traypak of 6 (NDC 0002-7014-16).

(℞) *Redi Vial® (dual compartment vial, Lilly) Kefzol® (Sterile Cefazolin Sodium, USP): No. 7082,* 500 mg (equivalent to cefazolin), and *No. 7083,* 1 g (equivalent to cefazolin), in singles (NDC 0002-7082-01 and NDC 0002-7083-01) (10/carton) and in Traypak of 10 (NDC 0002-7082-10 and NDC 0002-7083-10).

(℞) *Faspak® (flexible plastic bag, Lilly) Kefzol® (Sterile Cefazolin Sodium, USP), No. 7201,* 500 mg (equivalent to cefazolin), and *No. 7202,* 1 g (equivalent to cefazolin), in Faspak of 96 (NDC 0002-7201-74 and NDC 0002-7202-74).

(℞) *ADD-Vantage® (vials and diluent containers, Abbott) Vials: No. 7265,* 500 mg (equivalent to cefazolin), in Traypak of 25 (NDC 0002-7265-25); *No. 7266,* 1 g (equivalent to cefazolin), in Traypak of 25 (NDC 0002-7266-25).

The above ADD-Vantage Vials are to used only with Abbott Laboratories' Diluent Containers.

Instructions for use of the ADD-Vantage Vials are enclosed in the package.

[020486]

No. 767, 500 mg, 1's and 25's —6505-01-010-0833
No. 768, 1 g, 1's and 25's —6505-01-010-0832
No. 7014, 10 g, 6's—6505-01-008-3408
No. 7014, 10 g, 10's—6505-01-184-1574

LENTE® ILETIN® I

[*lĕn'tā' ĭ'lĕ-tĭn*]

(insulin zinc suspension, Lilly), *see under* Iletin® (insulin, Lilly).

MANDOL® ℞

[*măn'dōl*]

(cefamandole nafate)
For Injection
USP

DESCRIPTION

Mandol® (cefamandole nafate, Lilly) is a semisynthetic broad-spectrum cephalosporin antibiotic for parenteral administration. It is the sodium salt of 7-D-mandelamido-3-[[(1-methyl-1*H*-tetrazol-5-yl)-thio]methyl] -3-cephem-4-carboxylic acid, formate (ester). Mandol also contains 63 mg sodium carbonate/g of cefamandole activity. The total sodium content is approximately 77 mg (3.3 mEq sodium ion) per g of cefamandole activity. After addition of diluent, cefamandole nafate rapidly hydrolyzes to cefamandole, and both compounds have microbiologic activity in vivo. Solutions of Mandol range from light yellow to amber, depending on concentration and diluent used. The *p*H of freshly reconstituted solutions usually ranges from 6.0 to 8.5.

CLINICAL PHARMACOLOGY

After intramuscular administration of a 500-mg dose of cefamandole to normal volunteers, the mean peak serum concentration was 13 mcg/ml. After a 1-g dose, the mean peak concentration was 25 mcg/ml. These peaks occurred at 30 to 120 minutes. Following intravenous doses of 1, 2, and 3 g, serum concentrations were 139, 240, and 533 mcg/ml respectively at ten minutes. These concentrations declined to 0.8, 2.2, and 2.9 mcg/ml at four hours. Intravenous administration of 4-g doses every six hours produced no evidence of accumulation in the serum. The half-life after an intravenous dose is 32 minutes; after intramuscular administration, the half-life is 60 minutes.

Sixty-five to 85 percent of cefamandole is excreted by the kidneys over an eight-hour period, resulting in high urinary concentrations. Following intramuscular doses of 500 mg and 1 g, urinary concentrations averaged 254 and 1357 mcg/ml respectively. Intravenous doses of 1 and 2 g produced urinary levels averaging 750 and 1380 mcg/ml respectively. Probenecid slows tubular excretion and doubles the peak serum level and the duration of measurable serum concentrations.

The antibiotic reaches therapeutic levels in pleural and joint fluids and in bile and bone.

Microbiology—The bactericidal action of cefamandole results from inhibition of cell-wall synthesis. Cephalosporins have in vitro activity against a wide range of gram-positive and gram-negative organisms. Cefamandole is usually active against the following organisms in vitro and in clinical infections:

Gram-positive
- *Staphylococcus aureus,* including penicillinase and non-penicillinase-producing strains
- *S. epidermidis*
- Beta-hemolytic and other streptococci (Most strains of enterococci, e.g., *Streptococcus faecalis,* are resistant.)
- *S. pneumoniae* (formerly *Diplococcus pneumoniae*)

Gram-negative
- *Escherichia coli*
- *Klebsiella* species
- *Enterobacter* species (Initially susceptible organisms occasionally may become resistant during therapy.)
- *Haemophilus influenzae*
- *Proteus mirabilis*
- *P. rettgeri*
- *P. morganii*
- *P. vulgaris* (Some strains of *P. vulgaris* have been shown by in vitro tests to be resistant to cefamandole and other cephalosporins.)

Anaerobic organisms
- Gram-positive and gram-negative cocci (including *Peptococcus* and *Peptostreptococcus* species)
- Gram-positive bacilli (including *Clostridium* species)
- Gram-negative bacilli (including *Bacteroides* and *Fusobacterium* species). Most strains of *Bacteroides fragilis* are resistant.

Pseudomonas, Acinetobacter calcoaceticus (formerly *Mima* and *Herellea* species), and most *Serratia* strains are resistant to cephalosporins. Cefamandole is resistant to degradation by beta-lactamases from certain members of the *Enterobacteriaceae.*

Susceptibility Tests—Quantitative methods that require measurement of zone diameters give the most precise estimates of antibiotic susceptibility. One such procedure[1] has been recommended for use with discs to test susceptibility to cefamandole. Interpretation involves correlation of the diameters obtained in the disc test with minimum inhibitory concentration (MIC) values for cefamandole.

Reports from the laboratory giving results of the standardized single-disc susceptibility test[1] using a 30-mcg cefamandole disc should be interpreted according to the following criteria:

Susceptible organisms produce zones of 18 mm or greater, indicating that the tested organism is likely to respond to therapy.

Organisms of intermediate susceptibility produce zones of 15 to 17 mm, indicating that the tested organism would be susceptible if high dosage is used or if the infection is confined to tissues and fluids (e.g., urine), in which high antibiotic levels are attained.

Resistant organisms produce zones of 14 mm or less, indicating that other therapy should be selected.

For gram-positive isolates, the test may be performed with either the cephalosporin-class disc (30 mcg cephalothin) or the cefamandole disc (30 mcg cefamandole), and a zone of 18 mm is indicative of a cefamandole-susceptible organism.

Gram-negative organisms should be tested with the cefamandole disc (using the above criteria), since cefamandole has been shown by in vitro tests to have activity against certain strains of *Enterobacteriaceae* found resistant when tested with the cephalosporin-class disc. Gram-negative organisms having zones of less than 18 mm around the cephalothin disc are not necessarily of intermediate susceptibility or resistant to cefamandole.

The cefamandole disc should not be used for testing susceptibility to other cephalosporins.

A bacterial isolate may be considered susceptible if the MIC value for cefamandole[2] is not more than 16 mcg/ml. Organisms are considered resistant if the MIC is greater than 32 mcg/ml.

INDICATIONS AND USAGE

Mandol® (cefamandole nafate, Lilly) is indicated for the treatment of serious infections caused by susceptible strains of the designated microorganisms in the diseases listed below:

Lower respiratory infections, including pneumonia caused by *S. pneumoniae (D. pneumoniae), H. influenzae, Klebsiella* species, *S. aureus* (penicillinase and non-penicillinase-producing), beta-hemolytic streptococci, and *P. mirabilis*

Urinary tract infections caused by *E. coli, Proteus* species (both indole-negative and indole-positive), *Enterobacter* species, *Klebsiella* species, group D streptococci (*Note:* Most enterococci, e.g., *S. faecalis,* are resistant), and *S. epidermidis*

Peritonitis caused by *E. coli* and *Enterobacter* species

Septicemia caused by *E. coli, S. aureus* (penicillinase and non-penicillinase-producing), *S. pneumoniae, S. pyogenes* (group A beta-hemolytic streptococci), *H. influenzae,* and *Klebsiella* species

Skin and skin-structure infections caused by *S. aureus* (penicillinase and non-penicillinase-producing), *S. pyogenes* (group A beta-hemolytic streptococci), *H. influenzae, E. coli, Enterobacter* species, and *P. mirabilis*

Bone and joint infections caused by *S. aureus* (penicillinase and non-penicillinase-producing)

Clinical microbiologic studies in nongonococcal pelvic inflammatory disease in females, lower respiratory infections, and skin infections frequently reveal the growth of susceptible strains of both aerobic and anaerobic organisms. Mandol has been used successfully in these infections in which several organisms have been isolated. Most strains of *B. fragilis* are resistant in vitro; however, infections caused by susceptible strains have been treated successfully.

Specimens for bacteriologic cultures should be obtained in order to isolate and identify causative organisms and to determine their susceptibilities to cefamandole. Therapy may be instituted before results of susceptibility studies are known; however, once these results become available, the antibiotic treatment should be adjusted accordingly.

In certain cases of confirmed or suspected gram-positive or gram-negative sepsis or in patients with other serious infections in which the causative organism has not been identified, Mandol may be used concomitantly with an aminoglycoside (*see* PRECAUTIONS). The recommended doses of both antibiotics may be given, depending on the severity of the infection and the patient's condition. The renal function of the patient should be carefully monitored, especially if higher dosages of the antibiotics are to be administered.

Antibiotic therapy of beta-hemolytic streptococcal infections should continue for at least ten days.

Preventive Therapy—The administration of Mandol preoperatively, intraoperatively, and postoperatively may reduce the incidence of certain postoperative infections in patients undergoing surgical procedures that are classified as contaminated or potentially contaminated (e.g., gastrointestinal surgery, cesarean section, vaginal hysterectomy, or cholecystectomy in high-risk patients such as those with acute cholecystitis, obstructive jaundice, or common-bile-duct stones).

In major surgery in which the risk of postoperative infection is low but serious (cardiovascular surgery, neurosurgery, or prosthetic arthroplasty), Mandol may be effective in preventing such infections.

The perioperative use of Mandol should be discontinued after 24 hours; however, in prosthetic arthroplasty, it is recommended that administration be continued for 72 hours. If signs of infection occur, specimens for culture should be obtained for identification of the causative organism so that appropriate antibiotic therapy may be instituted.

CONTRAINDICATION

Mandol® (cefamandole nafate, Lilly) is contraindicated in patients with known allergy to the cephalosporin group of antibiotics.

WARNINGS

BEFORE THERAPY WITH MANDOL® (cefamandole nafate, Lilly) IS INSTITUTED, CAREFUL INQUIRY SHOULD BE MADE TO DETERMINE WHETHER THE PATIENT HAS HAD PREVIOUS HYPERSENSITIVITY REACTIONS TO CEPHALOSPORINS, PENICILLINS, OR OTHER DRUGS. THIS PRODUCT SHOULD BE GIVEN CAUTIOUSLY TO PENICILLIN-SENSITIVE PATIENTS. ANTIBIOTICS SHOULD BE ADMINISTERED WITH CAUTION TO ANY PATIENT WHO HAS DEMONSTRATED SOME FORM OF ALLERGY, PARTICULARLY TO DRUGS. SERIOUS ACUTE HYPERSENSITIVITY REACTIONS MAY REQUIRE EPINEPHRINE AND OTHER EMERGENCY MEASURES.

In newborn infants, accumulation of other cephalosporin-class antibiotics (with resulting prolongation of drug half-life) has been reported.

Pseudomembranous colitis has been reported with virtually all broad-spectrum antibiotics (including macrolides, semisynthetic penicillins, and cephalosporins); therefore, it is important to consider its diagnosis in patients who develop diarrhea in association with the use of antibiotics. Such colitis may range in severity from mild to life-threatening.

Treatment with broad-spectrum antibiotics alters the normal flora of the colon and may permit overgrowth of clostridia. Studies indicate that a toxin produced by *Clostridium difficile* is one primary cause of antibiotic-associated colitis. Mild cases of pseudomembranous colitis usually respond to drug discontinuance alone. In moderate to severe cases, management should include sigmoidoscopy, appropriate bacteriologic studies, and fluid, electrolyte, and protein supplementation. When the colitis does not improve after the drug has been discontinued, or when it is severe, oral vancomycin is the drug of choice for antibiotic-associated pseudomembranous colitis produced by *C. difficile*. Other causes of colitis should be ruled out.

PRECAUTIONS

General Precautions—Although Mandol® (cefamandole nafate, Lilly) rarely produces alteration in kidney function, evaluation of renal status is recommended, especially in seriously ill patients receiving maximum doses.

Prolonged use of Mandol may result in the overgrowth of nonsusceptible organisms. Careful observation of the patient is essential. If superinfection occurs during therapy, appropriate measures should be taken.

Nephrotoxicity has been reported following concomitant administration of aminoglycoside antibiotics and cephalosporins.

A false-positive reaction for glucose in the urine may occur with Benedict's or Fehling's solution or with Clinitest® tablets but not with Tes-Tape® (Glucose Enzymatic Test Strip, USP, Lilly). There may be a false-positive test for proteinuria with acid and denaturization-precipitation tests.

As with other broad-spectrum antibiotics, hypoprothrombinemia, with or without bleeding, has been reported rarely, but it has been promptly reversed by administration of vitamin K. Such episodes usually have occurred in elderly, debilitated, or otherwise compromised patients with deficient stores of vitamin K. Treatment of such individuals with antibiotics possessing significant gram-negative and/or anaerobic activity is thought to alter the number and/or type of intestinal bacterial flora, with consequent reduction in synthesis of vitamin K. Prophylactic administration of vitamin K may be indicated in such patients, especially when intestinal sterilization and surgical procedures are performed.

In a few patients receiving Mandol, nausea, vomiting, and vasomotor instability with hypotension and peripheral vasodilatation occurred following the ingestion of ethanol. Cefamandole inhibits the enzyme acetaldehyde dehydrogenase in laboratory animals. This causes accumulation of acetaldehyde when ethanol is administered concomitantly.

Broad-spectrum antibiotics should be prescribed with caution in individuals with a history of gastrointestinal disease, particularly colitis.

Carcinogenesis, Mutagenesis, Impairment of Fertility—Certain beta-lactam antibiotics containing the N-methylthiotetrazole side chain have been reported to cause delayed maturity of the testicular germinal epithelium when given to neonatal rats during initial spermatogenic development (6 to 36 days of age). In animals that were treated from 6 to 36 days of age with 1000 mg/kg/day of cefamandole (approximately 5 times the maximum clinical dose), the delayed maturity was pronounced and was associated with decreased testicular weights and a reduced number of germinal cells in the leading waves of spermatogenic development. The effect was slight in rats given 50 or 100 mg/kg/day. Some animals that were given 1000 mg/kg/day during days 6 to 36 were infertile after becoming sexually mature. No adverse effects have been observed in rats exposed in utero, in neonatal rats (4 days of age or younger) treated prior to the initiation of spermatogenesis, or in older rats (more than 36 days of age) after exposure for up to six months. The significance to man of these findings in rats is unknown because of differences in the time of initiation of spermatogenesis, rate of spermatogenic development, and duration of puberty.

Usage in Pregnancy—Pregnancy Category B—Reproduction studies have been performed in rats given doses of 500 or 1000 mg/kg/day and have revealed no evidence of impaired fertility or harm to the fetus due to Mandol. There are, however, no adequate and well-controlled studies in pregnant women. Because animal reproduction studies are not always predictive of human response, this drug should be used during pregnancy only if clearly needed.

Nursing Mothers—Caution should be exercised when Mandol is administered to a nursing woman.

Usage in Infancy—Mandol has been effectively used in this age group, but all laboratory parameters have not been extensively studied in infants between one and six months of age; safety of this product has not been established in prematures and infants under one month of age. Therefore, if Mandol is administered to infants, the physician should determine whether the potential benefits outweigh the possible risks involved.

ADVERSE REACTIONS

Gastrointestinal—Symptoms of pseudomembranous colitis may appear either during or after antibiotic treatment. Nausea and vomiting have been reported rarely. As with some penicillins and some other cephalosporins, transient hepatitis and cholestatic jaundice have been reported rarely.

Hypersensitivity—Anaphylaxis, maculopapular rash, urticaria, eosinophilia, and drug fever have been reported. These reactions are more likely to occur in patients with a history of allergy, particularly to penicillin.

Blood—Thrombocytopenia has been reported rarely. Neutropenia has been reported, especially in long courses of treatment. Some individuals have developed positive direct Coombs' tests during treatment with the cephalosporin antibiotics.

Liver—Transient rise in SGOT, SGPT, and alkaline phosphatase levels has been noted.

Kidney—Decreased creatinine clearance has been reported in patients with prior renal impairment. As with some other cephalosporins, transitory elevations of BUN have occasionally been observed with Mandol® (cefamandole nafate, Lilly); their frequency increases in patients over 50 years of age. In some of these cases, there was also a mild increase in serum creatinine.

Local Reactions—Pain on intramuscular injection is infrequent. Thrombophlebitis occurs rarely.

DOSAGE AND ADMINISTRATION

Dosage—Adults: The usual dosage range for cefamandole is 500 mg to 1 g every four to eight hours.

In infections of skin structures and in uncomplicated pneumonia, a dosage of 500 mg every six hours is adequate.

In uncomplicated urinary tract infections, a dosage of 500 mg every eight hours is sufficient. In more serious urinary tract infections, a dosage of 1 g every eight hours may be needed.

In severe infections, 1-g doses may be given at four to six-hour intervals.

In life-threatening infections or infections due to less susceptible organisms, doses up to 2 g every four hours (i.e., 12 g/day) may be needed.

Infants and Children: Administration of 50 to 100 mg/kg/day in equally divided doses every four to eight hours has been effective for most infections susceptible to Mandol® (cefamandole nafate, Lilly). This may be increased to a total daily dose of 150 mg/kg (not to exceed the maximum adult dose) for severe infections. (*See* WARNINGS AND PRECAUTIONS for this age group.)

Note: As with antibiotic therapy in general, administration of Mandol should be continued for a minimum of 48 to 72 hours after the patient becomes asymptomatic or after evidence of bacterial eradication has been obtained; a minimum of ten days of treatment is recommended in infections caused by group A beta-hemolytic streptococci in order to guard against the risk of rheumatic fever or glomerulonephritis; frequent bacteriologic and clinical appraisal is necessary during therapy of chronic urinary tract infection and may be required for several months after therapy has been completed; persistent infections may require treatment for several weeks; and doses smaller than those indicated above should not be used.

For perioperative use of Mandol, the following dosages are recommended:

Adults—1 or 2 g intravenously or intramuscularly one-half to one hour prior to the surgical incision followed by 1 or 2 g every six hours for 24 to 48 hours.

Children (three months of age and older)—50 to 100 mg/kg/day in equally divided doses by the routes and schedule designated above.

Note: In patients undergoing prosthetic arthroplasty, administration is recommended for as long as 72 hours.

In patients undergoing cesarean section, the initial dose may be administered just prior to surgery or immediately after the cord has been clamped.

Impaired Renal Function—When renal function is impaired, a reduced dosage must be employed and the serum levels closely monitored. After an initial dose of 1 to 2 g (depending on the severity of infection), a maintenance dosage schedule should be followed (see chart). Continued dosage should be determined by degree of renal impairment, severity of infection, and susceptibility of the causative organism.

[See table on next page].

When only serum creatinine is available, the following formula (based on sex, weight, and age of the patient) may be used to convert this value into creatinine clearance. The serum creatinine should represent a steady state of renal function.

$$\text{Males:} \quad \frac{\text{Weight (kg)} \times (140 - \text{age})}{72 \times \text{serum creatinine}}$$

$$\text{Females:} \quad 0.9 \times \text{above value}$$

Modes of Administration—Mandol® (cefamandole nafate, Lilly) may be given intravenously or by deep intramuscular injection into a large muscle mass (such as the gluteus or lateral part of the thigh) to minimize pain.

Intramuscular Administration—Each g of Mandol should be diluted with 3 ml of one of the following diluents: Sterile Water for Injection, Bacteriostatic Water for Injection, 0.9% Sodium Chloride Injection, or Bacteriostatic Sodium Chloride Injection. Shake well until dissolved.

Intravenous Administration—The intravenous route may be preferable for patients with bacterial septicemia, localized parenchymal abscesses (such as intra-abdominal abscess), peritonitis, or other severe or life-threatening infections when they may be poor risks because of lowered resistance. In those with normal renal function, the intravenous dosage for such infections is 3 to 12 g of Mandol daily. In conditions such as bacterial septicemia, 6 to 12 g/day may be given initially by the intravenous route for several days, and dosage may then be gradually reduced according to clinical response and laboratory findings.

Continued on next page

• **Identi-Code® symbol.**

Lilly—Cont.

If combination therapy with Mandol and an aminoglycoside is indicated, each of these antibiotics should be administered in different sites. *Do not mix an aminoglycoside with Mandol in the same intravenous fluid container.*

A SOLUTION OF 1 G MANDOL IN 22 ML OF STERILE WATER FOR INJECTION IS ISOTONIC.

The choice of saline, dextrose, or electrolyte solution and the volume to be employed are dictated by fluid and electrolyte management.

For direct intermittent intravenous administration, each g of cefamandole should be reconstituted with 10 ml of Sterile Water for Injection, 5% Dextrose Injection, or 0.9% Sodium Chloride Injection. Slowly inject the solution into the vein over a period of three to five minutes, or give it through the tubing of an administration set while the patient is also receiving one of the following intravenous fluids: 0.9% Sodium Chloride Injection; 5% Dextrose Injection; 10% Dextrose Injection; 5% Dextrose and 0.9% Sodium Chloride Injection; 5% Dextrose and 0.45% Sodium Chloride Injection; 5% Dextrose and 0.2% Sodium Chloride Injection; or Sodium Lactate Injection (M/6).

Intermittent intravenous infusion with a Y-type administration set or volume control set can also be accomplished while any of the above-mentioned intravenous fluids are being infused. However, during infusion of the solution containing Mandol® (cefamandole nafate, Lilly), it is desirable to discontinue the other solution. When this technique is employed, careful attention should be paid to the volume of the solution containing Mandol so that the calculated dose will be infused. When a Y-tube hookup is used, 100 ml of the appropriate diluent should be added to the 1 or 2-g piggyback (100-ml) vial. If Sterile Water for Injection is used as the diluent, reconstitute with approximately 20 ml/g to avoid a hypotonic solution.

For continuous intravenous infusion, each g of cefamandole should be diluted with 10 ml of Sterile Water for Injection. An appropriate quantity of the resulting solution may be added to an IV bottle containing one of the following fluids: 0.9% Sodium Chloride Injection; 5% Dextrose Injection; 10% Dextrose Injection; 5% Dextrose and 0.9% Sodium Chloride Injection; 5% Dextrose and 0.45% Sodium Chloride Injection; 5% Dextrose and 0.2% Sodium Chloride Injection; or Sodium Lactate Injection (M/6).

STABILITY

Reconstituted Mandol® (cefamandole nafate, Lilly) is stable for 24 hours at room temperature (25°C) and for 96 hours if stored under refrigeration (5°C). *During storage at room temperature, carbon dioxide develops inside the vial after reconstitution. This pressure may be dissipated prior to withdrawal of the vial contents, or it may be used to aid withdrawal if the vial is inverted over the syringe needle and the contents are allowed to flow into the syringe.*

Solutions of Mandol in Sterile Water for Injection, 5% Dextrose Injection, or 0.9% Sodium Chloride Injection that are frozen immediately after reconstitution in the original container are stable for six months when stored at −20°C. If the product is warmed (to a maximum of 37°C), care should be taken to avoid heating it after the thawing is complete. Once thawed, the solution should not be refrozen.

HOW SUPPLIED

℞ *Vials Mandol ® (Cefamandole Nafate for Injection, USP),* rubber-stoppered (Dry Powder): *No. 7060,* 500 mg (equivalent to cefamandole activity) (NDC 0002-7060-25), and *No. 7061,* 1 g (equivalent to cefamandole activity) (NDC 0002-7061-25), 10-ml size, in Traypak™ (multivial carton, Lilly) of 25; *No. 7068,* 1 g (equivalent to cefamandole activity), 100-ml size (NDC 0002-7068-10), *No. 7064,* 2 g (equivalent to cefamandole activity), 20-ml size (NDC 0002-7064-10), and *No. 7069,* 2 g (equivalent to cefamandole activity), 100-ml size (NDC 0002-7069-10), in Traypak of 10; No. 7072, 10 g (equivalent to cefamandole activity), 100-ml size (NDC 0002-7072-16), in Traypak of 6.

℞ *Faspak ® (flexible plastic bag, Lilly) Mandol ® (Cefamandole Nafate for Injection, USP): No. 7208,* 1 g (equivalent to cefamandole activity) (NDC 0002-7208-74), and *No. 7209,* 2 g (equivalent to cefamandole activity) (NDC 0002-7209-74), in packages of 96.

℞ *ADD-Vantage® (vials and diluent containers, Abbott) Vials: No. 7268,* 1 g (equivalent to cefamandole activity), in Traypak of 25 (NDC 0002-7268-25); *No. 7269,* 2 g (equivalent to cefamandole activity), in Traypak of 10 (NDC 0002-7269-10).

The above ADD-Vantage® Vials are to be used only with Abbott Laboratories' Add-Vantage Diluent Containers. Instructions for use of the ADD-Vantage Vials are enclosed in the package.

No. 7061, 1 g, 25's—6505-01-074-6598
No. 7064, 2 g, 10's—6505-01-074-5601

[040986]

1. Bauer, A. W., Kirby, W. M. M., Sherris, J. C., and Turck, M.: Antibiotic Susceptibility Testing by a Standardized Single Disk Method, Am. J. Clin. Pathol., *45*:493, 1966; Standardized Disc Susceptibility Test, Federal Register, *39*:19182-19184, 1974. National Committee for Clinical Laboratory Standards. Approved Standard: ASM-2, Performance Standards for Antimicrobial Disc Susceptibility Tests, July, 1975.
2. Determined by the ICS agar-dilution method (Ericsson, H. M., and Sherris, J. C.: Acta Pathol. Microbiol. Scand. [B], Supplement No. 217, 1971) or any other method that has been shown to give equivalent results.

MANDOL® (CEFAMANDOLE NAFATE)—MAINTENANCE DOSAGE GUIDE FOR PATIENTS WITH RENAL IMPAIRMENT

Creatinine Clearance (ml/min./1.73 m^2)	Renal Function	Life-Threatening Infections—Maximum Dosage	Less Severe Infections
>80	Normal	2 g q. 4 h.	1–2 g q. 6 h.
80–50	Mild Impairment	1.5 g q. 4 h. OR 2 g q. 6 h.	0.75–1.5 g q. 6 h.
50–25	Moderate Impairment	1.5 g q. 6 h. OR 2 g q. 8 h.	0.75–1.5 g q. 8 h.
25–10	Severe Impairment	1 g q. 6 h. OR 1.25 g q. 8 h.	0.5–1 g q. 8 h.
10–2	Marked Impairment	0.67 g q. 8 h. OR 1 g q. 12 h.	0.5–0.75 g q. 12 h.
<2	None	0.5 g q. 8 h. OR 0.75 g q. 12 h.	0.25–0.5 g q. 12 h.

METHADONE HYDROCHLORIDE ⓒ

[*měth 'a-dōn hī-drō- klō-rīd*]

DISKETS® (dispersible tablets, Lilly)
Tablets, USP
(*See also* Dolophine® Hydrochloride)

CONDITIONS FOR DISTRIBUTION AND USE OF METHADONE PRODUCTS:

Code of Federal Regulations,

Title 21, Sec. 291.505

METHADONE PRODUCTS, WHEN USED FOR THE TREATMENT OF NARCOTIC ADDICTION IN DETOXIFICATION OR MAINTENANCE PROGRAMS, SHALL BE DISPENSED ONLY BY APPROVED HOSPITAL PHARMACIES, APPROVED COMMUNITY PHARMACIES, AND MAINTENANCE PROGRAMS APPROVED BY THE FOOD AND DRUG ADMINISTRATION AND THE DESIGNATED STATE AUTHORITY.

APPROVED MAINTENANCE PROGRAMS SHALL DISPENSE AND USE METHADONE IN ORAL FORM ONLY AND ACCORDING TO THE TREATMENT REQUIREMENTS STIPULATED IN THE FEDERAL METHADONE REGULATIONS (21 CFR 291.505).

FAILURE TO ABIDE BY THE REQUIREMENTS IN THESE REGULATIONS MAY RESULT IN CRIMINAL PROSECUTION, SEIZURE OF THE DRUG SUPPLY, REVOCATION OF THE PROGRAM APPROVAL, AND INJUNCTION PRECLUDING OPERATION OF THE PROGRAM.

DESCRIPTION

Methadone Hydrochloride, USP (4,4-diphenyl -6-dimethylamino - heptanone-3 hydrochloride), is a white crystalline material which is water soluble. However, the Disket preparation of methadone hydrochloride has been specially formulated with insoluble excipients to deter the use of this drug by injection.

Each Disket contains 40 mg methadone hydrochloride. Each tablet also contains cellulose, FD&C Yellow No. 6, flavors, magnesium stearate, potassium phosphate, silicon dioxide, starch, and stearic acid.

ACTIONS

Methadone hydrochloride is a synthetic narcotic analgesic with multiple actions quantitatively similar to those of morphine, the most prominent of which involve the central nervous system and organs composed of smooth muscle. The principal actions of therapeutic value are analgesia and sedation and detoxification or maintenance in narcotic addiction. The methadone abstinence syndrome, although qualitatively similar to that of morphine, differs in that the onset is slower, the course is more prolonged, and the symptoms are less severe.

When administered orally, methadone is approximately one-half as potent as when given parenterally. Oral administration results in a delay of the onset, a lowering of the peak, and an increase in the duration of analgesic effect.

INDICATIONS

1. Detoxification treatment of narcotic addiction (heroin or other morphine-like drugs).
2. Maintenance treatment of narcotic addiction (heroin or other morphine-like drugs), in conjunction with appropriate social and medical services.

NOTE

If methadone is administered for treatment of heroin dependence for more than three weeks, the procedure passes from treatment of the acute withdrawal syndrome (detoxification) to maintenance therapy. Maintenance treatment is permitted to be undertaken only by approved methadone programs. This does not preclude the maintenance treatment of an addict who is hospitalized for medical conditions other than addiction and who requires temporary maintenance during the critical period of his stay or whose enrollment has been verified in a program which has approval for maintenance treatment with methadone.

CONTRAINDICATION

Hypersensitivity to methadone.

WARNINGS

Diskets Methadone Hydrochloride are for oral administration only. This preparation contains insoluble excipients and therefore *must not* be injected. It is recommended that Diskets Methadone Hydrochloride, if dispensed, be packaged in child-resistant containers to prevent accidental ingestion.

Methadone hydrochloride, a narcotic, is a Schedule II controlled substance under the Federal Controlled Substances Act. Appropriate security measures should be taken to safeguard stocks of methadone against diversion.

DRUG DEPENDENCE—**METHADONE CAN PRODUCE DRUG DEPENDENCE OF THE MORPHINE TYPE AND, THEREFORE, HAS THE POTENTIAL FOR BEING ABUSED. PSYCHIC DEPENDENCE, PHYSICAL DEPENDENCE, AND TOLERANCE MAY DEVELOP UPON REPEATED ADMINISTRATION OF METHADONE, AND IT SHOULD BE PRESCRIBED AND ADMINISTERED WITH THE SAME DEGREE OF CAUTION APPROPRIATE TO THE USE OF MORPHINE.**

Interaction with Other Central-Nervous-System Depressants —Methadone should be used with caution and in reduced dosage in patients who are concurrently receiving other narcotic analgesics, general anesthetics, phenothiazines, other tranquilizers, sedative-hypnotics, tricyclic antidepressants, and other CNS depressants (including alcohol). Respiratory depression, hypotension, and profound sedation or coma may result.

Anxiety —Since methadone, as used by tolerant subjects at a constant maintenance dosage, is not a tranquilizer, patients who are maintained on this drug will react to life problems and stresses with the same symptoms of anxiety as do other individuals. The physician should not confuse such symptoms with those of narcotic abstinence and should not attempt to treat anxiety by increasing the dosage of methadone. The action of methadone in maintenance treatment is limited to the control of narcotic symptoms and is ineffective for relief of general anxiety.

Head Injury and Increased Intracranial Pressure—The respiratory depressant effects of methadone and its capacity to elevate cerebrospinal-fluid pressure may be markedly exaggerated in the presence of increased intracranial pressure. Furthermore, narcotics produce side effects that may obscure the clinical course of patients with head injuries. In such patients, methadone must be used with caution and only if it is deemed essential.

Asthma and Other Respiratory Conditions— Methadone should be used with caution in patients having an acute asthmatic attack, in those with chronic obstructive pulmonary disease or cor pulmonale, and in individuals with a substantially decreased respiratory reserve, preexisting respiratory depression, hypoxia, or hypercapnia. In such patients, even usual therapeutic doses of narcotics may decrease respiratory drive while simultaneously increasing airway resistance to the point of apnea.

Hypotensive Effect—The administration of methadone may result in severe hypotension in an individual whose ability to maintain his blood pressure has already been compromised by a depleted blood volume or concurrent administration of such drugs as the phenothiazines or certain anesthetics.

Use in Ambulatory Patients—Methadone may impair the mental and/or physical abilities required for the performance of potentially hazardous tasks, such as driving a car or operating machinery. The patient should be cautioned accordingly.

Methadone, like other narcotics, may produce orthostatic hypotension in ambulatory patients.

Use in Pregnancy—Safe use in pregnancy has not been established in relation to possible adverse effects on fetal development. Therefore, methadone should not be used in pregnant women unless, in the judgment of the physician, the potential benefits outweigh the possible hazards.

PRECAUTIONS

***Interaction with Pentazocine*— Patients who are addicted to heroin or who are on the methadone maintenance program may experience withdrawal symptoms when given pentazocine.**

Interaction with Rifampin—The concurrent administration of rifampin may possibly reduce the blood concentration of methadone to a degree sufficient to produce withdrawal symptoms. The mechanism by which rifampin may decrease blood concentrations of methadone is not fully understood, although enhanced microsomal drug-metabolized enzymes may influence drug disposition.

Acute Abdominal Conditions—The administration of methadone or other narcotics may obscure the diagnosis or clinical course in patients with acute abdominal conditions.

Interaction with Monoamine Oxidase (MAO) Inhibitors—Therapeutic doses of meperidine have precipitated severe reactions in patients concurrently receiving monoamine oxidase inhibitors or those who have received such agents within 14 days. Similar reactions thus far have not been reported with methadone; but if the use of methadone is necessary in such patients, a sensitivity test should be performed in which repeated small incremental doses are administered over the course of several hours while the patient's condition and vital signs are under careful observation.

Special-Risk Patients—Methadone should be given with caution and the initial dose should be reduced in certain patients, such as the elderly or debilitated and those with severe impairment of hepatic or renal function, hypothyroidism, Addison's disease, prostatic hypertrophy, or urethral stricture.

ADVERSE REACTIONS

Heroin Withdrawal—During the induction phase of methadone maintenance treatment, patients are being withdrawn from heroin and may therefore show typical withdrawal symptoms, which should be differentiated from methadone-induced side effects. They may exhibit some or all of the following symptoms associated with acute withdrawal from heroin or other opiates: lacrimation, rhinorrhea, sneezing, yawning, excessive perspiration, gooseflesh, fever, chilliness alternating with flushing, restlessness, irritability, "sleepy yen," weakness, anxiety, depression, dilated pupils, tremors, tachycardia, abdominal cramps, body aches, involuntary twitching and kicking movements, anorexia, nausea, vomiting, diarrhea, intestinal spasms, and weight loss.

Initial Administration—Initially, the dosage of methadone should be carefully titrated to the individual. Induction too rapid for the patient's sensitivity is more likely to produce the following effects.

THE MAJOR HAZARDS OF METHADONE, AS OF OTHER NARCOTIC ANALGESICS, ARE RESPIRATORY DEPRESSION AND, TO A LESSER DEGREE, CIRCULATORY DEPRESSION. RESPIRATORY ARREST, SHOCK, AND CARDIAC ARREST HAVE OCCURRED.

The most frequently observed adverse reactions include lightheadedness, dizziness, sedation, nausea, vomiting, and sweating. These effects seem to be more prominent in ambulatory patients and in those who are not suffering severe pain. In such individuals, lower doses are advisable. Some adverse reactions may be alleviated in the ambulatory patient if he lies down.

Other adverse reactions include the following:

Central Nervous System—Euphoria, dysphoria, weakness, headache, insomnia, agitation, disorientation, and visual disturbances.

Gastrointestinal—Dry mouth, anorexia, constipation, and biliary tract spasm.

Cardiovascular—Flushing of the face, bradycardia, palpitation, faintness, and syncope.

Genitourinary—Urinary retention or hesitancy, antidiuretic effect, and reduced libido and/or potency.

Allergic—Pruritus, urticaria, other skin rashes, edema, and, rarely, hemorrhagic urticaria.

Maintenance on a Stabilized Dose—During prolonged administration of methadone, as in a methadone maintenance treatment program, there is a gradual, yet progressive, disappearance of side effects over a period of several weeks. However, constipation and sweating often persist.

DOSAGE AND ADMINISTRATION

For Detoxification Treatment—THE DRUG SHALL BE ADMINISTERED DAILY UNDER CLOSE SUPERVISION AS FOLLOWS:

A detoxification treatment course shall not exceed 21 days and may not be repeated earlier than four weeks after completion of the preceding course.

In detoxification, the patient may receive methadone when there are significant symptoms of withdrawal. The dosage schedules indicated below are recommended but could be varied in accordance with clinical judgment. Initially, a single oral dose of 15 to 20 mg of methadone will often be sufficient to suppress withdrawal symptoms. Additional methadone may be provided if withdrawal symptoms are not suppressed or if symptoms reappear. When patients are physically dependent on high doses, it may be necessary to exceed these levels. Forty mg/day in single or divided doses will usually constitute an adequate stabilizing dosage level. Stabilization can be continued for two to three days, and then the amount of methadone normally will be gradually decreased. The rate at which methadone is decreased will be determined separately for each patient. The dose of methadone can be decreased on a daily basis or at two-day intervals, but the amount of intake shall always be sufficient to keep withdrawal symptoms at a tolerable level. In hospitalized patients, a daily reduction of 20 percent of the total daily dose may be tolerated and may cause little discomfort. In ambulatory patients, a somewhat slower schedule may be needed. If methadone is administered for more than three weeks, the procedure is considered to have progressed from detoxification or treatment of the acute withdrawal syndrome to maintenance treatment, even though the goal and intent may be eventual total withdrawal.

For Maintenance Treatment—In maintenance treatment, the initial dosage of methadone should control the abstinence symptoms that follow withdrawal of narcotic drugs but should not be so great as to cause sedation, respiratory depression, or other effects of acute intoxication. It is important that the initial dosage be adjusted on an individual basis to the narcotic tolerance of the new patient. If such a patient has been a heavy user of heroin up to the day of admission, he may be given 20 mg four to eight hours later or 40 mg in a single oral dose. If he enters treatment with little or no narcotic tolerance (e.g., if he has recently been released from jail or other confinement), the initial dosage may be one-half these quantities. When there is any doubt, the smaller dose should be used initially. The patient should then be kept under observation, and, if symptoms of abstinence are distressing, additional 10-mg doses may be administered as needed. Subsequently, the dosage should be adjusted individually, as tolerated and required, up to a level of 120 mg daily. The patient will initially ingest the drug under observation daily, or at least six days a week, for the first three months. After demonstrating satisfactory adherence to the program regulations for at least three months, the patient may be permitted to reduce to three times weekly the occasions when he must ingest the drug under observation. He shall receive no more than a two-day take-home supply. With continuing adherence to the program's requirements for at least two years, he may then be permitted twice-weekly visits to the program for drug ingestion under observation, with a three-day take-home supply. A daily dose of 120 mg or more shall be justified in the medical record. Prior approval from state authority and the Food and Drug Administration is required for any dose above 120 mg administered at the clinic and for any dose above 100 mg to be taken at home. A regular review of dosage level should be made by the responsible physician, with careful consideration given to reduction of dosage as indicated on an individual basis. A new dosage level is only a test level until stability is achieved.

Special Considerations for a Pregnant Patient—Caution shall be taken in the maintenance treatment of pregnant patients. Dosage levels shall be kept as low as possible if continued methadone treatment is deemed necessary. It is the responsibility of the program sponsor to assure that each female patient be fully informed concerning the possible risks to a pregnant woman or her unborn child from the use of methadone.

Special Limitations—

Treatment of Patients under Age 18

1. The safety and effectiveness of methadone for use in the treatment of adolescents have not been proved by adequate clinical study. Special procedures are therefore necessary to assure that patients under age 16 will not be admitted to a program and that patients between 16 and 18 years of age will be admitted to maintenance treatment only under limited conditions.

2. Patients between 16 and 18 years of age who were enrolled and under treatment in approved programs on December 15, 1972, may continue in maintenance treatment. No new patients between 16 and 18 years of age may be admitted to a maintenance treatment program after March 15, 1973, unless a parent, legal guardian, or responsible adult designated by the state authority completes and signs Form FD 2635, "Consent for Methadone Treatment."

Methadone treatment of new patients between the ages of 16 and 18 years will be permitted after December 15, 1972, only with a documented history of two or more unsuccessful attempts at detoxification and a documented history of dependence on heroin or other morphine-like drugs beginning two years or more prior to application for treatment. No patient under age 16 may be continued or started on methadone treatment after December 15, 1972, but these patients may be detoxified and retained in the program in a drug-free state for follow-up and aftercare.

3. Patients under age 18 who are not placed on maintenance treatment may be detoxified. Detoxification may not exceed three weeks. A repeat episode of detoxification may not be initiated until four weeks after the completion of the previous detoxification.

OVERDOSAGE

Symptoms—Serious overdosage of methadone is characterized by respiratory depression (a decrease in respiratory rate and/ or tidal volume, Cheyne-Stokes respiration, cyanosis), extreme somnolence progressing to stupor or coma, maximally constricted pupils, skeletal-muscle flaccidity, cold and clammy skin, and, sometimes, bradycardia and hypotension. In severe overdosage, particularly by the intravenous route, apnea, circulatory collapse, cardiac arrest, and death may occur.

Treatment—Primary attention should be given to the reestablishment of adequate respiratory exchange through provision of a patent airway and institution of assisted or controlled ventilation. If a nontolerant person, especially a child, takes a large dose of methadone, effective narcotic antagonists are available to counteract the potentially lethal respiratory depression. **The physician must remember, however, that methadone is a long-acting depressant (36 to 48 hours), whereas the antagonists act for much shorter periods (one to three hours).** The patient must, therefore, be monitored continuously for recurrence of respiratory depression and treated repeatedly with the narcotic antagonist as needed. If the diagnosis is correct and respiratory depression is due only to overdosage of methadone, the use of respiratory stimulants is not indicated.

An antagonist should not be administered in the absence of clinically significant respiratory or cardiovascular depression. Intravenously administered narcotic antagonists (naloxone, nalorphine, and levallorphan) are the drugs of choice to reverse signs of intoxication. These agents should be given repeatedly until the patient's status remains satisfactory. The hazard that the narcotic antagonist will further depress respiration is less likely with the use of naloxone.

Oxygen, intravenous fluids, vasopressors, and other supportive measures should be employed as indicated.

NOTE: IN AN INDIVIDUAL PHYSICALLY DEPENDENT ON NARCOTICS, THE ADMINISTRATION OF THE USUAL DOSE OF A NARCOTIC ANTAGONIST WILL PRECIPITATE AN ACUTE WITHDRAWAL SYNDROME. THE SEVERITY OF THIS SYNDROME WILL DEPEND ON THE DEGREE OF PHYSICAL DEPENDENCE AND THE DOSE OF THE ANTAGONIST ADMINISTERED. THE USE OF A NARCOTIC ANTAGONIST IN SUCH A PERSON SHOULD BE AVOIDED IF POSSIBLE. IF IT MUST BE USED TO TREAT SERIOUS RESPIRATORY DEPRESSION IN

Continued on next page

• Identi-Code® symbol.

Lilly—Cont.

THE PHYSICALLY DEPENDENT PATIENT, THE ANTAGONIST SHOULD BE ADMINISTERED WITH EXTREME CARE AND BY TITRATION WITH SMALLER THAN USUAL DOSES OF THE ANTAGONIST.

HOW SUPPLIED

(©) *Diskets No. 1, Methadone Hydrochloride Tablets, USP, U53,** 40 mg, Peach-Colored (cross-scored), in bottles of 100 (NDC 0002-2153-02). [052085]

Shown in Product Identification Section, page 415

METUBINE® IODIDE ℞

[*mĕ-tū ′bēn ī-ō-dīd*]

(metocurine iodide)

Injection, USP

THIS DRUG SHOULD BE ADMINISTERED ONLY BY ADEQUATELY TRAINED INDIVIDUALS WHO ARE FAMILIAR WITH ITS ACTIONS, CHARACTERISTICS, AND HAZARDS.

DESCRIPTION

Metubine® Iodide (metocurine iodide, Lilly) is a nondepolarizing muscle relaxant and is presented as a sterile isotonic solution for intravenous injection.

Each ml contains 2 mg metocurine iodide and sodium chloride, 0.9 percent, with 0.5 percent phenol as a preservative. Sodium carbonate and/or hydrochloric acid may have been added during manufacture to adjust the *p* H in the range of 4 to 4.3.

The empirical formula is $C_{40}H_{48}I_2N_2O_6$, and the molecular weight is 906.64.

CLINICAL PHARMACOLOGY

Metubine® Iodide (metocurine iodide, Lilly) is a methyl analogue of tubocurarine which produces nondepolarizing (competitive) neuromuscular blockade at the myoneural junction. Recent animal studies suggest that Metubine Iodide does not produce the autonomic ganglionic blockade seen with other nondepolarizing muscle relaxants. Recent clinical findings suggest that Metubine Iodide reaches the neuromuscular junction more rapidly than does tubocurarine. After intravenous injection, there is rapid onset (one to four minutes) of muscle relaxation with maximum twitch inhibition (96 percent) in 1.5 to ten minutes. The maximum effect lasts 35 to 60 minutes. The time for recovery to 50 percent of control twitch response is in excess of three hours. Following bolus injection of 0.05 mg/kg, the mean terminal half-life of Metubine Iodide was 3.6 hours (217 minutes). Approximately 50 percent of the dose was excreted as unchanged drug in the urine over 48 hours, and 2 percent was excreted unchanged in the bile. Approximately 35 percent is protein bound, mainly to the beta and gamma globulins.

The use of repeated doses may be accompanied by a cumulative effect. The duration of action and degree of muscle relaxation may be altered by dehydration, body temperature changes, hypocalcemia, excess magnesium, or acid-base imbalance. Concurrently administered general anesthetics, certain antibiotics, and neuromuscular disease may potentiate the neuromuscular blocking action of Metubine Iodide.

Histamine release with Metubine Iodide occurs less frequently than with *d* -tubocurarine and is related to dosage and rapidity of administration. Effects on the cardiovascular system (e.g., changes in pulse rate, hypotension) are less than those reported with equipotent doses of *d* -tubocurarine and gallamine.

Because the main excretory pathway for Metubine Iodide is through the kidneys, severe renal disease or conditions associated with poor renal perfusion (shock states) may result in prolonged neuromuscular blockade.

Following intravenous injection in the mother, placental transfer of Metubine Iodide occurs rapidly, and, after six minutes, the fetal plasma concentration is approximately one-tenth the maternal level.

INDICATIONS AND USAGE

Metubine® Iodide (metocurine iodide, Lilly) is indicated as an adjunct to anesthesia to induce skeletal-muscle relaxation. It may be employed to reduce the intensity of muscle contractions in pharmacologically or electrically induced convulsions. It may also be employed to facilitate the management of patients undergoing mechanical ventilation.

CONTRAINDICATIONS

Metubine® Iodide (metocurine iodide, Lilly) is contraindicated in those persons with known hypersensitivity to the drug or to its iodide content.

WARNINGS

METUBINE® IODIDE (METOCURINE IODIDE, LILLY) SHOULD BE ADMINISTERED IN CAREFULLY ADJUSTED DOSES BY OR UNDER THE SUPERVISION OF EXPERIENCED CLINICIANS WHO ARE FAMILIAR WITH THE COMPLICATIONS WHICH MAY OCCUR WITH THE USE OF THIS DRUG. Metubine Iodide should not be administered unless facilities for intubation, artificial ventilation, oxygen therapy, and reversal agents are immediately available. The clinician must be prepared to assist or control respiration.

Metubine Iodide should be used with extreme caution in patients with myasthenia gravis. In such patients, a peripheral nerve stimulator may be valuable in assessing the effects of administration.

PRECAUTIONS

General Precautions —Metubine® Iodide (metocurine iodide, Lilly) should be used with caution in patients with poor renal perfusion or severe renal disease (*see* CLINICAL PHARMACOLOGY).

Rapid administration of large doses of Metubine Iodide may produce changes in blood pressure or heart rate or signs of histamine release.

Metubine Iodide has no effect on consciousness, pain threshold, or cerebration; therefore, it should be used with adequate anesthesia.

Drug Interactions —Synergistic or antagonistic effects may result when depolarizing and nondepolarizing muscle relaxants are administered simultaneously or sequentially.

Parenteral administration of high doses of certain antibiotics may intensify or resemble the neuroblocking action of muscle relaxants. These include neomycin, streptomycin, bacitracin, kanamycin, gentamicin, dihydrostreptomycin, polymyxin B, colistin, sodium colistimethate, and tetracyclines. If muscle relaxants and antibiotics must be administered simultaneously, the patient should be observed closely for any unexpected prolongation of respiratory depression.

Certain general anesthetics have a synergistic action with neuromuscular blocking agents. Diethyl ether, halothane, and isoflurane potentiate the neuromuscular blocking action of other nondepolarizing agents and may be presumed to do so with Metubine Iodide.

Administration of quinidine shortly after recovery may produce recurrent paralysis.

The effect of diazepam on neuromuscular blockade by Metubine Iodide is not clear. Until more information is available, patients should be carefully monitored for unexpected drug response and prolongation of action.

The use of magnesium sulfate in preeclamptic patients potentiates the effects of both depolarizing and nondepolarizing muscle relaxants.

Usage in Pregnancy—Pregnancy Category C —Intrauterine growth retardation and limb deformities resembling clubfoot were produced by *d* -tubocurarine chloride and succinylcholine chloride when administered to the rat fetus between the sixteenth and nineteenth days of gestation or when injected in chick embryos from the fifth to the fifteenth day of incubation. When *d* -tubocurarine was injected intramuscularly into the interscapular region of the fetuses on the sixteenth to the nineteenth day of gestation, the incidence of growth retardation and limb deformity ranged from 21 to 23 percent and 7 to 8 percent respectively.

There are no adequate and well-controlled studies of Metubine Iodide in pregnant women. Metubine Iodide should be used during pregnancy only if the potential benefit justifies the risk to the fetus.

Labor and Delivery —It is not known whether the use of muscle relaxants during labor or delivery has immediate or delayed adverse effects on the fetus, prolongs the duration of labor, or increases the likelihood that forceps delivery, obstetric intervention, or resuscitation of the newborn will be necessary.

Nursing Mothers —It is not known whether Metubine Iodide is excreted in human milk. Because many drugs are excreted in human milk, caution should be excercised when Metubine Iodide is administered to a nursing woman.

Usage in Children —A clinical study has shown that Metubine Iodide is twice as potent as *d* -tubocurarine in children, but the rate of recovery is the same. There may be a slight increase in heart rate, but no change occurs in blood pressure or ECG. Doses calculated on the basis of body weight or body surface area may be applicable when the advantages of nondepolarizing neuromuscular blockade are desired.

ADVERSE REACTIONS

The most frequently noted adverse reaction is prolongation of the drug's pharmacologic action. Neuromuscular effects may range from skeletal-muscle weakness to a profound relaxation that produces respiratory insufficiency or apnea.

Possible adverse reactions include allergic or hypersensitivity reactions to the drug or its iodide content and histamine release when large doses are administered rapidly. Signs of histamine release include erythema, edema, flushing, tachycardia, arterial hypotension, bronchospasm, and circulatory collapse.

Prolonged apnea and respiratory depression have occurred following the use of muscle relaxants. Many physiologic factors, drug interactions, and individual sensitivities may contribute to the development of respiratory paralysis (*see* CLINICAL PHARMACOLOGY and PRECAUTIONS).

OVERDOSAGE

An overdose of Metubine® Iodide (metocurine iodide, Lilly) may result in prolonged apnea, cardiovascular collapse, and sudden release of histamine.

Massive doses of metocurarine are not reversible by the antagonists edrophonium or neostigmine and atropine.

Overdosage may be avoided by the careful monitoring of response by means of a peripheral nerve stimulator.

The primary treatment for residual neuromuscular blockade with respiratory paralysis or inadequate ventilation is maintenance of the patient's airway and manual or mechanical ventilation.

Accompanying derangements of blood pressure, electrolyte imbalance, or circulating blood volume should be determined and corrected by appropriate fluid and electrolyte therapy.

Residual neuromuscular blockade following surgery may be reversed by the use of anticholinesterase inhibitors such as neostigmine or pyridostigmine bromide and atropine. Prescribing information should be consulted for the appropriate drug selection based on dosage and desired duration of action.

DOSAGE AND ADMINISTRATION

Metubine® Iodide (metocurine iodide, Lilly) should be administered intravenously as a sustained injection over a period of 30 to 60 seconds. INTRAMUSCULAR ADMINISTRATION OF METUBINE IODIDE IS NOT RECOMMENDED. Care must be taken to avoid overdosage. The use of a peripheral nerve stimulator to monitor response will minimize the risk of overdosage. The type of anesthetic used and nature of the surgical procedure will influence the amount of Metubine Iodide required. Doses of 0.2 to 0.4 mg/kg have been found satisfactory for endotracheal intubation. Relaxation following the initial dose may be expected to be effective for periods of 25 to 90 minutes, with an average of approximately 60 minutes. Supplemental administration may be made as indicated to provide needed surgical relaxation. Supplemental doses average 0.5 to 1 mg. The use of strong anesthetics that potentiate the effect of neuromuscular blocking drugs such as halothane, diethyl ether, isoflurane, or enflurane reduces the requirement for Metubine Iodide. Incremental doses should be reduced by approximately one-third to one-half.

Recommended Doses for Use during Electroshock Therapy —Doses required for satisfactory relaxation range from 1.75 to 5.5 mg. When the patient is treated for the first time, the drug is administered slowly by the intravenous route as a sustained injection until a head-drop response ensues. After dosage has been established, subsequent injections are completed in 15 to 50 seconds. The average dose ranges from 2 to 3 mg.

Drug Incompatibilities —Metubine Iodide is unstable in alkaline solutions. When it is combined with barbiturate solutions, precipitation may occur. Solutions of barbiturates, meperidine, and morphine sulfate should not be administered from the same syringe.

HOW SUPPLIED

(℞) *Vials (Multiple Dose) No. 586, Metubine® Iodide (Metocurine Iodide Injection, USP),* 2 mg/ml, 20 ml, rubber-stoppered, in singles (10/carton) (NDC 0002-1421-01). Store at controlled room temperature, 59° to 86°F (15° to 30°C). [032984]

MOXAM® ℞

[*mŏks ′ăm*]

(moxalactam disodium)

For Injection, USP

DESCRIPTION

Moxam® (moxalactam disodium, Lilly) is a semisynthetic broad-spectrum β-lactam antibiotic for parenteral administration. It is the disodium salt of (6R, 7R)-7-[[carboxy (4-hydroxyphenyl) acetyl] amino] -7-methoxy-3-[[(1-methyl-1*H* -tetrazol-5-yl)thio] methyl]-8-oxo-5-oxa-1-azabicyclo[4.2.0] oct-2-ene-2-carboxylic acid.

Moxam is a sterile dry powder which contains 150 mg mannitol/g of moxalactam activity. The total sodium content is approximately 88 mg (3.8 mEq sodium ion)/g of moxalactam activity. Sodium bicarbonate and/or sodium hydroxide may have been added during manufacture for neutralization. The *p* H of freshly reconstituted solutions usually ranges from 5.5 to 6.5.

CLINICAL PHARMACOLOGY

After rapid intravenous infusion (two minutes) of 500-mg and 1-g doses of moxalactam in normal adult volunteers, mean peak serum levels of 57 mcg/ml and 94 mcg/ml respectively were achieved.

Average serum concentrations following intravenous doses of 0.25, 0.5, 1, 2, 3, and 4 g infused over a 20-minute period in adult volunteers are listed in Table 1. Intravenous administration of 4-g doses every eight hours for seven doses produced no evidence of accumulation in the serum. The half-life after an intravenous dose is approximately 1.9 hours (114 minutes).

TABLE 1. MOXALACTAM SERUM LEVELS IN ADULTS (MCG/ML)

IV Dose	20 Minutes*	4 Hours*	8 Hours*
0.25 g	24	4	1
0.5 g	48	7	2
1 g	101	13	3
2 g	204	31	8
3 g	262	40	9
4 g	443	61	13

* Time after beginning of infusion.

Following intramuscular administration of 250-mg, 500-mg, and 1-g doses of moxalactam to normal adult volunteers, the mean peak serum concentrations were 10, 16, and 27 mcg/ml respectively. These peaks occurred at 60 to 120 minutes. After intramuscular administration, the half-life is approximately 2.1 hours (126 minutes).

Sixty to 90 percent of an intramuscular or intravenous dose is excreted by the kidneys over a 24-hour period, which results in high urinary concentrations. No metabolite of moxalactam has been detected in the urine. Following intravenous doses of 250 mg, 500 mg, 1 g, and 2 g, urinary concentrations were highest during the first two hours and were 170, 446, 1820, and 4220 mcg/ml respectively. These levels decreased at ten to 12 hours to 14, 59, 96, and 156 mcg/ml respectively.

The mean renal clearance of moxalactam was approximately 78 ml/min, with a calculated mean total body clearance of 99.3 ml/min for a man weighing 70 kg.

In patients with reduced renal function, the serum half-life of moxalactam is significantly prolonged. Although serum concentrations in patients with normal renal function declined to 0 within 24 to 48 hours after a 1-g intravenous dose, serum concentrations in patients with severe renal impairment were approximately 25 and 10 percent of peak levels at 24 and 48 hours respectively.

Therapeutic levels of moxalactam are achieved in the following fluids: pleural fluid, interstitial fluid, aqueous humor, and the cerebrospinal fluid of patients with normal and inflamed meninges.

Microbiology—The bactericidal activity of moxalactam results from inhibition of cell-wall synthesis. Moxalactam has in vitro activity against a wide range of gram-negative and certain gram-positive organisms. Moxalactam has a high degree of stability in the presence of β-lactamases, both penicillinases and cephalosporinases produced by gram-negative and gram-positive bacteria. Because of its unique chemical structure, moxalactam is also a potent inhibitor of β-lactamases from certain gram-negative bacteria, e.g., *Enterobacter cloacae* and *Pseudomonas aeruginosa*. Moxalactam is usually active against the following microorganisms in vitro and in clinical infections (*see* INDICATIONS AND USAGE).

Aerobes, gram-negative: *Haemophilus influenzae*, including ampicillin-resistant strains; *Escherichia coli; Klebsiella* species, including *Klebsiella pneumoniae; Proteus mirabilis; P. vulgaris; Providencia rettgeri* (formerly *Proteus rettgeri*); *Morganella morganii* (formerly *Proteus morganii*); *Enterobacter* species; *P. aeruginosa* (some strains are resistant); *Serratia* species.

Note.: Many strains of the above organisms that are multiply resistant to other antibiotics, e.g., penicillins, cephalosporins, and aminoglycosides, are susceptible to moxalactam.

Aerobes, gram-positive: staphylococci, including penicillinase-producing strains (*Note:* Methicillin-resistant staphylococci as well as some strains of *Staphylococcus epidermidis* are resistant to moxalactam); *Streptococcus pyogenes* (group A β-hemolytic streptococci); *S. agalactiae* (group B streptococci); *S. pneumoniae* (formerly *Diplococcus pneumoniae*) (*Note:* Most strains of enterococci, e.g., *S. faecalis*, are resistant).

Anaerobes: *Bacteroides* species, including *Bacteroides fragilis; Fusobacterium* species; *Clostridium* species (*Note:* Most strains of *Clostridium difficile* are resistant); *Eubacterium* species; *Peptococcus* species; *Peptostreptococcus* species; *Veillonella* species.

Moxalactam also demonstrates in vitro activity against the following microorganisms, although its clinical significance is unknown: *Neisseria gonorrhoeae; N. meningitidis; Providencia* species; *Salmonella* species, including *Salmonella typhi; Shigella* species.

Moxalactam is highly resistant to hydrolysis by β-lactamases of Richmond Types I, II, III, IV, and V. These enzymes are frequently produced by strains of *Enterobacteriaceae, P. aeruginosa, Acinetobacter* species, *H. influenzae*, and *Neisseria* species. Furthermore, moxalactam is stable to some β-lactamases not classified as Richmond types, such as those produced by strains of *S. aureus* and *B. fragilis*.

Moxalactam and aminoglycosides have been shown to be synergistic in vitro against some strains of *Enterobacteriaceae* and *P. aeruginosa*.

Disc Susceptibility Tests—Quantitative methods that require measurement of zone diameters give the most precise estimate of antibiotic susceptibility. One such procedure[1] has been recommended for use with discs to test susceptibility to moxalactam.

Reports from the laboratory giving results of the standard single-disc susceptibility test with a 30-mcg moxalactam disc should be interpreted according to the following criteria:

Susceptible organisms produce zones of 20 mm or greater, indicating that the test organism is likely to respond to therapy.

Organisms that produce zones of 15 to 19 mm are expected to be susceptible if high dosage is used or if the infection is confined to tissues and fluids (e.g., urine) in which high antibiotic levels are attained.

Resistant organisms produce zones of 14 mm or less, indicating that other therapy should be selected.

Organisms should be tested with the moxalactam disc, since moxalactam has been shown by in vitro tests to be active against certain strains found resistant when other β-lactam discs are used.

In other susceptibility testing procedures, e.g., ICS agar dilution[2] or the equivalent, a bacterial isolate may be considered susceptible if the MIC value for moxalactam is not more than 16 mcg/ml. Organisms are considered resistant to moxalactam if the MIC is equal to or greater than 64 mcg/ml. Organisms having an MIC value of less than 64 mcg/ml but greater than 16 mcg/ml are expected to be susceptible if high dosage is used or if the infection is confined to tissues and fluids (e.g., urine) in which high antibiotic levels are attained.

INDICATIONS AND USAGE

Moxam® (moxalactam disodium, Lilly) is indicated for the treatment of infections caused by susceptible strains of the designated microorganisms in the diseases listed below:

Lower respiratory infections, including pneumonia, caused by *S. pneumoniae, H. influenzae, Klebsiella* species, *Enterobacter* species, *S. aureus* (penicillin-sensitive and penicillin-resistant strains), *E. coli*, and *P. mirabilis*.

Urinary tract infections caused by *E. coli, Klebsiella* species, *Enterobacter* species, *Proteus* species (indole-positive and indole-negative), and *Serratia* species.

Intra-abdominal infections, such as peritonitis, endometritis, and pelvic cellulitis, caused by *E. coli; Peptostreptococcus* species; *Bacteroides* species, including *B. fragilis;* mixed aerobic and anaerobic organisms, such as *K. pneumoniae, S. agalactiae* (group B streptococci), *P. mirabilis, Enterobacter* species, *P. aeruginosa, Peptococcus* species, *Clostridium* species, *Fusobacterium* species, and *Eubacterium* species.

Bacterial septicemia caused by *S. aureus, E. coli, S. pneumoniae, Klebsiella* species, *Serratia* species, *Pseudomonas* species, and *B. fragilis*.

Central-nervous-system infections, e.g., meningitis and ventriculitis, caused by *E. coli* and *Klebsiella* species. Moxam has been used successfully in the treatment of a limited number of patients with meningitis and ventriculitis caused by other *Enterobacteriaceae* and *H. influenzae*.

Skin and skin-structure infections caused by *S. aureus* (penicillinase and non-penicillinase-producing); *S. pyogenes* (group A β-hemolytic streptococci); *E. coli; Serratia* species; mixed aerobic and anaerobic organisms, such as *Proteus* species, *Klebsiella* species, *Enterobacter* species, *Peptococcus* species, *Peptostreptococcus* species, *Bacteroides* species, and *Clostridium* species.

Bone and joint infections caused by *S. aureus* (penicillinase and non-penicillinase-producing), *P. aeruginosa*, and *Serratia* species.

Because of the serious nature of infections due to *P. aeruginosa* and because many strains of *Pseudomonas* species are moderately susceptible to moxalactam, higher dosage is recommended in serious systemic infections caused by this organism (*see* DOSAGE AND ADMINISTRATION). Moxam has been used successfully in the treatment of some patients with serious lower respiratory tract infections caused by *P. aeruginosa* and *Serratia* species. In such cases, higher dosage is recommended, and other therapy should be instituted if the response is not prompt.

Moxam has been used successfully in surgical infections in cases where concomitant therapy with other antibiotics may be used.

Specimens for bacteriologic cultures should be obtained in order to isolate and identify causative organisms and to determine their susceptibilities to moxalactam. Therapy may be instituted before results of susceptibility studies are known; however, once these results become available, the antibiotic treatment should be adjusted accordingly.

In certain cases of confirmed or suspected gram-positive or gram-negative sepsis or in patients with other serious infections in which the causative organism has not been identified, Moxam may be used concomitantly with an aminoglycoside. The dosage recommended in the labeling of both antibiotics may be given and depends on the severity of the infection and the patient's condition. Renal function should be carefully monitored, especially if higher dosages of the aminoglycosides are to be administered or if therapy is prolonged, because of the potential nephrotoxicity and ototoxicity of aminoglycosidic antibiotics. Some β-lactam antibiotics also have a certain degree of nephrotoxicity. Although, to date, this has not been noted when Moxam was given alone, it is possible that nephrotoxicity may be potentiated if Moxam is used concomitantly with an aminoglycoside.

CONTRAINDICATION

Moxam® (moxalactam disodium, Lilly) is contraindicated in patients with known allergy to the drug.

WARNINGS

Moxalactam can interfere with hemostasis through three different mechanisms: hypoprothrombinemia, platelet dysfunction, and very rarely, immune-mediated thrombocytopenia. Bleeding can be associated with these induced abnormalities. A total of 2.5 percent of clinical trial patients treated for four or more days experienced a bleeding event, most of which were serious.

Bleeding associated with hypoprothrombinemia can be prevented by the use of vitamin K. It is recommended that patients who receive moxalactam be given 10 mg of vitamin K per week prophylactically. The inhibition of platelet function, which may be accompanied by a prolonged bleeding time, is dose-dependent and can generally be avoided by limiting dosage to 4 g per day. It is recommended that the bleeding time be monitored in patients with normal renal function who receive more than 4 g of moxalactam per day for more than three days. All patients with significantly impaired renal function should have appropriate dosage reduction (*see* DOSAGE AND ADMINISTRATION) and should be monitored periodically with bleeding times. If the bleeding time becomes unduly prolonged, moxalactam should be discontinued.

If bleeding occurs in a patient receiving moxalactam and if the prothrombin time is prolonged, vitamin K should be given. Administration of fresh frozen plasma, packed red cells, and platelet concentrates may be indicated. Moxalactam should be discontinued if bleeding is due to platelet dysfunction. If moxalactam is discontinued because of platelet dysfunction, other beta-lactam antibiotics that are known to be associated with this phenomenon should be used with caution. See current prescribing information for alternative therapy.

Bleeding during moxalactam therapy may also be related to complications of underlying diseases (e.g., sepsis, malignancy, renal and hepatic dysfunction) or may result from the combined effects of underlying diseases and moxalactam therapy. When bleeding occurs, it is important to rule out disseminated intravascular coagulation (DIC) through appropriate laboratory tests since DIC occurs frequently in patients with sepsis, malignancy, or hepatic disease.

Hepatic and renal dysfunction, poor alimentation, thrombocytopenia, and the concomitant use of "high dose" heparin (more than 20,000 units/day), oral anticoagulants, and other drugs that affect hemostasis (e.g., aspirin) are factors that may increase the risk of bleeding during moxalactam therapy.

BEFORE THERAPY WITH MOXAM® (MOXALACTAM DISODIUM, LILLY) IS INSTITUTED, CAREFUL INQUIRY SHOULD BE MADE FOR A HISTORY OF HYPERSENSITIVITY REACTIONS TO MOXALACTAM DISODIUM, CEPHALOSPORINS, PENICILLINS, OR OTHER DRUGS. THIS PRODUCT SHOULD BE GIVEN WITH CAUTION TO PATIENTS WITH TYPE 1 HYPERSENSITIVITY REACTIONS TO PENICILLIN. ANTIBIOTICS SHOULD BE GIVEN WITH CAUTION TO ANY PATIENT WHO HAS HAD SOME FORM OF ALLERGY, PARTICULARLY TO DRUGS. IF AN ALLERGIC REACTION TO MOXALACTAM OCCURS, DISCONTINUE THE DRUG. SERIOUS HYPERSENSITIVITY REACTIONS MAY REQUIRE EPINEPHRINE AND OTHER EMERGENCY MEASURES.

Pseudomembranous colitis has been reported with virtually all broad-spectrum antibiotics (including macrolides, semisynthetic penicillins, and cephalosporins); therefore, it is important to consider its diagnosis in patients who develop diarrhea in association with the use of antibiotics. Such colitis may range in severity from mild to life-threatening.

Treatment with broad-spectrum antibiotics alters the normal flora of the colon and may permit overgrowth of clostridia. Studies indicate that a toxin produced by *Clostridium difficile* is one primary cause of antibiotic-associated colitis. Mild cases of pseudomembranous colitis usually respond to drug discontinuance alone. In moderate to severe cases, management should include sigmoidoscopy, appropriate bacteriologic studies, and fluid, electrolyte, and protein supplementation. When the colitis does not improve after the drug has been discontinued, or when it is severe, oral vancomycin is

Continued on next page

• **Identi-Code® symbol.**

Lilly—Cont.

the drug of choice for antibiotic-associated pseudomembranous colitis produced by *C. difficile.* Other causes of colitis should be ruled out.

PRECAUTIONS

A disulfiram-like reaction, i.e., nausea, vomiting, and vasomotor instability with hypotension and peripheral vasodilatation, has occurred following the ingestion of ethanol. The timing of the ingestion of alcohol is an important factor. When alcohol was ingested prior to the first dose of Moxam® (moxalactam disodium, Lilly), this syndrome was not observed. It has been reported only when ethanol ingestion followed the administration of Moxam. This has been observed as late as 48 hours after the last dose of Moxam. Moxalactam inhibits the enzyme acetaldehyde dehydrogenase in laboratory animals. This causes accumulation of acetaldehyde when ethanol is administered concomitantly.

Prolonged use of Moxam may result in the overgrowth of nonsusceptible organisms (e.g., enterococci). Careful observation of the patient is essential. If superinfection occurs during therapy, appropriate measures should be taken.

Broad-spectrum antibiotics should be prescribed with caution in individuals with a history of gastrointestinal disease, particularly colitis.

Carcinogenesis, Mutagenesis, Impairment of Fertility—Certain beta-lactam antibiotics containing the N-methylthiotetrazole side chain have been reported to cause delayed maturity of the testicular germinal epithelium when given to neonatal rats during initial spermatogenic development (6 to 40 days of age). In animals that were treated from 6 to 40 days of age with 1000 mg/kg/day of moxalactam (approximately 5 times the maximum clinical dose), the delayed maturity was pronounced and was associated with decreased testicular weights and a reduced number of germinal cells in the leading waves of spermatogenic development. The effect was slight in rats given 30 or 100 mg/kg/day. No adverse effects have been observed in rats exposed in utero or in older rats (more than 40 days of age) after exposure for up to 6 months. The significance to man of these findings in rats in unknown because of differences in the time of initiation of spermatogenesis, rate of spermatogenic development, and duration of puberty.

Usage in Pregnancy—Pregnancy Category C—Reproduction studies have been performed in mice, rats, rabbits, and ferrets. Administration of Moxam® (moxalactam disodium, Lilly) at ten to 20 times the usual human dose has resulted in an increased incidence of birth defects or embryotoxicity in the ferret. Since the incidence of birth defects and embryotoxicity in control ferrets was high and variable, its significance in ferrets after the administration of Moxam is unknown. Studies in mice and rats at doses up to 20 times the usual human dose (eight times the maximum dose) have revealed no evidence of impaired fertility or teratogenicity. A decrease in offspring viability was noted in rats, perhaps due to drug-related growth depression and decrease in food consumption by the pregnant dams. There are no adequate and well-controlled studies in pregnant women. Moxam should be used during pregnancy only if the potential benefit justifies the potential risk to the fetus.

Nursing Mothers—It is not known whether this drug is excreted in human milk. Studies have shown that it is excreted in the milk of rats. Because many drugs are excreted in human milk, caution should be exercised when Moxam is administered to a nursing woman.

ADVERSE REACTIONS

In clinical studies, adverse effects considered related to moxalactam therapy or of uncertain etiology are listed below:

Hematopoietic abnormalities, half of which were of uncertain etiology, occurred in about 5 percent of patients and included eosinophilia (1 in 35), disturbances in vitamin K-dependent clotting function (decreased prothrombin), increased bleeding time, thrombocytopenia (1 in 276) (*see* PRECAUTIONS), and reversible leukopenia (1 in 145). Reversible neutropenia has been reported in children who were three years of age or younger (1 in 23).

Local effects were reported in less than 4 percent of patients and included pain at the site of injection (1 in 70) and phlebitis (1 in 50).

Hypersensitivity reactions were reported in about 3 percent of patients and included morbilliform eruptions (1 in 60), fever (1 in 155), and positive Coombs' test (1 in 180). Two-thirds of the occurrences were considered related to therapy. Anaphylaxis occurred in one patient.

Gastrointestinal symptoms occurred in less than 3 percent of patients, the most frequent being diarrhea (1 in 60). Symptoms of pseudomembranous colitis may appear either during or after antibiotic treatment. Nausea and vomiting have been reported rarely.

Hepatic enzyme elevations (SGOT, SGPT, alkaline phosphatase) occurred in about 1 in 25 patients. Ninety percent of the abnormalities were of uncertain etiology.

Causal Relationship Uncertain—Although of uncertain etiology, the following transient abnormalities in clinical laboratory renal function test results are listed to serve as alerting information for the physician:

Elevated BUN (1 in 150), pyuria and hematuria (1 of each in 250), and elevated serum creatinine (1 in 300).

DOSAGE AND ADMINISTRATION

Dosage: Adults—The usual daily dose of Moxam® (moxalactam disodium, Lilly) is 2 to 4 g administered in divided doses every eight to 12 hours for five to ten days or up to 14 days. Most mild to moderate infections can be expected to respond to a dosage of 500 mg to 2 g every 12 hours.

In mild skin and skin-structure infections and in uncomplicated pneumonia, a dosage of 500 mg every eight hours is recommended.

In mild, uncomplicated urinary tract infections, a dosage of 250 mg every 12 hours is adequate. In urinary tract infections that are more difficult to treat, a dosage of 500 mg every 12 hours may be needed. In serious urinary tract infections, the dosage frequency may be increased to every eight hours.

In life-threatening infections or infections due to less susceptible organisms (e.g., *P. aeruginosa*), doses up to 4 g every eight hours (i.e., 12 g/day) may be needed. It is recommended that the bleeding time should be monitored in patients who receive more than 4 g of moxalactam/day for more than three days.

Prophylactic vitamin K, 10 mg/week, should be given to patients treated with Moxam.

Neonates, Infants, and Children—The following dosage schedule is recommended:

PEDIATRIC DOSAGE SCHEDULE

Neonates	
0–1 week of age	50 mg/kg q. 12 h.
1–4 weeks of age	50 mg/kg q. 8 h.
Infants	50 mg/kg q. 6 h.
Children	50 mg/kg q. 6 h. or q. 8 h.

This may be increased to a total daily dose of 200 mg/kg (not to exceed the maximum adult dose) for serious infections.

In pediatric gram-negative meningitis, an initial loading dose of 100 mg/kg is recommended prior to the utilization of the above dosage schedule.

Impaired Renal Function—When renal function is impaired, a reduced dose must be employed and the serum levels closely monitored. After an intial dose of 1 to 2 g (depending on the severity of the infection), a maintenance dosage schedule should be followed. Continued dosage should be determined by the degree of renal impairment, the severity of infection, and the susceptibility of the causative organism.

When only serum creatinine is available, the following formula (based on sex, weight, and age of the patient) may be used to convert this value into creatinine clearance. The serum creatinine should represent a steady state of renal function.

$$\text{Males: } \frac{\text{Weight (kg)} \times (140 - \text{age})}{72 \times \text{serum creatinine}}$$

$$\text{Females: } 0.9 \times \text{male value}$$

[See table below].

The serum half-life of moxalactam during hemodialysis has ranged from two to five hours. Maintenance doses of Moxam should be repeated following regular hemodialysis.

Administration: Moxam® (moxalactam disodium, Lilly) may be given intravenously or by deep intramuscular injection into a large muscle mass (such as the upper outer quadrant of the gluteus maximus or lateral part of the thigh).

Intramuscular Administration—Moxam should be diluted with one of the following diluents according to the table below: Sterile Water for Injection, Bacteriostatic Water for Injection, 0.9% Sodium Chloride Injection, Bacteriostatic Sodium Chloride Injection, or 0.5% or 1% Lidocaine Hydrochloride Injection.

[See table above].

IM Dilution Table for Moxam® (moxalactam disodium)

Vial Size	Volume Diluent to Be Added (ml)	Approximate Available Volume (ml)	Approximate Average Concentration (mg/ml)
1 g	3	3.7	270

Shake well until dissolved.

Individual IM doses of 2 g or more of Moxam at one site are not recommended.

Intravenous Administration—The intravenous route may be preferable for patients with bacterial septicemia, localized parenchymal abscesses (such as intra-abdominal abscess), peritonitis, meningitis, or other severe or life-threatening infections. In those with normal renal function, the intravenous dosage for such infections is 3 to 12 g of Moxam daily. In conditions such as septicemia, 6 to 12 g/day may be given initially by the intravenous route for several days, and the dosage may then be gradually reduced according to clinical response and laboratory findings.

A solution of 1 g of Moxam in 20 ml of Sterile Water for Injection is isotonic.

Solutions of Moxam, like those of most β-lactam antibiotics should not be added directly to aminoglycoside solutions (e.g., tobramycin sulfate, gentamicin sulfate, amikacin sulfate) because of potential interaction. However, Moxam and aminoglycosides may be administered sequentially by intermittent intravenous infusion to the same patient. After the administration of one of the two drugs, flush the tubing with an approved diluent and then administer the other drug solution.

For direct intermittent intravenous administration, add 10 ml of Sterile Water for Injection, 5% Dextrose Injection, or 0.9% Sodium Chloride Injection/g of moxalactam. Slowly inject directly into the vein over a period of three to five minutes or give through the tubing of an administration set while the patient is also receiving one of the approved *intravenous* diluents outlined in the COMPATIBILITY AND STABILITY section.

Intravenous solutions containing alcohol should be avoided (*see* PRECAUTIONS).

Intermittent intravenous infusion with a Y-type administration set or volume control set can also be accomplished while any of the approved intravenous fluids are being infused. However, during infusion of the solution containing Moxam, it is desirable to discontinue the other solution. When this technique is employed, careful attention should be paid to the volume of the solution containing moxalactam so that the calculated dose will be infused. When a Y-tube hookup is used, 50 to 100 ml of an appropriate intravenous diluent should be added to the 1 or 2-g piggyback (100-ml) vial. If Sterile Water for Injection is used as the diluent, reconstitute with approximately 20 ml to avoid a hypotonic solution.

For continuous intravenous infusion, each g of moxalactam should be diluted with 10 ml of Sterile Water for Injection. An appropriate quantity of the resulting solution may be added to an IV bottle containing one of the approved intravenous diluents outlined below under COMPATIBILITY AND STABILITY.

COMPATIBILITY AND STABILITY

Intramuscular—One g of Moxam® (moxalactam disodium, Lilly) reconstituted with 3 ml of Sterile Water for Injection, Bacteriostatic Water for Injection, 0.9% Sodium Chloride Injection, Bacteriostatic Sodium Chloride Injection, or 0.5% or 1% Lidocaine Hydrochloride Injection (without epinephrine) maintains satisfactory potency for 24 hours at room

MOXAM® (MOXALACTAM DISODIUM)—
MAINTENANCE DOSAGE GUIDE FOR PATIENTS
WITH RENAL IMPAIRMENT

Creatinine Clearance (ml/min./1.73 m²)	Renal Function	Life-Threatening Infections—Maximum Dosage	Less Severe Infections
>80	Normal	4 g q. 8 h.	0.5–2 g q. 8–12 h.
50–80	Mild Impairment	3 g q. 8 h.	0.5–1 g q. 8 h.
25–50	Moderate Impairment	2 g q. 8 h. OR 3 g q. 12 h.	0.25–1 g q. 12 h.
2–25	Severe Impairment	1 g q. 8 h. OR 1.25 g q. 12 h.	0.25–0.5 g q. 8 h
<2	0	1 g q. 24 h.	0.25–0.5 g q. 12 h.

temperature (25°C) or for 96 hours under refrigeration (5°C) when stored in the original glass containers.

One g of Moxam reconstituted with 3 ml of Sterile Water for Injection, 0.9% Sodium Chloride Injection, or 5% Dextrose Injection maintains potency for at least six months in the frozen state at −20°C when stored in the original glass containers.

Intravenous—The following diluents as constituted with Moxam to 1 g with 50 ml maintain potency for 24 hours at room temperature (25°C) or 96 hours under refrigeration (5°C) when stored in the original glass container: 5% Dextrose Injection, 10% Dextrose Injection, 0.9% Sodium Chloride Injection, 5% Dextrose and 0.2% Sodium Chloride Injection, 5% Dextrose and 0.45% Sodium Chloride Injection, 5% Dextrose and 0.9% Sodium Chloride Injection, Ringer's Injection, Lactated Ringer's Injection, Lactated Ringer's and 5% Dextrose Injection, Acetated Ringer's Injection, 5% Dextrose and 0.15% (20 mEq/L) Potassium Chloride Injection, 5% Dextrose and 0.2% Sodium Bicarbonate Injection, 10% Fructose Injection, Sodium Lactate Injection (M/6 Sodium Lactate), Plasma-Lyte® M in 5% Dextrose Injection, 5% Osmitrol® in Water for Injection, 6% Gentran® 75 Injection and 10% Travert®, Normosol®-M in D5-W Injection, and Ionosol®-B in D5-W Injection.

The following diluents as constituted with Moxam to 1 g with 50 ml and stored in Viaflex® intravenous containers maintain potency for 24 hours at room temperature (25°C) or 96 hours under refrigeration: 5% Dextrose Injection, 0.9% Sodium Chloride Injection, and Lactated Ringer's and 5% Dextrose Injection.

One g of Moxam reconstituted with 50 ml 5% Dextrose Injection or 0.9% Sodium Chloride Injection maintains potency for at least six months when stored in the frozen state at −20°C in either the original glass or Viaflex plastic containers.

Note: After the reconstitution periods mentioned above, any unused solutions or frozen material should be discarded. Do not refreeze.

Moxam in the dry state should be stored below 78°F (26°C). The dry material as well as solutions tend to darken with age, depending on storage conditions. Product potency, however, is not adversely affected.

HOW SUPPLIED

(℞) *Vials Moxam® (Moxalactam Disodium for Injection, USP): No. 7152,* 1 g (equivalent to moxalactam activity), 10-ml size (NDC 0002-7152-10), and *No. 7154,* 2 g (equivalent to moxalactam activity), 20-ml size (NDC 0002-7154-10), in Traypak™ (multivial carton, Lilly) of 10; *No. 7162,* 10 g (equivalent to moxalactam activity), 100-ml size (NDC 0002-7162-16), in Traypak of 6.

[040486]

1. Am. J. Clin. Pathol., *45:* 493, 1966; Federal Register, *39:* 19182–19184, 1974.
2. Ericsson, H. M., and Sherris, J. C.: Acta Pathol. Microbiol. Scand. [B], Supplement No. 217, 1971.

Vials No. 7154, 2 g, 10's—6505-01-142-2291

NEBCIN® ℞

[*nĕb'sin*]

(tobramycin sulfate)

Injection, USP

WARNINGS

Patients treated with Nebcin® (Tobramycin Sulfate Injection, USP, Lilly) and other aminoglycosides should be under close clinical observation, because these drugs have an inherent potential for causing ototoxicity and nephrotoxicity.

Neurotoxicity, manifested as both auditory and vestibular ototoxicity, can occur. The auditory changes are irreversible, are usually bilateral, and may be partial or total. Eighth-nerve impairment and nephrotoxicity may develop, primarily in patients having preexisting renal damage and in those with normal renal function to whom aminoglycosides are administered for longer periods or in higher doses than those recommended. Other manifestations of neurotoxicity may include numbness, skin tingling, muscle twitching, and convulsions. The risk of aminoglycoside-induced hearing loss increases with the degree of exposure to either high peak or high trough serum concentrations. Patients who develop cochlear damage may not have symptoms during therapy to warn them of eighth-nerve toxicity, and partial or total irreversible bilateral deafness may continue to develop after the drug has been discontinued. Rarely, nephrotoxicity may not become manifest until the first few days after cessation of therapy. Aminoglycoside-induced nephrotoxicity usually is reversible.

Renal and eighth-nerve function should be closely monitored in patients with known or suspected renal impairment and also in those whose renal function is initially normal but who develop signs of renal dysfunction during therapy. Peak and trough serum concentrations of aminoglycosides should be monitored periodically during therapy to assure adequate levels and to avoid potentially toxic levels. Prolonged serum concentrations above 12 mcg/ml should be avoided. Rising trough levels (above 2 mcg/ml) may indicate tissue accumulation. Such accumulation, excessive peak concentrations, advanced age, and cumulative dose may contribute to ototoxicity and nephrotoxicity (*see* PRECAUTIONS). Urine should be examined for decreased specific gravity and increased excretion of protein, cells, and casts. Blood urea nitrogen, serum creatinine, and creatinine clearance should be measured periodically. When feasible, it is recommended that serial audiograms be obtained in patients old enough to be tested, particularly high-risk patients. Evidence of impairment of renal, vestibular, or auditory function requires discontinuation of the drug or dosage adjustment.

Nebcin should be used with caution in premature and neonatal infants because of their renal immaturity and the resulting prolongation of serum half-life of the drug.

Concurrent and sequential use of other neurotoxic and/or nephrotoxic antibiotics, particularly other aminoglycosides (e.g., amikacin, streptomycin, neomycin, kanamycin, gentamicin, and paromomycin), cephaloridine, viomycin, polymyxin B, colistin, cisplatin, and vancomycin, should be avoided. Other factors that may increase patient risk are advanced age and dehydration.

Aminoglycosides should not be given concurrently with potent diuretics, such as ethacrynic acid and furosemide. Some diuretics themselves cause ototoxicity, and intravenously administered diuretics enhance aminoglycoside toxicity by altering antibiotic concentrations in serum and tissue.

Aminoglycosides can cause fetal harm when administered to a pregnant woman (*see* PRECAUTIONS).

DESCRIPTION

Tobramycin sulfate, a water-soluble antibiotic of the aminoglycoside group, is derived from the actinomycete *Streptomyces tenebrarius.* Nebcin® (tobramycin sulfate, Lilly), Injection, is a clear and colorless sterile aqueous solution for parenteral administration.

Each ml also contains 5 mg phenol as a preservative, 3.2 mg sodium bisulfite, 0.1 mg edetate disodium, and water for injection, q.s. Sulfuric acid and/or sodium hydroxide may have been added to adjust the pH. Tobramycin is 4-0-[2,6-diamino-2, 3, 6-trideoxy-α-D-glucopyranosyl]-6- 0- [3-amino -3- deoxy-α-D-glucopyranosyl] -2- deoxystreptamine.

CLINICAL PHARMACOLOGY

Tobramycin is rapidly absorbed following intramuscular administration. Peak serum concentrations of tobramycin occur between 30 and 90 minutes after intramuscular administration. Following an intramuscular dose of 1 mg/kg of body weight, maximum serum concentrations reach about 4 mcg/ml, and measurable levels persist for as long as eight hours. Therapeutic serum levels are generally considered to range from 4 to 6 mcg/ml. When Nebcin® (tobramycin sulfate, Lilly) is administered by intravenous infusion over a one-hour period, the serum concentrations are similar to those obtained by intramuscular administration. Nebcin is poorly absorbed from the gastrointestinal tract.

In patients with normal renal function, except neonates, Nebcin administered every eight hours does not accumulate in the serum. However, in those with reduced renal function and in neonates, the serum concentration of the antibiotic is usually higher and can be measured for longer periods of time than in normal adults. Dosage for such patients must, therefore, be adjusted accordingly (*see* DOSAGE AND ADMINISTRATION).

Following parenteral administration, little, if any, metabolic transformation occurs, and tobramycin is eliminated almost exclusively by glomerular filtration. Renal clearance is similar to that of endogenous creatinine. Ultrafiltration studies demonstrate that practically no serum protein binding occurs. In patients with normal renal function, up to 84 percent of the dose is recoverable from the urine in eight hours and up to 93 percent in 24 hours.

Peak urine concentrations ranging from 75 to 100 mcg/ml have been observed following the intramuscular injection of a single dose of 1 mg/kg. After several days of treatment, the amount of tobramycin excreted in the urine approaches the daily dose administered. When renal function is impaired, excretion of Nebcin is slowed, and accumulation of the drug may cause toxic blood levels.

The serum half-life in normal individuals is two hours. An inverse relationship exists between serum half-life and creatinine clearance, and the dosage schedule should be adjusted according to the degree of renal impairment (*see* DOSAGE AND ADMINISTRATION). In patients undergoing dialysis, 25 to 70 percent of the administered dose may be removed, depending on the duration and type of dialysis.

Tobramycin can be detected in tissues and body fluids after parenteral administration. Concentrations in bile and stools ordinarily have been low, which suggests minimum biliary excretion. Tobramycin has appeared in low concentration in the cerebrospinal fluid following parenteral administration, and concentrations are dependent on dose, rate of penetration, and degree of meningeal inflammation. It has also been found in sputum, peritoneal fluid, synovial fluid, and abscess fluids, and it crosses the placental membranes. Concentrations in the renal cortex are several times higher than the usual serum levels.

Probenecid does not affect the renal tubular transport of tobramycin.

Microbiology—In vitro tests demonstrate that tobramycin is bactericidal and that it acts by inhibiting the synthesis of protein in bacterial cells.

Tobramycin is usually active against most strains of the following organisms in vitro and in clinical infections:

- *Pseudomonas aeruginosa*
- *Proteus* species (indole-positive and indole-negative), including *Proteus mirabilis, P. morganii, P. rettgeri,* and *P. vulgaris*
- *Escherichia coli*
- *Klebsiella-Enterobacter-Serratia* group
- *Citrobacter* species
- *Providencia* species
- Staphylococci, including *Staphylococcus aureus* (coagulase-positive and coagulase-negative)

Aminoglycosides have a low order of activity against most gram-positive organisms, including *Streptococcus pyogenes, S. pneumoniae,* and enterococci.

Although most strains of group D streptococci demonstrate in vitro resistance, some strains in this group are susceptible. In vitro studies have shown that an aminoglycoside combined with an antibiotic which interferes with cell-wall synthesis affects some group D streptococcal strains synergistically. The combination of penicillin G and tobramycin results in a synergistic bactericidal effect in vitro against certain strains of *S. faecalis.* However, this combination is not synergistic against other closely related organisms, e.g., *S. faecium.* Speciation of group D streptococci alone cannot be used to predict susceptibility. Susceptibility testing and tests for antibiotic synergism are emphasized.

Cross-resistance between aminoglycosides occurs and depends largely on inactivation by bacterial enzymes.

Susceptibility Tests—If the FDA Standardized Disc Test method (formerly the Bauer-Kirby-Sherris-Turck method) of disc susceptibility testing is used, a disc containing 10 mcg tobramycin should give a zone of at least 15 mm when tested against a tobramycin-susceptible bacterial strain, a zone of 13 to 14 mm against strains of intermediate susceptibility, and a zone of 12 mm or less against resistant organisms. The minimum inhibitory concentration correlates are ≤ 4 mcg/ml for susceptibility and $\geq$ 8 mcg/ml for resistance.

INDICATIONS AND USAGE

Nebcin® (tobramycin sulfate, Lilly) is indicated for the treatment of serious bacterial infections caused by susceptible strains of the designated microorganisms in the diseases listed below:

Septicemia in the neonate, child, and adult caused by *P. aeruginosa, E. coli,* and *Klebsiella* species

Lower respiratory tract infections caused by *P. aeruginosa, Klebsiella* species, *Enterobacter* species, *Serratia* species, *E. coli,* and *S. aureus* (penicillinase and non-penicillinase-producing strains)

Serious central-nervous-system infections (meningitis) caused by susceptible organisms

Intra-abdominal infections, including peritonitis, caused by *E. coli, Klebsiella* species, and *Enterobacter* species.

Skin, bone, and skin-structure infections caused by *P. aeruginosa, Proteus* species, *E. coli, Klebsiella* species, *Enterobacter* species, and *S. aureus*

Complicated and recurrent urinary tract infections caused by *P. aeruginosa, Proteus* species (indole-positive and indole-negative), *E. coli, Klebsiella* species, *Enterobacter* species, *Serratia* species, *S. aureus, Providencia* species, and *Citrobacter* species

Aminoglycosides, including Nebcin, are not indicated in uncomplicated initial episodes of urinary tract infections unless the causative organisms are not susceptible to antibiotics having less potential toxicity. Nebcin may be considered in serious staphylococcal infections when penicillin or other potentially less toxic drugs are contraindicated and when bacterial susceptibility testing and clinical judgment indicate its use.

Bacterial cultures should be obtained prior to and during treatment to isolate and identify etiologic organisms and to test their susceptibility to tobramycin. If susceptibility tests show that the causative organisms are resistant to tobramycin, other appropriate therapy should be instituted. In pa-

Continued on next page

• **Identi-Code® symbol.**

Lilly—Cont.

tients in whom a serious life-threatening gram-negative infection is suspected, including those in whom concurrent therapy with a penicillin or cephalosporin and an aminoglycoside may be indicated, treatment with Nebcin may be initiated before the results of susceptibility studies are obtained. The decision to continue therapy with Nebcin® (tobramycin sulfate, Lilly) should be based on the results of susceptibility studies, the severity of the infection, and the important additional concepts discussed in the WARNINGS box above.

CONTRAINDICATIONS

A hypersensitivity to any aminoglycoside is a contraindication to the use of tobramycin. A history of hypersensitivity or serious toxic reactions to aminoglycosides may also contraindicate the use of any other aminoglycoside because of the known cross-sensitivity of patients to drugs in this class.

WARNINGS

See WARNINGS box above.

PRECAUTIONS

Serum and urine specimens for examination should be collected during therapy, as recommended in the WARNINGS box. Serum calcium, magnesium, and sodium should be monitored.

Peak and trough serum levels should be measured periodically during therapy. Prolonged concentrations above 12 mcg/ml should be avoided. Rising trough levels (above 2 mcg/ml) may indicate tissue accumulation. Such accumulation, advanced age, and cumulative dosage may contribute to ototoxicity and nephrotoxicity. It is particularly important to monitor serum levels closely in patients with known renal impairment.

A useful guideline would be to perform serum level assays after two or three doses, so that the dosage could be adjusted if necessary, and also at three to four-day intervals during therapy. In the event of changing renal function, more frequent serum levels should be obtained and the dosage or dosage interval adjusted according to the guidelines provided in the DOSAGE AND ADMINISTRATION section.

In order to measure the peak level, a serum sample should be drawn about 30 minutes following intravenous infusion or one hour after an intramuscular injection. Trough levels are measured by obtaining serum samples at eight hours or just prior to the next dose of Nebcin®(tobramycin sulfate, Lilly). These suggested time intervals are intended only as guidelines and may vary according to institutional practices. It is important, however, that there be consistency within the individual patient program unless computerized pharmacokinetic dosing programs are available in the institution. These serum-level assays may be especially useful for monitoring the treatment of severely ill patients with changing renal function or of those infected with less sensitive organisms or those receiving maximum dosage.

Neuromuscular blockade and respiratory paralysis have been reported in cats receiving very high doses of tobramycin (40 mg/kg). The possibility that prolonged or secondary apnea may occur should be considered if tobramycin is administered to anesthetized patients who are also receiving neuromuscular blocking agents, such as succinylcholine, tubocurarine, or decamethonium, or to patients receiving massive transfusions of citrated blood. If neuromuscular blockade occurs, it may be reversed by the administration of calcium salts.

Cross-allergenicity among aminoglycosides has been demonstrated.

In patients with extensive burns, altered pharmacokinetics may result in reduced serum concentrations of aminoglycosides. In such patients treated with Nebcin, measurement of serum concentration is especially recommended as a basis for determination of appropriate dosage.

Elderly patients may have reduced renal function that may not be evident in the results of routine screening tests, such an BUN or serum creatinine. A creatinine clearance determination may be more useful. Monitoring of renal function during treatment with aminoglycosides is particularly important in such patients.

An increased incidence of nephrotoxicity has been reported following concomitant administration of aminoglycoside antibiotics and cephalosporins.

Aminoglycosides should be used with caution in patients with muscular disorders, such as myasthenia gravis or parkinsonism, since these drugs may aggravate muscle weakness because of their potential curare-like effect on neuromuscular function.

Aminoglycosides may be absorbed in significant quantities from body surfaces after local irrigation or application and may cause neurotoxicity and nephrotoxicity.

See WARNINGS box regarding concurrent use of potent diuretics and concurrent and sequential use of other neurotoxic or nephrotoxic drugs.

The inactivation of tobramycin and other aminoglycosides by beta-lactam-type antibiotics (penicillins or cephalosporins) has been demonstrated in vitro and in patients with severe renal impairment. Such inactivation has not been found in patients with normal renal function who have been given the drugs by separate routes of administration.

Therapy with tobramycin may result in overgrowth of nonsusceptible organisms. If overgrowth of nonsusceptible organisms occurs, appropriate therapy should be initiated.

Pregnancy Category D—Aminoglycosides can cause fetal harm when administered to a pregnant woman. Aminoglycoside antibiotics cross the placenta, and there have been several reports of total irreversible bilateral congenital deafness in children whose mothers received streptomycin during pregnancy. Serious side effects to mother, fetus, or newborn have not been reported in the treatment of pregnant women with other aminoglycosides. If tobramycin is used during pregnancy or if the patient becomes pregnant while taking tobramycin, she should be apprised of the potential hazard to the fetus.

Usage in Children—See INDICATIONS and USAGE and DOSAGE AND ADMINISTRATION.

ADVERSE REACTIONS

Neurotoxicity—Adverse effects on both the vestibular and auditory branches of the eighth nerve have been noted, especially in patients receiving high doses or prolonged therapy, in those given previous courses of therapy with an ototoxin, and in cases of dehydration. Symptoms include dizziness, vertigo, tinnitus, roaring in the ears, and hearing loss. Hearing loss is usually irreversible and is manifested initially by diminution of high-tone acuity. Tobramycin and gentamicin sulfates closely parallel each other in regard to ototoxic potential.

Nephrotoxicity—Renal function changes, as shown by rising BUN, NPN, and serum creatinine and by oliguria, cylindruria, and increased proteinuria, have been reported, especially in patients with a history of renal impairment who are treated for longer periods or with higher doses than those recommended. Adverse renal effects can occur in patients with initially normal renal function.

Clinical studies and studies in experimental animals have been conducted to compare the nephrotoxic potential of tobramycin and gentamicin. In some of the clinical studies and in the animal studies, tobramycin caused nephrotoxicity significantly less frequently than gentamicin. In some other clinical studies, no significant difference in the incidence of nephrotoxicity between tobramycin and gentamicin was found.

Other reported adverse reactions possibly related to Nebcin® (tobramycin sulfate, Lilly) include anemia, granulocytopenia, and thrombocytopenia; and fever, rash, itching, urticaria, nausea, vomiting, headache, lethargy, pain at the injection site, mental confusion, and disorientation. Laboratory abnormalities possibly related to Nebcin include increased serum transaminases (SGOT, SGPT); increased serum LDH and bilirubin; decreased serum calcium, magnesium, sodium, and potassium; and leukopenia, leukocytosis, and eosinophilia.

OVERDOSAGE

In the event of overdosage or toxic reaction, hemodialysis or peritoneal dialysis will reduce serum levels. Hemodialysis is preferable because it is more efficient in reducing serum levels.

DOSAGE AND ADMINISTRATION

Nebcin® (tobramycin sulfate, Lilly) may be given intramuscularly or intravenously. Recommended dosages are the same for both routes. The patient's pretreatment body weight should be obtained for calculation of correct dosage. It is desirable to measure both peak and trough serum concentrations (*see* WARNINGS box and PRECAUTIONS).

Administration for Patients with Normal Renal Function—*Adults with Serious Infections:* 3 mg/kg/day in three equal doses every eight hours (*see* Table 1).

Adults with Life-Threatening Infections: Up to 5 mg/kg/day may be administered in three or four equal doses (*see* Table 1). The dosage should be reduced to 3 mg/kg/day as soon as clinically indicated. To prevent increased toxicity due to excessive blood levels, dosage should not exceed 5 mg/kg/day unless serum levels are monitored.
[See table below left].

Children: 6 to 7.5 mg/kg/day in three or four equally divided doses (2 to 2.5 mg/kg every eight hours or 1.5 to 1.89 mg/kg every six hours).

Premature or Full-Term Neonates One Week of Age or Less: Up to 4 mg/kg/day may be administered in two equal doses every 12 hours.

It is desirable to limit treatment to a short term. The usual duration of treatment is seven to ten days. A longer course of therapy may be necessary in difficult and complicated infections. In such cases, monitoring of renal, auditory, and vestibular functions is advised, because neurotoxicity is more likely to occur when treatment is extended longer than ten days.

Administration for Patients with Impaired Renal Function—Whenever possible, serum tobramycin concentrations should be monitored during therapy.

Following a loading dose of 1 mg/kg, subsequent dosage in these patients must be adjusted, either with reduced doses administered at eight-hour intervals or with normal doses given at prolonged intervals. Both of these methods are suggested as guides to be used when serum levels of tobramycin cannot be measured directly. They are based on either the creatinine clearance or the serum creatinine of the patient, because these values correlate with the half-life of tobramycin. The dosage schedules derived from either method should be used in conjunction with careful clinical and laboratory observations of the patient and should be modified as necessary. Neither method should be used when dialysis is being performed.

Reduced dosage at eight-hour intervals: When the creatinine clearance rate is 70 ml or less per minute or when the serum creatinine value is known, the amount of the reduced dose can be determined by multiplying the normal dose from Table 1 by the percent of normal dose from the accompanying nomogram.

TABLE 1. DOSAGE SCHEDULE GUIDE FOR NEBCIN® (TOBRAMYCIN SULFATE) IN ADULTS WITH NORMAL RENAL FUNCTION
(Dosage at Eight-Hour Intervals)

For Patient Weighing		Usual Dose for Serious Infections 1 mg/kg q. 8 h. (Total, 3 mg/kg/day)		Maximum Dose for Life-Threatening Infections (Reduce as soon as possible) 1.66 mg/kg q. 8 h. (Total, 5 mg/kg/day)	
kg	lb	mg/dose q. 8 h.	ml/dose*	mg/dose q. 8 h.	ml/dose*
120	264	120 mg	3 ml	200 mg	5 ml
115	253	115 mg	2.9 ml	191 mg	4.75 ml
110	242	110 mg	2.75 ml	183 mg	4.5 ml
105	231	105 mg	2.6 ml	175 mg	4.4 ml
100	220	100 mg	2.5 ml	166 mg	4.2 ml
95	209	95 mg	2.4 ml	158 mg	4 ml
90	198	90 mg	2.25 ml	150 mg	3.75 ml
85	187	85 mg	2.1 ml	141 mg	3.5 ml
80	176	80 mg	2 ml	133 mg	3.3 ml
75	165	75 mg	1.9 ml	125 mg	3.1 ml
70	154	70 mg	1.75 ml	116 mg	2.9 ml
65	143	65 mg	1.6 ml	108 mg	2.7 ml
60	132	60 mg	1.5 ml	100 mg	2.5 ml
55	121	55 mg	1.4 ml	91 mg	2.25 ml
50	110	50 mg	1.25 ml	83 mg	2.1 ml
45	99	45 mg	1.1 ml	75 mg	1.9 ml
40	88	40 mg	1 ml	66 mg	1.6 ml

*Applicable to all product forms except Nebcin, Pediatric, Injection (*see* HOW SUPPLIED).

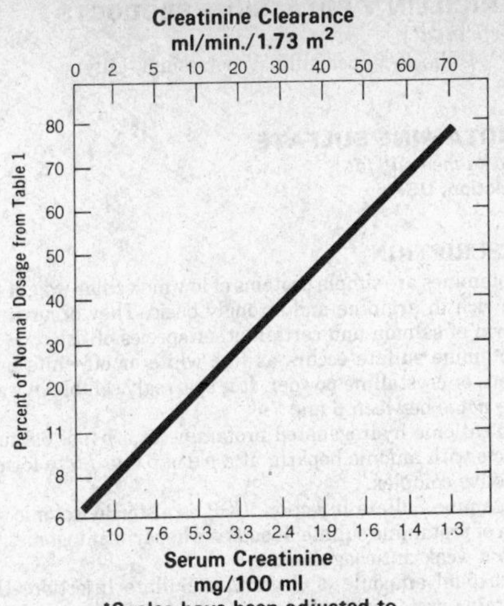

An alternate rough guide for determining reduced dosage at eight-hour intervals (for patients whose steady-state serum creatinine values are known) is to divide the normally recommended dose by the patient's serum creatinine.

Normal dosage at prolonged intervals: If the creatinine clearance rate is not available and the patient's condition is stable, a dosage frequency *in hours* for the dosage given in Table 1 can be determined by multiplying the patient's serum creatinine by six.

Dosage in Obese Patients—The appropriate dose may be calculated by using the patient's estimated lean body weight plus 40 percent of the excess as the basic weight on which to figure mg/kg.

Intramuscular Administration—Nebcin may be administered by withdrawing the appropriate dose directly from a vial or by using a prefilled Hyporet® (disposable syringe, Lilly).

Intravenous Administration—For intravenous administration, the usual volume of diluent (0.9% Sodium Chloride Injection or 5% Dextrose Injection) is 50 to 100 ml for adult doses. For children, the volume of diluent should be proportionately less than for adults. The diluted solution usually should be infused over a period of 20 to 60 minutes. Infusion periods of less than 20 minutes are not recommended, because peak serum levels may exceed 12 mcg/ml (*see* WARNINGS box).

Nebcin® (tobramycin sulfate, Lilly) should not be physically premixed with other drugs but should be administered separately according to the recommended dose and route.

HOW SUPPLIED

(℞) *Vials (Multiple Dose) Nebcin ® (Tobramycin Sulfate Injection, USP): No. 781,* 80 mg (equivalent to tobramycin) per 2 ml, 2 ml, rubber-stoppered, in singles (10 per carton) (NDC 0002-1499-01) and in Traypak™ (multivial carton, Lilly) of 25 (NDC 0002-1499-25); *No. 7090,* 1.2 g (equivalent to tobramycin) per 30 ml (Pharmacy Bulk Package), rubber-stoppered, in Traypak of 6 (NDC 0002-7090-16).

(℞) *Vials (Multiple Dose) No. 782, Nebcin ® (Tobramycin Sulfate Injection, USP), Pediatric,* 20 mg (equivalent to tobramycin) per 2 ml, 2 ml, rubber-stoppered, in singles (10 per carton) (NDC 0002-0501-01).

(℞) *Hyporets ® (disposable syringes, Lilly) Nebcin® (Tobramycin Sulfate Injection, USP): No. 55,* 60 mg (equivalent to tobramycin) per 1.5 ml, 1.5 ml, in packages of 24 (NDC 0002-0509-24), and *No. 42,* 80 mg (equivalent to tobramycin) per 2 ml, 2 ml, in packages of 24 (NDC 0002-0503-24). Each Hyporet is scored with a 10-mg (0.25-ml) fractional dose scale.

[111285]

Ampoules No. 751, 80 mg—1's—6505-01-010-3066

NEBCIN® ℞

[nĕb'sĭn]
(tobramycin sulfate)
Sterile

This vial is intended for use by the hospital pharmacist in the extemporaneous preparation of IV solutions.

WARNINGS

See under Nebcin, Injection, USP.

DESCRIPTION

Tobramycin sulfate, a water-soluble antibiotic of the aminoglycoside group, is derived from the actinomycete *Streptomyces tenebrarius.* Nebcin® (tobramycin sulfate, Lilly), Sterile, is supplied as a sterile dry powder and is intended for solution in Sterile Water for Injection, USP. Sulfuric acid and/or sodium hydroxide may have been added during manufacture to adjust the pH. Each vial contains 1200 mg of tobramycin activity. After dilution, the solution will contain 40 mg of tobramycin per ml. The product contains no preservative. *See also under* Nebcin, Injection, USP.

CLINICAL PHARMACOLOGY, INDICATIONS AND USAGE, CONTRAINDICATIONS, WARNINGS, PRECAUTIONS, ADVERSE REACTIONS, and OVERDOSAGE

See under Nebcin, Injection, USP.

DOSAGE AND ADMINISTRATION

The patient's pretreatment body weight should be obtained for calculation of correct dosage. It is desirable to measure both peak and trough serum concentrations (*see* WARNINGS box and PRECAUTIONS *under* Nebcin, Injection, USP).

Administration for Patients with Normal Renal Function-*—Adults with Serious Infections:* 3 mg/kg/day in three equal doses every eight hours (*see* Table 1 under Nebcin, Injection, USP).

Adults with Life-Threatening Infections: Up to 5 mg/kg/day may be administered in three or four equal doses (*see* Table 1). The dosage should be reduced to 3 mg/kg/day as soon as clinically indicated. To prevent increased toxicity due to excessive blood levels, dosage should not exceed 5 mg/kg/day unless serum levels are monitored.

Children: 6 to 7.5 mg/kg/day in three or four equally divided doses (2 to 2.5 mg/kg every eight hours or 1.5 to 1.89 mg/kg every six hours).

Premature or Full-Term Neonates One Week of Age or Less: Up to 4 mg/kg/day may be administered in two equal doses every 12 hours.

It is desirable to limit treatment to a short term. The usual duration of treatment is seven to ten days. A longer course of therapy may be necessary in difficult and complicated infections. In such cases, monitoring of renal, auditory, and vestibular functions is advised, because neurotoxicity is more likely to occur when treatment is extended longer than ten days.

Administration for Patients with Impaired Renal Function—Whenever possible, serum tobramycin concentrations should be monitored during therapy.

Following a loading dose of 1 mg/kg, subsequent dosage in these patients must be adjusted, either with reduced doses administered at eight-hour intervals or with normal doses given at prolonged intervals. Both of these methods are suggested as guides to be used when serum levels of tobramycin cannot be measured directly. They are based on either the creatinine clearance or the serum creatinine of the patient, because these values correlate with the half-life of tobramycin. The dosage schedules derived from either method should be used in conjunction with careful clinical and laboratory observations of the patient and should be modified as necessary. Neither method should be used when dialysis is being performed.

Reduced dosage at eight-hour intervals: When the creatinine clearance rate is 70 ml or less per minute or when the serum creatinine value is known, the amount of the reduced dose can be determined by multiplying the normal dose from Table 1 by the percent of normal dose from the nomogram *under* Nebcin, Injection, USP.

An alternate rough guide for determining reduced dosage at eight-hour intervals (for patients whose steady-state serum creatinine values are known) is to divide the normally recommended dose by the patient's serum creatinine.

Normal dosage at prolonged intervals: If the creatinine clearance rate is not available and the patient's condition is stable, a dosage frequency *in hours* for the dosage given in Table 1 can be determined by multiplying the patient's serum creatinine by six.

Dosage in Obese Patients—The appropriate dose may be calculated by using the patient's estimated lean body weight plus 40 percent of the excess as the basic weight on which to figure mg/kg.

Intravenous Administration—For intravenous administration, the usual volume of diluent (0.9% Sodium Chloride Injection or 5% Dextrose Injection) is 50 to 100 ml for adult doses. For children, the volume of diluent should be proportionately less than for adults. The diluted solution usually should be infused over a period of 20 to 60 minutes. Infusion periods of less than 20 minutes are not recommended, because peak serum levels may exceed 12 mcg/ml (*see* WARNINGS box).

Nebcin® (tobramycin sulfate, Lilly) should not be physically premixed with other drugs but should be administered separately according to the recommended dose and route.

PREPARATION AND STORAGE OF SOLUTION

Nebcin, Sterile, is supplied as a dry powder. The contents of the vial (No. 7040) should be diluted with 30 ml of Sterile Water for Injection, USP, to provide a solution containing 40 mg of tobramycin per ml. Prior to reconstitution, the vial should be stored at controlled room temperature, 59° to 86°F (15° to 30°C). After reconstitution, the solution should be kept in a refrigerator and used within 96 hours. If kept at room temperature, the solution must be used within 24 hours.

HOW SUPPLIED

(℞) *Vials No. 7040, Nebcin ® (tobramycin sulfate, Lilly), Sterile,* 1.2 g (equivalent to tobramycin), 40-ml size, rubber-stoppered (Dry Powder), in a Traypak™ (multivial carton, Lilly) of 6 (NDC 0002-7040-16).

[111285]

ONCOVIN® ℞

[ŏn'kō-vĭn]
(vincristine sulfate injection)
Solution

DESCRIPTION

Oncovin® (vincristine sulfate, Lilly) is the salt of an alkaloid obtained from a common flowering herb, the periwinkle plant (*Vinca rosea* Linn.). Originally known as leurocristine, it has also been referred to as LCR and VCR. The empirical formula for vincristine sulfate is $C_{46}H_{56}N_4O_{10} \cdot H_2SO_4$.

Each ml contains vincristine sulfate, 1 mg; mannitol, 100 mg; methylparaben, 1.3 mg; propylparaben, 0.2 mg; water for injection, q.s. Acetic acid and sodium acetate have been added for *p*H control. The *p*H of Oncovin Solution ranges from 3.5 to 5.5.

ACTION

The mode of action of Oncovin® (vincristine sulfate, Lilly) is unknown but is under investigation. Treatment of neoplastic cells in vitro with Oncovin demonstrated that it may cause an arrest of mitotic division at the stage of metaphase.

Central-nervous-system leukemia has been reported in patients undergoing otherwise successful therapy with Oncovin. This suggests that Oncovin does not penetrate well into the cerebrospinal fluid.

INDICATIONS

Oncovin® (vincristine sulfate, Lilly) is indicated in acute leukemia.

It has also been shown to be useful in combination with other oncolytic agents in Hodgkin's disease, lymphosarcoma, reticulum-cell sarcoma, rhabdomyosarcoma, neuroblastoma, and Wilms' tumor.

CONTRAINDICATIONS

Patients with the demyelinating form of Charcot-Marie-Tooth Syndrome should not be given Oncovin® (vincristine sulfate, Lilly). Careful attention should be given to those conditions listed under WARNINGS and PRECAUTIONS.

WARNINGS

This preparation is for intravenous use only. The intrathecal administration of Oncovin® (vincristine sulfate, Lilly) is uniformly fatal. Syringes containing this product should be labeled "ONCOVIN FOR INTRAVENOUS USE ONLY."

Oncovin can cause fetal harm when administered to a pregnant woman. When pregnant mice and hamsters were given doses of Oncovin that caused resorption of 23 to 85 percent of fetuses, fetal malformations were produced in those that survived. Five monkeys were given single doses of Oncovin between days 27 and 34 of their pregnancies; three of the fetuses were normal at term, and two viable fetuses at term had grossly evident malformations. In several animal species, Oncovin can induce teratogenic effects as well as embryolethality with doses which are nontoxic to the pregnant animal. There are no adequate and well-controlled studies in pregnant women. If this drug is used during pregnancy, or if the patient becomes pregnant while receiving this drug, she should be apprised of the potential hazard to the fetus. Women of childbearing potential should be advised to avoid becoming pregnant.

PRECAUTIONS

Acute uric acid nephropathy, which may occur after the administration of oncolytic agents, has also been reported with Oncovin® (vincristine sulfate, Lilly). In the presence of leukopenia or a complicating infection, administration of the next dose of Oncovin warrants careful consideration.

If central-nervous-system leukemia is diagnosed, additional agents may be required, since Oncovin does not appear to cross the blood-brain barrier in adequate amounts.

Particular attention should be given to dosage and neurologic side effects if Oncovin is administered to patients with preexisting neuromuscular disease and also when other drugs with neurotoxic potential are being used.

Acute shortness of breath and severe bronchospasm have been reported following the administration of vinca alkaloids. These reactions have been encountered most frequently when the vinca alkaloid was used in combination with mitomycin-C. The onset may be within minutes or several hours after the vinca is injected.

Care must be taken to avoid contamination of the eye with concentrations of Oncovin used clinically. If accidental contamination occurs, severe irritation (or, if the drug was delivered under pressure, even corneal ulceration) may result. The eye should be washed immediately and thoroughly.

Since dose-limiting clinical toxicity is manifested as neurotoxicity, clinical evaluation (history, physical examination) is necessary to detect the need for modification of dosage. Following administration of Oncovin, some individuals may have a fall in the white-blood-cell count or platelet count,

Continued on next page

• Identi-Code® symbol.

Lilly—Cont.

particularly when previous therapy or the disease itself has reduced bone-marrow function. Therefore, a complete blood count should be done before administration of each dose. Acute elevation of serum uric acid may also occur during induction of remission in acute leukemia; thus, such levels should be determined frequently during the first three to four weeks of treatment or appropriate measures taken to prevent uric acid nephropathy. The laboratory performing these tests should be consulted for its range of normal values. Laboratory tests both in vivo and in vitro have failed to demonstrate conclusively that this product is mutagenic. Fertility following treatment with Oncovin alone for malignant disease has not been studied in humans. Clinical reports of both male and female patients who received multiple-agent chemotherapy including Oncovin indicate that azoospermia and amenorrhea can occur in postpubertal patients. Recovery occurred many months after completion of chemotherapy in some, but not all, patients. When the same treatment is administered to prepubertal patients, it is much less likely to cause permanent azoospermia and amenorrhea.
Patients who received chemotherapy combinations including Oncovin with known carcinogens have developed second malignancies. The contributing role of Oncovin in this development has not been determined. No evidence of carcinogenicity was found following intraperitoneal administration of Oncovin in rats and mice, although this study was limited.
It is not known whether this drug is excreted in human milk. Because many drugs are excreted in human milk and because of the potential for serious adverse reactions from Oncovin in nursing infants, a decision should be made whether to discontinue nursing or the drug, taking into account the importance of the drug to the mother.

ADVERSE REACTIONS

In general, adverse reactions are reversible and are related to dosage. The most common adverse reaction is hair loss; the most troublesome are neuromuscular in origin.
When single weekly doses of the drug are employed, the adverse reactions of leukopenia, neuritic pain, and constipation are usually of short duration (i.e., less than seven days). When the dosage is reduced, these reactions may lessen or disappear. They seem to be increased when the calculated amount of drug is given in divided doses. Other adverse reactions, such as hair loss, sensory loss, paresthesia, difficulty in walking, slapping gait, loss of deep-tendon reflexes, and muscle wasting, may persist for at least as long as therapy is continued. Generalized sensorimotor dysfunction may become progressively more severe with continued treatment. In most instances, they have disappeared by about the sixth week after discontinuance of treatment, but in some patients the neuromuscular difficulties may persist for prolonged periods. Regrowth of hair may occur while maintenance therapy continues.
In addition to constipation (mentioned below), paralytic ileus may occur, particularly in young children. The ileus will reverse itself upon temporary discontinuance of Oncovin® (vincristine sulfate, Lilly) and with symptomatic care. It mimics the "surgical abdomen."
Frequently, there is a sequence in the development of neuromuscular side effects. Initially, only sensory impairment and paresthesias may be encountered. With continued treatment, neuritic pain may appear and, later, motor difficulties. No reports have yet been made of any agent that can reverse the neuromuscular manifestations accompanying therapy with Oncovin.
Convulsions, frequently with hypertension, have been reported in a few patients receiving Oncovin.
Rare occurrences of the syndrome attributed to inappropriate antidiuretic hormone secretion have been observed in patients treated with Oncovin. The syndrome has been described in association with several disease states. There is high urinary sodium excretion in the presence of hyponatremia; renal or adrenal disease, hypotension, dehydration, azotemia, and clinical edema are absent. With fluid deprivation, improvement occurs in the hyponatremia and in the renal loss of sodium.
Constipation may take the form of upper-colon impaction, and, on physical examination, the rectum may be found to be empty. Colicky abdominal pain coupled with an empty rectum may mislead the physician. A flat film of the abdomen is useful in demonstrating this condition. All cases have responded to high enemas and laxatives. A routine prophylactic regimen against constipation is recommended for all patients receiving Oncovin.
Other adverse reactions that have been reported are abdominal cramps, ataxia, foot drop, weight loss, hypertension, hypotension, rash, optic atrophy with blindness, transient cortical blindness, fever, paresthesia and numbness of the digits, oral ulceration, headache, vomiting, diarrhea, and intestinal necrosis and/or perforation. Polyuria, dysuria, and urinary retention due to bladder atony have occurred. Other drugs known to cause urinary retention particularly in the elderly should, if possible, be discontinued for the first few days following administration of Oncovin.
Cranial nerve manifestations including isolated paresis and/or paralysis of muscles controlled by cranial motor nerves may occur in absence of motor impairment elsewhere; extraocular muscles and laryngeal muscles are most commonly involved.
Jaw pain, pharyngeal pain, parotid gland pain, bone pain, back pain, limb pain, and myalgias have been reported; pain in these areas may be severe.
Oncovin does not appear to have any constant or significant effect on the platelets or the red blood cells.
Serious bone-marrow depression is usually not a major dose-limiting event. However, anemia, leukopenia, and thrombocytopenia have been reported. Thrombocytopenia, if present when therapy with Oncovin is begun, may actually improve before the appearance of marrow remission.

DOSAGE AND ADMINISTRATION

This preparation is for intravenous use only (*see* WARNINGS).

Neurotoxicity appears to be dose related. Extreme care must be used in calculating and administering the dose of Oncovin® (vincristine sulfate, Lilly), since overdosage may have a very serious or fatal outcome.

The concentration of vincristine is 1 mg/ml. Do not add extra fluid to the vial prior to removal of the dose. Withdraw the solution of Oncovin into an accurate dry syringe, measuring the dose of Oncovin carefully. Do not add extra fluid to the vial in an attempt to empty it completely.
The drug is administered intravenously *at weekly intervals.* The usual dose of Oncovin for children is 2 mg/m^2; for adults, 1.4 mg/m^2. Various dosage schedules have been used (see references in package insert).
The solution may be injected either directly into a vein or into the tubing of a running intravenous infusion. Injection of the Oncovin may be completed in about one minute.
Caution —It is extremely important that the needle be properly positioned in the vein before any vincristine is injected. If leakage into surrounding tissue should occur during intravenous administration of Oncovin, it may cause considerable irritation. The injection should be discontinued immediately, and any remaining portion of the dose should then be introduced into another vein. Local injection of hyaluronidase and the application of moderate heat to the area of leakage help disperse the drug and are thought to minimize discomfort and the possibility of cellulitis.
Parenteral drug products should be inspected visually for particulate matter and discoloration prior to administration, whenever solution and container permit.

OVERDOSAGE

Side effects following the use of Oncovin® (vincristine sulfate, Lilly) are dose related. Therefore, following administration of an overdose, patients can be expected to experience side effects in an exaggerated fashion. Supportive care should include the following: (1) prevention of side effects resulting from the syndrome of inappropriate secretion of antidiuretic hormone (this would include restriction of fluid intake and perhaps the administration of a diuretic affecting the function of the loop of Henle and the distal tubule); (2) administration of anticonvulsant doses of phenobarbital; (3) use of enemas to prevent ileus (in some instances, decompression of the gastrointestinal tract may be necessary); (4) monitoring the cardiovascular system; and (5) determining daily blood counts for guidance in transfusion requirements.
Folinic acid has been observed to have a protective effect in normal mice which were administered lethal doses of Oncovin (Cancer Res., *23:* 1390, 1963). Isolated case reports suggest that folinic acid may be helpful in treating humans who have received an overdose of Oncovin. A suggested schedule is to administer 15 mg of folinic acid intravenously every three hours for 24 hours and then every six hours for at least 48 hours. Theoretical tissue levels of Oncovin derived from pharmacokinetic data are predicted to remain significantly elevated for at least 72 hours. Treatment with folinic acid does not eliminate the need for the above-mentioned supportive measures.

HOW SUPPLIED

Multiple-Dose Vials:
1 mg/1 ml, 1 ml (No. 7194) (1's), NDC 0002-7194-01
2 mg/2 ml, 2 ml (No. 7195) (1's), NDC 0002-7195-01
5 mg/5 ml, 5 ml (No. 7196) (1's), NDC 0002-7196-01
Hyporets® (disposable syringes, Lilly), each scored with a 0.25-mg (0.25 ml) fractional dose scale:
1 mg/1 ml, 1 ml (No. 7198) (3s), NDC 0002-7198-09
2 mg/2 ml, 2 ml (No. 7199) (3s), NDC 0002-7199-09
No. 7194, 1mg/1ml—6505-01-150-4949
No. 7195, 2mg/2ml—6505-01-151-2341
This product should be refrigerated.

[101185]

PENICILLIN V POTASSIUM PRODUCTS

[*vē-sĭl'ĭn kā*]
see V-Cillin K® (penicillin V potassium, Lilly).

PROTAMINE SULFATE ℞

[*prō'ta-mēn sŭl'fāt*]
Injection, USP

DESCRIPTION

Protamines are simple proteins of low molecular weight that are rich in arginine and strongly basic. They occur in the sperm of salmon and certain other species of fish.
Protamine sulfate occurs as fine white or off-white amorphous or crystalline powder. It is sparingly soluble in water. The *p*H is between 6 and 7.
The cationic hydrogenated protamine at a *p*H of 6.8 to 7.1 reacts with anionic heparin at a *p*H of 5.0 to 7.5 to form an inactive complex.
Protamine Sulfate Injection, USP, is a sterile isotonic solution of protamine sulfate. It acts as a heparin antagonist. It is also a weak anticoagulant.
Each 5-ml ampoule of Protamine Sulfate Injection, USP, contains protamine sulfate equivalent to 50 mg of activity, and each 25-ml vial contains protamine sulfate equivalent to 250 mg of activity. Both products also contain 0.9 percent sodium chloride. Sodium phosphate and/or sulfuric acid may have been added during manufacture to adjust the *p*H. Contains no preservative.
Protamine sulfate is administered intravenously.

CLINICAL PHARMACOLOGY

When administered alone, protamine has an anticoagulant effect. However, when it is given in the presence of heparin (which is strongly acidic), a stable salt is formed which results in the loss of anticoagulant activity of both drugs.
Protamine sulfate has a rapid onset of action. Neutralization of heparin occurs within five minutes after intravenous administration. Although the metabolic fate of the heparin-protamine complex has not been elucidated, it has been postulated that protamine sulfate in the heparin-protamine complex may be partially metabolized or may be attacked by fibrinolysin, thus freeing heparin.

INDICATIONS AND USAGE

Protamine sulfate is indicated in the treatment of heparin overdosage.

CONTRAINDICATION

Protamine sulfate is contraindicated in patients who have shown previous intolerance to the drug.

WARNINGS

Hyperheparinemia or bleeding has been reported in experimental animals and in some patients 30 minutes to 18 hours after cardiac surgery (under cardiopulmonary bypass) in spite of complete neutralization of heparin by adequate doses of protamine sulfate at the end of the operation.
Therefore, it is important to keep the patient under close observation after cardiac surgery. Additional doses of protamine sulfate should be administered if indicated by coagulation studies, such as the heparin titration test with protamine and the determination of plasma thrombin time.
Too-rapid administration of protamine sulfate can cause severe hypotensive and anaphylactoid-like reactions (See DOSAGE AND ADMINISTRATION). Facilities to treat shock should be available.

PRECAUTIONS

Because of the anticoagulant effect of protamine, it is unwise to give more than 100 mg over a short period unless there is certain knowledge of a larger requirement.
Patients with a history of allergy to fish may develop hypersensitivity reactions to protamine, although to date no relationship has been established between allergic reactions to protamine and fish allergy.
Drug Interactions —Protamine sulfate has been shown to be incompatible with certain antibiotics, including several of the cephalosporins and penicillins (*see* DOSAGE AND ADMINISTRATION).
Carcinogenesis, Mutagenesis, Impairment of Fertility —Long-term or reproduction studies have not been performed in animals to evaluate carcinogenic potential, mutagenesis, or impairment of fertility.
Usage in Pregnancy —Pregnancy Category C —Animal reproduction studies have not been conducted with protamine sulfate. It is also not known whether protamine sulfate can cause fetal harm when administered to a pregnant woman or can affect reproduction capacity. Protamine sulfate should be given to a pregnant woman only if clearly needed.
Nursing Mothers —It is not known whether this drug is excreted in human milk. Because many drugs are excreted in human milk, caution should be exercised when protamine sulfate is administered to a nursing woman.
Usage in Children —Safety and effectiveness in children have not been established.

ADVERSE REACTIONS

Intravenous injections of protamine may cause a sudden fall in blood pressure, bradycardia, dyspnea, or transitory flushing and a feeling of warmth. There have been reports of anaphylaxis that resulted in respiratory embarrassment (*see* PRECAUTIONS). Other reported adverse reactions include nausea, vomiting, and lassitude.
Because fatal reactions often resembling anaphylaxis have been reported after administration of protamine sulfate, the drug should be given only when resuscitation techniques and treatment of anaphylactoid shock are readily available.

OVERDOSAGE

Because of the anticoagulant effect of protamine sulfate, overdosage of this drug may theoretically result in hemorrhage. However, in one study, overdosage of 600–800 mg of IV protamine sulfate had only minimal, transient effects on blood coagulation tests. The patient should be followed with coagulation studies and treated symptomatically.
The LD_{50} of protamine sulfate is 100 mg/kg in mice.

DOSAGE AND ADMINISTRATION

Each mg of protamine sulfate neutralizes approximately 90 USP units of heparin activity derived from lung tissue or about 115 USP units of heparin activity derived from intestinal mucosa.
Protamine Sulfate Injection should be given by very slow intravenous injection in doses not to exceed 50 mg of protamine sulfate in any ten-minute period (see WARNINGS).
Protamine sulfate is intended for injection without further dilution; however, if further dilution is desired, D5-W or normal saline may be used. Diluted solutions should not be stored since they contain no preservative.
Protamine sulfate should not be mixed with other drugs without knowledge of their compatibility, because protamine sulfate has been shown to be incompatible with certain antibiotics, including several of the cephalosporins and penicillins.
Because heparin disappears rapidly from the circulation, the dose of protamine sulfate required also decreases rapidly with the time elapsed following intravenous injection of heparin. For example, if the protamine sulfate is administered 30 minutes after the heparin, one-half the usual dose may be sufficient.
The dosage of protamine sulfate should be guided by blood coagulation studies (*see* WARNINGS).
Parenteral drug products should be inspected visually for particulate matter and discoloration prior to administration.

HOW SUPPLIED

(℞) *Protamine Sulfate Injection, USP: Ampoules No. 473,* 5 ml (equivalent to 50 mg of activity), in packages of 6 (NDC 0002-1691-16) and 25 (NDC 0002-1691-25); *Vials No. 735,* 25 ml (equivalent to 250 mg of activity), rubber-stoppered, in singles (10/carton) (NDC 0002-1462-01).
Both products should be stored in the refrigerator above freezing and below 50°F.
CAUTION—The total dose of protamine sulfate contained in Vials No. 735 (250 mg of activity in 25 ml) is five times greater than that in Ampoules No. 473 (50 mg of activity in 5 ml).
The large-size vials (No. 735) are designed only for antiheparin treatment in certain cases in which large doses of heparin have been given during surgery and are to be neutralized by large doses of protamine sulfate after surgical procedures.
[012086]
No. 473, 5 ml—6505-00-299-9667

REGULAR ILETIN® I

[*rĕg'ū-lĕr ĭ'lĕ-tĭn*]
(insulin injection, Lilly), *see under* Iletin® (insulin, Lilly).

SECONAL® SODIUM Ⓒ

[*sĕk'o'năl sō'dĭ-ŭm*]
(secobarbital sodium)
Capsules, USP

WARNING: MAY BE HABIT-FORMING

DESCRIPTION

The barbiturates are nonselective central-nervous-system (CNS) depressants that are primarily used as sedative-hypnotics. In subhypnotic doses, they are also used as anticonvulsants. The barbiturates and their sodium salts are subject to control under the Federal Controlled Substances Act. Seconal® Sodium (Secobarbital Sodium, USP, Lilly) is a barbituric acid derivative and occurs as a white, odorless, bitter powder that is very soluble in water, soluble in alcohol, and practically insoluble in ether.
Each Pulvule® contains 50 or 100 mg of secobarbital sodium. These products may also contain any or all of the following: D & C Yellow No. 10, F D & C Red No. 3, gelatin, magnesium stearate, silicone, starch, and other inactive ingredients.
Chemically, the drug is sodium 5-allyl-5-(1-methylbutyl)barbiturate, with the empirical formula $C_{12}H_{17}N_2NaO_3$.

CLINICAL PHARMACOLOGY

Seconal® Sodium (secobarbital sodium, Lilly), a short-acting barbiturate, is a CNS depressant. In ordinary doses, the drug acts as a sedative and hypnotic.
Barbiturates are capable of producing all levels of CNS mood alteration, from excitation to mild sedation, hypnosis, and deep coma. Overdosage can produce death. Barbiturates depress the sensory cortex, decrease motor activity, alter cerebellar function, and produce drowsiness, sedation, and hypnosis.
Barbiturate-induced sleep differs from physiologic sleep. Sleep laboratory studies have demonstrated that barbiturates reduce the amount of time spent in the rapid eye movement (REM) phase of sleep, or dreaming stage. Also, Stages III and IV sleep are decreased. Following abrupt cessation of barbiturates used regularly, patients may experience markedly increased dreaming, nightmares, and /or insomnia. Therefore, withdrawal of a single therapeutic dose over five or six days has been recommended to lessen the REM rebound and disturbed sleep which contribute to drug withdrawal syndrome (for example, decrease the dose from three to two doses a day for one week).
Seconal Sodium has been found to lose most of its effectiveness for both inducing and maintaining sleep by the end of 14 days of continued drug administration, even with the use of multiple doses.
Barbiturates have little analgesic action at subanesthetic doses. Rather, in subanesthetic doses these drugs may increase the reaction to painful stimuli. All barbiturates exhibit anticonvulsant activity in anesthetic doses. However, of the drugs in this class, only phenobarbital, mephobarbital, and metharbital are effective as oral anticonvulsants in subhypnotic doses.
Barbiturates are respiratory depressants, and the degree of depression is dependent on the dose. With hypnotic doses, respiratory depression is similar to that which occurs during physiologic sleep accompanied by a slight decrease in blood pressure and heart rate.
Barbiturates do not impair normal hepatic function but have been shown to induce liver microsomal enzymes, thus increasing and/or altering the metabolism of barbiturates and other drugs. (See PRECAUTIONS—*Drug Interactions.*)
Pharmacokinetics—Barbiturates are weak acids that are absorbed and rapidly distributed to all tissues and fluids, with high concentrations in the brain, liver, and kidneys. Lipid solubility of the barbiturates is the dominant factor in their distribution within the body. Barbiturates are bound to plasma and tissue proteins; the degree of binding increases as a function of lipid solubility. The onset of action of Seconal Sodium is from ten to 15 minutes, and the duration of action ranges from three to four hours. The plasma half-life of Seconal Sodium is 15 to 40 hours.
Secobarbital has a high lipid solubility, plasma protein binding, brain protein binding, a short delay in onset of activity, and a short duration of action.
Seconal Sodium is metabolized primarily by the hepatic microsomal enzyme system, and the metabolic products are excreted in the urine and, less commonly, in the feces. Seconal Sodium is detoxified in the liver.

INDICATIONS AND USAGE

Seconal® Sodium (secobarbital sodium, Lilly) is indicated for use as a hypnotic, for the short-term treatment of insomnia, since barbiturates appear to lose their effectiveness for sleep induction and sleep maintenance after two weeks (*see* CLINICAL PHARMACOLOGY above). It is also indicated for use as a preanesthetic agent.

CONTRAINDICATIONS

Seconal® Sodium (secobarbital sodium, Lilly) is contraindicated in patients who are hypersensitive to barbiturates. It is also contraindicated in patients with a history of manifest or latent porphyria, marked impairment of liver function, or respiratory disease in which dyspnea or obstruction is evident. It should not be administered to persons with known previous addiction to the sedative/hypnotic group, since ordinary doses may be ineffectual and may contribute to further addiction. Seconal Sodium should not be administered in the presence of acute or chronic pain, because paradoxical excitement may be induced or important symptoms may be masked.

WARNINGS

1. *Habit-Forming*—Seconal® Sodium (secobarbital sodium, Lilly) may be habit-forming. Tolerance and psychologic and physical dependence may occur with continued use (*see* DRUG ABUSE AND DEPENDENCE). Patients who have psychologic dependence on barbiturates may increase the dosage or decrease the dosage interval without consulting a physician and subsequently may develop a physical dependence on barbiturates. To minimize the possibility of overdosage or development of dependence, the prescribing and dispensing of Seconal Sodium should be limited to the amount required for the interval until the next appointment. The abrupt cessation after prolonged use of Seconal Sodium in a person who is dependent on the drug may result in withdrawal symptoms, including delirium, convulsions, and possibly death. Seconal Sodium should be withdrawn gradually from any patient known to be taking excessive doses over long periods (*see* DRUG ABUSE AND DEPENDENCE).
2. *Usage in Pregnancy*—Barbiturates may cause fetal damage when administered to a pregnant woman. Retrospective, case-controlled studies have suggested that there may be a relationship between the maternal consumption of barbiturates and a higher than expected incidence of fetal abnormalities. Seconal Sodium readily crosses the placental barrier and is distributed throughout fetal tissues; the highest concentrations are found in the placenta, liver, and brain. Withdrawal symptoms occur in infants born to women who receive Seconal Sodium throughout the last trimester of pregnancy (*see* DRUG ABUSE AND DEPENDENCE). If Seconal Sodium is used during pregnancy or if the patient becomes pregnant while taking this drug, the patient should be apprised of the potential hazard to the fetus.
3. *Synergistic Effects*—The concomitant use of alcohol or other CNS depressants may produce additive CNS depressant effects.

PRECAUTIONS

General Precautions—Barbiturates may be habit-forming. Tolerance and psychologic and physical dependence may occur with continuing use (*see* DRUG ABUSE AND DEPENDENCE below). Barbiturates should be administered with caution, if at all, to patients who are mentally depressed, have suicidal tendencies, or have a history of drug abuse.
Elderly or debilitated patients may react to barbiturates with marked excitement, depression, or confusion. In some persons, barbiturates repeatedly produce excitement rather than depression.
Barbiturates induce liver microsomal enzyme activity. This accelerates the biotransformation of various drugs and is probably part of the mechanism of the tolerance encountered with barbiturates. Seconal® Sodium (secobarbital sodium, Lilly) should, therefore, be used with caution in patients with decreased liver function. Seconal Sodium may decrease the potency of coumarin anticoagulants; therefore, patients receiving such concomitant therapy should have more frequent prothrombin determinations.
The systemic effects of exogenous hydrocortisone and endogenous hydrocortisone (cortisol) may be diminished by Seconal Sodium. Thus, this product should be administered with caution to patients with borderline hypoadrenal function, regardless of whether it is of pituitary or of primary adrenal origin.
Information for Patients—The following information should be given to patients receiving Seconal Sodium:
1. The use of Seconal Sodium carries with it an associated risk of psychologic and/or physical dependence. The patient should be warned against increasing the dose of the drug without consulting a physician.
2. Seconal Sodium may impair the mental and/or physical abilities required for the performance of potentially hazardous tasks, such as driving a car or operating machinery. The patient should be cautioned accordingly.
3. Alcohol should not be consumed while taking Seconal Sodium. The concurrent use of Seconal Sodium with other CNS depressants (e.g., alcohol, narcotics, tranquilizers, and antihistamines) may result in additional CNS depressant effects.
Laboratory Tests—Prolonged therapy with barbiturates should be accompanied by periodic evaluation of organic systems, including hematopoietic, renal and hepatic systems (*see General Precautions* and ADVERSE REACTIONS).
Drug Interactions—Seconal Sodium in combination with alcohol, tranquilizers, and other CNS depressants has additive depressant effects, and the patient should be so advised. Toxic effects and fatalities have occurred following overdoses of Seconal Sodium alone and in combination with other CNS depressants. Caution should be exercised in prescribing unnecessarily large amounts of Seconal Sodium for patients who have a history of emotional disturbances or suicidal ideation or who have misused alcohol and other CNS drugs (*see* OVERDOSAGE).
For information regarding concomitant administration of Seconal Sodium and coumarin anticoagulants or corticosteroids, *see General Precautions.*
Monoamine oxidase inhibitors prolong the effects of barbiturates, probably because the metabolism of the barbiturate is inhibited.
Usage in Pregnancy—1. *Teratogenic Effects. Pregnancy Category D. See* WARNINGS section—*Usage in Pregnancy.*
2. *Nonteratogenic Effects.* Reports of infants suffering from long-term barbiturate exposure in utero included the acute withdrawal syndrome of seizures and hyperirritability from

Continued on next page

• **Identi-Code® symbol.**

Lilly—Cont.

birth to a delayed onset of up to 14 days (*see* DRUG ABUSE AND DEPENDENCE).
Labor and Delivery—Hypnotic doses of barbiturates do not appear to impair uterine activity significantly during labor. Full anesthetic doses of barbiturates decrease the force and frequency of uterine contractions. Administration of sedative/ hypnotic barbiturates to the mother during labor may result in respiratory depression in the newborn. Premature infants are particularly susceptible to the depressant effects of barbiturates. If barbiturates are used during labor and delivery, resuscitation equipment should be available.
Data are not available to evaluate the effect of barbiturates when forceps delivery or other intervention is necessary or to determine the effect of barbiturates on the later growth, development, and functional maturity of the child.
Nursing Mothers—Caution should be exercised when Seconal Sodium is administered to a nursing woman, because small amounts of barbiturates are excreted in the milk.

ADVERSE REACTIONS

The following adverse reactions and their incidences were compiled from surveillance of thousands of hospitalized patients who received barbiturates. Because such patients may be less aware of certain of the milder adverse effects of barbiturates, the incidence of these reactions may be somewhat higher in fully ambulatory patients.

More than 1 in 100 Patients

The most common adverse reaction estimated to occur at a rate of one to three patients per 100 is the following:
Nervous System: Somnolence

Less than 1 in 100 Patients

Adverse reactions estimated to occur at a rate of less than one in 100 patients are listed below, grouped by organ system and by decreasing order of occurrence:
Nervous System: Agitation, confusion, hyperkinesia, ataxia, CNS depression, nightmares, nervousness, psychiatric disturbance, hallucinations, insomnia, anxiety, dizziness, abnormality in thinking
Respiratory System: Hypoventilation, apnea
Cardiovascular System: Bradycardia, hypotension, syncope
Digestive System: Nausea, vomiting, constipation
Other Reported Reactions: Headache, injection site reactions, hypersensitivity reactions (angioedema, skin rashes, exfoliative dermatitis), fever, liver damage

DRUG ABUSE AND DEPENDENCE

Controlled Substance—Seconal Sodium® (secobarbital sodium, Lilly) is a Schedule II drug.
Dependence—Barbiturates may be habit-forming; tolerance, psychologic dependence, and physical dependence may occur, especially following prolonged use of high doses of barbiturates. Daily administration in excess of 400 mg of secobarbital for approximately 90 days is likely to produce some degree of physical dependence. A dosage of 600 to 800 mg for at least 35 days is sufficient to produce withdrawal seizures. The average daily dose for the barbiturate addict is usually about 1.5 g. As tolerance to barbiturates develops, the amount needed to maintain the same level of intoxication increases; tolerance to a fatal dosage, however, does not increase more than twofold. As this occurs, the margin between intoxicating dosage and fatal dosage becomes smaller.
Symptoms of acute intoxication with barbiturates include unsteady gait, slurred speech, and sustained nystagmus. Mental signs of chronic intoxication include confusion, poor judgment, irritability, insomnia, and somatic complaints.
Symptoms of barbiturate dependence are similar to those of chronic alcoholism. If an individual appears to be intoxicated with alcohol to a degree that is radically disproportionate to the amount of alcohol in his or her blood, the use of barbiturates should be suspected. The lethal dose of a barbiturate is far less if alcohol is also ingested.
The symptoms of barbiturate withdrawal can be severe and may cause death. Minor withdrawal symptoms may appear eight to 12 hours after the last dose of a barbiturate. These symptoms usually appear in the following order: anxiety, muscle twitching, tremor of hands and fingers, progressive weakness, dizziness, distortion in visual perception, nausea, vomiting, insomnia, and orthostatic hypotension. Major withdrawal symptoms (convulsions and delirium) may occur within 16 hours and last up to five days after abrupt cessation of barbiturates. Intensity of withdrawal symptoms gradually declines over a period of approximately 15 days. Individuals susceptible to barbiturate abuse and dependence include alcoholics and opiate abusers as well as other sedative-hypnotic and amphetamine abusers.
Drug dependence on barbiturates arises from repeated administration on a continuous basis, generally in amounts exceeding therapeutic dose levels. The characteristics of drug dependence on barbiturates include the following: (a) a strong desire or need to continue taking the drug; (b) a tendency to increase the dose; (c) a psychic dependence on the effects of the drug related to subjective and individual appreciation of those effects; and (d) a physical dependence on the effects of the drug, requiring its presence for maintenance of homeostasis and resulting in a definite, characteristic, and self-limited abstinence syndrome when the drug is withdrawn.
Treatment of barbiturate dependence consists of cautious and gradual withdrawal of the drug.
Barbiturate-dependent patients can be withdrawn by using a number of different withdrawal regimens. In all cases, withdrawal takes an extended period. One method involves substituting a 30-mg dose of phenobarbital for each 100 to 200-mg dose of barbiturate that the patient has been taking. The total daily amount of phenobarbital is then administered in three or four divided doses, not to exceed 600 mg daily. Should signs of withdrawal occur on the first day of treatment, a loading dose of 200 to 300 mg of phenobarbital may be administered IM in addition to the oral dose. After stabilization on phenobarbital, the total daily dose is decreased by 30 mg a day as long as withdrawal is proceeding smoothly. A modification of this regimen involves initiating treatment at the patient's regular dosage level and decreasing the daily dosage by 10 percent if tolerated by the patient.
Infants that are physically dependent on barbiturates may be given phenobarbital, 3 to 10 mg/kg/day. After withdrawal symptoms (hyperactivity, disturbed sleep, tremors, and hyperreflexia) are relieved, the dosage of phenobarbital should be gradually decreased and completely withdrawn over a two-week period.

OVERDOSAGE

The toxic dose of barbiturates varies considerably. In general, an oral dose of 1 g of most barbiturates produces serious poisoning in an adult. Death commonly occurs after 2 to 10 g of ingested barbiturate. Barbiturate intoxication may be confused with alcoholism, bromide intoxication, and various neurologic disorders.
Symptoms—Acute overdosage with barbiturates is manifested by CNS and respiratory depression, which may progress to Cheyne-Stokes respiration, areflexia, constriction of the pupils to a slight degree (although in severe poisoning they may show paralytic dilation), oliguria, tachycardia, hypotension, lowered body temperature, and coma. Typical shock syndrome (apnea, circulatory collapse, respiratory arrest, and death) may occur.
In extreme overdose, all electrical activity in the brain may cease, in which case a "flat" EEG normally equated with clinical death cannot be accepted. This effect is fully reversible unless hypoxic damage occurs. Consideration should be given to the possibility of barbiturate intoxication even in situations that appear to involve trauma.
Complications such as pneumonia, pulmonary edema, cardiac arrhythmias, congestive heart failure, and renal failure may occur. Uremia may increase CNS sensitivity to barbiturates if renal function is impaired. Differential diagnosis should include hypoglycemia, head trauma, cerebrovascular accidents, convulsive states, and diabetic coma.
The sedated, therapeutic blood levels of secobarbital range between 0.5 to 5 mcg/ml; the usual lethal blood level ranges from 15 to 40 mcg/ml.
Treatment—Treatment of overdosage is mainly supportive and consists of the following:

1. Maintenance of an adequate airway, with assisted respiration and oxygen administration as necessary.
2. Monitoring of vital signs and fluid balance.
3. If the patient is conscious and has not lost the gag reflex, emesis may be induced with ipecac. Care should be taken to prevent pulmonary aspiration of vomitus. After completion of vomiting, 30 g activated charcoal in a glass of water may be administered.
4. If emesis is contraindicated, gastric lavage may be performed with a cuffed endotracheal tube in place with the patient in the face down position. Activated charcoal may be left in the emptied stomach and a saline cathartic administered.
5. Fluid therapy and other standard treatment for shock, if needed.
6. If renal function is normal, forced diuresis may aid in the elimination of the barbiturate. Alkalinization of the urine increases renal excretion of some barbiturates, especially phenobarbital, also aprobarbital, and mephobarbital (which is metabolized to phenobarbital).
7. Although not recommended as a routine procedure, hemodialysis may be used in severe barbiturate intoxications or if the patient is anuric or in shock.
8. Patient should be rolled from side to side every 30 minutes.
9. Antibiotics should be given if pneumonia is suspected.
10. Appropriate nursing care to prevent hypostatic pneumonia, decubiti, aspiration, and other complications of patients with altered states of consciousness.

DOSAGE AND ADMINISTRATION

Dosages of barbiturates must be individualized with full knowledge of their particular characteristics. Factors of consideration are the patient's age, weight, and condition.
Special Patient Population—Dosage should be reduced in the elderly or debilitated because these patients may be more sensitive to barbiturates. Dosage should be reduced for patients with impaired renal function or hepatic disease.
Adults—As a hypnotic, 100 mg at bedtime. Preoperatively, 200 to 300 mg one to two hours before surgery.
Children—Preoperatively, 2 to 6 mg/kg, with a maximum dosage of 100 mg.

HOW SUPPLIED

(Ⓒ) *Pulvules® Seconal® Sodium (Secobarbital Sodium Capsules, USP): No. 243, F42,** 50 mg (No. 4, Orange), in bottles of 100 (NDC 0002-0642-02); *No. 240, F40,** 100 mg (No. 3, Orange), in bottles of 100 (NDC 0002-0640-02) and 500 (NDC 0002-0640-03), and in 10 strips of 10 individually labeled blisters each containing 1 Pulvule (ID100) (NDC 0002-0640-33).
[073185]

Shown in Product Identification Section, page 415

SECONAL® SODIUM
[*sĕk ′ō-năl sō ′dĭ-um*]
(secobarbital sodium, Lilly) and
AMYTAL® SODIUM
[*ăm ′ĭ-tăl sō ′dĭ-ŭm*]
(amobarbital sodium, Lilly), *see* Tuinal® (secobarbital sodium and amobarbital sodium, Lilly).
SEMILENTE® ILETIN® I
[*sĕm ′ĭ-lĕn ′tā ĭ ′lĕ-tĭn*]
(prompt insulin zinc suspension, Lilly), *see under* Iletin® (insulin, Lilly).

SEROMYCIN® ℞
[*sĕr-ō-mī ′sĭn*]
(cycloserine)
Capsules, USP

DESCRIPTION

Seromycin® (cycloserine, Lilly), D-4-amino-3-isoxazolidinone, is a broad-spectrum antibiotic which is produced by a strain of *Streptomyces orchidaceus* and has also been synthesized. A white powder that is soluble in water and stable in alkaline solution, it is rapidly destroyed at neutral or acid *p*H.
Each Pulvule® contains cycloserine, 250 mg; D & C Yellow No. 10, F D & C Blue No. 1, F D & C Red No. 3, F D & C Yellow No. 6, gelatin, iron oxide, mineral oil, talc, titanium dioxide, and other inactive ingredients.

ACTIONS

Cycloserine inhibits cell-wall synthesis in susceptible strains of gram-positive and gram-negative bacteria and in *Mycobacterium tuberculosis.*

INDICATIONS

Seromycin® (cycloserine, Lilly) is indicated in the treatment of active pulmonary and extrapulmonary tuberculosis (including renal disease) when the organisms are susceptible to this drug and after failure of adequate treatment with the primary medications (streptomycin, isoniazid, and ethambutol). Like all antituberculosis drugs, Seromycin should be administered in conjunction with other effective chemotherapy and not as the sole therapeutic agent.
Seromycin may be effective in the treatment of acute urinary tract infections caused by susceptible strains of gram-positive and gram-negative bacteria, especially *Enterobacter* and *Escherichia coli.* It is generally no more and is usually less effective than other antimicrobial agents in the treatment of urinary tract infections caused by bacteria other than mycobacteria. Use of Seromycin in these infections should be considered only when the more conventional therapy has failed and when the organism has been demonstrated to be sensitive to the drug.

CONTRAINDICATIONS

Administration is contraindicated in patients with any of the following:
- Hypersensitivity to cycloserine
- Epilepsy
- Depression, severe anxiety, or psychosis
- Severe renal insufficiency
- Excessive concurrent use of alcoholic beverages

WARNINGS

Administration of Seromycin® (cycloserine, Lilly) should be discontinued or the dosage reduced if the patient develops allergic dermatitis or symptoms of central-nervous-system toxicity, such as convulsions, psychosis, somnolence, depression, confusion, hyperreflexia, headache, tremor, vertigo, paresis, or dysarthria.
The toxicity of Seromycin is closely related to excessive blood levels (above 30 mcg/ml), which are determined by high dosage or inadequate renal clearance. The ratio of toxic dose to effective dose in tuberculosis is small.
The risk of convulsions is increased in chronic alcoholics.
Patients should be monitored by hematologic, renal excretion, blood level, and liver function studies.

Usage in Pregnancy—The safety of the use of Seromycin during pregnancy has not been established.
Usage in Children—Safety and dosage have not been established for pediatric use.

PRECAUTIONS

Before treatment with Seromycin® (cycloserine, Lilly) is initiated, cultures should be taken and the organism's susceptibility to the drug should be established. In tuberculous infections, its sensitivity to the other antituberculosis agents in the regimen should also be demonstrated.
Blood levels should be determined at least weekly for patients having reduced renal function, for individuals receiving a daily dosage of more than 500 mg, and for those showing signs and symptoms suggestive of toxicity. The dosage should be adjusted to keep the blood level below 30 mcg/ml.
Anticonvulsant drugs or sedatives may be effective in controlling symptoms of central-nervous-system toxicity, such as convulsions, anxiety, and tremor. Patients receiving more than 500 mg of Seromycin daily should be closely observed for such symptoms. The value of pyridoxine in preventing CNS toxicity from cycloserine has not been proved.
Administration of Seromycin and other antituberculosis drugs has been associated in a few instances with vitamin B_{12} and/or folic acid deficiency, megaloblastic anemia, and sideroblastic anemia. If evidence of anemia develops during treatment, appropriate studies and therapy should be instituted.

ADVERSE REACTIONS

Most adverse reactions occurring during therapy with Seromycin® (cycloserine, Lilly) involve the nervous system or are manifestations of drug hypersensitivity. The following side effects have been observed in patients receiving Seromycin:
Nervous system symptoms (which appear to be related to higher dosages of drug, i.e., more than 500 mg daily)
- Convulsions
- Drowsiness and somnolence
- Headache
- Tremor
- Dysarthria
- Vertigo
- Confusion and disorientation with loss of memory
- Psychoses, possibly with suicidal tendencies
  - Character changes
  - Hyperirritability
  - Aggression
- Paresis
- Hyperreflexia
- Paresthesias
- Major and minor (localized) clonic seizures
- Coma

Allergic (apparently not related to dosage)
- Skin rash

Miscellaneous
- Elevated serum transaminase, especially in patients with preexisting liver disease

DOSAGE AND ADMINISTRATION

Seromycin® (cycloserine, Lilly) is effective orally and is currently administered only by this route. The usual dosage is 500 mg to 1 g daily in divided doses monitored by blood levels. The initial adult dosage most frequently given is 250 mg twice daily at 12-hour intervals for the first two weeks. The daily dosage of 1 g should not be exceeded.

HOW SUPPLIED

(℞) *Pulvules No. 12, Seromycin® (Cycloserine Capsules, USP), F04,** 250 mg (No. 1, Light-Gray Opaque Body, Red Opaque Cap), in bottles of 40 (NDC 0002-0604-40).

[072985]

TAZIDIME™ ℞
[*tă ʹzĭ-dēm*]
(ceftazidime)
for injection

DESCRIPTION

Tazidime™ (ceftazidime, Lilly) is a semisynthetic, broad-spectrum, beta-lactam antibiotic for parenteral administration. It is the pentahydrate of pyridinium, 1-[[7-[[(2-amino-4-thiazolyl) [(1-carboxy-1-methylethoxy) imino]acetyl]-amino]-2-carboxy -8- oxo-5-thia -1- azabicyclo[4.2.0]oct-2-en-3-yl]methyl]-, hydroxide, inner salt, [6R-[6α,7β(Z)]].
Tazidime is a sterile, dry powder. Tazidime also contains 118 mg sodium carbonate/g of ceftazidime activity. The total sodium content of the mixture is approximately 54 mg (2.3 mEq)/g of ceftazidime activity. Solutions of Tazidime range from light yellow to amber, depending on the diluent and concentration. The *p* H of freshly reconstituted solutions usually ranges from 5.0 to 8.0.

CLINICAL PHARMACOLOGY

After intravenous administration of a 500-mg or a 1-g dose of ceftazidime over 5 minutes to normal adult male volunteers, mean peak serum concentrations were 45 mcg/ml. and 90 mcg/ml, respectively. Following intravenous infusion of 500-mg, 1-g, and 2-g doses of ceftazidime over 20 to 30 minutes to normal adult male volunteers, mean peak serum concentrations of 42 mcg, 69 mcg, and 170 mcg/ml, respectively, were achieved. The average serum concentrations following intravenous infusion of 500-mg, 1-g, and 2-g doses to these volunteers over an 8-hour period are given in Table 1.

Table 1. Ceftazidime Concentration in Serum

Ceftazidime Dosage IV	Serum Concentrations (mcg/ml) ½ h	1 h	2 h	4 h	8 h
500 mg	42	25	12	6	2
1 g	60	39	23	11	3
2 g	129	75	42	13	5

The absorption and elimination of ceftazidime were directly proportional to the size of the dose. Following intravenous administration, the half-life was approximately 1.9 hours. Less than 10% of ceftazidime was protein bound. The degree of protein binding was independent of concentration. Following multiple intravenous doses of 1 g and 2 g every 8 hours for 10 days, there was no evidence of accumulation of ceftazidime in the serum in individuals with normal renal function.
Following intramuscular administration of 500-mg and 1-g doses of ceftazidime to normal adult volunteers, the mean peak serum concentrations were 17 mcg/ml and 39 mcg/ml, respectively, at approximately 1 hour. Serum concentrations remained above 4 mcg/ml for 6 and 8 hours after the intramuscular administration of 500-mg and 1-g doses, respectively. The half-life of ceftazidime in these volunteers was approximately 2 hours.
The presence of hepatic dysfunction had no effect on the pharmacokinetics of ceftazidime in individuals who received 2 g intravenously every 8 hours for 5 days. Therefore, dosage adjustment is not required for patients with hepatic dysfunction, unless renal function is impaired.
Approximately 80 to 90% of an intramuscular or intravenous dose of ceftazidime is excreted unchanged by the kidneys over a 24-hour period. After the intravenous administration of a single 500-mg or 1-g dose, approximately 50% of the dose appeared in the urine in the first 2 hours. An additional 20% was excreted 2 and 4 hours after administration, and approximately another 12% of the dose appeared in the urine 4 to 8 hours later. The elimination of ceftazidime by the kidneys resulted in high urinary concentrations.
The mean renal clearance of ceftazidime was approximately 100 ml/min. The calculated plasma clearance of approximately 115 ml/min. indicated nearly complete elimination of ceftazidime by the renal route. The administration of probenecid prior to administration of ceftazidime had no effect on the elimination kinetics of ceftazidime. This suggested that ceftazidime is eliminated by glomerular filtration and is not actively secreted by renal tubular mechanisms.
Since ceftazidime is eliminated almost solely by the kidneys, its serum half-life is significantly prolonged in patients with impaired renal function. Consequently, dosage for such patients must be adjusted (see DOSAGE AND ADMINISTRATION).
Therapeutic concentrations of ceftazidime are achieved in the following tissues and body fluids:
[See table above].

Table 2: Ceftazidime Concentrations in Tissues and Body Fluids

Tissue or Fluid	Dose/ Route	No. of Patients	Time of Sample Post-Dose	Average Tissue or Fluid Level (mcg/ml)
Urine	500 mg IM	6	0–2 hr	2,100.0
	2 g IV	6	0–2 hr	12,000.0
Bile	2 g IV	3	90 min.	36.4
Synovial fluid	2 g IV	13	2 hr	25.6
Peritoneal fluid	2 g IV	8	2 hr	48.6
Sputum	1 g IV	8	1 hr	9
Cerebrospinal fluid	2 g q 8 h IV	5	120 min.	9.8
(inflamed meninges)	2 g q 8 h IV	6	180 min.	9.4
Aqueous humor	2 g IV	13	1–3 hr	11
Blister fluid	1 g IV	7	2–3 hr	19.7
Lymphatic fluid	1 g IV	7	2–3 hr	23.4
Bone	2 g IV	8	0.67 hr	31.1
Heart muscle	2 g IV	35	30–280 min.	12.7
Skin	2 g IV	22	30–180 min.	6.6
Skeletal muscle	2 g IV	35	30–280 min.	9.4
Myometrium	2 g IV	31	1–2 hr	18.7

Microbiology: In vitro tests demonstrate that ceftazidime is bactericidal, exerting its effect by inhibition of enzymes responsible for cell-wall synthesis. Ceftazidime has in vitro activity against a wide range of gram-negative organisms, including strains resistant to gentamicin and other aminoglycosides. In addition, ceftazidime has been shown to be active against gram-positive organisms. It is highly stable to most clinically important beta-lactamases, plasmid or chromosomal, that are produced by gram-negative and gram-positive organisms and consequently is active against many strains resistant to ampicillin and other cephalosporins.
Ceftazidime has been shown to be active against the following organisms both in vitro and in clinical infections:

Gram-Negative —Pseudomonas species (including *Pseudomonas aeruginosa*); *Klebsiella* species (including *Klebsiella pneumoniae*); *Proteus mirabilis; Proteus vulgaris; Esherichia coli; Enterobacter* species (including *Enterobacter cloacae* and *Enterobacter aerogenes*); Citrobacter species (including *Citrobacter freundii* and *Citrobacter diversus*); Serratia species; *Haemophilus influenzae,* including ampicillin-resistant strains; and *Neisseria meningitidis.*

Gram-Positive —Staphylococcus aureus, including penicillinase- and non-penicillinase-producing strains; *Streptococcus pyogenes* (group A beta-hemolytic streptococci); *Streptococcus agalactiae* (group B streptococci); and *Streptococcus pneumoniae.*

Anaerobic Organisms —Bacteroides species (NOTE: most strains of *Bacteroides fragilis* are resistant).

Ceftazidime has also been shown to demonstrate in vitro activity against the following microorganisms, although its clinical significance is not known:

Staphylococcus epidermidis; Morganella morganii (formerly *Proteus morganii*); *Providencia* species (including *Providencia rettgeri,* formerly *Proteus rettgeri*); *Acinetobacter* species; *Salmonella* species; *Clostridium* species (not including *Clostridium difficile*); *Peptococcus* species; *Peptostreptococcus* species; *Neisseria gonorrhoeae; Haemophilus parainfluenzae; Yersinia enterocolitica;* and *Shigella* species.

Ceftazidime and the aminoglycosides have been shown to be synergistic in vitro against some strains of *P aeruginosa* and the *Enterobacteriaceae.* Ceftazidime and carbenicillin have also been shown to be synergistic in vitro against *P aeruginosa.*
Ceftazidime is not active in vitro against methicillin-resistant staphylococci; *Streptococcus faecalis* and many other enterococci; *Listeria monocytogenes; Campylobacter* species; or *C difficile.*
Susceptibility Tests—Quantitative methods that require measurement of zone diameters give the most precise estimates of antibiotic susceptibility. One such procedure[1–3] has been recommended for use with disks to test susceptibility to ceftazidime.
Reports from the laboratory giving results of the standard single-disk susceptibility test with a 30-mcg ceftazidime disk should be interpreted according to the following criteria:

Susceptible organisms produce zones of 18 mm or greater, indicating that the test organism is likely to respond to therapy.

Organisms of intermediate susceptibility produce zones of 15 to 17 mm, indicating that the tested organism would be susceptible if high dosage is used or if the infection is confined to tissues and fluids (eg, urine) in which high antibiotic levels are attained.

Resistant organisms produce zones of 14 mm or less, indicating that other therapy should be selected.

Organisms should be tested with the ceftazidime disk, since ceftazidime has been shown by in vitro tests to have activity

Continued on next page

* Identi-Code® symbol.

Lilly—Cont.

against certain strains found resistant when tested with other beta-lactam disks.

Standardized procedures require the use of laboratory control organisms. The 30-mcg ceftazidime disk should give zone diameters between 25 mm and 32 mm for *E coli* ATCC 25922, between 22 mm and 29 mm for *P. aeruginosa* ATCC 27853, and between 16 mm and 20 mm for *S. aureus* ATCC 25923.

In other susceptibility testing procedures, eg, ICS agar dilution or its equivalent, a bacterial isolate may be considered susceptible if the MIC value for ceftazidime is not more than 16 mcg/ml. Organisms are considered resistant if the MIC is equal to or greater than 64 mcg/ml. Organisms having an MIC value of less than 64 mcg/ml but greater than 16 mcg/ml are expected to be susceptible if high dosage is used or if the infection is confined to tissues and fluids (eg, urine) in which high antibiotic levels are attained.

As with standard diffusion methods, dilution procedures require the use of laboratory control organisms. Standard ceftazidime powder should give MIC values in the range of 4 mcg/ml and 16 mcg/ml for *S aureus* ATCC 25923, between 0.125 mcg/ml and 0.5 mcg/ml for *E coli* ATCC 25922, and between 0.5 mcg/ml and 2 mcg/ml for *P aeruginosa* ATCC 27853.

INDICATIONS AND USAGE

Tazidime™ (ceftazidime, Lilly) is indicated for the treatment of infections caused by susceptible strains of the designated organisms in the diseases listed below:

Lower respiratory tract infections, including pneumonia, caused by *P aeruginosa* and other *Pseudomonas* species; *H influenzae* (including ampicillin-resistant strains); *Klebsiella* species; *Enterobacter* species; *P mirabilis; E coli; Serratia* species; *Citrobacter* species; *S pneumoniae;* and *S aureus* (methicillin-susceptible strains)

Skin and skin-structure infections caused by *P aeruginosa; Klebsiella* species; *E coli; Proteus* species (including *P mirabilis* and indole-positive *Proteus); Enterobacter* species; *Serratia* species; *S aureus* (methicillin-susceptible strains); and *S pyogenes* (group A beta-hemolytic streptococci)

Urinary tract infections, both complicated and uncomplicated, caused by *P aeruginosa; Enterobacter* species; *Proteus* species (including *P. mirabilis* and indole-positive *Proteus); Klebsiella* species; and *E coli*

Bacterial septicemia caused by *P aeruginosa; Klebsiella* species. *H influenzae; E coli; Serratia* species; *S pneumoniae;* and *S aureus* (methicillin-susceptible strains)

Bone and joint infections caused by *P aeruginosa; Klebsiella* species; *Enterobacter* species; and *S aureus (methicillin-susceptible strains)*

Gynecologic infections, including endometritis, pelvic cellulitis, and other infections of the female genital tract, caused by *E coli*

Intra-abdominal infections, including peritonitis, caused by *E coli, Klebsiella* species, and *S aureus* (methicillin-susceptible strains) and polymicrobial infections caused by aerobic and anaerobic organisms and *Bacteroides* species (most strains of *B. fragilis* are resistant)

Central nervous system infections, including meningitis, caused by *H influenzae* and *Neisseria meningitidis.* Tazidime has also been used successfully in a limited number of cases of menigitis due to *P aeruginosa* and *S pneumoniae*

Specimens for bacterial cultures should be obtained prior to therapy in order to isolate and identify causative organisms and to determine their susceptibility to ceftazidime. Therapy may be instituted before results of susceptibility studies are known; however, once these results become available, the antibiotic treatment should be adjusted accordingly.

Tazidime may be used alone in cases of confirmed or suspected sepsis. Tazidime has been used successfully in clinical trials as empiric therapy in cases in which various concomitant therapies with other antibiotics have been used.

Tazidime may also be used concomitantly with other antibiotics, such as aminoglycosides, vancomycin, and clindamycin, in severe and life-threatening infections and in the immunocompromised patient. When such concomitant treatment is appropriate, prescribing information in the labeling for the other anitibiotics should be followed. The dose depends on the severity of the infection and the patient's condition.

CONTRAINDICATIONS

Tazidime™ (ceftazidime, Lilly) is contraindicated in patients who have shown hypersensitivity to ceftazidime or the cephalosporin group of antibiotics.

WARNINGS

BEFORE THERAPY WITH TAZIDIME™ (ceftazidime, Lilly) IS INSTITUTED, CAREFUL INQUIRY SHOULD BE MADE TO DETERMINE WHETHER THE PATIENT HAS HAD PREVIOUS HYPERSENSITIVITY REACTIONS TO CEFTAZIDIME, CEPHALOSPORINS, PENICILLINS, OR OTHER DRUGS. ANTIBIOTICS SHOULD BE ADMINISTERED WITH CAUTION TO ANY PATIENT WHO HAS DEMONSTRATED SOME FORM OF ALLERGY, PARTICULARLY TO DRUGS. THIS PRODUCT SHOULD BE GIVEN WITH CAUTION TO PATIENTS WITH TYPE 1 HYPERSENSITIVITY REACTIONS TO PENICILLIN. IF AN ALLERGIC REACTION TO TAZIDIME OCCURS, DISCONTINUE TREATMENT WITH THE DRUG. SERIOUS ACUTE HYPERSENSITIVITY REACTIONS MAY REQUIRE EPINEPHRINE AND OTHER EMERGENCY MEASURES.

Pseudomembranous colitis has been reported with virtually all broad-spectrum antibiotics (including macrolides, semisynthetic penicillins, and cephalosporins); therefore, it is important to consider its diagnosis in patients who develop diarrhea in association with the use of antibiotics.

Treatment with broad-spectrum antibiotics alters normal flora of the colon and may permit overgrowth of clostridia. Studies indicate a toxin produced by *C difficile* is one primary cause of antibiotic-associated colitis.

Mild cases of pseudomembraneous colitis responded to drug discontinuance alone. In moderate to severe cases, management should include fluid, electrolyte, and protein supplementation. When the colitis does not improve by drug discontinuance or when it is severe, oral vancomycin is the drug of choice for antibiotic-associated pseudomembranous colitis produced by *C difficile.* Other causes of colitis should be ruled out.

PRECAUTIONS

General—Tazidime™ (ceftazidime, Lilly) has not been shown to be nephrotoxic; however, because high and prolonged serum antibiotic concentrations can occur from usual doses in patients with transient or persistent reduction of urinary output because of renal insufficiency, the total daily dosage should be reduced when ceftazidime is administered to such patients (*see* DOSAGE AND ADMINISTRATION). Continued dosage should be determined by degree of renal impairment, severity of infection, and susceptibility of the causative organisms.

As with other antibiotics, prolonged use of Tazidime may result in overgrowth of nonsusceptible organisms. Repeated evaluation of the patient's condition is essential. If superinfection occurs during therapy, appropriate measures should be taken.

Tazidime should be prescribed with caution in individuals with a history of gastrointestinal disease, particularly colitis.

Drug Interactions—Nephrotoxicity has been reported following concomitant administration of cephalosporins and aminoglycoside antibiotics or potent diuretics, such as furosemide. Renal function should be carefully monitored, especially if higher dosages of the aminoglycosides are to be administered or if therapy is prolonged, because of the potential nephrotoxicity and ototoxicity of aminoglycosidic antibiotics. Nephrotoxicity and ototoxicity were not noted when Tazidime was given alone in clinical trials.

Carcinogenesis, Mutagenesis, Impairment of Fertility—Long-term studies in animals have not been performed to evaluate carcinogenic potential. However, a mouse micronucleus test and an Ames test were both negative for mutagenic effects.

Usage in Pregnancy—Pregnancy Category B—Reproduction studies have been performed in mice and rats at doses up to 40 times the human dose and have revealed no evidence of impaired fertility or harm to the fetus due to Tazidime. There are, however, no adequate and well-controlled studies in pregnant women. Because animal reproduction studies are not always predictive of human response, this drug should be used during pregnancy only if clearly needed.

Nursing Mothers—Ceftazidime is excreted in human milk in low concentrations. Caution should be exercised when Tazidime is administered to a nursing woman.

ADVERSE REACTIONS

Tazidime™ (ceftazidime, Lilly) is generally well tolerated. The incidence of adverse reactions associated with the administration of Tazidime was low in clinical trials. The most common were local reactions following intravenous injection and allergic and gastrointestinal reactions. Other adverse reactions were encountered infrequently. No disulfiram-like reactions were reported. The following adverse effects from clinical trials were considered to be either related to ceftazidime therapy or were of uncertain etiology:

Local effects, reported in less than 2% of patients, were phlebitis and inflammation at the site of injection (1 in 69 patients).

Hypersensitivity reactions, reported in 2% of patients, were pruritus, rash, and fever. Immediate hypersensitivity reactions occurred in 1 in 285 patients.

Gastrointestinal symptoms, reported in less than 2% of patients, were diarrhea (1 in 78), nausea (1 in 156), vomiting (1 in 500), and abdominal pain (1 in 416).

Less frequent adverse events (less than 1%) were candidiasis, vaginitis, and central nervous system events, which included headache, dizziness, and paresthesia.

Laboratory test changes noted during clinical trials with Tazidime were transient and included eosinophilia (1 in 13), positive Coombs' test without hemolysis (1 in 23), thrombocytosis (1 in 45), and slight elevations in one or more of the hepatic enzymes: SGOT (1 in 16), SGPT (1 in 15), LDH (1 in 18), and alkaline phosphatase (1 in 23). As with some other cephalosporins, transient elevations of blood urea, blood urea nitrogen, and/or serum creatinine were observed occasionally. Transient leukopenia, neutropenia, thrombocytopenia, and lymphocytosis were seen very rarely.

DOSAGE AND ADMINISTRATION

The usual adult dosage is 1 g administered intravenously or intramuscularly every 8 to 12 hours. The dosage and route should be determined by the susceptibility of the causative organisms, the severity of infection, and the condition and renal function of the patient.

The guidelines for dosage of Tazidime™ (ceftazidime, Lilly) are listed in Table 3. The following dosage schedule is recommended:

[See table at left].

Patients with Impaired Hepatic Function—No adjustment in dosage is required for patients with hepatic dysfunction.

Patients with Impaired Renal Function—Ceftazidime is excreted by the kidneys, almost exclusively by glomerular filtration. Therefore, in patients with impaired renal function (GFR < 50 ml/min.), it is recommended that the dose of Tazidime be reduced to compensate for its slower excretion. In patients with suspected renal insufficiency, an initial loading dose of 1 g of Tazidime may be given. An estimate of GFR should be made to determine the appropriate maintenance dose. The recommended dosage is presented in Table 4.

Table 3: Recommended Dosage Schedule for Ceftazidime

	Dose	Frequency
Adults		
Usual recommended dose	**1 g IV or IM**	**q8 or 12h**
Uncomplicated urinary tract infections	250 mg IV or IM	q12h
Bone and joint infections	2 g IV	q12h
Complicated urinary tract infections	500 mg IV or IM	q8 or 12h
Uncomplicated pneumonia; mild skin and skin structure infections	500 mg–1 g IV or IM	q8h
Serious gynecologic and intra-abdominal infections	2 g IV	q8h
Meningitis	2 g IV	q8h
Very severe life-threatening infections, especially in immunocompromised patients	2 g IV	q8h
Pseudomonal lung infections in patients with cystic fibrosis with normal renal function*	30–50 mg/kg IV to a maximum of 6 g/day	q8h
Neonates (0–4 weeks)	30 mg/kg IV	q12h
Infants and Children (1 month to 12 years)	30–50 mg/kg IV to a maximum of 6 g/day†	q8h

* Although clinical improvement has been shown, bacteriologic cures cannot be expected in patients with chronic respiratory disease and cystic fibrosis.

† The higher dose should be reserved for immunocompromised children or children with cystic fibrosis or meningitis.

Table 4. Recommended Maintenance Dosage of Tazidime™ (ceftazidime, Lilly) in Patients with Renal Insufficiency

Creatinine Clearance (ml/min.)	Recommended Dose of Tazidime	Frequency
50–31	1 g	q12h
30–16	1 g	q24h
15–6	500 mg	q24h
<5	500 mg	q48h

When only serum creatinine is available, the following formula (Cockcroft's equation)[4] may be used to estimate creatinine clearance. The serum creatinine should represent a steady state of renal function:

$$\text{Males: Creatinine Clearance (ml/min.)} = \frac{\text{Weight (kg)} \times (140 - \text{age})}{72 \times \text{serum creatinine (mg/dl)}}$$

$$\text{Females: } 0.85 \times \text{above value}$$

In patients with severe infections who would normally receive 6 g of Tazidime daily were it not for renal insufficiency, the dose given in the above table may be increased by 50% or the dosing frequency increased appropriately. Continued dosage should be determined by therapeutic monitoring, severity of the infection, and susceptibility of the causative organism.

In children, as for adults, the creatinine clearance should be adjusted for body surface area or lean body mass and the dosing frequency reduced in cases of renal insufficiency.

In patients undergoing hemodialysis, a loading dose of 1 g of Tazidime is recommended, followed by 1 g after each hemodialysis period.

Tazidime can also be used in patients undergoing intraperitoneal dialysis (IPD) and continuous ambulatory peritoneal dialysis (CAPD). In such patients, a loading dose of 1 g of Tazidime may be given, followed by 500 mg every 24 hours. In addition to intravenous use, Tazidime can be incorporated in the dialysis fluid at a concentration of 250 mg/2 L of dialysis fluid.

NOTE: Tazidime should generally be continued for 2 days after the signs and symptoms of infection have disappeared; however, in complicated infections, longer therapy may be required.

Administration—Tazidime™ (ceftazidime, Lilly) may be given intravenously or by deep intramuscular injection into a large muscle mass (such as the upper outer quadrant of the gluteus maximus or lateral part of the thigh).

Intramuscular Administration—For intramuscular administration, Tazidime should be reconstituted with one of the following diluents: Sterile Water for Injection, Bacteriostatic Water for Injection, or 0.5% or 1% Lidocaine Hydrochloride Injection. Refer to Table 5.

Intravenous Administration—The IV route is preferable for patients with bacterial septicemia, bacterial meningitis, peritonitis, or other severe or life-threatening infections or for patients who may be poor risks because of lowered resistance resulting from such debilitating conditions as malnutrition, trauma, surgery, diabetes, heart failure, or malignancy, particularly if shock is present or impending.

For direct intermittent intravenous administration, reconstitute Tazidime with Sterile Water for Injection (see Table 5). Slowly inject the solution directly into the vein over a period of 3 to 5 minutes or give through the tubing of an administration set while the patient is also receiving one of the compatible intravenous fluids (*see* COMPATIBILITY AND STABILITY).

For intravenous infusion, reconstitute the 1-g or 2-g piggyback (100-ml) vial with 100 ml Sterile Water for Injection or one of the compatible intravenous fluids listed in the COMPATIBILITY AND STABILITY section. Alternatively, reconstitute the 500-mg, 1-g, or 2-g vial and add an appropriate quantity of the resulting solution to an IV container with one of the compatible intravenous fluids.

Intermittent intravenous infusion with a Y-type administration set can be accomplished with compatible solutions. However, during infusion of a solution containing ceftazidime, it is desirable to discontinue the other solution.

ADD-Vantage vials are to be used only with Abbott ADD-Vantage diluent bags according to the printed tray card instructions included in each Traypak of vials.

Add-Vantage vials which have been joined to Abbott ADD-Vantage bags of diluent and activated to dissolve the drug are stable for 24 hours at room temperature and for 7 days under refrigeration. Joined vials which have not been activated may be used within a 14-day period; this period corresponds to that for use of Abbott ADD-Vantage containers following removal of the outer packaging (overwrap).

Freezing solutions of Tazidime in the ADD-Vantage system is not recommended.

[See table above].

Vials of Tazidime™ (ceftazidime, Lilly) may be supplied under reduced pressure. When Tazidime is dissolved, carbon dioxide is released and a positive pressure develops. For ease of use, please follow the recommended techniques of reconstitution described below.

Table 5: Preparation of Solutions of Tazidime™ (Ceftazidime)

	Amount of Diluent to Be Added (ml)	Approximate Available Volume (ml)	Approximate Ceftazidime Concentration (mg/ml)
Intramuscular			
500 mg, Vial No. 7230	1.5	1.8	280
1 g, Vial No. 7231	3.0	3.6	280
Intravenous			
500 mg, Vial No. 7230	5	5.3	100
1 g, Vial No. 7231	10	10.6	100
2 g, Vial No. 7234	10	11.2	180
Piggyback (100 ml)			
1 g, Vial No. 7238	100*	100	10
2 g, Vial No. 7239	100*	100	20
Pharmacy Bulk Package (100 ml)			
6 g, Vial No. 7241	26	30	200
	56	60	100

* Note: Addition should be in 2 stages (see Instructions for Reconstitution below).

Solutions of Tazidime, like those of most beta-lactam antibiotics, should not be added to solutions of aminoglycoside antibiotics because of potential interaction. However, if concurrent therapy with Tazidime and an aminoglycoside is indicated, each of these antibiotics should be administered in different sites.

Instructions for Reconstitution:

For 500-mg IM/IV, 1-g IM/IV, and 2-g IV vials

1. Inject the diluent and shake well to dissolve. The vials may contain a vacuum to assist injection of the diluent.
2. Carbon dioxide is released as the antibiotic dissolves, generating pressure within the vial. The solution will become clear within 1 to 2 minutes.
3. Invert the vial, and completely depress the syringe plunger prior to insertion.
4. Insert the needle through the vial stopper. Be sure the needle remains within the solution, and withdraw contents of the vial in the usual manner. Pressure in the vial may aid withdrawal.
5. The withdrawn solution may contain carbon dioxide bubbles which should be expelled from the syringe before injection.

For 1-g and 2-g piggyback vials

1. Inject 10 ml of the diluent and shake to dissolve. The vials may contain a vacuum to assist injection of the diluent.
2. Carbon dioxide is released as the antibiotic dissolves, generating pressure within the vial. The solution will become clear within 1 to 2 minutes.
3. Insert a vent needle to release pressure before adding additional diluent to the vial. Add diluent and then remove the vent needle.
4. Additional pressure that may develop in the vial, especially after storage, should be relieved prior to administration to the patient.

For a 6-g pharmacy bulk package

1. When diluent is being added, the vial must be vented to prevent buildup of pressure due to release of carbon dioxide formed as the antibiotic dissolves. Use standard venting procedures outlined in the venting card for Tazidime.
2. Inject 26 ml of diluent to provide a solution containing approximately 1 g of ceftazidime activity per 5 ml. Inject 56 ml of diluent to provide a solution contaning approximately 1 g of ceftazidime activity per 10 ml.
3. Dissolve the antibiotic by gently agitating the solution.
4. Allow sufficient time (1–2 minutes) for carbon dioxide to vent before dsipensing solution.
5. After storage, relieve any additional pressure which may develop in the vial before dispensing.

COMPATIBILITY AND STABILITY

Intramuscular—Vials of Tazidime™ (ceftazidime, Lilly), when reconstituted as directed with Sterile Water for Injection, Bacteriostatic Water for Injection, or 0.5% or 1% Lidocaine Hydrochloride Injection, maintain satisfactory potency for 24 hours at room temperature or for 7 days under refrigeration. Solutions in Sterile Water for Injection that are frozen immediately after reconstitution in the original container are stable for 3 months when stored at −20°C. Once thawed, solutions should not be refrozen. Thawed solutions may be stored for up to 24 hours at room temperature or for 4 days in a refrigerator.

Intravenous—Vials of Tazidime, when reconstituted as directed with Sterile Water for Injection, maintain satisfactory potency for 24 hours at room temperature or for 7 days under refrigeration. Solutions in Sterile Water for Injection in the original container or in 0.9% Sodium Chloride Injection or 5% Dextrose Injection in PVC small-volume containers that are frozen immediately after reconstitution are stable for 3 months when stored at −20°C. For larger volumes where it may be necessary to warm the frozen product (to a maximum of 40°C), care should be taken to avoid heating it after thawing is complete. Once thawed, solutions should not be refrozen. Thawed solutions may be stored for up to 24 hours at room temperature or for 4 days in a refrigerator.

Tazidime is compatible with the more commonly used intravenous infusion fluids. Solutions at concentrations between 1 mg/ml and 40 mg/ml in the following infusion fluids may be stored for up to 24 hours at room temperature or for 7 days if refrigerated: 0.9% Sodium Chloride Injection; M/6 Sodium Lactate Injection; Ringer's Injection, USP; Lactated Ringer's Injection, USP; 5% Dextrose Injection; 5% Dextrose and 0.225% Sodium Chloride Injection; 5% Dextrose and 0.45% Sodium Chloride Injection; 5% Dextrose and 0.9% Sodium Chloride Injection; 10% Dextrose Injection; 10% Invert Sugar in Water for Injection; and Normosol®-M in 5% Dextrose Injection.

When diluted with Abbott's ADD-Vantage diluents, 0.9% Sodium Chloride Injection and 5% Dextrose Injection, ADD-Vantage Tazidime may be stored for up to 24 hours at room temperature and up to 7 days if refrigerated.

Tazidime is less stable in Sodium Bicarbonate Injection than in other intravenous fluids. Sodium Bicarbonate Injection is not recommended as a diluent. Solutions of Tazidime in 5% Dextrose or 0.9% Sodium Chloride Injection are stable for at least 6 hours at room temperature in plastic tubing, drip chambers, and volume control devices of common intravenous infusion sets.

At a concentration of 4 mg/ml, Tazidime has been found compatible for 24 hours at room temperature or for 7 days under refrigeration in 0.9% Sodium Chloride Injection or 5% Dextrose Injection when admixed with cefuroxime sodium, 3 mg/ml; heparin, 10 units/ml or 50 units/ml; or potassium cloride, 10 mEq/L or 40 mEq/L.

Note: Parenteral drug products should be inspected visually for particulate matter whenever solution and container permit.

Tazidime powder and solutions will darken, depending on storage conditions. However, product potency is not adversely affected if storage conditions and storage periods are observed.

HOW SUPPLIED

(℞) *Vials* (Dry Powder) *Tazidime™ (ceftazidime, Lilly): No. 7230,* 500 mg,* 10-ml size, Traypak™ (multivial carton, Lilly) of 25 (NDC 0002-7230-25); *No. 7231,* 1 g,* 10-ml size, Traypak of 25 (NDC 0002-7231-25); *No. 7238,* 1 g,* 100-ml size, Traypak of 10 (NDC 0002-7238-10); *No. 7234,* 2 g,* 20-ml size, Traypak of 10 (NDC 0002-7234-10); *No. 7239,* 2 g,* 100-ml size, Traypak of 10 (NDC 0002-7239-10); *No. 7241,* 6 g,* 100-ml size (Pharmacy Bulk Package), Traypak of 6 (NDC 0002-7241-16).

(℞) *ADD-Vantage ® (vials and diluent containers, Abbott) Vials: No. 7290,* 1 g,* Traypak of 25 (NDC 0002-7290-25); *No. 7291,* 2 g,* Traypak of 10 (NDC 0002-7291-10).

The above ADD-Vantage™ Vials are to be used only with Abbott Laboratories' ADD-Vantage Diluent Containers.

*Equivalent to ceftazidime activity.

REFERENCES

1. Bauer A. W, Kirby W. M. M., Sherris J. C., *et al:* Antibiotic susceptibility testing by a standardized single disk method. Am J Clin Pathol, *45:* 493, 1966.
2. National Committee for Clinical Laboratory Standards, Approved Standard: Performance Standards for Antimicrobial Disc Susceptibility Tests (M2-A3), December, 1984.
3. Standardized disc susceptibility test, Federal Register *39* (May 30):19182–19184, 1974.

Continued on next page

* **Identi-Code® symbol.**

Lilly—Cont.

4. Cockcroft D. W., and Gault M. H.: Prediction of creatinine clearance from serum creatinine, Nephron. *16:* 31–41, 1978.

[040486]

TUINAL® (CII)

[*tōō'ĭ-năl*]

(secobarbital sodium and amobarbital sodium)
Capsules, USP

WARNING: MAY BE HABIT-FORMING

DESCRIPTION

Tuinal is a combination of equal parts of Seconal® Sodium (secobarbital sodium, Lilly) and Amytal® Sodium (amobarbital sodium, Lilly), barbituric acid derivatives that occur as white, odorless, bitter powders. They are very soluble in water, soluble in alcohol, and practically insoluble in ether and in chloroform.

Each Pulvule® No. 302 contains 25 mg Seconal Sodium and 25 mg Amytal Sodium.

Each Pulvule No. 303 contains 50 mg Seconal Sodium and 50 mg Amytal Sodium.

Each Pulvule No. 304 contains 100 mg Seconal Sodium and 100 mg Amytal Sodium.

Each Pulvule may also contain any or all of the following: D & C Yellow No. 10, F D & C Blue No. 1, F D & C Red No. 40, F D & C Yellow No. 6, gelatin, magnesium stearate, silicone, starch, and other inactive ingredients.

Chemically, Seconal Sodium is sodium 5-allyl-5-(1-methylbutyl)barbiturate, with the empirical formula $C_{12}H_{17}N_2NaO_3$.

Amytal Sodium is sodium 5-ethyl-5-isopentylbarbiturate, with the empirical formula $C_{11}H_{17}N_2NaO_3$.

CLINICAL PHARMACOLOGY

Tuinal, a moderately long-acting barbiturate, is a central-nervous-system depressant. In ordinary doses, the drug acts as a hypnotic. Its onset of action occurs in 15 to 30 minutes, and the duration of action ranges from three to 11 hours. It is detoxified in the liver.

INDICATIONS AND USAGE

For use whenever prompt and moderately sustained hypnotic effect is required. Not suitable for continuous daytime sedation. The prolonged administration of Tuinal is not recommended, since it has not been shown to be effective for a period of more than 14 days. If insomnia persists, drug-free intervals of one or more weeks should elapse before re-treatment is considered.

Attempts should be made to find alternative nondrug therapy for chronic insomnia.

CONTRAINDICATIONS

Tuinal is contraindicated in patients who are hypersensitive to barbiturates. It is also contraindicated in patients with a history of manifest or latent porphyria, marked impairment of liver function, or respiratory disease in which dyspnea or obstruction is evident. It should not be administered to persons with known previous addiction to the sedative/hypnotic group, since ordinary doses may be ineffectual and may contribute to further addiction. Tuinal should not be administered in the presence of acute or chronic pain, because paradoxical excitement may be induced or important symptoms may be masked.

WARNINGS

Prolonged, uninterrupted use of barbiturates (particularly the short-acting drugs), even in therapeutic doses, may result in psychic and physical dependence.

The central-nervous-system-depressant effect of secobarbital and amobarbital may be additive with that of other CNS depressants, including alcohol.

PRECAUTIONS

General Precautions—Barbiturates induce liver microsomal enzyme activity. This accelerates the biotransformation of various drugs and is probably part of the mechanism of the tolerance encountered with barbiturates. Tuinal should, therefore, be used with caution in patients with decreased liver function. This drug should also be administered cautiously to patients with a history of drug dependence or abuse (*see* DRUG ABUSE AND DEPENDENCE). Tuinal may decrease the potency of coumarin anticoagulants; therefore, patients receiving such concomitant therapy should have more frequent prothrombin determinations.

As with other sedatives and hypnotics, elderly or debilitated patients may react to barbiturates with marked excitement or depression.

The systemic effects of exogenous hydrocortisone and endogenous hydrocortisone (cortisol) may be diminished by Tuinal. Thus, this product should be administered with caution to patients with borderline hypoadrenal function, regardless of whether it is of pituitary or of primary adrenal origin.

Information for Patients—Tuinal may impair the mental and/or physical abilities required for the performance of potentially hazardous tasks, such as driving a car or operating machinery. The patient should be cautioned accordingly.

Drug Interactions—Tuinal in combination with alcohol, tranquilizers, and other central-nervous-system depressants has additive depressant effects, and the patient should be so advised. Patients taking this drug should be warned not to exceed the dosage recommended by their physician. Toxic effects and fatalities have occurred following overdoses of Tuinal alone and in combination with other central-nervous-system depressants. Caution should be exercised in prescribing unnecessarily large amounts of Tuinal for patients who have a history of emotional disturbances or suicidal ideation or who have misused alcohol and other CNS drugs (*see* OVERDOSAGE).

Usage in Pregnancy—Pregnancy Category B—Reproduction studies have been performed in animals and have revealed no evidence of impaired fertility or harm to the fetus due to Tuinal. There are, however, no adequate and well-controlled studies in pregnant women. Because animal reproduction studies are not always predictive of human response, this drug should be used during pregnancy only if clearly needed.

Labor and Delivery—Depression has been noted in infants born following the use of Tuinal during labor.

Nursing Mothers—Caution should be exercised when Tuinal is administered to a nursing woman.

Usage in Children—Safety and effectiveness in children have not been established.

ADVERSE REACTIONS

The following adverse reactions have been reported:

CNS Depression—Residual sedation or "hangover," drowsiness, and lethargy.

Respiratory/Circulatory—Respiratory depression, apnea, circulatory collapse.

Allergic—Hypersensitivity reactions, especially in individuals with asthma, urticaria, angioneurotic edema, or similar conditions; skin eruptions.

Other—Nausea and vomiting; headache.

DRUG ABUSE AND DEPENDENCE

Controlled Substance—Tuinal is a Schedule II drug.

Dependence—Prolonged, uninterrupted use of barbiturates (particularly the short-acting drugs), even in therapeutic doses, may result in psychic and physical dependence. Withdrawal symptoms due to physical dependence following chronic use of large doses of barbiturates may include delirium, convulsions, and death (*see* CONTRAINDICATIONS).

OVERDOSAGE

Symptoms—The manifestations of overdosage are early hypothermia followed by fever, sluggish or absent reflexes, respiratory depression, gradual appearance of circulatory collapse, pulmonary edema, and coma.

Treatment—General management should consist in symptomatic and supportive therapy, including gastric lavage, administration of intravenous fluids, and maintenance of blood pressure, body temperature, and adequate respiratory exchange. Dialysis will increase the rate of removal of barbiturates from the body fluids. Antibiotics may be required to control pulmonary complications.

DOSAGE AND ADMINISTRATION

50 to 200 mg at bedtime or one hour preoperatively.

HOW SUPPLIED

(CII) *Pulvules Tuinal® (Secobarbital Sodium and Amobarbital Sodium Capsules, USP), No. 302, F64,** 50 mg (No. 4, Blue Body, Orange Cap), in bottles of 100 (NDC 0002-0664-02); *No. 303, F65,** 100 mg (No. 3, Blue Body, Orange Cap), in bottles of 100 (NDC 0002-0665-02) and 1000 (NDC 0002-0665-04) and in strip packages of individually sealed Pulvules (DS1000) (NDC 0002-0665-35); *No. 304, F66,** 200 mg (No. 2, Blue Body, Orange Cap), in bottles of 100 (NDC 0002-0666-02) and 1000 (NDC 0002-0666-04) and in 10 strips of 10 individually labeled blisters each containing 1 Pulvule (ID100) (NDC 0002-0666-33).

[022486]

Shown in Product Identification Section, page 415

ULTRALENTE®ILETIN® I

[*ŭl'trá-lĕn'tā ī'lĕ-tĭn*]

(extended insulin zinc suspension, Lilly), *see under* Iletin® (insulin, Lilly).

VANCOCIN® HCL ℞

[*văn'kō-sĭn ăch'sē-ĕl*]

(vancomycin hydrochloride)
Sterile, USP
IntraVenous

DESCRIPTION

Vancocin® HCl (Sterile Vancomycin Hydrochloride, USP, Lilly), IntraVenous, is a tricyclic glycopeptide antibiotic derived from *Nocardia orientalis* (formerly *Streptomyces orientalis*) and has the chemical formula $C_{66}H_{75}Cl_2H_9O_{24}$. The formula weight is 1449; 500 mg of the base are equivalent to 0.35 mmol.

Sterile vials contain the equivalent of 500 mg of vancomycin base/10 ml of reconstituted solution. It is an off-white to buff-colored dry powder. When reconstituted in water, it is a clear, light-yellow to light-brown solution with a *p*H range of 2.5 to 4.5.

CLINICAL PHARMACOLOGY

Vancomycin is poorly absorbed after oral administration; it is given intravenously for therapy of systemic infections. Intramuscular injection is painful.

In subjects with normal kidney function, multiple intravenous dosing of 1 g of vancomycin (15 mg/kg) infused over 60 minutes produces mean plasma concentrations of approximately 63 mg/liter immediately at the completion of infusion, mean plasma concentrations of approximately 23 mg/liter 2 hours after infusion, and mean plasma concentrations of approximately 8 mg/liter 11 hours after the end of the infusion. Multiple dosing of 500 mg infused over 30 minutes produces mean plasma concentrations of about 49 mg/liter at the completion of infusion, mean plasma concentrations of about 19 mg/liter 2 hours after infusion, and mean plasma concentrations of about 10 mg/liter 6 hours after infusion. The plasma concentrations during multiple dosing are similar to those after a single dose.

The mean elimination half-life of vancomycin from plasma is 4 to 6 hours in subjects with normal renal function. In the first 24 hours, about 75% of an administered dose of vancomycin is excreted in urine by glomerular filtration. Mean plasma clearance is about 0.058 liter/kg/hr, and mean renal clearance is about 0.048 liter/kg/hr. Renal dysfunction slows excretion of vancomycin. In anephric patients, the average half-life of elimination is 7.5 days. The distribution coefficient is from 0.3 to 0.43 liter/kg. There is no apparent metabolism of the drug. About 60% of an intraperitoneal dose of vancomycin administered during peritoneal dialysis is absorbed systemically in 6 hours. Serum concentrations of about 10 mg/liter are achieved by intraperitoneal injection of 30 mg/kg of vancomycin. Vancomycin is not effectively removed by either hemodialysis or peritoneal dialysis; there have been no reports of vancomycin clearance with hemoperfusion.

Total systemic and renal clearance of vancomycin may be reduced in the elderly.

Vancomycin is approximately 55% serum protein bound as measured by ultrafiltration at vancomycin serum concentrations of 10 to 100 mg/liter. After IV administration of Vancocin® HCl (vancomycin hydrochloride, Lilly), inhibitory concentrations are present in pleural, pericardial, ascitic, and synovial fluids; in urine; in peritoneal dialysis fluid; and in atrial appendage tissue. Vancocin HCl does not readily diffuse across normal meninges into the spinal fluid; but, when the meninges are inflamed, penetration into the spinal fluid occurs.

Microbiology—The bactericidal action of vancomycin results primarily from inhibition of cell-wall biosynthesis. In addition, vancomycin alters bacterial-cell-membrane permeability and RNA synthesis. There is no cross-resistance between vancomycin and other antibiotics. Vancomycin is active against staphylococci, including *Staphylococcus aureus* and *Staphylococcus epidermidis* (including heterogeneous methicillin-resistant strains); streptococci, including *Streptococcus pyogenes, Streptococcus pneumoniae* (including penicillin-resistant strains), *Streptococcus agalactiae,* the viridans group, *Streptococcus bovis,* and enterococci (e.g., *Streptococcus faecalis*); *Clostridium difficile* (e.g., toxigenic strains implicated in pseudomembranous enterocolitis); and diphtheroids. Other organisms that are susceptible to varcomycin in vitro include *Listeria monocytogenes, Lactobacillus* species, *Actinomyces* species, *Clostridium* species, and *Bacillus* species.

Vancomycin is not active in vitro against gram-negative bacilli, mycobacteria, or fungi.

Synergy—The combination of vancomycin and an aminoglycoside acts synergistically in vitro against many strains of *S. aureus,* nonenterococcal group D streptococci, enterococci, and *Streptococcus* species (viridans group).

Disc Susceptibility Tests—The standardized method described by the National Committee for Clinical Laboratory Standards has been recommended for use with discs to test susceptibility to vancomycin. Results of standard single-dose susceptibility tests with a 30-mcg vancomycin hydrochloride disc should be interpreted according to the following criteria.

Susceptible organisms produce zones greater than or equal to 12 mm, indicating that the test organism is likely to respond to therapy. Organisms that produce zones of 10 or 11 mm are considered to be of intermediate susceptibility. Organisms in this category are likely to respond if the infection is confined to tissues or fluids in which high antibiotic concentrations are attained. Resistant organisms produce zones of 9 mm or less, indicating that other therapy should be selected.

With a standardized dilution method, a bacterial isolate may be considered susceptible if the MIC value for vancomycin is 4 mg/liter or less. Organisms are considered resistant to vancomycin if the MIC is greater than or equal to 16 mg/liter. Organisms having an MIC value of less than 16 mg/liter but greater than 4 mg/liter are considered to be of intermediate susceptibility.[1–3]

Standardized procedures require the use of laboratory control organisms. The 30-mcg vancomycin disc should give zone diameters between 15 and 19 mm for *S. aureus* ATCC 25923. As with the standard diffusion methods, dilution procedures require the use of laboratory control organisms. Standard vancomycin powder should give MIC values in the range of 0.5 mg/liter to 2.0 mg/liter for *S. aureus* ATCC 29213. For *S. faecalis* ATCC 29212, the MIC range should be 1.0 to 4.0 mg/liter.

INDICATIONS AND USAGE

Vancocin® HCl (vancomycin hydrochloride, Lilly) is indicated for the treatment of serious or severe infections caused by susceptible strains of methicillin-resistant (β-lactam-resistant) staphylococci. It is indicated for penicillin-allergic patients, for patients who cannot receive or who have failed to respond to other drugs, including the penicillins or cephalosporins, and for infections caused by vancomycin-susceptible organisms that are resistant to other antimicrobial drugs. Vancocin HCl is indicated for initial therapy when methicillin-resistant staphylococci are suspected, but after susceptibility data are available, therapy should be adjusted accordingly.

Vancocin HCl is effective in the treatment of staphylococcal endocarditis. Its effectiveness has been documented in other infections due to staphylococci, including septicemia, bone infections, lower respiratory tract infections, and skin and skin-structure infections. When staphylococcal infections are localized and purulent, antibiotics are used as adjuncts to appropriate surgical measures.

Vancocin HCl has been reported to be effective alone or in combination with an aminoglycoside for endocarditis caused by *S. viridans* or *S. bovis*. For endocarditis caused by enterococci (e.g., *S. faecalis*), Vancocin HCl has been reported to be effective only in combination with an aminoglycoside.

Vancocin HCl has been reported to be effective for the treatment of diphtheroid endocarditis. Vancocin HCl has been used successfully in combination with rifampin, an aminoglycoside, or both in early-onset prosthetic valve endocarditis caused by *S. epidermidis* or diphtheroids.

Specimens for bacteriologic cultures should be obtained in order to isolate and identify causative organisms and to determine their susceptibilities to Vancocin HCl.

The parenteral form of Vancocin HCl may be administered orally for treatment of antibiotic-associated pseudomembranous colitis produced by *C. difficile*. Parenteral administration of Vancocin HCl alone is of unproven benefit for this indication. Vancocin HCl is not effective by the oral route for other types of infection.

Although no controlled clinical efficacy studies have been conducted, intravenous vancomycin has been suggested by the American Heart Association and the American Dental Association for prophylaxis against bacterial endocarditis in patients allergic to penicillin who have congenital heart disease or rheumatic or other acquired valvular heart disease when these patients undergo dental procedures or surgical procedures of the upper respiratory tract.

Note: When selecting antibiotics for the prevention of bacterial endocarditis, the physician or dentist should read the full joint statement of the American Heart Association and the American Dental Association.[4]

CONTRAINDICATION

Vancocin® HCl (vancomycin hydrochloride, Lilly) is contraindicated in patients with known hypersensitivity to this antibiotic.

WARNINGS

Rapid bolus administration (e.g., over several minutes) may be associated with exaggerated hypotension and, rarely, cardiac arrest.

Vancocin® HCl (vancomycin hydrochloride, Lilly) should be administered in a dilute solution over a period of not less than 60 minutes to avoid rapid-infusion-related reactions. Stopping the infusion usually results in a prompt cessation of these reactions.

Ototoxicity has occurred in patients receiving Vancocin HCl. It may be transient or permanent. It has been reported mostly in patients who have been given excessive doses, who have an underlying hearing loss, or who are receiving concomitant therapy with another ototoxic agent, such as an aminoglycoside. Vancomycin should be used with caution in patients with renal insufficiency because the risk of toxicity is appreciably increased by high, prolonged blood concentrations.

Dosage of Vancocin HCl must be adjusted for patients with renal dysfunction (*see* PRECAUTIONS and DOSAGE AND ADMINISTRATION).

PRECAUTIONS

General—Clinically significant serum concentrations have been reported in some patients being treated for active *C. difficile*-induced pseudomembranous colitis after multiple oral doses of vancomycin.

In order to minimize the risk of nephrotoxicity when treating patients with underlying renal dysfunction or patients receiving concomitant therapy with an aminoglycoside, serial monitoring of renal function should be performed and particular care should be taken in following appropriate dosing schedules (*see* DOSAGE AND ADMINISTRATION).

Serial tests of auditory function may be helpful in order to minimize the risk of ototoxicity.

Reversible neutropenia has been reported in patients receiving Vancocin® HCl (vancomycin hydrochloride, Lilly) (*see* ADVERSE REACTIONS). Patients who will undergo prolonged therapy with Vancocin HCl or those who are receiving concomitant drugs which may cause neutropenia should have periodic monitoring of the leukocyte count.

Vancocin HCl is irritating to tissue and must be given by a secure intravenous route of administration. Pain, tenderness, and necrosis occur with intramuscular injection of Vancocin HCl or with inadvertent extravasation. Thrombophlebitis may occur, the frequency and severity of which can be minimized by administering the drug slowly as a dilute solution (2.5 to 5 g/liter) and by rotating the sites of infusion.

There have been reports that the frequency of infusion-related events (including hypotension, flushing, erythema, urticaria, and pruritus) increases with the concomitant administration of anesthetic agents. Infusion-related events may be minimized by the administration of Vancocin HCl as a 60-minute infusion prior to anesthetic induction.

The safety and efficacy of vancomycin administration by the intrathecal (intralumbar or intraventricular) route have not been assessed.

Concurrent and/or sequential systemic or topical use of other potentially neurotoxic and/or nephrotoxic drugs, such as amphotericin B, aminoglycosides, bacitracin, polymyxin B, colistin, viomycin, or cisplatin, requires careful monitoring.

Usage in Pregnancy—Pregnancy Category C—Animal reproduction studies have not been conducted with Vancocin HCl. It is also not known whether Vancocin HCl can cause fetal harm when administered to a pregnant woman or can affect reproduction capacity. Vancocin HCl should be given to a pregnant woman only if clearly needed.

Nursing Mothers—It is not known whether this drug is excreted in human milk. Because many drugs are excreted in human milk, caution should be exercised when Vancocin HCl is administered to a nursing woman. It is unlikely that a nursing infant can absorb a significant amount of vancomycin from the normal gastrointestinal tract.

Usage in Pediatrics—In premature neonates and young infants, it may be appropriate to confirm desired vancomycin serum concentrations. Concomitant administration of vancomycin and anesthetic agents has been associated with erythema and histamine-like flushing in children (*see* ADVERSE REACTIONS).

Geriatrics—The natural decrement of glomerular filtration with increasing age may lead to elevated vancomycin serum concentrations if dosage is not adjusted. Vancomycin dosage schedules should be adjusted in elderly patients (*see* DOSAGE AND ADMINISTRATION).

ADVERSE REACTIONS

Infusion-Related Events—During or soon after rapid infusion of Vancocin® HCl (vancomycin hydrochloride, Lilly), patients may develop anaphylactoid reactions, including hypotension, wheezing, dyspnea, urticaria, or pruritus. Rapid infusion may also cause flushing of the upper body ("red neck") or pain and muscle spasm of the chest and back. These reactions usually resolve within 20 minutes but may persist for several hours. Such events are infrequent if Vancocin HCl is given by a slow infusion over 60 minutes.

Nephrotoxicity—A few dozen cases of increased serum creatinine or BUN concentrations in patients given Vancocin HCl have been reported. Most of these have occurred in patients who were given aminoglycosides concomitantly or who had preexisting kidney dysfunction. When Vancocin HCl was discontinued, azotemia resolved in most patients.

Ototoxicity—A few dozen cases of hearing loss associated with Vancocin HCl have been reported. Most of these patients had kidney dysfunction, preexisting hearing loss, or concomitant treatment with an ototoxic drug. Vertigo, dizziness, and tinnitus have been reported rarely.

Hematopoietic—Reversible neutropenia, usually starting one week or more after onset of therapy with Vancocin HCl of after a total dose of more than 25 g, has been reported for several dozen patients. Neutropenia appears to be promptly reversible when Vancocin HCl is discontinued. Thrombocytopenia has rarely been reported.

Phlebitis—Inflammation at the injection site has been reporte.

Miscellaneous—Infrequently, patients have been reported to have had anaphylaxis, drug fever, chills, and rashes in association with Vancocin HCl.

OVERDOSAGE

Supportive care is advised, with maintenance of glomerular filtration, Vancomycin is poorly removed by dialysis. Hemoperfusion with Amberlite XAD-4 resin has been reported to be of limited benefit.

DOSAGE AND ADMINISTRATION

Patients with Normal Renal Function

Adults—The usual daily intravenous dose is 2 g divided either as 500 mg every 6 hours or 1 g every 12 hours. Each dose should be administered over a period of at least 60 minutes. Other patient factors, such as age or obesity, may call for modification of the usual daily dose.

Children—The total daily intravenous dosage of Vancocin® HCl (vancomycin hydrochloride, Lilly), calculated on the basis of 40 mg/kg of body weight, can be divided and incorporated into the child's 24-hour fluid requirement. Each dose should be administered over a period of at least 60 minutes.

Infants and Neonates—In neonates and young infants, the total daily intravenous dosage may be lower. In both neonates and infants, an initial dose of 15 mg/kg is suggested, followed by 10 mg/kg every 12 hours for neonates in the first week of life and every 8 hours thereafter up to the age of one month. Close monitoring of serum concentrations of vancomycin may be warranted in these patients.

Patients with Impaired Renal Function and Elderly Patients

Dosage adjustment must be made in patients with impaired renal function. In the elderly, dosage reduction may be necessary to a greater extent than expected because of decreasing renal function. Measurement of vancomycin serum concentrations can be helpful in optimizing therapy, especially in seriously ill patients with changing renal function. Vancomycin serum concentrations can be determined by use of microbiologic assay, radioimmunoassay, fluorescence polarization immunoassay, fluorescence immunoassay, or high-pressure liquid chromatography.

For most patients with renal impairment, the dosage can be calculated by using the following table if creatinine clearance can be measured or estimated accurately. The dosage of Vancocin HCl per day in mg is about 15 times the glomerular filtration rate in ml/min. (see table below).

DOSAGE TABLE FOR VANCOMYCIN
IN PATIENTS WITH IMPAIRED RENAL FUNCTION
(Adapted from Moellering *et al.*[5])

Creatinine Clearance ml/min.	Vancomycin Dose mg/24 h
100	1545
90	1390
80	1235
70	1080
60	925
50	770
40	620
30	465
20	310
10	155

The initial dose should be no less than 15 mg/kg, even in patients with mild to moderate renal insufficiency.

The table is not valid for functionally anephric patients. For such patients, an initial dose of 15 mg/kg of body weight should be given in order to achieve prompt therapeutic serum concentrations. The dose required to maintain stable concentrations is 1.9 mg/kg/24 h. Since individual maintenance doses of 250 to 1000 mg are convenient, one dose may be given every several days rather than on a daily basis in patients with marked renal impairment. In anuria, a dose of 1000 mg every 7 to 10 days has been recommended.

When only serum creatinine concentration is known, the following formula (based on sex, weight, and age of the patient) may be used to calculate creatinine clearance. Calculated creatinine clearances (ml/min.) are only estimates. The creatinine clearance should be measured promptly.

Men: $\frac{\text{Weight (kg)} \times (140 - \text{age in years})}{72 \times \text{serum creatinine concentration (mg/dl)}}$

Women: 0.85 × above value

The serum creatinine must represent a steady state of renal function. Otherwise, the estimated value for creatinine clearance is not valid. Such a calculated clearance is an overestimate of actual clearance in patients with conditions: (1) characterized by decreasing renal function, such as shock, severe heart failure, or oliguria; (2) in which a normal relationship between muscle mass and total body weight is not

Continued on next page

• **Identi-Code® symbol.**

Lilly—Cont.

present, such as in obese patients or those with liver disease, edema, or ascites; and (3) accompanied by debilitation, malnutrition, or inactivity.

PREPARATION AND STABILITY

At the time of use, reconstitute by adding 10 ml of Sterile Water for Injection to the 500-mg vial of dry, sterile vancomycin powder. FURTHER DILUTION IS REQUIRED.

After reconstitution, this 10-ml vial containing 500 mg of vancomycin may be stored in a refrigerator for 96 hours without significant loss of potency.

Intermittent infusion is the recommended method of administration. The reconstituted solution containing 500 mg of vancomycin can be added to 100 to 200 ml of diluent. The desired dose, diluted in this manner to a concentration of 2.5 to 5.0 g/liter, should be administered by intravenous infusion over a period of at least 60 minutes.

Compatibility with Other Drugs and Intravenous Fluids—The following diluents are physically and chemically compatible (with 4 g/liter of Vancocin® HCl [vancomycin hydrochloride, Lilly]):

- 5% Dextrose Injection, USP
- 5% Dextrose Injection and 0.9% Sodium Chloride Injection, USP
- Lactated Ringer's Injection, USP
- Lactated Ringer's and 5% Dextrose Injection
- Normosol®-M and 5% Dextrose
- 0.9% Sodium Chloride Injection, USP
- Isolyte® E
- Acetated Ringer's Injection

Vancomycin solution has a low pH and may cause physical instability of other compounds.

Parenteral drug products should be inspected visually for particulate matter and discoloration prior to administration, whenever solution or container permits.

For Oral Administration—The usual adult total daily dosage for antibiotic-associated pseudomembranous colitis produced by *C. difficile* is 500 mg to 2 g given in 3 or 4 divided doses for 7 to 10 days. The total daily dosage in chidren is 40 mg/kg of body weight in 3 or 4 divided doses. The total daily dosage should not exceed 2 g. The appropriate dose may be diluted in 1 oz of water and given to the patient to drink. The diluted material may be administered via nasogastric tube. Common flavoring syrups may be added to the solution to improve the taste for oral administration.

HOW SUPPLIED

(℞) *Vials No. 657, Vancocin® HCl (Sterile Vancomycin Hydrochloride, USP), IntraVenous,* equivalent to 500 mg vancomycin, 10-ml size, rubber-stoppered (Dry Powder), in singles (10/carton) (NDC 0002-1444-01).

REFERENCES

1. National Committee for Clinical Laboratory Standards, 1984. Performance Standards for Antimicrobial Disk Susceptibility Tests, MZ-A3, NCCLS, Villanova, PA 19805.
2. National Committee for Clinical Laboratory Standards, 1983. Methods for Dilution Antimicrobial Susceptibility Tests for Bacteria That Grow Aerobically, M7-T, NCCLS, Villanova, PA. 19805.
3. National Committee for Clinical Laboratory Standards, 1984. Reference Agar Dilution Procedure for Antimicrobial Susceptibility Testing of Anaerobic Bacteria, M11-A, NCCLS, Villanova, PA, 19805.
4. Shulman, S. T., Amren, D. P., Bisno, A. L., *et al.*: Prevention of Bacterial Endocarditis, Circulation, *70:* 1123A, 1984.
5. Moellering, R. C., Krogstad, D. J., and Greenblatt, D. J.: Vancomycin Therapy in Patients with Impaired Renal Function: A Nomogram for Dosage, Ann. Intern. Med., *94:* 343, 1981.

[021086]

6505-00-065-5220

VANCOCIN® HCl ℞

[*văn 'kō-sĭn ăch 'sē-ĕl*]
(vancomycin hydrochloride)
For Oral Solution, USP

This preparation is for oral use only. If parenteral vancomycin therapy is desired, use Vancocin® HCl (Sterile Vancomycin Hydrochloride, USP), IntraVenous, and consult package insert accompanying that preparation.

DESCRIPTION

Vancocin® HCl (vancomycin hydrochloride, Lilly) is a glycopeptide antibiotic derived from *Streptomyces orientalis* which is bactericidal against many gram-positive bacteria.

ACTIONS

Vancocin® HCl (vancomycin hydrochloride, Lilly) is poorly absorbed by mouth. Many strains of streptococci, staphylococci, *Clostridium difficile,* and other gram-positive bacteria are susceptible in vitro to concentrations of 0.5 to 5 mcg/ml. Staphylococci are generally susceptible to less than 5 mcg of Vancocin HCl per ml, but a small proportion of *Staphylococcus aureus* strains require 10 or 20 mcg/ml for inhibition. If the Bauer-Kirby method of disc susceptibility testing is used, a 30-mcg disc of Vancocin HCl should produce a zone of more than 11 mm when tested against a vancomycin-susceptible bacterial strain.

INDICATIONS

Vancocin® HCl (vancomycin hydrochloride, Lilly) may be administered orally for treatment of staphylococcal enterocolitis and antibiotic-associated pseudomembranous colitis produced by *C. difficile.* Parenteral antibiotic administration may be used concomitantly. Vancomycin is *not* effective by the oral route for other types of infection.

CONTRAINDICATION

Vancocin® HCl (vancomycin hydrochloride, Lilly) is contraindicated in patients with known hypersensitivity to this antibiotic.

WARNINGS

Because of its ototoxicity and nephrotoxicity, Vancocin® HCl (vancomycin hydrochloride, Lilly) should be used with care in patients with renal insufficiency. During parenteral therapy, the risk of toxicity is appreciably increased by high blood concentrations or prolonged treatment. If it is necessary to use Vancocin HCl parenterally in such patients, doses of less than 2 g/day usually will provide satisfactory blood levels.

Vancocin HCl should also be avoided in patients with previous hearing loss. If it is used in such patients, the dose of Vancocin HCl should be regulated, if possible, by periodic determination of the drug level in the blood. Deafness may be preceded by tinnitus. The elderly are more susceptible to auditory damage. Experience with other antibiotics suggests that deafness may be progressive despite cessation of treatment.

Concurrent and sequential use of other neurotoxic and/or nephrotoxic antibiotics, particularly streptomycin, neomycin, kanamycin, gentamicin, cephaloridine, paromomycin, viomycin, polymyxin B, colistin, tobramycin, and amikacin, requires careful monitoring.

PRECAUTIONS

Patients with borderline renal function and individuals over the age of 60 should be given serial tests of auditory function and of vancomycin blood levels. All patients receiving the drug should have periodic hematologic studies, urinalyses, and liver and renal function tests.

ADVERSE REACTIONS

Nausea, chills, fever, urticaria, and macular rashes have been associated with the administration of Vancocin HCl. It may also produce eosinophilia and anaphylactoid reactions. The use of Vancocin® HCl (vancomycin hydrochloride, Lilly) may result in overgrowth of nonsusceptible organisms. If new infections due to bacteria or fungi appear during therapy with this product, appropriate measures should be taken.

DOSAGE AND ADMINISTRATION

The contents of the 10-g vial may be mixed with distilled or deionized water (115 ml) for oral administration. When mixed with 115 ml of water, each 6 ml provide approximately 500 mg of vancomycin. The contents of the 1-g vial may be mixed with distilled or deionized water (20 ml). When reconstituted with 20 ml, each 5 ml contains approximately 250 mg of vancomycin. Mix thoroughly to dissolve. These mixtures may be kept for two weeks in a refrigerator without significant loss of potency.

Adults—The usual dose is 500 mg every six hours or 1 g every 12 hours.

The usual adult dosage for antibiotic-associated pseudomembranous colitis produced by *C. difficile* is 500 mg to 2 g of vancomycin orally/day in three or four divided doses administered for seven to ten days.

Children—The total daily dose is 20 mg/lb of body weight in divided doses.

HOW SUPPLIED

(℞) *Vancocin® HCl (Vancomycin Hydrochloride for Oral Solution, USP): M-5105,* 1 g (equivalent to vancomycin), in a Traypak™ (multivial carton, Lilly) of 6 (NDC 0002-5105-16); *M- 206,* 10 g (equivalent to vancomycin), in a screw-cap container (NDC 0002-2372-37).

M-206, 10 g—6505-01-178-7889

[072183]

VANCOMYCIN HYDROCHLORIDE,

[*văn 'kō-sĭn ăch 'sē-ĕl*]
see Vancocin® HCl (vancomycin hydrochloride, Lilly).

V-CILLIN K® ℞

[*vē-sĭl 'ĭn kā*]
(penicillin V potassium)
USP

DESCRIPTION

V-Cillin K® (Penicillin V Potassium, USP, Lilly) is the potassium salt of V- Cillin® (Penicillin V, USP, Lilly). This chemically improved form combines acid stability with immediate solubility and rapid absorption.

Each tablet contains penicillin V potassium equivalent to 125 mg (200,000 units), 250 mg (400,000 units), or 500 mg (800,000 units) penicillin V. The tablets also contain lactose, magnesium stearate, povidone, starch, stearic acid, and other inactive ingredients.

After being mixed as directed, each 5 ml of the oral solution will contain penicillin V potassium equivalent to 125 mg (200,000 units) or 250 mg (400,000 units) penicillin V. The suspensions also contain citric acid, FD&C Red No. 3, FD&C Red No. 40, FD&C Yellow No. 6, flavors, saccharin, sodium citrate, and sucrose.

ACTIONS AND PHARMACOLOGY

V-Cillin K® (penicillin V potassium, Lilly) is bactericidal against penicillin-sensitive microorganisms during the stage of active multiplication. It produces its effect by inhibiting biosynthesis of cell-wall mucopeptide. It is not active against the penicillinase-producing bacteria, which include many strains of staphylococci. The drug exerts high in vitro activity against staphylococci (except penicillinase-producing strains), streptococci (groups A, C, G, H, L, and M), and pneumococci. Other organisms sensitive in vitro to penicillin V are *Corynebacterium diphtheriae, Bacillus anthracis,* clostridia, *Actinomyces bovis, Streptobacillus moniliformis, Listeria monocytogenes, Leptospira,* and *Neisseria gonorrhoeae. Treponema pallidum* is extremely sensitive.

V-Cillin K has the distinct advantage over penicillin G in being resistant to inactivation by gastric acid. It may be given with meals; however, blood levels are slightly higher when the drug is given on an empty stomach. Average blood levels are two to five times higher than those following the same dose of oral penicillin G and also show much less individual variation.

Once absorbed, about 80 percent of V-Cillin K is bound to serum protein. Tissue levels are highest in the kidneys, and lesser amounts appear in the liver, skin, and intestines. Small concentrations are found in all other body tissues and the cerebrospinal fluid. The drug is excreted as rapidly as it is absorbed in individuals with normal kidney function; however, recovery of the drug from the urine indicates that only about 25 percent of the dose given is absorbed. In neonates, young infants, and individuals with impaired kidney function, excretion is considerably delayed.

INDICATIONS

V-Cillin K® (penicillin V potassium, Lilly) is indicated in the treatment of mild to moderately severe infections due to microorganisms whose sensitivity to penicillin G is within the range of serum levels common to this particular dosage form. Therapy should be guided by bacteriologic studies (including susceptibility tests) and by clinical response.

NOTE: Severe pneumonia, empyema, bacteremia, pericarditis, meningitis, and arthritis should not be treated with penicillin V during the acute stage.

Indicated surgical procedures should be performed.

The following infections will usually respond to adequate dosage of penicillin V:

Streptococcal Infections (without Bacteremia)—Mild to moderate infections of the upper respiratory tract, scarlet fever, and mild erysipelas.

NOTE: Streptococci in groups A, C, G, H, L, and M are very sensitive to penicillin. Other groups, including group D (enterococcus), are resistant.

Pneumococcal Infections—Mild to moderately severe infections of the respiratory tract.

Staphylococcal Infections Sensitive to Penicillin G—Mild infections of the skin and soft tissues.

NOTE: Reports indicate an increasing number of strains of staphylococci resistant to penicillin G, which emphasizes the need for culture and susceptibility studies in treating suspected staphylococcal infections.

Fusospirochetosis (Vincent's Gingivitis and Pharyngitis)—Mild to moderately severe infections of the oropharynx usually respond to therapy with oral penicillin.

NOTE: Necessary dental care should be accomplished in infections involving the gum tissue.

Medical Conditions in Which Oral Penicillin Therapy Is Indicated as Prophylaxis—To prevent recurrence following rheumatic fever and/or chorea. Prophylaxis with oral penicillin on a continuing basis has proved effective in preventing recurrence of these conditions.

Although no controlled clinical efficacy studies have been conducted, penicillin V has been suggested by the American Heart Association and the American Dental Association for use as part of a parenteral/oral regimen and as an alternative oral regimen for prophylaxis against bacterial endocarditis in patients with congenital heart disease or rheumatic or other acquired valvular heart disease when they undergo dental procedures and surgical procedures of the respiratory tract.[1] Since alpha-hemolytic streptococci relatively resistant to penicillin may be found when patients are receiving continuous oral penicillin for secondary prevention of rheumatic fever, prophylactic agents other than penicillin may be chosen for these patients and prescribed in addition to their continuous prophylactic regimen for rheumatic fever. Oral penicillin should not be used as adjunctive prophylaxis for genitourinary instrumentation or surgery, lower intestinal tract surgery, sigmoidoscopy, and childbirth.

Note: When selecting antibiotics for the prevention of bacterial endocarditis, the physician or dentist should read the full joint statement of the American Heart Association and the American Dental Association.[1]

CONTRAINDICATION

A previous hypersensitivity reaction to any penicillin is a contraindication.

WARNINGS

Serious and occasionally fatal hypersensitivity (anaphylactoid) reactions have been reported in patients receiving penicillin therapy. Although anaphylaxis is more frequent following parenteral therapy, it has occurred in patients given oral penicillins. These reactions are more likely in individuals with a history of sensitivity to multiple allergens.

There have been well-documented reports of individuals with a history of penicillin hypersensitivity who have experienced severe reactions when treated with a cephalosporin. Before therapy with a penicillin, careful inquiry should be made concerning previous hypersensitivity reactions to penicillins, cephalosporins, and other allergens. If an allergic reaction occurs, the drug should be discontinued and the patient treated with the usual agents (e.g., epinephrine or other pressor amines, antihistamines, or corticosteroids).

PRECAUTIONS

Penicillin should be used with caution in individuals with histories of significant allergies and/or asthma.

The oral route of administration should not be relied on in patients with severe illness or with nausea, vomiting, gastric dilatation, cardiospasm, or intestinal hypermotility.

Occasional patients will not absorb therapeutic amounts of orally administered penicillin. In streptococcal infections, therapy must be sufficient to eliminate the organism (a minimum of ten days); otherwise, the sequelae of streptococcal disease may occur. Cultures should be taken following completion of treatment to determine whether streptococci have been eradicated.

Prolonged use of antibiotics may promote the overgrowth of nonsusceptible organisms, including fungi. If superinfection occurs, appropriate measures should be taken.

ADVERSE REACTIONS

Although reactions have been reported much less frequently after oral than after parenteral penicillin therapy, it should be remembered that all degrees of hypersensitivity, including fatal anaphylaxis, have been observed with oral penicillin.

The most common reactions to oral penicillin are nausea, vomiting, epigastric distress, diarrhea, and black, hairy tongue. The hypersensitivity reactions noted are skin eruptions (ranging from maculopapular to exfoliative dermatitis); urticaria; reactions resembling serum sickness, including chills, fever, edema, arthralgia, and prostration; laryngeal edema; and anaphylaxis. Fever and eosinophilia may frequently be the only reactions observed. Hemolytic anemia, leukopenia, thrombocytopenia, neuropathy, and nephropathy are infrequent reactions and are usually associated with high doses of parenteral penicillin.

DOSAGE AND ADMINISTRATION

The dosage of V-Cillin K® (penicillin V potassium, Lilly) should be determined according to the sensitivity of the causative microorganism and the severity of infection and should be adjusted to the clinical response of the patient.

The usual dosage recommendations for adults and children 12 years and over are as follows:

Streptococcal Infections—Mild to moderately severe infections of the upper respiratory tract, including scarlet fever and mild erysipelas: 200,000 to 500,000 units every six to eight hours for ten days.

Pneumococcal Infections—Mild to moderately severe infections of the respiratory tract, including otitis media: 400,000 to 500,000 units every six hours until the patient has been afebrile for at least two days.

Staphylococcal Infections—Mild infections of skin and soft tissue (culture and susceptibility tests should be performed): 400,000 to 500,000 units every six to eight hours.

Fusospirochetosis (Vincent's Infection) of the Oropharynx—Mild to moderately severe infections: 400,000 to 500,000 units every six to eight hours.

Prophylaxis in the Following Conditions—To prevent recurrence following rheumatic fever and/or chorea: 200,000 to 250,000 units twice daily on a continuing basis.

For prophylaxis against bacterial endocarditis[1] in patients with congenital heart disease or rheumatic or other acquired valvular heart disease when undergoing dental procedures or surgical procedures of the upper respiratory tract, one of two regimens may be selected:

(1) For the oral regimen, the usual adult dosage is 2 g of penicillin V (1 g for children under 30 kg) one-half to one hour before the procedure and then 500 mg (250 mg for children under 30 kg) every six hours for eight doses; or
(2) For the combined parenteral/oral regimen, the dosage schedule is 1,000,000 units of aqueous crystalline penicillin G (30,000 units/kg for children) intramuscularly mixed with 600,000 units procaine penicillin G (600,000 units for children) one-half to one hour before the procedure and then oral penicillin V, 500 mg for adults or 250 mg for children less than 30 kg, every six hours for eight doses. Doses for children should not exceed recommendations for adults for a single dose or for a 24-hour period.

NOTE: Therapy for children under 12 years of age is calculated on the basis of body weight. For infants and small children, the suggested daily dose is 25,000 to 90,000 units (15 to 50 mg)/kg in three to six divided doses.

HOW SUPPLIED

(℞) *For Oral Solution, V-Cillin K® (Penicillin V Potassium for Oral Solution, USP): M-126, W07,** 125 mg (200,000 units) (equivalent to penicillin V) per 5 ml of solution, in 100 (NDC 0002-2307-48), 150 (NDC 0002-2307-68), and 200-ml-size (NDC 0002-2307-89) packages; *M-142, W16,** 250 mg (400,000 units) (equivalent to penicillin V) per 5 ml of solution, in 100 (NDC 0002-2316-48), 150 (NDC 0002-2316-68), and 200-ml-size (NDC 0002-2316-89) packages.

Each package consists of a bottle containing penicillin V potassium equivalent to penicillin V in a dry, pleasantly flavored mixture, buffered with sodium citrate and citric acid.

After being mixed, the solution should be stored in a refrigerator. It may be kept for 14 days without significant loss of potency. *Shake well before using. Keep tightly closed.*

(℞) *Tablets V-Cillin K® (Penicillin V Potassium Tablets, USP),* Specially Coated: *No. 1830, C27,** 125 mg (200,000 units) (equivalent to penicillin V), in bottles of 100 (NDC 0002-0327-02); *No. 1831, C29,** 250 mg (400,000 units) (equivalent to penicillin V), in bottles of 100 (NDC 0002-0329-02), and 500 (NDC 0002-0329-03); and *No. 1832, C46,** 500 mg (800,000 units) (equivalent to penicillin V) in bottles of 24 (NDC 0002-0346-24), 100 (NDC 0002-0346-02), and 500 (NDC 0002-0346-03).

[110185]

REFERENCE

1. American Heart Association: Prevention of Bacterial Endocarditis, Circulation, *56*:139A, 1977.

VELBAN® ℞

[vĕl′băn]
(vinblastine sulfate)
Sterile, USP

DESCRIPTION

Velban® (Vinblastine Sulfate, USP, Lilly) is the salt of an alkaloid extracted from *Vinca rosea* Linn., a common flowering herb known as the periwinkle (more properly known as *Catharanthus roseus* G. Don). Previously, the generic name was vincaleukoblastine, abbreviated VLB.

Chemical and physical evidence indicates that Velban has the empirical formula $C_{46}H_{58}O_9N_4 \cdot H_2SO_4$ and that it is a dimeric alkaloid containing both indole and dihydroindole moieties.

Vials of Velban contain 10 mg of sterile vinblastine sulfate, in the form of a lyophilized plug, without excipients. When sodium chloride solution is added prior to injection, the pH of the resulting solution lies in the range of 3.5 to 5.

ACTIONS

Velban® (vinblastine sulfate, Lilly) has been used for the palliative treatment of a variety of malignant neoplastic conditions. In susceptible clinical cases, Velban has produced temporary reduction in the size or temporary disappearance of some tumors. It has relieved pain and other symptoms and allowed some patients to regain appetite and weight.

Experimental data indicate that the action of Velban is different from that of other recognized antineoplastic agents. Tissue-culture studies suggest an interference with metabolic pathways of amino acids leading from glutamic acid to the citric acid cycle and to urea. In vivo experiments tend to confirm the in vitro results. A number of studies in vitro and in vivo have demonstrated that Velban produces a stathmokinetic effect and various atypical mitotic figures. The therapeutic responses, however, are not fully explained by the cytologic changes, since these changes are sometimes observed clinically and experimentally in the absence of any oncolytic effects.

Reversal of the antitumor effect of Velban by glutamic acid or tryptophan has been observed. In addition, glutamic acid and aspartic acid have protected mice from lethal doses of Velban. Aspartic acid was relatively ineffective in reversing the antitumor effect.

Other studies indicate that Velban has an effect on cell-energy production required for mitosis and interferes with nucleic acid synthesis.

Hematologic Effects—Clinically, leukopenia is an expected effect of Velban® (vinblastine sulfate, Lilly), and the level of the leukocyte count is an important guide to therapy with this drug. In general, the larger the dose employed, the more profound and longer lasting the leukopenia will be. The fact that the white-blood-cell count returns to normal levels after drug-induced leukopenia is an indication that the white-cell-producing mechanism is not permanently depressed. Usually, the white count has completely returned to normal after the virtual disappearance of white cells from the peripheral blood.

Following therapy with Velban, the nadir in white-blood-cell count may be expected to occur five to ten days after the last day of drug administration. Recovery of the white blood count is fairly rapid thereafter and is usually complete within another seven to 14 days. With the smaller doses employed for maintenance therapy, leukopenia may not be a problem.

Although the thrombocyte count ordinarily is not significantly lowered by therapy with Velban, patients whose bone marrow has been recently impaired by prior therapy with radiation or with other oncolytic drugs may show thrombocytopenia (less than 200,000 platelets/mm^3). When other chemotherapy or radiation has not been employed previously, thrombocyte reduction below the level of 200,000/mm^3 is rarely encountered, even when Velban may be causing significant leukopenia. Rapid recovery from thrombocytopenia within a few days is the rule.

The effect of Velban upon the red-cell count and hemoglobin is usually insignificant when other therapy does not complicate the picture. It should be remembered, however, that patients with malignant disease may exhibit anemia even in the absence of any therapy.

INDICATIONS

Vinblastine sulfate is indicated in the palliative treatment of the following:

I. *Frequently Responsive Malignancies*—
   - Generalized Hodgkin's disease (Stages III and IV, Ann Arbor modification of Rye staging system)
   - Lymphocytic lymphoma (nodular and diffuse, poorly and well differentiated)
   - Histiocytic lymphoma
   - Mycosis fungoides (advanced stages)
   - Advanced carcinoma of the testis
   - Kaposi's sarcoma
   - Letterer-Siwe disease (histiocytosis X)

II. *Less Frequently Responsive Malignancies*—
   - Choriocarcinoma resistant to other chemotherapeutic agents
   - Carcinoma of the breast, unresponsive to appropriate endocrine surgery and hormonal therapy

Current principles of chemotherapy for many types of cancer include the concurrent administration of several antineoplastic agents. For enhanced therapeutic effect without additive toxicity, agents with different dose-limiting clinical toxicities and different mechanisms of action are generally selected. Therefore, although Velban® (vinblastine sulfate, Lilly) is effective as a single agent in the aforementioned indications, it is usually administered in combination with other antineoplastic drugs. Such combination therapy produces a greater percentage of response than does a single-agent regimen. These principles have been applied, for example, in the chemotherapy of Hodgkin's disease.

Hodgkin's Disease—Velban has been shown to be one of the most effective single agents for the treatment of Hodgkin's disease. Advanced Hodgkin's disease has also been successfully treated with several multiple-drug regimens that included Velban. Patients who had relapses after treatment with the MOPP program—mechlorethamine hydrochloride (nitrogen mustard), vincristine sulfate (Oncovin® [vincristine sulfate, Lilly]), prednisone, and procarbazine—have likewise responded to combination-drug therapy that included Velban. A protocol using cyclophosphamide in place of nitrogen mustard and Velban instead of Oncovin is an alternative therapy for previously untreated patients with advanced Hodgkin's disease.

Advanced testicular germinal-cell cancers (embryonal carcinoma, teratocarcinoma, and choriocarcinoma) are sensitive to Velban alone, but better clinical results are achieved when Velban is administered concomitantly with other antineoplastic agents. The effect of bleomycin is significantly enhanced if Velban is administered six to eight hours prior to the administration of bleomycin; this schedule permits

Continued on next page

* Identi-Code® symbol.

Lilly—Cont.

more cells to be arrested during metaphase, the stage of the cell cycle in which bleomycin is active.

CONTRAINDICATIONS

Velban® (vinblastine sulfate, Lilly) is contraindicated in patients who are leukopenic. It should not be used in the presence of bacterial infection. Such infections must be brought under control prior to the initiation of therapy with Velban.

WARNINGS

Usage in Pregnancy—Caution is necessary with the administration of all oncolytic drugs during pregnancy. Information on the use of Velban® (vinblastine sulfate, Lilly) during pregnancy is very limited. Although no abnormalities of the human fetus have been reported thus far, animal studies with Velban suggest that teratogenic effects may occur.

Aspermia has been reported in man. Animal studies show metaphase arrest and degenerative changes in germ cells.

PRECAUTIONS

If leukopenia with less than 2000 white blood cells/mm^3 occurs following a dose of Velban® (vinblastine sulfate, Lilly), the patient should be watched carefully for evidence of infection until the white-blood-cell count has returned to a safe level.

When cachexia or ulcerated areas of the skin surface are present, there may be a more profound leukopenic response to the drug; therefore, its use should be avoided in older persons suffering from either of these conditions.

In patients with malignant-cell infiltration of the bone marrow, the leukocyte and platelet counts have sometimes fallen precipitously after moderate doses of Velban. Further use of the drug in such patients is inadvisable.

Acute shortness of breath and severe bronchospasm have been reported following the administration of vinca alkaloids. These reactions have been encountered most frequently when vinca alkaloid was used in combination with mitomycin-C. The onset may be within minutes or several hours after the vinca is injected.

The use of small amounts of Velban daily for long periods is not advised, even though the resulting total weekly dosage may be similar to that recommended. Little or no added therapeutic effect has been demonstrated when such regimens have been used. *Strict adherence to the recommended dosage schedule is very important.* When amounts equal to several times the recommended weekly dosage were given in seven daily installments for long periods, convulsions, severe and permanent central-nervous-system damage, and even death occurred.

Care must be taken to avoid contamination of the eye with concentrations of Velban used clinically. If accidental contamination occurs, severe irritation (or, if the drug was delivered under pressure, even corneal ulceration) may result. The eye should be washed with water immediately and thoroughly.

ADVERSE REACTIONS

Prior to the use of the drug, patients should be advised of the possibility of untoward symptoms.

In general, the incidence of adverse reactions attending the use of Velban® (vinblastine sulfate, Lilly) appears to be related to the size of the dose employed. With the exception of epilation, leukopenia, and neurologic side effects, adverse reactions generally have not persisted for longer than 24 hours. Neurologic side effects are not common; but when they do occur, they often last for more than 24 hours. Leukopenia, the most common adverse reaction, is usually the dose-limiting factor.

The following are manifestations which have been reported as adverse reactions:

Gastrointestinal—Nausea, vomiting, constipation, vesiculation of the mouth, ileus, diarrhea, anorexia, abdominal pain, rectal bleeding, pharyngitis, hemorrhagic enterocolitis, bleeding from an old peptic ulcer

Neurologic—Numbness, paresthesias, peripheral neuritis, mental depression, loss of deep-tendon reflexes, headache, convulsions

Miscellaneous—Malaise, weakness, dizziness, pain in tumor site, vesiculation of the skin

Nausea and vomiting usually may be controlled with ease by antiemetic agents. When epilation develops, it frequently is not total; and, in some cases, hair regrows while maintenance therapy continues.

Extravasation during intravenous injection may lead to cellulitis and phlebitis. If the amount of extravasation is great, sloughing may occur.

DOSAGE AND ADMINISTRATION

There are variations in the depth of the leukopenic response which follows therapy with Velban® (vinblastine sulfate, Lilly). For this reason, it is recommended that the drug be given no more frequently than *once every seven days*. It is wise to initiate therapy for adults by administering a single intravenous dose of 3.7 mg/m^2 of body surface area (bsa). Thereafter, white-blood-cell counts should be made to determine the patient's sensitivity to Velban.

A simplified and conservative incremental approach to dosage *at weekly intervals* may be outlined as follows:

	Adults	Children
First dose	3.7 mg/m^2 bsa	2.5 mg/m^2 bsa
Second dose	5.5 mg/m^2 bsa	3.75 mg/m^2 bsa
Third dose	7.4 mg/m^2 bsa	5.0 mg/m^2 bsa
Fourth dose	9.25 mg/m^2 bsa	6.25 mg/m^2 bsa
Fifth dose	11.1 mg/m^2 bsa	7.5 mg/m^2 bsa

The above-mentioned increases may be used until a maximum dose (not exceeding 18.5 mg/m^2 bsa for adults and 12.5 mg/m^2 bsa for children) is reached. The dose should not be increased after that dose which reduces the white-cell count to approximately 3000 cells/mm^3. In some adults, 3.7 mg/m^2 bsa may produce this leukopenia; other adults may require more than 11.1 mg/m^2 bsa; and, very rarely, as much as 18.5 mg/m^2 bsa may be necessary. For most adult patients, however, the weekly dosage will prove to be 5.5 to 7.4 mg/m^2 bsa.

When the dose of Velban which will produce the above degree of leukopenia has been established, a dose *one increment smaller* than this should be administered at weekly intervals for maintenance. Thus, the patient is receiving the maximum dose that does not cause leukopenia. *It should be emphasized that, even though seven days have elapsed, the next dose of Velban should not be given until the white-cell count has returned to at least 4000/mm^3.* In some cases, oncolytic activity may be encountered before leukopenic effect. When this occurs, there is no need to increase the size of subsequent doses.

The duration of maintenance therapy varies according to the disease being treated and the combination of antineoplastic agents being used. There are differences of opinion regarding the duration of maintenance therapy with the same protocol for a particular disease; for example, various durations have been used with the MOPP program in treating Hodgkin's disease. Prolonged chemotherapy for maintaining remissions involves several risks, among which are life-threatening infectious diseases, sterility, and possibly the appearance of other cancers through suppression of immune surveillance. In some disorders, survival following complete remission may not be as prolonged as that achieved with shorter periods of maintenance therapy. On the other hand, failure to provide maintenance therapy in some patients may lead to unnecessary relapse; complete remissions in patients with testicular cancer, unless maintained for at least two years, often result in early relapse.

To prepare a solution containing 1 mg of Velban/ml, add 10 ml of Sodium Chloride Injection (preserved with phenol or benzyl alcohol) to the 10 mg of Velban in the sterile vial. Other solutions are not recommended. The drug dissolves instantly to give a clear solution. After a solution has been made in this way and a portion of it has been removed from a vial, the remainder of the vial's contents may be stored in a refrigerator for future use for 30 days without significant loss of potency.

The dose of Velban (calculated to provide the desired amount) may be injected either into the tubing of a running intravenous infusion or directly into a vein. The latter procedure is readily adaptable to outpatient therapy. In either case, the injection may be completed in about one minute. If care is taken to insure that the needle is securely within the vein and that no solution containing Velban is spilled extravascularly, cellulitis and/or phlebitis will not occur. To minimize further the possibility of extravascular spillage, it is suggested that the syringe and needle be rinsed with venous blood before withdrawal of the needle. The dose should not be diluted in large volumes of diluent (i.e., 100 to 250 ml) or given intravenously for prolonged periods (ranging from 30 to 60 minutes or more), since this frequently results in irritation of the vein and increases the chance of extravasation.

Because of the enhanced possibility of thrombosis, it is considered inadvisable to inject a solution of Velban into an extremity in which the circulation is impaired or potentially impaired by such conditions as compressing or invading neoplasm, phlebitis, or varicosity.

CAUTION

If leakage into surrounding tissue should occur during intravenous administration of Velban® (vinblastine sulfate, Lilly), it may cause considerable irritation. The injection should be discontinued immediately, and any remaining portion of the dose should then be introduced into another vein. Local injection of hyaluronidase and the application of moderate heat to the area of leakage help disperse the drug and are thought to minimize discomfort and the possibility of cellulitis.

Parenteral drug products should be inspected visually for particulate matter and discoloration prior to administration, whenever solution and container permit.

Procedures for proper handling and disposal of anticancer drugs should be considered. Several guidelines on this subject have been published. There is no general agreement that all of the procedures recommended in the guidelines are necessary or appropriate.

References are available on request.

HOW SUPPLIED

(℞) *Vials No. 687, Velban® (Sterile Vinblastine Sulfate, USP)*, 10 mg, 10-ml size, rubber-stoppered (Dry Powder), in singles (10 per carton) (NDC 0002-1452-01). *The vials should be stored in a refrigerator (2° to 8°C, or 36° to 46°F) to assure extended stability.*

[012786]

ZINC-INSULIN CRYSTALS
[*ĭ'lĕ-tĭn*]
see under Iletin® (insulin, Lilly).

LyphoMed, Inc.
10401 WEST TOUHY
ROSEMONT, IL 60018

PENTAM™ 300 ℞
(Sterile Pentamidine Isethionate)

DESCRIPTION

PENTAM™ 300 (Sterile Pentamidine Isethionate), an antiprotozoal agent, is a nonpyrogenic lyophilized product. After reconstitution, it should be administered by parenteral (IM or IV) routes. For full prescribing information see package insert.

HOW SUPPLIED

Product No.	
113-15	PENTAM™ 300 (Sterile Pentamidine Isethionate) 300 mg, lyophilized product in single dose vials, packaged in boxes of 7's. (NDC 0469-1130-90)

Store the dry product between 2° and 8°C. Protect the dry product from light. Discard unused portion.

Macsil, Inc.
1326 FRANKFORD AVENUE
PHILADELPHIA, PA 19125

BALMEX® BABY POWDER

(See PDR For Nonprescription Drugs)

BALMEX® EMOLLIENT LOTION

(See PDR For Nonprescription Drugs)

BALMEX® OINTMENT

(See PDR For Nonprescription Drugs)

Mallard Incorporated
3021 WABASH AVE.
DETROIT, MI 48216-9986

ALLERSONE OINTMENT ℞
[*ăl 'er-sōne*]

COMPOSITION

Hydrocortisone	0.5%
Diperodon Hydrochloride	0.5%
Zinc Oxide	5.0%

HOW SUPPLIED

15 gm. tubes and 1 lb. jars.

ANOQUAN ℞
[*an 'o-kwan*]

DESCRIPTION

Each capsule contains:

Butalbital	50 mg.
Caffeine	40 mg.
Acetaminophen	325 mg.

HOW SUPPLIED

Bottles of 1000's and 100's.

PHENATE
[fe'nate]

DESCRIPTION
Each timed release tablet contains:
Acetaminophen .... 325 mg.
Chlorpheniramine Maleate .... 4 mg
Phenylpropanolamine HCl .... 40 mg.

HOW SUPPLIED
Bottles of 1000 and 100 tablets.

Marion Laboratories, Inc.
Pharmaceutical Products Division
MARION INDUSTRIAL PARK
MARION PARK DRIVE
KANSAS CITY, MO 64137

PRODUCT IDENTIFICATION NUMERICAL SUMMARY SOLID ORAL DOSAGE FORMS

Marion Laboratories, Inc.
Kansas City, MO 64137
To provide quick and positive identification of Marion Laboratories prescription drug products, we have imprinted an identifying number and the name MARION on the following tablets or capsules.

1375 DITROPAN® Tablets (oxybutynin chloride)
1550 NITRO-BID® Capsules, 2.5 mg (nitroglycerin)
1551 NITRO-BID® Capsules, 6.5 mg (nitroglycerin)
1553 NITRO-BID® Capsules, 9 mg (nitroglycerin)
1555 PAVABID® Capsules, 150 mg (papaverine hydrochloride)*
1712 CARAFATE® Tablets, 1 gm (sucralfate)
1771 CARDIZEM® Tablets, 30 mg (diltiazem hydrochloride)
1772 CARDIZEM® Tablets, 60 mg (diltiazem hydrochloride)

PAVABID® HP Capsulets, 300 mg (papaverine hydrochloride) is identified by the name MARION on one side and PAVABID HP on the reverse side.
*PAVABID Capsules, 150 mg (papaverine hydrochloride) also bear the brand name PAVABID.

CARAFATE® Tablets ℞
[kar'af-āt]
(sucralfate) 1 gm

DESCRIPTION
CARAFATE® (sucralfate) is α-D-Glucopyranoside, β-D-fructofuranosyl-, octakis-(hydrogen sulfate), aluminum complex.
Tablets for oral administration contain 1 gm of sucralfate.
Also contains: D&C Red # 30 Lake, FD&C Blue # 1 Lake, magnesium stearate, microcrystalline cellulose, and starch.
Therapeutic category: antiulcer

CLINICAL PHARMACOLOGY
Sucralfate is only minimally absorbed from the gastrointestinal tract. The small amounts of the sulfated disaccharide that are absorbed are excreted primarily in the urine.
Although the mechanism of sucralfate's ability to accelerate healing of duodenal ulcers remains to be fully defined, it is known that it exerts its effect through a local, rather than systemic, action. The following observations also appear pertinent:
1. Studies in human subjects and with animal models of ulcer disease have shown that sucralfate forms an ulcer-adherent complex with proteinaceous exudate at the ulcer site.
2. In vitro, a sucralfate-albumin film provides a barrier to diffusion of hydrogen ions.
3. In human subjects, sucralfate given in doses recommended for ulcer therapy inhibits pepsin activity in gastric juice by 32%.
4. In vitro, sucralfate adsorbs bile salts.

These observations suggest that sucralfate's antiulcer activity is the result of formation of an ulcer-adherent complex that covers the ulcer site and protects it against further attack by acid, pepsin, and bile salts. Sucralfate has negligible acid-neutralizing capacity, and its antiulcer effects cannot be attributed to neutralization of gastric acid.

CLINICAL TRIALS
Over 600 patients have participated in well-controlled clinical trials worldwide. Multicenter trials conducted in the United States, both of them placebo-controlled studies with endoscopic evaluation at 2 and 4 weeks, showed:

STUDY 1

Treatment Groups	Ulcer Healing/No. Patients	
	2 wk	4 wk [Overall]
Sucralfate	37/105 (35.2%)	82/109 (75.2%)
Placebo	26/106 (24.5%)	68/107 (63.6%)

STUDY 2

Treatment Groups	Ulcer Healing/No. Patients	
	2 wk	4 wk [Overall]
Sucralfate	8/24 (33%)	22/24 (92%)
Placebo	4/31 (13%)	18/31 (58%)

The sucralfate-placebo differences were statistically significant in both studies at 4 weeks but not at 2 weeks. The poorer result in the first study may have occurred because sucralfate was given two hours after meals and at bedtime rather than one hour before meals and at bedtime, the regimen used in international studies and in the second United States study. In addition, in the first study liquid antacid was utilized as needed, whereas in the second study antacid tablets were used.

INDICATIONS AND USAGE
CARAFATE (sucralfate) is indicated in the short-term (up to 8 weeks) treatment of duodenal ulcer.
Antacids may be prescribed as needed for relief of pain.

CONTRAINDICATIONS
There are no known contraindications to the use of sucralfate.

PRECAUTIONS
Duodenal ulcer is a chronic, recurrent disease. While short-term treatment with sucralfate can result in complete healing of the ulcer, a successful course of treatment with sucralfate should not be expected to alter the post-healing frequency or severity of duodenal ulceration.
Drug Interactions: Animal studies have shown that simultaneous administration of CARAFATE (sucralfate) with tetracycline, phenytoin, digoxin, or cimetidine will result in a statistically significant reduction in the bioavailability of these agents. The bioavailability of these agents may be restored simply by separating the administration of these agents from that of CARAFATE by two hours. This interaction appears to be nonsystemic in origin, presumably resulting from these agents being bound by CARAFATE in the gastrointestinal tract. The clinical significance of these animal studies is yet to be defined. However, because of the potential of CARAFATE to alter the absorption of some drugs from the gastrointestinal tract, the separate administration of CARAFATE from that of other agents should be considered when alterations in bioavailability are felt to be critical for concomitantly administered drugs.
Carcinogenesis, Mutagenesis, Impairment of Fertility: Chronic oral toxicity studies of 24 months' duration were conducted in mice and rats at doses up to 1 gm/kg (12 times the human dose). There was no evidence of drug-related tumorigenicity. A reproduction study in rats at doses up to 38 times the human dose did not reveal any indication of fertility impairment. Mutagenicity studies were not conducted.
Pregnancy: Teratogenic effects. Pregnancy Category B. Teratogenicity studies have been performed in mice, rats, and rabbits at doses up to 50 times the human dose and have revealed no evidence of harm to the fetus due to sucralfate. There are, however, no adequate and well-controlled studies in pregnant women. Because animal reproduction studies are not always predictive of human response, this drug should be used during pregnancy only if clearly needed.
Nursing Mothers: It is not known whether this drug is excreted in human milk. Because many drugs are excreted in human milk, caution should be exercised when sucralfate is administered to a nursing woman.
Pediatric Use: Safety and effectiveness in children have not been established.

ADVERSE REACTIONS
Adverse reactions to sucralfate in clinical trials were minor and only rarely led to discontinuation of the drug. In studies involving over 2,500 patients treated with sucralfate, adverse effects were reported in 121 (4.7%).
Constipation was the most frequent complaint (2.2%). Other adverse effects, reported in no more than one of every 350 patients, were diarrhea, nausea, gastric discomfort, indigestion, dry mouth, rash, pruritus, back pain, dizziness, sleepiness, and vertigo.

OVERDOSAGE
There is no experience in humans with overdosage. Acute oral toxicity studies in animals, however, using doses up to 12 gm/kg body weight, could not find a lethal dose. Risks associated with overdosage should, therefore, be minimal.

DOSAGE AND ADMINISTRATION
The recommended adult oral dosage for duodenal ulcer is 1 gm four times a day on an empty stomach.
Antacids may be prescribed as needed for relief of pain but should not be taken within one-half hour before or after sucralfate.
While healing with sucralfate may occur during the first week or two, treatment should be continued for 4 to 8 weeks unless healing has been demonstrated by x-ray or endoscopic examination.

HOW SUPPLIED
CARAFATE (sucralfate) 1-gm tablets are supplied in bottles of 100 (NDC 0088-1712-47) and in Unit Dose Identification Paks of 100 (NDC 0088-1712-49). Light-pink 1-gm tablets are embossed with MARION/1712.

Issued 9/85

Shown in Product Identification Section, page 415

CARDIZEM® Tablets ℞
[kar'diz-em]
(diltiazem HCl)
30 mg and 60 mg

DESCRIPTION
CARDIZEM® (diltiazem hydrochloride) is a calcium ion influx inhibitor (slow channel blocker or calcium antagonist). Chemically, diltiazem hydrochloride is 1,5-Benzothiazepin-4(5H)one,3- (acetyloxy) -5-[2-(dimethylamino)ethyl]-2,3-dihydro-2-(4-methoxyphenyl)-,monohydrochloride,(+) -cis-.
Diltiazem hydrochloride is a white to off-white crystalline powder with a bitter taste. It is soluble in water, methanol, and chloroform. It has a molecular weight of 450.98. Each tablet of CARDIZEM contains either 30 mg or 60 mg diltiazem hydrochloride.
Also contains: acetylated monoglyceride, D&C Yellow #10, ethylcellulose, FD&C Yellow #6 (60 mg) or FD&C Blue #1 (30 mg), hydroxypropyl methylcellulose, lactose, magnesium stearate, talc, and other ingredients.
For oral administration.

CLINICAL PHARMACOLOGY
The therapeutic benefits achieved with CARDIZEM are believed to be related to its ability to inhibit the influx of calcium ions during membrane depolarization of cardiac and vascular smooth muscle.
Mechanisms of Action. Although precise mechanisms of its antianginal actions are still being delineated, CARDIZEM is believed to act in the following ways:
1. Angina Due to Coronary Artery Spasm: CARDIZEM has been shown to be a potent dilator of coronary arteries both epicardial and subendocardial. Spontaneous and ergonovine-induced coronary artery spasm are inhibited by CARDIZEM.
2. Exertional Angina: CARDIZEM has been shown to produce increases in exercise tolerance, probably due to its ability to reduce myocardial oxygen demand. This is accomplished via reductions in heart rate and systemic blood pressure at submaximal and maximal exercise work loads.

In animal models, diltiazem interferes with the slow inward (depolarizing) current in excitable tissue. It causes excitation-contraction uncoupling in various myocardial tissues without changes in the configuration of the action potential. Diltiazem produces relaxation of coronary vascular smooth muscle and dilation of both large and small coronary arteries at drug levels which cause little or no negative inotropic effect. The resultant increases in coronary blood flow (epicardial and subendocardial) occur in ischemic and nonischemic models and are accompanied by dose-dependent decreases in systemic blood pressure and decreases in peripheral resistance.
Hemodynamic and Electrophysiologic Effects: Like other calcium antagonists, diltiazem decreases sinoatrial and atrioventricular conduction in isolated tissues and has a negative inotropic effect in isolated preparations. In the intact animal, prolongation of the AH interval can be seen at higher doses.
In man, diltiazem prevents spontaneous and ergonovine-provoked coronary artery spasm. It causes a decrease in peripheral vascular resistance and a modest fall in blood pressure and, in exercise tolerance studies in patients with ischemic heart disease, reduces the heart rate-blood pressure product for any given work load. Studies to date, primarily in patients with good ventricular function, have not revealed evidence of a negative inotropic effect; cardiac output, ejection fraction, and left ventricular end diastolic pressure have not been affected. There are as yet few data on the interaction of diltiazem and beta-blockers. Resting heart rate is usually unchanged or slightly reduced by diltiazem.
Intravenous diltiazem in doses of 20 mg prolongs AH conduction time and AV node functional and effective refractory periods approximately 20%. In a study involving single oral doses of 300 mg of CARDIZEM in six normal volunteers, the average maximum PR prolongation was 14% with no instances of greater than first-degree AV block. Diltiazem-associated prolongation of the AH interval is not more pronounced in patients with first-degree heart block. In patients with sick sinus syndrome, diltiazem significantly prolongs sinus cycle length (up to 50% in some cases).

Continued on next page

Marion—Cont.

Chronic oral administration of CARDIZEM in doses of up to 240 mg/day has resulted in small increases in PR interval, but has not usually produced abnormal prolongation. There were, however, three instances of second-degree AV block and one instance of third-degree AV block in a group of 959 chronically treated patients.

Pharmacokinetics and Metabolism. Diltiazem is absorbed from the tablet formulation to about 80% of a reference capsule and is subject to an extensive first pass effect, giving an absolute bioavailability (compared to intravenous dosing) of about 40%. CARDIZEM undergoes extensive hepatic metabolism in which 2% to 4% of the unchanged drug appears in the urine. In vitro binding studies show CARDIZEM is 70% to 80% bound to plasma proteins. Competitive ligand binding studies have also shown CARDIZEM binding is not altered by therapeutic concentrations of digoxin, hydrochlorothiazide, phenylbutazone, propranolol, salicylic acid, or warfarin. Single oral doses of 30 to 120 mg of CARDIZEM result in detectable plasma levels within 30 to 60 minutes and peak plasma levels two to three hours after drug administration. The plasma elimination half-life following single or multiple drug administration is approximately 3.5 hours. Desacetyl diltiazem is also present in the plasma at levels of 10% to 20% of the parent drug and is 25% to 50% as potent as a coronary vasodilator as diltiazem. Therapeutic blood levels of CARDIZEM appear to be in the range of 50–200 ng/ml. There is a departure from dose-linearity when single doses above 60 mg are given; a 120-mg dose gave blood levels three times that of the 60-mg dose. There is no information about the effect of renal or hepatic impairment on excretion or metabolism of diltiazem.

INDICATIONS AND USAGE

1. **Angina Pectoris Due to Coronary Artery Spasm.** CARDIZEM is indicated in the treatment of angina pectoris due to coronary artery spasm. CARDIZEM has been shown effective in the treatment of spontaneous coronary artery spasm presenting as Prinzmetal's variant angina (resting angina with ST-segment elevation occurring during attacks).
2. **Chronic Stable Angina [Classic Effort-Associated Angina].** CARDIZEM is indicated in the management of chronic stable angina in patients who cannot tolerate therapy with beta-blockers and/or nitrates or who remain symptomatic despite adequate doses of these agents. CARDIZEM has been effective in short-term controlled trials in reducing angina frequency and increasing exercise tolerance, but confirmation of sustained effectiveness is incomplete.

There are few controlled studies of the effectiveness of the concomitant use of diltiazem and beta-blockers or of the safety of this combination in patients with impaired ventricular function or conduction abnormalities.

CONTRAINDICATIONS

CARDIZEM is contraindicated in (1) patients with sick sinus syndrome except in the presence of a functioning ventricular pacemaker, (2) patients with second- or third-degree AV block except in the presence of a functioning ventricular pacemaker, and (3) patients with hypotension (less than 90 mm Hg systolic).

WARNINGS

1. **Cardiac Conduction.** CARDIZEM prolongs AV node refractory periods without significantly prolonging sinus node recovery time, except in patients with sick sinus syndrome. This effect may rarely result in abnormally slow heart rates (particularly in patients with sick sinus syndrome) or second- or third-degree AV block (six of 1,243 patients for 0.48%). Concomitant use of diltiazem with beta-blockers or digitalis may result in additive effects on cardiac conduction. A patient with Prinzmetal's angina developed periods of asystole (2 to 5 seconds) after a single dose of 60 mg of diltiazem.
2. **Congestive Heart Failure.** Although diltiazem has a negative inotropic effect in isolated animal tissue preparations, hemodynamic studies in humans with normal ventricular function have not shown a reduction in cardiac index nor consistent negative effects on contractility (dp/dt). Experience with the use of CARDIZEM alone or in combination with beta-blockers in patients with impaired ventricular function is very limited. Caution should be exercised when using the drug in such patients.
3. **Hypotension.** Decreases in blood pressure associated with CARDIZEM therapy may occasionally result in symptomatic hypotension.
4. **Acute Hepatic Injury.** In rare instances, significant elevations in enzymes such as alkaline phosphatase, CPK, LDH, SGOT, SGPT, and other symptoms consistent with acute hepatic injury have been noted. These reactions have been reversible upon discontinuation of drug therapy. The relationship to CARDIZEM is uncertain in most cases, but probable in some. (See PRECAUTIONS.)

PRECAUTIONS

General. CARDIZEM (diltiazem hydrochloride) is extensively metabolized by the liver and excreted by the kidneys and in bile. As with any new drug given over prolonged periods, laboratory parameters should be monitored at regular intervals. The drug should be used with caution in patients with impaired renal or hepatic function. In subacute and chronic dog and rat studies designed to produce toxicity, high doses of diltiazem were associated with hepatic damage. In special subacute hepatic studies, oral doses of 125 mg/kg and higher in rats were associated with histological changes in the liver which were reversible when the drug was discontinued. In dogs, doses of 20 mg/kg were also associated with hepatic changes; however, these changes were reversible with continued dosing.

Drug Interaction. Pharmacologic studies indicate that there may be additive effects in prolonging AV conduction when using beta-blockers or digitalis concomitantly with CARDIZEM. (See WARNINGS.)

Controlled and uncontrolled domestic studies suggest that concomitant use of CARDIZEM and beta-blockers or digitalis is usually well tolerated. Available data are not sufficient, however, to predict the effects of concomitant treatment, particularly in patients with left ventricular dysfunction or cardiac conduction abnormalities. In healthy volunteers, diltiazem has been shown to increase serum digoxin levels up to 20%.

Carcinogenesis, Mutagenesis, Impairment of Fertility. A 24-month study in rats and a 21-month study in mice showed no evidence of carcinogenicity. There was also no mutagenic response in in vitro bacterial tests. No intrinsic effect on fertility was observed in rats.

Pregnancy. Category C. Reproduction studies have been conducted in mice, rats, and rabbits. Administration of doses ranging from five to ten times greater (on a mg/kg basis) than the daily recommended therapeutic dose has resulted in embryo and fetal lethality. These doses, in some studies, have been reported to cause skeletal abnormalities. In the perinatal/postnatal studies there was some reduction in early individual pup weights and survival rates. There was an increased incidence of stillbirths at doses of 20 times the human dose or greater.

There are no well-controlled studies in pregnant women; therefore, use CARDIZEM in pregnant women only if the potential benefit justifies the potential risk to the fetus.

Nursing Mothers. Diltiazem is excreted in human milk. One report suggests that concentrations in breast milk may approximate serum levels. If use of CARDIZEM is deemed essential, an alternative method of infant feeding should be instituted.

Pediatric Use. Safety and effectiveness in children have not been established.

ADVERSE REACTIONS

Serious adverse reactions have been rare in studies carried out to date, but it should be recognized that patients with impaired ventricular function and cardiac conduction abnormalities have usually been excluded.

In domestic placebo-controlled trials, the incidence of adverse reactions reported during CARDIZEM therapy was not greater than that reported during placebo therapy.

The following represent occurrences observed in clinical studies which can be at least reasonably associated with the pharmacology of calcium influx inhibition. In many cases, the relationship to CARDIZEM has not been established. The most common occurrences as well as their frequency of presentation are: edema (2.4%), headache (2.1%), nausea (1.9%), dizziness (1.5%), rash (1.3%), asthenia (1.2%). In addition, the following events were reported infrequently (less than 1%):

Cardiovascular: Angina, arrhythmia, AV block (first degree), AV block (second or third degree—see conduction warning), bradycardia, congestive heart failure, flushing, hypotension, palpitations, syncope.

Nervous System: Amnesia, gait abnormality, hallucinations, insomnia, nervousness, paresthesia, personality change, somnolence, tinnitus, tremor.

Gastrointestinal: Anorexia, constipation, diarrhea, dysgeusia, dyspepsia, mild elevations of alkaline phosphatase, SGOT, SGPT, and LDH (see hepatic warnings), vomiting, weight increase.

Dermatologic: Petechiae, pruritus, photosensitivity, urticaria.

Other: Amblyopia, dyspnea, epistaxis, eye irritation, hyperglycemia, nasal congestion, nocturia, osteoarticular pain, polyuria, sexual difficulties.

The following postmarketing events have been reported infrequently in patients receiving CARDIZEM: alopecia, gingival hyperplasia, erythema multiforme, and leukopenia. However, a definitive cause and effect between these events and CARDIZEM therapy is yet to be established.

Overdosage or Exaggerated Response: Overdosage experience with oral diltiazem has been limited. Single oral doses of 300 mg of CARDIZEM have been well tolerated by healthy volunteers. In the event of overdosage or exaggerated response, appropriate supportive measures should be employed in addition to gastric lavage. The following measures may be considered:

Bradycardia: Administer atropine (0.60 to 1.0 mg). If there is no response to vagal blockade, administer isoproterenol cautiously.

High-Degree AV Block: Treat as for bradycardia above. Fixed high-degree AV block should be treated with cardiac pacing.

Cardiac Failure: Administer inotropic agents (isoproterenol, dopamine, or dobutamine) and diuretics.

Hypotension: Vasopressors (eg, dopamine or levarterenol bitartrate).

Actual treatment and dosage should depend on the severity of the clinical situation and the judgment and experience of the treating physician.

The oral LD_{50}'s in mice and rats range from 415 to 740 mg/kg and from 560 to 810 mg/kg, respectively. The intravenous LD_{50}'s in these species were 60 and 38 mg/kg, respectively. The oral LD_{50} in dogs is considered to be in excess of 50 mg/kg, while lethality was seen in monkeys at 360 mg/kg. The toxic dose in man is not known, but blood levels in excess of 800 ng/ml have not been associated with toxicity.

DOSAGE AND ADMINISTRATION

Exertional Angina Pectoris Due to Atherosclerotic Coronary Artery Disease or Angina Pectoris at Rest Due to Coronary Artery Spasm. Dosage must be adjusted to each patient's needs. Starting with 30 mg four times daily, before meals and at bedtime, dosage should be increased gradually (given in divided doses three or four times daily) at one- to two-day intervals until optimum response is obtained. Although individual patients may respond to any dosage level, the average optimum dosage range appears to be 180 to 360 mg/day. There are no available data concerning dosage requirements in patients with impaired renal or hepatic function. If the drug must be used in such patients, titration should be carried out with particular caution.

Concomitant Use With Other Antianginal Agents.

1. **Sublingual NTG** may be taken as required to abort acute anginal attacks during CARDIZEM therapy.
2. **Prophylactic Nitrate Therapy**—CARDIZEM may be safely coadministered with short- and long-acting nitrates, but there have been no controlled studies to evaluate the antianginal effectiveness of this combination.
3. **Beta-blockers.** (See WARNINGS and PRECAUTIONS.)

HOW SUPPLIED

CARDIZEM 30-mg tablets are supplied in bottles of 100 (NDC 0088-1771-47) and in Unit Dose Identification Paks of 100 (NDC 0088-1771-49). Each green tablet is engraved with MARION on one side and 1771 engraved on the other. CARDIZEM 60-mg scored tablets are supplied in bottles of 100 (NDC 0088-1772-47) and in Unit Dose Identification Paks of 100 (NDC 0088-1772-49). Each yellow tablet is engraved with MARION on one side and 1772 on the other.

Issued 7/86

Shown in Product Identification Section, page 415

DEBROX® Drops — OTC

[de'brox]

DESCRIPTION

Carbamide peroxide 6.5%. Also contains citric acid, glycerin, propylene glycol, sodium stannate, water, and other ingredients.

ACTIONS

DEBROX®, used as directed, cleanses the ear with sustained microfoam. DEBROX Drops foam on contact with earwax due to the release of oxygen.

INDICATIONS

DEBROX Drops provide a safe, nonirritating method of softening and removing earwax.

DIRECTIONS

Use directly from bottle. Tilt head sideways and squeeze bottle gently so that 5 to 10 drops flow into ear. Tip of bottle should not enter ear canal. Keep drops in ear for several minutes while head remains tilted or by inserting cotton. Repeat twice daily for up to four days if needed or as directed by physician. Any remaining wax may be removed by flushing with warm water, using a soft rubber bulb ear syringe. Avoid excessive pressure.

WARNINGS

Do not use if you have ear drainage or discharge, ear pain, irritation or rash in the ear, or are dizzy, unless directed by a physician. Do not use if you have an injury or perforation (hole) of the eardrum or after ear surgery, unless directed by a physician. Do not use for more than four consecutive days. If excessive earwax remains after use of this product, consult a physician. Consult a physician prior to use in children under 12.

CAUTIONS

Avoid exposing bottle to excessive heat and direct sunlight. Keep color tip on bottle when not in use. Avoid contact with eyes. Keep this and all drugs out of the reach of children. In case of accidental ingestion, seek professional assistance or contact a poison control center immediately.

HOW SUPPLIED

DEBROX Drops are available in ½- or 1-fl-oz plastic squeeze bottles with applicator spouts.

Issued 2/86

DITROPAN® Tablets and Syrup ℞

[*di 'tro-pan*]

(oxybutynin chloride)

DESCRIPTION

Each scored biconvex, engraved blue DITROPAN® Tablet contains 5 mg of oxybutynin chloride. Each 5 ml of DITROPAN® Syrup contains 5 mg of oxybutynin chloride. Chemically, oxybutynin chloride is the *dl*-(racemic) form of 4-diethylamino-2-butynyl phenylcyclohexylglycolate hydrochloride. The empirical formula of oxybutynin chloride is $C_{22}H_{32}Cl\ NO_3$.

Oxybutynin chloride is a white crystalline solid with a molecular weight of 393.9. It is readily soluble in water and acids, but relatively insoluble in alkalis.

DITROPAN® Tablets

Also contains: calcium stearate, FD&C Blue #1 Lake, lactose, and microcrystalline cellulose.

DITROPAN® Syrup

Also contains citric acid, FD&C Green #3, glycerin, methylparaben, flavor, sodium citrate, sorbitol, sucrose, and water.

ACTION

DITROPAN® (oxybutynin chloride) exerts direct antispasmodic effect on smooth muscle and inhibits the muscarinic action of acetylcholine on smooth muscle. DITROPAN exhibits only one fifth of the anticholinergic activity of atropine on the rabbit detrusor muscle, but four to ten times the antispasmodic activity. No blocking effects occur at skeletal neuromuscular junctions or autonomic ganglia (antinicotinic effects).

In patients with uninhibited neurogenic and reflex neurogenic bladder, cystometric studies have demonstrated that DITROPAN increases vesical capacity, diminishes the frequency of uninhibited contractions of the detrusor muscle and delays the initial desire to void. These effects are more consistently improved in patients with uninhibited neurogenic bladder.

DITROPAN was well tolerated in patients administered the drug in controlled studies of 30 days' duration and in uncontrolled studies in which some of the patients received the drug for two years.

INDICATIONS

DITROPAN® (oxybutynin chloride) is indicated for the relief of symptoms associated with voiding in patients with uninhibited neurogenic and reflex neurogenic bladder.

Pretreatment examination should include cystometry and other appropriate diagnostic procedures.

Cystometry should be repeated at appropriate intervals to evaluate response to therapy. The appropriate antimicrobial therapy should be instituted in the presence of infection.

CONTRAINDICATIONS

DITROPAN® (oxybutynin chloride) is contraindicated in patients with glaucoma. It is also contraindicated in partial or complete obstruction of the gastrointestinal tract, paralytic ileus, intestinal atony of the elderly or debilitated patient, megacolon, toxic megacolon complicating ulcerative colitis, severe colitis, and myasthenia gravis. It is contraindicated in patients with obstructive uropathy and in patients with unstable cardiovascular status in acute hemorrhage.

WARNINGS

DITROPAN® (oxybutynin chloride), when administered in the presence of high environmental temperature, can cause heat prostration (fever and heat stroke due to decreased sweating).

Diarrhea may be an early symptom of incomplete intestinal obstruction, especially in patients with ileostomy or colostomy. In this instance treatment with DITROPAN would be inappropriate and possibly harmful.

DITROPAN may produce drowsiness or blurred vision. The patient should be cautioned regarding activities requiring mental alertness such as operating a motor vehicle or other machinery or performing hazardous work while taking this drug.

PREGNANCY

Reproduction studies in the hamster, rabbit, rat, and mouse have shown no definite evidence of impaired fertility or harm to the animal fetus. The safety of DITROPAN administered to women who are or who may become pregnant has not been established. Therefore, DITROPAN should not be given to pregnant women unless, in the judgment of the physician, the probable clinical benefits outweigh the possible hazards.

USAGE IN CHILDREN

The safety and efficacy of DITROPAN administration have been demonstrated for children five years of age and older (see DOSAGE AND ADMINISTRATION). However, as there is insufficient clinical data for children under age five, DITROPAN is not recommended for this age group.

PRECAUTIONS

DITROPAN® (oxybutynin chloride) should be used with caution in the elderly and in all patients with autonomic neuropathy, hepatic or renal disease. Administration of DITROPAN in large doses to patients with ulcerative colitis may suppress intestinal motility to the point of producing a paralytic ileus and precipitate or aggravate toxic megacolon, a serious complication of the disease.

The symptoms of hyperthyroidism, coronary heart disease, congestive heart failure, cardiac arrhythmias, tachycardia, hypertension, and prostatic hypertrophy may be aggravated following administration of DITROPAN. DITROPAN should be administered with caution to patients with hiatal hernia associated with reflux esophagitis, since anticholinergic drugs may aggravate this condition.

ADVERSE REACTIONS

Following administration of DITROPAN® (oxybutynin chloride), the symptoms that can be associated with the use of other anticholinergic drugs may occur: dry mouth, decreased sweating, urinary hesitance and retention, blurred vision, tachycardia, palpitations, dilatation of the pupil, cycloplegia, increased ocular tension, drowsiness, weakness, dizziness, insomnia, nausea, vomiting, constipation, bloated feeling, impotence, suppression of lactation, severe allergic reactions or drug idiosyncrasies including urticaria and other dermal manifestations.

DOSAGE AND ADMINISTRATION

Tablets

Adults: The usual dose is one 5-mg tablet two to three times a day. The maximum recommended dose is one 5-mg tablet four times a day.

Children over 5 years of age: The usual dose is one 5-mg tablet two times a day. The maximum recommended dose is one 5-mg tablet three times a day.

Syrup

Adults: The usual dose is one teaspoon (5 mg/5 ml) syrup two to three times a day. The maximum recommended dose is one teaspoon (5 mg/5 ml) syrup four times a day.

Children over 5 years of age: The usual dose is one teaspoon (5 mg/5 ml) two times a day. The maximum recommended dose is one teaspoon (5 mg/5 ml) three times a day.

OVERDOSAGE

The symptoms of overdosage with DITROPAN® (oxybutynin chloride) progress from an intensification of the usual side effects of CNS disturbance (from restlessness and excitement to psychotic behavior), circulatory changes (flushing, fall in blood pressure, circulatory failure), respiratory failure, paralysis, and coma.

Measures to be taken are (1) immediate lavage of the stomach and (2) injection of physostigmine 0.5 to 2 mg intravenously, and repeated as necessary up to a total of 5 mg. Fever may be treated symptomatically (alcohol sponging, ice packs). Excitement of a degree which demands attention may be managed with sodium thiopental 2% solution given slowly intravenously or chloral hydrate (100 to 200 ml of a 2% solution) by rectal infusion. In the event of progression of the curare-like effect to paralysis of the respiratory muscles, artificial respiration is required.

HOW SUPPLIED

DITROPAN® (oxybutynin chloride) tablets are supplied in bottles of 100 tablets (NDC 0088-1375-47) and 1,000 tablets (NDC 0088-1375-58) and in Unit Dose Identification Paks of 100 tablets (NDC 0088-1375-49). Blue scored tablets are engraved with Marion on one side and 1375 on the other side.

DITROPAN® Syrup is supplied in bottles of 16 fluid ounces (473 ml) (NDC 0088-1373-18).

Pharmacist: Dispense in tight, light-resistant container as defined in the USP.

Store at controlled room temperature (59°–86°F).

Issued 9/85

Shown in Product Identification Section, page 415

GAVISCON® Antacid Tablets OTC

[*gav 'is-kon*]

COMPOSITION

Each chewable tablet contains the following active ingredients:

Aluminum hydroxide dried gel .... 80 mg
Magnesium trisilicate .... 20 mg

and the following inactive ingredients: alginic acid, calcium stearate, flavor, sodium bicarbonate, starch (may contain cornstarch), and sucrose.

INDICATIONS

GAVISCON is specifically formulated for the temporary relief of heartburn (acid indigestion) due to acid reflux. GAVISCON is not indicated for the treatment of peptic ulcers.

DIRECTIONS

Chew two to four tablets four times a day or as directed by a physician. Tablets should be taken after meals and at bedtime or as needed. For best results follow by a half glass of water or other liquid. Do not swallow whole.

WARNINGS

Do not take more than 16 tablets in a 24-hour period or 16 tablets daily for more than 2 weeks, except under the advice and supervision of a physician. Do not use this product except under the advice and supervision of a physician if you are on a sodium-restricted diet. Each GAVISCON Tablet contains approximately 0.8 mEq sodium.

DRUG INTERACTION PRECAUTIONS

Do not take this product if you are presently taking a prescription antibiotic drug containing any form of tetracycline.

Store at a controlled room temperature in a dry place.

Keep this and all drugs out of the reach of children.

In case of accidental overdose, seek professional assistance or contact a poison control center immediately.

HOW SUPPLIED

Available in bottle of 100 tablets and in foil-wrapped 2's in box of 30 tablets.

Issued 5/85

Shown in Product Identification Section, page 415

GAVISCON® Liquid Antacid OTC

[*gav 'is-kon*]

COMPOSITION

Each tablespoonful (15 ml) contains the following active ingredients:

Aluminum hydroxide .... 95 mg
Magnesium carbonate .... 412 mg

And the following inactive ingredients: D&C Yellow #10, edetate disodium, FD&C Blue #1, flavor, glycerin, paraben preservatives, saccharin sodium, sodium alginate, sorbitol solution, water, and xanthan gum.

INDICATIONS

For the relief of heartburn, sour stomach and/or acid indigestion, and upset stomach associated with heartburn, sour stomach and/or acid indigestion.

DIRECTIONS

Shake well before using. Take 1 or 2 tablespoonfuls four times a day or as directed by a physician. GAVISCON Liquid should be taken after meals and at bedtime, followed by half a glass of water.

Dispense product only by spoon or other measuring device.

WARNINGS

Except under the advice and supervision of a physician, do not take more than 8 tablespoonfuls in a 24-hour period or 8 tablespoonfuls daily for more than 2 weeks. May have laxative effect. Do not use this product if you have a kidney disease; do not use this product if you are on a sodium-restricted diet. Each tablespoonful of GAVISCON Liquid contains approximately 1.7 mEq sodium.

DRUG INTERACTION PRECAUTIONS

Do not take this product if you are presently taking a prescription antibiotic drug containing any form of tetracycline.

Keep tightly closed. Avoid freezing. Store at a controlled room temperature.

Keep this and all drugs out of the reach of children.

In case of accidental overdose, seek professional assistance or contact a poison control center immediately.

HOW SUPPLIED

Bottles of 12 fluid ounces (355 ml) and 6 fluid ounces (177 ml).

Issued 4/86

GAVISCON®-2 Antacid Tablets OTC

[*gav 'is-kon*]

COMPOSITION

Each chewable tablet contains the following active ingredients:

Aluminum hydroxide dried gel .... 160 mg
Magnesium trisilicate .... 40 mg

and the following inactive ingredients: alginic acid, calcium stearate, flavor, sodium bicarbonate, starch (may contain cornstarch), and sucrose.

Continued on next page

Marion—Cont.

INDICATIONS
GAVISCON is specifically formulated for the temporary relief of heartburn (acid indigestion) due to acid reflux. GAVISCON is not indicated for the treatment of peptic ulcers.

DIRECTIONS
Chew one to two tablets four times a day or as directed by a physician. Tablets should be taken after meals and at bedtime or as needed. For best results follow by a half glass of water or other liquid. Do not swallow whole.

WARNINGS
Do not take more than 8 tablets in a 24-hour period or 8 tablets daily for more than 2 weeks, except under the advice and supervision of a physician. Do not use this product except under the advice and supervision of a physician if you are on a sodium-restricted diet. Each GAVISCON-2 Tablet contains approximately 1.6 mEq sodium.

DRUG INTERACTION PRECAUTIONS
Do not take this product if you are presently taking a prescription antibiotic drug containing any form of tetracycline.
Store at a controlled room temperature in a dry place.
Keep this and all drugs out of the reach of children.
In case of accidental overdose, seek professional assistance or contact a poison control center immediately.

HOW SUPPLIED
Box of 48 foil-wrapped tablets.

Issued 5/85

Shown in Product Identification Section, page 415

GLY-OXIDE® Liquid — OTC
[*gli 'ok-sīd*]

DESCRIPTION
GLY-OXIDE® Liquid contains carbamide peroxide 10%, citric acid, flavor, glycerin, propylene glycol, sodium stannate, water, and other ingredients.

ACTIONS
GLY-OXIDE® Liquid has an oxygen-rich formula that works to relieve the pain of canker sores by cleaning and debriding damaged tissue so natural healing can occur.

INDICATIONS
For local treatment and hygienic prevention of minor oral inflammation such as canker sores, denture irritation, and postdental procedure irritation, place several drops on affected area four times daily, after meals and at bedtime, or as directed by a dentist or physician; expectorate after two or three minutes. Or place 10 drops onto tongue, mix with saliva, swish for several minutes, and expectorate.
As an adjunct to oral hygiene (orthodontics, dental appliances) after regular brushing, swish 10 or more drops vigorously. Continue for two to three minutes; expectorate.
When normal oral hygiene is inadequate or impossible (total care geriatrics, etc), swish 10 or more drops vigorously after meals and expectorate.

PRECAUTIONS
Severe or persistent oral inflammation, denture irritation, or gingivitus may be serious. If these conditions or unexpected side effects occur, consult a dentist or physician immediately.

DOSAGE AND ADMINISTRATION
Do not dilute. Apply directly from bottle. Replace color tip on bottle when not in use. Place several drops on affected area four times daily, after meals and at bedtime, or as directed by a dentist or physician; expectorate after two or three minutes. Or place 10 drops onto tongue, mix with saliva, swish for several minutes, and expectorate.
Avoid contact with eyes. Protect from heat and direct light. Keep this and all drugs out of the reach of children. In case of accidental overdose, seek professional assistance or contact a poison control center immediately.

HOW SUPPLIED
GLY-OXIDE® Liquid is available in ½-fl-oz and 2-fl-oz nonspill, plastic squeeze bottles with applicator spouts.

Issued 2/86

NITRO-BID® Plateau CAPS® — ℞
[*ni 'tro-bid*]
(nitroglycerin) 2.5 mg, 6.5 mg, 9 mg

DESCRIPTION
Each NITRO-BID® Controlled-Release Capsule contains:
2.5 mg nitroglycerin: Light purple and clear capsule with white beads; identification imprint MARION/1550.
6.5 mg nitroglycerin: Dark blue and yellow capsule with white beads; identification imprint MARION/1551.
9 mg nitroglycerin: Green and yellow capsule with white beads; identification imprint MARION/1553.
Also contains: calcium stearate, lactose, silica gel, starch, sucrose, talc, and other ingredients.

ACTION
The mechanism of action of nitroglycerin in the relief of angina pectoris is not as yet known. However, its main pharmacologic action is to relax smooth muscle, principally in the smaller blood vessels, thus dilating arterioles and capillaries, especially in the coronary circulation. In therapeutic doses, nitroglycerin is thought to increase the blood supply to the myocardium which may, in turn, relieve myocardial ischemia, the possible functional basis for the pain of angina pectoris. The sublingual administration of nitroglycerin is normally rapid and transient, but nitroglycerin in controlled-release NITRO-BID® 2.5, NITRO-BID® 6.5, and NITRO-BID® 9 produces a prolonged action.

INDICATIONS
Based on a review of this drug and a related drug by the National Academy of Sciences-National Research Council and/or other information, FDA has classified the indications as follows:
"Possibly" effective:
For the management, prophylaxis, or treatment of anginal attacks.
Final classification of the less-than-effective indications requires further investigation.

CONTRAINDICATIONS
Acute or recent myocardial infarction, severe anemia, closed-angle glaucoma, postural hypotension, increased intracranial pressure, and idiosyncrasy to the drug.

WARNINGS
Capsules must be swallowed. FOR ORAL, NOT SUBLINGUAL, USE. NITRO-BID® 2.5, NITRO-BID® 6.5, and NITRO-BID® 9 Controlled-Release Capsules are not intended for immediate relief of anginal attacks.

PRECAUTIONS
Intraocular pressure may be increased; therefore, caution is required in administering to patients with glaucoma. Tolerance to this drug and cross-tolerance to other organic nitrites and nitrates may occur. If blurring of vision, dryness of mouth, or lack of benefit occurs, the drug should be discontinued.

ADVERSE REACTIONS
Severe and persistent headaches, cutaneous flushing, dizziness, and weakness. Occasionally, drug rash or exfoliative dermatitis and nausea and vomiting may occur; these responses may disappear with a decrease in dosage. Adverse effects are enhanced by ingestion of alcohol, which appears to increase absorption from the gastrointestinal tract.

DOSAGE AND ADMINISTRATION
Administer the smallest effective dose two or three times daily at 8- to 12-hour intervals, unless clinical response suggests a different regimen. Patient should be titrated to anginal relief or hemodynamic response. Hemodynamic response can be measured by drop in systolic blood pressure. Discontinue if not effective.

HOW SUPPLIED
NITRO-BID® (nitroglycerin) 2.5, 6.5, and 9 Controlled-Release Capsules are available in 60- and 100-count bottles.

CAUTION
Federal law prohibits dispensing without prescription.

STORAGE
Store at a controlled room temperature. Dispense only in the original unopened container.

Issued 9/85

Shown in Product Identification Section, page 415

NITRO-BID® IV — ℞
[*ni 'tro-bid*]
(nitroglycerin)
FOR INTRAVENOUS USE ONLY

NOT FOR DIRECT INTRAVENOUS INJECTION. NITRO-BID IV MUST BE DILUTED IN DEXTROSE (5.0%) INJECTION, USP OR SODIUM CHLORIDE (0.9%) INJECTION, USP BEFORE INTRAVENOUS ADMINISTRATION. THE ADMINISTRATION SET USED FOR INFUSION MAY AFFECT THE AMOUNT OF NITRO-BID IV DELIVERED TO THE PATIENT. (SEE **WARNINGS** AND **DOSAGE AND ADMINISTRATION** SECTIONS.)
CAUTION: SEVERAL PREPARATIONS OF NITROGLYCERIN FOR INJECTION ARE AVAILABLE. THEY DIFFER IN CONCENTRATION AND/OR VOLUME PER VIAL. WHEN SWITCHING FROM ONE PRODUCT TO ANOTHER, ATTENTION MUST BE PAID TO THE DILUTION AND DOSAGE AND ADMINISTRATION INSTRUCTIONS.

DESCRIPTION
NITRO-BID IV (nitroglycerin) is a clear, practically colorless additive solution for intravenous infusion after dilution. Each milliliter contains 5 mg nitroglycerin and 45 mg propylene glycol dissolved in 70% ethanol.
The solution is sterile, nonpyrogenic, and nonexplosive. NITRO-BID IV, an organic nitrate, is a vasodilator. The chemical name for nitroglycerin is 1,2,3 propanetriol trinitrate.

CLINICAL PHARMACOLOGY
Relaxation of vascular smooth muscle is the principal pharmacologic action of NITRO-BID IV (nitroglycerin). Although venous effects predominate, nitroglycerin produces, in a dose-related manner, dilation of both arterial and venous beds. Dilation of the postcapillary vessels, including large veins, promotes peripheral pooling of blood and decreases venous return to the heart, reducing left ventricular end-diastolic pressure (preload). Arteriolar relaxation reduces systemic vascular resistance and arterial pressure (afterload). Myocardial oxygen consumption or demand (as measured by the pressure-rate product, tension-time index, and stroke-work index) is decreased by both the arterial and venous effects of nitroglycerin, and a more favorable supply-demand ratio can be achieved.
Therapeutic doses of intravenous nitroglycerin reduce systolic, diastolic, and mean arterial blood pressures. Effective coronary perfusion pressure is usually maintained, but can be compromised if blood pressure falls excessively or increased heart rate decreases diastolic filling time.
Elevated central venous and pulmonary capillary wedge pressures, pulmonary vascular resistance, and systemic vascular resistance are also reduced by nitroglycerin therapy.
Heart rate is usually slightly increased, presumably a reflex response to the fall in blood pressure. Cardiac index may be increased, decreased, or unchanged. Patients with elevated left ventricular filling pressure and systemic vascular resistance values in conjunction with a depressed cardiac index are likely to experience an improvement in cardiac index. On the other hand, when filling pressures and cardiac index are normal, cardiac index may be slightly reduced by intravenous nitroglycerin.
Nitroglycerin is widely distributed in the body with an apparent volume of distribution of approximately 200 liters in adult male subjects, and is rapidly metabolized to dinitrates and mononitrates, with a short half-life, estimated at one to four minutes. This results in a low plasma concentration after intravenous infusion. At plasma concentrations of between 50 and 100 ng/ml, the binding of nitroglycerin to plasma proteins is approximately 60%, while that of 1,2 dinitroglycerin and 1,3 dinitroglycerin is 60% and 30%, respectively. The activity and half-life of the dinitroglycerins are not well characterized. The mononitrate is not active.

INDICATIONS AND USAGE
NITRO-BID IV (nitroglycerin) is indicated for:

1. **Control of blood pressure in perioperative hypertension,** ie, hypertension associated with surgical procedures, especially cardiovascular procedures, such as the hypertension seen during intratracheal intubation, anesthesia, skin incision, sternotomy, cardiac bypass, and in the immediate postsurgical period.
2. **Congestive heart failure associated with acute myocardial infarction.**
3. **Treatment of angina pectoris** in patients who have not responded to recommended doses of organic nitrates and/or a beta-blocker.
4. **Production of controlled hypotension during surgical procedures.**

CONTRAINDICATIONS
NITRO-BID IV (nitroglycerin) should not be administered to individuals with:

1. A known hypersensitivity to nitroglycerin or a known idiosyncratic reaction to organic nitrates.
2. Hypotension or uncorrected hypovolemia, as the use of NITRO-BID IV in such states could produce severe hypotension or shock.
3. Increased intracranial pressure (eg, head trauma or cerebral hemorrhage).
4. Inadequate cerebral circulation, constrictive pericarditis, and pericardial tamponade.

WARNINGS

1. Nitroglycerin readily migrates into many plastics. To avoid absorption of nitroglycerin into plastic parenteral solution containers, the dilution and storage of nitroglycerin for intravenous infusion should be made only in glass parenteral solution bottles.
2. Some filters also absorb nitroglycerin; they should be avoided.
3. Forty percent to 80% of the total amount of nitroglycerin in the final diluted solution for infusion is absorbed by the polyvinyl chloride (PVC) tubing of the intravenous administration sets currently in general use. The higher rates of absorption occur when flow rates are low,

nitroglycerin concentrations are high, and tubing is long. Although the rate of loss is highest during the early phase of administration (when flow rates are lowest), the loss is neither constant nor self-limiting; consequently, no simple calculation or correction can be performed to convert the theoretical infusion rate (based on the concentration of the infusion solution) to the actual delivery rate. Because of this problem, Marion Laboratories recommends the use of the least absorptive infusion tubing available for infusions of NITRO-BID IV. DOSING INSTRUCTIONS MUST BE FOLLOWED WITH CARE. IT SHOULD BE NOTED THAT WHEN THESE INFUSION SETS ARE USED, THE CALCULATED DOSE WILL BE DELIVERED TO THE PATIENT DEPENDENT UPON THE LOSS OF NITROGLYCERIN DUE TO ABSORPTIVE TUBING. NOTE THAT THE DOSAGES COMMONLY USED IN PUBLISHED STUDIES UTILIZED GENERAL-USE PVC TUBING, AND RECOMMENDED DOSES BASED ON THIS EXPERIENCE ARE TOO HIGH IF NEW, LESS ABSORPTIVE INFUSION TUBING IS USED.

4. PROTECT FROM LIGHT UNTIL READY FOR USE.
5. NITRO-BID IV VIALS ARE INTENDED FOR SINGLE-DOSE ONLY. PROPERLY DISCARD ANY UNUSED PORTION.

PRECAUTIONS

NITRO-BID IV (nitroglycerin) should be used with caution in patients who have severe hepatic or renal disease.

Excessive hypotension, especially for prolonged periods of time, must be avoided because of possible deleterious effects on the brain, heart, liver, and kidney from poor perfusion and the attendant risk of ischemia, thrombosis, and altered function of these organs. Patients with normal or low pulmonary capillary wedge pressure are especially sensitive to the hypotensive effects of NITRO-BID IV. If pulmonary capillary wedge pressure is being monitored, it will be noted that a fall in wedge pressure precedes the onset of arterial hypotension, and the pulmonary capillary wedge pressure is thus a useful guide to safe titration of the drug.

Carcinogenesis, Mutagenesis, Impairment of Fertility: No long-term studies in animals were performed to evaluate carcinogenic potential of NITRO-BID IV (nitroglycerin).

Pregnancy: Category C. Animal reproduction studies have not been conducted with NITRO-BID IV. It is also not known whether NITRO-BID IV can cause fetal harm when administered to a pregnant woman or can affect reproduction capacity. NITRO-BID IV should be given to a pregnant woman only if clearly needed.

Nursing Mothers: It is not known whether nitroglycerin is excreted in human milk. Because many drugs are excreted in human milk, caution should be exercised when NITRO-BID IV is administered to a nursing woman.

Pediatric Use: The safety and effectiveness of NITRO-BID IV in children have not been established.

NITRO-BID IV contains alcohol and propylene glycol; safety for intracoronary injection has not been shown.

ADVERSE REACTIONS

The most frequent adverse reaction in patients treated with nitroglycerin is headache, which occurs in approximately 2% of patients. Other adverse reactions occurring in less than 1% of patients are the following: tachycardia, nausea, vomiting, apprehension, restlessness, muscle twitching, retrosternal discomfort, palpitations, dizziness, and abdominal pain. Paradoxical bradycardia and increased angina pectoris may accompany nitroglycerin-induced hypotension. The following additional adverse reactions have been reported with the oral and/or topical use of nitroglycerin: cutaneous flushing, weakness, and, occasionally, drug rash or exfoliative dermatitis.

OVERDOSAGE

Accidental overdosage of nitroglycerin may result in severe hypotension and reflex tachycardia which can be treated by elevating the legs and decreasing or temporarily terminating the infusion until the patient's condition stabilizes. Since the duration of the hemodynamic effects following nitroglycerin administration is quite short, additional corrective measures are usually not required. However, if further therapy is indicated, administration of an intravenous alpha-adrenergic agonist (eg, methoxamine or phenylephrine) should be considered.

DOSAGE AND ADMINISTRATION

NOT FOR DIRECT INTRAVENOUS INJECTION.

NITRO-BID IV (NITROGLYCERIN) IS A CONCENTRATED, POTENT DRUG WHICH MUST BE DILUTED IN DEXTROSE (5.0%) INJECTION, USP OR SODIUM CHLORIDE (0.9%) INJECTION, USP PRIOR TO ITS INFUSION. NITRO-BID IV SHOULD NOT BE ADMIXED WITH OTHER DRUGS.

NITRO-BID IV Administration Table

Each 1-ml vial = 5 mg nitroglycerin
Each 5-ml vial = 25 mg nitroglycerin
Each 10-ml vial = 50 mg nitroglycerin

Mixing Instructions	1 ml in 100 ml 5 ml in 500 ml 10 ml in 1000 ml	1 ml in 50 ml 5 ml in 250 ml 10 ml in 500 ml 20 ml in 1000 ml	2 ml in 50 ml 10 ml in 250 ml 20 ml in 500 ml 40 ml in 1000 ml	FLOW RATE milliliters/hour microdrops/minute
Concentration	50 mcg/ml	100 mcg/ml	200 mcg/ml	
Dosage	mcg/min	mcg/min	mcg/min	microdrops/min
	2.5	5	10	3
	5	10	20	6
	10	20	40	12
	20	40	80	24
	40	80	160	48
	60	120	240	72
	80	160	320	96

Dilution: It is important to consider the fluid requirements of the patient as well as the expected duration of infusion in selecting the appropriate dilution of NITRO-BID IV. [See table above].

Dosage: Dosage is affected by the type of infusion set used (see **WARNINGS**). Although the usual starting adult dose range reported in clinical studies was 25 mcg/min or more, those studies used PVC TUBING. **The use of nonabsorbing tubing will result in the need to use reduced doses.**

The dosage for NITRO-BID IV (nitroglycerin) infusion should initially be 5 mcg/min delivered through an infusion pump capable of exact and constant delivery of the drug. Subsequent titration must be adjusted to the clinical situation, with dose increments becoming more cautious as partial response is seen. Initial titration should be in 5-mcg/min increments, with increases every three to five minutes until some response is noted. If no response is seen at 20 mcg/min, increments of 10 and later 20 mcg/min can be used. Once a partial blood pressure response is observed, the dose increase should be reduced and the interval between increments should be lengthened. Patients with normal or low left ventricular filling pressure or pulmonary capillary wedge pressure (eg, angina patients without other complications) may be hypersensitive to the effects of NITRO-BID IV and may respond fully to doses as small as 5 mcg/min. These patients require especially careful titration and monitoring.

There is no fixed optimum dose of NITRO-BID IV. Due to variations in the responsiveness of individual patients to the drug, each patient must be titrated to the desired level of hemodynamic function. Therefore, continuous monitoring of physiologic parameters (eg, blood pressure, heart rate, and pulmonary capillary wedge pressure) MUST BE PERFORMED to achieve the correct dose. Adequate systemic blood pressure and coronary perfusion pressure must be maintained.

HOW SUPPLIED

NITRO-BID® IV is supplied in boxes of ten 1-ml vials (NDC 0088-1800-31), each vial containing 5 mg of nitroglycerin (5 mg/ml); ten 5-ml vials (NDC 0088-1800-32), each vial containing 25 mg nitroglycerin (5 mg/ml); and five 10-ml vials (NDC 0088-1800-33), each vial containing 50 mg nitroglycerin (5 mg/ml).

Mfd for
Marion Laboratories, Inc.
Mfd by
Taylor Pharmacal Co.
Decatur, IL 62525

Issued 3/85

NITRO-BID® Ointment ℞

[ni'tro-bid]
(nitroglycerin 2%)

DESCRIPTION

NITRO-BID® Ointment contains 2% nitroglycerin and lactose in a special absorptive lanolin and white petrolatum base formulated to provide a controlled release of the active ingredient. Each inch, as squeezed from the tube, or the contents squeezed from the pouch, contains approximately 15 mg nitroglycerin.

ACTIONS

When the ointment is spread on the skin, nitroglycerin is absorbed continuously into the systemic circulation. Nitroglycerin ointment reduces the work load of the heart by virtue of its smooth-muscle relaxation. This results predominantly in peripheral venous dilatation which reduces preload, but also to a lesser degree in peripheral arteriolar dilatation which reduces afterload. These hemodynamic effects have been advanced as explanations for the beneficial actions of nitroglycerin ointment in angina pectoris.

Computerized digital plethysmographic studies have shown the duration of action of nitroglycerin ointment (2 inches applied to the chest) to be eight hours in comparison to placebo; the onset of action occurred within 30 minutes of administration. Controlled clinical studies have demonstrated that nitroglycerin ointment increased measured exercise tolerance in patients with angina pectoris up to three hours after application (the maximal time interval studied).

INDICATIONS

This drug product has been conditionally approved by the FDA for the prevention and treatment of angina pectoris due to coronary artery disease. The conditional approval reflects a determination that the drug may be marketed while further investigation of its effectiveness is undertaken. A final evaluation of the effectiveness of the product will be announced by the FDA.

CONTRAINDICATIONS

In patients known to be intolerant of the organic nitrate drugs.

WARNINGS

In acute myocardial infarction or congestive heart failure, nitroglycerin ointment should be used under careful clinical and/or hemodynamic monitoring.

PRECAUTIONS

Nitroglycerin ointment should not be used for treatment of acute anginal attacks. Symptoms of hypotension, particularly when suddenly arising from the recumbent position, are signs of overdosage. When they occur, the dosage should be reduced.

ADVERSE REACTIONS

Transient headaches are the most common side effect, especially at higher dosages. Headaches should be treated with mild analgesics, and nitroglycerin ointment continued. Only with untreatable headaches should the dosage be reduced. Although uncommon, hypotension, an increase in heart rate, faintness, flushing, dizziness, and nausea may occur. These all are attributable to the pharmacologic effects of nitroglycerin on the cardiovascular system, but are symptoms of overdosage. When they occur and persist, the dosage should be reduced.

Occasionally, contact dermatitis has been reported with continuous use of topical nitroglycerin. Such incidence may be reduced by changing the site of application or by using topical corticosteroids.

DOSAGE AND ADMINISTRATION

When applying the ointment, place the specially designed Dose Measuring Applicator, supplied with the package, printed side down and squeeze the necessary amount of ointment from the tube or pouch onto the applicator. Then place the applicator with the ointment side down onto the desired area of the skin, usually the chest (although other areas can be used). Spread the ointment over a 6x6-inch (150x150-mm) area in a thin, uniform layer using the applicator. Cover the area with plastic wrap which can be held in place by adhesive tape. The applicator allows the patient to measure the necessary amount of ointment and to spread it without its being absorbed through the fingers while applying it to the skin surface.

The usual therapeutic dose is 2 inches (50 mm) applied every eight hours, although some patients may require as much as 4 to 5 inches (100 to 125 mm) and/or application every four hours.

Tube: Start at 1/2 inch (12.5 mm) every eight hours and increase the dose by 1/2 inch (12.5 mm) with each successive application to achieve the desired clinical effects. The optimal dosage should be selected based upon the clinical response, side effects, and the effects of therapy upon blood pressure. The greatest attainable decrease in resting blood pressure which is not associated with clinical symptoms of hypotension, especially during orthostasis, indicates the optimal dosage. To decrease adverse reactions, the dose and

Continued on next page

Marion—Cont.

frequency of application should be tailored to the individual patient's needs.
Keep the tube tightly closed and store at room temperature 59° to 86° F (15° to 30° C).
Foil Pouch: The 1-gm foil pouch is approximately equivalent to one inch as squeezed from a tube and is designed to be used in increments of one inch. Apply the ointment by squeezing the contents of the pouch onto a specially designed Dose Measuring Applicator, supplied with the package, printed side down.
Patient Instructions for Application: Information furnished with Dose Measuring Applicators.

HOW SUPPLIED

NITRO-BID® Ointment (nitroglycerin 2%) is available in 20-gm and 60-gm tubes and in Unit Dose Identification Paks of 100 1-gm foil pouches.

Issued 1/85

OS-CAL® 250 Tablets — OTC

[ahs'kal]
calcium supplement with vitamin D

Each tablet contains:
625 mg of calcium carbonate from oyster shell which provides:
Elemental calcium ... 250 mg
Vitamin D ... 125 USP Units
Ingredients: Oyster shell powder, corn syrup solids, talc, cornstarch, hydroxypropyl methylcellulose, calcium stearate, polysorbate 80, titanium dioxide, methyl propyl paraben, polyethylene glycol, pharmaceutical glaze, vitamin D, polyvinylpyrrolidone, carnauba wax, D&C Yellow #10, acetylated monoglyceride, FD&C Blue #1, simethicone emulsion, and edible gray ink.

INDICATIONS

OS-CAL® 250 Tablets provide a source of calcium when it is desired to increase the dietary intake of this mineral. OS-CAL 250 also contains vitamin D to aid in the absorption of calcium.

DIRECTIONS

Take one tablet three times a day at mealtime.
Three tablets daily provide:

	Quantity	%U.S. RDA* for Adults
Calcium	750 mg	75%
Vitamin D	375 units	94%

*Percent U.S. Recommended Daily Allowance.
Store at room temperature.
Keep out of reach of children.

HOW SUPPLIED

Bottles of 100, 240, 500, and 1000 tablets.

Issued 11/83

Shown in Product Identification Section, page 415

OS-CAL® 500 Chewable Tablets — OTC

[ahs'kal]
calcium supplement

Each tablet contains:
1,250 mg of calcium carbonate.
Elemental calcium ... 500 mg
Ingredients: Calcium carbonate, dextrose monohydrate, maltodextrin, microcrystalline cellulose, sodium chloride, Bavarian cream flavor, magnesium stearate, coconut flavor.

INDICATIONS

OS-CAL 500 Chewable Tablets provide a source of calcium when it is desired, or recommended by a physician, to increase the dietary intake of this mineral.

DIRECTIONS

One tablet 2 to 3 times a day with meals, or as recommended by your physician.
Two tablets provide: 1,000 mg calcium, 100% of U.S. RDA for adults and children 12 or more years of age.
Three tablets provide: 1,500 mg calcium, 115% of U.S. RDA for pregnant and lactating women.
Store at room temperature.
Keep out of reach of children.

HOW SUPPLIED

OS-CAL® 500 Chewable Tablets are available in bottles of 60 tablets.

Issued 8/85

Shown in Product Identification Section, page 415

OS-CAL® 500 Tablets — OTC

[ahs'kal]
calcium supplement

Each tablet contains:
1,250 mg of calcium carbonate from oyster shell which provides:
Elemental calcium ... 500 mg
Ingredients: Oyster shell powder, corn syrup solids, talc, hydroxypropyl methylcellulose, cornstarch, sodium starch glycolate, calcium stearate, polysorbate 80, pharmaceutical glaze, titanium dioxide, methyl propyl paraben, polyethylene glycol, polyvinylpyrrolidone, carnauba wax, D&C Yellow #10, acetylated monoglyceride, edetate disodium, FD&C Blue #1, and simethicone emulsion.

INDICATIONS

OS-CAL 500 Tablets provide a source of calcium when it is desired or recommended by a physician to increase the dietary intake of this mineral.

DIRECTIONS

Take one tablet 2 to 3 times a day at mealtime or as directed.
Two tablets daily provide:

	Quantity	%U.S. RDA†
Calcium	1,000 mg	100%*
		77%**

Three tablets daily provide:

	Quantity	%U.S. RDA†
Calcium	1,500 mg	150%*
		115%**

†Percent U.S. Recommended Daily Allowance.
*For adults and children 12 or more years of age.
**For pregnant and lactating women.
Store at room temperature.
Keep out of reach of children.

HOW SUPPLIED

Bottles of 60 and 120 tablets.

Issued 5/84

Shown in Product Identification Section, page 415

OS-CAL FORTE® Tablets — OTC

[ahs'kal for'ta]
multivitamin and mineral supplement

Each tablet contains:
Vitamin A (palmitate) ... 1668 USP Units
Vitamin D ... 125 USP Units
Thiamine mononitrate (vitamin B_1) ... 1.7 mg
Riboflavin (vitamin B_2) ... 1.7 mg
Pyridoxine hydrochloride (vitamin B_6) ... 2.0 mg
Cyanocobalamin (vitamin B_{12}) ... 1.6 mcg
Ascorbic acid (vitamin C) ... 50 mg
dl-alpha-tocopherol acetate (vitamin E) ... 0.8 IU
Niacinamide ... 15 mg
Calcium (from oyster shell) ... 250 mg
Iron (as ferrous fumarate) ... 5 mg
Magnesium (as oxide) ... 1.6 mg
Manganese (as sulfate) ... 0.3 mg
Zinc (as sulfate) ... 0.5 mg
Ingredients: Oyster shell powder, ascorbic acid, corn syrup solids, niacinamide, D&C Yellow #10 Aluminum Lake, ferrous fumarate, calcium stearate, FD&C Blue #1 Aluminum Lake, cornstarch, vitamin A palmitate, polysorbate 80, magnesium oxide, pyridoxine, thiamine, riboflavin, cyanocobalamin, vitamin E, pharmaceutical glaze, methyl paraben, zinc sulfate, manganese sulfate, propylparaben, povidone, vitamin D, hydroxypropyl methylcellulose, carnauba wax, titanium dioxide, ethylcellulose, and acetylated monoglyceride.

INDICATION

Multivitamin and mineral supplement.

DOSAGE

One tablet three times daily or as directed by physician.
Store at room temperature.
Keep out of the reach of children. In case of accidental overdose, seek professional assistance or contact a poison control center immediately.

HOW SUPPLIED

Bottles of 100 tablets.

Issued 3/86

Shown in Product Identification Section, page 415

OS-CAL® Plus Tablets — OTC

[ahs'kal]
multivitamin and multimineral supplement

Each tablet contains:
Elemental calcium (from oyster shell) ... 250 mg
Vitamin D ... 125 USP Units
Vitamin A (palmitate) ... 1666 USP Units
Vitamin C (ascorbic acid) ... 33 mg
Vitamin B_2 (riboflavin) ... 0.66 mg
Vitamin B_1 (thiamine mononitrate) ... 0.5 mg
Vitamin B_6 (pyridoxine HCl) ... 0.5 mg
Niacinamide ... 3.33 mg
Iron (as ferrous fumarate) ... 16.6 mg
Zinc (as the sulfate) ... 0.75 mg
Manganese (as the sulfate) ... 0.75 mg
Ingredients: Oyster shell powder, corn syrup solids, ferrous fumarate, ascorbic acid, calcium stearate, cornstarch, hydroxypropyl methylcellulose, polysorbate 80, titanium dioxide, vitamin A palmitate, niacinamide, ethylcellulose, manganese sulfate, methyl-propyl paraben, zinc sulfate, pharmaceutical glaze, acetylated monoglyceride, riboflavin, thiamine mononitrate, pyridoxine hydrochloride, povidone, vitamin D, carnauba wax, and D&C Red #33.

INDICATIONS

As a multivitamin and multimineral supplement.

DOSAGE

One (1) tablet three times a day before meals or as directed by a physician. For children under 4 years of age, consult a physician.
Store at room temperature.
Keep out of reach of children. In case of accidental overdose, seek professional assistance or contact a poison control center immediately.

HOW SUPPLIED

Bottles of 100 tablets.

Issued 3/86

Shown in Product Identification Section, page 415

PAVABID® Plateau CAPS® — ℞

[pav'uh-bid]
(papaverine hydrochloride) 150 mg

COMPOSITION

Each capsule contains:
Papaverine hydrochloride ... 150 mg
in a specially prepared base to provide prolonged activity.
Also contains: calcium stearate, starch, stearic acid, sucrose, talc, and other ingredients.

ACTION AND USES

The main actions of papaverine are exerted on cardiac and smooth muscle. Like quinidine, papaverine acts directly on the heart muscle to depress conduction and prolong the refractory period. Papaverine relaxes various smooth muscles. This relaxation may be prominent if spasm exists. The muscle cell is not paralyzed by papaverine and still responds to drugs and other stimuli causing contraction. The antispasmodic effect is a direct one, and unrelated to muscle innervation. Papaverine is practically devoid of effects on the central nervous system.
Papaverine relaxes the smooth musculature of the larger blood vessels, especially coronary, systemic peripheral, and pulmonary arteries. Perhaps by its direct vasodilating action on cerebral blood vessels, papaverine increases cerebral blood flow and decreases cerebral vascular resistance in normal subjects; oxygen consumption is unaltered. These effects may explain the benefit reported from the drug in cerebral vascular encephalopathy.
The direct actions of papaverine on the heart to depress conduction and irritability and to prolong the refractory period of the myocardium provide the basis for its clinical trial in abrogating atrial and ventricular premature systoles and ominous ventricular arrhythmias. The coronary vasodilator action could be an additional factor of therapeutic value when such rhythms are secondary to insufficiency or occlusion of the coronary arteries.
In patients with acute coronary thrombosis, the occurrence of ventricular rhythms is serious and requires measures designed to decrease myocardial irritability. Papaverine may have advantages over quinidine, used for a similar purpose, in that it may be given in an emergency by the intravenous route, does not depress myocardial contraction or cause cinchonism, and produces coronary vasodilation.

INDICATIONS

For the relief of cerebral and peripheral ischemia associated with arterial spasm and myocardial ischemia complicated by arrhythmias.

PRECAUTIONS

Use with caution in patients with glaucoma. Hepatic hypersensitivity has been reported with gastrointestinal symptoms, jaundice, eosinophilia, and altered liver function tests. Discontinue medication if these occur.

ADVERSE REACTIONS

Although occurring rarely, the reported side effects of papaverine include nausea, abdominal distress, anorexia, constipation, malaise, drowsiness, vertigo, sweating, headache, diarrhea, and skin rash.

DOSAGE AND ADMINISTRATION
One capsule every 12 hours. In difficult cases administration may be increased to one capsule every 8 hours, or two capsules every 12 hours.

HOW SUPPLIED
PAVABID® (papaverine hydrochloride) Capsules are available in bottles of 100, 250, 1000, and in Unit Dose Identification Paks of 100 capsules. Capsules are imprinted with MARION/1555.

CAUTION
Federal law prohibits dispensing without prescription.

Issued 11/85

Shown in Product Identification Section, page 415

PAVABID® HP Capsulets ℞

[pav 'uh-bid]
(papaverine hydrochloride) 300 mg

COMPOSITION
Each capsulet contains:
Papaverine hydrochloride .... 300 mg
Also contains: calcium stearate, FD&C Yellow, #6, FD&C Yellow #6 Lake, lactose, microcrystalline cellulose, starch, and other ingredients.

ACTION AND USES
The main actions of papaverine are exerted on cardiac and smooth muscle. Like quinidine, papaverine acts directly on the heart muscle to depress conduction and prolong the refractory period. Papaverine relaxes various smooth muscles. This relaxation may be prominent if spasm exists. The muscle cell is not paralyzed by papaverine, and still responds to drugs and other stimuli causing contraction. The antispasmodic effect is a direct one, and unrelated to muscle innervation. Papaverine is practically devoid of effects on the central nervous system.
Papaverine relaxes the smooth musculature of the larger blood vessels, especially coronary, systemic peripheral, and pulmonary arteries. Perhaps by its direct vasodilating action on cerebral blood vessels, papaverine increases cerebral blood flow and decreases cerebral vascular resistance in normal subjects; oxygen consumption is unaltered. These effects may explain the benefit reported from the drug in cerebral vascular encephalopathy.
The direct actions of papaverine on the heart to depress conduction and irritability and to prolong the refractory period of the myocardium provide the basis for its clinical trial in abrogating atrial and ventricular premature systoles and ominous ventricular arrhythmias. The coronary vasodilator action could be an additional factor of therapeutic value when such rhythms are secondary to insufficiency or occlusion of the coronary arteries.
In patients with acute coronary thrombosis, the occurrence of ventricular rhythms is serious and requires measures designed to decrease myocardial irritablilty. Papaverine may have advantages over quinidine, used for a similar purpose, in that it may be given in an emergency by the intravenous route, does not depress myocardial contraction or cause cinchonism, and produces coronary vasodilation.

INDICATIONS
For the relief of cerebral and peripheral ischemia associated with arterial spasm and myocardial ischemia complicated by arrhythmias.

PRECAUTIONS
Use with caution in patients with glaucoma. Hepatic hypersensitivity has been reported with gastrointestinal symptoms, jaundice, eosinophilia, and altered liver function tests. Discontinue medication if these occur.

ADVERSE REACTIONS
Although occurring rarely, the reported side effects of papaverine include nausea, abdominal distress, anorexia, constipation, malaise, drowsiness, vertigo, sweating, headache, diarrhea, and skin rash.

DOSAGE AND ADMINISTRATION
Dosage should be started at 150 mg (one-half capsulet) two to three times daily and titrated upward to the desired level. The 300-mg capsulet breaks into two separate half capsulets. To break: place capsulet on a hard surface with the embossed MARION M facing up, press down on the embossed M.

HOW SUPPLIED
PAVABID® (papaverine hydrochloride) HP Capsulets are available in 60-count bottles. Each light-orange capsulet is embossed with a raised M stamped MARION on one side and PAVABID HP on the other side.

CAUTION
Federal law prohibits dispensing without prescription.

Issued 11/85

Shown in Product Identification Section, page 415

SILVADENE® Cream ℞

[sil 'vuh-dēn]
(1% silver sulfadiazine)

DESCRIPTION
SILVADENE Cream is a soft, white, water-miscible cream containing the antimicrobial agent, silver sulfadiazine in micronized form. Each gram of SILVADENE Cream contains 10 mg of micronized silver sulfadiazine. The cream vehicle consists of white petrolatum, stearyl alcohol, isopropyl myristate, sorbitan monooleate, polyoxyl 40 stearate, propylene glycol, and water, with methylparaben 0.3% as a preservative.

ACTIONS
SILVADENE Cream (silver sulfadiazine) spreads easily and can be washed off readily with water.
Silver sulfadiazine has broad antimicrobial activity. It is bactericidal for many gram-negative and gram-positive bacteria as well as being effective against yeast. Results from in vitro testing are listed below.
Sufficient data have been obtained to demonstrate that silver sulfadiazine will inhibit bacteria that are resistant to other antimicrobial agents and that the compound is superior to sulfadiazine.

Genus & Species	No. of Sensitive Strains/Total Strains Tested Concentration of silver sulfadiazine 50 μg/ml	100 μg/ml
Pseudomonas aeruginosa	130/130	130/130
Pseudomonas maltophilia	7/7	7/7
Enterobacter species	48/50	50/50
Enterobacter cloacae	24/24	24/24
Klebsiella	53/54	54/54
Escherichia coli	63/63	63/63
Serratia	27/28	28/28
Proteus mirabilis	53/53	53/53
Proteus morganii	10/10	10/10
Proteus rettgeri	2/2	2/2
Proteus vulgaris	2/2	2/2
Providencia	1/1	1/1
Citrobacter	10/10	10/10
Herellea	8/9	9/9
Mima	2/2	2/2
Staphylococcus aureus	100/101	101/101
Staphylococcus epidermidis	51/51	51/51
β-hemolytic Streptococcus	4/4	4/4
Enterococcus (Group D *Streptococcus)*	52/53	53/53
Corynebacterium diphtheriae	2/2	2/2
Clostridium perfringens	0/2	2/2
Candida albicans	43/50	50/50

Studies utilizing radioactive micronized silver sulfadiazine, electron microscopy, and elaborate biochemical techniques have revealed that the mechanism of action of silver sulfadiazine on bacteria differs from silver nitrate and sodium sulfadiazine. SILVADENE Cream (silver sulfadiazine) acts only on the cell membrane and cell wall to produce its bactericidal effect.
Silver sulfadiazine by its chemical nature is not a carbonic anhydrase inhibitor. **Acidosis in patients treated with SILVADENE Cream has not been reported.** Since it is not a carbonic anhydrase inhibitor, SILVADENE Cream may be particularly of value in treating pediatric burn patients.

INDICATIONS
SILVADENE Cream (silver sulfadiazine) is a topical antimicrobial drug indicated as an adjunct for the prevention and treatment of wound sepsis in patients with second- and third-degree burns.

CONTRAINDICATIONS
Because sulfonamide therapy is known to increase the possibility of kernicterus, SILVADENE Cream should not be used at term pregnancy, on premature infants, or on newborn infants during the first month of life.

WARNINGS
SILVADENE Cream should be administered with great caution to patients with history of hypersensitivity to SILVADENE Cream. It is not known whether there is cross-sensitivity to other sulfonamides. If allergic reactions attributable to treatment with SILVADENE Cream occur, discontinuation of SILVADENE Cream must be considered. The use of SILVADENE Cream in some cases of glucose-6-phosphate dehydrogenase deficient individuals may be hazardous, as hemolysis may occur.

USE IN PREGNANCY
Safe use of SILVADENE Cream during pregnancy has not been established. Therefore, the preparation is not recommended for the treatment of women of childbearing potential, unless the burned area covers more than 20 percent of the total body surface area or the need for therapeutic benefit of SILVADENE Cream is, in the physician's judgment, greater than the possible risk to the fetus.
Fungal colonization in and below the eschar may occur concomitantly with reduction of bacterial growth in the burn wound. However, fungal dissemination is rare.
In the treatment of burn wounds involving extensive areas of the body, the serum sulfa concentration may approach adult therapeutic levels (8 to 12 mg%). Therefore, in these patients it would be advisable to monitor serum sulfa concentrations. Renal function should be carefully monitored and the urine should be checked for sulfa crystals.

PRECAUTIONS
If hepatic and renal functions become impaired and elimination of drug decreases, accumulation may occur and discontinuation of SILVADENE Cream should be weighed against the therapeutic benefit being achieved.
In considering the use of topical proteolytic enzymes in conjunction with SILVADENE Cream, the possibility should be noted that silver may inactivate such enzymes.

ADVERSE REACTIONS
It is frequently difficult to distinguish between an adverse reaction due to SILVADENE Cream (silver sulfadiazine) and reactions that may occur due to the concomitant use of other therapeutic agents used in the treatment of a patient having a severe burn wound. In the aggregate of 2,297 patients treated with SILVADENE Cream, there were 59 drug-related reactions (2.5%). Of these there were 51 cases of burning, 5 of rash, 2 of itching, and 1 of interstitial nephritis. However, SILVADENE Cream therapy was discontinued in only 0.9% of the patient population.
Since significant quantities of silver sulfadiazine are absorbed, it is possible that any of the adverse reactions attributable to sulfonamides may occur.

DOSAGE AND ADMINISTRATION
Prompt institution of appropriate regimens for care of the burned patient is of prime importance and includes the control of shock and pain. The burn wounds are then cleansed and debrided and SILVADENE Cream (silver sulfadiazine) is applied with sterile, gloved hand. The burn areas should be covered with SILVADENE Cream at all times. The cream should be applied once to twice daily to a thickness of approximately $\frac{1}{16}$ inch. Whenever necessary, the cream should be reapplied to any areas from which it has been removed by patient activity. Administration may be accomplished in minimal time because dressings are not required. However, if individual patient requirements make dressings necessary, they may be used.
When feasible, the patient should be bathed daily. This is an aid in debridement. A whirlpool bath is particularly helpful, but the patient may be bathed in bed or in a shower.
Reduction in bacterial growth after application of topical antibacterial agents has been reported to permit spontaneous healing of deep partial-thickness burns by preventing conversion of the partial thickness to full thickness by sepsis. However, reduction in bacterial colonization has caused delayed separation, in some cases necessitating escharotomy in order to prevent contracture.
Treatment with SILVADENE Cream should be continued until satisfactory healing has occurred or until the burn site is ready for grafting. **The drug should not be withdrawn from the therapeutic regimen while there remains the possibility of infection except if a significant adverse reaction occurs.**

HOW SUPPLIED
SILVADENE Cream (silver sulfadiazine) is available in 50-gm, 400-gm, and 1000-gm jars; and 20-gm tubes.
U.S. Patent 3,761,590.

Issued 3/82

Shown in Product Identification Section, page 415

THROAT DISCS® OTC

[thrōt disks]
Throat Lozenges

DESCRIPTION
Each lozenge contains sucrose, starch (may contain cornstarch), acacia, glycyrrhiza extract (licorice), gum traga-

Continued on next page

Marion—Cont.

canth, anethole, linseed, cubeb oleoresin, anise oil, peppermint oil, capsicum, and mineral oil.

INDICATIONS
Effective for soothing, temporary relief of minor throat irritations from hoarseness and coughs due to colds.

PRECAUTIONS
For severe or persistent cough or sore throat, or sore throat accompanied by high fever, headache, nausea, and vomiting, consult physician promptly. Not recommended for children under 3 years of age.

DOSAGE
Allow lozenge to dissolve slowly in mouth. One or two should give the desired relief. Do not use more than four lozenges per hour.

HOW SUPPLIED
Box of 60 lozenges.

Issued 5/85

Marlyn Company, Inc.
350 PAUMA PLACE
ESCONDIDO, CA 92025

HEP-FORTE®
[hep-for'tay]

DESCRIPTION
Hep Forte is a comprehensive formulation of protein, B factors and other nutritional factors which can be important in maintenance and support of normal hepatic function.

COMPOSITION
Each capsule contains:

Vitamin A (Palmitate)	1,200 I.U.
Vitamin E (d-Alpha Tocopherol)	10 I.U.
Vitamin C (Ascorbic Acid)	10 mg.
Folic Acid	0.06 mg.
Vitamin B1 (Thiamine Mononitrate)	1 mg.
Vitamin B2 (Riboflavin)	1 mg.
Niacinamide	10 mg.
Vitamin B6 (Pyridoxine HCl)	0.5 mg.
Vitamin B12 (Cobalamin)	1 mcg.
Biotin	3.3 mg.
Pantothenic Acid	2 mg.
Choline Bitartrate	21 mg.
Zinc (Zinc Sulfate)	2 mg.
Desiccated Liver	194.4 mg.
Liver Concentrate	64.8 mg.
Liver Fraction Number 2	64.8 mg.
Yeast (Dried)	64.8 mg.
dl-Methionine	10 mg.
Inositol	10 mg.

INDICATIONS
Hep Forte is of value as supportive or adjunctive treatment in cases of: alcoholism, hepatic dysfunction due to hepatotoxic drugs and liver poisons, male and female infertility due to hormonal imbalance caused by hepatic dysfunction.

CONTRAINDICATIONS
There are no known contraindications to Hep Forte.

DOSAGE
Three to six capsules daily.

HOW SUPPLIED
Bottles of 100, 300 or 500 capsules.
Literature Available.

MARLYN® FORMULA 50®

COMPOSITION
Each capsule contains:

Amino Acids	0.3 Gm*
Vitamin B6 (pyridoxine HCl)	1.0 mg.

*Approximate analysis of the amino acids: indispensable amino acids (lysine, tryptophan, phenylalanine, methionine, threonine, leucine, isoleucine, valine), 35.30%; semi-dispensable amino acids (arginine, histidine, tyrosine, cystine, glycine), 19.18%; dispensable amino acids (glutamic acid, alanine, aspartic acid, serine, proline), 45.56%.
Amino acids: Protein "building blocks" important to growth and development of all protein containing tissue including nails, hair, and skin.

DOSAGE AND ADMINISTRATION
The recommended daily dose is 6 capsules daily.

SUPPLY
Bottles of 100, 250 and 1000 capsules.

MARLYN PMS®

(See PDR For Nonprescription Drugs)

Mason Pharmaceuticals, Inc.
1201 DOVE STREET
SUITE #520
NEWPORT BEACH, CA 92660

DAMACET-P® Ⓒ℞
[dā"mă-set-p]
Hydrocodone and Acetominophen Tablets

DESCRIPTION
Each blue tablet contains:

Hydrocodone Bitartrate*	5 mg.
*WARNING: May be habit forming.	
Acetaminophen	500 mg.

Narcotic analgesic tablet for oral administration.

HOW SUPPLIED
DAMACET-P is supplied as 7/16", round, blue mottled tablets with an "M" logo on one side and "D-C" on the other.
Supplied in bottles of 100, NDC 12758-066-01
bottles of 500, NDC 12758-066-05

Storage: DAMACET-P should be stored at 59°–86°F, 15°–30°C.

Manufactured by:
Pharmaceutical Basics, Inc.
Denver, CO 80209
Manufactured expressly for
Mason Pharmaceuticals, Inc.
Newport Beach, CA 92660
5915-Revised May, 1985
Shown in Product Identification Section, page 415

DAMASON-P Ⓒ℞
(Hydrocodone Bitartrate 5mg, USP, Aspirin 224mg, Caffeine 32mg)

DESCRIPTION
Each pink tablet of DAMASON-P contains:

ACTIVE INGREDIENTS

Hydrocodone Bitartrate	5 mg
(Warning: May be habit forming)	
Aspirin	224 mg
Caffeine	32 mg

INACTIVE INGREDIENTS
Cellulose
Corn Starch
Stearic Acid
Color, Red #7 Lake

Narcotic analgesic tablet for oral administration.
Hydrocodone is a hydrogenated ketone of codeine available as bitartrate salt. Hydrocodone bitartrate is an opioid analgesic and antitussive and occurs as fine, white crystals or as a crystalline powder. It is affected by light.

CLINICAL PHARMACOLOGY
Hydrocodone is a semisynthetic narcotic analgesic with multiple actions similar to those of codeine. Most of these actions involve the central nervous system and smooth muscle. The precise mechanism of action of hydrocodone and other opiates is not known, although it is believed to relate to the existence of opiate receptors in the central nervous system. In addition to analgesia, narcotics may produce drowsiness, changes in mood and mental clouding No history of hepatic toxicity.
Radioimmunoassay techniques have recently been developed for the analysis of hydrocodone in human plasma. After a 10 mg. oral dose of hydrocodone bitartrate, a mean peak serum drug level of 23.6 ng/ml and an elimination half-life of 3.8 hours were found. DAMASON-P also contains the non-narcotic, anti-inflammatory, antipyretic analgesic, aspirin and caffeine.

INDICATIONS AND USAGE
For the relief of moderate to moderately severe pain.

CONTRAINDICATIONS
Hypersensitivity to aspirin, caffeine or hydrocodone.

WARNINGS
Reye Syndrome: This is a rare but serious disease which can follow flue or chicken pox in children and teenagers. While the cause of the Reye Syndrome is unknown, some reports claim aspirin (or salicylates) may increase the risk of developing this disease. Consult a doctor before use in children or teenagers with flue or chicken pox.
Acute Abdominal Conditions: The administration of narcotics may obscure the diagnosis or clinical course of patients with acute abdominal conditions.
Head Injury and Increased Intracranial Pressure: The respiratory depressant effects of narcotics and their capacity to elevate cerebrospinal fluid pressure may be markedly exaggerated in the presence of head injury, other intracranial lesions or a preexisting increase in intracranial pressure. Furthermore, narcotics produce adverse reactions which may obscure the clinical course of patients with head injuries.
Respiratory Depression: At high doses or in sensitive patients, hydrocodone may produce dose-related respiratory depression by acting directly on brain stem respiratory centers. Hydrocodone also affects centers that control respiratory rhythm, and may produce irregular and periodic breathing.
Other: Salicylates should be used with extreme caution in the presence of peptic ulcer or coagulation abnormalities.

PRECAUTIONS
Special Risk Patients: As with any narcotic analgesic agent, DAMASON-P should be used with caution in elderly or debilitated patients and those with severe impairment of hepatic or renal functions, hypothyroidism, Addison's disease, prostatic hypertrophy or urethral stricture. The usual precautions should be observed and the possibility of respiratory depression should be kept in mind.
Information for Patients: DAMASON-P, like all narcotics, may impair the mental and/or physical abilities required for the performance of potentially hazardous tasks such as driving a car or operating machinery; patients should be cautioned accordingly. DAMASON-P should be taken after meals or with a full glass of water.
Cough Reflex: Hydrocodone suppresses the cough reflex; as with all narcotics, caution should be exercised when DAMASON-P is used postoperatively and in patients with pulmonary disease.
Drug Interactions: Patients receiving other narcotic analgesics, general anesthetics, phenothiazines, other tranquilizers, sedative-hypnotics or other CNS depressants (including alcohol) concomitantly with DAMASON-P may exhibit an additive CNS depression. When such combined therapy is contemplated, the dose of one or both agents should be reduced. Aspirin may enhance the effects of anti-coagulants and inhibit the uricosuric effects of uricosuric agents.
The concurrent use of anticholinergics with hydrocodone may produce paralytic ileus.
The use of MAO inhibitors or tricyclic antidepressants with hydrocodone preparations may increase the effect of either the antidepressant or hydrocodone.
Usage In Pregnancy: "Pregnancy Category C." Hydrocodone has been shown to be teratogenic in hamsters when given in doses 700 times the human dose. There are no adequate and well-controlled studies in pregnant women. DAMASON-P should be used during pregnancy only if the potential benefit justifies the potential risk to the fetus.
Nonteratogenic Effects: Babies born to mothers who have been taking opioids regularly prior to delivery will be physically dependent. The withdrawal signs include irritability and excessive crying, tremors, hyperactive reflexes, increased respiratory rate, increased stools, sneezing, yawning, vomiting, and fever. The intensity of the syndrome does not always correlate with the duration of maternal opioid use or dose. There is no consensus on the best method of managing withdrawal.
Chlorpromazine 0.7 to 1.0 mg/kg q6h, and paregoric 2 to 4 drops/kg q4h, have been used to treat withdrawal symptoms in infants. The duration of therapy is 4 to 28 days, with the dosage decreased as tolerated.
Labor and Delivery: As with all narcotics, administration of DAMASON-P to the mother shortly before delivery may result in some degree of respiratory depression in the newborn, especially if higher doses are used.
Nursing Mothers: It is not known whether this drug is excreted in human milk. Because many drugs are excreted in human milk and because of the potential for serious adverse reactions in nursing infants from DAMASON-P, a decision should be made whether to discontinue nursing or to discontinue the drug, taking into account the importance of the drug to the mother. Hydrocodone is almost completely excreted within 72 hours.
Pediatric Use: Safety and efficacy in children have not been established.

ADVERSE REACTIONS
Central Nervous System: As with all narcotics, sedation, drowsiness, mental clouding, lethargy, impairment of mental and physical performance, anxiety, fear, dysphoria, dizziness, psychic dependence and mood changes may occur.
Gastrointestinal System: Nausea and vomiting occur infrequently; they are more frequent in ambulatory than in recumbent patients. Administration with meals may help reduce this problem. The antiemetic phenothiazines are useful in suppressing these effects; however, some phenothiazine derivatives seem to be antianalgesic and to increase the

amount of narcotic required to produce a given level of analgesia. Prolonged administration of DAMASON-P may produce constipation.

Genitourinary System: Ureteral spasm, spasm of vesical sphincters and urinary retention have been reported with codeine and its derivatives.

Drug Abuse and Dependence: DAMASON-P is subject to the Federal Controlled Substance Act (Schedule III). Psychic dependence, physical dependence, and tolerance may develop upon repeated administration of narcotics; therefore, DAMASON-P Tablets should be prescribed and administered with caution. However, psychic dependence is unlikely to develop when DAMASON-P Tablets are used for a short time for the treatment of pain.

Physical dependence, the condition in which continued administration of the drug is required to prevent the appearance of a withdrawal syndrome, assumes clinically significant proportions only after several weeks of continued narcotic use, although some mild degree of physical dependence may develop after a few days of narcotic therapy. Tolerance, in which increasingly larger doses are required in order to produce the same degree of analgesia, is manifested initially by a shortened duration of analgesic effect, and subsequently by decreases in the intensity of analgesia. The rate of development of tolerance varies among patients.

OVERDOSAGE

Aspirin:

Signs and Symptoms: Respiratory alkalosis is characteristic of the early phase in intoxication with aspirin while hyperventilation is occurring, and is quickly followed by metabolic acidosis in most people with severe intoxication. This occurs more readily in children. Hypoglycemia may occur in children who have taken large overdoses. Other laboratory findings associated with aspirin intoxication include ketonuria, hyponatremia, hypokalemia, and occasionally proteinuria. A slight rise in lactic dehydrogenase and hydroxybutyric dehydrogenase may occur.

Methemoglobin and sulfhemoglobin formation are seldom clinically significant in adults but may contribute to general toxicity. When prominent, they appear as a grayish cyanosis seen most clearly in the lips and nailbeds. Definitive diagnosis is made by spectroscopic analysis of water-diluted (1:100) blood specimen, which shows an abnormal band at 630 nm for methamoglobin and at 618 nm for sulfhemoglobin.

Concentrations of aspirin in plasma above 30 mg/100 ml are associated with toxicity. The single lethal dose of aspirin in adults is probably about 25–30 gm, but is not known with certainty.

Hydrocodone:

Signs and Symptoms: Serious overdose with hydrocodone is characterized by respiratory depression (a decrease in respiratory rate and/or tidal volume, Cheyne-Stokes respiration, cyanosis), extreme somnolence progressing to stupor or coma, skeletal muscle flaccidity, cold and clammy skin, and sometimes bradycardia and hypotension. In severe overdosage, apnea, circulatory collapse, cardiac arrest and death may occur.

Treatment: Primary attention should be given to the reestablishment of adequate respiratory exchange through provision of a patent airway and the institution of assisted or controlled ventilation. The narcotic antagonist naloxone hydrochloride is a specific antidote against respiratory depression which may result from overdosage or unusual sensitivity to narcotics, including hydrocodone. Therefore, an appropriate dose of naloxone hydrochloride, 0.55 mg/kgm, should be administered intravenously, (see package insert), simultaneously with efforts at respiratory resuscitation. Since the duration of action of hydrocodone may exceed that of the antagonist, the patient should be kept under continued surveillance and repeated doses of the antagonist should be administered as needed to maintain adequate respiration. An antagonist should not be administered in the absence of clinically significant respiratory or cardiovascular depression. Oxygen, intravenous fluids, vasopressors and other supportive measures should be employed as indicated.

Gastric emptying may be useful in removing unabsorbed drug.

DOSAGE AND ADMINISTRATION

Given orally, the dosage should be adjusted according to the severity of the pain and the response of the patient. However, it should be kept in mind that tolerance to hydrocodone can develop with continued use and that the incidence of untoward effects may be dose-related.

The usual dose is one tablet, orally, every six hours as needed for pain, with water or other liquids. If necessary, this dose may be repeated at four hour intervals. In cases of more severe pain, two tablets every six hours (up to 8 tablets in 24 hours) may be required.

CAUTION

Federal Law prohibits dispensing without prescription.

DAMASON-P has a schedule III classification which permits prescription refill up to six months or five times on physician's specification.

HOW SUPPLIED

DAMASON-P is supplied as 7/16", round, pink mottled tablets with an "M" logo on one side and "D-P" on the other. Supplied in bottles of 100, NDC 12758-055-01, bottles of 500, NDC 12758-055-05, and in hospital packs of 100, NDC 12758-055-25.

Storage: DAMASON-P should be stored at 59°-86°F, 15°-30°C.

Manufactured by:
Anabolic Inc.
Irvine, CA 92712
and:
Pharmaceutical Basics, Inc.
Denver, CO 80209
Manufactured expressly for:
Mason Pharmaceuticals, Inc.
Newport Beach, CA 92660
5815E-Revised May, 1986

Shown in Product Identification Section, page 415

Mayrand, Inc.
P. O. BOX 8869
FOUR DUNDAS CIRCLE
GREENSBORO, NC 27419

B–A–C TABLETS ℞

DESCRIPTION

Each yellow and white tablet for oral administration contains:

Butalbital* 50 mg.
*WARNING: May be habit forming.
Aspirin 650 mg.
Caffeine 40 mg.

Butalbital, 5-allyl-5-isobutyl-barbituric acid, a white odorless crystalline powder, is a short to intermediate-acting barbiturate.

ACTIONS

Pharmacologically, B-A-C TABLETS combines the analgesic properties of aspirin-caffeine with the anxiolytic and muscle relaxant properties of butalbital.

$CH_2{=}CHCH_2$ / CH_3 / CH_3CHCH_2 [structural formula]

BUTALBITAL

INDICATIONS

B-A-C TABLETS is indicated for the relief of the symptom complex of tension (or muscle contraction) headache.

CONTRAINDICATIONS

Hypersensitivity to aspirin, caffeine or barbiturates. Patients with porphyria.

PRECAUTIONS

1. General:
B-A-C TABLETS should be used with caution in patients with certain medical problems, including those with a history of asthma, allergies and nasal polyps. Also, the drug must be prescribed carefully for patients with hemophilia or other bleeding problems, peptic ulcer, renal impairment, or a history of drug abuse or dependence.

2. Information for Patients:
B-A-C TABLETS may impair the mental and/or physical abilities required for the performance of potentially hazardous tasks, such as driving a car or operating machinery. The patient should be cautioned accordingly.

3. Drug Interactions:
Patients receiving narcotic analgesics, antipsychotics, antianxiety agents, or other CNS depressants (including alcohol) concommitantly with B-A-C TABLETS may exhibit additive CNS depressant effects. When combined therapy is contemplated, the dose of one or both agents should be reduced.

DRUGS	EFFECT
Aspirin w/anti-inflammatory agents	Increased ulcerogenic effects
Butalbital w/coumarin anti-coagulants	Decreased effect of anticoagulant because of increased metabolism resulting from enzyme induction.
Butalbital w/tricyclic antidepressants	Decreased blood levels of the antidepressant.

4. Usage in Pregnancy:
Adequate studies have not been performed in animals to determine whether this drug effects fertility in males or females, has teratogenic potential or has other adverse effects on the fetus. While there are no well-controlled studies in pregnant women, over twenty years of marketing and clinical experience does not include any positive evidence of adverse effects on the fetus. Although there is no clearly defined risk, such experience cannot exclude the possibility of infrequent or subtle damage to the human fetus. B-A-C TABLETS should be used in pregnant women only when clearly needed.

5. Nursing Mothers:
The effects of B-A-C TABLETS on infants of nursing mothers are not known. Salicylates and barbiturates are excreted in the breast milk of nursing mothers. The serum levels in infants are believed to be insignificant with therapeutic doses.

6. Pediatric Use:
Safety and effectiveness in children below the age of 12 have not been established.

ADVERSE REACTIONS

The most frequent adverse reactions are drowsiness and dizziness. Less frequent adverse reactions are lightheadedness and gastrointestinal disturbances including nausea, vomiting and flatulence. Mental confusion or depression can occur due to intolerance or overdosage of butalbital.

DRUG ABUSE AND DEPENDENCE

Prolonged use of barbiturates can produce drug dependence, characterized by psychic dependence, and less frequently, physical dependence and tolerance. The abuse liability of B-A-C TABLETS is similar to that of other barbiturate-containing drug combinations. Caution should be exercised when prescribing medication for patients with a known propensity for taking excessive quantities of drugs, which is not uncommon in patients with chronic tension headache.

OVERDOSAGE

The toxic effects of acute overdosage of B-A-C TABLETS are attributable mainly to its barbiturate component, and, to a lesser extent, aspirin. Because toxic effects of caffeine occur in very high dosagees only, the possibility of significant caffeine toxicity from B-A-C TABLETS overdosage is unlikely. Symptoms attributable to acute barbiturate poisoning include drowsiness, confusion, and coma; respiratory depression; hypotension; shock. Symptoms of salicylate overdosage include central nausea and vomiting, tinnitus and deafness, vertigo and headaches, mental dullness and confusion, diaphoresis, rapid pulse and increased respiration and respiratory alkalosis. Treatment consists primarily of management of barbiturate intoxication and the correction of the acid-base imbalance due to salicylism. Vomiting should be induced mechanically or with emetics in the conscious patient. Gastric lavage may be used if the pharyngeal and laryngeal reflexes are present and if less than four hours have elapsed since ingestion. A cuffed endotracheal tube should be inserted before gastric lavage of the unconscious patient and when necessary to provide assisted respiration. Diuresis, alkalinization of the urine, and correction of electrolyte disturbances should be accomplished through administration of intravenous fluids such as sodium bicarbonate in 5% dextrose in water. Meticulous attention should be given to maintaining adequate pulmonary ventilation. Exchange transfusion is most feasible for a small infant, intermittent peritoneal dialysis is useful for cases of moderate severity in adults. Hemodialysis with the artificial kidney is the most effective means of removing salicylate and is indicated for the very severe cases of salicylate intoxication. Hypoprothrombinemia should be treated with intravenous Vitamin K (phytonadione).

DOSAGE AND ADMINISTRATION

Oral: One tablet every four hours as needed. Do not exceed 6 tablets per day.

Medication should be taken with food or a full glass of water or milk to lessen gastric irritation caused by aspirin.

HOW SUPPLIED

Available as yellow and white scored capsule-shaped tablets imprinted "M/R" in bottles of 100's, NDC #0259-1256-01.

B-A-C #3 Tablets Ⓒ III

DESCRIPTION

Each tablet contains:

Aspirin ......(5 gr.) 325 mg.
Butalbital ......50 mg
(Warning: May be habit forming.)
Caffeine ......40 mg.
Codeine Phosphate ......30 mg.
(Warning: May be habit forming.)

HOW SUPPLIED

B-A-C #3 Tablets are supplied in bottles of 100.

Continued on next page

Mayrand—Cont.

ELDERCAPS ℞

DESCRIPTION
Each capsule contains: Vitamin A Acetate, 4000 I.U.; Vitamin D_2, 400 I.U.; Vitamin E, 25 I.U.; Ascorbic Acid, 200 mg.; Thiamine Mononitrate, 10 mg.; Riboflavin, 5 mg.; Pyridoxine HCl, 2 mg.; Niacinamide, 25 mg.; d-Calcium Pantothenate, 10 mg.; Zinc Sulfate, 110 mg.; Magnesium Sulfate, 70 mg.; Manganese Sulfate, 5 mg.; Folic Acid, 1 mg.

INDICATIONS
ELDERCAPS are indicated for the prophylaxis or treatment of vitamin and mineral deficiencies associated with restricted diets, improper food intake, and decreased absorption or utilization. ELDERCAPS are also indicated in patients with increased requirements for vitamins and minerals due to chronic disease, infection or the stress of surgery.

WARNINGS
Folic acid alone is improper therapy in the treatment of pernicious anemia and other megaloblastic anemias where vitamin B_{12} is deficient.

PRECAUTIONS
Folic acid, especially in doses above 0.1 mg. daily, may obscure pernicious anemia, that is, hematological remission may occur while neurologic manifestations remain progressive.

DOSAGE
One capsule daily or as directed by the physician.

HOW SUPPLIED
Bottles of 100 capsules.

ELDERTONIC

DESCRIPTION
Each 45 ml. contains: Thiamine HCl, 1.5 mg.; Riboflavin, 1.7 mg.; Pyridoxine HCl, 2.0 mg.; Cyanocobalamin, 6.0 mcg.; Dexpanthenol, 10.0 mg.; Niacinamide, 20.0 mg.; Zinc, 15 mg. (as zinc sulfate); Manganese, 2.0 mg. (as manganese sulfate); Magnesium (minimum content as added magnesium), 2.0 mg. (as magnesium sulfate); Alcohol, 13.5%.
In a special sherry wine base.

INDICATIONS
B-complex vitamins with minerals for nutritional supplementation.

DOSAGE
Adults: one tablespoonful three times a day with meals.

WARNING
Do not exceed recommended dosage unless directed by a physician.

USAGE IN PREGNANCY
Safe use of this product in pregnancy has not been established.

CAUTION
Keep out of the reach of children.

HOW SUPPLIED
8 fl. oz.; Pints; Gallons

MAY–VITA ELIXIR ℞

DESCRIPTION
Each 45 ml. contains: Dexpanthenol, 10 mg; Niacinamide, 40 mg.; Pyridoxine HCl (B-6), 4 mg.; Cyanocobalamin (B-12), 12 mcg.; Folic Acid, 1 mg.; Iron, 36 mg. (as polysaccharide iron complex); Zinc, 15 mg. (as zinc sulfate); Manganese, 4 mg. (as manganese sulfate); Alcohol, 13%.

INDICATIONS
For vitamin and mineral replacement therapy in deficiency states and for treatment of iron deficiency anemia and/or nutritional megaloblastic anemias due to inadequate diet.

WARNINGS
Folic acid alone is improper therapy in the treatment of pernicious anemia and other megaloblastic anemias where vitamin B_{12} is deficient.

PRECAUTIONS
Folic acid, especially in doses above 0.1 mg. daily, may obscure pernicious anemia, in that hematologic remission may occur while neurological manifestations remain progressive.

ADVERSE REACTIONS
Allergic sensitization has been reported following both oral and parenteral administration of folic acid.

USE IN PREGNANCY
Safe use of this product in pregnancy has not been established.

DOSAGE
Usual adult dosage is one tablespoonful three times daily with meals. Do not exceed recommended dosage unless directed by a physician.

HOW SUPPLIED
Pint bottles.

NU-IRON 150 CAPS
NU-IRON Elixir (polysaccharide-iron complex)
Sugar Free

DESCRIPTION
NU-IRON is a highly water soluble complex of iron and a low molecular weight polysaccharide.
Each NU-IRON 150 Capsule contains:
Iron (elemental) .... 150 mg.
(as polysaccharide Iron Complex)
Each 5 ml. of NU-IRON Elixir contains:
Iron (elemental) .... 100 mg.
(as Polysaccharide Iron Complex)

ACTION AND USES
NU-IRON is a non-ionic, easily assimilated, relatively nontoxic form of iron. Full therapeutic doses may be achieved with virtually no gastrointestinal side effects. There is no metallic aftertaste and no staining of teeth.

INDICATIONS
For treatment of uncomplicated iron deficiency anemia.

CONTRAINDICATIONS
Hemochromatosis, hemosiderosis or a known hypersensitivity to any of the ingredients.

DOSAGE
ADULTS; One or two NU-IRON 150 Caps daily, or one or two teaspoonfuls NU-IRON Elixir daily. CHILDREN; 6 to 12 years old; one teaspoonful NU-IRON Elixir daily; 2 to 6 years old: ½ teaspoonful daily; under 2 years: ¼ teaspoonful daily.

HOW SUPPLIED
NU-IRON 150 Caps in bottles of 100. NU-IRON Elixir in 8 fl. oz. bottles.

SEDAPAP #3 CAPSULES Ⓒ III

DESCRIPTION
Each red and white capsule contains:
Acetaminophen .... 500 mg.
Butalbital .... 50 mg.
(Warning: May be habit forming.)
Codeine Phosphate .... 30 mg.
(Warning: May be habit forming.)

HOW SUPPLIED
Bottles of 100.

SEDAPAP-10 TABLETS ℞

DESCRIPTION
Each white capsule-shaped tablet for oral administration contains:
Acetaminophen .... 650 mg.
Butalbital .... 50 mg.
(WARNING: May be habit forming)

ACETAMINOPHEN BUTALBITAL

Acetaminophen is a non-salicylate analgesic-antipyretic which occurs as a white, odorless crystalline powder, possessing a slightly bitter taste.
Butalbital, 5-allyl-5-isobutyl-barbituric acid, a white odorless crystalline powder, is a short to intermediate-acting barbiturate.

ACTIONS
Pharmacologically, SEDAPAP-10 TABLETS combines the analgesic properties of acetaminophen with the anxiolytic and muscle relaxant properties of butalbital.

INDICATIONS
SEDAPAP-10 TABLETS is indicated for the relief of the symptom complex of tension (or muscle contraction) headache.

CONTRAINDICATIONS
Hypersensitivity to acetaminophen, or barbiturates. Patients with porphyria.

PRECAUTIONS
1. **General:**
SEDAPAP-10 TABLETS should be used with caution in patients with severe impairment of hepatic or renal function, or a history of drug abuse or dependence.
2. **Information for Patients:**
SEDAPAP-10 TABLETS may impair the mental and/or physical abilities required for the performance of potentially hazardous tasks, such as driving a car or operating machinery. The patient should be cautioned accordingly.
3. **Drug Interactions:**
Patients receiving narcotic analgesics, antipsychotics, antianxiety agents, or other CNS depressants (including alcohol) concommitantly with SEDAPAP-10 TABLETS may exhibit additive CNS depressant effects. When combined therapy is contemplated, the dose of one or both agents should be reduced.

DRUGS	EFFECT
Butalbital with coumarin anticoagulants	Decreased effect of anticoagulant because of increased metabolism resulting from enzyme induction.
Butalbital with tricyclic antidepressants	Decreased blood levels of the antidepressant.

4. **Usage in Pregnancy:**
Adequate studies have not been performed in animals to determine whether this drug effects fertility in males or females, has teratogenic potential or has other adverse effects on the fetus. SEDAPAP-10 TABLETS should be used only when, in the physician's opinion, the possible benefits outweigh the potential risks to both mother and child.
5. **Nursing Mothers:**
The effects of SEDAPAP-10 TABLETS on infants of nursing mothers is not known. Barbiturates are excreted in the breast milk of nursing mothers. The serum levels in infants are believed to be insignificant with therapeutic doses.
6. **Pediatric Use:**
Safety and effectiveness in children below the age of twelve have not been established.

ADVERSE REACTIONS
The most frequent adverse reactions are drowsiness and dizziness. Less frequent adverse reactions are lightheadedness and gastrointestinal disturbances including nausea and vomiting. Mental confusion or depression can occur due to intolerance or overdosage of butalbital.

DRUG ABUSE AND DEPENDENCE
Prolonged use of barbiturates can produce drug dependence, charcterized by psychic dependence, and less frequently, physical dependence and tolerance. The abuse liability of SEDAPAP-10 TABLETS is similar to that of other barbiturate-containing drug combinations. Caution should be exercised when prescribing medication for patients with a known propensity for taking excessive quantities of drugs, which is not uncommon in patients with chronic tension headache.

OVERDOSAGE
Acetaminophen: In massive overdosage, acetaminophen may cause hepatic toxicity. Early symptoms of a potentially hepatotoxic dose may include nausea, vomiting, diaphoresis, and general malaise. Clinical and laboratory evidence of hepatic toxicity may not be apparent until 48 to 72 hours post ingestion. IN ALL CASES OF SUSPECTED OVERDOSE, IMMEDIATELY CALL YOUR LOCAL POISON CONTROL CENTER OR THE ROCKY MOUNTAIN POISON CENTER'S TOLL FREE NUMBER (800-525-6115) for assistance in diagnosis and for directions in the use of N-acetylcysteine as an antidote.
Butalbital: Symptoms attributable to acute barbiturate poisoning include drowsiness, confusion, and coma; respiratory depression; hypotension; and shock. Vomiting should be induced mechanically or with emetics in the conscious patient. Gastric lavage may be used if the pharyngeal and laryngeal reflexes are present and if less than four hours have elapsed since ingestion. A cuffed endotracheal tube should be inserted before gastric lavage of the unconscious patient and when necessary to provide assisted respiration. Meticulous attention should be given to maintaining adequate pulmonary ventilation.

DOSAGE AND ADMINISTRATION
Oral: One tablet every four hours as needed. Do not exceed six tablets per day.

HOW SUPPLIED
Available as white capsule-shaped tablets imprinted "M/R" in bottles of 100's, NDC #0259-1278-01.

McGregor Pharmaceuticals Inc.

32580 GRAND RIVER AVENUE
FARMINGTON, MI 48024

ALL McGREGOR PRODUCTS ARE COMPLETELY DYE FREE.

Full prescribing information for all McGregor Pharmaceuticals products is available from your McGregor Pharmaceuticals representative.

Product Identification Codes

To provide quick and positive identification of McGregor Pharmaceuticals products, we have had imprinted the product identification number on our capsules. In order that you may quickly identify a product by its code number, we provide the following list of code numbers:

Product	Code Number
Rhindecon™ (Phenylpropanolamine HCl, 75 mg) Sustained Release Capsules ℞	**MCG 215**
Rhinolar™ (Phenylpropanolamine HCl 75 mg, Chlorpheniramine Maleate 8 mg, Methscopolamine Nitrate 2.5 mg) Sustained Release Capsule ℞	**MCG 219**
Rhinolar-EX™ (Phenylpropanolamine HCl 75 mg, Chlorpheniramine Maleate 8 mg) Sustained Release Capsule ℞	**MCG 210**
Rhinolar-EX 12™ (Phenylpropanolamine HCl 75 mg, Chlorpheniramine Maleate 12 mg) Sustained Release Capsule ℞	**MCG 211**

EDUCATIONAL MATERIAL

Samples: Starter samples on above products available upon request.

McNeil Consumer Products Company

McNEILAB, INC.
FORT WASHINGTON, PA 19034

CoTYLENOL® Cold Medication Tablets and Caplets — OTC

DESCRIPTION

Each CoTYLENOL Tablet or Caplet contains acetaminophen 325 mg., chlorpheniramine maleate 2 mg., pseudoephedrine hydrochloride 30 mg. and dextromethorphan hydrobromide 15 mg.

ACTIONS

CoTYLENOL Cold Medication Tablets and Caplets contain a clinically proven analgesic-antipyretic, decongestant, cough suppressant and antihistamine. Acetaminophen produces analgesia by elevation of the pain threshold and antipyresis through action on the hypothalamic heat-regulating center. Pseudoephedrine hydrochloride is a sympathomimetic amine which provides temporary relief of nasal congestion. Dextromethorphan is a cough suppressant which provides temporary relief of coughs due to minor throat irritations that may occur with the common cold. Chlorpheniramine is an antihistamine which helps provide temporary relief of runny nose, sneezing and watery and itchy eyes.

INDICATIONS

CoTYLENOL provides effective temporary relief of the symptoms associated with common colds and other upper respiratory infections including: fever, aches, pains, general discomfort, nasal and sinus congestion, cough, runny nose, sneezing, minor sore throat pain, headache, watery eyes.

ADVERSE REACTIONS

While the acetaminophen component is equal to aspirin in analgesic and antipyretic effectiveness, it is unlikely to produce many of the side effects associated with aspirin and aspirin-containing products. Although pseudoephedrine is virtually without pressor effect in normotensive patients, it should be used with caution in hypertensives.

USUAL DOSAGE

Adults: Two tablets or caplets every 6 hours, not to exceed 8 tablets or caplets in 24 hours. Children (6–12 years): One caplet or tablet every 6 hours, not to exceed 4 tablets or caplets in 24 hours for 5 days.

NOTE

Since CoTYLENOL Cold Medication Tablets and Caplets are available without prescription, the following appears on the package label: "WARNING: Do not administer to children under 6 or exceed the recommended dosage because nervousness, dizziness or sleeplessness may occur. May cause excitability especially in children. A persistent cough may be a sign of a serious condition. If fever persists for more than three days, or if symptoms do not improve or new ones occur within five days or are accompanied by high fever, rash, excessive mucus, persistent cough or headache, consult a physician before continuing use. This preparation may cause drowsiness; alcohol may increase the drowsiness effect. Avoid alcoholic beverages when taking this product. Use caution when driving a motor vehicle or operating machinery. Do not take this product if you have heart disease, high blood pressure, thyroid disease, diabetes, asthma, glaucoma, emphysema, chronic pulmonary disease, shortness of breath, difficulty in breathing, or difficulty in urination due to enlargement of the prostate gland or are taking a prescription drug for high blood pressure or depression, unless directed by a doctor. **Do not use if carton is opened, or if printed green neck wrap or printed foil inner seal is broken. Keep this and all medication out of the reach of children. As with any drug, if you are pregnant or nursing a baby, seek the advice of a health professional before using this product. In case of accidental overdosage, contact a physician or poison control center immediately.**"

OVERDOSAGE

Acetaminophen in massive overdosage may cause hepatic toxicity in some patients. In adults and adolescents, hepatic toxicity has rarely been reported following ingestion of acute overdosage of less than 10 grams. Fatalities are infrequent (less than 3–4% of untreated cases) and have rarely been reported with overdoses of less than 15 grams. In children, an acute overdosage of less than 150 mg/kg has not been associated with hepatic toxicity.

Early symptoms following a potentially hepatotoxic overdose may include: nausea, vomiting, diaphoresis and general malaise. Clinical and laboratory evidence of hepatic toxicity may not be apparent until 48 to 72 hours postingestion.

In adults and adolescents, regardless of the quantity of acetaminophen reported to have been ingested, administer MUCOMYST® acetylcysteine immediately if 24 hours or less have elapsed from the reported time of ingestion. For full prescribing information, refer to the MUCOMYST package insert. Do not await results of assays for acetaminophen level before initiating treatment with MUCOMYST acetylcysteine. The following additional procedures are recommended: The stomach should be emptied promptly by lavage or by induction of emesis with syrup of ipecac. A serum acetaminophen assay should be obtained as early as possible, but no sooner than four hours following ingestion. Liver function studies should be obtained initially and repeated at 24-hour intervals.

Serious toxicity or fatalities are extremely infrequent in children, possibly due to differences in the way they metabolize acetaminophen. In children, the maximum potential amount ingested can be more easily estimated. If more than 150 mg/kg or an unknown amount was ingested, obtain an acetaminophen plasma level. The acetaminophen plasma level should be obtained as soon as possible, but no sooner than 4 hours following the ingestion. Induce emesis using syrup of ipecac. If the plasma level is obtained and falls above the broken line on the nomogram, the MUCOMYST acetylcysteine therapy should be initiated and continued for a full course of therapy. If acetaminophen plasma assay capability is not available, and the estimated acetaminophen ingestion exceeds 150 mg/kg, MUCOMYST acetylcysteine therapy should be initiated and continued for a full course of therapy.

For additional emergency information, call your regional poison center or toll-free (1-800-525-6115) to the Rocky Mountain Poison Center for assistance in diagnosis and for directions in the use of MUCOMYST acetylcysteine as an antidote.

Chlorpheniramine toxicity should be treated as you would an antihistamine/anticholinergic overdose and is likely to be present within a few hours after acute ingestion.

Symptoms from pseudoephedrine overdose consist most often of mild anxiety, tachycardia and/or mild hypertension. Symptoms usually appear within 4 to 8 hours of ingestion and are transient, usually requiring no treatment.

Acute dextromethorphan overdose usually does not result in serious signs and symptoms unless massive amounts have been ingested. Signs and symptoms of a substantial overdose may include nausea and vomiting, visual disturbances, CNS disturbances, and urinary retention.

INACTIVE INGREDIENTS

Tablets: cellulose, starch, magnesium stearate, yellow #6 and yellow #10. Caplets: cellulose, glyceryl, triacetate, hydroxypropyl, methylcellulose, magnesium stearate, polyethylene glycol, sodium starch glycolate, starch, titanium dioxide, blue #1 and yellow #6 & #10.

HOW SUPPLIED

Tablets (colored yellow, imprinted "CoTYLENOL")—blister packs of 24, tamper-resistant bottles of 50 and 100. Caplets (light yellow, imprinted "CoTYLENOL")—blister packs of 24 and tamper-resistant bottles of 50.

Shown in Product Identification Section, page 416

CoTYLENOL® Cold Medication Liquid — OTC

DESCRIPTION

Each 30 ml (1 fl. oz.) contains acetaminophen 650 mg., chlorpheniramine maleate 4 mg., pseudoephedrine hydrochloride 60 mg., and dextromethorphan hydrobromide 30 mg. (alcohol 7%).

ACTIONS

CoTYLENOL Liquid Cold Medication contains a clinically proven analgesic-antipyretic, decongestant, cough suppressant and antihistamine. Acetaminophen produces analgesia by elevation of the pain threshold and antipyresis through action on the hypothalamic heat-regulating center. Pseudoephedrine hydrochloride is a sympathomimetic amine which provides temporary relief of nasal congestion. Dextromethorphan is a cough suppressant which provides temporary relief of coughs due to minor throat irritations that may occur with the common cold. Chlorpheniramine is an antihistamine which helps provide temporary relief of runny nose, sneezing and watery and itchy eyes.

INDICATIONS

CoTYLENOL provides effective temporary relief of the symptoms associated with common colds and other upper respiratory infections including: fever, aches, pains, general discomfort, nasal and sinus congestion, cough, runny nose, sneezing, minor sore throat pain, headache, watery eyes.

ADVERSE REACTIONS

While the acetaminophen component is equal to aspirin in analgesic and antipyretic effectiveness, it is unlikely to produce many of the side effects associated with aspirin and aspirin-containing products. Although pseudoephedrine is virtually without pressor effect in normotensive patients, it should be used with caution in hypertensives.

USUAL DOSAGE

Measuring cup is provided and marked for accurate dosing. Adults: 1 fluid ounce (2 tbsp.) every 6 hours as needed, not to exceed 4 doses in 24 hours. Children (6–12 yrs): ½ the adult dose (1 tbsp.) as indicated on the measuring cup provided, not to exceed 4 doses in 24 hours.

Note: Since CoTYLENOL Liquid Cold Medication is available without a prescription, the following appears on the package label: "WARNING: Do not administer to children under 6 or exceed the recommended dosage because nervousness, dizziness or sleeplessness may occur. May cause excitability especially in children. A persistent cough may be a sign of a serious condition. If fever persists for more than three days, or if symptoms do not improve or new ones occur within five days or are accompanied by high fever, rash, excessive mucus, persistent cough or headache, consult a physician before continuing use. This preparation may cause drowsiness; alcohol may increase the drowsiness effect. Avoid alcoholic beverages when taking this product. Use caution when driving a motor vehicle or operating machinery. Do not take this product if you have heart disease, high blood pressure, thyroid disease, diabetes, asthma, glaucoma, emphysema, chronic pulmonary disease, shortness of breath, difficulty in breathing, or difficulty in urination due to enlargement of the prostrate gland or are taking a prescription drug for high blood pressure or depression, unless directed by a doctor. **Do not use if carton is opened, or if printed plastic overwrap or printed foil inner seal is broken. Keep this and all medication out of the reach of children. As with any drug, if you are pregnant or nursing a baby, seek the advice of a health professional before using this product. In case of accidental overdosage, contact a physician or poison control center immediately.**"

OVERDOSAGE

Acetaminophen in massive overdosage may cause hepatic toxicity in some patients. In adults and adolescents, hepatic toxicity has rarely been reported following ingestion of acute overdosage of less than 10 grams. Fatalities are infrequent (less than 3–4% of untreated cases) and have rarely been reported with overdoses of less than 15 grams. In children, an acute overdosage of less than 150 mg/kg has not been associated with hepatic toxicity.

Continued on next page

McNeil Consumer—Cont.

Early symptoms following a potentially hepatotoxic overdose may include: nausea, vomiting, diaphoresis and general malaise. Clinical and laboratory evidence of hepatic toxicity may not be apparent until 48 to 72 hours postingestion.
In adults and adolescents, regardless of the quantity of acetaminophen reported to have been ingested, administer MUCOMYST® acetylcysteine immediately if 24 hours or less have elapsed from the reported time of ingestion. For full prescribing information, refer to the MUCOMYST package insert. Do not await results of assays for acetaminophen level before initiating treatment with MUCOMYST acetylcysteine. The following additional procedures are recommended: The stomach should be emptied promptly by lavage or by induction of emesis with syrup of ipecac. A serum acetaminophen assay should be obtained as early as possible, but no sooner than four hours following ingestion. Liver function studies should be obtained initially and repeated at 24-hour intervals.
Serious toxicity or fatalities are extremely infrequent in children, possibly due to differences in the way they metabolize acetaminophen. In children, the maximum potential amount ingested can be more easily estimated. If more than 150 mg/kg or an unknown amount was ingested, obtain an acetaminophen plasma level. The acetaminophen plasma level should be obtained as soon as possible, but no sooner than 4 hours following the ingestion. Induce emesis using syrup of ipecac. If the plasma level is obtained and falls above the broken line on the nomogram, the MUCOMYST acetylcysteine therapy should be initiated and continued for a full course of therapy. If acetaminophen plasma assay capability is not available, and the estimated acetaminophen ingestion exceeds 150 mg/kg, MUCOMYST acetylcysteine therapy should be initiated and continued for a full course of therapy.
For additional emergency information, call your regional poison center or toll-free (1-800-525-6115) to the Rocky Mountain Poison Center for assistance in diagnosis and for directions in the use of MUCOMYST acetylcysteine as an antidote.
Chlorpheniramine toxicity should be treated as you would an antihistamine/anticholinergic overdose and is likely to be present within a few hours after acute ingestion.
Symptoms from pseudoephedrine overdose consist most often of mild anxiety, tachycardia and/or mild hypertension. Symptoms usually appear within 4 to 8 hours of ingestion and are transient, usually requiring no treatment.
Acute dextromethorphan overdose usually does not result in serious signs and symptoms unless massive amounts have been ingested. Signs and symptoms of a substantial overdose may include nausea and vomiting, visual disturbances, CNS disturbances, and urinary retention.

INACTIVE INGREDIENTS

Alcohol (7%), citric acid, flavors, glycerin, polyethylene, glycol, saccharin, sodium benzoate, sorbitol, sucrose, purified water, yellow #6 and blue #1.

HOW SUPPLIED

Cherry/mint mentholated flavored (colored amber) in 5 oz. bottles with child-resistant safety cap, special dosage cup graded in ounces and tablespoons, and tamper-resistant packaging.

Shown in Product Identification Section, page 416

CHILDREN'S CoTYLENOL® OTC

Chewable Cold Tablets and Liquid Cold Formula

DESCRIPTION

Each Children's CoTYLENOL Chewable Cold Tablet contains acetaminophen 80 mg, chlorpheniramine maleate 0.5 mg and pseudoephedrine hydrochloride 7.5 mg. Children's CoTYLENOL Liquid Cold Formula is stable, cherry-flavored, red in color and contains no alcohol. Each teaspoon (5 ml) contains acetaminophen 160 mg, chlorpheniramine maleate 1 mg, and pseudoephedrine hydrochloride 15 mg.

ACTIONS AND INDICATIONS

Children's CoTYLENOL Chewable Cold Tablets and Liquid Cold Formula combine the nonsalicylate analgesic-antipyretic acetaminophen with the decongestant pseudoephedrine hydrochloride and the antihistamine chlorpheniramine maleate to help relieve nasal congestion, dry runny noses and prevent sneezing as well as to relieve the fever, aches, pains and general discomfort associated with colds and upper respiratory infections.
While the acetaminophen component is equal to aspirin in analgesic and antipyretic effectiveness, it is unlikely to produce the following side effects often associated with aspirin or aspirin-containing products: allergic reactions, even in aspirin-sensitive children or those with a history of allergy in general; "therapeutic toxicity" in feverish children, since electrolyte imbalance and acid-base changes are not likely to occur; gastric irritation even in children with an already upset stomach.

DOSAGE

Administer to children under 6 years only on the advice of a physician. Children's CoTYLENOL Chewable Cold Tablets: 2–5 years—2 tablets, 6–11 years—4 tablets.
Children's CoTYLENOL Liquid Cold Formula: 2–5 years—1 teaspoonful; 6–11 years—2 teaspoonsful. Measuring cup is provided and marked for accurate dosing.
Doses may be repeated every 4-6 hours as needed, not to exceed 4 doses in 24 hours.
Note: Since Children's CoTYLENOL Chewable Cold Tablets and Liquid Cold Formula are available without prescription, the following information appears on the package labels. The Warnings are identical for the two dosage forms except the Liquid Cold Formula does not contain the phenylketonurics statement since the product does not contain aspartame.

WARNING

Keep this and all medication out of the reach of children. In case of accidental overdosage, contact a physician or poison control center immediately. Phenylketonurics: contains phenylalanine. Do not exceed the recommended dosage because nervousness, dizziness or sleeplessness may occur. If fever persists for more than three days, or if symptoms do not improve or new ones occur within five days or are accompanied by high fever, consult a physician before continuing use. This preparation may cause drowsiness, or in some cases, excitability. Do not give this product to children who have heart disease, high blood pressure, thyroid disease, diabetes, glaucoma or asthma or are taking a prescription drug for high blood pressure or depression, except under the advice and supervision of a physician.

OVERDOSAGE

Acetaminophen in massive overdosage may cause hepatic toxicity in some patients. In adults and adolescents, hepatic toxicity has rarely been reported following ingestion of acute overdosage of less than 10 grams. Fatalities are infrequent (less than 3–4% of untreated cases) and have rarely been reported with overdoses of less than 15 grams. In children, an acute overdosage of less than 150 mg/kg has not been associated with hepatic toxicity.
Early symptoms following a potentially hepatotoxic overdose may include: nausea, vomiting, diaphoresis and general malaise. Clinical and laboratory evidence of hepatic toxicity may not be apparent until 48 to 72 hours postingestion.
In adults and adolescents, regardless of the quantity of acetaminophen reported to have been ingested, administer MUCOMYST® acetylcysteine immediately if 24 hours or less have elapsed from the reported time of ingestion. For full prescribing information, refer to the MUCOMYST package insert. Do not await the results of assays for acetaminophen level before initiating treatment with MUCOMYST acetylcysteine. The following additional procedures are recommended: The stomach should be emptied promptly by lavage or by induction of emesis with syrup of ipecac. A serum acetaminophen assay should be obtained as early as possible, but no sooner than four hours following ingestion. Liver function studies should be obtained initially and repeated at 24-hour intervals.
Serious toxicity or fatalities are extremely infrequent in children, possibly due to differences in the way they metabolize acetaminophen. In children, the maximum potential amount ingested can be more easily estimated. If more than 150 mg/kg or an unknown amount was ingested, obtain an acetaminophen plasma level. The acetaminophen plasma level should be obtained as soon as possible, but no sooner than 4 hours following the ingestion. Induce emesis using syrup of ipecac. If the plasma level is obtained and falls above the broken line on the nomogram, the MUCOMYST acetylcysteine therapy should be initiated and continued for a full course of therapy. If acetaminophen plasma assay capability is not available, and the estimated acetaminophen ingestion exceeds 150 mg/kg, MUCOMYST acetylcysteine therapy should be initiated and continued for a full course of therapy.
For additional emergency information, call your regional poison center or toll-free (1-800-525-6115) to the Rocky Mountain Poison Center for assistanece in diagnosis and for directions in the use of MUCOMYST acetylcysteine as an antidote.
Chlorpheniramine toxicity should be treated as you would an antihistamine/anticholinergic overdose and is likely to be present within a few hours after acute ingestion.
Pseudoephedrine may produce central nervous system stimulation and sympathomimetic effects on the cardiovascular system which are likely to be manifested within a few hours following ingestion.

INACTIVE INGREDIENTS

Chewable Tablets—Aspartame, cellulose, citric acid, ethylcellulose, flavors, magnesium stearate, mannitol, starch, sucrose and Yellow #6.
Liquid—Benzoic acid, citric acid, flavors, glycerin, polyethylene glycol, propylene glycol, sodium benzoate, sorbitol, sucrose, purified water and Red #40.

HOW SUPPLIED

Chewable Tablets (colored orange, scored, imprinted "CoTYLENOL")—bottles of 24. Cold Formula—bottles (colored red) of 4 fl. oz.

Shown in Product Identification Section, page 416

DELSYM® OTC

[del'sim]
(dextromethorphan polistirex)

DESCRIPTION

Provides 12-hour relief of coughs due to minor throat and bronchial irritation. Each teaspoonful (5 ml) contains dextromethorphan polistirex equivalent to 30 mg dextromethorphan hydrobromide.

INDICATIONS

For temporary relief of cough due to minor throat and bronchial irritation as may occur with the common cold or with inhaled irritants.

CONTRAINDICATIONS

Hypersensitivity to dextromethrophan.
Note: Since DELSYM dextromethorphan polistirex syrup is available without prescription, the following appears on the package labels.

WARNINGS

Do not give this product to children under 2 years except under the advice and supervision of a physician. Do not take this product for persistent or chronic cough such as occurs with smoking, asthma, or emphysema, or where cough is accompanied by excessive phlegm (mucus) unless directed by a physician.
As with any drug, if you are pregnant or nursing a baby, seek the advice of a health professional before using this product.

CAUTION

A persistent cough may be a sign of a serious condition. If cough persists for more than 1 week, tends to recur or is accompanied by a high fever, rash or persistent headache, consult a physician. Keep this and all drugs out of reach of children. In case of accidental overdose, seek professional assistance or contact a Poison Control Center immediately. Do not use if carton is opened, or red ring is disconnected from cap.

DIRECTIONS

Shake well before using. Adults: 2 teaspoonsful every 12 hours; do not exceed 4 teaspoonsful in 24 hours. Children 6–12: 1 teaspoonful every 12 hours; do not exceed 2 teaspoonsful in 24 hours. Children 2–5: ½ teaspoonful every 12 hours: do not exceed 1 teaspoonful in 24 hours. Children under 2: Use only under the advice and supervision of a physician.

OVERDOSAGE

Acute dextromethorphan overdose usually does not result in serious signs and symptoms unless a massive amount has been ingested. Signs and symptoms of a substantial overdose may include nausea and vomiting, visual disturbance, CNS disturbances, and urinary retention. Because of the sustained action of DELSYM, the onset of symptoms may be delayed, and the duration of symptoms may be prolonged.

HOW SUPPLIED

3 fl. oz. bottles (NDC 0045-0288-03)

INACTIVE INGREDIENTS

Citric Acid; Dye, Yellow No. 6; Ethylcellulose; Flavor; High Fructose Corn Syrup; Methylparaben; Polyethylene Glycol 3350; Polysorbate 80; Propylene Glycol; Propylparaben; Sucrose; Tragacanth; Vegetable Oil; Water; Xanthan Gum.

Shown in Product Identification Section, page 416

MEDIPREN® OTC

Ibuprofen Caplets and Tablets
Pain Reliever/Fever Reducer

WARNING

ASPIRIN SENSITIVE PATIENTS. Do not take this product if you have had a severe allergic reaction to aspirin (e.g., asthma, swelling, shock or hives) because even though this product contains no aspirin or salicylates, cross-reactions may occur in patients allergic to aspirin.

DESCRIPTION

Each MEDIPREN Caplet or Tablet contains ibuprofen 200 mg.

INDICATIONS

For the temporary relief of minor aches and pains associated with the common cold, headache, toothaches, muscular aches, backache, for the minor pain of arthritis, for the pain of menstrual cramps, and for reduction of fever.

Age Group	0–3 mos	4–11 mos	12–23 mos	2–3 yrs	4–5 yrs	6–8 yrs	9–10 yrs	11 yrs	Dosage
Weight (lbs)	6–11 lb	12–17 lb	18–23 lb	24–35 lb	36–47 lb	48–59 lb	60–71 lb	72–95 lb	
PEDIACARE Infants' Drops*	½ dropper (0.4 ml)	1 dropper (0.8 ml)	1½ droppers (1.2 ml)	2 droppers (1.6 ml)					q4–6h
PEDIACARE 1 Liquid				1 tsp	1½ tsp	2 tsp	2½ tsp	3 tsp	q4h
PEDIACARE 2 Liquid**				1 tsp	1½ tsp	2 tsp	2½ tsp	3 tsp	q4–6h
PEDIACARE 3 Liquid**				1 tsp	1½ tsp	2 tsp	2½ tsp	3 tsp	q4–6h
Chewable Tablets**				2 tabs	3 tabs	4 tabs	5 tabs	6 tabs	q4–6h

* administer to children under 2 years only on the advice of a physician
** administer to children under 6 years only on the advice of a physician

USUAL DOSAGE

Adults: One Caplet or Tablet every 4 to 6 hours while symptoms persist. If pain or fever does not respond to 1 Caplet or Tablet, 2 Caplets or Tablets may be used but do not exceed 6 Caplets or Tablets in 24 hours, unless directed by a doctor. The smallest effective dose should be used. Take with food or milk if occasional and mild heartburn, upset stomach, or stomach pain occurs with use. Consult a doctor if these symptoms are more than mild or if they persist.

Children: Do not give this product to children under 12 except under the advice and supervision of a doctor.

WARNINGS

Do not take for pain for more than 10 days or for fever for more than 3 days unless directed by a doctor. If pain or fever persists or gets worse, if new symptoms occur, or if the painful area is red or swollen, consult a doctor. These could be signs of serious illness. If you are under a doctor's care for any serious condition, consult a doctor before taking this product. As with aspirin and acetaminophen, if you have any condition which requires you to take prescription drugs or if you have had any problems or serious side effects from taking any non-prescription pain reliever, do not take this product without first discussing it with your doctor. If you experience any symptoms which are unusual or seem unrelated to the condition for which you took ibuprofen, consult a doctor before taking any more of it. Although ibuprofen is indicated for the same conditions as aspirin and acetaminophen, it should not be taken with them except under a doctor's direction. Do not combine this product with any other ibuprofen containing product. As with any drug, if you are pregnant or nursing a baby, seek the advice of a health professional before using this product. IT IS ESPECIALLY IMPORTANT NOT TO USE IBUPROFEN DURING THE LAST 3 MONTHS OF PREGNANCY UNLESS SPECIFICALLY DIRECTED TO DO SO BY A DOCTOR BECAUSE IT MAY CAUSE PROBLEMS IN THE UNBORN CHILD OR COMPLICATIONS DURING DELIVERY. Keep this and all drugs out of the reach of children.

OVERDOSAGE

In case of accidental overdose, contact a physician or poison control center.

STORAGE

Store at room temperature; avoid excessive heat 40°C (104°F).

INACTIVE INGREDIENTS

Colloidal silicon dioxide, glyceryl triacetate, hydroxypropyl methylcellulose, microcrystalline cellulose, pregelatinized starch, sodium lauryl sulfate, sodium starch glycolate, titanium dioxide, FD&C blue #1 and D&C yellow #10.

HOW SUPPLIED

Coated Caplets (colored white, imprinted "MEDIPREN")—bottles of 24's, 50's, 100's. Coated Tablets (colored white, imprinted "MEDIPREN")—bottles of 24's, 50's, 100's.

Shown in Product Identification Section, page 416

PEDIACARE™ 1 Children's Cough Relief Liquid OTC
PEDIACARE™ 2 Children's Cold Relief Liquid
PEDIACARE™ 3 Children's Cold Relief Liquid and Chewable Tablets
PEDIACARE™ Infants' Cold Relief Decongestant Oral Drops

DESCRIPTION

Each 5 ml (teaspoon) of PEDIACARE 1 Children's Cough Relief Liquid contains dextromethorphan hydrobromide 5 mg. Each 5 ml of PEDIACARE 2 Children's Cold Relief Liquid contains pseudoephedrine hydrochloride 15 mg and chlorpheniramine maleate 1 mg. Each 5 ml of PEDIACARE 3 Children's Cold Relief Liquid contains pseudoephedrine hydrochloride 15 mg, chlorpheniramine maleate 1 mg and dextromethorphan hydrobromide 5 mg. Each PEDIACARE 3 Cold Relief Chewable Tablet contains pseudoephedrine hydrochloride 7.5 mg, chlorpheniramine maleate 0.5 mg and dextromethorphan hydrobromide 2.5 mg. Each 0.8 ml oral dropper of PEDIACARE Infants' Drops contains pseudoephedrine hydrochloride 7.5 mg. PEDIACARE Liquid Products and Infants' Drops are stable, cherry flavored and red in color. PEDIACARE 3 Chewable Tablets are fruit flavored and pink in color.

ACTIONS AND INDICATIONS

PEDIACARE Cold Products are available in four different formulas, allowing you to select the ideal cold product to temporarily relieve the patient's particular cold symptoms. PEDIACARE 1 Liquid contains a cough suppressant, dextromethorphan hydrobromide, to provide temporary relief of coughs due to minor throat irritations that may occur with the common cold. PEDIACARE 2 Liquid contains a decongestant, pseudoephedrine hydrochloride, and an antihistamine, chlorpheniramine maleate, to provide temporary relief of nasal congestion, runny nose and sneezing due to the common cold, hay fever or other upper respiratory allergies. PEDIACARE 3 Liquid and Chewable Tablets contain all three of the above ingredients to provide temporary relief of nasal congestion, runny nose, sneezing and coughing due to the common cold, hay fever or other upper respiratory allergies. PEDIACARE Infants' Drops contain a decongestant, pseudoephedrine hydrochloride, to provide temporary relief of nasal congestion due to the common cold, hay fever or other upper respiratory allergies.

Professional Dosage: A calibrated dosage cup is provided for accurate dosing of the PEDIACARE Liquid formulas. A calibrated oral dropper is provided for accurate dosing of PEDIACARE Infants' Drops. All PEDIACARE 1 Liquid doses may be repeated every 4 hours, not to exceed 6 doses in 24 hours. All doses of PEDIACARE 2 Liquid, PEDIACARE 3 Liquid and Chewable Tablets and PEDIACARE Infants' Drops may be repeated every 4–6 hours, not to exceed 4 doses in 24 hours.

[See table above].

Note: Since PEDIACARE cold products are available without prescription, the following information appears on the package labels: "WARNINGS: Do not use if carton is opened, or if printed plastic bottle wrap or foil inner seal is broken. Keep this and all medication out of the reach of children. In case of accidental overdosage, contact a physician or poison control center immediately."

The following information appears on the appropriate package labels:

PEDIACARE 1 Children's Cough Relief Liquid: "Do not take for persistent or chronic cough such as occurs with asthma or where cough is accompanied by excessive mucus except under the advice and supervision of a physician. A persistent cough may be a sign of serious condition. If cough persists for more than seven days, tends to recur or is accompanied by high fever, rash or persistent headache, consult a physician."

"Inactive Ingredients: Benzoic acid, citric acid, flavors, glycerin, polyethylene glycol, propylene glycol, sodium benzoate, sorbitol, sucrose, purified water, Red #33, Blue #1 and Red #40."

PEDIACARE 2 Children's Cold Relief Liquid: "Do not exceed the recommended dosage because nervousness, dizziness or sleeplessness may occur. If symptoms do not improve within seven days or are accompanied by high fever, consult a physician before continuing use. This preparation may cause drowsiness, or in some cases, excitability. Do not give this product to children who have heart disease, high blood pressure, thyroid disease, diabetes, glaucoma or asthma, or are taking a prescription drug for high blood pressure or depression, except under the advise and supervision of a physician."

"Inactive Ingredients: Benzoic acid, citric acid, flavors, glycerin, polyethylene glycol, propylene glycol, sodium benzoate, sorbitol, sucrose, purified water, Red #33, Blue #1 and Red #40.

PEDIACARE 3 Children's Cold Relief Liquid and Chewable Tablets: "Do not exceed the recommended dosage because nervousness, dizziness or sleeplessness may occur. A persistent cough may be a sign of a serious condition. If symptoms do not improve within seven days, tend to recur, or are accompanied by high fever, rash, excessive mucus, persistent cough or headache, consult a physician before continuing use. This preparation may cause drowsiness or, in some cases, excitability. Do not give this product to children who have heart disease, high blood pressure, thyroid disease, diabetes, glaucoma or asthma, or are taking a prescription drug for high blood pressure or depression, except under the advice and supervision of a physician."

PEDIACARE 3 Liquid: Inactive Ingredients: Benzoic acid, citric acid, flavors, glycerin, polyethylene glycol, propylene glycol, sodium benzoate, sorbitol, sucrose, purified water, Red #33, Blue #1 and Red #40.

PEDIACARE 3 Chewable Tablets also contain the warning, "Phenylketonurics: contains phenylanine", and the inactive ingredient listing, "Inactive Ingredients: Aspartame, cellulose, citric acid, dextrose, flavors, magnésium stearate, magnesium trisilicate, mannitol, starch, sucrose and Red #3."

PEDIACARE Infants' Cold Relief Decongestant Oral Drops: "Do not exceed the recommended dosage because at higher doses nervousness, dizziness or sleeplessness may occur. Do not give this product to children who have heart disease, high blood pressure, thyroid disease or diabetes unless directed by a physician. Do not give this product to children for more than seven days. If symptoms do not improve or are accompanied by fever, consult a physician.

DRUG INTERACTION PRECAUTION

Do not give this product to children who are taking a prescription drug for high blood pressure or depression without first consulting a physician. Take by mouth only. Not for nasal use."

"Inactive Ingredients: Benzoic acid, citric acid, flavors, glycerin, polyethylene glycol, propylene glycol, purified water, sodium benzoate, sorbitol, sucrose and Red #40."

OVERDOSAGE

Acute dextromethorphan overdose usually does not result in serious signs and symptoms unless massive amounts have been ingested. Signs and symptoms of a substantial overdose may include nausea and vomiting, visual disturbances, CNS disturbances, and urinary retention. Symptoms from pseudoephedrine overdose consist most often of mild anxiety, tachycardia and/or mild hypertension. Symptoms usually appear within 4 to 8 hours of ingestion and are transient, usually requiring no treatment. Chlorpheniramine toxicity should be treated as you would an antihistamine/anticholinergic overdose and is likely to be present within a few hours after acute ingestion.

HOW SUPPLIED

PEDIACARE Liquid products (colored red)—bottles of 4 fl. oz with child-resistant safety cap and calibrated dosage cup. PEDIACARE 3 Chewable Tablets (pink, scored)—bottles of 24 with child-resistant safety cap. PEDIACARE Infants' Drops (colored red)—bottles of ½ fl. oz with calibrated dropper.

Shown in Product Identification Section, page 416

SINE-AID® OTC
Sinus Headache Tablets

DESCRIPTION

Each SINE-AID® Tablet contains acetaminophen 325 mg and pseudoephedrine hydrochloride 30 mg.

ACTIONS

SINE-AID® Tablets contain a clinically proven analgesic-antipyretic and a decongestant. Acetaminophen produces analgesia by elevation of the pain threshold and antipyresis through action on the hypothalamic heat-regulating center. Pseudoephedrine hydrochloride is a sympathomimetic amine which promotes sinus cavity drainage by reducing nasopharyngeal mucosal congestion.

INDICATIONS

SINE-AID® Tablets provide effective symptomatic relief from sinus headache pain and pressure caused by sinusitis.

ADVERSE REACTIONS

While the acetaminophen component is equal to aspirin in analgesic and antipyretic effectiveness, it is unlikely to produce many of the side effects associated with aspirin and aspirin-containing products. Since the product contains no antihistamine, SINE-AID® Tablets will not produce the drowsiness that may interfere with work, driving an automobile or operating dangerous machinery. SINE-AID® is particularly well-suited in patients with aspirin allergy, hemostatic disturbances (including anticoagulant therapy), and bleeding diatheses (e.g. hemophilia) and upper gastrointestinal disease (e.g. ulcer, gastritis, hiatus hernia). If a rare sensitivity occurs, the drug should be discontinued. Although pseudoephedrine is virtually without pressor effect in nor-

Continued on next page

McNeil Consumer—Cont.

motensive patients, it should be used with caution in hypertensives.

USUAL DOSAGE

Adult dosage: Two tablets every four to six hours. Do not exceed eight tablets in any 24 hour period. **Note:** Since SINE-AID® tablets are available without a prescription, the following appears on the package labels: "**WARNING:** Do not exceed the recommended dosage because at higher doses nervousness, dizziness or sleeplessness may occur. Do not administer to children under 12. If you have high blood pressure, heart disease, diabetes, thyroid disease, difficulty in urination due to enlargement of the prostate gland, or are presently taking a prescription drug for the treatment of high blood pressure or depression, do not take except under the advice and supervision of a physician. Do not take this product for more than 7 days. If symptoms do not improve or are accompanied by high fever, consult a physician. **Do not use if carton is opened, or printed foil inner seal is broken. Keep this and all medication out of the reach of children. As with any drug, if you are pregnant or nursing a baby, seek the advice of a health professional before using this product. In case of accidental overdosage, contact a physician or poison control center.**"

OVERDOSAGE

Acetaminophen in massive overdosage may cause hepatic toxicity in some patients. In adults and adolescents, hepatic toxicity has rarely been reported following ingestion of acute overdoses of less than 10 grams. Fatalities are infrequent (less than 3–4% of untreated cases) and have rarely been reported with overdoses of less than 15 grams. In children, an acute overdosage of less than 150 mg/kg has not been associated with hepatic toxicity.

Early symptoms following a potentially hepatotoxic overdose may include: nausea, vomiting, diaphoresis and general malaise. Clinical and laboratory evidence of hepatic toxicity may not be apparent until 48 to 72 hours postingestion.

In adults and adolescents, regardless of the quantity of acetaminophen reported to have been ingested, administer MUCOMYST® acetylcysteine immediately if 24 hours or less have elapsed from the reported time of ingestion. For full prescribing information, refer to the MUCOMYST package insert. Do not await results of assays for acetaminophen level before initiating treatment with MUCOMYST acetylcysteine. The following additional procedures are recommended: The stomach should be emptied promptly by lavage or by induction of emesis with syrup of ipecac. A serum acetaminophen assay should be obtained as early as possible, but no sooner than four hours following ingestion. Liver function studies should be obtained initially and repeated at 24-hour intervals.

Serious toxicity or fatalities are extremely infrequent in children, possibly due to differences in the way they metabolize acetaminophen. In children, the maximum potential amount ingested can be more easily estimated. If more than 150 mg/kg or an unknown amount was ingested, obtain an acetaminophen plasma level. The acetaminophen plasma level should be obtained as soon as possible, but no sooner than 4 hours following the ingestion. Induce emesis using syrup of ipecac. If the plasma level is obtained and falls above the broken line on the nomogram, the MUCOMYST acetylcysteine therapy should be initiated and continued for a full course of therapy. If acetaminophen plasma assay capability is not available, and the estimated acetaminophen ingestion exceeds 150 mg/kg, MUCOMYST acetylcysteine therapy should be initiated and continued for a full course of therapy.

For additional emergency information, call your regional poison center or toll-free (1-800-525-6115) to the Rocky Mountain Poison Center for assistance in diagnosis and for directions in the use of MUCOMYST acetylcysteine as an antidote.

INACTIVE INGREDIENTS

Cellulose, Sodium Lauryl Sulfate, Starch, Magneisum Stearate.

HOW SUPPLIED

Tablets (colored white, imprinted "SINE-AID®")—tamper-resistant bottles of 24, 50 and 100.

Shown in Product Identification Section, page 416

EXTRA STRENGTH SINE-AID® OTC

Sinus Headache Caplets

DESCRIPTION

Each EXTRA STRENGTH SINE-AID® Caplet contains acetaminophen 500 mg and pseudoephedrine hydrochloride 30 mg.

ACTIONS

EXTRA-STRENGTH SINE-AID® Caplets contain a clinically proven analgesic-antipyretic and a decongestant. Maximum allowable non-prescription levels of acetaminophen and pseudophedrine provide temporary relief of sinus congestion and pain. Acetaminophen produces analgesia by elevation of the pain threshold and antipyresis through action on the hypothalamic heat-regulating center. Pseudoephedrine hydrochloride is a sympathomimetic amine which promotes sinus cavity drainage by reducing nasopharyngeal mucosal congestion.

INDICATIONS

EXTRA STRENGTH SINE-AID® Caplets provide effective symptomatic relief from sinus headache pain and pressure caused by sinusitis.

ADVERSE REACTIONS

While the acetaminophen component is equal to aspirin in analgesic and antipyretic effectiveness, it is unlikely to produce many of the side effects associated with aspirin and aspirin-containing products. Since the product contains no antihistamine, EXTRA-STRENGTH SINE-AID® Caplets will not produce the drowsiness that may interfere with work, driving an automobile or operating dangerous machinery. SINE-AID® is particularly well-suited in patients with aspirin allergy, hemostatic disturbances (including anticoagulant therapy), and bleeding diatheses (e.g. hemophilia) and upper gastrointestinal disease (e.g. ulcer, gastritis, hiatus hernia). If a rare sensitivity occurs, the drug should be discontinued. Although pseudoephedrine is virtually without pressor effect in normotensive patients, it should be used with caution in hypertensives.

USUAL DOSAGE

Adult dosage: Two caplets every four to six hours. Do not exceed eight caplets in any 24 hour period. **Note:** Since EXTRA STRENGTH SINE-AID® Caplets are available without a prescription, the following appears on the package labels: "**WARNING:** Do not exceed the recommended dosage because at higher doses nervousness, dizziness or sleeplessness may occur. Do not administer to children under 12. If you have high blood pressure, heart disease, diabetes, thyroid disease, difficulty in urination due to enlargement of the prostate gland, or are presently taking a prescription drug for the treatment of high blood pressure or depression, do not take except under the advice and supervision of a physician. Do not take this product for more than 7 days. If symptoms do not improve or are accompanied by high fever, consult a physician. **Do not use if carton is opened, or if printed red-neck wrap or printed foil inner seal is broken. Keep this and all medication out of the reach of children. As with any drug, if you are pregnant or nursing a baby, seek the advice of a health professional before using this product. In case of accidental overdosage, contact a physician or poison control center.**"

OVERDOSAGE

Acetaminophen in massive overdosage may cause hepatic toxicity in some patients. In adults and adolescents, hepatic toxicity has rarely been reported following ingestion of acute overdoses of less than 10 grams. Fatalities are infrequent (less than 3–4% of untreated cases) and have rarely been reported with overdoses of less than 15 grams. In children, an acute overdosage of less than 150 mg/kg has not been associated with hepatic toxicity.

Early symptoms following a potentially hepatotoxic overdose may include: nausea, vomiting, diaphoresis and general malaise. Clinical and laboratory evidence of hepatic toxicity may not be apparent until 48 to 72 hours postingestion.

In adults and adolescents, regardless of the quantity of acetaminophen reported to have been ingested, administer MUCOMYST® acetylcysteine immediately if 24 hours or less have elapsed from the reported time of ingestion. For full prescribing information, refer to the MUCOMYST package insert. Do not await results of assays for acetaminophen level before initiating treatment with MUCOMYST acetylcysteine. The following additional procedures are recommended: The stomach should be emptied promptly by lavage or by induction of emesis with syrup of ipecac. A serum acetaminophen assay should be obtained as early as possible, but no sooner than four hours following ingestion. Liver function studies should be obtained initially and repeated at 24-hour intervals.

Serious toxicity or fatalities are extremely infrequent in children, possibly due to differences in the way they metabolize acetaminophen. In children, the maximum potential amount ingested can be more easily estimated. If more than 150 mg/kg or an unknown amount was ingested, obtain an acetaminophen plasma level. The acetaminophen plasma level should be obtained as soon as possible, but no sooner than 4 hours following the ingestion. Induce emesis using syrup of ipecac. If the plasma level is obtained and falls above the broken line on the nomogram, the MUCOMYST acetylcysteine therapy should be initiated and continued for a full course of therapy. If acetaminophen plasma assay capability is not available, and the estimated acetaminophen ingestion exceeds 150 mg/kg, MUCOMYST acetylcysteine therapy should be initiated and continued for a full course of therapy.

For additional emergency information, call your regional poison center or toll-free (1-800-525-6115) to the Rocky Mountain Poison Center for assistance in diagnosis and for directions in the use of MUCOMYST acetylcysteine as an antidote.

Symptoms from pseudoephedrine overdose consist most often of mild anxiety, tachycardia and/or mild hypertension. Symptoms usually appear within 4 to 8 hours of ingestion and are transient, usually requiring no treatment.

INACTIVE INGREDIENTS

Cellulose, hydroxypropyl methylcellulose, magnesium stearate, polyethylene glycol, sodium starch glycolate, starch, titanium dioxide, Blue #1 and Red #40.

HOW SUPPLIED

Caplets (colored white imprinted "Extra Strength SINE-AID")—tamper-resistant bottles of 24 and 50.

Shown in Product Identification Section, page 416

CHILDREN'S TYLENOL® OTC

acetaminophen

Chewable Tablets, Elixir, Drops

DESCRIPTION

Each Children's TYLENOL Chewable Tablet contains 80 mg. acetaminophen in a fruit flavored tablet. Children's TYLENOL acetaminophen Elixir is stable, cherry flavored, red in color and is alcohol free. Infants' TYLENOL Drops are stable, fruit flavored, orange in color and are alcohol free.

Children's TYLENOL Elixir: Each 5 ml. contains 160 mg. acetaminophen.

Infant's TYLENOL Drops: Each 0.8 ml. (one calibrated dropperful) contains 80 mg. acetaminophen.

ACTIONS

TYLENOL acetaminophen is an effective antipyretic /analgesic. It produces antipyresis through action on the hypothalamic heat-regulating center and analgesia by elevation of the pain threshold.

INDICATIONS

Children's TYLENOL Chewable Tablets, Elixir and Drops are designed for treatment of infants and children with conditions requiring reduction of fever or relief of pain—such as mild upper respiratory infections (tonsillitis, common cold, "grippe"), headache, myalgia, post-immunization reactions, post-tonsillectomy discomfort and gastroenteritis. TYLENOL acetaminophen is useful as an analgesic and antipyretic in many bacterial or viral infections, such as bronchitis, pharyngitis, tracheobronchitis, sinusitis, pneumonia, otitis media, and cervical adenitis.

PRECAUTIONS AND ADVERSE REACTIONS

TYLENOL acetaminophen has rarely been found to produce any side effects. If a rare sensitivity reaction occurs, the drug should be stopped. It is usually well tolerated by aspirin-sensitive patients.

USUAL DOSAGE

Doses may be repeated 4 or 5 times daily, but not to exceed 5 doses in 24 hours. Administer to children under 2 years only on the advice of a physician. Children's TYLENOL Chewable Tablets: 1–2 years: one and one half tablets. 2–3 years: two tablets. 4–5 years: three tablets, 6–8 years: four tablets. 9–10 years: five tablets. 11–12 years: six tablets.

Children's TYLENOL Elixir: (special cup for measuring dosage is provided) 4–11 months: one-half teaspoon. 12–23 months: three-quarters teaspoon, 2–3 years: one teaspoon. 4–5 years: one and one-half teaspoons. 6–8 years: 2 teaspoons. 9–10 years: two and one-half teaspoons. 11–12 years: three teaspoons.

Infants' TYLENOL Drops: 0–3 months: 0.4 ml. 4–11 months: 0.8 ml. 12–23 months: 1.2 ml. 2–3 years: 1.6 ml. 4–5 years: 2.4 ml.

Note: Since Children's TYLENOL acetaminophen Chewable Tablets, Elixir and Drops are available without prescription as an analgesic, the following appears on the package labels: "**WARNING: Do not use if carton is opened, or if printed foil inner seal is broken. Keep this and all medication out of the reach of children. In case of accidental overdosage, contact a physician or poison control center immediately. Phenylketonurics: contains phenylalanine.** Consult your physician if fever persists for more than three days or if pain continues for more than five days."

Note: Phenylketonurics warning applies to Children's TYLENOL Chewable Tablets only.

OVERDOSAGE

Acetaminophen in massive overdosage may cause hepatic toxicity in some patients. In adults and adolescents, hepatic toxicity has rarely been reported following ingestion of acute overdoses of less than 10 grams. Fatalities are infrequent (less than 3–4% of untreated cases) and have rarely been reported with overdoses of less than 15 grams. In children, an acute overdosage of less than 150 mg/kg has not been associated with hepatic toxicity.

Early symptoms following a potentially hepatotoxic overdose may include: nausea, vomiting, diaphoresis and general malaise. Clinical and laboratory evidence of hepatic toxicity may not be apparent until 48 to 72 hours postingestion.
In adults and adolescents, regardless of the quantity of acetaminophen reported to have been ingested, administer MUCOMYST® acetylcysteine immediately if 24 hours or less have elapsed from the reported time of ingestion. For full prescribing information, refer to the MUCOMYST package insert. Do not await results of assays for acetaminophen level before initiating treatment with MUCOMYST acetylcysteine. The following additional procedures are recommended: The stomach should be emptied promptly by lavage or by induction of emesis with syrup of ipecac. A serum acetaminophen assay should be obtained as early as possible, but no sooner than four hours following ingestion. Liver function studies should be obtained initially and repeated at 24-hour intervals.
Serious toxicity or fatalities are extremely infrequent in children, possibly due to differences in the way they metabolize acetaminophen. In children, the maximum potential amount ingested can be more easily estimated. If more than 150 mg/kg or an unknown amount was ingested, obtain an acetaminophen plasma level. The acetaminophen plasma level should be obtained as soon as possible, but no sooner than 4 hours following the ingestion. Induce emesis using syrup of ipecac. If the plasma level is obtained and falls above the broken line on the nomogram, the MUCOMYST acetylcysteine therapy should be initiated and continued for a full course of therapy. If acetaminophen plasma assay capability is not available, and the estimated acetaminophen ingestion exceeds 150 mg/kg, MUCOMYST acetylcysteine therapy should be initiated and continued for a full course of therapy.
For additional emergency information, call your regional poison center or toll-free (1-800-525-6115) to the Rocky Mountain Poison Center for assistance in diagnosis and for directions in the use of MUCOMYST acetylcysteine as an antidote.

INACTIVE INGREDIENTS

Children's Tylenol Chewable Tablets—Aspartame, Cellulose, Citric Acid, Ethylcellulose, Flavors, Hydroxypropyl Methylcellulose, Mannitol, Starch, Magnesium Stearate, Red #7.
Children's Tylenol Elixir—Benzoic Acid, Citric Acid, Flavors, Glycerin, Polyethylene Glycol, Propylene Glycol, Sodium Benzoate, Sorbitol, Sucrose, Purified Water, Red #33 and Red #40.
Infant's Tylenol Drops—Flavors, Propylene Glycol, Saccharin, Purified Water, Yellow #6.

HOW SUPPLIED

Chewable Tablets (colored pink, scored, imprinted "TYLENOL")—Bottles of 30 and child resistant blister packs of 48. Elixir (colored red)—bottles of 2 and 4 fl. oz. Drops (colored orange)—bottles of ½ oz. (15 ml.) with calibrated plastic dropper.
All packages listed above have child-resistant safety caps.

Shown in Product Identification Section, page 416

Junior Strength TYLENOL® OTC
acetaminophen
Coated Caplets

DESCRIPTION

Each Junior Strength Caplet contains 160mg acetaminophen in a small, coated, capsule shaped tablet.

ACTIONS

TYLENOL acetaminophen is an effective antipyretic/analgesic. It produces antipyresis through action on the hypothalmic heat-regulating center and analgesia by elevation of the pain threshold.

INDICATIONS

Junior Strength TYLENOL Caplets are designed for older children and young adults with conditions requiring reduction of fever or relief of pain—such as mild upper respiratory infections (tonsillitis, common cold, "grippe"), headache, myalgia, post-immunization reactions, post-tonsillectomy discomfort and gastroenteritis. TYLENOL acetaminophen is useful as an analgesic and antipyretic in many bacterial or viral infections, such as bronchitis, pharyngitis, tracheobronchitis, sinusitis, pneumonia, otitis media and cervical adenitis.

PRECAUTIONS AND ADVERSE REACTIONS

TYLENOL acetaminophen has rarely been found to produce any side effects. If a rare sensitivity reaction occurs, the drug should be stopped. It is usually well tolerated by aspirin-sensitive patients.

USUAL DOSAGE

Doses may be repeated 4 or 5 times daily, but not to exceed 5 doses in 24 hours each. For ages: 6–8 years: two caplets 9–10 years: two and one-half caplets, 11 years: three caplets, 12–14 years: four caplets.
Note: Since Junior Strength TYLENOL acetaminophen Caplets are available without a prescription as an analgesic, the following appears on the package labels:

WARNINGS

Do not use if carton is opened or if a blister unit is broken. Keep this and all medications out of the reach of children. In case of accidental overdosage, contact a physician or poison control center immediately. Consult your physician if fever persists for more than three days or if pain continues for more than five days. As with any drugs, if you are pregnant or nursing a baby, seek the advice of a health professional before using this product. Not for children who have difficulty swallowing tablets.

OVERDOSAGE

Acetaminophen in massive overdosage may cause hepatic toxicity in some patients. In adults and adolescents, hepatic toxicity has rarely been reported following ingestion of acute overdosage of less than 10 grams. Fatalities are infrequent (less than 3–4% of untreated cases) and have rarely been reported with overdoses of less than 15 grams. In children, an acute overdosage of less than 150 mg/kg has not been associated with hepatic toxicity.
Early symptoms following a potentially hepatotoxic overdose may include: nausea, vomiting, diaphoresis and general malaise. Clinical and laboratory evidence of hepatic toxicity may not be apparent until 48 to 72 hours postingestion.
In adults and adolescents, regardless of the quantity of acetaminophen reported to have been ingested, administer MUCOMYST® acetylcysteine immediately if 24 hours or less have elapsed from the reported time of ingestion. For full prescribing information, refer to the MUCOMYST package insert. Do not await the results of assays for acetaminophen level before initiating treatment with MUCOMYST acetylcysteine. The following additional procedures are recommended: The stomach should be emptied promptly by lavage or by induction of emesis with syrup of ipecac. A serum acetaminophen assay should be obtained as early as possible, but no sooner than four hours following ingestion. Liver function studies should be obtained initially and repeated at 24-hour intervals.
Serious toxicity or fatalities are extremely infrequent in children, possibly due to differences in the way they metabolize acetaminophen. In children, the maximum potential amount ingested can be more easily estimated. If more than 150 mg/kg or an unknown amount was ingested, obtain an acetaminophen plasma level. The acetaminophen plasma level should be obtained as soon as possible, but no sooner than 4 hours following the ingestion. Induce emesis using syrup of ipecac. If the plasma level is obtained and falls above the broken line on the nomogram, the MUCOMYST acetylcysteine therapy should be initiated and continued for a full course of therapy. If acetaminophen plasma assay capability is not available, and the estimated acetaminophen ingestion exceeds 150 mg/kg, MUCOMYST acetylcysteine therapy should be initiated and continued for a full course of therapy.
For additional emergency information, call your regional poison center or toll-free (1-800-525-6115) to the Rocky Mountain Poison Center for assistance in diagnosis and for directions in the use of MUCOMYST acetylcysteine as an antidote.

INACTIVE INGREDIENTS

Cellulose, Ethylcellulose, Magnesium Stearate, Sodium Lauryl Sulfate, Sodium Starch Glycolate, Starch.

HOW SUPPLIED

Coated Caplets, (colored white, coated, scored, imprinted "TYLENOL"). Package of 30. All packages are safety sealed and use child resistant blister packaging.

Shown in Product Identification Section, page 416

Regular Strength TYLENOL® acetaminophen Tablets and Caplets OTC

DESCRIPTION

Each Regular Strength TYLENOL Tablet or Caplet contains acetaminophen 325 mg.

ACTIONS

TYLENOL acetaminophen is a clinically proven analgesic and antipyretic. TYLENOL acetaminophen produces analgesia by elevation of the pain threshold and antipyresis through action on the hypothalamic heat-regulating center.

INDICATIONS

TYLENOL acetaminophen provides effective analgesia in a wide variety of arthritic and rheumatic conditions involving musculoskeletal pain, as well as in other painful disorders such as headache, dysmenorrhea, myalgias and neuralgias. In addition, TYLENOL acetaminophen is indicated as an analgesic and antipyretic in diseases accompanied by discomfort and fever, such as the common cold and other viral infections. TYLENOL acetaminophen is particularly well suited as an analgesic-antipyretic in the presence of aspirin allergy, hemostatic disturbances (including anticoagulant therapy), and bleeding diatheses (e.g., hemophilia) and upper gastrointestinal disease (e.g., ulcer, gastritis, hiatus hernia).
Precautions and Adverse Reactions: If a rare sensitivity reaction occurs, the drug should be stopped. TYLENOL acetaminophen has rarely been found to produce any side effects. It is usually well tolerated by aspirin-sensitive patients.

USUAL DOSAGE

Adults: One to two tablets or caplets every 4–6 hours. Not to exceed 12 tablets or caplets per day. Children (6 to 12): One-half to one tablet 3 or 4 times daily. (Junior Strength TYLENOL acetaminophen Coated Caplets, Chewable Tablets, Elixir and Drops are available for greater convenience in younger patients).
Note: Since TYLENOL acetaminophen tablets and caplets are available without prescription as an analgesic, the following appears on the package labels: "Caution: If pain persists for more than 10 days, or redness is present, or in arthritic or rheumatic conditions affecting children under 12 years, consult a physician immediately."
"WARNING: Do not use if printed red neck wrap or printed foil inner seal is broken. Keep this and all medications out of the reach of children. As with any drug, if you are pregnant or nursing a baby, seek the advice of a health professional before using this product. In case of accidental overdosage, contact a physician or poison control center immediately."

OVERDOSAGE

Acetaminophen in massive overdosage may cause hepatic toxicity in some patients. In adults and adolescents, hepatic toxicity has rarely been reported following ingestion of acute overdoses of less than 10 grams. Fatalities are infrequent (less than 3–4% of untreated cases) and have rarely been reported with overdoses of less than 15 grams. In children, an acute overdosage of less than 150 mg/kg has not been associated with hepatic toxicity.
Early symptoms following a potentially hepatotoxic overdose may include: nausea, vomiting, diaphoresis and general malaise. Clinical and laboratory evidence of hepatic toxicity may not be apparent until 48 to 72 hours postingestion.
In adults and adolescents, regardless of the quantity of acetaminophen reported to have been ingested, administer MUCOMYST® acetylcysteine immediately if 24 hours or less have elapsed from the reported time of ingestion. For full prescribing information, refer to the MUCOMYST package insert. Do not await results of assays for acetaminophen level before initiating treatment with MUCOMYST acetylcysteine. The following additional procedures are recommended: The stomach should be emptied promptly by lavage or by induction of emesis with syrup of ipecac. A serum acetaminophen assay should be obtained as early as possible, but no sooner than four hours following ingestion. Liver function studies should be obtained initially and repeated at 24-hour intervals.
Serious toxicity or fatalities are extremely infrequent in children, possibly due to differences in the way they metabolize acetaminophen. In children, the maximum potential amount ingested can be more easily estimated. If more than 150 mg/kg or an unknown amount was ingested, obtain an acetaminophen plasma level. The acetaminophen plasma level should be obtained as soon as possible, but no sooner than 4 hours following the ingestion. Induce emesis using syrup of ipecac. If the plasma level is obtained and falls above the broken line on the nomogram, the MUCOMYST acetylcysteine therapy should be initiated and continued for a full course of therapy. If acetaminophen plasma assay capability is not available, and the estimated acetaminophen ingestion exceeds 150 mg/kg, MUCOMYST acetylcysteine therapy should be initiated and continued for a full course of therapy.
For additional emergency information, call your regional poison center or toll-free (1-800-525-6115) to the Rocky Mountain Poison Center for assistance in diagnosis and for directions in the use of MUCOMYST acetylcysteine as an antidote.

INACTIVE INGREDIENTS

Tablets—Calcium Stearate or Magnesium Stearate, Cellulose, Docusate Sodium and Sodium Benzoate or Sodium Lauryl Sulfate, and Starch. Caplets—Cellulose, Hydroxypropyl Methylcellulose, Magnesium Stearate, Polyethylene Glycol, Sodium Starch Glycolate and Starch.

HOW SUPPLIED

Tablets (colored white, scored, imprinted "TYLENOL")—tins and vials of 12, and tamper-resistant bottles of 24, 50, 100 and 200. Caplets (colored white, "TYLENOL")—tamper-resistant bottles of 24, 50, 100.

Continued on next page

McNeil Consumer—Cont.

ALSO AVAILABLE

For additional pain relief, Extra-Strength TYLENOL® Tablets and Caplets, 500 mg, and Extra-Strength TYLENOL® Adult Liquid Pain Reliever (colored green; 1 fl. oz. = 1000 mg.)

Shown in Product Identification Section, page 416

Extra-Strength TYLENOL® acetaminophen Tablets and Caplets OTC

DESCRIPTION

Each Extra-Strength TYLENOL Tablet or Caplet contains acetaminophen 500 mg.

ACTIONS

TYLENOL acetaminophen is a clinically proven analgesic and antipyretic. Acetaminophen produces analgesia by elevation of the pain threshold and antipyresis through action on the hypothalamic heat-regulating center.

INDICATIONS

For relief of pain and fever Extra-Strength TYLENOL acetaminophen provides increased analgesic strength for minor conditions when the usual doses of mild analgesics are insufficient.

Precautions and Adverse Reactions: If a rare sensitivity reaction occurs, the drug should be stopped. TYLENOL acetaminophen has rarely been found to produce any side effects. It is usually well tolerated by aspirin-sensitive patients.

USUAL DOSAGE

Adults: Two Tablets or Caplets 3 or 4 times daily. No more than a total of eight Tablets or Caplets in any 24-hour period.

Note: Since Extra-Strength TYLENOL acetaminophen is available without a prescription, the following appears on the package labels: "Severe or recurrent pain or high or continued fever may be indicative of serious illness. Under these conditions, consult a physician. **WARNING: Do not use if printed red neck wrap or printed foil inner seal is broken. Keep this and all medication out of the reach of children. As with any drug, if you are pregnant or nursing a baby, seek the advice of a health professional before using this product. In case of accidental overdosage, contact a physician or poison control center immediately.**"

OVERDOSAGE

Acetaminophen in massive overdosage may cause hepatic toxicity in some patients. In adults and adolescents, hepatic toxicity has rarely been reported following ingestion of acute overdosage of less than 10 grams. Fatalities are infrequent (less than 3–4% of untreated cases) and have rarely been reported with overdoses of less than 15 grams. In children, an acute overdosage of less than 150 mg/kg has not been associated with hepatic toxicity.

Early symptoms following a potentially hepatotoxic overdose may include: nausea, vomiting, diaphoresis and general malaise. Clinical and laboratory evidence of hepatic toxicity may not be apparent until 48 to 72 hours postingestion.

In adults and adolescents, regardless of the quantity of acetaminophen reported to have been ingested, administer MUCOMYST® acetylcysteine immediately if 24 hours or less have elapsed from the reported time of ingestion. For full prescribing information, refer to the MUCOMYST package insert. Do not await the results of assays for acetaminophen level before initiating treatment with MUCOMYST acetylcysteine. The following additional procedures are recommended: The stomach should be emptied promptly by lavage or by induction of emesis with syrup of ipecac. A serum acetaminophen assay should be obtained as early as possible, but no sooner than four hours following ingestion. Liver function studies should be obtained initially and repeated at 24-hour intervals.

Serious toxicity or fatalities are extremely infrequent in children, possibly due to differences in the way they metabolize acetaminophen. In children, the maximum potential amount ingested can be more easily estimated. If more than 150 mg/kg or an unknown amount was ingested, obtain an acetaminophen plasma level. The acetaminophen plasma level should be obtained as soon as possible, but no sooner than 4 hours following the ingestion. Induce emesis using syrup of ipecac. If the plasma level is obtained and falls above the broken line on the nomogram, the MUCOMYST acetylcysteine therapy should be initiated and continued for a full course of therapy. If acetaminophen plasma assay capability is not available, and the estimated acetaminophen ingestion exceeds 150 mg/kg, MUCOMYST acetylcysteine therapy should be initiated and continued for a full course of therapy.

For additional emergency information, call your regional poison center or toll-free (1-800-525-6115) to the Rocky Mountain Poison Center for assistance in diagnosis and for directions in the use of MUCOMYST acetylcysteine as an antidote.

INACTIVE INGREDIENTS

Tablets—Calcium Stearate or Magnesium Stearate, Cellulose, Docusate Sodium and Sodium Benzoate or Sodium Lauryl Sulfate and Starch. Caplets—Cellulose, Hydroxypropyl Methylcellulose, Magnesium Stearate, Polyethylene Glycol, Sodium Starch Glycolate, Starch and Red #40.

HOW SUPPLIED

Tablets (colored white, imprinted "TYLENOL" and "500")—vials of 10 and tamper-resistant bottles of 30, 60, 100, and 200. Caplets (colored white, imprinted "TYLENOL 500 mg")—vials of 10 and tamper-resistant bottles of 24, 50, 100 and 175.

ALSO AVAILABLE

For adults who prefer liquids or can't swallow solid medication, Extra-Strength TYLENOL® Adult Liquid Pain Reliever (colored green; 1 fl. oz. = 1000 mg.).

Shown in Product Identification Section, page 416

Extra-Strength TYLENOL® acetaminophen Adult Liquid Pain Reliever OTC

DESCRIPTION

Each 15 ml. (½ fl. oz. or one tablespoonful) contains 500 mg. acetaminophen (alcohol 7%).

ACTIONS

TYLENOL acetaminophen is a clinically proven analgesic and antipyretic. Acetaminophen produces analgesia by elevation of the pain threshold and antipyresis through action on the hypothalamic heat-regulating center.

INDICATIONS

TYLENOL acetaminophen provides fast, effective relief of pain and/or fever for adults who prefer liquids or can't swallow solid medication, e.g., the aged, patients with easily triggered gag reflexes, extremely sore throats, or those on liquid diets.

Precautions and Adverse Reactions: If a rare sensitivity reaction occurs, the drug should be stopped. TYLENOL acetaminophen has rarely been found to produce any side effects. It is usually well tolerated by aspirin-sensitive patients.

USUAL DOSAGE

Extra-Strength TYLENOL Adult Liquid Pain Reliever is an adult preparation. Not for use in children under 12. Measuring cup is marked for accurate dosage. Extra-Strength Dose—1 fl. oz. (30 ml or 2 tablespoonsful, 1000 mg), which is equivalent to two 500 mg Extra-Strength TYLENOL Tablets or Caplets. Take every 4–6 hours, no more than 4 doses in any 24-hour period.

NOTE

Since Extra-Strength TYLENOL Adult Liquid Pain Reliever is available without a prescription, the following appears on the package labels: "Severe or recurrent pain or high or continued fever may be indicative of serious illness. Under these conditions, consult a physician. **WARNING: Do not use if printed plastic overwrap or printed foil inner seal is broken. Keep this and all medication out of the reach of children. As with any drug, if you are pregnant or nursing a baby, seek the advice of a health professional before using this product. In case of accidental overdosage, contact a physician or poison control center immediately.**"

OVERDOSAGE

Acetaminophen in massive overdosage may cause hepatic toxicity in some patients. In adults and adolescents, hepatic toxicity has rarely been reported following ingestion of acute overdosage of less than 10 grams. Fatalities are infrequent (less than 3–4% of untreated cases) and have rarely been reported with overdoses of less than 15 grams. In children, an acute overdosage of less than 150 mg/kg has not been associated with hepatic toxicity.

Early symptoms following a potentially hepatotoxic overdose may include: nausea, vomiting, diaphoresis and general malaise. Clinical and laboratory evidence of hepatic toxicity may not be apparent until 48 to 72 hours postingestion.

In adults and adolescents, regardless of the quantity of acetaminophen reported to have been ingested, administer MUCOMYST® acetylcysteine immediately if 24 hours or less have elapsed from the reported time of ingestion. For full prescribing information, refer to the MUCOMYST package insert. Do not await the results of assays for acetaminophen level before initiating treatment with MUCOMYST acetylcysteine. The following additional procedures are recommended: The stomach should be emptied promptly by lavage or by induction of emesis with syrup of ipecac. A serum acetaminophen assay should be obtained as early as possible, but no sooner than four hours following ingestion. Liver function studies should be obtained initially and repeated at 24-hour intervals.

Serious toxicity or fatalities are extremely infrequent in children, possibly due to differences in the way they metabolize acetaminophen. In children, the maximum potential amount ingested can be more easily estimated. If more than 150 mg/kg or an unknown amount was ingested, obtain an acetaminophen plasma level. The acetaminophen plasma level should be obtained as soon as possible, but no sooner than 4 hours following the ingestion. Induce emesis using syrup of ipecac. If the plasma level is obtained and falls above the broken line on the nomogram, the MUCOMYST acetylcysteine therapy should be initiated and continued for a full course of therapy. If acetaminophen plasma assay capability is not available, and the estimated acetaminophen ingestion exceeds 150 mg/kg, MUCOMYST acetylcysteine therapy should be initiated and continued for a full course of therapy.

For additional emergency information, call your regional poison center or toll-free (1-800-525-6115) to the Rocky Mountain Poison Center for assistance in diagnosis and for directions in the use of MUCOMYST acetylcysteine as an antidote.

INACTIVE INGREDIENTS

Alcohol, Citric Acid, Flavors, Glycerin, Polyethylene Glycol, Purified Water, Saccharin, Sodium Benzoate, Sorbitol, Sucrose, Yellow #6, Yellow #10 and Blue #1.

HOW SUPPLIED

Mint-flavored liquid (colored green), 8 fl. oz. tamper-resistant bottle with child resistent safety cap and special dosage cup.

Maximum-Strength TYLENOL® Sinus Medication Tablets and Caplets OTC

DESCRIPTION

Each Maximum-Strength TYLENOL® Sinus Medication tablet or caplet contains acetaminophen 500 mg and pseudoephedrine hydrochloride 30 mg.

ACTIONS

TYLENOL Sinus Medication contains a clinically proven analgesic-antipyretic and a decongestant. Maximum allowable non-prescription levels of acetaminophen and pseudoephedrine provide temporary relief of sinus congestion and pain.

TYLENOL® Acetaminophen produces analgesia by elevation of the pain threshold and antipyresis through action on the hypothalamic heat-regulating center. Pseudoephedrine hydrochloride is a sympathomimetic amine which promotes sinus cavity drainage by reducing nasopharyngeal mucosal congestion.

INDICATIONS

Maximum-Strength TYLENOL Sinus Medication provides effective symptomatic relief from sinus headache pain and pressure caused by sinusitis.

ADVERSE REACTIONS

While Maximum-Strength TYLENOL Sinus Medication's acetaminophen component is equal to aspirin in analgesic and antipyretic effectiveness, it is unlikely to produce many of the side effects associated with aspirin and aspirin-containing products. Since it contains no antihistamine, TYLENOL Sinus Medication will not produce the drowsiness that may interfere with work, driving an automobile or operating dangerous machinery. Maximum-Strength TYLENOL Sinus Medication is particularly well-suited in patients with aspirin allergy, hemostatic disturbances (including anticoagulant therapy), and bleeding diatheses (e.g. hemophilia) and upper gastrointestinal disease (e.g. ulcer, gastritis, hiatus hernia). If a rare sensitivity occurs, the drug should be discontinued. Although pseudoephedrine is virtually without pressor effect in normotensive patients, it should be used with caution in hypertensives.

USUAL DOSAGE

Adult dosage: Two tablets or caplets every four to six hours. Do not exceed eight tablets or caplets in any 24 hour period.

Note: Since TYLENOL Sinus Medication tablets and caplets are available without a prescription, the following appears on the package labels: "WARNING: Do not exceed the recommended dosage or administer to children under 12. Reduce dosage if nervousness, or sleeplessness occurs. If you have high blood pressure, heart disease, diabetes, or thyroid disease, or are presently taking a prescription drug for the treatment of high blood pressure or emotional disorders, do not take except under the advice and supervision of a physician. If symptoms persist for 7 days or are accompanied by high fever, consult a physician." **Do not use if carton is opened or if printed green neck wrap or printed foil inner seal is broken. Keep this and all medication out of the reach of children. As with any drug, if you are pregnant or nursing a baby, seek the advice of a health professional before using this product. In case of accidental overdosage, contact a physician or poison control center.**

OVERDOSAGE

Acetaminophen in massive overdosage may cause hepatic toxicity in some patients. In adults and adolescents, hepatic toxicity has rarely been reported following ingestion of acute overdosage of less than 10 grams. Fatalities are infrequent (less than 3–4% of untreated cases) and have rarely been reported with overdoses of less than 15 grams. In children, an acute overdosage of less than 150 mg/kg has not been associated with hepatic toxicity.
Early symptoms following a potentially hepatotoxic overdose may include: nausea, vomiting, diaphoresis and general malaise. Clinical and laboratory evidence of hepatic toxicity may not be apparent until 48 to 72 hours postingestion.
In adults and adolescents, regardless of the quantity of acetaminophen reported to have been ingested, administer MUCOMYST® acetylcysteine immediately if 24 hours or less have elapsed from the reported time of ingestion. For full prescribing information, refer to the MUCOMYST package insert. Do not await the results of assays for acetaminophen level before initiating treatment with MUCOMYST acetylcysteine. The following additional procedures are recommended: The stomach should be emptied promptly by lavage or by induction of emesis with syrup of ipecac. A serum acetaminophen assay should be obtained as early as possible, but no sooner than four hours following ingestion. Liver function studies should be obtained initially and repeated at 24-hour intervals.
Serious toxicity or fatalities are extremely infrequent in children, possibly due to differences in the way they metabolize acetaminophen. In children, the maximum potential amount ingested can be more easily estimated. If more than 150 mg/kg or an unknown amount was ingested, obtain an acetaminophen plasma level. The acetaminophen plasma level should be obtained as soon as possible, but no sooner than 4 hours following the ingestion. Induce emesis using syrup of ipecac. If the plasma level is obtained and falls above the broken line on the nomogram, the MUCOMYST acetylcysteine therapy should be initiated and continued for a full course of therapy. If acetaminophen plasma assay capability is not available, and the estimated acetaminophen ingestion exceeds 150 mg/kg, MUCOMYST acetylcysteine therapy should be initiated and continued for a full course of therapy.
For additional emergency information, call your regional poison center or toll-free (1-800-525-6115) to the Rocky Mountain Poison Center for assistance in diagnosis and for directions in the use of MUCOMYST acetylcysteine as an antidote.
Symptoms from pseudoephedrine overdose consist most often of mild anxiety, tachycardia and/or mild hypertension. Symptoms usually appear within 4 to 8 hours of ingestion and are transient, usually requiring no treatment.

INACTIVE INGREDIENTS

Caplets—Cellulose, hydroxypropyl methylcellulose, magnesium stearate, polyethylene glycol, polysorbate 80, sodium starch glycolate, starch, titanium dioxide, Blue #1, Red #40 and Yellow #10. Tablets—Cellulose, Magnesium Stearate, Sodium Lauryl Sulfate, Starch, Yellow #6, Yellow #10 and Blue #1.

HOW SUPPLIED

Tablets (colored light green, imprinted "Maximum-Strength TYLENOL Sinus")—tamper-resistant bottles of 24 and 50. Caplets (light green coating, printed "TYLENOL Sinus" in dark green) tamper resistant bottles of 24 and 50.
Shown in Product Identification Section, page 416

McNeil Pharmaceutical

McNEILAB, INC.
SPRING HOUSE, PA 19477

HALDOL® brand of haloperidol ℞
[hal'dawl]
tablets, concentrate, injection
1 mg (1000's):
Military NSN 6505-01-003-2415
VA NSN 6505-01-003-2415A
2 mg (1000's):
Military NSN 6505-00-876-7239
VA NSN 6505-00-876-7239A
5 mg (1000's):
Military NSN 6505-01-003-2416
VA NSN 6505-01-003-2416A
10 mg (1000's):
Military NSN 6505-01-003-2417
VA NSN 6505-01-003-2417A
Concentrate 120 mL:
Military NSN 6505-01-003-5341
VA NSN 6505-01-003-5341A
Injection 1 mL:
VA NSN 6505-00-268-8530A

DESCRIPTION

Haloperidol is the first of the butyrophenone series of major tranquilizers. The chemical designation is 4-[4-(p-chlorophenyl)-4- hydroxy-piperidino]-4'-fluorobutyrophenone and it has the following structural formula:

O OH
F- -C-CH_2-CH_2-CH_2-N
Cl

HALDOL haloperidol dosage forms include: tablets (½, 1*, 2, 5*, 10* and 20 mg); a concentrate with 2 mg per mL haloperidol (as the lactate); and a sterile parenteral form for intramuscular injection. The injection provides 5 mg haloperidol (as the lactate) with 1.8 mg methylparaben and 0.2 mg propylparaben per mL, and lactic acid for pH adjustment between 3.0–3.6.
Inactive ingredients: tablets—calcium phosphate, calcium stearate, corn starch, natural flavor—1.0 mg contains FD&C Yellow No. 5*; 2.0 mg contains D&C Red No. 33 and FD&C Blue No. 2; 5.0 mg contains FD&C Blue No. 1 and FD&C Yellow No. 5*; 10 mg contains FD&C Blue No. 1 and FD&C Yellow No. 5*; and 20 mg contains FD&C Red No. 40; concentrate—lactic acid and methylparaben.
* See Precautions

ACTIONS

The precise mechanism of action has not been clearly established.

INDICATIONS

HALDOL haloperidol is indicated for use in the management of manifestations of psychotic disorders.
HALDOL is indicated for the control of tics and vocal utterances of Tourette's Disorder in children and adults.
HALDOL is effective for the treatment of severe behavior problems in children of combative, explosive hyperexcitability (which cannot be accounted for by immediate provocation). HALDOL is also effective in the short-term treatment of hyperactive children who show excessive motor activity with accompanying conduct disorders consisting of some or all of the following symptoms: impulsivity, difficulty sustaining attention, aggressivity, mood lability and poor frustration tolerance. HALDOL should be reserved for these two groups of children only after failure to respond to psychotherapy or medications other than neuroleptics.

CONTRAINDICATIONS

HALDOL haloperidol is contraindicated in severe toxic central nervous system depression or comatose states from any cause and in individuals who are hypersensitive to this drug or have Parkinson's disease.

WARNINGS

Tardive Dyskinesia—A syndrome consisting of potentially irreversible, involuntary, dyskinetic movements may develop in patients treated with neuroleptic (antipsychotic) drugs. Although the prevalence of the syndrome appears to be highest among the elderly, especially elderly women, it is impossible to rely upon prevalence estimates to predict, at the inception of neuroleptic treatment, which patients are likely to develop the syndrome. Whether neuroleptic drug products differ in their potential to cause tardive dyskinesia is unknown.
Both the risk of developing the syndrome and the likelihood that it will become irreversible are believed to increase as the duration of treatment and the total cumulative dose of neuroleptic drugs administered to the patient increase. However, the syndrome can develop, although much less commonly, after relatively brief treatment periods at low doses.
There is no known treatment for established cases of tardive dyskinesia, although the syndrome may remit, partially or completely, if neuroleptic treatment is withdrawn. Neuroleptic treatment, itself, however, may suppress (or partially suppress) the signs and symptoms of the syndrome and thereby may possibly mask the underlying process. The effect that symptomatic suppression has upon the long-term course of the syndrome is unknown.
Given these considerations, neuroleptics should be prescribed in a manner that is most likely to minimize the occurrence of tardive dyskinesia. Chronic neuroleptic treatment should generally be reserved for patients who suffer from a chronic illness that, 1) is known to respond to neuroleptic drugs, and, 2) for whom alternative, equally effective, but potentially less harmful treatments are **not** available or appropriate. In patients who do require chronic treatment, the smallest dose and the shortest duration of treatment producing a satisfactory clinical response should be sought. The need for continued treatment should be reassessed periodically.
If signs and symptoms of tardive dyskinesia appear in a patient on neuroleptics, drug discontinuation should be considered. However, some patients may require treatment despite the presence of the syndrome. (For further information about the description of tardive dyskinesia and its clinical detection, please refer to ADVERSE REACTIONS.)
Usage in Pregnancy—Rodents given 2 to 20 times the usual maximum human dose of haloperidol by oral or parenteral routes showed an increase in incidence of resorption, reduced fertility, delayed delivery and pup mortality. No teratogenic effect has been reported in rats, rabbits or dogs at dosages within this range, but cleft palate has been observed in mice given 15 times the usual maximum human dose. Cleft palate in mice appears to be a non-specific response to stress or nutritional imbalance as well as to a variety of drugs, and there is no evidence to relate this phenomenon to predictable human risk for most of these agents.
There are no well controlled studies with HALDOL haloperidol in pregnant women. There are reports, however, of cases of limb malformations observed following maternal use of HALDOL along with other drugs which have suspected teratogenic potential during the first trimester of pregnancy. Causal relationships were not established in these cases. Since such experience does not exclude the possibility of fetal damage due to HALDOL, this drug should be used during pregnancy or in women likely to become pregnant only if the benefit clearly justifies a potential risk to the fetus. Infants should not be nursed during drug treatment.
Combined Use of HALDOL and Lithium—An encephalopathic syndrome (characterized by weakness, lethargy, fever, tremulousness and confusion, extrapyramidal symptoms, leukocytosis, elevated serum enzymes, BUN, and FBS) followed by irreversible brain damage has occurred in a few patients treated with lithium plus HALDOL. A causal relationship between these events and the concomitant administration of lithium and HALDOL has not been established; however, patients receiving such combined therapy should be monitored closely for early evidence of neurological toxicity and treatment discontinued promptly if such signs appear.
General—A number of cases of bronchopneumonia, some fatal, have followed the use of major tranquilizers, including HALDOL. It has been postulated that lethargy and decreased sensation of thirst due to central inhibition may lead to dehydration, hemoconcentration and reduced pulmonary ventilation. Therefore, if the above signs and symptoms appear, especially in the elderly, the physician should institute remedial therapy promptly.
Although not reported with HALDOL, decreased serum cholesterol and/or cutaneous and ocular changes have been reported in patients receiving chemically-related drugs.
HALDOL may impair the mental and/or physical abilities required for the performance of hazardous tasks such as operating machinery or driving a motor vehicle. The ambulatory patient should be warned accordingly.
The use of alcohol with this drug should be avoided due to possible additive effects and hypotension.

PRECAUTIONS

HALDOL haloperidol should be administered cautiously to patients:

— with severe cardiovascular disorders, because of the possibility of transient hypotension and/or precipitation of anginal pain. Should hypotension occur and a vasopressor be required, epinephrine should not be used since HALDOL may block its vasopressor activity and paradoxical further lowering of the blood pressure may occur.
— receiving anticonvulsant medications, with a history of seizures or EEG abnormalities, because HALDOL may lower the convulsive threshold. If indicated, adequate

Continued on next page

McNeil Pharm.—Cont.

anticonvulsant therapy should be concomitantly maintained.
— with known allergies, or with a history of allergic reactions to drugs.
— receiving anticoagulants, since an isolated instance of interference occurred with the effects of one anticoagulant (phenindione).

If concomitant antiparkinson medication is required, it may have to be continued after HALDOL is discontinued because of the difference in excretion rates. If both are discontinued simultaneously, extrapyramidal symptoms may occur. The physician should keep in mind the possible increase in intraocular pressure when anticholinergic drugs, including antiparkinson agents, are administered concomitantly with HALDOL.
When HALDOL is used to control mania in cyclic disorders, there may be a rapid mood swing to depression.
Severe neurotoxicity (rigidity, inability to walk or talk) may occur in patients with thyrotoxicosis who are also receiving antipsychotic medication, including HALDOL.
Carcinogenicity studies using oral haloperidol were conducted in Wistar rats (dosed at up to 5 mg/kg daily for 24 months) and in Albino Swiss mice (dosed at up to 5 mg/kg daily for 18 months). In the rat study survival was less than optimal in all dose groups, reducing the number of rats at risk for developing tumors. However, although a relatively greater number of rats survived to the end of the study in high dose male and female groups, these animals did not have a greater incidence of tumors than control animals. Therefore, although not optimal, this study does suggest the absence of a haloperidol related increase in the incidence of neoplasia in rats at doses up to 20 times the usual daily human dose for chronic or resistant patients.
In female mice at 5 and 20 times the highest initial daily dose for chronic or resistant patients, there was a statistically significant increase in mammary gland neoplasia and total tumor incidence; at 20 times the same daily dose there was a statistically significant increase in pituitary gland neoplasia. In male mice, no statistically significant differences in incidences of total tumors or specific tumor types were noted.
Neuroleptic drugs elevate prolactin levels; the elevation persists during chronic administration. Tissue culture experiments indicate that approximately one-third of human breast cancers are prolactin dependent *in vitro*, a factor of potential importance if the prescription of these drugs is contemplated in a patient with a previously detected breast cancer. Although disturbances such as galactorrhea, amenorrhea, gynecomastia, and impotence have been reported, the clinical significance of elevated serum prolactin levels is unknown for most patients. An increase in mammary neoplasms has been found in rodents after chronic administration of neuroleptic drugs. Neither clinical studies nor epidemiologic studies conducted to date, however, have shown an association between chronic administration of these drugs and mammary tumorigenesis; the available evidence is considered too limited to be conclusive at this time.
FD&C Yellow No. 5 (tartrazine) may cause allergic-type reactions (including bronchial asthma) in certain susceptible individuals. Although the overall incidence of FD&C Yellow No. 5 (tartrazine) sensitivity in the general population is low, it is frequently seen in patients who also have aspirin hypersensitivity.

ADVERSE REACTIONS

CNS Effects:
Extrapyramidal Reactions—Neuromuscular (extrapyramidal) reactions during the administration of HALDOL haloperidol have been reported frequently, often during the first few days of treatment. In most patients, these reactions involved Parkinson-like symptoms which, when first observed, were usually mild to moderately severe and usually reversible. Other types of neuromuscular reactions (motor restlessness, dystonia and tardive dystonia, akathisia, hyperreflexia, opisthotonos, oculogyric crises) have been reported far less frequently, but were often more severe. Severe extrapyramidal reactions have been reported to occur at relatively low doses. Generally the occurrence and severity of most extrapyramidal symptoms are dose related since they occur at relatively high doses and have been shown to disappear or become less severe when the dose is reduced. Administration of antiparkinson drugs such as benztropine mesylate U.S.P. or trihexyphenidyl hydrochloride U.S.P. may be required for control of such reactions. It should be noted that persistent extrapyramidal reactions have been reported and that the drug may have to be discontinued in such cases.
Withdrawal Emergent Neurological Signs— Generally, patients receiving short term therapy experience no problems with abrupt discontinuation of antipsychotic drugs. However, some patients on maintenance treatment experience transient dyskinetic signs after abrupt withdrawal. In certain of these cases the dyskinetic movements are indistinguishable from the syndrome described below under "Tardive Dyskinesia" except for duration. It is not known whether gradual withdrawal of antipsychotic drugs will reduce the rate of occurrence of withdrawal emergent neurological signs but until further evidence becomes available, it seems reasonable to gradually withdraw use of HALDOL.
Tardive Dyskinesia—As with all antipsychotic agents HALDOL has been associated with persistent dyskinesias. Tardive dyskinesia, a syndrome consisting of potentially irreversible, involuntary, dyskinetic movements, may appear in some patients on long-term therapy or may occur after drug therapy has been discontinued. The risk appears to be greater in elderly patients on high-dose therapy, especially females. The symptoms are persistent and in some patients appear irreversible. The syndrome is characterized by rhythmical involuntary movements of tongue, face, mouth or jaw (e.g., protrusion of tongue, puffing of cheeks, puckering of mouth, chewing movements). Sometimes these may be accompanied by involuntary movements of extremities.
There is no known effective treatment for tardive dyskinesia; antiparkinson agents usually do not alleviate the symptoms of this syndrome. It is suggested that all antipsychotic agents be discontinued if these symptoms appear. Should it be necessary to reinstitute treatment, or increase the dosage of the agent, or switch to a different antipsychotic agent, this syndrome may be masked.
It has been reported that fine vermicular movement of the tongue may be an early sign of the syndrome and if the medication is stopped at that time the syndrome may not develop.
Other CNS Effects—Insomnia, restlessness, anxiety, euphoria, agitation, drowsiness, depression, lethargy, headache, confusion, vertigo, grand mal seizures, exacerbation of psychotic symptoms including hallucinations, and catatonic-like behavorial states which may be responsive to drug withdrawal and/or treatment with anticholinergic drugs.
Body as a Whole:
Neuroleptic Malignant Syndrome—As with other neuroleptic drugs, a symptom complex sometimes referred to as neuroleptic malignant syndrome (NMS) has been reported. Cardinal features of NMS are hyperpyrexia, muscle rigidity, altered mental status (including catatonic signs), and evidence of autonomic instability (irregular pulse or blood pressure). Additional signs may include elevated CPK, myoglobinuria (rhabdomyolysis), and acute renal failure. NMS is potentially fatal, requires intensive symptomatic treatment and immediate discontinuation of neuroleptic treatment.
Hyperpyrexia and heat stroke, not associated with the above symptom complex, have also been reported.
Cardiovascular Effects: Tachycardia, hypotension, hypertension and ECG changes.
Hematologic Effects: Reports have appeared citing the occurrence of mild and usually transient leukopenia and leukocytosis, minimal decreases in red blood cell counts, anemia, or a tendency toward lymphomonocytosis. Agranulocytosis has rarely been reported to have occurred with the use of HALDOL, and then only in association with other medication.
Liver Effects: Impaired liver function and/or jaundice have been reported.
Dermatologic Reactions: Maculopapular and acneiform skin reactions and isolated cases of photosensitivity and loss of hair.
Endocrine Disorders: Lactation, breast engorgement, mastalgia, menstrual irregularities, gynecomastia, impotence, increased libido, hyperglycemia, hypoglycemia and hyponatremia.
Gastrointestinal Effects: Anorexia, constipation, diarrhea, hypersalivation, dyspepsia, nausea and vomiting.
Autonomic Reactions: Dry mouth, blurred vision, urinary retention and diaphoresis.
Respiratory Effects: Laryngospasm, bronchospasm and increased depth of respiration.
Special Senses: Cataracts, retinopathy and visual disturbances.
Other: Cases of sudden and unexpected death have been reported in association with the administration of HALDOL. The nature of the evidence makes it impossible to determine definitively what role, if any, HALDOL played in the outcome of the reported cases. The possibility that HALDOL caused death cannot, of course, be excluded, but it is to be kept in mind that sudden and unexpected death may occur in psychotic patients when they go untreated or when they are treated with other neuroleptic drugs.

OVERDOSAGE

Manifestations—In general, the symptoms of overdosage would be an exaggeration of known pharmacologic effects and adverse reactions, the most prominent of which would be: 1) severe extrapyramidal reactions, 2) hypotension, or 3) sedation. The patient would appear comatose with respiratory depression and hypotension which could be severe enough to produce a shock-like state. The extrapyramidal reaction would be manifest by muscular weakness or rigidity and a generalized or localized tremor as demonstrated by the akinetic or agitans types respectively. With accidental overdosage, hypertension rather than hypotension occurred in a two-year old child.
Treatment—Gastric lavage or induction of emesis should be carried out immediately followed by administration of activated charcoal. Since there is no specific antidote, treatment is primarily supportive. A patent airway must be established by use of an oropharyngeal airway or endotracheal tube or, in prolonged cases of coma, by tracheostomy. Respiratory depression may be counteracted by artificial respiration and mechanical respirators. Hypotension and circulatory collapse may be counteracted by use of intravenous fluids, plasma, or concentrated albumin, and vasopressor agents such as norepinephrine. Epinephrine should not be used. In case of severe extrapyramidal reactions, antiparkinson medication should be administered.

DOSAGE AND ADMINISTRATION

There is considerable variation from patient to patient in the amount of medication required for treatment. As with all neuroleptic drugs, dosage should be individualized according to the needs and response of each patient. Dosage adjustments, either upward or downward, should be carried out as rapidly as practicable to achieve optimum therapeutic control.
To determine the initial dosage, consideration should be given to the patient's age, severity of illness, previous response to other neuroleptic drugs, and any concomitant medication or disease state. Children, debilitated or geriatric patients, as well as those with a history of adverse reactions to neuroleptic drugs, may require less HALDOL haloperidol. The optimal response in such patients is usually obtained with more gradual dosage adjustments and at lower dosage levels, as recommended below.
Clinical experience suggests the following recommendations:

Oral Administration
Initial Dosage Range
Adults

Moderate Symptomatology	0.5 mg to 2.0 mg b.i.d. or t.i.d.
Severe Symptomatology	3.0 mg to 5.0 mg b.i.d. or t.i.d.

To achieve prompt control, higher doses may be required in some cases.

Geriatric or Debilitated Patients	0.5 mg to 2.0 mg b.i.d. or t.i.d.
Chronic or Resistant Patients	3.0 mg to 5.0 mg b.i.d. or t.i.d.

Patients who remain severely disturbed or inadequately controlled may require dosage adjustment. Daily dosages up to 100 mg may be necessary in some cases to achieve an optimal response. Infrequently, HALDOL has been used in doses above 100 mg for severely resistant patients; however, the limited clinical usage has not demonstrated the safety of prolonged administration of such doses.

Children
The following recommendations apply to children between the ages of 3 and 12 years (weight range 15 to 40 kg). HALDOL is not intended for children under 3 years old. Therapy should begin at the lowest dose possible (0.5 mg per day). If required, the dose should be increased by an increment of 0.5 mg at 5 to 7 day intervals until the desired therapeutic effect is obtained. (See chart below).
The total dose may be divided, to be given b.i.d. or t.i.d.

Psychotic Disorders	0.05 mg/kg/day to 0.15 mg/kg/day
Non-Psychotic Behavior Disorders and Tourette's Disorder	0.05 mg/kg/day to 0.075 mg/kg/day

Severely disturbed psychotic children may require higher doses.
In severely disturbed, non-psychotic children or in hyperactive children with accompanying conduct disorders, who have failed to respond to psychotherapy or medications other than neuroleptics, it should be noted that since these behaviors may be short-lived, short-term administration of HALDOL may suffice. There is no evidence establishing a maximum effective dosage. There is little evidence that behavior improvement is further enhanced in dosages beyond 6 mg per day.

Maintenance Dosage
Upon achieving a satisfactory therapeutic response, dosage should then be gradually reduced to the lowest effective maintenance level.

Intramuscular Administration

Adults

Parenteral medication, administered intramuscularly in doses of 2 to 5 mg, is utilized for prompt control of the acutely agitated patient with moderately severe to very severe symptoms. Depending on the response of the patient, subsequent doses may be given, administered as often as every hour, although 4 to 8 hour intervals may be satisfactory.

Controlled trials to establish the safety and effectiveness of intramuscular administration in children have not been conducted.

Parenteral drug products should be inspected visually for particulate matter and discoloration prior to administration, whenever solution and container permit.

Switchover Procedure

The oral form should supplant the injectable as soon as practicable. In the absence of bioavailability studies establishing bioequivalence between these two dosage forms the following guidelines for dosage are suggested. For an initial approximation of the total daily dose required, the parenteral dose administered in the preceeding 24 hours may be used. Since this dose is only an initial estimate, it is recommended that careful monitoring of clinical signs and symptoms, including clinical efficacy, sedation, and adverse effects, be carried out periodically for the first several days following the initiation of switchover. In this way, dosage adjustments, either upward or downward, can be quickly accomplished. Depending on the patient's clinical status, the first oral dose should be given within 12–24 hours following the last parenteral dose.

HOW SUPPLIED

HALDOL* brand of haloperidol Tablets Scored, Imprinted "McNEIL" and "HALDOL"

[See table above].

		Bottles Containing 100	Bottles Containing 1000	Unit Dose Blister Pack 10 × 10
½mg, white	NDC 0045-0240	x	x	x
1mg, yellow	NDC 0045-0241	x	x	x
2mg, pink	NDC 0045-0242	x	x	x
5mg, green	NDC 0045-0245	x	x	x
10mg, aqua	NDC 0045-0246	x	x	x
20mg, salmon	NDC 0045-0248	x		x

HALDOL® brand of haloperidol Concentrate 2 mg, per mL (as the lactate) Colorless, Odorless, and Tasteless Solution—NDC 0045-0250-15, bottles of 15 mL and NDC 0045-0250-04, bottles of 120 mL.

HALDOL® brand of haloperidol Injection 5 mg, per mL (as the lactate)—NDC 0045-0255-01, units of 10 × 1 mL ampuls; NDC 0045-0255-49, 10 mL multiple-dose vial; NDC 0045-0255-31 units of 10 × 1 mL disposable Pre-filled Syringe.

Dispense HALDOL haloperidol tablets and concentrate in a tight, light-resistant container as defined in the official compendium.

Revised 4/23/86

Shown in Product Identification Section, page 416

HALDOL® Decanoate ℞

[hal'dawl dek"ah-nō'āt]

(haloperidol decanoate)

injection

DESCRIPTION

HALDOL® (haloperidol) Decanoate is the decanoate ester of the butyrophenone, HALDOL haloperidol. It has a markedly extended duration of effect. It is available in sesame oil in sterile form for intramuscular injection. The structural formula of haloperidol decanoate, 4-(4-chlorophenyl)-1-[4-(4-fluorophenyl)-4-oxobutyl]-4 piperidinyl decanoate, is:

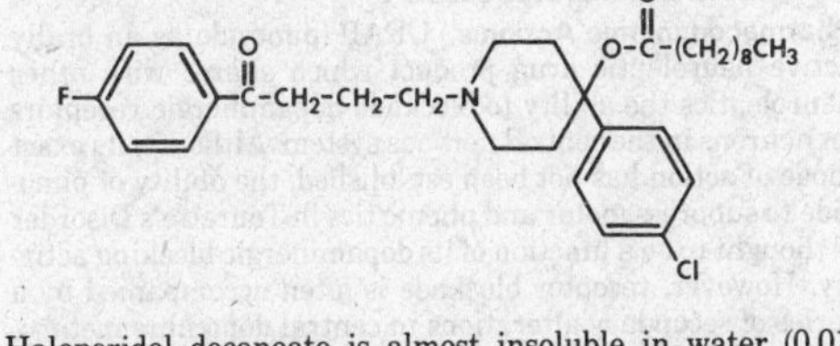

Haloperidol decanoate is almost insoluble in water (0.01 mg/mL), but is soluble in most organic solvents. Each mL contains 50 mg haloperidol (present as haloperidol decanoate 70.52 mg) in a sesame oil vehicle, with 1.2% (w/v) benzyl alcohol as a preservative.

CLINICAL PHARMACOLOGY

HALDOL (haloperidol) Decanoate is a long-acting form of HALDOL. The basic effects of HALDOL Decanoate are no different from those of HALDOL with the exception of duration of action. Haloperidol blocks the effects of dopamine and increases its turnover rate; however, the precise mechansim of action is unknown.

Administration of haloperidol decanoate in sesame oil results in slow and sustained release of haloperidol. The plasma concentrations of haloperidol gradually rise, reaching a peak at about 6 days after the injection, and falling thereafter, with an apparent half-life of about 3 weeks. Steady state plasma concentrations are achieved after the third or fourth dose. The relationship between dose of haloperidol decanoate and plasma haloperidol concentration is roughly linear for doses below 450 mg. It should be noted, however, that the pharmacokinetics of haloperidol decanoate following intramuscular injections can be quite variable between subjects.

INDICATIONS AND USAGE

HALDOL Decanoate is a long-acting parenteral antipsychotic drug intended for use in the management of patients requiring prolonged parenteral neuroleptic therapy (e.g., chronic schizophrenics).

CONTRAINDICATIONS

Since the pharmacologic and clinical actions of HALDOL (haloperidol) Decanoate are attributed to HALDOL as the active medication, Contraindications, Warnings, and additional information are those of HALDOL, modified only to reflect the prolonged action.

HALDOL is contraindicated in severe toxic central nervous system depression or comatose states from any cause and in individuals who are hypersensitive to this drug or have Parkinson's disease.

WARNINGS

Tardive Dyskinesia—A syndrome consisting of potentially irreversible, involuntary, dyskinetic movements may develop in patients treated with neuroleptic (antipsychotic) drugs. Although the prevalence of the syndrome appears to be highest among the elderly, especially elderly women, it is impossible to rely upon prevalence estimates to predict, at the inception of neuroleptic treatment, which patients are likely to develop the syndrome. Whether neuroleptic drug products differ in their potential to cause tardive dyskinesia is unknown.

Both the risk of developing the syndrome and the likelihood that it will become irreversible are believed to increase as the duration of treatment and the total cumulative dose of neuroleptic drugs administered to the patient increase. However, the syndrome can develop, although much less commonly, after relatively brief treatment periods at low doses.

There is no known treatment for established cases of tardive dyskinesia, although the syndrome may remit, partially or completely, if neuroleptic treatment is withdrawn. Neuroleptic treatment, itself, however, may suppress (or partially suppress) the signs and symptoms of the syndrome and thereby may possibly mask the underlying process. The effect that symptomatic suppression has upon the long-term course of the syndrome is unknown.

Given these considerations, neuroleptics should be prescribed in a manner that is most likely to minimize the occurrence of tardive dyskinesia. Chronic neuroleptic treatment should generally be reserved for patients who suffer from a chronic illness that 1) is known to respond to neuroleptic drugs, and 2) for whom alternative, equally effective, but potentially less harmful treatments are **not** available or appropriate. In patients who do require chronic treatment, the smallest dose and the shortest duration of treatment producing a satisfactory clinical response should be sought. The need for continued treatment should be reassessed periodically.

If signs and symptoms of tardive dyskinesia appear in a patient on neuroleptics, drug discontinuation should be considered. However, some patients may require treatment despite the presence of the syndrome. (For further information about the description of tardive dyskinesia and its clinical detection, please refer to ADVERSE REACTIONS.)

General—A number of cases of bronchopneumonia, some fatal, have followed the use of major tranquilizers, including HALDOL (haloperidol). It has been postulated that lethargy and decreased sensation of thirst due to central inhibition may lead to dehydration, hemoconcentration and reduced pulmonary ventilation. Therefore, if the above signs and symptoms appear, especially in the elderly, the physician should institute remedial therapy promptly.

Although not reported with HALDOL, decreased serum cholesterol and/or cutaneous and ocular changes have been reported in patients receiving chemically-related drugs.

PRECAUTIONS

HALDOL (haloperidol) Decanoate should be administered cautiously to patients:

—with severe cardiovascular disorders, because of the possibility of transient hypotension and/or precipitation of anginal pain. Should hypotension occur and a vasopressor be required, epinephrine should not be used since HALDOL may block its vasopressor activity, and paradoxical further lowering of the blood pressure may occur.

—receiving anticonvulsant medications, with a history of seizures, or with EEG abnormalities, because HALDOL may lower the convulsive threshold. If indicated, adequate anticonvulsant therapy should be concomitantly maintained.

—with known allergies, or with a history of allergic reactions to drugs.

—receiving anticoagulants, since an isolated instance of interference occurred with the effects of one anticoagulant (phenindione).

If concomitant antiparkinson medication is required, it may have to be continued after HALDOL Decanoate is discontinued because of the prolonged action of HALDOL Decanoate. If both drugs are discontinued simultaneously, extrapyramidal symptoms may occur. The physician should keep in mind the possible increase in intraocular pressure when anticholinergic drugs, including antiparkinson agents, are administered concomitantly with HALDOL Decanoate.

In patients with thyrotoxicosis who are also receiving antipsychotic medication, including HALDOL Decanoate, severe neurotoxicity (rigidity, inability to walk or talk) may occur.

When HALDOL is used to control mania in bipolar disorders, there may be a rapid mood swing to depression.

Information for Patients: HALDOL Decanoate may impair the mental and/or physical abilities required for the performance of hazardous tasks such as operating machinery or driving a motor vehicle. The ambulatory patient should be warned accordingly.

The use of alcohol with this drug should be avoided due to possible additive effects and hypotension.

Drug Interactions: An encephalopathic syndrome (characterized by weakness, lethargy, fever, tremulousness and confusion, extrapyramidal symtpoms, leukocytosis, elevated serum enzymes, BUN, and FBS) followed by irreversible brain damage has occurred in a few patients treated with lithium plus HALDOL. A causal relationship between these events and the concomitant administration of lithium and HALDOL has not been established; however, patients receiving such combined therapy should be monitored closely for early evidence of neurological toxicity and treatment discontinued promptly if such signs appear.

Carcinogenesis, Mutagenesis, and Impairment of Fertility: No mutagenic potential of haloperidol decanoate was found in the Ames Salmonella microsomal activation assay. Carcinogenicity studies using oral haloperidol were conducted in Wistar rats (dosed at up to 5 mg/kg daily for 24 months) and in Albino Swiss mice (dosed at up to 5 mg/kg daily for 18 months). In the rat study survival was less than optimal in all dose groups, reducing the number of rats at risk for developing tumors. However, although a relatively greater number of rats survived to the end of the study in high dose male and female groups, these animals did not have a greater incidence of tumors than control animals. Therefore, although not optimal, this study does suggest the absence of a haloperidol related increase in the incidence of neoplasia in rats at doses up to 20 times the usual daily human dose for chronic or resistant patients.

In female mice at 5 and 20 times the highest initial daily dose for chronic or resistant patients, there was a statistically significant increase in mammary gland neoplasia and total tumor incidence; at 20 times the same daily dose there was a statistically significant increase in pituitary gland neoplasia. In male mice, no statistically significant differences in incidences of total tumors or specific tumor types were noted.

Neuroleptic drugs elevate prolactin levels; the elevation persists during chronic administration. Tissue culture experiments indicate that approximately one-third of human breast cancers are prolactin dependent *in vitro*, a factor of potential importance if the prescription of these drugs is contemplated in a patient with a previously detected breast cancer. Although disturbances such as galactorrhea, amenorrhea, gynecomastia, and impotence have been reported, the clinical significance of elevated serum prolactin levels is unknown for most patients. An increase in mammary neoplasms has been found in rodents after chronic administration of neuroleptic drugs. Neither clinical studies nor epidemiologic studies conducted to date, however, have shown an association between chronic administration of these drugs and mammary tumorigenesis; the available evidence is considered too limited to be conclusive at this time.

Usage in Pregnancy: Pregnancy Category C. Rodents given up to 3 times the usual maximum human dose of haloperidol decanoate showed an increase in incidence of resorption, fetal mortality, and pup mortality. No fetal abnormalities were observed.

Continued on next page

McNeil Pharm.—Cont.

Cleft palate has been observed in mice given oral haloperidol at 15 times the usual maximum human dose. Cleft palate in mice appears to be a non-specific response to stress or nutritional imbalance as well as to a variety of drugs, and there is no evidence to relate this phenomenon to predictable human risk for most of these agents.

There are no adequate and well-controlled studies in pregnant women. There are reports, however, of two cases of limb malformations observed following maternal use of HALDOL along with other drugs which have suspected teratogenic potential during the first trimester of pregnancy. Causal relationships were not established with these cases. Since such experience does not exclude the possibility of fetal damage due to HALDOL, HALDOL Decanoate should be used during pregnancy or in women likely to become pregnant only if the benefit clearly justifies a potential risk to the fetus.

Nursing Mothers: Since haloperidol is excreted in human breast milk, infants should not be nursed during drug treatment with HALDOL Decanoate.

Pediatric Use: Safety and effectiveness of HALDOL Decanoate in children have not been established.

ADVERSE REACTIONS

Adverse reactions following the administration of HALDOL (haloperidol) Decanoate are those of HALDOL. Since vast experience has accumulated with HALDOL, the adverse reactions are reported for that compound as well as for HALDOL Decanoate. As with all injectable medications, local tissue reactions have been reported with HALDOL Decanoate.

CNS Effects: *Extrapyramidal Reactions*—Neuromuscular (extrapyramidal) reactions during the administration of HALDOL have been reported frequently, often during the first few days of treatment. These have also been reported with HALDOL Decanoate. In most patients, these reactions involved Parkinson-like symptoms which, when first observed, were usually mild to moderately severe and usually reversible. Other types of neuromuscular reactions (motor restlessness, dystonia and tardive dystonia, akathisia, hyperreflexia, opisthotonos, oculogyric crises) have been reported far less frequently, but were often more severe. Severe extrapyramidal reactions have been reported to occur at relatively low doses. Generally the occurrence and severity of most extrapyramidal symptoms are dose-related since they occur at relatively high doses and have been shown to disappear or become less severe when the dose is reduced. Administration of antiparkinson drugs such as benztropine mesylate U.S.P. or trihexyphenidyl hydrochloride U.S.P. may be required for control of such reactions. It should be noted that persistent extrapyramidal reactions have been reported and that the drug may have to be discontinued in such cases.

Withdrawal Emergent Neurological Signs—Generally, patients receiving short term therapy experience no problems with abrupt discontinuation of antipsychotic drugs. However, some patients on maintenance treatment experience transient dyskinetic signs after abrupt withdrawal. In certain of these cases the dyskinetic movements are indistinguishable from the syndrome described below under "Tardive Dyskinesia" except for duration. Although the long acting properties of HALDOL Decanoate provide gradual withdrawal, it is not known whether gradual withdrawal of antipsychotic drugs will reduce the rate of occurrence of withdrawal emergent neurological signs.

Tardive Dyskinesia—As with all antipsychotic agents HALDOL has been associated with persistent dyskinesias. Tardive dyskinesia, a syndrome consisting of potentially irreversible, involuntary, dyskinetic movements, may appear in some patients on long-term therapy with HALDOL Decanoate or may occur after drug therapy has been discontinued. The risk appears to be greater in elderly patients on high-dose therapy, especially females. The symptoms are persistent and in some patients appear irreversible. The syndrome is characterized by rhythmical involuntary movements of tongue, face, mouth, or jaw (e.g., protrusion of tongue, puffing of cheeks, puckering of mouth, chewing movements). Sometimes these may be accompanied by involuntary movements of extremities.

There is no known effective treatment for tardive dyskinesia; antiparkinson agents usually do not alleviate the symptoms of this syndrome. It is suggested that all antipsychotic agents be discontinued if these symptoms appear. Should it be necessary to reinstitute treatment, or increase the dosage of the agent, or switch to a different antipsychotic agent, this syndrome may be masked.

It has been reported that fine vermicular movement of the tongue may be an early sign of the syndrome and if the medication is stopped at that time the syndrome may not develop.

Other CNS effects—Insomnia, restlessness, anxiety, euphoria, agitation, drowsiness, depression, lethargy, headache, confusion, vertigo, grand mal seizures, exacerbation of psychotic symptoms including hallucinations, and catatonic-like behavioral states which may be responsive to drug withdrawal and/or treatment with anticholinergic drugs.

Body as a Whole: As with other neuroleptic drugs, a symptom complex sometimes referred to as neuroleptic malignant syndrome (NMS) has been reported. Cardinal features of NMS are hyperpyrexia, muscle rigidity, altered mental status (including catatonic signs), and evidence of autonomic instability (irregular pulse or blood pressure). Additional signs may include elevated CPK, myoglobinuria (rhabdomyolysis), and acute renal failure. NMS is potentially fatal, requires intensive symptomatic treatment and discontinuation of neuroleptic treatment.

Hyperpyrexia and heat stroke, not associated with the above symptom complex, have also been reported with HALDOL.

Cardiovascular Effects: Tachycardia, hypotension, hypertension and ECG changes.

Hematologic Effects: Reports have appeared citing the occurrence of mild and usually transient leukopenia and leukocytosis, minimal decreases in red blood cell counts, anemia, or a tendency toward lymphomonocytosis. Agranulocytosis has rarely been reported to have occurred with the use of HALDOL, and then only in association with other medication.

Liver Effects: Impaired liver function and/or jaundice have been reported.

Dermatologic Reactions: Maculopapular and acneiform skin reactions and isolated cases of photosensitivity and loss of hair.

Endocrine Disorders: Lactation, breast engorgement, mastalgia, menstrual irregularities, gynecomastia, impotence, increased libido, hyperglycemia, hypoglycemia and hyponatremia.

Gastrointestinal Effects: Anorexia, constipation, diarrhea, hypersalivation, dyspepsia, nausea and vomiting.

Autonomic Reactions: Dry mouth, blurred vision, urinary retention and diaphoresis.

Respiratory Effects: Laryngospasm, bronchospasm and increased depth of respiration.

Special Senses: Cataracts, retinopathy and visual disturbances.

Other: Cases of sudden and unexpected death have been reported in association with the administration of HALDOL. The nature of the evidence makes it impossible to determine definitively what role if any, HALDOL played in the outcome of the reported cases. The possibility that HALDOL caused death cannot, of course, be excluded, but it is to be kept in mind that sudden and unexpected death may occur in psychotic patients when they go untreated or when they are treated with other neuroleptic drugs.

OVERDOSAGE

While overdosage is less likely to occur with a parenteral than with an oral medication, information pertaining to HALDOL (haloperidol) is presented, modified only to reflect the extended duration of action of HALDOL Decanoate.

Manifestations—In general, the symptoms of overdosage would be an exaggeration of known pharmacologic effects and adverse reactions, the most prominent of which would be: 1) severe extrapyramidal reactions, 2) hypotension, or 3) sedation. The patient would appear comatose with respiratory depression and hypotension which could be severe enough to produce a shock-like state. The extrapyramidal reactions would be manifested by muscular weakness or rigidity and a generalized or localized tremor, as demonstrated by the akinetic or agitans types, respectively. With accidental overdosage, hypertension rather than hypotension occurred in a two-year old child.

Treatment—Since there is no specific antidote, treatment is primarily supportive. A patent airway must be established by use of an oropharyngeal airway or endotracheal tube or, in prolonged cases of coma, by tracheostomy. Respiratory depression may be counteracted by artificial respiration and mechanical respirators. Hypotension and circulatory collapse may be counteracted by use of intravenous fluids, plasma, or concentrated albumin, and vasopressor agents such as norepinephrine. Epinephrine should not be used. In case of severe extrapyramidal reactions, antiparkinson medication should be administered, and should be continued for several weeks, and then withdrawn very cautiously as extrapyramidal symptoms may emerge.

DOSAGE AND ADMINISTRATION

HALDOL (haloperidol) Decanoate should be administered by deep intramuscular injection into the gluteal region. A 2″ long 21 gauge needle is recommended. The maximum volume per injection site should not exceed 3 mL. The recommended interval between doses is 4 weeks. DO NOT ADMINISTER INTRAVENOUSLY.

Parenteral drug products should be inspected visually for particulate matter and discoloration prior to administration, whenever solution and container permit.

HALDOL Decanoate is intended for use in chronic psychotic patients who require prolonged parenteral neuroleptic therapy. These patients should be previously stabilized on antipsychotic medication before considering a conversion to Haldol Decanoate. Furthermore, it is recommended that patients being considered for Haldol Decanoate therapy be initially converted to oral haloperidol (from whatever other neuroleptic they are taking) in order to exclude the possibility of an unexpected adverse sensitivity to haloperidol. Close clinical supervision is required during the initial period of dose adjustment in order to minimize the risk of overdosage or reappearance of psychotic symptoms before the next injection. During dose adjustment or episodes of exacerbation of psychotic symptoms, Haldol Decanoate therapy can be supplemented with short-acting forms of haloperidol.

The starting dose of Haldol Decanoate should be based on the patient's clinical history, physical condition, and response to previous antipsychotic therapy. The preferred approach to determining the minimum effective dose is to begin with lower initial doses and to adjust the dose upward as needed. It is recommended that the initial dose of Haldol Decanoate be 10–15 times the previous daily dose in oral haloperidol equivalents, but no more than a maximum initial dose of 100 mg (2 mL). Haldol Decanoate has been effectively administered at monthly intervals in several clinical studies. However, variation in patient response may dictate a need for adjustment of the dosing interval as well as the dose.

Lower initial doses and more gradual adjustment are recommended for elderly or debilitated patients.

Clinical experience with HALDOL Decanoate at doses greater than 300 mg (6 mL) per month has been limited.

HOW SUPPLIED

HALDOL® (haloperidol) Decanoate contains 50 mg haloperidol as 70.5 mg per mL haloperidol decanoate for IM use only. NDC 0045-0253-01, 10×1 mL and 3 × 1 mL ampuls.

Store below 40° C (104° F). Do not refrigerate or freeze. Protect from light.

Revised 7/11/86

Shown in Product Identification Section, page 416

ORAP® ℞

[or 'ap]

(pimozide)

Tablets

DESCRIPTION

ORAP (pimozide) is an orally active neuroleptic agent of the diphenyl-butylpiperidine series. The structural formula of pimozide, 1-(1-(4,4- bis(4-fluorophenyl)-butyl)-4-piperidinyl)-1,3-dihydro-2*H*-benzimidazol-2-one is:

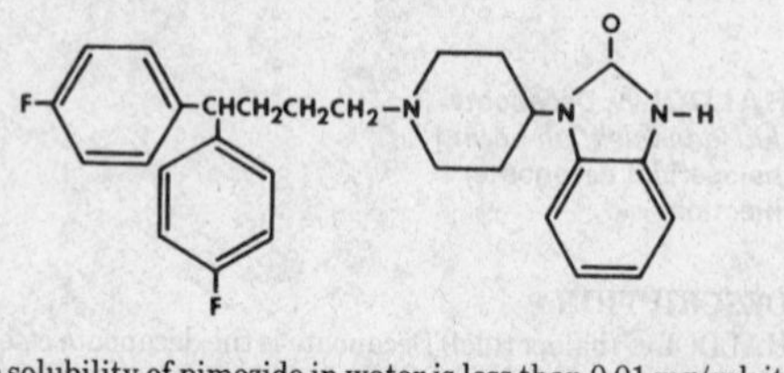

The solubility of pimozide in water is less than 0.01 mg/ml; it is slightly soluble in most organic solvents.

Each white ORAP tablet contains 2 mg of pimozide and the following inactive ingredients: calcium stearate, cellulose, lactose and corn starch.

CLINICAL PHARMACOLOGY

Pharmacodynamic Actions: ORAP (pimozide) is an orally active neuroleptic drug product which shares with other neuroleptics the ability to blockade dopaminergic receptors on neurons in the central nervous system. Although its exact mode of action has not been established, the ability of pimozide to suppress motor and phonic tics in Tourette's Disorder is thought to be a function of its dopaminergic blocking activity. However, receptor blockade is often accompanied by a series of secondary alterations in central dopamine metabolism and function which may contribute to both pimozide's therapeutic and untoward effects. In addition, pimozide, in common with other neuroleptic drugs, has various effects on other central nervous system receptor systems which are not fully characterized.

Metabolism and Pharmacokinetics: More than 50% of a dose of pimozide is absorbed after oral administration. Based on the pharmacokinetic and metabolic profile, pimozide appears to undergo significant first pass metabolism. Peak serum levels occur generally six to eight hours (range 4–12 hours) after dosing. Pimozide is extensively metabolized, primarily by N-dealkylation in the liver. Two major metabolites have been identified, 1-(4-piperidyl)-2-benzimidazolinone and 4,4-bis(4-fluorophenyl) butyric acid. The neuroleptic activity of these metabolites is undetermined. The major route of elimination of pimozide and its metabolites is through the kidney.

The mean serum elimination half-life of pimozide in schizophrenic patients was approximately 55 hours. There was a 13-fold interindividual difference in the area under the serum pimozide level-time curve and an equivalent degree of variation in peak serum levels among patients studied. The

significance of this is unclear since there are few correlations between plasma levels and clinical findings.
Effects of food, disease or concomitant medication upon the absorption, distribution, metabolism and elimination of pimozide are not known.

INDICATIONS AND USAGE

ORAP (pimozide) is indicated for the suppression of motor and phonic tics in patients with Tourette's Disorder who have failed to respond satisfactorily to standard treatment. ORAP is not intended as a treatment of first choice nor is it intended for the treatment for tics that are merely annoying or cosmetically troublesome. ORAP should be reserved for use in Tourette's Disorder patients whose development and /or daily life function is severely compromised by the presence of motor and phonic tics.
Evidence supporting approval of pimozide for use in Tourette's Disorder was obtained in two controlled clinical investigations which enrolled patients between the ages of 8 and 53 years. Most subjects in the two trials were 12 or older.

CONTRAINDICATIONS

1. ORAP (pimozide) is contraindicated in the treatment of simple tics or tics other than those associated with Tourette's Disorder.
2. ORAP should not be used in patients taking drugs that may, themselves, cause motor and phonic tics (e.g., pemoline, methylphenidate and amphetamines) until such patients have been withdrawn from these drugs to determine whether or not the drugs, rather than Tourette's Disorder, are responsible for the tics.
3. Because ORAP prolongs the QT interval of the electrocardiogram it is contraindicated in patients with congenital long QT syndrome, patients with a history of cardiac arrhythmias, or patients taking other drugs which prolong the QT interval of the electrocardiogram (see DRUG INTERACTIONS).
4. ORAP is contraindicated in patients with severe toxic central nervous system depression or comatose states from any cause.
5. ORAP is contraindicated in patients with hypersensitivity to it. As it is not known whether cross-sensitivity exists among the neuroleptics, pimozide should be used with appropriate caution in patients who have demonstrated hypersensitivity to other neuroleptic drugs.

WARNINGS

The use of ORAP (pimozide) in the treatment of Tourette's Disorder involves different risk/benefit considerations than when neuroleptic drugs are used to treat other conditions. Consequently, a decision to use ORAP should take into consideration the following (see also PRECAUTIONS—Information for Patients).
Tardive Dyskinesia: A syndrome consisting of potentially irreversible, involuntary, dyskinetic movements may develop in patients treated with neuroleptic (antipsychotic) drugs. Although the prevalence of the syndrome appears to be highest among the elderly, especially elderly women, it is impossible to rely upon prevalence estimates to predict, at the inception of neuroleptic treatment, which patients are likely to develop the syndrome. Whether neuroleptic drug products differ in their potential to cause tardive dyskinesia is unknown.
Both the risk of developing the syndrome and the likelihood that it will become irreversible are believed to increase as the duration of treatment and the total cumulative dose of neuroleptic drugs administered to the patient increase. However, the syndrome can develop, although much less commonly, after relatively brief treatment periods at low doses. There is no known treatment for established cases of tardive dyskinesia, although the syndrome may remit, partially or completely, if neuroleptic treatment is withdrawn. Neuroleptic treatment, itself, however, may suppress (or partially suppress) the signs and symptoms of the syndrome and thereby may possibly mask the underlying process. The effect that symptomatic suppression has upon the long-term course of the syndrome is unknown.
Given these considerations, neuroleptics should be prescribed in a manner that is most likely to minimize the occurrence of tardive dyskinesia. Chronic neuroleptic treatment should generally be reserved for patients who suffer from a chronic illness that, 1) is known to respond to neuroleptic drugs, and 2) for whom alternative, equally effective, but potentially less harmful treatments are not available or appropriate. In patients who do require chronic treatment, the smallest dose and the shortest duration of treatment producing a satisfactory clinical response should be sought. The need for continued treatment should be reassessed periodically.
If signs and symptoms of tardive dyskinesia appear in a patient on neuroleptics, drug discontinuation should be considered. However, some patients may require treatment despite the presence of the syndrome.
(For further information about the description of tardive dyskinesia and its clinical detection, please refer to ADVERSE REACTIONS and PRECAUTIONS—Information for Patients.)
Other: Sudden, unexpected deaths have occurred in experimental studies of conditions other than Tourette's Disorder. These deaths occurred while patients were receiving dosages in the range of 1 mg per kg. One possible mechanism for such deaths is prolongation of the QT interval predisposing patients to ventricular arrhythmia. An electrocardiogram should be performed before ORAP treatment is initiated and periodically thereafter, especially during the period of dose adjustment.
ORAP may have a tumorigenic potential. Based on studies conducted in mice, it is known that pimozide can produce a dose related increase in pituitary tumors. The full significance of this finding is not known, but should be taken into consideration in the physician's and patient's decisions to use this drug product. This finding should be given special consideration when the patient is young and chronic use of pimozide is anticipated. (see PRECAUTIONS—Carcinogenesis, Mutagenesis. Impairment of Fertility).

PRECAUTIONS

General: ORAP (pimozide) may impair the mental and/or physical abilities required for the performance of potentially hazardous tasks, such as driving a car or operating machinery, especially during the first few days of therapy.
ORAP produces anticholinergic side effects and should be used with caution in individuals whose conditions may be aggravated by anticholinergic activity.
ORAP should be administered cautiously to patients with impairment of liver or kidney function, because it is metabolized by the liver and excreted by the kidneys.
Neuroleptics should be administered with caution to patients receiving anticonvulsant medication, with a history of seizures, or EEG abnormalities, because they may lower the convulsive threshold. If indicated, adequate anticonvulsant therapy should be maintained concomitantly.
Information for Patients: Treatment with ORAP exposes the patient to serious risks. A decision to use ORAP chronically in Tourette's Disorder is one that deserves full consideration by the patient (or patient's family) as well as by the treating physician. Because the goal of treatment is symptomatic improvement, the patient's view of the need for treatment and assessment of response are critical in evaluating the impact of therapy and weighing its benefits against the risks. Since the physician is the primary source of information about the use of a drug in any disease, it is recommended that the following information be discussed with patients and/or their families.
ORAP is intended only for use in patients with Tourette's Disorder whose symptoms are severe and who cannot tolerate, or who do not respond to HALDOL® (haloperidol).
Given the likelihood that a proportion of patients exposed chronically to neuroleptics will develop tardive dyskinesia, it is advised that all patients in whom chronic use is contemplated be given, if possible, full information about this risk. The decision to inform patients and/or their guardians must obviously take into account the clinical circumstances and the competency of the patient to understand the information provided.
There is *very* little information available on the use of ORAP in children under 12 years of age.
The information available on ORAP from foreign marketing experience and from U.S. clinical trials indicate that ORAP has a side effect profile similar to that of other neuroleptic drugs. Patients should be informed that all types of side effects associated with the use of neuroleptics may be associated with the use of ORAP.
In addition, sudden, unexpected deaths have occurred in patients taking high doses of ORAP for conditions other than Tourette's Disorder. These deaths may have been the result of an effect of ORAP upon the heart. Therefore, patients should be instructed not to exceed the prescribed dose of ORAP and they should realize the need for the initial ECG and for follow-up ECGs during treatment.
Also, pimozide, at a dose about 15 times that given humans, caused an increase in the number of benign tumors of the pituitary gland in female mice. It is not possible to say how important this is. Similar tumors were not seen in rats given pimozide, nor at lower doses in mice, which is reassuring. However, any such finding must be considered to suggest a possible risk of long term use of the drug.
Laboratory tests: An ECG should be done at baseline and periodically thereafter throughout the period of dose adjustment. Any indication of prolongation of the QT, interval beyond an absolute limit of 0.47 seconds (children) or 0.52 seconds (adults), or more than 25% above the patient's original baseline should be considered a basis for stopping further dose increase (see CONTRAINDICATIONS) and considering a lower dose.
Since hypokalemia has been associated with ventricular arrhythmias, potassium insufficiency, secondary to diuretics, diarrhea, or other cause, should be corrected before ORAP therapy is initiated and normal potassium maintained during therapy.
Drug Interactions: Because ORAP prolongs the QT interval of the electrocardiogram, an additive effect on QT interval would be anticipated if administered with other drugs, such as phenothiazines, tricyclic antidepressants or antiarrhythmic agents, which prolong the QT interval. Such concomitant administration should not be undertaken (see CONTRAINDICATIONS).
ORAP may be capable of potentiating CNS depressants, including analgesics, sedatives, anxiolytics, and alcohol.
Carcinogenesis, Mutagenesis, Impairment of Fertility: Carcinogenicity studies were conducted in mice and rats. In mice, pimozide causes a dose-related increase in pituitary and mammary tumors.
When mice were treated for up to 18 monthss with pimozide, pituitary gland changes developed in females only. These changes were characterized as hyperplasia at doses approximating the human dose and adenoma at doses about fifteen times the maximum recommended human dose on a mg per kg basis. The mechanism for the induction of pituitary tumors in mice is not known.
Mammary gland tumors in female mice were also increased, but these tumors are expected in rodents treated with neuroleptic drugs which elevate prolactin levels. Chronic administration of a neuroleptic also causes elevated prolactin levels in humans. Tissue culture experiments indicate that approximately one-third of human breast cancers are prolactin-dependent *in vitro*, a factor of potential importance if the prescription of these drugs is contemplated in a patient with a previously detected breast cancer. Although disturbances such as galactorrhea, amenorrhea, gynecomastia, and impotence have been reported with neuroleptic drugs, the clinical significance of elevated serum prolactin levels is unknown for most patients. Neither clinical studies nor epidemiologic studies conducted to date have shown an association between chronic administration of these drugs and mammary tumorigenesis. The available evidence, however, is considered too limited to be conclusive at this time.
In a 24 month carcinogenicity study in rats, animals received up to 50 times the maximum recommended human dose. No increased incidence of overall tumors or tumors at any site was observed in either sex. Because of the limited number of animals surviving this study, the meaning of these results is unclear.
Pimozide did not have mutagenic activity in the Ames test with four bacterial test strains, in the mouse dominant lethal test or in the micronucleus test in rats.
Reproduction studies in animals were not adequate to assess all aspects of fertility. Nevertheless, female rats administered pimozide had prolonged estrus cycles, an effect also produced by other neuroleptic drugs.
Pregnancy: *Category C.* Reproduction studies performed in rats and rabbits at oral doses up to 8 times the maximum human dose did not reveal evidence of teratogenicity. In the rat, however, this multiple of the human dose resulted in decreased pregnancies and in the retarded development of fetuses. These effects are thought to be due to an inhibition or delay in implantation which is also observed in rodents administered other neuroleptic drugs. In the rabbit, maternal toxicity, mortality, decreased weight gain, and embryotoxicity including increased resorptions were dose related. Because animal reproduction studies are not always predictive of human response, pimozide should be given to a pregnant woman only if the potential benefits of treatment clearly outweight the potential risks.
Labor and Delivery: This drug has no recognized use in labor or delivery.
Nursing Mothers: It is not known whether pimozide is excreted in human milk. Because many drugs are excreted in human milk and because of the potential for tumorigenicity and unknown cardiovascular effects in the infant, a decision should be made whether to discontinue nursing or to discontinue the drug, taking into account the importance of the drug to the mother.
Pediatric Use: Although Tourette's Disorder most often has its onset between the ages of 2 and 15 years, information on the use and efficacy of ORAP in patients less than 12 years of age is limited. Because its use and safety have not been evaluated in other childhood disorders, ORAP is not recommended for use in any condition other than Tourette's Disorder.

ADVERSE REACTIONS

General: *Extrapyramidal reactions:* Neuromuscular (extrapyramidal) reactions during the administration of ORAP (pimozide) have been reported frequently, often during the first few days of treatment. In most patients, these reactions involved Parkinson-like symptoms which, when first observed, were usually mild to moderately severe and usually reversible.
Other types of neuromuscular reactions (motor restlessness, dystonia, akathisia, hyperreflexia, opisthotonos, oculogyric crises) have been reported far less frequently. Severe extrapyramidal reactions have been reported to occur at relatively low doses. Generally the occurrence and severity of most extrapyramidal symptoms are dose related since they occur at relatively high doses and have been shown to disappear or become less severe when the dose is reduced. Admin-

Continued on next page

McNeil Pharm.—Cont.

istration of antiparkinson drugs such as benztropine mesylate or trihexyphenidyl hydrochloride may be required for control of such reactions. It should be noted that persistent extrapyramidal reactions have been reported and that the drug may have to be discontinued in such cases.

Withdrawal Emergent Neurological Signs: Generally, patients receiving short term therapy experience no problems with abrupt discontinuation of neuroleptic drugs. However, some patients on maintenance treatment experience transient dyskinetic signs after abrupt withdrawal. In certain of these cases the dyskinetic movements are indistinguishable from the syndrome described below under "Tardive Dyskinesia" except for duration. It is not known whether gradual withdrawal of neuroleptic drugs will reduce the rate of occurrence of withdrawal emergent neurological signs but until further evidence becomes available, it seems reasonable to gradually withdraw use of ORAP.

Tardive Dyskinesia: ORAP may be associated with persistent dyskinesias. Tardive dyskinesia may appear in some patients on long-term therapy or may occur after drug therapy has been discontinued. The risk appears to be greater in elderly patients on high-dose therapy, especially females. The symptoms are persistent and in some patients appear irreversible. The syndrome is characterized by rhythmical involuntary movements of tongue, face, mouth or jaw (e.g., protrusion of tongue, puffing of cheeks, puckering of mouth, chewing movements). Sometimes these may be accompanied by involuntary movements of extremities.

There is no known effective treatment for tardive dyskinesia; antiparkinson agents usually do not alleviate the symptoms of this syndrome. It is suggested that all neuroloptic agents be discontinued if these symptoms appear. Should it be necessary to reinstitute treatment, or increase the dosage of the agent, or switch to a different neuroleptic agent, this syndrome may be masked.

It has been reported that fine vermicular movement of the tongue may be an early sign of the syndrome and if the medication is stopped at that time the syndrome may not develop.

Electrocardiographic Changes: Electrocardiographic changes have been observed in clinical trials of ORAP In Tourette's Disorder and schizophrenia. These have included prolongation of the QT interval, flattening, notching and inversion of the T wave and the appearance of U waves. Sudden, unexpected deaths and grand mal seizure have occurred at doses above 20 mg/day.

Neuroleptic Malignant Syndrome: As with other neuroleptic drugs, a symptom complex sometimes referred to as neuroleptic malignant syndrome (NMS) has been reported. Cardinal features of NMS are hyperpyrexia, muscle rigidity, altered mental status (including catatonic signs), and evidence of autonomic instability (irregular pulse or blood pressure). Additional signs may include elevated CPK, myoglobinuria (rhabdomyolysis), and acute renal failure. NMS is potentially fatal, requires intensive symptomatic treatment, and immediate discontinuation of neuroleptic treatment.

Hyperpyrexia: Hyperpyrexia, not associated with the above symptom complex, has been reported with other neuroleptic drugs.

Clinical Trials: The following adverse reaction tabulation was derived from 20 patients in a 6 week long placebo controlled clinical trial of ORAP in Tourette's Disorder.

Body System/ Adverse Reaction	Pimozide (N = 20)	Placebo N = 20)
Body as a Whole		
Headache	1	2
Gastrointestinal		
Dry mouth	5	1
Diarrhea	1	0
Nausea	0	2
Vomiting	0	1
Constipation	4	2
Eructations	0	1
Thirsty	1	0
Appetite increase	1	0
Endocrine		
Menstrual disorder	0	1
Breast secretions	0	1
Musculoskeletal		
Muscle cramps	0	1
Muscle tightness	3	0
Stooped posture	2	0
CNS		
Drowsiness	7	3
Sedation	14	5
Insomnia	2	2
Dizziness	0	1
Akathisia	8	0
Rigidity	2	0
Speech disorder	2	0
Handwriting change	1	0
Akinesia	8	0
Psychiatric		
Depression	2	3
Excitement	0	1
Nervous	1	0
Adverse behavior effect	5	0
Special Senses		
Visual disturbance	4	0
Taste change	1	0
Sensitivity of eyes to light	1	0
Decreased accommodation	4	1
Spots before eyes	0	1
Urogenital		
Impotence	3	0

Because clinical investigational experience with ORAP in Tourette's Disorder is limited, uncommon adverse reactions may not have been detected. The physician should consider that other adverse reactions associated with neuroleptics may occur.

Other Adverse Reactions: In addition to the adverse reactions listed above, those listed below have been reported in U.S. clinical trials of ORAP in conditions other than Tourette's Disorder.

Body as a Whole: Asthenia, chest pain, periorbital edema

Cardiovascular/Respiratory: Postural hypotension, hypotension, hypertension, tachycardia, palpitations

Gastrointestinal: Increased salivation, nausea, vomiting, anorexis, GI distress

Endocrine: Loss of libido

Metabolic/Nurtritional: Weight gain, weight loss

Central Nervous System: Dizziness, tremor, parkinsonism, fainting, dyskinesia

Psychiatric: Excitement

Skin: Rash, sweating, skin irritation

Special Senses: Blurred vision, cataracts

Urogenital: Nocturia, urinary frequency

OVERDOSAGE

In general, the signs and symptoms of overdosage with ORAP (pimozide) would be an exaggeration of known pharmacologic effects and adverse reactions, the most prominent of which would be: 1) electrocardiographic abnormalities, 2) severe extrapyramidal reactions, 3) hypotension, 4) a comatose state with respiratory depression.

In the event of overdosage, gastric lavage, establishment of a patent airway and, if necessary, mechanically-assisted respiration are advised. Electrocardiographic monitoring should commence immediately and continue until the ECG parameters are within the normal range. Hypotension and circulatory collapse may be counteracted by use of intravenous fluids, plasma, or concentrated albumin, and vasopressor agents such as norepinephrine. Epinephrine should not be used. In case of severe extrapyramidal reactions, antiparkinson medication should be administered. Because of the long half-life of pimozide, patients who take an overdose should be observed for at least 4 days. As with all drugs, the physician should consider contacting a poison control center for additional information on the treatment of overdose.

DOSAGE AND ADMINISTRATION

Reliable dose response data for the effects of ORAP (pimozide) on tic manifestations in Tourette's Disorder patients below the age of twelve are not available. Consequently, the suppression of tics by ORAP requires a slow and gradual introduction of the drug. The patient's dose should be carefully adjusted to a point where the suppression of tics and the relief afforded is balanced against the untoward side effects of the drug.

An ECG should be done at baseline and periodically thereafter especially during the period of dose adjustment (see WARNINGS and PRECAUTIONS-Laboratory Tests).

In general, treatment with ORAP should be initiated with a dose of 1 to 2 mg a day in divided doses. The dose may be increased thereafter every other day. Most patients are maintained at less than 0.2 mg/kg per day, or 10 mg/day, whichever is less. In no case should a dose of 0.3 mg/kg/day or 20 mg/day be exceeded.

Periodic attempts should be made to reduce the dosage of ORAP to see whether or not tics persist at the level and extent first identified. In attempts to reduce the dosage of ORAP, consideration should be given to the possibility that increases of tic intensity and frequency may represent a transient, withdrawal related phenomenon rather than a return of disease symptoms. Specifically, one to two weeks should be allowed to elapse before one concludes that an increase in tic manifestations is a function of the underlying disease syndrome rather than a response to drug withdrawal. A gradual withdrawal is recommended in any case.

ANIMAL PHARMACOLOGY

A chronic study in dogs indicated that pimozide caused gingival hyperplasia when administered for several months at about 5 times the maximum recommended human dose. This condition was reversible after withdrawal. This condition has not been observed following chronic administration of ORAP to man.

HOW SUPPLIED

ORAP® pimozide tablets, white, scored, imprinted "McNEIL" and "ORAP"—2 mg (white) NDC 0045-0352-60, bottles of 100.

Dispense in tight, light-resistant containers as defined in the official compendium.

Made in Canada 6/24/85

PANCREASE® ℞

[pan'kre-ace]

(pancrelipase) capsules

ENTERIC COATED MICROSPHERES

DESCRIPTION

PANCREASE pancrelipase is a white, dye-free, orally administered capsule containing enteric coated microspheres of porcine pancreatic enzyme concentrate, predominately steapsin (pancreatic lipase), amylase and protease. Each capsule contains no less than:

Lipase	4,000 U.S.P. Units
Amylase	20,000 U.S.P. Units
Protease	25,000 U.S.P. Units

Inactive ingredients include cellulose acetate phthalate, diethyl phthalate, gelatin, povidone, sodium starch glycollate, corn starch, sugar, talc and titanium dioxide.

CLINICAL PHARMACOLOGY

PANCREASE pancrelipase capsules resist gastric inactivation and deliver predictable, high levels of biologically active enzymes into the duodenum. The enzymes catalyze the hydrolysis of fats into glycerol and fatty acids, protein into proteoses and derived substances, and starch into dextrins and sugars. PANCREASE capsules are effective in controlling steatorrhea and its consequences at low daily dosage levels.

INDICATIONS AND USAGE

PANCREASE pancrelipase capsules are indicated for patients with exocrine pancreatic enzyme deficiency as in but not limited to:

- cystic fibrosis
- chronic pancreatitis
- post-pancreatectomy
- post-gastrointestinal bypass surgery (e.g. Billroth II gastroenterostomy)
- ductal obstruction from neoplasm (e.g. of the pancreas or common bile duct).

CONTRAINDICATIONS

PANCREASE pancrelipase capsules are contraindicated in patients known to be hypersensitive to pork protein.

WARNINGS

Should hypersensitivity occur, discontinue medication and treat symptomatically.

PRECAUTIONS

TO PROTECT ENTERIC COATING, MICROSPHERES SHOULD NOT BE CRUSHED OR CHEWED.

Where swallowing of capsules is difficult, they may be opened and the microspheres shaken onto a small quantity of a soft food (e.g. applesauce, gelatin, etc.), which does not require chewing, and swallowed immediately. Contact of the microspheres with foods having a pH greater than 5.5 can dissolve the protective enteric shell.

Pregnancy Category C. Diethyl phthalate, an enteric coating component of PANCREASE pancrelipase capsules has been shown with high intraperitoneal dosing to be tetratogenic in rats. However, when this coating was administered orally to rats up to 100 times the human dose, no teratogenic or embryocidal effects were observed. There were no adequate and well-controlled studies in pregnant women. PANCREASE capsules should be used in pregnancy only if the potential benefit justifies the potential risk to the fetus.

ADVERSE REACTIONS

The most frequently reported adverse reactions to PANCREASE pancrelipase capsules are gastrointestinal in nature. Less frequently, allergic-type reactions have also been observed. Extremely high doses of exogenous pancreatic enzymes have been associated with hyperuricosuria and hyperuricemia.

DOSAGE AND ADMINISTRATION

Usual dosage: One or two capsules during each meal and one capsule with snacks. Occasionally a third capsule with meals may be required depending upon individual requirements for control of steatorrhea.

HOW SUPPLIED

PANCREASE® pancrelipase capsules (white, dye-free, imprinted "McNeil" and "Pancrease") in bottles of:

100 ....NDC 0045-0095-60
250 ....NDC 0045-0095-69

Keep bottle tightly closed. Store at controlled room temperature (15°-30°C, 59°-86°F), in a dry place. Do not refrigerate.

4/18/85

Shown in Product Identification Section, page 416

PARAFLEX® (chlorzoxazone) tablets ℞
[par'a-flex]

DESCRIPTION
Each tablet contains chlorzoxazone *250 mg.
*5-chlorobenzoxazolinone
Inactive ingredients: calcium phosphate, calcium stearate, corn starch, wheat gluten, FD&C Red No. 3 and FD&C Yellow No. 6.

ACTIONS
Chlorzoxazone is a centrally-acting agent for painful musculoskeletal conditions. Data available from animal experiments as well as human study indicate that chlorzoxazone acts primarily at the level of the spinal cord and subcortical areas of the brain where it inhibits multisynaptic reflex arcs involved in producing and maintaining skeletal muscle spasm of varied etiology. The clinical result is a reduction of the skeletal muscle spasm with relief of pain and increased mobility of the involved muscles. Blood levels of chlorzoxazone can be detected in man during the first hour after administration and reach peak levels in the third and fourth hours. Chlorzoxazone is rapidly metabolized and is excreted in the urine, primarily in a conjugated form as the glucuronide. Less than one percent of a dose of chlorzoxazone is excreted unchanged in the urine in 24 hours.

INDICATIONS
PARAFLEX chlorzoxazone is indicated as an adjunct to rest, physical therapy, and other measures for the relief of discomfort associated with acute, painful musculoskeletal conditions. The mode of action of this drug has not been clearly identified, but may be related to its sedative properties. Chlorzoxazone does not directly relax tense skeletal muscles in man.

CONTRAINDICATIONS
PARAFLEX chlorzoxazone is contraindicated in patients with known intolerance to the drug.

WARNINGS
The concomitant use of alcohol or other central nervous system depressants may have an additive effect.
Usage in Pregnancy: The safe use of PARAFLEX chlorzoxazone has not been established with respect to the possible adverse effects upon fetal development. Therefore, it should be used in women of childbearing potential only when, in the judgment of the physician, the potential benefits outweigh the possible risks.

PRECAUTIONS
PARAFLEX chlorzoxazone should be used with caution in patients with known allergies or with a history of allergic reactions to drugs. If a sensitivity reaction occurs such as urticaria, redness, or itching of the skin, the drug should be stopped.
If any symptoms suggestive of liver dysfunction are observed, the drug should be discontinued.

ADVERSE REACTIONS
After more than twenty-six years of extensive clinical use of PARAFLEX chlorzoxazone and other chlorzoxazone-containing products in an estimated thirty-two million patients, it is apparent that the drug is well tolerated and seldom produces undesirable side effects. Occasional patients may develop gastrointestinal disturbances. It is possible in rare instances that PARAFLEX chlorzoxazóne may have been associated with gastrointestinal bleeding. Drowsiness, dizziness, lightheadedness, malaise, or overstimulation may be noted by an occasional patient. Rarely, allergic-type skin rashes, petechiae, or ecchymoses may develop during treatment. Angioneurotic edema or anaphylactic reactions are extremely rare. There is no evidence that the drug will cause renal damage. Rarely, a patient may note discoloration of the urine resulting from a phenolic metabolite of chlorzoxazone. This finding is of no known clinical significance.
Approximately thirty-six patients have been reported in whom the administration of PARAFLEX chlorzoxazone or other chlorzoxazone-containing products was suspected as being the cause of liver damage. In one case, the jaundice was subsequently considered to be due to a carcinoma of the head of the pancreas rather than to the drug. In a second case, there was no jaundice but an elevated alkaline phosphatase and BSP retention. In this patient there was a malignancy with bony and liver metastases. The role of the drug was difficult to determine. A third and fourth case had cholelithiasis. Diagnosis in a fifth case was submassive hepatic necrosis possibly due to abusive use of the drug for approximately one year. The remaining cases had a clinical picture compatible with either a viral hepatitis or a drug-induced hepatitis. In all these latter cases the drug was stopped, and, with one exception, the patients recovered. It is not possible to state that the hepatitis in these patients was or was not drug-induced.

DOSAGE AND ADMINISTRATION
Usual Adult Dosage: One tablet (250 mg) three or four times daily. Initial dosage for *painful musculoskeletal conditions* should be two tablets (500 mg) three or four times daily. If adequate response is not obtained with this dose, it may be increased to three tablets (750 mg) three or four times daily. As improvement occurs dosage can usually be reduced.
Usual Child's Dosage: One-half to two tablets (125 mg to 500 mg) three or four times daily given according to age and weight. The tablets may be crushed and mixed with food or a suitable vehicle for administration to children.

OVERDOSAGE
Symptoms: Initially, gastrointestinal disturbances such as nausea, vomiting, or diarrhea together with drowsiness, dizziness, lightheadedness or headache may occur. Early in the course there may be malaise or sluggishness followed by marked loss of muscle tone, making voluntary movement impossible. The deep tendon reflexes may be decreased or absent. The sensorium remains intact, and there is no peripheral loss of sensation. Respiratory depression may occur with rapid, irregular respiration and intercostal and substernal retraction. The blood pressure is lowered, but shock has not been observed.
Treatment: Gastric lavage or induction of emesis should be carried out, followed by administration of activated charcoal. Thereafter, treatment is entirely supportive. If respirations are depressed, oxygen and artificial respiration should be employed and a patent airway assured by use of an oropharyngeal airway or endotracheal tube. Hypotension may be counteracted by use of dextran, plasma, concentrated albumin or a vasopressor agent such as norepinephrine. Cholinergic drugs or analeptic drugs are of no value and should not be used.

HOW SUPPLIED
PARAFLEX® (chlorzoxazone) 250 mg tablets (colored orange, scored, imprinted "PARAFLEX" "McNEIL") —bottles of 100 **NDC** 0045-0317-60.
Dispense in tight container as defined in the official compendium.
7/18/85

PARAFON FORTE® ℞
[par'a-fahn for'ta]
(chlorzoxazone and acetaminophen) tablets

DESCRIPTION
Each tablet contains chlorzoxazone 250 mg and acetaminophen 300 mg.
Inactive ingredients: cellulose, docusate sodium, magnesium stearate, sodium benzoate, sodium metabisulfite*, corn starch, FD&C Blue No. 1, and FD&C Yellow No. 5†.
*See Warnings
†See Precautions

ACTIONS
PARAFON FORTE tablets provide symptomatic relief of pain, stiffness, and limitation of motion associated with most musculoskeletal disorders through (a) relaxation of muscle spasm by chlorzoxazone, an effective and well-tolerated centrally-acting agent; and (b) analgesia by acetaminophen, a nonsalicylate analgesic useful in skeletal muscle pain.
Data available from animal experiments, as well as human study, indicate that chlorzoxazone acts primarily at the level of the spinal cord and subcortical areas of the brain where it inhibits multisynaptic reflex arcs involved in producing and maintaining skeletal muscle spasm of varied etiology. Blood levels of chlorzoxazone can be detected in man during the first hour after administration and reach peak levels by the third to fourth hour. Chlorzoxazone is rapidly metabolized and is excreted in the urine, primarily in a conjugated form as the glucuronide. Less than one percent of a dose of chlorzoxazone is excreted unchanged in the urine in 24 hours.
Acetaminophen provides analgesic action to supplement that which results secondarily from muscle relaxation. Acetaminophen is rapidly absorbed after oral administration, with peak plasma levels occurring in one to two hours. After eight hours, only negligible amounts remain in the blood. Only 4 percent is excreted unchanged; 85 percent of the ingested dose is recovered in the urine in conjugated form as the glucuronide.

INDICATIONS
Based on a review of this drug by the National Academy of Sciences-National Research Council and/or other information, FDA has classified the indications as follows:
"Probably" effective as an adjunct to the rest and physical therapy for the relief of the discomfort associated with acute, painful musculoskeletal conditions. The mode of action of this drug has not been clearly identified, but may be related to its sedative properties. Chlorzoxazone does not directly relax tense skeletal muscles in man.

CONTRAINDICATIONS
PARAFON FORTE tablets are contraindicated in patients sensitive to either component.

WARNINGS
The concomitant use of alcohol or other central nervous system depressants may have an additive effect.
Usage in Pregnancy: The safe use of PARAFON FORTE tablets has not been established with respect to the possible adverse effects upon fetal development. Therefore, it should be used in women of childbearing potential only when, in the judgment of the physician, the potential benefits outweigh the possible risks.
Special Risk Patients: PARAFON FORTE tablets contain sodium metabisulfite, a sulfite that may cause allergic-type reactions (e.g. hives, itching, wheezing, anaphylaxis) in certain susceptible persons. Although the overall prevalence of sulfite sensitivity in the general population is probably low, it is seen more frequently in asthmatics or in atopic nonasthmatic persons.

PRECAUTIONS
PARAFON FORTE tablets should be used with caution in patients with known allergies or with a history of allergic reactions to drugs. If a sensitivity reaction occurs such as urticaria, redness, or itching of the skin, the drug should be stopped.
If any signs or symptoms suggestive of liver dysfunction are observed, the drug should be discontinued.
This product contains FD&C Yellow No. 5 (tartrazine) which may cause allergic-type reactions (including bronchial asthma) in certain susceptible individuals. Although the overall incidence of FD&C Yellow No. 5 (tartrazine) sensitivity in the general population is low, it is frequently seen in patients who also have aspirin hypersensitivity.

ADVERSE REACTIONS
After more than twenty-six years of extensive clinical use of PARAFLEX® (chlorzoxazone) tablets and other chlorzoxazone-containing products in an estimated thirty-two million patients, it is apparent that the drug is well tolerated and seldom produces undesirable side effects. Occasional patients may develop gastrointestinal disturbances. It is possible in rare instances that chlorzoxazone may have been associated with gastrointestinal bleeding. Drowsiness, dizziness, lightheadedness, malaise, or overstimulation may be noted by an occasional patient. Rarely, allergic-type skin rashes, petechiae, or ecchymoses may develop during treatment. Angioneurotic edema or anaphylactic reactions are extremely rare. There is no evidence that the drug will cause renal damage. Rarely, a patient may note discoloration of the urine resulting from a phenolic metabolite of chlorzoxazone. This finding is of no known clinical significance.
Approximately thirty-six patients have been reported in whom the administration of PARAFLEX chlorzoxazone or other chlorzoxazone-containing products was suspected as being the cause of liver damage. In one case, the jaundice was subsequently considered to be due to a carcinoma of the head of the pancreas rather than to the drug. In a second case, there was no jaundice but an elevated alkaline phosphatase and BSP retention. In this patient there was a malignancy with bony and liver metastases. The role of the drug was difficult to determine. A third and fourth case had cholelithiasis. Diagnosis in a fifth case was submassive hepatic necrosis possibly due to abusive use of the drug for approximately one year. The remaining cases had a clinical picture compatible with either a viral hepatitis or a drug-induced hepatitis. In all these latter cases the drug was stopped, and, with one exception, the patients recovered. It is not possible to state that the hepatitis in these patients was or was not drug induced.
Acetaminophen has rarely been found to produce any side effects.

DOSAGE AND ADMINISTRATION
Usual Adult Dosage: Two tablets 4 times daily.

OVERDOSAGE
Acetaminophen
Acetaminophen in massive overdosage may cause hepatic toxicity in some patients. In adults, hepatic toxicity has rarely been reported with less than 10 grams and fatalities with less than 15 grams, taken as single, massive overdoses. Importantly, for reasons not fully understood, young children seem to be more resistant than adults to the hepatotoxic effect of acetaminophen overdose.
Early symptoms following a potentially hepatotoxic overdose may include: nausea, vomiting, diaphoresis and general malaise. Clinical and laboratory evidence of hepatic toxicity usually are not apparent until 48 to 72 hours post-ingestion. Following recovery there are no residual, structural or functional hepatic abnormalities.

Continued on next page

McNeil Pharm.—Cont.

Since patients' estimates of the quantity of a drug ingested are notoriously unreliable, if an acetaminophen overdose is suspected a serum acetaminophen assay should be obtained as early as possible, but no sooner than four hours following ingestion. Liver function studies should be obtained initially and repeated at 24 hour intervals.
Antidotal therapy with N-acetylcysteine appears effective in preventing and/or minimizing the toxic effects of acetaminophen. For optimal results, the antidote should be administered within 16 hours of ingestion of the overdose.
The Rocky Mountain Poison Center (800-525-6115) should be contacted for assistance in interpreting plasma levels and for directions on the administration of N-acetylcysteine as an antidote.

Chlorzoxazone

Symptoms: Initially, gastrointestinal distur-bances such as nausea, vomiting, or diarrhea together with drowsiness, dizziness, lightheadedness or headache may occur. Early in the course there may be malaise or sluggishness followed by marked loss of muscle tone, making voluntary movement impossible. The deep tendon reflexes may be decreased or absent. The sensorium remains intact, and there is no peripheral loss of sensation. Respiratory depression may occur with rapid, irregular respiration and intercostal and substernal retraction. The blood pressure is lowered, but shock has not been observed.
Treatment: Gastric lavage or induction of emesis should be carried out, followed by administration of activated charcoal. Thereafter, treatment is entirely supportive. If respirations are depressed, oxygen and artificial respiration should be employed and a patent airway assured by use of an oropharyngeal airway or endotracheal tube. Hypotension may be counteracted by use of dextran, plasma, concentrated albumin or a vasopressor agent such as norepinephrine. Cholinergic drugs or analeptic drugs are of no value and should not be used.

HOW SUPPLIED

PARAFON FORTE® Tablets (colored green, imprinted "McNEIL"and "PARAFON FORTE")—bottles of 100 **NDC** 0045-0322-60 and 500 **NDC** 0045-0322-70; Unit dose of 200 **NDC** 0045-0322-58.
Dispense in a tight container as defined in the official compendium.

1/15/86

Shown in Product Identification Section, page 416

SUPROL® ℞

[su 'prōl]
(suprofen) capsules

DESCRIPTION

SUPROL® (suprofen) Capsules for oral administration each contain 200 mg of suprofen, a substituted arylacetic acid. The chemical name of suprofen is (αmethyl-4-]2-thienylcarbonyl) benzene acetic acid. It has the following structure:

[Structure: thiophene ring–C(=O)–benzene ring–CHCOOH with CH$_3$]

Inactive ingredients: silicon dioxide, gelatin, lactose, magnesium stearate, povidone, sodium lauryl sulfate, corn starch, FDC Blue No. 1, D & C Yellow No. 10, titanium dioxide.
SUPROL (suprofen) is a white microcrystalline powder, slightly soluble in water with an aqueous pKa of 3.95 and readily soluble in organic solvents such as ethanol and acetone.

CLINICAL PHARMACOLOGY

SUPROL (suprofen) is a nonsteroidal anti-inflammatory agent which has been developed as an analgesic. It also possesses antipyretic properties. The mechanism of action of SUPROL is uncertain, although it has been shown to be an inhibitor of prostaglandin biosynthesis. It has also been shown to block the contractile action of prostaglandin ($PGF_2\alpha$) and bradykinin on uterine tissue. SUPROL is a peripherally acting analgesic. It is not a narcotic and has no central analgesic activity.
After oral administration, SUPROL (suprofen) is rapidly and completely absorbed from the gastrointestinal tract. Peak plasma levels of 14–23 mcg/ml are found approximately 1 hour (0.5–2.0) after oral administration of 200 mg SUPROL. The elimination half-life of SUPROL ranges from 2–4 hours, with clearance of 80–100 ml/kg/hr following 200 mg doses. More than 99% of SUPROL in plasma is reversibly bound to proteins. SUPROL does not accumulate to any significant extent during multiple dose administration of 200 mg q.i.d. for five days.
SUPROL is metabolized by the liver in man. The primary route of excretion of SUPROL and its metabolites is renal. Approximately 85–95% of a 200 mg oral dose of SUPROL is recovered in the urine in 48 hours and 5–10% of the dose is found in feces in 72 hours. In the urine, less than 15% of the dose is excreted as unmetabolized suprofen while at least 50% appears as a glucuronide conjugate. The remaining 20–30% of the dose is excreted as 3 other minor metabolites and/or possibly some of their conjugates. In animal models, the conjugated major metabolite is inactive. The activities of the minor metabolites are unknown.
Concomitant administration of SUPROL with an antacid (aluminum and magnesium hydroxides) does not affect the bioavailability of SUPROL. Administration of SUPROL with food, however, decreases both the rate and extent of absorption. The rate is more affected, as indicated by lower peak plasma drug levels (peaks decrease 50–55% with food and 25–30% with milk), than the extent (AUC decreases 20% after food and 10% after milk).
In gastrointestinal blood loss studies utilizing ^{51}Cr tagged erythrocytes in normal volunteers, the normally recommended analgesic dose of SUPROL, 200 mg q.i.d., administered over 7–14 days caused significantly less fecal blood loss than 650 to 1000 mg q.i.d. of aspirin administered over the same period of time and was not significantly different from placebo.
SUPROL prolongs bleeding time by decreasing platelet adhesiveness and platelet aggregation. These effects of SUPROL, unlike aspirin, disappear within 24 hours after the drug is discontinued.
Comparative single-dose studies in patients with mild to moderate pain have established the analgesic properties of SUPROL (suprofen) Capsules 200 mg. SUPROL 200 mg is comparable in analgesic efficacy to aspirin 650 mg. Pain relief was generally evident within 1 to 2 hours following oral administration and persisted for 4 to 6 hours.
In long-term studies, approximately 20% of patients treated with SUPROL (800–1600 mg/day) or aspirin (2600–4000 mg/day) discontinued therapy due to adverse reactions. SUPROL had a similar incidence of upper gastrointestinal side effects including nausea and dyspepsia. Suprofen had more loose stools/diarrhea, however, particularly at 1600 mg/day. Patients taking suprofen experienced less tinnitus than patients taking aspirin.
In studies on dysmenorrhea, SUPROL (suprofen) 800 mg/day for 2–3 days/month was shown to be comparable to ibuprofen 1600 mg/day for 2–3 days/month.

INDICATIONS AND USAGE

SUPROL (suprofen) is indicated for the relief of mild to moderate pain. SUPROL is also indicated for the treatment of primary dysmenorrhea.

CONTRAINDICATIONS

SUPROL should not be used in patients who have previously exhibited intolerance to the drug. As with other nonsteroidal anti-inflammatory drugs, SUPROL should not be given to patients in whom aspirin and /or other nonsteroidal anti-inflammatory drugs induce bronchospasm, rhinitis, urticaria or other sensitivity reactions. Rare anaphylactic reactions to suprofen have been reported, although the aspirin sensitivity history of the patients is unknown.

WARNINGS

There have been reports of the abrupt onset of flank pain associated with generally reversible renal insufficiency, sometimes with abnormal urinary sediment, in patients who have taken as few as one to two doses of SUPROL (suprofen). If flank pain occurs, SUPROL should be discontinued and renal function monitored.
SUPROL (suprofen) should be given under close supervision to patients with a history of upper gastrointestinal tract disease and only after consulting the ADVERSE REACTIONS section. Peptic ulceration and/or gastrointestinal bleeding have been reported in 1% of patients receiving SUPROL Capsules at 800–1600 mg/day.

PRECAUTIONS

General—*Renal Toxicity:* As with other nonsteroidal anti-inflammatory drugs, (NSAID's), long-term administration of suprofen to animals has resulted in renal papillary necrosis and other abnormal renal pathology. In humans, there have been reports of acute nephritis with hematuria, proteinuria, and occasionally nephrotic syndrome.
Another form of renal toxicity has been seen in patients with prerenal conditions leading to a reduction in renal blood flow or blood volume, where the renal prostaglandins have a supportive role in the maintenance of renal perfusion. In these patients administration of an NSAID may cause a dose-dependent reduction in prostaglandin formation and may precipitate overt renal deocmpensation. Patients at greatest risk of this reaction are those with heart failure, liver dysfunction, those taking diuretics, and the elderly. Discontinuation of NSAID therapy is typically followed by recovery to the pretreatment state.
Since SUPROL and its metabolites are eliminated primarily by the kidneys, patients with impaired renal function should be closely monitored, and it should be anticipated that they will require lower doses.
Anemia: In long-term studies, decreases in hemoglobin and hematocrit have been reported in patients taking SUPROL. Appropriate tests should be performed if signs or symptoms of anemia are evident.
Liver Chemistry Abnormalities: As with other nonsteroidal anti-inflammatory drugs, borderline elevations of one or more liver tests may occur in up to 15% of patients. These abnormalities may progress, may remain essentially unchanged, or may be transient with continued therapy. The SGPT (ALT) test is probably the most sensitive indicator of liver dysfunction. Meaningful (three times the upper limit of normal) elevations of SGPT or SGOT (AST) occurred in controlled clinical trials in approximately 1% of patients. A patient with symptoms and/or signs suggesting liver dysfunction, or in whom an abnormal liver test has occurred, should be evaluated for evidence of the development of more severe hepatic reactions while on therapy with SUPROL. Severe hepatic reactions, including jaundice, have been reported with SUPROL as well as with other nonsteroidal anti-inflammatory drugs. Although such reactions are rare, if abnormal liver tests persist or worsen, if clinical signs and symptoms consistent with liver disease develop, or if systemic manifestations occur (e.g., eosinophilia, rash, etc.), SUPROL should be discontinued, since liver reactions can be fatal.
Peripheral Edema: Peripheral edema has been observed in 5% of patients receiving long-term therapy. Therefore, SUPROL should be used with caution in patients with fluid retention, heart failure or hypertension.
Ophthalmic Symptoms: Ophthalmologic examinations performed on long-term patients both prior to initiation and after discontinuation of therapy failed to show any drug-related eye changes. Three to 9% of patients reported changes in visual acuity, however, and because of reports of adverse eye findings in animals, i.e., attenuated retinal vasculature, retinal degeneration and cortical opacities in rats treated with 25 or 35 mg/kg/day (approximately the human dose) for 24 months (life-time treatment), it is recommended that patients who develop visual complaints during treatment with SUPROL have an ophthalmologic evaluation.
Drug Interactions: Although suprofen is highly protein bound (see CLINICAL PHARMACOLOGY), *in vitro* studies have shown that SUPROL does not displace phenytoin, warfarin or tolbutamide from their plasma protein-binding sites. As a result, the concomitant administration of SUPROL (suprofen) with highly protein-bound, weakly acidic therapeutic agents would not be expected to influence the efficacy or safety of these compounds. However, as prostaglandins are directly involved in the regulatory mechanisms of hemostasis and glucose metabolism, patients on anticoagulant or hypoglycemic therapy should be carefully observed while on SUPROL, as with other nonsteroidal anti-inflammatory drugs.
Patients taking diuretics are at greater risk of developing renal failure secondary to a decrease in renal blood flow caused by prostaglandin inhibition by nonsteroidal anti-inflammatory drugs, including suprofen. (See PRECAUTIONS—General.)
Drug/Laboratory Test Interactions: The drug has been shown to inhibit platelet aggregation and prolong template bleeding time *in vivo*, but the platelet function begins to normalize within 4 hours after dosing and approaches normal within 24 hours after the last dose of SUPROL. Therefore, patients who are taking anticoagulant therapy should be carefully observed while SUPROL is administered.
Carcinogenesis, Mutagenesis, Impairment of Fertility: Two 2-year studies in rats and an 18 month study in mice were performed to evaluate the carcinogenic potential of the drug. The initial rat study had inadequate survival. In mice, an increased incidence of benign liver tumors occurred in females at a dose of 40 mg/kg/day (approximately three times the human dose). Treated male mice (doses of 2.5, 10, and 40 mg/kg/day) also had an increased incidence of hepatomas (not dose related) when compared to control animals. No evidence of carcinogenicity was found in doses as high as 40 mg/kg/day in the rat and mouse. Based on a battery of mutagenicity tests (Ames, Micronucleus and dominant lethal) suprofen does not appear to have mutagenic potential.
Reproductive studies in rats at a dose of up to 40 mg/kg/day (approximately three times the human dose) revealed no impairment of fertility and only slight reductions of fertility at doses of 80 mg/kg/day (approximately 6 times the clnical dose). However, testicular atrophy/hypoplasia was observed in a six-month dog study (at 80 mg/kg/day) and a 12-month rat study (at 40 mg/kg/day).
Teratogenic Effects: Pregnancy Category B. Reproductive studies have been performed in rabbits at doses up to 200 mg/kg/day (approximately 15 times the human dose) and in rats at doses up to 80 mg/kg/day (approximately six times the human dose). In rats, doses of 40 mg/kg/day and above, and in rabbits, doses of 80 mg/kg/day and above, resulted in an increased incidence of fetal resorption associated with maternal toxicity. There was an increase in stillbirths and a decrease in postnatal survival in pregnant rats treated with suprofen at 2.5 mg/kg/day and above. As with other drugs

known to inhibit prostaglandin synthesis, an increased incidence of delayed parturition occurred in rats. As there are no adequate and well-controlled studies in pregnant women, this drug should be used during pregnancy only if clearly needed. Because of the known effect of drugs of this class on the fetal cardiovascular system (closure of ductus arteriosus), use during late pregnancy should be avoided.

Nursing Mothers: The excretion of SUPROL in milk after a single dose to nursing mothers has been measured. Peak concentrations of SUPROL in milk, 0.12 to 0.23 mcg/ml at one to two hours, were approximately 1% of the peak plasma concentrations and fell to 0.024–0.107 mcg/ml four hours after drug administration.

The maximum total daily exposure of a nursing infant to SUPROL (assuming nursing at time of peak concentration) was calculated from this study to be 0.03–0.06 mg/kg/day which represents 0.015% to 0.03% of the usual daily adult dose. Caution is advised in the use of SUPROL in nursing women since the safety of SUPROL in human neonates has not been established.

Pediatric Use: Safety and effectiveness in children have not been established.

ADVERSE REACTIONS

Those adverse reactions listed below were reported in controlled clinical trials in over 800 patients who received treatment in studies for one week or longer, of whom 537 were treated for at least three months, 331 treated for at least six months, and 103 for at least one year.

Gastrointestinal symptoms were the most frequently reported adverse experiences, ranging from 10 to 20%, in SUPROL long-term studies (see below).

Fifteen to 20% of patients dropped out of long-term studies because of adverse effects.

The incidence of adverse reactions in approximately 2,000 patients receiving short-term therapy for mild to moderate pain or dysmenorrhea was, in nearly all cases, lower than those listed below.

Incidence Greater Than 1%

Gastrointestinal: The most frequent adverse reaction occurring with SUPROL administration was nausea which occurred in about 15% of the patients. Reported less frequently were: Dyspepsia, 13%, loose stools/diarrhea, 10%, gastrointestinal distress*, abdominal pain*, constipation*, vomiting*, flatulence*, gastrointestinal bleeding, stomatitis, and other bowel changes.

Central Nervous System: Headache*, dizziness*, sedation*, mood changes*, sleep disturbances*, and paresthesia.

Body as a Whole: Pain* and asthenia.

Cardiovascular/Respiratory: Edema*, congestion (upper respiratory)*, hypertension and palpitation.

Dermatological: Dermatitis*, pruritus*, and skin irritation.

Hematologic: Purpura and bleeding.

Genitourinary: Urinary frequency, dysuria, and pyuria.

Musculoskeletal: Muscle cramps*, bursitis.

Special Senses: Changes in vision, conjunctivitis, and tinnitus.

* Reactions occurring in 3% to 9% of patients treated with SUPROL.

Reactions occurring in fewer than 3% of the patients are unmarked.

Incidence Less Than 1%
(Causal Relationship Probable)

The following adverse reactions, some of which have been reported during post-marketing use abroad, occurred less frequently than 1 in 100. The probability exists that there is a causal relationship between SUPROL and these adverse reactions.

Body as a Whole: Acute allergic reactions with dyspnea and epiglottal and/or laryngeal edema, anemia.

Gastrointestinal: Peptic ulcers, gastroenteritis.

Cardiovascular: Epistaxis.

Dermatologic: Rash.

Central Nervous System: Appetite changes.

Urogenital: Acute nephritis, acute flank pain with renal insufficiency (see WARNINGS).

Incidence Less Than 1%
(Causal Relationship Unknown)

Other adverse reactions reported during clinical trials or post-marketing use with a frequency of less than 1 in 100, but under circumstances in which a causal relationship between SUPROL and the reaction could not be determined. These rarely reported reactions are being listed as alerting information for the physician since the possibility of a causal relationship cannot be excluded.

Gastrointestinal: Jaundice.

Cardiovascular/Respiratory: Tachycardia.

Hematological: Thrombocytopenia, acute hemolytic anemia, leukopenia.

Genitourinary: Lime green urine.

DRUG ABUSE AND DEPENDENCE

SUPROL (suprofen) is a nonsteroidal anti-inflammatory agent and, therefore, is a non-narcotic, non-addicting analgesic drug.

Patients receiving SUPROL for up to six months have not developed tolerance to the drug.

OVERDOSAGE

The absence of experience with acute overdosage precludes characterization of sequelae and assessment of antidotal efficacy at this time. It is reasonable to assume, however, that the standard practices of gastric evacuation, activated charcoal administration and general supportive therapy would apply.

In mice, rats, guinea pigs and dogs, the oral LD_{50} values were found to be 590, 353, 280 and 160 mg/kg, respectively.

DOSAGE AND ADMINISTRATION

Mild to Moderate Pain or Dysmenorrhea: The recommended oral dose of SUPROL (suprofen) Capsules is 200 mg every four to six hours as required. Although studies at doses greater than 200 mg q.i.d. (800 mg/day) have been conducted, there is insufficient clinical experience to adequately evaluate the efficacy, and there was a higher incidence of gastrointestinal and CNS side effects at the higher doses. Therefore, doses exceeding 800 mg/day are not recommended (see CLINICAL PHARMACOLOGY).

Patients who receive long-term treatment should be observed for clinical signs of gastric irritation, anemia, or elevated liver enzymes (see PRECAUTIONS).

HOW SUPPLIED

SUPROL® (suprofen) Capsules 200 mg (colored blue and yellow, imprinted "SUPROL® 200 mg" and "McNEIL"), NDC 0045-1500-60, bottles of 100 and NDC 0045-1500-10, unit dose of 100's.

Store at room temperature.

Dispense in tight container as defined in the compendium.

4/24/86

Shown in Product Identification Section, page 416

TOLECTIN® DS (tolmetin sodium) ℞

[to-lek'tin]

capsules

TOLECTIN® 200 (tolmetin sodium) tablets

200 mg tablets—100's:

DESCRIPTION

TOLECTIN DS (tolmetin sodium) capsules for oral administration contain tolmetin sodium as the dihydrate in an amount equivalent to 400 mg of tolmetin. Each capsule contains 36 mg (1.568 mEq) of sodium and the following inactive ingredients: gelatin, magnesium stearate, corn starch, talc, FD&C Red No. 3, FD&C Yellow No. 6 and titanium dioxide.

TOLECTIN 200 (tolmetin sodium) tablets for oral administration contain tolmetin sodium as the dihydrate in an amount equivalent to 200 mg of tolmetin (scored for 100 mg). Each tablet contains 18 mg (0.784 mEq) of sodium and the following inactive ingredients: cellulose, magnesium stearate, silicon dioxide, corn starch and talc.

The pKa of tolmetin is 3.5 and tolmetin sodium is freely soluble in water.

Tolmetin sodium is a nonsteroidal anti-inflammatory agent. The structural formula is:

CH_3–C₆H₄–C(=O)–(pyrrole, N–CH_3)–CH_2–COONa·$2H_2O$

Sodium 1-methyl-5-(4-methylbenzoyl)-1*H*-pyrrole-2-acetate dihydrate.

CLINICAL PHARMACOLOGY

Studies in animals have shown TOLECTIN (tolmetin sodium) to possess anti-inflammatory, analgesic and antipyretic activity. In the rat, TOLECTIN prevents the development of experimentally induced polyarthritis and also decreases established inflammation.

The mode of action of TOLECTIN is not known. However, studies in laboratory animals and man have demonstrated that the anti-inflammatory action of TOLECTIN is *not* due to pituitary-adrenal stimulation. TOLECTIN inhibits prostaglandin synthetase *in vitro* and lowers the plasma level of prostaglandin E in man. This reduction in prostaglandin synthesis may be responsible for the anti-inflammatory action. TOLECTIN does not appear to alter the course of the underlying disease in man.

In patients with rheumatoid arthritis and in normal volunteers, tolmetin sodium is rapidly and almost completely absorbed with peak plasma levels being reached within 30–60 minutes after an oral therapeutic dose. Tolmetin displays a biphasic elimination from the plasma consisting of a rapid phase with a half-life of one to 2 hours followed by a slower phase with a half-life of about 5 hours. Peak plasma levels of approximately 40 μg/ml are obtained with a 400 mg oral dose. Essentially all of the administered dose is recovered in the urine in 24 hours either as an inactive oxidative metabolite or as conjugates of tolmetin. An 18-day multiple dose study demonstrated no accumulation of tolmetin when compared with a single dose.

In two fecal blood loss studies of 4 to 6 days duration involving 15 subjects each, TOLECTIN did not induce an increase in blood loss over that observed during a 4-day drug-free control period. In the same studies, aspirin produced a greater blood loss than occurred during the drug-free control period, and a greater blood loss than occurred during the TOLECTIN treatment period. In one of the two studies, indomethacin produced a greater fecal blood loss than occurred during the drug-free control period; in the second study, indomethacin did not induce a significant increase in blood loss.

TOLECTIN is effectve in treating both the acute flares and in the long-term management of the symptoms of rheumatoid arthritis, osteoarthritis and juvenile rheumatoid arthritis.

In patients with either rheumatoid arthritis or osteaoarthritis, TOLECTIN is as effective as aspirin and indomethacin in controlling disease activity, but the frequency of the milder gastrointestinal adverse effects and tinnitus was less than in aspirin-treated patients, and the incidence of central nervous system adverse effects was less than in indomethacin-treated patients.

In patients with juvenile rheumatoid arthritis, TOLECTIN is as effective as aspirin in controlling disease activity, with a similar incidence of adverse reactions. Mean SGOT values, initially elevated in patients on previous aspirin therapy, remained elevated in the aspirin group and decreased in the TOLECTIN group.

TOLECTIN has produced additional therapeutic benefit when added to a regimen of gold salts and, to a lesser extent, with corticosteroids. TOLECTIN should not be used in conjunction with salicylates since greater benefit from the combination is not likely, but the potential for adverse reactions is increased.

INDICATIONS AND USAGE

TOLECTIN (tolmetin sodium) is indicated for the relief of signs and symptoms of rheumatoid arthritis and osteoarthritis. TOLECTIN is indicated in the treatment of acute flares and the long-term management of the chronic disease.

TOLECTIN is also indicated for treatment of juvenile rheumatoid arthritis. The safety and effectiveness of TOLECTIN have not been established in children under 2 years of age (See PRECAUTIONS—Pediatric Use and DOSAGE AND ADMINISTRATION).

CONTRAINDICATIONS

Anaphylactoid reactions have been reported with TOLECTIN as with other nonsteroidal anti-inflammatory drugs. Because of the possibility of cross-sensitivity to other nonsteroidal anti-inflammatory drugs, particularly zomepirac sodium, anaphylactoid reactions may be more likely to occur in patients who have exhibited allergic reactions to these compounds. For this reason, TOLECTIN should not be given to patients in whom aspirin and other nonsteroidal anti-inflammatory drugs induce symptoms of asthma, rhinitis, urticaria and other symptoms of allergic or anaphylactoid reactions. Patients experiencing anaphylactoid reactions on TOLECTIN should be treated with conventional therapy, such as epinephrine, antihistamines and/or steroids.

WARNINGS

TOLECTIN (tolmetin sodium) should be given under close supervision to patients with a history of upper gastrointestinal tract disease and only after consulting the "Adverse Reactions" section. Peptic ulceration and gastrointestinal bleeding, sometimes severe, have been reported in patients receiving TOLECTIN.

In patients with active peptic ulcer, attempts should be made to treat the arthritis with non-ulcerogenic drugs, such as gold. If TOLECTIN must be given, the patient should be under close supervision for signs of ulcer perforation or severe gastrointestinal bleeding.

PRECAUTIONS

General: Because of ocular changes observed in animals and reports of adverse eye findings with nonsteroidal anti-inflammatory agents, it is recommended that patients who develop visual disturbances during treatment with TOLECTIN have ophthalmologic evaluations.

As with other nonsteroidal anti-inflammatory drugs, long-term administration of tolmetin to animals has resulted in renal papillary necrosis and other abnormal renal pathology. In humans, there have been reports of acute interstitial nephritis with hematuria, proteinuria, and occasionally nephrotic syndrome.

A second form of renal toxicity has been seen in patients with prerenal conditions leading to a reduction in renal blood flow or blood volume, where the renal prostaglandins have a supportive role in the maintenance of renal perfusion. In these patients administration of an NSAID may cause a dose dependent reduction in prostaglandin formation and may precipitate overt renal decompensation. Patients at greatest risk of this reaction are those with heart failure,

Continued on next page

McNeil Pharm.—Cont.

liver dysfunction, those taking diuretics, and the elderly. Discontinuation of NSAID therapy is typically followed by recovery to the pretreatment state.
Since TOLECTIN and its metabolites are eliminated primarily by the kidneys, patients with impaired renal function should be closely monitored, and its should be anticipated that they will require lower doses.
TOLECTIN prolongs bleeding time. Patients who may be adversely affected by prolongation of bleeding time should be carefully observed when TOLECTIN is administered.
In patients receiving concomitant TOLECTIN-steroid therapy, any reduction in steroid dosage should be gradual to avoid the possible complications of sudden steroid withdrawal.
Peripheral edema has been reported in some patients receiving TOLECTIN therapy. Therefore, as with other nonsteroidal anti-inflammatory drugs, TOLECTIN should be used with caution in patients with compromised cardiac function, hypertension, or other conditions predisposing to fluid retention.
As with other nonsteroidal anti-inflammatory drugs, borderline elevations of one or more liver tests may occur in up to 15% of patients. These abnormalities may progress, may remain essentially unchanged, or may be transient with continued therapy. The SGPT (ALT) test is probably the most sensitive indicator of liver dysfunction. Meaningful (3 times the upper limit of normal) elevations of SGPT or SGOT (AST) occurred in controlled clinical trials in less than 1% of patients. A patient with symptoms and/or signs suggesting liver dysfunction, or in whom an abnormal liver test has occurred, should be evaluated for evidence of the development of more severe hepatic reaction while on therapy with TOLECTIN. Severe hepatic reactions, including jaundice and fatal hepatitis, have been reported with TOLECTIN as with other nonsteroidal anti-inflammatory drugs. Although such reactions are rare, if abnormal liver tests persist or worsen, if clinical signs and symptoms consistent with liver disease develop, or if systemic manifestations occur (e.g. eosinophilia, rash, etc.), TOLECTIN should be discontinued.
Carcinogenesis, Mutagenesis, Impairment of Fertility: Tolmetin sodium did not possess any carcinogenic liability in the following long-term studies: a 24-month study in rats at doses as high as 75 mg/kg/day, and an 18-month study in mice at doses as high as 50 mg/kg/day.
No mutagenic potential of tolmetin sodium was found in the Ames Salmonella-Microsomal Activation Test.
Reproductive studies revealed no impairment of fertility in animals. Effects on parturition have been shown, however, as with other prostaglandin inhibitors. This information is detailed in the Pregnancy section below.
Pregnancy: Pregnancy Category C. Reproduction studies in rats and rabbits at doses up to 50 mg/kg (1.5 times the maximum clinical dose based on a body weight of 60 kg) revealed no evidence of teratogenesis or impaired fertility due to TOLECTIN. However, TOLECTIN is an inhibitor of prostaglandin synthetase. Drugs in this class have known effects on the fetal cardiovascular system which may cause constriction of the ductus arteriosus *in utero* during the third trimester of pregnancy, which may result in persistent pulmonary hypertension of the newborn.
There are no adequate and well-controlled studies in pregnant women. TOLECTIN should be used during pregnancy only if the potential benefit justifies the potential risk to the fetus.
Non-Teratogenic Effects: Prostaglandin inhibitors have also been shown to increase the incidence of dystocia and delayed parturition in animals.
Nursing Mothers: TOLECTIN has been shown to be secreted in human milk. Because of the possibility of the adverse effects of prostaglandin inhibiting drugs on neonates, use in nursing mothers should be avoided.
Pediatric Use: The safety and effectiveness of TOLECTIN in children under 2 years of age have not been established.
Drug Interactions: The *in vitro* binding of warfarin to human plasma proteins is unaffected by tolmetin, and tolmetin does not alter the prothrombin time of normal volunteers. However, increased prothrombin time and bleeding have been reported in patients on concomitant TOLECTIN and warfarin therapy. Therefore, caution should be exercised when administering TOLECTIN to patients on anticoagulants.
In adult diabetic patients under treatment with either sulfonylureas or insulin there is no change in the clinical effects of either TOLECTIN or the hypoglycemic agents.
Drug/Laboratory Test Interaction: The metabolites of tolmetin sodium in urine have been found to give positive tests for proteinuria using tests which rely on acid precipitation as their endpoint (e.g. sulfosalicylic acid). No interference is seen in the tests for proteinuria using dye-impregnated commercially available reagent strips (e.g. Albustix®, Uristix®, etc.).
Drug-Food Interaction: In a controlled single dose study, administration of TOLECTIN with milk had no effect on peak plasma tolmetin concentrations, but decreased total tolmetin bioavailability by 16%. When TOLECTIN was taken immediately after a meal, peak plasma tolmetin concentrations were reduced by 50% while total bioavailability was again decreased by 16%.

ADVERSE REACTIONS

The adverse reactions which have been observed in clinical trials encompass observations in about 4370 patients treated with TOLECTIN (tolmetin sodium), over 800 of whom have undergone at least one year of therapy. These adverse reactions, reported below by body system, are among those typical of nonsteroidal anti-inflammatory drugs and, as expected, gastrointestinal complaints were most frequent. In clinical trials with TOLECTIN, about 10% of patients dropped out because of adverse reactions, mostly gastrointestinal in nature.

Incidence Greater Than 1%

The following adverse reactions which occurred more frequently than 1 in 100 were reported in controlled clinical trials.
Gastrointestinal: Nausea (11%), dyspepsia,* gastrointestinal distress,* abdominal pain,* diarrhea,* flatulence,* vomiting,* constipation, gastritis, and peptic ulcer. Forty percent of the ulcer patients had a prior history of peptic ulcer disease and/or were receiving concomitant anti-inflammatory drugs including corticosteroids, which are known to produce peptic ulceration.
Body as a Whole: Headache,* asthenia,* chest pain
Cardiovascular: Elevated blood pressure,* edema*
Central Nervous System: Dizziness,* drowsiness, depression
Metabolic/Nutritional: Weight gain,* weight loss*
Dermatologic: Skin irritation
Special Senses: Tinnitus, visual disturbance
Hematologic: Small and transient decreases in hemoglobin and hematocrit not associated with gastrointestinal bleeding have occurred. These are similar to changes reported with other nonsteroidal anti-inflammatory drugs.
Urogenital: Elevated BUN, urinary tract infection
*Reactions occurring in 3% to 9% of patients treated with TOLECTIN. Reactions occurring in fewer than 3% of the patients are unmarked.

Incidence Less Than 1%
(Causal Relationship Probable)

The following adverse reactions were reported less frequently than 1 in 100 in controlled clinical trials or were reported since marketing. The probability exists that there is a causal relationship between TOLECTIN and these adverse reactions.
Gastrointestinal: Gastrointestinal bleeding with or without evidence of peptic ulcer, glossitis, stomatitis, hepatitis, liver function abnormalities
Body as a Whole: Anaphylactoid reactions, fever, lymphadenopathy, serum sickness
Hematologic: Hemolytic anemia, thrombocytopenia, granulocytopenia, agranulocytosis
Cardiovascular: Congestive heart failure in patients with marginal cardiac function
Dermatologic: Urticaria, purpura, erythema multiforme, toxic epidermal necrolysis
Urogenital: Hematuria, proteinuria, dysuria, renal failure

Incidence Less Than 1%
(Causal Relationship Unknown)

Other adverse reactions were reported less frequently than 1 in 100 in controlled clinical trials or were reported since marketing, but a causal relationship between TOLECTIN and the reaction could not be determined. These rarely reported reactions are being listed as alerting information for the physician since the possibility of a causal relationship cannot be excluded.
Body as Whole: Epistaxis
Special Senses: Optic neuropathy, retinal and macular changes

MANAGEMENT OF OVERDOSAGE

In the event of overdosage, the stomach should be emptied by inducing vomiting or by gastric lavage followed by the administration of activated charcoal.

DOSAGE AND ADMINISTRATION

In adults, the recommended starting dose for rheumatoid arthritis and osteoarthritis is 400 mg three times daily (1200 mg daily), preferably including a dose on arising and a dose at bedtime. To achieve optimal therapeutic effect the dose should be adjusted according to the patient's response. For rheumatoid arthritis control is usually achieved at doses of 600–1800 mg daily in divided doses (t.i.d. or q.i.d.). For osteoarthritis control is usually achieved at doses of 600–1600 mg daily in divided doses (t.i.d. or q.i.d.). Doses larger than 2000 mg/day for rheumatoid arthritis and 1600 mg/day for osteoarthritis have not been studied and therefore are not recommended.
The recommended starting dose for children (2 years and older) is 20 mg/kg/day in divided doses (t.i.d. or q.i.d.). When control has been achieved the usual dose ranges from 15 to 30 mg/kg/day. Doses higher than 30 mg/kg/day have not been studied and therefore are not recommended.
A therapeutic response to TOLECTIN (tolmetin sodium) can be expected in a few days to a week. Progressive improvement can be anticipated during succeeding weeks of therapy. If gastrointestinal symptoms occur, TOLECTIN can be administered with antacids other than sodium bicarbonate. TOLECTIN bioavailability and pharmacokinetics are not significantly affected by acute or chronic administration of magnesium and aluminum hydroxides; however, bioavailability is affected by food or milk (see PRECAUTIONS—Drug-Food Interaction).

HOW SUPPLIED

TOLECTIN® DS (tolmetin sodium) capsules 400 mg (colored orange opaque, with contrasting parallel bands imprinted "TOLECTIN DS" and "McNEIL"), NDC 0045-0414, bottles of 100 and unit dose of 100's.
TOLECTIN® 200 (tolmetin sodium) tablets 200 mg (white, scored, imprinted "TOLECTIN," "200" and "McNEIL"), NDC 0045-0412, bottles of 100.
Dispense in tight container as defined in the official compendium.

Revised 11/20/85
Shown in Product Identification Section, page 416

TYLENOL® with Codeine ℞
[*ti 'len-awl co 'dēn*]
tablets Ⓒ III, capsules Ⓒ III and elixir Ⓒ V

DESCRIPTION

Each TYLENOL with Codeine tablet contains:

No. 1 Codeine Phosphate*	7.5 mg
Acetaminophen	300 mg
No. 2 Codeine Phosphate*	15 mg
Acetaminophen	300 mg
No. 3 Codeine Phosphate*	30 mg
Acetaminophen	300 mg
No. 4 Codeine Phosphate*	60 mg
Acetaminophen	300 mg

Each TYLENOL with Codeine capsule contains:

No. 3 Codeine Phosphate*	30 mg
Acetaminophen	300 mg
No. 4 Codeine Phosphate*	60 mg
Acetaminophen	300 mg

Each 5 ml TYLENOL with Codeine elixir contains:

Codeine Phosphate*	12 mg
Acetaminophen	120 mg
Alcohol 7%	

**Warning*—May be habit forming.
Inactive ingredients: tablets—powdered cellulose, magnesium stearate, sodium metabisulfite*, pregelatinized starch, starch (corn); capsules—powdered cellulose, gelatin, magnesium stearate, sodium metabisulfite*, pregelatinized starch, starch (corn), titanium dioxide, No. 4 may contain FD&C Blue No. 1, FD&C Red No. 3, FD&C Red No. 40; elixir—alcohol, citric acid, propylene glycol, sodium benzoate, saccharin sodium, sucrose, natural and artificial flavors, FD&C Yellow No. 6.
Acetaminophen is a non-salicylate analgesic-antipyretic which occurs as a white, odorless crystalline powder, possessing a slightly bitter taste.
Codeine is an opioid analgesic-antitussive. Codeine is an alkaloid obtained from opium or prepared from morphine by methylation. Codeine occurs as colorless or white crystals, effloresces slowly in dry air and is affected by light.
*See Warnings

CLINICAL PHARMACOLOGY

TYLENOL with Codeine tablets, capsules and elixir combine the analgesic effects of a centrally acting analgesic, codeine, with a peripherally acting analgesic, acetaminophen. Both ingredients of TYLENOL with Codeine are well absorbed orally. Following oral administration of two TYLENOL with Codeine No. 3 tablets, a peak plasma codeine concentration of 173 ng/ml is reached at 75 minutes. After 6 hours, 27 percent of this remains in plasma. A peak plasma acetaminophen concentration of 7.3 μg/ml is reached 42 minutes after administration of two TYLENOL with Codeine No. 3 tablets. After 6 hours, 16 percent of the acetaminophen remains in plasma. The plasma elimination half-life is 2.3 hours for acetaminophen and 2.5 hours for codeine.
Codeine retains at least one-half of its analgesic activity when administered orally. A reduced first-pass metabolism of codeine by the liver accounts for the greater oral efficacy of codeine when compared to most other morphine-like narcotics. Following absorption, codeine is metabolized by the liver and metabolic products are excreted in the urine. Approximately 10 percent of the administered codeine is demethylated to morphine, which may account for its analgesic activity.
Acetaminophen is distributed throughout most tissues of the body. Acetaminophen is metabolized primarily in the liver. Little unchanged drug is excreted in the urine, but most metabolic products appear in the urine within 24 hours.

INDICATIONS AND USAGE

TYLENOL with Codeine tablets and capsules are indicated for the relief of mild to moderately severe pain.
TYLENOL with Codeine elixir is indicated for the relief of mild to moderate pain.

CONTRAINDICATIONS

TYLENOL with Codeine tablets, capsules or elixir should not be administered to patients who have previously exhibited hypersensitivity to codeine or acetaminophen.

WARNINGS

Special Risk Patients: TYLENOL with Codeine tablets and capsules contain sodium metabisulfite, a sulfite that may cause allergic-type reactions (e.g. hives, itching, wheezing, anaphylaxis) in certain susceptible persons. Although the overall prevalence of sulfite sensitivity in the general population is probably low, it is seen more frequently in asthmatics or in atopic nonasthmatic persons.
Drug Dependence: (See DRUG ABUSE AND DEPENDENCE)

PRECAUTIONS

General
Head Injury and Increased Intracranial Pressure: The respiratory depressant effects of narcotics and their capacity to elevate cerebrospinal fluid pressure may be markedly exaggerated in the presence of head injury, other intracranial lesions or a pre-existing increase in intracranial pressure. Furthermore, narcotics produce adverse reactions which may obscure the clinical course of patients with head injuries.
Acute Abdominal Conditions: The administration of this product or other narcotics may obscure the diagnosis or clinical course of patients with acute abdominal conditions.
Special Risk Patients: This drug should be given with caution to certain patients such as the elderly or debilitated, and those with severe impairment of hepatic or renal function, hypothyroidism, Addison's disease, and prostatic hypertrophy or urethral stricture.
Information for Patients
Codeine may impair the mental and/or physical abilities required for the performance of potentially hazardous tasks such as driving a car or operating machinery. The patient using this drug should be cautioned accordingly.
Drug Interactions
Patients receiving other narcotic analgesics, antipsychotics, anti-anxiety agents, or other CNS depressants (including alcohol) concomitantly with this drug may exhibit an additive CNS depression. When such combined therapy is contemplated, the dose of one or both agents should be reduced. The use of MAO inhibitors or tricyclic antidepressants with codeine preparations may increase the effect of either the antidepressant or codeine.
The concurrent use of anticholinergics with codeine may produce paralytic ileus.
Carcinogenesis, Mutagenesis, Impairment of Fertility
No long-term studies in animals have been performed with acetaminophen or codeine to determine carcinogenic potential or effects on fertility.
Acetaminophen and codeine have been found to have no mutagenic potential using the Ames Salmonella-Microsomal Activation test, the Basc test on Drosophila germ cells, and the Micronucleus test on mouse bone marrow.
Teratogenic Effects
Pregnancy Category C. Codeine has been shown to be teratogenic in mice when given in doses 17 times the maximum human daily dose. There are no adequate and well controlled studies in pregnant women. TYLENOL with Codeine should be used during pregnancy only if the potential benefit justifies the potential risk to the fetus.
Nursing Mothers
It is not known whether the components of this drug are excreted in human milk. Because many drugs are excreted in human milk, caution should be exercised when TYLENOL with Codeine is administered to a nursing woman.
Pediatric Use
Safe dosage of the elixir has not been established in children below the age of three; tablets and capsules should not be administered to children under 12.

ADVERSE REACTIONS

The most frequently observed adverse reactions include lightheadedness, dizziness, sedation, shortness of breath, nausea and vomiting. These effects seem to be more prominent in ambulatory than in non-ambulatory patients, and some of these adverse reactions may be alleviated if the patient lies down. Other adverse reactions include allergic reactions, euphoria, dysphoria, constipation, and pruritus.
At higher doses codeine has most of the disadvantages of morphine including respiratory depression.

DRUG ABUSE AND DEPENDENCE

TYLENOL with Codeine tablets and capsules are Schedule III controlled substances.
TYLENOL with Codeine elixir is a Schedule V controlled substance.
Codeine can produce drug dependence of the morphine type, and therefore has the potential for being abused. Psychic dependence, physical dependence and tolerance may develop upon repeated adminstration of this drug, and it should be prescribed and administered with the same degree of caution appropriate to the use of other oral narcotic-containing medications.

OVERDOSAGE

Acetaminophen
Signs and Symptoms: Acetaminophen in massive overdosage may cause hepatic toxicity in some patients. **In all cases of suspected overdose, immediately call your regional poison center or the Rocky Mountain Poison Center's toll-free number** (800-525-6115) for assistance in diagnosis and for directions in the use of N-acetylcysteine as an antidote.
In adults, hepatic toxicity has rarely been reported with acute overdoses of less than 10 grams and fatalities with less than 15 grams. Importantly, young children seem to be more resistant than adults to the hepatotoxic effect of an acetaminophen overdose. Despite this, the measures outlined below should be initiated in any adult or child suspected of having ingested an acetaminophen overdose.
Early symptoms following a potentially hepatotoxic overdose may include: nausea, vomiting, diaphoresis and general malaise. Clinical and laboratory evidence of hepatic toxicity may not be apparent until 48 to 72 hours post-ingestion.
Treatment: The stomach should be emptied promptly by lavage or by induction of emesis with syrup of ipecac. Patients' estimates of the quantity of a drug ingested are notoriously unreliable. Therefore, if an acetaminophen overdose is suspected, a serum acetaminophen assay should be obtained as early as possible, but no sooner than four hours following ingestion. Liver function studies should be obtained initially and repeated at 24 hour intervals.
The antidote, N-acetylcysteine, should be administered as early as possible, and within 16 hours of the overdose ingestion for optimal results, but in any case, within 24 hours. Following recovery, there are no residual, structural or functional hepatic abnormalities.
Codeine
Signs and Symptoms: Serious overdose with codeine is characterized by respiratory depression (a decrease in respiratory rate and/or tidal volume, Cheyne-Stokes respiration, cyanosis), extreme somnolence progressing to stupor or coma, skeletal muscle flaccidity, cold and clammy skin, and sometimes bradycardia and hypotension. In severe overdosage, apnea, circulatory collapse, cardiac arrest and death may occur.
Treatment: Primary attention should be given to the reestablishment of adequate respiratory exchange through provision of a patent airway and the institution of assisted or controlled ventilation. The narcotic antagonist naloxone is a specific antidote against respiratory depression which may result from overdosage or unusual sensitivity to narcotics, including codeine. Therefore, an appropriate dose of naloxone (see package insert) should be administered, preferably by the intravenous route, and simultaneously with efforts at respiratory resuscitation. Since the duration of action of codeine may exceed that of the antagonist, the patient should be kept under continued surveillance and repeated doses of the antagonist should be administered as needed to maintain adequate respiration.
An antagonist should not be administered in the absence of clinically significant respiratory or cardiovascular depression. Oxygen, intravenous fluids, vasopressors and other supportive measures should be employed as indicated.
Gastric emptying may be useful in removing unabsorbed drug.

DOSAGE AND ADMINISTRATION

Dosage should be adjusted according to severity of pain and response of the patient. However, it should be kept in mind that tolerance to codeine can develop with continued use and that the incidence of untoward effects is dose related Adult dose of codeine higher than 60 mg fail to give commensurate relief of pain but merely prolong analgesia and are associated with an appreciably increased incidence of undesirable side effects. Equivalently high doses in children would have similar effects.
TYLENOL with Codeine tablets and capsules are given orally. The usual adult dose is: Tablets No. 1, No. 2, and No. 3 and Capsules No. 3: One or two every four hours as required. Tablets and Capsules No. 4: One every four hours as required.
The recommended dose of codeine in children is 0.5 mg/kg body weight.
TYLENOL with Codeine elixir contains 12 mg of codeine/5 ml teaspoon and is given orally. The usual doses are:
Children (3 to 6 years): 1 teaspoonful (5 ml) 3 or 4 times daily; *(7 to 12 years):* 2 teaspoonfuls (10 ml) 3 or 4 times daily; *(under 3 years):* safe dosage has not been established.
Adults: 1 tablespoonful (15 ml) every 4 hours as needed.

HOW SUPPLIED

TYLENOL® with Codeine tablets (white, imprinted "McNEIL", "TYLENOL CODEINE" and either "1", "2", "3", "4") No. 1—NDC 0045-0510, bottles of 100; No. 2—NDC 0045-0511, bottles of 100 and 500; No. 3—NDC 0045-0513, bottles of 100, 500, and 1000; and No. 4—NDC 0045-0515—bottles of 100 and 500. No. 2, No. 3, and No. 4 also available in a Unit Dose Dispensit (20 × 25).
TYLENOL® with Codeine capsules No. 3 (colored white with red bands, imprinted "McNEIL" and "TYLENOL 3 CODEINE")—NDC 0045-0521, bottles of 100 and unit dose of 100's; TYLENOL® with Codeine capsules No. 4 (colored red with white bands, imprinted "McNEIL" and "TYLENOL 4 CODEINE")—NDC 0045-0522, bottles of 100 and unit dose of 100's.
TYLENOL® with Codeine elixir (colored amber, cherry flavored)—NDC 0045-0508, bottles of 1 pint, unit dose cup (10 × 5 ml) and unit dose cup (10 × 15 ml).
Dispense in tight, light-resistant container as defined in the official compendium.

5/7/86

Shown in Product Identification Section, page 416

TYLOX® capsules ℂ ℞

[*ti 'lox*]
(oxycodone and acetaminophen)
100's
Military NSN 6505-01-053-8621
Unit Dose (100's) 6505-01-053-8622

DESCRIPTION

Each capsule contains:

Oxycodone Hydrochloride	5 mg
Warning—May be habit forming.	
Acetaminophen	500 mg

Inactive ingredients: docusate sodium, gelatin, magnesium stearate, sodium benzoate, sodium metabisulfite*, corn starch, FD&C Blue No. 1, FD&C Red No. 3, FD&C Red No. 40, and titanium dioxide.
Oxycodone, a semisynthetic narcotic, is a white, odorless crystalline powder having a saline, bitter taste. It is derived from the opium alkaloid, thebaine.
TYLOX capsules also contain the nonsalicylate analgesic-antipyretic acetaminophen.
Acetaminophen occurs as a white, odorless crystalline powder possessing a slightly bitter taste.
*See Warnings

CLINICAL PHARMACOLOGY

The principal analgesic ingredient, oxycodone, is a semisynthetic narcotic with multiple actions qualitatively similar to those of morphine; the most prominent of these involve the central nervous system and organs composed of smooth muscle. The principal actions of therapeutic value of the oxycodone in this drug are analgesia and sedation.
Oxycodone is similar to codeine and methadone in that it retains at least one half of its analgesic activity when administered orally.
Acetaminophen is a nonopiate, non-salicylate analgesic and antipyretic.

INDICATIONS AND USAGE

TYLOX capsules are indicated for the relief of moderate to moderately severe pain.

CONTRAINDICATIONS

TYLOX capsules should not be administered to patients who have previously exhibited hypersensitivity to oxycodone or acetaminophen.

WARNINGS

TYLOX capsules contain sodium metabisulfite, a sulfite that may cause allergic-type reactions (e.g., hives, itching, wheezing, anaphylaxis) in certain susceptible persons. Although the overall prevalence of sulfite sensitivity in the general population is probably low, it is seen more frequently in asthmatics or in atopic nonasthmatic persons.

PRECAUTIONS

General
Head Injury and Increased Intracranial Pressure: The respiratory depressant effects of narcotics and their capacity to elevate cerebrospinal fluid pressure may be markedly exaggerated in the presence of head injury, other intracranial lesions, or a pre-existing increase in intracranial pressure. Furthermore, narcotics produce adverse reactions which may obscure the clinical course of patients with head injuries.
Acute Abdominal Conditions: The administration of TYLOX capsules or other narcotics may obscure the diagnosis or clinical course in patients with acute abdominal conditions.
Special Risk Patients: TYLOX capsules should be given with caution to certain patients such as the elderly or debilitated, and those with severe impairment of hepatic or renal function, hypothyroidism, Addison's disease, and prostatic hypertrophy or urethral stricture.

Continued on next page

McNeil Pharm.—Cont.

Information for Patients

Oxycodone may impair the mental and/or physical abilities required for the performance of potentially hazardous tasks such as driving a car or operating machinery. The patient using TYLOX capsules should be cautioned accordingly.

Drug Interactions

Patients receiving other narcotic analgesics, antipsychotics, antianxiety agents, or other CNS depressants, including alcohol, concomitantly with TYLOX capsules, may exhibit additive CNS depression due to the oxycodone component. When such combined therapy is contemplated, the dose of one or both agents should be reduced.

The use of MAO inhibitors or tricyclic antidepressants with oxycodone preparations may increase the effect of either the antidepressant or oxycodone.

The concurrent use of anticholinergics with oxycodone may produce paralytic ileus.

Carcinogenesis, Mutagenesis, Impairment of Fertility

No long-term studies in animals have been performed with oxycodone to determine carcinogenic and mutagenic potential, or effects on fertility. Acetaminophen has been found to have no mutagenic potential using the Ames Salmonella-Microsomal Activation test, the Basc test on Drosophila germ cells, and the Micronucleus test on mouse bone marrow. In animals, acetaminophen has not been evaluated for carcinogenic potential or for effects on fertility.

Pregnancy Category C. Animal reproductive studies have not been conducted with TYLOX. It is also not known whether TYLOX can cause fetal harm when administered to a pregnant woman or can affect reproductive capacity. TYLOX should not be given to a pregnant woman unless in the judgment of the physician, the potential benefits outweigh the possible hazards.

Nonteratogenic Effects: Use of narcotics during pregnancy may produce physical dependence in the neonate.

Nursing Mothers

It is not known whether the components of this drug are excreted in human milk. Because many drugs are excreted in human milk, caution should be exercised when TYLOX is administered to a nursing woman.

Pediatric Use

TYLOX capsules should not be administered to children.

ADVERSE REACTIONS

The most frequently observed adverse reactions include lightheadedness, dizziness, sedation, nausea, and vomiting. These effects seem to be more prominent in ambulatory patients than in non-ambulatory patients, and some of these adverse reactions may be alleviated if the patient lies down. Other adverse reactions include allergic reactions, euphoria, dysphoria, constipation, skin rash, and pruritus.

At higher doses oxycodone has most of the disadvantages of morphine including respiratory depression.

DRUG ABUSE AND DEPENDENCE

TYLOX capsules are a Schedule II controlled substance.

Oxycodone can produce drug dependence of the morphine type and, therefore, has the potential for being abused. Psychic dependence, physical dependence, and tolerance may develop upon repeated administration of TYLOX capsules, and they should be prescribed and administered with the same degree of caution appropriate to the use of other oral narcotic-containing medications.

OVERDOSAGE

Acetaminophen

Signs and Symptoms: Acetaminophen in massive overdosage may cause hepatic toxicity in some patients. In all cases of suspected overdose, immediately call your regional poison center or the Rocky Mountain Poison Center's toll-free number (800-525-6115) for assistance in diagnosis and for directions in the use of N-acetylcysteine as an antidote.

In adults, hepatic toxicity has rarely been reported with acute overdoses of less than 10 grams and fatalities with less than 15 grams. Importantly, young children seem to be more resistant than adults to the hepatotoxic effect of an acetaminophen overdose. Despite this, the measures outlined below should be initiated in any adult or child suspected of having ingested an acetaminophen overdose.

Early symptoms following a potentially hepatotoxic overdose may include: nausea, vomiting, diaphoresis, and general malaise. Clinical and laboratory evidence of hepatic toxicity may not be apparent until 48 to 72 hours post-ingestion.

Treatment: The stomach should be emptied promptly by lavage or by induction of emesis with syrup of ipecac. Patients' estimates of the quantity of a drug ingested are notoriously unreliable. Therefore, if an acetaminophen overdose is suspected, a serum acetaminophen assay should be obtained as early as possible, but no sooner than four hours following ingestion. Liver function studies should be obtained initially and repeated at 24-hour intervals.

The antidote, N-acetylcysteine, should be administered as early as possible, and within 16 hours of the overdose ingestion for optimal results, but in any case, within 24 hours. Following recovery, there are no residual, structural, or functional hepatic abnormalities.

Oxycodone

Signs and symptoms: Serious overdosage with oxycodone is characterized by respiratory depression (a decrease in respiratory rate and/or tidal volume, Cheyne-Stokes respiration, cyanosis), extreme somnolence progressing to stupor or coma, skeletal muscle flaccidity, cold and clammy skin, and sometimes bradycardia and hypotension. In severe overdosage, apnea, circulatory collapse, cardiac arrest, and death may occur.

Treatment: Primary attention should be given to the reestablishment of adequate respiratory exchange through provision of a patent airway and the institution of assisted or controlled ventilation. The narcotic antagonist naloxone is a specific antidote against respiratory depression which may result from overdosage or unusual sensitivity to narcotics, including oxycodone. Therefore, an appropriate dose of naloxone should be administered (see package insert) preferably by the intravenous route and simultaneously with efforts at respiratory resuscitation. Since the duration of action of oxycodone may exceed that of the antagonist, the patient should be kept under continued surveillance, and repeated doses of the antagonist should be administered as needed to maintain adequate respiration.

An antagonist should not be administered in the absence of clinically significant respiratory or cardiovascular depression.

Oxygen, intravenous fluids, vasopressors, and other supportive measures should be employed as indicated.

Gastric emptying may be useful in removing unabsorbed drug.

DOSAGE AND ADMINISTRATION

Dosage should be adjusted according to the severity of the pain and the response of the patient. However, it should be kept in mind that tolerance to oxycodone can develop with continued use and that the incidence of untoward effects is dose related. This product is inappropriate even in high doses for severe or intractable pain.

TYLOX capsules are given orally. The usual adult dose is one TYLOX capsule every 6 hours as needed for pain.

HOW SUPPLIED

TYLOX® capsules (colored red, imprinted "TYLOX McNEIL") NDC 0045-0526—bottles of 100 and unit dose 25's.

Dispense in tight container as defined in the official compendium.

6/18/86

Shown in Product Identification Section, page 416

EDUCATIONAL MATERIAL

Haldol® (haloperidol)
"Question and Answer Brochure"
"Haldol® Films Available" Brochure
Both are available free to physicians and pharmacists through McNeil representatives.

Parafon Forte® (chlorzoxazone and acetaminophen)
"Remedial Exercises for Low Back Pain" (English & Spanish)
"Remedial Exercises for Cervical Sprain" (English & Spanish)
Both are available free to physicians and pharmacists through McNeil representatives.

Tolectin® (tolmetin sodium)
"Six Steps to Control Your Arthritis Symptoms" (English & Spanish)
Juvenile Arthritis Film & Brochure
Both are available free to physicians and pharmacists through McNeil representatives.

Tylenol ® with Codeine (acetaminophen and codeine)
"Oral Analgesics and Pain Management" Film (16mm & MPO) and Brochure, featuring A. Sunshine, M.D., and S. Cooper, D.M.D., Ph.D.
Available free to physicians and pharmacists through McNeil representatives.

Mead Johnson Laboratories

Mead Johnson & Company
2404 W. PENNSYLVANIA ST.
EVANSVILLE, INDIANA 47721

IDENTIFICATION MARKINGS
SOLID ORAL DOSE FORMS

[See table below left].

Product	Strengths	Capsules	Tablets One Side
Estrace® (estradiol)	1mg		MJ755
Estrace®	2mg		MJ756
Natalins® Rx (multivitamin/multimineral supplement)			702
Ovcon®-35 (norethindrone & ethinyl estradiol)			583
inert green tabs in 28-day regimen			850
Ovcon®-50			584
inert green tabs in 28-day regimen			850
Quibron® (theophylline-guaifenesin) capsules		MJ516	
Quibron®-T Dividose® (theophylline anhydrous) tablets			MJ512 & trisect score lines Bisect score lines on each edge of the two long edges of tablet
Quibron®-T/SR Dividose® (tablets)			MJ519 & trisect score lines Bisect score lines on each edge of the two long edges of tablet

ESTRACE® ℞

[es'trās]
(Estradiol)

WARNING

1. ESTROGENS HAVE BEEN REPORTED TO INCREASE THE RISK OF ENDOMETRIAL CARCINOMA.

Three independent case control studies have shown an increased risk of endometrial cancer in postmenopausal women exposed to exogenous estrogens for prolonged periods.[1-3] This risk was independent of the other known risk factors for endometrial cancer. These studies are further supported by the finding that incidence rates of endometrial cancer have increased sharply since 1969 in eight different areas of the United States with population based cancer reporting systems, an increase which may be related to the rapidly expanding use of estrogens during the last decade.[4]

The three case control studies reported that the risk of endometrial cancer in estrogen users was about 4.5 to 13.9 times greater than in nonusers. The risk appears to depend on both duration of treatment[1] and on estrogen dose.[3] In view of these findings, when estrogens are used for the treatment of menopausal symptoms, the lowest dose that will control symptoms should be utilized and medication should be discontinued as soon as possible. When prolonged treatment is medically indicated, the patient should be reassessed on at least a semiannual basis to determine the need for continued therapy. Although the evidence must be considered preliminary, one study suggests that cyclic administration of low doses of estrogen may carry less risk than continuous administration;[3] it therefore appears prudent to utilize such a regimen.

Close clinical surveillance of all women taking estrogens is important. In all cases of undiagnosed persistent or recurring abnormal vaginal bleeding, adequate diagnostic measures should be undertaken to rule out malignancy.

There is no evidence at present that "natural" estrogens are more or less hazardous than "synthetic" estrogens at equiestrogenic doses.

2. ESTROGENS SHOULD NOT BE USED DURING PREGNANCY.

The use of female sex hormones, both estrogens and progestogens, during early pregnancy may seriously damage the offspring. It has been shown that females exposed *in utero* to diethylstilbestrol, a non-steroidal estrogen, have an increased risk of developing in later life a form of vaginal or cervical cancer that is ordinarily extremely rare.[5,6] This risk has been estimated as not greater than 4 per 1,000 exposures.[7] Furthermore, a high percentage of such exposed women (from 30 to 90 percent) have been found to have vaginal adenosis,[8-12] epithelial changes of the vagina and cervix. Although these changes are histologically benign, it is not known whether they are precursors of malignancy. Although similar data are not available with the use of other estrogens, it cannot be presumed they would not induce similar changes.

Several reports suggest an association between intrauterine exposure to female sex hormones and congenital anomalies, including congenital heart defects and limb reduction defects.[13-16] One case control study[16] estimated a 4.7-fold increased risk of limb reduction defects in infants exposed *in utero* to sex hormones (oral contraceptives, hormone withdrawal tests for pregnancy, or attempted treatment for threatened abortion). Some of these exposures were very short and involved only a few days of treatment. The data suggest that the risk of limb reduction defects in exposed fetuses is somewhat less than 1 per 1,000.

In the past, female sex hormones have been used during pregnancy in an attempt to treat threatened or habitual abortion. There is considerable evidence that estrogens are ineffective for these indications, and there is no evidence from well controlled studies that progestogens are effective for these uses.

If Estrace® is used during pregnancy, or if the patient becomes pregnant while taking this drug, she should be apprised of the potential risks to the fetus and the advisability of pregnancy continuation.

DESCRIPTION

Estrace® oral tablets contain 1 or 2 mg of micronized estradiol. Estradiol (17β-estradiol) is a white, crystalline solid, chemically described as estra-1,3,5(10)-triene-3,17β-diol. Estrace® oral tablets provide estrogen replacement therapy. The structural formula is:

CH_3 OH HO

Estrace Tablets, 1 mg, contain the following active ingredients: acacia, D&C Red No. 27 (aluminum lake), dibasic calcium phosphate, FD&C Blue No. 1 (aluminum lake), lactose, magnesium stearate, colloidal silicon dioxide, starch (corn), and talc.

Estrace Tablets, 2 mg, contain the following inactive ingredients: acacia, dibasic calcium phosphate, FD&C Blue No. 1 (aluminum lake), FD&C Yellow No. 5 (tartrazine) (aluminum lake), lactose, magnesium stearate, colloidal silicon dioxide, starch (corn), and talc.

Clinical Pharmacology

17β-Estradiol is the most potent physiologic estrogen and, in fact, is the major estrogenic hormone secreted by the human. Estradiol in Estrace® has been micronized and demonstrated to be rapidly and effectively absorbed from the gastrointestinal tract.[17]

INDICATIONS

Estrace® affords effective treatment of:

1. Moderate to severe *vasomotor* symptoms associated with the menopause. (There is no evidence that estrogens are effective for nervous symptoms or depression which might occur during menopause, and they should not be used to treat these conditions.)
2. Atrophic vaginitis.
3. Kraurosis vulvae.
4. Female hypogonadism.
5. Female castration.
6. Primary ovarian failure.
7. Breast cancer (for palliation only) in appropriately selected women and men with metastatic disease.
8. Prostatic carcinoma—palliative therapy of advanced disease.

ESTRACE® HAS NOT BEEN SHOWN TO BE EFFECTIVE FOR ANY PURPOSE DURING PREGNANCY AND ITS USE MAY CAUSE SEVERE HARM TO THE FETUS (SEE BOXED WARNING).

CONTRAINDICATIONS

Estrogens should not be used in women (or men) with any of the following conditions:

1. Known or suspected cancer of the breast except in appropriately selected patients being treated for metastatic disease.
2. Known or suspected estrogen-dependent neoplasia.
3. Known or suspected pregnancy (See Boxed Warning).
4. Undiagnosed abnormal genital bleeding.
5. Active thrombophlebitis or thromboembolic disorders.
6. A past history of thrombophlebitis, thrombosis or thromboembolic disorders associated with previous estrogen use (except when used in treatment of breast or prostatic malignancy).

WARNINGS

1. **Induction of malignant neoplasms.** Long term continuous administration of natural and synthetic estrogens in certain animal species increases the frequency of carcinomas of the breast, cervix, vagina, and liver. There is now evidence that estrogens increase the risk of carcinoma of the endometrium in humans. (See Boxed Warning).

At the present time there is no satisfactory evidence that estrogens given to postmenopausal women increase the risk of cancer of the breast,[18] although a recent long-term followup of a single physician's practice has raised this possibility.[19] Because of the animal data there is a need for caution in prescribing estrogens for women with a strong family history of breast cancer or who have breast nodules, fibrocystic disease, or abnormal mammograms.

2. **Gallbladder disease.** A recent study has reported a 2- to 3-fold increase in the risk of surgically confirmed gallbladder disease in women receiving postmenopausal estrogens,[18] similar to the 2-fold increase previously noted in users of oral contraceptives.[20,34] In the case of oral contraceptives, the increased risk appeared after two years of use.[34]

3. **Effects similar to those caused by estrogen-progestogen oral contraceptives.** There are several serious adverse effects of oral contraceptives, most of which have not, up to now, been documented as consequences of postmenopausal estrogen therapy. This may reflect the comparatively low doses of estrogen used in postmenopausal women. It would be expected that the larger doses of estrogen used to treat prostatic or breast cancer or postpartum breast engorgement are more likely to result in these adverse effects, and, in fact, it has been shown that there is an increased risk of thrombosis in men receiving estrogens for prostatic cancer and women for postpartum breast engorgement.[21-24]

a. **Thromboembolic disease.** It is now well established that users of oral contraceptives have an increased risk of various thromboembolic and thrombotic vascular diseases, such as thrombophlebitis, pulmonary embolism, stroke, and myocardial infarction.[25-32] Cases of retinal thrombosis, mesenteric thrombosis, and optic neuritis have been reported in oral contraceptive users. There is evidence that the risk of several of these adverse reactions is related to the dose of the drug.[33,34] An increased risk of post-surgery thromboembolic complications has also been reported in users of oral contraceptives.[35,36] If feasible, estrogen should be discontinued at least 4 weeks before surgery of the type associated with an increased risk of thromboembolism, or during periods of prolonged immobilization.

While an increased rate of thromboembolic and thrombotic disease in postmenopausal users of estrogens has not been found,[19,37] this does not rule out the possibility that such an increase may be present or that subgroups of women who have underlying risk factors or who are receiving relatively large doses of estrogens may have increased risk. Therefore, estrogens should not be used in persons with active thrombophlebitis or thromboembolic disorders, and they should not be used (except in treatment of malignancy) in persons with a history of such disorders in association with estrogen use. They should be used with caution in patients with cerebral vascular or coronary artery disease and only for those in whom estrogens are clearly needed.

Large doses of estrogen (5 mg conjugated estrogens per day), comparable to those used to treat cancer of the prostate and breast, have been shown in a large prospective clinical trial in men[38] to increase the risk of nonfatal myocardial infarction, pulmonary embolism and thrombophlebitis. When estrogen doses of this size are used, any of the thromboembolic and thrombotic adverse effects associated with oral contraceptive use should be considered a clear risk.

b. **Hepatic adenoma.** Hepatic adenomas appear to be associated with the use of oral contraceptives.[39-41] Although rare, these may rupture and may cause death through intraabdominal hemorrhage. Such lesions have not yet been reported in association with other estrogen or progestogen preparations but should be considered in estrogen users having abdominal pain and tenderness, abdominal mass, or hypovolemic shock. Hepatocellular carcinoma has also been reported in women taking estrogen-containing oral contraceptives.[40] The relationship of this malignancy to these drugs is not known at this time.

c. **Elevated blood pressure.** Increased blood pressure is not uncommon in women using oral contraceptives. There is now a report that this may occur with use of estrogens in the menopause[42] and blood pressure should be monitored with estrogen use, especially if high doses are used.

d. **Glucose tolerance.** A worsening of glucose tolerance has been observed in a significant percentage of patients on estrogen-containing oral contraceptives. For this reason, diabetic patients should be carefully observed while receiving estrogen.

4. **Hypercalcemia.** Administration of estrogens may lead to severe hypercalcemia in patients with breast cancer and bone metastases. If this occurs, the drug should be stopped and appropriate measures taken to reduce the serum calcium level.

PRECAUTIONS

A. General Precautions.

1. A complete medical and family history should be taken prior to the initiation of any estrogen therapy. The pretreatment and periodic physical examinations should include special reference to blood pressure, breasts, abdomen, and pelvic organs, and should include a Papanicolaou smear. As a general rule, estrogen should not be prescribed for longer than one year without another physical examination being performed.
2. Fluid retention—Because estrogens may cause some degree of fluid retention, conditions which might be influenced by this factor such as epilepsy, migraine, and cardiac or renal dysfunction, require careful observation.
3. Certain patients may develop undesirable manifestations of excessive estrogenic stimulation, such as abnormal or excessive uterine bleeding, mastodynia, etc.
4. Oral contraceptives appear to be associated with an increased incidence of mental depression. Although it is not clear whether this is due to the estrogenic or progestogenic component of the contraceptive, patients with a history of depression should be carefully observed.
5. Preexisting uterine leiomyomata may increase in size during estrogen use.
6. The pathologist should be advised of estrogen therapy when relevant specimens are submitted.
7. Patients with a past history of jaundice during pregnancy have an increased risk of recurrence of jaundice while receiving estrogen-containing oral contraceptive therapy. If jaundice develops in any patient receiving estrogen, the medication should be discontinued while the cause is investigated.
8. Estrogens may be poorly metabolized in patients with impaired liver function and they should be administered with caution in such patients.
9. Because estrogens influence the metabolism of calcium and phosphorus, they should be used with caution in patients with metabolic bone diseases that are associated with hypercalcemia or in patients with renal insufficiency.
10. Because of the effects of estrogens on epiphyseal closure, they should be used judiciously in young patients in whom bone growth is not complete.
11. Certain endocrine and liver function tests may be affected by estrogen-containing oral contraceptives. The following similar changes may be expected with larger doses of estrogen:

a. Increased sulfobromophthalein retention.
b. Increased prothrombin and factors VII and VIII, IX, and X; decreased antithrombin 3; increased norepinephrine-induced platelet aggregability.
c. Increased thyroid binding globulin (TBG) leading to increased circulating total thyroid hormone, as measured by PBI, T4 by column, or T4 by radioimmunoassay. Free T3 resin uptake is decreased, reflecting the elevated TBG; free T4 concentration is unaltered.
d. Impaired glucose tolerance.
e. Decreased pregnanediol excretion.
f. Reduced response to metyrapone test.
g. Reduced serum folate concentration.
h. Increased serum triglyceride and phospholipid concentration.

B. Information for the Patient. See text of Patient Package Insert on reverse side.

C. Pregnancy Category X. See Contraindications and Boxed Warning.

D. Nursing Mothers. As a general principle, the administration of any drug to nursing mothers should be done only when clearly necessary since many drugs are excreted in human milk.

Estrace 2 mg tablets contain FD&C Yellow No. 5 (tartrazine) which may cause allergic-type reactions (including bronchial asthma) in certain susceptible individuals. Although the overall incidence of FD&C Yellow No. 5 (tartrazine) sensitivity in the general population is low, it is frequently seen in patients who also have aspirin hypersensitivity.

Continued on next page

Mead Johnson Labs.—Cont.

ADVERSE REACTIONS

(See Warnings regarding induction of neoplasia, adverse effects on the fetus, increased incidence of gallbladder disease, and adverse effects similar to those of oral contraceptives, including thromboembolism.) The following additional adverse reactions have been reported with estrogenic therapy, including oral contraceptives:

1. **Genitourinary system.**
   Breakthrough bleeding, spotting, change in menstrual flow.
   Dysmenorrhea.
   Premenstrual-like syndrome.
   Amenorrhea during and after treatment.
   Increase in size of uterine fibromyomata.
   Vaginal candidiasis.
   Change in cervical eversion and in degree of cervical secretion.
   Cystitis-like syndrome.
2. **Breast.**
   Tenderness, enlargement, secretion.
3. **Gastrointestinal.**
   Nausea, vomiting.
   Abdominal cramps, bloating.
   Cholestatic jaundice.
4. **Skin.**
   Chloasma or melasma which may persist when drug is discontinued.
   Erythema multiforme.
   Erythema nodosum.
   Hemorrhagic eruption.
   Loss of scalp hair.
   Hirsutism.
5. **Eyes.**
   Steepening of corneal curvature.
   Intolerance to contact lenses.
6. **CNS.**
   Headache, migraine, dizziness.
   Mental depression.
   Chorea.
7. **Miscellaneous.**
   Increase or decrease in weight.
   Reduced carbohydrate tolerance.
   Aggravation of porphyria.
   Edema.
   Changes in libido.

OVERDOSAGE

Numerous reports of ingestion of large doses of estrogen-containing oral contraceptives by young children indicate that serious ill effects do not occur. Overdosage of estrogen may cause nausea, and withdrawal bleeding may occur in females.

DOSAGE AND ADMINISTRATION

1. **Given cyclically for short term use only:**
   For treatment of moderate to severe *vasomotor* symptoms, atrophic vaginitis, or kraurosis vulvae associated with the menopause. The lowest dose that will control symptoms should be chosen and medication should be discontinued as promptly as possible. Administration should be cyclic (e.g., 3 weeks on and 1 week off). Attempts to discontinue or taper medication should be made at 3 to 6 month intervals. The usual initial dosage range is 1 or 2 mg daily of micronized estradiol adjusted as necessary to control presenting symptoms. The minimal effective dose for maintenance therapy should be determined by titration.
2. **Given cyclically:**
   Female hypogonadism.
   Female castration.
   Primary ovarian failure.
   Treatment is usually initiated with a dose of 1 or 2 mg daily of micronized estradiol, adjusted as necessary to control presenting symptoms; the minimal effective dose for maintenance therapy should be determined by titration.
3. **Given chronically:**
   Inoperable progressing prostatic cancer—Suggested dosage is 1 to 2 mg three times daily. The effectiveness of therapy can be judged by phosphatase determinations as well as by symptomatic improvement of the patient.
   Inoperable progressing breast cancer in appropriately selected men and postmenopausal women (see INDICATIONS)—Suggested dosage is 10 mg three times daily for a period of at least three months.
   Treated patients with an intact uterus should be monitored closely for signs of endometrial cancer and appropriate diagnostic measures should be taken to rule out malignancy in the event of persistent or recurring abnormal vaginal bleeding.

HOW SUPPLIED

Estrace 1 mg; lavender scored tablets

NDC 0087-0755-01	Bottles of 100
NDC 0087-0755-44	Compacts of 25

Estrace 2 mg; turquoise scored tablets

NDC 0087-0756-01	Bottles of 100
NDC 0087-0756-44	Compacts of 25

PATIENT LABELING

WHAT YOU SHOULD KNOW ABOUT ESTROGENS

Estrogens are female hormones produced principally by the ovaries. The ovaries make several different kinds of estrogens. In addition, scientists have been able to make a variety of synthetic estrogens. As far as we know, all these estrogens have the same properties and therefore much the same usefulness, side effects, and risks. This leaflet is intended to help you understand what estrogens are used for, the risks involved in their use, and how to use them as safely as possible. This leaflet includes important information about Estrace® (estradiol) and estrogens in general, but not all the information. If you want to know more you can ask your doctor or pharmacist to let you read the professional package insert.

USES OF ESTROGEN

Estrogens are prescribed by doctors for a number of purposes, including:

1. To provide estrogen during a period of adjustment when a woman's ovaries no longer produce it, in order to prevent certain uncomfortable symptoms of estrogen deficiency. (All women normally experience a decrease in the production of estrogens, generally between 45–55; this is called the menopause.)
2. To prevent symptoms of estrogen deficiency when a woman's ovaries have been removed surgically before the natural menopause.
3. To prevent pregnancy. (Some estrogens are given along with a progestogen, another female hormone; these combinations are called oral contraceptives or birth control pills. They will not be discussed in this leaflet.) However, Estrace is not intended for this use.
4. To treat certain cancers in women and men.
5. To prevent painful swelling of the breasts after pregnancy in women who choose not to nurse their babies.

THERE IS NO PROPER USE OF ESTROGENS IN A PREGNANT WOMAN.

ESTROGENS IN THE MENOPAUSE

In the natural course of their lives, all women eventually experience a decrease in estrogen production. This usually occurs between ages 45 and 55 but may occur earlier or later. Sometimes the ovaries may need to be removed before natural menopause by an operation, producing a "surgical menopause."

When the amount of estrogen in the blood begins to decrease, many women may develop typical symptoms: feelings of warmth in the face, neck, and chest or sudden intense episodes of heat and sweating throughout the body (called "hot flashes" or "hot flushes"). These symptoms are sometimes very uncomfortable. A few women eventually develop changes in the vagina (called "atrophic vaginitis") which cause discomfort, especially during and after intercourse.

Estrogens can be prescribed to treat these symptoms of the menopause. It is estimated that considerably more than half of all women undergoing the menopause have only mild symptoms or no symptoms at all and therefore do not need estrogens. Other women may need estrogens for a few months, while their bodies adjust to lower estrogen levels. Sometimes the need will be for periods longer than six months. In an attempt to avoid over-stimulation of the uterus (womb), estrogens are usually given cyclically during each month of use, that is three weeks of pills followed by one week without pills.

Sometimes women experience nervous symptoms or depression during menopause. There is no evidence that estrogens are effective for such symptoms and they should not be used to treat them, although other treatment may be needed.

You may have heard that taking estrogens for long periods (years) after the menopause will keep your skin soft and supple and keep you feeling young. There is no evidence that this is so, however, and such long-term treatment carries additional risks.

ESTROGENS TO PREVENT SWELLING OF THE BREASTS AFTER PREGNANCY

If you do not breast feed your baby after delivery, your breasts may fill up with milk and become painful and engorged. This usually begins about three to four days after delivery and may last for a few days to up to a week or more. Sometimes the discomfort is severe, but usually it is not and can be controlled by pain-relieving drugs such as aspirin and by binding the breasts up tightly. Estrogens can sometimes be used successfully to try to prevent the breasts from filling up. While this treatment is sometimes successful, in many cases the breasts fill up to some degree in spite of treatment. The dose of estrogens needed to prevent pain and swelling of the breasts is much larger than the dose needed to treat symptoms of the menopause and this may increase your chances of developing blood clots in the legs or lungs or other parts of the body (see below, 4. Abnormal Blood Clotting). Therefore, it is important that you discuss the benefits and the risks of estrogen use with your doctor, before using estrogen, if you have decided not to breast feed your baby.

THE DANGERS OF ESTROGENS

1. **Cancer of the uterus.** If estrogens are used in the postmenopausal period for more than a year, there is an increased risk of **cancer of the endometrium** (uterine lining). Women taking estrogens have roughly 5 to 15 times as great a chance of getting this cancer as women who take no estrogens. To put this another way, while a postmenopausal woman not taking estrogens has one chance in 1,000 each year of getting cancer of the uterus, a woman taking estrogens has 5 to 15 chances in 1,000 each year. For this reason it **is important to take estrogens only when you really need them.**

The risk of this cancer is greater the longer estrogens are used and also seems to be greater when larger doses are taken. For this reason **it is important to take the lowest dose of estrogen that will control symptoms and to take it only as long as it is needed.** If estrogens are needed for longer periods of time, your doctor will want to reevaluate your need for estrogens at least every six months.

Women using estrogens should report any irregular vaginal bleeding to their doctors; such bleeding may be of no importance, but it can be an early warning of cancer of the uterus. If you have undiagnosed vaginal bleeding, you should not use estrogens until a diagnosis is made and you are certain there is no cancer of the uterus. If you have had your uterus completely removed (total hysterectomy), there is no danger of developing cancer of the uterus.

2. **Other possible cancers.** Estrogens can cause development of other tumors in animals, such as tumors of the breast, cervix, vagina, or liver, when given for a long time. At present, there is no satisfactory evidence that women using estrogens in the menopause have an increased risk of such tumors, but there is no way yet to be sure they do not; and one study raises the possibility that use of estrogens in the menopause may increase the risk of breast cancer many years later. This is a further reason to use estrogens only when clearly needed. While you are taking estrogens, it is important that you go to your doctor at least once a year for a physical examination. Also, if members of your family have had breast cancer or if you have breast nodules or abnormal mammograms (breast x-rays), your doctor may wish to carry out more frequent examinations.

3. **Gallbladder disease.** Women who use estrogens after menopause are two or three times more likely to develop gallbladder disease needing surgery than women who do not use estrogens. Birth control pills have a similar effect.

4. **Abnormal blood clotting.** Oral contraceptives increase the risk of blood clotting in various parts of the body. This can occur in different parts of the circulatory system causing thrombophlebitis (clot in the legs or pelvis), retinal thrombosis or optic neuritis (clots affecting vision, including blindness), mesenteric thrombosis (clots in the intestinal blood vessels), stroke (clot in the brain), heart attack (clot in a vessel of the heart) or a pulmonary embolism (clot which eventually lodges in the lungs). These can be fatal.

At this time use of estrogens in the menopause is not known to cause increased blood clotting, this has not been fully studied and there could still prove to be such a risk. It is recommended that if you have had clotting in the legs or lungs or a heart attack or stroke while you were using estrogens or birth control pills, you should not use estrogens (unless they are being used to treat cancer of the breast or prostate). If you have had a stroke or heart attack or if you have angina pectoris, estrogens should be used with great caution and only if clearly needed (for example, if you have severe symptoms of the menopause).

The larger doses of estrogen used to prevent swelling of the breasts after pregnancy have been reported to cause abnormal blood clotting as indicated above.

SPECIAL WARNING ABOUT PREGNANCY

You should not receive estrogen if you are pregnant. If this should occur, there is a greater than usual chance that the developing child will be born with a birth defect, although the possibility remains fairly small. A female child may have an increased risk of developing cancer of the vagina or cervix later in life (in the teens or twenties). Every possible effort should be made to avoid exposure to estrogens during pregnancy. If exposure occurs, see your doctor.

OTHER EFFECTS OF ESTROGENS

In addition to the serious known risks of estrogens described above, estrogens have the following side effects and potential risks which, if occurring, should be discussed promptly with your doctor.

1. **Nausea and vomiting.** The most common side effect of estrogen therapy is nausea. Vomiting is less common.
2. **Effects on breasts.** Estrogens may cause breast tenderness or enlargement and may cause the breasts to secrete a liquid.
3. **Effects on the uterus.** Estrogens may cause benign fibroid tumors of the uterus to get larger. Some women will have menstrual bleeding when estrogens are stopped. But if

the bleeding occurs on days you are still taking estrogens, you should report this to your doctor.

4. **Effects on liver.** Women taking oral contraceptives develop on rare occasions a tumor of the liver which can rupture, bleed into the abdomen, and cause death. So far, these tumors have not been reported in women using estrogens in the menopause, but you should report any swelling or unusual pain or tenderness in the abdomen to your doctor immediately.

Women with a past history of jaundice (yellowing of the skin and white parts of the eyes) may get jaundice again during estrogen use. If this occurs, stop taking estrogens and see your doctor.

5. **Other effects.** Estrogens may cause excess fluid to be retained in the body. This may make some conditions worse, such as epilepsy, migraine, heart disease, or kidney disease. Mental depression or high blood pressure may occur. A spotty darkening of the skin, particularly of the face, is possible and may persist.

SUMMARY

Estrogens have important uses, and they may have serious risks as well. You must decide, with your doctor, whether the risks are acceptable to you in view of the benefits of treatment. Except where your doctor has prescribed estrogens for use in special cases of cancer of the breast or prostate, you should not use estrogens if you have cancer of the breast or uterus, are pregnant, have undiagnosed abnormal vaginal bleeding, clotting in the legs or lungs or have had a stroke, heart attack or angina, or clotting in the legs or lungs in the past while you were taking estrogens.

You can use estrogens as safely as possible by understanding that your doctor will require regular physical examinations while you are taking them and will try to discontinue the drug as soon as possible and use the smallest dose possible. Be alert for signs of trouble including:

1. Abnormal bleeding from the vagina.
2. Pains in the calves or chest or sudden shortness of breath, or coughing blood (indicating possible clots in the legs, heart, or lungs).
3. Severe headache, dizziness, faintness, or changes in vision (indicating possible developing clots in the brain or eye).
4. Breast lumps (you should ask your doctor how to examine your own breasts).
5. Jaundice (yellowing of the skin).
6. Mental depression.

Based on his or her assessment of your medical needs, your doctor has prescribed this drug for you. Do not give the drug to anyone else.

REFERENCES

1. Ziel HK, Finkel WD: Increased risk of endometrial carcinoma among users of conjugated estrogens. New Eng J Med 293:1167–1170, 1975.
2. Smith DC, Prentice R, Thompson DJ, Herrmann WL: Association of exogenous estrogen and endometrial carcinoma. New Eng J Med 293:1164–1167, 1975.
3. Mack TM, Pike MC, Henderson BE, *et al:* Estrogens and endometrial cancer in a retirement community. New Eng J Med 294:1262–1267, 1976.
4. Weiss NS, Szekely DR, Austin DF: Increasing incidence of endometrial cancer in the United States. New Eng J Med 294:1259–1262, 1976.
5. Herbst AL, Ulfelder H, Poskanzer DC: Adenocarcinoma of vagina. New Eng J Med 284:878–881, 1971.
6. Greenwald P, Barlow J, Nasca P, Burnett W: Vaginal cancer after maternal treatment with synthetic estrogens. New Eng J Med 285:390–392, 1971.
7. Lanier A, Noller K, Decker D, *et al:* Cancer and stilbestrol. A follow-up of 1719 persons exposed to estrogens *in utero* and born 1943–1959. Mayo Clin Proceedings 48:793–799, 1973.
8. Herbst A, Kurman R, Scully R: Vaginal and cervical abnormalities after exposure to stilbestrol *in utero.* Obstet and Gynec 40:287–298, 1972.
9. Herbst A, Robboy S, Macdonald G, Scully R: The effects of local progesterone on stilbestrol-associated vaginal adenosis. Am J Obstet Gynec 118:607–615, 1974.
10. Herbst A, Poskanzer D, Robboy S, *et al:* Prenatal exposure to stilbestrol, a prospective comparison of exposed female offspring with unexposed controls. New Eng J Med 292:334–339, 1975.
11. Stafl A, Mattingly R, Foley D, Fetherston W: Clinical diagnosis of vaginal adenosis. Obstet and Gynec 43:118–128, 1974.
12. Sherman AI, Goldrath M, Berlin A, *et al:* Cervical-vaginal adenosis after *in utero* exposure to synthetic estrogens. Obstet Gynec 44:531–545, 1974.
13. Gal I, Kirman B, Stern J: Hormone pregnancy tests and congenital malformation. Nature 216:83, 1967.
14. Levy EP, Cohen A, Fraser FC: Hormone treatment during pregnancy and congenital heart defects. Lancet 1:611, 1973.
15. Nora J, Nora A: Birth defects and oral contraceptives. Lancet 1:941–942, 1973.
16. Janerich DT, Piper JM, Glebatis DM: Oral contraceptives and congenital limb-reduction defects. New Eng J Med 291:697–700, 1974.
17. Yen SSC, Martin PL, Burnier AM, et al: Circulating estradiol, estrone and gonadotropin levels following the administration of orally active 17β-estradiol in postmenopausal women. J Clin Endocrinol Metab 40:518–521, 1975.
18. Boston Collaborative Drug Surveillance Program: Surgically confirmed gallbladder disease, venous thromboembolism and breast tumors in relation to post-menopausal estrogen therapy. New Eng J Med 290:15–19, 1974.
19. Hoover R, Gray LA Sr, Cole P, MacMahon B: Menopausal estrogens and breast cancer. New Eng J Med 295:15–19, 1974.
20. Boston Collaborative Drug Surveillance Program: Oral contraceptives and venous thromboembolic disease, surgically confirmed gallbladder disease, and breast tumors. Lancet 1:1399–1404, 1973.
21. Daniel DG, Campbell H, Turnbull AC: Puerperal thromboembolism and suppression of lactation. Lancet 2:287–289, 1967.
22. The Veterans Administration Cooperative Urological Research Group: Carcinoma of the prostate: treatment comparisons. J Urol 98:516–522, 1967.
23. Bailar JC: Thromboembolism and oestrogen therapy. Lancet 2:560, 1967.
24. Blackard C, Doe R, Mellinger G, Byar D: Incidence of cardiovascular disease and death in patients receiving diethylstilbestrol for carcinoma of the prostate. Cancer 26:249–256, 1970.
25. Royal College of General Practitioners: Oral contraception and thromboembolic disease. J Roy Coll Gen Pract 13:267–279, 1967.
26. Inman WHW, Vessey MP: Investigation of deaths from pulmonary, coronary, and cerebral thrombosis and embolism in women of child-bearing age. Brit M J 2:193–199, 1968.
27. Vessey MP, Doll R: Investigation of relation between use of oral contraceptives and thromboembolic disease. A further report. Brit M J 2:651–657, 1969.
28. Sartwell PE, Masi AT, Arthes FG, *et al:* Thromboembolism and oral contraceptives: an epidemiological case control study. Am J Epidemiol 90:365–380, 1969.
29. Collaborative Group for the Study of Stroke in Young Women: Oral contraception and increased risk of cerebral ischemia or thrombosis. New Eng J Med 288:871–878, 1973.
30. Collaborative Group for the Study of Stroke in Young Women: Oral contraceptives and stroke in young women: Associated risk factors. JAMA 231:718–722, 1975.
31. Mann JI, Inman WHW: Oral contraceptives and death from myocardial infarction. Brit M J 2:245–248, 1975.
32. Mann JI, Vessey MP, Thorogood M, Doll R: Myocardial infarction in young women with special reference to oral contraceptive practice. Brit M J 2:241–245, 1975.
33. Inman WHW, Vessey VP, Westerholm B, Engelund A: Thromboembolic disease and the steroidal content of oral contraceptives. Brit M J 2:203–209, 1970.
34. Stolley PD, Tonascia JA, Tockman MS, *et al:* Thrombosis with low-estrogen oral contraceptives. Am J Epidemiol 102:197–208, 1975.
35. Vessey MP, Doll R, Fairbairn AS, Glober G: Post-operative thromboembolism and the use of the oral contraceptives. Brit M J 3:123–126, 1970.
36. Greene GR, Sartwell PE: Oral contraceptive use in patients with thromboembolism following surgery, trauma or infection. Am J Pub Health 62:680–685, 1972.
37. Rosenberg L, Armstrong MB, Jick H: Myocardial infarction and estrogen therapy in postmenopausal women. New Eng J Med 294:1256–1259, 1976.
38. Coronary Drug Project Research Group: The coronary drug project: initial findings leading to modifications of its research protocol. JAMA 214:1303–1313, 1970.
39. Baum J, Holtz F, Bookstein JJ, Klein EW: Possible association between benign hepatomas and oral contraceptives. Lancet 2:926–928, 1973.
40. Mays ET, Christopherson WM, Mahr MM, Williams HC: Hepatic changes in young women ingesting contraceptive steroids, hepatic hemorrhage and primary hepatic tumors. JAMA 235:730–732, 1976.
41. Edmondson HA, Henderson B, Benton B: Liver cell adenomas associated with the use of oral contraceptives. New Eng J Med 294:470–472, 1976.
42. Pfeffer RI, Van Den Noort S: Estrogen use and stroke risk in postmenopausal women. Am J Epidemiol 103:445–456, 1976.

Shown in Product Identification Section, page 416

ESTRACE® ℞

[ĕs ′trace]

(Estradiol Vaginal Cream 0.01%)

WARNING

1. ESTROGENS HAVE BEEN REPORTED TO INCREASE THE RISK OF ENDOMETRIAL CARCINOMA.

Three independent case control studies have shown an increased risk of endometrial cancer in postmenopausal women exposed to exogenous estrogens for prolonged periods.[1–3] This risk was independent of the other known risk factors for endometrial cancer. These studies are further supported by the finding that incidence rates of endometrial cancer have increased sharply since 1969 in eight different areas of the United States with population-based cancer reporting systems, an increase which may be related to the rapidly expanding use of estrogens during the last decade.[4]

The three case control studies reported that the risk of endometrial cancer in estrogen users was about 4.5 to 13.9 times greater than in nonusers. The risk appears to depend on both duration of treatment[1] and on estrogen dose.[3] In view of these findings, when estrogens are used for the treatment of menopausal symptoms, the lowest dose that will control symptoms should be utilized and medication should be discontinued as soon as possible. When prolonged treatment is medically indicated, the patient should be reassessed on at least a semiannual basis to determine the need for continued therapy. Although the evidence must be considered preliminary, one study suggests that cyclic administration of low doses of estrogen may carry less risk than continuous administration,[3] it therefore appears prudent to utilize such a regimen.

Close clinical surveillance of all women taking estrogens is important. In all cases of undiagnosed persistent or recurring abnormal vaginal bleeding, adequate diagnostic measures should be undertaken to rule out malignancy.

There is no evidence at present that "natural" estrogens are more or less hazardous than "synthetic" estrogens at equiestrogenic doses.

2. ESTROGENS SHOULD NOT BE USED DURING PREGNANCY.

The use of female sex hormones, both estrogens and progestogens, during early pregnancy may seriously damage the offspring. It has been shown that females exposed *in utero* to diethylstilbestrol, a non-steroidal estrogen, have an increased risk of developing in later life a form of vaginal or cervical cancer that is ordinarily extremely rare.[5,6] This risk has been estimated as not greater than 4 per 1,000 exposures.[7] Furthermore, a high percentage of such exposed women (from 30 to 90 percent) have been found to have vaginal adenosis,[9–12] epithelial changes of the vagina and cervix. Although these changes are histologically benign, it is not known whether they are precursors of malignancy. Although similar data are not available with the use of other estrogens, it cannot be presumed they would not induce similar changes.

Several reports suggest an association between intrauterine exposure to female sex hormones and congenital anomalies, including congenital heart defects and limb reduction defects.[13–16] One case control study[16] estimated a 4.7-fold increased risk of limb reduction defects in infants exposed *in utero* to sex hormones (oral contraceptives, hormone withdrawal tests for pregnancy, or attempted treatment for threatened abortion). Some of these exposures were very short and involved only a few days of treatment. The data suggest that the risk of limb reduction defects in exposed fetuses is somewhat less than 1 per 1,000.

In the past, female sex hormones have been used during pregnancy in an attempt to treat threatened or habitual abortion. There is considerable evidence that estrogens are ineffective for these indications, and there is no evidence from well controlled studies that progestogens are effective for these uses.

If Estrace® is used during pregnancy, or if the patient becomes pregnant while taking this drug, she should be apprised of the potential risks to the fetus and the advisability of pregnancy continuation.

DESCRIPTION

Each gram of Estrace® (17β-estradiol) Vaginal Cream contains 0.1 mg 17β-estradiol in a nonliquefying base containing purified water, propylene glycol, stearyl alcohol, white ceresin wax, glyceryl monostearate, hydroxypropyl methylcellulose, 2208 4000 cps, sodium lauryl sulfate, methylparaben, edetate disodium and tertiary-butylhydroquinone. Estradiol is chemically described as estra-1, 3, 5(10)-triene-3, 17β-diol. The structural formula is:

[See Chemical Formula at top of next page].

CLINICAL PHARMACOLOGY

Estrogens are important in the development and maintenance of the female reproductive system and secondary sex characteristics. They promote growth and development of the vagina, uterus, and fallopian tubes, and enlargement of the breasts. Indirectly, they contribute to the shaping of the

Continued on next page

Mead Johnson Labs.—Cont.

skeleton, maintenance of tone and elasticity or urogenital structures, changes in the epiphyses of the long bones that allow for the pubertal growth spurt and its termination, growth of axillary and pubic hair, and pigmentation of the nipples and genitals. Decline of estrogenic activity at the end of the menstrual cycle can bring on menstruation, although the cessation of progesterone secretion is the most important factor in the mature ovulatory cycle. However, in the pre-ovulatory or non-ovulatory cycle, estrogen is the primary determinant in the onset of menstruation. Estrogens also affect the release of pituitary gonadotropins.

Micronized 17β-estradiol achieves its pharmacologic effect in estrogen-responsive target tissues via anabolic stimulus at the cellular level. Micronized 17β-estradiol in Estrace Vaginal Cream is readily absorbed from mucosal surfaces.

In responsive tissues (female genital organs, breasts, hypothalamus, pituitary) estrogens enter the cell and are transported into the nucleus. As a result of estrogen action, specific RNA and protein synthesis occurs.

Metabolism and inactivation occur primarily in the liver. Some estrogens are excreted into the bile; however, they are reabsorbed from the intestine and returned to the liver through the portal venous system. Water-soluble estrogen conjugates are strongly acidic and are ionized in body fluids, which favor excretion through the kidneys since tubular reabsorption is minimal.

INDICATIONS

Estrace Vaginal Cream is indicated in the treatment of atrophic vaginitis and kraurosis vulvae.

ESTRACE® HAS NOT BEEN SHOWN TO BE EFFECTIVE FOR ANY PURPOSE DURING PREGNANCY AND ITS USE MAY CAUSE SEVERE HARM TO THE FETUS (SEE BOXED WARNING).

CONTRAINDICATIONS

Estrogens should not be used in women (or men) with any of the following conditions:

1. Known or suspected cancer of the breast, except in appropriately selected patients being treated for metastatic disease.
2. Known or suspected estrogen-dependent neoplasia.
3. Known or suspected pregnancy (See Boxed Warning).
4. Undiagnosed abnormal genital bleeding.
5. Active thrombophlebitis or thromboembolic disorders.
6. A past history of thrombophlebitis, thrombosis or thromboembolic disorders associated with previous estrogen use (except when used in treatment of breast or prostatic malignancy).

WARNINGS

1. **Induction of malignant neoplasms.** Long-term continuous administration of natural and synthetic estrogens in certain animal species increases the frequency of carcinomas of the breast, cervix, vagina, and liver. There is now evidence that estrogens increase the risk of carcinoma of the endometrium in humans. (See Boxed Warning).

At the present time there is no satisfactory evidence that estrogens given to postmenopausal women increase the risk of cancer of the breast,[17] although a recent long-term follow-up of a single physician's practice has raised this possibility.[18] Because of the animal data there is a need for caution in prescribing estrogens for women with a strong family history of breast cancer or who have breast nodules, fibrocystic disease, or abnormal mammograms.

2. **Gallbladder disease.** A recent study has reported a 2- to 3-fold increase in the risk of surgically confirmed gallbladder disease in women receiving postmenopausal estrogens,[17] similar to the 2-fold increase previously noted in users of oral contraceptives.[18,24a]

3. **Effects similar to those caused by estrogen-progestogen oral contraceptives.** There are several serious adverse effects of oral contraceptives, most of which have not, up to now, been documented as consequences of postmenopausal estrogen therapy. This may reflect the comparatively low doses of estrogen used in postmenopausal women. It would be expected that the larger doses of estrogen used to treat prostatic or breast cancer or postpartum breast engorgement are more likely to result in these adverse effects, and, in fact, it has been shown that there is an increased risk of thrombosis in men receiving estrogens for prostatic cancer and women for postpartum breast engorgement.[20-23]

a. **Thromboembolic disease.** It is now well established that users of oral contraceptives have an increased risk of various thromboembolic and thrombotic vascular diseases, such as thrombophlebitis, pulmonary embolism, stroke, and myocardial infarction.[24-31] Cases of retinal thrombosis, mesenteric thrombosis, and optic neuritis have been reported in oral contraceptive users. There is evidence that the risk of several of these adverse reactions is related to the dose of the drug.[32,33] An increased risk of post-surgery thromboembolic complications has also been reported in users of oral contraceptives.[34,35] If feasible, estrogen should be discontinued at least 4 weeks before surgery of the type associated with an increased risk of thromboembolism, or during periods of prolonged immobilization.

While an increased rate of thromboembolic and thrombotic disease in postmenopausal users of estrogens has not been found,[17-36] this does not rule out the possibility that such an increase may be present or that subgroups of women who have underlying risk factors or who are receiving relatively large doses of estrogens may have increased risk. Therefore, estrogens should not be used in persons with active thrombophlebitis or thromboembolic disorders, and they should not be used (except in treatment of malignancy) in persons with a history of such disorders in association with estrogen use. They should be used with caution in patients with cerebral vascular or coronary artery disease and only for those in whom estrogens are clearly needed.

Large doses of estrogen (5 mg conjugated estrogens per day), comparable to those used to treat cancer of the prostate and breast, have been shown in a large prospective clinical trial in men[37] to increase the risk of nonfatal myocardial infarction, pulmonary embolism and thrombophlebitis. When estrogen doses of this size are used, any of the thromboembolic and thrombotic adverse effects associated with oral contraceptive use should be considered a clear risk.

b. **Hepatic adenoma.** Hepatic adenomas appear to be associated with the use of oral contraceptives.[38-40] Although rare, these may rupture and may cause death through intraabdominal hemorrhage. Such lesions have not yet been reported in association with other estrogen or progestogen preparations but should be considered in estrogen users having abdominal pain and tenderness, abdominal mass, or hypovolemic shock. Hepatocellular carcinoma has also been reported in women taking estrogen-containing oral contraceptives.[36] The relationship of this malignancy to these drugs is not known at this time.

c. **Elevated blood pressure.** Increased blood pressure is not uncommon in women using oral contraceptives. There is now a report that this may occur with use of estrogens in the menopause[41] and blood pressure should be monitored with estrogen use, especially if high doses are used.

d. **Glucose tolerance.** A worsening of glucose tolerance has been observed in a significant percentage of patients on estrogen-containing oral contraceptives. For this reason, diabetic patients should be carefully observed while receiving estrogen.

4. **Hypercalcemia.** Administration of estrogens may lead to severe hypercalcemia in patients with breast cancer and bone metastases. If this occurs, the drug should be stopped and appropriate measures taken to reduce the serum calcium level.

PRECAUTIONS

A. General Precautions.

1. A complete medical and family history should be taken prior to the initiation of any estrogen therapy. The pretreatment and periodic physical examinations should include special reference to blood pressure, breasts, abdomen, and pelvic organs, and should include a Papanicolaou smear. As a general rule, estrogen should not be prescribed for longer than one year without another physical examination being performed.
2. Fluid retention — Because estrogens may cause some degree of fluid retention, conditions which might be influenced by this factor such as epilepsy, migraine, and cardiac or renal dysfunction, require careful observation.
3. Certain patients may develop undesirable manifestations of excessive estrogenic stimulation, such as abnormal or excessive uterine bleeding, mastodynia, etc.
4. Oral contraceptives appear to be associated with an increased incidence of mental depression.[24a] Although it is not clear whether this is due to the estrogenic or progestogenic component of the contraceptive, patients with a history of depression should be carefully observed.
5. Pre-existing uterine leiomyomata may increase in size during estrogen use.
6. The pathologist should be advised of estrogen therapy when relevant specimens are submitted.
7. Patients with a past history of jaundice during pregnancy have an increased risk of recurrence of jaundice while receiving estrogen-containing oral contraceptive therapy. If jaundice develops in any patient receiving estrogen, the medication should be discontinued while the cause is investigated.
8. Estrogens may be poorly metabolized in patients with impaired liver function and they should be administered with caution in such patients.
9. Because estrogens influence the metabolism of calcium and phosphorus, they should be used with caution in patients with metabolic bone diseases that are associated with hypercalcemia or in patients with renal insufficiency.
10. Because of the effects of estrogens on epiphyseal closure, they should be used judiciously in young patients in whom bone growth is not complete.
11. Certain endocrine and liver function tests may be affected by estrogen-containing oral contraceptives. The following similar changes may be expected with larger doses of estrogen:

a. Increased sulfobromophthalein retention.
b. Increased prothrombin and factors VII and VIII, IX, and X; decreased antithyrombin 3; increased norepinephrine-induced platelet aggregability.
c. Increased thyroid binding globulin (TBG) leading to increased circulating total thyroid hormone, as measured by PBI, T4 by volume, or T4 by radioimmunoassay, free T3 resin uptake is decreased, reflecting the elevated TBG; free T4 concentration is unaltered.
d. Impaired glucose tolerance.
e. Decreased pregnanediol excretion.
f. Reduced response to metyrapone test.
g. Reduced serum folate concentration.
h. Increased serum triglyceride and phospholipid concentration.

B. Information for the Patient. See text which appears after the physician References.

C. Pregnancy Category X. See Contraindications and Boxed Warning.

D. Nursing Mothers. As a general principle, the administration of any drug to nursing mothers should be done only when clearly necessary since many drugs are excreted in human milk.

ADVERSE REACTIONS

(See Warnings regarding induction of neoplasia, adverse effects on the fetus, increased incidence of gall bladder disease, and adverse effects similar to those of oral contraceptives, including thromboembolism.) The following additional adverse reactions have been reported with estrogenic therapy, including oral contraceptives:

1. **Genitourinary system.**
   Breakthrough bleeding, spotting, change in menstrual flow.
   Dysmenorrhea.
   Premenstrual-like syndrome.
   Amenorrhea during and after treatment.
   Increase in size of uterine fibromyomata.
   Vaginal candidiasis.
   Change in cervical eversion and in degree of cervical secretion.
   Cystitis-like syndrome.
2. **Breast.**
   Tenderness, enlargement, secretion.
3. **Gastrointestinal.**
   Nausea, vomiting.
   Abdominal cramps, bloating.
   Cholestatic jaundice.
4. **Skin.**
   Chloasma or melasma which may persist when drug is discontinued.
   Erythema multiforme
   Hemorrhagic eruption
   Hirsutism
   Erythema nodosum
   Loss of scalp hair
5. **Eyes.**
   Steepening of corneal curvature.
   Intolerance to contact lenses.
6. **CNS.**
   Headache, migraine, dizziness.
   Mental depression.
   Chorea.
7. **Miscellaneous.**
   Increase or decrease in weight.
   Reduced carbohydrate tolerance.
   Aggravation of porphyria.
   Edema.
   Changes in libido.

OVERDOSAGE

Numerous reports of ingestion of large doses of estrogen-containing oral contraceptives by young children indicate that serious ill effects do not occur. Overdosage of estrogen may cause nausea, and withdrawal bleeding may occur in females.

DOSAGE AND ADMINISTRATION

Given cyclically for short term use only.

For treatment of atrophic vaginitis or kraurosis vulvae.

The lowest dose that will control symptoms should be chosen and medication should be discontinued as promptly as possible. Administration should be cyclic (e.g., 3 weeks on and 1 week off).

Attempts to discontinue or taper medication should be made at 3 to 6 month intervals.

Usual Dosage: The usual dosage range is 2 to 4 g (marked on the applicator) daily for one or two weeks, then gradually reduced to one half initial dosage for a similar period. A maintenance dosage of 1 g. one to three times a week, may be used after restoration of the vaginal mucosa has been achieved.

Patients with an intact uterus should be monitored closely for signs of endometrial cancer and appropriate diagnostic measures should be taken to rule out malignancy in eventual persistent or recurring abnormal vaginal bleeding.

HOW SUPPLIED

Estrace (estradiol) Vaginal Cream.

NDC 0087-0754-42 42.5 g Tube with applicator.

INFORMATION FOR THE PATIENT

WHAT YOU SHOULD KNOW ABOUT ESTROGENS

Estrogens are female hormones produced principally by the ovaries. The ovaries make several different kinds of estrogens. In addition, scientists have been able to make a variety of synthetic estrogens. As far as we know, all these estrogens have the same properties and therefore much the same usefulness, side effects, and risks. This leaflet is intended to help you understand what estrogens are used for, the risks involved in their use, and how to use them as safely as possible. This leaflet includes important information about Estrace® (estradiol) and estrogens in general, but not all the information. If you want to know more, you can ask your doctor or pharmacist to let you read the professional package insert.

USES OF ESTROGEN

Estrogens are prescribed by doctors for a number of purposes, including:

1. To provide estrogen during a period of adjustment when a woman's ovaries no longer produce it, in order to prevent certain uncomfortable symptoms of estrogen deficiency. (All women normally experience a decrease in the production of estrogens, generally between 45–55; this is called the menopause).
2. To prevent symptoms of estrogen deficiency when a woman's ovaries have been removed surgically before the natural menopause.
3. To prevent pregnancy. (Some estrogens are given along with a progestogen, another female hormone; these combinations are called oral contraceptives or birth control pills. They will not be discussed in this leaflet.) However, Estrace is not intended for this use.
4. To treat certain cancers in women and men.
5. To prevent painful swelling of the breasts after pregnancy in women who choose not to nurse their babies.

THERE IS NO PROPER USE OF ESTROGENS IN A PREGNANT WOMAN.

ESTROGENS IN THE MENOPAUSE

In the natural course of their lives, all women eventually experience a decrease in estrogen production. This usually occurs between ages 45 and 55 but may occur earlier or later. Sometimes the ovaries may need to be removed before natural menopause by an operation, producing a "surgical menopause."

When the amount of estrogen in the blood begins to decrease, many women may develop typical symptoms: feelings of warmth in the face, neck, and chest or sudden intense episodes of heat and sweating throughout the body (called "hot flashes" or "hot flushes"). These symptoms are sometimes very uncomfortable. A few women eventually develop changes in the vagina (called "atrophic vaginitis") which cause discomfort, especially during and after intercourse.

Estrogens can be prescribed to treat these symptoms of the menopause. It is estimated that considerably more than half of all women undergoing the menopause have only mild symptoms or no symptoms at all and therefore do not need estrogens. Other women may need estrogens for a few months, while their bodies adjust to lower estrogen levels. Sometimes the need will be for periods longer than six months. In an attempt to avoid over-stimulation of the uterus (womb), estrogens are usually given cyclically during each month of use, that is three weeks of therapy followed by one week without therapy.

Sometimes women experience nervous symptoms or depression during menopause. There is no evidence that estrogens are effective for such symptoms and they should not be used to treat them, although other treatment may be needed.

You may have heard that taking estrogens for long periods (years) after the menopause will keep your skin soft and supple and keep you feeling young. There is no evidence that this is so, however, and such long-term treatment carries additional risks.

ESTROGENS TO PREVENT SWELLING OF THE BREASTS AFTER PREGNANCY

If you do not breast feed your baby after delivery, your breasts may fill up with milk and become painful and engorged. This usually begins about three to four days after delivery and may last for a few days to up to a week or more. Sometimes the discomfort is severe, but usually it is not and can be controlled by pain-relieving drugs such as aspirin and by binding the breasts up tightly. Estrogens can sometimes be used successfully to try to prevent the breasts from filling up. While this treatment is sometimes successful, in many cases the breasts fill up to some degree in spite of treatment. The dose of estrogens needed to prevent pain and swelling of the breasts is much larger than the dose needed to treat symptoms of the menopause and this may increase your chances of developing blood clots in the legs or lungs or other parts of the body (see below, 4. **Abnormal Blood Clotting**). Therefore, it is important that you discuss the benefits and the risks of estrogen use with your doctor, before using estrogen, if you have decided not to breast feed your baby.

THE DANGERS OF ESTROGENS

1. **Cancer of the uterus.** If estrogens are used in the postmenopausal period for more than a year, there is an increased risk of cancer of the endometrium (uterine lining). Women taking estrogens have roughly 5 to 15 times as great a chance of getting this cancer as women who take no estrogens. To put this another way, while a postmenopausal woman not taking estrogens has one chance in 1,000 each year of getting cancer of the uterus, a woman taking estrogens has 5 to 15 chances in 1,000 each year. For this reason **it is important to take estrogens only when you really need them.**

   The risk of this cancer is greater the longer estrogens are used and also seems to be greater when larger doses are taken. For this reason **it is important to take the lowest dose of estrogen that will control symptoms and to take it only as long as it is needed.** If estrogens are needed for longer periods of time, your doctor will want to reevaluate your need for estrogens at least every six months.

   Women using estrogens should report any irregular vaginal bleeding to their doctors; such bleeding may be of no importance, but it can be an early warning of cancer of the uterus. If you have undiagnosed vaginal bleeding, you should not use estrogens until a diagnosis is made and you are certain there is no cancer of the uterus.

   NOTE: If you have had your uterus completely removed (total hysterectomy), there is no danger of developing cancer of the uterus.
2. **Other possible cancers.** Estrogens can cause development of other tumors in animals, such as tumors of the breast, cervix, vagina, or liver, when given for a long time. At present, there is no satisfactory evidence that women using estrogens in the menopause have an increased risk of such tumors, but there is no way yet to be sure they do not; and one study raises the possibility that use of estrogens in the menopause may increase the risk of breast cancer many years later. This is a further reason to use estrogens only when clearly needed. While you are taking estrogens, it is important that you go to your doctor at least once a year for a physical examination. Also, if members of your family have had breast cancer or if you have breast nodules or abnormal mammograms (breast x-rays), your doctor may wish to carry out more frequent examinations.
3. **Gallbladder disease.** Women who use estrogens after menopause are two or three times more likely to develop gallbladder disease needing surgery than women who do not use estrogens. Birth control pills have a similar effect.
4. **Abnormal blood clotting.** Oral contraceptives increase the risk of blood clotting in various parts of the body. This can occur in different parts of the circulatory system causing thrombophlebitis (clot in the legs or pelvis), retinal thrombosis or optic neuritis (clots affecting vision, including blindness), mesenteric thrombosis (clots in the intestinal blood vessels), stroke (clot in the brain), heart attack (clot in a vessel of the heart) or a pulmonary embolism (clot which eventually lodges in the lungs). These can be fatal.

   At this time, use of estrogens in the menopause is not known to cause increased blood clotting; this has not been fully studied and there could still prove to be such a risk. It is recommended that if you have had clotting in the legs or lungs or a heart attack or stroke while you were using estrogens or birth control pills, you should not use estrogens (unless they are being used to treat cancer of the breast or prostate). If you have had a stroke or heart attack or if you have angina pectoris, estrogens should be used with great caution and only if clearly needed (for example, if you have severe symptoms of the menopause). The larger doses of estrogen used to prevent swelling of the breasts after pregnancy have been reported to cause abnormal blood clotting as indicated above.

SPECIAL WARNING ABOUT PREGNANCY

You should not receive estrogen if you are pregnant. If this should occur, there is a greater than usual chance that the developing child will be born with a birth defect, although the possibility remains fairly small. A female child may have an increased risk of developing cancer of the vagina or cervix later in life (in the teens or twenties). Every possible effort should be made to avoid exposure to estrogens during pregnancy. If exposure occurs, see your doctor.

OTHER EFFECTS OF ESTROGENS

In addition to the serious known risks of estrogens described above, estrogens have the following side effects and potential risks which, if occurring, should be discussed promptly with your doctor.

1. **Nausea and vomiting.** The most common side effect of estrogen therapy is nausea. Vomiting is less common.
2. **Effects on breasts.** Estrogens may cause breast tenderness or enlargement and may cause the breasts to secrete a liquid.
3. **Effects on the uterus.** Estrogens may cause benign fibroid tumors of the uterus to get larger. Some women will have menstrual bleeding when estrogens are stopped. But if the bleeding occurs on days you are still taking estrogens, you should report this to your doctor.
4. **Effects on liver.** Women taking oral contraceptives develop on rare occasions a tumor of the liver which can rupture, bleed into the abdomen, and cause death. So far, these tumors have not been reported in women using estrogens in the menopause, but you should report any swelling or unusual pain or tenderness in the abdomen to your doctor immediately.

   Women with a past history of jaundice (yellowing of the skin and white parts of the eyes) may get jaundice again during estrogen use. If this occurs, stop taking estrogens and see your doctor.
5. **Other effects.** Estrogens may cause excess fluid to be retained in the body. This may make some conditions worse, such as epilepsy, migraine, heart disease, or kidney disease. Mental depression or high blood pressure may occur. A spotty darkening of the skin, particularly of the face, is possible and may persist.

SUMMARY

Estrogens have important uses, and they may have serious risks as well. You must decide, with your doctor, whether the risks are acceptable to you in view of the benefits of treatment. Except where your doctor has prescribed estrogens for use in special cases of cancer of the breast or prostate, you should not use estrogens if you have cancer of the breast or uterus, are pregnant, have undiagnosed abnormal vaginal bleeding, clotting in the legs or lungs or have had a stroke, heart attack or angina, or clotting in the legs or lungs in the past while you were taking estrogens.

You can use estrogens as safely as possible by understanding that your doctor will require regular physical examinations while you are taking them and will try to discontinue the drug as soon as possible and use the smallest dose possible. Be alert for signs of trouble including:

1. Abnormal bleeding from the vagina.
2. Pains in the calves or chest or sudden shortness of breath, or coughing blood (indicating possible clots in the legs, heart, or lungs).
3. Severe headache, dizziness, faintness, or changes in vision (indicating possible developing clots in the brain or eye).
4. Breast lumps (you should ask your doctor how to examine your own breasts).
5. Jaundice (yellowing of the skin).
6. Mental depression.

Your doctor has prescribed this drug for you. Do not give this drug to anyone else.

REFERENCES

1. Ziel HK, Finkel WD: Increased risk of endometrial carcinoma among users of conjugated estrogens. New Eng J Med 293:1167–1170, 1975.

2. Smith, DC, Prentice R, Thompson DJ, Herrmann WL: Association of exogenous estrogen and endometrial carcinoma. New Eng J Med 293:1164–1167, 1975.

3. Mack TM, Pike MC, Henderson BE, *et al:* Estrogens and the endometrial cancer in a retirement community. New Eng J Med 294:1262–1267, 1976.

4. Weiss, NS, Szekely DR, Austin DF: Increasing incidence of endometrial cancer in the United States. New Eng J Med 294:1259–1262, 1976.

5. Herbst AL, Ulfelder H, Poskanzer DC: Adenocarcinoma of vagina. New Eng J Med 284:878–881, 1971.

6. Greenwald P, Barlow J, Nasca P, Burnett W: Vaginal cancer after maternal treatment with synthetic estrogens. New Eng J Med 285:390–392, 1971.

7. Lanier A, Noller K, Decker D, *et al:* Cancer and stilbestrol. A follow-up of 1719 persons exposed to estrogens *in utero* and born 1943–1959. Mayo Clin Proceedings 48:793–799, 1973.

8. Herbst A, Kurman R, Scully R: Vaginal and cervical abnormalities after exposure to stilbestrol *in utero.* Obstet and Gynec 40:287–298, 1972.

9. Herbst A, Robboy S, MacDonald G, Scully R: The effects of local progesterone on stilbestrol-associated vaginal adenosis. Am J Obstet Gynec 118:607–615, 1974.

10. Herbst A, Poskanzer D, Robboy S, *et al:* Prenatal exposure to stilbestrol, a prospective comparison of exposed fe-

Continued on next page

Mead Johnson Labs.—Cont.

male offspring with unexposed controls. New Eng J Med 292:334–339, 1975.
11. Stafl A, Mattingly R, Foley D, Fetherston W: Clinical diagnosis of vaginal adenosis. Obstet and Gynec 43:118–128, 1974.
12. Sherman Al, Goldrath M, Berlin A, *et al:* Cervical-vaginal adenosis after *in utero* exposure to synthetic estrogens. Obstet Gynec 44:531–545, 1974.
13. Gal I, Kirman B, Stern J: Hormone pregnancy tests and congenital malformation. Nature 216:83, 1967.
14. Levy EP, Cohen A, Fraser FC: Hormone treatment during pregnancy and congenital heart defects. Lancet 1:611, 1973.
15. Nora J, Nora A: Birth defects and oral contraceptives. Lancet 1:941–942, 1973.
16. Janerich DT, Piper JM, Glebatis DM: Oral contraceptives and congenital limb-reduction defects. New Engl J Med 291:697–700, 1974.
17. Boston Collaborative Drug Surveillance Program: Surgically confirmed gallbladder disease, venous thromboembolism and breast tumors in relation to post-menopausal estrogen therapy. New Eng J Med 290:15–19, 1974.
18. Hoover R, Gray LA Sr, Cole P, MacMahon B: Menopausal estrogens and breast cancer. New Eng J Med 295:15–19, 1974.
19. Boston Collaborative Drug Surveillance Program: Oral contraceptives and venous thromboembolic disease, surgically confirmed gall bladder disease, and breast tumors. Lancet 1:1399–1404, 1973.
20. Daniel DG, Campbell H, Turnbull AC: Puerperal thromboembolism and suppression of lactation. Lancet 2:287–289, 1967.
21. The Veterans Administration Cooperative Urological Research Group: Carcinoma of the prostate; treatment comparisons. J Urol 98:516–522, 1967.
22. Bailar JC: Thromboembolism and oestrogen therapy. Lancet 2:560, 1967.
23. Blackard C, Doe R, Mellinger G, Byar D: Incidence of cardiovascular disease and death in patients receiving diethylstilbestrol for carcinoma of the prostate. Cancer 26:249–256, 1970.
24. Royal College of General Practitioners: Oral contraception and thromboembolic disease. J Roy Coll Gen Pract 13:267–279, 1967.
24a. Royal College of General Practitioners: Oral Contraceptives and Health, New York, Pitman Corp, 1974.
25. Inman WHW, Vessey MP: Investigation of deaths from pulmonary, coronary, and cerebral thrombosis and embolism in women of childbearing age. Brit M J 2:193–199, 1968.
26. Vessey MP, Doll R: Investigation of relation between use of oral contraceptives and thromboembolic disease. A further report. Brit M J 2:651–657, 1969.
27. Sartwell PE, Masi AT, Arthes FG, *et al:* Thromboembolism and oral contraceptives: an epidemiological case control study. Am J Epidemiol 90:365–380, 1969.
28. Collaborative Group for the Study of Stroke in Young Women: Oral contraception and increased risk of cerebral ischemia or thrombosis. New Eng J Med 288:871–878, 1973.
29. Collaborative Group for the Study of Stroke in Young Women: Oral contraceptives and stroke in young women: Associated risk factors. JAMA 231:718–722, 1975.
30. Mann JI, Inman WHW: Oral contraceptives and death from myocardial infarction. Brit M J 2:245–248, 1975.
31. Mann JI, Vessey MP, Thorogood M, Doll R: Myocardial infarction in young women with special reference to oral contraceptive practice. Brit M J 2:241–245, 1975.
32. Inman WHW, Vessey MP, Westerholm B, Engelund A: Thromboembolic disease and the steroidal content of oral contraceptives. Brit M J 2:203–209, 1970.
33. Stolley PD, Tonascia JA, Tockman MS, *et al:* Thrombosis with low-estrogen oral contraceptives. Am J Epidemiol 102:197–208, 1975.
34. Vessey MP, Doll R, Fairbairn AS, Glober G: Post-operative thromboembolism and the use of the oral contraceptives. Brit M J 3:123–126, 1970.
35. Greene GR, Sartwell PE: Oral contraceptive use in patients with thromboembolism following surgery, trauma or infection. Am J Pub Health 62:680–685, 1972.
36. Rosenberg L, Armstrong MB, Jick H: Myocardial infarction and estrogen therapy in postmenopausal women. New Eng J Med 294:1256–1259, 1976.
37. Coronary Drug Project Research Group: The coronary drug project: initial findings leading to modifications of its research protocol. JAMA 214:1303–1313, 1970.
38. Baum J, Holtz F, Bookstein JJ, Klein EW: Possible association between benign hepatomas and oral contraceptives. Lancet 2:926–928, 1973.
39. Mays ET, Christopherson WM, Mahr MM, Williams HC: Hepatic changes in young women ingesting contraceptive steroids, hepatic hemorrhage and primary hepatic tumors. JAMA 235:730–732, 1976.
40. Edmondson HA, Henderson B, Benton B: Liver cell adenomas associated with the use of oral contraceptives. New Eng J Med 294:470–472, 1976.
41. Pfeffer RI, Van Den Noort S: Estrogen use and stroke risk in postmenopausal women. Am J Epidemiol 103:445–456, 1976.

Shown in Product Identification Section, page 416

K-LYTE® ℞
[k' līt]
Effervescent Tablets

Each tablet in solution provides 25 mEq (978 mg) potassium as bicarbonate and citrate.

K-LYTE® DS ℞
Effervescent Tablets
Each tablet in solution provides 50 mEq (1955 mg) potassium as bicarbonate and citrate.

K-LYTE/CL® ℞
Effervescent Tablets and Powder
Each tablet in solution and each dose of powder in solution provide the equivalent of 25 mEq (1865 mg) potassium chloride.

K-LYTE/CL® 50 ℞
Effervescent Tablets
Each tablet in solution provides the equivalent of 50 mEq (3730 mg) potassium chloride.

DESCRIPTION

[See table below].

Inactive Ingredients: All of the K-Lyte line effervescent tablets contain docusate sodium, natural and/or artificial flavors, light mineral oil, saccharin and talc.

K-Lyte® and K-Lyte® DS lime tablets, and K-Lyte/Cl® and K-Lyte/Cl® 50 citrus tablets have D&C Yellow No. 10. K-Lyte® and K-Lyte® DS orange tablets and K-Lyte/Cl® and K-Lyte/Cl® 50 fruit punch tablets have FD&C Yellow No. 6. K-Lyte orange and lime tablets have dextrose, and K-Lyte DS orange and lime tablets have lactose.

K-Lyte/Cl® powder contains the following inactive ingredients: adipic acid, FD&C Red No. 40, FD&C Yellow No. 6 (aluminum lake), flavors (natural and artificial), saccharin calcium, and sucrose.

Note: This listing of inactive ingredients is a voluntary action of Pharmaceutical Manufacturers Association members.

CLINICAL PHARMACOLOGY

Potassium ion is the principal intracellular cation of most body tissues and participates in a number of essential physiological processes. These include numerous enzymatic reactions in intermediary metabolism, the maintenance of intracellular tonicity, the transmission of nerve impulses, and the function of cardiac, skeletal, and smooth muscle. Disturbances in potassium metabolism may, therefore, elicit a broad range of clinical disorders. The normal serum potassium level is maintained principally by close renal regulation of potassium balance.

Potassium depletion may occur whenever potassium loss through renal excretion and/or loss from the gastrointestinal tract exceeds the potassium intake. Such depletion usually develops slowly as a consequence of prolonged therapy with oral diuretics, primary or secondary hyperaldosteronism, diabetic ketoacidosis, severe vomiting and diarrhea, or inadequate replacement of potassium in patients on prolonged parenteral nutrition. Potassium depletion may be accompanied by hypokalemia as well as hypochloremia and metabolic alkalosis.

Potassium deficiency may be manifested by generalized weakness, drowsiness, anorexia, and nausea; oliguria, edema, and chronic ileus with distention; shallow and infrequent respirations; low blood pressure, altered cardiac rhythms, and systolic murmurs; hypokalemia and such ECG changes as prominent U wave, lengthening of the Q-T interval, depression of the S-T segment, and depression or inversion of the T wave.

INDICATIONS AND USAGE

All K-LYTE® products are used for therapy or prophylaxis of potassium deficiency. They are useful when thiazide diuretics, corticosteroids, or vomiting and diarrhea cause excessive potassium loss; and when dietary potassium is low. These products may also be useful when potassium therapy is indicated in digitalis intoxication. K-LYTE/Cl and K-LYTE/Cl 50 are recommended in the management of hypokalemia accompanied by metabolic alkalosis and hypochloremia, e.g. as induced by vomiting.

CONTRAINDICATIONS

Potassium supplements are contraindicated in patients with hyperkalemia since a further increase in serum potassium concentration in such patients can produce cardiac arrest. Hyperkalemia may complicate any of the following conditions: chronic renal impairment, metabolic acidosis such as diabetic acidosis, acute dehydration, extensive tissue breakdown as in severe burns or adrenal insufficiency. Hypokalemia should not be treated by the concomitant administration of potassium salts and a potassium-sparing diuretic (e.g., spironolactone or triamterene), since the simultaneous administration of these agents can produce severe hyperkalemia.

WARNINGS

In patients with impaired mechanisms for excreting potassium, the administration of potassium salts can produce hyperkalemia and cardiac arrest. This occurs most commonly in patients given potassium by the intravenous route but may also occur in patients given potassium orally. Potentially fatal hyperkalemia can develop rapidly and may be asymptomatic. The use of potassium salts in patients with chronic renal disease, or any other condition which impairs potassium excretion, requires particularly careful monitoring of the serum potassium concentration and appropriate dosage adjustment.

PRECAUTIONS

General precautions—The diagnosis of potassium depletion is ordinarily made by demonstrating hypokalemia in a patient with a clinical history suggesting some cause for potassium depletion. When interpreting the serum potassium level, the physician should bear in mind that acute alkalosis *per se* can produce hypokalemia in the absence of a deficit in total body potassium, while acute acidosis *per se* can increase the serum potassium concentration into the normal range even in the presence of a reduced total body potassium. Therefore, the treatment of potassium depletion requires careful attention to acid-base balance and appropriate monitoring of serum electrolytes, the ECG, and the clinical status of the patient.

Information for patients—To minimize the possibility of gastrointestinal irritation associated with the oral ingestion of concentrated potassium salt preparations, patients should be carefully directed to dissolve each dose completely in the stated amount of water.

Laboratory tests—Frequent clinical evaluation of the patient should include ECG and serum potassium determinations.

Drug interactions—The simultaneous administration of potassium supplements and a potassium-sparing diuretic can produce severe hyperkalemia (see Contraindications). Potassium supplements should be used cautiously in patients who are using salt substitutes because most of the latter contain substantial amounts of potassium. Such concomitant use could result in hyperkalemia.

Usage in Pregnancy—Pregnancy Category C —Animal reproduction studies have not been conducted with any of the K-LYTE products. It is also not known whether these products can cause fetal harm when administered to a pregnant woman or can affect reproduction capacity. They should be given to a pregnant woman only if clearly needed.

Nursing Mothers—Many drugs are excreted in human milk and because of the potential for serious adverse reactions in nursing infants from oral potassium supplements, a decision

	K-LYTE	K-LYTE DS	K-LYTE/CL	K-LYTE/CL POWDER	K-LYTE/CL 50
Potassium Chloride	—	—	1.5 gm	1.86 gm	2.24 gm
Potassium Bicarbonate	2.5 gm	2.5 gm	0.5 gm	—	2.0 gm
Potassium Citrate	—	2.7 gm	—	—	—
L-lysine Monohydrochloride	—	—	0.91 gm	—	3.65 gm
Citric Acid	2.1 gm	2.1 gm	0.55 gm	—	1.0 gm

should be made whether to discontinue nursing or discontinue the drug, taking into account the importance of the drug to the mother.

Usage in Children—Safety and effectiveness in children have not been established.

ADVERSE REACTIONS

The most common adverse reactions to oral potassium supplements are nausea, vomiting, diarrhea and abdominal discomfort. These side effects occur more frequently when the medication is not taken with food or is not diluted properly or dissolved completely.

Hyperkalemia occurs only rarely in patients with normal renal function receiving potassium supplements orally. Signs and symptoms of hyperkalemia are cardiac arrhythmias, mental confusion, unexplained anxiety, numbness or tingling in hands, feet or lips, shortness of breath or difficult breathing, unusual tiredness or weakness and weakness or heaviness of legs (see Contraindications, Warnings and Overdosage).

OVERDOSAGE

The administration of oral potassium salts to persons with normal renal function rarely causes serious hyperkalemia. However, in patients with chronic renal disease, or any other condition which impairs potassium excretion or if potassium is administered too rapidly intravenously, potentially fatal hyperkalemia can result (see Contraindications and Warnings). The earliest clinical manifestations of this condition may be only increased serum potassium levels and characteristic ECG changes such as peaking of T-waves, loss of P-wave, depression of S-T segment and prolongation of the QT interval. These changes in the ECG usually appear when serum potassium concentration reaches 7 to 8 mEq per liter. Other clinical manifestations occurring at a concentration of 9 to 10 mEq per liter may include muscle paralysis and death from cardiac arrest.

The treatment of severe hyperkalemia should focus on reducing the serum potassium concentration by promoting the transfer of potassium from the extracellular to the intracellular space. The measures taken may include the following: a) intravenous administration of 1 liter of a 10 percent glucose solution containing 30-40 units of insulin; b) in the acidotic patient, intravenous administration of 150 mEq to 300 mEq of sodium bicarbonate. Other measures should include the elimination of potassium-containing medications and potassium-sparing diuretics and frequently the oral administration of a cation exchange resin (such as sodium polystyrene sulfonate) to remove gastrointestinal potassium. To assure rapid movement of the resin through the gastrointestinal tract, a nonabsorbable polyhydric alcohol (e.g., sorbitol) should be given in quantities sufficient to induce a soft to semiliquid bowel movement every few hours.

Hemodialysis is an effective alternative means of removing excess potassium.

DOSAGE AND ADMINISTRATION

Adults—One (1) K-LYTE/Cl 50 tablet (50 mEq potassium and chloride) or K-LYTE DS tablet (50 mEq potassium) completely dissolved in 6 to 8 ounces of cold or ice water, 1 to 2 times daily, depending on the requirements of the patient. One (1) K-LYTE/Cl tablet (25 mEq potassium and chloride) or one (1) K-LYTE tablet (25 mEq potassium) completely dissolved in 3 to 4 ounces of cold or ice water, 2 to 4 times daily, depending on the requirements of the patient. One dose (25 mEq potassium chloride) of K-LYTE/Cl powder completely dissolved in 6 ounces of cold or ice water, 2 to 4 times daily, depending on the requirements of the patient.

Note: It is suggested that all K-LYTE products be taken with meals and sipped slowly over a 5 to 10 minute period.

HOW SUPPLIED

K-LYTE® Effervescent Tablets. Each tablet in solution provides 25 mEq (978 mg) potassium.

NDC 0087-0760-01 Lime flavor, Boxes of 30
NDC 0087-0760-43 Lime flavor, Boxes of 100
NDC 0087-0760-02 Lime flavor, Boxes of 250
NDC 0087-0761-01 Orange flavor, Boxes of 30
NDC 0087-0761-43 Orange flavor, Boxes of 100
NDC 0087-0761-02 Orange flavor, Boxes of 250
VA 6505-00-934-3477 (Box of 30) Lime
6505-00-934-3477 (Box of 30) Defense

K-LYTE® DS Effervescent Tablets. Each tablet provides 50 mEq (1955 mg) potassium.

NDC 0087-0772-41 Lime flavor, Boxes of 30
NDC 0087-0772-42 Lime flavor, Boxes of 100
NDC 0087-0771-41 Orange flavor, Boxes of 30
NDC 0087-0771-42 Orange flavor, Boxes of 100

K-LYTE/CL® Effervescent Tablets. Each tablet in solution provides the equivalent of 25 mEq (1865 mg) potassium chloride.

NDC 0087-0766-41 Citrus flavor, Boxes of 30
NDC 0087-0766-43 Citrus flavor, Boxes of 100
NDC 0087-0766-42 Citrus flavor, Boxes of 250
NDC 0087-0767-41 Fruit Punch flavor, Boxes of 30
NDC 0087-0767-43 Fruit Punch flavor, Boxes of 100
NDC 0087-0767-42 Fruit Punch flavor, Boxes of 250

K-LYTE/CL® Powder. Each dose in solution provides the equivalent of 25 mEq (1865 mg) potassium chloride.

NDC 0087-0763-01 Fruit Punch flavor, 234 g can (30 measured doses with scoop)

K-LYTE/CL® 50 mEq Effervescent Tablets. Each tablet in solution provides the equivalent of 50 mEq (3730 mg) potassium chloride.

NDC 0087-0757-41 Fruit Punch flavor, Boxes of 30
NDC 0087-0757-42 Fruit Punch flavor, Boxes of 100
NDC 0087-0758-41 Citrus flavor, Boxes of 30
NDC 0087-0758-42 Citrus flavor, Boxes of 100

Store Below 86°F (30°C).

Shown in Product Identification Section, page 416

NATALINS® tablets

[*nā-tă-lins*]

Multivitamin and multimineral supplement

COMPOSITION

Each Natalins tablet supplies:

		% U.S. RDA Pregnant or Lactating Women
Vitamins		
Vitamin A, IU	8,000	100
Vitamin D, IU	400	100
Vitamin E, IU	30	100
Vitamin C (Ascorbic acid), mg	90	150
Folic acid, mg	0.8	100
Thiamine (Vitamin B_1), mg	1.7	100
Riboflavin (Vitamin B_2), mg	2	100
Niacin, mg	20	100
Vitamin B_6, mg	4	160
Vitamin B_{12}, mcg	8	100
Minerals		
Calcium, mg	200	15
Iodine, mcg	150	100
Iron, mg	45	250
Magnesium, mg	100	22

INGREDIENTS

Calcium carbonate, magnesium hydroxide, ferrous fumarate, sodium ascorbate, povidone, dl-alpha-tocopheryl acetate, acacia, niacinamide, vitamin A acetate, hydroxypropyl methylcellulose, polacrilin potassium, magnesium stearate, pyridoxine hydrochloride, ethylcellulose, riboflavin (color), titanium dioxide (color), silicon dioxide, thiamine mononitrate, glycerin, folic acid, vitamin D_3, calcium iodate, vitamin B_{12}.

INDICATIONS AND USAGE

Diet supplementation during pregnancy or lactation.

DOSAGE AND ADMINISTRATION

One tablet a day or as indicated.

HOW SUPPLIED

Natalins® tablets

NDC 0087-0700-01 Bottles of 100
NDC 0087-0700-06 Bottles of 1000

Shown in Product Identification Section, page 416

NATALINS® RX ℞

[*nā-tă-lins*]

Multivitamin and Multimineral Supplement Tablets with 1 mg folic acid and 60 mg Iron

Natalins Rx tablets provide twelve vitamins and six minerals to supplement the diet during pregnancy or lactation with no artificial flavor or color from synthetic sources.

COMPOSITION

Each Natalins Rx tablet supplies:

		% U.S. RDA Pregnant Or Lactating Women
Vitamins		
Vitamin A, IU	8,000	100
Vitamin D, IU	400	100
Vitamin E, IU	30	100
Vitamin C (Ascorbic acid), mg.	90	150
Folic acid (Folacin), mg.	1	125
Thiamine (Vitamin B_1), mg.	2.55	150
Riboflavin (Vitamin B_2), mg.	3	150
Niacin, mg.	20	100
Vitamin B_6, mg.	10	400
Vitamin B_{12}, mcg.	8	100
Biotin, mg.	0.05	16
Pantothenic acid, mg.	15	150
Minerals		
Calcium, mg.	200	15
Iodine, mcg.	150	100
Iron, mg.	60	333
Magnesium, mg.	100	22
Copper, mg.	2	100
Zinc, mg.	15	100

ACTIVE INGREDIENT

Each tablet contains 1.0 mg folic acid.

OTHER INGREDIENTS

Acacia, biotin, calcium carbonate, calcium iodate, calcium pantothenate, cholecalciferol, colloidal silicon dioxide, cupric oxide, cyanocobalamin, ethylcellulose, ferrous fumarate, glycerin, hydroxypropyl methylcellulose 2910, magnesium hydroxide, magnesium stearate, niacinamide, polacrilin potassium, povidone, pyridoxine hydrochloride, riboflavin, sodium ascorbate, thiamine mononitrate, titanium dioxide, dl-alpha-tocopheryl acetate, vitamin A acetate, zinc oxide.

INDICATIONS AND USAGE

Natalins Rx tablets help assure an adequate intake of the vitamins and minerals listed above.

Folic acid helps prevent the development of megaloblastic anemia during pregnancy.

CONTRAINDICATIONS

Supplemental vitamins and minerals should not be prescribed for patients with hemochromatosis or Wilson's disease.

WARNING

Keep Natalins Rx tablets out of the reach of children.

PRECAUTIONS

General—pernicious anemia should be excluded before using this product since folic acid may mask the symptoms of pernicious anemia. The calcium content should be considered before prescribing for patients with kidney stones. Do not exceed the recommended dose.

ADVERSE REACTIONS

No adverse reactions or undesirable side effects have been attributed to the use of Natalins Rx tablets.

DOSAGE AND ADMINISTRATION

One tablet daily, or as prescribed.

HOW SUPPLIED

Natalins® Rx Tablets: (Available on prescription.)

NDC 0087-0702-01 Bottles of 100
NDC 0087-0702-02 Bottles of 1000

Shown in Product Identification Section, page 417

OVCON®-50 ℞

[*äv'kăn*]

21 tablets of norethindrone 1 mg and ethinyl estradiol 0.05 mg. Each green tablet in the 28 day regimen contains inert ingredients.

OVCON®-35 ℞

21 tablets of norethindrone 0.4 mg and ethinyl estradiol 0.035 mg. Each green tablet in the 28 day regimen contains inert ingredients.

Oral contraceptives

DESCRIPTION

28-Day OVCON®-50 and OVCON®-35 tablets provide a continuous regimen for oral contraception derived from 21 tablets composed of norethindrone and ethinyl estradiol to be followed by 7 green tablets of inert ingredients.

21-Day OVCON®-50 and OVCON®-35 tablets provide a regimen for oral contraception derived from 21 tablets composed of norethindrone and ethinyl estradiol. The chemical name for norethindrone is 17-hydroxy-19-nor-17α-pregn-4-en-20-yn-3-one and for ethinyl estradiol the chemical name is 19-nor-17α-pregna-1,3,5 (10)-trien-20-yne-3, 17-diol. The structural formulas are:

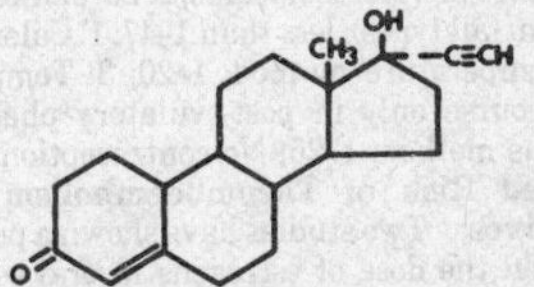

NORETHINDRONE

[See Chemical Formula at top of next page].

The active OVCON-50 tablets contain 1 mg norethindrone and 50 mcg ethinyl estradiol. The active OVCON-35 tablets contain 0.4 mg norethindrone and 35 mcg ethinyl estradiol.

Continued on next page

Mead Johnson Labs.—Cont.

ETHINYL ESTRADIOL

The green tablets contain inert ingredients.

OVCON-50, 21-Day contains the following inactive ingredients: dibasic calcium phosphate, D&C Yellow No. 10 (aluminum lake), FD&C Yellow No. 6 (aluminum lake), lactose, magnesium stearate, povidone, and sodium starch glycolate.

OVCON-50 contains the following inactive ingredients: acacia, dibasic calcium phosphate, D&C Yellow No. 10 (aluminum lake), FD&C Blue No. 1 (aluminum lake), FD&C Yellow No. 6 (aluminum lake), lactose, magnesium stearate, povidone, sodium starch glycolate, starch (corn), and talc.

OVCON-35, 21-Day contains the following inactive ingredients: dibasic calcium phosphate, FD&C Yellow No. 6 (aluminum lake), lactose, magnesium stearate, povidone, and sodium starch glycolate.

OVCON-35 contains the following inactive ingredients: acacia, dibasic calcium phosphate, D&C Yellow No. 10 (aluminum lake), FD&C Blue No. 1 (aluminum lake), FD&C Yellow No. 6 (aluminum lake), lactose, magnesium stearate, povidone, sodium starch glycolate, starch (corn), and talc.

CLINICAL PHARMACOLOGY

Combination oral contraceptives act primarily through the mechanism of gonadotropin suppression due to the estrogenic and progestational activity of the ingredients. Although the primary mechanism of action is inhibition of ovulation, alterations in the genital tract including changes in the cervical mucus (which increase the difficulty of sperm penetration) and the endometrium (which reduce the likelihood of implantation) may also contribute to contraceptive effectiveness.

INDICATIONS AND USAGE

OVCON is indicated for the prevention of pregnancy in women who elect to use oral contraceptives as a method of contraception.

Oral contraceptives are highly effective. The pregnancy rate in women using conventional combination oral contraceptives (containing 35 mcg or more of ethinyl estradiol or 50 mcg or more of mestranol) is generally reported as less than one pregnancy per 100 woman-years of use. Slightly higher rates (somewhat more than 1 pregnancy per 100 woman-years of use) are reported for some combination products containing 35 mcg or less of ethinyl estradiol, and rates on the order of 3 pregnancies per 100 woman-years are reported for the progestin-only oral contraceptives.

These rates are derived from separate studies conducted by different investigators in several population groups and cannot be compared precisely. Furthermore, pregnancy rates tend to be lower as clinical studies are continued, possibly due to selective retention in the longer studies of those patients who accept the treatment regimen and do not discontinue as a result of adverse reactions, pregnancy, or other reasons.

In clinical trials with OVCON-50, 1,126 patients completed 9,558 cycles and a total of 7 pregnancies were reported. This represents a pregnancy rate of 0.88 per 100 woman-years.

In clinical trials with OVCON-35, 2493 patients completed 35,881 cycles and a total of 33 pregnancies were reported. This represents a pregnancy rate of 1.10 per 100 woman-years.

The following table gives ranges of pregnancy rates reported in a standard textbook[1] for other means of contraception. An individual patient may achieve higher or lower rates with any given method (except the IUD), depending upon the degree of adherence to the method.

Pregnancies per 100 Woman-Years: IUD, less than 1–6; Diaphragm with spermicidal product (creams or jellies), 2–20; Condom, 3–36; Aerosol foams, 2–29; Jellies and creams, 4–36; Rhythm (all types), less than 1–47: 1. Calendar method, 14–47; 2. Temperature method, 1–20; 3. Temperature method—intercourse only in post-ovulatory phase, less than 1–7; 4. Mucus method, 1–25; No contraception, 60–80.

Dose-Related Risk of Thromboembolism from Oral Contraceptives: Two studies have shown a positive association between the dose of estrogens in oral contraceptives and the risk of thromboembolism.[2,3] For this reason, it is prudent and in keeping with good principles of therapeutics to minimize exposure to estrogen. The oral contraceptive product prescribed for any given patient should be that product which contains the least amount of estrogen that is compatible with an acceptable pregnancy rate and patient acceptance. It is recommended that new acceptors of oral contraceptives be started on preparations containing 50 mcg or less of estrogen.

CONTRAINDICATIONS

Oral contraceptives should not be used in women with any of the following conditions:

1. Thrombophlebitis or thromboembolic disorders.
2. A past history of deep vein thrombophlebitis or thromboembolic disorders.
3. Cerebral vascular or coronary artery disease.
4. Known or suspected carcinoma of the breast.
5. Known or suspected estrogen dependent neoplasia.
6. Undiagnosed abnormal genital bleeding.
7. Known or suspected pregnancy (see warning No. 5).
8. Benign or malignant liver tumor which developed during the use of oral contraceptives or other estrogen containing products.

WARNINGS

Cigarette smoking increases the risk of serious cardiovascular side effects from oral contraceptive use. This risk increases with age and with heavy smoking (15 or more cigarettes per day) and is quite marked in women over 35 years of age. Women who use oral contraceptives should be strongly advised not to smoke.

The use of oral contraceptives is associated with increased risk of several serious conditions including thromboembolism, stroke, myocardial infarction, hepatic adenoma, gall bladder disease, hypertension. Practitioners prescribing oral contraceptives should be familiar with the following information relating to these risks.

1. *Thromboembolic Disorders and Other Vascular Problems*

An increased risk of thromboembolic and thrombotic disease associated with the use of oral contraceptives is well established. Three principal studies in Great Britain[4-6] and three in the United States[7-10] have demonstrated an increased risk of fatal and nonfatal venous thromboembolism and stroke, both hemorrhagic and thrombotic. These studies estimate that users of oral contraceptives are 4 to 11 times more likely than nonusers to develop these diseases without evident cause (Table 2).

Cerebrovascular Disorders: In a collaborative American study[9,10] of cerebrovascular disorders in women with and without predisposing causes, it was estimated that the risk of hemorrhagic stroke was 2.0 times greater in users than nonusers and the risk of thrombotic stroke was 4 to 9.5 times greater in users than in nonusers (Table 2).

TABLE 2

SUMMARY OF RELATIVE RISK OF THROMBOEMBOLIC DISORDERS AND OTHER VASCULAR PROBLEMS IN ORAL CONTRACEPTIVE USERS COMPARED TO NONUSERS

	Relative risk, times greater
Idiopathic thromboembolic disease	4–11
Post surgery thromboembolic complications	4–6
Thrombotic stroke	4–9.5
Hemorrhagic stroke	2
Myocardial infarction	2–12

Myocardial Infarction: An increased risk of myocardial infarction associated with the use of oral contraceptives has been reported[11-13] confirming a previously suspected association. These studies, conducted in the United Kingdom, found, as expected, that the greater the number of underlying risk factors for coronary artery disease (cigarette smoking, hypertension, hypercholesterolemia, obesity, diabetes, history of preeclamptic toxemia) the higher the risk of developing myocardial infarction, regardless of whether the patient was an oral contraceptive user or not. Oral contraceptives, however, were found to be a clear additional risk factor.

In terms of relative risk, it has been estimated[52] that oral contraceptive users who do not smoke (smoking is considered a major predisposing condition to myocardial infarction) are about twice as likely to have a fatal myocardial infarction as nonusers who do not smoke. Oral contraceptive users who are also smokers have about a 5-fold increased risk of fatal infarction compared to users who do not smoke, but about a 10- to 12-fold increased risk compared to nonusers who do not smoke. Furthermore, the amount of smoking is also an important factor. In determining the importance of these relative risks, however, the baseline rates for various age groups, as shown in Table 3, must be given serious consideration. The importance of other predisposing conditions mentioned above in determining relative and absolute risks has not as yet been quantified; it is quite likely that the same synergistic action exists, but perhaps to a lesser extent.

TABLE 3

ESTIMATED ANNUAL MORTALITY RATE PER 100,000 WOMEN FROM MYOCARDIAL INFARCTION BY USE OF ORAL CONTRACEPTIVES, SMOKING HABITS, AND AGE (IN YEARS)

	Myocardial infarction			
	Women aged 30–39		Women aged 40–44	
Smoking habits	Users	Non Users	Users	Non Users
All smokers	10.2	2.6	62.0	15.9
Heavy[1]	13.0	5.1	78.7	31.3
Light	4.7	.9	28.6	5.7
Nonsmokers	1.8	1.2	10.7	7.4
Smokers and nonsmokers	5.4	1.9	32.8	11.7

[1]Heavy smoker: 15 or more cigarettes per day. From Jain, A.K., Studies in Family Planning, 8:50, 1977.

RISK OF DOSE

In an analysis of data derived from several national adverse reaction reporting systems,[2] British investigators concluded that the risk of thromboembolism including coronary thrombosis is directly related to the dose of estrogen used in oral contraceptives. Preparations containing 100 mcg or more of estrogen were associated with a higher risk of thromboembolism than those containing 50–80 mcg of estrogen. Their analysis did suggest, however, that the quantity of estrogen may not be the sole factor involved. This finding has been confirmed in the United States.[3] Careful epidemiological studies to determine the degree of thromboembolic risk associated with progestogen-only oral contraceptives have not been performed. Cases of thromboembolic disease have been reported in women using these products, and they should not be presumed to be free of excess risk.

PERSISTENCE OF RISK

Persistence of risk after discontinuation of oral contraceptive use has been reported for circulatory disease in general,[53,54] for non-rheumatic heart disease[54,55] and for cerebrovascular disease[54,56] including subarachnoid hemorrhage,[53,54,57] cerebral thrombosis,[56] and transient ischemic attacks.[56]

[See figure 1 next page].

Estimate of Excess Mortality from Circulatory Diseases: A large prospective study[53] carried out in the U.K. estimated the mortality rate per 100,000 women per year from diseases of the circulatory system for users and nonusers of oral contraceptives according to age, smoking habits, and duration of use. The overall excess death rate annually from circulatory diseases for oral contraceptive users was estimated to be 20 per 100,000 (ages 15–34—5/100,000; ages 35–44—33/100,000; ages 45–49—140/100,000), the risk being concentrated in older women, in those with a long duration of use, and in cigarette smokers. It was not possible, however, to examine the interrelationships of age, smoking and duration of use, nor to compare the effects of continuous versus intermittent use. Although the study showed a 10-fold increase in death due to circulatory diseases in users for 5 or more years, all of these deaths occurred in women 35 or older. Until larger numbers of women under 35 with continuous use for 5 or more years are available, it is not possible to assess the magnitude of the relative risk for this younger age group.

The available data from a variety of sources have been analyzed[14] to estimate the risk of death associated with various methods of contraception. The estimates of risk of death for each method include the combined risk of the contraceptive method (e.g., thromboembolic and thrombotic disease in the case of oral contraceptives) plus the risk attributable to pregnancy or abortion in the event of method failure. This latter risk varies with the effectiveness of the contraceptive method. The findings of this analysis are shown in Figure 2 below.[14] The study concluded that the mortality associated with all methods of birth control is low and below that associated with childbirth, with the exception of oral contraceptives in women over 40 who smoke. (The rates given for pill only/smokers for each age group are for smokers as a class. For "heavy" smokers [more than 15 cigarettes a day], the rates given would be about double; for "light" smokers [less than 15 cigarettes a day], about 50 percent.) The lowest mortality is associated with the condom or diaphragm backed up by early abortion.

[See figure 2 next page]

The risk of thromboembolic and thrombotic disease associated with oral contraceptives increases with age after approximately age 30 and, for myocardial infarction, is further increased by hypertension, hypercholesterolemia, obesity, diabetes, or history of preeclamptic toxemia and especially by cigarette smoking.

Based on the data currently available, the following chart gives a gross estimate of the risk of death from circulatory disorders associated with the use of oral contraceptives:

SMOKING HABITS AND OTHER PREDISPOSING CONDITIONS—RISK ASSOCIATED WITH USE OF ORAL CONTRACEPTIVES

Age	Below 30	30–39	40+
Heavy smokers	C	B	A
Light smokers	D	C	B
Nonsmokers (no predisposing conditions)	D	C,D	C
Nonsmokers (other predisposing conditions)	C	C,B	B,A

A—Use associated with very high risk.
B—Use associated with high risk.
C—Use associated with moderate risk.
D—Use associated with low risk.

The physician and the patient should be alert to the earliest manifestations of thromboembolic and thrombotic disorders (e.g., thrombophlebitis, pulmonary embolism, cerebrovascular insufficiency, coronary occlusion, retinal thrombosis, and mesenteric thrombosis). Should any of these occur or be suspected, the drug should be discontinued immediately.

A four- to six-fold increased risk of post surgery thromboembolic complications has been reported in oral contraceptive users.[15,16] If feasible, oral contraceptives should be discontinued at least 4 weeks before surgery of a type associated with an increased risk of thromboembolism or prolonged immobilization.

2. *Ocular Lesions.* There have been reports of neuro-ocular lesions such as optic neuritis or retinal thrombosis associated with the use of oral contraceptives. Discontinue oral contraceptive medication if there is unexplained, sudden or gradual, partial or complete loss of vision; onset of proptosis or diplopia; papilledema; or retinal vascular lesions and institute appropriate diagnostic and therapeutic measures.

3. *Carcinoma.* Long-term continuous administration of either natural or synthetic estrogen in certain animal species increases the frequency of carcinoma of the breast, cervix, vagina, and liver. Certain synthetic progestogens, none currently contained in oral contraceptives, have been noted to increase the incidence of mammary nodules, benign and malignant, in dogs.

In humans, three case control studies have reported an increased risk of endometrial carcinoma associated with the prolonged use of exogenous estrogen in post menopausal women.[17-19] One publication[20] reported on the first 21 cases submitted by physicians to a registry of cases of adenocarcinoma of the endometrium in women under 40 on oral contraceptives. Of the cases found in women without predisposing risk factors for adenocarcinoma of the endometrium (e.g., irregular bleeding at the time oral contraceptives were first given, polycystic ovaries), nearly all occurred in women who

Figure 1

Statistically Significant Findings	Interim Report	Later Report	Most Recent Report
• Royal College of Gen. Practitioners	Higher rate of reporting of cerebrovascular accidents in users[26]		Increased incidence of cerebrovascular disease among users[56]
• British Family Planning Association	Association between O.C. user and occurrence stroke[58]		
• Walnut Creek Study			
Degree of Risk			
• Royal College of Gen. Practitioners		4-fold increase in mortality from circulatory disease in users[54]	
• British Family Planning Association		4-fold increase (associated with age and smoking) in venous thrombosis and pulmonary embolism in users[58]	
• Walnut Creek Study			Risk of subarachnoid hemorrhage associated with O.C. use, heavy smoking and age.[57,59]
Persistence of Risk			
• Royal College of Gen. Practitioners	Rate of circulatory disease increased with duration of use, may persist after discontinuation[53]		Cerebrovascular disease significantly greater in former users (up to six years) than in controls[56]
• Walnut Creek Study			Significant association between past O.C. use and risk of subarachnoid hemorrhage[57]
• U S Hospital-Based Study			2–3 fold increase in rate of myocardial infarction in former users of more than 10 years[55]

had used a sequential oral contraceptive. These products are no longer marketed. No evidence has been reported suggesting an increased risk of endometrial cancer in users of conventional combination or progestogen-only oral contraceptives.

Several studies[8,21-24] have found no increase in breast cancer in women taking oral contraceptives or estrogens. One study[25] however, while also noting no overall increased risk of breast cancer in women treated with oral contraceptives, found an excess risk in the subgroups of oral contraceptive users with documented benign breast disease. A reduced occurrence of benign breast tumors in users of oral contraceptives has been well-documented.[8,21,25-27]

In summary, there is at present no confirmed evidence from human studies of an increased risk of cancer associated with oral contraceptives. Close clinical surveillance of all women taking oral contraceptives is, nevertheless, essential. In all cases of undiagnosed persistent or recurrent abnormal vaginal bleeding, appropriate diagnostic measures should be taken to rule out malignancy. Women with a strong family history of breast cancer or who have breast nodules, fibrocystic disease or abnormal mammograms should be monitored with particular care if they elect to use oral contraceptives instead of other methods of contraception.

4. *Hepatic Tumors.* Benign hepatic adenomas have been found to be associated with the use of oral contraceptives.[28-30,46] One study[46] showed that oral contraceptive formulations with high hormonal potency were associated with a higher risk than lower potency formulations. Although benign, hepatic adenomas may rupture and may cause death through intra-abdominal hemorrhage. This has been reported in short-term as well as long-term users of oral contraceptives. Two studies relate risk with duration of use of the contraceptive, the risk being much greater after 4 or more years of oral contraceptive use.[30,46] While hepatic adenoma is a rare lesion, it should be considered in women presenting abdominal pain and tenderness, abdominal mass or shock.

A few cases of hepatocellular carcinoma have been reported in women taking oral contraceptives. The relationship of these drugs to this type of malignancy is not known at this time.

5. *Use in or Immediately Preceding Pregnancy, Birth Defects in Offspring, and Malignancy in Female Offspring.* The use of female sex hormones—both estrogenic and progestational agents—during early pregnancy may seriously damage the offspring. It has been shown that females exposed **in utero** to diethylstilbestrol, a nonsteroidal estrogen, have an increased risk of developing in later life a form of vaginal or cervical cancer that is ordinarily extremely rare.[31,32] This risk has been estimated to be of the order of 1 in 1,000 exposures or less.[33,47] Although there is no evidence at the present time that oral contraceptives further enhance the risk of developing this type of malignancy, such patients should be monitored with particular care if they elect to use oral contraceptives instead of other methods of contraception. Furthermore, a high percentage of such exposed women (from 30 to 90%) have been found to have epithelial changes of the vagina and cervix.[34-38] Although these changes are histologically benign, it is not known whether this condition is a precursor of vaginal malignancy. Male children so exposed may develop abnormalities of the urogenital tract.[48-50] Although similar data are not available with the use of other

OVCON-50, -35

Figure 2

Estimated annual number of deaths associated with control of fertility and no control per 100,000 nonsterile women, by regimen of control and age of women.

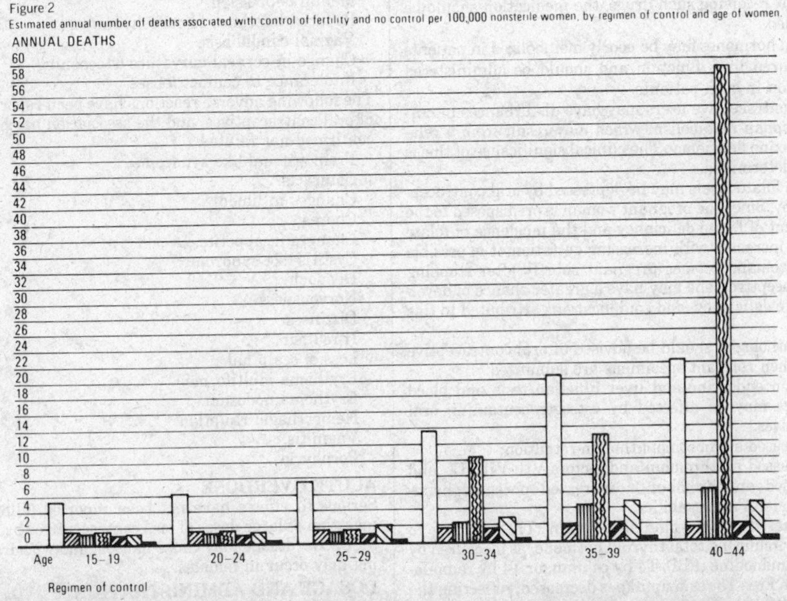

Continued on next page

Mead Johnson Labs.—Cont.

estrogens, it cannot be presumed that they would not induce similar changes.

An increased risk of congenital anomalies, including heart defects and limb defects, has been reported with the use of sex hormones, including oral contraceptives, in pregnancy.[39-42,51] One case control study[42] has estimated a 4.7-fold increase in risk of limb-reduction defects in infants exposed **in utero** to sex hormones (oral contraceptives, hormonal withdrawal tests for pregnancy or attempted treatment for threatened abortion). Some of these exposures were very short and involved only a few days of treatment. The data suggest that the risk of limb-reduction defects in exposed fetuses is somewhat less than one in 1,000 live births. In the past, female sex hormones have been used during pregnancy in an attempt to treat threatened or habitual abortion. There is considerable evidence that estrogens are ineffective for these indications, and there is no evidence from well controlled studies that progestogens are effective for these uses.

There is some evidence that triploidy and possibly other types of polyploidy are increased among abortuses from women who become pregnant soon after ceasing oral contraceptives.[43] Embryos with these anomalies are virtually always aborted spontaneously. Whether there is an overall increase in spontaneous abortion of pregnancies conceived soon after stopping oral contraceptives is unknown.

It is recommended that for any patient who has missed two consecutive periods, pregnancy should be ruled out before continuing the contraceptive regimen. If the patient has not adhered to the prescribed schedule, the possibility of pregnancy should be considered at the time of the first missed period (or after 45 days from the last menstrual period if the progestogen-only oral contraceptives are used), and further use of oral contraceptives should be withheld until pregnancy has been ruled out. If pregnancy is confirmed, the patient should be apprised of the potential risks to the fetus and the advisability of continuation of the pregnancy should be discussed in the light of these risks.

It is also recommended that women who discontinue oral contraceptives with the intent of becoming pregnant use an alternate form of contraception for a period of time before attempting to conceive. Many clinicians recommend 3 months although no precise information is available on which to base this recommendation.

The administration of progestogen-only or progestogen-estrogen combinations to induce withdrawal bleeding should not be used as a test of pregnancy.

6. *Gallbladder Disease.*

Studies[8,23,26] report an increased risk of surgically confirmed gallbladder disease in users of oral contraceptives and estrogens. In one study, an increased risk appeared after 2 years of use and doubled after 4 or 5 years of use. In one of the other studies, an increased risk was apparent between 6 and 12 months of use.

7. *Carbohydrate and Lipid Metabolic Effects.*

A decrease in glucose tolerance has been observed in a significant percentage of patients on oral contraceptives. For this reason, prediabetic and diabetic patients should be carefully observed while receiving oral contraceptives.

An increase in triglycerides and total phospholipids has been observed in patients receiving oral contraceptives.[44] The clinical significance of this finding remains to be defined.

8. *Elevated Blood Pressure.*

An increase in blood pressure has been reported in patients receiving oral contraceptives.[26] In some women, hypertension may occur within a few months of beginning oral contraceptive use. In the first year of use, the prevalence of women with hypertension is low in users and may be no higher than that of a comparable group of nonusers. The prevalence in users increases, however, with longer exposure, and in the fifth year of use is two and a half to three times the reported prevalence in the first year. Age is also strongly correlated with the development of hypertension in oral contraceptive users. Women who previously have had hypertension during pregnancy may be more likely to develop elevation of blood pressure when given oral contraceptives. Hypertension that develops as a result of taking oral contraceptives usually returns to normal after discontinuing the drug.

9. *Headache.*

The onset or exacerbation of migraine or development of headache of a new pattern which is recurrent, persistent, or severe, requires discontinuation of oral contraceptives and evaluation of the cause.

10. *Bleeding Irregularities.*

Breakthrough bleeding, spotting, and amenorrhea are frequent reasons for patients discontinuing oral contraceptives. In breakthrough bleeding, as in all cases of irregular bleeding from the vagina, nonfunctional causes should be borne in mind. In undiagnosed persistent or recurrent abnormal bleeding from the vagina, adequate diagnostic measures are indicated to rule out pregnancy or malignancy. If pathology has been excluded, time or a change to another formulation may solve the problem. Changing to an oral contraceptive with a higher estrogen content, while potentially useful in minimizing menstrual irregularity, should be done only if necessary since this may increase the risk of thromboembolic disease.

Women with a past history of oligomenorrhea or secondary amenorrhea or young women without regular cycles may have a tendency to remain anovulatory or to become amenorrheic after discontinuation of oral contraceptives. Women with these pre-existing problems should be advised of this possibility and encouraged to use other contraceptive methods. Post-use anovulation, possibly prolonged, may also occur in women without previous irregularities.

11. *Ectopic Pregnancy.*

Ectopic as well as intrauterine pregnancy may occur in contraceptive failures. However, in progestogen-only oral contraceptive failures, the ratio of ectopic to intrauterine pregnancies is higher than in women who are not receiving oral contraceptives, since the drugs are more effective in preventing intrauterine than ectopic pregnancies.

12. *Breast Feeding.*

Oral contraceptives given in the postpartum period may interfere with lactation. There may be a decrease in the quantity and quality of the breast milk. Furthermore, a small fraction of the hormonal agents in oral contraceptives has been identified in the milk of mothers receiving these drugs.[45] The effects, if any, on the breast-fed child have not been determined. If feasible, the use of oral contraceptives should be deferred until the infant has been weaned.

PRECAUTIONS

General

1. A complete medical and family history should be taken prior to the initiation of oral contraceptives. The pretreatment and periodic physical examinations should include special reference to blood pressure, breasts, abdomen and pelvic organs, including Papanicolaou smear and relevant laboratory tests. As a general rule, oral contraceptives should not be prescribed for longer than 1 year without another physical examination being performed.
2. Under the influence of estrogen-progestogen preparations, pre-existing uterine leiomyomata may increase in size.
3. Patients with a history of psychic depression should be carefully observed and the drug discontinued if depression recurs to a serious degree. Patients becoming significantly depressed while taking oral contraceptives should stop the medication and use an alternate method of contraception in an attempt to determine whether the symptom is drug related.
4. Oral contraceptives may cause some degree of fluid retention. They should be prescribed with caution, and only with careful monitoring, in patients with conditions which might be aggravated by fluid retention, such as convulsive disorders, migraine syndrome, asthma, or cardiac or renal insufficiency.
5. Patients with a past history of jaundice during pregnancy have an increased risk of recurrence of jaundice while receiving oral contraceptive therapy. If jaundice develops in any patient receiving such drugs, the medication should be discontinued.
6. Steroid hormones may be poorly metabolized in patients with impaired liver function and should be administered with caution in such patients.
7. Oral contraceptive users may have disturbances in normal tryptophan metabolism which may result from a relative pyridoxine deficiency. The clinical significance of this is yet to be determined.
8. Serum folate levels may be depressed by oral contraceptive therapy. Since the pregnant woman is predisposed to the development of folate deficiency and the incidence of folate deficiency increases with increasing gestation, it is possible that if a woman becomes pregnant shortly after stopping oral contraceptives, she may have a greater chance of developing folate deficiency, and complications attributed to this deficiency.
9. The pathologist should be advised of oral contraceptive therapy when relevant specimens are submitted.
10. Certain endocrine and liver function tests and blood components may be affected by estrogen-containing oral contraceptives:
    a. Increased sulfobromophthalein-retention.
    b. Increased prothrombin and factors VII, VIII, IX, and X; decreased antithrombin 3; increased norepinephrine-induced platelet aggregability.
    c. Increased thyroid binding globulin (TBG) leading to increased circulating total thyroid hormone, as measured by protein-bound iodine (PBI), T4 by column, or T4 by radioimmunoassay. Free T3 resin uptake is decreased, reflecting the elevated TBG, free T4 concentration is unaltered.
    d. Decreased pregnanediol excretion.
    e. Reduced response to metyrapone test.

INFORMATION FOR THE PATIENT

See Patient Labeling printed below

DRUG INTERACTIONS

Reduced efficacy and increased incidence of breakthrough bleeding have been associated with concomitant use of rifampin. A similar association has been suggested with barbiturates, phenylbutazone, phenytoin sodium, ampicillin, and tetracycline.

CARCINOGENESIS

See Warning section for information on the carcinogenic potential of oral contraceptives.

PREGNANCY

Pregnancy category X. See Contraindications and Warnings.

NURSING MOTHERS

See Warnings.

ADVERSE REACTIONS

An increased risk of the following serious adverse reactions has been associated with the use of oral contraceptives (see Warnings):

Thrombophlebitis.
Pulmonary embolism.
Coronary thrombosis.
Cerebral thrombosis.
Cerebral hemorrhage.
Hypertension.
Gallbladder disease.
Benign hepatomas.
Congenital anomalies.

There is evidence of an association between the following conditions and the use of oral contraceptives, although additional confirmatory studies are needed:

Mesenteric thrombosis.
Neuro-ocular lesions, e.g., retinal thrombosis and optic neuritis.

The following adverse reactions have been reported in patients receiving oral contraceptives and are believed to be drug related:

Nausea and/or vomiting, usually the most common adverse reactions, occur in approximately 10% or less of patients during the first cycle. Other reactions, as a general rule, are seen much less frequently or only occasionally.

Gastrointestinal symptoms (such as abdominal cramps and bloating).
Breakthrough bleeding.
Spotting.
Change in menstrual flow.
Dysmenorrhea.
Amenorrhea during and after treatment.
Temporary infertility after discontinuance of treatment.
Edema.
Chloasma or melasma which may persist.
Breast changes: tenderness, enlargement, and secretion.
Change in weight (increase or decrease).
Change in cervical erosion and cervical secretion.
Possible diminution in lactation when given immediately postpartum.
Cholestatic jaundice.
Migraine.
Increase in size of uterine leiomyomata.
Rash (allergic).
Mental depression.
Reduced tolerance to carbohydrates.
Vaginal candidiasis.
Change in corneal curvature (steepening).
Intolerance to contact lenses.

The following adverse reactions have been reported in users of oral contraceptives, and the association has been neither confirmed nor refuted:

Premenstrual-like syndrome.
Cataracts.
Changes in libido.
Chorea.
Changes in appetite.
Cystitis-like syndrome.
Headache.
Nervousness.
Dizziness.
Hirsutism.
Loss of scalp hair.
Erythema multiforme.
Erythema nodosum.
Hemorrhagic Eruption.
Vaginitis.
Porphyria.

ACUTE OVERDOSE

Serious ill effects have not been reported following acute ingestion of large doses of oral contraceptives by young children. Overdosage may cause nausea, and withdrawal bleeding may occur in females.

DOSAGE AND ADMINISTRATION

Note:

To achieve maximum contraceptive effectiveness, OVCON®-35 or OVCON®-50 must be taken exactly as directed and at intervals not exceeding 24 hours. For the initial cycle of OVCON-35 or OVCON-50 therapy, contraceptive efficacy should not be assumed until after the first seven consecutive days of administration. The possibility of ovulation and conception prior to initiation of medication should be considered.

In subsequent cycles where more than seven days elapse from the first day of menstruation until the first pill containing active contraceptive medication is taken, an additional method of birth control should be used until the oral contraceptive has been taken for seven consecutive days.

28-DAY REGIMEN

Sunday Start:

IF THIS IS YOUR FIRST PACKAGE, start taking the yellow or peach tablets on the first Sunday after your period begins, unless your period begins on Sunday. **If your period begins on Sunday, start taking the tablets that very same day.**

Continue to take one tablet each day.

After the last tablet in row 3 has been taken, start taking the green tablets in row 4 the very next day (Sunday).

After the last green tablet in row 4 has been taken, **start your new packet the following day** (Sunday) in the manner described above.

TAKE a tablet every day, without interruption. DO NOT MISS A TABLET. Your period will usually begin while you are taking the green tablets. It may continue during the first few tablets of the next packet.

Should you begin menstrual-like bleeding at another time, or if you do not have a period at all, **continue to take your one tablet daily** and notify your doctor. Your doctor should be informed promptly of any unusual changes in your general health.

Day Five Start:

IF THIS IS YOUR FIRST PACKAGE, count the first day of your menstrual bleeding as Day 1. Take your first yellow or peach tablet on Day 5.

CONTINUE to take one tablet daily, preferably in the evening or at bedtime. Take the tablets in order—first the yellow or peach, then the green ones.

TAKE a tablet every day, without interruption. DO NOT MISS A TABLET. Your period will usually begin while you are taking the green tablets. It may continue during the first few yellow or peach tablets.

Should you begin menstrual-like bleeding at another time, or if you do not have a period at all, **continue to take your one tablet daily** and notify your doctor. Your doctor should be informed promptly of any unusual changes in your general health.

If you miss a tablet, take it as soon as remembered. Also take the usual tablet for that day. Then resume your tablet-a-day schedule. Each missed tablet increases the possibility that the medication may not work. To reduce this possibility, use an additional method of protection until your next period. Because you are to take a tablet every day, without interruption, always have a new supply of tablets ready to take.

21-DAY REGIMEN

Sunday Start:

IF THIS IS YOUR FIRST PACKAGE, start taking the yellow or peach tablets on the first Sunday after your period begins, unless your period begins on Sunday. **If your period begins on Sunday, start taking the tablets that very same day.**

Continue to take one tablet each day.

After the last tablet in row 3 has been taken (on a Saturday), **stop for one week** before starting to take the tablets in your next package. Start your new packet on Sunday in the manner described above.

TAKE a tablet every day, without interruption. DO NOT MISS A TABLET. Your period will usually begin during your week off therapy.It may continue during the first few tablets of the next packet.

Should you begin menstrual-like bleeding at another time, or if you do not have a period at all, **continue to take your one tablet daily** and notify your doctor. Your doctor should be informed promptly of any unusual changes in your general health.

Day Five Start:

IF THIS IS YOUR FIRST PACKAGE, count the first day of your menstrual bleeding as Day 1. Take your first yellow or peach tablet on Day 5.

CONTINUE to take one tablet daily, preferably in the evening or at bedtime—take the tablets in order.

AFTER you have taken the last tablet, wait seven days and then begin your next package of tablets. You should begin again on the same day of the week. Thus, three weeks on, one week off tablets.

TAKE a tablet every day, without interruption. DO NOT MISS A TABLET. Your period will usually begin within four days after you have taken your last yellow or peach tablet.

Should you begin menstrual-like bleeding at another time, or if you do not have a period at all, **continue to take your tablets as directed** and notify your doctor. Your doctor should be informed promptly of any unusual changes in your general health.

If you miss a tablet, take it as soon as remembered. Also take the usual tablet for that day. Then resume your tablet-a-day schedule. Each missed tablet increases the possibility that the medication may not work. To reduce this possibility, use an additional method of protection until your next period. Because you are to take a tablet every day for three weeks, without interruption, always have a new supply of tablets ready to take.

Patients should be cautioned to follow the dosage schedule strictly.

Evening administration is suggested. If the regimen is interrupted, an additional contraceptive method is recommended for the rest of the cycle. Should spotting or breakthrough bleeding occur, it is recommended that the patient continue medication. If bleeding is persistent or recurrent, the patient should consult her physician.

Use of oral contraceptives in the event of a missed menstrual period:

1. If the patient has not adhered to the prescribed dosage regimen, the possibility of pregnancy should be considered after the first missed period and oral contraceptives should be withheld until pregnancy has been ruled out.
2. If the patient has adhered to the prescribed regimen and misses two consecutive periods, pregnancy should be ruled out before continuing the contraceptive regimen.

HOW SUPPLIED

OVCON®-50 is available in 21 and 28 day regimens. Each compact contains 21 yellow tablets of 1.0 mg. norethindrone and 0.05 mg. ethinyl estradiol. Each green tablet in the 28 day regimen contains inert ingredients.

	Compact of 21 tablets
NDC 0087-0584-42	Carton of 6 compacts
	Compact of 28 tablets
NDC 0087-0579-41	Carton of 6 compacts

OVCON®-35 is available in 21 and 28 day regimens. Each compact contains 21 peach tablets of 0.4 mg. norethindrone and 0.035 mg. ethinyl estradiol. Each green tablet in the 28 day regimen contains inert ingredients.

	Compact of 21 tablets
NDC 0087-0583-42	Carton of 6 compacts
	Compact of 28 tablets
NDC 0087-0578-41	Carton of 6 compacts

REFERENCES

1. "Population Reports," Series H, Number 2, May 1974; Series I, Number 1, June 1974; Series B, Number 2, Jan 1975; Series H, Number 3, 1975; Series H, Number 4, Jan 1976 (published by the Population Information Program, The George Washington University Medical Center, 2001 S St. NW Washington, DC).
2. Inman WHW, *et al.*: Brit M J 2:203, 1970.
3. Stolley PD, *et al.*: Am J Epidemiol 102:197, 1975.
4. Royal College of General Practitioners, J Coll Gen Pract 13:267, 1967.
5. Inman WHW, *et al.*: Brit M J 2:193, 1968.
6. Vessey MP, Doll R: Brit M J 2:651, 1969.
7. Sartwell PE, *et al.*: Am J Epidemiol 90:365, 1969.
8. Boston Collaborative Drug Surveillance Program: Lancet 1:1399, 1973.
9. Collaborative Group for the Study of Stroke in Young Women: N Eng J Med 288:871, 1973.
10. Collaborative Group for the Study of Stroke in Young Women: JAMA 231:871, 1975.
11. Mann JI, Inman WHW: Brit M J 2:245, 1975.
12. Mann JI, *et al.*: Brit M J 2:445, 1976.
13. Mann JI, *et al.*: Brit M J 2:241, 1975.
14. Tietze C: Family Planning Perspectives 9:74, 1977.
15. Vessey MP, *et al.*: Brit M J 3:123, 1970.
16. Greene GR, Sartwell PE: Am J Pub Health 62:680, 1972.
17. Smith DC, *et al.*: N Eng J Med 293:1164, 1975.
18. Ziel HK, Finkle WD: N Eng J Med 293:1167, 1975.
19. Mack TN, *et al.*: New Eng J Med 294:1262, 1976.
20. Silverberg SG, Makowski EL: Ob Gyn 46:503, 1975.
21. Vessey MP, *et al.*: Brit M J 3:719, 1972.
22. Vessey MP, *et al.*: Lancet 1:941, 1975.
23. Boston Collaborative Drug Surveillance Program: New Eng J Med 290:15, 1974.
24. Arthes FG, *et al.*: Cancer 28:1391, 1971.
25. Fasal E, Paffenbarger RS: J Natl Cancer Inst 55:767, 1975.
26. Royal College of General Practitioners: Oral Contraceptives and Health, London, Pitman, 1974.
27. Ory H, *et al.*: , New Eng J Med 294:419, 1976.
28. Baum J, *et al.*: Lancet 2:926, 1973.
29. Mays ET, *et al.*: JAMA 235:730, 1976.
30. Edmondson HA, *et al.*: New Eng J Med 294:470, 1976.
31. Herbst AL, *et al.*: New Eng J Med 284:878, 1971.
32. Greenwald P, *et al.*: New Eng J Med 285:390, 1971.
33. Lanier AP, *et al.*: Mayo Clin Proc 48:793, 1973.
34. Herbst AL, *et al.*: Ob Gyn 40:287, 1972.
35. Herbst AL, *et al.*: Am J Ob Gyn 118:607, 1974.
36. Herbst AL, *et al.*: New Eng J Med 292:334, 1975.
37. Stafl A, *et al.*: Ob Gyn 43:118, 1974.
38. Sherman AI, *et al.*: Ob Gyn 44:531, 1974.
39. Gal I, *et al.*: Nature 216:83, 1967.
40. Levy EP, *et al.*: Lancet 1:611, 1973.
41. Nora JJ, Nora AH: Lancet 1:941, 1973.
42. Janerich DT, *et al.*: New Eng J Med 291:697, 1974.
43. Carr DH: Canadian Med Assoc J 103:343, 1970.
44. Wynn V, *et al.*: Lancet 2:720, 1966.
45. Laumas KR, *et al.*: Am J Ob Gyn 98:411, 1967.
46. Center for Disease Control, Morbidity and Mortality Weekly Report, 26:293, 1977.
47. Herbst AL, *et al.*: Am J Ob Gyn 128:43, 1977.
48. Bibbo M, *et al.*: J Reprod Med 15:29, 1975.
49. Gill WB, *et al.*: J Reprod Med 16:147, 1976.
50. Henderson BE, *et al.*: Pediatrics 58:505, 1976.
51. Heinonen OP, *et al.*: New Eng J Med 296:67, 1977.
52. Jain AK: Studies in Family Planning 8:50, 1977.
53. Beral V: Lancet 2:727, 1977.
54. Layde PM, *et al.*: Lancet 1:541, 1981
55. Slone D, *et al.*: N Eng J Med 305:420, 1981.
56. Layde PM, *et al.*: J R Coll Gen Pract 33:75, 1983.
57. Petitti DB, *et al.*: Lancet 2:234, 1978.
58. Vessey M, *et al.*: J Biosoc Sci 8:373, 1976.
59. Ramcharan S, *et al.*: The Walnut Creek Contraceptive Drug Study, Vol. 3, US. Govt. Ptg. Off. J Reprod Med 25:346, 1980.

The Patient Labeling for oral contraceptive drug products is set forth below:

BRIEF SUMMARY
PATIENT PACKAGE INSERT

WARNING

Cigarette smoking increases the risk of serious adverse effects on the heart and blood vessels from oral contraceptive use. This risk increases with age and with heavy smoking (15 or more cigarettes per day) and is quite marked in women over 35 years of age. Women who use oral contraceptives should not smoke.

Oral contraceptives taken as directed are about 99% effective in preventing pregnancy. (The mini-pill, however, is somewhat less effective.) Forgetting to take your pills increases the chance of pregnancy. Various drugs, such as antibiotics, may also decrease the effectiveness of oral contraceptives.

Women who have or have had clotting disorders, cancer of the breast or sex organs, unexplained vaginal bleeding, a stroke, heart attack, angina pectoris, or who suspect they may be pregnant should not use oral contraceptives.

Most side effects of the pill are not serious. The most common side effects are nausea, vomiting, bleeding between menstrual periods, weight gain, and breast tenderness. However, proper use of oral contraceptives requires that they be taken under your doctor's continuous supervision, because they can be associated with serious side effects which may be fatal. Fortunately, these occur very infrequently. The serious side effects are:

1. Blood clots in the legs, lungs, brain, heart or other organs and hemorrhage into the brain due to bursting of a blood vessel.
2. Liver tumors, which may rupture and cause severe bleeding.
3. Birth defects if the pill is taken while you are pregnant.
4. High blood pressure.
5. Gallbladder disease.

The symptoms associated with these serious side effects are discussed in the detailed leaflet given you with your supply of pills. Notify your doctor if you notice any unusual physical disturbance while taking the pill.

The estrogen in oral contraceptives has been found to cause breast cancer and other cancers in certain animals. These findings suggest that oral contraceptives may also cause cancer in humans. However, studies to date in women taking currently marketed oral contraceptives have not confirmed that oral contraceptives cause cancer in humans.

The detailed leaflet describes more completely the benefits and risks of oral contraceptives. It also provides information on other forms of contraception. Read it carefully. If you have any questions, consult your doctor.

Caution: Oral contraceptives are of no value in the prevention or treatment of venereal disease.

Detailed Patient Labeling

What You Should Know About Oral Contraceptives:

Oral contraceptives ("the pill") are the most effective way (except for sterilization) to prevent pregnancy. They are also convenient and, for most women, free of serious or unpleasant side effects. Oral contraceptives must always be taken under the continuous supervision of a physician.

It is important that any woman who considers using an oral contraceptive understand the risks involved. Although the oral contraceptives have important advantages over other methods of contraception, they have certain risks that no other method has. Only you can decide whether the advantages are worth these risks. This leaflet will tell you about the most important risks. It will explain how you can help your doctor prescribe the pill as safely as possible by telling him about yourself and being alert for the earliest signs of

Continued on next page

Mead Johnson Labs.—Cont.

trouble. And it will tell you how to use the pill properly, so that it will be as effective as possible. There is more detailed information available in the leaflet prepared for doctors. Your pharmacist can show you a copy; you may need your doctor's help in understanding parts of it.

Who Should Not Use Oral Contraceptives:

A. If you have any of the following conditions you should not use the pill:

1. Clots in the legs or lungs.
2. Angina pectoris.
3. Known or suspected cancer of the breast or sex organs.
4. Unusual vaginal bleeding that has not yet been diagnosed.
5. Known or suspected pregnancy.

B. If you have had any of the following conditions you should not use the pill:

1. Heart attack or stroke.
2. Clots in the legs or lungs.

WARNING

> **C. Cigarette smoking increases the risk of serious adverse effects on the heart and blood vessels from oral contraceptive use. This risk increases with age and with heavy smoking (15 or more cigarettes per day) and is quite marked in women over 35 years of age. Women who use oral contraceptives should not smoke.**

D. If you have scanty or irregular periods or are a young woman without a regular cycle, you should use another method of contraception because, if you use the pill, you may have difficulty becoming pregnant or may fail to have menstrual periods after discontinuing the pill.

Deciding to Use Oral Contraceptives: If you do not have any of the conditions listed above and are thinking about using oral contraceptives, to help you decide, you need information about the advantages and risks of oral contraceptives and of other contraceptive methods as well. This leaflet describes the advantages and risks of oral contraceptives. Except for sterilization, the IUD and abortion, which have their own exclusive risks, the only serious risks of other methods of contraception are those due to pregnancy should the method fail. Your doctor can answer questions you may have with respect to other methods of contraception. He can also answer any questions you may have after reading this leaflet on oral contraceptives.

1. What Oral Contraceptives Are and How They Work. Oral Contraceptives are of two types. The most common, often simply called "the pill" is a combination of an estrogen and a progestogen, the two kinds of female hormones. The amount of estrogen and progestogen can vary, but the amount of estrogen is most important because both the effectiveness and some of the dangers of oral contraceptives are related to the amount of estrogen. This kind of oral contraceptive works principally by preventing release of an egg from the ovary. When the amount of estrogen is 50 micrograms or more of mestranol or 35 micrograms or more of ethinyl estradiol and the pill is taken as directed, oral contraceptives are more than 99% effective (i.e., there would be less than one pregnancy if 100 women used the pill for 1 year). Pills that contain 20 to 35 micrograms of estrogen vary slightly in effectiveness, ranging from 98% to more than 99% effective.

The second type of oral contraceptive, often called the "mini-pill", contains only a progestogen. It works in part by preventing release of an egg from the ovary but also by keeping sperm from reaching the egg and by making the uterus (womb) less receptive to any fertilized egg that reaches it. The mini-pill is less effective than the combination oral contraceptive, about 97% effective. In addition, the progestogen-only pill has a tendency to cause irregular bleeding which may be quite inconvenient, or cessation of bleeding entirely. The progestogen-only pill is used despite its lower effectiveness in the hope that it will prove not to have some of the serious side effects of the estrogen-containing pill (see below) but it is not yet certain that the mini-pill does in fact have fewer serious side effects. The discussion below, while based mainly on information about the combination pills, should be considered to apply as well to the mini-pill.

2. Other Nonsurgical Ways to Prevent Pregnancy. As this leaflet will explain, oral contraceptives have several serious risks. Other methods of contraception have lesser risks or none at all. They are also less effective than oral contraceptives, but, used properly, may be effective enough for many women. The following table gives reported pregnancy rates (the number of women out of 100 who would become pregnant in 1 year) for these methods:

Pregnancies per 100 Women per year:

Intrauterine device (IUD), less than 1–6;
Diaphragm with spermicidal products (creams or jellies), 2–20;
Condom (rubber), 3–36;
Aerosol foams, 2–29;
Jellies and creams, 4–36;
Periodic abstinence (rhythm) all types, less than 1–47:

1. Calendar method, 14–47;
2. Temperature method, 1–20;
3. Temperature method—intercourse only in post-ovulatory phase, less than 1–7;
4. Mucus method, 1–25;

No contraception, 60–80.

The figures (except for the IUD) vary widely because people differ in how well they use each method. Very faithful users of the various methods obtain very good results, except for users of the calendar method of periodic abstinence (rhythm). Except for the IUD, effective use of these methods requires somewhat more effort than simply taking a single pill every morning, but it is an effort that many couples undertake successfully. Your doctor can tell you a great deal more about these methods of contraception.

3. The Dangers of Oral Contraceptives.

a. Circulatory disorders (abnormal blood clotting and stroke due to hemorrhage). Blood clots (in various blood vessels of the body) are the most common of the serious side effects of oral contraceptives. A clot can result in a stroke (if the clot is in the brain), a heart attack (if the clot is in a blood vessel of the heart), or a pulmonary embolus (a clot which forms in the legs or pelvis, then breaks off and travels to the lungs). Any of these can be fatal. Clots also occur rarely in the blood vessels of the eye, resulting in blindness or impairment of vision in that eye. There is evidence that the risk of clotting increases with higher estrogen doses. It is therefore important to keep the dose of estrogen as low as possible, so long as the oral contraceptive used has an acceptable pregnancy rate and doesn't cause unacceptable changes in the menstrual pattern. Furthermore, cigarette smoking by oral contraceptive users increases the risk of serious adverse effects on the heart and blood vessels. This risk increases with age and with heavy smoking (15 or more cigarettes per day) and begins to become quite marked in women over 35 years of age. For this reason women who use oral contraceptives should not smoke.

The risk of abnormal clotting increases with age in both users and nonusers of oral contraceptives, but the increased risk from the contraceptive appears to be present at all ages. For oral contraceptive users in general, it has been estimated that in women between the ages of 15 and 34 the risk of death due to a circulatory disorder is about 1 in 12,000 per year, whereas for nonusers the rate is about 1 in 50,000 per year. In the age group 35 to 44, the risk is estimated to be about 1 in 2,500 per year for oral contraceptive users and about 1 in 10,000 per year for nonusers.

Even without the pill the risk of having a heart attack increases with age and is also increased by such heart attack risk factors as high blood pressure, high cholesterol, obesity, diabetes, and cigarette smoking. Without any risk factors present, the use of oral contraceptives alone may double the risk of heart attack. However, the combination of cigarette smoking, especially heavy smoking, and oral contraceptive use greatly increases the risk of heart attack. Oral contraceptive users who smoke are about 5 times more likely to have a heart attack than users who do not smoke and about 10 times more likely to have a heart attack than nonusers who do not smoke. It has been estimated that users between the ages of 30 and 39 who smoke have about a 1 in 10,000 chance each year of having a fatal heart attack compared to about a 1 in 50,000 chance in users who do not smoke, and about a 1 in 100,000 chance in nonusers who do not smoke. In the age group 40 to 44, the risk is about 1 in 1,700 per year for users who smoke compared to about 1 in 10,000 for users who do not smoke and to about 1 in 14,000 per year for nonusers who do not smoke. Heavy smoking (about 15 cigarettes or more a day) further increases the risk. If you do not smoke and have none of the other heart attack risk factors described above, you will have a smaller risk than listed. If you have several heart attack risk factors, the risk may be considerably greater than listed.

In addition to blood-clotting disorders, it has been estimated that women taking oral contraceptives are twice as likely as nonusers to have a stroke due to rupture of a blood vessel in the brain.

b. Formation of tumors. Studies have found that when certain animals are given the female sex hormone estrogen, which is an ingredient of oral contraceptives, continuously for long periods, cancers may develop in the breast, cervix, vagina, and liver.

These findings suggest that oral contraceptives may cause cancer in humans. However, studies to date in women taking currently marketed oral contraceptives have not confirmed that oral contraceptives cause cancer in humans. Several studies have found no increase in breast cancer in users, although one study suggested oral contraceptives might cause an increase in breast cancer in women who already have benign breast disease.

Women with a strong family history of breast cancer or who have breast nodules, fibrocystic disease, or abnormal mammograms or who were exposed to DES (diethylstilbestrol), an estrogen, during their mother's pregnancy must be followed very closely by their doctors if they choose to use oral contraceptives instead of another method of contraception. Many studies have shown that women taking oral contraceptives have less risk of getting benign breast disease than those who have not used oral contraceptives. Recently, strong evidence has emerged that estrogens (one component of oral contraceptives), when given for periods of more than one year to women after the menopause, increase the risk of cancer of the uterus (womb). There is also some evidence that a kind of oral contraceptive which is no longer marketed, the sequential oral contraceptive, may increase the risk of cancer of the uterus. There remains no evidence, however, that the oral contraceptives now available increase the risk of this cancer.

Oral contraceptives do cause, although rarely, a benign (nonmalignant) tumor of the liver. These tumors do not spread, but they may rupture and cause internal bleeding, which may be fatal. A few cases of cancer of the liver have been reported in women using oral contraceptives, but it is not yet known whether the drug caused them.

c. Dangers to a developing child if oral contraceptives are used in or immediately preceding pregnancy. Oral contraceptives should not be taken by pregnant women because they may damage the developing child. An increased risk of birth defects, including heart defects and limb defects, has been associated with the use of sex hormones, including oral contraceptives, in pregnancy. In addition, the developing female child whose mother has received DES (diethylstilbestrol), an estrogen, during pregnancy has a risk of getting cancer of the vagina or cervix in her teens or young adulthood. This risk is estimated to be about 1 in 1,000 exposures or less. Abnormalities of the urinary and sex organs have been reported in male offspring so exposed. It is possible that other estrogens, such as the estrogens in oral contraceptives, could have the same effect in the child if the mother takes them during pregnancy.

If you stop taking oral contraceptives to become pregnant, your doctor may recommend that you use another method of contraception for a short while. The reason for this is that there is evidence from studies in women who have had "miscarriages" soon after stopping the pill that the lost fetuses are more likely to be abnormal. Whether there is an overall increase in "miscarriage" in women who become pregnant soon after stopping the pill as compared with women who do not use the pill is not known, but it is possible that there may be. If, however, you do become pregnant soon after stopping oral contraceptives, and do not have a miscarriage, there is no evidence that the baby has an increased risk of being abnormal.

d. Gallbladder disease. Women who use oral contraceptives have a greater risk than nonusers of having gallbladder disease requiring surgery. The increased risk may first appear within 1 year of use and may double after 4 or 5 years of use.

e. Other side effects of oral contraceptives. Some women using oral contraceptives experience unpleasant side effects that are not dangerous and are not likely to damage their health. Some of these may be temporary. Your breasts may feel tender, nausea and vomiting may occur, you may gain or lose weight and your ankles may swell. A spotty darkening of the skin, particularly of the face, is possible and may persist. You may notice unexpected vaginal bleeding or changes in your menstrual period. Irregular bleeding is frequently seen when using the mini-pill or combination oral contraceptives containing less than 50 micrograms of estrogen.

More serious side effects include worsening of migraine, asthma, epilepsy, and kidney or heart disease because of a tendency for water to be retained in the body when oral contraceptives are used. Other side effects are growth of preexisting fibroid tumors of the uterus; mental depression; and liver problems with jaundice (yellowing of the skin). Your doctor may find that levels of sugar and fatty substances in your blood are elevated; the long-term effects of these changes are not known. While taking oral contraceptives some women develop high blood pressure which may persist after discontinuation.

Other reactions, although not proved to be caused by oral contraceptives, are occasionally reported. These include more frequent urination and some discomfort when urinating, nervousness, dizziness, some loss of scalp hair, an increase in body hair, an increase or decrease in sex drive, appetite changes, cataracts, and a need for a change in contact lens prescription or inability to use contact lenses.

After you stop using oral contraceptives there may be a delay before you are able to become pregnant or before you resume having menstrual periods. This is especially true of women who had irregular menstrual cycles prior to the use of oral contraceptives. As discussed previously, your doctor may recommend that you wait a short while after stopping the pill before you try to become pregnant. During this time, use another form of contraception. You should consult your physician before resuming use of oral contraceptives after childbirth, especially if you plan to nurse your baby. Drugs in oral contraceptives are known to appear in the milk, and the long-range effects on infants is not known at this time. Furthermore, oral contraceptives may cause a decrease in your milk supply as well as in the quality of the milk.

4. Comparison of the Risks of Oral Contraceptives and Other Contraceptive Methods. The many studies on the risks and effectiveness of oral contraceptives and other methods of contraception have been analyzed to estimate the risk of death associated with various methods of contraception. This risk has two parts: (a) the risk of the method itself (e.g., the risk that oral contraceptives will cause death due to abnormal clotting), and (b) the risk of death due to pregnancy or abortion in the event the method fails. The results of this analysis are shown in the bar graph below. The height of the bars is the number of deaths per 100,000 women each year. There are six sets of bars, each set referring to specific age groups of women. Within each set of bars there is a single bar for each of the different contraceptive methods. For oral contraceptives, there are two bars—one for smokers and the other for nonsmokers. The analysis is based on present knowledge and new information could, of course, alter it. The analysis shows that the risk of death from all methods of birth control is low and below that associated with child birth, except for oral contraceptives in women over 40 who smoke. It shows that the lowest risk of death is associated with the condom or diaphragm (traditional contraception) backed up by early abortion in case of failure of the condom or diaphragm to prevent pregnancy. Also, at any age the risk of death (due to unexpected pregnancy) from the use of traditional contraception, even without a backup of abortion, is generally the same as or less than that from use of oral contraceptives. (See Figure 1)

OVCON-50, -35

How to Use Oral Contraceptives as Safely and Effectively as Possible, Once You Have Decided to Use Them:

NOTE:

Reduced effectiveness and an increased incidence of breakthrough bleeding have been associated with the use of oral contraceptives with antibiotics such as rifampicin, ampicillin, and tetracycline or with certain other drugs, such as barbiturates, phenylbutazone or phenytoin sodium. You should use an additional means of contraception during any cycle in which any of these drugs are taken.

1. What to Tell your Doctor.

You can make use of the pill as safe as possible by telling your doctor if you have any of the following:

a. Conditions that mean you should not use oral contraceptives:

Clots in the legs or lungs.

Clots in the legs or lungs in the past.

A stroke, heart attack, or angina pectoris.

Known or suspected cancer of the breast or sex organs.

Unusual vaginal bleeding that has not yet been diagnosed.

Known or suspected pregnancy.

b. Conditions that your doctor will want to watch closely or which might cause him to suggest another method of contraception:

A family history of breast cancer.

Breast nodules, fibrocystic disease of the breast, or an abnormal mammogram.

Diabetes.

High blood pressure.

High cholesterol.

Cigarette smoking.

Migraine headaches.

Heart or kidney disease.

Epilepsy.

Mental depression.

Fibroid tumors of the uterus.

Gallbladder disease.

c. Once you are using oral contraceptives, you should be alert for signs of a serious adverse effect and call your doctor if they occur:

Sharp pain in the chest, coughing blood, or sudden shortness of breath (indicating possible clots in the lungs).

Pain in the calf (possible clot in the leg).

Crushing chest pain or heaviness (indicating possible heart attack).

Sudden severe headache or vomiting, dizziness or fainting, disturbance of vision or speech or weakness or numbness in an arm or leg (indicating a possible stroke).

Sudden partial or complete loss of vision (indicating a possible clot in the eye).

Breast lumps (you should ask your doctor to show you how to examine your own breasts).

Severe pain in the abdomen (indicating a possible ruptured tumor of the liver).

Severe depression.

Yellowing of the skin (jaundice).

2. How to Take the Pill So That It Is Most Effective. To achieve maximum contraceptive effectiveness, OVCON-50 or OVCON-35 must be taken exactly as directed and at intervals not exceeding 24 hours.

For Dosage and Administration see "DOSAGE AND ADMINISTRATION" section of professional labeling.

3. Use of oral contraceptives in the event of a missed menstrual period:

OVCON-50, -35

Figure 1.
Estimated annual number of deaths associated with control of fertility and no control per 100,000 nonsterile women, by regimen of control and age of women.

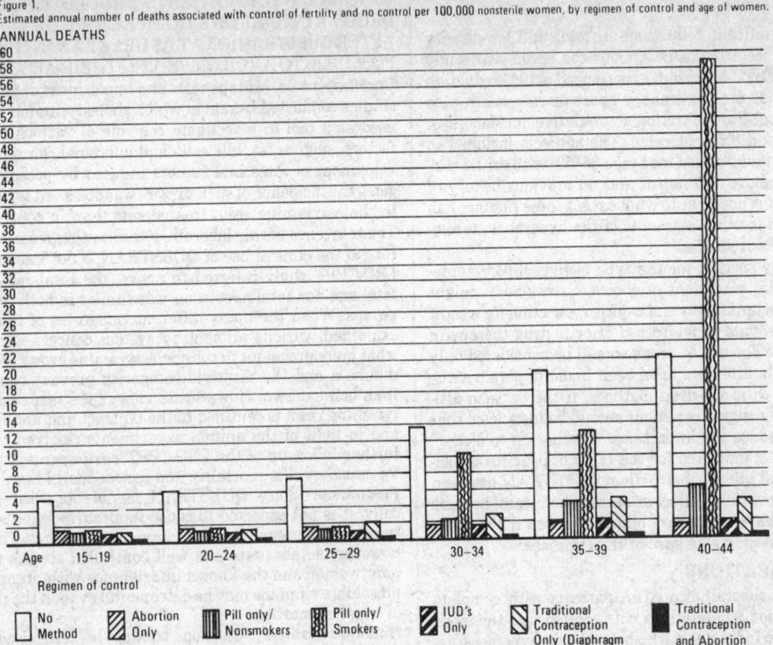

a. If the patient has not adhered to the prescribed dosage regimen, the possibility of pregnancy should be considered after the first missed period and oral contraceptives should be withheld until pregnancy has been ruled out.

b. If the patient has adhered to the prescribed regimen and misses two consecutive periods, pregnancy should be ruled out before continuing the contraceptive regimen.

c. At times there may be no menstrual period after a cycle of pills. Therefore, if you miss one menstrual period but have taken the pills **exactly as you were supposed to,** continue as usual into the next cycle. If you have not taken the pills correctly and miss a menstrual period, you may be pregnant and should stop taking oral contraceptives until your doctor determines whether or not you are pregnant. Until you can get to your doctor, use another form of contraception. If two consecutive menstrual periods are missed, you should stop taking pills until it is determined whether you are pregnant. If you do become pregnant while using oral contraceptives, you should discuss the risks to the developing child with your doctor.

4. Periodic Examination.

Your doctor will take a complete medical and family history before prescribing oral contraceptives. At that time and about once a year thereafter, he will generally examine your blood pressure, breasts, abdomen, and pelvic organs (including a Papanicolaou smear, i.e., test for cancer).

5. Note.

Each Ovcon-50 tablet (both yellow and green tablets) and the green tablets in the 28-day Ovcon-35 contain FD&C Yellow No. 5 (tartrazine) which may cause allergic type reactions (such as asthma symptoms) in a small number of women. Although the overall incidence of this allergy is very low, it may occur in persons who are also allergic to aspirin.

SUMMARY

Oral contraceptives are the most effective method, except sterilization, for preventing pregnancy. Other methods, when used conscientiously, are also very effective and have fewer risks. The serious risks of oral contraceptives are uncommon and the "pill" is a very convenient method of preventing pregnancy.

If you have certain conditions or have had these conditions in the past, you should not use oral contraceptives because the risk is too great. These conditions are listed in the leaflet. If you do not have these conditions, and decide to use the "pill," please read the leaflet carefully so that you can use the "pill" most safely and effectively.

Based on his or her assessment of your medical needs, your doctor has prescribed this drug for you. Do not give the drug to anyone else.

Shown in Product Identification Section, page 417

QUESTRAN® POWDER ℞
[kwest 'răn]
(Cholestyramine Resin Powder)

DESCRIPTION

QUESTRAN Powder (cholestyramine resin powder), the chloride salt of a basic anion exchange resin, a cholesterol lowering agent, is intended for oral administration. Cholestyramine resin is quite hydrophilic, but insoluble in water. The cholestyramine resin in QUESTRAN is not absorbed from the digestive tract. Nine grams of QUESTRAN Powder contain 4 grams of anhydrous cholestyramine resin. It is represented by the following structural formula:

Representation of structure of main polymeric groups

This product contains the following inactive ingredients: acacia, citric acid, FD&C Yellow No. 5 (tartrazine), FD&C Yellow No. 6, flavor (natural and artificial), polysorbate 80, propylene glycol alginate, and sucrose.

CLINICAL PHARMACOLOGY

Cholesterol is probably the sole precursor of bile acids. During normal digestion, bile acids are secreted into the intestines. A major portion of the bile acids is absorbed from the intestinal tract and returned to the liver via the enterohepatic circulation. Only very small amounts of bile acids are found in normal serum.

QUESTRAN resin adsorbs and combines with the bile acids in the intestine to form an insoluble complex which is excreted in the feces. This results in a partial removal of bile acids from the enterohepatic circulation by preventing their absorption.

The increased fecal loss of bile acids due to QUESTRAN administration leads to an increased oxidation of cholesterol to bile acids, a decrease in beta lipoprotein or low density lipoprotein plasma levels and a decrease in serum cholesterol levels. Although in man QUESTRAN (cholestyramine resin) produces an increase in hepatic synthesis of cholesterol, plasma cholesterol levels fall.

In patients with partial biliary obstruction, the reduction of serum bile acid levels by QUESTRAN reduces excess bile acids deposited in the dermal tissue with resultant decrease in pruritus.

INDICATIONS AND USAGE

1) QUESTRAN is indicated as adjunctive therapy to diet for the reduction of elevated serum cholesterol in patients with primary hypercholesterolemia (elevated low density lipoprotein [LDL] cholesterol) who do not respond adequately to diet. QUESTRAN may be useful to lower LDL cholesterol in patients who also have hypertriglyceridemia, but it is not indicated where hypertriglyceridemia is the abnormality of most concern.

In a large, placebo-controlled, multi-clinic study, the LRC-CPPT[a], hypercholesterolemic subjects treated with QUES-

Continued on next page

Mead Johnson Labs.—Cont.

TRAN had significant reductions in total and low-density lipoprotein cholesterol (LDL-C). Over the seven-year study period the QUESTRAN group experienced a 19% reduction in the combined rate of coronary heart disease death plus non-fatal myocardial infarction (cumulative incidences of 7% Questran and 8.6% placebo). The subjects included in the study were middle-aged men (age 35–59) with serum cholesterol levels above 265 mg/dl and no previous history of heart disease. It is not clear to what extent these findings can be extrapolated to other segments of the hypercholesterolemic population not studied.
Dietary therapy specific for the type of hyperlipoproteinemia is the initial treatment of choice. Excess body weight may be an important factor and caloric restriction for weight normalization should be addressed prior to drug therapy in the overweight. The use of drugs should be considered only when reasonable attempts have been made to obtain satisfactory results with non-drug methods. If the decision ultimately is to use drugs, the patient should be instructed that this does not reduce the importance of adhering to diet.
2) QUESTRAN is indicated for the relief of pruritus associated with partial biliary obstruction. QUESTRAN has been shown to have a variable effect on serum cholesterol in these patients. Patients with primary biliary cirrhosis may exhibit an elevated cholesterol as part of their disease.

CONTRAINDICATIONS

QUESTRAN is contraindicated in patients with complete biliary obstruction where bile is not secreted into the intestine and in those individuals who have shown hypersensitivity to any of its components.

PRECAUTIONS

General: Before instituting therapy with QUESTRAN (cholestyramine resin), diseases contributing to increased blood cholesterol such as hypothyroidism, diabetes mellitus, nephrotic syndrome, dysproteinemias and obstructive liver disease should be looked for and specifically treated. A favorable trend in cholesterol reduction should occur during the first month of QUESTRAN therapy. The therapy should be continued to sustain cholesterol reduction. If adequate cholesterol reduction is not attained, QUESTRAN therapy should be discontinued.
Chronic use of QUESTRAN may be associated with increased bleeding tendency due to hypoprothrombinemia associated with Vitamin K deficiency. This will usually respond promptly to parenteral Vitamin K_1 and recurrences can be prevented by oral administration of Vitamin K_1. Reduction of serum or red cell folate has been reported over long term administration of QUESTRAN. Supplementation with folic acid should be considered in these cases.
There is a possibility that prolonged use of QUESTRAN, since it is a chloride form of anion exchange resin, may produce hyperchloremic acidosis. This would especially be true in younger and smaller patients where the relative dosage may be higher.
QUESTRAN may produce or worsen pre-existing constipation. Dosage should be reduced or discontinued in such cases. Fecal impaction and aggravation of hemorrhoids may occur. Every effort should be made to avert severe constipation and its inherent problems in those patients with clinically symptomatic coronary artery disease.
This product contains FD&C Yellow No. 5 (tartrazine) which may cause allergic-type reactions (including bronchial asthma) in certain susceptible individuals. Although the overall incidence of FD&C Yellow No. 5 (tartrazine) sensitivity in the general population is low, it is frequently seen in patients who also have aspirin hypersensitivity.
Information for Patients: Inform your physician if you are pregnant or plan to become pregnant or are breast feeding. Drink plenty of fluids and mix each 9-gram dose of QUESTRAN Powder in at least 2 to 6 ounces of fluid before taking.
Laboratory Tests: Serum cholesterol levels should be determined frequently during the first few months of therapy and periodically thereafter. Serum triglyceride levels should be measured periodically to detect whether significant changes have occurred.
Drug Interactions: QUESTRAN may delay or reduce the absorption of concomitant oral medication such as phenylbutazone, warfarin, chlorothiazide (acidic) or propranolol (basic), as well as tetracycline, penicillin G, phenobarbital, thyroid and thyroxine preparations, and digitalis. The discontinuance of QUESTRAN (cholestyramine resin) could pose a hazard to health if a potentially toxic drug such as digitalis has been titrated to a maintenance level while the patient was taking QUESTRAN.
Because cholestyramine binds bile acids, QUESTRAN may interfere with normal fat digestion and absorption and thus may prevent absorption of fat soluble vitamins such as A, D and K. When QUESTRAN is given for long periods of time, concomitant supplementation with water-miscible (or parenteral) form of vitamins A and D should be considered.)
SINCE QUESTRAN MAY BIND OTHER DRUGS GIVEN CONCURRENTLY, PATIENTS SHOULD TAKE OTHER DRUGS AT LEAST ONE HOUR BEFORE OR 4–6 HOURS AFTER QUESTRAN (OR AT AS GREAT AN INTERVAL AS POSSIBLE) TO AVOID IMPEDING THEIR ABSORPTION.
Carcinogenesis, Mutagenesis and Impairment of Fertility: In studies conducted in rats in which cholestyramine resin was used as a tool to investigate the role of various intestinal factors, such as fat, bile salts and microbial flora, in the development of intestinal tumors induced by potent carcinogens, the incidence of such tumors was observed to be greater in cholestyramine resin treated rats than in control rats.
The relevance of this laboratory observation from studies in rats to the clinical use of QUESTRAN is not known. In the LRC-CPPT study referred to above, the total incidence of fatal and non-fatal neoplasms was similar in both treatment groups. When the many different categories of tumors are examined, various alimentary system cancers were somewhat more prevalent in the cholestyramine group. The small numbers and the multiple categories prevent conclusions from being drawn. However, in view of the fact that cholestyramine resin is confined to the GI tract and not absorbed, and in light of the animal experiments referred to above, further follow-up of the LRC-CPPT participants is planned for cause-specific mortality and cancer morbidity.
Pregnancy: Since QUESTRAN is not absorbed systemically, it is not expected to cause fetal harm when administered during pregnancy in recommended dosages. There are, however, no adequate and well controlled studies in pregnant women and the known interference with absorption of fat soluble vitamins may be detrimental even in the presence of supplementation.
Nursing Mothers: Caution should be exercised when QUESTRAN is administered to a nursing mother. The possible lack of proper vitamin absorption described in the "Pregnancy" section may have an effect on nursing infants.
Pediatric Use: As experience in infants and children is limited, a practical dosage schedule has not been established. In calculating pediatric dosage, 44.4 mg of anhydrous cholestyramine resin are contained in 100 mg of QUESTRAN.
The effects of long term drug administration, as well as its effect in maintaining lowered cholesterol levels in pediatric patients, are unknown.

ADVERSE REACTIONS

The most common adverse reaction is constipation. When used as a cholesterol lowering agent predisposing factors for most complaints of constipation are high dose and increased age (more than 60 years old). Most instances of constipation are mild, transient, and controlled with conventional therapy. Some patients require a temporary decrease in dosage or discontinuation of therapy.
Less Frequent Adverse Reactions: Abdominal discomfort, flatulence, nausea, vomiting, diarrhea, heartburn, anorexia, indigestive feeling and steatorrhea, bleeding tendencies due to hypoprothrombinemia (Vitamin K deficiency) as well as Vitamin A (one case of night blindness reported) and D deficiencies, hyperchloremic acidosis in children, osteoporosis, rash and irritation of the skin, tongue and perianal area.
One ten month old baby with biliary atresia had an impaction presumed to be due to QUESTRAN (cholestyramine resin) after three days administration of 9 grams daily. She developed acute intestinal sepsis and died.
Occasional calcified material has been observed in the biliary tree, including calcification of the gall bladder, in patients to whom cholestyramine resin has been given. However, this may be a manifestation of the liver disease and not drug related.
One patient experienced biliary colic on each of three occasions on which he took QUESTRAN. One patient diagnosed as acute abdominal symptom complex was found to have a "pasty mass" in the transverse colon on x-ray.
Other events (not necessarily drug-related) reported in patients taking QUESTRAN include:
Gastrointestinal—GI-rectal bleeding, black stools, hemorrhoidal bleeding, bleeding from known duodenal ulcer, dysphagia, hiccups, ulcer attack, sour taste, pancreatitis, rectal pain, diverticulitis.
Hematologic—Increased prothrombin time, ecchymosis, anemia.
Hypersensitivity—Urticaria, asthma, wheezing, shortness of breath.
Musculoskeletal—Backache, muscle and joint pains, arthritis.
Neurologic—Headache, anxiety, vertigo, dizziness, fatigue, tinnitus, syncope, drowsiness, femoral nerve pain, paresthesia.
Eye—Uveitis.
Renal—Hematuria, dysuria, burnt odor to urine, diuresis.
Miscellaneous—Weight loss, weight gain, increased libido, swollen glands, edema, dental bleeding.

OVERDOSAGE

Overdosage of QUESTRAN has not been reported. Should overdosage occur, however, the chief potential harm would be obstruction of the gastrointestinal tract. The location of such potential obstruction, the degree of obstruction, and the presence or absence of normal gut motility would determine treatment.

DOSAGE AND ADMINISTRATION

The recommended adult dose is one packet or one scoopful (9 grams of QUESTRAN Powder contain 4 grams of anhydrous cholestyramine resin) one to six times daily. Dosage may be adjusted as required to meet the patient's needs.
QUESTRAN should not be taken in its dry form. Always mix QUESTRAN Powder with water or other fluids before ingesting. See Preparation Instructions.

PREPARATION

The color of QUESTRAN (cholestyramine resin) may vary somewhat from batch to batch, but this variation does not affect the performance of the product. Place the contents of one packet or one level scoopful of QUESTRAN in a glass or cup. Add 2–6 ounces of water or the noncarbonated beverage of your choice. Stir to a uniform consistency.
QUESTRAN may also be mixed with highly fluid soups or pulpy fruits with a high moisture content such as applesauce or crushed pineapple.

HOW SUPPLIED

QUESTRAN is available in cartons of fifty 9-gram packets and in cans containing 378 grams. Nine grams of QUESTRAN Powder contain 4 grams of anhydrous cholestyramine resin.
NDC 0087-0580-01 Cartons of 50 packets
NDC 0087-0580-05 Cans, 378 gm

CLINICAL STUDIES

The NIH has concluded a 10-year randomized double-blind placebo-controlled study[a] in 12 lipid research clinics on the effect of lowering plasma cholesterol on coronary heart disease (CHD) risk (the risk of either coronary death or non-fatal myocardial infarction). Plasma cholesterol was lowered by a combination of a modest cholesterol-lowering diet and QUESTRAN. The dose response relationship between the amount of QUESTRAN ingested daily, the lowering of total plasma cholesterol, and the reduction in CHD risk is summarized below:

RELATION OF REDUCTION IN CHOLESTEROL TO REDUCTON IN CORONARY HEART DISEASE RISK

Packet Count	No.	Total Cholesterol Lowering	Reduction in CHD Risk
0–2	439	4.4%	10.9%
2–5	496	11.5%	26.1%
5–6	965	19.0%	39.3%

REFERENCE

[a]Anon: The Lipid Research Clinics Coronary Primary Prevention Trial Results: (I) Reduction in Incidence of Coronary Heart Disease; (II) The Relationship of Reduction in Incidence of Coronary Heart Disease to Cholesterol Lowering. JAMA 1984; 251:351–374.
Revised: January, 1985

QUIBRON® ℞
[kwi'bron]
(Theophylline-Guaifenesin)

DESCRIPTION

Each Quibron® soft gelatin capsule or tablespoon (15 ml) of liquid contains 150 mg of theophylline (anhydrous) and 90 mg of guaifenesin, as an oral bronchodilator-expectorant. Quibron Liquid contains no alcohol and is dye-free.

QUIBRON®-300 ℞
(Theophylline-Guaifenesin)

DESCRIPTION

Each Quibron®-300 soft gelatin capsule contains 300 mg of theophylline (anhydrous) and 180 mg of guaifenesin, as an oral bronchodilator-expectorant. The structural formulae for the active ingredients of Quibron and Quibron–300 are presented below:

Theophylline
(1*H*-Purine-2,6-Dione, 3,7-Dihydro-1,3-Dimethyl-)

H_3C O H N N N O N CH_3 — OCH_3 — $OCH_2CHOH-CH_2OH$

Guaifenesin
[3-(o-Methoxy phenoxy)-1,2-propanediol]

Theophylline, a xanthine compound, is a white, odorless crystalline powder, having a bitter taste.
Guaifenesin, a guaiacol compound, is a white to slightly yellow crystalline powder with a bitter, aromatic taste.

INACTIVE INGREDIENTS

QUIBRON and QUIBRON-300 Capsules contain: D&C Yellow No. 10, non-porcine gelatin, glycerin, edible ink, polyethylene glycol, and titanium dioxide.
QUIBRON Liquid contains: flavors, propylene glycol, sodium hydroxide, sorbitol solution, sucrose, and purified water.

CLINICAL PHARMACOLOGY

Theophylline

Mode of Action

Theophylline acts as a bronchodilator by direct relaxation of bronchial smooth muscle. Theophylline is a competitive inhibitor of cyclic nucleotide phosphodiesterase resulting in increased intracellular levels of cAMP which mediates smooth muscle relaxation. Like some other xanthines, theophylline acts as a coronary vasodilator, cardiac stimulant, skeletal muscle stimulant, central nervous system stimulant and diuretic.

Pharmacokinetics

As theophylline is released from the formulation it is, under usual conditions, absorbed completely and fairly rapidly. Excretion, principally as inactive metabolites, occurs primarily via the kidney. The half-life of theophylline varies among individuals with a wide range having been documented. Theophylline half-life is shortened in cigarette smokers. Half-life is prolonged in alcoholism, reduced hepatic or renal function, congestive heart failure and in patients receiving antibiotics such as troleandomycin or erythromycin. High fever for prolonged periods may decrease theophylline elimination. The theophylline half-life is generally shorter in children.

Representative Theophylline Serum Half-lives

	Half-life (hours) Mean	Range
Adults		
non-smokers	8.7	6.1–12.8
smokers	5.5	4.0– 7.7
congestive heart failure	22.9	3.1–82.0
Children (6–16 yrs)	3.7	1.4– 7.9

Therapeutic serum theophylline levels are usually 10–20 μg/ml.
Binding to plasma proteins is not extensive and theophylline is not preferentially taken up by any particular organ.
Theophylline-containing products may increase the plasma levels of free fatty acids and the urinary levels of epinephrine and norepinephrine.
Apparently no development of tolerance occurs with chronic use of theophylline.

CLINICAL PHARMACOLOGY

Guaifenesin

Mode of Action

Guaifenesin increases respiratory tract secretions, possibly by stimulating the goblet cells.

Pharmacokinetics

Guaifenesin appears to be well absorbed, but its pharmacokinetics has not been well studied.

INDICATIONS AND USAGE

Quibron and Quibron–300 are indicated for the symptomatic treatment of bronchospasm associated with such conditions as bronchial asthma, chronic bronchitis and pulmonary emphysema.

CONTRAINDICATIONS

Quibron products are contraindicated in individuals who have shown hypersensitivity to any of their components or xanthine derivatives.

WARNINGS

Excessive theophylline doses may be associated with toxicity; thus serum theophylline levels should be monitored to assure maximal benefit without excessive risk.
Serum levels of theophylline above the accepted therapeutic range (10–20 μg/ml) are associated with an increased incidence of toxicity. Such levels may be reached with customary doses in individuals who metabolize the drug slowly, especially patients (1) with lowered body plasma clearance (2) with liver dysfunction or chronic obstructive pulmonary disease or (3) older than 55 years of age, particularly males.
Serious toxicity, such as seizure or ventricular arrhythmias, is not necessarily preceded by less serious side-effects such as nausea, irritability or restlessness.
Many patients who have higher (greater than 20 μg/ml) theophylline serum levels exhibit tachycardia. Theophylline products may exacerbate pre-existing arrhythmias.

PRECAUTIONS

General

Use with caution in patients with severe cardiac disease, hypertension, acute myocardial injury, congestive heart failure, cor pulmonale, severe hypoxemia, hyperthyroidism, hepatic impairment, history of peptic ulcer, alcoholism and in the elderly. Concurrent administration with certain antibiotics (see DRUG INTERACTIONS section) may result in increased serum theophylline levels.
A decrease in serum half-life is seen in smokers (see Clinical Pharmacology/Pharmacokinetics).
Particular caution should be used in administering theophylline to patients in congestive heart failure. Reduced theophylline clearance in these patients may cause theophylline blood levels to persist long after discontinuing the drug.
Theophylline should not be administered concurrently with other xanthine medications.

Usage in Pregnancy

Teratogenic effects: Pregnancy Category C. Animal reproduction studies have not been conducted with Quibron products. It is also not known whether Quibron products can cause fetal harm when administered to a pregnant woman or can affect reproduction capacity. Quibron products should be given to a pregnant woman only if clearly indicated.
Nonteratogenic effects: It is not known whether use of this drug during labor or delivery has immediate or delayed adverse effects on the fetus, or whether it prolongs the duration of labor or increases the possibility of forceps delivery or other obstetrical intervention.

Nursing Mothers

Theophylline has been reported to be excreted in human milk and to have caused irritability in a nursing infant. Because of the potential for serious adverse reactions, a decision should be made whether to discontinue nursing or to discontinue Quibron or Quibron–300, taking into account the importance of this drug to the mother.

Drug Interactions

Drug	Effect
Theophylline with lithium carbonate	Increased renal excretion of lithium
Theophylline with propranolol	Mutual antagonism of therapeutic effects
Theophylline with furosemide	Increased diuresis
Theophylline with reserpine	Tachycardia
Theophylline with chlordiazepoxide	Fatty acid mobilization
Theophylline with troleandomycin or erythromycin	Increased theophylline plasma levels

Drug/Laboratory Test Interactions

Theophylline may interfere with the assay of uric acid, especially the phosphotungstate method. Thus, serum uric acid levels may be overestimated. Metabolites of guaifenesin may contribute to increased 5–hydroxyindoleacetic acid readings when determined with nitrosonaphthol reagent.

ADVERSE REACTIONS

The frequency of adverse reactions is related to serum theophylline levels and is usually not a problem at levels below 20 μg/ml. The most consistent adverse reactions are usually due to overdosage and, while all have not been reported with Quibron or Quibron–300, the following reactions may be considered when theophylline is administered. Central nervous system: clonic and tonic generalized convulsions, muscle twitching, reflex hyperexcitability, headaches, insomnia, restlessness, and irritability. Cardiovascular: circulatory failure, ventricular arrhythmias, hypotension, extrasystoles, tachycardia, palpitation, and flushing. Gastrointestinal: hematemesis, vomiting, diarrhea, epigastric pain, and nausea. Renal: increased excretion of renal tubular cells and red blood cells, albuminuria, and diuresis. Respiratory: tachypnea. Others: hyperglycemia and inappropriate ADH syndrome.

OVERDOSAGE

Symptoms

Nervousness, agitation, headache, insomnia, vomiting, tachycardia, extrasystoles, hyperreflexia, fasciculations and clonic and tonic convulsions. Children may be particularly prone to restlessness and hyperactivity that can proceed to convulsions.

Management

If potential oral overdose is established and seizure has **not** occurred.

1. Induce vomiting.
2. Administer a cathartic (this is particularly important if sustained release preparations have been taken).
3. Administer activated charcoal.
4. Monitor vital signs, maintain blood pressure and provide adequate hydration.

If patient is having seizure

1. Establish an airway.
2. Administer O_2.
3. Treat the seizure with intravenous diazepam 0.1 to 0.3 mg/kg up to 10 mg.
4. Monitor vital signs, maintain blood pressure and provide adequate hydration.

Post-Seizure Coma

1. Maintain airway and oxygenation.
2. If a result of oral medication, follow above recommendations to prevent absorption of drug, but intubation and lavage will have to be performed instead of inducing emesis and the cathartic and charcoal will need to be introduced via a large bore gastric lavage tube.
3. Continue to provide full supportive care and adequate hydration while waiting for drug to be metabolized. In general, the drug is metabolized rapidly enough so as to not warrant consideration of dialysis.

General

The oral LD_{50} of theophylline in mice is 350 mg/kg. The oral LD_{50} of guaifenesin in mice is 1725 mg/kg. In humans, adverse reactions often occur when serum theophylline levels exceed 20 μg/ml. Information on physiological variables which influence excretion of theophylline can be found under the heading "Clinical Pharmacology."

DOSAGE AND ADMINISTRATION

General

Therapeutic serum levels associated with optimal likelihood for benefit and minimal risk of toxicity are considered to be between 10 and 20 μg/ml, although levels of 5-10 μg/ml are reported to be effective for some patients. Levels above 20 μg/ml may produce toxic effects. There is great variation from patient to patient and dosage must be individualized because there is a relatively narrow range between therapeutic and toxic levels of theophylline. Monitoring of serum theophylline levels is highly recommended. Since theophylline does not distribute into fatty tissue, dosage should be calculated on the basis of ideal body weight.
Giving theophylline with food may prevent the rare case of stomach irritation and, although absorption may be slower, it is still complete.

Quibron

Treatment should be *initiated* at a dose of 16 mg/kg/day or 400 mg/day, whichever is smaller. The usual adjusted dosages are—Adults: 1–2 capsules or 1–2 tablespoons (15 ml) liquid every 6–8 hours. Children 9 to 12: 4–5 mg theophylline/kg body weight every 6–8 hours. Children under 9: 4–6 mg theophylline/kg body weight every 6–8 hours.
Approximate mg/kg dosage by TEASPOON (5 ml) of Quibron Liquid may be determined from the following table:

BODY WEIGHT		AVERAGE DOSAGE IN TEASPOONS (5 ml) TO PROVIDE THE FOLLOWING MG OF THEOPHYLLINE/ KG BODY WEIGHT/DOSE		
Lbs	Kgs	4 mg/kg	5 mg/kg	6 mg/kg
20	9	3/4	1	1
30	14	1	1½	1¾
40	18	1½	2	2¼
50	23	1¾	2¼	2¾
60	27	2	2¾	3¼
70	32	2½	3	3¾
80	36	3	3½	4¼
90	41	3¼	4	5
100	46	3½	4½	5½

If the desired response is not achieved with the recommended initial dose, and there are no adverse reactions, the dose may be cautiously adjusted upward in increments of no more than 25 percent at 2–3 day intervals until the following MAXIMUM DOSE WITHOUT MEASUREMENT OF SERUM CONCENTRATION or a maximum of 900 mg in any 24 hour period (whichever is less) is attained:

MAXIMUM DAILY DOSE WITHOUT MEASUREMENT OF SERUM CONCENTRATION	mg per kg Body Weight*
Children (under 9)	24
Children (9–12)	20
Adolescents (12–16)	18
Adults	13

*Use ideal body weight for obese patients

Do not attempt to maintain any dose that is not tolerated. If doses higher than those contained in the above MAXIMUM DOSE WITHOUT MEASUREMENT OF SERUM CONCENTRATION are necessary, it is recommended that serum theophylline levels be monitored. For therapeutic levels, draw blood sample just before next dose is due; for toxic levels, draw blood sample when last dose peaks (~2 hours after dosing). It is important that the patient has missed no doses during the previous 72 hours and that dosing intervals have been reasonably typical with no added doses during that period of time. DOSAGE ADJUSTMENT BASED ON SERUM THEOPHYLLINE MEASUREMENTS WHEN THESE INSTRUCTIONS HAVE **NOT** BEEN FOLLOWED, MAY RESULT IN RECOMMENDATIONS THAT PRESENT RISK OF TOXICITY TO THE PATIENT.

Quibron–300 Capsules

Quibron–300 is appropriate therapy when higher theophylline dosages are required. The usual recommended dosages for Quibron–300 are **Adults:** 1 capsule every 6–8 hours for

Continued on next page

Mead Johnson Labs.—Cont.

patients whose dosage has been adjusted upward to achieve therapeutic serum levels.

HOW SUPPLIED

Quibron® Capsules (yellow) in bottles of 100 (NDC 0087-0516-01); and 1000 (NDC 0087-0516-02). Unit Dose 100's (NDC 0087-0516-03).

Quibron® Liquid in 1 pint (NDC 0087-0510-03) and 1 gallon (NDC 0087-0510-01).

Quibron®–300 Capsules (yellow and white) in bottles of 100 (NDC 0087-0515-41).

Store at controlled room temperature of 59°–86°F (15°–30°C).

Shown in Product Identification Section, page 417

QUIBRON®–T ℞

[kwĭ'bran]

(Theophylline Anhydrous)

DIVIDOSE® TABLETS

DESCRIPTION

QUIBRON®-T tablets provide 300 mg of anhydrous theophylline as an oral bronchodilator in an immediate release formulation combined with the convenience of the unique DIVIDOSE® tablet design. With functional trisects and bisects, QUIBRON-T tablets can be conveniently and accurately divided into 100, 150, and 200 mg segments to provide a variety of dosing increments, as required.

QUIBRON-T tablets

One-third tablet	= 100 mg
One-half tablet	= 150 mg
Two-thirds tablet	= 200 mg
One tablet	= 300 mg

The product contains the following inactive ingredients: microcrystalline cellulose, yellow ferric oxide, hydroxypropyl methylcellulose 2910, lactose, magnesium stearate, colloidal silicon dioxide, and sodium starch glycolate.

Theophylline is a white, odorless, crystalline powder which has a bitter taste. It is chemically related to caffeine and its structure is shown below:

H_3C O H N N N O N CH_3

Theophylline

(1*H*-Purine-2,6-dione, 3,7-dihydro-1,3,-dimethyl-)

CLINICAL PHARMACOLOGY

Mode of Action

Theophylline acts as a bronchodilator by direct relaxation of bronchial smooth muscle. Theophylline is a competitive inhibitor of cyclic nucleotide phosphodiesterase resulting in increased intracellular levels of cAMP which mediates smooth muscle relaxation. Like some other xanthines, theophylline acts as a coronary vasodilator, cardiac stimulant, skeletal muscle stimulant, cerebral stimulant and diuretic. *In vitro*, theophylline has been shown to act synergistically with beta agonists that increase intracellular cyclic AMP through the stimulation of adenyl cyclase, but synergism has not been demonstrated in patient studies. More data are needed to determine if theophylline and beta agonists have a clinically important additive effect *in vivo*. Apparently, no development of tolerance occurs with chronic use of theophylline.

Pharmacokinetics

Theophylline excretion, principally as inactive metabolites, occurs primarily via the kidney. The half-life of theophylline varies among individuals with a wide range having been documented. Theophylline half-life is shortened in cigarette smokers. Half-life is prolonged in alcoholism, reduced hepatic or renal function, congestive heart failure, and patients receiving macrolide antibiotics (troleandomycin and erythromycin) or cimetidine. High fever for prolonged periods may decrease theophylline elimination. Older adults (over age 55) and patients with chronic obstructive pulmonary disease, with or without cor pulmonale, may also have much slower clearance rates. For such patients, the theophylline half-life may exceed 24 hours. The theophylline half-life is generally shorter in children.

It appears that between three months and two years of cessation of smoking may be necessary for elimination of the effect of smoking on theophylline pharmacokinetics.

Representative Theophylline Serum Half-Lives

	Half-life (hours)	
	Mean	Range
Adults		
non-smokers	8.7	6.1–12.8
smokers	5.5	4.0–7.7
congestive heart failure	22.9	3.1–82.0
Children (6–16 years)	3.7	1.4–7.9

Binding to plasma proteins is not extensive and theophylline is not preferentially taken up by any particular organ.

Theophylline-containing products may increase the plasma levels of free fatty acids and the urinary levels of epinephrine and norepinephrine.

INDICATIONS AND USAGE

QUIBRON-T is indicated for relief and/or prevention of symptoms from asthma and reversible bronchospasm associated with chronic bronchitis and emphysema.

CONTRAINDICATIONS

QUIBRON-T is contraindicated in individuals who have shown hypersensitivity to any of its components or xanthine derivatives.

WARNINGS

Status asthmaticus should be considered a medical emergency and is defined as that degree of bronchospasm which is not rapidly responsive to usual doses of conventional bronchodilators. Optional therapy for such patients frequently requires both ADDITIONAL MEDICATION, parenterally administered, and CLOSE MONITORING, preferably in an intensive care setting.

Although increasing the dose of theophylline may bring about relief, such treatment may be associated with toxicity. The likelihood of the development of such toxicity increases significantly when the serum theophylline concentration exceeds 20 μg/ml. Therefore, determination of serum theophylline levels is recommended to assure maximal benefit without excessive risk.

Serum levels above 20 μg/ml are rarely found after appropriate administration of the recommended doses. However, in individuals in whom theophylline plasma clearance is reduced for any reason, even conventional doses may result in increased serum levels and potential toxicity. Reduced theophylline clearance has been documented in the following readily identifiable groups: 1) patients with impaired renal or liver function; 2) patients over 55 years of age, particularly males and those with chronic lung disease; 3) those with cardiac failure from any cause; 4) neonates; and 5) those patients taking certain drugs (macrolide antibiotics and cimetidine). Decreased clearance of theophylline may be associated with either influenza immunization or active influenza infection. Reduction in dosage and laboratory monitoring are especially appropriate in the above individuals.

Less serious signs of theophylline toxicity (i.e., nausea and restlessness) may occur frequently when initiating therapy, but are usually transient; when such signs are persistent during therapy, they are often associated with serum concentrations above 20 mcg/ml. Unfortunately, however, serious side effects such as ventricular arrhythmias, convulsions, or even death may appear as the first sign of toxicity without any previous warning. Stated differently: SERIOUS TOXICITY IS NOT RELIABLY PRECEDED BY LESS SEVERE SIDE EFFECTS.

Many patients who require theophylline may exhibit tachycardia due to their underlying disease process so that the cause/effect relationship to elevated serum theophylline concentrations may not be appreciated.

Theophylline products may cause dysrhythmia and/or worsen pre-existing arrhythmias; any significant change in rate and/or rhythm warrants monitoring and further investigation.

The occurrence of arrhythmias and sudden death (with histological evidence of necrosis of the myocardium) has been recorded in laboratory animals (minipigs, rodents, and dogs) when theophylline and beta agonists were administered concomitantly, although not when either was administered alone. The significance of these findings when applied to human usage is currently unknown.

PRECAUTIONS

General: Theophylline half-life is shorter in smokers than in non-smokers. Therefore, smokers may require larger or more frequent doses.

Morphine and curare should be used with caution in patients with airway obstruction as they may suppress respiration and stimulate histamine release. Alternative drugs should be used when possible.

Use with caution in neonates, the elderly (especially males), and in patients with severe cardiac disease, hypertension, acute myocardial injury, congestive heart failure, cor pulmonale, severe hypoxemia, hyperthyroidism, hepatic impairment, history of peptic ulcer, or alcoholism. Concurrent administration with certain antibiotics (see DRUG INTERACTIONS section) may result in increased serum theophylline levels.

Particular caution should be used in administering theophylline to patients in congestive heart failure. Reduced theophylline clearance in these patients may cause theophylline blood levels to persist long after discontinuing the drug.

Theophylline should not be administered concurrently with other xanthine medications.

Use theophylline cautiously in patients with a history of peptic ulcer. Theophylline may occasionally act as a local irritant to the GI tract, although gastrointestinal symptoms are more commonly centrally mediated and associated with serum drug concentrations over 20 μg/ml.

Information for Patients: Patients should be instructed carefully on how to divide QUIBRON-T tablets along the appropriate tablet score.

The physician should reinforce the importance of taking only the prescribed dose and observing the correct time interval between doses.

Patients should be instructed to alert their physician if symptoms occur repeatedly, especially near the end of a dosing interval.

Drug Interactions: Toxic synergism with ephedrine has been documented and may occur with some other sympathomimetic bronchodilators. In addition, the following drug interactions have been demonstrated:

Drug	Effect
Theophylline with lithium carbonate	Increased renal excretion of lithium
Theophylline with propranolol	Mutual antagonism of therapeutic effects
Theophylline with cimetidine	Increased serum theophylline levels
Theophylline with troleandomycin or erythromycin	Increased serum theophylline levels

Drug/Laboratory Test Interactions: Spectrophotometric determination of theophylline is affected by coffee, tea, cola beverages, chocolate, and acetaminophen, which contribute to falsely high values.

Carcinogenesis, Mutagenesis, and Impairment of Fertility: Long-term animal studies have not been performed to evaluate the carcinogenic potential, mutagenic potential, or the effect on fertility of xanthine compounds.

Usage in Pregnancy: Pregnancy Category C. Animal reproduction studies have not been conducted with QUIBRON products. It is also not known whether QUIBRON products can cause fetal harm when administered to a pregnant woman or can affect reproduction capacity. QUIBRON products should be given to a pregnant woman only if clearly indicated.

Nursing Mothers: Theophylline has been reported to be excreted in human milk and to have caused irritability in a nursing infant. Because of the potential for serious adverse reactions, a decision should be made whether to discontinue nursing or to discontinue QUIBRON-T, taking into account the importance of this drug to the mother.

Pediatric Use: Due to the marked variation in theophylline metabolism in infants under 1 year old, this drug is not recommended for this age group.

ADVERSE REACTIONS

The frequency of adverse reactions is related to serum theophylline levels and is usually not a problem at levels below 20 μg/ml. The most consistent adverse reactions are usually due to overdosage and, while not all have been reported with QUIBRON-T, the following reactions may be considered when theophylline is administered. Central nervous system: clonic and tonic generalized convulsions, muscle twitching, reflex hyperexcitability, headaches, insomnia, restlessness, and irritability. Cardiovascular: circulatory failure, ventricular arrhythmias, hypotension, extrasystoles, tachycardia, palpitation, and flushing. Gastrointestinal: hematemesis, vomiting, diarrhea, epigastric pain, and nausea. Renal: increased excretion of renal tubular cells and red blood cells, albuminuria, and potentiation of diuresis. Respiratory: tachypnea. Others: hyperglycemia and inappropriate ADH syndrome, rash.

OVERDOSAGE

Symptoms: Nervousness, agitation, headache, insomnia, vomiting, tachycardia, extrasystoles, hyperreflexia, fasciculations, and clonic and tonic convulsions. Children may be particularly prone to restlessness and hyperactivity that can proceed to convulsions.

Management: If potential oral overdose is established and seizure has not occurred:

1. Induce vomiting.
2. Administer a cathartic (this is particularly important if sustained-release preparations have been taken).
3. Administer activated charcoal.
4. Monitor vital signs, maintain blood pressure and provide adequate hydration.

If patient is having seizure:

1. Establish an airway.
2. Administer O_2.
3. Treat the seizure with intravenous diazepam 0.1 to 0.3 mg/kg up to 10 mg.
4. Monitor vital signs, maintain blood pressure and provide adequate hydration.

Post-seizure coma:

1. Maintain airway and oxygenation.
2. If a result of oral medication, follow above recommendations to prevent absorption of drug, but intubation and lavage will have to be performed instead of inducing emesis, and the cathartic and charcoal will need to be introduced via a large bore gastric lavage tube.
3. Continue to provide full supportive care and adequate hydration while waiting for drug to be metabolized. In general, the drug is metabolized rapidly enough so as to not warrant consideration of dialysis; however, if serum levels exceed 50 μg/ml, charcoal hemoperfusion may be indicated.

General: The oral LD_{50} of theophylline in mice is 350 mg/kg. In humans, adverse reactions often occur when serum theophylline levels exceed 20 μg/ml. Information on physiological variables which influence excretion of theophylline can be found under the heading, "Clinical Pharmacology."

DOSAGE AND ADMINISTRATION

General: For most patients, effective use of theophylline, i.e., associated with optimal likelihood of benefit combined with minimal risk of toxicity, is considered to occur when serum levels are maintained between 10 and 20 μg/ml. Levels above 20 μg/ml may produce toxicity and, in a small number of patients, toxicity may even be seen with serum levels between 15–20 μg/ml, particularly during initiation of therapy.

There is considerable variation from patient to patient in the dosage required to achieve and maintain therapeutic and safe levels, primarily due to variable rates of elimination. Therefore, it is essential that not only must dosage be individualized, but titration and monitoring of serum levels be utilized where available. When serum concentration cannot be obtained, restriction of dosage to the amounts and intervals recommended in the guidelines listed below becomes essential. Dosage should be calculated on the basis of lean (ideal) body weight where mg/kg doses are presented. Theophylline does not distribute into fatty tissue. Giving theophylline with food may prevent some local gastric irritation and, though absorption is slower, it is still complete.

Dosing Frequency: When immediate-release products with rapid absorption (such as QUIBRON-T Tablets) are used, dosing to maintain serum levels generally requires administration every six hours. This is particularly true in children, but dosing intervals up to eight hours may be satisfactory in adults since they eliminate the drug at a slower rate. Some children, and adults requiring higher-than-average doses (those having rapid rates of clearance, e.g., half-lives of under six hours), may benefit and be more effectively controlled during chronic therapy when given a product with sustained-release characteristics (such as QUIBRON-T/SR), since these provide longer dosing intervals and/or less fluctuation in serum concentration between dosing. Those sustained-release products which provide flexibility in dosage through formulations of varying strengths are also helpful in controlling serum levels.

Dosing guidelines are approximations only and the wide range of theophylline clearance between individuals (particularly those with concomitant disease) makes indiscriminate usage hazardous.

As a practical consideration, it is not always possible to obtain serum level determinations. Under such conditions, restriction of the daily dose (in otherwise healthy adults) to not greater than 13 mg/kg/day (of anhydrous theophylline) in divided doses will result in relatively few patients exceeding serum levels of 20 μg/ml and the resultant risk of toxicity.

DOSAGE GUIDELINES

I. Acute symptoms of asthma requiring rapid theophyllinization

	Oral Loading	Followed by:	Maintenance:
Children 1 to 9 years	6 mg/kg	4 mg/kg q 4h × 3 doses	4 mg/kg q 6 h
Children age 9–16 years and young adult smokers	6 mg/kg	3 mg/kg q 4h × 3 doses	3 mg/kg q 6 h
Otherwise healthy, non-smoking adults	6 mg/kg	3 mg/kg q 6h × 2 doses	3 mg/kg q 8 h
Older patients and patients with cor pulmonale	6 mg/kg	2 mg/kg q 6h × 2 doses	2 mg/kg q 8 h
Patients with congestive heart failure	6 mg/kg	2 mg/kg q 8h × 2 doses	1–2 mg/kg q 12 h

A. Patients not currently receiving theophylline products (dosage recommendations are for anhydrous theophylline)

[See table above].

B. Patients currently receiving theophylline products: Determine, where possible, the time, amount, dosage form, and route of administration of the patient's last dose.

The loading dose for theophylline is based on the principle that each 0.5 mg/kg of theophylline administered as a loading dose will result in a 1.0 μg/ml increase in serum theophylline concentration. Ideally, the loading dose should be deferred if a serum theophylline concentration can be obtained rapidly.

If this is not possible, the clinician must exercise his judgment in selecting a dose based on the potential for benefit and risk. When there is sufficient respiratory distress to warrant a small risk, then 2.5 mg/kg of theophylline administered in rapidly-absorbed form is likely to increase serum concentration by approximately 5 μg/ml. If the patient is not experiencing theophylline toxicity, this is unlikely to result in dangerous adverse effects.

Subsequent to the decision regarding modification of the loading dose for this group of patients, the maintenance dosage recommendations are the same as those described above.

II. Chronic Therapy: Theophylline administration is a treatment of first choice for the management of chronic asthma (to prevent symptoms and maintain patent airways). Slow clinical titration is generally preferred to assure acceptance and safety of the medications.

Initial Dose: 16 mg/kg/24 hours or 400 mg/24 hours (whichever is less) of anhydrous theophylline in divided doses at 6- or 8-hour intervals.

Increasing Dose: The above dosage may be increased in approximately 25% increments at 2–3 day intervals so long as the drug is tolerated, until the maximum dose indicated in Section III (below) is reached.

III. Maximum Dose of Theophylline Where the Serum Concentration is Not Measured: If the desired response is not achieved with the recommended initial dose and there are no adverse reactions, the dose may be cautiously adjusted upward in increments of no more than 25% at 2–3 day intervals until the following maximum dose without measurement of serum concentration or a maximum of 900 mg in any 24-hour period (whichever is less) is attained:

WARNING: DO NOT ATTEMPT TO MAINTAIN ANY DOSE THAT IS NOT TOLERATED.

Not to exceed the following:

Age ≤ 9 years	24 mg/kg/day
Age 9–12 years	20 mg/kg/day
Age 12–16 years	18 mg/kg/day
Age ≥ 16 years	13 mg/kg/day OR 900 mg WHICHEVER IS LESS

IV. Measurement of Serum Theophylline Concentrations During Chronic Therapy: If the above maximum doses are to be maintained or exceeded, serum theophylline measurement is recommended. The serum sample should be obtained at the time of peak absorption (1–2 hours after administration for immediate-release products; 4 hours after dosing for most sustained-release formulations). It is important that the patient will have missed no doses during the previous 48 hours and that dosing intervals will have been reasonably typical, with no added doses during that period of time. DOSAGE ADJUSTMENT BASED ON SERUM THEOPHYLLINE MEASUREMENTS WHEN THESE INSTRUCTIONS HAVE NOT BEEN FOLLOWED MAY RESULT IN RECOMMENDATIONS THAT PRESENT RISK OF TOXICITY TO THE PATIENT.

V. Final Adjustment of Dosage

[See table below].

If serum theophylline is:		Directions:
Within normal limits	10 to 20 μg/ml	Maintain dosage if tolerated. Recheck serum theophylline concentration at 6-to 12-month intervals.*
Too high	20 to 25 μg/ml	Decrease doses by about 10%. Recheck serum theophylline concentration at 6-to 12-month intervals.*
	25 to 30 μg/ml	Skip next dose and decrease subsequent doses by about 25%.
	Over 30 μg/ml	Skip next 2 doses and decrease subsequent doses by 50%. Recheck serum theophylline.
Too low	7.5 to 10 μg/ml	Increase dose by about 25%. ** Recheck serum theophylline concentration at 6- to 12-month intervals.*
	5 to 7.5 μg/ml	Increase dose by about 25% to the nearest dose increment and recheck serum theophylline for guidance in further dosage adjustment. (Another increase will probably be needed, but this provides a safety check.)

* Finer adjustments in dosage may be needed for some patients.

** The total daily dose may need to be administered at more frequent intervals if symptoms occur repeatedly at the end of a dosing interval.

From **The Journal of Respiratory Diseases** 2(7):16, 1981.

Caution should be exercised for younger children who cannot complain of minor side effects. Older adults, those with cor pulmonale, congestive heart failure, and/or liver disease may have unusually low dosage requirements and, thus, may experience toxicity at the maximal dosage recommended above.

It is important that no patient be maintained on any dosage that is not tolerated. In instructing patients to increase dosage according to the schedule above, they should be instructed not to take a subsequent dose if apparent side effects occur and to resume therapy at a lower dose once adverse effects have disappeared.

DOSAGE OF THEOPHYLLINE TO PROVIDE mg ANHYDROUS THEOPHYLLINE/kg BODY WEIGHT*/DOSE

Body Weight* Lbs.	Kg	Approximate Dose in mg 3 mg/kg	4 mg/kg	6 mg/kg
20	9	27	36	54
30	14	42	56	84
40	18	54	72	109
50	23	69	92	138
60	27	81	108	162
70	32	96	128	192
80	36	108	144	216
90	41	123	164	246
100	46	138	184	276
120	55	165	220	330
140	64	192	256	384
160	73	219	292	438
180	82	246	328	492
200	91	273	364	546
220	100	300	400	600

*For obese patients, use lean (i.e., ideal) body weight.

HOW SUPPLIED

QUIBRON-T Tablets: Ivory, in the DIVIDOSE® tablet design with debossed "MJ" logo and "512" containing 300 mg anhydrous theophylline, in bottles of 100 (NDC 0087-0512-41). Store below 86°F (30°C).

Shown in Product Identification Section, page 417

QUIBRON®-T/SR ℞

[kwĭ'bran]

(Theophylline Anhydrous)

DIVIDOSE® TABLETS

PRODUCT OVERVIEW

KEY FACTS

Quibron®-T/SR tablets provide 300 mg of anhydrous theophylline in sustained release form as an oral bronchodilator. The unique Dividose® tablet design offers convenience and flexibility in dosage titration with 100, 150, and 200 mg segments.

MAJOR USES

Quibron-T/SR tablets are indicated for the symptomatic treatment of bronchospasm associated with such conditions as bronchial asthma, chronic bronchitis and pulmonary emphysema.

SAFETY INFORMATION

Excessive theophylline doses may be associated with toxicity; thus, serum theophylline levels should be monitored to assure maximal benefit without excessive risk. Quibron-T/SR tablets should not be crushed or chewed.

Continued on next page

Mead Johnson Labs.—Cont.

PRESCRIBING INFORMATION

QUIBRON®-T/SR ℞

[*kwĭ'bran*]

(Theophylline Anhydrous)

DIVIDOSE® TABLETS

DESCRIPTION

Quibron®-T/SR tablets provide 300 mg of anhydrous theophylline as an oral bronchodilator in a sustained release formulation combined with the convenience of the unique Dividose® tablet design. With functional trisects and bisects. Quibron-T/SR tablets can be conveniently and accurately divided into 100, 150, and 200 mg segments to provide a variety of dosing increments, as required.

QUIBRON-T/SR tablets

One-third tablet	= 100 mg
One-half tablet	= 150 mg
Two-thirds tablet	= 200 mg
One tablet	= 300 mg

Theophylline is a white odorless crystalline powder which has a bitter taste. It is chemically related to caffeine and its structure is shown below:

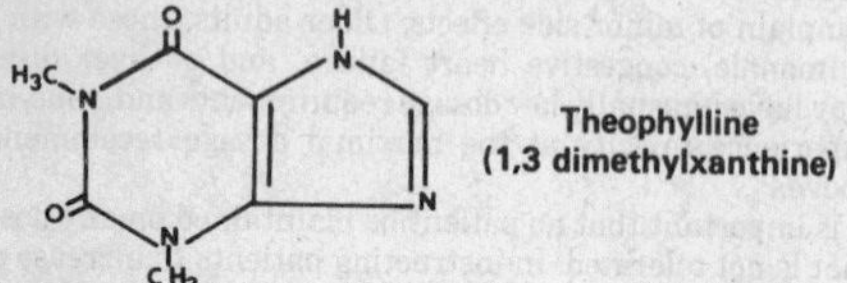

This product contains the following inactive ingredient: magnesium stearate.

CLINICAL PHARMACOLOGY

Mode of Action: Theophylline acts as a bronchodilator by direct relaxation of bronchial smooth muscle. Theophylline is a competitive inhibitor of cyclic nucleotide phosphodiesterase resulting in increased intracellular levels of cAMP which mediates smooth muscle relaxation. Like some other xanthines, theophylline acts as a coronary vasodilator, cardiac stimulant, skeletal muscle stimulant, central nervous system stimulant and diuretic.

Pharmacokinetics: Theophylline is, under usual conditions, absorbed completely and fairly rapidly. Excretion, principally as inactive metabolites, occurs primarily via the kidney. The half-life of theophylline varies among individuals with a wide range having been documented. Theophylline half-life is shorter in cigarette smokers. Half life is prolonged in alcoholism, reduced hepatic or renal function, congestive heart failure, and in patients receiving antibiotics such as troleandomycin and erythromycin. High fever for prolonged periods may decrease theophylline elimination. The theophylline half-life is generally shorter in children.

Representative Theophylline Serum Half-lives

	Half-life (hours) Mean	Range
Adults		
non-smokers	8.7	6.1–12.8
smokers	5.5	4.0–7.7
congestive heart failure	22.9	3.1–82.0
Children (6–16 years)	3.7	1.4–7.9

Therapeutic serum theophylline levels are usually 10–20 μg/ml.

Binding to plasma proteins is not extensive and theophylline is not preferentially taken up by any particular organ.

Theophylline-containing products may increase the plasma levels of free fatty acids and the urinary levels of epinephrine and norepinephrine.

Apparently no development of tolerance occurs with chronic use of theophylline.

INDICATIONS AND USAGE

Quibron-T/SR tablets are indicated for the symptomatic treatment of bronchospasm associated with such conditions as bronchial asthma, chronic bronchitis and pulmonary emphysema.

CONTRAINDICATIONS

Quibron-T/SR tablets are contraindicated in individuals who have shown hypersensitivity to any of its components or xanthine derivatives.

WARNINGS

Excessive theophylline doses may be associated with toxicity; thus serum theophylline levels should be monitored to assure maximal benefit without excessive risk.

Serum levels of theophylline above the accepted therapeutic range (10–20 μg/ml) are associated with an increased incidence of toxicity. Such levels may be reached with customary doses in individuals who metabolize the drug slowly, especially patients (1) with lowered body plasma clearance, (2) with liver dysfunction or chronic obstructive pulmonary disease, or (3) older than 55 years of age, particularly males. Serious toxicity, such as seizure, ventricular arrhythmias, is not necessarily preceded by less serious side-effects such as nausea, irritability or restlessness. Many patients who have higher (greater than 20 μg/ml) theophylline serum levels exhibit tachycardia. Theophylline products may exacerbate pre-existing arrhythmias.

PRECAUTIONS

General: Quibron T/SR tablets should not be chewed or crushed.

Use with caution in patients with severe cardiac disease, hypertension, acute myocardial injury, congestive heart failure, cor pulmonale, severe hypoxemia, hyperthyroidism, hepatic impairment, history of peptic ulcer, alcoholism, and in the elderly. Concurrent administration with certain antibiotics (see DRUG INTERACTIONS section) may result in increased serum theophylline levels.

A decrease in serum half-life is seen in smokers (see Clinical Pharmacology/Pharmacokinetics).

Particular caution should be used in administering theophylline to patients in congestive heart failure. Reduced theophylline clearance in these patients may cause theophylline blood levels to persist long after discontinuing the drug.

Theophylline should not be administered concurrently with other xanthine medications.

Patients should be instructed carefully on how to divide Quibron-T/SR tablets along the appropriate tablet score.

Sustained release theophylline is not useful in status asthmaticus.

Usage in Pregnancy: Teratogenic effects: Pregnancy Category C. Animal reproduction studies have not been conducted with Quibron-T/SR tablets. it is also not known whether Quibron-T/SR tablets can cause fetal harm when administered to a pregnant woman or can affect reproduction capacity. Quibron-T/SR tablets should be given to a pregnant woman only if clearly indicated.

Nonteratogenic effects: It is not known whether use of this drug during labor or delivery has immediate or delayed adverse effects on the fetus, or whether it prolongs the duration of labor or increases the possibility of forceps delivery or other obstetrical intervention.

Nursing Mothers: Theophylline has been reported to be excreted in human milk and to have caused irritability in a nursing infant. Because of the potential for serious adverse reactions, a decision should be made whether to discontinue nursing or to discontinue Quibron-T/SR tablets, taking into account the importance of this drug to the mother.

Drug Interactions

Drug	Effect
Theophylline with lithium carbonate	Increased renal excretion of lithium
Theophylline with propranolol	Mutual antagonism of therapeutic effects
Theophylline with cimetidine	Increased serum theophylline levels
Theophylline with clindamycin	Increased serum theophylline levels
Theophylline with lincomycin	Increased serum theophylline levels
Theophylline with troleandomycin or erythromycin	Increased serum theophylline levels

Drug/Laboratory Test Interactions: Theophylline may interfere with the assay of uric acid, especially the phosphotungstate method. Thus, serum uric acid levels may be overestimated.

ADVERSE REACTIONS

The frequency of adverse reactions is related to serum theophylline levels and is usually not a problem at levels below 20 μg/ml. The most consistent adverse reactions are usually due to overdosage and, while not all have not been reported with Quibron-T and/or with Quibron-T/SR tablets, the following reactions may be considered when theophylline is administered. Central nervous system: clonic and tonic generalized convulsions, muscle twitching, reflex hyperexcitability, headaches, insomnia, restlessness, and irritability. Cardiovascular: circulatory failure, ventricular arrhythmias, hypotension, extrasystoles, tachycardia, palpitation, and flushing. Gastrointestinal: hematemesis, vomiting, diarrhea, epigastric pain, and nausea. Renal: increased excretion of renal tubular cells and red blood cells, albuminuria, and diuresis. Respiratory: tachypnea. Others: hyperglycemia and inappropriate ADH syndrome.

OVERDOSAGE

Symptoms: Nervousness, agitation, headache, insomnia, nausea, vomiting, tachycardia, extrasystoles, hyperreflexia, fasciculations and clonic and tonic convulsions. Children may be particularly prone to restlessness and hyperactivity that can proceed to convulsions.

Management: If potential oral overdose is established and seizure has *not* occurred

1. Induce vomiting.
2. Administer a cathartic (this is particularly important if a sustained release preparation has been taken).
3. Administer activated charcoal.
4. Monitor vital signs, maintain blood pressure and provide adequate hydration.

If patient is having seizure

1. Establish an airway.
2. Administer O_2.
3. Treat the seizure with intravenous diazepam 0.1 to 0.3 mg/kg up to a total dose of 10 mg.
4. Monitor vital signs, maintain blood pressure and provide adequate hydration.

Post-seizure Coma

1. Maintain airway and oxygenation.
2. If the reaction occurs after oral medication, follow above recommendations to prevent absorption of drug, but intubation and lavage will have to be performed instead of inducing emesis and the cathartic and charcoal will need to be introduced via a large bore gastric lavage tube.
3. Continue to provide full supportive care and adequate hydration while waiting for drug to be metabolized. In general, the drug is metabolized sufficiently rapidly enough so as to not warrant consideration of dialysis.

General: The oral LD_{50} of theophylline in mice is 350 mg/kg. In humans, adverse reactions often occur when serum theophylline levels exceed 20 μg/ml. Information on physiological variables which influence excretion of theophylline can be found under the heading "Clinical Pharmacology."

DOSAGE AND ADMINISTRATION

General: Therapeutic serum levels associated with optimal likelihood for benefit and minimal risk of toxicity are considered to be between 10 μg/ml and 20 μg/ml although levels of 5–10 μg/ml have been reported to be effective for some patients. Levels above 20 μg/ml may produce toxic effects. Because of the variable rates of theophylline elimination among patients the dose necessary to achieve the desired serum level of 10–20 μg theophylline per ml varies from patient to patient. Thus, dosage must be individualized (see CLINICAL PHARMACOLOGY and WARNINGS sections) because there is a relatively narrow range between therapeutic and toxic levels of theophylline. Monitoring of serum theophylline levels is highly recommended.

Since theophylline does not distribute into fatty tissue, dosage should be calculated on the basis of ideal body weight.

Giving theophylline with food may prevent the rare case of stomach irritation and, although absorption may be slower, it is still complete.

The average initial dose for children (under 9 years of age) is one-third (100 mg) of a Quibron-T/SR tablet q 12 h.

The average initial dose for children (ages 9–12) is one half (150 mg) of a Quibron-T/SR tablet q 12 h.

The average initial dose for adolescents (ages 12–16) is two thirds (200 mg) of a Quibron-T/SR tablet q 12 h.

The average initial dose for adults is two thirds (200 mg) of a Quibron-T/SR tablet q 12 h.

If the desired response is not achieved with the recommended initial dose, and there are no adverse reactions, the dose may be cautiously adjusted upward in increments of no more than 25 percent at 2–3 day intervals until the following MAXIMUM DOSE WITHOUT MEASUREMENT OF SERUM CONCENTRATION or, in the case of adults, a maximum of 900 mg in any 24 hour period (whichever is less) is attained:

MAXIMUM DOSE WITHOUT MEASUREMENT OF SERUM CONCENTRATION

	mg per kg Body Weight* per day**
Children (under 9)	24
Children (9–12)	20
Adolescents (12–16)	18
Adults	13

*Use ideal body weight for obese patients.

**Some patients who clear theophylline more rapidly (e.g., children and heavy smokers) may require dosing at intervals more frequent than 12 hours.

Do not attempt to maintain any dose that is not tolerated. If doses higher than those contained in the above MAXIMUM DOSE WITHOUT MEASUREMENT OF SERUM CONCENTRATION are necessary, it is recommended that serum theophylline levels be monitored. For therapeutic levels draw blood sample when last dose peaks (4–5 hours after dosing). It is important that the patient has missed no doses during the previous 72 hours and that dosing intervals have been reasonably typical with no doses added during that period of time. DOSE ADJUSTMENT BASED ON SERUM THEOPHYLLINE MEASUREMENTS MADE WHEN THESE INSTRUCTIONS HAVE NOT BEEN FOLLOWED MAY RESULT IN RECOMMENDATIONS THAT PRESENT RISK OF TOXICITY TO THE PATIENT.

HOW SUPPLIED

Quibron-T/SR (white, in the Dividose® tablet design) containing 300 mg anhydrous theophylline.

NDC-0087-0519-41 Bottles of 100
NDC 0087-0519-44 Bottles of 500

Store below 86°F(30°C).

Shown in Product Identification Section, page 417

Mead Johnson Nutritional Division
Mead Johnson & Company
2404 W. PENNSYLVANIA ST.
EVANSVILLE, INDIANA 47721

b-CAPSA® I VACCINE ℞
(Haemophilus b Polysaccharide Vaccine)

DESCRIPTION

b-CAPSA® I Vaccine (Haemophilus b Polysaccharide Vaccine) is a sterile, lyophilized vaccine for intramuscular or subcutaneous administration. It is the capsular polysaccharide purified from the bacterium, Haemophilus influenzae type b, strain Eag and is a polymer of ribose, ribitol, and phosphate.

b-CAPSA® I Vaccine is manufactured according to methods developed by Praxis Biologics, Inc. Following growth in a unique, chemically defined, protein-free liquid medium, the bacteria are inactivated and separated. The polysaccharide is isolated from the culture supernatant by membrane filtration and precipitation with hexadecyltrimethylammonium bromide, and then purified from bacterial protein, nucleic acid, and endotoxin by physicochemical techniques.[1] The resulting high molecular weight polysaccharide is dissolved in lactose solution, sterilized by filtration, filled into vials, and lyophilized. Lactose is included in the vaccine at a concentration of 2.5 mg per 0.5 ml dose to improve product stability.[2] The lyophilized vaccine contains 25 μg of purified Haemophilus b polysaccharide per dose. The reconstituted vaccine contains thimerosal (mercurial derivative) 1:10,000 and sodium chloride for isotonicity. When reconstituted, *b*-CAPSA® I Vaccine is a clear, colorless liquid.

CLINICAL PHARMACOLOGY

Haemophilus influenzae type b is the most common cause of bacterial meningitis and a leading cause of serious, systemic bacterial diseases in young children in the United States. This vaccine will not stimulate protection against other types of Haemophilus influenzae or other microorganisms that cause meningitis or septic disease.

Several population-based studies conducted within the last 10 years in the U.S. indicate that a child's cumulative risk of developing systemic Haemophilus influenzae b (Hib) disease at some time during the first 5 years of life is about 1 in 200.[3] About 60% of the children have meningitis and 40% other systemic diseases, such as cellulitis, epiglottitis, pericarditis, pneumonia, sepsis, or septic arthritis.[3] In these U.S. studies, about 35–40% of systemic Hib disease has occurred in children 18 months of age or older. In contrast, a recent prospective, five-year analysis of all children in Finland indicated that 60% of bacteremic Hib disease occurred in children 18 months of age or older and 45% in those 2 or more years of age.[4]

The incidence of systemic Hib disease is increased in certain children, e.g., Eskimo[5] and American Indian[6] children, patients with asplenia, sickle cell disease,[7] and antibody deficiency syndromes.[8] Recent studies also indicate that Haemophilus influenzae b can cause outbreaks of systemic disease among previously healthy children attending nursery school or day care, and that attendance at day care significantly increases the risk of developing systemic Hib disease.[9–11] Furthermore, the risk of acquiring systemic Hib disease for a child in intimate contact with one who has developed such a disease is up to 400 times that of a child in the general population.[9]

Hib diseases usually can be treated successfully. Even with appropriate antibiotic therapy, however, the mortality rate of Hib meningitis[12] and other bacteremic diseases can be 5%, and serious, long-term neurologic sequelae have been observed in 19–45% of survivors of meningitis.[3,13] Up to 20% of Haemophilus influenzae b isolated in the USA from patients with systemic disease are resistant to ampicillin,[12,14] and the mortality rate of meningitis is significantly greater when it is caused by ampicillin-resistant than by ampicillin-sensitive Haemophilus influenzae b.[12] Moreover, resistance to chloramphenicol and to multiple antibiotics has emerged.[14] When properly administered, rifampin can prevent bacteremic Hib disease among contacts at risk,[15] and its use for this purpose has been recommended by health authorities.[15,16] Implementation of those recommendations can be difficult, however, especially in the setting of a large group. Thus, the strategy of controlling Hib disease by antibiotics has deficiencies.

The capsular polysaccharide of Haemophilus influenzae b (Haemophilus b polysaccharide) is its principal virulence factor. Anti-Haemophilus b polysaccharide antibody mediates complement-dependent bacteriolysis and opsonization in vitro and protects experimentally infected animals. Hyperimmune animal serum was used successfully to treat invasive human Hib diseases in the pre-antibiotic era, and antibody to the capsular polysaccharide was reported to be the protective component of that serum.[17]

For these reasons, Haemophilus b polysaccharide has been purified for use as a vaccine to prevent Hib diseases. More than 60,000 children and several hundred adults have been vaccinated with Haemophilus b polysaccharide in studies conducted in multiple centers.[4,18–23] Adverse reactions have been mild and transient. Adults and older children uniformly produce a long-lived, non-boostable antibody response.[4,18–20] Children respond variably and inversely to their age: infants respond less frequently with less antibody.[4,18–22] The percent of responding individuals increases significantly between 12 and 24 months of age.[4,18,20,22] Approximately 90% of children 24 months of age or older produce a significant antibody response to Haemophilus b polysaccharide vaccination, and most of the non-responders have high pre-vaccination titers.[4] The amount of antibody produced by children is also affected by the molecular size of the vaccine: vaccines containing high molecular weight capsular polysaccharide generate more antibody than those with low molecular weight polysaccharide.[24]

The efficacy of Haemophilus b polysaccharide vaccine was evaluated in a double-blind, controlled field trial conducted in Finland in children of 3 months to 5 years of age.[4,23] Approximately 98,000 children, half of whom received Haemophilus b polysaccharide vaccine, were followed for 4 years. In children 18–71 months of age, 90% protective efficacy (95% confidence limits, 55%–98%) in prevention of all forms of invasive Hib disease was demonstrated for the 4-year follow-up period. Of more than 4,000 children who were 18–23 months old when vaccinated, none who received Haemophilus b polysaccharide vaccine developed bacteremic Hib disease during the four years of follow-up. However, the number of cases of bacteremic Hib disease in the control group was too small to permit a meaningful assessment of Haemophilus b polysaccharide vaccine efficacy in that age group. Children younger than 18 months of age had little immunologic response to the vaccine and were not protected.

Administration of Haemophilus b polysaccharide vaccine has been recommended by the U.S. Public Health Services' Immunization Practices Advisory Committee (ACIP). The ACIP recommended that all children be immunized at 24 months of age and that immunization may be considered at 18 months of age for those in known high risk groups.[25]

Considerable evidence correlates the immunogenicity of bacterial polysaccharide vaccines with their physicochemical properties and the side effects with trace contaminants, especially endotoxin. The properties of *b*-CAPSA® I Vaccine are equivalent to those of the Haemophilus b polysaccharide vaccine used in the Finnish field trial. The unique, protein-free, chemically defined bacterial growth medium and purification procedures used in the preparation of *b*-CAPSA® I Vaccine minimize the content of protein, nucleic acids, and endotoxin and guarantee a large molecular weight.

The precise protective level of anti-Haemophilus b polysaccharide antibody has not been established. Titers associated with protection of agammaglobulinemic children[18,20] and experimentally infected animals by passively administered gamma globulin suggest that 0.15 μg/ml is protective. In a controlled field trial, levels ≥ 1 μg/ml in 3 week post-vaccination serum as determined by the Finnish antibody assay were correlated with clinical protection[26]; approximately 75% of tested 18–23 month old and 85% of 24–29 month old children achieved that level following Haemophilus b polysaccharide vaccination.[23]

Variability has been observed in the antibody results obtained by various laboratories using radioimmunoassays for measurement of anti-Hib polysaccharide antibodies. For this reason, seventy-four (74) pairs of sera from 24 to 26-month-old children were randomly selected from Haemophilus b polysaccharide vaccine immunization studies conducted in several centers. When these sera were analyzed by one radioimmunoassay, antibody responses of children from the different studies were not significantly different (ref: OBRR Study).[27]

A limited number of children have been reported to have received DTP and Haemophilus b polysaccharide vaccines at the same time.[22,24,28,29] No impairment of the immune response to individual antigens occurred. The incidence and type of associated reactions[22,24,28,29] approximated those reported for DTP vaccine.[30]

INDICATIONS AND USAGE

b-CAPSA® I Vaccine is indicated for immunization of childen 24 months to five years of age against diseases caused by Haemophilus influenzae b.

Children of 24 months of age and older have a high rate of seroconversion, and clinical studies indicate that they will be protected against bacteremic Hib diseases following a single vaccination with *b*-CAPSA® I Vaccine.

b-CAPSA® I Vaccine may be given to children 18–23 months of age known to be at high risk of systemic Hib disease, e.g., children who attend day care. A controlled field trial suggested that many children in this age group will be protected by a single vaccination, although the rate of seroconversion is not as high as with older children. Parents should be informed that the vaccine is not likely to be completely effective in this age group.

Studies are ongoing to determine the need and timing for revaccination, particularly for children vaccinated at 18–23 months of age.

b-CAPSA® I Vaccine will not protect children younger than 18 months of age and will not protect against Haemophilus influenzae other than type b or other microorganisms that cause meningitis or septic disease.

Physicians administering *b*-CAPSA® I Vaccine should recognize that antibody production by young children is a complex immunologic process and is not immediate.

CONTRAINDICATIONS

Hypersensitivity to any component of the vaccine, including thimerosal.

WARNINGS

If the vaccine is used in persons deficient in producing antibody, whether due to genetic defect or to immunosuppressive therapy, the expected immune response may not be obtained.

PRECAUTIONS

General

As with the injection of any biological material, epinephrine injection (1:1000) should be available for immediate use should an anaphylactoid reaction occur.

Any febrile illness or active infection is reason for delaying use of *b*-CAPSA® I Vaccine.

The vaccine should not be injected intradermally or intravenously, since the safety and immunogenicity of these routes of administration have not been evaluated. The vaccine should be given intramuscularly or subcutaneously.

It is important to use a separate sterile syringe and needle for each individual patient to prevent transmission of hepatitis viruses and other infectious agents from one person to another.

Pregnancy

Pregnancy Category C

Animal reproductive studies have not been conducted with *b*-CAPSA® I Vaccine. It is not known whether *b*-CAPSA® I Vaccine can cause fetal harm when administered to a pregnant woman or can affect reproductive capacity. Data are not available to support the use of this product during pregnancy at this time, regardless of benefits.

Nursing Mothers

There is no indication for using this product in nursing mothers.

Pediatric Use

b-CAPSA® I Vaccine is not recommended for infants younger than 18 months of age. See comments above about vaccine use in children older than 18 months of age.

ADVERSE REACTIONS

Different preparations of Haemophilus b polysaccharide produced by different procedures and administered at different doses have been evaluated in several field studies. Objectively observed side effects, e.g., erythema and induration at the injection site and fever, have generally been minor and lasted 24 hours or less.[18,21–23] The incidence of local side effects reported in the Finnish field trial was 51%. In all other reported trials, the incidence of these reactions was 4–9%.[18,21,22] Temperatures > 38.3°C (101°F) at 24 hours post-vaccination have occurred in up to 13% of vaccinated children. In the Finnish field trial, one child had a possible anaphylactoid reaction; following an injection of epinephrine, the child recovered rapidly and without complications.

Side effects associated with the use of *b*-CAPSA® I Vaccine were evaluated in a study conducted in physicians' offices that used 10 different lots of vaccine administered intramuscularly to 807 children of 18–60 months of age.[24] At 24 hours post-vaccination, objective local reactions (swelling, erythema) were observed in 0.6% of vaccinated children, and temperature > 38.3°C (101°F) in 0.5%.

Based on estimates with the first 2.3 million doses of *b*-CAPSA® I Vaccine administered, there were only 48 reported episodes of side effects at 24 hours or less. These were reported spontaneously by physicians to the manufacturer as follows: rash (14), vomiting/diarrhea (10), hives (9), seizures (9), and other (6). A cause and effect relationship between these side effects and the vaccination has not been established.

DOSAGE AND ADMINISTRATION

Parenteral drug products should be inspected visually for particulate matter and discoloration prior to administration whenever solution and container permit.

Continued on next page

Mead Johnson Nutr.—Cont.

Reconstitute *b*-CAPSA® I Vaccine with a sterile needle and syringe free of preservatives, antiseptics, and detergents. Use only diluent provided. The sterile diluent for reconstitution of the vaccine contains thimerosal (mercurial derivative) 1:10,000 added as the preservative and sodium chloride for isotonicity.

The lyophilized vaccine dissolves rapidly and, when reconstituted, is a clear, colorless liquid.

10 Dose Vial: Inject 6.0 ml of diluent into one vial of lyophilized *b*-CAPSA® I Vaccine. Mix to dissolve contents. The vial will deliver ten 0.5 ml doses of 25 μg Polysaccharide.

5 Dose Vial: Inject 3.0 ml of diluent into one vial of lyophilized *b*-CAPSA® I Vaccine. Mix to dissolve contents. The vial will deliver five 0.5 ml doses of 25 μg Polysaccharide.

DO NOT INJECT INTRAVENOUSLY.

The immunizing dose is a single injection of 0.5 ml of reconstituted *b*-CAPSA® I Vaccine given intramuscularly or subcutaneously. Studies to determine the need and timing of revaccination, particularly for children vaccinated at 18–23 months of age, are being conducted.

HOW SUPPLIED

No. 4001: Haemophilus b Polysaccharide *b*-CAPSA® I Vaccine contains one 10 dose vial of lyophilized vaccine and one vial containing 6.5 ml of diluent in a single package, NDC 0087-4004-41.

No. 4005: Haemophilus b Polysaccharide *b*-CAPSA® I Vaccine contains one 5 dose vial of lyophilized vaccine and one vial containing 3.3 ml of diluent in a single package, NDC 0087-4005-41.

STORAGE

b-CAPSA® I Vaccine may be shipped unrefrigerated. However, lyophilized *b*-CAPSA® I Vaccine should be refrigerated on receipt and stored, when not in use, at 2°–8°C (35°–46°F). Reconstituted *b*-CAPSA® I Vaccine is stable for 30 days when stored refrigerated at 2°–8°C (35°–46°F) as directed. The date of reconstitution should be recorded on the label of the vaccine vial. DO NOT FREEZE.

b-CAPSA® I Vaccine is manufactured by Praxis Biologics, Inc., Rochester, New York and distributed by Mead Johnson Nutritional Division, Evansville, Indiana 47721.

For information contact: MEAD JOHNSON NUTRITIONAL DIVISION at (812) 426-7480.

REFERENCES

1. Anderson, P., and Smith, D.H. Isolation of the capsular polysaccharide from the culture supernatant of **Haemophilus influenzae** b. Infect Immun 1977;15:472–477.
2. Tiesjema, R.H., Beuvery, E.C., and tePas, B.J. Enhanced stability of meningococcal polysaccharide vaccines by using lactose as a menstruum for lyophilization. Bull World Health Organ 1977;56:43–48.
3. Cochi, S.L., Broome, C.V., and Hightower, A.W. Assessment of strategies for immunization of U.S. children with **Haemophilus influenzae** type b polysaccharide vaccine: A cost-effectiveness model.
4. Peltola, H., Kayhty, H., Virtanen, M., and Makela, P.H. Prevention of **Haemophilus influenzae** type b bacteremic infections with the capsular polysaccharide vaccine. New Engl J Med 1984;310:1561–1566.
5. Ward, J.I., Margolis, H.S., Lum, M.K., Fraser, D.W., and Bender, T.R. **Haemophilus influenzae** disease in Alaskan Eskimos. Lancet 1981;i:1281–1285.
6. Coulehan, J.L., Michaels, R.H., Williams, K.E., Lemley, D.K., North, C.Q., Welty, T.K., and Rogers, K.D. Bacterial meningitis in Navajo Indians. Public Health Rep 1976;91:464–468.
7. Ward, J., and Smith, A.L. **Haemophilus influenzae** bacteremia in children with sickle cell disease. J Pediatr 1976;88:261–263.
8. Stiehm, E.R., and Fulginitti, V.A. (Eds.). Immunologic Disorders of Infants and Children. New York, W.B. Saunders, 1980.
9. Granoff, D.M. and Daum, R.S. Spread of **Haemophilus influenzae** type b: Recent epidemiologic and therapeutic considerations. J Pediatr 1980;97:854–860.
10. Redmond, S.R. and Pichichero, M.E. **Haemophilus influenzae** type b disease: An epidemiologic study with special reference to day care centers. JAMA 1984;252:2581–2584.
11. Istre, G., Conner, J., Hopkins, R., Hightower, A., and Broome, C.V. A Case Control Study of Systemic **Haemophilus influenzae** (HI) Infections: An Increased Risk from Daycare Attendance. Program and Abstracts of the Twenty-third Interscience Conference on Antimicrobial Agents and Chemotherapy 1983; Abstract No. 787, p. 229.
12. Istre, G.R., Conner, J.S., Glode, M.P., and Hopkins, R.S. Increasing ampicillin-resistance rates in **Haemophilus influenzae** meningitis. Am J Dis Child 1984;138:366–369.
13. Ferry, P.C., Culbertson, J.L., Cooper, J.A., Sitton, A.B., and Sell, S.H. Sequelae of **Haemophilus influenzae** meningitis. In: Sell, S.H., Wright, P.F., Eds. **Haemophilus influenzae,** New York. Elsevier Science Publishing Co., 1982:111–116.
14. Ampicillin and Chloramphenicol Resistance in Systemic **Haemophilus influenzae** Disease. Morbidity, Mortality Weekly Report, NCDC 1984 (Jan. 27);33:35–37.
15. Band, J.D., Fraser, D.W., and Ajello, G. Prevention of **Haemophilus influenzae** type b disease. JAMA 1984;251:2381–2384.
16. American Academy of Pediatrics, Committee on Infectious Diseases. Revision of recommendation for use of rifampin prophylaxis of contacts of patients with **Haemophilus influenzae** infection. Pediatr 1984;74:301–302.
17. Alexander, H.E., Heidelberger, M., and Leidy, G. The productive or curative element in type b **H. influenzae** rabbit serum. Yale J Biol Med 1944;16:425–434.
18. Smith, D.H., Peter, G., Ingram, D.L., Harding, A.L., and Anderson, P. Responses of children immunized with the capsular polysaccharide of **Haemophilus influenzae** type b. Pediatr 1973;52:637–645.
19. Anderson, P., Peter, G., Johnston, R.B.J., Wetterlow, L.H., and Smith, D.H. Immunization of humans with polyribophosphate, the capsular antigen of **Hemophilus influenzae** type b. J Clin Inves 1972;51:39–44.
20. Robbins, J.B., Parke, J.C., Schneerson, R., and Whisnant, J.K. Quantitative measurement of "natural" and immunization-induced **Haemophilus influenzae** type b capsular polysaccharide antibodies. Pediatr Res 1973;7:103–110.
21. Parke, J.C., Schneerson, R., Robbins, J.B., and Schlesselman, J.J. Interim report of a controlled field trial of immunization with capsular polysaccharides of **Haemophilus influenzae** type b and group C **Neisseria meningitidis** in Mecklenburg County, North Carolina. J Infect Dis 1977;136:551–556.
22. Pincus, D.J., Morrison, D., Andrews, C., et al. Age-related response of two **Haemophilus influenzae** type b vaccines. J Pediatr 1982;100:197–201.
23. Peltola, H., Kayhty, H., Sivonen, A., and Makela, H. **Haemophilus influenzae** type b capsular polysaccharide vaccine in children: A double-blind field study of 100,000 vaccinees 3 months to 5 years of age in Finland. Pediatr 1977;60:730–737.
24. Data on file at Praxis Biologics.
25. Recommendations of the Immunization Practices Advisory Committee. Polysaccharide vaccine for prevention of Haemophilus influenzae type b disease. Morbidity and Mortality Weekly Report 1985 (April 19); 34(15):201–205.
26. Kayhty, H., Peltola, H., Karanko, V., and Makela, P.H. The protective level of serum antibodies to the capsular polysaccharide of **Haemophilus influenzae** type b. J Infect Dis 1983;147:1100.
27. Data on file at Office of Biologics Research and Review (OBRR).
28. Coulehan, J.L., Hallowell, C., Michaels, R.H., Welty, T.K., Lui, N., and Kuo, J.S.C. Immunogenicity of a **Haemophilus influenzae** type b vaccine in combination with diphtheria-pertussis-tetanus vaccine in infants. J Infect Dis 1983;148:530–534.
29. Lepow, M.L., Peter, G., Glode, M.P., Daum, R.S., Calnen, G., Knight, K.M., Mayer, D., Kuo, J.S.C., and Lui, N.S.T. Response of infants to **Haemophilus influenzae** type b polysaccharide and diphtheria-tetanus-pertussis vaccines in combination. J Infect Dis 1984;149:950-955.
30. Cody, C.L., Baraff, L.J., Cherry, J.D., Marcy, S.M., and Manclark, C.R. Nature and rates of adverse reactions associated with DTP and DT immunizations in infants and children. Pediatr 1981;68:650–660.

Manufactured by
PRAXIS
BIOLOGICS
Distributed by
MEAD JOHNSON
NUTRITIONAL DIVISION

CASEC® powder
[*kā'sek*]
Calcium caseinate
Protein supplement

(See PDR For Nonprescription Drugs)

CE-VI-SOL®
[*se'vi-sahl"*]
Vitamin C supplement drops

(See PDR For Nonprescription Drugs)

CRITICARE HN®
[*cri'tĭ-care"*]
Ready to Use High Nitrogen Elemental Diet

(See PDR For Nonprescription Drugs)

ENFAMIL® concentrated liquid • powder
[*en'fah-mĭl"*]
Infant formula

(See PDR For Nonprescription Drugs)

ENFAMIL® with Iron
[*en'fah-mĭl"*]
concentrated liquid • powder
Infant formula

(See PDR For Nonprescription Drugs)

ENFAMIL NURSETTE®
[*en'fah-mĭl"*]
Infant formula

(See PDR For Nonprescription Drugs)

ENFAMIL® ready-to-use
[*en'fah-mĭl"*]
Infant formula

(See PDR For Nonprescription Drugs)

ENFAMIL® with Iron ready-to-use
[*en'fah-mĭl"*]
Infant formula

(See PDR For Nonprescription Drugs)

FER-IN-SOL®
[*fair'ĭn-sahl"*]
Iron supplement
- **drops**
- **syrup**
- **capsules**

Ferrous sulfate, Mead Johnson

(See PDR For Nonprescription Drugs)

ISOCAL®
[*ī'sō-cal"*]
Complete liquid diet

(See PDR For Nonprescription Drugs)

ISOCAL® HCN
[*ī'sō-cal"*]
High Calorie and Nitrogen Nutritionally Complete Liquid Tube Feeding Formula

(See PDR For Nonprescription Drugs)

LOFENALAC® powder
[*lō-fen'ah-lak"*]
Low phenylalanine food

(See PDR For Nonprescription Drugs)

LONALAC® powder
[*lōn'ah-lak"*]
Low sodium, high protein beverage mix

(See PDR For Nonprescription Drugs)

LYTREN®
[*lī'tren*]
Oral electrolyte solution

(See PDR For Nonprescription Drugs)

MCT Oil
Medium chain triglycerides oil

(See PDR For Nonprescription Drugs)

MODUCAL® Dietary Carbohydrate
[*mah'dju-cal"*]

(See PDR For Nonprescription Drugs)

NATURACIL®

[natch 'er-ah-sil ″]

A natural-fiber laxative

DESCRIPTION

Naturacil is a unique non-powdered, chewable form of bulk laxative. It is a safe and effective natural-fiber bulking agent that promotes evacuation through normal physiological mechanisms.

Active Ingredient: Each adult dose (2 pieces) contains 3.4 g of psyllium seed husks, an excellent natural grain source of dietary fiber.

Inactive Ingredients: Chocolate flavor (artificial), corn syrup, FD&C Blue No. 2 (aluminum lake), FD&C Red No. 40 (aluminum lake), FD&C Yellow No. 6 (aluminum lake), glycerin, nonfat milk, partially hydrogenated vegetable oil (soybean and cottonseed oil), and sucrose. Naturacil contains no cocoa or chocolate derivative.

Each adult dose (2 pieces) contains 54 Calories, 9.6 g of available carbohydrate and 11 mg sodium.

CLINICAL PHARMACOLOGY

One of the most important causes of constipation is lack of adequate fiber in the diet. The psyllium seed husks in Naturacil provide an excellent source of dietary fiber because they contain a mucilage which has a high water-holding capacity. Known chemically as an arabinoxylan, this mucilage, when mixed with intestinal fluid, forms a gel which increases the bulk and water content of the stool. Because of this action, Naturacil, when taken with liquid, promotes the gentle, natural evacuation of the sigmoid colon and rectum.

INDICATIONS AND USAGE

Naturacil is indicated for the relief and prevention of simple constipation, for restoring regularity, and for the bowel management of patients with:

- Functional Constipation
- Diverticulosis
- Hemorrhoids
- Irritable Bowel Syndrome/Spastic Colon
- Postsurgical Bowel Requirements

Naturacil is a non-habit-forming bulking agent that may be used when long-term therapy is indicated. Diabetic patients should take into consideration that Naturacil contains 38.4 Calories from carbohydrates per dose.

CONTRAINDICATIONS

Naturacil or any bulk-forming laxative is contraindicated in cases of intestinal obstruction or fecal impaction. May cause allergic reaction in people sensitive to inhaled or ingested psyllium.

DOSAGE AND ADMINISTRATION

The usual adult dosage is two pieces, one to three times daily; the dosage for children 6 to 12 years of age is one piece, one to three times daily. Doses should be accompanied by 8 fluid ounces of any liquid the patient prefers. Results may occur within 24 hours, but continued use for two to three days may be necessary for optimal effect.

STORAGE

Store at room temperature.

HOW SUPPLIED

Cartons of 24 pieces (12 adult doses) and 40 pieces (20 adult doses). Each piece is individually wrapped in foil.

Naturacil 24's: NDC #0087-0444-01

Naturacil 40's: NDC #0087-0444-02

IS THIS PRODUCT OTC

Yes. See also PDR for Nonprescription Drugs.

NUTRAMIGEN®

[nū-tram 'ĭ-jen ″]

Protein hydrolysate formula with added amino acids

- **powder**
- **ready-to-feed, 8 fl oz Nursette® bottles**
- **ready-to-feed, 32 fl oz cans**

(See PDR For Nonprescription Drugs)

POLY-VI-FLOR® ℞

[pahl-ē-vī 'flōr ″]

- **1.0 mg**
- **0.5 mg**
- **0.25 mg**

Multivitamin and fluoride supplement chewable tablets

DESCRIPTION

[See table above].

Active ingredient for caries prophylaxis: Fluoride as sodium fluoride.

Other ingredients: Ascorbic acid, cholecalciferol, colloidal silicon dioxide, cyanocobalamin, dextrates, FD&C Blue No. 2 (aluminum lake), FD&C Red No. 40 (aluminum lake), FD&C Yellow No. 6 (aluminum lake), folic acid, fruit flavors (artificial), lactose, magnesium stearate, niacinamide, pyridoxine hydrochloride, riboflavin, silica gel, sodium ascorbate, sodium chloride, sucrose, thiamine mononitrate, dl-alpha-tocopheryl acetate, vitamin A acetate.

	Poly-Vi-Flor chewable tablets			Percentage of U.S. Recommended Daily Allowance	
	1.0mg	0.5mg	0.25mg	Children 2–4	Adults & Children 4 or More
Each tablet supplies:					
Vitamin A, IU	2500	2500	2500	100	50
Vitamin D, IU	400	400	400	100	100
Vitamin E, IU	15	15	15	150	50
Vitamin C, mg	60	60	60	150	100
Folic acid, mg	0.3	0.3	0.3	150	75
Thiamine, mg	1.05	1.05	1.05	150	70
Riboflavin, mg	1.2	1.2	1.2	150	70
Niacin, mg	13.5	13.5	13.5	150	68
Vitamin B_6, mg	1.05	1.05	1.05	150	53
Vitamin B_{12}, mcg	4.5	4.5	4.5	150	75
Fluoride, mg	1	0.5	0.25	*	*

* U.S. Recommended Daily Allowance has not been established.

CLINICAL PHARMACOLOGY

It is well established that fluoridation of the water supply (1 ppm fluoride) during the period of tooth development leads to a significant decrease in the incidence of dental caries. Poly-Vi-Flor chewable tablets provide sodium fluoride, and ten essential vitamins in a chewable tablet. Because the tablets are chewable, they provide a *topical* as well as *systemic* source of fluoride.[1,2]

Hydroxyapatite is the principal crystal for all calcified tissue in the human body. The fluoride ion reacts with the *hydroxyapatite* in the tooth as it is formed to produce the more caries-resistant crystal, *fluorapatite*. The reaction may be expressed by the equation:[3]

$$Ca_{10}(PO_4)_6(OH)_2 + 2F^- \rightarrow Ca_{10}(PO_4)_6F_2 + 2OH^-$$

(Hydroxyapatite) (Fluorapatite)

Three stages of fluoride deposition in tooth enamel can be distinguished.[3]

1. Small amounts (reflecting the low levels of fluoride in tissue fluids) are incorporated into the enamel crystals while they are being formed.
2. After enamel has been laid down, fluoride deposition continues in the surface enamel. Diffusion of fluoride from the surface inward is apparently restricted.
3. After eruption, the surface enamel acquires fluoride from water, food, supplementary fluoride and smaller amounts from saliva.

INDICATIONS AND USAGE

Supplementation of the diet with ten essential vitamins.

Supplementation of the diet with the fluoride for caries prophylaxis.

Poly-Vi-Flor 1.0 mg chewable tablets provide fluoride in tablet form for children over 3 years in areas where the water fluoride level is less than 0.3 ppm.[4]

Poly-Vi-Flor 0.5 mg chewable tablets provide fluoride in tablet form for children 2-3 years of age where the drinking water has a fluoride content of 0.3 ppm or less, and for children 3 years of age and above where the drinking water has a fluoride level greater than 0.3 ppm and not more than 0.7 ppm.[4]

Poly-Vi-Flor 0.25 mg chewable tablets provide fluoride in tablet form for children 2–3 years of age where the drinking water has a fluoride level greater than 0.3 ppm and not more than 0.7 ppm.[4]

Poly-Vi-Flor chewable tablets supply significant amounts of vitamins A, D, E, C, thiamine, riboflavin, niacin, pyridoxine, cyanocobalamin and folic acid to supplement the diet, and to help assure that nutritional deficiencies of these vitamins will not develop. Thus, in a single easy-to-use preparation, children over three years of age obtain ten essential vitamins and the important mineral, fluoride.

The American Academy of Pediatrics recommends that children up to age 16, in areas where drinking water contains less than optimal levels of fluoride, receive daily fluoride supplementation.

Children using Poly-Vi-Flor chewable tablets regularly should receive semiannual dental examinations. The regular brushing of teeth and attention to good oral hygiene practices are also essential.

WARNINGS

As in the case of all medications, keep out of the reach of children.

PRECAUTIONS

The suggested dose *should not be exceeded*, since dental fluorosis may result from continued ingestion of large amounts of fluoride.

Before prescribing Vi-Flor® products:

1. determine the fluoride content of the drinking water.
2. make sure the child is not receiving significant amounts of fluoride from other medications.
3. periodically check to make sure that the child does not develop significant dental fluorosis.

ADVERSE REACTIONS

Allergic rash and other idiosyncrasies have been rarely reported.

DOSAGE AND ADMINISTRATION

One tablet daily or as prescribed.

HOW SUPPLIED

Poly-Vi-Flor 1.0 mg (multivitamin and fluoride supplement) chewable tablets are available in 100- and 1000-tablet bottles.

NDC 0087-0474-02 Bottles of 100

NDC 0087-0474-03 Bottles of 1000

Poly-Vi-Flor 0.5 mg (multivitamin and fluoride supplement) chewable tablets are available in 100 tablet bottles.

NDC 0087-0468-41 Bottles of 100

Poly-Vi-Flor 0.25 mg (multivitamin and fluoride supplement) chewable tablets are available in 100-tablet bottles.

NDC 0087-0487-41 Bottles of 100

LITERATURE AVAILABLE

Yes.

REFERENCES

1. Hennon, D.K.; Stookey, G.K., and Muhler, J.C.: The Clinical Anticariogenic Effectiveness of Supplementary Fluoride-Vitamin Preparations— Results at the End of Three Years, J. Dentistry for Children 33:3–12 (Jan.) 1966.
2. Hennon, D.K.; Stookey, G.K., and Muhler, J.C.: The Clinical Anticariogenic Effectiveness of Supplementary Fluoride-Vitamin Preparations— Results at the End of Four Years, J. Dentistry for Children 34:439–443 (Nov.) 1967.
3. Brudevold, F., and McCann, H.G.: Fluoride and Caries Control—Mechanism of Action, in Nizel, A.E.: The Science of Nutrition and Its Application in Clinical Dentistry, Philadelphia, W.B. Saunders Company, 1966, pp. 331–347.
4. American Academy of Pediatrics Committee on Nutrition: Fluoride Supplementation: Revised Dosage Schedule. Pediatrics 63:150, 1979.

POLY-VI-FLOR® ℞

[pahl-ē-vī 'flōr ″]

- **0.5 mg**
- **0.25 mg**

Multivitamin and fluoride supplement drops

DESCRIPTION

[See table on bottom next page].

See INDICATIONS AND USAGE section below for use by infants and children under two years of age.

This product does not contain the essential vitamin folic acid.

Active ingredient for caries prophylaxis: Fluoride as sodium fluoride.

Other ingredients: Ascorbic acid, caramel color, cholecalciferol, cyanocobalamin, ferrous sulfate, fruit flavor (artificial), glycerin, niacinamide, polysorbate 80, pyridoxine hydrochloride, riboflavin-5-phosphate sodium, thiamine hydrochloride, d-alpha-tocopheryl acid succinate, vitamin A palmitate, water, and other ingredients.

CLINICAL PHARMACOLOGY

For information on fluoridation see Poly-Vi-Flor chewable tablets.

INDICATIONS AND USAGE

Supplementation of the diet with nine essential vitamins.

Supplementation of the diet with fluoride for caries prophylaxis.

The American Academy of Pediatrics recommends that children up to age 16, in areas where drinking water contains

Continued on next page

Mead Johnson Nutr.—Cont.

less than optimal levels of fluoride, receive daily fluoride supplementation.

Poly-Vi-Flor 0.5 mg (multivitamin and fluoride supplement) drops provide fluoride in drop form for children ages 2–3 years in areas where the drinking water contains less than 0.3 ppm fluoride; and for children over 3 years in areas where the drinking water contains 0.3 thru 0.7 ppm of fluoride.[2] Each 1.0 ml provides sodium fluoride (0.5 mg fluoride) plus nine essential vitamins.

Poly-Vi-Flor 0.25 mg (multivitamin and fluoride supplement) drops provide fluoride in drop form for infants and young children from birth to 2 years of age in areas where the drinking water contains less than 0.3 ppm of fluoride and for children ages 2–3 years in areas where the drinking water contains 0.3 thru 0.7 ppm of fluoride. Each 1.0 ml supplies sodium fluoride (0.25 mg fluoride) plus nine essential vitamins.

The American Academy of Pediatrics[2] and the American Dental Association[3] currently recommend that infants and children under 2 years of age, in areas where drinking water contains less than 0.3 ppm of fluoride, and children 2-3, in areas where the drinking water contains 0.3 through 0.7 ppm of fluoride, receive 0.25 mg of supplemental fluoride daily which is provided in a full dose (1 ml) of Poly-Vi-Flor® 0.25 mg drops. A half dose (0.5 ml) of Poly-Vi-Flor 0.5 mg drops could also provide a daily fluoride intake of 0.25 mg; however, this dosage reduces vitamin supplementation by half.

Poly-Vi-Flor 0.5 mg drops and 0.25 mg drops supply significant amounts of vitamins A, D, E, C, thiamine, riboflavin, niacin, pyridoxine, and cyanocobalamin to supplement the diet, and to help assure that nutritional deficiencies of these vitamins will not develop. Thus in a single easy-to-use preparation, infants and children obtain nine essential vitamins and fluoride.

A comprehensive 5½ year series of studies of the effectiveness of Tri-Vi-Flor® and Poly-Vi-Flor® products in caries protection has been published.[4-7] Children in this continuing study lived in an area where the water supply contained only 0.05 ppm fluoride. The subjects were divided into two groups, one which used only nonfluoridated Vi-Sol® vitamin products and the other Tri-Vi-Flor and Poly-Vi-Flor vitamin-fluoride products.

The three-year interim report showed 63% fewer carious surfaces in primary teeth and 43% fewer carious surfaces in permanent teeth of the children taking Vi-Flor® vitamin-fluoride products.[4]

After four years the studies continued to support the effectiveness of Tri-Vi-Flor and Poly-Vi-Flor, showing a reduction in carious surfaces of 68% in primary teeth and 46% in permanent teeth.[5]

Results at the end of 5½ years further confirmed the previous findings and indicated that significant reductions in dental caries are apparent with the continued use of Vi-Flor vitamin-fluoride products.[6]

WARNINGS

As in the case of all medications, keep out of the reach of children.

PRECAUTIONS

The suggested dose should not be exceeded since dental fluorosis may result from continued ingestion of large amounts of fluoride.

When prescribing Vi-Flor products:

1. determine the fluoride content of the drinking water.
2. make sure the child is not receiving significant amounts of fluoride from other medications.
3. periodically check to make sure that the child does not develop significant dental fluorosis.

Poly-Vi-Flor 0.5 mg drops and 0.25 mg drops should be dispensed in the original plastic container, since contact with glass leads to instability and precipitation. (The amount of sodium fluoride in both the 30- and 50-ml sizes (0.5 mg drops) and in the 50 ml size (0.25 mg drops) is well below the maximum to be dispensed at one time according to recommendations of the American Dental Association.)

ADVERSE REACTIONS

Allergic rash and other idiosyncrasies have been rarely reported.

DOSAGE AND ADMINISTRATION

1.0 ml daily or as prescribed.

Drops may be dropped directly into mouth with 'Safti-Dropper', or mixed with cereal, fruit juice or other food.

HOW SUPPLIED

Poly-Vi-Flor 0.5 mg (multivitamin and fluoride supplement) drops are available on prescription only in bottles of 30 and 50 ml.

NDC 0087-0472-01 Bottles of 1 fl oz (30 ml)
NDC 0087-0472-02 Bottles of 1⅔ fl oz (50 ml)
FSN 6505-080-0967 (50 ml)

Poly-Vi-Flor 0.25 mg (multivitamin and fluoride supplement) drops are available on prescription only in bottles of 50 ml.

NDC 0087-0451-41 Bottles of 50 ml.

LITERATURE AVAILABLE

Yes.

REFERENCES

1. Brudevold, F., and McCann, H.G.: Fluoride and Caries Control—Mechanism of Action, in Nizel, A.E.: The Science of Nutrition and its Application in Clinical Dentistry, Philadelphia, W. B. Saunders Company, 1966, pp. 331–347.
2. American Academy of Pediatrics, Committee on Nutrition: Fluoride Supplementation: Revised Dosage Schedule, Pediatrics 63:150, 1979.
3. Accepted Dental Therapeutics, Ed. 38, Chicago, American Dental Association, 1979, p. 321.
4. Hennon, D.K.; Stookey, G.K., and Muhler, J.C.: The Clinical Anticariogenic Effectiveness of Supplementary Fluoride-Vitamin Preparations— Results at the End of Three Years, J. Dentistry for Children 33:3–12 (Jan.) 1966.
5. Hennon, D.K.; Stookey, G.K., and Muhler, J.C.: The Clinical Anticariogenic Effectiveness of Supplementary Fluoride-Vitamin Preparations— Results at the End of Four Years, J. Dentistry for Children 24:439–443 (Nov.) 1967.
6. Hennon, D.K.; Stookey, G.K., and Muhler, J.C.: The Clinical Anticariogenic Effectiveness of Supplementary Fluoride-Vitamin Preparations— Results at the End of Five and a Half Years, Phar. and Ther. In Dent. 1:1, 1970.
7. Hennon, D.K.; Stookey, G.K., and Beiswanger, B.B.: Fluoride vitamin supplements: Effects on dental caries and fluorosis when used in areas with suboptimum fluoride in the water supply. J.Am.Dent.Assoc. 95:965, 1977.

Each 1.0 ml supplies:	Poly-Vi-Flor drops 0.5mg	0.25mg	Percentage of U.S. Recommended Daily Allowance: Infants	Children Under 4
Vitamin A, IU	1500	1500	100	60
Vitamin D, IU	400	400	100	100
Vitamin E, IU	5	5	100	50
Vitamin C, mg	35	35	100	88
Thiamine, mg	0.5	0.5	100	71
Riboflavin, mg	0.6	0.6	100	75
Niacin, mg	8	8	100	89
Vitamin B_6, mg	0.4	0.4	100	57
Vitamin B_{12}, mcg	2	2	100	67
Fluoride, mg	0.5	0.25	*	*

* U.S. Recommended Daily Allowance has not been established.

Each tablet supplies:	Poly-Vi-Flor w/Iron chewable tablets 1.0 mg	0.5 mg	0.25 mg	Percentage of U.S. Recommended Daily Allowance: Children 2-4	Adults & Children 4 or More
Vitamin A, IU	2500	2500	2500	100	50
Vitamin D, IU	400	400	400	100	100
Vitamin E, IU	15	15	15	150	50
Vitamin C, mg	60	60	60	150	100
Folic acid, mg	0.3	0.3	0.3	150	75
Thiamine, mg	1.05	1.05	1.05	150	70
Riboflavin, mg	1.2	1.2	1.2	150	70
Niacin, mg	13.5	13.5	13.5	150	68
Vitamin B_6, mg	1.05	1.05	1.05	150	53
Vitamin B_{12}, mcg	4.5	4.5	4.5	150	75
Iron, mg	12	12	12	120	67
Copper, mg	1	1	1	100	50
Zinc, mg	10	10	10	125	67
Fluoride, mg	1	0.5	0.25	*	*

*U.S. Recommended Daily Allowance has not been established.

POLY–VI–FLOR® with Iron ℞

[*pahl-ē-vī 'flōr"*]

- 1.0 mg
- 0.5 mg
- 0.25 mg

Multivitamin, mineral and fluoride supplement chewable tablets

DESCRIPTION

[See table above].

Active ingredient for caries prophylaxis: Fluoride as sodium fluoride.

Other ingredients: Ascorbic acid, cholecalciferol, colloidal silicon dioxide, cupric oxide, cyanocobalamin, dextrates, FD&C Red No. 40 (aluminum lake), ferrous fumarate, folic acid, fruit flavors (artificial), lactose, magnesium stearate, niacinamide, pyridoxine hydrochloride, riboflavin, silica gel, sodium ascorbate, sodium chloride, stearic acid, sucrose, thiamine mononitrate, dl-alpha-tocopheryl acetate, vitamin A acetate, zinc oxide.

CLINICAL PHARMACOLOGY

For information on fluoridation see Poly-Vi-Flor chewable tablets.

Poly-Vi-Flor with Iron chewable tablets provide sodium fluoride, iron, copper, zinc and ten essential vitamins in a chewable tablet. Because the tablets are chewable, they provide a *topical* as well as *systemic* source of fluoride.[1,2]

INDICATIONS AND USAGE

Supplementation of the diet with ten essential vitamins, iron, copper and zinc.

Supplementation of the diet with fluoride, for caries prophylaxis.

The American Academy of Pediatrics recommends that children up to age 16, in areas where drinking water contains less than optimal levels of fluoride, receive daily fluoride supplementation.

Poly-Vi-Flor 1.0 mg chewable tablets with Iron were developed to provide fluoride in tablet form for children over 3 years in areas where the water fluoride level is less than 0.3 ppm.[3]

Poly-Vi-Flor 0.5 mg with Iron chewable tablets provides fluoride for children 2–3 years of age where the drinking water has fluoride content of 0.3 ppm or less, and for children 3 years of age and above where the drinking water has a fluoride level greater than 0.3 ppm and not more than 0.7 ppm.[3]

Poly-Vi-Flor 0.25 mg with Iron chewable tablets provide fluoride in tablet form for children 2–3 years of age where the drinking water has a fluoride level greater than 0.3 ppm and not more than 0.7 ppm.[3]

Poly-Vi-Flor with Iron chewable tablets supply significant amounts of vitamins A, D, E, C, thiamine, riboflavin, niacin, pyridoxine, cyanocobalamin, folic acid, iron, copper and zinc to supplement the diet, and to help assure that deficiencies of these nutrients will not develop. Thus, in a single easy-to-use preparation, children over three years of age obtain ten essential vitamins, iron, and fluoride.

Children using Poly-Vi-Flor with Iron chewable tablets regularly should receive semiannual dental examinations. The regular brushing of teeth and attention to good oral hygiene practices are also essential.

WARNINGS

As in the case of all medications, keep out of the reach of children.

PRECAUTIONS

The suggested dose of Poly-Vi-Flor with Iron chewable tablets *should not be exceeded,* since dental fluorosis may result from continued ingestion of large amounts of fluoride.

Before prescribing Vi-Flor® products:

1. determine the fluoride content of the drinking water.
2. make sure the child is not receiving significant amounts of fluoride from other medications.
3. periodically check to make sure that the child does not develop significant dental fluorosis.

The toxicity of ferrous fumarate is not established. However, to prevent possible serious harmful effects in the event of accidental overdosage, it is recommended that no more than 100 tablets be dispensed at one time.

ADVERSE REACTIONS

Allergic rash and other idiosyncrasies have been rarely reported.

DOSAGE AND ADMINISTRATION

One tablet daily or as prescribed.

HOW SUPPLIED

Poly-Vi-Flor 1.0 mg with Iron (multivitamin, mineral and fluoride supplement) chewable tablets are available in 100- and 1000-tablet bottles.
NDC 0087-0476-03 Bottles of 100
NDC 0087-0476-04 Bottles of 1000
Poly-Vi-Flor 0.5 mg with Iron (multivitamin, mineral and fluoride supplement) chewable tablets are available only in 100-tablet bottles.
NDC 0087-0482-41 Bottles of 100
Poly-Vi-Flor 0.25 mg with Iron (multivitamin, mineral and fluoride supplement) chewable tablets are available in 100-tablet bottles.
NDC 0087-0488-41 Bottles of 100

LITERATURE AVAILABLE

Yes.

REFERENCES

1. Hennon, D.K.; Stookey, G.K., and Muhler, J.C.: The Clinical Anticariogenic Effectiveness of Supplementary Fluoride-Vitamin Preparations— Results at the End of Three Years, J. Dentistry for Children 33:3–12 (Jan.) 1966.
2. Hennon, D.K.; Stookey, G.K., and Muhler, J.C.: The Clinical Anticariogenic Effectiveness of Supplementary Fluoride-Vitamin Preparations— Results at the End of Four Years, J. Dentistry for Children 34:439–443 (Nov.) 1967.
3. American Academy of Pediatrics Committee on Nutrition: Fluoride Supplementation: Revised Dosage Schedule. Pediatrics 63:150, 1979.

POLY-VI-FLOR® with Iron ℞
[*pahl-ē-vī 'flōr"*]
● 0.5 mg
● 0.25 mg
Multivitamin, iron and fluoride supplement drops

DESCRIPTION

[See table above].
See INDICATIONS AND USAGE section below for use by infants and children under two years of age.
This product does not contain the essential vitamins folic acid and B_{12}.
Active ingredient for caries prophylaxis: Fluoride as sodium fluoride.
Other ingredients: Ascorbic acid, caramel color, cholecalciferol, ferrous sulfate, fruit flavor (artificial), glycerin, niacinamide, polysorbate 80, pyridoxine hydrochloride, riboflavin-5-phosphate sodium, thiamine hydrochloride, d-alpha-tocopheryl acid succinate, vitamin A palmitate, water, and other ingredients.

CLINICAL PHARMACOLOGY

For information on fluoridation see Poly-Vi-Flor chewable tablets.

INDICATIONS AND USAGE

Supplementation of the diet with eight essential vitamins and iron.
Supplementation of the diet with fluoride for caries prophylaxis.
The American Academy of Pediatrics recommends that children up to age 16, in areas where drinking water contains less than optimal levels of fluoride, receive daily fluoride supplementation.
Poly-Vi-Flor 0.5 mg with Iron (multivitamin, iron, and fluoride supplement) drops provide fluoride in drop form for children ages 2–3 years in areas where the drinking water contains less than 0.3 ppm fluoride; and for children over 3 years in areas where the drinking water contains 0.3 thru 0.7 ppm of fluoride.[1] Each 1.0 ml provides sodium fluoride (0.5 mg fluoride) plus eight essential vitamins and iron.
Poly-Vi-Flor 0.25 mg with Iron drops provide fluoride in drop form for infants and young children from birth to 2 years of age in areas where the drinking water contains less than 0.3 ppm of fluoride and for children ages 2-3 years in areas where the drinking water contains 0.3 thru 0.7 ppm of fluoride. Each 1.0 ml supplies sodium fluoride (0.25 mg fluoride) plus eight essential vitamins and iron.

Each 1.0 ml supplies:	Poly-Vi-Flor w/Iron drops 0.5 mg	0.25 mg	Percentage of U.S. Recommended Daily Allowance: Infants	Children Under 4
Vitamin A, IU	1500	1500	100	60
Vitamin D, IU	400	400	100	100
Vitamin E, IU	5	5	100	50
Vitamin C, mg	35	35	100	88
Thiamine, mg	0.5	0.5	100	71
Riboflavin, mg	0.6	0.6	100	75
Niacin, mg	8	8	100	89
Vitamin B_6, mg	0.4	0.4	100	57
Iron, mg	10	10	67	100
Fluoride, mg	0.5	0.25	*	*

*U.S. Recommended Daily Allowance has not been established.

The American Academy of Pediatrics[1] and the American Dental Association[2] currently recommend that infants and children under 2 years of age, in areas where drinking water contains less than 0.3 ppm of fluoride, and children 2-3, in areas where the drinking water contains 0.3 through 0.7 ppm of fluoride, receive 0.25 mg of supplemental fluoride daily which is provided in a full dose (1 ml) of Poly-Vi-Flor® 0.25 mg with Iron drops. A half dose (0.5 ml) of Poly-Vi-Flor 0.5 mg with Iron drops could also provide a daily fluoride intake of 0.25 mg; however, this dosage reduces vitamin supplementation by half.
Poly-Vi-Flor with Iron drops supply significant amounts of vitamins A, D, E, C, thiamine, riboflavin, niacin, pyridoxine, and ferrous sulfate to supplement the diet, and to help assure that deficiencies of these nutrients will not develop. Thus, in a single easy-to-use preparation, infants and children obtain eight essential vitamins and iron, plus fluoride.
A comprehensive 5½ year series of studies of the effectiveness of Tri-Vi-Flor® and Poly-Vi-Flor® products in caries protection has been published.[3-6] Children in this continuing study lived in an area where the water supply contained only 0.05 ppm fluoride. The subjects were divided into two groups, one which used only nonfluoridated Vi-Sol® vitamin products and the other Tri-Vi-Flor and Poly-Vi-Flor vitamin-fluoride products.
The three-year interim report showed 63% fewer carious surfaces in primary teeth and 43% fewer carious surfaces in permanent teeth of the children taking Vi-Flor® vitamin-fluoride products.[3]
After four years the studies continued to support the effectiveness of Tri-Vi-Flor and Poly-Vi-Flor, showing a reduction in carious surfaces of 68% in primary teeth and 46% in permanent teeth.[4]
Results at the end of 5½ years further confirmed the previous findings and indicated that significant reductions in dental caries are apparent with the continued use of Vi-Flor vitamin-fluoride products.[5]

WARNINGS

As in the case of all medications, keep out of the reach of children.

PRECAUTIONS

The suggested dose should not be exceeded since dental fluorosis may result from continued ingestion of large amounts of fluoride.
When prescribing Vi-Flor products:

1. determine the fluoride content of the drinking water.
2. make sure the child is not receiving significant amounts of fluoride from other medications.
3. periodically check to make sure that the child does not develop significant dental fluorosis.

Poly-Vi-Flor with Iron drops should be dispensed in the original plastic container, since contact with glass leads to instability and precipitation. (The amount of sodium fluoride in the 50-ml. size is well below the maximum to be dispensed at one time according to recommendations of the American Dental Association.)

ADVERSE REACTIONS

Allergic rash and other idiosyncrasies have been reported rarely.

DOSAGE AND ADMINISTRATION

1.0 ml daily or as prescribed.
May be dropped directly into mouth with 'Safti-Dropper,' or mixed with cereal, fruit juice or other foods.

HOW SUPPLIED

Poly-Vi-Flor 0.5 mg (multivitamin, fluoride and iron supplement) with Iron drops are available in bottles of 50 ml.
NDC 0087-0469-41 Bottles of 1⅔ fl oz (50 ml)
Poly-Vi-Flor 0.25 mg (multivitamin, fluoride and iron supplement) with Iron drops are available in bottles of 50 ml.
NDC 0087-0483-41 Bottles of 1⅔ fl oz (50 ml)

LITERATURE AVAILABLE

Yes.

REFERENCES

1. American Academy of Pediatrics, Committee on Nutrition: Fluoride Supplementation: Revised Dosage Schedule, Pediatrics 63:150, 1979.
2. Accepted Dental Therapeutics, Ed. 38, Chicago, American Dental Association, 1979, p. 321.
3. Hennon, D.K.; Stookey, G.K., and Muhler, J.C.: The Clinical Anticariogenic Effectiveness of Supplementary Fluoride-Vitamin Preparations— Results at the End of Three Years, J. Dentistry for Children 33:3–12 (Jan.) 1966.
4. Hennon, D.K.; Stookey, G.K., and Muhler, J.C.: The Clinical Anticariogenic Effectiveness of Supplementary Fluoride-Vitamin Preparations— Results at the End of Four Years, J. Dentistry for Children 34:439–443 (Nov.) 1967.
5. Hennon, D.K.; Stookey, G.K., and Muhler, J.C.: The Clinical Anticariogenic Effectiveness of Supplementary Fluoride-Vitamin Preparations— Results at the End of Five and a Half Years, Phar. and Ther. In Dent. 1:1, 1970.
6. Hennon, D.K.; Stookey, G.K., and Beiswanger, B.B.: Fluoride-vitamin supplements: Effects on Dental Caries and Fluorosis When Used in Areas With Suboptimum Fluoride in the Water Supply. J. Am. Dent. Assoc. 95:965, 1977.

POLY-VI-SOL®
[*pahl-ē-vī 'sahl"*]
Vitamins
drops ● chewable tablets

(See PDR For Nonprescription Drugs)

POLY-VI-SOL® with Iron
[*pahl-ē-vī 'sahl"*]
Chewable vitamins and minerals

(See PDR For Nonprescription Drugs)

POLY-VI-SOL® with Iron
[*pahl-ē-vī 'sahl"*]
Multivitamin and Iron supplement drops

(See PDR For Nonprescription Drugs)

PORTAGEN®
[*port 'ă-jen*]
Nutritionally complete powder with Medium Chain Triglycerides
U.S. Patent No. 3,450,819

(See PDR For Nonprescription Drugs)

PREGESTIMIL®
[*prē-jest 'ĭ-mĭl"*]
Protein hydrolysate formula with medium chain triglycerides and added amino acids

(See PDR For Nonprescription Drugs)

PROSOBEE® concentrated liquid ● ready-to-use ● powder
[*prō-sō 'be*]
Milk-free, sucrose-free formula with soy protein isolate

(See PDR For Nonprescription Drugs)

Continued on next page

Mead Johnson Nutr.—Cont.

SMURF™
[smerf]
Chewable vitamins

(See PDR For Nonprescription Drugs)

SMURF™
[smerf]
Chewable vitamins with iron and zinc

(See PDR For Nonprescription Drugs)

SUSTACAL®
[sŭs 'tă-cal"]
- **liquid (ready to use)**
- **powder (mix with milk)**
- **pudding (ready-to-eat)**

Nutritionally complete food

(See PDR For Nonprescription Drugs)

SUSTACAL® HC
[sŭs 'tă-cal"]
High Calorie Nutritionally Complete Food

(See PDR For Nonprescription Drugs)

SUSTAGEN® powder
[sus 'tă-jen]
Nutritional supplement

(See PDR For Nonprescription Drugs)

TEMPRA® drops, syrup, and chewable tablets
[tem 'prah]
Acetaminophen

(See PDR For Nonprescription Drugs)

TRAUMACAL®
[tră 'mă-cal"]
Nutritionally Complete Liquid for Traumatized Patients

(See PDR For Nonprescription Drugs)

TRIND® liquid
[trĭnd]
nasal decongestant • antihistamine

(See PDR For Nonprescription Drugs)

TRIND-DM® liquid
[trĭnd]
antitussive • nasal decongestant • antihistamine

(See PDR For Nonprescription Drugs)

TRI-VI-FLOR® 1.0 mg ℞
[trī 'vī-flōr"]
Vitamins A, D, C and fluoride chewable tablets

DESCRIPTION
[See table below].
Active ingredient for caries prophylaxis: Fluoride as sodium fluoride.
Other ingredients: Ascorbic acid, cholecalciferol, dextrates, FD&C Blue No. 2 (aluminum lake), FD&C Red No. 40 (aluminum lake), FD&C Yellow No. 6 (aluminum lake), fruit flavors (artificial), magnesium stearate, sodium chloride, sodium ascorbate, stearic acid, surcrose, vitamin A acetate.

Each tablet supplies:		Percentage of U.S. Recommended Daily Allowance: Children 2-4	Adults & Children 4 or More
Vitamin A, IU	2500	100	50
Vitamin D, IU	400	100	100
Vitamin C, mg	60	150	100
Fluoride, mg	1.0	*	*

*U.S. Recommended Daily Allowance has not been established.

CLINICAL PHARMACOLOGY
For information of fluoridation see Poly-Vi-Flor® chewable tablets.
Tri-Vi-Flor tablets provide sodium fluoride (1 mg fluoride) and three basic vitamins in a chewable tablet. Because the tablets are chewable, they provide a *topical* as well as *systemic* source of fluoride.[1,2]

INDICATIONS AND USAGE
Supplementation of the diet with vitamins A, D, and C.
Supplementation of the diet with fluoride for caries prophylaxis.
The American Academy of Pediatrics recommends that children up to age 16, in areas where drinking water contains less than optimal levels of fluoride, receive daily fluoride supplementation.
Tri-Vi-Flor 1.0 mg (vitamins A, D, C and fluoride) chewable tablets provide fluoride in tablet form for children 3 years of age and older where the drinking water contains less than 0.3 ppm of fluoride.[3]
Tri-Vi-Flor 1.0 mg chewable tablets supply vitamins A, D and C to help assure that nutritional deficiencies of these vitamins will not develop.
Tri-Vi-Flor 1.0 mg chewable tablets also provide the important mineral fluoride for caries prophylaxis. Thus in a single easy-to-use preparation, children over 3 years of age obtain three basic vitamins and the important mineral fluoride.
A study of fluoride tablets given to 121 children revealed the efficacy of sodium fluoride in tablet form. The authors concluded that the caries reduction was comparable to that previously reported for children drinking fluoridated water.[4]
A comprehensive 5½ year series of studies of the effectiveness of Tri-Vi-Flor® and Poly-Vi-Flor® products in caries protection has been published.[1,2,5] Children in this continuing study lived in an area where the water supply contained only 0.05 ppm fluoride. The subjects were divided into two groups, one which used only non-fluoridated Vi-Sol® vitamin products and the other Tri-Vi-Flor and Poly-Vi-Flor vitamin-fluoride products.
The three-year interim report showed 63% fewer carious surfaces in primary teeth and 43% fewer carious surfaces in permanent teeth of the children taking Vi-Flor® vitamin-fluoride products.[1]
After four years the studies continued to support the effectiveness of Tri-Vi-Flor and Poly-Vi-Flor, showing a reduction in carious surfaces of 68% in primary teeth and 46% in permanent teeth.[2]
Results at the end of 5½ years further confirmed the previous findings and indicated that significant reductions in dental caries are apparent with the continued use of Vi-Flor vitamin-fluoride products.[5]

WARNINGS
As in the case of all medications, keep out of the reach of children.

PRECAUTIONS
The suggested dose of Tri-Vi-Flor 1.0 mg chewable tablets *should not be exceeded,* since dental fluorosis may result from continued ingestion of large amounts of fluoride.
When prescribing Vi-Flor products:
1. determine the fluoride content of the drinking water.
2. make sure the child is not receiving significant amounts of fluoride from other medications.
3. periodically check to make sure that the child does not develop significant dental fluorosis.

ADVERSE REACTIONS
Allergic rash and other idiosyncrasies have been rarely reported.

DOSAGE AND ADMINISTRATION
One chewable tablet daily or as prescribed.

HOW SUPPLIED
Tri-Vi-Flor 1.0 mg (vitamins A, D, C and fluoride) chewable tablets are available in 100- and 1000-tablet bottles.
NDC 0087-0477-01 Bottles of 100
NDC 0087-0477-02 Bottles of 1000

LITERATURE AVAILABLE
Yes.

REFERENCES

1. Hennon, D.K., Stookey, G.K. and Muhler, J.C.: The Clinical Anticariogenic Effectiveness of Supplementary Fluoride-Vitamin Preparations—Results at the End of Three Years. J Dent for Children 33:3–12 (Jan.) 1966.
2. Hennon, D.K., Stookey, G.K. and Muhler, J.C.: The Clinical Anticariogenic Effectiveness of Supplementary Fluoride-Vitamin Preparations—Results at the End of Four Years, J Dent for Children 34:439–443 (Nov.) 1967.
3. American Academy of Pediatrics, Committee on Nutrition: Fluoride supplementation: Revised Dosage Schedule. Pediatrics 63:150, 1979.
4. Arnold, F.A., Jr., McClure, F.J. and White, C.L.: Sodium Fluoride Tablets for Children, Dental Progress 1:12–16 (Oct.) 1960.
5. Hennon, D.K., Stookey, G.K. and Muhler, J.C.: The Clinical Anticariogenic Effectiveness of Supplementary Fluoride-Vitamin Preparations—Results at the End of Five and a Half Years, Phar. and Ther. in Dent. 1:1, 1970.

TRI-VI-FLOR® ℞
[trī 'vī-flōr"]
- **0.5 mg**
- **0.25 mg**

Vitamins A, D, C and fluoride drops

DESCRIPTION
[See table above].
See INDICATIONS AND USAGE section below for use by infants and children under two years of age.
Active ingredient for caries prophylaxis: Fluoride as sodium fluoride.
Other ingredients: Ascorbic acid, caramel color, cholecalciferol, fruit flavor (artificial), glycerin, polysorbate 80, sodium hydroxide, vitamin A palmitate, water.

Each 1.0 ml supplies:	Tri-Vi-Flor Drops 0.5mg	Tri-Vi-Flor Drops 0.25mg	Percentage of U.S. Recommended Daily Allowance: Infants	Children Under 4
Vitamin A, IU	1500	1500	100	60
Vitamin D, IU	400	400	100	100
Vitamin C, mg	35	35	100	100
Fluoride, mg	0.5	0.25	*	*

*U.S. Recommended Daily Allowance has not been established.

CLINICAL PHARMACOLOGY
For information on fluoridation see Poly-Vi-Flor® chewable tablets.

INDICATIONS AND USAGE
Supplementation of the diet with vitamins A, D and C.
Tri-Vi-Flor drops also provide fluoride for caries prophylaxis.
The American Academy of Pediatrics recommends that children up to age 16, in areas where drinking water contains less than optimal levels of fluoride, receive daily fluoride supplementation.
Tri-Vi-Flor 0.5 mg (vitamins A, D, C and fluoride) drops provide fluoride in drop form for children ages 2-3 years in areas where the drinking water contains less than 0.3 ppm fluoride; and for children over 3 years in areas where the drinking water contains 0.3 thru 0.7 ppm of fluoride.[1] Each 1.0 ml provides sodium fluoride (0.5 mg fluoride) plus three basic vitamins.
Tri-Vi-Flor 0.25 mg (vitamins A, D, C and fluoride) drops provide fluoride in drop form for infants and young children from birth to 2 years of age in areas where the drinking water contains less than 0.3 ppm of fluoride; and for children ages 2-3 years in areas where the drinking water contains 0.3 thru 0.7 ppm of fluoride. Each 1.0 ml supplies sodium fluoride (0.25 mg fluoride) plus three basic vitamins.
The American Academy of Pediatrics[1] and the American Dental Association[6] currently recommend that infants and children under 2 years of age, in areas where drinking water contains less than 0.3 ppm of fluoride, and children 2-3, in areas where the drinking water contains 0.3 through 0.7 ppm of fluoride, receive 0.25 mg of supplemental fluoride daily which is provided in a full dose (1 ml) of Tri-Vi-Flor® 0.25 mg drops. A half dose (0.5 ml) of Tri-Vi-Flor 0.5 mg drops could also provide a daily fluoride intake of 0.25 mg; however, this dosage reduces vitamin supplementation by half.

A comprehensive 5½ year series of studies of the effectiveness of Tri-Vi-Flor® and Poly-Vi-Flor® products in caries protection has been published.[2-5] Children in this continuing study lived in an area where the water supply contained only 0.05 ppm fluoride. The subjects were divided into two groups, one which used only nonfluoridated Vi-Sol® vitamin products and the other Tri-Vi-Flor and Poly-Vi-Flor vitamin-fluoride products.

The three-year interim report showed 63% fewer carious surfaces in primary teeth and 43% fewer carious surfaces in permanent teeth of the children taking Vi-Flor® vitamin-fluoride products.[2]

After four years the studies continued to support the effectiveness of Tri-Vi-Flor and Poly-Vi-Flor, showing a reduction in carious surfaces of 68% in primary teeth and 46% in permanent teeth.[3]

Results at the end of 5½ years further confirmed the previous findings and indicated that significant reductions in dental caries are apparent with the continued use of Vi-Flor vitamin-fluoride products.[4]

WARNINGS

As in the case of all medications, keep out of the reach of children.

PRECAUTIONS

The suggested dose should not be exceeded since dental fluorosis may result from continued ingestion of large amounts of fluoride.

When prescribing Vi-Flor products:

1. determine the fluoride content of the drinking water.
2. make sure the child is not receiving significant amounts of fluoride from other medications.
3. periodically check to make sure that the child does not develop significant dental fluorosis.

Tri-Vi-Flor drops should be dispensed in the original plastic container, since contact with glass leads to instability and precipitation. (The amount of sodium fluoride in both the 30- and 50-ml sizes is well below the maximum to be dispensed at one time acccording to recommendations of the American Dental Association.)

ADVERSE REACTIONS

Allergic rash and other idiosyncrasies have been rarely reported.

DOSAGE AND ADMINISTRATION

1.0 ml daily, or as prescribed.

May be dropped directly into mouth with 'Safti-Dropper,' or mixed with cereal, fruit juice or other food.

HOW SUPPLIED

Tri-Vi-Flor 0.5 mg (vitamins A,D,C, and fluoride) drops are available in bottles of 30 and 50 ml.

NDC 0087-0473-01 Bottles of 1 fl oz (30 ml)
NDC 0087-0473-02 Bottles of 1⅔ fl oz (50 ml)

Tri-Vi-Flor 0.25 mg (vitamins A, D, C and fluoride) drops are available in bottles of 50 ml.

NDC 0087-0452-41 Bottles of 50 ml.

LITERATURE AVAILABLE

Yes.

REFERENCES

1. American Academy of Pediatrics, Committee on Nutrition: Fluoride Supplementation: Revised Dosage Schedule, Pediatrics 63:150, 1979.
2. Hennon, D.K.; Stookey, G.K., and Muhler, J.C.: The Clinical Anticariogenic Effectiveness of Supplementary Fluoride-Vitamin Preparations— Results at the End of Three Years, J. Dentistry for Children 33:3–12 (Jan.) 1966.
3. Hennon, D.K.; Stookey, G.K., and Muhler, J.C.: The Clinical Anticariogenic Effectiveness of Supplementary Fluoride-Vitamin Preparations— Results at the End of Four Years, J. Dentistry for Children 34:439–443 (Nov.) 1967.
4. Hennon, D.K.; Stookey, G.K., and Muhler, J.C.: The Clinical Anticariogenic Effectiveness of Supplementary Fluoride-Vitamin Preparations— Results at the End of Five and a Half Years, Phar. and Ther. in Dent. 1:1, 1970.
5. Hennon, D.K.; Stookey, G.K., and Beiswanger, B.B.: Fluoride-vitamin supplements: Effects on dental caries and fluorosis when used in areas with suboptimum fluoride in the water supply. J. Am. Dent. Assoc. 95:965, 1977.
6. Accepted Dental Therapeutics, Ed. 38, Chicago, American Dental Association, 1979, p. 321.

Product	Strength	Capsules	Tablets One Side
Desyrel® (trazodone HCl)	50mg		Desyrel MJ775
Desyrel®	100mg		Desyrel MJ776
Duricef® (cefadroxil) capsules	500mg	MJ784	
Duricef® (cefadroxil) tablets	1g		MJ785 & score line
Klotrix® (potassium chloride)			Klotrix MJ770 10mEq

TRI-VI-FLOR® 0.25 mg with Iron ℞

[*trī'vī-flōr"*]

Vitamins A, D, C, iron and fluoride drops

DESCRIPTION

Each 1.0 ml supplies:		Percentage of U.S. Recommended Daily Allowance: Infants	Children Under 4
Vitamin A, IU	1500	100	60
Vitamin D, IU	400	100	100
Vitamin C, mg	35	100	88
Iron, mg	10	67	100
Fluoride, mg	0.25	*	*

* U.S. Recommended Daily Allowance has not been established.

Active ingredients for caries prophylaxis: Fluoride as sodium fluoride.

Other ingredients: Ascorbic acid, caramel color, cholecalciferol, ferrous sulfate, fruit flavor (artificial), glycerin, polysorbate 80, propylene glycol, sodium hydroxide, vitamin A palmitate, water, and other ingredients.

CLINICAL PHARMACOLOGY

For information on fluoridation see Poly-Vi-Flor® chewable tablets.

INDICATIONS AND USAGE

Supplementation of the diet with vitamins A, D, C and iron.

Supplementation of the diet with fluoride for caries prophylaxis.

The American Academy of Pediatrics recommends that children up to age 16, in areas where drinking water contains less than optimal levels of fluoride, receive daily fluoride supplementation.

Tri-Vi-Flor 0.25 mg with Iron (vitamins A, D, C, iron and fluoride) drops provide fluoride in drop form for infants and young children from birth to 2 years of age in areas where the drinking water contains less than 0.3 ppm of fluoride; and for children ages 2-3 years in areas where the drinking water contains 0.3 thru 0.7 ppm of fluoride.[2] Each 1.0 ml supplies sodium fluoride (0.25 mg fluoride) plus three basic vitamins and iron.

WARNINGS

As in the case of all medications, keep out of the reach of children.

PRECAUTIONS

The suggested dose should not be exceeded since dental fluorosis may result from continued ingestion of large amounts of fluoride.

When prescribing Vi-Flor® products:

1. determine the fluoride content of the drinking water.
2. make sure the child is not receiving significant amounts of fluoride from other medications.
3. periodically check to make sure that the child does not develop significant dental fluorosis.

TRI-VI-FLOR 0.25 mg with Iron drops should be dispensed in the original plastic container, since contact with glass leads to instability and precipitation. (The amount of sodium fluoride in the 50-ml size is well below the maximum to be dispensed at one time according to recommendations of the American Dental Association.)

ADVERSE REACTIONS

Allergic rash and other idiosyncrasies have been rarely reported.

DOSAGE AND ADMINISTRATION

1.0 ml daily, or as prescribed. May be dropped directly into mouth with 'Safti-Dropper', or mixed with cereal, fruit juice or other food.

USE FULL DOSAGE.

HOW SUPPLIED

Tri-Vi-Flor 0.25 mg with Iron (vitamins A, D, C, iron and fluoride) drops are available in bottles of 50 ml.

REFERENCES

1. Brudevold, F. and McCann, H.G.: Fluoride and caries control—mechanism of action, in Nizel, A.E.: The Science of Nutrition and its Application in Clinical Dentistry, Philadelphia, WB Saunders Company, 1966, pp 332–347.
2. American Academy of Pediatrics, Committee on Nutrition: Fluoride Supplementation: Revised Dosage Schedule, Pediatrics 63:150, 1979.

TRI-VI-SOL®

[*trī'vī-sahl"*]

Vitamin A, D and C Supplement drops

(See PDR For Nonprescription Drugs)

TRI-VI-SOL® with Iron

[*trī'vī-sahl"*]

Vitamins A, D, C and Iron drops

(See PDR For Nonprescription Drugs)

Mead Johnson Pharmaceutical Division

Mead Johnson & Company
2404 W. PENNSYLVANIA ST.
EVANSVILLE, INDIANA 47721

IDENTIFICATION MARKINGS SOLID ORAL DOSE FORMS

[See table above].

COLACE®

[*kō'lās*]

Docusate sodium, Mead Johnson capsules • syrup • liquid (drops)

PRODUCT OVERVIEW

KEY FACTS

Colace is a stool softener. This surface-active agent helps keep stools soft for easy, natural passage. Colace is not a laxative; thus, not habit forming. It is available in three forms: capsules, 50 mg and 100 mg; syrup; liquid (drops, 1% solution).

MAJOR USES

Colace is useful in constipation due to hard stools in painful anorectal conditions, in cardiac and other conditions in which maximum ease of passage is desirable to avoid difficult or painful defecation, and when peristaltic stimulants are contraindicated.

SAFETY INFORMATION

There are no known contraindications to Colace. The incidence of side effects—none of a serious nature—is exceedingly small.

PRESCRIBING INFORMATION

COLACE®

[*kō' lās*]

Docusate sodium, Mead Johnson capsules • syrup • liquid (drops)

DESCRIPTION

Colace (Docusate sodium) is a stool softener.

Colace Capsules, 50 mg, contain the following inactive ingredients: citric acid, D&C Red No. 33, FD&C Red No. 40, non-porcine gelatin, edible ink, polyethylene glycol, propylene glycol, and purified water.

Colace Capsules, 100 mg, contain the following inactive ingredients: citric acid, D&C Red No. 33, FD&C Red No. 40, FD&C Yellow No. 6, non-porcine gelatin, edible ink, polyethylene glycol, propylene glycol, titanium dioxide, and purified water.

Colace Liquid, 1%, contains the following inactive ingredients: citric acid, D&C Red No. 33, methylparaben, poloxamer, polyethylene glycol, propylene glycol, propylparaben, sodium citrate, vanillin, and purified water.

Colace Syrup contains the following inactive ingredients: alcohol, citric acid, D&C Red No. 33, FD&C Red No. 40, flavor (natural), menthol, methylparaben, peppermint oil, poloxamer, polyethylene glycol, propylparaben, sodium citrate, sucrose, and purified water.

ACTIONS AND USES

Colace, a surface-active agent, helps to keep stools soft for easy, natural passage. Not a laxative, thus not habit forming. Useful in constipation due to hard stools, in painful anorectal conditions, in cardiac and other conditions in which maximum ease of passage is desirable to avoid difficult or painful defecation, and when peristaltic stimulants are contraindi-

Continued on next page

Mead Johnson Pharm.—Cont.

cated. *Note:* When peristaltic stimulation is needed due to inadequate bowel motility, see Peri-Colace® (laxative and stool softener).

CONTRAINDICATIONS

There are no known contraindications to Colace.

SIDE EFFECTS

The incidence of side effects—none of a serious nature—is exceedingly small. Bitter taste, throat irritation, and nausea (primarily associated with the use of the syrup and liquid) are the main side effects reported. Rash has occurred.

ADMINISTRATION AND DOSAGE

Orally—Suggested daily Dosage: *Adults and older children:* 50 to 200 mg. *Children 6 to 12:* 40 to 120 mg. *Children 3 to 6:* 20 to 60 mg. *Infants and children under 3:* 10 to 40 mg. The higher doses are recommended for initial therapy. Dosage should be adjusted to individual response. The effect on stools is usually apparent one to three days after the first dose. Give Colace liquid in half a glass of milk or fruit juice or in infant formula, to mask bitter taste. *In enemas*—Add 50 to 100 mg. Colace (5 to 10 ml. Colace liquid) to a retention or flushing enema.

WARNING

As with any drug, if you are pregnant or nursing a baby, seek the advice of a health professional before using this product.

HOW SUPPLIED

Colace® capsules, 50 mg.
NDC 0087-0713-01 Bottles of 30
NDC 0087-0713-02 Bottles of 60
NDC 0087-0713-03 Bottles of 250
NDC 0087-0713-05 Bottles of 1000
NDC 0087-0713-07 Cartons of 100 single unit packs
Colace® capsules, 100 mg.
NDC 0087-0714-43 Cartons of 10 single unit packs
NDC 0087-0714-01 Bottles of 30
NDC 0087-0714-02 Bottles of 60
NDC 0087-0714-03 Bottles of 250
NDC 0087-0714-05 Bottles of 1000
NDC 0087-0714-07 Cartons of 100 single unit packs
Note: Colace capsules should be stored at controlled room temperature (59°–86°F. or 15°–30°C.)
Colace® liquid, 1% solution; 10 mg./ml. (with calibrated dropper)
NDC 0087-0717-04 Bottles of 16 fl. oz.
NDC 0087-0717-02 Bottles of 30 ml.
6505-00-045-7786 (Bottle of 30 ml) Defense
Colace® syrup, 20 mg./5-ml. teaspoon; contains not more than 1% alcohol
NDC 0087-0720-01 Bottles of 8 fl. oz.
NDC 0087-0720-02 Bottles of 16 fl. oz.
Shown in Product Identification Section, page 417

DESYREL® ℞

[des 'ē-rel]
(Trazodone HCl)

DESCRIPTION

DESYREL®, trazodone hydrochloride, is an antidepressant chemically unrelated to tricyclic, tetracyclic, or other known antidepressant agents. It is a triazolopyridine derivative designated as 2-[3-[4-(3-chlorophenyl)-1-piperazinyl] propyl]-1,2,4-triazolo[4, 3-a]pyridin-3(2H)-one hydrochloride. DESYREL is a white odorless crystalline powder which is freely soluble in water. Its molecular weight is 408.3. The empirical formula is $C_{19}H_{22}ClN_5O \cdot HCl$ and the structural formula is represented as follows:

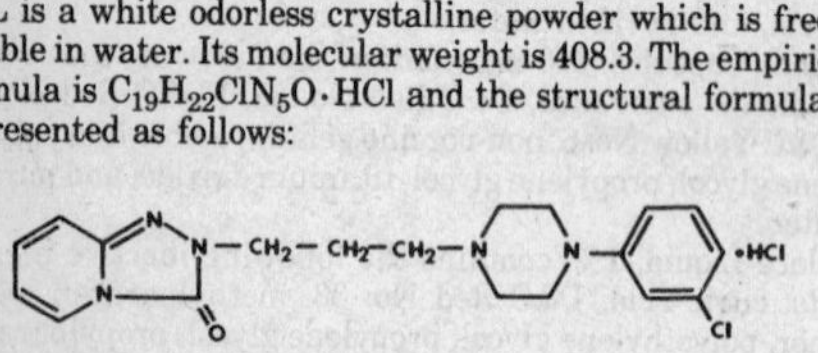

DESYREL is supplied for oral administration in 50 mg, 100 mg and 150 mg tablets.
DESYREL® Tablets, 50 mg, contain the following inactive ingredients: dibasic calcium phosphate, castor oil, microcrystalline cellulose, ethylcellulose, FD&C Yellow No. 6 (aluminum lake), lactose, magnesium stearate, povidone, sodium starch glycolate, and starch (corn).
DESYREL® Tablets, 100 mg, contain the following inactive ingredients: dibasic calcium phosphate, castor oil, microcrystalline cellulose, ethylcellulose, lactose, magnesium stearate, povidone, sodium starch glycolate, and starch (corn).
DESYREL® Tablets, 150 mg, contain the following inactive ingredients: microcrystalline cellulose, FD&C Yellow No. 6 (aluminum lake), magnesium stearate, pregelatinized starch, and stearic acid.

CLINICAL PHARMACOLOGY

The mechanism of DESYREL's antidepressant action in man is not fully understood. In animals, DESYREL selectively inhibits serotonin uptake by brain synaptosomes and potentiates the behavioral changes induced by the serotonin precursor, 5-hydroxytryptophan. Cardiac conduction effects of DESYREL in the anesthetized dog are qualitatively dissimilar and quantitatively less pronounced than those seen with tricyclic antidepressants. DESYREL is not a monoamine oxidase inhibitor and, unlike amphetamine-type drugs, does not stimulate the central nervous system.
In man, DESYREL is well absorbed after oral administration without selective localization in any tissue. When DESYREL is taken shortly after ingestion of food, there may be an increase in the amount of drug absorbed, a decrease in maximum concentration and a lengthening in the time to maximum concentration. Peak plasma levels occur approximately one hour after dosing when DESYREL is taken on an empty stomach or two hours after dosing when taken with food. Elimination of DESYREL is biphasic, consisting of an initial phase (half-life 3–6 hours) followed by a slower phase (half-life 5–9 hours), and is unaffected by the presence or absence of food. Since the clearance of DESYREL from the body is sufficiently variable, in some patients DESYREL may accumulate in the plasma.
For those patients who responded to DESYREL, one-third of the inpatients and one-half of the outpatients had a significant therapeutic response by the end of the first week of treatment. Three-fourths of all responders demonstrated a significant therapeutic effect by the end of the second week. One-fourth of responders required 2–4 weeks for a significant therapeutic response.

INDICATIONS AND USAGE

DESYREL is indicated for the treatment of depression. The efficacy of DESYREL has been demonstrated in both inpatient and outpatient settings and for depressed patients with and without prominent anxiety. The depressive illness of patients studied corresponds to the Major Depressive Episode criteria of the American Psychiatric Association's Diagnostic and Statistical Manual, III.[a]
Major Depressive Episode implies a prominent and relatively persistent (nearly every day for at least two weeks) depressed or dysphoric mood that usually interferes with daily functioning, and includes at least four of the following eight symptoms: change in appetite, change in sleep, psychomotor agitation or retardation, loss of interest in usual activities or decrease in sexual drive, increased fatigability, feelings of guilt or worthlessness, slowed thinking or impaired concentration, and suicidal ideation or attempts.

CONTRAINDICATIONS

DESYREL is contraindicated in patients hypersensitive to DESYREL.

WARNINGS

TRAZODONE HAS BEEN ASSOCIATED WITH THE OCCURRENCE OF PRIAPISM. IN APPROXIMATELY 1/3 OF THE CASES REPORTED, SURGICAL INTERVENTION WAS REQUIRED AND, IN A PORTION OF THESE CASES, PERMANENT IMPAIRMENT OF ERECTILE FUNCTION OR IMPOTENCE RESULTED. MALE PATIENTS WITH PROLONGED OR INAPPROPRIATE ERECTIONS SHOULD IMMEDIATELY DISCONTINUE THE DRUG AND CONSULT THEIR PHYSICIAN.
Recent clinical studies in patients with pre-existing cardiac disease indicate that DESYREL may be arrhythmogenic in some patients in that population. Arrhythmias identified include isolated PVC's, ventricular couplets, and in two patients short episodes (3–4 beats) of ventricular tachycardia. Until the results of prospective studies are available, patients with pre-existing cardiac disease should be closely monitored particularly for cardiac arrhythmias. There have also been post-introduction reports of arrhythmias in DESYREL-treated patients, some of whom did not have pre-existing cardiac disease.
DESYREL is not recommended for use during the initial recovery phase of myocardial infarction.

PRECAUTIONS

General: The possibility of suicide in seriously depressed patients is inherent in the illness and may persist until significant remission occurs. Therefore, prescriptions should be written for the smallest number of tablets consistent with good patient management.
Hypotension, including orthostatic hypotension and syncope, has been reported to occur in patients receiving DESYREL. Concomitant administration of antihypertensive therapy with DESYREL may require a reduction in the dose of the antihypertensive drug.
Little is known about the interaction between DESYREL and general anesthetics; therefore, prior to elective surgery, DESYREL should be discontinued for as long as clinically feasible.
As with all antidepressants, the use of DESYREL should be based on the consideration of the physician that the expected benefits of therapy outweigh potential risk factors.

Information for Patients: Because priapism has been reported to occur in patients receiving DESYREL, patients with prolonged or inappropriate penile erection should immediately discontinue the drug and consult with the physician.
Antidepressants may impair the mental and/or physical abilities required for the performance of potentially hazardous tasks, such as operating an automobile or machinery; the patient should be cautioned accordingly.
DESYREL may enhance the response to alcohol, barbiturates, and other CNS depressants.
DESYREL should be given shortly after a meal or light snack. Within any individual patient, total drug absorption may be up to 20% higher when the drug is taken with food rather than on an empty stomach. The risk of dizziness/lightheadedness may increase under fasting conditions.

Laboratory Tests: Occasional low white blood cell and neutrophil counts have been noted in patients receiving DESYREL. These were not considered clinically significant and did not necessitate discontinuation of the drug; however, the drug should be discontinued in any patient whose white blood cell count or absolute neutrophil count falls below normal levels. White blood cell and differential counts are recommended for patients who develop fever and sore throat (or other signs of infection) during therapy.

Drug Interactions: Increased serum digoxin or phenytoin levels have been reported to occur in patients receiving DESYREL concurrently with either of those two drugs.
It is not known whether interactions will occur between monoamine oxidase (MAO) inhibitors and DESYREL. Due to the absence of clinical experience, if MAO inhibitors are discontinued shortly before or are to be given concomitantly with DESYREL, therapy should be initiated cautiously with gradual increase in dosage until optimum response is achieved.

Therapeutic Interactions: Concurrent administration with electroshock therapy should be avoided because of the absence of experience in this area.

Carcinogenesis, Mutagenesis, Impairment of Fertility: No drug- or dose-related occurrence of carcinogenesis was evident in rats receiving DESYREL in daily oral doses up to 300 mg/kg for 18 months.

Pregnancy Category C: DESYREL has been shown to cause increased fetal resorption and other adverse effects on the fetus in two studies using the rat when given at dose levels approximately 30–50 times the proposed maximum human dose. There was also an increase in congenital anomalies in one of three rabbit studies at approximately 15–50 times the maximum human dose. There are no adequate and well-controlled studies in pregnant women. DESYREL should be used during pregnancy only if the potential benefit justifies the potential risk to the fetus.

Nursing Mothers: DESYREL and/or its metabolites have been found in the milk of lactating rats, suggesting that the drug may be secreted in human milk. Caution should be exercised when DESYREL is administered to a nursing woman.

Pediatric Use: Safety and effectiveness in children below the age of 18 have not been established.

ADVERSE REACTIONS

Because the frequency of adverse drug effects is affected by diverse factors (e.g., drug dose, method of detection, physician judgment, disease under treatment, etc.) a single meaningful estimate of adverse event incidence is difficult to obtain. This problem is illustrated by the variation in adverse event incidence observed and reported from the inpatients and outpatients treated with DESYREL. It is impossible to determine precisely what accounts for the differences observed.

Clinical Trial Reports: The table below is presented solely to indicate the relative frequency of adverse events reported in representative controlled clinical studies conducted to evaluate the safety and efficacy of DESYREL. [See table on next page].
The figures cited cannot be used to predict precisely the incidence of untoward events in the course of usual medical practice where patient characteristics and other factors often differ from those which prevailed in the clinical trials. These incidence figures, also, cannot be compared with those obtained from other clinical studies involving related drug products and placebo as each group of drug trials is conducted under a different set of conditions.
Occasional sinus bradycardia has occurred in long-term studies.
In addition to the relatively common (i.e., greater than 1%) untoward events enumerated above, the following adverse events have been reported to occur in association with the use of DESYREL in the controlled clinical studies: akathisia, allergic reaction, anemia, chest pain, delayed urine flow, early menses, flatulence, hallucinations/delusions, hematuria, hypersalivation, hypomania, impaired speech, impotence, increased appetite, increased libido, increased urinary frequency, missed periods, muscle twitches, numbness, and retrograde ejaculation.

Post Introduction Reports: Voluntary reports received since market introduction include the following: agitation, apnea, diplopia, edema, grand mal seizures, hallucinations, hemolytic anemia, liver enzyme alterations, methemoglobinemia, nausea/vomiting (most frequently), paresthesia, priapism (see PRECAUTIONS, Information for Patients; some patients have required surgical intervention), rash, and weakness.

Cardiovascular system effects which have been reported are the following: Orthostatic hypotension and syncope, palpitations, bradycardia, atrial fibrillation, myocardial infarction, cardiac arrest, arrhythmia, and ventricular ectopic activity, including ventricular tachycardia (see WARNINGS).

OVERDOSE

Animal Oral LD_{50}

The oral LD_{50} of the drug is 610 mg/kg in mice, 486 mg/kg in rats, and 560 mg/kg in rabbits.

Signs and Symptoms: Death from overdose has occurred in patients ingesting DESYREL and other drugs concurrently (namely, alcohol; alcohol + chloral hydrate + diazepam; amobarbital; chlordiazepoxide; or meprobamate).

The most severe reactions reported to have occurred with overdose of DESYREL alone have been priapism, respiratory arrest, seizures, and EKG changes. The reactions reported most frequently have been drowsiness and vomiting. Overdosage may cause an increase in incidence or severity of any of the reported adverse reactions (see ADVERSE REACTIONS).

Treatment: There is no specific antidote for DESYREL. Treatment should be symptomatic and supportive in the case of hypotension or excessive sedation. Any patient suspected of having taken an overdose should have the stomach emptied by gastric lavage. Forced diuresis may be useful in facilitating elimination of the drug.

DOSAGE AND ADMINISTRATION

The dosage should be initiated at a low level and increased gradually, noting the clinical response and any evidence of intolerance. Occurrence of drowsiness may require the administration of a major portion of the daily dose at bedtime or a reduction of dosage. DESYREL should be taken shortly after a meal or light snack. Symptomatic relief may be seen during the first week, with optimal antidepressant effects typically evident within two weeks. Twenty-five percent of those who respond to DESYREL require more than two weeks (up to four weeks) of drug administration.

Usual Adult Dosage: An initial dose of 150 mg/day in divided doses is suggested. The dose may be increased by 50 mg/day every three to four days. The maximum dose for outpatients usually should not exceed 400 mg/day in divided doses. Inpatients (i.e. more severely depressed patients) may be given up to but not in excess of 600 mg/day in divided doses.

Maintenance: Dosage during prolonged maintenance therapy should be kept at the lowest effective level. Once an adequate response has been achieved, dosage may be gradually reduced, with subsequent adjustment depending on therapeutic response.

HOW SUPPLIED

DESYREL® (trazodone hydrochloride)

Tablets, 50 mg—round, orange/scored, film-sealed (imprinted with MJ logo)

NDC 0087-0775-41 Bottles of 100

NDC 0087-0775-43 Bottles of 1000

NDC 0087-0775-42 Cartons of 100 Unit Doses

Tablets, 100 mg—round, white/scored, film-sealed (imprinted with MJ logo)

NDC 0087-0776-41 Bottles of 100

NDC 0087-0776-43 Bottles of 1000

NDC 0087-0776-42 Cartons of 100 Unit Doses

Tablets, 150 mg—orange, in the Dividose® tablet design (imprinted with MJ logo)

NDC 0087-0778-43 Bottles of 100

U.S. Patent No. 4,215,104

Store at room temperature. Protect from temperatures above 104°F (40°C).

Dispense in tight, light-resistant container (USP).

REFERENCES

a. Williams JBW, Ed: Diagnostic and Statistical Manual of Mental Disorders-III, American Psychiatric Association, May, 1980.

Shown in Product Identification Section, page 417

	Treatment Emergent Symptom Incidence			
	Inpts.		Outpts.	
	D	P	D	P
Number of Patients	142	95	157	158
% of Patients Reporting				
Allergic				
Skin Condition/Edema	2.8	1.1	7.0	1.3
Autonomic				
Blurred Vision	6.3	4.2	14.7	3.8
Constipation	7.0	4.2	7.6	5.7
Dry Mouth	14.8	8.4	33.8	20.3
Cardiovascular				
Hypertension	2.1	1.1	1.3	*
Hypotension	7.0	1.1	3.8	0.0
Shortness of Breath	*	1.1	1.3	0.0
Syncope	2.8	2.1	4.5	1.3
Tachycardia/Palpitations	0.0	0.0	7.0	7.0
CNS				
Anger/Hostility	3.5	6.3	1.3	2.5
Confusion	4.9	0.0	5.7	7.6
Decreased Concentration	2.8	2.1	1.3	0.0
Disorientation	2.1	0.0	*	0.0
Dizziness/Lightheadedness	19.7	5.3	28.0	15.2
Drowsiness	23.9	6.3	40.8	19.6
Excitement	1.4	1.1	5.1	5.7
Fatigue	11.3	4.2	5.7	2.5
Headache	9.9	5.3	19.8	15.8
Insomnia	9.9	10.5	6.4	12.0
Impaired Memory	1.4	0.0	*	*
Nervousness	14.8	10.5	6.4	8.2
Gastrointestinal				
Abdominal/Gastric Disorder	3.5	4.2	5.7	4.4
Bad Taste in Mouth	1.4	0.0	0.0	0.0
Diarrhea	0.0	1.1	4.5	1.9
Nausea/Vomiting	9.9	1.1	12.7	9.5
Musculoskeletal				
Musculoskeletal Aches/Pains	5.6	3.2	5.1	2.5
Neurological				
Incoordination	4.9	0.0	1.9	0.0
Paresthesia	1.4	0.0	0.0	*
Tremors	2.8	1.1	5.1	3.8
Sexual Function				
Decreased Libido	*	1.1	1.3	*
Other				
Decreased Appetite	3.5	5.3	0.0	*
Eyes Red/Tired/Itching	2.8	0.0	0.0	0.0
Head Full-Heavy	2.8	0.0	0.0	0.0
Malaise	2.8	0.0	0.0	0.0
Nasal/Sinus Congestion	2.8	0.0	5.7	3.2
Nightmares/Vivid Dreams	*	1.1	5.1	5.7
Sweating/Clamminess	1.4	1.1	*	*
Tinnitus	1.4	0.0	0.0	*
Weight Gain	1.4	0.0	4.5	1.9
Weight Loss	*	3.2	5.7	2.5

*Incidence less than 1%.

D = DESYREL P = Placebo

DURICEF® ℞

[dur'ĭ-sef]

(Cefadroxil)

DESCRIPTION

DURICEF® (cefadroxil) is a semisynthetic cephalosporin antibiotic intended for oral administration. It is a white to yellowish-white crystalline powder. It is soluble in water and it is acid-stable. It is chemically designated as 7- [[D-2-amino-2-(4-hydroxyphenyl) acetyl] amino]-3- methyl-8-oxo -5- thia-1-azabicyclo [4.2.0] oct-2- ene-2-carboxylic acid monohydrate. It has the following structural formula:

DURICEF® tablets, 1 g, contain the following inactive ingredients: microcrystalline cellulose and magnesium stearate.

DURICEF® for Oral Suspension contains the following inactive ingredients: FD&C Yellow No. 6, flavors (natural and artificial), polysorbate 80, sodium benzoate, sucrose, and xanthan gum.

DURICEF® capsules contain the following inactive ingredients: D&C Red No. 28, FD&C Blue No. 1, FD&C Red No. 40, gelatin, magnesium stearate, and titanium dioxide.

Clinical Pharmacology—DURICEF (cefadroxil) is rapidly absorbed after oral administration. Following single doses of 500 and 1000 mg., average peak serum concentrations were approximately 16 and 28 mcg./ml., respectively. Measurable levels were present 12 hours after administration. Over 90 percent of the drug is excreted unchanged in the urine within twenty-four hours. Peak urine concentrations are approximately 1800 mcg./ml. during the period following a single 500 mg. oral dose. Increases in dosage generally produce a proportionate increase in DURICEF urinary concentration. The urine antibiotic concentration, following a 1 gm. dose, was maintained well above the MIC of susceptible urinary pathogens for 20 to 22 hours.

Microbiology: *In vitro* tests demonstrate that the cephalosporins are bactericidal because of their inhibition of cell-wall synthesis. DURICEF is active against the following organisms *in vitro:*

Beta-hemolytic streptococci

Staphylococci, including coagulase-positive, coagulase-negative, and penicillinase-producing strains

Streptococcus (Diplococcus) pneumoniae

Escherichia coli.

Proteus mirabilis

Klebsiella species

Note:—Most strains of *Enterococci (Streptococcus faecalis* and *S. faecium)* are resistant to DURICEF. It is not active against most strains of *Enterobacter species, P. morganii,* and *P. vulgaris,* It has no activity against *Pseudomonas* sp. and *Acinetobacter calcoaceticus* (formerly *Mima* and *Herellea* sp.)

Disc Susceptibility Tests.—Quantitative methods that require measurement of zone diameters give the most precise estimates of antibiotic susceptibility. One recommended procedure (CFR Section 460.1) uses cephalosporin class disc for testing susceptibility; interpretations correlate zone diameters of this disc test with MIC values for DURICEF. With this procedure, a report from the laboratory of "resistant" indicates that the infecting organism is not likely to respond to therapy. A report of "intermediate susceptibility" suggests that the organism would be susceptible if the infection is confined to the urinary tract, as DURICEF produces high antibiotic levels in the urine.

Continued on next page

Mead Johnson Pharm.—Cont.

INDICATIONS

DURICEF (cefadroxil) is indicated for the treatment of the following infections when caused by susceptible strains of the designated microorganisms:

Urinary tract infections caused by *E. coli*, *P. mirabilis*, and *Klebsiella* species

Skin and skin structure infections caused by staphylococci and/or streptococci

Pharyngitis and tonsillitis caused by Group A beta-hemolytic streptococci (Penicillin is the usual drug of choice in the treatment and prevention of streptococcal infections, including the prophylaxis of rheumatic fever. DURICEF is generally effective in the eradication of streptococci from the nasopharynx; however substantial data establishing the efficacy of DURICEF in the subsequent prevention of rheumatic fever are not available at present.)

Note: Culture and susceptibility tests should be initiated prior to and during therapy. Renal function studies should be performed when indicated.

CONTRAINDICATIONS

DURICEF (cefadroxil) is contraindicated in patients with known allergy to the cephalosporin group of antibiotics.

WARNING

IN PENICILLIN-ALLERGIC PATIENTS, CEPHALOSPORIN ANTIBIOTICS SHOULD BE USED WITH GREAT CAUTION. THERE IS CLINICAL AND LABORATORY EVIDENCE OF PARTIAL CROSS-ALLERGENICITY OF THE PENICILLINS AND THE CEPHALOSPORINS, AND THERE ARE INSTANCES OF PATIENTS WHO HAVE HAD REACTIONS TO BOTH DRUGS (INCLUDING FATAL ANAPHYLAXIS AFTER PARENTERAL USE).

Any patient who has demonstrated a history of some form of allergy, particularly to drugs, should receive antibiotics cautiously and then only when absolutely necessary. No exception should be made with regard to DURICEF (cefadroxil).

Pseudomembranous colitis has been reported with the use of cephalosporins (and other broad spectrum antibiotics); therefore, it is important to consider its diagnosis in patients who develop diarrhea in association with antibiotic use.

Treatment with broad spectrum antibiotics alters normal flora of the colon and may permit overgrowth of clostridia. Studies indicate a toxin produced by *Clostridium difficile* is one primary cause of antibiotic-associated colitis. Cholestyramine and colestipol resins have been shown to bind the toxin *in vitro*.

Mild cases of colitis may respond to drug discontinuance alone.

Moderate to severe cases should be managed with fluid, electrolyte and protein supplementation as indicated.

When the colitis is not relieved by drug discontinuance or when it is severe, oral vancomycin is the treatment of choice for antibiotic-associated pseudomembranous colitis produced by *C. difficile*. Other causes of colitis should also be considered.

PRECAUTIONS

Patients should be followed carefully so that any side-effects or unusual manifestations of drug idiosyncrasy may be detected. If a hypersensitivity reaction occurs, the drug should be discontinued and the patient treated with the usual agents (e.g., epinephrine or other pressor amines, antihistamines, or corticosteroids).

DURICEF (cefadroxil) should be used with caution in the presence of markedly impaired renal function (creatinine clearance rate of less than 50 ml/min/1.73 M²). (See Dosage and Administration.) In patients with known or suspected renal impairment, careful clinical observation and appropriate laboratory studies should be made prior to and during therapy.

Prolonged use of DURICEF may result in the overgrowth of nonsusceptible organisms. Careful observation of the patient is essential. If superinfection occurs during therapy, appropriate measures should be taken.

Positive direct Coombs tests have been reported during treatment with the cephalosporin antibiotics. In hematologic studies or in transfusion cross-matching procedures when antiglobulin tests are performed on the minor side or in Coombs testing of newborns whose mothers have received cephalosporin antibiotics before parturition, it should be recognized that a positive Coombs test may be due to the drug.

DURICEF should be prescribed with caution in individuals with a history of gastrointestinal disease, particularly colitis.

Usage in Pregnancy: Pregnancy Category B: Reproduction studies have been performed in mice and rats at doses up to 11 times the human dose and have revealed no evidence of impaired fertility or harm to the fetus due to cefadroxil. There are, however, no adequate and well controlled studies in pregnant women. Because animal reproduction studies are not always predictive of human response, this drug should be used during pregnancy only if clearly needed.

Nursing Mothers: Caution should be exercised when cefadroxil is administered to a nursing mother.

ADVERSE REACTIONS

Gastrointestinal—Symptoms of pseudomembranous colitis can appear during antibiotic treatment. Nausea and vomiting have been reported rarely.

Hypersensitivity—Allergies (in the form of rash, urticaria, and angioedema) have been observed. These reactions usually subsided upon discontinuation of the drug.

Other reactions have included genital pruritus, genital moniliasis, vaginitis, and moderate transient neutropenia.

DOSAGE AND ADMINISTRATION

DURICEF (cefadroxil) is acid stable and may be administered orally without regard to meals. Administration with food may be helpful in diminishing potential gastrointestinal complaints occasionally associated with oral cephalosporin therapy.

Adults—

Urinary Tract Infections

For uncomplicated lower urinary tract infections (i.e. cystitis) the usual dosage is one or two grams per day in single (q.d.) or divided doses (b.i.d.).

For all other urinary tract infections the usual dosage is two grams per day in divided doses (b.i.d.).

Skin and Skin Structure Infections

For skin and skin structure infections the usual dosage is one gram per day in single (q.d.) or divided doses (b.i.d.).

Pharyngitis and Tonsillitis

Treatment of Group A beta hemolytic streptococcal pharyngitis and tonsillitis—One gram per day in divided doses (b.i.d.) for ten days.

Children—

The recommended daily dosage for children is 30 mg/kg/day in divided doses every 12 hours as indicated: [See table below].

In the treatment of beta-hemolytic streptococcal infections, a therapeutic dosage of Duricef should be administered for at least ten days.

In patients with renal impairment, the dosage of cefadroxil should be adjusted according to creatinine clearance rates to prevent drug accumulation. The following schedule is suggested. In adults, the initial dose is 1000 mg of DURICEF (cefadroxil) and the maintenance dose (based on the creatinine clearance rate [ml/min/1.73M²]) is 500 mg at the time intervals listed below.

Creatinine Clearances	Dosage Interval
0/10 ml/min	36 hours
10–25 ml/min	24 hours
25–50 ml/min	12 hours

Patients with creatinine clearance rates over 50 ml/min may be treated as if they were patients having normal renal function.

HOW SUPPLIED

DURICEF® (cefadroxil) for Oral Suspension

125 mg/5 ml	50 ml size	(NDC 0087-0786-42)
	100 ml size	(NDC 0087-0786-41)
250 mg/5 ml	50 ml size	(NDC 0087-0782-42)
	100 ml size	(NDC 0087-0782-41)
500 mg/5 ml	100 ml size	(NDC 0087-0783-41)

All with orange-pineapple flavor. Directions for mixing are included on the label. Shake well before using. Keep container tightly closed. After mixing, store in refrigerator. Discard unused portion after 14 days.

DURICEF (cefadroxil) capsules, 500 mg, in bottles of 50 (NDC 0087-0784-46), 100 (NDC 0087-0784-42) and in 10 strips of 10 individually labeled blisters each containing 1 capsule (NDC 0087-0784-44).

DURICEF (cefodroxil) tablets, 1 gm, in bottles of 24 (NDC 0087-0785-41), 100 (NDC 0087-0785-42) and in 10 strips of 10 individually labeled blisters each containing 1 tablet (NDC 0087-0785-44).

U.S. Patent 4,504,657

Shown in Product Identification Section, page 417

Child's Weight lbs	kg	Duricef Suspension 125 mg/5 ml	250 mg/5 ml	500 mg/5 ml
10	4.5	½ tsp b.i.d.		
20	9.1	1 tsp b.i.d.	½ tsp b.i.d.	
30	13.6	1½ tsp b.i.d.	¾ tsp b.i.d.	
40	18.2	2 tsp b.i.d.	1 tsp b.i.d.	½ tsp b.i.d.
50	22.7	2½ tsp b.i.d.	1¼ tsp b.i.d.	¾ tsp b.i.d.
60	27.3	3 tsp b.i.d.	1½ tsp b.i.d.	¾ tsp b.i.d.
70 and above	31.8+	—	—	1 tsp b.i.d.

KLOTRIX® ℞

[*klō'trix*]

(Potassium Chloride)

Slow-Release Tablets 10 mEq

PRODUCT OVERVIEW

KEY FACTS

Klotrix is a film-coated (not enteric-coated) tablet containing 750 mg potassium chloride (equivalent to 10 mEq) in a wax matrix. Klotrix is formulated to provide a controlled release of potassium from the matrix to minimize the likelihood of producing high localized concentrations of potassium within the gastrointentinal tract.

MAJOR USES

Klotrix is suggested for therapeutic use in patients with hypokalemia with or without metabolic alkalosis; in digitalis intoxication and in patients with hypokalemic familial periodic paralysis. It also can be used for prevention of potassium depletion when the dietary intake of potassium is inadequate.

SAFETY INFORMATION

Potassium supplements are contraindicated in patients with hyperkalemia. Because of reports of intestinal and gastric ulceration and bleeding with slow release potassium chloride preparations, these drugs should be reserved for those patients who cannot tolerate or refuse to take liquid or effervescent potassium preparations or for patients in whom there is a problem of compliance with these preparations.

PRESCRIBING INFORMATION

KLOTRIX® ℞

[*klō'trix*]

(Potassium Chloride)

Slow-Release Tablets 10 mEq

DESCRIPTION

KLOTRIX is a film-coated (not enteric-coated) tablet containing 750 mg potassium chloride (equivalent to 10 mEq) in a wax matrix. This formulation is intended to provide a controlled release of potassium from the matrix to minimize the likelihood of producing high localized concentrations of potassium within the gastrointestinal tract.

This product contains the following inactive ingredients: ethylcellulose, FD&C Yellow No. 6 (aluminum lake), glycerin, hydroxypropyl methylcellulose 2910, edible ink, magnesium stearate, povidone, colloidal silicon dioxide, stearic acid, and titanium dioxide.

ACTIONS

Potassium ion is the principal intracellular cation of most body tissues. Potassium ions participate in a number of essential physiological processes, including the maintenance of intracellular tonicity, the transmission of nerve impulses, the contraction of cardiac, skeletal, and smooth muscle and the maintenance of normal renal function.

Potassium depletion may occur whenever the rate of potassium loss through renal excretion and/or loss from the gastrointestinal tract exceeds the rate of potassium intake. Such depletion usually develops slowly as a consequence of prolonged therapy with oral diuretics, primary or secondary hyperaldosteronism, diabetic ketoacidosis, severe diarrhea, or inadequate replacement of potassium in patients on prolonged parenteral nutrition.

Potassium depletion due to these causes is usually accompanied by a concomitant deficiency of chloride and is manifested by hypokalemia and metabolic alkalosis. Potassium depletion may produce weakness, fatigue, disturbances of cardiac rhythm (primarily ectopic beats), prominent U-waves in the electrocardiogram, and in advanced cases flaccid paralysis and/or impaired ability to concentrate urine.

Potassium depletion associated with metabolic alkalosis is managed by correcting the fundamental causes of the deficiency whenever possible and administering supplemental potassium chloride, in the form of high potassium food or potassium chloride solution or tablets.

In rare circumstances (e.g., patients with renal tubular acidosis) potassium depletion may be associated with metabolic acidosis and hyperchloremia. In such patients potassium replacement should be accomplished with potassium salts other than the chloride, such as potassium bicarbonate, potassium citrate, or potassium acetate.

INDICATIONS

BECAUSE OF REPORTS OF INTESTINAL AND GASTRIC ULCERATION AND BLEEDING WITH SLOW RELEASE POTASSIUM CHLORIDE PREPARATIONS, THESE DRUGS SHOULD BE RESERVED FOR THOSE PATIENTS WHO CANNOT TOLERATE OR REFUSE TO TAKE LIQUID OR EFFERVESCENT POTASSIUM PREPARATIONS OR FOR

PATIENTS IN WHOM THERE IS A PROBLEM OF COMPLIANCE WITH THESE PREPARATIONS.

1. For therapeutic use in patients with hypokalemia with or without metabolic alkalosis; in digitalis intoxication and in patients with hypokalemic familial periodic paralysis.
2. For prevention of potassium depletion when the dietary intake of potassium is inadequate in the following conditions: Patients receiving digitalis and diuretics for congestive heart failure; hepatic cirrhosis with ascites; states of aldosterone excess with normal renal function; potassium-losing nephropathy, and certain diarrheal states.
3. The use of potassium salts in patients receiving diuretics for uncomplicated essential hypertension is often unnecessary when such patients have a normal dietary pattern. Serum potassium should be checked periodically, however, and, if hypokalemia occurs, dietary supplementation with potassium-containing foods may be adequate to control milder cases. In more severe cases supplementation with potassium salts may be indicated.

CONTRAINDICATIONS

Potassium supplements are contraindicated in patients with hyperkalemia since a further increase in serum potassium concentration in such patients can produce cardiac arrest. Hyperkalemia may complicate any of the following conditions: chronic renal failure, systemic acidosis such as diabetic acidosis, acute dehydration, extensive tissue breakdown as in severe burns, adrenal insufficiency, or the administration of a potassium-sparing diuretic (e.g., spironolactone, triamterene).
Wax-matrix potassium chloride preparations have produced esophageal ulceration in certain cardiac patients with esophageal compression due to an enlarged left atrium.
All solid forms of potassium supplements are contraindicated in any patient in whom there is cause for arrest or delay in tablet passage through the gastrointestinal tract. In these instances, potassium supplementation should be with a liquid preparation.

WARNINGS

Hyperkalemia
In patients with impaired mechanisms for excreting potassium, the administration of potassium salts can produce hyperkalemia and cardiac arrest. This occurs most commonly in patients given potassium by the intravenous route but may also occur in patients given potassium orally. Potentially fatal hyperkalemia can develop rapidly and be asymptomatic.
The use of potassium salts in patients with chronic renal disease, or any other condition which impairs potassium excretion, requires particularly careful monitoring of the serum potassium concentration and appropriate dosage adjustment.

Interaction with Potassium-Sparing Diuretics
Hypokalemia should not be treated by the concomitant administration of potassium salts and a potassium-sparing diuretic (e.g., spironolactone or triamterene), since the simultaneous administration of these agents can produce severe hyperkalemia.

Gastrointestinal lesions
Potassium chloride tablets have produced stenotic and/or ulcerative lesions of the small bowel and deaths. These lesions are caused by a high localized concentration of potassium ion in the region of a rapidly dissolving tablet, which injures the bowel wall and thereby produces obstruction, hemorrhage, or perforation. Klotrix is a wax-matrix tablet formulated to provide a controlled rate of release of potassium chloride and thus to minimize the possibility of a high local concentration of potassium ion near the bowel wall. While the reported frequency of small-bowel lesions is much less with wax-matrix tablets (less than one per 100,000 patient-years) than with enteric-coated potassium chloride tablets (40–50 per 100,000 patient-years) cases associated with wax-matrix tablets have been reported both in foreign countries and in the United States. In addition, perhaps because the wax-matrix preparations are not enteric-coated and release potassium in the stomach, there have been reports of upper gastrointestinal bleeding associated with these products. The total number of gastrointestinal lesions remains less than one per 100,000 patient-years. Klotrix should be discontinued immediately and the possibility of bowel obstruction or perforation considered if severe vomiting, abdominal pain, distention, or gastrointestinal bleeding occurs.

Metabolic acidosis
Hypokalemia in patients with metabolic acidosis should be treated with an alkalinizing potassium salt such as potassium bicarbonate, potassium citrate, or potassium acetate.

PRECAUTIONS

The diagnosis of potassium depletion is ordinarily made by demonstrating hypokalemia in a patient with a clinical history suggesting some cause for potassium depletion. In interpreting the serum potassium level, the physician should bear in mind that acute alkalosis *per se* can produce hypokalemia in the absence of a deficit in total body potassium, while acute acidosis *per se* can increase the serum potassium concentration into the normal range even in the presence of a reduced total body potassium. The treatment of potassium depletion, particularly in the presence of cardiac disease, renal disease, or acidosis, requires careful attention to acid-base balance and appropriate monitoring of serum electrolytes, the electrocardiogram, and the clinical status of the patient.

ADVERSE REACTIONS

The most common adverse reactions to oral potassium salts are nausea, vomiting, abdominal discomfort, and diarrhea. These symptoms are due to irritation of the gastrointestinal tract and are best managed by diluting the preparation further, taking the dose with meals, or reducing the dose.
One of the most severe adverse effects is hyperkalemia (see Contraindications, Warnings and Overdosage). There also have been reports of upper and lower gastrointestinal conditions including obstruction, bleeding, ulceration and perforation (see Contraindications and Warnings); other factors known to be associated with such conditions were present in many of these patients. Skin rash has been reported rarely.

OVERDOSAGE

The administration of oral potassium salts to persons with normal excretory mechanisms for potassium rarely causes serious hyperkalemia. However, if excretory mechanisms are impaired or if potassium is administered too rapidly intravenously, potentially fatal hyperkalemia can result (see Contraindications and Warnings). It is important to recognize that hyperkalemia is usually asymptomatic and may be manifested only by an increased serum potassium concentration and characteristic electrocardiographic changes (peaking of T-waves, loss of P-wave, depression of S-T segment, and prolongation of the QT interval). Late manifestations include muscle paralysis and cardiovascular collapse from cardiac arrest. Treatment measures for hyperkalemia include the following: (1) elimination of foods and medications containing potassium and of potassium-sparing diuretics: (2) intravenous administration of 300 to 500 ml/hr of 10% dextrose solution containing 10–20 units of insulin per 1,000 ml; (3) correction of acidosis, if present, with intravenous sodium bicarbonate; (4) use of exchange resins, hemodialysis, or peritoneal dialysis.
In treating hyperkalemia, it should be recalled that in patients who have been stabilized on digitalis, too rapid a lowering of the serum potassium concentration can produce digitalis toxicity.

DOSAGE AND ADMINISTRATION

The usual dietary intake of potassium by the average adult is 40 to 80 mEq per day. Potassium depletion sufficient to cause hypokalemia usually requires the loss of 200 or more mEq of potassium from the total body store. Dosage must be adjusted to the individual needs of each patient but is typically in the range of 20 mEq per day for the prevention of hypokalemia to 40–100 mEq per day or more for the treatment of potassium depletion.
Note: Klotrix slow-release tablets must be swallowed whole and never crushed or chewed.
Following release of the potassium chloride, the expended wax matrix, which is not absorbed, may be observed in the stool.

HOW SUPPLIED

Tablets (light orange, film-coated) each containing 750 mg potassium chloride (equivalent to 10 mEq each of potassium and chloride).

NDC 0087-0770-41	Bottles of 100
NDC 0087-0770-42	Bottles of 1000
NDC 0087-0770-43	Unit Dose Cartons of 100
VA6505-01-103-0211B	(1000's)

U.S. Pat. No. 4,140,756
Shown in Product Identification Section, page 417

MUCOMYST® ℞
[*mū'co-mist*]
(Acetylcysteine)

DESCRIPTION

Acetylcysteine is the nonproprietary name for the N-acetyl derivative of the naturally occurring amino acid, L-cysteine. Chemically, it is N-acetyl-L-cysteine.
The compound is a white crystalline powder which melts at 104–110°C and has a very slight odor. It has a molecular weight of 163.2. The agent is supplied in vials containing a 10% or 20% solution of acetylcysteine as the sodium salt. This product contains the following inactive ingredients: disodium edetate, sodium hydroxide, and purified water.

MUCOMYST (acetylcysteine) As A Mucolytic Agent

ACTIONS

(Mucolytic) The viscosity of pulmonary mucous secretions depends on the concentrations of mucoprotein and to a lesser extent deoxyribonucleic acid (DNA). The latter increases with increasing purulence owing to cellular debris. The mucolytic action of acetylcysteine is related to the sulfhydryl group in the molecule. This group probably "opens" disulfide linkages in mucus thereby lowering the viscosity. The mucolytic activity of acetylcysteine is unaltered by the presence of DNA, and increases with increasing pH. Significant mucolysis occurs between pH 7 and 9.

INDICATIONS

Mucomyst (acetylcysteine) is indicated as adjuvant therapy for patients with abnormal, viscid, or inspissated mucous secretions in such conditions as:

- Chronic bronchopulmonary disease (chronic emphysema, emphysema with bronchitis, chronic asthmatic bronchitis, tuberculosis, bronchiectasis and primary amyloidosis of the lung)
- Acute bronchopulmonary disease (pneumonia, bronchitis, tracheobronchitis)
- Pulmonary complications of cystic fibrosis
- Tracheostomy care
- Pulmonary complications associated with surgery
- Use during anesthesia
- Post-traumatic chest conditions
- Atelectasis due to mucous obstruction
- Diagnostic bronchial studies (bronchograms, bronchospirometry, and bronchial wedge catheterization)

CONTRAINDICATIONS

Mucomyst (acetylcysteine) is contraindicated in those patients who are sensitive to it.

WARNINGS

After proper administration of acetylcysteine, an increased volume of liquefied bronchial secretions may occur. When cough is inadequate, the open airway must be maintained by mechanical suction if necessary. When there is a large mechanical block due to foreign body or local accumulation, the airway should be cleared by endotracheal aspiration, with or without bronchoscopy.
Asthmatics under treatment with Mucomyst (acetylcysteine) should be watched carefully. If bronchospasm progresses, this medication should be immediately discontinued.

PRECAUTIONS

With the administration of acetylcysteine, the patient may initially notice a slight disagreeable odor which soon is not noticeable. With a face mask there may be stickiness on the face after nebulization which is easily removed by washing with water.
Under certain conditions, a color change may take place in the solution of acetylcysteine in the opened bottle. The light purple color is the result of a chemical reaction which does not significantly impair the safety or mucolytic efficacy of acetylcysteine.
Continued nebulization of an acetylcysteine solution with a dry gas will result in an increased concentration of the drug in the nebulizer because of evaporation of the solvent. Extreme concentration may impede nebulization and efficient delivery of the drug. Dilution of the nebulizing solution with Sterile Water for Injection, U.S.P., as concentration occurs, will obviate this problem.

ADVERSE EFFECTS

Adverse effects have included stomatitis, nausea and rhinorrhea. Sensitivity and sensitization to Mucomyst have been reported very rarely. A few susceptible patients, particularly asthmatics (see Warnings), may experience varying degrees of bronchospasm associated with the administration of nebulized acetylcysteine. Most patients with bronchospasm are quickly relieved by the use of a bronchodilator given by nebulization.

DOSAGE AND ADMINISTRATION

Mucomyst (acetylcysteine) is available in plastic stoppered glass vials containing 4 ml, 10 ml or 30 ml. The 20% solution may be diluted to a lesser concentration with either sterile normal saline or Sterile Water for Injection, U.S.P. The 10% solution may be used undiluted.

Nebulization—face mask, mouth piece, tracheostomy
When nebulized into a face mask, mouth piece, or tracheostomy, 1–10 ml of the 20% solution or 2–20 ml of the 10% solution may be given every 2–6 hours; the recommended dose for most patients is 3–5 ml of the 20% solution or 6–10 ml of the 10% solution 3 to 4 times a day.

Nebulization—tent, Croupette
In special circumstances it may be necessary to nebulize into a tent or Croupette, and this method of use must be individualized to take into account the available equipment and the patient's particular needs. This form of administration requires very large volumes of the solution, occasionally as much as 300 ml during a single treatment period. If a tent or Croupette must be used, the recommended dose is the vol-

Continued on next page

Mead Johnson Pharm.—Cont.

ume of solution (using 10% or 20% acetylcysteine) that will maintain a very heavy mist in the tent or Croupette for the desired period. Administration for intermittent or continuous prolonged periods, including overnight, may be desirable.

Direct Instillation

When used by direct instillation, 1–2 ml of a 10 to 20% solution may be given as often as every hour.

When used for the routine nursing care of patients with tracheostomy, 1 to 2 ml of a 10 to 20% solution may be given every 1 to 4 hours by instillation into the tracheostomy.

Acetylcysteine may be introduced directly into a particular segment of the bronchopulmonary tree by inserting (under local anesthesia and direct vision) a small plastic catheter into the trachea. Two to 5 ml of the 20% solution may then be instilled by means of a syringe connected to the catheter.

Acetylcysteine may also be given through a percutaneous intratracheal catheter. One to 2 ml of the 20% or 2–4 ml of the 10% solution every 1 to 4 hours may then be given by a syringe attached to the catheter.

Diagnostic Bronchograms

For diagnostic bronchial studies, 2 or 3 administrations of 1 to 2 ml of the 20% solution or 2–4 ml of the 10% solution should be given by nebulization or by instillation intratracheally, prior to the procedure.

ADMINISTRATION OF AEROSOL

Materials

Mucomyst may be administered using conventional nebulizers made of plastic or glass. Certain materials used in nebulization equipment react with acetylcysteine. The most reactive of these are certain metals (notably iron and copper) and rubber. Where materials may come into contact with acetylcysteine solution, parts made of the following acceptable materials should be used: glass, plastic, aluminum, anodized aluminum, chromed metal, tantalum, sterling silver, or stainless steel. Silver may become tarnished after exposure, but this is not harmful to the drug action nor to the patient.

Nebulizing Gases

Compressed tank gas (air) or an air compressor should be used to provide pressure for nebulizing the solution. Oxygen may also be used but should be used with usual caution in patients with severe respiratory disease and CO_2 retention.

APPARATUS

Mucomyst (acetylcysteine) is usually administered as a fine nebulae for its local effect, and the nebulizer used should be capable of providing optimal quantities of a suitable range of particle sizes.

The selection of apparatus for nebulization depends upon the desired particle size and rate of administration. Commercially available nebulizers will produce nebulae of acetylcysteine satisfactory for retention in the respiratory tract. Most of the nebulizers tested will supply a high proportion of the drug solution as particles of less than 10 microns in diameter. Mitchell[a] has shown that a range of particle size up to 10 microns should be satisfactorily retained in the respiratory tract.

Units that nebulized acetylcysteine with a satisfactory efficiency were the Maxi-Myst Nebulizer (Mead Johnson Pharmaceutical Division, Evansville, Indiana), Mist-O_2-Gette ET-I-T (Mist O_2 Gen Equipment Co., 2711 Adeline St., Oakland, Calif), De Vilbiss 42 (The De Vilbiss Co., Somerset Pa.), and Vaponefrin Standard Plastic Nebulizer (Vaponefrin Co., Division U.S. Vitamin & Pharmaceutical Corporation, 800 Second Avenue, New York, New York). Other units tested performed with equivalent or lesser efficiency of nebulization.

Hand bulbs may be used but are not recommended for routine use for nebulizing Mucomyst (acetylcysteine) because their output is generally too small. Some hand-operated nebulizers deliver particles that are larger than optimum for inhalation therapy.

Heated (hot pot) Nebulizer

Mucomyst should not be placed directly into the chamber of a heated (hot pot) nebulizer. A heated nebulizer may be part of the nebulization assembly to provide a warm saturated atmosphere if the Mucomyst aerosol is introduced by means of a separate unheated nebulizer. Usual precautions for administration of warm saturated nebulae should be observed.

The nebulized solution may be breathed directly from the nebulizer. Nebulizers may also be attached to plastic face masks, plastic face tents, plastic mouth pieces, conventional plastic oxygen tents, or head tents. Suitable nebulizers may also be fitted for use with the various intermittent positive pressure breathing (IPPB) machines.

The nebulizing equipment should be cleaned immediately after use; the residues may occlude the fine orifices or corrode metal parts.

Prolonged Nebulization

When three-fourths of the initial volume of acetylcysteine solution has been nebulized, a quantity of Sterile Water for Injection, U.S.P. (approximately equal to the volume of solution remaining) should be added to the nebulizer. This obviates any concentration of the agent in the residual solvent remaining after prolonged nebulization.

Storage of Opened Vials

If only a portion of the solution in the vial is used, to minimize contamination the remainder should be stored in the refrigerator and used within 96 hours.

[See table below and on next page].

COMPATIBILITY

The physical and chemical compatibility of acetylcysteine solutions with other drugs commonly administered by nebulization, direct instillation, or topical application, has been studied.

Acetylcysteine should not be mixed with all antibiotics. For example, the antibiotics tetracycline hydrochloride, oxytetracycline hydrochloride, and erythromycin lactobionate were found to be incompatible when mixed in the same solution. These agents may be administered from separate solutions if administration of these agents is desirable.

The supplying of these data should not be interpreted as a recommendation for combining Mucomyst with other drugs. The table is not presented as positive assurance that no incompatibility will be present, since these data are based only on short-term compatibility studies done in the Mead Johnson Research Center. Manufacturers of drug products may change formulations. This could alter compatibilities. These data are intended to serve only as a guide for predicting compounding problems.

If it is deemed advisable to prepare an admixture, it should be administered as soon as possible after preparation. Do not store unused mixtures.

MUCOMYST (acetylcysteine) As An Antidote For Acetaminophen Overdose

ACTIONS

(Antidotal) Acetaminophen is rapidly absorbed from the upper gastrointestinal tract with peak plasma levels occurring between 30 and 60 minutes after therapeutic doses and usually within 4 hours following an overdose. The parent compound, which is nontoxic, is extensively metabolized in the liver to form principally the sulfate and glucuronide conjugates which are also nontoxic and are rapidly excreted in the urine. A small fraction of an ingested dose is metabolized in the liver by the cytochrome P-450 mixed function oxidase enzyme system to form a reactive, potentially toxic, intermediate metabolite which preferentially conjugates with hepatic glutathione to form the nontoxic cysteine and mercapturic acid derivatives which are then excreted by the kidney. Therapeutic doses of acetaminophen do not saturate the glucuronide and sulfate conjugation pathways and do not result in the formation of sufficient reactive metabolite to deplete glutathione stores. However, following ingestion of a large overdose (150 mg/kg or greater) the glucuronide and sulfate conjugation pathways are saturated resulting in a larger fraction of the drug being metabolized via the P-450 pathway. The increased formation of reactive metabolite may deplete the hepatic stores of glutathione with subsequent binding of the metabolite to protein molecules within the hepatocyte resulting in cellular necrosis. Acetylcysteine has been shown to reduce the extent of liver injury following acetaminophen overdose. Its effectiveness depends on early administration, with benefit seen principally in patients treated within 16 hours of the overdose. Acetylcysteine probably protects the liver by maintaining or restoring the glutathione levels, or by acting as an alternate substrate for conjugation with, and thus detoxification of, the reactive metabolite.

IN VITRO COMPATIBILITY[1] TESTS OF MUCOMYST

PRODUCT AND/OR AGENTS	MANUFACTURER (TRADEMARK)	COMPATIBILITY RATING	RATIO TESTED[6]	
			ACETYLCYSTEINE	PRODUCT OR AGENT
ANESTHETIC, GAS				
Halothane U.S.P.	Ayerst (Halothane)	Compatible	20%	Infinite
Nitrous Oxide U.S.P.	National Cylinder Gas Company	Compatible	20%	Infinite
ANESTHETIC LOCAL				
Cocaine HCl	Merck	Compatible	10%	5%
Lidocaine HCl	Astra (Xylocaine HCl)	Compatible	10%	2%
Tetracaine HCl	Winthrop (Pontocaine HCl)	Compatible	10%	1%
ANTIBACTERIALS (A parenteral form of each antibiotic was used)				
Bacitracin[2,3] (mix and use at once)	Upjohn	Compatible	10%	5,000 U/ml
Cephaloridine[2,4]	Lilly (Loridine)	Compatible	10%	46 mg/ml
Chloramphenicol Sodium Succinate	Parke, Davis (Chloromycetin)	Compatible	20%	20 mg/ml
Disodium Carbenicillin[2] (mix and use at once)	Roerig (Geopen)	Compatible	10%	125 mg/ml
Gentamicin Sulfate[2]	Schering (Garamycin)	Compatible	10%	20 mg/ml
Kanamycin Sulfate[2] (mix and use at once)	Bristol (Kantrex)	Compatible	10%	167 mg/ml
		Compatible	17%	85 mg/ml
Lincomycin HCl[2]	Upjohn (Lincocin)	Compatible	10%	150 mg/ml
Neomycin Sulfate[2]	Upjohn (Mycifradin Sulfate)	Compatible	10%	100 mg/ml
Novobiocin Sodium[2]	Upjohn (Albamycin)	Compatible	10%	25 mg/ml
Pencillin G Potassium[2] (mix and use at once)	Lilly (Buffered Potassium Pencillin G)	Compatible	10%	25,000 U/ml
		Compatible	10%	100,000 U/ml
Polymyxin B Sulfate[2]	Burroughs Wellcome (Aerosporin)	Compatible	10%	50,000 U/ml
Rolitetracycline[2] (mix and use at once)	Bristol (Syntetrin-IM)	Compatible	10%	87.5 mg/ml
Sodium Cephalothin	Lilly (Keflin)	Compatible	10%	110 mg/ml
Sodium Colistimethate[2] (mix and use at once)	Warner-Chilcott (Coly-Mycin M)	Compatible	10%	37.5 mg/ml
Vancomycin HCl[2]	Lilly (Vancocin HCl)	Compatible	10%	25 mg/ml
Amphotericin B	Squibb (Fungizone Intravenous)	Incompatible	4–15%	1.0–4.0 mg/ml
Chlortetracycline HCl[2]	Lederle (Aureomycin HCl)	Incompatible	10%	12.5 mg/ml
Erythromycin Lactobionate	Abbott (Erythrocin Lactobionate-IV)	Incompatible	10%	15 mg/ml
Oxytetracycline HCl	Pfizer (Terramycin IV)	Incompatible	10%	12.5 mg/ml
Sodium Ampicillin	Bristol (Polycillin-N)	Incompatible	10%	50 mg/ml
Tetracycline HCl	Lederle (Achromycin)	Incompatible	10%	12.5 mg/ml

IN VITRO COMPATIBILITY[1] TESTS OF MUCOMYST

PRODUCT AND/OR AGENTS	MANUFACTURER (TRADEMARK)	COMPATIBILITY RATING	RATIO TESTED[6]	
			ACETYLCYSTEINE	PRODUCT OR AGENT
BRONCHODILATORS				
Isoproterenol HCl[2]		Compatible	3.0%	0.5%
Isoproterenol HCl[2]		Compatible	10%	0.05%
Isoproterenol HCl[2]		Compatible	20%	0.05%
Isoproterenol HCl	Winthrop (Isuprel 1%)	Compatible	13.3% (2 parts)	.33% (1 part)
Aerolone Compound	Lilly	Compatible	13.3% (2 parts)	(1 part)
Bronkosol	Breon	Compatible	13.3% (2 parts)	(1 part)
Epinephrine HCl	Parke, Davis (Adrenalin HCl 1:100)	Compatible	13.3% (2 parts)	.33% (1 part)
CONTRAST MEDIA				
Iodized Oil U.S.P.	Fougera (Lipiodol)	Incompatible	20%/20 ml	40%/10 ml
DECONGESTANTS				
Phenylephrine HCl[2]		Compatible	3.0%	.25%
Phenylephrine HCl	Winthrop (Neo-Synephrine HCl Nasal Solution, 0.5%)	Compatible	13.3% (2 parts)	.17% (1 part)
ENZYMES				
Pancreatic Dornase (mix and use at once)	Merck (Dornavac)	Compatible	16.7%	8,000 U/ml
Chymotrypsin	Armour	Incompatible	5%	400 γ/ml
Trypsin	Armour	Incompatible	5%	400 γ/ml
SOLVENTS				
Alcohol		Compatible	12%	10–20%
Propylene Glycol		Compatible	3%	10%
STEROIDS				
Dexamethasone 21-Phosphate	Merck (Decadron Phosphate)	Compatible	16%	0.8 mg/ml
Prednisolone 21-Phosphate[5]	Merck (Hydeltrasol)	Compatible	16.7%	3.3 mg/ml
OTHER AGENTS				
Hydrogen Peroxide		Incompatible	(All ratios)	
Sodium Bicarbonate, U.S.P.		Compatible	20% (1 part)	4.2% (1 part)

[1] The rating, **Incompatible**, is based on the formation of a precipitate, a change in clarity, immiscibility, or a rapid loss of potency of acetylcysteine or the active ingredient of the PRODUCT AND/OR AGENT in the admixture.
The rating **Compatible**, means that there was no significant physical change in the admixture when compared with a control solution of the PRODUCT AND/OR AGENT, and that there was no predicted chemical incompatibility. All of the admixtures have been tested for short-term chemical compatibility by assaying for the concentration of acetylcysteine after mixing.

[2] The active ingredient in the PRODUCT AND/OR AGENT was also assayed after mixing. Some of the admixtures developed minor physical changes which were considered to be insufficient to rate the admixture **Incompatible.** These are listed in footnotes 3, 4, and 5.

[3] A strong odor developed after storage for 24 hours at room temperature.

[4] The admixture was a slightly darker shade of yellow than a control solution of the PRODUCT AND/OR AGENT.

[5] A light tan color developed after storage for 24 hours at room temperature.

[6] Entries are final concentrations. Values in parentheses relate volumes of Mucomyst® solutions to volumes of test solutions.

INDICATIONS

Acetylcysteine, administered orally, is indicated as an antidote to prevent or lessen hepatic injury which may occur following the ingestion of a potentially hepatotoxic quantity of acetaminophen.

It is essential to initiate treatment as soon as possible after the overdose and, in any case, within 24 hours of ingestion.

CONTRAINDICATIONS

There are no contraindications to oral administration of acetylcysteine in the treatment of acetaminophen overdose.

WARNINGS

Generalized urticaria has been observed rarely in patients receiving oral acetylcysteine for acetaminophen overdose. If this occurs or other allergic symptoms appear, treatment with acetylcysteine should be discontinued unless it is deemed essential and the allergic symptoms can be otherwise controlled.

If encephalopathy due to hepatic failure becomes evident, acetylcysteine treatment should be discontinued to avoid further administration of nitrogenous substances. There are no data indicating that acetylcysteine adversely influences hepatic failure, but this remains a theoretical possibility.

PRECAUTIONS

Occasionally severe and persistent vomiting occurs as a symptom of acute acetaminophen overdose. Treatment with oral acetylcysteine may aggravate the vomiting. Patients at risk of gastric hemorrhage (e.g., esophageal varices, peptic ulcers, etc.) should be evaluated concerning the risk of upper gastrointestinal hemorrhage versus the risk of developing hepatic toxicity, and treatment with acetylcysteine given accordingly.

Dilution of the acetylcysteine (SEE PREPARATION OF MUCOMYST (acetylcysteine) FOR ORAL ADMINISTRATION) minimizes the propensity of oral acetylcysteine to aggravate vomiting.

ADVERSE REACTIONS

Oral administration of acetylcysteine, especially in the large doses needed to treat acetaminophen overdose, may result in nausea, vomiting and other gastrointestinal symptoms. Rash with or without mild fever has been observed rarely.

DOSAGE AND ADMINISTRATION

Regardless of the quantity of acetaminophen reported to have been ingested, administer MUCOMYST (acetylcysteine) immediately if 24 hours or less have elapsed from the reported time of ingestion of an overdose of acetaminophen. Do not await results of assays for acetaminophen level before initiating treatment with MYCOMYST. The following procedures are recommended:

1. The stomach should be emptied promptly by lavage or by inducing emesis with syrup of ipecac. Syrup of ipecac should be given in a dose of 15 to 30 ml for children and 30 to 45 ml for adults accompanied by drinking copious quantities of water. The dose should be repeated if emesis does not occur in 20 minutes.
2. In the case of a mixed drug overdose activated charcoal may be indicated. However, if activated charcoal has been administered, lavage before administering acetylcysteine treatment. Activated charcoal adsorbs acetylcysteine *in vitro* and may do so in patients and thereby may reduce its effectiveness.
3. Draw blood for acetaminophen plasma assay and for baseline SGOT, SGPT, bilirubin, prothrombin time, creatinine, BUN, blood sugar and electrolytes. The acetaminophen assay provides a basis for determining the need for continuing with the maintenance doses of acetylcysteine treatment. If an assay cannot be obtained or if the acetaminophen level is clearly in the toxic range (above the dashed line of the nomogram) dosing with acetylcysteine should be continued for the full course of therapy. The laboratory measurements are used to monitor hepatic and renal function and electrolyte and fluid balance.
4. Administer the loading dose of acetylcysteine, 140 mg per kg of body weight. (Prepare MUCOMYST for oral administration as described in the Dosage Guide and Preparation table.)
5. Four hours after the loading dose administer the first maintenance dose (70 mg of acetylcysteine per kg of body weight). The maintenance dose is then repeated at 4 hour intervals for a total of 17 doses unless the acetaminophen assay reveals a nontoxic level as discussed below.
6. If the patient vomits the loading dose or any maintenance dose within one hour of administration, repeat that dose.
7. In the occasional instances where the patient is persistently unable to retain the orally administered acetylcysteine, the antidote may be administered by duodenal intubation.
8. Repeat SGOT, SGPT, bilirubin, prothrombin time, creatinine, BUN, blood sugar and electrolytes daily if the acetaminophen plasma level is in the potentially toxic range as discussed below.

PREPARATION OF MUCOMYST (acetylcysteine) FOR ORAL ADMINISTRATION—Oral administration requires dilution of the 20% solution with cola drinks, Fresca® or other soft drinks, to a final concentration of 5% (see Dosage Guide and Preparation table). If administered via gastric tube or Miller-Abbott tube, water may be used as the diluent. The dilutions should be freshly prepared and utilized within one hour. Remaining undiluted solutions in opened vials can be stored in the refrigerator up to 96 hours. **MUCOMYST IS NOT APPROVED FOR PARENTERAL INJECTION.**

ACETAMINOPHEN ASSAYS—INTERPRETATION AND METHODOLOGY: The acute ingestion of acetaminophen in quantities of 150 mg/kg or greater may result in hepatic toxicity. However, the reported history of the quantity of a drug ingested as an overdose is often inaccurate and is not a reliable guide to therapy of the overdose. **THEREFORE, PLASMA OR SERUM ACETAMINOPHEN CONCENTRATIONS, DETERMINED AS EARLY AS POSSIBLE, BUT NO SOONER THAN FOUR HOURS FOLLOWING AN ACUTE OVERDOSE, ARE ESSENTIAL IN ASSESSING THE POTENTIAL RISK OF HEPATOTOXICITY. IF AN ASSAY FOR ACETAMINOPHEN CANNOT BE OBTAINED, IT IS NECESSARY TO ASSUME THAT THE OVERDOSE IS POTENTIALLY TOXIC.**

Interpretation of Acetaminophen Assays:

1. When results of the plasma acetaminophen assay are available refer to the nomogram below to determine if plasma concentration is in the potentially toxic range. Values above the solid line connecting 200 mcg/ml at 4 hours with 50 mcg/ml at 12 hours are associated with a possibility of hepatic toxicity if an antidote is not administered. (Do not wait for assay results to begin acetylcysteine treatment).

Continued on next page

Mead Johnson Pharm.—Cont.

2. If the plasma level is above the broken line continue with maintenance doses of acetylcysteine. It is better to err on the safe side and thus the broken line is plotted 25% below the solid line which defines possible toxicity.
3. If the plasma level is below the broken line described above, there is minimal risk of hepatic toxicity and acetylcysteine treatment can be discontinued.

Acetaminophen Assay Methodology:
Assay procedures most suitable for determining acetaminophen concentrations utilize high pressure liquid chromatography (HPLC) or gas liquid chromatography (GLC). The assay should measure only parent acetaminophen and not conjugated. The assay procedures listed below fulfill this requirement:

Selected techniques (non-inclusive)
HPLC:
1. Blair, D and Rumack, BH, *Clin Chem* 23(4):743–745 (April) 1977.
2. Howie, D, Andriaenssens, PI and Prescott, LF, *Journ Pharm and Pharmacol* 29(4)235–237 (April) 1977.

GLC:
3. Prescott, LF, *Journ Pharm and Pharmacol* 23(10):807–808 (October) 1971.

Colorimetric:
4. Glynn, JP and Kendal, SE, *The Lancet 1:* 1147–1148 (May 17) 1975.

SUPPORTIVE TREATMENT OF ACETAMINOPHEN OVERDOSE
1. Maintain fluid and electrolyte balance based on clinical evaluation of state of hydration and serum electrolytes.
2. Treat as necessary for hypoglycemia.
3. Administer vitamin K_1 if prothrombin time ratio exceeds 1.5 or fresh frozen plasma if the prothrombin time ratio exceeds 3.0.
4. Diuretics and forced diuresis should be avoided

[See table below].

Estimating potential for hepatotoxicity:
The following nomogram has been developed to estimate the probability that plasma levels in relation to intervals post ingestion will result in hepatotoxicity.
[See nomogram next column]

HOW SUPPLIED

Mucomyst®20% acetylcysteine solution (200 mg Acetylcysteine per ml). Sterile, Not for injection

NDC 0087-0570-03	Cartons of three 10 ml vials, 1 plastic dropper
VA 6505-00-767-9111A 6505-00-767-9111	Defense
NDC 0087-0570-09	Cartons of three 30 ml vials
VA 6505-00-782-2688A 6505-00-782-2688	Defense
NDC 0087-0570-07	Cartons of twelve 4 ml vials

Mucomyst®-10, 10% acetylcysteine solution. (100 mg Acetylcysteine per ml). Sterile, Not for injection

NDC 0087-0572-01	Cartons of three 10 ml vials, 1 plastic dropper
NDC 0087-0572-02	Cartons of three 30 ml vials
NDC 0087-0572-03	Cartons of twelve 4 ml vials

Plasma or Serum Acetaminophen Concentration vs Time Post Acetaminophen Ingestion

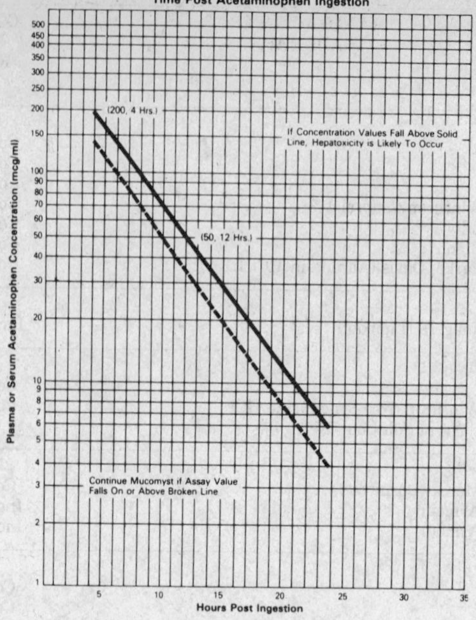

Plasma or Serum Acetaminophen Concentration (mcg/ml)

(200, 4 Hrs.)

If Concentration Values Fall Above Solid Line, Hepatoxicity is Likely To Occur

(50, 12 Hrs.)

Continue Mucomyst if Assay Value Falls On or Above Broken Line

Hours Post Ingestion

*Adapted from Rumack and Matthews, *Pediatrics* 55:871–876, 1975.

[a]Amer. Rev. Resp. Dis. *82* : 627–639, 1960.

PERI–COLACE® capsules • syrup
[peri-kō'lās]
Casanthranol and docusate sodium

PRODUCT OVERVIEW

KEY FACTS
Peri-Colace is a combination of the mild stimulant laxative casanthronal and the stool softener Colace (docusate sodium). This product provides gentle peristaltic stimulation and helps to keep stools soft for easier passage. It is available in two forms: capsules and syrup.

MAJOR USES
Peri-Colace is useful in the management of chronic or temporary constipation.

SAFETY INFORMATION
Do not use Peri-Colace when abdominal pain, nausea, or vomiting are present. Frequent or prolonged use of this preparation may result in dependence on laxatives.

PRESCRIBING INFORMATION

PERI-COLACE® capsules • syrup
[peri-kō'las]
Casanthranol and docusate sodium

DESCRIPTION
Peri-Colace is a combination of the mild stimulant laxative casanthranol and the stool-softener Colace (docusate sodium). Each capsule contains 30 mg of casanthranol and 100 mg of Colace; the syrup contains 30 mg of casanthranol and 60 mg of Colace per 15-ml tablespoon (10 mg of casanthranol and 20 mg of Colace per 5-ml teaspoon) and 10% alcohol.
Peri-Colace Capsules contain the following inactive ingredients: D&C Red No. 33, FD&C Red No. 40, non-porcine gelatin, edible ink, polyethylene glycol, propylene glycol, titanium dioxide, and purified water.
Peri-Colace Syrup contains the following inactive ingredients: alcohol, citric acid, flavors, methyl salicylate, methylparaben, poloxamer, polyethylene glycol, propylparaben, sodium citrate, sorbitol solution, sucrose, and purified water.

ACTION AND USES
Peri-Colace provides gentle peristaltic stimulation and helps to keep stools soft for easier passage. Bowel movement is induced gently—usually overnight or in 8 to 12 hours. Nausea, griping, abnormally loose stools, and constipation rebound are minimized. Useful in management of chronic or temporary constipation.
Note: To prevent hard stools when laxative stimulation is not needed or undesirable, see Colace (stool softener).

SIDE EFFECTS
The incidence of side effects—none of a serious nature—is exceedingly small. Nausea, abdominal cramping or discomfort, diarrhea, and rash are the main side effects reported.

ADMINISTRATION AND DOSAGE
Adults —1 or 2 capsules, or 1 or 2 tablespoons syrup at bedtime, or as indicated. In severe cases, dosage may be increased to 2 capsules or 2 tablespoons twice daily, or 3 capsules at bedtime. *Children* —1 to 3 teaspoons of syrup at bedtime, or as indicated.

WARNINGS
Do not use when abdominal pain, nausea, or vomiting are present. Frequent or prolonged use of this preparation may result in dependence on laxatives.
As with any drug, if you are pregnant or nursing a baby, seek the advice of a health professional before using this product.

OVERDOSAGE
In addition to symptomatic treatment, gastric lavage, if timely, is recommended in cases of large overdosage.

HOW SUPPLIED
Peri-Colace® Capsules
NDC 0087-0715-43 Cartons of 10 single unit packs
NDC 0087-0715-01 Bottles of 30
NDC 0087-0715-02 Bottles of 60
NDC 0087-0715-03 Bottles of 250
NDC 0087-0715-05 Bottles of 1000
NDC 0087-0715-07 Cartons of 100 single unit packs
Note: Peri-Colace capsules should be stored at controlled room temperatures (59°–86°F or 15°– 30°C).
Peri-Colace® Syrup
NDC 0087-0721-01 Bottles of 8 fl. oz.
NDC 0087-0721-02 Bottles of 16 fl. oz.

Shown in Product Identification Section, page 417

Doses in relation to body weight are:

DOSAGE GUIDE AND PREPARATION

Body Weight (kg)	Body Weight (lb)	Loading Dose of MUCOMYST® (acetylcysteine)** grams Acetylcysteine	ml of 20% MUCOMYST	ml of Diluent	Total ml of 5% Solution
100–109	220–240	15	75	225	300
90– 99	198–218	14	70	210	280
80– 89	176–196	13	65	195	260
70– 79	154–174	11	55	165	220
60– 69	132–152	10	50	150	200
50– 59	110–130	8	40	120	160
40– 49	88–108	7	35	105	140
30– 39	66– 86	6	30	90	120
20– 29	44– 64	4	20	60	80
		Maintenance Dose **			
(kg)	(lb)				
100–109	220–240	7.5	37	113	150
90– 99	198–218	7	35	105	140
80– 89	176–196	6.5	33	97	130
70– 79	154–174	5.5	28	82	110
60– 69	132–152	5	25	75	100
50– 59	110–130	4	20	60	80
40– 49	88–108	3.5	18	52	70
30– 39	66– 86	3	15	45	60
20– 29	44– 64	2	10	30	40

**If patient weighs less than 20 kg (usually patients younger than 6 years), calculate the dose of MUCOMYST. Each ml of 20% MUCOMYST contains 200 mg of acetylcysteine. The loading dose is 140 mg per kilogram of body weight. The maintenance dose is 70 mg/kg. Three (3) mls of diluent are added to each ml of 20% MUCOMYST. Do not decrease the proportion of diluent.

Medical Market Specialties Inc.
P.O. BOX 307
CEDAR GROVE, NJ 07009

PROGLYCEM ℞
[*pro-gli 'sem*]
brand of diazoxide
CAPSULES
SUSPENSION, USP
FOR ORAL ADMINISTRATION

DESCRIPTION
Diazoxide is 7-chloro-3-methyl-2H-1,2,4-benzothiadiazine 1,1-diazoxide. It is a white powder practically insoluble to sparingly soluble in water.

CLINICAL PHARMACOLOGY
Diazoxide administered orally produces a prompt dose-related increase in blood glucose level, due primarily to an inhibition of insulin release from the pancreas and also to an extrapancreatic effect. The hyperglycemic effect begins within an hour and generally lasts no more than eight hours in the presence of normal renal function.
PROGLYCEM decreases the excretion of sodium chloride and water resulting in fluid retention which may be clinically significant.
The hypotensive effect of diazoxide on blood pressure is usually not marked with the oral preparation.
Other pharmacologic actions of PROGLYCEM include increased pulse rate, increased serum uric acid levels due to decreased excretion, increased serum levels of free fatty acids, decreased para-aminohippuric acid (PAH) clearance with no appreciable effect on glomerular filtration rate.
PROGLYCEM-induced hyperglycemia is reversed by the administration of insulin or tolbutamide. The inhibition of insulin release by PROGLYCEM is antagonized by alpha-adrenergic blocking agents.
PROGLYCEM is extensively bound (more than 90%) to serum proteins, and is excreted in the kidneys. The plasma half-life 28±8.3 hours. In four children aged four and six years, the plasma half-life varied from 9.5 to 24 hours. The half-life may be prolonged following overdosage, and in patients with impaired renal function.

INDICATIONS AND USAGE
PROGLYCEM (oral diazoxide) is useful in the management of hypoglycemia due to hyperinsulinism associated with the following conditions when surgery or other therapy is unsuccessful.
ADULTS: inoperable islet cell adenoma or carcinoma, or extrapancreatic malignancy.
INFANTS AND CHILDREN: leucine sensitivity, islet cell hyperplasia, nesidioblastosis, extrapancreatic malignancy, islet cell adenoma, or adenomatosis. PROGYLCEM may be used preoperatively as a temporary measure, and postoperatively, if hypoglycemia persists.

CONTRAINDICATIONS
The use of PROGLYCEM for functional hypoglycemia is contraindicated. The drug should not be used in patients hypersensitive to diazoxide or to other thiazides unless the potential benefits outweigh the possible risks.

WARNINGS
Diazoxide may lead to significant fluid retention which in patients with a compromised cardiac reserve, may precipitate congestive heart failure. The fluid retention will respond to conventional therapy with diuretics. It should be noted that concomitently administered thiazides may potentiate the hyperglycemic and hyperuricemic actions of diazoxide.
Ketoacidosis and nonketotic hyperosmolar coma have been reported in patients treated with recommended doses of PROGLYCEM usually during intercurrent illness. Prompt recognition and treatment are essential (see OVERDOSAGE), and prolonged surveillance following the acute episode is necessary because of the long drug half-life.
Transient cataracts occur in association with hyperosmolar coma in an infant, and subsided on correction of the hyperosmolarity. Cataracts have been observed in several animals receiving daily doses of intravenous or oral diazoxide.

PRECAUTIONS
General: Treatment with PROGLYCEM should be initiated under close clinical supervision, with careful monitoring of blood glucose and clinical response until the patient's condition has stabilized. This usually requires several days. If not effective in two to three weeks, the drug should be discontinued.
Prolonged treatment requires regular monitoring of the urine for sugar and ketones, especially under stress conditions, with prompt reporting of any abnormalities to the physician. Additionally, blood sugar levels should be monitored periodically by the physician to determine the need or dose adjustment.
In some patients, higher blood levels have been observed with the oral suspension than with the capsule formulation of PROGLYCEM. Dosage should be adjusted as necessary in individual patients if changed from one formulaton to the other.
The antihypertensive effect of other drugs may be enhanced by PROGLYCEM.

DRUG INTERACTIONS
Since diazoxide is highly bound to serum proteins, it may displace other substances which are also bound to protein, such as bilirubin or coumarin and its derivatives, resulting in higher blood levels of these substances. Concomitant administration of oral diazoxide and diphenylhydantoin may result in a loss of seizure control. The concomitant administration of thiazides or other commonly used diuretics may potentiate the hyperglycemic and other hyperglycemic effects of diazoxide.
Pregnancy Category C: Reproduction studies in rats and rabbits have revealed increased fetal resorptions and delayed parturition, as well as fetal skeletal and cardiac anomalies. The drug has also been demonstrated to cross the placental barrier in animals and to cause degeneration of the fetal pancreatic beta cells. Since there are no adequate data on fetal effects of this drug when given to pregnant women, safety in pregnancy has not been estblished. When the use of PROGLYCEM is considered, the indications should be limited to those specified for adults and the potential benefits to the mother must be weighed against possible harmful effects to the fetus.
Non-Teratogenic Effects: Diazoxide crosses the placental barrier and appears in cord blood. When given to the mother prior to delivery of the infant, the drug may produce fetal or neonatal hyperbilirubinemia, thrombocytopenia, altered carbohydrate metabolism or possibly other side effects that have occurred in adults. Alopecia and hypertrichosis lanuginosa have occurred in infants whose mothers received oral diazoxide during the last 19 to 60 days of pregnancy.

LABOR AND DELIVERY
Since intravenous administration of the drug during labor may cause cesation of uterine contractions, and administration of oxytocic agents may be required to reinstate labor, caution is advised in administering PROGLYCEM at that time.

ADVERSE REACTIONS
Frequent and Serious: Sodium and fluid retention is most common in young infants and in adults and may precipitate congestive heart failure in patients with compromised cardiac reserve. It usually responds to diuretic therapy. INFREQUENT AND SERIOUS: Diabetic ketoacidosis and hyperosmolar non-ketotic coma may develop very rapidly (see OVERDOSAGE and WARNING).
Other Frequent Adverse Reactions: Hirsutism of the lanugo type, mainly on the forehead, back and limbs subsides on discontinuation of the drug. HYPERGLYCEMIA OR GLYCOSURIA may require reduction in dosage in order to avoid progression towards ketoacidosis or hyperosmolar coma. GASTROINTESTINAL INTOLERANCE may include anorexia, nausea, vomiting, abdominal pain, illeus, diarrhea, transient loss of taste. Tachycardia, palpitations, increased levels of serum uric acid are common. THROMBOCYTOPENIA with or without purpura may require discontinuation of the drug. Neutropenia is transient, is not associated with increased susceptibility to infection, and ordinarily does not require discontinuation of the drug. Skin rash, headache, weakness, and malaise may also occur.
Other adverse reactions which have been observed are: CARDIOVASCULAR—hypotension and transient hypertension. Chest pain has been reported rarely. HEMATOLOGIC—eosinophilia, decreased hemoglobin/hemocrit, excessive bleeding, decreased IgG. HEPATO-RENAL—increased AST, alkaline phosphatase, azotemia, decreased creatinine clearance, reversible nephrotic syndrome, decreased urinary output, hematuria, albuminuria. NEUROLOGIC—anxiety, dizziness, insomnia, polyneuritis, paresthesia, pruritus, extrapyramidal signs. OPHTHALOMOLOGIC—transient cataracts, subconjunctival hemorrhage, ring scotoma, blurred vision, diplopia, lacrimation. SKELETAL, INTEGUMENTARY—monilial dermatitis, herpes, advance in bone-age, loss of scalp hair. SYSTEMIC—fever, lymphadenopathy. OTHER—gout, acute pancreatitis, pancreatic necrosis, galactorraga, enlargement of lump in breast.

OVERDOSAGE
An overdosage of PROGLYCEM causes marked hyperglycemia which may be associated with ketoacidosis. It will respond to prompt insulin administration and restoration of fluid and electrolyte balance. Because of the drug's long half-life (approximately 30 hours), the symptoms of overdosage require prolonged surveillance for periods of up to seven days, until the blood sugar level stabilizes with the normal range. Peritoneal dialysis and hemodialysis have lowered diazoxide blood levels in two patients.

DOSAGE AND ADMINISTRATION
The dosage of PROGLYCEM must be individualized based on the severity of the hypoglycemic condition and the blood glucose level and clinical response of the patient. The dosage should be adjusted until the desired clinical and laboratory effects are produced with the least amount of the drug. Special care should be taken to assure accuracy of dosage in infants and young children.
ADULTS AND CHILDREN: The usual daily dosage is 3 to 8 mg/kg, divided into two or three equal doses every 8 to 12 hours. In certain instances, patients with refractory hypoglycemia may require higher dosages.
INFANTS AND NEWBORNS: The usual daily dosage is 8 to 15 mg/kg, divided into two or three equal doses every 8 to 12 hours.

HOW SUPPLIED
PROGLYCEM **Capsules,** 50 mg, half opaque orange and half clear capsules, branded in black with MMS and either product identification letters, PBA, or numbers, 830, bottle of 100 (NDC #52891-830-05).
PROGLYCEM **Suspension,** 50 mg/ml, a chocolate-mint flavored suspension, bottle of 30 ml (NDC #52891-426-04), with dropper calibrated to deliver 10, 20, 30, 40, and 50 mg diazoxide. **Shake well before each use: Protect from light. Store in carton until contents are used. Store PROGLYCEM Capsules and Suspension between 2° and 30° C (36° and 86° F).**

Medical Products Panamericana, Inc.
P.O. BOX 771
CORAL GABLES, FL 33134

VG CAPSULES™ ℞

COMPOSITION
Each capsule contains: Vitamin C (Ascorbic Acid) 500 mg.; Vitamin B1 (Thiamine) 15 mg.; Vitamin B2 (Riboflavin) 15 mg.; Niacinamide 100 mg.; Vitamin B6 (Pyridoxine) 5 mg.; Vitamin B12 5 mcg.; Calcium Pantothenate 20 mg.; Folic Acid 0.5 mg.; Vitamin E (d-alpha tocopheryl acetate) 30 I.U.; 1-lysine Hydrochloride (need in human nutrition established, but no U.S. RDA established) 25 mg.; Manganese Sulfate 4 mg.; Magnesium Sulfate 35 mg. (equivalent to 25 mg. dried $MgSO_4$); Zinc Sulfate 80 mg. (equivalent to 25 mg. dried $ZnSO_4$).

INDICATIONS
Indicated in the treatment of patients with deficiencies of, or increased requirements for Vitamin C and/or B-Complex Vitamins including Folic Acid, Zinc, Magnesium and/or Manganese.

ADMINISTRATION AND DOSAGE
One Capsule Daily or as directed by a physician.

PRECAUTIONS
Folic Acid may obscure pernicious anemia; the peripheral blood picture may revert to normal while neurological manifestations remain progressive.

CAUTION
Federal Law prohibits dispensing without prescription.

SUPPLIED
NDC 0576-0506-30 Bottle of 30 Capsules.

Medicone Company
225 VARICK ST.
NEW YORK, NY 10014

MEDICONE® DERMA Ointment

(See 1987 PDR For Nonprescription Drugs)

MEDICONE® DERMA-HC Ointment ℞

COMPOSITION
Each gram contains:

Hydrocortisone acetate	10.0 mg.
Benzocaine	19.8 mg.
8-Hydroxyquinoline sulfate	10.4 mg.
Ephedrine hydrochloride	1.1 mg.
Menthol	4.8 mg.
Ichthammol	9.9 mg.
Zinc oxide	135.8 mg.
Petrolatum, Lanolin, perfume	q.s.

Continued on next page

Medicone—Cont.

ACTION AND USES

Offers the advantage of quick, lasting comfort during treatment of severely inflamed dermatoses by affording prompt temporary local anesthetic action, inhibiting pain, burning, itching and controlling the scratch reflex. The hydrocortisone acetate reduces inflammation and swelling, aiding the normal healing process. The non-drying base will not disintegrate or liquefy at body temperature and is not washed off by exudate, perspiration or urine. Effectively suppresses inflammation, pain, swelling, burning and itching in contact dermatitis, eczematoid dermatitis, atopic dermatitis, neurodermatitis, seborrheic dermatitis, allergic dermatitis, rhus dermatitis, pruritus ani and pruritus vulvae.

ADMINISTRATION AND DOSAGE

Apply to affected area 2 to 4 times daily. When adequate improvement is noted, reduce frequency of application or continue maintenance control with regular Medicone Derma ointment.

PRECAUTIONS

Observe the usual adrenocorticosteroid precautions. Exercise care if the patient is on other corticosteroid therapy or if infection is present or if rash or irritation develops. Do not use in the eyes.

CONTRAINDICATIONS

Do not use in the presence of tuberculosis of the skin.

HOW SUPPLIED

7 gram and 20 gram tubes.

Shown in Product Identification Section, page 417

MEDICONE® DRESSING Cream

(See 1987 PDR For Nonprescription Drugs)

MEDICONE® Rectal Ointment

(See 1987 PDR For Nonprescription Drugs)

MEDICONE® Rectal Suppositories

(See 1987 PDR For Nonprescription Drugs)
Shown in Product Identification Section, page 417

MEDICONET®
(medicated rectal wipes)

(See 1987 PDR For Nonprescription Drugs)

Products are listed alphabetically in the **PINK SECTION.**

Products are cross-indexed by product classifications in the **BLUE SECTION**

Products are cross-indexed by generic and chemical names in the **YELLOW SECTION**

Merck Sharp & Dohme

DIVISION OF MERCK & CO., INC.
WEST POINT, PA 19486

Product Identification Codes

To provide quick and positive identification of Merck Sharp & Dohme products, we have imprinted a code number on tablet and capsule products. In order that you may identify a product by its code number, we have compiled below a numerical list of code numbers with their corresponding product names. We are also listing the code numbers by alphabetical listing of products as a cross reference.
The code number as it appears on tablets and capsules bears the letters MSD plus the numerical code. Decadron® (Dexamethasone, MSD) tablets 0.25 mg is identified MSD 20.

Numerical Listing

MSD Code No.	Product	Product No.
20	Decadron® (Dexamethasone, MSD) Tablets 0.25 mg	7592
21	Cogentin® (Benztropine Mesylate, MSD) Tablets 0.5 mg	3297
23	Elavil® (Amitriptyline HCl, MSD) Tablets 10 mg	3287
25	Indocin® (Indomethacin, MSD) Capsules 25 mg	3316
26	Vivactil® (Protriptyline HCl, MSD) Tablets 5 mg	3313
41	Decadron® (Dexamethasone, MSD) Tablets 0.5 mg	7598
42	HydroDIURIL® (Hydrochlorothiazide, MSD) Tablets 25 mg	3263
43	Mephyton® (Phytonadione, MSD) Tablets 5 mg	7776
45	Elavil® (Amitriptyline HCl, MSD) Tablets 25 mg	3288
47	Vivactil® (Protriptyline HCl, MSD) Tablets 10 mg	3314
49	Daranide® (Dichlorphenamide, MSD) Tablets 50 mg	3256
50	Indocin® (Indomethacin, MSD) Capsules 50 mg	3317
52	Inversine® (Mecamylamine HCl, MSD) Tablets 2.5 mg	3219
53	Hydropres® 25 (Reserpine-Hydrochlorothiazide, MSD) Tablets	3265
59	Blocadren® (Timolol Maleate, MSD) Tablets 5 mg	3343
60	Cogentin® (Benztropine Mesylate, MSD) Tablets 2 mg	3172
62	Periactin® (Cyproheptadine HCl, MSD) Tablets 4 mg	3276
63	Decadron® (Dexamethasone, MSD) Tablets 0.75 mg	7601
65	Edecrin® (Ethacrynic Acid, MSD) Tablets 25 mg	3321
67	Timolide® 10-25 (Timolol Maleate-Hydrochlorothiazide, MSD) Tablets	3373
90	Edecrin® (Ethacrynic Acid, MSD) Tablets 50 mg	3322
92	Midamor® (Amiloride HCl, MSD) Tablets 5 mg	3381
95	Decadron® (Dexamethasone, MSD) Tablets 1.5 mg	7638
97	Decadron® (Dexamethasone, MSD) Tablets 4 mg	7645
102	Elavil® (Amitriptyline HCl, MSD) Tablets 50 mg	3320
105	HydroDIURIL® (Hydrochlorothiazide, MSD) Tablets 50 mg	3264
127	Hydropres® 50 (Reserpine-Hydrochlorothiazide, MSD) Tablets	3266
135	Aldomet® (Methyldopa, MSD) Tablets 125 mg	3341
136	Blocadren® (Timolol Maleate, MSD) Tablets 10 mg	3344
147	Decadron® (Dexamethasone, MSD) Tablets 6 mg	7648
150	Indocin® (Indomethacin, MSD) Suppositories 50 mg	3354
214	Diuril® (Chlorothiazide, MSD) Tablets 250 mg	3244
219	Cortone® (Cortisone Acetate, MSD) Tablets 25 mg	7063
230	Diupres-250® Tablets	3261
401	Aldomet® (Methyldopa, MSD) Tablets 250 mg	3290
403	Urecholine® (Bethanechol Chloride, MSD) Tablets 5 mg	7785
405	Diupres-500® Tablets	3262
410	HydroDIURIL® (Hydrochlorothiazide, MSD) Tablets 100 mg	3340
412	Urecholine® (Bethanechol Chloride, MSD) Tablets 10 mg	7787
423	Aldoril® 15 (Methyldopa-Hydrochlorothiazide, MSD) Tablets	3294
430	Elavil® (Amitriptyline HCl, MSD) Tablets 75 mg	3348
432	Diuril® (Chlorothiazide, MSD) Tablets 500 mg	3245
435	Elavil® (Amitriptyline HCl, MSD) Tablets 100 mg	3349
437	Blocadren® (Timolol Maleate, MSD) Tablets 20 mg	3371
456	Aldoril® 25 (Methyldopa-Hydrochlorothiazide, MSD) Tablets	3295
457	Urecholine® (Bethanechol Chloride, MSD) Tablets 25 mg	7788
460	Urecholine® (Bethanechol Chloride, MSD) Tablets 50 mg	7790
501	Benemid® (Probenecid, MSD) Tablets 0.5 g	3337
516	Aldomet® (Methyldopa, MSD) Tablets 500 mg	3292
517	Triavil® 4-50 Tablets	3364
602	Cuprimine® (Penicillamine, MSD) Capsules 250 mg	3299
612	Aldoclor® 150 Tablets	3318
614	ColBENEMID® (Probenecid-Colchicine, MSD) Tablets	3283
619	Hydrocortone® (Hydrocortisone, MSD) Tablets 10 mg	7604
625	Hydrocortone® (Hydrocortisone, MSD) Tablets 20 mg	7602
634	Aldoclor® 250 Tablets	3319
635	Cogentin® (Benztropine Mesylate, MSD) Tablets 1 mg	3334
647	Sinemet® 10-100 (Carbidopa-Levodopa, MSD) Tablets	3346
650	Sinemet® 25-100 (Carbidopa-Levodopa, MSD) Tablets	3365
654	Sinemet® 25-250 (Carbidopa-Levodopa, MSD) Tablets	3347
672	Cuprimine® (Penicillamine, MSD) Capsules 125 mg	3350
673	Elavil® (Amitriptyline HCl, MSD) Tablets 150 mg	3351
675	Dolobid® (Diflunisal, MSD) Tablets 250 mg	3390
679	Cuprid® (Trientine Hydrochloride, MSD) Capsules 250 mg	3511
690	Demser® (Metyrosine, MSD) Capsules 250 mg	3355
693	Indocin® SR (Indomethacin, MSD) Capsules 75 mg	3370
694	Aldoril® D30 (Methyldopa-Hydrochlorothiazide, MSD) Tablets	3362
697	Dolobid® (Diflunisal, MSD) Tablets 500 mg	3392
707	Tonocard® (Tocainide HCl, MSD) Tablets 400 mg	3409
709	Tonocard® (Tocainide HCl, MSD) Tablets 600 mg	3410
712	Vasotec® (Enalapril Maleate, MSD) Tablets 5 mg	3412
713	Vasotec® (Enalapril Maleate, MSD) Tablets 10 mg	3413
714	Vasotec® (Enalapril Maleate, MSD) Tablets 20 mg	3414
907	Mintezol® (Thiabendazole, MSD) Chewable Tablets 500 mg	3332
914	Triavil® 2-10 Tablets	3328
917	Moduretic® (Amiloride HCl-Hydrochlorothiazide, MSD) Tablets	3385
921	Triavil® 2-25 Tablets	3311
931	Flexeril® (Cyclobenzaprine HCl, MSD) Tablets 10 mg	3358
934	Triavil® 4-10 Tablets	3310
935	Aldoril® D50 (Methyldopa-Hydrochlorothiazide, MSD) Tablets	3363
941	Clinoril® (Sulindac, MSD) Tablets 150 mg	3360
942	Clinoril® (Sulindac, MSD) Tablets 200 mg	3353
946	Triavil® 4-25 Tablets	3312

Alphabetical Listing

MSD Code No.	Product	Product No.
612	Aldoclor® 150, Tablets	3318
634	Aldoclor® 250 Tablets	3319
135	Aldomet® (Methyldopa, MSD) Tablets 125 mg	3341
401	Aldomet® (Methyldopa, MSD) Tablets 250 mg	3290
516	Aldomet® (Methyldopa, MSD) Tablets 500 mg	3292
423	Aldoril® 15 (Methyldopa-Hydrochlorothiazide, MSD) Tablets	3294
456	Aldoril® 25 (Methyldopa-Hydrochlorothiazide, MSD) Tablets	3295
694	Aldoril® D30 (Methyldopa-Hydrochlorothiazide, MSD) Tablets	3362
935	Aldoril® D50 (Methyldopa-Hydrochlorothiazide, MSD) Tablets	3363
501	Benemid® (Probenecid, MSD) Tablets 0.5 g	3337
59	Blocadren® (Timolol Maleate, MSD) Tablets 5 mg	3343
136	Blocadren® (Timolol Maleate, MSD) Tablets 10 mg	3344
437	Blocadren® (Timolol Maleate, MSD) Tablets 20 mg	3371
941	Clinoril® (Sulindac, MSD) Tablets 150 mg	3360
942	Clinoril® (Sulindac, MSD) Tablets 200 mg	3353
21	Cogentin® (Benztropine Mesylate, MSD) Tablets 0.5 mg	3297
635	Cogentin® (Benztropine Mesylate, MSD) Tablets 1 mg	3334
60	Cogentin® (Benztropine Mesylate, MSD) Tablets 2 mg	3172
614	ColBENEMID® (Probenecid-Colchicine, MSD) Tablets	3283
219	Cortone® (Cortisone Acetate, MSD) Tablets 25 mg	7063
679	Cuprid® (Trientine Hydrochloride, MSD) Capsules 250 mg	3511
672	Cuprimine® (Penicillamine, MSD) Capsules 125 mg	3350
602	Cuprimine® (Penicillamine, MSD) Capsules 250 mg	3299
49	Daranide® (Dichlorphenamide, MSD) Tablets 50 mg	3256
20	Decadron® (Dexamethasone, MSD) Tablets 0.25 mg	7592
41	Decadron® (Dexamethasone, MSD) Tablets 0.5 mg	7598
63	Decadron® (Dexamethasone, MSD) Tablets 0.75 mg	7601
95	Decadron® (Dexamethasone, MSD) Tablets 1.5 mg	7638
97	Decadron® (Dexamethasone, MSD) Tablets 4 mg	7645
147	Decadron® (Dexamethasone, MSD) Tablets 6 mg	7648
690	Demser® (Metyrosine, MSD) Capsules 250 mg	3355
230	Diupres-250® Tablets	3261
405	Diupres-500® Tablets	3262
214	Diuril® (Chlorothiazide, MSD) Tablets 250 mg	3244
432	Diuril® (Chlorothiazide, MSD) Tablets 500 mg	3245
675	Dolobid® (Diflunisal, MSD) Tablets 250 mg	3390
697	Dolobid® (Diflunisal, MSD) Tablets 500 mg	3392
65	Edecrin® (Ethacrynic Acid, MSD) Tablets 25 mg	3321
90	Edecrin® (Ethacrynic Acid, MSD) Tablets 50 mg	3322
23	Elavil® (Amitriptyline HCl, MSD) Tablets 10 mg	3287
45	Elavil® (Amitriptyline HCl, MSD) Tablets 25 mg	3288
102	Elavil® (Amitriptyline HCl, MSD) Tablets 50 mg	3320
430	Elavil® (Amitriptyline HCl, MSD) Tablets 75 mg	3348
435	Elavil® (Amitriptyline HCl, MSD) Tablets 100 mg	3349
673	Elavil® (Amitriptyline HCl, MSD) Tablets 150 mg	3351
931	Flexeril® (Cyclobenzaprine HCl, MSD) Tablets 10 mg	3358
619	Hydrocortone® (Hydrocortisone, MSD) Tablets 10 mg	7604
625	Hydrocortone® (Hydrocortisone, MSD) Tablets 20 mg	7602
42	HydroDIURIL® (Hydrochlorothiazide, MSD) Tablets 25 mg	3263
105	HydroDIURIL® (Hydrochlorothiazide, MSD) Tablets 50 mg	3264
410	HydroDIURIL® (Hydrochlorothiazide, MSD) Tablets 100 mg	3340
53	Hydropres® 25 (Reserpine-Hydrochlorothiazide, MSD) Tablets	3265
127	Hydropres® 50 (Reserpine-Hydrochlorothiazide, MSD) Tablets	3266
25	Indocin® (Indomethacin, MSD) Capsules 25 mg	3316
50	Indocin® (Indomethacin, MSD) Capsules 50 mg	3317
693	Indocin® SR (Indomethacin, MSD) Capsules 75 mg	3370
150	Indocin® (Indomethacin, MSD) Suppositories 50 mg	3354
52	Inversine® (Mecamylamine HCl, MSD) Tablets 2.5 mg	3219
43	Mephyton® (Phytonadione, MSD) Tablets 5 mg	7776
92	Midamor® (Amiloride HCl, MSD) Tablets 5 mg	3381
907	Mintezol® (Thiabendazole, MSD) Chewable Tablets 500 mg	3332
917	Moduretic® (Amiloride HCl-Hydrochlorothiazide, MSD) Tablets	3385
62	Periactin® (Cyproheptadine HCl, MSD) Tablets 4 mg	3276
647	Sinemet® 10-100 (Carbidopa-Levodopa, MSD) Tablets	3346
650	Sinemet® 25-100 (Carbidopa-Levodopa, MSD) Tablets	3365
654	Sinemet® 25-250 (Carbidopa-Levodopa, MSD) Tablets	3347
67	Timolide® 10-25 (Timolol Maleate-Hydrochlorothiazide, MSD) Tablets	3373
707	Tonocard® (Tocainide HCl, MSD) Tablets 400 mg	3409
709	Tonocard® (Tocainide HCl, MSD) Tablets 600 mg	3410
914	Triavil® 2-10 Tablets	3328
921	Triavil® 2-25 Tablets	3311
934	Triavil® 4-10 Tablets	3310
946	Triavil® 4-25 Tablets	3312
517	Triavil® 4-50 Tablets	3364
403	Urecholine® (Bethanechol Chloride, MSD) Tablets 5 mg	7785
412	Urecholine® (Bethanechol Chloride, MSD) Tablets 10 mg	7787
457	Urecholine® (Bethanechol Chloride, MSD) Tablets 25 mg	7788
460	Urecholine® (Bethanechol Chloride, MSD) Tablets 50 mg	7790
712	Vasotec® (Enalapril Maleate, MSD) Tablets 5 mg	3412
713	Vasotec® (Enalapril Maleate, MSD) Tablets 10 mg	3413
714	Vasotec® (Enalapril Maleate, MSD) Tablets 20 mg	3414
26	Vivactil® (Protriptyline HCl, MSD) Tablets 5 mg	3313
47	Vivactil® (Protriptyline HCl, MSD) Tablets 10 mg	3314

ALDOCLOR® Tablets ℞

Antihypertensive

WARNING

This fixed combination drug is not indicated for initial therapy of hypertension. Hypertension requires therapy titrated to the individual patient. If the fixed combination represents the dosage so determined, its use may be more convenient in patient management. The treatment of hypertension is not static, but must be reevaluated as conditions in each patient warrant.

DESCRIPTION

ALDOCLOR® is a combination of methyldopa and chlorothiazide. The chemical name for methyldopa is levo-3-(3,4-dihydroxyphenyl)-2-methylalanine. Chlorothiazide is 6-chloro-2*H*-1, 2, 4-benzothiadiazine-7-sulfonamide 1, 1-dioxide.

ALDOCLOR is supplied as tablets in two strengths for oral use:

ALDOCLOR 150, contains 250 mg of methyldopa and 150 mg of chlorothiazide.

ALDOCLOR 250, contains 250 mg of methyldopa and 250 mg of chlorothiazide.

Each tablet contains the following inactive ingredients: calcium disodium edetate, cellulose, citric acid, D&C Yellow 10, ethylcellulose, FD&C Yellow 6, gelatin, glycerin, guar gum, hydroxypropyl methylcellulose, magnesium stearate, starch, talc, and titanium dioxide. ALDOCLOR 150 also contains iron oxides, ALDOCLOR 250 also contains FD&C Blue 2.

ACTIONS

ALDOMET® (Methyldopa, MSD)

Methyldopa, a unique antihypertensive, is an aromatic-amino-acid decarboxylase inhibitor in animals and in man. Although the mechanism of action has yet to be conclusively demonstrated, the antihypertensive effect of methyldopa probably is due to its metabolism to alpha-methylnorepinephrine, which then lowers arterial pressure by stimulation of central inhibitory alpha-adrenergic receptors, false neurotransmission, and/or reduction of plasma renin activity. Methyldopa has been shown to cause a net reduction in the tissue concentration of serotonin, dopamine, norepinephrine, and epinephrine.

Only methyldopa, the *L*-isomer of alpha-methyldopa, has the ability to inhibit dopa decarboxylase and to deplete animal tissues of norepinephrine. In man, the antihypertensive activity appears to be due solely to the *L*-isomer. About twice the dose of the racemate (*DL*-alpha-methyldopa) is required for equal antihypertensive effect.

Methyldopa has no direct effect on cardiac function and usually does not reduce glomerular filtration rate, renal blood flow, or filtration fraction. Cardiac output usually is maintained without cardiac acceleration. In some patients the heart rate is slowed.

Normal or elevated plasma renin activity may decrease in the course of methyldopa therapy.

Methyldopa reduces both supine and standing blood pressure. It usually produces highly effective lowering of the supine pressure with infrequent symptomatic postural hypotension. Exercise hypotension and diurnal blood pressure variations rarely occur.

DIURIL® (Chlorothiazide, MSD)

Chlorothiazide is a diuretic and antihypertensive. It affects the renal tubular mechanism of electrolyte reabsorption. At maximal therapeutic dosage all thiazides are approximately equal in their diuretic efficacy.

Chlorothiazide increases excretion of sodium and chloride in approximately equivalent amounts. Natriuresis may be accompanied by some loss of potassium and bicarbonate.

The mechanism of the antihypertensive effect of thiazides is unknown. Chlorothiazide does not affect normal blood pressure.

Chlorothiazide is eliminated rapidly by the kidney.

ALDOCLOR

The concomitant use of methyldopa and chlorothiazide, as provided in ALDOCLOR, frequently produces a more pronounced antihypertensive response than when either compound is the sole therapeutic agent. Particularly in those cases of hypertensive vascular disease where sodium and water retention is a problem, the coadministration of these two drugs in the form of ALDOCLOR will help control the fluid imbalance.

In severe essential hypertension and in malignant hypertension, ALDOCLOR may achieve effective lowering of blood pressure with fewer side effects than occur with other compounds used for this purpose.

ALDOCLOR reduces both supine and standing blood pressure; more effective lowering of the supine pressure with less frequent symptomatic postural hypotension can be obtained with ALDOCLOR than with most other antihypertensive agents. In patients treated with ALDOCLOR, exercise hypotension and diurnal blood pressure variations rarely occur.

INDICATION

Hypertension (see box warning).

CONTRAINDICATIONS

Active hepatic disease, such as acute hepatitis and active cirrhosis.

If previous methyldopa therapy has been associated with liver disorders (see WARNINGS).

Anuria.

Hypersensitivity to methyldopa, or to chlorothiazide or other sulfonamide-derived drugs.

Continued on next page

Information on the Merck Sharp & Dohme products listed on these pages is the full prescribing information from product circulars in use August 31, 1986.

Merck Sharp & Dohme—Cont.

WARNINGS

Methyldopa

It is important to recognize that a positive Coombs test, hemolytic anemia, and liver disorders may occur with methyldopa therapy. The rare occurrences of hemolytic anemia or liver disorders could lead to potentially fatal complications unless properly recognized and managed. Read this section carefully to understand these reactions.

With prolonged methyldopa therapy, 10 to 20 percent of patients develop a positive direct Coombs test which usually occurs between 6 and 12 months of methyldopa therapy. Lowest incidence is at daily dosage of 1 g or less. This on rare occasions may be associated with hemolytic anemia, which could lead to potentially fatal complications. One cannot predict which patients with a positive direct Coombs test may develop hemolytic anemia.

Prior existence or development of a positive direct Coombs test is not in itself a contraindication to use of methyldopa. If a positive Coombs test develops during methyldopa therapy, the physician should determine whether hemolytic anemia exists and whether the positive Coombs test may be a problem. For example, in addition to a positive direct Coombs test there is less often a positive indirect Coombs test which may interfere with cross matching of blood.

At the start of methyldopa therapy, it is desirable to do a blood count (hematocrit, hemoglobin, or red cell count) for a baseline or to establish whether there is anemia. Periodic blood counts should be done during therapy to detect hemolytic anemia. It may be useful to do a direct Coombs test before therapy and at 6 and 12 months after the start of therapy.

If Coombs-positive hemolytic anemia occurs, the cause may be methyldopa and the drug should be discontinued. Usually the anemia remits promptly. If not, corticosteroids may be given and other causes of anemia should be considered. If the hemolytic anemia is related to methyldopa, the drug should not be reinstituted.

When methyldopa causes Coombs positivity alone or with hemolytic anemia, the red cell is usually coated with gamma globulin of the IgG (gamma G) class only. The positive Coombs test may not revert to normal until weeks to months after methyldopa is stopped.

Should the need for transfusion arise in a patient receiving methyldopa, both a direct and an indirect Coombs test should be performed on his blood. In the absence of hemolytic anemia, usually only the direct Coombs test will be positive. A positive direct Coombs test alone will not interfere with typing or cross matching. If the indirect Coombs test is also positive, problems may arise in the major cross match and the assistance of a hematologist or transfusion expert will be needed.

Occasionally, fever has occurred within the first three weeks of methyldopa therapy, associated in some cases with eosinophilia or abnormalities in one or more liver function tests, such as serum alkaline phosphatase, serum transaminases (SGOT, SGPT), bilirubin, cephalin cholesterol flocculation, prothrombin time, and bromsulphalein retention. Jaundice, with or without fever, may occur with onset usually within the first two to three months of therapy. In some patients the findings are consistent with those of cholestasis.

Rarely fatal hepatic necrosis has been reported after use of methyldopa. These hepatic changes may represent hypersensitivity reactions. Periodic determination of hepatic function should be done particularly during the first 6 to 12 weeks of therapy or whenever an unexplained fever occurs. If fever, abnormalities in liver function tests, or jaundice appear, stop therapy with methyldopa. If caused by methyldopa, the temperature and abnormalities in liver function characteristically have reverted to normal when the drug was discontinued. Methyldopa should not be reinstituted in such patients.

Rarely, a reversible reduction of the white blood cell count with a primary effect on the granulocytes has been seen. The granulocyte count returned promptly to normal on discontinuance of the drug. Rare cases of granulocytopenia have been reported. In each instance, upon stopping the drug, the white cell count returned to normal. Reversible thrombocytopenia has occurred rarely.

When methyldopa is used with other antihypertensive drugs, potentiation of antihypertensive effect may occur. Patients should be followed carefully to detect side reactions or unusual manifestations of drug idiosyncrasy.

Chlorothiazide

Use with caution in severe renal disease. In patients with renal disease, thiazides may precipitate azotemia. Cumulative effects of the drug may develop in patients with impaired renal function.

Thiazides should be used with caution in patients with impaired hepatic function or progressive liver disease, since minor alterations of fluid and electrolyte balance may precipitate hepatic coma.

Thiazides may add to or potentiate the action of other antihypertensive drugs.

Sensitivity reactions may occur in patients with or without a history of allergy or bronchial asthma.

The possibility of exacerbation or activation of systemic lupus erythematosus has been reported.

Lithium generally should not be given with diuretics because they reduce its renal clearance and add a high risk of lithium toxicity. Read circulars for lithium preparations before use of such concomitant therapy.

PREGNANCY AND NURSING

Use of any drug in women who are or may become pregnant requires that anticipated benefits be weighed against possible risks.

Methyldopa crosses the placental barrier and appears in cord blood. No unusual adverse reactions have been reported in association with the use of methyldopa during pregnancy. Though no obvious teratogenic effects have been reported, the possibility of fetal injury cannot be excluded.

Thiazides also cross the placental barrier and appear in cord blood. Hazards include fetal or neonatal jaundice, thrombocytopenia, and possibly other adverse reactions which have occurred in the adult.

Methyldopa and thiazides appear in breast milk. Patients taking ALDOCLOR should not nurse.

PRECAUTIONS

Methyldopa

Methyldopa should be used with caution in patients with a history of previous liver disease or dysfunction (see WARNINGS).

Methyldopa may interfere with measurement of: urinary uric acid by the phosphotungstate method, serum creatinine by the alkaline picrate method, and SGOT by colorimetric methods. Interference with spectrophotometric methods for SGOT analysis has not been reported.

Since methyldopa causes fluorescence in urine samples at the same wave lengths as catecholamines, falsely high levels of urinary catecholamines may be reported. This will interfere with the diagnosis of pheochromocytoma. It is important to recognize this phenomenon before a patient with a possible pheochromocytoma is subjected to surgery. Methyldopa does not interfere with measurement of VMA (vanillylmandelic acid), a test for pheochromocytoma, by those methods which convert VMA to vanillin. Methyldopa is not recommended for the treatment of patients with pheochromocytoma. Rarely, when urine is exposed to air after voiding, it may darken because of breakdown of methyldopa or its metabolites.

Rarely, involuntary choreoathetotic movements have been observed during therapy with methyldopa in patients with severe bilateral cerebrovascular disease. Should these movements occur, stop therapy.

Patients may require reduced doses of anesthetics when on methyldopa. If hypotension does occur during anesthesia, it usually can be controlled by vasopressors. The adrenergic receptors remain sensitive during treatment with methyldopa.

Hypertension has recurred occasionally after dialysis in patients given methyldopa because the drug is removed by this procedure.

Chlorothiazide

Periodic determination of serum electrolytes to detect possible electrolyte imbalance should be performed at appropriate intervals.

All patients receiving diuretic therapy should be observed for evidence of fluid or electrolyte imbalance: namely, hyponatremia, hypochloremic alkalosis, and hypokalemia. Serum and urine electrolyte determinations are particularly important when the patient is vomiting excessively or receiving parenteral fluids. Warning signs or symptoms of fluid and electrolyte imbalance include dryness of mouth, thirst, weakness, lethargy, drowsiness, restlessness, muscle pains or cramps, muscular fatigue, hypotension, oliguria, tachycardia, and gastrointestinal disturbances such as nausea and vomiting.

Hypokalemia may develop, especially with brisk diuresis, when severe cirrhosis is present, during concomitant use of corticosteroids or ACTH, or after prolonged therapy.

Interference with adequate oral electrolyte intake will also contribute to hypokalemia. Hypokalemia can sensitize or exaggerate the response of the heart to the toxic effects of digitalis (e.g., increased ventricular irritability). Hypokalemia may be avoided or treated by use of potassium supplements such as foods with a high potassium content.

Although any chloride deficit is generally mild and usually does not require specific treatment except under extraordinary circumstances (as in liver disease or renal disease), chloride replacement may be required in the treatment of metabolic alkalosis.

Dilutional hyponatremia may occur in edematous patients in hot weather; appropriate therapy is water restriction, rather than administration of salt, except in rare instances when the hyponatremia is life threatening. In actual salt depletion, appropriate replacement is the therapy of choice.

Hyperuricemia may occur or acute gout may be precipitated in certain patients receiving thiazides.

Insulin requirements in diabetic patients may be increased, decreased, or unchanged. Latent diabetes mellitus may become manifest during thiazide therapy.

Thiazides may increase the responsiveness to tubocurarine.

In some patients, the administration of a non-steroidal anti-inflammatory agent can reduce the diuretic, natriuretic, and antihypertensive effects of loop, potassium-sparing and thiazide diuretics. Therefore, when ALDOCLOR and non-steroidal anti-inflammatory agents are used concomitantly, the patient should be observed closely to determine if the desired effect of the diuretic is obtained.

The antihypertensive effects of the drug may be enhanced in the postsympathectomy patient. Thiazides may decrease arterial responsiveness to norepinephrine. This diminution is not sufficient to preclude effectiveness of the pressor agent for therapeutic use.

If progressive renal impairment becomes evident, consider withholding or discontinuing diuretic therapy.

Thiazides may decrease serum PBI levels without signs of thyroid disturbance.

Thiazides have been shown to increase the urinary excretion of magnesium; this may result in hypomagnesemia.

Thiazides may decrease urinary calcium excretion. Thiazides may cause intermittent and slight elevation of serum calcium in the absence of known disorders of calcium metabolism. Marked hypercalcemia may be evidence of hidden hyperparathyroidism. Thiazides should be discontinued before carrying out tests for parathyroid function.

ADVERSE REACTIONS

Methyldopa

Sedation, usually transient, may occur during the initial period of therapy or whenever the dose is increased. Headache, asthenia, or weakness may be noted as early and transient symptoms. However, significant adverse effects due to methyldopa have been infrequent and this agent usually is well tolerated.

Nervous System/Psychiatric: Sedation, headache, asthenia or weakness, dizziness, lightheadedness, symptoms of cerebrovascular insufficiency, paresthesias, parkinsonism, Bell's palsy, decreased mental acuity, involuntary choreoathetotic movements. Psychic disturbances including nightmares and reversible mild psychoses or depression.

Cardiovascular: Bradycardia, prolonged carotid sinus hypersensitivity, aggravation of angina pectoris. Orthostatic hypotension (decrease daily dosage). Edema (and weight gain) usually relieved by use of a diuretic. (Discontinue methyldopa if edema progresses or signs of heart failure appear.)

Digestive: Nausea, vomiting, distention, constipation, flatus, diarrhea, colitis, mild dryness of mouth, sore or "black" tongue, pancreatitis, sialadenitis.

Hepatic: Abnormal liver function tests, jaundice, liver disorders.

Hematologic: Positive Coombs test, hemolytic anemia. Bone marrow depression, leukopenia, granulocytopenia, thrombocytopenia. Positive tests for antinuclear antibody, LE cells, and rheumatoid factor.

Allergic: Drug-related fever, lupus-like syndrome, myocarditis, pericarditis.

Skin: Rash as in eczema or lichenoid eruption; toxic epidermal necrolysis.

Respiratory: Nasal stuffiness.

Metabolic: Rise in BUN.

Urogenital: Breast enlargement, gynecomastia, lactation, amenorrhea, impotence, decreased libido.

Endocrine: Hyperprolactinemia.

Musculoskeletal: Mild arthralgia, with or without joint swelling; myalgia.

Chlorothiazide

Body as a Whole: Weakness.

Cardiovascular: Orthostatic hypotension (may be aggravated by alcohol, barbiturates, or narcotics).

Digestive: Anorexia, gastric irritation, nausea, vomiting, cramping, diarrhea, constipation, jaundice (intrahepatic cholestatic jaundice), pancreatitis, sialadenitis.

Hematologic: Leukopenia, agranulocytosis, thrombocytopenia, aplastic anemia, hemolytic anemia.

Metabolic: Hyperglycemia, glycosuria, hyperuricemia, electrolyte imbalance (see PRECAUTIONS).

Musculoskeletal: Muscle spasm.

Nervous System/Psychiatric: Dizziness, vertigo, paresthesias, headache, restlessness.

Special Senses: Transient blurred vision, xanthopsia.

Hypersensitivity: Purpura, photosensitivity, rash, urticaria, necrotizing angiitis (vasculitis and cutaneous vasculitis), fever, respiratory distress including pneumonitis and pulmonary edema, anaphylactic reactions.

Whenever adverse reactions are moderate or severe, thiazide dosage should be reduced or therapy withdrawn.

DOSAGE AND ADMINISTRATION

Dosage: As determined by individual titration (see box warning).

The usual starting dosage is 1 tablet of ALDOCLOR 150 or 1 tablet of ALDOCLOR 250 two or three times a day in the first 48 hours. The daily dosage then may be increased or decreased, preferably at intervals of not less than two days, until an adequate response is achieved. To minimize the sedation associated with methyldopa, start dosage increases in the evening. By adjustment of dosage, morning hypotension may be prevented without sacrificing control of afternoon blood pressure.

When ALDOCLOR is given to patients on other antihypertensives, the dose of these agents may need to be adjusted to effect a smooth transition. When ALDOCLOR is given with antihypertensives other than thiazides, the initial dosage of methyldopa should be limited to 500 mg daily in divided doses.

Although occasional patients have responded to higher doses, the maximum recommended daily dosage is 3.0 g of methyldopa and 1.0 to 2.0 g of chlorothiazide. Once an effective dosage range is attained, a smooth blood pressure response occurs in most patients in 12 to 24 hours. If ALDOCLOR alone does not adequately control blood pressure, additional methyldopa may be given separately to obtain the maximum blood pressure response.

Since both components of ALDOCLOR have a relatively short duration of action, withdrawal is followed by return of hypertension usually within 48 hours. This is not complicated by an overshoot of blood pressure.

Occasionally tolerance may occur, usually between the second and third month of therapy. Increasing the dosage of either methyldopa or chlorothiazide separately or together frequently will restore effective control of blood pressure.

Methyldopa is largely excreted by the kidney and patients with impaired renal function may respond to smaller doses of ALDOCLOR. Syncope in older patients may be related to an increased sensitivity and advanced arteriosclerotic vascular disease. This may be avoided by lower doses.

HOW SUPPLIED

No. 3318—Tablets ALDOCLOR 150 are beige, oval, film coated tablets coded MSD 612. Each tablet contains 250 mg of methyldopa and 150 mg of chlorothiazide. They are supplied as follows:

NDC 0006-0612-68 bottles of 100.

Shown in Product Identification Section, page 417

No. 3319—Tablets ALDOCLOR 250 are green, oval, film coated tablets coded MSD 634. Each tablet contains 250 mg of methyldopa and 250 mg of chlorothiazide. They are supplied as follows:

NDC 0006-0634-68 bottles of 100.

Shown in Product Identification Section, page 417

A.H.F.S. Category: 24:08

DC 7059827 Issued October 1985

ALDOMET® Tablets (Methyldopa, MSD), U.S.P. ℞

ALDOMET® Oral Suspension (Methyldopa, MSD), U.S.P. ℞

DESCRIPTION

Methyldopa is the *L*-isomer of alpha-methyldopa. Its chemical name is levo-3-(3,4 - dihydroxyphenyl) -2-methylalanine. Its structural formula is:

[Structural formula: 3,4-dihydroxyphenyl ring (HO, HO) –CH_2–C(CH_3)(NH_2)–CO_2H]

ALDOMET is supplied as tablets, in three strengths, each containing 125 mg, 250 mg, or 500 mg of methyldopa per tablet. Inactive ingredients in the tablets are calcium disodium edetate, cellulose, citric acid, colloidal silicon dioxide, D&C Yellow 10, ethylcellulose, guar gum, hydroxypropyl methylcellulose, iron oxide, magnesium stearate, propylene glycol, talc, and titanium dioxide.

Oral Suspension ALDOMET is supplied as a white to off-white preparation; each 5 mL contains 250 mg of methyldopa and alcohol 1 percent, with benzoic acid 0.1 percent and sodium bisulfite 0.2 percent added as preservatives. Inactive ingredients in the oral suspension are artificial and natural flavors, cellulose, citric acid, confectioner's sugar, disodium edetate, glycerin, polysorbate, purified water, and sodium carboxymethylcellulose.

ACTIONS

ALDOMET® (Methyldopa, MSD), a unique antihypertensive, is an aromatic-amino-acid decarboxylase inhibitor in animals and in man. Although the mechanism of action has yet to be conclusively demonstrated, the antihypertensive effect of methyldopa probably is due to its metabolism to alpha-methylnorepinephrine, which then lowers arterial pressure by stimulation of central inhibitory alpha-adrenergic receptors, false neurotransmission, and/or reduction of plasma renin activity. Methyldopa has been shown to cause a net reduction in the tissue concentration of serotonin, dopamine, norepinephrine, and epinephrine.

Only methyldopa, the *L*-isomer of alpha-methyldopa, has the ability to inhibit dopa decarboxylase and to deplete animal tissues of norepinephrine. In man the antihypertensive activity appears to be due solely to the *L*-isomer. About twice the dose of the racemate (*DL*-alpha-methyldopa) is required for equal antihypertensive effect.

Methyldopa has no direct effect on cardiac function and usually does not reduce glomerular filtration rate, renal blood flow, or filtration fraction. Cardiac output usually is maintained without cardiac acceleration. In some patients the heart rate is slowed.

Normal or elevated plasma renin activity may decrease in the course of methyldopa therapy.

ALDOMET reduces both supine and standing blood pressure. Methyldopa usually produces highly effective lowering of the supine pressure with infrequent symptomatic postural hypotension. Exercise hypotension and diurnal blood pressure variations rarely occur.

INDICATION

Hypertension.

CONTRAINDICATIONS

Active hepatic disease, such as acute hepatitis and active cirrhosis.

If previous methyldopa therapy has been associated with liver disorders (see WARNINGS).

Hypersensitivity to any component of these products, including sulfites. Oral Suspension ALDOMET contains sodium bisulfite. Tablets ALDOMET contain no sulfites. (see PRECAUTIONS).

WARNINGS

It is important to recognize that a positive Coombs test, hemolytic anemia, and liver disorders may occur with methyldopa therapy. The rare occurrences of hemolytic anemia or liver disorders could lead to potentially fatal complications unless properly recognized and managed. Read this section carefully to understand these reactions.

With prolonged methyldopa therapy, 10 to 20 percent of patients develop a positive direct Coombs test which usually occurs between 6 and 12 months of methyldopa therapy. Lowest incidence is at daily dosage of 1 g or less. This on rare occasions may be associated with hemolytic anemia, which could lead to potentially fatal complications. One cannot predict which patients with a positive direct Coombs test may develop hemolytic anemia.

Prior existence or development of a positive direct Coombs test is not in itself a contraindication to use of methyldopa. If a positive Coombs test develops during methyldopa therapy, the physician should determine whether hemolytic anemia exists and whether the positive Coombs test may be a problem. For example, in addition to a positive direct Coombs test there is less often a positive indirect Coombs test which may interfere with cross matching of blood.

At the start of methyldopa therapy, it is desirable to do a blood count (hematocrit, hemoglobin, or red cell count) for a baseline or to establish whether there is anemia. Periodic blood counts should be done during therapy to detect hemolytic anemia. It may be useful to do a direct Coombs test before therapy and at 6 and 12 months after the start of therapy.

If Coombs-positive hemolytic anemia occurs, the cause may be methyldopa and the drug should be discontinued. Usually the anemia remits promptly. If not, corticosteroids may be given and other causes of anemia should be considered. If the hemolytic anemia is related to methyldopa, the drug should not be reinstituted.

When methyldopa causes Coombs positivity alone or with hemolytic anemia, the red cell is usually coated with gamma globulin of the IgG (gamma G) class only. The positive Coombs test may not revert to normal until weeks to months after methyldopa is stopped.

Should the need for transfusion arise in a patient receiving methyldopa, both a direct and an indirect Coombs test should be performed on his blood. In the absence of hemolytic anemia, usually only the direct Coombs test will be positive. A positive direct Coombs test alone will not interfere with typing or cross matching. If the indirect Coombs test is also positive, problems may arise in the major cross match and the assistance of a hematologist or transfusion expert will be needed.

Occasionally, fever has occurred within the first 3 weeks of methyldopa therapy, associated in some cases with eosinophilia or abnormalities in one or more liver function tests, such as serum alkaline phosphatase, serum transaminases (SGOT, SGPT), bilirubin, cephalin cholesterol flocculation, prothrombin time, and bromsulphalein retention. Jaundice, with or without fever, may occur with onset usually within the first 2 to 3 months of therapy. In some patients the findings are consistent with those of cholestasis.

Rarely, fatal hepatic necrosis has been reported after use of methyldopa. These hepatic changes may represent hypersensitivity reactions. Periodic determinations of hepatic function should be done particularly during the first 6 to 12 weeks of therapy or whenever an unexplained fever occurs. If fever, abnormalities in liver function tests, or jaundice appear, stop therapy with methyldopa. If caused by methyldopa, the temperature and abnormalities in liver function characteristically have reverted to normal when the drug was discontinued. Methyldopa should not be reinstituted in such patients.

Rarely, a reversible reduction of the white blood cell count with a primary effect on the granulocytes has been seen. The granulocyte count returned promptly to normal on discontinuance of the drug. Rare cases of granulocytopenia have been reported. In each instance, upon stopping the drug, the white cell count returned to normal. Reversible thrombocytopenia has occurred rarely.

When methyldopa is used with other antihypertensive drugs, potentiation of antihypertensive effect may occur. Patients should be followed carefully to detect side reactions or unusual manifestations of drug idiosyncrasy.

Pregnancy and Nursing

Use of any drug in women who are or may become pregnant or intend to nurse requires that anticipated benefits be weighed against possible risks.

Methyldopa crosses the placental barrier, appears in cord blood, and appears in breast milk.

No unusual adverse reactions have been reported in association with the use of methyldopa during pregnancy. Though no obvious teratogenic effects have been reported, the possibility of fetal injury cannot be excluded. Also, the possibility of injury to a nursing infant cannot be excluded.

PRECAUTIONS

Methyldopa should be used with caution in patients with a history of previous liver disease or dysfunction (see WARNINGS).

Sulfites have been reported to cause severe allergic reactions in certain susceptible individuals, particularly patients with asthma. Oral Suspension ALDOMET contains sodium bisulfite. Tablets ALDOMET contain no sulfites.

Methyldopa may interfere with measurement of: urinary uric acid by the phosphotungstate method, serum creatinine by the alkaline picrate method, and SGOT by colorimetric methods. Interference with spectrophotometric methods for SGOT analysis has not been reported.

Since methyldopa causes fluorescence in urine samples at the same wave lengths as catecholamines, falsely high levels of urinary catecholamines may be reported. This will interfere with the diagnosis of pheochromocytoma. It is important to recognize this phenomenon before a patient with a possible pheochromocytoma is subjected to surgery. Methyldopa does not interfere with measurement of VMA (vanillylmandelic acid), a test for pheochromocytoma, by those methods which convert VMA to vanillin. Methyldopa is not recommended for the treatment of patients with pheochromocytoma. Rarely, when urine is exposed to air after voiding, it may darken because of breakdown of methyldopa or its metabolites.

Rarely, involuntary choreoathetotic movements have been observed during therapy with methyldopa in patients with severe bilateral cerebrovascular disease. Should these movements occur, stop therapy.

Patients may require reduced doses of anesthetics when on methyldopa. If hypotension does occur during anesthesia, it usually can be controlled by vasopressors. The adrenergic receptors remain sensitive during treatment with methyldopa.

Hypertension has recurred occasionally after dialysis in patients given methyldopa because the drug is removed by this procedure.

Continued on next page

Information on the Merck Sharp & Dohme products listed on these pages is the full prescribing information from product circulars in use August 31, 1986.

Merck Sharp & Dohme—Cont.

ADVERSE REACTIONS

Sedation, usually transient, may occur during the initial period of therapy or whenever the dose is increased. Headache, asthenia, or weakness may be noted as early and transient symptoms. However, significant adverse effects due to ALDOMET have been infrequent and this agent usually is well tolerated.
Nervous System/Psychiatric: Sedation, headache, asthenia or weakness, dizziness, lightheadedness, symptoms of cerebrovascular insufficiency, paresthesias, parkinsonism, Bell's palsy, decreased mental acuity, involuntary choreoathetotic movements. Psychic disturbances including nightmares and reversible mild psychoses or depression.
Cardiovascular: Bradycardia, prolonged carotid sinus hypersensitivity, aggravation of angina pectoris. Orthostatic hypotension (decrease daily dosage). Edema (and weight gain) usually relieved by use of a diuretic. (Discontinue methyldopa if edema progresses or signs of heart failure appear.)
Digestive: Nausea, vomiting, distention, constipation, flatus, diarrhea, colitis, mild dryness of mouth, sore or "black" tongue, pancreatitis, sialadenitis.
Hepatic: Abnormal liver function tests, jaundice, liver disorders.
Hematologic: Positive Coombs test, hemolytic anemia. Bone marrow depression, leukopenia, granulocytopenia, thrombocytopenia. Positive tests for antinuclear antibody, LE cells, and rheumatoid factor.
Allergic: Drug-related fever, lupus-like syndrome, myocarditis, pericarditis.
Skin: Rash as in eczema or lichenoid eruption; toxic epidermal necrolysis.
Respiratory: Nasal stuffiness.
Metabolic: Rise in BUN.
Urogenital: Breast enlargement, gynecomastia, lactation, amenorrhea, impotence, decreased libido.
Endocrine: Hyperprolactinemia.
Musculoskeletal: Mild arthralgia, with or without joint swelling; myalgia.

DOSAGE AND ADMINISTRATION

ADULTS

Initiation of Therapy
The usual starting dosage of ALDOMET is 250 mg two or three times a day in the first 48 hours. The daily dosage then may be increased or decreased, preferably at intervals of not less than two days, until an adequate response is achieved. To minimize the sedation, start dosage increases in the evening. By adjustment of dosage, morning hypotension may be prevented without sacrificing control of afternoon blood pressure.
When methyldopa is given to patients on other antihypertensives, the dose of these agents may need to be adjusted to effect a smooth transition. When ALDOMET is given with antihypertensives other than thiazides, the initial dosage of ALDOMET should be limited to 500 mg daily in divided doses; when ALDOMET is added to a thiazide, the dosage of thiazide need not be changed.

Maintenance Therapy
The usual daily dosage of ALDOMET is 500 mg to 2 g in two to four doses. Although occasional patients have responded to higher doses, the maximum recommended daily dosage is 3 g. Once an effective dosage range is attained, a smooth blood pressure response occurs in most patients in 12 to 24 hours. Since methyldopa has a relatively short duration of action, withdrawal is followed by return of hypertension usually within 48 hours. This is not complicated by an overshoot of blood pressure.
Occasionally tolerance may occur, usually between the second and third month of therapy. Adding a diuretic or increasing the dosage of methyldopa frequently will restore effective control of blood pressure. A thiazide may be added at any time during methyldopa therapy and is recommended if therapy has not been started with a thiazide or if effective control of blood pressure cannot be maintained on 2 g of methyldopa daily.
Methyldopa is largely excreted by the kidney and patients with impaired renal function may respond to smaller doses. Syncope in older patients may be related to an increased sensitivity and advanced arteriosclerotic vascular disease. This may be avoided by lower doses.

CHILDREN

Initial dosage is based on 10 mg/kg of body weight daily in two to four doses. The daily dosage then is increased or decreased until an adequate response is achieved. The maximum dosage is 65 mg/kg or 3 g daily, whichever is less.

HOW SUPPLIED

No. 3341—Tablets ALDOMET, 125 mg, are yellow, film coated, round tablets, coded MSD 135. They are supplied as follows:
NDC 0006-0135-68 bottles of 100.
Shown in Product Identification Section, page 417
No. 3290—Tablets ALDOMET, 250 mg, are yellow, film coated, round tablets, coded MSD 401. They are supplied as follows:
NDC 0006-0401-68 bottles of 100
(6505-00-890-1856, 250 mg 100's)
NDC 0006-0401-28 unit dose packages of 100
(6505-00-149-0090, 250 mg individually sealed 100's)
NDC 0006-0401-78 unit of use bottles of 100
NDC 0006-0401-82 bottles of 1000
(6505-00-931-6646, 250 mg 1000's).
Shown in Product Identification Section, page 417
No. 3292—Tablets ALDOMET, 500 mg, are yellow, film coated, round tablets, coded MSD 516. They are supplied as follows:
NDC 0006-0516-54 unit of use bottles of 60
NDC 0006-0516-68 bottles of 100
NDC 0006-0516-28 unit dose packages of 100
NDC 0006-0516-78 unit of use bottles of 100
NDC 0006-0516-74 bottles of 500.
Shown in Product Identification Section, page 417
No. 3382—Oral Suspension ALDOMET, 250 mg per 5 mL, is an off-white, creamy suspension with a citric orange-pineapple flavor. It is supplied as follows:
NDC 0006-3382-74 bottles of 473 mL.
Storage
Store Oral Suspension ALDOMET below 26°C (78°F) in a tight, light-resistant container. Protect from freezing.
A.H.F.S. Category: 24:08
DC 6649719 Issued May 1985

ALDOMET® Ester HCl Injection ℞
(Methyldopate Hydrochloride, MSD), U.S.P.

DESCRIPTION

Injection ALDOMET® ester hydrochloride (Methyldopate Hydrochloride, MSD) is an antihypertensive agent for intravenous use, each 5 mL of which contains:

Methyldopate hydrochloride	250.0 mg
Inactive ingredients:	
Citric acid anhydrous	25.0 mg
Disodium edetate	2.5 mg
Monothioglycerol	10.0 mg
Sodium hydroxide to adjust pH	
Water for Injection, q.s. to	5.0 mL

Methylparaben 7.5 mg, propylparaben 1.0 mg, and sodium bisulfite 16.0 mg added as preservatives.
Methyldopate hydrochloride [levo-3-(3,4-dihydroxyphenyl)-2-methylalanine, ethyl ester hydrochloride] is the ethyl ester of methyldopa, supplied as the hydrochloride salt. Methyldopate hydrochloride is more soluble and stable in solution than methyldopa and is the preferred form for intravenous use.

The structural formula for methyldopate hydrochloride is:

HO, HO — (benzene ring) — CH_2—C(CH_3)($NH_2 \cdot HCl$)—$CO_2C_2H_5$

ACTIONS

ALDOMET® (Methyldopa, MSD), a unique antihypertensive, is an aromatic-amino-acid decarboxylase inhibitor in animals and in man. Although the mechanism of action has yet to be conclusively demonstrated, the antihypertensive effect of methyldopa probably is due to its metabolism to alpha-methyl-norepinephrine, which then lowers arterial pressure by stimulation of central inhibitory alpha-adrenergic receptors, false neurotransmission, and/or reduction of plasma renin activity. Methyldopa has been shown to cause a net reduction in the tissue concentration of serotonin, dopamine, norepinephrine, and epinephrine.
Only methyldopa, the *L*-isomer of alpha-methyldopa, has the ability to inhibit dopa decarboxylase and to deplete animal tissues of norepinephrine. In man the antihypertensive activity appears to be due solely to the *L*-isomer. About twice the dose of the racemate (*DL*-alpha-methyldopa) is required for equal antihypertensive effect.
Methyldopa has no direct effect on cardiac function and usually does not reduce glomerular filtration rate, renal blood flow, or filtration fraction. Cardiac output usually is maintained without cardiac acceleration. In some patients the heart rate is slowed.
Normal or elevated plasma renin activity may decrease in the course of methyldopa therapy.
Methyldopa reduces both supine and standing blood pressure. It usually produces highly effective lowering of the supine pressure with infrequent symptomatic postural hypotension. Exercise hypotension and diurnal blood pressure variations rarely occur.
Methyldopate hydrochloride is the ethyl ester of methyldopa hydrochloride and possesses the same pharmacologic attributes.

INDICATION

Hypertension, when parenteral medication is indicated.
The treatment of hypertensive crises may be initiated with injection ALDOMET ester hydrochloride.

CONTRAINDICATIONS

Active hepatic disease, such as acute hepatitis and active cirrhosis.
If previous methyldopa therapy has been associated with liver disorders (see WARNINGS).
Hypersensitivity to any component of this product, including sulfites (see PRECAUTIONS).

WARNINGS

It is important to recognize that a positive Coombs test, hemolytic anemia, and liver disorders may occur with methyldopa therapy. The rare occurrences of hemolytic anemia or liver disorders could lead to potentially fatal complications unless properly recognized and managed. Read this section carefully to understand these reactions.
With prolonged methyldopa therapy, 10 to 20 percent of patients develop a positive direct Coombs test which usually occurs between 6 and 12 months of methyldopa therapy. Lowest incidence is at daily dosage of 1 g or less. This on rare occasions may be associated with hemolytic anemia, which could lead to potentially fatal complications. One cannot predict which patients with a positive direct Coombs test may develop hemolytic anemia.
Prior existence or development of a positive direct Coombs test is not in itself a contraindication to use of methyldopa. If a positive Coombs test develops during methyldopa therapy, the physician should determine whether hemolytic anemia exists and whether the positive Coombs test may be a problem. For example, in addition to a positive direct Coombs test there is less often a positive indirect Coombs test which may interfere with cross matching of blood.
At the start of methyldopa therapy, it is desirable to do a blood count (hematocrit, hemoglobin, or red cell count) for a baseline or to establish whether there is anemia. Periodic blood counts should be done during therapy to detect hemolytic anemia. It may be useful to do a direct Coombs test before therapy and at 6 and 12 months after the start of therapy.
If Coombs-positive hemolytic anemia occurs, the cause may be methyldopa and the drug should be discontinued. Usually the anemia remits promptly. If not, corticosteroids may be given and other causes of anemia should be considered. If the hemolytic anemia is related to methyldopa, the drug should not be reinstituted.
When methyldopa causes Coombs positivity alone or with hemolytic anemia, the red cell is usually coated with gamma globulin of the IgG (gamma G) class only. The positive Coombs test may not revert to normal until weeks to months after methyldopa is stopped.
Should the need for transfusion arise in a patient receiving methyldopa, both a direct and an indirect Coombs test should be performed on his blood. In the absence of hemolytic anemia, usually only the direct Coombs test will be positive. A positive direct Coombs test alone will not interfere with typing or cross matching. If the indirect Coombs test is also positive, problems may arise in the major cross match and the assistance of a hematologist or transfusion expert will be needed.
Occasionally, fever has occurred within the first three weeks of methyldopa therapy, associated in some cases with eosinophilia or abnormalities in one or more liver function tests, such as serum alkaline phosphatase, serum transaminases (SGOT, SGPT), bilirubin, cephalin cholesterol flocculation, prothrombin time, and bromsulphalein retention. Jaundice, with or without fever, may occur with onset usually within the first two to three months of therapy. In some patients the findings are consistent with those of cholestasis.
Rarely fatal hepatic necrosis has been reported after use of methyldopa. These hepatic changes may represent hypersensitivity reactions. Periodic determination of hepatic function should be done particularly during the first 6 to 12 weeks of therapy or whenever an unexplained fever occurs. If fever, abnormalities in liver function tests, or jaundice appear, stop therapy with methyldopa. If caused by methyldopa, the temperature and abnormalities in liver function characteristically have reverted to normal when the drug

was discontinued. Methyldopa should not be reinstituted in such patients.

Rarely, a reversible reduction of the white blood cell count with a primary effect on the granulocytes has been seen. The granulocyte count returned promptly to normal on discontinuance of the drug. Rare cases of granulocytopenia have been reported. In each instance, upon stopping the drug, the white cell count returned to normal. Reversible thrombocytopenia has occurred rarely.

When methyldopa is used with other antihypertensive drugs, potentiation of antihypertensive effect may occur. Patients should be followed carefully to detect side reactions or unusual manifestations of drug idiosyncrasy.

Pregnancy and Nursing

Use of any drug in women who are or may become pregnant or intend to nurse requires that anticipated benefits be weighed against possible risks.

Methyldopa crosses the placental barrier, appears in cord blood, and appears in breast milk.

No unusual adverse reactions have been reported in association with the use of methyldopa during pregnancy. Though no obvious teratogenic effects have been reported, the possibility of fetal injury cannot be excluded. Also, the possibility of injury to a nursing infant cannot be excluded.

PRECAUTIONS

Methyldopa should be used with caution in patients with a history of previous liver disease or dysfunction (see WARNINGS).

Sulfites have been reported to cause severe allergic reactions in certain susceptible individuals, particularly patients with asthma.

Methyldopa may interfere with measurement of: urinary uric acid by the phosphotungstate method, serum creatinine by the alkaline picrate method, and SGOT by colorimetric methods. Interference with spectrophotometric methods for SGOT analysis has not been reported.

A paradoxical pressor response has been reported with intravenous administration of ALDOMET ester hydrochloride.

Since methyldopa causes fluorescence in urine samples at the same wave lengths as catecholamines, falsely high levels of urinary catecholamines may be reported. This will interfere with the diagnosis of pheochromocytoma. It is important to recognize this phenomenon before a patient with a possible pheochromocytoma is subjected to surgery. Methyldopa does not interfere with measurement of VMA (vanillylmandelic acid), a test for pheochromocytoma, by those methods which convert VMA to vanillin. Methyldopa is not recommended for the treatment of patients with pheochromocytoma. Rarely, when urine is exposed to air after voiding, it may darken because of breakdown of methyldopa or its metabolites.

Rarely involuntary choreoathetotic movements have been observed during therapy with methyldopa in patients with severe bilateral cerebrovascular disease. Should these movements occur, stop therapy.

Patients may require reduced doses of anesthetics when on methyldopa. If hypotension does occur during anesthesia, it usually can be controlled by vasopressors. The adrenergic receptors remain sensitive during treatment with methyldopa.

Hypertension has recurred occasionally after dialysis in patients given methyldopa because the drug is removed by this procedure.

ADVERSE REACTIONS

Sedation, usually transient, may occur during the initial period of therapy or whenever the dose is increased. Headache, asthenia, or weakness may be noted as early and transient symptoms. However, significant adverse effects due to methyldopa have been infrequent and this agent usually is well tolerated.

Nervous System/Psychiatric: Sedation, headache, asthenia or weakness, dizziness, lightheadedness, symptoms of cerebrovascular insufficiency, paresthesias, parkinsonism, Bell's palsy, decreased mental acuity, involuntary choreoathetotic movements. Psychic disturbances including nightmares and reversible mild psychoses or depression.

Cardiovascular: Bradycardia, prolonged carotid sinus hypersensitivity, aggravation of angina pectoris. Paradoxical pressor response with intravenous use. Orthostatic hypotension (decrease daily dosage). Edema (and weight gain) usually relieved by use of a diuretic. (Discontinue methyldopa if edema progresses or signs of heart failure appear.)

Digestive: Nausea, vomiting, distention, constipation, flatus, diarrhea, colitis, mild dryness of mouth, sore or "black" tongue, pancreatitis, sialadenitis.

Hepatic: Abnormal liver function tests, jaundice, liver disorders.

Hematologic: Positive Coombs test, hemolytic anemia. Bone marrow depression, leukopenia, granulocytopenia, thrombocytopenia. Positive tests for antinuclear antibody, LE cells, and rheumatoid factor.

Allergic: Drug-related fever, lupus-like syndrome, myocarditis, pericarditis.

Skin: Rash as in eczema or lichenoid eruption; toxic epidermal necrolysis.

Respiratory: Nasal stuffiness.

Metabolic: Rise in BUN.

Urogenital: Breast enlargement, gynecomastia, lactation, amenorrhea, impotence, decreased libido.

Endocrine: Hyperprolactinemia.

Musculoskeletal: Mild arthralgia, with or without joint swelling; myalgia.

DOSAGE AND ADMINISTRATION

Injection ALDOMET ester hydrochloride, when given intravenously in effective doses, causes a decline in blood pressure that may begin in four to six hours and last 10 to 16 hours after injection.

Add the desired dose of injection ALDOMET ester hydrochloride to 100 mL of 5 percent Dextrose Injection U.S.P. Alternatively the desired dose may be given in 5% dextrose in water in a concentration of 100 mg/10 mL. Give this intravenous infusion slowly over a period of 30 to 60 minutes.

ADULTS

The usual adult dosage intravenously is 250 to 500 mg at six hour intervals as required. The maximum recommended intravenous dose is 1.0 g every six hours.

When control has been obtained, oral therapy with tablets ALDOMET (Methyldopa, MSD) may be substituted for intravenous therapy, starting with the same dosage schedule used for the parenteral route. The effectiveness and anticipated responses are described in the circular for tablets ALDOMET (Methyldopa, MSD).

Since methyldopa has a relatively short duration of action, withdrawal is followed by return of hypertension usually within 48 hours. This is not complicated by an overshoot of blood pressure.

Occasionally tolerance may occur, usually between the second and third month of therapy. Adding a diuretic or increasing the dosage of methyldopa frequently will restore effective control of blood pressure. A thiazide may be added at any time during methyldopa therapy and is recommended if therapy has not been started with a thiazide or if effective control of blood pressure cannot be maintained on 2.0 g of methyldopa daily.

Methyldopa is largely excreted by the kidney and patients with impaired renal function may respond to smaller doses. Syncope in older patients may be related to an increased sensitivity and advanced arteriosclerotic vascular disease. This may be avoided by lower doses.

CHILDREN

The recommended daily dosage is 20 to 40 mg/kg of body weight in divided doses every six hours. The maximum dosage is 65 mg/kg or 3.0 g daily, whichever is less. When the blood pressure is under control, continue with oral therapy using tablets ALDOMET (Methyldopa, MSD) in the same dosage as for the parenteral route.

HOW SUPPLIED

No. 3293—Injection ALDOMET ester hydrochloride, 250 mg per 5 mL, is a clear, colorless solution and is supplied as follows:

NDC 0006-3293-05 in 5 mL vials.

A.H.F.S. Category: 24:08

DC 6112027 Issued December 1984

ALDORIL® Tablets (Methyldopa-Hydrochlorothiazide, MSD), U.S.P. ℞

WARNING

This fixed combination drug is not indicated for initial therapy of hypertension. Hypertension requires therapy titrated to the individual patient. If the fixed combination represents the dosage so determined, its use may be more convenient in patient management. The treatment of hypertension is not static, but must be reevaluated as conditions in each patient warrant.

DESCRIPTION

ALDORIL® (Methyldopa-Hydrochlorothiazide, MSD) is a combination of two antihypertensive agents methyldopa and hydrochlorothiazide. The chemical name for methyldopa is levo-3-(3,4-dihydroxyphenyl)-2-methylalanine. Hydrochlorothiazide is 6-chloro-3,4-dihydro- 2*H* -1,2,4-benzothiadiazine-7- sulfonamide 1,1-dioxide.

ALDORIL is supplied as tablets in four strengths for oral use:

ALDORIL 15, contains 250 mg of methyldopa and 15 mg of hydrochlorothiazide.

ALDORIL 25, contains 250 mg of methyldopa and 25 mg of hydrochlorothiazide.

ALDORIL D30, contains 500 mg of methyldopa and 30 mg of hydrochlorothiazide.

ALDORIL D50, contains 500 mg of methyldopa and 50 mg of hydrochlorothiazide.

Each tablet contains the following inactive ingredients: calcium disodium edetate, calcium phosphate, cellulose, citric acid, colloidal silicon dioxide, ethylcellulose, guar gum, hydroxypropyl methylcellulose, magnesium stearate, propylene glycol, talc, and titanium dioxide. ALDORIL 15 and ALDORIL D30 also contain iron oxide and FD&C Red 3.

ACTIONS

ALDOMET® (Methyldopa, MSD)

Methyldopa, a unique antihypertensive, is an aromatic-amino-acid decarboxylase inhibitor in animals and in man. Although the mechanism of action has yet to be conclusively demonstrated, the antihypertensive effect of methyldopa probably is due to its metabolism to alpha-methylnorepinephrine, which then lowers arterial pressure by stimulation of central inhibitory alpha-adrenergic receptors, false neurotransmission, and/or reduction of plasma renin activity. Methyldopa has been shown to cause a net reduction in the tissue concentration of serotonin, dopamine, norepinephrine, and epinephrine.

Only methyldopa, the *L*-isomer of alpha-methyldopa, has the ability to inhibit dopa decarboxylase and to deplete animal tissues of norepinephrine. In man, the antihypertensive activity appears to be due solely to the *L*-isomer. About twice the dose of the racemate (*DL*-alpha-methyldopa) is required for equal antihypertensive effect.

Methyldopa has no direct effect on cardiac function and usually does not reduce glomerular filtration rate, renal blood flow, or filtration fraction. Cardiac output usually is maintained without cardiac acceleration. In some patients the heart rate is slowed.

Normal or elevated plasma renin activity may decrease in the course of methyldopa therapy.

Methyldopa reduces both supine and standing blood pressure. It usually produces highly effective lowering of the supine pressure with infrequent symptomatic postural hypotension. Exercise hypotension and diurnal blood pressure variations rarely occur.

HydroDIURIL®
(Hydrochlorothiazide, MSD)

Hydrochlorothiazide is a diuretic and antihypertensive. It affects the renal tubular mechanism of electrolyte reabsorption. At maximal therapeutic dosage all thiazides are approximately equal in their diuretic efficacy.

Hydrochlorothiazide increases excretion of sodium and chloride in approximately equivalent amounts. Natriuresis may be accompanied by some loss of potassium and bicarbonate. The mechanism of the antihypertensive effect of thiazides is unknown. Hydrochlorothiazide does not affect normal blood pressure.

Hydrochlorothiazide is eliminated rapidly by the kidney.

ALDORIL (Methyldopa-Hydrochlorothiazide, MSD)

The concomitant use of methyldopa and hydrochlorothiazide, as provided in ALDORIL, frequently produces a more pronounced antihypertensive response than when either compound is the sole therapeutic agent. Particularly in those cases of hypertensive vascular disease where sodium and water retention is a problem, the coadministration of these two drugs in the form of ALDORIL will help control the fluid imbalance.

In severe essential hypertension and in malignant hypertension ALDORIL may achieve effective lowering of blood pressure with fewer side effects than occur with other compounds used for this purpose.

ALDORIL reduces both supine and standing blood pressure; more effective lowering of the supine pressure with less frequent symptomatic postural hypotension can be obtained with ALDORIL than with most other antihypertensive agents. In patients treated with ALDORIL, exercise hypotension and diurnal blood pressure variations rarely occur.

INDICATION

Hypertension (see box warning).

CONTRAINDICATIONS

Active hepatic disease, such as acute hepatitis and active cirrhosis.

Continued on next page

Information on the Merck Sharp & Dohme products listed on these pages is the full prescribing information from product circulars in use August 31, 1986.

Merck Sharp & Dohme—Cont.

If previous methyldopa therapy has been associated with liver disorders (see WARNINGS).
Anuria.
Hypersensitivity to methyldopa, or to hydrochlorothiazide or other sulfonamide-derived drugs.

WARNINGS

Methyldopa
It is important to recognize that a positive Coombs test, hemolytic anemia, and liver disorders may occur with methyldopa therapy. The rare occurrences of hemolytic anemia or liver disorders could lead to potentially fatal complications unless properly recognized and managed. Read this section carefully to understand these reactions.
With prolonged methyldopa therapy, 10 to 20 percent of patients develop a positive direct Coombs test which usually occurs between 6 and 12 months of methyldopa therapy. Lowest incidence is at daily dosage of 1 g or less. This on rare occasions may be associated with hemolytic anemia, which could lead to potentially fatal complications. One cannot predict which patients with a positive direct Coombs test may develop hemolytic anemia.
Prior existence or development of a positive direct Coombs test is not in itself a contraindication to use of methyldopa. If a positive Coombs test develops during methyldopa therapy, the physician should determine whether hemolytic anemia exists and whether the positive Coombs test may be a problem. For example, in addition to a positive direct Coombs test there is less often a positive indirect Coombs test which may interfere with cross matching of blood.
At the start of methyldopa therapy, it is desirable to do a blood count (hematocrit, hemoglobin, or red cell count) for a baseline or to establish whether there is anemia. Periodic blood counts should be done during therapy to detect hemolytic anemia. It may be useful to do a direct Coombs test before therapy and at 6 and 12 months after the start of therapy.
If Coombs-positive hemolytic anemia occurs, the cause may be methyldopa and the drug should be discontinued. Usually the anemia remits promptly. If not, corticosteroids may be given and other causes of anemia should be considered. If the hemolytic anemia is related to methyldopa, the drug should not be reinstituted.
When methyldopa causes Coombs positivity alone or with hemolytic anemia, the red cell is usually coated with gamma globulin of the IgG (gamma G) class only. The positive Coombs test may not revert to normal until weeks to months after methyldopa is stopped.
Should the need for transfusion arise in a patient receiving methyldopa, both a direct and an indirect Coombs test should be performed on his blood. In the absence of hemolytic anemia, usually only the direct Coombs test will be positive. A positive direct Coombs test alone will not interfere with typing or cross matching. If the indirect Coombs test is also positive, problems may arise in the major cross match and the assistance of a hematologist or transfusion expert will be needed.
Occasionally, fever has occurred within the first three weeks of methyldopa therapy, associated in some cases with eosinophilia or abnormalities in one or more liver function tests, such as serum alkaline phosphatase, serum transaminases (SGOT, SGPT), bilirubin, cephalin cholesterol flocculation, prothrombin time, and bromsulphalein retention. Jaundice, with or without fever, may occur with onset usually within the first two to three months of therapy. In some patients the findings are consistent with those of cholestasis.
Rarely fatal hepatic necrosis has been reported after use of methyldopa. These hepatic changes may represent hypersensitivity reactions. Periodic determination of hepatic function should be done particularly during the first 6 to 12 weeks of therapy or whenever an unexplained fever occurs. If fever, abnormalities in liver function tests, or jaundice appear, stop therapy with methyldopa. If caused by methyldopa, the temperature and abnormalities in liver function characteristically have reverted to normal when the drug was discontinued. Methyldopa should not be reinstituted in such patients.
Rarely, a reversible reduction of the white blood cell count with a primary effect on the granulocytes has been seen. The granulocyte count returned promptly to normal on discontinuance of the drug. Rare cases of granulocytopenia have been reported. In each instance, upon stopping the drug, the white cell count returned to normal. Reversible thrombocytopenia has occurred rarely.
When methyldopa is used with other antihypertensive drugs, potentiation of antihypertensive effect may occur. Patients should be followed carefully to detect side reactions or unusual manifestations of drug idiosyncrasy.
Hydrochlorothiazide
Use with caution in severe renal disease. In patients with renal disease, thiazides may precipitate azotemia. Cumulative effects of the drug may develop in patients with impaired renal function.
Thiazides should be used with caution in patients with impaired hepatic function or progressive liver disease, since minor alterations of fluid and electrolyte balance may precipitate hepatic coma.
Thiazides may add to or potentiate the action of other antihypertensive drugs.
Sensitivity reactions may occur in patients with or without a history of allergy or bronchial asthma.
The possibility of exacerbation or activation of systemic lupus erythematosus has been reported.
Lithium generally should not be given with diuretics because they reduce its renal clearance and add a high risk of lithium toxicity. Read circulars for lithium preparations before use of such concomitant therapy.

PREGNANCY AND NURSING

Use of any drug in women who are or may become pregnant requires that anticipated benefits be weighed against possible risks.
Methyldopa crosses the placental barrier and appears in cord blood. No unusual adverse reactions have been reported in association with the use of methyldopa during pregnancy. Though no obvious teratogenic effects have been reported, the possibility of fetal injury cannot be excluded.
Thiazides also cross the placental barrier and appear in cord blood. Hazards include fetal or neonatal jaundice, thrombocytopenia, and possibly other adverse reactions which have occurred in the adult.
Methyldopa and thiazides appear in breast milk. Patients taking ALDORIL should not nurse.

PRECAUTIONS

Methyldopa
Methyldopa should be used with caution in patients with a history of previous liver disease or dysfunction (see WARNINGS).
Methyldopa may interfere with measurement of: urinary uric acid by the phosphotungstate method, serum creatinine by the alkaline picrate method, and SGOT by colorimetric methods. Interference with spectrophotometric methods for SGOT analysis has not been reported.
Since methyldopa causes fluorescence in urine samples at the same wave lengths as catecholamines, falsely high levels of urinary catecholamines may be reported. This will interfere with the diagnosis of pheochromocytoma. It is important to recognize this phenomenon before a patient with a possible pheochromocytoma is subjected to surgery. Methyldopa does not interfere with measurement of VMA (vanillylmandelic acid), a test for pheochromocytoma, by those methods which convert VMA to vanillin. Methyldopa is not recommended for the treatment of patients with pheochromocytoma. Rarely, when urine is exposed to air after voiding, it may darken because of breakdown of methyldopa or its metabolites.
Rarely, involuntary choreoathetotic movements have been observed during therapy with methyldopa in patients with severe bilateral cerebrovascular disease. Should these movements occur, stop therapy.
Patients may require reduced doses of anesthetics when on methyldopa. If hypotension does occur during anesthesia, it usually can be controlled by vasopressors. The adrenergic receptors remain sensitive during treatment with methyldopa.
Hypertension has recurred occasionally after dialysis in patients given methyldopa because the drug is removed by this procedure.
Hydrochlorothiazide
Periodic determination of serum electrolytes to detect possible electrolyte imbalance should be performed at appropriate intervals.
All patients receiving diuretic therapy should be observed for evidence of fluid or electrolyte imbalance: namely, hyponatremia, hypochloremic alkalosis, and hypokalemia. Serum and urine electrolyte determinations are particularly important when the patient is vomiting excessively or receiving parenteral fluids. Warning signs or symptoms of fluid and electrolyte imbalance include dryness of mouth, thirst, weakness, lethargy, drowsiness, restlessness, muscle pains or cramps, muscular fatigue, hypotension, oliguria, tachycardia, and gastrointestinal disturbances such as nausea and vomiting.
Hypokalemia may develop, especially with brisk diuresis, when severe cirrhosis is present, during concomitant use of corticosteroids or ACTH, or after prolonged therapy.
Interference with adequate oral electrolyte intake will also contribute to hypokalemia. Hypokalemia can sensitize or exaggerate the response of the heart to the toxic effects of digitalis (e.g., increased ventricular irritability). Hypokalemia may be avoided or treated by use of potassium supplements such as foods with a high potassium content.
Although any chloride deficit is generally mild and usually does not require specific treatment except under extraordinary circumstances (as in liver disease or renal disease), chloride replacement may be required in the treatment of metabolic alkalosis.
Dilutional hyponatremia may occur in edematous patients in hot weather; appropriate therapy is water restriction, rather than administration of salt, except in rare instances when the hyponatremia is life threatening. In actual salt depletion, appropriate replacement is the therapy of choice.
Hyperuricemia may occur or acute gout may be precipitated in certain patients receiving thiazides.
Insulin requirements in diabetic patients may be increased, decreased, or unchanged. Latent diabetes mellitus may become manifest during thiazide therapy.
Thiazides may increase the responsiveness to tubocurarine.
In some patients, the administration of a non-steroidal anti-inflammatory agent can reduce the diuretic, natriuretic, and antihypertensive effects of loop, potassium-sparing and thiazide diuretics. Therefore, when ALDORIL and non-steroidal anti-inflammatory agents are used concomitantly, the patient should be observed closely to determine if the desired effect of the diuretic is obtained.
The antihypertensive effects of the drug may be enhanced in the postsympathectomy patient. Thiazides may decrease arterial responsiveness to norepinephrine. This diminution is not sufficient to preclude effectiveness of the pressor agent for therapeutic use.
If progressive renal impairment becomes evident, consider withholding or discontinuing diuretic therapy.
Thiazides may decrease serum PBI levels without signs of thyroid disturbance.
Thiazides have been shown to increase the urinary excretion of magnesium; this may result in hypomagnesemia.
Thiazides may decrease urinary calcium excretion. Thiazides may cause intermittent and slight elevation of serum calcium in the absence of known disorders of calcium metabolism. Marked hypercalcemia may be evidence of hidden hyperparathyroidism. Thiazides should be discontinued before carrying out tests for parathyroid function.

ADVERSE REACTIONS

Methyldopa
Sedation, usually transient, may occur during the initial period of therapy or whenever the dose is increased. Headache, asthenia, or weakness may be noted as early and transient symptoms. However, significant adverse effects due to methyldopa have been infrequent and this agent usually is well tolerated.
Nervous System/Psychiatric: Sedation, headache, asthenia or weakness, dizziness, lightheadedness, symptoms of cerebrovascular insufficiency, paresthesias, parkinsonism, Bell's palsy, decreased mental acuity, involuntary choreoathetotic movements. Psychic disturbances including nightmares and reversible mild psychoses or depression.
Cardiovascular: Bradycardia, prolonged carotid sinus hypersensitivity, aggravation of angina pectoris. Orthostatic hypotension (decrease daily dosage). Edema (and weight gain) usually relieved by use of a diuretic. (Discontinue methyldopa if edema progresses or signs of heart failure appear.)
Digestive: Nausea, vomiting, distention, constipation, flatus, diarrhea, colitis, mild dryness of mouth, sore or "black" tongue, pancreatitis, sialadenitis.
Hepatic: Abnormal liver function tests, jaundice, liver disorders.
Hematologic: Positive Coombs test, hemolytic anemia. Bone marrow depression, leukopenia, granulocytopenia, thrombocytopenia. Positive tests for antinuclear antibody, LE cells, and rheumatoid factor.
Allergic: Drug-related fever, lupus-like syndrome, myocarditis, pericarditis.
Skin: Rash as in eczema or lichenoid eruption; toxic epidermal necrolysis.
Respiratory: Nasal stuffiness.
Metabolic: Rise in BUN.
Urogenital: Breast enlargement, gynecomastia, lactation, amenorrhea, impotence, decreased libido.
Endocrine: Hyperprolactinemia.
Musculoskeletal: Mild arthralgia, with or without joint swelling; myalgia.
Hydrochlorothiazide
Body as a Whole: Weakness.
Cardiovascular: Orthostatic hypotension (may be aggravated by alcohol, barbiturates, or narcotics).
Digestive: Anorexia, gastric irritation, nausea, vomiting, cramping, diarrhea, constipation, jaundice (intrahepatic cholestatic jaundice), pancreatitis, sialadenitis.
Hematologic: Leukopenia, agranulocytosis, thrombocytopenia, aplastic anemia, hemolytic anemia.
Metabolic: Hyperglycemia, glycosuria, hyperuricemia, electrolyte imbalance (see PRECAUTIONS).

Musculoskeletal: Muscle spasm.
Nervous System/Psychiatric: Dizziness, vertigo, paresthesias, headache, restlessness.
Special Senses: Transient blurred vision, xanthopsia.
Hypersensitivity: Purpura, photosensitivity, rash, urticaria, necrotizing angiitis (vasculitis and cutaneous vasculitis), fever, respiratory distress including pneumonitis and pulmonary edema, anaphylactic reactions.
Whenever adverse reactions are moderate or severe, thiazide dosage should be reduced or therapy withdrawn.

DOSAGE AND ADMINISTRATION

Dosage: As determined by individual titration (see box warning).
The usual dosage is 1 tablet of ALDORIL 15, ALDORIL 25, ALDORIL D30, or ALDORIL D50 two or three times a day in the first 48 hours. The daily dosage then may be increased or decreased, preferably at intervals of not less than two days, until an adequate response is achieved. To minimize the sedation associated with methyldopa, start dosage increases in the evening. By adjustment of dosage, morning hypotension may be prevented without sacrificing control of afternoon blood pressure.
When ALDORIL is given to patients on other antihypertensives, the dose of these agents may need to be adjusted to effect a smooth transition. When ALDORIL is given with antihypertensives other than thiazides, the initial dosage of methyldopa should be limited to 500 mg daily in divided doses.
Although occasional patients have responded to higher doses, the maximum recommended daily dosage is 3.0 g of methyldopa and 100 to 200 mg of hydrochlorothiazide. Once an effective dosage range is attained, a smooth blood pressure response occurs in most patients in 12 to 24 hours. If ALDORIL alone does not adequately control blood pressure, additional methyldopa may be given separately to obtain the maximum blood pressure response.
Since both components of ALDORIL have a relatively short duration of action, withdrawal is followed by return of hypertension usually within 48 hours. This is not complicated by an overshoot of blood pressure.
Occasionally tolerance may occur, usually between the second and third month of therapy. Increasing the dosage of either methyldopa or hydrochlorothiazide separately or together frequently will restore effective control of blood pressure.
Methyldopa is largely excreted by the kidney and patients with impaired renal function may respond to smaller doses of ALDORIL. Syncope in older patients may be related to an increased sensitivity and advanced arteriosclerotic vascular disease. This may be avoided by lower doses.

HOW SUPPLIED

No. 3294—Tablets ALDORIL 15 are salmon, round, film coated tablets, coded MSD 423. Each tablet contains 250 mg of methyldopa and 15 mg of hydrochlorothiazide. They are supplied as follows:
NDC 0006-0423-68 bottles of 100
NDC 0006-0423-28 unit dose packages of 100
NDC 0006-0423-82 bottles of 1000.
Shown in Product Identification Section, page 417
No. 3295—Tablets ALDORIL 25 are white, round, film coated tablets, coded MSD 456. Each tablet contains 250 mg of methyldopa and 25 mg of hydrochlorothiazide. They are supplied as follows:
NDC 0006-0456-68 bottles of 100
NDC 0006-0456-28 unit dose packages of 100
NDC 0006-0456-82 bottles of 1000.
Shown in Product Identification Section, page 417
No. 3362—Tablets ALDORIL D30 are salmon, oval, film coated tablets, coded MSD 694. Each tablet contains 500 mg of methyldopa and 30 mg of hydrochlorothiazide. They are supplied as follows:
NDC 0006-0694-68 bottles of 100.
Shown in Product Identification Section, page 417
No. 3363—Tablets ALDORIL D50 are white, oval, film coated tablets, coded MSD 935. Each tablet contains 500 mg of methyldopa and 50 mg of hydrochlorothiazide. They are supplied as follows:
NDC 0006-0935-68 bottles of 100.
Shown in Product Identification Section, page 417
A.H.F.S. Category: 24:08
DC 6086034 Issued October 1985

alphaREDISOL® Injection ℞
(Hydroxocobalamin, MSD) Crystalline, U.S.P.

DESCRIPTION

Hydroxocobalamin Injection is a sterile solution of hydroxocobalamin.
Hydroxocobalamin appears as dark red orthorhombic needles or as an amorphous or crystalline red powder. It is very hygroscopic in the anhydrous form, and moderately soluble in water. It has a molecular weight of 1346.37. The vitamin B_{12} coenzymes are very unstable in light. Hydroxocobalamin shares the cobalamin molecular structure with cyanocobalamin.
The chemical name is Cobinamide hydroxide phosphate 3′-ester with 5,6-dimethyl-1-α-D-ribofuranosylbenzimidazole inner salt. The empirical formula is $C_{62}H_{89}CoN_{13}O_{15}P$. The cobalt content is 4.38%. The structural formula is:

Each ml of alphaREDISOL® (Hydroxocobalamin, MSD) contains:

Crystalline hydroxocobalamin	1,000 mcg
Inactive ingredients:	
Sodium chloride	0.82%
Anhydrous sodium acetate	0.02%
Acetic acid	to adjust pH
Water for Injection q.s.	1 ml
Added as preservatives:	
Methylparaben	0.15%
Propylparaben	0.02%

The pH is 3.5–5.0.

CLINICAL PHARMACOLOGY

Vitamin B_{12} is essential to growth, cell reproduction, hematopoiesis, nucleoprotein and myelin synthesis.
Fifty percent of the administered dose of hydroxocobalamin disappears from the injection site in 2.5 hours. Hydroxocobalamin is bound to plasma proteins and stored in the liver. It is excreted in the bile and undergoes some enterohepatic recycling. Within 72 hours after injection of 500 to 1000 mcg of hydroxocobalamin 16 to 66 percent of the injected dose may appear in the urine. The major portion is excreted within the first 24 hours.

INDICATIONS AND USAGE

I. Pernicious anemia, both uncomplicated and accompanied by nervous system involvement.
II. Dietary deficiency of vitamin B_{12}, occurring in strict vegetarians and in their breast-fed infants. (Isolated vitamin B_{12} deficiency is very rare.)
III. Malabsorption of vitamin B_{12}, resulting from structural or functional damage to the stomach, where intrinsic factor is secreted or to the ileum, where intrinsic factor facilitates vitamin B_{12} absorption. These conditions include tropical sprue, and nontropical sprue (idiopathic steatorrhea, gluten-induced enteropathy). Folate deficiency in these patients is usually more severe than vitamin B_{12} deficiency.
IV. Inadequate secretion of intrinsic factor, resulting from lesions that destroy the gastric mucosa (ingestion of corrosives, extensive neoplasia), and a number of conditions associated with a variable degree of gastric atrophy (such as multiple sclerosis, certain endocrine disorders, iron deficiency, and subtotal gastrectomy). Total gastrectomy always produces vitamin B_{12} deficiency.
Structural lesions leading to vitamin B_{12} deficiency include regional ileitis, ileal resections, malignancies, etc.
V. Competition for vitamin B_{12} by intestinal parasites or bacteria.
The fish tapeworm (Diphyllobothrium latum) absorbs huge quantities of vitamin B_{12} and infested patients often have associated gastric atrophy. The blind-loop syndrome may produce deficiency of vitamin B_{12} or folate.
VI. Inadequate utilization of vitamin B_{12}. This may occur if antimetabolites for the vitamin are employed in the treatment of neoplasia.
VII. For the Schilling Test.

CONTRAINDICATIONS

Hypersensitivity to any component of this medication.

WARNINGS

Avoid the intravenous route.
Folic acid is not a substitute for vitamin B_{12} although it may improve vitamin B_{12} deficient megaloblastic anemia. Exclusive use of folic acid in treating vitamin B_{12} deficient megaloblastic anemia could result in progressive and irreversible neurologic damage.
Blunted or impeded therapeutic response to vitamin B_{12} may be due to such conditions as infection, uremia, drugs having bone marrow suppressant properties such as chloramphenicol, and concurrent iron or folic acid deficiency.

PRECAUTIONS

General
The validity of diagnostic vitamin B_{12} or folic acid blood assays could be compromised by medications, and this should be considered before relying on such tests for therapy.
Vitamin B_{12} is not a substitute for folic acid and since it might improve folic acid deficient megaloblastic anemia, indiscriminate use of vitamin B_{12} could mask the true diagnosis.
Hypokalemia and thrombocytosis could occur upon conversion of severe megaloblastic to normal erythropoiesis with B_{12} therapy. Therefore, serum potassium levels and the platelet count should be monitored carefully during therapy.
Vitamin B_{12} deficiency may suppress the signs of polycythemia vera. Treatment with vitamin B_{12} may unmask this condition.
Carcinogenesis, Mutagenesis, Impairment of Fertility
Studies of carcinogenicity, mutagenesis, or impairment of fertility have not been performed with alphaREDISOL.
Pregnancy
Pregnancy Category C: Animal reproduction studies have not been conducted with alphaREDISOL. It is also not known whether alphaREDISOL can cause fetal harm when administered to a pregnant woman or can affect reproduction capacity. AlphaREDISOL should be given to a pregnant woman only if clearly needed.

ADVERSE REACTIONS

Mild transient diarrhea, itching, transitory exanthema, feeling of swelling of entire body, and anaphylaxis.
A few patients may experience pain after injection of alphaREDISOL.

OVERDOSAGE

The intravenous LD_{50} of alphaREDISOL in mice is greater than 50 ml/kg.

DOSAGE AND ADMINISTRATION

Protect from light.
Parenteral drug products should be inspected visually for particulate matter and discoloration prior to administration, whenever solution and container permit.
AlphaREDISOL injection should be given only intramuscularly.
In patients with Addisonian Pernicious Anemia, parenteral therapy with vitamin B_{12} is the recommended method of treatment and will be required for the remainder of the patient's life. Oral therapy is not dependable. In other patients with vitamin B_{12} deficiency, the duration of therapy and route of administration will depend upon the cause and whether or not it is reversible.
Confirmatory diagnostic studies should be performed prior to initiating therapy, if possible, and the patient should be followed with appropriate studies to demonstrate hematologic improvement (Hgb, hematocrit, RBC, reticulocyte count). A diagnostic trial utilizing physiologic doses of vitamin B_{12} (1 mcg daily) and observing daily reticulocyte counts after establishing a baseline may also be performed. The observation of reticulocytosis which usually occurs between the third and tenth day of therapy confirms the diagnosis of vitamin B_{12} deficiency.
In seriously ill patients it may be advisable to administer both vitamin B_{12} and folic acid while awaiting the results of distinguishing laboratory studies. It is not necessary to withold vitamin B_{12} therapy until the precise cause of B_{12}

Continued on next page

Information on the Merck Sharp & Dohme products listed on these pages is the full prescribing information from product circulars in use August 31, 1986.

Merck Sharp & Dohme—Cont.

deficiency is established since absorption studies can be performed at any time.
Serum potassium should be closely observed the first 48 hours and potassium should be administered if necessary.
Treatment of Vitamin B_{12} Deficiency:
Thirty mcg daily for 5 to 10 days followed by 100 to 200 mcg monthly injected intramuscularly. If the patient is critically ill, or has neurologic disease, an infectious disease or hyperthyroidism, considerably higher doses may be indicated. However, current data indicate that the optimum obtainable neurologic response may be expected with a dosage of vitamin B_{12} sufficient to produce good hematologic response. Children may be given a total of 1 to 5 mg over a period of 2 or more weeks in doses of 100 mcg, then 30 to 50 mcg every 4 weeks for maintenance.
Patients who have normal intestinal absorption may be treated with an oral therapeutic multivitamin preparation, containing 15 mcg vitamin B_{12} daily.
Schilling Test:
The flushing dose is 1000 mcg.

HOW SUPPLIED

No. 3285X—Injection alphaREDISOL, 1000 mcg per ml, is a clear solution having a deep red color, and is supplied as follows:
NDC 0006-3285-10 in 10 ml vials.
A.H.F.S. Category: 88:08
DC 6234507 Issued January 1982

AMINOHIPPURATE SODIUM, MSD "PAH" ℞
Injection, U.S.P.

DESCRIPTION

Aminohippurate sodium, MSD is the para-amino analog of hippuric acid, commonly abbreviated "PAH". It is water soluble, lipid-insoluble, and has a pKa of 3.83.
It is provided as a sterile 20 percent aqueous solution. Each 10 ml contains: Aminohippurate sodium 2 g. Inactive ingredients: Sodium hydroxide to adjust pH, water for injection, q.s.

ACTIONS

PAH is used as a diagnostic agent to measure effective renal plasma flow (ERPF). In addition to being filtered by the glomeruli it is actively secreted by the proximal tubules. At low plasma concentrations (1.0 to 2.0 mg/100 ml), an average of 90 percent of this compound is cleared by the kidneys from the renal blood stream in a single circulation. It is ideally suited for measurement of ERPF since it has a high clearance, is essentially nontoxic at the plasma concentrations reached with recommended doses, and its analytical determination is relatively simple and accurate.
PAH is also used in research procedures for measurement of the functional capacity of the renal tubular secretory mechanism or transport maximum (Tm_{PAH}). This is accomplished by elevating the plasma concentration to saturation levels (40 to 60 mg/100 ml) where the maximal capacity of the tubular cells to secrete PAH is reached. Inulin clearance is generally measured during Tm_{PAH} determinations since glomerular filtration rate (GFR) must be known before calculations involving secretory Tm measurements can be made (See CALCULATIONS).

INDICATIONS

For the estimation of effective renal plasma flow.
For the measurement of the functional capacity of the renal tubular secretory mechanism.

PRECAUTIONS

Intravenous solutions must be administered with caution in patients with low cardiac reserve, since a rapid increase in plasma volume can precipitate congestive heart failure.
For measurement of effective renal plasma flow small doses of PAH are used. However, in research procedures for Tm_{PAH} determinations high plasma levels are required to saturate the capacity of the tubular cells. During these procedures the intravenous administration of PAH solutions should be carried out slowly and with caution. The patient should be continuously observed for any adverse reactions.
Renal clearance measurements of PAH cannot be made with any significant accuracy in patients receiving sulfonamides, procaine, or thiazolesulfone. These compounds interfere with chemical color development essential to the analytical procedures.
Probenecid depresses tubular secretion of certain weak acids such as PAH. Therefore, patients receiving probenecid will have erroneously low ERPF and Tm_{PAH} values.

ADVERSE REACTIONS

The following adverse reactions may occur:
Vasomotor disturbances, flushing, tingling, nausea, vomiting, and cramps.
Patients may have a sensation of warmth or the desire to defecate or urinate during or shortly following the administration of a primary dose.

DOSAGE AND ADMINISTRATION

For intravenous use only
Clearance measurements using single injection technics are generally inaccurate, particularly in the measurement of effective renal plasma flow. For this reason, intravenous infusions at fixed rates are used to sustain the plasma PAH concentration at the desired level.
For the measurement of effective renal plasma flow the concentration of PAH in the plasma is maintained at 2 mg per 100 ml.
As a research procedure for the measurement of Tm_{PAH}, the plasma level of PAH must be sufficient to saturate the capacity of the tubular secretory cells. Concentrations of from 40 to 60 mg per 100 ml are usually necessary.
Technical details of these tests may be found in Smith[1]; Wesson[2]; Bauer[3]; and Pitts[4].

CALCULATIONS

Effective Renal Plasma Flow (ERPF)
The clearance of PAH, which is extracted almost completely from the plasma during its passage through the renal circulation, constitutes a measure of ERPF. Hence:

$$ERPF = \frac{U_{PAH}V}{P_{PAH}}$$

Where U_{PAH} = concentration of PAH (mg/ml) in the urine
V = rate of urine excretion (ml/min), and
P_{PAH} = plasma concentration of PAH (mg/ml).

Example: U_{PAH} = 8.0 mg/ml
V = 1.5 ml/min
P_{PAH} = 0.02 mg/ml

$$ERPF = \frac{8.0 \times 1.5}{0.02} = 600 \text{ ml/min}$$

Based on PAH clearance studies, the ERPF for normal men is 675 ± 150 ml/min and for normal women 595 ± 125 ml/min.
Maximum Tubular Secretory Mechanism (Tm_{PAH})
The quantity of PAH secreted by the tubules (Tm_{PAH}) is given by the difference between the total rate of excretion ($U_{PAH}V$) and the quantity filtered by the glomeruli (GFR × P_{PAH}). Hence:

$$Tm_{PAH} = U_{PAH}V - (GFR \times P_{PAH} \times 0.83)$$

0.83 is a correction factor that takes into account that portion of PAH which is bound to plasma protein and hence is unfilterable.

Example: U_{PAH} = 9.55 mg/ml
V = 16.68 ml/min
GFR = 120 ml/min
P_{PAH} = 0.60 mg/ml

Then $Tm_{PAH} = 9.55 \times 16.68 - (120 \times 0.60 \times 0.83) =$ 100 mg/min.
Average normal values of Tm_{PAH} are 80–90 mg/min.
Notes
The value of the expression $U_{PAH}V$, used in calculations of ERPF and Tm_{PAH}, may be found by determining the amount of PAH in a measured volume of urine excreted within a specific period of time.
The above calculations are based on a body surface area of 1.73 m^2. Corrections for variations in surface area are made by multiplying the values obtained for ERPF and Tm_{PAH} by 1.73/A, where A represents the body surface area of the patient.

HOW SUPPLIED

No. 95—Aminohippurate Sodium, 20 percent sterile solution for intravenous injection, is supplied as follows:
NDC 0006-3395-10 in 10 ml ampuls.

REFERENCES

1. Smith, H. W.: Lectures on the kidney, University Extension Division, University of Kansas, Lawrence, Kansas, 1943.
2. Wesson, L. G., Jr.: "Physiology of the Human Kidney," New York, Grune & Stratton, 1969, pp. 632–655.
3. Bauer, J. D.; Ackermann, P. G.; Toro, G.: "Brays Clinical Laboratory Methods," ed. 7, St. Louis, Mosby, 1968.
4. Pitts, R. F.: "Physiology of the Kidney and Body Fluids," ed. 2, Chicago, Year Book Medical Publishers, 1968.

A.H.F.S. Category: 36:40
DC 6505415 Issued September 1976

ANTIVENIN ℞
(Latrodectus mactans), MSD, U.S.P.
Black Widow Spider Antivenin
Equine Origin

DESCRIPTION

Antivenin (Latrodectus mactans), MSD is a sterile, non-pyrogenic preparation derived by drying a frozen solution of specific venom-neutralizing globulins obtained from the blood serum of healthy horses immunized against venom of black widow spiders (Latrodectus mactans). It is standardized by biological assay on mice, in terms of one dose of antivenin neutralizing the venom in not less than 6000 mouse LD_{50} of Latrodectus mactans. Thimerosal (mercury derivative) 1:10,000 is added as a preservative. When constituted as specified, it is opalescent and contains not more than 20.0 percent of solids.
Each vial contains not less than 6000 Antivenin units. One unit of Antivenin will neutralize one average mouse lethal dose of black widow spider venom when the Antivenin and the venom are injected simultaneously in mice under suitable conditions.

CLINICAL PHARMACOLOGY

The pharmacological mode of action is unknown and metabolic and pharmacokinetic data in humans are unavailable.

INDICATIONS AND USAGE

Antivenin (Latrodectus mactans), MSD is used to treat patients with symptoms due to bites by the black widow spider (Latrodectus mactans). Early use of the Antivenin is emphasized for prompt relief.
Local muscular cramps begin from 15 minutes to several hours after the bite which usually produces a sharp pain similar to that caused by puncture with a needle. The exact sequence of symptoms depends somewhat on the location of the bite. The venom acts on the myoneural junctions or on the nerve endings, causing an ascending motor paralysis or destruction of the peripheral nerve endings. The groups of muscles most frequently affected at first are those of the thigh, shoulder, and back. After a varying length of time, the pain becomes more severe, spreading to the abdomen, and weakness and tremor usually develop. The abdominal muscles assume a boardlike rigidity, but tenderness is slight. Respiration is thoracic. The patient is restless and anxious. Feeble pulse, cold, clammy skin, labored breathing and speech, light stupor, and delirium may occur. Convulsions also may occur, particularly in small children. The temperature may be normal or slightly elevated. Urinary retention, shock, cyanosis, nausea and vomiting, insomnia, and cold sweats also have been reported. The syndrome following the bite of the black widow spider may be confused easily with any medical or surgical condition with acute abdominal symptoms.
The symptoms of black widow spider bite increase in severity for several hours, perhaps a day, and then very slowly become less severe, gradually passing off in the course of two or three days except in fatal cases. Residual symptoms such as general weakness, tingling, nervousness, and transient muscle spasm may persist for weeks or months after recovery from the acute stage.
If possible, the patient should be hospitalized. Other additional measures giving greatest relief are prolonged warm baths and intravenous injection of 10 mL of 10 percent solution of calcium gluconate repeated as necessary to control muscle pain. Morphine also may be required to control pain. Barbiturates may be used for extreme restlessness. However, as the venom is a neurotoxin, it can cause respiratory paralysis. This must be borne in mind when considering use of morphine or a barbiturate. Adrenocorticosteroids have been used with varying degrees of success. Supportive therapy is indicated by the condition of the patient. Local treatment of the site of the bite is of no value. Nothing is gained by applying a tourniquet or by attempting to remove venom from the site of the bite by incision and suction.
In otherwise healthy individuals between the ages of 16 and 60, the use of Antivenin may be deferred and treatment with muscle relaxants may be considered.

WARNINGS

Prior to treatment with any product prepared from horse serum, a careful review of the patient's history should be taken emphasizing prior exposure to horse serum or any

allergies. Serious sickness and even death could result from the use of horse serum in a sensitive patient. A skin or conjunctival test should be performed prior to administration of Antivenin.
Skin test: Inject into (not under) the skin not more than 0.02 mL of the test material (1:10 dilution of normal horse serum in physiologic saline). Evaluate result in 10 minutes. A positive reaction is an urticarial wheal surrounded by a zone of erythema. A control test using Sodium Chloride Injection facilitates interpretation of the results.
Conjunctival test: For adults instill into the conjunctival sac one drop of a 1:10 dilution of horse serum and for children one drop of 1:100 dilution. Itching of the eye and reddening of the conjunctiva indicate a positive reaction, usually within 10 minutes.
Patients should be observed for serum sickness for an average of 8 to 12 days following administration of Antivenin.
Desensitization should be attempted only when the administration of Antivenin is considered necessary to save life. Epinephrine must be available in case of untoward reaction.
Desensitization: If the history is positive or the results of the sensitivity tests are mildly or questionably positive, Antivenin should be administered as follows to reduce the risk of an immediate severe allergic reaction:

1. In separate sterile vials or syringes prepare 1:10 or 1:100 dilutions of Antivenin in Sodium Chloride for Injection.
2. Allow at least 15 but preferably 30 minutes between injections and only proceed with the next dose if no reactions occurred following the previous dose.
3. Using a tuberculin syringe, inject subcutaneously 0.1, 0.2 and 0.5 mL of the 1:100 dilution at 15 or 30 minute intervals; repeat with the 1:10 dilution, and finally the undiluted Antivenin.
4. If there is a reaction after any of the injections, place a tourniquet proximal to the sites of injection and administer epinephrine, 1:1000 (0.3 to 1.0 mL subcutaneously, 0.05 to 0.1 mL intravenously), proximal to the tourniquet or into another extremity. Wait at least 30 minutes before giving another injection of Antivenin, the amount of which should be the same as the last one not evoking a reaction.
5. If no reaction has occurred after 0.5 mL of undiluted Antivenin has been given, it is probably safe to continue the dose at 15 minute intervals until the entire dose has been injected.

PRECAUTIONS

Carcinogenesis, Mutagenesis, Impairment of Fertility
No long term studies in animals have been performed to evaluate the potential for carcinogenesis, mutagenesis, or impairment of fertility.
Pregnancy
Pregnancy Category C. Animal reproduction studies have not been conducted with Black Widow Spider Antivenin. It is also not known whether Black Widow Spider Antivenin can cause fetal harm when administered to a pregnant woman or can affect reproduction capacity. Black Widow Spider Antivenin should be given to a pregnant woman only if clearly needed.
Nursing Mothers
It is not known whether this drug is excreted in human milk. Because many drugs are excreted in human milk, caution should be exercised when Black Widow Spider Antivenin is administered to a nursing woman.
Pediatric Use
Controlled clinical studies for safety and effectiveness in children have not been conducted; however, there have been virtually no adverse effects reported in those children who have received the product.

ADVERSE REACTIONS

Anaphylaxis and serum sickness have been reported following use of Antivenin.

DOSAGE AND ADMINISTRATION

Using a sterile syringe, remove from the accompanying vial 2.5 mL of Sterile Diluent for Antivenin and inject into the vial of Antivenin. With the needle still in the rubber stopper, shake the vial to dissolve the contents completely.
Parenteral drug products should be inspected visually for particulate matter and discoloration prior to administration, whenever solution and container permit.
The dose for adults and children is the entire contents of a restored vial (2.5 mL) of Antivenin. It may be given intramuscularly, preferably in the region of the anterolateral thigh so that a tourniquet may be applied in the event of a systemic reaction. Symptoms usually subside in 1 to 3 hours. Although one dose of Antivenin usually is adequate, a second dose may be necessary in some cases.
Antivenin also may be given intravenously in 10 to 50 mL of saline solution over a 15 minute period. It is the preferred route in severe cases, or when the patient is under 12, or in shock. One restored vial usually is enough.

HOW SUPPLIED

No. 4084—Antivenin (Latrodectus mactans), MSD equine origin is a white to grey crystalline powder, each vial containing not less than 6000 Antivenin units. Thimerosal (mercury derivative) 1:10,000 is added as preservative, **NDC** 0006-4084-00. A 2.5 mL vial of Sterile Diluent for Antivenin is included. Also supplied is a 1 mL vial of normal horse serum (1:10 dilution) for sensitivity testing. Thimerosal (mercury derivative) 1:10,000 is added as preservative.

A.H.F.S. Category: 80:04
DC 6145212 Issued March 1985

AquaMEPHYTON® Injection ℞
(Phytonadione, MSD), U.S.P.
Aqueous Colloidal Solution of Vitamin K_1

WARNING—INTRAVENOUS USE

Severe reactions, including fatalities, have occurred during and immediately after INTRAVENOUS injection of AquaMEPHYTON® (Phytonadione, MSD), even when precautions have been taken to dilute the AquaMEPHYTON and to avoid rapid infusion. Typically these severe reactions have resembled hypersensitivity or anaphylaxis, including shock and cardiac and/or respiratory arrest. Some patients have exhibited these severe reactions on receiving AquaMEPHYTON for the first time. Therefore the INTRAVENOUS route should be restricted to those situations where other routes are not feasible and the serious risk involved is considered justified.

DESCRIPTION

AquaMEPHYTON injection is a yellow, sterile, aqueous colloidal solution of vitamin K_1, available for injection by the intravenous, intramuscular, and subcutaneous routes.
Each milliliter contains:

Phytonadione	2 mg or 10 mg
Inactive ingredients:	
Polyoxyethylated fatty acid derivative	70 mg
Dextrose	37.5 mg
Water for Injection, q.s.	1 ml
Added as preservative:	
Benzyl alcohol	0.9%

ACTIONS

AquaMEPHYTON aqueous colloidal solution of vitamin K_1 for parenteral injection, possesses the same type and degree of activity as does naturally-occurring vitamin K, which is necessary for the production via the liver of active prothrombin (factor II), proconvertin (factor VII), plasma thromboplastin component (factor IX), and Stuart factor (factor X). The prothrombin test is sensitive to the levels of three of these four factors—II, VII, and X. The mechanism by which vitamin K promotes formation of these clotting factors in the liver is not known.
The action of the aqueous colloidal solution, when administered intravenously, is generally detectable within an hour or two and hemorrhage is usually controlled within 3 to 6 hours. A normal prothrombin level may often be obtained in 12 to 14 hours.
In the prophylaxis and treatment of hemorrhagic disease of the newborn, phytonadione has demonstrated a greater margin of safety than that of the water-soluble vitamin K analogues.

INDICATIONS

AquaMEPHYTON is indicated in the following coagulation disorders which are due to faulty formation of factors II, VII, IX and X when caused by vitamin K deficiency or interference with vitamin K activity.
AquaMEPHYTON injection is indicated in:
- anticoagulant-induced prothrombin deficiency;
- prophylaxis and therapy of hemorrhagic disease of the newborn;
- hypoprothrombinemia due to antibacterial therapy;
- hypoprothrombinemia secondary to factors limiting absorption or synthesis of vitamin K, e.g., obstructive jaundice, biliary fistula, sprue, ulcerative colitis, celiac disease, intestinal resection, cystic fibrosis of the pancreas, and regional enteritis;
- other drug-induced hypoprothrombinemia where it is definitely shown that the result is due to interference with vitamin K metabolism, e.g., salicylates.

CONTRAINDICATION

Hypersensitivity to any component of this medication.

WARNINGS

Benzyl alcohol as a preservative in Bacteriostatic Sodium Chloride Injection has been associated with toxicity in newborns. Data are unavailable on the toxicity of other preservatives in this age group. There is no evidence to suggest that the small amount of benzyl alcohol contained in AquaMEPHYTON, when used as recommended, is associated with toxicity.
An immediate coagulant effect should not be expected after administration of phytonadione. It takes a minimum of 1 to 2 hours for measurable improvement in the prothrombin time. Whole blood or component therapy may also be necessary if bleeding is severe.
Phytonadione will not counteract the anticoagulant action of heparin.
When vitamin K_1 is used to correct excessive anticoagulant-induced hypoprothrombinemia, anticoagulant therapy still being indicated, the patient is again faced with the clotting hazards existing prior to starting the anticoagulant therapy. Phytonadione is not a clotting agent, but overzealous therapy with vitamin K_1 may restore conditions which originally permitted thromboembolic phenomena. Dosage should be kept as low as possible, and prothrombin time should be checked regularly as clinical conditions indicate.
Repeated large doses of vitamin K are not warranted in liver disease if the response to initial use of the vitamin is unsatisfactory. Failure to respond to vitamin K may indicate that the condition being treated is inherently unresponsive to vitamin K.
Reproduction studies have not been performed in animals. There is no adequate information of whether this drug may affect fertility in human males or females or have a teratogenic potential or other adverse effect on the fetus.

PRECAUTIONS

Protect from light at all times.
Temporary resistance to prothrombin-depressing anticoagulants may result, especially when larger doses of phytonadione are used. If relatively large doses have been employed, it may be necessary when reinstituting anticoagulant therapy to use somewhat larger doses of the prothrombin-depressing anticoagulant, or to use one which acts on a different principle, such as heparin sodium.

ADVERSE REACTIONS

Deaths have occurred after intravenous administration. (See Box Warning at beginning of circular.)
Transient "flushing sensations" and "peculiar" sensations of taste have been observed, as well as rare instances of dizziness, rapid and weak pulse, profuse sweating, brief hypotension, dyspnea, and cyanosis.
Pain, swelling, and tenderness at the injection site may occur. The possibility of allergic sensitivity, including an anaphylactoid reaction, should be kept in mind.
Rarely, after repeated injections, reactions resembling erythema perstans have been reported.
Hyperbilirubinemia has been observed in the newborn following administration of phytonadione. This has occurred rarely and primarily with doses above those recommended.

DOSAGE AND ADMINISTRATION

Whenever possible, AquaMEPHYTON should be given by the subcutaneous or intramuscular route. When intravenous administration is considered unavoidable, the drug should be injected very slowly, not exceeding 1 mg per minute.
The human minimum daily requirements for vitamin K have not been established officially but they have been estimated to be 1 to 5 mcg/kg of body weight for infants and 0.03 mcg/kg for adults. Usually, the dietary abundance of vitamin K will satisfy these requirements, except during the first five to eight days of the neonatal period.
Anticoagulant-Induced Prothrombin Deficiency
To correct excessively prolonged prothrombin time caused by oral anticoagulant therapy—2.5 to 10 mg or up to 25 mg initially is recommended. In rare instances 50 mg may be required. Frequency and amount of subsequent doses should be determined by prothrombin time response or clinical condition. If in 6 to 8 hours after parenteral administration the prothrombin time has not been shortened satisfactorily, the dose should be repeated.

Continued on next page

Information on the Merck Sharp & Dohme products listed on these pages is the full prescribing information from product circulars in use August 31, 1986.

Merck Sharp & Dohme—Cont.

In the event of shock or excessive blood loss, the use of whole blood or component therapy is indicated.
Smaller doses are recommended for patients being treated with the shorter-acting anticoagulants, and for those in need of continued anticoagulant therapy. The smallest effective dose should be sought to obviate the possibility of temporary refractoriness to further anticoagulant therapy, and to avoid lowering the prothrombin time too far below that indicating an effective level of anticoagulant activity.
Larger doses are recommended for patients on the longer-acting anticoagulants, for those with severe bleeding, and for those not needing further anticoagulant therapy. Although more than 25 mg may be necessary and a dose may need to be repeated, these courses of action are indicated *only rarely.*
Prophylaxis and Treatment
of Hemorrhagic Disease of the Newborn
Prophylaxis
The Committee on Nutrition of the American Academy of Pediatrics recommends that vitamin K_1 be given to the newborn. A single intramuscular dose of AquaMEPHYTON 0.5 to 1.0 mg is recommended. Although less desirable, AquaMEPHYTON 1 to 5 mg may be given to the mother 12 to 24 hours before delivery.
Treatment
AquaMEPHYTON 1.0 mg should be given either subcutaneously or intramuscularly. Higher doses may be necessary if the mother has been receiving oral anticoagulants.
Empiric administration of vitamin K_1 should not replace proper laboratory evaluation of the coagulation mechanism. A prompt response (shortening of the prothrombin time in 2 to 4 hours) following administration of vitamin K_1 is usually diagnostic of hemorrhagic disease of the newborn, and failure to respond indicates another diagnosis or coagulation disorder.
Whole blood or component therapy may be indicated if bleeding is excessive. This therapy, however, does not correct the underlying disorder and AquaMEPHYTON should be given concurrently.
Hypoprothrombinemia Due to Other Causes
A dosage of 2.5 to 25 mg or more (rarely up to 50 mg) is recommended, the amount and route of administration depending upon the severity of the condition and response obtained.
If possible, discontinuation or reduction of the dosage of drugs interfering with coagulation mechanisms (such as salicylates, antibiotics) is suggested as an alternative to administering concurrent AquaMEPHYTON. The severity of the coagulation disorder should determine whether the immediate administration of AquaMEPHYTON is required in addition to discontinuation or reduction of interfering drugs.

DIRECTIONS FOR DILUTION

AquaMEPHYTON may be diluted with 0.9% Sodium Chloride Injection, 5% Dextrose Injection, or 5% Dextrose and Sodium Chloride Injection. Benzyl alcohol as a preservative has been associated with toxicity in newborns. *Therefore, all of the above diluents should be preservative-free* (See WARNINGS). *Other diluents should not be used.* When dilutions are indicated, administration should be started immediately after mixture with the diluent, and unused portions of the dilution should be discarded, as well as unused contents of the ampul.

HOW SUPPLIED

Injection AquaMEPHYTON is a yellow, sterile, aqueous colloidal solution and is supplied in the following concentrations:
No. 7780—10 mg of vitamin K_1 per ml
NDC 0006-7780-64 boxes of 6–1 ml ampuls (6505-00-854-2499 10 mg 1.0 ml 6's)
NDC 0006-7780-66 boxes of 25–1 ml ampuls.
No. 7782—10 mg of vitamin K_1 per ml
NDC 0006-7782-30 in 2.5 ml multiple dose vials
NDC 0006-7782-03 in 5 ml multiple dose vials.
No. 7784—1 mg of vitamin K_1 per 0.5 ml
NDC 0006-7784-33 boxes of 25–0.5 ml ampuls (6505-00-180-6372 1 mg 0.5 ml 25's).
A.H.F.S. Category: 88:24
DC 6136713 Issued June 1982

ARAMINE® Injection ℞
(Metaraminol Bitartrate, MSD), U.S.P.

DESCRIPTION

Injection ARAMINE® (Metaraminol Bitartrate, MSD) is a sterile solution, each mL of which contains:
Metaraminol bitartrate equivalent to metaraminol...10.0 mg
Inactive ingredients:
Sodium chloride....4.4 mg
Water for Injection q.s. ad ....1.0 mL
Methylparaben 0.15%, propylparaben 0.02%, and sodium bisulfite 0.2% added as preservatives.
Metaraminol bitartrate is the generic name for levo-1-(m-hydroxyphenyl)-2-amino-1-propanol hydrogen D-tartrate. The structural formula for metaraminol bitartrate is:

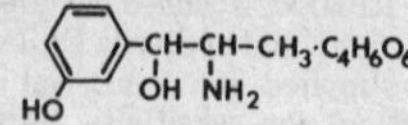

Metaraminol bitartrate is a white, crystalline powder, freely soluble in water, slightly soluble in alcohol, and practically insoluble in chloroform and in ether.

ACTIONS

ARAMINE is a potent sympathomimetic amine that increases both systolic and diastolic blood pressure.
The pressor effect of ARAMINE begins in 1 to 2 minutes after intravenous infusion, in about 10 minutes after intramuscular injection, and in 5 to 20 minutes after subcutaneous injection. The effect lasts from about 20 minutes to one hour. ARAMINE has a positive inotropic effect on the heart and a peripheral vasoconstrictor action.
Renal, coronary, and cerebral blood flow are a function of perfusion pressure and regional resistance. In most instances of cardiogenic shock, the beneficial effect of sympathomimetic amines is attributable to their positive inotropic effect. In patients with insufficient or failing vasoconstriction, there is additional advantage to the peripheral action of ARAMINE, but in most patients with shock, vasoconstriction is adequate and any further increase is unnecessary. Therefore, blood flow to vital organs may decrease with ARAMINE if regional resistance increases excessively.
The pressor effect of ARAMINE is decreased but not reversed by alpha-adrenergic blocking agents. Primary or secondary fall in blood pressure and tachyphylactic response to repeated use are uncommon.

INDICATIONS

Based on a review of this drug by the National Academy of Sciences-National Research Council and/or other information, FDA has classified the indications as follows:
Effective: ARAMINE is indicated for prevention and treatment of the acute hypotensive state occurring with spinal anesthesia. Adjunctive treatment of hypotension due to hemorrhage; reactions to medications; surgical complications; and shock associated with brain damage due to trauma or tumor.
"Probably" effective: It may also be useful as an adjunct in the treatment of hypotension due to cardiogenic shock or septicemia.
Final classification of the less-than-effective indications requires further investigation.

CONTRAINDICATIONS

Use of ARAMINE with cyclopropane or halothane anesthesia should be avoided, unless clinical circumstances demand such use.
Hypersensitivity to any component of this product, including sulfites (see PRECAUTIONS).

PRECAUTIONS

Sulfites have been reported to cause severe allergic reactions in certain susceptible individuals, particularly patients with asthma.
Caution should be used to avoid excessive blood pressure response. Rapidly induced hypertensive responses have been reported to cause acute pulmonary edema, arrhythmias, and cardiac arrest. ARAMINE should be used with caution in digitalized patients, since the combination of digitalis and sympathomimetic amines is capable of causing ectopic arrhythmic activity.
Patients with cirrhosis should be treated with caution, with adequate restoration of electrolytes if diuresis ensues. Fatal ventricular arrhythmia has been reported in one patient with Laennec's cirrhosis while receiving metaraminol bitartrate. In several instances, ventricular extrasystoles that appeared during infusion of this vasopressor subsided promptly when the rate of infusion was reduced.
With the prolonged action of ARAMINE, a cumulative effect is possible, and with an excessive vasopressor response there may be a prolonged elevation of blood pressure even with discontinuation of therapy. Monoamine oxidase inhibitors have been reported to potentiate the action of sympathomimetic amines.
When vasopressor amines are used for long periods, the resulting vasoconstriction may prevent adequate expansion of circulating volume and may cause perpetuation of the shock state. There is evidence that plasma volume may be reduced in all types of shock, and that the measurement of central venous pressure is useful in assessing the adequacy of the circulating blood volume. Therefore, blood or plasma volume expanders should be employed when the principal reason for hypotension or shock is decreased circulating volume.
Because of its vasoconstrictor effect ARAMINE should be given with caution in heart or thyroid disease, hypertension, or diabetes. Sympathomimetic amines may provoke a relapse in patients with a history of malaria.

ADVERSE REACTIONS

Sympathomimetic amines, including ARAMINE, may cause sinus or ventricular tachycardia, or other arrhythmias, especially in patients with myocardial infarction. See also PRECAUTIONS.
Also, in patients with a history of malaria, these compounds may provoke a relapse.
Abscess formation, tissue necrosis, or sloughing rarely may follow the use of ARAMINE. In choosing the site of injection, it is important to avoid those areas recognized as *not* suitable for use of any pressor agent and to discontinue the infusion immediately if infiltration or thrombosis occurs. Although the physician may be forced by the urgent nature of the patient's condition to choose injection sites that are not recognized as suitable, he should, when possible, use the preferred areas of injection. The larger veins of the antecubital fossa or the thigh are preferred to veins in the dorsum of the hand or ankle veins, particularly in patients with peripheral vascular disease, diabetes mellitus, Buerger's disease, or conditions with coexistent hypercoagulability.

DOSAGE AND ADMINISTRATION

ARAMINE may be given intramuscularly, subcutaneously, or intravenously, the route depending on the nature and severity of the indication.
Allow at least 10 minutes to elapse before increasing the dose because the maximum effect is not immediately apparent.
When the vasopressor is discontinued, observe the patient carefully as the effect of the drug tapers off, so that therapy can be reinitiated promptly if the blood pressure falls too rapidly. The response to vasopressors may be poor in patients with coexistent shock and acidosis. Established methods of shock management, such as blood or fluid replacement when indicated, and other measures directed to the specific cause of the shock state also should be used.
Intramuscular or Subcutaneous Injection (for prevention of hypotension—see INDICATIONS):
The recommended dose is 2 to 10 mg (0.2 to 1 mL). As with other agents given subcutaneously, only the preferred sites of injection, as set forth in standard texts, should be used.
Intravenous Infusion (for adjunctive treatment of hypotension—see INDICATIONS):
The recommended dose is 15 to 100 mg (1.5 to 10 mL) in 500 mL of Sodium Chloride Injection or 5% Dextrose Injection, adjusting the rate of infusion to maintain the blood pressure at the desired level. Higher concentrations of ARAMINE, 150 to 500 mg per 500 mL of infusion fluid, have been used. If the patient needs more saline or dextrose solution at a rate of flow that would provide an excessive dose of the vasopressor, the recommended volume of infusion fluid (500 mL) should be increased accordingly. ARAMINE may also be added to *less* than 500 mL of infusion fluid if a smaller volume is desired.
Compatibility Information
In addition to Sodium Chloride Injection and Dextrose Injection 5%, the following infusion solutions were found physically and chemically compatible with injection ARAMINE when 5 mL of injection ARAMINE, 10 mg/mL (metaraminol equivalent), was added to 500 mL of infusion solution: Ringer's Injection, Lactated Ringer's Injection, Dextran 6% in Saline†, Normosol®-R pH 7.4†, and Normosol®-M in D5-W†.
When injection ARAMINE is mixed with an infusion solution, sterile precautions should be observed. Since infusion solutions generally do not contain preservatives, mixtures should be used within 24 hours.
Direct Intravenous Injection: In severe shock, where time is of great importance, this agent should be given by direct intravenous injection. The suggested dose is 0.5 to 5 mg (0.05 to 0.5 mL), followed by an infusion of 15 to 100 mg (1.5 to 10 mL) in 500 mL of infusion fluid as described previously.
If necessary, vials may be sterilized by autoclaving or by immersion in a sterilizing solution.

HOW SUPPLIED

No. 3222X—Injection ARAMINE 1%, containing metaraminol bitartrate equivalent to 10 mg of metaraminol per mL, is a clear, colorless solution and is supplied as follows:
NDC 0006-3222-10 in 10 mL vials (6505-00-753-9601 10 mL vial).

†Product of Abbott Laboratories
A.H.F.S. Category: 12:12
DC 6019020 Issued December 1984

ATTENUVAX® ℞

(Measles Virus Vaccine Live, MSD), U.S.P.
(More Attenuated Enders' Strain)

DESCRIPTION

ATTENUVAX® (Measles Virus Vaccine Live, MSD) is a live virus vaccine for immunization against measles (rubeola).
ATTENUVAX is a sterile lyophilized preparation of a more attenuated line of measles virus derived from Enders' attenuated Edmonston strain. The further modification of the virus in ATTENUVAX was achieved in the Merck Institute for Therapeutic Research by multiple passage of Edmonston strain virus in cell cultures of chick embryo at low temperature.
The reconstituted vaccine is for subcutaneous administration. When reconstituted as directed, the dose for injection is 0.5 mL and contains not less than the equivalent of 1,000 $TCID_{50}$ (tissue culture infectious doses) of the U.S. Reference Measles Virus. Each dose also contains approximately 25 mcg of neomycin. The product contains no preservative. Sorbitol and hydrolized gelatin are added as stabilizers.

CLINICAL PHARMACOLOGY

ATTENUVAX produces a modified measles infection in susceptible persons. Fever and rash may appear. Extensive clinical trials have demonstrated that ATTENUVAX is highly immunogenic and generally well tolerated. A single injection of the vaccine has been shown to induce measles hemagglutination-inhibiting (HI) antibodies in 97 percent or more of susceptible persons. Vaccine-induced antibody levels have been shown to persist for at least 13 years without substantial decline. If the present pattern continues, it will provide a basis for the expectation that immunity following vaccination will be permanent. However, continued surveillance will be required to demonstrate this point.

INDICATIONS AND USAGE

ATTENUVAX is indicated for immunization against measles (rubeola) in persons 15 months of age or older. A booster is not needed. Infants who are less than 15 months of age may fail to respond to the vaccine due to presence in the circulation of residual measles antibody of maternal origin; the younger the infant, the lower the likelihood of seroconversion. In geographically isolated or other relatively inaccessible populations for whom immunization programs are logistically difficult, and in population groups in which natural measles infection may occur in a significant proportion of infants before 15 months of age, it may be desirable to give the vaccine to infants at an earlier age. Infants vaccinated under these conditions at less than 12 months of age should be revaccinated after reaching 15 months of age. There is some evidence to suggest that infants immunized at less than one year of age may not develop sustained antibody levels when later reimmunized. The advantage of early protection must be weighed against the chance for failure to respond adequately on reimmunization.
According to ACIP recommendations, most persons born in 1956 or earlier are likely to have been infected naturally and generally need not be considered susceptible. All children, adolescents, and adults born after 1956 are considered susceptible and should be vaccinated, if there are no contraindications. This includes persons who may be immune to measles but who lack adequate documentation of immunity as evidenced by: (1) physician-diagnosed measles, (2) laboratory evidence of measles immunity, or (3) adequate immunization with live measles vaccine on or after the first birthday.
ATTENUVAX given immediately after exposure to natural measles may provide some protection. If, however, the vaccine is given a few days before exposure, substantial protection may be provided.
Revaccination: Children vaccinated when younger than 12 months of age should be revaccinated, particularly if vaccine was administered with immune serum globulin or measles immune globulin, a standardized globulin preparation. Based on available evidence, there is no reason to routinely revaccinate persons who were vaccinated originally when 12 months of age or older. However, persons should be revaccinated if there is evidence to suggest that initial immunization was ineffective.
Despite the risk of reactions (see ADVERSE REACTIONS), persons born since 1956 who have previously been given inactivated vaccine alone or followed by live vaccine within 3 months should be revaccinated with live vaccine to reduce the risk of the severe atypical form of natural measles that may occur.
Use with other Vaccines
Routine administration of DTP (diphtheria, tetanus, pertussis) and/or OPV (oral poliovirus vaccine) concomitantly with measles, mumps and rubella vaccines is not recommended because there are insufficient data relating to the simultaneous administration of these antigens. However, the American Academy of Pediatrics has noted that in some circumstances, particularly when the patient may not return, some practitioners prefer to administer all these antigens on a single day. If done, separate sites and syringes should be used for DTP and ATTENUVAX.
ATTENUVAX should not be given less than one month before or after administration of other virus vaccines.

CONTRAINDICATIONS

Do not give ATTENUVAX to pregnant females; the possible effects of the vaccine on fetal development are unknown at this time. If vaccination of postpubertal females is undertaken, pregnancy should be avoided for three months following vaccination (see PRECAUTIONS, *Pregnancy*).
Anaphylactoid reaction to neomycin (each dose of reconstituted vaccine contains approximately 25 mcg of neomycin).
History of anaphylactoid reaction to eggs (see HYPERSENSITIVITY TO EGGS below).
Any febrile respiratory illness or other active febrile infection.
Active untreated tuberculosis.
Patients receiving immunosuppressive therapy. This contraindication does not apply to patients who are receiving corticosteroids as replacement therapy, e.g., for Addison's disease.
Individuals with blood dyscrasias, leukemia, lymphomas of any type, or other malignant neoplasms affecting the bone marrow or lymphatic systems.
Primary immunodeficiency states, including cellular immune deficiencies, hypogammaglobulinemic and dysgammaglobulinemic states.
Individuals with a family history of congenital or hereditary immunodeficiency, until the immune competence of the potential vaccine recipient is demonstrated.

HYPERSENSITIVITY TO EGGS

Live measles vaccine is produced in chick embryo cell culture. Persons with a history of anaphylactoid or other immediate reactions (e.g., hives, swelling of the mouth and throat, difficulty breathing, hypotension and shock) subsequent to egg ingestion should not be vaccinated. Evidence indicates that persons are not at increased risk if they have egg allergies that are not anaphylactoid in nature. Such persons should be vaccinated in the usual manner. There is no evidence to indicate that persons with allergies to chickens or feathers are at increased risk of reaction to the vaccine.

PRECAUTIONS

General
Adequate treatment provisions including epinephrine, should be available for immediate use should an anaphylactoid reaction occur.
Due caution should be employed in administration of measles vaccine to persons with a history of febrile convulsions, or cerebral injury, or of any other condition in which stress due to fever should be avoided. The physician should be alert to the temperature elevation which may occur following vaccination. (See ADVERSE REACTIONS).
Vaccination should be deferred for at least 3 months following blood or plasma transfusions, or administration of human immune serum globulin.
There are no reports of transmission of live attenuated measles virus from vaccinees to susceptible contacts.
It has been reported that attenuated measles virus vaccine, live, may result in a temporary depression of tuberculin skin sensitivity. Therefore, if a tuberculin test is to be done, it should be administered either before or simultaneously with ATTENUVAX.
Children under treatment for tuberculosis have not experienced exacerbation of the disease when immunized with live measles virus vaccine; no studies have been reported to date of the effect of measles virus vaccines on untreated tuberculous children.
As for any vaccine, vaccination with ATTENUVAX may not result in seroconversion in 100% of susceptible persons given the vaccine.
Pregnancy
Pregnancy Category C
Animal reproduction studies have not been conducted with ATTENUVAX. It is also not known whether ATTENUVAX can cause fetal harm when administered to a pregnant woman or can affect reproduction capacity. Therefore, the vaccine should not be administered to pregnant females; furthermore, pregnancy should be avoided for three months following vaccination (see CONTRAINDICATIONS).
Reports have indicated that contracting of natural measles during pregnancy enhances fetal risk. Increased rates of spontaneous abortion, stillbirth, congenital defects and prematurity have been observed subsequent to natural measles during pregnancy. There are no adequate studies of the attenuated (vaccine) strain of measles virus in pregnancy. However, it would be prudent to assume that the vaccine strain of virus is also capable of inducing adverse fetal effects for up to three months following vaccination.
Vaccine administration to postpubertal females entails a potential for inadvertent immunization during pregnancy. Theoretical risks involved should be weighed against the risks that measles poses to the unimmunized adolescent or adult. Advisory committees reviewing this matter have recommended vaccination of postpubertal females who are presumed to be susceptible to measles and not known to be pregnant. If a measles exposure occurs during pregnancy, one should consider the possibility of providing temporary passive immunity through the administration of immune globulin (human).
Nursing Mothers
It is not known whether measles vaccine virus is secreted in human milk. Therefore, because many drugs are excreted in human milk, caution should be exercised when ATTENUVAX is administered to a nursing woman.

ADVERSE REACTIONS

Because of the slightly acidic pH (6.2–6.6) of the vaccine, patients may complain of burning and/or stinging of short duration at the injection site.
Occasional
Moderate fever [101–102.9°F (38.3–39.4°C)] may occur during the month after vaccination. Generally, fever, rash, or both appear between the 5th and the 12th days. Rash, when it occurs, is usually minimal, but rarely may be generalized.
Less Common
High fever [over 103°F (39.4°C)].
Rare
Reactions at injection site. Allergic reactions such as wheal and flare at the injection site or urticaria have been reported.
Children developing fever may, on rare occasions, exhibit febrile convulsions.
Thrombocytopenia and purpura have occurred rarely.
Forms of optic neuritis, including retrobulbar neuritis, papillitis, and retinitis may infrequently follow viral infections, and have been reported to occur 1 to 3 weeks following inoculation with some live virus vaccines.
Experience from more than 80 million doses of all live measles vaccines given in the U.S. through 1975 indicates that significant central nervous system reactions such as encephalitis and encephalopathy, occurring within 30 days after vaccination, have been temporally associated with measles vaccine approximately once for every million doses. In no case has it been shown that reactions were actually caused by vaccine. The Center for Disease Control has pointed out that "a certain number of cases of encephalitis may be expected to occur in a large childhood population in a defined period of time even when no vaccines are administered". However, the data suggest the possibility that some of these cases may have been caused by measles vaccines. The risk of such serious neurological disorders following live measles virus vaccine administration remains far less than that for encephalitis and encephalopathy with natural measles (one per two thousand reported cases).
There have been isolated reports of ocular palsies and Guillain-Barre syndrome occurring after immunization with vaccines containing live attenuated measles virus. The ocular palsies have occurred approximately 3–24 days following vaccination. No definite causal relationship has been established between either of these events and vaccination.
There have been reports of subacute sclerosing panencephalitis (SSPE) in children who did not have a history of natural measles but did receive measles vaccine. Some of these cases may have resulted from unrecognized measles in the first year of life or possibly from the measles vaccination. Based on estimated nationwide measles vaccine distribution, the association of SSPE cases to measles vaccination is about one case per million vaccine doses distributed. This is far less than the association with natural measles, 6–22 cases of SSPE per million cases of measles. The results of a retrospective case-controlled study conducted by the Center for Disease Control suggest that the overall effect of measles vaccine has been to protect against SSPE by preventing measles with its inherent higher risk of SSPE.
Local reactions characterized by marked swelling, redness and vesiculation at the injection site of attenuated live virus measles vaccines, and systemic reactions including atypical

Continued on next page

Information on the Merck Sharp & Dohme products listed on these pages is the full prescribing information from product circulars in use August 31, 1986.

Merck Sharp & Dohme—Cont.

measles, have occurred in persons who have previously received killed measles vaccine. Rarely, more severe reactions that require hospitalization, including prolonged high fevers, panniculitis, and extensive local reactions, have been reported.

DOSAGE AND ADMINISTRATION

FOR SUBCUTANEOUS ADMINISTRATION
Do not inject intravenously
The dosage of vaccine is the same for all persons. Inject the total volume of the single dose vial (about 0.5 mL) or 0.5 mL of the multiple dose vial of reconstituted vaccine subcutaneously, preferably into the outer aspect of upper arm. *Do not give immune globulin (IG) concurrently with* ATTENUVAX.
During shipment, to insure that there is no loss of potency, the vaccine must be maintained at a temperature of 10°C (50°F) or less.
Before reconstitution, store ATTENUVAX at 2–8°C (35.6–46.4°F). *Protect from light.*
CAUTION: A sterile syringe free of preservatives, antiseptics, and detergents should be used for each injection and/or reconstitution of the vaccine because these substances may inactivate the live virus vaccine. A 25 gauge, ⅝″ needle is recommended.
To reconstitute, use only the diluent supplied, since it is free of preservatives or other antiviral substances which might inactivate the vaccine.

Single Dose Vial—First withdraw the entire volume of diluent into the syringe to be used for reconstitution. Inject all the diluent in the syringe into the vial of lyophilized vaccine, and agitate to mix thoroughly. Withdraw the entire contents into a syringe and inject the total volume of restored vaccine subcutaneously.
It is important to use a separate sterile syringe and needle for each individual patient to prevent transmission of hepatitis B and other infectious agents from one person to another.

10 Dose Vial (available only to government agencies/institutions)—Withdraw the entire contents (7 mL) of the diluent vial into the sterile syringe to be used for reconstitution, and introduce into the 10 dose vial of lyophilized vaccine. Agitate to ensure thorough mixing. The outer labeling suggests "For Jet Injector or Syringe Use". Use with separate sterile syringes is permitted for containers of 10 doses or less. The vaccine and diluent do not contain preservatives; therefore, the user must recognize the potential contamination hazards and exercise special precautions to protect the sterility and potency of the product. The use of aseptic techniques and proper storage prior to and after restoration of the vaccine and subsequent withdrawal of the individual doses is essential. Use 0.5 mL of the reconstituted vaccine for subcutaneous injection.
It is important to use a separate sterile syringe and needle for each individual patient to prevent transmission of hepatitis B and other infectious agents from one person to another.

50 Dose Vial (available only to government agencies/institutions)—Withdraw the entire contents (30 mL) of diluent vial into the sterile syringe to be used for reconstitution and introduce into the 50 dose vial of lyophilized vaccine. Agitate to ensure thorough mixing. With full aseptic precautions, attach the vial to the sterilized multidose jet injector apparatus. Use 0.5 mL of the reconstituted vaccine for subcutaneous injection.

Each dose of ATTENUVAX contains not less than 1,000 $TCID_{50}$ (tissue culture infectious doses) of measles virus vaccine expressed in terms of the assigned titer of the U.S. Reference Measles Virus.
Parenteral drug products should be inspected visually for particulate matter and discoloration prior to administration. ATTENUVAX, when reconstituted, is clear yellow.

HOW SUPPLIED

No. 4709—ATTENUVAX is supplied as a single-dose vial of lyophilized vaccine, **NDC** 0006-4709-00, and a vial of diluent.
No. 4589X/4309—ATTENUVAX is supplied as follows: (1) a box of 10 single-dose vials of lyophilized vaccine (package A), **NDC** 0006-4589-00; and (2) a box of 10 vials of diluent (package B). To conserve refrigerator space, the diluent may be stored separately at room temperature.
Available only to government agencies/institutions:
No. 4614X—ATTENUVAX is supplied as one 10 dose vial of lyophilized vaccine, **NDC** 0006-4614-00, and one 7 mL vial of diluent.
No. 4591X—ATTENUVAX is supplied as one 50 dose vial of lyophilized vaccine, **NDC** 0006-4591-00, and one 30 mL vial of diluent.
Storage
It is recommended that the vaccine be used as soon as possible after reconstitution. Protect vaccine from light at all times, since such exposure may inactivate the virus. Store reconstituted vaccine in the vaccine vial in a dark place at 2–8°C (35.6–46.4°F) and discard if not used within 8 hours.

A.H.F.S. Category: 80:12
DC 7075508 Issued September 1985

BENEMID® Tablets (Probenecid, MSD), U.S.P. ℞

DESCRIPTION

Probenecid is the generic name for 4-[(dipropylamino) sulfonyl] benzoic acid (molecular weight 285.36). It has the following structural formula:

$$(CH_3CH_2CH_2)_2N{-}SO_2{-}C_6H_4{-}COOH$$

Probenecid is a white or nearly white, fine, crystalline powder. Probenecid is soluble in dilute alkali, in alcohol, in chloroform, and in acetone; it is practically insoluble in water and in dilute acids.
Each tablet contains 0.5 g probenecid and the following inactive ingredients: calcium stearate, D&C Yellow 10, gelatin, hydroxypropyl methylcellulose, iron oxide, magnesium carbonate, polyethylene glycol, starch, talc, and titanium dioxide.

ACTIONS

BENEMID® (Probenecid, MSD) is a uricosuric and renal tubular blocking agent. It inhibits the tubular reabsorption of urate, thus increasing the urinary excretion of uric acid and decreasing serum urate levels. Effective uricosuria reduces the miscible urate pool, retards urate deposition, and promotes resorption of urate deposits.
BENEMID inhibits the tubular secretion of penicillin and usually increases penicillin plasma levels by any route the antibiotic is given. A 2-fold to 4-fold elevation has been demonstrated for various penicillins.
BENEMID also has been reported to inhibit the renal transport of many other compounds including aminohippuric acid (PAH), aminosalicylic acid (PAS), indomethacin, sodium iodomethamate and related iodinated organic acids, 17-ketosteroids, pantothenic acid, phenolsulfonphthalein (PSP), sulfonamides, and sulfonylureas. See also DRUG INTERACTIONS.
BENEMID decreases both hepatic and renal excretion of sulfobromophthalein (BSP). The tubular reabsorption of phosphorus is inhibited in hypoparathyroid but not in euparathyroid individuals.
BENEMID does not influence plasma concentrations of salicylates, nor the excretion of streptomycin, chloramphenicol, chlortetracycline, oxytetracycline, or neomycin.

INDICATIONS

For treatment of the hyperuricemia associated with gout and gouty arthritis.
As an adjuvant to therapy with penicillin or with ampicillin, methicillin, oxacillin, cloxacillin, or nafcillin, for elevation and prolongation of plasma levels by whatever route the antibiotic is given.

CONTRAINDICATIONS

Hypersensitivity to this product.
Children under 2 years of age.
Not recommended in persons with known blood dyscrasias or uric acid kidney stones.
Therapy with BENEMID should not be started until an acute gouty attack has subsided.

WARNINGS

Exacerbation of gout following therapy with BENEMID may occur; in such cases colchicine or other appropriate therapy is advisable.
BENEMID increases plasma concentrations of methotrexate in both animals and humans. In animal studies, increased methotrexate toxicity has been reported. If BENEMID is given with methotrexate, the dosage of methotrexate should be reduced and serum levels may need to be monitored.
In patients on BENEMID the use of salicylates in either small or large doses is contraindicated because it antagonizes the uricosuric action of BENEMID. The biphasic action of salicylates in the renal tubules accounts for the so-called "paradoxical effect" of uricosuric agents. In patients on BENEMID who require a mild analgesic agent the use of acetaminophen rather than small doses of salicylates would be preferred.
Rarely, severe allergic reactions and anaphylaxis have been reported with the use of BENEMID. Most of these have been reported to occur within several hours after readministration following prior usage of the drug.
The appearance of hypersensitivity reactions requires cessation of therapy with BENEMID.
Use in Pregnancy: BENEMID crosses the placental barrier and appears in cord blood. The use of any drug in women of childbearing potential requires that the anticipated benefit be weighed against possible hazards.

PRECAUTIONS

General
Hematuria, renal colic, costovertebral pain, and formation of uric acid stones associated with the use of BENEMID in gouty patients may be prevented by alkalization of the urine and a liberal fluid intake (*see* DOSAGE AND ADMINISTRATION). In these cases when alkali is administered, the acid-base balance of the patient should be watched.
Use with caution in patients with a history of peptic ulcer.
BENEMID has been used in patients with some renal impairment but dosage requirements may be increased. BENEMID may not be effective in chronic renal insufficiency particularly when the glomerular filtration rate is 30 mL/minute or less. Because of its mechanism of action, BENEMID is not recommended in conjunction with a penicillin in the presence of *known* renal impairment.
A reducing substance may appear in the urine of patients receiving BENEMID. This disappears with discontinuance of therapy. Suspected glycosuria should be confirmed by using a test specific for glucose.
Drug Interactions
When BENEMID is used to elevate plasma concentrations of penicillin or other beta-lactams, or when such drugs are given to patients taking BENEMID therapeutically, high plasma concentrations of the other drug may increase the incidence of adverse reactions associated with that drug. In the case of penicillin or other beta-lactams, psychic disturbances have been reported.
The use of salicylates antagonizes the uricosuric action of BENEMID (*see* WARNINGS). The uricosuric action of BENEMID is also antagonized by pyrazinamide.
BENEMID produces an insignificant increase in free sulfonamide plasma concentrations but a significant increase in total sulfonamide plasma levels. Since BENEMID decreases the renal excretion of conjugated sulfonamides, plasma concentrations of the latter should be determined from time to time when a sulfonamide and BENEMID are coadministered for prolonged periods. BENEMID may prolong or enhance the action of oral sulfonylureas and thereby increase the risk of hypoglycemia.
It has been reported that patients receiving BENEMID require significantly less thiopental for induction of anesthesia. In addition, ketamine and thiopental anesthesia were significantly prolonged in rats receiving probenecid.
When BENEMID is given to patients receiving indomethacin, the plasma levels of indomethacin are likely to be increased. Therefore, a lower dosage of indomethacin may be required to produce a therapeutic effect, and increases in the dosage of indomethacin should be made cautiously and in small increments. BENEMID may increase plasma levels of rifampin. The clinical significance of this is not known.
In animals and in humans, BENEMID has been reported to increase plasma concentrations of methotrexate (*see* WARNINGS).
Falsely high readings for theophylline have been reported in an *in vitro* study, using the Schack and Waxler technic, when therapeutic concentrations of theophylline and BENEMID were added to human plasma.

ADVERSE REACTIONS

The following adverse reactions have been observed and within each category are listed in order of decreasing severity.
Central Nervous System: headache, dizziness.
Metabolic: precipitation of acute gouty arthritis.
Gastrointestinal: hepatic necrosis, vomiting, nausea, anorexia, sore gums.
Genitourinary: nephrotic syndrome, uric acid stones with or without hematuria, renal colic, costovertebral pain, urinary frequency.
Hypersensitivity: anaphylaxis, fever, urticaria, pruritus.
Hematologic: aplastic anemia, leukopenia, hemolytic anemia which could be related to genetic deficiency of glucose-6-phosphate dehydrogenase in red blood cells, anemia.
Integumentary: dermatitis, alopecia, flushing.

DOSAGE AND ADMINISTRATION

Gout
Therapy with BENEMID should not be *started* until an acute gouty attack has subsided. However, if an acute attack is precipitated *during* therapy, BENEMID may be continued

BENEMID® (Probenecid, MSD) Penicillin Therapy (Gonorrhea)*

	Recommended Regimens**	Remarks
Uncomplicated gonococcal infection in men and women (urethral, cervical, rectal)	4.8 million units of aqueous procaine penicillin G† I.M., in at least 2 doses injected at different sites at one visit + 1 g of BENEMID (Probenecid, MSD) orally just before injections *or* 3.5 g of ampicillin† orally + 1 g of BENEMID orally given simultaneously.	Follow-up: Obtain urethral and other appropriate cultures from men, and cervical, anal, and other appropriate cultures from women, 7 to 14 days after completion of treatment. Treatment of sexual partners: Persons with known recent exposure to gonorrhea should receive same treatment as those known to have gonorrhea. Examination and treatment of male sex partners of persons with gonorrhea are essential because of high prevalence of nonsymptomatic urethral gonococcal infection in such men.
Pharyngeal gonococcal infection in men and women	4.8 million units of aqueous procaine penicillin G† I.M., in at least 2 doses injected at different sites at one visit + 1 g of BENEMID orally just before injections	Pharyngeal gonococcal infections may be more difficult to treat than anogenital gonorrhea. Posttreatment cultures are essential.
Uncomplicated gonorrhea in pregnant patients	4.8 million units of aqueous procaine penicillin G† I.M., in at least 2 doses injected at different sites at one visit *or* 3.5 g of ampicillin† orally + 1 g of BENEMID orally given simultaneously	
Acute gonococcal salpingitis	*Outpatients:* Aqueous procaine penicillin G† or ampicillin† with BENEMID as for gonorrhea in pregnancy, followed by 500 mg of ampicillin 4 times a day for 10 days *Hospitalized patients:* See details in CDC recommendations	Follow-up of patients with acute salpingitis is essential. All patients should receive repeat pelvic examinations and cultures for *Neisseria gonorrhoeae* after treatment. Examination and appropriate treatment of male sex partners are essential because of high prevalence of nonsymptomatic urethral gonorrhea in such men.
Disseminated gonococcal infection (arthritis-dermatitis syndrome)	10 million units of aqueous crystalline penicillin G† I.V. a day for 3 days or till significant clinical improvement occurs. May be followed with 500 mg of ampicillin† 4 times a day orally to complete 7 days of treatment *or* 3.5 g of ampicillin† orally with 1 g of BENEMID, followed by 500 mg of ampicillin† 4 times a day for at least 7 days	
Gonococcal infection in children	For postpubertal children and/or those weighing over 45 kg (100 lb) use the dosage regimens given above for adults Uncomplicated vulvovaginitis and urethritis: aqueous procaine penicillin G† 75,000—100,000 units/kg I.M., with BENEMID 23 mg/kg orally	See CDC recommendations for detailed information about prevention and treatment of neonatal gonococcal infection and gonococcal ophthalmia.

Note: Before treating gonococcal infections in patients with suspected primary or secondary syphilis, perform proper diagnostic procedures including darkfield examinations. If concomitant syphilis is suspected, perform monthly serological tests for at least 4 months.

* Recommended by Venereal Disease Control Advisory Committee, Center for Disease Control, U.S. Department of Health, Education, and Welfare, Public Health Service (Morbidity and Mortality Weekly Report, Vol. *23:* 341, 342, 347, 348, Oct. 11, 1974).

** See CDC recommendations for definition of regimens of choice, alternative regimens, treatment of hypersensitive patients, and other aspects of therapy.

† See package circulars of manufacturers for detailed information about contraindications, warnings, precautions, and adverse reactions.

without changing the dosage, and full therapeutic dosage of colchicine or other appropriate therapy should be given to control the acute attack.

The recommended adult dosage is 0.25 g (1/2 tablet of BENEMID) twice a day for one week, followed by 0.5 g (1 tablet) twice a day thereafter.

Some degree of renal impairment may be present in patients with gout. A daily dosage of 1 g may be adequate. However, if necessary, the daily dosage may be increased by 0.5 g increments every 4 weeks within tolerance (and usually not above 2 g per day) if symptoms of gouty arthritis are not controlled or the 24 hour uric acid excretion is not above 700 mg. As noted, BENEMID may not be effective in chronic renal insufficiency particularly when the glomerular filtration rate is 30 mL/minute or less.

Gastric intolerance may be indicative of overdosage, and may be corrected by decreasing the dosage.

As uric acid tends to crystallize out of an acid urine, a liberal fluid intake is recommended, as well as sufficient sodium bicarbonate (3 to 7.5 g daily) or potassium citrate (7.5 g daily) to maintain an alkaline urine (*see* PRECAUTIONS).

Alkalization of the urine is recommended until the serum urate level returns to normal limits and tophaceous deposits disappear, i.e., during the period when urinary excretion of uric acid is at a high level. Thereafter, alkalization of the urine and the usual restriction of purine-producing foods may be somewhat relaxed.

BENEMID should be continued at the dosage that will maintain normal serum urate levels. When acute attacks have been absent for 6 months or more and serum urate levels remain within normal limits, the daily dosage may be decreased by 0.5 g every 6 months. The maintenance dosage should not be reduced to the point where serum urate levels tend to rise.

BENEMID and Penicillin Therapy (General)

Adults:

The recommended dosage is 2 g (4 tablets of BENEMID) daily in divided doses. This dosage should be reduced in older patients in whom renal impairment may be present.

Children 2-14 years of age:

Initial dose: 25 mg/kg body weight (*or* 0.7 g/square meter body surface).

Maintenance dose: 40 mg/kg body weight (*or* 1.2 g/square meter body surface) per day, divided into 4 doses.

For children weighing more than 50 kg (110 lb) the adult dosage is recommended.

BENEMID is contraindicated in children under 2 years of age.

The PSP excretion test may be used to determine the effectiveness of BENEMID in retarding penicillin excretion and maintaining therapeutic levels. The renal clearance of PSP is reduced to about one-fifth the normal rate when dosage of BENEMID is adequate.

Penicillin Therapy (Gonorrhea)

[See table above].

HOW SUPPLIED

No. 3337—Tablets BENEMID, 0.5 g, are yellow, capsule shaped, scored, film coated tablets, coded MSD 501. They are supplied as follows:

NDC 0006-0501-68 bottles of 100
(6505-00-104-9735 100's)
NDC 0006-0501-28 unit dose packages of 100
NDC 0006-0501-82 bottles of 1000
(6505-00-181-8387 1000's).

Shown in Product Identification Section, page 417

A.H.F.S. Category: 40:40
DC 6103918 Issued April 1985

BIAVAX®$_{II}$ ℞

(Rubella and Mumps Virus Vaccine Live, MSD), U.S.P.

DESCRIPTION

BIAVAX® II (Rubella and Mumps Virus Vaccine Live, MSD) is a live virus vaccine for immunization against rubella (German measles) and mumps.

BIAVAX II is a sterile lyophilized preparation of the Wistar RA 27/3 strain of live attenuated rubella virus grown in human diploid cell (WI-38) culture; and the Jeryl Lynn (B level) strain of mumps virus grown in cell cultures of chick embryo. The vaccine viruses are the same as those used in the manufacture of MERUVAX® II (Rubella Virus Vaccine Live, MSD) and MUMPSVAX® (Mumps Virus Vaccine Live, MSD). The two viruses are mixed before being lyophilized. The reconstituted vaccine is for subcutaneous administration. When reconstituted as directed, the dose for injection is 0.5 mL and contains not less than the equivalent of 1,000 $TCID_{50}$ of the U.S. Reference Rubella Virus and 5,000 $TCID_{50}$ of the U.S. Reference Mumps Virus. Each dose contains approximately 25 mcg of neomycin. The product contains no preservative. Sorbitol and hydrolized gelatin are added as stabilizers.

CLINICAL PHARMACOLOGY

Clinical studies of 73 double seronegative children 12 months to 2 years of age demonstrated that BIAVAX II is

Continued on next page

Information on the Merck Sharp & Dohme products listed on these pages is the full prescribing information from product circulars in use August 31, 1986.

Merck Sharp & Dohme—Cont.

highly immunogenic and generally well tolerated. In these studies, a single injection of the vaccine induced rubella hemagglutination-inhibition (HI) antibodies in 100 percent, and mumps neutralizing antibodies in 97 percent of the susceptible children.

The RA 27/3 rubella strain in BIAVAX II elicits higher immediate post-vaccination HI, complement-fixing and neutralizing antibody levels than other strains of rubella vaccine and has been shown to induce a broader profile of circulating antibodies including anti-theta and anti-iota precipitating antibodies. The RA 27/3 rubella strain immunologically simulates natural infection more closely than other rubella vaccine viruses. The increased levels and broader profile of antibodies produced by RA 27/3 strain rubella virus vaccine appear to correlate with greater resistance to subclinical reinfection with the wild virus, and provide greater confidence for lasting immunity.

Vaccine induced antibody levels following administration of BIAVAX II have been shown to persist for at least two years without substantial decline. Antibody levels after immunization with BIAVAX (Rubella and Mumps Virus Vaccine Live, MSD), containing the HPV-77 strain of rubella, have persisted for 10.5 years without substantial decline. If the present pattern continues, it will provide a basis for the expectation that immunity following vaccination will be permanent. However, continued surveillance will be required to demonstrate this point.

INDICATIONS AND USAGE

BIAVAX II is indicated for simultaneous immunization against rubella and mumps in persons 12 months of age or older. A booster is not needed.

The vaccine is not recommended for infants younger than 12 months because they may retain maternal rubella and mumps neutralizing antibodies which may interfere with the immune response.

Previously unimmunized children of susceptible pregnant women should receive live attenuated rubella vaccine, because an immunized child will be less likely to acquire natural rubella and introduce the virus into the household.

Non-Pregnant Adolescent and Adult Females

Immunization of susceptible non-pregnant adolescent and adult females of childbearing age with live attenuated rubella virus vaccine is indicated if certain precautions are observed (see below and PRECAUTIONS). Vaccinating susceptible postpubertal females confers individual protection against subsequently acquiring rubella infection during pregnancy, which in turn prevents infection of the fetus and consequent congenital rubella injury.

Women of childbearing age should be advised not to become pregnant for three months after vaccination and should be informed of the reasons for this precaution.*

It is recommended that rubella susceptibility be determined by serologic testing prior to immunization.** If immune, as evidenced by a specific rubella antibody titer of 1:8 or greater (hemagglutination-inhibition test), vaccination is unnecessary. Congenital malformations do occur in up to seven percent of all live births. Their chance appearance after vaccination could lead to misinterpretation of the cause, particularly if the prior rubella-immune status of vaccinees is unknown.

Postpubertal females should be informed of the frequent occurrence of self-limited arthralgia and possible arthritis beginning 2 to 4 weeks after vaccination (see ADVERSE REACTIONS).

Postpartum Women

It has been found convenient in many instances to vaccinate rubella-susceptible women in the immediate postpartum period. (See *Nursing Mothers*).

* NOTE: The Immunization Practices Advisory Committee (ACIP) has recommended "In view of the importance of protecting this age group against rubella, reasonable precautions in a rubella immunization program include asking females if they are pregnant, excluding those who say they are, and explaining the theoretical risks to the others."

** NOTE: The Immunization Practices Advisory Committee (ACIP) has stated "When practical, and when reliable laboratory services are available, potential vaccinees of childbearing age can have serologic tests to determine susceptibility to rubella. . . . However, routinely performing serologic tests for all females of childbearing age to determine susceptibility so that vaccine is given only to proven susceptibles is expensive and has been ineffective in some areas. Accordingly, the ACIP believes that rubella vaccination of a woman who is not known to be pregnant and has no history of vaccination is justifiable without serologic testing."

Revaccination: Children vaccinated when younger than 12 months of age should be revaccinated. Based on available evidence, there is no reason to routinely revaccinate persons who were vaccinated originally when 12 months of age or older. However, persons should be revaccinated if there is evidence to suggest that initial immunization was ineffective.

Use with other Vaccines

Routine administration of DTP (diphtheria, tetanus, pertussis) and/or OPV (oral poliovirus vaccine) concomitantly with measles, mumps and rubella vaccines is not recommended because there are insufficient data relating to the simultaneous administration of these antigens. However, the American Academy of Pediatrics has noted that in some circumstances, particularly when the patient may not return, some practitioners prefer to administer all these antigens on a single day. If done, separate sites and syringes should be used for DTP and BIAVAX II.

BIAVAX II should not be given less than one month before or after administration of other virus vaccines.

CONTRAINDICATIONS

Do not give BIAVAX II to pregnant females; the possible effects of the vaccine on fetal development are unknown at this time. If vaccination of postpubertal females is undertaken, pregnancy should be avoided for three months following vaccination. (See PRECAUTIONS, *Pregnancy*).

Anaphylactoid reaction to neomycin (each dose of reconstituted vaccine contains approximately 25 mcg of neomycin).

History of anaphylactoid reaction to eggs (see HYPERSENSITIVITY TO EGGS below).

Any febrile respiratory illness or other active febrile infection.

Active untreated tuberculosis.

Patients receiving immunosuppressive therapy. This contraindication does not apply to patients who are receiving corticosteroids as replacement therapy, e.g., for Addison's disease.

Individuals with blood dyscrasias, leukemia, lymphomas of any type, or other malignant neoplasms affecting the bone marrow or lymphatic systems.

Primary immunodeficiency states, including cellular immune deficiencies, hypogammaglobulinemic and dysgammaglobulinemic states.

Individuals with a family history of congenital or hereditary immunodeficiency, until the immune competence of the potential vaccine recipient is demonstrated.

HYPERSENSITIVITY TO EGGS

Live mumps vaccine is produced in chick embryo cell culture. Persons with a history of anaphylactic or other immediate reactions (e.g., hives, swelling of the mouth and throat, difficulty breathing, hypotension, or shock) subsequent to egg ingestion should not be vaccinated. Evidence indicates that persons are not at increased risk if they have egg allergies that are not anaphylactic in nature. Such persons may be vaccinated in the usual manner. There is no evidence to indicate that persons with allergies to chickens or feathers are at increased risk of reaction to the vaccine.

PRECAUTIONS

General

Adequate treatment provisions including epinephrine, should be available for immediate use should an anaphylactoid reaction occur.

Vaccination should be deferred for at least 3 months following blood or plasma transfusions, or administration of human immune serum globulin.

Excretion of small amounts of the live attenuated rubella virus from the nose and throat has occurred in the majority of susceptible individuals 7–28 days after vaccination. There is no confirmed evidence to indicate that such virus is transmitted to susceptible persons who are in contact with the vaccinated individuals. Consequently, transmission through close personal contact, while accepted as a theoretical possibility, is not regarded as a significant risk. However, transmission of the rubella vaccine virus to infants via breast milk has been documented (see *Nursing Mothers*).

There are no reports of transmission of live attenuated mumps virus from vaccinees to susceptible contacts.

It has been reported that live attenuated rubella and mumps virus vaccines given individually may result in a temporary depression of tuberculin skin sensitivity. Therefore, if a tuberculin test is to be done, it should be administered either before or simultaneously with BIAVAX II.

As for any vaccine, vaccination with BIAVAX II may not result in seroconversion in 100% of susceptible persons given the vaccine.

Pregnancy

Pregnancy Category C

Animal reproduction studies have not been conducted with BIAVAX II. It is also not known whether BIAVAX II can cause fetal harm when administered to a pregnant woman or can affect reproduction capacity. Therefore, the vaccine should not be administered to pregnant females; furthermore, pregnancy should be avoided for three months following vaccination (see CONTRAINDICATIONS).

In counseling women who are inadvertently vaccinated when pregnant or who become pregnant within 3 months of vaccination, the physician should be aware of the following: (1) In a 10 year survey involving over 700 pregnant women who received rubella vaccine within 3 months before or after conception, (of whom 189 received the Wistar RA 27/3 strain) none of the newborns had abnormalities compatible with congenital rubella syndrome; and (2) although mumps virus is capable of infecting the placenta and fetus, there is no good evidence that it causes congenital malformations in humans. Mumps vaccine virus also has been shown to infect the placenta, but the virus has not been isolated from the fetal tissues from susceptible women who were vaccinated and underwent elective abortions.

Nursing Mothers

It is not known whether mumps vaccine virus is secreted in human milk. Recent studies have shown that lactating postpartum women immunized with live attenuated rubella vaccine may secrete the virus in breast milk and transmit it to breast-fed infants. In the infants with serological evidence of rubella infection, none exhibited severe disease; however, one exhibited mild clinical illness typical of acquired rubella. Caution should be exercised when BIAVAX II is administered to a nursing woman.

ADVERSE REACTIONS

Because of the slightly acidic pH (6.2–6.6) of the vaccine, patients may complain of burning and/or stinging of short duration at the injection site.

The adverse clinical reactions associated with the use of BIAVAX II are those expected to follow administration of the monovalent vaccines given separately. These may include malaise, sore throat, headache, fever, and rash; mild local reactions such as erythema, induration, tenderness and regional lymphadenopathy; parotitis; orchitis; nerve deafness; thrombocytopenia and purpura; allergic reactions such as wheal and flare at the injection site or urticaria; and arthritis, arthralgia and polyneuritis.

Moderate fever [101–102.9°F (38.3–39.4°C)] occurs occasionally, and high fever [above 103°F (39.4°C)] occurs less commonly. On rare occasions, children developing fever may exhibit febrile convulsions. Rash occurs infrequently and is usually minimal, but rarely may be generalized.

Forms of optic neuritis, including retrobulbar neuritis and papillitis may infrequently follow viral infections, and have been reported to occur 1 to 3 weeks following inoculation with some live virus vaccines.

Isolated reports of polyneuropathy including Guillain-Barré syndrome have been reported after immunization with rubella containing vaccines.

Clinical experience with live attenuated rubella and mumps virus vaccines given individually indicates that encephalitis and other nervous system reactions have occurred very rarely. These might occur also with BIAVAX II.

Transient arthritis, arthralgia and polyneuritis are features of natural rubella and vary in frequency and severity with age and sex, being greatest in adult females and least in prepubertal children. This type of involvement as well as myalgia have also been reported following administration of MERUVAX II (Rubella Virus Vaccine Live, MSD). In children, joint reactions are rare and of brief duration if they do occur. In women, incidence rates for arthritis and arthralgia are generally higher than those seen in children (children: 0–3%; women: 12–20%), and the reactions tend to be more marked and of longer duration. Symptoms may persist for a matter of months or on rare occasions for years. In adolescent girls, the reactions appear to be intermediate in incidence between those seen in children and in adult women. Even in older women (35–45 years), these reactions are generally well tolerated and rarely interfere with normal activities.

DOSAGE AND ADMINISTRATION

FOR SUBCUTANEOUS ADMINISTRATION

Do not inject intravenously.

The dosage of vaccine is the same for all persons. Inject the total volume (about 0.5 mL) of reconstituted vaccine subcutaneously, preferably into the outer aspect of upper arm. *Do not give immune globulin (IG) concurrently with* BIAVAX II.

During shipment, to insure that there is no loss of potency, the vaccine must be maintained at a temperature of 10°C (50°F) or less.

Before reconstitution, store BIAVAX II at 2–8°C (35.6–46.4°F). *Protect from light.*

CAUTION: A sterile syringe free of preservatives, antiseptics, and detergents should be used for each injection of the vaccine because these substances may inactivate the live virus vaccine. A 25 gauge, ⅝″ needle is recommended.

To reconstitute, use only the diluent supplied, since it is free of preservatives or other antiviral substances which might inactivate the vaccine. First withdraw the entire volume of diluent into the syringe to be used for reconstitution. Inject all the diluent in the syringe into the vial of lyophilized vaccine, and agitate to mix thoroughly. Withdraw the entire contents into a syringe and inject the total volume of restored vaccine subcutaneously.

It is important to use a separate sterile syringe and needle for each individual patient to prevent transmission of hepatitis B virus and other infectious agents from one person to another.

Each dose of BIAVAX II contains not less than the equivalent of 1,000 $TCID_{50}$ of the U.S. Reference Rubella Virus and 5,000 $TCID_{50}$ of the U.S. Reference Mumps Virus.

Parenteral drug products should be inspected visually for particulate matter and discoloration prior to administration. BIAVAX II, when reconstituted, is clear yellow.

HOW SUPPLIED

No. 4746—BIAVAX II is supplied as a single-dose vial of lyophilized vaccine, **NDC** 0006-4746-00, and a vial of diluent.

No. 4669/4309—BIAVAX II is supplied as follows: (1) a box of 10 single-dose vials of lyophilized vaccine (package A), **NDC** 0006-4669-00; and (2) a box of 10 vials of diluent (package B). To conserve refrigerator space, the diluent may be stored separately at room temperature.

Storage

It is recommended that the vaccine be used as soon as possible after reconstitution. Protect the vaccine from light at all times, since such exposure may inactivate the virus. Store reconstituted vaccine in the vaccine vial in a dark place at 2–8°C (35.6–46.4°F) and discard if not used within eight hours.

A.H.F.S. Category: 80:12

DC 7032310 Issued January 1986

BLOCADREN® Tablets ℞

(Timolol Maleate, MSD), U.S.P.

DESCRIPTION

BLOCADREN® (Timolol Maleate, MSD) is a non-selective beta-adrenergic receptor blocking agent. The chemical name for timolol maleate is (S)-1-[(1, 1-dimethylethyl) amino] -3-[[4-(4-morpholinyl)- 1, 2, 5-thiadiazol-3-yl]oxy]-2-propanol, (Z)-butenedioate (1:1) salt. It possesses an asymmetric carbon atom in its structure and is provided as the levoisomer. Its empirical formula is $C_{13}H_{24}N_4O_3S \cdot C_4H_4O_4$ and its structural formula is:

Timolol maleate has a molecular weight of 432.49. It is a white, odorless, crystalline powder which is soluble in water, methanol, and alcohol.

BLOCADREN is supplied as tablets in three strengths containing 5 mg, 10 mg or 20 mg timolol maleate for oral administration. Inactive ingredients are cellulose, FD&C Blue 2, magnesium stearate, and starch.

CLINICAL PHARMACOLOGY

BLOCADREN is a $beta_1$ and $beta_2$ (non-selective) adrenergic receptor blocking agent that does not have significant intrinsic sympathomimetic, direct myocardial depressant, or local anesthetic activity.

Pharmacodynamics

Clinical pharmacology studies have confirmed the beta-adrenergic blocking activity as shown by (1) changes in resting heart rate and response of heart rate to changes in posture; (2) inhibition of isoproterenol-induced tachycardia; (3) alteration of the response to the Valsalva maneuver and amyl nitrite administration; and (4) reduction of heart rate and blood pressure changes on exercise.

BLOCADREN decreases the positive chronotropic, positive inotropic, bronchodilator, and vasodilator responses caused by beta-adrenergic receptor agonists. The magnitude of this decreased response is proportional to the existing sympathetic tone and the concentration of BLOCADREN at receptor sites.

In normal volunteers, the reduction in heart rate response to a standard exercise was dose dependent over the test range of 0.5 to 20 mg, with a peak reduction at 2 hours of approximately 30% at higher doses.

Beta-adrenergic receptor blockade reduces cardiac output in both healthy subjects and patients with heart disease. In patients with severe impairment of myocardial function beta-adrenergic receptor blockade may inhibit the stimulatory effect of the sympathetic nervous system necessary to maintain adequate cardiac function.

Beta-adrenergic receptor blockade in the bronchi and bronchioles results in increased airway resistance from unopposed parasympathetic activity. Such an effect in patients with asthma or other bronchospastic conditions is potentially dangerous.

Clinical studies indicate that BLOCADREN at a dosage of 20–60 mg/day reduces blood pressure without causing postural hypotension in most patients with essential hypertension. Administration of BLOCADREN to patients with hypertension results initially in a decrease in cardiac output, little immediate change in blood pressure, and an increase in calculated peripheral resistance. With continued administration of BLOCADREN blood pressure decreases within a few days, cardiac output usually remains reduced, and peripheral resistance falls toward pretreatment levels. Plasma volume may decrease or remain unchanged during therapy with BLOCADREN. In the majority of patients with hypertension BLOCADREN also decreases plasma renin activity. Dosage adjustment to achieve optimal antihypertensive effect may require a few weeks. When therapy with BLOCADREN is discontinued, the blood pressure tends to return to pretreatment levels gradually. In most patients the antihypertensive activity of BLOCADREN is maintained with long-term therapy and is well tolerated.

The mechanism of the antihypertensive effects of beta-adrenergic receptor blocking agents is not established at this time. Possible mechanisms of action include reduction in cardiac output, reduction in plasma renin activity, and a central nervous system sympatholytic action.

A Norwegian multi-center, double-blind study compared the effects of timolol maleate with placebo in 1,884 patients who had survived the acute phase of a myocardial infarction. Patients with systolic blood pressure below 100 mm Hg, sick sinus syndrome and contraindications to beta blockers, including uncontrolled heart failure, second or third degree AV block and bradycardia (<50 beats per minute), were excluded from the multi-center trial. Therapy with BLOCADREN, begun 7 to 28 days following infarction, was shown to reduce overall mortality; this was primarily attributable to a reduction in cardiovascular mortality. BLOCADREN significantly reduced the incidence of sudden deaths (deaths occurring without symptoms or within 24 hours of the onset of symptoms), including those occurring within one hour, and particularly instantaneous deaths (those occurring without preceding symptoms). The protective effect of BLOCADREN was consistent regardless of age, sex or site of infarction. The effect was clearest in patients with a first infarction who were considered at a high risk of dying, defined as those with one or more of the following characteristics during the acute phase: transient left ventricular failure, cardiomegaly, newly appearing atrial fibrillation or flutter, systolic hypotension, or SGOT (ASAT) levels greater than four times the upper limit of normal. Therapy with BLOCADREN also reduced the incidence of non-fatal reinfarction. The mechanism of the protective effect of BLOCADREN is unknown.

Pharmacokinetics and Metabolism

BLOCADREN is rapidly and nearly completely absorbed (about 90%) following oral ingestion. Detectable plasma levels of timolol occur within one-half hour and peak plasma levels occur in about one to two hours. The drug half-life in plasma is approximately 4 hours and this is essentially unchanged in patients with moderate renal insufficiency. Timolol is partially metabolized by the liver and timolol and its metabolites are excreted by the kidney. Timolol is not extensively bound to plasma proteins; i.e., <10% by equilibrium dialysis and approximately 60% by ultrafiltration. An *in vitro* hemodialysis study, using ^{14}C timolol added to human plasma or whole blood, showed that timolol was readily dialyzed from these fluids; however, a study of patients with renal failure showed that timolol did not dialyze readily.

Plasma levels following oral administration are about half those following intravenous administration indicating approximately 50% first pass metabolism. The level of beta sympathetic activity varies widely among individuals, and no simple correlation exists between the dose or plasma level of timolol maleate and its therapeutic activity. Therefore, objective clinical measurements such as reduction of heart rate and/or blood pressure should be used as guides in determining the optimal dosage for each patient.

INDICATIONS AND USAGE

Hypertension

BLOCADREN is indicated for the treatment of hypertension. It may be used alone or in combination with other antihypertensive agents, especially thiazide-type diuretics.

Myocardial Infarction

BLOCADREN is indicated in patients who have survived the acute phase of a myocardial infarction, and are clinically stable, to reduce cardiovascular mortality and the risk of reinfarction.

CONTRAINDICATIONS

BLOCADREN is contraindicated in patients with bronchial asthma or with a history of bronchial asthma, or severe chronic obstructive pulmonary disease (see WARNINGS); sinus bradycardia; second and third degree atrioventricular block; overt cardiac failure (see WARNINGS); cardiogenic shock; hypersensitivity to this product.

WARNINGS

Cardiac Failure

Sympathetic stimulation may be essential for support of the circulation in individuals with diminished myocardial contractility, and its inhibition by beta-adrenergic receptor blockade may precipitate more severe failure. Although beta blockers should be avoided in overt congestive heart failure, they can be used, if necessary, with caution in patients with a history of failure who are well-compensated, usually with digitalis and diuretics. Both digitalis and timolol maleate slow AV conduction. If cardiac failure persists, therapy with BLOCADREN should be withdrawn.

In Patients Without a History of Cardiac Failure continued depression of the myocardium with beta-blocking agents over a period of time can, in some cases, lead to cardiac failure. At the first sign or symptom of cardiac failure, patients receiving BLOCADREN should be digitalized and/or be given a diuretic, and the response observed closely. If cardiac failure continues, despite adequate digitalization and diuretic therapy, BLOCADREN should be withdrawn.

Exacerbation of Ischemic Heart Disease Following Abrupt Withdrawal—Hypersensitivity to catecholamines has been observed in patients withdrawn from beta blocker therapy; exacerbation of angina and, in some cases, myocardial infarction have occurred after *abrupt* discontinuation of such therapy. When discontinuing chronically administered timolol maleate, particularly in patients with ischemic heart disease, the dosage should be gradually reduced over a period of one to two weeks and the patient should be carefully monitored. If angina markedly worsens or acute coronary insufficiency develops, timolol maleate administration should be reinstituted promptly, at least temporarily, and other measures appropriate for the management of unstable angina should be taken. Patients should be warned against interruption or discontinuation of therapy without the physician's advice. Because coronary artery disease is common and may be unrecognized, it may be prudent not to discontinue timolol maleate therapy abruptly even in patients treated only for hypertension.

Obstructive Pulmonary Disease

PATIENTS WITH CHRONIC OBSTRUCTIVE PULMONARY DISEASE (e.g., CHRONIC BRONCHITIS, EMPHYSEMA) OF MILD OR MODERATE SEVERITY, BRONCHOSPASTIC DISEASE OR A HISTORY OF BRONCHOSPASTIC DISEASE (OTHER THAN BRONCHIAL ASTHMA OR A HISTORY OF BRONCHIAL ASTHMA, IN WHICH 'BLOCADREN' IS CONTRAINDICATED, see CONTRAINDICATIONS), SHOULD IN GENERAL NOT RECEIVE BETA BLOCKERS, INCLUDING 'BLOCADREN'. However, if BLOCADREN is necessary in such patients, then the drug should be administered with caution since it may block bronchodilation produced by endogenous and exogenous catecholamine stimulation of $beta_2$ receptors.

Major Surgery

The necessity or desirability of withdrawal of beta-blocking therapy prior to major surgery is controversial. Beta-adrenergic receptor blockade impairs the ability of the heart to respond to beta-adrenergically mediated reflex stimuli. This may augment the risk of general anesthesia in surgical procedures. Some patients receiving beta-adrenergic receptor blocking agents have been subject to protracted severe hypotension during anesthesia. Difficulty in restarting and maintaining the heartbeat has also been reported. For these reasons, in patients undergoing elective surgery, some authorities recommend gradual withdrawal of beta-adrenergic receptor blocking agents.

If necessary during surgery, the effects of beta-adrenergic blocking agents may be reversed by sufficient doses of such agonists as isoproterenol, dopamine, dobutamine or levarterenol (see OVERDOSAGE).

Diabetes Mellitus

BLOCADREN should be administered with caution in patients subject to spontaneous hypoglycemia or to diabetic

Continued on next page

Information on the Merck Sharp & Dohme products listed on these pages is the full prescribing information from product circulars in use August 31, 1986.

Merck Sharp & Dohme—Cont.

patients (especially those with labile diabetes) who are receiving insulin or oral hypoglycemic agents. Beta-adrenergic receptor blocking agents may mask the signs and symptoms of acute hypoglycemia.

Thyrotoxicosis

Beta-adrenergic blockade may mask certain clinical signs (e.g., tachycardia) of hyperthyroidism. Patients suspected of developing thyrotoxicosis should be managed carefully to avoid abrupt withdrawal of beta blockade which might precipitate a thyroid storm.

PRECAUTIONS

General

Impaired Hepatic or Renal Function: Since BLOCADREN is partially metabolized in the liver and excreted mainly by the kidneys, dosage reductions may be necessary when hepatic and/or renal insufficiency is present.

Dosing in the Presence of Marked Renal Failure: Although the pharmacokinetics of BLOCADREN are not greatly altered by renal impairment, marked hypotensive responses have been seen in patients with marked renal impairment undergoing dialysis after 20 mg doses. Dosing in such patients should therefore be especially cautious.

Muscle Weakness: Beta-adrenergic blockade has been reported to potentiate muscle weakness consistent with certain myasthenic symptoms (e.g., diplopia, ptosis, and generalized weakness). Timolol has been reported rarely to increase muscle weakness in some patients with myasthenia gravis or myasthenic symptoms.

Cerebrovascular Insufficiency: Because of potential effects of beta-adrenergic blocking agents relative to blood pressure and pulse, these agents should be used with caution in patients with cerebrovascular insufficiency. If signs or symptoms suggesting reduced cerebral blood flow are observed, consideration should be given to discontinuing these agents.

Drug Interactions

Close observation of the patient is recommended when BLOCADREN is administered to patients receiving catecholamine-depleting drugs such as reserpine, because of possible additive effects and the production of hypotension and/or marked bradycardia, which may produce vertigo, syncope, or postural hypotension.

Blunting of the antihypertensive effect of beta-adrenoceptor blocking agents by non-steroidal anti-inflammatory drugs has been reported. When using these agents concomitantly, patients should be observed carefully to confirm that the desired therapeutic effect has been obtained.

Literature reports suggest that oral calcium antagonists may be used in combination with beta-adrenergic blocking agents when heart function is normal, but should be avoided in patients with impaired cardiac function. Hypotension, AV conduction disturbances, and left ventricular failure have been reported in some patients receiving beta-adrenergic blocking agents when an oral calcium antagonist was added to the treatment regimen. Hypotension was more likely to occur if the calcium antagonist were a dihydropyridine derivative, e.g. nifedipine, while left ventricular failure and AV conduction disturbances were more likely to occur with either verapamil or diltiazem.

Intravenous calcium antagonists should be used with caution in patients receiving beta-adrenergic blocking agents.

The concomitant use of beta-adrenergic blocking agents with digitalis and either diltiazem or verapamil may have additive effects in prolonging AV conduction time.

Carcinogenesis, Mutagenesis, Impairment of Fertility

In a two-year study of timolol maleate in rats, there was a statistically significant ($P \leq 0.05$) increase in the incidence of adrenal pheochromocytomas in male rats administered 300 times the maximum recommended human dose (1 mg/kg/day). Similar differences were not observed in rats administered doses equivalent to 25 or 100 times the maximum recommended human dose. In a lifetime study in mice, there were statistically significant ($P \leq 0.05$) increases in the incidence of benign and malignant pulmonary tumors and benign uterine polyps in female mice at 500 mg/kg/day, but not at 5 or 50 mg/kg/day. There was also a significant increase in mammary adenocarcinomas at the 500 mg/kg/day dose. This was associated with elevations in serum prolactin which occurred in female mice administered timolol at 500 mg/kg, but not at doses of 5 or 50 mg/kg/day. An increased incidence of mammary adenocarcinomas in rodents has been associated with administration of several other therapeutic agents which elevate serum prolactin, but no correlation between serum prolactin levels and mammary tumors has been established in man. Furthermore, in adult human female subjects who received oral dosages of up to 60 mg of timolol maleate, the maximum recommended human oral dosage, there were no clinically meaningful changes in serum prolactin.

There was a statistically significant increase ($P \leq 0.05$) in the overall incidence of neoplasms in female mice at the 500 mg/kg/day dosage level.

Timolol maleate was devoid of mutagenic potential when evaluated *in vivo* (mouse) in the micronucleus test and cytogenetic assay (doses up to 800 mg/kg) and *in vitro* in a neoplastic cell transformation assay (up to 100 μg/mL). In Ames tests the highest concentrations of timolol employed, 5000 or 10,000 μg/plate, were associated with statistically significant elevations ($P \leq 0.05$) of revertants observed with tester strain TA100 (in seven replicate assays), but not in the remaining three strains. In the assays with tester strain TA100, no consistent dose response relationship was observed, nor did the ratio of test to control revertants reach 2. A ratio of 2 is usually considered the criterion for a positive Ames test.

Reproduction and fertility studies in rats showed no adverse effect on male or female fertility at doses up to 150 times the maximum recommended human dose.

Pregnancy

Pregnancy Category C. Teratogenicity studies with timolol in mice and rabbits at doses up to 50 mg/kg/day (50 times the maximum recommended human dose) showed no evidence of fetal malformations. Although delayed fetal ossification was observed at this dose in rats, there were no adverse effects on postnatal development of offspring. Doses of 1000 mg/kg/day (1,000 times the maximum recommended human dose) were maternotoxic in mice and resulted in an increased number of fetal resorptions. Increased fetal resorptions were also seen in rabbits at doses of 100 times the maximum recommended human dose, in this case without apparent maternotoxicity. There are no adequate and well-controlled studies in pregnant women. BLOCADREN should be used during pregnancy only if the potential benefit justifies the potential risk to the fetus.

Nursing Mothers

Because of the potential for serious adverse reactions from timolol in nursing infants, a decision should be made whether to discontinue nursing or to discontinue the drug, taking into account the importance of the drug to the mother.

Pediatric Use

Safety and effectiveness in children have not been established.

ADVERSE REACTIONS

BLOCADREN is usually well tolerated in properly selected patients. Most adverse effects have been mild and transient. In a multicenter (12-week) clinical trial comparing timolol maleate and placebo, the following adverse reactions were reported spontaneously and considered to be causally related to timolol maleate:

BLOCADREN	Adverse Reaction†		Withdrawal‡	
	Timolol (n = 945) %	Placebo (n = 939) %	Timolol (n = 945) %	Placebo (n = 939) %
Asthenia or Fatigue	5	1	<1	<1
Heart Rate <40 beats/minute	5	<1	4	<1
Cardiac Failure—Nonfatal	8	7	3	2
Hypotension	3	2	3	1
Pulmonary Edema—Nonfatal	2	<1	<1	<1
Claudication	3	3	1	<1
AV Block 2nd or 3rd degree	<1	<1	<1	<1
Sinoatrial Block	<1	<1	<1	<1
Cold Hands and Feet	8	<1	<1	0
Nausea or Digestive Disorders	8	6	1	<1
Dizziness	6	4	1	0
Bronchial Obstruction	2	<1	1	<1

† When an adverse reaction recurred in a patient, it is listed only once.
‡ Only principal reason for withdrawal in each patient is listed.
These adverse reactions can also occur in patients treated for hypertension.

	Timolol Maleate (n = 176) %	Placebo (n = 168) %
BODY AS A WHOLE		
fatigue/tiredness	3.4	0.6
headache	1.7	1.8
chest pain	0.6	0
asthenia	0.6	0
CARDIOVASCULAR		
bradycardia	9.1	0
arrhythmia	1.1	0.6
syncope	0.6	0
edema	0.6	1.2
DIGESTIVE		
dyspepsia	0.6	0.6
nausea	0.6	0
SKIN		
pruritus	1.1	0
NERVOUS SYSTEM		
dizziness	2.3	1.2
vertigo	0.6	0
paresthesia	0.6	0
PSYCHIATRIC		
decreased libido	0.6	0
RESPIRATORY		
dyspnea	1.7	0.6
bronchial spasm	0.6	0
rales	0.6	0
SPECIAL SENSES		
eye irritation	1.1	0.6
tinnitus	0.6	0

These data are representative of the incidence of adverse effects that may be observed in a properly selected hypertensive patient population, e.g., a group excluding patients with bronchospastic disease, congestive heart failure or other contraindications to beta blocker therapy. These adverse reactions can also occur in patients with coronary artery disease.

In a different population, the coronary artery disease population, studied in the Norwegian multi-center trial (see CLINICAL PHARMACOLOGY), the frequency of the principal adverse reactions and the frequency with which these resulted in discontinuation of therapy in the timolol and placebo groups were:

[See table below].

The following additional adverse effects have been reported in clinical experience with the drug: *Body as a Whole:* extremity pain, decreased exercise tolerance, weight loss; *Cardiovascular:* cardiac arrest, cardiac failure, cerebral vascular accident, worsening of angina pectoris, worsening of arterial insufficiency, Raynaud's phenomenon, palpitations, vasodilatation; *Digestive:* gastrointestinal pain, hepatomegaly, vomiting, diarrhea, dyspepsia; *Hematologic:* nonthrombocytopenic purpura; *Endocrine:* hyperglycemia, hypoglycemia; *Skin:* rash, skin irritation, increased pigmentation, sweating; *Musculoskeletal:* arthralgia; *Nervous System:* local weakness, increase in signs and symptoms of myasthenia gravis; *Psychiatric:* depression, nightmares, somnolence, insomnia, nervousness, diminished concentration, hallucinations; *Respiratory:* cough; *Special Senses:* visual disturbances, diplopia, ptosis, dry eyes; *Urogenital:* impotence, urination difficulties.

There have been reports of retroperitoneal fibrosis in patients receiving timolol maleate and in patients receiving other beta-adrenergic blocking agents. A causal relationship between this condition and therapy with beta-adrenergic blocking agents has not been established.

Potential Adverse Effects: In addition, a variety of adverse effects not observed in clinical trials with BLOCADREN, but reported with other beta-adrenergic blocking agents, should be considered potential adverse effects of BLOCADREN: *Nervous System:* Reversible mental depression progressing to catatonia; an acute reversible syndrome characterized by disorientation for time and place, short-term memory loss, emotional lability, slightly clouded sensorium, and decreased performance on neuropsychometrics; *Cardiovascular:* Intensification of AV block (see CONTRAINDICATIONS); *Digestive:* Mesenteric arterial thrombosis, ischemic colitis; *Hematologic:* Agranulocytosis, thrombocytopenic purpura; *Allergic:* Erythematous rash, fever combined with aching and sore throat, laryngospasm with respiratory distress; *Miscellaneous:* Reversible alopecia, Peyronie's disease.

There have been reports of a syndrome comprising psoriasiform skin rash, conjunctivitis sicca, otitis, and sclerosing serositis attributed to the beta-adrenergic receptor blocking agent, practolol. This syndrome has not been reported with BLOCADREN.

Clinical Laboratory Test Findings: Clinically important changes in standard laboratory parameters were rarely associated with the administration of BLOCADREN. Slight increases in blood urea nitrogen, serum potassium, and serum uric acid, and slight decreases in hemoglobin and hematocrit occurred, but were not progressive or associated with clinical manifestations.

OVERDOSAGE

No data are available in regard to overdosage in humans. The oral LD_{50} of the drug is 1190 and 900 mg/kg in female mice and female rats, respectively.

An *in vitro* hemodialysis study, using ^{14}C timolol added to human plasma or whole blood, showed that timolol was readily dialyzed from these fluids; however, a study of patients with renal failure showed that timolol did not dialyze readily.

The most common signs and symptoms to be expected with overdosage with a beta-adrenergic receptor blocking agent are symptomatic bradycardia, hypotension, bronchospasm, and acute cardiac failure. Therapy with BLOCADREN should be discontinued and the patient observed closely. The following additional therapeutic measures should be considered:

(1) *Gastric lavage*

(2) *Symptomatic bradycardia:* Use atropine sulfate intravenously in a dosage of 0.25 mg to 2 mg to induce vagal blockade. If bradycardia persists, intravenous isoproterenol hydrochloride should be administered cautiously. In refractory cases the use of a transvenous cardiac pacemaker may be considered.

(3) *Hypotension:* Use sympathomimetic pressor drug therapy, such as dopamine, dobutamine or levarterenol. In refractory cases the use of glucagon hydrochloride has been reported to be useful.

(4) *Bronchospasm:* Use isoproterenol hydrochloride. Additional therapy with aminophylline may be considered.

(5) *Acute cardiac failure:* Conventional therapy with digitalis, diuretics, and oxygen should be instituted immediately. In refractory cases the use of intravenous aminophylline is suggested. This may be followed if necessary by glucagon hydrochloride which has been reported to be useful.

(6) *Heart block (second or third degree):* Use isoproterenol hydrochloride or a transvenous cardiac pacemaker.

DOSAGE AND ADMINISTRATION

Hypertension

The usual initial dosage of BLOCADREN is 10 mg twice a day, whether used alone or added to diuretic therapy. Dosage may be increased or decreased depending on heart rate and blood pressure response. The usual total maintenance dosage is 20–40 mg per day. Increases in dosage to a maximum of 60 mg per day divided into two doses may be necessary. There should be an interval of at least seven days between increases in dosages.

BLOCADREN may be used with a thiazide diuretic or with other antihypertensive agents. Patients should be observed carefully during initiation of such concomitant therapy.

Myocardial Infarction

The recommended dosage for long-term prophylactic use in patients who have survived the acute phase of a myocardial infarction is 10 mg given twice daily (see CLINICAL PHARMACOLOGY).

HOW SUPPLIED

No. 3343—Tablets BLOCADREN, 5 mg, are light blue, round, compressed tablets, with code MSD 59 on one side and BLOCADREN on the other. They are supplied as follows:

NDC 0006-0059-68 bottles of 100.

Shown in Product Identification Section, page 417

No. 3344—Tablets BLOCADREN, 10 mg, are light blue, round, scored, compressed tablets, with code MSD 136 on one side and BLOCADREN on the other. They are supplied as follows:

NDC 0006-0136-68 bottles of 100

NDC 0006-0136-28 unit dose packages of 100.

Shown in Product Identification Section, page 417

No. 3371—Tablets BLOCADREN, 20 mg, are light blue, capsule shaped, scored, compressed tablets, with code MSD 437 on one side and BLOCADREN on the other. They are supplied as follows:

NDC 0006-0437-68 bottles of 100.

Shown in Product Identification Section, page 417

Storage

Store in a well-closed container, protected from light.

A.H.F.S. Categories: 24:04, 24:08

DC 7117621 Issued April 1985

CLINORIL® Tablets ℞
(Sulindac, MSD), U.S.P.

DESCRIPTION

Sulindac is a non-steroidal, anti-inflammatory indene derivative designated chemically as (Z)-5-fluoro-2-methyl-1-[[*p*-(methylsulfinyl) phenyl]methylene]-1*H*-indene-3-acetic acid. It is not a salicylate, pyrazolone or propionic acid derivative. Its empirical formula is $C_{20}H_{17}FO_3S$, with a molecular weight of 356.42. Sulindac, a yellow crystalline compound, is a weak organic acid practically insoluble in water below pH 4.5, but very soluble as the sodium salt or in buffers of pH 6 or higher.

CLINORIL® (Sulindac, MSD) is available in 150 and 200 mg tablets for oral administration. Each tablet contains the following inactive ingredients: cellulose, magnesium stearate, starch.

Following absorption, sulindac undergoes two major biotransformations—reversible reduction to the sulfide metabolite, and irreversible oxidation to the sulfone metabolite. Available evidence indicates that the biological activity resides with the sulfide metabolite.

The structural formulas of sulindac and its metabolites are:

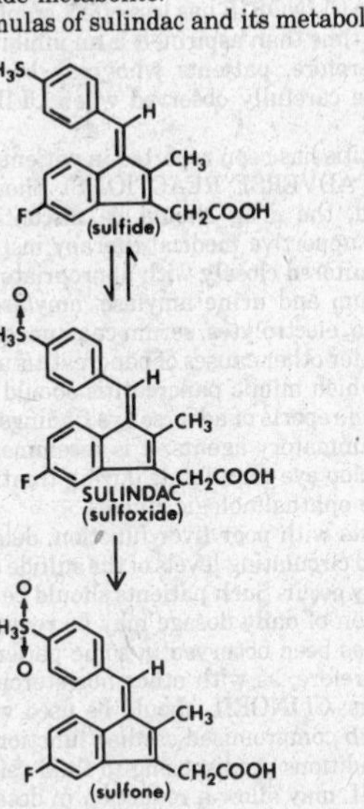

CLINICAL PHARMACOLOGY

CLINORIL is a non-steroidal anti-inflammatory drug, also possessing analgesic and antipyretic activities. Its mode of action, like that of other non-steroidal, anti-inflammatory agents, is not known; however, its therapeutic action is not due to pituitary-adrenal stimulation. Inhibition of prostaglandin synthesis by the sulfide metabolite may be involved in the anti-inflammatory action of CLINORIL.

Sulindac is approximately 90% absorbed in man after oral administration. The peak plasma concentrations of the biologically active sulfide metabolite are achieved in about two hours when sulindac is administered in the fasting state, and in about three to four hours when sulindac is administered with food. The mean half-life of sulindac is 7.8 hours while the mean half-life of the sulfide metabolite is 16.4 hours. Sustained plasma levels of the sulfide metabolite are consistent with a prolonged anti-inflammatory action which is the rationale for a twice per day dosage schedule.

Sulindac and its sulfone metabolite undergo extensive enterohepatic circulation relative to the sulfide metabolite in animals. Similar enterohepatic circulation together with the reversible metabolism are probably major contributors to sustained plasma levels of the active drug in man.

The primary route of excretion in man is via the urine as both sulindac and its sulfone metabolite (free and glucuronide conjugates). Approximately 50% of the administered dose is excreted in the urine, with the conjugated sulfone metabolite accounting for the major portion. Less than 1% of the administered dose of sulindac appears in the urine as the sulfide metabolite. Approximately 25% is found in the feces, primarily as the sulfone and sulfide metabolites.

The bioavailability of sulindac, as assessed by urinary excretion, was not changed by concomitant administration of an antacid containing magnesium and aluminum hydroxides (MAALOX®, William H. Rorer, Inc.).

Because CLINORIL is excreted in the urine primarily as biologically inactive forms, it may possibly affect renal function to a lesser extent than other non-steroidal anti-inflammatory drugs, however, renal adverse experiences have been reported with CLINORIL (see ADVERSE REACTIONS). In a study of patients with chronic glomerular disease treated with therapeutic doses of CLINORIL, no effect was demonstrated on renal blood flow, glomerular filtration rate, or urinary excretion of prostaglandin E_2 and the primary metabolite of prostacyclin, 6-keto-$PGF_{1}\alpha$. However, in other studies in healthy volunteers and patients with liver disease, CLINORIL was found to blunt the renal responses to intravenous furosemide, i.e., the diuresis, natriuresis, increments in plasma renin activity and urinary excretion of prostaglandins. These observations may represent a differentiation of the effects of CLINORIL on renal functions based on differences in pathogenesis of the renal prostaglandin dependence associated with differing dose-response relationships of different NSAIDS to the various renal functions influenced by prostaglandins. These observations need further clarification and in the interim, sulindac should be used with caution in patients whose renal function may be impaired (see PRECAUTIONS).

In healthy men, the average fecal blood loss, measured over a two-week period during administration of 400 mg per day of CLINORIL, was similar to that for placebo, and was statistically significantly less than that resulting from 4800 mg per day of aspirin.

In controlled clinical studies CLINORIL was evaluated in the following five conditions:

1. *Osteoarthritis*

In patients with osteoarthritis of the hip and knee, the anti-inflammatory and analgesic activity of CLINORIL was demonstrated by clinical measurements that included: assessments by both patient and investigator of overall response; decrease in disease activity as assessed by both patient and investigator; improvement in ARA Functional Class; relief of night pain; improvement in overall evaluation of pain, including pain on weight bearing and pain on active and passive motion; improvement in joint mobility, range of motion, and functional activities; decreased swelling and tenderness; and decreased duration of stiffness following prolonged inactivity.

In clinical studies in which dosages were adjusted according to patient needs, CLINORIL 200 to 400 mg daily was shown to be comparable in effectiveness to aspirin 2400 to 4800 mg daily. CLINORIL was generally well tolerated, and patients on it had a lower overall incidence of total adverse effects, of milder gastrointestinal reactions, and of tinnitus than did patients on aspirin. (See ADVERSE REACTIONS.)

2. *Rheumatoid Arthritis*

In patients with rheumatoid arthritis, the anti-inflammatory and analgesic activity of CLINORIL was demonstrated by clinical measurements that included: assessments by both patient and investigator of overall response; decrease in disease activity as assessed by both patient and investigator; reduction in overall joint pain; reduction in duration and severity of morning stiffness; reduction in day and night pain; decrease in time required to walk 50 feet; decrease in general pain as measured on a visual analog scale; improvement in the Ritchie articular index; decrease in proximal interphalangeal joint size; improvement in ARA Functional Class; increase in grip strength; reduction in painful joint count and score; reduction in swollen joint count and score; and increased flexion and extension of the wrist.

In clinical studies in which dosages were adjusted according to patient needs, CLINORIL 300 to 400 mg daily was shown to be comparable in effectiveness to aspirin 3600 to 4800 mg daily. CLINORIL was generally well tolerated, and patients on it had a lower overall incidence of total adverse effects, of milder gastrointestinal reactions, and of tinnitus than did patients on aspirin. (See ADVERSE REACTIONS.)

In patients with rheumatoid arthritis, CLINORIL may be used in combination with gold salts at usual dosage levels. In clinical studies, CLINORIL added to the regimen of gold salts usually resulted in additional symptomatic relief but did not alter the course of the underlying disease.

3. *Ankylosing spondylitis*

In patients with ankylosing spondylitis, the anti-inflammatory and analgesic activity of CLINORIL was demonstrated by clinical measurements that included: assessments by both patient and investigator of overall response; decrease in disease activity as assessed by both patient and investigator; improvement in ARA Functional Class; improvement in patient and investigator evaluation of spinal pain, tenderness and/or spasm; reduction in the duration of morning stiffness; increase in the time to onset of fatigue; relief of night pain; increase in chest expansion; and increase in spinal mobility evaluated by fingers-to-floor distance, occiput to wall distance, the Schober Test, and the Wright Modification of the Schober Test. In a clinical study in which dosages were adjusted according to patient need, CLINORIL 200 to 400 mg daily was as effective as indomethacin 75 to 150 mg daily. In a second study, CLINORIL 300 to 400 mg daily was comparable in effectiveness to phenylbutazone 400 to 600 mg daily. CLINORIL was better tolerated than phenylbutazone. (See ADVERSE REACTIONS.)

4. *Acute painful shoulder (Acute subacromial bursitis/supraspinatus tendinitis)*

In patients with acute painful shoulder (acute subacromial bursitis/supraspinatus tendinitis), the anti-inflammatory and analgesic activity of CLINORIL was demonstrated by clinical measurements that included: assessments by both patient and investigator of overall response; relief of night

Continued on next page

Information on the Merck Sharp & Dohme products listed on these pages is the full prescribing information from product circulars in use August 31, 1986.

Merck Sharp & Dohme—Cont.

pain, spontaneous pain, and pain on active motion; decrease in local tenderness; and improvement in range of motion measured by abduction, and internal and external rotation. In clinical studies in acute painful shoulder, CLINORIL 300 to 400 mg daily and oxyphenbutazone 400 to 600 mg daily were shown to be equally effective and well tolerated.

5. *Acute gouty arthritis*

In patients with acute gouty arthritis, the anti-inflammatory and analgesic activity of CLINORIL was demonstrated by clinical measurements that included: assessments by both the patient and investigator of overall response; relief of weight-bearing pain; relief of pain at rest and on active and passive motion; decrease in tenderness; reduction in warmth and swelling; increase in range of motion; and improvement in ability to function. In clinical studies, CLINORIL at 400 mg daily and phenylbutazone at 600 mg daily were shown to be equally effective. In these short-term studies in which reduction of dosage was permitted according to response, both drugs were equally well tolerated.

INDICATIONS AND USAGE

CLINORIL is indicated for acute or long-term use in the relief of signs and symptoms of the following:

1. Osteoarthritis
2. Rheumatoid arthritis*
3. Ankylosing spondylitis
4. Acute painful shoulder (Acute subacromial bursitis/supraspinatus tendinitis)
5. Acute gouty arthritis

CONTRAINDICATIONS

CLINORIL should not be used in:

Patients who are hypersensitive to this product.

Patients in whom acute asthmatic attacks, urticaria, or rhinitis are precipitated by aspirin or other non-steroidal anti-inflammatory agents.

WARNINGS

Peptic ulceration and gastrointestinal bleeding have been reported in patients receiving CLINORIL. Fatalities have occurred. Gastrointestinal bleeding is associated with higher morbidity and mortality in labile patients such as the elderly, patients with hemorrhagic disorders, etc. In patients with active gastrointestinal bleeding or an active peptic ulcer, an appropriate ulcer regimen should be instituted, and the physician must weigh the benefits of therapy with CLINORIL against possible hazards, and carefully monitor the patient's progress. When CLINORIL is given to patients with a history of either upper or lower gastrointestinal tract disease, it should be given under close supervision and only after consulting the ADVERSE REACTIONS section.

Rarely, fever and other evidence of hypersensitivity (see ADVERSE REACTIONS) including abnormalities in one or more liver function tests and severe skin reactions have occurred during therapy with CLINORIL. Fatalities have occurred in these patients. Hepatitis, jaundice, or both, with or without fever, may occur usually within the first one to three months of therapy. Determinations of liver function should be considered whenever a patient on therapy with CLINORIL develops unexplained fever, rash or other dermatologic reactions or constitutional symptoms. If unexplained fever or other evidence of hypersensitivity occurs, therapy with CLINORIL should be discontinued. The elevated temperature and abnormalities in liver function caused by CLINORIL characteristically have reverted to normal after discontinuation of therapy. Administration of CLINORIL should not be reinstituted in such patients.

In addition to hypersensitivity reactions involving the liver, in some patients the findings are consistent with those of cholestatic hepatitis. As with other non-steroidal anti-inflammatory drugs, borderline elevations of one or more liver tests without any other signs and symptoms may occur in up to 15% of patients. These abnormalities may progress, may remain essentially unchanged, or may be transient with continued therapy. The SGPT (ALT) test is probably the most sensitive indicator of liver dysfunction. Meaningful (3 times the upper limit of normal) elevations of SGPT or SGOT (AST) occurred in controlled clinical trials in less than 1% of patients. A patient with symptoms and/or signs suggesting liver dysfunction, or in whom an abnormal liver test has occurred, should be evaluated for evidence of the development of more severe hepatic reaction while on therapy with CLINORIL. Although such reactions as described above are rare, if abnormal liver tests persist or worsen, if clinical signs and symptoms consistent with liver disease develop, or if systemic manifestations occur (e.g. eosinophilia, rash, etc.), CLINORIL should be discontinued.

In clinical trials with CLINORIL, the use of doses of 600 mg/day has been associated with an increased incidence of mild liver test abnormalities (see DOSAGE AND ADMINISTRATION for maximum dosage recommendation).

PRECAUTIONS

General

Although CLINORIL has less effect on platelet function and bleeding time than aspirin, it is an inhibitor of platelet function; therefore, patients who may be adversely affected should be carefully observed when CLINORIL is administered.

Pancreatitis has been reported in patients receiving CLINORIL (see ADVERSE REACTIONS). Should pancreatitis be suspected, the drug should be discontinued and not restarted, supportive medical therapy instituted, and the patient monitored closely with appropriate laboratory studies (e.g., serum and urine amylase, amylase/creatinine clearance ratio, electrolytes, serum calcium, glucose, lipase, etc.). A search for other causes of pancreatitis as well as those conditions which mimic pancreatitis should be conducted.

Because of reports of adverse eye findings with non-steroidal anti-inflammatory agents, it is recommended that patients who develop eye complaints during treatment with CLINORIL have ophthalmologic studies.

In patients with poor liver function, delayed, elevated and prolonged circulating levels of the sulfide and sulfone metabolites may occur. Such patients should be monitored closely; a reduction of daily dosage may be required.

Edema has been observed in some patients taking CLINORIL. Therefore, as with other non-steroidal anti-inflammatory drugs, CLINORIL should be used with caution in patients with compromised cardiac function, hypertension, or other conditions predisposing to fluid retention.

CLINORIL may allow a reduction in dosage or the elimination of chronic corticosteroid therapy in some patients with rheumatoid arthritis. However, it is generally necessary to reduce corticosteroids gradually over several months in order to avoid an exacerbation of disease or signs and symptoms of adrenal insufficiency. Abrupt withdrawal of chronic corticosteroid treatment is generally not recommended even when patients have had a serious complication of chronic corticosteroid therapy.

Renal Effects

As with other non-steroidal anti-inflammatory drugs, long term administration of sulindac to animals has resulted in renal papillary necrosis and other abnormal renal pathology. In humans, there have been reports of acute interstitial nephritis with hematuria, proteinuria, and occasionally nephrotic syndrome.

A second form of renal toxicity has been seen in patients with prerenal and renal conditions leading to a reduction in renal blood flow or blood volume, where the renal prostaglandins have a supportive role in the maintenance of renal perfusion. In these patients administration of an NSAID may cause a dose dependent reduction in prostaglandin formation and may precipitate overt renal decompensation. CLINORIL may affect renal function less than other NSAIDs in patients with chronic glomerular renal disease (see CLINICAL PHARMACOLOGY). Until these observations are better understood and clarified, however, and because renal adverse experiences have been reported with CLINORIL (see ADVERSE REACTIONS), caution should be exercised when administering the drug to patients with conditions associated with increased risk of the effects of non-steroidal anti-inflammatory drugs on renal function, such as those with renal or hepatic dysfunction, complications associated with advanced age, extracellular volume depletion from any cause, congestive heart failure, sepsis, or concomitant use of any nephrotoxic drug. Discontinuation of NSAID therapy is typically followed by recovery to the pretreatment state.

Since CLINORIL is eliminated primarily by the kidneys, patients with significantly impaired renal function should be closely monitored; a lower daily dosage should be anticipated to avoid excessive drug accumulation.

Use in Pregnancy

CLINORIL is not recommended for use in pregnant women, since safety for use has not been established, and because of the known effect of drugs of this class on the human fetal cardiovascular system (closure of the ductus arteriosus) during the third trimester of pregnancy. In reproduction studies in the rat, a decrease in average fetal weight and an increase in numbers of dead pups were observed on the first day of the postpartum period at dosage levels of 20 and 40 mg/kg/day ($2\frac{1}{2}$ and 5 times the usual maximum daily dose in humans), although there was no adverse effect on the survival and growth during the remainder of the postpartum period. CLINORIL prolongs the duration of gestation in rats, as do other compounds of this class which also may cause dystocia and delayed parturition in pregnant animals. Visceral and skeletal malformations observed in low incidence among rabbits in some teratology studies did not occur at the same dosage levels in repeat studies, nor at a higher dosage level in the same species.

Nursing Mothers

Nursing should not be undertaken while a patient is on CLINORIL. It is not known whether sulindac is secreted in human milk; however, it is secreted in the milk of lactating rats.

Use in Children

Pediatric indications and dosage have not been established, but studies in juvenile rheumatoid arthritis are in progress.

Drug Interactions

DMSO should not be used with sulindac. Concomitant administration has been reported to reduce the plasma levels of the active sulfide metabolite and potentially reduce efficacy. In addition, this combination has been reported to cause peripheral neuropathy.

Although sulindac and its sulfide metabolite are highly bound to protein, studies, in which CLINORIL was given at a dose of 400 mg daily, have shown no clinically significant interaction with oral anticoagulants or oral hypoglycemic agents. However, patients should be monitored carefully until it is certain that no change in their anticoagulant or hypoglycemic dosage is required. Special attention should be paid to patients taking higher doses than those recommended and to patients with renal impairment or other metabolic defects that might increase sulindac blood levels.

The concomitant administration of aspirin with sulindac significantly depressed the plasma levels of the active sulfide metabolite. A double-blind study compared the safety and efficacy of CLINORIL 300 or 400 mg daily given alone or with aspirin 2.4 g/day for the treatment of osteoarthritis. The addition of aspirin did not alter the types of clinical or laboratory adverse experiences for CLINORIL; however, the combination showed an increase in the incidence of gastrointestinal adverse experiences. Since the addition of aspirin did not have a favorable effect on the therapeutic response to CLINORIL, the combination is not recommended.

The concomitant administration of CLINORIL and diflunisal in normal volunteers resulted in lowering of the plasma levels of the active sulindac sulfide metabolite by approximately one-third.

Probenecid given concomitantly with sulindac had only a slight effect on plasma sulfide levels, while plasma levels of sulindac and sulfone were increased. Sulindac was shown to produce a modest reduction in the uricosuric action of probenecid, which probably is not significant under most circumstances.

Neither propoxyphene hydrochloride nor acetaminophen had any effect on the plasma levels of sulindac or its sulfide metabolite.

ADVERSE REACTIONS

The following adverse reactions were reported in clinical trials or have been reported since the drug was marketed. The probability exists of a causal relationship between CLINORIL and these adverse reactions. The adverse reactions which have been observed in clinical trials encompass observations in 1,865 patients, including 232 observed for at least 48 weeks.

Incidence Greater Than 1%

Gastrointestinal

The most frequent types of adverse reactions occurring with CLINORIL are gastrointestinal; these include gastrointestinal pain (10%), dyspepsia*, nausea* with or without vomiting, diarrhea*, constipation*, flatulence, anorexia and gastrointestinal cramps.

Dermatologic

Rash*, pruritus.

Central Nervous System

Dizziness*, headache*, nervousness.

Special Senses

Tinnitus.

Miscellaneous

Edema (see PRECAUTIONS).

Incidence Less Than 1 in 100

Gastrointestinal

Gastritis or gastroenteritis. Peptic ulcer and gastrointestinal bleeding have been reported. GI perforation has been reported rarely.

Liver function abnormalities; jaundice, sometimes with fever; cholestasis; hepatitis.

Pancreatitis (see PRECAUTIONS).

Dermatologic

Stomatitis, sore or dry mucous membranes, alopecia, photosensitivity.

---

* The safety and effectiveness of CLINORIL have not been established in rheumatoid arthritis patients who are designated in the American Rheumatism Association classification as Functional Class IV (incapacitated, largely or wholly bedridden, or confined to wheelchair; little or no self-care).

* Incidence between 3% and 9%. Those reactions occurring in 1 to 3% of patients are not marked with an asterisk.

Erythema multiforme, toxic epidermal necrolysis, Stevens-Johnson syndrome, and exfoliative dermatitis have been reported.

Cardiovascular

Congestive heart failure, especially in patients with marginal cardiac function; palpitation; hypertension.

Hematologic

Thrombocytopenia; ecchymosis; purpura; leukopenia; agranulocytosis; neutropenia; bone marrow depression, including aplastic anemia; hemolytic anemia; increased prothrombin time in patients on oral anticoagulants (see PRECAUTIONS).

Genitourinary

Urine discoloration; vaginal bleeding; hematuria; proteinuria; renal impairment, including renal failure; interstitial nephritis; nephrotic syndrome.

Psychiatric

Depression; psychic disturbances including acute psychosis.

Nervous System

Vertigo; insomnia; paresthesia; convulsions; syncope; aseptic meningitis.

Special Senses

Blurred vision; decreased hearing; metallic or bitter taste.

Respiratory

Epistaxis.

Hypersensitivity Reactions

Anaphylaxis and angioneurotic edema.

A potentially fatal apparent hypersensitivity syndrome has been reported. This syndrome may include constitutional symptoms (fever, chills), cutaneous findings (rash or other dermatologic reactions—see above), involvement of major organs (changes in liver function, jaundice, pancreatitis, pneumonitis, leukopenia, eosinophilia, anemia, renal impairment, including renal failure), and other less specific findings (adenitis, arthralgia, fatigue, chest pain).

Causal Relationship Unknown

Other reactions have been reported in clinical trials or since the drug was marketed, but occurred under circumstances where a causal relationship could not be established. However, in these rarely reported events, that possibility cannot be excluded. Therefore, these observations are listed to serve as alerting information to physicians.

Metabolic

Hyperglycemia.

Nervous System

Neuritis.

Special Senses

Transient visual disturbances.

Miscellaneous.

Gynecomastia.

MANAGEMENT OF OVERDOSAGE

Cases of overdosage have been reported and rarely, deaths have occurred. The following signs and symptoms may be observed following overdosage: stupor, coma, diminished urine output and hypotension.

In the event of overdosage, the stomach should be emptied by inducing vomiting or by gastric lavage, and the patient carefully observed and given symptomatic and supportive treatment.

Animal studies show that absorption is decreased by the prompt administration of activated charcoal and excretion is enhanced by alkalinization of the urine.

DOSAGE AND ADMINISTRATION

CLINORIL should be administered orally twice a day with food. The maximum dosage is 400 mg per day. Dosages above 400 mg per day are not recommended.

In osteoarthritis, rheumatoid arthritis, and ankylosing spondylitis, the recommended starting dosage is 150 mg twice a day. The dosage may be lowered or raised depending on the response.

A prompt response (within one week) can be expected in about one-half of patients with osteoarthritis, ankylosing spondylitis, and rheumatoid arthritis. Others may require longer to respond.

In acute painful shoulder (acute subacromial bursitis/supraspinatus tendinitis) and acute gouty arthritis, the recommended dosage is 200 mg twice a day. After a satisfactory response has been achieved, the dosage may be reduced according to the response. In acute painful shoulder, therapy for 7–14 days is usually adequate. In acute gouty arthritis, therapy for 7 days is usually adequate.

HOW SUPPLIED

No. 3360—Tablets CLINORIL 150 mg are yellow, hexagon-shaped, compressed tablets, coded MSD 941. They are supplied as follows:

NDC 0006-0941-54 unit of use bottles of 60
NDC 0006-0941-68 in bottles of 100
NDC 0006-0941-78 unit of use bottles of 100
NDC 0006-0941-28 unit dose packages of 100.

Shown in Product Identification Section, page 417

No. 3353—Tablets CLINORIL 200 mg are yellow, hexagon-shaped, scored, compressed tablets, coded MSD 942. They are supplied as follows:

NDC 0006-0942-54 unit of use bottles of 60
NDC 0006-0942-68 in bottles of 100
NDC 0006-0942-78 unit of use bottles of 100
NDC 0006-0942-28 unit dose packages of 100.

Shown in Product Identification Section, page 417

A.H.F.S. Category: 28:08
DC 7020021 Issued August 1985

COGENTIN® Tablets ℞
(Benztropine Mesylate, MSD), U.S.P.
COGENTIN® Injection ℞
(Benztropine Mesylate, MSD), U.S.P.

DESCRIPTION

Benztropine mesylate is a synthetic compound resulting from the combination of the active portions of atropine and diphenhydramine.

It is a crystalline white powder, very soluble in water, with the following structural formula:

COGENTIN® (Benztropine Mesylate, MSD) is supplied as tablets in three strengths (0.5 mg, 1 mg, and 2 mg per tablet), and as an injection for intravenous and intramuscular use.

Tablets COGENTIN contain 0.5, 1 or 2 mg of benztropine mesylate. Each tablet contains the following inactive ingredients: calcium phosphate, cellulose, lactose, magnesium stearate and starch.

Each milliliter of the injection contains:

Benztropine mesylate	1.0 mg
Sodium chloride	9.0 mg
Water for injection q.s.	1.0 mL

ACTIONS

COGENTIN possesses both anticholinergic and antihistaminic effects, although only the former have been established as therapeutically significant in the management of parkinsonism.

In the isolated guinea pig ileum, the anticholinergic activity of this drug is about equal to that of atropine; however, when administered orally to unanesthetized cats, it is only about half as active as atropine.

In laboratory animals, its antihistaminic activity and duration of action approach those of pyrilamine maleate.

INDICATIONS

For use as an adjunct in the therapy of all forms of parkinsonism.

Useful also in the control of extrapyramidal disorders (except tardive dyskinesia—see PRECAUTIONS) due to neuroleptic drugs (e.g., phenothiazines).

CONTRAINDICATIONS

Hypersensitivity to COGENTIN tablets or to any component of COGENTIN injection.

Because of its atropine-like side effects, this drug is contraindicated in children under three years of age, and should be used with caution in older children.

WARNINGS

Safe use in pregnancy has not been established.

COGENTIN may impair mental and/or physical abilities required for performance of hazardous tasks, such as operating machinery or driving a motor vehicle.

When COGENTIN is given concomitantly with phenothiazines or other drugs with anticholinergic activity, patients should be advised to report gastrointestinal complaints promptly. Paralytic ileus, sometimes fatal, has occurred in patients taking anticholinergic-type antiparkinsonism drugs, including COGENTIN, in combination with phenothiazines and/or tricyclic antidepressants.

Since COGENTIN contains structural features of atropine, it may produce anhidrosis. For this reason, it should be administered with caution during hot weather, especially when given concomitantly with other atropine-like drugs to the chronically ill, the alcoholic, those who have central nervous system disease, and those who do manual labor in a hot environment. Anhidrosis may occur more readily when some disturbance of sweating already exists. If there is evidence of anhidrosis, the possibility of hyperthermia should be considered. Dosage should be decreased at the discretion of the physician so that the ability to maintain body heat equilibrium by perspiration is not impaired. Severe anhidrosis and fatal hyperthermia have occurred.

PRECAUTIONS

Since COGENTIN has cumulative action, continued supervision is advisable. Patients with a tendency to tachycardia and patients with prostatic hypertrophy should be observed closely during treatment.

Dysuria may occur, but rarely becomes a problem. Urinary retention has been reported with COGENTIN.

The drug may cause complaints of weakness and inability to move particular muscle groups, especially in large doses. For example, if the neck has been rigid and suddenly relaxes, it may feel weak, causing some concern. In this event, dosage adjustment is required.

Mental confusion and excitement may occur with large doses, or in susceptible patients. Visual hallucinations have been reported occasionally. Furthermore, in the treatment of extrapyramidal disorders due to neuroleptic drugs (e.g., phenothiazines), in patients with mental disorders, occasionally there may be intensification of mental symptoms. In such cases, antiparkinsonian drugs can precipitate a toxic psychosis. Patients wiith mental disorders should be kept under careful observation, especially at the beginning of treatment or if dosage is increased.

Tardive dyskinesia may appear in some patients on long-term therapy with phenothiazines and related agents, or may occur after therapy with these drugs has been discontinued. Antiparkinsonism agents do not alleviate the symptoms of tardive dyskinesia, and in some instances may aggravate them. COGENTIN is not recommended for use in patients with tardive dyskinesia.

The physician should be aware of the possible occurrence of glaucoma. Although the drug does not appear to have any adverse effect on simple glaucoma, it probably should not be used in angle-closure glaucoma.

ADVERSE REACTIONS

The adverse reactions below, most of which are anticholinergic in nature, have been reported and within each category are listed in order of decreasing severity.

Cardiovascular

Tachycardia.

Digestive

Constipation, dry mouth, nausea, vomiting.

If dry mouth is so severe that there is difficulty in swallowing or speaking, or loss of appetite and weight, reduce dosage, or discontinue the drug temporarily.

Slight reduction in dosage may control nausea and still give sufficient relief of symptoms. Vomiting may be controlled by temporary discontinuation, followed by resumption at a lower dosage.

Nervous System

Toxic psychosis, including confusion, disorientation, memory impairment, visual hallucinations; exacerbation of pre-existing psychotic symptoms; nervousness; depression; listlessness; numbness of fingers.

Special Senses

Blurred vision, dilated pupils.

Urogenital

Urinary retention, dysuria.

Metabolic/Immune or Skin

Occasionally, an allergic reaction, e.g., skin rash, develops. If this can not be controlled by dosage reduction, the medication should be discontinued.

DOSAGE AND ADMINISTRATION

COGENTIN tablets should be used when patients are able to take oral medication.

The injection is especially useful for psychotic patients with acute dystonic reactions or other reactions that make oral medication difficult or impossible. It is recommended also when a more rapid response is desired than can be obtained with the tablets.

Since there is no significant difference in onset of effect after intravenous or intramuscular injection, usually there is no need to use the intravenous route. The drug is quickly effective after either route, with improvement sometimes notice-

Continued on next page

Information on the Merck Sharp & Dohme products listed on these pages is the full prescribing information from product circulars in use August 31, 1986.

Merck Sharp & Dohme—Cont.

able a few minutes after injection. In emergency situations, when the condition of the patient is alarming, 1 to 2 mL of the injection normally will provide quick relief. If the parkinsonian effect begins to return, the dose can be repeated.
Because of cumulative action, therapy should be initiated with a low dose which is increased gradually at five or six-day intervals to the smallest amount necessary for optimal relief. Increases should be made in increments of 0.5 mg, to a maximum of 6 mg, or until optimal results are obtained without excessive adverse reactions.

Postencephalitic and
Idiopathic Parkinsonism—
The usual daily dose is 1 to 2 mg, with a range of 0.5 to 6 mg orally or parenterally.
As with any agent used in parkinsonism, dosage must be individualized according to age and weight, and the type of parkinsonism being treated. Generally, older patients and thin patients cannot tolerate large doses. Most patients with postencephalitic parkinsonism need fairly large doses and tolerate them well. Patients with a poor mental outlook are usually poor candidates for therapy.
In idiopathic parkinsonism, therapy may be initiated with a single daily dose of 0.5 to 1 mg at bedtime. In some patients, this will be adequate; in others 4 to 6 mg a day may be required.
In postencephalitic parkinsonism, therapy may be initiated in most patients with 2 mg a day in one or more doses. In highly sensitive patients, therapy may be initiated with 0.5 mg at bedtime, and increased as necessary.
Some patients experience greatest relief by taking the entire dose at bedtime; others react more favorably to divided doses, two to four times a day. Frequently, one dose a day is sufficient, and divided doses may be unnecessary or undesirable.
The long duration of action of this drug makes it particularly suitable for bedtime medication when its effects may last throughout the night, enabling patients to turn in bed during the night more easily, and to rise in the morning.
When COGENTIN is started, do not terminate therapy with other antiparkinsonian agents abruptly. If the other agents are to be reduced or discontinued, it must be done gradually. Many patients obtain greatest relief with combination therapy.
COGENTIN may be used concomitantly with SINEMET® (Carbidopa-Levodopa, MSD), or with levodopa, in which case periodic dosage adjustment may be required in order to maintain optimum response.

Drug-Induced Extrapyramidal Disorders—In treating extrapyramidal disorders due to neuroleptic drugs (e.g., phenothiazines), the recommended dosage is 1 to 4 mg once or twice a day orally or parenterally. Dosage must be individualized according to the need of the patient. Some patients require more than recommended; others do not need as much.
In acute dystonic reactions, 1 to 2 mL of the injection usually relieves the condition quickly. After that, the tablets, 1 to 2 mg twice a day, usually prevent recurrence.
When extrapyramidal disorders develop soon after initiation of treatment with neuroleptic drugs (e.g., phenothiazines), they are likely to be transient. One to 2 mg of COGENTIN tablets two or three times a day usually provides relief within one or two days. After one or two weeks, the drug should be withdrawn to determine the continued need for it. If such disorders recur, COGENTIN can be reinstituted.
Certain drug-induced extrapyramidal disorders that develop slowly may not respond to COGENTIN.

OVERDOSAGE

Manifestations—May be any of those seen in atropine poisoning or antihistamine overdosage: CNS depression, preceded or followed by stimulation; confusion; nervousness; listlessness; intensification of mental symptoms or toxic psychosis in patients with mental illness being treated with neuroleptic drugs (e.g., phenothiazines); hallucinations (especially visual); dizziness; muscle weakness; ataxia; dry mouth; mydriasis; blurred vision; palpitations; tachycardia; nausea; vomiting; dysuria; numbness of fingers; dysphagia; allergic reactions, e.g., skin rash; headache; hot, dry, flushed skin; delirium; coma; shock; convulsions; respiratory arrest; anhidrosis; hyperthermia; glaucoma; constipation.
Treatment—Physostigmine salicylate, 1 to 2 mg, SC or IV, reportedly will reverse symptoms of anticholinergic intoxication (Duvoisin, R.C.; Katz, R.: J. Amer. Med. Ass. *206*:1963-1965, Nov. 25, 1968). A second injection may be given after 2 hours if required. Otherwise treatment is symptomatic and supportive. Induce emesis or perform gastric lavage (contraindicated in precomatose, convulsive, or psychotic states). Maintain respiration. A short-acting barbiturate may be used for CNS excitement, but with caution to avoid subsequent depression; supportive care for depression (avoid convulsant stimulants such as picrotoxin, pentylenetetrazol, or bemegride); artificial respiration for severe respiratory depression; a local miotic for mydriasis and cycloplegia; ice bags or other cold applications and alcohol sponges for hyperpyrexia, a vasopressor and fluids for circulatory collapse. Darken room for photophobia.

HOW SUPPLIED

No. 3297—Tablets COGENTIN, 0.5 mg, are white, round, scored, compressed tablets, coded MSD 21. They are supplied as follows:
NDC 0006-0021-68 in bottles of 100.
Shown in Product Identification Section, page 417
No. 3334—Tablets COGENTIN, 1 mg, are white, oval shaped, scored, compressed tablets, coded MSD 635. They are supplied as follows:
NDC 0006-0635-68 in bottles of 100
NDC 0006-0635-28 unit dose packages of 100.
Shown in Product Identification Section, page 417
No. 3172—Tablets COGENTIN, 2 mg, are white, round, scored, compressed tablets, coded MSD 60. They are supplied as follows:
NDC 0006-0060-68 in bottles of 100
(6505-00-680-1907, 2 mg 100's)
NDC 0006-0060-28 unit dose packages of 100
NDC 0006-0060-82 in bottles of 1000.
Shown in Product Identification Section, page 417
No. 3275—Injection COGENTIN, 1 mg per mL, is a clear, colorless solution and is supplied as follows:
NDC 0006-3275-16 in boxes of 6×2 mL ampuls.
A.H.F.S. Category: 12:08
DC 6460715 Issued July 1985

ColBENEMID® Tablets ℞
(Probenecid-Colchicine, MSD), U.S.P.

DESCRIPTION

ColBENEMID® (Probenecid-Colchicine, MSD) contains BENEMID® (Probenecid, MSD) and colchicine.
Probenecid is the generic name for 4-[(dipropylamino) sulfonyl] benzoic acid (molecular weight 285.36). It has the following structural formula:

$$(CH_3CH_2CH_2)_2NSO_2-C_6H_4-COOH$$

Probenecid is a white or nearly white, fine, crystalline powder. It is soluble in dilute alkali, in alcohol, in chloroform, and in acetone; it is practically insoluble in water and in dilute acids.
Colchicine is an alkaloid obtained from various species of Colchicum. The chemical name for colchicine is (*S*)-*N*-(5,6,7,9-tetrahydro-1,2,3,10-tetramethoxy-9-oxobenzo [*a*] heptalen-7-yl) acetamide (molecular weight 399.43). It has the following structural formula:

[Structural formula: CH_3O, CH_3O, CH_3O, $NHCOCH_3$, O, OCH_3]

Colchicine consists of pale yellow scales or powder; it darkens on exposure to light. Colchicine is soluble in water, freely soluble in alcohol and in chloroform, and slightly soluble in ether.
Each tablet contains 0.5 g probenecid and 0.5 mg colchicine and the following inactive ingredients: calcium stearate, gelatin, magnesium carbonate, starch.

ACTIONS

Probenecid is a uricosuric and renal tubular blocking agent. It inhibits the tubular reabsorption of urate, thus increasing the urinary excretion of uric acid and decreasing serum urate levels. Effective uricosuria reduces the miscible urate pool, retards urate deposition, and promotes resorption of urate deposits.
Probenecid inhibits the tubular secretion of penicillin and usually increases penicillin plasma levels by any route the antibiotic is given. A 2-fold to 4-fold elevation has been demonstrated for various penicillins.
Probenecid also has been reported to inhibit the renal transport of many other compounds including aminohippuric acid (PAH), aminosalicylic acid (PAS), indomethacin, sodium iodomethamate and related iodinated organic acids, 17-ketosteroids, pantothenic acid, phenolsulfonphthalein (PSP), sulfonamides, and sulfonylureas. See also DRUG INTERACTIONS.
Probenecid decreases both hepatic and renal excretion of sulfobromophthalein (BSP). The tubular reabsorption of phosphorus is inhibited in hypoparathyroid but not in euparathyroid individuals.
Probenecid does not influence plasma concentrations of salicylates, nor the excretion of streptomycin, chloramphenicol, chlortetracycline, oxytetracycline, or neomycin.
The mode of action of colchicine in gout is unknown. It is not an analgesic, though it relieves pain in acute attacks of gout. It is not a uricosuric agent and will not prevent progression of gout to chronic gouty arthritis. It does have a prophylactic, suppressive effect that helps to reduce the incidence of acute attacks and to relieve the residual pain and mild discomfort that patients with gout occasionally feel.
In man and certain other animals, colchicine can produce a temporary leukopenia that is followed by leukocytosis.
Colchicine has other pharmacologic actions in animals: It alters neuromuscular function, intensifies gastrointestinal activity by neurogenic stimulation, increases sensitivity to central depressants, heightens response to sympathomimetic compounds, depresses the respiratory center, constricts blood vessels, causes hypertension by central vasomotor stimulation, and lowers body temperature.

INDICATIONS

For the treatment of chronic gouty arthritis when complicated by frequent, recurrent acute attacks of gout.

CONTRAINDICATIONS

Hypersensitivity to this product or to probenecid or colchicine.
Children under 2 years of age.
Not recommended in persons with known blood dyscrasias or uric acid kidney stones.
Therapy with ColBENEMID should not be started until an acute gouty attack has subsided.
Pregnancy: Probenecid crosses the placental barrier and appears in cord blood. Colchicine can arrest cell division in animals and plants. In certain species of animal under certain conditions, colchicine has produced teratogenic effects. The possibility of such effects in humans also has been reported. Because of the colchicine component, ColBENEMID is contraindicated in pregnant patients. The use of any drug in women of childbearing potential requires that the anticipated benefit be weighed against possible hazards.

WARNINGS

Exacerbation of gout following therapy with ColBENEMID may occur; in such cases additional colchicine or other appropriate therapy is advisable.
Probenecid increases plasma concentrations of methotrexate in both animals and humans. In animal studies, increased methotrexate toxicity has been reported. If ColBENEMID is given with methotrexate, the dosage of methotrexate should be reduced and serum levels may need to be monitored.
In patients on ColBENEMID the use of salicylates in either small or large doses is contraindicated because it antagonizes the uricosuric action of probenecid. The biphasic action of salicylates in the renal tubules accounts for the so-called "paradoxical effect" of uricosuric agents. In patients on ColBENEMID who require a mild analgesic agent the use of acetaminophen rather than small doses of salicylates would be preferred.
Rarely, severe allergic reactions and anaphylaxis have been reported with the use of ColBENEMID. Most of these have been reported to occur within several hours after readministration following prior usage of the drug.
The appearance of hypersensitivity reactions requires cessation of therapy with ColBENEMID.
Colchicine has been reported to adversely affect spermatogenesis in animals. Reversible azoospermia has been reported in one patient.

PRECAUTIONS

General
Hematuria, renal colic, costovertebral pain, and formation of uric acid stones associated with the use of ColBENEMID in gouty patients may be prevented by alkalization of the urine and a liberal fluid intake (*see* DOSAGE AND ADMINISTRATION). In these cases when alkali is administered, the acid-base balance of the patient should be watched.
Use with caution in patients with a history of peptic ulcer.
ColBENEMID has been used in patients with some renal impairment but dosage requirements may be increased. ColBENEMID may not be effective in chronic renal insufficiency particularly when the glomerular filtration rate is 30 mL/minute or less.
A reducing substance may appear in the urine of patients receiving probenecid. This disappears with discontinuance of therapy. Suspected glycosuria should be confirmed by using a test specific for glucose.
Adequate animal studies have not been conducted to determine the carcinogenicity potential of probenecid or this drug combination. Since colchicine is an established mutagen, its

ability to act as a carcinogen must be suspected and administration of ColBENEMID should involve a weighing of the benefit-vs-risk when long-term administration is contemplated.

Drug Interactions

When probenecid is used to elevate plasma concentrations of penicillin, or other beta-lactams, or when such drugs are given to patients taking probenecid therapeutically, high plasma concentrations of the other drug may increase the incidence of adverse reactions associated with that drug. In the case of penicillin, or other beta-lactams, psychic disturbances have been reported.

The use of salicylates antagonizes the uricosuric action of probenecid (*see* WARNINGS). The uricosuric action of probenecid is also antagonized by pyrazinamide.

Probenecid produces an insignificant increase in free sulfonamide plasma concentrations but a significant increase in total sulfonamide plasma levels. Since probenecid decreases the renal excretion of conjugated sulfonamides, plasma concentrations of the latter should be determined from time to time when a sulfonamide and ColBENEMID are coadministered for prolonged periods. Probenecid may prolong or enhance the action of oral sulfonylureas and thereby increase the risk of hypoglycemia.

It has been reported that patients receiving probenecid require significantly less thiopental for induction of anesthesia. In addition, ketamine and thiopental anesthesia were significantly prolonged in rats receiving probenecid.

When probenecid is given to patients receiving indomethacin, the plasma levels of indomethacin are likely to be increased. Therefore, a lower dosage of indomethacin may be required to produce a therapeutic effect, and increases in the dosage of indomethacin should be made cautiously and in small increments. Probenecid may increase plasma levels of rifampin. The clinical significance of this is not known.

In animals and in humans, probenecid has been reported to increase plasma concentrations of methotrexate (*see* WARNINGS).

Falsely high readings for theophylline have been reported in an *in vitro* study, using the Schack and Waxler technic, when therapeutic concentrations of theophylline and probenecid were added to human plasma.

ADVERSE REACTIONS

The following adverse reactions have been observed and within each category are listed in order of decreasing severity.

Probenecid

Central Nervous System: headache, dizziness.
Metabolic: precipitation of acute gouty arthritis.
Gastrointestinal: hepatic necrosis, vomiting, nausea, anorexia, sore gums.
Genitourinary: nephrotic syndrome, uric acid stones with or without hematuria, renal colic, costovertebral pain, urinary frequency.
Hypersensitivity: anaphylaxis, fever, urticaria, pruritus.
Hematologic: aplastic anemia, leukopenia, hemolytic anemia which could be related to genetic deficiency of glucose-6-phosphate dehydrogenase in red blood cells, anemia.
Integumentary: dermatitis, alopecia, flushing.

Colchicine

Side effects due to colchicine appear to be a function of dosage. The possibility of increased colchicine toxicity in the presence of hepatic dysfunction should be considered. The appearance of any of the following symptoms may require reduction of dosage or discontinuance of the drug.
Central Nervous System: peripheral neuritis.
Musculoskeletal: muscular weakness.
Gastrointestinal: nausea, vomiting, abdominal pain, or diarrhea may be particularly troublesome in the presence of peptic ulcer or spastic colon.
Hypersensitivity: urticaria.
Hematologic: aplastic anemia, agranulocytosis.
Integumentary: dermatitis, purpura, alopecia.
At toxic doses, colchicine may cause severe diarrhea, generalized vascular damage, and renal damage with hematuria and oliguria.

DOSAGE AND ADMINISTRATION

Therapy with ColBENEMID should not be *started* until an acute gouty attack has subsided. However, if an acute attack is precipitated *during* therapy, ColBENEMID may be continued without changing the dosage, and additional colchicine or other appropriate therapy should be given to control the acute attack.

The recommended adult dosage is 1 tablet of ColBENEMID daily for one week, followed by 1 tablet twice a day thereafter.

Some degree of renal impairment may be present in patients with gout. A daily dosage of 2 tablets may be adequate. However, if necessary, the daily dosage may be increased by 1 tablet every four weeks within tolerance (and usually not above 4 tablets per day) if symptoms of gouty arthritis are not controlled or the 24 hour uric acid excretion is not above 700 mg. As noted, probenecid may not be effective in chronic renal insufficiency particularly when the glomerular filtration rate is 30 mL/minute or less.

Gastric intolerance may be indicative of overdosage, and may be corrected by decreasing the dosage.

As uric acid tends to crystallize out of an acid urine, a liberal fluid intake is recommended, as well as sufficient sodium bicarbonate (3 to 7.5 g daily) or potassium citrate (7.5 g daily) to maintain an alkaline urine (*see* PRECAUTIONS).

Alkalization of the urine is recommended until the serum urate level returns to normal limits and tophaceous deposits disappear, i.e., during the period when urinary excretion of uric acid is at a high level. Thereafter, alkalization of the urine and the usual restriction of purine-producing foods may be somewhat relaxed.

ColBENEMID (or probenecid) should be continued at the dosage that will maintain normal serum urate levels. When acute attacks have been absent for six months or more and serum urate levels remain within normal limits, the daily dosage of ColBENEMID may be decreased by 1 tablet every six months. The maintenance dosage should not be reduced to the point where serum urate levels tend to rise.

HOW SUPPLIED

No. 3283—Tablets ColBENEMID are white to off-white, capsule-shaped, scored tablets, coded MSD 614. Each tablet contains 0.5 g of probenecid and 0.5 mg of colchicine. They are supplied as follows:
NDC 0006-0614-68 bottles of 100.

Shown in Product Identification Section, page 417

Storage

Protect from light. Store container in carton until contents have been used.

A.H.F.S. Category: 40:40
DC 6213022 Issued April 1985

CORTONE® Acetate Saline Suspension (Cortisone Acetate, MSD), U.S.P. ℞

For intramuscular injection only

DESCRIPTION

Cortisone acetate, a synthetic adrenocortical steroid, is a white or practically white, odorless, crystalline powder. It is stable in air. It is insoluble in water. The molecular weight is 402.49. It is designated chemically as 21-(acetyloxy)-17-hydroxypregn-4-ene-3,11,20-trione. The empirical formula is $C_{23}H_{30}O_6$ and the structural formula is:

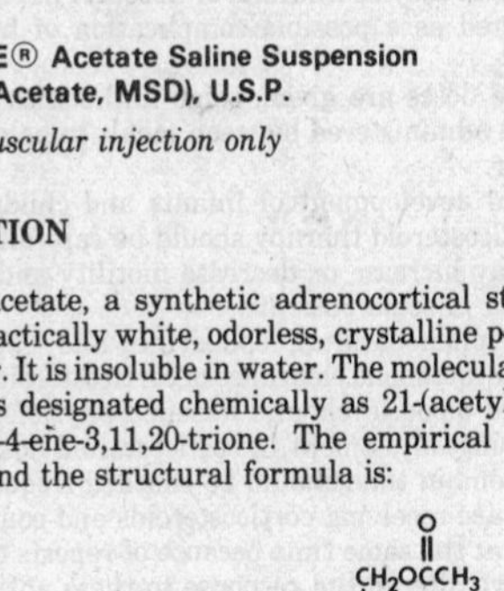

CORTONE® Acetate (Cortisone Acetate, MSD) saline suspension is a sterile suspension of cortisone acetate in an aqueous medium (pH 5.0 to 7.0). It is supplied in two strengths, one containing 25 mg of cortisone acetate per milliliter, the other containing 50 mg per milliliter. Inactive ingredients per mL: sodium chloride, 9 mg; polysorbate 80, 4 mg; sodium carboxymethylcellulose, 5 mg; Water for Injection q.s. 1 mL. Benzyl alcohol, 9 mg, added as preservative. No attempt should be made to alter CORTONE Acetate saline suspension. Diluting it or mixing it with other substances may affect the state of suspension or change the rate of absorption and reduce its effectiveness.

ACTIONS

CORTONE Acetate saline suspension has a slow onset but long duration of action when compared with more soluble preparations. When daily corticosteroid therapy is required and oral therapy is not feasible, the required daily dosage may be given in a single intramuscular injection of this preparation.

Naturally occurring glucocorticoids (hydrocortisone and cortisone), which also have salt-retaining properties, are used as replacement therapy in adrenocortical deficiency states. They are also used for their potent anti-inflammatory effects in disorders of many organ systems.

Glucocorticoids cause profound and varied metabolic effects. In addition, they modify the body's immune responses to diverse stimuli.

INDICATIONS

When oral therapy is not feasible:

1. *Endocrine disorders*

Primary or secondary adrenocortical insufficiency (hydrocortisone or cortisone is the drug of choice; synthetic analogs may be used in conjunction with mineralocorticoids where applicable; in infancy, mineralocorticoid supplementation is of particular importance)

Acute adrenocortical insufficiency (hydrocortisone or cortisone is the drug of choice; mineralocorticoid supplementation may be necessary, particularly when synthetic analogs are used)

Preoperatively, and in the event of serious trauma or illness, in patients with known adrenal insufficiency or when adrenocortical reserve is doubtful

Shock unresponsive to conventional therapy if adrenocortical insufficiency exists or is suspected

Congenital adrenal hyperplasia
Nonsuppurative thyroiditis
Hypercalcemia associated with cancer

2. *Rheumatic disorders*

As adjunctive therapy for short-term administration (to tide the patient over an acute episode or exacerbation) in:

Post-traumatic osteoarthritis
Synovitis of osteoarthritis
Rheumatoid arthritis, including juvenile rheumatoid arthritis (selected cases may require low-dose maintenance therapy)
Acute and subacute bursitis
Epicondylitis
Acute nonspecific tenosynovitis
Acute gouty arthritis
Psoriatic arthritis
Ankylosing spondylitis

3. *Collagen diseases*

During an exacerbation or as maintenance therapy in selected cases of:

Systemic lupus erythematosus
Acute rheumatic carditis
Systemic dermatomyositis (polymyositis)

4. *Dermatologic diseases*

Pemphigus
Severe erythema multiforme (Stevens-Johnson syndrome)
Exfoliative dermatitis
Bullous dermatitis herpetiformis
Severe seborrheic dermatitis
Severe psoriasis
Mycosis fungoides

5. *Allergic states*

Control of severe or incapacitating allergic conditions intractable to adequate trials of conventional treatment in:

Bronchial asthma
Contact dermatitis
Atopic dermatitis
Serum sickness
Seasonal or perennial allergic rhinitis
Drug hypersensitivity reactions
Urticarial transfusion reactions
Acute noninfectious laryngeal edema (epinephrine is the drug of first choice)

6. *Ophthalmic diseases*

Severe acute and chronic allergic and inflammatory processes involving the eye, such as:

Herpes zoster ophthalmicus
Iritis, iridocyclitis
Chorioretinitis
Diffuse posterior uveitis and choroiditis
Optic neuritis
Sympathetic ophthalmia
Anterior segment inflammation
Allergic conjunctivitis
Keratitis
Allergic corneal marginal ulcers

7. *Gastrointestinal diseases*

To tide the patient over a critical period of the disease in:

Ulcerative colitis (Systemic therapy)
Regional enteritis (Systemic therapy)

8. *Respiratory diseases*

Symptomatic sarcoidosis
Berylliosis
Fulminating or disseminated pulmonary tuberculosis when used concurrently with appropriate antituberculous chemotherapy
Loeffler's syndrome not manageable by other means
Aspiration pneumonitis

9. *Hematologic disorders*

Acquired (autoimmune) hemolytic anemia
Erythroblastopenia (RBC anemia)
Congenital (erythroid) hypoplastic anemia

Continued on next page

Information on the Merck Sharp & Dohme products listed on these pages is the full prescribing information from product circulars in use August 31, 1986.

Merck Sharp & Dohme—Cont.

10. *Neoplastic diseases*
For palliative management of:
Leukemias and lymphomas in adults
Acute leukemia of childhood
11. *Edematous states*
To induce diuresis or remission of proteinuria in the nephrotic syndrome, without uremia, of the idiopathic type, or that due to lupus erythematosus
12. *Miscellaneous*
Tuberculous meningitis with subarachnoid block or impending block when used concurrently with appropriate antituberculous chemotherapy
Trichinosis with neurologic or myocardial involvement.

CONTRAINDICATIONS

Systemic fungal infections
Hypersensitivity to any component of this product

WARNINGS

In patients on corticosteroid therapy subjected to any unusual stress, increased dosage of rapidly acting corticosteroids before, during, and after the stressful situation is indicated.
Drug-induced secondary adrenocortical insufficiency may result from too rapid withdrawal of corticosteroids and may be minimized by gradual reduction of dosage. This type of relative insufficiency may persist for months after discontinuation of therapy; therefore, in any situation of stress occurring during that period, hormone therapy should be reinstituted. If the patient is receiving steroids already, dosage may have to be increased. Since mineralocorticoid secretion may be impaired, salt and/or a mineralocorticoid should be administered concurrently.
Corticosteroids may mask some signs of infection, and new infections may appear during their use. There may be decreased resistance and inability to localize infection when corticosteroids are used. Moreover, corticosteroids may affect the nitroblue-tetrazolium test for bacterial infection and produce false negative results.
In cerebral malaria, a double-blind trial has shown that the use of corticosteroids is associated with prolongation of coma and a higher incidence of pneumonia and gastrointestinal bleeding.
Corticosteroids may activate latent amebiasis. Therefore, it is recommended that latent or active amebiasis be ruled out before initiating corticosteroid therapy in any patient who has spent time in the tropics or any patient with unexplained diarrhea.
Prolonged use of corticosteroids may produce posterior subcapsular cataracts, glaucoma with possible damage to the optic nerves, and may enhance the establishment of secondary ocular infections due to fungi or viruses.
Usage in pregnancy. Since adequate human reproduction studies have not been done with corticosteroids, use of these drugs in pregnancy or in women of childbearing potential requires that the anticipated benefits be weighed against the possible hazards to the mother and embryo or fetus. Infants born of mothers who have received substantial doses of corticosteroids during pregnancy should be carefully observed for signs of hypoadrenalism.
Corticosteroids appear in breast milk and could suppress growth, interfere with endogenous corticosteroid production, or cause other unwanted effects. Mothers taking pharmacologic doses of corticosteroids should be advised not to nurse.
Average and large doses of cortisone or hydrocortisone can cause elevation of blood pressure, salt and water retention, and increased excretion of potassium. These effects are less likely to occur with the synthetic derivatives except when used in large doses. Dietary salt restriction and potassium supplementation may be necessary. All corticosteroids increase calcium excretion.
Administration of live virus vaccines, including smallpox, is contraindicated in individuals receiving immunosuppressive doses of corticosteroids. If inactivated viral or bacterial vaccines are administered to individuals receiving immunosuppressive doses of corticosteroids, the expected serum antibody response may not be obtained.
The use of CORTONE Acetate saline suspension in active tuberculosis should be restricted to those cases of fulminating or disseminated tuberculosis in which the corticosteroid is used for the management of the disease in conjunction with an appropriate antituberculous regimen.
If corticosteroids are indicated in patients with latent tuberculosis or tuberculin reactivity, close observation is necessary as reactivation of the disease may occur. During prolonged corticosteroid therapy, these patients should receive chemoprophylaxis.
Because rare instances of anaphylactoid reactions have occurred in patients receiving parenteral corticosteroid therapy, appropriate precautionary measures should be taken prior to administration, especially when the patient has a history of allergy to any drug.

PRECAUTIONS

CORTONE Acetate saline suspension, like many other steroid formulations, is sensitive to heat. Therefore, it should not be autoclaved when it is desirable to sterilize the exterior of the vial.
Following prolonged therapy, withdrawal of corticosteroids may result in symptoms of the corticosteroid withdrawal syndrome including fever, myalgia, arthralgia, and malaise. This may occur in patients even without evidence of adrenal insufficiency.
There is an enhanced effect of corticosteroids in patients with hypothyroidism and in those with cirrhosis.
Corticosteroids should be used cautiously in patients with ocular herpes simplex for fear of corneal perforation.
The lowest possible dose of corticosteroid should be used to control the condition under treatment, and when reduction in dosage is possible, the reduction must be gradual.
Psychic derangements may appear when corticosteroids are used, ranging from euphoria, insomnia, mood swings, personality changes, and severe depression to frank psychotic manifestations. Also, existing emotional instability or psychotic tendencies may be aggravated by corticosteroids.
Aspirin should be used cautiously in conjunction with corticosteroids in hypoprothrombinemia.
Steroids should be used with caution in nonspecific ulcerative colitis, if there is a probability of impending perforation, abscess, or other pyogenic infection, also in diverticulitis, fresh intestinal anastomoses, active or latent peptic ulcer, renal insufficiency, hypertension, osteoporosis, and myasthenia gravis. Signs of peritoneal irritation following gastrointestinal perforation in patients receiving large doses of corticosteroids may be minimal or absent. Fat embolism has been reported as a possible complication of hypercortisonism.
When large doses are given, some authorities advise that antacids be administered between meals to help to prevent peptic ulcer.
Growth and development of infants and children on prolonged corticosteroid therapy should be carefully followed.
Steroids may increase or decrease motility and number of spermatozoa in some patients.
Phenytoin, phenobarbital, ephedrine, and rifampin may enhance the metabolic clearance of corticosteroids, resulting in decreased blood levels and lessened physiologic activity, thus requiring adjustment in corticosteroid dosage.
The prothrombin time should be checked frequently in patients who are receiving corticosteroids and coumarin anticoagulants at the same time because of reports that corticosteroids have altered the response to these anticoagulants. Studies have shown that the usual effect produced by adding corticosteroids is inhibition of response to coumarins, although there have been some conflicting reports of potentiation not substantiated by studies.
When corticosteroids are administered concomitantly with potassium-depleting diuretics, patients should be observed closely for development of hypokalemia.
Injection of a steroid into an infected site is to be avoided.

ADVERSE REACTIONS

Fluid and electrolyte disturbances
Sodium retention
Fluid retention
Congestive heart failure in susceptible patients
Potassium loss
Hypokalemic alkalosis
Hypertension
Musculoskeletal
Muscle weakness
Steroid myopathy
Loss of muscle mass
Osteoporosis
Vertebral compression fractures
Aseptic necrosis of femoral and humeral heads
Pathologic fracture of long bones
Tendon rupture
Gastrointestinal
Peptic ulcer with possible subsequent perforation and hemorrhage
Perforation of the small and large bowel, particularly in patients with inflammatory bowel disease
Pancreatitis
Abdominal distention
Ulcerative esophagitis
Dermatologic
Impaired wound healing
Thin fragile skin
Petechiae and ecchymoses
Erythema
Increased sweating
May suppress reactions to skin tests
Other cutaneous reactions, such as allergic dermatitis, urticaria, angioneurotic edema
Neurologic
Convulsions
Increased intracranial pressure with papilledema (pseudotumor cerebri) usually after treatment
Vertigo
Headache
Endocrine
Menstrual irregularities
Development of cushingoid state
Suppression of growth in children
Secondary adrenocortical and pituitary unresponsiveness, particularly in times of stress, as in trauma, surgery, or illness
Decreased carbohydrate tolerance
Manifestations of latent diabetes mellitus
Increased requirements for insulin or oral hypoglycemic agents in diabetics
Hirsutism
Ophthalmic
Posterior subcapsular cataracts
Increased intraocular pressure
Glaucoma
Exophthalmos
Metabolic
Negative nitrogen balance due to protein catabolism
Other
Anaphylactoid or hypersensitivity reactions
Thromboembolism
Weight gain
Increased appetite
Nausea
Malaise
Psychic disturbances
The following *additional* adverse reactions are related to parenteral corticosteroid therapy:
Rare instances of blindness associated with intralesional therapy around the face and head
Hyperpigmentation or hypopigmentation
Subcutaneous and cutaneous atrophy
Sterile abscess

DOSAGE AND ADMINISTRATION

For intramuscular injection only
DOSAGE REQUIREMENTS ARE VARIABLE AND MUST BE INDIVIDUALIZED ON THE BASIS OF THE DISEASE AND THE RESPONSE OF THE PATIENT.
The initial dosage varies from 20 to 300 mg a day depending on the disease being treated. In less severe diseases doses lower than 20 mg may suffice, while in severe diseases doses higher than 300 mg may be required. The initial dosage should be maintained or adjusted until the patient's response is satisfactory. If a satisfactory clinical response does not occur after a reasonable period of time, discontinue CORTONE Acetate saline suspension and transfer the patient to other therapy.
After a favorable initial response, the proper maintenance dosage should be determined by decreasing the initial dosage in small amounts to the lowest dosage that maintains an adequate clinical response.
Patients should be observed closely for signs that might require dosage adjustment, including changes in clinical status resulting from remissions or exacerbations of the disease, individual drug responsiveness, and the effect of stress (e.g., surgery, infection, trauma). During stress it may be necessary to increase dosage temporarily.
If the drug is to be stopped after more than a few days of treatment, it usually should be withdrawn gradually.

HOW SUPPLIED

No. 7062 —Saline Suspension CORTONE Acetate is a white, mobile suspension, each mL containing 25 mg cortisone acetate, and is supplied as follows:
NDC 0006-7062-20 in 20 mL vials.
No. 7069—Saline Suspension CORTONE Acetate is a white, mobile suspension, each mL containing 50 mg cortisone acetate, and is supplied as follows:
NDC 0006-7069-10 in 10 mL vials.
Storage
Sensitive to heat. Do not autoclave.
Protect from freezing.

A.H.F.S. Category: 68:04
DC 6599312 Issued April 1985

CORTONE® Acetate Tablets (Cortisone Acetate, MSD), U.S.P. ℞

DESCRIPTION

Glucocorticoids are adrenocortical steroids, both naturally occurring and synthetic, which are readily absorbed from the gastrointestinal tract.

Cortisone acetate is a white or practically white, odorless, crystalline powder. It is stable in air. It is insoluble in water. The molecular weight is 402.49. It is designated chemically as 21-(acetyloxy)-17-hydroxypregn-4-ene-3,11,20-trione. The empirical formula is $C_{23}H_{30}O_6$ and the structural formula is:

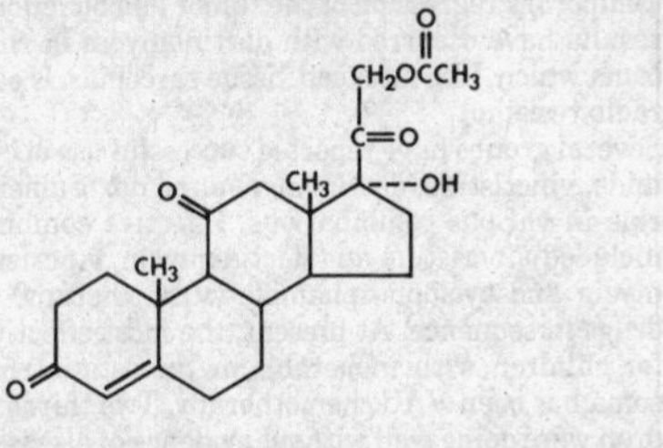

CORTONE® Acetate (Cortisone Acetate, MSD) tablets contain 25 mg of cortisone acetate in each tablet.
Inactive ingredients are lactose, magnesium stearate, and starch.

ACTIONS

Naturally occurring glucocorticoids (hydrocortisone and cortisone), which also have salt-retaining properties, are used as replacement therapy in adrenocortical deficiency states. They are also used for their potent anti-inflammatory effects in disorders of many organ systems.
Glucocorticoids cause profound and varied metabolic effects. In addition, they modify the body's immune responses to diverse stimuli.

INDICATIONS

1. *Endocrine Disorders*
Primary or secondary adrenocortical insufficiency (hydrocortisone or cortisone is the first choice; synthetic analogs may be used in conjunction with mineralocorticoids where applicable; in infancy mineralocorticoid supplementation is of particular importance).
  Congenital adrenal hyperplasia
  Nonsuppurative thyroiditis
  Hypercalcemia associated with cancer
2. *Rheumatic Disorders*
As adjunctive therapy for short-term administration (to tide the patient over an acute episode or exacerbation) in:
  Psoriatic arthritis
  Rheumatoid arthritis, including juvenile rheumatoid arthritis (selected cases may require low-dose maintenance therapy)
  Ankylosing spondylitis
  Acute and subacute bursitis
  Acute nonspecific tenosynovitis
  Acute gouty arthritis
  Post-traumatic osteoarthritis
  Synovitis of osteoarthritis
  Epicondylitis
3. *Collagen Diseases*
During an exacerbation or as maintenance therapy in selected cases of—
  Systemic lupus erythematosus
  Acute rheumatic carditis
  Systemic dermatomyositis (polymyositis)
4. *Dermatologic Diseases*
  Pemphigus
  Bullous dermatitis herpetiformis
  Severe erythema multiforme (Stevens-Johnson syndrome)
  Exfoliative dermatitis
  Mycosis fungoides
  Severe psoriasis
  Severe seborrheic dermatitis
5. *Allergic States*
Control of severe or incapacitating allergic conditions intractable to adequate trials of conventional treatment:
  Seasonal or perennial allergic rhinitis
  Bronchial asthma
  Contact dermatitis
  Atopic dermatitis
  Serum sickness
  Drug hypersensitivity reactions
6. *Ophthalmic Diseases*
Severe acute and chronic allergic and inflammatory processes involving the eye and its adnexa, such as—
  Allergic conjunctivitis
  Keratitis
  Allergic corneal marginal ulcers
  Herpes zoster ophthalmicus
  Iritis and iridocyclitis
  Chorioretinitis
  Anterior segment inflammation
  Diffuse posterior uveitis and choroiditis
  Optic neuritis
  Sympathetic ophthalmia
7. *Respiratory Diseases*
  Symptomatic sarcoidosis
  Loeffler's syndrome not manageable by other means
  Berylliosis
  Fulminating or disseminated pulmonary tuberculosis when used concurrently with appropriate antituberculous chemotherapy
  Aspiration pneumonitis
8. *Hematologic Disorders*
  Idiopathic thrombocytopenic purpura in adults
  Secondary thrombocytopenia in adults
  Acquired (autoimmune) hemolytic anemia
  Erythroblastopenia (RBC anemia)
  Congenital (erythroid) hypoplastic anemia
9. *Neoplastic Diseases*
For palliative management of:
  Leukemias and lymphomas in adults
  Acute leukemia of childhood
10. *Edematous States*
To induce a diuresis or remission of proteinuria in the nephrotic syndrome, without uremia, of the idiopathic type or that due to lupus erythematosus
11. *Gastrointestinal Diseases*
To tide the patient over a critical period of the disease in:
  Ulcerative colitis
  Regional enteritis
12. *Miscellaneous*
Tuberculous meningitis with subarachnoid block or impending block when used concurrently with appropriate antituberculous chemotherapy
Trichinosis with neurologic or myocardial involvement

CONTRAINDICATIONS

Systemic fungal infections
Hypersensitivity to this product

WARNINGS

In patients on corticosteroid therapy subjected to unusual stress, increased dosage of rapidly acting corticosteroids before, during, and after the stressful situation is indicated.
Drug-induced secondary adrenocortical insufficiency may result from too rapid withdrawal of corticosteroids and may be minimized by gradual reduction of dosage. This type of relative insufficiency may persist for months after discontinuation of therapy; therefore, in any situation of stress occurring during that period, hormone therapy should be reinstituted. If the patient is receiving steroids already, dosage may have to be increased. Since mineralocorticoid secretion may be impaired, salt and/or a mineralocorticoid should be administered concurrently.
Corticosteroids may mask some signs of infection, and new infections may appear during their use. There may be decreased resistance and inability to localize infection when corticosteroids are used. Moreover, corticosteroids may affect the nitroblue-tetrazolium test for bacterial infection and produce false negative results.
In cerebral malaria, a double-blind trial has shown that the use of corticosteroids is associated with prolongation of coma and a higher incidence of pneumonia and gastrointestinal bleeding.
Corticosteroids may activate latent amebiasis. Therefore, it is recommended that latent or active amebiasis be ruled out before initiating corticosteroid therapy in any patient who has spent time in the tropics or any patient with unexplained diarrhea.
Prolonged use of corticosteroids may produce posterior subcapsular cataracts, glaucoma with possible damage to the optic nerves, and may enhance the establishment of secondary ocular infections due to fungi or viruses.
Usage in pregnancy: Since adequate human reproduction studies have not been done with corticosteroids, use of these drugs in pregnancy or in women of childbearing potential requires that the anticipated benefits be weighed against the possible hazards to the mother and embryo or fetus. Infants born of mothers who have received substantial doses of corticosteroids during pregnancy should be carefully observed for signs of hypoadrenalism.
Corticosteroids appear in breast milk and could suppress growth, interfere with endogenous corticosteroid production, or cause other unwanted effects. Mothers taking pharmacologic doses of corticosteroids should be advised not to nurse.
Average and large doses of hydrocortisone or cortisone can cause elevation of blood pressure, salt and water retention, and increased excretion of potassium. These effects are less likely to occur with the synthetic derivatives except when used in large doses. Dietary salt restriction and potassium supplementation may be necessary. All corticosteroids increase calcium excretion.
Administration of live virus vaccines, including smallpox, is contraindicated in individuals receiving immunosuppressive doses of corticosteroids. If inactivated viral or bacterial vaccines are administered to individuals receiving immunosuppressive doses of corticosteroids, the expected serum antibody response may not be obtained. However, immunization procedures may be undertaken in patients who are receiving corticosteroids as replacement therapy, e.g., for Addison's disease.
The use of CORTONE Acetate tablets in active tuberculosis should be restricted to those cases of fulminating or disseminated tuberculosis in which the corticosteroid is used for the management of the disease in conjunction with an appropriate antituberculous regimen.
If corticosteroids are indicated in patients with latent tuberculosis or tuberculin reactivity, close observation is necessary as reactivation of the disease may occur. During prolonged corticosteroid therapy, these patients should receive chemoprophylaxis.

PRECAUTIONS

Following prolonged therapy, withdrawal of corticosteroids may result in symptoms of the corticosteroid withdrawal syndrome including fever, myalgia, arthralgia, and malaise. This may occur in patients even without evidence of adrenal insufficiency.
There is an enhanced effect of corticosteroids in patients with hypothyroidism and in those with cirrhosis.
Corticosteroids should be used cautiously in patients with ocular herpes simplex because of possible corneal perforation.
The lowest possible dose of corticosteroid should be used to control the condition under treatment, and when reduction in dosage is possible, the reduction should be gradual.
Psychic derangements may appear when corticosteroids are used, ranging from euphoria, insomnia, mood swings, personality changes, and severe depression, to frank psychotic manifestations. Also, existing emotional instability or psychotic tendencies may be aggravated by corticosteroids.
Aspirin should be used cautiously in conjunction with corticosteroids in hypoprothrombinemia.
Steroids should be used with caution in nonspecific ulcerative colitis, if there is a probability of impending perforation, abscess, or other pyogenic infection, diverticulitis, fresh intestinal anastomoses, active or latent peptic ulcer, renal insufficiency, hypertension, osteoporosis, and myasthenia gravis. Signs of peritoneal irritation following gastrointestinal perforation in patients receiving large doses of corticosteroids may be minimal or absent. Fat embolism has been reported as a possible complication of hypercortisonism.
When large doses are given, some authorities advise that corticosteroids be taken with meals and antacids taken between meals to help to prevent peptic ulcer.
Growth and development of infants and children on prolonged corticosteroid therapy should be carefully observed.
Steroids may increase or decrease motility and number of spermatozoa in some patients.
Phenytoin, phenobarbital, ephedrine, and rifampin may enhance the metabolic clearance of corticosteroids, resulting in decreased blood levels and lessened physiologic activity, thus requiring adjustment in corticosteroid dosage.
The prothrombin time should be checked frequently in patients who are receiving corticosteroids and coumarin anticoagulants at the same time because of reports that corticosteroids have altered the response to these anticoagulants. Studies have shown that the usual effect produced by adding corticosteroids is inhibition of response to coumarins, although there have been some conflicting reports of potentiation not substantiated by studies.
When corticosteroids are administered concomitantly with potassium-depleting diuretics, patients should be observed closely for development of hypokalemia.

ADVERSE REACTIONS

Fluid and Electrolyte Disturbances
  Sodium retention
  Fluid retention
  Congestive heart failure in susceptible patients
  Potassium loss
  Hypokalemic alkalosis
  Hypertension
Musculoskeletal
  Muscle weakness
  Steroid myopathy
  Loss of muscle mass
  Osteoporosis
  Vertebral compression fractures
  Aseptic necrosis of femoral and humeral heads
  Pathologic fracture of long bones
  Tendon rupture

Continued on next page

Information on the Merck Sharp & Dohme products listed on these pages is the full prescribing information from product circulars in use August 31, 1986.

Merck Sharp & Dohme—Cont.

Gastrointestinal
Peptic ulcer with possible perforation and hemorrhage
Perforation of the small and large bowel, particularly in patients with inflammatory bowel disease
Pancreatitis
Abdominal distention
Ulcerative esophagitis
Dermatologic
Impaired wound healing
Thin fragile skin
Petechiae and ecchymoses
Erythema
Increased sweating
May suppress reactions to skin tests
Other cutaneous reactions, such as allergic dermatitis, urticaria, angioneurotic edema
Neurologic
Convulsions
Increased intracranial pressure with papilledema (pseudotumor cerebri), usually after treatment
Vertigo
Headache
Endocrine
Menstrual irregularities
Development of cushingoid state
Suppression of growth in children
Secondary adrenocortical and pituitary unresponsiveness, particularly in times of stress, as in trauma, surgery, or illness
Decreased carbohydrate tolerance
Manifestations of latent diabetes mellitus
Increased requirements for insulin or oral hypoglycemic agents in diabetics
Hirsutism
Ophthalmic
Posterior subcapsular cataracts
Increased intraocular pressure
Glaucoma
Exophthalmos
Metabolic
Negative nitrogen balance due to protein catabolism
Other
Hypersensitivity
Thromboembolism
Weight gain
Increased appetite
Nausea
Malaise
Psychic disturbances

DOSAGE AND ADMINISTRATION

For oral administration
DOSAGE REQUIREMENTS ARE VARIABLE AND MUST BE INDIVIDUALIZED ON THE BASIS OF THE DISEASE AND THE RESPONSE OF THE PATIENT.
The initial dosage varies from 25 to 300 mg a day depending on the disease being treated. In less severe diseases doses lower than 25 mg may suffice, while in severe diseases doses higher than 300 mg may be required. The initial dosage should be maintained or adjusted until the patient's response is satisfactory. If satisfactory clinical response does not occur after a reasonable period of time, discontinue CORTONE Acetate tablets and transfer the patient to other therapy.
After a favorable initial response, the proper maintenance dosage should be determined by decreasing the initial dosage in small amounts to the lowest dosage that maintains an adequate clinical response.
Patients should be observed closely for signs that might require dosage adjustment, including changes in clinical status resulting from remissions or exacerbations of the disease, individual drug responsiveness, and the effect of stress (e.g., surgery, infection, trauma). During stress it may be necessary to increase dosage temporarily.
If the drug is to be stopped after more than a few days of treatment, it usually should be withdrawn gradually.

HOW SUPPLIED

No. 7063—Tablets Cortone Acetate, 25 mg each, are white, round, scored, compressed tablets, coded MSD 219. They are supplied as follows:
NDC 0006-0219-68 in bottles of 100.
A.H.F.S. Category: 68:04
DC 6014427 Issued April 1985

COSMEGEN® Injection ℞
(Dactinomycin, MSD), U.S.P.

WARNING

Dactinomycin is extremely corrosive to soft tissue. If extravasation occurs during intravenous use, severe damage to soft tissues will occur. In at least one instance, this has led to contracture of the arms.

DOSAGE

The dosage of COSMEGEN® (Dactinomycin, MSD) is calculated in micrograms (mcg). The usual adult dosage is 500 micrograms (0.5 mg) daily intravenously for a maximum of five days. The dosage for adults or children should not exceed 15 mcg/kg or 400–600 mcg/square meter of body surface daily intravenously for five days. Calculation of the dosage for obese or edematous patients should be on the basis of surface area in an effort to relate dosage to lean body mass.

DESCRIPTION

Dactinomycin is one of the actinomycins, a group of antibiotics produced by various species of *Streptomyces*. Dactinomycin is the principal component of the mixture of actinomycins produced by *Streptomyces parvullus*. Unlike other species of *Streptomyces*, this organism yields an essentially pure substance that contains only traces of similar compounds differing in the amino acid content of the peptide side chains. The empirical formula is $C_{62}H_{86}N_{12}O_{16}$ and the structural formula is:

CH(CH3)2 / CH / NCH3 / Sarcosine / L-Proline / D-Valine / CO / CH / NH / CO — CH(CH3)2 / CH / NCH3 / Sarcosine / L-Proline / D-Valine / CO / CH / NH / CO; O; OC; CO; CH / CH3; CH / CH3; N; NH2; =O; O; CH3; CH3

COSMEGEN is a sterile, yellow lyophilized powder for injection by the intravenous route or by regional perfusion after reconstitution. Each vial contains 0.5 mg (500 mcg) of dactinomycin and 20.0 mg of mannitol.

CLINICAL PHARMACOLOGY

Action
Generally, the actinomycins exert an inhibitory effect on gram-positive and gram-negative bacteria and on some fungi. However, the toxic properties of the actinomycins (including dactinomycin) in relation to antibacterial activity are such as to preclude their use as antibiotics in the treatment of infectious diseases.
Because the actinomycins are cytotoxic, they have an antineoplastic effect which has been demonstrated in experimental animals with various types of tumor implant. This cytotoxic action is the basis for their use in the palliative treatment of certain types of cancer.
Pharmacokinetics and Metabolism
Results of a study in patients with malignant melanoma indicate that dactinomycin (^{3}H actinomycin D) is minimally metabolized, is concentrated in nucleated cells, and does not penetrate the blood brain barrier. Approximately 30% of the dose was recovered in urine and feces in one week. The terminal plasma half-life for radioactivity was approximately 36 hours.

INDICATIONS AND USAGE

Wilms' Tumor
The neoplasm responding most frequently to COSMEGEN is Wilms' tumor. With low doses of both dactinomycin and radiotherapy, temporary objective improvement may be as good as and may last longer than with higher doses of each given alone. In the National Wilms' Tumor study, combination therapy with dactinomycin and vincristine together with surgery and radiotherapy, was shown to have significantly improved the prognosis of patients in groups II and III. Dactinomycin and vincristine were given for a total of seven cycles, so that maintenance therapy continued for approximately 15 months.
Postoperative radiotherapy in group I patients and optimal combination chemotherapy for those in group IV are unsettled issues. About 70 percent of lung metastases have disappeared with an appropriate combination of radiation, dactinomycin and vincristine.
Rhabdomyosarcoma
Temporary regression of the tumor and beneficial subjective results have occurred with dactinomycin in rhabdomyosarcoma which, like most soft tissue sarcomas, is comparatively radio-resistant.
Several groups have reported successful use of cyclophosphamide, vincristine, dactinomycin and doxorubicin hydrochloride in various combinations. Effective combinations have included vincristine and dactinomycin; vincristine, dactinomycin and cyclophosphamide (VAC therapy) and all four drugs in sequence. At present, the most effective treatment for children with inoperable or metastatic rhabdomyosarcoma has been VAC chemotherapy. Two thirds of these children were doing well without evidence of disease at a median time of three years after diagnosis.
Carcinoma of Testis and Uterus
The sequential use of dactinomycin and methotrexate, along with meticulous monitoring of human chorionic gonadotropin levels until normal, has resulted in survival in the majority of women with metastatic choriocarcinoma. Sequential therapy is used if there is:
1. Stability in gonadotropin titers following two successive courses of an agent.
2. Rising gonadotropin titers during treatment.
3. Severe toxicity preventing adequate therapy.

In patients with nonmetastatic choriocarcinoma, dactinomycin or methotrexate or both, have been used successfully, with or without surgery.
Dactinomycin has been beneficial as a single agent in the treatment of metastatic nonseminomatour testicular carcinoma when used in cycles of 500 mcg/day for five consecutive days, every 6–8 weeks for periods of four months or longer.
Other Neoplasms
Dactinomycin has been given intravenously or by regional perfusion, either alone or with other antineoplastic compounds or x-ray therapy, in the palliative treatment of Ewing's sarcoma and sarcoma botryoides. For nonmetastatic Ewing's sarcoma, promising results were obtained when dactinomycin (45 mcg/m^2) and cyclophosphamide (1200 mg/m^2) were given sequentially and with radiotherapy, over an 18 month period. Those with metastatic disease remain the subject of continued investigation with a more aggressive chemotherapeutic regimen employed initially.
Temporary objective improvement and relief of pain and discomfort have followed the use of dactinomycin usually in conjunction with radiotherapy for sarcoma botryoides. This palliative effect ranges from transitory inhibition of tumor growth to a considerable but temporary regression in tumor size.
COSMEGEN (Dactinomycin, MSD) and Radiation Therapy
Much evidence suggests that dactinomycin potentiates the effects of x-ray therapy. The converse also appears likely; i.e., dactinomycin may be more effective when radiation therapy also is given.
With combined dactinomycin-radiation therapy, the normal skin, as well as the buccal and pharyngeal mucosa, show early erythema. A smaller than usual x-ray dose when given with dactinomycin causes erythema and vesiculation, which progress more rapidly through the stages of tanning and desquamation. Healing may occur in four to six weeks rather than two to three months. Erythema from previous x-ray therapy may be reactivated by dactinomycin alone, even when irradiation occurred many months earlier, and especially when the interval between the two forms of therapy is brief. This potentiation of radiation effect represents a special problem when the irradiation treatment area includes the mucous membrane. When irradiation is directed toward the nasopharynx, the combination may produce severe oropharyngeal mucositis. *Severe reactions may ensue if high doses of both dactinomycin and radiation therapy are used or if the patient is particularly sensitive to such combined therapy.*
Because of this potentiating effect, dactinomycin may be tried in radio-sensitive tumors not responding to doses of x-ray therapy that can be tolerated. Objective improvement in tumor size and activity may be observed when lower, better tolerated doses of both types of therapy are employed.
COSMEGEN (Dactinomycin, MSD) and Perfusion Technic
Dactinomycin alone or with other antineoplastic agents has also been given by the isolation-perfusion technic, either as palliative treatment or as an adjunct to resection of a tumor. Some tumors considered resistant to chemotherapy and radiation therapy may respond when the drug is given by the perfusion technic. Neoplasms in which dactinomycin has been tried by this technic include various types of sarcoma, carcinoma, and adenocarcinoma.
In some instances tumors regressed, pain was relieved for variable periods, and surgery made possible. On other occa-

sions, however, the outcome has been less favorable. Nevertheless, in selected cases, the drug by perfusion may provide more effective palliation than when given systemically.
Dactinomycin by the isolation-perfusion technic offers certain advantages, provided leakage of the drug through the general circulation into other areas of the body is minimal. By this technic the drug is in continuous contact with the tumor for the duration of treatment. The dose may be increased well over that used by the systemic route, usually without adding to the danger of toxic effects. If the agent is confined to an isolated part, it should not interfere with the patient's defense mechanism. Systemic absorption of toxic products from neoplastic tissue can be minimized by removing the perfusate when the procedure is finished.

CONTRAINDICATIONS

If dactinomycin is given at or about the time of infection with chicken pox or herpes zoster, a severe generalized disease, which may result in death, may occur.

PRECAUTIONS

General
COSMEGEN should be administered only under the supervision of a physician who is experienced in the use of cancer chemotherapeutic agents.
This drug is highly toxic and both powder and solution must be handled and administered with care. Inhalation of dust or vapors and contact with skin or mucous membranes, especially those of the eyes, must be avoided. Should accidental eye contact occur, copious irrigation with water should be instituted immediately, followed by prompt ophthalmologic consultation. Should accidental skin contact occur, the affected part must be irrigated immediately with copious amounts of water for at least 15 minutes.
As with all antineoplastic agents, dactinomycin is a toxic drug and very careful and frequent observation of the patient for adverse reactions is necessary. These reactions may involve any tissue of the body. The possibility of an anaphylactoid reaction should be borne in mind.
Increased incidence of gastrointestinal toxicity and marrow suppression has been reported when dactinomycin was given with x-ray therapy.
Particular caution is necessary when administering dactinomycin in the first two months after irradiation for the treatment of right-sided Wilms' tumor, since hepatomegaly and elevated SGOT levels have been noted.
Nausea and vomiting due to dactinomycin make it necessary to give this drug intermittently. It is extremely important to observe the patient daily for toxic side effects when multiple chemotherapy is employed, since a full course of therapy occasionally is not tolerated. If stomatitis, diarrhea, or severe hemopoietic depression appear during therapy, these drugs should be discontinued until the patient has recovered.
Recent reports indicate an increased incidence of second primary tumors following treatment with radiation and anti-neoplastic agents, such as dactinomycin. Multi-modal therapy creates the need for careful, long-term observation of cancer survivors.
Laboratory Tests
Many abnormalities of renal, hepatic, and bone marrow function have been reported in patients with neoplastic disease and receiving dactinomycin. It is advisable to check renal, hepatic, and bone marrow functions frequently.
Drug/Laboratory Test Interactions
It has been reported that dactinomycin may interfere with bioassay procedures for the determination of antibacterial drug levels.
Carcinogenesis, Mutagenesis, Impairment of Fertility
The International Agency on Research on Cancer has judged that dactinomycin is a positive carcinogen in animals. Local sarcomas were produced in mice and rats after repeated subcutaneous or intraperitoneal injection. Mesenchymal tumors occurred in male F344 rats given intraperitoneal injections of 0.05 mg/kg, 2 to 5 times per week for 18 weeks. The first tumor appeared at 23 weeks.
Dactinomycin has been shown to be mutagenic in a number of test systems *in vitro* and *in vivo* including human fibroblasts and leucocytes, and HELA cells. DNA damage and cytogenetic effects have been demonstrated in the mouse and the rat.
Adequate fertility studies have not been reported.
Pregnancy
Pregnancy Category C. COSMEGEN has been shown to cause malformations and embryotoxicity in the rat, rabbit and hamster when given in doses of 50–100 mcg/kg intravenously (3–7 times the maximum recommended human dose). There are no adequate and well-controlled studies in pregnant women. COSMEGEN should be used during pregnancy only if the potential benefit justifies the potential risk to the fetus.
Nursing Mothers
It is not known whether this drug is excreted in human milk. Because many drugs are excreted in human milk and because of the potential for serious adverse reactions in nursing infants from COSMEGEN, a decision should be made whether to discontinue nursing or to discontinue the drug, taking into account the importance of the drug to the mother.
Pediatric Use
The greater frequency of toxic effects of dactinomycin in infants suggest that this drug should be given to infants only over the age of 6 to 12 months.

ADVERSE REACTIONS

Toxic effects (excepting nausea and vomiting) usually do not become apparent until two to four days after a course of therapy is stopped, and may not be maximal before one to two weeks have elapsed. Deaths have been reported. However, adverse reactions are usually reversible on discontinuance of therapy. They include the following:
Miscellaneous (malaise, fatigue, lethargy, fever, myalgia, proctitis, hypocalcemia).
Oral (cheilitis, dysphagia, esophagitis, ulcerative stomatitis, pharyngitis).
Gastrointestinal (anorexia, nausea, vomiting, abdominal pain, diarrhea, gastrointestinal ulceration). Nausea and vomiting, which occur early during the first few hours after administration, may be alleviated by giving antiemetics.
Hematologic (anemia, even to the point of aplastic anemia, agranulocytosis, leukopenia, thrombopenia, pancytopenia, reticulopenia). Platelet and white cell counts should be done *daily* to detect severe hemopoietic depression. If either count markedly decreases, the drug should be withheld to allow marrow recovery. This often takes up to three weeks.
Dermatologic (alopecia, skin eruptions, acne, flare-up of erythema or increased pigmentation of previously irradiated skin).
Soft tissues. Dactinomycin is extremely corrosive. If extravasation occurs during intravenous use, severe damage to soft tissues will occur. In at least one instance, this has led to contracture of the arms.

OVERDOSAGE

The intravenous LD_{50} of COSMEGEN in the rat is 460 mcg/kg.

DOSAGE AND ADMINISTRATION

Toxic reactions due to dactinomycin are frequent and may be severe (see ADVERSE REACTIONS), thus limiting in many instances the amount that may be given. However, the severity of toxicity varies markedly and is only partly dependent on the dose employed. The drug must be given in short courses.
Intravenous Use
The dosage of dactinomycin varies depending on the tolerance of the patient, the size and location of the neoplasm, and the use of other forms of therapy. It may be necessary to decrease the usual dosages suggested below when other chemotherapy or x-ray therapy is used concomitantly or has been used previously.
The dosage for adults or children should not exceed 15 mcg/kg or 400–600 mcg/square meter of body surface daily intravenously for five days. Calculation of the dosage for obese or edematous patients should be on the basis of surface area in an effort to relate dosage to lean body mass.
Adults: The usual adult dosage is 500 mcg (0.5 mg) daily intravenously for a maximum of five days.
Children: In children 15 mcg (0.015 mg) per kilogram of body weight is given intravenously daily for five days. An alternative schedule is a total dosage of 2500 mcg (2.5 mg) per square meter of body surface given intravenously over a one week period.
In both adults and children, a second course may be given after at least three weeks have elapsed, provided all signs of toxicity have disappeared.
Reconstitute COSMEGEN by adding 1.1 ml of **Sterile Water for Injection (without preservative)** using aseptic precautions. The resulting solution of dactinomycin will contain approximately 500 mcg or 0.5 mg per ml.
Parenteral drug products should be inspected visually for particulate matter and discoloration prior to administration, whenever solution and container permit. When reconstituted, COSMEGEN is a clear, gold-colored solution.
Once reconstituted, the solution of dactinomycin can be added to infusion solutions of Dextrose Injection 5 percent or Sodium Chloride Injection either directly or to the tubing of a running intravenous infusion.
Although reconstituted COSMEGEN is chemically stable, the product does not contain a preservative and accidental microbial contamination might result. Any unused portion should be discarded. Use of water containing preservatives (benzyl alcohol or parabens) to reconstitute COSMEGEN for injection, results in the formation of a precipitate.
Partial removal of dactinomycin from intravenous solutions by cellulose ester membrane filters used in some intravenous in-line filters has been reported.
Since dactinomycin is extremely corrosive to soft tissue, precautions for materials of this nature should be observed.
If the drug is given directly into the vein without the use of an infusion, the "two-needle technic" should be used. Reconstitute and withdraw the calculated dose from the vial with one sterile needle. Use another sterile needle for direct injection into the vein.
Discard any unused portion of the dactinomycin solution.
Isolation-Perfusion Technic
The dosage schedules and the technic itself vary from one investigator to another; the published literature, therefore, should be consulted for details. In general, the following doses are suggested:
- 50 mcg (0.05 mg) per kilogram of body weight for lower extremity or pelvis.
- 35 mcg (0.035 mg) per kilogram of body weight for upper extremity.

It may be advisable to use lower doses in obese patients, or when previous chemotherapy or radiation therapy has been employed.
Complications of the perfusion technic are related mainly to the amount of drug that escapes into the systemic circulation and may consist of hemopoietic depression, absorption of toxic products from massive destruction of neoplastic tissue, increased susceptibility to infection, impaired wound healing, and superficial ulceration of the gastric mucosa. Other side effects may include edema of the extremity involved, damage to soft tissues of the perfused area, and (potentially) venous thrombosis.

HOW SUPPLIED

No. 3298—Injection COSMEGEN is a lyophilized powder and is supplied as follows: **NDC** 0006-3298-22 in vials containing 0.5 mg (500 micrograms) of dactinomycin and 20.0 mg of mannitol. In the dry form the compound is an amorphous yellow powder. The solution is clear and gold-colored.
Special Handling
Due to the drug's toxic and mutagenic properties, appropriate precautions including the use of appropriate safety equipment are recommended for the preparation of COSMEGEN for parenteral administration. The National Institutes of Health presently recommends that the preparation of injectable antineoplastic drugs should be performed in a Class II laminar flow biological safety cabinet and that personnel preparing drugs of this class should wear surgical gloves and a closed front surgical-type gown with knit cuffs.
A.H.F.S. Category: 10:00
DC 6059221 Issued September 1983

CUPRID® Capsules ℞
(Trientine Hydrochloride, MSD)

DESCRIPTION

Trientine hydrochloride is *N,N'*-bis (2-aminoethyl)-1,2-ethanediamine dihydrochloride. It is a white to pale yellow crystalline hygroscopic powder. It is freely soluble in water, soluble in methanol, slightly soluble in ethanol, and insoluble in chloroform and ether.
The empirical formula is $C_6H_{18}N_4 \cdot 2HCl$ with a molecular weight of 219.2. The structural formula is:
$NH_2(CH_2)_2NH(CH_2)_2NH(CH_2)_2NH_2 \cdot 2HCl$
Trientine hydrochloride is a chelating compound for removal of excess copper from the body. CUPRID® (Trientine Hydrochloride, MSD) is available as 250 mg capsules for oral administration. Capsules CUPRID contain stearic acid as an inactive ingredient.

CLINICAL PHARMACOLOGY

Introduction
Wilson's disease (hepatolenticular degeneration) is an autosomal inherited metabolic defect resulting in an inability to maintain a near-zero balance of copper. Excess copper accumulates possibly because the liver lacks the mechanism to excrete free copper into the bile. Hepatocytes store excess copper but when their capacity is exceeded copper is released into the blood and is taken up into extrahepatic sites. This condition is treated with a low copper diet and the use of che-

Continued on next page

Information on the Merck Sharp & Dohme products listed on these pages is the full prescribing information from product circulars in use August 31, 1986.

Merck Sharp & Dohme—Cont.

lating agents that bind copper to facilitate its excretion from the body.

Clinical Summary

Forty-one patients (18 male and 23 female) between the ages of 6 and 54 with a diagnosis of Wilson's disease and who were intolerant of d-penicillamine were treated in two separate studies with trientine hydrochloride. The dosage varied from 450 to 2400 mg per day. The average dosage required to achieve an optimal clinical response varied between 1000 mg and 2000 mg per day. The mean duration of trientine hydrochloride therapy was 48.7 months (range 2–164 months). Thirty-four of the 41 patients improved, 4 had no change in clinical global response, 2 were lost to follow-up and one showed deterioration in clinical condition. One of the patients who improved while on therapy with trientine hydrochloride experienced a recurrence of the symptoms of systemic lupus erythematosus which had appeared originally during therapy with penicillamine. Therapy with trientine hydrochloride was discontinued. No other adverse reactions, except iron deficiency, were noted among any of these 41 patients.

One investigator treated 13 patients with trientine hydrochloride following their development of intolerance to d-penicillamine. Retrospectively, he compared these patients to an additional group of 12 patients with Wilson's disease who were both tolerant of and controlled with d-penicillamine therapy, but who failed to continue any copper chelation therapy. The mean age at onset of disease of the latter group was 12 years as compared to 21 years for the former group. The trientine hydrochloride group received d-penicillamine for an average of 4 years as compared to an average of 10 years for the non-treated group.

Various laboratory parameters showed changes in favor of the patients treated with trientine hydrochloride. Free and total serum copper, SGOT, and serum bilirubin all showed mean increases over baseline in the untreated group which were significantly larger than with the patients treated with trientine hydrochloride. In the 13 patients treated with trientine hydrochloride, previous symptoms and signs relating to d-penicillamine intolerance disappeared in 8 patients, improved in 4 patients, and remained unchanged in one patient. The neurological status in the trientine hydrochloride group was unchanged or improved over baseline, whereas in the untreated group, 6 patients remained unchanged and 6 worsened. Kayser-Fleischer rings improved significantly during trientine hydrochloride treatment.

The clinical outcome of the two groups also differed markedly. Of the 13 patients on therapy with trientine hydrochloride (mean duration of therapy 4.1 years; range 1 to 13 years), all were alive at the data cutoff date, and in the non-treated group (mean years with no therapy 2.7 years; range 3 months to 9 years), 9 of the 12 died of hepatic disease.

Chelating Properties

Preclinical Studies

Studies in animals have shown that trientine hydrochloride has cupriuretic activities in both normal and copper-loaded rats. In general, the effects of trientine hydrochloride on urinary copper excretion are similar to those of equimolar doses of penicillamine, although in one study they were significantly smaller.

Human Studies

Renal clearance studies were carried out with penicillamine and trientine hydrochloride on separate occasions in selected patients treated with penicillamine for at least one year. Six-hour excretion rates of copper were determined off treatment and after a single dose of 500 mg of penicillamine or 1.2 g of trientine hydrochloride. The mean urinary excretion rates of copper were as follows:

No. of Patients	Single Dose Treatment	Basal Excretion Rate ($\mu g\ Cu^{++}/6hr$)	Test-dose Excretion Rate ($\mu g\ Cu^{++}/6hr$)
6	Trientine, 1.2 g	19	234
4	Penicillamine, 500 mg	17	320

In patients *not* previously treated with chelating agents, a similar comparison was made:

No. of Patients	Single Dose Treatment	Basal Excretion Rate ($\mu g\ Cu^{++}/6hr$)	Test-dose Excretion Rate ($\mu g\ Cu^{++}/6hr$)
8	Trientine, 1.2 g	71	1326
7	Penicillamine, 500 mg	68	1074

These results demonstrate that CUPRID is effective as a cupriuretic agent in patients with Wilson's disease although on a molar basis it appears to be less potent or less effective than penicillamine. Evidence from a radio-labelled copper study indicates that the different cupriuretic effect between these two drugs could be due to a difference in selectivity of the drugs for different copper pools within the body.

Pharmacokinetics

Data on the pharmacokinetics of trientine hydrochloride are not available. Dosage adjustment recommendations are based upon clinical use of the drug (see DOSAGE AND ADMINISTRATION).

INDICATIONS AND USAGE

CUPRID is indicated in the treatment of patients with Wilson's disease who are intolerant of penicillamine. Clinical experience with CUPRID is limited and alternate dosing regimens have not been well-characterized; all endpoints in determining an individual patient's dose have not been well defined. CUPRID and penicillamine cannot be considered interchangeable. CUPRID should be used when continued treatment with penicillamine is no longer possible because of intolerable or life endangering side effects.

Unlike penicillamine, CUPRID is not recommended in cystinuria or rheumatoid arthritis. The absence of a sulfhydryl moiety renders it incapable of binding cystine and, therefore, it is of no use in cystinuria. In 15 patients with rheumatoid arthritis, CUPRID was reported not to be effective in improving any clinical or biochemical parameter after 12 weeks of treatment.

CUPRID is not indicated for treatment of biliary cirrhosis.

CONTRAINDICATIONS

Hypersensitivity to this product.

WARNINGS

Patient experience with trientine hydrochloride is limited (see CLINICAL PHARMACOLOGY). Patients receiving CUPRID should remain under regular medical supervision throughout the period of drug administration. Patients (especially women) should be closely monitored for evidence of iron deficiency anemia.

PRECAUTIONS

General

There are no reports of hypersensitivity in patients who have been administered trientine hydrochloride for Wilson's disease. However, there have been reports of asthma, bronchitis and dermatitis occurring after prolonged environmental exposure in workers who use trientine hydrochloride as a hardener of epoxy resins. Patients should be observed closely for signs of possible hypersensitivity.

Information for Patients

Patients should be directed to take CUPRID on an empty stomach, at least one hour before meals or two hours after meals and at least one hour apart from any other drug, food, or milk. The capsules should be swallowed whole with water and should not be opened or chewed. Because of the potential for contact dermatitis, any site of exposure to the capsule contents should be washed with water promptly. For the first month of treatment, the patient should have his temperature taken nightly, and he should be asked to report any symptom such as fever or skin eruption.

Laboratory Tests

The most reliable index for monitoring treatment is the determination of free copper in the serum, which equals the difference between quantitatively determined total copper and ceruloplasmin-copper. Adequately treated patients will usually have less than 10 mcg free copper/dL of serum.

Therapy may be monitored with a 24 hour urinary copper analysis periodically (i.e., every 6–12 months). Urine must be collected in copper-free glassware. Since a low copper diet should keep copper absorption down to less than one milligram a day, the patient probably will be in the desired state of negative copper balance if 0.5 to 1.0 milligram of copper is present in a 24-hour collection of urine.

Drug Interactions

In general, mineral supplements should not be given since they may block the absorption of CUPRID. However, iron deficiency may develop, especially in children and menstruating or pregnant women, or as a result of the low copper diet recommended for Wilson's disease. If necessary, iron may be given in short courses, but since iron and CUPRID each inhibit absorption of the other, two hours should elapse between administration of CUPRID and iron.

It is important that CUPRID be taken on an empty stomach, at least one hour before meals or two hours after meals and at least one hour apart from any other drug, food, or milk. This permits maximum absorption and reduces the likelihood of inactivation of the drug by metal binding in the gastrointestinal tract.

Carcinogenesis, Mutagenesis, Impairment of Fertility

Data on carcinogenesis, mutagenesis, and impairment of fertility are not available.

Pregnancy

Pregnancy Category C. Trientine hydrochloride was teratogenic in rats at doses similar to the human dose. The frequencies of both resorptions and fetal abnormalities, including hemorrhage and edema, increased while fetal copper levels decreased when trientine hydrochloride was given in the maternal diets of rats. There are no adequate and well-controlled studies in pregnant women. CUPRID should be used during pregnancy only if the potential benefit justifies the potential risk to the fetus.

Nursing Mothers

It is not known whether this drug is excreted in human milk. Because many drugs are excreted in human milk, caution should be exercised when CUPRID is administered to a nursing mother.

Pediatric Use

Controlled studies of the safety and effectiveness of CUPRID in children have not been conducted. It has been used clinically in children as young as 6 years with no reported adverse experiences.

ADVERSE REACTIONS

Clinical experience with CUPRID has been limited. The following adverse reactions have been reported in patients with Wilson's disease who were on therapy with trientine hydrochloride: iron deficiency, systemic lupus erythematosus (see CLINICAL PHARMACOLOGY).

CUPRID is not indicated for treatment of biliary cirrhosis, but in one study of 4 patients treated with trientine hydrochloride for primary biliary cirrhosis, the following adverse reactions were reported: heartburn; epigastric pain and tenderness; thickening, fissuring and flaking of the skin; hypochromic microcytic anemia; acute gastritis; aphthoid ulcers; abdominal pain; melena; anorexia; malaise; cramps; muscle pain; weakness; rhabdomyolysis. A causal relationship of these reactions to drug therapy could not be rejected or established.

OVERDOSAGE

There is a report of an adult woman who ingested 30 grams of trientine hydrochloride without apparent ill effects. No other data on overdosage are available.

DOSAGE AND ADMINISTRATION

Systemic evaluation of dose and/or interval between dose has not been done. However, on limited clinical experience, the recommended initial dose of CUPRID is 500–750 mg/day for children and 750–1250 mg/day for adults given in divided doses two, three or four times daily. This may be increased to a maximum of 2000 mg/day for adults or 1500 mg/day for children age 12 or under. The daily dose of CUPRID should be increased only when the clinical response is not adequate or the concentration of free serum copper is persistently above 20 mcg/dL. Optimal long-term maintenance dosage should be determined at 6–12 month intervals (see PRECAUTIONS, *Laboratory Tests*).

It is important that CUPRID be given on an empty stomach, at least one hour before meals or two hours after meals and at least one hour apart from any other drug, food, or milk. The capsules should be swallowed whole with water and should not be opened or chewed.

HOW SUPPLIED

No. 3511—Capsules CUPRID, 250 mg, are light brown opaque capsules and are coded MSD 679. They are supplied as follows:

NDC 0006-0679-68 in bottles of 100.

Shown in Product Identification Section, page 417

Storage

Keep container tightly closed.

Store at 2°–8°C (35.6°–46.4°F).

A.H.F.S. Category: 12:20

DC 7325101 Issued November 1985

CUPRIMINE® Capsules ℞
(Penicillamine, MSD), U.S.P.

Physicians planning to use penicillamine should thoroughly familiarize themselves with its toxicity, special dosage considerations, and therapeutic benefits. Penicillamine should never be used casually. Each patient should remain constantly under the close supervision of the physician. Patients should be warned to report promptly any symptoms suggesting toxicity.

DESCRIPTION

Penicillamine is 3-mercapto-D-valine. It is a white or practically white, crystalline powder, freely soluble in water, slightly soluble in alcohol, and insoluble in ether, acetone, benzene, and carbon tetrachloride. Although its configuration is D, it is levorotatory as usually measured:

$[\alpha]^{25°}_{D} = -63° \pm 5°$ (C = 1, 1N NaOH).

The empirical formula is $C_5H_{11}NO_2S$, giving it a molecular weight of 149.21. The structural formula is:

SH NH₂ on $(CH_3)_2C—CHCOOH$

It reacts readily with formaldehyde or acetone to form a thiazolidine-carboxylic acid.

Capsules CUPRIMINE® (Penicillamine, MSD) for oral administration contain either 125 mg or 250 mg of penicillamine. Each capsule contains the following inactive ingredients: D & C Yellow 10, gelatin, lactose, magnesium stearate, and titanium dioxide. The 125 mg capsule also contains iron oxide.

CLINICAL PHARMACOLOGY

Penicillamine is a chelating agent recommended for the removal of excess copper in patients with Wilson's disease. From *in vitro* studies which indicate that one atom of copper combines with two molecules of penicillamine, it would appear that one gram of penicillamine should be followed by the excretion of about 200 milligrams of copper; however, the actual amount excreted is about one percent of this.

Penicillamine also reduces excess cystine excretion in cystinuria. This is done, at least in part, by disulfide interchange between penicillamine and cystine, resulting in formation of penicillamine-cysteine disulfide, a substance that is much more soluble than cystine and is excreted readily.

Penicillamine interferes with the formation of cross-links between tropocollagen molecules and cleaves them when newly formed.

The mechanism of action of penicillamine in rheumatoid arthritis is unknown although it appears to suppress disease activity. Unlike cytotoxic immunosuppressants, penicillamine markedly lowers IgM rheumatoid factor but produces no significant depression in absolute levels of serum immunoglobulins. Also unlike cytotoxic immunosuppressants which act on both, penicillamine *in vitro* depresses T-cell activity but not B-cell activity.

In vitro, penicillamine dissociates macroglobulins (rheumatoid factor) although the relationship of the activity to its effect in rheumatoid arthritis is not known.

In rheumatoid arthritis, the onset of therapeutic response to CUPRIMINE may not be seen for two or three months. In those patients who respond, however, the first evidence of suppression of symptoms such as pain, tenderness, and swelling is generally apparent within three months. The optimum duration of therapy has not been determined. If remissions occur, they may last from months to years, but usually require continued treatment (see DOSAGE AND ADMINISTRATION).

In all patients receiving penicillamine, it is important that CUPRIMINE be given on an empty stomach, at least one hour before meals or two hours after meals, and at least one hour apart from any other drug, food, or milk. This permits maximum absorption and reduces the likelihood of inactivation by metal binding in the gastrointestinal tract.

Methodology for determining the bioavailability of penicillamine is not available; however, penicillamine is known to be a very soluble substance.

INDICATIONS

CUPRIMINE is indicated in the treatment of Wilson's disease, cystinuria, and in patients with severe, active rheumatoid arthritis who have failed to respond to an adequate trial of conventional therapy. Available evidence suggests that CUPRIMINE is not of value in ankylosing spondylitis.

Wilson's Disease—Wilson's disease (hepatolenticular degeneration) results from the interaction of an inherited defect and an abnormality in copper metabolism. The metabolic defect, which is the consequence of the autosomal inheritance of one abnormal gene from each parent, manifests itself in a greater positive copper balance than normal. As a result, copper is deposited in several organs and appears eventually to produce pathologic effects most prominently seen in the brain, where degeneration is widespread; in the liver, where fatty infiltration, inflammation, and hepatocellular damage progress to postnecrotic cirrhosis; in the kidney, where tubular and glomerular dysfunction results; and in the eye, where characteristic corneal copper deposits are known as Kayser-Fleischer rings.

Two types of patients require treatment for Wilson's disease: (1) the symptomatic, and (2) the asymptomatic in whom it can be assumed the disease will develop in the future if the patient is not treated.

Diagnosis, suspected on the basis of family or individual history, physical examination, or a low serum concentration of ceruloplasmin*, is confirmed by the demonstration of Kayser-Fleischer rings or, particularly in the asymptomatic patient, by the quantitative demonstration in a liver biopsy specimen of a concentration of copper in excess of 250 mcg/g dry weight.

Treatment has two objectives:

(1) to minimize dietary intake and absorption of copper.
(2) to promote excretion of copper deposited in tissues.

The first objective is attained by a daily diet that contains no more than one or two milligrams of copper. Such a diet should exclude, most importantly, chocolate, nuts, shellfish, mushrooms, liver, molasses, broccoli, and cereals enriched with copper, and be composed to as great an extent as possible of foods with a low copper content. Distilled or demineralized water should be used if the patient's drinking water contains more than 0.1 mg of copper per liter.

For the second objective, a copper chelating agent is used. Penicillamine is the only one of these agents that is orally effective.

In symptomatic patients this treatment usually produces marked neurologic improvement, fading of Kayser-Fleischer rings, and gradual amelioration of hepatic dysfunction and psychic disturbances.

Clinical experience to date suggests that life is prolonged with the above regimen.

Noticeable improvement may not occur for one to three months. Occasionally, neurologic symptoms become worse during initiation of therapy with CUPRIMINE. Despite this, the drug should not be discontinued permanently, although temporary interruption may result in clinical improvement of the neurological symptoms but it carries an increased risk of developing a sensitivity reaction upon resumption of therapy (see WARNINGS).

Treatment of asymptomatic patients has been carried out for over ten years. Symptoms and signs of the disease appear to be prevented indefinitely if daily treatment with CUPRIMINE can be continued.

Cystinuria—Cystinuria is characterized by excessive urinary excretion of the dibasic amino acids, arginine, lysine, ornithine, and cystine, and the mixed disulfide of cysteine and homocysteine. The metabolic defect that leads to cystinuria is inherited as an autosomal, recessive trait. Metabolism of the affected amino acids is influenced by at least two abnormal factors: (1) defective gastrointestinal absorption and (2) renal tubular dysfunction.

Arginine, lysine, ornithine, and cysteine are soluble substances, readily excreted. There is no apparent pathology connected with their excretion in excessive quantities.

Cystine, however, is so slightly soluble at the usual range of urinary pH that it is not excreted readily, and so crystallizes and forms stones in the urinary tract. Stone formation is the only known pathology in cystinuria.

Normal daily output of cystine is 40 to 80 mg. In cystinuria, output is greatly increased and may exceed 1 g/day. At 500 to 600 mg/day, stone formation is almost certain. When it is more than 300 mg/day, treatment is indicated.

Conventional treatment is directed at keeping urinary cystine diluted enough to prevent stone formation, keeping the urine alkaline enough to dissolve as much cystine as possible, and minimizing cystine production by a diet low in methionine (the major dietary precursor of cystine). Patients must drink enough fluid to keep urine specific gravity below 1.010, take enough alkali to keep urinary pH at 7.5 to 8, and maintain a diet low in methionine. This diet is not recommended in growing children and probably is contraindicated in pregnancy because of its low protein content (see PRECAUTIONS).

When these measures are inadequate to control recurrent stone formation, CUPRIMINE may be used as additional therapy. When patients refuse to adhere to conventional treatment, CUPRIMINE may be a useful substitute. It is capable of keeping cystine excretion to near normal values, thereby hindering stone formation and the serious consequences of pyelonephritis and impaired renal function that develop in some patients.

Bartter and colleagues depict the process by which penicillamine interacts with cystine to form penicillamine-cysteine mixed disulfide as:

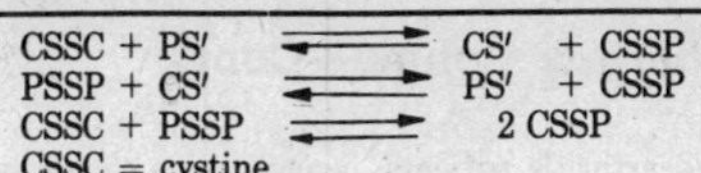

CSSC + PS′ ⇌ CS′ + CSSP
PSSP + CS′ ⇌ PS′ + CSSP
CSSC + PSSP ⇌ 2 CSSP

CSSC = cystine
CS′ = deprotonated cysteine
PSSP = penicillamine
PS′ = deprotonated penicillamine sulfhydryl
CSSP = penicillamine-cysteine mixed disulfide

In this process, it is assumed that the deprotonated form of penicillamine, PS′, is the active factor in bringing about the disulfide interchange.

Rheumatoid Arthritis—Because CUPRIMINE can cause severe adverse reactions, its use in rheumatoid arthritis should be restricted to patients who have severe, active disease and who have failed to respond to an adequate trial of conventional therapy. Even then, benefit-to-risk ratio should be carefully considered. Other measures, such as rest, physiotherapy, salicylates, and corticosteroids should be used, when indicated, in conjunction with CUPRIMINE (see PRECAUTIONS).

CONTRAINDICATIONS

Except for the treatment of Wilson's disease or certain cases of cystinuria, use of penicillamine during pregnancy is contraindicated (see PRECAUTIONS).

Although breast milk studies have not been reported in animals or humans, mothers on therapy with penicillamine should not nurse their infants.

Patients with a history of penicillamine-related aplastic anemia or agranulocytosis should not be restarted on penicillamine (see WARNINGS and ADVERSE REACTIONS).

Because of its potential for causing renal damage, penicillamine should not be administered to rheumatoid arthritis patients with a history or other evidence of renal insufficiency.

WARNINGS

The use of penicillamine has been associated with fatalities due to certain diseases such as aplastic anemia, agranulocytosis, thrombocytopenia, Goodpasture's syndrome, and myasthenia gravis.

Because of the potential for serious hematological and renal adverse reactions to occur at any time, routine urinalysis, white and differential blood cell count, hemoglobin determination, and direct platelet count must be done every two weeks for at least the first six months of penicillamine therapy and monthly thereafter. Patients should be instructed to report promptly the development of signs and symptoms of granulocytopenia and/or thrombocytopenia such as fever, sore throat, chills, bruising or bleeding. The above laboratory studies should then be promptly repeated.

Leukopenia and thrombocytopenia have been reported to occur in up to five percent of patients during penicillamine therapy. Leukopenia is of the granulocytic series and may or may not be associated with an increase in eosinophils. A confirmed reduction in WBC below 3500 per cubic mL mandates discontinuance of penicillamine therapy. Thrombocytopenia may be on an idiosyncratic basis, with decreased or absent megakaryocytes in the marrow, when it is part of an aplastic anemia. In other cases the thrombocytopenia is presumably on an immune basis since the number of megakaryocytes in the marrow has been reported to be normal or sometimes increased. The development of a platelet count below 100,000 per cubic mL, even in the absence of clinical bleeding, requires at least temporary cessation of penicillamine therapy. A progressive fall in either platelet count or WBC in three successive determinations, even though values are still within the normal range, likewise requires at least temporary cessation.

Proteinuria and/or hematuria may develop during therapy and may be warning signs of membranous glomerulopathy which can progress to a nephrotic syndrome. Close observation of these patients is essential. In some patients the proteinuria disappears with continued therapy; in others, penicillamine must be discontinued. When a patient develops proteinuria or hematuria the physician must ascertain whether it is a sign of drug-induced glomerulopathy or is unrelated to penicillamine.

Rheumatoid arthritis patients who develop moderate degrees of proteinuria may be continued cautiously on penicillamine therapy, provided that quantitative 24-hour urinary protein determinations are obtained at intervals of one to two weeks. Penicillamine dosage should not be increased under these circumstances. Proteinuria which exceeds 1 g/24 hours, or proteinuria which is progressively increasing, requires either discontinuance of the drug or a reduction in the dosage. In some patients, proteinuria has been reported to clear following reduction in dosage.

Continued on next page

* For quantitative test for serum ceruloplasmin see: Morell, A.G.; Windsor, J.; Sternlieb, I.; Scheinberg, I.H.: Measurement of the concentration of ceruloplasmin in serum by determination of its oxidase activity, in "Laboratory Diagnosis of Liver Disease", F.W. Sunderman; F.W. Sunderman, Jr. (eds.), St. Louis, Warren H. Green, Inc., 1968, pp. 193-195.

Information on the Merck Sharp & Dohme products listed on these pages is the full prescribing information from product circulars in use August 31, 1986.

Merck Sharp & Dohme—Cont.

In rheumatoid arthritis patients, penicillamine should be discontinued if unexplained gross hematuria or persistent microscopic hematuria develops.

In patients with Wilson's disease or cystinuria the risks of continued penicillamine therapy in patients manifesting potentially serious urinary abnormalities must be weighed against the expected therapeutic benefits.

When penicillamine is used in cystinuria, an annual x-ray for renal stones is advised. Cystine stones form rapidly, sometimes in six months.

Up to one year or more may be required for any urinary abnormalities to disappear after penicillamine has been discontinued.

Because of rare reports of intrahepatic cholestasis and toxic hepatitis, liver function tests are recommended every six months for the duration of therapy.

Goodpasture's syndrome has occurred rarely. The development of abnormal urinary findings associated with hemoptysis and pulmonary infiltrates on x-ray requires immediate cessation of penicillamine.

Obliterative bronchiolitis has been reported rarely. The patient should be cautioned to report immediately pulmonary symptoms such as exertional dyspnea, unexplained cough or wheezing. Pulmonary function studies should be considered at that time.

Myasthenic syndrome sometimes progressing to myasthenia gravis has been reported. In the majority of cases, symptoms of myasthenia have receded after withdrawal of penicillamine.

Pemphigoid-type reactions characterized by bullous lesions clinically indistinguishable from pemphigus have occurred and have required discontinuation of penicillamine and treatment with corticosteroids.

Once instituted for Wilson's disease or cystinuria, treatment with penicillamine should, as a rule, be continued on a daily basis. Interruptions for even a few days have been followed by sensitivity reactions after reinstitution of therapy.

Use in Pregnancy —Penicillamine has been shown to be teratogenic in rats when given in doses 10 times higher than the highest dose recommended for human use. Skeletal defects, cleft palates and fetal toxicity (resorptions) have been reported.

There are no controlled studies on the use of penicillamine in pregnant women. Although normal outcomes have been reported, characteristic congenital cutis laxa and associated birth defects have been reported in infants born of mothers who received therapy with penicillamine during pregnancy. Penicillamine should be used in women of childbearing potential only when the expected benefits outweigh the possible hazards. Women on therapy with penicillamine who are of childbearing potential should be apprised of this risk and followed closely for early recognition of pregnancy.

Wilson's Disease—Reported experience* shows that continued treatment with penicillamine throughout pregnancy protects the mother against relapse of the Wilson's disease, and that discontinuation of penicillamine has deleterious effects on the mother.

If penicillamine is administered during pregnancy to patients with Wilson's disease, it is recommended that the daily dosage be limited to 1 g. If cesarean section is planned, the daily dosage should be limited to 250 mg during the last six weeks of pregnancy and postoperatively until wound healing is complete.

Cystinuria —If possible, penicillamine should not be given during pregnancy to women with cystinuria (see CONTRAINDICATIONS). There are reports of women with cystinuria on therapy with penicillamine who gave birth to infants with generalized connective tissue defects who died following abdominal surgery. If stones continue to form in these patients, the benefits of therapy to the mother must be evaluated against the risk to the fetus.

Rheumatoid Arthritis—Penicillamine should not be administered to rheumatoid arthritis patients who are pregnant (see CONTRAINDICATIONS) and should be discontinued promptly in patients in whom pregnancy is suspected or diagnosed.

There is a report that a woman with rheumatoid arthritis treated with less than one gram a day of penicillamine during pregnancy gave birth (cesarean delivery) to an infant with growth retardation, flattened face with broad nasal bridge, low set ears, short neck with loose skin folds, and unusually lax body skin.

PRECAUTIONS

Some patients may experience drug fever, a marked febrile response to penicillamine, usually in the second to third week following initiation of therapy. Drug fever may sometimes be accompanied by a macular cutaneous eruption.

*Scheinberg, I.H., Sternlieb, I.: N. Engl. J. Med. *293*: 1300-1302, Dec. 18, 1975.

In the case of drug fever in patients with Wilson's disease or cystinuria, because no alternative treatment is available, penicillamine should be temporarily discontinued until the reaction subsides. Then penicillamine should be reinstituted with a small dose that is gradually increased until the desired dosage is attained. Systemic steroid therapy may be necessary, and is usually helpful, in such patients in whom toxic reactions develop a second or third time.

In the case of drug fever in rheumatoid arthritis patients, because other treatments are available, penicillamine should be discontinued and another therapeutic alternative tried since experience indicates that the febrile reaction will recur in a very high percentage of patients upon readministration of penicillamine.

The skin and mucous membranes should be observed for allergic reactions. Early and late rashes have occurred. Early rash occurs during the first few months of treatment and is more common. It is usually a generalized pruritic, erythematous, maculopapular or morbilliform rash and resembles the allergic rash seen with other drugs. Early rash usually disappears within days after stopping penicillamine and seldom recurs when the drug is restarted at a lower dosage. Pruritus and early rash may often be controlled by the concomitant administration of antihistamines. Less commonly, a late rash may be seen, usually after six months or more of treatment, and requires discontinuation of penicillamine. It is usually on the trunk, is accompanied by intense pruritus, and is usually unresponsive to topical corticosteroid therapy. Late rash may take weeks to disappear after penicillamine is stopped and usually recurs if the drug is restarted.

The appearance of a drug eruption accompanied by fever, arthralgia, lymphadenopathy or other allergic manifestations usually requires discontinuation of penicillamine.

Certain patients will develop a positive antinuclear antibody (ANA) test and some of these may show a lupus erythematosus-like syndrome similar to drug-induced lupus associated with other drugs. The lupus erythematosus-like syndrome is not associated with hypocomplementemia and may be present without nephropathy. The development of a positive ANA test does not mandate discontinuance of the drug; however, the physician should be alerted to the possibility that a lupus erythematosus-like syndrome may develop in the future.

Some patients may develop oral ulcerations which in some cases have the appearance of aphthous stomatitis. The stomatitis usually recurs on rechallenge but often clears on a lower dosage. Although rare, cheilosis, glossitis and gingivostomatitis have also been reported. These oral lesions are frequently dose-related and may preclude further increase in penicillamine dosage or require discontinuation of the drug.

Hypogeusia (a blunting or diminution in taste perception) has occurred in some patients. This may last two to three months or more and may develop into a total loss of taste; however, it is usually self-limited despite continued penicillamine treatment. Such taste impairment is rare in patients with Wilson's disease.

Penicillamine should not be used in patients who are receiving concurrently gold therapy, antimalarial or cytotoxic drugs, oxyphenbutazone or phenylbutazone because these drugs are also associated with similar serious hematologic and renal adverse reactions. Patients who have had gold salt therapy discontinued due to a major toxic reaction may be at greater risk of serious adverse reactions with penicillamine but not necessarily of the same type.

Patients who are allergic to penicillin may theoretically have cross-sensitivity to penicillamine. The possibility of reactions from contamination of penicillamine by trace amounts of penicillin has been eliminated now that penicillamine is being produced synthetically rather than as a degradation product of penicillin.

Because of their dietary restrictions, patients with Wilson's disease and cystinuria should be given 25 mg/day of pyridoxine during therapy, since penicillamine increases the requirement for this vitamin. Patients also may receive benefit from a multivitamin preparation, although there is no evidence that deficiency of any vitamin other than pyridoxine is associated with penicillamine. In Wilson's disease, multivitamin preparations must be copper-free.

Rheumatoid arthritis patients whose nutrition is impaired should also be given a daily supplement of pyridoxine. Mineral supplements should not be given, since they may block the response to penicillamine.

Iron deficiency may develop, especially in children and in menstruating women. In Wilson's disease, this may be a result of adding the effects of the low copper diet, which is probably also low in iron, and the penicillamine to the effects of blood loss or growth. In cystinuria, a low methionine diet may contribute to iron deficiency, since it is necessarily low in protein. If necessary, iron may be given in short courses, but a period of two hours should elapse between administration of penicillamine and iron, since orally administered iron has been shown to reduce the effects of penicillamine.

Penicillamine causes an increase in the amount of soluble collagen. In the rat this results in inhibition of normal healing and also a decrease in tensile strength of intact skin. In man this may be the cause of increased skin friability at sites especially subject to pressure or trauma, such as shoulders, elbows, knees, toes, and buttocks. Extravasations of blood may occur and may appear as purpuric areas, with external bleeding if the skin is broken, or as vesicles containing dark blood. Neither type is progressive. There is no apparent association with bleeding elsewhere in the body and no associated coagulation defect has been found. Therapy with penicillamine may be continued in the presence of these lesions. They may not recur if dosage is reduced. Other reported effects probably due to the action of penicillamine on collagen are excessive wrinkling of the skin and development of small, white papules at venipuncture and surgical sites.

The effects of penicillamine on collagen and elastin make it advisable to consider a reduction in dosage to 250 mg/day, when surgery is contemplated. Reinstitution of full therapy should be delayed until wound healing is complete.

Carcinogenesis—Long-term animal carcinogenicity studies have not been done with penicillamine. There is a report that five of ten autoimmune disease-prone NZB hybrid mice developed lymphocytic leukemia after 6 months' intraperitoneal treatment with a dose of 400 mg/kg penicillamine 5 days per week.

Nursing Mothers —See CONTRAINDICATIONS.

Usage in Children —The efficacy of CUPRIMINE in juvenile rheumatoid arthritis has not been established.

ADVERSE REACTIONS

Penicillamine is a drug with a high incidence of untoward reactions, some of which are potentially fatal. Therefore, it is mandatory that patients receiving penicillamine therapy remain under close medical supervision throughout the period of drug administration (see WARNINGS and PRECAUTIONS).

Reported incidences (%) for the most commonly occurring adverse reactions in rheumatoid arthritis patients are noted, based on 17 representative clinical trials reported in the literature (1270 patients).

Allergic—Generalized pruritus, early and late rashes (5%), pemphigoid-type reactions, and drug eruptions which may be accompanied by fever, arthralgia, or lymphadenopathy have occurred (see WARNINGS and PRECAUTIONS). Some patients may show a lupus erythematosus-like syndrome similar to drug-induced lupus produced by other pharmacological agents (see PRECAUTIONS).

Urticaria and exfoliative dermatitis have occurred.

Thyroiditis has been reported; hypoglycemia in association with anti-insulin antibodies has been reported. These reactions are extremely rare.

Some patients may develop a migratory polyarthralgia, often with objective synovitis (see DOSAGE AND ADMINISTRATION).

Gastrointestinal—Anorexia, epigastric pain, nausea, vomiting, or occasional diarrhea may occur (17%).

Isolated cases of reactivated peptic ulcer have occurred, as have hepatic dysfunction and pancreatitis. Intrahepatic cholestasis and toxic hepatitis have been reported rarely. There have been a few reports of increased serum alkaline phosphatase, lactic dehydrogenase, and positive cephalin flocculation and thymol turbidity tests.

Some patients may report a blunting, diminution, or total loss of taste perception (12%); or may develop oral ulcerations. Although rare, cheilosis, glossitis, and gingivostomatitis have been reported (see PRECAUTIONS).

Gastrointestinal side effects are usually reversible following cessation of therapy.

Hematological—Penicillamine can cause bone marrow depression (see WARNINGS). Leukopenia (2%) and thrombocytopenia (4%) have occurred. Fatalities have been reported as a result of thrombocytopenia, agranulocytosis, and aplastic anemia.

Thrombotic thrombocytopenic purpura, hemolytic anemia, red cell aplasia, monocytosis, leukocytosis, eosinophilia, and thrombocytosis have also been reported.

Renal—Patients on penicillamine therapy may develop proteinuria (6%) and/or hematuria which, in some, may progress to the development of the nephrotic syndrome as a result of an immune complex membranous glomerulopathy (see WARNINGS).

Central Nervous System—Tinnitus, optic neuritis and peripheral sensory and motor neuropathies (including polyradiculoneuropathy, i.e., Guillain-Barre Syndrome) have been reported. Muscular weakness may or may not occur with the peripheral neuropathies.

Neuromuscular—Myasthenia gravis (see WARNINGS).

Other—Adverse reactions that have been reported rarely include thrombophlebitis; hyperpyrexia (see PRECAUTIONS); falling hair or alopecia; lichen planus; polymyositis; dermatomyositis; mammary hyperplasia; elastosis perforans serpiginosa; toxic epidermal necrolysis; anetoderma (cutaneous macular atrophy); and Goodpasture's syndrome, a severe and ultimately fatal glomerulonephritis associated with intra-alveolar hemorrhage (see WARNINGS). Fatal renal

vasculitis has also been reported. Allergic alveolitis, obliterative bronchiolitis, interstitial pneumonitis and pulmonary fibrosis have been reported in patients with severe rheumatoid arthritis, some of whom were receiving penicillamine. Bronchial asthma also has been reported.
Increased skin friability, excessive wrinkling of skin, and development of small white papules at venipuncture and surgical sites have been reported (see PRECAUTIONS).
The chelating action of the drug may cause increased excretion of other heavy metals such as zinc, mercury and lead.
There have been reports associating penicillamine with leukemia. However, circumstances involved in these reports are such that a cause and effect relationship to the drug has not been established.

DOSAGE AND ADMINISTRATION

In all patients receiving penicillamine, it is important that CUPRIMINE be given on an empty stomach, at least one hour before meals or two hours after meals, and at least one hour apart from any other drug, food, or milk.
Wilson's Disease—Optimal dosage can be determined only by measurement of urinary copper excretion. The urine must be collected in copper-free glassware, and should be quantitatively analyzed for copper before and soon after initiation of therapy with CUPRIMINE. Continued therapy should be monitored by doing a 24-hour urinary copper analysis every three months or so for the duration of therapy. Since a low copper diet should keep copper absorption down to less than one milligram a day, the patient probably will be in negative copper balance if 0.5 to one milligram of copper is present in a 24-hour collection of urine.
To achieve this, the suggested initial dosage of CUPRIMINE in the treatment of Wilson's disease is 1 g/day for children or adults. This may be increased, as indicated by the urinary copper analyses, but it is seldom necessary to exceed a dosage of 2 g/day.
In patients who cannot tolerate as much as 1 g/day initially, initiating dosage with 250 mg/day, and increasing gradually to the requisite amount, gives closer control of the effects of the drug and may help to reduce the incidence of adverse reactions.
Cystinuria—It is recommended that CUPRIMINE be used along with conventional therapy. By reducing urinary cystine, it decreases crystalluria and stone formation. In some instances, it has been reported to decrease the size of, and even to dissolve, stones already formed.
The usual dosage of CUPRIMINE in the treatment of cystinuria is 2 g/day for adults, with a range of 1 to 4 g/day. For children, dosage can be based on 30 mg/kg/day. The total daily amount should be divided into four doses. If four equal doses are not feasible, give the larger portion at bedtime. If adverse reactions necessitate a reduction in dosage, it is important to retain the bedtime dose.
Initiating dosage with 250 mg/day, and increasing gradually to the requisite amount, gives closer control of the effects of the drug and may help to reduce the incidence of adverse reactions.
In addition to taking CUPRIMINE, patients should drink copiously. It is especially important to drink about a pint of fluid at bedtime and another pint once during the night when urine is more concentrated and more acid than during the day. The greater the fluid intake, the lower the required dosage of CUPRIMINE.
Dosage must be individualized to an amount that limits cystine excretion to 100–200 mg/day in those with no history of stones, and below 100 mg/day in those who have had stone formation and/or pain. Thus, in determining dosage, the inherent tubular defect, the patient's size, age, and rate of growth, and his diet and water intake all must be taken into consideration.
The standard nitroprusside cyanide test has been reported useful as a qualitative measure of the effective dose*: Add 2 mL of freshly prepared 5 percent sodium cyanide to 5 mL of a 24-hour aliquot of protein-free urine and let stand ten minutes. Add 5 drops of freshly prepared 5 percent sodium nitroprusside and mix. Cystine will turn the mixture magenta. If the result is negative, it can be assumed that cystine excretion is less than 100 mg/g creatinine.
Although penicillamine is rarely excreted unchanged, it also will turn the mixture magenta. If there is any question as to which substance is causing the reaction, a ferric chloride test can be done to eliminate doubt: Add 3 percent ferric chloride dropwise to the urine. Penicillamine will turn the urine an immediate and quickly fading blue. Cystine will not produce any change in appearance.
Rheumatoid Arthritis—The principal rule of treatment with CUPRIMINE in rheumatoid arthritis is patience. The onset of therapeutic response is typically delayed. Two or three months may be required before the first evidence of a clinical response is noted (see CLINICAL PHARMACOLOGY).

*Lotz, M., Potts, J.T. and Bartter, F.C.: Brit. Med. J. *2*:521, Aug. 28, 1965 (in Medical Memoranda).

When treatment with CUPRIMINE has been interrupted because of adverse reactions or other reasons, the drug should be reintroduced cautiously by starting with a lower dosage and increasing slowly.
Initial Therapy—The currently recommended dosage regimen in rheumatoid arthritis begins with a single daily dose of 125 mg or 250 mg which is thereafter increased at one to three month intervals, by 125 mg or 250 mg/day, as patient response and tolerance indicate. If a satisfactory remission of symptoms is achieved, the dose associated with the remission should be continued (see *Maintenance Therapy*). If there is no improvement and there are no signs of potentially serious toxicity after two to three months of treatment with doses of 500–750 mg/day, increases of 250 mg/day at two to three month intervals may be continued until a satisfactory remission occurs (see *Maintenance Therapy*) or signs of toxicity develop (see WARNINGS and PRECAUTIONS). If there is no discernible improvement after three to four months of treatment with 1000 to 1500 mg of penicillamine/day, it may be assumed the patient will not respond and CUPRIMINE should be discontinued.
Maintenance Therapy—The maintenance dosage of CUPRIMINE must be individualized, and may require adjustment during the course of treatment. Many patients respond satisfactorily to a dosage within the 500–750 mg/day range. Some need less.
Changes in maintenance dosage levels may not be reflected clinically or in the erythrocyte sedimentation rate for two to three months after each dosage adjustment.
Some patients will subsequently require an increase in the maintenance dosage to achieve maximal disease suppression. In those patients who do respond, but who evidence incomplete suppression of their disease after the first six to nine months of treatment, the daily dosage of CUPRIMINE may be increased by 125 mg or 250 mg/day at three-month intervals. It is unusual in current practice to employ a dosage in excess of 1 g/day, but up to 1.5 g/day has sometimes been required.
Management of Exacerbations—During the course of treatment some patients may experience an exacerbation of disease activity following an initial good response. These may be self-limited and can subside within twelve weeks. They are usually controlled by the addition of nonsteroidal anti-inflammatory drugs, and only if the patient has demonstrated a true "escape" phenomenon (as evidenced by failure of the flare to subside within this time period) should an increase in the maintenance dose ordinarily be considered.
In the rheumatoid patient, migratory polyarthralgia due to penicillamine is extremely difficult to differentiate from an exacerbation of the rheumatoid arthritis. Discontinuance or a substantial reduction in dosage of CUPRIMINE for up to several weeks will usually determine which of these processes is responsible for the arthralgia.
Duration of Therapy—The optimum duration of therapy with CUPRIMINE in rheumatoid arthritis has not been determined. If the patient has been in remission for six months or more, a gradual, stepwise dosage reduction in decrements of 125 mg or 250 mg/day at approximately three month intervals may be attempted.
Concomitant Drug Therapy—CUPRIMINE should not be used in patients who are receiving gold therapy, antimalarial or cytotoxic drugs, oxyphenbutazone, or phenylbutazone (see PRECAUTIONS). Other measures, such as salicylates, other nonsteroidal anti-inflammatory drugs, or systemic corticosteroids, may be continued when penicillamine is initiated. After improvement commences, analgesic and anti-inflammatory drugs may be slowly discontinued as symptoms permit. Steroid withdrawal must be done gradually, and many months of treatment with CUPRIMINE may be required before steroids can be completely eliminated.
Dosage Frequency—Based on clinical experience dosages up to 500 mg/day can be given as a single daily dose. Dosages in excess of 500 mg/day should be administered in divided doses.

HOW SUPPLIED

No. 3299—Capsules CUPRIMINE, 250 mg, are ivory-colored capsules containing a white or nearly white powder, and are coded MSD 602. They are supplied as follows:
NDC 0006-0602-68 in bottles of 100.
Shown in Product Identification Section, page 417
No. 3350—Capsules CUPRIMINE, 125 mg, are opaque yellow and gray capsules containing a white or nearly white powder, and are coded MSD 672. They are supplied as follows:
NDC 0006-0672-68 in bottles of 100.
Shown in Product Identification Section, page 417
Storage
Keep container tightly closed.
A.H.F.S. Category: 64:00
DC 6177835 Issued March 1985

DARANIDE® Tablets ℞
(Dichlorphenamide, MSD), U.S.P.

DESCRIPTION

DARANIDE® (Dichlorphenamide, MSD) is an oral carbonic anhydrase inhibitor. Dichlorphenamide, a dichlorinated benzenedisulfonamide, is known chemically as 4,5-dichloro-1,3-benzenedisulfonamide. Its empirical formula is $C_6H_6Cl_2N_2O_4S_2$ and its structural formula is:

Dichlorphenamide is a white or practically white, crystalline compound with a molecular weight of 305.16. It is very slightly soluble in water but soluble in dilute solutions of sodium carbonate and sodium hydroxide. Dilute alkaline solutions of dichlorphenamide are stable at room temperature.
DARANIDE is supplied as tablets, for oral administration, each containing 50 mg dichlorphenamide. Inactive ingredients are D&C Yellow 10, lactose, magnesium stearate, and starch.

ACTIONS

Carbonic anhydrase inhibitors reduce intraocular pressure by partially suppressing the secretion of aqueous humor (inflow), although the mechanism by which they do this is not fully understood. Evidence suggests that HCO_3^- ions are produced in the ciliary body by hydration of carbon dioxide under the influence of carbonic anhydrase and diffuse into the posterior chamber with Na^+ ions. The aqueous fluid contains more Na^+ and HCO_3^- ions than does plasma and consequently is hypertonic. Water is attracted to the posterior chamber by osmosis. Systemic administration of a carbonic anhydrase inhibitor has been shown to inactivate carbonic anhydrase in the ciliary body of the rabbit's eye and to reduce the high concentration of HCO_3^- ions in ocular fluids. As is the case with all carbonic anhydrase inhibitors, DARANIDE in high doses causes some decrease in renal blood flow and glomerular filtration rate.
In man, DARANIDE begins to act within an hour and maximal effect is observed in two to four hours. The lowered intraocular tension may be maintained for approximately 6 to 12 hours.

INDICATIONS

For adjunctive treatment of: chronic simple (open-angle) glaucoma, secondary glaucoma, and preoperatively in acute angle-closure glaucoma where delay of surgery is desired in order to lower intraocular pressure.

CONTRAINDICATIONS

DARANIDE is contraindicated in hepatic insufficiency, renal failure, adrenocortical insufficiency, hyperchloremic acidosis, or in conditions in which serum levels of sodium or potassium are depressed. DARANIDE should not be used in patients with severe pulmonary obstruction who are unable to increase their alveolar ventilation since their acidosis may be increased.
DARANIDE is contraindicated in patients who are hypersensitive to this product.

WARNING

Use in Pregnancy: Studies with dichlorphenamide in rats have demonstrated teratogenic effects (skeletal anomalies) at high doses. There is no evidence of these effects in human beings; however, DARANIDE should not be used in women of childbearing age or in pregnancy, especially during the first trimester, unless the benefits to be expected outweigh potential adverse effects.

PRECAUTIONS

Potassium excretion is increased by DARANIDE and hypokalemia may develop with brisk diuresis, when severe cir-

Continued on next page

Information on the Merck Sharp & Dohme products listed on these pages is the full prescribing information from product circulars in use August 31, 1986.

Merck Sharp & Dohme—Cont.

rhosis is present, or during concomitant use of steroids or ACTH.
Interference with adequate oral electrolyte intake will also contribute to hypokalemia. Hypokalemia can sensitize or exaggerate the response of the heart to the toxic effects of digitalis (e.g., increased ventricular irritability). Hypokalemia may be avoided or treated by use of potassium supplements such as foods with a high potassium content. DARANIDE should be used with caution in patients with severe degrees of respiratory acidosis.

ADVERSE REACTIONS

Certain side effects characteristic of carbonic anhydrase inhibitors may occur with DARANIDE. These effects may include gastrointestinal disturbances (anorexia, nausea, and vomiting), loss of weight, constipation, urinary frequency, renal colic, renal calculi, skin eruptions, pruritus, leukopenia, agranulocytosis, thrombocytopenia, headache, weakness, nervousness, globus hystericus, sedation, lassitude, depression, confusion, disorientation, dizziness, ataxia, tremor, tinnitus, and paresthesias of the hands, feet, and tongue.

DOSAGE AND ADMINISTRATION

DARANIDE is usually most successful when given in conjunction with miotics such as isoflurophate, demecarium bromide, pilocarpine, physostigmine, or carbachol. In acute angle-closure glaucoma, it may be used together with miotics and osmotic agents in an attempt to reduce intraocular tension rapidly. If this is not quickly relieved, surgery may be mandatory.
Dosage must be adjusted carefully to meet the requirements of the individual patient. A priming dose of 100 to 200 mg of DARANIDE (2 to 4 tablets) is suggested for adults, followed by 100 mg (2 tablets) every 12 hours until the desired response has been obtained. The recommended maintenance dosage for adults is 25 to 50 mg (½ to 1 tablet) once to three times daily.

HOW SUPPLIED

No. 3256—Tablets DARANIDE, 50 mg each, are yellow, round, scored, compressed tablets, coded MSD 49. They are supplied as follows:
NDC 0006-0049-68 bottles of 100.
Shown in Product Identification Section, page 417
A.H.F.S. Category: 52:10
DC 6010115 Issued May 1985

DECADERM® 0.1% Topical ℞
(Dexamethasone, MSD)
in ESTERGEL®
(Isopropyl Myristate Gel, MSD)

DESCRIPTION

DECADERM® (Dexamethasone, MSD) is a topical steroid preparation containing 0.1% of dexamethasone. The topical corticosteroids constitute a class of primarily synthetic steroids used as anti-inflammatory and anti-pruritic agents. Dexamethasone is 9-fluoro-11β,17,21-trihydroxy-16α-methylpregna-1,4-diene-3,20-dione.
Its empirical formula is $C_{22}H_{29}FO_5$ and its structural formula is:

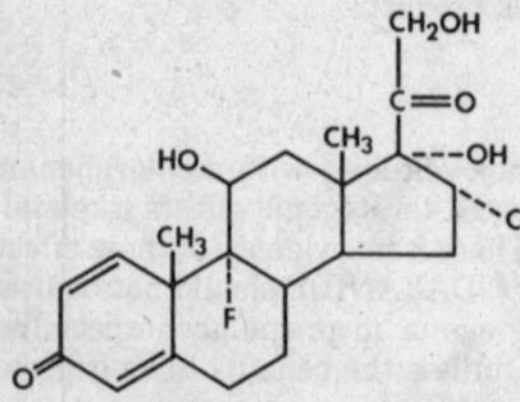

Dexamethasone has a molecular weight of 392.47.
Dexamethasone is slightly soluble both in isopropyl myristate (.23 mg/ml) and in water (.11 mg/ml) at 37°C.
Each gram of DECADERM contains 1 mg dexamethasone in ESTERGEL®, a specially formulated vehicle consisting of gelled isopropyl myristate, wool alcohols B.P., refined lanolin alcohol, microcrystalline wax, anhydrous citric acid, and anhydrous sodium phosphate dibasic.
This emollient gel vehicle is anhydrous, lipophilic, hydrophilic, and moisture-retentive. The base largely disappears when rubbed on the skin.

CLINICAL PHARMACOLOGY

Topical corticosteroids share anti-inflammatory, anti-pruritic and vasoconstrictive actions.
The mechanism of anti-inflammatory activity of the topical corticosteroids is unclear. Various laboratory methods, including vasoconstrictor assays, are used to compare and predict potencies and/or clinical efficacies of the topical corticosteroids. There is some evidence to suggest that a recognizable correlation exists between vasoconstrictor potency and therapeutic efficacy in man.
Pharmacokinetics
The extent of percutaneous absorption of topical corticosteroids is determined by many factors including the vehicle, the integrity of the epidermal barrier, and the use of occlusive dressings.
Topical corticosteroids can be absorbed from normal intact skin. Inflammation and/or other disease processes in the skin increase percutaneous absorption. Occlusive dressings substantially increase the percutaneous absorption of topical corticosteroids. Thus, occlusive dressings may be a valuable therapeutic adjunct for treatment of resistant dermatoses. (See DOSAGE AND ADMINISTRATION)
Once absorbed through the skin, topical corticosteroids are handled through pharmacokinetic pathways similar to systemically administered corticosteroids. Corticosteroids are bound to plasma proteins in varying degrees. Corticosteroids are metabolized primarily in the liver and are then excreted by the kidneys. Some of the topical corticosteroids and their metabolites are also excreted into the bile.

INDICATIONS AND USAGE

DECADERM is indicated for relief of the inflammatory and pruritic manifestations of corticosteroid-responsive dermatoses.

CONTRAINDICATIONS

Topical corticosteroids are contraindicated in those patients with a history of hypersensitivity to any of the components of the preparation.

PRECAUTIONS

General
Systemic absorption of topical corticosteroids has produced reversible hypothalamic-pituitary-adrenal (HPA) axis suppression, manifestations of Cushing's syndrome, hyperglycemia, and glycosuria in some patients.
Conditions which augment systemic absorption include the application of the more potent corticosteroids, use over large surface areas, prolonged use, and the addition of occlusive dressings.
Therefore, patients receiving a large dose of a potent topical corticosteroid applied to a large surface area or under an occlusive dressing should be evaluated periodically for evidence of HPA axis suppression by using urinary free cortisol and ACTH stimulation tests. If HPA axis suppression is noted, an attempt should be made to withdraw the drug, to reduce the frequency of application, or to substitute a less potent corticosteroid.
Recovery of HPA axis function is generally prompt and complete upon discontinuation of the drug. Infrequently, signs and symptoms of corticosteroid withdrawal may occur, requiring supplemental systemic corticosteroids.
Children may absorb proportionally larger amounts of topical corticosteroids and thus be more susceptible to systemic toxicity (See PRECAUTIONS, *Pediatric Use*).
If irritation develops, topical corticosteroids should be discontinued and appropriate therapy instituted.
In the presence of dermatological infections, the use of an appropriate antifungal or antibacterial agent should be instituted. If a favorable response does not occur promptly, the corticosteroid should be discontinued until the infection has been adequately controlled.
This product is not for ophthalmic use. However, if applied to the eyelids or skin near the eyes, the drug may enter the eyes. In patients with a history of herpes simplex keratitis, ocular exposure to corticosteroids may lead to a recurrence. Prolonged ocular exposure may cause steroid glaucoma.
Generally, occlusive dressings should not be used on weeping or exudative lesions.
If occlusive dressing therapy is used, inspect lesions between dressings for development of infection. If infection develops, the technique should be discontinued and appropriate antimicrobial therapy instituted.
When large areas of the body are covered with an occlusive dressing, thermal homeostasis may be impaired. If elevation of body temperature occurs, use of the occlusive dressing should be discontinued.
Information for the Patient
Patients using topical corticosteroids should receive the following information and instructions:

1. This medication is to be used as directed by the physician. It is for external use only. Avoid contact with the eyes.
2. Patients should be advised not to use this medication for any disorder other than that for which it was prescribed.
3. The treated skin area should not be bandaged or otherwise covered or wrapped so as to be occlusive unless directed by the physician.
4. Patients should report any signs of local adverse reactions, especially under occlusive dressing.
5. Parents of pediatric patients should be advised not to use tight-fitting diapers or plastic pants on a child being treated in the diaper area, as these garments may constitute occlusive dressings.

Laboratory Tests
The following tests may be helpful in evaluating the HPA axis suppression:
- Urinary free cortisol test
- ACTH stimulation test

Carcinogenesis, Mutagenesis, and Impairment of Fertility
Long-term animal studies have not been performed to evaluate the carcinogenic potential or the effect on fertility of topical corticosteroids.
Studies to determine mutagenicity with prednisolone and hydrocortisone have revealed negative results.
Pregnancy
Pregnancy Category C: Corticosteroids are generally teratogenic in laboratory animals when administered systemically at relatively low dosage levels. The more potent corticosteroids have been shown to be teratogenic after dermal application in laboratory animals. There are no adequate and well-controlled studies in pregnant women on teratogenic effects from topically applied corticosteroids. Therefore, topical corticosteroids should be used during pregnancy only if the potential benefit justifies the potential risk to the fetus. Drugs of this class should not be used extensively on pregnant patients, in large amounts, or for prolonged periods of time.
Nursing Mothers
It is not known whether topical administration of corticosteroids could result in sufficient systemic absorption to produce detectable quantities in breast milk. Systemically administered corticosteroids are secreted into breast milk in quantities *not* likely to have a deleterious effect on the infant. Nevertheless, caution should be exercised when topical corticosteroids are administered to a nursing woman.
Pediatric Use
Pediatric patients may demonstrate greater susceptibility to topical corticosteroid-induced HPA axis suppression and Cushing's syndrome than mature patients because of a larger skin surface area to body weight ratio.
Hypothalamic-pituitary-adrenal (HPA) axis suppression, Cushing's syndrome, and intracranial hypertension have been reported in children receiving topical corticosteroids. Manifestations of adrenal suppression in children include linear growth retardation, delayed weight gain, low plasma cortisol levels, and absence of response to ACTH stimulation. Manifestations of intracranial hypertension include bulging fontanelles, headaches, and bilateral papilledema.
Administration of topical corticosteroids to children should be limited to the least amount compatible with an effective therapeutic regimen. Chronic corticosteroid therapy may interfere with the growth and development of children.

ADVERSE REACTIONS

The following adverse reactions are reported infrequently with topical corticosteroids, but may occur more frequently with the use of occlusive dressings. These reactions are listed in an approximate decreasing order of occurrence:
Burning
Itching
Irritation
Dryness
Folliculitis
Hypertrichosis
Acneiform eruptions
Hypopigmentation
Perioral dermatitis
Allergic contact dermatitis
Maceration of the skin
Secondary infection
Skin atrophy
Striae
Miliaria

OVERDOSAGE

Topically applied corticosteroids can be absorbed in sufficient amounts to produce systemic effects (See PRECAUTIONS).

DOSAGE AND ADMINISTRATION

Apply to the affected area as a thin film three or four times daily.

Occlusive dressings may be used for the management of psoriasis or recalcitrant conditions.
Before using this preparation in the ear, clean the aural canal thoroughly and sponge dry. Confirm that the eardrum is intact. With a cotton-tipped applicator, apply a thin coating of the cream to the affected canal area three or four times a day.

HOW SUPPLIED

No. 7631—0.1% Topical DECADERM is pale yellow in color, and is supplied as follows:
NDC 0006-7631-24 in 30 g tubes.

A.H.F.S. Category: 84:06
DC 6822406 Issued April 1983

DECADRON® Elixir ℞
(Dexamethasone, MSD), U.S.P.

DESCRIPTION

Glucocorticoids are adrenocortical steroids, both naturally occurring and synthetic, which are readily absorbed from the gastrointestinal tract.
Dexamethasone, a synthetic adrenocortical steroid, is a white to practically white, odorless, crystalline powder. It is stable in air. It is practically insoluble in water. The molecular weight is 392.47. It is designated chemically as 9-fluoro-11β,17,21-trihydroxy-16α-methylpregna -1, 4-diene-3,20-dione. The empirical formula is $C_{22}H_{29}FO_5$ and the structural formula is:

DECADRON® (Dexamethasone, MSD) elixir contains 0.5 mg of dexamethasone in each 5 mL. Benzoic acid, 0.1%, is added as a preservative. It also contains alcohol 5%. Inactive ingredients are FD&C Red 40, flavors, glycerin, purified water, and sodium saccharin.

ACTIONS

Naturally occurring glucocorticoids (hydrocortisone and cortisone), which also have salt-retaining properties, are used as replacement therapy in adrenocortical deficiency states. Their synthetic analogs, including dexamethasone, are primarily used for their potent anti-inflammatory effects in disorders of many organ systems.
Glucocorticoids cause profound and varied metabolic effects. In addition, they modify the body's immune responses to diverse stimuli.
At equipotent anti-inflammatory doses, dexamethasone almost completely lacks the sodium-retaining property of hydrocortisone and closely related derivatives of hydrocortisone.

INDICATIONS

1. *Endocrine Disorders*
Primary or secondary adrenocortical insufficiency (hydrocortisone or cortisone is the first choice; synthetic analogs may be used in conjunction with mineralocorticoids where applicable; in infancy mineralocorticoid supplementation is of particular importance)
   - Congenital adrenal hyperplasia
   - Nonsuppurative thyroiditis
   - Hypercalcemia associated with cancer
2. *Rheumatic Disorders*
As adjunctive therapy for short-term administration (to tide the patient over an acute episode or exacerbation) in:
   - Psoriatic arthritis
   - Rheumatoid arthritis, including juvenile rheumatoid arthritis (selected cases may require low-dose maintenance therapy)
   - Ankylosing spondylitis
   - Acute and subacute bursitis
   - Acute nonspecific tenosynovitis
   - Acute gouty arthritis
   - Post-traumatic osteoarthritis
   - Synovitis of osteoarthritis
   - Epicondylitis
3. *Collagen Diseases*
During an exacerbation or as maintenance therapy in selected cases of—
   - Systemic lupus erythematosus
   - Acute rheumatic carditis
4. *Dermatologic Diseases*
   - Pemphigus
   - Bullous dermatitis herpetiformis
   - Severe erythema multiforme (Stevens-Johnson syndrome)
   - Exfoliative dermatitis
   - Mycosis fungoides
   - Severe psoriasis
   - Severe seborrheic dermatitis
5. *Allergic States*
Control of severe or incapacitating allergic conditions intractable to adequate trials of conventional treatment:
   - Seasonal or perennial allergic rhinitis
   - Bronchial asthma
   - Contact dermatitis
   - Atopic dermatitis
   - Serum sickness
   - Drug hypersensitivity reactions
6. *Ophthalmic Diseases*
Severe acute and chronic allergic and inflammatory processes involving the eye and its adnexa, such as—
   - Allergic conjunctivitis
   - Keratitis
   - Allergic corneal marginal ulcers
   - Herpes zoster ophthalmicus
   - Iritis and iridocyclitis
   - Chorioretinitis
   - Anterior segment inflammation
   - Diffuse posterior uveitis and choroiditis
   - Optic neuritis
   - Sympathetic ophthalmia
7. *Respiratory Diseases*
   - Symptomatic sarcoidosis
   - Loeffler's syndrome not manageable by other means
   - Berylliosis
   - Fulminating or disseminated pulmonary tuberculosis when used concurrently with appropriate antituberculous chemotherapy
   - Aspiration pneumonitis
8. *Hematologic Disorders*
   - Idiopathic thrombocytopenic purpura in adults
   - Secondary thrombocytopenia in adults
   - Acquired (autoimmune) hemolytic anemia
   - Erythroblastopenia (RBC anemia)
   - Congenital (erythroid) hypoplastic anemia
9. *Neoplastic Diseases*
For palliative management of:
   - Leukemias and lymphomas in adults
   - Acute leukemia of childhood
10. *Edematous States*
To induce a diuresis or remission of proteinuria in the nephrotic syndrome, without uremia, of the idiopathic type or that due to lupus erythematosus
11. *Gastrointestinal Diseases*
To tide the patient over a critical period of the disease in:
   - Ulcerative colitis
   - Regional enteritis
12. *Miscellaneous*
Tuberculous meningitis with subarachnoid block or impending block when used concurrently with appropriate antituberculous chemotherapy
Trichinosis with neurologic or myocardial involvement
13. *Diagnostic testing of adrenocortical hyperfunction.*

CONTRAINDICATIONS

Systemic fungal infections
Hypersensitivity to this product

WARNINGS

In patients on corticosteroid therapy subjected to unusual stress, increased dosage of rapidly acting corticosteroids before, during, and after the stressful situation is indicated.
Drug-induced secondary adrenocortical insufficiency may result from too rapid withdrawal of corticosteroids and may be minimized by gradual reduction of dosage. This type of relative insufficiency may persist for months after discontinuation of therapy; therefore, in any situation of stress occurring during that period, hormone therapy should be reinstituted. If the patient is receiving steroids already, dosage may have to be increased. Since mineralocorticoid secretion may be impaired, salt and/or a mineralocorticoid should be administered concurrently.
Corticosteroids may mask some signs of infection, and new infections may appear during their use. There may be decreased resistance and inability to localize infection when corticosteroids are used. Moreover, corticosteroids may affect the nitroblue-tetrazolium test for bacterial infection and produce false negative results.
In cerebral malaria, a double-blind trial has shown that the use of corticosteroids is associated with prolongation of coma and a higher incidence of pneumonia and gastrointestinal bleeding.
Corticosteroids may activate latent amebiasis. Therefore, it is recommended that latent or active amebiasis be ruled out before initiating corticosteroid therapy in any patient who has spent time in the tropics or any patient with unexplained diarrhea.
Prolonged use of corticosteroids may produce posterior subcapsular cataracts, glaucoma with possible damage to the optic nerves, and may enhance the establishment of secondary ocular infections due to fungi or viruses.
Usage in pregnancy: Since adequate human reproduction studies have not been done with corticosteroids, use of these drugs in pregnancy or in women of childbearing potential requires that the anticipated benefits be weighed against the possible hazards to the mother and embryo or fetus. Infants born of mothers who have received substantial doses of corticosteroids during pregnancy should be carefully observed for signs of hypoadrenalism.
Corticosteroids appear in breast milk and could suppress growth, interfere with endogenous corticosteroid production, or cause other unwanted effects. Mothers taking pharmacologic doses of corticosteroids should be advised not to nurse.
Average and large doses of hydrocortisone or cortisone can cause elevation of blood pressure, salt and water retention, and increased excretion of potassium. These effects are less likely to occur with the synthetic derivatives except when used in large doses. Dietary salt restriction and potassium supplementation may be necessary. All corticosteroids increase calcium excretion.
Administration of live virus vaccines, including smallpox, is contraindicated in individuals receiving immunosuppressive doses of corticosteroids. If inactivated viral or bacterial vaccines are administered to individuals receiving immunosuppressive doses of corticosteroids, the expected serum antibody response may not be obtained. However, immunization procedures may be undertaken in patients who are receiving corticosteroids as replacement therapy, e.g., for Addison's disease.
The use of DECADRON elixir in active tuberculosis should be restricted to those cases of fulminating or disseminated tuberculosis in which the corticosteroid is used for the management of the disease in conjunction with an appropriate antituberculous regimen.
If corticosteroids are indicated in patients with latent tuberculosis or tuberculin reactivity, close observation is necessary as reactivation of the disease may occur. During prolonged corticosteroid therapy, these patients should receive chemoprophylaxis.

PRECAUTIONS

Following prolonged therapy, withdrawal of corticosteroids may result in symptoms of the corticosteroid withdrawal syndrome including fever, myalgia, arthralgia, and malaise. This may occur in patients even without evidence of adrenal insufficiency.
There is an enhanced effect of corticosteroids in patients with hypothyroidism and in those with cirrhosis.
Corticosteroids should be used cautiously in patients with ocular herpes simplex because of possible corneal perforation.
The lowest possible dose of corticosteroid should be used to control the condition under treatment, and when reduction in dosage is possible, the reduction should be gradual.
Psychic derangements may appear when corticosteroids are used, ranging from euphoria, insomnia, mood swings, personality changes, and severe depression, to frank psychotic manifestations. Also, existing emotional instability or psychotic tendencies may be aggravated by corticosteroids.
Aspirin should be used cautiously in conjunction with corticosteroids in hypoprothrombinemia.
Steroids should be used with caution in nonspecific ulcerative colitis, if there is a probability of impending perforation, abscess, or other pyogenic infection, diverticulitis, fresh intestinal anastomoses, active or latent peptic ulcer, renal insufficiency, hypertension, osteoporosis, and myasthenia gravis. Signs of peritoneal irritation following gastrointestinal perforation in patients receiving large doses of corticosteroids may be minimal or absent. Fat embolism has been reported as a possible complication of hypercortisonism.
When large doses are given, some authorities advise that corticosteroids be taken with meals and antacids taken between meals to help to prevent peptic ulcer.
Growth and development of infants and children on prolonged corticosteroid therapy should be carefully observed.
Steroids may increase or decrease motility and number of spermatozoa in some patients.
Phenytoin, phenobarbital, ephedrine, and rifampin may enhance the metabolic clearance of corticosteroids, resulting in decreased blood levels and lessened physiologic activity, thus requiring adjustment in corticosteroid dosage. These

Continued on next page

Information on the Merck Sharp & Dohme products listed on these pages is the full prescribing information from product circulars in use August 31, 1986.

Merck Sharp & Dohme—Cont.

interactions may interfere with dexamethasone suppression tests which should be interpreted with caution during administration of these drugs.
The prothrombin time should be checked frequently in patients who are receiving corticosteroids and coumarin anticoagulants at the same time because of reports that corticosteroids have altered the response to these anticoagulants. Studies have shown that the usual effect produced by adding corticosteroids is inhibition of response to coumarins, although there have been some conflicting reports of potentiation not substantiated by studies.
When corticosteroids are administered concomitantly with potassium-depleting diuretics, patients should be observed closely for development of hypokalemia.

ADVERSE REACTIONS

Fluid and Electrolyte Disturbances
- Sodium retention
- Fluid retention
- Congestive heart failure in susceptible patients
- Potassium loss
- Hypokalemic alkalosis
- Hypertension

Musculoskeletal
- Muscle weakness
- Steroid myopathy
- Loss of muscle mass
- Osteoporosis
- Vertebral compression fractures
- Aseptic necrosis of femoral and humeral heads
- Pathologic fracture of long bones
- Tendon rupture

Gastrointestinal
- Peptic ulcer with possible perforation and hemorrhage
- Perforation of the small and large bowel, particularly in patients with inflammatory bowel disease
- Pancreatitis
- Abdominal distention
- Ulcerative esophagitis

Dermatologic
- Impaired wound healing
- Thin fragile skin
- Petechiae and ecchymoses
- Erythema
- Increased sweating
- May suppress reactions to skin tests
- Other cutaneous reactions, such as allergic dermatitis, urticaria, angioneurotic edema

Neurologic
- Convulsions
- Increased intracranial pressure with papilledema (pseudotumor cerebri) usually after treatment
- Vertigo
- Headache

Endocrine
- Menstrual irregularities
- Development of cushingoid state
- Suppression of growth in children
- Secondary adrenocortical and pituitary unresponsiveness, particularly in times of stress, as in trauma, surgery, or illness
- Decreased carbohydrate tolerance
- Manifestations of latent diabetes mellitus
- Increased requirements for insulin or oral hypoglycemic agents in diabetics
- Hirsutism

Ophthalmic
- Posterior subcapsular cataracts
- Increased intraocular pressure
- Glaucoma
- Exophthalmos

Metabolic
- Negative nitrogen balance due to protein catabolism

Other
- Hypersensitivity
- Thromboembolism
- Weight gain
- Increased appetite
- Nausea
- Malaise
- Psychic disturbances

DOSAGE AND ADMINISTRATION

For oral administration
DOSAGE REQUIREMENTS ARE VARIABLE AND MUST BE INDIVIDUALIZED ON THE BASIS OF THE DISEASE AND THE RESPONSE OF THE PATIENT.
The initial dosage varies from 0.75 to 9 mg a day depending on the disease being treated. In less severe diseases doses lower than 0.75 mg may suffice, while in severe diseases doses higher than 9 mg may be required. The initial dosage should be maintained or adjusted until the patient's response is satisfactory. If satisfactory clinical response does not occur after a reasonable period of time, discontinue DECADRON elixir and transfer the patient to other therapy.
After a favorable initial response, the proper maintenance dosage should be determined by decreasing the initial dosage in small amounts to the lowest dosage that maintains an adequate clinical response.
Patients should be observed closely for signs that might require dosage adjustment, including changes in clinical status resulting from remissions or exacerbations of the disease, individual drug responsiveness, and the effect of stress (e.g., surgery, infection, trauma). During stress it may be necessary to increase dosage temporarily.
If the drug is to be stopped after more than a few days of treatment, it usually should be withdrawn gradually.
The following milligram equivalents facilitate changing to DECADRON from other glucocorticoids:

DECADRON	Methylprednisolone and Triamcinolone	Prednisolone and Prednisone	Hydrocortisone	Cortisone
0.75 mg =	4 mg =	5 mg =	20 mg =	25 mg

Dexamethasone suppression tests

1. Tests for Cushing's syndrome
   Give 1.0 mg of DECADRON orally at 11:00 p.m. Blood is drawn for plasma cortisol determination at 8:00 a.m. the following morning.
   For greater accuracy, give 0.5 mg of DECADRON orally every 6 hours for 48 hours. Twenty-four hour urine collections are made for determination of 17-hydroxycorticosteroid excretion.
2. Test to distinguish Cushing's syndrome due to pituitary ACTH excess from Cushing's syndrome due to other causes
   Give 2.0 mg of DECADRON orally every 6 hours for 48 hours. Twenty-four hour urine collections are made for determination of 17-hydroxycorticosteroid excretion.

HOW SUPPLIED

No. 7622—Elixir DECADRON, 0.5 mg dexamethasone per 5 mL, is a clear, red liquid and is supplied as follows:
NDC 0006-7622-55 bottles of 100 mL with calibrated dropper assembly.
NDC 0006-7622-66 bottles of 237 mL without dropper assembly.
Storage
Store in a container which is kept tightly closed.
A.H.F.S. Category: 68:04
DC 6030725 Issued April 1985

DECADRON® Tablets ℞
(Dexamethasone, MSD), U.S.P.

DESCRIPTION

Glucocorticoids are adrenocortical steroids, both naturally occurring and synthetic, which are readily absorbed from the gastrointestinal tract.
Dexamethasone, a synthetic adrenocortical steroid, is a white to practically white, odorless, crystalline powder. It is stable in air. It is practically insoluble in water. The molecular weight is 392.47. It is designated chemically as 9-fluoro-11β, 17, 21-trihydroxy-16α-methylpregna-1, 4-diene-3,20-dione. The empirical formula is $C_{22}H_{29}FO_5$ and the structural formula is:

DECADRON® (Dexamethasone, MSD) tablets are supplied in six potencies, 0.25 mg, 0.5 mg, 0.75 mg, 1.5 mg, 4 mg, and 6 mg. Inactive ingredients are calcium phosphate, lactose, magnesium stearate, and starch. Tablets DECADRON 0.25 mg also contain FD&C Yellow 6. Tablets DECADRON 0.5 mg also contain D&C Yellow 10 and FD&C Yellow 6. Tablets DECADRON 0.75 mg also contain FD&C Blue 1. Tablets DECADRON 1.5 mg also contain FD&C Red 40. Tablets DECADRON 6 mg also contain FD&C Blue 1 and iron oxide.

ACTIONS

Naturally occurring glucocorticoids (hydrocortisone and cortisone), which also have salt-retaining properties, are used as replacement therapy in adrenocortical deficiency states. Their synthetic analogs including dexamethasone are primarily used for their potent anti-inflammatory effects in disorders of many organ systems.
Glucocorticoids cause profound and varied metabolic effects. In addition, they modify the body's immune responses to diverse stimuli.
At equipotent anti-inflammatory doses, dexamethasone almost completely lacks the sodium-retaining property of hydrocortisone and closely related derivatives of hydrocortisone.

INDICATIONS

1. *Endocrine Disorders*
   Primary or secondary adrenocortical insufficiency (hydrocortisone or cortisone is the first choice; synthetic analogs may be used in conjunction with mineralocorticoids where applicable; in infancy mineralocorticoid supplementation is of particular importance)
   - Congenital adrenal hyperplasia
   - Nonsuppurative thyroiditis
   - Hypercalcemia associated with cancer
2. *Rheumatic Disorders*
   As adjunctive therapy for short-term administration (to tide the patient over an acute episode or exacerbation) in:
   - Psoriatic arthritis
   - Rheumatoid arthritis, including juvenile rheumatoid arthritis (selected cases may require low-dose maintenance therapy)
   - Ankylosing spondylitis
   - Acute and subacute bursitis
   - Acute nonspecific tenosynovitis
   - Acute gouty arthritis
   - Post-traumatic osteoarthritis
   - Synovitis of osteoarthritis
   - Epicondylitis
3. *Collagen Diseases*
   During an exacerbation or as maintenance therapy in selected cases of—
   - Systemic lupus erythematosus
   - Acute rheumatic carditis
4. *Dermatologic Diseases*
   - Pemphigus
   - Bullous dermatitis herpetiformis
   - Severe erythema multiforme (Stevens-Johnson syndrome)
   - Exfoliative dermatitis
   - Mycosis fungoides
   - Severe psoriasis
   - Severe seborrheic dermatitis
5. *Allergic States*
   Control of severe or incapacitating allergic conditions intractable to adequate trials of conventional treatment:
   - Seasonal or perennial allergic rhinitis
   - Bronchial asthma
   - Contact dermatitis
   - Atopic dermatitis
   - Serum sickness
   - Drug hypersensitivity reactions
6. *Ophthalmic Diseases*
   Severe acute and chronic allergic and inflammatory processes involving the eye and its adnexa, such as—
   - Allergic conjunctivitis
   - Keratitis
   - Allergic corneal marginal ulcers
   - Herpes zoster ophthalmicus
   - Iritis and iridocyclitis
   - Chorioretinitis
   - Anterior segment inflammation
   - Diffuse posterior uveitis and choroiditis
   - Optic neuritis
   - Sympathetic ophthalmia
7. *Respiratory Diseases*
   - Symptomatic sarcoidosis
   - Loeffler's syndrome not manageable by other means
   - Berylliosis
   - Fulminating or disseminated pulmonary tuberculosis when used concurrently with appropriate antituberculous chemotherapy
   - Aspiration pneumonitis
8. *Hematologic Disorders*
   - Idiopathic thrombocytopenic purpura in adults
   - Secondary thrombocytopenia in adults
   - Acquired (autoimmune) hemolytic anemia
   - Erythroblastopenia (RBC anemia)
   - Congenital (erythroid) hypoplastic anemia

9. *Neoplastic Diseases*
For palliative management of:
Leukemias and lymphomas in adults
Acute leukemia of childhood
10. *Edematous States*
To induce a diuresis or remission of proteinuria in the nephrotic syndrome, without uremia, of the idiopathic type or that due to lupus erythematosus
11. *Gastrointestinal Diseases*
To tide the patient over a critical period of the disease in:
Ulcerative colitis
Regional enteritis
12. *Cerebral Edema* associated with primary or metastatic brain tumor, craniotomy, or head injury. Use in cerebral edema is not a substitute for careful neurosurgical evaluation and definitive management such as neurosurgery or other specific therapy.
13. *Miscellaneous*
Tuberculous meningitis with subarachnoid block or impending block when used concurrently with appropriate antituberculous chemotherapy
Trichinosis with neurologic or myocardial involvement
14. *Diagnostic testing of adrenocortical hyperfunction.*

CONTRAINDICATIONS

Systemic fungal infections
Hypersensitivity to this drug

WARNINGS

In patients on corticosteroid therapy subjected to unusual stress, increased dosage of rapidly acting corticosteroids before, during, and after the stressful situation is indicated.
Drug-induced secondary adrenocortical insufficiency may result from too rapid withdrawal of corticosteroids and may be minimized by gradual reduction of dosage. This type of relative insufficiency may persist for months after discontinuation of therapy; therefore, in any situation of stress occurring during that period, hormone therapy should be reinstituted. If the patient is receiving steroids already, dosage may have to be increased. Since mineralocorticoid secretion may be impaired, salt and/or a mineralocorticoid should be administered concurrently.
Corticosteroids may mask some signs of infection, and new infections may appear during their use. There may be decreased resistance and inability to localize infection when corticosteroids are used. Moreover, corticosteroids may affect the nitroblue-tetrazolium test for bacterial infection and produce false negative results.
In cerebral malaria, a double-blind trial has shown that the use of corticosteroids is associated with prolongation of coma and a higher incidence of pneumonia and gastrointestinal bleeding.
Corticosteroids may activate latent amebiasis. Therefore, it is recommended that latent or active amebiasis be ruled out before initiating corticosteroid therapy in any patient who has spent time in the tropics or any patient with unexplained diarrhea.
Prolonged use of corticosteroids may produce posterior subcapsular cataracts, glaucoma with possible damage to the optic nerves, and may enhance the establishment of secondary ocular infections due to fungi or viruses.
Usage in pregnancy: Since adequate human reproduction studies have not been done with corticosteroids, use of these drugs in pregnancy or in women of childbearing potential requires that the anticipated benefits be weighed against the possible hazards to the mother and embryo or fetus. Infants born of mothers who have received substantial doses of corticosteroids during pregnancy should be carefully observed for signs of hypoadrenalism.
Corticosteroids appear in breast milk and could suppress growth, interfere with endogenous corticosteroid production, or cause other unwanted effects. Mothers taking pharmacologic doses of corticosteroids should be advised not to nurse.
Average and large doses of hydrocortisone or cortisone can cause elevation of blood pressure, salt and water retention, and increased excretion of potassium. These effects are less likely to occur with the synthetic derivatives except when used in large doses. Dietary salt restriction and potassium supplementation may be necessary. All corticosteroids increase calcium excretion.
Administration of live virus vaccines, including smallpox, is contraindicated in individuals receiving immunosuppressive doses of corticosteroids. If inactivated viral or bacterial vaccines are administered to individuals receiving immunosuppressive doses of corticosteroid the expected serum antibody response may not be obtained. However, immunization procedures may be undertaken in patients who are receiving corticosteroids as replacement therapy, e.g., for Addison's disease.
The use of DECADRON tablets in active tuberculosis should be restricted to those cases of fulminating or disseminated tuberculosis in which the corticosteroid is used for the management of the disease in conjunction with an appropriate antituberculous regimen.
If corticosteroids are indicated in patients with latent tuberculosis or tuberculin reactivity, close observation is necessary as reactivation of the disease may occur. During prolonged corticosteroid therapy, these patients should receive chemoprophylaxis.

PRECAUTIONS

Following prolonged therapy, withdrawal of corticosteroids may result in symptoms of the corticosteroid withdrawal syndrome including fever, myalgia, arthralgia, and malaise. This may occur in patients even without evidence of adrenal insufficiency.
There is an enhanced effect of corticosteroids in patients with hypothyroidism and in those with cirrhosis.
Corticosteroids should be used cautiously in patients with ocular herpes simplex because of possible corneal perforation.
The lowest possible dose of corticosteroids should be used to control the condition under treatment, and when reduction in dosage is possible, the reduction should be gradual.
Psychic derangements may appear when corticosteroids are used, ranging from euphoria, insomnia, mood swings, personality changes, and severe depression, to frank psychotic manifestations. Also, existing emotional instability or psychotic tendencies may be aggravated by corticosteroids.
Aspirin should be used cautiously in conjunction with corticosteroids in hypoprothrombinemia.
Steroids should be used with caution in nonspecific ulcerative colitis, if there is a probability of impending perforation, abscess, or other pyogenic infection, diverticulitis, fresh intestinal anastomoses, active or latent peptic ulcer, renal insufficiency, hypertension, osteoporosis, and myasthenia gravis. Signs of peritoneal irritation following gastrointestinal perforation in patients receiving large doses of corticosteroids may be minimal or absent. Fat embolism has been reported as a possible complication of hypercortisonism.
When large doses are given, some authorities advise that corticosteroids be taken with meals and antacids taken between meals to help to prevent peptic ulcer.
Growth and development of infants and children on prolonged corticosteroid therapy should be carefully observed.
Steroids may increase or decrease motility and number of spermatozoa in some patients.
Phenytoin, phenobarbital, ephedrine, and rifampin may enhance the metabolic clearance of corticosteroids, resulting in decreased blood levels and lessened physiologic activity, thus requiring adjustment in corticosteroid dosage. These interactions may interfere with dexamethasone suppression tests which should be interpreted with caution during administration of these drugs.
The prothrombin time should be checked frequently in patients who are receiving corticosteroids and coumarin anticoagulants at the same time because of reports that corticosteroids have altered the response to these anticoagulants. Studies have shown that the usual effect produced by adding corticosteroids is inhibition of response to coumarins, although there have been some conflicting reports of potentiation not substantiated by studies.
When corticosteroids are administered concomitantly with potassium-depleting diuretics, patients should be observed closely for development of hypokalemia.

ADVERSE REACTIONS

Fluid and Electrolyte Disturbances
Sodium retention
Fluid retention
Congestive heart failure in susceptible patients
Potassium loss
Hypokalemic alkalosis
Hypertension
Musculoskeletal
Muscle weakness
Steroid myopathy
Loss of muscle mass
Osteoporosis
Vertebral compression fractures
Aseptic necrosis of femoral and humeral heads
Pathologic fracture of long bones
Tendon rupture
Gastrointestinal
Peptic ulcer with possible perforation and hemorrhage
Perforation of the small and large bowel, particularly in patients with inflammatory bowel disease
Pancreatitis
Abdominal distention
Ulcerative esophagitis
Dermatologic
Impaired wound healing
Thin fragile skin
Petechiae and ecchymoses
Erythema
Increased sweating
May suppress reactions to skin tests
Other cutaneous reactions, such as allergic dermatitis, urticaria, angioneurotic edema
Neurologic
Convulsions
Increased intracranial pressure with papilledema (pseudotumor cerebri) usually after treatment
Vertigo
Headache
Endocrine
Menstrual irregularities
Development of cushingoid state
Suppression of growth in children
Secondary adrenocortical and pituitary unresponsiveness, particularly in times of stress, as in trauma, surgery, or illness
Decreased carbohydrate tolerance
Manifestations of latent diabetes mellitus
Increased requirements for insulin or oral hypoglycemic agents in diabetics
Hirsutism
Ophthalmic
Posterior subcapsular cataracts
Increased intraocular pressure
Glaucoma
Exophthalmos
Metabolic
Negative nitrogen balance due to protein catabolism
Other
Hypersensitivity
Thromboembolism
Weight gain
Increased appetite
Nausea
Malaise
Psychic disturbances

DOSAGE AND ADMINISTRATION

For oral administration
DOSAGE REQUIREMENTS ARE VARIABLE AND MUST BE INDIVIDUALIZED ON THE BASIS OF THE DISEASE AND THE RESPONSE OF THE PATIENT.
The initial dosage varies from 0.75 to 9 mg a day depending on the disease being treated. In less severe diseases doses lower than 0.75 mg may suffice, while in severe diseases doses higher than 9 mg may be required. The initial dosage should be maintained or adjusted until the patient's response is satisfactory. If satisfactory clinical response does not occur after a reasonable period of time, discontinue DECADRON tablets and transfer the patient to other therapy.
After a favorable initial response, the proper maintenance dosage should be determined by decreasing the initial dosage in small amounts to the lowest dosage that maintains an adequate clinical response.
Patients should be observed closely for signs that might require dosage adjustment, including changes in clinical status resulting from remissions or exacerbations of the disease, individual drug responsiveness, and the effect of stress (e.g., surgery, infection, trauma). During stress it may be necessary to increase dosage temporarily.
If the drug is to be stopped after more than a few days of treatment, it usually should be withdrawn gradually.
The following milligram equivalents facilitate changing to DECADRON from other glucocorticoids:

DECADRON	Methylprednisolone and Triamcinolone	Prednisolone and Prednisone	Hydrocortisone	Cortisone
0.75 mg =	4 mg =	5 mg =	20 mg =	25 mg

In *acute, self-limited allergic disorders or acute exacerbations of chronic allergic disorders*, the following dosage schedule combining parenteral and oral therapy is suggested:

Continued on next page

Information on the Merck Sharp & Dohme products listed on these pages is the full prescribing information from product circulars in use August 31, 1986.

Merck Sharp & Dohme—Cont.

DECADRON® Phosphate (Dexamethasone Sodium Phosphate, MSD) injection, 4 mg per mL:
First Day
1 or 2 mL, intramuscularly
DECADRON tablets, 0.75 mg:
Second Day
4 tablets in two divided doses
Third Day
4 tablets in two divided doses
Fourth Day
2 tablets in two divided doses
Fifth Day
1 tablet
Sixth Day
1 tablet
Seventh Day
No treatment
Eighth Day
Follow-up visit

This schedule is designed to ensure adequate therapy during acute episodes, while minimizing the risk of overdosage in chronic cases.

In *cerebral edema*, DECADRON Phosphate (Dexamethasone Sodium Phosphate, MSD) injection is generally administered initially in a dosage of 10 mg intravenously followed by 4 mg every six hours intramuscularly until the symptoms of cerebral edema subside. Response is usually noted within 12 to 24 hours and dosage may be reduced after two to four days and gradually discontinued over a period of five to seven days. For palliative management of patients with recurrent or inoperable brain tumors, maintenance therapy with either DECADRON Phosphate (Dexamethasone Sodium Phosphate, MSD) injection or DECADRON tablets in a dosage of two mg two or three times daily may be effective.

Dexamethasone suppression tests

1. Tests for Cushing's syndrome
   Give 1.0 mg of DECADRON orally at 11:00 p.m. Blood is drawn for plasma cortisol determination at 8:00 a.m. the following morning.
   For greater accuracy, give 0.5 mg of DECADRON orally every 6 hours for 48 hours. Twenty-four hour urine collections are made for determination of 17-hydroxycorticosteroid excretion.
2. Test to distinguish Cushing's syndrome due to pituitary ACTH excess from Cushing's syndrome due to other causes
   Give 2.0 mg of DECADRON orally every 6 hours for 48 hours. Twenty-four hour urine collections are made for determination of 17-hydroxycorticosteroid excretion.

HOW SUPPLIED

Tablets DECADRON are compressed, pentagonal-shaped tablets, colored to distinguish potency. They are scored and coded on one side and are available as follows:
No. 7648—6 mg, green in color and coded MSD 147.
NDC 0006-0147-50 bottles of 50
NDC 0006-0147-28 single unit packages of 100.
Shown in Product Identification Section, page 417
No. 7645—4 mg, white in color and coded MSD 97.
NDC 0006-0097-50 bottles of 50
NDC 0006-0097-28 single unit packages of 100.
Shown in Product Identification Section, page 417
No. 7638—1.5 mg, pink in color and coded MSD 95.
NDC 0006-0095-50 bottles of 50
NDC 0006-0095-28 single unit packages of 100.
Shown in Product Identification Section, page 417
No. 7601—0.75 mg, bluish-green in color and coded MSD 63.
NDC 0006-0063-12 5-12 PAK® (package of 12)
NDC 0006-0063-68 bottles of 100
NDC 0006-0063-28 single unit packages of 100
NDC 0006-0063-82 bottles of 1000.
Shown in Product Identification Section, page 417
No. 7598—0.5 mg, yellow in color and coded MSD 41.
NDC 0006-0041-68 bottles of 100
(6505-00-687-8482 0.5 mg 100's)
NDC 0006-0041-28 single unit packages of 100
NDC 0006-0041-82 bottles of 1000.
Shown in Product Identification Section, page 417
No. 7592—0.25 mg, orange in color and coded MSD 20.
NDC 0006-0020-68 bottles of 100.
Shown in Product Identification Section, page 417
A.H.F.S. Category: 68:04
DC 6025243 Issued June 1985

DECADRON® Phosphate Injection (Dexamethasone Sodium Phosphate, MSD), U.S.P. ℞

DESCRIPTION

Dexamethasone sodium phosphate, a synthetic adrenocortical steroid, is a white or slightly yellow, crystalline powder. It is freely soluble in water and is exceedingly hygroscopic. The molecular weight is 516.41. It is designated chemically as 9-fluoro-11β, 17-dihydroxy-16α-methyl-21-(phosphonooxy)pregna-1, 4-diene-3, 20-dione disodium salt. The empirical formula is $C_{22}H_{28}FNa_2O_8P$ and the structural formula is:

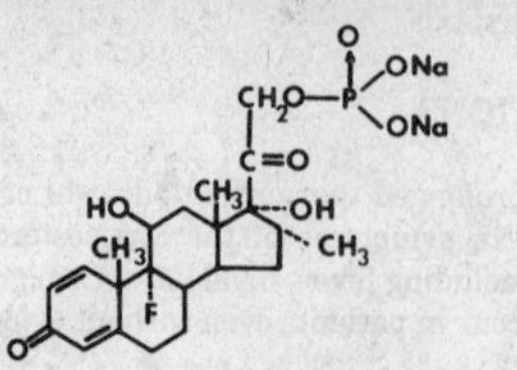

DECADRON® Phosphate (Dexamethasone Sodium Phosphate, MSD) injection is a sterile solution (pH 7.0 to 8.5) of dexamethasone sodium phosphate, and is supplied in two concentrations: 4 mg/mL and 24 mg/mL. The 24 mg/mL concentration offers the advantage of less volume in indications where high doses of corticosteroids by the intravenous route are needed.

Each milliliter of DECADRON Phosphate injection, 4 mg/mL, contains dexamethasone sodium phosphate equivalent to 4 mg dexamethasone phosphate or 3.33 mg dexamethasone. Inactive ingredients per mL: 8 mg creatinine, 10 mg sodium citrate, sodium hydroxide to adjust pH, and Water for Injection q.s., with 1 mg sodium bisulfite, 1.5 mg methylparaben, and 0.2 mg propylparaben added as preservatives.

Each milliliter of DECADRON Phosphate injection, 24 mg/mL, contains dexamethasone sodium phosphate equivalent to 24 mg dexamethasone phosphate or 20 mg dexamethasone. Inactive ingredients per mL: 8 mg creatinine, 10 mg sodium citrate, 0.5 mg disodium edetate, sodium hydroxide to adjust pH, and Water for Injection q.s., with 1 mg sodium bisulfite, 1.5 mg methylparaben, and 0.2 mg propylparaben added as preservatives.

ACTIONS

DECADRON Phosphate injection has a rapid onset but short duration of action when compared with less soluble preparations. Because of this, it is suitable for the treatment of acute disorders responsive to adrenocortical steroid therapy.

Naturally occurring glucocorticoids (hydrocortisone and cortisone), which also have salt-retaining properties, are used as replacement therapy in adrenocortical deficiency states. Their synthetic analogs, including dexamethasone, are primarily used for their potent anti-inflammatory effects in disorders of many organ systems.

Glucocorticoids cause profound and varied metabolic effects. In addition, they modify the body's immune responses to diverse stimuli.

At equipotent anti-inflammatory doses, dexamethasone almost completely lacks the sodium-retaining property of hydrocortisone and closely related derivatives of hydrocortisone.

INDICATIONS

A. By intravenous or intramuscular injection when oral therapy is not feasible:

1. *Endocrine disorders*
Primary or secondary adrenocortical insufficiency (hydrocortisone or cortisone is the drug of choice; synthetic analogs may be used in conjunction with mineralocorticoids where applicable; in infancy, mineralocorticoid supplementation is of particular importance)
Acute adrenocortical insufficiency (hydrocortisone or cortisone is the drug of choice; mineralocorticoid supplementation may be necessary, particularly when synthetic analogs are used)
Preoperatively, and in the event of serious trauma or illness, in patients with known adrenal insufficiency or when adrenocortical reserve is doubtful
Shock unresponsive to conventional therapy if adrenocortical insufficiency exists or is suspected
Congenital adrenal hyperplasia
Nonsuppurative thyroiditis
Hypercalcemia associated with cancer

2. *Rheumatic disorders*
As adjunctive therapy for short-term administration (to tide the patient over an acute episode or exacerbation) in:
Post-traumatic osteoarthritis
Synovitis of osteoarthritis
Rheumatoid arthritis, including juvenile rheumatoid arthritis (selected cases may require low-dose maintenance therapy)
Acute and subacute bursitis
Epicondylitis
Acute nonspecific tenosynovitis
Acute gouty arthritis
Psoriatic arthritis
Ankylosing spondylitis

3. *Collagen diseases*
During an exacerbation or as maintenance therapy in selected cases of:
Systemic lupus erythematosus
Acute rheumatic carditis

4. *Dermatologic diseases*
Pemphigus
Severe erythema multiforme (Stevens-Johnson syndrome)
Exfoliative dermatitis
Bullous dermatitis herpetiformis
Severe seborrheic dermatitis
Severe psoriasis
Mycosis fungoides

5. *Allergic states*
Control of severe or incapacitating allergic conditions intractable to adequate trials of conventional treatment in:
Bronchial asthma
Contact dermatitis
Atopic dermatitis
Serum sickness
Seasonal or perennial allergic rhinitis
Drug hypersensitivity reactions
Urticarial transfusion reactions
Acute noninfectious laryngeal edema (epinephrine is the drug of first choice)

6. *Ophthalmic diseases*
Severe acute and chronic allergic and inflammatory processes involving the eye, such as:
Herpes zoster ophthalmicus
Iritis, iridocyclitis
Chorioretinitis
Diffuse posterior uveitis and choroiditis
Optic neuritis
Sympathetic ophthalmia
Anterior segment inflammation
Allergic conjunctivitis
Keratitis
Allergic corneal marginal ulcers

7. *Gastrointestinal diseases*
To tide the patient over a critical period of the disease in:
Ulcerative colitis (Systemic therapy)
Regional enteritis (Systemic therapy)

8. *Respiratory diseases*
Symptomatic sarcoidosis
Berylliosis
Fulminating or disseminated pulmonary tuberculosis when used concurrently with appropriate antituberculous chemotherapy
Loeffler's syndrome not manageable by other means
Aspiration pneumonitis

9. *Hematologic disorders*
Acquired (autoimmune) hemolytic anemia
Idiopathic thrombocytopenic purpura in adults (I.V. only; I.M. administration is contraindicated)
Secondary thrombocytopenia in adults
Erythroblastopenia (RBC anemia)
Congenital (erythroid) hypoplastic anemia

10. *Neoplastic diseases*
For palliative management of:
Leukemias and lymphomas in adults
Acute leukemia of childhood

11. *Edematous states*
To induce diuresis or remission of proteinuria in the nephrotic syndrome, without uremia, of the idiopathic type, or that due to lupus erythematosus

12. *Miscellaneous*
Tuberculous meningitis with subarachnoid block or impending block when used concurrently with appropriate antituberculous chemotherapy
Trichinosis with neurologic or myocardial involvement

13. *Diagnostic testing of adrenocortical hyperfunction*

14. *Cerebral Edema* associated with primary or metastatic brain tumor, craniotomy, or head injury. Use in cerebral edema is not a substitute for careful neurosurgical evaluation and definitive management such as neurosurgery or other specific therapy.

B. By intra-articular or soft tissue injection:
As adjunctive therapy for short-term administration (to tide the patient over an acute episode or exacerbation) in:
Synovitis of osteoarthritis
Rheumatoid arthritis
Acute and subacute bursitis
Acute gouty arthritis
Epicondylitis
Acute nonspecific tenosynovitis
Post-traumatic osteoarthritis.

C. By intralesional injection:
Keloids
Localized hypertrophic, infiltrated, inflammatory lesions of: lichen planus, psoriatic plaques, granuloma annulare, and lichen simplex chronicus (neurodermatitis)

Discoid lupus erythematosus
Necrobiosis lipoidica diabeticorum
Alopecia areata
May also be useful in cystic tumors of an aponeurosis or tendon (ganglia).

CONTRAINDICATIONS

Systemic fungal infections. (See WARNINGS regarding amphotericin B)
Hypersensitivity to any component of this product, including sulfites (See WARNINGS regarding sodium bisulfite).

WARNINGS

Sodium bisulfite has been reported to cause severe allergic reactions in certain susceptible individuals, particularly patients with asthma. Anaphylactoid and hypersensitivity reactions have been reported for injection DECADRON Phosphate (see ADVERSE REACTIONS). Since Injection DECADRON Phosphate contains sodium bisulfite, this product should not be used in patients allergic to sulfites.
Corticosteroids may exacerbate systemic fungal infections and therefore should not be used in the presence of such infections unless they are needed to control drug reactions due to amphotericin B. Moreover, there have been cases reported in which concomitant use of amphotericin B and hydrocortisone was followed by cardiac enlargement and congestive failure.
In patients on corticosteroid therapy subjected to any unusual stress, increased dosage of rapidly acting corticosteroids before, during, and after the stressful situation is indicated.
Drug-induced secondary adrenocortical insufficiency may result from too rapid withdrawal of corticosteroids and may be minimized by gradual reduction of dosage. This type of relative insufficiency may persist for months after discontinuation of therapy; therefore, in any situation of stress occurring during that period, hormone therapy should be reinstituted. If the patient is receiving steroids already, dosage may have to be increased. Since mineralocorticoid secretion may be impaired, salt and/or a mineralocorticoid should be administered concurrently.
Corticosteroids may mask some signs of infection, and new infections may appear during their use. There may be decreased resistance and inability to localize infection when corticosteroids are used. Moreover, corticosteroids may affect the nitroblue-tetrazolium test for bacterial infection and produce false negative results.
In cerebral malaria, a double-blind trial has shown that the use of corticosteroids is associated with prolongation of coma and a higher incidence of pneumonia and gastrointestinal bleeding.
Corticosteroids may activate latent amebiasis. Therefore, it is recommended that latent or active amebiasis be ruled out before initiating corticosteroid therapy in any patient who has spent time in the tropics or any patient with unexplained diarrhea.
Prolonged use of corticosteroids may produce posterior subcapsular cataracts, glaucoma with possible damage to the optic nerves, and may enhance the establishment of secondary ocular infections due to fungi or viruses.
Usage in pregnancy. Since adequate human reproduction studies have not been done with corticosteroids, use of these drugs in pregnancy or in women of childbearing potential requires that the anticipated benefits be weighed against the possible hazards to the mother and embryo or fetus. Infants born of mothers who have received substantial doses of corticosteroids during pregnancy should be carefully observed for signs of hypoadrenalism.
Corticosteroids appear in breast milk and could suppress growth, interfere with endogenous corticosteroid production, or cause other unwanted effects. Mothers taking pharmacologic doses of corticosteroids should be advised not to nurse.
Average and large doses of cortisone or hydrocortisone can cause elevation of blood pressure, salt and water retention, and increased excretion of potassium. These effects are less likely to occur with the synthetic derivatives except when used in large doses. Dietary salt restriction and potassium supplementation may be necessary. All corticosteroids increase calcium excretion.
Administration of live virus vaccines, including smallpox, is contraindicated in individuals receiving immunosuppressive doses of corticosteroids. If inactivated viral or bacterial vaccines are administered to individuals receiving immunosuppressive doses of corticosteroids, the expected serum antibody response may not be obtained. However, immunization procedures may be undertaken in patients who are receiving corticosteroids as replacement therapy, e.g., for Addison's disease.
The use of DECADRON Phosphate injection in active tuberculosis should be restricted to those cases of fulminating or disseminated tuberculosis in which the corticosteroid is used for the management of the disease in conjunction with an appropriate antituberculous regimen.
If corticosteroids are indicated in patients with latent tuberculosis or tuberculin reactivity, close observation is necessary as reactivation of the disease may occur. During prolonged corticosteroid therapy, these patients should receive chemoprophylaxis.
Because rare instances of anaphylactoid reactions have occurred in patients receiving parenteral corticosteroid therapy, appropriate precautionary measures should be taken prior to administration, especially when the patient has a history of allergy to any drug.

PRECAUTIONS

This product, like many other steroid formulations, is sensitive to heat. Therefore, it should not be autoclaved when it is desirable to sterilize the exterior of the vial.
Following prolonged therapy, withdrawal of corticosteroids may result in symptoms of the corticosteroid withdrawal syndrome including fever, myalgia, arthralgia, and malaise. This may occur in patients even without evidence of adrenal insufficiency.
There is an enhanced effect of corticosteroids in patients with hypothyroidism and in those with cirrhosis.
Corticosteroids should be used cautiously in patients with ocular herpes simplex for fear of corneal perforation.
The lowest possible dose of corticosteroid should be used to control the condition under treatment, and when reduction in dosage is possible, the reduction must be gradual.
Psychic derangements may appear when corticosteroids are used, ranging from euphoria, insomnia, mood swings, personality changes, and severe depression to frank psychotic manifestations. Also, existing emotional instability or psychotic tendencies may be aggravated by corticosteroids.
Aspirin should be used cautiously in conjunction with corticosteroids in hypoprothrombinemia.
Steroids should be used with caution in nonspecific ulcerative colitis, if there is a probability of impending perforation, abscess, or other pyogenic infection, also in diverticulitis, fresh intestinal anastomoses, active or latent peptic ulcer, renal insufficiency, hypertension, osteoporosis, and myasthenia gravis. Signs of peritoneal irritation following gastrointestinal perforation in patients receiving large doses of corticosteroids may be minimal or absent. Fat embolism has been reported as a possible complication of hypercortisonism.
When large doses are given, some authorities advise that antacids be administered between meals to help to prevent peptic ulcer.
Growth and development of infants and children on prolonged corticosteroid therapy should be carefully followed.
Steroids may increase or decrease motility and number of spermatozoa in some patients.
Phenytoin, phenobarbital, ephedrine, and rifampin may enhance the metabolic clearance of corticosteroids resulting in decreased blood levels and lessened physiologic activity, thus requiring adjustment in corticosteroid dosage. These interactions may interfere with dexamethasone suppression tests which should be interpreted with caution during administration of these drugs.
The prothrombin time should be checked frequently in patients who are receiving corticosteroids and coumarin anticoagulants at the same time because of reports that corticosteroids have altered the response to these anticoagulants. Studies have shown that the usual effect produced by adding corticosteroids is inhibition of response to coumarins, although there have been some conflicting reports of potentiation not substantiated by studies.
When corticosteroids are administered concomitantly with potassium-depleting diuretics, patients should be observed closely for development of hypokalemia.
Intra-articular injection of a corticosteroid may produce systemic as well as local effects.
Appropriate examination of any joint fluid present is necessary to exclude a septic process.
A marked increase in pain accompanied by local swelling, further restriction of joint motion, fever, and malaise is suggestive of septic arthritis. If this complication occurs and the diagnosis of sepsis is confirmed, appropriate antimicrobial therapy should be instituted.
Injection of a steroid into an infected site is to be avoided.
Corticosteroids should not be injected into unstable joints.
Patients should be impressed strongly with the importance of not overusing joints in which symptomatic benefit has been obtained as long as the inflammatory process remains active.
Frequent intra-articular injection may result in damage to joint tissues.
The slower rate of absorption by intramuscular administration should be recognized.

ADVERSE REACTIONS

Fluid and electrolyte disturbances
Sodium retention
Fluid retention
Congestive heart failure in susceptible patients
Potassium loss
Hypokalemic alkalosis
Hypertension
Musculoskeletal
Muscle weakness
Steroid myopathy
Loss of muscle mass
Osteoporosis
Vertebral compression fractures
Aseptic necrosis of femoral and humeral heads
Pathologic fracture of long bones
Tendon rupture
Gastrointestinal
Peptic ulcer with possible subsequent perforation and hemorrhage
Perforation of the small and large bowel, particularly in patients with inflammatory bowel disease
Pancreatitis
Abdominal distention
Ulcerative esophagitis
Dermatologic
Impaired wound healing
Thin fragile skin
Petechiae and ecchymoses
Erythema
Increased sweating
May suppress reactions to skin tests
Burning or tingling, especially in the perineal area (after I.V. injection)
Other cutaneous reactions, such as allergic dermatitis, urticaria, angioneurotic edema
Neurologic
Convulsions
Increased intracranial pressure with papilledema (pseudotumor cerebri) usually after treatment
Vertigo
Headache
Endocrine
Menstrual irregularities
Development of cushingoid state
Suppression of growth in children
Secondary adrenocortical and pituitary unresponsiveness, particularly in times of stress, as in trauma, surgery, or illness
Decreased carbohydrate tolerance
Manifestations of latent diabetes mellitus
Increased requirements for insulin or oral hypoglycemic agents in diabetics
Hirsutism
Ophthalmic
Posterior subcapsular cataracts
Increased intraocular pressure
Glaucoma
Exophthalmos
Metabolic
Negative nitrogen balance due to protein catabolism
Other
Anaphylactoid or hypersensitivity reactions
Thromboembolism
Weight gain
Increased appetite
Nausea
Malaise
Psychic disturbances
The following *additional* adverse reactions are related to parenteral corticosteroid therapy:
Rare instances of blindness associated with intralesional therapy around the face and head
Hyperpigmentation or hypopigmentation
Subcutaneous and cutaneous atrophy
Sterile abscess
Postinjection flare (following intra-articular use)
Charcot-like arthropathy

DOSAGE AND ADMINISTRATION

DECADRON Phosphate injection, 4 mg/mL—*For intravenous, intramuscular, intra-articular, intralesional, and soft tissue injection.*
DECADRON Phosphate injection, 24 mg/mL—*For intravenous injection only.*
DECADRON Phosphate injection can be given directly from the vial or the disposable syringe, or it can be added to Sodium Chloride Injection or Dextrose Injection and administered by intravenous drip.

Continued on next page

Information on the Merck Sharp & Dohme products listed on these pages is the full prescribing information from product circulars in use August 31, 1986.

Merck Sharp & Dohme—Cont.

Solutions used for intravenous administration or further dilution of this product should be preservative-free when used in the neonate, especially the premature infant.
When it is mixed with an infusion solution, sterile precautions should be observed. Since infusion solutions generally do not contain preservatives, mixtures should be used within 24 hours.
DOSAGE REQUIREMENTS ARE VARIABLE AND MUST BE INDIVIDUALIZED ON THE BASIS OF THE DISEASE AND THE RESPONSE OF THE PATIENT.

Intravenous and Intramuscular Injection

The initial dosage of DECADRON Phosphate injection varies from 0.5 to 9 mg a day depending on the disease being treated. In less severe diseases doses lower than 0.5 mg may suffice, while in severe diseases doses higher than 9 mg may be required.
The initial dosage should be maintained or adjusted until the patient's response is satisfactory. If a satisfactory clinical response does not occur after a reasonable period of time, discontinue DECADRON Phosphate injection and transfer the patient to other therapy.
After a favorable initial response, the proper maintenance dosage should be determined by decreasing the initial dosage in small amounts to the lowest dosage that maintains an adequate clinical response.
Patients should be observed closely for signs that might require dosage adjustment, including changes in clinical status resulting from remissions or exacerbations of the disease, individual drug responsiveness, and the effect of stress (e.g., surgery, infection, trauma). During stress it may be necessary to increase dosage temporarily.
If the drug is to be stopped after more than a few days of treatment, it usually should be withdrawn gradually.
When the intravenous route of administration is used, dosage usually should be the same as the oral dosage. In certain overwhelming, acute, life-threatening situations, however, administration in dosages exceeding the usual dosages may be justified and may be in multiples of the oral dosages. The slower rate of absorption by intramuscular administration should be recognized.

Shock

There is a tendency in current medical practice to use high (pharmacologic) doses of corticosteroids for the treatment of unresponsive shock. The following dosages of DECADRON phosphate injection have been suggested by various authors:

*Author**	*Dosage*
Cavanagh[1]	3 mg/kg of body weight per 24 hours by constant intravenous infusion after an initial intravenous injection of 20 mg
Dietzman[2]	2 to 6 mg/kg of body weight as a single intravenous injection
Frank[3]	40 mg initially followed by repeat intravenous injection every 4 to 6 hours while shock persists
Oaks[4]	40 mg initially followed by repeat intravenous injection every 2 to 6 hours while shock persists
Schumer[5]	1 mg/kg of body weight as a single intravenous injection

Administration of high dose corticosteroid therapy should be continued only until the patient's condition has stabilized and usually not longer than 48 to 72 hours.
Although adverse reactions associated with high dose, short term corticosteroid therapy are uncommon, peptic ulceration may occur.

Cerebral Edema

DECADRON Phosphate injection is generally administered initially in a dosage of 10 mg intravenously followed by 4 mg every six hours intramuscularly until the symptoms of cerebral edema subside. Response is usually noted within 12 to 24 hours and dosage may be reduced after two to four days and gradually discontinued over a period of five to seven days. For palliative management of patients with recurrent or inoperable brain tumors, maintenance therapy with two mg two or three times a day may be effective.

*1. Cavanagh, D.; Singh, K. B.: Endotoxin shock in pregnancy and abortion, in "Corticosteroids in the Treatment of Shock", Schumer, W.; Nyhus, L. M., Editors, Urbana, University of Illinois Press, 1970, pp. 86-96.
2. Dietzman, R. H.; Ersek, R. A.; Bloch, J. M.; Lillehei, R. C.: High-output, low-resistance gram-negative septic shock in man, Angiology *20:* 691-700, Dec. 1969.
3. Frank, E.: Clinical observations in shock and management (In: Shields, T. F., ed.: Symposium on current concepts and management of shock), J. Maine Med. Ass. *59:* 195-200, Oct. 1968.
4. Oaks, W. W.; Cohen, H. E.: Endotoxin shock in the geriatric patient, Geriat. *22:* 120-130, Mar. 1967.
5. Schumer, W.; Nyhus, L. M.: Corticosteroid effect on biochemical parameters of human oligemic shock, Arch. Surg. *100:* 405-408, Apr. 1970.

Acute Allergic Disorders

In acute, self-limited allergic disorders or acute exacerbations of chronic allergic disorders, the following dosage schedule combining parenteral and oral therapy is suggested:
DECADRON Phosphate injection, 4 mg/mL: *first day,* 1 or 2 mL (4 or 8 mg), intramuscularly.
DECADRON® (Dexamethasone, MSD) tablets, 0.75 mg: *second and third days,* 4 tablets in two divided doses each day; *fourth day,* 2 tablets in two divided doses; *fifth and sixth days,* 1 tablet each day; *seventh day,* no treatment; *eighth day,* follow-up visit.
This schedule is designed to ensure adequate therapy during acute episodes, while minimizing the risk of overdosage in chronic cases.

Intra-articular, Intralesional, and Soft Tissue Injection

Intra-articular, intralesional, and soft tissue injections are generally employed when the affected joints or areas are limited to one or two sites. Dosage and frequency of injection varies depending on the condition and the site of injection. The usual dose is from 0.2 to 6 mg. The frequency usually ranges from once every three to five days to once every two to three weeks. Frequent intra-articular injection may result in damage to joint tissues.
Some of the usual single doses are:

Site of Injection	Amount of Dexamethasone Phosphate (mg)
Large Joints (e.g., Knee)	2 to 4
Small Joints (e.g., Interphalangeal, Temporomandibular)	0.8 to 1
Bursae	2 to 3
Tendon Sheaths	0.4 to 1
Soft Tissue Infiltration	2 to 6
Ganglia	1 to 2

DECADRON Phosphate injection is particularly recommended for use in conjunction with one of the less soluble, longer-acting steroids for intra-articular and soft tissue injection.

HOW SUPPLIED

No. 7628X—Injection DECADRON Phosphate, 4 mg per mL, is a clear, colorless solution, and is available in 1 mL and 2.5 mL disposable syringes and in 1 mL, 5 mL, and 25 mL vials as follows:
NDC 0006-7628-01, 1 mL single dose disposable syringe (6505-00-935-4117, 1 mL syringe)
NDC 0006-7628-66, boxes of 25 × 1 mL vials
NDC 0006-7628-30, 2.5 mL single dose disposable syringe
NDC 0006-7628-03, 5 mL vial (6505-00-963-5355, 5 mL vial)
NDC 0006-7628-25, 25 mL vial

FOR INTRAVENOUS USE ONLY:

No. 7646—Injection DECADRON Phosphate, 24 mg per mL, is a clear, colorless to light yellow solution and is available in 5 mL and 10 mL vials as follows:
NDC 0006-7646-03, 5 mL vial
NDC 0006-7646-10, 10 mL vial.

Storage

Sensitive to heat. Do not autoclave.
Protect from freezing.
Protect from light. Store container in carton until contents have been used.

A.H.F.S. Category: 68:04
DC 6597122 Issued April 1985

DECADRON® Phosphate with XYLOCAINE® Injection ℞
(Dexamethasone Sodium Phosphate-Lidocaine Hydrochloride)

For local injection only

DESCRIPTION

Dexamethasone sodium phosphate is a white or slightly yellow, crystalline powder. It is freely soluble in water and is exceedingly hygroscopic. The molecular weight is 516.41. It is designated chemically as 9-fluoro-11β, 17-dihydroxy-16α-methyl-21-(phosphonooxy)pregna-1,4-diene-3,20-dione disodium salt. The empirical formula is $C_{22}H_{28}FNa_2O_8P$ and the structural formula is:

Lidocaine hydrochloride is a white, crystalline powder that is very soluble in water and alcohol, soluble in chloroform, and insoluble in ether. The molecular weight is 288.82. It is designated chemically as 2-(diethylamino)-*N*-(2,6- dimethylphenyl)acetamide, monohydrochloride, monohydrate. The empirical formula is $C_{14}H_{22}N_2O \cdot HCl \cdot H_2O$ and the structural formula is:

DECADRON® Phosphate with XYLOCAINE* (Dexamethasone Sodium Phosphate-Lidocaine Hydrochloride) Injection is provided as a sterile solution (pH 6.5 to 6.9) for the convenience of physicians who prefer to treat patients with simultaneous administration of a corticosteroid and a local anesthetic.
Each milliliter contains dexamethasone sodium phosphate equivalent to dexamethasone phosphate, 4 mg; and lidocaine hydrochloride, 10 mg. Inactive ingredients per mL: citric acid anhydrous, 10 mg; creatinine, 8 mg; sodium bisulfite, 0.5 mg; disodium edetate, 0.5 mg; sodium hydroxide to adjust pH; and Water for Injection, q.s., 1 mL.
Methylparaben, 1.5 mg, and propylparaben, 0.2 mg, added as preservatives.

ACTIONS

DECADRON Phosphate (Dexamethasone Sodium Phosphate, MSD) is a synthetic glucocorticoid used primarily for its potent anti-inflammatory effects in disorders of many organ systems. Glucocorticoids cause profound and varied metabolic effects. In addition, they modify the body's immune responses to diverse stimuli.
XYLOCAINE (Lidocaine Hydrochloride) is a local anesthetic with a rapid onset and moderate duration of action.
Local anesthesia appears within a few minutes after injection of DECADRON Phosphate with XYLOCAINE and lasts 45 minutes to one hour. By the time the anesthesia wears off, steroid activity usually has begun. If the anesthesia wears off before full steroid effect appears, there may be some discomfort beginning about an hour after injection and relief of pain may be delayed for a short time.

INDICATIONS

Acute and subacute bursitis
Acute and subacute nonspecific tenosynovitis

CONTRAINDICATIONS

Hypersensitivity to any component of this product, including sulfites (see WARNINGS).
Dexamethasone Sodium Phosphate
Systemic fungal infections
Lidocaine Hydrochloride
Patients with known history of hypersensitivity to local anesthetics of the amide type (e.g., mepivacaine, prilocaine)
Severe shock
Heart block

WARNINGS

Sodium bisulfite has been reported to cause severe allergic reactions in certain susceptible individuals, particularly patients with asthma. Anaphylactoid and hypersensitivity reactions have been reported for Injection DECADRON Phosphate with XYLOCAINE (see ADVERSE REACTIONS). Since Injection DECADRON Phosphate with XY-

*Registered trademark of Astra Pharmaceutical Products, Inc.

LOCAINE contains sodium bisulfite, this product should not be used in patients allergic to sulfites.

Lidocaine Hydrochloride

RESUSCITATIVE EQUIPMENT AND DRUGS SHOULD BE IMMEDIATELY AVAILABLE WHEN ANY LOCAL ANESTHETIC IS USED.

Usage in pregnancy: The safe use of lidocaine hydrochloride has not been established with respect to adverse effects upon fetal development. Careful consideration should be given to this fact before administering this drug to women of childbearing potential, particularly during early pregnancy.

Dexamethasone Sodium Phosphate

In patients on corticosteroid therapy subjected to unusual stress, increased dosage of rapidly acting corticosteroids before, during, and after the stressful situation is indicated.

Drug-induced secondary adrenocortical insufficiency may result from too rapid withdrawal of corticosteroids and may be minimized by gradual reduction of dosage. This type of relative insufficiency may persist for months after discontinuation of therapy: therefore, in any situation of stress occurring during that period, hormone therapy should be reinstituted. If the patient is receiving steroids already, dosage may have to be increased. Since mineralocorticoid secretion may be impaired, salt and/or a mineralocorticoid should be administered concurrently.

Corticosteroids may mask some signs of infection, and new infections may appear during their use. There may be decreased resistance and inability to localize infection when corticosteroids are used. Moreover, corticosteroids may affect the nitroblue-tetrazolium test for bacterial infection and produce false negative results.

Corticosteroids may activate latent amebiasis. Therefore, it is recommended that latent or active amebiasis be ruled out before initiating corticosteroid therapy in any patient who has spent time in the tropics or any patient with unexplained diarrhea.

Prolonged use of corticosteroids may produce posterior subcapsular cataracts, glaucoma with possible damage to the optic nerves, and may enhance the establishment of secondary ocular infections due to fungi or viruses.

Usage in pregnancy: Since adequate human reproduction studies have not been done with corticosteroids, use of these drugs in pregnancy or in women of childbearing potential requires that the anticipated benefits be weighed against the possible hazards to the mother and embryo or fetus. Infants born of mothers who have received substantial doses of corticosteroids during pregnancy should be carefully observed for signs of hypoadrenalism.

Corticosteroids appear in breast milk and could suppress growth, interfere with endogenous corticosteroid production, or cause other unwanted effects. Mothers taking pharmacologic doses of corticosteroids should be advised not to nurse.

Average and large doses of cortisone or hydrocortisone can cause elevation of blood pressure, salt and water retention, and increased excretion of potassium. These effects are less likely to occur with the synthetic derivatives except when used in large doses. Dietary salt restriction and potassium supplementation may be necessary. All corticosteroids increase calcium excretion.

Administration of live virus vaccines, including smallpox, is contraindicated in individuals receiving immunosuppressive doses of corticosteroids. If inactivated viral or bacterial vaccines are administered to individuals receiving immunosuppressive doses of corticosteroids, the expected serum antibody response may not be obtained.

If corticosteroids are indicated in patients with latent tuberculosis or tuberculin reactivity, close observation is necessary as reactivation of the disease may occur. During prolonged corticosteroid therapy, these patients should receive chemoprophylaxis.

Because rare instances of anaphylactoid reactions have occurred in patients receiving parenteral corticosteroid therapy, appropriate precautionary measures should be taken prior to administration, especially when the patient has a history of allergy to any drug.

PRECAUTIONS

This product, like many other steroid formulations, is sensitive to heat. Therefore, it should not be autoclaved when it is desirable to sterilize the exterior of the vial.

Therapy with this preparation does not eliminate the need for conventional supportive measures. Although capable of ameliorating symptoms, and even suppressing them completely in some patients, it is not a cure. Neither the hormone nor the anesthetic has any effect on the basic cause of inflammation.

Supportive measures, such as analgesics, pertinent orthopedic procedures, heat or cold, rest, rehabilitation, and physiotherapy must be used as applicable. If physiotherapy is applied immediately following injection, it may cause severe pain.

In some patients, a single injection fully restores mobility. Patients should be strongly impressed with the importance of not overusing the affected part as long as the inflammatory process remains active.

Injection into an infected site is to be avoided.

Dexamethasone Sodium Phosphate

Following prolonged therapy, withdrawal of corticosteroids may result in symptoms of the corticosteroid withdrawal syndrome including fever, myalgia, arthralgia, and malaise. This may occur in patients even without evidence of adrenal insufficiency.

There is an enhanced effect of corticosteroids in patients with hypothyroidism and in those with cirrhosis.

Corticosteroids should be used cautiously in patients with ocular herpes simplex for fear of corneal perforation.

Psychic derangements may appear when corticosteroids are used, ranging from euphoria, insomnia, mood swings, personality changes, and severe depression to frank psychotic manifestations. Also, existing emotional instability or psychotic tendencies may be aggravated by corticosteroids.

Aspirin should be used cautiously in conjunction with corticosteroids in hypoprothrombinemia.

Steroids should be used with caution in non-specific ulcerative colitis, if there is a probability of impending perforation, abscess, or other pyogenic infection, also in diverticulitis, fresh intestinal anastomoses, active or latent peptic ulcer, renal insufficiency, hypertension, osteoporosis, and myasthenia gravis. Signs of peritoneal irritation folllowing gastrointestinal perforation in patients receiving large doses of corticosteroids may be minimal or absent. Fat embolism has been reported as a possible complication of hypercortisonism.

When large doses are given, some authorities advise that antacids be administered between meals to help to prevent peptic ulcer.

Growth and development of infants and children on prolonged corticosteroid therapy should be carefully followed.

Steroids may increase or decrease motility and number of spermatozoa in some patients.

Phenytoin, phenobarbital, ephedrine, and rifampin may enhance the metabolic clearance of corticosteroids, resulting in decreased blood levels and lessened physiologic activity, thus requiring adjustment in corticosteroid dosage.

The prothrombin time should be checked frequently in patients who are receiving corticosteroids and coumarin anticoagulants at the same time because of reports that corticosteroids have altered the response to these anticoagulants. Studies have shown that the usual effect produced by adding corticosteroids is inhibition of response to coumarins, although there have been some conflicting reports of potentiation not substantiated by studies.

When corticosteroids are administered concomitantly with potassium-depleting diuretics, patients should be observed closely for development of hypokalemia.

Lidocaine Hydrochloride

The safety and effectiveness of lidocaine hydrochloride depend on proper dosage, correct technique, adequate precautions, and readiness for emergencies.

Injection of repeated doses may cause significant increases in blood levels with each repeated dose due to slow accumulation of the drug or its metabolites. Tolerance varies with the status of the patient. Debilitated, elderly patients, acutely ill patients, and children should be given reduced doses commensurate with their age and physical status. INJECTIONS SHOULD ALWAYS BE MADE SLOWLY AND WITH FREQUENT ASPIRATIONS. Aspiration is advisable since it reduces the possibility of intravascular injection, thereby keeping the incidence of side effects and anesthetic failures to a minimum. Consult standard textbooks for specific techniques and precautions for various local anesthetic procedures.

Lidocaine hydrochloride should be used with caution in persons with known drug sensitivities. Patients allergic to para-aminobenzoic acid derivatives (procaine, tetracaine, benzocaine, etc.) have not shown cross sensitivity to lidocaine hydrochloride.

Local anesthetics react with certain metals and cause the release of their respective ions which, if injected, may cause severe local irritation. Adequate precaution should be taken to avoid this type of interaction.

ADVERSE REACTIONS

Dexamethasone Sodium Phosphate

Fluid and electrolyte disturbances

- Sodium retention
- Fluid retention
- Congestive heart failure in susceptible patients
- Potassium loss
- Hypokalemic alkalosis
- Hypertension

Musculoskeletal

- Muscle weakness
- Steroid myopathy
- Loss of muscle mass
- Osteoporosis
- Vertebral compression fractures
- Aseptic necrosis of femoral and humeral heads
- Pathologic fracture of long bones
- Tendon rupture

Gastrointestinal

- Peptic ulcer with possible subsequent perforation and hemorrhage
- Perforation of the small and large bowel, particularly in patients with inflammatory bowel disease
- Pancreatitis
- Abdominal distention
- Ulcerative esophagitis

Dermatologic

- Impaired wound healing
- Thin fragile skin
- Petechiae and ecchymoses
- Erythema
- Increased sweating
- May suppress reactions to skin tests
- Other cutaneous reactions, such as allergic dermatitis, urticaria, angioneurotic edema

Neurologic

- Convulsions
- Increased intracranial pressure with papilledema (pseudotumor cerebri) usually after treatment
- Vertigo
- Headache

Endocrine

- Menstrual irregularities
- Development of cushingoid state
- Suppression of growth in children
- Secondary adrenocortical and pituitary unresponsiveness, particularly in times of stress, as in trauma, surgery, or illness
- Decreased carbohydrate tolerance
- Manifestations of latent diabetes mellitus
- Increased requirements for insulin or oral hypoglycemic agents in diabetics

Ophthalmic

- Posterior subcapsular cataracts
- Increased intraocular pressure
- Glaucoma
- Exophthalmos

Metabolic

- Negative nitrogen balance due to protein catabolism

Other

- Anaphylactoid or hypersensitivity reactions
- Thromboembolism
- Weight gain
- Increased appetite
- Nausea
- Malaise
- Psychic disturbances

The following *additional* adverse reactions are related to parenteral corticosteroid therapy:

- Rare instances of blindness associated with intralesional therapy around the face and head
- Hyperpigmentation or hypopigmentation
- Subcutaneous and cutaneous atrophy
- Sterile abscess
- Charcot-like arthropathy

Lidocaine Hydrochloride

Adverse reactions may result from high plasma levels due to excessive dosage, rapid absorption or inadvertent intravascular injection, or may result from a hypersensitivity, idiosyncrasy or diminished tolerance on the part of the patient. Such reactions are systemic in nature and involve the central nervous system and/or the cardiovascular system.

CNS reactions are excitatory and/or depressant, and may be characterized by nervousness, dizziness, blurred vision, and tremors followed by drowsiness, convulsions, unconsciousness, and possibly respiratory arrest. The excitatory reactions may be very brief or may not occur at all, in which case the first manifestations of toxicity may be drowsiness merging into unconsciousness and respiratory arrest.

Cardiovascular reactions are depressant, and may be characterized by hypotension, myocardial depression, bradycardia and possibly cardiac arrest.

Treatment of a patient with toxic manifestations consists of assuring and maintaining a patent airway and supporting ventilation using oxygen and assisted or controlled respiration as required. This usually will be sufficient in the management of most reactions. Should circulatory depression occur, vasopressors, such as ephedrine or metaraminol, and intravenous fluids may be used. Should a convulsion persist despite oxygen therapy, small increments of an ultra-short acting barbiturate (thiopental or thiamylal) or a short acting barbiturate (pentobarbital or secobarbital) may be given intravenously.

Continued on next page

Information on the Merck Sharp & Dohme products listed on these pages is the full prescribing information from product circulars in use August 31, 1986.

Merck Sharp & Dohme—Cont.

Allergic reactions are characterized by cutaneous lesions, urticaria, edema or anaphylactoid reactions. The detection of sensitivity by skin testing is of doubtful value.

DOSAGE AND ADMINISTRATION

For local injection only

DOSAGE AND FREQUENCY OF INJECTION ARE VARIABLE AND MUST BE INDIVIDUALIZED ON THE BASIS OF THE DISEASE AND THE RESPONSE OF THE PATIENT.

Injections should always be made slowly and with frequent aspiration.

The initial dose ranges from 0.1 to 0.75 mL depending on the disease being treated and the size of the area to be injected. Frequency of injection depends on symptomatic response. In some patients, acute conditions are controlled adequately by a single injection. In others, additional injections are required, usually at intervals of four to seven days. If satisfactory clinical response does not occur after a reasonable period of time, discontinue DECADRON Phosphate with XYLOCAINE Injection and transfer the patient to other therapy.

Patients should be observed closely for signs that might require dosage adjustment, including changes in clinical status resulting from remissions or exacerbations of the disease, and individual drug responsiveness.

The usual doses are:

	Acute and Subacute Bursitis	Acute and Subacute Nonspecific Tenosynovitis
Amount of injection (mL)	0.5 to 0.75	0.1 to 0.25
Amount of dexamethasone sodium phosphate (mg)	2 to 3	0.4 to 1
Amount of lidocaine hydrochloride (mg)	5 to 7.5	1 to 2.5

DECADRON Phosphate with XYLOCAINE may be given undiluted directly from the vial, or it may be diluted with Sterile Water for Injection or Sodium Chloride Injection, using up to five parts of diluent to each part of injection. Dilutions should be used within one hour, since there is a possibility of change in pH, and this may adversely affect the stability or activity of the components.

HOW SUPPLIED

No. 7625X—Injection DECADRON Phosphate with XYLOCAINE, containing 4 mg dexamethasone phosphate equivalent and 10 mg lidocaine hydrochloride per mL, is a clear, colorless solution, and is available as follows:

NDC 0006-7625-03 in 5 mL vials.

Storage

Sensitive to heat. Do not autoclave.

Protect from freezing.

A.H.F.S. Categories: 68:04-72:00

DC 7349314 Issued April 1985

DECADRON® Phosphate ℞

(Dexamethasone Sodium Phosphate, MSD), U.S.P.
0.05% Dexamethasone Phosphate Equivalent
Sterile Ophthalmic Ointment

DESCRIPTION

Sterile Ophthalmic Ointment DECADRON® Phosphate (Dexamethasone Sodium Phosphate, MSD) is a topical steroid ointment containing dexamethasone sodium phosphate equivalent to 0.5 mg (0.05%) dexamethasone phosphate in each gram. Inactive ingredients: white petrolatum and mineral oil.

Dexamethasone sodium phosphate is an inorganic ester of dexamethasone.

ACTION

Inhibition of inflammatory response to inciting agents of mechanical, chemical or immunological nature. No generally accepted explanation of this steroid property has been advanced.

INDICATIONS

For the treatment of the following conditions:

Steroid responsive inflammatory conditions of the palpebral and bulbar conjunctiva, cornea, and anterior segment of the globe, such as allergic conjunctivitis, acne rosacea, superficial punctate keratitis, herpes zoster keratitis, iritis, cyclitis, selected infective conjunctivitis when the inherent hazard of steroid use is accepted to obtain an advisable diminution in edema and inflammation; corneal injury from chemical or thermal burns, or penetration of foreign bodies.

CONTRAINDICATIONS

Acute superficial herpes simplex keratitis.
Fungal diseases of ocular structures.
Acute infectious stages of vaccinia, varicella and most other viral diseases of the cornea and conjunctiva.
Tuberculosis of the eye.
Hypersensitivity to a component of this medication.

WARNINGS

Employment of steroid medication in the treatment of stromal herpes simplex requires great caution; frequent slit-lamp microscopy is mandatory.

Prolonged use may result in elevated intraocular pressure and/or glaucoma, damage to the optic nerve, defects in visual acuity and fields of vision, posterior subcapsular cataract formation, or may result in secondary ocular infections.

Viral, bacterial, and fungal infections of the cornea may be exacerbated by the application of steroids.

Acute purulent untreated infection of the eye may be masked or activity enhanced by the presence of steroid medication.

In those diseases causing thinning of the cornea or sclera, perforation has been known to occur with the use of topical steroids.

Usage in Pregnancy

Safety of intensive or protracted use of topical steroids during pregnancy has not been substantiated.

PRECAUTIONS

As fungal infections of the cornea are particularly prone to develop coincidentally with long-term local steroid applications, fungus invasion must be considered in any persistent corneal ulceration where a steroid has been used or is in use. Intraocular pressure should be checked frequently.

ADVERSE REACTIONS

Glaucoma with optic nerve damage, visual acuity and field defects, posterior subcapsular cataract formation, secondary ocular infection from pathogens including herpes simplex, perforation of the globe.

Rarely, filtering blebs have been reported when topical steroids have been used following cataract surgery.

Rarely, stinging or burning may occur.

DOSAGE AND ADMINISTRATION

The duration of treatment will vary with the type of lesion and may extend from a few days to several weeks, according to therapeutic response. Relapses, more common in chronic active lesions than in self-limited conditions, usually respond to retreatment.

Apply a thin coating of ointment three or four times a day. When a favorable response is observed, reduce the number of daily applications to two, and later to one a day as a maintenance dose if this is sufficient to control symptoms.

Ophthalmic ointment DECADRON phosphate is particularly convenient when an eye pad is used. It may also be the preparation of choice for patients in whom therapeutic benefit depends on prolonged contact of the active ingredients with ocular tissues.

HOW SUPPLIED

No. 7615—0.05% Sterile Ophthalmic Ointment DECADRON phosphate is a clear unctuous ointment and is supplied as follows:

NDC 0006-7615-04 in 3.5 g tubes.

A.H.F.S. Category: 52:08

DC 6033125 Issued May 1981

DECADRON® Phosphate ℞

(Dexamethasone Sodium Phosphate, MSD), U.S.P.
0.1% Dexamethasone Phosphate Equivalent
Sterile Ophthalmic Solution

DESCRIPTION

Ophthalmic Solution DECADRON® Phosphate (Dexamethasone Sodium Phosphate, MSD) in the 5 mL OCUMETER® ophthalmic dispenser is a topical steroid solution containing dexamethasone sodium phosphate equivalent to 1 mg (0.1%) dexamethasone phosphate in each milliliter of buffered solution. Inactive ingredients: creatinine, sodium citrate, sodium borate, polysorbate 80, disodium edetate, hydrochloric acid to adjust pH, and water for injection. Sodium bisulfite 0.1%, phenylethanol 0.25% and benzalkonium chloride 0.02% added as preservatives.

Dexamethasone sodium phosphate is a water soluble, inorganic ester of dexamethasone. It is approximately three thousand times more soluble in water at 25°C than hydrocortisone.

ACTION

Inhibition of inflammatory response to inciting agents of mechanical, chemical or immunological nature. No generally accepted explanation of this steroid property has been advanced.

INDICATIONS

For the treatment of the following conditions:

Ophthalmic:

Steroid responsive inflammatory conditions of the palpebral and bulbar conjunctiva, cornea, and anterior segment of the globe, such as allergic conjunctivitis, acne rosacea, superficial punctate keratitis, herpes zoster keratitis, iritis, cyclitis, selected infective conjunctivitis when the inherent hazard of steroid use is accepted to obtain an advisable diminution in edema and inflammation; corneal injury from chemical or thermal burns, or penetration of foreign bodies.

Otic:

Steroid responsive inflammatory conditions of the external auditory meatus, such as allergic otitis externa, selected purulent and nonpurulent infective otitis externa when the hazard of steroid use is accepted to obtain an advisable diminution in edema and inflammation.

CONTRAINDICATIONS

Acute superficial herpes simplex keratitis.
Fungal diseases of ocular or auricular structures.
Acute infectious stages of vaccinia, varicella and most other viral diseases of the cornea and conjunctiva.
Tuberculosis of the eye.
Hypersensitivity to any component of this product, including sulfites (see PRECAUTIONS).
Perforation of a drum membrane.

WARNINGS

Employment of steroid medication in the treatment of stromal herpes simplex requires great caution; frequent slit-lamp microscopy is mandatory.

Prolonged use may result in elevated intraocular pressure and/or glaucoma, damage to the optic nerve, defects in visual acuity and fields of vision, posterior subcapsular cataract formation, or may result in secondary ocular infections.

Viral, bacterial, and fungal infections of the cornea may be exacerbated by the application of steroids.

Acute purulent untreated infection of the eye or ear may be masked or activity enhanced by the presence of steroid medication.

In those diseases causing thinning of the cornea or sclera, perforation has been known to occur with the use of topical steroids.

Usage in Pregnancy

Safety of intensive or protracted use of topical steroids during pregnancy has not been substantiated.

PRECAUTIONS

As fungal infections of the cornea are particularly prone to develop coincidentally with long-term local steroid applications, fungus invasion must be considered in any persistent corneal ulceration where a steroid has been used or is in use. Intraocular pressure should be checked frequently.

Sulfites have been reported to cause severe allergic reactions in certain susceptible individuals, particularly patients with asthma.

ADVERSE REACTIONS

Glaucoma with optic nerve damage, visual acuity and field defects, posterior subcapsular cataract formation, secondary ocular infection from pathogens including herpes simplex, perforation of the globe.
Rarely, filtering blebs have been reported when topical steroids have been used following cataract surgery.
Rarely, stinging or burning may occur.

DOSAGE AND ADMINISTRATION

The duration of treatment will vary with the type of lesion and may extend from a few days to several weeks, according to therapeutic response. Relapses, more common in chronic active lesions than in self-limited conditions, usually respond to retreatment.
Eye—Instill one or two drops of solution into the conjunctival sac every hour during the day and every two hours during the night as initial therapy. When a favorable response is observed, reduce dosage to one drop every four hours. Later, further reduction in dosage to one drop three or four times daily may suffice to control symptoms.
Ear—Clean the aural canal thoroughly and sponge dry. Instill the solution directly into the aural canal. A suggested initial dosage is three or four drops two or three times a day. When a favorable response is obtained, reduce dosage gradually and eventually discontinue.
If preferred, the aural canal may be packed with a gauze wick saturated with solution. Keep the wick moist with the preparation and remove from the ear after 12 to 24 hours. Treatment may be repeated as often as necessary at the discretion of the physician.

HOW SUPPLIED

Sterile ophthalmic solution DECADRON Phosphate is a clear, colorless to pale yellow solution.
No. 7643—Ophthalmic solution DECADRON Phosphate is supplied as follows:
NDC 0006-7643-03 in 5 mL white, opaque, plastic OCUMETER ophthalmic dispenser with a controlled drop tip.
(6505-00-007-4536 0.1% 5 mL).

A.H.F.S. Category: 52:08
DC 6460013 Issued December 1984

DECADRON® Phosphate RESPIHALER® ℞
(Dexamethasone Sodium Phosphate, MSD), U.S.P.

DESCRIPTION

RESPIHALER® DECADRON® Phosphate (Dexamethasone Sodium Phosphate, MSD) is an aerosol for oral inhalation which contains dexamethasone sodium phosphate, an inorganic ester of dexamethasone, a synthetic adrenocortical steroid with basic glucocorticoid actions and effects.
Each RESPIHALER DECADRON Phosphate contains an amount sufficient to deliver at least 170 sprays. The metering valve of the aerosol-mechanism of the RESPIHALER dispenses dexamethasone sodium phosphate equivalent to approximately 0.1 mg of dexamethasone phosphate or approximately 0.084 mg of dexamethasone with each activation. On a regimen of 12 inhalations daily, it has been determined that the patient absorbs approximately 0.4-0.6 mg of dexamethasone. The inactive ingredients are fluorochlorohydrocarbons included as propellants. Alcohol 2%.
Dexamethasone sodium phosphate, a synthetic adrenocortical steroid, is a white or slightly yellow, crystalline powder. It is freely soluble in water and is exceedingly hygroscopic. It is prepared by a special process to produce particles in the range of 0.5 to 4 microns in size. The molecular weight is 516.41. It is designated chemically as 9-fluoro-11β, 17-dihydroxy-16α-methyl-21-(phosphono-oxy)pregna-1, 4-diene-3, 20-dione disodium salt. The empirical formula is $C_{22}H_{28}FNa_2O_8P$ and the structural formula is:

ACTIONS

Because of the high water solubility of dexamethasone sodium phosphate, the aerosolized particles dissolve readily in the secretions of the bronchial and bronchiolar mucous membrane.

INDICATIONS

RESPIHALER DECADRON Phosphate is indicated for the treatment of bronchial asthma and related corticosteroid responsive bronchospastic states intractable to adequate trial of conventional therapy.

CONTRAINDICATIONS

Systemic fungal infections.
Hypersensitivity to any component of this medication.
Persistently positive cultures of the sputum for *Candida albicans.*

WARNINGS

Rare instances of laryngeal and pharyngeal fungal infections have been observed in patients using RESPIHALER DECADRON Phosphate. These have usually responded promptly to discontinuation of therapy and institution of antifungal treatment.
In patients on therapy with RESPIHALER DECADRON Phosphate subjected to unusual stress, increased dosage of rapidly acting corticosteroids before, during, and after the stressful situation is indicated.
Drug-induced secondary adrenocortical insufficiency may result from too rapid withdrawal of corticosteroids and may be minimized by gradual reduction of dosage. This type of relative insufficiency may persist for months after discontinuation of therapy; therefore, in any situation of stress occurring during that period, hormone therapy should be reinstituted. If the patient is receiving steroids already, dosage may have to be increased. Since mineralocorticoid secretion may be impaired, salt and/or a mineralocorticoid should be administered concurrently.
Dexamethasone may mask some signs of infection, and new infections may appear during its use. There may be decreased resistance and inability to localize infection when corticosteroids are used. Moreover, dexamethasone may affect the nitroblue-tetrazolium test for bacterial infection and produce false negative results.
Corticosteroids may activate latent amebiasis. Therefore, it is recommended that latent or active amebiasis be ruled out before initiating corticosteroid therapy in any patient who has spent time in the tropics or any patient with unexplained diarrhea.
Prolonged use of RESPIHALER DECADRON Phosphate may produce posterior subcapsular cataracts, glaucoma with possible damage to the optic nerves, and may enhance the establishment of secondary ocular infections due to fungi or viruses.
Usage in pregnancy: Since adequate human reproduction studies have not been done with RESPIHALER DECADRON Phosphate, use of this drug in pregnancy or in women of childbearing potential requires that the anticipated benefits be weighed against the possible hazards to the mother and embryo or fetus. Infants born of mothers who have received substantial doses of dexamethasone during pregnancy, should be carefully observed for signs of hypoadrenalism.
Dexamethasone appears in breast milk and could suppress growth, interfere with endogenous corticosteroid production, or cause other unwanted effects. Mothers taking pharmacologic doses of dexamethasone should be advised not to nurse.
Average and large doses of hydrocortisone or cortisone can cause elevation of blood pressure, salt and water retention, and increased excretion of potassium. These effects are less likely to occur with the synthetic derivatives and with RESPIHALER DECADRON Phosphate, except when used in large doses. Dietary salt restriction and potassium supplementation may be necessary. All corticosteroids increase calcium excretion.
Administration of live virus vaccines, including smallpox, is contraindicated in individuals receiving immunosuppressive doses of corticosteroids. If inactivated viral or bacterial vaccines are administered to individuals receiving immunosuppressive doses of corticosteroids, the expected serum antibody response may not be obtained.
If RESPIHALER DECADRON Phosphate is indicated in patients with latent tuberculosis or tuberculin reactivity, close observation is necessary as reactivation of the disease may occur. During prolonged therapy with RESPIHALER DECADRON Phosphate, these patients should receive chemoprophylaxis.

PRECAUTIONS

RESPIHALER DECADRON Phosphate is *not* indicated for relief of the occasional mild and isolated attack of asthma which is readily responsive to the immediate, though shortlived, action of epinephrine, isoproterenol, aminophylline, etc. Nor should it be employed for the treatment of severe status asthmaticus where intensive measures are required.
RESPIHALER DECADRON Phosphate should be considered only for the following classes of patients: patients not on corticosteroid therapy who have not responded adequately to other treatment; patients already on systemic corticosteroid therapy—in an attempt to reduce or eliminate systemic administration.
Although systemic absorption is low when RESPIHALER DECADRON Phosphate is used in the recommended dosage, adrenal suppression may occur. In addition, other systemic effects of steroid administration must be considered as a possibility.
Following prolonged therapy, withdrawal of corticosteroids may result in symptoms of the corticosteroid withdrawal syndrome including fever, myalgia, arthralgia, and malaise. This may occur in patients even without evidence of adrenal insufficiency.
There is an enhanced effect of dexamethasone in patients with hypothyroidism and in those with cirrhosis.
RESPIHALER DECADRON Phosphate should be used cautiously in patients with ocular herpes simplex for fear of corneal perforation.
The lowest possible dose of RESPIHALER DECADRON Phosphate should be used to control the condition under treatment, and when reduction in dosage is possible, the reduction must be gradual.
Psychic derangements may appear when dexamethasone is used, ranging from euphoria, insomnia, mood swings, personality changes, and severe depression, to frank psychotic manifestations. Also, existing emotional instability or psychotic tendencies may be aggravated.
Aspirin should be used cautiously in conjunction with RESPIHALER DECADRON Phosphate in hypoprothrombinemia.
RESPIHALER DECADRON Phosphate should be used with caution in nonspecific ulcerative colitis, if there is a probability of impending perforation, abscess or other pyogenic infection; also in diverticulitis; fresh intestinal anastomoses; active or latent peptic ulcer; renal insufficiency; hypertension; osteoporosis; and myasthenia gravis. Signs of peritoneal irritation following gastrointestinal perforation in patients receiving large doses of corticosteroids may be minimal or absent. Fat embolism has been reported as a possible complication of hypercortisonism.
Growth and development of infants and children on prolonged therapy with RESPIHALER DECADRON Phosphate should be carefully followed.
Dexamethasone may increase or decrease motility and number of spermatozoa in some patients.
Phenytoin, phenobarbital, ephedrine and rifampin may enhance the metabolic clearance of dexamethasone, resulting in decreased blood levels and lessened physiologic activity, thus requiring adjustment in dexamethasone dosage.
The prothrombin time should be checked frequently in patients who are receiving RESPIHALER DECADRON Phosphate and coumarin anticoagulants at the same time because of reports that corticosteroids have altered the response to these anticoagulants. Studies have shown that the usual effect produced by adding corticosteroids is inhibition of response to coumarins, although there have been some conflicting reports of potentiation, not substantiated by studies.
When RESPIHALER DECADRON Phosphate is used concomitantly with potassium-depleting diuretics, patients should be observed closely for development of hypokalemia.
Since the contents of RESPIHALER DECADRON Phosphate are under pressure, the container should not be broken, stored in extreme heat, or incinerated. It should be stored at a temperature below 120°F.

ADVERSE REACTIONS

Side effects which may occur in patients treated with RESPIHALER DECADRON Phosphate include throat irritation, hoarseness, coughing, and laryngeal and pharyngeal fungal infections.
Patients should be observed for the hormonal effects described below:
Fluid and Electrolyte Disturbances
- Sodium retention
- Fluid retention
- Congestive heart failure in susceptible patients
- Potassium loss
- Hypokalemic alkalosis
- Hypertension

Musculoskeletal
- Muscle weakness
- Steroid myopathy
- Loss of muscle mass
- Osteoporosis
- Vertebral compression fractures
- Aseptic necrosis of femoral and humeral heads
- Pathologic fracture of long bones
- Tendon rupture

Continued on next page

Information on the Merck Sharp & Dohme products listed on these pages is the full prescribing information from product circulars in use August 31, 1986.

Merck Sharp & Dohme—Cont.

Gastrointestinal
Peptic ulcer with possible subsequent perforation and hemorrhage
Perforation of the small and large bowel, particularly in patients with inflammatory bowel disease
Pancreatitis
Abdominal distention
Ulcerative esophagitis
Dermatologic
Impaired wound healing
Thin fragile skin
Petechiae and ecchymoses
Erythema
Increased sweating
May suppress reactions to skin tests
Other cutaneous reactions, such as allergic dermatitis, urticaria, angioneurotic edema
Neurologic
Convulsions
Increased intracranial pressure with papilledema (pseudo-tumor cerebri) usually after treatment
Vertigo
Headache
Endocrine
Menstrual irregularities
Development of cushingoid state
Suppression of growth in children
Secondary adrenocortical and pituitary unresponsiveness, particularly in times of stress, as in trauma, surgery, or illness
Decreased carbohydrate tolerance
Manifestations of latent diabetes mellitus
Increased requirements for insulin or oral hypoglycemic agents in diabetics
Ophthalmic
Posterior subcapsular cataracts
Increased intraocular pressure
Glaucoma
Exophthalmos
Metabolic
Negative nitrogen balance due to protein catabolism
Other
Hypersensitivity
Thromboembolism
Weight gain
Increased appetite
Nausea
Malaise
Psychic disturbances

DOSAGE AND ADMINISTRATION

Recommended *initial dosage:*
Adults —3 inhalations 3 or 4 times per day.
Children —2 inhalations 3 or 4 times per day.
Maximum dosage:
Adults — 3 inhalations *per dose;* 12 inhalations *per day.*
Children — 2 inhalations *per dose;* 8 inhalations *per day.*

When a favorable response is attained, the dose may be gradually reduced. In patients on systemic corticosteroids, it is recommended that systemic therapy be reduced or eliminated before reduction of RESPIHALER dosage is begun. Gradual reduction of systemic corticosteroid therapy must be emphasized to avoid withdrawal symptoms.

HOW SUPPLIED

No. 7626X—RESPIHALER DECADRON Phosphate, aerosol for oral inhalation, is supplied as follows: **NDC** 0006-7626-13 in a pressurized container, and includes a plastic adapter.
Storage
Store at a temperature below 120°F.

A.H.F.S. Category: 68:04
DC 6055715 Issued April 1985

DECADRON® Phosphate Topical Cream ℞
(Dexamethasone Sodium Phosphate, MSD), U.S.P.
0.1% Dexamethasone Phosphate Equivalent

DESCRIPTION

DECADRON® Phosphate (Dexamethasone Sodium Phosphate, MSD) Topical Cream is a topical steroid preparation.

The topical corticosteroids constitute a class of primarily synthetic steroids used as anti-inflammatory and anti-pruritic agents.

Dexamethasone sodium phosphate is 9-fluoro-11β,17-dihydroxy-16α-methyl-21-(phosphonooxy)pregna-1,4-diene-3,20-dione disodium salt. Its empirical formula is $C_{22}H_{28}FNa_2O_8P$ and its structural formula is:

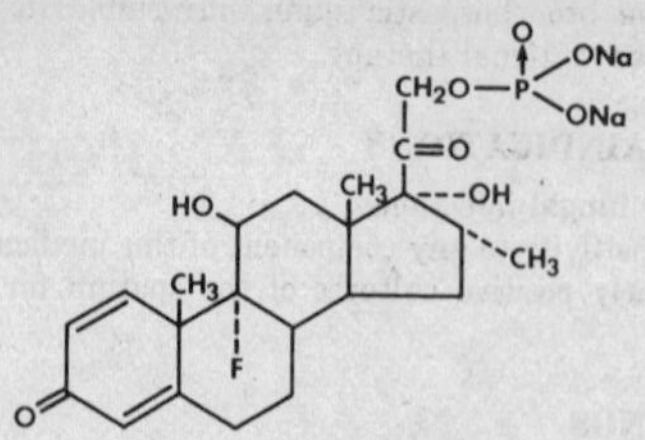

Dexamethasone sodium phosphate has a molecular weight of 516.41.

DECADRON Phosphate Topical Cream contains in each gram: dexamethasone sodium phosphate equivalent to 1 mg (0.1%) dexamethasone phosphate in a greaseless bland base. Inactive ingredients: stearyl alcohol, cetyl alcohol, mineral oil, polyoxyl 40 stearate, sorbitol solution, methyl polysilicone emulsion, creatinine, sodium citrate, disodium edetate, sodium hydroxide to adjust pH, and purified water. Methylparaben, 0.15%, and sorbic acid, 0.1% added as preservatives.

CLINICAL PHARMACOLOGY

Topical corticosteroids share anti-inflammatory, anti-pruritic and vasoconstrictive actions.

The mechanism of anti-inflammatory activity of the topical corticosteroids is unclear. Various laboratory methods, including vasoconstrictor assays, are used to compare and predict potencies and/or clinical efficacies of the topical corticosteroids. There is some evidence to suggest that a recognizable correlation exists between vasoconstrictor potency and therapeutic efficacy in man.

Pharmacokinetics
The extent of percutaneous absorption of topical corticosteroids is determined by many factors including the vehicle, the integrity of the epidermal barrier, and the use of occlusive dressings.

Topical corticosteroids can be absorbed from normal intact skin. Inflammation and/or other disease processes in the skin increase percutaneous absorption. Occlusive dressings substantially increase the percutaneous absorption of topical corticosteroids. Thus, occlusive dressings may be a valuable therapeutic adjunct for treatment of resistant dermatoses. (See DOSAGE AND ADMINISTRATION)

Once absorbed through the skin, topical corticosteroids are handled through pharmacokinetic pathways similar to systemically administered corticosteroids. Corticosteroids are bound to plasma proteins in varying degrees. Corticosteroids are metabolized primarily in the liver and are then excreted by the kidneys. Some of the topical corticosteroids and their metabolites are also excreted into the bile.

INDICATIONS AND USAGE

DECADRON Phosphate Topical Cream is indicated for relief of the inflammatory and pruritic manifestations of corticosteroid-responsive dermatoses.

CONTRAINDICATIONS

Topical corticosteroids are contraindicated in those patients with a history of hypersensitivity to any of the components of the preparation.

PRECAUTIONS

General
Systemic absorption of topical corticosteroids has produced reversible hypothalamic-pituitary-adrenal (HPA) axis suppression, manifestations of Cushing's syndrome, hyperglycemia, and glycosuria in some patients.

Conditions which augment systemic absorption include the application of the more potent corticosteroids, use over large surface areas, prolonged use, and the addition of occlusive dressings.

Therefore, patients receiving a large dose of a potent topical corticosteroid applied to a large surface area or under an occlusive dressing should be evaluated periodically for evidence of HPA axis suppression by using urinary free cortisol and ACTH stimulation tests. If HPA axis suppression is noted, an attempt should be made to withdraw the drug, to reduce the frequency of application, or to substitute a less potent corticosteroid.

Recovery of HPA axis function is generally prompt and complete upon discontinuation of the drug. Infrequently, signs and symptoms of corticosteroid withdrawal may occur, requiring supplemental systemic corticosteroids.

Children may absorb proportionally larger amounts of topical corticosteroids and thus be more susceptible to systemic toxicity (See PRECAUTIONS, *Pediatric Use*).

If irritation develops, topical corticosteroids should be discontinued and appropriate therapy instituted.

In the presence of dermatological infections, the use of an appropriate antifungal or antibacterial agent should be instituted. If a favorable response does not occur promptly, the corticosteroid should be discontinued until the infection has been adequately controlled.

This product is not for ophthalmic use. However, if applied to the eyelids or skin near the eyes, the drug may enter the eyes. In patients with a history of herpes simplex keratitis, ocular exposure to corticosteroids may lead to a recurrence. Prolonged ocular exposure may cause steroid glaucoma.

Generally, occlusive dressings should not be used on weeping or exudative lesions.

If occlusive dressing therapy is used, inspect lesions between dressings for development of infection. If infection develops, the technique should be discontinued and appropriate antimicrobial therapy instituted.

When large areas of the body are covered with an occlusive dressing, thermal homeostasis may be impaired. If elevation of body temperature occurs, use of the occlusive dressing should be discontinued.

Information for the Patient
Patients using topical corticosteroids should receive the following information and instructions:

1. This medication is to be used as directed by the physician. It is for external use only. Avoid contact with the eyes.
2. Patients should be advised not to use this medication for any disorder other than that for which it was prescribed.
3. The treated skin area should not be bandaged or otherwise covered or wrapped so as to be occlusive unless directed by the physician.
4. Patients should report any signs of local adverse reactions, especially under occlusive dressing.
5. Parents of pediatric patients should be advised not to use tight-fitting diapers or plastic pants on a child being treated in the diaper area, as these garments may constitute occlusive dressings.

Laboratory Tests
The following tests may be helpful in evaluating the HPA axis suppression:

- Urinary free cortisol test
- ACTH stimulation test

Carcinogenesis, Mutagenesis, and Impairment of Fertility
Long-term animal studies have not been performed to evaluate the carcinogenic potential or the effect on fertility of topical corticosteroids.

Studies to determine mutagenicity with prednisolone and hydrocortisone have revealed negative results.

Pregnancy
Pregnancy Category C: Corticosteroids are generally teratogenic in laboratory animals when administered systemically at relatively low dosage levels. The more potent corticosteroids have been shown to be teratogenic after dermal application in laboratory animals. There are no adequate and well-controlled studies in pregnant women on teratogenic effects from topically applied corticosteroids. Therefore, topical corticosteroids should be used during pregnancy only if the potential benefit justifies the potential risk to the fetus. Drugs of this class should not be used extensively on pregnant patients, in large amounts, or for prolonged periods of time.

Nursing Mothers
It is not known whether topical administration of corticosteroids could result in sufficient systemic absorption to produce detectable quantities in breast milk. Systemically administered corticosteroids are secreted into breast milk in quantities *not* likely to have a deleterious effect on the infant. Nevertheless, caution should be exercised when topical corticosteroids are administered to a nursing woman.

Pediatric Use
Pediatric patients may demonstrate greater susceptibility to topical corticosteroid-induced HPA axis suppression and Cushing's syndrome than mature patients because of a larger skin surface area to body weight ratio.

Hypothalamic-pituitary-adrenal (HPA) axis suppression, Cushing's syndrome, and intracranial hypertension have been reported in children receiving topical corticosteroids. Manifestations of adrenal suppression in children include linear growth retardation, delayed weight gain, low plasma cortisol levels, and absence of response to ACTH stimulation. Manifestations of intracranial hypertension include bulging fontanelles, headaches, and bilateral papilledema.

Administration of topical corticosteroids to children should be limited to the least amount compatible with an effective therapeutic regimen. Chronic corticosteroid therapy may interfere with the growth and development of children.

ADVERSE REACTIONS

The following adverse reactions are reported infrequently with topical corticosteroids, but may occur more frequently with the use of occlusive dressings. These reactions are listed in an approximate decreasing order of occurrence:

Burning
Itching
Irritation
Dryness
Folliculitis
Hypertrichosis
Acneiform eruptions
Hypopigmentation
Perioral dermatitis
Allergic contact dermatitis
Maceration of the skin
Secondary infection
Skin atrophy
Striae
Miliaria

OVERDOSAGE

Topically applied corticosteroids can be absorbed in sufficient amounts to produce systemic effects (See PRECAUTIONS).

DOSAGE AND ADMINISTRATION

Apply to the affected area as a thin film three or four times daily.
Occlusive dressings may be used for the management of psoriasis or recalcitrant conditions.
Before using this preparation in the *ear*, clean the aural canal thoroughly and sponge dry. Confirm that the eardrum is intact. With a cotton-tipped applicator, apply a thin coating of the cream to the affected canal area three or four times a day.

HOW SUPPLIED

No. 7616X — 0.1% Topical Cream DECADRON Phosphate is a white cream, and is supplied as follows:
NDC 0006-7616-12 in 15 g tubes
NDC 0006-7616-24 in 30 g tubes.

A.H.F.S. Category: 84:06
DC 6005423 Issued April 1983

DECADRON® Phosphate ℞
TURBINAIRE®
(Dexamethasone Sodium Phosphate, MSD), U.S.P.

DESCRIPTION

TURBINAIRE® DECADRON® Phosphate (Dexamethasone Sodium Phosphate, MSD) is an aerosol for intranasal application. The inactive ingredients are fluorochlorohydrocarbons as propellants and alcohol 2%. One cartridge delivers an amount sufficient to ensure delivery of 170 metered sprays, each containing dexamethasone sodium phosphate equivalent to approximately 0.1 mg dexamethasone phosphate or to approximately 0.084 mg dexamethasone. Twelve sprays deliver a theoretical maximum of 1.0 mg dexamethasone.
Dexamethasone sodium phosphate, a synthetic adrenocortical steroid, is a white or slightly yellow, crystalline powder. It is freely soluble in water and is exceedingly hygroscopic. The molecular weight is 516.41. It is designated chemically as 9-fluoro-11β, 17-dihydroxy-16α-methyl-21-(phosphonooxy) pregna-1, 4-diene-3, 20-dione disodium salt. The empirical formula is $C_{22}H_{28}FNa_2O_8P$ and the structural formula is:

ACTION

Inhibition of inflammatory response to inciting agents of mechanical, chemical or immunological nature.

INDICATIONS

Allergic or inflammatory nasal conditions, and nasal polyps (excluding polyps originating within the sinuses).

CONTRAINDICATIONS

Systemic fungal infections.
Hypersensitivity to components.
Tuberculous, viral and fungal nasal conditions, ocular herpes simplex.

WARNINGS

In patients on therapy with TURBINAIRE DECADRON Phosphate subjected to unusual stress, increased dosage of rapidly acting corticosteroids before, during, and after the stressful situation is indicated.
Drug-induced secondary adrenocortical insufficiency may result from too rapid withdrawal of corticosteroids and may be minimized by gradual reduction of dosage. This type of relative insufficiency may persist for months after discontinuation of therapy; therefore, in any situation of stress occurring during that period, hormone therapy should be reinstituted. If the patient is receiving steroids already, dosage may have to be increased. Since mineralocorticoid secretion may be impaired, salt and/or a mineralocorticoid should be administered concurrently.
Dexamethasone may mask some signs of infection, and new infections may appear during its use. There may be decreased resistance and inability to localize infection when corticosteroids are used. Therefore, patients with bacterial infections should also be given appropriate antibiotic therapy if TURBINAIRE DECADRON Phosphate is used. Moreover, dexamethasone may affect the nitroblue-tetrazolium test for bacterial infection and produce false negative results.
Corticosteroids may activate latent amebiasis. Therefore, it is recommended that latent or active amebiasis be ruled out before initiating corticosteroid therapy in any patient who has spent time in the tropics or any patient with unexplained diarrhea.
Prolonged use of TURBINAIRE DECADRON Phosphate may produce posterior subcapsular cataracts, glaucoma with possible damage to the optic nerves, and may enhance the establishment of secondary ocular infections due to fungi or viruses.
Usage in pregnancy: Since adequate human reproduction studies have not been done with TURBINAIRE DECADRON Phosphate, use of this drug in pregnancy or in women of childbearing potential requires that the anticipated benefits be weighed against the possible hazards to the mother and embryo or fetus. Infants born of mothers who have received substantial doses of dexamethasone during pregnancy, should be carefully observed for signs of hypoadrenalism.
Dexamethasone appears in breast milk and could suppress growth, interfere with endogenous corticosteroid production, or cause other unwanted effects. Mothers taking pharmacologic doses of dexamethasone should be advised not to nurse.
Average and large doses of hydrocortisone or cortisone can cause elevation of blood pressure, salt and water retention, and increased excretion of potassium. These effects are less likely to occur with the synthetic derivatives and with TURBINAIRE DECADRON Phosphate, except when used in large doses. Dietary salt restriction and potassium supplementation may be necessary. All corticosteroids increase calcium excretion.
Administration of live virus vaccines, including smallpox, is contraindicated in individuals receiving immunosuppressive doses of corticosteroids. If inactivated viral or bacterial vaccines are administered to individuals receiving immunosuppressive doses of corticosteroids, the expected serum antibody response may not be obtained.
If TURBINAIRE DECADRON Phosphate is indicated in patients with latent tuberculosis or tuberculin reactivity, close observation is necessary as reactivation of the disease may occur. During prolonged therapy with TURBINAIRE DECADRON Phosphate, these patients should receive chemoprophylaxis.

PRECAUTIONS

During local corticosteroid therapy, the possibility of pharyngeal candidiasis should be kept in mind.
Although systemic absorption is low when TURBINAIRE DECADRON Phosphate is used in the recommended dosage, adrenal suppression may occur. In addition, other systemic effects of steroid administration must be considered as a possibility.
Following prolonged therapy, withdrawal of corticosteroids may result in symptoms of the corticosteroid withdrawal syndrome including fever, myalgia, arthralgia, and malaise. This may occur in patients even without evidence of adrenal insufficiency. Replacement of systemic steroid with TURBINAIRE DECADRON Phosphate should be gradual and carefully monitored by the physician.
There is an enhanced effect of dexamethasone in patients with hypothyroidism and in those with cirrhosis.
TURBINAIRE DECADRON Phosphate should be used cautiously in patients with ocular herpes simplex for fear of corneal perforation.
The lowest possible dose of TURBINAIRE DECADRON Phosphate should be used to control the condition under treatment, and when reduction in dosage is possible, the reduction must be gradual. If beneficial effect is not evident within 7 days after initiation of therapy, the patient should be re-evaluated.
Psychic derangements may appear when dexamethasone is used, ranging from euphoria, insomnia, mood swings, personality changes, and severe depression, to frank psychotic manifestations. Also, existing emotional instability or psychotic tendencies may be aggravated.
Aspirin should be used cautiously in conjunction with TURBINAIRE DECADRON Phosphate in hypoprothrombinemia.
TURBINAIRE DECADRON Phosphate should be used with caution in patients with nonspecific ulcerative colitis, if there is a probability of impending perforation, abscess or other pyogenic infection; also in diverticulitis; fresh intestinal anastomoses; active or latent peptic ulcer; renal insufficiency; hypertension; osteoporosis; and myasthenia gravis.
Signs of peritoneal irritation following gastrointestinal perforation in patients receiving large doses of corticosteroids may be minimal or absent. Fat embolism has been reported as a possible complication of hypercortisonism.
Because clinical studies have not been done, the use of this product in children under the age of 6 years is not recommended. Growth and development of children 6 years of age or older on prolonged therapy with TURBINAIRE DECADRON Phosphate should be carefully followed.
Dexamethasone may increase or decrease motility and number of spermatozoa in some patients.
Phenytoin, phenobarbital, ephedrine and rifampin may enhance the metabolic clearance of dexamethasone, resulting in decreased blood levels and lessened physiologic activity, thus requiring adjustment in dexamethasone dosage.
The prothrombin time should be checked frequently in patients who are receiving TURBINAIRE DECADRON Phosphate and coumarin anticoagulants at the same time because of reports that corticosteroids have altered the response to these anticoagulants. Studies have shown that the usual effect produced by adding corticosteroids is inhibition of response to coumarins, although there have been some conflicting reports of potentiation, not substantiated by studies.
When TURBINAIRE DECADRON Phosphate is used concomitantly with potassium-depleting diuretics, patients should be observed closely for development of hypokalemia.
Since the contents of TURBINAIRE DECADRON Phosphate are under pressure, the container should not be broken, stored in extreme heat, or incinerated. It should be stored at a temperature below 120°F.

ADVERSE REACTIONS

Nasal irritation and dryness are the most common adverse reactions. The following have been reported: headache, lightheadedness, urticaria, nausea, epistaxis, rebound congestion, bronchial asthma, perforation of the nasal septum, and anosmia. Signs of adrenal hypercorticism may occur in some patients, especially with overdosage.
Systemic effects from therapy with TURBINAIRE DECADRON Phosphate are less likely to occur than with oral or parenteral corticosteroid therapy because of a lower total dose administered. Nevertheless, patients should be observed for the hormonal effects described below because of absorption of dexamethasone from the nasal mucosa.

Fluid and Electrolyte Disturbances
Sodium retention
Fluid retention
Congestive heart failure in susceptible patients
Potassium loss
Hypokalemic alkalosis
Hypertension

Musculoskeletal
Muscle weakness
Steroid myopathy
Loss of muscle mass
Osteoporosis
Vertebral compression fractures
Aseptic necrosis of femoral and humeral heads
Pathologic fracture of long bones
Tendon rupture

Gastrointestinal
Peptic ulcer with possible subsequent perforation and hemorrhage
Perforation of the small and large bowel, particularly in patients with inflammatory bowel disease

Continued on next page

Information on the Merck Sharp & Dohme products listed on these pages is the full prescribing information from product circulars in use August 31, 1986.

Merck Sharp & Dohme—Cont.

Pancreatitis
Abdominal distention
Ulcerative esophagitis
Dermatologic
Impaired wound healing
Thin fragile skin
Petechiae and ecchymoses
Erythema
Increased sweating
May suppress reactions to skin tests
Other cutaneous reactions, such as allergic dermatitis, urticaria, angioneurotic edema.
Neurologic
Convulsions
Increased intracranial pressure with papilledema (pseudotumor cerebri) usually after treatment
Vertigo
Headache
Endocrine
Menstrual irregularities
Development of cushingoid state
Suppression of growth in children
Secondary adrenocortical and pituitary unresponsiveness, particularly in times of stress, as in trauma, surgery, or illness
Decreased carbohydrate tolerance
Manifestations of latent diabetes mellitus
Increased requirements for insulin or oral hypoglycemic agents in diabetics
Ophthalmic
Posterior subcapsular cataracts
Increased intraocular pressure
Glaucoma
Exophthalmos
Metabolic
Negative nitrogen balance due to protein catabolism
Other
Hypersensitivity
Thromboembolism
Weight gain
Increased appetite
Nausea
Malaise
Psychic disturbances

DOSAGE AND ADMINISTRATION

DO NOT EXCEED THE RECOMMENDED DOSAGE.
The usual initial dosage of TURBINAIRE DECADRON Phosphate is:
Adults—2 sprays in each nostril 2 or 3 times a day.
Children (6 to 12 years of age)—1 or 2 sprays in each nostril 2 times a day depending on age.
See accompanying instructions on the proper use of TURBINAIRE.
When improvement occurs the dosage should be gradually reduced. Some patients will be symptom-free on one spray in each nostril 2 times a day. The maximum daily dosage for adults is 12 sprays, and for children, 8 sprays. Therapy should be discontinued as soon as feasible. It may be reinstituted if recurrence of symptoms occurs.

HOW SUPPLIED

No. 7634—TURBINAIRE DECADRON Phosphate, aerosol for intranasal application, is supplied as follows: **NDC** 0006-7634-13 in a pressurized container and includes a plastic adapter.
(6505-00-885-6302, 12.6 Grams, 170 Metered Doses)
No. 7642—Refill unit for TURBINAIRE DECADRON Phosphate aerosol for intranasal application is supplied as follows: **NDC** 0006-7642-13 in a pressurized container.
Storage
Store at a temperature below 120°F.
A.H.F.S. Category: 52:08
DC 6006420 Issued April 1985

DECADRON-LA® Suspension
(Dexamethasone Acetate, MSD), U.S.P. ℞

NOT FOR INTRAVENOUS USE

DESCRIPTION

Dexamethasone acetate, a synthetic adrenocortical steroid, is a white to practically white, odorless powder. It is a practically insoluble ester of dexamethasone. The structural formula is:
[See Chemical Formula at top of next column].
Dexamethasone acetate is present in DECADRON-LA® (Dexamethasone Acetate, MSD) suspension as the monohydrate, with the empirical formula, $C_{24}H_{31}FO_6 \cdot H_2O$, and molecular weight, 452.52. Dexamethasone acetate is designated chemically as 21-(acetyloxy)-9-fluoro-11β,17-dihydroxy-16α-methylpregna-1,4-diene-3,20-dione.
DECADRON-LA suspension is a sterile white suspension (pH 5.0 to 7.5) that settles on standing, but is easily resuspended by mild shaking.
Each milliliter contains dexamethasone acetate equivalent to 8 mg dexamethasone. Inactive ingredients per mL: 6.67 mg sodium chloride; 5 mg creatinine; 0.5 mg disodium edetate; 5 mg sodium carboxymethylcellulose; 0.75 mg polysorbate 80; sodium hydroxide to adjust pH; and Water for Injection, q.s. 1 mL, with 9 mg benzyl alcohol, and 1 mg sodium bisulfite added as preservatives.

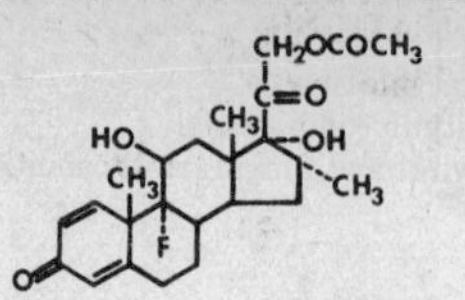

ACTIONS

DECADRON-LA suspension is a long-acting, repository adrenocorticosteroid preparation with a prompt onset of action. It is suitable for intramuscular or local injection, but not when an immediate effect of short duration is desired.
Naturally occurring glucocorticoids (hydrocortisone and cortisone), which also have salt-retaining properties, are used as replacement therapy in adrenocortical deficiency states. Their synthetic analogs, including dexamethasone, are primarily used for their potent anti-inflammatory effects in disorders of many organ systems.
Glucocorticoids cause profound and varied metabolic effects. In addition, they modify the body's immune responses to diverse stimuli.
At equipotent anti-inflammatory doses, dexamethasone almost completely lacks the sodium-retaining property of hydrocortisone.

INDICATIONS

A. By intramuscular injection when oral therapy is not feasible:
1. *Endocrine disorders*
Congenital adrenal hyperplasia
Nonsuppurative thyroiditis
Hypercalcemia associated with cancer
2. *Rheumatic disorders*
As adjunctive therapy for short-term administration (to tide the patient over an acute episode or exacerbation) in:
Post-traumatic osteoarthritis
Synovitis of osteoarthritis
Rheumatoid arthritis, including juvenile rheumatoid arthritis (selected cases may require low-dose maintenance therapy)
Acute and subacute bursitis
Epicondylitis
Acute nonspecific tenosynovitis
Acute gouty arthritis
Psoriatic arthritis
Ankylosing spondylitis
3. *Collagen diseases*
During an exacerbation or as maintenance therapy in selected cases of:
Systemic lupus erythematosus
Acute rheumatic carditis
4. *Dermatologic diseases*
Pemphigus
Severe erythema multiforme (Stevens-Johnson syndrome)
Exfoliative dermatitis
Bullous dermatitis herpetiformis
Severe seborrheic dermatitis
Severe psoriasis
Mycosis fungoides
5. *Allergic states*
Control of severe or incapacitating allergic conditions intractable to adequate trials of conventional treatment in:
Bronchial asthma
Contact dermatitis
Atopic dermatitis
Serum sickness
Seasonal or perennial allergic rhinitis
Drug hypersensitivity reactions
Urticarial transfusion reactions
6. *Ophthalmic diseases*
Severe acute and chronic allergic and inflammatory processes involving the eye, such as:
Herpes zoster ophthalmicus
Iritis, Iridocyclitis
Chorioretinitis
Diffuse posterior uveitis and choroiditis
Optic neuritis
Sympathetic ophthalmia
Anterior segment inflammation
Allergic conjunctivitis
Keratitis
Allergic corneal marginal ulcers
7. *Gastrointestinal diseases*
To tide the patient over a critical period of the disease in:
Ulcerative colitis (Systemic therapy)
Regional enteritis (Systemic therapy)
8. *Respiratory diseases*
Symptomatic sarcoidosis
Berylliosis
Loeffler's syndrome not manageable by other means
Aspiration pneumonitis
9. *Hematologic disorders*
Acquired (autoimmune) hemolytic anemia
Secondary thrombocytopenia in adults
Erythroblastopenia (RBC anemia)
Congenital (erythroid) hypoplastic anemia
10. *Neoplastic diseases*
For palliative management of:
Leukemias and lymphomas in adults
Acute leukemia of childhood
11. *Edematous states*
To induce diuresis or remission of proteinuria in the nephrotic syndrome, without uremia, of the idiopathic type, or that due to lupus erythematosus
12. *Miscellaneous*
Trichinosis with neurologic or myocardial involvement.
B. By intra-articular or soft tissue injection as adjunctive therapy for short-term administration (to tide the patient over an acute episode or exacerbation) in:
Synovitis of osteoarthritis
Rheumatoid arthritis
Acute and subacute bursitis
Acute gouty arthritis
Epicondylitis
Acute nonspecific tenosynovitis
Post-traumatic osteoarthritis.
C. By intralesional injection in:
Keloids
Localized hypertrophic, infiltrated, inflammatory lesions of: lichen planus, psoriatic plaques, granuloma annulare, and lichen simplex chronicus (neurodermatitis)
Discoid lupus erythematosus
Necrobiosis lipoidica diabeticorum
Alopecia areata
May also be useful in cystic tumors of an aponeurosis or tendon (ganglia).

CONTRAINDICATIONS

Systemic fungal infections
Hypersensitivity to any component of this product, including sulfites (see WARNINGS).

WARNINGS

DO NOT INJECT INTRAVENOUSLY
Sodium bisulfite has been reported to cause severe allergic reactions in certain susceptible individuals, particularly patients with asthma. Anaphylactoid and hypersensitivity reactions have been reported for Suspension DECADRON-LA (see ADVERSE REACTIONS). Since Suspension DECADRON-LA contains sodium bisulfite, this product should not be used in patients allergic to sulfites.
In patients on corticosteroid therapy subjected to any unusual stress, increased dosage of rapidly acting corticosteroids before, during, and after the stressful situation is indicated.
Drug-induced secondary adrenocortical insufficiency may result from too rapid withdrawal of corticosteroids and may be minimized by gradual reduction of dosage. This type of relative insufficiency may persist for months after discontinuation of therapy; therefore, in any situation of stress occurring during that period, hormone therapy should be reinstituted. If the patient is receiving steroids already, dosage may have to be increased. Since mineralocorticoid secretion may be impaired, salt and/or a mineralocorticoid should be administered concurrently.
Corticosteroids may mask some signs of infection, and new infections may appear during their use. There may be decreased resistance and inability to localize infection when corticosteroids are used. Moreover, corticosteroids may affect the nitroblue-tetrazolium test for bacterial infection and produce false negative results.
In cerebral malaria, a double-blind trial has shown that the use of corticosteroids is associated with prolongation of coma and a higher incidence of pneumonia and gastrointestinal bleeding.
Corticosteroids may activate latent amebiasis. Therefore, it is recommended that latent or active amebiasis be ruled out before initiating corticosteroid therapy in any patient who has spent time in the tropics or any patient with unexplained diarrhea.

Prolonged use of corticosteroids may produce posterior subcapsular cataracts, glaucoma with possible damage to the optic nerves, and may enhance the establishment of secondary ocular infections due to fungi or viruses.
Usage in pregnancy. Since adequate human reproduction studies have not been done with corticosteroids, use of these drugs in pregnancy or in women of childbearing potential requires that the anticipated benefits be weighed against the possible hazards to the mother and embryo or fetus. Infants born of mothers who have received substantial doses of corticosteroids during pregnancy should be carefully observed for signs of hypoadrenalism.
Corticosteroids appear in breast milk and could suppress growth, interfere with endogenous corticosteroid production, or cause other unwanted effects. Mothers taking pharmacologic doses of corticosteroids should be advised not to nurse.
Average and large doses of cortisone or hydrocortisone can cause elevation of blood pressure, salt and water retention, and increased excretion of potassium. These effects are less likely to occur with the synthetic derivatives except when used in large doses. Dietary salt restriction and potassium supplementation may be necessary. All corticosteroids increase calcium excretion.
Administration of live virus vaccines, including smallpox, is contraindicated in individuals receiving immunosuppressive doses of corticosteroids. If inactivated viral or bacterial vaccines are administered to individuals receiving immunosuppressive doses of corticosteroids, the expected serum antibody response may not be obtained.
If corticosteroids are indicated in patients with latent tuberculosis or tuberculin reactivity, close observation is necessary as reactivation of the disease may occur. During prolonged corticosteroid therapy, these patients should receive chemoprophylaxis.
Because rare instances of anaphylactoid reactions have occurred in patients receiving parenteral corticosteroid therapy, appropriate precautionary measures should be taken prior to administration, especially when the patient has a history of allergy to any drug.
Repository adrenocorticosteroid preparations may cause atrophy at the site of injection. To minimize the likelihood and/or severity of atrophy, do not inject subcutaneously, avoid injection into the deltoid muscle, and avoid repeated intramuscular injections into the same site if possible.
Dosage in children under 12 has not been established.

PRECAUTIONS

DECADRON-LA suspension is not recommended as initial therapy in acute, life-threatening situations.
This product, like many other steroid formulations, is sensitive to heat. Therefore, it should not be autoclaved when it is desirable to sterilize the exterior of the vial.
Following prolonged therapy, withdrawal of corticosteroids may result in symptoms of the corticosteroid withdrawal syndrome including fever, myalgia, arthralgia, and malaise. This may occur in patients even without evidence of adrenal insufficiency.
There is an enhanced effect of corticosteroids in patients with hypothyroidism and in those with cirrhosis.
Corticosteroids should be used cautiously in patients with ocular herpes simplex for fear of corneal perforation.
Psychic derangements may appear when corticosteroids are used, ranging from euphoria, insomnia, mood swings, personality changes, and severe depression to frank psychotic manifestations. Also, existing emotional instability or psychotic tendencies may be aggravated by corticosteroids.
Aspirin should be used cautiously in conjunction with corticosteroids in hypoprothrombinemia.
Steroids should be used with caution in nonspecific ulcerative colitis, if there is a probability of impending perforation, abscess, or other pyogenic infection, also in diverticulitis, fresh intestinal anastomoses, active or latent peptic ulcer, renal insufficiency, hypertension, osteoporosis, and myasthenia gravis. Signs of peritoneal irritation following gastrointestinal perforation in patients receiving large doses of corticosteroids may be minimal or absent. Fat embolism has been reported as a possible complication of hypercortisonism.
When large doses are given, some authorities advise that antacids be administered between meals to help to prevent peptic ulcer.
Growth and development of infants and children on prolonged corticosteroid therapy should be carefully followed.
Steroids may increase or decrease motility and number of spermatozoa in some patients.
Phenytoin, phenobarbital, ephedrine, and rifampin may enhance the metabolic clearance of corticosteroids, resulting in decreased blood levels and lessened physiologic activity, thus requiring adjustment in corticosteroid dosage.
The prothrombin time should be checked frequently in patients who are receiving corticosteroids and coumarin anticoagulants at the same time because of reports that corticosteroids have altered the response to these anticoagulants. Studies have shown that the usual effect produced by adding corticosteroids is inhibition of response to coumarins, although there have been some conflicting reports of potentiation not substantiated by studies.
When corticosteroids are administered concomitantly with potassium-depleting diuretics, patients should be observed closely for development of hypokalemia.
Intra-articular injection of a corticosteroid may produce systemic as well as local effects.
Appropriate examination of any joint fluid present is necessary to exclude a septic process.
A marked increase in pain accompanied by local swelling, further restriction of joint motion, fever, and malaise is suggestive of septic arthritis. If this complication occurs and the diagnosis of sepsis is confirmed, appropriate antimicrobial therapy should be instituted.
Injection of a steroid into an infected site is to be avoided.
Corticosteroids should not be injected into unstable joints.
Patients should be impressed strongly with the importance of not overusing joints in which symptomatic benefit has been obtained as long as the inflammatory process remains active.
Frequent intra-articular injection may result in damage to joint tissues.

ADVERSE REACTIONS

Fluid and electrolyte disturbances
Sodium retention
Fluid retention
Congestive heart failure in susceptible patients
Potassium loss
Hypokalemic alkalosis
Hypertension
Musculoskeletal
Muscle weakness
Steroid myopathy
Loss of muscle mass
Osteoporosis
Vertebral compression fractures
Aseptic necrosis of femoral and humeral heads
Pathologic fracture of long bones
Tendon rupture
Gastrointestinal
Peptic ulcer with possible subsequent perforation and hemorrhage
Perforation of the small and large bowel, particularly in patients with inflammatory bowel disease
Pancreatitis
Abdominal distention
Ulcerative esophagitis
Dermatologic
Impaired wound healing
Thin fragile skin
Petechiae and ecchymoses
Erythema
Increased sweating
May suppress reactions to skin tests
Other cutaneous reactions, such as allergic dermatitis, urticaria, angioneurotic edema
Neurologic
Convulsions
Increased intracranial pressure with papilledema (pseudotumor cerebri) usually after treatment
Vertigo
Headache
Endocrine
Menstrual irregularities
Development of cushingoid state
Suppression of growth in children
Secondary adrenocortical and pituitary unresponsiveness, particularly in times of stress, as in trauma, surgery, or illness
Decreased carbohydrate tolerance
Manifestations of latent diabetes mellitus
Increased requirements for insulin or oral hypoglycemic agents in diabetics
Hirsutism
Ophthalmic
Posterior subcapsular cataracts
Increased intraocular pressure
Glaucoma
Exophthalmos
Metabolic
Negative nitrogen balance due to protein catabolism
Other
Anaphylactoid or hypersensitivity reactions
Thromboembolism
Weight gain
Increased appetite
Nausea
Malaise
Psychic disturbances

The following *additional* adverse reactions are related to parenteral corticosteroid therapy:
Rare instances of blindness associated with intralesional therapy around the face and head
Hyperpigmentation or hypopigmentation
Subcutaneous and cutaneous atrophy
Sterile abscess
Postinjection flare (following intra-articular use)
Charcot-like arthropathy
Scarring
Induration
Inflammation
Paresthesia
Delayed pain or soreness
Muscle twitching, ataxia, hiccups, and nystagmus have been reported in low incidence after injection of DECADRON-LA suspension.

DOSAGE AND ADMINISTRATION

For intramuscular, intralesional, intra-articular, and soft tissue injection.
Dosage Requirements Are Variable and Must Be Individualized on the Basis of the Disease and the Response of the Patient.
Dosage in children under 12 has not been established.
Intramuscular Injection
Dosage ranges from 1 to 2 mL, equivalent to 8 to 16 mg of dexamethasone. If further treatment is needed, dosage may be repeated at intervals of 1 to 3 weeks.
Intralesional Injection
The usual dose is 0.1 to 0.2 mL, equivalent to 0.8 to 1.6 mg of dexamethasone, per injection site.
Intra-articular and Soft Tissue Injection
The dose varies, depending on the location and the severity of inflammation. The usual dose is 0.5 to 2 mL, equivalent to 4 to 16 mg of dexamethasone. If further treatment is needed, dosage may be repeated at intervals of 1 to 3 weeks. Frequent intra-articular injection may result in damage to joint tissues.

HOW SUPPLIED

No. 7644—Suspension DECADRON-LA, 8 mg dexamethasone equivalent per mL, is a sterile white suspension, and is supplied as follows:
NDC 0006-7644-01 in 1 mL vials
NDC 0006-7644-03 in 5 mL vials.
Storage
Sensitive to heat. Do not autoclave.
Protect from freezing.

A.H.F.S. Category: 68:04
DC 6626715 Issued April 1985

DECASPRAY® Topical Aerosol (Dexamethasone, MSD), U.S.P. ℞

DESCRIPTION

Topical Aerosol DECASPRAY® (Dexamethasone, MSD) is a topical steroid preparation, each 25 g of which contains 10 mg of dexamethasone. The topical corticosteroids constitute a class of primarily synthetic steroids used as anti-inflammatory and anti-pruritic agents.
Dexamethasone is 9-fluoro-11β, 17, 21-trihydroxy-16α-methylpregna-1, 4-diene-3, 20 dione. Its empirical formula is $C_{22}H_{29}FO_5$ and its structural formula is:

Dexamethasone has a molecular weight of 392.47.
The inactive ingredients are isopropyl myristate, and isobutane. Each second of spray dispenses approximately 0.075 mg of dexamethasone.

CLINICAL PHARMACOLOGY

Topical corticosteroids share anti-inflammatory, anti-pruritic, and vasoconstrictive actions.
The mechanism of anti-inflammatory activity of the topical corticosteroids is unclear. Various laboratory methods, including vasoconstrictor assays, are used to compare and predict potencies and/or clinical efficacies of the topical cortico-

Continued on next page

Information on the Merck Sharp & Dohme products listed on these pages is the full prescribing information from product circulars in use August 31, 1986.

Merck Sharp & Dohme—Cont.

steroids. There is some evidence to suggest that a recognizable correlation exists between vasoconstrictor potency and therapeutic efficacy in man.

Pharmacokinetics

The extent of percutaneous absorption of topical corticosteroids is determined by many factors including the vehicle, the integrity of the epidermal barrier, and the use of occlusive dressings.

Topical corticosteroids can be absorbed from normal intact skin. Inflammation and/or other disease processes in the skin increase percutaneous absorption. Occlusive dressings substantially increase the percutaneous absorption of topical corticosteroids. Thus, occlusive dressings may be a valuable therapeutic adjunct for treatment of resistant dermatoses. (See DOSAGE AND ADMINISTRATION.)

Once absorbed through the skin, topical corticosteroids are handled through pharmacokinetic pathways similar to systemically administered corticosteroids. Corticosteroids are bound to plasma proteins in varying degrees. Corticosteroids are metabolized primarily in the liver and are then excreted by the kidneys. Some of the topical corticosteroids and their metabolites are also excreted into the bile.

INDICATIONS AND USAGE

DECASPRAY Topical Aerosol is indicated for relief of the inflammatory and pruritic manifestations of corticosteroid-responsive dermatoses.

CONTRAINDICATIONS

Topical corticosteroids are contraindicated in those patients with a history of hypersensitivity to any of the components of the preparation.

WARNINGS

Avoid spraying in eyes or nose. Contents under pressure. Do not puncture or burn. Keep out of reach of children. Use only as directed. Intentional misuse by deliberately concentrating and inhaling the contents can be harmful or fatal.

PRECAUTIONS

General

Systemic absorption of topical corticosteroids has produced reversible hypothalamic-pituitary-adrenal (HPA) axis suppression, manifestations of Cushing's syndrome, hyperglycemia, and glycosuria in some patients.

Conditions which augment systemic absorption include the application of the more potent corticosteroids, use over large surface areas, prolonged use, and the addition of occlusive dressings.

Therefore, patients receiving a large dose of a potent topical corticosteroid applied to a large surface area or under an occlusive dressing should be evaluated periodically for evidence of HPA axis suppression by using urinary free cortisol and ACTH stimulation tests. If HPA axis suppression is noted, an attempt should be made to withdraw the drug, to reduce the frequency of application, or to substitute a less potent corticosteroid.

Recovery of HPA axis function is generally prompt and complete upon discontinuation of the drug. Infrequently, signs and symptoms of corticosteroid withdrawal may occur, requiring supplemental systemic corticosteroids.

Children may absorb proportionally larger amounts of topical corticosteroids and thus be more susceptible to systemic toxicity (See PRECAUTIONS, *Pediatric Use*).

If irritation develops, topical corticosteroids should be discontinued and appropriate therapy instituted.

In the presence of dermatological infections, the use of an appropriate antifungal or antibacterial agent should be instituted. If a favorable response does not occur promptly, the corticosteroid should be discontinued until the infection has been adequately controlled.

The product is not for ophthalmic use. However, if applied to the eyelids or skin near the eyes, the drug may enter the eyes. In patients with a history of herpes simplex keratitis ocular exposure to corticosteroids may lead to a recurrence. Prolonged ocular exposure may cause steroid glaucoma.

A few individuals may be sensitive to one or more of the components of this product. If any reaction indicating sensitivity is observed, discontinue use.

Generally, occlusive dressings should not be used on weeping or exudative lesions.

If occlusive dressing therapy is used, inspect lesions between dressings for development of infection. If infection develops, the technique should be discontinued and appropriate antimicrobial therapy instituted.

When large areas of the body are covered with an occlusive dressing, thermal homeostasis may be impaired. If elevation of body temperature occurs, use of the occlusive dressing should be discontinued.

CAUTION: Flammable. Do not use around open flame or while smoking.

Information for the Patient

Patients using topical corticosteroids should receive the following information and instructions:

1. This medication is to be used as directed by the physician. It is for external use only. Avoid contact with the eyes.
2. Patients should be advised not to use this medication for any disorder other than that for which it was prescribed.
3. The treated skin area should not be bandaged or otherwise covered or wrapped so as to be occlusive unless directed by the physician.
4. Patients should report any signs of local adverse reactions, especially under occlusive dressing.
5. Parents of pediatric patients should be advised not to use tight-fitting diapers or plastic pants on a child being treated in the diaper area, as these garments may constitute occlusive dressings.

Laboratory Tests

The following tests may be helpful in evaluating the HPA axis suppression:

- Urinary free cortisol test
- ACTH stimulation test

Carcinogenesis, Mutagenesis, and Impairment of Fertility

Long-term animal studies have not been performed to evaluate the carcinogenic potential or the effect on fertility of topical corticosteroids.

Studies to determine mutagenicity with prednisolone and hydrocortisone have revealed negative results.

Pregnancy

Pregnancy Category C: Corticosteroids are generally teratogenic in laboratory animals when administered systemically at relatively low dosage levels. The more potent corticosteroids have been shown to be teratogenic after dermal application in laboratory animals. There are no adequate and well-controlled studies in pregnant women on teratogenic effects from topically applied corticosteroids. Therefore, topical corticosteroids should be used during pregnancy only if the potential benefit justifies the potential risk to the fetus. Drugs of this class should not be used extensively on pregnant patients, in large amounts, or for prolonged periods of time.

Nursing Mothers

It is not known whether topical administration of corticosteroids could result in sufficient systemic absorption to produce detectable quantities in breast milk. Systemically administered corticosteroids are secreted into breast milk in quantities *not* likely to have a deleterious effect on the infant. Nevertheless, caution should be exercised when topical corticosteroids are administered to a nursing woman.

Pediatric Use

Pediatric patients may demonstrate greater susceptibility to topical corticosteroid-induced HPA axis suppression and Cushing's syndrome than mature patients because of a larger skin surface area to body weight ratio.

Hypothalamic-pituitary-adrenal (HPA) axis suppression, Cushing's syndrome, and intracranial hypertension have been reported in children receiving topical corticosteroids. Manifestations of adrenal suppression in children include linear growth retardation, delayed weight gain, low plasma cortisol levels, and absence of response to ACTH stimulation. Manifestations of intracranial hypertension include bulging fontanelles, headaches, and bilateral papilledema.

Administration of topical corticosteroids to children should be limited to the least amount compatible with an effective therapeutic regimen. Chronic corticosteroid therapy may interfere with the growth and development of children.

ADVERSE REACTIONS

The following adverse reactions are reported infrequently with topical corticosteroids, but may occur more frequently with the use of occlusive dressings. These reactions are listed in an approximate decreasing order of occurrence:

Burning
Itching
Irritation
Dryness
Folliculitis
Hypertrichosis
Acneiform eruptions
Hypopigmentation
Perioral dermatitis
Allergic contact dermatitis
Maceration of the skin
Secondary infection
Skin atrophy
Striae
Miliaria

OVERDOSAGE

Topically applied corticosteroids can be absorbed in sufficient amounts to produce systemic effects (See PRECAUTIONS).

DOSAGE AND ADMINISTRATION

Patients should be instructed in the correct way to use DECASPRAY. The preparation is readily applied, even on hairy areas. It does not have to be rubbed into the skin. Optimal effects will be obtained with DECASPRAY when these directions are followed:

1. Keep the affected area clean to reduce the possibility of infection.
2. Shake the container *gently* once or twice each time before using. Hold it about six inches from the area to be treated. Effective medication may be obtained with the container held either upright or inverted, since it is fitted with a special valve that dispenses approximately the same dosage in either position.
3. Spray each four inch square of affected area for one or two seconds three or four times a day, depending on the nature of the condition and the response to therapy.
4. When a favorable response is obtained, reduce dosage gradually and eventually discontinue.
5. Occlusive dressings may be used for the management of psoriasis or recalcitrant conditions.

HOW SUPPLIED

No. 7623X—DECASPRAY is supplied as follows:
NDC 0006-7623-25 in a 25 g pressurized container.
A.H.F.S. Category: 84:06
DC 6005318 Issued April 1983

DEMSER® Capsules
(Metyrosine, MSD), U.S.P. ℞

DESCRIPTION

DEMSER® (Metyrosine, MSD) is (−)-α-methyl-*L*-tyrosine or (α-MPT). It has the following structural formula:

$$HO-C_6H_4-CH_2-C(CH_3)(NH_2)-COOH$$

Metyrosine is a white, crystalline compound of molecular weight 195. It is very slightly soluble in water, acetone, and methanol, and insoluble in chloroform and benzene. It is soluble in acidic aqueous solutions. It is also soluble in alkaline aqueous solutions, but is subject to oxidative degradation under these conditions.

DEMSER is supplied as capsules, for oral administration. Each capsule contains 250 mg metyrosine. Inactive ingredients are colloidal silicon dioxide, gelatin, hydroxypropyl cellulose, magnesium stearate, and titanium dioxide. The capsules may also contain any combination of D&C Red 33, D&C Yellow 10, FD&C Blue 1, and FD&C Blue 2.

CLINICAL PHARMACOLOGY

DEMSER inhibits tyrosine hydroxylase, which catalyzes the first transformation in catecholamine biosynthesis, i.e., the conversion of tyrosine to dihydroxyphenylalanine (DOPA). Because the first step is also the rate-limiting step, blockade of tyrosine hydroxylase activity results in decreased endogenous levels of catecholamines, usually measured as decreased urinary excretion of catecholamines and their metabolites.

In patients with pheochromocytoma, who produce excessive amounts of norepinephrine and epinephrine, administration of one to four grams of DEMSER per day has reduced catecholamine biosynthesis from about 35 to 80 percent as measured by the total excretion of catecholamines and their metabolites (metanephrine and vanillylmandelic acid). The maximum biochemical effect usually occurs within two to three days, and the urinary concentration of catecholamines and their metabolites usually returns to pretreatment levels within three to four days after DEMSER is discontinued. In some patients the total excretion of catecholamines and catecholamine metabolites may be lowered to normal or near normal levels (less than 10 mg/24 hours). In most patients the duration of treatment has been two to eight weeks, but several patients have received DEMSER for periods of one to 10 years.

Most patients with pheochromocytoma treated with DEMSER experience decreased frequency and severity of hypertensive attacks with their associated headache, nausea, sweating, and tachycardia. In patients who respond, blood pressure decreases progressively during the first two days of therapy with DEMSER; after withdrawal, blood pres-

sure usually increases gradually to pretreatment values within two to three days.
Metyrosine is well absorbed from the gastrointestinal tract. From 53 to 88 percent (mean 69 percent) was recovered in the urine as unchanged drug following maintenance oral doses of 600 to 4000 mg/24 hours in patients with pheochromocytoma or essential hypertension. Less than 1% of the dose was recovered as catechol metabolites. These metabolites are probably not present in sufficient amounts to contribute to the biochemical effects of metyrosine. The quantities excreted, however, are sufficient to interfere with accurate determination of urinary catecholamines determined by routine techniques.
Plasma half-life of metyrosine determined over an 8-hour period after single oral doses was 3.4–3.7 hours in three patients.
For further information, refer to: Sjoerdsma, A.; Engelman, K.; Waldman, T. A.; Cooperman, L. H.; Hammond, W. G.: Pheochromocytoma: Current concepts of diagnosis and treatment, Ann. Intern. Med. *65:* 1302–1326, Dec. 1966.

INDICATIONS AND USAGE

DEMSER is indicated in the treatment of patients with pheochromocytoma for:
1. Preoperative preparation of patients for surgery
2. Management of patients when surgery is contraindicated
3. Chronic treatment of patients with malignant pheochromocytoma.

DEMSER is not recommended for the control of essential hypertension.

CONTRAINDICATIONS

DEMSER is contraindicated in persons known to be hypersensitive to this compound.

WARNINGS

Maintain Fluid Volume During and After Surgery
When DEMSER is used preoperatively, alone or especially in combination with alpha-adrenergic blocking drugs, adequate intravascular volume must be maintained intraoperatively (especially after tumor removal) and postoperatively to avoid hypotension and decreased perfusion of vital organs resulting from vasodilatation and expanded volume capacity. Following tumor removal, large volumes of plasma may be needed to maintain blood pressure and central venous pressure within the normal range.
In addition, life-threatening arrhythmias may occur during anesthesia and surgery, and may require treatment with a beta blocker or lidocaine. During surgery, patients should have continuous monitoring of blood pressure and electrocardiogram.
Intraoperative Effects
While the preoperative use of DEMSER in patients with pheochromocytoma is thought to decrease intraoperative problems with blood pressure control, DEMSER does not eliminate the danger of hypertensive crises or arrhythmias during manipulation of the tumor, and the alpha-adrenergic blocking drug, phentolamine, may be needed.
Interaction with Alcohol
DEMSER may add to the sedative effects of alcohol and other CNS depressants, e.g., hypnotics, sedatives, and tranquilizers. (See PRECAUTIONS, *Information for Patients and Drug Interactions.)*

PRECAUTIONS

General
Metyrosine Crystalluria: **Crystalluria and urolithiasis have been found in dogs treated with DEMSER (Metyrosine, MSD) at doses similar to those used in humans, and crystalluria has also been observed in a few patients. To minimize the risk of crystalluria, patients should be urged to maintain water intake sufficient to achieve a daily urine volume of 2000 mL or more, particularly when doses greater than 2 g per day are given. Routine examination of the urine should be carried out. Metyrosine will crystallize as needles or rods. If metyrosine crystalluria occurs, fluid intake should be increased further. If crystalluria persists, the dosage should be reduced or the drug discontinued.**
Relatively Little Data Regarding Long-term Use: The total human experience with the drug is quite limited and few patients have been studied long-term. Chronic animal studies have not been carried out. Therefore, suitable laboratory tests should be carried out periodically in patients requiring prolonged use of DEMSER and caution should be observed in patients with impaired hepatic or renal function.
Information for Patients
When receiving DEMSER, patients should be warned about engaging in activities requiring mental alertness and motor coordination, such as driving a motor vehicle or operating machinery. DEMSER may have additive sedative effects with alcohol and other CNS depressants, e.g., hypnotics, sedatives, and tranquilizers.
Patients should be advised to maintain a liberal fluid intake. (See PRECAUTIONS, *General.*)
Drug Interactions
Caution should be observed in administering DEMSER to patients receiving phenothiazines or haloperidol because the extrapyramidal effects of these drugs can be expected to be potentiated by inhibition of catecholamine synthesis.
Concurrent use of DEMSER with alcohol or other CNS depressants can increase their sedative effects. (See WARNINGS and PRECAUTIONS, *Information for Patients.*)
Laboratory Test Interference
Spurious increases in urinary catecholamines may be observed in patients receiving DEMSER due to the presence of metabolites of the drug.
Carcinogenesis, Mutagenesis, Impairment of Fertility
Long-term carcinogenic studies in animals and studies on mutagenesis and impairment of fertility have not been performed with metyrosine.
Pregnancy
Pregnancy Category C. Animal reproduction studies have not been conducted with DEMSER. It is also not known whether DEMSER can cause fetal harm when administered to a pregnant woman or can affect reproduction capacity. DEMSER should be given to a pregnant woman only if clearly needed.
Nursing Mothers
It is not known whether DEMSER is excreted in human milk. Because many drugs are excreted in human milk, caution should be exercised when DEMSER is administered to a nursing woman.
Pediatric Use
Safety and effectiveness in children under 12 years of age have not been established.

ADVERSE REACTIONS

Central Nervous System
Sedation: The most common adverse reaction to DEMSER is moderate to severe sedation, which has been observed in almost all patients. It occurs at both low and high dosages. Sedative effects begin within the first 24 hours of therapy, are maximal after two to three days, and tend to wane during the next few days. Sedation usually is not obvious after one week unless the dosage is increased, but at dosages greater than 2000 mg/day some degree of sedation or fatigue may persist.
In most patients who experience sedation, temporary changes in sleep pattern occur following withdrawal of the drug. Changes consist of insomnia that may last for two or three days and feelings of increased alertness and ambition. Even patients who do not experience sedation while on DEMSER may report symptoms of psychic stimulation when the drug is discontinued.
Extrapyramidal Signs: Extrapyramidal signs such as drooling, speech difficulty, and tremor have been reported in approximately 10 percent of patients. These occasionally have been accompanied by trismus and frank parkinsonism.
Anxiety and Psychic Disturbances: Anxiety and psychic disturbances such as depression, hallucinations, disorientation, and confusion may occur. These effects seem to be dose-dependent and may disappear with reduction of dosage.
Diarrhea
Diarrhea occurs in about 10 percent of patients and may be severe. Anti-diarrheal agents may be required if continuation of DEMSER is necessary.
Miscellaneous
Infrequently, slight swelling of the breast, galactorrhea, nasal stuffiness, decreased salivation, dry mouth, headache, nausea, vomiting, abdominal pain, and impotence or failure of ejaculation may occur. Crystalluria (see PRECAUTIONS) and transient dysuria and hematuria have been observed in a few patients. Hematologic disorders (including eosinophilia, anemia, thrombocytopenia, and thrombocytosis), increased SGOT levels, peripheral edema, and hypersensitivity reactions such as urticaria and pharyngeal edema have been reported rarely.

OVERDOSAGE

Signs of metyrosine overdosage include those central nervous system effects observed in some patients even at low dosages.
At doses exceeding 2000 mg/day, some degree of sedation or feeling of fatigue may persist. Doses of 2000–4000 mg/day can result in anxiety or agitated depression, neuromuscular effects (including fine tremor of the hands, gross tremor of the trunk, tightening of the jaw with trismus), diarrhea, and decreased salivation with dry mouth.
Reduction of drug dose or cessation of treatment results in the disappearance of these symptoms.
The acute toxicity of metyrosine was 442 mg/kg and 752 mg/kg in the female mouse and rat respectively.

DOSAGE AND ADMINISTRATION

The recommended initial dosage of DEMSER for adults and children 12 years of age and older is 250 mg orally four times daily. This may be increased by 250 mg to 500 mg every day to a maximum of 4.0 g/day in divided doses. When used for preoperative preparation, the optimally effective dosage of DEMSER should be given for at least five to seven days.
Optimally effective dosages of DEMSER usually are between 2.0 and 3.0 g/day, and the dose should be titrated by monitoring clinical symptoms and catecholamine excretion. In patients who are hypertensive, dosage should be titrated to achieve normalization of blood pressure and control of clinical symptoms. In patients who are usually normotensive, dosage should be titrated to the amount that will reduce urinary metanephrines and/or vanillylmandelic acid by 50 percent or more.
If patients are not adequately controlled by the use of DEMSER, an alpha-adrenergic blocking agent (phenoxybenzamine) should be added.
Use of DEMSER in children under 12 years of age has been limited and a dosage schedule for this age group cannot be given.

HOW SUPPLIED

No. 3355—Capsules DEMSER, 250 mg, are opaque, two-toned blue capsules coded MSD 690 on one side and DEMSER on the other. They are supplied as follows:
NDC 0006-0690-68 bottles of 100.
Shown in Product Identification Section, page 417
A.H.F.S. Category: 92:00
DC 7111505 Issued September 1985

DIUPRES® Tablets ℞
Antihypertensive

WARNING

This fixed combination drug is not indicated for initial therapy of hypertension. Hypertension requires therapy titrated to the individual patient. If the fixed combination represents the dosage so determined, its use may be more convenient in patient management. The treatment of hypertension is not static, but must be reevaluated as conditions in each patient warrant.

DESCRIPTION

DIUPRES® combines two antihypertensive agents: DIURIL® (Chlorothiazide, MSD) and reserpine. The chemical name for chlorothiazide is 6-chloro-2*H*-1,2,4-benzothiadiazine-7-sulfonamide 1,1-dioxide. Reserpine (11,17α-dimethoxy-18β-[(3,4,5-trimethoxybenzoyl)oxy]-3β, 20α-yohimban-16β-carboxylic acid methyl ester) is a crystalline alkaloid derived from Rauwolfia serpentina.
DIUPRES is supplied as tablets in two strengths for oral use:
DIUPRES-250, contains 250 mg of chlorothiazide and 0.125 mg of reserpine.
DIUPRES-500, contains 500 mg of chlorothiazide and 0.125 mg of reserpine.
Each tablet contains the following inactive ingredients: FD&C Red 3, gelatin, lactose, magnesium stearate, starch and talc.

ACTIONS

Chlorothiazide
Chlorothiazide is a diuretic and antihypertensive. It affects the renal tubular mechanism of electrolyte reabsorption. At maximal therapeutic dosage all thiazides are approximately equal in their diuretic efficacy.
Chlorothiazide increases excretion of sodium and chloride in approximately equivalent amounts. Natriuresis may be accompanied by some loss of potassium and bicarbonate.
The mechanism of the antihypertensive effect of thiazides is unknown. Chlorothiazide does not affect normal blood pressure.
Chlorothiazide is eliminated rapidly by the kidney.
Reserpine
Reserpine has antihypertensive, bradycardic, and tranquilizing properties. It lowers arterial blood pressure by deple-

Continued on next page

Information on the Merck Sharp & Dohme products listed on these pages is the full prescribing information from product circulars in use August 31, 1986.

Merck Sharp & Dohme—Cont.

tion of catecholamines. Reserpine is beneficial in relieving anxiety, tension, and headache in the hypertensive patient. It acts at the hypothalamic level of the central nervous system to promote relaxation without hypnosis or analgesia. The sleep pattern shown by the electroencephalogram following barbiturates does not occur with this drug. In laboratory animals spontaneous activity and response to external stimuli are decreased, but confusion or difficulty of movement is not evident.
The bradycardic action of reserpine promotes relaxation and may eliminate sinus tachycardia. It is most pronounced in subjects with sinus tachycardia and usually is not prominent in persons with a normal pulse rate.
Miosis, relaxation of the nictitating membrane, ptosis, hypothermia, and increased gastrointestinal activity are noted in animals given reserpine, sometimes in subclinical doses. None of these effects, except increased gastrointestinal activity, has been found to be clinically significant in man with therapeutic doses.

INDICATION

Hypertension (see box warning).

CONTRAINDICATIONS

Chlorothiazide is contraindicated in anuria.
DIUPRES is contraindicated in hypersensitivity to chlorothiazide or other sulfonamide-derived drugs or to reserpine.
Electroshock therapy should not be given to patients while on reserpine, as severe and even fatal reactions have been reported with minimal convulsive electroshock dosage. After discontinuing reserpine, allow at least seven days before starting electroshock therapy.
Active peptic ulcer, ulcerative colitis, and active mental depression, especially suicidal tendencies, are contraindications to reserpine therapy.

WARNINGS

Chlorothiazide
Use with caution in severe renal disease. In patients with renal disease, thiazides may precipitate azotemia. Cumulative effects of the drug may develop in patients with impaired renal function.
Thiazides should be used with caution in patients with impaired hepatic function or progressive liver disease, since minor alterations of fluid and electrolyte balance may precipitate hepatic coma.
Thiazides may add to or potentiate the action of other antihypertensive drugs.
Sensitivity reactions may occur in patients with or without a history of allergy or bronchial asthma.
The possibility of exacerbation or activation of systemic lupus erythematosus has been reported.
Lithium generally should not be given with diuretics because they reduce its renal clearance and add a high risk of lithium toxicity. Read circulars for lithium preparations before use of such concomitant therapy.
Reserpine
The occurrence of mental depression due to reserpine in doses of 0.25 mg daily or less is unusual. In any event, DIUPRES should be discontinued at the first sign of depression.
Use in Pregnancy
Reserpine has been demonstrated to cross the placental barrier in guinea pigs with depression of adrenal catecholamine stores in the newborn. There is some evidence that side effects such as nasal congestion, lethargy, depressed Moro reflex, and bradycardia may appear in infants born of reserpine-treated mothers.
Thiazides cross the placental barrier and appear in cord blood. The use of thiazides in pregnancy requires that the anticipated benefit be weighed against possible hazards to the fetus. These hazards include fetal or neonatal jaundice, thrombocytopenia, and possibly other adverse reactions which have occurred in the adult.
Nursing Mothers
Thiazides and reserpine appear in breast milk. If use of the drug is deemed essential, the patient should stop nursing.

PRECAUTIONS

Chlorothiazide
Periodic determination of serum electrolytes to detect possible electrolyte imbalance should be performed at appropriate intervals.
All patients receiving diuretic therapy should be observed for evidence of fluid or electrolyte imbalance: namely, hyponatremia, hypochloremic alkalosis, and hypokalemia. Serum and urine electrolyte determinations are particularly important when the patient is vomiting excessively or receiving parenteral fluids. Warning signs or symptoms of fluid and electrolyte imbalance include dryness of mouth, thirst, weakness, lethargy, drowsiness, restlessness, muscle pains or cramps, muscular fatigue, hypotension, oliguria, tachycardia, and gastrointestinal disturbances such as nausea and vomiting.
Hypokalemia may develop, especially with brisk diuresis, when severe cirrhosis is present, during concomitant use of corticosteroids or ACTH, or after prolonged therapy.
Interference with adequate oral electrolyte intake will contribute to hypokalemia. Hypokalemia can sensitize or exaggerate the response of the heart to the toxic effects of digitalis (e.g., increased ventricular irritability). Hypokalemia may be avoided or treated by use of potassium supplements such as foods with a high potassium content.
Although any chloride deficit is generally mild and usually does not require specific treatment except under extraordinary circumstances (as in liver disease or renal disease), chloride replacement may be required in the treatment of metabolic alkalosis.
Dilutional hyponatremia may occur in edematous patients in hot weather. Appropriate therapy is water restriction, rather than administration of salt, except in rare instances when the hyponatremia is life threatening. In actual salt depletion, appropriate replacement is the therapy of choice.
Hyperuricemia may occur or acute gout may be precipitated in certain patients receiving thiazides.
Insulin requirements in diabetic patients may be increased, decreased, or unchanged. Latent diabetes mellitus may become manifest during thiazide therapy.
Thiazides may increase the responsiveness to tubocurarine.
In some patients, the administration of a non-steroidal anti-inflammatory agent can reduce the diuretic, natriuretic, and antihypertensive effects of loop, potassium-sparing and thiazide diuretics. Therefore, when DIUPRES and non-steroidal anti-inflammatory agents are used concomitantly, the patient should be observed closely to determine if the desired effect of the diuretic is obtained.
The antihypertensive effect of the drug may be enhanced in the postsympathectomy patient. Thiazides may decrease arterial responsiveness to norepinephrine. This diminution is not sufficient to preclude effectiveness of the pressor agent for therapeutic use.
If progressive renal impairment becomes evident, consider withholding or discontinuing diuretic therapy.
Thiazides may decrease serum PBI levels without signs of thyroid disturbance.
Thiazides have been shown to increase the urinary excretion of magnesium; this may result in hypomagnesemia.
Thiazides may decrease urinary calcium excretion. Thiazides may cause intermittent and slight elevation of serum calcium in the absence of known disorders of calcium metabolism. Marked hypercalcemia may be evidence of hidden hyperparathyroidism. Thiazides should be discontinued before carrying out tests for parathyroid function.
Reserpine
Since reserpine may increase gastric secretion and motility, it should be used cautiously in patients with a history of peptic ulcer, ulcerative colitis, or other gastrointestinal disorder. This compound may precipitate biliary colic in patients with gallstones, or bronchial asthma in susceptible persons.
Reserpine may cause hypotension including orthostatic hypotension.
In hypertensive patients on reserpine therapy significant hypotension and bradycardia may develop during surgical anesthesia. The anesthesiologist should be aware that reserpine has been taken, since it may be necessary to give vagal blocking agents parenterally to prevent or reverse hypotension and/or bradycardia.
Anxiety or depression, as well as psychosis, may develop during reserpine therapy. If depression is present when therapy is begun, it may be aggravated. Mental depression is unusual with reserpine doses of 0.25 mg daily or less. In any case, DIUPRES should be discontinued at the first sign of depression. Extreme caution should be used in treating patients with a history of mental depression, and the possibility of suicide should be kept in mind.
As with most antihypertensive therapy, caution should be exercised when treating hypertensive patients with renal insufficiency, since they adjust poorly to lowered blood pressure levels. Use reserpine cautiously with digitalis and quinidine; cardiac arrhythmias have occurred with reserpine preparations.
When two or more antihypertensives are given, the individual dosages may have to be reduced to prevent excessive drop in blood pressure. In hypertensive patients with coronary artery disease, it is important to avoid a precipitous drop in blood pressure.
Animal tumorigenicity: Rodent studies have shown that reserpine is an animal tumorigen, causing an increased incidence of mammary fibroadenomas in female mice, malignant tumors of the seminal vesicles in male mice, and malignant adrenal medullary tumors in male rats. These findings arose in 2 year studies in which the drug was administered in the feed at concentrations of 5 and 10 ppm—about 100 to 300 times the usual human dose. The breast neoplasms are thought to be related to reserpine's prolactin-elevating effect. Several other prolactin-elevating drugs have also been associated with an increased incidence of mammary neoplasia in rodents.
The extent to which these findings indicate a risk to humans is uncertain. Tissue culture experiments show that about one-third of human breast tumors are prolactin-dependent *in vitro,* a factor of considerable importance if the use of the drug is contemplated in a patient with previously detected breast cancer. The possibility of an increased risk of breast cancer in reserpine users has been studied extensively; however, no firm conclusion has emerged. Although a few epidemiologic studies have suggested a slightly increased risk (less than twofold in all studies except one) in women who have used reserpine, other studies of generally similar design have not confirmed this. Epidemiologic studies conducted using other drugs (neuroleptic agents) that, like reserpine, increase prolactin levels and therefore would be considered rodent mammary carcinogens, have not shown an association between chronic administration of the drug and human mammary tumorigenesis. While long-term clinical observation has not suggested such an association, the available evidence is considered too limited to be conclusive at this time. An association of reserpine intake with pheochromocytoma or tumors of the seminal vesicles has not been explored.

ADVERSE REACTIONS

Chlorothiazide
Body as a Whole: Weakness.
Cardiovascular: Orthostatic hypotension (may be aggravated by alcohol, barbiturates, or narcotics).
Digestive: Anorexia, gastric irritation, nausea, vomiting, cramping, diarrhea, constipation, jaundice (intrahepatic cholestatic jaundice), pancreatitis, sialadenitis.
Hematologic: Leukopenia, agranulocytosis, thrombocytopenia, aplastic anemia, hemolytic anemia.
Metabolic: Hyperglycemia, glycosuria, hyperuricemia, electrolyte imbalance (see PRECAUTIONS).
Musculoskeletal: Muscle spasm.
Nervous System/Psychiatric: Dizziness, vertigo, paresthesias, headache, restlessness.
Special Senses: Transient blurred vision, xanthopsia.
Hypersensitivity: Purpura, photosensitivity, rash, urticaria, necrotizing angiitis (vasculitis and cutaneous vasculitis), fever, respiratory distress including pneumonitis and pulmonary edema, anaphylactic reactions.
Whenever adverse reactions are moderate or severe, thiazide dosage should be reduced or therapy withdrawn.
Reserpine
Cardiovascular: Bradycardia, angina pectoris, arrhythmia, premature ventricular contractions, and other direct cardiac effects (e.g., fluid retention, congestive failure).
Digestive: Hypersecretion and increased motility, nausea, vomiting, anorexia, diarrhea, dryness of mouth, increased salivation.
Hematologic: Excessive bleeding following prostatic surgery, thrombocytopenic purpura.
Metabolic: Weight gain.
Musculoskeletal: Muscular aches.
Nervous System/Psychiatric: Excessive sedation, mental depression, nightmares, headache, dizziness, syncope, nervousness, paradoxical anxiety, central nervous system sensitization (dull sensorium, deafness, glaucoma, uveitis, optic atrophy), parkinsonism (usually reversible with decreased dosage or discontinuance of therapy).
Respiratory: Nasal congestion, dyspnea, epistaxis, enhanced susceptibility to colds.
Hypersensitivity: Flushing of skin, pruritus, rash.
Urogenital: Dysuria, nonpuerperal lactation, impotence, decreased libido.

DOSAGE AND ADMINISTRATION

The initial dosage of DIUPRES should conform to the dosages of the individual components established during titration (see box warning).
The usual adult dosage of DIUPRES-250® is 1 or 2 tablets once or twice a day; that of DIUPRES-500® is 1 tablet once or twice a day. Dosage may require adjustment according to the blood pressure response of the patient.
Careful observations for changes in blood pressure must be made when DIUPRES is used with other antihypertensive drugs.

HOW SUPPLIED

No. 3261—Tablets DIUPRES-250 are pink, round, scored, compressed tablets, coded MSD 230. Each tablet contains 250 mg of chlorothiazide and 0.125 mg of reserpine. They are supplied as follows:
NDC 0006-0230-68 in bottles of 100
NDC 0006-0230-82 in bottles of 1000.
Shown in Product Identification Section, page 417
No. 3262—Tablets DIUPRES-500 are pink, round, scored, compressed tablets, coded MSD 405. Each tablet contains 500

mg of chlorothiazide and 0.125 mg of reserpine. They are supplied as follows:
NDC 0006-0405-68 in bottles of 100
NDC 0006-0405-82 in bottles of 1000.

Shown in Product Identification Section, page 417

A.H.F.S. Category: 24:08
DC 6053133 Issued October 1985

DIURIL® Intravenous Sodium ℞
(Chlorothiazide Sodium, MSD), U.S.P.

DESCRIPTION

DIURIL® (Chlorothiazide, MSD) is 6-chloro-2*H*-1,2,4-benzothiadiazine-7-sulfonamide 1,1- dioxide. Its structural formula is:

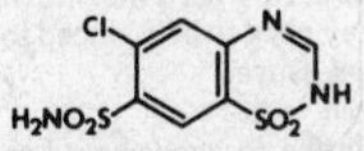

It is a white, or practically white, crystalline compound very slightly soluble in water, but readily soluble in dilute aqueous sodium hydroxide. It is soluble in urine to the extent of about 150 mg per 100 mL at pH 7.
Intravenous Sodium DIURIL® (Chlorothiazide Sodium, MSD) is supplied in a vial containing:

Chlorothiazide sodium equivalent
to chlorothiazide .... 0.5 g
Inactive ingredients:
Mannitol .... 0.25 g
Sodium hydroxide to adjust pH, with 0.4 mg thimerosal (mercury derivative) added as preservative.

ACTIONS

DIURIL is a diuretic and antihypertensive.
DIURIL affects the renal tubular mechanism of electrolyte reabsorption. At maximal therapeutic dosage all thiazides are approximately equal in their diuretic efficacy.
DIURIL increases excretion of sodium and chloride in approximately equivalent amounts. Natriuresis may be accompanied by some loss of potassium and bicarbonate.
After oral use diuresis begins within 2 hours, peaks in about 4 hours and lasts about 6 to 12 hours. Following intravenous use of Sodium DIURIL, onset of the diuretic action occurs in 15 minutes and the maximal action in 30 minutes. DIURIL is eliminated rapidly by the kidney.
The mechanism of the antihypertensive effect of thiazides is unknown. DIURIL does not affect normal blood pressure.

INDICATIONS

Intravenous Sodium DIURIL is indicated as adjunctive therapy in edema associated with congestive heart failure, hepatic cirrhosis, and corticosteroid and estrogen therapy.
Intravenous Sodium DIURIL has also been found useful in edema due to various forms of renal dysfunction such as nephrotic syndrome, acute glomerulonephritis, and chronic renal failure.
Use in Pregnancy. Routine use of diuretics during normal pregnancy is inappropriate and exposes mother and fetus to unnecessary hazard. Diuretics do not prevent development of toxemia of pregnancy and there is no satisfactory evidence that they are useful in the treatment of toxemia.
Edema during pregnancy may arise from pathologic causes or from the physiologic and mechanical consequences of pregnancy. Thiazides are indicated in pregnancy when edema is due to pathologic causes, just as they are in the absence of pregnancy (however, see WARNINGS). Dependent edema in pregnancy, resulting from restriction of venous return by the gravid uterus, is properly treated through elevation of the lower extremities and use of support stockings. Use of diuretics to lower intravascular volume in this instance is illogical and unnecessary. During normal pregnancy there is hypervolemia which is not harmful to the fetus or the mother in the absence of cardiovascular disease. However, it may be associated with edema, rarely generalized edema. If such edema causes discomfort, increased recumbency will often provide relief. Rarely this edema may cause extreme discomfort which is not relieved by rest. In these instances, a short course of diuretic therapy may provide relief and be appropriate.

CONTRAINDICATIONS

Anuria.
Hypersensitivity to any component of this product or to other sulfonamide-derived drugs.

WARNINGS

Intravenous use in infants and children has been limited and is not generally recommended.
Use with caution in severe renal disease. In patients with renal disease, thiazides may precipitate azotemia. Cumulative effects of the drug may develop in patients with impaired renal function.
Thiazides should be used with caution in patients with impaired hepatic function or progressive liver disease, since minor alterations of fluid and electrolyte balance may precipitate hepatic coma.
Thiazides may add to or potentiate the action of other antihypertensive drugs.
Sensitivity reactions may occur in patients with or without a history of allergy or bronchial asthma.
The possibility of exacerbation or activation of systemic lupus erythematosus has been reported.
Lithium generally should not be given with diuretics because they reduce its renal clearance and add a high risk of lithium toxicity. Read circulars for lithium preparations before use of such concomitant therapy.

Use in Pregnancy. Thiazides cross the placental barrier and appear in cord blood. The use of thiazides in pregnancy requires that the anticipated benefit be weighed against possible hazards to the fetus. These hazards include fetal or neonatal jaundice, thrombocytopenia, and possibly other adverse reactions which have occurred in the adult.

Nursing Mothers. Thiazides appear in breast milk. If use of the drug is deemed essential, the patient should stop nursing.

PRECAUTIONS

Periodic determination of serum electrolytes to detect possible electrolyte imbalance should be performed at appropriate intervals.
All patients receiving diuretic therapy should be observed for evidence of fluid or electrolyte imbalance: namely, hyponatremia, hypochloremic alkalosis, and hypokalemia. Serum and urine electrolyte determinations are particularly important when the patient is vomiting excessively or receiving parenteral fluids. Warning signs or symptoms of fluid and electrolyte imbalance include dryness of mouth, thirst, weakness, lethargy, drowsiness, restlessness, muscle pains or cramps, muscular fatigue, hypotension, oliguria, tachycardia, and gastrointestinal disturbances such as nausea and vomiting.
Hypokalemia may develop especially with brisk diuresis, when severe cirrhosis is present, during concomitant use of corticosteroids or ACTH, or after prolonged therapy.
Interference with adequate oral electrolyte intake will also contribute to hypokalemia. Hypokalemia can sensitize or exaggerate the response of the heart to the toxic effects of digitalis (e.g., increased ventricular irritability). Hypokalemia may be avoided or treated by use of potassium supplements such as foods with a high potassium content.
Although any chloride deficit is generally mild and usually does not require specific treatment except under extraordinary circumstances (as in liver disease or renal disease), chloride replacement may be required in the treatment of metabolic alkalosis.
Dilutional hyponatremia may occur in edematous patients in hot weather; appropriate therapy is water restriction, rather than administration of salt, except in rare instances when the hyponatremia is life threatening. In actual salt depletion, appropriate replacement is the therapy of choice.
Hyperuricemia may occur or acute gout may be precipitated in certain patients receiving thiazides.
Insulin requirements in diabetic patients may be increased, decreased, or unchanged. Latent diabetes mellitus may become manifest during thiazide therapy.
Thiazides may increase the responsiveness to tubocurarine.
In some patients, the administration of a non-steroidal anti-inflammatory agent can reduce the diuretic, natriuretic, and antihypertensive effects of loop, potassium-sparing and thiazide diuretics. Therefore, when Sodium DIURIL and non-steroidal anti-inflammatory agents are used concomitantly, the patient should be observed closely to determine if the desired effect of the diuretic is obtained.
The antihypertensive effects of the drug may be enhanced in the postsympathectomy patient. Thiazides may decrease arterial responsiveness to norepinephrine. This diminution is not sufficient to preclude effectiveness of the pressor agent for therapeutic use.
If progressive renal impairment becomes evident, consider withholding or discontinuing diuretic therapy.
Thiazides may decrease serum PBI levels without signs of thyroid disturbance.
Thiazides have been shown to increase the urinary excretion of magnesium; this may result in hypomagnesemia.
Thiazides may decrease urinary calcium excretion. Thiazides may cause intermittent and slight elevation of serum calcium in the absence of known disorders of calcium metabolism. Marked hypercalcemia may be evidence of hidden hyperparathyroidism. Thiazides should be discontinued before carrying out tests for parathyroid function.

ADVERSE REACTIONS

Body as a Whole: Weakness.
Cardiovascular: Orthostatic hypotension (may be aggravated by alcohol, barbiturates, or narcotics).
Digestive: Anorexia, gastric irritation, nausea, vomiting, cramping, diarrhea, constipation, jaundice (intrahepatic cholestatic jaundice), pancreatitis, sialadenitis.
Hematologic: Leukopenia, agranulocytosis, thrombocytopenia, aplastic anemia, hemolytic anemia.
Metabolic: Hyperglycemia, glycosuria, hyperuricemia, electrolyte imbalance (see PRECAUTIONS).
Musculoskeletal: Muscle spasm.
Nervous System/Psychiatric: Dizziness, vertigo, paresthesias, headache, restlessness.
Special Senses: Transient blurred vision, xanthopsia.
Urogenital: Hematuria (one case following intravenous use).
Hypersensitivity: Purpura, photosensitivity, rash, urticaria, necrotizing angiitis (vasculitis and cutaneous vasculitis), fever, respiratory distress including pneumonitis and pulmonary edema, anaphylactic reactions.
Whenever adverse reactions are moderate or severe, thiazide dosage should be reduced or therapy withdrawn.

DOSAGE AND ADMINISTRATION

Intravenous Sodium DIURIL should be reserved for patients unable to take oral medication or for emergency situations.
Therapy should be individualized according to patient response. Use the smallest dosage necessary to achieve the required response.
Intravenous use in infants and children has been limited and is not generally recommended.
When medication can be taken orally, therapy with DIURIL tablets or oral suspension may be substituted for intravenous therapy, using the same dosage schedule as for the parenteral route.
Add 18 mL of Sterile Water for Injection to the vial to form an isotonic solution for intravenous injection. Never add less than 18 mL. Unused solution may be stored at room temperature for 24 hours, after which it must be discarded. The solution is compatible with dextrose or sodium chloride solutions for intravenous infusion. Avoid simultaneous administration of solutions of chlorothiazide with whole blood or its derivatives.
Extravasation must be rigidly avoided. Do not give subcutaneously or intramuscularly.
The usual adult dosage is 0.5 to 1.0 g once or twice a day. Many patients with edema respond to intermittent therapy, i.e., administration on alternate days or on three to five days each week. With an intermittent schedule, excessive response and the resulting undesirable electrolyte imbalance are less likely to occur.

HOW SUPPLIED

No. 3250—Intravenous Sodium DIURIL is a dry, white powder usually in plug form, supplied in vials containing chlorothiazide sodium equivalent to 0.5 g of chlorothiazide.
NDC 0006-3250-32.

A.H.F.S. Category: 40:28
DC 7413522 Issued October 1985

DIURIL® Tablets ℞
(Chlorothiazide, MSD), U.S.P.
DIURIL® Oral Suspension ℞
(Chlorothiazide, MSD), U.S.P.

DESCRIPTION

DIURIL® (Chlorothiazide, MSD) is 6-chloro-2*H*-1,2,4-benzothiadiazine-7-sulfonamide 1,1-dioxide. Its structural formula is:

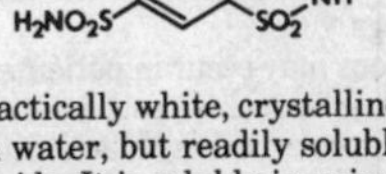

It is a white, or practically white, crystalline compound very slightly soluble in water, but readily soluble in dilute aqueous sodium hydroxide. It is soluble in urine to the extent of about 150 mg per 100 mL at pH 7.

Continued on next page

Information on the Merck Sharp & Dohme products listed on these pages is the full prescribing information from product circulars in use August 31, 1986.

Merck Sharp & Dohme—Cont.

DIURIL is supplied as 250 mg and 500 mg tablets for oral use. Each tablet contains the following inactive ingredients: gelatin, magnesium stearate, starch and talc. The 250 mg tablet also contains lactose.
Oral Suspension DIURIL contains 250 mg per 5 mL, alcohol 0.5 percent, with methylparaben 0.12 percent, propylparaben 0.02 percent, and benzoic acid 0.1 percent added as preservatives. The inactive ingredients are D&C Yellow 10, flavors, glycerin, purified water, sodium saccharin, sucrose and tragacanth.

ACTIONS

DIURIL is a diuretic and antihypertensive.
DIURIL affects the renal tubular mechanism of electrolyte reabsorption. At maximal therapeutic dosage all thiazides are approximately equal in their diuretic efficacy.
DIURIL increases excretion of sodium and chloride in approximately equivalent amounts. Natriuresis may be accompanied by some loss of potassium and bicarbonate.
After oral use diuresis begins within 2 hours, peaks in about 4 hours and lasts about 6 to 12 hours. DIURIL is eliminated rapidly by the kidney.
The mechanism of the antihypertensive effect of thiazides is unknown. DIURIL does not affect normal blood pressure.

INDICATIONS

DIURIL is indicated as adjunctive therapy in edema associated with congestive heart failure, hepatic cirrhosis, and corticosteroid and estrogen therapy.
DIURIL has also been found useful in edema due to various forms of renal dysfunction such as nephrotic syndrome, acute glomerulonephritis, and chronic renal failure.
DIURIL is indicated in the management of hypertension either as the sole therapeutic agent or to enhance the effectiveness of other antihypertensive drugs in the more severe forms of hypertension.
Use in Pregnancy. Routine use of diuretics during normal pregnancy is inappropriate and exposes mother and fetus to unnecessary hazard. Diuretics do not prevent development of toxemia of pregnancy and there is no satisfactory evidence that they are useful in the treatment of toxemia.
Edema during pregnancy may arise from pathologic causes or from the physiologic and mechanical consequences of pregnancy. Thiazides are indicated in pregnancy when edema is due to pathologic causes, just as they are in the absence of pregnancy (however, see WARNINGS, below).
Dependent edema in pregnancy, resulting from restriction of venous return by the gravid uterus, is properly treated through elevation of the lower extremities and use of support stockings. Use of diuretics to lower intravascular volume in this instance is illogical and unnecessary. During normal pregnancy there is hypervolemia which is not harmful to the fetus or the mother in the absence of cardiovascular disease. However, it may be associated with edema, rarely generalized edema. If such edema causes discomfort, increased recumbency will often provide relief. Rarely this edema may cause extreme discomfort which is not relieved by rest. In these instances, a short course of diuretic therapy may provide relief and be appropriate.

CONTRAINDICATIONS

Anuria.
Hypersensitivity to this product or to other sulfonamide-derived drugs.

WARNINGS

Use with caution in severe renal disease. In patients with renal disease, thiazides may precipitate azotemia. Cumulative effects of the drug may develop in patients with impaired renal function.
Thiazides should be used with caution in patients with impaired hepatic function or progressive liver disease, since minor alterations of fluid and electrolyte balance may precipitate hepatic coma.
Thiazides may add to or potentiate the action of other antihypertensive drugs.
Sensitivity reactions may occur in patients with or without a history of allergy or bronchial asthma.
The possibility of exacerbation or activation of systemic lupus erythematosus has been reported.
Lithium generally should not be given with diuretics because they reduce its renal clearance and add a high risk of lithium toxicity. Read circulars for lithium preparations before use of such concomitant therapy.
Use in Pregnancy. Thiazides cross the placental barrier and appear in cord blood. The use of thiazides in pregnancy requires that the anticipated benefit be weighed against possible hazards to the fetus. These hazards include fetal or neonatal jaundice, thrombocytopenia, and possibly other adverse reactions which have occurred in the adult.
Nursing Mothers. Thiazides appear in breast milk. If use of the drug is deemed essential, the patient should stop nursing.

PRECAUTIONS

Periodic determination of serum electrolytes to detect possible electrolyte imbalance should be performed at appropriate intervals.
All patients receiving diuretic therapy should be observed for evidence of fluid or electrolyte imbalance: namely, hyponatremia, hypochloremic alkalosis, and hypokalemia. Serum and urine electrolyte determinations are particularly important when the patient is vomiting excessively or receiving parenteral fluids. Warning signs or symptoms of fluid and electrolyte imbalance include dryness of mouth, thirst, weakness, lethargy, drowsiness, restlessness, muscle pains or cramps, muscular fatigue, hypotension, oliguria, tachycardia, and gastrointestinal disturbances such as nausea and vomiting.
Hypokalemia may develop, especially with brisk diuresis, when severe cirrhosis is present, during concomitant use of corticosteroids or ACTH, or after prolonged therapy.
Interference with adequate oral electrolyte intake will also contribute to hypokalemia. Hypokalemia can sensitize or exaggerate the response of the heart to the toxic effects of digitalis (e.g., increased ventricular irritability). Hypokalemia may be avoided or treated by use of potassium supplements such as foods with a high potassium content.
Although any chloride deficit is generally mild and usually does not require specific treatment except under extraordinary circumstances (as in liver disease or renal disease), chloride replacement may be required in the treatment of metabolic alkalosis.
Dilutional hyponatremia may occur in edematous patients in hot weather; appropriate therapy is water restriction, rather than administration of salt, except in rare instances when the hyponatremia is life threatening. In actual salt depletion, appropriate replacement is the therapy of choice.
Hyperuricemia may occur or acute gout may be precipitated in certain patients receiving thiazides.
Insulin requirements in diabetic patients may be increased, decreased, or unchanged. Latent diabetes mellitus may become manifest during thiazide therapy.
Thiazides may increase the responsiveness to tubocurarine.
In some patients, the administration of a non-steroidal anti-inflammatory agent can reduce the diuretic, natriuretic, and antihypertensive effects of loop, potassium-sparing and thiazide diuretics. Therefore, when DIURIL and non-steroidal anti-inflammatory agents are used concomitantly, the patient should be observed closely to determine if the desired effect of the diuretic is obtained.
The antihypertensive effects of the drug may be enhanced in the postsympathectomy patient. Thiazides may decrease arterial responsiveness to norepinephrine. This diminution is not sufficient to preclude effectiveness of the pressor agent for therapeutic use.
If progressive renal impairment becomes evident, consider withholding or discontinuing diuretic therapy.
Thiazides may decrease serum PBI levels without signs of thyroid disturbance.
Thiazides have been shown to increase the urinary excretion of magnesium; this may result in hypomagnesemia.
Thiazides may decrease urinary calcium excretion. Thiazides may cause intermittent and slight elevation of serum calcium in the absence of known disorders of calcium metabolism. Marked hypercalcemia may be evidence of hidden hyperparathyroidism. Thiazides should be discontinued before carrying out tests for parathyroid function.

ADVERSE REACTIONS

Body as a Whole: Weakness.
Cardiovascular: Orthostatic hypotension (may be aggravated by alcohol, barbiturates, or narcotics).
Digestive: Anorexia, gastric irritation, nausea, vomiting, cramping, diarrhea, constipation, jaundice (intrahepatic cholestatic jaundice), pancreatitis, sialadenitis.
Hematologic: Leukopenia, agranulocytosis, thrombocytopenia, aplastic anemia, hemolytic anemia.
Metabolic: Hyperglycemia, glycosuria, hyperuricemia, electrolyte imbalance (see PRECAUTIONS).
Musculoskeletal: Muscle spasm.
Nervous System/Psychiatric: Dizziness, vertigo, paresthesias, headache, restlessness.
Special Senses: Transient blurred vision, xanthopsia.
Hypersensitivity: Purpura, photosensitivity, rash, urticaria, necrotizing angiitis (vasculitis and cutaneous vasculitis), fever, respiratory distress including pneumonitis and pulmonary edema, anaphylactic reactions.
Whenever adverse reactions are moderate or severe, thiazide dosage should be reduced or therapy withdrawn.

DOSAGE AND ADMINISTRATION

Therapy should be individualized according to patient response. Use the smallest dosage necessary to achieve the required response.
Adults
For Diuresis
The usual adult dosage is 0.5 to 1.0 g once or twice a day. Many patients with edema respond to intermittent therapy, i.e., administration on alternate days or on three to five days each week. With an intermittent schedule, excessive response and the resulting undesirable electrolyte imbalance are less likely to occur.
For Control of Hypertension
The usual adult starting dosage is 0.5 or 1.0 g a day as a single or divided dose. Dosage is increased or decreased according to blood pressure response. Rarely some patients may require up to 2.0 g a day in divided doses.
When thiazides are used with other antihypertensives, the dose of the latter may need to be reduced to prevent excessive decrease in blood pressure.
Infants and Children
The usual oral pediatric dosage is based on 10 mg of DIURIL per pound of body weight per day in two doses. Infants under 6 months of age may require up to 15 mg per pound per day in two doses.
On this basis, infants up to 2 years of age may be given 125 to 375 mg daily in two doses (2.5 to 7.5 mL, or ½ to 1½ teaspoonfuls of the oral suspension daily). Children from 2 to 12 years of age may be given 375 mg to 1.0 g daily in two doses (7.5 to 20 mL, or 1½ to 4 teaspoonfuls of oral suspension daily). Dosage in both age groups should be based on body weight.

HOW SUPPLIED

No. 3244—Tablets DIURIL, 250 mg, are white, round, scored, compressed tablets, coded MSD 214. They are supplied as follows:
NDC 0006-0214-68 bottles of 100
NDC 0006-0214-28 unit dose packages of 100
NDC 0006-0214-82 bottles of 1000.
Shown in Product Identification Section, page 417
No. 3245—Tablets DIURIL, 500 mg, are white, round, scored, compressed tablets, coded MSD 432. They are supplied as follows:
NDC 0006-0432-68 bottles of 100
NDC 0006-0432-28 unit dose packages of 100
NDC 0006-0432-82 bottles of 1000
NDC 0006-0432-86 bottles of 5000.
Shown in Product Identification Section, page 417
No. 3239—Oral Suspension DIURIL, 250 mg per 5 mL, is a yellow, creamy suspension, and is supplied as follows:
NDC 0006-3239-66 bottles of 237 mL.
A.H.F.S. Category: 40:28
DC 6020745 Issued October 1985

DOLOBID® Tablets ℞
(Diflunisal, MSD)

DESCRIPTION

Diflunisal is 2′, 4′-difluoro-4-hydroxy-3-biphenylcarboxylic acid. Its empirical formula is $C_{13}H_8F_2O_3$ and its structural formula is:

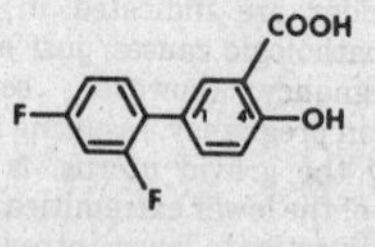

Diflunisal has a molecular weight of 250.20. It is a stable, white, crystalline compound with a melting point of 211–213°C. It is practically insoluble in water at neutral or acidic pH. Because it is an organic acid, it dissolves readily in dilute alkali to give a moderately stable solution at room temperature. It is soluble in most organic solvents including ethanol, methanol, and acetone.
DOLOBID® (Diflunisal, MSD) is available in 250 and 500 mg tablets for oral administration. Tablets DOLOBID contain the following inactive ingredients: cellulose, FD&C Yellow 6 hydroxypropyl cellulose, hydroxypropyl methylcellulose, magnesium stearate, starch, talc, and titanium dioxide.

CLINICAL PHARMACOLOGY

Action
DOLOBID is a non-steroidal drug with analgesic, anti-inflammatory and antipyretic properties. It is a peripherally-acting non-narcotic analgesic drug. Habituation, tolerance and addiction have not been reported.

Diflunisal is a difluorophenyl derivative of salicylic acid. Chemically, diflunisal differs from aspirin (acetylsalicylic acid) in two respects. The first of these two is the presence of a difluorophenyl substituent at carbon 1. The second difference is the removal of the 0-acetyl group from the carbon 4 position. Diflunisal is not metabolized to salicylic acid, and the fluorine atoms are not displaced from the difluorophenyl ring structure.

The precise mechanism of the analgesic and anti-inflammatory actions of diflunisal is not known. Diflunisal is a prostaglandin synthetase inhibitor. In animals, prostaglandins sensitize afferent nerves and potentiate the action of bradykinin in inducing pain. Since prostaglandins are known to be among the mediators of pain and inflammation, the mode of action of diflunisal may be due to a decrease of prostaglandins in peripheral tissues.

Pharmacokinetics and Metabolism

DOLOBID is rapidly and completely absorbed following oral administration with peak plasma concentrations occurring between 2 to 3 hours. The drug is excreted in the urine as two soluble glucuronide conjugates accounting for about 90% of the administered dose. Little or no diflunisal is excreted in the feces. Diflunisal appears in human milk in concentrations of 2–7% of those in plasma. More than 99% of diflunisal in plasma is bound to proteins.

As is the case with salicylic acid, concentration-dependent pharmacokinetics prevail when DOLOBID is administered; a doubling of dosage produces a greater than doubling of drug accumulation. The effect becomes more apparent with repetitive doses. Following single doses, peak plasma concentrations of 41 ± 11 μg/mL (mean ± S.D.) were observed following 250 mg doses, 87 ± 17 μg/mL were observed following 500 mg and 124 ± 11 μg/mL following single 1000 mg doses. However, following administration of 250 mg b.i.d., a mean peak level of 56 ± 14 μg/mL was observed on day 8, while the mean peak level after 500 mg b.i.d. for 11 days was 190 ± 33 μg/mL. In contrast to salicylic acid which has a plasma half-life of 2½ hours, the plasma half-life of diflunisal is 3 to 4 times longer (8 to 12 hours), because of a difluorophenyl substituent at carbon 1. Because of its long half-life and nonlinear pharmacokinetics, several days are required for diflunisal plasma levels to reach steady state following multiple doses. For this reason, an initial loading dose is necessary to shorten the time to reach steady state levels, and 2 to 3 days of observation are necessary for evaluating changes in treatment regimens if a loading dose is not used.

Studies in baboons to determine passage across the blood-brain barrier have shown that only small quantities of diflunisal, under normal or acidotic conditions are transported into the cerebrospinal fluid (CSF). The ratio of blood/CSF concentrations after intravenous doses of 50 mg/kg or oral doses of 100 mg/kg of diflunisal was 100:1. In contrast, oral doses of 500 mg/kg of aspirin resulted in a blood/CSF ratio of 5:1.

Mild to Moderate Pain

DOLOBID is a peripherally-acting analgesic agent with a long duration of action. DOLOBID produces significant analgesia within 1 hour and maximum analgesia within 2 to 3 hours.

Consistent with its long half-life, clinical effects of DOLOBID mirror its pharmacokinetic behavior, which is the basis for recommending a loading dose when instituting therapy. Patients treated with DOLOBID, on the first dose, tend to have a slower onset of pain relief when compared with drugs achieving comparable peak effects. However, DOLOBID produces longer-lasting responses than the comparative agents.

Comparative single dose clinical studies have established the analgesic efficacy of DOLOBID at various dose levels relative to other analgesics. Analgesic effect measurements were derived from hourly evaluations by patients during eight and twelve-hour postdosing observation periods. The following information may serve as a guide for prescribing DOLOBID.

DOLOBID 500 mg was comparable in analgesic efficacy to aspirin 650 mg, acetaminophen 600 mg or 650 mg, and acetaminophen 650 mg with propoxyphene napsylate 100 mg. Patients treated with DOLOBID had longer lasting responses than the patients treated with the comparative analgesics.

DOLOBID 1000 mg was comparable in analgesic efficacy to acetaminophen 600 mg with codeine 60 mg. Patients treated with DOLOBID had longer lasting responses than the patients who received acetaminophen with codeine.

A loading dose of 1000 mg provides faster onset of pain relief, shorter time to peak analgesic effect, and greater peak analgesic effect than an initial 500 mg dose.

In contrast to the comparative analgesics, a significantly greater proportion of patients treated with DOLOBID did not remedicate and continued to have a good analgesic effect eight to twelve hours after dosing. Seventy-five percent (75%) of patients treated with DOLOBID continued to have a good analgesic response at four hours. When patients having a good analgesic response at four hours were followed, 78% of these patients continued to have a good analgesic response at eight hours and 64% at twelve hours.

Osteoarthritis

The effectiveness of DOLOBID for the treatment of osteoarthritis was studied in patients with osteoarthritis of the hip and/or knee. The activity of DOLOBID was demonstrated by clinical improvement in the signs and symptoms of disease activity.

In a double-blind multicenter study of 12 weeks' duration in which dosages were adjusted according to patient response, DOLOBID, 500 or 750 mg daily, was shown to be comparable in effectiveness to aspirin, 2000 or 3000 mg daily. Patients treated with DOLOBID had a lower overall incidence of digestive system adverse experiences, and of dizziness, edema, and tinnitus. In open-label extensions of this study to 24 or 48 weeks, DOLOBID continued to show similar effectiveness and generally was well tolerated.

Rheumatoid Arthritis

In controlled clinical trials, the effectiveness of DOLOBID was established for both acute exacerbations and long-term management of rheumatoid arthritis. The activity of DOLOBID was demonstrated by clinical improvement in the signs and symptoms of disease activity.

In a double-blind multicenter study of 12 weeks' duration in which dosages were adjusted according to patient response, DOLOBID 500 or 750 mg daily was comparable in effectiveness to aspirin 2,600 or 3,900 mg daily. Patients on DOLOBID had a lower incidence of dyspepsia, gastrointestinal pain and tinnitus. In open-label extensions of this study to 52 weeks, DOLOBID continued to be effective and was generally well tolerated. Patients treated with DOLOBID had a lower incidence of tinnitus and a lower overall incidence of gastrointestinal adverse experiences.

DOLOBID 500, 750, or 1000 mg daily was compared with aspirin 2000, 3000, or 4000 mg daily in a multicenter study of 8 weeks' duration in which dosages were adjusted according to patient response. In this study, DOLOBID was comparable in efficacy to aspirin. Patients receiving DOLOBID had a lower incidence of gastrointestinal adverse effects than did patients treated with aspirin. Patients treated with DOLOBID also had a lower incidence of tinnitus and hearing loss.

In a double-blind multicenter study of 12 weeks' duration in which dosages were adjusted according to patient needs, DOLOBID 500 or 750 mg daily and ibuprofen 1600 or 2400 mg daily were comparable in effectiveness and tolerability.

In a double-blind multicenter study of 12 weeks' duration, DOLOBID 750 mg daily was comparable in efficacy to naproxen 750 mg daily. The incidence of gastrointestinal adverse effects and tinnitus was comparable for both drugs. This study was extended to 48 weeks on an open-label basis. DOLOBID continued to be effective and generally well tolerated.

In patients with rheumatoid arthritis, DOLOBID and gold salts may be used in combination at their usual dosage levels. In clinical studies, DOLOBID added to the regimen of gold salts usually resulted in additional symptomatic relief but did not alter the course of the underlying disease.

Antipyretic Activity

DOLOBID is not recommended for use as an antipyretic agent. In single 250 mg, 500 mg, or 750 mg doses, DOLOBID produced measurable but not clinically useful decreases in temperature in patients with fever; however, the possibility that it may mask fever in some patients, particularly with chronic or high doses, should be considered.

Uricosuric Effect

In normal volunteers, an increase in the renal clearance of uric acid and a decrease in serum uric acid was observed when DOLOBID was administered at 500 mg or 750 mg daily in divided doses. Patients on long-term therapy taking DOLOBID at 500 mg to 1000 mg daily in divided doses showed a prompt and consistent reduction across studies in mean serum uric acid levels, which were lowered as much as 1.4 mg%. It is not known whether DOLOBID interferes with the activity of other uricosuric agents.

Effect on Platelet Function

As an inhibitor of prostaglandin synthetase, DOLOBID has a dose-related effect on platelet function and bleeding time. In normal volunteers, 250 mg b.i.d. for 8 days had no effect on platelet function, and 500 mg b.i.d., the usual recommended dose, had a slight effect. At 1000 mg b.i.d., which exceeds the maximum recommended dosage, however, DOLOBID inhibited platelet function. In contrast to aspirin, these effects of DOLOBID were reversible, because of the absence of the chemically labile and biologically reactive 0-acetyl group at the carbon 4 position. Bleeding time was not altered by a dose of 250 mg b.i.d., and was only slightly increased at 500 mg b.i.d. At 1000 mg b.i.d., a greater increase occurred, but was not statistically significantly different from the change in the placebo group.

Effect on Fecal Blood Loss

When DOLOBID was given to normal volunteers at the usual recommended dose of 500 mg twice daily, fecal blood loss was not significantly different from placebo. Aspirin at 1000 mg four times daily produced the expected increase in fecal blood loss. DOLOBID at 1000 mg twice daily (NOTE: exceeds the recommended dosage) caused a statistically significant increase in fecal blood loss, but this increase was only one-half as large as that associated with aspirin 1300 mg twice daily.

Effect on Blood Glucose

DOLOBID did not affect fasting blood sugar in diabetic patients who were receiving tolbutamide or placebo.

INDICATIONS AND USAGE

DOLOBID is indicated for acute or long-term use for symptomatic treatment of the following:

1. Mild to moderate pain
2. Osteoarthritis
3. Rheumatoid arthritis

CONTRAINDICATIONS

Patients who are hypersensitive to this product.

Patients in whom acute asthmatic attacks, urticaria, or rhinitis are precipitated by aspirin or other non-steroidal anti-inflammatory drugs.

WARNINGS

Peptic ulceration and gastrointestinal bleeding have been reported in patients receiving DOLOBID. Fatalities have occurred rarely. In patients with active gastrointestinal bleeding or an active peptic ulcer, the physician must weigh the benefits of therapy with DOLOBID against possible hazards, institute an appropriate ulcer regimen, and carefully monitor the patient's progress. When DOLOBID is given to patients with a history of either upper or lower gastrointestinal tract disease, it should be given only after consulting the ADVERSE REACTIONS section and under close supervision.

PRECAUTIONS

General

Although DOLOBID has less effect on platelet function and bleeding time than aspirin, at higher doses it is an inhibitor of platelet function; therefore, patients who may be adversely affected should be carefully observed when DOLOBID is administered (see CLINICAL PHARMACOLOGY).

Because of reports of adverse eye findings with agents of this class, it is recommended that patients who develop eye complaints during treatment with DOLOBID have ophthalmologic studies.

Peripheral edema has been observed in some patients taking DOLOBID. Therefore, as with other drugs in this class, DOLOBID should be used with caution in patients with compromised cardiac function, hypertension, or other conditions predisposing to fluid retention.

Renal Effects

As with other non-steroidal anti-inflammatory drugs, long term administration of diflunisal to animals has resulted in renal papillary necrosis and other abnormal renal pathology. In humans, there have been reports of acute interstitial nephritis with hematuria and proteinuria. Occasionally nephrotic syndrome has been observed with other NSAIDs.

A second form of renal toxicity has been seen in patients with prerenal and renal conditions leading to a reduction in renal blood flow or blood volume, where the renal prostaglandins have a supportive role in the maintenance of renal perfusion. In these patients administration of an NSAID may cause a dose dependent reduction in prostaglandin formation and may precipitate overt renal decompensation. Patients at greatest risk of this reaction are those with conditions such as renal or hepatic dysfunction, complications associated with advanced age, extracellular volume depletion from any cause, congestive heart failure, sepsis, or concomitant use of any nephrotoxic drug. DOLOBID or other NSAIDs should be given with caution and renal function should be monitored in any patient who may have reduced renal reserve. Discontinuation of NSAID therapy is typically followed by recovery to the pretreatment state.

Since DOLOBID is eliminated primarily by the kidneys, patients with significantly impaired renal function should be closely monitored; a lower daily dosage should be anticipated to avoid excessive drug accumulation.

Laboratory Tests

As with other non-steroidal anti-inflammatory drugs, borderline elevations of one or more liver tests may occur in up to 15% of patients. These abnormalities may progress, may remain essentially unchanged, or may be transient with continued therapy. The SGPT (ALT) test is probably the

Continued on next page

Merck Sharp & Dohme—Cont.

most sensitive indicator of liver dysfunction. Meaningful (3 times the upper limit of normal) elevations of SGPT or SGOT (AST) occurred in controlled clinical trials in less than 1% of patients. A patient with symptoms and/or signs suggesting liver dysfunction, or in whom an abnormal liver test has occurred, should be evaluated for evidence of the development of more severe hepatic reactions while on therapy with DOLOBID. Severe hepatic reactions, including jaundice, have been reported with DOLOBID as well as with other non-steroidal anti-inflammatory drugs. Although such reactions are rare, if abnormal liver tests persist or worsen, if clinical signs and symptoms consistent with liver disease develop, or if systemic manifestations occur (e.g., eosinophilia, rash, etc.), DOLOBID should be discontinued, since liver reactions can be fatal.

Drug Interactions

DOLOBID prolongs the prothrombin time in patients who are on oral anticoagulants. DOLOBID has not been shown to interact with tolbutamide. DOLOBID interacts with hydrochlorothiazide, furosemide, acetaminophen, aspirin, indomethacin, sulindac and naproxen (see below).

Oral Anticoagulants: In some normal volunteers, the concomitant administration of DOLOBID and warfarin, acenocoumarol, or phenprocoumon resulted in prolongation of prothrombin time. This may occur because diflunisal competitively displaces coumarins from protein binding sites. Accordingly, when DOLOBID is administered with oral anticoagulants, the prothrombin time should be closely monitored during and for several days after concomitant drug administration. Adjustment of dosage of oral anticoagulants may be required.

Tolbutamide: In diabetic patients receiving DOLOBID and tolbutamide, no significant effects were seen on tolbutamide plasma levels or fasting blood glucose.

Hydrochlorothiazide: In normal volunteers, concomitant administration of DOLOBID and hydrochlorothiazide resulted in significantly increased plasma levels of hydrochlorothiazide. DOLOBID decreased the hyperuricemic effect of hydrochlorothiazide.

Furosemide: In normal volunteers, the concomitant administration of DOLOBID and furosemide had no effect on the diuretic activity of furosemide. DOLOBID decreased the hyperuricemic effect of furosemide.

Antacids: Concomitant administration of antacids may reduce plasma levels of DOLOBID. This effect is small with occasional doses of antacids, but may be clinically significant when antacids are used on a continuous schedule.

Acetaminophen: In normal volunteers, concomitant administration of DOLOBID and acetaminophen resulted in an approximate 50% increase in plasma levels of acetaminophen. Acetaminophen had no effect on plasma levels of DOLOBID. Since acetaminophen in high doses has been associated with hepatotoxicity, concomitant administration of DOLOBID and acetaminophen should be used cautiously, with careful monitoring of patients.

Concomitant administration of DOLOBID and acetaminophen in dogs, but not in rats, at approximately 2 times the recommended maximum human therapeutic dose of each (40-52 mg/kg/day of DOLOBID/acetaminophen), resulted in greater gastrointestinal toxicity than when either drug was administered alone. The clinical significance of these findings has not been established.

Drug Interactions: Non-steroidal Anti-inflammatory Drugs

The administration of diflunisal to normal volunteers receiving indomethacin decreased the renal clearance and significantly increased the plasma levels of indomethacin. In some patients the combined use of indomethacin and DOLOBID has been associated with fatal gastrointestinal hemorrhage. Therefore, indomethacin and DOLOBID should not be used concomitantly.

Since no further clinical data are available about the safety and effectiveness of DOLOBID when used in combination with other non-steroidal anti-inflammatory drugs, no recommendation for their concomitant use can be made. The following information was obtained from studies in normal volunteers.

Aspirin: In normal volunteers, a small decrease in diflunisal levels was observed when multiple doses of DOLOBID and aspirin were administered concomitantly.

Sulindac: The concomitant administration of DOLOBID and sulindac in normal volunteers resulted in lowering of the plasma levels of the active sulindac sulfide metabolite by approximately one-third.

Naproxen: The concomitant administration of DOLOBID and naproxen in normal volunteers had no effect on the plasma levels of naproxen, but significantly decreased the urinary excretion of naproxen and its glucuronide metabolite. Naproxen had no effect on plasma levels of DOLOBID.

Carcinogenesis, Mutagenesis, Impairment of Fertility

In a two-year study in the mouse, there was an apparent but not statistically significant increase in the incidence of pulmonary adenoma and hepatocellular adenoma. Since findings were inconclusive, the study is being repeated.

Diflunisal did not affect the type or incidence of neoplasia in a 105-week study in the rat.

Diflunisal passes the placental barrier to a minor degree in the rat. Diflunisal had no mutagenic activity after oral administration in the dominant lethal assay, in the Ames microbial mutagen test or in the V-79 Chinese hamster lung cell assay.

No evidence of impaired fertility was found in reproduction studies in rats at doses up to 50 mg/kg/day.

Pregnancy

Pregnancy Category C. A dose of 60 mg/kg/day of diflunisal (equivalent to two times the maximum human dose) was maternotoxic, embryotoxic, and teratogenic in rabbits. In three of six studies in rabbits, evidence of teratogenicity was observed at doses ranging from 40 to 50 mg/kg/day. Teratology studies in mice, at doses up to 45 mg/kg/day, and in rats at doses up to 100 mg/kg/day, revealed no harm to the fetus due to diflunisal. Aspirin and other salicylates have been shown to be teratogenic in a wide variety of species, including the rat and rabbit, at doses ranging from 50 to 400 mg/kg/day (approximately one to eight times the human dose). There are no adequate and well controlled studies with diflunisal in pregnant women. DOLOBID should be used during the first two trimesters of pregnancy only if the potential benefit justifies the potential risk to the fetus. Because of the known effect of drugs of this class on the human fetal cardiovascular system (closure of ductus arteriosus), use during the third trimester of pregnancy is not recommended.

In rats at a dose of one and one-half times the maximum human dose, there was an increase in the average length of gestation. Similar increases in the length of gestation have been observed with aspirin, indomethacin, and phenylbutazone, and may be related to inhibition of prostaglandin synthetase. Drugs of this class may cause dystocia and delayed parturition in pregnant animals.

Nursing Mothers

Diflunisal is excreted in human milk in concentrations of 2–7% of those in plasma. Because of the potential for serious adverse reactions in nursing infants from DOLOBID, a decision should be made whether to discontinue nursing or to discontinue the drug, taking into account the importance of the drug to the mother.

Pediatric Use

The adverse effects observed following diflunisal administration to neonatal animals appear to be species, age, and dose-dependent. At dose levels approximately 3 times the usual human therapeutic dose, both aspirin (200 to 400 mg/kg/day) and diflunisal (80 mg/kg/day) resulted in death, leukocytosis, weight loss, and bilateral cataracts in neonatal (4 to 5-day-old) beagle puppies after 2 to 10 doses. Administration of an 80 mg/kg/day dose of diflunisal to 25-day-old puppies resulted in lower mortality, and did not produce cataracts. In newborn rats, a 400 mg/kg/day dose of aspirin resulted in increased mortality and some cataracts, whereas the effects of diflunisal administration at doses up to 140 mg/kg/day were limited to a decrease in average body weight gain.

Safety and effectiveness in infants and children have not been established, and use of the drug in children below the age of 12 years is not recommended.

ADVERSE REACTIONS

The adverse reactions observed in controlled clinical trials encompass observations in 2,427 patients.

Listed below are the adverse reactions reported in the 1,314 of these patients who received treatment in studies of two weeks or longer. Five hundred thirteen patients were treated for at least 24 weeks, 255 patients were treated for at least 48 weeks, and 46 patients were treated for 96 weeks. In general, the adverse reactions listed below were 2 to 14 times less frequent in the 1,113 patients who received short-term treatment for mild to moderate pain.

Incidence Greater Than 1%

Gastrointestinal

The most frequent types of adverse reactions occurring with DOLOBID are gastrointestinal: these include nausea*, vomiting, dyspepsia*, gastrointestinal pain*, diarrhea*, constipation, and flatulence.

Psychiatric

Somnolence, insomnia.

Central Nervous System

Dizziness.

Special Senses

Tinnitus.

Dermatologic

Rash*.

Miscellaneous

Headache*, fatigue/tiredness.

*Incidence between 3% and 9%. Those reactions occurring in 1% to 3% are not marked with an asterisk.

Incidence Less Than 1 in 100

The following adverse reactions, occurring less frequently than 1 in 100, were reported in clinical trials or since the drug was marketed. The probability exists of a causal relationship between DOLOBID and these adverse reactions.

Dermatologic

Erythema multiforme, exfoliative dermatitis, Stevens-Johnson syndrome, toxic epidermal necrolysis, urticaria, pruritus, sweating, dry mucous membranes, stomatitis, photosensitivity.

Gastrointestinal

Peptic ulcer, gastrointestinal bleeding, anorexia, eructation, gastrointestinal perforation.

Liver function abnormalities; jaundice, sometimes with fever; cholestasis; hepatitis.

Hematologic

Thrombocytopenia.

Genitourinary

Dysuria; renal impairment, including renal failure; interstitial nephritis; hematuria; proteinuria.

Psychiatric

Nervousness, depression, hallucinations, confusion, disorientation.

Central Nervous System

Vertigo; light-headedness; paresthesias.

Special Senses

Transient visual disturbances including blurred vision.

Hypersensitivity Reactions

Acute anaphylactic reaction with bronchospasm.

A potentially life-threatening, apparent hypersensitivity syndrome has been reported. This multisystem syndrome includes constitutional symptoms (fever, chills), and cutaneous findings (see *Dermatologic*). It may also include involvement of major organs (changes in liver function, jaundice, leukopenia, thrombocytopenia, eosinophilia, renal impairment, including renal failure), and less specific findings (adenitis, arthralgia, arthritis, malaise, anorexia, disorientation).

Miscellaneous

Asthenia, edema.

Causal Relationship Unknown

Other reactions have been reported in clinical trials or since the drug was marketed, but occurred under circumstances where a causal relationship could not be established. However, in these rarely reported events, that possibility cannot be excluded. Therefore, these observations are listed to serve as alerting information to physicians.

Respiratory

Dyspnea.

Cardiovascular

Palpitation, syncope.

Musculoskeletal

Muscle cramps.

Miscellaneous

Chest pain.

Potential Adverse Effects

In addition, a variety of adverse effects not observed with DOLOBID in clinical trials or in marketing experience, but reported with other non-steroidal analgesic/anti-inflammatory agents, should be considered potential adverse effects of DOLOBID.

OVERDOSAGE

Cases of overdosage have occurred and deaths have been reported. Most patients recovered without evidence of permanent sequelae. The most common signs and symptoms observed with overdosage were drowsiness, vomiting, nausea, diarrhea, hyperventilation, tachycardia, sweating, tinnitus, disorientation, stupor and coma. Diminished urine output and cardiorespiratory arrest have also been reported. The lowest dosage of DOLOBID at which a death has been reported was 15 grams without the presence of other drugs. In a mixed drug overdose, ingestion of 7.5 grams of DOLOBID resulted in death.

In the event of overdosage, the stomach should be emptied by inducing vomiting or by gastric lavage, and the patient carefully observed and given symptomatic and supportive treatment. Because of the high degree of protein binding, hemodialysis may not be effective.

DOSAGE AND ADMINISTRATION

Concentration-dependent pharmacokinetics prevail when DOLOBID is administered; a doubling of dosage produces a greater than doubling of drug accumulation. The effect becomes more apparent with repetitive doses.

For mild to moderate pain, an initial dose of 1000 mg followed by 500 mg every 12 hours is recommended for most patients. Following the initial dose, some patients may require 500 mg every 8 hours.

A lower dosage may be appropriate depending on such factors as pain severity, patient response, weight, or advanced age; for example, 500 mg initially, followed by 250 mg every 8–12 hours.

For osteoarthritis and rheumatoid arthritis, the suggested dosage range is 500 mg to 1000 mg daily in two divided doses. The dosage of DOLOBID may be increased or decreased according to patient response.
Maintenance doses higher than 1500 mg a day are not recommended.
DOLOBID may be administered with water, milk or meals. Tablets should be swallowed whole, not crushed or chewed.

HOW SUPPLIED

Tablets DOLOBID are capsule-shaped, film-coated tablets supplied as follows:
No. 3390—250 mg peach colored, coded MSD 675
NDC 0006-0675-28 unit dose package of 100
NDC 0006-0675-61 unit of use bottles of 60.
Shown in Product Identification Section, page 417
No. 3392—500 mg orange colored, coded MSD 697
NDC 0006-0697-28 unit dose package of 100
NDC 0006-0697-61 unit of use bottles of 60.
Shown in Product Identification Section, page 417
A.H.F.S. Category: 28:08
DC 7170717 Issued October 1985

EDECRIN® Tablets ℞
(Ethacrynic Acid, MSD), U.S.P.
Intravenous
SODIUM EDECRIN® ℞
(Ethacrynate Sodium, MSD), U.S.P.

EDECRIN® (Ethacrynic Acid, MSD) is a potent diuretic which, if given in excessive amounts, may lead to profound diuresis with water and electrolyte depletion. Therefore, careful medical supervision is required, and dose and dose schedule must be adjusted to the individual patient's needs (see DOSAGE AND ADMINISTRATION).

DESCRIPTION

Ethacrynic acid is an unsaturated ketone derivative of an aryloxyacetic acid. It is designated chemically as [2,3-dichloro-4-(2-methylene-1-oxobutyl)phenoxy] acetic acid, and has a molecular weight of 303.14. Ethacrynic acid is a white, or practically white, crystalline powder, very slightly soluble in water, but soluble in most organic solvents such as alcohols, chloroform, and benzene. Its empirical formula is $C_{13}H_{12}Cl_2O_4$ and its structural formula is:

OCH_2COOH / Cl / Cl / $COCCH_2CH_3$ / CH_2

Ethacrynate sodium, the sodium salt of ethacrynic acid, is soluble in water at 25°C to the extent of about 7 percent. Solutions of the sodium salt are relatively stable at about pH 7 at room temperature for short periods, but as the pH or temperature increases the solutions are less stable. The molecular weight of ethacrynate sodium is 325.12. Its empirical formula is $C_{13}H_{11}Cl_2NaO_4$ and its structural formula is:

OCH_2COONa / Cl / Cl / $COCCH_2CH_3$ / CH_2

EDECRIN is supplied as 25 mg and 50 mg tablets for oral use. Each tablet contains the following inactive ingredients: colloidal silicon dioxide, lactose, magnesium stearate, starch and talc. The 50 mg tablet also contains D&C Yellow 10, FD&C Blue 1 and FD&C Yellow 6. Intravenous SODIUM EDECRIN® (Ethacrynate Sodium, MSD) is a sterile freeze-dried powder and is supplied in a vial containing:
Ethacrynate sodium equivalent to ethacrynic acid ..... 50.0 mg
Inactive ingredients:
Mannitol ..... 62.5 mg
with 0.1 mg thimerosal (mercury derivative) added as preservative.

CLINICAL PHARMACOLOGY

Pharmacokinetics and Metabolism
EDECRIN acts on the ascending limb of the loop of Henle and on the proximal and distal tubules. Urinary output is usually dose dependent and related to the magnitude of fluid accumulation. Water and electrolyte excretion may be increased several times over that observed with thiazide diuretics, since EDECRIN inhibits reabsorption of a much greater proportion of filtered sodium than most other diuretic agents. Therefore, EDECRIN is effective in many patients who have significant degrees of renal insufficiency (see WARNINGS concerning deafness). EDECRIN has little or no effect on glomerular filtration or on renal blood flow, except following pronounced reductions in plasma volume when associated with rapid diuresis.
The electrolyte excretion pattern of ethacrynic acid varies from that of the thiazides and mercurial diuretics. Initial sodium and chloride excretion is usually substantial and chloride loss exceeds that of sodium. With prolonged administration, chloride excretion declines, and potassium and hydrogen ion excretion may increase. EDECRIN is effective whether or not there is clinical acidosis or alkalosis.
Although EDECRIN, in carefully controlled studies in animals and experimental subjects, produces a more favorable sodium/potassium excretion ratio than the thiazides, in patients with increased diuresis excessive amounts of potassium may be excreted.
Onset of action is rapid, usually within 30 minutes after an oral dose of EDECRIN or within 5 minutes after an intravenous injection of SODIUM EDECRIN. After oral use, diuresis peaks in about 2 hours and lasts about 6 to 8 hours.
The sulfhydryl binding propensity of ethacrynic acid differs somewhat from that of the organomercurials. Its mode of action is not by carbonic anhydrase inhibition.
Ethacrynic acid does not cross the blood-brain barrier.

INDICATIONS AND USAGE

EDECRIN is indicated for treatment of edema when an agent with greater diuretic potential than those commonly employed is required.
1. Treatment of the edema associated with congestive heart failure, cirrhosis of the liver, and renal disease, including the nephrotic syndrome.
2. Short-term management of ascites due to malignancy, idiopathic edema, and lymphedema.
3. Short-term management of hospitalized pediatric patients, other than infants, with congenital heart disease or the nephrotic syndrome.
4. Intravenous SODIUM EDECRIN is indicated when a rapid onset of diuresis is desired, e.g., in acute pulmonary edema, or when gastrointestinal absorption is impaired or oral medication is not practicable.

CONTRAINDICATIONS

All diuretics, including ethacrynic acid, are contraindicated in anuria. If increasing electrolyte imbalance, azotemia, and/or oliguria occur during treatment of severe, progressive renal disease, the diuretic should be discontinued.
In a few patients this diuretic has produced severe, watery diarrhea. If this occurs, it should be discontinued and not used again.
Until further experience in infants is accumulated, therapy with oral and parenteral EDECRIN is contraindicated.
Hypersensitivity to any component of this product.

WARNINGS

The effects of EDECRIN on electrolytes are related to its renal pharmacologic activity and are dose dependent. The possibility of profound electrolyte and water loss may be avoided by weighing the patient throughout the treatment period, by careful adjustment of dosage, by initiating treatment with small doses, and by using the drug on an intermittent schedule when possible. When excessive diuresis occurs, the drug should be withdrawn until homeostasis is restored. When excessive electrolyte loss occurs, the dosage should be reduced or the drug temporarily withdrawn.
Initiation of diuretic therapy with EDECRIN in the cirrhotic patient with ascites is best carried out in the hospital. When maintenance therapy has been established, the individual can be satisfactorily followed as an outpatient.
EDECRIN should be given with caution to patients with advanced cirrhosis of the liver, particularly those with a history of previous episodes of electrolyte imbalance or hepatic encephalopathy. Like other diuretics it may precipitate hepatic coma and death.
Too vigorous a diuresis, as evidenced by rapid and excessive weight loss, may induce an acute hypotensive episode. In elderly cardiac patients, rapid contraction of plasma volume and the resultant hemoconcentration should be avoided to prevent the development of thromboembolic episodes, such as cerebral vascular thromboses and pulmonary emboli which may be fatal. Excessive loss of potassium in patients receiving digitalis glycosides may precipitate digitalis toxicity. Care should also be exercised in patients receiving potassium-depleting steroids.
A number of possibly drug-related deaths have occurred in critically ill patients refractory to other diuretics. These generally have fallen into two categories: (1) patients with severe myocardial disease who have been receiving digitalis and presumably developed acute hypokalemia with fatal arrhythmia; (2) patients with severely decompensated hepatic cirrhosis with ascites, with or without accompanying encephalopathy, who were in electrolyte imbalance and died because of intensification of the electrolyte defect.
Deafness, tinnitus, and vertigo with a sense of fullness in the ears have occurred, most frequently in patients with severe impairment of renal function. These symptoms have been associated most often with intravenous administration and with doses in excess of those recommended. The deafness has usually been reversible and of short duration (one to 24 hours). However, in some patients the hearing loss has been permanent. A number of these patients were also receiving drugs known to be ototoxic. EDECRIN may increase the ototoxic potential of other drugs (see PRECAUTIONS, subsection *Drug Interactions*).
Lithium generally should not be given with diuretics (see PRECAUTIONS, subsection *Drug Interactions*).

PRECAUTIONS

General
Weakness, muscle cramps, paresthesias, thirst, anorexia, and signs of hyponatremia, hypokalemia, and/or hypochloremic alkalosis may occur following vigorous or excessive diuresis and these may be accentuated by rigid salt restriction. Rarely tetany has been reported following vigorous diuresis. *During therapy with ethacrynic acid, liberalization of salt intake and supplementary potassium chloride are often necessary.*
When a metabolic alkalosis may be anticipated, e.g., in cirrhosis with ascites, the use of potassium chloride or a potassium-sparing agent before and during therapy with EDECRIN may mitigate or prevent the hypokalemia.
Loop diuretics have been shown to increase the urinary excretion of magnesium; this may result in hypomagnesemia.
The safety and efficacy of ethacrynic acid in hypertension have not been established. However, the dosage of coadministered antihypertensive agents may require adjustment.
Orthostatic hypotension may occur in patients receiving other antihypertensive agents when given ethacrynic acid.
EDECRIN has little or no effect on glomerular filtration or on renal blood flow, except following pronounced reductions in plasma volume when associated with rapid diuresis. A transient increase in serum urea nitrogen may occur. Usually, this is readily reversible when the drug is discontinued.
As with other diuretics used in the treatment of renal edema, hypoproteinemia may reduce responsiveness to ethacrynic acid and the use of salt-poor albumin should be considered.
A number of drugs, including ethacrynic acid, have been shown to displace warfarin from plasma protein; a reduction in the usual anticoagulant dosage may be required in patients receiving both drugs.
EDECRIN may increase the risk of gastric hemorrhage associated with corticosteroid treatment.
Laboratory Tests
Frequent serum electrolyte, CO_2 and BUN determinations should be performed early in therapy and periodically thereafter during active diuresis. Any electrolyte abnormalities should be corrected or the drug temporarily withdrawn.
Increases in blood glucose and alterations in glucose tolerance tests have been observed in patients receiving EDECRIN.
Drug Interactions
Lithium generally should not be given with diuretics because they reduce its renal clearance and add a high risk of lithium toxicity. Read circulars for lithium preparations before use of such concomitant therapy.
EDECRIN may increase the ototoxic potential of other drugs such as aminoglycoside and some cephalosporin antibiotics. Their concurrent use should be avoided.
A number of drugs, including ethacrynic acid, have been shown to displace warfarin from plasma protein; a reduction in the usual anticoagulant dosage may be required in patients receiving both drugs.
In some patients, the administration of a non-steroidal anti-inflammatory agent can reduce the diuretic, natriuretic, and antihypertensive effects of loop, potassium-sparing and thiazide diuretics. Therefore, when EDECRIN and non-steroidal anti-inflammatory agents are used concomitantly, the patient should be observed closely to determine if the desired effect of the diuretic is obtained.

Continued on next page

Information on the Merck Sharp & Dohme products listed on these pages is the full prescribing information from product circulars in use August 31, 1986.

Merck Sharp & Dohme—Cont.

Carcinogenesis, Mutagenesis, Impairment of Fertility
There was no evidence of a tumorigenic effect in a 79-week oral chronic toxicity study in rats at doses up to 45 times the human dose.
Ethacrynic acid had no effect on fertility in a two-litter study in rats or a two-generation study in mice at 10 times the human dose.
Pregnancy
Pregnancy Category B: Reproduction studies in the mouse and rabbit at doses up to 50 times the human dose showed no evidence of external abnormalities of the fetus due to EDECRIN.
In a two-litter study in the dog and rat, oral doses of 5 or 20 mg/kg/day (2½ or 10 times the human dose), respectively, did not interfere with pregnancy or with growth and development of the pups. Although there was reduction in the mean body weights of the fetuses in a teratogenic study in the rat at a dose level of 100 mg/kg (50 times the human dose), there was no effect on mortality or postnatal development. Functional and morphologic abnormalities were not observed.
There are, however, no adequate and well-controlled studies in pregnant women. Since animal reproduction studies are not always predictive of human response, EDECRIN should be used during pregnancy only if clearly needed.
Nursing Mothers
It is not known whether this drug is excreted in human milk. Because many drugs are excreted in human milk and because of the potential for serious adverse reactions in nursing infants from EDECRIN, a decision should be made whether to discontinue nursing or to discontinue the drug, taking into account the importance of the drug to the mother.
Pediatric Use
For information on oral use in pediatrics, other than infants, see INDICATIONS AND USAGE and DOSAGE AND ADMINISTRATION.
Safety and effectiveness in infants have not been established (see CONTRAINDICATIONS).
Safety and effectiveness of intravenous use in children have not been established (see DOSAGE AND ADMINISTRATION, *Intravenous Use*).

ADVERSE REACTIONS

Gastrointestinal
Anorexia, malaise, abdominal discomfort or pain, dysphagia, nausea, vomiting, and diarrhea have occurred. These are more frequent with large doses or after one to three months of continuous therapy. A few patients have had sudden onset of profuse, watery diarrhea. Discontinue EDECRIN if diarrhea is severe and do not give it again. Gastrointestinal bleeding has occurred in some patients. Rarely, acute pancreatitis has been reported.
Metabolic
Reversible hyperuricemia and acute gout have been reported. Acute symptomatic hypoglycemia with convulsions occurred in two uremic patients who received doses above those recommended. Hyperglycemia has been reported. Rarely, jaundice and abnormal liver function tests have been reported in seriously ill patients receiving multiple drug therapy, including EDECRIN.
Hematologic
Agranulocytosis or severe neutropenia has been reported in a few critically ill patients also receiving agents known to produce this effect. Thrombocytopenia has been reported rarely. Henoch-Schönlein purpura has been reported rarely in patients with rheumatic heart disease receiving multiple drug therapy, including EDECRIN.
Special Senses (See WARNINGS)
Deafness, tinnitus and vertigo with a sense of fullness in the ears, and blurred vision have occurred.
Central Nervous System
Headache, fatigue, apprehension, confusion.
Miscellaneous
Skin rash, fever, chills, hematuria.
SODIUM EDECRIN occasionally has caused local irritation and pain after intravenous use.

OVERDOSAGE

Overdosage may lead to excessive diuresis with electrolyte depletion and dehydration.
In the event of overdosage, symptomatic and supportive measures should be employed. Emesis should be induced or gastric lavage performed. Correct dehydration, electrolyte imbalance, hepatic coma, and hypotension by established procedures. If required, give oxygen or artificial respiration for respiratory impairment.
In the mouse, the oral LD_{50} of ethacrynic acid is 627 mg/kg and the intravenous LD_{50} of ethacrynate sodium is 175 mg/kg.

DOSAGE AND ADMINISTRATION

Dosage must be regulated carefully to prevent a more rapid or substantial loss of fluid or electrolyte than is indicated or necessary. The magnitude of diuresis and natriuresis is largely dependent on the degree of fluid accumulation present in the patient. Similarly, the extent of potassium excretion is determined in large measure by the presence and magnitude of aldosteronism.
Oral Use
EDECRIN is available for oral use as 25 mg and 50 mg tablets.
Dosage: To Initiate Diuresis
In Adults: The smallest dose required to produce gradual weight loss (about 1 to 2 pounds per day) is recommended. Onset of diuresis usually occurs at 50 to 100 mg for adults. After diuresis has been achieved, the minimally effective dose (usually from 50 to 200 mg daily) may be given on a continuous or intermittent dosage schedule. Dosage adjustments are usually in 25 to 50 mg increments to avoid derangement of water and electrolyte excretion.
The patient should be weighed under standard conditions before and during the institution of diuretic therapy with this compound. Small alterations in dose should effectively prevent a massive diuretic response. The following schedule may be helpful in determining the smallest effective dose.
Day 1—50 mg (single dose) after a meal
Day 2—50 mg twice daily after meals, if necessary
Day 3—100 mg in the morning and 50 to 100 mg following the afternoon or evening meal, depending upon response to the morning dose
A few patients may require initial and maintenance doses as high as 200 mg twice daily. These higher doses, which should be achieved gradually, are most often required in patients with severe, refractory edema.
In children (excluding infants, see CONTRAINDICATIONS): The initial dose should be 25 mg. Careful stepwise increments in dosage of 25 mg should be made to achieve effective maintenance.
Maintenance Therapy
It is usually possible to reduce the dosage and frequency of administration once dry weight has been achieved.
EDECRIN (Ethacrynic Acid, MSD) may be given intermittently after an effective diuresis is obtained with the regimen outlined above. Dosage may be on an alternate daily schedule or more prolonged periods of diuretic therapy may be interspersed with rest periods. Such an intermittent dosage schedule allows time for correction of any electrolyte imbalance and may provide a more efficient diuretic response.
The chloruretic effect of this agent may give rise to retention of bicarbonate and a metabolic alkalosis. This may be corrected by giving chloride (ammonium chloride or arginine chloride). Ammonium chloride should not be given to cirrhotic patients.
EDECRIN has additive effects when used with other diuretics. For example, a patient who is on maintenance dosage of an oral diuretic may require additional intermittent diuretic therapy, such as an organomercurial, for the maintenance of basal weight. The intermittent use of EDECRIN orally may eliminate the need for injections of organomercurials. Small doses of EDECRIN may be added to existing diuretic regimens to maintain basal weight. This drug may potentiate the action of carbonic anhydrase inhibitors, with augmentation of natriuresis and kaliuresis. Therefore, when adding EDECRIN the initial dose and changes of dose should be in 25 mg increments, to avoid electrolyte depletion. Rarely, patients who failed to respond to ethacrynic acid have responded to older established agents.
While many patients do not require supplemental potassium, the use of potassium chloride or potassium-sparing agents, or both, during treatment with EDECRIN is advisable, especially in cirrhotic or nephrotic patients and in patients receiving digitalis.
Salt liberalization usually prevents the development of hyponatremia and hypochloremia. During treatment with EDECRIN, salt may be liberalized to a greater extent than with other diuretics. Cirrhotic patients, however, usually require at least moderate salt restriction concomitant with diuretic therapy.
Intravenous Use
Intravenous SODIUM EDECRIN is for intravenous use when oral intake is impractical or in urgent conditions, such as acute pulmonary edema.
The usual intravenous dose for the average sized adult is 50 mg, or 0.5 to 1.0 mg per kg of body weight. Usually only one dose has been necessary; occasionally a second dose at a new injection site, to avoid possible thrombophlebitis, may be required. A single intravenous dose not exceeding 100 mg has been used in critical situations.
Insufficient pediatric experience precludes recommendation for this age group.
To reconstitute the dry material, add 50 mL of 5 percent Dextrose Injection, or Sodium Chloride Injection to the vial. Occasionally, some 5 percent Dextrose Injection solutions may have a low pH (below 5). The resulting solution with such a diluent may be hazy or opalescent. Intravenous use of such a solution is not recommended. Inspect the vial containing Intravenous SODIUM EDECRIN for particulate matter and discoloration before use.
The solution may be given slowly through the tubing of a running infusion or by direct intravenous injection over a period of several minutes. Do not mix this solution with whole blood or its derivatives. Discard unused reconstituted solution after 24 hours.
SODIUM EDECRIN should not be given subcutaneously or intramuscularly because of local pain and irritation.

HOW SUPPLIED

No. 3321—Tablets EDECRIN, 25 mg, are white, capsule shaped, scored tablets, coded MSD 65. They are supplied as follows:
NDC 0006-0065-68 in bottles of 100.
Shown in Product Identification Section, page 417
No. 3322—Tablets EDECRIN, 50 mg, are green, capsule shaped, scored tablets, coded MSD 90. They are supplied as follows:
NDC 0006-0090-68 in bottles of 100.
Shown in Product Identification Section, page 417
No. 3330—Intravenous SODIUM EDECRIN is a dry white material either in a plug form or as a powder. It is supplied in vials containing ethacrynate sodium equivalent to 50 mg of ethacrynic acid, **NDC** 0006-3330-50.
A.H.F.S. Category: 40:28
DC 7413624 Issued October 1985

ELAVIL® Tablets ℞
(Amitriptyline HCl, MSD), U.S.P.
ELAVIL® Injection ℞
(Amitriptyline HCl, MSD), U.S.P.

DESCRIPTION

Amitriptyline HCl, a dibenzocycloheptadiene derivative, is a white or practically white, crystalline compound that is freely soluble in water.
It is designated chemically as 10,11-dihydro-*N,N*-dimethyl-5*H*-dibenzo [*a,d*] cycloheptene- Δ^5,γ-propylamine hydrochloride. The molecular weight is 313.87. The empirical formula is $C_{20}H_{23}N \cdot HCl$, and the structural formula is:

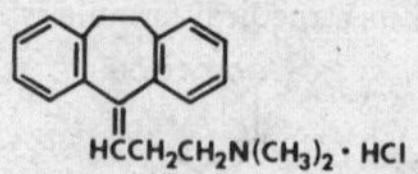

ELAVIL® (Amitriptyline HCl, MSD) is supplied as 10 mg, 25 mg, 50 mg, 75 mg, 100 mg, and 150 mg tablets and as a sterile solution for intramuscular use. Inactive ingredients of the tablets are calcium phosphate, cellulose, colloidal silicon dioxide, hydroxypropyl cellulose, hydroxypropyl methylcellulose, lactose, magnesium stearate, starch, stearic acid, talc, and titanium dioxide. Tablets ELAVIL 10 mg also contain FD&C Blue 1. Tablets ELAVIL 25 mg also contain D&C Yellow 10, FD&C Blue 1, and FD&C Yellow 6. Tablets ELAVIL 50 mg also contain D&C Yellow 10, FD&C Yellow 6 and iron oxide. Tablets ELAVIL 75 mg also contain FD&C Yellow 6. Tablets ELAVIL 100 mg also contain FD&C Blue 2 and FD&C Red 40. Tablets ELAVIL 150 mg also contain FD&C Blue 2 and FD&C Yellow 6. Each milliliter of the sterile solution contains:
Amitriptyline hydrochloride .... 10 mg
Dextrose .... 44 mg
Water for Injection, q.s. .... 1 mL
Added as preservatives:
Methylparaben .... 1.5 mg
Propylparaben .... 0.2 mg

ACTIONS

ELAVIL is an antidepressant with sedative effects. Its mechanism of action in man is not known. It is not a monoamine oxidase inhibitor and it does not act primarily by stimulation of the central nervous system.
Amitriptyline inhibits the membrane pump mechanism responsible for uptake of norepinephrine and serotonin in adrenergic and serotonergic neurons. Pharmacologically this action may potentiate or prolong neuronal activity since reuptake of these biogenic amines is important physiologically in terminating transmitting activity. This interference with the reuptake of norepinephrine and/or serotonin is believed by some to underlie the antidepressant activity of amitriptyline.

INDICATIONS

For the relief of symptoms of depression. Endogenous depression is more likely to be alleviated than are other depressive states.

CONTRAINDICATIONS

ELAVIL is contraindicated in patients who have shown prior hypersensitivity to it.
It should not be given concomitantly with monoamine oxidase inhibitors. Hyperpyretic crises, severe convulsions, and deaths have occurred in patients receiving tricyclic antidepressant and monoamine oxidase inhibiting drugs simultaneously. When it is desired to replace a monoamine oxidase inhibitor with ELAVIL, a minimum of 14 days should be allowed to elapse after the former is discontinued. ELAVIL should then be initiated cautiously with gradual increase in dosage until optimum response is achieved.
This drug is not recommended for use during the acute recovery phase following myocardial infarction.

WARNINGS

ELAVIL may block the antihypertensive action of guanethidine or similarly acting compounds.
It should be used with caution in patients with a history of seizures and, because of its atropine-like action, in patients with a history of urinary retention, angle-closure glaucoma or increased intraocular pressure. In patients with angle-closure glaucoma, even average doses may precipitate an attack.
Patients with cardiovascular disorders should be watched closely. Tricyclic antidepressant drugs, including ELAVIL, particularly when given in high doses, have been reported to produce arrhythmias, sinus tachycardia, and prolongation of the conduction time. Myocardial infarction and stroke have been reported with drugs of this class.
Close supervision is required when ELAVIL is given to hyperthyroid patients or those receiving thyroid medication.
ELAVIL may enhance the response to alcohol and the effects of barbiturates and other CNS depressants. In patients who may use alcohol excessively, it should be borne in mind that the potentiation may increase the danger inherent in any suicide attempt or overdosage. Delirium has been reported with concurrent administration of amitriptyline and disulfiram.
Usage in Pregnancy—Safe use of ELAVIL during pregnancy and lactation has not been established; therefore, in administering the drug to pregnant patients, nursing mothers, or women who may become pregnant, the possible benefits must be weighed against the possible hazards to mother and child.
Animal reproduction studies have been inconclusive and clinical experience has been limited.
Usage in Children—In view of the lack of experience with the use of this drug in children, it is not recommended at the present time for patients under 12 years of age.

PRECAUTIONS

Schizophrenic patients may develop increased symptoms of psychosis; patients with paranoid symptomatology may have an exaggeration of such symptoms. Depressed patients, particularly those with known manic-depressive illness, may experience a shift to mania or hypomania. In these circumstances the dose of amitriptyline may be reduced or a major tranquilizer such as perphenazine may be administered concurrently.
When ELAVIL is given with anticholinergic agents or sympathomimetic drugs, including epinephrine combined with local anesthetics, close supervision and careful adjustment of dosages are required.
Paralytic ileus may occur in patients taking tricyclic antidepressants in combination with anticholinergic-type drugs.
Cimetidine is reported to reduce hepatic metabolism of certain tricyclic antidepressants, thereby delaying elimination and increasing steady-state concentrations of these drugs. Clinically significant effects have been reported with the tricyclic antidepressants when used concomitantly with cimetidine.
Increases in plasma levels of tricyclic antidepressants, and in the frequency and severity of side effects, particularly anticholinergic, have been reported when cimetidine was added to the drug regimen. Discontinuation of cimetidine in well-controlled patients receiving tricyclic antidepressants and cimetidine may decrease the plasma levels and efficacy of the antidepressants.
Caution is advised if patients receive large doses of ethchlorvynol concurrently. Transient delirium has been reported in patients who were treated with one gram of ethchlorvynol and 75-150 mg of ELAVIL.
The possibility of suicide in depressed patients remains until significant remission occurs. Potentially suicidal patients should not have access to large quantities of this drug. Prescriptions should be written for the smallest amount feasible.
Concurrent administration of ELAVIL and electroshock therapy may increase the hazards associated with such therapy. Such treatment should be limited to patients for whom it is essential.
When possible, the drug should be discontinued several days before elective surgery.
Both elevation and lowering of blood sugar levels have been reported.
ELAVIL should be used with caution in patients with impaired liver function.
Information for Patients
While on therapy with ELAVIL, patients should be advised as to the possible impairment of mental and/or physical abilities required for performance of hazardous tasks, such as operating machinery or driving a motor vehicle.

ADVERSE REACTIONS

Note: Included in the listing which follows are a few adverse reactions which have not been reported with this specific drug. However, pharmacological similarities among the tricyclic antidepressant drugs require that each of the reactions be considered when amitriptyline is administered.
Cardiovascular: Hypotension, particularly orthostatic hypotension; hypertension; tachycardia; palpitation; myocardial infarction; arrhythmias; heart block; stroke.
CNS and Neuromuscular: Confusional states; disturbed concentration; disorientation; delusions; hallucinations; excitement; anxiety; restlessness; insomnia; nightmares; numbness, tingling, and paresthesias of the extremities; peripheral neuropathy; incoordination; ataxia; tremors; seizures; alteration in EEG patterns; extrapyramidal symptoms; tinnitus; syndrome of inappropriate ADH (antidiuretic hormone) secretion.
Anticholinergic: Dry mouth, blurred vision, disturbance of accommodation, increased intraocular pressure, constipation, paralytic ileus, urinary retention, dilatation of urinary tract.
Allergic: Skin rash, urticaria, photosensitization, edema of face and tongue.
Hematologic: Bone marrow depression including agranulocytosis, leukopenia, eosinophilia, purpura, thrombocytopenia.
Gastrointestinal: Nausea, epigastric distress, vomiting, anorexia, stomatitis, peculiar taste, diarrhea, parotid swelling, black tongue. Rarely hepatitis (including altered liver function and jaundice).
Endocrine: Testicular swelling and gynecomastia in the male, breast enlargement and galactorrhea in the female, increased or decreased libido, elevation and lowering of blood sugar levels.
Other: Dizziness, weakness, fatigue, headache, weight gain or loss, edema, increased perspiration, urinary frequency, mydriasis, drowsiness, alopecia.
Withdrawal Symptoms: After prolonged administration, abrupt cessation of treatment may produce nausea, headache, and malaise. Gradual dosage reduction has been reported to produce, within two weeks, transient symptoms including irritability, restlessness, and dream and sleep disturbance. These symptoms are not indicative of addiction. Rare instances have been reported of mania or hypomania occurring within 2–7 days following cessation of chronic therapy with tricyclic antidepressants.

DOSAGE AND ADMINISTRATION

Oral Dosage
Dosage should be initiated at a low level and increased gradually, noting carefully the clinical response and any evidence of intolerance.
Initial Dosage for Adults—For outpatients 75 mg of amitriptyline HCl a day in divided doses usually is satisfactory. If necessary, this may be increased to a total of 150 mg per day. Increases are made preferably in the late afternoon and/or bedtime doses. A sedative effect may be apparent before the antidepressant effect is noted, but an adequate therapeutic effect may take as long as 30 days to develop.
An alternate method of initiating therapy in outpatients is to begin with 50 to 100 mg amitriptyline HCl at bedtime. This may be increased by 25 or 50 mg as necessary in the bedtime dose to a total of 150 mg per day.
Hospitalized patients may require 100 mg a day initially. This can be increased gradually to 200 mg a day if necessary. A small number of hospitalized patients may need as much as 300 mg a day.
Adolescent and Elderly Patients—In general, lower dosages are recommended for these patients. Ten mg 3 times a day with 20 mg at bedtime may be satisfactory in adolescent and elderly patients who do not tolerate higher dosages.
Maintenance—The usual maintenance dosage of amitriptyline HCl is 50 to 100 mg per day. In some patients 40 mg per day is sufficient. For maintenance therapy the total daily dosage may be given in a single dose preferably at bedtime. When satisfactory improvement has been reached, dosage should be reduced to the lowest amount that will maintain relief of symptoms. It is appropriate to continue maintenance therapy 3 months or longer to lessen the possibility of relapse.
Intramuscular Dosage
Initially, 20 to 30 mg (2 to 3 mL) four times a day.
When ELAVIL injection is administered intramuscularly, the effects may appear more rapidly than with oral administration.
When ELAVIL injection is used for initial therapy in patients unable or unwilling to take ELAVIL tablets, the tablets should replace the injection as soon as possible.
Usage in Children
In view of the lack of experience with the use of this drug in children, it is not recommended at the present time for patients under 12 years of age.
Plasma Levels
Because of the wide variation in the absorption and distribution of tricyclic antidepressants in body fluids, it is difficult to directly correlate plasma levels and therapeutic effect. However, determination of plasma levels may be useful in identifying patients who appear to have toxic effects and may have excessively high levels, or those in whom lack of absorption or noncompliance is suspected. Adjustments in dosage should be made according to the patient's clinical response and not on the basis of plasma levels.*

OVERDOSAGE

Manifestations—High doses may cause temporary confusion, disturbed concentration, or transient visual hallucinations. Overdosage may cause drowsiness; hypothermia; tachycardia and other arrhythmic abnormalities, such as bundle branch block; ECG evidence of impaired conduction; congestive heart failure; dilated pupils; disorders of ocular motility; convulsions; severe hypotension; stupor; and coma. Other symptoms may be agitation, hyperactive reflexes, muscle rigidity, vomiting, hyperpyrexia, or any of those listed under ADVERSE REACTIONS.
All patients suspected of having taken an overdosage should be admitted to a hospital as soon as possible. *Treatment* is symptomatic and supportive. Empty the stomach as quickly as possible by emesis followed by gastric lavage upon arrival at the hospital. Following gastric lavage, activated charcoal may be administered. Twenty to 30 g of activated charcoal may be given every four to six hours during the first 24 to 48 hours after ingestion. An ECG should be taken and close monitoring of cardiac function instituted if there is any sign of abnormality. Maintain an open airway and adequate fluid intake; regulate body temperature.
The intravenous administration of 1–3 mg of physostigmine salicylate is reported to reverse the symptoms of tricyclic antidepressant poisoning. Because physostigmine is rapidly metabolized, the dosage of physostigmine should be repeated as required particularly if life threatening signs such as arrhythmias, convulsions, and deep coma recur or persist after the initial dosage of physostigmine. Because physostigmine itself may be toxic, it is not recommended for routine use.
Standard measures should be used to manage circulatory shock and metabolic acidosis. Cardiac arrhythmias may be treated with neostigmine, pyridostigmine, or propranolol. Should cardiac failure occur, the use of digitalis should be considered. Close monitoring of cardiac function for not less than five days is advisable.
Anticonvulsants may be given to control convulsions. Amitriptyline increases the CNS depressant action but not the anticonvulsant action of barbiturates; therefore, an inhalation anesthetic, diazepam, or paraldehyde is recommended for control of convulsions.
Dialysis is of no value because of low plasma concentrations of the drug.
Since overdosage is often deliberate, patients may attempt suicide by other means during the recovery phase.
Deaths by deliberate or accidental overdosage have occurred with this class of drugs.

HOW SUPPLIED

No. 3287—Tablets ELAVIL, 10 mg, are blue, round, film coated tablets, coded MSD 23. They are supplied as follows:
NDC 0006-0023-68 bottles of 100
(6505-00-079-7453, 10 mg 100's)
NDC 0006-0023-28 unit dose packages of 100
NDC 0006-0023-82 bottles of 1000
NDC 0006-0023-86 bottles of 5000.
Shown in Product Identification Section, page 417

*Hollister, L. E., J. Amer. Med. Ass. *241:* 2530–2533, June 8, 1979.

Continued on next page

Information on the Merck Sharp & Dohme products listed on these pages is the full prescribing information from product circulars in use August 31, 1986.

Merck Sharp & Dohme—Cont.

No. 3288—Tablets ELAVIL, 25 mg, are yellow, round, film coated tablets, coded MSD 45. They are supplied as follows:
NDC 0006-0045-68 bottles of 100
(6505-00-082-2659, 25 mg 100's)
NDC 0006-0045-28 unit dose packages of 100
(6505-00-118-2509, 25 mg individually sealed 100's)
NDC 0006-0045-82 bottles of 1000
(6505-00-724-6358, 25 mg 1000's)
NDC 0006-0045-86 bottles of 5000.
Shown in Product Identification Section, page 417
No. 3320—Tablets ELAVIL, 50 mg, are beige, round, film coated tablets, coded MSD 102. They are supplied as follows:
NDC 0006-0102-68 bottles of 100
NDC 0006-0102-28 unit dose packages of 100
NDC 0006-0102-82 bottles of 1000.
Shown in Product Identification Section, page 417
No. 3348—Tablets ELAVIL, 75 mg, are orange, round, film coated tablets, coded MSD 430. They are supplied as follows:
NDC 0006-0430-68 bottles of 100
NDC 0006-0430-28 unit dose packages of 100.
Shown in Product Identification Section, page 417
No. 3349—Tablets ELAVIL, 100 mg, are mauve, round, film coated tablets, coded MSD 435. They are supplied as follows:
NDC 0006-0435-68 bottles of 100
NDC 0006-0435-28 unit dose packages of 100.
Shown in Product Identification Section, page 417
No. 3351—Tablets ELAVIL, 150 mg, are blue, capsule shaped, film coated tablets, coded MSD 673. They are supplied as follows:
NDC 0006-0673-30 bottles of 30
NDC 0006-0673-68 bottles of 100
NDC 0006-0673-28 unit dose packages of 100.
Shown in Product Identification Section, page 417
No. 3286—Injection ELAVIL, 10 mg/mL, is a clear, colorless solution, and is supplied as follows:
NDC 0006-3286-10 in 10 mL vials.

METABOLISM

Studies in man following oral administration of ^{14}C-labeled drug indicated that amitriptyline is rapidly absorbed and metabolized. Radioactivity of the plasma was practically negligible, although significant amounts of radioactivity appeared in the urine by 4 to 6 hours and one-half to one-third of the drug was excreted within 24 hours.
Amitriptyline is metabolized by N-demethylation and bridge hydroxylation in man, rabbit, and rat. Virtually the entire dose is excreted as glucuronide or sulfate conjugate of metabolites, with little unchanged drug appearing in the urine. Other metabolic pathways may be involved.

A.H.F.S. Category: 28:16:04
DC 6613126 Issued October 1985

ELSPAR®
(Asparaginase, MSD) ℞

WARNING

IT IS RECOMMENDED THAT ASPARAGINASE BE ADMINISTERED TO PATIENTS ONLY IN A HOSPITAL SETTING UNDER THE SUPERVISION OF A PHYSICIAN WHO IS QUALIFIED BY TRAINING AND EXPERIENCE TO ADMINISTER CANCER CHEMOTHERAPEUTIC AGENTS, BECAUSE OF THE POSSIBILITY OF SEVERE REACTIONS, INCLUDING ANAPHYLAXIS AND SUDDEN DEATH. THE PHYSICIAN MUST BE PREPARED TO TREAT ANAPHYLAXIS AT EACH ADMINISTRATION OF THE DRUG.
IN THE TREATMENT OF EACH PATIENT THE PHYSICIAN MUST WEIGH CAREFULLY THE POSSIBILITY OF ACHIEVING THERAPEUTIC BENEFIT VERSUS THE RISK OF TOXICITY. THE FOLLOWING DATA SHOULD BE THOROUGHLY REVIEWED BEFORE ADMINISTERING THE COMPOUND.

DESCRIPTION

ELSPAR® (Asparaginase, MSD) contains the enzyme L-asparagine amidohydrolase, type EC-2, derived from *Escherichia coli.* It is a white crystalline powder that is freely soluble in water and practically insoluble in methanol, acetone and chloroform. Its activity is expressed in terms of International Units (I.U.) according to the recommendation of the International Union of Biochemistry. The specific activity of ELSPAR is at least 225 I.U. per milligram of protein and each vial contains 10,000 I.U. of asparaginase and 80 mg of mannitol, an inactive ingredient, as a sterile, white lyophilized plug or powder for intravenous or intramuscular injection after reconstitution.

CLINICAL PHARMACOLOGY

Action
In a significant number of patients with acute leukemia, particularly lymphocytic, the malignant cells are dependent on an exogenous source of asparagine for survival. Normal cells, however, are able to synthesize asparagine and thus are affected less by the rapid depletion produced by treatment with the enzyme asparaginase. This is a unique approach to therapy based on a metabolic defect in asparagine synthesis of some malignant cells. ELSPAR, derived from *Escherichia coli,* is effective in inducing remissions in some patients with acute lymphocytic leukemia.

Asparagine Dependence Test
An asparagine dependence test has been utilized during the investigational studies. In this test leukemic cells obtained from some marrow cultures could be shown to require asparagine in *vitro,* suggesting sensitivity to asparaginase therapy in *vivo.* However, present data indicate that the correlation between asparagine dependence in such tests and the final response to therapy is sufficiently poor that the test is not recommended as a basis for selection of patients for treatment.
Pharmacokinetics and Metabolism
In a study in patients with metastatic cancer and leukemia, initial plasma levels of L-asparaginase following intravenous administration were correlated to dose. Daily administration resulted in a cumulative increase in plasma levels. Plasma half-life varied from 8 to 30 hours; it did not appear to be influenced by dosage, either single or repetitive, and could not be correlated with age, sex, surface area, renal or hepatic function, diagnosis or extent of disease. Apparent volume of distribution was approximately 70–80% of estimated plasma volume. There was some slow movement of asparaginase from vascular to extravascular, extracellular space. L-asparaginase was detected in the lymph. Cerebrospinal fluid levels were less than 1% of concurrent plasma levels. Only trace amounts appeared in the urine.
In a study in which patients with leukemia and metastatic cancer received intramuscular L-asparaginase, peak plasma levels of asparaginase were reached 14 to 24 hours after dosing. Plasma half-life was 39 to 49 hours. No asparaginase was detected in the urine.

INDICATIONS AND USAGE

ELSPAR is indicated in the therapy of patients with acute lymphocytic leukemia. This agent is useful primarily in combination with other chemotherapeutic agents in the induction of remissions of the disease in children. ELSPAR should not be used as the sole induction agent unless combination therapy is deemed inappropriate. ELSPAR is not recommended for maintenance therapy.

CONTRAINDICATIONS

ELSPAR is contraindicated in patients with pancreatitis or a history of pancreatitis. Acute hemorrhagic pancreatitis, in some instances fatal, has been reported following asparaginase administration. Asparaginase is also contraindicated in patients who have had previous anaphylactic reactions to it.

WARNINGS

Allergic reactions to asparaginase are frequent and may occur during the primary course of therapy. They are not completely predictable on the basis of the intradermal skin test. Anaphylaxis and death have occurred even in a hospital setting with experienced observers.
Once a patient has received ELSPAR as part of a treatment regimen, retreatment with this agent at a later time is associated with increased risk of hypersensitivity reactions. In patients found by skin testing to be hypersensitive to asparaginase, and in any patient who has received a previous course of therapy with asparaginase, therapy with this agent should be instituted or reinstituted only after successful desensitization, and then only if in the judgement of the physician the possible benefit is greater than the increased risk. Desensitization itself may be hazardous. (See DOSAGE AND ADMINISTRATION, *Intradermal Skin Test.*)
In view of the unpredictability of the adverse reactions to asparaginase, it is recommended that this product be used in a hospital setting. Asparaginase has an adverse effect on liver function in the majority of patients. Therapy with asparaginase may increase pre-existing liver impairment caused by prior therapy or the underlying disease. Because of this there is a possibility that asparaginase may increase the toxicity of other medications.
The administration of ELSPAR *intravenously concurrently with or immediately before* a course of vincristine and prednisone may be associated with increased toxicity. (See DOSAGE AND ADMINISTRATION, *Recommended Induction Regimens.*)

PRECAUTIONS

General
This drug may be a contact irritant and both powder and solution must be handled and administered with care. Inhalation of dust or vapors and contact with skin or mucous membranes, especially those of the eyes, must be avoided. In case of contact, wash with copious amounts of water for at least 15 minutes.
Asparaginase has been reported to have immunosuppressive activity in animal experiments. Accordingly, the possibility that use of the drug in man may predispose to infection should be considered.
Asparaginase toxicity is reported to be greater in adults than in children.
Laboratory Tests
The fall in circulating lymphoblasts often is quite marked; normal or below normal leukocyte counts are noted frequently within the first several days after initiating therapy. This may be accompanied by a marked rise in serum uric acid. The possible development of uric acid nephropathy should be borne in mind. Appropriate preventive measures should be taken, e.g., allopurinol, increased fluid intake, alkalization of urine. As a guide to the effects of therapy, the patient's peripheral blood count and bone marrow should be monitored frequently.
Frequent serum amylase determinations should be obtained to detect early evidence of pancreatitis. If pancreatitis occurs, therapy should be stopped and not reinstituted.
Blood sugar should be monitored during therapy with ELSPAR because hyperglycemia may occur.
Drug Interactions
Tissue culture and animal studies indicate that ELSPAR can diminish or abolish the effect of methotrexate on malignant cells. This effect on methotrexate activity persists as long as plasma asparagine levels are suppressed. These results would seem to dictate against the clinical use of methotrexate with ELSPAR, or during the period following ELSPAR therapy when plasma asparagine levels are below normal.
Drug/Laboratory Test Interactions
L-asparaginase has been reported to interfere with the interpretation of thyroid function tests by producing a rapid and marked reduction in serum concentrations of thyroxine-binding globulin within two days after the first dose. Serum concentrations of thyroxine-binding globulin returned to pretreatment values within four weeks of the last dose of L-asparaginase.
Animal Toxicology
A one-month intravenous toxicity study of ELSPAR in dogs at doses of 250, 1000, and 2000 I.U./kg/day revealed reduced serum total protein and albumin with loss of body weight at the highest dose level and anorexia, emesis, and diarrhea at all dosage levels. A similar study in monkeys at doses of 100, 300, and 1000 I.U./kg/day also revealed reduction of serum total protein and albumin and body weight loss at all dosage levels. Bromsulfalein retention and fatty changes in the liver were noted in monkeys that were given 300 and 1000 I.U./kg/day. The rabbit was unusually sensitive to ELSPAR since a single intravenous dose of 1000 I.U./kg caused hypocalcemia associated with necrosis of the parathyroid cells, convulsions, and death in about one third of the animals. Some rabbits that died showed small thymic and lymph node hemorrhages and necrosis of the germinal centers in the lymph nodes and spleen. The intravenous administration of calcium gluconate alleviated or prevented the adverse effects.
Changes in the pancreatic islets (not pancreatitis) ranging from edema to necrosis were observed in the rabbits in the acute intravenous toxicity studies (doses of 12,500 to 50,000 I.U./kg) but not in rabbits that received 1000 I.U./kg. The anatomical changes and the hypocalcemia found in the rabbits were not observed in the subacute intravenous studies in the dogs and monkeys.
Carcinogenesis, Mutagenesis, Impairment of Fertility
The intraperitoneal injection of 2500 I.U./kg/ day for 4 days in newborn Swiss mice resulted in a small increase in pulmonary adenomas; lymphatic leukemia was not increased.
L-asparaginase at concentrations of 152-909 I.U./plate was not mutagenic in the Ames microbial mutagen test with or without metabolic activation.
There are no adequate studies on the effects of asparaginase on fertility.
Pregnancy
Pregnancy Category C. In mice and rats ELSPAR has been shown to retard the weight gain of mothers and fetuses when given in doses of more than 1000 I.U./kg (the recommended human dose). Resorptions, gross abnormalities and skeletal abnormalities were observed. The intravenous administration of 50 or 100 I.U./kg (one-twentieth or one-tenth of the human dose) to pregnant rabbits on Day 8 and 9 of gestation resulted in dose dependent embryotoxicity and gross abnormalities. There are no adequate and well-controlled studies in pregnant women. ELSPAR should be used during pregnancy only if the potential benefit justifies the potential risk to the fetus.

Nursing Mothers
It is not known whether this drug is secreted in human milk. Because many drugs are secreted in human milk and because of the potential for serious adverse reactions in nursing infants from ELSPAR, a decision should be made whether to discontinue nursing or to discontinue the drug, taking into account the importance of the drug to the mother.

ADVERSE REACTIONS

Allergic reactions, including skin rashes, urticaria, arthralgia, respiratory distress, and acute anaphylaxis have been reported. (See WARNINGS.) Acute reactions have occurred in the absence of a positive skin test and during continued maintenance of therapeutic serum levels of ELSPAR.
In children with advanced leukemia, a lower incidence of anaphylaxis has been reported with intramuscular administration, although there was a higher incidence of milder hypersensitivity reactions than with intravenous administration.
Fatal hyperthermia has been reported.
Pancreatitis, sometimes fulminant and fatal, has occurred during or following therapy with ELSPAR.
Hyperglycemia with glucosuria and polyuria has been reported in low incidence. Serum and urine acetone usually have been absent or negligible in these patients; this syndrome thus resembles hyperosmolar, nonketotic, hyperglycemia induced by a variety of other agents. This complication usually responds to discontinuance of ELSPAR, judicious use of intravenous fluid, and insulin, but may be fatal on occasion.
In addition to hypofibrinogenemia, depression of various other clotting factors has been reported. Most marked has been a decrease in plasma levels of factors V and VIII with a variable decrease in factors VII and IX. A decrease in circulating platelets has occurred in low incidence which, together with the increased levels of fibrin degradation products in the serum, may indicate development of a consumption coagulopathy. Bleeding has been a problem in only a minority of patients with demonstrable coagulopathy. However, intracranial hemorrhage and fatal bleeding associated with low fibrinogen levels have been reported. Increased fibrinolytic activity, apparently compensatory in nature, also has occurred.
Some patients have shown central nervous system effects consisting of depression, somnolence, fatigue, coma, confusion, agitation, and hallucinations varying from mild to severe. Rarely, a Parkinson-like syndrome has occurred, with tremor and a progressive increase in muscular tone. These side effects usually have reversed spontaneously after treatment was stopped. Therapy with ELSPAR is associated with an increase in blood ammonia during the conversion of asparagine to asparatic acid by the enzyme. No clear correlation exists between the degree of elevation of blood ammonia levels and the appearance of CNS changes. Chills, fever, nausea, vomiting, anorexia, abdominal cramps, weight loss, headache, and irritability may occur and usually are mild.
Azotemia, usually pre-renal, occurs frequently. Acute renal shut down and fatal renal insufficiency have been reported during treatment. Proteinuria has occurred infrequently.
A variety of liver function abnormalities have been reported, including elevations of SGOT, SGPT, alkaline phosphatase, bilirubin (direct and indirect), and depression of serum albumin, cholesterol (total and esters), and plasma fibrinogen. Increases and decreases of total lipids have occurred. Marked hypoalbuminemia associated with peripheral edema has been reported. However, these abnormalities usually are reversible on discontinuance of therapy and some reversal may occur during the course of therapy. Fatty changes in the liver have been documented by biopsy. Malabsorption syndrome has been reported.
Rarely, transient bone marrow depression has been observed, as evidenced by a delay in return of hemoglobin or hematocrit levels to normal in patients undergoing hematologic remission of leukemia. Marked leukopenia has been reported.

OVERDOSAGE

The acute intravenous LD_{50} of ELSPAR for mice was about 500,000 I.U./kg and for rabbits about 22,000 I.U./kg.

DOSAGE AND ADMINISTRATION

As a component of selected multiple agent induction regimens, ELSPAR may be administered by either the intravenous or the intramuscular route. When administered intravenously this enzyme should be given over a period of not less than thirty minutes through the side arm of an already running infusion of Sodium Chloride Injection or Dextrose Injection 5% (D_5W). ELSPAR has little tendency to cause phlebitis when given intravenously. Anaphylactic reactions require the immediate use of epinephrine, oxygen, and intravenous steroids.
When administering ELSPAR intramuscularly, the volume at a single injection site should be limited to 2 ml. If a volume greater than 2 ml is to be administered, two injection sites should be used.
Unfavorable interactions of ELSPAR with some antitumor agents have been demonstrated. It is recommended therefore, that ELSPAR be used in combination regimens only by physicians familiar with the benefits and risks of a given regimen. During the period of its inhibition of protein synthesis and cell replication ELSPAR may interfere with the action of drugs such as methotrexate which require cell replication for their lethal effect. ELSPAR may interfere with the enzymatic detoxification of other drugs, particularly in the liver.
Recommended Induction Regimens:
When using chemotherapeutic agents in combination for the induction of remissions in patients with acute lymphocytic leukemia, regimens are sought which provide maximum chance of success while avoiding excessive cumulative toxicity or negative drug interactions.
One of the following combination regimens incorporating ELSPAR is recommended for acute lymphocytic leukemia in children:
In the regimens below, Day 1 is considered to be the first day of therapy.
Regimen I
Prednisone 40 mg/square meter of body surface area per day orally in three divided doses for 15 days, followed by tapering of the dosage as follows:
20 mg/square meter for 2 days, 10 mg/square meter for 2 days, 5 mg/square meter for 2 days, 2.5 mg/square meter for 2 days and then discontinue.
Vincristine sulfate 2 mg/square meter of body surface area intravenously once weekly on Days 1, 8, and 15 of the treatment period. The maximum single dose should not exceed 2.0 mg.
Asparaginase 1,000 I.U./kg/day intravenously for ten successive days beginning on Day 22 of the treatment period.
Regimen II
Prednisone 40 mg/square meter of body surface area per day orally in three divided doses for 28 days (the total daily dose should be to the nearest 2.5 mg), following which the dosage of prednisone should be discontinued gradually over a 14 day period.
Vincristine sulfate 1.5 mg/square meter of body surface area intravenously weekly for four doses, on Days 1, 8, 15, and 22 of the treatment period. The maximum single dose should not exceed 2.0 mg.
Asparaginase 6,000 I.U./square meter of body surface area intramuscularly on Days 4, 7, 10, 13, 16, 19, 22, 25, and 28 of the treatment period. When a remission is obtained with either of the above regimens, appropriate maintenance therapy must be instituted. ELSPAR should not be used as part of a maintenance regimen. The above regimens do not preclude a need for special therapy directed toward the prevention of central nervous system leukemia.
It should be noted that ELSPAR has been used in combination regimens other than those recommended above. It is important to keep in mind that ELSPAR administered intravenously concurrently with or immediately before a course of vincristine and prednisone may be associated with increased toxicity. Physicians using a given regimen should be thoroughly familiar with its benefits and risks. Clinical data are insufficient for a recommendation concerning the use of combination regimens in adults. Asparaginase toxicity is reported to be greater in adults than in children.
Use of ELSPAR as the sole induction agent should be undertaken only in an unusual situation when a combined regimen is inappropriate because of toxicity or other specific patient-related factors, or in cases refractory to other therapy. When ELSPAR is to be used as the sole induction agent for children or adults the recommended dosage regimen is 200 I.U./kg/ day intravenously for 28 days. When complete remissions were obtained with this regimen, they were of short duration, 1 to 3 months. ELSPAR has been used as the sole induction agent in other regimens. Physicians using a given regimen should be thoroughly familiar with its benefits and risks.
Patients undergoing induction therapy must be carefully monitored and the therapeutic regimen adjusted according to response and toxicity.
Such adjustments should always involve decreasing dosages of one or more agents or discontinuation depending on the degree of toxicity. Patients who have received a course of ELSPAR, if retreated, have an increased risk of hypersensitivity reactions. Therefore, retreatment should be undertaken only when the benefit of such therapy is weighed against the increased risk.
Intradermal Skin Test:
Because of the occurrence of allergic reactions, an intradermal skin test should be performed prior to the initial administration of ELSPAR and when ELSPAR is given after an interval of a week or more has elapsed between doses. The skin test solution may be prepared as follows: Reconstitute the contents of a 10,000 I.U. vial with 5.0 ml of diluent. From this solution (2,000 I.U./ml) withdraw 0.1 ml and inject it into another vial containing 9.9 ml of diluent, yielding a skin test solution of approximately 20.0 I.U./ml. Use 0.1 ml of this solution (about 2.0 I.U.) for the intradermal skin test. The skin test site should be observed for at least one hour for the appearance of a wheal or erythema either of which indicates a positive reaction. An allergic reaction even to the skin test dose in certain sensitized individuals may rarely occur. A negative skin test reaction does not preclude the possibility of the development of an allergic reaction.

Desensitization:
Desensitization should be performed before administering the first dose of ELSPAR on initiation of therapy in positive reactors, and on retreatment of any patient in whom such therapy is deemed necessary after carefully weighing the increased risk of hypersensitivity reactions. Rapid desensitization of the patient may be attempted with progressively increasing amounts of intravenously administered ELSPAR provided adequate precautions are taken to treat an acute allergic reaction should it occur. One reported schedule begins with a total of 1 I.U. given intravenously and doubles the dose every 10 minutes, provided no reaction has occurred, until the accumulated total amount given equals the planned doses for that day.
For convenience the following table is included to calculate the number of doses necessary to reach the patient's total dose for that day:

Injection Number	ELSPAR Dose in I.U.	Accumulated Total Dose
1	1	1
2	2	3
3	4	7
4	8	15
5	16	31
6	32	63
7	64	127
8	128	255
9	256	511
10	512	1023
11	1024	2047
12	2048	4095
13	4096	8191
14	8192	16383
15	16384	32767
16	32768	65535
17	65536	131071
18	131072	262143

For example: A patient weighing 20 kg who is to receive 200 I.U./kg (total dose 4000 I.U.) would receive injections 1 through 12 during desensitization.

DIRECTIONS FOR RECONSTITUTION

Parenteral drug products should be inspected visually for particulate matter and discoloration prior to administration whenever solution and container permit. When reconstituted, ELSPAR should be a clear, colorless solution. If the solution becomes cloudy, discard.
For Intravenous Use
Reconstitute with Sterile Water for Injection or with Sodium Chloride Injection. The volume recommended for reconstitution is 5 ml for the 10,000 unit vials. Ordinary shaking during reconstitution does not inactivate the enzyme. This solution may be used for direct intravenous administration within an eight hour period following restoration. For administration by infusion, solutions should be diluted with the isotonic solutions, Sodium Chloride Injection or Dextrose Injection 5%. These solutions should be infused within eight hours and only if clear.
Occasionally, a very small number of gelatinous fiber-like particles may develop on standing. Filtration through a 5.0 micron filter during administration will remove the particles with no resultant loss in potency. Some loss of potency has been observed with the use of a 0.2 micron filter.
For Intramuscular Use
When ELSPAR is administered intramuscularly according to the schedule cited in the induction regimen, reconstitution is carried out by adding 2 ml Sodium Chloride Injection to the 10,000 unit vial. The resulting solution should be used within eight hours and only if clear.

HOW SUPPLIED

No. 4612 — ELSPAR is a white lyophilized plug or powder supplied as follows:
NDC 0006-4612-00 in a sterile 10 ml vial containing 10,000 I.U. of asparaginase and 80 mg mannitol, an inactive ingredient.

Continued on next page

Information on the Merck Sharp & Dohme products listed on these pages is the full prescribing information from product circulars in use August 31, 1986.

Merck Sharp & Dohme—Cont.

Personnel preparing ELSPAR should avoid drug contact with skin, mucous membranes, or eyes and avoid inhaling the dust or vapor.

Store at 2–8°C (36–46°F). ELSPAR does not contain a preservative. Unused, reconstituted solution should be stored at 2 to 8°C (36 to 46°F) and discarded after eight hours, or sooner if it becomes cloudy.

A.H.F.S. Category: 44:00
DC 7407109 Issued September 1983

FLEXERIL® Tablets ℞
(Cyclobenzaprine HCl, MSD), U.S.P.

DESCRIPTION

Cyclobenzaprine hydrochloride is a white, crystalline tricyclic amine salt with the empirical formula $C_{20}H_{21}N \cdot HCl$ and a molecular weight of 311.9. It has a melting point of 217°C, and a pK_a of 8.47 at 25°C. It is freely soluble in water and alcohol, sparingly soluble in isopropanol, and insoluble in hydrocarbon solvents. If aqueous solutions are made alkaline, the free base separates. Cyclobenzaprine HCl is designated chemically as 3-(5*H*-dibenzo[*a,d*]cyclohepten-5-ylidene)-*N, N*-dimethyl-1-propanamine hydrochloride, and has the following structural formula:

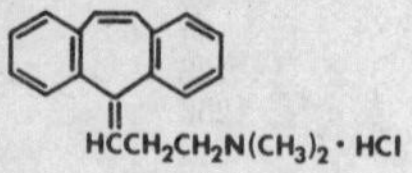

$HCCH_2CH_2N(CH_3)_2 \cdot HCl$

FLEXERIL® (Cyclobenzaprine HCl, MSD) is supplied as 10 mg tablets for oral administration.

Tablets FLEXERIL contain the following inactive ingredients: hydroxypropyl cellulose, hydroxypropyl methylcellulose, iron oxide, lactose, magnesium stearate, starch, and titanium dioxide.

CLINICAL PHARMACOLOGY

Cyclobenzaprine HCl relieves skeletal muscle spasm of local origin without interfering with muscle function. It is ineffective in muscle spasm due to central nervous system disease.

Cyclobenzaprine reduced or abolished skeletal muscle hyperactivity in several animal models. Animal studies indicate that cyclobenzaprine does not act at the neuromuscular junction or directly on skeletal muscle. Such studies show that cyclobenzaprine acts primarily within the central nervous system at brain stem as opposed to spinal cord levels, although its action on the latter may contribute to its overall skeletal muscle relaxant activity. Evidence suggests that the net effect of cyclobenzaprine is a reduction of tonic somatic motor activity, influencing both gamma (γ) and alpha (α) motor systems.

Pharmacological studies in animals showed a similarity between the effects of cyclobenzaprine and the structurally related tricyclic antidepressants, including reserpine antagonism, norepinephrine potentiation, potent peripheral and central anticholinergic effects, and sedation. Cyclobenzaprine caused slight to moderate increase in heart rate in animals.

Cyclobenzaprine is well absorbed after oral administration, but there is a large intersubject variation in plasma levels. Cyclobenzaprine is eliminated quite slowly with a half-life as long as one to three days. It is highly bound to plasma proteins, is extensively metabolized primarily to glucuronide-like conjugates, and is excreted primarily via the kidneys.

No significant effect on plasma levels or bioavailability of FLEXERIL or aspirin was noted when single or multiple doses of the two drugs were administered concomitantly. Concomitant administration of FLEXERIL and aspirin is usually well tolerated and no unexpected or serious clinical or laboratory adverse effects have been observed. No studies have been performed to indicate whether FLEXERIL enhances the clinical effect of aspirin or other analgesics, or whether analgesics enhance the clinical effect of FLEXERIL in acute musculoskeletal conditions.

Clinical Studies

Controlled clinical studies show that FLEXERIL significantly improves the signs and symptoms of skeletal muscle spasm as compared with placebo. The clinical responses include improvement in muscle spasm as determined by palpation, reduction in local pain and tenderness, increased range of motion, and less restriction in activities of daily living. When daily observations were made, clinical improvement was observed as early as the first day of therapy.

Eight double-blind controlled clinical studies were performed in 642 patients comparing FLEXERIL, diazepam*, and placebo. Muscle spasm, local pain and tenderness, limitation of motion, and restriction in activities of daily living were evaluated. In three of these studies there was a significantly greater improvement with FLEXERIL than with diazepam, while in the other studies the improvement following both treatments was comparable.

Although the frequency and severity of adverse reactions observed in patients treated with FLEXERIL were comparable to those observed in patients treated with diazepam, dry mouth was observed more frequently in patients treated with FLEXERIL and dizziness more frequently in those treated with diazepam. The incidence of drowsiness, the most frequent adverse reaction, was similar with both drugs.

Analysis of the data from controlled studies shows that FLEXERIL produces clinical improvement whether or not sedation occurs.

Surveillance Program

A post-marketing surveillance program was carried out in 7607 patients with acute musculoskeletal disorders, and included 297 patients treated for 30 days or longer. The overall effectiveness of FLEXERIL was similar to that observed in the double-blind controlled studies; the overall incidence of adverse effects was less (see ADVERSE REACTIONS).

INDICATIONS AND USAGE

FLEXERIL is indicated as an adjunct to rest and physical therapy for relief of muscle spasm associated with acute, painful musculoskeletal conditions.

Improvement is manifested by relief of muscle spasm and its associated signs and symptoms, namely, pain, tenderness, limitation of motion, and restriction in activities of daily living.

FLEXERIL (Cyclobenzaprine HCl, MSD) should be used only for short periods (up to two or three weeks) because adequate evidence of effectiveness for more prolonged use is not available and because muscle spasm associated with acute, painful musculoskeletal conditions is generally of short duration and specific therapy for longer periods is seldom warranted.

FLEXERIL has not been found effective in the treatment of spasticity associated with cerebral or spinal cord disease, or in children with cerebral palsy.

CONTRAINDICATIONS

Hypersensitivity to the drug.

Concomitant use of monoamine oxidase inhibitors or within 14 days after their discontinuation.

Acute recovery phase of myocardial infarction, and patients with arrhythmias, heart block or conduction disturbances, or congestive heart failure.

Hyperthyroidism.

WARNINGS

Cyclobenzaprine is closely related to the tricyclic antidepressants, e.g., amitriptyline and imipramine. In short term studies for indications other than muscle spasm associated with acute musculoskeletal conditions, and usually at doses somewhat greater than those recommended for skeletal muscle spasm, some of the more serious central nervous system reactions noted with the tricyclic antidepressants have occurred (see WARNINGS, below, and ADVERSE REACTIONS).

FLEXERIL may interact with monoamine oxidase (MAO) inhibitors. Hyperpyretic crisis, severe convulsions, and deaths have occurred in patients receiving tricyclic antidepressants and MAO inhibitor drugs.

Tricyclic antidepressants have been reported to produce arrhythmias, sinus tachycardia, prolongation of the conduction time leading to myocardial infarction and stroke.

FLEXERIL may enhance the effects of alcohol, barbiturates, and other CNS depressants.

PRECAUTIONS

General

Because of its atropine-like action, FLEXERIL should be used with caution in patients with a history of urinary retention, angle-closure glaucoma, increased intraocular pressure, and in patients taking anticholinergic medication.

Information for Patients

FLEXERIL may impair mental and/or physical abilities required for performance of hazardous tasks, such as operating machinery or driving a motor vehicle.

Drug Interactions

FLEXERIL may enhance the effects of alcohol, barbiturates, and other CNS depressants.

Tricyclic antidepressants may block the antihypertensive action of guanethidine and similarly acting compounds.

*VALIUM® (diazepam, Roche)

Carcinogenesis, Mutagenesis, Impairment of Fertility

In rats treated with FLEXERIL for up to 67 weeks at doses of approximately 5 to 40 times the maximum recommended human dose, pale, sometimes enlarged, livers were noted and there was a dose-related hepatocyte vacuolation with lipidosis. In the higher dose groups this microscopic change was seen after 26 weeks and even earlier in rats which died prior to 26 weeks; at lower doses, the change was not seen until after 26 weeks.

Cyclobenzaprine did not affect the onset, incidence or distribution of neoplasia in an 81-week study in the mouse or in a 105-week study in the rat.

At oral doses of up to 10 times the human dose, cyclobenzaprine did not adversely affect the reproductive performance or fertility of male or female rats. Cyclobenzaprine did not demonstrate mutagenic activity in the male mouse at dose levels of up to 20 times the human dose.

Pregnancy

Pregnancy Category B: Reproduction studies have been performed in rats, mice and rabbits at doses up to 20 times the human dose, and have revealed no evidence of impaired fertility or harm to the fetus due to FLEXERIL. There are, however, no adequate and well-controlled studies in pregnant women. Because animal reproduction studies are not always predictive of human response, this drug should be used during pregnancy only if clearly needed.

Nursing Mothers

It is not known whether this drug is excreted in human milk. Because cyclobenzaprine is closely related to the tricyclic antidepressants, some of which are known to be excreted in human milk, caution should be exercised when FLEXERIL is administered to a nursing woman.

Pediatric Use

Safety and effectiveness of FLEXERIL in children below the age of 15 have not been established.

ADVERSE REACTIONS

The following list of adverse reactions is based on the experience in 473 patients treated with FLEXERIL in controlled clinical studies, 7607 patients in the post-marketing surveillance program, and reports received since the drug was marketed. The overall incidence of adverse reactions among patients in the surveillance program was less than the incidence in the controlled clinical studies.

The adverse reactions reported most frequently with FLEXERIL were drowsiness, dry mouth and dizziness. The incidence of these common adverse reactions was lower in the surveillance program than in the controlled clinical studies:

	Clinical Studies	*Surveillance Program*
drowsiness	39%	16%
dry mouth	27%	7%
dizziness	11%	3%

Among the less frequent adverse reactions, there was no appreciable difference in incidence in controlled clinical studies or in the surveillance program. Adverse reactions which were reported in 1% to 3% of the patients were: fatigue/tiredness, asthenia, nausea, constipation, dyspepsia, unpleasant taste, blurred vision, headache, nervousness, and confusion.

Incidence Less Than 1 in 100

The following adverse reactions have been reported at an incidence of less than 1 in 100:

Body as a Whole: Syncope; facial edema; malaise.

Cardiovascular: Tachycardia; arrhythmia; vasodilatation; palpitation; hypotension.

Digestive: Vomiting; anorexia; diarrhea; gastrointestinal pain; gastritis; thirst; flatulence; edema of the tongue; abnormal liver function and rare reports of hepatitis, jaundice and cholestasis.

Musculoskeletal: Local weakness.

Nervous System and Psychiatric: Ataxia; vertigo; dysarthria; tremors; hypertonia; convulsions; muscle twitching; disorientation; insomnia; depressed mood; abnormal sensations; anxiety; agitation; abnormal thinking and dreaming; hallucinations; excitement; paresthesia.

Skin: Sweating; skin rash; urticaria.

Special Senses: Ageusia; tinnitus.

Urogenital: Urinary frequency and/or retention.

Causal Relationship Unknown

Other reactions, reported rarely for FLEXERIL under circumstances where a causal relationship could not be established or reported for other tricyclic drugs, are listed to serve as alerting information to physicians:

Body as a Whole: Chest pain; edema.

Cardiovascular: Hypertension; myocardial infarction; heart block; stroke.

Digestive: Paralytic ileus; tongue discoloration; stomatitis; parotid swelling.

Endocrine: Inappropriate ADH syndrome.

Hematic and Lymphatic: Purpura; bone marrow depression; leukopenia; eosinophilia; thrombocytopenia.

Metabolic, Nutritional and Immune: Elevation and lowering of blood sugar levels; weight gain or loss.

Musculoskeletal: Myalgia.
Nervous System and Psychiatric: Decreased or increased libido; abnormal gait; delusions; peripheral neuropathy; alteration in EEG patterns; extrapyramidal symptoms.
Respiratory: Dyspnea.
Skin: Pruritus; photosensitization; alopecia.
Urogenital: Impaired urination; dilatation of urinary tract; impotence; testicular swelling; gynecomastia; breast enlargement; galactorrhea.

DRUG ABUSE AND DEPENDENCE

Pharmacologic similarities among the tricyclic drugs require that certain withdrawal symptoms be considered when FLEXERIL is administered, even though they have not been reported to occur with this drug. Abrupt cessation of treatment after prolonged administration may produce nausea, headache, and malaise. These are not indicative of addiction.

OVERDOSAGE

Manifestations: High doses may cause temporary confusion, disturbed concentration, transient visual hallucinations, agitation, hyperactive reflexes, muscle rigidity, vomiting, or hyperpyrexia, in addition to anything listed under ADVERSE REACTIONS. Based on the known pharmacologic actions of the drug, overdosage may cause drowsiness, hypothermia, tachycardia and other cardiac rhythm abnormalities such as bundle branch block, ECG evidence of impaired conduction, and congestive heart failure. Other manifestations may be dilated pupils, convulsions, severe hypotension, stupor, and coma.
The acute oral LD_{50} of FLEXERIL is approximately 338 and 425 mg/kg in mice and rats, respectively.
Treatment: Treatment is symptomatic and supportive. Empty the stomach as quickly as possible by emesis, followed by gastric lavage. After gastric lavage, activated charcoal may be administered. Twenty to 30 g of activated charcoal may be given every four to six hours during the first 24 to 48 hours after ingestion. An ECG should be taken and close monitoring of cardiac function must be instituted if there is any evidence of dysrhythmia. Maintenance of an open airway, adequate fluid intake, and regulation of body temperature are necessary.
The intravenous administration of 1-3 mg of physostigmine salicylate is reported to reverse symptoms of poisoning by atropine and other drugs with anticholinergic activity. Physostigmine may be helpful in the treatment of cyclobenzaprine overdose. Because physostigmine is rapidly metabolized, the dosage of physostigmine should be repeated as required, particularly if life-threatening signs such as arrhythmias, convulsions, and deep coma recur or persist after the initial dosage of physostigmine. Because physostigmine itself may be toxic, it is not recommended for routine use.
Standard medical measures should be used to manage circulatory shock and metabolic acidosis. Cardiac arrhythmias may be treated with neostigmine, pyridostigmine, or propranolol. When signs of cardiac failure occur, the use of a short-acting digitalis preparation should be considered. Close monitoring of cardiac function for not less than five days is advisable.
Anticonvulsants may be given to control seizures.
Dialysis is probably of no value because of low plasma concentrations of the drug.
Since overdosage is often deliberate, patients may attempt suicide by other means during the recovery phase. Deaths by deliberate or accidental overdosage have occurred with this class of drugs.

DOSAGE AND ADMINISTRATION

The usual dosage of FLEXERIL is 10 mg three times a day, with a range of 20 to 40 mg a day in divided doses. Dosage should not exceed 60 mg a day. Use of FLEXERIL for periods longer than two or three weeks is not recommended. (See INDICATIONS AND USAGE).

HOW SUPPLIED

No. 3358—Tablets FLEXERIL, 10 mg, are butterscotch yellow, D-shaped, film coated tablets, coded MSD 931. They are supplied as follows:
NDC 0006-0931-68 in bottles of 100
NDC 0006-0931-28 unit dose packages of 100
NDC 0006-0931-30 BACK-PACK® unit-of-use package of 30.

Shown in Product Identification Section, page 417
A.H.F.S. Category: 12:20
DC 6919209 Issued May 1985

FLOROPRYL® Sterile Ophthalmic Ointment (Isoflurophate, MSD), U.S.P. ℞
For Topical Application into the Conjunctival Sac Only

DESCRIPTION

FLOROPRYL® (Isoflurophate, MSD) is available as 0.025 per cent sterile ophthalmic ointment in polyethylene-mineral oil gel. Isoflurophate is known chemically as diisopropyl fluorophosphate.

ACTIONS

FLOROPRYL is a cholinesterase inhibitor with sustained activity. Application to the eye produces intense miosis and ciliary muscle contraction due to inhibition of cholinesterase.
FLOROPRYL *irreversibly* inactivates cholinesterase. Thus, following use of FLOROPRYL in the eye, cholinesterase must be either regenerated or supplied from depots elsewhere in the body before ophthalmic action dependent on cholinesterase returns.
If given systemically in sufficient amounts, FLOROPRYL reduces plasma cholinesterase to zero. However, when applied locally to the eye, plasma cholinesterase is reduced only slightly.

INDICATIONS

Open-angle glaucoma
Conditions obstructing aqueous outflow, such as synechial formation, that are amenable to miotic therapy
Following iridectomy
Accommodative esotropia (accommodative convergent strabismus)

CONTRAINDICATIONS

Active uveal inflammation
Most cases of angle-closure (narrow-angle) glaucoma or patients with narrow angles, due to possibility of producing pupillary block and increasing angle blockage
Glaucoma associated with iridocyclitis
Hypersensitivity to the active or inactive ingredients

WARNINGS

Succinylcholine should be administered with extreme caution before or during general anesthesia to patients receiving cholinesterase inhibitors because of possible respiratory and cardiovascular collapse.
Because of possible adverse additive effects, FLOROPRYL should be administered only with extreme caution to patients with myasthenia gravis who are receiving systemic anticholinesterase therapy; conversely, extreme caution should be exercised in the use of an anticholinesterase drug for the treatment of myasthenia gravis patients who are already undergoing topical therapy with cholinesterase inhibitors.
Use in pregnancy: The safe use of anticholinesterase drugs in pregnancy has not been established, nor has the absence of adverse effects on the fetus or on respiration of the neonate. Therefore, the use of FLOROPRYL during pregnancy requires that its potential benefits be weighed against its possible hazards.

PRECAUTIONS

Except in aphakic patients, FLOROPRYL should be used in glaucoma only when shorter-acting miotics have proved inadequate.
Gonioscopy is recommended prior to medication with FLOROPRYL.
When an intraocular inflammatory process is present, the intensity and persistence of miosis and ciliary muscle contraction that result from anticholinesterase therapy require abstention from, or cautious use of, FLOROPRYL.
Systemic effects are infrequent when FLOROPRYL is applied carefully. The hands should be washed immediately following application.
Discontinue FLOROPRYL if salivation, urinary incontinence, diarrhea, profuse sweating, muscle weakness, respiratory difficulties, shock, or cardiac irregularities occur.
Persons receiving cholinesterase inhibitors who are exposed to organophosphate-type insecticides and pesticides (gardeners, organophosphate plant or warehouse workers, farmers, residents of communities which are undergoing insecticide spraying or dusting, etc.) should be warned of the added systemic effects possible from absorption through the respiratory tract or skin. Wearing of respiratory masks, frequent washing, and clothing changes may be advisable.
Anticholinesterase drugs should be used with extreme caution, if at all, in patients with marked vagotonia, bronchial asthma, spastic gastrointestinal disturbances, peptic ulcer, pronounced bradycardia and hypotension, recent myocardial infarction, epilepsy, parkinsonism, and other disorders that may respond adversely to vagotonic effects.
After long-term use of FLOROPRYL, dilation of blood vessels and resulting greater permeability increase the possibility of hyphema during ophthalmic surgery. Therefore, this drug should be discontinued immediately before operation.
Despite observance of all precautions and the use of only the recommended dose, there is some evidence that repeated administration may cause depression of the concentration of cholinesterase in the serum and erythrocytes, with resultant systemic effects.

ADVERSE REACTIONS

Stinging, burning, lacrimation, lid muscle twitching, conjunctival and ciliary redness, brow ache, headache, and induced myopia with visual blurring may occur.
Retinal detachment has been reported occasionally.
Activation of latent iritis or uveitis may occur.
Iris cysts may form, enlarge, and obscure vision. Occurrence is more frequent in children. The iris cyst usually shrinks upon discontinuance of the miotic. Rarely, the cyst may rupture or break free into the aqueous. Frequent examination for this occurrence is advisable.
Prolonged use may cause conjunctival thickening and obstruction of nasolacrimal canals.
Should systemic effects occur, manifested by nausea, vomiting, abdominal cramps, diarrhea, urinary incontinence, salivation, difficulty in breathing, bradycardia, or cardiac irregularities, parenteral administration of atropine sulfate is indicated, 0.4 mg. to 0.6 mg. or more for adults, proportionately less for children. Pralidoxime chloride in addition to atropine may be considered. Artificial respiration may be required.
Lens opacities have been reported in patients on anticholinesterase therapy. Routine slit-lamp examinations, including the lens, should accompany prolonged use.
Paradoxical increase in intraocular pressure may follow anticholinesterase application. This may be alleviated by pupil-dilating medication.

DOSAGE AND ADMINISTRATION

FLOROPRYL *is intended solely for topical use in the conjunctival sac.*
Isoflurophate hydrolyzes in the presence of water to form hydrofluoric acid. To prevent absorption of moisture and loss of potency, the ointment tube should be kept tightly closed; the tip of the tube should not be washed or allowed to touch the eyelid or other moist surface.
Whenever possible, FLOROPRYL should be applied at night before retiring to lessen blurring of vision. As it is an extremely potent drug, it should be used with great care and only by those familiar with its use and thoroughly indoctrinated in the technic of application.
The required dose is applied in the conjunctival sac, with the patient supine, care being taken not to touch the cornea with the tip of the tube. *Wash the hands immediately after administration.*
FLOROPRYL *should not be used more often than directed. Caution is necessary to avoid overdosage.*
Keep frequency of use to a minimum in all patients, but especially in children, to reduce the chance of iris cyst development (see ADVERSE REACTIONS). If tolerance develops, another miotic should be used. FLOROPRYL may be resumed later.
Glaucoma
For initial therapy ¼ inch strip of ophthalmic ointment FLOROPRYL 0.025 per cent is placed in the glaucomatous eye every 8 to 72 hours. A decrease in intraocular pressure should occur within a few hours. During this period, keep the patient under supervision and make tonometric examinations at least hourly for 3 or 4 hours to be sure that no immediate rise in pressure occurs (see ADVERSE REACTIONS).
Strabismus
Essentially equal visual acuity of both eyes is prerequisite to successful treatment. For initial evaluation FLOROPRYL may be used as a diagnostic aid to determine if an accommodative factor exists. This is especially useful preoperatively in young children and in patients with normal hypermetropic refractive errors. Not more than ¼ inch strip of ointment is administered every night for 2 weeks. If the eyes become straighter, an accommodative factor is demonstrated. This technic may supplement or complement standard testing with atropine and trial with glasses for the accommodative factor.

Continued on next page

Information on the Merck Sharp & Dohme products listed on these pages is the full prescribing information from product circulars in use August 31, 1986.

Merck Sharp & Dohme—Cont.

In esotropia uncomplicated by amblyopia or anisometropia, ophthalmic ointment FLOROPRYL may be used in both eyes, not more than 1/4 inch strip at a time every night for 2 weeks, as too severe a degree of miosis may interfere with vision. The dosage is then reduced to from 1/4 inch strip every other day to 1/4 inch strip once a week for 2 months, after which the patient's status should be re-evaluated.
If benefit can not be maintained with a dosage interval of at least 48 hours, therapy with FLOROPRYL should be stopped. Frequency of administration and duration of maintenance therapy depend on how long the eyes remain straight without medication. Intervals between administration should be gradually increased to the greatest length compatible with good results. Therapy may need to be continued indefinitely. Occasionally, however, the miotic may be needed only when the eyes begin to turn in. In a few instances, it has been possible to discontinue therapy entirely after several months.

TREATMENT OF ADVERSE EFFECTS

If FLOROPRYL is taken systemically by accident, or if systemic effects occur after topical application in the eye or from accidental skin contact, atropine sulfate in a dose (for adults) of 0.4 to 0.6 mg. or more should be given parenterally (intravenously if necessary). A proportionately smaller amount should be given to children.
The use of much larger doses of atropine in treating anticholinesterase intoxication in adults has been reported (Gordon, A.S.; Frye, C. W., J. Amer. Med. Ass. *159*:1181, Nov. 19, 1955; Grob, D., Arch. Intern. Med. *98*:221, Aug. 1956; Richards, A. G., Can. Med. Ass. J. *91*:82, July 11, 1964; Taylor, W. J. R., et al., Can. Med. Ass. J. *93*:966, Oct. 30, 1965). Initially 2 to 6 mg. may be given followed by 2 mg. every hour or more often, as long as muscarinic effects continue. The greater possibility of atropinization with large doses, particularly in sensitive individuals, should be borne in mind.
Pralidoxime* chloride has been reported to be useful in treatment of systemic effects due to cholinesterase inhibitors. However, its use is recommended in addition to and not as a substitute for atropine.
A short-acting barbiturate is indicated if convulsions occur that are not entirely relieved by atropine. Barbiturate dosage should be carefully adjusted to avoid central respiratory depression. Marked weakness or paralysis of muscles of respiration should be treated promptly by artificial respiration and maintenance of a clear airway.

HOW SUPPLIED

No. 7742—Sterile ophthalmic ointment FLOROPRYL 0.025 per cent is an opaque white, smooth, unctuous ointment and is supplied as follows:
NDC 0006-7742-04 in a 3.5 g. tube.

*PROTOPAM® Chloride (Pralidoxime Chloride). Ayerst Laboratories.

A.H.F.S. Category: 52:20
DC 6024019 Issued January 1974

HEP–B–GAMMAGEE® ℞
(Hepatitis B Immune Globulin [Human], MSD), U.S.P.

DESCRIPTION

HEP-B-GAMMAGEE® [Hepatitis B Immune Globulin (Human), MSD] is a sterile solution of human immunoglobulin (10–18% protein) prepared by a patented process from the pooled plasma of a small group of well-monitored individuals who were hyperimmunized with hepatitis B vaccine to produce high levels of antibody to the hepatitis B surface antigen (anti-HBs). HEP-B-GAMMAGEE is prepared from human plasma that was nonreactive when tested for hepatitis B surface antigen (HBsAg). The pooled plasma is processed by MSD and/or Armour Pharmaceutical Company using Cohn cold ethanol fractionation procedures. The product is dissolved in 0.3 molar glycine and contains thimerosal (mercury derivative) 1:10,000 added as a preservative. The solution has a pH of 6.8 ± 0.4 adjusted with hydrochloric acid or sodium hydroxide. Each vial of HEP-B-GAMMAGEE contains anti-HBs equivalent to or exceeding the potency of anti-HBs in a U.S. reference Hepatitis B Immune Globulin (Bureau of Biologics, FDA).

CLINICAL PHARMACOLOGY

Hepatitis B Immune Globulin (Human) provides passive immunization for individuals exposed to the hepatitis B virus (HBV) as evidenced by a reduction in the attack rate of hepatitis B following its use. The administration of the usual recommended dose of HEP-B-GAMMAGEE generally results in a detectable level of circulating antibody to hepatitis B surface antigen (anti-HBs) which persists for approximately 2 months or longer. The possibility of hepatitis B transmission is remote, as it is with other immune globulins prepared by the cold ethanol process.

INDICATIONS AND USAGE

HEP-B-GAMMAGEE is indicated for post-exposure prophylaxis following either parenteral exposure, direct mucous membrane contact, or oral ingestion involving HBsAg-positive materials such as blood, plasma or serum. Such exposures might occur by accidental "needle-stick", accidental splash, or a pipetting accident. HEP-B-GAMMAGEE is also indicated for post-exposure prophylaxis in infants born to hepatitis B-positive (HBsAg-positive) mothers.
Use of Hepatitis B Immune Globulin (Human) has been and continues to be evaluated in other situations which include nonparenteral exposure to hepatitis B, in dialysis patients and among hospital staffs. In addition, it has been tested as a prophylactic measure for susceptible individuals in close association with HBsAg-positive persons. These studies are still in progress and there are insufficient data at present on effectiveness, dosage and schedule for any of these uses to be included as definite indications.

CONTRAINDICATIONS

None known.

WARNINGS

Persons with isolated immunoglobulin A deficiency have the potential for developing antibodies to immunoglobulin A and could have anaphylactic reactions to subsequent administration of blood products that contain immunoglobulin A. Therefore, as with any immune globulin preparation, Hepatitis B Immune Globulin (Human) should be given to such persons only if the expected benefits outweigh the potential risks.
In patients who have severe thrombocytopenia or any coagulation disorder that would contraindicate intramuscular injections, Hepatitis B Immune Globulin (Human) should be given only if the expected benefits outweigh the potential risks.

PRECAUTIONS

General
HEP-B-GAMMAGEE should be given with caution to patients with a history of prior systemic allergic reactions following the administration of human immune globulin preparations. Hypersensitivity reactions to injections of immune serum globulin occur rarely. The incidence of these reactions may be increased in patients receiving large intramuscular doses or in patients receiving repeated injections of immune serum globulin.
HEP-B-GAMMAGEE *must not be administered intravenously* because of the potential for serious reactions. Injections should be made intramuscularly. Care should be taken to draw back on the plunger of the syringe before injection in order to be certain that the needle is not in a blood vessel. Epinephrine should be available for treatment of acute allergic symptoms.

Drug Interactions
Antibodies present in immune globulin preparations may interfere with the immune response to live virus vaccines such as measles, mumps, and rubella. Therefore, vaccination with live virus vaccines should be deferred until approximately three months after administration of Hepatitis B Immune Globulin. It may be necessary to revaccinate persons who received Hepatitis B Immune Globulin shortly after live virus vaccination.

Pregnancy
Pregnancy Category C. Animal reproduction studies have not been conducted with HEP-B-GAMMAGEE. Clinical experience with other immunoglobulin preparations administered during pregnancy suggests that there are no known adverse effects on the fetus from immune globulins per se. However, it is not known whether HEP-B-GAMMAGEE can cause fetal harm when administered to a pregnant woman or can affect reproduction capacity. HEP-B-GAMMAGEE should be given to a pregnant woman only if clearly needed.

Nursing Mothers
It is not known whether this drug is excreted in human milk. Because many drugs are excreted in human milk, caution should be exercised when HEP-B-GAMMAGEE is administered to a nursing woman.

ADVERSE REACTIONS

Local pain and tenderness at the injection site, urticaria and angioedema may occur. Anaphylactic reactions, although rare, have been reported following the injection of human immune globulin preparations. Anaphylaxis is more likely to occur if Hepatitis B Immune Globulin (Human) is given intravenously; therefore, Hepatitis B Immune Globulin (Human) must be administered *only* intramuscularly. In highly allergic individuals, repeated injections may lead to anaphylactic shock.

OVERDOSAGE

Although no data are available, clinical experience with other immunoglobulin preparations suggests that the only manifestations would be pain and tenderness at the injection site.

DOSAGE AND ADMINISTRATION

Parenteral drug products should be inspected visually for particulate matter and discoloration prior to administration, whenever solution and container permit. HEP-B-GAMMAGEE is a clear, very slightly amber, moderately viscous liquid.
HEP-B-GAMMAGEE is administered *intramuscularly. It must not be injected intravenously.*
It is important to use a separate sterile syringe and needle for each individual patient to prevent transmission of hepatitis B and other infectious agents from one person to another.

Adults
The recommended dose is 0.06 ml per kilogram of body weight; the usual adult dose is 3 to 5 ml administered intramuscularly, preferably in the gluteal or deltoid region. The appropriate dose should be administered as soon after exposure as possible (preferably within 7 days) and repeated 28–30 days after exposure.

Newborns
The immunization regimen for infants born to hepatitis B-positive (HBsAg-positive) mothers consists of three doses. A dose of 0.5 ml should be administered intramuscularly in the anterolateral thigh as soon after birth as possible and repeated at 3 months and 6 months of age. Administration of the first dose later than 24 hours after birth results in a progressive loss of efficacy.

HOW SUPPLIED

No. 4692—HEP-B-GAMMAGEE is supplied as follows:
NDC 0006-4692-00 in 5 ml vials.
Store at 2–8° C (35.6–46.4° F). Do not freeze. Do not use after expiration date.

A.H.F.S. Category: 80:04
DC 7062006 Issued November 1982

HEPTAVAX–B® ℞
(Hepatitis B Vaccine, MSD)

DESCRIPTION

HEPTAVAX-B® (Hepatitis B Vaccine, MSD) is a non-infectious formalin-inactivated subunit viral vaccine derived from surface antigen (HBsAg or Australia antigen) of hepatitis B virus. The antigen is harvested and purified from the plasma of human carriers of hepatitis B virus according to methods developed by Merck Sharp and Dohme Research Laboratories.
The starting plasma from which the antigen is extracted is obtained from a small, closely monitored population of asymptomatic HBsAg-positive donors. Periodically each donor is required to undergo a health examination, and appropriate laboratory tests are performed prior to each plasmapheresis.
The vaccine production process uses purification and inactivation steps which are known to remove or inactivate not only infectious hepatitis B virus particles, but also representatives of all known groups of animal viruses. Such groups include rhabdo-, pox-, toga-, reo-, herpes-, corona-, myxo-, picorna-, parvo-, and retrovirus; delta agent, and slow viruses.
Initial purification is accomplished by double ultracentrifugation. This is followed by an inactivation process consisting of three sequential treatments using pepsin, 8 Molar urea, and formalin. Each of these treatments alone has been shown to inactivate 10^5 or more infectious doses of hepatitis B virus/mL, and one or more of the treatments also has been shown to inactivate members of many other virus groups, including those listed above. In addition, studies in chimpanzees and humans show that hepatitis B vaccine produced according to this process does not transmit the agent(s) of non-A/non-B hepatitis. Follow-up data from clinical trials of HEPTAVAX-B provide no evidence to suggest transmission

of Acquired Immune Deficiency Syndrome (AIDS) by this vaccine, even when the vaccine has been used routinely in infants in Alaska. Each of the three sequential treatments, pepsin, urea, and formalin, have been shown to inactivate retroviruses, including HTLV-I, HTLV-II, HTLV-III and LAV, which have been associated with AIDS. Other studies have shown that individuals who have received this vaccine showed no rise in antibodies to HTLV-I, HTLV-II, HTLV-III or LAV. Other studies have shown no detectable HTLV DNA in this vaccine.

Each lot of hepatitis B vaccine is tested for sterility and is inoculated into cell cultures and several species of animals including chimpanzees, to rule out the presence of adventitious viruses.

HEPTAVAX-B is a sterile suspension for intramuscular injection; however, it may be administered subcutaneously to persons at risk of hemorrhage following intramuscular injections (see DOSAGE AND ADMINISTRATION). Each 1.0 mL dose of the adult formulation vaccine contains 20 mcg of hepatitis B surface antigen formulated in an alum adjuvant, and thimerosal (mercury derivative) 1:20,000 added as a preservative. Each 0.5 mL dose of the pediatric formulation vaccine contains 10 mcg of hepatitis B surface antigen formulated in an alum adjuvant, and thimerosal (mercury derivative) 1:20,000 added as a preservative. The vaccine is prepared without regard to subtype. HEPTAVAX-B is indicated for immunization of persons at risk of infection from hepatitis B virus including all known subtypes.

CLINICAL PHARMACOLOGY

Hepatitis B virus is one of at least three hepatitis viruses that cause a systemic infection, with a major pathology in the liver. The others are hepatitis A virus, and non-A, non-B hepatitis viruses.

Hepatitis B virus is an important cause of viral hepatitis. There is no specific treatment for this disease. The incubation period for type B hepatitis is relatively long; six weeks to six months may elapse between exposure and the onset of clinical symptoms. The prognosis following infection with hepatitis B virus is variable and dependent on at least three factors: (1) Age—Infants and younger children usually experience milder initial disease than older persons; (2) Dose of Virus—The higher the dose, the more likely acute icteric hepatitis B will result; and, (3) Severity of Associated Underlying Disease—Underlying malignancy or pre-existing hepatic disease predisposes to increased mortality and morbidity.

Persistence of viral infection (the chronic hepatitis B virus carrier state) occurs in 5–10% of persons following acute hepatitis B, and occurs more frequently after initial anicteric hepatitis B than after initial icteric disease. Consequently, carriers of hepatitis B surface antigen (HBsAg) frequently give no history of recognized acute hepatitis. It has been estimated that more than 170 million people in the world today are persistently infected with hepatitis B virus. The Centers for Disease Control (CDC) estimates that there are approximately 0.7 to 1.0 million chronic carriers of hepatitis B virus in the USA and that this pool of carriers grows by 2%–3% (8,000 to 16,000 individuals) annually. Chronic carriers represent the largest human reservoir of hepatitis B virus.

The serious complications and sequelae of hepatitis B virus infection include massive hepatic necrosis, cirrhosis of the liver, chronic active hepatitis, and hepatocellular carcinoma. Chronic carriers of HBsAg appear to be at increased risk of developing hepatocellular carcinoma, which accounts for 80 to 90 percent of primary liver carcinomas. Although a number of etiologic factors are associated with development of hepatocellular carcinoma, the single most important etiologic factor appears to be active infection with the hepatitis B virus.

There is also evidence that several diseases other than hepatitis have been associated with hepatitis B virus infection through an immunologic mechanism involving antigen antibody complexes. Such diseases include a syndrome with rash, urticaria, and arthralgia resembling serum sickness; polyarteritis nodosa; membranous glomerulonephritis; and infantile papular acrodermatitis.

Although the vehicles for transmission of the virus are predominantly blood and blood products, viral antigen has also been found in tears, saliva, breast milk, urine, semen and vaginal secretions. Hepatitis B virus is quite stable and capable of surviving for days on environmental surfaces. Infection may occur when hepatitis B virus, transmitted by infected body fluids, is implanted via mucous surfaces or percutaneously introduced through accidental or deliberate breaks in the skin.

Transmission of hepatitis B virus infection is often associated with close interpersonal contact with an infected individual and with crowded living conditions. In such circumstances, transmission by inoculation via routes other than overt parenteral ones may be quite common. Infection in infancy by the hepatitis B virus usually leads to the chronic carrier state. Perinatal transmission of hepatitis B infection from infected mother to child, at or shortly after birth, can occur if the mother is a hepatitis B surface antigen (HBsAg) carrier or if the mother has an acute hepatitis B infection in the third trimester. Among infants born to women in whom sera are positive for both the hepatitis B surface antigen and the e antigen, 85–90% are infected and become chronic carriers.

Hepatitis B is endemic throughout the world and is a serious medical problem in population groups at increased risk. (Refer to INDICATIONS AND USAGE)

Numerous epidemiological studies have shown that persons who develop anti-HBs following active infection with the hepatitis B virus are protected against the disease on re-exposure to the virus.

Clinical studies established that HEPTAVAX-B when injected into the deltoid muscle induced protective levels of antibody in greater than 90% of healthy individuals who received the recommended 3 dose regimen. A lower response rate (81%) to vaccine may be obtained if the vaccine is administered as a buttock injection. A protective antibody (anti-HBs) level has been defined by the Immunization Practices Advisory Committee as 1) 10 or more sample ratio units (SRU) as determined by radioimmunoassay or 2) a positive result as determined by enzyme immunoassay.

Responsiveness to the vaccine is age dependent. The seroconversion rate for children 1–10 years of age was 100%. In contrast, seroconversion rates for adults ranged from 92 to 96% for those 20 to 49 years of age and 77% for those 50 years of age or older. Immunocompromised and immunosuppressed persons respond less well than do healthy individuals. Studies among hemodialysis patients show that approximately 60 percent of those who receive three 40 μg doses of the vaccine develop anti-HBs.

These studies show that vaccine-induced levels of anti-HBs also are lower and tend to remain at protective levels for shorter periods in hemodialysis patients than do levels in healthy adults. Protective efficacy of the vaccine was not demonstrated in hemodialysis patients in a large double-blind clinical study in which the overall attack rate for hepatitis B was low. Nevertheless, the Immunization Practices Advisory Committee (ACIP) in reviewing these data recommended that the vaccine continue to be used in hemodialysis patients as an adjunctive measure to reduce the rate of transmission of hepatitis B.

The protective efficacy of HEPTAVAX-B has been demonstrated in adults at high risk of contracting hepatitis B infection.

In two clinical trials efficacy was 98% for individuals whose anti-HBs titers were equal to or greater than 10 SRU after the recommended 3 doses of vaccine. These individuals were protected against acute hepatitis B, chronic antigenemia and asymptomatic infections (excluding seroconversion for anti-HBc). Efficacy among all vaccine recipients without regard to the level of antibody response was 82–87%.

In one of the above studies involving individuals at high risk of contracting hepatitis B infection, there was evidence of protective immunity in approximately 78% of vaccinated subjects following 2 doses of the 3 dose regimen. However, the third dose was required to raise the proportion of seroconverters to 92%, induce higher titers, and provide an extended period of protection.

In a third study, conducted in medical staff at hemodialysis units, protective antibody developed in 96% of vaccine recipients after administration of three doses of vaccine. Additionally, this study demonstrated the subtype cross-protection of HEPTAVAX-B. A lot of the vaccine selected to contain only the *ad* antigenic subtype induced protection against infection from the *ay* subtype hepatitis B virus. These results confirm that monovalent HBsAg/*ad* vaccine can provide protection in populations at high risk of infection with the *ay* subtype virus (e.g., patients and staff in hemodialysis units and users of illicit injectable drugs).

A protective level of anti-HBs (≥ 10 SRU) is produced in greater than 90% of healthy individuals when the 3 dose regimen of HEPTAVAX-B is administered in the deltoid muscle. In regard to serologic confirmation of post-vaccination immunity and revaccination of nonresponders, the Immunization Practices Advisory Committee has issued the following recommendations:

> Testing for immunity following vaccination is not recommended routinely but is advised for persons whose subsequent management depends on knowing their immune status, such as dialysis patients and staff, and for persons in whom a suboptimal response may be anticipated, such as those who have received vaccine in the buttock.
>
> Revaccination of persons who do not respond to the primary series (nonresponders) produces adequate antibody in only one-third when the primary vaccination has been given in the deltoid. Therefore, revaccination of non-responders to deltoid injection is not recommended routinely. For persons who did not respond to a primary vaccine series given in the buttock, preliminary data from two small studies suggest that revaccination in the arm induces adequate antibody in over 75%. Revaccination should be strongly considered for such persons.

Adverse reactions in individuals who have received a fourth or fifth injection have been similar in type and severity to those of the initial three dose series (see ADVERSE REACTIONS).

The duration of protection and need for booster doses are not yet defined. Studies have shown that anti-HBs levels may fall below 10 SRU in some vaccinees over a period of 3–4 years. In one study, 71% of adults who initially responded to the vaccine with protective levels of anti-HBs retained levels of ≥ 10 SRU over $4\frac{1}{2}$ years. Among those in this population who lost antibody, protection against chronic antigenemia and hepatitis appeared to persist. Individuals who remain at high risk of exposure to hepatitis B virus may wish to periodically determine their anti-HBs level. If antibody levels fall below 10 SRU, administration of an additional dose of HEPTAVAX-B should be considered.

Recent studies have established the relative efficacies of immune globulin and/or hepatitis B vaccine in infants born to HBsAg-positive, HBeAg-positive mothers; following accidental percutaneous or permucosal exposure to HBsAg positive blood, or sexual exposure to HBsAg-positive persons (See DOSAGE AND ADMINISTRATION).

It has been demonstrated that Hepatitis B Immune Globulin, when administered simultaneously with HEPTAVAX-B at separate body sites, did not interfere with the induction of protective antibodies against hepatitis B virus elicited by the vaccine.

Reports in the literature describe a more virulent form of hepatitis B (case fatality rates of up to 12%) associated with superinfections or coinfections by delta virus, an incomplete RNA virus. Delta virus can only infect and cause illness in persons infected with hepatitis B virus since the delta agent requires a coat of HBsAg in order to become infectious. Therefore, persons immune to hepatitis B virus infection should also be immune to delta virus infection.

INDICATIONS AND USAGE

HEPTAVAX-B is indicated for immunization against infection caused by all known subtypes of hepatitis B virus.

HEPTAVAX-B will not prevent hepatitis caused by other agents, such as hepatitis A virus, non-A, non-B hepatitis viruses, or other viruses known to infect the liver.

Vaccination is recommended in persons of all ages, especially those who are or will be at increased risk of infection with hepatitis B virus, for example:

- *Health Care Personnel*
  Dentists and oral surgeons.
  Physicians and surgeons.
  Nurses.
  Paramedical personnel and custodial staff who may be exposed to the virus via blood or other patient specimens.
  Dental hygienists and dental nurses.
  Laboratory personnel handling blood, blood products and other patient specimens.
  Dental, medical and nursing students.
- *Selected Patients and Patient Contacts*
  Patients and staff in hemodialysis units and hematology/oncology units.
  Patients requiring frequent and/or large volume blood transfusions or clotting factor concentrates (e.g., persons with hemophilia, thalassemia).
  Clients (residents) and staff of institutions for the mentally handicapped.
  Classroom contacts of deinstitutionalized mentally handicapped persons who have persistent hepatitis B antigenemia and who show aggressive behavior.
  Household and other intimate contacts of persons with persistent hepatitis B antigenemia.
- *Infants Born to HBsAg Positive Mothers* (See DOSAGE AND ADMINISTRATION)
- *Populations with high incidence of the disease,* such as:
  Alaskan Eskimos.
  Indochinese refugees.
  Haitian refugees.
- *Military Personnel identified as being at increased risk*
- *Morticians and Embalmers*
- *Blood bank and plasma fractionation workers*
- *Persons at Increased Risk of the Disease Due to Their Sexual Practices,* such as:
  Persons who repeatedly contract sexually transmitted diseases.
  Homosexually active males.
  Female prostitutes.
- *Prisoners*
- *Users of illicit injectable drugs*

Continued on next page

Information on the Merck Sharp & Dohme products listed on these pages is the full prescribing information from product circulars in use August 31, 1986.

Merck Sharp & Dohme—Cont.

Revaccination
See CLINICAL PHARMACOLOGY

CONTRAINDICATIONS

Hypersensitivity to any component of the vaccine.

WARNINGS

Persons with immuno-deficiency or those receiving immunosuppressive therapy require larger vaccine doses and respond less well than do healthy individuals. Refer to DOSAGE AND ADMINISTRATION for use in such individuals.
Because of the long incubation period for hepatitis B, it is possible for unrecognized infection to be present at the time HEPTAVAX-B is given. HEPTAVAX-B may not prevent hepatitis B in such patients.
Patients who develop symptoms suggestive of hypersensitivity after an injection should not receive further injections of HEPTAVAX-B (see CONTRAINDICATIONS).

PRECAUTIONS

General
As with any parenteral vaccine, epinephrine should be available for immediate use should an anaphylactoid reaction occur.
Any serious active infection is reason for delaying use of HEPTAVAX-B, except when, in the opinion of the physician, withholding the vaccine entails a greater risk.
Caution and appropriate care should be exercised in administering HEPTAVAX-B to individuals with severely compromised cardiopulmonary status or to others in whom a febrile or systemic reaction could pose a significant risk.
Pregnancy
Pregnancy Category C. Animal reproduction studies have not been conducted with HEPTAVAX-B. It is also not known whether HEPTAVAX-B can cause fetal harm when administered to a pregnant woman or can affect reproductive capacity. HEPTAVAX-B should be given to a pregnant woman only if clearly needed.
Nursing Mothers
Studies in 12 lactating women have failed to reveal evidence of this vaccine being secreted in breast milk.
Pediatric Use
HEPTAVAX-B has been shown to be well-tolerated and highly immunogenic in infants and children of all ages. Newborns also respond well; maternally transferred antibodies do not interfere with the active immune response to the vaccine. See DOSAGE AND ADMINISTRATION for recommended pediatric dosage and for recommended dosage for infants born to HBsAg positive mothers.

ADVERSE REACTIONS

HEPTAVAX-B is generally well tolerated. No serious adverse reactions attributable to vaccination were reported during the course of clinical trials involving administration of HEPTAVAX-B to over 19,000 individuals. There was no tendency towards increasing frequency or severity of complaints with successive doses of the vaccine. As with any vaccine, there is the possibility that broad use of the vaccine could reveal rare adverse reactions not observed in clinical trials.
In three double-blind placebo-controlled studies among 3,350 persons, the overall rates of adverse reactions reported by vaccine recipients (24.3%, 21.5% and 22.8%) did not differ significantly from those of placebo recipients (21.4%, 18.7% and 21.9%). Approximately half of all reported reactions were injection site soreness, which occurred somewhat more frequently among vaccine recipients.
In another group of studies, 3,516 doses of vaccine were administered to 1,255 healthy adults. Vaccinees were monitored for 5 days after each dose, and the following adverse reactions were reported:

	% of doses
BODY AS A WHOLE	
Injection site reactions, consisting principally of soreness, and including erythema, swelling, warmth and induration	12.3
Fatigue/asthenia	1.9
Malaise	0.8
Fever (≥100°F)	1.8
Chills	0.4
Sensation of warmth	0.4
Irritability	0.1
Diaphoresis	0.1
DIGESTIVE SYSTEM	
Gastrointestinal illness including anorexia, nausea, vomiting, abdominal pain and diarrhea	2.0
Abdominal cramps	0.3
HEMATOLOGIC AND LYMPHATIC SYSTEM	
Adenitis	0.1
MUSCULOSKELETAL SYSTEM	
Myalgia	1.2
Arthralgia	0.7
NERVOUS SYSTEM	
Headache	3.1
Dizziness	0.5
Disturbed sleep	0.2
Paresthesia	0.2
RESPIRATORY SYSTEM	
Upper respiratory illness	2.5
INTEGUMENTARY SYSTEM	
Rash (non-specific)	0.3

In a double-blind, placebo-controlled, clinical trial of 1,330 health-care workers, the frequency of elevations in SGPT (ALT) in vaccine recipients was not significantly different from that in placebo recipients. In marketed use of the vaccine, non-specific abnormalities in SGPT (ALT) and other liver function tests have been reported, but no causal relationship has been established.
The following additional adverse reactions have been reported with use of the marketed vaccine:
Hypersensitivity Reactions
Symptoms of immediate hypersensitivity including urticaria, angioedema, and pruritus have been reported rarely within the first few hours after vaccination. An apparent hypersensitivity syndrome of delayed onset has been reported rarely, days to weeks after vaccination. This has included the following findings: arthritis (usually transient), fever, and dermatologic reactions such as urticaria, erythema multiforme, or ecchymoses.
Nervous System
Neurological disorders such as paresthesias, optic neuritis, myelitis including transverse myelitis, and acute radiculoneuropathy including Guillain-Barré syndrome have been rarely reported in temporal association with administration of HEPTAVAX-B.

DOSAGE AND ADMINISTRATION

Do not inject intravenously or intradermally.
HEPTAVAX-B is for intramuscular injection. The deltoid muscle is the preferred site for intramuscular injection in adults. Data suggest that injections given in the buttocks frequently are given into fatty tissue instead of into muscle. Such injections may result in a lower seroconversion rate than is expected. The anterolateral thigh is the recommended site for intramuscular injection in infants and children.
HEPTAVAX-B may be administered subcutaneously to persons at risk of hemorrhage following intramuscular injections. The immune responses and clinical reactions following intramuscular and subcutaneous administration of HEPTAVAX-B have been shown to be comparable. However, when other aluminum-adsorbed vaccines have been administered subcutaneously, an increased incidence of local reactions including subcutaneous nodules has been observed. Therefore, subcutaneous administration should be used only in persons (e.g., hemophiliacs) at risk of hemorrhage following intramuscular injections.

Shake well before withdrawal and use. Thorough agitation at the time of administration is necessary to maintain suspension of the vaccine.
Parenteral drug products should be inspected visually for particulate matter and discoloration prior to administration. After thorough agitation, HEPTAVAX-B is a slightly opaque, white suspension.
The immunization regimen consists of 3 doses of vaccine given according to the following schedule:

1st dose: at elected date
2nd dose: 1 month later
3rd dose: 6 months after the first dose

The volume of vaccine to be given on each occasion is as follows:
[See table below].

HEPTAVAX-B Group	Formulation	Initial	1 month	6 months
Younger Children (Birth to 10 years of age)	Pediatric 10 mcg/0.5 mL	0.5 mL	0.5 mL	0.5 mL
Adults and Older Children	Adult 20 mcg/1.0 mL	1.0 mL	1.0 mL	1.0 mL
Dialysis Patients and Immunocompromised Patients	Adult 20 mcg/1.0 mL	2.0 mL*	2.0 mL*	2.0 mL*

*Two 1.0 mL doses given at different sites.

Revaccination—(see CLINICAL PHARMACOLOGY).
Dosage For Infants Born of HBsAg Positive Mothers
Infants born to HBsAg positive mothers are at high risk of becoming chronic carriers of hepatitis B virus and of developing the chronic sequelae of hepatitis B virus infection. Well-controlled studies have shown that administration of three 0.5 mL doses of Hepatitis B Immune Globulin starting at birth is 75% effective in preventing establishment of the chronic carrier state in these infants during the first year of life. Protection can be transient, whereupon the effectiveness of the Hepatitis B Immune Globulin would decline thereafter. Results from clinical studies indicate that administration of one 0.5 mL dose of Hepatitis B Immune Globulin at birth and three 20 mcg (1.0 mL) doses of HEPTAVAX-B, the first dose given within one week after birth, was 85–93% effective in preventing establishment of the chronic carrier state in infants born to HBsAg and HBeAg positive mothers. Preliminary data from studies using one 0.5 mL dose of Hepatitis B Immune Globulin and three 10 mcg (0.5 mL) doses of HEPTAVAX-B in the same type of population indicate that this lower dose of vaccine is equally effective.
Testing for HBsAg and anti-HBs is recommended at 12–15 months. If HBsAg is not detectable, and anti-HBs is present, the child has been protected.
The recommended dosage for infants born to HBsAg positive mothers is as follows:

Treatment	Birth	Within 7 days	1 month	6 months
HEPTAVAX-B pediatric formulation 10 mcg/0.5 mL		0.5 mL*	0.5 mL	0.5 mL
HEPATITIS B IMMUNE GLOBULIN	0.5 mL	—	—	—

*The first dose of HEPTAVAX-B may be given at birth at the same time as Hepatitis B Immune Globulin, but should be administered in the opposite anterolateral thigh. This procedure may be preferable to ensure absorption of the vaccine.

Known or Presumed Exposure to HBsAg
There are no prospective studies directly testing the efficacy of a combination of Hepatitis B Immune Globulin and HEPTAVAX-B in preventing clinical hepatitis B following percutaneous, ocular or mucous membrane exposure to hepatitis B virus. However, since most persons with such exposures (e.g., health care workers) are candidates for the hepatitis B vaccine and since combined hepatitis B Immune Globulin plus vaccine is more efficacious than Hepatitis B Immune Globulin alone in perinatal exposures, the following guidelines are recommended for persons who have been exposed to hepatitis B virus such as through (1) percutaneous (needlestick), ocular, mucous membrane exposure to blood known or presumed to contain HBsAg, (2) human bites by known or presumed HBsAg carriers, that penetrate the skin, or (3) following intimate sexual contact with known or presumed HBsAg carriers:

Hepatitis B Immune Globulin (0.06 mL/kg) should be given as soon as possible after exposure and within 24 hours if possible. Hepatitis B vaccine 1.0 mL (20 mcg/1.0 mL) should be given intramuscularly within 7 days of exposure and second and third doses given one and six months, respectively, after the first dose.

The vaccine is used as supplied; no dilution or reconstitution is necessary. It is important to use a separate sterile syringe and needle for each individual patient to prevent transmission of hepatitis and other infectious agents from one person to another.
3.0 mL Vial
For Syringe Use Only: Withdraw the recommended dose from the vial using a sterile needle and syringe free of preservatives, antiseptics, and detergents.

HOW SUPPLIED

No. 4720—HEPTAVAX-B, Adult Formulation, is supplied as a multi-dose vial of vaccine, 20 mcg/1.0 mL, NDC 0006-4720-00 in 3 mL vials.
No. 4736—HEPTAVAX-B, Pediatric Formulation, is supplied as a one dose vial of vaccine, 10 mcg/0.5 mL, NDC 0006-4736-00 in 0.5 mL vials.
Storage
Store unopened and opened vials at 2–8°C (35.6–46.4°F). Storage above or below the recommended temperature may reduce potency.
Do not freeze since freezing destroys potency.
A.H.F.S. Category: 80:12
DC 7409206 Issued December 1985

HUMORSOL® Ophthalmic Solution ℞
(Demecarium Bromide, MSD), U.S.P.
For Topical Application into the Conjunctival Sac Only

DESCRIPTION

Ophthalmic Solution HUMORSOL® (Demecarium Bromide, MSD) is a sterile solution supplied in two dosage strengths: 0.125 percent and 0.25 percent. The inactive ingredients are sodium chloride and water for injection; benzalkonium chloride 1:5000 is added as preservative. Demecarium bromide is a quaternary ammonium compound. Its chemical name is decamethylenebis (m-dimethyl-aminophenyl-N-methylcarbamate) dimethobromide.

ACTIONS

HUMORSOL is a cholinesterase inhibitor with sustained activity. It acts mainly on true (erythrocyte) cholinesterase. Application of HUMORSOL to the eye produces intense miosis and ciliary muscle contraction due to inhibition of cholinesterase. These effects are accompanied by increased capillary permeability of the ciliary body and iris, increased permeability of the blood-aqueous barrier, and vasodilation. Myopia may be induced or, if present, may be augmented by the increased refractive power of the lens that results from the accommodative effect of the drug. HUMORSOL indirectly produces some of the muscarinic and nicotinic effects of acetylcholine as quantities of the latter accumulate.

INDICATIONS

Open-angle glaucoma
Conditions obstructing aqueous outflow, such as synechial formation, that are amenable to miotic therapy
Following iridectomy
Accommodative esotropia (accommodative convergent strabismus)

CONTRAINDICATIONS

Active uveal inflammation
Most cases of angle-closure (narrow-angle) glaucoma or patients with narrow angles, due to the possibility of producing pupillary block and increasing angle blockage
Glaucoma associated with iridocyclitis
Hypersensitivity to the active or inactive ingredients

WARNINGS

Succinylcholine should be administered with extreme caution before or during general anesthesia to patients receiving cholinesterase inhibitors because of possible respiratory and cardiovascular collapse.
Because of possible adverse additive effects, HUMORSOL should be administered only with extreme caution to patients with myasthenia gravis who are receiving systemic anticholinesterase therapy; conversely, extreme caution should be exercised in the use of an anticholinesterase drug for the treatment of myasthenia gravis patients who are already undergoing topical therapy with cholinesterase inhibitors.
Use in pregnancy: The safe use of anticholinesterase drugs in pregnancy has not been established, nor has the absence of adverse effects on the fetus or on respiration of the neonate. Therefore, the use of HUMORSOL during pregnancy requires that its potential benefits be weighed against its possible hazards.

PRECAUTIONS

Except in aphakic patients, HUMORSOL should be used in glaucoma only when shorter-acting miotics have proved inadequate.
Gonioscopy is recommended prior to medication with HUMORSOL.
When an intraocular inflammatory process is present, the intensity and persistence of miosis and ciliary muscle contraction that result from anticholinesterase therapy require abstention from, or cautious use of, HUMORSOL.
Systemic effects are infrequent when HUMORSOL is instilled carefully. Compression of the lacrimal sac during and following instillation for a minute or two minimizes drainage into the nasal chamber with its extensive absorption surface. Wash the hands immediately after instillation.
Discontinue HUMORSOL if salivation, urinary incontinence, diarrhea, profuse sweating, muscle weakness, respiratory difficulties, shock, or cardiac irregularities occur.
Persons receiving cholinesterase inhibitors who are exposed to organophosphate-type insecticides and pesticides (gardeners, organophosphate plant or warehouse workers, farmers, residents of communities which are undergoing insecticide spraying or dusting, etc.) should be warned of the added systemic effects possible from absorption through the respiratory tract or skin. Wearing of respiratory masks, frequent washing, and clothing changes may be advisable.
Anticholinesterase drugs should be used with extreme caution, if at all, in patients with marked vagotonia, bronchial asthma, spastic gastrointestinal disturbances, peptic ulcer, pronounced bradycardia and hypotension, recent myocardial infarction, epilepsy, parkinsonism, and other disorders that may respond adversely to vagotonic effects.
After long-term use of HUMORSOL, dilation of blood vessels and resulting greater permeability increase the possibility of hyphema during ophthalmic surgery. Therefore, this drug should be discontinued before surgery.
Despite observance of all precautions and the use of only the recommended dose, there is some evidence that repeated administration may cause depression of the concentration of cholinesterase in the serum and erythrocytes, with resultant systemic effects.

ADVERSE REACTIONS

Stinging, burning, lacrimation, lid muscle twitching, conjunctival and ciliary redness, brow ache, headache, and induced myopia with visual blurring may occur.
Activation of latent iritis or uveitis may occur.
Retinal detachment has been reported occasionally.
Iris cysts may form, enlarge, and obscure vision. Occurrence is more frequent in children. The iris cyst usually shrinks upon discontinuance of the miotic. Rarely, the cyst may rupture or break free into the aqueous. Frequent examination for this occurrence is advisable.
Prolonged use may cause conjunctival thickening and obstruction of nasolacrimal canals.
Should systemic effects occur, manifested by nausea, vomiting, abdominal cramps, diarrhea, urinary incontinence, salivation, difficulty in breathing, bradycardia, or cardiac irregularities, parenteral administration of atropine sulfate is indicated: 0.4 to 0.6 mg or more for adults, proportionately less for children. Pralidoxime chloride in addition to atropine may be considered. Artificial respiration may be required.
Lens opacities have been reported in patients on anticholinesterase therapy. Routine slit-lamp examinations, including the lens, should accompany prolonged use.
Paradoxical increase in intraocular pressure may follow anticholinesterase instillation. This may be alleviated by pupil-dilating medication.

DOSAGE AND ADMINISTRATION

HUMORSOL *is intended solely for topical use in the conjunctival sac.*
As HUMORSOL is an extremely potent drug, the physician should thoroughly familiarize himself with its use and the technic of instillation.
The required dose is applied in the conjunctival sac, with the patient supine, care being taken not to touch the cornea with the tip of the OCUMETER® ophthalmic dispenser. *The patient or person administering the medication should apply continuous gentle pressure on the lacrimal sac with the index finger for a minute or two following instillation of the drops. This prevents overflow of solution into the nasal and pharyngeal spaces, which might cause systemic absorption. Wash the hands immediately after administration.*
HUMORSOL *should not be used more often than directed. Caution is necessary to avoid overdosage.*
Initial titration and dosage adjustments with HUMORSOL must be individualized to obtain maximal therapeutic effect. The patient must be closely observed during the initial period. If the response is not adequate within the first 24 hours, other measures should be considered.
Keep frequency of use to a minimum in all patients, but especially in children, to reduce the chance of iris cyst development (see ADVERSE REACTIONS).
Glaucoma
For initial therapy with HUMORSOL place 1 drop (children) or 1 or 2 drops (adults) in the glaucomatous eye. A decrease in intraocular pressure should occur within a few hours. During this period, keep the patient under supervision and make tonometric examinations at least hourly for 3 or 4 hours to be sure that no immediate rise in pressure occurs (see ADVERSE REACTIONS).
If necessary, the dosage may be increased from 1 or 2 drops twice a week to 1 or 2 drops twice a day. Duration of effect varies with the individual. The 0.125 percent strength used twice a day usually results in smooth control of the physiologic diurnal variation in intraocular pressure. This is probably the preferred dosage for most wide (open) angle glaucoma patients.
Strabismus
Essentially equal visual acuity of both eyes is prerequisite to the successful treatment of esotropia with HUMORSOL. For initial evaluation it may be used as a diagnostic aid to determine if an accommodative factor exists. This is especially useful preoperatively in young children and in patients with normal hypermetropic refractive errors. One drop is given daily for 2 weeks, then 1 drop every 2 days for 2 to 3 weeks. If the eyes become straighter, an accommodative factor is demonstrated. This technic may supplement or complement standard testing with atropine and trial with glasses for the accommodative factor.
In esotropia uncomplicated by amblyopia or anisometropia, HUMORSOL may be instilled in both eyes, *not more than 1 drop at a time every day for 2 to 3 weeks,* as too severe a degree of miosis may interfere with vision. Then reduce the dosage to 1 drop every other day for 3 to 4 weeks and reevaluate the patient's status.
HUMORSOL may be continued in a dosage of 1 drop every 2 days to 1 drop twice a week. (The latter dosage may be maintained for several months.) Evaluate the patient's condition every 4 to 12 weeks. If improvement continues, change the schedule to 1 drop once a week and eventually to a trial without medication. However, if after 4 months, control of the condition still requires 1 drop every 2 days, therapy with HUMORSOL should be stopped.

TREATMENT OF ADVERSE EFFECTS

If HUMORSOL is taken systemically by accident, or if systemic effects occur after topical application in the eye or from accidental skin contact, administer atropine sulfate parenterally (intravenously if necessary) in a dose (for adults) of 0.4 to 0.6 mg or more. Give a proportionately smaller amount to children.
The use of much larger doses of atropine in treating anticholinesterase intoxication in adults has been reported (Gordon, A. S.; Frye, C. W., J. Amer. Med. Ass. *159:* 1181, Nov. 19, 1955; Grob. D., Arch. Intern. Med. *98:* 221, Aug. 1956; Richards, A. G., Can. Med. Ass. J. *91:* 82, July 11, 1964; Taylor, W. J. R., et al., Can. Med. Ass. J. *93:* 966, Oct. 30, 1965). Initially 2 to 6 mg may be given followed by 2 mg every hour or more often, as long as muscarinic effects continue. The greater possibility of atropinization with large doses, particularly in sensitive individuals, should be borne in mind.
Pralidoxime* chloride has been reported to be useful in treating systemic effects due to cholinesterase inhibitors. However, its use is recommended in addition to and not as a substitute for atropine.
A short-acting barbiturate is indicated if convulsions occur that are not entirely relieved by atropine. Barbiturate dosage should be carefully adjusted to avoid central respiratory depression. Marked weakness or paralysis of muscles of respiration should be treated promptly by artificial respiration and maintenance of a clear airway.

HOW SUPPLIED

Ophthalmic Solution HUMORSOL is a clear, colorless, sterile, aqueous solution and is supplied in a 5 ml white, opaque, plastic OCUMETER ophthalmic dispenser with a controlled-drop tip:

No. 3255—0.125 percent solution.
NDC 0006-3255-03.
No. 3267—0.25 percent solution.
NDC 0006-3267-03.
A.H.F.S. Category: 52:20
DC 6378210 Issued May 1975

*PROTOPAM® Chloride (Pralidoxime Chloride) Ayerst Laboratories

Continued on next page

Information on the Merck Sharp & Dohme products listed on these pages is the full prescribing information from product circulars in use August 31, 1986.

Merck Sharp & Dohme—Cont.

HYDELTRASOL® Injection ℞
(Prednisolone Sodium Phosphate, MSD), U.S.P.

DESCRIPTION

Prednisolone sodium phosphate, a synthetic adrenocortical steroid, is a white or slightly yellow powder that is slightly hygroscopic and is freely soluble in water. The molecular weight is 484.39. It is designated chemically as 11β, 17-dihydroxy-21-(phosphonooxy) pregna-1,4-diene-3,20-dione disodium salt. The empirical formula is $C_{21}H_{27}Na_2O_8P$ and the structural formula is:

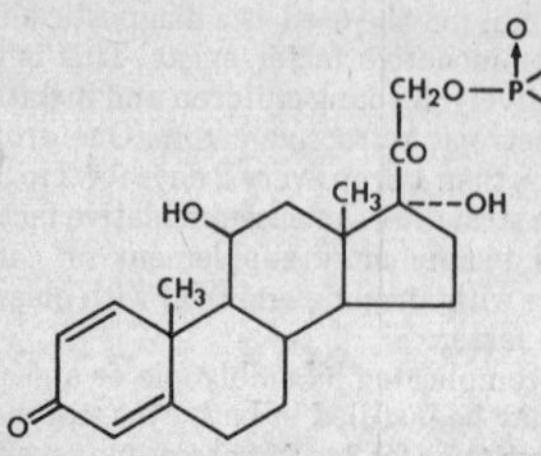

HYDELTRASOL® (Prednisolone Sodium Phosphate, MSD) injection is a sterile solution (pH 7.0 to 8.0) for intravenous, intramuscular, intra-articular, intralesional, and soft tissue administration.
Each milliliter contains prednisolone sodium phosphate equivalent to 20 mg prednisolone phosphate. Inactive ingredients per mL: niacinamide, 25 mg; sodium hydroxide to adjust pH; disodium edetate, 0.5 mg; Water for Injection, q.s. 1 mL. Sodium bisulfite, 1 mg, and phenol, 5 mg, added as preservatives.

ACTIONS

HYDELTRASOL injection has a rapid onset but short duration of action when compared with less soluble preparations. Because of this, it is suitable for the treatment of acute disorders responsive to adrenocortical steroid therapy.
Naturally occurring glucocorticoids (hydrocortisone and cortisone), which also have salt-retaining properties, are used as replacement therapy in adrenocortical deficiency states. Their synthetic analogs, including prednisolone, are primarily used for their potent anti-inflammatory effects in disorders of many organ systems.
Glucocorticoids cause profound and varied metabolic effects. In addition, they modify the body's immune responses to diverse stimuli.
At equipotent anti-inflammatory doses, prednisolone has less tendency to cause salt and water retention than either hydrocortisone or cortisone.

INDICATIONS

A. By intravenous or intramuscular injection when oral therapy is not feasible:
1. *Endocrine disorders*
Primary or secondary adrenocortical insufficiency (hydrocortisone or cortisone is the drug of choice; synthetic analogs may be used in conjunction with mineralocorticoids where applicable; in infancy, mineralocorticoid supplementation is of particular importance)
Acute adrenocortical insufficiency (hydrocortisone or cortisone is the drug of choice; mineralocorticoid supplementation may be necessary, particularly when synthetic analogs are used)
Preoperatively, and in the event of serious trauma or illness, in patients with known adrenal insufficiency or when adrenocortical reserve is doubtful
Congenital adrenal hyperplasia
Nonsuppurative thyroiditis
Hypercalcemia associated with cancer
2. *Rheumatic disorders*
As adjunctive therapy for short-term administration (to tide the patient over an acute episode or exacerbation) in:
Post-traumatic osteoarthritis
Synovitis of osteoarthritis
Rheumatoid arthritis, including juvenile rheumatoid arthritis (selected cases may require low-dose maintenance therapy)
Acute and subacute bursitis
Epicondylitis
Acute nonspecific tenosynovitis
Acute gouty arthritis
Psoriatic arthritis
Ankylosing spondylitis
3. *Collagen diseases*
During an exacerbation or as maintenance therapy in selected cases of:
Systemic lupus erythematosus
Acute rheumatic carditis
Systemic dermatomyositis (polymyositis)
4. *Dermatologic diseases*
Pemphigus
Severe erythema multiforme (Stevens-Johnson syndrome)
Exfoliative dermatitis
Bullous dermatitis herpetiformis
Severe seborrheic dermatitis
Severe psoriasis
Mycosis fungoides
5. *Allergic states*
Control of severe or incapacitating allergic conditions intractable to adequate trials of conventional treatment in:
Bronchial asthma
Contact dermatitis
Atopic dermatitis
Serum sickness
Seasonal or perennial allergic rhinitis
Drug hypersensitivity reactions
Urticarial transfusion reactions
Acute noninfectious laryngeal edema (epinephrine is the drug of first choice)
6. *Ophthalmic diseases*
Severe acute and chronic allergic and inflammatory processes involving the eye, such as:
Herpes zoster ophthalmicus
Iritis, iridocyclitis
Chorioretinitis
Diffuse posterior uveitis and choroiditis
Optic neuritis
Sympathetic ophthalmia
Anterior segment inflammation
Allergic conjunctivitis
Keratitis
Allergic corneal marginal ulcers
7. *Gastrointestinal diseases*
To tide the patient over a critical period of the disease in:
Ulcerative colitis (Systemic therapy)
Regional enteritis (Systemic therapy)
8. *Respiratory diseases*
Symptomatic sarcoidosis
Berylliosis
Fulminating or disseminated pulmonary tuberculosis when used concurrently with appropriate antituberculous chemotherapy
Loeffler's syndrome not manageable by other means
Aspiration pneumonitis
9. *Hematologic disorders*
Acquired (autoimmune) hemolytic anemia
Idiopathic thrombocytopenic purpura in adults (I.V. only; I.M. administration is contraindicated)
Secondary thrombocytopenia in adults
Erythroblastopenia (RBC anemia)
Congenital (erythroid) hypoplastic anemia
10. *Neoplastic diseases*
For palliative management of:
Leukemias and lymphomas in adults
Acute leukemia of childhood
11. *Edematous states*
To induce diuresis or remission of proteinuria in the nephrotic syndrome, without uremia, of the idiopathic type, or that due to lupus erythematosus
12. *Miscellaneous*
Tuberculous meningitis with subarachnoid block or impending block when used concurrently with appropriate antituberculous chemotherapy
Trichinosis with neurologic or myocardial involvement.
B. By intra-articular or soft tissue injection:
As adjunctive therapy for short-term administration (to tide the patient over an acute episode or exacerbation) in:
Synovitis of osteoarthritis
Rheumatoid arthritis
Acute and subacute bursitis
Acute gouty arthritis
Epicondylitis
Acute nonspecific tenosynovitis
Post-traumatic osteoarthritis.
C. By intralesional injection:
Keloids
Localized hypertrophic, infiltrated, inflammatory lesions of: lichen planus, psoriatic plaques, granuloma annulare, and lichen simplex chronicus (neurodermatitis)
Discoid lupus erythematosus
Necrobiosis lipoidica diabeticorum
Alopecia areata
May also be useful in cystic tumors of an aponeurosis or tendon (ganglia).

CONTRAINDICATIONS

Systemic fungal infections (see WARNINGS regarding amphotericin B)
Hypersensitivity to any component of this product, including sulfites (see WARNINGS regarding sodium bisulfite).

WARNINGS

Sodium bisulfite has been reported to cause severe allergic reactions in certain susceptible individuals, particularly patients with asthma. Anaphylactoid and hypersensitivity reactions have been reported for Injection HYDELTRASOL (see ADVERSE REACTIONS). Since Injection HYDELTRASOL contains sodium bisulfite, this product should not be used in patients allergic to sulfites.
Corticosteroids may exacerbate systemic fungal infections and therefore should not be used in the presence of such infections unless they are needed to control drug reactions due to amphotericin B. Moreover, there have been cases reported in which concomitant use of amphotericin B and hydrocortisone was followed by cardiac enlargement and congestive failure.
In patients on corticosteroid therapy subjected to any unusual stress, increased dosage of rapidly acting corticosteroids before, during, and after the stressful situation is indicated.
Drug-induced secondary adrenocortical insufficiency may result from too rapid withdrawal of corticosteroids and may be minimized by gradual reduction of dosage. This type of relative insufficiency may persist for months after discontinuation of therapy; therefore, in any situation of stress occurring during that period, hormone therapy should be reinstituted. If the patient is receiving steroids already, dosage may have to be increased. Since mineralocorticoid secretion may be impaired, salt and/or a mineralocorticoid should be administered concurrently.
Corticosteroids may mask some signs of infection, and new infections may appear during their use. There may be decreased resistance and inability to localize infection when corticosteroids are used. Moreover, corticosteroids may affect the nitroblue-tetrazolium test for bacterial infection and produce false negative results.
In cerebral malaria, a double-blind trial has shown that the use of corticosteroids is associated with prolongation of coma and a higher incidence of pneumonia and gastrointestinal bleeding.
Corticosteroids may activate latent amebiasis. Therefore, it is recommended that latent or active amebiasis be ruled out before initiating corticosteroid therapy in any patient who has spent time in the tropics or any patient with unexplained diarrhea.
Prolonged use of corticosteroids may produce posterior subcapsular cataracts, glaucoma with possible damage to the optic nerves, and may enhance the establishment of secondary ocular infections due to fungi or viruses.
Usage in pregnancy. Since adequate human reproduction studies have not been done with corticosteroids, use of these drugs in pregnancy or in women of childbearing potential requires that the anticipated benefits be weighed against the possible hazards to the mother and embryo or fetus. Infants born of mothers who have received substantial doses of corticosteroids during pregnancy should be carefully observed for signs of hypoadrenalism.
Corticosteroids appear in breast milk and could suppress growth, interfere with endogenous corticosteroid production, or cause other unwanted effects. Mothers taking pharmacologic doses of corticosteroids should be advised not to nurse.
Average and large doses of cortisone or hydrocortisone can cause elevation of blood pressure, salt and water retention, and increased excretion of potassium. These effects are less likely to occur with the synthetic derivatives except when used in large doses. Dietary salt restriction and potassium supplementation may be necessary. All corticosteroids increase calcium excretion.
Administration of live virus vaccines, including smallpox, is contraindicated in individuals receiving immunosuppressive doses of corticosteroids. If inactivated viral or bacterial vaccines are administered to individuals receiving immunosuppressive doses of corticosteroids, the expected serum antibody response may not be obtained. However, immunization procedures may be undertaken in patients who are receiving corticosteroids as replacement therapy, e.g., for Addison's disease.
The use of HYDELTRASOL injection in active tuberculosis should be restricted to those cases of fulminating or disseminated tuberculosis in which the corticosteroid is used for the management of the disease in conjunction with appropriate antituberculous regimen.
If corticosteroids are indicated in patients with latent tuberculosis or tuberculin reactivity, close observation is necessary as reactivation of the disease may occur. During prolonged corticosteroid therapy, these patients should receive chemoprophylaxis.
Because rare instances of anaphylactoid reactions have occurred in patients receiving parenteral corticosteroid therapy, appropriate precautionary measures should be taken prior to administration, especially when the patient has a history of allergy to any drug.

PRECAUTIONS

This product, like many other steroid formulations, is sensitive to heat. Therefore, it should not be autoclaved when it is desirable to sterilize the exterior of the vial.
Following prolonged therapy, withdrawal of corticosteroids may result in symptoms of the corticosteroid withdrawal

syndrome including fever, myalgia, arthralgia, and malaise. This may occur in patients even without evidence of adrenal insufficiency.
There is an enhanced effect of corticosteroids in patients with hypothyroidism and in those with cirrhosis.
Corticosteroids should be used cautiously in patients with ocular herpes simplex for fear of corneal perforation.
The lowest possible dose of corticosteroid should be used to control the condition under treatment, and when reduction in dosage is possible, the reduction must be gradual.
Psychic derangements may appear when corticosteroids are used, ranging from euphoria, insomnia, mood swings, personality changes, and severe depression to frank psychotic manifestations. Also, existing emotional instability or psychotic tendencies may be aggravated by corticosteroids.
Aspirin should be used cautiously in conjunction with corticosteroids in hypoprothrombinemia.
Steroids should be used with caution in nonspecific ulcerative colitis, if there is a probability of impending perforation, abscess, or other pyogenic infection, also in diverticulitis, fresh intestinal anastomoses, active or latent peptic ulcer, renal insufficiency, hypertension, osteoporosis, and myasthenia gravis. Signs of peritoneal irritation following gastrointestinal perforation in patients receiving large doses of corticosteroids may be minimal or absent. Fat embolism has been reported as a possible complication of hypercortisonism.
When large doses are given, some authorities advise that antacids be administered between meals to help to prevent peptic ulcer.
Growth and development of infants and children on prolonged corticosteroid therapy should be carefully followed.
Steroids may increase or decrease motility and number of spermatozoa in some patients.
Phenytoin, phenobarbital, ephedrine, and rifampin may enhance the metabolic clearance of corticosteroids, resulting in decreased blood levels and lessened physiologic activity, thus requiring adjustment in corticosteroid dosage.
The prothrombin time should be checked frequently in patients who are receiving corticosteroids and coumarin anticoagulants at the same time because of reports that corticosteroids have altered the response to these anticoagulants. Studies have shown that the usual effect produced by adding corticosteroids is inhibition of response to coumarins, although there have been some conflicting reports of potentiation not substantiated by studies.
When corticosteroids are administered concomitantly with potassium-depleting diuretics, patients should be observed closely for development of hypokalemia.
Intra-articular injection of a corticosteroid may produce systemic as well as local effects.
Appropriate examination of any joint fluid present is necessary to exclude a septic process.
A marked increase in pain accompanied by local swelling, further restriction of joint motion, fever, and malaise is suggestive of septic arthritis. If this complication occurs and the diagnosis of sepsis is confirmed, appropriate antimicrobial therapy should be instituted.
Injection of a steroid into an infected site is to be avoided.
Corticosteroids should not be injected into unstable joints.
Patients should be impressed strongly with the importance of not overusing joints in which symptomatic benefit has been obtained as long as the inflammatory process remains active.
Frequent intra-articular injection may result in damage to joint tissues.
The slower rate of absorption by intramuscular administration should be recognized.

ADVERSE REACTIONS

Fluid and electrolyte disturbances
Sodium retention
Fluid retention
Congestive heart failure in susceptible patients
Potassium loss
Hypokalemic alkalosis
Hypertension
Musculoskeletal
Muscle weakness
Steroid myopathy
Loss of muscle mass
Osteoporosis
Vertebral compression fractures
Aseptic necrosis of femoral and humeral heads
Pathologic fracture of long bones
Tendon rupture
Gastrointestinal
Peptic ulcer with possible subsequent perforation and hemorrhage
Perforation of the small and large bowel, particularly in patients with inflammatory bowel disease
Pancreatitis
Abdominal distention
Ulcerative esophagitis
Dermatologic
Impaired wound healing
Thin fragile skin
Petechiae and ecchymoses
Erythema
Increased sweating
May suppress reactions to skin tests
Burning or tingling, especially in the perineal area (after I.V. injection)
Other cutaneous reactions, such as allergic dermatitis, urticaria, angioneurotic edema
Neurologic
Convulsions
Increased intracranial pressure with papilledema (pseudotumor cerebri) usually after treatment
Vertigo
Headache
Endocrine
Menstrual irregularities
Development of cushingoid state
Suppression of growth in children
Secondary adrenocortical and pituitary unresponsiveness, particularly in times of stress, as in trauma, surgery, or illness
Decreased carbohydrate tolerance
Manifestations of latent diabetes mellitus
Increased requirements for insulin or oral hypoglycemic agents in diabetics
Hirsutism
Ophthalmic
Posterior subcapsular cataracts
Increased intraocular pressure
Glaucoma
Exophthalmos
Metabolic
Negative nitrogen balance due to protein catabolism
Other
Anaphylactoid or hypersensitivity reactions
Thromboembolism
Weight gain
Increased appetite
Nausea
Malaise
Psychic disturbances
The following *additional* adverse reactions are related to parenteral corticosteroid therapy:
Rare instances of blindness associated with intralesional therapy around the face and head
Hyperpigmentation or hypopigmentation
Subcutaneous and cutaneous atrophy
Sterile abscess
Postinjection flare (following intra-articular use)
Charcot-like arthropathy.

DOSAGE AND ADMINISTRATION

For intravenous, intramuscular, intra-articular, intralesional, and soft tissue injection.
DOSAGE REQUIREMENTS ARE VARIABLE AND MUST BE INDIVIDUALIZED ON THE BASIS OF THE DISEASE AND THE RESPONSE OF THE PATIENT.
Intravenous and Intramuscular Injection
HYDELTRASOL injection can be given directly from the vial, or it can be added to Sodium Chloride Injection or Dextrose Injection and given by intravenous drip.
Benzyl alcohol as a preservative has been associated with toxicity in premature infants. Solutions used for intravenous administration or further dilution of this product should be preservative-free when used in the neonate, especially the premature infant.
When it is mixed with an infusion solution, sterile precautions should be observed. Since infusion solutions generally do not contain preservatives, mixtures should be used within 24 hours.
The initial dosage varies from 4 to 60 mg a day depending on the disease being treated. In less severe diseases doses lower than 4 mg may suffice, while in severe diseases doses higher than 60 mg may be required. Usually the daily parenteral dose of HYDELTRASOL injection is the same as the daily oral dose of prednisolone and the dosage interval is every 4 to 8 hours.
The initial dosage should be maintained or adjusted until the patient's response is satisfactory. If a satisfactory clinical response does not occur after a reasonable period of time, discontinue HYDELTRASOL injection and transfer the patient to other therapy.
After a favorable initial response, the proper maintenance dosage should be determined by decreasing the initial dosage in small amounts to the lowest dosage that maintains an adequate clinical response.
Patients should be observed closely for signs that might require dosage adjustment, including changes in clinical status resulting from remissions or exacerbations of the disease, individual drug responsiveness, and the effect of stress (e.g., surgery, infection, trauma). During stress it may be necessary to increase dosage temporarily.
If the drug is to be stopped after more than a few days of treatment, it usually should be withdrawn gradually.
Intra-articular, Intralesional, and Soft Tissue Injection
Intra-articular, intralesional, and soft tissue injections are generally employed when the affected joints or areas are limited to one or two sites. Dosage and frequency of injection vary depending on the condition being treated and the site of injection. The usual dose is from 2 to 30 mg. The frequency usually ranges from once every three to five days to once every two to three weeks. Frequent intra-articular injection may result in damage to joint tissues.
Some of the usual single doses are:
[See table above].

	Doses	
Site of Injection	Amount of Injection (mL)	Amount of Prednisolone Phosphate (mg)
Large Joints (e.g., Knee)	0.5 to 1	10 to 20
Small Joints (e.g., Interphalangeal, Temporomandibular)	0.2 to 0.25	4 to 5
Bursae	0.5 to 0.75	10 to 15
Tendon Sheaths	0.1 to 0.25	2 to 5
Soft Tissue Infiltration	0.5 to 1.5	10 to 30
Ganglia	0.25 to 0.5	5 to 10

HYDELTRASOL injection is particularly recommended for use in conjunction with one of the less soluble, longer-acting steroids, such as HYDELTRA-T.B.A.® (Prednisolone Tebutate, MSD) suspension or HYDROCORTONE® Acetate (Hydrocortisone Acetate, MSD) saline suspension, available for intra-articular and soft tissue injection.

HOW SUPPLIED

No. 7577X—Injection HYDELTRASOL, 20 mg prednisolone phosphate equivalent per mL, is a clear, colorless to slightly yellow solution, and is supplied as follows:
NDC 0006-7577-02 in 2 mL vials
NDC 0006-7577-03 in 5 mL vials.
(6505-00-890-1496 20 mg/mL 5 mL vial)
Storage
Sensitive to heat. Do not autoclave.
Protect from light. Store container in carton until contents have been used.

A.H.F.S. Category: 68:04
DC 6026223 Issued April 1985

HYDELTRA–T.B.A.® Suspension (Prednisolone Tebutate, MSD), U.S.P. ℞

For intra-articular, intralesional, and soft tissue injection only.

DESCRIPTION

Prednisolone tebutate, a synthetic adrenocortical steroid, is a white to slightly yellow powder sparingly soluble in alco-

Continued on next page

Information on the Merck Sharp & Dohme products listed on these pages is the full prescribing information from product circulars in use August 31, 1986.

Merck Sharp & Dohme—Cont.

hol, freely soluble in chloroform, and very slightly soluble in water. The molecular weight is 476.61 (monohydrate). It is designated chemically as 11β,17- dihydroxy - 21 - [(3,3-dimethyl-1-oxobutyl)oxy] pregna-1,4-diene-3,20-dione. The empirical formula is $C_{27}H_{38}O_6$ and the structural formula is:

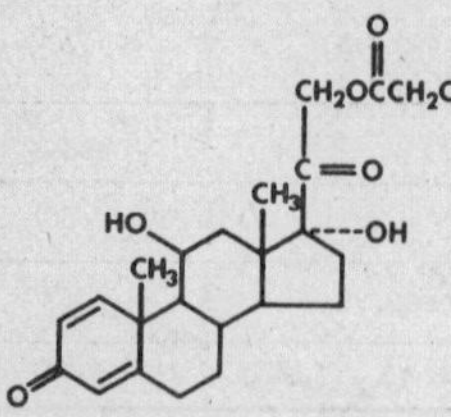

HYDELTRA-T.B.A.® (Prednisolone Tebutate, MSD) suspension is a white to slightly yellow suspension (pH 6.0 to 8.0) that settles upon standing. Each mL contains prednisolone tebutate, 20 mg. Inactive ingredients per mL: sodium citrate, 1 mg; polysorbate 80, 1 mg; sorbitol solution, 0.5 mL (equal to 450 mg d-sorbitol); Water for Injection, q.s., 1 mL. Benzyl alcohol, 9 mg, added as preservative.

ACTIONS

HYDELTRA-T.B.A. has a slow onset but long duration of action when compared with more soluble preparations. Because of its slight solubility, it is suitable for intra-articular, intralesional, and soft tissue injection where its anti-inflammatory effects are confined mainly to the area in which it has been injected, although it is capable of producing systemic hormonal effects.

Naturally occurring glucocorticoids (hydrocortisone and cortisone), which also have salt-retaining properties, are used as replacement therapy in adrenocortical deficiency states. Their synthetic analogs, including prednisolone, are primarily used for their potent anti-inflammatory effects in disorders of many organ systems.

Glucocorticoids cause profound and varied metabolic effects. In addition, they modify the body's immune responses to diverse stimuli.

INDICATIONS

A. By intra-articular or soft tissue injection:

As adjunctive therapy for short-term administration (to tide the patient over an acute episode or exacerbation) in:

- Synovitis of osteoarthritis
- Rheumatoid arthritis
- Acute and subacute bursitis
- Acute gouty arthritis
- Epicondylitis
- Acute nonspecific tenosynovitis
- Post-traumatic osteoarthritis

B. By intralesional injection:

May be useful in cystic tumors of an aponeurosis or tendon (ganglia).

CONTRAINDICATIONS

Systemic fungal infections

Hypersensitivity to any component of this product

WARNINGS

In patients on corticosteroid therapy subjected to any unusual stress, increased dosage of rapidly acting corticosteroids before, during, and after the stressful situation is indicated.

Drug-induced secondary adrenocortical insufficiency may result from too rapid withdrawal of corticosteroids and may be minimized by gradual reduction of dosage. This type of relative insufficiency may persist for months after discontinuation of therapy; therefore, in any situation of stress occurring during that period, hormone therapy should be reinstituted. If the patient is receiving steroids already, dosage may have to be increased. Since mineralocorticoid secretion may be impaired, salt and/or a mineralocorticoid should be administered concurrently.

Corticosteroids may mask some signs of infection, and new infections may appear during their use. There may be decreased resistance and inability to localize infection when corticosteroids are used. Moreover, corticosteroids may affect the nitroblue-tetrazolium test for bacterial infection and produce false negative results.

In cerebral malaria, a double-blind trial has shown that the use of corticosteroids is associated with prolongation of coma and a higher incidence of pneumonia and gastrointestinal bleeding.

Corticosteroids may activate latent amebiasis. Therefore, it is recommended that latent or active amebiasis be ruled out before initiating corticosteroid therapy in any patient who has spent time in the tropics or any patient with unexplained diarrhea.

Prolonged use of corticosteroids may produce posterior subcapsular cataracts, glaucoma with possible damage to the optic nerves, and may enhance the establishment of secondary ocular infections due to fungi or viruses.

Usage in pregnancy. Since adequate human reproduction studies have not been done with corticosteroids, use of these drugs in pregnancy or in women of childbearing potential requires that the anticipated benefits be weighed against the possible hazards to the mother and embryo or fetus. Infants born of mothers who have received substantial doses of corticosteroids during pregnancy should be carefully observed for signs of hypoadrenalism.

Corticosteroids appear in breast milk and could suppress growth, interfere with endogenous corticosteroid production, or cause other unwanted effects. Mothers taking pharmacologic doses of corticosteroids should be advised not to nurse.

Average and large doses of cortisone or hydrocortisone can cause elevation of blood pressure, salt and water retention, and increased excretion of potassium. These effects are less likely to occur with the synthetic derivatives except when used in large doses. Dietary salt restriction and potassium supplementation may be necessary. All corticosteroids increase calcium excretion.

Administration of live virus vaccines, including smallpox, is contraindicated in individuals receiving immunosuppressive doses of corticosteroids. If inactivated viral or bacterial vaccines are administered to individuals receiving immunosuppressive doses of corticosteroids, the expected serum antibody response may not be obtained.

If corticosteroids are indicated in patients with latent tuberculosis or tuberculin reactivity, close observation is necessary as reactivation of the disease may occur. During prolonged corticosteroid therapy, these patients should receive chemoprophylaxis.

Because rare instances of anaphylactoid reactions have occurred in patients receiving parenteral corticosteroid therapy, appropriate precautionary measures should be taken prior to administration, especially when the patient has a history of allergy to any drug.

PRECAUTIONS

This product, like many other steroid formulations, is sensitive to heat. Therefore, it should not be autoclaved when it is desirable to sterilize the exterior of the vial.

Following prolonged therapy, withdrawal of corticosteroids may result in symptoms of the corticosteroid withdrawal syndrome including fever, myalgia, arthralgia, and malaise. This may occur in patients even without evidence of adrenal insufficiency.

There is an enhanced effect of corticosteroids in patients with hypothyroidism and in those with cirrhosis.

Corticosteroids should be used cautiously in patients with ocular herpes simplex for fear of corneal perforation.

Psychic derangements may appear when corticosteroids are used, ranging from euphoria, insomnia, mood swings, personality changes, and severe depression to frank psychotic manifestations. Also, existing emotional instability or psychotic tendencies may be aggravated by corticosteroids.

Aspirin should be used cautiously in conjunction with corticosteroids in hypoprothrombinemia.

Steroids should be used with caution in nonspecific ulcerative colitis, if there is a probability of impending perforation, abscess, or other pyogenic infection, also in diverticulitis, fresh intestinal anastomoses, active or latent peptic ulcer, renal insufficiency, hypertension, osteoporosis, and myasthenia gravis. Signs of peritoneal irritation following gastrointestinal perforation in patients receiving large doses of corticosteroids may be minimal or absent. Fat embolism has been reported as a possible complication of hypercortisonism.

When large doses are given, some authorities advise that antacids be administered between meals to help to prevent peptic ulcer.

Growth and development of infants and children on prolonged corticosteroid therapy should be carefully followed.

Steroids may increase or decrease motility and number of spermatozoa in some patients.

Phenytoin, phenobarbital, ephedrine, and rifampin may enhance the metabolic clearance of corticosteroids, resulting in decreased blood levels and lessened physiologic activity, thus requiring adjustment in corticosteroid dosage.

The prothrombin time should be checked frequently in patients who are receiving corticosteroids and coumarin anticoagulants at the same time because of reports that corticosteroids have altered the response to these anticoagulants. Studies have shown that the usual effect produced by adding corticosteroids is inhibition of response to coumarins, although there have been some conflicting reports of potentiation not substantiated by studies.

When corticosteroids are administered concomitantly with potassium-depleting diuretics, patients should be observed closely for development of hypokalemia.

Intra-articular injection of a corticosteroid may produce systemic as well as local effects.

Appropriate examination of any joint fluid present is necessary to exclude a septic process.

A marked increase in pain accompanied by local swelling, further restriction of joint motion, fever, and malaise is suggestive of septic arthritis. If this complication occurs and the diagnosis of sepsis is confirmed, appropriate antimicrobial therapy should be instituted.

Injection of a steroid into an infected site is to be avoided.

Corticosteroids should not be injected into unstable joints.

Patients should be impressed strongly with the importance of not overusing joints in which symptomatic benefit has been obtained as long as the inflammatory process remains active.

Frequent intra-articular injection may result in damage to joint tissues.

ADVERSE REACTIONS

Fluid and electrolyte disturbances
- Sodium retention
- Fluid retention
- Congestive heart failure in susceptible patients
- Potassium loss
- Hypokalemic alkalosis
- Hypertension

Musculoskeletal
- Muscle weakness
- Steroid myopathy
- Loss of muscle mass
- Osteoporosis
- Vertebral compression fractures
- Aseptic necrosis of femoral and humeral heads
- Pathologic fracture of long bones
- Tendon rupture

Gastrointestinal
- Peptic ulcer with possible subsequent perforation and hemorrhage
- Perforation of the small and large bowel, particularly in patients with inflammatory bowel disease
- Pancreatitis
- Abdominal distention
- Ulcerative esophagitis

Dermatologic
- Impaired wound healing
- Thin fragile skin
- Petechiae and ecchymoses
- Erythema
- Increased sweating
- May suppress reactions to skin tests
- Other cutaneous reactions, such as allergic dermatitis, urticaria, angioneurotic edema

Neurologic
- Convulsions
- Increased intracranial pressure with papilledema (pseudotumor cerebri) usually after treatment
- Vertigo
- Headache

Endocrine
- Menstrual irregularities
- Development of cushingoid state
- Suppression of growth in children
- Secondary adrenocortical and pituitary unresponsiveness, particularly in times of stress, as in trauma, surgery, or illness
- Decreased carbohydrate tolerance
- Manifestations of latent diabetes mellitus
- Increased requirements for insulin or oral hypoglycemic agents in diabetics
- Hirsutism

Ophthalmic
- Posterior subcapsular cataracts
- Increased intraocular pressure
- Glaucoma
- Exophthalmos

Metabolic
- Negative nitrogen balance due to protein catabolism

Other
- Anaphylactoid or hypersensitivity reactions
- Thromboembolism
- Weight gain
- Increased appetite
- Nausea
- Malaise
- Psychic disturbances

Foreign body granulomatous reactions involving the synovium have been reported with repeated injections of HYDELTRA-T.B.A.
Localized pain and swelling, sometimes distal to the site of injection and persisting for several days, have been reported.
The following *additional* adverse reactions are related to injection of corticosteroids:
Rare instances of blindness associated with intralesional therapy around the face and head
Hyperpigmentation or hypopigmentation
Subcutaneous and cutaneous atrophy
Sterile abscess
Postinjection flare (following intra-articular use)
Charcot-like arthropathy

DOSAGE AND ADMINISTRATION

For intra-articular, intralesional, and soft tissue injection only.

DOSAGE AND FREQUENCY OF INJECTION ARE VARIABLE AND MUST BE INDIVIDUALIZED ON THE BASIS OF THE DISEASE AND THE RESPONSE OF THE PATIENT.

The initial dose varies from 4 to 40 mg depending on the disease being treated and the size of the area to be injected. Frequency of injection depends on symptomatic response, and usually is once every two or three weeks. Severe conditions may require injection once a week. Frequent intra-articular injection may result in damage to joint tissues. If satisfactory clinical response does not occur after a reasonable period of time, discontinue HYDELTRA-T.B.A. suspension and transfer the patient to other therapy.
Patients should be observed closely for signs that might require dosage adjustment, including changes in clinical status resulting from remissions or exacerbations of the disease, and individual drug responsiveness.
For rapid onset of action, a soluble adrenocortical hormone preparation, such as DECADRON® Phosphate (Dexamethasone Sodium Phosphate, MSD) injection or HYDELTRASOL® (Prednisolone Sodium Phosphate, MSD) injection, may be given with HYDELTRA-T.B.A.
If desired, a local anesthetic may be used, and may be injected before HYDELTRA-T.B.A., or mixed in a syringe with HYDELTRA-T.B.A. and given simultaneously.
If used prior to intra-articular injection of the steroid, inject most of the anesthetic into the soft tissues of the surrounding area and instill a small amount into the joint.
If given together, mixing should be done in the injection syringe by drawing the steroid in *first*, then the anesthetic. In this way, the anesthetic will not be introduced inadvertently into the vial of steroid. *The mixture must be used immediately and any unused portion discarded.*
Some of the usual single doses are:

Large Joints (e.g., Knee)	20 mg (1 mL), occasionally 30 mg (1.5 mL). Doses over 40 mg (2 mL) not recommended.
Small Joints (e.g., Interphalangeal, Temporomandibular)	8 to 10 mg (0.4 to 0.5 mL).
Bursae	20 to 30 mg (1 to 1.5 mL).
Tendon Sheaths	4 to 10 mg (0.2 to 0.5 mL).
Ganglia	10 to 20 mg (0.5 to 1 mL).

HOW SUPPLIED

No. 7572—Suspension HYDELTRA-T.B.A., 20 mg per mL, is a white, milky suspension, and is supplied as follows:
NDC 0006-7572-01 in 1 mL vials
(6505-00-225-7499 1 mL vial)
NDC 0006-7572-03 in 5 mL vials
(6505-00-890-1353 5 mL vial).
Storage
Sensitive to heat. Do not autoclave.
Protect from freezing.
Protect from light. Store container in carton until contents have been used.

A.H.F.S. Category: 68:04
DC 6138623 Issued April 1985

HYDROCORTONE® ℞

Acetate Saline Suspension
(Hydrocortisone Acetate, MSD), U.S.P.

For intra-articular, intralesional, and soft tissue injection only.

DESCRIPTION

Hydrocortisone acetate, a synthetic adrenocortical steroid, is a white to practically white, odorless, crystalline powder. It is insoluble in water and slightly soluble in alcohol and chloroform. The molecular weight is 404.50. It is designated chemically as 21-(acetyloxy)-11β,17-dihydroxypregn-4-ene-3,20-dione. The empirical formula is $C_{23}H_{32}O_6$ and the structural formula is:

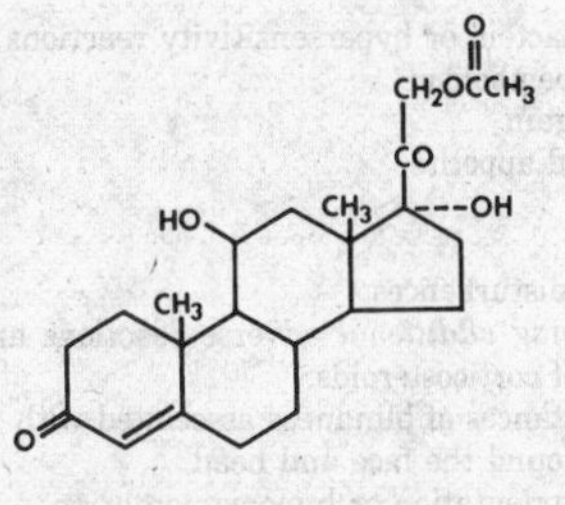

HYDROCORTONE® Acetate (Hydrocortisone Acetate, MSD) saline suspension is a sterile suspension of hydrocortisone acetate (pH 5.0 to 7.0) in a suitable aqueous medium. It is supplied in two strengths, one containing 25 mg hydrocortisone acetate per milliliter, the other containing 50 mg per milliliter. Inactive ingredients per mL: sodium chloride, 9 mg; polysorbate 80, 4 mg; sodium carboxymethylcellulose, 5 mg; and Water for Injection, q.s., 1 mL. Benzyl alcohol, 9 mg, added as preservative.

ACTIONS

HYDROCORTONE Acetate saline suspension has a slow onset but long duration of action when compared with more soluble preparations. Because of its insolubility, it is suitable for intra-articular, intralesional, and soft tissue injection where its anti-inflammatory effects are confined mainly to the area in which it has been injected, although it is capable of producing systemic hormonal effects.
Naturally occurring glucocorticoids (hydrocortisone and cortisone), which also have salt-retaining properties, are used as replacement therapy in adrenocortical deficiency states. They are also used for their potent anti-inflammatory effect in disorders of many organ systems.
Glucocorticoids cause profound and varied metabolic effects. In addition, they modify the body's immune responses to diverse stimuli.

INDICATIONS

A. By intra-articular or soft tissue injection:
As adjunctive therapy for short-term administration (to tide the patient over an acute episode or exacerbation) in:
Synovitis of osteoarthritis
Rheumatoid arthritis
Acute and subacute bursitis
Acute gouty arthritis
Epicondylitis
Acute nonspecific tenosynovitis
Post-traumatic osteoarthritis
B. By intralesional injection:
Keloids
Localized hypertrophic, infiltrated, inflammatory lesions of: lichen planus, psoriatic plaques, granuloma annulare, and lichen simplex chronicus (neurodermatitis)
Discoid lupus erythematosus
Necrobiosis lipoidica diabeticorum
Alopecia areata
May also be useful in cystic tumors of an aponeurosis or tendon (ganglia).

CONTRAINDICATIONS

Systemic fungal infections
Hypersensitivity to any component of this product

WARNINGS

In patients on corticosteroid therapy subjected to any unusual stress, increased dosage of rapidly acting corticosteroids before, during, and after the stressful situation is indicated.
Drug-induced secondary adrenocortical insufficiency may result from too rapid withdrawal of corticosteroids and may be minimized by gradual reduction of dosage. This type of relative insufficiency may persist for months after discontinuation of therapy; therefore, in any situation of stress occurring during that period, hormone therapy should be reinstituted. If the patient is receiving steroids already, dosage may have to be increased. Since mineralocorticoid secretion may be impaired, salt and/or a mineralocorticoid should be administered concurrently.
Corticosteroids may mask some signs of infection, and new infections may appear during their use. There may be decreased resistance and inability to localize infection when corticosteroids are used. Moreover, corticosteroids may affect the nitroblue-tetrazolium test for bacterial infection and produce false negative results.
In cerebral malaria, a double-blind trial has shown that the use of corticosteroids is associated with prolongation of coma and a higher incidence of pneumonia and gastrointestinal bleeding.
Corticosteroids may activate latent amebiasis. Therefore, it is recommended that latent or active amebiasis be ruled out before initiating corticosteroid therapy in any patient who has spent time in the tropics or any patient with unexplained diarrhea.
Prolonged use of corticosteroids may produce posterior subcapsular cataracts, glaucoma with possible damage to the optic nerves, and may enhance the establishment of secondary ocular infections due to fungi or viruses.
Usage in pregnancy: Since adequate human reproduction studies have not been done with corticosteroids, use of these drugs in pregnancy or in women of childbearing potential requires that the anticipated benefits be weighed against the possible hazards to the mother and embryo or fetus. Infants born of mothers who have received substantial doses of corticosteroids during pregnancy should be carefully observed for signs of hypoadrenalism.
Corticosteroids appear in breast milk and could suppress growth, interfere with endogenous corticosteroid production, or cause other unwanted effects. Mothers taking pharmacologic doses of corticosteroids should be advised not to nurse.
Average and large doses of cortisone or hydrocortisone can cause elevation of blood pressure, salt and water retention, and increased excretion of potassium. These effects are less likely to occur with the synthetic derivatives except when used in large doses. Dietary salt restriction and potassium supplementation may be necessary. All corticosteroids increase calcium excretion.
Administration of live virus vaccines, including smallpox, is contraindicated in individuals receiving immunosuppressive doses of corticosteroids. If inactivated viral or bacterial vaccines are administered to individuals receiving immunosuppressive doses of corticosteroids, the expected serum antibody response may not be obtained.
If corticosteroids are indicated in patients with latent tuberculosis or tuberculin reactivity, close observation is necessary as reactivation of the disease may occur. During prolonged corticosteroid therapy, these patients should receive chemoprophylaxis.
Because rare instances of anaphylactoid reactions have occurred in patients receiving parenteral corticosteroid therapy, appropriate precautionary measures should be taken prior to administration, especially when the patient has a history of allergy to any drug.

PRECAUTIONS

This product, like many other steroid formulations, is sensitive to heat. Therefore, it should not be autoclaved when it is desirable to sterilize the exterior of the vial.
Following prolonged therapy, withdrawal of corticosteroids may result in symptoms of the corticosteroid withdrawal syndrome including fever, myalgia, arthralgia, and malaise. This may occur in patients even without evidence of adrenal insufficiency.
There is an enhanced effect of corticosteroids in patients with hypothyroidism and in those with cirrhosis.
Corticosteroids should be used cautiously in patients with ocular herpes simplex for fear of corneal perforation.
Psychic derangements may appear when corticosteroids are used, ranging from euphoria, insomnia, mood swings, personality changes, and severe depression to frank psychotic manifestations. Also, existing emotional instability or psychotic tendencies may be aggravated by corticosteroids.
Aspirin should be used cautiously in conjunction with corticosteroids in hypoprothrombinemia.
Steroids should be used with caution in nonspecific ulcerative colitis, if there is a probability of impending perfora-

Continued on next page

Information on the Merck Sharp & Dohme products listed on these pages is the full prescribing information from product circulars in use August 31, 1986.

Merck Sharp & Dohme—Cont.

tion, abscess, or other pyogenic infection, also in diverticulitis, fresh intestinal anastomoses, active or latent peptic ulcer, renal insufficiency, hypertension, osteoporosis, and myasthenia gravis. Signs of peritoneal irritation following gastrointestinal perforation in patients receiving large doses of corticosteroids may be minimal or absent. Fat embolism has been reported as a possible complication of hypercortisonism.
When large doses are given, some authorities advise that antacids be administered between meals to help to prevent peptic ulcer.
Growth and development of infants and children on prolonged corticosteroid therapy should be carefully followed.
Steroids may increase or decrease motility and number of spermatozoa in some patients.
Phenytoin, phenobarbital, ephedrine, and rifampin may enhance the metabolic clearance of corticosteroids resulting in decreased blood levels and lessened physiologic activity, thus requiring adjustment in corticosteroid dosage.
The prothrombin time should be checked frequently in patients who are receiving corticosteroids and coumarin anticoagulants at the same time because of reports that corticosteroids have altered the response to these anticoagulants. Studies have shown that the usual effect produced by adding corticosteroids is inhibition of response to coumarins, although there have been some conflicting reports of potentiation not substantiated by studies.
When corticosteroids are administered concomitantly with potassium-depleting diuretics, patients should be observed closely for development of hypokalemia.
Intra-articular injection of a corticosteroid may produce systemic as well as local effects.
Appropriate examination of any joint fluid present is necessary to exclude a septic process.
A marked increase in pain accompanied by local swelling, further restriction of joint motion, fever, and malaise is suggestive of septic arthritis. If this complication occurs and the diagnosis of sepsis is confirmed, appropriate antimicrobial therapy should be instituted.
Injection of a steroid into an infected site is to be avoided.
Corticosteroids should not be injected into unstable joints.
Patients should be impressed strongly with the importance of not overusing joints in which symptomatic benefit has been obtained as long as the inflammatory process remains active.
Frequent intra-articular injection may result in damage to joint tissues.

ADVERSE REACTIONS

Fluid and electrolyte disturbances
Sodium retention
Fluid retention
Congestive heart failure in susceptible patients
Potassium loss
Hypokalemic alkalosis
Hypertension
Musculoskeletal
Muscle weakness
Steroid myopathy
Loss of muscle mass
Osteoporosis
Vertebral compression fractures
Aseptic necrosis of femoral and humeral heads
Pathologic fracture of long bones
Tendon rupture
Gastrointestinal
Peptic ulcer with possible subsequent perforation and hemorrhage
Perforation of the small and large bowel, particularly in patients with inflammatory bowel disease
Pancreatitis
Abdominal distention
Ulcerative esophagitis
Dermatologic
Impaired wound healing
Thin fragile skin
Petechiae and ecchymoses
Erythema
Increased sweating
May suppress reactions to skin tests
Other cutaneous reactions, such as allergic dermatitis, urticaria, angioneurotic edema
Neurologic
Convulsions
Increased intracranial pressure with papilledema (pseudotumor cerebri) usually after treatment
Vertigo
Headache
Endocrine
Menstrual irregularities
Development of cushingoid state
Suppression of growth in children
Secondary adrenocortical and pituitary unresponsiveness, particularly in times of stress, as in trauma, surgery, or illness
Decreased carbohydrate tolerance
Manifestations of latent diabetes mellitus
Increased requirements for insulin or oral hypoglycemic agents in diabetics
Hirsutism
Ophthalmic
Posterior subcapsular cataracts
Increased intraocular pressure
Glaucoma
Exophthalmos
Metabolic
Negative nitrogen balance due to protein catabolism
Other
Anaphylactoid or hypersensitivity reactions
Thromboembolism
Weight gain
Increased appetite
Nausea
Malaise
Psychic disturbances
The following *additional* adverse reactions are related to injection of corticosteroids:
Rare instances of blindness associated with intralesional therapy around the face and head
Hyperpigmentation or hypopigmentation
Subcutaneous and cutaneous atrophy
Sterile abscess
Postinjection flare (following intra-articular use)
Charcot-like arthropathy.

DOSAGE AND ADMINISTRATION

For intra-articular, intralesional, and soft tissue injection only
DOSAGE AND FREQUENCY OF INJECTION ARE VARIABLE AND MUST BE INDIVIDUALIZED ON THE BASIS OF THE DISEASE AND THE RESPONSE OF THE PATIENT.
The initial dose varies from 5 to 75 mg depending on the disease being treated and the size of the area to be injected. Frequency of injection depends on symptomatic response, and usually is once every two or three weeks. Severe conditions may require injection once a week. Frequent intra-articular injection may result in damage to joint tissues. If satisfactory clinical response does not occur after a reasonable period of time, discontinue HYDROCORTONE Acetate saline suspension and transfer the patient to other therapy.
Patients should be observed closely for signs that might require dosage adjustment, including changes in clinical status resulting from remissions or exacerbations of the disease, and individual drug responsiveness.
Some of the usual single doses are:

Large Joints (e.g., Knee)	25 mg, occasionally 37.5 mg. Doses over 50 mg not recommended
Small Joints (e.g, Interphalangeal, Temporomandibular)	10 to 25 mg
Bursae	25 to 37.5 mg
Tendon Sheaths	5 to 12.5 mg
Soft Tissue Infiltration	25 to 50 mg, occasionally 75 mg
Ganglia	12.5 to 25 mg

For rapid onset of action, a soluble adrenocortical hormone preparation, such as DECADRON® Phosphate (Dexamethasone Sodium Phosphate, MSD) injection or HYDELTRASOL® (Prednisolone Sodium Phosphate, MSD) injection, may be given with HYDROCORTONE Acetate saline suspension.
If desired, a local anesthetic may be used, and may be injected before HYDROCORTONE Acetate saline suspension or mixed in a syringe with HYDROCORTONE Acetate saline suspension and given simultaneously.
If used prior to intra-articular injection of the steroid, inject most of the anesthetic into the soft tissues of the surrounding area and instill a small amount into the joint.
If given together, mixing should be done in the injection syringe by drawing the steroid in *first*, then the anesthetic. In this way, the anesthetic will not be introduced inadvertently into the vial of steroid. *The mixture must be used immediately and any unused portion discarded.*

HOW SUPPLIED

No. 7501—Saline suspension HYDROCORTONE Acetate is a white, mobile suspension, containing 25 mg hydrocortisone acetate in each mL, and is supplied as follows:
NDC 0006-7501-03 in 5 mL vials.
No. 7519—Saline suspension HYDROCORTONE Acetate is a white, mobile suspension, containing 50 mg hydrocortisone acetate in each mL, and is supplied as follows:
NDC 0006-7519-03 in 5 mL vials.
Storage
Sensitive to heat. Do not autoclave.
Protect from freezing.
A.H.F.S. Category: 68:04
DC 7348725 Issued April 1985

HYDROCORTONE® Phosphate Injection (Hydrocortisone Sodium Phosphate, MSD), U.S.P. ℞

DESCRIPTION

Hydrocortisone sodium phosphate, a synthetic adrenocortical steroid, is a white to light yellow, odorless or practically odorless powder. It is freely soluble in water and is exceedingly hygroscopic. The molecular weight is 486.41. It is designated chemically as 11β, 17-dihydroxy-21-(phosphonooxy) pregn-4-ene-3,20-dione disodium salt. The empirical formula is $C_{21}H_{29}Na_2O_8P$ and the structural formula is:

HYDROCORTONE® Phosphate (Hydrocortisone Sodium Phosphate, MSD) injection is a sterile solution (pH 7.5 to 8.5) for intravenous, intramuscular, and subcutaneous administration.
Each milliliter contains hydrocortisone sodium phosphate equivalent to 50 mg hydrocortisone. Inactive ingredients per mL: 8 mg creatinine, 10 mg sodium citrate, sodium hydroxide to adjust pH, and Water for Injection, q.s. 1 mL, with 3.2 mg sodium bisulfite, 1.5 mg methylparaben, and 0.2 mg propylparaben added as preservatives.

ACTIONS

HYDROCORTONE Phosphate injection has a rapid onset but short duration of action when compared with less soluble preparations. Because of this, it is suitable for the treatment of acute disorders responsive to adrenocortical steroid therapy.
Naturally occurring glucocorticoids (hydrocortisone and cortisone), which also have salt-retaining properties, are used as replacement therapy in adrenocortical deficiency states. They are also used for their potent anti-inflammatory effects in disorders of many organ systems.
Glucocorticoids cause profound and varied metabolic effects. In addition, they modify the body's immune responses to diverse stimuli.

INDICATIONS

When oral therapy is not feasible:
1. *Endocrine disorders*
Primary or secondary adrenocortical insufficiency (hydrocortisone or cortisone is the drug of choice; synthetic analogs may be used in conjunction with mineralocorticoids where applicable; in infancy, mineralocorticoid supplementation is of particular importance)
Acute adrenocortical insufficiency (hydrocortisone or cortisone is the drug of choice; mineralocorticoid supplementation may be necessary, particularly when synthetic analogs are used)
Preoperatively, and in the event of serious trauma or illness, in patients with known adrenal insufficiency or when adrenocortical reserve is doubtful
Shock unresponsive to conventional therapy if adrenocortical insufficiency exists or is suspected
Congenital adrenal hyperplasia
Nonsuppurative thyroiditis
Hypercalcemia associated with cancer
2. *Rheumatic disorders*
As adjunctive therapy for short-term administration (to tide the patient over an acute episode or exacerbation) in:

Post-traumatic osteoarthritis
Synovitis of osteoarthritis
Rheumatoid arthritis, including juvenile rheumatoid arthritis (selected cases may require low-dose maintenance therapy)
Acute and subacute bursitis
Epicondylitis
Acute nonspecific tenosynovitis
Acute gouty arthritis
Psoriatic arthritis
Ankylosing spondylitis

3. *Collagen diseases*
During an exacerbation or as maintenance therapy in selected cases of:
Systemic lupus erythematosus
Acute rheumatic carditis
Systemic dermatomyositis (polymyositis)

4. *Dermatologic diseases*
Pemphigus
Severe erythema multiforme (Stevens-Johnson syndrome)
Exfoliative dermatitis
Bullous dermatitis herpetiformis
Severe seborrheic dermatitis
Severe psoriasis
Mycosis fungoides

5. *Allergic states*
Control of severe or incapacitating allergic conditions intractable to adequate trials of conventional treatment in:
Bronchial asthma
Contact dermatitis
Atopic dermatitis
Serum sickness
Seasonal or perennial allergic rhinitis
Drug hypersensitivity reactions
Urticarial transfusion reactions
Acute noninfectious laryngeal edema (epinephrine is the drug of first choice)

6. *Ophthalmic diseases*
Severe acute and chronic allergic and inflammatory processes involving the eye, such as:
Herpes zoster ophthalmicus
Iritis, iridocyclitis
Chorioretinitis
Diffuse posterior uveitis and choroiditis
Optic neuritis
Sympathetic ophthalmia
Anterior segment inflammation
Allergic conjunctivitis
Keratitis
Allergic corneal marginal ulcers

7. *Gastrointestinal diseases*
To tide the patient over a critical period of the disease in:
Ulcerative colitis (Systemic therapy)
Regional enteritis (Systemic therapy)

8. *Respiratory diseases*
Symptomatic sarcoidosis
Berylliosis
Fulminating or disseminated pulmonary tuberculosis when used concurrently with appropriate antituberculous chemotherapy
Loeffler's syndrome not manageable by other means
Aspiration pneumonitis

9. *Hematologic disorders*
Acquired (autoimmune) hemolytic anemia
Idiopathic thrombocytopenic purpura in adults (I.V. only; I.M. administration is contraindicated)
Secondary thrombocytopenia in adults
Erythroblastopenia (RBC anemia)
Congenital (erythroid) hypoplastic anemia

10. *Neoplastic diseases*
For palliative management of:
Leukemias and lymphomas in adults
Acute leukemia of childhood

11. *Edematous states*
To induce diuresis or remission of proteinuria in the nephrotic syndrome, without uremia, of the idiopathic type, or that due to lupus erythematosus

12. *Miscellaneous*
Tuberculous meningitis with subarachnoid block or impending block when used concurrently with appropriate antituberculous chemotherapy
Trichinosis with neurologic or myocardial involvement

CONTRAINDICATIONS

Systemic fungal infections (see WARNINGS regarding amphotericin B)
Hypersensitivity to any component of this product, including sulfites (see WARNINGS regarding sodium bisulfite)

WARNINGS

Sodium bisulfite has been reported to cause severe allergic reactions in certain susceptible individuals, particularly patients with asthma. Anaphylactoid and hypersensitivity reactions have been reported for Injection HYDROCORTONE Phosphate (see ADVERSE REACTIONS). Since Injection HYDROCORTONE Phosphate contains sodium bisulfite, this product should not be used in patients allergic to sulfites.

Corticosteroids may exacerbate systemic fungal infections and therefore should not be used in the presence of such infections unless they are needed to control drug reactions due to amphotericin B. Moreover, there have been cases reported in which concomitant use of amphotericin B and hydrocortisone was followed by cardiac enlargement and congestive failure.

In patients on corticosteroid therapy subjected to any unusual stress, increased dosage of rapidly acting corticosteroids before, during, and after the stressful situation is indicated.

Drug-induced secondary adrenocortical insufficiency may result from too rapid withdrawal of corticosteroids and may be minimized by gradual reduction of dosage. This type of relative insufficiency may persist for months after discontinuation of therapy; therefore, in any situation of stress occurring during that period, hormone therapy should be reinstituted. If the patient is receiving steroids already, dosage may have to be increased. Since mineralocorticoid secretion may be impaired, salt and/or a mineralocorticoid should be administered concurrently.

Corticosteroids may mask some signs of infection, and new infections may appear during their use. There may be decreased resistance and inability to localize infection when corticosteroids are used. Moreover, corticosteroids may affect the nitroblue-tetrazolium test for bacterial infection and produce false negative results.

In cerebral malaria, a double-blind trial has shown that the use of corticosteroids is associated with prolongation of coma and a higher incidence of pneumonia and gastrointestinal bleeding.

Corticosteroids may activate latent amebiasis. Therefore, it is recommended that latent or active amebiasis be ruled out before initiating corticosteroid therapy in any patient who has spent time in the tropics or any patient with unexplained diarrhea.

Prolonged use of corticosteroids may produce posterior subcapsular cataracts, glaucoma with possible damage to the optic nerves, and may enhance the establishment of secondary ocular infections due to fungi or viruses.

Usage in pregnancy. Since adequate human reproduction studies have not been done with corticosteroids, use of these drugs in pregnancy or in women of childbearing potential requires that the anticipated benefits be weighed against the possible hazards to the mother and embryo or fetus. Infants born of mothers who have received substantial doses of corticosteroids during pregnancy should be carefully observed for signs of hypoadrenalism.

Corticosteroids appear in breast milk and could suppress growth, interfere with endogenous corticosteroid production, or cause other unwanted effects. Mothers taking pharmacologic doses of corticosteroids should be advised not to nurse.

Average and large doses of cortisone or hydrocortisone can cause elevation of blood pressure, salt and water retention, and increased excretion of potassium. These effects are less likely to occur with the synthetic derivatives except when used in large doses. Dietary salt restriction and potassium supplementation may be necessary. All corticosteroids increase calcium excretion.

Administration of live virus vaccines, including smallpox, is contraindicated in individuals receiving immunosuppressive doses of corticosteroids. If inactivated viral or bacterial vaccines are administered to individuals receiving immunosuppressive doses of corticosteroids, the expected serum antibody response may not be obtained. However, immunization procedures may be undertaken in patients who are receiving corticosteroids as replacement therapy, e.g., for Addison's disease.

The use of HYDROCORTONE Phosphate injection in active tuberculosis should be restricted to those cases of fulminating or disseminated tuberculosis in which the corticosteroid is used for the management of the disease in conjunction with an appropriate antituberculous regimen.

If corticosteroids are indicated in patients with latent tuberculosis or tuberculin reactivity, close observation is necessary as reactivation of the disease may occur. During prolonged corticosteroid therapy, these patients should receive chemoprophylaxis.

Because rare instances of anaphylactoid reactions have occurred in patients receiving parenteral corticosteroid therapy, appropriate precautionary measures should be taken prior to administration, especially when the patient has a history of allergy to any drug.

PRECAUTIONS

This product, like many other steroid formulations, is sensitive to heat. Therefore, it should not be autoclaved when it is desirable to sterilize the exterior of the vial.

Following prolonged therapy, withdrawal of corticosteroids may result in symptoms of the corticosteroid withdrawal syndrome including fever, myalgia, arthralgia, and malaise. This may occur in patients even without evidence of adrenal insufficiency.

There is an enhanced effect of corticosteroids in patients with hypothyroidism and in those with cirrhosis.

Corticosteroids should be used cautiously in patients with ocular herpes simplex for fear of corneal perforation.

The lowest possible dose of corticosteroid should be used to control the condition under treatment, and when reduction in dosage is possible, the reduction must be gradual.

Psychic derangements may appear when corticosteroids are used, ranging from euphoria, insomnia, mood swings, personality changes, and severe depression to frank psychotic manifestations. Also, existing emotional instability or psychotic tendencies may be aggravated by corticosteroids.

Aspirin should be used cautiously in conjunction with corticosteroids in hypoprothrombinemia.

Steroids should be used with caution in nonspecific ulcerative colitis, if there is a probability of impending perforation, abscess, or other pyogenic infection, also in diverticulitis, fresh intestinal anastomoses, active or latent peptic ulcer, renal insufficiency, hypertension, osteoporosis, and myasthenia gravis. Signs of peritoneal irritation following gastrointestinal perforation in patients receiving large doses of corticosteroids may be minimal or absent. Fat embolism has been reported as a possible complication of hypercortisonism.

When large doses are given, some authorities advise that antacids be administered between meals to help to prevent peptic ulcer.

Growth and development of infants and children on prolonged corticosteroid therapy should be carefully followed.

Steroids may increase or decrease motility and number of spermatozoa in some patients.

Phenytoin, phenobarbital, ephedrine, and rifampin may enhance the metabolic clearance of corticosteroids, resulting in decreased blood levels and lessened physiologic activity, thus requiring adjustment in corticosteroid dosage.

The prothrombin time should be checked frequently in patients who are receiving corticosteroids and coumarin anticoagulants at the same time because of reports that corticosteroids have altered the response to these anticoagulants. Studies have shown that the usual effect produced by adding corticosteroids is inhibition of response to coumarins, although there have been some conflicting reports of potentiation not substantiated by studies.

When corticosteroids are administered concomitantly with potassium-depleting diuretics, patients should be observed closely for development of hypokalemia.

Injection of a steroid into an infected site is to be avoided.

The slower rate of absorption by intramuscular administration should be recognized.

ADVERSE REACTIONS

Fluid and electrolyte disturbances
Sodium retention
Fluid retention
Congestive heart failure in susceptible patients
Potassium loss
Hypokalemic alkalosis
Hypertension

Musculoskeletal
Muscle weakness
Steroid myopathy
Loss of muscle mass
Osteoporosis
Vertebral compression fractures
Aseptic necrosis of femoral and humeral heads
Pathologic fracture of long bones
Tendon rupture

Gastrointestinal
Peptic ulcer with possible subsequent perforation and hemorrhage
Perforation of the small and large bowel, particularly in patients with inflammatory bowel disease
Pancreatitis
Abdominal distention
Ulcerative esophagitis

Dermatologic
Impaired wound healing
Thin fragile skin
Petechiae and ecchymoses
Erythema

Continued on next page

Information on the Merck Sharp & Dohme products listed on these pages is the full prescribing information from product circulars in use August 31, 1986.

Merck Sharp & Dohme—Cont.

Increased sweating
May suppress reactions to skin tests
Burning or tingling, especially in the perineal area (after I.V. injection)
Other cutaneous reactions, such as allergic dermatitis, urticaria, angioneurotic edema
Neurologic
Convulsions
Increased intracranial pressure with papilledema (pseudotumor cerebri) usually after treatment
Vertigo
Headache
Endocrine
Menstrual irregularities
Development of cushingoid state
Suppression of growth in children
Secondary adrenocortical and pituitary unresponsiveness, particularly in times of stress, as in trauma, surgery, or illness
Decreased carbohydrate tolerance
Manifestations of latent diabetes mellitus
Increased requirements for insulin or oral hypoglycemic agents in diabetics
Hirsutism
Ophthalmic
Posterior subcapsular cataracts
Increased intraocular pressure
Glaucoma
Exophthalmos
Metabolic
Negative nitrogen balance due to protein catabolism
Other
Anaphylactoid or hypersensitivity reactions
Thromboembolism
Weight gain
Increased appetite
Nausea
Malaise
Psychic disturbances

The following *additional* adverse reactions are related to parenteral corticosteroid therapy:
Rare instances of blindness associated with intralesional therapy around the face and head
Hyperpigmentation or hypopigmentation
Subcutaneous and cutaneous atrophy
Sterile abscess

DOSAGE AND ADMINISTRATION

For intravenous, intramuscular, and subcutaneous injection.
HYDROCORTONE Phosphate injection can be given directly from the vial or the disposable syringe, or it can be added to Sodium Chloride Injection or Dextrose Injection and administered by intravenous drip.
Benzyl alcohol as a preservative has been associated with toxicity in premature infants. Solutions used for intravenous administration or further dilution of this product should be preservative-free when used in the neonate, especially the premature infant.
When it is mixed with an infusion solution, sterile precautions should be observed. Since infusion solutions generally do not contain preservatives, mixtures should be used within 24 hours.
DOSAGE REQUIREMENTS ARE VARIABLE AND MUST BE INDIVIDUALIZED ON THE BASIS OF THE DISEASE AND THE RESPONSE OF THE PATIENT.
The initial dosage varies from 15 to 240 mg a day depending on the disease being treated. In less severe diseases doses lower than 15 mg may suffice, while in severe diseases doses higher than 240 mg may be required. Usually the parenteral dosage ranges are one-third to one-half the oral dose given every 12 hours. However, in certain overwhelming, acute, life-threatening situations, administration in dosages exceeding the usual dosages may be justified and may be in multiples of the oral dosages.
The initial dosage should be maintained or adjusted until the patient's response is satisfactory. If a satisfactory clinical response does not occur after a reasonable period of time, discontinue HYDROCORTONE Phosphate injection and transfer the patient to other therapy.
After a favorable initial response, the proper maintenance dosage should be determined by decreasing the initial dosage in small amounts to the lowest dosage that maintains an adequate clinical response.
Patients should be observed closely for signs that might require dosage adjustment, including changes in clinical status resulting from remissions or exacerbations of the disease, individual drug responsiveness, and the effect of stress (e.g., surgery, infection, trauma). During stress it may be necessary to increase dosage temporarily.
If the drug is to be stopped after more than a few days of treatment, it usually should be withdrawn gradually.

HOW SUPPLIED

No. 7633—Injection HYDROCORTONE Phosphate, 50 mg hydrocortisone equivalent per mL, is a clear, light yellow solution, and is supplied as follows:
NDC 0006-7633-04 in 2 mL multiple dose vials
NDC 0006-7633-10 in 10 mL multiple dose vials
NDC 0006-7633-02 in 2 mL single dose disposable syringes.
Storage
Sensitive to heat. Do not autoclave.
A.H.F.S. Category: 68:04
DC 6521918 Issued April 1985

HYDROCORTONE® Tablets ℞
(Hydrocortisone, MSD), U.S.P.

DESCRIPTION

Glucocorticoids are adrenocortical steroids, both naturally occurring and synthetic, which are readily absorbed from the gastrointestinal tract.
Hydrocortisone is a white to practically white, odorless, crystalline powder, very slightly soluble in water. The molecular weight is 362.47. It is designated chemically as 11β,17,21-trihydroxypregn-4-ene-3,20-dione. The empirical formula is $C_{21}H_{30}O_5$ and the structural formula is:

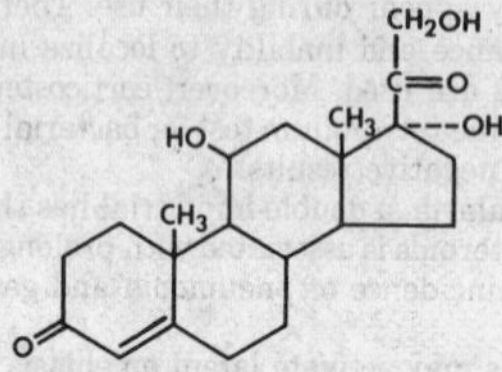

Hydrocortisone is believed to be the principal hormone secreted by the adrenal cortex.
HYDROCORTONE® (Hydrocortisone, MSD) tablets are supplied in two potencies, 10 mg and 20 mg.
Inactive ingredients are lactose, magnesium stearate, and starch.

ACTIONS

Naturally occurring glucocorticoids (hydrocortisone and cortisone), which also have salt-retaining properties, are used as replacement therapy in adrenocortical deficiency states. They are also used for their potent anti-inflammatory effects in disorders of many organ systems.
Glucocorticoids cause profound and varied metabolic effects. In addition, they modify the body's immune responses to diverse stimuli.

INDICATIONS

1. *Endocrine Disorders*
Primary or secondary adrenocortical insufficiency (hydrocortisone or cortisone is the first choice; synthetic analogs may be used in conjunction with mineralocorticoids where applicable; in infancy mineralocorticoid supplementation is of particular importance)
Congenital adrenal hyperplasia
Nonsuppurative thyroiditis
Hypercalcemia associated with cancer
2. *Rheumatic Disorders*
As adjunctive therapy for short-term administration (to tide the patient over an acute episode or exacerbation) in:
Psoriatic arthritis
Rheumatoid arthritis, including juvenile rheumatoid arthritis (selected cases may require low-dose maintenance therapy)
Ankylosing spondylitis
Acute and subacute bursitis
Acute nonspecific tenosynovitis
Acute gouty arthritis
Post-traumatic osteoarthritis
Synovitis of osteoarthritis
Epicondylitis
3. *Collagen Diseases*
During an exacerbation or as maintenance therapy in selected cases of—
Systemic lupus erythematosus
Acute rheumatic carditis
Systemic dermatomyositis (polymyositis)
4. *Dermatologic Diseases*
Pemphigus
Bullous dermatitis herpetiformis
Severe erythema multiforme (Stevens-Johnson syndrome)
Exfoliative dermatitis
Mycosis fungoides
Severe psoriasis
Severe seborrheic dermatitis
5. *Allergic States*
Control of severe or incapacitating allergic conditions intractable to adequate trials of conventional treatment:
Seasonal or perennial allergic rhinitis
Bronchial asthma
Contact dermatitis
Atopic dermatitis
Serum sickness
Drug hypersensitivity reactions
6. *Ophthalmic Diseases*
Severe acute and chronic allergic and inflammatory processes involving the eye and its adnexa, such as—
Allergic conjunctivitis
Keratitis
Allergic corneal marginal ulcers
Herpes zoster ophthalmicus
Iritis and iridocyclitis
Chorioretinitis
Anterior segment inflammation
Diffuse posterior uveitis and choroiditis
Optic neuritis
Sympathetic ophthalmia
7. *Respiratory Diseases*
Symptomatic sarcoidosis
Loeffler's syndrome not manageable by other means
Berylliosis
Fulminating or disseminated pulmonary tuberculosis when used concurrently with appropriate antituberculous chemotherapy
Aspiration pneumonitis
8. *Hematologic Disorders*
Idiopathic thrombocytopenic purpura in adults
Secondary thrombocytopenia in adults
Acquired (autoimmune) hemolytic anemia
Erythroblastopenia (RBC anemia)
Congenital (erythroid) hypoplastic anemia
9. *Neoplastic Diseases*
For palliative management of:
Leukemias and lymphomas in adults
Acute leukemia of childhood
10. *Edematous States*
To induce a diuresis or remission of proteinuria in the nephrotic syndrome, without uremia, of the idiopathic type or that due to lupus erythematosus
11. *Gastrointestinal Diseases*
To tide the patient over a critical period of the disease in:
Ulcerative colitis
Regional enteritis
12. *Miscellaneous*
Tuberculous meningitis with subarachnoid block or impending block when used concurrently with appropriate antituberculous chemotherapy
Trichinosis with neurologic or myocardial involvement

CONTRAINDICATIONS

Systemic fungal infections
Hypersensitivity to this product

WARNINGS

In patients on corticosteroid therapy subjected to unusual stress, increased dosage of rapidly acting corticosteroids before, during, and after the stressful situation is indicated.
Drug-induced secondary adrenocortical insufficiency may result from too rapid wthdrawal of corticosteroids and may be minimized by gradual reduction of dosage. This type of relative insufficiency may persist for months after discontinuation of therapy; therefore, in any situation of stress occurring during that period, hormone therapy should be reinstituted. If the patient is receiving steroids already, dosage may have to be increased. Since mineralocorticoid secretion may be impaired, salt and/or a mineralocorticoid should be administered concurrently.
Corticosteroids may mask some signs of infection, and new infections may appear during their use. There may be decreased resistance and inability to localize infection when corticosteroids are used. Moreover, corticosteroids may affect the nitroblue-tetrazolium test for bacterial infection and produce false negative results.
In cerebral malaria, a double-blind trial has shown that the use of corticosteroids is associated with prolongation of coma and a higher incidence of pneumonia and gastrointestinal bleeding.
Corticosteroids may activate latent amebiasis. Therefore, it is recommended that latent or active amebiasis be ruled out before initiating corticosteroid therapy in any patient who has spent time in the tropics or any patient with unexplained diarrhea.
Prolonged use of corticosteroids may produce posterior subcapsular cataracts, glaucoma with possible damage to the optic nerves, and may enhance the establishment of secondary ocular infections due to fungi or viruses.

Usage in pregnancy: Since adequate human reproduction studies have not been done with corticosteroids, use of these drugs in pregnancy or in women of childbearing potential requires that the anticipated benefits be weighed against the possible hazards to the mother and embryo or fetus. Infants born of mothers who have received substantial doses of corticosteroids during pregnancy should be carefully observed for signs of hypoadrenalism.
Corticosteroids appear in breast milk and could suppress growth, interfere with endogenous corticosteroid production, or cause other unwanted effects. Mothers taking pharmacologic doses of corticosteroids should be advised not to nurse.
Average and large doses of hydrocortisone or cortisone can cause elevation of blood pressure, salt and water retention, and increased excretion of potassium. These effects are less likely to occur with the synthetic derivatives except when used in large doses. Dietary salt restriction and potassium supplementation may be necessary. All corticosteroids increase calcium excretion.
Administration of live virus vaccines, including smallpox, is contraindicated in individuals receiving immunosuppressive doses of corticosteroids. If inactivated viral or bacterial vaccines are administered to individuals receiving immunosuppressive doses of corticosteroids, the expected serum antibody response may not be obtained. However, immunization procedures may be undertaken in patients who are receiving corticosteroids as replacement therapy, e.g., for Addison's disease.
The use of HYDROCORTONE tablets in active tuberculosis should be restricted to those cases of fulminating or disseminated tuberculosis in which the corticosteroid is used for the management of the disease in conjunction with an appropriate antituberculous regimen.
If corticosteroids are indicated in patients with latent tuberculosis or tuberculin reactivity, close observation is necessary as reactivation of the disease may occur. During prolonged corticosteroid therapy, these patients should receive chemoprophylaxis.

PRECAUTIONS

Following prolonged therapy, withdrawal of corticosteroids may result in symptoms of the corticosteroid withdrawal syndrome including fever, myalgia, arthralgia, and malaise. This may occur in patients even without evidence of adrenal insufficiency.

There is an enhanced effect of corticosteroids in patients with hypothyroidism and in those with cirrhosis.
Corticosteroids should be used cautiously in patients with ocular herpes simplex because of possible corneal perforation.

The lowest possible dose of corticosteroid should be used to control the condition under treatment, and when reduction in dosage is possible, the reduction should be gradual.
Psychic derangements may appear when corticosteroids are used, ranging from euphoria, insomnia, mood swings, personality changes, and severe depression, to frank psychotic manifestations. Also, existing emotional instability or psychotic tendencies may be aggravated by corticosteroids.
Aspirin should be used cautiously in conjunction with corticosteroids in hypoprothrombinemia.

Steroids should be used with caution in nonspecific ulcerative colitis, if there is a probability of impending perforation, abscess, or other pyogenic infection, diverticulitis, fresh intestinal anastomoses, active or latent peptic ulcer, renal insufficiency, hypertension, osteoporosis, and myasthenia gravis. Signs of peritoneal irritation following gastrointestinal perforation in patients receiving large doses of corticosteroids may be minimal or absent. Fat embolism has been reported as a possible complication of hypercortisonism.

When large doses are given, some authorities advise that corticosteroids be taken with meals and antacids taken between meals to help to prevent peptic ulcer.
Growth and development of infants and children on prolonged corticosteroid therapy should be carefully observed.
Steroids may increase or decrease motility and number of spermatozoa in some patients.

Phenytoin, phenobarbital, ephedrine, and rifampin may enhance the metabolic clearance of corticosteroids, resulting in decreased blood levels and lessened physiologic activity, thus requiring adjustment in corticosteroid dosage.
The prothrombin time should be checked frequently in patients who are receiving corticosteroids and coumarin anticoagulants at the same time because of reports that corticosteroids have altered the response to these anticoagulants. Studies have shown that the usual effect produced by adding corticosteroids is inhibition of response to coumarins, although there have been some conflicting reports of potentiation not substantiated by studies.

When corticosteroids are administered concomitantly with potassium-depleting diuretics, patients should be observed closely for development of hypokalemia.

ADVERSE REACTIONS

Fluid and Electrolyte Disturbances
Sodium retention
Fluid retention
Congestive heart failure in susceptible patients
Potassium loss
Hypokalemic alkalosis
Hypertension
Musculoskeletal
Muscle weakness
Steroid myopathy
Loss of muscle mass
Osteoporosis
Vertebral compression fractures
Aseptic necrosis of femoral and humeral heads
Pathologic fracture of long bones
Tendon rupture
Gastrointestinal
Peptic ulcer with possible perforation and hemorrhage
Perforation of the small and large bowel, particularly in patients with inflammatory bowel disease
Pancreatitis
Abdominal distention
Ulcerative esophagitis
Dermatologic
Impaired wound healing
Thin fragile skin
Petechiae and ecchymoses
Erythema
Increased sweating
May suppress reactions to skin tests
Other cutaneous reactions, such as allergic dermatitis, urticaria, angioneurotic edema
Neurologic
Convulsions
Increased intracranial pressure with papilledema (pseudotumor cerebri) usually after treatment
Vertigo
Headache
Endocrine
Menstrual irregularities
Development of cushingoid state
Suppression of growth in children
Secondary adrenocortical and pituitary unresponsiveness, particularly in times of stress, as in trauma, surgery, or illness
Decreased carbohydrate tolerance
Manifestations of latent diabetes mellitus
Increased requirements for insulin or oral hypoglycemic agents in diabetics
Hirsutism
Ophthalmic
Posterior subcapsular cataracts
Increased intraocular pressure
Glaucoma
Exophthalmos
Metabolic
Negative nitrogen balance due to protein catabolism
Other
Hypersensitivity
Thromboembolism
Weight gain
Increased appetite
Nausea
Malaise
Psychic disturbances

DOSAGE AND ADMINISTRATION

For oral administration
DOSAGE REQUIREMENTS ARE VARIABLE AND MUST BE INDIVIDUALIZED ON THE BASIS OF THE DISEASE AND THE RESPONSE OF THE PATIENT.
The initial dosage varies from 20 to 240 mg a day depending on the disease being treated. In less severe diseases doses lower than 20 mg may suffice, while in severe diseases doses higher than 240 mg may be required. The initial dosage should be maintained or adjusted until the patient's response is satisfactory. If satisfactory clinical response does not occur after a reasonable period of time, discontinue HYDROCORTONE tablets and transfer the patient to other therapy.
After a favorable initial response, the proper maintenance dosage should be determined by decreasing the initial dosage in small amounts to the lowest dosage that maintains an adequate clinical response.
Patients should be observed closely for signs that might require dosage adjustment, including changes in clinical status resulting from remissions or exacerbations of the disease, individual drug responsiveness, and the effect of stress (e.g, surgery, infection, trauma). During stress it may be necessary to increase dosage temporarily.
If the drug is to be stopped after more than a few days of treatment, it usually should be withdrawn gradually.

HOW SUPPLIED

No. 7604—Tablets HYDROCORTONE, 10 mg each, are white, oval shaped compressed tablets, scored on one side, coded MSD 619, and are supplied as follows:
NDC 0006-0619-68 in bottles of 100.
No. 7602—Tablets HYDROCORTONE, 20 mg each, are white, oval shaped compressed tablets, scored on one side, coded MSD 625, and are supplied as follows:
NDC 0006-0625-68 in bottles of 100.

A.H.F.S. Category: 68:04
DC 6367323 Issued April 1985

HydroDIURIL® Tablets ℞
(Hydrochlorothiazide, MSD), U.S.P.

DESCRIPTION

HydroDIURIL® (Hydrochlorothiazide, MSD) is the 3,4-dihydro derivative of chlorothiazide. Its chemical name is 6-chloro-3,4-dihydro-2*H*-1, 2, 4-benzothiadiazine-7-sulfonamide 1,1-dioxide and its structural formula is:

It is a white, or practically white, crystalline compound slightly soluble in water, but freely soluble in sodium hydroxide solution.
HydroDIURIL is supplied as 25 mg, 50 mg and 100 mg tablets for oral use. Each tablet contains the following inactive ingredients: calcium phosphate, D&C Yellow 6, gelatin, lactose, magnesium stearate, starch and talc.

ACTIONS

HydroDIURIL is a diuretic and antihypertensive.
HydroDIURIL affects the renal tubular mechanism of electrolyte reabsorption. At maximal therapeutic dosage all thiazides are approximately equal in their diuretic efficacy.
HydroDIURIL increases excretion of sodium and chloride in approximately equivalent amounts. Natriuresis may be accompanied by some loss of potassium and bicarbonate.
After oral use diuresis begins within 2 hours, peaks in about 4 hours and lasts about 6 to 12 hours. HydroDIURIL is eliminated rapidly by the kidney.
The mechanism of the antihypertensive effect of thiazides is unknown. HydroDIURIL does not affect normal blood pressure.

INDICATIONS

HydroDIURIL is indicated as adjunctive therapy in edema associated with congestive heart failure, hepatic cirrhosis, and corticosteroid and estrogen therapy.
HydroDIURIL has also been found useful in edema due to various forms of renal dysfunction such as nephrotic syndrome, acute glomerulonephritis, and chronic renal failure.
HydroDIURIL is indicated in the management of hypertension either as the sole therapeutic agent or to enhance the effectiveness of other antihypertensive drugs in the more severe forms of hypertension.
Use in Pregnancy. Routine use of diuretics during normal pregnancy is inappropriate and exposes mother and fetus to unnecessary hazard. Diuretics do not prevent development of toxemia of pregnancy and there is no satisfactory evidence that they are useful in the treatment of toxemia.
Edema during pregnancy may arise from pathologic causes or from the physiologic and mechanical consequences of pregnancy. Thiazides are indicated in pregnancy when edema is due to pathologic causes, just as they are in the absence of pregnancy (however, see WARNINGS). Dependent edema in pregnancy, resulting from restriction of venous return by the gravid uterus, is properly treated through elevation of the lower extremities and use of support stockings. Use of diuretics to lower intravascular volume in this instance is illogical and unnecessary. During normal pregnancy there is hypervolemia which is not harmful to the fetus or the mother in the absence of cardiovascular disease. However, it may be associated with edema, rarely generalized edema. If such edema causes discomfort, increased recumbency will often provide relief. Rarely this edema may cause extreme discomfort which is not relieved by rest. In

Continued on next page

Information on the Merck Sharp & Dohme products listed on these pages is the full prescribing information from product circulars in use August 31, 1986.

Merck Sharp & Dohme—Cont.

these instances, a short course of diuretic therapy may provide relief and be appropriate.

CONTRAINDICATIONS

Anuria.
Hypersensitivity to this product or to other sulfonamide-derived drugs.

WARNINGS

Use with caution in severe renal disease. In patients with renal disease, thiazides may precipitate azotemia. Cumulative effects of the drug may develop in patients with impaired renal function.
Thiazides should be used with caution in patients with impaired hepatic function or progressive liver disease, since minor alterations of fluid and electrolyte balance may precipitate hepatic coma.
Thiazides may add to or potentiate the action of other antihypertensive drugs.
Sensitivity reactions may occur in patients with or without a history of allergy or bronchial asthma.
The possibility of exacerbation or activation of systemic lupus erythematosus has been reported.
Lithium generally should not be given with diuretics because they reduce its renal clearance and add a high risk of lithium toxicity. Read circulars for lithium preparations before use of such concomitant therapy.
Use in Pregnancy. Thiazides cross the placental barrier and appear in cord blood. The use of thiazides in pregnancy requires that the anticipated benefit be weighed against possible hazards to the fetus. These hazards include fetal or neonatal jaundice, thrombocytopenia, and possibly other adverse reactions which have occurred in the adult.
Nursing Mothers. Thiazides appear in breast milk. If use of the drug is deemed essential, the patient should stop nursing.

PRECAUTIONS

Periodic determination of serum electrolytes to detect possible electrolyte imbalance should be performed at appropriate intervals.
All patients receiving diuretic therapy should be observed for evidence of fluid or electrolyte imbalance: namely, hyponatremia, hypochloremic alkalosis, and hypokalemia. Serum and urine electrolyte determinations are particularly important when the patient is vomiting excessively or receiving parenteral fluids. Warning signs or symptoms of fluid and electrolyte imbalance include dryness of mouth, thirst, weakness, lethargy, drowsiness, restlessness, muscle pains or cramps, muscular fatigue, hypotension, oliguria, tachycardia, and gastrointestinal disturbances such as nausea and vomiting.
Hypokalemia may develop, especially with brisk diuresis, when severe cirrhosis is present, during concomitant use of corticosteroids or ACTH, or after prolonged therapy.
Interference with adequate oral electrolyte intake will also contribute to hypokalemia. Hypokalemia can sensitize or exaggerate the response of the heart to the toxic effects of digitalis (e.g., increased ventricular irritability). Hypokalemia may be avoided or treated by use of potassium supplements such as foods with a high potassium content.
Although any chloride deficit is generally mild and usually does not require specific treatment except under extraordinary circumstances (as in liver disease or renal disease), chloride replacement may be required in the treatment of metabolic alkalosis.
Dilutional hyponatremia may occur in edematous patients in hot weather; appropriate therapy is water restriction, rather than administration of salt, except in rare instances when the hyponatremia is life threatening. In actual salt depletion, appropriate replacement is the therapy of choice.
Hyperuricemia may occur or acute gout may be precipitated in certain patients receiving thiazides.
Insulin requirements in diabetic patients may be increased, decreased, or unchanged. Latent diabetes mellitus may become manifest during thiazide therapy.
Thiazides may increase the responsiveness to tubocurarine.
In some patients, the administration of a non-steroidal anti-inflammatory agent can reduce the diuretic, natriuretic, and antihypertensive effects of loop, potassium-sparing and thiazide diuretics. Therefore, when HydroDIURIL and non-steroidal anti-inflammatory agents are used concomitantly, the patient should be observed closely to determine if the desired effect of the diuretic is obtained.
The antihypertensive effects of the drug may be enhanced in the postsympathectomy patient. Thiazides may decrease arterial responsiveness to norepinephrine. This diminution is not sufficient to preclude effectiveness of the pressor agent for therapeutic use.
If progressive renal impairment becomes evident, consider withholding or discontinuing diuretic therapy.
Thiazides may decrease serum PBI levels without signs of thyroid disturbance.
Thiazides have been shown to increase the urinary excretion of magnesium; this may result in hypomagnesemia.
Thiazides may decrease urinary calcium excretion. Thiazides may cause intermittent and slight elevation of serum calcium in the absence of known disorders of calcium metabolism. Marked hypercalcemia may be evidence of hidden hyperparathyroidism. Thiazides should be discontinued before carrying out tests for parathyroid function.

ADVERSE REACTIONS

Body as a Whole: Weakness.
Cardiovascular: Orthostatic hypotension (may be aggravated by alcohol, barbiturates, or narcotics).
Digestive: Anorexia, gastric irritation, nausea, vomiting, cramping, diarrhea, constipation, jaundice (intrahepatic cholestatic jaundice), pancreatitis, sialadenitis.
Hematologic: Leukopenia, agranulocytosis, thrombocytopenia, aplastic anemia, hemolytic anemia.
Metabolic: Hyperglycemia, glycosuria, hyperuricemia, electrolyte imbalance (see PRECAUTIONS).
Musculoskeletal: Muscle spasm.
Nervous System/Psychiatric: Dizziness, vertigo, paresthesias, headache, restlessness.
Special Senses: Transient blurred vision, xanthopsia.
Hypersensitivity: Purpura, photosensitivity, rash, urticaria, necrotizing angiitis (vasculitis and cutaneous vasculitis), fever, respiratory distress including pneumonitis and pulmonary edema, anaphylactic reactions.
Whenever adverse reactions are moderate or severe, thiazide dosage should be reduced or therapy withdrawn.

DOSAGE AND ADMINISTRATION

Therapy should be individualized according to patient response. Use the smallest dosage necessary to achieve the required response.

Adults
For Diuresis
The usual adult dosage is 50 to 100 mg once or twice a day. Many patients with edema respond to intermittent therapy, i.e., administration on alternate days or on three to five days each week. With an intermittent schedule, excessive response and the resulting undesirable electrolyte imbalance are less likely to occur.
For Control of Hypertension
The usual adult starting dosage is 50 or 100 mg a day as a single or divided dose. Dosage is increased or decreased according to blood pressure response. Rarely some patients may require up to 200 mg a day in divided doses.
When thiazides are used with other antihypertensives, the dose of the latter may need to be reduced to prevent excessive decrease in blood pressure.

Infants and Children
The usual pediatric dosage is based on 1.0 mg of HydroDIURIL per pound of body weight per day in two doses. Infants under 6 months of age may require up to 1.5 mg per pound per day in two doses.
On this basis, infants up to 2 years of age may be given 12.5 to 37.5 mg daily in two doses. Children from 2 to 12 years of age may be given 37.5 to 100 mg daily in two doses. Dosage in both age groups should be based on body weight.

HOW SUPPLIED

No. 3263—Tablets HydroDIURIL, 25 mg, are peach-colored, round, scored, compressed tablets, coded MSD 42. They are supplied as follows:
NDC 0006-0042-68 bottles of 100
NDC 0006-0042-28 unit dose packages of 100
NDC 0006-0042-82 bottles of 1000.
Shown in Product Identification Section, page 417
No. 3264—Tablets HydroDIURIL, 50 mg, are peach-colored, round, scored, compressed tablets, coded MSD 105. They are supplied as follows:
NDC 0006-0105-68 bottles of 100
NDC 0006-0105-28 unit dose packages of 100
NDC 0006-0105-82 bottles of 1000
NDC 0006-0105-86 bottles of 5000.
Shown in Product Identification Section, page 417
No. 3340—Tablets HydroDIURIL, 100 mg, are peach-colored, round, scored, compressed tablets, coded MSD 410. They are supplied as follows:
NDC 0006-0410-68 bottles of 100.
Shown in Product Identification Section, page 417
A.H.F.S. Category: 40:28
DC 7398036 Issued October 1985

HYDROPRES® Tablets ℞
(Reserpine-Hydrochlorothiazide, MSD), U.S.P.

WARNING

This fixed combination drug is not indicated for initial therapy of hypertension. Hypertension requires therapy titrated to the individual patient. If the fixed combination represents the dosage so determined, its use may be more convenient in patient management. The treatment of hypertension is not static, but must be re-evaluated as conditions in each patient warrant.

DESCRIPTION

HYDROPRES® (Reserpine-Hydrochlorothiazide, MSD) combines two antihypertensive agents: HydroDIURIL® (Hydrochlorothiazide, MSD) and reserpine. The chemical name for hydrochlorothiazide is 6-chloro-3, 4-dihydro-2*H*-1,2,4-benzothiadiazine-7-sulfonamide 1,1-dioxide. Reserpine (11, 17α-dimethoxy -18β- [(3,4,5-trimethoxybenzoyl) oxy]-3β, 20α-yohimban-16β-carboxylic acid methyl ester) is a crystalline alkaloid derived from Rauwolfia serpentina.
HYDROPRES is supplied as tablets in two strengths for oral use:
HYDROPRES 25, contains 25 mg of hydrochlorothiazide and 0.125 mg of reserpine.
HYDROPRES 50, contains 50 mg of hydrochlorothiazide and 0.125 mg of reserpine.
Each tablet contains the following inactive ingredients: calcium phosphate, D&C Yellow 10, FD&C Blue 1, FD&C Yellow 6, lactose, magnesium stearate, starch and talc.

ACTIONS

Hydrochlorothiazide
Hydrochlorothiazide is a diuretic and antihypertensive. It affects the renal tubular mechanism of electrolyte reabsorption. At maximal therapeutic dosage all thiazides are approximately equal in their diuretic efficacy.
Hydrochlorothiazide increases excretion of sodium and chloride in approximately equivalent amounts. Natriuresis may be accompanied by some loss of potassium and bicarbonate.
The mechanism of the antihypertensive effect of thiazides is unknown. Hydrochlorothiazide does not affect normal blood pressure.
Hydrochlorothiazide is eliminated rapidly by the kidney.
Reserpine
Reserpine has antihypertensive, bradycardic, and tranquilizing properties. It lowers arterial blood pressure by depletion of catecholamines. Reserpine is beneficial in relieving anxiety, tension, and headache in the hypertensive patient. It acts at the hypothalamic level of the central nervous system to promote relaxation without hypnosis or analgesia. The sleep pattern shown by the electroencephalogram following barbiturates does not occur with this drug. In laboratory animals spontaneous activity and response to external stimuli are decreased, but confusion or difficulty of movement is not evident.
The bradycardic action of reserpine promotes relaxation and may eliminate sinus tachycardia. It is most pronounced in subjects with sinus tachycardia and usually is not prominent in persons with a normal pulse rate.
Miosis, relaxation of the nictitating membrane, ptosis, hypothermia, and increased gastrointestinal activity are noted in animals given reserpine, sometimes in subclinical doses. None of these effects, except increased gastrointestinal activity, has been found to be clinically significant in man with therapeutic doses.

INDICATION

Hypertension (see box warning).

CONTRAINDICATIONS

Hydrochlorothiazide is contraindicated in anuria.
HYDROPRES is contraindicated in hypersensitivity to hydrochlorothiazide or other sulfonamide-derived drugs or to reserpine.
Electroshock therapy should not be given to patients while on reserpine, as severe and even fatal reactions have been reported with minimal convulsive electroshock dosage. After discontinuing reserpine, allow at least seven days before starting electroshock therapy.
Active peptic ulcer, ulcerative colitis, and active mental depression, especially suicidal tendencies, are contraindications to reserpine therapy.

WARNINGS

Hydrochlorothiazide
Use with caution in severe renal disease. In patients with

renal disease, thiazides may precipitate azotemia. Cumulative effects of the drug may develop in patients with impaired renal function.
Thiazides should be used with caution in patients with impaired hepatic function or progressive liver disease, since minor alterations of fluid and electrolyte balance may precipitate hepatic coma.
Thiazides may add to or potentiate the action of other antihypertensive drugs.
Sensitivity reactions may occur in patients with or without a history of allergy or bronchial asthma.
The possibility of exacerbation or activation of systemic lupus erythematosus has been reported.
Lithium generally should not be given with diuretics because they reduce its renal clearance and add a high risk of lithium toxicity. Read circulars for lithium preparations before use of such concomitant therapy.

Reserpine
The occurrence of mental depression due to reserpine in doses of 0.25 mg daily or less is unusual. In any event, HYDROPRES should be discontinued at the first sign of depression.

Use in Pregnancy
Reserpine has been demonstrated to cross the placental barrier in guinea pigs with depression of adrenal catecholamine stores in the newborn. There is some evidence that side effects such as nasal congestion, lethargy, depressed Moro reflex, and bradycardia may appear in infants born of reserpine-treated mothers.
Thiazides cross the placental barrier and appear in cord blood. The use of thiazides in pregnancy requires that the anticipated benefit be weighed against possible hazards to the fetus. These hazards include fetal or neonatal jaundice, thrombocytopenia, and possibly other adverse reactions which have occurred in the adult.

Nursing Mothers
Thiazides and reserpine appear in breast milk. If use of the drug is deemed essential, the patient should stop nursing.

PRECAUTIONS

Hydrochlorothiazide
Periodic determination of serum electrolytes to detect possible electrolyte imbalance should be performed at appropriate intervals.
All patients receiving diuretic therapy should be observed for evidence of fluid or electrolyte imbalance: namely, hyponatremia, hypochloremic alkalosis, and hypokalemia. Serum and urine electrolyte determinations are particularly important when the patient is vomiting excessively or receiving parenteral fluids. Warning signs or symptoms of fluid and electrolyte imbalance include dryness of mouth, thirst, weakness, lethargy, drowsiness, restlessness, muscle pains or cramps, muscular fatigue, hypotension, oliguria, tachycardia, and gastrointestinal disturbances such as nausea and vomiting.
Hypokalemia may develop, especially with brisk diuresis, when severe cirrhosis is present, during concomitant use of corticosteroids or ACTH, or after prolonged therapy.
Interference with adequate oral electrolyte intake will contribute to hypokalemia. Hypokalemia can sensitize or exaggerate the response of the heart to the toxic effects of digitalis (e.g., increased ventricular irritability). Hypokalemia may be avoided or treated by use of potassium supplements such as foods with a high potassium content.
Although any chloride deficit is generally mild and usually does not require specific treatment except under extraordinary circumstances (as in liver disease or renal disease), chloride replacement may be required in the treatment of metabolic alkalosis.
Dilutional hyponatremia may occur in edematous patients in hot weather. Appropriate therapy is water restriction, rather than administration of salt, except in rare instances when the hyponatremia is life threatening. In actual salt depletion, appropriate replacement is the therapy of choice.
Hyperuricemia may occur or acute gout may be precipitated in certain patients receiving thiazides.
Insulin requirements in diabetic patients may be increased, decreased, or unchanged. Latent diabetes mellitus may become manifest during thiazide therapy.
Thiazides may increase the responsiveness to tubocurarine.
In some patients, the administration of a non-steroidal anti-inflammatory agent can reduce the diuretic, natriuretic, and antihypertensive effects of loop, potassium-sparing and thiazide diuretics. Therefore, when HYDROPRES and non-steroidal anti-inflammatory agents are used concomitantly, the patient should be observed closely to determine if the desired effect of the diuretic is obtained.
The antihypertensive effect of the drug may be enhanced in the postsympathectomy patient. Thiazides may decrease arterial responsiveness to norepinephrine. This diminution is not sufficient to preclude effectiveness of the pressor agent for therapeutic use.
If progressive renal impairment becomes evident, consider withholding or discontinuing diuretic therapy.
Thiazides may decrease serum PBI levels without signs of thyroid disturbance.
Thiazides have been shown to increase the urinary excretion of magnesium; this may result in hypomagnesemia.
Thiazides may decrease urinary calcium excretion. Thiazides may cause intermittent and slight elevation of serum calcium in the absence of known disorders of calcium metabolism. Marked hypercalcemia may be evidence of hidden hyperparathyroidism. Thiazides should be discontinued before carrying out tests for parathyroid function.

Reserpine
Since reserpine may increase gastric secretion and motility, it should be used cautiously in patients with a history of peptic ulcer, ulcerative colitis, or other gastrointestinal disorder. This compound may precipitate biliary colic in patients with gallstones, or bronchial asthma in susceptible persons.
Reserpine may cause hypotension including orthostatic hypotension.
In hypertensive patients on reserpine therapy significant hypotension and bradycardia may develop during surgical anesthesia. The anesthesiologist should be aware that reserpine has been taken, since it may be necessary to give vagal blocking agents parenterally to prevent or reverse hypotension and/or bradycardia.
Anxiety or depression, as well as psychosis, may develop during reserpine therapy. If depression is present when therapy is begun, it may be aggravated. Mental depression is unusual with reserpine doses of 0.25 mg daily or less. In any case, HYDROPRES should be discontinued at the first sign of depression. Extreme caution should be used in treating patients with a history of mental depression, and the possibility of suicide should be kept in mind.
As with most antihypertensive therapy, caution should be exercised when treating hypertensive patients with renal insufficiency, since they adjust poorly to lowered blood pressure levels. Use reserpine cautiously with digitalis and quinidine; cardiac arrhythmias have occurred with reserpine preparations.
When two or more antihypertensives are given, the individual dosages may have to be reduced to prevent excessive drop in blood pressure. In hypertensive patients with coronary artery disease, it is important to avoid a precipitous drop in blood pressure.
Animal tumorigenicity: Rodent studies have shown that reserpine is an animal tumorigen, causing an increased incidence of mammary fibroadenomas in female mice, malignant tumors of the seminal vesicles in male mice, and malignant adrenal medullary tumors in male rats. These findings arose in 2 year studies in which the drug was administered in the feed at concentrations of 5 and 10 ppm—about 100 to 300 times the usual human dose. The breast neoplasms are thought to be related to reserpine's prolactin-elevating effect. Several other prolactin-elevating drugs have also been associated with an increased incidence of mammary neoplasia in rodents.
The extent to which these findings indicate a risk to humans is uncertain. Tissue culture experiments show that about one-third of human breast tumors are prolactin-dependent *in vitro*, a factor of considerable importance if the use of the drug is contemplated in a patient with previously detected breast cancer. The possibility of an increased risk of breast cancer in reserpine users has been studied extensively; however, no firm conclusion has emerged. Although a few epidemiologic studies have suggested a slightly increased risk (less than twofold in all studies except one) in women who have used reserpine, other studies of generally similar design have not confirmed this. Epidemiologic studies conducted using other drugs (neuroleptic agents) that, like reserpine, increase prolactin levels and therefore would be considered rodent mammary carcinogens, have not shown an association between chronic administration of the drug and human mammary tumorigenesis. While long-term clinical observation has not suggested such an association, the available evidence is considered too limited to be conclusive at this time. An association of reserpine intake with pheochromocytoma or tumors of the seminal vesicles has not been explored.

ADVERSE REACTIONS

Hydrochlorothiazide
Body as a Whole: Weakness.
Cardiovascular: Orthostatic hypotension (may be aggravated by alcohol, barbiturates, or narcotics).
Digestive: Anorexia, gastric irritation, nausea, vomiting, cramping, diarrhea, constipation, jaundice (intrahepatic cholestatic jaundice), pancreatitis, sialadenitis.
Hematologic: Leukopenia, agranulocytosis, thrombocytopenia, aplastic anemia, hemolytic anemia.
Metabolic: Hyperglycemia, glycosuria, hyperuricemia, electrolyte imbalance (see PRECAUTIONS).
Musculoskeletal: Muscle spasm.
Nervous System/Psychiatric: Dizziness, vertigo, paresthesias, headache, restlessness.
Special Senses: Transient blurred vision, xanthopsia.
Hypersensitivity: Purpura, photosensitivity, rash, urticaria, necrotizing angiitis (vasculitis and cutaneous vasculitis), fever, respiratory distress including pneumonitis and pulmonary edema, anaphylactic reactions.
Whenever adverse reactions are moderate or severe, thiazide dosage should be reduced or therapy withdrawn.
Reserpine
Cardiovascular: Bradycardia, angina pectoris, arrhythmia, premature ventricular contractions, and other direct cardiac effects (e.g., fluid retention, congestive failure).
Digestive: Hypersecretion and increased motility, nausea, vomiting, anorexia, diarrhea, dryness of mouth, increased salivation.
Hematologic: Excessive bleeding following prostatic surgery, thrombocytopenic purpura.
Metabolic: Weight gain.
Musculoskeletal: Muscular aches.
Nervous System/Psychiatric: Excessive sedation, mental depression, nightmares, headache, dizziness, syncope, nervousness, paradoxical anxiety, central nervous system sensitization (dull sensorium, deafness, glaucoma, uveitis, optic atrophy), parkinsonism (usually reversible with decreased dosage or discontinuance of therapy).
Respiratory: Nasal congestion, dyspnea, epistaxis, enhanced susceptibility to colds.
Hypersensitivity: Flushing of skin, pruritus, rash.
Urogenital: Dysuria, nonpuerperal lactation, impotence, decreased libido.

DOSAGE AND ADMINISTRATION

The initial dosage of HYDROPRES should conform to the dosages of the individual components established during titration (see box warning).
The usual adult dosage of HYDROPRES 25 is 1 or 2 tablets once or twice a day; that of HYDROPRES 50 is 1 tablet once or twice a day. Dosage may require adjustment according to the blood pressure response of the patient.
Careful observations for changes in blood pressure must be made when HYDROPRES is used with other antihypertensive drugs.

HOW SUPPLIED

No. 3265—Tablets HYDROPRES 25 are green, round, scored, compressed tablets, coded MSD 53. Each tablet contains 25 mg of hydrochlorothiazide and 0.125 mg of reserpine. They are supplied as follows:
NDC 0006-0053-68 in bottles of 100
NDC 0006-0053-82 in bottles of 1000.
Shown in Product Identification Section, page 417
No. 3266—Tablets HYDROPRES 50 are green, round, scored, compressed tablets, coded MSD 127. Each tablet contains 50 mg of hydrochlorothiazide and 0.125 mg of reserpine. They are supplied as follows:
NDC 0006-0127-68 in bottles of 100
NDC 0006-0127-82 in bottles of 1000.
Shown in Product Identification Section, page 417
A.H.F.S. Category: 24:08
DC 7414633 Issued October 1985

INDOCIN® Capsules, Oral Suspension and Suppositories ℞
(Indomethacin, MSD), U.S.P.
INDOCIN® SR Capsules ℞
(Indomethacin, MSD), U.S.P.

DESCRIPTION

INDOCIN® (Indomethacin, MSD) cannot be considered a simple analgesic and should not be used in conditions other than those recommended under INDICATIONS.
INDOCIN is supplied in four dosage forms. Capsules INDOCIN for oral administration contain either 25 mg or 50 mg of indomethacin and the following inactive ingredients: colloidal silicon dioxide, FD & C Blue 1, FD & C Red 3, gelatin, lactose, lecithin, magnesium stearate, and titanium dioxide. Capsules INDOCIN SR for sustained release oral administration contain 75 mg of indomethacin and the following inactive ingredients: cellulose, confectioner's sugar, FD & C Blue 1, FD & C Blue 2, FD & C Red 3, gelatin, hydroxypropyl methylcellulose, magnesium stearate, polyvinyl acetate-crotonic acid copolymer, starch, and titanium dioxide. Suspension INDOCIN for oral use contains 25 mg of indometha-

Continued on next page

Information on the Merck Sharp & Dohme products listed on these pages is the full prescribing information from product circulars in use August 31, 1986.

Merck Sharp & Dohme—Cont.

cin per 5 mL, alcohol 1%, and sorbic acid 0.1% added as a preservative and the following inactive ingredients: antifoam AF emulsion, flavors, purified water, sodium hydroxide or hydrochloric acid to adjust pH, sorbitol solution, tragacanth. Suppositories INDOCIN for rectal use contain 50 mg of indomethacin and the following inactive ingredients: glycerin, polyethylene glycol 8000, polyethylene glycol 3350, sodium chloride, edetic acid, butylated hydroxyanisole and butylated hydroxytoluene. Indomethacin is a non-steroidal anti-inflammatory indole derivative designated chemically as 1-(4-chlorobenzoyl)-5-methoxy-2-methyl-1*H*-indole-3-acetic acid. Indomethacin is practically insoluble in water and sparingly soluble in alcohol. It has a pKa of 4.5 and is stable in neutral or slightly acidic media and decomposes in strong alkali. The suspension has a pH of 4.0–5.0. The structural formula is:

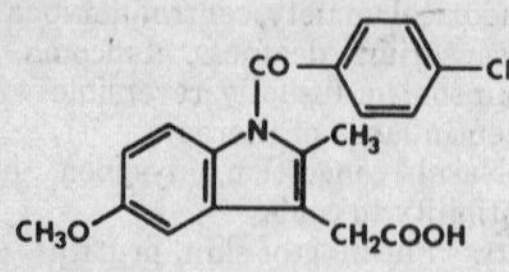

CLINICAL PHARMACOLOGY

INDOCIN is a non-steroidal drug with anti-inflammatory, antipyretic and analgesic properties. Its mode of action, like that of other anti-inflammatory drugs, is not known. However, its therapeutic action is not due to pituitary-adrenal stimulation.
INDOCIN is a potent inhibitor of prostaglandin synthesis *in vitro*. Concentrations are reached during therapy which have been demonstrated to have an effect *in vivo* as well. Prostaglandins sensitize afferent nerves and potentiate the action of bradykinin in inducing pain in animal models. Moreover, prostaglandins are known to be among the mediators of inflammation. Since indomethacin is an inhibitor of prostaglandin synthesis, its mode of action may be due to a decrease of prostaglandins in peripheral tissues.
INDOCIN has been shown to be an effective anti-inflammatory agent, appropriate for long-term use in rheumatoid arthritis, ankylosing spondylitis, and osteoarthritis.
INDOCIN affords relief of symptoms; it does not alter the progressive course of the underlying disease.
INDOCIN suppresses inflammation in rheumatoid arthritis as demonstrated by relief of pain, and reduction of fever, swelling and tenderness. Improvement in patients treated with INDOCIN for rheumatoid arthritis has been demonstrated by a reduction in joint swelling, average number of joints involved, and morning stiffness; by increased mobility as demonstrated by a decrease in walking time; and by improved functional capability as demonstrated by an increase in grip strength.
Capsules INDOCIN have been found effective in relieving the pain, reducing the fever, swelling, redness, and tenderness of acute gouty arthritis. Capsules INDOCIN rather than Capsules INDOCIN SR are recommended for treatment of acute gouty arthritis—see INDICATIONS.
Following single oral doses of Capsules INDOCIN 25 mg or 50 mg, indomethacin is readily absorbed, attaining peak plasma concentrations of about 1 and 2 mcg/mL, respectively, at about 2 hours. Orally administered Capsules INDOCIN are virtually 100% bioavailable, with 90% of the dose absorbed within 4 hours. A single 50 mg dose of Oral Suspension INDOCIN was found to be bioequivalent to a 50 mg INDOCIN Capsule when each was administered with food.
Capsules INDOCIN SR 75 mg are designed to release 25 mg of the drug initially and the remaining 50 mg over approximately 12 hours (90% of dose absorbed by 12 hours). When measured over a 24-hour period, the cumulative amount and time-course of indomethacin absorption from a single Capsule INDOCIN SR are comparable to those of 3 doses of 25 mg Capsules INDOCIN given at 4–6 hour intervals.
Plasma concentrations of indomethacin fluctuate less and are more sustained following administration of Capsules INDOCIN SR than following administration of 25 mg Capsules INDOCIN given at 4–6 hour intervals. In multiple-dose comparisons, the mean daily steady-state plasma level of indomethacin attained with daily administration of Capsules INDOCIN SR 75 mg was indistinguishable from that following Capsules INDOCIN 25 mg given at 0, 6 and 12 hours daily. However, there was a significant difference in indomethacin plasma levels between the two dosage regimens especially after 12 hours.
Controlled clinical studies of safety and efficacy in patients with osteoarthritis have shown that one Capsule INDOCIN SR was clinically comparable to one 25 mg Capsule INDOCIN t.i.d.; and in controlled clinical studies in patients with rheumatoid arthritis, one Capsule INDOCIN SR taken in the morning and one in the evening were clinically indistinguishable from one 50 mg Capsule INDOCIN t.i.d.
Indomethacin is eliminated via renal excretion, metabolism, and biliary excretion. Indomethacin undergoes appreciable enterohepatic circulation. The mean half-life of indomethacin is estimated to be about 4.5 hours. With a typical therapeutic regimen of 25 or 50 mg t.i.d., the steady-state plasma concentrations of indomethacin are an average 1.4 times those following the first dose.
The rate of absorption is more rapid from the rectal suppository than from Capsules INDOCIN. Ordinarily, therefore, the total amount absorbed from the suppository would be expected to be at least equivalent to the capsule. In controlled clinical trials, however, the amount of indomethacin absorbed was found to be somewhat less (80–90%) than that absorbed from Capsules INDOCIN. This is probably because some subjects did not retain the material from the suppository for the one hour necessary to assure complete absorption. Since the suppository dissolves rather quickly rather than melting slowly, it is seldom recovered in recognizable form if the patient retains the suppository for more than a few minutes.
Indomethacin exists in the plasma as the parent drug and its desmethyl, desbenzoyl, and desmethyl-desbenzoyl metabolites, all in the unconjugated form. About 60 percent of an oral dosage is recovered in urine as drug and metabolites (26 percent as indomethacin and its glucuronide), and 33 percent is recovered in feces (1.5 percent as indomethacin).
About 90% of indomethacin is bound to protein in plasma over the expected range of therapeutic plasma concentrations.
In a gastroscopic study in 45 healthy subjects, the number of gastric mucosal abnormalities was significantly higher in the group receiving Capsules INDOCIN than in the group taking Suppositories INDOCIN or placebo.
In a double-blind comparative clinical study involving 175 patients with rheumatoid arthritis, however, the incidence of upper gastrointestinal adverse effects with Suppositories or Capsules INDOCIN was comparable. The incidence of lower gastrointestinal adverse effects was greater in the suppository group.

INDICATIONS

Because of its potential to cause adverse reactions, particularly at high dose levels, the use of INDOCIN in rheumatoid arthritis and osteoarthritis in adults should be carefully considered for active disease unresponsive to adequate trial with salicylates and other measures of established value, such as appropriate rest.
In accord with this important concept indomethacin has been found effective in active stages of the following:
1. Moderate to severe rheumatoid arthritis including acute flares of chronic disease.
2. Moderate to severe ankylosing spondylitis.
3. Moderate to severe osteoarthritis.
4. Acute painful shoulder (bursitis and/or tendinitis).
5. Acute gouty arthritis.

Capsules INDOCIN SR are recommended for all of the indications for Capsules INDOCIN except acute gouty arthritis.
INDOCIN may enable the reduction of steroid dosage in patients receiving steroids for the more severe forms of rheumatoid arthritis. In such instances the steroid dosage should be reduced slowly and the patients followed very closely for any possible adverse effects.
The use of INDOCIN in conjunction with aspirin or other salicylates is not recommended. Controlled clinical studies have shown that the combined use of INDOCIN and aspirin does not produce any greater therapeutic effect than the use of INDOCIN alone. Furthermore, in one of these clinical studies, the incidence of gastrointestinal side effects was significantly increased with combined therapy (see DRUG INTERACTIONS).

CONTRAINDICATIONS

INDOCIN should not be used in:
Patients who are hypersensitive to this product.
Patients in whom acute asthmatic attacks, urticaria, or rhinitis are precipitated by aspirin or other non-steroidal anti-inflammatory agents.
Suppositories INDOCIN are contraindicated in patients with a history of proctitis or recent rectal bleeding.

WARNINGS

General:
Because of the variability of the potential of INDOCIN to cause adverse reactions in the individual patient, the following are strongly recommended:
1. The lowest possible effective dose for the individual patient should be prescribed. Increased dosage tends to increase adverse effects, particularly in doses over 150–200 mg/day, without corresponding increase in clinical benefits.
2. Careful instructions to, and observations of, the individual patient are essential to the prevention of serious adverse reactions. As advancing years appear to increase the possibility of adverse reactions, INDOCIN should be used with greater care in the aged.
3. Effectiveness of INDOCIN in children has not been established. INDOCIN should not be prescribed for children 14 years of age and younger unless toxicity or lack of efficacy associated with other drugs warrants the risk.
   In experience with more than 900 children reported in the literature or to Merck Sharp and Dohme who were treated with Capsules INDOCIN, side effects in children were comparable to those reported in adults. Experience in children has been confined to the use of Capsules INDOCIN.
   If a decision is made to use indomethacin for children two years of age or older, such patients should be monitored closely and periodic assessment of liver function is recommended. There have been cases of hepatotoxicity reported in children with juvenile rheumatoid arthritis, including fatalities.
   If indomethacin treatment is instituted, a suggested starting dose is 2 mg/kg/day given in divided doses. Maximum daily dosage should not exceed 4 mg/kg/day or 150–200 mg/day, whichever is less. As symptoms subside, the total daily dosage should be reduced to the lowest level required to control symptoms, or the drug should be discontinued.
4. If Capsules INDOCIN SR are used for initial therapy or during dosage adjustment, observe the patient closely (see DOSAGE AND ADMINISTRATION).

Gastrointestinal Effects:
Single or multiple ulcerations, including perforation and hemorrhage of the esophagus, stomach, duodenum or small and large intestine, have been reported to occur with INDOCIN. Fatalities have been reported in some instances. Rarely, intestinal ulceration has been associated with stenosis and obstruction.
Gastrointestinal bleeding without obvious ulcer formation and perforation of pre-existing sigmoid lesions (diverticulum, carcinoma, etc.) have occurred. Increased abdominal pain in ulcerative colitis patients or the development of ulcerative colitis and regional ileitis have been reported to occur rarely.
Because of the occurrence, and at times severity, of gastrointestinal reactions to INDOCIN, the prescribing physician must be continuously alert for any sign or symptom signaling a possible gastrointestinal reaction. The risks of continuing therapy with INDOCIN in the face of such symptoms must be weighed against the possible benefits to the individual patient.
INDOCIN should not be given to patients with active gastrointestinal lesions or with a history of recurrent gastrointestinal lesions except under circumstances which warrant the very high risk and where patients can be monitored very closely.
The gastrointestinal effects may be reduced by giving Capsules INDOCIN or Capsules INDOCIN SR immediately after meals, with food, or with antacids.
Renal Effects:
As with other non-steroidal anti-inflammatory drugs, long term administration of indomethacin to animals has resulted in renal papillary necrosis and other abnormal renal pathology. In humans, there have been reports of acute interstitial nephritis with hematuria, proteinuria, and occasionally nephrotic syndrome.
A second form of renal toxicity has been seen in patients with prerenal and renal conditions leading to a reduction in renal blood flow or blood volume, where the renal prostaglandins have a supportive role in the maintenance of renal perfusion. In these patients administration of an NSAID may cause a dose dependent reduction in prostaglandin formation and may precipitate overt renal decompensation. Patients at greatest risk of this reaction are those with conditions such as renal or hepatic dysfunction, complications associated with advanced age, extracellular volume depletion from any cause, congestive heart failure, sepsis, or concomitant use of any nephrotoxic drug. INDOCIN or other NSAIDs should be given with caution and renal function should be monitored in any patient who may have reduced renal reserve. Discontinuation of NSAID therapy is typically followed by recovery to the pretreatment state.
Increases in serum potassium concentration, including hyperkalemia, have been reported, even in some patients without renal impairment. In patients with normal renal function, these effects have been attributed to a hyporeninemic-hypoaldosteronism state (see PRECAUTIONS, *Drug Interactions*).
Since INDOCIN is eliminated primarily by the kidneys, patients with significantly impaired renal function should be closely monitored; a lower daily dosage should be anticipated to avoid excessive drug accumulation.
Ocular Effects:
Corneal deposits and retinal disturbances, including those of the macula, have been observed in some patients who had received prolonged therapy with INDOCIN. The prescribing physician should be alert to the possible association between the changes noted and INDOCIN. It is advisable to discontinue therapy if such changes are observed. Blurred vision may be a significant symptom and warrants a thorough oph-

thalmological examination. Since these changes may be asymptomatic, ophthalmologic examination at periodic intervals is desirable in patients where therapy is prolonged.

Central Nervous System Effects:

INDOCIN may aggravate depression or other psychiatric disturbances, epilepsy, and parkinsonism, and should be used with considerable caution in patients with these conditions. If severe CNS adverse reactions develop, INDOCIN should be discontinued.

INDOCIN may cause drowsiness; therefore, patients should be cautioned about engaging in activities requiring mental alertness and motor coordination, such as driving a car. INDOCIN may also cause headache. Headache which persists despite dosage reduction requires cessation of therapy with INDOCIN.

Use in Pregnancy and the Neonatal Period

INDOCIN is not recommended for use in pregnant women, since safety for use has not been established, and because of the known effect of drugs of this class on the human fetal cardiovascular system (closure of the ductus arteriosus) during the third trimester of pregnancy.

Teratogenic studies were conducted in mice and rats at dosages of 0.5, 1.0, 2.0, and 4.0 mg/kg/day. Except for retarded fetal ossification at 4 mg/kg/day considered secondary to the decreased average fetal weights, no increase in fetal malformations was observed as compared with control groups. Other studies in mice reported in the literature using higher doses (5 to 15 mg/kg/day) have described maternal toxicity and death, increased fetal resorptions, and fetal malformations. Comparable studies in rodents using high doses of aspirin have shown similar maternal and fetal effects.

As with other non-steroidal anti-inflammatory agents which inhibit prostaglandin synthesis, indomethacin has been found to delay parturition in rats.

In rats and mice, 4.0 mg/kg/day given during the last three days of gestation caused a decrease in maternal weight gain and some maternal and fetal deaths. An increased incidence of neuronal necrosis in the diencephalon in the live-born fetuses was observed. At 2.0 mg/kg/day, no increase in neuronal necrosis was observed as compared to the control groups. Administration of 0.5 or 4.0 mg/kg/day during the first three days of life did not cause an increase in neuronal necrosis at either dose level.

Use in Nursing Mothers

INDOCIN is excreted in the milk of lactating mothers. INDOCIN is not recommended for use in nursing mothers.

PRECAUTIONS

INDOCIN may mask the usual signs and symptoms of infection. Therefore, the physician must be continually on the alert for this and should use the drug with extra care in the presence of existing controlled infection.

Fluid retention and peripheral edema have been observed in some patients taking INDOCIN. Therefore, as with other non-steroidal anti-inflammatory drugs, INDOCIN should be used with caution in patients with cardiac dysfunction, hypertension, or other conditions predisposing to fluid retention.

In a study of patients with severe heart failure and hyponatremia, INDOCIN was associated with significant deterioration of circulatory hemodynamics, presumably due to inhibition of prostaglandin dependent compensatory mechanisms.

INDOCIN, like other non-steroidal anti-inflammatory agents, can inhibit platelet aggregation. This effect is of shorter duration than that seen with aspirin and usually disappears within 24 hours after discontinuation of INDOCIN. INDOCIN has been shown to prolong bleeding time (but within the normal range) in normal subjects. Because this effect may be exaggerated in patients with underlying hemostatic defects, INDOCIN should be used with caution in persons with coagulation defects.

As with other non-steroidal anti-inflammatory drugs, borderline elevations of one or more liver tests may occur in up to 15% of patients. These abnormalities may progress, may remain essentially unchanged, or may be transient with continued therapy. The SGPT (ALT) test is probably the most sensitive indicator of liver dysfunction. Meaningful (3 times the upper limit of normal) elevations of SGPT or SGOT (AST) occurred in controlled clinical trials in less than 1% of patients. A patient with symptoms and/or signs suggesting liver dysfunction, or in whom an abnormal liver test has occurred, should be evaluated for evidence of the development of more severe hepatic reaction while on therapy with INDOCIN. Severe hepatic reactions, including jaundice and cases of fatal hepatitis, have been reported with INDOCIN as with other non-steroidal anti-inflammatory drugs. Although such reactions are rare, if abnormal liver tests persist or worsen, if clinical signs and symptoms consistent with liver disease develop, or if systemic manifestations occur (e.g., eosinophilia, rash, etc.), INDOCIN should be discontinued.

Carcinogenesis, Mutagenesis, Impairment of Fertility

In an 81-week chronic oral toxicity study in the rat at doses up to 1 mg/kg/day, indomethacin had no tumorigenic effect. Indomethacin produced no neoplastic or hyperplastic changes related to treatment in lifetime carcinogenic studies in the rat and mouse at maximally tolerated doses (up to 1.5 mg/kg/day).

Indomethacin did not have any mutagenic effect in *in vitro* bacterial tests (Ames test and *E. coli* with or without metabolic activation) and a series of *in vivo* tests including the host-mediated assay, sex-linked recessive lethals in *Drosophila*, and the micronucleus test in mice.

Indomethacin had no effect on fertility in mice in a two generation reproduction study or a two litter reproduction study in rats.

Drug Interactions

In normal volunteers receiving indomethacin, the administration of diflunisal decreased the renal clearance and significantly increased the plasma levels of indomethacin. In some patients, combined use of INDOCIN and diflunisal has been associated with fatal gastrointestinal hemorrhage. Therefore, diflunisal and INDOCIN should not be used concomitantly.

In a study in normal volunteers, it was found that chronic concurrent administration of 3.6 g of aspirin per day decreases indomethacin blood levels approximately 20%.

Clinical studies have shown that INDOCIN does not influence the hypoprothrombinemia produced by anticoagulants. However, when any additional drug, including INDOCIN, is added to the treatment of patients on anticoagulant therapy, the patients should be observed for alterations of the prothrombin time.

When INDOCIN is given to patients receiving probenecid, the plasma levels of indomethacin are likely to be increased. Therefore, a lower total daily dosage of INDOCIN may produce a satisfactory therapeutic effect. When increases in the dose of INDOCIN are made, they should be made carefully and in small increments.

Capsules INDOCIN 50 mg t.i.d. produced a clinically relevant elevation of plasma lithium and reduction in renal lithium clearance in psychiatric patients and normal subjects with steady state plasma lithium concentrations. This effect has been attributed to inhibition of prostaglandin synthesis. As a consequence, when INDOCIN and lithium are given concomitantly, the patient should be carefully observed for signs of lithium toxicity. (Read circulars for lithium preparations before use of such concomitant therapy.) In addition, the frequency of monitoring serum lithium concentration should be increased at the outset of such combination drug treatment.

In some patients, the administration of INDOCIN can reduce the diuretic, natriuretic, and, antihypertensive effects of loop, potassium-sparing, and thiazide diuretics. Therefore, when INDOCIN and diuretics are used concomitantly, the patient should be observed closely to determine if the desired effect of the diuretic is obtained.

INDOCIN reduces basal plasma renin activity (PRA), as well as those elevations of PRA induced by furosemide administration, or salt or volume depletion. These facts should be considered when evaluating plasma renin activity in hypertensive patients.

It has been reported that the addition of triamterene to a maintenance schedule of INDOCIN resulted in reversible acute renal failure in two of four healthy volunteers. INDOCIN and triamterene should not be administered together.

INDOCIN and potassium-sparing diuretics each may be associated with increased serum potassium levels. The potential effects of INDOCIN and potassium-sparing diuretics on potassium kinetics and renal function should be considered when these agents are administered concurrently.

Most of the above effects concerning diuretics have been attributed, at least in part, to mechanisms involving inhibition of prostaglandin synthesis by INDOCIN.

Blunting of the antihypertensive effect of beta-adrenoceptor blocking agents by non-steroidal anti-inflammatory drugs including INDOCIN has been reported. Therefore, when using these blocking agents to treat hypertension, patients should be observed carefully in order to confirm that the desired therapeutic effect has been obtained. There are reports that INDOCIN can reduce the antihypertensive effect of captopril in some patients.

Pediatric Use

Effectiveness in children 14 years of age and younger has not been established (see WARNINGS).

ADVERSE REACTIONS

The adverse reactions for Capsules INDOCIN listed in the following table have been arranged into two groups: (1) incidence greater than 1%; and (2) incidence less than 1%. The incidence for group (1) was obtained from 33 double-blind controlled clinical trials reported in the literature (1,092 patients). The incidence for group (2) was based on reports in clinical trials, in the literature, and on voluntary reports since marketing. The probability of a causal relationship exists between INDOCIN and these adverse reactions, some of which have been reported only rarely.

In controlled clinical trials, the incidence of adverse reactions to Capsules INDOCIN SR and equal 24-hour doses of Capsules INDOCIN were similar.

The adverse reactions reported with Capsules INDOCIN may occur with use of the suppositories. In addition, rectal irritation and tenesmus have been reported in patients who have received the suppositories.

The adverse reactions reported with Capsules INDOCIN may also occur with use of the suspension.

[See table on next page].

Causal relationship unknown: Other reactions have been reported but occurred under circumstances where a causal relationship could not be established. However, in these rarely reported events, the possibility cannot be excluded. Therefore, these observations are being listed to serve as alerting information to physicians:

Hematologic: Although there have been several reports of leukemia, the supporting information is weak.

Genitourinary: Urinary frequency.

OVERDOSAGE

The following symptoms may be observed following overdosage: nausea, vomiting, intense headache, dizziness, mental confusion, disorientation, or lethargy. There have been reports of paresthesias, numbness, and convulsions.

Treatment is symptomatic and supportive. The stomach should be emptied as quickly as possible if the ingestion is recent. If vomiting has not occurred spontaneously, the patient should be induced to vomit with syrup of ipecac. If the patient is unable to vomit, gastric lavage should be performed. Once the stomach has been emptied, 25 or 50 g of activated charcoal may be given. Depending on the condition of the patient, close medical observation and nursing care may be required. The patient should be followed for several days because gastrointestinal ulceration and hemorrhage have been reported as adverse reactions of indomethacin. Use of antacids may be helpful.

The oral LD_{50} of indomethacin in mice and rats (based on 14 day mortality response) was 50 and 12 mg/kg, respectively.

DOSAGE AND ADMINISTRATION

INDOCIN is available as 25 and 50 mg Capsules INDOCIN, 75 mg Capsules INDOCIN SR for oral use, Oral Suspension INDOCIN, containing 25 mg of indomethacin per 5 mL, and 50 mg Suppositories INDOCIN for rectal use. Capsules INDOCIN SR 75 mg once a day can be substituted for Capsules INDOCIN 25 mg t.i.d. However, there will be significant differences between the two dosage regimens in indomethacin blood levels, especially after 12 hours (see CLINICAL PHARMACOLOGY). In addition, Capsules INDOCIN SR 75 mg b.i.d. can be substituted for Capsules INDOCIN 50 mg t.i.d. Capsules INDOCIN SR may be substituted for all the indications for Capsules INDOCIN except acute gouty arthritis.

Adverse reactions appear to correlate with the size of the dose of INDOCIN in most patients but not all. Therefore, every effort should be made to determine the smallest effective dosage for the individual patient.

Always give Capsules INDOCIN, Capsules INDOCIN SR, or Oral Suspension INDOCIN with food, immediately after meals, or with antacids to reduce gastric irritation.

Pediatric Use

INDOCIN ordinarily should not be prescribed for children 14 years of age and under (see WARNINGS).

Dosage Recommendations for Active Stages of the Following:

1. Moderate to severe rheumatoid arthritis including acute flares of chronic disease; moderate to severe ankylosing spondylitis; and moderate to severe osteoarthritis.

   Suggested Dosage:

   Capsules INDOCIN 25 mg b.i.d. or t.i.d. If this is well tolerated, increase the daily dosage by 25 or by 50 mg, if required by continuing symptoms, at weekly intervals until a satisfactory response is obtained or until a total daily dose of 150–200 mg is reached. DOSES ABOVE THIS AMOUNT GENERALLY DO NOT INCREASE THE EFFECTIVENESS OF THE DRUG.

In patients who have persistent night pain and/or morning stiffness, the giving of a large portion, up to a maximum of 100 mg, of the total daily dose at bedtime, either orally or by rectal suppositories, may be helpful in affording relief. The total daily dose should not exceed 200 mg. In acute flares of chronic rheumatoid arthritis, it may be necessary to increase the dosage by 25 mg or, if required, by 50 mg daily.

If Capsules INDOCIN SR 75 mg are used for initiating indomethacin treatment, one capsule daily should be the usual

Continued on next page

Information on the Merck Sharp & Dohme products listed on these pages is the full prescribing information from product circulars in use August 31, 1986.

Merck Sharp & Dohme—Cont.

starting dose in order to observe patient tolerance since 75 mg per day is the maximum recommended starting dose for indomethacin (see above). If Capsules INDOCIN SR are used to increase the daily dose, patients should be observed for possible signs and symptoms of intolerance since the daily increment will exceed the daily increment recommended for the other dosage forms. For patients who require 150 mg of INDOCIN per day and have demonstrated acceptable tolerance, INDOCIN SR may be prescribed as one capsule twice daily.

If minor adverse effects develop as the dosage is increased, reduce the dosage rapidly to a tolerated dose and OBSERVE THE PATIENT CLOSELY.

If severe adverse reactions occur, STOP THE DRUG. After the acute phase of the disease is under control, an attempt to reduce the daily dose should be made repeatedly until the patient is receiving the smallest effective dose or the drug is discontinued.

Careful instructions to, and observations of, the individual patient are essential to the prevention of serious, irreversible, including fatal, adverse reactions.
As advancing years appear to increase the possibility of adverse reactions, INDOCIN should be used with greater care in the aged.

2. Acute painful shoulder (bursitis and/or tendinitis).
   Initial Dose:
   75–150 mg daily in 3 or 4 divided doses.
   The drug should be discontinued after the signs and symptoms of inflammation have been controlled for several days. The usual course of therapy is 7–14 days.

3. Acute gouty arthritis.
   Suggested Dosage:
   Capsules INDOCIN 50 mg t.i.d. until pain is tolerable. The dose should then be rapidly reduced to complete cessation of the drug. Definite relief of pain has been reported within 2 to 4 hours. Tenderness and heat usually subside in 24 to 36 hours, and swelling gradually disappears in 3 to 5 days.

HOW SUPPLIED

No. 3316—Capsules INDOCIN, 25 mg are opaque blue and white capsules, coded MSD 25. They are supplied as follows:
NDC 0006-0025-68 bottles of 100
(6505-00-926-2154, 25 mg 100's)
NDC 0006-0025-78 unit of use bottles of 100
NDC 0006-0025-28 unit dose packages of 100
(6505-00-118-2776, 25 mg individually sealed 100's)
NDC 0006-0025-82 bottles of 1000
(6505-00-931-0680, 25 mg 1000's).
Shown in Product Identification Section, page 417
No. 3317—Capsules INDOCIN, 50 mg are opaque blue and white capsules, coded MSD 50. They are supplied as follows:
NDC 0006-0050-54 unit of use bottles of 60
NDC 0006-0050-68 bottles of 100
NDC 0006-0050-78 unit of use bottles of 100
NDC 0006-0050-28 unit dose packages of 100.
Shown in Product Identification Section, page 417
No. 3376—Oral Suspension INDOCIN, 25 mg per 5 mL, is an off-white suspension with a pineapple coconut mint flavor. It is supplied as follows:
NDC 0006-3376-66 in bottles of 237 mL.
Storage
Store below 30°C (86°F). Avoid temperatures above 50°C (122°F). Protect from freezing.
No. 3370—Capsules INDOCIN SR, 75 mg each, are capsules with an opaque blue cap and clear body containing a mixture of blue and white pellets, coded MSD 693. They are supplied as follows:
NDC 0006-0693-31 unit of use bottles of 30
NDC 0006-0693-61 unit of use bottles of 60.
Shown in Product Identification Section, page 417
No. 3354—Suppositories INDOCIN, 50 mg each, are white, opaque, rectal suppositories and are supplied as follows:
NDC 0006-0150-30, boxes of 30.
Shown in Product Identification Section, page 417

Suppositories INDOCIN are distributed by:
MERCK SHARP & DOHME, Division of Merck & Co., Inc.
West Point, Pa. 19486

Incidence greater than 1%	*Incidence less than 1%*	
GASTROINTESTINAL		
nausea* with or without vomiting dyspepsia* (including indigestion, heartburn and epigastric pain) diarrhea abdominal distress or pain constipation	anorexia bloating (includes distention) flatulence peptic ulcer gastroenteritis rectal bleeding proctitis single or multiple ulcerations, including perforation and hemorrhage of the esophagus, stomach, duodenum or small and large intestines intestinal ulceration associated with stenosis and obstruction	gastrointestinal bleeding without obvious ulcer formation and perforation of pre-existing sigmoid lesions (diverticulum, carcinoma, etc.) development of ulcerative colitis and regional ileitis ulcerative stomatitis toxic hepatitis and jaundice (some fatal cases have been reported)
CENTRAL NERVOUS SYSTEM		
headache** dizziness* vertigo somnolence depression and fatigue (including malaise and listlessness)	anxiety (includes nervousness) muscle weakness involuntary muscle movements insomnia muzziness psychic disturbances including psychotic episodes mental confusion drowsiness	light-headedness syncope paresthesia aggravation of epilepsy and parkinsonism depersonalization coma peripheral neuropathy convulsions
SPECIAL SENSES		
tinnitus	ocular—corneal deposits and retinal disturbances, including those of the macula, have been reported in some patients on prolonged therapy with INDOCIN	blurred vision hearing disturbances, deafness

[Continued following page]

Manufactured by:
MERCK SHARP & DOHME
(Italia) S.p.A.
27100—Pavia, Italy
Capsules and Oral Suspension INDOCIN® and INDOCIN® SR are distributed and manufactured by:
MERCK SHARP & DOHME, Division of Merck & Co., Inc.
West Point, Pa. 19486
A.H.F.S. Category: 28:08
DC 7342910 Issued January 1986

INDOCIN® I.V. ℞
(Indomethacin Sodium Trihydrate, MSD)

DESCRIPTION

Sterile INDOCIN® I.V. (Indomethacin Sodium Trihydrate, MSD) for intravenous administration is lyophilized indomethacin sodium trihydrate. Each vial contains indomethacin sodium trihydrate equivalent to 1.0 mg indomethacin. Indomethacin sodium trihydrate is designated chemically as 1-(4-chlorobenzoyl) -5- methoxy-2-methyl-1*H* -indole-3-acetic acid, sodium salt, trihydrate. Its molecular weight is 433.8. Its empirical formula is $C_{19}H_{15}ClNNaO_4 \cdot 3H_2O$ and its structural formula is:

CLINICAL PHARMACOLOGY

Although the exact mechanism of action through which indomethacin causes closure of a patent ductus arteriosus is not known, it is believed to be through inhibition of prostaglandin synthesis. Indomethacin has been shown to be a potent inhibitor of prostaglandin synthesis, both *in vitro* and *in vivo.* In human newborns with certain congenital heart malformations, PGE 1 dilates the ductus arteriosus. In fetal and newborn lambs, E type prostaglandins have also been shown to maintain the patency of the ductus, and as in human newborns, indomethacin causes its constriction.
In double-blind placebo-controlled studies of INDOCIN I.V. in 460 small pre-term infants, weighing 1750 g or less, the infants treated with placebo had a ductus closure rate after 48 hours of 25 to 30 percent, whereas those treated with INDOCIN I.V. had a 75 to 80 percent closure rate. In one of these studies, a multicenter study, involving 405 pre-term infants, later re-opening of the ductus arteriosus occurred in 26 percent of infants treated with INDOCIN I.V., however, 70 percent of these closed subsequently without the need for surgery or additional indomethacin.
Pharmacokinetics and Metabolism
The disposition of indomethacin following intravenous administration (0.2 mg/kg) in pre-term neonates with patent ductus arteriosus has not been extensively evaluated. Even though the plasma half-life of indomethacin was variable among premature infants, it was shown to vary inversely with postnatal age and weight. In one study, of 28 evaluable infants, the plasma half-life in those infants less than 7 days old averaged 20 hours (range: 3–60 hours, n = 18). In infants older than 7 days, the mean plasma half-life of indomethacin was 12 hours (range: 4–38 hours, n = 10). Grouping the infants by weight, mean plasma half-life in those weighing less than 1000 g was 21 hours (range: 9–60 hours, n = 10); in those infants weighing more than 1000 g, the mean plasma half-life was 15 hours (range: 3–52 hours, n = 18).
Following intravenous administration in adults, indomethacin is eliminated via renal excretion, metabolism, and biliary excretion. Indomethacin undergoes appreciable enterohepatic circulation. The mean plasma half-life of indomethacin is 4.5 hours. In the absence of enterohepatic circulation, it is 90 minutes.
In adults, about 99 percent of indomethacin is bound to protein in plasma over the expected range of therapeutic plasma concentrations. The percent bound in neonates has not been studied. In controlled trials in premature infants, however, no evidence of bilirubin displacement has been observed as evidenced by increased incidence of bilirubin encephalopathy (kernicterus).

INDICATIONS AND USAGE

INDOCIN I.V. is indicated to close a hemodynamically significant patent ductus arteriosus in premature infants weighing between 500 and 1750 g when after 48 hours usual medical management (e.g., fluid restriction, diuretics, digitalis, respiratory support, etc.) is ineffective. Clear-cut clinical evidence of a hemodynamically significant patent ductus arteriosus should be present, such as respiratory distress, a continuous murmur, a hyperactive precordium, cardiomegaly and pulmonary plethora on chest x-ray.

CARDIOVASCULAR		
none	hypertension hypotension tachycardia chest pain	congestive heart failure arrhythmia; palpitations
METABOLIC		
none	edema weight gain fluid retention flushing or sweating	hyperglycemia glycosuria hyperkalemia
INTEGUMENTARY		
none	pruritus rash; urticaria petechiae or ecchymosis	exfoliative dermatitis erythema nodosum loss of hair Stevens-Johnson syndrome erythema multiforme toxic epidermal necrolysis
HEMATOLOGIC		
none	leukopenia bone marrow depression anemia secondary to obvious or occult gastrointestinal bleeding	aplastic anemia hemolytic anemia agranulocytosis thrombocytopenic purpura
HYPERSENSITIVITY		
none	acute anaphylaxis acute respiratory distress rapid fall in blood pressure resembling a shock-like state angioedema	dyspnea asthma purpura angiitis pulmonary edema
GENITOURINARY		
none	hematuria vaginal bleeding proteinuria nephrotic syndrome interstitial nephritis	BUN elevation renal insufficiency, including renal failure
MISCELLANEOUS		
none	epistaxis breast changes, including enlargement and tenderness, or gynecomastia	

*Reactions occurring in 3% to 9% of patients treated with INDOCIN. (Those reactions occurring in less than 3% of the patients are unmarked.)

**Reactions occurring in over 10% of patients treated with INDOCIN.

CONTRAINDICATIONS

INDOCIN I.V. is contraindicated in: infants with proven or suspected infection that is untreated; infants who are bleeding, especially those with active intracranial hemorrhage or gastrointestinal bleeding; infants with thrombocytopenia; infants with coagulation defects; infants with or who are suspected of having necrotizing enterocolitis; infants with significant impairment of renal function; infants with congenital heart disease in whom patency of the ductus arteriosus is necessary for satisfactory pulmonary or systemic blood flow (e.g., pulmonary atresia, severe tetralogy of Fallot, severe coarctation of the aorta).

WARNINGS

Gastrointestinal Effects:
In the collaborative study, major gastrointestinal bleeding was no more common in those infants receiving indomethacin than in those infants on placebo. However, minor gastrointestinal bleeding (i.e. chemical detection of blood in the stool) was more commonly noted in those infants treated with indomethacin. Severe gastrointestinal effects have been reported in adults with various arthritic disorders treated chronically with oral indomethacin. [For further information, see package circular for Capsules INDOCIN® (Indomethacin, MSD)].

Central Nervous System Effects:
Prematurity per se, is associated with an increased incidence of spontaneous intraventricular hemorrhage. Because indomethacin may inhibit platelet aggregation, the potential for intraventricular bleeding may be increased. However, in the large multi-center study of INDOCIN I.V. (see CLINICAL PHARMACOLOGY), the incidence of intraventricular hemorrhage in babies treated with INDOCIN I.V. was not significantly higher than in the control infants.

Renal Effects:
INDOCIN I.V. may cause significant reduction in urine output (50 percent or more) with concomitant elevations of blood urea nitrogen and creatinine, and reductions in glomerular filtration rate and creatinine clearance. These effects in most infants are transient, disappearing with cessation of therapy with INDOCIN I.V. However, because adequate renal function can depend upon renal prostaglandin synthesis, INDOCIN I.V. may precipitate renal insufficiency, including acute renal failure, especially in infants with other conditions that may adversely affect renal function (e.g., extracellular volume depletion from any cause, congestive heart failure, sepsis, concomitant use of any nephrotoxic drug, hepatic dysfunction). When significant suppression of urine volume occurs after a dose of INDOCIN I.V., no additional dose should be given until the urine output returns to normal levels.

INDOCIN I.V. in pre-term infants may suppress water excretion to a greater extent than sodium excretion. When this occurs, a significant reduction in serum sodium values (i.e. hyponatremia) may result. Infants should have serum electrolyte determinations done during therapy with INDOCIN I.V. Renal function and serum electrolytes should be monitored (see PRECAUTIONS, *Drug Interactions* and DOSAGE AND ADMINISTRATION).

PRECAUTIONS

General
INDOCIN (Indomethacin, MSD) may mask the usual signs and symptoms of infection. Therefore, the physician must be continually on the alert for this and should use the drug with extra care in the presence of existing controlled infection.

Severe hepatic reactions have been reported in adults treated chronically with oral indomethacin for arthritic disorders. [For further information, see package circular for Capsules INDOCIN (Indomethacin, MSD)]. If clinical signs and symptoms consistent with liver disease develop in the neonate, or if systemic manifestations occur, INDOCIN I.V. should be discontinued.

INDOCIN I.V. may inhibit platelet aggregation. In one small study, platelet aggregation was grossly abnormal after indomethacin therapy (given orally to premature infants to close the ductus arteriosus). Platelet aggregation returned to normal by the tenth day. Premature infants should be observed for signs of bleeding.

The drug should be administered carefully to avoid extravascular injection or leakage as the solution may be irritating to tissue.

Drug Interactions
Pre-term infants with patent ductus arteriosus and associated cardiac failure are frequently treated with digitalis. The half-life of digitalis in pre-term infants may be further prolonged, due to reduced renal function during therapy with indomethacin. Where both drugs are used concomitantly, the infant should be observed closely; frequent ECGs and serum digitalis levels may be required to prevent or to detect digitalis toxicity early.

Therapy with indomethacin may blunt the natriuretic effect of furosemide. This response has been attributed to inhibition of prostaglandin synthesis by non-steroidal anti-inflammatory drugs. In a study of 19 premature infants with patent ductus arteriosus treated with either INDOCIN I.V. alone or a combination of INDOCIN I.V. and furosemide, results showed that infants receiving both INDOCIN I.V. and furosemide had significantly higher urinary output, higher levels of sodium and chloride excretion, and higher glomerular filtration rates than did those infants receiving INDOCIN I.V. alone. In this study, the data suggested that therapy with furosemide helped to maintain renal function in the premature infant when INDOCIN I.V. was added to the treatment of patent ductus arteriosus.

Neonatal Effects
In rats and mice, oral indomethacin 4.0 mg/kg/day given during the last three days of gestation caused a decrease in maternal weight gain and some maternal and fetal deaths. An increased incidence of neuronal necrosis in the diencephalon in the live-born fetuses was observed. At 2.0 mg/kg/day, no increase in neuronal necrosis was observed as compared to the control groups. Administration of 0.5 or 4.0 mg/kg/day during the first three days of life did not cause an increase in neuronal necrosis at either dose level.

Pregnant rats, given 2.0 mg/kg/day and 4.0 mg/kg/day during the last trimester of gestation, delivered offspring whose pulmonary blood vessels were both reduced in number and excessively muscularized. These findings are similar to those observed in the syndrome of persistent pulmonary hypertension of the newborn.

ADVERSE REACTIONS

In a double-blind placebo-controlled trial of 405 premature infants weighing less than or equal to 1750 g with evidence of large ductal shunting, in those infants treated with indomethacin (n = 206), there was a statistically significantly greater incidence of bleeding problems, including gross or microscopic bleeding into the gastrointestinal tract, oozing from the skin after needle stick, pulmonary hemorrhage, and disseminated intravascular coagulopathy. There was no statistically significant difference between treatment groups with reference to intracranial hemorrhage.

The infants treated with indomethacin sodium trihydrate also had a significantly higher incidence of transient oliguria and elevations of serum creatinine (greater than or equal to 1.8 mg/dL) than did the infants treated with placebo.

The incidences of retrolental fibroplasia (grades III and IV) and pneumothorax in infants treated with INDOCIN I.V. were no greater than in placebo controls and were statistically significantly lower than in surgically-treated infants.

The following additional adverse reactions in infants have been reported from the collaborative study, anecdotal case reports, and from other studies using rectal, oral, or intravenous indomethacin for treatment of patent ductus arteriosus. The rates are based on the experience of 849 indomethacin-treated infants reported in the medical literature, regardless of the route of administration. One year follow-up is available on 175 infants and shows no long-term sequelae which could be attributed to indomethacin. In the collaborative study, only electrolyte imbalance and renal dysfunction (of the reactions listed below) occurred statistically significantly more frequently after INDOCIN I.V. than after placebo.

Renal: renal dysfunction in 41 percent of infants, including one or more of the following: reduced urinary output; reduced urine sodium, chloride, or potassium, urine osmolality, free water clearance, or glomerular filtration rate; elevated serum creatinine or BUN; uremia.

Gastrointestinal: gastrointestinal bleeding*, vomiting, abdominal distention, transient ileus.

Metabolic: hyponatremia*, elevated serum potassium*, reduction in blood sugar, including hypoglycemia, increased weight gain (fluid retention).

Coagulation: decreased platelet aggregation (see PRECAUTIONS).

*Incidence 3–9 percent. Those reactions which are unmarked occurred in 1–3 percent of patients.

Continued on next page

Information on the Merck Sharp & Dohme products listed on these pages is the full prescribing information from product circulars in use August 31, 1986.

Merck Sharp & Dohme—Cont.

The following adverse reactions have also been reported in infants treated with indomethacin, however, a causal relationship to therapy with INDOCIN I.V. has not been established:

Cardiovascular: intracranial bleeding**, bradycardia.
Respiratory: apnea, exacerbation of pre-existing pulmonary infection.
Metabolic: acidosis/alkalosis.
Gastrointestinal: necrotizing enterocolitis.
Ophthalmic: retrolental fibroplasia.**

A variety of additional adverse experiences have been reported in adults treated with oral indomethacin for moderate to severe rheumatoid arthritis, osteoarthritis, ankylosing spondylitis, acute painful shoulder and acute gouty arthritis (see section ADDITIONAL ADVERSE REACTIONS—ADULTS). Their relevance to the pre-term neonate receiving indomethacin for patent ductus arteriosus is unknown, however, the possibility exists that these experiences may be associated with the use of INDOCIN I.V. in pre-term neonates.

DOSAGE AND ADMINISTRATION

FOR INTRAVENOUS ADMINISTRATION ONLY.
Dosage recommendations for closure of the ductus arteriosus depends on the age of the infant at the time of therapy. A course of therapy is defined as three intravenous doses of INDOCIN I.V. given at 12–24 hour intervals, with careful attention to urinary output. If anuria or marked oliguria (urinary output < 0.6 mL/kg/hr) is evident at the scheduled time of the second or third dose of INDOCIN I.V., no additional doses should be given until laboratory studies indicate that renal function has returned to normal (see WARNINGS, *Renal Effects*).
Dosage according to age is as follows:

AGE at 1st dose	DOSAGE (mg/kg)		
	1st	2nd	3rd
Less than 48 hours	0.2	0.1	0.1
2–7 days	0.2	0.2	0.2
over 7 days	0.2	0.25	0.25

If the ductus arteriosus closes or is significantly reduced in size after an interval of 48 hours or more from completion of the first course of INDOCIN I.V., no further doses are necessary. If the ductus arteriosus re-opens, a second course of 1–3 doses may be given, each dose separated by a 12–24 hour interval as described above.

If the infant remains unresponsive to therapy with INDOCIN I.V. after 2 courses, surgery may be necessary for closure of the ductus arteriosus. If severe adverse reactions occur, STOP THE DRUG.

Directions for Use
Parenteral drug products should be inspected visually for particulate matter and discoloration prior to administration whenever solution and container permit.

The solution may be prepared with 1 to 2 mL of preservative-free sterile sodium chloride injection 0.9 percent or sterile, preservative-free water for injection. Benzyl alcohol as a preservative has been associated with toxicity in newborns. Therefore, all diluents should be preservative-free. If 1 mL of diluent is used, the concentration of indomethacin in the solution will equal approximately 0.1 mg/0.1 mL; if 2 mL of diluent are used, the concentration of the solution will equal approximately 0.05 mg/0.1 mL. Any unused portion of the solution should be discarded because there is no preservative contained in the vial. A fresh solution should be prepared just prior to each administration. Once reconstituted, the indomethacin solution may be injected intravenously over 5–10 seconds.

Further dilution with intravenous infusion solutions is not recommended. INDOCIN I.V. is not buffered, and reconstitution with solutions at pH values below 6.0 may result in precipitation of the insoluble indomethacin free acid moiety.

HOW SUPPLIED

No. 3406—Sterile INDOCIN I.V. is a lyophilized white to yellow powder or plug supplied as single dose vials containing indomethacin sodium trihydrate, equivalent to 1.0 mg indomethacin.

**Incidence in both indomethacin and placebo-treated infants 3–9 percent. Those reactions which are unmarked occurred in less than 3 percent.

NDC 0006-3406-17.
Storage
Store below 30°C (86°F). *Protect from light.* Store container in carton until contents have been used.

ADDITIONAL ADVERSE REACTIONS—ADULTS

The following adverse reactions have been reported in adults treated with oral indomethacin for moderate to severe rheumatoid arthritis, osteoarthritis, ankylosing spondylitis, acute painful shoulder and acute gouty arthritis. Complaints not of relevance in the treatment of the premature infant, such as anorexia, psychic disturbances, and blurred vision, are not listed.

Incidence 1% to 3%	***Incidence less than 1%***	
GASTROINTESTINAL		
diarrhea constipation	bloating (includes distention) flatulence peptic ulcer gastroenteritis rectal bleeding proctitis perforation and hemorrhage of the esophagus, stomach, duodenum or small intestines intestinal ulceration associated with stenosis and obstruction	gastrointestinal bleeding without obvious ulcer formation and perforation of pre-existing sigmoid lesions development of ulcerative stomatitis toxic hepatitis and jaundice (some fatal cases have been reported)
CENTRAL NERVOUS SYSTEM		
none	involuntary muscle movements	aggravation of epilepsy coma peripheral neuropathy convulsions
SPECIAL SENSES		
none	hearing disturbances, deafness	
CARDIOVASCULAR		
none	hypertension tachycardia	arrhythmia congestive heart failure
METABOLIC		
none	edema weight gain flushing	hyperglycemia glycosuria hyperkalemia
INTEGUMENTARY		
none	rash; urticaria petechiae or ecchymosis	exfoliative dermatitis erythema nodosum loss of hair Stevens-Johnson syndrome erythema multiforme toxic epidermal necrolysis
HEMATOLOGIC		
none	leukopenia bone marrow depression anemia secondary to obvious or occult gastrointestinal bleeding	aplastic anemia hemolytic anemia agranulocytosis thrombocytopenic purpura
HYPERSENSITIVITY		
none	acute respiratory distress rapid fall in blood pressure resembling a shock-like state	dyspnea asthma purpura angiitis pulmonary edema
GENITOURINARY		
none	hematuria vaginal bleeding	renal insufficiency, including renal failure
MISCELLANEOUS		
none	epistaxis breast changes, including enlargement and tenderness, or gynecomastia	

See package circular for Capsules INDOCIN (Indomethacin, MSD) for additional information concerning adverse reactions and other cautionary statements.

A.H.F.S. Category: 28:08
DC 7287002 Issued March 1985

INVERSINE® Tablets ℞
(Mecamylamine HCl, MSD), U.S.P.

DESCRIPTION

INVERSINE® (Mecamylamine HCl, MSD) is a potent, oral antihypertensive agent and ganglion blocker, and is a secondary amine. It is *N*,2,3,3-tetramethylbicyclo[2.2.1] heptan-2-amine hydrochloride. Its empirical formula is $C_{11}H_{21}N \cdot HCl$ and its structural formula is:

It is a white, odorless, or practically odorless, crystalline powder, is highly stable, soluble in water and has a molecular weight of 203.75.
INVERSINE is supplied as tablets for oral use, each containing 2.5 mg mecamylamine HCl. Inactive ingredients are acacia, calcium phosphate, D&C Yellow 10, FD&C Yellow 6, lactose, magnesium stearate, starch, and talc.

CLINICAL PHARMACOLOGY

Mecamylamine reduces blood pressure in both normotensive and hypertensive individuals. It has a gradual onset of action (½ to 2 hours) and a long-lasting effect (usually 6 to 12 hours or more). A small oral dosage often produces a smooth and predictable reduction of blood pressure. Although this antihypertensive effect is predominantly orthostatic, the supine blood pressure is also significantly reduced.
Pharmacokinetics and Metabolism
Mecamylamine is almost completely absorbed from the gastrointestinal tract, resulting in consistent lowering of blood pressure in most patients with hypertensive cardiovascular disease. Mecamylamine is excreted slowly in the urine in the unchanged form. The rate of its renal elimination is influenced markedly by urinary pH. Alkalinization of the urine reduces, and acidification promotes, renal excretion of mecamylamine.
Mecamylamine crosses the blood-brain and placental barriers.

INDICATIONS AND USAGE

For the management of moderately severe to severe essential hypertension and in uncomplicated cases of malignant hypertension.

CONTRAINDICATIONS

INVERSINE should not be used in mild, moderate, labile hypertension and may prove unsuitable in uncooperative patients. It is contraindicated in coronary insufficiency or recent myocardial infarction.
INVERSINE should be given with great discretion, if at all, when renal insufficiency is manifested by a rising or elevated BUN. The drug is contraindicated in uremia. Patients receiving antibiotics and sulfonamides should generally not be treated with ganglion blockers. Other contraindications are glaucoma, organic pyloric stenosis or hypersensitivity to the product.

WARNINGS

Mecamylamine, a secondary amine, readily penetrates into the brain and thus may produce central nervous sytem effects. Tremor, choreiform movements, mental aberrations, and convulsions may occur rarely. These have occurred most often when large doses of INVERSINE were used, especially in patients with cerebral or renal insufficiency.
When ganglion blockers or other potent antihypertensive drugs are discontinued suddenly, hypertensive levels return. In patients with malignant hypertension and others, this may occur abruptly and may cause fatal cerebral vascular accidents or acute congestive heart failure. When INVERSINE is withdrawn, this should be done gradually and other antihypertensive therapy usually must be substituted. On the other hand, the effects of INVERSINE sometimes may last from hours to days after therapy is discontinued.

PRECAUTIONS

General
The patient's condition should be evaluated carefully, particularly as to renal and cardiovascular function. When renal, cerebral, or coronary blood flow is deficient, any additional impairment, which might result from added hypotension, must be avoided. The use of INVERSINE in patients with marked cerebral and coronary arteriosclerosis or after a recent cerebral accident requires caution.

The action of INVERSINE may be potentiated by excessive heat, fever, infection, hemorrhage, pregnancy, anesthesia, surgery, vigorous exercise, other antihypertensive drugs, alcohol, and salt depletion as a result of diminished intake or increased excretion due to diarrhea, vomiting, excessive sweating, or diuretics.
During therapy with INVERSINE, sodium intake should not be restricted but, if necessary, the dosage of the ganglion blocker must be adjusted.
Since urinary retention may occur in patients on ganglion blockers, caution is required in patients with prostatic hypertrophy, bladder neck obstruction, and urethral stricture.
Frequent loose bowel movements with abdominal distention and decreased borborygmi may be the first signs of paralytic ileus. If these are present, INVERSINE should be discontinued immediately and remedial steps taken.
Information for Patients
INVERSINE may cause dizziness, lightheadedness, or fainting, especially when rising from a lying or sitting position. This effect may be increased by alcoholic beverages, exercise, or during hot weather. Getting up slowly may help alleviate such a reaction.
Drug Interactions
Patients receiving antibiotics and sulfonamides generally should not be treated with ganglion blockers.
The action of INVERSINE may be potentiated by anesthesia, other antihypertensive drugs and alcohol.
Carcinogenesis, Mutagenesis, Impairment of Fertility
Long-term studies in animals have not been performed to evaluate the effects upon fertility, mutagenic or carcinogenic potential of INVERSINE.
Pregnancy
Pregnancy Category C. Animal reproduction studies have not been conducted with INVERSINE. It is not known whether INVERSINE can cause fetal harm when given to a pregnant woman or can affect reproductive capacity. INVERSINE should be given to a pregnant woman only if clearly needed.
Nursing Mothers
Because of the potential for serious adverse reactions in nursing infants from INVERSINE, a decision should be made whether to discontinue nursing or to discontinue the drug, taking into account the importance of the drug to the mother.

ADVERSE REACTIONS

The following adverse reactions have been reported and within each category are listed in order of decreasing severity.
Gastrointestinal: Ileus, constipation (sometimes preceded by small, frequent liquid stools), vomiting, nausea, anorexia, glossitis and dryness of mouth.
Cardiovascular: Orthostatic dizziness and syncope, postural hypotension.
Nervous System/Psychiatric: Convulsions, choreiform movements, mental aberrations, tremor, and paresthesias (see WARNINGS).
Respiratory: Interstitial pulmonary edema and fibrosis.
Urogenital: Urinary retention, impotence, decreased libido.
Special Senses: Blurred vision, dilated pupils.
Miscellaneous: Weakness, fatigue, sedation.

OVERDOSAGE

Signs of overdosage include: hypotension (which may progress to peripheral vascular collapse), postural hypotension, nausea, vomiting, diarrhea, constipation, paralytic ileus, urinary retention, dizziness, anxiety, dry mouth, mydriasis, blurred vision, or palpitations. A rise in intraocular pressure may occur.
Pressor amines may be used to counteract excessive hypotension. Since patients being treated with ganglion blockers are more than normally reactive to pressor amines, small doses of the latter are recommended to avoid excessive response.
The oral LD_{50} of mecamylamine in the mouse is 92 mg/kg.

DOSAGE AND ADMINISTRATION

Therapy is usually started with one 2.5 mg tablet of INVERSINE twice a day. This initial dosage should be modified by increments of one 2.5 mg tablet at intervals of not less than 2 days until the desired blood pressure response occurs (the criterion being a dosage just under that which causes signs of mild postural hypotension).
The average total daily dosage of INVERSINE is 25 mg, usually in three divided doses. However, as little as 2.5 mg daily may be sufficient to control hypertension in some patients. A range of two to four or even more doses may be required in severe cases when smooth control is difficult to obtain. In severe or urgent cases, larger increments at smaller intervals may be needed. Partial tolerance may develop in certain patients, requiring an increase in the daily dosage of INVERSINE.
Administration of INVERSINE after meals may cause a more gradual absorption and smoother control of excessively high blood pressure. The timing of doses in relation to meals should be consistent. Since the blood pressure response to antihypertensive drugs is increased in the early morning, the larger dose should be given at noontime and perhaps in the evening. The morning dose, as a rule, should be relatively small and in some instances may even be omitted.
The *initial regulation of dosage* should be determined by blood pressure readings in the erect position at the time of maximal effect of the drug, as well as by other signs and symptoms of orthostatic hypertension.
The *effective maintenance dosage* should be regulated by blood pressure readings in the erect position and by limitation of dosage to that which causes slight faintness or dizziness in this position. If the patient or a relative can use a sphygmomanometer, instructions may be given to reduce or omit a dose if readings fall below a designated level or if faintness or lightheadedness occurs. *However, no change should be instituted without the knowledge of the physician.*
Close supervision and education of the patient, as well as critical adjustment of dosage, are essential to successful therapy.
Other Antihypertensive Agents
When INVERSINE is given with other antihypertensive drugs, the dosage of these other agents, as well as that of INVERSINE, should be reduced to avoid excessive hypotension. However, thiazides should be continued in their usual dosage, while that of INVERSINE is decreased by at least 50 percent.

HOW SUPPLIED

No. 3219—Tablets INVERSINE, 2.5 mg, are yellow, round, scored, compressed tablets, coded MSD 52. They are supplied as follows:
NDC 0006-0052-68 in bottles of 100.
A.H.F.S. Category: 24:08
DC 6041721 Issued September 1985

LACRISERT® Sterile Ophthalmic Insert ℞
(Hydroxypropyl Cellulose Ophthalmic Insert, MSD)

DESCRIPTION

LACRISERT® (Hydroxypropyl Cellulose Ophthalmic Insert, MSD) is a rod-shaped, water soluble, ophthalmic preparation made of hydroxypropyl cellulose, 5 mg. LACRISERT contains no preservatives or other ingredients. It is about 1.27 mm in diameter by about 3.5 mm long.
LACRISERT is supplied in packages of 60 units, together with illustrated instructions and a special applicator for removing LACRISERT from the unit dose blister and inserting it into the eye. A spare applicator is included in each package.

ACTIONS

LACRISERT acts to stabilize and thicken the precorneal tear film and prolong the tear film breakup time which is usually accelerated in patients with dry eye states. LACRISERT also acts to lubricate and protect the eye. LACRISERT usually reduces the signs and symptoms resulting from moderate to severe dry eye syndromes.

INDICATIONS

LACRISERT is indicated in patients with moderate to severe dry eye syndromes, including keratoconjunctivitis sicca.
LACRISERT is indicated especially in patients who remain symptomatic after an adequate trial of therapy with artificial tear solutions.
LACRISERT is also indicated for patients with:
Exposure keratitis
Decreased corneal sensitivity
Recurrent corneal erosions
LACRISERT usually reduces the signs and symptoms resulting from moderate to severe dry eye syndromes, such as conjunctival hyperemia, corneal and conjunctival staining with rose bengal, exudation, itching, burning, foreign body sensation, smarting, photophobia, dryness and blurred or cloudy vision. Progressive visual deterioration which occurs in some patients may be retarded, halted, or sometimes reversed.
In a multicenter crossover study the 5 mg LACRISERT administered once a day during the waking hours was compared to artificial tears used four or more times daily. There was a significant prolongation of tear film breakup time and a significant decrease in foreign body sensation associated with dry eye syndrome in patients during treatment with inserts as compared to artificial tears. Improvement, as measured by amelioration of symptoms, by slit lamp examination and by rose bengal staining of the cornea and conjunctiva, was greater in most patients with moderate to severe symptoms during treatment with LACRISERT. Patient comfort was usually better with LACRISERT than with artificial tears solution, and most patients preferred LACRISERT.
In most patients treated with LACRISERT for over one year, improvement was observed as evidenced by amelioration of symptoms generally associated with keratoconjunctivitis sicca such as burning, tearing, foreign body sensation, itching, photophobia and blurred or cloudy vision.
During studies in healthy volunteers, a thickened precorneal tear film was usually observed through the slit lamp while LACRISERT was present in the conjunctival sac.

CONTRAINDICATIONS

LACRISERT is contraindicated in patients who are hypersensitive to hydroxypropyl cellulose.

WARNINGS

Instructions for inserting and removing LACRISERT should be carefully followed.

PRECAUTIONS

Because this product may produce transient blurring of vision, patients should be instructed to exercise caution when operating hazardous machinery or driving a motor vehicle.
If improperly placed in the inferior cul-de-sac, LACRISERT may result in corneal abrasion (see DOSAGE AND ADMINISTRATION).

ADVERSE REACTIONS

The following adverse reactions have been reported in patients treated with LACRISERT, but were in most instances mild and transient:
Transient blurring of vision (See PRECAUTIONS)
Ocular discomfort or irritation
Matting or stickiness of eyelashes
Photophobia
Hypersensitivity
Edema of the eyelids
Hyperemia

DOSAGE AND ADMINISTRATION

One LACRISERT ophthalmic insert in each eye once daily is usually sufficient to relieve the symptoms associated with moderate to severe dry eye syndromes. Individual patients may require more flexibility in the use of LACRISERT; some patients may require twice daily use for optimal results.
Clinical experience with LACRISERT indicates that in some patients several weeks may be required before satisfactory improvement of symptoms is achieved.
LACRISERT is inserted into the inferior cul-de-sac of the eye beneath the base of the tarsus, not in apposition to the cornea. Illustrated instructions are included in each package.
While in the licensed practitioner's office, the patient should read the instructions, then practice insertion and removal of LACRISERT until proficiency is achieved.
NOTE: Occasionally LACRISERT is inadvertently expelled from the eye, especially in patients with shallow conjunctival fornices. The patient should be cautioned against rubbing the eye(s) containing LACRISERT, especially upon awakening, so as not to dislodge or expel the insert. If required, another LACRISERT ophthalmic insert may be inserted. If experience indicates that transient blurred vision develops in an individual patient, the patient may want to remove LACRISERT a few hours after insertion to avoid this. Another LACRISERT ophthalmic insert may be inserted if needed.
If LACRISERT causes worsening of symptoms, the patient should be instructed to inspect the conjunctival sac to make certain LACRISERT is in the proper location, deep in the inferior cul-de-sac of the eye beneath the base of the tarsus. If these symptoms persist, LACRISERT should be removed and the patient should contact the practitioner.

HOW SUPPLIED

No. 3380—LACRISERT, a rod-shaped, water-soluble, ophthalmic preparation made of hydroxypropyl cellulose, 5 mg, is supplied as follows:
NDC 0006-3380-60 in packages containing 60 unit doses, two reusable applicators and a storage container.
Store below 30°C (86°F).
DC 7189405 Issued November 1984

Continued on next page

Information on the Merck Sharp & Dohme products listed on these pages is the full prescribing information from product circulars in use August 31, 1986.

Merck Sharp & Dohme—Cont.

M-M-R®$_{II}$ ℞
(Measles, Mumps, and Rubella Virus Vaccine Live, MSD), U.S.P.

DESCRIPTION

M-M-R® II (Measles, Mumps, and Rubella Virus Vaccine Live, MSD) is a live virus vaccine for immunization against measles (rubeola), mumps and rubella (German measles).
M-M-R II is a sterile lyophilized preparation of (1) ATTENUVAX® (Measles Virus Vaccine Live, MSD), a more attenuated line of measles virus, derived from Enders' attenuated Edmonston strain and grown in cell cultures of chick embryo; (2) MUMPSVAX® (Mumps Virus Vaccine Live, MSD), the Jeryl Lynn (B level) strain of mumps virus grown in cell cultures of chick embryo; and (3) MERUVAX® II (Rubella Virus Vaccine Live, MSD), the Wistar RA 27/3 strain of live attenuated rubella virus grown in human diploid cell (WI-38) culture. The vaccine viruses are the same as those used in the manufacture of ATTENUVAX (Measles Virus Vaccine Live, MSD), MUMPSVAX (Mumps Virus Vaccine Live, MSD) and MERUVAX II (Rubella Virus Vaccine Live, MSD). The three viruses are mixed before being lyophilized. The product contains no preservative.
The reconstituted vaccine is for subcutaneous administration. When reconstituted as directed, the dose for injection is 0.5 mL and contains not less than the equivalent of 1,000 $TCID_{50}$ (tissue culture infectious doses) of the U.S. Reference Measles Virus; 5,000 $TCID_{50}$ of the U.S. Reference Mumps Virus; and 1,000 $TCID_{50}$ of the U.S. Reference Rubella Virus. Each dose contains approximately 25 mcg of neomycin. The product contains no preservative. Sorbitol and hydrolized gelatin are added as stabilizers.

CLINICAL PHARMACOLOGY

Clinical studies of 279 triple seronegative children, 11 months to 7 years of age, demonstrated that M-M-R II is highly immunogenic and generally well tolerated. In these studies, a single injection of the vaccine induced measles hemagglutination-inhibition (HI) antibodies in 95 percent, mumps neutralizing antibodies in 96 percent, and rubella HI antibodies in 99 percent of susceptible persons.
The RA 27/3 rubella strain in M-M-R II elicits higher immediate post-vaccination HI, complement-fixing and neutralizing antibody levels than other strains of rubella vaccine and has been shown to induce a broader profile of circulating antibodies including anti-theta and anti-iota precipitating antibodies. The RA 27/3 rubella strain immunologically simulates natural infection more closely than other rubella vaccine viruses. The increased levels and broader profile of antibodies produced by RA 27/3 strain rubella virus vaccine appear to correlate with greater resistance to subclinical reinfection with the wild virus, and provide greater confidence for lasting immunity.
Vaccine induced antibody levels following administration of M-M-R II have been shown to persist for at least two years without substantial decline. Antibody levels after immunization with M-M-R (Measles, Mumps, and Rubella Virus Vaccine Live, MSD), containing the HPV-77 strain of rubella, have persisted for 10.5 years without substantial decline. If the present pattern continues, it will provide a basis for the expectation that immunity following vaccination will be permanent. However, continued surveillance will be required to demonstrate this point.

INDICATIONS AND USAGE

M-M-R II is indicated for simultaneous immunization against measles, mumps, and rubella in persons 15 months of age or older. A booster is not needed.
Infants who are less than 15 months of age may fail to respond to the measles component of the vaccine due to presence in the circulation of residual measles antibody of maternal origin, the younger the infant, the lower the likelihood of seroconversion. In geographically isolated or other relatively inaccessible populations for whom immunization programs are logistically difficult, and in population groups in which natural measles infection may occur in a significant proportion of infants before 15 months of age, it may be desirable to give the vaccine to infants at an earlier age. Infants vaccinated under these conditions at less than 12 months of age should be revaccinated after reaching 15 months of age. There is some evidence to suggest that infants immunized at less than one year of age may not develop sustained antibody levels when later reimmunized. The advantage of early protection must be weighed against the chance for failure to respond adequately on reimmunization.
Previously unimmunized children of susceptible pregnant women should receive live attenuated rubella vaccine, because an immunized child will be less likely to acquire natural rubella and introduce the virus into the household.

Non-Pregnant Adolescent and Adult Females
Immunization of susceptible non-pregnant adolescent and adult females of childbearing age with live attenuated rubella virus vaccine is indicated if certain precautions are observed (see below and PRECAUTIONS). Vaccinating susceptible postpubertal females confers individual protection against subsequently acquiring rubella infection during pregnancy, which in turn prevents infection of the fetus and consequent congenital rubella injury.
Women of childbearing age should be advised not to become pregnant for three months after vaccination and should be informed of the reasons for this precaution.*
It is recommended that rubella susceptibility be determined by serologic testing prior to immunization.** If immune, as evidenced by a specific rubella antibody titer of 1:8 or greater (hemagglutination-inhibition test), vaccination is unnecessary. Congenital malformations do occur in up to seven percent of all live births. Their chance appearance after vaccination could lead to misinterpretation of the cause, particularly if the prior rubella-immune status of vaccinees is unknown.
Postpubertal females should be informed of the frequent occurrence of self-limited arthralgia and possible arthritis beginning 2 to 4 weeks after vaccination (see ADVERSE REACTIONS).
Postpartum Women
It has been found convenient in many instances to vaccinate rubella-susceptible women in the immediate postpartum period. (See *Nursing Mothers*).
Revaccination: Children vaccinated when younger than 12 months of age should be revaccinated. Based on available evidence, there is no reason to routinely revaccinate persons who were vaccinated originally when 12 months of age or older. However, persons should be revaccinated if there is evidence to suggest that initial immunization was ineffective.
Use with other Vaccines
Routine administration of DTP (diphtheria, tetanus, pertussis) and/or OPV (oral poliovirus vaccine) concomitantly with measles, mumps and rubella vaccines is not recommended because there are insufficient data relating to the simultaneous administration of these antigens. However, the American Academy of Pediatrics has noted that in some circumstances, particularly when the patient may not return, some practitioners prefer to administer all these antigens on a single day. If done, separate sites and syringes should be used for DTP and M-M-R II.
M-M-R II should not be given less than one month before or after administration of other virus vaccines.

CONTRAINDICATIONS

Do not give M-M-R II to pregnant females; the possible effects of the vaccine on fetal development are unknown at this time. If vaccination of postpubertal females is undertaken, pregnancy should be avoided for three months following vaccination. (See PRECAUTIONS, *Pregnancy*).
Anaphylactoid reaction to neomycin (each dose of reconstituted vaccine contains approximately 25 mcg of neomycin).
History of anaphylactoid reaction to eggs (see HYPERSENSITIVITY TO EGGS below).
Any febrile respiratory illness or other active febrile infection.
Active untreated tuberculosis.
Patients receiving immunosuppressive therapy. This contraindication does not apply to patients who are receiving corticosteroids as replacement therapy, e.g., for Addison's disease.
Individuals with blood dyscrasias, leukemia, lymphomas of any type, or other malignant neoplasms affecting the bone marrow or lymphatic systems.
Primary immunodeficiency states, including cellular immune deficiencies, hypogammaglobulinemic and dysgammaglobulinemic states.

*NOTE: The Immunization Practices Advisory Committee (ACIP) has recommended "In view of the importance of protecting this age group against rubella, reasonable precautions in a rubella immunization program include asking females if they are pregnant, excluding those who say they are, and explaining the theoretical risks to the others."

**NOTE: The Immunization Practices Advisory Committee (ACIP) has stated "When practical, and when reliable laboratory services are available, potential vaccinees of childbearing age can have serologic tests to determine susceptibility to rubella. . . . However, routinely performing serologic tests for all females of childbearing age to determine susceptibility so that vaccine is given only to proven susceptibles is expensive and has been ineffective in some areas. Accordingly, the ACIP believes that rubella vaccination of a woman who is not known to be pregnant and has no history of vaccination is justifiable without serologic testing."

Individuals with a family history of congenital or hereditary immunodeficiency, until the immune competence of the potential vaccine recipient is demonstrated.

HYPERSENSITIVITY TO EGGS

Live measles vaccine and live mumps vaccine are produced in chick embryo cell culture. Persons with a history of anaphylactic or other immediate reactions (e.g., hives, swelling of the mouth and throat, difficulty breathing, hypotension, or shock) subsequent to egg ingestion should not be vaccinated. Evidence indicates that persons are not at increased risk if they have egg allergies that are not anaphylactic in nature. Such persons may be vaccinated in the usual manner. There is no evidence to indicate that persons with allergies to chickens or feathers are at increased risk of reaction to the vaccine.

PRECAUTIONS

General
Adequate treatment provisions including epinephrine, should be available for immediate use should an anaphylactoid reaction occur.
Due caution should be employed in administration of M-M-R II to persons with a history of febrile convulsions, cerebral injury or any other condition in which stress due to fever should be avoided. The physician should be alert to the temperature elevation which may occur following vaccination. (See ADVERSE REACTIONS).
Vaccination should be deferred for at least 3 months following blood or plasma transfusions, or administration of human immune serum globulin.
Excretion of small amounts of the live attenuated rubella virus from the nose or throat has occurred in the majority of susceptible individuals 7–28 days after vaccination. There is no confirmed evidence to indicate that such virus is transmitted to susceptible persons who are in contact with the vaccinated individuals. Consequently, transmission through close personal contact, while accepted as a theoretical possibility, is not regarded as a significant risk. However, transmission of the rubella vaccine virus to infants via breast milk has been documented (see *Nursing Mothers*).
There are no reports of transmission of live attenuated measles or mumps viruses from vaccinees to susceptible contacts.
It has been reported that live attenuated measles, mumps and rubella virus vaccines given individually may result in a temporary depression of tuberculin skin sensitivity. Therefore, if a tuberculin test is to be done, it should be administered either before or simultaneously with M-M-R II.
As for any vaccine, vaccination with M-M-R II may not result in seroconversion in 100% of susceptible persons given the vaccine.
Pregnancy
Pregnancy Category C
Animal reproduction studies have not been conducted with M-M-R II. It is also not known whether M-M-R II can cause fetal harm when administered to a pregnant woman or can affect reproduction capacity. Therefore, the vaccine should not be administered to pregnant females; furthermore, pregnancy should be avoided for three months following vaccination (see CONTRAINDICATIONS).
In counseling women who are inadvertently vaccinated when pregnant or who become pregnant within 3 months of vaccination, the physician should be aware of the following: (1) In a 10 year survey involving over 700 pregnant women who received rubella vaccine within 3 months before or after conception (of whom 189 received the Wistar RA 27/3 strain), none of the newborns had abnormalities compatible with congenital rubella syndrome; (2) Although mumps virus is capable of infecting the placenta and fetus, there is no good evidence that it causes congenital malformations in humans. Mumps vaccine virus also has been shown to infect the placenta, but the virus has not been isolated from the fetal tissues from susceptible women who were vaccinated and underwent elective abortions; and (3) Reports have indicated that contracting of natural measles during pregnancy enhances fetal risk. Increased rates of spontaneous abortion, stillbirth, congenital defects and prematurity have been observed subsequent to natural measles during pregnancy. There are no adequate studies of the attenuated (vaccine) strain of measles virus in pregnancy. However, it would be prudent to assume that the vaccine strain of virus is also capable of inducing adverse fetal effects.
Nursing Mothers
It is not known whether measles or mumps vaccine virus is secreted in human milk. Recent studies have shown that lactating postpartum women immunized with live attenuated rubella vaccine may secrete the virus in breast milk and transmit it to breast-fed infants. In the infants with serological evidence of rubella infection, none exhibited severe disease; however, one exhibited mild clinical illness typical of acquired rubella. Caution should be exercised when M-M-R II is administered to a nursing woman.

ADVERSE REACTIONS

Because of the slightly acidic pH (6.2–6.6) of the vaccine, patients may complain of burning and/or stinging of short duration at the injection site.

The adverse clinical reactions associated with the use of M-M-R II are those expected to follow administration of the monovalent vaccines given separately. These may include malaise, sore throat, headache, fever, and rash; mild local reactions such as erythema, induration, tenderness and regional lymphadenopathy; parotitis; orchitis; nerve deafness; thrombocytopenia and purpura; allergic reactions such as wheal and flare at the injection site or urticaria; and arthritis, arthralgia and polyneuritis.

Moderate fever [101–102.9°F (38.3–39.4°C)] occurs occasionally, and high fever [above 103°F (39.4°C)] occurs less commonly. On rare occasions, children developing fever may exhibit febrile convulsions. Rash occurs infrequently and is usually minimal, but rarely may be generalized.

Forms of optic neuritis, including retrobulbar neuritis, papillitis, and retinitis may infrequently follow viral infections, and have been reported to occur 1 to 3 weeks following inoculation with some live virus vaccines.

Clinical experience with live attenuated measles, mumps and rubella virus vaccines given individually indicates that encephalitis and other nervous system reactions have occurred very rarely. These might occur also with M-M-R II.

Experience from more than 80 million doses of all live measles vaccines given in the U.S. through 1975 indicates that significant central nervous system reactions such as encephalitis and encephalopathy, occurring within 30 days after vaccination, have been temporally associated with measles vaccine approximately once for every million doses. In no case has it been shown that reactions were actually caused by vaccine. The Center for Disease Control has pointed out that "a certain number of cases of encephalitis may be expected to occur in a large childhood population in a defined period of time even when no vaccines are administered". However, the data suggest the possibility that some of these cases may have been caused by measles vaccines. The risk of such serious neurological disorders following live measles virus vaccine administration remains far less than that for encephalitis and encephalopathy with natural measles (one per two thousand reported cases).

There have been isolated reports of ocular palsies and Guillain-Barre syndrome occurring after immunization with vaccines containing live attenuated measles virus. The ocular palsies have occurred approximately 3–24 days following vaccination. No definite causal relationship has been established between either of these events and vaccination. Isolated reports of polyneuropathy including Guillain-Barré syndrome have also been reported after immunization with rubella containing vaccines.

There have been reports of subacute sclerosing panencephalitis (SSPE) in children who did not have a history of natural measles but did receive measles vaccine. Some of these cases may have resulted from unrecognized measles in the first year of life or possibly from the measles vaccination. Based on estimated nationwide measles vaccine distribution, the association of SSPE cases to measles vaccination is about one case per million vaccine doses distributed. This is far less than the association with natural measles, 6–22 cases of SSPE per million cases of measles. The results of a retrospective case-controlled study conducted by the Center for Disease Control suggest that the overall effect of measles vaccine has been to protect against SSPE by preventing measles with its inherent higher risk of SSPE.

Local reactions characterized by marked swelling, redness and vesiculation at the injection site of attenuated live measles virus vaccines, and systemic reactions including atypical measles, have occurred in persons who received killed measles vaccine previously. M-M-R II was not given under this condition in clinical trials. Rarely, more severe reactions that require hospitalization, including prolonged high fevers and extensive local reactions, have been reported. Panniculitis has been reported rarely following administration of measles vaccine.

Transient arthritis, arthralgia and polyneuritis are features of natural rubella and vary in frequency and severity with age and sex, being greatest in adult females and least in prepubertal children. This type of involvement as well as myalgia have also been reported following administration of MERUVAX II (Rubella Virus Vaccine Live, MSD). In children, joint reactions are rare and of brief duration if they do occur. In women, incidence rates for arthritis and arthralgia are generally higher than those seen in children (children: 0–3%; women: 12–20%), and the reactions tend to be more marked and of longer duration. Symptoms may persist for a matter of months or on rare occasions for years. In adolescent girls, the reactions appear to be intermediate in incidence between those seen in children and in adult women. Even in older women (35–45 years), these reactions are generally well tolerated and rarely interfere with normal activities.

DOSAGE AND ADMINISTRATION

FOR SUBCUTANEOUS ADMINISTRATION
Do not inject intravenously.

The dosage of vaccine is the same for all persons. Inject the total volume of the single dose vial (about 0.5 mL) or 0.5 mL of the 10 dose vial of reconstituted vaccine subcutaneously, preferably into the outer aspect of upper arm. *Do not give immune globulin (IG) concurrently with* M-M-R II.

During shipment, to insure that there is no loss of potency, the vaccine must be maintained at a temperature of 10°C (50°F) or less.

Before reconstitution, store M-M-R II at 2–8°C (35.6–46.4°F). *Protect from light.*

CAUTION: A sterile syringe free of preservatives, antiseptics, and detergents should be used for each injection and/or reconstitution of the vaccine because these substances may inactivate the live virus vaccine. A 25 gauge, 5/8″ needle is recommended.

To reconstitute, use only the diluent supplied, since it is free of preservatives or other antiviral substances which might inactivate the vaccine.

Single Dose Vial—First withdraw the entire volume of diluent into the syringe to be used for reconstitution. Inject all the diluent in the syringe into the vial of lyophilized vaccine, and agitate to mix thoroughly. Withdraw the entire contents into a syringe and inject the total volume of restored vaccine subcutaneously.

It is important to use a separate sterile syringe and needle for each individual patient to prevent transmission of hepatitis B and other infectious agents from one person to another.

10 Dose Vial (available only to government agencies/institutions)

Withdraw the entire contents (7 mL) of the diluent vial into the sterile syringe to be used for reconstitution, and introduce into the 10 dose vial of lyophilized vaccine. Agitate to ensure thorough mixing. The outer labeling suggests "For Jet Injector or Syringe Use". Use with separate sterile syringes is permitted for containers of 10 doses or less. The vaccine and diluent do not contain preservatives; therefore, the user must recognize the potential contamination hazards and exercise special precautions to protect the sterility and potency of the product. The use of aseptic techniques and proper storage prior to and after restoration of the vaccine and subsequent withdrawal of the individual doses is essential. Use 0.5 mL of the reconstituted vaccine for subcutaneous injection.

It is important to use a separate sterile syringe and needle for each individual patient to prevent transmission of hepatitis B and other infectious agents from one person to another.

Each dose contains not less than the equivalent of 1,000 $TCID_{50}$ of the U.S. Reference Measles Virus, 5,000 $TCID_{50}$ of the U.S. Reference Mumps Virus and 1,000 $TCID_{50}$ of the U.S. Reference Rubella Virus.

Parenteral drug products should be inspected visually for particulate matter and discoloration prior to administration. M-M-R II, when reconstituted, is clear yellow.

HOW SUPPLIED

No. 4749—M-M-R II is supplied as a single-dose vial of lyophilized vaccine, **NDC** 0006-4749-00, and a vial of diluent.

No. 4681/4309—M-M-R II is supplied as follows: (1) a box of 10 single-dose vials of lyophilized vaccine (package A), **NDC** 0006-4681-00; and (2) a box of 10 vials of diluent (package B). To conserve refrigerator space, the diluent may be stored separately at room temperature.

Available only to government agencies/institutions

No. 4682X—M-M-R II is supplied as one 10 dose vial of lyophilized vaccine, **NDC** 0006-4682-00, and one 7 mL vial of diluent.

Storage

It is recommended that the vaccine be used as soon as possible after reconstitution. Protect vaccine from light at all times, since such exposure may inactivate the virus. Store reconstituted vaccine in the vaccine vial in a dark place at 2–8°C (35.6–46.4°F) and discard if not used within 8 hours.

A.H.F.S. Category: 80:12

DC 7034409 Issued January 1986

M-R-VAX® II ℞
(Measles and Rubella Virus Vaccine Live, MSD), U.S.P.

DESCRIPTION

M-R-VAX® II (Measles and Rubella Virus Vaccine Live, MSD) is a live virus vaccine for immunization against measles (rubeola) and rubella (German measles).

M-R-VAX II is a sterile lyophilized preparation of (1) ATTENUVAX® (Measles Virus Vaccine Live, MSD), a more attenuated line of measles virus, derived from Enders' attenuated Edmonston strain and grown in cell cultures of chick embryo; and (2) MERUVAX® II (Rubella Virus Vaccine Live, MSD), the Wistar RA 27/3 strain of live attenuated rubella virus grown in human diploid cell (WI-38) culture. The vaccine viruses are the same as those used in the manufacture of ATTENUVAX (Measles Virus Vaccine Live, MSD) and MERUVAX II (Rubella Virus Vaccine Live, MSD). The two viruses are mixed before being lyophilized. The product contains no preservative.

The reconstituted vaccine is for subcutaneous administration. When reconstituted as directed, the dose for injection is 0.5 mL and contains not less than the equivalent of 1,000 $TCID_{50}$ (tissue culture infectious doses) of the U.S. Reference Measles Virus; and 1,000 $TCID_{50}$ of the U.S. Reference Rubella Virus. Each dose contains approximately 25 mcg of neomycin. The product contains no preservative. Sorbitol and hydrolized gelatin are added as stabilizers.

CLINICAL PHARMACOLOGY

Clinical studies of 237 double seronegative children, 10 months to 10 years of age, demonstrated that M-R-VAX II is highly immunogenic and generally well tolerated. In these studies, a single injection of the vaccine induced measles hemagglutination-inhibition (HI) antibodies in 95 percent and rubella HI antibodies in 99 percent of susceptible persons.

The RA 27/3 rubella strain in M-R-VAX II elicits higher immediate post-vaccination HI, complement-fixing and neutralizing antibody levels than other strains of rubella vaccine and has been shown to induce a broader profile of circulating antibodies including anti-theta and anti-iota precipitating antibodies. The RA 27/3 rubella strain immunologically simulates natural infection more closely than other rubella vaccine viruses. The increased levels and broader profile of antibodies produced by RA 27/3 strain rubella virus vaccine appear to correlate with greater resistance to subclinical reinfection with the wild virus, and provide greater confidence for lasting immunity.

Vaccine induced antibody levels following administration of M-R-VAX II have been shown to persist for at least two years without substantial decline. Antibody levels after immunization with M-R-VAX (Measles and Rubella Virus Vaccine Live, MSD), containing the HPV-77 strain of rubella, have persisted for 9 years without substantial decline. If the present pattern continues, it will provide a basis for the expectation that immunity following vaccination will be permanent. However, continued surveillance will be required to demonstrate this point.

INDICATIONS AND USAGE

M-R-VAX II is indicated for simultaneous immunization against measles and rubella in persons 15 months of age or older. A booster is not needed.

Infants who are less than 15 months of age may fail to respond to the measles component of the vaccine due to presence in the circulation of residual measles antibody of maternal origin; the younger the infant, the lower the likelihood of seroconversion. In geographically isolated or other relatively inaccessible populations for whom immunization programs are logistically difficult, and in population groups in which natural measles infection may occur in a significant proportion of infants before 15 months of age, it may be desirable to give the vaccine to infants at an earlier age. Infants vaccinated under these conditions at less than 12 months of age should be revaccinated after reaching 15 months of age. There is some evidence to suggest that infants immunized at less than one year of age may not develop sustained antibody levels when later reimmunized. The advantage of early protection must be weighed against the chance for failure to respond adequately on reimmunization.

Previously unimmunized children of susceptible pregnant women should receive live attenuated rubella vaccine, because an immunized child will be less likely to acquire natural rubella and introduce the virus into the household.

Non-Pregnant Adolescent and Adult Females

Immunization of susceptible non-pregnant adolescent and adult females of childbearing age with live attenuated rubella virus vaccine is indicated if certain precautions are observed (see below and PRECAUTIONS). Vaccinating susceptible postpubertal females confers individual protection against subsequently acquiring rubella infection during pregnancy, which in turn prevents infection of the fetus and consequent congenital rubella injury.

Continued on next page

Information on the Merck Sharp & Dohme products listed on these pages is the full prescribing information from product circulars in use August 31, 1986.

Merck Sharp & Dohme—Cont.

Women of childbearing age should be advised not to become pregnant for three months after vaccination and should be informed of the reason for this precaution.*

It is recommended that rubella susceptibility be determined by serologic testing prior to immunization.** If immune, as evidenced by a specific rubella antibody titer of 1:8 or greater (hemagglutination-inhibition test), vaccination is unnecessary. Congenital malformations do occur in up to seven percent of all live births. Their chance appearance after vaccination could lead to misinterpretation of the cause, particularly if the prior rubella-immune status of vaccinees is unknown.

Postpubertal females should be informed of the frequent occurrence of self-limited arthralgia and possible arthritis beginning 2 to 4 weeks after vaccination (see ADVERSE REACTIONS).

Postpartum Women

It has been found convenient in many instances to vaccinate rubella-susceptible women in the immediate postpartum period. (See *Nursing Mothers*).

Revaccination: Children vaccinated when younger than 12 months of age should be revaccinated. Based on available evidence, there is no reason to routinely revaccinate persons who were vaccinated originally when 12 months of age or older. However, persons should be revaccinated if there is evidence to suggest that initial immunization was ineffective.

Use with other Vaccines

Routine administration of DTP (diphtheria, tetanus, pertussis) and/or OPV (oral poliovirus vaccine) concomitantly with measles, mumps and rubella vaccines is not recommended because there are insufficient data relating to the simultaneous administration of these antigens. However, the American Academy of Pediatrics has noted that in some circumstances, particularly when the patient may not return, some practitioners prefer to administer all these antigens on a single day. If done, separate sites and syringes should be used for DTP and M-R-VAX II.

M-R-VAX II should not be given less than one month before or after administration of other virus vaccines.

CONTRAINDICATIONS

Do not give M-R-VAX II to pregnant females; the possible effects of the vaccine on fetal development are unknown at this time. If vaccination of postpubertal females is undertaken, pregnancy should be avoided for three months following vaccination. (See PRECAUTIONS, *Pregnancy*).

Anaphylactoid reaction to neomycin (each dose of reconstituted vaccine contains approximately 25 mcg of neomycin).

History of anaphylactoid reaction to eggs (see HYPERSENSITIVITY TO EGGS below).

Any febrile respiratory illness or other active febrile infection.

Active untreated tuberculosis.

Patients receiving immunosuppressive therapy. This contraindication does not apply to patients who are receiving corticosteroids as replacement therapy, e.g., for Addison's disease.

Individuals with blood dyscrasias, leukemia, lymphomas of any type, or other malignant neoplasms affecting the bone marrow or lymphatic systems.

Primary immunodeficiency states, including cellular immune deficiencies, hypogammaglobulinemic and dysgammaglobulinemic states.

Individuals with a family history of congenital or hereditary immunodeficiency, until the immune competence of the potential vaccine recipient is demonstrated.

---

*NOTE: The Immunization Practices Advisory Committee (ACIP) has recommended "In view of the importance of protecting this age group against rubella, reasonable precautions in a rubella immunization program include asking females if they are pregnant, excluding those who say they are, and explaining the theoretical risks to the others."

**NOTE: The Immunization Practices Advisory Committee (ACIP) has stated "When practical, and when reliable laboratory services are available, potential vaccinees of childbearing age can have serologic tests to determine susceptibility to rubella. . . . However, routinely performing serologic tests for all females of childbearing age to determine susceptibility so that vaccine is given only to proven susceptibles is expensive and has been ineffective in some areas. Accordingly, the ACIP believes that rubella vaccination of a woman who is not known to be pregnant and has no history of vaccination is justifiable without serologic testing."

HYPERSENSITIVITY TO EGGS

Live measles vaccine is produced in chick embryo cell culture. Persons with a history of anaphylactic or other immediate reactions (e.g., hives, swelling of the mouth and throat, difficulty breathing, hypotension, or shock) subsequent to egg ingestion should not be vaccinated. Evidence indicates that persons are not at increased risk if they have egg allergies that are not anaphylactic in nature. Such persons may be vaccinated in the usual manner. There is no evidence to indicate that persons with allergies to chickens or feathers are at increased risk of reaction to the vaccine.

PRECAUTIONS

General

Adequate treatment provisions including epinephrine, should be available for immediate use should an anaphylactoid reaction occur.

Due caution should be employed in administration of M-R-VAX II to persons with a history of febrile convulsions, cerebral injury or any other condition in which stress due to fever should be avoided. The physician should be alert to the temperature elevation which may occur following vaccination. (See ADVERSE REACTIONS).

Vaccination should be deferred for at least 3 months following blood or plasma transfusions, or administration of human immune serum globulin.

Excretion of small amounts of the live attenuated rubella virus from the nose or throat has occurred in the majority of susceptible individuals 7–28 days after vaccination. There is no confirmed evidence to indicate that such virus is transmitted to susceptible persons who are in contact with the vaccinated individuals. Consequently, transmission through close personal contact, while accepted as a theoretical possibility, is not regarded as a significant risk. However, transmission of the rubella vaccine virus to infants via breast milk has been documented (see *Nursing Mothers*).

There are no reports of transmission of live attenuated measles virus from vaccinees to susceptible contacts.

It has been reported that live attenuated measles and rubella virus vaccines given individually may result in a temporary depression of tuberculin skin sensitivity. Therefore, if a tuberculin test is to be done, it should be administered either before or simultaneously with M-R-VAX II.

As for any vaccine, vaccination with M-R-VAX II may not result in seroconversion in 100% of susceptible persons given the vaccine.

Pregnancy

Pregnancy Category C

Animal reproduction studies have not been conducted with M-R-VAX II. It is also not known whether M-R-VAX II can cause fetal harm when administered to a pregnant woman or can affect reproduction capacity. Therefore, the vaccine should not be administered to pregnant females; futhermore, pregnancy should be avoided for three months following vaccination (see CONTRAINDICATIONS).

In counseling women who are inadvertently vaccinated when pregnant or who become pregnant within 3 months of vaccination, the physician should be aware of the following: (1) In a 10 year survey involving over 700 pregnant women who received rubella vaccine within 3 months before or after conception, (of whom 189 received the Wistar RA 27/3 strain), none of the newborns had abnormalities compatible with congenital rubella syndrome; (2) Reports have indicated that contracting of natural measles during pregnancy enhances fetal risk. Increased rates of spontaneous abortion, stillbirth, congenital defects and prematurity have been observed subsequent to natural measles during pregnancy. There are no adequate studies of the attenuated (vaccine) strain of measles virus in pregnancy. However, it would be prudent to assume that the vaccine strain of virus is also capable of inducing adverse fetal effects.

Nursing Mothers

It is not known whether measles vaccine virus is secreted in human milk. Recent studies have shown that lactating postpartum women immunized with live attenuated rubella vaccine may secrete the virus in breast milk and transmit it to breast-fed infants. In the infants with serological evidence of rubella infection, none exhibited severe disease; however, one exhibited mild clinical illness typical of acquired rubella. Caution should be exercised when M-R-VAX II is administered to a nursing woman.

ADVERSE REACTIONS

Because of the slightly acidic pH (6.2–6.6) of the vaccine, patients may complain of burning and/or stinging of short duration at the injection site.

The adverse clinical reactions associated with the use of M-R-VAX II are those expected to follow administration of the monovalent vaccines given separately. These may include malaise, sore throat, headache, fever and rash; mild local reactions such as erythema, induration, tenderness and regional lymphadenopathy; thrombocytopenia and purpura; allergic reactions such as wheal and flare at the injection site or urticaria; and arthritis, arthralgia and polyneuritis.

Moderate fever [101–102.9°F (38.3–39.4°C)] occurs occasionally, and high fever [above 103°F (39.4°C)] occurs less commonly. On rare occasions, children developing fever may exhibit febrile convulsions. Rash occurs infrequently and is usually minimal, but rarely may be generalized.

Forms of optic neuritis, including retrobulbar neuritis, papillitis, and retinitis may infrequently follow viral infections, and have been reported to occur 1 to 3 weeks following inoculation with some live virus vaccines.

Clinical experience with live attenuated measles and rubella virus vaccines given individually indicates that encephalitis and other nervous system reactions have occurred very rarely. These might occur also with M-R-VAX II.

Experience from more than 80 million doses of all live measles vaccines given in the U.S. through 1975 indicates that significant central nervous system reactions such as encephalitis and encephalopathy, occurring within 30 days after vaccination, have been temporally associated with measles vaccine approximately once for every million doses. In no case has it been shown that reactions were actually caused by vaccine. The Center for Disease Control has pointed out that "a certain number of cases of encephalitis may be expected to occur in a large childhood population in a defined period of time even when no vaccines are administered". However, the data suggest the possibility that some of these cases may have been caused by measles vaccines. The risk of such serious neurological disorders following live measles virus vaccine administration remains far less than that for encephalitis and encephalopathy with natural measles (one per two thousand reported cases).

There have been isolated reports of ocular palsies and Guillain-Barré syndrome occurring after immunization with vaccines containing live attenuated measles virus. The ocular palsies have occurred approximately 3–24 days following vaccination. No definite causal relationship has been established between either of these events and vaccination. Isolated reports of polyneuropathy including Guillain-Barré syndrome have also been reported after immunization with rubella containing vaccines.

There have been reports of subacute sclerosing panencephalitis (SSPE) in children who did not have a history of natural measles but did receive measles vaccine. Some of these cases may have resulted from unrecognized measles in the first year of life or possibly from the measles vaccination. Based on estimated nationwide measles vaccine distribution, the association of SSPE cases to measles vaccination is about one case per million vaccine doses distributed. This is far less than the association with natural measles, 6–22 cases of SSPE per million cases of measles. The results of a retrospective case-controlled study conducted by the Center for Disease Control suggest that the overall effect of measles vaccine has been to protect against SSPE by preventing measles with its inherent higher risk of SSPE.

Local reactions characterized by marked swelling, redness and vesiculation at the injection site of attenuated live measles virus vaccines, and systemic reactions including atypical measles, have occurred in persons who received killed measles vaccine previously. M-R-VAX II was not given under this condition in clinical trials. Rarely, more severe reactions that require hospitalization, including prolonged high fevers and extensive local reactions, have been reported. Panniculitis has been reported rarely following administration of measles vaccine.

Transient arthritis, arthralgia and polyneuritis are features of natural rubella and vary in frequency and severity with age and sex, being greatest in adult females and least in prepubertal children. This type of involvement as well as myalgia have also been reported following administration of MERUVAX II (Rubella Virus Vaccine Live, MSD). In children, joint reactions are rare and of brief duration if they do occur. In women, incidence rates for arthritis and arthralgia are generally higher than those seen in children (children: 0–3%; women: 12–20%), and the reactions tend to be more marked and of longer duration. Symptoms may persist for a matter of months or on rare occasions for years. In adolescent girls, the reactions appear to be intermediate in incidence between those seen in children and in adult women. Even in older women (35–45 years), these reactions are generally well tolerated and rarely interfere with normal activities.

DOSAGE AND ADMINISTRATION

FOR SUBCUTANEOUS ADMINISTRATION

Do not inject intravenously

The dosage of vaccine is the same for all persons. Inject the total volume of the single dose vial (about 0.5 mL) or 0.5 mL of the multiple dose vial of reconstituted vaccine subcutaneously, preferably into the outer aspect of upper arm. *Do not give immune globulin (IG) concurrently with* M-R-VAX II.

During shipment, to insure that there is no loss of potency, the vaccine must be maintained at a temperature of 10°C (50°F) or less.

Before reconstitution, store M-R-VAX II at 2–8°C (35.6–46.4°F). *Protect from light.*

CAUTION: A sterile syringe free of preservatives, antiseptics, and detergents should be used for each injection and/or reconstitution of the vaccine because these substances may inactivate the live virus vaccine. A 25 gauge, 5/8″ needle is recommended.

To reconstitute, use only the diluent supplied, since it is free of preservatives or other antiviral substances which might inactivate the vaccine.

Single Dose Vial—First withdraw the entire volume of diluent into the syringe to be used for reconstitution. Inject all the diluent in the syringe into the vial of lyophilized vaccine, and agitate to mix thoroughly. Withdraw the entire contents into a syringe and inject the total volume of restored vaccine subcutaneously.

It is important to use a separate sterile syringe and needle for each individual patient to prevent transmission of hepatitis B and other infectious agents from one person to another.

10 Dose Vial (available only to government agencies/institutions)—Withdraw the entire contents (7 mL) of the diluent vial into the sterile syringe to be used for reconstitution, and introduce into the 10 dose vial of lyophilized vaccine. Agitate to ensure thorough mixing. The outer labeling suggests "For Jet Injector or Syringe Use". Use with separate sterile syringes is permitted for containers of 10 doses or less. The vaccine and diluent do not contain preservatives; therefore, the user must recognize the potential contamination hazards and exercise special precautions to protect the sterility and potency of the product. The use of aseptic techniques and proper storage prior to and after restoration of the vaccine and subsequent withdrawal of the individual doses is essential. Use 0.5 mL of the reconstituted vaccine for subcutaneous injection.

It is important to use a separate sterile syringe and needle for each individual patient to prevent transmission of hepatitis B and other infectious agents from one person to another.

50 Dose Vial (available only to government agencies/institutions)—Withdraw the entire contents (30 mL) of diluent vial into the sterile syringe to be used for reconstitution and introduce into the 50 dose vial of lyophilized vaccine. Agitate to ensure thorough mixing. With full aseptic precautions, attach the vial to the sterilized multidose jet injector apparatus. Use 0.5 mL of the reconstituted vaccine for subcutaneous injection.

Each dose contains not less than the equivalent of 1,000 $TCID_{50}$ of the U.S. Reference Measles Virus and 1,000 $TCID_{50}$ of the U.S. Reference Rubella Virus.

Parenteral drug products should be inspected visually for particulate matter and discoloration prior to administration. M-R-VAX II, when reconstituted, is clear yellow.

HOW SUPPLIED

No. 4751—M-R-VAX II is supplied as a single-dose vial of lyophilized vaccine, **NDC** 0006-4751-00, and a vial of diluent.

No. 4677/4309—M-R-VAX II is supplied as follows: (1) a box of 10 single-dose vials of lyophilized vaccine (package A), **NDC** 0006-4677-00; and (2) a box of 10 vials of diluent (package B). To conserve refrigerator space, the diluent may be stored separately at room temperature.

Available only to government agencies/institutions:

No. 4678—M-R-VAX II is supplied as one 10 dose vial of lyophilized vaccine, **NDC** 0006-4678-00, and one 7 mL vial of diluent.

No. 4679—M-R-VAX II is supplied as one 50 dose vial of lyophilized vaccine, **NDC** 0006-4679-00, and one 30 mL vial of diluent.

Storage

It is recommended that the vaccine be used as soon as possible after reconstitution. Protect vaccine from light at all times, since such exposure may inactivate the virus. Store reconstituted vaccine in the vaccine vial in a dark place at 2–8°C (35.6–46.4°F) and discard if not used within 8 hours.

A.H.F.S. Category: 80:12

DC 7032911 Issued January 1986

MEFOXIN® ℞

(Cefoxitin Sodium, MSD), U.S.P.

DESCRIPTION

MEFOXIN® (Sterile Cefoxitin Sodium, MSD) is a semi-synthetic, broad-spectrum cepha antibiotic for parenteral administration. It is derived from cephamycin C, which is produced by *Streptomyces lactamdurans*. It is the sodium salt of 3-(hydroxymethyl)-7α-methoxy-8-oxo-7-[2-(2-thienyl) acetamido]-5-thia-1-azabicyclo [4.2.0] oct-2-ene-2-carboxylate carbamate (ester). The empirical formula is $C_{16}H_{16}N_3NaO_7S_2$, and the structural formula is:

[See Chemical Formula at top of next column].

MEFOXIN contains approximately 53.8 mg (2.3 milliequivalents) of sodium per gram of cefoxitin activity. Solutions of MEFOXIN range from clear to light amber in color. The pH of freshly constituted solutions usually ranges from 4.2 to 7.0.

CLINICAL PHARMACOLOGY

Clinical Pharmacology

After intramuscular administration of a 1 gram dose of MEFOXIN to normal volunteers, the mean peak serum concentration was 24 mcg/mL. The peak occurred at 20 to 30 minutes. Following an intravenous dose of 1 gram, serum concentrations were 110 mcg/mL at 5 minutes, declining to less than 1 mcg/mL at 4 hours. The half-life after an intravenous dose is 41 to 59 minutes; after intramuscular administration, the half-life is 64.8 minutes. Approximately 85 percent of cefoxitin is excreted unchanged by the kidneys over a 6-hour period, resulting in high urinary concentrations. Following an intramuscular dose of 1 gram, urinary concentrations greater than 3000 mcg/mL were observed. Probenecid slows tubular excretion and produces higher serum levels and increases the duration of measurable serum concentrations.

Cefoxitin passes into pleural and joint fluids and is detectable in antibacterial concentrations in bile.

Clinical experience has demonstrated that MEFOXIN can be administered to patients who are also receiving carbenicillin, kanamycin, gentamicin, tobramycin, or amikacin (see PRECAUTIONS and ADMINISTRATION).

Microbiology

The bactericidal action of cefoxitin results from inhibition of cell wall synthesis. Cefoxitin has *in vitro* activity against a wide range of gram-positive and gram-negative organisms. The methoxy group in the 7α position provides MEFOXIN with a high degree of stability in the presence of beta-lactamases, both penicillinases and cephalosporinases, of gram-negative bacteria. Cefoxitin is usually active against the following organisms *in vitro* and in clinical infections:

Gram-positive

Staphylococcus aureus, including penicillinase and non-penicillinase producing strains.
Staphylococcus epidermidis
Beta-hemolytic and other streptococci (most strains of enterococci, e.g., *Streptococcus faecalis,* are resistant)
Streptococcus pneumoniae (formerly *Diplococcus pneumoniae*)

Gram-negative

Escherichia coli
Klebsiella species (including *K. pneumoniae*)
Hemophilus influenzae
Neisseria gonorrhoeae, including penicillinase and non-penicillinase producing strains
Proteus mirabilis
Morganella morganii (formerly *Proteus morganii*)
Proteus vulgaris
Providencia species, including *Providencia rettgeri* (formerly *Proteus rettgeri*)

Anaerobic organisms

Peptococcus species
Peptostreptococcus species
Clostridium species
Bacteroides species, including the *B. fragilis* group (includes *B. fragilis, B. distasonis, B. ovatus, B. thetaiotaomicron, B. vulgatus*)

MEFOXIN is inactive *in vitro* against most strains of *Pseudomonas aeruginosa* and enterococci and many strains of *Enterobacter cloacae.*

Methicillin-resistant staphylococci are almost uniformly resistant to MEFOXIN.

Susceptibility Tests

For fast-growing aerobic organisms, quantitative methods that require measurements of zone diameters give the most precise estimates of antibiotic susceptibility. One such procedure* has been recommended for use with discs to test susceptibility to cefoxitin. Interpretation involves correlation of the diameters obtained in the disc test with minimal inhibitory concentration (MIC) values for cefoxitin.

Reports from the laboratory giving results of the standardized single disc susceptibility test* using a 30 mcg cefoxitin disc should be interpreted according to the following criteria: Organisms producing zones of 18 mm or greater are considered susceptible, indicating that the tested organism is likely to respond to therapy.

Organisms of intermediate susceptibility produce zones of 15 to 17 mm, indicating that the tested organism would be susceptible if high dosage is used or if the infection is confined to tissues and fluids (e.g., urine) in which high antibiotic levels are attained.

Resistant organisms produce zones of 14 mm or less, indicating that other therapy should be selected.

The cefoxitin disc should be used for testing cefoxitin susceptibility.

Cefoxitin has been shown by *in vitro* tests to have activity against certain strains of *Enterobacteriaceae* found resistant when tested with the cephalosporin class disc. For this reason, the cefoxitin disc should not be used for testing susceptibility to cephalosporins, and cephalosporin discs should not be used for testing susceptibility to cefoxitin.

Dilution methods, preferably the agar plate dilution procedure, are most accurate for susceptibility testing of obligate anaerobes.

A bacterial isolate may be considered susceptible if the MIC value for cefoxitin† is not more than 16 mcg/mL. Organisms are considered resistant if the MIC is greater than 32 mcg/mL.

INDICATIONS AND USAGE

Treatment

MEFOXIN is indicated for the treatment of serious infections caused by susceptible strains of the designated microorganisms in the diseases listed below.

(1) Lower respiratory tract infections, including pneumonia and lung abscess, caused by *Streptococcus pneumoniae* (formerly *Diplococcus pneumoniae*), other streptococci (excluding enterococci, e.g., *Streptococcus faecalis*), *Staphylococcus aureus* (penicillinase and non-penicillinase producing), *Escherichia coli, Klebsiella* species, *Hemophilus influenzae,* and *Bacteroides* species.

(2) Genitourinary infections. Urinary tract infections caused by *Escherichia coli, Klebsiella* species, *Proteus mirabilis,* indole-positive Proteus (i.e., *Proteus morganii, rettgeri,* and *vulgaris*), and *Providencia* species. Uncomplicated gonorrhea due to *Neisseria gonorrhoeae* (penicillinase and non-penicillinase producing).

(3) Intra-abdominal infections, including peritonitis and intra-abdominal abscess, caused by *Escherichia coli, Klebsiella* species, *Bacteroides* species including the *Bacteroides fragilis* group**, and *Clostridium* species.

(4) Gynecological infections, including endometritis, pelvic cellulitis, and pelvic inflammatory disease caused by *Escherichia coli, Neisseria gonorrhoeae* (penicillinase and non-penicillinase producing), *Bacteroides* species including the *Bacteroides fragilis* group**, *Clostridium* species, *Peptococcus* species, *Peptostreptococcus* species, and Group B streptococci.

(5) Septicemia caused by *Streptococcus pneumoniae* (formerly *Diplococcus pneumoniae*), *Staphylococcus aureus* (penicillinase and non-penicillinase producing), *Escherichia coli, Klebsiella* species, and *Bacteroides* species including the *Bacteroides fragilis* group.**

(6) Bone and joint infections caused by *Staphylococcus aureus* (penicillinase and non-penicillinase producing).

(7) Skin and skin structure infections caused by *Staphylococcus aureus* (penicillinase and non-penicillinase producing), *Staphylococcus epidermidis,* streptococci (excluding enterococci, e.g., *Streptococcus faecalis*), *Escherichia coli, Proteus mirabilis, Klebsiella* species, *Bacteroides* species including the *Bacteroides fragilis* group**, *Clostridium* species, *Peptococcus* species, and *Peptostreptococcus* species.

Appropriate culture and susceptibility studies should be performed to determine the susceptibility of the causative organisms to MEFOXIN. Therapy may be started while awaiting the results of these studies.

In randomized comparative studies, MEFOXIN and cephalothin were comparably safe and effective in the management of infections caused by gram-positive cocci and gram-negative rods susceptible to the cephalosporins. MEFOXIN has a

* Bauer, A. W.; Kirby, W. M. M.; Sherris, J. C.; Turck, M.: Antibiotic susceptibility testing by a standardized single disc method, Amer. J. Clin. Path. 45: 493–496, Apr. 1966. Standardized disc susceptibility test, Federal Register 37: 20527–20529, 1972. National Committee for Clinical Laboratory Standards: Approved Standard: ASM-2, Performance Standards for Antimicrobial Disc Susceptibility Tests, July 1975.

† Determined by the ICS agar dilution method (Ericsson and Sherris, Acta Path. Microbiol. Scand. (B) Suppl. No. 217, 1971) or any other method that has been shown to give equivalent results.

** *B. fragilis, B. distasonis, B. ovatus, B. thetaiotaomicron, B. vulgatus.*

Continued on next page

Information on the Merck Sharp & Dohme products listed on these pages is the full prescribing information from product circulars in use August 31, 1986.

Merck Sharp & Dohme—Cont.

high degree of stability in the presence of bacterial beta-lactamases, both penicillinases and cephalosporinases.
Many infections caused by aerobic and anaerobic gram-negative bacteria resistant to some cephalosporins respond to MEFOXIN. Similarly, many infections caused by aerobic and anaerobic bacteria resistant to some penicillin antibiotics (ampicillin, carbenicillin, penicillin G) respond to treatment with MEFOXIN. Many infections caused by mixtures of susceptible aerobic and anaerobic bacteria respond to treatment with MEFOXIN.

Prevention

When compared to placebo in randomized controlled studies in patients undergoing gastrointestinal surgery, vaginal hysterectomy, abdominal hysterectomy and cesarean section, the prophylactic use of MEFOXIN resulted in a significant reduction in the number of postoperative infections.
The prophylactic administration of MEFOXIN perioperatively (preoperatively, intraoperatively, and postoperatively) may reduce the incidence of certain postoperative infections in patients undergoing surgical procedures (e.g., hysterectomy, gastrointestinal surgery and transurethral prostatectomy) that are classified as contaminated or potentially contaminated.
The perioperative use of MEFOXIN may be effective in surgical patients in whom infection at the operative site would present a serious risk, e.g., prosthetic arthroplasty.
In patients undergoing cesarean section, intraoperative (after clamping the umbilical cord) and postoperative use of MEFOXIN may reduce the incidence of certain postoperative infections.
Effective prophylactic use depends on the time of administration. MEFOXIN usually should be given one-half to one hour before the operation, which is sufficient time to achieve effective levels in the wound during the procedure. Prophylactic administration should usually be stopped within 24 hours since continuing administration of any antibiotic increases the possibility of adverse reactions but, in the majority of surgical procedures, does not reduce the incidence of subsequent infection. However, in patients undergoing prosthetic arthroplasty, it is recommended that MEFOXIN be continued for 72 hours after the surgical procedure.
If there are signs of infection, specimens for culture should be obtained for identification of the causative organism so that appropriate therapy may be instituted.

CONTRAINDICATIONS

MEFOXIN is contraindicated in patients who have shown hypersensitivity to cefoxitin and the cephalosporin group of antibiotics.

WARNINGS

BEFORE THERAPY WITH MEFOXIN IS INSTITUTED, CAREFUL INQUIRY SHOULD BE MADE TO DETERMINE WHETHER THE PATIENT HAS HAD PREVIOUS HYPERSENSITIVITY REACTIONS TO CEFOXITIN, CEPHALOSPORINS, PENICILLINS, OR OTHER DRUGS. THIS PRODUCT SHOULD BE GIVEN WITH CAUTION TO PENICILLIN-SENSITIVE PATIENTS. ANTIBIOTICS SHOULD BE ADMINISTERED WITH CAUTION TO ANY PATIENT WHO HAS DEMONSTRATED SOME FORM OF ALLERGY, PARTICULARLY TO DRUGS. IF AN ALLERGIC REACTION TO MEFOXIN OCCURS, DISCONTINUE THE DRUG. SERIOUS HYPERSENSITIVITY REACTIONS MAY REQUIRE EPINEPHRINE AND OTHER EMERGENCY MEASURES.

Pseudomembranous colitis has been reported with virtually all antibiotics (including cephalosporins); therefore, it is important to consider its diagnosis in patients who develop diarrhea in association with antibiotic use. This colitis may range from mild to life threatening in severity.

Table 1—Guidelines for Dosage of MEFOXIN

Type of Infection	Daily Dosage	Frequency and Route
Uncomplicated forms* of infections such as pneumonia, urinary tract infection, cutaneous infection	3–4 grams	1 gram every 6–8 hours IV or IM
Moderately severe or severe infections	6–8 grams	1 gram every 4 hours *or* 2 grams every 6–8 hours IV
Infections commonly needing antibiotics in higher dosage (e.g., gas gangrene)	12 grams	2 grams every 4 hours *or* 3 grams every 6 hours IV

*Including patients in whom bacteremia is absent or unlikely

Table 2—Maintenance Dosage of MEFOXIN in Adults with Reduced Renal Function

Renal Function	Creatinine Clearance (mL/min)	Dose (grams)	Frequency
Mild impairment	50–30	1–2	every 8–12 hours
Moderate impairment	29–10	1–2	every 12–24 hours
Severe impairment	9–5	0.5–1	every 12–24 hours
Essentially no function	<5	0.5–1	every 24–48 hours

Treatment with broad-spectrum antibiotics alters normal flora of the colon and may permit overgrowth of clostridia. Studies indicate a toxin produced by *Clostridium difficile* is one primary cause of antibiotic-associated colitis.
Mild cases of pseudomembranous colitis may respond to drug discontinuance alone. In more severe cases, management may include sigmoidoscopy, appropriate bacteriological studies, fluid, electrolyte and protein supplementation, and the use of a drug such as oral vancomycin as indicated. Isolation of the patient may be advisable. Other causes of colitis should also be considered.

PRECAUTIONS

General

The total daily dose should be reduced when MEFOXIN is administered to patients with transient or persistent reduction of urinary output due to renal insufficiency (see DOSAGE), because high and prolonged serum antibiotic concentrations can occur in such individuals from usual doses.
Antibiotics (including cephalosporins) should be prescribed with caution in individuals with a history of gastrointestinal disease, particularly colitis.
As with other antibiotics, prolonged use of MEFOXIN may result in overgrowth of nonsusceptible organisms. Repeated evaluation of the patient's condition is essential. If superinfection occurs during therapy, appropriate measures should be taken.

Drug Interactions

Increased nephrotoxicity has been reported following concomitant administration of cephalosporins and aminoglycoside antibiotics.

Drug/Laboratory Test Interactions

As with cephalothin, high concentrations of cefoxitin (>100 micrograms/mL) may interfere with measurement of serum and urine creatinine levels by the Jaffé reaction, and produce false increases of modest degree in the levels of creatinine reported. Serum samples from patients treated with cefoxitin should not be analyzed for creatinine if withdrawn within 2 hours of drug administration.
High concentrations of cefoxitin in the urine may interfere with measurement of urinary 17-hydroxy-corticosteroids by the Porter-Silber reaction, and produce false increases of modest degree in the levels reported.
A false-positive reaction for glucose in the urine may occur. This has been observed with CLINITEST* reagent tablets.

Carcinogenesis, Mutagenesis, Impairment of Fertility

Long-term studies in animals have not been performed with cefoxitin to evaluate carcinogenic or mutagenic potential. Studies in rats treated intravenously with 400 mg/kg of cefoxitin (approximately three times the maximum recommended human dose) revealed no effects on fertility or mating ability.

Pregnancy

Pregnancy Category B. Reproduction studies performed in rats and mice at parenteral doses of approximately one to seven and one-half times the maximum recommended human dose did not reveal teratogenic or fetal toxic effects, although a slight decrease in fetal weight was observed.
There are, however, no adequate and well-controlled studies in pregnant women. Because animal reproduction studies are not always predictive of human response, this drug should be used during pregnancy only if clearly needed.
In the rabbit, cefoxitin was associated with a high incidence of abortion and maternal death. This was not considered to be a teratogenic effect but an expected consequence of the rabbit's unusual sensitivity to antibiotic-induced changes in the population of the microflora of the intestine.

Nursing Mothers

MEFOXIN is excreted in human milk in low concentrations. Caution should be exercised when MEFOXIN is administered to a nursing woman.

Pediatric Use

Safety and efficacy in infants from birth to three months of age have not yet been established. In children three months of age and older, higher doses of MEFOXIN have been associated with an increased incidence of eosinophilia and elevated SGOT.

* Registered trademark of Ames Company, Division of Miles Laboratories, Inc.

ADVERSE REACTIONS

MEFOXIN is generally well tolerated. The most common adverse reactions have been local reactions following intravenous or intramuscular injection. Other adverse reactions have been encountered infrequently.

Local Reactions

Thrombophlebitis has occurred with intravenous administration. Pain, induration, and tenderness after intramuscular injections have been reported.

Allergic Reactions

Rash (including exfoliative dermatitis), pruritus, eosinophilia, fever, and other allergic reactions including anaphylaxis have been noted.

Cardiovascular

Hypotension

Gastrointestinal

Diarrhea, including documented pseudomembranous colitis which can appear during or after antibiotic treatment. Nausea and vomiting have been reported rarely.

Blood

Eosinophilia, leukopenia, including granulocytopenia, neutropenia, anemia, including hemolytic anemia, thrombocytopenia, and bone marrow depression. A positive direct Coombs test may develop in some individuals, especially those with azotemia.

Liver Function

Transient elevations in SGOT, SGPT, serum LDH, and serum alkaline phosphatase have been reported.

Renal Function

Elevations in serum creatinine and/or blood urea nitrogen levels have been observed. As with the cephalosporins, acute renal failure has been reported rarely. The role of MEFOXIN in changes in renal function tests is difficult to assess, since factors predisposing to prerenal azotemia or to impaired renal function usually have been present.

OVERDOSAGE

The acute intravenous LD_{50} in the adult female mouse and rabbit was about 8.0 g/kg and greater than 1.0 g/kg respectively. The acute intraperitoneal LD_{50} in the adult rat was greater than 10.0 g/kg.

DOSAGE

TREATMENT

Adults

The usual adult dosage range is 1 gram to 2 grams every six to eight hours. Dosage and route of administration should be determined by susceptibility of the causative organisms, severity of infection, and the condition of the patient (see Table 1 for dosage guidelines).
[See table left].
MEFOXIN may be used in patients with reduced renal function with the following dosage adjustments:
In adults with renal insufficiency, an initial loading dose of 1 gram to 2 grams may be given. After a loading dose, the recommendations for *maintenance dosage* (Table 2) may be used as a guide.
[See table above].
When only the serum creatinine level is available, the following formula (based on sex, weight, and age of the patient) may be used to convert this value into creatinine clearance. The serum creatinine should represent a steady state of renal function.

Males: $\frac{\text{Weight (kg)} \times (140 - \text{age})}{72 \times \text{serum creatinine (mg/100 mL)}}$

Females: 0.85 × above value

In patients undergoing hemodialysis, the loading dose of 1 to 2 grams should be given after each hemodialysis, and the maintenance dose should be given as indicated in Table 2.

Antibiotic therapy for group A beta-hemolytic streptococcal infections should be maintained for at least 10 days to guard against the risk of rheumatic fever or glomerulonephritis. In staphylococcal and other infections involving a collection of pus, surgical drainage should be carried out where indicated.

The recommended dosage of MEFOXIN **for uncomplicated gonorrhea** is 2 grams intramuscularly, with 1 gram of BENEMID® (Probenecid, MSD) given by mouth at the same time or up to ½ hour before MEFOXIN.

Infants and Children

The recommended dosage in children three months of age and older is 80 to 160 mg/kg of body weight per day divided into four to six equal doses. The higher dosages should be used for more severe or serious infections. The total daily dosage should not exceed 12 grams.

At this time no recommendation is made for children from birth to three months of age (See PRECAUTIONS).

In children with renal insufficiency the dosage and frequency of dosage should be modified consistent with the recommendations for adults (see Table 2).

PREVENTION

For prophylactic use, the following doses are recommended:

Adults:

1) 2 grams administered intravenously or intramuscularly just prior to surgery (approximately one-half to one hour before the initial incision).
2) 2 grams every 6 hours after the first dose for no more than 24 hours (continued for 72 hours after prosthetic arthroplasty).

Children (3 months and older):

30 to 40 mg/kg doses may be given at the times designated above.

Cesarean section patients:

The first dose of 2.0 grams is administered intravenously as soon as the umbilical cord is clamped. The second and third doses should be given as 2.0 grams intravenously or intramuscularly 4 hours and 8 hours after the first dose. Subsequent doses may be given every 6 hours for no more than 24 hours.

Transurethral prostatectomy patients:

One gram administered just prior to surgery; 1 gram every 8 hours for up to five days.

PREPARATION OF SOLUTION

Table 3 is provided for convenience in constituting MEFOXIN for both intravenous and intramuscular administration.

[See table above].

For intravenous use, 1 gram should be constituted with at least 10 mL of Sterile Water for Injection, and 2 grams, with 10 or 20 mL. The 10 gram bulk package should be constituted with 50 or 100 mL of Sterile Water for Injection or any of the solutions listed under the *Intravenous* portion of the COMPATIBILITY AND STABILITY section. CAUTION: NOT FOR DIRECT INFUSION. One or 2 grams of MEFOXIN for infusion may be constituted with 50 or 100 mL of 0.9 percent Sodium Chloride Injection, 5 percent or 10 percent Dextrose Injection, or any of the solutions listed under the *Intravenous* portion of the COMPATIBILITY AND STABILITY section.

Benzyl alcohol as a preservative has been associated with toxicity in neonates. While toxicity has not been demonstrated in infants greater than three months of age, in whom use of MEFOXIN may be indicated, small infants in this age range may also be at risk for benzyl alcohol toxicity. Therefore, diluent containing benzyl alcohol should not be used when MEFOXIN is constituted for administration to infants.

For intramuscular use, each gram of MEFOXIN may be constituted with 2 mL of Sterile Water for Injection, *or*—

For intramuscular use ONLY: each gram of MEFOXIN may be constituted with 2 mL of 0.5 percent lidocaine hydrochloride solution* (without epinephrine) to minimize the discomfort of intramuscular injection.

ADMINISTRATION

MEFOXIN may be administered intravenously or intramuscularly after constitution.

Parenteral drug products should be inspected visually for particulate matter and discoloration prior to administration whenever solution and container permit.

* See package circular of manufacturer for detailed information concerning contraindications, warnings, precautions, and adverse reactions.

Table 3—Preparation of Solution

MEFOXIN

Strength	Amount of Diluent to be Added (mL)*	Approximate Withdrawable Volume (mL)	Approximate Average Concentration (mg/mL)
1 gram Vial	2 (Intramuscular)	2.5	400
2 gram Vial	4 (Intramuscular)	5	400
1 gram Vial	10 (IV)	10.5	95
2 gram Vial	10 or 20 (IV)	11.1 or 21.0	180 or 95
1 gram Infusion Bottle	50 or 100 (IV)	50 or 100	20 or 10
2 gram Infusion Bottle	50 or 100 (IV)	50 or 100	40 or 20
10 gram Bulk	50 or 100 (IV)	55 or 105	180 or 95

*Shake to dissolve and let stand until clear.

Intravenous Administration

The intravenous route is preferable for patients with bacteremia, bacterial septicemia, or other severe or life-threatening infections, or for patients who may be poor risks because of lowered resistance resulting from such debilitating conditions as malnutrition, trauma, surgery, diabetes, heart failure, or malignancy, particularly if shock is present or impending.

For intermittent intravenous administration, a solution containing 1 gram or 2 grams in 10 mL of Sterile Water for Injection can be injected over a period of three to five minutes. Using an infusion system, it may also be given over a longer period of time through the tubing system by which the patient may be receiving other intravenous solutions. However, during infusion of the solution containing MEFOXIN, it is advisable to temporarily discontinue administration of any other solutions at the same site.

For the administration of higher doses by continuous intravenous infusion, a solution of MEFOXIN may be added to an intravenous bottle containing 5 percent Dextrose Injection, 0.9 percent Sodium Chloride Injection, 5 percent Dextrose and 0.9 percent Sodium Chloride Injection, or 5 percent Dextrose Injection with 0.02 percent sodium bicarbonate solution. BUTTERFLY** or scalp vein-type needles are preferred for this type of infusion.

Solutions of MEFOXIN, like those of most beta-lactam antibiotics, should not be added to aminoglycoside solutions (e.g., gentamicin sulfate, tobramycin sulfate, amikacin sulfate) because of potential interaction. However, MEFOXIN and aminoglycosides may be administered separately to the same patient.

** Registered trademark of Abbott Laboratories.

Intramuscular Administration

As with all intramuscular preparations, MEFOXIN should be injected well within the body of a relatively large muscle such as the upper outer quadrant of the buttock (i.e., gluteus maximus); aspiration is necessary to avoid inadvertent injection into a blood vessel.

COMPATIBILITY AND STABILITY

Intravenous

MEFOXIN, as supplied in vials or the bulk package and constituted to 1 gram/10 mL with Sterile Water for Injection, Bacteriostatic Water for Injection (see PREPARATION OF SOLUTION), 0.9 percent Sodium Chloride Injection, or 5 percent Dextrose Injection, maintains satisfactory potency for 24 hours at room temperature, for one week under refrigeration (below 5°C), and for at least 30 weeks in the frozen state.

These primary solutions may be further diluted in 50 to 1000 mL of the following solutions and maintain potency for 24 hours at room temperature and at least 48 hours under refrigeration:

Sterile Water for Injection‡
0.9 percent Sodium Chloride Injection
5 percent or 10 percent Dextrose Injection‡
5 percent Dextrose and 0.9 percent Sodium Chloride Injection
5 percent Dextrose Injection with 0.02 percent sodium bicarbonate solution
5 percent Dextrose Injection with 0.2 percent or 0.45 percent saline solution
Ringer's Injection
Lactated Ringer's Injection‡
5 percent dextrose in Lactated Ringer's Injection‡
5 percent or 10 percent invert sugar in water
10 percent invert sugar in saline solution
5 percent Sodium Bicarbonate Injection
Neut (sodium bicarbonate)*‡
M/6 sodium lactate solution
AMINOSOL* 5 percent Solution
NORMOSOL-M in D5-W*‡
IONOSOL B w/Dextrose 5 percent*‡
POLYONIC M 56 in 5 percent Dextrose**
Mannitol 5% and 2.5%
Mannitol 10%‡
ISOLYTE*** E
ISOLYTE*** E with 5% dextrose

* Registered trademark of Abbott Laboratories.
** Registered trademark of Cutter Laboratories, Inc.
*** Registered trademark of American Hospital Supply Corporation.
‡ In these solutions, MEFOXIN has been found to be stable for a period of one week under refrigeration.
† Travenol Laboratories, Inc.

MEFOXIN, as supplied in infusion bottles and constituted with 50 to 100 mL of 0.9 percent Sodium Chloride Injection, or 5 percent or 10 percent Dextrose Injection, maintains satisfactory potency for 24 hours at room temperature or for 1 week under refrigeration (below 5°C).

Limited studies with solutions of MEFOXIN in 0.9 percent Sodium Chloride Injection, Lactated Ringer's Injection, and 5 percent Dextrose Injection in VIAFLEX† intravenous bags show stability for 24 hours at room temperature, 48 hours under refrigeration, 26 weeks in the frozen state, and 24 hours at room temperature thereafter. Also, solutions of MEFOXIN in 0.9 percent Sodium Chloride Injection show similar stability in plastic tubing, drip chambers, and volume control devices of common intravenous infusion sets.

After constitution with Sterile Water for Injection and subsequent storage in disposable plastic syringes, MEFOXIN is stable for 24 hours at room temperature and 48 hours under refrigeration.

After the periods mentioned above, any unused solutions or frozen material should be discarded. Do not refreeze.

Intramuscular

MEFOXIN, as constituted with Sterile Water for Injection, Bacteriostatic Water for Injection, or 0.5 percent or 1 percent lidocaine hydrochloride solution (without epinephrine), maintains satisfactory potency for 24 hours at room temperature, for one week under refrigeration (below 5°C), and for at least 30 weeks in the frozen state.

After the periods mentioned above, any unused solutions or frozen material should be discarded. Do not refreeze.

MEFOXIN has also been found compatible when admixed in intravenous infusions with the following:

Heparin 0.1 units/mL at room temperature—8 hours
Heparin 100 units/mL at room temperature—24 hours
M.V.I.†† concentrate at room temperature 24 hours; under refrigeration 48 hours
BEROCCA††† C-500 at room temperature 24 hours; under refrigeration 48 hours
Insulin in Normal Saline at room temperature 24 hours; under refrigeration 48 hours
Insulin in 10% invert sugar at room temperature 24 hours; under refrigeration 48 hours

HOW SUPPLIED

Sterile MEFOXIN is a dry white to off-white powder supplied in vials and infusion bottles containing cefoxitin sodium as follows:

No. 3356—1 gram cefoxitin equivalent
NDC 0006-3356-71 in trays of 10 vials.
NDC 0006-3356-45 in trays of 25 vials.
No. 3368—1 gram cefoxitin equivalent
NDC 0006-3368-71 in trays of 10 infusion bottles.
No. 3357—2 gram cefoxitin equivalent
NDC 0006-3357-73 in trays of 10 vials.
NDC 0006-3357-53 in trays of 25 vials.
No. 3369—2 gram cefoxitin equivalent
NDC 0006-3369-73 in trays of 10 infusion bottles.
No. 3388—10 gram cefoxitin equivalent

†† Registered trademark of USV Pharmaceutical Corp.
††† Registered trademark of Roche Laboratories.

Continued on next page

Information on the Merck Sharp & Dohme products listed on these pages is the full prescribing information from product circulars in use August 31, 1986.

Merck Sharp & Dohme—Cont.

NDC 0006-3388-10 in bulk bottles.
Special storage instructions
MEFOXIN in the dry state should be stored below 30°C. Avoid exposure to temperatures above 50°C. The dry material as well as solutions tend to darken, depending on storage conditions; product potency, however, is not adversely affected.

A.H.F.S. Category: 8:12.28
DC 7057120 Issued July 1985

MEPHYTON® Tablets ℞
(Phytonadione, MSD), U.S.P.
Vitamin K_1

DESCRIPTION

MEPHYTON® (Phytonadione, MSD) tablets containing 5 mg of phytonadione are yellow, compressed tablets, scored on one side. Inactive ingredients are acacia, calcium phosphate, colloidal silicon dioxide, lactose, magnesium stearate, starch, and talc.

ACTIONS

MEPHYTON tablets possess the same type and degree of activity as does naturally-occurring vitamin K, which is necessary for the production via the liver of active prothrombin (factor II), proconvertin (factor VII), plasma thromboplastin component (factor IX), and Stuart factor (factor X). The prothrombin test is sensitive to the levels of three of these four factors—II, VII, and X. The mechanism by which vitamin K promotes formation of these clotting factors in the liver is not known.
The tablets generally exert their effect within 6 to 10 hours.

INDICATIONS

MEPHYTON is indicated in the following coagulation disorders which are due to faulty formation of factors II, VII, IX and X when caused by vitamin K deficiency or interference with vitamin K activity.
Mephyton tablets are indicated in:
—anticoagulant-induced prothrombin deficiency;
—hypoprothrombinemia secondary to antibacterial therapy;
—hypoprothrombinemia secondary to administration of salicylates;
—hypoprothrombinemia secondary to obstructive jaundice or biliary fistulas but only if bile salts are administered concurrently, since otherwise the oral vitamin K will not be absorbed.

CONTRAINDICATION

Hypersensitivity to any component of this medication.

WARNINGS

An immediate coagulant effect should not be expected after administration of phytonadione.
Phytonadione will not counteract the anticoagulant action of heparin.
When vitamin K_1 is used to correct excessive anticoagulant-induced hypoprothrombinemia, anticoagulant therapy still being indicated, the patient is again faced with the clotting hazards existing prior to starting the anticoagulant therapy. Phytonadione is not a clotting agent, but overzealous therapy with vitamin K_1 may restore conditions which originally permitted thromboembolic phenomena. Dosage should be kept as low as possible, and prothrombin time should be checked regularly as clinical conditions indicate.
Repeated large doses of vitamin K are not warranted in liver disease if the response to initial use of the vitamin is unsatisfactory. Failure to respond to vitamin K may indicate a congenital coagulation defect or that the condition being treated is unresponsive to vitamin K.
Reproduction studies have not been performed in animals. There is no adequate information of whether this drug may affect fertility in human males or females or have a teratogenic potential or other adverse effect on the fetus.

PRECAUTIONS

Protect from light at all times.
Temporary resistance to prothrombin-depressing anticoagulants may result, especially when larger doses of phytonadione are used. If relatively large doses have been employed, it may be necessary when reinstituting anticoagulant therapy to use somewhat larger doses of the prothrombin-depressing anticoagulant, or to use one which acts on a different principle, such as heparin sodium.

ADVERSE REACTIONS

Transient "flushing sensations" and "peculiar" sensations of taste have been observed with parenteral phytonadione, as well as rare instances of dizziness, rapid and weak pulse, profuse sweating, brief hypotension, dyspnea, and cyanosis. Hyperbilirubinemia has been observed in the newborn following administration of parenteral phytonadione. This has occurred rarely and primarily with doses above those recommended.

DOSAGE AND ADMINISTRATION

The human minimum daily requirements for vitamin K have not been established officially but they have been estimated to be 1 to 5 mcg/kg of body weight for infants and 0.03 mcg/kg for adults. Usually, the dietary abundance of vitamin K will satisfy these requirements, except during the first five to eight days of the neonatal period.
Anticoagulant-Induced Prothrombin Deficiency
To correct excessively prolonged prothrombin times caused by oral anticoagulant therapy—2.5 to 10 mg or up to 25 mg initially is recommended. In rare instances 50 mg may be required. Frequency and amount of subsequent doses should be determined by prothrombin time response or clinical condition. If, in 12 to 48 hours after oral administration, the prothrombin time has not been shortened satisfactorily, the dose should be repeated.
Hypoprothrombinemia Due to Other Causes
If possible, discontinuation or reduction of the dosage of drugs interfering with coagulation mechanisms (such as salicylates, antibiotics) is suggested as an alternative to administering concurrent MEPHYTON. The severity of the coagulation disorder should determine whether the immediate administration of MEPHYTON is required in addition to discontinuation or reduction of interfering drugs.
A dosage of 2.5 to 25 mg or more (rarely up to 50 mg) is recommended, the amount and route of administration depending upon the severity of the condition and response obtained.
The oral route should be avoided when the clinical disorder would prevent proper absorption. Bile salts must be given with the tablets when the endogenous supply of bile to the gastrointestinal tract is deficient.

HOW SUPPLIED

No. 7776—Tablets MEPHYTON, 5 mg vitamin K_1, are yellow, round, scored, compressed tablets, coded MSD 43. They are supplied as follows:
NDC 0006-0043-68 bottles of 100.

A.H.F.S. Category: 88:24
DC 6597709 Issued July 1985

MERUVAX®$_{II}$ ℞
(Rubella Virus Vaccine Live, MSD), U.S.P.
(Wistar RA 27/3 Strain)

DESCRIPTION

MERUVAX® II (Rubella Virus Vaccine Live, MSD) is a live virus vaccine for immunization against rubella (German measles).
MERUVAX II is a sterile lyophilized preparation of the Wistar Institute RA 27/3 strain of live attenuated rubella virus. The virus was adapted to and propagated in human diploid cell (WI-38) culture.
The reconstituted vaccine is for subcutaneous administration. When reconstituted as directed, the dose for injection is 0.5 mL and contains not less than the equivalent of 1,000 $TCID_{50}$ (tissue culture infectious doses) of the U.S. Reference Rubella Virus. Each dose also contains approximately 25 mcg of neomycin. The product contains no preservative. Sorbitol and hydrolized gelatin are added as stabilizers.

CLINICAL PHARMACOLOGY

MERUVAX II produces a modified, non-communicable rubella infection in susceptible persons.
Extensive clinical trials of rubella virus vaccines, prepared using RA 27/3 strain rubella virus, have been carried out in more than 28,000 human subjects (approximately 11,000 with MERUVAX II) in the U.S.A. and more than 20 additional countries. A single injection of the vaccine has been shown to induce rubella hemagglutination-inhibiting (HI) antibodies in 97% or more of susceptible persons. The RA 27/3 rubella strain elicits higher immediate post-vaccination HI, complement-fixing and neutralizing antibody levels than other strains of rubella vaccine and has been shown to induce a broader profile of circulating antibodies including anti-theta and anti-iota precipitating antibodies. The RA 27/3 rubella strain immunologically simulates natural infection more closely than other rubella vaccine viruses. The increased levels and broader profile of antibodies produced by RA 27/3 strain rubella virus vaccine appear to correlate with greater resistance to subclinical reinfection with the wild virus, and provide greater confidence for lasting immunity.
Vaccine-induced antibody levels have been shown to persist for at least 10 years without substantial decline. If the present pattern continues, it will provide a basis for the expectation that immunity following vaccination will be permanent. However, continued surveillance will be required to demonstrate this point.

INDICATIONS AND USAGE†

1. *Children Between 12 Months of Age and Puberty*
MERUVAX II is indicated for immunization against rubella (German measles) in persons from 12 months of age to puberty. A booster is not needed. It is not recommended for infants younger than 12 months because they may retain maternal rubella neutralizing antibodies that may interfere with the immune response. Children in kindergarten and the first grades of elementary school deserve priority for vaccination because often they are epidemiologically the major source of virus dissemination in the community. A history of rubella illness is usually not reliable enough to exclude children from immunization.
Previously unimmunized children of susceptible pregnant women should receive live attenuated rubella vaccine, because an immunized child will be less likely to acquire natural rubella and introduce the virus into the household.
2. *Adolescent and Adult Males*
Vaccination of adolescent or adult males may be a useful procedure in preventing or controlling outbreaks of rubella in circumscribed population groups (e.g., military bases and schools).
3. *Non-Pregnant Adolescent and Adult Females*
Immunization of susceptible non-pregnant adolescent and adult females of childbearing age with live attenuated rubella virus vaccine is indicated if certain precautions are observed (see below and PRECAUTIONS). Vaccinating susceptible postpubertal females confers individual protection against subsequently acquiring rubella infection during pregnancy, which in turn prevents infection of the fetus and consequent congenital rubella injury.
Women of childbearing age should be advised not to become pregnant for three months after vaccination and should be informed of the reason for this precaution.*
It is recommended that rubella susceptibility be determined by serologic testing prior to immunization.** If immune, as evidenced by a specific rubella antibody titer of 1:8 or greater (hemagglutination-inhibition test), vaccination is unnecessary. Congenital malformations do occur in up to seven percent of all live births. Their chance appearance after vaccination could lead to misinterpretation of the cause, particularly if the prior rubella-immune status of vaccinees is unknown.
Postpubertal females should be informed of the frequent occurrence of self-limited arthralgia and possible arthritis beginning 2 to 4 weeks after vaccination (see ADVERSE REACTIONS).
4. *Postpartum Women*
It has been found convenient in many instances to vaccinate rubella-susceptible women in the immediate postpartum period (see *Nursing Mothers*).
Revaccination:
Children vaccinated when younger than 12 months of age should be revaccinated. Based on available evidence, there is no reason to routinely revaccinate persons who were vaccinated originally when 12 months of age or older. However,

† Based in part on the recommendation for rubella vaccine use of the Immunization Practices Advisory Committee (ACIP), Morbidity and Mortality Weekly Report: 33 (22): 301–310, 315–318, June 8, 1984.

*NOTE: The Immunization Practices Advisory Committee (ACIP) has recommended "In view of the importance of protecting this age group against rubella, reasonable precautions in a rubella immunization program include asking females if they are pregnant, excluding those who say they are, and explaining the theoretical risks to the others."

**NOTE: The Immunization Practices Advisory Committee (ACIP) has stated "When practical, and when reliable laboratory services are available, potential vaccinees of childbearing age can have serologic tests to determine susceptibility to rubella. . . . However, routinely performing serologic tests for all females of childbearing age to determine susceptibility so that vaccine is given only to proven susceptibles is expensive and has been ineffective in some areas. Accordingly, the ACIP believes that rubella vaccination of a woman who is not known to be pregnant and has no history of vaccination is justifiable without serologic testing."

persons should be revaccinated if there is evidence to suggest that initial immunization was ineffective.

Use with Other Vaccines

Routine administration of DTP (diphtheria, tetanus, pertussis) and/or OPV (oral poliovirus vaccine) concomitantly with measles, mumps and rubella vaccines is not recommended because there are insufficient data relating to the simultaneous administration of these antigens. However, the American Academy of Pediatrics has noted that in some circumstances, particularly when the patient may not return, some practitioners prefer to administer all these antigens on a single day. If done, separate sites and syringes should be used for DTP and MERUVAX II.

MERUVAX II should not be given less than one month before or after administration of other virus vaccines.

CONTRAINDICATIONS

Do not give MERUVAX II to pregnant females; the possible effects of the vaccine on fetal development are unknown at this time. If vaccination of postpubertal females is undertaken, pregnancy should be avoided for three months following vaccination. (See PRECAUTIONS, *Pregnancy*).

Anaphylactoid reaction to neomycin (each dose of reconstituted vaccine contains approximately 25 mcg of neomycin).

Any febrile respiratory illness or other active febrile infection.

Active untreated tuberculosis.

Patients receiving immunosuppressive therapy. This contraindication does not apply to patients who are receiving corticosteroids as replacement therapy, e.g., for Addison's disease.

Individuals with blood dyscrasias, leukemia, lymphomas of any type, or other malignant neoplasms affecting the bone marrow or lymphatic systems.

Primary immunodeficiency states, including cellular immune deficiencies, hypogammaglobulinemic and dysgammaglobulinemic states.

Individuals with a family history of congenital or hereditary immunodeficiency, until the immune competence of the potential vaccine recipient is demonstrated.

PRECAUTIONS

General

Adequate treatment provisions including epinephrine, should be available for immediate use should an anaphylactoid reaction occur.

Excretion of small amounts of the live attenuated rubella virus from the nose or throat has occurred in the majority of susceptible individuals 7–28 days after vaccination. There is no confirmed evidence to indicate that such virus is transmitted to susceptible persons who are in contact with the vaccinated individuals. Consequently, transmission through close personal contact, while accepted as a theoretical possibility, is not regarded as a significant risk. However, transmission of the vaccine virus to infants via breast milk has been documented (see *Nursing Mothers*).

There is no evidence that live rubella virus vaccine given after exposure to natural rubella virus will prevent illness. There is, however, no contraindication to vaccinating children already exposed to natural rubella.

Vaccination should be deferred for at least three months following blood or plasma transfusions, or administration of human immune serum globulin. However, susceptible postpartum patients who received blood products may receive MERUVAX II prior to discharge provided that a repeat HI titer is drawn 6–8 weeks after vaccination to insure seroconversion. Similarly, although studies with other live rubella virus vaccines suggest that MERUVAX II may be given in the immediate postpartum period to those non-immune women who have received anti-Rho (D) globulin (human) without interfering with vaccine effectiveness, a follow-up post-vaccination HI titer should also be determined.

It has been reported that attenuated rubella virus vaccine, live, may result in a temporary depression of tuberculin skin sensitivity. Therefore, if a tuberculin test is to be done, it should be administered either before or simultaneously with MERUVAX II.

As for any vaccine, vaccination with MERUVAX II may not result in seroconversion in 100% of susceptible persons given the vaccine.

Pregnancy

Pregnancy Category C

Animal reproduction studies have not been conducted with MERUVAX II. It is also not known whether MERUVAX II can cause fetal harm when administered to a pregnant woman or can affect reproduction capacity. There is evidence suggesting transmission of rubella vaccine viruses to products of conception. Therefore, rubella vaccine should not be administered to pregnant females (see CONTRAINDICATIONS).

In counseling women who are inadvertently vaccinated when pregnant or who become pregnant within 3 months of vaccination, the physician should be aware of the following: In a 10 year survey involving over 700 pregnant women who received rubella vaccine within 3 months before or after conception, (of whom 189 received the Wistar RA 27/3 strain) none of the newborns had abnormalities compatible with congenital rubella syndrome.

Nursing Mothers

Recent studies have shown that lactating postpartum women immunized with live attenuated rubella vaccine may secrete the virus in breast milk and transmit it to breast-fed infants. In the infants with serological evidence of rubella infection, none exhibited severe disease; however, one exhibited mild clinical illness typical of acquired rubella. Caution should be exercised when MERUVAX II is administered to a nursing woman.

ADVERSE REACTIONS

Because of the slightly acidic pH (6.2–6.6) of the vaccine, patients may complain of burning and/or stinging of short duration at the injection site.

Symptoms of the same kind as those seen following natural rubella may occur after vaccination. These include regional lymphadenopathy, urticaria, rash, malaise, sore throat, fever, headache, polyneuritis, and occasionally temporary arthralgia that is infrequently associated with signs of inflammation. Local pain, wheal and flare, induration, and erythema may occur at the site of injection. Reactions are usually mild and transient.

Moderate fever [101–102.9°F (38.3–39.4°C)] occurs occasionally, and high fever [over 103°F (39.4°C)] occurs less commonly.

In children, joint reactions are uncommon and of brief duration if they do occur. In women, incidence rates for arthritis and arthralgia are generally higher than those seen in children (children: 0–3%; women: 12–20%) and the reactions tend to be more marked and of longer duration. Symptoms may persist for a matter of months or on rare occasions for years. In adolescent girls, the reactions appear to be intermediate in incidence between those seen in children and in adult women. Even in older women (35–45 years), these reactions are generally well tolerated and rarely interfere with normal activities. Myalgia has been reported rarely after administration of MERUVAX II.

Forms of optic neuritis, including retrobulbar neuritis and papillitis may infrequently follow viral infections, and have been reported to occur 1 to 3 weeks following inoculation with some live virus vaccines.

Isolated reports of polyneuropathy including Guillain-Barré syndrome have been reported after immunization with rubella containing vaccines.

Clinical experience with live rubella vaccines thus far indicates that encephalitis and other nervous system reactions have occurred very rarely in subjects who were given the vaccines, but a cause and effect relationship has not been established.

In view of the decreases in platelet counts that have been reported, thrombocytopenic purpura is a theoretical hazard.

DOSAGE AND ADMINISTRATION

FOR SUBCUTANEOUS ADMINISTRATION

Do not inject intravenously

The dosage of vaccine is the same for all persons. Inject the total volume of the single dose vial (about 0.5 mL) or 0.5 mL of the multiple dose vial of reconstituted vaccine subcutaneously, preferably into the outer aspect of upper arm. *Do not give immune globulin (IG) concurrently with* MERUVAX II.

To insure that there is no loss of potency during shipment, the vaccine must be maintained at a temperature of 10°C (50°F) or less.

Before reconstitution, store MERUVAX II at 2–8°C (35.6–46.4°F). *Protect from light.*

CAUTION: A sterile syringe free of preservatives, antiseptics, and detergents should be used for each injection and/or reconstitution of the vaccine because these substances may inactivate the live virus vaccine. A 25 gauge, 5/8″ needle is recommended.

To reconstitute, use only the diluent supplied, since it is free of preservatives or other antiviral substances which might inactivate the vaccine.

Single Dose Vial—First withdraw the entire volume of diluent into the syringe to be used for reconstitution. Inject all the diluent in the syringe into the vial of lyophilized vaccine, and agitate to mix thoroughly. Withdraw the entire contents into a syringe and inject the total volume of restored vaccine subcutaneously.

It is important to use a separate sterile syringe and needle for each individual patient to prevent transmission of hepatitis B and other infectious agents from one person to another.

10 Dose Vial (available only to government agencies/institutions)—Withdraw the entire contents (7 mL) of the diluent vial into the sterile syringe to be used for reconstitution, and introduce into the 10 dose vial of lyophilized vaccine. Agitate to ensure thorough mixing. The outer labeling suggests "For Jet Injector or Syringe Use". Use with separate sterile syringes is permitted for containers of 10 doses or less. The vaccine and diluent do not contain preservatives; therefore, the user must recognize the potential contamination hazards and exercise special precautions to protect the sterility and potency of the product. The use of aseptic techniques and proper storage prior to and after restoration of the vaccine and subsequent withdrawal of the individual doses is essential. Use 0.5 mL of the reconstituted vaccine for subcutaneous injection.

It is important to use a separate sterile syringe and needle for each individual patient to prevent transmission of hepatitis B and other infectious agents from one person to another.

50 Dose Vial (available only to government agencies/institutions)—Withdraw the entire contents (30 mL) of diluent vial into the sterile syringe to be used for reconstitution and introduce into the 50 dose vial of lyophilized vaccine. Agitate to ensure thorough mixing. With full aseptic precautions, attach the vial to the sterilized multidose jet injector apparatus. Use 0.5 mL of the reconstituted vaccine for subcutaneous injection.

Each dose contains not less than the equivalent of 1,000 $TCID_{50}$ of the U.S. Reference Rubella Virus.

Parenteral drug products should be inspected visually for particulate matter and discoloration prior to administration. MERUVAX II, when reconstituted, is clear yellow.

HOW SUPPLIED

No. 4747—MERUVAX II is supplied as a single-dose vial of lyophilized vaccine, **NDC** 0006-4747-00, and a vial of diluent.

No. 4673/4309—MERUVAX II is supplied as follows: (1) a box of 10 single-dose vials of lyophilized vaccine (package A), **NDC** 0006-4673-00; and (2) a box of 10 vials of diluent (package B). To conserve refrigerator space, the diluent may be stored separately at room temperature.

Available only to government agencies/institutions:

No. 4674—MERUVAX II is supplied as one 10 dose vial of lyophilized vaccine, **NDC** 0006-4674-00, and one 7 mL vial of diluent.

No. 4675—MERUVAX II is supplied as one 50 dose vial of lyophilized vaccine, **NDC** 0006-4675-00, and one 30 mL vial of diluent.

Storage

It is recommended that the vaccine be used as soon as possible after reconstitution. Protect vaccine from light at all times, since such exposure may inactivate the virus. Store reconstituted vaccine in the vaccine vial in a dark place at 2–8°C (35.6–46.4°F) and discard if not used within 8 hours.

A.H.F.S. Category: 80:12

DC 7030811 Issued January 1986

MIDAMOR® Tablets ℞
(Amiloride HCl, MSD), U.S.P.

DESCRIPTION

Amiloride HCl, an antikaliuretic-diuretic agent, is a pyrazine-carbonyl-guanidine that is unrelated chemically to other known antikaliuretic or diuretic agents. It is the salt of a moderately strong base (pKa 8.7). It is designated chemically as 3,5-diamino-6-chloro-*N*-(diaminomethylene) pyrazinecarboxamide monohydrochloride, dihydrate and has a molecular weight of 302.14. Its empirical formula is $C_6H_8ClN_7O \cdot HCl \cdot 2H_2O$ and its structural formula is:

[structural formula: Cl, N, C(=O)—N=C(NH₂)—NH₂ • HCl • 2H₂O; H₂N, N, NH₂]

MIDAMOR® (Amiloride HCl, MSD) is available for oral use as tablets containing 5 mg of anhydrous amiloride HCl. Each tablet contains the following inactive ingredients: calcium phosphate, D&C Yellow 10, iron oxide, lactose, magnesium stearate and starch.

CLINICAL PHARMACOLOGY

MIDAMOR is a potassium-conserving (antikaliuretic) drug that possesses weak (compared with thiazide diuretics) natriuretic, diuretic, and antihypertensive activity. These effects have been partially additive to the effects of thiazide diuretics in some clinical studies. When administered with a thia-

Continued on next page

Information on the Merck Sharp & Dohme products listed on these pages is the full prescribing information from product circulars in use August 31, 1986.

Merck Sharp & Dohme—Cont.

zide or loop diuretic, MIDAMOR has been shown to decrease the enhanced urinary excretion of magnesium which occurs when a thiazide or loop diuretic is used alone. MIDAMOR has potassium-conserving activity in patients receiving kaliuretic-diuretic agents.

MIDAMOR is not an aldosterone antagonist and its effects are seen even in the absence of aldosterone.

MIDAMOR usually begins to act within 2 hours after an oral dose. Its effect on electrolyte excretion reaches a peak between 6 and 10 hours and lasts about 24 hours. Peak plasma levels are obtained in 3 to 4 hours and the plasma half-life varies from 6 to 9 hours. Effects on electrolytes increase with single doses of amiloride HCl up to approximately 15 mg.

Amiloride HCl is not metabolized by the liver but is excreted unchanged by the kidneys. About 50 percent of a 20 mg dose of MIDAMOR is excreted in the urine and 40 percent in the stool within 72 hours. MIDAMOR has little effect on glomerular filtration rate or renal blood flow. Because amiloride HCl is not metabolized by the liver, drug accumulation is not anticipated in patients with hepatic dysfunction, but accumulation can occur if the hepatorenal syndrome develops.

INDICATIONS AND USAGE

MIDAMOR is indicated as adjunctive treatment with thiazide diuretics or other kaliuretic-diuretic agents in congestive heart failure or hypertension to:

a. help restore normal serum potassium levels in patients who develop hypokalemia on the kaliuretic diuretic
b. prevent development of hypokalemia in patients who would be exposed to particular risk if hypokalemia were to develop, e.g., digitalized patients or patients with significant cardiac arrhythmias.

The use of potassium-conserving agents is often unnecessary in patients receiving diuretics for uncomplicated essential hypertension when such patients have a normal diet. MIDAMOR has little additive diuretic or antihypertensive effect when added to a thiazide diuretic.

MIDAMOR should rarely be used alone. It has weak (compared with thiazides) diuretic and antihypertensive effects. Used as single agents, potassium sparing diuretics, including MIDAMOR, result in an increased risk of hyperkalemia (approximately 10% with amiloride). MIDAMOR should be used alone only when persistent hypokalemia has been documented and only with careful titration of the dose and close monitoring of serum electrolytes.

CONTRAINDICATIONS

Hyperkalemia

MIDAMOR should not be used in the presence of elevated serum potassium levels (greater than 5.5 mEq per liter).

Antikaliuretic Therapy or Potassium Supplementation

MIDAMOR should not be given to patients receiving other potassium-conserving agents, such as spironolactone or triamterene. Potassium supplementation in the form of medication or a potassium-rich diet should not be used with MIDAMOR except in severe and/or refractory cases of hypokalemia. Such concomitant therapy can be associated with rapid increases in serum potassium levels. If potassium supplementation is used, careful monitoring of the serum potassium level is necessary.

Impaired Renal Function

Anuria, acute or chronic renal insufficiency, and evidence of diabetic nephropathy are contraindications to the use of MIDAMOR. Patients with evidence of renal functional impairment (blood urea nitrogen [BUN] levels over 30 mg per 100 mL or serum creatinine levels over 1.5 mg per 100 mL) or diabetes mellitus should not receive the drug without careful, frequent and continuing monitoring of serum electrolytes, creatinine, and BUN levels. Potassium retention associated with the use of an antikaliuretic agent is accentuated in the presence of renal impairment and may result in the rapid development of hyperkalemia.

Hypersensitivity

MIDAMOR is contraindicated in patients who are hypersensitive to this product.

WARNINGS

Hyperkalemia

Like other potassium-conserving agents, amiloride may cause hyperkalemia (serum potassium levels greater than 5.5 mEq per liter) which, if uncorrected, is potentially fatal. Hyperkalemia occurs commonly (about 10%) when amiloride is used without a kaliuretic diuretic. This incidence is greater in patients with renal impairment, diabetes mellitus (with or without recognized renal insufficiency), and in the elderly. When MIDAMOR is used concomitantly with a thiazide diuretic in patients without these complications, the risk of hyperkalemia is reduced to about 1–2%. It is thus essential to monitor serum potassium levels carefully in any patient receiving amiloride, particularly when it is first introduced, at the time of diuretic dosage adjustments, and during any illness that could affect renal function.

Warning signs or symptoms of hyperkalemia include paresthesias, muscular weakness, fatigue, flaccid paralysis of the extremities, bradycardia, shock, and ECG abnormalities. Monitoring of the serum potassium level is essential because mild hyperkalemia is not usually associated with an abnormal ECG.

When abnormal, the ECG in hyperkalemia is characterized primarily by tall, peaked T waves or elevations from previous tracings. There may also be lowering of the R wave and increased depth of the S wave, widening and even disappearance of the P wave, progressive widening of the QRS complex, prolongation of the PR interval, and ST depression.

Treatment of hyperkalemia: If hyperkalemia occurs in patients taking MIDAMOR, the drug should be discontinued immediately. If the serum potassium level exceeds 6.5 mEq per liter, active measures should be taken to reduce it. Such measures include the intravenous administration of sodium bicarbonate solution or oral or parenteral glucose with a rapid-acting insulin preparation. If needed, a cation exchange resin such as sodium polystyrene sulfonate may be given orally or by enema. Patients with persistent hyperkalemia may require dialysis.

Diabetes Mellitus

In diabetic patients, hyperkalemia has been reported with the use of all potassium-conserving diuretics, including MIDAMOR, even in patients without evidence of diabetic nephropathy. Therefore, MIDAMOR should be avoided, if possible, in diabetic patients and, if it is used, serum electrolytes and renal function must be monitored frequently.

MIDAMOR should be discontinued at least 3 days before glucose tolerance testing.

Metabolic or Respiratory Acidosis

Antikaliuretic therapy should be instituted only with caution in severely ill patients in whom respiratory or metabolic acidosis may occur, such as patients with cardiopulmonary disease or poorly controlled diabetes. If MIDAMOR is given to these patients, frequent monitoring of acid-base balance is necessary. Shifts in acid-base balance alter the ratio of extracellular/intracellular potassium, and the development of acidosis may be associated with rapid increases in serum potassium levels.

PRECAUTIONS

General

Electrolyte Imbalance and BUN Increases

Hyponatremia and hypochloremia may occur when MIDAMOR is used with other diuretics and increases in BUN levels have been reported. These increases usually have accompanied vigorous fluid elimination, especially when diuretic therapy was used in seriously ill patients, such as those who had hepatic cirrhosis with ascites and metabolic alkalosis, or those with resistant edema. Therefore, when MIDAMOR is given with other diuretics to such patients, careful monitoring of serum electrolytes and BUN levels is important. In patients with pre-existing severe liver disease, hepatic encephalopathy, manifested by tremors, confusion, and coma, and increased jaundice, have been reported in association with diuretics, including amiloride HCl.

Drug Interactions

Lithium generally should not be given with diuretics because they reduce its renal clearance and add a high risk of lithium toxicity. Read circulars for lithium preparations before use of such concomitant therapy.

In some patients, the administration of a non-steroidal anti-inflammatory agent can reduce the diuretic, natriuretic, and antihypertensive effects of loop, potassium-sparing and thiazide diuretics. Therefore, when MIDAMOR and non-steroidal anti-inflammatory agents are used concomitantly, the patient should be observed closely to determine if the desired effect of the diuretic is obtained. Since indomethacin and potassium-sparing diuretics, including MIDAMOR, each may be associated with increased serum potassium levels, the potential effects on potassium kinetics and renal function should be considered when these agents are administered concurrently.

Carcinogenicity, Mutagenicity, Impairment of Fertility

There was no evidence of a tumorigenic effect when amiloride HCl was administered for 92 weeks to mice at doses up to 10 mg/kg/day (25 times the maximum daily human dose). Amiloride HCl has also been administered for 104 weeks to male and female rats at doses up to 6 and 8 mg/kg/day (15 and 20 times the maximum daily dose for humans, respectively) and showed no evidence of carcinogenicity.

Amiloride HCl was devoid of mutagenic activity in various strains of *Salmonella typhimurium* with or without a mammalian liver microsomal activation system (Ames test).

Pregnancy

Pregnancy Category B. Teratogenicity studies with amiloride HCl in rabbits and mice given 20 and 25 times the maximum human dose, respectively, revealed no evidence of harm to the fetus, although studies showed that the drug crossed the placenta in modest amounts. Reproduction studies in rats at 20 times the expected maximum daily dose for humans showed no evidence of impaired fertility. At approximately 5 or more times the expected maximum daily dose for humans, some toxicity was seen in adult rats and rabbits and a decrease in rat pup growth and survival occurred.

There are, however, no adequate and well-controlled studies in pregnant women. Because animal reproduction studies are not always predictive of human response, this drug should be used during pregnancy only if clearly needed.

Nursing Mothers

Studies in rats have shown that amiloride is excreted in milk in concentrations higher than that found in blood, but it is not known whether MIDAMOR is excreted in human milk. Because many drugs are excreted in human milk and because of the potential for serious adverse reactions in nursing infants from MIDAMOR, a decision should be made whether to discontinue nursing or to discontinue the drug, taking into account the importance of the drug to the mother.

Pediatric Use

Safety and effectiveness in children have not been established.

ADVERSE REACTIONS

MIDAMOR is usually well tolerated and, except for hyperkalemia (serum potassium levels greater than 5.5 mEq per liter—see WARNINGS), significant adverse effects have been reported infrequently. Minor adverse reactions were reported relatively frequently (about 20%) but the relationship of many of the reports to amiloride HCl is uncertain and the overall frequency was similar in hydrochlorothiazide treated groups. Nausea/anorexia, abdominal pain, flatulence, and mild skin rash have been reported and probably are related to amiloride. Other adverse experiences that have been reported with amiloride are generally those known to be associated with diuresis, or with the underlying disease being treated.

The adverse reactions for MIDAMOR listed in the following table have been arranged into two groups: (1) incidence greater than one percent; and (2) incidence one percent or less. The incidence for group (1) was determined from clinical studies conducted in the United States (837 patients treated with MIDAMOR). The adverse effects listed in group (2) include reports from the same clinical studies and voluntary reports since marketing. The probability of a causal relationship exists between MIDAMOR and these adverse reactions, some of which have been reported only rarely.

Incidence $> 1\%$	*Incidence* $\leq 1\%$
Body as a Whole	
Headache*	Back pain
Weakness	Chest pain
Fatigability	Neck/shoulder ache
	Pain, extremities
Cardiovascular	
None	Angina pectoris
	Orthostatic hypotension
	Arrhythmia
	Palpitation
Digestive	
Nausea/anorexia*	Jaundice
Diarrhea*	GI bleeding
Vomiting*	Abdominal fullness
Abdominal pain	GI disturbance
Gas pain	Thirst
Appetite changes	Heartburn
Constipation	Flatulence
	Dyspepsia
Metabolic	
Elevated serum potassium levels (> 5.5 mEq per liter)†	None
Integumentary	
None	Skin rash
	Itching
	Dryness of mouth
	Pruritus
	Alopecia
Musculoskeletal	
Muscle cramps	Joint pain
	Leg ache
Nervous	
Dizziness	Paresthesia
Encephalopathy	Tremors
	Vertigo
Psychiatric	
None	Nervousness
	Mental confusion
	Insomnia
	Decreased libido
	Depression
	Somnolence

Respiratory

Cough	Shortness of breath
Dyspnea	

Special Senses

None	Visual disturbances
	Nasal congestion
	Tinnitus
	Increased intraocular pressure

Urogenital

Impotence	Polyuria
	Dysuria
	Urinary frequency
	Bladder spasms

* Reactions occurring in 3% to 8% of patients treated with MIDAMOR. (Those reactions occurring in less than 3% of the patients are unmarked.)
† See WARNINGS.

Causal Relationship Unknown
Other reactions have been reported but occurred under circumstances where a causal relationship could not be established. However, in these rarely reported events, that possibility cannot be excluded. Therefore, these observations are listed to serve as alerting information to physicians.
Activation of probable pre-existing peptic ulcer
Aplastic anemia
Neutropenia
Abnormalities of liver function tests

OVERDOSAGE

No data are available in regard to overdosage in humans.
The oral LD_{50} of amiloride hydrochloride (calculated as the base) is 56 mg/kg in mice and 36 to 85 mg/kg in rats, depending on the strain.
It is not known whether the drug is dialyzable.
The most likely signs and symptoms to be expected with overdosage are dehydration and electrolyte imbalance. These can be treated by established procedures. Therapy with MIDAMOR should be discontinued and the patient observed closely. There is no specific antidote. Emesis should be induced or gastric lavage performed. Treatment is symptomatic and supportive. If hyperkalemia occurs, active measures should be taken to reduce the serum potassium levels.

DOSAGE AND ADMINISTRATION

MIDAMOR should be administered with food.
MIDAMOR, one 5 mg tablet daily, should be added to the usual antihypertensive or diuretic dosage of a kaliuretic diuretic. The dosage may be increased to 10 mg per day, if necessary. More than two 5 mg tablets of MIDAMOR daily usually are not needed, and there is little controlled experience with such doses. If persistent hypokalemia is documented with 10 mg, the dose can be increased to 15 mg, then 20 mg, with careful monitoring of electrolytes.
In treating patients with congestive heart failure after an initial diuresis has been achieved, potassium loss may also decrease and the need for MIDAMOR should be reevaluated. Dosage adjustment may be necessary. Maintenance therapy may be on an intermittent basis.
If it is necessary to use MIDAMOR alone (see INDICATIONS), the starting dosage should be one 5 mg tablet daily. This dosage may be increased to 10 mg per day, if necessary. More than two 5 mg tablets usually are not needed, and there is little controlled experience with such doses. If persistent hypokalemia is documented with 10 mg, the dose can be increased to 15 mg, then 20 mg, with careful monitoring of electrolytes.

HOW SUPPLIED

No. 3381—Tablets MIDAMOR, 5 mg, are yellow, diamond-shaped, compressed tablets, coded MSD 92. They are supplied as follows:
NDC 0006-0092-68 bottles of 100.

Shown in Product Identification Section, page 417

A.H.F.S. Category: 40:28
DC 7130010 Issued October 1985

MINTEZOL® Chewable Tablets ℞
(Thiabendazole, MSD)

MINTEZOL® Suspension ℞
(Thiabendazole, MSD), U.S.P.

DESCRIPTION

MINTEZOL® (Thiabendazole, MSD) is an anthelmintic provided as 500 mg chewable tablets, and as a suspension, containing 500 mg thiabendazole per 5 mL. The suspension also contains sorbic acid 0.1% added as a preservative. Inactive ingredients in the tablets are acacia, calcium phosphate, flavors, lactose, magnesium stearate, mannitol, methylcellulose, and sodium saccharin. Inactive ingredients in the suspension are an antifoam agent, flavors, polysorbate, purified water, sorbitol solution, and tragacanth.
Thiabendazole is a white to off-white odorless powder with a molecular weight of 201.26, which is practically insoluble in water but readily soluble in dilute acid and alkali. Its chemical name is 2-(4-thiazolyl)-1*H*-benzimidazole. The empirical formula is $C_{10}H_7N_3S$ and the structural formula is:

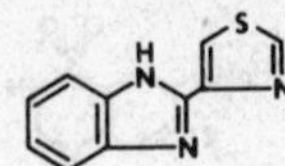

CLINICAL PHARMACOLOGY

In man, thiabendazole is rapidly absorbed and peak plasma concentration is reached within 1 to 2 hours after the oral administration of a suspension. It is metabolized almost completely to the 5-hydroxy form which appears in the urine as glucuronide or sulfate conjugates. In 48 hours, about 5% of the administered dose is recovered from the feces and about 90% from the urine. Most is excreted in the first 24 hours.

Mechanism of Action
The precise mode of action of thiabendazole on the parasite is unknown, but it may inhibit the helminth-specific enzyme fumarate reductase.
Thiabendazole is vermicidal and/or vermifugal against *Ascaris lumbricoides* ("common roundworm"), *Strongyloides stercoralis* (threadworm), *Necator americanus*, and *Ancylostoma duodenale* (hookworm), *Trichuris trichiura* (whipworm), *Ancylostoma braziliense* (dog and cat hookworm), *Toxocara canis* and *Toxocara cati* (ascarids), and *Enterobius vermicularis* (pinworm).
Its effect on larvae of *Trichinella spiralis* that have migrated to muscle is questionable.
Thiabendazole also suppresses egg and/or larval production and may inhibit the subsequent development of those eggs or larvae which are passed in the feces.

INDICATIONS AND USAGE

MINTEZOL is indicated for the treatment of:
Strongyloidiasis (threadworm)
Cutaneous larva migrans (creeping eruption)
Visceral larva migrans
Trichinosis: Relief of symptoms and fever and a reduction of eosinophilia have followed the use of MINTEZOL during the invasion stage of the disease.

Although not indicated as primary therapy, when enterobiasis (pinworm) occurs with any of the conditions listed above, additional therapy is not required for most patients. MINTEZOL should be used only in the following infestations when more specific therapy is not available or cannot be used or when further therapy with a second agent is desirable: Uncinariasis (hookworm: *Necator americanus* and *Ancylostoma duodenale*); Trichuriasis (whipworm); Ascariasis (large roundworm).

CONTRAINDICATION

Hypersensitivity to this product.

WARNINGS

If hypersensitivity reactions occur, the drug should be discontinued immediately and not be resumed. Erythema multiforme has been associated with thiabendazole therapy; in severe cases (Stevens-Johnson syndrome), fatalities have occurred.
Because CNS side effects may occur quite frequently, activities requiring mental alertness should be avoided.

PRECAUTIONS

General
MINTEZOL is not suitable for the treatment of mixed infections with ascaris because it may cause these worms to migrate.
Ideally, supportive therapy is indicated for anemic, dehydrated or malnourished patients prior to initiation of the anthelmintic therapy.
In the presence of hepatic or renal dysfunction, patients should be carefully monitored.
MINTEZOL should be used only in patients in whom susceptible worm infestation has been diagnosed and should not be used prophylactically.

Information for Patients
Because CNS side effects may occur quite frequently, activities requiring mental alertness should be avoided.

Laboratory Tests
Rarely, a transient rise in cephalin flocculation and SGOT has occurred in patients receiving MINTEZOL.

Drug Interactions
Thiabendazole may compete with other drugs, such as theophylline, for sites of metabolism in the liver, thus elevating the serum levels of such compounds to potentially toxic levels. Therefore, when concomitant use of thiabendazole and xanthine derivatives is anticipated, it may be necessary to monitor blood levels and/or reduce the dosage of such compounds. Such concomitant use should be administered under careful medical supervision.

Carcinogenesis, Mutagenesis, Impairment of Fertility
Thiabendazole has been used in numerous short- and long-term studies in animals at doses up to 15 times the usual human dose and was without carcinogenic effects. It did not adversely affect fertility in the mouse at 2½ times the usual human dose or in the rat at a dose equivalent to the usual human dose. Thiabendazole had no mutagenic activity in *in vitro* microbial mutagen test, the micronucleus test and the host mediated assay *in vivo.*

Pregnancy
Pregnancy Category C: Reproduction and teratogenic studies done in the rabbit at a dose up to 15 times the usual human dose, in the rat at a dose equivalent to the human dose, and in the mouse at a dose up to 2½ times the usual human dose, revealed no evidence of harm to the fetus. In an additional study in the mouse, no defects were observed when thiabendazole was given in an aqueous suspension, at a dose 10 times the usual human dose; however, cleft palate and axial skeletal defects were observed when thiabendazole was suspended in olive oil and given at the same dose. There are no adequate and well controlled studies in pregnant women. MINTEZOL should be used during pregnancy only if the potential benefit justifies the potential risk to the fetus.

Nursing Mothers
It is not known whether this drug is excreted in human milk. Because of the potential for serious adverse reactions in nursing infants from MINTEZOL, a decision should be made whether to discontinue nursing or to discontinue the drug, taking into account the importance of the drug to the mother.

Pediatric Use
The safety and effectiveness of thiabendazole for the treatment of Strongyloidiasis, Ascariasis, Uncinariasis, Trichuriasis and Trichinosis in children weighing less than 30 lbs has been limited.

ADVERSE REACTIONS

Gastrointestinal: anorexia, nausea, vomiting, diarrhea, epigastric distress, jaundice, cholestasis and parenchymal liver damage.
Central Nervous System: dizziness, weariness, drowsiness, giddiness, headache, numbness, hyperirritability, convulsions, collapse, psychic disturbances.
Special Senses: tinnitus, abnormal sensation in eyes, xanthopsia, blurring of vision, drying of mucous membranes (mouth, eyes, etc.).
Cardiovascular: hypotension.
Metabolic: hyperglycemia.
Hematologic: transient leukopenia.
Genitourinary: hematuria, enuresis, malodor of the urine, crystalluria.
Hypersensitivity: pruritus, fever, facial flush, chills, conjunctival injection, angioedema, anaphylaxis, skin rashes (including perianal), erythema multiforme (including Stevens-Johnson syndrome), and lymphadenopathy.
Miscellaneous: appearance of live Ascaris in the mouth and nose.

OVERDOSAGE

Overdosage may be associated with transient disturbances of vision and psychic alterations.
There is no specific antidote in the event of overdosage. Therefore, symptomatic and supportive measures should be employed. Emesis should be induced or gastric lavage performed carefully.
The oral LD_{50} of MINTEZOL is 3.6 g/kg, 3.1 g/kg and 3.8 g/kg in the mouse, rat, and rabbit respectively.

DOSAGE AND ADMINISTRATION

The recommended maximum daily dose of MINTEZOL *is 3 grams.*

Continued on next page

Information on the Merck Sharp & Dohme products listed on these pages is the full prescribing information from product circulars in use August 31, 1986.

Merck Sharp & Dohme—Cont.

MINTEZOL should be given after meals if possible. Tablets MINTEZOL should be chewed before swallowing. Dietary restriction, complementary medications and cleansing enemas are not needed.
The usual dosage schedule for all conditions is two doses per day. The dosage is determined by the patient's weight.
A weight-dose chart follows:

Weight	Each Dose g	Each Dose mL
30 lb	0.25 (½ tablet)	2.5 (½ teaspoon)
50 lb	0.5 (1 tablet)	5.0 (1 teaspoon)
75 lb	0.75 (1½ tablets)	7.5 (1½ teaspoons)
100 lb	1.0 (2 tablets)	10.0 (2 teaspoons)
125 lb	1.25 (2½ tablets)	12.5 (2½ teaspoons)
150 lb & over	1.5 (3 tablets)	15.0 (3 teaspoons)

The regimen for each indication follows:
[See table below].

HOW SUPPLIED

No. 3331 — MINTEZOL Suspension, 500 mg per 5 mL, is white to off-white and is supplied as follows:
NDC 0006-3331-60 in bottles of 120 mL
(6505-00-935-5858 0.5 g/5 mL 120 mL).
No. 3332 — MINTEZOL Chewable Tablets, 500 mg, are white to off-white, orange-flavored, round, scored, compressed tablets, coded MSD 907. They are supplied as follows:
NDC 0006-0907-36 in boxes of 36 strip packaged, individually foil-wrapped tablets.

Shown in Product Identification Section, page 417

A.H.F.S. Category: 8:08
DC 6857709 Issued June 1985

MODURETIC® Tablets ℞
(Amiloride HCl-Hydrochlorothiazide, MSD), U.S.P.

DESCRIPTION

MODURETIC® (Amiloride HCl-Hydrochlorothiazide, MSD) combines the potassium-conserving action of amiloride HCl with the natriuretic action of hydrochlorothiazide.
Amiloride HCl is designated chemically as 3,5-diamino-6-chloro-*N*-(diaminomethylene) pyrazinecarboxamide monohydrochloride, dihydrate and has a molecular weight of 302.14. Its empirical formula is $C_6H_8ClN_7O \cdot HCl \cdot 2H_2O$ and its structural formula is:
[See Chemical Formula at top of next column].

Hydrochlorothiazide is designated chemically as 6-chloro-3,4-dihydro-2*H*-1,2,4-benzothiadiazine-7-sulfonamide 1,1-dioxide and has a molecular weight of 297.72. Its empirical formula is $C_7H_8ClN_3O_4S_2$ and its structural formula is:

MODURETIC is available for oral use as tablets containing 5 mg of anhydrous amiloride HCl and 50 mg of hydrochlorothiazide. Each tablet contains the following inactive ingredients: calcium phosphate, FD&C Yellow 6, guar gum, lactose, magnesium stearate and starch.

CLINICAL PHARMACOLOGY

MODURETIC provides diuretic and antihypertensive activity (principally due to the hydrochlorothiazide component), while acting through the amiloride component to prevent the excessive potassium loss that may occur in patients receiving a thiazide diuretic. Due to its amiloride component, the urinary excretion of magnesium is less with MODURETIC than with a thiazide or loop diuretic used alone (see PRECAUTIONS). The onset of the diuretic action of MODURETIC is within 1 to 2 hours and this action appears to be sustained for approximately 24 hours.

Amiloride HCl
Amiloride HCl is a potassium-conserving (antikaliuretic) drug that possesses weak (compared with thiazide diuretics) natriuretic, diuretic, and antihypertensive activity. These effects have been partially additive to the effects of thiazide diuretics in some clinical studies. Amiloride HCl has potassium-conserving activity in patients receiving kaliuretic-diuretic agents.
Amiloride HCl is not an aldosterone antagonist and its effects are seen even in the absence of aldosterone.
Amiloride HCl usually begins to act within 2 hours after an oral dose. Its effect on electrolyte excretion reaches a peak between 6 and 10 hours and lasts about 24 hours. Peak plasma levels are obtained in 3 to 4 hours and the plasma half-life varies from 6 to 9 hours. Effects on electrolytes increase with single doses of amiloride HCl up to approximately 15 mg.
Amiloride HCl is not metabolized by the liver but is excreted unchanged by the kidneys. About 50 percent of a 20 mg dose of amiloride HCl is excreted in the urine and 40 percent in the stool within 72 hours. Amiloride HCl has little effect on glomerular filtration rate or renal blood flow. Because amiloride HCl is not metabolized by the liver, drug accumulation is not anticipated in patients with hepatic dysfunction, but accumulation can occur if the hepatorenal syndrome develops.

Therapeutic Regimens

Indication	*Regimen*	*Comments*
•STRONGYLOIDIASIS	2 doses per day for 2 successive days.	A single dose of 20 mg/lb or 50 mg/kg may be employed as an alternative schedule, but a higher incidence of side effects should be expected.
CUTANEOUS LARVA MIGRANS (Creeping Eruption)	2 doses per day for 2 successive days.	If active lesions are still present 2 days after completion of therapy, a second course is recommended.
VISCERAL LARVA MIGRANS	2 doses per day for 7 successive days.	Safety and efficacy data on the seven-day treatment course are limited.
•TRICHINOSIS	2 doses per day for 2–4 successive days according to the response of the patient.	The optimal dosage for the treatment of trichinosis has not been established.
Other Indications		
• Intestinal roundworms (including Ascariasis, Uncinariasis and Trichuriasis)	2 doses per day for 2 successive days.	A single dose of 20 mg/lb or 50 mg/kg may be employed as an alternative schedule, but a higher incidence of side effects should be expected.

• Clinical experience with thiabendazole for treatment of each of these conditions in children weighing less than 30 lbs has been limited.

Hydrochlorothiazide
Hydrochlorothiazide is a diuretic and antihypertensive agent. It affects the renal tubular mechanism of electrolyte reabsorption.
Hydrochlorothiazide increases excretion of sodium and chloride in approximately equivalent amounts. Natriuresis may be accompanied by some loss of potassium and bicarbonate. The onset of the diuretic action of hydrochlorothiazide occurs in 2 hours and the peak action in about 4 hours. Diuretic activity lasts about 6 to 12 hours. Hydrochlorothiazide is eliminated rapidly by the kidney.
The mechanism of the antihypertensive effect of thiazides may be related to the excretion and redistribution of body sodium. Hydrochlorothiazide usually does not cause clinically important changes in normal blood pressure.

INDICATIONS AND USAGE

MODURETIC is indicated in those patients with hypertension or with congestive heart failure who develop hypokalemia when thiazides or other kaliuretic diuretics are used alone, or in whom maintenance of normal serum potassium levels is considered to be clinically important, e.g., digitalized patients, or patients with significant cardiac arrhythmias.
The use of potassium-conserving agents is often unnecessary in patients receiving diuretics for uncomplicated essential hypertension when such patients have a normal diet.
MODURETIC may be used alone or as an adjunct to other antihypertensive drugs, such as methyldopa or beta blockers. Since MODURETIC enhances the action of these agents, dosage adjustments may be necessary to avoid an excessive fall in blood pressure and other unwanted side effects.
This fixed combination drug is not indicated for initial therapy of edema or hypertension. If the fixed combination represents the dose titrated to an individual patient's needs, it may be more convenient than the separate components.

CONTRAINDICATIONS

Hyperkalemia
MODURETIC should not be used in the presence of elevated serum potassium levels (greater than 5.5 mEq per liter).
Antikaliuretic Therapy or Potassium Supplementation
MODURETIC should not be given to patients receiving other potassium-conserving agents, such as spironolactone or triamterene. Potassium supplementation in the form of medication or a potassium-rich diet should not be used with MODURETIC except in severe and/or refractory cases of hypokalemia. Such concomitant therapy can be associated with rapid increases in serum potassium levels. If potassium supplementation is used, careful monitoring of the serum potassium level is necessary.
Impaired Renal Function
Anuria, acute or chronic renal insufficiency, and evidence of diabetic nephropathy are contraindications to the use of MODURETIC. Patients with evidence of renal functional impairment (blood urea nitrogen [BUN] levels over 30 mg per 100 mL or serum creatinine levels over 1.5 mg per 100 mL) or diabetes mellitus should not receive the drug without careful, frequent and continuing monitoring of serum electrolytes, creatinine, and BUN levels. Potassium retention associated with the use of an antikaliuretic agent is accentuated in the presence of renal impairment and may result in the rapid development of hyperkalemia.
Hypersensitivity
MODURETIC is contraindicated in patients who are hypersensitive to this product, or to other sulfonamide-derived drugs.

WARNINGS

Hyperkalemia

Like other potassium-conserving diuretic combinations, MODURETIC may cause hyperkalemia (serum potassium levels greater than 5.5 mEq per liter). In patients without renal impairment or diabetes mellitus, the risk of hyperkalemia with MODURETIC is about 1-2%. This risk is higher in patients with renal impairment or diabetes mellitus (even without recognized diabetic nephropathy). Since hyperkalemia, if uncorrected, is potentially fatal, it is essential to monitor serum potassium levels carefully in any patient receiving MODURETIC, particularly when it is first introduced, at the time of dosage adjustments, and during any illness that could affect renal function.

Warning signs or symptoms of hyperkalemia include paresthesias, muscular weakness, fatigue, flaccid paralysis of the extremities, bradycardia, shock, and ECG abnormalities. Monitoring of the serum potassium level is essential because mild hyperkalemia is not usually associated with an abnormal ECG.
When abnormal, the ECG in hyperkalemia is characterized primarily by tall, peaked T waves or elevations from previous tracings. There may also be lowering of the R wave and

increased depth of the S wave, widening and even disappearance of the P wave, progressive widening of the QRS complex, prolongation of the PR interval, and ST depression.

Treatment of hyperkalemia: If hyperkalemia occurs in patients taking MODURETIC, the drug should be discontinued immediately. If the serum potassium level exceeds 6.5 mEq per liter, active measures should be taken to reduce it. Such measures include the intravenous administration of sodium bicarbonate solution or oral or parenteral glucose with a rapid-acting insulin preparation. If needed, a cation exchange resin such as sodium polystyrene sulfonate may be given orally or by enema. Patients with persistent hyperkalemia may require dialysis.

Diabetes Mellitus

In diabetic patients, hyperkalemia has been reported with the use of all potassium-conserving diuretics, including amiloride HCl, even in patients without evidence of diabetic nephropathy. Therefore, MODURETIC should be avoided, if possible, in diabetic patients and, if it is used, serum electrolytes and renal function must be monitored frequently.

MODURETIC should be discontinued at least 3 days before glucose tolerance testing.

Metabolic or Respiratory Acidosis

Antikaliuretic therapy should be instituted only with caution in severely ill patients in whom respiratory or metabolic acidosis may occur, such as patients with cardiopulmonary disease or poorly controlled diabetes. If MODURETIC is given to these patients, frequent monitoring of acid-base balance is necessary. Shifts in acid-base balance alter the ratio of extracellular/intracellular potassium, and the development of acidosis may be associated with rapid increases in serum potassium levels.

PRECAUTIONS

General

Electrolyte Imbalance and BUN Increases

Determination of serum electrolytes to detect possible electrolyte imbalance should be performed at appropriate intervals.

Patients should be observed for clinical signs of fluid or electrolyte imbalance: i.e., hyponatremia, hypochloremic alkalosis, and hypokalemia. Serum and urine electrolyte determinations are particularly important when the patient is vomiting excessively or receiving parenteral fluids. Warning signs or symptoms of fluid and electrolyte imbalance include dryness of mouth, thirst, weakness, lethargy, drowsiness, restlessness, muscle pains or cramps, muscular fatigue, hypotension, oliguria, tachycardia, and gastrointestinal disturbances such as nausea and vomiting.

Hyponatremia and hypochloremia may occur during the use of thiazides and other diuretics. Any chloride deficit during thiazide therapy is generally mild and may be lessened by the amiloride HCl component of MODURETIC. Hypochloremia usually does not require specific treatment except under extraordinary circumstances (as in liver disease or renal disease). Dilutional hyponatremia may occur in edematous patients in hot weather; appropriate therapy is water restriction, rather than administration of salt, except in rare instances when the hyponatremia is life threatening. In actual salt depletion, appropriate replacement is the therapy of choice.

Hypokalemia may develop during thiazide therapy, especially with brisk diuresis, when severe cirrhosis is present, during concomitant use of corticosteroids or ACTH, or after prolonged therapy. However, this usually is prevented by the amiloride HCl component of MODURETIC.

Interference with adequate oral electrolyte intake will also contribute to hypokalemia. Hypokalemia can sensitize or exaggerate the response of the heart to the toxic effects of digitalis (e.g., increased ventricular irritability).

Thiazides have been shown to increase the urinary excretion of magnesium; this may result in hypomagnesemia. Amiloride HCl, a component of MODURETIC, has been shown to decrease the enhanced urinary excretion of magnesium which occurs when a thiazide or loop diuretic is used alone.

Increases in BUN levels have been reported with amiloride HCl and with hydrochlorothiazide. These increases usually have accompanied vigorous fluid elimination, especially when diuretic therapy was used in seriously ill patients, such as those who had hepatic cirrhosis with ascites and metabolic alkalosis, or those with resistant edema. Therefore, when MODURETIC is given to such patients, careful monitoring of serum electrolyte and BUN levels is important. In patients with pre-existing severe liver disease, hepatic encephalopathy, manifested by tremors, confusion, and coma, and increased jaundice, have been reported in association with diuretic therapy including amiloride HCl and hydrochlorothiazide.

In patients with renal disease, diuretics may precipitate azotemia. Cumulative effects of the components of MODURETIC may develop in patients with impaired renal function. If renal impairment becomes evident, MODURETIC should be discontinued (see CONTRAINDICATIONS and WARNINGS).

Drug Interactions

Thiazides may add to or potentiate the action of other antihypertensive drugs.

Thiazides may increase the responsiveness to tubocurarine.

Lithium generally should not be given with diuretics because they reduce its renal clearance and add a high risk of lithium toxicity. Read circulars for lithium preparations before use of such concomitant therapy.

In some patients, the administration of a non-steroidal anti-inflammatory agent can reduce the diuretic, natriuretic, and antihypertensive effects of loop, potassium-sparing and thiazide diuretics. Therefore, when MODURETIC and non-steroidal anti-inflammatory agents are used concomitantly, the patient should be observed closely to determine if the desired effect of the diuretic is obtained. Since indomethacin and potassium-sparing diuretics, including MODURETIC, each may be associated with increased serum potassium levels, the potential effects on potassium kinetics and renal function should be considered when these agents are administered concurrently.

Metabolic and Endocrine Effects

Thiazides may decrease serum PBI levels without signs of thyroid disturbance.

In diabetic patients, insulin requirements may be increased, decreased, or unchanged due to the hydrochlorothiazide component. Diabetes mellitus that has been latent may become manifest during administration of thiazide diuretics.

Because calcium excretion is decreased by thiazides, MODURETIC should be discontinued before carrying out tests for parathyroid function. Pathologic changes in the parathyroid glands, with hypercalcemia and hypophosphatemia have been observed in a few patients on prolonged thiazide therapy; however, the common complications of hyperparathyroidism such as renal lithiasis, bone resorption, and peptic ulceration have not been seen.

Hyperuricemia may occur or acute gout may be precipitated in certain patients receiving thiazide therapy.

Other Precautions

In patients receiving thiazides, sensitivity reactions may occur with or without a history of allergy or bronchial asthma. The possibility of exacerbation or activation of systemic lupus erythematosus has been reported with the use of thiazides.

Carcinogenicity, Mutagenicity, Impairment of Fertility

There was no evidence of a tumorigenic effect when amiloride HCl was administered for 92 weeks to mice at doses up to 10 mg/kg/day (25 times the maximum daily human dose). Amiloride HCl has also been administered for 104 weeks to male and female rats at doses up to 6 and 8 mg/kg/day (15 and 20 times the maximum daily dose for humans, respectively) and showed no evidence of carcinogenicity.

Amiloride HCl was devoid of mutagenic activity in various strains of *Salmonella typhimurium* with or without a mammalian liver microsomal activation system (Ames test).

Pregnancy

Pregnancy Category B. Teratogenicity studies have been performed with combinations of amiloride HCl and hydrochlorothiazide in rabbits and mice at doses up to 25 times the expected maximum daily dose for humans and have revealed no evidence of harm to the fetus. No evidence of impaired fertility in rats was apparent at dosage levels up to 25 times the expected maximum human daily dose. A perinatal and postnatal study in rats showed a reduction in maternal body weight gain during and after gestation at a daily dose of 25 times the expected maximum daily dose for humans. The body weights of alive pups at birth and at weaning were also reduced at this dose level. There are no adequate and well controlled studies in pregnant women. Because animal reproduction studies are not always predictive of human responses, and because of the data listed below with the individual components, this drug should be used during pregnancy only if clearly needed.

Amiloride HCl: Teratogenicity studies with amiloride HCl in rabbits and mice given 20 and 25 times the maximum human dose, respectively, revealed no evidence of harm to the fetus, although studies showed that the drug crossed the placenta in modest amounts. Reproduction studies in rats at 20 times the expected maximum daily dose for humans showed no evidence of impaired fertility. At approximately 5 or more times the expected maximum daily dose for humans, some toxicity was seen in adult rats and rabbits and a decrease in rat pup growth and survival occurred.

Hydrochlorothiazide: Thiazides cross the placental barrier and appear in cord blood. The possible hazards to the fetus include fetal or neonatal jaundice, thrombocytopenia, and possibly other adverse reactions which have occurred in the adult.

Nursing Mothers

Studies in rats have shown that amiloride is excreted in milk in concentrations higher than that found in blood, but it is not known whether amiloride HCl is excreted in human milk. However, thiazides appear in breast milk. Because of the potential for serious adverse reactions in nursing infants, a decision should be made whether to discontinue nursing or to discontinue the drug, taking into account the importance of the drug to the mother.

Pediatric Use

Safety and effectiveness in children have not been established.

ADVERSE REACTIONS

MODURETIC is usually well tolerated and significant clinical adverse effects have been reported infrequently. The risk of hyperkalemia (serum potassium levels greater than 5.5 mEq per liter) with MODURETIC is about 1–2% in patients without renal impairment or diabetes mellitus (see WARNINGS). Minor adverse reactions to amiloride HCl have been reported relatively frequently (about 20%) but the relationship of many of the reports to amiloride HCl is uncertain and the overall frequency was similar in hydrochlorothiazide treated groups. Nausea/anorexia, abdominal pain, flatulence, and mild skin rash have been reported and probably are related to amiloride. Other adverse experiences that have been reported with MODURETIC are generally those known to be associated with diuresis, thiazide therapy, or with the underlying disease being treated. Clinical trials have not demonstrated that combining amiloride and hydrochlorothiazide increases the risk of adverse reactions over those seen with the individual components.

The adverse reactions for MODURETIC listed in the following table have been arranged into two groups: (1) incidence greater than one percent; and (2) incidence one percent or less. The incidence for group (1) was determined from clinical studies conducted in the United States (607 patients treated with MODURETIC). The adverse effects listed in group (2) include reports from the same clinical studies and voluntary reports since marketing. The probability of a causal relationship exists between MODURETIC and these adverse reactions, some of which have been reported only rarely.

Incidence > 1%	*Incidence ≤ 1%*
Body as a Whole	
Headache*	Malaise
Weakness*	Chest pain
Fatigue/tiredness	Back pain
	Syncope
Cardiovascular	
Arrhythmia	Tachycardia
	Digitalis toxicity
	Orthostatic hypotension
	Angina pectoris
Digestive	
Nausea/anorexia*	Constipation
Diarrhea	GI bleeding
Gastrointestinal pain	GI disturbance
	Appetite changes
Abdominal pain	Abdominal fullness
	Hiccups
	Thirst
	Vomiting
	Anorexia
	Flatulence
Metabolic	
Elevated serum potassium levels (>5.5 mEq per liter)†	Gout
	Dehydration
Integumentary	
Rash*	Flushing
Pruritus	
Musculoskeletal	
Leg ache	Muscle cramps/spasm
	Joint pain
Nervous	
Dizziness*	Paresthesia/numbness
	Stupor
	Vertigo
Psychiatric	
None	Insomnia
	Nervousness
	Depression
	Sleepiness
	Mental confusion
Respiratory	
Dyspnea	None
Special Senses	
None	Bad taste
	Visual disturbance
	Nasal congestion

Continued on next page

Information on the Merck Sharp & Dohme products listed on these pages is the full prescribing information from product circulars in use August 31, 1986.

Merck Sharp & Dohme—Cont.

Urogenital	
None	Impotence
	Nocturia
	Dysuria
	Incontinence
	Renal dysfunction including renal failure

* Reactions occurring in 3% to 8% of patients treated with MODURETIC. (Those reactions occurring in less than 3% of the patients are unmarked.)

† See WARNINGS.

Other adverse reactions that have been reported with the individual components are listed below:

Amiloride—Body as a Whole: Fatigability, neck/shoulder ache, painful extremities; *Cardiovascular:* Palpitation; *Digestive:* Abnormal liver function, jaundice, activation of probable pre-existing peptic ulcer, heartburn, dyspepsia; *Integumentary:* Itching, alopecia, dry mouth; *Nervous System/Psychiatric:* Encephalopathy, tremors, decreased libido; *Respiratory:* Cough, shortness of breath; *Special Senses:* Tinnitus, increased intraocular pressure; *Hematologic:* Aplastic anemia, neutropenia; *Urogenital:* Polyuria, urinary frequency, bladder spasms.

Hydrochlorothiazide—Digestive: Cramping, gastric irritation, jaundice (intrahepatic cholestatic jaundice), pancreatitis, sialadenitis; *Metabolic:* Glycosuria, hyperglycemia, hyperuricemia, electrolyte imbalance (see PRECAUTIONS); *Nervous System/Psychiatric:* Restlessness; *Special Senses:* Transient blurred vision, xanthopsia; *Hematologic:* Agranulocytosis, aplastic anemia, hemolytic anemia, leukopenia, thrombocytopenia; *Hypersensitivity:* Purpura, photosensitivity, urticaria, necrotizing angiitis (vasculitis, cutaneous vasculitis), fever, respiratory distress including pneumonitis and pulmonary edema, anaphylactic reactions.

OVERDOSAGE

No data are available in regard to overdosage in humans.
The oral LD_{50} of the combination drug is 189 and 422 mg/kg for female mice and female rats, respectively.
It is not known whether the drug is dialyzable.
No specific information is available on the treatment of overdosage with MODURETIC, and no specific antidote is available. Treatment is symptomatic and supportive. Therapy with MODURETIC should be discontinued and the patient observed closely. Suggested measures include induction of emesis and/or gastric lavage.
Amiloride HCl: No data are available in regard to overdosage in humans.
The oral LD_{50} of amiloride HCl (calculated as the base) is 56 mg/kg in mice and 36 to 85 mg/kg in rats, depending on the strain.
The most common signs and symptoms to be expected with overdosage are dehydration and electrolyte imbalance. If hyperkalemia occurs, active measures should be taken to reduce the serum potassium levels.
Hydrochlorothiazide: The oral LD_{50} of hydrochlorothiazide is greater than 10.0 g/kg in both mice and rats.
The most common signs and symptoms observed are those caused by electrolyte depletion (hypokalemia, hypochloremia, hyponatremia) and dehydration resulting from excessive diuresis. If digitalis has also been administered, hypokalemia may accentuate cardiac arrhythmias.

DOSAGE AND ADMINISTRATION

MODURETIC should be administered with food.
The usual starting dosage is 1 tablet a day. The dosage may be increased to 2 tablets a day, if necessary. More than 2 tablets of MODURETIC daily usually are not needed and there is no controlled experience with such doses. The daily dose is usually given as a single dose but may be given in divided doses. Once an initial diuresis has been achieved, dosage adjustment may be necessary. Maintenance therapy may be on an intermittent basis.

HOW SUPPLIED

No. 3385—Tablets MODURETIC are peach-colored, diamond-shaped, scored, compressed tablets, coded MSD 917. Each tablet contains 5 mg of anhydrous amiloride HCl and 50 mg of hydrochlorothiazide. They are supplied as follows:
NDC 0006-0917-68 in bottles of 100
NDC 0006-0917-28 unit dose packages of 100.

Shown in Product Identification Section, page 417

A.H.F.S. Category: 40:28
DC 7168011 Issued October 1985

MUMPSVAX® ℞

(Mumps Virus Vaccine Live, MSD), U.S.P.
Jeryl Lynn Strain

DESCRIPTION

MUMPSVAX® (Mumps Virus Vaccine Live, MSD) is a live virus vaccine for immunization against mumps.
MUMPSVAX is a sterile lyophilized preparation of the Jeryl Lynn (B level) strain of mumps virus. The virus was adapted to and propagated in cell cultures of chick embryo free of avian leukosis virus and other adventitious agents.
The reconstituted vaccine is for subcutaneous administration. When reconstituted as directed, the dose for injection is 0.5 mL and contains not less than the equivalent of 5,000 $TCID_{50}$ (tissue culture infectious doses) of the U.S. Reference Mumps Virus. Each dose contains approximately 25 mcg of neomycin. The product contains no preservative. Sorbitol and hydrolized gelatin are added as stabilizers.

CLINICAL PHARMACOLOGY

MUMPSVAX produces a modified, non-communicable mumps infection in susceptible persons. Extensive clinical trials have demonstrated that MUMPSVAX is highly immunogenic and well tolerated. A single injection of the vaccine has been shown to induce mumps neutralizing antibodies in approximately 97 percent of susceptible children and approximately 93 percent of susceptible adults. The pattern of antibody response closely resembles that observed for natural mumps. Although the antibody level is significantly lower than that following natural infection, it is protective and long lasting. Vaccine-induced antibody levels have been shown to persist for at least 15 years with a rate of decline comparable to that seen in natural infection. If the present pattern continues, it will provide a basis for the expectation that immunity following vaccination will be permanent. However, continued surveillance will be required to demonstrate this point.

INDICATIONS AND USAGE

MUMPSVAX is indicated for immunization against mumps in persons 12 months of age or older. Most adults are likely to have been infected naturally and generally may be considered immune, even if they did not have clinically recognizable disease. A booster is not needed. It is not recommended for infants younger than 12 months because they may retain maternal mumps neutralizing antibodies which may interfere with the immune response.
Evidence indicates that the vaccine will not offer protection when given after exposure to natural mumps. Passively acquired antibody can interfere with the response to live, attenuated-virus vaccines. Therefore, administration of mumps virus vaccine should be deferred until approximately three months after passive immunization.
Revaccination: Children vaccinated when younger than 12 months of age should be revaccinated. Based on available evidence, there is no reason to routinely revaccinate persons who were vaccinated originally when 12 months of age or older. However, persons should be revaccinated if there is evidence to suggest that initial immunization was ineffective.
Use with other Vaccines
Routine administration of DTP (diphtheria, tetanus, pertussis) and/or OPV (oral poliovirus vaccine) concomitantly with measles, mumps and rubella vaccines is not recommended because there are insufficient data relating to the simultaneous administration of these antigens. However, the American Academy of Pediatrics has noted that in some circumstances, particularly when the patient may not return, some practitioners prefer to administer all these antigens on a single day. If done, separate sites and syringes should be used for DTP and MUMPSVAX.
MUMPSVAX should not be given less than one month before or after administration of other virus vaccines.

CONTRAINDICATIONS

Do not give MUMPSVAX to pregnant females; the possible effects of the vaccine on fetal development are unknown at this time. If vaccination of postpubertal females is undertaken, pregnancy should be avoided for three months following vaccination (see PRECAUTIONS, *Pregnancy*).
Anaphylactoid reaction to neomycin (each dose of reconstituted vaccine contains approximately 25 mcg of neomycin).
History of anaphylactoid reaction to eggs (see HYPERSENSITIVITY TO EGGS below).
Any febrile respiratory illness or other active febrile infection.
Active untreated tuberculosis.
Patients receiving immunosuppressive therapy. This contraindication does not apply to patients who are receiving corticosteroids as replacement therapy, e.g., for Addison's disease.
Individuals with blood dyscrasias, leukemia, lymphomas of any type, or other malignant neoplasms affecting the bone marrow or lymphatic systems.
Primary immunodeficiency states, including cellular immune deficiencies, hypogammaglobulinemic and dysgammaglobulinemic states.
Individuals with a family history of congenital or hereditary immunodeficiency, until the immune competence of the potential vaccine recipient is demonstrated.

HYPERSENSITIVITY TO EGGS

Live mumps vaccine is produced in chick embryo cell culture. Persons with a history of anaphylactic or other immediate reactions (e.g., hives, swelling of the mouth and throat, difficulty breathing, hypotension, or shock) subsequent to egg ingestion should be vaccinated only with extreme caution. Evidence indicates that persons are not at increased risk if they have egg allergies that are not anaphylactic in nature. Such persons may be vaccinated in the usual manner. There is no evidence to indicate that persons with allergies to chickens or feathers are at increased risk of reaction to the vaccine.

PRECAUTIONS

General
Adequate treatment provisions including epinephrine, should be available for immediate use should an anaphylactoid reaction occur.
Vaccination should be deferred for at least 3 months following blood or plasma transfusions, or administration of human immune serum globulin.
There are no reports of transmission of live mumps virus from vaccinees to susceptible contacts.
It has been reported that mumps virus vaccine, live, may result in a temporary depression of tuberculin skin sensitivity. Therefore, if a tuberculin test is to be done, it should be administered either before or simultaneously with MUMPSVAX.
As for any vaccine, vaccination with MUMPSVAX may not result in seroconversion in 100% of susceptible persons given the vaccine.
Pregnancy
Pregnancy Category C
Animal reproduction studies have not been conducted with MUMPSVAX. It is also not known whether MUMPSVAX can cause fetal harm when administered to a pregnant woman or can affect reproduction capacity. Therefore, mumps virus vaccine should not be given to persons known to be pregnant; furthermore, pregnancy should be avoided for three months following vaccination. Although mumps virus is capable of infecting the placenta and fetus, there is no good evidence that it causes congenital malformations in humans. Mumps vaccine virus also has been shown to infect the placenta, but the virus has not been isolated from the fetal tissues from susceptible women who were vaccinated and underwent elective abortions.
Nursing Mothers
It is not known whether mumps vaccine virus is secreted in human milk. Therefore, because many drugs are excreted in human milk, caution should be exercised when MUMPSVAX is administered to a nursing woman.

ADVERSE REACTIONS

Because of the slightly acidic pH (6.2–6.6) of the vaccine, patients may complain of burning and/or stinging of short duration at the injection site.
Mild fever occurs occasionally. Fever above 103°F (39.4°C) is uncommon.
Parotitis has been reported to occur in very low incidence, and orchitis rarely, in persons who were vaccinated. In most instances investigated, prior exposure to natural mumps was established. In other instances, whether or not this was due to vaccine or to prior natural mumps exposure or to other causes has not been established.
Reports of purpura and allergic reactions such as wheal and flare at the injection site or urticaria have been extremely rare.
Forms of optic neuritis, including retrobulbar neuritis and papillitis may infrequently follow viral infections, and have been reported to occur 1 to 3 weeks following inoculation with some live virus vaccines.
Very rarely encephalitis, febrile seizures, nerve deafness and other nervous system reactions have occurred in vaccinees. A cause-effect relationship has not been established.

DOSAGE AND ADMINISTRATION

FOR SUBCUTANEOUS ADMINISTRATION
Do not inject intravenously
The dosage of vaccine is the same for all persons. Inject the total volume (about 0.5 mL) of reconstituted vaccine subcutaneously, preferably into the outer aspect of upper arm. *Do*

not give immune serum globulin (ISG) concurrently with MUMPSVAX.
During shipment, to insure that there is no loss of potency, the vaccine must be maintained at a temperature of 10°C (50°F) or less.
Before reconstitution, store MUMPSVAX at 2–8°C (35.6–46.4°F). *Protect from light.*
CAUTION: A sterile syringe free of preservatives, antiseptics, and detergents should be used for each injection and/or reconstitution of the vaccine because these substances may inactivate the live virus vaccine. A 25 gauge, ⅝" needle is recommended.
To reconstitute, use only the diluent supplied, since it is free of preservatives or other antiviral substances which might inactivate the vaccine.

Single Dose Vial—First withdraw the entire volume of diluent into the syringe to be used for reconstitution. Inject all the diluent in the syringe into the vial of lyophilized vaccine, and agitate to mix thoroughly. Withdraw the entire contents into a syringe and inject the total volume of restored vaccine subcutaneously.
It is important to use a separate sterile syringe and needle for each individual patient to prevent transmission of hepatitis B and other infectious agents from one person to another.

10 Dose Vial (available only to government agencies/institutions)—Withdraw the entire contents (7 mL) of the diluent vial into the sterile syringe to be used for reconstitution, and introduce into the 10 dose vial of lyophilized vaccine. Agitate to ensure thorough mixing. The outer labeling suggests "For Jet Injector or Syringe Use". Use with separate sterile syringes is permitted for containers of 10 doses or less. The vaccine and diluent do not contain preservatives; therefore, the user must recognize the potential contamination hazards and exercise special precautions to protect the sterility and potency of the product. The use of aseptic techniques and proper storage prior to and after restoration of the vaccine and subsequent withdrawal of the individual doses is essential. Use 0.5 mL of the reconstituted vaccine for subcutaneous injection.
It is important to use a separate sterile syringe and needle for each individual patient to prevent transmission of hepatitis B and other infectious agents from one person to another.

50 Dose Vial (available only to government agencies/institutions)—Withdraw the entire contents (30 mL) of the diluent vial into the sterile syringe to be used for reconstitution and introduce into the 50 dose vial of lyophilized vaccine. Agitate to ensure thorough mixing. With full aseptic precautions, attach the vial to the sterilized multidose jet injector apparatus. Use 0.5 mL of the reconstituted vaccine for subcutaneous injection.

Each dose of MUMPSVAX contains not less than the equivalent of 5,000 $TCID_{50}$ of the U.S. Reference Mumps Virus.
Parenteral drug products should be inspected visually for particulate matter and discoloration prior to administration. MUMPSVAX, when reconstituted, is clear yellow.

HOW SUPPLIED

No. 4753—MUMPSVAX is supplied as a single-dose vial of lyophilized vaccine, **NDC** 0006-4753-00, and a vial of diluent.
No. 4584X/4309—MUMPSVAX is supplied as follows: (1) a box of 10 single-dose vials of lyophilized vaccine (package A), **NDC** 0006-4584-00; and (2) a box of 10 vials of diluent (package B). To conserve refrigerator space, the diluent may be stored separately at room temperature.
Available only to government agencies/institutions:
No. 4664X—MUMPSVAX is supplied as one 10 dose vial of lyophilized vaccine, **NDC** 0006-4664-00, and one 7 mL vial of diluent.
No. 4593X—MUMPSVAX is supplied as one 50 dose vial of lyophilized vaccine, **NDC** 0006-4593-00, and one 30 mL vial of diluent.

Storage
It is recommended that the vaccine be used as soon as possible after reconstitution. Protect vaccine from light at all times, since such exposure may inactivate the virus. Store reconstituted vaccine in the vaccine vial in a dark place at 2–8°C (35.6–46.4°F) and discard if not used within 8 hours.

A.H.F.S. Category: 80:12
DC 7075407 Issued October 1984

MUSTARGEN®, Trituration of (Mechlorethamine HCl for Injection, MSD), U.S.P. ℞

DESCRIPTION

MUSTARGEN® (Mechlorethamine HCl, MSD) a nitrogen mustard also known as HN2 hydrochloride, is a nitrogen analog of sulfur mustard. It is a white, crystalline, hygroscopic powder that is very soluble in water and also soluble in alcohol.

Mechlorethamine hydrochloride is designated chemically as 2-chloro- *N* -(2-chloroethyl)- *N* -methylethanamine hydrochloride. The molecular weight is 192.52 and the melting point is 108–111°C. The empirical formula is $C_5H_{11}Cl_2N \cdot HCl$, and the structural formula is: $CH_3N(CH_2CH_2Cl)_2 \cdot HCl$.
Trituration of MUSTARGEN is a white crystalline powder. Each vial of MUSTARGEN contains 10 mg of mechlorethamine hydrochloride triturated with sodium chloride q.s. 100 mg.

ACTIONS

Mechlorethamine, a biologic alkylating agent, has a cytotoxic action which inhibits rapidly proliferating cells.

INDICATIONS

Before using MUSTARGEN *see Contraindications, Warnings, Precautions, Adverse Reactions, and Dosage and Administration.*
MUSTARGEN, administered intravenously, is indicated for the palliative treatment of Hodgkin's disease (Stages III and IV), lymphosarcoma, chronic myelocytic or chronic lymphocytic leukemia, polycythemia vera, mycosis fungoides, and bronchogenic carcinoma.
MUSTARGEN, administered intrapleurally, intraperitoneally, or intrapericardially, is indicated for the palliative treatment of metastatic carcinoma resulting in effusion.

CONTRAINDICATIONS

Because of the toxicity of MUSTARGEN, and the unpleasant side effects following its use, the potential risk and discomfort from the use of this drug in patients with inoperable neoplasms or in the terminal stage of the disease must be balanced against the limited gain obtainable. These gains will vary with the nature and the status of the disease under treatment. The routine use of MUSTARGEN in all cases of widely disseminated neoplasms is to be discouraged.
The use of MUSTARGEN in patients with leukopenia, thrombocytopenia, and anemia, due to invasion of the bone marrow by tumor carries a greater risk. In such patients a good response to treatment with disappearance of the tumor from the bone marrow may be associated with improvement of bone marrow function. However, in the absence of a good response or in patients who have been previously treated with chemotherapeutic agents, hematopoiesis may be further compromised, and leukopenia, thrombocytopenia and anemia may become more severe and lead to the demise of the patient.
Tumors of bone and nervous tissue have responded poorly to therapy. Its use is contraindicated in the presence of known infectious diseases. Results are unpredictable in disseminated and malignant tumors of different types.

WARNINGS

> Extravasation of the drug into subcutaneous tissues results in a painful inflammation. The area usually becomes indurated and sloughing may occur. If leakage of drug is obvious, prompt infiltration of the area with sterile isotonic sodium thiosulfate (⅙ molar) and application of an ice compress for 6 to 12 hours may minimize the local reaction. For a ⅙ molar solution of sodium thiosulfate use 4.14 g of sodium thiosulfate per 100 ml of Sterile Water for Injection or 2.64 g of anhydrous sodium thiosulfate per 100 ml, or dilute 4 ml of Sodium Thiosulfate Injection (10%) with 6 ml of Sterile Water for Injection.

Before using MUSTARGEN, *an accurate histologic diagnosis of the disease, a knowledge of its natural course, and an adequate clinical history are important. The hematologic status of the patient must first be determined. It is essential to understand the hazards and therapeutic effects to be expected. Careful clinical judgment must be exercised in selecting patients. If the indication for its use is not clear, the drug should not be used.*
As nitrogen mustard therapy may contribute to extensive and rapid development of amyloidosis, it should be used only if foci of acute and chronic suppurative inflammation are absent.

Usage in Pregnancy
There is evidence that the nitrogen mustards have induced fetal abnormalities particularly when used early in pregnancy. The possible benefits of administration of MUSTARGEN in women of childbearing potential must be weighed against the considered risks; patients should be apprised of the risks involved. In pregnant patients requiring treatment for a life-threatening progressive tumor, use of MUSTARGEN should be avoided at least until the third trimester.

Nursing Mothers
Although breast milk studies have not been performed in animals or humans, breast feeding should be stopped before beginning treatment with MUSTARGEN.

PRECAUTIONS

This drug is highly toxic and both powder and solution must be handled and administered with care. Since MUSTARGEN is a powerful vesicant, it is intended primarily for intravenous use, and in most instances is given by this route. Inhalation of dust or vapors and contact with skin or mucous membranes, especially those of the eyes, must be avoided. Should accidental eye contact occur, copious irrigation with water, normal saline or a balanced salt ophthalmic irrigating solution should be instituted immediately, followed by prompt ophthalmologic consultation. Should accidental skin contact occur, the affected part must be irrigated immediately with copious amounts of water, for at least 15 minutes, followed by 2 percent sodium thiosulfate solution. (See also box warning.)
Do not use if the solution is discolored or if droplets of water are visible within the vial. Prepare fresh solution for injection and dispose of the unused portion after neutralization. (See DOSAGE AND ADMINISTRATION.)
Precautions must be observed with the use of MUSTARGEN and x-ray therapy or other chemotherapy in alternating courses. Hematopoietic function is characteristically depressed by either form of therapy, and neither MUSTARGEN following x-ray therapy nor x-ray therapy subsequent to the drug should be given until bone marrow function has recovered. In particular, irradiation of such areas as sternum, ribs, and vertebrae shortly after a course of nitrogen mustard may lead to hematologic complications.
Therapy with alkylating agents such as MUSTARGEN may be associated with an increased incidence of a second malignant tumor, especially when such therapy is combined with other antineoplastic agents or radiation therapy.
Hyperuricemia may develop during therapy with MUSTARGEN. The problem of urate precipitation should be anticipated, particularly in the treatment of the lymphomas, and adequate methods for control of hyperuricemia should be instituted and careful attention directed toward adequate fluid intake before treatment.
Since drug toxicity, especially sensitivity to bone marrow failure, seems to be more common in chronic lymphatic leukemia than in other conditions, the drug should be given in this condition with great caution, if at all.

ADVERSE REACTIONS

Clinical use of MUSTARGEN *usually is accompanied by toxic manifestations.*

Local Toxicity
Thrombosis and thrombophlebitis may result from direct contact of the drug with the intima of the injected vein. Avoid high concentration and prolonged contact with the drug, especially in cases of elevated pressure in the antebrachial vein (e.g., in mediastinal tumor compression from severe vena cava syndrome).

Systemic Toxicity
Nausea, vomiting and depression of formed elements in the circulating blood are dose-limiting side effects and usually occur with the use of full doses of MUSTARGEN. Jaundice, alopecia, vertigo, tinnitus and diminished hearing may occur infrequently. Rarely, hemolytic anemia associated with such diseases as the lymphomas and chronic lymphocytic leukemia may be precipitated by treatment with alkylating agents including MUSTARGEN. Also, various chromosomal abnormalities have been reported in association with nitrogen mustard therapy.
MUSTARGEN is given preferably at night in case sedation for side effects is required. Nausea and vomiting usually occur 1 to 3 hours after use of the drug. Emesis may disappear in the first 8 hours, but nausea may persist for 24 hours. Nausea and vomiting may be so severe as to precipitate vascular accidents in patients with a hemorrhagic tendency. Premedication with antiemetics, in addition to sedatives, may help control severe nausea and vomiting. Anorexia, weakness and diarrhea may also occur.
The usual course of MUSTARGEN (total dose of 0.4 mg/kg either given as a single intravenous dose or divided into two or four daily doses of 0.2 or 0.1 mg/kg respectively) generally produces a lymphocytopenia within 24 hours after the first injection; significant granulocytopenia occurs within 6 to 8 days and lasts for 10 days to 3 weeks. Agranulocytosis appears to be relatively infrequent and recovery from leukopenia in most cases is complete within two weeks of the maxi-

Continued on next page

Information on the Merck Sharp & Dohme products listed on these pages is the full prescribing information from product circulars in use August 31, 1986.

Merck Sharp & Dohme—Cont.

mum reduction. Thrombocytopenia is variable but the time course of the appearance and recovery from reduced platelet counts generally parallels the sequence of granulocyte levels. In some cases severe thrombocytopenia may lead to bleeding from the gums and gastrointestinal tract, petechiae, and small subcutaneous hemorrhages; these symptoms appear to be transient and in most cases disappear with return to a normal platelet count. However, a severe and even uncontrollable depression of the hematopoietic system occasionally may follow the usual dose of MUSTARGEN, particularly in patients with widespread disease and debility and in patients previously treated with other antineoplastic agents or x-ray. Persistent pancytopenia has been reported. In rare instances, hemorrhagic complications may be due to hyperheparinemia. Erythrocyte and hemoglobin levels may decline during the first 2 weeks after therapy but rarely significantly. Depression of the hematopoietic system may be found up to 50 days or more after starting therapy.
MUSTARGEN has been reported to have immunosuppressive activity. Therefore, it should be borne in mind that use of the drug may predispose the patient to bacterial, viral or fungal infection. This is more likely to occur when concomitant steroid therapy is employed.
Occasionally, a maculopapular skin eruption occurs, but this may be idiosyncratic and does not necessarily recur with subsequent courses of the drug. In one patient erythema multiforme has been observed. Herpes zoster, a common complicating infection in patients with lymphomas, may first appear after therapy is instituted and on occasion may be precipitated by treatment. Further treatment should be discontinued during the acute phase of this illness to avoid progression to generalized herpes zoster.
Since the gonads are susceptible to MUSTARGEN, treatment may be followed by delayed catamenia, oligomenorrhea, or temporary or permanent amenorrhea. Impaired spermatogenesis, azoospermia, and total germinal aplasia have been reported in male patients treated with alkylating agents, especially in combination with other drugs. In some instances spermatogenesis may return in patients in remission, but this may occur only several years after intensive chemotherapy has been discontinued. Patients should be warned of the potential risk to their reproductive capacity.
With total doses exceeding 0.4 mg/kg of body weight for a single course, severe leukopenia, anemia, thrombocytopenia and a hemorrhagic diathesis with subsequent delayed bleeding may develop. Death may follow. The only treatment in instances of excessive dosage appears to be repeated blood product transfusions, antibiotic treatment of complicating infections and general supportive measures. *Extreme caution must be used in exceeding the average recommended dose.*

DOSAGE AND ADMINISTRATION

Intravenous Administration
The dosage of MUSTARGEN varies with the clinical situation, the therapeutic response and the magnitude of hematologic depression. A total dose of 0.4 mg/kg of body weight for each course usually is given either as a single dose or in divided doses of 0.1 to 0.2 mg/kg per day. Dosage should be based on ideal dry body weight. The presence of edema or ascites must be considered so that dosage will be based on actual weight unaugmented by these conditions.
Within a few minutes after intravenous injection, MUSTARGEN undergoes chemical transformation, combines with reactive compounds, and is no longer present in its active form in the blood stream. Subsequent courses should not be given until the patient has recovered hematologically from the previous course; this is best determined by repeated studies of the peripheral blood elements awaiting their return to normal levels. It is often possible to give repeated courses of MUSTARGEN as early as three weeks after treatment.
The margin of safety in therapy with MUSTARGEN *is narrow and considerable care must be exercised in the matter of dosage.* Repeated examinations of blood are *mandatory* as a guide to subsequent therapy.
Preparation of Solution and Intravenous Administration
Each vial of MUSTARGEN contains 10 mg of mechlorethamine hydrochloride triturated with sodium chloride q.s. 100 mg. In neutral or alkaline aqueous solution it undergoes rapid chemical transformation and is highly unstable. Although solutions prepared according to instructions are acidic and do not decompose as rapidly, they should be prepared immediately before each injection since they will decompose on standing.
Using a sterile 10 ml syringe, inject 10 ml of Sterile Water for Injection or 10 ml Sodium Chloride Injection into a vial of MUSTARGEN. With the needle still in the rubber stopper, shake the vial several times to dissolve the drug completely. The resultant solution contains 1 mg of mechlorethamine hydrochloride per ml.
Withdraw into the syringe the calculated volume of solution required for a single injection. *Dispose of any remaining solution after neutralization* (see below). Although the drug may be injected directly into any suitable vein, it is injected preferably into the rubber or plastic tubing of a flowing intravenous infusion set. This reduces the possibility of severe local reactions due to extravasation or high concentration of the drug. Injecting the drug into the tubing rather than adding it to the entire volume of the infusion fluid minimizes a chemical reaction between the drug and the solution. The rate of injection apparently is not critical provided it is completed within a few minutes.

Intracavitary Administration
Nitrogen mustard has been used by intracavitary administration with varying success in certain malignant conditions for the control of pleural, peritoneal, and pericardial effusions caused by malignant cells.
The technic and the dose used by any of these routes varies. Therefore, if MUSTARGEN is given by the intracavitary route, the published articles concerning such use should be consulted. *Because of the inherent risks involved, the physician should be experienced in the appropriate injection technics, and be thoroughly aware of the indications, dosages, hazards, and precautions as set forth in the published literature. When using* MUSTARGEN *by the intracavitary route, the general precautions concerning this agent should be borne in mind.*
As a general guide, reference is made especially to the technics of Weisberger et al. Intracavitary use is indicated in the presence of pleural, peritoneal, or pericardial effusion due to metastatic tumors. Local therapy with nitrogen mustard is used only when malignant cells are demonstrated in the effusion. Intracavitary injection is not recommended when the accumulated fluid is chylous in nature, since results are likely to be poor.
Paracentesis is first performed with most of the fluid being removed from the pleural or peritoneal cavity. The intracavitary use of MUSTARGEN may exert at least some of its effect through production of a chemical poudrage. Therefore, the removal of excess fluid allows the drug to more easily contact the peritoneal and pleural linings. For intrapleural or intrapericardial injection nitrogen mustard is introduced directly through the thoracentesis needle. For intraperitoneal injection it is given through a rubber catheter inserted into the trocar used for paracentesis or through a No. 18 gauge needle inserted at another site. This drug should be injected slowly, with frequent aspiration to ensure that a free flow of fluid is present. If fluid cannot be aspirated, pain and necrosis due to injection of solution outside the cavity may occur. Free flow of fluid also is necessary to prevent injection into a loculated pocket and to ensure adequate dissemination of nitrogen mustard.
The usual dose of nitrogen mustard for intracavitary injection is 0.4 mg/kg of body weight, though 0.2 mg/kg (or 10 to 20 mg) has been used by the intrapericardial route. The solution is prepared, as previously described for intravenous injection, by adding 10 ml of Sterile Water for Injection or 10 ml of Sodium Chloride Injection to the vial containing 10 mg of mechlorethamine hydrochloride. (Amounts of diluent of 50 to 100 ml of normal saline have also been used.) The position of the patient should be changed every 5 to 10 minutes for an hour after injection to obtain more uniform distribution of the drug throughout the serous cavity. The remaining fluid may be removed from the pleural or peritoneal cavity by paracentesis 24 to 36 hours later. The patient should be followed carefully by clinical and x-ray examination to detect reaccumulation of fluid.
Pain occurs rarely with intrapleural use; it is common with intraperitoneal injection and is often associated with nausea, vomiting, and diarrhea of 2 to 3 days duration. Transient cardiac irregularities may occur with intrapericardial injection. Death, possibly accelerated by nitrogen mustard, has been reported following the use of this agent by the intracavitary route. Although absorption of MUSTARGEN when given by the intracavitary route is probably not complete because of its rapid deactivation by body fluids, the systemic effect is unpredictable. The acute side effects such as nausea and vomiting are usually mild. Bone marrow depression is generally milder than when the drug is given intravenously. Care should be taken to avoid use by the intracavitary route when other agents which may suppress bone marrow function are being used systemically.

Neutralization of Equipment and Unused Solution
To clean rubber gloves, tubing, glassware, etc., after giving MUSTARGEN, soak them in an aqueous solution containing equal volumes of sodium thiosulfate (5%) and sodium bicarbonate (5%) for 45 minutes. Excess reagents and reaction products are washed away easily with water. Any unused injection solution should be neutralized by mixing with an equal volume of sodium thiosulfate/sodium bicarbonate solution. Allow the mixture to stand for 45 minutes. Vials that have contained MUSTARGEN should be treated in the same way with thiosulfate/bicarbonate solution before disposal.

HOW SUPPLIED

No. 7753—Trituration of MUSTARGEN is a white crystalline powder, each vial containing 10 mg mechlorethamine hydrochloride with sodium chloride q.s. 100 mg, and is supplied as follows:
NDC 0006-7753-31 in treatment sets of 4 vials.
Special Handling
Due to the drug's toxic and mutagenic properties, appropriate precautions including the use of appropriate safety equipment are recommended for the preparation of MUSTARGEN for parenteral administration. The National Institutes of Health presently recommends that the preparation of injectable antineoplastic drugs should be performed in a Class II laminar flow biological safety cabinet and that personnel preparing drugs of this class should wear surgical gloves and a closed front surgical-type gown with knit cuffs.
A.H.F.S. Category: 10:00
DC 6382424 Issued September 1983

MYOCHRYSINE® Injection ℞
(Gold Sodium Thiomalate, MSD), U.S.P.

Physicians planning to use MYOCHRYSINE® *(Gold Sodium Thiomalate, MSD) should thoroughly familiarize themselves with its toxicity and its benefits. The possibility of toxic reactions should always be explained to the patient before starting therapy. Patients should be warned to report promptly any symptoms suggesting toxicity. Before each injection of* MYOCHRYSINE, *the physician should review the results of laboratory work, and see the patient to determine the presence or absence of adverse reactions since some of these can be severe or even fatal.*

DESCRIPTION

MYOCHRYSINE is a sterile aqueous solution of gold sodium thiomalate. It contains 0.5 percent benzyl alcohol added as a preservative. The pH of the product is 5.8–6.5.
Gold sodium thiomalate is a mixture of the mono- and disodium salts of gold thiomalic acid. The structural formula is:

$$\begin{array}{l} \quad\;\; CH_2COO^- \\ \quad\;\; | \\ Au{-}S{-}CHCOO^- \end{array} \cdot\; xNa^+ \;\cdot\; (2-x)H^+$$

mercaptobutanedioic acid, monogold (1+) sodium salt
The molecular weight for $C_4H_3AuNa_2O_4S$ (the disodium salt) is 390.07 and for $C_4H_4AuNaO_4S$ (the monosodium salt) is 368.09.
MYOCHRYSINE is supplied as a solution for intramuscular injection containing 10 mg, 25 mg, or 50 mg of gold sodium thiomalate per mL.

CLINICAL PHARMACOLOGY

The mode of action of gold sodium thiomalate is unknown. The predominant action appears to be a suppressive effect on the synovitis of active rheumatoid disease.

INDICATIONS AND USAGE

MYOCHRYSINE is indicated in the treatment of selected cases of active rheumatoid arthritis— both adult and juvenile type. The greatest benefit occurs in the early active stage. In late stages of the illness when cartilage and bone damage have occurred, gold can only check the progression of rheumatoid arthritis and prevent further structural damage to joints. It cannot repair damage caused by previously active disease.
MYOCHRYSINE should be used only as *one part* of a complete program of therapy; alone it is not a complete treatment.

CONTRAINDICATIONS

Severe toxicity resulting from previous exposure to gold or other heavy metals.
Severe debilitation.
Systemic lupus erythematosus.

WARNINGS

Before treatment is started, the patient's hemoglobin, erythrocyte, white blood cell, differential and platelet counts should be determined, and urinalysis should be done to serve as basic reference. Urine should be analyzed for protein and sediment changes prior to each injection. Complete blood counts including platelet estimation should be made before every second injection throughout treatment. The occurrence of purpura or ecchymoses at any time always requires a platelet count.

Danger signals of possible gold toxicity include: rapid reduction of hemoglobin, leukopenia below 4000 WBC/cu mL, eosinophilia above 5 percent, platelet decrease below 100,000/cu mL, albuminuria, hematuria, pruritus, skin eruption, stomatitis, or persistent diarrhea. No additional injections of MYOCHRYSINE should be given unless further studies show these abnormalities to be caused by conditions other than gold toxicity.

PRECAUTIONS

General
Gold salts should not be used concomitantly with penicillamine.
The safety of coadministration with cytotoxic drugs has not been established.
Caution is indicated in the use of MYOCHRYSINE in patients with the following:
1. a history of blood dyscrasias such as granulocytopenia or anemia caused by drug sensitivity,
2. allergy or hypersensitivity to medications,
3. skin rash,
4. previous kidney or liver disease,
5. marked hypertension,
6. compromised cerebral or cardiovascular circulation.

Diabetes mellitus or congestive heart failure should be under control before gold therapy is instituted.
Carcinogenicity
Renal adenomas have been reported in long-term toxicity studies of rats receiving MYOCHRYSINE at high dose levels (2 mg/kg weekly for 45 weeks, followed by 6 mg/kg daily for 47 weeks), approximately 2 to 42 times the usual human dose. These adenomas are histologically similar to those produced in rats by chronic administration of experimental gold compounds and other heavy metals, such as lead. No reports have been received of renal adenomas in man in association with the use of MYOCHRYSINE.
Pregnancy
Pregnancy Category C.
MYOCHRYSINE has been shown to be teratogenic during the organogenetic period in rats and rabbits when given in doses, respectively, of 140 and 175 times the usual human dose. Hydrocephaly and microphthalmia were the malformations observed in rats when MYOCHRYSINE was administered subcutaneously at a dose of 25 mg/kg/day from day 6 through day 15 of gestation. In rabbits, limb malformations and gastroschisis were the malformations observed when MYOCHRYSINE was administered subcutaneously at doses of 20–45 mg/kg/day from day 6 through day 18 of gestation. There are no adequate and well-controlled studies in pregnant women. MYOCHRYSINE should be used during pregnancy only if the potential benefit to the mother justifies the potential risk to the fetus.
Nursing Mothers
The presence of gold has been demonstrated in the milk of lactating mothers. In addition, gold has been found in the serum and red blood cells of a nursing infant. In view of the above findings and because of the potential for serious adverse reactions in nursing infants from MYOCHRYSINE, a decision should be made whether to discontinue nursing or to discontinue the drug, taking into account the importance of the drug to the mother. The slow excretion and persistence of gold in the mother, even after therapy is discontinued, must also be kept in mind.

ADVERSE REACTIONS

A variety of adverse reactions may develop during the initial phase (weekly injections) of therapy or during maintenance treatment. Adverse reactions are observed most frequently when the cumulative dose of MYOCHRYSINE administered is between 400 and 800 mg. Very uncommonly, complications occur days to months after cessation of treatment.
Cutaneous reactions: Dermatitis is the most common reaction. *Any eruption, especially if pruritic, that develops during treatment with* MYOCHRYSINE *should be considered a reaction to gold until proven otherwise.* Pruritus often exists before dermatitis becomes apparent, and therefore should be considered a warning signal of impending cutaneous reaction. The most serious form of cutaneous reaction is generalized exfoliative dermatitis which may lead to alopecia and shedding of nails. Gold dermatitis may be aggravated by exposure to sunlight or an actinic rash may develop.
Mucous membrane reactions: Stomatitis is the second most common adverse reaction. Shallow ulcers on the buccal membranes, on the borders of the tongue, and on the palate or in the pharynx may occur as the only adverse reaction, or along with dermatitis. Sometimes diffuse glossitis or gingivitis develops. A metallic taste may precede these oral mucous membrane reactions and should be considered a warning signal.
Conjunctivitis is a rare reaction.
Renal reactions: Gold may be toxic to the kidney and produce a nephrotic syndrome or glomerulitis with hematuria. These renal reactions are usually relatively mild and subside completely if recognized early and treatment is discontinued. They may become severe and chronic if treatment is continued after onset of the reaction. Therefore, it is important to perform a *urinalysis before every injection,* and to discontinue treatment promptly if proteinuria or hematuria develops.
Hematologic reactions: Blood dyscrasia due to gold toxicity is rare, but because of the potential serious consequences it must be constantly watched for and recognized early by frequent blood examinations done throughout treatment. Granulocytopenia; thrombocytopenia, with or without purpura; hypoplastic and aplastic anemia; and eosinophilia have all been reported. These hematologic disorders may occur separately or in combinations.
Nitritoid and allergic reactions: Reactions of the "nitritoid type" which may resemble anaphylactoid effects have been reported. Flushing, fainting, dizziness and sweating are most frequently reported. Other symptoms that may occur include: nausea, vomiting, malaise and weakness.
More severe, but less common effects include: anaphylactic shock, syncope, bradycardia, thickening of the tongue, difficulty in swallowing and breathing, and angioneurotic edema. These effects may occur almost immediately after injection or as late as 10 minutes following injection. They may occur at any time during the course of therapy and if observed, treatment with MYOCHRYSINE should be discontinued.
Miscellaneous reactions: Gastrointestinal reactions have been reported, including nausea, vomiting, anorexia, abdominal cramps and diarrhea. Ulcerative enterocolitis, which can be severe or even fatal, has been reported rarely.
There have been rare reports of reactions involving the eye such as iritis, corneal ulcers, and gold deposits in ocular tissues. Peripheral and central nervous system complications have been reported rarely. Peripheral neuropathy, with or without fasciculations, sensorimotor effects (including Guillain-Barré syndrome) and elevated spinal fluid protein have been reported. Central nervous system complications have included confusion, hallucinations and seizures. Usually these signs and symptoms cleared upon discontinuation of gold therapy.
Hepatitis, jaundice, with or without cholestasis, gold bronchitis, pulmonary injury manifested by interstitial pneumonitis and fibrosis, partial or complete hair loss and fever have also been reported.
Sometimes arthralgia occurs for a day or two after an injection of MYOCHRYSINE; this reaction usually subsides after the first few injections.

MANAGEMENT OF ADVERSE REACTIONS

Treatment with MYOCHRYSINE should be discontinued immediately when toxic reactions occur. Minor complications such as localized dermatitis, mild stomatitis, or slight proteinuria generally require no other therapy and resolve spontaneously with suspension of MYOCHRYSINE. Moderately severe skin and mucous membrane reactions often benefit from topical corticosteroids, oral antihistaminics, and soothing or anesthetic lotions.
If stomatitis or dermatitis becomes severe or more generalized, systemic corticosteroids (generally, prednisone 10 to 40 mg daily in divided doses) may provide symptomatic relief.
For serious renal, hematologic, pulmonary, and enterocolitic complications, high doses of systemic corticosteroids (prednisone 40 to 100 mg daily in divided doses) are recommended. The optimum duration of corticosteroid treatment varies with the response of the individual patient. Therapy may be required for many months when adverse effects are unusually severe or progressive.
In patients whose complications do not improve with high-dose corticosteroid treatment, or who develop significant steroid-related adverse reactions, a chelating agent may be given to enhance gold excretion. Dimercaprol (BAL) has been used successfully, but patients must be monitored carefully as numerous untoward reactions may attend its use. Corticosteroids and a chelating agent may be used concomitantly.
MYOCHRYSINE *should not be reinstituted after severe or idiosyncratic reactions.*
MYOCHRYSINE may be readministered following resolution of mild reactions, using a reduced dosage schedule. If an initial test dose of 5 mg MYOCHRYSINE is well-tolerated, progressively larger doses (5 to 10 mg increments) may be given at weekly to monthly intervals until a dose of 25 to 50 mg is reached.

DOSAGE AND ADMINISTRATION

MYOCHRYSINE should be administered only by intramuscular injection, preferably intragluteally. It should be given with the patient lying down. He should remain recumbent for approximately 10 minutes after the injection.
Therapeutic effects from MYOCHRYSINE occur slowly. Early improvement, often limited to a reduction in morning stiffness, may begin after six to eight weeks of treatment, but beneficial effects may not be observed until after months of therapy.
Parenteral drug products should be inspected visually for particulate matter and discoloration prior to administration. Do not use if material has darkened. Color should not exceed pale yellow.
For the adult of average size the following dosage schedule is suggested:

Weekly Injections
1st injection .... 10 mg
2nd injection .... 25 mg
3rd and subsequent injections, 25 to 50 mg

until there is toxicity or major clinical improvement, or, in the absence of either of these, the cumulative dose of MYOCHRYSINE reaches one gram.
MYOCHRYSINE is continued until the cumulative dose reaches one gram unless toxicity or major clinical improvement occurs. If significant clinical improvement occurs before a cumulative dose of one gram has been administered, the dose may be decreased or the interval between injections increased as with maintenance therapy. Maintenance doses of 25 to 50 mg every other week for two to 20 weeks are recommended. If the clinical course remains stable, injections of 25 to 50 mg may be given every third and subsequently every fourth week indefinitely. Some patients may require maintenance treatment at intervals of one to three weeks. Should the arthritis exacerbate during maintenance therapy, weekly injections may be resumed temporarily until disease activity is suppressed.
Should a patient fail to improve during initial therapy (cumulative dose of one gram), several options are available:
1— the patient may be considered to be unresponsive and MYOCHRYSINE is discontinued
2— the same dose (25 to 50 mg) of MYOCHRYSINE may be continued for approximately ten additional weeks
3— the dose of MYOCHRYSINE may be increased by increments of 10 mg every one to four weeks, not to exceed 100 mg in a single injection.

If significant clinical improvement occurs using option 2 or 3, the maintenance schedule described above should be initiated. If there is no significant improvement or if toxicity occurs, therapy with MYOCHRYSINE should be stopped. The higher the individual dose of MYOCHRYSINE, the greater the risk of gold toxicity. Selection of one of these options for chrysotherapy should be based upon a number of factors, including the physician's experience with gold salt therapy, the course of the patient's condition, the choice of alternative treatments, and the availability of the patient for the close supervision required.
Juvenile Rheumatoid Arthritis
The pediatric dose of MYOCHRYSINE is proportional to the adult dose on a weight basis. After the initial test dose of 10 mg, the recommended dose for children is one mg per kilogram body weight, not to exceed 50 mg for a single injection. Otherwise, the guidelines given above for administration to adults also apply to children.
Concomitant Drug Therapy—Gold salts should not be used concomitantly with penicillamine.
The safety of coadministration with cytotoxic drugs has not been established. Other measures, such as salicylates, other non-steroidal anti-inflammatory drugs, or systemic corticosteroids, may be continued when MYOCHRYSINE is initiated. After improvement commences, analgesic and anti-inflammatory drugs may be discontinued slowly as symptoms permit.

HOW SUPPLIED

Injection MYOCHRYSINE is a clear colorless to light yellow solution, depending on potency, which must be protected from light. It is supplied as follows:
No. 7763—10 mg of gold sodium thiomalate per mL as
NDC 0006-7763-64 in boxes of 6 x 1 mL ampuls.
No. 7764—25 mg of gold sodium thiomalate per mL as
NDC 0006-7764-64 in boxes of 6 x 1 mL ampuls.
No. 7762—50 mg of gold sodium thiomalate per mL as
NDC 0006-7762-64 in boxes of 6 x 1 mL ampuls.
NDC 0006-7762-10 in 10 mL vials.

A.H.F.S. Category: 60:00
DC 6015524 Revised August 1985

Continued on next page

Information on the Merck Sharp & Dohme products listed on these pages is the full prescribing information from product circulars in use August 31, 1986.

Merck Sharp & Dohme—Cont.

NEODECADRON® Sterile Ophthalmic Ointment ℞
(Neomycin Sulfate-Dexamethasone Sodium Phosphate, MSD), U.S.P.

DESCRIPTION

Sterile ophthalmic ointment NEODECADRON® (Neomycin Sulfate-Dexamethasone Sodium Phosphate, MSD) is a topical corticosteroid-antibiotic ointment for use in certain disorders of the anterior segment of the eye.
Ophthalmic ointment NEODECADRON contains in each gram: dexamethasone sodium phosphate equivalent to 0.5 mg (0.05%) dexamethasone phosphate and neomycin sulfate equivalent to 3.5 mg neomycin base. Inactive ingredients: white petrolatum and mineral oil.
Dexamethasone sodium phosphate is an inorganic ester of dexamethasone. Its empirical formula is $C_{22}H_{28}FNa_2O_8P$.
Neomycin sulfate is the sulfate salt of neomycin, an antibacterial substance produced by the growth of *Streptomyces fradiae* Waksman (Fam. Streptomycetaceae).

CLINICAL PHARMACOLOGY

Dexamethasone sodium phosphate, a corticosteroid, suppresses the inflammatory response to a variety of agents, and it probably delays or slows healing. Since corticosteroids may inhibit the body's defense mechanism against infection, a concomitant antimicrobial drug may be used when this inhibition is considered to be clinically significant in a particular case.
Neomycin sulfate, the anti-infective component in the combination, is included to provide action against specific organisms susceptible to it. Neomycin sulfate is considered active mainly against gram-negative organisms, except *Bacteroides* spp. and *Pseudomonas aeruginosa,* which are resistant. Gram-positive organisms except for *Staphylococcus aureus* are usually resistant.
When a decision to administer both a corticosteroid and an antimicrobial is made, the administration of such drugs in combination has the advantage of greater patient compliance and convenience, with the added assurance that the appropriate dosage of both drugs is administered, plus assured compatibility of ingredient when both types of drug are in the same formulation and, particularly, that the correct volume of drug is delivered and retained.
The relative potency of corticosteroids depends on the molecular structure, concentration, and release from the vehicle.

INDICATIONS AND USAGE

For steroid-responsive inflammatory ocular conditions for which a corticosteroid is indicated and where bacterial infection or a risk of bacterial ocular infection exists.
Ocular steroids are indicated in inflammatory conditions of the palpebral and bulbar conjunctiva, cornea, and anterior segment of the globe where the inherent risk of steroid use in certain infective conjunctivitides is accepted to obtain a diminution in edema and inflammation. They are also indicated in chronic anterior uveitis and corneal injury from chemical, radiation, or thermal burns, or penetration of foreign bodies.
The use of a combination drug with an anti-infective component is indicated where the risk of infection is high or where there is an expectation that potentially dangerous numbers of bacteria will be present in the eye.
The particular anti-infective drug in this product is active against the following common bacterial eye pathogens:
Staphylococcus aureus
Escherichia coli
Haemophilus influenzae
Klebsiella/Enterobacter species
Neisseria species
The product does not provide adequate coverage against:
Pseudomonas aeruginosa
Serratia marcescens
Streptococci, including *Streptococcus pneumoniae*

CONTRAINDICATIONS

Epithelial herpes simplex keratitis (dendritic keratitis), acute infectious stages of vaccinia, varicella, and many other viral diseases of the cornea and conjunctiva. Mycobacterial infection of the eye. Fungal diseases of ocular structures. Hypersensitivity to a component of the medication (hypersensitivity to the antibiotic component occurs at a higher rate than for other components).
The use of these combinations is always contraindicated after uncomplicated removal of a corneal foreign body.

WARNINGS

Prolonged use may result in glaucoma, with damage to the optic nerve, defects in visual acuity and fields of vision, and posterior subcapsular cataract formation. Prolonged use may suppress the host response and thus increase the hazard of secondary ocular infections. In those diseases causing thinning of the cornea or sclera, perforations have been known to occur with the use of topical corticosteroids. In acute purulent conditions of the eye, corticosteroids may mask infection or enhance existing infection. If these products are used for 10 days or longer, intraocular pressure should be routinely monitored even though it may be difficult in children and uncooperative patients.
Employment of corticosteroid medication in the treatment of herpes simplex requires great caution: periodic slit-lamp microscopy is recommended.
Any substance (e.g. neomycin sulfate) may occasionally cause cutaneous sensitization. If any reaction indicating such sensitivity is observed, discontinue use.

PRECAUTIONS

The initial prescriptions and renewal of the medication order beyond 8 grams should be made by a physician only after examination of the patient with the aid of magnification, such as slit-lamp biomicroscopy and, where appropriate, fluorescein staining.
The possibility of persistent fungal infections of the cornea should be considered after prolonged corticosteroid dosing.
Usage in Pregnancy
Safety of intensive or protracted use of topical corticosteroids during pregnancy has not been substantiated.

ADVERSE REACTIONS

Adverse reactions have occurred with corticosteroid/anti-infective combination drugs which can be attributed to the corticosteroid component, the anti-infective component, or the combination. Exact incidence figures are not available since no denominator of treated patients is available.
Reactions occurring most often from the presence of the anti-infective ingredient are allergic sensitizations. The reactions due to the corticosteroid component in decreasing order of frequency are: elevation of intraocular pressure (IOP) with possible development of glaucoma, and infrequent optic nerve damage; posterior subcapsular cataract formation; and delayed wound healing.
Secondary Infection: The development of secondary infection has occurred after use of combinations containing corticosteroids and antimicrobials. Fungal infections of the cornea are particularly prone to develop coincidentally with long-term applications of corticosteroid. The possibility of fungal invasion must be considered in any persistent corneal ulceration where corticosteroid treatment has been used.
Secondary bacterial ocular infection following suppression of host responses also occurs.

DOSAGE AND ADMINISTRATION

The duration of treatment will vary with the type of lesion and may extend from a few days to several weeks, according to therapeutic response. Relapses, more common in chronic active lesions than in self-limited conditions, usually respond to retreatment.
Apply a thin coating of ophthalmic ointment NEODECADRON three or four times a day. When a favorable response is observed, reduce the number of daily applications to two, and later to one a day as maintenance dose if this is sufficient to control symptoms.
Not more than 8 grams should be prescribed initially and the prescription should not be refilled without further evaluation as outlined in PRECAUTIONS above.
Ophthalmic ointment NEODECADRON is particularly convenient when an eye pad is used. It may also be the preparation of choice for patients in whom therapeutic benefit depends on prolonged contact of the active ingredients with ocular tissues.

HOW SUPPLIED

No. 7617—Sterile Ophthalmic Ointment NEODECADRON is a clear, unctuous ointment, and is supplied as follows:
NDC 0006-7617-04 in 3.5 g tubes
(6505-00-823-7956 0.05% 3.5 g)

A.H.F.S. Category: 52:08
DC 6167722 Issued June 1982

NEODECADRON® Sterile Ophthalmic Solution ℞
(Neomycin Sulfate-Dexamethasone Sodium Phosphate, MSD), U.S.P.

DESCRIPTION

Ophthalmic solution NEODECADRON® (Neomycin Sulfate-Dexamethasone Sodium Phosphate, MSD) is a topical corticosteroid-antibiotic solution for use in certain disorders of the anterior segment of the eye.
Each milliliter of buffered ophthalmic solution NEODECADRON in the OCUMETER® ophthalmic dispenser contains: dexamethasone sodium phosphate equivalent to 1 mg (0.1%) dexamethasone phosphate, and neomycin sulfate equivalent to 3.5 mg neomycin base. Inactive ingredients: creatinine, sodium citrate, sodium borate, polysorbate 80, disodium edetate, hydrochloric acid to adjust pH to 6.6–7.2, and water for injection. Benzalkonium chloride 0.02% and sodium bisulfite 0.1% added as preservatives.
Dexamethasone sodium phosphate is a water soluble, inorganic ester of dexamethasone. Its empirical formula is $C_{22}H_{28}FNa_2O_8P$. It is approximately three thousand times more soluble in water at 25°C than hydrocortisone.
Neomycin sulfate is the sulfate salt of neomycin, an antibacterial substance produced by the growth of *Streptomyces fradiae* Waksman (Fam. Streptomycetaceae).

CLINICAL PHARMACOLOGY

Dexamethasone sodium phosphate, a corticosteroid, suppresses the inflammatory response to a variety of agents, and it probably delays or slows healing. Since corticosteroids may inhibit the body's defense mechanism against infection, a concomitant antimicrobial drug may be used when this inhibition is considered to be clinically significant in a particular case. Neomycin sulfate, the anti-infective component in the combination, is included to provide action against specific organisms susceptible to it. Neomycin sulfate is considered active mainly against gram-negative organisms, except *Bacteroides* spp. and *Pseudomonas aeruginosa,* which are resistant. Gram-positive organisms except for *Staphylococcus aureus* are usually resistant.
When a decision to administer both a corticosteroid and an antimicrobial is made, the administration of such drugs in combination has the advantage of greater patient compliance and convenience, with the added assurance that the appropriate dosage of both drugs is administered, plus assured compatibility of ingredients when both types of drug are in the same formulation and, particularly, that the correct volume of drug is delivered and retained.
The relative potency of corticosteroids depends on the molecular structure, concentration, and release from the vehicle.

INDICATIONS AND USAGE

For steroid-responsive inflammatory ocular conditions for which a corticosteroid is indicated and where bacterial infection or a risk of bacterial ocular infection exists.
Ocular steroids are indicated in inflammatory conditions of the palpebral and bulbar conjunctiva, cornea, and anterior segment of the globe where the inherent risk of steroid use in certain infective conjunctivitides is accepted to obtain a diminution in edema and inflammation. They are also indicated in chronic anterior uveitis and corneal injury from chemical, radiation, or thermal burns, or penetration of foreign bodies.
The use of a combination drug with an anti-infective component is indicated where the risk of infection is high or where there is an expectation that potentially dangerous numbers of bacteria will be present in the eye.
The particular anti-infective drug in this product is active against the following common bacterial eye pathogens:
Staphylococcus aureus
Escherichia coli
Haemophilus influenzae
Klebsiella/Enterobacter species
Neisseria species
The product does not provide adequate coverage against:
Pseudomonas aeruginosa
Serratia marcescens
Streptococci, including *Streptococcus pneumoniae*

CONTRAINDICATIONS

Epithelial herpes simplex keratitis (dendritic keratitis), acute infectious stages of vaccinia, varicella, and many other viral diseases of the cornea and conjunctiva. Mycobacterial infection of the eye. Fungal diseases of ocular structures. Hypersensitivity to any component of the medication, including sulfites (see PRECAUTIONS). (Hypersensitivity to the antibiotic component occurs at a higher rate than for other components).
The use of these combinations is always contraindicated after uncomplicated removal of a corneal foreign body.

WARNINGS

Prolonged use may result in glaucoma, with damage to the optic nerve, defects in visual acuity and fields of vision, and posterior subcapsular cataract formation. Prolonged use may suppress the host response and thus increase the hazard of secondary ocular infections. In those diseases causing thinning of the cornea or sclera, perforations have been known to occur with the use of topical corticosteroids. In

acute purulent conditions of the eye, corticosteroids may mask infection or enhance existing infection. If these products are used for 10 days or longer, intraocular pressure should be routinely monitored even though it may be difficult in children and uncooperative patients.
Employment of corticosteroid medication in the treatment of herpes simplex requires great caution: periodic slit-lamp microscopy is recommended.
Any substance (e.g. neomycin sulfate) may occasionally cause cutaneous sensitization. If any reaction indicating such sensitivity is observed, discontinue use.

PRECAUTIONS

The initial prescription and renewal of the medication order beyond 20 milliliters should be made by a physician only after examination of the patient with the aid of magnification, such as slit-lamp biomicroscopy and, where appropriate, fluorescein staining.
The possibility of persistent fungal infections of the cornea should be considered after prolonged corticosteroid dosing.
Sulfites have been reported to cause severe allergic reactions in certain susceptible individuals, particularly patients with asthma.
Usage in Pregnancy
Safety of intensive or protracted use of topical corticosteroids during pregnancy has not been substantiated.

ADVERSE REACTIONS

Adverse reactions have occurred with corticosteroid/anti-infective combination drugs which can be attributed to the corticosteroid component, the anti-infective component, or the combination. Exact incidence figures are not available since no denominator of treated patients is available.
Reactions occurring most often from the presence of the anti-infective ingredient are allergic sensitizations. The reactions due to the corticosteroid component in decreasing order of frequency are: elevation of intraocular pressure (IOP) with possible development of glaucoma, and infrequent optic nerve damage; posterior subcapsular cataract formation; and delayed wound healing.
Secondary Infection: The development of secondary infection has occurred after use of combinations containing corticosteroids and antimicrobials. Fungal infections of the cornea are particularly prone to develop coincidentally with long-term applications of corticosteroid. The possibility of fungal invasion must be considered in any persistent corneal ulceration where corticosteroid treatment has been used. Secondary bacterial ocular infection following suppression of host responses also occurs.

DOSAGE AND ADMINISTRATION

The duration of treatment will vary with the type of lesion and may extend from a few days to several weeks, according to therapeutic response. Relapses, more common in chronic active lesions than in self-limited conditions, usually respond to retreatment.
Instill one or two drops of ophthalmic solution NEODECADRON into the conjunctival sac every hour during the day and every two hours during the night as initial therapy. When a favorable response is observed, reduce dosage to one drop every four hours. Later, further reduction in dosage to one drop three or four times daily may suffice to control symptoms.
Not more than 20 milliliters should be prescribed initially and the prescription should not be refilled without further evaluation as outlined in PRECAUTIONS above.

HOW SUPPLIED

Sterile ophthalmic solution NEODECADRON is a clear, colorless to pale yellow solution.
No. 7639—Ophthalmic solution NEODECADRON is supplied as follows:
NDC 0006-7639-03 in 5 mL white opaque, plastic OCUMETER ophthalmic dispenser with a controlled drop tip.
(6505-01-039-4352 0.1% 5 mL).

A.H.F.S. Category: 52:08
DC 6361418 Issued December 1984

NEODECADRON® Topical Cream ℞
(Neomycin Sulfate-Dexamethasone Sodium Phosphate, MSD)

DESCRIPTION

NEODECADRON® (Neomycin Sulfate-Dexamethasone Sodium Phosphate, MSD) Topical Cream is a topical steroid-antibiotic preparation.
NEODECADRON Topical Cream contains in each gram: dexamethasone sodium phosphate equivalent to 1 mg (0.1%) dexamethasone phosphate, and neomycin sulfate equivalent to 3.5 mg neomycin base, in a greaseless bland base. Inactive ingredients: stearyl alcohol, cetyl alcohol, mineral oil, polyoxyl 40 stearate, sorbitol solution, methyl polysilicone emulsion, creatinine, disodium edetate, sodium citrate, sodium hydroxide to adjust pH, and purified water. Methylparaben 0.15%, sodium bisulfite 0.25%, and sorbic acid 0.1% added as preservatives.
Dexamethasone sodium phosphate is 9-fluoro-11β,17-dihydroxy-16α-methyl-21-(phosphonooxy)pregna-1,4-diene-3,20-dione disodium salt. Its empirical formula is $C_{22}H_{28}FNa_2O_8P$ and its structural formula is:

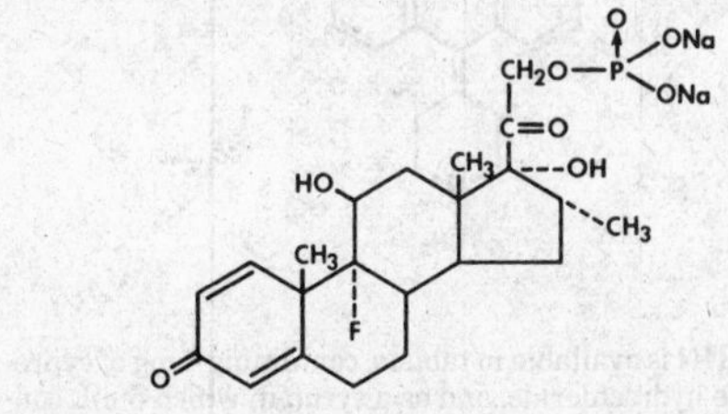

Dexamethasone sodium phosphate has a molecular weight of 516.41.
Glucocorticoids are adrenocortical steroids, both naturally occurring and synthetic. Dexamethasone is a synthetic analog of naturally occurring glucocorticoids (hydrocortisone and cortisone).
Neomycin sulfate is the sulfate salt of neomycin, an antibacterial substance produced by the growth of *Streptomyces fradiae* Waksman (Fam. Streptomycetaceae).

CLINICAL PHARMACOLOGY

Topical corticosteroids share anti-inflammatory, anti-pruritic, and vasoconstrictive actions.
The mechanism of anti-inflammatory activity of the topical corticosteroids is unclear. Various laboratory methods, including vasoconstrictor assays, are used to compare and predict potencies and/or clinical efficacies of the topical corticosteroids. There is some evidence to suggest that a recognizable correlation exists between vasoconstrictor potency and therapeutic efficacy in man.
Pharmacokinetics
The extent of percutaneous absorption of topical corticosteroids is determined by many factors including the vehicle, the integrity of the epidermal barrier, and the use of occlusive dressings.
Topical corticosteroids can be absorbed from normal intact skin. Inflammation and/or other disease processes in the skin increase percutaneous absorption. Occlusive dressings substantially increase the percutaneous absorption of topical corticosteroids. Thus, occlusive dressings may be a valuable therapeutic adjunct for treatment of resistant dermatoses. (See DOSAGE AND ADMINISTRATION.)
Once absorbed through the skin, topical corticosteroids are handled through pharmacokinetic pathways similar to systemically administered corticosteroids. Corticosteroids are bound to plasma proteins in varying degrees. Corticosteroids are metabolized primarily in the liver and are then excreted by the kidneys. Some of the topical corticosteroids and their metabolites are also excreted into the bile.
The antibiotic component, neomycin, is bactericidal to many gram-positive and gram-negative bacteria.

INDICATIONS AND USAGE

For the treatment of corticosteroid-responsive dermatoses with secondary infection. It has not been demonstrated that this steroid-antibiotic combination provides greater benefit than the steroid component alone after 7 days of treatment (see WARNINGS).

CONTRAINDICATIONS

Topical corticosteroids are contraindicated in those patients with a history of hypersensitivity to any of the components of the preparation, including sulfites (see PRECAUTIONS).

WARNINGS

Because of the concern of nephrotoxicity and ototoxicity associated with neomycin, this combination product should not be used over a wide area or for extended periods of time.

PRECAUTIONS

General
Sulfites have been reported to cause severe allergic reactions in certain susceptible individuals, particularly patients with asthma.
Systemic absorption of topical corticosteroids has produced reversible hypothalamic-pituitary-adrenal (HPA) axis suppression, manifestations of Cushing's syndrome, hyperglycemia, and glycosuria in some patients.
Conditions which augment systemic absorption include the application of the more potent corticosteroids, use over large surface areas, prolonged use, and the addition of occlusive dressings.
Therefore, patients receiving a large dose of a potent topical corticosteroid applied to a large surface area or under an occlusive dressing should be evaluated periodically for evidence of HPA axis suppression by using urinary free cortisol and ACTH stimulation tests. If HPA axis suppression is noted, an attempt should be made to withdraw the drug, to reduce the frequency of application, or to substitute a less potent corticosteroid.
Recovery of HPA axis function is generally prompt and complete upon discontinuation of the drug. Infrequently, signs and symptoms of corticosteroid withdrawal may occur, requiring supplemental systemic corticosteroids.
Children may absorb proportionally larger amounts of topical corticosteroids and thus be more susceptible to systemic toxicity (See PRECAUTIONS, *Pediatric Use*).
If irritation develops, topical corticosteroids should be discontinued and appropriate therapy instituted.
In the presence of dermatological infections, the use of an appropriate antifungal or antibacterial agent should be instituted. If a favorable response does not occur promptly, the corticosteroid should be discontinued until the infection has been adequately controlled.
This product is not for ophthalmic use. However, if applied to the eyelids or skin near the eyes, the drug may enter the eyes. In patients with a history of herpes simplex keratitis, ocular exposure to corticosteroids may lead to a recurrence. Prolonged ocular exposure may cause steroid glaucoma.
A few individuals may be sensitive to one or more of the components of this product. Sensitivity to neomycin may occasionally develop, especially when it is applied to abraded skin. If any reaction indicating sensitivity is observed, discontinue use. There are reports in the current medical literature that indicate an increase in the prevalence of persons sensitive to neomycin.
Generally, occlusive dressings should not be used on weeping or exudative lesions.
If the occlusive dressing technique is employed, caution should be exercised with regard to the use of plastic films which are often inflammable and may pose a suffocation hazard for children.
When large areas of the body are covered with an occlusive dressing, thermal homeostasis may be impaired. If elevation of body temperature occurs, use of the occlusive dressing should be discontinued.
Information for the Patient
Patients using topical corticosteroids should receive the following information and instructions:

1. This medication is to be used as directed by the physician. It is for external use only. Avoid contact with the eyes.
2. Patients should be advised not to use this medication for any disorder other than that for which it was prescribed.
3. The treated skin area should not be bandaged or otherwise covered or wrapped so as to be occlusive unless directed by the physician.
4. Patients should report any signs of local adverse reactions, especially under occlusive dressings.
5. Parents of pediatric patients should be advised not to use tight-fitting diapers or plastic pants on a child being treated in the diaper area, as these garments may constitute occlusive dressings.

Laboratory Tests
The following tests may be helpful in evaluating the HPA axis suppression:

- Urinary free cortisol test
- ACTH stimulation test

Carcinogenesis, Mutagenesis and Impairment of Fertility
Long-term animal studies have not been performed to evaluate the carcinogenic potential or the effect on fertility of Topical Cream NEODECADRON.
Studies to determine mutagenicity with prednisolone and hydrocortisone have revealed negative results.
Pregnancy
Pregnancy Category C: Corticosteroids are generally teratogenic in laboratory animals when administered systemically at relatively low dosage levels. The more potent corticosteroids have been shown to be teratogenic after dermal application in laboratory animals. There are no adequate and well controlled studies in pregnant women on teratogenic effects from topically applied corticosteroids. Therefore, topical corticosteroids should be used during pregnancy only if the potential benefit justifies the potential risk to the fetus. Drugs of this class should not be used extensively on preg-

Continued on next page

Information on the Merck Sharp & Dohme products listed on these pages is the full prescribing information from product circulars in use August 31, 1986.

Merck Sharp & Dohme—Cont.

nant patients, in large amounts, or for prolonged periods of time.

Nursing Mothers

It is not known whether topical administration of corticosteroids could result in sufficient systemic absorption to produce detectable quantities in breast milk. Systemically administered corticosteroids are secreted into breast milk in quantities *not* likely to have a deleterious effect on the infant. Nevertheless, caution should be exercised when topical corticosteroids are administered to a nursing woman.

Pediatric Use

Pediatric patients may demonstrate greater susceptibility to topical corticosteroid-induced HPA axis suppression and Cushing's syndrome than mature patients bcause of a larger skin surface area to body weight ratio.

Hypothalamic-pituitary-adrenal (HPA) axis suppression, Cushing's syndrome, and intracranial hypertension have been reported in children receiving topical corticosteroids. Manifestations of adrenal suppression in children include linear growth retardation, delayed weight gain, low plasma cortisol levels, and absence of response to ACTH stimulation. Manifestations of intracranial hypertension include bulging fontanelles, headaches, and bilateral papilledema.

Administration of topical corticosteroids to children should be limited to the least amount compatible with an effective therapeutic regimen. Chronic corticosteroid therapy may interfere with the growth and development of children.

ADVERSE REACTIONS

The following adverse reactions are reported infrequently with topical corticosteroids, but may occur more frequently with the use of occlusive dressings. These reactions are listed in an approximate decreasing order of occurrence:

Burning
Itching
Irritation
Dryness
Folliculitis
Hypertrichosis
Acneiform eruptions
Hypopigmentation
Perioral dermatitis
Allergic contact dermatitis
Maceration of the skin
Secondary infection
Skin atrophy
Striae
Miliaria

Prevalence of neomycin hypersensitivity is increasing. Ototoxicity and nephrotoxicity have been reported with prolonged use or use of large amounts of topical neomycin preparations.

OVERDOSAGE

Topically applied corticosteroids can be absorbed in sufficient amounts to produce systemic effects (see PRECAUTIONS).

DOSAGE AND ADMINISTRATION

Apply to the affected area as a thin film three or four times daily.

Before using NEODECADRON Topical Cream in the *ear*, clean the aural canal thoroughly and sponge dry. Confirm that the eardrum is intact. With a cotton-tipped applicator, apply a thin coating of the cream to the affected canal area two or three times a day. When a favorable response is obtained, reduce the number of daily applications to one or two, and eventually discontinue.

HOW SUPPLIED

No. 7607—Topical Cream NEODECADRON is a white cream, and is supplied as follows:

NDC 0006-7607-12 in 15 g tubes
NDC 0006-7607-24 in 30 g tubes

A.H.F.S. Category: 84:06

DC 6005623 Issued December 1984

PERIACTIN® Tablets ℞
(Cyproheptadine HCl, MSD), U.S.P.
PERIACTIN® Syrup ℞
(Cyproheptadine HCl, MSD), U.S.P.

DESCRIPTION

PERIACTIN® (Cyproheptadine HCl, MSD) is an antihistaminic and antiserotonergic agent.

Cyproheptadine hydrochloride is a white to slightly yellowish, crystalline solid, with a molecular weight of 350.89, which is soluble in water, freely soluble in methanol, sparingly soluble in ethanol, soluble in chloroform, and practically insoluble in ether. It is the sesquihydrate of 4-(5*H*-dibenzo [*a,d*] cyclohepten-5-ylidene)-1-methylpiperidine hydrochloride. The empirical formula of the anhydrous salt is $C_{21}H_{21}N \cdot HCl$ and the structural formula of the anhydrous salt is:

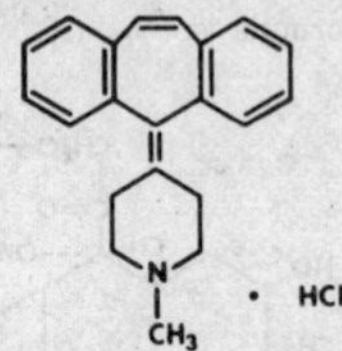

PERIACTIN is available in tablets, containing 4 mg of cyproheptadine hydrochloride, and as a syrup in which 5 mL contains 2 mg of cyproheptadine hydrochloride.

The tablets also contain the following inactive ingredients: calcium phosphate, lactose, magnesium stearate, and starch. The syrup contains the following inactive ingredients: D & C Yellow 10, artificial flavors, glycerin, purified water, sodium saccharin, and sucrose.

CLINICAL PHARMACOLOGY

PERIACTIN is a serotonin and histamine antagonist with anticholinergic and sedative effects. Antiserotonin and antihistamine drugs appear to compete with serotonin and histamine, respectively, for receptor sites.

Pharmacokinetics and Metabolism

After a single 4 mg oral dose of ^{14}C-labelled cyproheptadine HCl in normal subjects, given as tablets or syrup, 2-20% of the radioactivity was excreted in the stools. Only about 34% of the stool radioactivity was unchanged drug, corresponding to less than 5.7% of the dose. At least 40% of the administered radioactivity was excreted in the urine. No significant difference in the mean urinary excretion exists between the tablet and syrup formulations. No detectable amounts of unchanged drug were present in the urine of patients on chronic 12-20 mg daily doses of PERIACTIN Syrup. The principle metabolite found in human urine has been identified as a quaternary ammonium glucuronide conjugate of cyproheptadine. Elimination is diminished in renal insufficiency.

INDICATIONS AND USAGE

Perennial and seasonal allergic rhinitis
Vasomotor rhinitis
Allergic conjunctivitis due to inhalant allergens and foods
Mild, uncomplicated allergic skin manifestations of urticaria and angioedema
Amelioration of allergic reactions to blood or plasma
Cold urticaria
Dermatographism
As therapy for anaphylactic reactions *adjunctive* to epinephrine and other standard measures after the acute manifestations have been controlled

CONTRAINDICATIONS

Newborn or Premature Infants

This drug should *not* be used in newborn or premature infants.

Nursing Mothers

Because of the higher risk of antihistamines for infants generally and for newborns and prematures in particular, antihistamine therapy is contraindicated in nursing mothers.

Lower Respiratory Disease

Antihistamines should not be used to treat lower respiratory tract symptoms including asthma.

Other Conditions

Hypersensitivity to cyproheptadine and other drugs of similar chemical structure:

Monoamine oxidase inhibitor therapy
(see DRUG INTERACTIONS)
Angle-closure glaucoma
Stenosing peptic ulcer
Symptomatic prostatic hypertrophy
Bladder neck obstruction
Pyloroduodenal obstruction
Elderly, debilitated patients

WARNINGS

Children

Overdosage of antihistamines, particularly in infants and children, may produce hallucinations, central nervous system depression, convulsions, and death.

Antihistamines may diminish mental alertness; conversely, particularly, in the young child, they may occasionally produce excitation.

CNS Depressants

Antihistamines may have additive effects with alcohol and other CNS depressants, e.g., hypnotics, sedatives, tranquilizers, antianxiety agents.

Activities Requiring Mental Alertness

Patients should be warned about engaging in activities requiring mental alertness and motor coordination, such as driving a car or operating machinery.

Antihistamines are more likely to cause dizziness, sedation, and hypotension in elderly patients.

PRECAUTIONS

General

Cyproheptadine has an atropine-like action and, therefore, should be used with caution in patients with:

History of bronchial asthma
Increased intraocular pressure
Hyperthyroidism
Cardiovascular disease
Hypertension

Information for Patients

Antihistamines may diminish mental alertness; conversely, particularly, in the young child, they may occasionally produce excitation.

Patients should be warned about engaging in activities requiring mental alertness and motor coordination, such as driving a car or operating machinery.

Drug Interactions

MAO Inhibitors prolong and intensify the anticholinergic effects of antihistamines.

Antihistamines may have additive effects with alcohol and other CNS depressants, e.g., hypnotics, sedatives, tranquilizers, antianxiety agents.

Carcinogenesis, Mutagenesis, Impairment of Fertility

Long-term carcinogenic studies have not been done with cyproheptadine.

Cyproheptadine had no effect on fertility in a two-litter study in rats or a two generation study in mice at about 10 times the human dose.

Cyproheptadine did not produce chromosome damage in human lymphocytes or fibroblasts *in vitro;* high doses (10^{-4} M) were cytotoxic. Cyproheptadine did not have any mutagenic effect in the Ames microbial mutagen test; concentrations of above 500 mcg/plate inhibited bacterial growth.

Pregnancy

Pregnancy Category B: Reproduction studies have been performed in rabbits, mice, and rats at doses up to 32 times the human dose and have revealed no evidence of impaired fertility or harm to the fetus due to cyproheptadine. There are, however, no adequate and well-controlled studies in pregnant women. Because animal reproduction studies are not always predictive of human response, this drug should be used during pregnancy only if clearly needed.

Nursing Mothers

It is not known whether this drug is excreted in human milk. Because many drugs are excreted in human milk, and because of the potential for serious adverse reactions in nursing infants from PERIACTIN, a decision should be made whether to discontinue nursing or to discontinue the drug, taking into account the importance of the drug to the mother (see CONTRAINDICATIONS).

Pediatric Use

Safety and effectiveness in children below the age of two have not been established. See CONTRAINDICATIONS, *Newborn Premature Infants,* and WARNINGS, *Children.*

ADVERSE REACTIONS

Adverse reactions which have been reported with the use of antihistamines are as follows:

Central Nervous System: Sedation and sleepiness (often transient), dizziness, disturbed coordination, confusion, restlessness, excitation, nervousness, tremor, irritability, insomnia, paresthesias, neuritis, convulsions, euphoria, hallucinations, hysteria, faintness.

Integumentary: Allergic manifestation of rash and edema, excessive perspiration, urticaria, photosensitivity.

Special Senses: Acute labyrinthitis, blurred vision, diplopia, vertigo, tinnitus.

Cardiovascular: Hypotension, palpitation, tachycardia, extrasystoles, anaphylactic shock.

Hematologic: Hemolytic anemia, leukopenia, agranulocytosis, thrombocytopenia.

Digestive System: Dryness of mouth, epigastric distress, anorexia, nausea, vomiting, diarrhea, constipation, jaundice.

Genitourinary: Urinary frequency, difficult urination, urinary retention, early menses.

Respiratory: Dryness of nose and throat, thickening of bronchial secretions, tightness of chest and wheezing, nasal stuffiness.

Miscellaneous: Fatigue, chills, headache.

OVERDOSAGE

Antihistamine overdosage reactions may vary from central nervous system depression to stimulation especially in children. Also, atropine-like signs and symptoms (dry mouth; fixed, dilated pupils; flushing, etc.) as well as gastrointestinal symptoms may occur.
If vomiting has not occurred spontaneously the patient should be induced to vomit with syrup of ipecac.
If the patient is unable to vomit, perform gastric lavage followed by activated charcoal. Isotonic or ½ isotonic saline is the lavage of choice. Precautions against aspiration must be taken especially in infants and children.
When life threatening CNS signs and symptoms are present, intravenous physostigmine salicylate may be considered. Dosage and frequency of administration are dependent on age, clinical response, and recurrence after response. (See package circulars for physostigmine products.)
Saline cathartics, as milk of magnesia, by osmosis draw water into the bowel and, therefore, are valuable for their action in rapid dilution of bowel content.
Stimulants should *not* be used.
Vasopressors may be used to treat hypotension.
The oral LD_{50} of cyproheptadine is 123 mg/kg, and 295 mg/kg in the mouse and rat, respectively.

DOSAGE AND ADMINISTRATION

DOSAGE SHOULD BE INDIVIDUALIZED ACCORDING TO THE NEEDS AND THE RESPONSE OF THE PATIENT.
Each PERIACTIN tablet contains 4 mg of cyproheptadine hydrochloride. Each 5 mL of PERIACTIN syrup contains 2 mg of cyproheptadine hydrochloride.
Although intended primarily for administration to children, the syrup is also useful for administration to adults who cannot swallow tablets.
Children
The total daily dosage for children may be calculated on the basis of body weight or body area using approximately 0.25 mg/kg/day (0.11 mg/lb/day) or 8 mg per square meter of body surface (8 mg/M^2). In small children for whom the calculation of dosage based upon body size is most important, it may be necessary to use PERIACTIN syrup to permit accurate dosage.
Age 2 to 6 years
The usual dose is 2 mg (½ tablet or 1 teaspoon) two or three times a day, adjusted as necessary to the size and response of the patient. The dose is not to exceed 12 mg a day.
Age 7 to 14 years
The usual dose is 4 mg (1 tablet or 2 teaspoons) two or three times a day, adjusted as necessary to the size and response of the patient. The dose is not to exceed 16 mg a day.
Adults
The total daily dose for adults should not exceed 0.5 mg/kg/day (0.23 mg/lb/day).
The therapeutic range is 4 to 20 mg a day, with the majority of patients requiring 12 to 16 mg a day. An occasional patient may require as much as 32 mg a day for adequate relief. It is suggested that dosage be initiated with 4 mg (1 tablet or 2 teaspoons) three times a day and adjusted according to the size and response of the patient.

HOW SUPPLIED

No. 3276—Tablets PERIACTIN, containing 4 mg of cyproheptadine hydrochloride each, are white, round, scored compressed tablets, coded MSD 62. They are supplied as follows:
NDC 0006-0062-68 bottles of 100.
(6505-00-890-1884 4 mg 100's)
Shown in Product Identification Section, page 418
No. 3289X—Syrup PERIACTIN, 2 mg per 5 mL is a clear, yellow, syrupy liquid. Contains alcohol 5%, with sorbic acid 0.1% added as preservative and is supplied as follows:
NDC 0006-3289-74 bottles of 473 mL.
Storage
Store Tablets PERIACTIN in a well-closed container.
Store Syrup PERIACTIN in a container which is kept tightly closed.

23 Pneumococcal Capsular Types Included in PNEUMOVAX 23

Nomenclature	Pneumococcal Types																						
Danish	1	2	3	4	5	6B	7F	8	9N	9V	10A	11A	12F	14	15B	17F	18C	19F	19A	20	22F	23F	33F
U.S.	1	2	3	4	5	26	51	8	9	68	34	43	12	14	54	17	56	19	57	20	22	23	70

A.H.F.S. Category: 4:00
DC 6589615 Issued March 1985

PNEUMOVAX® 23 ℞
(Pneumococcal Vaccine, Polyvalent, MSD)

DESCRIPTION

PNEUMOVAX® 23 (Pneumococcal Vaccine, Polyvalent, MSD), is a sterile, liquid vaccine for intramuscular or subcutaneous injection. It consists of a mixture of highly purified capsular polysaccharides from the 23 most prevalent or invasive pneumococcal types accounting for at least 90% of pneumococcal blood isolates and at least 85% of all pneumococcal isolates from sites which are generally sterile as determined by ongoing surveillance of U.S. data.
PNEUMOVAX 23 is manufactured according to methods developed by the MERCK SHARP & DOHME Research Laboratories. Each 0.5 ml dose of vaccine contains 25 μg of each polysaccharide type dissolved in isotonic saline solution containing 0.25% phenol as preservative.
Type 6B pneumococcal polysaccharide exhibits somewhat greater stability in purified form than does Type 6A. A high degree of cross-reactivity between the two types has been demonstrated in adult volunteers. Therefore, Type 6B has replaced Type 6A, which had been used in the 14-valent vaccine. Although contained in the 14-valent vaccine, Type 25 is not included in PNEUMOVAX 23 because it has recently become a rare isolate in many parts of the world including the United States, Canada and Europe.
[See table above].

CLINICAL PHARMACOLOGY

Pneumococcal infection is a leading cause of death throughout the world and a major cause of pneumonia, meningitis, and otitis media. The emergence of strains of pneumococci with increased resistance to one or more of the common antibiotics and recent isolations of pneumococci with multiple antibiotic resistance emphasize the importance of vaccine prophylaxis against pneumococcal disease. Based on projection from limited observations in the United States, it has been estimated that 400,000 to 500,000 cases of pneumococcal pneumonia may occur annually. The overall case fatality rate ranges from 5–10%. Populations at high risk are the elderly; individuals with immune deficiencies; patients with asplenia or splenic deficiencies, including sickle cell anemia and other severe hemoglobinopathies; alcoholics; and patients with the following diseases: Hodgkin's disease, multiple myeloma and nephrotic syndrome. About 25% of all persons with pneumococcal pneumonia develop bacteremia. Death occurs in about 28% of these bacteremic patients over 50 years of age. Of all patients with pneumococcal bacteremia who died despite treatment with penicillin or tetracycline, as many as 60% died within five days of onset of the illness.
The annual incidence of pneumococcal meningitis is approximately 1.5 to 2.5 per 100,000 population. One-half of the cases occur in children, in whom the fatality rate is about 40%. Children with sickle cell disease have been estimated to have a risk of pneumococcal meningitis nearly 600 times greater than normal children. Within the first two years of life, about 15 to 20% of all children develop otitis media caused by pneumococci, and 50% of all children develop such illness within the first 10 years of life (see under INDICATIONS AND USAGE). Other illnesses caused by pneumococci include acute exacerbations of chronic bronchitis, sinusitis, arthritis and conjunctivitis.
Invasive pneumococcal disease causes high morbidity and mortality in spite of effective antimicrobial control by antibiotics. These effects of pneumococcal disease appear due to irreversible physiologic damage caused by the bacteria during the first 5 days following onset of illness, and occur irrespective of antimicrobial therapy. Vaccination offers an effective means of further reducing the mortality and morbidity of this disease.
Pneumococci can be isolated from 38–55% of all cases of acute otitis media and from two-thirds of those in which pathogenic bacteria are cultured from the middle-ear fluid (MEF). The demonstration of soluble pneumococcal antigens in many MEF samples that are negative by bacteriological culture methods points to an even greater role of pneumococci in otitis media.
At present, there are 83 known pneumococcal capsular types. However, the preponderance of pneumococcal diseases is caused by only some capsular types. For example, a 10-year (1952–1962) surveillance at a New York medical center, showed that 56% of all deaths due to pneumococcal pneumonia were caused by 6 capsular types and that approximately 78% of all pneumococcal pneumonias were caused by 12 capsular types. Such unequal distribution of pneumococcal capsular types causing disease has been shown throughout the world. It is on the basis of this information that the pneumococcal vaccine is composed of 23 capsular types, designed to provide coverage of approximately 90% of the most frequently reported types.
It has been established that the purified pneumococcal capsular polysaccharides induce antibody production and that such antibody is effective in preventing pneumococcal disease. Studies in humans have demonstrated the immunogenicity (antibody-stimulating capability) of each of the 23 capsular types when tested in polyvalent vaccines. Adults of all ages responded immunologically to the vaccines. Earlier studies with 12- and 14-valent pneumococcal vaccines in children two years of age and older and in adults showed immunogenic responses. Protective capsular type-specific antibody levels develop by the third week following vaccination.
The protective efficacy of pneumococcal vaccines containing 6 and 12 capsular polysaccharides was investigated in controlled studies of gold miners in South Africa, in whom there is a high attack rate for pneumococcal pneumonia. Capsular type-specific attack rates for pneumococcal pneumonia were observed for the period from 2 weeks through about 1 year after vaccination. The rates for pneumonia caused by the same capsular types represented in the vaccines are given in the table. Protective efficacy was 76% and 92%, respectively, in the two studies for the capsular types represented.
[See table below left].
In similar studies carried out by Dr. R. Austrian and associates using similar pneumococcal vaccines prepared for the National Institute of Allergy and Infectious Diseases, the reduction in pneumonias caused by the capsular types contained in the vaccines was 79%. Reduction in type-specific pneumococcal bacteremia was 82%. A preliminary report suggests that in patients with sickle cell anemia and/or anatomical or functional asplenia, the vaccine was highly effective in persons over two years of age in preventing severe pneumococcal disease and bacteremia.
In a controlled study conducted in Finland among 455 children 2 to 6 years of age with one or more prior episodes of acute otitis media, PNEUMOVAX (Pneumococcal Vaccine, Polyvalent, MSD) (14-valent) was found to effect a significant reduction in the number of clinical cases of pneumococcal otitis media during a six-month postvaccination period of analysis. There was an overall 73% reduction in the frequency of cases caused by serotypes in the vaccine other than type 6. No protection was found for type 6.
Another trial conducted in Sweden among children attending day-care nurseries showed a 30% reduction in visits for acute otitis media of all causes in children over 2 years of age. This reduction was noted over a one-year follow-up and was seen both in children with a history of otitis prior to vaccination and in those children with no such history.
The duration of protective effect of PNEUMOVAX 23 is presently unknown, but it has been shown in previous studies with other pneumococcal vaccines that antibody induced by the vaccine may persist for as long as 5 years. Type-specific antibody levels induced by PNEUMOVAX (Pneumococcal Vaccine, Polyvalent, MSD) (14-valent) have been observed to decline over a 42-month period of observation, but remain significantly above prevaccination levels in almost all recipients who manifest an initial response.

Continued on next page

PNEUMOVAX 23

Number of Capsular Types in Pneumococcal Vaccine	Rate/1000 for Pneumonia Caused by Homologous Capsular Types		Protective Efficacy
	Vaccinated Group	Control Group	
6	9.2	38.3	76%
12	1.8	22.0	92%

Information on the Merck Sharp & Dohme products listed on these pages is the full prescribing information from product circulars in use August 31, 1986.

Merck Sharp & Dohme—Cont.

INDICATIONS AND USAGE

PNEUMOVAX 23 is indicated for immunization against pneumococcal disease caused by those pneumococcal types included in the vaccine. Effectiveness of the vaccine in the prevention of pneumococcal pneumonia and pneumococcal bacteremia has been demonstrated in controlled trials.

PNEUMOVAX 23 *will not immunize against capsular types of pneumococcus other than those contained in the vaccine.*

Use in selected individuals over 2 years of age as follows: (1) patients who have anatomical asplenia or who have splenic dysfunction due to sickle cell disease or other causes; (2) persons with chronic illnesses in which there is an increased risk of pneumococcal disease, such as functional impairment of cardiorespiratory, hepatic and renal systems; (3) persons 50 years of age or older; (4) patients with other chronic illnesses who may be at greater risk of developing pneumococcal infection or experiencing more severe pneumococcal illness as a result of alcohol abuse or coexisting diseases including diabetes mellitus, chronic cerebrospinal fluid leakage, or conditions associated with immunosuppression; (5) patients with Hodgkin's disease if immunization can be given at least 10 days prior to treatment. For maximal antibody response immunization should be given at least 14 days prior to the start of treatment with radiation or chemotherapy. Immunization of patients less than 10 days prior to or during treatment is not recommended. (see CONTRAINDICATIONS.)

Use in communities. Persons over 2 years of age as follows: (1) closed groups such as those in residential schools, nursing homes and other institutions. (To decrease the likelihood of acute outbreaks of pneumococcal disease in closed institutional populations where there is increased risk that the disease may be severe, vaccination of the entire closed population should be considered where there are no other contraindications.); (2) groups epidemiologically at risk in the community when there is a generalized outbreak in the population due to a single pneumococcal type included in the vaccine; (3) patients at high risk of influenza complications, particularly pneumonia.

Use in preventing pneumococcal otitis media. Children 2 years of age or older who, in the judgment of the physician, are at risk for developing middle ear infections. See CLINICAL PHARMACOLOGY for results of clinical studies.

PNEUMOVAX 23 may not be effective in preventing infection resulting from basilar skull fracture or from external communication with cerebrospinal fluid.

Simultaneous administration of pneumococcal polysaccharide vaccine and whole-virus influenza vaccine gives satisfactory antibody response without increasing the occurrence of adverse reactions. Simultaneous administration of the pneumococcal vaccine and split-virus influenza vaccine may also be expected to yield satisfactory results.

Revaccination

Revaccination of adults is not recommended. Adults previously immunized with any polyvalent pneumococcal vaccine should not receive PNEUMOVAX 23 or PNEUMOVAX (Pneumococcal Vaccine, Polyvalent, MSD) (14-valent) since an increased incidence and severity of adverse reactions among healthy adults receiving such reinjections have been noted, most likely due to sustained high antibody levels.

Certain groups of children at very high risk for pneumococcal disease (e.g., children with sickle cell disease or nephrotic syndrome) may have lower peak levels of antibody response and/or more rapid rates of decline in antibody levels than do healthy adults. However, insufficient data are available at this time to permit formulation of guidelines for reimmunization of high-risk children.

CONTRAINDICATIONS

Hypersensitivity to any component of the vaccine. Epinephrine injection (1:1000) must be immediately available should an acute anaphylactoid reaction occur due to any component of the vaccine.

Revaccination of adults is contraindicated. Adults previously immunized with any polyvalent pneumococcal vaccine should not receive PNEUMOVAX 23 or PNEUMOVAX (Pneumococcal Vaccine, Polyvalent, MSD) (14-valent) since an increased incidence and severity of adverse reactions among healthy adults receiving such reinjections have been noted, most likely due to sustained high antibody levels.

Patients with Hodgkin's disease immunized less than 7 to 10 days prior to immunosuppressive therapy have in some instances been found to have post-immunization antibody levels below their pre-immunization levels. Because of these results, immunization less than 10 days prior to or during treatment is contraindicated.

Patients with Hodgkin's disease who have received extensive chemotherapy and/or nodal irradiation have been shown to have an impaired antibody response to a 12-valent pneumococcal vaccine. Because, in some intensively treated patients, administration of that vaccine depressed pre-existing levels of antibody to some pneumococcal types, PNEUMOVAX 23 is not recommended at this time for patients who have received these forms of therapy for Hodgkin's disease.

WARNINGS

If the vaccine is used in persons receiving immunosuppressive therapy, the expected serum antibody response may not be obtained.

Intradermal administration may cause severe local reactions.

PRECAUTIONS

General

Caution and appropriate care should be exercised in administering PNEUMOVAX 23 to individuals with severely compromised cardiac and/or pulmonary function in whom a systemic reaction would pose a significant risk.

Any febrile respiratory illness or other active infection is reason for delaying use of PNEUMOVAX 23, except when, in the opinion of the physician, withholding the agent entails even greater risk.

In patients who require penicillin (or other antibiotic) prophylaxis against pneumococcal infection, such prophylaxis should not be discontinued after vaccination with PNEUMOVAX 23.

Pregnancy

Pregnancy Category C: Animal reproduction studies have not been conducted with PNEUMOVAX 23. It is also not known whether PNEUMOVAX 23 can cause fetal harm when administered to a pregnant woman or can affect reproduction capacity. PNEUMOVAX 23 should be given to a pregnant woman only if clearly needed.

Nursing Mothers

It is not known whether this drug is excreted in human milk. Because many drugs are excreted in human milk, caution should be exercised when PNEUMOVAX 23 is administered to a nursing woman.

Pediatric Use

Children less than 2 years of age do not respond satisfactorily to the capsular types of PNEUMOVAX 23 that are most often the cause of pneumococcal disease in this age group. Safety and effectiveness in children below the age of 2 years have not been established. Accordingly, PNEUMOVAX 23 is not recommended in this age group.

ADVERSE REACTIONS

Local erythema and soreness at the injection site, usually of less than 48 hours duration, occurs commonly; local induration occurs less commonly. In a study of PNEUMOVAX 22 (containing 22 capsular types) in 29 adults, 21 (71%) showed local reaction characterized principally by local soreness and/or induration at the injection site within 2 days after vaccination.

Rash and arthralgia have been reported rarely.

Low grade fever (less than 100.9°F) occurs occasionally and is usually confined to the 24-hour period following vaccination. Although rare, fever over 102°F has been reported.

Patients with otherwise stabilized idiopathic thrombocytopenic purpura have, on rare occasions, experienced a relapse in their thrombocytopenia, occurring 2 to 14 days after vaccination, and lasting up to 2 weeks.

Reactions of greater severity, duration, or extent are unusual. Neurological disorders such as paresthesias and acute radiculoneuropathy including Guillain-Barré syndrome have been rarely reported in temporal association with administration of pneumococcal vaccine. No cause and effect relationship has been established. Rarely, anaphylactoid reactions have been reported.

DOSAGE AND ADMINISTRATION

Do not inject intravenously. Intradermal administration should be avoided.

Parenteral drug products should be inspected visually for particulate matter and discoloration prior to administration, whenever solution and container permit. PNEUMOVAX 23 is a clear, colorless solution.

Administer a single 0.5 ml dose of PNEUMOVAX 23 subcutaneously or intramuscularly (preferably in the deltoid muscle or lateral mid-thigh), with appropriate precautions to avoid intravascular administration.

Single-Dose and 5-Dose Vials

For Syringe Use Only: Withdraw 0.5 ml from the vial using a sterile needle and syringe free of preservatives, antiseptics and detergents.

It is important to use a separate sterile syringe and needle for each individual patient to prevent transmission of hepatitis B and other infectious agents from one person to another.

Store unopened and opened vials at 2–8°C (35.6– 46.4°F). The vaccine is used directly as supplied. No dilution or reconstitution is necessary. Phenol 0.25% added as preservative. All vaccine must be discarded after the expiration date.

HOW SUPPLIED

No. 4739—PNEUMOVAX 23 contains one 5-dose vial of liquid vaccine, **NDC** 0006-4739-00. For use with syringe only.

No. 4741—PNEUMOVAX 23 is supplied as follows: **NDC** 0006-4741-00. A box of 5 individual cartons, each containing a single-dose vial of vaccine.

A.H.F.S. Category: 80:12

DC 7267001 Issued May 1983

PRIMAXIN® ℞

(Imipenem-Cilastatin Sodium, MSD)

DESCRIPTION

PRIMAXIN® (Imipenem-Cilastatin Sodium, MSD) is a formulation of imipenem, a thienamycin antibiotic, and cilastatin sodium, the inhibitor of the renal dipeptidase, dehydropeptidase I, with sodium bicarbonate added as a buffer. PRIMAXIN is a potent broad spectrum antibacterial agent for intravenous administration.

Imipenem (N-formimidoylthienamycin monohydrate) is a crystalline derivative of thienamycin, which is produced by *Streptomyces cattleya*. Its chemical name is [5*R*-[5α, 6α (*R* *)]]-6-(1-hydroxyethyl)-3-[[2-[(iminomethyl)amino] ethyl] thio]-7-oxo-1-azabicyclo [3.2.0] hept-2-ene-2-carboxylic acid monohydrate. It is an off-white, nonhygroscopic crystalline compound with a molecular weight of 317.37. It is sparingly soluble in water, and slightly soluble in methanol. Its empirical formula is $C_{12}H_{17}N_3O_4S \cdot H_2O$, and its structural formula is:

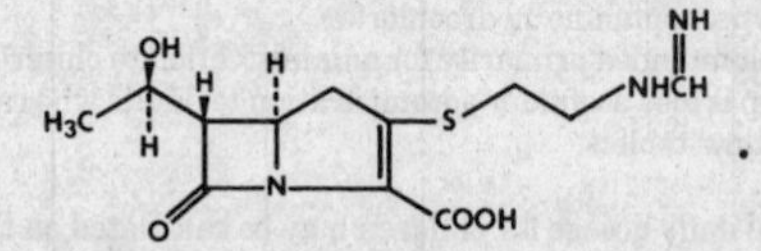

Cilastatin sodium is the sodium salt of a derivatized heptenoic acid. Its chemical name is [*Z*, 7(*R*),2(*S*)]-7-[(2-amino-2-carboxyethyl)thio]-2-[[(2,2-dimethyl-cyclopropyl)carbonyl] amino]-2-heptenoic acid monosodium salt. It is an off-white to yellowish-white, hygroscopic, amorphous compound with a molecular weight of 380.43. It is very soluble in water and in methanol. Its empirical formula is $C_{16}H_{25}N_2O_5S$ Na, and its structural formula is:

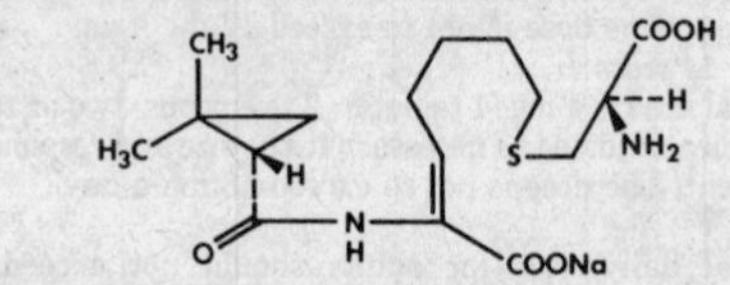

PRIMAXIN is buffered to provide solutions in the pH range of 6.5 to 7.5. There is no significant change in pH when solutions are prepared and used as directed. (See COMPATIBILITY AND STABILITY.) PRIMAXIN 250 contains 18.8 mg of sodium (0.8 mEq) and PRIMAXIN 500 contains 37.5 mg of sodium (1.6 mEq). Solutions of PRIMAXIN range from colorless to yellow. Variations of color within this range do not affect the potency of the product.

CLINICAL PHARMACOLOGY

Intravenous Administration

Intravenous infusion of PRIMAXIN over 20 minutes results in peak plasma levels of imipenem antimicrobial activity that range from 14 to 24 mcg/mL for the 250 mg dose, from 21 to 58 mcg/mL for the 500 mg dose and from 41 to 83 mcg/mL for the 1000 mg dose. At these doses, plasma levels of imipenem antimicrobial activity decline to below 1 mcg/mL or less in 4 to 6 hours. Peak plasma levels of cilastatin following a 20-minute intravenous infusion of PRIMAXIN, range from 15 to 25 mcg/mL for the 250 mg dose, from 31 to 49 mcg/mL for the 500 mg dose and from 56 to 88 mcg/mL for the 1000 mg dose.

General

The plasma half-life of each component is approximately 1 hour. The binding of imipenem to human serum proteins is approximately 20% and that of cilastatin is approximately 40%. Approximately 70% of the administered imipenem is recovered in the urine within 10 hours after which no further urinary excretion is detectable. Urine concentrations of imipenem in excess of 10 mcg/mL can be maintained for up to 8 hours with PRIMAXIN at the 500 mg dose. Approximately 70% of the cilastatin sodium dose is recovered in the urine within 10 hours of administration of PRIMAXIN.

No accumulation of PRIMAXIN in plasma or urine is observed with regimens administered as frequently as every 6 hours in patients with normal renal function.

Imipenem, when administered alone, is metabolized in the kidneys by dehydropeptidase I resulting in relatively low levels in urine. Cilastatin sodium, an inhibitor of this enzyme, effectively prevents renal metabolism of imipenem so that when imipenem and cilastatin sodium are given concomitantly fully adequate antibacterial levels of imipenem are achieved in the urine.

After a 1 gram dose, the following average levels of imipenem were measured (usually at 1 hour post-dose) in the tissues and fluids listed:

sputum	2.1 mcg/mL
pleural	22.0 mcg/mL
peritoneal	3.9 mcg/mL
bile	2.5 mcg/mL
aqueous humor	1.8 mcg/mL
interstitial fluid	16.0 mcg/mL
CSF (uninflamed meninges)	0.8 mcg/mL
reproductive organs	4.3 mcg/g (2½ hours post-dose)
bone	2.4 mcg/g

Microbiology

The bactericidal activity of imipenem results from the inhibition of cell wall synthesis. Its greatest affinity is for penicillin binding proteins (PBP) 1A, 1B, 2, 4, 5, and 6 of *Escherichia coli*, and 1A, 1B, 2, 4 and 5 of *Pseudomonas aeruginosa*. The lethal effect is related to binding to PBP 2 and PBP 1B. Imipenem has *in vitro* activity against a wide range of gram-positive and gram-negative organisms.

Imipenem has a high degree of stability in the presence of beta-lactamases, both penicillinases and cephalosporinases produced by gram-negative and gram-positive bacteria. It is a potent inhibitor of beta-lactamases from certain gram-negative bacteria which are inherently resistant to most beta-lactam antibiotics, e.g., *Pseudomonas aeruginosa*, *Serratia* spp., and *Enterobacter* spp.

In vitro, imipenem is active against most strains of clinical isolates of the following microorganisms:

Gram-positive:

Group D streptococci (including enterococci e.g., *Streptococcus faecalis*)

NOTE: Imipenem is inactive against *Streptococcus faecium.*

Streptococcus pyogenes (Group A streptococci)
Streptococcus agalactiae (Group B streptococci)
Group C streptococci
Group G streptococci
Viridans streptococci
Streptococcus pneumoniae (formerly *Diplococcus pneumoniae*)
Staphylococcus aureus including penicillinase producing strains
Staphylococcus epidermidis including penicillinase producing strains

NOTE: Many strains of methicillin-resistant staphylococci are resistant to imipenem.

Gram-negative:

Escherichia coli
Proteus mirabilis
Proteus vulgaris
Morganella morganii
Providencia rettgeri
Providencia stuartii
Citrobacter spp.
Klebsiella spp. including *K. pneumoniae* and *K. oxytoca*
Enterobacter spp.
Hafnia spp. including *H. alvei*
Serratia marcescens
Serratia spp. including *S. liquefaciens*
Haemophilus parainfluenzae
H. influenzae
Gardnerella vaginalis
Acinetobacter spp.
Pseudomonas aeruginosa

NOTE: Imipenem is inactive against *P. maltophilia* and some strains of *P. cepacia*

Anaerobes:

Bacteroides spp. including *Bacteroides bivius, Bacteroides fragilis, Bacteroides melaninogenicus*
Clostridium spp. including *C. perfringens*
Eubacterium spp.
Fusobacterium spp.
Peptococcus spp.
Peptostreptococcus spp.
Propionibacterium spp. including *P. acnes*
Actinomyces spp.
Veillonella spp.

Imipenem has been shown to be active *in vitro* against the following microorganisms; however, clinical efficacy has not yet been established.

Gram-positive:

Listeria monocytogenes
Nocardia spp.

Gram-negative:

Salmonella spp.
Shigella spp.
Yersinia spp. including *Yersinia enterocolitica, Yersinia pseudotuberculosis*
Bordetella bronchiseptica
Campylobacter spp.
Achromobacter spp.
Alcaligenes spp.
Moraxella spp.
Pasteurella multocida
Aeromonas hydrophila
Plesiomonas shigelloides
Neisseria gonorrhoeae (including penicillinase-producing strains)

Anaerobes:

Bacteroides asaccharolyticus
Bacteroides disiens
Bacteroides distasonis
Bacteroides ovatus
Bacteroides thetaiotaomicron
Bacteroides vulgatus

In vitro tests show imipenem to act synergistically with aminoglycoside antibiotics against some isolates of *Pseudomonas aeruginosa.*

Susceptibility Testing

Quantitative methods that require measurement of zone diameters give the most precise estimate of antibiotic susceptibility. One such procedure has been recommended for use with discs to test susceptibility to imipenem.

Reports from the laboratory giving results of the standard single-disc susceptibility test with a 10 mcg imipenem disc should be interpreted according to the following criteria.

Susceptible organisms produce zones of 16 mm or greater, indicating that the test organism is likely to respond to therapy.

Organisms that produce zones of 14 to 15 mm are expected to be susceptible if high dosage is used or if the infection is confined to tissues and fluids in which high antibiotic levels are attained.

Resistant organisms produce zones of 13 mm or less, indicating that other therapy should be selected.

A bacterial isolate may be considered susceptible if the MIC value for imipenem is equal to or less than 8 mcg/mL. Organisms are considered resistant if the MIC is equal to or greater than 16 mcg/mL.

The standardized quality control procedure requires use of control organisms. The 10 mcg imipenem disc should give the zone diameters listed below for the quality control strains.

Organism	ATCC	Zone Size Range
E. coli	25922	27–31 mm
Ps. aeruginosa	27853	20–28 mm

Dilution susceptibility tests should give MICs between the ranges listed below for the quality control strains.

Organism	ATCC	MIC (mcg/mL)
E. coli	25922	0.06–0.25
S. aureus	29213	0.008–0.03
S. faecalis	29212	0.25–1.0
Ps. aeruginosa	27853	1.0–4.0

Based on blood levels of imipenem achieved in man, breakpoint criteria have been established for imipenem.

Category	Zone Diameter (mm)	Recommended MIC Breakpoint (mcg/mL)
Susceptible	≥16	≤8
Moderately Susceptible	14–15	
Resistant	≤13	≥16

INDICATIONS AND USAGE

PRIMAXIN is indicated for the treatment of serious infections caused by susceptible strains of the designated microorganisms in the diseases listed below:

(1) **Lower respiratory tract infections.** *Staphylococcus aureus* (penicillinase producing strains)*, *Escherichia coli, Klebsiella* species, *Enterobacter* species, *Haemophilus influenzae, Haemophilus parainfluenzae*, Acinetobacter* species*, *Serratia marcescens*.*

(2) **Urinary tract infections** (Complicated and uncomplicated). *Staphylococcus aureus* (penicillinase producing strains)*, Group D streptococci (enterococci), *Escherichia coli, Klebsiella* species, *Enterobacter* species, *Proteus vulgaris*, Providencia rettgeri*, Morganella morganii*, Pseudomonas aeruginosa.*

(3) **Intra-abdominal infections.** *Staphylococcus aureus* (penicillinase producing strains)*, *Staphylococcus epidermidis**, Group D streptococci (enterococci), *Escherichia coli, Klebsiella* species, *Enterobacter* species, *Proteus* species (indole positive and indole negative), *Morganella morganii*, Pseudomonas aeruginosa, Citrobacter* species*, *Clostridium* species, Gram-positive anaerobes, including *Peptococcus* species*, *Peptostreptococcus* species*, *Eubacterium* species, *Propionibacterium* species*, *Bifidobacterium* species, *Bacteroides* species, including *B. fragilis, Fusobacterium* species*.

(4) **Gynecologic infections.** *Staphylococcus aureus* (penicillinase producing strains)*, *Staphylococcus epidermidis,* Group B streptococci, Group D streptococci (enterococci), *Escherichia coli, Klebsiella* species*, *Proteus* species (indole positive and indole negative)*, *Enterobacter* species*, Gram-positive anaerobes, including *Peptococcus* species*, *Peptostreptococcus* species*, *Propionibacterium* species*, *Bifidobacterium* species*, *Bacteroides* species, *B. fragilis*, Gardnerella vaginalis*.*

(5) **Bacterial septicemia.** *Staphylococcus aureus* (penicillinase producing strains), Group D streptococci (enterococci)*, *Escherichia coli, Klebsiella* species*, *Pseudomonas aeruginosa*, Serratia* species*, *Enterobacter* species*, *Bacteroides* species, *B. fragilis*.*

(6) **Bone and joint infections.** *Staphylococcus aureus* (penicillinase producing strains), *Staphylococcus epidermidis**, Group D streptococci (enterococci)*, *Enterobacter* species*, *Pseudomonas aeruginosa.*

(7) **Skin and skin structure infections.** *Staphylococcus aureus* (penicillinase producing strains), *Staphylococcus epidermidis,* Group D streptococci (enterococci), *Escherichia coli, Klebsiella* species, *Enterobacter* species, *Proteus vulgaris*, Providencia rettgeri*, Morganella morganii, Pseudomonas aeruginosa, Serratia* species, *Citrobacter* species*, *Acinetobacter* species*, Gram-positive anaerobes, including *Peptococcus* species and *Peptostreptococcus* species, *Bacteroides* species, including *B. fragilis, Fusobacterium* species*.

(8) **Endocarditis.** *Staphylococcus aureus* (penicillinase producing strains).

(9) **Polymicrobic infections.** PRIMAXIN is indicated for polymicrobic infections including those in which *S. pneumoniae* (pneumonia, septicemia), Group A beta-hemolytic streptococcus (skin and skin structure), or non-penicillinase-producing *S. aureus* is one of the causative organisms. However monobacterial infections due to these organisms are usually treated with narrower spectrum antibiotics, such as penicillin G.

Although clinical improvement has been observed in patients with cystic fibrosis, chronic pulmonary disease, and lower respiratory tract infections caused by *Pseudomonas aeruginosa*, bacterial eradication may not necessarily be achieved.

As with other beta-lactam antibiotics, some strains of *Pseudomonas aeruginosa* may develop resistance fairly rapidly on treatment with PRIMAXIN. When clinically appropriate during therapy of *Pseudomonas aeruginosa* infections, periodic susceptibility testing should be done.

Infections resistant to other antibiotics, for example, cephalosporins, penicillin, and aminoglycosides, have been shown to respond to treatment with PRIMAXIN.

CONTRAINDICATIONS

PRIMAXIN is contraindicated in patients who have shown hypersensitivity to any component of this product.

WARNINGS

SERIOUS AND OCCASIONALLY FATAL HYPERSENSITIVITY (anaphylactic) REACTIONS HAVE BEEN REPORTED IN PATIENTS RECEIVING THERAPY WITH BETA-LACTAMS. THESE REACTIONS ARE MORE APT TO OCCUR IN PERSONS WITH A HISTORY OF SENSITIVITY TO MULTIPLE ALLERGENS.

THERE HAVE BEEN REPORTS OF PATIENTS WITH A HISTORY OF PENICILLIN HYPERSENSITIVITY WHO HAVE EXPERIENCED SEVERE HYPERSENSITIVITY REACTIONS WHEN TREATED WITH ANOTHER BETA-LACTAM. BEFORE INITIATING THERAPY WITH PRIMAXIN, CAREFUL INQUIRY SHOULD BE MADE CONCERNING PREVIOUS HYPERSENSITIVITY REACTIONS TO PENICILLINS, CEPHALOSPORINS, OTHER BETA-LACTAMS, AND OTHER ALLERGENS. IF AN ALLERGIC REACTION TO PRIMAXIN OCCURS, DISCONTINUE THE DRUG. SERIOUS HYPERSENSITIVITY REACTIONS MAY REQUIRE EPINEPHRINE AND OTHER EMERGENCY MEASURES.

* Efficacy for this organism in this organ system was demonstrated in less than 10 infections.

Continued on next page

Information on the Merck Sharp & Dohme products listed on these pages is the full prescribing information from product circulars in use August 31, 1986.

Merck Sharp & Dohme—Cont.

Pseudomembranous colitis has been reported with virtually all antibiotics, including PRIMAXIN; therefore it is important to consider its diagnosis in patients who develop diarrhea in association with antibiotic use. This colitis may range in severity from mild to life threatening.
Mild cases of pseudomembranous colitis may respond to drug discontinuance alone. In more severe cases, management may include sigmoidoscopy, appropriate bacteriological studies, fluid, electrolyte and protein supplementation, and the use of a drug such as oral vancomycin, as indicated. Isolation of the patient may be advisable. Other causes of colitis should also be considered.

PRECAUTIONS

General
CNS adverse experiences such as myoclonic activity, confusional states, or seizures have been reported with PRIMAXIN. These experiences have occurred most commonly in patients with CNS disorders (e.g., brain lesions or history of seizures) who also have compromised renal function. However, there were rare reports in which there was no recognized or documented underlying CNS disorder. Close adherence to recommended dosage schedules is urged especially in patients with known factors that predispose to seizures (see DOSAGE AND ADMINISTRATION). Anticonvulsant therapy should be continued in patients with a known seizure disorder. If focal tremors, myoclonus, or seizures occur, patients should be placed on anticonvulsant therapy. If CNS symptoms continue, the dosage of PRIMAXIN should be decreased or discontinued.
As with other antibiotics, prolonged use of PRIMAXIN may result in overgrowth of nonsusceptible organisms. Repeated evaluation of the patient's condition is essential. If superinfection occurs during therapy, appropriate measures should be taken.
While PRIMAXIN possesses the characteristic low toxicity of the beta-lactam group of antibiotics, periodic assessment of organ system function during prolonged therapy is advisable.
Drug Interactions
Since concomitant administration of PRIMAXIN and probenecid results in only minimal increases in plasma levels of imipenem and plasma half-life, it is not recommended that probenecid be given with PRIMAXIN.
PRIMAXIN should not be mixed with or physically added to other antibiotics. However, PRIMAXIN may be administered concomitantly with other antibiotics, such as aminoglycosides.
Carcinogenesis, Mutagenesis, Impairment of Fertility
Gene toxicity studies were performed in a variety of bacterial and mammalian tests *in vivo* and *in vitro*. The tests were: V79 mammalian cell mutation assay (PRIMAXIN alone and imipenem alone), Ames test (cilastatin sodium alone), unscheduled DNA synthesis assay (PRIMAXIN) and *in vivo* mouse cytogenicity test (PRIMAXIN). None of these tests showed any evidence of genetic damage.
Reproduction tests in male and female rats were performed with PRIMAXIN at dosage levels up to 8 times the usual human dose. Slight decreases in live fetal body weight were restricted to the highest dosage level. No other adverse effects were observed on fertility, reproductive performance, fetal viability, growth or postnatal development of pups. Similarly, no adverse effects on the fetus or on lactation were observed when PRIMAXIN was administered to rats late in gestation.
Pregnancy
Pregnancy Category C. Teratogenicity studies with cilastatin sodium in rabbits and rats at 10 and 33 times the usual human dose, respectively, showed no evidence of adverse effect on the fetus. No evidence of teratogenicity or adverse effect on postnatal growth or behavior was observed in rats given imipenem at dosage levels up to 30 times the usual human dose. Similarly, no evidence of adverse effect on the fetus was observed in teratology studies in rabbits with imipenem at dosage levels at the usual human dose.
Teratology studies with PRIMAXIN at doses up to 11 times the usual human dose in pregnant mice and rats during the period of major organogenesis revealed no evidence of teratogenicity.
Data from preliminary studies suggests an apparent intolerance to PRIMAXIN (including emesis, inappetence, body weight loss, diarrhea and death) at doses equivalent to the average human dose in pregnant rabbits and cynomolgus monkeys that is not seen in non-pregnant animals in these or other species. In other studies, PRIMAXIN was well tolerated in equivalent or higher doses (up to 11 times the average human dose) in pregnant rats and mice. Further studies are underway to evaluate these findings.
There are, however, no adequate and well-controlled studies in pregnant women. PRIMAXIN should be used during pregnancy only if the potential benefit justifies the potential risk to the fetus.
Nursing Mothers
It is not known whether this drug is excreted in human milk. Because many drugs are excreted in human milk, caution should be exercised when PRIMAXIN is administered to a nursing woman.
Pediatric Use
Safety and effectiveness in infants and children below 12 years of age have not yet been established.

ADVERSE REACTIONS

PRIMAXIN is generally well tolerated. Many of the 1,723 patients treated in clinical trials were severely ill and had multiple background diseases and physiological impairments, making it difficult to determine causal relationship of adverse experiences to therapy with PRIMAXIN.
Local Adverse Reactions
Adverse local clinical reactions that were reported as possibly, probably or definitely related to therapy with PRIMAXIN were:
Phlebitis/thrombophlebitis—3.1%
Pain at the injection site—0.7%
Erythema at the injection site—0.4%
Vein induration—0.2%
Infused vein infection—0.1%
Systemic Adverse Reactions
The most frequently reported systemic adverse clinical reactions that were reported as possibly, probably, or definitely related to PRIMAXIN were nausea (2.0%), diarrhea (1.8%), vomiting (1.5%), rash (0.9%), fever (0.5%), hypotension (0.4%), seizures (0.4%) (see *PRECAUTIONS*), dizziness (0.3%), pruritus (0.3%), urticaria (0.2%), somnolence (0.2%).
Additional adverse systemic clinical reactions reported as possibly, probably or definitely drug related occurring in less than 0.2% of the patients are listed within each body system in order of decreasing severity: *Gastrointestinal*—pseudomembranous colitis (see WARNINGS), hemorrhagic colitis, gastroenteritis, abdominal pain, glossitis, tongue papillar hypertrophy, heartburn, pharyngeal pain, increased salivation; *CNS*—encephalopathy, confusion, myoclonus, paresthesia, vertigo, headache; *Special Senses*—transient hearing loss in patients with impaired hearing, tinnitus; *Respiratory*—chest discomfort, dyspnea, hyperventilation, thoracic spine pain; *Cardiovascular*—palpitations, tachycardia; *Renal*—oliguria/anuria, polyuria; *Skin*—erythema multiforme, facial edema, flushing, cyanosis, hyperhidrosis, skin texture changes, candidiasis, pruritis vulvae; *Body as a whole*—polyarthralgia, asthenia/weakness.
Adverse Laboratory Changes
Adverse laboratory changes without regard to drug relationship that were reported during clinical trials were:
Hepatic: Increased SGPT, SGOT, alkaline phosphatase, bilirubin and LDH.
Hemic: Increased eosinophils, positive Coombs test, decreased WBC and neutrophils, increased WBC, increased platelets, decreased platelets, decreased hemoglobin and hematocrit, increased monocytes, abnormal prothrombin time, increased lymphocytes, increased basophils.
Electrolytes: Decreased serum sodium, increased potassium, increased chloride.
Renal: Increased BUN, creatinine.
Urinalysis: Presence of urine protein, urine red blood cells, urine white blood cells, urine casts, urine bilirubin, and urine urobilinogen.

OVERDOSAGE

The intravenous LD_{50} of imipenem is greater than 2000 mg/kg in the rat and approximately 1500 mg/kg in the mouse.
The intravenous LD_{50} of cilastatin sodium is approximately 5000 mg/kg in the rat and approximately 8700 mg/kg in the mouse.
The intravenous LD_{50} of PRIMAXIN is approximately 1000 mg/kg/day in the rat and approximately 1100 mg/kg/day in the mouse.
Information on overdosage in humans is not available.

DOSAGE AND ADMINISTRATION

The dosage recommendations for PRIMAXIN represent the quantity of imipenem to be administered. An equivalent amount of cilastatin is also present in the solution.
Initially, the total daily dosage for PRIMAXIN should be based on the type or severity of infection and given in equally divided doses. Subsequent dosing must be based on consideration of severity of illness, degree of susceptibility of the pathogen(s), age, weight, and creatinine clearance.
Serum creatinine alone may not be a sufficiently accurate measure of renal function. Creatinine clearance (T_{cc}) may be estimated from the following equation:

$$T_{cc}\ (\text{Males}) = \frac{(\text{wt. in kg})\ (140 - \text{age})}{(72)\ (\text{creatinine in mg/dL})}$$

$$T_{cc}\ (\text{Female}) = 0.85 \times \text{above value}$$

Each 250 mg or 500 mg dose should be given by intravenous infusion over twenty to thirty minutes. Each 1000 mg dose should be infused over forty to sixty minutes. In patients who develop nausea during the infusion, the rate of infusion may be slowed.

INTRAVENOUS DOSING SCHEDULE FOR ADULTS WITH NORMAL RENAL FUNCTION

Type or severity of infection	Gram-positive organisms Anaerobes Highly susceptible gram-negative organisms	Other gram-negative organisms
Mild	250 mg q6h	500 mg q6h
Moderate	500 mg q8h–500 mg q6h	500 mg q6h–1 g q8h
Severe, life threatening	500 mg q6h	1 g q8h–1 g q6h
Uncomplicated urinary tract infection	250 mg q6h	250 mg q6h
Complicated urinary tract infection	500 mg q6h	500 mg q6h

Due to the high antimicrobial activity of PRIMAXIN, it is recommended that the maximum total daily dosage not exceed 50 mg/kg/day or 4.0 g/day, whichever is lower. There is no evidence that higher doses provide greater efficacy.

INTRAVENOUS DOSING SCHEDULE FOR ADULTS WITH IMPAIRED RENAL FUNCTION

Patients with creatinine clearance of ≤ 70 mL/min/1.73 m² require adjustment of the dosage of PRIMAXIN as indicated in the table below. Doses cited are in every case the imipenem component of a 1:1 ratio of imipenem:cilastatin Na and are based on a body weight of 70 kg. Proportionate reduction in dose administered should be made for patients with reduced body weight.
[See table left].

Intravenous Dosage of PRIMAXIN in Adults With Impaired Renal Function

Creatinine Clearance (mL/min/1.73 m²)	Renal Function	Less Severe Infections or Presence of Highly Susceptible Organisms	Life Threatening Infections—Maximum Dosage
30–70	Mild Impairment	500 mg q8h	500 mg q6h
20–30	Moderate Impairment	500 mg q12h	500 mg q8h
5–20	Severe to Marked Impairment	250 mg q12h	500 mg q12h
0–5	None, but on hemodialysis	250 mg q12h	500 mg q12h

PRIMAXIN is cleared by hemodialysis. In patients undergoing hemodialysis, a supplemental dose of PRIMAXIN should be given after hemodialysis unless the next dose is scheduled within four hours. The benefits versus the risks should be considered in patients on hemodialysis. Dialysis patients, especially those with CNS background diseases, should be carefully monitored (see PRECAUTIONS).

PREPARATION OF SOLUTION

120 mL Infusion Bottles
Contents of the 120 mL infusion bottles of PRIMAXIN Powder should be restored with 100 mL of diluent (see list of diluents under COMPATIBILITY AND STABILITY) and shaken until a clear solution is obtained.
13 mL Vials
Contents of the 13 mL vials must be suspended and transferred to 100 mL of an appropriate infusion solution.
A suggested procedure is to add approximately 10 mL from the appropriate infusion solution (see list of diluents under COMPATIBILITY AND STABILITY) to the vial. Shake well and transfer the resulting suspension to the infusion solution container.
CAUTION: THE SUSPENSION IS NOT FOR DIRECT INFUSION.
Repeat with an additional 10 mL of infusion solution to ensure complete transfer of vial contents to the infusion solution. **The resulting mixture should be agitated until clear.**

COMPATIBILITY AND STABILITY

Before reconstitution:
The dry powder should be stored at a temperature below 30°C.
Reconstituted solutions:
Solutions of PRIMAXIN range from colorless to yellow. Variations of color within this range do not affect the potency of the product.
PRIMAXIN, as supplied in infusion bottles and vials and reconstituted as above with the following diluents, maintains satisfactory potency for four hours at room temperature and for 24 hours under refrigeration (4°C) (note exception below). Solutions of PRIMAXIN should not be frozen.

- 0.9% Sodium Chloride Injection*
- 5% or 10% Dextrose Injection
- 5% Dextrose Injection with 0.02% sodium bicarbonate solution
- 5% Dextrose and 0.9% Sodium Chloride Injection
- 5% Dextrose Injection with 0.225% or 0.45% saline solution
- NORMOSOL†-M in D5-W
- 5% Dextrose Injection with 0.15% potassium chloride solution
- Mannitol 2.5%, 5% and 10%

PRIMAXIN should not be mixed with or physically added to other antibiotics. However, PRIMAXIN may be administered concomitantly with other antibiotics, such as aminoglycosides.

HOW SUPPLIED

PRIMAXIN is supplied as a sterile powder mixture in vials and infusion bottles containing imipenem (anhydrous equivalent) and cilastatin sodium as follows:
No. 3514—250 mg imipenem equivalent and 250 mg cilastatin equivalent and 10 mg sodium bicarbonate as a buffer
NDC 0006-3514-74 in trays of 10 vials.
No. 3516—500 mg imipenem equivalent and 500 mg cilastatin equivalent and 20 mg sodium bicarbonate as a buffer
NDC 0006-3516-75 in trays of 10 vials.
No. 3515—250 mg imipenem equivalent and 250 mg cilastatin equivalent and 10 mg sodium bicarbonate as a buffer
NDC 0006-3515-74 in trays of 10 infusion bottles.
No. 3517—500 mg imipenem equivalent and 500 mg cilastatin equivalent and 20 mg sodium bicarbonate as a buffer
NDC 0006-3517-75 in trays of 10 infusion bottles.

A.H.F.S. Category: 8:12.28
DC 7362400 Issued November 1985

REDISOL® Injectable ℞
(Cyanocobalamin, MSD), U.S.P.
Crystalline Vitamin B_{12}

DESCRIPTION

Cyanocobalamin Injection is a sterile solution of cyanocobalamin.
Cyanocobalamin appears as dark red crystals or as an amorphous or crystalline red powder. It is very hygroscopic in the anhydrous form, and sparingly soluble in water (about 1:80). It has a molecular weight of 1355.38. It is stable to autoclaving for short periods at 121°C. The vitamin B_{12} coenzymes are very unstable in light. Hydroxocobalamin is equally effective and shares the cobalamin molecular structure with cyanocobalamin.
The chemical name is 5,6-dimethylbenzimidazolyl cyanocobamide. The cobalt content is 4.34%. The pH is 4.5–7.0. The empirical formula is: $C_{63}H_{88}Co\ N_{14}O_{14}P$. Its structural formula is:

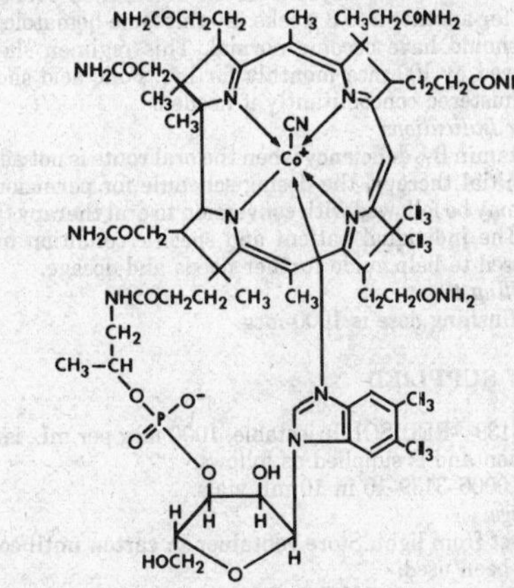

$NH_2COCH_2CH_2$ CH_3 $CH_3CH_2CONH_2$
NH_2COCH_2 CH_3 CH_3 $CH_2CH_2CONH_2$
CN Co+
NH_2COCH_2 CH_3 CH_3
$NHCOCH_2CH_2$ CH_3 CH_3 $CH_2CH_2CONH_2$
CH_2
CH_3–CH
O P O OH
$HOCH_2$ H H

Each mL of REDISOL® (Cyanocobalamin, MSD) Injectable contains:
Crystalline Cyanocobalamin USP .... 1000 mcg
Inactive ingredients:
Sodium chloride 0.83%
Water for Injection q.s. .... 1 mL
Added as preservatives:
Methylparaben 0.15%
Propylparaben 0.02%

CLINICAL PHARMACOLOGY

Vitamin B_{12} is essential to growth, cell reproduction, hematopoiesis, nucleoprotein and myelin synthesis.
Cyanocobalamin is quantitatively and rapidly absorbed from intramuscular and subcutaneous sites of injection; the plasma level of the compound reaches its peak within 1 hour after intramuscular injection. Fifty percent of the dose disappears from the injection site in 40 minutes. Absorbed vitamin B_{12} is transported via specific B_{12} binding proteins, transcobalamin I and II to the various tissues. The liver is the main organ for vitamin B_{12} storage.
Within 48 hours after injection of 100 or 1000 mcg of vitamin B_{12}, 50 to 98% of the injected dose may appear in the urine. The major portion is excreted within the first eight hours. Intravenous administration results in even more rapid excretion with little opportunity for liver storage.
Gastrointestinal absorption of vitamin B_{12} depends on the presence of sufficient intrinsic factor and calcium ions. Intrinsic factor deficiency causes pernicious anemia, which may be associated with subacute combined degeneration of the spinal cord. Prompt parenteral administration of vitamin B_{12} prevents progression of neurologic damage.
The average diet supplies about 5 to 15 mcg/day of vitamin B_{12} in a protein-bound form that is available for absorption after normal digestion. Vitamin B_{12} is not present in foods of plant origin, but is abundant in foods of animal origin. In people with normal absorption, deficiencies have been reported only in strict vegetarians who consume no products of animal origin (including no milk products or eggs).
Vitamin B_{12} is bound to intrinsic factor during transit through the stomach; separation occurs in the terminal ileum in the presence of calcium, and vitamin B_{12} enters the mucosal cell for absorption. It is then transported by the transcobalamin binding proteins. A small amount (approximately 1% of the total amount ingested) is absorbed by simple diffusion, but this mechanism is adequate only with very large doses. Oral absorption is considered too undependable to rely on in patients with pernicious anemia or other conditions resulting in malabsorption of vitamin B_{12}.
Cyanocobalamin is the most widely used form of vitamin B_{12} and has hematopoietic activity apparently identical to that of the antianemia factor in purified liver extract.
Colchicine, para-aminosalicylic acid and heavy alcohol intake for longer than 2 weeks may produce malabsorption of vitamin B_{12}.

INDICATIONS AND USAGE

I. Pernicious anemia, both uncomplicated and accompanied by nervous system involvement.
II. Dietary deficiency of vitamin B_{12}, occurring in strict vegetarians and in their breast-fed infants. (Isolated vitamin B_{12} deficiency is very rare.)
III. Malabsorption of vitamin B_{12}, resulting from structural or functional damage to the stomach, where intrinsic factor is secreted, or to the ileum, where intrinsic factor facilitates vitamin B_{12} absorption. These conditions include tropical sprue, and nontropical sprue (idiopathic steatorrhea, gluten-induced enteropathy). Folate deficiency in these patients is usually more severe than vitamin B_{12} deficiency.
IV. Inadequate secretion of intrinsic factor, resulting from lesions that destroy the gastric mucosa (ingestion of corrosives, extensive neoplasia), and a number of conditions associated with a variable degree of gastric atrophy (such as multiple sclerosis, certain endocrine disorders, iron deficiency, and subtotal gastrectomy). Total gastrectomy always produces vitamin B_{12} deficiency.
Structural lesions leading to vitamin B_{12} deficiency include regional ileitis, ileal resections, malignancies, etc.
V. Competition for vitamin B_{12} by intestinal parasites or bacteria.
The fish tapeworm (Diphyllobothrium latum) absorbs huge quantities of vitamin B_{12} and infested patients often have associated gastric atrophy. The blind-loop syndrome may produce deficiency of vitamin B_{12} or folate.
VI. Inadequate utilization of vitamin B_{12}.
This may occur if antimetabolites for the vitamin are employed in the treatment of neoplasia.
VII. For the Schilling Test.

CONTRAINDICATIONS

Hypersensitivity to any component of this medication.

WARNINGS

Folic acid is not a substitute for vitamin B_{12} therapy. Exclusive use of folic acid in treating vitamin B_{12} deficient megaloblastic anemia could result in progressive and irreversible neurologic damage.
Blunted or impeded therapeutic response to vitamin B_{12} may be due to such conditions as infection, uremia, drugs having bone marrow suppressant properties such as chloramphenicol, and concurrent iron or folic acid deficiency.
Anaphylactic shock and death have been reported after parenteral vitamin B_{12} administration. An intradermal test dose is recommended before cyanocobalamin injection is administered to patients suspected of being sensitive to this drug.
Hypokalemia and sudden death have been reported to occur in severe megaloblastic anemia which is treated intensely (see PRECAUTIONS, *Laboratory Tests*).
A rapid onset of severe and swift optic nerve atrophy has been reported in patients with Leber's disease (hereditary optic nerve atrophy) who have been treated with cyanocobalamin.

PRECAUTIONS

General
Vitamin B_{12} deficiency that is allowed to progress for longer than 3 months may produce permanent degenerative lesions of the spinal cord. Doses of folic acid greater than 0.1 mg per day may result in hematologic remission in patients with vitamin B_{12} deficiency. Neurologic manifestations of vitamin B_{12} deficiency will not be prevented with folic acid, and if not treated concomitantly with vitamin B_{12}, irreversible damage will result.
Doses of cyanocobalamin exceeding 10 mcg daily may produce hematologic response in patients with folate deficiency. Indiscriminate administration may mask the true diagnosis.
Information for patients:
Patients with pernicious anemia should be informed that they will require monthly injections of vitamin B_{12} for the remainder of their lives. Failure to do so will result in return of the anemia and in development of incapacitating and irreversible damage to the nerves of the spinal cord. Also, patients should be warned about the danger of taking folic acid in place of vitamin B_{12}, because the former may prevent anemia but allow progression of subacute combined degeneration.
A vegetarian diet which contains no animal products (including milk products or eggs) does not supply any vitamin B_{12}. Patients following such a diet, should be advised to take oral vitamin B_{12} regularly. The need for vitamin B_{12} is increased by pregnancy and lactation. Deficiency has been recognized in infants of vegetarian mothers who were breast fed, even though the mothers had no symptoms of deficiency at the time.

Continued on next page

*PRIMAXIN has been found to be stable in 0.9% Sodium Chloride Injection for 10 hours at room temperature and 48 hours under refrigeration.
†Registered trademark of Abbott Laboratories, Inc.

Merck Sharp & Dohme—Cont.

Laboratory Tests
Specific confirmatory diagnostic tests should be performed prior to initiating therapy. These should include hemoglobin, hematocrit, red blood cell count, reticulocyte count, folic acid, potassium, and platelet count.
With vitamin B_{12} therapy, hypokalemia and thrombocytosis could occur upon conversion of severe megaloblastic erythropoiesis to normal. Therefore, serum potassium levels and platelet count should be monitored carefully during therapy. Serum potassium should be closely monitored during the first 48 hours and potassium administered if necessary.
The patient should be followed with appropriate studies to demonstrate hematologic improvement (hemoglobin, hematocrit, red blood cell count, reticulocyte count). A diagnostic trial utilizing physiologic doses of vitamin B_{12} (1 mcg daily) and observing daily reticulocyte counts after establishing a baseline may also be performed. The occurrence of reticulocytosis, usually seen between the third and tenth day of therapy, confirms the diagnosis of vitamin B_{12} deficiency.
Drug/Laboratory Test Interactions
Persons taking most antibiotics, methotrexate and pyrimethamine invalidate folic acid and vitamin B_{12} diagnostic blood assays.
Carcinogenesis, Mutagenesis, Impairment of Fertility
Studies of carcinogenicity, mutagenesis or impairment of fertility have not been conducted with REDISOL.
Pregnancy
Pregnancy Category C: Animal reproduction studies have not been conducted with REDISOL. It is also not known whether REDISOL can cause fetal harm when administered to a pregnant woman or can affect reproduction capacity. REDISOL should be given to a pregnant woman only if clearly needed.
Nursing Mothers:
Vitamin B_{12} is known to be excreted in human milk. Amounts of vitamin B_{12} that are recommended by the Food and Nutrition Board, National Academy of Science—National Research Council for lactating women (4 mcg daily) should be consumed during lactation.
Vitamin B_{12} appears in the milk of nursing mothers in concentrations which approximates the mother's vitamin B_{12} blood level.
Pediatric use:
Intake in children should be in the amount (0.5 to 3 mcg daily) recommended by the Food and Nutrition Board, National Academy of Science—National Research Council.

ADVERSE REACTIONS

Generalized: Anaphylactic shock and death (see WARNINGS).
Cardiovascular: Pulmonary edema and congestive heart failure early in treatment; peripheral vascular thrombosis.
Hematological: Polycythemia.
Gastrointestinal: Mild transient diarrhea.
Dermatological: Itching; transitory exanthema.
Miscellaneous: Feeling of swelling of entire body; pain after injection.

OVERDOSAGE

No overdosage in humans has been reported with this drug. The intravenous LD_{50} of REDISOL in mice is greater than 50 mL/kg.

DOSAGE AND ADMINISTRATION

Avoid using the intravenous route. Use of this product intravenously will result in almost all of the vitamin being lost in the urine.
Parenteral drug products should be inspected visually for particulate matter and discoloration prior to administration, whenever solution and container permit.
In seriously ill patients it may be advisable to administer both vitamin B_{12} and folic acid while awaiting the results of distinguishing laboratory studies. It is not necessary to withhold vitamin B_{12} therapy until the precise cause of B_{12} deficiency is established since absorption studies can be performed at any time.
Treatment of Vitamin B_{12} Deficiency:
Thirty mcg daily for 5 to 10 days followed by 100–200 mcg monthly, injected intramuscularly or subcutaneously. If the patient is critically ill, or has neurologic disease, an infectious disease or hyperthyroidism, considerably higher doses may be indicated. However, current data indicate that the optimum obtainable neurologic response may be expected with a dosage of vitamin B_{12} sufficient to produce good hematologic response.
Children may be given a total dosage of 1 to 5 mg over a period of 2 or more weeks in doses of 100 mcg; maintenance dosage is 30 to 50 mcg every 4 weeks.

Pernicious Anemia
Parenteral vitamin B_{12} is the recommended treatment and will be required for the remainder of the patient's life. The oral form is not dependable. A dose of 100 mcg daily for 6 or 7 days should be administered by intramuscular or deep subcutaneous injection. If there is clinical improvement and if a reticulocyte response is observed, the same amount may be given on alternate days for seven doses, then every 3 to 4 days for another 2 to 3 weeks. By this time hematologic values should have become normal. This regimen should be followed by 100 mcg monthly for life. Folic acid should be administered concomitantly if needed.
Other Indications
In vitamin B_{12} deficiency when the oral route is not adequate for initial therapy, the dosing schedule for pernicious anemia may be followed with conversion to oral therapy thereafter. The individual patient and specific condition must be assessed to help guide further needs and dosage.
Schilling test:
The flushing dose is 1000 mcg.

HOW SUPPLIED

No. 3139—REDISOL Injectable, 1000 mcg per mL, is a pink solution and is supplied as follows:
NDC 0006-3139-10 in 10 mL vials.
Storage
Protect from light. Store container in carton until contents have been used.

A.H.F.S. Category: 88:08
DC 6361015 Issued April 1985

SINEMET® Tablets ℞
(Carbidopa-Levodopa, MSD), U.S.P.

DESCRIPTION

When SINEMET® (Carbidopa-Levodopa, MSD) is to be given to patients who are being treated with levodopa, levodopa must be discontinued at least eight hours before therapy with SINEMET is started. In order to reduce adverse reactions, it is necessary to individualize therapy. See the WARNINGS and DOSAGE AND ADMINISTRATION sections before initiating therapy.
Carbidopa, an inhibitor of aromatic amino acid decarboxylation, is a white, crystalline compound, slightly soluble in water, with a molecular weight of 244.3. It is designated chemically as (—)-L-α-hydrazino-α-methyl-β-(3, 4-dihydroxybenzene) propanoic acid monohydrate, and has the following structural formula:

OH
CH_3
HO–⟨ring⟩–$CH_2CCOOH \cdot H_2O$
$NHNH_2$

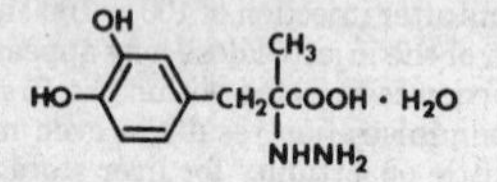

Tablet content is expressed in terms of anhydrous carbidopa which has a molecular weight of 226.3.
Levodopa, an aromatic amino acid, is a white, crystalline compound, slightly soluble in water, with a molecular weight of 197.2. It is designated chemically as (—)-L-α-amino-β-(3,4-dihydroxybenzene) propanoic acid, and has the following structural formula:

OH
HO–⟨ring⟩–$CH_2CHCOOH$
NH_2

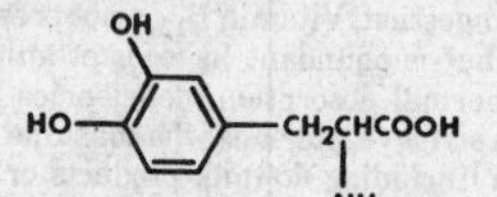

SINEMET is supplied as tablets in three strengths:
SINEMET 10-100, containing 10 mg of carbidopa and 100 mg of levodopa
SINEMET 25-100, containing 25 mg of carbidopa and 100 mg of levodopa
SINEMET 25-250, containing 25 mg of carbidopa and 250 mg of levodopa.
Inactive ingredients are cellulose, magnesium stearate, and starch. Tablets SINEMET 10-100 and 25-250 also contain FD&C Blue 2. Tablets SINEMET 25-100 also contain D&C Yellow 10 and FD&C Yellow 6.

ACTIONS

Current evidence indicates that symptoms of Parkinson's disease are related to depletion of dopamine in the corpus striatum. Administration of dopamine is ineffective in the treatment of Parkinson's disease apparently because it does not cross the blood-brain barrier. However, levodopa, the metabolic precursor of dopamine, does cross the blood-brain barrier, and presumably is converted to dopamine in the basal ganglia. This is thought to be the mechanism whereby levodopa relieves symptoms of Parkinson's disease.

When levodopa is administered orally it is rapidly converted to dopamine in extracerebral tissues so that only a small portion of a given dose is transported unchanged to the central nervous system. For this reason, large doses of levodopa are required for adequate therapeutic effect and these may often be attended by nausea and other adverse reactions, some of which are attributable to dopamine formed in extracerebral tissues.
Since levodopa competes with certain amino acids, the absorption of levodopa may be impaired in some patients on a high protein diet.
Carbidopa inhibits decarboxylation of peripheral levodopa. It does not cross the blood-brain barrier and does not affect the metabolism of levodopa within the central nervous system.
Since its decarboxylase inhibiting activity is limited to extracerebral tissues, administration of carbidopa with levodopa makes more levodopa available for transport to the brain. In dogs, reduced formation of dopamine in extracerebral tissues, such as the heart, provides protection against the development of dopamine-induced cardiac arrhythmias. Clinical studies tend to support the hypothesis of a similar protective effect in humans although controlled data are too limited at the present time to draw firm conclusions.
Carbidopa reduces the amount of levodopa required by about 75 percent and, when administered with levodopa, increases both plasma levels and the plasma half-life of levodopa, and decreases plasma and urinary dopamine and homovanillic acid.
In clinical pharmacologic studies, simultaneous administration of carbidopa and levodopa produced greater urinary excretion of levodopa in proportion to the excretion of dopamine than administration of the two drugs at separate times.
Pyridoxine hydrochloride (vitamin B_6), in oral doses of 10 mg to 25 mg, may reverse the effects of levodopa by increasing the rate of aromatic amino acid decarboxylation. Carbidopa inhibits this action of pyridoxine.

INDICATIONS

SINEMET is indicated in the treatment of the symptoms of idiopathic Parkinson's disease (paralysis agitans), postencephalitic parkinsonism, and symptomatic parkinsonism which may follow injury to the nervous system by carbon monoxide intoxication and manganese intoxication. SINEMET is indicated in these conditions to permit the administration of lower doses of levodopa with reduced nausea and vomiting, with more rapid dosage titration, with a somewhat smoother response, and with supplemental pyridoxine (vitamin B_6).

The incidence of levodopa-induced nausea and vomiting is less with SINEMET than with levodopa. In many patients this reduction in nausea and vomiting will permit more rapid dosage titration.

In some patients a somewhat smoother antiparkinsonian effect results from therapy with SINEMET than with levodopa. However, patients with markedly irregular ("on-off") responses to levodopa have not been shown to benefit from SINEMET.

Since carbidopa prevents the reversal of levodopa effects caused by pyridoxine, SINEMET can be given to patients receiving supplemental pyridoxine (vitamin B_6).

Although the administration of carbidopa permits control of parkinsonism and Parkinson's disease with much lower doses of levodopa, there is no conclusive evidence at present that this is beneficial other than in reducing nausea and vomiting, permitting more rapid titration, and providing a somewhat smoother response to levodopa. *Carbidopa does not decrease adverse reactions due to central effects of levodopa. By permitting more levodopa to reach the brain, particularly when nausea and vomiting is not a dose-limiting factor, certain adverse CNS effects, e.g., dyskinesias, may occur at lower dosages and sooner during therapy with SINEMET than with levodopa.*

Certain patients who responded poorly to levodopa have improved when SINEMET was substituted. This is most likely due to decreased peripheral decarboxylation of levodopa which results from administration of carbidopa rather than to a primary effect of carbidopa on the nervous system. Carbidopa has not been shown to enhance the intrinsic efficacy of levodopa in parkinsonian syndromes.

In considering whether to give SINEMET to patients already on levodopa who have nausea and /or vomiting, the practitioner should be aware that, while many patients may be expected to improve, some do not. Since one cannot predict which patients are likely to improve, this can only be determined by a trial of therapy. It should be further noted that in controlled trials comparing SINEMET with levodopa, about half of the patients with nausea and/or vomiting on levodopa improved spontaneously despite being retained on the same dose of levodopa during the controlled portion of the trial.

CONTRAINDICATIONS

Monoamine oxidase inhibitors and SINEMET should not be given concomitantly. These inhibitors must be discontinued at least two weeks prior to initiating therapy with SINEMET.
SINEMET is contraindicated in patients with known hypersensitivity to this drug, and in narrow angle glaucoma.
Because levodopa may activate a malignant melanoma, it should not be used in patients with suspicious, undiagnosed skin lesions or a history of melanoma.

WARNINGS

When patients are receiving levodopa, it must be discontinued at least eight hours before SINEMET is started. SINEMET should be substituted at a dosage that will provide approximately 25 percent of the previous levodopa dosage (see DOSAGE AND ADMINISTRATION). Patients who are taking SINEMET should be instructed not to take additional levodopa unless it is prescribed by the physician.
As with levodopa, SINEMET may cause involuntary movements and mental disturbances. These reactions are thought to be due to increased brain dopamine following administration of levodopa. All patients should be observed carefully for the development of depression with concomitant suicidal tendencies. Patients with past or current psychoses should be treated with caution. *Because carbidopa permits more levodopa to reach the brain and, thus, more dopamine to be formed, dyskinesias may occur at lower dosages and sooner with* SINEMET *than with levodopa.* The occurrence of dyskinesias may require dosage reduction.
SINEMET should be administered cautiously to patients with severe cardiovascular or pulmonary disease, bronchial asthma, renal, hepatic or endocrine disease.
Care should be exercised in administering SINEMET, as with levodopa, to patients with a history of myocardial infarction who have residual atrial, nodal, or ventricular arrhythmias. In such patients, cardiac function should be monitored with particular care during the period of initial dosage adjustment, in a facility with provisions for intensive cardiac care.
As with levodopa there is a possibility of upper gastrointestinal hemorrhage in patients with a history of peptic ulcer.
A symptom complex resembling the neuroleptic malignant syndrome including muscular rigidity, elevated body temperature, mental changes, and increased serum creatinine phosphokinase has been reported when antiparkinsonian agents were withdrawn abruptly. Therefore, patients should be observed carefully when the dosage of SINEMET is reduced abruptly or discontinued, especially if the patient is receiving neuroleptics.
Usage in Pregnancy and Lactation: Although the effects of SINEMET on human pregnancy and lactation are unknown, both levodopa and combinations of carbidopa and levodopa have caused visceral and skeletal malformations in rabbits. Use of SINEMET in women of childbearing potential requires that the anticipated benefits of the drug be weighed against possible hazards to mother and child. SINEMET should not be given to nursing mothers.
Usage in Children: The safety of SINEMET in patients under 18 years of age has not been established.

PRECAUTIONS

As with levodopa, periodic evaluations of hepatic, hematopoietic, cardiovascular, and renal function are recommended during extended therapy.
Patients with chronic wide angle glaucoma may be treated cautiously with SINEMET provided the intraocular pressure is well controlled and the patient is monitored carefully for changes in intraocular pressure during therapy.
Laboratory Tests
Abnormalities in laboratory tests may include elevations of liver function tests such as alkaline phosphatase, SGOT (ALT), SGPT (AST), lactic dehydrogenase, and bilirubin. Abnormalities in protein-bound iodine, blood urea nitrogen and positive Coombs test have also been reported. Commonly, levels of blood urea nitrogen, creatinine, and uric acid are lower during administration of SINEMET than with levodopa.
SINEMET may cause a false-positive reaction for urinary ketone bodies when a test tape is used for determination of ketonuria. This reaction will not be altered by boiling the urine specimen. False-negative tests may result with the use of glucose-oxidase methods of testing for glucosuria.
Drug Interactions
Caution should be exercised when the following drugs are administered concomitantly with SINEMET:
Symptomatic postural hypotension can occur when SINEMET is added to the treatment of a patient receiving antihypertensive drugs. Therefore, when therapy with SINEMET is started, dosage adjustment of the antihypertensive drug may be required. For patients receiving monoamine oxidase inhibitors, see CONTRAINDICATIONS.
There have been rare reports of adverse reactions, including hypertension and dyskinesia, resulting from the concomitant use of tricyclic antidepressants and SINEMET.
Phenothiazines and butyrophenones may reduce the therapeutic effects of levodopa. In addition, the beneficial effects of levodopa in Parkinson's disease have been reported to be reversed by phenytoin and papaverine. Patients taking these drugs with SINEMET should be carefully observed for loss of therapeutic response.

ADVERSE REACTIONS

The most common serious adverse reactions occurring with SINEMET are choreiform, dystonic, and other involuntary movements. Other serious adverse reactions are mental changes including paranoid ideation and psychotic episodes, depression with or without development of suicidal tendencies, and dementia. Convulsions also have occurred; however, a causal relationship with SINEMET has not been established.
A common but less serious effect is nausea.
Less frequent adverse reactions are cardiac irregularities and/or palpitations, orthostatic hypotensive episodes, bradykinetic episodes (the "on-off" phenomenon), anorexia, vomiting, and dizziness.
Rarely, gastrointestinal bleeding, development of duodenal ulcer, hypertension, phlebitis, hemolytic and non-hemolytic anemia, thrombocytopenia, leukopenia, and agranulocytosis have occurred.
Laboratory tests which have been reported to be abnormal are alkaline phosphatase, SGOT (ALT), SGPT (AST), lactic dehydrogenase, bilirubin, blood urea nitrogen, protein-bound iodine, and Coombs test.
Other adverse reactions that have been reported with levodopa are:
Nervous System: ataxia, numbness, increased hand tremor, muscle twitching, muscle cramps, blepharospasm (which may be taken as an early sign of excess dosage, consideration of dosage reduction may be made at this time), trismus, activation of latent Horner's syndrome.
Psychiatric: confusion, sleepiness, insomnia, nightmares, hallucinations, delusions, agitation, anxiety, euphoria.
Gastrointestinal: dry mouth, bitter taste, sialorrhea, dysphagia, bruxism, hiccups, abdominal pain and distress, constipation, diarrhea, flatulence, burning sensation of tongue.
Metabolic: weight gain or loss, edema.
Integumentary: flushing, increased sweating, dark sweat, skin rash, loss of hair.
Genitourinary: urinary retention, urinary incontinence, dark urine, priapism.
Special Senses: diplopia, blurred vision, dilated pupils, oculogyric crises.
Miscellaneous: weakness, faintness, fatigue, headache, hoarseness, malaise, hot flashes, sense of stimulation, bizarre breathing patterns, neuroleptic malignant syndrome.

DOSAGE AND ADMINISTRATION

The optimum daily dosage of SINEMET must be determined by careful titration in each patient. SINEMET tablets are available in a 1:4 ratio of carbidopa to levodopa (SINEMET 25-100) as well as a 1:10 ratio (SINEMET 25-250 and SINEMET 10-100). Tablets of the two ratios may be given separately or combined as needed to provide the optimum dosage.
Studies show that peripheral dopa decarboxylase is saturated by carbidopa at approximately 70 to 100 mg a day. Patients receiving less than this amount of carbidopa are more likely to experience nausea and vomiting.
Usual Initial Dosage
Dosage is best initiated with one tablet of SINEMET 25-100 three times a day. This dosage schedule provides 75 mg of carbidopa per day. Dosage may be increased by one tablet every day or every other day, as necessary, until a dosage of six tablets of SINEMET 25-100 a day is reached. If SINEMET 10-100 is used, dosage may be initiated with one tablet three or four times a day and increased by one tablet every day or every other day until a total of eight tablets (2 tablets q.i.d.) is reached.
How to Transfer Patients from Levodopa
Levodopa must be discontinued at least eight hours before starting SINEMET (Carbidopa-Levodopa, MSD). A daily dosage of SINEMET should be chosen that will provide approximately 25 percent of the previous levodopa dosage. Patients who are taking less than 1500 mg of levodopa a day should be started on one tablet of SINEMET 25-100 three or four times a day. The suggested starting dosage for most patients taking more than 1500 mg of levodopa is one tablet of SINEMET 25-250 three or four times a day.
Maintenance
Therapy should be individualized and adjusted according to the desired therapeutic response. When a greater proportion of carbidopa is required, one tablet of SINEMET 25-100 may be substituted for each tablet of SINEMET 10-100. When more levodopa is required, SINEMET 25-250 should be substituted at a dosage of one tablet three or four times a day. If necessary, the dosage may be increased by one-half or one tablet every day or every other day to a maximum of eight tablets a day. Experience with total daily dosages of carbidopa greater than 200 mg is limited.
Because both therapeutic and adverse responses occur more rapidly with SINEMET than with levodopa alone, patients should be monitored closely during the dose adjustment period. Specifically, involuntary movements will occur more rapidly with SINEMET than with levodopa. The occurrence of involuntary movements may require dosage reduction. Blepharospasm may be a useful early sign of excess dosage in some patients.
Current evidence indicates that other standard drugs for Parkinson's disease (except levodopa) may be continued while SINEMET is being administered, although their dosage may have to be adjusted.
If general anesthesia is required, SINEMET may be continued as long as the patient is permitted to take fluids and medication by mouth. If therapy is interrupted temporarily, the usual daily dosage may be administered as soon as the patient is able to take oral medication.

OVERDOSAGE

Management of acute overdosage with SINEMET is basically the same as management of acute overdosage with levodopa; however, pyridoxine is not effective in reversing the actions of SINEMET.
General supportive measures should be employed, along with immediate gastric lavage. Intravenous fluids should be administered judiciously and an adequate airway maintained. Electrocardiographic monitoring should be instituted and the patient carefully observed for the development of arrhythmias; if required, appropriate antiarrhythmic therapy should be given. The possibility that the patient may have taken other drugs as well as SINEMET should be taken into consideration. To date, no experience has been reported with dialysis; hence, its value in overdosage is not known.

HOW SUPPLIED

No. 3346—Tablets SINEMET 10-100 are dark dapple-blue, oval, scored, uncoated tablets, coded MSD 647. They are supplied as follows:
NDC 0006-0647-68 bottles of 100
(6505-01-020-8280 100's)
NDC 0006-0647-28 unit dose packages of 100.
Shown in Product Identification Section, page 418
No. 3365—Tablets SINEMET 25-100 are yellow, oval, scored tablets, coded MSD 650. They are supplied as follows:
NDC 0006-0650-68 bottles of 100
(6505-01-097-1233 100's)
NDC 0006-0650-28 unit dose packages of 100.
Shown in Product Identification Section, page 418
No. 3347—Tablets SINEMET 25-250 are light dapple-blue, oval, scored, uncoated tablets, coded MSD 654. They are supplied as follows:
NDC 0006-0654-68 bottles of 100
(6505-01-020-8279 100's)
NDC 0006-0654-28 unit dose packages of 100.
Shown in Product Identification Section, page 418
Storage
Tablets SINEMET 10-100 and Tablets SINEMET 25-250 must be protected from light.
A.H.F.S. Category: 92:00
DC 6834815 Issued October 1985

TIMOLIDE® Tablets ℞
(Timolol Maleate-Hydrochlorothiazide, MSD), U.S.P.

DESCRIPTION

TIMOLIDE® (Timolol Maleate-Hydrochlorothiazide, MSD) is for the treatment of hypertension. It combines the antihypertensive activity of two agents: a non-selective beta-adrenergic receptor blocking agent (timolol maleate) and a diuretic (hydrochlorothiazide).
Timolol maleate is (S)-1-[(1, 1-dimethylethyl) amino]-3-[[4- (4-morpholinyl)-1, 2, 5-thiadiazol -3- yl] oxy]-2-propanol, (Z)-butenedioate (1:1) salt. Its empirical formula is $C_{13}H_{24}N_4O_3S \cdot C_4H_4O_4$ and its structural formula is:
[See Chemical Formula at top of next page].
Timolol maleate has a molecular weight of 432.49. It is a white, odorless, crystalline powder which is soluble in water, methanol, and alcohol.

Continued on next page

Information on the Merck Sharp & Dohme products listed on these pages is the full prescribing information from product circulars in use August 31, 1986.

Merck Sharp & Dohme—Cont.

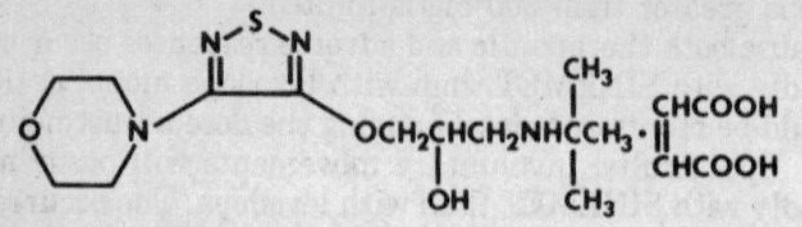

Hydrochlorothiazide is 6-chloro-3,4-dihydro-2*H*-1,2,4-benzothiadiazine-7-sulfonamide 1, 1- dioxide. Its empirical formula is $C_7H_8ClN_3O_4S_2$ and its structural formula is:

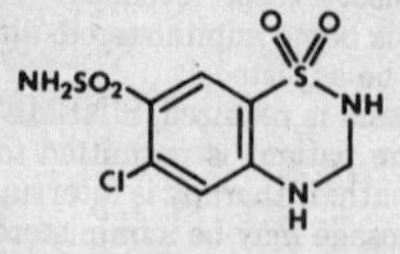

Hydrochlorothiazide has a molecular weight of 297.72. It is a white, or practically white, crystalline powder which is slightly soluble in water, but freely soluble in sodium hydroxide solution.

TIMOLIDE is supplied as tablets containing 10 mg of timolol maleate and 25 mg of hydrochlorothiazide for oral administration. Inactive ingredients are cellulose, FD&C Blue 2, magnesium stearate, and starch.

CLINICAL PHARMACOLOGY

TIMOLIDE

Timolol maleate and hydrochlorothiazide have been used singly and concomitantly for the treatment of hypertension. The antihypertensive effects of these agents are additive. The two components of TIMOLIDE have similar dosage schedules, and studies have shown that there is no interference with bioavailability when these agents are given together in the single combination tablet. Therefore, this combination provides a convenient formulation for the concomitant administration of these two entities.

In controlled clinical trials with TIMOLIDE in selected patients with mild to moderate essential hypertension, about 90 percent had a good to excellent response. In patients with more severe hypertension, TIMOLIDE may be administered with other antihypertensives such as ALDOMET® (Methyldopa, MSD) or a vasodilator.

Although the mechanisms of action of timolol maleate and hydrochlorothiazide in the treatment of hypertension have not been established, they are thought to be different; for example, hydrochlorothiazide increases plasma renin activity while timolol maleate reduces plasma renin activity.

Timolol Maleate

Timolol maleate is a $beta_1$ and $beta_2$ (non-selective) adrenergic receptor blocking agent that does not have significant intrinsic sympathomimetic, direct myocardial depressant, or local anesthetic activity.

Pharmacodynamics

Clinical pharmacology studies have confirmed the beta-adrenergic blocking activity as shown by (1) changes in resting heart rate and response of heart rate to changes in posture; (2) inhibition of isoproterenol-induced tachycardia; (3) alteration of the response to the Valsalva maneuver and amyl nitrite administration; and (4) reduction of heart rate and blood pressure changes on exercise.

Timolol maleate decreases the positive chronotropic, positive inotropic, bronchodilator, and vasodilator responses caused by beta-adrenergic receptor agonists. The magnitude of this decreased response is proportional to the existing sympathetic tone and the concentration of timolol maleate at receptor sites.

In normal volunteers, the reduction in heart rate response to a standard exercise was dose dependent over the test range of 0.5 to 20 mg, with a peak reduction at 2 hours of approximately 30% at higher doses.

Beta-adrenergic receptor blockade reduces cardiac output in both healthy subjects and patients with heart disease. In patients with severe impairment of myocardial function beta-adrenergic receptor blockade may inhibit the stimulatory effect of the sympathetic nervous system necessary to maintain adequate cardiac function.

Beta-adrenergic receptor blockade in the bronchi and bronchioles results in increased airway resistance from unopposed parasympathetic activity. Such an effect in patients with asthma or other bronchospastic conditions is potentially dangerous.

Clinical studies indicate that timolol maleate at a dosage of 20–60 mg/day reduces blood pressure without causing postural hypotension in most patients with essential hypertension. Administration of timolol maleate to patients with hypertension results initially in a decrease in cardiac output, little immediate change in blood pressure, and an increase in calculated peripheral resistance. With continued administration of timolol maleate blood pressure decreases within a few days, cardiac output usually remains reduced, and peripheral resistance falls toward pretreatment levels. Plasma volume may decrease or remain unchanged during therapy with timolol maleate. In the majority of patients with hypertension timolol maleate also decreases plasma renin activity. Dosage adjustment to achieve optimal antihypertensive effect may require a few weeks. When therapy with timolol maleate is discontinued, the blood pressure tends to return to pretreatment levels gradually. In most patients the antihypertensive activity of timolol maleate is maintained with long-term therapy and is well tolerated.

The mechanism of the antihypertensive effects of beta-adrenergic receptor blocking agents is not established at this time. Possible mechanisms of action include reduction in cardiac output, reduction in plasma renin activity, and a central nervous system sympatholytic action.

Pharmacokinetics and Metabolism

Timolol maleate is rapidly and nearly completely absorbed (about 90%) following oral ingestion. Detectable plasma levels of timolol occur within one-half hour and peak plasma levels occur in about one to two hours. The drug half-life in plasma is approximately 4 hours and this is essentially unchanged in patients with moderate renal insufficiency. Timolol is partially metabolized by the liver and timolol and its metabolites are excreted by the kidney. Timolol is not extensively bound to plasma proteins; i.e., $<10\%$ by equilibrium dialysis and approximately 60% by ultrafiltration. An *in vitro* hemodialysis study, using ^{14}C timolol added to human plasma or whole blood, showed that timolol was readily dialyzed from these fluids; however, a study of patients with renal failure showed that timolol did not dialyze readily. Plasma levels following oral administration are about half those following intravenous administration indicating approximately 50% first pass metabolism. The level of beta sympathetic activity varies widely among individuals, and no simple correlation exists between the dose or plasma level of timolol maleate and its therapeutic activity. Therefore, objective clinical measurements such as reduction of heart rate and/or blood pressure should be used as guides in determining the optimal dosage for each patient.

Hydrochlorothiazide

Hydrochlorothiazide is a diuretic and antihypertensive agent. It affects the renal tubular mechanism of electrolyte reabsorption. Hydrochlorothiazide increases excretion of sodium and chloride in approximately equivalent amounts. Natriuresis may be accompanied by some loss of potassium and bicarbonate. The mechanism of the antihypertensive effect of thiazides may be related to the excretion and redistribution of body sodium. Hydrochlorothiazide usually does not cause clinically important changes in normal blood pressure.

INDICATIONS AND USAGE

TIMOLIDE is indicated for the treatment of hypertension. **This fixed combination drug is not indicated for initial therapy of hypertension. If the fixed combination represents the dose titrated to an individual patient's needs, it may be more convenient than the separate components.**

CONTRAINDICATIONS

TIMOLIDE is contraindicated in patients with bronchial asthma or with a history of bronchial asthma, or severe chronic obstructive pulmonary disease (see WARNINGS); sinus bradycardia; second and third degree atrioventricular block; overt cardiac failure (see WARNINGS); cardiogenic shock; anuria; hypersensitivity to this product or to sulfonamide-derived drugs.

WARNINGS

Cardiac Failure

Sympathetic stimulation may be essential for support of the circulation in individuals with diminished myocardial contractility, and its inhibition by beta-adrenergic receptor blockade may precipitate more severe failure. Although beta blockers should be avoided in overt congestive heart failure, they can be used, if necessary, with caution in patients with a history of failure who are well-compensated, usually with digitalis and diuretics. Both digitalis and timolol maleate slow AV conduction. If cardiac failure persists, therapy with TIMOLIDE should be withdrawn.

In Patients Without a History of Cardiac Failure continued depression of the myocardium with beta-blocking agents over a period of time can, in some cases, lead to cardiac failure. At the first sign or symptom of cardiac failure, patients receiving TIMOLIDE should be digitalized and/or be given additional diuretic therapy. Observe the patient closely. If cardiac failure continues, despite adequate digitalization and diuretic therapy, TIMOLIDE should be withdrawn.

Renal and Hepatic Disease and Electrolyte Disturbances

Since timolol maleate is partially metabolized in the liver and excreted mainly by the kidneys, dosage reductions may be necessary when hepatic and/or renal insufficiency is present.

Although the pharmacokinetics of timolol maleate are not greatly altered by renal impairment, marked hypotensive responses have been seen in patients with marked renal impairment undergoing dialysis after 20 mg doses. Dosing in such patients should therefore be especially cautious.

In patients with renal disease, thiazides may precipitate azotemia, and cumulative effects may develop in the presence of impaired renal function. If progressive renal impairment becomes evident, TIMOLIDE should be discontinued.

In patients with impaired hepatic function or progressive liver disease, even minor alterations in fluid and electrolyte balance may precipitate hepatic coma. Hepatic encephalopathy, manifested by tremors, confusion, and coma, has been reported in association with diuretic therapy including hydrochlorothiazide.

Exacerbation of Ischemic Heart Disease Following Abrupt Withdrawal—Hypersensitivity to catecholamines has been observed in patients withdrawn from beta blocker therapy; exacerbation of angina and, in some cases, myocardial infarction have occurred after *abrupt* discontinuation of such therapy. When discontinuing chronically administered timolol maleate, particularly in patients with ischemic heart disease, the dosage should be gradually reduced over a period of one to two weeks and the patient should be carefully monitored. If angina markedly worsens or acute coronary insufficiency develops, timolol maleate administration should be reinstituted promptly, at least temporarily, and other measures appropriate for the management of unstable angina should be taken. Patients should be warned against interruption or discontinuation of therapy without the physician's advice. Because coronary artery disease is common and may be unrecognized, it may be prudent not to discontinue timolol maleate therapy abruptly even in patients treated only for hypertension.

Obstructive Pulmonary Disease

PATIENTS WITH CHRONIC OBSTRUCTIVE PULMONARY DISEASE (e.g., CHRONIC BRONCHITIS, EMPHYSEMA) OF MILD OR MODERATE SEVERITY, BRONCHOSPASTIC DISEASE OR A HISTORY OF BRONCHOSPASTIC DISEASE (OTHER THAN BRONCHIAL ASTHMA OR A HISTORY OF BRONCHIAL ASTHMA, IN WHICH 'TIMOLIDE' IS CONTRAINDICATED, see CONTRAINDICATIONS), SHOULD IN GENERAL NOT RECEIVE BETA BLOCKERS, INCLUDING 'TIMOLIDE'. However, if TIMOLIDE is necessary in such patients, then the drug should be administered with caution since it may block bronchodilation produced by endogenous and exogenous catecholamine stimulation of $beta_2$ receptors.

Major Surgery

The necessity or desirability of withdrawal of beta-blocking therapy prior to major surgery is controversial. Beta-adrenergic receptor blockade impairs the ability of the heart to respond to beta-adrenergically mediated reflex stimuli. This may augment the risk of general anesthesia in surgical procedures. Some patients receiving beta-adrenergic receptor blocking agents have been subject to protracted severe hypotension during anesthesia. Difficulty in restarting and maintaining the heartbeat has also been reported. For these reasons, in patients undergoing elective surgery, some authorities recommend gradual withdrawal of beta-adrenergic receptor blocking agents.

If necessary during surgery, the effects of beta-adrenergic blocking agents may be reversed by sufficient doses of such agonists as isoproterenol, dopamine, dobutamine or levarterenol (see OVERDOSAGE).

Metabolic and Endocrine Effects

Beta-adrenergic blockade may mask certain clinical signs (e.g., tachycardia) of hyperthyroidism. Patients suspected of developing thyrotoxicosis should be managed carefully to avoid abrupt withdrawal of beta blockade which might precipitate a thyroid storm. Thiazides may decrease serum PBI levels without signs of thyroid disturbance.

Beta-adrenergic receptor blocking agents may mask the signs and symptoms of acute hypoglycemia. Therefore, TIMOLIDE should be administered with caution to patients subject to spontaneous hypoglycemia, or to diabetic patients (especially those with labile diabetes) who are receiving insulin or oral hypoglycemic agents. Insulin requirements in diabetic patients may be increased, decreased, or unchanged by thiazides. Diabetes mellitus which has been latent may become manifest during administration of thiazide diuretics.

Because calcium excretion is decreased by thiazides, TIMOLIDE should be discontinued before carrying out tests for parathyroid function. Pathologic changes in the parathyroid glands, with hypercalcemia and hypophosphatemia, have been observed in a few patients on prolonged thiazide therapy; however, the common complications of hyperparathyroidism such as renal lithiasis, bone resorption, and peptic ulceration have not been seen.

Hyperuricemia may occur or acute gout may be precipitated in certain patients receiving thiazide therapy.

PRECAUTIONS

General

Electrolyte and Fluid Balance Status: Periodic determination of serum electrolytes to detect possible electrolyte imbalance should be performed at appropriate intervals.

Patients should be observed for clinical signs of fluid or electrolyte imbalance, i.e., hyponatremia, hypochloremic alkalosis, and hypokalemia. Serum and urine electrolyte determinations are particularly important when the patient is vomiting excessively or receiving parenteral fluids. Warning signs or symptoms of fluid and electrolyte imbalance include dryness of the mouth, thirst, weakness, lethargy, drowsiness, restlessness, muscle pains or cramps, muscular fatigue, hypotension, oliguria, tachycardia, and gastrointestinal disturbances such as nausea and vomiting.

Hypokalemia may develop, especially with brisk diuresis, when severe cirrhosis is present, or during concomitant use of corticosteroids or ACTH.

Interference with adequate oral electrolyte intake will also contribute to hypokalemia. Hypokalemia can sensitize or exaggerate the response of the heart to the toxic effects of digitalis (e.g., increased ventricular irritability). Hypokalemia may be avoided or treated by use of potassium supplements or foods with a high potassium content.

Any chloride deficit during thiazide therapy is generally mild and usually does not require specific treatment except under extraordinary circumstances (as in liver disease or renal disease). Dilutional hyponatremia may occur in edematous patients in hot weather; appropriate therapy is water restriction rather than administration of salt except in rare instances when the hyponatremia is life threatening. In actual salt depletion, appropriate replacement is the therapy of choice.

Thiazides have been shown to increase urinary excretion of magnesium, which may result in hypomagnesemia.

Muscle Weakness: Beta-adrenergic blockade has been reported to potentiate muscle weakness consistent with certain myasthenic symptoms (e.g., diplopia, ptosis, and generalized weakness). Timolol has been reported rarely to increase muscle weakness in some patients with myasthenia gravis or myasthenic symptoms.

Cerebrovascular Insufficiency: Because of potential effects of beta-adrenergic blocking agents relative to blood pressure and pulse, these agents should be used with caution in patients with cerebrovascular insufficiency. If signs or symptoms suggesting reduced cerebral blood flow are observed, consideration should be given to discontinuing these agents.

Drug Interactions

TIMOLIDE may potentiate the action of other antihypertensive agents used concomitantly. Close observation of the patient is recommended when TIMOLIDE is administered to patients receiving catecholamine-depleting drugs such as reserpine, because of possible additive effects and the production of hypotension and/or marked bradycardia, which may produce vertigo, syncope, or postural hypotension.

Blunting of the antihypertensive effect of beta-adrenoceptor blocking agents by non-steroidal anti-inflammatory drugs has been reported. In some patients, the administration of a non-steroidal anti-inflammatory agent can reduce the diuretic, natriuretic, and antihypertensive effects of loop, potassium-sparing and thiazide diuretics. Therefore, when TIMOLIDE and non-steroidal anti-inflammatory agents are used concomitantly, the patient should be observed closely to determine if the desired therapeutic effect has been obtained.

Literature reports suggest that oral calcium antagonists may be used in combination with beta-adrenergic blocking agents when heart function is normal, but should be avoided in patients with impaired cardiac function. Hypotension, AV conduction disturbances, and left ventricular failure have been reported in some patients receiving beta-adrenergic blocking agents when an oral calcium antagonist was added to the treatment regimen. Hypotension was more likely to occur if the calcium antagonist were a dihydropyridine derivative, e.g., nifedipine, while left ventricular failure and AV conduction disturbances were more likely to occur with either verapamil or diltiazem.

Intravenous calcium antagonists should be used with caution in patients receiving beta-adrenergic blocking agents.

The concomitant use of beta-adrenergic blocking agents with digitalis and either diltiazem or verapamil may have additive effects in prolonging AV conduction time.

Thiazides may decrease arterial responsiveness to norepinephrine. This diminution is not sufficient to preclude the therapeutic effectiveness of norepinephrine. Thiazides may increase the responsiveness to tubocurarine.

Lithium generally should not be given with diuretics because they reduce its renal clearance and add a high risk of lithium toxicity. Read circulars for lithium preparations before use of such preparations with TIMOLIDE.

Other Precautions

In patients receiving thiazides, sensitivity reactions may occur with or without a history of allergy or bronchial asthma. The possible exacerbation or activation of systemic lupus erythematosus has been reported. The antihypertensive effects of thiazides may be enhanced in the post-sympathectomy patient.

Carcinogenesis, Mutagenesis, Impairment of Fertility

In a two-year study of timolol maleate in rats, there was a statistically significant ($P \leq 0.05$) increase in the incidence of adrenal pheochromocytomas in male rats administered 300 times the maximum recommended human dose (1 mg/kg/day). Similar differences were not observed in rats administered doses equivalent to 25 or 100 times the maximum recommended human dose. In a lifetime study in mice, there were statistically significant ($P \leq 0.05$) increases in the incidence of benign and malignant pulmonary tumors and benign uterine polyps in female mice at 500 mg/kg/day, but not at 5 or 50 mg/kg/day. There was also a significant increase in mammary adenocarcinomas at the 500 mg/kg/day dose. This was associated with elevations in serum prolactin which occurred in female mice administered timolol at 500 mg/kg, but not at doses of 5 or 50 mg/kg/day. An increased incidence of mammary adenocarcinomas in rodents has been associated with administration of several other therapeutic agents which elevate serum prolactin, but no correlation between serum prolactin levels and mammary tumors has been established in man. Furthermore, in adult human female subjects who received oral dosages of up to 60 mg of timolol maleate, the maximum recommended human oral dosage, there were no clinically meaningful changes in serum prolactin.

There was a statistically significant increase ($P \leq 0.05$) in the overall incidence of neoplasms in female mice at the 500 mg/kg/day dosage level.

Timolol maleate was devoid of mutagenic potential when evaluated *in vivo* (mouse) in the micronucleus test and cytogenetic assay (doses up to 800 mg/kg) and *in vitro* in a neoplastic cell transformation assay (up to 100 µg /mL). In Ames tests the highest concentrations of timolol employed, 5000 or 10,000 µg/plate, were associated with statistically significant elevations ($P \leq 0.05$) of revertants observed with tester strain TA100 (in seven replicate assays), but not in the remaining three strains. In the assays with tester strain TA100, no consistent dose response relationship was observed, nor did the ratio of test to control revertants reach 2. A ratio of 2 is usually considered the criterion for a positive Ames test.

Reproduction and fertility studies in rats showed no adverse effect on male or female fertility at doses up to 150 times the maximum recommended human dose.

Pregnancy

Pregnancy Category C. Combinations of timolol maleate and hydrochlorothiazide were studied for teratogenic potential in the mouse and rabbit. The timolol maleate/hydrochlorothiazide combinations were administered orally to pregnant mice and pregnant rabbits at dosage levels of 1/2.5, 4/10, or 8/10 mg/kg/day. No teratogenic, embryotoxic, fetotoxic, or maternotoxic effects attributable to treatment were observed in either species. There are no adequate and well-controlled studies in pregnant women with TIMOLIDE. Because of the data listed below with the individual components, TIMOLIDE should be used during pregnancy only if the potential benefit justifies the potential risk to the fetus.

Timolol Maleate: Teratogenicity studies with timolol maleate in mice and rabbits at doses up to 50 mg/kg/day (50 times the maximum recommended human dose) showed no evidence of fetal malformations. Although delayed fetal ossification was observed at this dose in rats, there were no adverse effects on postnatal development of offspring. Doses of 1000 mg/kg/day (1,000 times the maximum recommended human dose) were maternotoxic in mice and resulted in an increased number of fetal resorptions. Increased fetal resorptions were also seen in rabbits at doses of 100 times the maximum recommended human dose, in this case without apparent maternotoxicity.

Hydrochlorothiazide: TIMOLIDE contains hydrochlorothiazide. Thiazides cross the placental barrier and appear in cord blood. The possible hazards to the fetus include fetal or neonatal jaundice, thrombocytopenia, and possibly other adverse reactions which have occurred in the adult.

Nursing Mothers

Because of the potential for serious adverse reactions from timolol and hydrochlorothiazide in nursing infants, a decision should be made whether to discontinue nursing or to discontinue the drug, taking into account the importance of the drug to the mother.

Pediatric Use

Safety and effectiveness in children have not been established.

ADVERSE REACTIONS

TIMOLIDE is usually well tolerated in properly selected patients. Most adverse effects have been mild and transient. The adverse reactions listed in the following table were spontaneously reported and have been arranged into two groups: (1) incidence greater than 1%; and (2) incidence less than 1%. The incidence was obtained from clinical studies conducted in the United States (257 patients treated with TIMOLIDE).

Incidence Greater Than 1%	*Incidence Less Than 1%*
BODY AS A WHOLE	
fatigue/tiredness (1.9%)	chest pain
asthenia (1.9%)	headache
CARDIOVASCULAR	
hypotension (1.6%)	arrhythmia
bradycardia (1.2%)	syncope
	cardiac failure
DIGESTIVE SYSTEM	
none	diarrhea
	dyspepsia
	nausea
	gastrointestinal pain
	constipation
INTEGUMENTARY	
none	rash
	increased pigmentation
	dry mucous membranes
MUSCULOSKELETAL	
none	myalgia
NERVOUS SYSTEM	
dizziness (1.2%)	none
PSYCHIATRIC	
none	insomnia
	decreased libido
	nervousness
	confusion
	trouble concentrating
	somnolence
RESPIRATORY	
bronchial spasm (1.6%)	rales
dyspnea (1.2%)	
UROGENITAL	
none	renal colic

The following additional adverse effects have been reported in clinical experience with the drug: cerebral ischemia, cerebral vascular accident, gout, muscle cramps, oculogyric crisis, worsening of chronic obstructive pulmonary disease, earache, and impotence.

Other adverse reactions that have been reported with the individual components are listed below:

Timolol Maleate—Body as a Whole: extremity pain, decreased exercise tolerance, weight loss; *Cardiovascular:* cardiac arrest, cerebral vascular accident, worsening of angina pectoris, sinoatrial block, AV block, worsening of arterial insufficiency, Raynaud's phenomenon, claudication, palpitations, vasodilitation, cold hands and feet, edema; *Digestive:* hepatomegaly, vomiting; *Hematologic:* nonthrombocytopenic purpura; *Endocrine:* hyperglycemia, hypoglycemia; *Skin:* skin irritation, pruritus, sweating; *Musculoskeletal:* arthralgia; *Nervous System:* local weakness, vertigo, paresthesia, increase in signs and symptoms of myasthenia gravis; *Psychiatric:* depression, nightmares, hallucinations; *Respiratory:* cough; *Special Senses:* visual disturbances, diplopia, ptosis, eye irritation, dry eyes, tinnitus; *Urogenital:* urination difficulties.

There have been reports of retroperitoneal fibrosis in patients receiving timolol maleate and in patients receiving other beta-adrenergic blocking agents. A causal relationship between this condition and therapy with beta-adrenergic blocking agents has not been established.

Hydrochlorothiazide—Body as a Whole: weakness; *Digestive:* anorexia, gastric irritation, vomiting, cramping, jaundice (intrahepatic cholestatic jaundice), pancreatitis, sialadenitis; *Nervous System/ Psychiatric:* vertigo, paresthesias, restlessness; *Hematologic:* Leukopenia, agranulocytosis, thrombocytopenia, aplastic anemia, hemolytic anemia; *Cardiovascular:* orthostatic hypotension (may be aggravated by alcohol, barbiturates, or narcotics); *Hypersensitivity:* purpura, photosensitivity, urticaria, necrotizing angiitis (vasculitis, cutaneous vasculitis), fever, respiratory distress including pneumonitis and pulmonary edema, anaphylactic reactions; *Metabolic:* hyperglycemia, glycosuria, hyperuricemia, electrolyte imbalance (see PRECAUTIONS); *Musculoskeletal:* muscle spasm; *Special Senses:* transient blurred vision, xanthopsia.

Potential Adverse Effects: In addition, a variety of adverse effects not observed in clinical trials with timolol maleate, but reported with other beta-adrenergic blocking agents, should be considered potential adverse effects of timolol maleate: *Nervous System:* Reversible mental depression progres-

Continued on next page

Information on the Merck Sharp & Dohme products listed on these pages is the full prescribing information from product circulars in use August 31, 1986.

Merck Sharp & Dohme—Cont.

sing to catatonia; an acute reversible syndrome characterized by disorientation for time and place, short-term memory loss, emotional lability, slightly clouded sensorium, and decreased performance on neuropsychometrics; *Cardiovascular:* Intensification of AV block (see CONTRAINDICATIONS); *Digestive:* Mesenteric arterial thrombosis, ischemic colitis; *Hematologic:* Agranulocytosis, thrombocytopenic purpura; *Allergic:* Erythematous rash, fever combined with aching and sore throat, laryngospasm with respiratory distress; *Miscellaneous:* Reversible alopecia, Peyronie's disease.
There have been reports of a syndrome comprising psoriasiform skin rash, conjunctivitis sicca, otitis, and sclerosing serositis attributed to the beta-adrenergic receptor blocking agent, practolol. This syndrome has not been reported with TIMOLIDE or BLOCADREN® (Timolol Maleate, MSD).
Clinical Laboratory Test Findings: Clinically important changes in standard laboratory parameters were rarely associated with the administration of TIMOLIDE. The changes in laboratory parameters were not progressive and usually were not associated with clinical manifestations. The most common changes were increases in serum triglycerides and uric acid and decreases in serum potassium and chloride.

OVERDOSAGE

No data are available in regard to overdosage in humans. Pretreatment of mice with hydrochlorothiazide (5 mg/kg) did not alter the LD_{50} of timolol (1320 mg/kg compared to 1300 mg/kg without pretreatment).
No specific information is available on the treatment of overdosage with TIMOLIDE, and no specific antidote is available. Treatment is symptomatic and supportive. Therapy with TIMOLIDE should be discontinued and the patient observed closely. Suggested measures include induction of emesis and/or gastric lavage, and correction of dehydration, electrolyte imbalance, and hypotension by established procedures.
Timolol Maleate
No data are available in regard to overdosage in humans. The oral LD_{50} of the drug is 1190 and 900 mg/kg in female mice and female rats, respectively.
An *in vitro* hemodialysis study, using ^{14}C timolol added to human plasma or whole blood, showed that timolol was readily dialyzed from these fluids; however, a study of patients with renal failure showed that timolol did not dialyze readily.
The most common signs and symptoms to be expected with overdosage with a beta-adrenergic receptor blocking agent are symptomatic bradycardia, hypotension, bronchospasm, and acute cardiac failure. If overdosage occurs the following therapeutic measures should be considered:
(1) *Gastric lavage.*
(2) *Symptomatic bradycardia:* Use atropine sulfate intravenously in a dosage of 0.25 mg to 2 mg to induce vagal blockade. If bradycardia persists, intravenous isoproterenol hydrochloride should be administered cautiously. In refractory cases the use of a transvenous cardiac pacemaker may be considered.
(3) *Hypotension:* Use sympathomimetic pressor drug therapy, such as dopamine, dobutamine or levarterenol. In refractory cases the use of glucagon hydrochloride has been reported to be useful.
(4) *Bronchospasm:* Use isoproterenol hydrochloride. Additional therapy with aminophylline may be considered.
(5) *Acute cardiac failure:* Conventional therapy with digitalis, diuretics, and oxygen should be instituted immediately. In refractory cases the use of intravenous aminophylline is suggested. This may be followed, if necessary, by glucagon hydrochloride which has been reported to be useful.
(6) *Heart block (second or third degree):* Use isoproterenol hydrochloride or a transvenous cardiac pacemaker.
Hydrochlorothiazide
The most common signs and symptoms observed with hydrochlorothiazide overdosage are those caused by electrolyte depletion (hypokalemia, hypochloremia, hyponatremia) and dehydration resulting from excessive diuresis. If digitalis has also been administered, hypokalemia may accentuate cardiac arrhythmias.

DOSAGE AND ADMINISTRATION

The recommended starting and maintenance dosage is 1 tablet twice a day. If the antihypertensive response is not satisfactory, another antihypertensive agent may be added.

HOW SUPPLIED

No. 3373—Tablets TIMOLIDE 10-25 are light blue, flat, hexagonal-shaped, compressed tablets, with MSD 67 code on one side and TIMOLIDE on the other. Each tablet contains 10 mg of timolol maleate and 25 mg of hydrochlorothiazide. They are supplied as follows:
NDC 0006-0067-68 bottles of 100.
Shown in Product Identification Section, page 418

Storage
Store in a well-closed container, protected from light.
A.H.F.S. Category: 24:08
DC 7244221 Issued October 1985

TIMOPTIC® Sterile Ophthalmic Solution (Timolol Maleate, MSD), U.S.P. ℞

DESCRIPTION

TIMOPTIC® (Timolol Maleate, MSD) Ophthalmic Solution is a non-selective beta-adrenergic receptor blocking agent. Its chemical name is (S)- 1- [(1, 1-dimethylethyl)amino] -3- [[4- (4- morpholinyl) -1, 2, 5-thiadiazol-3-yl]oxy] -2- propanol, (Z)- butenedioate (1:1) salt. Timolol maleate possesses an asymmetric carbon atom in its structure and is provided as the levo isomer. The nominal optical rotation of timolol maleate is

$[\alpha]^{25°}_{405\ nm}$ in 0.1N HCl (C = 5%) = −12.2°.

Its empirical formula is $C_{13}H_{24}N_4O_3S \cdot C_4H_4O_4$ and its structural formula is:

Timolol maleate has a molecular weight of 432.49. It is a white, odorless, crystalline powder which is soluble in water, methanol, and alcohol. TIMOPTIC is stable at room temperature.
TIMOPTIC Ophthalmic Solution is supplied as a sterile, isotonic, buffered, aqueous solution of timolol maleate in two dosage strengths: Each mL of TIMOPTIC 0.25% contains 2.5 mg of timolol (3.4 mg of timolol maleate). Each mL of TIMOPTIC 0.5% contains 5.0 mg of timolol (6.8 mg of timolol maleate). Inactive ingredients: monobasic and dibasic sodium phosphate, sodium hydroxide to adjust pH, and water for injection. Benzalkonium chloride 0.01% is added as preservative.

CLINICAL PHARMACOLOGY

Timolol maleate is a $beta_1$ and $beta_2$ (non-selective) adrenergic receptor blocking agent that does not have significant intrinsic sympathomimetic, direct myocardial depressant, or local anesthetic (membrane-stabilizing) activity.
Beta-adrenergic receptor blockade reduces cardiac output in both healthy subjects and patients with heart disease. In patients with severe impairment of myocardial function beta-adrenergic receptor blockade may inhibit the stimulatory effect of the sympathetic nervous system necessary to maintain adequate cardiac function.
Beta-adrenergic receptor blockade in the bronchi and bronchioles results in increased airway resistance from unopposed para-sympathetic activity. Such an effect in patients with asthma or other bronchospastic conditions is potentially dangerous.
TIMOPTIC Ophthalmic Solution, when applied topically in the eye, has the action of reducing elevated as well as normal intraocular pressure, whether or not accompanied by glaucoma. Elevated intraocular pressure is a major risk factor in the pathogenesis of glaucomatous visual field loss. The higher the level of intraocular pressure, the greater the likelihood of glaucomatous visual field loss and optic nerve damage.
The onset of reduction in intraocular pressure following administration of TIMOPTIC can usually be detected within one-half hour after a single dose. The maximum effect usually occurs in one to two hours and significant lowering of intraocular pressure can be maintained for periods as long as 24 hours with a single dose. Repeated observations over a period of one year indicate that the intraocular pressure-lowering effect of TIMOPTIC is well maintained.
The precise mechanism of the ocular hypotensive action of TIMOPTIC is not clearly established at this time. Tonography and fluorophotometry studies in man suggest that its predominant action may be related to reduced aqueous formation. However, in some studies a slight increase in outflow facility was also observed. Unlike miotics, TIMOPTIC reduces intraocular pressure with little or no effect on accommodation or pupil size. Thus, changes in visual acuity due to increased accommodation are uncommon, and dim or blurred vision and night blindness produced by miotics are not evident. In addition, in patients with cataracts the inability to see around lenticular opacities when the pupil is constricted is avoided.
In the clinical studies which are reported below, ocular pressure reductions to less than 22 mmHg were used as a reasonable reference point to allow comparisons between treatments. Reduction of ocular pressure to just below 22 mmHg may not be optimal for all patients; therapy should be individualized.
In controlled multiclinic studies in patients with untreated intraocular pressures of 22 mmHg or greater, TIMOPTIC 0.25 percent or 0.5 percent administered twice a day produced a greater reduction in intraocular pressure than 1, 2, 3, or 4 percent pilocarpine solution administered four times a day or 0.5, 1, or 2 percent epinephrine hydrochloride solution administered twice a day.
In the multiclinic studies comparing TIMOPTIC with pilocarpine, 61 percent of patients treated with TIMOPTIC had intraocular pressure reduced to less than 22 mmHg compared to 32 percent of patients treated with pilocarpine. For patients completing these studies, the mean reduction in pressure at the end of the study from pretreatment was 30.7 percent for patients treated with TIMOPTIC and 21.7 percent for patients treated with pilocarpine.
In the multiclinic studies comparing TIMOPTIC with epinephrine, 69 percent of patients treated with TIMOPTIC had intraocular pressure reduced to less than 22 mmHg compared to 42 percent of patients treated with epinephrine. For patients completing these studies, the mean reduction in pressure at the end of the study from pretreatment was 33.2 percent for patients treated with TIMOPTIC and 28.1 percent for patients treated with epinephrine.
In these studies, TIMOPTIC was generally well tolerated and produced fewer and less severe side effects than either pilocarpine or epinephrine. A slight reduction of resting heart rate in some patients receiving TIMOPTIC (mean reduction 2.9 beats/minute standard deviation 10.2) was observed.
TIMOPTIC has also been used in patients with glaucoma wearing conventional (PMMA) hard contact lenses, and has generally been well tolerated. TIMOPTIC has not been studied in patients wearing lenses made with materials other than PMMA.

INDICATIONS AND USAGE

TIMOPTIC Ophthalmic Solution has been shown to be effective in lowering intraocular pressure and may be used in:
Patients with chronic open-angle glaucoma
Patients with aphakic glaucoma
Some patients with secondary glaucoma
Other patients with elevated intraocular pressure who are at sufficient risk to require lowering of the ocular pressure.
Clinical trials have also shown that in patients who respond inadequately to multiple antiglaucoma drug therapy the addition of TIMOPTIC may produce a further reduction of intraocular pressure.

CONTRAINDICATIONS

TIMOPTIC is contraindicated in patients with bronchial asthma or with a history of bronchial asthma, or severe chronic obstructive pulmonary disease (see WARNINGS); sinus bradycardia; second and third degree atrioventricular block; overt cardiac failure (see WARNINGS); cardiogenic shock; hypersensitivity to any component of this product.

WARNINGS

As with other topically applied ophthalmic drugs, this drug may be absorbed systemically.
The same adverse reactions found with systemic administration of beta-adrenergic blocking agents may occur with topical administration. For example, severe respiratory reactions and cardiac reactions, including death due to bronchospasm in patients with asthma, and rarely death in association with cardiac failure, have been reported following administration of TIMOPTIC (see CONTRAINDICATIONS).
Cardiac Failure
Sympathetic stimulation may be essential for support of the circulation in individuals with diminished myocardial contractility, and its inhibition by beta-adrenergic receptor blockade may precipitate more severe failure.
In Patients Without a History of Cardiac Failure continued depression of the myocardium with beta-blocking agents over a period of time can, in some cases, lead to cardiac failure. At the first sign or symptom of cardiac failure TIMOPTIC should be discontinued.
Obstructive Pulmonary Disease
PATIENTS WITH CHRONIC OBSTRUCTIVE PULMONARY DISEASE (e.g., CHRONIC BRONCHITIS, EMPHYSEMA) OF MILD OR MODERATE SEVERITY, BRONCHOSPASTIC DISEASE OR A HISTORY OF BRONCHOSPASTIC DISEASE (OTHER THAN BRONCHIAL ASTHMA OR A HISTORY OF BRONCHIAL ASTHMA, IN WHICH 'TIMOPTIC' IS CONTRAINDICATED, see CONTRAINDICATIONS), SHOULD IN GENERAL NOT RECEIVE BETA BLOCKERS, INCLUDING 'TIMOPTIC'. However, if

TIMOPTIC is necessary in such patients, then the drug should be administered with caution since it may block bronchodilation produced by endogenous and exogenous catecholamine stimulation of $beta_2$ receptors.

Major Surgery

The necessity or desirability of withdrawal of beta-adrenergic blocking agents prior to major surgery is controversial. Beta-adrenergic receptor blockade impairs the ability of the heart to respond to beta-adrenergically mediated reflex stimuli. This may augment the risk of general anesthesia in surgical procedures. Some patients receiving beta-adrenergic receptor blocking agents have been subject to protracted severe hypotension during anesthesia. Difficulty in restarting and maintaining the heartbeat has also been reported. For these reasons, in patients undergoing elective surgery, some authorities recommend gradual withdrawal of beta-adrenergic receptor blocking agents.

If necessary during surgery, the effects of beta-adrenergic blocking agents may be reversed by sufficient doses of such agonists as isoproterenol, dopamine, dobutamine or levarterenol (see OVERDOSAGE).

Diabetes Mellitus

Beta-adrenergic blocking agents should be administered with caution in patients subject to spontaneous hypoglycemia or to diabetic patients (especially those with labile diabetes) who are receiving insulin or oral hypoglycemic agents. Beta-adrenergic receptor blocking agents may mask the signs and symptoms of acute hypoglycemia.

Thyrotoxicosis

Beta-adrenergic blocking agents may mask certain clinical signs (e.g., tachycardia) of hyperthyroidism. Patients suspected of developing thyrotoxicosis should be managed carefully to avoid abrupt withdrawal of beta-adrenergic blocking agents which might precipitate a thyroid storm.

PRECAUTIONS

General

Patients who are receiving a beta-adrenergic blocking agent orally and TIMOPTIC should be observed for a potential additive effect either on the intraocular pressure or on the known systemic effects of beta blockade.

Because of potential effects of beta-adrenergic blocking agents relative to blood pressure and pulse, these agents should be used with caution in patients with cerebrovascular insufficiency. If signs or symptoms suggesting reduced cerebral blood flow develop following initiation of therapy with TIMOPTIC, alternative therapy should be considered.

Muscle Weakness: Beta-adrenergic blockade has been reported to potentiate muscle weakness consistent with certain myasthenic symptoms (e.g., diplopia, ptosis, and generalized weakness). Timolol has been reported rarely to increase muscle weakness in some patients with myasthenia gravis or myasthenic symptoms.

In patients with angle-closure glaucoma, the immediate objective of treatment is to reopen the angle. This requires constricting the pupil with a miotic. TIMOPTIC has little or no effect on the pupil. When TIMOPTIC is used to reduce elevated intraocular pressure in angle-closure glaucoma, it should be used with a miotic and not alone.

As with the use of other antiglaucoma drugs, diminished responsiveness to TIMOPTIC after prolonged therapy has been reported in some patients. However, in one long-term study in which 96 patients have been followed for at least 3 years, no significant difference in mean intraocular pressure has been observed after initial stabilization.

Drug Interactions

Although TIMOPTIC used alone has little or no effect on pupil size, mydriasis resulting from concomitant therapy with TIMOPTIC and epinephrine has been reported occasionally.

Close observation of the patient is recommended when a beta blocker is administered to patients receiving catecholamine-depleting drugs such as reserpine, because of possible additive effects and the production of hypotension and/or marked bradycardia, which may produce vertigo, syncope, or postural hypotension.

Caution should be used in the coadministration of beta-adrenergic blocking agents, such as TIMOPTIC, and oral or intravenous calcium antagonists, because of possible atrioventricular conduction disturbances, left ventricular failure, and hypotension. In patients with impaired cardiac function, coadministration should be avoided.

The concomitant use of beta-adrenergic blocking agents with digitalis and calcium antagonists may have additive effects in prolonging atrioventricular conduction time.

Animal Studies

No adverse ocular effects were observed in rabbits and dogs administered TIMOPTIC topically in studies lasting one and two years respectively.

Carcinogenesis, Mutagenesis, Impairment of Fertility

In a two-year oral study of timolol maleate in rats, there was a statistically significant ($P \leq 0.05$) increase in the incidence of adrenal pheochromocytomas in male rats administered 300 times the maximum recommended human oral dose* (1 mg/kg/day). Similar differences were not observed in rats administered oral doses equivalent to 25 or 100 times the maximum recommended human oral dose. In a lifetime oral study in mice, there were statistically significant ($P \leq 0.05$) increases in the incidence of benign and malignant pulmonary tumors and benign uterine polyps in female mice at 500 mg/kg/day, but not at 5 or 50 mg/kg/day. There was also a significant increase in mammary adenocarcinomas at the 500 mg/kg/day dose. This was associated with elevations in serum prolactin which occurred in female mice administered timolol at 500 mg/kg, but not at doses of 5 or 50 mg/kg/day. An increased incidence of mammary adenocarcinomas in rodents has been associated with administration of several other therapeutic agents which elevate serum prolactin, but no correlation between serum prolactin levels and mammary tumors has been established in man. Furthermore, in adult human female subjects who received oral dosages of up to 60 mg of timolol maleate, the maximum recommended human oral dosage, there were no clinically meaningful changes in serum prolactin.

There was a statistically significant increase ($P \leq 0.05$) in the overall incidence of neoplasms in female mice at the 500 mg/kg/day dosage level.

Timolol maleate was devoid of mutagenic potential when evaluated *in vivo* (mouse) in the micronucleus test and cytogenetic assay (doses up to 800 mg/kg) and *in vitro* in a neoplastic cell transformation assay (up to 100 μg/mL). In Ames tests the highest concentrations of timolol employed, 5000 or 10,000 μg/plate, were associated with statistically significant elevations ($P \leq 0.05$) of revertants observed with tester strain TA100 (in seven replicate assays), but not in the remaining three strains. In the assays with tester strain TA100, no consistent dose response relationship was observed, nor did the ratio of test to control revertants reach 2. A ratio of 2 is usually considered the criterion for a positive Ames test.

Reproduction and fertility studies in rats showed no adverse effect on male or female fertility at doses up to 150 times the maximum recommended human oral dose.

Pregnancy

Pregnancy Category C. Teratogenicity studies with timolol in mice and rabbits at doses up to 50 mg/kg/day (50 times the maximum recommended human oral dose) showed no evidence of fetal malformations. Although delayed fetal ossification was observed at this dose in rats, there were no adverse effects on postnatal development of offspring. Doses of 1000 mg/kg/day (1,000 times the maximum recommended human oral dose) were maternotoxic in mice and resulted in an increased number of fetal resorptions. Increased fetal resorptions were also seen in rabbits at doses of 100 times the maximum recommended human oral dose, in this case without apparent maternotoxicity. There are no adequate and well-controlled studies in pregnant women. TIMOPTIC should be used during pregnancy only if the potential benefit justifies the potential risk to the fetus.

Nursing Mothers

Because of the potential for serious adverse reactions from timolol in nursing infants, a decision should be made whether to discontinue nursing or to discontinue the drug, taking into account the importance of the drug to the mother.

Pediatric Use

Safety and effectiveness in children have not been established by adequate and well-controlled studies.

ADVERSE REACTIONS

TIMOPTIC Ophthalmic Solution is usually well tolerated. The following adverse reactions have been reported either in clinical trials of up to 3 years duration prior to release in 1978 or since the drug has been marketed.

BODY AS A WHOLE

Headache, asthenia.

CARDIOVASCULAR

Bradycardia, arrhythmia, hypotension, syncope, heart block, cerebral vascular accident, cerebral ischemia, congestive heart failure, palpitation, cardiac arrest.

DIGESTIVE

Nausea.

NERVOUS SYSTEM/PSYCHIATRIC

Dizziness, depression, increase in signs and symptoms of myasthenia gravis.

SKIN

Hypersensitivity, including localized and generalized rash; urticaria.

RESPIRATORY

Bronchospasm (predominantly in patients with pre-existing bronchospastic disease), respiratory failure, dyspnea.

ENDOCRINE

Masked symptoms of hypoglycemia in insulin-dependent diabetics (See WARNINGS).

SPECIAL SENSES

Signs and symptoms of ocular irritation, including conjunctivitis, blepharitis, keratitis, blepharoptosis, decreased corneal sensitivity, visual disturbances including refractive changes (due to withdrawal of miotic therapy in some cases), diplopia, ptosis.

Causal Relationship Unknown: The following adverse effects have been reported, and a causal relationship to therapy with TIMOPTIC has not been established: *Body as a Whole:* Fatigue; *Cardiovascular:* Hypertension, chest pain; *Digestive:* Dyspepsia, anorexia, dry mouth; *Nervous System/Psychiatric:* Behavioral changes including confusion, hallucinations, anxiety, disorientation, nervousness, somnolence, and other psychic disturbances; *Skin:* Alopecia; *Special Senses:* Aphakic cystoid macular edema; *Urogenital:* Retroperitoneal fibrosis, impotence.

The following additional adverse effects have been reported in clinical experience with oral timolol maleate, and may be considered potential effects of ophthalmic timolol maleate: *Body as a Whole:* Extremity pain, decreased exercise tolerance, weight loss; *Cardiovascular:* Edema, pulmonary edema (non-fatal), cardiac failure, heart rate <40 beats/minute, worsening of angina pectoris, worsening of arterial insufficiency, AV block, sinoatrial block, Raynaud's phenomenon, vasodilatation; *Digestive:* Gastrointestinal pain, hepatomegaly, vomiting, diarrhea; *Hematologic:* Nonthrombocytopenic purpura; *Endocrine:* Hyperglycemia, hypoglycemia; *Skin:* Pruritus, skin irritation, increased pigmentation, sweating, cold hands and feet; *Musculoskeletal:* Arthralgia, claudication; *Nervous System/Psychiatric:* Vertigo, paresthesia, local weakness, decreased libido, nightmares, insomnia, diminished concentration; *Respiratory:* Rales, cough, bronchial obstruction; *Special Senses:* Tinnitus, dry eyes; *Urogenital:* Urination difficulties.

Potential Adverse Effects: In addition, a variety of adverse effects have been reported with other beta-adrenergic blocking agents and may be considered potential effects of ophthalmic timolol maleate: *Digestive:* Mesenteric arterial thrombosis, ischemic colitis; *Hematologic:* Agranulocytosis, thrombocytopenic purpura; *Nervous System:* Reversible mental depression progressing to catatonia; an acute reversible syndrome characterized by disorientation for time and place, short-term memory loss, emotional lability, slightly clouded sensorium, and decreased performance on neuropsychometrics; *Allergic:* Erythematous rash, fever combined with aching and sore throat, laryngospasm with respiratory distress; *Urogenital:* Peyronie's disease.

There have been reports of a syndrome comprising psoriasiform skin rash, conjunctivitis sicca, otitis and sclerosing serositis attributed to the beta- adrenergic receptor blocking agent, practolol. This syndrome has not been reported with timolol maleate.

OVERDOSAGE

No data are available in regard to overdosage in humans. The oral LD_{50} of the drug is 1190 and 900 mg/kg in female mice and female rats, respectively.

An *in vitro* hemodialysis study, using ^{14}C timolol added to human plasma or whole blood, showed that timolol was readily dialyzed from these fluids; however, a study of patients with renal failure showed that timolol did not dialyze readily.

The most common signs and symptoms to be expected with overdosage with administration of a systemic beta-adrenergic receptor blocking agent are symptomatic bradycardia, hypotension, bronchospasm, and acute cardiac failure. The following therapeutic measures should be considered:

(1) *Gastric lavage:* If ingested.

(2) *Symptomatic bradycardia:* Use atropine sulfate intravenously in a dosage of 0.25 mg to 2 mg to induce vagal blockade. If bradycardia persists, intravenous isoproterenol hydrochloride should be administered cautiously. In refractory cases the use of a transvenous cardiac pacemaker may be considered.

(3) *Hypotension:* Use sympathomimetic pressor drug therapy, such as dopamine, dobutamine or levarterenol. In refractory cases the use of glucagon hydrochloride has been reported to be useful.

(4) *Bronchospasm:* Use isoproterenol hydrochloride. Additional therapy with aminophylline may be considered.

(5) *Acute cardiac failure:* Conventional therapy with digitalis, diuretics, and oxygen should be instituted immediately. In refractory cases the use of intravenous aminophylline is suggested. This may be followed if necessary by glucagon hydrochloride which has been reported to be useful.

(6) *Heart block (second or third degree):* Use isoproterenol hydrochloride or a transvenous cardiac pacemaker.

Continued on next page

*The maximum recommended single oral dose is 30 mg of timolol. One drop of TIMOPTIC 0.5% contains about 1/150 of this dose which is about 0.2 mg.

Information on the Merck Sharp & Dohme products listed on these pages is the full prescribing information from product circulars in use August 31, 1986.

Merck Sharp & Dohme—Cont.

DOSAGE AND ADMINISTRATION

TIMOPTIC Ophthalmic Solution is available in concentrations of 0.25 and 0.5 percent. The usual starting dose is one drop of 0.25 percent TIMOPTIC in the affected eye(s) twice a day. If the clinical response is not adequate, the dosage may be changed to one drop of 0.5 percent solution in the affected eye(s) twice a day.

Since in some patients the pressure-lowering response to TIMOPTIC may require a few weeks to stabilize, evaluation should include a determination of intraocular pressure after approximately 4 weeks of treatment with TIMOPTIC.

If the intraocular pressure is maintained at satisfactory levels, the dosage schedule may be changed to one drop once a day in the affected eye(s). Because of diurnal variations in intraocular pressure, satisfactory response to the once-a-day dose is best determined by measuring the intraocular pressure at different times during the day.

Dosages above one drop of 0.5 percent TIMOPTIC twice a day generally have not been shown to produce further reduction in intraocular pressure. If the patient's intraocular pressure is still not at a satisfactory level on this regimen, concomitant therapy with pilocarpine and other miotics, and/or epinephrine, and/or systemically administered carbonic anhydrase inhibitors, such as acetazolamide, can be instituted.

When a patient is transferred from a single antiglaucoma agent, continue the agent already being used and add one drop of 0.25 percent TIMOPTIC in the affected eye(s) twice a day. On the following day, discontinue the previously used antiglaucoma agent completely and continue with TIMOPTIC. If a higher dosage of TIMOPTIC is required, substitute one drop of 0.5 percent solution in the affected eye(s) twice a day.

When a patient is transferred from several concomitantly administered antiglaucoma agents, individualization is required. Adjustments should involve one agent at a time and usually should be made at intervals of not less than one week. A recommended approach is to continue the agents being used and to add one drop of 0.25 percent TIMOPTIC in the affected eye(s) twice a day. On the following day, discontinue one of the other antiglaucoma agents. The remaining antiglaucoma agents may be decreased or discontinued according to the patient's response to treatment. If a higher dosage of TIMOPTIC is required, substitute one drop of 0.5 percent solution in the affected eye(s) twice a day. The physician may be able to discontinue some or all of the other antiglaucoma agents.

HOW SUPPLIED

Sterile Ophthalmic Solution TIMOPTIC is a clear, colorless to light yellow solution.

No. 3366—TIMOPTIC Ophthalmic Solution, 0.25% timolol equivalent, is supplied in a white, opaque, plastic OCUMETER® ophthalmic dispenser with a controlled drop tip as follows:

NDC 0006-3366-03, 5 mL
NDC 0006-3366-10, 10 mL
NDC 0006-3366-12, 15 mL.

No. 3367—TIMOPTIC Ophthalmic Solution, 0.5% timolol equivalent, is supplied in a white, opaque, plastic OCUMETER ophthalmic dispenser with a controlled drop tip as follows:

NDC 0006-3367-03, 5 mL
NDC 0006-3367-10, 10 mL
NDC 0006-3367-12, 15 mL.

Storage

Protect from light. Store at room temperature.

A.H.F.S. Category: 52:36
DC 7046021 Issued April 1985

TONOCARD® Tablets (Tocainide HCl, MSD) ℞

DESCRIPTION

TONOCARD* (Tocainide HCl, MSD) is a primary amine analog of lidocaine with antiarrhythmic properties useful in the treatment of ventricular arrhythmias. The chemical name for tocainide hydrochloride is 2-amino-*N*-(2,6-dimethylphenyl) propanamide hydrochloride. Its empirical formula is $C_{11}H_{16}N_2O \cdot HCl$, with a molecular weight of 228.72. The structural formula is:

CH_3
$-NHCOCHCH_3 \cdot HCl$
NH_2
CH_3

Tocainide hydrochloride is a white crystalline powder with a bitter taste and is freely soluble in water. It is supplied as 400 mg and 600 mg tablets for oral administration. Each tablet contains the following inactive ingredients: hydroxypropyl methylcellulose, iron oxide, magnesium stearate, methylcellulose, polyethylene glycol, and titanium dioxide.

* Registered trademark of Astra Pharmaceutical Products, Inc.

CLINICAL PHARMACOLOGY

Action

Tocainide, like lidocaine, produces dose dependent decreases in sodium and potassium conductance, thereby decreasing the excitability of myocardial cells. In experimental animal models, the dose-related depression of sodium current is more pronounced in ischemic tissue than in normal tissue.

Electrophysiology

Tocainide is a Class I antiarrhythmic compound with electrophysiologic properties in man similar to those of lidocaine, but dissimilar from quinidine, procainamide, and disopyramide.

In studies of isolated dog Purkinje fibers, tocainide in concentrations of 1–50 mcg/mL had no significant effect on resting membrane potential, but reduced the amplitude and rate of depolarization (dv/dt) of the action potential. Tocainide decreased the effective refractory period (ERP) to a lesser extent than the action potential duration (APD) resulting in an increase in the ERP/APD ratio.

In patients with cardiac disease, TONOCARD produced no clinically significant changes in sinus nodal function, effective refractory periods, or intracardiac conduction times when studied under electrophysiologic testing procedures.

Tocainide, like lidocaine, characteristically does not prolong ventricular depolarization (QRS duration) or repolarization (QT intervals) as measured by electrocardiography. Theoretically, therefore, TONOCARD may be useful in the treatment of ventricular arrhythmias associated with a prolonged QT interval.

Patients who respond to lidocaine also respond to TONOCARD in a majority of cases. Failure to respond to lidocaine usually predicts failure to respond to TONOCARD, but there are exceptions to this.

Pharmacokinetics

Following oral administration of tocainide, peak plasma concentrations occur within 0.5 to 2 hours. The average plasma half-life in patients is approximately 15 hours. Although the effective plasma concentration may vary from patient to patient, the usual therapeutic plasma range (as defined by 50–80 percent PVC suppression) is 4–10 mcg/mL (18–45 micromole/L), expressed as tocainide hydrochloride. Tocainide is approximately 10 percent bound to plasma protein.

In contrast to lidocaine, tocainide undergoes negligible first pass hepatic degradation. Following oral administration, the bioavailability of TONOCARD approaches 100 percent. The extent of its bioavailability is unaffected by food. Tocainide has no cardioactive metabolites. Approximately 40 percent of the administered dose of tocainide is excreted unchanged in the urine. Acidification of the urine has not been shown to significantly alter tocainide excretion in the urine, but alkalinization of the urine results in a significant decrease in the percent of tocainide excreted unchanged in the urine. Animal data indicate that tocainide crosses the blood-brain barrier; however, it has less lipid solubility than lidocaine.

Hemodynamics

Cardiac catheterization studies in man utilizing intravenous tocainide infusions (0.5–0.75 mg/kg/min over 15 min) have shown that tocainide usually produces a small degree of depression of parameters of left ventricular function, such as left ventricular dP/dt, and left ventricular end diastolic pressure. There were usually no changes in cardiac output or clinical evidence of increasing congestive heart failure in the well-compensated patients studied. Small but statistically significant increases in aortic and pulmonary arterial pressures have been consistently observed and are probably related to small increases in vascular resistance. When used concomitantly with a beta-blocking drug, tocainide further reduced cardiac index and left ventricular dP/dt and further increased pulmonary wedge pressure.

No clinically significant changes in heart rate, blood pressure, or signs of myocardial depression were observed in a study of 72 post-myocardial infarction patients receiving long-term therapy with oral TONOCARD at usual doses (400 mg q8h). When tocainide was administered orally at a dose of 120 mg/kg to anesthetized dogs (14 times the initial maximum dose recommended for humans), a negative inotropic effect was observed: the rate of change of left ventricular pressure decreased by up to 29 percent of control at 3 hours after administration. This effect was not observed at lower doses (60 mg/kg). Tocainide has been used safely in patients with acute myocardial infarction and various degrees of congestive heart failure. It has, however, a small negative inotropic effect and can increase peripheral resistance slightly. It therefore should be used cautiously in patients with known heart failure, particularly if a beta blocker is given as well. (See PRECAUTIONS).

INDICATIONS AND USAGE

TONOCARD is indicated for the suppression of symptomatic ventricular arrhythmias, including frequent premature ventricular contractions, unifocal or multifocal, couplets, and ventricular tachycardia.

In a controlled comparison with quinidine, 600 mg b.i.d. of TONOCARD produced a mean reduction of 42 percent in PVC count, compared to a 54 percent reduction by quinidine 300 mg every 6 hours. Among all patients entered into the study, about one-fifth of tocainide recipients and one-third of quinidine recipients had 75 percent or greater reductions in PVC count or had elimination of ventricular tachycardia.

Like other antiarrhythmics, tocainide has not been shown to prevent sudden death in patients with serious ventricular ectopic activity, and also, like other antiarrhythmics, it has potentially serious adverse effects, including the ability to worsen arrhythmias. It is therefore essential that each patient given tocainide be evaluated electrocardiographically and clinically prior to, and during, tocainide therapy to determine whether the response to tocainide supports continued treatment.

CONTRAINDICATIONS

Patients who are hypersensitive to this product or to local anesthetics of the amide type.

Patients with second or third degree atrioventricular block in the absence of an artificial ventricular pacemaker.

WARNINGS

Blood Dyscrasias: Agranulocytosis, bone marrow depression, leukopenia, hypoplastic anemia and thrombocytopenia have been reported in patients receiving TONOCARD. Many of these events occurred in patients who were seriously ill and who were receiving concomitant drugs; fatalities have occurred. Since most of these events have been noted during the first 12 weeks of therapy, it is recommended that blood counts, including differential and platelet counts, be performed at least once within the first two to three weeks of therapy; and periodically thereafter, particularly within the first three months of therapy. Blood counts should be performed promptly if the patient develops any signs of infection (such as fever, chills, sore throat, or stomatitis), bruising, or bleeding. If any of these hematologic disorders is identified, TONOCARD should be discontinued and appropriate treatment should be instituted if necessary. Blood counts usually return to normal within one month of discontinuation. Caution should be used in patients with pre-existing marrow failure or cytopenia of any type. (See ADVERSE REACTIONS).

Acceleration of Ventricular Rate: Acceleration of ventricular rate occurs infrequently when antiarrhythmics are administered to patients with atrial flutter or fibrillation (see ADVERSE REACTIONS).

PRECAUTIONS

General

Pulmonary Fibrosis: Pulmonary fibrosis, interstitial pneumonitis, fibrosing alveolitis, pulmonary edema, and pneumonia, possibly drug related, have been reported in patients receiving TONOCARD. Many of these events occurred in patients who were seriously ill. The experiences are usually characterized by bilateral infiltrates on x-ray and are frequently associated with dyspnea and cough. Fever may or may not be present. Patients should be instructed to promptly report the development of any pulmonary symptoms such as exertional dyspnea, cough or wheezing. Chest x-rays are advisable at that time. If these pulmonary disorders develop, TONOCARD should be discontinued. (See ADVERSE REACTIONS).

In patients with known heart failure or minimal cardiac reserve, TONOCARD should be used with caution because of the potential for aggravating the degree of heart failure.

Caution should be used in the institution or continuation of antiarrhythmic therapy in the presence of signs of increasing depression of cardiac conductivity.

In patients with severe liver or kidney disease, the rate of drug elimination may be significantly decreased (see DOSAGE AND ADMINISTRATION).

Since antiarrhythmic drugs may be ineffective in patients with hypokalemia, the possibility of a potassium deficit should be explored and, if present, the deficit should be corrected.

Like all other oral antiarrhythmics, TONOCARD has been reported to increase arrhythmias in some patients (see ADVERSE REACTIONS).

Information for Patients

Patients should be instructed to promptly report the development of bruising or bleeding; any signs of infections such as fever, chills, sore throat, or soreness and ulcers in the mouth; or any pulmonary symptoms, such as exertional dyspnea, cough, or wheezing.

Laboratory Tests

As with other antiarrhythmics, abnormal liver function tests, particularly in the early stages of therapy, have been reported. Periodic monitoring of liver function should be considered. Hepatitis and jaundice have been reported in some patients.

Drug Interactions

Specific interaction studies with digoxin and metoprolol have been conducted, no clinically significant interaction was seen with digoxin, but tocainide and metoprolol had additive effects on wedge pressure and cardiac index. TONOCARD has also been used in open studies with digitalis, beta-blocking agents, other antiarrhythmic agents, anticoagulants, and diuretics, without evidence of clinically significant interactions. Nevertheless, caution should be exercised in the use of multiple drug therapy.

TONOCARD is equally effective in digitalized and non-digitalized patients. In 17 patients with refractory ventricular arrhythmias on concomitant therapy, serum digoxin levels (1.1 ± 0.4 ng/mL) remained in the expected normal range (0.5–2.5 ng/mL) during tocainide administration.

Carcinogenesis, Mutagenesis, Impairment of Fertility

The carcinogenic potential of tocainide was studied in mice using oral doses up to 300 mg/kg/day (about 6 times the maximum recommended human dose) for up to 94 weeks in males and 102 weeks in females and in rats at doses up to 200 mg/kg/day for 24 months. Tocainide did not affect the type or incidence of neoplasia in the two studies.

Tocainide did not show any mutagenic effect when evaluated *in vivo* in the micronucleus test using mice at oral doses up to 187.5 mg/kg/day (about 7 times the usual human dose). Also, no mutagenic activity was seen *in vitro* in the Ames microbial mutagen test or in the mouse lymphoma forward mutation assay.

Reproduction and fertility studies in rats showed no adverse effects on male or female fertility at oral doses up to 200 mg/kg/day (about 8 times the usual human dose).

Pregnancy

Pregnancy Category C. In a teratogenicity study in rabbits, tocainide was administered orally at doses of 25, 50, and 100 mg/kg/day (about 1 to 4 times the usual human dose). No evidence of a drug-related teratogenic effect was noted; however, these doses were maternotoxic and produced a dose-related increase in abortions and stillbirths. In a teratogenicity study in rats, an oral dose of 300 mg/kg/day (about 12 times the usual human dose) showed no evidence of treatment-related fetal malformations, but maternotoxicity and an increase in fetal resorptions were noted. An oral dose of 30 mg/kg/day (about twice the usual human dose) did not produce any adverse effects.

In reproduction studies in rats at maternotoxic oral doses of 200 and 300 mg/kg/day (about 8 and 12 times the usual human dose, respectively), dystocia, and delayed parturition occurred which was accompanied by an increase in stillbirths and decreased survival in offspring during the first week postpartum. Growth and viability of surviving offspring were not affected for the remainder of the lactation period.

There are no adequate and well-controlled studies in pregnant women. TONOCARD should be used during pregnancy only if the potential benefit justifies the potential risk to the fetus.

Nursing Mothers

It is not known whether tocainide is secreted in human milk. Because many drugs are secreted in human milk and because of the potential for serious adverse reactions in nursing infants from TONOCARD, a decision should be made whether to discontinue nursing or to discontinue the drug, taking into account the importance of the drug to the mother.

Pediatric Use

Safety and effectiveness in children have not been established.

ADVERSE REACTIONS

TONOCARD commonly produces minor, transient, nervous system and gastrointestinal adverse reactions, but is otherwise generally well tolerated. TONOCARD has been evaluated in both short-term (n = 1,358) and long-term (n = 262) controlled studies as well as a compassionate use program. Dosages were lower in most of the controlled studies (1200 mg/day) and higher in the compassionate use program (1800 mg and more). In long-term (2–6 months) controlled studies, the most frequent adverse reactions were lightheadedness/dizziness (15.3 percent), nausea (14.5 percent), paresthesia/numbness (9.2 percent), and tremor (8.4 percent). These reactions were generally mild, transient, dose-related and reversible with a reduction in dosage, by taking the drug with food, or by therapy discontinuation. Tremor, when present, may be useful as a clinical indicator that the maximum dose is being approached. Adverse reactions leading to therapy discontinuation occurred in 21 percent of patients in long-term controlled trials and were usually related to the nervous system or gastrointestinal system.

Adverse reactions occurring in greater than one percent of patients from the short-term and long-term controlled studies appear in the following table:

	Percent of Patients Controlled Studies Short-Term (n = 1,358)	Long-Term (n = 262)
NERVOUS SYSTEM		
Lightheadedness/dizziness/vertigo/giddiness	8.0	15.3
Paresthesia/numbness	3.5	9.2
Tremor/quivering/tremulousness	2.9	8.4
Confusion/disorientation/hallucinations	2.1	2.7
Altered mood/awareness	1.5	3.4
Restlessness/shakiness/nervousness	1.5	0.4
Blurred vision/visual disturbances	1.3	1.5
Discoordination/unsteadiness/walking disturbances	1.2	0.0
Anxiety	1.1	1.5
Tinnitus/hearing loss	0.4	1.5
Ataxia	0.2	3.0
Nystagmus	0.0	1.1
GASTROINTESTINAL SYSTEM		
Nausea	15.2	14.5
Vomiting	8.3	4.6
Anorexia	1.2	1.9
Diarrhea/loose stools	0.0	3.8
CARDIOVASCULAR SYSTEM		
Hypotension	3.4	2.7
Bradycardia	1.8	0.4
Palpitations	1.8	0.4
Chest pain	1.6	0.4
Conduction disturbances	1.5	0.0
Left ventricular failure	1.4	0.0
OTHER		
Sweating/cold sweat/night sweats/clammy	5.1	2.3
Headache	2.1	4.6
Tiredness/drowsiness/fatigue/lethargy/lassitude/sleepiness	1.6	0.8
Hot/cold feelings	0.5	1.5
Rash/skin lesion	0.4	8.4

An additional group of about 2,000 patients has been treated in a program allowing for the use of TONOCARD under compassionate use circumstances. These patients were seriously ill with the large majority on multiple drug therapy, and comparatively high doses of TONOCARD were used. Fifty-four percent of the patients continued in the program for one year or longer, and 12 percent were treated for longer than three years, with the longest duration of therapy being nine years. Adverse reactions leading to therapy discontinuation occurred in 12 percent of patients (usually central nervous system effects or rash). A tabulation of adverse reactions occurring in one percent or more of patients follows:

	Percent of Patients Compassionate Use (n = 1,927)
NERVOUS SYSTEM	
Lightheadedness/dizziness/vertigo/giddiness	25.3
Tremor/quivering/tremulousness	21.6
Restlessness/shakiness/nervousness	11.5
Confusion/disorientation/hallucinations	11.2
Altered mood/awareness	11.0
Ataxia	10.8
Blurred vision/visual disturbances	10.0
Paresthesia/numbness	9.2
Nystagmus	1.1
GASTROINTESTINAL SYSTEM	
Nausea	24.6
Anorexia	11.3
Vomiting	9.0
Diarrhea/loose stools	6.8
CARDIOVASCULAR SYSTEM	
Increased ventricular arrhythmias/PVCs	10.9
CHF/progression of CHF	4.0
Tachycardia	3.2
Hypotension	1.8
Conduction disturbances	1.3
Bradycardia	1.0
OTHER	
Rash/skin lesion	12.2
Sweating/cold sweat/night sweats/clammy	8.3
Arthritis/arthralgia	4.7
Myalgia	1.7
Lupus	1.6

Adverse reactions occurring in less than one percent of patients in either the controlled studies or the compassionate use program or since the drug was marketed are as follows:

Nervous System: Coma, convulsions/seizures, depression, psychosis, mental change, agitation, altered taste/smell, difficulty concentrating, diplopia, dysarthria, impaired memory, increased stuttering/slurred speech, insomnia/sleeping disturbance, local anesthesia, nightmares, thirst, weakness, myasthenia gravis.

Gastrointestinal System: Abnormal liver function tests, hepatitis, jaundice, (see PRECAUTIONS); stomatitis; abdominal pain/discomfort; constipation; dysphagia; gastrointestinal symptoms (including dyspepsia).

Cardiovascular System: Ventricular fibrillation, extension of acute myocardial infarction, cardiogenic shock, angina, AV block, hypertension, increased QRS duration, pleurisy/pericarditis, prolonged QT interval, right bundle branch block, syncope, vaso-vagal episodes, cardiomegaly, sinus arrest.

Pulmonary System: Respiratory arrest, pulmonary edema, pulmonary embolism, pulmonary fibrosis, fibrosing alveolitis, interstitial pneumonitis, pneumonia, dyspnea.

Other: Hematologic disorder (agranulocytosis, bone marrow depression, hypoplastic anemia, anemia, leukopenia, thrombocytopenia), increased ANA, urinary retention, polyuria/increased diuresis, alopecia, cinchonism, claudication, cold extremities, dry mouth, earache, edema, fever, hiccups, itching, leg cramps, malaise, metallic/menthol taste, muscle twitching/spasm, neck pain, pain radiating from neck, pallor/flushed face, pressure on shoulder, yawning.

Agranulocytosis, bone marrow depression, leukopenia, hypoplastic anemia, and thrombocytopenia have been reported (0.18 percent) in patients receiving TONOCARD in controlled trials and the compassionate use program. Many of these events occurred in patients who were seriously ill or who were receiving concomitant drugs; fatalities have occurred. Most of these events have been noted during the first 12 weeks of therapy. (See WARNINGS).

Pulmonary fibrosis, interstitial pneumonitis, fibrosing alveolitis, pulmonary edema, and pneumonia, possibly drug related, have been reported in patients receiving TONOCARD. The incidence of pulmonary fibrosis (including interstitial pneumonitis and fibrosing alveolitis) was 0.11 percent in controlled trials and the compassionate use program. These events usually occurred in seriously ill patients. Symptoms of these pulmonary disorders and/or x-ray changes usually occurred following 3–18 weeks of therapy and two patients died. (See PRECAUTIONS).

DRUG ABUSE AND DEPENDENCE

Drug withdrawal after chronic treatment has not shown any indication of psychological or physical dependence.

Continued on next page

Information on the Merck Sharp & Dohme products listed on these pages is the full prescribing information from product circulars in use August 31, 1986.

Merck Sharp & Dohme—Cont.

OVERDOSAGE

The initial and most important signs and symptoms of overdosage would be expected to be related to the central nervous system. Other adverse reactions, such as gastrointestinal disturbances, may follow. (See ADVERSE REACTIONS).
Should convulsions or respiratory depression or arrest develop, the patency of the airway and adequacy of ventilation must be assured immediately. Should convulsions persist despite ventilatory therapy with oxygen, small increments of anticonvulsive agents may be given intravenously. Examples of such agents include a benzodiazepine (e.g., diazepam), an ultra-short-acting barbiturate (e.g., thiopental or thiamylal), or a short-acting barbiturate (e.g., pentobarbital or secobarbital).
The oral LD_{50} of tocainide was calculated to be about 800 mg/kg in mice, 1000 mg/kg in rats, and 230 mg/kg in guinea pigs; deaths were usually preceded by convulsions.
Studies in normal individuals to date indicate that tocainide has a hemodialysis clearance approximately equivalent to its renal clearance.

DOSAGE AND ADMINISTRATION

The dosage of TONOCARD must be individualized on the basis of antiarrhythmic response and tolerance, both of which are dose related. Clinical and electrocardiographic evaluation (including Holter monitoring if necessary for evaluation) are needed to determine whether the desired antiarrhythmic response has been obtained and to guide titration and dose adjustment. Adverse effects appearing shortly after dosing, for example, suggest a need for dividing the dose further with a shorter dose-interval. Loss of arrhythmia control prior to the next dose suggests use of a shorter dose interval and/or a dose increase. Absence of a clear response suggests reconsideration of therapy.
The recommended initial dosage is 400 mg every 8 hours. The usual adult dosage is between 1200 and 1800 mg/day in a three dose daily divided regimen. Doses beyond 2400 mg per day have been administered infrequently. Patients who tolerate the t.i.d. regimen may be tried on a twice daily regimen with careful monitoring.
Some patients, particularly those with renal or hepatic impairment, may be adequately treated with less than 1200 mg/day.

HOW SUPPLIED

No. 3409—Tablets TONOCARD, 400 mg, are oval, yellow, scored, film-coated tablets, coded MSD 707. They are supplied as follows:
NDC 0006-0707-68 bottles of 100
(6505-01-203-6240 100's)
NDC 0006-0707-28 unit dose packages of 100.
Shown in Product Identification Section, page 418
No. 3410—Tablets TONOCARD, 600 mg, are oblong, yellow, scored, film-coated tablets, coded MSD 709. They are supplied as follows:
NDC 0006-0709-68 bottles of 100
(6505-01-206-0273 100's)
NDC 0006-0709-28 unit dose packages of 100.
Shown in Product Identification Section, page 418
A.H.F.S. Category:24:04
DC 7369905 Issued July 1985

TRIAVIL® Tablets ℞
Tranquilizer-antidepressant

DESCRIPTION

TRIAVIL®, a broad-spectrum psychotherapeutic agent for the management of outpatients and hospitalized patients with psychoses or neuroses characterized by mixtures of anxiety or agitation with symptoms of depression, is a combination of perphenazine and ELAVIL® (Amitriptyline HCl, MSD). Since such mixed syndromes can occur in patients with various degrees of intensity of mental illness, TRIAVIL tablets are provided in multiple combinations to afford dosage flexibility for optimum management.
TRIAVIL tablets are provided as:
TRIAVIL 2-10, containing 2 mg of perphenazine and 10 mg of amitriptyline HCl.
TRIAVIL 2-25, containing 2 mg of perphenazine and 25 mg of amitriptyline HCl.
TRIAVIL 4-10, containing 4 mg of perphenazine and 10 mg of amitriptyline HCl.
TRIAVIL 4-25, containing 4 mg of perphenazine and 25 mg of amitriptyline HCl.
TRIAVIL 4-50, containing 4 mg of perphenazine and 50 mg of amitriptyline HCl.
Inactive ingredients are calcium phosphate, cellulose, hydroxypropyl cellulose, hydroxypropyl methylcellulose, lactose, magnesium stearate, starch, talc, and titanium dioxide. TRIAVIL 2-10 also contains FD&C Blue 1. TRIAVIL 2-25 and 4-50 also contain FD&C Yellow 6. TRIAVIL 4-10 also contains iron oxide. TRIAVIL 4-25 also contains D&C Yellow 10 and FD&C Yellow 6.

ACTIONS

Perphenazine—In common with all members of the piperazine group of phenothiazine derivatives, perphenazine has greater behavioral potency than phenothiazine derivatives of other groups without a corresponding increase in autonomic, hematologic, or hepatic side effects.
Extrapyramidal effects, however, may occur more frequently. These effects are interpreted as neuropharmacologic. They usually regress after discontinuation of the drug.
Perphenazine is a potent tranquilizer and also a potent antiemetic. Orally, its milligram potency is about five or six times that of chlorpromazine with respect to behavorial effects. It is capable of alleviating symptoms of anxiety, tension, psychomotor excitement, and other manifestations of emotional stress without apparent dulling of mental acuity.
ELAVIL (Amitriptyline HCl, MSD) is an antidepressant with sedative effects. Its mechanism of action in man is not known. It is not a monoamine oxidase inhibitor and it does not act primarily by stimulation of the central nervous system.

INDICATIONS

TRIAVIL is recommended for treatment of (1) patients with *moderate to severe anxiety and/or agitation and depressed mood,* (2) patients with *depression in whom anxiety and/or agitation are severe,* and (3) patients with *depression and anxiety in association with chronic physical disease.* In many of these patients anxiety masks the depressive state so that, although therapy with a tranquilizer appears to be indicated, the administration of a tranquilizer alone will not be adequate.
Schizophrenic patients who have associated depressive symptoms should be considered for therapy with TRIAVIL.
Many patients presenting symptoms such as agitation, anxiety, insomnia, psychomotor retardation, functional somatic complaints, a feeling of tiredness, loss of interest, and anorexia have responded well to therapy with TRIAVIL.

CONTRAINDICATIONS

TRIAVIL is contraindicated in depression of the central nervous system from drugs (barbiturates, alcohol, narcotics, analgesics, antihistamines); in the presence of evidence of bone marrow depression; and in patients known to be hypersensitive to phenothiazines or amitriptyline.
It should not be given concomitantly with monoamine oxidase inhibitors. Hyperpyretic crises, severe convulsions, and deaths have occurred in patients receiving tricyclic antidepressants and monoamine oxidase inhibitors simultaneously. When it is desired to replace a monoamine oxidase inhibitor with TRIAVIL, a minimum of 14 days should be allowed to elapse after the former is discontinued. TRIAVIL should then be initiated cautiously with gradual increase in dosage until optimum response is achieved.
Amitriptyline HCl is not recommended for use during the acute recovery phase following myocardial infarction.

WARNINGS

Tardive dyskinesia
Tardive dyskinesia, a syndrome consisting of potentially irreversible, involuntary dyskinetic movements may develop in patients treated with neuroleptic (antipsychotic) drugs. Although the prevalence of the syndrome appears to be highest among the elderly, especially elderly women, it is impossible to rely upon prevalence estimates to predict, at the inception of neuroleptic treatment, which patients are likely to develop the syndrome. Whether neuroleptic drug products differ in their potential to cause tardive dyskinesia is unknown.
Both the risk of developing the syndrome and the likelihood that it will become irreversible are believed to increase as the duration of treatment and the total cumulative dose of neuroleptic drugs administered to the patient increase. However, the syndrome can develop, although much less commonly, after relatively brief treatment periods at low doses.
There is no known treatment for established cases of tardive dyskinesia, although the syndome may remit, partially or completely, if neuroleptic treatment is withdrawn. Neuroleptic treatment, itself, however, may suppress (or partially suppress) the signs and symptoms of the syndrome and thereby may possibly mask the underlying disease process. The effect that symptomatic suppression has upon the long-term course of the syndrome is unknown.
Given these considerations, neuroleptics should be prescribed in a manner that is most likely to minimize the occurrence of tardive dyskinesia. Chronic neuroleptic treatment should generally be reserved for patients who suffer from a chronic mental illness that, 1) is known to respond to neuroleptic drugs, and, 2) for whom alternative, equally effective, but potentially less harmful treatments are *not* available or appropriate. In patients who do require chronic treatment, the smallest dose and the shortest duration of treatment producing a satisfactory clinical response should be sought. The need for continued treatment should be reassessed periodically.
If signs and symptoms of tardive dyskinesia appear in a patient on neuroleptics, drug discontinuation should be considered. However, some patients may require treatment despite the presence of the syndrome.
(For further information about the description of tardive dyskinesia and its clinical detection, please refer to the section on ADVERSE REACTIONS).
General
TRIAVIL should not be given concomitantly with guanethidine or similarly acting compounds, since amitriptyline, like other tricyclic antidepressants, may block the antihypertensive effect of these compounds.
Because of the atropine-like activity of amitriptyline, TRIAVIL should be used with caution in patients with a history of urinary retention, or with angle-closure glaucoma or increased intraocular pressure. In patients with angle-closure glaucoma, even average doses may precipitate an attack.
It should be used with caution also in patients with convulsive disorders. Dosage of anticonvulsive agents may have to be increased.
Patients with cardiovascular disorders should be watched closely. Tricyclic antidepressants, including amitriptyline HCl, particularly when given in high doses, have been reported to produce arrhythmias, sinus tachycardia, and prolongation of the conduction time. Myocardial infarction and stroke have been reported with drugs of this class.
Close supervision is required when amitriptyline HCl is given to hyperthyroid patients or those receiving thyroid medication.
TRIAVIL may enhance the response to alcohol and the effects of barbiturates and other CNS depressants. In patients who may use alcohol excessively, it should be borne in mind that the potentiation may increase the danger inherent in any suicide attempt or overdosage. Delirium has been reported with concurrent administration of amitriptyline and disulfiram.
Usage in Pregnancy—TRIAVIL is not recommended for use in pregnant patients or in nursing mothers at this time. Reproduction studies in rats have shown no fetal abnormalities; however, clinical experience and follow-up in pregnancy have been limited, and the possibility of adverse effects on fetal development must be considered.
Usage in Children—Since dosage for children has not been established, TRIAVIL is not recommended for use in children.

PRECAUTIONS

General
The possibility of suicide in depressed patients remains during treatment and until significant remission occurs. Such patients should not have access to large quantities of this drug.

Perphenazine
As with all phenothiazine compounds, perphenazine should not be used indiscriminately. Caution should be observed in giving it to patients who have previously exhibited severe adverse reactions to other phenothiazines.
Some of the untoward actions of perphenazine tend to appear more frequently when high doses are used. However, as with other phenothiazine compounds, patients receiving perphenazine in any dosage should be kept under close supervision.
The antiemetic effect of perphenazine may obscure signs of toxicity due to overdosage of other drugs, or render more difficult the diagnosis of disorders such as brain tumors or intestinal obstruction.
A significant, not otherwise explained, rise in body temperature may suggest individual intolerance to perphenazine, in which case TRIAVIL should be discontinued.
Neuroleptic drugs elevate prolactin levels; the elevation persists during chronic administration. Tissue culture experiments indicate that approximately one third of human breast cancers are prolactin dependent *in vitro*, a factor of potential importance if the prescription of these drugs is contemplated in a patient with a previously detected breast cancer. Although disturbances such as galactorrhea, amenorrhea, gynecomastia, and impotence have been reported, the clinical significance of elevated serum prolactin levels is unknown for most patients. An increase in mammary neoplasms has been found in rodents after chronic administra-

tion of neuroleptic drugs. Neither clinical studies nor epidemiologic studies conducted to date, however, have shown an association between chronic administration of these drugs and mammary tumorigenesis; the available evidence is considered too limited to be conclusive at this time.

ELAVIL (Amitriptyline HCl, MSD)
Depressed patients, particularly those with known manic depressive illness, may experience a shift to mania or hypomania. Patients with paranoid symptomatology may have an exaggeration of such symptoms. The tranquilizing effect of TRIAVIL seems to reduce the likelihood of these effects.
Concurrent administration of amitriptyline HCl and electroshock therapy may increase the hazards associated with such therapy. Such treatment should be limited to patients for whom it is essential.
Discontinue the drug several days before elective surgery if possible.
Both elevation and lowering of blood sugar levels have been reported.
ELAVIL (Amitriptyline HCl, MSD) should be used with caution in patients with impaired liver function.
Information for Patients
While on therapy with TRIAVIL, patients should be advised as to the possible impairment of mental and/or physical abilities required for performance of hazardous tasks, such as operating machinery or driving a motor vehicle.
Drug Interactions
Perphenazine
If hypotension develops, epinephrine should not be employed, as its action is blocked and partially reversed by perphenazine.
Phenothiazines may potentiate the action of central nervous system depressants (opiates, analgesics, antihistamines, barbiturates, alcohol) and atropine. In concurrent therapy with any of these, TRIAVIL should be given in reduced dosage. Phenothiazines also may potentiate the action of heat and phosphorous insecticides.
ELAVIL (Amitriptyline HCl, MSD)
When ELAVIL (Amitriptyline HCl, MSD) is given with anticholinergic agents or sympathomimetic drugs, including epinephrine combined with local anesthetics, close supervision and careful adjustment of dosages are required.
Paralytic ileus may occur in patients taking tricyclic antidepressants in combination with anticholinergic-type drugs.
Cimetidine is reported to reduce hepatic metabolism of certain tricyclic antidepressants, thereby delaying elimination and increasing steady-state concentrations of these drugs. Clinically significant effects have been reported with the tricyclic antidepressants when used concomitantly with cimetidine. Increases in plasma levels of tricyclic antidepressants, and in the frequency and severity of side effects, particularly anticholinergic, have been reported when cimetidine was added to the drug regimen. Discontinuation of cimetidine in well-controlled patients receiving tricyclic antidepressants and cimetidine may decrease the plasma levels and efficacy of the antidepressants.
Caution is advised if patients receive large doses of ethchlorvynol concurrently. Transient delirium has been reported in patients who were treated with 1 g of ethchlorvynol and 75-150 mg of ELAVIL (Amitriptyline HCl, MSD).

ADVERSE REACTIONS

To date, clinical evaluation of TRIAVIL has not revealed any adverse reactions peculiar to the combination. The adverse reactions that occurred were limited to those that have been reported previously for perphenazine and amitriptyline.
Treatment with TRIAVIL is commonly associated with sedation, hypotension, neurological impairments, and dry mouth.
Perphenazine
The common acute neurological effects of neuroleptic drugs, including perphenazine, consist of dystonia, akathisia or motor restlessness, and pseudoparkinsonism.
More chronic use of neuroleptics may be associated with the development of tardive dyskinesia. The salient features of this syndrome are described in the WARNINGS section and below.
Neurological:
Tardive dyskinesia:
The syndrome is characterized by involuntary choreoathetoid movements which variously involve the tongue, face, mouth, lips, or jaw (e.g., protrusion of the tongue, puffing of cheeks, puckering of the mouth, chewing movements), trunk and extremities. The severity of the syndrome and the degree of impairment produced vary widely.
The syndrome may become clinically recognizable either during treatment, upon dosage reduction, or upon withdrawal of treatment. Movements may decrease in intensity and may disappear altogether if further treatment with neuroleptics is withheld. It is generally believed that reversibility is more likely after short rather than long term neuroleptic exposure. Consequently, early detection of tardive dyskinesia is important. To increase the likelihood of detecting the syndrome at the earliest possible time, the dosage of neuroleptic drug should be reduced periodically (if clinically possible) and the patient observed for signs of the disorder. It has been suggested that fine vermicular movements of the tongue may be an early sign of the syndrome, and that the full-blown syndrome may not develop if medication is stopped when lingual vermiculation appears.
1. Dystonia
This may present as acute, reversible torticollis, opisthotonos, carpopedal spasm, trismus, dysphagia, respiratory difficulty, oculogyric crisis, and protrusion of the tongue. Treatment consists of the parenteral administration of either an anticholinergic antiparkinsonian agent or diphenhydramine.
2. Akathisia
Akathisia presents as constant motor restlessness. The patient with akathisia often complains, *when asked*, about his/her inability to stop moving. Akathisia should *not* be treated with an increased dose of neuroleptic; rather, the dose of antipsychotic may be lowered until the motor restlessness has subsided. The efficacy of anticholinergic treatment of this side effect is unestablished.
3. Pseudoparkinsonism
Pseudoparkinsonism refers to a drug-induced state similar to the classic syndrome. Generally, anticholinergic antiparkinsonian agents (i.e., benztropine, biperiden, procyclidine, or trihexphenidyl) and amantadine are helpful in alleviating symptoms that cannot be managed by neuroleptic dose reduction. The value of prophylactic antiparkinsonian drug therapy has not been established. The need for continued use of antiparkinsonian medication should be re-evaluated periodically.
Cardiovascular: Hypotension, hypertension, tachycardia, peripheral edema, occasional change in pulse rate, ECG abnormalities (quinidine-like effect), reversed epinephrine effect.
CNS and Neuromuscular: Extrapyramidal symptoms, including acute dyskinesia (see *Neurological*), hyperflexia, ataxia, reactivation of psychoses and production of catatonic-like states, muscle weakness, paradoxical excitement, hypnotic effects, mild insomnia, lassitude, headache, altered cerebrospinal fluid proteins.
Autonomic: Urinary frequency or incontinence, dry mouth or salivation, nasal congestion.
Allergic: Anaphylactoid reactions, laryngeal edema, asthma, angioneurotic edema.
Hematologic: Blood dyscrasias including pancytopenia, agranulocytosis, leukopenia, thrombocytopenic purpura, eosinophilia.
Gastrointestinal: Liver damage (jaundice, biliary stasis), obstipation, vomiting, nausea, constipation, anorexia.
Dermatologic: Eczema up to exfoliative dermatitis, urticaria, erythema, itching, photosensitivity.
Ophthalmic: Pigmentation of the cornea and lens, blurred vision.
Endocrine: Lactation, galactorrhea, hyperglycemia, gynecomastia, disturbances in menstrual cycle.
Other: False-positive pregnancy tests, including immunologic.
Other adverse reactions that should be considered because they have been reported with various phenothiazine compounds, but not with perphenazine, include:
CNS and Neuromuscular: Grand mal convulsions, cerebral edema.
Gastrointestinal: Polyphagia.
Dermatologic: Photophobia, pigmentation.
Ophthalmic: Pigmentary retinopathy.
Endocrine: Failure of ejaculation.
ELAVIL (Amitriptyline HCl, MSD)
Note: Included in the listing which follows are a few adverse reactions which have not been reported with this specific drug. However, pharmacological similarities among the tricyclic antidepressant drugs require that each of the reactions be considered when amitriptyline is administered.
Cardiovascular: Hypotension, particularly orthostatic hypotension; hypertension; tachycardia; palpitation; myocardial infarction; arrhythmias; heart block; stroke.
CNS and Neuromuscular: Confusional states; disturbed concentration; disorientation; delusions; hallucinations; excitement; anxiety; restlessness; insomnia; nightmares; numbness, tingling, and paresthesias of the extremities; peripheral neuropathy; incoordination; ataxia; tremors; seizures; alteration in EEG patterns; extrapyramidal symptoms; tinnitus; syndrome of inappropriate ADH (antidiuretic hormone) secretion.
Anticholinergic: Dry mouth, blurred vision, disturbance of accommodation, increased intraocular pressure, constipation, paralytic ileus, urinary retention, dilatation of urinary tract.
Allergic: Skin rash, urticaria, photosensitization, edema of face and tongue.
Hematologic: Bone marrow depression including agranulocytosis, leukopenia, eosinophilia, purpura, thrombocytopenia.
Gastrointestinal: Nausea, epigastric distress, vomiting, anorexia, stomatitis, peculiar taste, diarrhea, parotid swelling, black tongue. Rarely hepatitis (including altered liver function and jaundice).
Endocrine: Testicular swelling and gynecomastia in the male, breast enlargement and galactorrhea in the female, increased or decreased libido, elevation and lowering of blood sugar levels.
Other: Dizziness, weakness, fatigue, headache, weight gain or loss, edema, increased perspiration, urinary frequency, mydriasis, drowsiness, alopecia.
Withdrawal Symptoms: After prolonged administration, abrupt cessation of treatment may produce nausea, headache, and malaise. Gradual dosage reduction has been reported to produce, within two weeks, transient symptoms including irritability, restlessness, and dream and sleep disturbance. These symptoms are not indicative of addiction. Rare instances have been reported of mania or hypomania occurring within 2-7 days following cessation of chronic therapy wih tricyclic antidepressants.

DOSAGE AND ADMINISTRATION

Since dosage for children has not been established, TRIAVIL is not recommended for use in children.
The total daily dose of TRIAVIL should not exceed four tablets of the 4-50 or eight tablets of any other dosage strength.

Initial Dosage
In psychoneurotic patients when anxiety and depression are of such a degree as to warrant combined therapy, one tablet of TRIAVIL 2-25 or TRIAVIL 4-25 three or four times a day or one tablet of TRIAVIL 4-50 twice a day is recommended.
In more severely ill patients with schizophrenia, TRIAVIL 4-25 is recommended in an initial dose of two tablets three times a day. If necessary, a fourth dose may be given at bedtime.
In elderly patients and adolescents, and some other patients in whom anxiety tends to predominate, TRIAVIL 4-10 may be administered three or four times a day initially, then adjusted as required for subsequent adequate therapy.

Maintenance Dosage
Depending on the condition being treated, therapeutic response may take from a few days to a few weeks or even longer. After a satisfactory response is noted, dosage should be reduced to the smallest amount necessary to obtain relief from the symptoms for which TRIAVIL is being administered. A useful maintenance dosage is one tablet of TRIAVIL 2-25 or 4-25 two to four times a day or one tablet of TRIAVIL 4-50 twice a day. TRIAVIL 2-10 and 4-10 can be used to increase flexibility in adjusting maintenance dosage to the lowest amount consistent with relief of symptoms. In some patients, maintenance dosage is required for many months.

OVERDOSAGE

Manifestations—High doses may cause temporary confusion, disturbed concentration, or transient visual hallucinations. Overdosage may cause drowsiness; hypothermia; tachycardia and other arrhythmic abnormalities, such as bundle branch block; ECG evidence of impaired conduction; congestive heart failure; dilated pupils; disorders of ocular motility; convulsions; severe hypotension; stupor; and coma. Other symptoms may be agitation, hyperactive reflexes, muscle rigidity, vomiting, hyperpyrexia, or any of the adverse reactions listed for perphenazine or amitriptyline.
Levarterenol (norepinephrine) may be used to treat hypotension, but not epinephrine.
All patients suspected of having taken an overdosage should be admitted to a hospital as soon as possible. *Treatment* is symptomatic and supportive. Empty the stomach as quickly as possible by emesis followed by gastric lavage upon arrival at the hospital. Saline emetics should not be used as the antiemetic effect of perphenazine may cause retention of the saline load and subsequent hypernatremia. Following gastric lavage, activated charcoal may be administered. Twenty to 30 g of activated charcoal may be given every four to six hours during the first 24 to 48 hours after ingestion. An ECG should be taken and close monitoring of cardiac function instituted if there is any sign of abnormality. Maintain an open airway and adequate fluid intake; regulate body temperature.
The intravenous administration of 1–3 mg of physostigmine salicylate is reported to reverse the symptoms of tricyclic antidepressant poisoning. Because physostigmine is rapidly metabolized, the dosage of physostigmine should be repeated as required particularly if life threatening signs such as arrhythmias, convulsions, and deep coma recur or persist after the initial dosage of physostigmine. On this basis, in severe overdosage with perphenazine-amitriptyline combinations,

Continued on next page

Information on the Merck Sharp & Dohme products listed on these pages is the full prescribing information from product circulars in use August 31, 1986.

Merck Sharp & Dohme—Cont.

symptomatic treatment of central anticholinergic effects with physostigmine salicylate should be considered. Because physostigmine itself may be toxic, it is not recommended for routine use.
Standard measures should be used to manage circulatory shock and metabolic acidosis. Cardiac arrhythmias may be treated with neostigmine, pyridostigmine, or propranolol. Should cardiac failure occur, the use of digitalis should be considered. Close monitoring of cardiac function for not less than five days is advisable.
Anticonvulsants may be given to control convulsions. Amitriptyline and perphenazine increase the CNS depressant action but not the anticonvulsant action of barbiturates; therefore, an inhalation anesthetic, diazepam, or paraldehyde is recommended for control of convulsions. The management of acute symptoms of parkinsonism resulting from perphenazine intoxication may be treated with appropriate doses of COGENTIN® (Benztropine Mesylate, MSD) or diphenhydramine hydrochloride.*
Dialysis is of no value because of low plasma concentrations of the drug.
Since overdosage is often deliberate, patients may attempt suicide by other means during the recovery phase.
Deaths by deliberate or accidental overdosage have occurred with this class of drugs.

HOW SUPPLIED

No. 3328—Tablets TRIAVIL 2–10 are blue, triangular, film coated tablets, coded MSD 914. They are supplied as follows:
NDC 0006-0914-68 bottles of 100
NDC 0006-0914-28 unit dose package of 100
NDC 0006-0914-74 bottles of 500.
Shown in Product Identification Section, page 418
No. 3311—Tablets TRIAVIL 2–25 are orange, triangular, film coated tablets, coded MSD 921. They are supplied as follows:
NDC 0006-0921-68 bottles of 100
NDC 0006-0921-28 unit dose package of 100
NDC 0006-0921-74 bottles of 500.
(6505-00-931-4303 500's)
Shown in Product Identification Section, page 418
No. 3310—Tablets TRIAVIL 4–10 are salmon, triangular, film coated tablets, coded MSD 934. They are supplied as follows:
NDC 0006-0934-68 bottles of 100
NDC 0006-0934-28 unit dose package of 100
NDC 0006-0934-74 bottles of 500.
Shown in Product Identification Section, page 418
No. 3312—Tablets TRIAVIL 4–25 are yellow, triangular, film coated tablets, coded MSD 946. They are supplied as follows:
NDC 0006-0946-68 bottles of 100
(6505-01-012-7558 100's)
NDC 0006-0946-28 unit dose package of 100
NDC 0006-0946-74 bottles of 500.
Shown in Product Identification Section, page 418
No. 3364—Tablets TRIAVIL 4-50 are orange, diamond shaped, film coated tablets, coded MSD 517. They are supplied as follows:
NDC 0006-0517-60 bottles of 60
NDC 0006-0517-68 bottles of 100
NDC 0006-0517-28 unit dose package of 100.
Shown in Product Identification Section, page 418
A.H.F.S. Categories: 28:16:04, 28:16:08
DC 6613226 Issued October 1985

TURBINAIRE®—see under DECADRON® Phosphate, TURBINAIRE® (Dexamethasone Sodium Phosphate, MSD)

URECHOLINE® Tablets ℞
(Bethanechol Chloride, MSD), U.S.P.
URECHOLINE® Injection ℞
(Bethanechol Chloride, MSD), U.S.P.

DESCRIPTION

URECHOLINE® (Bethanechol Chloride, MSD), a cholinergic agent, is a synthetic ester which is structurally and pharmacologically related to acetylcholine.
It is designated chemically as 2-[(aminocarbonyl)oxy]-*N, N, N*-trimethyl-1-propanaminium chloride. Its empirical formula is $C_7H_{17}ClN_2O_2$ and its structural formula is:
[See Chemical Formula at top of next column].

*BENADRYL® (Diphenhydramine Hydrochloride), Parke, Davis & Co.

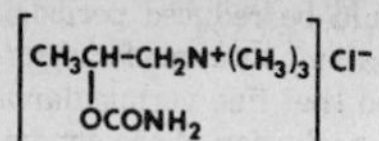

It is a white, hygroscopic crystalline compound having a slight amine-like odor, freely soluble in water, and has a molecular weight of 196.68.
URECHOLINE is supplied as 5 mg, 10 mg, 25 mg, and 50 mg tablets for oral use. Inactive ingredients in the tablets are calcium phosphate, lactose, magnesium stearate, and starch. Tablets URECHOLINE 10 mg also contain FD&C Red 3 and FD&C Red 40. Tablets URECHOLINE 25 mg and 50 mg also contain D&C Yellow 10 and FD&C Yellow 6.
URECHOLINE is also supplied as a sterile solution for subcutaneous use only. The sterile solution is essentially neutral. Each milliliter contains bethanechol chloride, 5 mg, and Water for Injection, q.s., 1 mL. It may be autoclaved at 120° C for 20 minutes without discoloration or loss of potency.

CLINICAL PHARMACOLOGY

Bethanechol chloride acts principally by producing the effects of stimulation of the parasympathetic nervous system. It increases the tone of the detrusor urinae muscle, usually producing a contraction sufficiently strong to initiate micturition and empty the bladder. It stimulates gastric motility, increases gastric tone, and often restores impaired rhythmic peristalsis.
Stimulation of the parasympathetic nervous system releases acetylcholine at the nerve endings. When spontaneous stimulation is reduced and therapeutic intervention is required, acetylcholine can be given, but it is rapidly hydrolyzed by cholinesterase, and its effects are transient. Bethanechol chloride is not destroyed by cholinesterase and its effects are more prolonged than those of acetylcholine.
Effects on the GI and urinary tracts sometimes appear within 30 minutes after oral administration of bethanechol chloride, but more often 60–90 minutes are required to reach maximum effectiveness. Following oral administration, the usual duration of action of bethanechol is one hour, although large doses (300–400 mg) have been reported to produce effects for up to six hours. Subcutaneous injection produces a more intense action on bladder muscle than does oral administration of the drug.
Because of the selective action of bethanechol, nicotinic symptoms of cholinergic stimulation are usually absent or minimal when orally or subcutaneously administered in therapeutic doses, while muscarinic effects are prominent. Muscarinic effects usually occur within 5–15 minutes after subcutaneous injection, reach a maximum in 15–30 minutes, and disappear within two hours. Doses that stimulate micturition and defecation and increase peristalsis do not ordinarily stimulate ganglia or voluntary muscles. Therapeutic test doses in normal human subjects have little effect on heart rate, blood pressure, or peripheral circulation.
Bethanechol chloride does not cross the blood-brain barrier because of its charged quaternary amine moiety. The metabolic fate and mode of excretion of the drug have not been elucidated.
A clinical study* was conducted on the relative effectiveness of oral and subcutaneous doses of bethanechol chloride on the stretch response of bladder muscle in patients with urinary retention. Results showed that 5 mg of the drug given subcutaneously stimulated a response that was more rapid in onset and of larger magnitude than an oral dose of 50 mg, 100 mg, or 200 mg. All the oral doses, however, had a longer duration of effect than the subcutaneous dose. Although the 50 mg oral dose caused little change in intravesical pressure in this study, this dose has been found in other studies to be clinically effective in the rehabilitation of patients with decompensated bladders.

INDICATIONS AND USAGE

For the treatment of acute postoperative and postpartum nonobstructive (functional) urinary retention and for neurogenic atony of the urinary bladder with retention.

CONTRAINDICATIONS

Hypersensitivity to URECHOLINE tablets or to any component of URECHOLINE injection, hyperthyroidism, peptic ulcer, latent or active bronchial asthma, pronounced bradycardia or hypotension, vasomotor instability, coronary artery disease, epilepsy, and parkinsonism.
URECHOLINE should not be employed when the strength or integrity of the gastrointestinal or bladder wall is in question, or in the presence of mechanical obstruction; when increased muscular activity of the gastrointestinal tract or urinary bladder might prove harmful, as following recent urinary bladder surgery, gastrointestinal resection and anastomosis, or when there is possible gastrointestinal obstruction; in bladder neck obstruction, spastic gastrointestinal disturbances, acute inflammatory lesions of the gastrointestinal tract, or peritonitis; or in marked vagotonia.

*Diokno, A. C.; Lapides, J., Urol. *10:* 23–24, July 1977.

WARNING

The sterile solution is for subcutaneous use only. It should never be given intramuscularly or intravenously. Violent symptoms of cholinergic over-stimulation, such as circulatory collapse, fall in blood pressure, abdominal cramps, bloody diarrhea, shock, or sudden cardiac arrest are likely to occur if the drug is given by either of these routes. Although rare, these same symptoms have occurred after subcutaneous injection, and may occur in cases of hypersensitivity or overdosage.

PRECAUTIONS

General
In urinary retention, if the sphincter fails to relax as URECHOLINE contracts the bladder, urine may be forced up the ureter into the kidney pelvis. If there is bacteriuria, this may cause reflux infection.
Information for Patients
URECHOLINE tablets should preferably be taken one hour before or two hours after meals to avoid nausea or vomiting. Dizziness, lightheadedness or fainting may occur, especially when getting up from a lying or sitting position.
Drug Interactions
Special care is required if this drug is given to patients receiving ganglion blocking compounds because a critical fall in blood pressure may occur. Usually, severe abdominal symptoms appear before there is such a fall in the blood pressure.
Carcinogenesis, Mutagenesis, Impairment of Fertility
Long-term studies in animals have not been performed to evaluate the effects upon fertility, mutagenic or carcinogenic potential of URECHOLINE.
Pregnancy
Pregnancy Category C. Animal reproduction studies have not been conducted with URECHOLINE. It is also not known whether URECHOLINE can cause fetal harm when administered to a pregnant woman or can affect reproduction capacity. URECHOLINE should be given to a pregnant woman only if clearly needed.
Nursing Mothers
It is not known whether this drug is secreted in human milk. Because many drugs are secreted in human milk and because of the potential for serious adverse reactions from URECHOLINE in nursing infants, a decision should be made whether to discontinue nursing or to discontinue the drug, taking into account the importance of the drug to the mother.
Pediatric Use
Safety and effectiveness in children have not been established.

ADVERSE REACTIONS

Adverse reactions are rare following oral administration of bethanechol, but are more common following subcutaneous injection. Adverse reactions are more likely to occur when dosage is increased.
The following adverse reactions have been observed: *Body as a Whole:* malaise; *Digestive:* abdominal cramps or discomfort, colicky pain, nausea and belching, diarrhea, borborygmi, salivation; *Renal:* urinary urgency; *Nervous System:* headache; *Cardiovascular:* a fall in blood pressure with reflex tachycardia, vasomotor response; *Skin:* flushing producing a feeling of warmth, sensation of heat about the face, sweating; *Respiratory:* bronchial constriction, asthmatic attacks; *Special Senses:* lacrimation, miosis.

OVERDOSAGE

Early signs of overdosage are abdominal discomfort, salivation, flushing of the skin ("hot feeling"), sweating, nausea and vomiting.
Atropine is a specific antidote. The recommended dose for adults is 0.6 mg (1/100 grain). Repeat doses can be given every two hours, according to clinical response. The recommended dosage in infants and children up to 12 years of age is 0.01 mg/kg (to a maximum single dose of 0.4 mg) repeated every two hours as needed until the desired effect is obtained, or adverse effects of atropine preclude further usage. Subcutaneous injection of atropine is preferred except in emergencies when the intravenous route may be employed.
When URECHOLINE is administered subcutaneously, a syringe containing a dose of atropine sulfate should always be available to treat symptoms of toxicity.
The oral LD_{50} of bethanechol chloride is 1510 mg/kg in the mouse.

DOSAGE AND ADMINISTRATION

Dosage and route of administration must be individualized, depending on the type and severity of the condition to be treated.

Preferably give the drug when the stomach is empty. If taken soon after eating, nausea and vomiting may occur.

Oral—The usual adult dosage is 10 to 50 mg three or four times a day. The minimum effective dose is determined by giving 5 or 10 mg initially and repeating the same amount at hourly intervals until satisfactory response occurs or until a maximum of 50 mg has been given. The effects of the drug sometimes appear within 30 minutes and usually within 60 to 90 minutes. They persist for about an hour.

Subcutaneous—The usual dose is 1 mL (5 mg), although some patients respond satisfactorily to as little as 0.5 mL (2.5 mg). The minimum effective dose is determined by injecting 0.5 mL (2.5 mg) initially and repeating the same amount at 15 to 30 minute intervals to a maximum of four doses until satisfactory response is obtained, unless disturbing reactions appear. The minimum effective dose may be repeated thereafter three or four times a day as required.

Rarely, single doses up to 2 mL (10 mg) may be required. Such large doses may cause severe reactions and should be used only after adequate trial of single doses of 0.5 to 1 mL (2.5 to 5 mg) has established that smaller doses are not sufficient.

URECHOLINE is usually effective in 5 to 15 minutes after subcutaneous injection.

If necessary, the effects of the drug can be abolished promptly by atropine (see OVERDOSAGE).

Parenteral drug products should be inspected visually for particulate matter and discoloration prior to administration, whenever solution and container permit.

HOW SUPPLIED

Tablets URECHOLINE are round, compressed tablets, scored on one side. They are supplied as follows:

No. 7785—5 mg, white in color, coded MSD 403.
NDC 0006-0403-68 in bottles of 100
NDC 0006-0403-28 unit dose packages of 100.
Shown in Product Identification Section, page 418

No. 7787—10 mg, pink in color, coded MSD 412.
NDC 0006-0412-68 in bottles of 100
(6505-00-616-7856 10 mg 100's)
NDC 0006-0412-28 unit dose packages of 100.
Shown in Product Identification Section, page 418

No. 7788—25 mg, yellow in color, coded MSD 457.
NDC 0006-0457-68 in bottles of 100
NDC 0006-0457-28 unit dose packages of 100.
Shown in Product Identification Section, page 418

No. 7790 — 50 mg, yellow in color, coded MSD 460.
NDC 0006-0460-68 in bottles of 100
NDC 0006-0460-28 in unit dose packages of 100.
Shown in Product Identification Section, page 418

No. 7786—Injection URECHOLINE, 5 mg per mL, is a clear, colorless solution, and is supplied as follows:
NDC 0006-7786-29 in box of 6 × 1 mL vials
(6505-00-616-8947 in box of 6 × 1 mL vials).

Storage
Store Tablets URECHOLINE in a tightly-closed container.

A.H.F.S. Category: 12:04
DC 6208429 Issued June 1985

VASOTEC® Tablets ℞
(Enalapril Maleate, MSD)

DESCRIPTION

VASOTEC® (Enalapril Maleate, MSD) is the maleate salt of enalapril, the ethyl ester of a long-acting angiotension converting enzyme inhibitor, enalaprilat. Enalapril maleate is chemically described as (*S*)-1-[*N*-[1-(ethoxycarbonyl)-3-phenylpropyl]-L-alanyl]-L-proline, (*Z*)-2-butenedioate salt (1:1). Its empirical formula is $C_{20}H_{28}N_2O_5 \bullet C_4H_4O_4$, and its structural formula is:

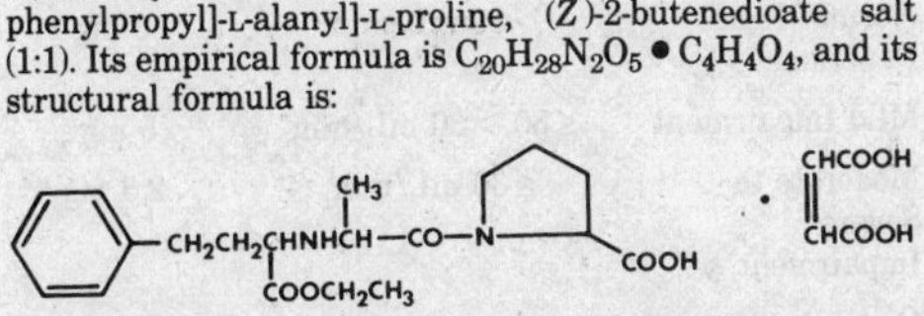

Enalapril maleate is a white to off-white, crystalline powder with a molecular weight of 492.53. It is sparingly soluble in water, soluble in ethanol, and freely soluble in methanol.

Enalapril is a pro-drug; following oral administration, it is bioactivated by hydrolysis of the ethyl ester to enalaprilat which is the active angiotensin converting enzyme inhibitor.

Enalapril maleate is supplied as 5 mg, 10 mg, and 20 mg tablets for oral administration. In addition to the active ingredient enalapril maleate, each tablet contains the following inactive ingredients: iron oxides, lactose, magnesium stearate, starch, and other ingredients.

CLINICAL PHARMACOLOGY

Mechanism of Action

Enalapril, after hydrolysis to enalaprilat, inhibits angiotensin-converting enzyme (ACE) in human subjects and animals. ACE is a peptidyl dipeptidase that catalyzes the conversion of angiotensin I to the vasoconstrictor substance, angiotensin II. Angiotensin II also stimulates aldosterone secretion by the adrenal cortex. Inhibition of ACE results in decreased plasma angiotensin II which leads to decreased vasopressor activity and to decreased aldosterone secretion. Although the latter decrease is small, it results in small increases of serum potassium. In hypertensive patients treated with VASOTEC alone for up to 48 weeks, mean increases in serum potassium of approximately 0.2 mEq/L were observed. In patients treated with VASOTEC plus a thiazide diuretic, there was essentially no change in serum potassium. (See PRECAUTIONS.) Removal of angiotensin II negative feedback on renin secretion leads to increased plasma renin activity.

ACE is identical to kininase the enzyme that degrades bradykinin. Whether increased levels of bradykinin, a potent vasodepressor peptide, play a role in the therapeutic effects of VASOTEC remains to be elucidated.

While the mechanism through which VASOTEC lowers blood pressure is believed to be primarily suppression of the renin-angiotensin-aldosterone system, VASOTEC is antihypertensive even in patients with low-renin hypertension. Although VASOTEC was antihypertensive in all races studied, black hypertensive patients (usually a low-renin hypertensive population) had a smaller average response to enalapril monotherapy than non-black patients.

Pharmacokinetics and Metabolism

Following oral administration of VASOTEC, peak serum concentrations of enalapril occur within about one hour. Based on urinary recovery, the extent of absorption of enalapril is approximately 60 percent. Enalapril absorption is not influenced by the presence of food in the gastrointestinal tract. Following absorption, enalapril is hydrolyzed to enalaprilat, which is a more potent angiotensin converting enzyme inhibitor than enalapril; enalaprilat is poorly absorbed when administered orally. Peak serum concentrations of enalaprilat occur three to four hours after an oral dose of enalapril maleate. Excretion of VASOTEC is primarily renal. Approximately 94 percent of the dose is recovered in the urine and feces as enalaprilat or enalapril. The principal components in urine are enalaprilat, accounting for about 40 percent of the dose, and intact enalapril. There is no evidence of metabolites of enalapril, other than enalaprilat.

The serum concentration profile of enalaprilat exhibits a prolonged terminal phase, apparently representing a small fraction of the administered dose that has been bound to ACE. The amount bound does not increase with dose, indicating a saturable site of binding. The effective half-life for accumulation of enalaprilat following multiple doses of enalapril maleate is 11 hours.

The disposition of enalapril and enalaprilat in patients with renal insufficiency is similar to that in patients with normal renal function until the glomerular filtration rate is 30 mL/min or less. With renal function ≤ 30 mL/min, peak and trough enalaprilat levels increase, time to peak concentration increases and time to steady state may be delayed. The effective half-life of enalaprilat following multiple doses of enalapril maleate is prolonged at this level of renal insufficiency. (See DOSAGE AND ADMINISTRATION.) Enalaprilat is dialyzable at the rate of 62 mL/min.

Studies in dogs indicate that enalapril crosses the blood-brain barrier poorly, if at all; enalaprilat does not enter the brain. Multiple doses of enalapril maleate in rats do not result in accumulation in any tissues. Milk of lactating rats contains radioactivity following administration of ^{14}C enalapril maleate. Radioactivity was found to cross the placenta following administration of labeled drug to pregnant hamsters.

Pharmacodynamics

Administration of VASOTEC to patients with hypertension of severity ranging from mild to severe results in a reduction of both supine and standing blood pressure usually with no orthostatic component. Symptomatic postural hypotension is therefore infrequent, although it might be anticipated in volume-depleted patients. (See WARNINGS.)

In most patients studied, after oral administration of an individual dose of enalapril, onset of antihypertensive activity was seen at one hour with peak reduction of blood pressure achieved by four to six hours.

At recommended doses, antihypertensive effects have been maintained for at least 24 hours. In some patients the effects may diminish toward the end of the dosing interval (see DOSAGE AND ADMINISTRATION).

In some patients achievement of optimal blood pressure reduction may require several weeks of therapy.

The antihypertensive effects of VASOTEC have continued during long term therapy. Abrupt withdrawal of VASOTEC has not been associated with a rapid increase in blood pressure.

In hemodynamic studies in patients with essential hypertension, blood pressure reduction was accompanied by a reduction in peripheral arterial resistance with an increase in cardiac output and little or no change in heart rate. Following administration of VASOTEC, there is an increase in renal blood flow; glomerular filtration rate is usually unchanged. The effects appear to be similar in patients with renovascular hypertension.

When given together with thiazide-type diuretics, the blood pressure lowering effects of VASOTEC are approximately additive.

INDICATIONS AND USAGE

VASOTEC is indicated for the treatment of hypertension.

In using VASOTEC, consideration should be given to the fact that another angiotensin converting enzyme inhibitor, captopril, has caused agranulocytosis, particularly in patients with renal impairment or collagen vascular disease, and that available data are insufficient to show that VASOTEC does not have a similar risk. (See WARNINGS.)

VASOTEC is effective alone or in combination with other antihypertensive agents, especially thiazide-type diuretics. The blood pressure lowering effects of VASOTEC and thiazides are approximately additive.

CONTRAINDICATIONS

VASOTEC is contraindicated in patients who are hypersensitive to this product.

WARNINGS

Angioedema

Angioedema has been reported in patients treated with angiotensin converting enzyme inhibitors, including VASOTEC. Angioedema associated with laryngeal edema and/or shock may be fatal. **If laryngeal stridor or angioedema of the face, tongue or glottis occurs, treatment with VASOTEC should be discontinued and appropriate therapy instituted immediately.** (See ADVERSE REACTIONS.)

Hypotension

Excessive hypotension was rarely seen in uncomplicated hypertensive patients but is a possible consequence of enalapril use in severely salt/volume depleted persons such as those treated vigorously with diuretics or patients on dialysis. (See PRECAUTIONS, *Drug Interactions* and ADVERSE REACTIONS.) In patients with severe congestive heart failure, with or without associated renal insufficiency, excessive hypotension has been observed and may be associated with oliguria and/or progressive azotemia, and rarely with acute renal failure and/or death. Because of the potential fall in blood pressure in these patients, therapy should be started under very close medical supervision. Such patients should be followed closely for the first two weeks of treatment and whenever the dose of enalapril and/or diuretic is increased.

If hypotension occurs, the patient should be placed in supine position and, if necessary, receive an intravenous infusion of normal saline. A transient hypotensive response is not a contraindication to further doses which usually can be given without difficulty once the blood pressure has increased after volume expansion.

Neutropenia/Agranulocytosis

Another angiotensin converting enzyme inhibitor has been shown to cause agranulocytosis and bone marrow depression, rarely in uncomplicated patients but more frequently in patients with renal impairment especially if they also have a collagen vascular disease. Available data from clinical trials of enalapril are insufficient to show that enalapril does not cause agranulocytosis at similar rates. Foreign marketing experience has revealed several cases of neutropenia or agranulocytosis in which a causal relationship to enalapril cannot be excluded. Periodic monitoring of white blood cell counts in patients with collagen vascular disease and renal disease should be considered.

PRECAUTIONS

General

Impaired Renal Function: In clinical studies in hypertensive patients with unilateral or bilateral renal artery stenosis, increases in blood urea nitrogen and serum creatinine were observed in 20 percent of patients. These increases were almost always reversible upon discontinuation of enalapril and/or diuretic therapy. In such patients renal

Continued on next page

Information on the Merck Sharp & Dohme products listed on these pages is the full prescribing information from product circulars in use August 31, 1986.

Merck Sharp & Dohme—Cont.

function should be monitored during the first few weeks of therapy.

Some hypertensive patients with no apparent pre-existing renal vascular disease have developed increases in blood urea and serum creatinine, usually minor and transient, especially when VASOTEC has been given concomitantly with a diuretic. This is more likely to occur in patients with pre-existing renal impairment. Dosage reduction of VASOTEC and/or discontinuation of the diuretic may be required.

Hyperkalemia: Elevated serum potassium (greater than 5.7 mEq/L) was observed in approximately one percent of hypertensive patients in clinical trials. In most cases these were isolated values which resolved despite continued therapy. Hyperkalemia was a cause of discontinuation of therapy in 0.28 percent of hypertensive patients. Risk factors for the development of hyperkalemia may include renal insufficiency, diabetes mellitus, and the concomitant use of agents to treat hypokalemia. (See *Drug Interactions.*)

Surgery/Anesthesia: In patients undergoing major surgery or during anesthesia with agents that produce hypotension, enalapril may block angiotensin II formation secondary to compensatory renin release. If hypotension occurs and is considered to be due to this mechanism, it can be corrected by volume expansion.

Information for Patients

Angioedema: Angioedema, including laryngeal edema, may occur especially following the first dose of enalapril. Patients should be so advised and told to report immediately any signs or symptoms suggesting angioedema (swelling of face, eyes, lips, tongue, difficulty in breathing) and to take no more drug until they have consulted with the prescribing physician.

Hypotension: Patients should be cautioned to report lightheadedness especially during the first days of therapy. If actual syncope occurs, the patients should be told to discontinue the drug until they have consulted with the prescribing physician.

All patients should be cautioned that excessive perspiration and dehydration may lead to an excessive fall in blood pressure because of reduction in fluid volume. Other causes of volume depletion such as vomiting or diarrhea may also lead to a fall in blood pressure; patients should be advised to consult with the physician.

Neutropenia: Patients should be told to report promptly any indication of infection (e.g., sore throat, fever) which may be a sign of neutropenia.

NOTE: As with many other drugs, certain advice to patients being treated with enalapril is warranted. This information is intended to aid in the safe and effective use of this medication. It is not a disclosure of all possible adverse or intended effects.

Drug Interactions

Hypotension—Patients on Diuretic Therapy: Patients on diuretics and especially those in whom diuretic therapy was recently instituted, may occasionally experience an excessive reduction of blood pressure after initiation of therapy with enalapril. The possibility of hypotensive effects with enalapril can be minimized by either discontinuing the diuretic or increasing the salt intake prior to initiation of treatment with enalapril. (See WARNINGS, and DOSAGE AND ADMINISTRATION.)

Agents Causing Renin Release: The antihypertensive effect of VASOTEC is augmented by antihypertensive agents that cause renin release (e.g., diuretics).

Other Cardiovascular Agents: VASOTEC has been used concomitantly with beta adrenergic-blocking agents, methyldopa, nitrates, calcium-blocking agents, hydralazine and prazosin without evidence of clinically significant adverse interactions.

Agents Increasing Serum Potassium: VASOTEC may attenuate potassium loss caused by thiazide-type diuretics. Potassium-sparing diuretics (e.g., spironolactone, triamterene, or amiloride), potassium supplements, or potassium containing salt substitutes may lead to significant increases in serum potassium. Therefore, if concomitant use of these agents is indicated, they should be used with caution and with frequent monitoring of serum potassium.

Carcinogenesis, Mutagenesis, Impairment of Fertility

There was no evidence of a tumorigenic effect when enalapril was administered for 106 weeks to rats at a dose up to 90 mg/kg/day (150 times the maximum daily human dose). Enalapril has also been administered for 94 weeks to male and female mice at doses up to 90 and 180 mg/kg/day, respectively, (150 and 300 times the maximum daily dose for humans), and showed no evidence of carcinogenicity.

Neither enalapril maleate nor the active diacid was mutagenic in the Ames microbial mutagen test with or without metabolic activation. Enalapril was also negative in the following genotoxicity studies: rec-assay, reverse mutation assay with E. coli, sister chromatid exchange with cultured mammalian cells, and the micronucleus test with mice, as well as in an *in vivo* cytogenic study using mouse bone marrow.

There were no adverse effects on reproductive performance in male and female rats treated with 10 to 90 mg/kg/day of enalapril.

Pregnancy

Pregnancy Category C. There was no fetotoxicity or teratogenicity in rats treated with up to 200 mg/kg/day of enalapril (333 times the maximum human dose). Fetotoxicity, expressed as a decrease in average fetal weight, occurred in rats given 1200 mg/kg/day of enalapril, but did not occur when these animals were supplemented with saline. Enalapril was not teratogenic in rabbits. However, maternal and fetal toxicity occurred in some rabbits at doses of 1 mg/kg/day or more. Saline supplementation prevented the maternal and fetal toxicity seen at doses of 3 and 10 mg/kg/day, but not at 30 mg/kg/day (50 times the maximum human dose).

There are no adequate and well-controlled studies in pregnant women. VASOTEC should be used during pregnancy only if the potential benefit justifies the potential risk to the fetus.

Nursing Mothers

It is not known whether this drug is secreted in human milk. Because many drugs are secreted in human milk, caution should be exercised when VASOTEC is given to a nursing mother.

Pediatric Use

Safety and effectiveness in children have not been established.

ADVERSE REACTIONS

VASOTEC has been evaluated for safety in more than 10,000 patients, including over 1000 patients treated for one year or more. VASOTEC has been found to be generally well tolerated in controlled clinical trials involving 2677 patients.

The most frequent clinical adverse experiences in controlled trials were: headache (4.8 percent), dizziness (4.6 percent) and fatigue (2.8 percent). For the most part, adverse experiences were mild and transient in nature. Discontinuation of therapy was required in 6.0 percent of patients. In clinical trials, the overall frequency of adverse experiences was not related to total daily dosage within the range of 10 to 40 mg. The overall percentage of patients treated with VASOTEC reporting adverse experiences was comparable to placebo.

Adverse experiences occurring in greater than one percent of patients treated with VASOTEC in controlled clinical trials are shown below.

	Percent of Patients in Controlled Studies	
	VASOTEC* (n = 2677) Incidence (discontinuation)	Placebo (n = 230) Incidence
Headache	4.8 (0.3)	9.1
Dizziness	4.6 (0.4)	4.3
Fatigue	2.8 (<0.1)	2.6
Diarrhea	1.6 (0.2)	1.7
Rash	1.5 (0.3)	0.4
Hypotension	1.4 (0.3)	0.4
Cough	1.3 (0.2)	0.9
Nausea	1.3 (0.2)	1.7
Orthostatic Effects	1.3 (<0.1)	0.0

*Includes 363 patients treated for congestive heart failure receiving concomitant digoxin and diuretic therapy.

Clinical adverse experiences occurring in 0.5 to 1.0 percent of patients in the controlled trials included:

Cardiovascular: Syncope, orthostatic hypotension, palpitations, chest pain.

Nervous System: Insomnia, nervousness, paresthesia, somnolence.

Gastrointestinal System: Abdominal pain, vomiting, dyspepsia.

Other: Dyspnea, muscle cramps, hyperhydrosis, impotence, pruritus, asthenia.

Angioedema: Angioedema has been reported in patients receiving VASOTEC (0.2 percent). Angioedema associated with laryngeal edema and/or shock may be fatal. If angioedema of the face, tongue or glottis occurs, treatment with VASOTEC should be discontinued and appropriate therapy instituted immediately. (See WARNINGS.)

Hypotension: Combining the results of clinical trials in patients with hypertension or congestive heart failure, hypotension (including postural hypotension, and other orthostatic effects) was reported in 2.3 percent of patients following the initial dose of enalapril or during extended therapy. In the hypertensive patients, hypotension occurred in 0.9 percent and syncope occurred in 0.5 percent of patients. Hypotension or syncope was a cause for discontinuation of therapy in 0.1 percent of hypertensive patients. (See WARNINGS.)

Clinical Laboratory Test Findings

Hyperkalemia: (See PRECAUTIONS.)

Creatinine, Blood Urea Nitrogen: Minor increases in blood urea nitrogen and serum creatinine, reversible upon discontinuation of therapy, were observed in about 0.2 percent of patients with essential hypertension treated with VASOTEC alone. Increases are more likely to occur in patients receiving concomitant diuretics or in patients with renal artery stenosis. (See PRECAUTIONS.)

Hemoglobin and Hematocrit: Small decreases in hemoglobin and hematocrit (mean decreases of approximately 0.3 g percent and 1.0 vol percent, respectively) occur frequently in hypertensive patients treated with VASOTEC but are rarely of clinical importance unless another cause of anemia coexists. In clinical trials, less than 0.1 percent of patients discontinued therapy due to anemia.

Other (Causal Relationship Unknown): Rarely, elevations of liver enzymes and/or serum bilirubin have occurred.

In overseas marketing experience, rare cases of neutropenia, thrombocytopenia, and bone marrow depression have been reported.

OVERDOSAGE

Limited data are available in regard to overdosage in humans.

The oral LD_{50} of enalapril is 2000 mg/kg in mice and rats. The most likely manifestation of overdosage would be hypotension, for which the usual treatment would be intravenous infusion of normal saline solution.

Enalaprilat may be removed from general circulation by hemodialysis.

DOSAGE AND ADMINISTRATION

In patients who are currently being treated with a diuretic, symptomatic hypotension occasionally may occur following the initial dose of VASOTEC. The diuretic should, if possible, be discontinued for two to three days before beginning therapy with VASOTEC to reduce the likelihood of hypotension. (See WARNINGS.) If the patient's blood pressure is not controlled with VASOTEC alone, diuretic therapy may be resumed.

If the diuretic cannot be discontinued an initial dose of 2.5 mg (break the 5 mg tablet) should be used to determine whether excess hypotension will occur.

The recommended initial dose in patients not on diuretics is 5 mg once a day. Dosage should be adjusted according to blood pressure response. The usual dosage range is 10 to 40 mg per day administered in a single dose or two divided doses. In some patients treated once daily, the antihypertensive effect may diminish toward the end of the dosing interval. In such patients, an increase in dosage or twice daily administration should be considered. If blood pressure is not controlled with VASOTEC alone, a diuretic may be added.

Concomitant administration of VASOTEC with potassium supplements, potassium salt substitutes, or potassium-sparing diuretics may lead to increases of serum potassium (see PRECAUTIONS).

Dosage Adjustment in Renal Impairment

The usual dose of enalapril is recommended for patients with a creatinine clearance > 30 mL/min (serum creatinine of up to approximately 3 mg/dL). For patients with creatinine clearance ≤ 30 mL/min (serum creatinine ≥ 3 mg/dL), the first dose is 2.5 mg once daily. The dosage may be titrated upward until blood pressure is controlled or to a maximum of 40 mg daily.

Renal Status	Creatinine-Clearance mL/min	Initial Dose mg/day
Normal Renal Function	>80 mL/min	5 mg
Mild Impairment	≤80 >30 mL/min	5 mg
Moderate to Severe Impairment	≤30 mL/min	2.5 mg
Dialysis Patients	—	2.5 mg on dialysis days*

*Dosage on nondialysis days should be adjusted depending on the blood pressure response.

HOW SUPPLIED

No. 3412—Tablets VASOTEC, 5 mg, are white, barrel shaped, scored, compressed tablets, with code MSD 712 on one side and VASOTEC on the other. They are supplied as follows:

NDC 0006-0712-68 bottles of 100 (with desiccant)
NDC 0006-0712-28 unit dose packages of 100.
Shown in Product Identification Section, page 418
No. 3413—Tablets VASOTEC, 10 mg, are red, barrel shaped, compressed tablets, with code MSD 713 on one side and VASOTEC on the other. They are supplied as follows:
NDC 0006-0713-68 bottles of 100 (with desiccant)
NDC 0006-0713-28 unit dose packages of 100.
Shown in Product Identification Section, page 418
No. 3414—Tablets VASOTEC, 20 mg, are peach, barrel shaped, compressed tablets, with code MSD 714 on one side and VASOTEC on the other. They are supplied as follows:
NDC 0006-0714-68 bottles of 100 (with desiccant)
NDC 0006-0714-28 unit dose packages of 100.
Shown in Product Identification Section, page 418

Storage
Store below 30°C (86°F) and avoid transient temperatures above 50°C (122°F). Keep container tightly closed. Protect from moisture.

A.H.F.S. Category: 24:08
DC 7358403 Issued December 1985

VIVACTIL® Tablets ℞
(Protriptyline HCl, MSD), U.S.P.

DESCRIPTION

Protriptyline HCl, a dibenzocycloheptene derivative, is a white to yellowish powder freely soluble in water.
It is designated chemically as *N*-methyl-5*H*-dibenzo[a,d]cycloheptene-5-propylamine hydrochloride.
The molecular weight is 299.8. The empirical formula is $C_{19}H_{21}N \cdot HCl$, and the structural formula is:

H CH₂CH₂CH₂NHCH₃ · HCl

VIVACTIL® (Protriptyline HCl, MSD) is supplied as 5 mg and 10 mg film coated tablets. Inactive ingredients are calcium phosphate, cellulose, guar gum, hydroxypropyl cellulose, hydroxypropyl methylcellulose, lactose, magnesium stearate, starch, talc, and titanium dioxide. Tablets VIVACTIL 5 mg and 10 mg also contain FD&C Yellow 6. Tablets VIVACTIL 10 mg also contain D&C Yellow 10.

ACTIONS

VIVACTIL is an antidepressant agent. The mechanism of its antidepressant action in man is not known. It is not a monoamine oxidase inhibitor, and it does not act primarily by stimulation of the central nervous system.
VIVACTIL has been found in some studies to have a more rapid onset of action than imipramine or amitriptyline. The initial clinical effect may occur within one week. Sedative and tranquilizing properties are lacking. The rate of excretion is slow.

INDICATIONS

VIVACTIL is indicated for the treatment of symptoms of mental depression in patients who are under close medical supervision. Its activating properties make it particularly suitable for withdrawn and anergic patients.

CONTRAINDICATIONS

VIVACTIL is contraindicated in patients who have shown prior hypersensitivity to it.
It should not be given concomitantly with a monoamine oxidase inhibiting compound. Hyperpyretic crises, severe convulsions, and deaths have occurred in patients receiving tricyclic antidepressant and monoamine oxidase inhibiting drugs simultaneously. When it is desired to substitute VIVACTIL for a monoamine oxidase inhibitor, a minimum of 14 days should be allowed to elapse after the latter is discontinued. VIVACTIL should then be initiated cautiously with gradual increase in dosage until optimum response is achieved.
This drug should not be used during the acute recovery phase following myocardial infarction.

WARNINGS

VIVACTIL may block the antihypertensive effect of guanethidine or similarly acting compounds.
VIVACTIL should be used with caution in patients with a history of seizures, and, because of its autonomic activity, in patients with a tendency to urinary retention, or increased intraocular tension.
Tachycardia and postural hypotension may occur more frequently with VIVACTIL than with other antidepressant drugs. VIVACTIL should be used with caution in elderly patients and patients with cardiovascular disorders; such patients should be observed closely because of the tendency of the drug to produce tachycardia, hypotension, arrhythmias, and prolongation of the conduction time. Myocardial infarction and stroke have occurred with drugs of this class.
On rare occasions, hyperthyroid patients or those receiving thyroid medication may develop arrhythmias when this drug is given.
In patients who may use alcohol excessively, it should be borne in mind that the potentiation may increase the danger inherent in any suicide attempt or overdosage.

Usage in Children
This drug is not recommended for use in children because safety and effectiveness in the pediatric age group have not been established.

Usage in Pregnancy
Safe use in pregnancy and lactation has not been established; therefore, use in pregnant women, nursing mothers or women who may become pregnant requires that possible benefits be weighed against possible hazards to mother and child.
In mice, rats, and rabbits, doses about ten times greater than the recommended human doses had no apparent adverse effects on reproduction.

PRECAUTIONS

When protriptyline HCl is used to treat the depressive component of schizophrenia, psychotic symptoms may be aggravated. Likewise, in manic-depressive psychosis, depressed patients may experience a shift toward the manic phase if they are treated with an antidepressant drug. Paranoid delusions, with or without associated hostility, may be exaggerated. In any of these circumstances, it may be advisable to reduce the dose of VIVACTIL or to use a major tranquilizing drug concurrently.
Symptoms, such as anxiety or agitation, may be aggravated in overactive or agitated patients.
When VIVACTIL is given with anticholinergic agents or sympathomimetic drugs, including epinephrine combined with local anesthetics, close supervision and careful adjustment of dosages are required.
Cimetidine is reported to reduce hepatic metabolism of certain tricyclic antidepressants, thereby delaying elimination and increasing steady-state concentrations of these drugs. Clinically significant effects have been reported with the tricyclic antidepressants when used concomitantly with cimetidine. Increases in plasma levels of tricyclic antidepressants, and in the frequency and severity of side effects, particularly anticholinergic, have been reported when cimetidine was added to the drug regimen. Discontinuation of cimetidine in well-controlled patients receiving tricyclic antidepressants and cimetidine may decrease the plasma levels and efficacy of the antidepressants.
It may enhance the response to alcohol and the effects of barbiturates and other CNS depressants.
The possibility of suicide in depressed patients remains during treatment and until significant remission occurs. This type of patient should not have access to large quantities of the drug.
Concurrent administration of VIVACTIL and electroshock therapy may increase the hazards of therapy. Such treatment should be limited to patients for whom it is essential.
Discontinue the drug several days before elective surgery, if possible.
Both elevation and lowering of blood sugar levels have been reported.
Information for Patients
While on therapy with VIVACTIL, patients should be advised as to the possible impairment of mental and/or physical abilities required for performance of hazardous tasks, such as operating machinery or driving a motor vehicle.

ADVERSE REACTIONS

Note: Included in the listing which follows are a few adverse reactions which have not been reported with this specific drug. However, the pharmacological similarities among the tricyclic antidepressant drugs require that each of the reactions be considered when protriptyline is administered. VIVACTIL is more likely to aggravate agitation and anxiety and produce cardiovascular reactions such as tachycardia and hypotension.
Cardiovascular: hypotension, particularly orthostatic hypotension; hypertension; tachycardia; palpitation; myocardial infarction; arrhythmias; heart block; stroke.
Psychiatric: confusional states (especially in the elderly) with hallucinations, disorientation, delusions, anxiety, restlessness, agitation; insomnia, panic, and nightmares; hypomania; exacerbation of psychosis.
Neurological: numbness, tingling, and paresthesias of extremities; incoordination, ataxia, tremors, peripheral neuropathy; extrapyramidal symptoms; seizures; alteration in EEG patterns, tinnitus; syndrome of inappropriate ADH (antidiuretic hormone) secretion.
Anticholinergic: dry mouth and rarely associated sublingual adenitis; blurred vision, disturbance of accommodation, increased intraocular pressure, mydriasis; constipation, paralytic ileus; urinary retention, delayed micturition, dilatation of the urinary tract.
Allergic: skin rash, petechiae, urticaria, itching, photosensitization (avoid excessive exposure to sunlight), edema (general, or of face and tongue), drug fever.
Hematologic: bone marrow depression; agranulocytosis; leukopenia; eosinophilia; purpura; thrombocytopenia.
Gastrointestinal: nausea and vomiting, anorexia, epigastric distress, diarrhea, peculiar taste, stomatitis, abdominal cramps, black tongue.
Endocrine: gynecomastia in the male; breast enlargement and galactorrhea in the female; increased or decreased libido, impotence; testicular swelling; elevation or depression of blood sugar levels.
Other: jaundice (simulating obstructive); altered liver function; weight gain or loss; perspiration; flushing; urinary frequency, nocturia; drowsiness, dizziness, weakness and fatigue; headache; parotid swelling; alopecia.
Withdrawal Symptoms: Though not indicative of addiction, abrupt cessation of treatment after prolonged therapy may produce nausea, headache, and malaise.

DOSAGE AND ADMINISTRATION

Dosage should be initiated at a low level and increased gradually, noting carefully the clinical response and any evidence of intolerance.
Usual Adult Dosage—Fifteen to 40 mg a day divided into 3 or 4 doses. If necessary, dosage may be increased to 60 mg a day. Dosages above this amount are not recommended. Increases should be made in the morning dose.
Adolescent and Elderly Patients—In general, lower dosages are recommended for these patients. Five mg 3 times a day may be given initially, and increased gradually if necessary. In elderly patients, the cardiovascular system must be monitored closely if the daily dose exceeds 20 mg.
When satisfactory improvement has been reached, dosage should be reduced to the smallest amount that will maintain relief of symptoms.
Minor adverse reactions require reduction in dosage. Major adverse reactions or evidence of hypersensitivity require prompt discontinuation of the drug.
Usage in Children—This drug is not recommended for use in children because safety and effectiveness in the pediatric age group have not been established.

OVERDOSAGE

Manifestations—High doses may cause temporary confusion, disturbed concentration, or transient visual hallucinations. Overdosage may cause drowsiness; hypothermia; tachycardia and other arrhythmic abnormalities, for example, bundle branch block; ECG evidence of impaired conduction; congestive heart failure; dilated pupils; convulsions; severe hypotension; stupor; and coma. Other symptoms may be agitation, hyperactive reflexes, muscle rigidity, vomiting, hyperpyrexia, or any of those listed under ADVERSE REACTIONS.
Experience in the management of overdosage with protriptyline is limited. The following recommendations are based on the management of overdosage with other tricyclic antidepressants.
All patients suspected of having taken an overdosage should be admitted to a hospital as soon as possible. *Treatment* is symptomatic and supportive. Empty the stomach as quickly as possible by emesis followed by gastric lavage upon arrival at the hospital. Following gastric lavage, activated charcoal may be administered. Twenty to 30 g of activated charcoal may be given every four to six hours during the first 24 to 48 hours after ingestion. An ECG should be taken and close monitoring of cardiac function instituted if there is any sign of abnormality. Maintain an open airway and adequate fluid intake; regulate body temperature.
The intravenous administration of 1-3 mg of physostigmine salicylate is reported to reverse the symptoms of other tricyclic antidepressant poisoning in humans. Because physostigmine is rapidly metabolized, the dosage of physostigmine should be repeated as required particularly if life threatening signs such as arrhythmias, convulsions, and deep coma recur or persist after the initial dosage of physostigmine.

Continued on next page

Information on the Merck Sharp & Dohme products listed on these pages is the full prescribing information from product circulars in use August 31, 1986.

Merck Sharp & Dohme—Cont.

Because physostigmine itself may be toxic, it is not recommended for routine use.
Standard measures should be used to manage circulatory shock and metabolic acidosis. Cardiac arrhythmias may be treated with neostigmine, pyridostigmine, or propranolol. Should cardiac failure occur, the use of digitalis should be considered. Close monitoring of cardiac function for not less than five days is advisable.
Anticonvulsants may be given to control convulsions.
Dialysis is of no value because of low plasma concentrations of the drug.
Since overdosage is often deliberate, patients may attempt suicide by other means during the recovery phase.
Deaths by deliberate or accidental overdosage have occurred with this class of drugs.

HOW SUPPLIED

No. 3313—Tablets VIVACTIL, 5 mg, are orange, oval, film coated tablets, coded MSD 26. They are supplied as follows:
NDC 0006-0026-68 bottles of 100.
Shown in Product Identification Section, page 418
No. 3314—Tablets VIVACTIL, 10 mg, are yellow, oval, film coated tablets, coded MSD 47. They are supplied as follows:
NDC 0006-0047-68 bottles of 100
NDC 0006-0047-28 unit dose packages of 100.
Shown in Product Identification Section, page 418

METABOLISM

Metabolic studies indicate that protriptyline is well absorbed from the gastrointestinal tract and is rapidly sequestered in tissues. Relatively low plasma levels are found after administration, and only a small amount of unchanged drug is excreted in the urine of dogs and rabbits. Preliminary studies indicate that demethylation of the secondary amine moiety occurs to a significant extent, and that metabolic transformation probably takes place in the liver. It penetrates the brain rapidly in mice and rats, and moreover that which is present in the brain is almost all unchanged drug.
Studies on the disposition of radioactive protriptyline in human test subjects showed significant plasma levels within 2 hours, peaking at 8 to 12 hours, then declining gradually.
Urinary excretion studies in the same subjects showed significant amounts of radioactivity in 2 hours. The rate of excretion was slow. Cumulative urinary excretion during 16 days accounted for approximately 50% of the drug. The fecal route of excretion did not seem to be important.
A.H.F.S. Category: 28:16:04
DC 6380618 Issued October 1985

Information on the Merck Sharp & Dohme products listed on these pages is the full prescribing information from product circulars in use August 31, 1986.

Mericon Industries, Inc.
8819 N. PIONEER ROAD
PEORIA, IL 61615

ORAZINC CAPSULES OTC
(zinc sulfate USP)

(See PDR For Nonprescription Drugs)

ORAZINC LOZENGES OTC
(zinc gluconate)

(See PDR For Nonprescription Drugs)

Merieux Institute, Inc.
P. O. BOX 52-3980
MIAMI, FL 33152-3980

IMOGAM® RABIES ℞
[*ĭm 'o-găm*]
(Rabies Immune Globulin-Human)

NDC 50361-180-20 2ml (300IU) pediatric vial
NDC 50361-180-10 10ml (1500IU) adult vial
Supplied in tamper proof plastic box.

IMOVAX® RABIES ℞
[*ĭm 'o-vak*]
(Rabies Vaccine Human Diploid Cell)

NDC 50361-250-10 1ml IM pre-exposure/post-exposure single dose vial
Supplied in tamper proof unit dose plastic box containing disposable syringe with 1 ml of Sterile Water for Injection U.S.P. for reconstitution and sterile disposable needles for reconstitution and administration, and 1 ml vial of lyophilized vaccine.

IMOVAX® RABIES I.D.
[*im 'o-vak I.D.*]
(Rabies Vaccine Human Diploid Cell)

NDC 50361-250-20 0.1ml I.D. pre-exposure immunization only intradermal syringe.
Supplied in a box containing tamperproof vacuum sealed glass tube holding syringe that contains 0.1ml of lyophilized Rabies Vaccine; a vial of Sterile Water for Injection U.S.P. for reconstitution of the vaccine.
The potency of IMOVAX® RABIES I.D. is equal to or greater than 2.5 I.U./ml of rabies antigen. A 0.1ml intradermal dose contains at least 0.25 I.U. Three 0.1ml I.D. are required for pre-exposure immunization.

MONO-VACC® TEST (O.T.) ℞
[*mon 'ō-vak*]
TUBERCULIN, MONO-VACC®TEST (O.T.)
(old tuberculin)
Multiple Puncture Device

NDC 50361-770-40 25 test per box.
Supplied in plastic tamper proof box of 25 test/box. Also available test reading cards in English or Spanish.

MULTITEST® CMI™ ℞
[*mul 'tĭ-test*]
(Skin Test Antigens for Cellular Hypersensitivity)

NDC 50361-780-80
DESCRIPTION
Skin Test Antigens for Cellular Hypersensitivity, MULTITEST® CMI™ is a disposable, plastic applicator consisting of eight sterile test heads preloaded with the following seven delayed hypersensitivity skin test antigens and glycerin negative control for precutaneous administration: Tetanus Toxoid Antigen, Diphtheria Toxoid Antigen, Streptococcus Antigen, Old Tuberculin, Candida Antigen, Trichophyton Antigen, and Proteus Antigen.
MULTITEST® CMI™ provides a quick, convenient and uniform procedure for delayed cutaneous hypersensitivity testing.
Supplied in box of 10 individual cartons containing one preloaded MULTITEST® CMI™ per carton.

EDUCATIONAL MATERIAL

Booklets
"Rabies Concepts for the Medical Professional", Daniel Fishbein, Leigh Sawyer, William G. Winkler, Editors. Chapters dealing with rabies in humans, animals, diagnosis, pre and post-exposure prophylaxis, etiology, glossary and bibliography. 1 each free to: Physicians, Pharmacists, Public Health Officials and Veterinarians. For additional quantities and prices, please write or call.
Newsletter
"IMMUNEWS", Merieux Institute, Inc., Editor. Quarterly newsletter on recently published articles on rabies, coverage of rabies conferences and rabies enzootic and epizootic updates. Free by subscription only (no charge). 1 copy each to: Physicians, Pharmacists, Public Health Officials and Veterinarians.
Video Cassettes
"Play it Safe", Merieux Institute, Inc., Editor. A 30 second Public Service Announcement available for Professional Organization, ie, State or County Medical Societies for commercial. T.V. broadcast warning about rabies danger and prophylaxis available in ½" or ¾" V.H.S. Suitable for duplication for T.V. broadcast and with space available to identify Medical or Pharmaceutical Society, Public Health Agency or Veterinary Society. Available on a No Charge loan basis for duplication. Call or write for additional information.
"Rabies/LaRage", Institut Merieux, Editor. A 30 minute ½" or ¾" V.H.S. cassette color film on rabies and its treatment in humans.
"Rabies 100 Years After Pasteur", Institut Merieux, Editor. A 20 minute ½" or ¾" V.H.S. cassette color film on progress made in rabies prevention and treatment since Pasteur's first vaccination in 1885. This, and "Rabies/LaRage" are available free of charge for showing at group functions, society meetings, etc. Allow 7 weeks (minimum) prior to desired date. Call or write for additional information.
Charts
"Rabies-What to do in an Emergency", Merieux Institute, Inc., Editor. Wall chart and pocket chart with ACIP/CDC recommendations on what to do in rabies exposure. Free to: Physicians, Pharmacists, Public Health Officials and Veterinarians.

Merrell Dow Pharmaceuticals Inc.

Subsidiary of The Dow Chemical Company
CINCINNATI, OH 45242-9553

AVC™ Cream/Suppositories ℞

AVAILABLE ONLY ON PRESCRIPTION

DESCRIPTION
AVC Cream
Each tube contains:
Sulfanilamide 15.0%
Aminacrine hydrochloride 0.2%
Allantoin 2.0%
with lactose, in a water-miscible base made from propylene glycol, stearic acid, diglycol stearate, and trolamine; buffered with lactic acid to an acid pH.
AVC Suppositories
Each suppository contains:
Sulfanilamide .... 1.05 g
Aminacrine hydrochloride .... 0.014 g
Allantoin .... 0.14 g
with lactose, in a base made from polyethylene glycol 400, polysorbate 80, polyethylene glycol 4000, and glycerin; buffered with lactic acid to an acid pH. AVC Suppositories have an inert covering, which dissolves promptly in the vagina. The covering is composed of gelatin, glycerin, water, methylparaben, and propylparaben. Contains color additives including FD&C Yellow No. 5 (tartrazine).

ACTIONS
AVC is a vaginal preparation combining aminacrine hydrochloride and sulfanilamide. Sulfanilamide is believed to block certain metabolic processes essential for the growth of susceptible bacteria. Aminacrine hydrochloride, a highly ionized acridine derivative, is thought to act by interfering or competing with certain hydrogen ions in microbial enzyme systems.
These ingredients are combined in a specially compounded base buffered to the pH of the normal vagina to encourage the presence of the normally occurring Döderlein's bacilli of the vagina.

INDICATIONS
Based on a review of AVC by the National Academy of Sciences—National Research Council and/or other information, FDA has classified the indications as follows:
"Probably" effective: For the relief of symptoms of vulvovaginitis where isolation of the specific organism responsible (usually *Trichomonas vaginalis, Candida albicans,* or *Hemophilus vaginalis*) is not possible.
NOTE: When the offending organism is known, treatment with a specific agent known to be active against that microorganism is preferred.
"Possibly" effective: For the treatment of trichomoniasis, vulvovaginal candidiasis, and vaginitis due to *Hemophilus vaginalis* or other susceptible bacteria.
Final classification of the less-than-effective indications requires further investigation.

CONTRAINDICATIONS
AVC should not be used in patients known to be sensitive to the sulfonamides.

PRECAUTIONS

As with all sulfonamides, the usual precautions apply. Patients should be observed for manifestations such as skin rash or other evidence of systemic toxicity, and if these develop, the medication should be discontinued.

AVC Suppositories contain FD&C Yellow No. 5 (tartrazine), which may cause allergic-type reactions (including bronchial asthma) in certain susceptible individuals. Although the overall incidence of FD&C Yellow No. 5 (tartrazine) sensitivity in the general population is low, it is frequently seen in patients who also have aspirin hypersensitivity.

ADVERSE REACTIONS

Although some absorption of sulfanilamide may occur through the vaginal mucosa, systemic manifestations attributable to this drug are infrequent. Local sensitivity reactions such as increased discomfort or a burning sensation have occasionally been reported following the use of topical sulfonamides. Treatment should be discontinued if either local or systemic manifestations of sulfonamide toxicity or sensitivity occur.

DOSAGE AND ADMINISTRATION

1 applicatorful (about 6 g) or 1 suppository intravaginally once or twice daily. Improvements in symptoms should occur within a few days, but treatment should be continued through one complete menstrual cycle unless a definite diagnosis is made and specific therapy initiated.

If there is no response within a few days or if symptoms recur, AVC should be discontinued and another attempt made by appropriate laboratory methods to isolate the organism responsible (*Trichomonas vaginalis, Candida albicans, Hemophilus vaginalis*) and institute specific therapy.

Douching with a suitable solution before insertion may be recommended for hygienic purposes. A pad may be used to prevent staining of clothing.

HOW SUPPLIED

AVC Cream
0068-0110-13: 4 oz. tube with applicator
AVC Suppositories
0068-0111-16: Box of 16 suppositories with inserter

Product Information as of August, 1979

Suppositories are
Manufactured by
R. P. Scherer, North America
Clearwater, Florida 33518 for
MERRELL DOW PHARMACEUTICALS INC.
Subsidiary of The Dow Chemical Company
Cincinnati, Ohio 45215, U.S.A.

ACCURBRON® ℞

[*ăk 'ĕr-brŏn*]
(theophylline)

CAUTION: Federal law prohibits dispensing without prescription.

DESCRIPTION

Each 15 mL tablespoonful of Accurbron (theophylline) syrup for oral use contains theophylline (anhydrous) 150 mg. Also contains as inactive ingredients: alcohol (7.5%), flavors, invert sugar, propylene glycol, saccharin sodium, sodium gluconate, sorbitol, and water.

Theophylline, a xanthine bronchodilator, is chemically 1*H*-Purine-2,6-dione, 3,7-dihydro-1,3-dimethyl-, with the following structure:

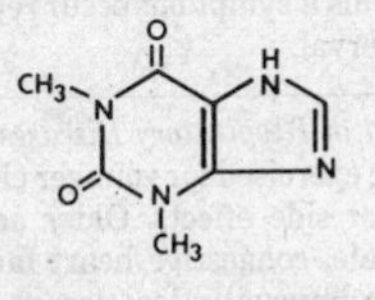

Theophylline anhydrous is a white, odorless, crystalline powder having a bitter taste.

CLINICAL PHARMACOLOGY

Theophylline directly relaxes the smooth muscle of the bronchial airways and pulmonary blood vessels thus acting mainly as a bronchodilator and smooth muscle relaxant. It also produces other actions typical of the xanthine derivatives: coronary vasodilation, cardiac stimulation, diuresis, cerebral stimulation, and skeletal muscle stimulation. The actions of theophylline may be mediated through inhibition of phosphodiesterase and a resultant increase in intracellular cyclic AMP.

In vitro, theophylline has been shown to act synergistically with beta agonists that increase intracellular cyclic AMP through the stimulation of adenyl cyclase, but synergism has not been demonstrated in patient studies. More data are needed to determine if theophylline and beta agonists have a clinically important additive effect *in vivo*. Apparently, no development of tolerance occurs with chronic use of theophylline.

Pharmacokinetics

The half-life of theophylline is influenced by a number of known variables. It is prolonged in patients suffering from chronic alcoholism, impaired hepatic or renal function, congestive heart failure, and in patients receiving macrolide antibiotics and cimetidine. Older adults (over age 55) and patients with chronic obstructive pulmonary disease, with or without cor pulmonale, may also have much slower clearance rates. For such patients, the theophylline half-life may exceed 24 hours.

Newborns and neonates have extremely slow clearance rates compared to older infants (over 6 months) and children, and may also have a theophylline half-life of over 24 hours. High fever for prolonged periods may also reduce the rate of theophylline elimination.

THEOPHYLLINE ELIMINATION CHARACTERISTICS

	Theophylline Clearance Rates mL/kg/min (mean ± S.D.)	Half-life Average Hours mean ± S.D.)
Children (over 6 months of age)	1.45 ± 0.58	3.7 ± 1.1
Adult nonsmokers uncomplicated asthma	0.65 ± 0.19	8.7 ± 2.2

The half-life of theophylline in smokers (1 to 2 packs/day) averages 4–5 hours, much shorter than the half-life in nonsmokers which averages 7–9 hours. The increase in theophylline clearance caused by smoking is probably the result of induction of drug-metabolizing enzymes that do not readily normalize after cessation of smoking. It appears that between 3 months and 2 years may be necessary for normalization of the effect of smoking on theophylline pharmacokinetics.

INDICATIONS

For relief and/or prevention of symptoms from asthma and reversible bronchospasm associated with chronic bronchitis and emphysema.

CONTRAINDICATIONS

This product is contraindicated in individuals who have shown hypersensitivity to its components.

WARNINGS

Status asthmaticus should be considered a medical emergency and is defined as that degree of bronchospasm which is not rapidly responsive to usual doses of conventional bronchodilators. Optimal therapy for such patients frequently requires both *additional medication*, parenterally administered, and *close monitoring*, preferably in an intensive care setting.

Although increasing the dose of theophylline may bring about relief, such treatment may be associated with toxicity. The likelihood of such toxicity developing increases significantly when the serum theophylline concentration exceeds 20 mcg/mL. Therefore, determination of serum theophylline levels is recommended to assure maximal benefit without excessive risk.

Serum levels above 20 mcg/mL are rarely found after appropriate administration of the recommended doses. However, in individuals in whom theophylline plasma clearance is reduced *for any reason*, even conventional doses may result in increased serum levels and potential toxicity. Reduced theophylline clearance has been documented in the following readily identifiable groups: 1) patients with impaired renal or liver function; 2) patients over 55 years of age, particularly males and those with chronic lung disease; 3) those with cardiac failure from any cause; 4) neonates; and 5) those patients taking certain drugs (macrolide antibiotics and cimetidine). Also, decreased clearance of theophylline may be associated with either influenza immunization or active infection with influenza. Reduction of dosage and laboratory monitoring is especially appropriate in any of these groups.

Less serious signs of theophylline toxicity, i.e., nausea and restlessness, may appear in up to 50% of patients. However, serious side effects such as ventricular arrhythmias, convulsions or even death may appear as the first sign of toxicity without any previous warning. Stated differently, *serious toxicity is not reliably preceded by less severe side effects*.

Many patients who require theophylline may exhibit tachycardia due to their underlying disease process so that the cause/effect relationship of elevated serum theophylline concentrations may not be appreciated.

Theophylline products may cause dysrhythmia and/or worsen pre-existing arrhythmias; any significant change in rate and/or rhythm warrants monitoring and further investigation.

The occurrence of arrhythmias and sudden death (with histological evidence of necrosis of the myocardium) has been recorded in laboratory animals (minipigs, rodents and dogs) when theophylline and beta agonists were administered concomitantly, although not when either was administered alone. The significance of these findings when applied to human usage is currently unknown.

PRECAUTIONS

General

Theophylline half-life is shorter in smokers than in nonsmokers. Therefore, smokers may require larger or more frequent doses. Morphine and curare should be used with caution in patients with airway obstruction as they may suppress respiration and stimulate histamine release. Alternative drugs should be used when possible. Theophylline should not be administered concurrently with other xanthine medications. Use with caution in patients with severe cardiac disease, severe hypoxemia, hypertension, hyperthyroidism, acute myocardial injury, cor pulmonale, congestive heart failure, liver disease, in the elderly (especially males), and in neonates. In particular, great caution should be used in giving theophylline to patients with congestive heart failure. Frequently, such patients have markedly prolonged theophylline serum levels with theophylline persisting in serum for long periods following discontinuation of the drug. Use theophylline cautiously in patients with history of peptic ulcer. Theophylline may occasionally act as a local irritant to the GI tract although gastrointestinal symptoms are more commonly centrally mediated and associated with serum drug concentrations over 20 mcg/mL.

Information for Patients

The physician should reinforce the importance of taking only the prescribed dose and the appropriate time interval between doses. If necessary, taking the drug with food will help avoid local irritation of the GI tract.

Drug Interactions

Toxic synergism with ephedrine has been documented and may occur with some other sympathomimetic bronchodilators. In addition, the following drug interactions have been reported:

DRUG	EFFECT
Aminophylline with lithium carbonate	Increased excretion of lithium carbonate.
Aminophylline with propranolol	Antagonism of propranolol effect.
Theophylline with cimetidine	Increased theophylline blood levels. A single dose of cimetidine may increase theophylline levels. Seizures have been reported in patients using this drug combination.
Theophylline with troleandomycin, erythromycin	Increased theophylline blood levels.
Theophylline with allopurinol	When used long term in high doses (i.e., 600 mg allopurinol per day) allopurinol may increase theophylline blood levels.
Theophylline with influenza vaccine	Theophylline blood levels may increase significantly following vaccination and may remain elevated for longer than 24 hours.
Theophylline with phenytoin	Decreased theophylline and phenytoin levels.

Other drug interactions have been reported but are not fully substantiated.

Drug—Laboratory Test Interactions

When plasma levels of theophylline are measured by spectrophotometric methods, coffee, tea, cola beverages, chocolate, and acetaminophen may contribute to falsely high values.

Carcinogenesis, Mutagenesis, and Impairment of Fertility

Long-term animal studies have not been performed to evaluate the carcinogenic potential, mutagenic potential, or the effect on fertility of xanthine compounds.

Pregnancy

Category C—Animal reproduction studies have not been conducted with theophylline. It is not known whether theophylline can cause fetal harm when administered to a pregnant woman or can affect reproduction capacity. Xanthines should be given to a pregnant woman only if clearly needed.

Nursing Mothers

It has been reported that theophylline distributes readily into breast milk and may cause adverse effects in the infant. Caution must be used if prescribing xanthines to a mother who is nursing, taking into account the risk-benefit of this therapy.

Pediatric Use

Due to the marked variation in theophylline metabolism in infants under 6 months of age, this drug is not recommended for this age group.

Continued on next page

Information on Merrell Dow products is based on labeling in effect in May, 1986.

Merrell Dow—Cont.

ADVERSE REACTIONS

The most consistent adverse reactions are usually due to overdose and are:

1. *Gastrointestinal:* nausea, vomiting, epigastric pain, hematemesis, diarrhea.
2. *Central nervous system:* headaches, irritability, restlessness, insomnia, reflex hyperexcitability, muscle twitching, clonic and tonic generalized convulsions.
3. *Cardiovascular:* palpitation, tachycardia, extrasystoles, flushing, hypotension, circulatory failure, ventricular arrhythmias.
4. *Respiratory:* tachypnea.
5. *Renal:* albuminuria, increased excretion of renal tubular and red blood cells, potentiation of diuresis.
6. *Others:* hyperglycemia and inappropriate ADH syndrome; rash.

OVERDOSAGE

Management

If potential oral overdose is established and seizure has not occurred:

A. Induce vomiting.
B. Administer a cathartic.
C. Administer activated charcoal.

If patient is having a seizure:

A. Establish an airway.
B. Administer oxygen.
C. Treat the seizure with intravenous diazepam, 0.1 to 0.3 mg/kg up to 10 mg.
D. Monitor vital signs, maintain blood pressure and provide adequate hydration.

Post seizure coma:

A. Maintain airway and oxygenation.
B. Follow above recommendations to prevent absorption of the drug, but intubation and lavage will have to be performed instead of inducing emesis. The cathartic and charcoal should be introduced via a large bore gastric lavage tube.
C. Continue to provide full supportive care and adequate hydration while waiting for drug to be metabolized. In general, the drug is metabolized sufficiently rapid so as to not warrant consideration of dialysis. However, if serum levels exceed 50 mcg/mL, charcoal hemoperfusion may be indicated.

DOSAGE AND ADMINISTRATION

For most patients *effective use* of theophylline, i.e., optimal likelihood of benefit combined with minimal risk of toxicity, is considered to occur when serum levels are maintained between 10 and 20 mcg/mL. Levels above 20 mcg/mL may produce toxicity, and in a small number of patients toxicity may even be seen with serum levels between 15–20 mcg/mL, particularly during initiation of therapy.

There is considerable variation from patient to patient in the dosage required to achieve and maintain therapeutic and safe levels, primarily due to variable rates of elimination. Therefore, it is not only essential to individualize the dosage, but also to titrate and monitor serum levels whenever possible. Serum theophylline concentration should be obtained at the times of peak and trough concentrations. When serum concentration cannot be obtained, restriction of dosage to the amounts and intervals recommended in the guidelines listed below becomes essential.

Dosage should be calculated on the basis of lean (ideal) body weight where mg/kg doses are presented. Theophylline does not distribute into fatty tissue. Giving theophylline with food may prevent some local gastric irritation and though absorption is slower, it is still complete.

Frequency of Dosing: Dosing to maintain serum levels generally requires administration every 6 hours. This is particularly true in children, but dosing intervals up to 8 hours may be satisfactory in adults since they eliminate the drug at a slower rate. Some children and adults require higher than average doses, i.e., those having rapid rates of clearance and half-lives of under 6 hours.

Dosage guidelines are approximations only and the wide range of theophylline clearance between individuals (particularly those with concomitant disease) makes indiscriminate usage hazardous.

As a practical consideration, it is not always possible to obtain serum level determinations. Under such conditions, restriction of the daily dose (in otherwise healthy adults) to not greater than 16 mg/kg/day (of anhydrous theophylline) in divided doses will result in relatively few patients exceeding serum levels of 20 mcg/mL and reduce the risk of toxicity.

Dosage Guidelines

NOTE: Accurbron Syrup contains 150 mg/15 mL (10 mg/mL) of anhydrous theophylline.

1. Acute Symptoms of Asthma Requiring Rapid Theophyllinazation

   A. Patients not currently receiving theophylline products. Dosage recommendations are for theophylline anhydrous.

[See table below].

   B. Patients currently receiving theophylline products.

   Whenever possible, determine the time, amount, dosage form, and route of administration of the patient's last dose.

   The loading dose for theophylline is based on the principle that each 0.5 mg/kg of theophylline administered as a loading dose will result in a 1.0 mcg/mL increase in serum theophylline concentration.

   Ideally, the loading dose should be deferred if a serum theophylline concentration can be obtained rapidly. If this is not possible, the clinician must exercise his judgment in selecting a dose based on the potential for benefit and risk.

   When there is sufficient respiratory distress to warrant a small risk, 2.5 mg/kg of theophylline administered in rapidly absorbed form is likely to increase serum concentration by approximately 5 mcg/mL. If the patient is not experiencing theophylline toxicity, this is unlikely to result in dangerous adverse effects.

   After modifying the loading dose for this group of patients, the maintenance dosage recommendations are the same as those described in TABLE I.

II. Chronic Therapy

   Theophylline administration is a treatment of first choice for the management of chronic asthma (to prevent symptoms and maintain patent airways). Slow clinical titration is generally preferred to increase the likelihood of acceptance and to remain within effective and safe therapeutic levels for each specific patient.

   Initial Dose

   16 mg/kg/24 hours or 400 mg/24 hours (whichever is less) of anhydrous theophylline in divided doses at 6 or 8 hour intervals.

   Increasing Dose

   The above dosage may be increased in approximately 25 percent increments at 2-3 day intervals so long as the drug is tolerated, until the maximum dose indicated in Section III (below) is reached.

III. Maximum Dose of Theophylline When the Serum Concentration is Not Measured

TABLE II

WARNING: DO NOT ATTEMPT TO MAINTAIN ANY DOSE THAT IS NOT TOLERATED.

Not to exceed the following:

Age		
< 9 years	24 mg/kg/day	(2.4 mL Accurbron/kg/day)
9-12 years	20 mg/kg/day	(2.0 mL Accurbron/kg/day)
12-16 years	18 mg/kg/day	(1.8 mL Accurbron/kg/day)
> 16 years	13 mg/kg/day *or* 900 mg *whichever is less*	

Note: Use ideal body weight for obese patients.

IV. Measurement of Serum Theophylline Concentrations During Chronic Therapy

   If the above maximum doses are to be maintained or exceeded, serum theophylline measurement is recommended. The serum sample should be obtained at the time of peak absorption, 1 to 2 hours after administration. It is important that the patient will not have missed any doses during the previous 48 hours and that dosing intervals will have been reasonably typical with no added doses during that period of time. **IF THESE INSTRUCTIONS HAVE NOT BEEN FOLLOWED, DOSAGE ADJUSTMENT BASED ON SERUM THEOPHYLLINE MEASUREMENTS MAY RESULT IN RECOMMENDATIONS THAT PRESENT RISK OF TOXICITY TO THE PATIENT.**

V. Final Adjustment of Dosage After Serum Theophylline Measurement

TABLE III

If serum theophylline is		*Directions*
Within normal limits	10 to 20 mcg/mL	Maintain dosage if tolerated. Recheck serum theophylline concentration at 6- to 12-month intervals.*
Too high	20 to 25 mcg/mL	Decrease doses by about 10%. Recheck serum theophylline concentration at 6-to 12-month intervals.*
	25 to 30 mcg/mL	Skip next dose and decrease subsequent doses by about 25%.
	Over 30 mcg/mL	Skip next 2 doses and decrease subsequent doses by 50%. Recheck serum theophylline.
Too low	7.5 to 10 mcg/mL	Increase dose by about 25%.** Recheck serum theophylline concentration at 6- to 12-month intervals.*
	5 to 7.5 mcg/mL	Increase dose by about 25% to the nearest dose increment and recheck serum theophylline for guidance in further dosage adjustment (another increase will probably be needed, but this provides a safety check).

*Finer adjustments in dosage may be needed for some patients

**The total daily dose may need to be administered at more frequent intervals if symptoms occur repeatedly at the end of a dosing interval.

From the *Journal of Respiratory Diseases* 2(7):16, 1981

Caution should be exercised for younger children who cannot complain of minor side effects. Older adults and patients with cor pulmonale, congestive heart failure, and/or liver disease may have unusually low dosage requirements and thus may experience toxicity at the maximal dosage recommended above.

It is important that no patient be maintained on any dosage that is not tolerated. Patients increasing dosage according to the schedule in TABLE III should be instructed not to take a subsequent dose if apparent side effects occur, and to resume therapy at a lower dose once adverse effects have disappeared.

TABLE I

	Oral Loading	*Followed by*	*Maintenance*
1. Children 6 months to 9 years	6 mg/kg	4 mg/kg q4 hrs × 3 doses	4 mg/kg q6 hrs
2. Children age 9-16 years and young adult smokers	6 mg/kg	3 mg/kg q4 hrs × 3 doses	3 mg/kg q6 hrs
3. Otherwise healthy nonsmoking adults	6 mg/kg	3 mg/kg q6 hrs × 2 doses	3 mg/kg q8 hrs
4. Older patients and patients with cor pulmonale	6 mg/kg	2 mg/kg q6 hrs × 2 doses	2 mg/kg q8 hrs
5. Patients with congestive heart failure	6 mg/kg	2 mg/kg q8 hrs × 2 doses	1-2 mg/kg q12 hrs

HOW SUPPLIED

Accurbron Syrup is a dye-free, pleasant tasting liquid available in pint bottles containing 150 mg theophylline (anhydrous) in each 15 mL (10 mg per mL). The package includes a 15 mL graduated measuring spoon marked in 1 mL increments. Store at controlled room temperature 15°–30°C (59°–86°F). Avoid freezing. Protect from excessive heat and light.

Product Information as of March, 1985

MERRELL DOW PHARMACEUTICALS INC.
Subsidiary of The Dow Chemical Company
Cincinnati, Ohio 45215, U.S.A.

CANTIL® ℞

[*kăn'tĭl*]
(mepenzolate bromide USP)
Tablets

CAUTION: Federal law prohibits dispensing without prescription.

DESCRIPTION

Cantil (mepenzolate bromide USP) chemically is 3-[(hydroxydiphenylacetyl) oxy]-1,1- dimethylpiperidinium bromide and has the following structure:

Mepenzolate bromide occurs as a white or light cream-colored powder, which is freely soluble in methanol, slightly soluble in water and chloroform, and practically insoluble in ether.
Each yellow tablet contains 25 mg mepenzolate bromide USP. This tablet also contains inactive ingredients: corn starch, FD&C Yellow No. 5 (tartrazine, See PRECAUTIONS), glucose, lactose, magnesium stearate, microcrystalline cellulose, and sucrose.

CLINICAL PHARMACOLOGY

Cantil diminishes gastric acid and pepsin secretion. Cantil also suppresses spontaneous contractions of the colon. Pharmacologically, it is a post-ganglionic parasympathetic inhibitor.
Radiotracer studies in which Cantil-^{14}C was used in animals and humans indicate that absorption following oral administration, as with other quaternary ammonium compounds, is low. Between 3 and 22% of an orally administered dose is excreted in the urine over a 5-day period, with the majority of the radioactivity appearing on Day 1. The remainder appears in the next 5 days in the feces and presumably has not been absorbed.

INDICATION

Cantil is indicated for use as adjunctive therapy in the treatment of peptic ulcer. Cantil has not been shown to be effective in contributing to the healing of peptic ulcer, decreasing the rate of recurrence or preventing complications.

CONTRAINDICATIONS

Glaucoma, obstructive uropathy (for example, bladder neck obstruction due to prostatic hypertrophy), obstructive disease of the gastrointestinal tract (for example, pyloroduodenal stenosis, achalasia), paralytic ileus, intestinal atony of the elderly or debilitated patient, unstable cardiovascular status in acute hemorrhage, severe ulcerative colitis, toxic megacolon complicating ulcerative colitis, myasthenia gravis, allergic or idiosyncratic reactions to Cantil or related compounds.

WARNINGS

In the presence of high environmental temperature, heat prostration (fever and heat stroke due to decreased sweating) can occur with use of Cantil.
Cantil may produce drowsiness or blurred vision. The patient should be cautioned regarding activities requiring mental alertness such as operating a motor vehicle or other machinery or performing hazardous work while taking this drug.
With overdosage, a curare-like action may occur, i.e., neuromuscular blockade leading to muscular weakness and possible paralysis.
It should be noted that the use of anticholinergic drugs in the treatment of gastric ulcer may produce a delay in gastric emptying time and may complicate such therapy (antral stasis).

Pregnancy

Reproduction studies in rats and rabbits have shown no evidence of impaired fertility or harm to the animal fetus. Information on possible adverse effects in the pregnant female is limited to uncontrolled data derived from marketing experience. Such experience has revealed no reports of the effect of Cantil on human pregnancies. No controlled studies to establish the safety of the drug in pregnancy have been performed.

Pediatric Use

Since there is no adequate experience in children who have received this drug, safety and efficacy in children have not been established. Newborn animal studies have been undertaken that show that younger animals are more sensitive to the toxic effects of mepenzolate bromide than are older animals.

PRECAUTIONS

Use Cantil with caution in the elderly and in all patients with:

Autonomic neuropathy
Hepatic or renal disease
Ulcerative colitis. Large doses may suppress intestinal motility to the point of producing a paralytic ileus and for this reason precipitate or aggravate "toxic megacolon," a serious complication of the disease.

Hyperthyroidism, coronary heart disease, congestive heart failure, "cardiac tachyarrhythmias," tachycardia, hypertension, and prostatic hypertrophy.
Hiatal hernia associated with reflux esophagitis, since anticholinergic drugs may aggravate this condition.
This product contains FD&C Yellow No. 5 (tartrazine), which may cause allergic-type reactions (including bronchial asthma) in certain susceptible individuals. Although the overall incidence of FD&C Yellow No. 5 (tartrazine) sensitivity in the general population is low, it is frequently seen in patients who also have aspirin hypersensitivity.

Nursing Mothers

It is not known whether this drug is secreted in human milk. As a general rule, nursing should not be undertaken while a patient is on a drug since many drugs are excreted in human milk.

ADVERSE REACTIONS

Xerostomia, decreased sweating, urinary hesitancy and retention, blurred vision, tachycardia, palpitations, dilatation of the pupil, cycloplegia, increased ocular tension, loss of taste, headaches, nervousness, mental confusion, drowsiness, weakness, dizziness, insomnia, nausea, vomiting, constipation, bloated feeling, impotence, suppression of lactation, severe allergic reaction or drug idiosyncrasies including anaphylaxis, urticaria and other dermal manifestations.

OVERDOSAGE

The symptoms of overdosage with Cantil progress from an intensification of the usual adverse effects to CNS disturbances (from restlessness and excitement to psychotic behavior), circulatory changes (flushing, fall in blood pressure, circulatory failure), respiratory failure, paralysis, and coma. Measures to be taken are (1) immediate lavage of the stomach and (2) injection of physostigmine 0.5 to 2 mg intravenously, repeated as necessary up to a total of 5 mg. Fever may be treated symptomatically (alcohol sponging, ice packs). Excitement of a degree that demands attention may be managed with sodium thiopental 2% solution given slowly intravenously or chloral hydrate (100–200 ml of a 2% solution) by rectal infusion. In the event of progression of the curare-like effect to paralysis of the respiratory muscles, artificial respiration should be instituted and maintained until effective respiratory action returns.

DOSAGE AND ADMINISTRATION

Usual Adult Dose: 1 or 2 tablets three times a day preferably with meals and 1 or 2 tablets at bedtime. Begin with the lower dosage when possible and adjust subsequently according to the patient's response.
Since there is no adequate experience in children who have received this drug, safety and efficacy in children have not been established.

DRUG INTERACTIONS

Concomitant administration of anticholinergic drugs and any other drugs which would increase the anticholinergic effects of Cantil is to be avoided.

HOW SUPPLIED

Tablets (25 mg) debossed MERRELL 37: bottles of 100.

Product Information as of April, 1985
Shown in Product Identification Section, page 418

CEPHULAC® (lactulose) Syrup ℞

[*sĕf'ū-lăk*]
FOR ORAL OR RECTAL ADMINISTRATION

CAUTION: Federal law prohibits dispensing without prescription.

DESCRIPTION

Lactulose is 4-O-β-D-galacto-pyranosyl-D-fructofuranose. The structural formula is:
[See Chemical Formula at top of next column].
The molecular formula is $C_{12}H_{22}O_{11}$ and the molecular weight is 342.30. Each 15 ml of Cephulac contains: 10 g lactulose (and less than 2.2 g galactose, less than 1.2 g lactose, and 1.2 g or less of other sugars). Also contains FD&C Blue No. 1, FD&C Yellow No. 6, water and flavoring. A minimal quantity of sodium hydroxide is used to adjust pH when necessary.

CLINICAL PHARMACOLOGY

Lactulose causes a decrease in blood ammonia concentration and reduces the degree of portal-systemic encephalopathy. These actions are considered to be results of the following:

Bacterial degradation of lactulose in the colon acidifies the colonic contents.

This acidification of colonic contents results in the retention of ammonia in the colon as the ammonium ion. Since the colonic contents are then more acid than the blood, ammonia can be expected to migrate from the blood into the colon to form the ammonium ion.
The acid colonic contents convert NH_3 to the ammonium ion $[NH_4]^+$, trapping it and preventing its absorption.
The laxative action of the metabolites of lactulose then expels the trapped ammonium ion from the colon.

Experimental data indicate that lactulose is poorly absorbed. Lactulose given orally to man and experimental animals resulted in only small amounts reaching the blood. Urinary excretion has been determined to be 3% or less and is essentially complete within 24 hours.
When incubated with extracts of human small intestinal mucosa, lactulose was not hydrolyzed during a 24-hour period and did not inhibit the activity of these extracts on lactose. Lactulose reaches the colon essentially unchanged. There it is metabolized by bacteria with the formation of low molecular weight acids that acidify the colonic contents.

INDICATIONS

For the prevention and treatment of portal-systemic encephalopathy, including the stages of hepatic pre-coma and coma. Controlled studies have shown that lactulose syrup therapy reduces the blood ammonia levels by 25–50%; this is generally paralleled by an improvement in the patients' mental state and by an improvement in EEG patterns. The clinical response has been observed in about 75% of patients, which is at least as satisfactory as that resulting from neomycin therapy. An increase in patients' protein tolerance is also frequently observed with lactulose therapy. In the treatment of chronic portal-systemic encephalopathy, Cephulac has been given for over 2 years in controlled studies.

CONTRAINDICATIONS

Since Cephulac contains galactose (less than 2.2 g/15 ml), it is contraindicated in patients who require a low galactose diet.

WARNINGS

A theoretical hazard may exist for patients being treated with lactulose syrup who may be required to undergo electrocautery procedures during proctoscopy or colonoscopy. Accumulation of H_2 gas in significant concentration in the presence of an electrical spark may result in an explosive reaction. Although this complication has not been reported with lactulose, patients on lactulose therapy undergoing such procedures should have a thorough bowel cleansing with a non-fermentable solution. Insufflation of CO_2 as an additional safeguard may be pursued but is considered to be a redundant measure.
Use in Pregnancy
Studies in laboratory animals have not revealed a teratogenic potential of lactulose. The safety of lactulose syrup during pregnancy and its effect on the mother or the fetus have not been evaluated in humans. The physician and patient should understand that the possibility that lactulose syrup might cause damage to the human fetus cannot be excluded. Lactulose syrup should not be given during pregnancy unless, in the opinion of the physician, the possible benefits outweigh the possible risks.

PRECAUTIONS

Lactulose syrup contains galactose (less than 2.2 g/15 ml) and lactose (less than 1.2 g/15 ml) and it should be used with caution in diabetics.
There have been conflicting reports about the concomitant use of neomycin and lactulose syrup. Theoretically, the elimination of certain colonic bacteria by neomycin and possibly other anti-infective agents may intefere with the desired degradation of lactulose and thus prevent the acidification of

Continued on next page

Information on Merrell Dow products is based on labeling in effect in May, 1986.

Merrell Dow—Cont.

colonic contents. Thus the status of the lactulose-treated patient should be closely monitored in the event of concomitant oral anti-infective therapy.

Other laxatives should not be used especially during the initial phase of therapy for portal-systemic encephalopathy because the loose stools resulting from their use may falsely suggest that adequate Cephulac dosage has been achieved.

In the overall management of portal-systemic encephalopathy it should be recognized that there is serious underlying liver disease with complications such as electrolyte disturbance (e.g., hypokalemia) for which other specific therapy may be required.

ADVERSE REACTIONS

Cephulac may produce gaseous distention with flatulence or belching and abdominal discomfort such as cramping in about 20% of patients. Excessive dosage can lead to diarrhea. Nausea and vomiting have been reported infrequently.

OVERDOSAGE

There have been no reports of accidental overdosage. In the event of overdosage it is expected that diarrhea and abdominal cramps would be the major symptoms.

DOSAGE AND ADMINISTRATION

Oral

Adult: The usual adult, oral dosage is 2 to 3 tablespoonfuls (30 to 45 ml, containing 20 g to 30 g of lactulose) three or four times daily. The dosage may be adjusted every day or two to produce 2 or 3 soft stools daily.

Hourly doses of 30 to 45 ml of Cephulac may be used to induce the rapid laxation indicated in the initial phase of the therapy of portal-systemic encephalopathy. When the laxative effect has been achieved, the dose of Cephulac may then be reduced to the recommended daily dose. Improvement in the patient's condition may occur within 24 hours but may not begin before 48 hours or even later.

Continuous long-term therapy is indicated to lessen the severity and prevent the recurrence of portal-systemic encephalopathy. The dose of Cephulac for this purpose is the same as the recommended daily dose.

Pediatric: Very little information on the use of lactulose in young children and adolescents has been recorded. As with adults, the subjective goal in proper treatment is to produce 2 or 3 soft stools daily. On the basis of information available, the recommended initial daily oral dose in infants is 2.5 to 10 ml in divided doses. For older children and adolescents the total daily dose is 40 to 90 ml. If the initial dose causes diarrhea, the dose should be reduced immediately. If diarrhea persists, lactulose should be discontinued.

Rectal

When the adult patient is in the impending coma or coma stage of portal-systemic encephalopathy and the danger of aspiration exists, or when the necessary endoscopic or intubation procedures physically interfere with the administration of the recommended oral doses, Cephulac may be given as a retention enema via a rectal balloon catheter. Cleansing enemas containing soap suds or other alkaline agents should not be used.

Three hundred ml of Cephulac should be mixed with 700 ml of water or physiologic saline and retained for 30 to 60 minutes. Cephulac enema may be repeated every 4 to 6 hours. If the enema is inadvertently evacuated too promptly, it may be repeated immediately.

The goal of treatment is reversal of the coma stage in order that the patient may be able to take oral medication. Reversal of coma may take place within 2 hours of the first enema in some patients. Cephulac given orally in the recommended doses should be started before Cephulac by enema is stopped entirely.

HOW SUPPLIED

1 pint (473 ml containing 315 g of lactulose)
2 quarts (1.89 liters containing 1260 g or 1.26 kg of lactulose)
30 ml (containing 20 g of lactulose) unit dose containers

Product Information as of March, 1985

Store at room temperature, below 86°F (30°C). Do not freeze. Under recommended storage conditions, a normal darkening of color may occur. Such darkening is characteristic of sugar solutions and does not affect therapeutic action. Prolonged exposure to temperatures above 86°F (30°C) or to direct light may cause extreme darkening and turbidity which may be pharmaceutically objectionable. If this condition develops do not use.

Prolonged exposure to freezing temperatures may cause change to a semisolid, too viscous to pour. Viscosity will return to normal upon warming to room temperature.

Shown in Product Identification Section, page 418

CHRONULAC® ℞

[*krŏn'ū-lăk*]
(lactulose)
Syrup

CAUTION: Federal law prohibits dispensing without a prescription.

DESCRIPTION

Chronulac is 4-O-β-D-galac-topyranosyl-D-fructofuranose. The structural formula is:

[structural formula: CH₂OH, CH₂OH, OH, HO, OH, HO, O, CH₂OH, OH, OH]

The molecular formula is $C_{12}H_{22}O_{11}$ and the molecular weight is 342.30. Each 15 ml of Chronulac contains: 10 g lactulose (and less than 2.2 g galactose, less than 1.2 g lactose, and 1.2 g or less of other sugars). Also contains FD&C Blue No. 1, FD&C Yellow No. 6, water and flavoring. A minimal quantity of sodium hydroxide is used to adjust pH when necessary.

CLINICAL PHARMACOLOGY

Chronulac is poorly absorbed from the gastrointestinal tract and no enzyme capable of hydrolysis of this disaccharide is present in human gastrointestinal tissue. As a result, oral doses of Chronulac reach the colon virtually unchanged. In the colon, Chronulac is broken down primarily to lactic acid, and also to small amounts of formic and acetic acids, by the action of colonic bacteria, which results in an increase in osmotic pressure and slight acidification of the colonic contents. This in turn causes an increase in stool water content and softens the stool.

Since Chronulac does not exert its effect until it reaches the colon, and since transit time through the colon may be slow, 24 to 48 hours may be required to produce a normal bowel movement.

Chronulac given orally to man and experimental animals resulted in only small amounts reaching the blood. Urinary excretion has been determined to be 3% or less and is essentially complete within 24 hours.

INDICATION

For the treatment of constipation. In patients with a history of chronic constipation, lactulose syrup (Chronulac) therapy increases the number of bowel movements per day and the number of days on which bowel movements occur.

CONTRAINDICATIONS

Since Chronulac contains galactose (less than 2.2 g/15 ml), it is contraindicated in patients who require a low galactose diet.

WARNINGS

A theoretical hazard may exist for patients being treated with lactulose syrup who may be required to undergo electrocautery procedures during proctoscopy or colonoscopy. Accumulation of H_2 gas in significant concentration in the presence of an electrical spark may result in an explosive reaction. Although this complication has not been reported with lactulose, patients on lactulose therapy undergoing such procedures should have a thorough bowel cleansing with a non-fermentable solution. Insufflation of CO_2 as an additional safeguard may be pursued but is considered to be a redundant measure.

Use in Pregnancy

Studies in laboratory animals (mice, rats, rabbits) have not revealed a teratogenic potential of Chronulac. The safety of Chronulac syrup during pregnancy and its effect on the mother or the fetus have not been evaluated in humans.

The physician and patient should understand that the possibility that Chronulac might cause damage to the human fetus cannot be excluded. Chronulac should not be given during pregnancy unless, in the opinion of the physician, the possible benefits outweigh the possible risks.

Use in Nursing Mothers

There are no data on secretion of Chronulac in human milk or effect on the nursing infant.

Use in Children

There is insufficient experience to recommend a dose of Chronulac that is safe and effective for treatment of constipation in children.

PRECAUTIONS

Elderly, debilitated patients who receive Chronulac for more than six months should have serum electrolytes (potassium, chloride, carbon dioxide) measured periodically. Also, since Chronulac contains galactose (less than 2.2 g/15 ml) and lactose (less than 1.2 g/15 ml), it should be used with caution in diabetics.

ADVERSE REACTIONS

Initial dosing may produce flatulence and intestinal cramps, which are usually transient. Excessive dosage can lead to diarrhea. Nausea has been reported.

OVERDOSAGE

There have been no reports of accidental overdosage. In the event of overdosage it is expected that diarrhea and abdominal cramps would be the major symptoms. Medication should be terminated.

DOSAGE AND ADMINISTRATION

The usual dose is 1 to 2 tablespoonfuls (15 to 30 ml, containing 10 g to 20 g of lactulose) daily. The dose may be increased to 60 ml daily if necessary. Twenty-four to 48 hours may be required to produce a normal bowel movement.

Note: Some patients have found that Chronulac may be more acceptable when mixed with fruit juice, water, or milk.

HOW SUPPLIED

8 fl. oz. bottles (237 ml)
30 ml unit dose cups (containing 20 g of lactulose) in trays of 10 cups
1 quart bottles (946 ml)

Product Information as of March, 1985

Store at room temperature, below 86°F (30°C). Do not freeze. Under recommended storage conditions, a normal darkening of color may occur. Such darkening is characteristic of sugar solutions and does not affect therapeutic action. Prolonged exposure to temperatures above 86°F (30°C) or to direct light may cause extreme darkening and turbidity which may be pharmaceutically objectionable. If this condition develops do not use.

Prolonged exposure to freezing temperatures may cause change to a semisolid, too viscous to pour. Viscosity will return to normal upon warming to room temperature.

Shown in Product Identification Section, page 418

CLOMID® ℞

[*klăhm'ĭd*]
(clomiphene citrate)

For prescribing information, write to:
Professional Relations Manager
MERRELL DOW PHARMACEUTICALS INC.
Subsidiary of The Dow Chemical Company
Cincinnati, Ohio 45242-9553, U.S.A.

Shown in Product Identification Section, page 418

DV®

(dienestrol cream USP)

CAUTION: Federal law prohibits dispensing without prescription.

WARNINGS

1. ESTROGENS HAVE BEEN REPORTED TO INCREASE THE RISK RATIO FOR ENDOMETRIAL CARCINOMA.

Three independent case control studies have reported an increased risk ratio of endometrial cancer in postmenopausal women exposed to exogenous estrogens for prolonged periods.[1–3] This reported risk was independent of the other risk factors studied. Additionally, the incidence rates of endometrial cancer have increased since 1969 in 8 different areas of the United States with population-based cancer reporting systems, an increase that may [or may not] be related to the expanded use of estrogens during the last decade.[4]

The 3 case control studies reported that the estimated risk ratio for endometrial cancer in estrogen users was about 4.5 to 13.9 times greater than in nonusers. The risk appeared to depend on both duration of treatment[1] and on estrogen dose.[3] In view of these reports, when estrogens are used for the treatment of menopausal symptoms, the lowest dose that will control symptoms should be utilized and medication should be discontinued as soon as possible. When prolonged treatment is medically indicated, the patient should be reassessed on at least a semiannual basis to determine the need for continued therapy. Although the evidence must be considered preliminary, one study suggests that cyclic administration of low doses of estrogen may carry less risk than continuous administration;[3] it therefore appears prudent to utilize such a regimen.

Close clinical surveillance of all women taking estrogens is important. In all cases of undiagnosed persistent or recurring abnormal vaginal bleeding, adequate diagnostic measures should be undertaken to rule out malignancy.

There is no evidence at present that "natural" estrogens are more or less hazardous than "synthetic" estrogens at equiestrogenic doses.

2. ESTROGENS SHOULD NOT BE USED DURING PREGNANCY.

The use of exogenous estrogens and progestagens during early pregnancy has been reported to damage the offspring. An association has been reported between *in utero* exposure of the female fetus to diethylstilbestrol, a non-steroidal estrogen, and an increased risk of the post-pubertal development of an ordinarily rare form of vaginal or cervical cancer.[5,6] This risk for diethylstilbestrol was recently estimated to be in the range of 0.14 to 1.4 per 1000 exposures,[7] consistent with a previous risk estimate of not greater than 4 per 1000 exposures.[8] Furthermore, a high percentage of such females exposed *in utero* (30 to over 90%) has been reported to have vaginal adenosis, epithelial changes of the vagina and cervix.[9–12] Although these changes are histologically benign, it is not known whether they are precursors of adenocarcinoma. Although similar data are not available with the use of other estrogens, it cannot be presumed they would not induce similar changes.

Several reports suggest a possible association between fetal exposure to exogenous estrogens and progestagens and congenital anomalies, including congenital heart defects and limb defects.[13–16]

One case control study[16] estimated a 4.7 fold increased risk of limb reduction defects in infants exposed *in utero* to exogenous steroids (oral contraceptives, hormone withdrawal tests for pregnancy, or attempted treatment for threatened abortion). Some of these exposures were very short and involved only a few days of treatment. The data suggest that the risk of limb reduction defects in exposed fetuses is somewhat less than 1 per 1000.

This product is not for use in therapy of threatened or habitual abortion.

If DV (dienestrol cream USP) is used during pregnancy, or if the patient becomes pregnant while using this drug, she should be apprised of the potential risks to the fetus, and the advisability of pregnancy continuation.

DESCRIPTION

DV (dienestrol cream USP) is a synthetic estrogen in cream form suitable for vaginal administration. Each tube contains:

Dienestrol USP 0.01%

with lactose, in a water-miscible base made from propylene glycol, stearic acid, diglycol stearate, trolamine, benzoic acid, butylated hydroxytoluene, and disodium edetate; buffered with lactic acid to an acid pH.

Chemistry

Generic name: Dienestrol USP

Chemical name:

Phenol,4,4′-(1,2-diethylidene-1,2-ethanediyl)bis-,(*E,E*)-. 4,4′-(Diethylideneethylene)diphenol.

Structural Formula:

H—C—CH3

HO—⟨ ⟩—C—C—⟨ ⟩—OH

H3C—C—H

Dienestrol occurs as colorless, white, or practically white needlelike crystals or as a white or practically white crystalline powder. It is odorless. It is practically insoluble in water, is slightly soluble in chloroform and fatty oils, and is soluble in alcohol, acetone, ether, and propylene glycol.

INDICATIONS

For the treatment of atrophic vaginitis and kraurosis vulvae associated with the menopause.

DV (dienestrol cream USP) HAS NOT BEEN SHOWN TO BE EFFECTIVE FOR ANY PURPOSE DURING PREGNANCY AND THE USE MAY HAVE POTENTIAL RISKS TO THE FETUS. (SEE BOXED WARNING.)

CONTRAINDICATIONS

DV (dienestrol cream USP) should not be used in patients with any of the following conditions:

1. Known or suspected cancer of the breast except in appropriately selected patients being treated for metastatic disease.
2. Known or suspected estrogen-dependent neoplasia.
3. Known or suspected pregnancy. (See Boxed Warning.)
4. Undiagnosed abnormal genital bleeding.
5. Active thrombophlebitis or thromboembolic disorders.
6. A past history of thrombophlebitis, thrombosis, or thromboembolic disorders.
7. Hypersensitivity to the ingredients of the cream.

WARNINGS

1. *Induction of malignant neoplasms.* Long-term continuous administration of natural and synthetic estrogens in certain animal species increases the frequency of carcinomas of the breast, cervix, vagina, and liver. There are now reports that estrogens increase the risk of carcinoma of the endometrium in humans. (See Boxed Warning.)

At the present time there is no satisfactory evidence that estrogens given to postmenopausal women increase the risk of cancer of the breast,[17] although a recent long-term follow-up of a single physician's practice has raised this possibility.[18] Because of the animal data, there is a need for caution in prescribing estrogens for women with a strong family history of breast cancer or who have breast nodules, fibrocystic disease, or abnormal mammograms.

2. *Gallbladder disease.* A recent study has reported a two to threefold increase in the risk of surgically confirmed gallbladder disease in women receiving postmenopausal estrogens,[17] similar to the twofold increase previously noted in users of oral contraceptives.[19] In the case of oral contraceptives the increased risk appeared after a period of use.[19]

3. *Effects similar to those caused by estrogen-progestagen oral contraceptives.* There are several adverse effects reported in association with oral contraceptives, most of which have not been documented as consequences of postmenopausal estrogen therapy, although it has been reported that there is an increased risk of thrombosis in men receiving high doses of estrogens for prostatic cancer and in women receiving estrogens for postpartum breast engorgement.[20–23]

The possibility that the adverse effects reported in association with oral contraceptives may be associated with larger doses of estrogen cannot be excluded.

a. *Thromboembolic disease.* Studies have now shown that users of oral contraceptives have an increased risk of various thromboembolic, thrombotic, and vascular diseases, such as thrombophlebitis, pulmonary embolism, stroke, and myocardial infarction.[24–31] Cases of retinal thrombosis, mesenteric thrombosis, and optic neuritis have been reported in oral contraceptive users. There is evidence that the risk of several of these adverse reactions is related to the dose of the drug.[32,33] An increased risk of post-surgery thromboembolic complications has also been reported in users of oral contraceptives.[34,35] If feasible, estrogen should be discontinued at least 4 weeks before surgery of the type associated with an increased risk of thromboembolism, or during periods of prolonged immobilization.

While an increased rate of thromboembolic and thrombotic disease in postmenopausal users of estrogens has not been found,[17,36] this does not rule out the possibility that such an increase may be present, or that subgroups of women who have underlying risk factors, or who are receiving relatively large doses of estrogens may have an increased risk. Therefore, estrogens should not be used in persons with active thrombophlebitis or thromboembolic disorders, and they should not be used (except in treatment of malignancy) in persons with a history of such disorders. They should be used with caution in patients with cerebral vascular or coronary artery disease and only for those in whom estrogens are needed.

Doses of estrogen (5 mg conjugated estrogens per day), comparable to those used to treat cancer of the prostate and breast, have been reported in a large prospective clinical trial in men[37] to increase the risk of nonfatal myocardial infarction, pulmonary embolism, and thrombophlebitis. When estrogen doses of this size are used, any of the thromboembolic and thrombotic adverse effects associated with oral contraceptive use should be considered as a risk.

b. *Hepatic adenoma.* Benign hepatic adenomas have been reported to be associated with the use of oral contraceptives.[38–40] Although benign and rare, these may rupture and may cause death through intra-abdominal hemorrhage. Such lesions have not yet been reported in association with other estrogen or progestagen preparations but should be considered in estrogen users having abdominal pain and tenderness, abdominal mass, or hypovolemic shock. Hepatocellular carcinoma has also been reported in women taking estrogen-containing oral contraceptives.[39] The relationship of this malignancy to these drugs is not known at this time.

c. *Elevated blood pressure.* Increased blood pressure is not uncommon in women using oral contraceptives and there is now a report that this may occur with use of estrogens in the menopause[41] and blood pressure should be monitored with estrogen use, especially if high doses are used.

d. *Glucose tolerance.* A worsening of glucose tolerance has been observed in a significant percentage of patients on estrogen-containing oral contraceptives. For this reason diabetic patients should be carefully observed while receiving estrogen.

4. *Hypercalcemia.* Administration of estrogens may lead to hypercalcemia in patients with breast cancer and bone metastases. If this occurs, the drug should be stopped and appropriate measures taken to reduce the serum calcium level.

PRECAUTIONS

A. General Precautions

1. A complete medical and family history should be taken prior to the initiation of any estrogen therapy. The pretreatment and periodic physical examinations should include special reference to blood pressure, breasts, abdomen, and pelvic organs, and should include a Papanicolaou smear. As a general rule, estrogens should not be prescribed for longer than 1 year without another physical examination being performed.

2. For conditions due to infection with known organisms, specific treatment should be given for the organism responsible.

3. Fluid retention—Because estrogens may cause some degree of fluid retention, conditions that might be influenced by this factor such as epilepsy, migraine, and cardiac or renal dysfunction require careful observation.

4. Certain patients may develop undesirable manifestations of excessive estrogenic stimulation, such as abnormal or excessive uterine bleeding, mastodynia, etc. In order to avoid this, the dosage should be reduced or the estrogens should be administered intermittently in the menopausal or hypogonadal patient.

5. The age of the patient constitutes no absolute limiting factor, although treatment with estrogens may mask the onset of the climacteric.

6. Oral contraceptives have been reported to be associated with an increased incidence of mental depression. Although it is not clear whether this is possibly due to the estrogenic or progestagenic component of the contraceptive, patients with a history of depression should be carefully observed.

7. Patients having pre-existing uterine leiomyomata should be observed for increased growth of myomata during estrogen therapy.

8. The pathologist should be advised of estrogen therapy when relevant specimens are submitted.

9. Patients with a past history of jaundice during pregnancy have an increased risk of recurrence of jaundice while receiving estrogen-containing oral contraceptive therapy. If jaundice develops in any patient receiving estrogen, the medication should be discontinued while the cause is investigated.

10. Estrogens may be poorly metabolized in patients with impaired liver function and they should be administered with caution in such patients.

11. Because estrogens influence the metabolism of calcium and phosphorus, they should be used with caution in patients with metabolic bone diseases that are associated with hypercalcemia or in patients with renal insufficiency.

12. Because of the effects of estrogens on epiphyseal closure, they should be used judiciously in young patients in whom bone growth is not complete.

13. Judicious assessment of the following changes in certain endocrine and liver function tests is necessary for patients receiving large doses of estrogen:

a. Increased sulfobromophthalein retention.
b. Increased prothrombin and factors VII, VIII, IX, and X; decreased antithrombin 3; increased norepinephrine-induced platelet aggregability.
c. Increased thyroid binding globulin (TBG) leading to increased circulating total thyroid hormone, as measured by PBI, T4 by column, or T4 by radioimmunoassay. Free T3 resin uptake is decreased, reflecting the elevated TBG; free T4 concentration is unaltered.
d. Impaired glucose tolerance.
e. Decreased pregnanediol excretion.
f. Reduced response to metyrapone test.
g. Reduced serum folate concentration.
h. Increased serum triglyceride, phospholipid, or cholesterol.

B. Information For The Patient

A patient package insert accompanies this drug product, the text of which is reproduced below.

C. Pregnancy Category X

See Contraindications and Boxed Warning.

D. Nursing Mothers

As a general principle, the administration of any drug to nursing mothers should be done only when clearly necessary since many drugs are excreted in human milk.

ADVERSE REACTIONS

(See Warnings regarding reports of induction of neoplasia, adverse effects on the fetus, increased incidence of gallbladder disease, and adverse effects similar to those of oral contraceptives, including thromboembolism.)

Since there is a possibility of dienestrol absorption through the vaginal mucosa, uterine bleeding might be provoked by excessive administration of dienestrol in menopausal women. Cytologic study or D & C may be required to differentiate this uterine bleeding from carcinoma. Tenderness of the breasts and vaginal discharge due to mucus hypersecretion may result from excessive estrogenic stimulation; endometrial withdrawal bleeding may occur if use of dienestrol is suddenly discontinued. Such reactions indicate overdosage. Menstrual irregularity may be made worse by dienestrol if a sufficient amount is absorbed. Dienestrol may cause serious bleeding in a woman sterilized because of endometriosis and in whom remaining foci of endometrium could be activated.

Continued on next page

Information on Merrell Dow products is based on labeling in effect in May, 1986.

Merrell Dow—Cont.

The following additional adverse reactions have been reported with estrogenic therapy including oral contraceptives:

1. *Genitourinary system*
Breakthrough bleeding, spotting, change in menstrual flow and cycle.
Dysmenorrhea.
Premenstrual-like syndrome.
Amenorrhea during and after treatment.
Increase in size of uterine fibromyomata.
Vaginal candidiasis.
Change in cervical eversion and in degree of cervical secretion.
Cystitis-like syndrome.
2. *Breasts*
Tenderness, enlargement, secretion.
3. *Gastrointestinal*
Nausea, vomiting.
Abdominal cramps, bloating.
Cholestatic jaundice.
4. *Skin*
Chloasma or melasma which may persist when drug is discontinued.
Erythema multiforme.
Erythema nodosum.
Hemorrhagic eruption.
Loss of scalp hair.
Hirsutism.
Urticaria.
5. *Eyes*
Steepening of corneal curvature.
Intolerance to contact lenses.
6. *CNS*
Headache, migraine, dizziness.
Mental depression.
Chorea.
7. *Miscellaneous*
Increase or decrease in weight.
Reduced carbohydrate tolerance.
Aggravation of porphyria.
Edema.
Changes in libido and/or potency.

ACUTE OVERDOSAGE

Numerous reports of ingestion of large doses of estrogen-containing oral contraceptives by young children indicate that serious ill effects usually do not occur. Overdosage of estrogen may cause nausea, and withdrawal bleeding may occur in females.

DOSAGE AND ADMINISTRATION

For treatment of atrophic vaginitis, or kraurosis vulvae associated with the menopause. The lowest dose that will control symptoms should be chosen and medication should be discontinued as promptly as possible. Attempts to discontinue or taper medication should be made at 3 to 6 month intervals.
The usual dosage range is 1 applicatorful once or twice daily for 1 or 2 weeks, then reduced to one-half initial dosage for a similar period.
A maintenance dosage of 1 applicatorful 1 to 3 times a week may be used after restoration of the vaginal mucosa has been achieved.
Treated patients with an intact uterus should be monitored closely for signs of endometrial cancer and appropriate diagnostic measures should be taken to rule out malignancy in the event of persistent or recurring abnormal vaginal bleeding.

HOW SUPPLIED

DV Cream 0.01%
NDC 0068-0293-13: 3 oz. tube with applicator designed to deliver approximately 6 ml. Each applicatorful contains about 6 g of cream (equivalent to 0.60 mg of dienestrol)

REFERENCES

1. Ziel, H.K. and Finkel, W.D.: Increased risk of endometrial carcinoma among users of conjugated estrogens. New Eng. J. Med. 293:1167–1170, 1975.
2. Smith, D.C., Prentice, R., Thompson, D.J., and Hermann, W.L.: Association of exogenous estrogen and endometrial carcinoma. New Eng. J. Med. 293:1164–1167, 1975.
3. Mack, T.M., Pike, M.C., Henderson, B.E., Pfeffer, R.I., Gerkins, V.R., Arthur, M., and Brown, S.E.: Estrogens and endometrial cancer in a retirement community. New Eng. J. Med. 294:1262–1267, 1976.
4. Weiss, N.S., Szekely, D.R., and Austin, D.F.: Increasing incidence of endometrial cancer in the United States. New Eng. J. Med. 294:1259–1262, 1976.
5. Herbst, A.L., Ulfelder, H., and Poskanzer, D.C.: Adenocarcinoma of the vagina. New Eng. J. Med. 284:878–881, 1971.
6. Greenwald, P., Barlow, J.J., Nasca, P.C., and Burnett, W.S.: Vaginal cancer after maternal treatment with synthetic estrogens. New Eng. J. Med. 285:390–392, 1971.
7. Herbst, A.L., Cole, P., Colton, T., Robboy, S.J., and Scully, R.E.: Age-incidence and risk of diethylstilbestrol-related clear cell adenocarcinoma of the vagina and cervix. Amer. J. Obstet. Gynec. 128:43–50, 1977.
8. Lanier, A.P., Noller, K.L., Decker, D.G., Elveback, L.R., and Kurland, L.T.: Cancer and stilbestrol. A follow-up of 1719 persons exposed to estrogens in utero and born 1943–1959. Mayo Clin. Proc. 48:793–799, 1973.
9. Herbst, A.L., Kurman, R.J., and Scully, R.E.: Vaginal and cervical abnormalities after exposure to stilbestrol in utero. Obstet. Gynec. 40:287–298, 1972.
10. Herbst, A.L., Poskanzer, D.C., Robboy, S.J., Friedlander, L., and Scully, R.E.: Prenatal exposure to stilbestrol. A prospective comparison of exposed female offspring with unexposed controls. New Eng. J. Med. 292:334–339, 1975.
11. Stafl, A., Mattingly, R.F., Foley, D.V., and Fetherston, W.C.: Clinical diagnosis of vaginal adenosis. Obstet. Gynec. 43:118–128, 1974.
12. Sherman, A.I., Goldrath, M., Berlin, A., Vakhariya, V., Banooni, F., Michaels, W., Goodman, P., and Brown, S.: Cervical-vaginal adenosis after *in utero* exposure to synthetic estrogens. Obstet. Gynec. 44:531–545, 1974.
13. Gal, I., Kirman, B., and Stern, J.: Hormone pregnancy tests and congenital malformation. Nature 216:83, 1967.
14. Levy, E.P., Cohen, A., and Fraser, F.C.: Hormone treatment during pregnancy and congenital heart defects. Lancet 1:611, 1973.
15. Nora, J.J. and Nora, A.H.: Birth defects and oral contraceptives. Lancet 1:941–942, 1973.
16. Janerich, D.T., Piper, J.M., and Glebatis, D.M.: Oral contraceptives and congenital limb-reduction defects. New Eng. J. Med. 291:697–700, 1974.
17. Boston Collaborative Drug Surveillance Program: Surgically confirmed gall bladder disease, venous thromboembolism, and breast tumors in relation to post menopausal estrogen therapy. New Eng. J. Med. 290:15–19, 1974.
18. Hoover, R., Gray, L.A., Sr., Cole, P., and MacMahon, B.: Menopausal estrogens and breast cancer. New Eng. J. Med. 295:401–405, 1976.
19. Boston Collaborative Drug Surveillance Program: Oral contraceptives and venous thromboembolic disease, surgically confirmed gallbladder disease, and breast tumors. Lancet 1:1399–1404, 1973.
20. Daniel, D.G., Campbell, H., and Turnbull, A.C.: Puerperal thromboembolism and suppression of lactation. Lancet 2:287–289, 1967.
21. Bailer, J.C., III: Thromboembolism and oestrogen therapy. Lancet 2:560, 1967.
22. The Veterans Administration Cooperative Urological Research Group: Carcinoma of the prostate: Treatment comparisons. J. Urol. 98:516–522, 1967.
23. Blackard, C.E., Doe, R.P., Mellinger, G.T., and Byar, D.P.: Incidence of cardiovascular disease and death in patients receiving diethylstilbestrol for carcinoma of the prostate. Cancer 26:249–256, 1970.
24. Royal College of General Practitioners: Oral contraception and thromboembolic disease. J. Roy. Coll. Gen. Pract. 13:267–269, 1967.
25. Inman, W.H.W. and Vessey, M.P.: Investigation of deaths from pulmonary, coronary, and cerebral thrombosis and embolism in women of child-bearing age. Brit. Med. J. 2:193–199, 1968.
26. Vessey, M.P. and Doll, R.: Investigation of relation between use of oral contraceptives and thromboembolic disease. A further report. Brit. Med. J. 2:651–657, 1969.
27. Sartwell, P.E., Masi, A.T., Arthes, F.G., Greene, G.R., and Smith, H.E.: Thromboembolism and oral contraceptives: An epidemiological case-control study. Amer. J. Epidem. 90:365–380, 1969.
28. Collaborative Group for the Study of Stroke in Young Women: Oral contraception and increased risk of cerebral ischemia or thrombosis. New Eng. J. Med. 288:871–878, 1973.
29. Collaborative Group for the Study of Stroke in Young Women: Oral contraceptives and stroke in young women: Associated risk factors. J.A.M.A. 231:718–722, 1975.
30. Mann, J.I. and Inman, W.H.W.: Oral contraceptives and death from myocardial infarction. Brit. Med. J. 2:245–248, 1975.
31. Mann, J.I., Vessey, M.P., Thorogood, M., and Doll, R.: Myocardial infarction in young women with special reference in oral contraceptive practice. Brit. Med. J. 2:241–245, 1975.
32. Inman, W.H.W., Vessey, M.P., Westerholm, B., and Engelund, A.: Thromboembolic disease and the steroidal content of oral contraceptives. A report to the Committee on Safety of Drugs. Brit. Med. J. 2:203–209, 1970.
33. Stolley, P.D., Tonascia, J.A., Tockman, M.S., Sartwell, P.E., Rutledge, A.H., and Jacobs, M.P.: Thrombosis with low-estrogen oral contraceptives. Amer. J. Epidem. 102:197–208, 1975.
34. Vessey, M.P., Doll, R., Fairbairn, A.S., and Glober, G.: Postoperative thromboembolism and the use of the oral contraceptives. Brit. Med. J. 3:123–126, 1970.
35. Greene, G.R. and Sartwell, P.E.: Oral contraceptive use in patients with thromboembolism following surgery, trauma, or infection. Amer. J. Public Health 62:680–685, 1972.
36. Rosenberg, L., Armstrong, B., Phil, D., and Jick, H.: Myocardial infarction and estrogen therapy in post-menopausal women. New Eng. J. Med. 294:1256–1259, 1976.
37. Coronary Drug Project Research Group: The coronary drug project: Initial findings leading to modifications of its research protocol. J.A.M.A. 214:1303–1313, 1970.
38. Baum, J., Holtz, F., Bookstein, J.J., and Klein, E.W.: Possible association between benign hepatomas and oral contraceptives. Lancet 2:926–928, 1973.
39. Mays, E.T., Christopherson, W.M., Mahr, M.M., and Williams, H.C.: Hepatic changes in young women ingesting contraceptive steroids. Hepatic hemorrhage and primary hepatic tumors. J.A.M.A. 235:730–732, 1976.
40. Edmondson, H., Henderson, A.B., and Benton, B.: Liver-cell adenomas associated with the use of oral contraceptives. New Eng. J. Med. 294:470–472, 1976.
41. Pfeffer, R.I. and Van Den Noort, S.: Estrogen use and stroke risk in postmenopausal women. Amer. J. Epidem. 103:445–456, 1976.

PATIENT INFORMATION ABOUT ESTROGENS

DV® (dienestrol cream USP)

INFORMATION FOR PATIENTS

DV (dienestrol) is a synthetic estrogen in cream form suitable for vaginal administration.

What You Should Know About Estrogens:
Estrogens are female hormones produced by the ovaries. The ovaries make several different kinds of estrogens. In addition, scientists have been able to make a variety of synthetic estrogens. As far as we know, all these estrogens have many similar properties and therefore much the same usefulness, side effects, and risks. This leaflet is intended to help you understand what estrogens are sometimes used for, the risks involved in their use, and how to use them as safely as possible.
This leaflet includes important information about estrogens, but not all the information. If you want to know more, you can ask your doctor or pharmacist to let you read the package insert for this product prepared for the doctor.

USES OF ESTROGEN

Estrogens are prescribed by doctors for a number of purposes, including:

1. To provide estrogen during a period of adjustment when a woman's ovaries produce it in decreased amounts in order to prevent certain uncomfortable symptoms of estrogen deficiency. (All women normally produce less estrogen, generally between the ages of 45 and 55; this is called the menopause.)
2. To prevent symptoms of estrogen deficiency when a woman's ovaries have been removed surgically before the natural menopause.
3. To prevent pregnancy. (Estrogens are given along with a progestagen, another female hormone; these combinations are called oral contraceptives or birth control pills. Patient labeling is available to women taking oral contraceptives and they will not be discussed in this leaflet.) *This product is not intended to prevent pregnancy.*
4. To treat certain cancers in women and men. *This product is not intended to treat cancer.*
5. To prevent painful swelling of the breasts after pregnancy in women who choose not to nurse their babies. *This product is not for prevention of swelling of the breasts after pregnancy.*

THERE IS NO PROPER USE OF DV IN A PREGNANT WOMAN.

ESTROGENS IN THE MENOPAUSE

In the natural course of their lives, all women eventually experience a decrease in estrogen production. This usually occurs between ages 45 and 55 but may occur earlier or later. Sometimes the ovaries may need to be removed before or during natural menopause by an operation, producing a "surgical menopause."
When the amount of estrogen in the blood begins to decrease, many women may develop typical symptoms: feelings of warmth in the face, neck, and chest or sudden intense episodes of heat and sweating throughout the body (called "hot flashes" or "hot flushes"). These symptoms are sometimes very uncomfortable.
A few women eventually develop changes in the vagina (called "atrophic vaginitis") which cause discomfort, especially during and after intercourse. Estrogens can be prescribed to treat these symptoms of the menopause. It is estimated that considerably more than half of all women undergoing the menopause have only mild symptoms or no symptoms at all and therefore do not need estrogens. Other women may need estrogens for a few months, while their bodies adjust to lower estrogen levels. Sometimes the need will be for periods longer than six months. In an attempt to avoid over-stimulation of the uterus (womb), estrogens are

usually given cyclically during each month of use, that is, three weeks of pills followed by one week without pills.

Sometimes women experience nervous symptoms or depression during menopause. There is no well-documented evidence that estrogens are effective for such symptoms and they should not be used to treat them, although other treatment may be needed.

You may have heard that taking estrogens for long periods (years) after the menopause will keep your skin soft and supple and keep you feeling young. There is no evidence that this is so, however, and such long-term treatment carries important risks.

THE DANGERS OF ESTROGENS

1. *Cancer of the uterus.* Several independent studies have reported an increased risk ratio of endometrial cancer (cancer of the lining of the uterus) if estrogens are used in the postmenopausal period for more than a year. Women taking estrogens are reported to have roughly 5 to 10 times as great a chance of getting this cancer as women who take no estrogens. To put this another way, while a postmenopausal woman not taking estrogens has 1 chance in 1,000 each year of getting cancer of the uterus, a woman taking estrogens has 5 to 10 chances in 1,000 each year. For this reason *it is important to take estrogens only when you really need them.*

   The risk of this cancer is reported to be greater the longer estrogens are used and also seems to be greater when larger doses are taken. For this reason *it is important to take the lowest dose of estrogen that will control symptoms and to take it only as long as it is needed.* If estrogens are needed for longer periods of time, your doctor will want to reevaluate your need for estrogens at least every six months.

   Women using estrogens should report any irregular vaginal bleeding to their doctors; such bleeding may be of no importance, but it can be an early warning of cancer of the uterus. If you have undiagnosed vaginal bleeding, you should not use estrogens until a diagnosis is made that there is no cancer of the uterus.

   If you have had your uterus completely removed (total hysterectomy), there is no danger of developing cancer of the uterus.
2. *Other possible cancers.* Long-term continuous administration of estrogens in certain animal species increases the frequency of cancers of the breast, cervix, vagina, and liver. At present there is no satisfactory evidence that women using estrogen in the menopause have an increased risk of such tumors, but there is no way yet to be sure they do not; and one study raises the possibility that use of estrogens in the menopause may increase the risk of breast cancer many years later. This is a further reason to use estrogens only when clearly needed. While you are taking estrogens, it is important that you go to your doctor at least every six months for an examination. Also, if members of your family have had breast cancer or if you have breast nodules or abnormal mammograms (breast x-rays), your doctor may wish to carry out more frequent examinations of your breasts.
3. *Gallbladder disease.* Women who use estrogens after menopause are reported to be more likely to develop gallbladder disease needing surgery than women who do not use estrogens. Birth control pills have a similar effect.
4. *Abnormal blood clotting.* Oral contraceptives increase the risk of blood clotting in various parts of the body. This can result in a stroke (if the clot is in the brain), a heart attack (clot in a blood vessel of the heart), or a pulmonary embolus (a clot which forms in the legs or pelvis, then breaks off and travels to the lungs). Any of these can be fatal.

   At this time use of estrogens in the menopause is not known to cause such blood clotting, but the possibility that such clotting in association with oral contraceptives may be associated with larger doses of estrogen cannot be excluded. It is recommended that if you have had clotting in the legs or lungs or a heart attack or stroke while you were using estrogens or birth control pills, you should not use estrogens (unless they are being used to treat cancer of the breast or prostate). If you have had a stroke or heart attack or if you have angina pectoris, estrogens should be used with caution and only if clearly needed (for example, if you have severe symptoms of the menopause).

   The larger doses of estrogen used to prevent swelling of the breasts after pregnancy have been reported to increase the risk of clotting in the legs and lungs.

Special Warning About Pregnancy:

You should not receive estrogen if you are pregnant. It has been reported that there is a greater than usual chance that the developing child will be born with a birth defect, although the possibility remains fairly small. It is also reported that a female child may have an increased risk of developing cancer of the vagina or cervix later in life (in the teens or twenties). Every possible effort should be made to avoid exposure to DV during pregnancy. If exposure occurs, see your doctor.

Other Effects of Estrogens:

In addition to the serious reported risks of estrogens described above, estrogens have the following side effects and potential risks:

1. *Nausea and vomiting.* The most common side effect of estrogen therapy is nausea. Vomiting is less common.
2. *Effects on breasts.* Estrogens may cause breast tenderness or enlargement and may cause the breasts to secrete a liquid. These effects are not dangerous.
3. *Effects on the uterus.* Estrogens may cause benign fibroid tumors of the uterus to get larger.

   Some women will have menstrual bleeding when estrogens are stopped. But if the bleeding occurs on days you are still taking estrogens you should report this to your doctor.
4. *Effects on liver.* Women taking oral contraceptives develop on rare occasions a tumor of the liver which can rupture and bleed into the abdomen. So far, these tumors have not been reported in women using estrogens in the menopause, but you should report any swelling or unusual pain or tenderness in the abdomen to your doctor immediately.

   Women with a past history of jaundice (yellowing of the skin and white parts of the eyes) may get jaundice again during estrogen use. If this occurs, stop taking estrogens and see your doctor.
5. *Other effects.* Estrogens may cause excess fluid to be retained in the body. This may make some conditions worse, such as epilepsy, migraine, heart disease, or kidney disease.

SUMMARY

Estrogens have important uses, but they have reported risks of potentially serious conditions developing as well. You must decide, with your doctor, whether the risks are acceptable to you in view of the benefits of treatment. Except where your doctor has prescribed DV for use in special cases, you should not use DV if you have cancer of the breast or uterus, are pregnant, have undiagnosed abnormal vaginal bleeding, clotting in the legs or lungs, or have had a stroke, heart attack or angina, or clotting in the legs or lungs in the past while you were taking estrogens.

You can use DV as safely as possible by understanding that your doctor will require regular physical examinations while you are taking it and will try to discontinue the drug as soon as possible and use the smallest dose possible. Be alert for signs of trouble including:

1. Abnormal bleeding from the vagina.
2. Pains in the calves or chest or sudden shortness of breath, or coughing blood (indicating possible clots in the legs, heart, or lungs).
3. Severe headache, dizziness, faintness, or changes in vision (indicating possible developing clots in the brain or eye).
4. Breast lumps. (You should ask your doctor how to examine your own breasts.)
5. Jaundice (yellowing of the skin).
6. Mental depression.

Based on his or her assessment of your medical needs, your doctor has prescribed this drug for you. Do not give the drug to anyone else.

HOW SUPPLIED

DV (dienestrol cream USP) is a synthetic estrogen in cream form suitable for vaginal administration.

Each tube contains:

Dienestrol 0.01%

with lactose, in a water-miscible base made from propylene glycol, stearic acid, diglycol stearate, trolamine, benzoic acid, butylated hydroxytoluene, and disodium edetate; buffered with lactic acid to an acid pH.

Product Information as of May, 1985

HIPREX® ℞

[*hĭp′rĕx*]

(methenamine hippurate)

AVAILABLE ONLY ON PRESCRIPTION

DESCRIPTION

Each yellow capsule-shaped tablet contains 1 g methenamine hippurate which is the hippuric acid salt of methenamine (hexamethylenetetramine). The tablet also contains inactive ingredients: FD&C Yellow No. 5 (tartrazine, See PRECAUTIONS), magnesium stearate, povidone, and saccharin sodium.

ACTIONS

Microbiology: Hiprex (methenamine hippurate) has antibacterial activity because the methenamine component is hydrolyzed to formaldehyde in acid urine. Hippuric acid, the other component, has some antibacterial activity and also acts to keep the urine acid. The drug is generally active against *E. coli*, enterococci and staphylococci. *Enterobacter aerogenes* is generally resistant. The urine must be kept sufficiently acid for urea-splitting organisms such as *Proteus* and *Pseudomonas* to be inhibited.

Human Pharmacology: Within ½ hour after ingestion of a single 1-gram dose of Hiprex, antibacterial activity is demonstrable in the urine. Urine has continuous antibacterial activity when Hiprex is administered at the recommended dosage schedule of 1 gram twice daily. Over 90% of methenamine moiety is excreted in the urine within 24 hours after administration of a single 1-gram dose. Similarly, the hippurate moiety is rapidly absorbed and excreted, and it reaches the urine by both tubular secretion and glomerular filtration. This action may be important in older patients or in those with some degree of renal impairment.

INDICATIONS

Hiprex is indicated for prophylactic or suppressive treatment of frequently recurring urinary tract infections when long-term therapy is considered necessary. This drug should only be used after eradication of the infection by other appropriate antimicrobial agents.

CONTRAINDICATIONS

Hiprex (methenamine hippurate) is contraindicated in patients with renal insufficiency, severe hepatic insufficiency, or severe dehydration. Methenamine preparations should not be given to patients taking sulfonamides because some sulfonamides may form an insoluble precipitate with formaldehyde in the urine.

WARNINGS

Large doses of methenamine (8 grams daily for 3 to 4 weeks) have caused bladder irritation, painful and frequent micturition, albuminuria, and gross hematuria.

PRECAUTIONS

1. Care should be taken to maintain an acid pH of the urine, especially when treating infections due to urea-splitting organisms such as *Proteus* and strains of *Pseudomonas.*
2. In a few instances in one study, the serum transaminase levels were slightly elevated during treatment but returned to normal while the patients were still taking Hiprex. Because of this report, it is recommended that liver function studies be performed periodically on patients taking the drug, especially those with liver dysfunction.
3. *Use in pregnancy:* In early pregnancy the safe use of Hiprex is not established. In the last trimester, safety is suggested, but not definitely proved. No adverse effects on the fetus were seen in studies in pregnant rats and rabbits. Hiprex taken during pregnancy can interfere with laboratory tests of urine estriol (resulting in unmeasurably low values) when acid hydrolysis is used in the laboratory procedure. This interference is due to the presence in the urine of methenamine and/or formaldehyde. Enzymatic hydrolysis, in place of acid hydrolysis, will circumvent this problem.
4. This product contains FD&C Yellow No. 5 (tartrazine), which may cause allergic-type reactions (including bronchial asthma) in certain susceptible individuals. Although the overall incidence of FD&C Yellow No. 5 (tartrazine) sensitivity in the general population is low, it is frequently seen in patients who also have aspirin hypersensitivity.

ADVERSE REACTIONS

Minor adverse reactions have been reported in less than 3.5% of patients treated. These reactions have included nausea, upset stomach, dysuria, and rash.

DOSAGE AND ADMINISTRATION

1 tablet (1.0 g) twice daily (morning and night) for adults and children over 12 years of age.

½ to 1 tablet (0.5 to 1.0 g) twice daily (morning and night) for children 6 to 12 years of age.

Since the antibacterial activity of Hiprex is greater in acid urine, restriction of alkalinizing foods and medications is desirable. If necessary, as indicated by urinary pH and clinical response, supplemental acidification of the urine should be instituted. The efficacy of therapy should be monitored by repeated urine cultures.

HOW SUPPLIED

1-gram scored, capsule-shaped yellow tablets debossed MERRELL 277 in bottles of 100

Product Information as of April, 1985

Shown in Product Identification Section, page 418

LORELCO® Tablets ℞

[*lō-rĕl′cō*]

(probucol tablets)

CAUTION: Federal law prohibits dispensing without prescription.

DESCRIPTION

Lorelco (probucol) film-coated tablets for oral administration contain 250 mg of probucol per tablet. Each tablet also con-

Continued on next page

Information on Merrell Dow products is based on labeling in effect in May, 1986.

Merrell Dow—Cont.

tains as inactive ingredients: corn starch, ethylcellulose, glycerin, hydroxypropyl cellulose, hydroxypropyl methylcellulose 2910, iron oxide, lactose, magnesium stearate, microcrystalline cellulose, polysorbate 80, talc, and titanium dioxide. Lorelco is an agent for the reduction of elevated serum cholesterol. The chemical name is 4,4′-(isopropylidenedithio) bis (2,6-di-t-butylphenol). Its chemical structure does not resemble that of any other available cholesterol-lowering agent. It is lipophilic.

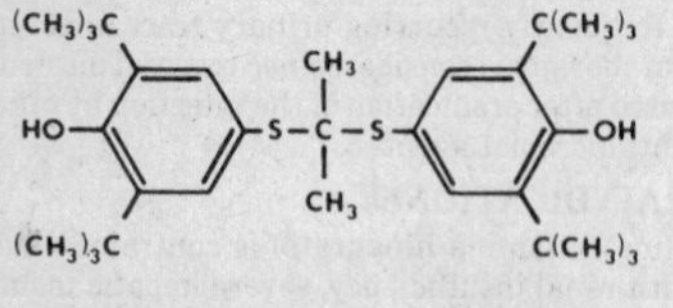

$(CH_3)_3C$ $C(CH_3)_3$
CH_3
HO— S—C—S —OH
CH_3
$(CH_3)_3C$ $C(CH_3)_3$

CLINICAL PHARMACOLOGY

Lorelco (probucol) lowers serum cholesterol and has relatively little effect on serum triglycerides. Patients responding to probucol exhibit a decrease in low density lipoprotein cholesterol. Cholesterol is reduced not only in the low density lipoprotein fraction, but also in some high density lipoprotein fractions with proportionately greater effect on the high density portion in some patients. Epidemiological studies have shown that both low HDL-cholesterol and high LDL-cholesterol are independent risk factors for coronary heart disease. The risk of lowering HDL-cholesterol while lowering LDL-cholesterol remains unknown. There is little or no effect reported on very low density lipoprotein.

Studies on the mode of action of Lorelco indicate that it increases the fractional rate of catabolism of low density lipoproteins. This effect may be linked to the observed increased excretion of fecal bile acids, a final metabolic pathway for the elimination of cholesterol from the body. Lorelco also exhibits inhibition of early stages of cholesterol synthesis and slight inhibition of absorption of dietary cholesterol. There is no increase in the cyclic precursors of cholesterol, namely desmosterol and 7-dehydrocholesterol. On this basis, it is concluded that Lorelco does not affect the later stages of cholesterol biosynthesis.

Absorption of Lorelco from the gastrointestinal tract is limited and variable. When it is administered with food, peak blood levels are higher and less variable. With continuous administration in a dosage of 500 mg b.i.d., the blood levels of an individual gradually increase over the first three to four months and thereafter remain fairly constant. In 116 patients treated with Lorelco for periods of three months to one year, the mean blood level was 23.6 ± 17.2 mcg/ml (± S.D.) ranging to 78.3 mcg/ml. Levels observed after seven years of treatment in 40 patients yielded an average value of 21.5 ± 16.5 mcg/ml (± S.D.) ranging to 62.0 mcg/ml.

At the end of 12 months of treatment in eight patients, blood levels averaged 19.0 mcg/ml. Six weeks after cessation of therapy, the average had fallen by 60 percent. After six months the average had fallen by 80 percent.

In December 1984 a National Institutes of Health Consensus Development Conference Panel[1] concluded that lowering definitely elevated blood cholesterol levels (specifically blood levels of low-density lipoprotein cholesterol) will reduce the risk of heart attacks due to coronary heart disease. The effect of probucol-induced reduction of serum cholesterol or triglyceride levels or alteration of HDL-cholesterol levels on morbidity or mortality due to coronary heart disease has not yet been established. Several years may be required before ongoing long-term investigations will resolve this question.

INDICATIONS AND USAGE

Serious animal toxicity has been encountered with probucol. See WARNINGS and ANIMAL PHARMACOLOGY AND TOXICOLOGY sections. Probucol is not an innocuous drug and strict attention should be paid to the INDICATIONS and WARNINGS.

Drug therapy should not be used for the routine treatment of elevated blood lipids for the prevention of coronary heart disease. Dietary therapy specific for the type of hyperlipidemia is the initial treatment of choice. Excess body weight may be an important factor and should be addressed prior to any drug therapy. Physical exercise can be an important ancillary measure. Contributory disease such as hypothyroidism or diabetes mellitus should be looked for and adequately treated. The use of drugs should be considered only when reasonable attempts have been made to obtain satisfactory results with non-drug methods. If the decision ultimately is to use drugs, the patient should be instructed that this does not reduce the importance of adhering to diet.

The selection of patients for cholesterol-lowering drug therapy should take into account other important coronary risk factors such as smoking, hypertension, and diabetes mellitus. Consideration should be given to the efficacy, safety, and compliance factors for each of the cholesterol-lowering drugs prior to selecting the one most appropriate for an individual patient.

Lorelco may be indicated for the reduction of elevated serum cholesterol in patients with primary hypercholesterolemia (elevated low density lipoproteins) who have not responded adequately to diet, weight reduction and control of diabetes mellitus. Lorelco may be useful to lower elevated cholesterol that occurs in patients with combined hypercholesterolemia and hypertriglyceridemia, but it is not indicated where hypertriglyceridemia is the abnormality of most concern.

It is not always possible to predict from the lipoprotein type or other factors which patients will exhibit favorable results. Lipid levels should be periodically assessed. Small or transient changes in high density lipoprotein cholesterol may be due to inaccuracies in the method of determination. Substantial changes are sometimes seen with diet.

The effect of probucol-induced reduction of serum cholesterol or triglyceride levels or alteration of HDL-cholesterol levels on morbidity or mortality due to coronary heart disease has not yet been established. Several years may be required before ongoing long-term investigations will resolve this question.

CONTRAINDICATIONS

(See also PRECAUTIONS.) Lorelco is contraindicated in patients who are known to have a hypersensitivity to it.

WARNINGS

SERIOUS ANIMAL TOXICITY HAS BEEN ENCOUNTERED WITH PROBUCOL IN RHESUS MONKEYS FED AN ATHEROGENIC DIET AND IN BEAGLE DOGS. (SEE ANIMAL PHARMACOLOGY AND TOXICOLOGY SECTION.)

Although Q-T prolongation can occur in patients on probucol, the arrhythmias observed in monkeys fed large doses of probucol added to an atherogenic diet have not been reported in man; nevertheless, the following precautions are deemed prudent:

1. At the start of treatment with Lorelco and throughout the treatment period, patients should be advised to adhere to a low cholesterol, low fat diet.
2. As part of an overall evaluation, a baseline, six month, and one year repeat ECG tracing should be considered. If marked prolongation of the Q-T interval (after correction for rate) occurs, the possible benefits and risks should be carefully considered before making the decision to continue the probucol administration.

Lorelco should not be used in patients with evidence of recent or progressive myocardial damage or findings suggestive of ventricular arrhythmias.

No instances of increase in ectopy attributed to Lorelco have been reported. However, patients with unexplained syncope while on Lorelco should have ECG surveillance.

PRECAUTIONS

General: Because Lorelco is intended for long-term administration, adequate baseline studies should be performed to determine that the patient has elevated serum cholesterol levels. Serum lipid levels should be determined before treatment and repeated during the first few months of treatment and periodically thereafter. A favorable trend in cholesterol reduction should be evident during the first three to four months of administration of Lorelco. Probucol lowers serum total and LDL cholesterol, and also lowers HDL-cholesterol in many patients with elevated LDL-cholesterol. Epidemiologic studies within hypercholesterolemic populations have shown that serum HDL-cholesterol is an independent, inversely correlated, risk factor for coronary heart disease (see CLINICAL PHARMACOLOGY). Animal or human studies which could confirm or deny the hypothesis that drug induced alteration in HDL-cholesterol affects cardiovascular risk have not been carried out. It is not known whether probucol-induced reduction of serum HDL-cholesterol will affect cardiovascular risk since no long-term, controlled clinical trials of probucol for the prevention of coronary heart disease, similar to the LRC-CPPT (See CLINICAL STUDIES), have been performed. The probable benefits obtained from LDL-cholesterol reduction must be weighed against the possible risk of a reduction in HDL-cholesterol when assessing the response of each patient receiving Lorelco treatment. If satisfactory lipid alteration is not achieved, the drug should be discontinued.

Information for Patients: The patient should be instructed to adhere to a prudent diet. Females should be cautioned against becoming pregnant for at least six months after discontinuing Lorelco and should not breast feed their infants during therapy with Lorelco.

Laboratory Tests: The physician should schedule periodic blood lipid determinations and should consider periodic electrocardiograms. (See WARNINGS.)

Elevations of the serum transaminases (glutamic-oxalacetic and glutamic-pyruvic), bilirubin, alkaline phosphatase, creatine phosphokinase, uric acid, blood urea nitrogen and blood glucose above the normal range were observed on one or more occasions in various patients treated with Lorelco. Most often these were transient and/or could have been related to the patient's clinical state or other modes of therapy. Although the basis for the relationship between probucol and these abnormalities is not firm, the possibility that some of these are drug-related cannot be excluded. In the controlled trials, the incidence of abnormal laboratory values was no higher in the patients treated with probucol than in the patients who received placebo. If abnormal laboratory tests persist or worsen, if clinical signs consistent with the abnormal laboratory tests develop, or if systemic manifestations occur, probucol should be discontinued.

Drug Interactions: The addition of clofibrate to probucol is not recommended since the lowering effect on mean serum levels of either LDL or total cholesterol is generally not significantly additive and, in some patients, there may be a pronounced lowering of HDL-cholesterol. Neither oral hypoglycemic agents nor oral anticoagulants alter the effect of Lorelco on serum cholesterol. The dosage of these agents is not usually modified when given with Lorelco. Monkeys fed a high fat, high cholesterol diet admixed with probucol exhibited serious toxicity. The toxicity observed in monkeys has not been reported in man. (See WARNINGS and ANIMAL PHARMACOLOGY AND TOXICOLOGY sections.)

Carcinogenesis, Mutagenesis, Impairment of Fertility: In chronic studies of two years duration in rats, no toxicity or carcinogenicity was observed. These results are consistent with the lack of any adverse effect on fertility and the negative findings in tests for mutagenic activity in rats.

Pregnancy:

Teratogenic Effects

Pregnancy—Category B: Reproduction studies have been performed in rats and rabbits at doses up to 50 times the human dose, and have revealed no evidence of impaired fertility or harm to the fetus due to probucol. There are, however, no adequate and well-controlled studies in pregnant women. Because animal reproduction studies are not always predictive of human response, this drug should be used during pregnancy only if clearly needed. Furthermore, if a patient wishes to become pregnant, it is recommended that the drug be withdrawn and birth control procedures be used for at least six months because of persistence of the drug in the body for prolonged periods. (See CLINICAL PHARMACOLOGY.)

Labor and Delivery: The effect of Lorelco on human labor and delivery is unknown.

Nursing Mothers: It is not known whether this drug is secreted in human milk, but it is likely to be since such excretion has been shown in animals. It is recommended that nursing not be undertaken while a patient is on Lorelco.

Pediatric Use: Safety and effectiveness in children have not been established.

ADVERSE REACTIONS

Gastrointestinal:
diarrhea or loose stools, flatulence, abdominal pain, nausea, vomiting, indigestion, gastrointestinal bleeding

Cardiovascular:
prolongation of the Q-T interval on ECG

Neurologic:
headache, dizziness, paresthesias, insomnia, tinnitus, peripheral neuritis

Hematologic:
eosinophilia, low hemoglobin and/or hematocrit, thrombocytopenia

Dermatologic:
rash, pruritus, ecchymosis, petechiae, hyperhidrosis, fetid sweat

Genitourinary:
impotency, nocturia

Ophthalmic:
conjunctivitis, tearing, blurred vision

Endocrine:
enlargement of multinodular goiter

Idiosyncrasies:
An idiosyncratic reaction observed with initiation of therapy and characterized by dizziness, palpitations, syncope, nausea, vomiting and chest pain has been observed.

Other:
diminished sense of taste and smell, anorexia, angioneurotic edema

DRUG ABUSE AND DEPENDENCE

No evidence of abuse potential has been associated with Lorelco, nor is there evidence of psychological or physical dependence in humans.

OVERDOSAGE

There is a single report of a 15 kg, three-year-old male child who ingested 5 gm of probucol. Emesis was induced by ipecac. The child remained well, apart from a brief episode of loose stools and flatulence. No specific information is available on the treatment of overdosage with Lorelco and no specific antidote is available. Probucol is not dialyzable. Treatment is symptomatic and supportive. Probucol has shown no identifiable acute toxicity in mice and rats. In these animals the LD_{50} (oral) is in excess of 5 gm/kg of body weight.

DOSAGE AND ADMINISTRATION

For adult use only. The recommended and maximal dose is 500 mg (two tablets of 250 mg each) twice daily with the morning and evening meals.

HOW SUPPLIED

Each white film-coated tablet contains 250 mg probucol and is imprinted with the DOW diamond trademark over the code number 51, or LORELCO 250.

Bottles of 120 tablets, a 30-day supply for one patient (NDC 0068-0051-52)

Keep well closed. Store in a dry place. Avoid excessive heat. Dispense in well closed light-resistant container with child-resistant closure.

ANIMAL PHARMACOLOGY AND TOXICOLOGY

In rhesus monkeys administration of probucol in diets containing unusually high amounts of cholesterol and saturated fat resulted in the death of four of eight animals after several weeks. Premonitory syncope was frequently observed and was associated with a pronounced prolongation of the Q-T intervals (30 to 50 percent longer than that observed in untreated monkeys). Serum levels of probucol greater than 20 mcg/ml were generally associated with some prolongation in the Q-T interval in the cholesterol-fed monkey. A 75 msec or greater increase in Q-T interval from control values was usually seen at 40 mcg/ml and above. Blood levels in humans receiving probucol average approximately 20 mcg/ml and not uncommonly reach levels of 40 mcg/ml and higher. Rhesus monkeys fed normal (low fat) chow and receiving probucol three to thirty times the human dose equivalent achieved blood levels only one-third those of many human subjects. No adverse effects were detected in these monkeys over an eight-year period of continuous drug administration. In another study in rhesus monkeys, an atherogenic diet was fed for two years and daily treatment with probucol, separated in time from the atherogenic meal, was carried out during the second year. Serum probucol levels ranged 20 to 50 mcg/ml in five of ten monkeys, and less in the remaining animals. Marked prolongation of the Q-T_c interval in the electrocardiogram or syncopal behavior was never observed over the entire one-year treatment period. Regression of gross aortic lesions comparable to that observed in a parallel group of monkeys receiving cholestyramine was seen in animals receiving probucol. It should be emphasized that both HDL-cholesterol and LDL-cholesterol were markedly reduced in this regression study. During the performance of a two-year chronic study involving 32 probucol-treated dogs (beagles) there were 12 fatalities. Subsequent experiments have indicated that probucol sensitizes the canine myocardium to epinephrine, resulting in ventricular fibrillation in many dogs. Among the animal species in which probucol has been studied, the dog is peculiar with respect to the phenomenon of sudden death due to the sensitization of the myocardium to epinephrine. In contrast to findings in the dog, injections of epinephrine to probucol-treated monkeys did not induce ventricular fibrillation.

In other studies, monkeys were given probucol either before and after, or only after myocardial infarction induced by coronary artery ligation. In these studies there was no difference between probucol- and placebo-treated groups with respect to either survival or detailed blind quantitation of myocardial changes (gross and histopathologic).

Probucol has shown no identifiable toxicity in mice and rats. In these animals the LD_{50} (oral) is in excess of five gm/kg of body weight. In chronic studies of two-year duration in rats, no toxicity or carcinogenicity was observed.

From studies in rats, dogs and monkeys, it is known that probucol accumulates slowly in adipose tissue. Approximately 90 percent of probucol administered orally is unabsorbed. For that which is absorbed, the biliary tract is the major pathway for clearance from the body and very little is excreted by way of the kidneys.

Myocardial injury was produced in various groups of rats by one of the following procedures: aortic coarctation, coronary ligation, or cobalt or isoproterenol injection. After probucol administration, no deleterious effects related to treatment occurred as measured by survival and microscopic examination of myocardial damage.

Probucol was administered to minipigs beginning ten days before ligation of coronary artery and continued for 60 days post surgery. Challenge with epinephrine at the end of 60 days failed to induce ventricular fibrillation in any of the coronary-ligated, probucol-treated minipigs.

CLINICAL STUDIES

In a multicenter, randomized, double-blind study, the LRC-CPPT[2], hypercholesterolemic patients treated with an oral bile acid sequestrant (cholestyramine) and a cholesterol lowering diet experienced average total and low-density lipoprotein cholesterol reductions greater than those obtained in the placebo group treated with diet alone. The cumulative seven-year incidence of the primary end point—combined incidence of definite CHD death and/or definite nonfatal myocardial infarction—was 7% in the cholestyramine group and 8.6% in the placebo group. This was a 19% reduction in risk (P less than 0.05, single-tail test) of the primary end point reflecting a 24% reduction in definite CHD death and a 19% reduction in nonfatal myocardial infarction.

The subjects included in the study were middle-aged men (35–59 years old) with serum cholesterol levels at least 265 mg/dl and no previous history of heart disease. It is not clear to what extent these findings can be extrapolated to other segments of the hypercholesterolemic population not studied.

The bile acid sequestrant, cholestyramine was used in the above trial. Caution should be exercised in extrapolating these results to probucol since it differs from cholestyramine with regard to its mode of action, spectrum of cholesterol-lowering potency, effect on HDL-cholesterol, and possible toxicity. The effect of probucol-induced reduction of serum cholesterol levels on morbidity or mortality due to coronary heart disease has not yet been established. Several years may be required before ongoing long-term investigations will resolve this question.

REFERENCES

1. Consensus Development Panel, Lowering blood cholesterol to prevent heart disease, *JAMA* 253: 2080–2086, 1985.
2. The Lipid Research Clinics Program; The Lipid Research Clinics coronary primary prevention trial results. I. Reduction in incidence of coronary heart disease, *JAMA* 251: 351–64, 1984.

Product Information as of April, 1986

MERRELL DOW PHARMACEUTICALS INC.
Subsidiary of The Dow Chemical Company
Cincinnati, Ohio 45215, U.S.A.

Shown in Product Identification Section, page 418

METAHYDRIN® ℞

[*mĕt″ăh-hī′drĭn*]
(trichlormethiazide USP)

AVAILABLE ONLY ON PRESCRIPTION

DESCRIPTION

Metahydrin is an oral diuretic and antihypertensive of the thiazide class. Differing from other thiazides by the inclusion of a dichloromethyl radical at the 3 position on the benzothiadiazine structure, it has the following formula:

Each pink tablet contains Metahydrin (trichlormethiazide USP) 2 mg. Tablets also contain as inactive ingredients: corn starch, D&C Red No. 33, FD&C Red No. 3, FD&C Yellow No. 5 (tartrazine, See PRECAUTIONS), FD&C Yellow No. 6, lactose, magnesium stearate, and pregelatinized corn starch.

Each aqua blue tablet contains Metahydrin (trichlormethiazide USP) 4 mg. Tablets also contain as inactive ingredients: corn starch, FD&C Blue No. 1, FD&C Yellow No. 5 (tartrazine, See PRECAUTIONS), lactose, magnesium stearate, and pregelatinized corn starch.

ACTION

The mechanism of action results in an interference with the renal tubular mechanism of electrolyte reabsorption. At maximal therapeutic dosage all thiazides are approximately equal in their diuretic potency. The mechanism whereby thiazides function in the control of hypertension is unknown.

INDICATIONS

Metahydrin is indicated as adjunctive therapy in edema associated with congestive heart failure, hepatic cirrhosis, and corticosteroid and estrogen therapy.

Metahydrin has also been found useful in edema due to various forms of renal dysfunction as:

Nephrotic syndrome;
Acute glomerulonephritis; and
Chronic renal failure.

Metahydrin is indicated in the management of hypertension either as the sole therapeutic agent or to enhance the effectiveness of other antihypertensive drugs in the more severe forms of hypertension.

Usage in Pregnancy. The routine use of diuretics in an otherwise healthy woman is inappropriate and exposes mother and fetus to unnecessary hazard. Diuretics do not prevent development of toxemia of pregnancy, and there is no satisfactory evidence that they are useful in the treatment of developed toxemia.

Edema during pregnancy may arise from pathologic causes or from the physiologic and mechanical consequences of pregnancy. Thiazides are indicated in pregnancy when edema is due to pathologic causes, just as they are in the absence of pregnancy. (However, see Warnings, below.) Dependent edema in pregnancy, resulting from restriction of venous return by the expanded uterus, is properly treated through elevation of the lower extremities and use of support hose; use of diuretics to lower intravascular volume in this case is illogical and unnecessary. There is hypervolemia during normal pregnancy, which is harmful to neither the fetus nor the mother (in the absence of cardiovascular disease), but which is associated with edema, including generalized edema, in the majority of pregnant women. If this edema produces discomfort, increased recumbency will often provide relief. In rare instances, this edema may cause extreme discomfort which is not relieved by rest. In these cases, a short course of diuretics may provide relief and may be appropriate.

CONTRAINDICATIONS

Anuria.

Hypersensitivity to this or other sulfonamide-derived drugs.

WARNINGS

Thiazides should be used with caution in severe renal disease. In patients with renal disease, thiazides may precipitate azotemia. Cumulative effects of the drug may develop in patients with impaired renal function.

Thiazides should be used with caution in patients with impaired hepatic function or progressive liver disease, since minor alterations of fluid and electrolyte balance may precipitate hepatic coma.

Thiazides may add to or potentiate the action of other antihypertensive drugs. Potentiation occurs with ganglionic or peripheral adrenergic blocking drugs.

Sensitivity reactions may occur in patients with a history of allergy or bronchial asthma.

The possibility of exacerbation or activation of systemic lupus erythematosus has been reported.

Usage in Pregnancy. Thiazides cross the placental barrier and appear in cord blood. The use of thiazides in pregnant women requires that the anticipated benefit be weighed against possible hazards to the fetus. These hazards include fetal or neonatal jaundice, thrombocytopenia, and possibly other adverse reactions which have occurred in the adult.

Nursing Mothers. Thiazides appear in the breast milk. If use of the drug is deemed essential, the patient should stop nursing.

PRECAUTIONS

Periodic determination of serum electrolytes to detect possible electrolyte imbalance should be performed at appropriate intervals.

All patients receiving thiazide therapy should be observed for clinical signs of fluid or electrolyte imbalance; namely, hyponatremia, hypochloremic alkalosis, and hypokalemia. Serum and urine electrolyte determinations are particularly important when the patient is vomiting excessively or receiving parenteral fluids. Medication such as digitalis may also influence serum electrolytes. Warning signs, irrespective of cause, are: dryness of mouth, thirst, weakness, lethargy, drowsiness, restlessness, muscle pains or cramps, muscular fatigue, hypotension, oliguria, tachycardia, and gastrointestinal disturbances such as nausea and vomiting.

Hypokalemia may develop with thiazides as with any other potent diuretic, especially with brisk diuresis, when severe cirrhosis is present, or during concomitant use of corticosteroids or ACTH.

Interference with adequate oral electrolyte intake will also contribute to hypokalemia. Digitalis therapy may exaggerate metabolic effects of hypokalemia especially with reference to myocardial activity.

Any chloride deficit is generally mild and usually does not require specific treatment except under extraordinary circumstances (as in liver disease or renal disease). Dilutional hyponatremia may occur in edematous patients in hot weather; appropriate therapy is water restriction, rather than administration of salt except in rare instances when the hyponatremia is life threatening. In actual salt depletion, appropriate replacement is the therapy of choice.

Hyperuricemia may occur or frank gout may be precipitated in certain patients receiving thiazide therapy.

Insulin requirements in diabetic patients may be increased, decreased, or unchanged. Latent diabetes mellitus may become manifest during thiazide administration.

Thiazide drugs may increase the responsiveness to tubocurarine.

The antihypertensive effects of the drug may be enhanced in the postsympathectomy patient.

Thiazides may decrease arterial responsiveness to norepinephrine. This diminution is not sufficient to preclude effectiveness of the pressor agent for therapeutic use.

If progressive renal impairment becomes evident, as indicated by a rising nonprotein nitrogen or blood urea nitrogen, a careful reappraisal of therapy is necessary with consideration given to withholding or discontinuing diuretic therapy.

Continued on next page

Merrell Dow—Cont.

Thiazides may decrease serum PBI levels without signs of thyroid disturbance.
This product contains FD&C Yellow No. 5 (tartrazine), which may cause allergic-type reactions (including bronchial asthma) in certain susceptible individuals. Although the overall incidence of FD&C Yellow No. 5 (tartrazine) sensitivity in the general population is low, it is frequently seen in patients who also have aspirin hypersensitivity.

ADVERSE REACTIONS

1. Gastrointestinal System Reactions: anorexia, gastric irritation, nausea, diarrhea, constipation, jaundice (intrahepatic cholestatic jaundice), vomiting, cramping, pancreatitis.
2. Central Nervous System Reactions: dizziness, vertigo, parasthesias, headache, xanthopsia.
3. Hematologic Reactions: leukopenia, agranulocytosis, thrombocytopenia, aplastic anemia.
4. Dermatologic-Hypersensitivity Reactions: purpura, photosensitivity, rash, urticaria, necrotizing angiitis (vasculitis) (cutaneous vasculitis).
5. Cardiovascular Reaction: orthostatic hypotension may occur and may be aggravated by alcohol, barbiturates, or narcotics.
6. Other: hyperglycemia, glycosuria, hyperuricemia, muscle spasm, weakness, restlessness.

Whenever adverse reactions are moderate or severe, Metahydrin dosage should be reduced or therapy withdrawn.

DOSAGE AND ADMINISTRATION

Therapy should be individualized according to patient response. This therapy should be titrated to gain maximal therapeutic response as well as the minimal dose possible to maintain that therapeutic response.
The usual daily doses of Metahydrin for antihypertensive and diuretic effect are as follows:
The usual dose is one 2 mg or 4 mg tablet once daily.
In initiating therapy, these doses may be given twice daily.

HOW SUPPLIED

2 mg pink tablets debossed MERRELL 62: bottles of 100
4 mg aqua blue tablets debossed MERRELL 63: bottles of 100

Product Information as of April, 1985
Shown in Product Identification Section, page 418

METATENSIN® ℞

[*mĕt″ăh-tĕn′sĭn*]
(trichlormethiazide USP and reserpine)

CAUTION: Federal law prohibits dispensing without prescription.

> **WARNING**
> This fixed combination drug is not indicated for initial therapy of hypertension. Hypertension requires therapy titrated to the individual patient. If the fixed combination represents the dosage so determined, its use may be more convenient in patient management. The treatment of hypertension is not static, but must be re-evaluated as conditions in each patient warrant.

DESCRIPTION

Each yellow tablet contains Metahydrin® (trichlormethiazide USP) and reserpine 0.1 mg. The tablet also contains inactive ingredients: corn starch, FD&C Yellow No. 5 (tartrazine, See PRECAUTIONS), lactose, magnesium stearate and pregelatinized corn starch.
Each lavender tablet contains Metahydrin (trichlormethiazide USP) 4 mg and reserpine 0.1 mg. The tablet also contains inactive ingredients: corn starch, D&C Red No. 33, FD&C Blue No. 1, lactose, magnesium stearate, and pregelatinized corn starch.
Metahydrin (trichlormethiazide USP) is an orally effective diuretic and antihypertensive of the thiazide class, differing from other thiazides by the inclusion of a dichloromethyl radical at the 3 position on the benzothiadiazine structure. It has the following formula:

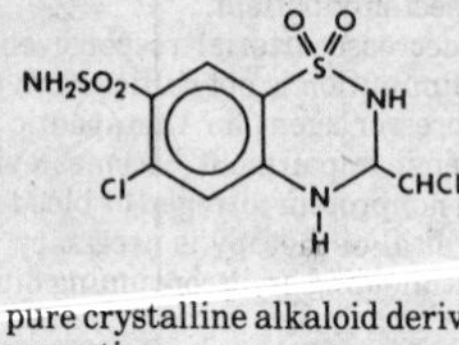

Reserpine is a pure crystalline alkaloid derived from the root of Rauwolfia serpentina.

ACTION

Trichlormethiazide
The mechanism of action results in an interference with the renal tubular mechanism of electrolyte reabsorption. At maximal therapeutic dosage all thiazides are approximately equal in their diuretic potency. The mechanism whereby thiazides function in the control of hypertension is unknown.

Reserpine
Reserpine probably produces its antihypertensive effects through depletion of tissue stores of epinephrine and norepinephrine from peripheral sites. By contrast, its sedative and tranquilizing properties are thought to be related to depletion of 5-hydroxytryptamine from the brain.
Reserpine is characterized by slow onset of action and sustained effect. Both its cardiovascular and central nervous system effects may persist following withdrawal of the drug.

INDICATIONS

Hypertension (See box Warning.)
Usage in Pregnancy. The routine use of diuretics in an otherwise healthy woman is inappropriate and exposes mother and fetus to unnecessary hazard. Diuretics do not prevent development of toxemia of pregnancy, and there is no satisfactory evidence that they are useful in the treatment of developed toxemia.
Edema during pregnancy may arise from pathologic causes or from the physiologic and mechanical consequences of pregnancy. Thiazides are indicated in pregnancy when edema is due to pathologic causes, just as they are in the absence of pregnancy. (However, see Warnings, below.) Dependent edema in pregnancy, resulting from restriction of venous return by the expanded uterus, is properly treated through elevation of the lower extremities and use of support hose; use of diuretics to lower intravascular volume in this case is illogical and unnecessary. There is hypervolemia during normal pregnancy, which is harmful to neither the fetus nor the mother (in the absence of cardiovascular disease), but which is associated with edema, including generalized edema, in the majority of pregnant women. If this edema produces discomfort, increased recumbency will often provide relief. In rare instances, this edema may cause extreme discomfort which is not relieved by rest. In these cases, a short course of diuretics may provide relief and may be appropriate.

CONTRAINDICATIONS

Trichlormethiazide
Trichlormethiazide is contraindicated in patients with anuria and in patients known to be hypersensitive to this or other sulfonamide derived drugs.

Reserpine
Hypersensitivity, mental depression especially with suicidal tendencies, active peptic ulcer and ulcerative colitis.

WARNINGS

Trichlormethiazide
Use with caution in severe renal disease. In patients with renal disease, thiazides may precipitate azotemia. Cumulative effects of the drug may develop in patients with impaired renal function.
Thiazides should be used with caution in patients with impaired hepatic function or progressive liver disease, since minor alterations of fluid and electrolyte balance may precipitate hepatic coma.
Thiazides may add to or potentiate the action of other antihypertensive drugs. Potentiation occurs with ganglionic or peripheral adrenergic blocking drugs. Sensitivity reactions may occur in patients with a history of allergy or bronchial asthma. Exacerbation or activation of systemic lupus erythematosis has been reported.

Reserpine
As suicide is always a possible result of mental depression, discontinue treatment if mood depression develops.
Reserpine may induce peptic ulceration; discontinue use if peptic ulcer develops.
Electroshock therapy should not be given to patients taking reserpine, since severe and even fatal reactions have been reported. The drug should be discontinued for two weeks before giving electroshock therapy.
MAO inhibitors should be avoided or used with extreme caution.
Usage in Pregnancy. Trichlormethiazide: Thiazides cross the placental barrier and appear in cord blood. The use of thiazides in pregnant women requires that the anticipated benefit be weighed against possible hazards to the fetus. These hazards include fetal or neonatal jaundice, thrombocytopenia, and possibly other adverse reactions which have occurred in the adult.
Reserpine: The safety of reserpine for use during pregnancy or lactation has not been established; therefore, the drug should be used in pregnant patients or in women of childbearing potential only when, in the judgment of the physician, it is essential to the welfare of the patient.
Increased respiratory secretions, nasal congestion, cyanosis, and anorexia may occur in infants born to reserpine-treated mothers, since reserpine crosses the placental barrier and appears in maternal breast milk.
Nursing Mothers. Thiazides and reserpine appear in breast milk. If use of Metatensin is deemed essential, the patient should stop nursing.

PRECAUTIONS

The #2 tablet contains FD&C Yellow No. 5 (tartrazine), which may cause allergic-type reactions (including bronchial asthma) in certain susceptible individuals. Although the overall incidence of FD&C Yellow No. 5 (tartrazine) sensitivity in the general population is low, it is frequently seen in patients who also have aspirin hypersensitivity.

Trichlormethiazide
Periodic determinations of serum electrolytes to detect possible electrolyte imbalance should be performed at appropriate intervals.
All patients receiving thiazide therapy should be observed for clinical signs of fluid or electrolyte imbalance; namely, hyponatremia, hypochloremic alkalosis, and hypokalemia. Serum and urine electrolyte determinations are particularly important when the patient is vomiting excessively or receiving parenteral fluids.
Medication such as digitalis may also influence serum electrolytes. Warning signs, irrespective of cause, are: dryness of mouth, thirst, weakness, lethargy, drowsiness, restlessness, muscle pains or cramps, muscular fatigue, hypotension, oliguria, tachycardia, and gastrointestinal disturbances such as nausea and vomiting.
Hypokalemia may develop with thiazides as with any other potent diuretic, especially with brisk diuresis, when severe cirrhosis is present, or during concomitant use of corticosteroids or ACTH.
Interference with adequate oral electrolyte intake will also contribute to hypokalemia. Digitalis therapy may exaggerate metabolic effects of hypokalemia especially with reference to myocardial activity.
Any chloride deficit is generally mild and usually does not require specific treatment except under extraordinary circumstances (as in liver disease or renal disease). Dilutional hyponatremia may occur in edematous patients in hot weather; appropriate therapy is water restriction, rather than administration of salt except in rare instances when the hyponatremia is life threatening. In actual salt depletion, appropriate replacement is the therapy of choice.
Hyperuricemia may occur or frank gout may be precipitated in certain patients receiving thiazide therapy.
Insulin requirements in diabetic patients may be increased, decreased, or unchanged. Latent diabetes mellitus may become manifest during thiazide administration.
Thiazide drugs may increase the responsiveness to tubocurarine.
The antihypertensive effects of the drug may be enhanced in the postsympathectomy patient.
Thiazides may decrease arterial responsiveness to norepinephrine. This diminution is not sufficient to preclude effectiveness of the pressor agent for therapeutic use.
If progressive renal impairment becomes evident, as indicated by a rising non-protein nitrogen or blood urea nitrogen, a careful reappraisal of therapy is necessary with consideration given to withholding or discontinuing diuretic therapy.
Thiazides may decrease serum PBI levels without signs of thyroid disturbance.

Reserpine
Caution should be used in treating hypertensive patients with renal insufficiency.
Cardiac arrhythmias have occurred in patients receiving digitalis and quinidine with reserpine.
Reserpine potentiates many anesthetic agents; hypotension and bradycardia have been noted during anesthesia. In addition, a relative sensitivity to norepinephrine or other pressor agents may exist due to the previous action of reserpine; thus usual amounts of the pressor agent may be excessive.
Use with caution in patients with a previous history of depression, peptic ulcer or other gastrointestinal disorders and in hypertensive patients with functionally severe coronary artery disease.
Animal tumorigenicity. Rodent studies have shown that reserpine is an animal tumorigen, causing an increased incidence of mammary fibroadenomas in female mice, malignant tumors of the seminal vesicles in male mice, and malignant adrenal medullary tumors in male rats. These findings arose in 2-year studies in which the drug was administered in the feed at concentrations of 5 and 10 ppm—about 100 to 300 times the usual human dose. The breast neoplasms are thought to be related to reserpine's prolactin-elevating effect. Several other prolactin-elevating drugs have also been associated with an increased incidence of mammary neoplasia in rodents.
The extent to which these findings indicate a risk to humans is uncertain. Tissue culture experiments show that about one-third of human breast tumors are prolactin-dependent in vitro, a factor of considerable importance if the use of the drug is contemplated in a patient with previously detected breast cancer. The possibility of an increased risk of breast cancer in reserpine users has been studied extensively; however, no firm conclusion has emerged. Although a few epidemiologic studies have suggested a slightly increased risk (less than twofold in all studies except one) in women who have used reserpine, other studies of generally similar design

have not confirmed this. Epidemiologic studies conducted using other drugs (neuroleptic agents) that, like reserpine, increase prolactin levels and therefore would be considered rodent mammary carcinogens, have not shown an association between chronic administration of the drug and human mammary tumorigenesis. While long-term clinical observation has not suggested such an association, the available evidence is considered too limited to be conclusive at this time. An association of reserpine intake with pheochromocytoma or tumors of the seminal vesicles has not been explored.

ADVERSE REACTIONS

Trichlormethiazide

1. Gastrointestinal System Reactions: anorexia, gastric irritation, nausea, diarrhea, constipation, jaundice (intrahepatic cholestatic jaundice), vomiting, cramping, pancreatitis.
2. Central Nervous System Reactions: dizziness, vertigo, paresthesias, headache, xanthopsia.
3. Hematologic Reactions: leukopenia, agranulocytosis, thrombocytopenia, aplastic anemia.
4. Dermatologic-Hypersensitivity Reactions: purpura, photosensitivity, rash, urticaria, necrotizing angiitis (vasculitis) (cutaneous vasculitis).
5. Cardiovascular Reaction: orthostatic hypotension may occur and may be aggravated by alcohol, barbiturates, or narcotics.
6. Other: hyperglycemia, glycosuria, hyperuricemia, muscle spasm, weakness, restlessness.

Reserpine

Gastric hypersecretion; vomiting; nervousness; paradoxical anxiety, CNS sensitization manifested by deafness, glaucoma, uveitis, and optic atrophy; purpura; nasal stuffiness; loose stools; reversible parkinsonism; muscular fatigue and weakness; and nightmares. Mental depression, particularly when doses of reserpine of over 1.0 mg daily are used, has been reported. Other side effects of reserpine reported include anorexia, nausea, dizziness, headaches, impotence, flushing of the skin, dryness of the mouth, biliary colic, blurring of vision, muscular aches and pruritus. Hypotension, including the orthostatic variety, may occur in some patients. Angina pectoris, arrhythmias and congestive heart failure have also been reported but are uncommon.

After the onset of therapy with reserpine, a turbulent phase of short duration may occur. Very rare additional adverse effects that have been observed in association with reserpine therapy include epistaxis, skin eruptions and edema due to sodium retention. Bradycardia may occur as an exaggerated response related to the pharmacodynamic effect of reserpine.

DOSAGE

As determined by individual titration. (See box Warning.)

In the stabilized hypertensive patient, administration may be continued on a once-daily basis administered in the morning. The maximum single effective dose of Metatensin is 8 mg (in some patients 4 mg). Doses in excess of 8 mg normally will not produce any increase in sodium and water excretion and in refractory patients may increase excretion of potassium.

HOW SUPPLIED

Metatensin #2
(trichlormethiazide 2.0 mg and reserpine 0.1 mg)
Bottles of 100 yellow tablets debossed MERRELL 64

Metatensin #4
(trichlormethiazide 4.0 mg and reserpine 0.1 mg)
Bottles of 100 and 1000 lavender tablets debossed MERRELL 65

Product Information as of April, 1985
Shown in Product Identification Section, page 418

NORPRAMIN® ℞

[nŏr'prăm-ĭn]
(desipramine hydrochloride tablets USP)

CAUTION: Federal law prohibits dispensing without prescription.

DESCRIPTION

Norpramin (desipramine hydrochloride USP) is an antidepressant drug of the tricyclic type, and is chemically: 5*H*-Dibenz[*b,f*] azepine-5-propanamine, 10, 11-dihydro-N-methyl-, monohydrochloride.

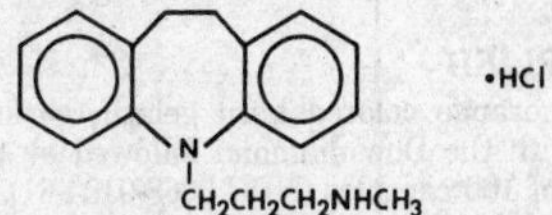

INACTIVE INGREDIENTS

The following inactive ingredients are contained in all dosage strengths: acacia, calcium carbonate, corn starch, FD&C Blue No. 1, FD&C Red No. 3, FD&C Yellow No. 6, hydrogenated soy oil, iron oxide, light mineral oil, magnesium stearate, mannitol, polyethylene glycol 8000, pregelatinized corn starch, sodium benzoate (except 150 mg), sucrose, talc, titanium dioxide and other ingredients. In addition, Norpramin 25, 50, 75, and 100 mg tablets contain FD&C Yellow No. 5 (tartrazine) (SEE PRECAUTIONS).

CLINICAL PHARMACOLOGY

Mechanism of Action

Available evidence suggests that many depressions have a biochemical basis in the form of a relative deficiency of neurotransmitters such as norepinephrine and serotonin. Norepinephrine deficiency may be associated with relatively low urinary 3-methoxy-4-hydroxyphenyl glycol (MHPG) levels, while serotonin deficiencies may be associated with low spinal fluid levels of 5-hydroxyindolacetic acid.

While the precise mechanism of action of the tricyclic antidepressants is unknown, a leading theory suggests that they restore normal levels of neurotransmitters by blocking the re-uptake of these substances from the synapse in the central nervous system. Evidence indicates that the secondary amine tricyclic antidepressants, including Norpramin, may have greater activity in blocking the re-uptake of norepinephrine. Tertiary amine tricyclic antidepressants, such as amitriptyline, may have greater effect on serotonin re-uptake.

Norpramin (desipramine hydrochloride) is not a monoamine oxidase (MAO) inhibitor and does not act primarily as a central nervous system stimulant. It has been found in some studies to have a more rapid onset of action than imipramine. Earliest therapeutic effects may occasionally be seen in 2 to 5 days, but full treatment benefit usually requires 2 to 3 weeks to obtain.

Metabolism

Tricyclic antidepressants, such as desipramine hydrochloride, are rapidly absorbed from the gastrointestinal tract. Tricyclic antidepressants or their metabolites are to some extent excreted through the gastric mucosa and re-absorbed from the gastrointestinal tract. Desipramine is metabolized in the liver and approximately 70% is excreted in the urine.

The rate of metabolism of tricyclic antidepressants varies widely from individual to individual, chiefly on a genetically determined basis. Up to a thirty-sixfold difference in plasma level may be noted among individuals taking the same oral dose of desipramine. In general, the elderly metabolize tricyclic antidepressants more slowly than do younger adults.

Certain drugs, particularly the psychostimulants and the phenothiazines, increase plasma levels of concomitantly administered tricyclic antidepressants through competition for the same metabolic enzyme systems. Concurrent administration of cimetidine and tricyclic antidepressants can produce clinically significant increases in the plasma concentrations of the tricyclic antidepressants. Conversely, decreases in plasma levels of the tricyclic antidepressants have been reported upon discontinuation of cimetidine which may result in the loss of the therapeutic efficacy of the tricyclic antidepressant. Other substances, particularly barbiturates and alcohol, induce liver enzyme activity and thereby reduce tricyclic antidepressant plasma levels. Similar effects have been reported with tobacco smoke.

Research on the relationship of plasma level to therapeutic response with the tricyclic antidepressants has produced conflicting results. While some studies report no correlation, many studies cite therapeutic levels for most tricyclics in the range of 50 to 300 nanograms per milliliter. The therapeutic range is different for each tricyclic antidepressant. For desipramine, an optimal range of therapeutic plasma levels has not been established.

INDICATIONS

Norpramin (desipramine hydrochloride) is indicated for relief of symptoms in various depressive syndromes, especially endogenous depression.

CONTRAINDICATIONS

Desipramine hydrochloride should not be given in conjunction with, or within 2 weeks of, treatment with an MAO inhibitor drug; hyperpyretic crises, severe convulsions, and death have occurred in patients taking MAO inhibitors and tricyclic antidepressants. When Norpramin (desipramine hydrochloride) is substituted for an MAO inhibitor, at least 2 weeks should elapse between treatments. Norpramin should then be started cautiously and should be increased gradually.

The drug is contraindicated in the acute recovery period following myocardial infarction. It should not be used in those who have shown prior hypersensitivity to the drug. Cross sensitivity between this and other dibenzazepines is a possibility.

WARNINGS

1. Extreme caution should be used when this drug is given in the following situations:

a. In patients with cardiovascular disease, because of the possibility of conduction defects, arrhythmias, tachycardias, strokes, and acute myocardial infarction.

b. In patients with a history of urinary retention or glaucoma, because of the anticholinergic properties of the drug.

c. In patients with thyroid disease or those taking thyroid medication, because of the possibility of cardiovascular toxicity, including arrhythmias.

d. In patients with a history of seizure disorder, because this drug has been shown to lower the seizure threshold.

2. This drug is capable of blocking the antihypertensive effect of guanethidine and similarly acting compounds.
3. USE IN PREGNANCY
Safe use of desipramine hydrochloride during pregnancy and lactation has not been established; therefore, if it is to be given to pregnant patients, nursing mothers, or women of childbearing potential, the possible benefits must be weighed against the possible hazards to mother and child. Animal reproductive studies have been inconclusive.
4. USE IN CHILDREN
Norpramin (desipramine hydrochloride) is not recommended for use in children since safety and effectiveness in the pediatric age group have not been established.
5. The patient should be cautioned that this drug may impair the mental and/or physical abilities required for the performance of potentially hazardous tasks such as driving a car or operating machinery.
6. In patients who may use alcohol excessively, it should be borne in mind that the potentiation may increase the danger inherent in any suicide attempt or overdosage.

PRECAUTIONS

1. It is important that this drug be dispensed in the least possible quantities to depressed outpatients, since suicide has been accomplished with this class of drug. Ordinary prudence requires that children not have access to this drug or to potent drugs of any kind; if possible this drug should be dispensed in containers with child-resistant safety closures. Storage of this drug in the home must be supervised responsibly.
2. If serious adverse effects occur, dosage should be reduced or treatment should be altered.
3. Norpramin (desipramine hydrochloride) therapy in patients with manic-depressive illness may induce a hypomanic state after the depressive phase terminates.
4. The drug may cause exacerbation of psychosis in schizophrenic patients.
5. Close supervision and careful adjustment of dosage are required when this drug is given concomitantly with anticholinergic or sympathomimetic drugs.
6. Patients should be warned that while taking this drug their reponse to alcoholic beverages may be exaggerated.
7. Clinical experience in the concurrent administration of ECT and antidepressant drugs is limited. Thus, if such treatment is essential, the possibility of increased risk relative to benefits should be considered.
8. If Norpramin (desipramine hydrochloride) is to be combined with other psychotropic agents such as tranquilizers or sedative/hypnotics, careful consideration should be given to the pharmacology of the agents employed since the sedative effects of Norpramin and benzodiazepines (e.g., chlordiazepoxide or diazepam) are additive. Both the sedative and anticholinergic effects of the major tranquilizers are also additive to those of Norpramin.
9. Concurrent administration of cimetidine and tricyclic antidepressants can produce clinically significant increases in the plasma levels of the tricyclic antidepressants (see CLINICAL PHARMACOLOGY, *Metabolism*). Conversely, decreases in plasma levels of the tricyclic antidepressants have been reported upon discontinuation of cimetidine which may result in the loss of the therapeutic efficacy of the tricyclic antidepressant.
10. This drug should be discontinued as soon as possible prior to elective surgery because of the possible cardiovascular effects. Hypertensive episodes have been observed during surgery in patients taking desipramine hydrochloride.
11. Both elevation and lowering of blood sugar levels have been reported.
12. Leukocyte and differential counts should be performed in any patient who develops fever and sore throat during therapy; the drug should be discontinued if there is evidence of pathologic neutrophil depression.
13. Norpramin 25, 50, 75, and 100 mg tablets contain FD&C Yellow No. 5 (tartrazine), which may cause allergic-type reactions (including bronchial asthma) in certain susceptible individuals. Although the overall incidence of FD&C Yellow No. 5 (tartrazine) sensitivity in the general population is low, it is frequently seen in patients who also have aspirin hypersensitivity.

Continued on next page

Information on Merrell Dow products is based on labeling in effect in May, 1986.

Merrell Dow—Cont.

ADVERSE REACTIONS

Note: Included in the following listing are a few adverse reactions that have not been reported with this specific drug. However, the pharmacologic similarities among the tricyclic antidepressant drugs require that each of the reactions be considered when Norpramin (desipramine hydrochloride) is given.

Cardiovascular: hypotension, hypertension, tachycardia, palpitation, arrhythmias, heart block, myocardial infarction, stroke.

Psychiatric: confusional states (especially in the elderly) with hallucinations, disorientation, delusions; anxiety, restlessness, agitation; insomnia and nightmares; hypomania; exacerbation of psychosis.

Neurologic: numbness, tingling, paresthesias of extremities; incoordination, ataxia, tremors; peripheral neuropathy; extrapyramidal symptoms; seizures; alteration in EEG patterns; tinnitus.

Anticholinergic: dry mouth, and rarely associated sublingual adenitis; blurred vision, disturbance of accommodation, mydriasis, increased intraocular pressure; constipation, paralytic ileus; urinary retention, delayed micturition, dilatation of urinary tract.

Allergic: skin rash, petechiae, urticaria, itching, photosensitization (avoid excessive exposure to sunlight), edema (of face and tongue or general), drug fever, cross sensitivity with other tricyclic drugs.

Hematologic: Bone marrow depressions including agranulocytosis, eosinophilia, purpura, thrombocytopenia.

Gastrointestinal: anorexia, nausea and vomiting, epigastric distress, peculiar taste, abdominal cramps, diarrhea, stomatitis, black tongue.

Endocrine: gynecomastia in the male, breast enlargement and galactorrhea in the female; increased or decreased libido, impotence, testicular swelling; elevation or depression of blood sugar levels; syndrome of inappropriate antidiuretic hormone secretion (SIADH).

Other: jaundice (simulating obstructive), altered liver function; weight gain or loss; perspiration, flushing; urinary frequency, nocturia; parotid swelling; drowsiness, dizziness, weakness and fatigue, headache; alopecia.

Withdrawal Symptoms: Though not indicative of addiction, abrupt cessation of treatment after prolonged therapy may produce nausea, headache, and malaise.

DOSAGE AND ADMINISTRATION

Not recommended for use in children.

Lower dosages are recommended for elderly patients and adolescents. Lower dosages are also recommended for outpatients compared to hospitalized patients, who are closely supervised. Dosage should be initiated at a low level and increased according to clinical response and any evidence of intolerance. Following remission, maintenance medication may be required for a period of time and should be at the lowest dose that will maintain remission.

Usual Adult Dose:

The usual adult dose is 100 to 200 mg per day. In more severely ill patients, dosage may be further increased gradually to 300 mg/day if necessary. Dosages above 300 mg/day are not recommended.

Dosage should be initiated at a lower level and increased according to tolerance and clinical response.

Treatment of patients requiring as much as 300 mg should generally be initiated in hospitals, where regular visits by the physician, skilled nursing care, and frequent electrocardiograms (ECG's) are available.

The best available evidence of impending toxicity from very high doses of Norpramin is prolongation of the QRS or QT intervals on the ECG. Prolongation of the PR interval is also significant, but less closely correlated with plasma levels. Clinical symptoms of intolerance, especially drowsiness, dizziness, and postural hypotension, should also alert the physician to the need for reduction in dosage. Plasma desipramine measurement would constitute the optimal guide to dosage monitoring.

Initial therapy may be administered in divided doses or a single daily dose.

Maintenance therapy may be given on a once-daily schedule for patient convenience and compliance.

Adolescent and Geriatric Dose:

The usual adolescent and geriatric dose is 25 to 100 mg daily. Dosage should be initiated at a lower level and increased according to tolerance and clinical response to a usual maximum of 100 mg daily. In more severely ill patients, dosage may be further increased to 150 mg/day. Doses above 150 mg/day are not recommended in these age groups.

Initial therapy may be administered in divided doses or a single daily dose.

Maintenance therapy may be given on a once-daily schedule for patient convenience and compliance.

OVERDOSAGE

There is no specific antidote for desipramine, nor are there specific phenomena of diagnostic value characterizing poisoning by the drug.

Within an hour of ingestion the patient may become agitated or stuporous and then comatose. Hypotension, shock, and renal shutdown may ensue. Grand mal seizures, both early and late after ingestion, have been reported. Hyperactive reflexes, hyperpyrexia, muscle rigidity, vomiting, and ECG evidence of impaired conduction may occur. Serious disturbances of cardiac rate, rhythm, and output can occur. The precepts of early evacuation of the ingested material and subsequent support of respiration (airway and movement), circulation, and renal output apply.

The principles of management of coma and shock by means of the mechanical respirator, cardiac pacemaker, monitoring of central venous pressure, and regulation of fluid and acid-base balance are well known in most medical centers and are not further discussed here.

Because CNS involvement, respiratory depression, and cardiac arrhythmia can occur suddenly, hospitalization and close observation are generally advisable, even when the amount ingested is thought to be small or the initial degree of intoxication appears slight or moderate. Most patients with ECG abnormalities should have continuous cardiac monitoring for at least 72 hours and be closely observed until well after cardiac status has returned to normal; relapses may occur after apparent recovery.

The slow intravenous administration of physostigmine salicylate has been reported to reverse most of the anticholinergic cardiovascular and CNS effects of overdose with tricyclic antidepressants. In adults, 1 to 3 mg has been reported to be effective. In children, the dose should be started with 0.5 mg and repeated at 5-minute intervals to determine the minimum effective dose; no more than 2 mg. should be given. Because of the short duration of action of physostigmine, the effective dose should be repeated at 30-minute to 60-minute intervals, as necessary. Rapid injection should be avoided to reduce the possibility of physostigmine-induced convulsions.

Other possible therapeutic considerations include:

(a) Dialysis: Desipramine is found in low concentration in the serum, even after a massive oral dose. *In vitro* experiments in which blood bank blood was used indicate that it is very poorly dialyzed. Because of indications that the drug is secreted in gastric juice, constant gastric lavage has been suggested.

(b) Pharmacologic treatment of shock: Since desipramine potentiates the action of such vasopressor agents as levarterenol and metaraminol, they should be used only with caution.

(c) Pharmacologic control of seizures: Intravenous barbiturates are the treatment of choice for the control of grand mal seizures. One may, alternately, consider the parenteral use of diphenylhydantoin, which has less central depressant effect but also has an effect on heart rhythm that has not yet been fully defined.

(d) Pharmacologic control of cardiac function: Severe disturbances of cardiac rate, rhythm, and output are probably the initiating events in shock. Intravascular volume must be maintained by i.v. fluids. Digitalization should be carried out early in view of the fact that a positive inotropic effect can be achieved without increase in cardiac work. Many of the cardiodynamic effects of digitalis are the exact opposite of those of massive doses of desipramine (animal studies).

HOW SUPPLIED

10 mg blue coated tablets imprinted 68-7
NDC 0068-0007-01: bottles of 100

25 mg yellow coated tablets imprinted MERRELL 11 or NORPRAMIN 25
NDC 0068-0011-01: bottles of 100
NDC 0068-0011-61: unit dose dispenser of 100
NDC 0068-0011-10: bottles of 1000

50 mg green coated tablets imprinted MERRELL 15 or NORPRAMIN 50
NDC 0068-0015-01: bottles of 100
NDC 0068-0015-61: unit dose dispenser of 100
NDC 0068-0015-10: bottles of 1000

75 mg orange coated tablets imprinted MERRELL 19 or NORPRAMIN 75
NDC 0068-0019-01: bottles of 100

100 mg peach coated tablets imprinted MERRELL 20 or NORPRAMIN 100
NDC 0068-0020-01: bottles of 100

150 mg white coated tablets imprinted MERRELL 21 or NORPRAMIN 150
NDC 0068-0021-50: bottles of 50

Norpramin tablets should be stored at room temperature, preferably below 86°F (30°C). Protect from excessive heat.

U.S. Patent Numbers 3,454,554 and 3,454,698

Product Information as of January, 1985

Shown in Product Identification Section, page 418

NOVAFED® Capsules ℞

[*nō 'vă-fĕd*]

pseudoephedrine hydrochloride

Controlled-Release Decongestant

CAUTION: Federal law prohibits dispensing without prescription.

DESCRIPTION

Each Novafed capsule contains 120 mg of pseudoephedrine hydrochloride in specially formulated pellets designed to provide continuous therapeutic effect for 12 hours. About one-half of the active ingredient is released soon after administration and the rest slowly over the remaining time period. Each capsule also contains as inactive ingredients; corn starch, FD&C Blue No. 1, FD&C Red No. 3, FD&C Yellow No. 6, gelatin, sucrose, titanium dioxide, and other ingredients.

ACTIONS

Pseudoephedrine (a sympathomimetic) is an orally effective nasal decongestant with peripheral effects similar to epinephrine and central effects similar to, but less intense than, amphetamines. It has the potential for excitatory side effects. At the recommended oral dosage, it has little or no pressor effect in normotensive adults. Patients have not been reported to experience the rebound congestion sometimes experienced with frequent, repeated use of topical decongestants.

INDICATIONS

Relief of nasal congestion or eustachian tube congestion. May be given concomitantly with analgesics, antihistamines, expectorants and antibiotics.

CONTRAINDICATIONS

Patients with severe hypertension, severe coronary artery disease, and patients on MAO inhibitor therapy. Also contraindicated in patients with hypersensitivity or idiosyncrasy to sympathomimetic amines which may be manifested by insomnia, dizziness, weakness, tremor or arrhythmias.

Children under 12: Should not be used by children under 12 years.

Nursing Mothers: Contraindicated because of the higher than usual risk for infants from sympathomimetic amines.

WARNINGS

Use judiciously and sparingly in patients with hypertension, diabetes mellitus, ischemic heart disease, increased intraocular pressure, hyperthyroidism or prostatic hypertrophy. See, however, Contraindications. Sympathomimetics may produce central nervous stimulation with convulsions or cardiovascular collapse with accompanying hypotension.

Do not exceed recommended dosage.

Use in Pregnancy: Safety in pregnancy has not been established.

Use in Elderly: The elderly (60 years and older) are more likely to have adverse reactions to sympathomimetics. Overdosage of sympathomimetics in this age group may cause hallucinations, convulsions, CNS depression, and death. Safe use of a short-acting sympathomimetic should be demonstrated in the individual elderly patient before considering the use of a sustained-action formulation.

PRECAUTIONS

Patients with diabetes, hypertension, cardiovascular disease and hyper-reactivity to ephedrine.

ADVERSE REACTIONS

Hyper-reactive individuals may display ephedrine-like reactions such as tachycardia, palpitations, headache, dizziness or nausea. Sympathomimetics have been associated with certain untoward reactions including fear, anxiety, tenseness, restlessness, tremor, weakness, pallor, respiratory difficulty, dysuria, insomnia, hallucinations, convulsions, CNS depression, arrhythmias, and cardiovascular collapse with hypotension.

DRUG INTERACTIONS

MAO inhibitors and beta adrenergic blockers increase the effects of pseudoephedrine. Sympathomimetics may reduce the antihypertensive effects of methyldopa, mecamylamine, reserpine and veratrum alkaloids.

DOSAGE AND ADMINISTRATION

One capsule every 12 hours. Do not give to children under 12 years of age.

HOW SUPPLIED

Brown and orange colored hard gelatin capsules, monogrammed with the Dow diamond followed by the number 104. Bottle of 100 capsules (NDC 0068-0104-61).

Product Information as of April, 1985

Manufactured by KV Pharmaceutical Company, St. Louis, MO 63144 for
MERRELL DOW PHARMACEUTICALS INC.
Subsidiary of The Dow Chemical Company
Cincinnati, Ohio 45215, U.S.A.

Shown in Product Identification Section, page 418

NOVAFED® A CAPSULES ℞

[nō′vă-fĕd]

Controlled-Release

Decongestant plus Antihistamine

CAUTION: Federal law prohibits dispensing without prescription.

DESCRIPTION

Each NOVAFED A capsule for oral use contains 120 mg pseudoephedrine hydrochloride, and 8 mg of chlorpheniramine maleate. The specially formulated pellets in each capsule are designed to provide continuous therapeutic effect for about 12 hours. About one-half of the active ingredients is released soon after administration and the remainder is released slowly over the remaining time period.

Each capsule also contains as inactive ingredients: calcium stearate, corn starch, FD&C Blue No. 1, FD&C Red No. 3, FD&C Yellow No. 6, gelatin, povidone, shellac, sucrose, talc, titanium dioxide and other ingredients.

Pseudoephedrine hydrochloride is a nasal decongestant. Chemically it is α-[1-(methyl-amino)ethyl]-[*S*-(*R**,*R**)]-benzenemethanol hydrochloride.

Chlorpheniramine maleate is an antihistamine. Chemically it is α-(4-chlorophenyl)-N,N-dimethyl-2-pyridinepropanamine.

CLINICAL PHARMACOLOGY

Pseudoephedrine is an orally active sympathomimetic amine and exerts a decongestant action on the nasal mucosa. Pseudoephedrine produces peripheral effects similar to those of ephedrine and central effects similar to, but less intense than amphetamines. It has the potential for excitatory side effects. At the recommended oral dosages it has little or no pressor effect in normotensive adults. The serum half-life (T-½) of pseudoephedrine is approximately 4 to 6 hours. T-½ is decreased with increased excretion of drug at urine pH lower than 6 and may be increased with decreased excretion at urine pH higher than 8.

Chlorpheniramine is an antihistaminic that possesses anticholinergic and sedative effects. It is considered one of the most effective and least toxic of the histamine antagonists. Chlorpheniramine is an H_1 receptor antagonist. It antagonizes many of the pharmacologic actions of histamine. It prevents released histamine from dilating capillaries and causing edema of the respiratory mucosa. Chlorpheniramine has a duration of action of 4 to 6 hours in clinical studies. Its half-life in serum, however, is 12 to 16 hours.

INDICATIONS AND USAGE

Relief of nasal congestion and eustachian tube congestion associated with the common cold, sinusitis and acute upper respiratory infections. It is also indicated for symptomatic relief of perennial and seasonal allergic rhinitis, vasomotor rhinitis, allergic conjunctivitis due to inhalant allergens and foods and mild, uncomplicated allergic skin manifestations of urticaria and angioedema. Decongestants in combination with antihistamines have been used for many years to relieve eustachian tube congestion associated with acute eustachian salpingitis, aerotitis media, acute otitis media and serous otitis media. May be given concomitantly with analgesics and antibiotics.

CONTRAINDICATIONS

Patients with severe hypertension, severe coronary artery disease, and in patients on MAO inhibitor therapy. Antihistamines are contraindicated in patients with narrow-angle glaucoma, urinary retention, peptic ulcer, during an asthmatic attack, and in patients receiving MAO inhibitors.

Hypersensitivity: Contraindicated in patients with hypersensitivity or idiosyncrasy to sympathomimetic amines or phenanthrene derivatives.

Nursing Mothers: Contraindicated because of the higher than usual risk for infants from sympathomimetic amines.

WARNINGS

Sympathomimetic amines should be used judiciously and sparingly in patients with hypertension, diabetes mellitus, ischemic heart disease, increased intraocular pressure, hyperthyroidism or prostatic hypertrophy (see CONTRAINDICATIONS). Sympathomimetics may produce CNS stimulation with convulsions or cardiovascular collapse with accompanying hypotension.

Chlorpheniramine maleate has an atropine-like action and should be used with caution in patients with increased intraocular pressure, cardiovascular disease, hypertension or in patients with a history of bronchial asthma (see CONTRAINDICATIONS). Do not exceed recommended dose.

Use in Elderly: The elderly (60 years and older) are more likely to have adverse reactions to sympathomimetics. Overdosage of sympathomimetics in this age group may cause hallucinations, convulsions, CNS depression and death.

PRECAUTIONS

General: Should be used with caution in patients with diabetes, hypertension, cardiovascular disease and hyperreactivity to ephedrine. The antihistaminic may cause drowsiness and ambulatory patients who operate machinery or motor vehicles should be cautioned accordingly.

Information for Patients: Antihistamines may impair mental and physical abilities required for the performance of potentially hazardous tasks, such as driving a vehicle or operating machinery, and mental alertness in children.

Drug Interactions: MAO inhibitors and beta adrenergic blockers increase the effect of sympathomimetics. Sympathomimetics may reduce the antihypertensive effects of methyldopa, mecamylamine, reserpine and veratrum alkaloids. Concomitant use of antihistamines with alcohol, tricyclic antidepressants, barbiturates and other CNS depressants may have an additive effect.

Pregnancy Category C: Animal reproduction studies have not been conducted with NOVAFED A capsules. It is also not known whether NOVAFED A capsules can cause fetal harm when administered to a pregnant woman or can affect reproduction capacity. NOVAFED A capsules may be given to a pregnant woman only if clearly needed.

Nursing Mothers: Pseudoephedrine is contraindicated in nursing mothers because of the higher than usual risk for infants from sympathomimetic amines.

ADVERSE REACTIONS

Hyperreactive individuals may display ephedrine-like reactions such as tachycardia, palpitations, headache, dizziness, or nausea. Patients sensitive to antihistamines may experience mild sedation. Sympathomimetic drugs have been associated with certain untoward reactions including fear, anxiety, tenseness, restlessness, tremor, weakness, pallor, respiratory difficulty, dysuria, insomnia, hallucinations, convulsions, CNS depression, arrhythmias, and cardiovascular collapse with hypotension.

Possible side effects of antihistamines are drowsiness, restlessness, dizziness, weakness, dry mouth, anorexia, nausea, headache, nervousness, blurring of vision , heartburn, dysuria and very rarely dermatitis. Patient idiosyncrasy to adrenergic agents may be manifested by insomnia, dizziness, weakness, tremor, or arrhythmias.

OVERDOSAGE

Acute overdosage with NOVAFED A capsules may produce clinical signs of CNS stimulation and variable cardiovascular effects. Pressor amines should be used with great caution in the presence of pseudoephedrine. Patients with signs of stimulation should be treated conservatively.

DOSAGE AND ADMINISTRATION

One capsule every 12 hours. Do not give to children under 12 years of age.

CAUTION

Federal law prohibits dispensing without prescription.

HOW SUPPLIED

NOVAFED A is supplied in red and orange colored hard gelatin capsules monogrammed with the Dow diamond followed by the number 106, or NOVAFED A in bottles of 100 capsules (NDC 0068-0106-61).

Product Information as of April, 1985

Manufactured by KV Pharmaceutical Company, St. Louis, MO 63144 for

MERRELL DOW PHARMACEUTICALS INC.

Subsidiary of The Dow Chemical Company

Cincinnati, Ohio 45215, U.S.A.

Shown in Product Identification Section, page 418

QUINAMM™ 260 mg

(quinine sulfate tablets)

CAUTION: Federal law prohibits dispensing without prescription.

DESCRIPTION

Quinamm is available as tablets for oral administration. Each tablet contains 260 mg quinine sulfate. Also contains, as inactive ingredients: corn starch, pregelatinized starch, sodium starch glycolate, sucrose, and zinc stearate.

Neuromuscular Agent

Quinine sulfate has the following structural formula:

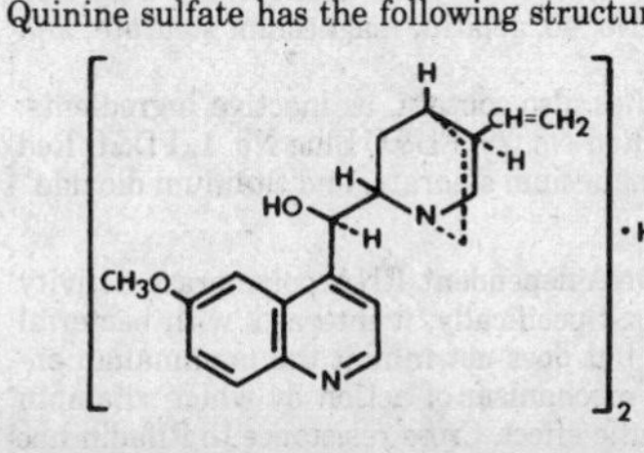

Quinine sulfate occurs as a white, crystalline powder, which darkens on exposure to light. It is odorless and has a persistent, very bitter taste. It is slightly soluble in water, alcohol, chloroform, and ether.

CLINICAL PHARMACOLOGY

Quinine, a cinchona alkaloid, acts on skeletal muscle by three mechanisms: it increases the refractory period by direct action on the muscle fiber, it decreases the excitability of the motor end-plate, an action similar to that of curare, and it affects the distribution of calcium within the muscle fiber.

Quinine is readily absorbed when given orally. Absorption occurs mainly from the upper part of the small intestine, and is almost complete even in patients with marked diarrhea.

The cinchona alkaloids in large measure are metabolically degraded in the body, especially in the liver; less than 5% of an administered dose is excreted unaltered in the urine. It is reported that there is no accumulation of the drugs in the body upon continued administration. The metabolic degradation products are excreted in the urine, where many of them have been identified as hydroxy derivatives, but small amounts also appear in the feces, gastric juice, bile, and saliva. Renal excretion of quinine is twice as rapid when the urine is acidic as when it is alkaline, due to the greater tubular reabsorption of the alkaloidal base that occurs in an alkaline media. Excretion is also limited by the binding of a large fraction of cinchona alkaloids to plasma proteins.

Peak plasma concentrations of cinchona alkaloids occur within 1 to 3 hours after a single oral dose. The half-life is 4 to 5 hours. After chronic administration of total daily doses of 1 g of drug, the average plasma quinine concentration is approximately 7μg/ml. After termination of quinine therapy, the plasma level falls rapidly and only a negligible concentration is detectable after 24 hours.

A large fraction (approximately 70%) of the plasma quinine is bound to proteins. This explains in part why the concentration of alkaloid in cerebrospinal fluid is only 2 to 5% of that in the plasma. However, it can traverse the placental membrane and readily reach fetal tissues.

Tinnitus and impairment of hearing rarely should occur at plasma quinine concentrations of less than 10 μg/ml. While this level would not be anticipated from use of 1 or 2 tablets of Quinamm daily, an occasional patient may have some evidence of cinchonism on this dosage, such as tinnitus. (See WARNINGS section.)

INDICATIONS AND USAGE

For the prevention and treatment of nocturnal recumbency leg muscle cramps.

CONTRAINDICATIONS

Quinamm may cause fetal harm when administered to a pregnant woman. Congenital malformations in the human have been reported with the use of quinine, primarily with large doses (up to 30 g) for attempted abortion. In about half of these reports, the malformation was deafness related to auditory nerve hypoplasia. Among the other abnormalities reported were limb anomalies, visceral defects, and visual changes. In animal tests, teratogenic effects were found in rabbits and guinea pigs and were absent in mice, rats, dogs, and monkeys. Quinamm is contraindicated in women who are or may become pregnant. If this drug is used during pregnancy, or if the patient becomes pregnant while taking this drug, the patient should be apprised of the potential hazard to the fetus.

Because of the quinine content, Quinamm is contraindicated in patients with known quinine hypersensitivity and in patients with glucose-6-phosphate dehydrogenase (G-6-PD) deficiency.

Since thrombocytopenic purpura may follow the administration of quinine in highly sensitive patients, a history of this occurrence associated with previous quinine ingestion contraindicates its further use. Recovery usually occurs following withdrawal of the medication and appropriate therapy.

This drug should not be used in patients with tinnitus or optic neuritis or in patients with a history of blackwater fever.

WARNINGS

Repeated doses or overdosage of quinine in some individuals may precipitate a cluster of symptoms referred to as cinchonism. Such symptoms, in the mildest form, include ringing in the ears, headache, nausea, and slightly disturbed vision; however, when medication is continued or after large single doses, symptoms also involve the gastrointestinal tract, the nervous and cardiovascular systems, and the skin.

Hemolysis (with the potential for hemolytic anemia) has been associated with a G-6-PD deficiency in patients taking quinine. Quinamm should be stopped immediately if evidence of hemolysis appears.

If symptoms occur, drug should be discontinued and supportive measures instituted. In case of overdosage, see OVERDOSAGE section of prescribing information.

Continued on next page

Information on Merrell Dow products is based on labeling in effect in May, 1986.

Merrell Dow—Cont.

PRECAUTIONS

General

Quinamm should be discontinued if there is any evidence of hypersensitivity. (See CONTRAINDICATIONS.) Cutaneous flushing, pruritus, skin rashes, fever, gastric distress, dyspnea, ringing in the ears, and visual impairment are the usual expressions of hypersensitivity, particularly if only small doses of quinine have been taken. Extreme flushing of the skin accompanied by intense, generalized pruritus is the most common form. Hemoglobinuria and asthma from quinine are rare types of idiosyncrasy.

In patients with atrial fibrillation, the administration of quinine requires the same precautions as those for quinidine. (See *Drug Interactions.*)

Drug Interactions

Increased plasma levels of digoxin have been demonstrated in individuals after concomitant quinine administration. Increased plasma levels of digitoxin have been demonstrated in individuals after concomitant quinidine administration. It is therefore recommended that plasma levels of digoxin or digitoxin be determined periodically for those individuals taking either of these glycosides and Quinamm concomitantly.

Concurrent use of aluminum-containing antacids may delay or decrease absorption of quinine.

Cinchona alkaloids, including quinine, have the potential to depress the hepatic enzyme system that synthesizes the vitamin K-dependent factors. The resulting hypoprothrombinemic effect may enhance the action of warfarin and other oral anticoagulants.

The effects of neuromuscular blocking agents (particularly pancuronium, succinylcholine, and tubocurarine) may be potentiated with quinine, and result in respiratory difficulties.

Urinary alkalizers (such as acetazolamide and sodium bicarbonate) may increase quinine blood levels with potential for toxicity.

Drug/Laboratory Interactions

Quinine may produce an elevated value for urinary 17-ketogenic steroids when the Zimmerman method is used.

Carcinogenesis, Mutagenesis, Impairment of Fertility

A study of quinine sulfate administered in drinking water (0.1%) to rats for periods up to 20 months showed no evidence of neoplastic changes.

Mutation studies of quinine (dihydrochloride) in male and female mice gave negative results by the micronucleus test. Intraperitoneal injections (0.5 mM/kg) were given twice, 24 hours apart. Direct *Salmonella typhimurium* tests were negative; when mammalian liver homogenate was added, positive results were found.

Mutation studies of quinine hydrochloride, 100 mg/kg, p.o. in Chinese hamsters showed no genotoxic activity in the sister chromatid exchange (SCE) test, micronucleus test, or chromosome aberration test. In mice given quinine hydrochloride, 100 mg/kg, p.o., the micronucleus test and chromosome aberration test were negative; the SCE test exhibited an increase of SCEs/cell. Tests were repeated in two inbred strains of mice using 55, 75, and 110 mg/kg p.o. The effect was more pronounced in these mice and the increase in SCEs/cell demonstrated a linear dose relationship. One of the inbred strains had positive micronucleus test findings. The chromosome aberration test also revealed an increase of chromatid breaks. The Ames test system results were negative for point mutation.

No information relating to the effect of quinine upon fertility in animal or in man has been found.

Pregnancy

Category X. See CONTRAINDICATIONS.

Nonteratogenic Effects

Because quinine crosses the placenta in humans, the potential for fetal effects is present. Stillbirths in mothers taking quinine have been reported in which no obvious cause for the fetal deaths was shown. Quinine in toxic amounts has been associated with abortion. Whether this action is always due to direct effect on the uterus is questionable.

Nursing Mothers

Caution should be exercised when Quinamm is given to nursing women because quinine is excreted in breast milk (in small amounts).

ADVERSE REACTIONS

The following adverse reactions have been reported with Quinamm in therapeutic or excessive dosage. (Individual or multiple symptoms may represent cinchonism or hypersensitivity.)

Hematologic: acute hemolysis, thrombocytopenic purpura, agranulocytosis, hypoprothrombinemia

CNS: visual disturbances, including blurred vision with scotomata, photophobia, diplopia, diminished visual fields, and disturbed color vision; tinnitus, deafness, and vertigo; headache, nausea, vomiting, fever, apprehension, restlessness, confusion, and syncope

Dermatologic/allergic: cutaneous rashes (urticarial, the most frequent type of allergic reaction, papular, or scarlatinal), pruritus, flushing of the skin, sweating, occasional edema of the face

Respiratory: asthmatic symptoms

Cardiovascular: anginal symptoms

Gastrointestinal: nausea and vomiting (may be CNS-related), epigastric pain, hepatitis

DRUG ABUSE AND DEPENDENCE

Tolerance, abuse, or dependence with Quinamm has not been reported.

OVERDOSAGE

The more common signs and symptoms of overdosage are tinnitus, dizziness, skin rash, and gastrointestinal disturbance (intestinal cramping). With higher doses, cardiovascular and CNS effects may occur, including headache, fever, vomiting, apprehension, confusion, and convulsions. Other effects are listed in the ADVERSE REACTIONS section.

Fatalities with quinine have been reported from single oral doses of 2 to 8 grams; a single fatality reported with a dose of 1.5 grams may reflect an idiosyncratic effect. Several cases of blindness following large overdoses of quinine, with partial recovery of vision in each instance, have been reported. Tinnitus and impaired hearing may occur at plasma quinine concentrations over 10 μg/ml. This level would not be normally attained with the use of 1 or 2 Quinamm tablets daily, but in a hypersensitive patient, as little as 0.3 g of quinine may produce tinnitus.

Treatment

Treatment for overdosage should include initially efforts to remove any residual Quinamm from the stomach by gastric lavage or by emesis induced with syrup of ipecac. The blood pressure should be supported and measures used to maintain renal function. Artificial respiration may be needed. Sedatives, oxygen, and other supportive measures should be used as necessary.

Fluid and electrolyte balance with intravenous fluids should be maintained. Acidification of the urine will promote renal excretion of quinine. In the presence of hemoglobinuria, however, acidification of the urine may augment renal blockade. Quinine should be readily dialyzable by hemodialysis and/or hemoperfusion procedures.

Evidence of angioedema or asthma may require the use of epinephrine, corticosteroids, and antihistamines. In the acute phase of toxic amaurosis caused by quinine, vasodilators administered intravenously may have a salutary effect. Stellate block has also been used effectively for quinine-associated blindness. Residual visual impairment occasionally yields to vasodilators.

DOSAGE AND ADMINISTRATION

1 tablet upon retiring. If needed, 2 tablets may be taken nightly —1 following the evening meal and 1 upon retiring. After several consecutive nights in which recumbency leg cramps do not occur, Quinamm may be discontinued in order to determine whether continued therapy is needed.

HOW SUPPLIED

NDC 0068-0547-15

260 mg tablets in bottles of 100. Tablets are round, white, debossed W one side, Merrell 547 other side.

Store at room temperature, below 86°F (30°C).

Product Information as of December, 1984

Shown in Product Identification Section, page 418

RIFADIN® ℞

[*rif'ă-dĭn*]

rifampin

CAUTION: Federal law prohibits dispensing without prescription.

DESCRIPTION

Rifadin (rifampin) is a semi-synthetic antibiotic derivative of rifamycin B. Specifically, Rifadin is the hydrazone, 3-(4-methylpiperazinyliminomethyl) rifamycin SV.

Available as 150 and 300 mg capsules for oral administration.

The 150 mg capsules also contain, as inactive ingredients: corn starch, edible white ink, FD&C Blue No. 1, FD&C Red No. 3, FD&C Red No. 40, gelatin, magnesium stearate, and titanium dioxide.

The 300 mg capsules also contain, as inactive ingredients: corn starch, D&C Red No. 28, FD&C Blue No. 1, FD&C Red No. 40, gelatin, magnesium stearate, and titanium dioxide.

ACTIONS

Rifadin inhibits DNA-dependent RNA polymerase activity in susceptible cells. Specifically, it interacts with bacterial RNA polymerase, but does not inhibit the mammalian enzyme. This is the mechanism of action by which rifampin exerts its therapeutic effect. Cross resistance to Rifadin has only been shown with other rifamycins.

Peak blood levels in normal adults vary widely from individual to individual. Peak levels occur between 2 and 4 hours following the oral administration of a 600 mg dose. The average peak value is 7 mcg/ml; however, the peak level may vary from 4 to 32 mcg/ml.

In normal subjects the $T\frac{1}{2}$ (biological half-life) of Rifadin in blood is approximately three hours. Elimination occurs mainly through the bile and, to a much lesser extent, the urine.

INDICATIONS

Pulmonary tuberculosis. In the initial treatment and in retreatment of patients with pulmonary tuberculosis Rifadin must be used in conjunction with at least one other antituberculosis drug. Frequently used regimens have been the following:

- isoniazid and Rifadin
- ethambutol and Rifadin
- isoniazid, ethambutol and Rifadin

Neisseria meningitidis carriers: Rifadin is indicated for the treatment of asymptomatic carriers of *N. meningitidis* to eliminate meningococci from the nasopharynx.

Rifadin is not indicated for the treatment of meningococcal infection.

To avoid the indiscriminate use of Rifadin, diagnostic laboratory procedures, including serotyping and susceptibility testing, should be performed to establish the carrier state and the correct treatment. In order to preserve the usefulness of Rifadin in the treatment of asymptomatic meningococcal carriers, it is recommended that the drug be reserved for situations in which the risk of meningococcal meningitis is high.

Both in the treatment of tuberculosis and in the treatment of meningococcal carriers, small numbers of resistant cells, present within large populations of susceptible cells, can rapidly become the predominating type. Since rapid emergence of resistance can occur, culture and susceptibility tests should be performed in the event of persistent positive cultures.

CONTRAINDICATIONS

A history of previous hypersensitivity reaction to any of the rifamycins.

WARNINGS

Rifampin has been shown to produce liver dysfunction. There have been fatalities associated with jaundice in patients with liver disease or receiving rifampin concomitantly with other hepatoxic agents. Since an increased risk may exist for individuals with liver disease, benefits must be weighed carefully against the risk of further liver damage. Periodic liver function monitoring is mandatory.

The possibility of rapid emergence of resistant meningococci restricts the use of Rifadin to short-term treatment of the asymptomatic carrier state. Rifadin is not to be used for the treatment of meningococcal disease.

Several studies of tumorigenicity potential have been done in rodents. In one strain of mice known to be particularly susceptible to the spontaneous development of hepatomas, rifampin given at a level 2–10 times the maximum dosage used clinically, resulted in a significant increase in the occurrence of hepatomas in female mice of this strain after one year of administration. There was no evidence of tumorigenicity in the males of this strain, in males or females of another mouse strain or in rats.

Usage in Pregnancy: Although rifampin has been reported to cross the placental barrier and appear in cord blood, the effect of Rifadin, alone or in combination with other antituberculosis drugs, on the human fetus is not known. An increase in congenital malformations, primarily spina bifida and cleft palate, has been reported in the offspring of rodents given oral doses of 150–250 mg/kg/day of rifampin during pregnancy.

The possible teratogenic potential in women capable of bearing children should be carefully weighed against the benefits of therapy.

PRECAUTIONS

Rifadin is not recommended for intermittent therapy; the patient should be cautioned against intentional or accidental interruption of the daily dosage regimen since rare renal hypersensitivity reactions have been reported when therapy was resumed in such cases.

Rifampin has been observed to increase the requirement for anticoagulant drugs of the coumarin type. The cause of this phenomenon is unknown. In patients receiving anticoagulants and rifampin concurrently, it is recommended that the prothrombin time be performed daily or as frequently as necessary to establish and maintain the required dose of anticoagulant.

Urine, feces, saliva, sputum, sweat and tears may be colored red-orange by rifampin and its metabolites. Soft contact lenses may be permanently stained. Individuals to be treated should be made aware of these possibilities.

It has been reported that the reliability of oral contraceptives may be affected in some patients being treated for tuberculosis with rifampin in combination with at least one other antituberculosis drug. In such cases, alternative contraceptive measures may need to be considered.

It has also been reported that rifampin given in combination with other antituberculosis drugs may decrease the pharmacologic activity of methadone, oral hypoglycemics, digitoxin, quinidine, disopyramide, dapsone and corticosteroids. In these cases, dosage adjustment of the interacting drugs is recommended.

Therapeutic levels of rifampin have been shown to inhibit standard microbiological assays for serum folate and vitamin B_{12}. Alternative methods must be considered when determining folate and vitamin B_{12} concentrations in the presence of rifampin.

Since rifampin has been reported to cross the placental barrier and appear in cord blood, neonates of rifampin-treated mothers should be carefully observed for any evidence of adverse effects.

ADVERSE REACTIONS

Gastrointestinal disturbances such as heartburn, epigastric distress, anorexia, nausea, vomiting, gas, cramps, and diarrhea have been noted in some patients. Headache, drowsiness, fatigue, menstrual disturbances, ataxia, dizziness, inability to concentrate, mental confusion, visual disturbances, muscular weakness, fever, pains in the extremities and generalized numbness have also been noted.

Hypersensitivity reactions have been reported. Encountered occasionally have been pruritus, urticaria, rash, pemphigoid reaction, eosinophilia, sore mouth, sore tongue and exudative conjunctivitis. Rarely, hepatitis or a shock-like syndrome with hepatic involvement and abnormal liver function tests have been reported. Transient abnormalities in liver function tests (e.g., elevations in serum bilirubin, BSP, alkaline phosphatase, serum transaminases) have also been observed.

Thrombocytopenia, transient leukopenia, hemolytic anemia and decreased hemoglobin have been observed. Thrombocytopenia has occurred when Rifadin and ethambutol were administered concomitantly according to an intermittent dose schedule twice weekly, and in high doses.

Elevations in BUN and serum uric acid have occurred. Rarely, hemolysis, hemoglobinuria, hematuria, renal insufficiency or acute renal failure have been reported and are generally considered to be hypersensitivity reactions. These have usually occurred during intermittent therapy or when treatment was resumed following intentional or accidental interruption of a daily dosage regimen and were reversible when rifampin was discontinued and appropriate therapy instituted.

Although rifampin has been reported to have an immunosuppressive effect in some animal experiments, available human data indicate that this has no clinical significance.

DOSAGE AND ADMINISTRATION

It is recommended that Rifadin be administered once daily, either one hour before, or two hours after a meal.

Data are not available for determination of dosage for children under 5.

Pulmonary tuberculosis:

Adults: 600 mg (two 300 mg or four 150 mg capsules) in a single daily administration.

Children: 10–20 mg/kg not to exceed 600 mg/day.

In the treatment of pulmonary tuberculosis, Rifadin must be used in conjunction with at least one other antituberculous agent. In general, therapy should be continued until bacterial conversion and maximal improvement have occurred.

Meningococcal carriers:

It is recommended that Rifadin be administered once daily for four consecutive days in the following doses:

Adults: 600 mg (two 300 mg or four 150 mg capsules) in a single daily administration.

Children: 10–20 mg/kg not to exceed 600 mg/day.

Preparation of Extemporaneous Oral Suspension:

For pediatric and adult patients, in whom capsule swallowing is difficult or where lower doses are needed, a liquid suspension may be prepared as follows.

Rifadin 1% w/v suspension (10 mg/ml) can be compounded using one of five syrups—Simple Syrup (Syrup NF), Simple Syrup (Humco Laboratories), Simple Syrup (Whiteworth Inc.), Wild Cherry Syrup (Eli Lilly and Company) and Syrpalta® Syrup (Emerson Laboratories).

1. Empty contents of four Rifadin 300 mg capsules or eight Rifadin 150 mg capsules onto a piece of weighing paper.
2. If necessary, gently crush the capsule contents with a spatula to produce a fine powder.
3. Transfer rifampin powder blend to a four-ounce amber glass prescription bottle.
4. Rinse the paper and spatula with 20 ml of one of the above recommended syrups and add the rinse to the bottle. Shake vigorously.
5. Add 100 ml of syrup to the bottle and shake vigorously.

This compounding procedure results in a 1% w/v suspension containing 10 mg rifampin/ml. Stability studies indicate that the suspension is stable for four weeks when stored at room temperature (25 ± 3°C) or in a refrigerator (2–8°C). This extemporaneously prepared suspension must be shaken well prior to administration.

Susceptibility testing: Pulmonary tuberculosis. Rifampin susceptibility powders are available for both direct and indirect methods of determining the susceptibility of strains of mycobacteria. The MIC's of susceptible clinical isolates when determined in 7H10 or other non-egg-containing media have ranged from 0.1 to 2 mcg/ml.

Meningococcal carriers: Susceptibility discs containing 5 mcg of rifampin are available for susceptibility testing of *N. meningitidis.*

Quantitative methods that require measurement of zone diameters give the most precise estimates of antibiotic susceptibility. One such procedure* has been recommended for use with discs for testing susceptibility to rifampin. Interpretations correlate zone diameters from the disc test with MIC (minimal inhibitory concentration) values for rifampin. A range of MIC's from 0.1 to 1 mcg/ml has been found *in vitro* for susceptible strains of *N. meningitidis.* With this procedure, a report from the laboratory of "resistant" indicates that the organism is not likely to be eradicated from the nasopharynx of asymptomatic carriers.

OVERDOSAGE

Signs and Symptoms:

Nausea, vomiting, and increasing lethargy will probably occur within a short time after ingestion; actual unconsciousness may occur with severe hepatic involvement. Brownish-red or orange discoloration of the skin, urine, sweat, saliva, tears, and feces is proportional to amount ingested.

Liver enlargement, possibly with tenderness, can develop within a few hours after severe overdosage and jaundice may develop rapidly. Hepatic involvement may be more marked in patients with prior impairment of hepatic function. Other physical findings remain essentially normal.

Direct and total bilirubin levels may increase rapidly with severe overdosage; hepatic enzyme levels may be affected, especially with prior impairment of hepatic function. A direct effect upon the hematopoietic system, electrolyte levels, or acid-base balance is unlikely.

Treatment:

Since nausea and vomiting are likely to be present, gastric lavage is probably preferable to induction of emesis. Activated charcoal slurry instilled into the stomach following evacuation of gastric contents can help absorb any remaining drug in the G.I. tract. Antiemetic medication may be required to control severe nausea/vomiting.

Active diuresis (with measured intake and output) will help promote excretion of the drug. Bile drainage may be indicated in presence of serious impairment of hepatic function lasting more than 24–48 hours; under these circumstances, extracorporeal hemodialysis may be required.

In patients with previously adequate hepatic function, reversal of liver enlargement and impaired hepatic excretory function probably will be noted within 72 hours, with rapid return toward normal thereafter.

HOW SUPPLIED

150 mg maroon and scarlet capsules imprinted with the Dow diamond trademark over the code number 510.

Bottles of 30 (NDC 0068-0510-30)

300 mg maroon and scarlet capsules imprinted with the Dow diamond trademark and the code number 508.

Bottles of 30 (NDC 0068-0508-30)
Bottles of 60 (NDC 0068-0508-60)
Bottles of 100 (NDC 0068-0508-61)

**Bauer, A.W., Kirby, W.M., Sherris, J.C., and Turck, M. Antibiotic susceptibility testing by a standardized single disk method. Am. J. Clin. Path. 45:493-496, 1966.*

Product Information as of April, 1985

Rifadin 150 mg capsules are
manufactured by
MERRELL DOW PHARMACEUTICALS (CANADA) INC.
Richmond Hill, Ontario, L4C 5H2
Canada for
MERRELL DOW PHARMACEUTICALS INC.
Subsidiary of The Dow Chemical Company
Cincinnati, Ohio 45215, U.S.A.

Shown in Product Identification Section, page 418

RIFAMATE® ℞

[rĭf'ăh-māt]
rifampin and isoniazid
Capsules

CAUTION: Federal law prohibits dispensing without prescription.

WARNING

Severe and sometimes fatal hepatitis associated with isoniazid therapy may occur and may develop even after many months of treatment. The risk of developing hepatitis is age related. Approximate case rates by age are: 0 per 1,000 for persons under 20 years of age, 3 per 1,000 for persons in the 20–34 year age group, 12 per 1,000 for persons in the 35–49 year age group, 23 per 1,000 for persons in the 50–64 year age group, and 8 per 1,000 for persons over 65 years of age. The risk of hepatitis is increased with daily consumption of alcohol. Precise data to provide a fatality rate for isoniazid-related hepatitis are not available; however, in a U.S. Public Health Service Surveillance Study of 13,838 persons taking isoniazid, there were 8 deaths among 174 cases of hepatitis.

Therefore, patients given isoniazid should be carefully monitored and interviewed at monthly intervals. Serum transaminase concentration becomes elevated in about 10–20 percent of patients, usually during the first few months of therapy, but it can occur at any time. Usually enzyme levels return to normal despite continuance of drug, but in some cases progressive liver dysfunction occurs. Patients should be instructed to report immediately any of the prodromal symptoms of hepatitis, such as fatigue, weakness, malaise, anorexia, nausea, or vomiting. If these symptoms appear or if signs suggestive of hepatic damage are detected, isoniazid should be discontinued promptly, since continued use of the drug in these cases has been reported to cause a more severe form of liver damage.

Patients with tuberculosis should be given appropriate treatment with alternative drugs. If isoniazid must be reinstituted, it should be reinstituted only after symptoms and laboratory abnormalities have cleared. The drug should be restarted in very small and gradually increasing doses and should be withdrawn immediately if there is any indication of recurrent liver involvement.

Treatment should be deferred in persons with acute hepatic diseases.

DESCRIPTION

Rifamate is a combination capsule containing 300 mg rifampin and 150 mg isoniazid. The capsules also contain as inactive ingredients: colloidal silicon dioxide, FD&C Blue No. 1, FD&C Red No. 40, gelatin, magnesium stearate, sodium starch glycolate, and titanium dioxide.

Rifampin is a semisynthetic antibiotic derivative of rifamycin B. Specifically, rifampin is the hydrazone, 3-(4-methyl-piperazinylimino-methyl) rifamycin SV.

Isoniazid is the hydrazide of isonicotinic acid. It exists as colorless or white crystals or as a white, crystalline powder that is water soluble, odorless, and slowly affected by exposure to air and light.

ACTIONS

Rifampin

Rifampin inhibits DNA-dependent RNA polymerase activity in susceptible cells. Specifically, it interacts with bacterial RNA polymerase but does not inhibit the mammalian enzyme. This is the mechanism of action by which rifampin exerts its therapeutic effect. Rifampin cross resistance has only been shown with other rifamycins.

In a study of 14 normal human adult males, peak blood levels of rifampin occured 1 ½ to 3 hours following oral administration of two Rifamate capsules. The peaks ranged from 6.9 to 14 mcg/ml with an average of 10 mcg/ml.

In normal subjects the $T_{1/2}$ (biological half-life) of rifampin in blood is approximately 3 hours. Elimination occurs mainly through the bile and, to a much lesser extent the urine.

Isoniazid

Isoniazid acts against actively growing tubercle bacilli.

After oral administration isoniazid produces peak blood levels within 1 to 2 hours which decline to 50% or less within 6 hours. It diffuses readily into all body fluids (cerebrospinal, pleural, and ascitic fluids), tissues, organs and excreta (saliva, sputum, and feces). The drug also passes through the placental barrier and into milk in concentrations comparable to those in the plasma. From 50 to 70% of a dose of isoniazid is excreted in the urine in 24 hours.

Isoniazid is metabolized primarily by acetylation and dehydrazination. The rate of acetylation is genetically determined. Approximately 50% of Blacks and Caucasians are "slow inactivators"; the majority of Eskimos and Orientals are "rapid inactivators."

The rate of acetylation does not significantly alter the effectiveness of isoniazid. However, slow acetylation may lead to higher blood levels of the drug, and thus an increase in toxic reactions.

Pyridoxine deficiency (B_6) is sometimes observed in adults with high doses of isoniazid and is considered probably due to its competition with pyridoxal phosphate for the enzyme apotryptophanase.

INDICATIONS

For pulmonary tuberculosis in which organisms are susceptible, and when the patient has been titrated on the individ-

Continued on next page

Merrell Dow—Cont.

ual components and it has therefore been established that this fixed dosage is therapeutically effective.
This fixed-dosage combination drug is not recommended for initial therapy of tuberculosis or for preventive therapy.
In the treatment of tuberculosis, small numbers of resistant cells, present within large populations of susceptible cells, can rapidly become the predominating type. Since rapid emergence of resistance can occur, culture and susceptibility tests should be performed in the event of persistent positive cultures.
This drug is *not* indicated for the treatment of meningococcal infections or asymptomatic carriers of *N. meningitidis* to eliminate meningococci from the nasopharynx.

CONTRAINDICATIONS

Previous isoniazid-associated hepatic injury; severe adverse reactions to isoniazid, such as drug fever, chills, and arthritis; acute liver disease of any etiology.
A history of previous hypersensitivity reaction to any of the rifamycins or to isoniazid, including drug-induced hepatitis.

WARNINGS

Rifamate (rifampin-isoniazid) is a combination of two drugs, each of which has been associated with liver dysfunction. Liver function tests should be performed prior to therapy with Rifamate and periodically during treatment.

Rifampin

Rifampin has been shown to produce liver dysfunction. There have been fatalities associated with jaundice in patients with liver disease or receiving rifampin concomitantly with other hepatoxic agents. Since an increased risk may exist for individuals with liver disease, benefits must be weighed carefully against the risk of further liver damage.
Several studies of tumorigenicity potential have been done in rodents. In one strain of mice known to be particularly susceptible to the spontaneous development of hepatomas, rifampin given at a level 2–10 times the maximum dosage used clinically, resulted in a significant increase in the occurrence of hepatomas in female mice of this strain after one year of administration. There was no evidence of tumorigenicity in the males of this strain, in males or females of another mouse strain, or in rats.

Isoniazid

See the boxed warning.

PRECAUTIONS

Rifampin

Rifampin is not recommended for intermittent therapy; the patient should be cautioned against intentional or accidental interruption of the daily dosage regimen since rare renal hypersensitivity reactions have been reported when therapy was resumed in such cases.
Rifampin has been observed to increase the requirements for anticoagulant drugs of the coumarin type. The cause of the phenomenon is unknown. In patients receiving anticoagulants and rifampin concurrently, it is recommended that the prothrombin time be performed daily or as frequently as necessary to establish and maintain the required dose of anticoagulant.
Urine, feces, saliva, sputum, sweat and tears may be colored red-orange by rifampin and its metabolites. Soft contact lenses may be permanently stained. Individuals to be treated should be made aware of these possibilities.
It has been reported that the reliability of oral contraceptives may be affected in some patients being treated for tuberculosis with rifampin in combination with at least one other antituberculosis drug. In such cases, alternative contraceptive measures may need to be considered.
It has also been reported that rifampin given in combination with other antituberculosis drugs may decrease the pharmacologic activity of methadone, oral hypoglycemics, digitoxin, quinidine, disopyramide, dapsone and corticosteroids. In these cases, dosage adjustment of the interacting drugs is recommended.
Therapeutic levels of rifampin have been shown to inhibit standard assays for serum folate and vitamin B_{12}. Alternative methods must be considered when determining folate and vitamin B_{12} concentrations in the presence of rifampin.
Since rifampin has been reported to cross the placental barrier and appear in cord blood and in maternal milk, neonates and newborns of rifampin-treated mothers should be carefully observed for any evidence of untoward effects.

Isoniazid

All drugs should be stopped and an evaluation of the patient should be made at the first sign of a hypersensitivity reaction.
Use of isoniazid should be carefully monitored in the following:
1. Patients who are receiving phenytoin (diphenylhydantoin) concurrently. Isoniazid may decrease the excretion of phenytoin or may enhance its effects. To avoid phenytoin intoxication, appropriate adjustment of the anticonvulsant dose should be made.
2. Daily users of alcohol. Daily ingestion of alcohol may be associated with a higher incidence of isoniazid hepatitis.
3. Patients with current chronic liver disease or severe renal dysfunction.

Periodic ophthalmoscopic examination during isoniazid therapy is recommended when visual symptoms occur.

Usage in Pregnancy and Lactation

Rifampin

Although rifampin has been reported to cross the placental barrier and appear in cord blood, the effect of rifampin, alone or in combination with other antituberculosis drugs, on the human fetus is not known. An increase in congenital malformations, primarily spina bifida and cleft palate, has been reported in the offspring of rodents given oral doses of 150–250 mg/kg/day of rifampin during pregnancy.
The possible teratogenic potential in women capable of bearing children should be carefully weighed against the benefits of therapy.

Isoniazid

It has been reported that in both rats and rabbits, isoniazid may exert an embryocidal effect when administered orally during pregnancy, although no isoniazid-related congenital anomalies have been found in reproduction studies in mammalian species (mice, rats, and rabbits). Isoniazid should be prescribed during pregnancy only when therapeutically necessary. The benefit of preventive therapy should be weighed against a possible risk to the fetus. Preventive treatment generally should be started after delivery because of the increased risk of tuberculosis for new mothers.
Since isoniazid is known to cross the placental barrier and to pass into maternal breast milk, neonates and breast-fed infants of isoniazid treated mothers should be carefully observed for any evidence of adverse effects.

Carcinogenesis:

Isoniazid has been reported to induce pulmonary tumors in a number of strains of mice.

ADVERSE REACTIONS

Rifampin

Nervous system reactions: headache, drowsiness, fatigue, ataxia, dizziness, inability to concentrate, mental confusion, visual disturbances, muscular weakness, pain in extremities and generalized numbness.
Gastrointestinal disturbances: in some patients heartburn, epigastric distress, anorexia, nausea, vomiting, gas, cramps, and diarrhea.
Hepatic reactions: transient abnormalities in liver function tests (e.g. elevations in serum bilirubin, BSP, alkaline phosphatase, serum transaminases) have been observed. Rarely, hepatitis or a shocklike syndrome with hepatic involvement and abnormal liver function tests.
Hematologic reactions: thrombocytopenia, transient leukopenia, hemolytic anemia, eosinophilia and decreased hemoglobin have been observed. Thrombocytopenia has occurred when rifampin and ethambutol were administered concomitantly according to an intermittent dose schedule twice weekly and in high doses.
Allergic and immunological reactions: occasionally pruritus, urticaria, rash, pemphigoid reaction, eosinophilia, sore mouth, sore tongue and exudative conjunctivitis. Rarely, hemolysis, hemoglobinuria, hematuria, renal insufficiency or acute renal failure have been reported which are generally considered to be hypersensitivity reactions. These have usually occurred during intermittent therapy or when treatment was resumed following intentional or accidental interruption of a daily dosage regimen and were reversible when rifampin was discontinued and appropriate therapy instituted.
Although rifampin has been reported to have an immunosuppressive effect in some animal experiments, available human data indicate that this has no clinical significance.
Metabolic reactions: elevations in BUN and serum uric acid have occurred.
Miscellaneous reactions: fever and menstrual disturbances have been noted.

Isoniazid

The most frequent reactions are those affecting the nervous system and the liver.
Nervous system reactions: Peripheral neuropathy is the most common toxic effect. It is dose-related, occurs most often in the malnourished and in those predisposed to neuritis (e.g., alcoholics and diabetics), and is usually preceded by paresthesias of the feet and hands. The incidence is higher in "slow inactivators".
Other neurotoxic effects, which are uncommon with conventional doses, are convulsions, toxic encephalopathy, optic neuritis and atrophy, memory impairment, and toxic psychosis.
Gastrointestinal reactions: Nausea, vomiting, and epigastric distress.
Hepatic reactions: Elevated serum transaminases (SGOT; SGPT), bilirubinemia, bilirubinuria, jaundice, and occasionally severe and sometimes fatal hepatitis. The common prodromal symptoms are anorexia, nausea, vomiting, fatigue, malaise, and weakness. Mild and transient elevation of serum transaminase levels occurs in 10 to 20 percent of persons taking isoniazid. The abnormality usually occurs in the first 4 to 6 months of treatment but can occur at any time during therapy. In most instances, enzyme levels return to normal with no necessity to discontinue medication. In occasional instances, progressive liver damage occurs, with accompanying symptoms. In these cases, the drug should be discontinued immediately. The frequency of progressive liver damage increases with age. It is rare in persons under 20, but occurs in up to 2.3 percent of those over 50 years of age.
Hematologic reactions: agranulocytosis, hemolytic sideroblastic or aplastic anemia, thrombocytopenia and eosinophilia.
Hypersensitivity reactions: fever, skin eruptions (morbilliform, maculopapular, purpuric, or exfoliative), lymphadenopathy and vasculitis.
Metabolic and endocrine reactions: pyridoxine deficiency, pellagra, hyperglycemia, metabolic acidosis, and gynecomastia.
Miscellaneous reactions: rheumatic syndrome and systemic lupus erythematosus-like syndrome.

OVERDOSAGE

Rifampin

Signs and Symptoms

Nausea, vomiting, and increasing lethargy will probably occur within a short time after ingestion; actual unconsciousness may occur with severe hepatic involvement. Brownish-red or orange discoloration of the skin, urine, sweat, saliva, tears, and feces is proportional to amount ingested.
Liver enlargement, possibly with tenderness, can develop within a few hours after severe overdosage and jaundice may develop rapidly. Hepatic involvement may be more marked in patients with prior impairment of hepatic function. Other physical findings remain essentially normal.
Direct and total bilirubin levels may increase rapidly with severe overdosage; hepatic enzyme levels may be affected, especially with prior impairment of hepatic function. A direct effect upon hemopoietic system, electrolyte levels or acid-base balance is unlikely.

Isoniazid

Signs and Symptoms

Isoniazid overdosage produces signs and symptoms within 30 minutes to 3 hours. Nausea, vomiting, dizziness, slurring of speech, blurring of vision, visual hallucinations (including bright colors and strange designs), are among the early manifestations. With marked overdosage, respiratory distress and CNS depression, progressing rapidly from stupor to profound coma, are to be expected, along with severe, intractable seizures. Severe metabolic acidosis, acetonuria, and hyperglycemia are typical laboratory findings.

Rifamate (rifampin and isoniazid capsules)

Treatment

The airway should be secured and adequate respiratory exchange established. Only then should gastric emptying (lavage-aspiration) be attempted; this may be difficult because of seizures. Since nausea and vomiting are likely to be present, gastric lavage is probably preferable to induction of emesis.
Activated charcoal slurry instilled into the stomach following evacuation of gastric contents can help absorb any remaining drug in the GI tract. Antiemetic medication may be required to control severe nausea and vomiting.
Blood samples should be obtained for immediate determination of gases, electrolytes, BUN, glucose, etc. Blood should be typed and crossmatched in preparation for possible hemodialysis.
Rapid control of metabolic acidosis is fundamental to management. Intravenous sodium bicarbonate should be given at once and repeated as needed, adjusting subsequent dosage on the basis of laboratory findings (i.e. serum sodium, pH, etc.). At the same time, anticonvulsants should be given intravenously (i.e. barbiturates, diphenylhydantoin, diazepam) as required, and large doses of intravenous pyridoxine.
Forced osmotic diuresis must be started early and should be continued for some hours after clinical improvement to hasten renal clearance of drug and help prevent relapse. Fluid intake and output should be monitored.
Bile drainage may be indicated in presence of serious impairment of hepatic function lasting more than 24–48 hours. Under these circumstances, and for severe cases extra-corporeal hemodialysis may be required; if this is not available, peritoneal dialysis can be used along with forced diuresis.
Along with measures based on initial and repeated determination of blood gases and other laboratory tests as needed, meticulous respiratory and other intensive care should be utilized to protect against hypoxia, hypotension, aspiration, pneumonitis, etc.
In patients with previously adequate hepatic function, reversal of liver enlargement and impaired hepatic excretory function probably will be noted within 72 hours, with rapid return toward normal thereafter.
Untreated or inadequately treated cases of gross isoniazid overdosage can terminate fatally, but good response has been reported in most patients brought under adequate treatment within the first few hours after drug ingestion.

DOSAGE AND ADMINISTRATION

In general, therapy should be continued until bacterial conversion and maximal improvement have occured.

Adults: Two Rifamate (rifampin-isoniazid) capsules (600 mg rifampin, 300 mg isoniazid) once daily, administered one hour before or two hours after a meal.

Concomitant administration of pyridoxine (B_6) is recommended in the malnourished, in those predisposed to neuropathy (e.g. diabetics) and in adolescents.

Susceptibility Testing

Rifampin

Rifampin susceptibility powders are available for both direct and indirect methods of determining the susceptibility of strains of mycobacteria. The MIC's of susceptible clinical isolates when determined in 7H10 or other non-egg-containing media have ranged from 0.1 to 2 mcg/ml.

Quantitative methods that require measurement of zone diameters give the most precise estimates of antibiotic susceptibility. One such procedure has been recommended for use with discs for testing susceptibility to rifampin. Interpretations correlate zone diameters from the disc test with MIC (minimal inhibitory concentration) values for rifampin.

HOW SUPPLIED

Capsules (opaque red), containing 300 mg rifampin and 150 mg isoniazid; bottles of 60 (NDC 0068-0509-60).

Product Information as of April, 1985

Shown in Product Identification Section, page 418

SELDANE® (terfenadine) ℞

[*sel'dān*]

60 mg Tablets

CAUTION: Federal law prohibits dispensing without prescription.

DESCRIPTION

Seldane (terfenadine) is available as tablets for oral administration. Each tablet contains 60 mg terfenadine. Tablets also contain, as inactive ingredients: corn starch, gelatin, lactose, magnesium stearate, and sodium bicarbonate.

Terfenadine is a histamine H_1-receptor antagonist with the chemical name α-[4-(1,1-Dimethylethyl)phenyl]-4-(hydroxydiphenylmethyl)-1-piperidinebutanol.

It has the following chemical structure:

Terfenadine occurs as a white to off-white crystalline powder. It is freely soluble in chloroform, soluble in ethanol, and very slightly soluble in water.

CLINICAL PHARMACOLOGY

Terfenadine is chemically and pharmacologically distinct from other antihistamines.

Histamine skin wheal studies have shown that Seldane in single and repeated doses of 60 mg in 64 subjects has an antihistaminic effect beginning at 1–2 hours, reaching its maximum at 3–4 hours, and lasting in excess of 12 hours.

Clinical trials of Seldane involved about 2,600 patients, most receiving either Seldane, another antihistamine and/or placebo in double-blind, randomized controlled comparisons. The four best controlled and largest trials each lasted 7 days and involved about 1,000 total patients in comparisons of Seldane (60 mg b.i.d.) with an active drug (chlorpheniramine, 4 mg t.i.d.; dexchlorpheniramine, 2 mg t.i.d.; or clemastine 1 mg b.i.d.). In the four trials, about 50–70% of Seldane or other antihistamine recipients had moderate to complete relief of symptoms, compared with 30–50% of placebo recipients, with a significant difference favoring the active drugs in each study. In these studies, Seldane was associated with less frequent drowsiness than the other antihistamines; the frequency of drowsiness with Seldane was similar to the frequency with placebo. None of these studies showed a difference between Seldane and other antihistamines in the frequency of anticholinergic effects. In studies which included 52 subjects in whom EEG assessments were made, no depressant effects have been observed.

Animal studies have demonstrated that terfenadine is a peripheral specific histamine H_1-receptor antagonist. In these animal studies, no sedative or anticholinergic effects were observed at effective antihistaminic doses. Radioactive disposition and autoradiographic studies in rats and radioligand binding studies with guinea pig brain H_1-receptors indicate that, at effective antihistamine doses, neither terfenadine nor its metabolites penetrate the blood brain barrier well.

Pharmacokinetic studies in 27 male subjects, using ^{14}C-labeled terfenadine, demonstrated that an oral dose of terfenadine is well absorbed from the gastrointestinal tract and rapidly and extensively biotransformed. Following administration of a single 60 mg Seldane tablet, detectable plasma levels were observed within one-half hour. Plasma levels peaked at about 2 hours after administration; a distribution half-life of 3.4 hours was followed by an elimination half-life of 20.25 hours. Terfenadine is extensively (97%) bound to human serum protein. Elimination studies in 6 male volunteers showed that fecal excretion accounted for 60% of the dose while 40% of the dose was eliminated via the urine. Almost all of the dose was eliminated in the form of metabolic products.

Following administration of single doses of 60 or 180 mg of Seldane, a linear response was observed in maximum plasma concentration. Area under the curve (AUC) calculations, however, indicate a nearly four-fold increase in response for a three-fold increase in dose.

INDICATIONS AND USAGE

Seldane is indicated for the relief of symptoms associated with seasonal allergic rhinitis such as sneezing, rhinorrhea, pruritus, and lacrimation.

CONTRAINDICATIONS

Seldane is contraindicated in patients with a known hypersensitivity to terfenadine or any of its ingredients.

PRECAUTIONS

Information for patients

Patients taking Seldane should receive the following information and instructions. Antihistamines are prescribed to reduce allergic symptoms. Patients should be questioned about pregnancy or lactation before starting Seldane therapy, since the drug should be used in pregnancy or lactation only if the potential benefit justifies the potential risk to fetus or baby. Patients should be instructed to take Seldane only as needed and not to exceed the prescribed dose. Patients should also be instructed to store this medication in a tightly closed container in a cool, dry place, away from heat or direct sunlight, and away from children.

Carcinogenesis, mutagenesis, impairment of fertility

Oral doses of terfenadine, corresponding to 63 times the recommended human daily dose, in mice for 18 months or in rats for 24 months, revealed no evidence of tumorigenicity. Microbial and micronucleus test assays with terfenadine have revealed no evidence of mutagenesis.

Reproduction and fertility studies in rats showed no effects on male or female fertility at oral doses of up to 21 times the human daily dose. At 63 times the human daily dose there was a small but significant reduction in implants and at 125 times the human daily dose reduced implants and increased post-implantation losses were observed, which were judged to be secondary to maternal toxicity.

Pregnancy Category C

There was no evidence of animal teratogenicity. Reproduction studies have been performed in rats at doses 63 times and 125 times the human daily dose and have revealed decreased pup weight gain and survival when terfenadine was administered throughout pregnancy and lactation. There are no adequate and well-controlled studies in pregnant women. Seldane should be used during pregnancy only if the potential benefit justifies the potential risk to the fetus.

Nonteratogenic effects

Seldane is not recommended for nursing women. The drug has caused decreased pup weight gain and survival in rats given doses 63 times and 125 times the human daily dose throughout pregnancy and lactation. Effects on pups exposed to Seldane only during lactation are not known, and there are no adequate and well-controlled studies in women during lactation.

Pediatric use

Safety and effectiveness of Seldane in children below the age of 12 years have not been established.

General

Consideration should be given to potential anticholinergic (drying) effects in patients with lower airway disease, including asthma.

ADVERSE REACTIONS

Experience from clinical studies, including both controlled and uncontrolled studies involving more than 2,400 patients who received Seldane, provides information on adverse experience incidence for periods of a few days up to six months. The usual dose in these studies was 60 mg twice daily, but in a small number of patients, the dose was as low as 20 mg twice a day, or as high as 600 mg daily.

In controlled clinical studies using the recommended dose of 60 mg b.i.d., the incidence of reported adverse effects in patients receiving Seldane was similar to that reported in patients receiving placebo.

[See table above].

ADVERSE EVENTS REPORTED IN CLINICAL TRIALS

Percent of Patients Reporting

Adverse Event	Controlled Studies* Seldane N = 781	Controlled Studies* Placebo N = 665	Controlled Studies* Control N = 626***	All Clinical Studies** Seldane N = 2462	All Clinical Studies** Placebo N = 1478
Central Nervous System					
Drowsiness	9.0	8.1	18.1	8.5	8.2
Headache	6.3	7.4	3.8	15.8	11.2
Fatigue	2.9	0.9	5.8	4.5	3.0
Dizziness	1.4	1.1	1.0	1.5	1.2
Nervousness	0.9	0.2	0.6	1.7	1.0
Weakness	0.9	0.6	0.2	0.6	0.5
Appetite increase	0.6	0.0	0.0	0.5	0.0
Gastrointestinal System					
Gastrointestinal Distress (Abdominal distress, Nausea, Vomiting, Change in Bowel habits)	4.6	3.0	2.7	7.6	5.4
Eye, Ear, Nose, and Throat					
Dry Mouth/Nose/Throat	2.3	1.8	3.5	4.8	3.1
Cough	0.9	0.2	0.5	2.5	1.7
Sore Throat	0.5	0.3	0.5	3.2	1.6
Epistaxis	0.0	0.8	0.2	0.7	0.4
Skin					
Eruption or itching	1.0	1.7	1.4	1.6	2.0

* Duration of treatment in "CONTROLLED STUDIES" was usually 7–14 DAYS.

** Duration of treatment in "ALL CLINICAL STUDIES" was up to 6 months.

*** CONTROL DRUGS: Chlorpheniramine (291 patients), d-Chlorpheniramine (189 patients), Clemastine (146 patients)

In addition to the more frequent side effects reported in clinical trials (See Table), adverse effects have been reported at a lower incidence in clinical trials and/or spontaneously during marketing of Seldane that warrant listing as possibly associated with drug administration. These include: alopecia, anaphylaxis, angioedema, bronchospasm, depression, galactorrhea, insomnia, menstrual disorders (including dysmenorrhea), musculoskeletal pain, nightmares, palpitation, paresthesia, sweating, tachycardia, tremor, urinary frequency, and visual disturbances. In clinical trials, several instances of mild, or in one case, moderate transaminase elevations were seen in patients receiving Seldane. Mild elevations were also seen in placebo treated patients. Foreign marketing experiences include isolated reports of jaundice, cholestatic hepatitis, and hepatitis; in most cases available information is incomplete. In neither the clinical trials nor foreign experience is a causal relationship of liver abnormalities to Seldane use clear.

OVERDOSAGE

One case of overdosage has been reported in a 16-year-old female who took 25 tablets (1500 mg). She was seen approximately one hour after ingestion and treated by gastric lavage. Her recovery was complete and uneventful except for a decrease in BP from 110/60 to 90/50 mmHg two hours after admission.

Continued on next page

Information on Merrell Dow products is based on labeling in effect in May, 1986.

Merrell Dow—Cont.

Treatment of overdosage would reasonably consist of emesis (ipecac syrup), except in patients with impaired consciousness, followed by the administration of activated charcoal to absorb any remaining drug. If vomiting is unsuccessful, or contraindicated, gastric lavage should be performed with normal saline. Saline cathartics may also be of value for rapid dilution of the bowel contents. It is not known if terfenadine is dialyzable.
Treatment of the signs and symptoms of overdosage should be symptomatic and supportive after the acute stage.
Oral LD_{50} values for terfenadine were greater than 5000 mg/kg in mature mice and rats. The oral LD_{50} was 438 mg/kg in newborn rats. Single doses as high as ten times (600 mg) the recommended therapeutic dose in adults have been well tolerated.

DOSAGE AND ADMINISTRATION

The usual dosage for adults and children 12 years and older is 60 mg (1 tablet) twice daily.

HOW SUPPLIED

NDC 0068-0723-61

60 mg tablets in bottles of 100. Tablets are round, white, and debossed "SELDANE". Store tablets at controlled room temperature (59°–86°F) (15°–30°C). Protect from exposure to temperatures above 104°F (40°C) and moisture.

Product Information as of May, 1985
Shown in Product Identification Section, page 418

TACE® ℞

[tās]
(CHLOROTRIANISENE USP)
12 mg and 25 mg
Capsules

AVAILABLE ONLY ON PRESCRIPTION

WARNINGS

1. ESTROGENS HAVE BEEN REPORTED TO INCREASE THE RISK RATIO FOR ENDOMETRIAL CARCINOMA.
Three independent case control studies have reported an increased risk ratio of endometrial cancer in postmenopausal women exposed to exogenous estrogens for prolonged periods.[1-3] This reported risk was independent of the other risk factors studied. Additionally, the incidence rates of endometrial cancer have increased since 1969 in 8 different areas of the United States with population-based cancer reporting systems, an increase that may [or may not] be related to the expanded use of estrogens during the last decade.[4]
The 3 case control studies reported that the estimated risk ratio for endometrial cancer in estrogen users was about 4.5 to 13.9 times greater than in nonusers. The risk appeared to depend on both duration of treatment[1] and on estrogen dose.[3] In view of these reports, when estrogens are used for the treatment of menopausal symptoms, the lowest dose that will control symptoms should be utilized and medication should be discontinued as soon as possible. When prolonged treatment is medically indicated, the patient should be reassessed on at least a semiannual basis to determine the need for continued therapy. Although the evidence must be considered preliminary, one study suggests that cyclic administration of low doses of estrogen may carry less risk than continuous administration;[3] it therefore appears prudent to utilize such a regimen.
Close clinical surveillance of all women taking estrogens is important. In all cases of undiagnosed persistent or recurring abnormal vaginal bleeding, adequate diagnostic measures should be undertaken to rule out malignancy.
There is no evidence at present that "natural" estrogens are more or less hazardous than "synthetic" estrogens at equiestrogenic doses.
2. ESTROGENS SHOULD NOT BE USED DURING PREGNANCY.
The use of exogenous estrogens and progestagens during early pregnancy has been reported to damage the offspring. An association has been reported between *in utero* exposure of the female fetus to diethylstilbestrol, a nonsteroidal estrogen, and an increased risk of the post-pubertal development of an ordinarily rare form of vaginal or cervical cancer.[5,6] This risk for diethylstilbestrol was recently estimated to be in the range of 0.14 to 1.4 per 1000 exposures,[7] consistent with a previous risk estimate of not greater than 4 per 1000 exposures.[8] Furthermore, a high percentage of such females exposed *in utero* (30 to over 90%) has been reported to have vaginal adenosis, epithelial changes of the vagina and cervix.[9-12] Although these changes are histologically benign, it is not known whether they are precursors of adenocarcinoma. Although similar data are not available with the use of other estrogens, it cannot be presumed they would not induce similar changes.
Several reports suggest a possible association between fetal exposure to exogenous estrogens and progestagens and congenital anomalies, including congenital heart defects and limb reduction defects.[13-16] One case control study[16] estimated a 4.7 fold increased risk of limb reduction defects in infants exposed *in utero* to exogenous steroids (oral contraceptives, hormone withdrawal tests for pregnancy, or attempted treatment for threatened abortion). Some of these exposures were very short and involved only a few days of treatment. The data suggest that the risk of limb reduction defects in exposed fetuses is somewhat less than 1 per 1000.
This product is not for use in therapy of threatened or habitual abortion.
If TACE (CHLOROTRIANISENE USP) is used during pregnancy, or if the patient becomes pregnant while taking this drug, she should be apprised of the potential risks to the fetus, and the advisability of pregnancy continuation.

DESCRIPTION

TACE (CHLOROTRIANISENE USP) is a long-acting, synthetic estrogen in capsule form suitable for oral administration.
Each green, soft gelatin capsule contains 12 mg of chlorotrianisene. This capsule also contains inactive ingredients: corn oil (solvent), FD&C Blue No. 1, FD&C Yellow No. 5 (tartrazine, See PRECAUTIONS), gelatin, glycerin, methylparaben, propylparaben, titanium dioxide, and water. Each two-tone green, hard gelatin capsule contains 25 mg of chlorotrianisene. This capsule also contains inactive ingredients: FD&C Blue No. 1 *or* FD&C Green No. 3, FD&C Blue No. 2, FD&C Red No. 40, FD&C Yellow No. 5 (tartrazine, See PRECAUTIONS), FD&C Yellow No. 6, gelatin, iron oxide, magnesium stearate, titanium oxide, and tristearin (solvent).
Chemistry
Generic name: Chlorotrianisene USP
Chemical name: Benzene, 1, 1′, 1″-(1-chloro - 1 - ethenyl - 2 - ylidene) tris [4 - methoxy]-. Chlorotris (*p* -methoxyphenyl) ethylene.
Chlorotrianisene occurs as small, white crystals or as a crystalline powder. It is odorless. It is slightly soluble in alcohol and very slightly soluble in water.

INDICATIONS

1. Postpartum breast engorgement—Although estrogens have been widely used for the prevention of postpartum breast engorgement, controlled studies have demonstrated that the incidence of significant painful engorgement in patients not receiving such hormonal therapy is low and usually responsive to appropriate analgesic or other supportive therapy. Consequently, the benefit to be derived from estrogen therapy for this indication must be carefully weighed against the potential risk of puerperal thromboembolism associated with the use of estrogens.[17]
2. Prostatic carcinoma—palliative therapy of advanced disease.
3. Moderate to severe *vasomotor* symptoms associated with the menopause. (There is no well-documented evidence that estrogens are effective for nervous symptoms or depression which might occur during menopause and they should not be used to treat these conditions.)
4. Atrophic vaginitis.
5. Kraurosis vulvae.
6. Female hypogonadism.

TACE (CHLOROTRIANISENE USP) HAS NOT BEEN SHOWN TO BE EFFECTIVE FOR ANY PURPOSE DURING PREGNANCY, AND ITS USE MAY HAVE POTENTIAL RISKS TO THE FETUS. (SEE BOXED WARNING.)

CONTRAINDICATIONS

TACE (CHLOROTRIANISENE USP) should not be used in women or men with any of the following conditions:
1. Known or suspected cancer of the breast except in appropriately selected patients being treated for metastatic disease.
2. Known or suspected estrogen-dependent neoplasia.
3. Known or suspected pregnancy (See Boxed Warning.)
4. Undiagnosed abnormal genital bleeding.
5. Active thrombophlebitis or thromboembolic disorders.
6. A past history of thrombophlebitis, thrombosis, or thromboembolic disorders (except when used in treatment of prostatic malignancy).

WARNINGS

1. *Induction of malignant neoplasms.* Long-term continuous administration of natural and synthetic estrogens in certain animal species increases the frequency of carcinomas of the breast, cervix, vagina, and liver. There are now reports that estrogens increase the risk of carcinoma of the endometrium in humans. (See Boxed Warning.)
At the present time there is no satisfactory evidence that estrogens given to postmenopausal women increase the risk of cancer of the breast,[18] although a recent long-term followup of a single physician's practice has raised this possibility.[19] Because of the animal data, there is a need for caution in prescribing estrogens for women with a strong family history of breast cancer or who have breast nodules, fibrocystic disease, or abnormal mammograms.
2. *Gallbladder disease.* A recent study has reported a two to threefold increase in the risk of surgically confirmed gallbladder disease in women receiving postmenopausal estrogens,[18] similar to the twofold increase previously noted in users of oral contraceptives.[20] In the case of oral contraceptives the increased risk appeared after a period of use.[20]
3. *Effects similar to those caused by estrogen-progestagen oral contraceptives.* There are several adverse effects reported in association with oral contraceptives, most of which have not been documented as consequences of postmenopausal estrogen therapy, although it has been reported that there is an increased risk of thrombosis in men receiving high doses of estrogens for prostatic cancer and in women receiving estrogens for postpartum breast engorgement.[17,21-23] The possibility that the adverse effects reported in association with oral contraceptives may be associated with larger doses of estrogen cannot be excluded.
a. *Thromboembolic disease.* Studies have now shown that users of oral contraceptives have an increased risk of various thromboembolic, thrombotic, and vascular diseases, such as thrombophlebitis, pulmonary embolism, stroke, and myocardial infarction.[24-31] Cases of retinal thrombosis, mesenteric thrombosis, and optic neuritis have been reported in oral contraceptive users. There is evidence that the risk of several of these adverse reactions is related to the dose of the drug.[32,33] An increased risk of post-surgery thromboembolic complications has also been reported in users of oral contraceptives.[34,35] If feasible, estrogen should be discontinued at least 4 weeks before surgery of the type associated with an increased risk of thromboembolism, or during periods of prolonged immobilization.
While an increased rate of thromboembolic and thrombotic disease in postmenopausal users of estrogens has not been found,[18,36] this does not rule out the possibility that such an increase may be present, or that subgroups of women who have underlying risk factors, or who are receiving relatively large doses of estrogens may have an increased risk. Therefore, estrogens should not be used in persons with active thrombophlebitis or thromboembolic disorders, and they should not be used (except in treatment of malignancy) in persons with a history of such disorders. They should be used with caution in patients with cerebral vascular or coronary artery disease and only for those in whom estrogens are needed.
Doses of estrogen (5 mg conjugated estrogens per day), comparable to those used to treat cancer of the prostate and breast, have been reported in a large prospective clinical trial in men[37] to increase the risk of nonfatal myocardial infarction, pulmonary embolism, and thrombophlebitis. When estrogen doses of this size are used, any of the thromboembolic and thrombotic adverse effects associated with oral contraceptive use should be considered as a risk.
b. *Hepatic adenoma.* Benign hepatic adenomas have been reported to be associated with the use of oral contraceptives.[38-40] Although benign and rare, these may rupture and may cause death through intra-abdominal hemorrhage. Such lesions have not yet been reported in association with other estrogen or progestagen preparations but should be considered in estrogen users having abdominal pain and tenderness, abdominal mass, or hypovolemic shock. Hepatocellular carcinoma has also been reported in women taking estrogen-containing oral contraceptives.[39] The relationship of this malignancy to these drugs is not known at this time.
c. *Elevated blood pressure.* Increased blood pressure is not uncommon in women using oral contraceptives and there is now a report that this may occur with use of estrogens in the menopause[41] and blood pressure should be monitored with estrogen use, especially if high doses are used.
d. *Glucose tolerance.* A worsening of glucose tolerance has been observed in a significant percentage of patients on estrogen-containing oral contraceptives. For this reason diabetic patients should be carefully observed while receiving estrogen.
4. *Hypercalcemia.* Administration of estrogens may lead to hypercalcemia in patients with breast cancer and bone metastases. If this occurs, the drug should be stopped and appropriate measures taken to reduce the serum calcium level.

PRECAUTIONS

A. General Precautions
1. A complete medical and family history should be taken prior to the initiation of any estrogen therapy. The pretreatment and periodic physical examinations should include special reference to blood pressure, breasts, abdomen, and pelvic organs, and should include a Papanicolaou smear. As a general rule, estrogen should not be prescribed for longer

than 1 year without another physical examination being performed.

2. Fluid retention—Because estrogens may cause some degree of fluid retention, conditions that might be influenced by this factor such as epilepsy, migraine, and cardiac or renal dysfunction require careful observation.

3. Certain patients may develop undesirable manifestations of excessive estrogenic stimulation, such as abnormal or excessive uterine bleeding, mastodynia, etc.

4. Oral contraceptives have been reported to be associated with an increased incidence of mental depression. Although it is not clear whether this is possibly due to the estrogenic or progestagenic component of the contraceptive, patients with a history of depression should be carefully observed.

5. Patients having pre-existing uterine leiomyomata should be observed for increased growth of myomata during estrogen therapy.

6. The pathologist should be advised of estrogen therapy when relevant specimens are submitted.

7. Patients with a past history of jaundice during pregnancy have an increased risk of recurrence of jaundice while receiving estrogen-containing oral contraceptive therapy. If jaundice develops in any patient receiving estrogen, the medication should be discontinued while the cause is investigated.

8. Estrogens may be poorly metabolized in patients with impaired liver function and they should be administered with caution in such patients.

9. Because estrogens influence the metabolism of calcium and phosphorus, they should be used with caution in patients with metabolic bone diseases that are associated with hypercalcemia or in patients with renal insufficiency.

10. Because of the effects of estrogens on epiphyseal closure, they should be used judiciously in young patients in whom bone growth is not complete.

11. Judicious assessment of the following changes in certain endocrine and liver function tests is necessary for patients receiving large doses of estrogen:

a. Increased sulfobromophthalein retention.

b. Increased prothrombin and factors VII, VIII, IX, and X; decreased antithrombin 3; increased norepinephrine-induced platelet aggregability.

c. Increased thyroid binding globulin (TBG) leading to increased circulating total thyroid hormone, as measured by PBI, T4 by column, or T4 by radioimmunoassay. Free T3 resin uptake is decreased, reflecting the elevated TBG; free T4 concentration is unaltered.

d. Impaired glucose tolerance.

e. Decreased pregnanediol excretion.

f. Reduced response to metyrapone test.

g. Reduced serum folate concentration.

h. Increased serum triglyceride, phospholipid, or cholesterol.

12. This product contains FD&C Yellow No. 5 (tartrazine), which may cause allergic-type reactions (including bronchial asthma) in certain susceptible individuals. Although the overall incidence of FD&C Yellow No. 5 (tartrazine) sensitivity in the general population is low, it is frequently seen in patients who also have aspirin hypersensitivity.

B. Information For The Patient

A patient package insert accompanies this drug product. This insert is available from pharmacists who carry this product and from the company upon request.

C. Pregnancy Category X

See Contraindications and Boxed Warning.

D. Nursing Mothers

As a general principle, the administration of any drug to nursing mothers should be done only when clearly necessary since many drugs are excreted in human milk.

ADVERSE REACTIONS

(See Warnings regarding reports of induction of neoplasia, adverse effects on the fetus, increased incidence of gallbladder disease, and adverse effects similar to those of oral contraceptives, including thromboembolism.) The following additional adverse reactions have been reported with estrogenic therapy including oral contraceptives:

1. *Genitourinary system*

Breakthrough bleeding, spotting, change in menstrual flow and cycle.

Dysmenorrhea.

Premenstrual-like syndrome.

Amenorrhea during and after treatment.

Increase in size of uterine fibromyomata.

Vaginal candidiasis.

Change in cervical eversion and in degree of cervical secretion.

Cystitis-like syndrome.

2. *Breasts*

Tenderness, enlargement, secretion.

3. *Gastrointestinal*

Nausea, vomiting.

Abdominal cramps, bloating.

Cholestatic jaundice.

4. *Skin*

Chloasma or melasma, which may persist when drug is discontinued.

Erythema multiforme.

Erythema nodosum.

Hemorrhagic eruption.

Loss of scalp hair.

Hirsutism.

Urticaria.

5. *Eyes*

Steepening of corneal curvature.

Intolerance to contact lenses.

6. *CNS*

Headache, migraine, dizziness.

Mental depression.

Chorea.

7. *Miscellaneous*

Increase or decrease in weight.

Reduced carbohydrate tolerance.

Aggravation of porphyria.

Edema.

Changes in libido and/or potency.

ACUTE OVERDOSAGE

Numerous reports of ingestion of large doses of estrogen-containing oral contraceptives by young children indicate that serious ill effects usually do not occur. Overdosage of estrogen may cause nausea, and withdrawal bleeding may occur in females.

DOSAGE AND ADMINISTRATION

Given for a few days

Prevention of postpartum breast engorgement.

The usual dosage is one 12 mg capsule four times daily for 7 days, or two 25 mg capsules every six hours for 6 doses. For immediate postpartum use, the first dose should be given within 8 hours after delivery.

Given chronically

Inoperable progressing prostatic cancer.

The usual dosage is 12 to 25 mg daily (one or two 12 mg capsules or one 25 mg capsule).

Given cyclically for short-term use only

For treatment of moderate to severe *vasomotor* symptoms, atrophic vaginitis, or kraurosis vulvae associated with the menopause.

The lowest dose that will control symptoms should be chosen and medication should be discontinued as promptly as possible.

Administration should be cyclic (*e.g.*, 3 weeks on and 1 week off).

Attempts to discontinue or taper medication should be made at 3-month to 6-month intervals.

The usual dosage range for vasomotor symptoms associated with the menopause is 12 to 25 mg daily (one or two 12 mg capsules or one 25 mg capsule) for 30 days; one or more courses may be prescribed.

The usual dosage range for atrophic vaginitis or kraurosis vulvae is 12 to 25 mg daily (one or two 12 mg capsules or one 25 mg capsule) for 30 to 60 days.

Given cyclically

For female hypogonadism.

The usual dosage is 12 to 25 mg daily (one or two 12 mg capsules or one 25 mg capsule) for 21 days. This course may, if desired, be followed immediately by the intramuscular injection of 100 mg of progesterone; alternatively, an oral progestogen such as medroxyprogesterone may be given during the last 5 days of TACE (CHLOROTRIANISENE USP) therapy. The next course may begin on the 5th day of the induced uterine bleeding.

Treated patients with an intact uterus should be monitored closely for signs of endometrial cancer, and appropriate diagnostic measures should be taken to rule out malignancy in the event of persistent or recurrent abnormal vaginal bleeding.

HOW SUPPLIED

TACE 12 mg (CHLOROTRIANISENE CAPSULES USP) green capsules imprinted MERRELL 690

NDC 0068-0690-61: bottles of 100

TACE 25 mg (CHLOROTRIANISENE CAPSULES USP) two-tone green capsules imprinted MERRELL 691

NDC 0068-0691-60: bottles of 60

REFERENCES

1. Ziel, H.K. and Finkel, W.D.: Increased risk of endometrial carcinoma among users of conjugated estrogens. New Eng. J. Med. 293:1167–1170, 1975.

2. Smith, D.C., Prentice, R., Thompson, D.J., and Hermann, W.L.: Association of exogenous estrogen and endometrial carcinoma. New Eng. J. Med. 293:1164–1167, 1975.

3. Mack, T.M., Pike, M.C., Henderson, B.E., Pfeffer, R. I., Gerkins, V.R., Arthur, M., and Brown, S.E.: Estrogens and endometrial cancer in a retirement community. New Eng. J. Med. 294:1262–1267, 1976.

4. Weiss, N.S., Szekely, D.R., and Austin, D.F.: Increasing incidence of endometrial cancer in the United States. New Eng. J. Med. 294:1259–1262, 1976.

5. Herbst, A.L., Ulfelder, H., and Poskanzer, D.C.: Adenocarcinoma of the vagina. New Eng. J. Med. 284:878–881, 1971.

6. Greenwald, P., Barlow, J.J., Nasca, P.C., and Burnett, W.S.: Vaginal cancer after maternal treatment with synthetic estrogens. New Eng. J. Med. 285: 390–392, 1971.

7. Herbst, A.L., Cole, P., Colton, T., Robboy, S.J., and Scully, R.E.: Age-incidence and risk of diethylstilbestrol-related clear cell adenocarcinoma of the vagina and cervix. Amer. J. Obstet. Gynec. 128:43–50, 1977.

8. Lanier, A.P., Noller, K.L., Decker, D.G., Elveback, L.R., and Kurland, L.T.: Cancer and Stilbestrol. A follow-up of 1719 persons exposed to estrogens in utero and born 1943–1959. Mayo Clin. Proc. 48:793–799, 1973.

9. Herbst, A.L., Kurman, R.J., and Scully, R.E.: Vaginal and cervical abnormalities after exposure to stilbestrol in utero. Obstet. Gynec. 40:287-298, 1972.

10. Herbst, A.L., Poskanzer, D.C., Robboy, S.J., Friedlander, L. and Scully, R.E.: Prenatal exposure to stilbestrol. A prospective comparison of exposed female offspring with unexposed controls. New Eng. J. Med. 292:334–339, 1975.

11. Stafl, A., Mattingly, R.F., Foley, D.V., and Fetherston, W.C.: Clinical diagnosis of vaginal adenosis. Obstet. Gynec. 43:118–128, 1974.

12. Sherman, A.I., Goldrath, M., Berlin A., Vakhariya, V., Banooni, F., Michaels, W., Goodman, P., and Brown, S.: Cervical-vaginal adenosis after *in utero* exposure to synthetic estrogens. Obstet. Gynec. 44:531–545, 1974.

13. Gal, I., Kirman, B., Stern, J.: Hormone pregnancy tests and congenital malformation. Nature 216:83, 1967.

14. Levy, E.P., Cohen, A., and Fraser, F.C.: Hormone treatment during pregnancy and congenital heart defects. Lancet 1:611, 1973.

15. Nora, J.J. and Nora, A.H.: Birth defects and oral contraceptives. Lancet 1:941–942, 1973.

16. Janerich, D.T., Piper, J.M., and Glebatis, D.M.: Oral contraceptives and congenital limb-reduction defects. New Eng. J. Med. 291:697–700, 1974.

17. Daniel, D.G., Campbell, H., and Turnbull, A.C.: Puerperal thromboembolism and suppression of lactation. Lancet 2:287–289, 1967.

18. Boston Collaborative Drug Surveillance Program: Surgically confirmed gall bladder disease, venous thromboembolism, and breast tumors in relation to post menopausal estrogen therapy. New Eng. J. Med. 290:15–19, 1974.

19. Hoover, R., Gray, L.A., Sr., Cole, P., and MacMahon, B.: Menopausal estrogens and breast cancer. New Eng. J. Med. 295:401–405, 1976.

20. Boston Collaborative Drug Surveillance Program: Oral contraceptives and venous thromboembolic disease, surgically confirmed gall-bladder disease, and breast tumors. Lancet 1:1399–1404, 1973.

21. Bailar, J.C., III: Thromboembolism and oestrogen therapy. Lancet 2:560, 1967.

22. The Veterans Administration Cooperative Urological Research Group: Carcinoma of the prostate: Treatment comparisons. J. Urol. 98:516–522, 1967.

23. Blackard, C.E., Doe, R.P., Mellinger, G.T., and Byar, D.P.: Incidence of cardiovascular disease and death in patients receiving diethylstilbestrol for carcinoma of the prostate. Cancer 26:249–256, 1970.

24. Royal College of General Practitioners: Oral contraception and thromboembolic disease. J. Roy. Coll. Gen. Pract. 13:267–269, 1967.

25. Inman, W.H.W. and Vessey, M.P.: Investigation of deaths from pulmonary, coronary, and cerebral thrombosis and embolism in women of child-bearing age. Brit. Med. J. 2:193–199, 1968.

26. Vessey, M.P. and Doll, R.: Investigation of relation between use of oral contraceptives and thromboembolic disease. A further report. Brit. Med. J. 2:651–657, 1969.

27. Sartwell, P.E., Masi, A.T., Arthes, F.G., Greene, G.R. and Smith, H.E.: Thromboembolism and oral contraceptives: An epidemiological case-control study. Amer. J. Epidem. 90:365-380, 1969.

28. Collaborative Group for the Study of Stroke in Young Women: Oral contraception and increased risk of cerebral ischemia or thrombosis. New Eng. J. Med. 288:871–878, 1973.

29. Collaborative Group for the Study of Stroke in Young Women: Oral contraceptives and stroke in young women: Associated risk factors. J.A.M.A. 231:718–722, 1975.

30. Mann, J.I. and Inman, W.H.W.: Oral contraceptives and death from myocardial infarction. Brit. Med. J. 2:245–248, 1975.

31. Mann, J.I., Vessey, M.P., Thorogood, M., and Doll, R.: Myocardial infarction in young women with special refer-

Continued on next page

Information on Merrell Dow products is based on labeling in effect in May, 1986.

Merrell Dow—Cont.

ence in oral contraceptive practice. Brit. Med. J. 2:241–245, 1975.

32. Inman, W.H.W., Vessey, M.P., Westerholm, B., and Engelund, A.: Thromboembolic disease and the steroidal content of oral contraceptives. A report to the Committee on Safety of Drugs. Brit. Med. J. 2:203–209, 1970.
33. Stolley, P.D., Tonascia, J.A., Tockman, M.S., Sartwell, P.E., Rutledge, A.H., and Jacobs, M.P.: Thrombosis with low-estrogen oral contraceptives. Amer. J. Epidem. 102:197–208, 1975.
34. Vessey, M.P., Doll, R., Fairbairn, A.S., and Glober, G.: Post-operative thromboembolism and the use of the oral contraceptives. Brit. Med. J. 3:123–126, 1970.
35. Greene, G.R. and Sartwell, P.E.: Oral contraceptive use in patients with thromboembolism following surgery, trauma, or infection. Amer. J. Public Health 62:680–685, 1972.
36. Rosenberg, L., Armstrong, B., Phil. D., and Jick H.: Myocardial infarction and estrogen therapy in post-menopausal women. New Eng. J. Med. 294:1256–1259, 1976.
37. Coronary Drug Project Research Group: The coronary drug project: initial findings leading to modifications of its research protocol. J.A.M.A. 214:1303–1313, 1970.
38. Baum, J., Holtz, F., Bookstein, J.J., and Klein, E.W.: Possible association between benign hepatomas and oral contraceptives. Lancet 2:926–928, 1973.
39. Mays, E.T., Christopherson, W.M., Mahr, M.M., and Williams, H.C.: Hepatic changes in young women ingesting contraceptive steroids. Hepatic hemorrhage and primary hepatic tumors. J.A.M.A. 235:730–732, 1976.
40. Edmondson, H., Henderson, A.B., and Benton, B.: Liver-cell adenomas associated with the use of oral contraceptives. New Eng. J. Med. 294:470–472, 1976.
41. Pfeffer, R.I. and Van Den Noort, S.: Estrogen use and stroke risk in postmenopausal women. Amer. J. Epidem. 103:445–456, 1976.

Product Information as of April, 1985

TACE 12 mg Capsules
Manufactured by
R. P. Scherer, North America
Clearwater, Florida 33518 for
MERRELL DOW PHARMACEUTICALS INC.
Subsidiary of The Dow Chemical Company
Cincinnati, Ohio 45215, U.S.A.

TACE® ℞
(CHLOROTRIANISENE)
12 mg and 25 mg
Capsules

INFORMATION FOR PATIENTS

TACE (CHLOROTRIANISENE) is a synthetic estrogen supplied in 12 mg, 25 mg, and 72 mg capsules.

What You Should Know About Estrogens: Estrogens are female hormones produced by the ovaries. The ovaries make several different kinds of estrogens. In addition, scientists have been able to make a variety of synthetic estrogens. As far as we know, all these estrogens have many similar properties and therefore much the same usefulness, side effects, and risks. This leaflet is intended to help you understand what estrogens are sometimes used for, the risks involved in their use, and how to use them as safely as possible.

This leaflet includes important information about estrogens, but not all the information. If you want to know more, you can ask your doctor or pharmacist to let you read the package insert for this product prepared for the doctor.

USES OF ESTROGEN

Estrogens are prescribed by doctors for a number of purposes, including:

1. To provide estrogen during a period of adjustment when a woman's ovaries produce it in decreased amounts in order to prevent certain uncomfortable symptoms of estrogen deficiency. (All women normally produce less estrogen, generally between the ages of 45 and 55; this is called the menopause.)
2. To prevent symptoms of estrogen deficiency when a woman's ovaries have been removed surgically before the natural menopause.
3. To prevent pregnancy. (Estrogens are given along with a progestagen, another female hormone; these combinations are called oral contraceptives or birth control pills. Patient labeling is available to women taking oral contraceptives and they will not be discussed in this leaflet.) *This product is not intended to prevent pregnancy.*
4. To treat certain cancers in women and men. *This product is not intended to treat cancers in women.*
5. To prevent painful swelling of the breasts after pregnancy in women who choose not to nurse their babies.

THERE IS NO PROPER USE OF TACE IN A PREGNANT WOMAN.

ESTROGENS IN THE MENOPAUSE

In the natural course of their lives, all women eventually experience a decrease in estrogen production. This usually occurs between ages 45 and 55 but may occur earlier or later. Sometimes the ovaries may need to be removed before or during natural menopause by an operation, producing a "surgical menopause."

When the amount of estrogen in the blood begins to decrease, many women may develop typical symptoms: feelings of warmth in the face, neck, and chest or sudden intense episodes of heat and sweating throughout the body (called "hot flashes" or "hot flushes"). These symptoms are sometimes very uncomfortable. A few women eventually develop changes in the vagina (called "atrophic vaginitis") which cause discomfort, especially during and after intercourse.

Estrogens can be prescribed to treat these symptoms of the menopause. It is estimated that considerably more than half of all women undergoing the menopause have only mild symptoms or no symptoms at all and therefore do not need estrogens. Other women may need estrogens for a few months, while their bodies adjust to lower estrogen levels. Sometimes the need will be for periods longer than six months. In an attempt to avoid overstimulation of the uterus (womb), estrogens are usually given cyclically during each month of use, that is, three weeks of pills followed by one week without pills.

Sometimes women experience nervous symptoms or depression during menopause. There is no well-documented evidence that estrogens are effective for such symptoms and they should not be used to treat them, although other treatment may be needed.

You may have heard that taking estrogens for long periods (years) after the menopause will keep your skin soft and supple and keep you feeling young. There is no evidence that this is so, however, and such long-term treatment carries important risks.

ESTROGENS TO PREVENT SWELLING OF THE BREASTS AFTER PREGNANCY

If you do not breast feed your baby after delivery, your breasts may fill up with milk and become engorged and painful. This usually begins about 3 to 4 days after delivery and may last for a few days to up to a week or more. Sometimes the discomfort is severe, but usually it is not and can be controlled by pain relieving drugs such as aspirin and by binding the breasts up tightly. Estrogens can be used to try to prevent the breasts from filling up.

While this treatment is usually successful in reducing amount of filling, in many cases the breasts fill up to some degree in spite of treatment. The daily dose of estrogens needed to prevent pain and swelling of the breasts is larger than the dose needed to treat symptoms of the menopause and this may increase your chances of developing blood clots in the legs or lungs. (See below.) Therefore, it is important that you discuss the benefits and the risks of estrogen use with your doctor if you have decided not to breast feed your baby.

THE DANGERS OF ESTROGENS

1. *Cancer of the uterus.* Several independent studies have reported an increased risk ratio of endometrial cancer (cancer of the lining of the uterus) if estrogens are used in the post-menopausal period for more than a year. Women taking estrogens are reported to have roughly 5 to 10 times as great a chance of getting this cancer as women who take no estrogens. To put this another way, while a postmenopausal woman not taking estrogens has 1 chance in 1,000 each year of getting cancer of the uterus, a woman taking estrogens has 5 to 10 chances in 1,000 each year. For this reason *it is important to take estrogens only when you really need them.*

The risk of this cancer is reported to be greater the longer estrogens are used and also seems to be greater when larger doses are taken. For this reason *it is important to take the lowest dose of estrogen that will control symptoms and to take it only as long as it is needed.* If estrogens are needed for longer periods of time, your doctor will want to reevaluate your need for estrogens at least every six months.

Women using estrogens should report any irregular vaginal bleeding to their doctors; such bleeding may be of no importance, but it can be an early warning of cancer of the uterus. If you have undiagnosed vaginal bleeding, you should not use estrogens until a diagnosis is made that there is no cancer of the uterus.

If you have had your uterus completely removed (total hysterectomy), there is no danger of developing cancer of the uterus.

2. *Other possible cancers.* Long-term continuous administration of estrogens in certain animal species increases the frequency of cancers of the breast, cervix, vagina, and liver. At present there is no satisfactory evidence that women using estrogen in the menopause have an increased risk of such tumors, but there is no way yet to be sure they do not; and one study raises the possibility that use of estrogens in the menopause may increase the risk of breast cancer many years later. This is a further reason to use estrogens only when clearly needed. While you are taking estrogens, it is important that you go to your doctor at least every six months for an examination. Also, if members of your family have had breast cancer or if you have breast nodules or abnormal mammograms (breast x-rays), your doctor may wish to carry out more frequent examinations of your breasts.

3. *Gall bladder disease.* Women who use estrogens after menopause are reported to be more likely to develop gall bladder disease needing surgery than women who do not use estrogens. Birth control pills have a similar effect.

4. *Abnormal blood clotting.* Oral contraceptives increase the risk of blood clotting in various parts of the body. This can result in a stroke (if the clot is in the brain), a heart attack (clot in a blood vessel of the heart), or a pulmonary embolus (a clot which forms in the legs or pelvis, then breaks off and travels to the lungs). Any of these can be fatal.

At this time use of estrogens in the menopause is not known to cause such blood clotting, but the possibility that such clotting in association with oral contraceptives may be associated with larger doses of estrogen cannot be excluded. It is recommended that if you have had clotting in the legs or lungs or a heart attack or stroke while you were using estrogens or birth control pills, you should not use estrogens (unless they are being used to treat cancer of the breast or prostate). If you have had a stroke or heart attack or if you have angina pectoris, estrogens should be used with caution and only if clearly needed (for example, if you have severe symptoms of the menopause).

The larger doses of estrogen used to prevent swelling of the breasts after pregnancy have been reported to increase the risk of clotting in the legs and lungs.

Special Warning About Pregnancy: You should not receive estrogen if you are pregnant. It has been reported that there is a greater than usual chance that the developing child will be born with a birth defect, although the possibility remains fairly small. It is also reported that a female child may have an increased risk of developing cancer of the vagina or cervix later in life (in the teens or twenties). Every possible effort should be made to avoid exposure to TACE during pregnancy. If exposure occurs, see your doctor.

Other Effects of Estrogens: In addition to the serious reported risks of estrogens described above, estrogens have the following side effects and potential risks:

1. *Nausea and vomiting.* The most common side effect of estrogen therapy is nausea. Vomiting is less common.
2. *Effects on breasts.* Estrogens may cause breast tenderness or enlargement and may cause the breasts to secrete a liquid. These effects are not dangerous.
3. *Effects on the uterus.* Estrogens may cause benign fibroid tumors of the uterus to get larger.

Some women will have menstrual bleeding when estrogens are stopped. But if the bleeding occurs on days you are still taking estrogens you should report this to your doctor.

4. *Effects on liver.* Women taking oral contraceptives develop on rare occasions a tumor of the liver which can rupture and bleed into the abdomen. So far, these tumors have not been reported in women using estrogens in the menopause, but you should report any swelling or unusual pain or tenderness in the abdomen to your doctor immediately.

Women with a past history of jaundice (yellowing of the skin and white parts of the eyes) may get jaundice again during estrogen use. If this occurs, stop taking estrogens and see your doctor.

5. *Other effects.* Estrogens may cause excess fluid to be retained in the body. This may make some conditions worse, such as epilepsy, migraine, heart disease, or kidney disease.

SUMMARY

Estrogens have important uses, but they have reported risks of potentially serious conditions developing as well. You must decide, with your doctor, whether the risks are acceptable to you in view of the benefits of treatment. Except where your doctor has prescribed TACE for use in special cases of cancer of the prostate, you should not use TACE if you have cancer of the breast or uterus, are pregnant, have undiagnosed abnormal vaginal bleeding, clotting in the legs or lungs, or have had a stroke, heart attack or angina, or clotting in the legs or lungs in the past while you were taking estrogens.

You can use TACE as safely as possible by understanding that your doctor will require regular physical examinations while you are taking it and will try to discontinue the drug as soon as possible and use the smallest dose possible. Be alert for signs of trouble including:

1. Abnormal bleeding from the vagina.
2. Pains in the calves or chest or sudden shortness of breath, or coughing blood (indicating possible clots in the legs, heart, or lungs).
3. Severe headache, dizziness, faintness, or changes in vision (indicating possible developing clots in the brain or eye).
4. Breast lumps. (You should ask your doctor how to examine your own breasts.)
5. Jaundice (yellowing of the skin).
6. Mental depression.

Based on his or her assessment of your medical needs, your doctor has prescribed this drug for you. Do not give this drug to anyone else.

HOW SUPPLIED

TACE (CHLOROTRIANISENE) is a long-acting synthetic estrogen in capsule form. The capsule is suitable for taking by mouth.

Each green, soft gelatin capsule imprinted MERRELL 690 contains 12 mg of chlorotrianisene. This capsule also contains inactive ingredients: corn oil (solvent), FD&C Blue No. 1, FD&C Yellow No. 5 (tartrazine) as a color additive, gelatin, glycerin, methylparaben, propylparaben, titanium dioxide, and water.

Each two-tone green, hard gelatin capsule imprinted MERRELL 691 contains 25 mg of chlorotrianisene. This capsule also contains inactive ingredients: FD&C Blue No. 1 *or* FD&C Green No. 3, FD&C Blue No. 2, FD&C Red No. 40, FD&C Yellow No. 5 (tartrazine) as a color additive, FD&C Yellow No. 6, gelatin, iron oxide, magnesium stearate, titanium dioxide, and tristearin (solvent).

Patient Information as of April, 1985
Shown in Product Identification Section, page 418

TACE® ℞
[*tās*]
(CHLOROTRIANISENE USP)
72 mg Capsules

AVAILABLE ONLY ON PRESCRIPTION

WARNINGS

1. ESTROGENS HAVE BEEN REPORTED TO INCREASE THE RISK RATIO FOR ENDOMETRIAL CARCINOMA.

Three independent case control studies have reported an increased risk ratio of endometrial cancer in postmenopausal women exposed to exogenous estrogens for prolonged periods.[1-3] This reported risk was independent of the other risk factors studied. Additionally, the incidence rates of endometrial cancer have increased since 1969 in 8 different areas of the United States with population-based cancer reporting systems, an increase that may [or may not] be related to the expanded use of estrogens during the last decade.[4]

The 3 case control studies reported that the estimated risk ratio for endometrial cancer in estrogen users was about 4.5 to 13.9 times greater than in nonusers. The risk appeared to depend on both duration of treatment[1] and on estrogen dose.[3] In view of these reports, when estrogens are used for the treatment of menopausal symptoms, the lowest dose that will control symptoms should be utilized and medication should be discontinued as soon as possible. When prolonged treatment is medically indicated, the patient should be reassessed on at least a semiannual basis to determine the need for continued therapy. Although the evidence must be considered preliminary, one study suggests that cyclic administration of low doses of estrogen may carry less risk than continuous administration;[3] it therefore appears prudent to utilize such a regimen.

Close clinical surveillance of all women taking estrogens is important. In all cases of undiagnosed persistent or recurring abnormal vaginal bleeding, adequate diagnostic measures should be undertaken to rule out malignancy.

There is no evidence at present that "natural" estrogens are more or less hazardous than "synthetic" estrogens at equiestrogenic doses.

2. ESTROGENS SHOULD NOT BE USED DURING PREGNANCY.

The use of exogenous estrogens and progestagens during early pregnancy has been reported to damage the offspring. An association has been reported between *in utero* exposure of the female fetus to diethylstilbestrol, a non-steroidal estrogen, and an increased risk of the post-pubertal development of an ordinarily rare form of vaginal or cervical cancer.[5,6] This risk for diethylstilbestrol was recently estimated to be in the range of 0.14 to 1.4 per 1000 exposures,[7] consistent with a previous risk estimate of not greater than 4 per 1000 exposures.[8] Furthermore, a high percentage of such females exposed *in utero* (30 to over 90%) has been reported to have vaginal adenosis, epithelial changes of the vagina and cervix.[9-12] Although these changes are histologically benign, it is not known whether they are precursors of adenocarcinoma. Although similar data are not available with the use of other estrogens, it cannot be presumed they would not induce similar changes.

Several reports suggest a possible association between fetal exposure to exogenous estrogens and progestagens and congenital anomalies, including congenital heart defects and limb reduction defects.[13-16] One case control study[16] estimated a 4.7 fold increased risk of limb reduction defects in infants exposed *in utero* to exogenous steriods (oral contraceptives, hormone withdrawal tests for pregnancy, or attempted treatment for threatened abortion). Some of these exposures were very short and involved only a few days of treatment. The data suggest that the risk of limb reduction defects in exposed fetuses is somewhat less than 1 per 1000.

This product is not for use in therapy of threatened or habitual abortion.

If TACE (CHLOROTRIANISENE USP) is used during pregnancy, or if the patient becomes pregnant while taking this drug, she should be apprised of the potential risks to the fetus, and the advisability of pregnancy continuation.

DESCRIPTION

TACE (CHLOROTRIANISENE USP) is a long-acting, synthetic estrogen in capsule form suitable for oral administration.

Each two-tone green and yellow soft gelatin capsule contains 72 mg of TACE (CHLOROTRIANISENE) in Dispex®, an emulsifiable vehicle containing corn oil, sorbitan trioleate, polysorbate 80, and benzyl benzoate. This capsule also contains other inactive ingredients: FD&C Blue No. 1, FD&C Yellow No. 5 (tartrazine, See PRECAUTIONS), gelatin, glycerin, iron oxide, methylparaben, propylparaben, sorbitol, titanium dioxide and water.

Chemistry

Generic name: Chlorotrianisene USP

Chemical name: Benzene, 1, 1′, 1″-(1-chloro-1-ethenyl-2-ylidene) tris [4-methoxy]-. Chlorotris (*p*-methoxyphenyl) ethylene.

Chlorotrianisene occurs as small, white crystals or as a crystalline powder. It is odorless. It is slightly soluble in alcohol and very slightly soluble in water.

INDICATIONS

Postpartum breast engorgement —Although estrogens have been widely used for the prevention of postpartum breast engorgement, controlled studies have demonstrated that the incidence of significant painful engorgement in patients not receiving such hormonal therapy is low and usually responsive to appropriate analgesic or other supportive therapy. Consequently, the benefit to be derived from estrogen therapy for this indication must be carefully weighed against the potential risk of puerperal thromboembolism associated with the use of estrogens.[17]

TACE (CHLOROTRIANISENE USP) HAS NOT BEEN SHOWN TO BE EFFECTIVE FOR ANY PURPOSE DURING PREGNANCY, AND ITS USE MAY HAVE POTENTIAL RISKS TO THE FETUS. (SEE BOXED WARNING.)

CONTRAINDICATIONS

TACE (CHLOROTRIANISENE USP) should not be used in women or men with any of the following conditions:

1. Known or suspected cancer of the breast except in appropriately selected patients being treated for metastatic disease.
2. Known or suspected estrogen-dependent neoplasia.
3. Known or suspected pregnancy. (See Boxed Warning.)
4. Undiagnosed abnormal genital bleeding.
5. Active thrombophlebitis or thromboembolic disorders.
6. A past history of thrombophlebitis, thrombosis, or thromboembolic disorders (except when used in treatment of prostatic malignancy).

WARNINGS

1. *Induction of malignant neoplasms.* Long-term continuous administration of natural and synthetic estrogens in certain animal species increases the frequency of carcinomas of the breast, cervix, vagina, and liver. There are now reports that estrogens increase the risk of carcinoma of the endometrium in humans. (See Boxed Warning.)

At the present time there is no satisfactory evidence that estrogens given to postmenopausal women increase the risk of cancer of the breast,[18] although a recent long-term followup of a single physician's practice has raised this possibility.[19] Because of the animal data, there is a need for caution in prescribing estrogens for women with a strong family history of breast cancer or who have breast nodules, fibrocystic disease, or abnormal mammograms.

2. *Gallbladder disease.* A recent study has reported a two to threefold increase in the risk of surgically confirmed gallbladder disease in women receiving postmenopausal estrogens,[18] similar to the twofold increase previously noted in users of oral contraceptives.[20] In the case of oral contraceptives the increased risk appeared after a period of use.[20]

3. *Effects similar to those caused by estrogen-progestagen oral contraceptives.* There are several adverse effects reported in association with oral contraceptives, most of which have not been documented as consequences of postmenopausal estrogen therapy, although it has been reported that there is an increased risk of thrombosis in men receiving high doses of estrogens for prostatic cancer and in women receiving estrogens for postpartum breast engorgement.[17,21-23] The possibility that the adverse effects reported in association with oral contraceptives may be associated with larger doses of estrogen cannot be excluded.

a. *Thromboembolic disease.* Studies have now shown that users of oral contraceptives have an increased risk of various thromboembolic, thrombotic, and vascular diseases, such as thrombophlebitis, pulmonary embolism, stroke, and myocardial infarction.[24-31] Cases of retinal thrombosis, mesenteric thrombosis, and optic neuritis have been reported in oral contraceptive users. There is evidence that the risk of several of these adverse reactions is related to the dose of the drug.[32, 33] An increased risk of post-surgery thromboembolic complications has also been reported in users of oral contraceptives.[34,35] If feasible, estrogen should be discontinued at least 4 weeks before surgery of the type associated with an increased risk of thromboembolism, or during periods of prolonged immobilization.

While an increased rate of thromboembolic and thrombotic disease in postmenopausal users of estrogens has not been found,[18, 36] this does not rule out the possibility that such an increase may be present, or that subgroups of women who have underlying risk factors, or who are receiving relatively large doses of estrogens may have an increased risk. Therefore, estrogens should not be used in persons with active thrombophlebitis or thromboembolic disorders, and they should not be used (except in treatment of malignancy) in persons with a history of such disorders. They should be used with caution in patients with cerebral vascular or coronary artery disease and only for those in whom estrogens are needed.

Doses of estrogen (5 mg conjungated estrogens per day), comparable to those used to treat cancer of the prostate and breast, have been reported in a large prospective clinical trial in men[37] to increase the risk of nonfatal myocardial infarction, pulmonary embolism, and thrombophlebitis. When estrogen doses of this size are used, any of the thromboembolic and thrombotic adverse effects associated with oral contraceptive use should be considered as a risk.

b. *Hepatic adenoma.* Benign hepatic adenomas have been reported to be associated with the use of oral contraceptives.[38-40] Although benign and rare, these may rupture and may cause death through intra-abdominal hemorrhage. Such lesions have not yet been reported in association with other estrogen or progestagen preparations but should be considered in estrogen users having abdominal pain and tenderness, abdominal mass, or hypovolemic shock. Hepatocellular carcinoma has also been reported in women taking estrogen-containing oral contraceptives.[39] The relationship of this malignancy to these drugs is not known at this time.

c. *Elevated blood pressure.* Increased blood pressure is not uncommon in women using oral contraceptives and there is now a report that this may occur with use of estrogens in the menopause[41] and blood pressure should be monitored with estrogen use, especially if high doses are used.

d. *Glucose tolerance.* A worsening of glucose tolerance has been observed in a significant percentage of patients on estrogen-containing oral contraceptives. For this reason diabetic patients should be carefully observed while receiving estrogen.

4. *Hypercalcemia.* Administration of estrogens may lead to hypercalcemia in patients with breast cancer and bone metastases. If this occurs, the drug should be stopped and appropriate measures taken to reduce the serum calcium level.

PRECAUTIONS

A. General Precautions

1. A complete medical and family history should be taken prior to the initiation of any estrogen therapy. The pretreatment and periodic physical examinations should include special reference to blood pressure, breasts, abdomen, and pelvic organs, and should include a Papanicolaou smear. As a general rule, estrogen should not be prescribed for longer than 1 year without another physical examination being performed.
2. Fluid retention—Because estrogens may cause some degree of fluid retention, conditions that might be influenced by this factor such as epilepsy, migraine, and cardiac or renal dysfunction require careful observation.
3. Certain patients may develop undesirable manifestations of excessive estrogenic stimulation, such as abnormal or excessive uterine bleeding, mastodynia, etc.
4. Oral contraceptives have been reported to be associated with an increased incidence of mental depression. Although it is not clear whether this is possibly due to the estrogenic or progestagenic component of the contraceptive, patients with a history of depression should be carefully observed.
5. Patients having pre-existing uterine leiomyomata should be observed for increased growth of myomata during estrogen therapy.
6. The pathologist should be advised of estrogen therapy when relevant specimens are submitted.
7. Patients with a past history of jaundice during pregnancy have an increased risk of recurrence of jaundice while

Continued on next page

Information on Merrell Dow products is based on labeling in effect in May, 1986.

Merrell Dow—Cont.

receiving estrogen-containing oral contraceptive therapy. If jaundice develops in any patient receiving estrogen, the medication should be discontinued while the cause is investigated.
8. Estrogens may be poorly metabolized in patients with impaired liver function and they should be administered with caution in such patients.
9. Because estrogens influence the metabolism of calcium and phosphorus, they should be used with caution in patients with metabolic bone diseases that are associated with hypercalcemia or in patients with renal insufficiency.
10. Because of the effects of estrogens on epiphyseal closure, they should be used judiciously in young patients in whom bone growth is not complete.
11. Judicious assessment of the following changes in certain endocrine and liver function tests is necessary for patients receiving large doses of estrogen:
a. Increased sulfobromophthalein retention.
b. Increased prothrombin and factors VII, VIII, IX and X; decreased antithrombin 3; increased norepinephrine-induced platelet aggregability.
c. Increased thyroid binding globulin (TBG) leading to increased circulating total thyroid hormone, as measured by PBI, T4 by column, or T4 by radioimmunoassay. Free T3 resin uptake is decreased, reflecting the elevated TBG; free T4 concentration is unaltered.
d. Impaired glucose tolerance.
e. Decreased pregnanediol excretion.
f. Reduced response to metyrapone test.
g. Reduced serum folate concentration.
h. Increased serum triglyceride, phospholipid, or cholesterol.
12. This product contains FD&C Yellow No. 5 (tartrazine), which may cause allergic-type reactions (including bronchial asthma) in certain susceptible individuals. Although the overall incidence of FD&C Yellow No. 5 (tartrazine) sensitivity in the general population is low, it is frequently seen in patients who also have aspirin hypersensitivity.
B. Information For The Patient
A patient package insert accompanies this drug product. This insert is available from pharmacists who carry this product and from the company upon request.
C. Pregnancy Category X
See Contraindications and Boxed Warning.
D. Nursing Mothers
As a general principle, the administration of any drug to nursing mothers should be done only when clearly necessary since many drugs are excreted in human milk.

ADVERSE REACTIONS

(See Warnings regarding reports of induction of neoplasia, adverse effects on the fetus, increased incidence of gallbladder disease, and adverse effects similar to those of oral contraceptives, including thromboembolism.) The following additional adverse reactions have been reported with estrogenic therapy including oral contraceptives:
1. *Genitourinary system*
Breakthrough bleeding, spotting, change in menstrual flow and cycle.
Dysmenorrhea.
Premenstrual-like syndrome.
Amenorrhea during and after treatment.
Increase in size of uterine fibromyomata.
Vaginal candidiasis.
Change in cervical eversion and in degree of cervical secretion.
Cystitis-like syndrome.
2. *Breasts*
Tenderness, enlargement, secretion.
3. *Gastrointestinal*
Nausea, vomiting.
Abdominal cramps, bloating.
Cholestatic jaundice.
4. *Skin*
Chloasma or melasma, which may persist when drug is discontinued.
Erythema multiforme.
Erythema nodosum.
Hemorrhagic eruption.
Loss of scalp hair.
Hirsutism.
Urticaria.
5. *Eyes*
Steepening of corneal curvature.
Intolerance to contact lenses.
6. *CNS*
Headache, migraine, dizziness.
Mental depression.
Chorea.
7. *Miscellaneous*
Increase or decrease in weight.
Reduced carbohydrate tolerance.
Aggravation of porphyria.
Edema.
Changes in libido and/or potency.

ACUTE OVERDOSAGE

Numerous reports of ingestion of large doses of estrogen-containing oral contraceptives by young children indicate that serious ill effects usually do not occur. Overdosage of estrogen may cause nausea, and withdrawal bleeding may occur in females.

DOSAGE AND ADMINISTRATION

Given for a few days
Prevention of postpartum breast engorgement.
The usual dosage is 1 TACE 72 mg capsule twice daily for 2 days. The first dose should be given as soon as possible after delivery but within 8 hours.

HOW SUPPLIED

TACE 72 mg (CHLOROTRIANISENE CAPSULES USP) green and yellow capsules imprinted MERRELL 692
NDC 0068-0692-48: packages of 48 capsules.

REFERENCES

1. Ziel, H. K. and Finkel, W. D.: Increased risk of endometrial carcinoma among users of conjugated estrogens. New Eng. J. Med. 293: 1167–1170, 1975.
2. Smith, D.C., Prentice, R., Thompson, D.J., and Hermann, W.L.: Association of exogenous estrogen and endometrial carcinoma. New Eng. J. Med. 293:1164–1167, 1975.
3. Mack, T.M., Pike, M.C., Henderson, B.E., Pfeffer, R.I., Gerkins, V.R., Arthur, M., and Brown, S.E.: Estrogens and endometrial cancer in a retirement community. New Eng. J. Med. 294:1262–1267, 1976.
4. Weiss, N.S., Szekely, D.R., and Austin, D.F.: Increasing incidence of endometrial cancer in the United States. New Eng. J. Med. 294:1259–1262, 1976.
5. Herbst, A.L., Ulfelder, H., and Poskanzer, D.C.: Adenocarcinoma of the vagina. New Eng. J. Med. 284:878–881, 1971.
6. Greenwald, P., Barlow, J.J., Nasca, P.C., and Burnett, W.S.: Vaginal cancer after maternal treatment with synthetic estrogens. New Eng. J. Med. 285:390–392, 1971.
7. Herbst, A.L., Cole, P., Colton, T., Robboy, S.J., and Scully, R.E.: Age-incidence and risk of diethylstilbestrol-related clear cell adenocarcinoma of the vagina and cervix. Amer. J. Obstet. Gynec. 128:43–50, 1977.
8. Lanier, A.P., Noller, K.L., Decker, D.G., Elveback, L.R., and Kurland, L.T.: Cancer and stilbestrol. A follow-up of 1719 persons exposed to estrogens in utero and born 1943-1959. Mayo Clin. Proc. 48:793–799, 1973.
9. Herbst, A.L., Kurman, R.J., and Scully, R.E.: Vaginal and cervical abnormalities after exposure to stilbestrol in utero. Obstet. Gynec. 40:287–298, 1972.
10. Herbst, A.L., Poskanzer, D.C., Robboy, S.J., Friedlander, L., and Scully, R.E.: Prenatal exposure to stilbestrol. A prospective comparison of exposed female offspring with unexposed controls. New Eng. J. Med. 292:334–339, 1975.
11. Stafl, A., Mattingly, R.F., Foley, D.V., and Fetherston, W.C.: Clincial diagnosis of vaginal adenosis. Obstet. Gynec. 43:118–128, 1974.
12. Sherman, A.I., Goldrath, M., Berlin, A., Vakhariya, V., Banooni, F., Michaels, W., Goodman, P., and Brown, S.: Cervical-vaginal adenosis after *in utero* exposure to synthetic estrogens. Obstet. Gynec. 44:531–545, 1974.
13. Gal, I., Kirman, B., and Stern. J.: Hormone pregnancy tests and congenital malformation, Nature 216:83, 1967.
14. Levy, E.P., Cohen, A., and Fraser, F.C.: Hormone treatment during pregnancy and congenital heart defects. Lancet 1:611, 1973.
15. Nora, J.J. and Nora, A.H.: Birth defects and oral contraceptives. Lancet 1:941–942, 1973.
16. Janerich, D.T., Piper, J.M., and Glebatis, D.M.: Oral contraceptives and congenital limb-reduction defects. New Eng. J. Med. 291:697–700, 1974.
17. Daniel, D.G., Campbell, H., and Turnbull, A.C.: Puerperal thromboembolism and suppression of lactation. Lancet 2:287–289, 1967.
18. Boston Collaborative Drug Surveillance Program: Surgically confirmed gall bladder disease, venous thromboembolism, and breast tumors in relation to post menopausal estrogen therapy. New Eng. J. Med. 290:15–19, 1974.
19. Hoover, R., Gray, L.A., Sr., Cole, P., and MacMahon, B.: Menopausal estrogens and breast cancer. New Eng. J. Med. 295:401–405, 1976.
20. Boston Collaborative Drug Surveillance Program: Oral contraceptives and venous thromboembolic disease, surgically confirmed gall-bladder disease, and breast tumors. Lancet 1:1399–1404, 1973.
21. Bailar, J.C., III: Thromboembolism and oestrogen therapy. Lancet 2:560, 1967.
22. The Veterans Administration Cooperative Urological Research Group: Carcinoma of the prostate: Treatment comparisons. J. Urol. 98:516–522, 1967.
23. Blackard, C.E., Doe, R.P., Mellinger, G.T., and Byar, D.P.: Incidence of cardiovascular disease and death in patients receiving diethylstilbestrol for carcinoma of the prostate. Cancer 26:249–256, 1970.
24. Royal College of General Practitioners: Oral contraception and thromboembolic disease. J. Roy. Coll. Gen. Pract. 13:267–269, 1967.
25. Inman, W.H.W. and Vessey, M.P.: Investigation of deaths from pulmonary, coronary, and cerebral thrombosis and embolism in women of child-bearing age. Brit. Med. J. 2:193–199, 1968.
26. Vessey, M.P. and Doll, R.: Investigation of relation between use of oral contraceptives and thromboembolic disease. A further report. Brit. Med. J. 2:651–657, 1969.
27. Sartwell, P.E., Masi, A.T., Arthes, F.G., Greene, G.R., and Smith, H.E.: Thromboembolism and oral contraceptives: An epidemiological case-control study. Amer. J. Epidem. 90:365–380, 1969.
28. Collaborative Group for the Study of Stroke in Young Women: Oral contraception and increased risk of cerebral ischemia or thrombosis. New Eng. J. Med. 288:871–878, 1973.
29. Collaborative Group for the Study of Stroke in Young Women: Oral contraceptives and stroke in young women: Associated risk factors. J.A.M.A. 231:718–722, 1975.
30. Mann, J.I. and Inman, W.H.W.: Oral contraceptives and death from myocardial infarction. Brit. Med. J. 2:245–248, 1975.
31. Mann, J.I., Vessey, M.P., Thorogood, M., and Doll, R.: Myocardial infarction in young women with special reference in oral contraceptive practice. Brit. Med. J. 2:241–245, 1975.
32. Inman, W.H.W., Vessey, M.P., Westerholm, B., and Engelund, A.: Thromboembolic disease and the steroidal content of oral contraceptives. A report to the Committee on Safety of Drugs. Brit. Med. J. 2:203–209, 1970.
33. Stolley, P.D., Tonascia, J.A., Tockman, M.S., Sartwell, P.E., Rutledge, A.H., and Jacobs, M.P.: Thrombosis with low-estrogen oral contraceptives. Amer. J. Epidem. 102:197–208, 1975.
34. Vessey, M.P., Doll, R., Fairbairn, A.S., and Glober, G.: Post-operative thromboembolism and the use of the oral contraceptives. Brit. Med. J. 3:123-126, 1970.
35. Greene, G.R. and Sartwell, P.E.: Oral contraceptive use in patients with thromboembolism following surgery, trauma, or infection. Amer. J. Public Health 62:680–685, 1972.
36. Rosenberg, L., Armstrong, B., Phil, D., and Jick, H.: Myocardial infarction and estrogen therapy in post-menopausal women. New Eng. J. Med. 294:1256–1259, 1976.
37. Coronary Drug Project Research Group: The coronary drug project: Initial findings leading to modifications of its research protocol. J.A.M.A. 214:1303–1313, 1970.
38. Baum, J., Holtz, F., Bookstein, J.J., and Klein, E.W.: Possible association between benign hepatomas and oral contraceptives. Lancet 2:926–928, 1973.
39. Mays, E.T., Christopherson, W.M., Mahr, M.M., and Williams, H.C.: Hepatic changes in young women ingesting contraceptive steroids. Hepatic hemorrhage and primary hepatic tumors. J.A.M.A. 235:730–732, 1976.
40. Edmondson, H., Henderson, A.B., and Benton, B.: Liver-cell adenomas associated with the use of oral contraceptives. New Eng. J. Med. 294:470–472, 1976.
41. Pfeffer, R.I. and Van Den Noort, S.: Estrogen use and stroke risk in postmenopausal women. Amer. J. Epidem. 103:445–456, 1976.

Product Information as of April, 1985
Manufactured by
R. P. Scherer, North America
Clearwater, Florida 33518 for
MERRELL DOW PHARMACEUTICALS INC.
Subsidiary of The Dow Chemical Company
Cincinnati, Ohio 45215, U.S.A.

TACE® ℞
(CHLOROTRIANISENE)
72 mg Capsules

INFORMATION FOR PATIENTS

TACE (CHLOROTRIANISENE) is a synthetic estrogen supplied in 12 mg, 25 mg, and 72 mg capsules.

What You Should Know About Estrogens: Estrogens are female hormones produced by the ovaries. The ovaries make several different kinds of estrogens. In addition, scientists have been able to make a variety of synthetic estrogens. As far as we know, all these estrogens have many similar properties and therefore much the same usefulness, side effects, and risks. This leaflet is intended to help you understand what estrogens are sometimes used for, the risks involved in their use, and how to use them as safely as possible.
This leaflet includes important information about estrogens, but not all the information. If you want to know more, you can ask your doctor or pharmacist to let you read the package insert for this product prepared for the doctor.

USES OF ESTROGEN

Estrogens are prescribed by doctors for a number of purposes, including:

1. To provide estrogen during a period of adjustment when a woman's ovaries produce it in decreased amounts in order to prevent certain uncomfortable symptoms of estrogen deficiency. (All women normally produce less estrogen, generally between the ages of 45 and 55; this is called the menopause.)
2. To prevent symptoms of estrogen deficiency when a woman's ovaries have been removed surgically before the natural menopause.
3. To prevent pregnancy. (Estrogens are given along with a progestagen, another female hormone; these combinations are called oral contraceptives or birth control pills. Patient labeling is available to women taking oral contraceptives and they will not be discussed in this leaflet.) *This product is not intended to prevent pregnancy.*
4. To treat certain cancers in women and men. *This product is not intended to treat cancers in women.*
5. To prevent painful swelling of the breasts after pregnancy in women who choose not to nurse their babies.

THERE IS NO PROPER USE OF TACE IN A PREGNANT WOMAN.

ESTROGENS IN THE MENOPAUSE

In the natural course of their lives, all women eventually experience a decrease in estrogen production. This usually occurs between ages 45 and 55 but may occur earlier or later. Sometimes the ovaries may need to be removed before or during natural menopause by an operation, producing a "surgical menopause."

When the amount of estrogen in the blood begins to decrease, many women may develop typical symptoms: feelings of warmth in the face, neck, and chest or sudden intense episodes of heat and sweating throughout the body (called "hot flashes" or "hot flushes"). These symptoms are sometimes very uncomfortable. A few women eventually develop changes in the vagina (called "atrophic vaginitis") which cause discomfort, especially during and after intercourse.

Estrogens can be prescribed to treat these symptoms of the menopause. It is estimated that considerably more than half of all women undergoing the menopause have only mild symptoms or no symptoms at all and therefore do not need estrogens. Other women may need estrogens for a few months, while their bodies adjust to lower estrogen levels. Sometimes the need will be for periods longer than six months. In an attempt to avoid overstimulation of the uterus (womb), estrogens are usually given cyclically during each month of use, that is, three weeks of pills followed by one week without pills.

Sometimes women experience nervous symptoms or depression during menopause. There is no well-documented evidence that estrogens are effective for such symptoms and they should not be used to treat them, although other treatment may be needed.

You may have heard that taking estrogens for long periods (years) after the menopause will keep your skin soft and supple and keep you feeling young. There is no evidence that this is so, however, and such long-term treatment carries important risks.

ESTROGENS TO PREVENT SWELLING OF THE BREASTS AFTER PREGNANCY

If you do not breast feed your baby after delivery, your breasts may fill up with milk and become engorged and painful. This usually begins about 3 to 4 days after delivery and may last for a few days to up to a week or more. Sometimes the discomfort is severe, but usually it is not and can be controlled by pain relieving drugs such as aspirin and by binding the breasts up tightly. Estrogens can be used to try to prevent the breasts from filling up.

While this treatment is usually successful in reducing amount of filling, in many cases the breasts fill up to some degree in spite of treatment. The daily dose of estrogens needed to prevent pain and swelling of the breasts is larger than the dose needed to treat symptoms of the menopause and this may increase your chances of developing blood clots in the legs or lungs. (See below.) Therefore, it is important that you discuss the benefits and the risks of estrogen use with your doctor if you have decided not to breast feed your baby.

THE DANGERS OF ESTROGENS

1. *Cancer of the uterus.* Several independent studies have reported an increased risk ratio of endometrial cancer (cancer of the lining of the uterus) if estrogens are used in the post-menopausal period for more than a year. Women taking estrogens are reported to have roughly 5 to 10 times as great a chance of getting this cancer as women who take no estrogens. To put this another way, while a postmenopausal woman not taking estrogens has 1 chance in 1,000 each year of getting cancer of the uterus, a woman taking estrogens has 5 to 10 chances in 1,000 each year. For this reason *it is important to take estrogens only when you really need them.*

The risk of this cancer is reported to be greater the longer estrogens are used and also seems to be greater when larger doses are taken. For this reason *it is important to take the lowest dose of estrogen that will control symptoms and to take it only as long as it is needed.* If estrogens are needed for longer periods of time, your doctor will want to reevaluate your need for estrogens at least every six months.

Women using estrogens should report any irregular vaginal bleeding to their doctors; such bleeding may be of no importance, but it can be an early warning of cancer of the uterus. If you have undiagnosed vaginal bleeding, you should not use estrogens until a diagnosis is made that there is no cancer of the uterus.

If you have had your uterus completely removed (total hysterectomy), there is no danger of developing cancer of the uterus.

2. *Other possible cancers.* Long-term continuous administration of estrogens in certain animal species increases the frequency of cancers of the breast, cervix, vagina, and liver. At present there is no satisfactory evidence that women using estrogen in the menopause have an increased risk of such tumors, but there is no way yet to be sure they do not; and one study raises the possibility that use of estrogens in the menopause may increase the risk of breast cancer many years later. This is a further reason to use estrogens only when clearly needed. While you are taking estrogens, it is important that you go to your doctor at least every six months for an examination. Also, if members of your family have had breast cancer or if you have breast nodules or abnormal mammograms (breast x-rays), your doctor may wish to carry out more frequent examinations of your breasts.
3. *Gall bladder disease.* Women who use estrogens after menopause are reported to be more likely to develop gall bladder disease needing surgery than women who do not use estrogens. Birth control pills have a similar effect.
4. *Abnormal blood clotting.* Oral contraceptives increase the risk of blood clotting in various parts of the body. This can result in a stroke (if the clot is in the brain), a heart attack (clot in a blood vessel of the heart), or a pulmonary embolus (a clot which forms in the legs or pelvis, then breaks off and travels to the lungs). Any of these can be fatal.

At this time use of estrogens in the menopause is not known to cause such blood clotting, but the possibility that such clotting in association with oral contraceptives may be associated with larger doses of estrogen cannot be excluded. It is recommended that if you have had clotting in the legs or lungs or a heart attack or stroke while you were using estrogens or birth control pills, you should not use estrogens (unless they are being used to treat cancer of the breast or prostate). If you have had a stroke or heart attack or if you have angina pectoris, estrogens should be used with caution and only if clearly needed (for example, if you have severe symptoms of the menopause).

The larger doses of estrogen used to prevent swelling of the breasts after pregnancy have been reported to increase the risk of clotting in the legs and lungs.

Special Warning About Pregnancy: You should not receive estrogen if you are pregnant. It has been reported that there is a greater than usual chance that the developing child will be born with a birth defect, although the possibility remains fairly small. It is also reported that a female child may have an increased risk of developing cancer of the vagina or cervix later in life (in the teens or twenties). Every possible effort should be made to avoid exposure to TACE during pregnancy. If exposure occurs, see your doctor.

Other Effects of Estrogens: In addition to the serious reported risks of estrogens described above, estrogens have the following side effects and potential risks:

1. *Nausea and vomiting.* The most common side effect of estrogen therapy is nausea. Vomiting is less common.
2. *Effects on breasts.* Estrogens may cause breast tenderness or enlargement and may cause the breasts to secrete a liquid. These effects are not dangerous.
3. *Effects on the uterus.* Estrogens may cause benign fibroid tumors of the uterus to get larger.

Some women will have menstrual bleeding when estrogens are stopped. But if the bleeding occurs on days you are still taking estrogens you should report this to your doctor.

4. *Effects on liver.* Women taking oral contraceptives develop on rare occasions a tumor of the liver which can rupture and bleed into the abdomen. So far, these tumors have not been reported in women using estrogens in the menopause, but you should report any swelling or unusual pain or tenderness in the abdomen to your doctor immediately.

Women with a past history of jaundice (yellowing of the skin and white parts of the eyes) may get jaundice again during estrogen use. If this occurs, stop taking estrogens and see your doctor.

5. *Other effects.* Estrogens may cause excess fluid to be retained in the body. This may make some conditions worse, such as epilepsy, migraine, heart disease, or kidney disease.

SUMMARY

Estrogens have important uses, but they have reported risks of potentially serious conditions developing as well. You must decide, with your doctor, whether the risks are acceptable to you in view of the benefits of treatment. Except where your doctor has prescribed TACE for use in special cases of cancer of the prostate, you should not use TACE if you have cancer of the breast or uterus, are pregnant, have undiagnosed abnormal vaginal bleeding, clotting in the legs or lungs, have had a stroke, heart attack or angina, or clotting in the legs or lungs in the past while you were taking estrogens.

You can use TACE as safely as possible by understanding that your doctor will require regular physical examinations while you are taking it and will try to discontinue the drug as soon as possible and use the smallest dose possible. Be alert for signs of trouble including:

1. Abnormal bleeding from the vagina.
2. Pains in the calves or chest or sudden shortness of breath, or coughing blood (indicating possible clots in the legs, heart, or lungs).
3. Severe headache, dizziness, faintness, or changes in vision (indicating possible developing clots in the brain or eye).
4. Breast lumps. (You should ask your doctor how to examine your own breasts.)
5. Jaundice (yellowing of the skin).
6. Mental depression.

Based on his or her assessment of your medical needs, your doctor has prescribed this drug for you. Do not give this drug to anyone else.

HOW SUPPLIED

TACE (CHLOROTRIANISENE) is a long-acting synthetic estrogen in capsule form. The capsule is suitable for taking by mouth.

Each two-tone green and yellow, soft gelatin capsule imprinted MERRELL 692 contains 72 mg of chlorotrianisene in Dispex®, an emulsifiable vehicle containing corn oil, sorbitan trioleate, polysorbate 80, and benzyl benzoate. This capsule also contains other inactive ingredients: FD&C Blue No. 1, FD&C Yellow No. 5 (tartrazine) as a color additive, gelatin, glycerin, iron oxide, methylparaben, propylparaben, sorbitol, titanium dioxide, and water.

Patient Information as of April, 1985

Shown in Product Identification Section, page 418

TUSSEND® Ⓒ ℞

[tŭs 'ĕnd]

Antitussive-Decongestant
Liquid and Tablets

DESCRIPTION

Each 5 ml teaspoonful or tablet of Tussend for oral use contains hydrocodone bitartrate, 5 mg (Warning: may be habit forming) and pseudoephedrine hydrochloride 60 mg. The tablets also contain as inactive ingredients: colloidal silicon dioxide, corn starch, ethylcellulose, FD&C Red No. 3, FD&C Yellow No. 6, glycerin, hydrogenated vegetable oil, hydroxypropyl cellulose, hydroxypropyl methylcellulose, pregelatinized corn starch, and titanium dioxide. The liquid also contains as inactive ingredients: alcohol 5%, caramel, FD&C Red No. 40, flavors, glycerin, invert sugar, saccharin sodium, sodium chloride, sorbitol, and water.

Hydrocodone bitartrate is an antitussive. Chemically it is 4,5α-epoxy-3-methoxy-17-methylmorphinan-6-one tartrate (1:1) hydrate (2:5) with the following structure:

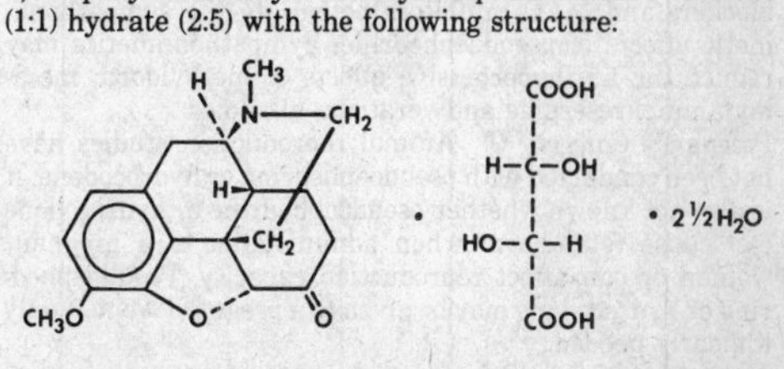

Pseudoephedrine hydrochloride is a nasal decongestant. Chemically it is α-[1-(methylamino)ethyl]-[*S*-(*R**,*R**)]-benzenemethanol hydrochloride with the following structure:

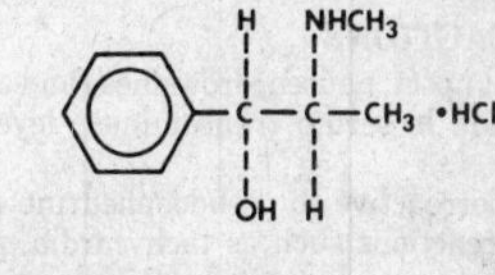

CLINICAL PHARMACOLOGY

Hydrocodone is a narcotic-analgesic chemically and pharmacologically related to codeine. Hydrocodone suppresses the cough reflex by depressing the medullary cough center. The duration of antitussive action of hydrocodone in man after oral administration is 4 to 8 hours. Hydrocodone is approxi-

Continued on next page

Merrell Dow—Cont.

mately three times more potent than codeine on a weight basis.

Pseudoephedrine is an orally active sympathomimetic amine and exerts a decongestant action on the nasal mucosa. Pseudoephedrine produces peripheral effects similar to those of ephedrine and central effects similar to, but less intense than amphetamines. It has the potential for excitatory side effects. At the recommended oral dosages it has little or no pressor effect in normotensive adults. The serum half-life ($T^1/_2$) of pseudoephedrine is approximately 4 to 6 hours. $T^1/_2$ is decreased with increased excretion of drug at a urine pH lower than 6 and may be increased with decreased excretion at urine pH higher than 8.

INDICATIONS AND USAGE

For exhausting cough spasms accompanying upper respiratory tract congestion associated with the common cold, influenza, bronchitis and sinusitis.

CONTRAINDICATIONS

Patients with severe hypertension, severe coronary artery disease, and in patients on MAO inhibitor therapy.

Hypersensitivity: Contraindicated in patients with hypersensitivity or idiosyncrasy to sympathomimetic amines, phenanthrene derivatives, or to any other formula ingredients.

Nursing Mothers: Contraindicated because of the higher than usual risk for infants from sympathomimetic amines.

WARNINGS

Hydrocodone should be prescribed and administered with the same degree of caution as all oral medications containing a narcotic-analgesic. Extreme caution should be exercised in the use of hydrocodone in patients with severe respiratory impairment or patients with impaired respiratory drive.

If sympathomimetic amines are used in patients with hypertension, diabetes mellitus, ischemic heart disease, hyperthyroidism, increased intraocular pressure or prostatic hypertrophy, judicious caution should be exercised (see CONTRAINDICATIONS).

Use in elderly: The elderly (60 years and older) are more likely to have adverse reactions to sympathomimetics. Overdosage of sympathomimetics in this age group may cause hallucinations, convulsions, CNS depression and death.

PRECAUTIONS

General: Caution should be exercised if used in patients with diabetes, hypertension, cardiovascular disease, hyperreactivity to ephedrine, or decreased respiratory drive (see CONTRAINDICATIONS).

Information for Patients: Hydrocodone may produce drowsiness. Persons who perform hazardous tasks requiring mental alertness or physical coordination should be cautioned accordingly. Concomitant use of hydrocodone with tranquilizers, alcohol or other depressants may produce additive depressant effects. Do not exceed the prescribed dosage.

Drug Interactions: Hydrocodone may potentiate the effects of other narcotics, general anesthetics, tranquilizers, sedatives and hypnotics, tricyclic antidepressants, MAO inhibitors, alcohol, and other CNS depressants. Beta adrenergic blockers and MAO inhibitors potentiate the sympathomimetic effects of pseudoephedrine. Sympathomimetics may reduce the antihypertensive effects of methyldopa, mecamylamine, reserpine and veratrum alkaloids.

Pregnancy Category C: Animal reproduction studies have not been conducted with pseudoephedrine or hydrocodone. It is also not known whether pseudoephedrine or hydrocodone can cause fetal harm when administered to a pregnant woman or can affect reproduction capacity. Pseudoephedrine or hydrocodone may be given to a pregnant woman only if clearly needed.

Nursing Mothers: Because of the potential for serious adverse reactions in nursing infants from sympathomimetic amines, pseudoephedrine is contraindicated in nursing mothers.

ADVERSE REACTIONS

Gastrointestinal upset, nausea, drowsiness and constipation. A slight elevation in serum transaminase levels has been noted.

Individuals hyperreactive to pseudoephedrine may display ephedrine-like reactions such as tachycardia, palpitations, headache, dizziness or nausea. Sympathomimetic drugs have been associated with certain untoward reactions including fear, anxiety, tenseness, restlessness, tremor, weakness, pallor, respiratory difficulty, dysuria, insomnia, hallucinations, convulsions, CNS depression, arrhythmias, and cardiovascular collapse with hypotension.

Patient idiosyncrasy to adrenergic agents may be manifested by insomina, dizziness, weakness, tremor or arrhythmias.

DRUG ABUSE AND DEPENDENCE

Controlled Substance: Hydrocodone in Tussend mixture is controlled by the Drug Enforcement Administration. Tussend is a Schedule III controlled substance.

Abuse: Human experience indicates that abuse of Tussend is uncommon. However, hydrocodone is a narcotic drug related to codeine with roughly three times the abuse potential of codeine on a weight basis.

Dependence: Hydrocodone can produce drug dependence of the morphine type. Psychic dependence, physical dependence and tolerance may develop if dosage recommendations are greatly exceeded over a prolonged period of time.

OVERDOSAGE

Acute overdosage with Tussend may produce variable clinical signs as hydrocodone produces CNS depression and cardiovascular depression while pseudoephedrine produces CNS stimulation and variable cardiovascular effects. Hydrocodone is likely to be responsible for most of the severe reactions from overdosage. Pressor amines should be used with great caution when taking pseudoephedrine. Patients with signs of stimulation should be treated conservatively and depressant medications should be avoided if possible because of potential drug interaction with hydrocodone.

DOSAGE AND ADMINISTRATION

Adults and children over 90 lbs, 1 tablet or one teaspoonful; children 50 to 90 lbs, 1/2 teaspoonful; children 25 to 50 lbs, 1/4 teaspoonful. May be given four times a day as needed. May be taken with meals.

CAUTION

Federal law prohibits dispensing without prescription.

HOW SUPPLIED

Tussend liquid is supplied in pints (NDC 0068-1018-16). Tussend tablets are supplied in bottles of 100 (NDC 0068-0042-61).

Product Information as of April, 1985

Shown in Product Identification Section, page 418

TUSSEND® EXPECTORANT ℞ ©

[*tŭs'ĕnd*]

Antitussive-Decongestant-Expectorant Liquid

DESCRIPTION

Each 5 ml teaspoonful of Tussend Expectorant liquid for oral use contains hydrocodone bitartrate, 5 mg (Warning: May be habit forming), pseudoephedrine hydrochloride 60 mg, guaifenesin (glyceryl guaiacolate) 200 mg. The expectorant also contains as inactive ingredients: alcohol 12.5%. FD&C Yellow No. 6, flavors, glycerin, hydrochoric acid, invert sugar, saccharin sodium, sodium chloride, sodium gluconate, sorbitol, and water.

Hydrocodone bitartrate is an antitussive. Chemically it is 4,5α-epoxy-3-methoxy-17-methylmorphinan-6-one tartrate (1:1) hydrate (2:5) with following structure:

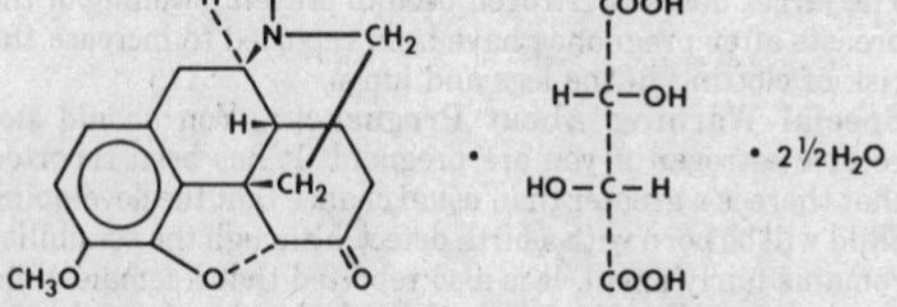

Pseudoephedrine hydrochloride is a nasal decongestant. Chemically it is α-[1-(methylamino)ethyl]-[S-(R*,R*)]-benzenemethanol hydrochloride with the following structure:

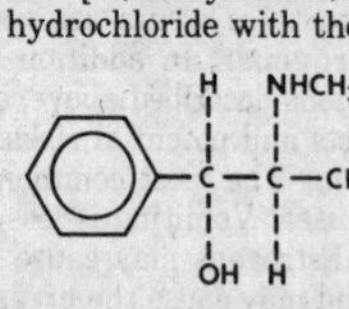

Guaifenesin is an expectorant. Chemically it is 3-(0-methoxyphenoxy)-1,2 propanediol with the following structure:

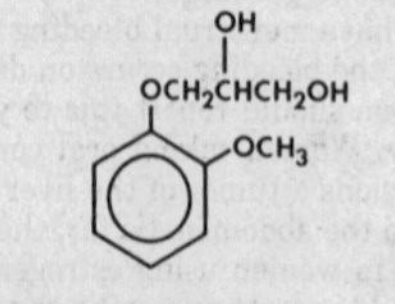

CLINICAL PHARMACOLOGY

Hydrocodone is a narcotic-analgesic chemically and pharmacologically related to codeine. Hydrocodone suppresses the cough reflex by depressing the medullary cough center. The duration of antitussive action of hydrocodone in man after oral administration is 4 to 8 hours. Hydrocodone is approximately three times more potent than codeine on a weight basis.

Pseudoephedrine is an orally active sympathomimetic amine and exerts a decongestant action on the nasal mucosa. Pseudoephedrine produces peripheral effects similar to those of ephedrine and central effects similar to, but less intense than amphetamines. It has the potential for excitatory side effects. At the recommended oral dosages it has little or no pressor effect in normotensive adults. The serum half-life (T-1/2) of pseudoephedrine is approximately 4 to 6 hours. T-1/2 is decreased with increased excretion of drug at a urine pH lower than 6 and may be increased with decreased excretion at urine pH higher than 8.

Guaifenesin is used as an expectorant. On the basis of studies in animals, guaifenesin is thought to increase mucus flow in the lung by stimulation of gastric mucosal reflexes. Objective human data are lacking.

INDICATIONS AND USAGE

For exhausting, nonproductive cough accompanying respiratory tract congestion associated with the common cold, influenza, sinusitis and bronchitis.

CONTRAINDICATIONS

Patients with severe hypertension, severe coronary artery disease, and in patients on MAO inhibitor therapy.

Hypersensitivity: Contraindicated in patients with hypersensitivity or idiosyncrasy to sympathomimetic amines, phenanthrene derivatives, or to any other formula ingredients.

Nursing Mothers: Contraindicated because of the higher than usual risk for infants for sympathomimetic amines.

WARNINGS

Hydrocodone should be prescribed and administered with the same degree of caution as all oral medications containing a narcotic analgesic. Extreme caution should be exercised in the use of hydrocodone in patients with severe respiratory impairment or patients with impaired respiratory drive.

If sympathomimetic amines are used in patients with hypertension, diabetes mellitus, ischemic heart disease, hyperthyroidism, increased intraocular pressure or prostatic hypertrophy, judicious caution should be exercised (see CONTRAINDICATIONS).

Use in Elderly: The elderly (60 years and older) are more likely to have adverse reactions to sympathomimetics. Overdosage of sympathomimetics in this age group may cause hallucinations, convulsions, CNS depression and death.

PRECAUTIONS

General: Caution should be exercised if used in patients with diabetes, hypertension, cardiovascular diseases, hyperreactivity to ephedrine, or decreased respiratory drive (see CONTRAINDICATIONS).

Information for Patients: Hydrocodone may produce drowsiness. Persons who perform hazardous tasks requiring mental alertness or physical coordination should be cautioned accordingly. Concomitant use of hydrocodone with tranquilizers, alcohol or other depressants may produce additive depressant effects. Do not exceed the prescribed dosage.

Drug Interactions: Hydrocodone may potentiate the effects of other narcotics, general anesthetics, tranquilizers, sedatives and hypnotics, tricyclic antidepressants, MAO inhibitors, alcohol, and other CNS depressants. Beta adrenergic blockers and MAO inhibitors potentiate the sympathomimetic effects of pseudoephedrine. Sympathomimetics may reduce the antihypertensive effects of methyldopa, mecamylamine, reserpine and veratrum alkaloids.

Laboratory Test Interactions: Guaifenesin interferes with the colorimetric determination of 5-hydroxyindoleacetic acid (5-HIAA) and vanilmandelic acid (VMA).

Pregnancy Category C: Animal reproduction studies have not been conducted with pseudoephedrine, guaifenesin, or hydrocodone. It is also not known whether pseudoephedrine, guaifenesin or hydrocodone can cause fetal harm when administered to a pregnant woman or can affect reproduction capacity. Pseudoephedrine or hydrocodone may be given to a pregnant woman only if clearly needed.

Nursing Mothers: Because of the potential for serious adverse reactions in nursing infants from sympathomimetic amines, pseudoephedrine is contraindicated in nursing mothers.

ADVERSE REACTIONS

Gastrointestinal upset, nausea, drowsiness and constipation. A slight elevation in serum transaminase levels has been noted.

Individuals hyperreactive to pseudoephedrine may display ephedrine-like reactions such as tachycardia, palpitations, headache, dizziness or nausea. Sympathomimetic drugs have been associated with certain untoward reactions including fear, anxiety, tenseness, restlessness, tremor, weakness, pallor, respiratory difficulty, dysuria, insomnia, hallucinations, convulsions, CNS depression, arrhythmias, and cardiovascular collapse with hypotension.

Patient idiosyncrasy to adrenergic agents may be manifested by insomnia, dizziness, weakness, tremor or arrhythmias.

DRUG ABUSE AND DEPENDENCE

Controlled Substance: Hydrocodone in Tussend Expectorant mixture is controlled by the Drug Enforcement Administration. Tussend Expectorant is a Schedule III controlled substance.

Abuse: Human experience indicates that abuse of Tussend Expectorant is uncommon. However, hydrocodone is a nar-

cotic drug related to codeine with roughly three times the abuse potential of codeine on a weight basis.
Dependence: Hydrocodone can produce drug dependence of the morphine type. Psychic dependence, physical dependence and tolerance may develop if dosage recommendations are greatly exceeded over a prolonged period of time.

OVERDOSAGE

Acute overdosage with Tussend Expectorant may produce variable clinical signs as hydrocodone produces CNS depression and cardiovascular depression while pseudoephedrine produces CNS stimulation and variable cardiovascular effects. Hydrocodone is likely to be responsible for most of the severe reactions from overdosage. Pressor amines should be used with great caution when taking pseudoephedrine. Patients with signs of stimulation should be treated conservatively and depressant medications should be avoided if possible because of potential drug interaction with hydrocodone.

DOSAGE AND ADMINISTRATION

Adults and children over 90 lbs, 1 teaspoonful; children 50 to 90 lbs, 1/2 teaspoonful; children 25 to 50 lbs, 1/4 teaspoonful. May be given four times a day as needed. May be taken with meals.

CAUTION

Federal law prohibits dispensing without prescription.

HOW SUPPLIED

Tussend Expectorant is supplied in pints (NDC 0068-1016-16).
Product Information as of April, 1985
Shown in Product Identification Section, page 418

Information on Merrell Dow products is based on labeling in effect in May, 1986.

Metro Med Inc.

2201 DENTON DRIVE
AUSTIN, TX 78758

ALPHA–PHED Capsules ℞
[ăl 'fa-fĕd]

DESCRIPTION

Each capsule contains:

Aspirin	400 mg.
Pseudoephedrine HCl	20 mg.
Caffeine	32 mg.

HOW SUPPLIED

Bottles of 100 (NDC 0454-3704-01).
For full prescribing information please see package insert.

BETA–PHED Capsules ℞
[bā 'tă-fĕd]

DESCRIPTION

Each capsule contains:

Acetaminophen	500 mg.
Pseudoephedrine HCl	20 mg.
Caffeine	32 mg.

HOW SUPPLIED

Bottles of 100 (NDC 0454-3905-01).
For full prescribing information please see package insert.

ESPROGYN Pack ℞
[ĕs 'pra-jan]

DESCRIPTION

Each pack contains 25 conjugated estrogen tablets, 0.625 mg. and 10 medroxyprogesterone tablets, 10 mg.

HOW SUPPLIED

Each (NDC 0454-8342-07).
For full prescribing information please see package insert.

FURONATAL FA® ℞
[fū 'rō-nā "tăl]

DESCRIPTION

Each tablet contains:		U.S.R.D.A.
Vitamin A	8000 IU	100%
Vitamin D	400 IU	100%
Vitamin E	30 IU	100%
Vitamin C	60 mg	100%
Folic Acid	1 mg	125%
Vitamin B-1	2 mg	100%
Vitamin B-2	2.8 mg	100%
Niacinamide	20 mg	100%
Vitamin B-6	2.5 mg	100%
Vitamin B-12	8 mcg	100%
Iron	65 mg	340%
Calcium	125 mg	10%

HOW SUPPLIED

Bottles of 100 (NDC 0454-2502-06)
Bottles of 1000 (NDC 0454-2502-10)
For full prescribing information please see package insert.

HISTAMIC® Capsules ℞
HISTAMIC® Tablets ℞
[hĭs-tă 'mĭc]

DESCRIPTION

Each orange and clear capsule contains: Phenylephrine HCl 25 mg.—
Phenylpropanolamine 50 mg.—Chlorpheniramine maleate 12 mg.—Phenyltoloxamine citrate 30 mg. Each sustained release tablet contains: Phenylpropanolamine HCl 40 mg.—Phenylephrine HCl 10 mg.—Phenyltoloxamine Citrate 15 mg.—Chlorpheniramine 5 mg.

HOW SUPPLIED

HISTAMIC Capsules	100-(NDC 0454-3603-01)
	1000-(NDC 0454-3603-10)
HISTAMIC Tablets	100-(NDC 0454-3703-01)

For full prescribing information please see package insert.

SPAN–FF® Capsules OTC
[spăn-ff]

DESCRIPTION

Each SPAN-FF® capsule contains 325 mg Ferrous Fumarate especially encased in bead form for optimal dispersion of the iron content, thereby minimizing the potential intolerance, while increasing the solubility and making available a maximum amount of solute iron. SPAN-FF® is tasteless, odorless, and will not stain the teeth. These properties, combined with the high availability of Elemental Iron, make SPAN-FF® unique in action and flexible in administration.

HOW SUPPLIED

SPAN-FF® capsules are available in bottles of 100 (NDC 0454-3002-01) and 1000 (NDC 0454-3002-10).
For full prescribing information please see package insert.

SPAN R/D® Capsules Ⓒ ℞
[spăn R/D]
(phentermine hydrochloride)

DESCRIPTION

Each capsules contains Phentermine Hydrochloride 37.5 mg.

HOW SUPPLIED

Bottles of 100 (NDC 0454-4354-01).
For full prescribing information please see package insert.

EDUCATIONAL MATERIAL

Samples available on all Metro Med products upon request by physician.

Miles Laboratories, Inc.

P. O. BOX 340
ELKHART, IN 46515

ALKA-SELTZER® Effervescent Pain Reliever & Antacid With Specially Buffered Aspirin
[al-kuh-selt-sir]

ACTIVE INGREDIENTS

Each tablet contains: aspirin 324 mg., heat treated sodium bicarbonate 1916 mg., citric acid 1000 mg. ALKA-SELTZER® in water contains principally the antacid sodium citrate and the analgesic sodium acetylsalicylate. Buffered pH is between 6 and 7.

INACTIVE INGREDIENTS

None

INDICATIONS

ALKA-SELTZER® Effervescent Pain Reliever & Antacid is an analgesic and an antacid and is indicated for relief of sour stomach, acid indigestion or heartburn with headache or body aches and pains. Also for fast relief of upset stomach with headache from overindulgence in food and drink—especially recommended for taking before bed and again on arising. Effective for pain relief alone: headache or body and muscular aches and pains.

ACTIONS

When the ALKA-SELTZER® Effervescent Pain Reliever & Antacid tablet is dissolved in water, the acetylsalicylate ion differs from acetylsalicylic acid chemically, physically and pharmacologically. Being fat insoluble, it is not absorbed by the gastric mucosal cells. Studies and observations in animals and man including radiochrome determinations of fecal blood loss, measurement of ion fluxes and direct visualization with gastrocamera, have shown that, as contrasted with acetylsalicylic acid, the acetylsalicylate ion delivered in the solution does not alter gastric mucosal permeability to permit back-diffusion of hydrogen ion, and gastric damage and acute gastric mucosal lesions are therefore not seen after administration of the product.
ALKA-SELTZER® Effervescent Pain Reliever & Antacid has the capacity to neutralize gastric hydrochloric acid quickly and effectively. In-vitro, 154 ml. of 0.1 N hydrochloric acid are required to decrease the pH of one tablet of ALKA-SELTZER® Effervescent Pain Reliever & Antacid in solution to 4.0. Measured against the in vitro standard established by the Food and Drug Administration one tablet neutralizes 17.2 mEq of acid. ALKA-SELTZER® Effervescent Pain Reliever & Antacid is able to resist pH changes caused by the continuing secretion of acid in the normal individual and to maintain an elevated pH until emptying occurs.
ALKA-SELTZER® Effervescent Pain Reliever & Antacid provides highly water soluble acetylsalicylate ions which are fat insoluble. Acetylsalicylate ions are not absorbed from the stomach. They empty from the stomach and thereby become available for absorption from the duodenum. Thus, fast drug absorption and high plasma acetylsalicylate levels are achieved. Plasma levels of salicylate following the administration of ALKA-SELTZER® Effervescent Pain Reliever & Antacid solution (acetylsalicylate equivalent to 648 mg. acetylsalicylic acid) can reach 29 mg./liter in 10 minutes and rise to peak levels as high as 55 mg./liter within 30 minutes.

WARNINGS

Children and teenagers should not use this medicine for chicken pox or flu symptoms before a doctor is consulted about Reye's Syndrome, a rare but serious illness. As with any drug, if you are pregnant or nursing a baby, seek the advice of a health professional before using this product. Except under the advice and supervision of a physician, do not take more than, Adults: 8 tablets in a 24 hour period. (60 years of age or older: 4 tablets in a 24 hour period), or use the maximum dosage for more than 10 days. Do not use if you are allergic to aspirin or have asthma, if you have a coagulation (bleeding) disease, or if you are on a sodium restricted diet. Each tablet contains 567 mg. of sodium.
Keep this and all drugs out of the reach of children.

DOSAGE AND ADMINISTRATION

ALKA-SELTZER® Effervescent Pain Reliever & Antacid is taken in solution, approximately three ounces of water per tablet is sufficient.
Adults: 2 tablets every 4 hours. CAUTION: If symptoms persist or recur frequently, or if you are under treatment for ulcer, consult your physician.

Professional Labeling:
ASPIRIN FOR MYOCARDIAL INFARCTION

INDICATION

The Aspirin contained in ALKA-SELTZER is indicated to reduce the risk of death and/or non-fatal myocardial infarction in patients with a previous infarction or unstable angina pectoris.

CLINICAL TRIALS

The indication is supported by the results of six, large, randomized multicenter, placebo-controlled studies[1–7] involving 10,816 predominantly male, post-myocardial infarction (MI) patients and one randomized placebo-controlled study of 1,266 men with unstable angina. Therapy with aspirin was begun at intervals after the onset of acute MI varying from less than 3 days to more than 5 years and continued for periods of from less than one year to four years. In the unstable angina study, treatment was started within 1 month after the onset of unstable angina and continued for 12 weeks and complicating conditions such as congestive heart failure were not included in the study.
Aspirin therapy in MI patients was associated with about a 20 percent reduction in the risk of subsequent death and/or non-fatal reinfarction, a median absolute decrease of 3 percent from the 12 to 22 percent event rates in the placebo groups. In aspirin-treated unstable angina patients the reduction in risk was about 50 percent, a reduction in event rate of 5 percent from the 10 percent rate in the placebo group over the 12 weeks of the study.
Daily dosage of aspirin in the post-myocardial infarction studies was 300 mg in one study and 900 to 1500 mg in five studies. A dose of 325 mg was used in the study of unstable angina.

Continued on next page

Miles Labs.—Cont.

ADVERSE REACTIONS

Gastrointestinal Reactions: Doses of 1000 mg per day of aspirin tablets caused gastrointestinal symptoms and bleeding that in some cases were clinically significant. In the largest post-infarction study (the Aspirin Myocardial Infarction Study (AMIS) with 4,500 people), the percentage incidences of gastrointestinal symptoms for the aspirin (1000 mg of a standard, solid-tablet formulation) and placebo-treated subjects, respectively, were: stomach pain (14.5%; 4.4%); heartburn (11.9%; 4.8%); nausea and/or vomiting (7.6%; 2.1%); hospitalization for gastrointestinal disorder (4.9%; 3.5%). In the AMIS and other trials, aspirin treated patients had increased rates of gross gastrointestinal bleeding. Symptoms and signs of gastrointestinal irritation were not significantly increased in subjects treated for unstable angina with buffered aspirin in solution. As with all aspirin products ALKA-SELTZER is contraindicated in patients with aspirin sensitivity, with asthma, or with coagulation disease.

CARDIOVASCULAR AND BIOCHEMICAL

In the AMIS trial, the dosage of 1000 mg per day of aspirin was associated with small increases in systolic blood pressure (BP) (average 1.5 to 2.1 mm) and diastolic BP (0.5 to 0.6 mm), depending upon whether maximal or last available readings were used. Blood urea nitrogen and uric acid levels were also increased, but by less than 1.0 mg%. Subjects with marked hypertension or renal insufficiency had been excluded from the trial so that the clinical importance of these observations for such subjects or for any subjects treated over more prolonged periods is not known. It is recommended that patients placed on long-term aspirin treatment, even at doses of 300 mg per day, be seen at regular intervals to assess changes in these measurements.

SODIUM IN BUFFERED ASPIRIN FOR SOLUTION FORMULATIONS

One tablet daily of buffered aspirin in solution adds 567 mg of sodium to that in the diet and may not be tolerated by patients with active sodium-retaining states such as congestive heart or renal failure. This amount of sodium adds about 30 percent to the 70 to 90 meq intake suggested as appropriate for dietary treatment of essential hypertension in the 1984 Report of the Joint National Committee on Detection, Evaluation, and Treatment of High Blood Pressure[8].

DOSAGE AND ADMINISTRATION

Although most of the studies used dosages exceeding 300 mg, daily, two trials used only 300 mg and pharmacologic data indicate that this dose inhibits platelet function fully. Therefore, 300 mg or a conventional 325 mg aspirin dose daily is a reasonable, routine dose that would minimize gastrointestinal adverse reactions. This use of aspirin applies to both solid, oral dosage forms (buffered and plain aspirin) and buffered aspirin in solution.

REFERENCES

(1) Elwood, P. C., et al., "A Randomized Controlled Trial of Acetysalicylic Acid in the Secondary Prevention of Mortality from Myocardial Infarction," *British Medical Journal* 1:436–440, 1974.

(2) The Coronary Drug Project Research Group, "Aspirin in Coronary Heart Disease," *Journal of Chronic Diseases,* 29:625–642, 1976.

(3) Breddin, K., et al., "Secondary Prevention of Myocardial Infarction: A Comparison of Acetylsalicylic Acid, Phenprocoumon or Placebo," Int. Congr. Series 470:263–268, 1979.

(4) Aspirin Myocardial Infarction Study Research Group, "A Randomized, Controlled Trial of Aspirin in Persons Recovered from Myocardial Infarction," *Journal American Medical Association* 245:661–669, 1980.

(5) Elwood, P. C., and P. M. Sweetnam, "Aspirin and Secondary Mortality after Myocardial Infarction." *Lancet* pp. 1313–1315, December 22–29, 1979.

(6) The Persantine-Aspirin Reinfarction Study Research Group, "Persantine and Aspirin in Coronary Heart Disease," *Circulation,* 62: 449–460, 1980.

(7) Lewis, H. D., et al., "Protective Effects of Aspirin Against Acute Myocardial Infarction and Death in Men with Unstable Angina, Results of a Veterans Administration Cooperative Study," *New England Journal of Medicine* 309:396–403, 1983.

(8) "1984 Report of the Joint National Committee on Detection, Evaluation, Treatment of High Blood Pressure," U.S. Department of Health and Human Services and United States Public Health Service, National Institutes of Health.

HOW SUPPLIED

Tablets: in bottles of 8 and 26; foil sealed; box of 12; dispenser boxes of 24 tablets in 12 foil twin packs and 36 tablets in 18 foil twin packs; 100 tablets in 50 foil twin packs; carton of 72 tablets in 36 foil twin packs.

Product Identification Mark:
"Alka-Seltzer" embossed on each tablet.

Flavored ALKA-SELTZER®

Effervescent Antacid & Pain Reliever

[al-kuh-selt-sir]

ACTIVE INGREDIENTS

Each tablet contains: Aspirin 324 mg, heat treated sodium bicarbonate 1710 mg, citric acid 1220 mg. Alka-Seltzer in water contains principally the antacid sodium citrate and the analgesic sodium acetylsalicylate.

INACTIVE INGREDIENTS

Flavors, Saccharin, Sodium.

INDICATIONS

SPARKLING FRESH TASTE!

Flavored Alka-Seltzer®

For speedy relief of ACID INDIGESTION, SOUR STOMACH or HEARTBURN with HEADACHE, or BODY ACHES AND PAINS. Also for fast relief of UPSET STOMACH with HEADACHE from overindulgence in food and drink—especially recommended for taking before bed and again on arising. EFFECTIVE FOR PAIN RELIEF ALONE: HEADACHE or BODY and MUSCULAR ACHES and PAINS.

WARNINGS

Children and teenagers should not use this medicine for chicken pox and flu symptoms before a doctor is consulted about Reye's Syndrome, a rare but serious illness.

As with any drug, if you are pregnant or nursing a baby, seek the advice of a health professional before using this product.

Except under the advice and supervision of a physician: Do not take more than, ADULTS: 6 tablets in a 24-hour period, (60 years of age or older: 4 tablets in a 24-hour period), or use the daily maximum dosage for more than 10 days. Do not use if you are allergic to aspirin or have asthma, if you have a coagulation (bleeding) disease, or if you are on a sodium restricted diet. Each tablet contains 506 mg of sodium.

KEEP this and all drugs out of the reach of children.

DIRECTIONS

Alka-Seltzer must be dissolved in water before taking. ADULTS: 2 tablets every 4 hours. CAUTION: If symptoms persist or recur frequently or if you are under treatment for ulcer, consult your physician.

PROFESSIONAL LABELING

ASPIRIN FOR MYOCARDIAL INFARCTION

INDICATION

The Aspirin contained in Alka-Seltzer is indicated to reduce the risk of death and/or non-fatal myocardial infarction in patients with a previous infarction or unstable angina pectoris.

CLINICAL TRIALS

The indication is supported by the results of six, large, randomized multicenter, placebo-controlled studies[1–7] involving 10,816, predominantly male, post-myocardial infarction (MI) patients and one randomized placebo-controlled study of 1,266 men with unstable angina. Therapy with aspirin was begun at intervals after the onset of acute MI varying from less than 3 days to more than 5 years and continued for periods of from less than one year to four years. In the unstable angina study, treatment was started within 1 month after the onset of unstable angina and continued for 12 weeks and complicating conditions such as congestive heart failure were not included in the study.

Aspirin therapy in MI patients was associated with about a 20 percent reduction in the risk of subsequent death and/or non-fatal reinfarction, a median absolute decrease of 3 percent from the 12 to 22 percent event rates in the placebo groups. In aspirin-treated unstable angina patients the reduction in risk was about 50 percent, a reduction in event rate of 5 percent from the 10 percent rate in the placebo group over the 12 week of the study.

Daily dosage of aspirin in the post-myocardial infarction studies was 300 mg in one study and 900 to 1500 mg in five studies. A dose of 325 mg was used in the study of unstable angina.

ADVERSE REACTIONS

Gastrointestinal Reactions: Doses of 1000 mg per day of aspirin tablets caused gastrointestinal symptoms and bleeding that in some cases were clinically significant. In the largest post-infarction study (the Aspirin Myocardial Infarction Study (AMIS) with 4,500 people), the percentage incidences of gastrointestinal symptoms for the aspirin (1000 mg of a standard, solid-tablet formulation) and placebo-treated subjects, respectively, were: stomach pain (14.5%; 4.4%); heartburn (11.9%; 4.8%); nausea and/or vomiting (7.6%; 2.1%); hospitalization for gastrointestinal disorder (4.9%; 3.5%). In the AMIS and other trials, aspirin treated patients had increased rates of gross gastrointestinal bleeding. Symptoms and signs of gastrointestinal irritation were not significantly increased in subjects treated for unstable angina with buffered aspirin in solution. As with all aspirin products Alka-Seltzer is contraindicated in patients with aspirin sensitivity, with asthma, or with coagulation disease.

Cardiovascular and Biochemical: In the AMIS trial, the dosage of 1000 mg per day of aspirin was associated with small increases in systolic blood pressure (BP) (average 1.5 to 2.1 mm) and diastolic BP (0.5 to 0.6 mm), depending upon whether maximal or last available readings were used. Blood urea nitrogen and uric acid levels were also increased, but by less than 1.0 mg%. Subjects with marked hypertension or renal insufficiency had been excluded from the trial so that the clinical importance of these observations for such subjects or for any subjects treated over more prolonged periods is not known. It is recommended that patients placed on long-term aspirin treatment, even at doses of 300 mg per day, be seen at regular intervals to assess changes in these measurements.

Sodium in Buffered Aspirin for Solution Formulations: One tablet daily of flavored buffered aspirin in solution adds 506 mg of sodium to that in the diet and may not be tolerated by patients with active sodium-retaining states such as congestive heart or renal failure. This amount of sodium adds about 30 percent to the 70 to 90 meq intake suggested as appropriate for dietary treatment of essential hypertension in the 1984 Report of the Joint National Committee on Detection, Evaluation, and Treatment of High Blood Pressure[8].

DOSAGE AND ADMINISTRATION

Although most of the studies used dosages exceeding 300 mg, daily, two trials used only 300 mg and pharmacologic data indicate that this dose inhibits platelet function fully. Therefore, 300 mg or a conventional 325 mg aspirin dose daily is a reasonable, routine dose that would minimize gastrointestinal adverse reactions. This use of aspirin applies to both solid, oral dosage forms (buffered and plain aspirin) and buffered aspirin in solution.

REFERENCES

(1) Elwood, P. C., et al., A Randomized Controlled Trial of Acetysalicylic Acid in the Secondary Prevention of Mortality from Myocardial Infarction," *British Medical Journal* 1:436–440, 1974.

(2) The Coronary Drug Project Research Group, "Aspirin in Coronary Heart Disease," *Journal of Chronic Diseases,* 29:625–642, 1976.

(3) Breddin K., et al., "Secondary Prevention of Myocardial Infarction: A Comparison of Acetylsalicylic Acid, Phenprocoumon or Placebo," *Int. Congr. Series* 470:263–268, 1979.

(4) Aspirin Myocardial Infarction Study Research Group, "A Randomized, Controlled Trial of Aspirin in Persons Recovered from Myocardial Infarction," *Journal American Medical Association* 245:661–669, 1980.

(5) Elwood, P. C., and P. M. Sweetnam, "Aspirin and Secondary Mortality after Myocardial Infarction," *Lancet* pp. 1313–1315, December 22–29, 1979.

(6) The Persantine-Aspirin Reinfarction Study Research Group, "Persantine and Aspirin in Coronary Heart Disease," *Circulation,* 62: 449–460, 1980.

(7) Lewis, H. D., et al., "Protective Effects of Aspirin Against Acute Myocardial Infarction and Death in Men with Unstable Angina, Results of a Veterans Administration Cooperative Study," *New England Journal of Medicine* 309:396–403, 1983.

(8) "1984 Report of the Joint National Committee on Detection, Evaluation, Treatment of High Blood Pressure," U.S. Department of Health and Human Services and United States Public Health Service, National Institutes of Health.

HOW SUPPLIED

Foil sealed effervescent tablets in cartons of 12's and 36's.

ALKA-SELTZER® Effervescent Antacid

[al-kuh-selt-sir]

ACTIVE INGREDIENTS

Each tablet contains heat treated sodium bicarbonate 958 mg., citric acid 832 mg., potassium bicarbonate 312 mg. ALKA-SELTZER® Effervescent Antacid in water contains principally the antacids sodium citrate and potassium citrate.

INACTIVE INGREDIENTS

A tableting aid.

INDICATIONS

ALKA-SELTZER® Effervescent Antacid is indicated for relief of acid indigestion, sour stomach or heartburn.

ACTIONS

The ALKA-SELTZER® Effervescent Antacid solution provides quick and effective neutralization of gastric acid. Measured by the in vitro standard established by the Food and Drug Administration one tablet will neutralize 10.6 mEq of acid.

WARNINGS

Except under the advice and supervision of a physician, do not take more than: Adults: 8 tablets in a 24 hour period (60 years of age or older: 7 tablets in a 24 hour period), Children 4 tablets in a 24 hour period; or use the maximum dosage of this product for more than 2 weeks.

Do not use this product if you are on a sodium restricted diet. Each tablet contains 311 mg. of sodium.

Keep this and all drugs out of the reach of children. As with any drug, if you are pregnant or nursing a baby, seek the advice of a health professional before using this product.

DOSAGE AND ADMINISTRATION

ALKA-SELTZER® Effervescent Antacid is taken in solution; approximately 3 oz. of water per tablet is sufficient. Adults: one or two tablets every 4 hours as needed. Children: ½ the adult dosage.

HOW SUPPLIED

Tablets: foil sealed, box of 12 in 6 foil twin packs; dispenser boxes of 20 tablets in 10 foil twin packs; 36 tablets in 18 foil twin packs.

ALKA-SELTZER PLUS® Cold Medicine

[*al-kuh-selt-sir*]

ACTIVE INGREDIENTS

Each dry ALKA-SELTZER PLUS® Cold Tablet contains the following active ingredients: Phenylpropanolamine bitartrate 24 mg., chlorpheniramine maleate 2 mg., aspirin 324 mg. The product is dissolved in water prior to ingestion and the aspirin is converted into its soluble ionic form, sodium acetylsalicylate.

INACTIVE INGREDIENTS

Citric acid, flavors, sodium bicarbonate

INDICATIONS

For relief of the symptoms of head colds, common flu, sinus congestion and hay fever.

ACTIONS

Each tablet contains: A decongestant which helps restore free breathing, shrink swollen nasal tissue and relieve sinus congestion due to head colds or hay fever. An antihistamine which helps relieve the runny nose, sneezing, sniffles, itchy watering eyes that accompany colds or hay fever. Specially buffered aspirin which relieves headache, scratchy sore throat, general body aches and the feverish feeling of a cold and common flu.

WARNINGS

Children and teenagers should not use this medicine for chicken pox or flu symptoms before a doctor is consulted about Reye's Syndrome, a rare but serious illness. Do not use if you are allergic to aspirin or have asthma, or if you have a coagulation (bleeding) disease. If symptoms do not improve in 7 days or are accompanied by high fever or if fever persists for more than 3 days consult a physician before continuing use. Do not take this product if you have glaucoma or difficulty in urination due to enlargement of the prostate gland except under the advice and supervision of a physician. Avoid alcoholic beverages while taking this product.

CAUTION

Individuals with high blood pressure, diabetes, heart or thyroid disease or on a sodium restricted diet should use only as directed by a physician. Each tablet contains 506 mg. of sodium. Product may cause drowsiness: use caution if operating heavy machinery or driving a vehicle. Keep this and all drugs out of the reach of children. As with any drug, if you are pregnant or nursing a baby, seek the advice of a health professional before using this product.

DOSAGE AND ADMINISTRATION

ALKA-SELTZER PLUS® is taken in solution; approximately 3 ounces of water per tablet is sufficient. Adults: two tablets every 4 hours up to 8 tablets in 24 hours.

HOW SUPPLIED

Tablets: carton of 12 tablets in 6 foil twin packs; carton of 20 tablets in 10 foil twin packs; carton of 36 tablets in 18 foil twin packs.

Product Identification Mark:

"Alka-Seltzer Plus" embossed on each tablet.

BACTINE® Antiseptic·Anesthetic First Aid Spray

[*bak-tēn*]

(See PDR For Nonprescription Drugs)

BACTINE® Hydrocortisone (0.5%) Skin Care Cream

[*bak-tēn*]

(See PDR For Nonprescription Drugs)

BIOCAL™ 250 mg Chewable Tablets

[*bī'ō-căl*]

Calcium Supplement

EACH TABLET CONTAINS

625 mg of calcium carbonate, U.S.P. which provides: 250 mg elemental calcium.

INDICATION

Calcium supplementation

DESCRIPTION

BIOCAL™ 250 mg Tablets are round, white, pleasant-tasting mint flavored chewable tablets containing pure calcium carbonate. No sugar, salt, preservatives, or artificial colors added.

DIRECTIONS

Four chewable tablets daily provide:

Elemental Calcium	For Adults and Children Over 4 % U.S. RDA	For Pregnant or Lactating Women
1000 mg	100%	77%

Chew 2 to 4 tablets daily or as recommended by a physician. Keep out of reach of children.

HOW SUPPLIED

Bottles of 60 tablets.

BIOCAL™ 500 mg Tablets

[*bī'ō-căl*]

Calcium Supplement

EACH TABLET CONTAINS

1250 mg of calcium carbonate, U.S.P. which provides: 500 mg elemental Calcium.

INDICATIONS

Calcium supplementation.

DESCRIPTION

BIOCAL™ 500 mg Tablets are white, capsule-shaped tablets containing pure calcium carbonate. No sugar, salt, preservatives, artificial colors or flavors added.

DIRECTIONS

Two tablets daily provide:

Elemental Calcium	For Adults % U.S. RDA	For Pregnant or Lactating Women % U.S. RDA
1000 mg	100%	77%

Take one or two tablets daily or as recommended by a physician.

Keep out of reach of children.

HOW SUPPLIED

Bottles of 60 tablets.

BUGS BUNNY® Children's Chewable Vitamins (Sugar Free)

(Multivitamin Supplement)

BUGS BUNNY® Children's Chewable Vitamins Plus Iron (Sugar Free)

(Multivitamin Supplement with Iron)

BUGS BUNNY® Vitamins Plus Minerals (Sugar Free)

FLINTSTONES® Children's Chewable Vitamins Plus Iron

(Multivitamin Supplement with Iron)

FLINTSTONES® Children's Chewable Vitamins

(Multivitamin Supplement)

FLINTSTONES® COMPLETE

With Iron, Calcium & Minerals Children's Chewable Vitamins

(See PDR For Nonprescription Drugs)

BUGS BUNNY® With Extra C (Sugar Free)

Multivitamin Supplement

(See PDR For Nonprescription Drugs)

FLINTSTONES® With Extra C

Multivitamin Supplement

(See PDR For Nonprescription Drugs)

MILES® NERVINE

NIGHTTIME SLEEP-AID

(See PDR For Nonprescription Drugs)

ONE-A-DAY® Essential

(Multivitamin Supplement)

Within™ from ONE-A-DAY®

(Multivitamin with Calcium and Extra Iron)

(See PDR For Nonprescription Drugs)

ONE-A-DAY® Maximum Formula

(Multivitamin/Multimineral Supplement for adults and teens)

(See PDR For Nonprescription Drugs)

ONE-A-DAY® Plus Extra C

High Potency 300 mg Vitamin C Plus 10 Essential Vitamins (For Adults and Teens)

(See PDR For Nonprescription Drugs)

ONE-A-DAY® STRESSGARD™

Vitamins (B Complex Plus C Stress Formula) High Potency Multivitamin/Multimineral Supplement For Adults

(See PDR For Nonprescription Drugs)

Miles Pharmaceuticals

Division of Miles Laboratories, Inc.
400 MORGAN LANE
WEST HAVEN, CT 06516

PRODUCT IDENTIFICATION CODES

To provide an accurate identification of Miles Pharmaceuticals products, each solid dosage form is coded with the name Miles and a 3 digit product identification number.

PRODUCT	PRODUCT IDENTIFICATION CODE NUMBER
ORAL DOSAGE FORMS	
Adalat Capsules 10 mg (nifedipine)	811
Decholin® Tablets 250 mg (dehydrocholic acid)	121
Lithane® Tablets 300 mg (lithium carbonate)	951
Mycelex® Troche 10 mg (clotrimazole)	095
Niclocide® Chewable Tablets 500 mg (niclosamide)	721
Stilphostrol® Tablets 50 mg (diethylstilbestrol diphosphate)	132
NON-ORAL DOSAGE FORMS	
Domeboro® Tablets (aluminum sulfate, calcium acetate)	411
Mycelex®-G Vaginal Tablets 100 mg (clotrimazole)	093
Mycelex®-G 500 mg Vaginal Tablets (clotrimazole)	097

ADALAT® ℞

Capsules
(nifedipine)
For Oral Use

PRODUCT OVERVIEW

KEY FACTS

Adalat (nifedipine) is a vasospecific antianginal drug of the calcium channel blocker class. The hemodynamic and electrophysiological actions of Adalat make it especially appropriate in patients with angina and coexisting cardiovascular conditions. (see Mechanism of Action section below.)

Continued on next page

Miles Pharm.—Cont.

MAJOR USES

Adalat can be used in patients with vasospastic angina and in angina suggestive of a vasospastic component, as well as in patients with chronic stable angina without vasospasm who are unresponsive or intolerant to beta blockers and/or organic nitrates.

SAFETY INFORMATION

Careful monitoring of blood pressure is suggested during initial administration and titration, since Adalat decreases peripheral vascular resistance. Patients only rarely discontinue Adalat therapy because of its adverse effects, and unwanted effects on the cardiovascular system are usually not serious.

PRESCRIBING INFORMATION

ADALAT® ℞

Capsules
(nifedipine)
For Oral Use

DESCRIPTION

ADALAT (nifedipine) is an antianginal drug belonging to a new class of pharmacological agents, the calcium channel blockers. Nifedipine is 3, 5-pyridinedicarboxylic acid, 1,4-dihydro-2, 6-dimethyl-4-(2-nitrophenyl)-, dimethyl ester, $C_{17}H_{18}N_2O_6$, and has the structural formula:

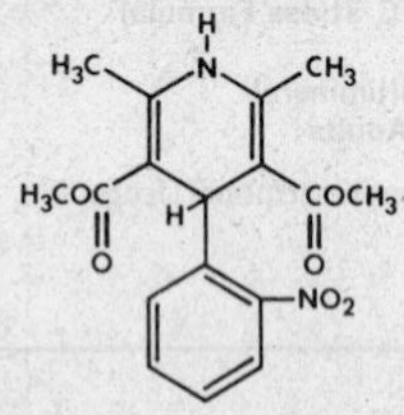

Nifedipine is a yellow crystalline substance, practically insoluble in water but soluble in ethanol. It has a molecular weight of 346.3. ADALAT CAPSULES are formulated as soft gelatin capsules for oral administration each containing 10 mg of nifedipine.

CLINICAL PHARMACOLOGY

ADALAT is a calcium ion influx inhibitor (slow channel blocker or calcium ion antagonist) and inhibits the transmembrane influx of calcium ions into cardiac muscle and smooth muscle. The contractile processes of cardiac muscle and vascular smooth muscle are dependent upon the movement of extracellular calcium ions into these cells through specific ion channels. ADALAT selectively inhibits calcium ion influx across the cell membrane of cardiac muscle and vascular smooth muscle without changing serum calcium concentrations.

Mechanism of Action

The precise means by which this inhibition relieves angina has not been fully determined, but includes at least the following two mechanisms:

1) Relaxation and prevention of coronary artery spasm

ADALAT dilates the main coronary arteries and coronary arterioles, both in normal and ischemic regions, and is a potent inhibitor of coronary artery spasm, whether spontaneous or ergonovine-induced. This property increases myocardial oxygen delivery in patients with coronary artery spasm, and is responsible for the effectiveness of ADALAT in vasospastic (Prinzmetal's or variant) angina. Whether this effect plays any role in classical angina is not clear, but studies of exercise tolerance have not shown an increase in the maximum exercise rate-pressure product, a widely accepted measure of oxygen utilization. This suggests that, in general, relief of spasm or dilation of coronary arteries is not an important factor in classical angina.

2) Reduction of oxygen utilization

ADLAT regularly reduces arterial pressure at rest and at a given level of exercise by dilating peripheral arterioles and reducing the total peripheral resistance (afterload) against which the heart works. This unloading of the heart reduces myocardial energy consumption and oxygen requirements and probably accounts for the effectiveness of ADALAT in chronic stable angina.

Pharmacokinetics and Metabolism

ADALAT is rapidly and fully absorbed after oral administration. The drug is detectable in serum 10 minutes after oral administration, and peak blood levels occur in approximately 30 minutes. It is highly bound by serum proteins. ADALAT® is extensively converted to inactive metabolites and approximately 80 percent of ADALAT and metabolites are eliminated via the kidneys. The half-life of nifedipine in plasma is approximately two hours. There is no information on the effects of renal or hepatic impairment on excretion or metabolism of ADALAT.

Hemodynamics

Like other slow channel blockers, ADALAT exerts a negative inotropic effect on isolated myocardial tissue. This is rarely, if ever, seen in intact animals or man, probably because of reflex responses to its vasodilating effects. In man, ADALAT causes decreased peripheral vascular resistance and a fall in systolic and diastolic pressure, usually modest (5–10mm Hg systolic), but sometimes larger. There is usually a small increase in heart rate, a reflex response to vasodilation. Measurements of cardiac function in patients with normal ventricular function have generally found a small increase in cardiac index without major effects on ejection fraction, left ventricular and diastolic pressure (LVEDP) or volume (LVEDV). In patients with impaired ventricular function, most acute studies have shown some increase in ejection fraction and reduction in left ventricular filing pressure.

Electrophysiologic Effects

Although like other members of its class, ADALAT decreases sinoatrial node function and atrioventricular conduction in isolated myocardial preparations, such effects have not been seen in studies in intact animals or in man. In formal electrophysiologic studies, predominantly in patients with normal conduction systems, ADALAT has had no tendency to prolong atrioventricular conduction, prolong sinus node recovery time, or slow sinus rate.

INDICATIONS AND USAGE

I. Vasospastic Angina

ADALAT (nifedipine) is indicated for the management of vasospastic angina confirmed by any of the following criteria: 1) classical pattern of angina at rest accompanied by ST segment elevation, 2) angina or coronary artery spasm provoked by ergonovine, or 3) angiographically demonstrated coronary artery spasm. In those patients who have had angiography, the presence of significant fixed obstructive disease is not incompatible with the diagnosis of vasospastic angina, provided that the above criteria are satisfied. ADALAT may also be used where the clinical presentation suggests a possible vasospastic component but where vasospasm has not been confirmed, e.g., where pain has a variable threshold on exertion or in unstable angina where electrocardiographic findings are compatible with intermittent vasospasm, or when angina is refractory to nitrates and/or adequate doses of beta blockers.

II. Chronic Stable Angina
(Classical Effort-Associated Angina)

ADALAT is indicated for the management of chronic stable angina (effort-associated angina) without evidence of vasospasm in patients who remain symptomatic despite adequate doses of beta blockers and/or organic nitrates or who cannot tolerate those agents.

In chronic stable angina (effort-associated angina) ADALAT has been effective in controlled trials of up to eight weeks duration in reducing angina frequency and increasing exercise tolerance, but confirmation of sustained effectiveness and evaluation of long term safety in these patients are incomplete.

Controlled studies in small numbers of patients suggest concomitant use of ADALAT® and beta blocking agents may be beneficial in patients with chronic stable angina, but available information is not sufficient to predict with confidence the effects of concurrent treatment, especially in patients with compromised left ventricular function or cardiac conduction abnormalities. When introducing such concomitant therapy, care must be taken to monitor blood pressure closely since severe hypotension can occur from the combined effects of the drugs. (See WARNINGS).

CONTRAINDICATIONS

Known hypersensitivity reaction to ADALAT.

WARNINGS

Excessive Hypotension

Although in most patients, the hypotensive effect of ADALAT is modest and well tolerated, occasional patients have had exessive and poorly tolerated hypotension. These responses have usually occurred during initial titration or at the time of subsequent upward dosage adjustment, and may be more likely in patients on concomitant beta blockers.

Severe hypotension and/or increased fluid volume requirements have been reported in patients receiving ADALAT together with a beta blocking agent who underwent coronary artery bypass surgery using high dose fentanyl anesthesia. The interaction with high dose fentanyl appears to be due to the combination of ADALAT and a beta blocker, but the possibility that it may occur with ADALAT alone, with low doses of fentanyl, in other surgical procedures, or with other narcotic analgesics can not be ruled out. In ADALAT treated patients where surgery using high dose fentanyl anesthesia is contemplated, the physician should be aware of these potential problems and, if the patient's condition permits, sufficient time (at least 36 hours) should be allowed for ADALAT to be washed out of the body prior to surgery.

Increased Angina

Occasional patients have developed well documented increased frequency, duration or severity of angina on starting ADALAT or at the time of dosage increases. The mechanism of this response is not established but could result from decreased coronary perfusion associated with decreased diastolic pressure with increased heart rate, or from increased demand resulting from increased heart rate alone.

Beta Blocker Withdrawal

Patients recently withdrawn from beta blockers may develop a withdrawal syndrome with increased angina, probably related to increased sensitivity to catecholamines. Initiation of ADALAT treatment will not prevent this occurrence and might be expected to exacerbate it by provoking reflex catecholamine release. There have been occasional reports of increased angina in a setting of beta blocker withdrawal and ADALAT initiation. It is important to taper beta blockers if possible rather than stopping them abruptly before beginning ADALAT.

Congestive Heart Failure

Rarely, patients, usually receiving a beta blocker, have developed heart failure after beginning ADALAT. Patients with tight aortic stenosis may be at greater risk for such an event, as the unloading effect of ADALAT® would be expected to be of less benefit to these patients, owing to their fixed impedance to flow across the aortic valve.

PRECAUTIONS

General: Hypotension: Because ADALAT decreases peripheral vascular resistance, careful monitoring of blood pressure during the initial administration and titration of ADALAT is suggested. Close observation is especially recommended for patients already taking medications that are known to lower blood pressure. (See WARNINGS).

Peripheral edema: Mild to moderate peripheral edema, typically associated with arterial vasodilation and not due to left ventricular dysfunction, occurs in about one in ten patients treated with ADALAT (nifedipine). This edema occurs primarily in the lower extremities and usually responds to diuretic therapy. With patients whose angina is complicated by congestive heart failure, care should be taken to differentiate this peripheral edema from the effects of increasing left ventricular dysfunction.

Laboratory tests: Rare, usually transient, but occasionally significant elevations of enzymes such as alkaline phosphatase, CPK, LDH, SGOT and SGPT have been noted. The relationship to ADALAT therapy is uncertain in most cases, but probable in some. These laboratory abnormalities have rarely been associated with clinical symptoms, however, cholestasis with or without jaundice has been reported. Rare instances of allergic hepatitis have been reported.

ADALAT, like other calcium channel blockers, decreases platelet aggregation *in vitro*. Limited clinical studies have demonstrated a moderate but statistically significant decrease in platelet aggregation and increase in bleeding time in some ADALAT patients. This is thought to be a function of inhibition of calcium transport across the platelet membrane. No clinical significance for these findings has been demonstrated.

Although ADALAT has been used safely in patients with renal dysfunction and has been reported to exert a beneficial effect in certain cases, rare, reversible elevations in BUN and serum creatinine have been reported in patients with pre-existing chronic renal insufficiency. The relationship to ADALAT therapy is uncertain in most cases, but probable in some.

Drug Interactions: Beta-adrenergic blocking agents: (See INDICATIONS and WARNINGS). Experience in over 1400 patients in a non-comparative clinical trial has shown that concomitant administration of ADALAT and beta-blocking agents is usually well tolerated, but there have been occasional literature reports suggesting that the combination may increase the likelihood of congestive heart failure, severe hypotension or exacerbation of angina.

Long acting nitrates: ADALAT may be safely co-administered with nitrates, but there have been no controlled studies to evaluate the antianginal effectiveness of this combination.

Digitalis: Administration of ADALAT with digoxin increased digoxin levels in nine of twelve normal volunteers. The average increase was 45%. Another investigator found no increase in digoxin levels in thirteen patients with coronary artery disease. In an uncontrolled study of over two hundred patients with congestive heart failure during which digoxin blood levels were not measured, digitalis toxicity was not observed. Since there have been isolated reports of patients with elevated digoxin levels, it is recommended that digoxin levels be monitored when initiating, adjusting, and discontinuing ADALAT to avoid possible over- or under-digitalization.

Coumarin anticoagulants: There have been rare reports of increased prothrombin time in patients taking coumarin anticoagulants to whom ADALAT® was administered. However, the relationship to ADALAT therapy is uncertain.

Cimetidine: A study in six healthy volunteers has shown a significant increase in peak nifedipine plasma levels (80%)

and area-under-the-curve (74%) after a one week course of cimetidine at 1000 mg per day and nifedipine at 40 mg per day. Ranitidine produced smaller, non-significant increases. The effect may be mediated by the known inhibition of cimetidine on hepatic cytochrome P-450, the enzyme system probably responsible for the first-pass metabolism of nifedipine. If nifedipine therapy is initiated in a patient currently receiving cimetidine, cautious titration is advised.

Carcinogenesis, mutagenesis, impairment of fertility: Nifedipine was administered orally to rats for two years and was not shown to be carcinogenic. When given to rats prior to mating, nifedipine caused reduced fertility at a dose approximately 30 times the maximum recommended human dose. *In vitro* mutagenicity studies were negative.

Pregnancy: Pregnancy category C. Nifedipine has been shown to be teratogenic in rats when given in doses 30 times the maximum recommended human dose. Nifedipine was embryotoxic (increased fetal resorptions, decreased fetal weight, increased stunted forms, increased fetal deaths, decreased neonatal survival) in rats, mice and rabbits at doses of from 3 to 10 times the maximum recommended human dose. In pregnant monkeys, doses ⅔ and twice the maximum recommended human dose resulted in small placentas and underdeveloped chorionic villi. In rats doses three times maximum human dose and higher caused prolongation of pregnancy. There are no adequate and well controlled studies in pregnant women. ADALAT should be used during pregnancy only if the potential benefit justifies the potential risk to the fetus.

ADVERSE REACTIONS

In multiple-dose U.S. and foreign controlled studies in which adverse reactions were reported spontaneously, adverse effects were frequent but generally not serious and rarely required discontinuation of therapy or dosage adjustment. Most were expected consequences of the vasodilator effects of ADALAT.

Adverse Reactions	ADALAT (%) (N = 226)	Placebo (%) (N = 235)
Dizziness, lightheadedness, giddiness	27	15
Flushing, heat sensation	25	8
Headache	23	20
Weakness	12	10
Nausea, heartburn	11	8
Muscle cramps, tremor	8	3
Peripheral edema	7	1
Nervousness, mood changes	7	4
Palpitation	7	5
Dyspnea, cough, wheezing	6	3
Nasal congestion, sore throat	6	8

There is also a large uncontrolled experience in over 2100 patients in the United States. Most of the patients had vasospastic or resistant angina pectoris, and about half had concomitant treatment with beta-adrenergic blocking agents. The most common adverse events were:

Incidence Approximately 10%

Cardiovascular: peripheral edema

Central Nervous System: dizziness or lightheadedness

Gastrointestinal: nausea

Systemic: headache and flushing, weakness

Incidence Approximately 5%

Cardiovascular: transient hypotension

Incidence 2% or Less

Cardiovascular: palpitation

Respiratory: nasal and chest congestion, shortness of breath

Gastrointestinal: diarrhea, constipation, cramps, flatulence

Musculoskeletal: inflammation, joint stiffness, muscle cramps

Central Nervous System: shakiness, nervousness, jitteriness, sleep disturbances, blurred vision, difficulties in balance

Other: dermatitis, pruritus, urticaria, fever, sweating, chills, sexual difficulties.

Incidence Approximately 0.5%

Cardiovascular: syncope. Syncopal episodes did not recur with reduction in the dose of ADALAT® or concomitant antianginal medication.

Incidence Less Than 0.5%

Hematologic: thrombocytopenia, anemia, leukopenia, purpura

Gastrointestinal: allergic hepatitis

Oral: gingival hyperplasia

Other: erythromelalgia

Several of these side effects appear to be dose related. Peripheral edema occurred in about one in 25 patients at doses less than 60 mg per day and in about one patient in eight at 120 mg per day or more. Transient hypotension, generally of mild to moderate severity and seldom requiring discontinuation of therapy, occurred in one of 50 patients at less than 60 mg per day and in one of 20 patients at 120 mg per day or more. Very rarely, introduction of ADALAT therapy was associated with an increase in anginal pain, possibly due to associated hypotension.

In addition, more serious adverse events were observed, not readily distinguishable from the natural history of the disease in these patients. It remains possible, however, that some or many of these events were drug related. Myocardial infarction occurred in about 4% of patients and congestive heart failure or pulmonary edema in about 2%. Ventricular arrhythmias or conduction disturbances each occurred in fewer than 0.5% of patients.

In a subgroup of over 1000 patients receiving ADALAT with concomitant beta blocker therapy, the pattern and incidence of adverse experiences was not different from that of the entire group of ADALAT treated patients (See PRECAUTIONS).

In a subgroup of approximately 250 patients with a diagnosis of congestive heart failure as well as angina, dizziness or lightheadedness, peripheral edema, headache or flushing each occurred in one in eight patients. Hypotension occurred in about one in 20 patients. Syncope occurred in approximately one patient in 250. Myocardial infarction or symptoms of congestive heart failure each occurred in about one patient in 15. Atrial or ventricular dysrhythmias each occurred in about one patient in 150.

OVERDOSAGE

Although there is no well documented experience with ADALAT® overdosage, available data suggest that gross overdosage could result in excessive peripheral vasodilation with subsequent marked and probably prolonged systemic hypotension. Clinically significant hypotension due to ADALAT overdosage calls for active cardiovascular support including monitoring of cardiac and respiratory function, elevation of extremities, and attention to circulating fluid volume and urine output. A vasoconstrictor (such as norepinephrine) may be helpful in restoring vascular tone and blood pressure, provided that there is no contraindication to its use. Clearance of ADALAT would be expected to be prolonged in patients with impaired liver function. Since ADALAT is highly protein-bound, dialysis is not likely to be of benefit.

DOSAGE AND ADMINISTRATION

The dosage of ADALAT needed to suppress angina and that can be tolerated by the patient must be established by titration. Excessive doses can result in hypotension. The starting dose is one 10 mg capsule, swallowed whole, 3 times/day. The usual effective dose range is 10–20 mg three times daily. Some patients, especially those with evidence of coronary artery spasm, respond only to higher doses, more frequent administration, or both. In such patients, doses of 20–30 mg three or four times daily may be effective. Doses above 120 mg daily are rarely necessary. More than 180 mg per day is not recommended.

In most cases, ADALAT titration should proceed over a 7–14 day period so that the physician can assess the response to each dose level and monitor the blood pressure before proceeding to higher doses.

If symptoms so warrant, titration may proceed more rapidly provided that the patient is assessed frequently. Based on the patient's physical activity level, attack frequency, and sublingual nitroglycerin consumption, the dose of ADALAT may be increased from 10 mg t.i.d. to 20 mg t.i.d. and then to 30 mg t.i.d. over a three-day period.

In hospitalized patients under close observation, the dose may be increased in 10 mg increments over four to six-hour periods as required to control pain and arrhythmias due to ischemia. A single dose should rarely exceed 30 mg.

No "rebound effect" has been observed upon discontinuation of ADALAT. However, if discontinuation of ADALAT is necessary, sound clinical practice suggests that the dosage should be decreased gradually with close physician supervision.

Co-Administration with Other Antianginal Drugs

Sublingual nitroglycerin may be taken as required for the control of acute manifestations of angina, particularly during ADALAT titration. See **Precautions, Drug Interactions,** for information on co-administration of ADALAT with beta blockers or long acting nitrates.

HOW SUPPLIED

Each orange, soft gelatin ADALAT CAPSULE contains 10 mg of nifedipine. The capsules are identified as follows: Miles 811. ADALAT CAPSULES are supplied in bottles of 100 (**NDC** 0026-8811-51), 300 (**NDC** 0026-8811-18), and unit dose (10 × 10) (**NDC** 0026-8811-48).

The capsules should be protected from light and moisture and stored at controlled room temperature 59° to 77°F (15° to 25°C) in the manufacturer's original container.

Encapsulated by
R.P. Scherer N.A.
Clearwater, FL 33518
Manufactured by
Miles Pharmaceuticals
PD 100631 Rev. 11/85

Shown in Product Identification Section, page 418

AZLIN® ℞
Sterile azlocillin sodium
for intravenous use.

PRODUCT OVERVIEW

KEY FACTS

AZLIN® is a semisynthetic broad spectrum penicillin antibiotic for parenteral administration. A bactericidal antibiotic, AZLIN® acts by interfering with cell wall synthesis. It is active against *Pseudomonas aeruginosa* and other *Pseudomonas* species, many of which are resistant to other broad spectrum antibiotics. AZLIN® is also active *in vitro* against many strains of the organisms listed below.

MAJOR USES

AZLIN® is primarily indicated for treatment of serious infections caused by susceptible strains of *P. aeruginosa.* It has been proven effective in treatment of infections of the lower respiratory tract, urinary tract, skin and skin structure, bones and joints, including osteomyelitis, and bacterial septicemia. In certain severe infections when the causative organisms are unknown and *Pseudomonas* is suspected, AZLIN® may be administered with an aminoglycoside or cephalosporin as initial therapy. As soon as results of culture and susceptibility tests become available, antimicrobial therapy should be adjusted as indicated.

SAFETY INFORMATION

AZLIN® is contraindicated in patients with a history of hypersensitivity reactions to any of the penicillins. Although AZLIN® shares with other penicillins the low potential for toxicity, as with any potent drug, periodic assessment of organ system functions, including renal, hepatic and hematopoietic, is advisable during prolonged therapy.

PRESCRIBING INFORMATION

AZLIN® ℞
Sterile azlocillin sodium
for intravenous use.

DESCRIPTION

AZLIN® (sterile azlocillin sodium) is a semisynthetic broad spectrum penicillin antibiotic for parenteral administration. It is the monosodium salt of 6-D-2 (2-OXO-imidazolidine-1-carboxamido) -2- phenyl- acetamido -penicillanic acid.

Structural Formula:

Empirical Formula: $C_{20}H_{22}N_5O_6S$ Na

AZLIN® has a molecular weight of 483.5 and contains 49.8 mg (2.17 mEq) of sodium per one gram of azlocillin activity. The dosage form is supplied as a sterile white to pale yellow powder, which is freely soluble in water. When reconstituted, aqueous solutions of AZLIN® are clear and range from colorless to pale yellow with a pH of 6.0 to 8.0.

CLINICAL PHARMACOLOGY

Intravenous Administration. In healthy adult volunteers, mean serum levels of azlocillin 30 minutes after a 5–10 minute intravenous injection of 1g, 2g, or 5g are 35, 106 and 256 mcg/ml, respectively. Serum levels, as noted below, lack dose proportionality:

[See first table on bottom next page].

After an intravenous infusion (30 min) of 2g or 3 g azlocillin, mean serum levels 5 minutes after dosing are 130 mcg/ml (73–189) and 180 mcg/ml (133–235), respectively.

[See second table on bottom next page].

Following intravenous infusion (30 min) of a 3g dose of azlocillin every 6 hours for 5 days, mean peak serum concentrations were higher than 150 mcg/ml; trough levels were between 4–12 mcg/ml. From the first to the last day of dosing, the serum half-life increased from 61 minutes to approximately 77 minutes.

General. As with other penicillins, azlocillin is excreted primarily by the kidney through glomerular filtration and tubular secretion. The rate of elimination is dose dependent and also related to the status of renal function. In patients with normal renal function, 50 to 70% of the administered dose is recovered from the urine within 24 hours after dosing. Two hours after an intravenous injection of 2g, concentrations of active drug in urine generally exceed 4000 mcg/ml. By 4–8 hours after injection, concentrations are still above 500 mcg/ml. The serum elimination half-life of azlocillin is dose dependent and ranges from approximately 55 minutes after an intravenous dose of 2g to about 70 minutes after intravenous dose of 5g. Probenecid interferes with the renal tubular secretion of azlocillin, thereby in-

Continued on next page

Miles Pharm.—Cont.

creasing serum concentrations and prolonging serum half-life of the antibiotic.

In patients with reduced renal function, the serum half-life of azlocillin is prolonged, depending on degree of renal impairment. Dosage adjustments are usually not necessary except in patients with moderate to severe renal impairment. (See Dosage and Administration). As with other penicillins, azlocillin is metabolized only slightly; less than 10% of the administered dose is found in the urine in the form of the penicilloate or penilloate. The drug is readily removed from the serum by hemodialysis.

Following an intravenous dose of 2g azlocillin, peak concentrations of active drug in bile generally exceed 1000 mcg/ml. The bile levels are approximately 15 times higher than the corresponding serum levels. Biliary excretion is reduced in patients with common bile duct obstruction.

Following parenteral administration, the apparent volume of distribution is approximately 20% of body weight. The drug is present in active form in the serum, urine, bile, bronchial and wound secretions, bone and other tissues. As with other penicillins, penetration into the cerebrospinal fluid (CSF) is generally poor, however, higher CSF concentrations are obtained in the presence of meningeal inflammation.

The serum level of uric acid has been noted to be depressed in some patients receiving azlocillin; this effect appears to be transient.

Protein binding studies indicate that the degree of azlocillin binding is low (25–45%) and depends upon testing methods and concentrations of drug studied.

Microbiology

Azlocillin is a bactericidal antibiotic which acts by interfering with synthesis of cell wall components. It is active against *Pseudomonas aeruginosa* and other species of Pseudomonas, many of which are resistant to other broad spectrum antibiotics. Azlocillin is also active *in vitro* against many strains of the following organisms, however, clinical efficacy for infections other than those included in the indication section has not been documented:

Gram-negative bacteria

Escherichia coli
Proteus mirabilis
Proteus vulgaris
Morganella morganii (formerly *P. morganii*)
Providencia rettgeri (formerly *P. rettgeri*)
Providencia stuartii
Enterobacter species
Shigella species
Haemophilus influenzae
Haemophilus parainfluenzae
Neisseria species
Citrobacter species

Some strains of *Klebsiella, Serratia, Salmonella,* and *Acinetobacter* are also susceptible.

Gram-positive bacteria

Staphylococcus aureus (non-penicillinase producing strains)
Beta-hemolytic streptococci (Groups A and B)
Streptococcus pneumoniae (formerly *Diplococcus pneumoniae*)
Streptococcus faecalis (enterococcus)
Listeria monocytogenes

Anaerobic Organisms

Peptococcus species
Peptostreptococcus species
Clostridium species
Bacteroides species (including *B. fragilis* group)
Fusobacterium species
Veillonella species
Eubacterium species

Azlocillin is inactive against penicillinase-producing strains of *Staphylococcus aureus* and is susceptible to inactivation by beta-lactamases produced by the Enterobacteriaceae.

In vitro studies have shown that azlocillin combined with an aminoglycoside (e.g., gentamicin, tobramycin, amikacin, sisomicin) acts synergistically against many strains of *Pseudomonas aeruginosa.*

Azlocillin is slightly more active when tested at alkaline pH and, as with other penicillins, has reduced activity when tested *in vitro* with increasing inoculum. The minimal bactericidal concentration (MBC) may exceed the minimal inhibitory concentration (MIC) by four-fold or more depending on medium used. Resistance to azlocillin *in vitro* develops slowly (multiple step mutation). Some strains of *Pseudomonas aeruginosa* have developed resistance fairly rapidly.

Susceptibility Tests

Quantitative methods that require measurement of zone diameters give good estimates of bacterial susceptibility. One such procedure* has been recommended for use with discs to test susceptibility to antimicrobials. When the causative organism is tested by the Kirby-Bauer disc diffusion method, a 75 mcg azlocillin disc should give a zone of 18 mm or greater to indicate susceptibility. Zone sizes of 14 mm or less indicate resistance. Zone sizes of 15 to 17 mm indicate intermediate susceptibility. With this procedure, a report from the laboratory of "Susceptible" indicates that the infecting organism is likely to respond to therapy. A report of "Resistant" indicates that the infecting organism is not likely to respond to therapy; other therapy should be selected. A report of "Intermediate Susceptibility" suggests that the organism may be susceptible if the infection is confined to tissues and fluids (e.g., urine), in which high antibiotic levels are attained. The azlocillin disc should be used for testing susceptibility to azlocillin. Standardized procedure requires use of control organisms. The 75 mcg azlocillin disc should give zone diameters between 24 and 30 mm for *P. aeruginosa* ATCC 27853. For *E. coli* ATCC 25922 the zone diameters should be between 21 and 24 mm.

* Bauer, A.W., Kirby, W.M., Sherris, J.C., and Turck, M.: Antibiotic Testing by a Standardized Single Disc Method, Am. J. Clin. Pathol., 45:493, 1966; Standardized Disc Susceptibility Test, FEDERAL REGISTER, 39: 19182–19184, 1974.

In certain conditions, it may be desirable to do additional susceptibility testing by broth or agar dilution techniques. Dilution methods, preferably the agar plate dilution procedure, are most accurate for susceptibility testing of obligate anaerobes. *Pseudomonas* species and the *Enterobacteriaceae* are considered susceptible if the MIC of azlocillin is no greater than 64 mcg/ml and are considered resistant if the MIC is greater than 128 mcg/ml. The MIC values of azlocillin for the control strains are the following:

P. aeruginosa ATCC 27853, 4–8 mcg/ml and
E. coli ATCC 25922, 8–16 mcg/ml.

Azlocillin standard is available for broth or agar dilution studies.

INDICATIONS AND USAGE

AZLIN® is indicated primarily for the treatment of serious infections caused by susceptible strains of *Pseudomonas aeruginosa* in the conditions listed below:

LOWER RESPIRATORY TRACT INFECTIONS including pneumonia and lung abscess.

URINARY TRACT INFECTIONS both complicated and uncomplicated of the lower and upper urinary tract.

SKIN AND SKIN STRUCTURE INFECTIONS including ulcers, abscesses, burns and severe external otitis.

BONE AND JOINT INFECTIONS including osteomyelitis.

BACTERIAL SEPTICEMIA

Azlocillin has also been shown to be effective for the treatment of Lower Respiratory Tract Infections caused by *Escherichia coli* and *Haemophilus influenzae;* Urinary Tract Infections and Skin Structure Infections caused by *Escherichia coli, Proteus mirabilis* or *Streptococcus faecalis;* and Septicemia caused by *Escherichia coli.*

Appropriate culture and susceptibility tests should be performed before treatment in order to isolate and identify organisms causing infections and to determine their susceptibility to azlocillin. Therapy with AZLIN® may be initiated before results of these tests are known; once results become available, appropriate therapy should be continued.

In certain severe infections, when the causative organisms are unknown and *Pseudomonas aeruginosa* is suspected, AZLIN® may be administered in conjunction with an aminoglycoside or a cephalosporin antibiotic as initial therapy. As soon as results of culture and susceptibility tests become available, antimicrobial therapy should be adjusted as indicated. Culture and susceptibility testing, performed periodically during therapy, will provide information on the therapeutic effect of the antimicrobial and will monitor for the possible emergence of bacterial resistance.

AZLIN® has been used effectively in combination with an aminoglycoside antibiotic for the treatment of life-threatening infections caused by *Pseudomonas aeruginosa* including acute pulmonary exacerbation in patients with cystic fibrosis. For the treatment of febrile episodes in immunosuppressed patients with granulocytopenia, AZLIN® should be combined with an aminoglycoside or a cephalosporin antibiotic.

CONTRAINDICATIONS

AZLIN® is contraindicated in patients with a history of hypersensitivity reactions to any of the penicillins.

WARNINGS

Serious and occasionally fatal hypersensitivity (anaphylactic) reactions have occurred in patients receiving a penicillin. These reactions are more apt to occur in individuals with a history of sensitivity to multiple allergens. There have been reports of individuals with a history of penicillin hypersensitivity reactions who have experienced severe hypersensitivity reactions when treated with a cephalosporin. Before therapy with azlocillin is instituted, careful inquiry should be made to determine whether the patient has had previous hypersensitivity reactions to penicillins, cephalosporins or other drugs. Antibiotics should be used with caution in any patient who has demonstrated some form of allergy, particularly to drugs.

If an allergic reaction occurs during therapy with azlocillin, the drug should be discontinued. SERIOUS ANAPHYLACTOID REACTIONS REQUIRE IMMEDIATE EMERGENCY TREATMENT WITH EPINEPHRINE. OXYGEN, INTRAVENOUS STEROIDS, AND AIRWAY MANAGEMENT, INCLUDING INTUBATION, SHOULD ALSO BE PROVIDED AS INDICATED.

PRECAUTIONS

Although AZLIN® shares with other penicillins the low potential for toxicity, as with any potent drug, periodic assessment of organ system functions, including renal, hepatic and hematopoietic, is advisable during prolonged therapy.

Bleeding manifestations have occurred in some patients receiving beta-lactam antibiotics. These reactions have been associated with abnormalities of coagulation tests, such as clotting time, platelet aggregation and prothrombin time and are more likely to occur in patients with renal impairment. Although AZLIN® has rarely been associated with any bleeding abnormalities, the possibility of this occurring should be kept in mind, particularly in patients with severe renal impairment receiving maximum doses of the drug.

AZLIN® has only rarely been reported to cause hypokalemia; however, the possibility of this occurring should also be kept in mind, particularly when treating patients with fluid and electrolyte imbalance. Periodic monitoring of serum potassium may be advisable in patients receiving prolonged therapy.

AZLIN® is a monosodium salt containing only 49.8 mg (2.17

AZLIN®

AZLOCILLIN SERUM LEVELS IN ADULTS (mcg/ml) 5–10 MIN IV INJECTION

DOSE	5 min	15 min	30 min	1 hr	2 hr	3 hr	4 hr	6 hr	8 hr
1g			**35** (29–41)	**22** (18–26)	**9.4** (7.2–14)	**4.3** (2.6–6.8)	**2.2** (1.2–4.0)		
2g	**239** (142–363)	**139** (85–188)	**106** (83–134)	**47** (30–60)	**19** (16–26)	**12** (8.7–13)	**7.4** (5.7–11)	**2.1** (1.8–2.9)	**0.5** (0–0.7)
5g	**527** (470–604)	**353** (258–440)	**256** (184–287)	**174** (116–231)	**85** (43–121)	**55** (26–91)	**33** (15–58)	**7.7** (1.6–19)	**4.1** (1.4–7.8)

AZLIN®

AZLOCILLIN SERUM LEVELS IN ADULTS (mcg/ml) 30 MIN IV INFUSION

DOSE	0	5 min	15 min	30 min	45 min	1 hr	1.5 hr	2 hr	3 hr	4 hr	6 hr	8 hr
2g	**165** (55–278)	**130** (73–189)	**104** (62–175)	**85** (42–121)	**62** (23–85)	**49** (27–82)	**36** (19–57)	**26** (13–48)	**13** (5–25)	**6** (2–11)	**2** (1–4)	**1** (1–4)
3g	**214** (155–273)	**180** (133–235)	**139** (119–186)	**104** (61–159)	**82** (58–121)	**68** (38–94)	**58** (35–74)	**39** (17–53)	**24** (9–36)	**10** (3–14)	**3** (1–5)	**1** (1–4)

mEq) of sodium per gram of azlocillin. This should be considered when treating patients requiring restricted salt intake.
As with any penicillin, an allergic reaction, including anaphylaxis, may occur during AZLIN® administration, particularly in a hypersensitive individual.
The rapid intravenous administration of AZLIN® has been associated with transient chest discomfort. Therefore, the drug should not be infused over a period of less than five minutes.
As with other antibiotics, prolonged use of AZLIN® may result in overgrowth of non-susceptible organisms. If this occurs, appropriate measures should be taken.

Interactions with Drugs and Laboratory Tests

As with other penicillins, the mixing of azlocillin with an aminoglycoside in solutions for parenteral administration can result in substantial inactivation of the aminoglycoside.
Probenecid interferes with the renal tubular secretion of azlocillin, thereby increasing serum concentrations and prolonging serum half-life of the antibiotic.
The serum level of uric acid has been noted to be depressed in some patients receiving azlocillin; this effect appears to be transient.
High urine concentrations of azlocillin may produce false positive protein reactions (pseudoproteinuria) with the following methods: sulfosalicylic acid and boiling test, acetic acid test, biuret reaction, and nitric acid test. The bromphenol blue (Multi-stix®) reagent strip test has been reported to be reliable.

Pregnancy Category B

Reproduction studies have been performed in rats and mice at doses up to 2 times the human dose, and have revealed no evidence of impaired fertility or harm to the fetus, due to AZLIN®. There are however no adequate and well controlled studies in pregnant women. Because animal reproductive studies are not always predictive of human response, this drug should be used during pregnancy only if clearly needed. Azlocillin crosses the placenta and is found in cord blood and amniotic fluid.

Nursing Mothers

Azlocillin is detected in low concentrations in the milk of nursing mothers, therefore caution should be exercised when AZLIN® is administered to a nursing woman.

Drug Abuse and Dependence

Neither AZLIN® abuse nor AZLIN® dependence has been reported.

ADVERSE REACTIONS

As with other penicillins, the following adverse reactions may occur:
Hypersensitivity reactions: skin rash, pruritus, urticaria, arthralgia, myalgia, drug fever, chills, chest discomfort, and anaphylactic reactions.
Central nervous system: headache, giddiness, neuromuscular hyperirritability or convulsive seizures.
Gastro-intestinal disturbances: disturbances of taste and smell, stomatitis, flatulence, nausea, vomiting and diarrhea, epigastric pain.
Hemic and Lymphatic Systems: thrombocytopenia, leukopenia, neutropenia, eosinophilia and reduction of hemoglobin or hematocrit. Prolongation of prothrombin time and bleeding time.
Abnormalities of hepatic and renal function tests: elevation of serum aspartate aminotransferase (SGOT), serum alanine aminotransferase (SGPT), serum alkaline phosphatase, serum LDH, serum bilirubin. Elevation of serum creatinine and/or BUN, hypernatremia. Reduction in serum potassium and uric acid.
Local reactions: pain and thrombophlebitis with intravenous administration.

OVERDOSAGE

As with other penicillins, AZLIN® in overdosage has the potential to cause neuromuscular hyperirritability or convulsive seizures. Hemodialysis, if necessary, will aid in removal of the drug from the blood.

DOSAGE AND ADMINISTRATION

AZLIN® (sterile azlocillin sodium) may be administered by slow intravenous injection (5 min or longer) or by intravenous infusion (30 min).
The recommended adult dosage for serious infections is 200–300 mg/kg per day given in 4 to 6 divided doses. The usual dose is 3g given every 4 hours (18g/day). For life-threatening infections, up to 350 mg/kg per day may be administered, but the total daily dosage should ordinarily not exceed 24g.
[See table above].

AZLIN® DOSAGE GUIDE (ADULTS)

Condition	Daily Dosage Range	Usual Daily Dosage	Frequency and Route of Administration
Urinary tract infection (uncomplicated)	100–125 mg/kg	8g	2g every 6 hours IV
Urinary tract infection (complicated)	150–200 mg/kg	12g	3g every 6 hours IV
Lower respiratory tract infection Skin & skin structure infection Bone & joint infection Septicemia	225–300 mg/kg	16–18g	3g every 4 hours or 4g every 6 hours IV

For patients with life-threatening infections, 4g may be administered every 4 hours (24g/day).
Dosage for any individual patient must take into consideration the site and severity of infection, the susceptibility of the organisms causing infection, and the status of the patient's host defense mechanisms.
The duration of therapy depends upon the severity of infection. Generally, AZLIN® should be continued for at least 2 days after the signs and symptoms of infection have disappeared. The usual duration is 10 to 14 days; however, in difficult and complicated infections, more prolonged therapy may be required (e.g., osteomyelitis).
In certain deep-seated infections, involving abscess formation, appropriate surgical drainage should be performed in conjunction with antimicrobial therapy.

Patients with Impaired Renal Function

The rate of elimination of azlocillin is dose dependent and related to the degree of renal function impairment. After an intravenous dose of 5g, the serum half-life is approximately 1 hour in patients with creatinine clearances above 80 ml/min, 2.0 hr in those with clearances of 30–79 ml/min, 4.0 hr in those with clearances of 10–29 ml/min and approximately 5.9 hr in patients with clearances of less than 10 ml/min. Dosage adjustments of AZLIN® are not required in patients with mild impairment of renal function. For patients with a creatinine clearance of ≤ 30 ml/min (serum creatinine of approximately 3.0 mg% or greater), the following dosage guide may be used.
[See table below].

AZLIN® DOSAGE GUIDE FOR PATIENTS WITH IMPAIRED RENAL FUNCTION

Creatinine Clearance ml/min	Urinary Tract Infection (Uncomplicated)	Urinary Tract Infection (Complicated)	Serious Systemic Infection
>30	Usual Recommended Dosage		
10–30	1.5 g every 12 hours	1.5g every 8 hours	2g every 8 hours
<10	1.5 g every 12 hours	2g every 12 hours	3g every 12 hours

For patients undergoing hemodialysis for renal failure, 3g may be administered after each dialysis and then every 12 hours.
For patients with renal failure, particularly those with concomitant hepatic insufficiency, measurement of serum levels of azlocillin will provide additional guidance for adjusting dosage.

Intravenous Administration

AZLIN® may be administered intravenously by intermittent infusion or by direct slow intravenous injection.
Infusion. Each gram of azlocillin should be reconstituted by vigorous shaking with at least 10 ml of Sterile Water for Injection, 5% Dextrose Injection or 0.9% Sodium Chloride Injection. The dissolved drug should be further diluted to desired volume (50-100 ml) with an appropriate intravenous solution. (See Compatibility and Stability section). The solution of reconstituted drug may then be administered over a period of 30 minutes by direct infusion or through a Y-type intravenous infusion set which may already be in place. If this method or the "piggyback" method of administration is used, it is advisable to discontinue temporarily the administration of any other solutions during the infusion of AZLIN®.
Injection. The reconstituted solution of AZLIN® may also be injected directly into a vein or into intravenous tubing; when administered in this way, the injection should be given slowly over a period of 5 minutes or longer. To minimize venous irritation, the concentration of drug should not exceed 10%.
When AZLIN® is given in combination with another antimicrobial, such as an aminoglycoside, each drug should be given separately in accordance with the recommended dosage and routes of administration for each drug.
After reconstitution and prior to administration, AZLIN® as with other parenteral drugs, should be inspected visually for particulate matter and discoloration.

Pediatric Use

Only limited data are available on the safety and effectiveness of AZLIN® in the treatment of infants with documented serious infection. Until further experience is gained, the drug should not be used in the newborn period.
In children with acute pulmonary exacerbation of cystic fibrosis, azlocillin may be administered at a dose of 75 mg/kg every 4 hours (450 mg/kg/day). The total daily dosage should not exceed 24g. The drug may be infused intravenously over a period of about 30 minutes.

COMPATIBILITY AND STABILITY

AZLIN® at concentrations of 10 mg/ml and 50 mg/ml is stable (loss of potency less than 10%) when stored at room temperature in the following intravenous solutions for the time periods stated. When stored under refrigeration (below 8°C), AZLIN® at concentrations up to 100 mg/ml is stable for the time periods stated:

INTRAVENOUS SOLUTION	STABILITY
Sterile Water for Injection, U.S.P.	24 hours
0.9% Sodium Chloride Injection, U.S.P.	24 hours
5% Dextrose Injection, U.S.P.	24 hours
5% Dextrose in 0.225% Sodium Chloride Injection, U.S.P.	24 hours
Lactated Ringer's Injection, U.S.P.	24 hours
5% Dextrose in 0.45% Sodium Chloride Injection, U.S.P.	24 hours

Unused portion must be discarded after the time period stated.

HOW SUPPLIED

AZLIN® (sterile azlocillin sodium) is a white to pale yellow powder supplied in vials and infusion bottles. Each vial contains azlocillin sodium equivalent to 2g, 3g or 4g azlocillin. Each infusion bottle contains azlocillin sodium equivalent to 2g, 3g or 4g azlocillin.
AZLIN® vials and infusion bottles should be stored at or below 30°C (86°F). The powder as well as the reconstituted solution of drug may darken slightly, depending upon storage conditions, but potency is not affected.
Issued: June, 1982 PD 100585 19230

BILTRICIDE® ℞
(praziquantel)

DESCRIPTION

BILTRICIDE (praziquantel) is a trematodicide provided in tablet form for the oral treatment of schistosome infections.
BILTRICIDE (praziquantel) is 2-(cyclohexylcarbonyl)-1,2,3,6,7,11b-hexahydro4H-pyrazino [2,1-a] isoquinolin-4-one with the molecular formula: $C_{19}H_{24}N_2O_2$.
The structural formula is as follows:

Praziquantel is a colorless crystalline powder of bitter taste. The compound is stable under normal conditions and melts at 136–140°C with decomposition. The active substance is hygroscopic. Praziquantel is easily soluble in chloroform and dimethylsulfoxide, soluble in ethanol and very slightly soluble in water.
BILTRICIDE lacquered tablets contain 600 mg of praziquantel.

Continued on next page

Miles Pharm.—Cont.

CLINICAL PHARMACOLOGY

BILTRICIDE induces a rapid contraction of schistosomes by a specific effect on the permeability of the cell membrane. The drug further causes vacuolization and disintegration of the schistosome tegument.

After oral administration BILTRICIDE is rapidly absorbed (80%), subjected to a first pass effect, metabolized and eliminated by the kidneys. Maximal serum concentration is achieved 1–3 hours after dosing. The half-life of praziquantel in serum is 0.8–1.5 hours.

INDICATIONS AND USAGE

BILTRICIDE® is indicated for the treatment of infections due to: *Schistosoma mekongi, Schistosoma japonicum, Schistosoma mansoni and Schistosoma hematobium.*

CONTRAINDICATIONS

BILTRICIDE should not be given to patients who previously have shown hypersensitivity to the drug. Since parasite destruction within the eye may cause irreparable lesions, ocular cysticercosis should not be treated with this compound.

PRECAUTIONS

Information for the patient: Patients should be warned not to drive a car and not to operate machinery on the day of BILTRICIDE treatment and the following day. Minimal increases in liver enzymes have been reported in some patients.

When schistosomiasis or fluke infection is found to be associated with cerebral cysticercosis it is advised to hospitalize the patient for the duration of treatment.

Drug Interactions: No data are available regarding interaction of BILTRICIDE with other drugs.

Mutagenesis, Carcinogenesis: Mutagenic effects in Salmonella tests found by one laboratory have not been confirmed in the same tested strain by other laboratories. Long term carcinogenicity studies in rats and golden hamsters did not reveal any carcinogenic effect.

Pregnancy Category B: Reproduction studies have been performed in rats and rabbits at doses up to 40 times the human dose and have revealed no evidence of impaired fertility or harm to the fetus due to BILTRICIDE. There are, however, no adequate and well-controlled studies in pregnant women. An increase of the abortion rate was found in rats at three times the single human therapeutic dose. While animal reproduction studies are not always predictive of human response this drug should be used during pregnancy only if clearly needed.

Nursing mothers: BILTRICIDE® appeared in the milk of nursing women at a concentration of about ¼ that of maternal serum. Women should not nurse on the day of BILTRICIDE treatment and during the subsequent 72 hours.

Pediatric use: Safety in children under 4 years of age has not been established.

ADVERSE EFFECTS

In general BILTRICIDE is very well tolerated. Side effects are usually mild and transient and do not require treatment. The following side effects were observed generally in order of severity: malaise, headache, dizziness, abdominal discomfort with or without nausea, rise in temperature and, rarely, urticaria. Such symptoms can, however, also result from the infection itself. Such side effects may be more frequent and/or serious in patients with a heavy worm burden. In patients with liver impairment caused by the infection, no adverse effects of BILTRICIDE have occurred which would necessitate restriction in use.

OVERDOSAGE

In rats and mice the acute LD_{50} was about 2,500 mg/kg. No data are available in humans. In the event of overdose a fast-acting laxative should be given.

DOSAGE AND ADMINISTRATION

The dosage recommended for the treatment of schistosomiasis is: 3 × 20 mg/kg bodyweight as a one day treatment. The tablets should be washed down unchewed with some liquid during meals. Keeping the tablets or segments thereof in the mouth can reveal a bitter taste which can promote gagging or vomiting. The interval between the individual doses should not be less than 4 and not more than 6 hours.

HOW SUPPLIED

BILTRICIDE is supplied as a 600 mg white, film-coated, oblong tablet with three scores. When broken each of the four segments contains 150 mg of active ingredient so that the dosage can be easily adjusted to the patient's bodyweight.

Segments are broken off by pressing the score (notch) with thumbnails. If ¼ of a tablet is required, this is best achieved by breaking the segment from the outer end.

BILTRICIDE® is available in bottles of 6.

STORAGE CONDITIONS

Store below 86°F (30°C).

PD100576 19253 April 1983

Shown in Product Identification Section, page 418

CORT-DOME® ℞
1%, ½% and ¼%
(hydrocortisone) creme **acid pH**

DESCRIPTION

Cort-Dome® Creme contains microdispersed hydrocortisone (the active ingredient) in a compatible vehicle buffered to the acid pH range of normal skin. Each gram of Cort-Dome® Creme contains 10.0mg/g (1%), 5.0mg/g (½%) or 2.5mg/g (¼%) of hydrocortisone. Cort-Dome® Creme is applied topically. Hydrocortisone is a corticosteroid. Chemically, hydrocortisone is Pregn-4-ene-3, 20-dione,11,17,21-trihydroxy-,(11β)-. with the following structural formula:

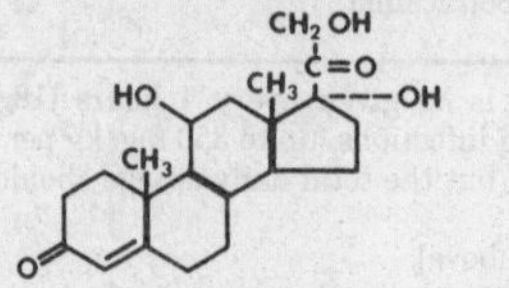

The vehicle for Cort-Dome® Creme 1%, ½%, and ¼% contains glycerin, calcium acetate, cetyl-stearyl alcohol-sodium lauryl sulfate, aluminum sulfate, purified water, synthetic beeswax (B-wax), white petrolatum, dextrin, and light mineral oil, preserved with methylparaben.

EMPIRICAL FORMULA	MOLECULAR WEIGHT	CAS REGISTRY NUMBER
$C_{21}H_{30}O_5$	362.47	50-23-7

CLINICAL PHARMACOLOGY

Topical corticosteroids share anti-inflammatory, anti-pruritic and vasoconstrictive actions.

The mechanism of anti-inflammatory activity of the topical corticosteroids is unclear. Various laboratory methods, including vasoconstrictor assays, are used to compare and predict potencies and/or clinical efficacies of the topical corticosteroids. There is some evidence to suggest that a recognizable correlation exists between vasoconstrictor potency and therapeutic efficacy in man.

Pharmacokinetics

The extent of percutaneous absorption of topical corticosteroids is determined by many factors including the vehicle, the integrity of the epidermal barrier, and the use of occlusive dressings.

Topical corticosteroids can be absorbed from normal intact skin. Inflammation and/or other disease processes in the skin increase percutaneous absorption. Occlusive dressings substantially increase the percutaneous absorption of topical corticosteroids. Thus, occlusive dressings may be a valuable therapeutic adjunct for treatment of resistant dermatoses. (See DOSAGE AND ADMINISTRATION).

Once absorbed through the skin, topical corticosteroids are handled through pharmacokinetic pathways similar to systemically administered corticosteroids. Corticosteroids are bound to plasma proteins in varying degrees. Corticosteroids are metabolized primarily in the liver and are then excreted by the kidneys. Some of the topical corticosteroids and their metabolites are also excreted into the bile.

INDICATIONS AND USAGE

Topical corticosteroids are indicated for the relief of the inflammatory and pruritic manifestations of corticosteroid-responsive dermatoses.

CONTRAINDICATIONS

Topical corticosteroids are contraindicated in those patients with a history of hypersensitivity to any of the components of the preparation.

PRECAUTIONS

General

Systemic absorption of topical corticosteroids has produced reversible hypothalamic-pituitary-adrenal (HPA) axis suppression, manifestations of Cushing's syndrome, hyperglycemia, and glucosuria in some patients.

Conditions which augment systemic absorption include the application of the more potent steroids, use over large surface areas, prolonged use, and the addition of occlusive dressings.

Therefore, patients receiving a large dose of a potent topical steroid applied to a large surface area or under an occlusive dressing should be evaluated periodically for evidence of HPA axis suppression by using the urinary free cortisol and ACTH stimulation tests. If HPA axis suppression is noted, an attempt should be made to withdraw the drug, to reduce the frequency of application, or to substitute a less potent steroid.

Recovery of HPA axis function is generally prompt and complete upon discontinuation of the drug. Infrequently, signs and symptoms of steroid withdrawal may occur, requiring supplemental systemic corticosteroids.

Children may absorb proportionally larger amounts of topical corticosteroids and thus be more susceptible to systemic toxicity. (See PRECAUTIONS—Pediatric Use).

If irritation develops, topical corticosteroids should be discontinued and appropriate therapy instituted.

In the presence of dermatological infections, the use of an appropriate antifungal or antibacterial agent should be instituted. If a favorable response does not occur promptly, the corticosteroid should be discontinued until the infection has been adequately controlled.

Information for the Patient

Patients using topical corticosteroids should receive the following information and instructions:

1. This medication is to be used as directed by the physician. It is for external use only. Avoid contact with the eyes.
2. Patients should be advised not to use this medication for any disorder other than for which it was prescribed.
3. The treated skin area should not be bandaged or otherwise covered or wrapped as to be occlusive unless directed by the physician.
4. Patients should report any signs of local adverse reactions especially under occlusive dressing.
5. Parents of pediatric patients should be advised not to use tight-fitting diapers or plastic pants on a child being treated in the diaper area, as these garments may constitute occlusive dressings.

Laboratory Tests

The following tests may be helpful in evaluating the HPA axis suppression:

Urinary free cortisol test

ACTH stimulation test

Carcinogenesis, Mutagenesis, and Impairment of Fertility

Long-term animal studies have not been performed to evaluate the carcinogenic potential or the effect on fertility of topical corticosteroids.

Studies to determine mutagenicity with prednisolone and hydrocortisone have revealed negative results.

Pregnancy Category C

Corticosteroids are generally teratogenic in laboratory animals when administered systemically at relatively low-dosage levels. The more potent corticosteroids have been shown to be teratogenic after dermal application in laboratory animals. There are no adequate and well-controlled studies in pregnant women on teratogenic effects from topically applied corticosteroids. Therefore, topical corticosteroids should be used during pregnancy only if the potential benefit justifies the potential risk to the fetus. Drugs of this class should not be used extensively on pregnant patients, in large amounts, or for prolonged periods of time.

Nursing Mothers

It is not known whether topical administration of corticosteroids could result in sufficient systemic absorption to produce detectable quantities in breast milk. Systemically administered corticosteroids are secreted into breast milk in quantities *not* likely to have a deleterious effect on the infant. Nevertheless, caution should be exercised when topical corticosteroids are administered to a nursing woman.

Pediatric Use

Pediatric patients may demonstrate greater susceptibility to topical corticosteroid-induced HPA axis suppression and Cushing's syndrome than mature patients because of a larger skin surface area to body weight ratio.

Hypothalamic-pituitary-adrenal (HPA) axis suppression, Cushing's syndrome, and intracranial hypertension have been reported in children receiving topical corticosteroids. Manifestations of adrenal suppression in children include linear growth retardation, delayed weight gain, low plasma cortisol levels, and absence of response to ACTH stimulation. Manifestations of intracranial hypertension include bulging fontanelles, headaches, and bilateral papilledema.

Administration of topical corticosteroids to children should be limited to the least amount compatible with an effective therapeutic regimen. Chronic corticosteroid therapy may interfere with the growth and development of children.

ADVERSE REACTIONS

The following local adverse reactions are reported infrequently with topical corticosteroids, but may occur more frequently with the use of occlusive dressings. These reactions are listed in an approximate decreasing order of occurrence:

Burning
Itching
Irritation
Dryness
Folliculitis
Hypertrichosis
Acneiform eruptions
Hypopigmentation
Perioral dermatitis
Allergic contact dermatitis
Maceration of the skin
Secondary infection
Skin atrophy
Striae
Miliaria

OVERDOSAGE

Topically applied corticosteroids can be absorbed in sufficient amounts to produce systemic effects. (See PRECAUTIONS).

DOSAGE AND ADMINISTRATION

Topical corticosteroids are generally applied to the affected area as a thin film from two to four times daily depending on the severity of the condition.
Occlusive dressings may be used for the management of psoriasis or recalcitrant conditions.
If an infection develops, the use of occlusive dressings should be discontinued and appropriate antimicrobial therapy instituted.

HOW SUPPLIED

Cort-Dome® Creme ¼%-1 oz. tube and 4 oz. dispensajar.
Cort-Dome® Creme ½%-½ oz. tube, 1 oz tube and 4 oz.
Cort-Dome® Creme 1%-½ oz. tube, 1 oz. tube.
Cort-Dome® Creme is a white semi-solid.
Store below 86°F (30°C), avoid freezing.

CAUTION

Federal (USA) law prohibits dispensing without a prescription.
Jan 1984 PD100596 19509

CORT-DOME® ℞
1%, ½%, ¼% and ⅛%
(hydrocortisone)
lotion **acid pH**

DESCRIPTION

Cort-Dome® Lotion contains microdispersed hydrocortisone (the active ingredient) in a compatible vehicle buffered to the acid pH range of normal skin. Each ml of Cort-Dome® Lotion contains 10.0mg/ml (1%). 5.0mg/ml(½%), 2.5mg/ml (¼%) or 1.25mg/ml (⅛%) of hydrocortisone. Cort-Dome® Lotion is applied topically. Hydrocortisone is a corticosteroid. Chemically, hydrocortisone is Pregn-4-ene-3,20-dione,11,17,21-trihydroxy-(11β)-. with the following structural formula:

The vehicle for Cort-Dome® Lotion 1%, ½%, ¼% and ⅛% is composed of glyceryl monostearyl, cetyl-stearyl alcohol-sodium lauryl sulfate, butyl stearate, aluminum sulfate, calcium acetate, dextrin, isopropyl myristate, polyoxyethylene sorbitan monolaurate, glycerin, and purified water preserved with methyl and propyl parabens.

EMPIRICAL FORMULA	MOLECULAR WEIGHT	CAS REGISTRY NUMBER
$C_{21}H_{30}O_5$	362.47	50-23-7

CLINICAL PHARMACOLOGY

Topical corticosteroids share anti-inflammatory, anti-pruritic and vasoconstrictive actions.
The mechanism of anti-inflammatory activity of the topical corticosteroids is unclear. Various laboratory methods, including vasoconstrictor assays, are used to compare and predict potencies and/or clinical efficacies of the topical corticosteroids. There is some evidence to suggest that a recognizable correlation exists between vasoconstrictor potency and therapeutic efficacy in man.

Pharmacokinetics

The extent of percutaneous absorption of topical corticosteroids is determined by many factors including the vehicle, the integrity of the epidermal barrier, and the use of occlusive dressings.
Topical corticosteroids can be absorbed from normal intact skin. Inflammation and/or other disease processes in the skin increase percutaneous absorption. Occlusive dressings substantially increase the percutaneous absorption of topical corticosteroids. Thus, occlusive dressings may be a valuable therapeutic adjunct for treatment of resistant dermatoses. (See DOSAGE AND ADMINISTRATION).
Once absorbed through the skin, topical corticosteroids are handled through pharmacokinetic pathways similar to systemically administered corticosteroids. Corticosteroids are bound to plasma proteins in varying degrees. Corticosteroids are metabolized primarily in the liver and are then excreted by the kidneys. Some of the topical corticosteroids and their metabolites are also excreted into the bile.

INDICATIONS AND USAGE

Topical corticosteroids are indicated for the relief of the inflammatory and pruritic manifestations of corticosteroid-responsive dermatoses.

CONTRAINDICATIONS

Topical corticosteroids are contraindicated in those patients with a history of hypersensitivity to any of the components of the preparation.

PRECAUTIONS

General

Systemic absorption of topical corticosteroids has produced reversible hypothalamic-pituitary-adrenal (HPA) axis suppression, manifestations of Cushing's syndrome, hyperglycemia, and glucosuria in some patients.
Conditions which augment systemic absorption include the application of the more potent steroids, use over large surface areas, prolonged use, and the addition of occlusive dressings.
Therefore, patients receiving a large dose of a potent topical steroid applied to a large surface area or under an occlusive dressing should be evaluated periodically for evidence of HPA axis suppression by using the urinary free cortisol and ACTH stimulation tests. If HPA axis suppression is noted, an attempt should be made to withdraw the drug, to reduce the frequency of application, or to substitute a less potent steroid.
Recovery of HPA axis function is generally prompt and complete upon discontinuation of the drug. Infrequently, signs and symptoms of steroid withdrawal may occur, requiring supplemental systemic corticosteroids.
Children may absorb proportionally larger amounts of topical corticosteroids and thus be more susceptible to systemic toxicity. (See PRECAUTIONS—Pediatric Use).
If irritation develops, topical corticosteroids should be discontinued and appropriate therapy instituted.
In the presence of dermatological infections, the use of an appropriate antifungal or antibacterial agent should be instituted. If a favorable response does not occur promptly, the corticosteroid should be discontinued until the infection has been adequately controlled.

Information for the Patient

Patients using topical corticosteroids should receive the following information and instructions:
1. This medication is to be used as directed by the physician. It is for external use only. Avoid contact with the eyes.
2. Patients should be advised not to use this medication for any disorder other than for which it was prescribed.
3. The treated skin area should not be bandaged or otherwise covered or wrapped as to be occlusive unless directed by the physician.
4. Patients should report any signs of local adverse reactions especially under occlusive dressing.
5. Parents of pediatric patients should be advised not to use tightfitting diapers or plastic pants on a child being treated in the diaper area, as these garments may constitute occlusive dressings.

Laboratory Tests

The following tests may be helpful in evaluating the HPA axis suppression:
Urinary free cortisol test
ACTH stimulation test

Carcinogenesis, Mutagenesis, and Impairment of Fertility

Long-term animal studies have not been performed to evaluate the carcinogenic potential or the effect on fertility of topical corticosteroids.
Studies to determine mutagenicity with prednisolone and hydrocortisone have revealed negative results.

Pregnancy Category C

Corticosteroids are generally teratogenic in laboratory animals when administered systemically at relatively low dosage levels. The more potent corticosteroids have been shown to be teratogenic after dermal application in laboratory animals. There are no adequate and well-controlled studies in pregnant women on teratogenic effects from topically applied corticosteroids. Therefore, topical corticosteroids should be used during pregnancy only if the potential benefit justifies the potential risk to the fetus. Drugs of this class should not be used extensively on pregnant patients, in large amounts, or for prolonged periods of time.

Nursing Mothers

It is not known whether topical administration of corticosteroids could result in sufficient systemic absorption to produce detectable quantities in breast milk. Systemically administered corticosteroids are secreted into breast milk in quantities *not* likely to have a deleterious effect on the infant. Nevertheless, caution should be exercised when topical corticosteroids are administered to a nursing woman.

Pediatric Use

Pediatric patients may demonstrate greater susceptibility to topical corticosteroid-induced HPA axis suppression and Cushing's syndrome than mature patients because of a larger skin surface area to body weight ratio.
Hypothalamic-pituitary-adrenal (HPA) axis suppression, Cushing's syndrome, and intracranial hypertension have been reported in children receiving topical corticosteroids. Manifestations of adrenal suppression in children include linear growth retardation, delayed weight gain, low plasma cortisol levels, and absence of response to ACTH stimulation.
Manifestations of intracranial hypertension include bulging fontaneiles, headaches, and bilateral papilledema.
Administration of topical corticosteroids to children should be limited to the least amount compatible with an effective therapeutic regimen. Chronic corticosteroid therapy may interfere with the growth and development of children.

ADVERSE REACTIONS

The following local adverse reactions are reported infrequently with topical corticosteroids, but may occur more frequently with the use of occlusive dressings. These reactions are listed in an approximate decreasing order of occurrence:
Burning
Itching
Irritation
Dryness
Folliculitis
Hypertrichosis
Acneiform eruptions
Hypopigmentation
Perioral dermatitis
Allergic contact dermatitis
Maceration of the skin
Secondary infection
Skin atrophy
Striae
Miliaria

OVERDOSAGE

Topically applied corticosteroids can be absorbed in sufficient amounts to produce systemic effects. (See PRECAUTIONS).

DOSAGE AND ADMINISTRATION

Topical corticosteroids are generally applied to the affected area as a thin film from two to four times daily depending on the severity of the condition.
Occlusive dressings may be used for the management of psoriasis or recalcitrant conditions.
In an infection develops, the use of occlusive dressings should be discontinued and appropriate antimicrobial therapy instituted.

HOW SUPPLIED

Cort-Dome® (hydrocortisone) Lotion ⅛%-6 fl. oz. bottle, Cort-Dome® Lotion ¼%-4 fl. oz. bottles. Cort-Dome® Lotion ½%-4 fl. oz. bottles. Cort-Dome® Lotion 1%-1 fl. oz. bottles.
Cort-Dome® Lotion is a white semi-fluid liquid.
Store below 86°F (30°C), avoid freezing.

CAUTION

Federal (USA) law prohibits dispensing without a prescription.
Aug 1983 PD100570 19384

CORT-DOME® ℞
(hydrocortisone acetate)
high potency suppositories

DESCRIPTION

Each Cort-Dome High Potency Suppository contains 25 mg hydrocortisone acetate in a monoglyceride base. Hydrocortisone acetate is a corticosteroid. Chemically, hydrocortisone acetate is pregn-4-ene-3, 20-dione, 21-(acetyloxy)-11, 17-dihydroxy-(11β)- with the following structural formula:

CLINICAL PHARMACOLOGY

In normal subjects, about 26 percent of hydrocortisone acetate is absorbed when the hydrocortisone acetate suppository is applied to the rectum. Absorption of hydrocortisone acetate may vary across abraded or inflamed surfaces.
Topical steroids are primarily effective because of their anti-inflammatory, anti-pruritic and vasoconstrictive action.

INDICATIONS AND USAGE

For use in inflamed hemorrhoids, post-irradiation (factitial) proctitis, as an adjunct in the treatment of chronic ulcerative colitis, cryptitis, other inflammatory conditions of the anorectum, and pruritis ani.

CONTRAINDICATION

Cort-Dome suppositories are contraindicated in those patients with a history of hypersensitivity to any of the components.

Continued on next page

Miles Pharm.—Cont.

PRECAUTIONS
Do not use unless adequate proctologic examination is made.
If irritation develops, the product should be discontinued and appropriate therapy instituted.
In the presence of an infection, the use of an appropriate antifungal or antibacterial agent should be instituted. If a favorable response does not occur promptly, the corticosteroids should be discontinued until the infection has been adequately controlled.
No long term studies in animals have been performed to evaluate the carcinogenic potential of corticosteroid suppositories.
Pregnancy Category C. In laboratory animals, topical steroids have been associated with an increase in the incidence of fetal abnormalities when gestating females have been exposed to rather low dosage levels. There are no adequate and well controlled studies in pregnant women. Cort-Dome High Potency Suppositories should only be used during pregnancy if the potential benefit justifies the risk to the fetus. Drugs of this class should not be used extensively on pregnant patients, in large amounts, or for prolonged periods of time.
It is not known whether this drug is excreted in human milk and because many drugs are excreted in human milk and because of the potential for serious adverse reactions in nursing infants from Cort-Dome High Potency Suppositories, a decision should be made whether to discontinue nursing or to discontinue the drug, taking into account the importance of the drug to the mother.

ADVERSE REACTIONS
The following local adverse reactions have been reported with corticosteroid suppositories.
1. Burning
2. Itching
3. Irritation
4. Dryness
5. Folliculitis
6. Hypopigmentation
7. Allergic Contact Dermatitis
8. Secondary infection

DRUG ABUSE AND DEPENDENCE
Drug abuse and dependence has not been reported in patients treated with Cort-Dome Suppositories.

OVERDOSAGE
If signs and symptoms of systemic overdosage occur discontinue use.

DOSAGE AND ADMINISTRATION
Usual dosage: One suppository in the rectum morning and night for two weeks, in non-specific proctitis. In more severe cases, one suppository three times daily; or two suppositories twice daily. In factitial proctitis, recommended therapy is six to eight weeks or less, according to response.

HOW SUPPLIED
Cort-Dome High Potency Suppository is yellowish-white, waxy, smooth surfaced rod shaped with one rounded end, approximately 38 mm. long by 9.5 mm. in diamter. Package of 12 suppositories.
Store below 86°F (30°C), avoid freezing.
March 1981 PD100536 16734

DECHOLIN® Tablets
(dehydrocholic acid)

DESCRIPTION
Each tablet contains 250 mg dehydrocholic acid.
Inactive Ingredients: Corn starch, gelatin, lactose, magnesium stearate, potato starch and talc.

INDICATIONS
For relief of occasional constipation (irregularity). This product generally produces bowel movement in 6–12 hours.

WARNINGS
Do not use laxative products when abdominal pain, nausea, or vomiting are present unless directed by a doctor.
If you have noticed a sudden change in bowel habits that persists over a period of 2 weeks, consult a doctor before using a laxative.
Laxative products should not be used for a period longer than 1 week unless directed by a doctor.
Rectal bleeding or failure to have a bowel movement after use of a laxative may indicate a serious condition. Discontinue use and consult your doctor.
KEEP THIS AND ALL MEDICATIONS OUT OF THE REACH OF CHILDREN.

WARNING
As with any drug, if you are pregnant or nursing a baby, seek the advice of a health professional before using this product.

DOSAGE AND ADMINISTRATION
Adults and children 12 years of age and over: oral dosage is 250 to 500 milligrams three times a day, not to exceed 1500 milligrams in 24 hours. Children under 12 years of age: consult a doctor.

HOW SUPPLIED
White tablets coded with number 121-Miles in bottles of 100 and 500.
Store at controlled room temperature (59°–86°F.).
Shown in Product Identification Section, page 418

DOMEBORO® Powder Packets, Effervescent Tablets (acid pH) Astringent Wet Dressing

One packet or tablet dissolved in a pint of water makes a modified Burow's Solution approximately equivalent to a 1:40 dilution, two packets or tablets a 1:20 dilution, and four packets or tablets a 1:10 dilution.
Buffered to an acid pH.

CONTAINS
Aluminum sulfate and calcium acetate.

INDICATIONS
A soothing wet dressing for relief of inflammatory conditions of the skin such as insect bites, poison ivy, swellings and bruises or athlete's foot.

DIRECTIONS
Dissolve one or two packets or tablets in a pint (large glass) of water and stir. When the powder disperses, shake resulting mixture. Do not strain or filter. Bandage the site of application loosely. Pour mixture on bandage every 15 to 30 minutes to keep dressing moist. Continue for 4 to 8 hours unless otherwise directed by physician. Do not use plastic or other impervious material to prevent evaporation without consulting your physician.

CAUTION
Keep away from eyes. For external use only. Store below 86°F. (30°C.), avoid freezing. Material in diluted form may be stored for 7 days at room temperature.

HOW SUPPLIED
Powder Packets: Boxes of 12 and 100. Each packet contains 2.2 gm. Individually foil-wrapped *Tablets:* Boxes of 12, 100 and 1000.
White tablets coded with number 411-Miles.
Shown in Product Identification Section, page 000

DOME-PASTE® Bandage
3″ and 4″ Bandages
(Medicated Bandage for Leg or Arm, Improved Unna's boot)

COMPOSITION
Each medicated bandage is impregnated with zinc oxide, calamine and gelatin. No heating or painting necessary.

INDICATIONS
For those conditions of the extremities (e.g. varicose veins and associated ulcers, stasis edema, thrombophlebitis, lymphangitis).

CAUTION
If skin sensitivity or irritation develops discontinue use and consult a physician.

ADMINISTRATION AND DOSAGE
Detailed instructions for application are supplied on each carton.

HOW SUPPLIED
3″ and 4″ cotton bandage by 360″ (10 yd.). Each carton contains one medicated bandage in polyethylene bag.

DOMOL® Bath and Shower Oil
(diisopropyl sebacate, isopropyl myristate)

COMPOSITION
Contains sebacate*, a special skin moisturizing agent, refined mineral oil and skin softener.
*Diisopropyl sebacate.

ACTION AND USES
Effective, pleasant way to lubricate skin and relieve itchy discomfort. It lubricates skin and restores the protective action of skin oils washed away by soaps and detergents. DOMOL helps maintain skin's normal condition by retarding evaporation of skin's moisture.

DIRECTIONS FOR USE
Bath—Add 1 or 2 capfuls to bathtub or water. Soak for 10-20 minutes.
Shower—Pour 1 capful on wet sponge or washcloth. Rub gently over body, rinse under shower.
Infant's Bath—Add 1 capful to basin or bathinette of water.
Sponge Bath—Add 1 or 2 capfuls to about a pint of water. Sponge body gently with washcloth or cellulose sponge. After bathing the skin should be patted dry rather than rubbed.

HOW SUPPLIED
8 fl. oz. unbreakable plastic bottle.

DTIC-Dome® ℞
(dacarbazine)
Sterile

WARNING
It is recommended that DTIC-Dome (dacarbazine) be administered under the supervision of a qualified physician experienced in the use of cancer chemotherapeutic agents.
1. Hemopoietic depression is the most common toxicity with DTIC-Dome (See Warnings).
2. Hepatic necrosis has been reported (See Warnings).
3. Studies have demonstrated this agent to have a carcinogenic and teratogenic effect when used in animals.
4. In treatment of each patient, the physician must weigh carefully the possibility of achieving therapeutic benefit against the risk of toxicity.

DESCRIPTION
DTIC-Dome Sterile (dacarbazine) is a colorless to an ivory colored solid which is light sensitive. Each vial contains 100mg of dacarbazine, or 200mg of dacarbazine (the active ingredient), anhydrous citric acid and mannitol. DTIC-Dome is reconstituted and administered intravenously (pH 3-4) DTIC-Dome is an anticancer agent. Chemically, DTIC-Dome is 5-(3, 3-dimethyl-l-triazeno)-imidazole-4-carboxamide (DTIC).

CLINICAL PHARMACOLOGY
After intravenous administration of DTIC-Dome, the volume of distribution exceeds total body water content suggesting localization in some body tissue, probably the liver. Its disappearance from the plasma is biphasic with initial half-life of 19 minutes and a terminal half-life of 5 hours. In a patient with renal and hepatic dysfunctions, the half-lives were lengthened to 55 minutes and 7.2 hours. The average cumulative excretion of unchanged DTIC in the urine is 40% of the injected dose in 6 hours. DTIC is subject to renal tubular secretion rather than glomerular filtration. At therapeutic concentrations DTIC is not appreciably bound to human plasma protein.
In man, DTIC is extensively degraded. Besides unchanged DTIC, 5-aminoimidazole -4 carboxamide (AIC) is a major metabolite of DTIC excreted in the urine. AIC is not derived endogenously but from the injected DTIC, because the administration of radioactive DTIC labeled with ^{14}C in the imidazole portion of the molecule (DTIC-2-^{14}C) gives rise to AIC-2-^{14}C.
Although the exact mechanism of action of DTIC-Dome is not known, three hypotheses have been offered:
1. inhibition of DNA synthesis by acting as a purine analog
2. action as an alkylating agent
3. interaction with SH groups

INDICATIONS AND USAGE
DTIC-Dome is indicated in the treatment of metastatic malignant melanoma. In addition, DTIC-Dome is also indicated for Hodgkin's disease as a secondary-line therapy when used in combination with other effective agents.

CONTRAINDICATIONS
DTIC-Dome is contraindicated in patients who have demonstrated a hypersensitivity to it in the past.

WARNINGS
Hemopoietic depression is the most common toxicity with DTIC-Dome and involves primarily the leukocytes and platelets, although, anemia may sometimes occur. Leukopenia and thrombocypenia may be severe enough to cause death. The possible bone marrow depression requires careful monitoring of white blood cells, red blood cells, and platelet levels. Hemopioetic toxicity may warrant temporary suspension or cessation of therapy with DTIC-Dome.
Hepatic toxicity accompanied by hepatic vein thrombosis and hepatocellular necrosis resulting in death, has been reported. The incidence of such reactions has been low; approximately 0.01% of patients treated. This toxicity has been observed mostly when DTIC-Dome has been administered concomitantly with other anti-neoplastic drugs; however, it has also been reported in some patients treated with DTIC-Dome alone.
Anaphylaxis can occur following the administration of DTIC-Dome.

PRECAUTIONS

Hospitalization is not always necessary but adequate laboratory study capability must be available. Extravasation of the drug subcutaneously during intravenous administration may result in tissue damage and severe pain. Local pain, burning sensation, and irritation at the site of injection may be relieved by locally applied hot packs.

Carcinogenicity of DTIC was studied in rats and mice. Proliferative endocardial lesions, including fibrosarcomas and sarcomas were induced by DTIC in rats. In mice, administration of DTIC resulted in the induction of angiosarcomas of the spleen.

Pregnancy Category C—DTIC-Dome has been shown to be teratogenic in rats when given in doses 20 times the human daily dose on day 12 of gestation. DTIC when administered in 10 times the human daily dose to male rats (twice weekly for 9 weeks) did not affect the male libido, although female rats mated to male rats had higher incidence of resorptions than controls. In rabbits, DTIC daily dose 7 times the human daily dose given on Days 6–15 of gestation resulted in fetal skeletal anomalies. There are no adequate and well controlled studies in pregnant women. DTIC-Dome should be used during pregnancy only if the potential benefit justifies the potential risk to the fetus.

It is not known whether this drug is excreted in human milk. Because many drugs are excreted in human milk and because of the potential for tumorigenicity shown for DTIC-Dome in animal studies, a decision should be made whether to discontinue nursing or to discontinue the drug, taking into account the importance of the drug to the mother.

ADVERSE REACTIONS

Symptoms of anorexia, nausea, and vomiting are the most frequently noted of all toxic reactions. Over 90% of patients are affected with the initial few doses. The vomiting lasts 1–12 hours and is incompletely and unpredictably palliated with phenobarbital and/or prochlorperazine. Rarely, intractable nausea and vomiting have necessitated discontinuance of therapy with DTIC-Dome. Rarely, DTIC-Dome has caused diarrhea. Some helpful suggestions include restricting the patient's oral intake of food for 4–6 hours prior to treatment. The rapid toleration of these symptoms suggests that a central nervous system mechanism may be involved, and usually these symptoms subside after the first 1 or 2 days.

There are a number of minor toxicities that are infrequently noted. Patients have experienced an influenza-like syndrome of fever to 39°C, myalgias and malaise. These symptoms occur usually after large single doses, may last for several days, and they may occur with successive treatments.

Alopecia has been noted as has facial flushing and facial paresthesia. There have been few reports of significant liver or renal function test abnormalities in man. However, these abnormalities have been observed more frequently in animal studies.

Erythematous and urticarial rashes have been observed infrequently after administration of DTIC-Dome. Rarely, photosensitivity reactions may occur.

OVERDOSAGE

Give supportive treatment and monitor blood cell counts.

DOSAGE AND ADMINISTRATION

MALIGNANT MELANOMA—The recommended dosage is 2 to 4.5mg/kg/day for 10 days. Treatment may be repeated at 4 week intervals.

An alternate recommended dosage is 250mg/square meter body surface/day I.V. for 5 days. Treatment may be repeated every 3 weeks.

HODGKIN'S DISEASE: The recommended dosage of DTIC-Dome in the treatment of Hodgkin's Disease is 150mg/square meter body surface/day for 5 days, in combination with other effective drugs. Treatment may be repeated every 4 weeks. An alternative recommended dosage is 375mg/square meter body surface on day 1, in combination with other effective drugs, to be repeated every 15 days.

DTIC-Dome (dacarbazine) 100mg/vial and 200mg/vial are reconstituted with 9.9 ml and 19.7 ml, respectively, of Sterile Water for Injection, U.S.P. The resulting solution contains 10mg/ml of dacarbazine having a pH of 3.0 to 4.0. The calculated dose of the resulting solution is drawn into a syringe and administered *only* intravenously.

The reconstituted solution may be further diluted with 5% dextrose injection, U.S.P. or sodium chloride injection, U.S.P. and administered as an intravenous infusion.

After reconstitution and prior to use, the solution in the vial may be stored at 4°C for up to 72 hours or at normal room conditions (temperature and light) for up to 8 hours. If the reconstituted solution is further diluted in 5% dextrose, injection, U.S.P. or sodium chloride injection, U.S.P., the resulting solution may be stored at 4°C for up to 24 hours or at normal room conditions for up to 8 hours.

Procedures for proper handling and disposal of anticancer drugs should be considered. Several guidelines on this subject have been published.[7–12] There is no general agreement that all of the procedures recommended in the guidelines are necessary or appropriate.

HOW SUPPLIED

10 ml vials containing 100mg or 20 ml vials containing 200 mg of DTIC-Dome as sterile dacarbazine in boxes of 12.

REFERENCES

1. Loo, T.J., *et al.*: Mechanism of action and pharmacology studies with DTIC (NSC-45388). Cancer Treatment Reports 60: 149–152, 1976.
2. Nathanson, L., *et al.*: Characteristics of prognosis and response to an imidazole carboxamide in malignant melanoma. Clinical Pharmacology and Therapeutics 12: 955–962, 1971.
3. Costanza, M.E., *et al.*: Therapy of malignant melanoma with an imidazole carboxamide and bischloroethyl nitrosourea. Cancer 30: 1457–1461, 1972.
4. Luce, J.K., *et al.*: Clinical trials with the antitumor agent 5-(3, 3-dimethyl-l-triazeno) imidazole-4-carboxamide (NSC-45388). Cancer Chemotherapy Reports 54: 119–124, 1970.
5. Bonadonna, G., *et al.*: Combined Chemotherapy (MOPP or ABVD)—radiotherapy approach in advanced Hodgkin's disease. Cancer Treatment Reports 61: 769–777, 1977.
6. Santoro, A., and Bonadonna, G.: Prolonged disease-free survival in MOPP-resistant Hodgkin's disease after treatment with adriamycin, bleomycin, vinblastine and decarbazine (ABVD). Cancer Chemotherapy Pharmacol. 2: 101–105, 1979.
7. Recommendations for the Safe Handling of Parenteral Antineoplastic Drugs. NIH Publication No. 83-2621. For sale by the Superintendent of Documents, U.S. Government Printing Office, Washington, D.C. 20402.
8. AMA Council Report. Guidelines for Handling Parenteral Antineoplastics. JAMA, March 15, 1985.
9. National Study Commission on Cytotoxic Exposure—Recommendations for Handling Cytotoxic Agents. Available from Louis P. Jeffrey, Sc. D., Director of Pharmacy Services, Rhode Island Hospital, 593 Eddy Street, Providence, Rhode Island 02902.
10. Clinical Oncological Society of Australia: Guidelines and recommendations for safe handling of antineoplastic agents. Med. J. Australia 1: 426–428, 1983.
11. Jones, R.B., *et al.*: Safe handling of chemotherapeutic agents: A report from the Mount Sinai Medical Center. Ca-A Cancer Journal for Clinicians Sept./Oct. 258–263, 1983.
12. American Society of Hospital Pharmacists technical assistance bulletin on handling cytotoxic drugs in hospitals. Am. J. Hosp. Pharm. 42: 131–137, 1985.

Manufactured by:
Ben Venue Laboratories
Bedford, Ohio 44146
Distributed by:
Miles Pharmaceuticals
Division of Miles Laboratories, Inc.
West Haven, Connecticut 06516 USA
PD100644 Feb 1986

LITHANE® ℞

(lithium carbonate)
TABLETS
For Control of Manic Episodes in Manic-Depressive Psychosis

Warning

Lithium toxicity is closely related to serum lithium levels, and can occur at doses close to therapeutic levels. Facilities for prompt and accurate serum lithium determinations should be available before initiating therapy.

DESCRIPTION

Lithium carbonate is a white, light, alkaline powder with molecular formula Li_2CO_3 and molecular weight 73.89. Lithium is an element of the alkali-metal group with atomic number 3, atomic weight 6.94, and an emission line at 671 nm on the flame photometer. Lithane® tablets contain the following inactive ingredients: Corn Starch, Dibasic Calcium Phosphate, FD & C Yellow No. 5 Dye, Lake, FD & C Blue No. 1 Dye, Lake, Magnesium Stearate, Polyethylene Glycol, Sodium Lauyl Sulfate.

ACTIONS

Preclinical studies have shown that lithium alters sodium transport in nerve and muscle cells and effects a shift toward intraneuronal metabolism of catecholamines, but the specific biochemical mechanism of lithium action in mania is unknown.

INDICATIONS

Lithium carbonate is indicated in the treatment of manic episodes of manic-depressive illness. Maintenance therapy prevents or diminishes the intensity of subsequent episodes in those manic-depressive patients with a history of mania.

Typical symptoms of mania include pressure of speech, motor hyperactivity, reduced need for sleep, flight of ideas, grandiosity, elation, poor judgment, aggressiveness, and possibly hostility. When given to a patient experiencing a manic episode, lithium may produce a normalization of symptomatology within 1 to 3 weeks.

WARNINGS

Lithium should generally not be given to patients with significant renal or cardiovascular disease, severe debilitation or dehydration, or sodium depletion, and to patients receiving diuretics, since the risk of lithium toxicity is very high in such patients. If the psychiatric indication is life-threatening, and if such a patient fails to respond to other measures, lithium treatment may be undertaken with extreme caution, including daily serum lithium determinations and adjustment to the usually low doses ordinarily tolerated by these individuals. In such instances, hospitalization is a necessity.

Chronic lithium therapy may be associated with diminution of renal concentrating ability, occasionally presenting as nephrogenic diabetes insipidus, with polyuria and polydipsia. Such patients should be carefully managed to avoid dehydration with resulting lithium retention and toxicity. This condition is usually reversible when lithium is discontinued.

Morphologic changes with glomerular and interstitial fibrosis and nephron atrophy have been reported in patients on chronic lithium therapy. Morphologic changes have also been seen in manic-depressive patients never exposed to lithium. The relationship between renal functional and morphologic changes and their association with lithium therapy have not been established.

When kidney function is assessed, for baseline data prior to starting lithium therapy or thereafter, routine urinalysis and other tests may be used to evaluate tubular function (e.g. urine specific gravity or osmolality following a period of water deprivation, or 24 hour urine volume) and glomerular function (e.g. serum creatinine or creatinine clearance). During lithium therapy, progressive or sudden changes in renal function, even within the normal range, indicate the need for reevaluation of treatment.

Lithium therapy has been reported in some cases to be associated with morphologic changes in the kidneys. The relationship between such changes and renal function has not been established.

An encephalopathic syndrome (characterized by weakness, lethargy, fever, tremulousness and confusion, extrapyramidal symptoms, leukocytosis, elevated serum enzymes, BUN and FBS) followed by irreversible brain damage has occurred in a few patients treated with lithium plus haloperidol. A causal relationship between these events and the concomitant administration of lithium and haloperidol has not been established; however, patients receiving such combined therapy should be monitored closely for early evidence of neurologic toxicity and treatment discontinued promptly if such signs appear. The possibility of similar adverse interactions with other antipsychotic medication exists.

Lithium toxicity is closely related to serum lithium levels, and can occur at doses close to therapeutic levels (see DOSAGE AND ADMINISTRATION).

Outpatients and their families should be warned that the patient must discontinue lithium carbonate therapy and contact his physician if such clinical signs of lithium toxicity as diarrhea, vomiting, tremor, mild ataxia, drowsiness, or muscular weakness occur.

Lithium carbonate may impair mental and/or physical abilities. Caution patients about activities requiring alertness (e.g., operating vehicles or machinery).

Lithium may prolong the effects of neuromuscular blocking agents. Therefore, neuromuscular blocking agents should be given with caution to patients receiving lithium.

Usage in Pregnancy: Adverse effects on nidation in rats, embryo viability in mice, and metabolism *in vitro* of rat testis and human spermatozoa have been attributed to lithium, as have teratogenicity in submammalian species and cleft palates in mice. Studies in rats, rabbits, and monkeys have shown no evidence of lithium-induced teratology.

In humans, lithium carbonate may cause fetal harm when administered to a pregnant woman. Data from lithium birth registries suggest an increase in cardiac and other anomalies, especially Ebstein' anomaly. If this drug is used during pregnancy, or if a patient becomes pregnant while taking this drug, the patient should be apprised of the potential hazard to the fetus.

There are lithium birth registries in the United States and elsewhere; however there is at the present time insufficient data to determine the effects of lithium carbonate on human fetuses. Therefore, at this point, lithium should not be used in pregnancy, especially the first trimester, unless in the opinion of the physician, the potential benefits outweigh the possible hazards.

Usage in Nursing Mothers: Lithium is excreted in human milk. Nursing should not be undertaken during lithium therapy except in rare and unusual circumstances where, in

Continued on next page

Miles Pharm.—Cont.

the view of the physician, the potential benefits to the mother outweigh possible hazards to the child.

Usage in Children: Since information regarding the safety and effectiveness of lithium carbonate in children under 12 years of age is not available, its use in such patients is not recommended at this time.

PRECAUTIONS

The ability to tolerate lithium is greater during the acute manic phase and decreases when manic symptoms subside (see DOSAGE AND ADMINISTRATION).

Caution should be used when lithium and diuretics are used concomitantly because diuretic-induced sodium loss may reduce the renal clearance of lithium and increase serum lithium levels with risk of lithium toxicity. Patients receiving such combined therapy should have serum lithium levels monitored closely and the lithium dosage adjusted if necessary.

The distribution space of lithium approximates that of total body water. Lithium is primarily excreted in urine with insignificant excretion in feces. Renal excretion of lithium is proportional to its plasma concentration. The half-life of elimination of lithium is approximately 24 hours. Lithium decreases sodium reabsorption by the renal tubules which could lead to sodium depletion. Therefore, it is essential for the patient to maintain a normal diet, including salt, and an adequate fluid intake (2500–3000 ml) at least during the initial stabilization period. Decreased tolerance to lithium has been reported to ensue from protracted sweating or diarrhea and, if such occur, supplemental fluid and salt should be administered.

In addition to sweating and diarrhea, concomitant infection with elevated temperatures may also necessitate a temporary reduction or cessation of medication.

Previously existing underlying thyroid disorders do not necessarily constitute a contraindication to lithium treatment; where hypothyroidism exists, careful monitoring of thyroid function during lithium stabilization and maintenance allows for correction of changing thyroid parameters, if any; where hypothroidism occurs during lithium stabilization and maintenance, supplemental thyroid treatment may be used.

This product contains FD&C Yellow No. 5 (tartrazine) which may cause allergic-type reactions (including bronchial asthma) in certain susceptible individuals. Although the over-all incidence of FD&C Yellow No. 5 (tartrazine) sensitivity in the general population is low, it is frequently seen in patients who also have aspirin hypersensitivity.

Indomethacin has been reported to increase steady state plasma lithium levels from 30 to 59 percent. There is also some evidence that other nonsteroidal anti-inflammatory agents may have a similar effect. When such combinations are used, increased plasma lithium level monitoring is recommended.

Indomethacin (50 mg t.i.d.) has been reported to increase steady state plasma lithium levels from 30 to 59 percent. There is also evidence that other nonsteroidal, anti-inflammatory may have a similar effect. When such combinations are used, increased plasma lithium level monitoring is recommended.

ADVERSE REACTIONS

Adverse reactions are seldom encountered at serum lithium levels below 1.5 mEq./l., except in the occasional patient sensitive to lithium. Mild to moderate toxic reactions may occur at levels from 1.5–2.5 mEq./l., and moderate to severe reactions may be seen at levels from 2.0–2.5 mEq./l., depending upon individual response to the drug.

Fine hand tremor, polyuria, and mild thirst may occur during initial therapy for the acute manic phase, and may persist throughout treatment. Transient and mild nausea and general discomfort may also appear during the first few days of lithium administration.

These side effects are an inconvenience rather than a disabling condition, and usually subside with continued treatment or a temporary reduction or cessation of dosage. If persistent, a cessation of dosage is indicated.

Diarrhea, vomiting, drowsiness, muscular weakness, and lack of coordination may be early signs of lithium intoxication, and can occur at lithium levels below 2.0 mEq./l. At higher levels, giddiness, ataxia, blurred vision, tinnitus, and a large output of dilute urine may be seen. Serum lithium levels above 3.0 mEq./l. may produce a complex clinical picture involving multiple organs and organ systems. Serum lithium levels should not be permitted to exceed 2.0 mEq./l, during the acute treatment phase.

The following reactions have been reported and appear to be related to serum lithium levels, including levels within the therapeutic range:

Neurological: Cases of pseudotumor cerebri (increased intracranial pressure and papilledema) have been reported with lithium use. If undetected, this condition may result in enlargement of the blind spot, constriction of visual fields and eventual blindness due to optic atrophy. Lithium should be discontinued, if clinically possible, if this syndrome occurs.

Neuromuscular: tremor, muscle hyperirritability (fasciculations, twitching, clonic movements of whole limbs), ataxia, choreo-athetotic movements, hyperactive deep tendon reflexes.

Central Nervous System: blackout spells, epileptiform seizures, slurred speech, dizziness, vertigo, incontinence of urine or feces, somnolence, psychomotor retardation, restlessness, confusion stupor, coma.

Cardiovascular: cardiac arrhythmia, hypotension, peripheral circulatory collapse.

Gastrointestinal: anorexia, nausea, vomiting, diarrhea.

Genitourinary: albuminuria, oliguria, polyuria, glycosuria.

Dermatologic: drying and thinning of hair, anesthesia of skin, chronic folliculitis, xerosis cutis, alopecia, and exacerbation of psoriasis.

Autonomic Nervous System: blurred vision, dry mouth.

Thyroid Abnormalities: Euthyroid goiter and/or hypothyroidism (including myxedema) accompanied by lower T_3 and T_4. I^{131} iodine uptake may be elevated. (See **Precautions.**) Paradoxically, rare cases of hyperthroidism have been reported.

EEG. Changes: diffuse slowing, widening of frequency spectrum, potentiation and disorganization of background rhythm.

EKG. Changes: reversible flattening, isoelectricity or inversion of T-waves.

Miscellaneous: fatigue, lethargy, tendency to sleep, dehydration, weight loss, transient scotomata.

Miscellaneous reactions unrelated to dosage are: transient electroencephalographic and electrocardiographic changes, leucocytosis, headache, diffuse non-toxic goiter with or without hypothyroidism, transient hyperglycemia, generalized pruritus with or without rash, cutaneous ulcers, albuminuria, worsening of organic brain syndromes, excessive weight gain, edematous swelling of ankles or wrists, and thirst or polyuria, sometimes resembling diabetes insipidus, and metallic taste. A single report has been received of the development of painful discoloration of fingers and toes and coldness of the extremities within one day of the starting of treatment of lithium. The mechanism through which these symptoms (resembling Raynaud's Syndrome) developed is not known. Recovery followed discontinuance.

DOSAGE AND ADMINISTRATION

Acute Mania: Optimal patient response to lithium carbonate usually can be established and maintained with 600 mg t.i.d. Such doses will normally produce an effective serum lithium level ranging between 1.0 and 1.5 mEq./l. Dosage must be individualized according to serum levels and clinical response. Regular monitoring of the patient's clinical state and of serum lithium levels is necessary. Serum levels should be determined twice per week during the acute phase, and until the serum level and clinical condition of the patient have been stabilized.

Long term Control: The desirable lithium levels are 0.6 to 1.2 mEq./l. Dosage will vary from one individual to another, but usually 300 mg t.i.d. or q.i.d. will maintain this level. Serum lithium levels in uncomplicated cases receiving maintenance therapy during remission should be monitored at least every two months.

Patients abnormally sensitive to lithium may exhibit toxic signs at serum levels of 1.0 to 1.5 mEq./l. Elderly patients often respond to reduced dosage, and may exhibit signs of toxicity at serum levels ordinarily tolerated by other patients.

N.B.: Blood samples for serum lithium determinations should be drawn immediately prior to the next dose when lithium concentrations are relatively stable (i.e., 8–12 hours after the previous dose). Total reliance must not be placed on serum levels alone. Accurate patient evaluation requires both clinical and laboratory analysis.

OVERDOSAGE

The toxic levels for lithium are close to the therapeutic levels. It is therefore important that patients and their families be cautioned to watch for early toxic symptoms and to discontinue the drug and inform the physician should they occur. Toxic symptoms are listed in detail under ADVERSE REACTIONS.

Treatment: No specific antidote for lithium poisoning is known. Early symptoms of lithium toxicity can usually be treated by reduction or cessation of dosage of the drug and resumption of the treatment at a lower dose after 24 to 48 hours. In severe cases of lithium poisoning, the first and foremost goal of treatment consists of elimination of this ion from the organism.

Treatment is essentially the same as that used in barbiturate poisoning: 1) lavage, 2) correction of fluid and electrolyte imbalance, and 3) regulation of kidney functioning. Urea, mannitol, and aminophylline all produce significant increases in lithium excretion. Hemodialysis is an effective and rapid means of removing the ion from the severely toxic patient. Infection prophylaxis, regular chest X-rays, and preservation of adequate respiration are essential.

HOW SUPPLIED

Lithane® (lithium carbonate) is available as round green scored tablets containing 300 mg of lithium carbonate embossed with the word "MILES" and the three digit code 951, in bottles of 100.

PD100591 Revised July 1983
Manufactured for
Miles Pharmaceuticals
Division of Miles Laboratories, Inc.
West Haven, Connecticut 06516 USA
by Pfizer, Inc., New York, N.Y. 10017
©1980, Miles Laboratories, Inc.

Shown in Product Identification Section, page 418

MEZLIN® ℞

(sterile mezlocillin sodium)
for intravenous or intramuscular use.

PRODUCT OVERVIEW

KEY FACTS

MEZLIN® is a semisynthetic broad spectrum penicillin antibiotic for parenteral administration. MEZLIN® is bactericidal against a wide range of gram-negative and gram-positive pathogens, including aerobic and anaerobic strains. It is particularly useful for treating mixed infections.

MAJOR USES

MEZLIN® has been proven effective for treatment of serious infections, including bacteremia, caused by susceptible strains of the microorganisms listed below. In certain severe infections when the causative organisms are unknown, MEZLIN® may be administered with an aminoglycoside or a cephalosporin as initial therapy. As soon as results of culture and susceptibility tests become available, antimicrobial therapy should be adjusted as indicated.

SAFETY INFORMATION

MEZLIN® is contraindicated in patients with a history of hypersensitivity reactions to any of the penicillins. Although MEZLIN® shares with other penicillins the low potential for toxicity, as with any potent drug, periodic assessment of organ system functions is advisable during prolonged therapy.

PRESCRIBING INFORMATION

MEZLIN® ℞

(sterile mezlocillin sodium)
for intravenous or intramuscular use.

DESCRIPTION

MEZLIN® (sterile mezlocillin sodium) is a semisynthetic broad spectrum penicillin antibiotic for parenteral administration. It is the monohydrate sodium salt of 6-{D-2 [3-(methyl-sulfonyl) -2- OXO-imidazolidine-1-carboxamido]-2- phenylacetamido} penicillanic acid.

Structural Formula:

Empirical Formula: $C_{21}H_{24}N_5O_8S_2Na \cdot H_2O$

MEZLIN® has a molecular weight of 579.6 and contains 42.6 mg (1.85 mEq) of sodium per one gram of mezlocillin activity. The dosage form is supplied as a sterile white to pale yellow crystalline powder, which is freely soluble in water. When reconstituted, solutions of MEZLIN® are clear and range from colorless to pale yellow with a pH of 4.5 to 8.0.

CLINICAL PHARMACOLOGY

Intravenous Administration. In healthy adult volunteers, mean serum levels of mezlocillin 5 minutes after a 5-minute intravenous injection of 1g, 2g, or 5g are 100, 253 or 411 mcg/ml, respectively. Serum levels, as noted below, lack dose proportionality.

[See table on top next page].
[See table on bottom next page].

Following intravenous infusion (2 hr) of a 3g dose of mezlocillin every 4 hours for 7 days, mean peak serum concentrations are higher than 100 mcg/ml, and levels above 50 mcg/ml are maintained throughout dosing.

Intramuscular Administration. MEZLIN® is rapidly absorbed after intramuscular injection. In healthy volunteers, the mean peak serum concentration occurs approximately 45 minutes after a single dose of 1g and is about 15 mcg/ml. The oral administration of 1g probenecid before injection produces an increase in mezlocillin serum levels of about 50%. After repetitive intramuscular doses of 1g mezlocillin every 6 hours, peak levels in the serum generally range between 35 and 45 mcg/ml. The relationship between the phar-

MEZLIN®

MEZLOCILLIN SERUM LEVELS IN ADULTS (mcg/ml) 5 MIN IV INJECTION

DOSE	0	5 min	10 min	20 min	30 min	1 hr	2 hr	3 hr	4 hr	6 hr	8 hr
1g	**149** (132–185)	**100** (64–143)	**66** (47–87)	**50** (31–87)	**40** (22–83)	**18** (8–31)	**5.3** (3.3–7.7)	**2.5** (1.7–3.7)	**1.7** (0.7–2.8)	**0.5** (0–1.2)	**0.1** (0–0.2)
2g	**314** (207–362)	**253** (161–364)	**161** (113–214)	**117** (76–174)	**82** (55–112)	**56** (23–88)	**20** (7.5–32)	**11** (3.8–16)	**4.4** (1.6–8.7)	**1.5** (0.5–2.6)	**0.6** (0.1–1.4)
5g	**547** (268–854)	**411** (199–597)	**357** (246–456)	**250** (203–353)	**226** (190–333)	**131** (104–193)	**76** (59–104)	**31** (20–40)	**13** (6.4–17)	**4.6** (2.1–9.4)	**1.9** (1.1–3.6)

After an intravenous infusion (15 min) of 3g, mean levels 15 minutes after dosing are 269 mcg/ml (170–280).
A 30-minute intravenous infusion of 3g produces mean peak concentrations of 263 mcg/ml; 1 hour and 4 hours later the concentrations are 57 mcg/ml and 4.4 mcg/ml, respectively:

MEZLIN®

MEZLOCILLIN SERUM LEVELS IN ADULTS (mcg/ml) 30 MIN IV INFUSION

DOSE	0	5 min	15 min	30 min	45 min	1 hr	2 hr	3 hr	4 hr	6 hr	8 hr
3g	**263** (87–489)	**170** (63–371)	**141** (75–301)	**109** (56–288)	**79** (41–135)	**57** (28–100)	**26** (14–55)	**12** (5.8–26)	**4.4** (2.2–6.5)	**1.6** (1.0–3.4)	<1

macokinetics of intramuscular and intravenous dosing has not yet been clearly established.

General. As with other penicillins, mezlocillin is excreted primarily by glomerular filtration and tubular secretion. The rate of elimination is dose dependent and related to the degree of renal functional impairment. In patients with normal renal function, approximately 55% of the administered dose is recovered from the urine within the first 6 hours after dosing. Two hours after an intravenous injection of 2g, concentrations of active drug in urine generally exceed 4000 mcg/ml. By 4–6 hours after injection, concentrations usually decline to a range of about 50 to 200 mcg/ml. The serum elimination half-life of mezlocillin after intravenous dosing is approximately 55 minutes.

In patients with reduced renal function, the half-life is only slightly prolonged. Dosage adjustments are usually not necessary except in patients with severe renal impairment. (See Dosage and Administration). As with other penicillins, mezlocillin is metabolized only slightly; less than 10% of the drug excreted in the urine is in the form of the penicilloate or penilloate. The drug is readily removed from the serum by hemodialysis and, to a lesser extent, by peritoneal dialysis.

Up to 26% of a dose of mezlocillin is recovered from the bile of patients with normal liver function. Following intravenous doses of 2 to 5g, concentrations of active drug in bile generally range from 500 to 2500 mcg/ml. The biliary excretion of mezlocillin is reduced in patients with common bile duct obstruction.

Mezlocillin is not appreciably absorbed when given orally. Following parenteral administration, the apparent volume of distribution is approximately equal to the extracellular fluid volume. The drug is present in active form in the serum, urine, bile, peritoneal fluid, pleural fluid, bronchial and wound secretions, bone and other tissues. As with other penicillins, penetration into the cerebrospinal fluid (CSF) is generally poor, however higher CSF concentrations are obtained in the presence of meningeal inflammation.

Protein binding studies indicate that the degree of mezlocillin binding is low (16–42%) and depends upon testing methods and concentrations of drug studied.

Microbiology

Mezlocillin is a bactericidal antibiotic which acts by interfering with synthesis of cell wall components. It is active against a variety of gram-negative and gram-positive bacteria, including aerobic and anaerobic strains. Mezlocillin is usually active *in vitro* against most strains of the following organisms:

Gram-negative bacteria

Escherichia coli	*Klebsiella* species (including *K. pneumoniae*)
Proteus mirabilis	*Enterobacter* species
Proteus vulgaris	*Shigella* species*
Morganella morganii (formerly *P. morganii*)	*Pseudomonas aeruginosa (and other species)*
Providencia rettgeri (formerly *Proteus rettgeri*)	*Haemophilus influenzae*
Providencia stuartii	*Haemophilus parainfluenzae*
Citrobacter species*	*Neisseria* species

Many strains of *Serratia, Salmonella**, and *Acinetobacter** are also susceptible.

Gram-positive bacteria

Staphylococcus aureus (non-penicillinase producing strains)
Beta-hemolytic *streptococci* (Groups A and B)
Streptococcus pneumoniae (formerly *Diplococcus pneumoniae*)
Streptococcus faecalis (enterococcus)

Anaerobic Organisms

Peptococcus species	*Fusobacterium* species*
Peptostreptococcus species	*Veillonella* species*
Clostridium species*	*Eubacterium* species*

Bacteroides species (including *B. fragilis* group)

*Mezlocillin has been shown to be active *in vitro* against these organisms, however clinical efficacy has not yet been established.

Noteworthy is mezlocillin's broadened spectrum of *in vitro* activity against important pathogenic aerobic gram-negative bacteria, including strains of *Pseudomonas, Klebsiella, Enterobacter, Serratia, Proteus, Escherichia* and *Haemophilus,* as well as *Bacteroides* and other anaerobes; and its excellent inhibitory effect against gram-positive organisms including *Streptococcus faecalis* (enterococcus). It is inactive against penicillinase-producing strains of *Staphylococcus aureus.*

In vitro studies have shown that mezlocillin combined with an aminoglycoside (e.g., gentamicin, tobramycin, amikacin, sisomicin) acts synergistically against strains of *Streptococcus faecalis* and *Pseudomonas aeruginosa.* In some instances, this combination also acts synergistically *in vitro* against other gram-negative bacteria such as *Serratia, Klebsiella* and *Acinetobacter* species.

Mezlocillin is slightly more active when tested at alkaline pH and, as with other penicillins, has reduced activity when tested *in vitro* with increasing inoculum. The minimum bactericidal concentration (MBC) generally exceeds the minimum inhibitory concentration (MIC) by a factor of 2 or 3. Resistance to mezlocillin *in vitro* develops slowly (multiple step mutation). Some strains of *Pseudomonas aeruginosa* have developed resistance fairly rapidly. Mezlocillin is not stable in the presence of penicillinase and strains of *Staphylococcus aureus* resistant to penicillin are also resistant to mezlocillin.

Susceptibility Tests

Quantitative methods that require measurement of zone diameters give good estimates of bacterial susceptibility. One such procedure* has been recommended for use with discs to test susceptibility to antimicrobials. When the causative organism is tested by the Kirby-Bauer method of disc susceptibility, a 75 mcg mezlocillin disc should give a zone of 18 mm or greater to indicate susceptibility. Zone sizes of 14 mm or less indicate resistance. Zone sizes of 15 to 17 mm indicate intermediate susceptibility. Susceptible strains of *Haemophilus* and *Neisseria* species give zones of ≥29 mm, resistant strains ≤28 mm. With this procedure, a report from the laboratory of "Susceptible" indicates that the infecting organism is likely to respond to therapy. A report of "Resistant" indicates that the infecting organism is not likely to respond to therapy; other therapy should be selected. A report of "Intermediate Susceptibility" suggests that the organism may be susceptible if the infection is confined to tissues and fluids (e.g., urine), in which high antibiotic levels are attained. The mezlocillin disc should be used for testing susceptibility to mezlocillin. In certain conditions, it may be desiriable to do additional susceptibility testing by broth or agar dilution techniques. Dilution methods, preferably the agar plate dilution procedure, are most accurate for susceptibility testing of obligate anaerobes. *Enterobacteriaceae, Pseudomonas* species and *Acinetobacter* species are considered susceptible if the MIC of mezlocillin is no greater than 64 mcg/ml and are considered resistant if the MIC is greater than 128 mcg/ml. *Haemophilus* species and *Neisseria* species are considered susceptible if the MIC of mezlocillin is less than or equal to 1 mcg/ml. Mezlocillin standard is available for broth or agar dilution studies.

*Bauer, A.W., Kirby, W.M., Sherris, J.C. and Turck, M.: Antibiotic Testing by a Standardized Single Disc Method, Am. J. Clin. Pathol., 45:493, 1966. Standardized Disc Susceptibility Test, FEDERAL REGISTER 39: 19182-19184, 1974.

INDICATIONS AND USAGE

MEZLIN® is indicated for the treatment of serious infections caused by susceptible strains of the designated microorganisms in the conditions listed below:

LOWER RESPIRATORY TRACT INFECTIONS including pneumonia and lung abscess caused by *Haemophilus influenzae, Klebsiella* species including *K. pneumoniae, Proteus mirabilis, Pseudomonas* species including *P. aeruginosa, E. coli,* and *Bacteroides* species including *B. fragilis.*

INTRA-ABDOMINAL INFECTIONS including acute cholecystitis, cholangitis, peritonitis, hepatic abscess and intra-abdominal abscess caused by susceptible *E. coli, Proteus mirabilis, Klebsiella* species, *Pseudomonas* species, *S. faecalis (enterococcus), Bacteroides* species, *Peptococcus* species, and *Peptostreptococcus* species.

URINARY TRACT INFECTIONS caused by susceptible *E. coli, Proteus mirabilis,* the indole positive *Proteus* species, *Morganella morganii; Klebsiella* species, *Enterobacter* species, *Serratia* species, *Pseudomonas* species, *S. faecalis* (enterococcus).

Uncomplicated gonorrhea due to susceptible *Neisseria gonorrhoeae.*

GYNECOLOGICAL INFECTIONS including endometritis, pelvic cellulitis, and pelvic inflammatory disease associated with susceptible *Neisseria gonorrhoeae, Peptococcus* species, *Peptostreptococcus* species, *Bacteroides* species, *E. coli, Proteus mirabilis, Klebsiella* species, and *Enterobacter* species.

SKIN AND SKIN STRUCTURE INFECTIONS caused by susceptible *S. faecalis* (enterococcus), *E. coli, Proteus mirabilis,* the indole positive *Proteus* species, *Proteus vulgaris,* and *Providencia rettgeri; Klebsiella* species, *Enterobacter* species, *Pseudomonas* species, *Peptococcus* species, and *Bacteroides* species.

SEPTICEMIA including bacteremia caused by susceptible *E. coli, Klebsiella* species, *Enterobacter* species, *Pseudomonas* species, *Bacteroides* species, and *Peptococcus* species.

Mezlocillin has also been shown to be effective for the treatment of infections caused by *Streptococcus* species including Group A Beta-hemolytic *Streptococcus* and *Streptococcus pneumoniae* (formerly *Diplococcus pneumoniae*) however, infections caused by these organisms are ordinarily treated with more narrow spectrum penicillins.

Appropriate culture and susceptibility tests should be performed before treatment in order to isolate and identify organisms causing infection and to determine their susceptibility to mezlocillin. Therapy with MEZLIN® may be initiated before results of these tests are known; once results become

Fifteen minutes after a 4g intravenous injection (2–5 min), the concentration in serum is 254 mcg/ml; 1 hour and 4 hours later levels are 93 mcg/ml and 9.1 mcg/ml, respectively:

MEZLIN®

MEZLOCILLIN SERUM LEVELS IN ADULTS (mcg/ml) 2–5 MIN IV INJECTION

DOSE	0	15 min	30 min	45 min	1 hr	2 hr	3 hr	4 hr	6 hr
4g	—	**254** (155–400)	**163** (99–260)	**122** (78–215)	**93** (67–133)	**47** (22–96)	**20** (8–45)	**9.1** (6–13)	**8.4** (5–17)

Continued on next page

Miles Pharm.—Cont.

available, appropriate therapy should be continued.
Mezlocillin's broad spectrum of activity makes it particularly useful for treating mixed infections caused by susceptible strains of both gram-negative and gram-positive aerobic or anaerobic bacteria. It is not effective, however, against infections caused by penicillinase-producing *Staphylococcus aureus.*
In certain severe infections, when the causative organisms are unknown, MEZLIN® may be administered in conjunction with an aminoglycoside or a cephalosporin antibiotic as initial therapy. As soon as results of culture and susceptibility tests become available, antimicrobial therapy should be adjusted if indicated. Culture and sensitivity testing, performed periodically during therapy, will provide information on the therapeutic effect of the antimicrobal and will monitor for the possible emergence of bacterial resistance.
MEZLIN® has been used effectively in combination with an aminoglycoside antibiotic for the treatment of life-threatening infections caused by *Pseudomonas aeruginosa.* For the treatment of febrile episodes in immunosuppressed patients with granulocytopenia, MEZLIN® should be combined with an aminoglycoside or a cephalosporin antibiotic.

CONTRAINDICATIONS

MEZLIN® is contraindicated in patients with a history of hypersensitivity reactions to any of the penicillins.

WARNINGS

Serious and occasionally fatal hypersensitivity (anaphylactic) reactions have occurred in patients receiving a penicillin. These reactions are more apt to occur in individuals with a history of sensitivity to multiple allergens. There have been reports of individuals with a history of penicillin hypersensitivity reactions who have experienced severe hypersensitivity reactions when treated with a cephalosporin. Before therapy with mezlocillin is instituted, careful inquiry should be made to determine whether the patient has had previous hypersensitivity reactions to penicillins, cephalosporins or other drugs. Antibiotics should be used with caution in any patient who has demonstrated some form of allergy, particularly to drugs.
If an allergic reaction occurs during therapy with mezlocillin, the drug should be discontinued. SERIOUS ANAPHYLACTOID REACTIONS REQUIRE IMMEDIATE EMERGENCY TREATMENT WITH EPINEPHRINE. OXYGEN, INTRAVENOUS STERIODS, AND AIRWAY MANAGEMENT, INCLUDING INTUBATION, SHOULD ALSO BE PROVIDED AS INDICATED.

PRECAUTIONS

Although MEZLIN® shares with other pencillins the low potential for toxicity as with any potent drug, periodic assessment of organ system functions, including renal, hepatic and hematopoietic, is advisable during prolonged therapy.
MEZLIN® has been reported rarely to cause acute interstitial nephritis.
Bleeding manifestations have occurred in some patients receiving beta-lactam antibiotics. These reactions have been associated with abnormalities of coagulation tests such as clotting time, platelet aggregation and prothrombin time and are more likely to occur in patients with renal impairment. Although MEZLIN® has rarely been associated with any bleeding abnormalities, the possibility of this occurring should be kept in mind, particularly in patients with severe renal impairment receiving maximum doses of the drug.
MEZLIN® has only rarely been reported to cause hypokalemia, however, the possibility of this occurring should also be kept in mind particularly when treating patients with fluid and electrolyte imbalance. Periodic monitoring of serum potassium may be advisable in patients receiving prolonged therapy.
MEZLIN® is a monosodium salt containing only 42.6 mg (1.85 mEq) of sodium per gram of mezlocillin. This should be considered when treating patients requiring restricted salt intake.
As with any penicillin, an allergic reaction, including anaphylaxis, may occur during MEZLIN® administration, particularly in a hypersensitive individual.
As with other antibiotics, prolonged use of MEZLIN® may result in overgrowth of non-susceptible organisms. If this occurs, appropriate measures should be taken.
Antimicrobials used in high doses for short periods to treat gonorrhea may mask or delay the symptoms of incubating syphilis. Therefore, prior to treatment, patients with gonorrhea should also be evaluated for syphilis. Specimens for dark field examination should be obtained from any suspected primary lesion and serologic tests should be performed. Patients treated with MEZLIN® should undergo follow-up serologic tests three months after therapy.

Interactions with Drugs and Laboratory Tests
As with other penicillins, the mixing of mezlocillin with a aminoglycoside in solutions for parenteral administration can result in substantial inactivation of the aminoglycoside.
Probenecid interferes with the renal tubular secretion of mezlocillin, thereby increasing serum concentrations and prolonging serum half-life of the antibiotic.
High urine concentrations of mezlocillin may produce false positive protein reactions (pseudoproteinuria) with the following methods sulfosalicyclic acid and boiling test, acetic acid test, biuret reaction, and nitric acid test. The bromphenol blue (Multi-stix®) reagent strip test has been reported to be reliable.

Pregnancy Category B
Reproduction studies have been performed in rats and mice at doses up to 2 times the human dose, and have revealed no evidence of impaired fertility or harm to the fetus, due to MEZLIN®. There are however no adequate and well controlled studies in pregnant women. Because animal reproductive studies are not always predictive of human response, this drug should be used during pregnancy only if clearly needed. Mezlocillin crosses the placenta and is found in low concentrations in cord blood and amniotic fluid.

Nursing Mothers
Mezlocillin is detected in low concentrations in the milk of nursing mothers, therefore caution should be exercised when MEZLIN® is administered to a nursing woman.

ADVERSE REACTIONS

As with other penicillins, the following adverse reactions may occur:
Hypersensitivity reactions: skin rash, pruritus, urticaria, drug fever, acute interstitial nephritis and anaphylactic reactions.
Gastro-intestinal distrubances: abnormal taste sensation, nausea, vomiting and diarrhea. If diarrhea persists, pseudomembranous colitis should be considered.
Hemic and Lymphatic Systems: thrombocytopenia, leukopenia, neutropenia, eosinophilia, reduction of hemoglobin or hematocrit, and positive Coombs' test.
Abnormalities of hepatic and renal function tests: elevation of serum aspartate aminotransferase (SGOT), serum alanine aminotransferase (SGPT), serum alkaline phosphatase, serum bilirubin. Elevation of serum creatinine and/or BUN. Reduction in serum potassium.
Central nervous system: convulsive seizures or neuromuscular hyperirritability.
Local reactions: thrombophlebitis with intravenous administration, pain with intramsucular injection.

OVERDOSAGE

As with other penicillins, MEZLIN® in overdosage has the potential to cause neuromuscular hyperirritability or convulsive seizures. Hemodialysis, if necessary, will aid in removal of the drug from the blood.

DOSAGE AND ADMINISTRATION

MEZLIN® (sterile mezlocillin sodium) may be administered intravenously or intramuscularly. For serious infections, the intravenous route of administration should be used. Intramuscular doses should not exceed 2g per injection.
The recommended adult dosage for serious infections is 200-300 mg/kg per day given in 4 to 6 divided doses. The usual dose is 3g given every 4 hours (18g/day) or 4g given every 6 hours (16g/day). For life-threatening infections, up to 350 mg/kg per day may be administered, but the total daily dosage should ordinarily not exceed 24g.
[See table above].

MEZLIN® DOSAGE GUIDE (ADULTS)

Condition	Daily Dosage Range	Usual Daily Dosage	Frequency and Route of Administration
Urinary tract infection (uncomplicated)	100–125 mg/kg	6-8g	1.5–2g every 6 hours IV or IM
Urinary tract infection (complicated)	150–200 mg/kg	12g	3g every 6 hours IV
Lower respiratory tract infection Intra-abdominal infection Gynecological infection Skin & skin structure infection Septicemia	225–300 mg/kg	16–18g	4g every 6 hours or 3g every 4 hours IV

For patients with life-threatening infections, 4g may be administered every 4 hours (24g/day).
Dosage for any individual patient must take into consideration the site and severity of infection, the susceptibility of the organisms causing infection, and the status of the patient's host defense mechanism.
The duration of therapy depends upon the severity of infection. Generally, MEZLIN® should be continued for at least 2 days after the signs and symptoms of infection have disappeared. The usual duration is 7 to 10 days; however, in difficult and complicated infections, more prolonged therapy may be required. Antibiotic therapy for Group A beta-hemolytic streptococcal infections should be maintained for at least 10 days to reduce the risk of rheumatic fever or glomerulonephritis.
In certain deep-seated infections, involving abscess formation, appropriate surgical drainage should be performed in conjunction with antimicrobial therapy.
For acute, uncomplicated gonococcal urethritis, the usual dose is 1–2g given once intravenously or by intramuscular injection. Probenecid 1g may be given orally at the time of dosing or up to ½-hour before. (For full prescribing information, refer to probenecid package insert).

Patients with Impaired Renal Function
The rate of elimination of mezlocillin is dose dependent and related to the degree of renal function impairment. After an intravenous dose of 3g the serum half-life is approximately 1 hour in patients with creatinine clearances above 60 ml/min, 1.3 hr in those with clearances of 30–59 ml/min, 1.6 hr in those with clearances of 10–29 ml/min and approximately 3.6 hr in patients with clearances of less than 10 ml/min. Dosage adjustments of MEZLIN® are not required in patients with mild impairment of renal function. For patients with a creatinine clearance of ≤30 ml/min (serum creatinine of approximately 3.0 mg% or greater), the following dosage guide may be used.
[See table below].

For life-threatening infections, 3g may be given every 6 hours to patients with creatinine clearances between 10–30 ml/min and 2g every 6 hours to those with clearances less than 10 ml/min.
For patients with serious systemic infection undergoing hemodialysis for renal failure, 3-4g may be administered after each dialysis and then every 12 hours. Patients undergoing peritoneal dialysis may receive 3g every 12 hours.
For patients with renal failure and hepatic insufficiency, measurement of serum levels of mezlocillin will provide additional guidance for adjusting dosage.

Intravenous Administration
MEZLIN® may be administered intravenously by intermittent infusion or by direct intravenous injection.
Infusion. Each gram of mezlocillin should be reconstituted by vigorous shaking with at least 10 ml of Sterile Water for Injection, 5% Dextrose Injection or 0.9% Sodium Chloride Injection. The dissolved drug should be further diluted to desired volume (50-100 ml) with an appropriate intravenous solution (See Compatibility and Stability section). The solution of reconstituted drug may then be administered over a period of 30 minutes by direct infusion or through a Y-type intravenous infusion set which may already be in place. If this method or the "piggyback" method of administration is used, it is advisable to discontinue temporarily the administration of any other solutions during the infusion of MEZLIN®.

MEZLIN® DOSAGE GUIDE FOR PATIENTS WITH IMPAIRED RENAL FUNCTION

Creatinine Clearance ml/min	Urinary Tract Infection (Uncomplicated)	Urinary Tract Infection (Complicated)	Serious Systemic Infection
>30	Usual Recommended Dosage		
10–30	1.5g every 8 hours	1.5g every 6 hours	3g every 8 hours
<10	1.5g every 8 hours	1.5g every 8 hours	2g every 8 hours

Injection. The reconstituted solution of MEZLIN® may also be injected directly into a vein or into intravenous tubing, when administered this way, the injection should be given slowly over a period of 3–5 minutes. To minimize venous irritation, the concentration of drug should not exceed 10%.

When MEZLIN® is given in combination with another antimicrobial, such as an aminoglycoside, each drug should be given separately in accordance with the recommended dosage and routes of administration for each drug.

Intramuscular Administration

Each gram of mezlocillin may be reconstituted by vigorous shaking with 3-4 ml of sterile water for injection or with 3-4 ml of 0.5 or 1.0% lidocaine hydrochloride solution (without epinephrine). (For Full prescribing information, refer to lidocaine package insert). Intramuscular doses of MEZLIN® should not exceed 2g per injection.

As with all intramuscular preparations, MEZLIN® should be injected well within the body of a relatively large muscle, such as the upper outer quadrant of the buttock (i.e., gluteus maximus), aspiration will help avoid unintentional injection into a blood vesel. Slow injection (12-15 sec) will minimize the discomfort associated with intramuscular administration.

Infants and Children

Only limited data are available on the safety and effectiveness of MEZLIN® in the treatment of infants and children with documented serious infection. In the event a child has an infection for which MEZLIN® may be judged particularly appropriate, the following dosage guide may be used: [See table above right]

For infants beyond one month of age and children up to the age of 12 years, 50 mg/kg may be administered every 4 hours (300 mg/kg/day).

The drug may be infused intravenously over 30-minutes or be given by intramuscular injection.

MEZLIN® DOSAGE GUIDE (NEWBORNS)

BODY WEIGHT (gm)	AGE ≤7 DAYS	AGE >7 DAYS
≤2000	75 mg/kg every 12 hours (150 mg/kg/day)	75 mg/kg every 8 hours (225 mg/kg/day)
>2000	75 mg/kg every 12 hours (150 mg/kg/day)	75 mg/kg every 6 hours (300 mg/kg/day)

COMPATIBILITY AND STABILITY

MEZLIN® at concentrations of 10 mg/ml and 100 mg/ml is stable (loss of potency less than 10%) in the following intravenous solutions for the time periods stated.
[See table below].

If precipitation should occur under refrigeration, the product should be warmed to 37°C for 20 minutes in a water bath and shaken well.

*This solution is stable from 10 mg/ml to 50 mg/ml under refrigeration.

MEZLIN® at concentrations up to 250 mg/ml is stable for 24 hours at room temperature in the following diluents:
- Sterile Water for Injection, USP
- 0.9% Sodium Chloride Injection, USP
- 0.5% and 1.0% Lidocaine Hydrochloride solution (without epinephrine)

MEZLIN® is stable for up to 28 days when frozen at -12 C at concentrations up to 100 mg/ml in the following diluents:
- Sterile Water for Injection, USP
- 0.9% Sodium Chloride Injection, USP or 5% Dextrose Injection, USP

HOW SUPPLIED

MEZLIN® (sterile mezlocillin sodium) is a white to pale yellow crystalline powder supplied in vials and infusion bottles.

Each vial contains mezlocillin sodium equivalent to 1g, 2g, 3g or 4g mezlocillin. Each infusion bottle contains mezlocillin sodium equivalent to 2g, 3g or 4g mezlocillin.

MEZLIN® vials and infusion bottles should be stored at or below 30°C (86°F). The powder as well as the reconstituted solution of drug may darken slightly, depending upon storage conditions, but potency is not affected.

Miles Pharmaceuticals
Division of Miles Laboratories, Inc.
West Haven, Connecticut 06516 USA
Sept 1985 PD100633 B502/2A 20267

MEZLIN — **STABILITY**

INTRAVENOUS SOLUTION	Controlled Room Temperature	Refrigeration
Sterile Water for Injection, USP	48 hours	7 days
0.9% Sodium Chloride Injection, USP	48 hours	7 days
5% Dextrose Injection, USP	48 hours	7 days
5% Dextrose in 0.225% Sodium Chloride Injection, USP	72 hours	7 days
Lactated Ringer's Injection, USP	72 hours	7 days
5% Dextrose in Electrolyte #75 Injection	72 hours	7 days
5% Dextrose in 0.45% Sodium Chloride Injection, USP	48 hours	48 hours
Ringer's Injection	24 hours	24 hours
10% Dextrose Injection	24 hours	24 hours
5% Fructose Injection	24 hours	24 hours

MITHRACIN® ℞
(plicamycin)
FOR INTRAVENOUS USE

WARNING

IT IS RECOMMENDED THAT MITHRACIN (plicamycin) BE ADMINISTERED ONLY TO HOSPITALIZED PATIENTS BY OR UNDER THE SUPERVISION OF A QUALIFIED PHYSICIAN WHO IS EXPERIENCED IN THE USE OF CANCER CHEMOTHERAPEUTIC AGENTS, BECAUSE OF THE POSSIBILITY OF SEVERE REACTIONS. FACILITIES FOR THE DETERMINATION OF NECESSARY LABORATORY STUDIES MUST BE AVAILABLE.

SEVERE THROMBOCYTOPENIA, A HEMORRHAGIC TENDENCY AND EVEN DEATH MAY RESULT FROM THE USE OF MITHRACIN. ALTHOUGH SEVERE TOXICITY IS MORE APT TO OCCUR IN PATIENTS WHO HAVE FAR-ADVANCED DISEASE OR ARE OTHERWISE CONSIDERED POOR RISKS FOR THERAPY, SERIOUS TOXICITY MAY ALSO OCCASIONALLY OCCUR EVEN IN PATIENTS WHO ARE IN RELATIVELY GOOD CONDITION.

IN THE TREATMENT OF EACH PATIENT, THE PHYSICIAN MUST WEIGH CAREFULLY THE POSSIBILITY OF ACHIEVING THERAPEUTIC BENEFIT VERSUS THE RISK OF TOXICITY WHICH MAY OCCUR WITH MITHRACIN THERAPY. THE FOLLOWING DATA CONCERNING THE USE OF MITHRACIN IN THE TREATMENT OF TESTICULAR TUMORS, HYPERCALCEMIC AND/OR HYPERCALCIURIC CONDITIONS ASSOCIATED WITH VARIOUS ADVANCED MALIGNANCIES, SHOULD BE THOROUGHLY REVIEWED BEFORE ADMINISTERING THIS COMPOUND.

DESCRIPTION

Mithracin is a yellow crystalline compound which is produced by a microorganism, *Streptomyces plicatus.* Mithracin is available in vials as a freeze-dried, sterile preparation for intravenous administration. Each vial contains 2500 mcg of Mithracin with 100 mg of mannitol and sufficient disodium phosphate to adjust to pH 7. After reconstitution with sterile water for injection, the solution has a pH of 7. The drug is unstable in acid solutions with a pH below 4.

Mithracin is an antineoplastic agent. It has an empirical formula of $C_{52}H_{76}O_{24}$. The following structural formula has been proposed for this compound.

CLINICAL PHARMACOLOGY

Although the exact mechanism by which Mithracin causes tumor inhibition is not yet known, studies have indicated that this compound forms a complex with deoxyribonucleic acid (DNA) and inhibits cellular ribonucleic acid (RNA) and enzymic RNA synthesis. The binding of Mithracin to DNA in the presence of Mg^{++} (or other divalent cations) is responsible for the inhibition of DNA-dependent or DNA-directed RNA synthesis. This action presumably accounts for the biological properties of Mithracin.

Mithracin shows potent cytotoxicity against malignant cells of human origin (Hela cells) growing in tissue culture. Mithracin is lethal to Hela cells in 48 hours at concentrations as low as 0.5 micrograms per milliliter of tissue culture medium. Mithracin has shown significant anti-tumor activity against experimental leukemia in mice when administered intraperitoneally.

Plicamycin may lower serum calcium levels; the exact mechanism (or mechanisms) by which the drug exerts this effect is unknown. It appears that plicamycin may block the hypercalcemic action of pharmacologic doses of vitamin D. It has also been suggested that plicamycin may lower calcium serum levels by inhibiting the effect of parathyroid hormone upon osteoclasts. Plicamycin's inhibition of DNA-dependent RNA synthesis appears to render osteoclasts unable to fully respond to parathyroid hormone with the biosynthesis necessary for osteolysis. Decreases in serum phosphate levels and urinary calcium excretion accompany the lowering of serum calcium concentrations.

Radioautography studies[1] with ^{3}H-labeled plicamycin in C3H mice slow that the greatest concentrations of the isotope are in the Kupffer cells of the liver and cells of the renal tubules. Plicamycin is rapidly cleared from the blood within the first 2 hours and excretion is also rapid. Sixty-seven percent of measured excretion occurs within 4 hours, 75% within 8 hours, and 90% is recovered in the first 24 hours after injection. There is no evidence of protein binding, nor is there any evidence of metabolism of the carbohydrate moiety of the drug to carbon dioxide and water with loss through respiration. Plicamycin crosses the blood-brain barrier; the concentration found in brain tissue is low but it persists longer than in other tissues. The experimental results in animals correlate closely with results achieved in man.[2]

INDICATIONS

Mithracin is a potent antineoplastic agent which has been shown to be useful in the treatment of carefully selected hospitalized patients with malignant tumors of the testis in whom successful treatment by surgery and/or radiation is impossible. Also, on the basis of limited clinical experience to date, it may be considered in the treatment of certain symptomatic patients with hypercalcemia and hypercalciuria associated with a variety of advanced neoplasms.

The use of Mithracin in other types of neoplastic disease is not recommended at the present time.

CONTRAINDICATIONS

Mithracin (plicamycin) is contraindicated in patients with thrombocytopenia, thrombocytopathy, coagulation disorder or an increased susceptibility to bleeding due to other causes. Mithracin should not be administered to any patient with impairment of bone marrow function.

Mithracin may cause fetal harm when administered to a pregnant woman. Mithracin is contraindicated in women who are or may become pregnant. If this drug is used during pregnancy or if the patient becomes pregnant while taking this drug, the patient should be apprised of the potential hazard to the fetus.

PRECAUTIONS

General: Mithracin should be administered only to patients who ar hospitalized and who can be observed carefully and frequently during and after therapy.

Severe thrombocytopenia, a hemorrhagic tendency and even death may result from the use of Mithracin. Although severe toxicity is more apt to occur in patients who have far-advanced disease or are otherwise considered poor risks for therapy, serious toxicity may also occasionally occur even in patients who are in relatively good condition.

Electrolyte imbalance, especially hypocalcemia, hypokalemia, and hypophosphatemia, should be corrected with appropriate electrolyte therapy prior to treatment with Mithracin.

Mithracin should be used with extreme caution in patients with significant impairment of renal or hepatic function.

Mithracin should not normally be administered to patients who are pregnant or to mothers who are breast feeding.

In the treatment of each patient, the physician must weigh carefully the possibility of achieving therapeutic benefit versus the risk of toxicity which may occur with Mithracin therapy.

Laboratory Tests: The following laboratory studies should be obtained frequently during therapy and for several days

Continued on next page

Miles Pharm.—Cont.

following the last dose: platelet count, prothrombin time, bleeding time. The occurrence of thrombocytopenia or a significant prolongation of prothrombin time or bleeding time is an indication for the termination of therapy.

Carcinogenesis, mutagenesis, impairment of fertility: No long-term studies in animals have been performed to evaluate the carcinogenic potential of Mithracin. Histologic evidence of inhibition of spermatogenesis was observed in a substantial number of male rats receiving doses of 0.6 mg/kg/day and above.

Pregnancy Category X: See "Contraindications" section.

Nursing Mothers: It is not known whether this drug is excreted in human milk. Because many drugs are excreted in human milk and because of the potential for serious adverse reactions in nursing infants from Mithracin, a decision should be made whether to discontinue nursing or to discontinue the drug, taking into account the importance of the drug to the mother.

ADVERSE REACTIONS

THE MOST IMPORTANT FORM OF TOXICITY ASSOCIATED WITH THE USE OF MITHRACIN CONSISTS OF A BLEEDING SYNDROME WHICH USUALLY BEGINS WITH AN EPISODE OF EPISTAXIS. This bleeding tendency may only consist of a single or several episodes of epistaxis and progress no further. However, in some cases, this hemorrhagic syndrome can start with an episode of hematemesis which may progress to more wide-spread hemorrhage in the gastrointestinal tract or to a more generalized bleeding tendency. This hemorrhagic diathesis is most likely due to abnormalities in multiple clotting factors.

A detailed analysis of the clinical data in 1,160 patients treated with Mithracin indicates that the hemorrhagic syndrome is dose related. With doses of 30 mcg/kg/day or less for 10 or fewer doses, the incidence of bleeding episodes has been 5.4% with an associated drug-related mortality rate of 1.6%. With doses greater than 30 mcg/kg/day and/or for more than 10 doses, a significantly larger number of bleeding episodes occurred (11.9%) and the associated drug-related mortality rate was also significantly higher (5.7%).

The most common side effects reported with the use of Mithracin consist of gastrointestinal symptoms: anorexia, nausea, vomiting, diarhea, and stomatitis. Other less frequently reported side effects include fever, drowsiness, weakness, lethargy, malaise, headache, depression, phlebitis, facial flushing, and skin rash.

The following laboratory abnormalities have been reported during therapy with Mithracin (plicamycin) and in most instances were reversible following cessation of treatment:

Hematologic Abnormalities: Depression of platelet count, white count, hemoglobin and prothrombin content; elevation of clotting time and bleeding time; abnormal clot retraction. Thrombocytopenia may be rapid in onset and may occur at any time during therapy or within several days following the last dose. With the occurrence of severe thrombocytopenia, the infusion of platelet concentrates of platelet-rich plasma may be helpful in elevating the platelet count.

The occurrence of leukopenia with the use of Mithracin is relatively uncommon, occurring only in approximately 6% of patients.

It has been uncommon for abnormalities in clotting time or clot retraction to be demonstrated prior to the onset of an overt bleeding episode noted in some patients treated with Mithracin. Nevertheless, the performance of these tests periodically is recommended because in a few instances, an abnormality in one of these studies may have served as a warning to terminate therapy because of impeding serious toxicity.

Abnormal Liver Function Tests: Increased levels of serum glutamic oxalacetic transaminase, serum glutamic pyruvic transaminase, lactic dehydrogenase, alkaline phosphatase, serum bilirubin, ornithine carbamyl transferase, isocitric dehydrogenase, and increased retention of bromsulphalein.

Abnormal Renal Function Tests: Increased blood urea nitrogen and serum creatinine; proteinuria.

Abnormalities in Electrolyte Concentrations: Depression of serum calcium, phosphorus, and potassium.

OVERDOSAGE

Generally, adverse effects following the use of Mithracin, especially the hemorrhagic syndrome, are dose related. Therefore, following administration of an overdose, patients can be expected to experience an exaggeration of the usual adverse effects. Close monitoring of the hematologic picture, including factors involved in the clotting mechanism, hepatic and renal functions, and serum electrolytes, is necessary. No specific antidote for Mithracin is known. Management of overdosage would include general supportive measures to sustain the patient through the period of toxicity.

DOSAGE

The daily dose of Mithracin is based on the patient's body weight. If a patient has abnormal fluid retention such as edema, hydrothorax or ascites, the patient's ideal weight rather than actual body weight should be used to calculate the dose.

Treatment of Testicular Tumors: In the treatment of patients with testicular tumors the recommended daily dose of Mithracin (plicamycin) is 25 to 30 MICROGRAMS per kilogram of body weight. Therapy should be continued for a period of 8 to 10 days unless significant side effects or toxicity occur during therapy. A course of therapy consisting of more than 10 daily doses is not recommended. Individual daily doses should not exceed 30 micrograms per kilogram of body weight.

In those patients with responsive tumors, some degree of tumor regression is usually evident within 3 or 4 weeks following the initial course of therapy. If tumor masses remain unchanged following an initial course of therapy, additional courses of therapy at monthly intervals are warranted.

When a significant tumor regression is obtained, it is suggested that additional courses of therapy be given at monthly intervals until a complete regression of tumor masses is achieved or until definite tumor progression or new tumor masses occur in spite of continued courses of therapy.

Treatment of Hypercalcemia and Hypercalciuria: Reversal of hypercalcemia and hypercalciuria can usually be achieved with Mithracin at doses considerably lower than those recommended for use in the treatment of testicular tumors.

In hypercalcemia and hypercalciuria associated with advanced malignancy the recommended course of treatment with Mithracin is 25 micrograms per kilogram of body weight per day for 3 or 4 days.

If the desired degree of reversal of hypercalcemia or hypercalciuria is not achieved with the initial course of therapy, additional courses of therapy may then be administered at intervals of one week or more to achieve the desired result or to maintain serum calcium and urinary calcium excretion at normal levels. It may be possible to maintain normal calcium balance with single, weekly doses or with a schedule of 2 or 3 doses per week.

NOTE: BECAUSE OF THE DRUG'S TOXICITY AND THE LIMITED CLINICAL EXPERIENCE TO DATE IN THESE INDICATIONS, THE FOLLOWING RECOMMENDATIONS SHOULD BE KEPT IN MIND BY THE PHYSICIAN.

1. **CONSIDER CASES OF HYPERCALCEMIA AND HYPERCALCIURIA NOT RESPONSIVE TO CONVENTIONAL TREATMENT.**
2. **APPLY SAME CONTRAINDICATIONS AND PRECAUTIONARY MEASURES AS IN ANTITUMOR TREATMENT.**
3. **RENAL FUNCTION SHOULD BE CAREFULLY MONITORED BEFORE, DURING, AND AFTER TREATMENT.**
4. **BENEFITS OF USE DURING PREGNANCY OR IN WOMEN OF CHILD-BEARING AGE SHOULD BE WEIGHED AGAINST POTENTIAL TOXICITY TO EMBRYO OR FETUS.**

ADMINISTRATION

By IV administration only. The appropriate daily dose of Mithracin should be diluted in one liter of 5% Dextrose Injection, USP or Sodium Chloride Injection, USP and administered by slow intravenous infusion over a period of 4 to 6 hours. Rapid direct intravenous injection of Mithracin should be avoided as it may be associated with a higher incidence and greater severity of gastrointestinal side effects. Extravasation of solutions of Mithracin may cause local irritation and cellulitis at injection sites. Should thrombophlebitis or perivascular cellulitis occur, the infusion should be terminated and reinstituted at another site. The application of moderate heat to the site of extravasation may help to disperse the compound and minimize discomfort and local tissue irritation. The use of antiemetic compounds prior to and during treatment with Mithracin may be helpful in relieving nausea and vomiting.

Procedures for proper handling and disposal of anti-cancer drugs should be considered. Several guidelines on this subject have been published.[3–8] There is no general agreement that all of the procedures recommended in the guidelines are necessary or appropriate.

HOW SUPPLIED

Mithracin is available in vials as a freeze-dried preparation for intravenous administration. Each vial contains 2500 mcg of Mithracin with 100 mg of mannitol and sufficient disodium phosphate to adjust to pH 7. These vials should be stored at refrigerator temperatures between 2°C. to 8°C. (36°F. to 46°F.).

To reconstitute, add aseptically 4.9 ml of Sterile Water for Injection to the contents of the vial and shake to dissolve. Each ml of the resulting solution will then contain 500 mcg of Mithracin. AFTER REMOVAL OF THE APPROPRIATE DOSE, THE REMAINING UNUSED SOLUTION MUST BE DISCARDED, FRESH SOLUTIONS MUST BE PREPARED IN THE ABOVE MANNER EACH DAY OF THERAPY.

ANIMAL PHARMACOLOGY AND TOXICOLOGY

In mice the average intravenous LD_{50} of Mithracin is 2,000 mcg/kg of body weight. When administered orally, it is not toxic to mice even at doses 100 times greater than the intravenous LD_{50}. In rats the average intravenous LD_{50} of Mithracin is 1,700 mcg/kg of body weight. It is not toxic to rats when administered orally at doses 17 times greater than the intravenous LD_{50}. In dogs and monkeys Mithracin is essentially non-toxic when administered intravenously for 24 days at daily doses as high as 50 and 24 mcg/kg of body weight, respectively. However, at higher doses of 100 mcg/kg/day intravenously it is lethal to dogs and monkeys. Signs of toxicity in dogs and monkeys included anorexia, vomiting, listlessness, nelena, anemia, lymphopenia, elevated alkaline phosphatase, serum glutamic oxalacetic transaminase, serum glutamic pyruvic transaminase values, hypochloremia, and azotemia. Dogs also showed marked thrombocytopenia, hyponatremia, hypokalemia, hypocalcemia, and decreased prothrombin consumption. Necropsy findings consisted of necrosis of lymphoid tissue and multiple generalized hemorrhages. Mithracin (plicamycin) was only mildly irritating when injected intramuscularly in rabbits and subcutaneously in guinea pigs. Histologic evidence of inhibition of spermatogenesis was observed in a substantial number of male rats receiving doses of 0.6 mg/kg/day and above. This preclinical finding of selective drug effect constituted the scientific rationale for clinical trials in testicular tumors.

Clinical Reports:

Treatment of Patients with Inoperable Testicular Tumors: In a combined series of 305 patients with inoperable testicular tumors treated with Mithracin, 33 patients (10.8%) showed a complete disappearance of tumor masses and an additional 80 patients (26.2%) responded with significant partial regression of tumor masses. The longest duration of a continuing complete response is now over 8½ years. The therapeutic responses in this series of patients have been summarized by type of testicular tumor in the accompanying table.

[See table above].

MITHRACIN

RESULTS IN 305 TESTICULAR TUMOR CASES BY TUMOR TYPE

TYPE OF TESTICULAR TUMOR	TOTAL	COMPLETE RESPONSE	PARTIAL RESPONSE	NO RESPONSE
EMBRYONAL CELL	173	26	42	105
TERATOMA	5	0	1	4
TERATOCARCINOMA	23	0	5	18
SEMINOMA	18	0	7	11
CHORIOCARCINOMA	13	1	6	6
MIXED TUMOR	73	6	19	48
TOTALS	305	33	80	192

Mithracin may be useful in the treatment of patients with testicular tumors which are resistant to other chemotherapeutic agents. Prior radiation therapy or prior chemotherapy did not alter the response rate with Mithracin. This suggests that there is no significant cross resistance between Mithracin (plicamycin) and other chemotherapeutic agents.

Treatment of Patients with Hypercalcemia and Hypercalciuria: A limited number of patients with hypercalcemia (range: 12.0–25.8 mg%) and patients with hypercalciuria (range 215–492 mg/day) associated with malignant disease were treated with Mithracin. Hypercalcemia and hypercalciuria were promptly reversed in all patients. In some patients, the primary malignancy was of non-testicular origin.

REFERENCES

1. Kennedy, B.D., et al: Cancer Res.27:1534, 1967.
2. Ransohoff, J., et al: Cancer Chemother. Rep. 49:51, 1965.
3. Recommendations for the Safe Handling of Parenteral Antineoplastic Drugs. NIH Publication No. 83-2621. For sale by the Superintendent of Documents, U.S. Government Printing Office, Washington, D.C. 20402.
4. AMA Council Report. Guidelines for Handling Parenteral Antineoplastics. JAMA, March 15, 1985.
5. National Study Commission on Cytotoxic Exposure—Recommendations for Handling Cytotoxic Agents. Available from Louis P. Jeffrey, Sc.D., Director of Pharmacy Services, Rhode Island Hospital, 593 Eddy Street, Providence, Rhode Island 02902.
6. Clinical Oncological Society of Australia: Guidelines and recommendations for safe handling of antineoplastic agents. Med J Australia 1:426–428, 1983.
7. Jones, R.B., et al: Safe handling of chemotherapeutic agents: A report from the Mount Sinai Medical Center. Ca—A Cancer Journal for Clinicians, Sept/Oct. 258–263, 1983.
8. American Society of Hospital Pharmacists technical assistance bulletin on handling cytotoxic drugs in hospitals. Am J Hosp Pharm 42:131–137, 1985.

Manufactured for
Miles Pharmaceuticals
Division of Miles Laboratories, Inc.
West Haven, Connecticut 06516 USA
by Pfizer Laboratories, New York, N.Y. 10017
PD100640 Revised February 1986

MYCELEX® 1% ℞
(clotrimazole) Cream
For dermatologic use only

PRODUCT OVERVIEW

KEY FACTS

Mycelex®-1% (dermatologic Cream) contains 10 mg clotrimazole in a vanishing cream base. Clotrimazole is a broad spectrum antifungal which exhibits fungicidal activity in vitro against *Candida albicans* and other species of the genus *Candida*. No single-step or multiple-step resistance to clotrimazole has developed during successive passages of *Candida albicans*.

MAJOR USES

Mycelex®-1% (Dermatologic Cream) is a clinically proven effective antifungal indicated for the topical treatment of the following dermal infections; tinea pedis, tinea cruris, and tinea corporis, due to *Trichophyton rubrum, Trichophyton mentagrophytes; Epidermophton floccosum* and *Microsporum canis;* candidiasis due to *Candida albicans;* and tinea versicolor due to *Malassezia furfur.*

SAFETY INFORMATION

Mycelex® Cream is contraindicated in individuals who have shown hypersensitivity to any of its components. Mycelex Cream is not for opthalmic use.

PRESCRIBING INFORMATION

MYCELEX® 1% ℞
(clotrimazole) Cream
For dermatologic use only

DESCRIPTION

Mycelex Cream 1% contains clotrimazole, a synthetic antifungal agent having the chemical name [1-(o-Chloro-*a,a*-diphenylbenzyl)imidazole]: the empirical formula $C_{22}H_{17}ClN_2$; a molecular weight of 344.84; and the chemical structure:

Clotrimazole is an odorless, white crystalline substance. It is practically insoluble in water, sparingly soluble in ether and very soluble in polyethylene glycol 400, ethanol and chloroform.

Each gram of Mycelex Cream contains 10 mg clotrimazole, dispersed in an emulsion vehicle composed of sorbitan monostearate, polysorbate 60, cetyl esters wax, cetostearyl alcohol, 2-octyldodecanol, purified water; benzyl alcohol (1%) as preservative.

CLINICAL PHARMACOLOGY

Clotrimazole is a broad-spectrum antifungal agent that is used for the treatment of dermal infections caused by various species of pathogenic dermatophytes, yeasts, and *Malassezia furfur*. The primary action of clotrimazole is against dividing and growing organisms.

In vitro, clotrimazole exhibits fungistatic and fungicidal activity against isolates of *Trichophyton rubrum, Trichophyton mentagrophytes, Epidermophyton floccosum, Microsporum canis,* and *Candida* species, including *Candida albicans*. In general, the *in vitro* activity of clotrimazole corresponds to that of tolnaftate and griseofulvin against the mycelia of dermatophytes (*Trichophyton, Microsporum,* and *Epidermophyton),* and to that of the polyenes (amphotericin B and nystatin) against budding fungi (*Candida*). Using an *in vivo* (mouse) and an *in vitro* (mouse kidney homogenate) testing system, clotrimazole and miconazole were equally effective in preventing the growth of the pseudomycelia and mycelia of *Candida albicans.*

Strains of fungi having a natural resistance to clotrimazole are rare. Only a single isolate of *Candida guilliermondi* has been reported to have primary resistance to clotrimazole.

No single-step or multiple-step resistance to clotrimazole has developed during successive passages of *Candida albicans* and *Trichophyton mentagrophytes*. No appreciable change in sensitivity was detected after successive passage of isolates of *C. albicans, C. krusei*, or *C. pseudotropicalis* in liquid or solid media containing clotrimazole. Also, resistance could not be developed in chemically induced mutant strains of polyene-resistant isolates of *C. albicans*. Slight, reversible resistance was noted in three isolates of *C. albicans* tested by one investigator. There is a single report that records the clinical emergence of a *C. albicans* strain with considerable resistance to flucytosine and miconazole, and with cross-resistance to clotrimazole, the strain remained sensitive to nystatin and amphotericin B.

In studies of the mechanism of action, the minimum fungicidal concentration of clotrimazole caused leakage of intracellular phosphorus compounds into the ambient medium with concomitant breakdown of cellular nucleic acids and accelerated potassium efflux. Both these events began rapidly and extensively after addition of the drug.

Clotrimazole appears to be well absorbed in humans following oral administration and is eliminated mainly as inactive metabolites. Following topical and vaginal administration, however, clotrimazole appears to be minimally absorbed.

Six hours after the application of radioactive clotrimazole 1% cream and 1% solution onto intact and acutely inflamed skin, the concentration of clotrimazole varied from 100 mcg/cm in the stratum corneum to 0.5 to 1 mcg/cm in the stratum reticulare, and 0.1 mcg/cm in the subcutis. No measurable amount of radioactivity ($\leq$ 0.001 mcg/ml) was found in the serum within 48 hours after application under occlusive dressing of 0.5 ml of the solution or 0.8 g of the cream. Only 0.5% or less of the applied radioactivity was excreted in the urine.

Following intravaginal administration of 100mg ^{14}C-clotrimazole vaginal tablets to nine adult females, an average peak serum level, corresponding to only 0.03 μg equivalents/ml of clotrimazole, was reached one to two days after application. After intravaginal administration of 5 g of 1% ^{14}C-clotrimazole vaginal cream, containing 50 mg active drug, to five subjects (one with candida colpitis), serum levels corresponding to approximately 0.01 μg equivalents/ml were reached between 8 and 24 hours after application.

INDICATIONS AND USAGE

Mycelex® Cream is indicated for the topical treatment of the following dermal infections: tinea pedis, tinea cruris, and tinea corporis due to *Trichophyton rubrum, Trichophyton mentagrophytes, Epidermophyton floccosum,* and *Microsporum canis;* candidiasis due to *Candida albicans,* and tinea versicolor due to *Malassezia furfur.*

CONTRAINDICATIONS

Mycelex® Cream is contraindicated in individuals sensitive to its components.

WARNINGS

Mycelex Cream is not for ophthalmic use.

PRECAUTIONS

General: If irritation or sensitivity develops with the use of Mycelex Cream, treatment should be discontinued and appropriate therapy instituted.

Information For Patients:

The patient should be advised to:

1. Use the medication for the full treatment time even though the symptoms may have improved. Notify the physician if there is no improvement after four weeks of treatment.
2. Inform the physician if the area of application shows signs of increased irritation (redness, itching, burning, blistering, swelling, oozing) indicative of possible sensitization.
3. Avoid the use of occlusive wrappings or dressings.
4. Avoid sources of infection or reinfection.

Laboratory Tests: If there is lack of response to Mycelex® Cream, appropriate microbiological studies should be repeated to confirm the diagnosis and rule out other pathogens before instituting another course of antimycotic therapy.

Drug Interactions: Synergism or antagonism between clotrimazole and nystatin, or amphotericin B, or flucytosine against strains of *C. albicans* has not been reported.

Carcinogenesis, mutagenesis, impairment of fertility: An 18-month oral dosing study with clotrimazole in rats has not revealed any carcinogenic effect.

In tests for mutagenesis, chromosomes of the spermatophores of Chinese hamsters which had been exposed to clotrimazole were examined for structural changes during the metaphase. Prior to testing, the hamsters had received five oral clotrimazole doses of 100 mg/kg body weight. The results of this study showed that clotrimazole had no mutagenic effect.

Usage in Pregnancy: Pregnancy Category B: The disposition of ^{14}C-clotrimazole has been studied in humans and animals. Clotrimazole is very poorly absorbed following dermal application or intravaginal administration to humans. (See Clinical Pharmacology.)

In clinical trials, use of vaginally applied clotrimazole in pregnant women in their second and third trimesters has not been associated with ill effects. There are, however, no adequate and well-controlled studies in pregnant women during the first trimester of pregnancy.

Studies in pregnant rats with intravaginal doses up to 100 mg/kg have revealed no evidence of harm to the fetus due to clotrimazole.

High oral doses of clotrimazole in rats and mice ranging from 50 to 120 mg/kg resulted in embryotoxicity (possibly secondary to maternal toxicity), impairment of mating, decreased litter size and number of viable young and decreased pup survival to weaning. However, clotrimazole was not teratogenic in mice, rabbits and rats at oral doses up to 200, 180 and 100 mg/kg, respectively. Oral absorption in the rat amounts to approximately 90% of the administered dose.

Because animal reproduction studies are not always predictive of human response, this drug should be used only if clearly indicated during the first trimester of pregnancy.

Nursing Mothers: It is not known whether this drug is excreted in human milk. Because many drugs are excreted in human milk, caution should be exercised when clotrimazole is used by a nursing woman.

Pediatric Use: Safety and effectiveness in children have been established for clotrimazole when used as indicated and in the recommended dosage.

ADVERSE REACTIONS

The following adverse reactions have been reported in connection with the use of the cream and solution forms of this product: erythema, stinging, blistering, peeling, edema, pruritus, urticaria, burning, and general irritation of the skin.

OVERDOSAGE

Acute overdosage with topical application of clotrimazole is unlikely and would not be expected to lead to a life-threatening situation.

DOSAGE AND ADMINISTRATION

Gently massage sufficient Mycelex® Cream into the affected and surrounding skin areas twice a day, in the morning and evening.

Clinical improvement, with relief of pruritus, usually occurs within the first week of treatment with Mycelex. If the patient shows no clinical improvement after four weeks of treatment with Mycelex, the diagnosis should be reviewed.

HOW SUPPLIED

Mycelex Cream 1% is supplied in 15, 30, and (2 × 45) gram tubes.

Store between 2° and 30°C [36° and 86°F].

U.S. Patents No. 3,660,577 and 3,705,172.

January, 1985 PD100609 20168

MYCELEX® 1% ℞
(clotrimazole) Solution
For dermatologic use only

PRODUCT OVERVIEW

KEY FACTS

Mycelex®-1% (Solution) contains 10 mg of clotrimazole per milliliter. Clotrimazole is a broad spectrum antifungal which exhibits fungicidal activity in vitro against *Candida albicans* and other species of the genus Candida. No single-step or multiple-step resistance to clotrimazole has developed during successive passages of *Candida albicans.*

MAJOR USES

Mycelex®-1% (Solution) is a clinically proven effective antifungal indicated for the topical treatment of the following dermal infections: tinea pedis, tinea cruris, and tinea corporis due to *Trichophyton rubrum, Trichophyton mentagrophytes; Epidermophyton floccosum* and Microsporum canis; candidiasis due to *Candida albicans;* and tinea versicolor due to *Malassezia furfur.*

Continued on next page

Miles Pharm.—Cont.

SAFETY INFORMATION

Mycelex®-1% (Solution) is contraindicated in individuals who have shown hypersensitivity to any of its components. Mycelex Cream is not for opthalmic use.

PRESCRIBING INFORMATION

MYCELEX® 1% ℞
(clotrimazole) Solution
For dermatologic use only

DESCRIPTION

Mycelex Solution 1% contains clotrimazole, a synthetic antifungal agent having the chemical name [1-(o-Chloro-α,α-diphenylbenzyl)imidazole]; the empirical formula $C_{22}H_{17}ClN_2$; a molecular weight of 344.84; and the chemical structure:

Clotrimazole is an odorless, white crystalline substance. It is practically insoluble in water, sparingly soluble in ether and very soluble in polyethylene glycol 400, ethanol and chloroform.
Mycelex Solution contains 10 mg/ml of clotrimazole (the active ingredient) in a non-aqueous vehicle of polyethylene glycol 400.

CLINICAL PHARMACOLOGY

Clotrimazole is a broad-spectrum antifungal agent that is used for the treatment of dermal infections caused by various species of pathogenic dermatophytes, yeasts, and *Malassezia furfur*. The primary action of clotrimazole is against dividing and growing organisms.
In vitro, clotrimazole exhibits fungistatic and fungicidal activity against isolates of *Trichophyton rubrum, Trichophyton mentagrophytes, Epidermophyton floccosum, Microsporum canis*, and *Candida* species, including *Candida albicans*. In general, the *in vitro* activity of clotrimazole corresponds to that of tolnaftate and griseofulvin against the mycelia of dermatophytes (*Trichophyton, Microsporum*, and *Epidermophyton*), and to that of the polyenes (amphotericin B and nystatin) against budding fungi (*Candida*). Using an *in vivo* (mouse) and an *in vitro* (mouse kidney homogenate) testing system, clotrimazole and miconazole were equally effective in preventing the growth of the pseudomycelia and mycelia of *Candida albicans*.
Strains of fungi having a natural resistance to clotrimazole are rare. Only a single isolate of *Candida guilliermondi* has been reported to have primary resistance to clotrimazole.
No single-step or multiple-step resistance to clotrimazole has developed during successive passages of *Candida albicans* and *Trichophyton mentagrophytes*. No appreciable change in sensitivity was detected after successive passage of isolates of *C. albicans, C. krusei*, or *C. pseudotropicalis* in liquid or solid media containing clotrimazole. Also, resistance could not be developed in chemically induced mutant strains of polyene-resistant isolates of *C. albicans*. Slight, reversible resistance was noted in three isolates of *C. albicans* tested by one investigator. There is a single report that records the clinical emergence of a *C. albicans* strain with considerable resistance to flucytosine and miconazole, and with cross-resistance to clotrimazole, the strain remained sensitive to nystatin and amphotericin B.
In studies of the mechanism of action, the minimum fungicidal concentration of clotrimazole caused leakage of intracellular phosphorus compounds into the ambient medium with concomitant breakdown of cellular nucleic acids and accelerated potassium efflux. Both these events began rapidly and extensively after addition of the drug.
Clotrimazole appears to be well absorbed in humans following oral administration and is eliminated mainly as inactive metabolities. Following topical and vaginal administration, however, clotrimazole appears to be minimally absorbed.
Six hours after the application of radioactive clotrimazole 1% cream and 1% solution onto intact and acutely inflamed skin, the concentration of clotrimazole varied from 100 mcg/cm in the stratum corneum to 0.5 to 1 mcg/cm in the stratum reticulare, and 0.1 mcg/cm in the subcutis. No measurable amount of radioactivity ($\geq$0.001 mcg/ml) was found in the serum within 48 hours after application under occlusive dressing of 0.5 ml of the solution or 0.8 g of the cream. Only 0.5% or less of the applied radioactivity was excreted in the urine.
Following intravaginal administration of 100 mg ^{14}C-clotrimazole vaginal tablets to nine adult females, an average peak serum level, corresponding to only 0.03 μg equivalents/ml of clotrimazole, was reached one to two days after application. After intravaginal administration of 5g of 1% ^{14}C-clotrimazole vaginal cream, containing 50 mg active drug, to five subjects (one with candida colpitis), serum levels corresponding to approximately 0.01 μg equivalents/ml were reached between 8 and 24 hours after application.

INDICATIONS AND USAGE

Mycelex Solution is indicated for the topical treatment of the following dermal infections; tinea pedis, tinea cruris, and tinea corporis due to *Trichophyton rubrum, Trichophyton mentagrophytes, Epidermophyton floccosum*, and *Microsporum canis;* candidiasis due to *Candida albicans*, and tinea versicolor due to *Malassezia furfur*.

CONTRAINDICATIONS

Mycelex® Solution is contraindicated in individuals sensitive to its components.

WARNINGS

Mycelex Solution is not for ophthalmic use.

PRECAUTIONS

General: If irritation or sensitivity develops with the use of Mycelex Solution, treatment should be discontinued and appropriate therapy instituted.
Information For Patients:
The patient should be advised to:
1. Use the medication for the full treatment time even though the symptoms may have improved. Notify the physician if there is no improvement after four weeks of treatment.
2. Inform the physician if the area of application shows signs of increased irritation (redness, itching, burning, blistering, swelling, oozing) indicative of possible sensitization.
3. Avoid the use of occlusive wrappings or dressings.
4. Avoid sources of infection or reinfection.

Laboratory Tests: If there is lack of response to Mycelex Solution, appropriate microbiological studies should be repeated to confirm the diagnosis and rule out other pathogens before instituting another course of antimycotic therapy.
Drug Interactions: Synergism or antagonism between clotrimazole and nystatin, or amphotericin B. or flucytosine against strains of *C. albicans* has not been reported.
Carcinogenesis, mutagenesis, impairment of fertility: An 18-month oral dosing study with clotrimazole in rats has not revealed any carcinogenic effect.
In tests for mutagenesis, chromosomes of the spermatophores of Chinese hamsters which had been exposed to clotrimazole were examined for structural changes during the metaphase. Prior to testing, the hamsters had received five oral clotrimazole doses of 100 mg/kg body weight. The results of this study showed that clotrimazole had no mutagenic effect.
Usage In Pregnancy: Pregnancy Category B: The disposition of ^{14}C-clotrimazole has been studied in humans and animals. Clotrimazole is very poorly absorbed following dermal application or intravaginal administration to humans. (See clinical Pharmacology.)
In clinical trials, use of vaginally applied clotrimazole in pregnant women in their second and third trimesters has not been associated with ill effects. There are, however, no adequate and well-controlled studies in pregnant women during the first trimester of pregnancy.
Studies in pregnant rats with intravaginal doses up to 100 mg/kg have revealed no evidence of harm to the fetus due to clotrimazole.
High oral doses of clotrimazole in rats and mice ranging from 50 to 120 mg/kg resulted in embryotoxicity (possibly secondary to maternal toxicity), impairment of mating, decreased litter size and number of viable young and decreased pup survival to weaning. However, clotrimazole was not teratogenic in mice, rabbits and rats at oral doses up to 200, 180 and 100 mg/kg, respectively. Oral absorption in the rat amounts to approximately 90% of the administered dose.
Because animal reproduction studies are not always predictive of human response, this drug should be used only if clearly indicated during the first trimester of pregnancy.
Nursing Mothers: It is not known whether this drug is excreted in human milk. Because many drugs are excreted in human milk, caution should be exercised when clotrimazole is used by a nursing woman.
Pediatric Use: Safety and effectiveness in children have been established for clotrimazole when used as indicated and in the recommended dosage.

ADVERSE REACTIONS

The following adverse reactions have been reported in connection with the use of the cream and solution forms of this product: erythema, stinging, blistering, peeling, edema, pruritus, urticaria, burning, and general irritation of the skin.

OVERDOSAGE

Acute overdosage with topical application of clotrimazole is unlikely and would not be expected to lead to a life-threatening situation.

DOSAGE AND ADMINISTRATION

Gently massage sufficient Mycelex Solution into the affected and surrounding skin areas twice a day, in the morning and evening.
Clinical improvement, with relief of pruritus, usually occurs within the first week of treatment with Mycelex. If the patient shows no clinical improvement after four weeks of treatment with Mycelex, the diagnosis should be reviewed.

HOW SUPPLIED

Mycelex Solution 1% is supplied in 10 ml and 30 ml plastic bottles.
Store between 2° and 30°C [36° and 86°F]. Shake well before using.
U. S. Patents No. 3,660,577 and 3,705,172
January, 1985 PD100608 19956

MYCELEX® ℞
(clotrimazole)
Troche

PRODUCT OVERVIEW

KEY FACTS

MYCELEX® Troche is a slow-dissolving tablet (lozenge) containing 10 mg of clotrimazole, a synthetic antifungal agent for topical use in the mouth. Clotrimazole is a broad-spectrum antifungal which exhibits fungicidal activity *in vitro* against *Candida albicans* and other species of the genus *Candida*. No single-step or multiple-step resistance to clotrimazole has developed during successive passages of *Candida albicans*.

MAJOR USES

MYCELEX® Troche has been proven effective in the treatment of oropharyngeal candidiasis (oral thrush) in patients over 3 years of age.

SAFETY INFORMATION

MYCELEX® Troches are contra-indicated in patients who are hypersensitive to any of its components. MYCELEX Troches are not indicated f or the treatment of systemic mycoses. Since elevated SGOT levels have been reported, periodic assessment of hepatic function is advisable, particularly, in patients with pre-existing hepatic impairment.

PRESCRIBING INFORMATION

MYCELEX® ℞
(clotrimazole)
Troche

DESCRIPTION

Each Mycelex® Troche contains 10 mg clotrimazole [1(o-chloro-α, α-diphenylbenzyl) imidazole], a synthetic antifungal agent, for topical use in the mouth.
Structural Formula:

Chemical Formula:
$C_{22}H_{17}ClN_2$
The troche dosage form is a large, slowly dissolving tablet (lozenge) containing 10 mg of clotrimazole dispersed in dextrose, microcrystalline cellulose, povidone, and magnesium stearate.

CLINICAL PHARMACOLOGY

Clotrimazole is a broad-spectrum antifungal agent that inhibits the growth of pathogenic yeasts by altering the permeability of cell membranes. It exhibits fungicidal activity *in vitro* against *Candida albicans* and other species of the genus *Candida*. No single-step or multiple-step resistance to clotrimazole has developed during successive passages of *Candida albicans* in the laboratory.
After oral administration of a 10 mg clotrimazole troche to healthy volunteers concentrations sufficient to inhibit most species of *Candida* persist in saliva for up to three hours following the approximately 30 minutes needed for a troche to dissolve. The long term effective concentration of drug in saliva appears to be related to the slow release of clotrimazole from the oral mucosa to which the drug is apparently bound. Repetitive dosing at three hour intervals maintains effective salivary levels above the minimum inhibitory concentration of most strains of *Candida*. In another study the mean serum concentrations were 4.98 $\pm$ 3.7 and 3.23 $\pm$ 1.4 nanograms/ml at 30 and 60 minutes respectively.

INDICATIONS AND USAGE

Mycelex Troches are indicated for the local treatment of oropharyngeal candidiasis. The diagnosis should be confirmed by a KOH smear and/or culture prior to treatment.

CONTRAINDICATIONS

Mycelex Troches are contraindicated in patients who are hypersensitive to any of its components.

WARNING

Mycelex Troches are not indicated for the treatment of systemic mycoses.

PRECAUTIONS

Abnormal liver function tests have been reported in patients treated with clotrimazole troches; elevated SGOT levels were reported in about 15% of patients in the clinical trials. In most cases the elevations were minimal and it was often impossible to distinguish effects of clotrimazole from those of other therapy and the underlying disease (malignancy in most cases). Periodic assessment of hepatic function is advisable particularly in patients with pre-existing hepatic impairment.

Since patients must be instructed to allow each troche to dissolve slowly in the mouth in order to achieve maximum effect of the medication, they must be of such an age and physical and/or mental condition to comprehend such instructions.

Carcinogenesis: An 18 month dosing study with clotrimazole in rats has not revealed any carcinogenic effect.

Usage in Pregnancy: Pregnancy Category C: Clotrimazole has been shown to be embryotoxic in rats and mice when given in doses 100 times the adult human dose (in mg/kg), possibly secondary to maternal toxicity. The drug was not teratogenic in mice, rabbits, and rats when given in doses up to 200, 180, and 100 times the human dose.

Clotrimazole given orally to mice from nine weeks before mating through weaning at a dose 120 times the human dose was associated with impairment of mating, decreased number of viable young, and decreased survival to weaning. No effects were observed at 60 times the human dose. When the drug was given to rats during a similar time period at 50 times the human dose, there was a slight decrease in the number of pups per litter and decreased pup viability.

There are no adequate and well controlled studies in pregnant women. Clotrimazole troches should be used during pregnancy only if the potential benefit justifies the potential risk to the fetus.

Pediatric Use: Safety and effectiveness of clotrimazole in children below the age of 3 years have not been established; therefore, its use in such patients is not recommended.

ADVERSE REACTIONS

Abnormal liver function tests have been reported in patients treated with clotrimazole troches; elevated SGOT levels were reported in about 15% of patients in the clinical trials (see **Precautions** section).

Nausea and vomiting was reported in about one in twenty patients.

OVERDOSE

No data available.

DRUG ABUSE AND DEPENDENCE

No data available.

DOSAGE AND ADMINISTRATION

Mycelex® Troches are administered only as a lozenge that must be dissolved slowly in the mouth. The recommended dose is one troche five times a day for fourteen consecutive days. Only limited data are available on the safety and effectiveness of the clotrimazole troche after prolonged administration; therefore, therapy should be limited to short term use, if possible.

HOW SUPPLIED

Mycelex® Troches, white discoid, uncoated tablets are supplied in bottles of 70 and 140. Each tablet will be identified with the following: Miles 095.

Store below 86°F (30°C), avoid freezing.

PD100613 20075 January, 1985

Shown in Product Identification Section, page 419

MYCELEX®-G 1% ℞

(clotrimazole) Vaginal Cream

PRODUCT OVERVIEW

KEY FACTS

Mycelex®-G-1% Vaginal Cream is an effective vaginal antifungal cream. Each applicatorful of Mycelex-G-1% Vaginal Cream contains approximately 50 mg of clotrimazole. Clotrimazole is a broad spectrum antifungal which exhibits fungicidal activity in vitro against *Candida albicans* and other species of the genus *Candida*. No single-step or multiple-step resistance to clotrimazole has developed during successive passages of *Candida albicans*.

MAJOR USES

Mycelex®-G-1% Vaginal Cream has been proven clinically effective for the local treatment of vulvovaginal candidiasis.

SAFETY INFORMATION

Mycelex®-G-1% Vaginal Cream is contraindicated in women who have shown hypersensitivity to any of the components. If there is a lack of response to treatment with Mycelex®-G-1% Vaginal Cream, appropriate microbiological studies should be repeated to confirm the diagnosis and rule out other pathogens before instituting another course of antimycotic therapy. No adequate and well-controlled studies in pregnany women during the first trimester of pregnancy.

PRESCRIBING INFORMATION

MYCELEX®-G 1% ℞

(clotrimazole) Vaginal Cream

DESCRIPTION

Mycelex-G is clotrimazole [1-(o-Chloro-α,α -diphenylbenzyl) imidazole], a synthetic antifungal agent having the chemical formula, $C_{22}H_{17}ClN_2$, and following chemical structure:

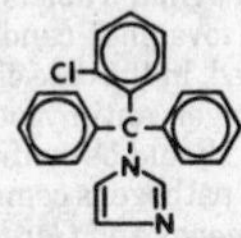

Each applicatorful of Mycelex-G Vaginal Cream contains approximately 50 mg. clotrimazole dispersed in sorbitan monostearate, polysorbate 60, cetyl esters wax, cetostearyl alcohol, 2-octyldodecanol, purified water, and as a preservative, benzyl alcohol (1%).

ACTIONS

Clotrimazole is a broad spectrum antifungal agent that inhibits the growth of pathogenic yeasts. Clotrimazole exhibits fungicidal activity *in vitro* against *Candida albicans* and other species of the genus *Candida*.

No single-step or multiple-step resistance to clotrimazole has developed during successive passages of *Candida albicans*.

INDICATIONS

Mycelex-G Vaginal Cream is indicated for the local treatment of patients with vulvovaginal candidiasis (moniliasis). As Mycelex-G Vaginal Cream has been shown to be effective only for candidal vulvovaginitis, the diagnosis should be confirmed by KOH smears and/or cultures. Other pathogens commonly associated with vulvovaginitis (*Trichomonas* and *Hemophilus vaginalis*) should be ruled out by appropriate laboratory methods.

Studies have shown that women taking oral contraceptives had a cure rate similar to those not taking oral contraceptives.

CONTRAINDICATIONS

Mycelex-G Vaginal Cream is contraindicated in women who have shown hypersensitivity to any of the components of the preparation.

PRECAUTIONS

Laboratory Tests: If there is a lack of response to Mycelex-G Vaginal Cream, appropriate microbiological studies should be repeated to confirm the diagnosis and rule out other pathogens before instituting another course of antimycotic therapy.

Usage in Pregnancy: While Mycelex-G Vaginal Cream has not been studied in the first trimester of pregnancy, use in the second and third trimesters has not been associated with ill effects.

Application of ^{14}C labeled clotrimazole has shown negligible absorption (peak serum level of 0.01 mcg/ml 24 hours after insertion of vaginal cream containing 50 mg. of active drug) from both normal and inflamed human vaginal mucosa.

ADVERSE REACTIONS

Three (0.5%) of the 653 patients treated with Mycelex-G Vaginal Cream reported complaints during therapy that were possibly drug related. Vaginal burning occurred in one patient; erythema, irritation and burning in another; intercurrent cystitis was reported in the third.

DOSAGE AND ADMINISTRATION

Mycelex-G Vaginal Cream has been found to be effective when used from seven to fourteen days; studies have shown that patients treated for fourteen days had a significantly higher cure rate. The recommended dose is one applicatorful a day for seven to fourteen consecutive days; using the applicator supplied, insert one applicatorful of cream (approximately 5 grams) intravaginally preferably at bedtime.

HOW SUPPLIED

Mycelex-G Vaginal Cream 1% is supplied in 45 and 90 gram tubes with a measured-dose applicator; for seven-day and for fourteen-day treatments.

Store between 35° and 86° F (2° and 30° C).

February, 1981 PD 100526

MYCELEX®-G 100 mg ℞

(clotrimazole) Vaginal Tablets

PRODUCT OVERVIEW

KEY FACTS

Mycelex®-G 100 mg is an effective vaginal antifungal tablet containing 100 mg of clotrimazole (the active ingredient). Clotrimazole is a broad spectrum antifungal which exhibits fungicidal activity in vitro against *Candida albicans* and other species of the genus *Candida*. No single-step or multiple-step resistance to clotrimazole has developed during successive passages of *Candida albicans*.

MAJOR USES

Mycelex®-G 100 Vaginal Tablet has been proven clinically effective for the local treatment of vulvovaginal candidiasis.

SAFETY INFORMATION

Mycelex®-G 100 mg Vaginal Tablet is contraindicated in women who have shown hypersensitivity to any of the components. If there is a lack of response to treatment with Mycelex-G 100 mg Vaginal Tablets, appropriate microbiological studies should be repeated to confirm the diagnosis and rule out other pathogens before instituting another course of antimycotic therapy. No adequate and well-controlled studies in pregnant women during the first trimester of pregnancy.

PRESCRIBING INFORMATION

MYCELEX®–G 100 mg ℞

(clotrimazole) Vaginal Tablets

DESCRIPTION

Mycelex-G is clotrimazole [1-(o-Chloro-α, α-diphenylbenzyl) imidazole], a synthetic antifungal agent having the chemical formula, $C_{22}H_{17}ClN_2$.

Each Mycelex-G Vaginal Tablet contains 100 mg clotrimazole dispersed in lactose, povidone, corn starch and magnesium stearate.

ACTIONS

Clotrimazole is a broad-spectrum antifungal agent that inhibits the growth of pathogenic yeasts. Clotrimazole exhibits fungicidal activity *in vitro* against *Candida albicans* and other species of the genus *Candida*.

No single-step or multiple-step resistance to clotrimazole has developed during successive passages of *Candida albicans*.

INDICATIONS

Mycelex-G Vaginal Tablets are indicated for the local treatment of vulvovaginal candidiasis. The diagnosis should be confirmed by KOH smears and/or cultures. Other pathogens commonly associated with vulvovaginitis *(Trichomonas* and *Hemophilus vaginalis)* should be ruled out by appropriate laboratory methods.

CONTRAINDICATIONS

Mycelex-G Vaginal Tablets are contraindicated in women who have shown hypersensitivity to any components of the preparation.

PRECAUTIONS

Laboratory Tests: If there is a lack of response to Mycelex-G Vaginal Tablets, appropriate microbiological studies should be repeated to confirm the diagnosis and rule out other pathogens before instituting another course of antimycotic therapy.

Application of ^{14}C-labeled clotrimazole has shown negligible absorption (peak of 0.03 mcg/ml of serum 24 hours after insertion of a 100 mg tablet) from both normal and inflammed human vaginal mucosa.

Usage in Pregnancy: While Mycelex-G Vaginal Tablets have not been studied in the first trimester of pregnancy, use in the second and third trimesters has not been associated with ill effects. Follow-up reports now available on 71 neonates of 117 pregnant patients reveal no adverse effects or complications attributable to Mycelex-G therapy.

ADVERSE REACTIONS

Eighteen (1.6%) of the 1116 patients treated with Mycelex-G in double-blind studies reported complaints during therapy that were possibly drug-related. Mild burning occured in six patients while other complaints, such as skin rash, itching, vulval irritation, lower abdominal cramps and bloating, slight cramping, slight urinary frequency, and burning or irritation in the sexual partner, occurred rarely.

DOSAGE AND ADMINISTRATION

The recommended dose is one tablet a day for seven consecutive days. Recent studies indicate that an alternative regimen of two tablets a day for three consecutive days is similarly effective in non-pregnant patients; however, in pregnant patients the three-day treatment course did not prove to be effective and is therefore not recommended. They should receive the seven-day treatment. Using the applica-

Continued on next page

Miles Pharm.—Cont.

tor supplied, insert one or two tablets intravaginally preferably at bedtime.
In the event of treatment failure, other pathogens commonly responsible for vaginitis should be ruled out before instituting another course of antimycotic therapy. There are no studies to show whether a second course of clotrimazole would be effective in patients who fail to respond to the initial course.

HOW SUPPLIED

Mycelex-G Vaginal Tablets 100 mg, white, bullet-shaped, uncoated tablets coded with number 093-Miles, supplied in a strip of seven tablets with plastic applicator and patient leaflet of instructions.
DPSC Stocked: NSN 6505-01-090-6795
Do not store above 35°C [95°F].
U.S. Patent No. 3,660,577 and 3,705,172
PD100606 Mar. 1984 19786

Shown in Product Identification Section, page 418

MYCELEX®-G 500 mg ℞
brand of clotrimazole
Vaginal Tablet

PRODUCT OVERVIEW

KEY FACTS

Mycelex®-G 500 mg is an effective antifungal containing 500 mg of clotrimazole (the active ingredient). Clotrimazole is a broad spectrum antifungal which exhibits fungicidal activity in vitro against *Candida albicans* and other species of the genus *Candida*. No single-step or multiple-step resistance to clotrimazole has developed during successive passages of *Candida albicans*.

MAJOR USES

Mycelex®-G 500 mg has proved to be clinically effective for local treatment of vulvovaginal candidiasis when one day therapy is felt warranted. In the case of severe vulvovaginal candidiasis longer antimycotic therapy such as Mycelex®-G 100 mg tablets or Mycelex®-G Cream is recommended.

SAFETY INFORMATION

Mycelex®-G 500 Vaginal Tablets are contraindicated in women who have shown hypersensitivity to any components of the compound. If there is a lack of response to treatment with Mycelex®-G 500 mg, appropriate microbiological studies should be repeated to confirm the diagnosis and rule out other pathogens before instituting another course of antimycotic therapy. No adequate and well-controlled studies in pregnant women during the first trimester of pregnancy.

PRESCRIBING INFORMATION

MYCELEX®-G 500mg ℞
brand of clotrimazole
Vaginal Tablet

DESCRIPTION

Each Mycelex®-G 500 mg Vaginal Tablet contains 500 mg clotrimazole (the active ingredient) dispersed in lactose, microcrystalline cellulose, lactic acid, corn starch, crospovidone, calcium lactate, magnesium stearate, silicon dioxide and hydroxypropyl methylcellulose. Chemically, clotrimazole is [1-(o-Chloro-α, α-diphenylbenzyl) imidazole], a synthetic antifungal agent having the chemical formual $C_{22}H_{17}ClN_2$; a molecular weight of 344.84; and the following chemical structure:

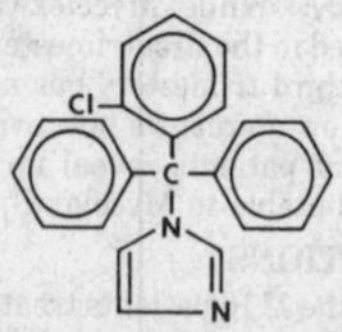

Clotrimazole is an odorless, white crystalline substance, practically insoluble in water, sparingly soluble in ether, soluble in carbon tetrachloride, and very soluble in ethanol and chloroform.

CLINICAL PHARMACOLOGY

Serum levels and levels in vaginal secretions of clotrimazole were measured in six healthy volunteers who had one 500 mg vaginal tablet inserted. Although serum levels of clotrimazole were higher than those in other volunteers given 100 mg and 200 mg vaginal tablets these levels did not exceed 10 nanograms/ml. It has been estimated that three to ten percent of a vaginal dose of clotrimazole may be absorbed, but the drug rapidly and efficiently degrades to microbiologically inactive metabolites. The clotrimazole concentrations remaining in vaginal secretions were still in the mg/ml range for 48 hours and in two of the six subjects at 72 hours.
The findings of high clotrimazole concentrations in vaginal secretions for up to 72 hours and low concentrations in the serum suggest that nearly all the clotrimazole given in the 500 mg vaginal tablet remains in the vagina for 48 hours, and in some cases 72 hours, in fungicidal concentrations.
Clotrimazole is a broad-spectrum antifungal agent. It has been postulated that the compound affects the permeability characteristics of the membrane allowing the leakage of essential intracellular components with a consequent inhibition of the synthesis of such macromolecules as protein, lipid, DNA, and polysaccharides.
At concentrations as low as 2–5 μg/ml, clotrimazole exhibits fungicidal activity *in vitro* against *Candida albicans* and other species of the genus *Candida.*
No single-step or multiple-step resistance to clotrimazole has developed during successive passages of *Candida albicans.*

INDICATIONS

Mycelex®-G 500 mg Vaginal Tablets are indicated for the local treatment of vulvovaginal candidiasis when one day therapy is felt warranted. In the case of severe vulvovaginitis due to candidiasis, longer antimycotic therapy is recommended. The diagnosis should be confirmed by KOH smears and/or cultures. Other pathogens commonly associated with vulvovaginitis, *Trichomonas* and *Gardnerella (Haemophilus) vaginalis* , should be ruled out by appropriate laboratory methods.

CONTRAINDICATIONS

Mycelex®-G 500 mg Vaginal Tablets are contraindicated in women who have shown hypersensitivity to any components of the preparation.

WARNINGS

None.

PRECAUTIONS

If there is a lack of response to Mycelex®-G 500 mg Vaginal Tablets, appropriate microbiological studies should be repeated to confirm the diagnosis and rule out other pathogens before instituting another course of antimycotic therapy.

CARCINOGENESIS

No long term studies in animals have been performed to evaluate the carcinogenic potential of Mycelex®-G 500 mg Vaginal Tablets intravaginally. A long term study in rats (Wistar strains) where clotrimazole was administered orally provided no indication of carcinogenicity.

USAGE IN PREGNANCY

Pregnancy Category B: The disposition of ^{14}C-clotrimazole has been studied in humans and animals. Clotrimazole is poorly absorbed following intravaginal administration to humans, whereas it is rather well absorbed after oral administration.
In clinical trials, use of vaginally applied clotrimazole in pregnant women in their second and third trimesters has not been associated with ill effects. There are, however, no adequate and well-controlled studies in pregnant women during the first trimester of pregnancy.
Studies in pregnant rats given repeated intravaginal doses up to 100 mg/kg/day have revealed no evidence of harm to the fetus due to clotrimazole.
Repeated high oral doses of clotrimazole in rats and mice ranging from 50 to 120 mg/kg resulted in embryotoxicity (possibly secondary to maternal toxicity), impairment of mating, decreased litter size and number of viable young and decreased pup survival to weaning. However, clotrimazole was not teratogenic in mice, rabbits and rats at oral doses up to 200, 180 and 100 mg/kg, respectively. Oral absorption in the rat amounts to approximately 90% of the administered dose.
Because animal reproduction studies are not always predictive of human response, this drug should be used only if clearly indicated during the first trimester of pregnancy.

ADVERSE REACTIONS

Of 297 patients in double-blind studies with the 500 mg vaginal tablet, 3 of 149 patients treated with active drug and 3 of 148 patients treated with placebo reported complaints during therapy that were possibly drug related. In the active drug group, vomiting occurred in one patient, vaginal soreness with coitus in another, and complaints of vaginal irritation, itching, burning and dyspareunia in the third patient. In the placebo group, clitoral irritation occurred in one patient and dysuria, described as remotely related to drug, in the other. A third patient in the placebo group developed bacterial vaginitis which the investigator classed as possibly related to drug.
Eighteen (1.6%) of the 1116 patients treated with Mycelex®-G in other formulations in double-blind studies reported complaints during therapy that were possibly drug-related. Mild burning occurred in six patients while other complaints such as skin rash, itching, vulval irritation, lower abdominal cramps and bloating, slight cramping, slight urinary frequency, and burning or irritation in the sexual partner, occurred rarely.

OVERDOSAGE

No data available.

DRUG ABUSE AND DEPENDENCE

Drug abuse and dependence with Mycelex®-G 500 mg Vaginal Tablets has not been reported.

DOSAGE AND ADMINISTRATION

The recommended dose is one tablet inserted intravaginally one time only, preferably at bedtime. In the event of treatment failure, that is, persistence of signs and symptoms of vaginitis after five days, other pathogens commonly responsible for vaginitis should be ruled out before instituting another course of antimycotic therapy.

HOW SUPPLIED

Mycelex®-G 500 mg Vaginal Tablets are white, bullet shaped, uncoated tablets, coded with Miles on one side and 097 on the other, supplied as a single 500 mg tablet with plastic applicator and patient instructions.
Store Below 30°C (86°F).
August, 1985 PD100620 20185

Shown in Product Identification Section, page 418

MYCELEX® Twin Pack ℞
(clotrimazole)
500 mg Vaginal Tablet and Topical Cream

PRODUCT OVERVIEW

KEY FACTS

Mycelex® Twin Pack is an effective vaginal antifungal product containing:

- Mycelex®-G 500 mg Vaginal Tablet
- Mycelex® Topical Cream

Clotrimazole is the active ingredient in both dosage forms. Clotrimazole is a broad spectrum antifungal which exhibits fungicidal activity in vitro against *Candida albicans* and other species of the genus Candida. No single-step or multiple-step resistance to clotrimazole has developed during successive passages of *Candida albicans*.

MAJOR USES

Mycelex® Twin Pack is indicated for local treatment of vulvovaginal candidiasis with pronounced vulvitis. In the case of severe vulvovaginal candidiasis longer antimycotic therapy, such as Mycelex-G 100mg tablets or Mycelex®-G Cream is recommended.

SAFETY INFORMATION

Mycelex® Twin Pack is contraindicated only in patients who have shown hypersensitivity to any components of the compound. If there is a lack of response to treatment with Mycelex® Twin Pack appropriate microbiological studies should be repeated to confirm the diagnosis and rule out other pathogens before instituting another course of antimycotic therapy. No adequate and well-controlled studies in pregnant women during the first trimester of pregnancy.

PRESCRIBING INFORMATION

MYCELEX® Twin Pack ℞
(clotrimazole)
500 mg Vaginal Tablet and Topical Cream

7 DAY THERAPY
MYCELEX® 1%
(Clotrimazole) Cream
For Dermatologic Use Only

DESCRIPTION

Mycelex Cream 1% contains clotrimazole, a synthetic antifungal agent having the chemical name [1-(o-Chloro-α,α-diphenylbenzyl)imidazole]: the empirical formula $C_{22}H_{17}ClN_2$; a molecular weight of 344.84; and the chemical structure:

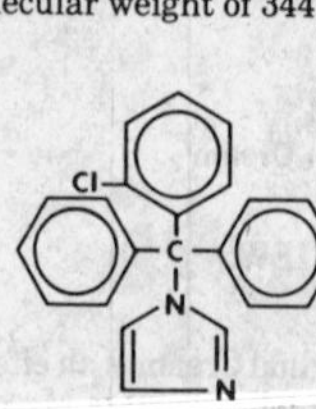

Clotrimazole is an odorless, white crystalline substance. It is practically insoluble in water, sparingly soluble in ether and very soluble in polyethylene glycol 400, ethanol and chloroform.
Each gram of Mycelex Cream contains 10 mg clotrimazole, dispersed in an emulsion vehicle composed of sorbitan monostearate, polysorbate 60, cetyl esters wax, cetostearyl alcohol, 2-octyldodecanol, purified water; benzyl alcohol (1%) as preservative.

CLINICAL PHARMACOLOGY

Clotrimazole is a broad-spectrum antifungal agent that is used for the treatment of dermal infections caused by various species of pathogenic dermatophytes, yeasts, and *Malassezia furfur.* The primary action of clotrimazole is against dividing and growing organisms.

In vitro, clotrimazole exhibits fungistatic and fungicidal activity against isolates of *Trichophyton rubrum, Tricophyton mentagrophytes, Epidermophyton floccosum, Microsporum canis,* and *Candida* species, including *Candida albicans.* In general, the *in vitro* activity of clotrimazole corresponds to that of tolnaftate and griseofulyin against the mycelia of dermatophytes *(Trichophyton, Microsporum,* and *Epidermophyton),* and to that of the polyenes (amphotericin B and nystatin) against budding fungi *(Candida).* Using an *in vivo* (mouse) and an *in vitro* (mouse kidney homogenate) testing system, clotrimazole and miconazole were equally effective in preventing the growth of the pseudomycelia and mycelia of *Candida albicans.*

Strains of fungi having a natural resistance to clotrimazole are rare. Only a single isolate of *Candida guilliermondi* has been reported to have primary resistance to clotrimazole. No single-step or multiple-step resistance to clotrimazole has devloped during successive passages of *Candida albicans* and *Trichophyton mentagrophytes.* No appreciable change in sensitivity was detected after successive passage of isolates of *C. albicans, C. krusei,* or *C. pseudotropicalis* in liquid or solid media containing clotrimazole. Also, resistance could not be developed in chemically induced mutant strains of polyene-resistant isolates of *C. albicans.* Sight, reversible resistance was noted in three isolates of *C. albicans* tested by one investigator. There is a single report that records the clinical emergence of a *C. albicans* strain with considerable resistance to flucytosine and miconazole, and with cross-resistance to clotrimazole, the strain remained sensitive to nystatin and amphotericin B.

In studies of the mechanism of action, the minimum fungicidal concentration of clotrimazole caused leakage of intracellular phosphorus compounds into the ambient medium with concomitant breakdown of cellular nucleic acids and accelerated potassium efflus. Both these events began rapidly and extensively after addition of the drug.

Clotrimazole appears to be well absorbed in humans following oral administration and is eliminated mainly as inactive metabolites. Following topical and vaginal administration, however, clotrimazole appears to be minimally absorbed.

Six hours after the application of radioactive clotrimazole 1% cream and 1% solution onto intact and acutely inflamed skin, the concentration of clotrimazole varied from 100 mcg/cm in the stratum corneum to 0.5 to 1 mcg/cm in the stratum reticulare, and 0.1 mcg/cm in the subcutis. No measurable amount of radioactivity (<0.001 mcg/ml) was found in the serum within 48 hours after application under occlusive dressing of 0.5 ml of the solution or 0.8 g of the cream. Only 0.5% or less of the applied radioactivity was excreted in the urine.

Following intravaginal administration of 100 mg ^{14}C-clotrimazole vaginal tablets to nine adult females, and average peak serum level, corresponding to only 0.03 μg equivalents/ml of clotrimazole, was reached one to two days after aplication. After intravaginal administration of 5 g of 1% ^{14}C-clotrimazole vaginal cream, containing 50 mg active drug, to five subjects (one with candida colpitis), serum levels corresponding to approximately 0.01 μg equivalents/ml were reached between 8 and 24 hours after application.

INDICATIONS AND USAGE

Mycelex Cream is indicated for the topical treatment of the following dermal infections; tinea pedis, tinea cruris, and tinea corporis due to *Trichophyton rubrum, Trichophyton metagrophytes, Epidermophyton floccosum,* and *Microsporum canis;* candidiasis due to *Candida albicans,* and tinea versicolor due to *Malassezia furfur.*

CONTRAINDICATIONS

Mycelex Cream is contraindicated in individuals sensitive to its components.

WARNINGS

Mycelex Cream is not for ophthalmic use.

PRECAUTIONS

General

If irritation or sensitivity develops with the use of Mycelex Cream, treatment should be discontinued and appropriate therapy instituted.

Information for Patients

The patient should be advised to:

1. Use the medication for the full treatment time even though the symptoms may have improved. Notify the physician if there is no improvement after four weeks of treatment.
2. Inform the physician if the area of application shows signs of increased irritation (redness, itching, burning, blistering, swelling, oozing) indicative of possible sensitization.
3. Avoid the use of occlusive wrappings or dressings.
4. Avoid sources of infection or reinfection.

Laboratory Tests

If there is lack of response to Mycelex Cream, appropriate microbiological studies should be repeated to confirm the diagnosis and rule out other pathogens before instituting another course of antimycotic therapy.

Drug Interactions

Synergism or antagonism between clotrimazole and nystatin, or amphotericin B. or flucytosine against strains of *C. albicans* has not been reported.

Carcinogenesis, mutagenesis, impairment of fertility

An 18-month oral dosing study with clotrimazole in rats has not revealed any carcinogenic effect.

In tests for mutagenesis, chromosomes of the spermatophores of Chinese hamsters which had been exposed to clotrimazole were examined for structural changes during the metaphase. Prior to testing the hamsters had received five oral clotrimazole doses of 100 mg/kg body weight. The results of this study showed that clotrimazole had no mutagenic effect.

Usage in Pregnancy: Pregnancy Category B

The disposition of ^{14}C-clotrimazole has been studied in humans and animals. Clotrimazole is very poorly absorbed following dermal application or intravaginal administration to humans. (See Clinical Pharmacology.)

In clinical trials, use of vaginally applied clotrimazole in pregnant women in their second and third trimesters has not been associated with ill effects. There are, however, no adequate and well-controlled studies in pregnant women during the first trimester of pregnancy.

Studies in pregnant rats with intravaginal doses up to 100 mg/kg have revealed no evidence of harm to the fetus due to clotrimazole.

High *oral* doses of clotrimazole in rats and mice ranging from 50 to 120 mg/kg resulted in embryotoxicity (possibly secondary to maternal toxicity), impairment of mating, decreased litter size and number of viable young and decreased pup survival to weaning. However, clotrimazole was *not* teratogenic in mice, rabbits and rats at oral doses of up to 200, 180 and 100 mg/kg, respectively. Oral absorption in the rat amounts to approximately 90% of the administered dose.

Because animal reproduction studies are not always predictive of human response, this drug should be used only if clearly indicated during the first trimester of pregnancy.

Nursing Mothers

It is not known whether this drug is excreted in human milk. Because many drugs are excreted in human milk, caution should be exercised when clotrimazole is used by a nursing woman.

Pediatric Use

Safety and effectiveness in children have been established for clotrimazole when used as indicated and in the recommended dosage.

ADVERSE REACTIONS

The following adverse reactions have been reported in connection with the use of the cream and solution forms of this product: erythema, stinging, blistering, peeling, edema, pruritis, urticaria, burning, and general irritation of the skin.

OVERDOSAGE

Active overdosage with topical application of clotrimazole is unlikely and would not be expected to lead to a life-threatening situation.

DOSAGE AND ADMINISTRATION

Gently massage sufficient Mycelex Cream into the affected and surrounding skin areas twice a day, in the morning and evening.

Clinical improvement, with relief of pruritus, usually occurs within the first week of treatment with Mycelex. If the patient shows no clinical improvement after four weeks of treatment with Mycelex, the diagnosis should be reviewed.

HOW SUPPLIED

Mycelex Cream 1% is supplied in 15, 30, and (2 + 45) gram tubes. A twin pack is also available containing one Mycelex Cream 1% 7 g tube with one Mycelex-G 500 mg tablet.

Store between 2° and 30°C (36° and 86° F).

U.S. Patents No. 3,660,577 and 3,705,172.

1 DAY THERAPY

MYCELEX®–G 500 mg

(Brand of Clotrimazole)

Vaginal Tablets

DESCRIPTION

Each Mycelex®-G 500 mg Vaginal Tablet contains 500 mg clotrimazole (the active ingredient) dispersed in lactose, microcrystalline cellulose, lactic acid, corn starch, corspovidone, calcium lactate, magnesium stearate, silicon dioxide and hydroxypropyl methylcellulose. Chemically, clotrimazole is [1-(o-Chloro-α, α-diphenylbenzyl) imidazole], a synthetic antifungal agent having the chemical formula $C_{22}H_{17}ClN_2$; a molecular weight of 344.84; and the following chemical structure:

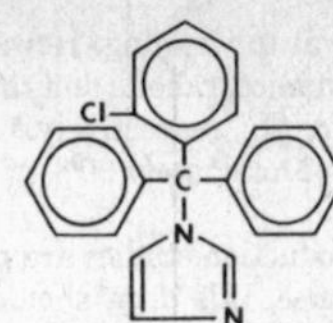

Clotrimazole is an odorless, white crystalline substance, practically insoluble in water, sparingly soluble in ether, soluble in carbon tertrachloride, and very soluble in ethanol and chloroform.

CLINICAL PHARMACOLOGY

Serum levels and levels in vaginal secretions of clotrimazole were measured in six healthy volunteers who had one 500 mg vaginal tablet inserted. Although serum levels of clotrimazole were higher than those in other volunteers given 100 mg and 200 mg vaginal tablets these levels did not exceed 10 nanograms/ml. It has been estimated that three to ten percent of a vaginal dose of clotrimazole may be absorbed, but the drug rapidly and efficiently degrades to microbiologically inactive metabolites. The clotrimazole concentrations remaining in vaginal secretions were still in the mg/ml range for 48 hours and in two of the six subjects at 72 hours.

The findings of high clotrimazole concentrations in vaginal secretions for up to 72 hours and low concentrations in the serum suggest that nearly all the clotrimazole given in the 500 mg vaginal tablet remains in the vagina for 48 hours, and in some cases 72 hours, in fungicidal concentrations.

Clotrimazole is a broad-spectrum antifungal agent. It has been postulated that the compound affects the permeability characteristics of the membrane allowing the leakage of essential intracellular components with a consequent inhibition of the synthesis of such macromolecules as protein, lipid, DNA, and polysaccharides.

At concentrations as low as 2–5 μ/ml, clotrimazole exhibits fungicidal activity *in vitro* against *Candida albicans* and other species of the genus *Candida.*

No single-step or multiple-step resistance to clotrimazole has developed during successive passages of *Candida albicans.*

INDICATIONS

Mycelex-G 500 mg Vaginal Tablets are indicated for the local treatment of vulvovaginal candidiasis when one day therapy is felt warranted. In the case of severe vulvovaginitis due to candidiasis, longer antimycotic therapy is recommended. The diagnosis should be confirmed by KOH smears and/or cultures. Other pathogens commonly associated with vulvovaginitis, *Trichomonas* and *Gardnerella (Haemophilus) vaginalis,* should be ruled out by appropriate laboratory methods.

CONTRAINDICATIONS

Mycelex-G 500 mg Vaginal Tablets are contraindicated in women who have shown hypersensitivity to any components of the preparation.

WARNINGS

None.

PRECAUTIONS

If there is a lack of response to Mycelex-G 500 mg Vaginal Tablets, appropriate microbiological studies should be repeated to confirm the diagnosis and rule out other pathogens before instituting another course of antimycotic therapy.

CARCINOGENESIS

No long term studies in animals have been performed to evaluate the carcinogenic potential of Mycelex-G 500 mg Vaginal Tablets intravaginally. A long term study in rats (Wistar strains) where clotrimazole was administered orally provided no indication of carcinogenicity.

USAGE IN PREGNANCY

Pregnancy Category B: The disposition of ^{14}C-clotrimazole has been studied in humans and animals. Clotrimazole is poorly absorbed following intravaginal administration to humans, whereas it is rather well absorbed after oral administration.

In clinical trials, use of vaginally applied clotrimazole in pregnant women in their second and third trimesters has not been associated with ill effects. There are, however, no adequate and well-controlled studies in pregnant women during the first trimester of pregnancy.

Studies in pregnant rats given repeated intravaginal doses up to 100 mg/kg/day have revealed no evidence of harm to the fetus due to clotrimazole.

Repeated high oral doses of clotrimazole in rats and mice ranging from 50 to 120 mg/kg resulted in embryotoxicity (possibly secondary to maternal toxicity), impairment of mating, decreased litter size and number of viable young and

Continued on next page

Miles Pharm.—Cont.

decreased pup survival to weaning. However, clotrimazole was not teratogenic in mice, rabbits and rats of oral doses up to 200, 180 and 100 mg/kg, respectively. Oral absorption in the rat amounts to approximately 90% of the administered dose.
Because animal reproduction studies are not always predictive of human response, this drug should be used only if clearly indicated during the first trimester of pregnancy.

ADVERSE REACTIONS

Of 297 patients in double-blind studies with the 500 mg vaginal tablet, 3 of 149 patients treated with active drug and 3 of 148 patients treated with placebo reported complaints during therapy that were possibly drug related. In the active drug group, vomiting occurred in one patient, vaginal soreness with coitus in another, and complaints of vaginal irritation, itching, burning and dyspareunia in the third patient. In the placebo group, clitoral irritation occurred in one patient and dysuria, described as remotely related to drug, in the other. A third patient in the placebo group developed bacterial vaginitis which the investigator classed as possibly related to the drug.
Eighteen (1.6%) of the 1116 patients treated with Mycelex-G in other formulations in double-blind studies reported complaints during therapy that were possibly drug-related. Mild burning occurred in six patients while other complaints such as skin rash, itching, vulval irritation, lower abdominal cramps and bloating, slight cramping, slight urinary frequency, and burning or irritation in the sexual partner, occurred rarely.

OVERDOSAGE

No data available.

DRUG ABUSE AND DEPENDENCE

Drug abuse and dependence with Mycelex-G 500 mg Vaginal Tablets has not been reported.

DOSAGE AND ADMINISTRATION

The recommended dose is one tablet inserted intravaginally one time only, preferably at bedtime. In the event of treatment failure, that is, persistence of signs and symptoms of vaginitis after five days, other pathogens commonly responsible for vaginitis should be ruled out before instituting another course of antimycotic therapy.

HOW SUPPLIED

Mycelex-G 500 mg Vaginal Tablets are white, bullet shaped, uncoated tablets, coded with Miles on one side and 097 on the other, supplied as a single 500 mg tablet with plastic applicator and patient instructions, or in twin pack with Mycelex 1% cream 7 g tube.
Store below 30°C (86°F).
U.S. Patent Numbers 3,660,577; 3,705,172; 3,839,573; 4,457,938.
PD Rev 2/86

NICLOCIDE® ℞
(niclosamide)
Chewable Tablets

DESCRIPTION

NICLOCIDE (niclosamide) is an anthelmintic provided in chewable tablet form at a strength of 500 mg per tablet. Niclosamide is 2′, 5-Dichloro-4′-nitrosalicylanilide. Inactive ingredients: corn starch, magnesium stearate, povidone, sodium lauryl sulfate, sodium saccharin, talc and vanillin. The empirical formula is $C_{13}H_8Cl_2N_2O_4$ with the following structural formula.

[structural formula: OH, Cl, CONH, Cl, NO_2]

CLINICAL PHARMACOLOGY

NICLOCIDE inhibits oxidative phosphorylation in the mitochondria of cestodes. Both *in vitro* and *in vivo*, the scolex and proximal segments are killed on contact with the drug. The scolex of the tapeworm, loosened from the gut wall, may be digested in the intestine, and thus may not be identified in the feces even after extensive purging.
The use of NICLOCIDE has not been associated with the development of anemia, leukopenia or thrombocytopenia nor have there been any effects on normal renal and hepatic functions.

INDICATIONS AND USAGE

NICLOCIDE (niclosamide) is indicated for the treatment of tapeworm infections by *Taenia saginata* (beef tapeworm), *Diphyllobothrium latum* (fish tapeworm) and *Hymenolepis nana* (dwarf tapeworm).

CONTRAINDICATIONS

NICLOCIDE™ Tablets are contraindicated in individuals who have shown hypersensitivity to any of its components.

PRECAUTIONS

NICLOCIDE affects the cestodes of the intestine only. It is without effect in cysticercosis.
Drug Interactions: No data are available regarding interaction of niclosamide with other drugs.
Carcinogenesis, mutagenesis, impairment of fertility:
Carcinogenicity Potential: Although carcinogenicity studies on niclosamide *per se* have not been done, long-term feeding studies on its ethanolamine salt in rats and mice did not show carcinogenicity. Mutagenicity tests have not been performed.
Pregnancy: Pregnancy Category B: Reproduction studies in rabbits and rats at doses of 25 times the human therapeutic dose and in mice at 12 times the human therapeutic dose, have revealed no evidence of impaired fertility or harm to the fetus due to niclosamide. There are, however, no adequate and well-controlled studies in pregnant women. Because animal studies are not always predictive of human response, the drug should be used during pregnancy only if clearly needed.
Nursing Mothers: No studies are available.
Pediatric Use: In children under 2 years of age, the safety of the drug has not been established.

ADVERSE REACTIONS

The incidence of side effects has been reported as follows: nausea/vomiting 4.1%, abdominal discomfort including loss of appetite 3.4%, diarrhea 1.6%, drowsiness, dizziness, and or headache 1.4%, and skin rash including pruritus ani 0.3%. Other side effects listed in decreasing order of frequency were: oral irritation, fever, rectal bleeding, weakness, bad taste in mouth, sweating, palpitations, constipation, alopecia, edema of an arm, backache and irritability. There was also one instance of a transient rise in SGOT in an i.v. narcotic addict. Two cases of urticaria reported may be related to the breakdown products of the tapeworm. All side effects were mild or moderate and transitory and did not necessitate discontinuation of the treatment.

OVERDOSAGE

Insufficient data are available. In the event of overdose a fast-acting laxative and enema should be given. Vomiting should not be induced.

DOSAGE AND ADMINISTRATION

1. *Taenia saginata* and *Diphyllobothrium latum*
   a. Adults: 4 tablets (2.0 g) chewed thoroughly in a single dose.
   b. Children weighing more than 34 kg (75 lbs): 3 tablets (1.5 g) chewed thoroughly in a single dose.
   c. Children weighing between 11 and 34 kg (25 to 75 lbs): 2 tablets (1.0 g) chewed thoroughly in a single dose.
2. *Hymenolepis nana*
   a. Adults: 4 tablets (2.0 g) chewed thoroughly as a single daily dose for 7 days.
   b. Children weighing more than 34 kg (75 lbs): 3 tablets (1.5g) chewed thoroughly on the first day, then 2 tablets (1.0 g) daily for next 6 days.
   c. Children weighing between 11 and 34 kg (25 to 75 lbs): 2 tablets (1.0 g) to be chewed thoroughly on the first day, then one tablet (0.5 g) daily for next 6 days.

   T. saginata and *D. latum* infections are usually due to a single adult worm and require an intermediate host in their life cycle. With *Hymenolepis nana* multiple infections are the rule. No intermediate host is required; both larval and adult stages of the worm may be found in the human intestine where the complete life cycle occurs. Since the drug is more effective against the mature than the larval stage, therapy must be extended over several days to cover all stages of maturation.
   Patients with *H. nana* must be instructed to observe strict personal and environmental hygiene to avoid autoinfection with this parasite.
3. NICLOCIDE™ must be thoroughly chewed and then swallowed with a little water. No special dietary restrictions are necessary before or after treatment. The best time to take the drug is after a light meal (e.g., breakfast). A mild laxative may be desirable in constipated patients to achieve a normal bowel movement. Young children should have the tablets crushed to a fine powder and mixed with a small amount of water to form a paste.
   NICLOCIDE has a vanilla taste which is not unpleasant to most persons.
   NICLOCIDE is suitable for administration on an ambulatory or outpatient basis.
4. Follow-up:
   As the vermicidal action of NICLOCIDE renders the tapeworm, especially the scolex and proximal segments, vulnerable to destruction during their passage through the gut, it is not always possible to identify the scolex in stools. The sooner the tapeworm is passed and examined after treatment, the better the chance of identification of the scolex. Segments and/or ova of beef or fish tapeworm may be present in the stool for up to 3 days after therapy. Persistent *T. saginata* or *D. latum* segments and/ or ova on the seventh day post therapy indicate failure. A second identical course of treatment may be given at that time.
   No patient should be considered cured unless the stool has been negative for a minimum of three months.

HOW SUPPLIED

NICLOCIDE is available as round, light yellow chewable tablets, scored on one side, coded with the word Miles and number 721, each containing 500 mg of niclosamide, and is supplied in boxes of 4 tablets.
Storage Conditions: Store below 86°F (30°C), avoid freezing.
Manufactured: by
Bayvet Division Cutter Laboratories, Inc.
Shawnee, Kansas 66201

Distributed by:
Miles Pharmaceuticals
Division of Miles Laboratories, Inc.
West Haven, Connecticut 06516
Shown in Product Identification Section, page 419
PD100614 20124 June 1985

Otic DOMEBORO® Solution (acid pH) ℞
(acetic acid 2%)

INGREDIENTS

Aluminum Sulfate, Boric Acid, Calcium Carbonate, Glacial Acetic Acid, Purified Water, and Sodium Hydroxide.

INDICATIONS

For the treatment of superficial infections of the external auditory canal caused by organisms susceptible to the action of the antimicrobial.

PRECAUTIONS

If undue irritation or sensitivity develops, discontinue treatment.

CAUTION

Federal (U.S.A.) law prohibits dispensing without prescription.
For external use only. Not for ophthalmic use. Store below 86°F (30°C), avoid freezing.

USUAL DOSAGE

Instill 4–6 drops in the ear every 2 to 3 hours.

HOW SUPPLIED

2 fl. oz. (60 cc.) plastic squeeze bottle with otic tip.

STILPHOSTROL® ℞
(diethylstilbestrol diphosphate)

DESCRIPTION

STILPHOSTROL (diethylstilbestrol diphosphate) is available as tablets containing 50 mg diethylstilbestrol diphosphate, colored white to off-white with grey to tan mottling. STILPHOSTROL is also available for intravenous administration as a sterile solution in 5 ml ampules containing 0.25 gram diethylstilbestrol diphosphate as its sodium salt. The solution is clear, colorless to light straw-colored, with a pH of 9.0 to 10.5, and may darken with age and exposure to heat and light.
STILPHOSTROL is a phosphoryiated, nonsteroidal estrogen with the chemical name: Diethylstilbestrol 4,4-Diphosphoric ester, an empirical formula of $C_{18}H_{22}O_8P_2$, and the following structural formula:

[structural formula: H_2O_3PO–, C_2H_5, C=C, C_2H_5, –OPO_3H_2]

CLINICAL PHARMACOLOGY

Putative receptor proteins for estrogens have been detected in estrogen-responsive tissues. Estrogens are first bound to a cytoplasmic receptor protein. Following modification, the estrogen-protein complex is translocated to the nucleus where ultimate binding of the estrogen containing complex occurs. As a result of such binding characteristic metabolic alterations ensue.
In the male patient with androgenic hormone dependent conditions such as metastatic carcinoma of the prostate gland, estrogens counter the androgenic influence by com-

peting for the receptor sites. As a result of treatment with estrogens, metastatic lesions in the bone may also show improvement.

It has been demonstrated in animal studies that diethylstilbestrol diphosphate is rapidly hydrolysed to diethylstilbestrol through phosphatase activity in the blood and tissues. When diethylstilbestrol diphosphate (92 mg/kg body wt.) was injected intravenously into rabbits over a period of 2 to 3 minutes, free diethylstilbestrol appeared in the blood stream as early as 5 minutes after termination of injection, and within 15 minutes had reached a concentration of 16.3 ug/ml of plasma. This was followed by a rapid decline in concentration, only 1.2 ug/ml remaining after 2 hours.[1] It is, therefore, expected that the high concentration of serum acid phosphate in patients with prostatic carcinoma will hydrolyse diethylstilbestrol diphosphate to free, active diethylstilbestrol.

Diethylstilbestrol is metabolized by the body in much the same manner as the endogenous hormones. Inactivation of estrogen is carried out mainly in the liver. A certain proportion of the estrogen reaching that organ is excreted into the bile, only to be reabsorbed from the intestine. During this enterohepatic circulation, degradation of estrogen occurs through conversion to less active products, through oxidation to nonestrogenic substances, and through conjugation with sulfuric and glucuronic acids. These water-soluble conjugates are strong acids and are thus fully ionized in the body fluids; penetration into cells is therefore limited, and excretion by the kidney is favored because little tubular reabsorption is possible.

INDICATION AND USAGE

STILPHOSTROL (diethylstilbestrol diphosphate) is indicated for the treatment of prostatic carcinoma—palliative therapy of advanced disease.

CONTRAINDICATIONS

Estrogens should not be used in men with any of the following conditions:

1. Known or suspected cancer of the breast except in appropriately selected patients being treated for metastatic disease.
2. Known or suspected estrogen-dependent neoplasia.
3. Active thrombophlebitis or thromboembolic disorders.

STILPHOSTROL IS NOT INDICATED IN THE TREATMENT OF ANY DISORDER IN WOMEN.

WARNINGS

1. Induction of malignant neoplasms: Long-term continuous administration of natural and synthetic estrogens in certain animal species increases the frequency of carcinomas of the breast, cervix, vagina, and liver.
2. Gallbladder disease: A study has reported a 2- to 3-fold increase in the risk of surgically confirmed gallbladder disease in women receiving postmenopausal estrogens,[2] similar to a 2-fold increase previously noted in users of oral contraceptives.[3,9]
3. Effects similar to those caused by estrogen-progestogen oral contraceptives: There are several serious adverse effects of oral contraceptives. It has been shown that there is an increased risk of thrombosis in men receiving estrogens for prostatic cancer and women for postpartum breast engorgement.[4–7]
   a. Thromboembolic disease: It is now well established that users of oral contraceptives have an increased risk of various thromboembolic and thrombotic vascular diseases, such as thrombophlebitis, pulmonary embolism, stroke, and myocardial infarction.[8–16] Cases of retinal thrombosis, mesenteric thrombosis, and optic neuritis have been reported in oral contraceptive users. There is evidence that the risk of several of these adverse reactions is related to the dose of the drug.[17,18] An increased risk of postsurgery thromboembolic complications has also been reported in users of oral contraceptives.[19,20] If feasible, estrogen should be discontinued at least 4 weeks before surgery of the type associated with an increased risk of thromboembolism or during periods of prolonged immobilization.
   Estrogens should not be used in persons with active thrombophlebitis or thromboembolic disorders. They should be used with caution in patients with cerebral vascular or coronary artery disease and only for those in whom estrogens are clearly indicated.
   Large doses of estrogen (5 mg conjugated estrogens per day), comparable to those used to treat cancer of the prostate, have been shown in a large prospective clinical trial in men[21] to increase the risk of nonfatal myocardial infarction, pulmonary embolism and thrombophlebitis. When estrogen doses of this size are used, any of the thromboembolic and thrombotic adverse effects associated with oral contraceptive use should be considered a clear risk.
   b. Hepatic adenoma: Benign hepatic adenomas appear to be associated with the use of oral contraceptives.[22–24] Although benign, and rare, these may rupture and may cause death through intra-abdominal hemorrhage. Such lesions have not yet been reported in association with other estrogen or progestogen preparations but should be considered in estrogen users having abdominal pain and tenderness, abdominal mass, or hypovolemic shock. Hepatocellular carcinoma has also been reported in women taking estrogen-containing oral contraceptives.[23] The relationship of this malignancy to these drugs is not known at this time.
   c. Elevated blood pressure: Women using oral contraceptives sometimes experience increased blood pressure which, in most cases, returns to normal on discontinuing the drug. There is now a report that this may occur with use of estrogens in the menopause[25] and blood pressure should be monitored with estrogen use, especially if high doses are used.
   d. Glucose tolerance: A worsening of glucose tolerance has been observed in a significant percentage of patients on estrogen-containing oral contraceptives. For this reason, diabetic patients should be carefully observed while receiving estrogen.
4. Hypercalcemia: Administration of estrogens may lead to severe hypercalcemia in patients with breast cancer and bone metastases. If this occurs, the drug should be stopped and appropriate measures taken to reduce the serum calcium level.

PRECAUTIONS

General:

1. A complete medical and family history should be taken prior to the initiation of any estrogen therapy. The pretreatment and periodic physical examinations should include special reference to blood pressure, breasts, abdomen and pelvic organs. As a general rule, estrogen should not be prescribed for longer than one year without another physical examination being performed.
2. Fluid retention—Because estrogens may cause some degree of fluid retention, conditions which might be influenced by this factor such as asthma, epilepsy, migraine, and cardiac or renal dysfunction, require careful observation.
3. Certain patients may develop undesirable manifestations of excessive estrogenic stimulation, such as gynecomastia.
4. Oral contraceptives appear to be associated with an increased incidence of mental depression. Although it is not clear whether this is due to the estrogenic or progestogenic component of the contraceptive, patients with a history of depression should be carefully observed.
5. If jaundice develops in any patient receiving estrogen, the medication should be discontinued while the cause is investigated.
6. Estrogens may be poorly metabolized in patients with impaired liver function and they should be administered with caution in such patients.
7. Because estrogens influence the metabolism of calcium and phosphorus, they should be used with caution in patients with metabolic bone diseases that are associated with hypercalcemia or in patients with renal insufficiency.

Information for Patients:

1. Stilphostrol should not be used by women.
2. The following side effects have been reported in patients being treated with Stilphostrol. If they occur they should be reported promptly to your physician:
   - Mood changes, depression
   - Nervousness, dizziness
   - Loss of appetite, nausea, vomiting, abdominal cramps, bloating
   - Skin rash
   - Chest pain and shortness of breath
   - Numbness or tingling about the nose or mouth
   - Fluid accumulation
   - Swelling or tenderness of breasts
   - Disturbances of vision
   - Frequent or uncomfortable urination
   - Painful swelling of extremities
3. The patient should consult a physician regularly for evaluation of blood pressure and heart rate.
4. Diabetic patients should monitor urines very carefully. Test of blood sugar may be necessary as well.
5. The following clinical problems are associated with the use of Stilphostrol:
   - Hepatic cutaneous prophyria
   - Erythema nodosum
   - Erythema multiforme

   A significant association has been shown between the use of estrogen containing drugs and the following serious reactions:
   1. Thrombophlebitis
   2. Pulmonary embolism
   3. Cerebral thrombosis
   4. There is suggestive evidence that there may be a relationship with coronary thrombosis.

The following adverse reactions are known to have occurred in patients receiving estrogens:

- Change in body weight
- Headache
- Loss of sex drive
- Post injection flare
- Aggravation of migraine headaches
- Loss of scalp hair
- Hemorrhagic eruption
- Fatigue
- Backache

Drug/Laboratory Test Interactions:

1. The pathologist should be advised of estrogen therapy when relevant specimens are submitted.
2. Certain endocrine and liver function tests may be affected by estrogen-containing oral contraceptives.

The following similar changes may be expected with larger doses of estrogen.

a. Increased sulfobromophthalein retention.
b. Increased prothrombin and factors VII, VIII, IX, and X; decreased antithrombin 3; incresed norepinephrine-induced platelet aggregability.
c. Increased thyroid binding globulin (TBG) leading to increased circulating total thyroid hormone, as measured by PBI, T4 by column, or T4 by radioimmunoassay. Free T3 resin uptake is decreased, reflecting the elevated TBG; free T4 concentration is unaltered.
d. Impaired glucose tolerance.
e. Reduced response to metyrapone test.
f. Reduced serum folate concentration.
g. Increased serum triglyceride and phospholipid concentration.

Carcinogenesis, mutagenesis, impairment of fertility: (See Warnings regarding induction of neoplasia.)

Pregnancy: Pregnancy Category X. STILPHOSTROL IS NOT INDICATED IN THE TREATMENT OF ANY DISORDER IN WOMEN.

Pediatric Use: Because of the effects of estrogen on epiphyseal closure, they should be used judiciously in young patients in whom bone growth is not complete.

ADVERSE REACTIONS

See Warnings regarding induction of neoplasia, increased incidence of gallbladder disease, and adverse effects similar to those of oral contraceptives, including thromboembolism.)

The following additional adverse reactions have been reported with estrogenic therapy, including oral contraceptives:

1. Breasts: Tenderness, enlargement, secretion.
2. Gastrointestinal: Nausea, vomiting; abdominal cramps, bloating; cholestatic jaundice.
3. Skin: Chloasma or melasma which may persist when drug is discontinued; erythema multiforme, erythema nodosum; hemorrhagic eruption; loss of scalp hair; hirsutism.
4. Eyes: Steepening of corneal curvature; intolerance to contact lenses.
5. CNS: Headache, migraine, dizziness, mental depression; chorea.
6. Miscellaneous: Increase or decrease in weight; reduced carbohydrate tolerance; aggravation of porphyria; edema; changes in libido; transient itching and burning sensation in the perineal region.

OVERDOSAGE

Numerous reports of ingestion of large doses of estrogen-containing oral contraceptives by young children indicate that acute serious ill effects do not occur. Overdosage of estrogen may cause nausea.

DOSAGE AND ADMINISTRATION

Inoperable, progressing prostatic cancer.

STILPHOSTROL Tablets 50 mg: Start with one tablet three times a day and increase this dose level to four or more tablets three times a day, depending on the tolerance of the patient. Maximum daily dose not to exceed one gram.

Alternatively, if relief is not obtained with high oral dosages, STILPHOSTROL may be administered intravenously. STILPHOSTROL solution must be diluted before intravenous infusion.

STILPHOSTROL Ampules 0.25 gram: It is recommended that 0.5 gram (2 amupules) dissolved in approximately 250 ml of normal saline for injection USP, or 5% dextrose for injection USP, be given intravenously the first day, and that each day thereafter one gram (4 ampules) be similarly administered in approximately 250 to 500 ml of normal saline for injection USP, or 5% dextrose for injection USP.

The infusion should be administered slowly (20–30 drops per minute) during the first 10–15 minutes and then the rate of flow adjusted so that the entire amount is given in a period of about one hour. This procedure should be followed for five days or more depending on the response of the patient. Following the first intensive course of therapy, 0.25–0.5 gram (1 or 2 ampules) may be administered in a similar manner once or twice weekly or maintenance obtained with STILPHOSTROL Tablets.

Stability of Solution: After reconstitution, if storage is desired, the solution should be kept at room temperature and away from direct light. Under these conditions the solution is stable for about 5 days, so long as cloudiness or evidence of a precipitate has not occurred.

Continued on next page

Miles Pharm.—Cont.

HOW SUPPLIED

STILPHOSTROL Tablets–Bottles of 50 tablets.

Each scored tablet, white to off-white with grey to tan mottling, contains diethylstilbestrol diphosphate 50 mg. Each tablet is identified with: Miles 132.

STORAGE: Store at controlled room temperature (59°–86°F), protect from light.

STILPHOSTROL Ampules—Boxes of 20 ampules.

Each 5 ml ampule contains diethylstilbestrol diphosphate 0.25 gram as a solution of its sodium salt.

STORAGE: Store at controlled room temperature (50°–86°F), protect from light.

REFERENCES

1. Johnson, W., et al: Proc. Soc. Exp. Biol. Med. 106:327–330, 1961.
2. Boston Collaborative Drug Surveillance Program: N. Eng. J. Med. 290:15–19, 1974.
3. Boston Collaborative Drug Surveillance Program: Lancet 1:1399–1404, 1973.
4. Daniel, D.G., et al: Lancet 2:287–289, 1967.
5. The Veterans Administration Cooperative Urological Research Group: J. Urol. 98:516–522, 1967.
6. Bailar, J.C.: Lancet 2-560, 1967.
7. Blackard, C., et al: Cancer 26:249–256, 1970.
8. Royal College of General Practitioners: R. Coll. Gen. Pract. 13:267–279, 1967.
9. Royal College of General Practitioners: Oral Contraceptives and Health, New York, Pitman Corp., 1974.
10. Inman, W.H.W., et al: Br. Med. J. 2:193–199, 1968.
11. Vessey, M.P., et al: Br. Med. J. 2:651–657, 1969.
12. Sartwell, P.E., et al: Am.J. Epidemiol. 90:365–380, 1969.
13. Collaborative Group for the Study of Stroke in Young Women: N. Eng. J. Med. 288:871–878, 1973.
14. Collaborative Group for the Study of Stroke in Young Women: J.A.M.A. 231:718–722, 1975.
15. Mann, J.I., et al: Br. Med. J. 2:245–248, 1975.
16. Mann, J.I., et al: Br. Med. J. 2:241–245, 1975.
17. Inman, W.H.W., et al: Br. Med. J. 2:203–209, 1970.
18. Stolley, P.D., et al: Am. J. Epidemiol. 102:197–208, 1975.
19. Vessey, M.P., et al: Br. Med. J. 3:123–126, 1970.
20. Greene, G.R., et al: Am. J. Public Health 62:680–685, 1972.
21. Coronary Drug Project Research Group: J.A.M.A. 214:1303–1313, 1970.
22. Baum, J., et al: Lancet 2:926–928, 1973.
23. Mays, E.T., et al: J.A.M.A. 235:730–732, 1976.
24. Edmonson, H.A., et al: N. Eng. J. Med. 294:470–472, 1976.
25. Pfeffer, R.I., et al: M. J. Epidemiol. 103:445–456, 1976.

PD 100611 Rev 2/86

Shown in Product Identification Section, page 419

TRIDESILON® 0.05% ℞
(desonide)
creme

DESCRIPTION

Tridesilon® Creme contains microdispersed desonide (the active ingredient) in a compatible vehicle buffered to the pH range of normal skin. Each gram of Tridesilon® Creme contains 0.5 milligrams of desonide. Tridesilon® Creme is applied topically.

Tridesilon® (desonide) is a non-fluorinated corticosteroid. Chemically, desonide is Pregna-1,4-diene-3,20-dione,11,21-dihydroxy-16,17-[(1-methylethylidene)bis(oxy)]-,(11β,16α)-with the following structural formula:

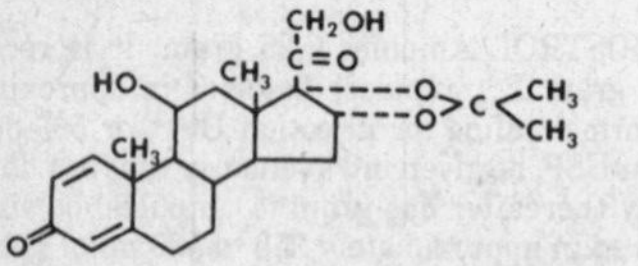

The vehicle for Tridesilon® Creme 0.05% contains glycerin, sodium lauryl sulfate, aluminum sulfate, calcium acetate, dextrin, purified water, cetyl stearyl alcohol, synthetic beeswax, (B-wax), white petrolatum, and light mineral oil. Preserved with methylparaben.

EMPIRICAL FORMULA	MOLECULAR WEIGHT	CAS REGISTRY NUMBER
$C_{24}H_{32}O_6$	416.51	638-94-8

CLINICAL PHARMACOLOGY

Topical corticosteroids share anti-inflammatory, anti-pruritic and vasoconstrictive actions.

The mechanism of anti-inflammatory activity of the topical corticosteroids is unclear. Various laboratory methods, including vasoconstrictor assays, are used to compare and predict potencies and/or clinical efficacies of the topical corticosteroids. There is some evidence to suggest that a recognizable correlation exists between vasoconstrictor potency and therapeutic efficacy in man.

Pharmacokinetics

The extent of percutaneous absorption of topical corticosteroids is determined by many factors including the vehicle, the integrity of the epidermal barrier, and the use of occlusive dressings.

Topical corticosteroids can be absorbed from normal intact skin. Inflammation and/or other disease processes in the skin increase percutaneous absorption. Occlusive dressings substantially increase the percutaneous absorption of topical corticosteroids. Thus, occlusive dressings may be a valuable therapeutic adjunct for treatment of resistant dermatoses. (See DOSAGE AND ADMINISTRATION).

Once absorbed through the skin, topical corticosteroids are handled through pharmacokinetic pathways similar to systemically administered corticosteroids. Corticosteroids are bound to plasma proteins in varying degrees. Corticosteroids are metabolized primarily in the liver and are then excreted by the kidneys. Some of the topical corticosteroids and their metabolites are also excreted into the bile.

INDICATIONS AND USAGE

Topical corticosteroids are indicated for the relief of the inflammatory and pruritic manifestations of corticosteroid-responsive dermatoses.

CONTRAINDICATIONS

Topical corticosteroids are contraindicated in those patients with a history of hypersensitivity to any of the components of the preparation.

PRECAUTIONS

General

Systemic absorption of topical corticosteroids has produced reversible hypothalmic-pituitary-adrenal (HPA) axis suppression, manifestations of Cushing's syndrome, hyperglycemia, and glucosuria in some patients.

Conditions which augment systemic absorption include the application of the more potent steroids, use over large surface areas, prolonged use, and the addition of occlusive dressings.

Therefore, patients receiving a large dose of a potent topical steroid applied to a large surface area or under an occlusive dressing should be evaluated periodically for evidence of HPA axis suppression by using the urinary free cortisol and ACTH stimulation tests. If HPA axis suppression is noted, an attempt should be made to withdraw the drug, to reduce the frequency of application, or to substitute a less potent steroid.

Recovery of HPA axis function is generally prompt and complete upon discontinuation of the drug. Infrequently, signs and symptoms of steroid withdrawal may occur, requiring supplemental systemic corticosteroids.

Children may absorb proportionally larger amounts of topical corticosteroids and thus be more susceptible to systemic toxicity. (See PRECAUTIONS—Pediatric Use).

If irritation develops, topical corticosteroids should be discontinued and appropriate therapy instituted.

In the presence of dermatological infections, the use of an appropriate antifungal or antibacterial agent should be instituted. If a favorable response does not occur promptly, the corticosteroid should be discontinued until the infection has been adequately controlled.

Information for the Patient

Patients using topical corticosteroids should receive the following information and instructions:

1. This medication is to be used as directed by the physician. It is for external use only. Avoid contact with eyes.
2. Patients should be advised not to use this medication for any disorder other than for which it was prescribed.
3. The treated skin area should not be bandaged or otherwise covered or wrapped as to be occlusive unless directed by the physician.
4. Patients should report any signs of local adverse reactions especially under occlusive dressing.
5. Parents of pediatric patients should be advised not to use tightfitting diapers or plastic pants on a child being treated in the diaper area, as these garments may constitute occlusive dressings.

Laboratory Tests

The following tests may be helpful in evaluating the HPA axis suppression:

Urinary free cortisol test
ACTH stimulation test

Carcinogenesis, Mutagenesis, and Impairment of Fertility

Long-term animal studies have not been performed to evaluate the carcinogenic potential or the effect on fertility of topical corticosteroids.

Studies to determine mutagenicity with prednisolone and hydrocortisone have revealed negative results.

Pregnancy Category C

Corticosteroids are generally teratogenic in laboratory animals when administered systemically at relatively low dosage levels. The more potent corticosteroids have been shown to be teratogenic after dermal application in laboratory animals. There are no adequate and well-controlled studies in pregnant women on teratogenic effects from topically applied corticosteroids. Therefore, topical corticosteroids should be used during pregnancy only if the potential benefit justifies the potential risk to the fetus. Drugs of this class should not be used extensively on pregnant patients, in large amounts, or for prolonged periods of time.

Nursing Mothers

It is not known whether topical administration of corticosteroids could result in sufficient systemic absorption to produce detectable quantities in breast milk. Systemically administered corticosteroids are secreted into breast milk in quantities *not* likely to have a deleterious effect on the infant. Nevertheless, caution should be exercised when topical corticosteroids are administered to a nursing woman.

Pediatric Use

Pediatric patients may demonstrate greater susceptibility to topical corticosteroid-induced HPA axis suppression and Cushing's syndrome than mature patients because of a larger skin surface area to body weight ratio.

Hypothalamic-pituitary-adrenal (HPA) axis suppression. Cushing's syndrome, and intracranial hypertension have been reported in children receiving topical corticosteroids. Manifestations of adrenal supression in children include linear growth retardation, delayed weight gain, low plasma cortisol levels, and absence of response to ACTH stimulation. Manifestations of intracranial hypertension include bulging fontanelles, headaches, and bilateral papilledema.

Administration of topical corticosteroids to children should be limited to the least amount compatible with an effective therapeutic regimen. Chronic corticosteroid therapy may interfere with the growth and development of children.

ADVERSE REACTIONS

The following local adverse reactions are reported infrequently with topical corticosteroids, but may occur more frequently with the use of occlusive dressings. These reactions are listed in an approximate decreasing order of occurrence:

Burning
Itching
Irritation
Dryness
Folliculitis
Hypertrichosis
Acneiform eruptions
Hypopigmentation
Perioral dermatitis
Allergic contact dermatitis
Maceration of the skin
Secondary infection
Skin atrophy
Striae
Miliaria

OVERDOSAGE

Topically applied corticosteroids can be absorbed in sufficient amounts to produce systemic effects. (See PRECAUTIONS).

DOSAGE AND ADMINISTRATION

Topical corticosteroids are generally applied to the affected area as a thin film from two to four times daily depending on the severity of the condition.

Occlusive dressings may be used for management of psoriasis or recalcitrant conditions.

If an infection develops, the use of occlusive dressings should be discontinued and appropriate antimicrobial therapy instituted.

HOW SUPPLIED

Tridesilon® (desonide) Creme 0.05% is supplied in 15 and 60 gram tubes and in 5 pound jars. It is a white semi-solid. **Store below 86°F (30°C), avoid freezing.**

CAUTION

Federal (USA) law prohibits dispensing without a prescription.

January, 1984 PD100597 19508

TRIDESILON® 0.05% ℞
(desonide)
ointment

DESCRIPTION

Tridesilon® Ointment contains microdispersed desonide (the active ingredient) in white petrolatum. Each gram of Tridesilon® Ointment contains 0.5 miligrams of desonide. Tridesilon® Ointment is applied topically.

Tridesilon® (desonide) is a non-fluorinated corticosteroid. Chemically, desonide is Pregna-1,4-diene-3,20-dione,11,21-dihydroxy-16,17-[(1-methylethylidene)bis(oxy)]-,11β,16α)-with the following structural formula:

[See Chemical Formula at top of next page].

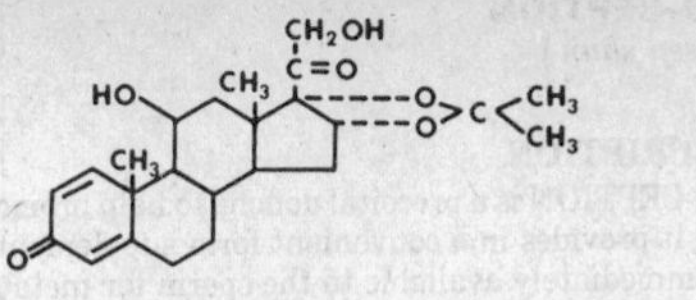

EMPIRICAL FORMULA	MOLECULAR WEIGHT	CAS REGISTRY NUMBER
$C_{24}H_{32}O_6$	416.51	638-94-8

CLINICAL PHARMACOLOGY

Topical corticosteroids share anti-inflammatory, anti-puritic and vasoconstrictive actions.

The mechanism of anti-inflammatory activity of the topical corticosteroids is unclear. Various laboratory methods, including vasoconstrictor assays, are used to compare and predict potencies and/or clinical efficacies of the topical corticosteroids. There is some evidence to suggest that a recognizable correlation exists between vasoconstrictor potency and therapeutic efficacy in man.

Pharmacokinetics

The extent of percutaneous absorption of topical corticosteroids is determined by many factors including the vehicle, the integrity of the epidermal barrier, and the use of occlusive dressings.

Topical corticosteroids can be absorbed from normal intact skin. Inflammation and/or other disease processes in the skin increase percutaneous absorption. Occlusive dressings substantially increase the percutaneous absorption of topical corticosteroids. Thus, occlusive dressings may be a valuable therapeutic adjunct for treatment of resistant dermatoses. (See DOSAGE AND ADMINISTRATION).

Once absorbed through the skin, topical corticosteroids are handled through pharmacokinetic pathways similar to systemically administered corticosteroids. Corticosteroids are bound to plasma proteins in varying degrees. Corticosteroids are metabolized primarily in the liver and are then excreted by the kidneys. Some of the topical corticosteroids and their metabolites are also excreted into the bile.

INDICATIONS AND USAGE

Topical corticosteroids are indicated for the relief of the inflammatory and pruritic manifestations of corticosteroid-responsive dermatoses.

CONTRAINDICATIONS

Topical corticosteroids are contraindicated in those patients with a history of hypersensitivity to any of the components of the preparation.

PRECAUTIONS

General

Systemic absorption of topical corticosteroids has produced reversible hypothalamic-pituitary-adrenal (HPA) axis suppression, manifestations of Cushing's syndrome, hyperglycemia, and glucosuria in some patients.

Conditions which augment systemic absorption include the application of the more potent steroids, use over large surface areas, prolonged use, and the addition of occlusive dressings.

Therefore, patients receiving a large dose of a potent topical steroid applied to a large surface area or under an occlusive dressing should be evaluated periodically for evidence of HPA axis suppression by using the urinary free cortisol and ACTH stimulation tests. If HPA axis suppression is noted, an attempt should be made to withdraw the drug, to reduce the frequency of application, or to substitute a less potent steroid.

Recovery of HPA axis functions is generally prompt and complete upon discontinuation of the drug. Infrequently, signs and symptoms of steroid withdrawal may occur, requiring supplemental systemic corticosteroids.

Children may absorb proportionally larger amounts of topical corticosteroids and thus be more susceptible to systemic toxicity. (See PRECAUTIONS—Pediatric Use).

If irritation develops, topical corticosteroids should be discontinued and appropriate therapy instituted.

In the presence of dermatological infections, the use of an appropriate antifungal or antibacterial agent should be instituted. If a favorable response does not occur promptly, the corticosteroid should be discontinued until the infection has been adequately controlled.

Information for the Patient

Patients using topical corticosteroids should receive the following information and instructions:

1. This medication is to be used as directed by the physician. It is for external use only. Avoid contact with the eyes.
2. Patients should be advised not to use this medication for any disorder other than for which it was prescribed.
3. The treated skin area should not be bandaged or otherwise covered or wrapped so as to be occlusive unless directed by the physician.
4. Patients should report any signs of local adverse reactions especially under occlusive dressing.
5. Parents of pediatric patients should be advised not to use tight-fitting diapers or plastic pants on a child being treated in the diaper area, as these garments may constitute occlusive dressings.

Laboratory Tests

The following tests may be helpful in evaluating the HPA axis suppression.

Urinary free cortisol test
ACTH stimulation test

Carcinogenesis, Mutagenesis, and Impairment of Fertility

Long-term animal studies have not been performed to evaluate the carcinogenic potential or the effect on fertility of topical corticosteroids.

Studies to determine mutagenicity with prednisolone and hydrocortisone have revealed negative results.

Pregnancy Category C

Corticosteroids are generally teratogenic in laboratory animals when administered systemically at relatively low dosage levels. The more potent corticosteroids have been shown to be teratogenic after dermal application in laboratory animals. There are no adequate and well-controlled studies in pregnant women on teratogenic effects from topically applied corticosteroids. Therefore, topical corticosteroids should be used during pregnancy only if the potential benefit justifies the potential risk to the fetus. Drugs of this class should not be used extensively on pregnant patients, in large amounts, or for prolonged periods of time.

Nursing Mothers

It is not known whether topical administration of corticosteroids could result in sufficient systemic absorption to produce detectable quantities in breast milk. Systemically administered corticosteroids are secreted into breast milk in quantities *not* likely to have a deleterious effect on the infant. Nevertheless, caution should be exercised when topical corticosteroids are administered to a nursing woman.

Pediatric Use

Pediatric patients may demonstrate greater susceptibility to topical corticosteroid-induced HPA axis and Cushing's syndrome than mature patients because of a larger skin surface area to body weight ratio.

Hypothalmic-pituitary-adrenal (HPA) axis suppression, Cushing's syndrome, and intracranial hypertension have been reported in children receiving topical corticosteroids. Manifestations of adrenal suppression in children include linear growth retardation, delayed weight gain, low plasma cortisol levels, and absence of response to ACTH stimulation. Manifestations of intracranial hypertension include bulging fontanelles, headaches, and bilateral papilledema.

Administration of topical costicosteroids to children should be limited to the least amount compatible with an effective therapeutic regimen. Chronic corticosteroid therapy may interfere with the growth and development of children.

ADVERSE REACTIONS

The following local adverse reactions are reported infrequently with topical corticosteroids, but may occur more frequently with the use of occlusive dressings. These reactions are listed in an approximate decreasing order of occurrence:

Burning
Itching
Irritation
Dryness
Folliculitis
Hypertrichosis
Acneiform eruptions
Hypopigmentation
Perioral dermatitis
Allergic contact dermatitis
Maceration of the skin
Secondary infection
Skin atrophy
Striae
Miliaria

OVERDOSAGE

Topically applied corticosteroids can be absorbed in sufficient amounts to produce systemic effects. (See PRECAUTIONS).

DOSAGE AND ADMINISTRATION

Topical corticosteroids are generally applied to the affected area as a thin film from two to four times daily depending on the severity of the condition.

Occlusive dressings may be used for the management of psoriasis or recalcitrant conditions.

If an infection develops, the use of occlusive dressings should be discontinued and appropriate antimicrobial therapy instituted.

HOW SUPPLIED

Tridesilon® (desonide) Ointment 0.05% is supplied in 15 and 60 gram tubes. It is white or faintly yellowish, transparent semi-solid.

Store below 86°F (30°C), avoid freezing.

CAUTION

Federal (USA) law prohibits dispensing without a prescription.

Dec 1985 PD100634 20275

TRIDESILON® 0.05% ℞
Otic
(desonide 0.05%–acetic acid 2%)
solution

DESCRIPTION

Otic Tridesilon® Solution contains desonide 0.05% and acetic acid 2% (the active ingredients) in a compatible vehicle buffered to the pH range of the normal ear. Otic Tridesilon® Solution is instilled into the external auditory canal. Tridesilon® (desonide) is a non-fluorinated corticosteroid. Chemically, desonide is Pregna-1,4-diene-3,20-dione,11,21-dihydroxy-16,17-[(1-methylethylidene)bis(oxy)]-,(11β,16α)- with the following structural formula:

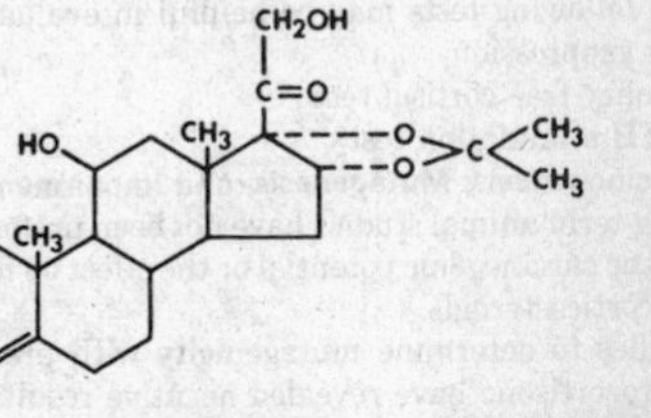

EMPIRICAL FORMULA	MOLECULAR WEIGHT	CAS REGISTRY NUMBER
$C_{24}H_{32}O_6$	416.51	638-94-8

Acetic acid is an astringent and antimicrobial agent. Chemically, it is $C_2H_4O_2$ with the following structural formula:

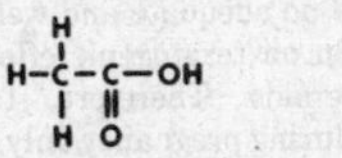

The base is composed of purified water, propylene glycol, sodium acetate, and citric acid.

CLINICAL PHARMACOLOGY

Topical corticosteroids share anti-inflammatory, anti-pruritic and vasoconstrictive actions.

The mechanism of anti-inflammatory activity of the topical corticosteroids is unclear. Various laboratory methods, including vasoconstrictor assays, are used to compare and predict potencies and/or clinical efficacies of the topical corticosteroids. There is some evidence to suggest that a recognizable correlation exists between vasoconstrictor potency and therapeutic efficacy in man.

Pharmacokinetics

The extent of percutaneous absorption of topical corticosteroids is determined by many factors including the vehicle, the integrity of the epidermal barrier, and the use of occlusive dressings.

Topical corticosteroids can be absorbed from normal intact skin. Inflammation and/or other disease processes in the skin increase percutaneous absorption. Occlusive dressings substantially increase the percutaneous absorption of topical corticosteroids.

Once absorbed through the skin, topical corticosteroids are handled through pharmacokinetic pathways similar to systemically administered corticosteroids. Corticosteroids are bound to plasma proteins in varying degrees. Corticosteroids are metabolized primarily in the liver and are then excreted by the kidneys. Some of the topical corticosteroids and their metabolites are also excreted into the bile.

INDICATIONS AND USAGE

Otic Tridesilon Solution is indicated for the treatment of superficial infections of the external auditory canal caused by organisms susceptible to the action of the antimicrobial and accompanied by inflammation.

CONTRAINDICATIONS

Otic Tridesilon Solution (desonide 0.05%-acetic acid 2%) is contraindicated in those patients who have shown hypersensitivity to any of the components of the preparation. Perforated tympanic membranes are frequently considered a contraindication to the use of external ear canal medication.

PRECAUTIONS

General

Systemic absorption of topical corticosteroids has produced reversible hypothalamic-pituitary-adrenal (HPA) axis suppression, manifestations of Cushing's syndrome, hyperglycemia, and glucosuria in some patients.

Conditions which augment systemic absorption include the application of the more potent steroids, use over large surface areas, prolonged use, and the addition of occlusive dressings.

Children may absorb proportionally larger amounts of topical corticosteroids and thus be more susceptible to systemic toxicity. (See PRECAUTIONS—Pediatric Use).

If irritation develops, the product should be discontinued and appropriate therapy instituted.

Continued on next page

Miles Pharm.—Cont.

If infection persists or new infection appears, appropriate therapy should be instituted. If a favorable response does not occur promptly, the corticosteroid should be discontinued until the infection has been adequately controlled.

Information for the Patient

Patients using topical corticosteroids should receive the following information and instructions:

1. This medication is to be used as directed by the physician. It is for external use only. Avoid contact with the eyes.
2. Patients should be advised not to use this medication for any disorder other than for which it was prescribed.

Laboratory Tests

The following tests may be helpful in evaluating the HPA axis suppression:

Urinary free cortisol test

ACTH stimulation test

Carcinogenesis, Mutagenesis, and Impairment of Fertility

Long-term animal studies have not been preformed to evaluate the carcinogenic potential or the effect on fertility of topical corticosteroids.

Studies to determine mutagenicity with prednisolone and hydrocortisone have revealed negative results.

Pregnancy Category C

Corticosteroids are generally teratogenic in laboratory animals when administered systemically at relatively low dosage levels. The more potent corticosteroids have been shown to be teratogenic after dermal application in laboratory animals. There are no adequate and well-controlled studies in pregnant women on teratogenic effects from topically applied corticosteroids. Therefore, topical corticosteroids should be used during pregnancy only if the potential benefit justifies the potential risk to the fetus. Drugs of this class should not be used extensively on pregnant patients, in large amounts, or for prolonged periods of time.

Nursing Mothers

It is not known whether topical administration of corticosteroids could result in sufficient systemic absorption to produce detectable quantities in breast milk. Systemically administered corticosteroids are secreted into breast milk in quantities *not* likely to have a deleterious effect on the infant. Nevertheless, caution should be exercised when topical corticosteroids are administered to a nursing woman.

Pediatric Use

Pediatric patients may demonstrate greater susceptibility to topical corticosteroid-induced HPA axis suppression and Cushing's syndrome than mature patients because of a larger skin surface area to body weight ratio.

Hypothalamic-pituitary-adrenal (HPA) axis suppression. Cushing's syndrome, and intracranial hypertension have been reported in children receiving topical corticosteroids. Manifestations of adrenal suppression in children include linear growth retardation, delayed weight gain, low plasma cortisol levels, and absence of response to ACTH stimulation. Manifestations of intracranial hypertension include bulging fontanelles, headaches, and bilateral papilledema.

Administration of topical corticosteroids to children should be limited to the least amount compatible with an effective therapeutic regimen.

Chronic corticosteroid therapy may interfere with the growth and development of children.

ADVERSE REACTIONS

The following local adverse reactions may occur infrequently with otic use of topical corticosteroids. These reactions are listed in an approximate decreasing order of occurrence.

Burning	Hypopigmentation
Itching	Allergic contact dermatitis
Irritation	Maceration of the skin
Dryness	Secondary infection
Folliculitis	Skin atrophy
Hypertrichosis	

OVERDOSAGE

Topically applied corticosteroids can be absorbed in sufficient amounts to produce systemic effects. (See PRECAUTIONS).

DOSAGE AND ADMINISTRATION

All ceruminous material and debris should be carefully removed to permit Otic Tridesilon® Solution (desonide 0.05%–acetic acid 2%) to contact the infected surfaces. Instill 3 to 4 drops into the ear 3 to 4 times daily. If preferred, a gauze or cotton wick saturated with the solution may be inserted in the ear canal and allowed to remain in situ. It should be kept moist by further addition of the solution, as required.

HOW SUPPLIED

Otic Tridesilon® Solution (desonide 0.05%–acetic acid 2%) is supplied in 10cc bottles with dropper.

Otic Tridesilon® is a clear colorless solution.

Store below 86°F (30°C), avoid freezing.

CAUTION

Federal (USA) law prohibits dispensing without a prescription. For external use only.

Aug., 1983 PD100572 19386

Milex Products, Inc.

5915 NORTHWEST HIGHWAY
CHICAGO, IL 60631

AMINO-CERV™ ℞

[*ah-me 'no-serv*]

pH 5.5 Cervical Creme

ACTIVE INGREDIENTS

Urea 8.34%, Sodium Propionate 0.50%, Methionine 0.83%, Cystine 0.35%, Inositol 0.83%, Benzalkonium Chloride 0.000004%. Buffered to pH of 5.5 in a water-miscible creme base.

DESCRIPTION

An AMINO-ACID and UREA creme specifically formulated for cervical treatment: Cervicitis (mild), postpartum cervicitis, postpartum cervical tears, post cauterization, post cryosurgery and post conization.

ADVANTAGES

METHIONINE and CYSTINE are amino-acids necessary for wound healing and forming of epithelial tissue. INOSITOL acts as an essential growth factor and promotes epithelialization.

UREA aids in debridement, dissolves the coagulum and promotes epithelialization. Its solvent action on fibroblasts prevents the formation of excessive tissue—thus preventing stenosis when used as directed.

BENZALKONIUM CHLORIDE serves to lower surface tension and thus aids in spreading the medication. Along with SODIUM PROPIONATE it also exerts a bacteriostatic effect.

AMINO-CERV is geared to the higher pH of the healthy cervix in contrast with pH 4 vaginal preparations. With its pH factor of 5.5 Amino-Cerv promotes faster healing of the cervix, yet will not adversely affect a healthy vagina.

DIRECTIONS

When immediate postpartum bleeding has subsided (usually from 24 to 48 hours after delivery), one Milex-Jector full of AMINO-CERV creme should be applied nightly for four weeks. In mild CERVICITIS (not requiring cautery or cryosurgery) one applicatorful of AMINO-CERV should be injected in the vagina nightly upon retiring for 2 weeks.

A small amount of AMINO-CERV should be applied immediately after HOT CAUTERIZATION, HOT CONIZATION and CRYOSURGERY. One applicatorful should be injected nightly upon retiring for 2 to 4 weeks (the duration of treatment depends on extent of cauterization or hot conization or cryosurgery). During the weekly office visit for (2 to 4 visits) the physician should again apply a small amount of AMINO-CERV with a probe or applicator. The canal is to be completely probed on the last visit.

After COLD CONING, one applicatorful should be injected upon retiring about 24 hours after surgery and nightly thereafter for four weeks. During the four weekly office visits following cold coning, a small amount of AMINO-CERV should be applied with a probe or applicator into the canal by the physician. The canal is to be completely probed on the last visit.

Reasons For Variation of Directions:

(1) After hot conization, cauterization and cryosurgery immediate use of AMINO-CERV is indicated to aid in dissolving dead or burned tissue.

(2) After cold coning, there is no dead tissue to slough off. Therefore, a wait of 24 hours or longer is desirable for normal healing to take place and for some fibroblasts to be laid down before applying the AMINO-CERV (which has a solvent action on both the fibroblasts and the absorbable sutures). When NONABSORBABLE sutures are used, AMINO-CERV can be used immediately.

CONTRAINDICATIONS

Deleterious side effects have not been a problem at the doses recommended. The usual precautions against allergic reactions should be observed.

STORAGE

Store at room temperature.

PACKAGING

$2\frac{3}{4}$ oz. tube with Milex-Jector (2 weeks supply, 14 applications).

Available only on hospital direct orders: $5\frac{1}{2}$ oz. tube with MILEX-JECTOR (4 weeks supply, 28 applications).

PRO-CEPTION

[*pro-sep 'shun*]

DESCRIPTION

PRO-CEPTION is a precoital douche to help promote conception. It provides in a convenient form supplementary nutrient immediately available to the sperm for metabolism and movement. Also effective for removal of a thick tenacious mucous plug of the cervix.

DIRECTIONS

The screw cap is used as a measuring device and filled level with the powder which is then dissolved in eight ounces of lukewarm water. The woman is told to douche while in a recumbent position and to retain the solution (10 to 15 minutes). Following coitus the patient should remain recumbent for two hours or more. May be used as a companion with Milex Oligospermia Cups. Frequently used in connection with PRO-CEPTION Basal Thermometers.

CONTRAINDICATIONS

None.

PACKAGING

Available in 12 douche container.

Mission Pharmacal Company

1325 E. DURANGO ST.
SAN ANTONIO, TX 78210

CALCET®

[*kăl 'cet*]

Calcium Supplement
NDC-0178-0251-01

COMPOSITION

Each tablet contains:

	% US RDA*	
Calcium Lactate		240 mg.
Calcium Gluconate		240 mg.
Calcium Carbonate		240 mg.
(Calcium	15	152.8 mg.)
Vitamin D2	25	100. Units

* Percent of U.S. Recommended Daily Allowance for adults and children 4 or more years of age.

INDICATIONS

CALCET® tablets are indicated as a daily supplement to provide a dietary source of calcium. CALCET® tablets are of particular value in people who have milk allergies, in people who have low calcium leg cramps or calcium deficiencies due to low dietary calcium.

DOSAGE

TWO CALCET® TABLETS AT BEDTIME as a general or prenatal supplement. In calcium deficiency states or in nocturnal leg cramping, dosage should be increased to TWO CALCET® TABLETS AT BEDTIME plus one tablet midmorning and one tablet mid-afternoon.

HOW SUPPLIED

CALCET® tablets are supplied as yellow, oval shaped, coated tablets in bottles of 100 tablets.

LITERATURE AVAILABLE

Yes.

CALCET PLUS™

[*kăl 'cet*]

Calcium-Iron-Zinc-Multivitamin
NDC 0178-0252-60

COMPOSITION

Each tablet contains:

		%USRDA*
Vitamin C (Calcium Ascorbate, Ascorbic Acid)	500 mg.	800
Vitamin B_1 (Thiamine Mononitrate)	2.25 mg.	150
Vitamin B_2 (Riboflavin)	2.55 mg.	150
Vitamin B_3 (Niacinamide)	30.0 mg.	150
Vitamin B_5 (d-Calcium Pantothenate)	15.0 mg.	150
Vitamin B_6 (Pyridoxine Hydrochloride)	3.0 mg.	150
Vitamin B_{12} (Crystalline on Resin)	9 mcg.	150
Folic Acid	0.8 mg.	200
Vitamin A (Vitamin A Acetate)	5000 USPU	100

Vitamin D	400	USPU	100
Vitamin E	30	USPU	100
(d-Alpha Tocopheryl Acid Succinate)			
Calcium	152.8	mg.	15
(Calcium Ascorbate, Calcium Carbonate)			
Iron	18.0	mg.	100
(Ferrous Fumarate)			
Zinc	15.0	mg.	100
(Zinc Sulfate, dried)			

* USRDA: U.S. recommended daily allowance for adults and children 4 or more years of age.

INDICATIONS

CALCET PLUS tablets are indicated as adjunctive therapy in osteoporosis, pre- and post-operative patients, low calcium leg cramping, for patients with milk allergies and nursing mothers.

DOSAGE

Two CALCET PLUS tablets at bedtime.

HOW SUPPLIED

CALCET PLUS tablets are supplied as white, oval shaped, coated tablets in bottles of 60's.

LITERATURE AVAILABLE

Yes.

CITRACAL®

[sit 'ra-cal]

Calcium Citrate

DESCRIPTION

Each tablet contains:
950 mg. Calcium Citrate,
200 mg. Calcium ....20% USRDA
USRDA: U.S. recommended daily allowance for adults and children 4 or more years of age.

Ingredients: Major: Calcium citrate.
Minor: (less than 45 mg) Magnesium stearate, cellulose gum; microcrystalline cellulose, talc, povidone, titanium dioxide, sugar.
Trace: Carnauba wax, bee's wax, food glaze.
Citracal™ tablets contain no lactose, salt, starch, nitrates, preservatives, artifical flavors or colors.

DIRECTIONS FOR USE

Take 2 to 4 tablets a day or as recommended by your physician.
STORE AT ROOM TEMPERATURE.
KEEP OUT OF THE REACH OF CHILDREN.

HOW SUPPLIED

CITRACAL™ NDC 0178-0800-01 is supplied as white, bolus shaped, sugar coated tablets in bottles of 100 tablets each.

COMPETE®

[kŏm 'pēt]

Multivitamins with Iron and Zinc
NDC-0178-0221-01

DESCRIPTION

COMPETE® is a multivitamin with iron and zinc formulated to provide an especially well tolerated group of nutritional components for the active, stressful lifestyle of the 1980's. COMPETE® provides 150% of the U.S.R.D.A. of all components except vitamins A and D, which have been maintained at a 100% level, and vitamin B_6 which is provided in a level of 1250% U.S.R.D.A. for the particular needs of today's active woman using birth control tablets.

Composition: Each tablet contains:

	Quantity/ Tablet	%USRDA
Vitamin A	5000 I.U.	100%
Vitamin D	400 I.U.	100%
Vitamin E	45 I.U.	150%
Vitamin C	90 mg	150%
Folic Acid	0.4 mg	150%
Thiamine Mononitrate	2.25 mg	150%
Riboflavin	2.6 mg	150%
Niacinamide	30 mg	150%
Pyridoxine HCl	25.0 mg	1250%
Vitamin B_{12}	9 mcg	150%
Iron (As Ferrous Gluconate 233 mg)	27 mg	150%
Zinc (As Zinc Sulfate)	22.5 mg	150%

DOSAGE

One tablet at bedtime as directed by your physician.

WARNING

KEEP THIS AND ALL MEDICATIONS OUT OF THE REACH OF CHILDREN.

In case of accidental overdose, seek professional assistance or contact a poison control center immediately.

PRECAUTION

Folic Acid, especially in doses above 0.1 mg. daily, may obscure pernicious anemia in that hematologic remission may occur while neurological manifestations remain progressive.

HOW SUPPLIED

COMPETE® is supplied as orange, football-shaped, sugar coated tablets in bottles of 100.

FERRALET®

[fer "a-lét]

Ferrous Gluconate
NDC-0178-0082-01

COMPOSITION

Each tablet contains:

		% US RDA*
Ferrous Gluconate	320 mg	
(Iron	37.0 mg.)	206.0

*Percent of U.S. recommended daily allowance for adults and children 4 or more years of age.

DESCRIPTION

The FERRALET® tablet contains only one active ingredient, iron, as ferrous gluconate. FERRALET® is particularly well tolerated in most patients because ferrous gluconate is non-astringent, non-irritating, and will not precipitate protein from aqueous media. FERRALET® provides a more efficient source of ferrous ion because of the low ionization constant of ferrous gluconate, coupled with high solubility and stability over the entire pH range of the gastrointestinal tract. FERRALET® provides utilizable iron throughout the entire length of the intestinal absorption bed. With FERRALET®, heavy iron loading is not necessary due to the superior efficiency of the iron component. The result of moderate ferrous ion dosage is usually improved patient acceptance and excellent dosage continuity. FERRALET® is manufactured in a unique, easy to swallow shape, to further enhance patient acceptance of the product. FERRALET® has a tailored disintegration rate to minimize gastric intoleration with a rapid dissolution rate to assure rapid availability for absorption.

INDICATIONS

Anemias amenable to iron therapy.

DOSAGE

One to three tablets a day depending upon the severity of the anemia and the particular toleration of the patient.

HOW SUPPLIED

FERRALET® is packaged in bottles of 100 tablets.

LITERATURE AVAILABLE

Yes.

FOSFREE®

[fos 'frē]

Calcium—Vitamins—Iron
NDC-0178-0031-01

COMPOSITION

Each tablet contains:

	One Tablet	% US RDA
Calcium Lactate	250.0 mg.	
Calcium Gluconate	250.0 mg.	
Calcium Carbonate	300.0 mg.	
(Calcium	175.7 mg.)	17
Ferrous Gluconate	125.0 mg.	
(Iron	14.5 mg.)	80
Vitamin D_2	150.0 USP U.	optional
Vitamin A Acetate	1500.0 USP U.	30
Ascorbic Acid (C)	50.0 mg.	83
Pyridoxine HCl (B_6)	3.0 mg.	150
Thiamine Mononitrate (B_1)	5.0 mg.	333
Riboflavin (B_2)	2.0 mg.	117
Niacinamide (B_3)	10.0 mg.	50
d-Calcium Pantothenate (B_5)	1.0 mg.	10
Vitamin B_{12} (Crystalline on resin)	2.0 mcg.	33

ACTION AND USES

FOSFREE® tablets are primarily indicated as a prenatal, postpartum or geriatric supplement particularly when soluble calcium salt supplementation is desired. FOSFREE® is a specific for hypocalcemic tetany (nocturnal leg cramping).

ADMINISTRATION AND DOSAGE

One or two FOSFREE® tablets at bedtime as a general or prenatal supplement. In calcium deficiency states or in nocturnal leg cramping, dosage should be increased to two FOSFREE® tablets at bedtime plus one tablet mid-morning and one tablet mid-afternoon.

HOW SUPPLIED

FOSFREE® is supplied as yellow capsule shaped coated tablets in bottles of 100 tablets.

LITERATURE AVAILABLE

Yes.

IROMIN–G®

[i 'rō-min]

Hematinic Supplement
NDC-0178-0081-01

COMPOSITION

Each tablet contains:

	% US RDA	
Ferrous Gluconate		260 mg.
(Iron	214	30 mg.)
Ascorbic Acid (C)	166	100.0 mg.
Thiamine Mononitrate (B_1)	333	5.0 mg.
Pyridoxine HCl (B_6)	1250	25.0 mg.
Riboflavin (B_2)	117	2.0 mg.
Niacinamide	50	10.0 mg.
Folic Acid	200	0.8 mg.
d-Calcium Pantothenate	10	1.0 mg.
Vitamin B_{12} (Crystalline on resin)	33	2.0 mcg.
Vitamin A Acetate	80	4000.0 USP U.
Vitamin D_2	Optional	400.0 USP U.
Calcium Carbonate		70.0 mg.
Calcium Gluconate		100.0 mg.
Calcium Lactate		100.0 mg.
(Calcium	5	50.0 mg.)

ACTION AND USES

Secondary anemias, and as a supplement for the prenatal, teenage and geriatric diet.

ADMINISTRATION AND DOSAGE

One to three tablets daily after meals or as directed by a physician.

PRECAUTION

Folic Acid, especially in doses above 0.1 mg. daily, may obscure pernicious anemia in that hematologic remission may occur while neurological manifestations remain progressive.

SIDE EFFECTS

IROMIN-G® is virtually free of side effects when given in the recommended dosage. The rare constipation, diarrhea, or gastric upset can usually be controlled by dosage adjustment.

HOW SUPPLIED

IROMIN-G® is supplied as red football shaped coated tablets in bottles of 100 tablets.

LITERATURE AVAILABLE

Yes.

MISSION PHARMACAL UROLOGICALS

CALCIBIND™ ℞

[kal 'sē-bīnd]

Cellulose Sodium Phosphate (CSP)

DESCRIPTION

Cellulose Sodium Phosphate (CSP), the active ingredient in CALCIBIND™, is a synthetic compound made by phosphorylation of cellulose and has the following structural formula:

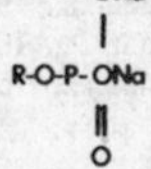

It has an inorganic phosphate content of approximately 34% and sodium content of approximately 11%. It is insoluble in water and non-absorbable. It has excellent ion exchange properties, the sodium ion exchanging for calcium. When taken orally, CSP binds calcium, the complex of calcium and cellulose phosphate being excreted in feces. The dosage of CALCIBIND™ is powder for oral administration.

HOW SUPPLIED

CALCIBIND™ NDC 0178-0255-90, is available for oral administration in boxes of 90 packets containing 2.5 grams of

Continued on next page

Mission—Cont.

CSP powder each. CALCIBIND™ NDC 0178-0255-30 is available for oral administration in bottles of 300 grams of CSP bulk powder.

LITHOSTAT® ℞
[*lith 'o-stat*]
Acetohydroxamic Acid (AHA)

DESCRIPTION
Acetohydroxamic acid (AHA) is a stable, synthetic compound derived from hydroxylamine and ethyl acetate. Its molecular structure is similar to urea:

ACETOHYDROXAMIC ACID (AHA)

AHA is weakly acidic, highly soluble in water, and chelates metals - notably iron. The molecular weight is 75.068. AHA has a PKA of 9.32 and a melting point of 89–91°C. Available as 250 mg tablets.

HOW SUPPLIED
LITHOSTAT®, NDC 0178-0500-01, is available for oral administration as 250 mg scored tablets, in unit of use packages of 100 tablets.

UROCIT®-K ℞
[*yu 'ro-cĭt kay*]
Potassium Citrate

DESCRIPTION
Urocit®-K is a citrate salt of potassium. Its empirical formula is $K_3C_6H_5O_7 \cdot H_2O$, and its structural formula is:

Potassium citrate is a white granular powder that is soluble in water at 154g/100 ml, almost insoluble in alcohol, and insoluble in organic solvents.
Urocit®-K is supplied as wax matrix tablets, containing 5 meq (540 mg) potassium citrate each, for oral administration.

HOW SUPPLIED
Urocit®-K (NDC 0178-0600-01) is available for oral administration in tablet form (5 meq potassium citrate/tablet), in bottles each containing 100 tablets.

MISSION PRENATAL SERIES

MISSION PRENATAL®
Vitamins—Iron—Calcium—.4 mg. Folic Acid
NDC 0178-132-01

MISSION PRENATAL® F.A.
Vitamins—Iron—Calcium—.8 mg. Folic Acid and Zinc
NDC 0178-0153-01

MISSION PRENATAL® H.P.
Vitamins—Iron—Calcium—0.8 mg. Folic Acid
NDC 0178-0161-01

COMPOSITION
Each tablet contains:

	%U.S.R.D.A.	
Ferrous Gluconate		260 mg.
(Iron	214	30 mg.)
Ascorbic Acid (C)	167	100.0 mg.
Thiamine Mononitrate (B_1)	270	5.0 mg.
*† Pyridoxine HCl (B_6)	99	3.0 mg.
Riboflavin (B_2)	100	2.0 mg.
Niacinamide	50	10.0 mg.
d-Calcium Pantothenate	9	1.0 mg.
Vitamin B_{12} (Crystalline on Resin)	25	2.0 mcg.
*† Folic Acid	50	0.4 mg.
Vitamin A Acetate	50	4000.0 USPU
Vitamin D_2	100	400.0 USPU
Calcium Carbonate		70.0 mg.
Calcium Gluconate		100.0 mg.
Calcium Lactate		100.0 mg.
(Calcium	4	50.0 mg.)
Zinc (as Zinc Sulfate)		15.0 mg.

*Pyridoxine HCL—Mission® Prenatal F.A. =10mg., 329%U.S.R.D.A.
*Folic Acid—Mission® Prenatal F.A. =.8mg., 100%U.S.R.D.A.
†Pyridoxine HCL—Mission®Prenatal H.P. =25 mg., 1250%U.S.R.D.A.
†Folic Acid—Mission® Prenatal H.P. =1.0 mg., 125%U.S.R.D.A.
Zinc—only in Mission® Prenatal F.A.

INDICATIONS
ALL MISSION® PRENATALS are prenatal and postpartum supplements.

DOSAGE
Take one tablet at bedtime or as directed by your physician. Keep this and all medications out of the reach of children.

PRECAUTION
Folic Acid, especially in doses above 0.1 mg. daily, may obscure pernicious anemia in that hematologic remission may occur while neurological manifestations remain progressive.

HOW SUPPLIED
MISSION® PRENATAL is supplied as pink, football-shaped, sugar-coated tablets in bottles of 100.
MISSION® PRENATAL F.A. is supplied as blue, football-shaped, sugar coated tablets in bottles of 100.
MISSION® PRENATAL H.P. is supplied as green, football-shaped, sugar-coated tablets in bottles of 100.

MISSION PRENATAL™ Rx ℞
Prenatal Supplement with Vitamins and Minerals
NDC 0178-0007-01

COMPOSITION
Each Tablet Contains:

			%USRDA*
Vitamin A (as Vitamin A Acetate)	8000	I.U.	100
Vitamin D	400	I.U.	100
Vitamin C (as Ascorbic Acid, Calcium Ascorbate)	240	mg.	400
Vitamin B_1 (as Thiamine Mononitrate)	4	mg.	235
Vitamin B_2 (as Riboflavin)	2	mg.	100
Vitamin B_3 (as Niacinamide)	20	mg.	100
Vitamin B_5 (as Calcium Pantothenate)	10	mg.	100
Vitamin B_6 (as Pyridoxine Hydrochloride)	20	mg.	800
Vitamin B_{12} (as Cyanocobalamine on resin)	8	mcg.	100
Folic Acid	1	mg.	125
Iron (as Ferrous Fumarate)	60	mg.	333
Calcium (as Calcium Carbonate and Calcium Ascorbate)	175	mg.	13.5
Iodine (as Potassium Iodide)	0.3	mg.	200
Zinc (as Zinc Sulfate, dried)	15	mg.	100
Copper (as Cupric Oxide)	2	mg.	100

* USRDA: U.S. recommended daily allowance for pregnant or lactating women.

INDICATIONS
MISSION PRENATAL Rx is a prenatal and postpartum supplement.

DOSAGE
Take one tablet at bedtime or as directed by your physician.

CAUTION
Federal law prohibits dispensing without a prescription.

HOW SUPPLIED
MISSION PRENATAL Rx is supplied as pink, football shape, film-coated tablets in bottles of 100.

LITERATURE AVAILABLE
Yes.

MISSION® SURGICAL SUPPLEMENT
A dietary supplement for pre-surgical and post-surgical patients. NDC 0178-0168-01

COMPOSITION
Each tablet contains:

		%USRDA*
Ascorbic Acid (C)	500.0 mg	833
Thiamine Mononitrate (B_1)	2.5 mg	150
Riboflavin(B_2)	2.6 mg	150
Niacinamide (B_3)	30.0 mg	150
Calcium Pantothenate (B_5)	16.3 mg	150
Pyridoxine Hydrochloride (B_6)	3.6 mg	150
Vitamin B_{12}	9.0 mcg	150
Vitamin A Acetate	5000 USPU	100
Vitamin D_2	400 USPU	100
Vitamin E Succinate	45 IU	150
Iron (as Ferrous Gluconate)	27.0 mg	150
Zinc (as Zinc Sulfate)	22.5 mg	150

*USRDA: U.S. Recoommended Daily Allowance for adults and children 4 or more years of age.

ACTION AND USES
A dietary supplement specifically designed to provide the vitamin and mineral nutritional assistance needed by the pre- and post-surgical patient for optimal recovery from the stress of surgery.

ADMINISTRATION AND DOSAGE
One tablet at bedtime or as directed by physician.

WARNING
KEEP THIS AND ALL MEDICATIONS OUT OF THE REACH OF CHILDREN. In case of accidental overdose, seek professional assistance or contact a poison control center immediately.

HOW SUPPLIED
MISSION® PRE-SURGICAL is supplied as a light green, bolus-shaped, sugar coated tablet in bottles of 100.

LITERATURE AVAILABLE
Yes.

PRULET®
[*prŭ-let'*]
White Phenolphthalein tablets N.F.
NDC 0178-0090-01

COMPOSITION
Each tablet contains:
White phenolphthalein N.F. .... 60 mg.

ACTION AND USES
PRULET® is a mild and gentle, effective laxative for patients with atonic or hypotonic bowel syndrome.
PRULET® is a chewable tablet in lemon—lime flavor.

ADMINISTRATION AND DOSAGE
Take one to three tablets administered at bedtime; then adjust to need.

CONTRAINDICATIONS
Not to be taken in the presence of nausea, vomiting, abdominal pains, or other symptoms of appendicitis.

PRECAUTIONS
Phenolphthalein is known to produce skin eruptions in sensitized individuals. If a skin rash or eruption appears, do not take this or any other preparation containing phenolphthalein. PRULET® may cause pink to red urine coloration in patients with an alkaline urine.

HOW SUPPLIED
PRULET® is supplied in green scored tablets in film strip packages of 12 and 40 tablets.

LITERATURE AVAILABLE
Yes.

SUPAC®
[*sŭ 'pac*]
Analgesic Compound
NDC-0178-0100-01

COMPOSITION
Each tablet contains:

Acetaminophen	160 mg.
Aspirin	230 mg.
Caffeine	33 mg.
Calcium Gluconate	60 mg.

ACTION AND USES
For temporary relief of pain accompanying simple head colds, temporary relief of pain accompanying menstruation, sinus and tension headache, minor traumatic pain, tooth extractions, arthritic and rheumatic pain syndromes.

ADMINISTRATION AND DOSAGE
Adults—One or two tablets. This dose may be repeated in 4 hours. Do not exceed 4 tablets at a single dose or 16 tablets in a 24 hour period. Children—6 to 12 years of age, ½ of the

maximum adult dose or dosage; 3 to 6 years of age, ⅓ of the maximum adult dose or dosage.

PRECAUTIONS

If pain persists for more than 10 days, or redness is present, or in conditions affecting children under 12 years of age, physicians should be alert to other possible complications.

HOW SUPPLIED

SUPAC® is supplied as white scored tablets in bottles of 100 and 1000 tablets.

LITERATURE AVAILABLE

Yes.

THERABID®

[thĕr'a-bid]
Therapeutic Multivitamin
NDC 0178-0171-01

COMPOSITION

Each Tablet Contains:

		% US RDA
Ascorbic Acid (Vitamin C)	500 mg.	833
Thiamine Mononitrate (Vitamin B_1)	15 mg.	1000
Riboflavin (Vitamin B_2)	10 mg.	588
Niacinamide (Vitamin B_3)	100 mg.	500
Calcium Pantothenate (Vitamin B_5)	20 mg.	200
Pyridoxine Hydrochloride (Vitamin B_6)	10 mg.	500
Vitamin B_{12}	5 mcg.	83
Vitamin A Acetate	5,000 U.	100
Vitamin D_2	200 U.	optional
Vitamin E (as a-tocopheryl acetate)	30 IU	100

ACTION AND USES

THERABID® is a therapeutic multivitamin preparation.

ADMINISTRATION AND DOSAGE

One to two tablets per day or at the discretion of the physician.

PRECAUTIONS

Do not exceed a dosage of four tablets per day.

HOW SUPPLIED

THERABID® is supplied as green capsule shaped sugar coated tablets in bottles of 100 tablets.

LITERATURE AVAILABLE

Yes.

THERA-GESIC®

[ther'a-jē-zik]
Analgesic Creme Balm
Methyl Salicylate and Menthol

DESCRIPTION

THERA-GESIC® contains Methyl Salicylate and Menthol in a rapidly absorbed greaseless base.

ACTIONS

Topical analgesic, counter irritant.

INDICATIONS

For the temporary relief of pain associated with musculoskeletal soreness and discomfort; additionally, as a topical adjunct in arthritis, rheumatism, and bursitis.

CONTRAINDICATIONS

Do not use in patients with Aspirin or Salicylate idiosyncrasy.

WARNINGS

Use only as directed. Keep away from children to avoid accidental poisoning. Keep away from eyes, mucous membranes, broken or irritated skin. If skin irritation develops, or if pain lasts 10 days or more, or if redness is present, discontinue use and consult a physician. DO NOT SWALLOW. If swallowed, induce vomiting, call a physician.

PRECAUTIONS

Do not use excessive amounts of THERA-GESIC® or occlude a fresh application of THERA-GESIC®. Do not heat pack THERA-GESIC® covered skin. For use by adults only.

ADVERSE REACTIONS

Adverse reactions related to the Salicylate and Menthol components are possible. These include excessive irritation, tinnitus, nausea or vomiting if excessive or extreme dosage is employed.

DOSAGE AND ADMINISTRATION

Gently massage THERA-GESIC® in thin applications into the sore or painful area as well as into the area immediately surrounding the painful area. The number of thin applications applied controls the intensity of the action of THERA-GESIC®. One application provides a mild effect, two provide a strong effect and three applications provide a very strong effect. Once THERA-GESIC® has penetrated the skin, the area may be washed, leaving the area dry, clean and free from the typical wintergreen odor without decreasing the effectiveness of the product. If you intend to bandage or wrap the area, the area should be washed first to avoid excessive irritation.

HOW SUPPLIED

NDC-0178-0320-03	Tubes–3 oz.
NDC-0178-0320-05	Tubes–5 oz.

Muro Pharmaceutical, Inc.
890 EAST STREET
TEWKSBURY, MA 01876-9987

BROMFED® CAPSULES ℞

[brōm'fĕd]

A light green and clear capsule containing white beads. Timed-Release.
Each capsule contains:
Brompheniramine maleate .... 12 mg.
Pseudoephedrine hydrochloride .... 120 mg.
in a specially prepared base to provide prolonged action.

BROMFED-PD® CAPSULES ℞

A dark green and clear capsule containing white beads. Timed-Release.
Each capsule contains:
Brompheniramine maleate .... 6 mg.
Pseudoephedrine hydrochloride .... 60 mg.
in a specially prepared base to provide prolonged action.

BROMFED® and **BROMFED-PD® CAPSULES** also contain inactive ingredients: benzyl alcohol, butyl paraben, carboxymethylcellulose sodium, D & C yellow #10, edetate calcium disodium, FD&C blue #1, FD&C yellow #6, gelatin, methyl paraben, pharmaceutical glaze, propyl paraben, sodium lauryl sulfate, sodium propionate, starch, sucrose and other ingredients.

BROMFED® TABLETS ℞

A white scored tablet.
Each tablet contains:
Brompheniramine maleate .... 4 mg.
Pseudoephedrine hydrochloride .... 60 mg.
Also contains as inactive ingredients colloidal silicon dioxide, lactose, magnesium stearate, microcrystalline cellulose and sodium glycolate.

BROMFED contains ingredients of the following therapeutic classes: antihistamine and decongestant.

CLINICAL PHARMACOLOGY

Brompheniramine maleate is an alkylamine type antihistamine. This group of antihistamines are among the most active histamine antagonists and are generally effective in relatively low doses. The drugs are not so prone to produce drowsiness and are among the most suitable agents for day time use; but again, a significant proportion of patients do experience this effect. Pseudoephedrine hydrochloride is a sympathomimetic which acts predominently on alpha receptors and has little action on beta receptors. It therefore functions as an oral nasal decongestant with minimal CNS stimulation.

INDICATIONS

For the temporary relief of symptoms of seasonal and perennial allergic rhinitis, and vasomotor rhinitis, including nasal obstruction (congestion).

CONTRAINDICATIONS

Hypersensitivity to any of the ingredients. Also contraindicated in patients with severe hypertension, severe coronary artery disease, patients on MAO inhibitor therapy, patients with narrow-angle glaucoma, urinary retention, peptic ulcer and during an asthmatic attack.

WARNINGS

Considerable caution should be exercised in patients with hypertension, diabetes mellitus, ischemic heart disease, hyperthyroidism, increased intraocular pressure and prostatic hypertrophy. The elderly (60 years or older) are more likely to exhibit adverse reactions.
Antihistamines may cause excitability, especially in children. At dosages higher than the recommended dose, nervousness, dizziness or sleeplessness may occur.

PRECAUTIONS

General: Caution should be exercised in patients with high blood pressure, heart disease, diabetes or thyroid disease. The antihistamine in this product may exhibit additive effects with other CNS depressants, including alcohol.
Information for Patients: Antihistamine may cause drowsiness and ambulatory patients who operate machinery or motor vehicles should be cautioned accordingly.
Drug Interactions: MAO inhibitors and beta adrenergic blockers increase the effects of sympathomimetics. Sympathomimetics may reduce the antihypertensive effects of methyldopa, mecamylamine, reserpine and veratrum alkaloids. Concomitant use of antihistamines with alcohol and other CNS depressants may have an additive effect.
Pregnancy: The safety of use of this product in pregnancy has not been established.

ADVERSE REACTIONS

Adverse reactions include drowsiness, lassitude, nausea, giddiness, dryness of mouth, blurred vision, cardiac palpitations, flushing, increased irritability or excitement (especially in children).

DOSAGE AND ADMINISTRATION

BROMFED® CAPSULES Adults and children over 12 years of age—1 capsule orally every 12 hours.
BROMFED-PD® CAPSULES Children 6 to 12 years of age—1 capsule orally every 12 hours.
BROMFED® TABLETS Adults and children 12 and over: One tablet every 4 hours not to exceed 6 doses in 24 hours. Children 6 to 12 years: One-half tablet every 4 hours not to exceed 6 doses in 24 hours. Do not give to children under 6 years except under the advice and supervision of a physician.

HOW SUPPLIED

BROMFED® CAPSULES. Bottle of 100 (NDC 0451-4000-50) and 500 (NDC 0451-4000-60). Each capsule is coded "BROMFED" "MURO 12-120".
BROMFED-PD® CAPSULES. Bottle of 100 (NDC 0451-4001-50) and 500 (NDC 0451-4001-60). Each capsule is coded "BROMFED-PD" "MURO 6-60".
BROMFED® TABLETS. Bottle of 100 (NDC 0451-4060-50). Each tablet is coded "MURO 4060" on one side and scored on the reverse side.
Dispense in tight containers as defined in USP. Store between 15°–30°C (59°–86°F).
CAUTION: FEDERAL (U.S.A.) LAW PROHIBITS DISPENSING WITHOUT A PRESCRIPTION.

GUAIFED® Capsule ℞

[gwi'ah-fĕd]

A white opaque and clear capsule containing white beads.
Each capsule contains:
Pseudoephedrine hydrochloride .... 120 mg.
in a specially prepared base to provide prolonged action.
Guaifenesin .... 250 mg.
designed for immediate release to provide rapid action.

GUAIFED®–PD CAPSULE ℞

A blue and clear capsule containing white beads.
Each capsule contains:
Pseudoephedrine hydrochloride .... 60 mg.
in a specially prepared base to provide prolonged action.
Guaifenesin .... 300 mg.
designed for immediate release to provide rapid action.

GUAIFED® and **GUAIFED®–PD CAPSULES** also contain as inactive ingredients: Benzyl Alcohol, Butyl Paraben, Edetate Calcium Disodium, Gelatin, Methyl Paraben, Pharmaceutical Glaze, Propyl Paraben, Sodium Lauryl Sulfate, Sodium Propionate, Starch, Sucrose, Titanium Dioxide, FD&C Blue #1 (GUAIFED-PD only) and other ingredients.

GUAIFED® and **GUAIFED®–PD** contains ingredients of the following therapeutic classes: nasal decongestant and expectorant.

CLINICAL PHARMACOLOGY

Pseudoephedrine hydrochloride is a sympathomimetic which acts predominantly on alpha adrenergic receptors in the mucosa of the respiratory tract, producing vasoconstriction and has little action on beta receptors. It therefore functions as an oral nasal decongestant with minimal CNS stimulation. Pseudoephedrine hydrochloride also increases sinus drainage and secretions. Guaifenesin is an expectorant which increases the output of phlegm (sputum) and bronchial secretions by reducing adhesiveness and surface tension. The increased flow of less viscid secretions promotes ciliary action and changes a dry, unproductive cough to one that is more productive and less frequent.

INDICATIONS

For temporary relief of nasal congestion and dry non-productive cough associated with the common cold and other respiratory allergies. Helps drainage of the bronchial tubes by thinning the mucus.

CONTRAINDICATIONS

This product is contraindicated in patients with a known hypersensitivity to any of its ingredients. Also contraindicated in patients with severe hypertension, severe coronary

Continued on next page

Muro—Cont.

artery disease and patients on MAO inhibitor therapy. Should not be used during pregnancy or in nursing mothers. Considerable caution should be exercised in patients with hypertension, diabetes mellitus, ischemic heart disease, hyperthyroidism, increased intraocular pressure and prostatic hypertrophy. The elderly (60 years or older) are more likely to exhibit adverse reactions. At dosages higher than the recommended dose, nervousness, dizziness or sleeplessness may occur.

PRECAUTIONS

General: Caution should be exercised in patients with high blood pressure, heart disease, diabetes or thyroid disease and in patients who exhibit difficulty in urination due to enlargement of the prostate gland. Check with a physician if symptoms do not improve within 7 days or if accompanied by high fever, rash or persistent headache.

Drug Interactions: Do not take this product if you are presently taking a prescription drug for high blood pressure or depression, without first consulting a physician. MAO inhibitors and beta adrenergic blockers may increase the effect of sympathomimetics. Sympathomimetics may reduce the antihypertensive effects of methyldopa, mecamylamine, reserpine and veratrum alkaloids. Pseudoephedrine hydrochloride may increase the possibility of cardiac arrhythmias in patients presently taking digitalis glycosides.

Pregnancy: Pregnancy Catagory B. It has been shown that pseudoephedrine hydrochloride can cause reduced average weight, length, and rate of skeletal ossification in the animal fetus.

Nursing Mothers: Pseudoephedrine is excreted in breast milk; use by nursing mother is not recommended because of the higher than usual risk of side effects from sympathomimetic amines for infants, especially newborn and premature infants.

Geriatrics: Pseudoephedrine should be used with caution in the elderly because they may be more sensitive to the effects of the sympathomimetics.

WARNINGS

Do not take this product for persistent or chronic cough such as occurs with smoking, asthma, or emphysema, or where cough is accompanied by excessive secretions except under the advice and supervision of a physician. This medication should be taken a few hours prior to bedtime to minimize the possibility of sleeplessness. Take this medication with a glass of water after each dose, to help loosen mucus in the lungs.

ADVERSE REACTIONS

Adverse reactions include nausea, cardiac palpitations, increased irritability or excitement, headache, dizziness, tachycardia, diarrhea, drowsiness, stomach pain, seizures, slowed heart rate, shortness of breath and/or troubled breathing.

OVERDOSAGE

KEEP THIS AND ALL DRUGS OUT OF THE REACH OF CHILDREN. IN CASE OF SUSPECTED OVERDOSE, IMMEDIATELY CALL YOUR REGIONAL POISON CONTROL CENTER and/or SEEK PROFESSIONAL ASSISTANCE.

Symptoms of overdosage may be caused by pseudoephedrine. Symptoms of overdosage with pseudoephedrine include anxiety, tenseness, respiratory difficulty, headache and awareness of the slow forceful heartbeat.

TREATMENT OF OVERDOSE

The stomach should be emptied promptly by emetics and/or gastric lavage. The installation of activated charcoal also should be considered. Cardiac function and serum electrolytes should be monitored and treatment instigated if indicated. If convulsions or marked CNS excitement occurs, diazepam may be used.

DOSAGE AND ADMINISTRATION

GUAIFED® CAPSULES Adults and children over 12 years of age: 1 capsule orally every 12 hours.

GUAIFED® PD CAPSULES Adults and children over 12 years of age: 1 or 2 capsules orally every 12 hours. Children 6 to 12 years of age—1 capsule orally every 12 hours.

HOW SUPPLIED

GUAIFED® CAPSULES Bottle of 100 (NDC 0451-4002-50). Each capsule is coded "GUAIFED" "MURO 120-250".

GUAIFED®-PD CAPSULES Bottle of 100 (NDC 0451-4003-50). Each capsule is coded "GUAIFED-PD" "MURO 60-300". Dispense in tight containers as defined in USP. Store at controlled room temperature, between 15°–30°C (59°–86°F). Dispense in child resistant container.

Keep this and all drugs out of reach of children.

CAUTION: FEDERAL (U.S.A.) LAW PROHIBITS DISPENSING WITHOUT A PRESCRIPTION.

LIQUID PRED® Syrup ℞

Each teaspoonful contains:
Prednisone 5mg/5ml

HOW SUPPLIED

NDC-0451-1201-04–4 fl. oz. (120 ml)
NDC-0451-1201-08–8 fl. oz. (240 ml)

PRELONE™ SYRUP ℞

(Prednisolone 15 mg per 5 mL)

PRELONE Syrup contains 15 mg prednisolone in each 5 mL. Benzoic acid, 0.1%, is added as a preservative. It also contains alcohol 5%, citric acid, edetate disodium, glycerin, Propylene glycol, Purified water, Sodium saccharin, Sucrose, artificial flavor, FD&C blue #1 and red #40.

HOW SUPPLIED

PRELONE Syrup is a cherry red liquid containing 15 mg of Prednisolone in each 5 mL (teaspoonful) and is supplied in 240 mL bottles. NDC #0451-1500-08.

SALINEX Nasal Mist and Drops

[sal 'i-nĕx]
(Buffered isotonic sodium chloride solution)

(See PDR for Nonprescription Drugs)

Nature's Bounty, Inc.

90 ORVILLE DRIVE
BOHEMIA, NY 11716

ENER-B™

Intra-nasal Vitamin B-12 Gel

DESCRIPTION

ENER-B™ is the first intra-nasal application for Vitamin B-12. Each delivery supplies 400 mcg. of Vitamin B-12. This method of delivery provides the highest Vitamin B-12 blood levels that can be obtained without a prescription. Clinical tests show that ENER-B produced 8.4 to 10 times more Vitamin B-12 in the blood than tablets.

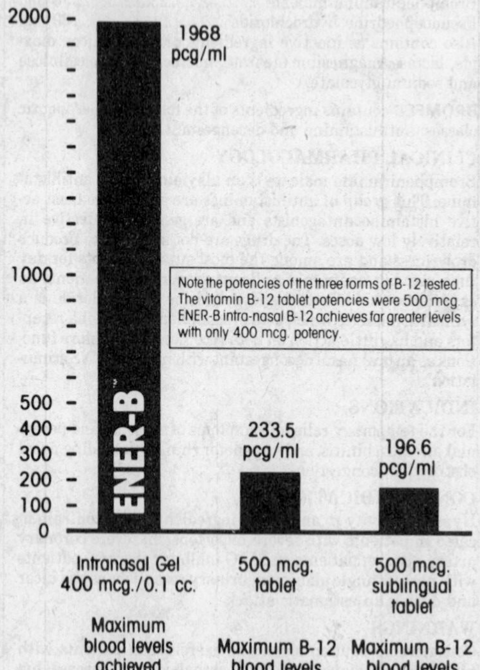

Clinical Test results are available by writing Nature's Bounty.

POTENCY AND ADMINISTRATION

Each nasal applicator delivers 1/10 cc of gel into the nose which adheres to the mucous membranes providing 400 mcg. of Vitamin B-12. Odorless and non-irritating to the nose.

HOW SUPPLIED

Packages of 12 unit doses. Supplies 400 mcg. of B-12 each.

Neutrogena Dermatologics

Division of
Neutrogena Corporation
5755 W. 96TH STREET
P.O. BOX 45036
LOS ANGELES, CA 90045

MELANEX® ℞

[mel 'an-ex]
(3% hydroquinone) Topical Solution

COMPOSITION

Melanex (3% hydroquinone) Topical Solution contains 30 mg hydroquinone per ml in a vehicle of 47.3% alcohol, purified water, laureth-4, isopropyl alcohol 4%, propylene glycol and ascorbic acid.

Pharmacological class: Depigmenting agent.

CLINICAL PHARMACOLOGY

It has been suggested that the primary action of hydroquinone is directed at tyrosinase. The selective inhibition of the enzyme affects melanogenesis in the melanocytes resulting in cessation of melanin formation and subsequent reduction in pigmentation. Additional studies indicate that hydroquinone acts on the essential subcellular metabolic processes of melanocytes with resultant cytolysis, i.e., nonenzyme-medicated depigmentation.

INDICATIONS AND USAGE

Melanex is indicated in the temporary bleaching of hyperpigmented skin conditions such as chloasma, melasma, freckles, senile lentigines, and other forms of melanin hyperpigmentation.

DOSAGE AND ADMINISTRATION

Apply to affected areas twice daily, in the morning and before bedtime. During the day, an effective broad spectrum sunscreen should be used and unnecessary solar exposure avoided, or protective clothing should be worn to cover bleached skin in order to prevent repigmentation from occurring.

CONTRAINDICATIONS

Melanex is contraindicated in persons who have shown hypersensitivity to hydroquinone or any of the other ingredients. The safety of topical treatment with hydroquinone during pregnancy has not been established.

PRECAUTIONS

Concurrent use of Melanex with benzoyl peroxide may result in transient dark staining of skin areas so treated. This is due to the oxidation of hydroquinone by the benzoyl peroxide. This transient staining can be removed by discontinuing concurrent usage and normal soap cleansing.

For external use only. Hydroquinone preparations may produce skin irritation in susceptible individuals and have a slight potential to produce an allergic response. Therefore, the physician should use appropriate caution. If rash or irritation develops, discontinue use and consult physician. Do not use on children under 12. If no improvement is seen after three months of treatment, use of product should be discontinued. Avoid contact with eyes. In case of accidental contact, patient should rinse eyes thoroughly with water and contact physician. A bitter taste and anesthetic effect may occur if applied to lips. Keep out of the reach of children. Use of Melanex in paranasal and infraorbital areas increases the chance of irritation (see Adverse Reactions). A Patient Instruction Sheet for using Melanex is provided (to the physician) to be given to the patient at the discretion of the physician.

ADVERSE REACTIONS

The following have been reported: dryness and fissuring of paranasal and infraorbital areas, erythema and stinging. Hydroquinone has been known to produce irritation and sensitization in susceptible individuals.

HOW SUPPLIED

1.0 fl oz (30 ml) bottle with Appliderm™ Applicator Unit and pinpoint rod applicator.

Note: Slight darkening of the Melanex solution is normal and will not affect potency. See expiration date on bottle.

For additional information, call Neutrogena Corporation, Technical Department, (800) 421-6857. In California, call (213) 642-1150, collect.

NDC #10812-9300-1

VEHICLE/N®
VEHICLE/N® MILD

COMPOSITION

Vehicle/N and Vehicle/N MILD are both versatile liquid vehicles for extemporaneous compounding of topical drugs. Both formulations solubilize selected dermatologic agents and provide astringent and drying actions.

The Appliderm™ Applicator Unit automatically filters the compounded drug and provides a convenient, spill-proof, self-contained unit for topical application.

Vehicle/N contains:

Alcohol	47.5%
Purified Water	
Laureth-4	
Isopropyl Alcohol	4.0%
Propylene Glycol	

Vehicle/N MILD contains:

Alcohol	41.5%
Purified Water	
Isopropyl Alcohol	6.0%
Laureth-4	

PRECAUTIONS

Do not use near fire or flame due to alcohol content. Both Neutrogena Vehicle/N and Vehicle/N MILD preparations contain substantial alcohol and are not suitable for use in acute dermatoses. Stinging may be noted if used on irritated or abraded skin. Avoid contact with eyes or eyelids. If the product accidentally comes in contact with eyes, rinse thoroughly with water and contact physician. For external use only. Keep out of reach of children.

CONTRAINDICATIONS

Vehicle/N and Vehicle/N MILD are contraindicated in persons who have shown hypersensitivity to any of their listed ingredients.

AVAILABILITY

50 ml in plastic bottle with applicator top. (Bottle filled to 3/4 capacity to ensure proper mixing.)

Note: Laboratory and clinical evaluations necessary to determine the safety and efficacy of the preparations resulting from the addition of any drugs to Neutrogena Vehicle/N and Vehicle/N MILD have not been conducted. Neutrogena Corporation makes no claims regarding the safety or efficacy of extemporaneously prepared products.

For additional information, call Neutrogena Corporation, Technical Department, (800) 421-6857. In California, call (213) 642-1150 collect.

Vehicle/N: NDC #10812-9100-1

Vehicle/N MILD: NDC #10812-9400-1

Patent Pending

Norcliff Thayer Inc.

303 SOUTH BROADWAY
TARRYTOWN, NY 10591

A-200 Pyrinate® Pediculicide Shampoo Liquid, Gel

A-200 Pyrinate® Liquid

DESCRIPTION

Active ingredients: pyrethrins 0.17%, piperonyl butoxide technical 2% (equivalent to 1.6% (butylcarbityl) (6-propylpiperonyl) ether and 0.4% related compounds).

Inert ingredients: benzyl alcohol, butyl stearate, fragrance, octoxynol-9, oleic acid, oleoresin parsley seed, petroleum distillate, water.

A-200 Pyrinate® Gel

DESCRIPTION

Active ingredients: pyrethrins 0.33%, piperonyl butoxide technical 4% (equivalent to 3.2% (butylcarbityl) (6-propylpiperonyl) ether and 0.8% related compounds).

Inert ingredients: benzyl alcohol, butyl stearate, carbomer 940, fragrance, octoxynol-9, oleic acid, oleoresin parsley seed, petroleum distillate, triisopropanolamine, water.

ACTIONS

A-200 Pyrinate is an effective pediculicide for control of head lice (Pediculus humanus capitis), pubic lice (Phthirus pubis) and body lice (Pediculus humanus corporis), and their nits.

INDICATIONS

A-200 Pyrinate Liquid and Gel are indicated for the treatment of human pediculosis—head lice, body lice and pubic lice, and their eggs. A-200 Pyrinate Gel is specially formulated for pubic lice and head lice in children, where control of application is desirable.

CONTRAINDICATIONS

A-200 Pyrinate is contraindicated in individuals hypersensitive to any of its ingredients or allergic to ragweed.

PRECAUTIONS

A-200 Pyrinate is for external use only. It is harmful if swallowed or inhaled. It may be irritating to the eyes and mucous membranes. In case of accidental contact with eyes, they should be immediately flushed with water. In order to prevent reinfestation with lice, all clothing and bedding must be sterilized or treated concurrent with the application of this preparation. If skin irritation or signs of infection are present, a physician should be consulted.

ADMINISTRATION AND DOSAGE

Apply sufficient A-200 Pyrinate to completely "wet" the hair and scalp or skin of any infested area. Allow application to remain no longer than 10 minutes. Wash and rinse with plenty of warm water. Remove dead lice and eggs from hair with fine comb. To restore body and luster to hair following scalp applications, follow with a good shampoo. If necessary, this treatment may be repeated, but should not exceed two applications within 24 hours.

HOW SUPPLIED

A-200 Pyrinate Liquid in 2 and 4 fl. oz. unbreakable plastic bottles with special comb. A-200 Pyrinate Gel in 1 oz. tubes.

LITERATURE AVAILABLE

Patient literature available upon request.

Shown in Product Identification Section, page 419

AVAIL™
Calcium Intensive Multivitamin and Minerals for Women

(See PDR For Nonprescription Drugs)

ESOTÉRICA® MEDICATED FADE CREAM
Regular
Facial
Fortified with Sunscreen Scented
Fortified with Sunscreen Unscented

(See PDR For Nonprescription Drugs)

LIQUIPRIN®
(acetaminophen)

(See PDR For Nonprescription Drugs)

NATURE'S REMEDY® Laxative

(See PDR For Nonprescription Drugs)

NoSalt®
Salt Alternative
Regular and Seasoned

(See PDR For Nonprescription Drugs)

OXY CLEAN® Lathering Facial Scrub

(See PDR For Nonprescription Drugs)

OXY CLEAN® MEDICATED
Cleanser
Pads
Soap

(See PDR For Nonprescription Drugs)

OXY-5® Lotion with Sorboxyl
OXY-10® Lotion and Cover with Sorboxyl
Benzoyl Peroxide Lotion 5% and 10%

(See PDR For Nonprescription Drugs)

OXY-10® WASH Antibacterial Skin Wash

(See PDR For Nonprescription Drugs)

TUMS® Antacid Tablets, Regular and Extra Strength

(See PDR For Nonprescription Drugs)

Nordisk-USA

6500 ROCK SPRING DRIVE
SUITE 304
BETHESDA, MD 20817

PURIFIED PORK INSULIN PRODUCTS

INSULATARD® NPH
[in 'sŭl-ă "tard nph]
U-100 Purified Pork, Purified Pork insulin isophane suspension.

PRODUCT OVERVIEW

KEY FACTS

Insulatard NPH insulin is produced from the pork insulin molecule and has low immunogenic potential. Insulatard NPH contains no excess protamine and can be mixed reliably with Nordisk Velosulin without altering the time course of either component insulin. The resultant mixtures (NPH & Regular) impose no usage restrictions on the mixer or user regarding the timing of the injection of the combination of insulins.

Insulatard NPH and Velosulin may be mixed in the same syringe without loss of effectiveness, whether used immediately or used over extended periods of time (five minutes, two days, two weeks).

MAJOR USES

Insulatard NPH is indicated in the treatment of insulin-requiring diabetes mellitus. The route of administration of Insulatard NPH is via subcutaneous injection.

SAFETY INFORMATION

Insulatard NPH is a safe and an appropriate insulin to use or dispense for the diabetic patient when NPH insulin is indicated. As with any insulin product in achieving glycemic control, careful monitoring and changes in daily dosage or timing of injections may be necessary.

PRESCRIBING INFORMATION

INSULATARD® NPH
[in 'sŭl-ă "tard nph]
U-100 Purified Pork, Purified Pork insulin isophane suspension.

WARNING

ANY CHANGE OF INSULIN SHOULD BE MADE CAUTIOUSLY ONLY UNDER MEDICAL SUPERVISION. WHEN CHANGING TO PURIFIED PORK INSULIN FROM ANY OTHER INSULIN A DOSAGE ADJUSTMENT, IF ANY, IS LIKELY TO BE A REDUCTION TO AVOID HYPOGLYCEMIA. CHANGES IN PURITY, STRENGTH (U-40, U-80, U-100), BRAND (MANUFACTURER), TYPE (LENTE, NPH, REGULAR, ETC.) AND/ OR SPECIES SOURCE (BEEF, PORK, BEEF/ PORK) MAY RESULT IN THE NEED FOR A CHANGE IN DOSAGE. IT IS NOT POSSIBLE TO IDENTIFY WHICH PATIENTS WILL REQUIRE A REDUCTION IN DOSAGE TO AVOID HYPOGLYCEMIA WHEN USING THIS INSULIN. ADJUSTMENT MAY BE NEEDED WITH THE FIRST DOSE OR OVER A PERIOD OF SEVERAL WEEKS. (SEE DOSAGE ADJUSTMENT SECTION). BE AWARE OF THE POSSIBILITY OF SYMPTOMS OF EITHER HYPOGLYCEMIA OR HYPERGLYCEMIA. SEE SECTIONS ENTITLED INSULIN REACTION AND HYPERGLYCEMIA.

DESCRIPTION

INSULATARD NPH is a suspension of protamine insulin crystals. It has a slower speed of action than VELOSULIN (Regular) and a shorter duration than Protamine Zinc Insulin. The effect on the blood sugar begins approximately 1½ hours after the injection and lasts up to approximately 24 hours, having its maximum effect between the 4th and 12th hour.

DIRECTIONS

Shake vial carefully to obtain a uniformly cloudy suspension of the crystals. Avoid heavy foaming. Do not use a vial if the insulin remains clear after it has been shaken. Also do not use it if you see lumps that float or stick to the sides.

INSULATARD NPH can be mixed with any other Nordisk insulin preparation. In the mixture the different insulins will keep their original effect (stable mixtures).

Keep INSULATARD NPH in a cold place (refrigerator) at 2 degrees to 10 degrees C (35–50 degrees F), but do not let it freeze or be exposed to direct sunlight. Do not use the insulin after the expiration date stamped on the label.

DOSAGE ADJUSTMENT

Reductions in dosage resulting from the switchover to this purified pork insulin from any other insulin have been observed to be in the neighborhood of 10–20% initially to maintain control.

Continued on next page

Nordisk-USA—Cont.

Adjustment may be needed either with the first dose or over a period of several weeks, and it is therefore recommended that the patient be monitored closely by a physician during the changeover and that dosage be adjusted downwards as necessary.
It is not possible to identify which patients will require a reduction in dose to avoid hypoglycemia when using purified pork insulins.
Be aware of the possibility of symptoms indicating the need for adjustment. See sections on Insulin Reaction or Hyperglycemia.
Use the Correct Syringe: INSULATARD NPH is available in the U-100 strength (100 units per ml). The patient must understand the markings on the syringe and use only a syringe marked for U-100.
Avoid contamination and possible infection by following these instructions:
Reusable syringes and needles must be sterile when used. The best method of sterilization is to boil the syringe, plunger and needle in water for 5 minutes. If this is not possible, as when travelling, the parts may be sterilized by immersion for at least 5 minutes in a sterilizing liquid like ethyl alcohol, 70%. Do not use bathing, rubbing or medicated alcohol for sterilization. Remove all liquid from the syringe by pushing the plunger in and out several times and leave it to dry if alcohol has been used for sterilization. To prepare the dose, clean the rubber cap with cotton dipped in alcohol such as ethyl alcohol, 70%. The rubber cap must never be removed. Air is drawn into the syringe corresponding in amount to the prescribed amount of insulin. The needle is plunged through the cap in a downward position and the vial and syringe then inverted so that the air may be pushed out of the syringe into the vial. The prescribed amount of insulin is drawn into the syringe, and this is best done by drawing up slightly more insulin than required and then pushing the piston back to the desired mark. In this way any air bubbles are forced out of the syringe. Withdraw the needle from the vial without changing the position of the plunger in the syringe and lay aside the syringe so that it will not come in contact with any object. Disinfect the skin with a cotton swab dipped in a suitable antiseptic, such as ethyl alcohol, 70%. Pinch up the skin that has been disinfected and push the needle at a right angle quickly into the tissue under the skin. Do not inject deeper into a muscle or a vein. Give each injection in a different place from the previous one. If instructed to mix two types of insulin in the syringe, air should be injected into each vial first.

WARNING

Patients who have been directed to mix two types of insulin should be aware that insulin hypodermic syringes may vary in amount of space between the bottom line and the needle. Because of this, the patient should not change:
1. The order of mixture prescribed, or
2. the model and brand of the syringe or needle.

Failure to heed this warning can result in a dosage error.
Insulin injections, a balanced diet, and regular exercise are required to secure proper control of diabetes. Urine should be tested regularly for sugar. Consistent presence of sugar in the urine indicates that diabetes is not properly controlled.
As with any drug, if you are pregnant or nursing a baby, seek professional advice before using this product.

ADVERSE REACTIONS

Insulin allergy occurs very rarely, but when it does, it may cause a serious reaction including a general skin rash over the body, shortness of breath, fast pulse, sweating, and a drop in blood pressure.
In a very few diabetics, the skin where insulin has been injected may become red, swollen and itchy. This local reaction may occur if the injection is not properly made, if the skin is sensitive to the cleansing solution or if the patient is allergic to insulin.
Patients with severe systemic reactions to insulin (i.e. generalized urticaria, angioedema, anaphylaxis) should be skin tested with <u>each</u> new preparation to be used prior to initiation of therapy.
Insulin Reaction: Insulin reaction (hypoglycemia) can occur if the patient takes too much insulin, misses a meal or exercises or works harder than normal. The symptoms, which usually come on suddenly, are hunger, dizziness, and sweating. Eating sugar or a sugar-sweetened product will normally correct the condition.
Hyperglycemia: Hyperglycemia can occur if the patient takes too little insulin, eats significantly more than usual, or develops a cold or other infection. The symptoms are thirst, frequent passing of urine, and in severe cases nausea and abdominal pain. These symptoms generally come on gradually.

HOW SUPPLIED

10 ml vials
100 units per ml.
NDC # 50445-200-01
Brochures, Time Action Profile Charts, Samples—Free to Physicians.

INSULATARD® NPH HUMAN

[in 'sŭl-ă "tard nph hyōō 'men]
U-100 Human, Human insulin isophane suspension (semi-synthetic)

PRODUCT OVERVIEW

KEY FACTS

Insulatard NPH Human insulin is produced semi-synthetically by enzymatic conversion of the pork insulin molecule and has low immunogenic potential. Insulatard NPH Human contains no excess protamine and can be mixed reliably with Velosulin Human without altering the time course of either component insulin. The resultant mixtures (NPH & Regular) impose no usage restrictions on the mixer or user regarding the timing of the injection of the combination of insulins. Insulatard NPH Human and Velosulin Human may be mixed in the same syringe without loss of effectiveness, whether used immediately or used over extended periods of time (five minutes, two days, two weeks).

MAJOR USES

Insulatard NPH Human is indicated in the treatment of insulin-requiring diabetes mellitus. The route of administration for Insulatard NPH Human is via subcutaneous injection.

SAFETY INFORMATION

Insulatard NPH Human is a safe and an appropriate insulin to use or dispense for the diabetic patient when human insulin is indicated. As with any insulin product in achieving maximum glycemic control, careful monitoring and changes in daily dosage or timing of injections may be necessary.

PRESCRIBING INFORMATION

INSULATARD® NPH HUMAN

[in 'sŭl-ă "tard nph hyōō 'men]
U-100 Human, Human insulin isophane suspension (semi-synthetic)

WARNING

This Nordisk human insulin is structurally identical to the insulin produced by the pancreas in the human body. This structural identity is obtained by enzymatic conversion of purified pork insulin. Any change of insulin should be made cautiously and only under medical supervision. Changes in purity, strength (U-40, U-100), brand (manufacturer), type (lente, NPH, regular) and/or species source (beef, pork, beef/pork, human) may result in the need for a change in dosage. Adjustment may be needed with the first dose or over a period of several weeks. Be aware of the possibility of symptoms of either hypoglycemia or hyperglycemia. See sections entitled insulin reaction and hyperglycemia.

DESCRIPTION

Insulatard® NPH Human is a suspension of protamine insulin crystals. It has a slower speed of action than Velosulin® Human (Regular) and a shorter duration than Protamine Zinc Insulin. The effect on the blood sugar begins approximately 1½ hours after the injection and lasts up to approximately 24 hours, having its maximum effect between the 4th and 12th hour.

DIRECTIONS

Shake vial carefully to obtain a uniformly cloudy suspension of the crystals. Avoid heavy foaming. Do not use a vial if the insulin remains clear after it has been shaken. Also do not use it if you see lumps that float or stick to the sides.
This preparation can be mixed with any other Nordisk human insulin preparation. In the mixture the different insulins will keep their original effects (stable mixtures).
Keep the insulin in a cold place (refrigerator), but do not let it freeze. Do not let it be exposed to direct sunlight. Do not use the insulin after the expiration date stamped on the label.
Use the correct syringe
The volume of the dose depends on the number of units of insulin per ml. Insulatard® NPH Human is only available in the U-100 strength (100 units per ml). Make sure of the markings on the syringe and use only a syringe marked for U-100.
Avoid contamination and possible infection by following below-mentioned instructions.
Reusable syringes and needles must be sterile when used. The best method of sterilization is to boil the syringe, plunger and needle in water for 5 minutes. If this is not possible, as when travelling, the parts may be sterilized by immersion for at least 5 minutes in a sterilizing liquid like ethyl alcohol, 70%. Do not use bathing, rubbing or medicated alcohol for sterilization. Remove all liquid from the syringe by pushing the plunger in and out several times and leave it to dry if alcohol has been used for sterilization. To prepare the dose, clean the rubber cap with cotton dipped in alcohol such as ethyl alcohol, 70%. The rubber cap must never be removed. Air is then drawn into the syringe corresponding in amount to the prescribed amount of insulin. The needle is plunger through the rubber cap in a downward position and the vial and syringe then inverted so that the air may be pushed out of the syringe into the vial. The prescribed amount of insulin is drawn into the syringe and this is best done by drawing up slightly more insulin than required and then pushing the piston back to the desired mark. In this way air bubbles are forced out of the syringe. Then withdraw the needle from the vial without changing the position of the plunger in the syringe and lay aside the syringe so that it will not come in contact with any object. Disinfect the skin with a cotton swab dipped in a suitable antiseptic, such as ethhyl alcohol, 70%. Pinch up the skin that has been disinfected and push the needle at a right angle quickly into the tissue under the skin. Do not inject deeper into a muscle or a vein. Give each injection in a different place from the previous one. If instructed to mix two types of insulin in the syringe, air should be injected into each vial first.
Usage in pregnancy
Pregnancy may make managing diabetes more difficult. Pregnant women or nursing mothers should be instructed to regularly consult their physician, pharmacist or nurse educator when using this product. Each case of diabetes is different and consequently an individual problem. Insulin injections, a balanced diet, regular exercise, and continuous cooperation with a physician are required to secure proper control. The patient should be told to do urine testing for sugar regulating. Consistent presence of sugar indicates the diabetes is not properly controlled.

WARNING

Patients who have been directed to mix two types of insulin should be aware that insulin hypodermic syringes may vary in amount of space between the bottom line and the needle. Because of this, patients should not change:
1. The order of mixture prescribed, or
2. The model and brand of the syringe or needle prescribed without first consulting a physician.

Failure to heed this warning can result in a dosage error.

ADVERSE REACTIONS

Insulin allergy occurs very rarely, but when it does, it may cause a serious reaction including a general skin rash over the body, shortness of breath, fast pulse, sweating, and a drop in blood pressure. If any of these symptoms develop the patient should seek immediate medical attention. In a very few diabetics, the skin where insulin has been injected may become red, swollen and itchy. It may occur if the injection is not properly made, if the skin is sensitive to the cleansing solution or if the patient is allergic to insulin. The patient should be instructed that if a local reaction occurs to notify a physician.
Patients with severe systemic allergic reactions to insulin (i.e. generalized urticaria, angioedema, anaphylaxis) should be skin tested with <u>each</u> new preparation to be used prior to initiation of therapy.
Insulin reaction
Insulin reaction (hypoglycemia) can occur if too much insulin is used, a meal is missed, or exercise or work is harder than normal. The symptoms, which usually come on suddenly, are hunger, dizziness, and sweating. Eating sugar or a sugar-sweetened product will normally correct the condition.
Hyperglycemia
Hyperglycemia can occur if a patient takes too little insulin, eats significantly more than usual, or develops a cold or other infection. The symptoms come on gradually. They are thirst, frequent passing of urine, and in severe cases nausea and abdominal pain.

HOW SUPPLIED

10 ml vials
100 units per ml
NDC #50445-222-01
Brochures, Time Action Profile Charts, Samples-Free to Physicians.

MIXTARD®

[mix ' tard]
U-100, Isophane purified pork insulin suspension and purified pork insulin injection

PRODUCT OVERVIEW

Mixtard is produced from the pork insulin molecule and has low immunogenic potential. Mixtard is a unique and stable premixture of 30% regular acting (Velosulin) and 70% intermediate acting (Insulatard NPH) purified pork insulins for more convenient and accurate insulin administration. Mixtard provides the rapid onset (½ hour) of Regular insulin and sustained duration (up to 24 hours) of NPH insulin.

MAJOR USES

Mixtard is indicated in the treatment of insulin-requiring diabetes mellitus. The route of administration for Mixtard is via subcutaneous injection. Mixtard is ideal for diabetic patients who have difficulty in mixing insulins. These patients include: elderly diabetics, diabetics with impaired vision or neurologic handicaps, or those diabetic patients simply unable to follow mixing instructions.

SAFETY INFORMATION

Mixtard insulin is a safe and an appropriate insulin to use or dispense for the diabetic patient when mixed insulin therapy is indicated. As with any insulin product in achieving maximum glycemic control, careful monitoring and changes in daily dosage or timing of injections may be necessary.

PRESCRIBING INFORMATION

MIXTARD®

[mix 'tard]

U-100 Pork, Isophane purified pork insulin suspension and purified pork insulin injection

WARNING

ANY CHANGE OF INSULIN SHOULD BE MADE CAUTIOUSLY ONLY UNDER MEDICAL SUPERVISION. WHEN CHANGING TO PURIFIED PORK INSULIN FROM ANY OTHER INSULIN A DOSAGE ADJUSTMENT, IF ANY, IS LIKELY TO BE A REDUCTION TO AVOID HYPOGLYCEMIA. CHANGES IN PURITY, STRENGTH (U-40, U-80, U-100), BRAND (MANUFACTURER), TYPE (LENTE, NPH, REGULAR, ETC.) AND/ OR SPECIES SOURCE (BEEF, PORK, BEEF/ PORK) MAY RESULT IN THE NEED FOR A CHANGE IN DOSAGE. IT IS NOT POSSIBLE TO IDENTIFY WHICH PATIENTS WILL REQUIRE A REDUCTION IN DOSAGE TO AVOID HYPOGLYCEMIA WHEN USING THIS INSULIN. ADJUSTMENT MAY BE NEEDED WITH THE FIRST DOSE OR OVER A PERIOD OF SEVERAL WEEKS. (SEE DOSAGE ADJUSTMENT SECTION). BE AWARE OF THE POSSIBILITY OF SYMPTOMS OF EITHER HYPOGLYCEMIA OR HYPERGLYCEMIA. SEE SECTIONS ENTITLED INSULIN REACTION AND HYPERGLYCEMIA.

DESCRIPTION

MIXTARD is a standard mixture of 30% VELOSULIN (corresponding to Regular insulin) and 70% INSULATARD NPH. The content of VELOSULIN gives the preparation a rapid onset of effect on the blood sugar, approximately $\frac{1}{2}$ hour after the injection. The content of INSULATARD NPH gives it a duration of up to 24 hours, depending on the size of the dose. The maximal effect lies between the 4th and the 8th hour after injection.

DIRECTIONS

Shake vial carefully to obtain a uniformly cloudy suspension of the crystals. Avoid heavy foaming. Do not use a vial if the insulin remains clear after it has been shaken. Also do not use it if you see lumps that float or stick to the sides.

MIXTARD can be mixed with any other Nordisk insulin preparation. In the mixture the different insulins will keep their original effect (stable mixtures).

Keep MIXTARD in a cold place (refrigerator) at 2 degrees to 10 degrees C (35–50 degrees F), but do not let it freeze or be exposed to direct sunlight. Do not use the insulin after the expiration date stamped on the label.

DOSAGE ADJUSTMENT

Reductions in dosage resulting from the switchover to this purified pork insulin from any other insulin have been observed to be in the neighborhood of 10–20% initially to maintain control. Adjustment may be needed either with the first dose or over a period of several weeks, and it is therefore recommended that the patient be monitored closely by a physician during the changeover and that dosage be adjusted downwards as necessary.

It is not possible to identify which patients will require a reduction in dose to avoid hypoglycemia when using purified pork insulins.

Be aware of the possibility of symptoms indicating the need for adjustment. See sections on Insulin Reaction or Hyperglycemia.

Use the Correct Syringe: MIXTARD is available in the U-100 strength (100 units per ml). The patient must understand the markings on the syringe and use only a syringe marked for U-100.

Avoid contamination and possible infection by following these instructions:

Reusable syringes and needles must be sterile when used. The best method of sterilization is to boil the syringe, plunger and needle in water for 5 minutes. If this is not possible, as when travelling, the parts may be sterilized by immersion for at least 5 minutes in a sterilizing liquid like ethyl alcohol, 70%. Do not use bathing, rubbing or medicated alcohol for sterilization. Remove all liquid from the syringe by pushing the plunger in and out several times and leave it to dry if alcohol has been used for sterilization. To prepare the dose, clean the rubber cap with cotton dipped in alcohol such as ethyl alcohol, 70%. The rubber cap must never be removed. Air is drawn into the syringe corresponding in amount to the prescribed amount of insulin. The needle is plunged through the cap in a downward position and the vial and syringe then inverted so that the air may be pushed out of the syringe into the vial. The prescribed amount of insulin is drawn into the syringe, and this is best done by drawing up slightly more insulin than required and then pushing the piston back to the desired mark. In this way any air bubbles are forced out of the syringe. Withdraw the needle from the vial without changing the position of the plunger in the syringe and lay aside the syringe so that it will not come in contact with any object. Disinfect the skin with a cotton swab dipped in a suitable antiseptic, such as ethyl alcohol, 70%. Pinch up the skin that has been disinfected and push the needle at a right angle quickly into the tissue under the skin. Do not inject deeper into a muscle or a vein. Give each injection in a different place from the previous one. If you instruct the patient to mix two types of insulin in the syringe, air should be injected into each vial first.

WARNING

Insulin injections, a balanced diet, and regular exercise are required to secure proper control of diabetes. Urine should be tested regularly for sugar. Consistent presence of sugar in the urine indicates that diabetes is not properly controlled. As with any drug, if you are pregnant or nursing a baby, seek professional advice before using this product.

ADVERSE REACTIONS

Insulin allergy occurs very rarely, but when it does, it may cause a serious reaction including a general skin rash over the body, shortness of breath, fast pulse, sweating, and a drop in blood pressure.

In a very few diabetics, the skin where insulin has been injected may become red, swollen and itchy. This local reaction may occur if the injection is not properly made, if the skin is sensitive to the cleansing solution or if the patient is allergic to insulin.

Patients with severe systemic reactions to insulin (i.e. generalized urticaria, angioedema, anaphylaxis) should be skin tested with <u>each</u> new preparation to be used prior to initiation of therapy with that preparation.

Insulin Reaction: Insulin reaction (hypoglycemia) can occur if the patient takes too much insulin, misses a meal or exercises or works harder than normal. The symptoms, which usually come on suddenly, are hunger, dizziness, and sweating. Eating sugar or a sugar-sweetened product will normally correct the condition.

Hyperglycemia: Hyperglycemia can occur if the patient takes too little insulin, eats significantly more than usual, or develops a cold or other infection. The symptoms are thirst, frequent passing of urine, and in severe cases nausea and abdominal pain. These symptoms generally come on gradually.

HOW SUPPLIED

10 ml vials
100 units per ml.
NDC #50445-300-01
Brochures, Time Action Profile Charts, Samples - Free to physicians.

VELOSULIN®

[vĕl"ō'sul"in]

U-100 Purified Pork, Purified Pork Injection (regular)

PRODUCT OVERVIEW

KEY FACTS

Velosulin is produced from the pork insulin molecule and has low immunogenic potential. Velosulin is the only buffered regular acting animal species insulin, making the product beneficial for insulin infusion pump therapy. Velosulin can be mixed with Nordisk Insulatard NPH reliably without usage restrictions and without loss of effectiveness over extended periods of time.

MAJOR USES

Velosulin is indicated in the treatment of insulin-requiring diabetes mellitus. The general route of administration for Velosulin is via subcutaneous injection although intramuscular or intravenous administration may be performed under the supervision of a physician. Velosulin has also proven beneficial for diabetic patients on insulin infusion pump therapy.

SAFETY INFORMATION

Velosulin is a safe and an appropriate insulin to use or dispense for the diabetic patient when regular insulin is indicated. As with any insulin product in achieving maximum glycemic control, careful monitoring and changes in daily dosage or timing of injections may be necessary.

PRESCRIBING INFORMATION

VELOSULIN®

[vĕl"ō'sul"in]

U-100 Purified Pork, Purified Pork Injection (regular)

WARNING

ANY CHANGE OF INSULIN SHOULD BE MADE CAUTIOUSLY ONLY UNDER MEDICAL SUPERVISION. WHEN CHANGING TO PURIFIED PORK INSULIN FROM ANY OTHER INSULIN A DOSAGE ADJUSTMENT, IF ANY, IS LIKELY TO BE A REDUCTION TO AVOID HYPOGLYCEMIA. CHANGES IN PURITY, STRENGTH (U-40, U-80, U-100), BRAND (MANUFACTURER), TYPE (LENTE, NPH, REGULAR, ETC.) AND/ OR SPECIES SOURCE (BEEF, PORK, BEEF/ PORK) MAY RESULT IN THE NEED FOR A CHANGE IN DOSAGE. IT IS NOT POSSIBLE TO IDENTIFY WHICH PATIENTS WILL REQUIRE A REDUCTION IN DOSAGE TO AVOID HYPOGLYCEMIA WHEN USING THIS INSULIN. ADJUSTMENT MAY BE NEEDED WITH THE FIRST DOSE OR OVER A PERIOD OF SEVERAL WEEKS. (SEE DOSAGE ADJUSTMENT SECTION). BE AWARE OF THE POSSIBILITY OF SYMPTOMS OF EITHER HYPOGLYCEMIA OR HYPERGLYCEMIA. SEE SECTIONS ENTITLED INSULIN REACTION AND HYPERGLYCEMIA.

DESCRIPTION

VELOSULIN is a clear solution of insulin obtained from pork pancreas. It has a rapid onset of effect on the blood sugar, approximately $\frac{1}{2}$ hour after the injection. The effect lasts up to approximately 8 hours with a maximal effect between the 1st and 3rd hour.

DIRECTIONS

Do not use the preparation if the color has become other than water clear or if the liquid has become viscous. VELOSULIN can be mixed with any other Nordisk insulin preparation. In the mixture the different insulins will keep their original effect (stable mixtures).

Keep VELOSULIN in a cold place (refrigerator) at 2 degrees to 10 degrees C (35–50 degrees F), but do not let it freeze or be exposed to direct sunlight. Do not use the insulin after the expiration date stamped on the label.

DOSAGE ADJUSTMENT

Reductions in dosage resulting from the switchover to this purified pork insulin from any other insulin have been observed to be in the neighborhood of 10–20% initially to maintain control.

Adjustment may be needed either with the first dose or over a period of several weeks, and it is therefore recommended that the patient be monitored closely by a physician during the changeover and that dosage be adjusted downwards as necessary.

It is not possible to identify which patients will require a reduction in dose to avoid hypoglycemia when using purified pork insulins.

Be aware of the possibility of symptoms indicating the need for adjustment. See sections on Insulin Reaction or Hyperglycemia.

Use the Correct Syringe: VELOSULIN is available in the U-100 strength (100 units per ml). The patient must understand the markings on the syringe and use only a syringe marked for U-100.

Avoid contamination and possible infection by following these instructions:

Reusable syringes and needles must be sterile when used. The best method of sterilization is to boil the syringe, plunger and needle in water for 5 minutes. If this is not possible, as when travelling, the parts may be sterilized by immersion for at least 5 minutes in a sterilizing liquid like ethyl alcohol, 70%. Do not use bathing, rubbing or medicated alcohol for sterilization. Remove all liquid from the syringe by pushing the plunger in and out several times and leave it to dry if alcohol has been used for sterilization. To prepare the dose, clean the rubber cap with cotton dipped in alcohol such as ethyl alcohol, 70%. The rubber cap must never be removed. Air is drawn into the syringe corresponding in amount to the prescribed amount of insulin. The needle is plunged through the cap in a downward position and the vial and syringe then inverted so that the air may be pushed out of the syringe into the vial. The prescribed amount of insulin is drawn into the syringe, and this is best done by drawing up slightly more insulin than required and then pushing the piston back to the desired mark. In this way any air bubbles are forced out of the syringe. Withdraw the needle from the vial without changing the position of the plunger in the syringe and lay aside the syringe so that it will not come in contact with any object. Disinfect the skin with a cotton swab dipped in a suitable antiseptic, such as ethyl alcohol, 70%. Pinch up the skin that has been disinfected and push the needle at a right angle quickly into the tissue under the skin. Do not inject deeper into a muscle or vein. Give each injection in a different place from the previous one. If instructed to mix two types of insulin in the syringe, air should be injected into each vial first.

Continued on next page

Nordisk-USA—Cont.

WARNING

Patients who have been directed to mix two types of insulin should be aware that insulin hypodermic syringes may vary in amount of space between the bottom line and the needle. Because of this, the patient should not change:

1. The order of mixture prescribed, or
2. The model and brand of the syringe or needle.

Failure to heed this warning can result in a dosage error. Insulin injections, a balanced diet, and regular exercise are required to secure proper control of diabetes. Urine should be tested regularly for sugar. Consistent presence of sugar in the urine indicates that diabetes is not properly controlled. As with any drug, if you are pregnant or nursing a baby, seek professional advice before using this product.

ADVERSE REACTIONS

Insulin allergy occurs very rarely, but when it does, it may cause a serious reaction including a general skin rash over the body, shortness of breath, fast pulse, sweating, and a drop in blood pressure.

In a very few diabetics, the skin where insulin has been injected may become red, swollen and itchy. This local reaction may occur if the injection is not properly made, if the skin is sensitive to the cleansing solution or if the patient is allergic to insulin.

Patients with severe systemic reactions to insulin (i.e. generalized urticaria, angioedema, anaphylaxis) should be skin tested with each new preparation to be used prior to initiation of therapy.

Insulin Reaction: Insulin reaction (hypoglycemia) can occur if the patient takes too much insulin, misses a meal or exercises or works harder than normal. The symptoms, which usually come on suddenly, are hunger, dizziness, and sweating. Eating sugar or a sugar-sweetened product will normally correct the condition.

Hyperglycemia: Hyperglycemia can occur if the patient takes too little insulin, eats significantly more than usual, or develops a cold or other infection. The symptoms are thirst, frequent passing of urine, and in severe cases nausea and abdominal pain. These symptoms generally come on gradually.

HOW SUPPLIED

10 ml vials
100 units per ml.
NDC # 50445-100-01
Brochures, Time Action Profile Charts, Samples—Free to Physicians.

VELOSULIN® HUMAN

[vĕl″ō′sul″in hyōō′men]
U-100 Human, Human insulin injection
(semi-synthetic)

PRODUCT OVERVIEW

KEY FACTS

Velosulin Human insulin is produced semi-synthetically by enzymatic conversion of the pork insulin molecule and has low immunogenic potential. Velosulin Human is the only buffered regular acting human insulin, making the product beneficial for insulin infusion pump therapy. Velosulin Human can be mixed with Nordisk Insulatard NPH Human reliably without usage restrictions, and without loss of effectiveness over extended periods of time.

MAJOR USES

Velosulin Human is indicated in the treatment of insulin-requiring diabetes mellitus. The general route of administration for Velosulin Human is via subcutaneous injection although intramuscular or intravenous administration may be performed under the supervision of a physician. Velosulin Human has also proven beneficial for diabetic patients on insulin infusion pump therapy.

SAFETY INFORMATION

Velosulin Human is a safe and an appropriate insulin to use or dispense for the diabetic patient when human insulin is indicated. As with any insulin product in achieving maximum glycemic control, careful monitoring and changes in daily dosage or timing of injections may be necessary.

PRESCRIBING INFORMATION

VELOSULIN® HUMAN

[vĕl″ō′sul″in hyōō′men]
U-100 Human, Human insulin injection
(semi-synthetic)

WARNING

This Nordisk human insulin is structurally identical to the insulin produced by the pancreas in the human body. This structural identity is obtained by enzymatic conversion of purified pork insulin. Any change of insulin should be made cautiously and only under medical supervision. Changes in purity, strength (U-40, U-100), brand (manufacturer), type (lente, NPH, regular) and/or species (beef, pork, beef/pork, human) may result in the need for a change in dosage. Adjustment may be needed with the first dose or over a period of several weeks. Be aware of the possibility of symptoms of either hypoglycemia or hyperglycemia. See sections entitled insulin reaction and hyperglycemia.

DESCRIPTION

Velosulin® Human is a clear solution of insulin. It has a rapid onset of effect on the blood sugar, approx. ½ hour after the injection. The effect lasts up to approximately 8 hours with a maximal effect between the 1st and 3rd hour. Do not use the preparation if the color has become other than water clear or if the liquid has become viscous.

DIRECTIONS

This preparation can be mixed with any other Nordisk human insulin preparation. In the mixture the different insulins will keep their original effects (stable mixtures).

Keep the insulin in a cold place (refrigerator), but do not let it freeze. Do not let it be exposed to direct sunlight. Do not use the insulin after the expiration date stamped on the label.

Use the correct syringe.

The volume of the dose depends on the number of units of insulin per ml.

Velosulin® Human is only available in the U-100 strength (100 units per ml).

Make sure of the markings on the syringe and use only a syringe marked for U-100.

Avoid contamination and possible infection by following below-mentioned instructions.

Reusable syringes and needles must be sterile when used. The best method of sterilization is to boil the syringe, plunger and needle in water for 5 minutes. If this is not possible, as when travelling, the parts may be sterilized by immersion for at least 5 minutes in sterilizing liquid like ethyl alcohol, 70%. Do not use bathing, rubbing or medicated alcohol for sterilization. Remove all liquid from the syringe by pushing plunger in and out several times and leave it to dry if alcohol has been used for sterilization. To prepare the dose, clean the rubber cap with cotton dipped in alcohol such as ethyl alcohol, 70%. The rubber cap must never be removed. Air is then drawn into the syringe corresponding in amount to the prescribed amount of insulin. The needle is plunged through the rubber cap in a downward position and the vial and syringe then inverted so that the air may be pushed out of the syringe into the vial. The prescribed amount of insulin is drawn into the syringe and this is best done by drawing up slightly more insulin than required and then pushing the piston back to the desired mark. In this way air bubbles are forced out of the syringe. Then withdraw the needle from the vial without changing the position of the plunger in the syringe and lay aside the syringe so that it will not come in contact with any object. Disinfect the skin with a cotton swab dipped in a suitable antiseptic, such as ethyl alcohol, 70%. Pinch up the skin that has been disinfected and push the needle at a right angle quickly into the tissue under the skin. Do not inject deeper into a muscle or a vein. Give each injection in a different place from the previous one. If instructed to mix two types of insulin in the syringe, air should be injected into each vial first.

Usage in Pregnancy

Pregnancy may make managing diabetes more difficult. Pregnant women or nursing mothers should be instructed to regularly consult a physician, pharmacist, or a nurse-educator when using this product.

Each case of diabetes is different and consequently an individual problem. Insulin injections, a balanced diet, regular exercise, and continuous cooperation with a physician are required to secure proper control. The patient should be instructed to do urine testing for sugar. Regular consistent presence of sugar indicates the diabetes is not properly controlled.

WARNING

Patients who have been directed to mix two types of insulin should be aware that insulin hypodermic syringes may vary in amount of space between the bottom line and the needle. Because of this, patients should not change:

1. The order of mixture prescribed, or
2. The model and brand of the syringe or needle prescribed without first consulting a physician.

Failure to heed this warning can result in a dosage error.

ADVERSE REACTIONS

Insulin allergy occurs very rarely, but when it does, it may cause a serious reaction including a general skin rash over the body, shortness of breath, fast pulse, sweating, and a drop in blood pressure. If any of these symptoms develop the patient should seek immediate medical attention.

In a very few diabetics, the skin where insulin has been injected may become red, swollen and itchy. It may occur if the injection is not properly made, if the skin is sensitive to the cleansing solution or if the patient is allergic to insulin. The patient should be instructed that if a local reaction occurs, to notify a physician.

Patients with severe systemic allergic reactions to insulin (i.e. generalized urticaria, angioedema, anaphylaxis) should be skin tested with each new preparation to be used prior to initiation of therapy.

Insulin Reaction

Insulin reaction (hypoglycemia) can occur if too much insulin is used, a meal is missed or exercise or work is harder than normal. The symptoms, which usually come on suddenly, are hunger, dizziness, and sweating. Eating sugar or a sugar- sweetened product will normally correct the condition.

Hyperglycemia

Hyperglycemia can occur if a patient takes too little insulin, eats significantly more than usual, or develops a cold or other infection. The symptoms come on gradually. They are thirst, frequent passing of urine, and in severe cases nausea and abdominal pain.

HOW SUPPLIED

10 ml vials
100 units per ml.
NDC #50445-111-01
Brochures, Time Action Profile Charts, Samples-Free to Physicians

Norwich Eaton Pharmaceuticals, Inc.

A Proctor & Gamble Company
(formerly Eaton Laboratories, Professional Products Group, Norwich Products or Consumer Products Group)
NORWICH, NY 13815-0231
(See also Procter & Gamble)

Literature on Norwich Eaton products sent to physicians on request.

Information on these Norwich Eaton products is based on labeling in effect July 25, 1986. Further information on these and other Norwich Eaton products may be obtained by direct inquiry to Medical Department,
Norwich Eaton Pharmaceuticals, Inc.
P.O. Box 191, Norwich, NY 13815-0191.

BUPRENEX® Ⓒ ℞

[būp′rĕn-ex]
(buprenorphine hydrochloride)
INJECTABLE

DESCRIPTION

BUPRENEX (buprenorphine hydrochloride), is a narcotic under the Controlled Substances Act due to its chemical deriviation from thebaine. Chemically, it is 17-(cyclopropylmethyl)-α-(1,1-dimethylethyl)-4, 5-epoxy-18, 19-dihydro-3-hydroxy-6-methoxy-α-methyl-6, 14-ethenomorphinan-7-methanol, hydrochloride [5α, 7α(S)]. Buprenorphine hydrochloride is a white powder, weakly acidic and with limited solubility in water. BUPRENEX is a clear, sterile, injectable agonist-antagonist analgesic intended for intravenous or intramuscular administration. Each ml of BUPRENEX contains 0.324 mg buprenorphine hydrochloride (equivalent to 0.3 mg buprenorphine), 50 mg anhydrous dextrose, water for injection and HCl to adjust pH. Buprenorphine hydrochloride has the molecular formula, $C_{29}H_{41}NO_4 \cdot HCl$, and the following structure:

Molecular weight: 504.09

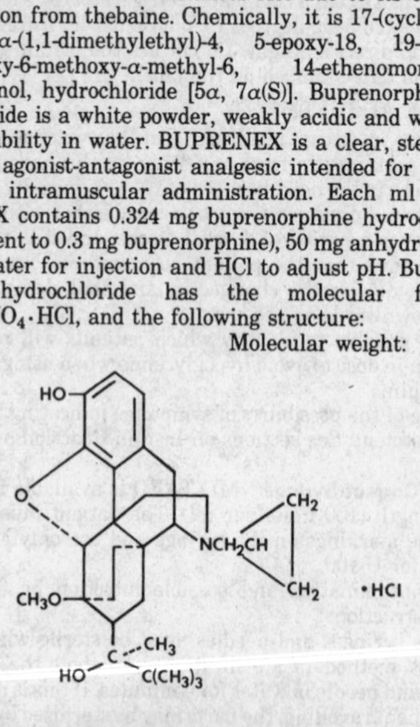

CLINICAL PHARMACOLOGY

BUPRENEX is a parenteral opiate analgesic approximately 30 times as potent as morphine sulfate. The onset of analgesic effect occurs 15 minutes after intramuscular injection and persists up to 6 hours. Peak analgesic activity usually is observed at 1 hour. When used intravenously, the time to onset and peak effect are shortened.

The limits of sensitivity of available analytical methodology precluded demonstration of bioequivalence between intramuscular and intravenous routes of administration. In postoperative patients, pharmacokinetic studies have shown elimination half-lives ranging from 1,2–7.2 hours (mean 2.2 hours) after intravenous administration of 0.3 mg of buprenorphine.
Buprenorphine, in common with morphine and other phenolic opiate analgesics, is metabolized by the liver and its clearance is related to hepatic blood flow. Studies in patients anesthetized with 0.5% halothane have shown that this anesthetic decreases hepatic blood flow by about 30%. This would lead to a decrease in buprenorphine clearance with a consequent small increase in plasma levels of buprenorphine. As such changes are unimportant clinically and do not persist in the postoperative phase, dosage adjustments are not required.

Mechanism of Analgesic Action: The exact mechanism of action of BUPRENEX has not been established. It has been proposed that BUPRENEX exerts its analgesic effect via high affinity binding to the opiate receptors in the central nervous system.
BUPRENEX is a partial agonist at one subclass of opiate receptors. *In vitro* and *in vivo* studies have shown that BUPRENEX has a high affinity for the μ subclass and dissociates from this receptor slowly. It is believed that these qualities of receptor binding contribute to the long duration of action and low level of physical dependence seen with BUPRENEX.

Narcotic Antagonist Activity: Buprenorphine demonstrates narcotic antagonist activity and has been shown to be equipotent with naloxone as an antagonist of morphine in the mouse tail flick test.

Cardiovascular Effects: BUPRENEX may cause a decrease or, rarely, an increase in pulse rate and blood pressure in some patients.

Effects on Respiration: A therapeutic dose of BUPRENEX (0.3 mg buprenorphine) can decrease respiratory rate in an equivalent manner to an equianalgesic dose of morphine (10 mg). One clinical study in normal volunteers indicated that the dose response curve for respiratory depression up to 1.2 mg was shallow. In another study in which BUPRENEX was administered in doses generally well in excess of those recommended, there was no clinically significant alteration in respiratory frequency, depth, and pattern, and in serial arterial blood gases. These data suggest that although the antagonist activity of buprenorphine becomes manifest at doses slightly above the recommended therapeutic range, doses in the recommended therapeutic range may produce severe respiratory depression in predisposed individuals (see WARNINGS).

INDICATIONS AND USAGE

BUPRENEX is indicated for the relief of moderate to severe pain.

CONTRAINDICATIONS

BUPRENEX should not be administered to patients who have been shown to be hypersensitive to the drug.

WARNINGS

Use in Narcotic-Dependent Patients: Because of the narcotic antagonist activity of BUPRENEX, use in the physically dependent individual may result in withdrawal effects.

Impaired Respiration: There have been occasional reports of clinically significant respiratory depression associated with buprenorphine. BUPRENEX should be used with caution in patients with either compromised respiratory function (e.g., chronic obstructive pulmonary disease, cor pulmonale, decreased respiratory reserve, hypoxia, hypercapnia, or preexisiting respiratory depression), or patients given other respiratory depressant drugs. In patients with respiratory depression naloxone or doxapram may be of some benefit, but in some patients these agents were not entirely effective. The use of assisted or controlled ventilation may be necessary. (See OVERDOSAGE.)

Use in Ambulatory Patients: BUPRENEX may impair the mental or physical abilities required for the performance of potentially dangerous tasks such as driving a car or operating machinery. Therefore, BUPRENEX should be administered with caution to ambulatory patients who should be warned to avoid such hazards.

Head Injury and Increased Intracranial Pressure: BUPRENEX, like other potent analgesics, may itself elevate cerebrospinal fluid pressure and should be used with caution in head injury, intracranial lesions and other circumstances where cerebrospinal pressure may be increased. BUPRENEX can produce miosis and changes in the level of consciousness which may interfere with patient evaluation.

Interaction with Other Central Nervous System Depressants: Patients receiving other narcotic analgesics, general anesthetics, phenothiazines, other tranquilizers, sedative hypnotics or other CNS depressants (including alcohol) concomitantly with BUPRENEX may exhibit an additive CNS depression. When such combined therapy is contemplated, the dose of one or both agents should be reduced.

PRECAUTIONS

General: BUPRENEX should be administered with caution in the elderly or debilitated and those with severe impairment of hepatic, pulmonary, or renal function; myxedema or hypothyroidism; adrenal cortical insufficiency (e.g., Addison's disease); CNS depression or coma; toxic psychoses; prostatic hypertrophy or urethral stricture; acute alcoholism; delirium tremens; or kyphoscoliosis. Naloxone is only partially effective in reversing the respiratory depression produced by BUPRENEX. Therefore, the primary management of BUPRENEX overdose should be mechanical assistance of respiration. (See **OVERDOSAGE Treatment** section).
Because BUPRENEX is metabolized by the liver, the activity of BUPRENEX may be altered in those individuals with impaired hepatic function.
BUPRENEX has been shown to increase intracholedochal pressure to a similar degree as other opiate analgesics, and thus should be administered with caution to patients with dysfunction of the biliary tract.

Information for Patients: The effects of BUPRENEX, particularly drowsiness, may be potentiated by other centrally acting agents such as alcohol or benzodiazepines. It is particularly important that in these circumstances patients must not drive or operate machinery. BUPRENEX has some pharmacologic effects similar to morphine which in susceptible patients may lead to self-administration of the drug when pain no longer exists. Patients must not exceed the dosage of BUPRENEX prescribed by their physician. Patients should be urged to consult their physician if other prescription medications are currently being used or are prescribed for future use.

Drug Interactions: Although specific information is not presently available, care should be taken when BUPRENEX is used in combination with central nervous system depressant drugs and MAO inhibitors. Drug interactions common to other potent opiate analgesics may also occur with BUPRENEX (see WARNINGS). There is one report of respiratory and cardiovascular collapse in a patient who received therapeutic doses of BUPRENEX and diazepam. There is another report of a suspected interaction between BUPRENEX and phenprocoumon in which a purpuric response was noted.

Impairment of Fertility: The effects of BUPRENEX on fertility and gestation indices were investigated in rats by the subcutaneous and intramuscular routes at doses 10 to 1,000 times the proposed human doses. Dystocia was noted in dams treated with 1,000 times the human dose. No effects on fertility or gestation were noted in these Segment I studies.

Pregnancy: Pregnancy Category C. Reproduction studies have been performed in the rat at doses which ranged from 10 to 1,000 times the proposed human dose by the subcutaneous and intramuscular routes and 160 times the proposed human dose by the intravenous route. By the intramuscular route, BUPRENEX produced mild but statistically significant ($p < 0.05$) post-implantation losses and early fetal deaths of 10 and 100 but not 1,000 times the proposed human dose. No fetal malformations were noted in rats at any dose when BUPRENEX was administered by subcutaneous, intramuscular, or intravenous routes. In rabbits, intramuscularly administered BUPRENEX produced a dose-related trend for extra rib formation which attained statistical significance ($p < 0.01$) at 1,000 times the proposed human dose. By the intravenous route, doses in rats of 40 and 160 times the proposed human dose of BUPRENEX caused a slight increase in post-implantation losses that may have been treatment-related. No major fetal malformations were noted in drug treated groups when administered by intramuscular or intravenous routes.
There are no adequate and well-controlled studies in pregnant women. BUPRENEX should be used during pregnancy only if the potential benefit justifies the potential risk to the fetus.

Labor and Delivery: The safety of BUPRENEX given during labor and delivery has not been established.

Nursing Mothers: An apparent lack of milk production during general reproduction studies with BUPRENEX in rats caused decreased viability and lactation indices. It is unknown at this time whether or not BUPRENEX is excreted in human milk. Despite the lack of specific knowledge on this issue, it is reasonable to assume that BUPRENEX will enter human milk and caution should be exercised in the use of BUPRENEX when it is administered to nursing mothers.

Pediatric Use: Safety and effectiveness in children have not been established.

ADVERSE REACTIONS

The most frequent side effect in clinical studies involving 1,133 patients was sedation which occurred in approximately two-thirds of the patients. Although sedated, these patients could easily be aroused to an alert state.

Other less frequent adverse reactions occurring in 5–10% of the patients were:

Nausea	Dizziness/Vertigo

Occurring in 1–5% of the patients:

Sweating	Headache
Hypotension	Nausea/Vomiting
Vomiting	Hypoventilation
Miosis	

The following adverse reactions were reported to have occurred in less than 1% of the patients:

CNS Effect: confusion, blurred vision, euphoria, weakness/fatigue, dry mouth, nervousness, depression, slurred speech, paresthesia.

Cardiovascular: hypertension, tachycardia, bradycardia.

Gastrointestinal: constipation.

Respiratory: dyspnea, cyanosis.

Dermatological: pruritus.

Ophthalmological: diplopia, visual abnormalities.

Miscellaneous: injection site reaction, urinary retention, dreaming, flushing/warmth, chills/cold, tinnitus, conjunctivitis, Wenckebach block, and psychosis.

Other effects observed infrequently include malaise, hallucinations, depersonalization, coma, dyspepsia, flatulence, apnea, rash, amblyopia, tremor, and pallor.
The following reaction has been reported to occur rarely: loss of appetite. In addition, single reports of dysphoria/agitation, diarrhea, urticaria, and convulsions/lack of muscle coordination have been reported.
In the United Kingdom, buprenorphine hydrochloride was made available under monitored release regulation during the first year of sale, and yielded data from 1,736 physicians or 9,123 patients (17,120 administrations). No important new adverse effects attributable to buprenorphine hydrochloride were observed.

DRUG ABUSE AND DEPENDENCE

Buprenorphine hydrochloride is a partial agonist of the morphine type; i.e., it has certain opioid properties which may lead to psychic dependence of the morphine type due to an opiate-like euphoric component of the drug. Direct dependence studies have shown little physical dependence upon withdrawal of the drug. However, caution should be used in prescribing to individuals who are known to be drug abusers or ex-narcotic addicts. The drug may not substitute in acutely dependent narcotic addicts due to its antagonist component.

OVERDOSAGE

Manifestations: Because of the antagonist properties of BUPRENEX at higher doses, its safety in acute overdosage is expected to be greater than that of other opioid analgesics. However, there is limited experience of accidental or intentional overdosage at the present time. Doses 10 to 20 times the normal 0.3 mg dose of BUPRENEX have been administered intravenously without producing clinically significant respiratory effects. Extrapolating from the animal pharmacology of the agent, large doses may produce CNS depression with manifestations in the respiratory and cardiovascular systems. In rodents, the lethal dose is at least 1,000 times the effective dose. The LD_{50} in mice was 26, 94, and 261 mg/kg for intravenous, intraperitoneal, and oral administration, respectively. The LD_{50} in the rat was 30, 243, and 600 mg/kg for intravenous, intraperitoneal, and oral administration, respectively.

Treatment: The respiratory and cardiac status of the patients should be monitored carefully. Primary attention should be given to the reestablishment of adequate respiratory exchange through provision of a patent airway and institution of assisted or controlled ventilation. Oxygen, intravenous fluids, vasopressors, and other supportive measures should be employed as indicated. Experience has shown that naloxone may be of value in the management of buprenorphine overdosage. Doxapram (a respiratory stimulant) also has been used.

DOSAGE AND ADMINISTRATION

The usual dosage for persons 13 years of age and over is 1 ml BUPRENEX (0.3 mg buprenorphine) given by intramuscular or slow intravenous injection at up to 6-hour intervals as needed.
Occasionally, it may be necessary to administer up to 0.6 mg depending on the severity of the pain and the response of the patient. At this time, there is insufficient data to recommend single doses greater than 0.6 mg for long-term use.
Parenteral drug products should be inspected visually for particulate matter and discoloration prior to administration, whenever solution and container permit.

HOW SUPPLIED

BUPRENEX (buprenorphine hydrochloride) is supplied in clear glass snap-ampuls of 1 ml (0.3 mg buprenorphine). **NDC** 0149-0757-01
Avoid excessive heat (over 104°F or 40°C). Protect from prolonged exposure to light.

Continued on next page

Norwich Eaton—Cont.

CAUTION
Federal law prohibits dispensing without prescription.

Manufactured by:
Reckitt & Colman Pharmaceutical Division
Kingston-upon-Hull
England HU8 7DS
Distributed by:
Norwich Eaton Pharmaceuticals, Inc.
Norwich, New York 13815
A Procter & Gamble Company
under license from Reckitt & Colman Products, Limited
Buprenex® is a trademark of Reckitt & Colman (Overseas) Limited.
REVISED JUNE 1985 BUP-P4

COMHIST® LA ℞
[*kŏm 'hist*]

DESCRIPTION
Each COMHIST LA yellow and clear capsule for oral administration contains:
chlorpheniramine maleate .... 4 mg
phenyltoloxamine citrate .... 50 mg
phenylephrine hydrochloride .... 20 mg
in a special base to provide a prolonged therapeutic effect. This product contains ingredients of the following therapeutic classes: antihistamine and decongestant.
Chlorpheniramine maleate is an antihistamine having the chemical name γ-(4-chlorophenyl)-N,N-dimethyl-2-pyridinepropanamine,(Z)-2-butenedioate(1:1) with the following structure:

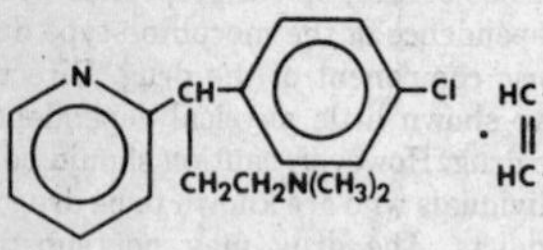

Phenyltoloxamine citrate is an antihistamine having the chemical name N,N-dimethyl-2-(α-phenyl-o-tolyloxy) ethylamine dihydrogen citrate with the following structure:

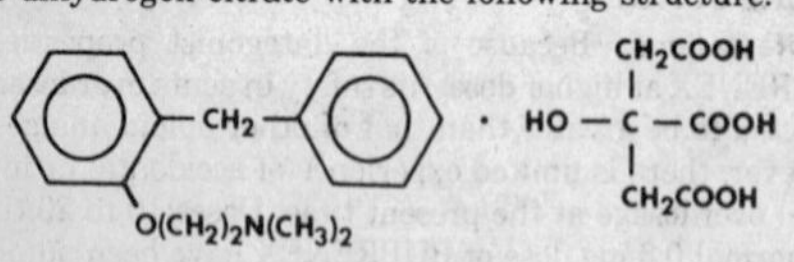

Phenylephrine hydrochloride is a decongestant having the chemical name 3-hydroxy-α[(methylamino)methyl]benzene-methanol hydrochloride with the following structure:

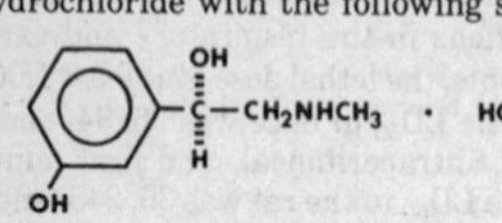

INACTIVE INGREDIENTS
Each capsule contains FD&C Blue #2, edible black ink, gelatin, sugar spheres, D&C Yellow #10, FD&C Yellow #6, and other ingredients.

CLINICAL PHARMACOLOGY
Chlorpheniramine maleate is an alkylamine-type antihistamine while phenyltoloxamine citrate belongs to the ethanolamine chemical class. The antihistamines in COMHIST LA act by competing with histamine for H_1 histamine receptor sites, thereby preventing the action of histamine on the cell. Clinically, chlorpheniramine and phenyltoloxamine suppress the histamine-mediated symptoms of allergic rhinitis, relieving sneezing, rhinorrhea, and itching of the eyes, nose, and throat.
Phenylephrine hydrochloride is an α-adrenergic receptor agonist (sympathomimetic) which produces vasoconstriction by stimulating α-receptors within the mucosa of the respiratory tract. Clinically, phenylephrine shrinks swollen mucous membranes, reduces tissue hyperemia, edema, and nasal congestion, and increases nasal airway patency.

INDICATIONS AND USAGE
COMHIST LA is indicated for the relief of rhinorrhea and congestion associated with seasonal and/or perennial allergic rhinitis and vasomotor rhinitis.

CONTRAINDICATIONS
COMHIST LA is contraindicated in persons hypersensitive to any of its components. It should not be administered to children under 12 years of age, patients with severe hypertension, narrow angle glaucoma, or asthmatic symptoms, or patients taking monoamine oxidase inhibitors.

WARNINGS
Chlorpheniramine maleate and phenyltoloxamine citrate should be used with extreme caution in patients with stenosing peptic ulcer, pyloroduodenal obstruction, prostatic hypertrophy, or bladder neck obstruction. These compounds have an atropine-like action and therefore should be used with caution in patients with a history of bronchial asthma, increased intraocular pressure, cardiovascular disease, or hypertension. Sympathomimetic amines should be used with caution in patients with hypertension, diabetes mellitus, heart disease, increased intraocular pressure, hyperthyroidism, or prostatic hypertrophy.

PRECAUTIONS
Information for Patients: This product may cause sedation. Patients should be cautioned against engaging in activities requiring mental alertness, such as driving a car or operating machinery.
Drug Interactions: The sedative effects of chlorpheniramine maleate and phenyltoloxamine citrate are additive to the CNS depressant effects of alcohol, hypnotics, sedatives, and tranquilizers. COMHIST LA should not be used in patients taking monoamine oxidase inhibitors.
Pregnancy: Pregnancy Category C. Animal reproduction studies have not been conducted with COMHIST LA. It is also not known whether COMHIST LA can cause fetal harm when administered to a pregnant woman or can affect reproduction capacity. COMHIST LA should be given to pregnant woman only if clearly needed.
Nursing Mothers: It is not known whether the drugs in COMHIST LA are excreted in human milk. Because many drugs are excreted in human milk and because of the potential for serious adverse reactions in nursing infants, a decision should be made whether to discontinue nursing or to discontinue the product, taking into account the importance of the drug to the mother.
Pediatric Use: Safety and effectiveness of COMHIST LA in children below the age of 12 have not been established.

ADVERSE REACTIONS
General: Urticaria, drug rash, dryness of mouth, nose, and throat.
Cardiovascular System: Hypotension, headache, palpitations.
Hematologic System: Thrombocytopenia, agranulocytosis, leukopenia.
Nervous System: Sedation, dizziness, excitation (especially in children), nervousness, insomnia, blurred vision, convulsions.
Gastrointestinal System: Epigastric distress, anorexia, nausea, vomiting, diarrhea, constipation.
Genitourinary System: Urinary frequency, urinary retention.
Respiratory System: Thickening of bronchial secretions, tightness of chest and wheezing, nasal stuffiness.

OVERDOSAGE
The treatment of overdosage should provide symptomatic and supportive care. If the amount ingested is considered dangerous or excessive, induce vomiting with ipecac syrup unless the patient is convulsing, comatose, or has lost the gag reflex, in which case perform gastric lavage using a large-bore tube. If indicated, follow with activated charcoal and a saline cathartic. Since the effects of COMHIST LA may last up to 12 hours, treatment should be continued for at least that length of time.

DOSAGE AND ADMINISTRATION
Adults and children 12 years of age and older—1 capsule every 8 to 12 hours; not recommended for children under 12 years of age.

HOW SUPPLIED
COMHIST LA is available as a yellow and clear capsule imprinted "COMHIST LA" and "01490446".
NDC 0149-0446-01 Bottle of 100

CAUTION
Federal law prohibits dispensing without prescription.
Manufactured for
Norwich Eaton Pharmaceuticals, Inc.
Norwich, New York 13815
A Procter & Gamble Company
by **KV Pharmaceutical Company**
St. Louis, Missouri 63144
REVISED SEPTEMBER 1985 COMLA-X7

DANTRIUM® ℞
[*dan 'trē-um*]
(dantrolene sodium)
CAPSULES

Dantrium (dantrolene sodium) has a potential for hepatotoxicity, and should not be used in conditions other than those recommended. Symptomatic hepatitis (fatal and non-fatal) has been reported at various dose levels of the drug. The incidence reported in patients taking up to 400 mg/day is much lower than in those taking doses of 800 mg or more per day. Even sporadic short courses of these higher dose levels within a treatment regimen markedly increased the risk of serious hepatic injury. Liver dysfunction as evidenced by blood chemical abnormalities alone (liver enzyme elevations) has been observed in patients exposed to Dantrium for varying periods of time. Overt hepatitis has occurred at varying intervals after initiation of therapy, but has been most frequently observed between the third and twelfth month of therapy. The risk of hepatic injury appears to be greater in females, in patients over 35 years of age, and in patients taking other medication(s) in addition to Dantrium (dantrolene sodium). Dantrium should be used only in conjunction with appropriate monitoring of hepatic function including frequent determination of SGOT or SGPT. If no observable benefit is derived from the administration of Dantrium after a total of 45 days, therapy should be discontinued. The lowest possible effective dose for the individual patient should be prescribed.

DESCRIPTION
The chemical formula of Dantrium (dantrolene sodium) is hydrated 1-[[[5-(4-nitrophenyl)-2-furanyl]methylene]amino]-2, 4-imidazolidinedione sodium salt. It is an orange powder, slightly soluble in water, but due to its slightly acidic nature the solubility increases somewhat in alkaline solution. The anhydrous salt has a molecular weight of 336. The hydrated salt contains approximately 15% water (3½ moles) and has a molecular weight of 399. The structural formula for the hydrated salt is:

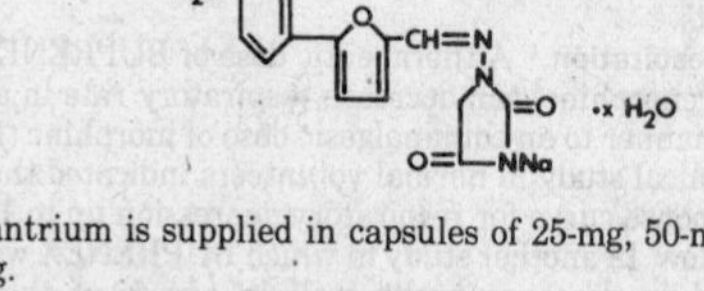

Dantrium is supplied in capsules of 25-mg, 50-mg, and 100-mg.

INACTIVE INGREDIENTS
Each capsule contains edible black ink, gelatin, lactose, magnesium stearate, FD&C Red #3, starch, talc, titanium dioxide, and may contain one or more of the following: D&C Blue #2, D&C Red #33, iron oxide red, D&C Yellow #10, FD&C Yellow #6, iron oxide yellow.

CLINICAL PHARMACOLOGY
In isolated nerve-muscle preparation, Dantrium has been shown to produce relaxation by affecting the contractile response of the skeletal muscle at a site beyond the myoneural junction, directly on the muscle itself. In skeletal muscle, Dantrium dissociates the excitation-contraction coupling, probably by interfering with the release of Ca^{++} from the sarcoplasmic reticulum. This effect appears to be more pronounced in fast muscle fibers as compared to slow ones, but generally affects both. A central nervous system effect occurs, with drowsiness, dizziness and generalized weakness occasionally present. Although Dantrium does not appear to directly affect the CNS, the extent of its indirect effect is unknown. The absorption of Dantrium after oral administration in humans is incomplete and slow but consistent, and dose-related blood levels are obtained. The duration and intensity of skeletal muscle relaxation is related to the dosage and blood levels. The mean biologic half-life of Dantrium in adults is 8.7 hours after a 100-mg dose. Specific metabolic pathways in the degradation and elimination of Dantrium in human subjects have been established. Metabolic patterns are similar in adults and children. In addition to the parent compound, dantrolene, which is found in measurable amounts in blood and urine, the major metabolites noted in body fluids are the 5-hydroxy analog and the acetamido analog. Since Dantrium is probably metabolized by hepatic microsomal enzymes, enhancement of its metabolism by other drugs is possible. However, neither phenobarbital nor diazepam appears to affect Dantrium metabolism.
Clinical experience in the management of fulminant human malignant hyperthermia, as well as experiments conducted in malignant hyperthermia susceptible swine, have revealed that the administration of intravenous dantrolene, combined with indicated supportive measures, is effective in reversing the hypermetabolic process of malignant hyperthermia. Known differences between human and swine malignant hyperthermia are minor. The prophylactic administration of oral or intravenous dantrolene to malignant hyperthermia susceptible swine will attenuate or prevent the development of signs of malignant hyperthermia in a manner dependent upon the dosage of dantrolene administered and the intensity of the malignant hyperthermia triggering stimulus. Limited clinical experience with the administration of oral dantrolene to patients judged malignant hyperthermia susceptible, when combined with clinical experi-

ence in the use of intravenous dantrolene for the treatment of malignant hyperthermia and data derived from the above cited animal model experiments, suggest that oral dantrolene will also attenuate or prevent the development of signs of human malignant hyperthermia, provided that currently accepted practices in the management of such patients are adhered to (see INDICATIONS AND USAGE); intravenous dantrolene should also be available for use should the signs of malignant hyperthermia appear.

INDICATIONS AND USAGE

In Chronic Spasticity:

Dantrium is indicated in controlling the manifestations of clinical spasticity resulting from upper motor neuron disorders (e.g. spinal cord injury, stroke, cerebral palsy, or multiple sclerosis). It is of particular benefit to the patient whose functional rehabilitation has been retarded by the sequelae of spasticity. Such patients must have presumably reversible spasticity where relief of spasticity will aid in restoring residual function. Dantrium is not indicated in the treatment of skeletal muscle spasm resulting from rheumatic disorders.

If improvement occurs, it will ordinarily occur within the dosage titration (see DOSAGE AND ADMINISTRATION), and will be manifested by a decrease in the severity of spasticity and the ability to resume a daily function not quite attainable without Dantrium.

Occasionally, subtle but meaningful improvement in spasticity may occur with Dantrium therapy. In such instances information regarding improvement should be solicited from the patient and those who are in constant daily contact and attendance with him. Brief withdrawal of Dantrium for a period of 2 to 4 days will frequently demonstrate exacerbation of the manifestations of spasticity and may serve to confirm a clinical impression.

A decision to continue the administration of Dantrium on a long-term basis is justified if introduction of the drug into the patient's regimen:

- produces a significant reduction in painful and/ or disabling spasticity such as clonus, or
- permits a significant reduction in the intensity and/or degree of nursing care required, or
- rids the patient of any annoying manifestation of spasticity considered important by the patient himself.

In Malignant Hyperthermia:

Oral Dantrium is also indicated preoperatively to prevent or attenuate the development of signs of malignant hyperthermia in known, or strongly suspect, malignant hyperthermia susceptible patients who require anesthesia and/or surgery. Currently accepted clinical practices in the management of such patients must still be adhered to (careful monitoring for early signs of malignant hyperthermia, minimizing exposure to triggering mechanisms and prompt use of intravenous dantrolene sodium and indicated supportive measures should signs of malignant hyperthermia appear); see also the package insert for Dantrium (dantrolene sodium) Intravenous.

Oral Dantrium should be administered following a malignant hyperthermic crisis to prevent recurrence of the signs of malignant hyperthermia.

CONTRAINDICATIONS

Active hepatic disease, such as hepatitis and cirrhosis, is a contraindication for use of Dantrium. Dantrium is contraindicated where spasticity is utilized to sustain upright posture and balance in locomotion or whenever spasticity is utilized to obtain or maintain increased function.

WARNINGS

It is important to recognize that fatal and non-fatal liver disorders of an idiosyncratic or hypersensitivity type may occur with Dantrium therapy.

At the start of Dantrium therapy, it is desirable to do liver function studies (SGOT, SGPT, alkaline phosphatase, total bilirubin) for a baseline or to establish whether there is preexisting liver disease. If baseline liver abnormalities exist and are confirmed, there is a clear possibility that the potential for Dantrium hepatotoxicity could be enhanced, although such a possibility has not yet been established.

Liver function studies (e.g. SGOT or SGPT) should be performed at appropriate intervals during Dantrium therapy. If such studies reveal abnormal values, therapy should generally be discontinued. Only where benefits of the drug have been of major importance to the patient, should reinitiation or continuation of therapy be considered. Some patients have revealed a return to normal laboratory values in the face of continued therapy while others have not.

If symptoms compatible with hepatitis, accompanied by abnormalities in liver functions tests or jaundice appear, Dantrium should be discontinued. If caused by Dantrium and detected early, the abnormalities in liver function characteristically have reverted to normal when the drug was discontinued.

Dantrium therapy has been reinstituted in a few patients who have developed clinical and/or laboratory evidence of hepatocellular injury. If such reinstitution of therapy is done, it should be attempted only in patients who clearly need Dantrium and only after previous symptoms and laboratory abnormalities have cleared. The patient should be hospitalized and the drug should be restarted in very small and gradually increasing doses. Laboratory monitoring should be frequent and the drug should be withdrawn immediately if there is any indication of recurrent liver involvement. Some patients have reacted with unmistakable signs of liver abnormality upon administration of a challenge dose, while others have not.

Dantrium should be used with particular caution in females and in patients over 35 years of age in view of apparent greater likelihood of drug-induced, potentially fatal, hepatocellular disease in these groups.

Long-term safety of Dantrium in humans has not been established. Chronic studies in rats, dogs and monkeys at dosages greater than 30 mg/kg/day showed growth or weight depression and signs of hepatopathy and possible occlusion nephropathy, all of which were reversible upon cessation of treatment. Sprague-Dawley female rats fed dantrolene sodium for 18 months at dosage levels of 15, 30 and 60 mg/kg/day showed an increased incidence of benign and malignant mammary tumors compared with concurrent controls and, at the highest dosage, an increase in the incidence of hepatic lymphangiomas and hepatic angiosarcomas. These effects were not seen in $2\frac{1}{2}$-year studies in Sprague-Dawley or Fischer 344 rats or in 2-year studies in mice of the HaM/ICR strain. Carcinogenicity in humans cannot be fully excluded, so that this possible risk of chronic administration must be weighed against the benefits of the drug (i.e., after a brief trial) for the individual patient.

Usage in Pregnancy: The safety of Dantrium for use in women who are or who may become pregnant has not been established. Dantrium should not be used in nursing mothers.

Usage in Children: The long-term safety of Dantrium in children under the age of 5 years has not been established. Because of the possibility that adverse effects of the drug could become apparent only after many years, a benefit-risk consideration of the long-term use of Dantrium is particularly important in pediatric patients.

Drug Interactions: While a definite drug interaction with estrogen therapy has not yet been established, caution should be observed if the two drugs are to be given concomitantly. Hepatotoxicity has occurred more often in women over 35 years of age receiving concomitant estrogen therapy.

PRECAUTIONS

Dantrium should be used with caution in patients with impaired pulmonary function, particularly those with obstructive pulmonary disease, and in patients with severely impaired cardiac function due to myocardial disease. It should be used with caution in patients with a history of previous liver disease or dysfunction (See WARNINGS).

Patients should be cautioned against driving a motor vehicle or participating in hazardous occupations while taking Dantrium. Caution should be exercised in the concomitant administration of tranquilizing agents.

Dantrium might possibly evoke a photosensitivity reaction; patients should be cautioned about exposure to sunlight while taking it.

ADVERSE REACTIONS

The most frequently occurring side effects of Dantrium have been drowsiness, dizziness, weakness, general malaise, fatigue, and diarrhea. These are generally transient, occurring early in treatment, and can often be obviated by beginning with a low dose and increasing dosage gradually until an optimal regimen is established. Diarrhea may be severe and may necessitate temporary withdrawal of Dantrium therapy. If diarrhea recurs upon readministration of Dantrium, therapy should probably be withdrawn permanently.

Other less frequent side effects, listed according to system are:

Gastrointestinal: Constipation, GI bleeding, anorexia, swallowing difficulty, gastric irritation, abdominal cramps.

Hepatobiliary: Hepatitis (See WARNINGS).

Neurologic: Speech disturbance, seizure, headache, lightheadedness, visual disturbance, diplopia, alteration of taste, insomnia.

Cardiovascular: Tachycardia, erratic blood pressure, phlebitis.

Psychiatric: Mental depression, mental confusion, increased nervousness.

Urogenital: Increased urinary frequency, crystalluria, hematuria, difficult erection, urinary incontinence and/or nocturia, difficult urination and/or urinary retention.

Integumentary: Abnormal hair growth, acne-like rash, pruritus, urticaria, eczematoid eruption, sweating.

Musculoskeletal: Myalgia, backache.

Respiratory: Feeling of suffocation.

Special Senses: Excessive tearing.

Hypersensitivity: Pleural effusion with pericarditis.

Other: Chills and fever.

DOSAGE AND ADMINISTRATION

For Use in Chronic Spasticity:

Prior to the administration of Dantrium, consideration should be given to the potential response to treatment. A decrease in spasticity sufficient to allow a daily function not otherwise attainable should be the therapeutic goal of treatment with Dantrium. Refer to INDICATIONS AND USAGE section for description of response to be anticipated.

It is important to establish a therapeutic goal (regain and maintain a specific function such as therapeutic exercise program, utilization of braces, transfer maneuvers, etc.) before beginning Dantrium therapy. Dosage should be increased until the maximum performance compatible with the dysfunction due to underlying disease is achieved. No further increase in dosage is then indicated.

Usual Dosage: It is important that the dosage be titrated and individualized for maximum effect. The lowest dose compatible with optimal response is recommended.

In view of the potential for liver damage in long-term Dantrium use, therapy should be stopped if benefits are not evident within 45 days.

Adults: Begin therapy with 25 mg once daily; increase to 25 mg two, three, or four times daily and then by increments of 25 mg up to as high as 100 mg two, three, or four times daily if necessary. As most patients will respond to a dose of 400 mg/day or less, rarely should doses higher than 400 mg/day be used (see Box Warning.)

Each dosage level should be maintained for four to seven days to determine the patient's response. The dose should not be increased beyond, and may even have to be reduced to, the amount at which the patient received maximal benefit without adverse effects.

Children: A similar approach should be utilized starting with 0.5 mg/kg of body weight twice daily; this is increased to 0.5 mg/kg three or four times daily and then by increments of 0.5 mg/kg up to as high as 3.0 mg/kg two, three, or four times daily, if necessary. Doses higher than 100 mg four times daily should not be used in children.

For Malignant Hyperthermia:

Preoperatively: Administer 4 to 8 mg/kg/day of oral Dantrium in 3 or 4 divided doses for one or two days prior to surgery, with the last dose being given approximately 3 to 4 hours before scheduled surgery with a minimum of water. This dosage will usually be associated with skeletal muscle weakness and sedation (sleepiness or drowsiness); adjustment can usually be made within the recommended dosage range to avoid incapacitation or excessive gastrointestinal irritation (including nausea and/or vomiting).

Post Crisis Follow-up:

Oral Dantrium should also be administered following a malignant hyperthermia crisis, in doses of 4 to 8 mg/kg per day in four divided doses, for a one to three day period to prevent recurrence of the manifestations of malignant hyperthermia.

OVERDOSAGE

For acute overdosage, general supportive measures should be employed along with immediate gastric lavage.

Intravenous fluids should be administered in fairly large quantities to avert the possibility of crystalluria. An adequate airway should be maintained and artificial resuscitation equipment should be at hand. Electrocardiographic monitoring should be instituted, and the patient carefully observed. To date, no experience has been reported with dialysis and its value in Dantrium overdosage is not known.

HOW SUPPLIED

Dantrium (dantrolene sodium) is available in:

25 mg opaque, orange and light brown capsules:

NDC 0149-0030-05 bottle of 100

NDC 0149-0030-66 bottle of 500

NDC 0149-0030-77 hospital unit-dose strips in boxes of 100.

50-mg opaque, orange and dark brown capsules:

NDC 0149-0031-05 bottle of 100.

100-mg opaque, orange and light brown capsules:

NDC 0149-0033-05 bottle of 100

NDC 0149-0033-77 hospital unit-dose strips in boxes of 100.

Address medical inquiries to Norwich Eaton Pharmaceuticals, Inc. Medical Department, Norwich, NY 13815.

Manufactured by

Eaton Laboratories, Inc.

Manati, Puerto Rico 00701

Distributed by

Norwich Eaton Pharmaceuticals, Inc.

Norwich, New York 13815

A Procter & Gamble Company

REVISED JANUARY 1985 DANCP-P8

Continued on next page

Norwich Eaton—Cont.

DANTRIUM® ℞
[*dan 'trē-um*]
(dantrolene sodium)
INTRAVENOUS

DESCRIPTION

Dantrium Intravenous is a sterile, lyophilized formulation of dantrolene sodium, and in this form provides a preparation for intravenous use. Each 70 ml vial contains 20 mg dantrolene sodium, 3000 mg mannitol, and sufficient sodium hydroxide to yield a pH of approximately 9.5 when reconstituted with 60 ml sterile water for injection U.S.P. (without a bacteriostatic agent).
Dantrolene sodium is classified as a direct-acting skeletal muscle relaxant. Chemically, dantrolene sodium is hydrated 1-[[[5-(4-nitrophenyl)-2-furanyl]methylene]amino] -2,4-imidazolidinedione sodium salt. The structural formula for the hydrated salt is:

O_2N–C₆H₄–(furan)–CH=NN–C=O / NNa / CH_2–C=O · $3\frac{1}{2}H_2O$

The hydrated salt contains approximately 15% water ($3\frac{1}{2}$ moles) and has a molecular weight of 399. The anhydrous salt (dantrolene) has a molecular weight of 336.

ACTIONS

Dantrolene sodium is a muscle relaxant acting specifically on skeletal muscle. It does not affect neuromuscular transmission nor does it have measurable effects on the electrically excitable surface membrane. Studies have shown that in the presence of dantrolene sodium, the responses of the muscle to caffeine are decreased or delayed.
In isolated muscle preparations, dantrolene sodium uncouples the excitation and contraction of skeletal muscle, probably by interfering with the release of calcium from the sarcoplasmic reticulum.
In the anesthetic-induced malignant hyperthermia syndrome, evidence points to an intrinsic abnormality of muscle tissue. In affected humans and swine, it has been postulated that "triggering agents" induce a sudden rise in myoplasmic calcium either by preventing the sarcoplasmic reticulum from accumulating calcium adequately, or by accelerating its release. This rise in myoplasmic calcium activates acute catabolic processes common to the malignant hyperthermia crisis.
Dantrolene sodium may prevent the increase in myoplasmic calcium and the acute catabolism within the muscle cell by interfering with the release of calcium from the sarcoplasmic reticulum to the myoplasm. Thus, the physiologic, metabolic, and biochemical changes associated with the crisis may be reversed or attenuated.
Specific metabolic pathways in the degradation and elimination of dantrolene sodium in humans have been established. Dantrolene is found in measurable amounts in blood and urine. In addition, its major metabolites in body fluids are the 5-hydroxy analog and the acetamido analog. Another metabolite with an unknown structure appears related to acetylaminodantrolene. Dantrolene sodium may also undergo hydrolysis and subsequent oxidation forming nitrophenylfuroic acid.
Since dantrolene sodium is metabolized by the liver, enhancement of its metabolism by other drugs is possible. However, neither phenobarbital nor diazepam appears to affect dantrolene sodium metabolism.
The mean biologic half-life of dantrolene sodium after intravenous administration is about 5 hours. Based on assays of whole blood and plasma, slightly greater amounts of dantrolene are associated with red blood cells than with the plasma fraction of blood. Significant amounts of dantrolene are bound to plasma proteins, mostly albumin, and this binding is readily reversible. Binding to plasma protein is not significantly altered by diazepam, diphenylhydantoin, or phenylbutazone. Binding to plasma proteins is reduced by warfarin and clofibrate and increased by tolbutamide.
In animals, dantrolene sodium given intravenously has no appreciable effect on the cardiovascular system or on respiratory function. A transient inconsistent effect on smooth muscles has been observed at high doses.
Because of the low drug concentration requiring the administration of large volumes of fluid, acute toxicity of a dantrolene sodium intravenous formulation could not be assessed. In 14-day (subacute) studies, the intravenous formulation of dantrolene sodium was relatively non-toxic to rats at doses of 10 mg/kg/day and 20 mg/kg/day. While 10 mg/kg/day in dogs for 14 days evoked little toxicity, 20 mg/kg/day for 14 days caused hepatic changes of questionable biologic significance.

INDICATIONS

Dantrium Intravenous is indicated, along with appropriate supportive measures, for the management of the fulminant hypermetabolism of skeletal muscle characteristic of malignant hyperthermia crisis. It should be administered by intravenous injection as soon as the malignant hyperthermia reaction is recognized (i.e. tachycardia, tachypnea, central venous desaturation, hypercarbia, metabolic acidosis, skeletal muscle rigidity, increased utilization of anesthesia circuit carbon dioxide absorber, cyanosis and mottling of the skin, and, in many cases, fever).

CONTRAINDICATIONS

None.

WARNINGS

The use of Dantrium Intravenous in the management of malignant hyperthermia crisis is not a substitute for previously known supportive measures. These measures must be individualized, but it will usually be necessary to discontinue the suspect triggering agents, attend to increased oxygen requirements, manage the metabolic acidosis, institute cooling when necessary, attend to urinary output and monitor for electrolyte imbalance.

PRECAUTIONS

a) Because of the high pH of the intravenous formulation of Dantrium, care must be taken to prevent extravasation of the intravenous solution into the surrounding tissues.
b) Pregnancy: The safety of Dantrium Intravenous in women who are or who may become pregnant has not been established; it should be given only when the potential benefits have been weighed against the possible risk to mother and child.
c) Drug Intractions: The combination of therapeutic doses of intravenous dantrolene sodium and verapamil in halothane/α-chloralose anesthetized swine has resulted in ventricular fibrillation and cardiovascular collapse in association with marked hyperkalemia. It is recommended that the combination of intravenous dantrolene sodium and calcium channel blockers, such as verapamil, not be used during reversal of a malignant hyperthermia crisis until the relevance of these findings to humans is established.

ADVERSE REACTIONS

The serious reactions reported with chronic oral Dantrium use have been hepatitis, seizures, and pleural effusion with pericarditis. Hypersensitivity with attendant skin reactions has been infrequently noted. None of the reactions reported in patients taking oral Dantrium have been reported in patients treated with short-term Dantrium Intravenous therapy for malignant hyperthermia.

DOSAGE AND ADMINISTRATION

As soon as the malignant hyperthermia reaction is recognized, all anesthetic agents should be discontinued. Dantrium Intravenous should be administered by continuous rapid intravenous push beginning at a minimum dose of 1 mg/kg, and continuing until symptoms subside or the maximum cumulative dose of 10 mg/kg has been reached. If the physiologic and metabolic abnormalities reappear, the regimen may be repeated. It is important to note that administration of Dantrium Intravenous should be continuous until symptoms subside. The effective dose to reverse the crisis is directly dependent upon the individual's degree of susceptibility to malignant hyperthermia, the amount and time of exposure to the triggering agent, and the time elapsed between onset of the crisis and initiation of treatment.
Children's Dose: Experience to date indicates that the dose for children is the same as for adults.
Preoperatively: Dantrium (dantrolene sodium) Capsules are indicated preoperatively as possible protection against the development of a malignant hyperthermia crisis in individuals thought to be susceptible.
Oral administration of Dantrium Capsules: Administer 4 to 8 mg/kg/day of oral dantrolene in 3 or 4 divided doses for one or two days prior to surgery, with the last dose being given approximately 3 to 4 hours before scheduled surgery with a minimum of water.
This dosage usually will be associated with skeletal muscle weakness and sedation (sleepiness or drowsiness); adjustment can usually be made within the recommended dosage range to avoid incapacitation or excessive gastrointestinal irritation (including nausea and/or vomiting). See also the package insert for oral dantrolene sodium (Dantrium Capsules).
Post Crisis Follow-up: Dantrium (dantrolene sodium) Capsules should also be administered following a malignant hyperthermia crisis in doses of 4 to 8 mg/kg per day in four divided doses, for a one to three day period to prevent recurrence of the manifestations of malignant hyperthermia.

PREPARATION

Each vial of Dantrium Intravenous should be reconstituted by adding 60 ml of sterile water for injection U.S.P. (without a bacteriostatic agent), and the vial shaken until the solution is clear. The contents of the vial must be *protected from direct light* and *used within 6 hours* after reconstitution. Store reconstituted solutions at controlled room temperature (59°F to 86°F or 15°C to 30°C).

HOW SUPPLIED

Dantrium Intravenous (NDC 0149-0734-02) is available in vials containing a sterile lyophilized mixture of 20 mg dantrolene sodium, 3000 mg mannitol, and sufficient sodium hydroxide to yield a pH of approximately 9.5 when reconstituted with 60 ml sterile water for injection U.S.P. (without a bacteriostatic agent).
Store unreconstituted product below 86°F (30°C) and avoid prolonged exposure to light.
Address medical inquiries to Norwich Eaton Pharmaceuticals Inc., Medical Department, Norwich, NY 13815.
Manufactured by
Eaton Laboratories, Inc.
Manati, Puerto Rico 00701
Distributed by
Norwich Eaton Pharmaceuticals, Inc.
Norwich, New York 13815
A Procter & Gamble Company
REVISED DECEMBER 1983 DANIV-P2

DIDRONEL® ℞
[*dī 'drō-nel*]
(etidronate disodium)

DESCRIPTION

DIDRONEL tablets contain 200 mg of etidronate disodium, the disodium salt of (1-hydroxyethylidene) diphosphonic acid, for oral administration. This compound, also known as EHDP, regulates bone metabolism. It is a white powder, highly soluble in water, with a molecular weight of 250 and the following structural formula:

HO—P(ONa)(=O)—C(OH)(CH_3)—P(ONa)(=O)—OH

INACTIVE INGREDIENTS

Each tablet contains magnesium stearate, microcrystalline cellulose, and starch.

CLINICAL PHARMACOLOGY

DIDRONEL acts primarily on bone. It can inhibit the formation, growth and dissolution of hydroxyapatite crystals and their amorphous percursors by chemisorption to calcium phosphate surfaces. Inhibition of crystal resorption occurs at lower doses than are required to inhibit crystal growth. Both effects increase as the dose increases.
DIDRONEL is not metabolized. Absorption averages about 1% of an oral dose of 5 mg/kg body weight/day. This increases to about 2.5% at 10 mg/kg/day and 6% at 20 mg/kg/day. Most of the absorbed drug is cleared from the blood within 6 hours. Within 24 hours about half of the absorbed dose is excreted in the urine. The remainder is chemically adsorbed to bone, especially to areas of elevated osteogenesis, and is slowly eliminated. Unabsorbed drug is excreted intact in the feces.
DIDRONEL therapy does not adversely affect serum levels of parathyroid hormone or calcium. Hyperphosphatemia has been observed in DIDRONEL patients, usually in association with doses of 10–20 mg/kg/day. No adverse effects have been traced to this, and it is not a contraindication for therapy. It is apparently due to drug-related increased tubular reabsorption of phosphate by the kidney. Serum phosphate levels generally return to normal 2–4 weeks posttherapy.

PAGET'S DISEASE

Paget's disease of bone (osteitis deformans) is an idiopathic, progressive disease characterized by abnormal and accelerated bone metabolism in one or more bones. Signs and symptoms may include bone pain and/or deformity, neurologic disorders, elevated cardiac output and other vascular disorders, and increased serum alkaline phosphatase and/or urinary hydroxyproline levels. Bone fractures are common in patients with Paget's disease.
DIDRONEL slows accelerated bone turnover (resorption and accretion) in pagetic lesions and, to a lesser extent, in normal bone. This has been demonstrated histologically, scintigraphically, biochemically, and through calcium kinetic and balance studies. Reduced bone turnover is often accompanied by symptomatic improvement, including reduced bone pain. Also, the incidence of pagetic fractures may be reduced, and elevated cardiac output and other vascular disorders may be improved by DIDRONEL therapy.

HETEROTOPIC OSSIFICATION

Heterotopic ossification, also referred to as myositis ossificans (circumscripta, progressiva or traumatica), ectopic calcification, periarticular ossification, or paraosteoarthropathy, is characterized by metaplastic osteogenesis. It usually presents with signs of localized inflammation or pain, elevated skin temperature, and redness. When tissues near joints are involved, functional loss may also be present. Heterotopic ossification may occur for no known reason as in myositis ossificans progressiva or may follow a wide variety of surgical, occupational, and sports trauma (e.g., hip arthroplasty, spinal cord injury, head injury, burns and severe thigh bruises). Heterotopic ossification has also been observed in non-traumatic conditions (e.g., infections of the central nervous system, peripheral neuropathy, tetanus, biliary cirrhosis, Peyronie's disease, as well as in association with a variety of benign and malignant neoplasms).

Clinical trials have demonstrated the efficacy of Didronel in heterotopic ossification following total hip replacement, or due to spinal cord injury.

—*Heterotopic ossification complicating total hip replacement* typically develops radiographically 3–8 weeks postoperatively in the pericapsular area of the affected hip joint. The overall incidence is about 50%; about one-third of these cases are clinically significant.

—*Heterotopic ossification due to spinal cord injury* typically develops radiographically 1–4 months after injury. It occurs below the level of injury, usually at major joints. The overall incidence is about 40%; about one-half of these cases are clinically significant.

DIDRONEL chemisorbs to calcium hydroxyapatite crystals and their amorphous precursors, blocking the aggregation, growth and mineralization of these crystals. This is thought to be the mechanism by which DIDRONEL presents or retards heterotopic ossification. There is no evidence DIDRONEL affects mature heterotopic bone.

INDICATIONS AND USAGE

PAGET'S DISEASE

DIDRONEL is indicated for the treatment of symptomatic Paget's disease of bone.

DIDRONEL therapy usually arrests or significantly impedes the disease process as evidenced by:

—Symptomatic relief, including decreased pain and/or increased mobility (experienced by 3 out of 5 patients).

—Reductions in serum alkaline phosphatase and urinary hydroxyproline levels (30% or more in 4 out of 5 patients).

—Histomorphometry showing reduced numbers of osteoclasts and osteoblasts, and more lamellar bone formation.

—Bone scans showing reduced radionuclide uptake at pagetic lesions.

In addition, reductions in pagetically elevated cardiac output and skin temperature have been observed in some patients. Also, the incidence of pagetic fractures may be reduced when DIDRONEL is administered intermittently over a period of years.

In many patients, the disease process will be suppressed for a period of at least one year following cessation of therapy. The upper limit of this period has not been determined.

DIDRONEL's effects have not been studied in patients with asymptomatic Paget's disease. However, DIDRONEL treatment of such patients may be warranted if extensive involvement threatens irreversible neurologic damage, major joints, or major weight-bearing bones.

HETEROTOPIC OSSIFICATION

DIDRONEL is indicated in the prevention and treatment of heterotopic ossification following total hip replacement or due to spinal cord injury.

DIDRONEL reduces the incidence of clinically important heterotopic bone by about two-thirds. Among those patients who form heterotopic bone, DIDRONEL retards the progression of immature lesions and reduces the severity by at least half. Follow-up data (at least nine months posttherapy) suggest these benefits persist.

In total hip replacement patients, DIDRONEL does not promote loosening of the prosthesis or impede trochanteric reattachment.

In spinal cord injury patients, DIDRONEL does not inhibit fracture healing or stabilization of the spine.

CONTRAINDICATIONS

None known.

WARNINGS

In Paget's patients the response to therapy may be of slow onset and continue for months after DIDRONEL therapy is discontinued. Dosage should not be increased prematurely. A 90-day drug-free interval should be provided between courses of therapy.

Heterotopic ossification: No specific warnings.

PRECAUTIONS

General. Patients should maintain an adequate nutritional status, particularly an adequate intake of calcium and vitamin D.

Therapy has been withheld from some patients with enterocolitis since diarrhea may be experienced, particularly at higher doses.

DIDRONEL is not metabolized and is excreted intact via the kidney. There is no experience to specifically guide treatment in patients with impaired renal function. DIDRONEL dosage should be reduced when reductions in glomerular filtration rates are present. Patients with renal impairment should be closely monitored. DIDRONEL suppresses bone turnover, and may retard mineralization of osteoid laid down during the bone accretion process. These effects are dose and time dependent. Osteoid, which may accumulate noticeably at doses of 10–20 mg/kg/day, mineralizes normally posttherapy. In patients with fractures, especially of long bones, it may be advisable to delay or interrupt treatment until callus is evident.

Carcinogenesis. Long-term studies in rats have indicated that DIDRONEL is not carcinogenic.

Pregnancy: Teratogenic Effects. Pregnancy Category B. Reproduction/teratology studies performed in rats and rabbits at doses up to five times the maximum human dose by the intended route of administration have revealed no evidence of impaired fertility or harm to the fetus due to DIDRONEL. At doses of twenty-two times the maximum human dose, a decrease in live fetuses were observed in rats. The only incidence of malformations occurred in rats at exaggerated doses following parenteral administration and were skeletal in nature. These malformations were deemed the result of the pharmacological action of the drug. There are no adequate, well-controlled studies in pregnant women. Because animal reproduction studies are not always predictive of human response, this drug should be used during pregnancy only if clearly needed.

Nursing Mothers. It is not known whether this drug is excreted in human milk. Because many drugs are excreted in human milk, caution should be exercised when DIDRONEL is administered to a nursing woman.

Pediatric Use. Safety and effectiveness in children have not been established.

ADVERSE REACTIONS

The incidence of gastrointestinal complaints (diarrhea, nausea) is the same for DIDRONEL at 5 mg/kg/day as for placebo, about 1 patient in 15. At 10–20 mg/kg/day the incidence may increase to 2 or 3 in 10. These complaints are often alleviated by dividing the total daily dose.

Hypersensitivity reactions including angioedema/urticaria, rash and/or pruritis have been reported rarely.

In Paget's patients increased or recurrent bone pain at pagetic sites, and/or the onset of pain at previously asymptomatic sites has been reported. At 5 mg/kg/day about 1 patient in 10 (verus 1 in 15 in the placebo group) report these phenomena. At higher doses the incidence rises to about 2 in 10. When therapy continues, pain resolves in some patients but persists in others.

Heterotopic ossification: No specific adverse reactions.

OVERDOSAGE

While there is no experience with acute overdosage, it is theoretically possible that enough DIDRONEL could be taken to result in hypocalcemia.

DOSAGE AND ADMINISTRATION

DIDRONEL should be taken as a single, oral dose. However, should gastrointestinal discomfort occur, the dose may be divided. To maximize absorption, patients should avoid taking the following items within two hours of dosing:

—Food, especially those high in calcium, such as milk or milk products.

—Vitamins with mineral supplements or antacids which are high in metals such as calcium, iron, magnesium or aluminum.

PAGET'S DISEASE

Initial Treatment Regimens:

5–10 mg/kg/day, not to exceed 6 months, or
11–20 mg/kg/day, not to exceed 3 months.

The recommended initial dose is 5 mg/kg/day for a period not to exceed six months. Doses above 10 mg/kg/day should be reserved for when 1) lower doses are ineffective or 2) there is an overriding need to suppress rapid bone turnover (especially when irreversible neurologic damage is possible) or reduce elevated cardiac output. Doses in excess of 20 mg/kg/day are not recommended.

Retreatment Guidelines. Retreatment should be initiated only after: 1) a DIDRONEL-free period of at least 90 days and 2) there is biochemical, symptomatic or other evidence of active disease process. It is advisable to monitor patients every 3–6 months although some patients may go drug free for extended periods. Retreatment regimens are the same as for initial treatment. For most patients the original dose will be adequate for retreatment. If not, consideration should be given to increasing the dose within the recommended guidelines.

HETEROTOPIC OSSIFICATION

The following treatment regimens have been shown to be effective:

—Total Hip Replacement Patients: 20 mg/kg/day for 1 month before and 3 months after surgery (4 months total).

—Spinal Cord Injured Patients: 20 mg/kg/day for 2 weeks followed by 10 mg/kg/day for 10 weeks (12 weeks total). DIDRONEL therapy should begin as soon as medically feasible following the injury, preferably prior to evidence of heterotopic ossification.

Retreatment has not been studied.

HOW SUPPLIED

Didronel is available as 200-mg, white, rectangular tablets with "P&G" on one face and "402" on the other.

NDC 0149-0405-60 bottle of 60

400-mg, white, scored, capsule-shaped tablets with "N E" on one face and "406" on the other.

NDC 0149-0406-60 bottle of 60

CAUTION

Federal law prohibits dispensing without prescription.

Shown in Product Identification Section, page 419

REVISED OCTOBER 1985 DID-P5

DUVOID® ℞

[*dū 'void*]
(bethanechol chloride—oral)

DESCRIPTION

Duvoid (bethanechol chloride), an ester of a choline-like compound, is 2-[(amino-carbonyl)oxy]-N,N,N-trimethyl-1-propanaminium chloride. Bethanechol chloride is a white, hygroscopic, crystalline powder having a slight amine-like odor and is freely soluble in water.

$$\left[\begin{array}{l} CH_3CH-CH_2N+(CH_3)_3 \\ \quad\; | \\ \quad O-CO-NH_2 \end{array}\right] Cl^-$$

Molecular weight: 196.68
Molecular formula: $C_7H_{17}ClN_2O_2$

Duvoid, a cholinergic agent, is available as 10-mg, 25-mg, and 50-mg tablets intended for oral administration.

INACTIVE INGREDIENTS

Each tablet contains calcium pyrophosphate, magnesium stearate, microcrystalline cellulose, starch, and may contain one or more of the following: FD&C Blue #2, FD&C Yellow #6.

CLINICAL PHARMACOLOGY

Duvoid acts principally by producing the effects of stimulation of the parasympathetic nervous system. It increases the tone of the detrusor urinae muscle, usually producing a contraction sufficiently strong to initiate micturition and empty the bladder. It stimulates gastric motility, increases gastric tone, and often restores impaired rhythmic peristalsis.

Stimulation of the parasympathetic nervous system releases acetylcholine at the nerve endings. When spontaneous stimulation is reduced and therapeutic intervention is required, acetylcholine can be given, but is rapidly hydrolyzed by cholinesterase, and its effects are transient. Bethanechol chloride is not destroyed by cholinesterase and its effects are more prolonged than those of acetylcholine.

It has predominant muscarinic action and only feeble nicotinic action. Doses that stimulate micturition and defecation and increase peristalsis do not ordinarily stimulate ganglia or voluntary muscles. Therapeutic test doses in normal human subjects have little effect on heart rate, blood pressure, or peripheral circulation.

INDICATIONS AND USAGE

Duvoid is indicated for the treatment of acute postoperative and postpartum nonobstructive (functional) urinary retention, and neurogenic atony of the urinary bladder with retention.

CONTRAINDICATIONS

Duvoid is contraindicated in the presence of mechanical obstruction of the gastrointestinal or urinary tracts, or in conditions where the integrity of the gastrointestinal or bladder wall is questionable. Also, it is contraindicated in spastic gastrointestinal disturbances, peptic ulcer, acute inflammatory conditions of the gastrointestinal tract, or peritonitis, or in marked vagotonia.

Duvoid is also contraindicated in latent or active asthma, hyperthyroidism, coronary occlusion, bradycardia, vasomotor instability, hypotension, coronary artery disease, epilepsy, and parkinsonism.

WARNINGS

Asthmatic attacks may be precipitated, especially in susceptible individuals. Substernal pressure or pain may occur; however, it is uncertain whether this is due to bronchoconstriction, or spasm of the esophagus. Myocardial hypoxia must be considered if a marked fall in blood pressure occurs. Transient syncope with cardiac arrest, transient complete heart block, dyspnea, and orthostatic hypotension may be associated with large doses. Patients with hypertension may react to the drug with a precipitous fall in blood pressure. Short periods of atrial fibrillation have been observed in hyperthyroid individuals following the administration of cholinergic drugs. Involuntary defecation and urinary urgency may occur after large doses.

PRECAUTIONS

General: In urinary retention, if the sphincter fails to relax as Duvoid contracts the bladder, urine may be forced up the ureter into the kidney pelvis. If there is bacteriuria, this may cause a reflux infection.

Continued on next page

Norwich Eaton—Cont.

Drug Interactions: Special care and consideration are required when Duvoid is administered to patients concomitantly being treated with other drugs with which pharmacologic interactions may occur. Examples of drugs with potential for such interactions are: quinidine and procainamide, which may antagonize cholinergic effects; cholinergic drugs, particularly cholinesterase inhibitors, where additive effects may occur. When administered to patients receiving ganglionic blocking compounds a critical fall in blood pressure may occur, usually preceded by severe abdominal symptoms.
Pregnancy: Pregnancy Category C. Animal reproduction studies have not been conducted with Duvoid. It is also not known whether Duvoid can cause fetal harm when administered to a pregnant woman or can affect reproduction capacity. Duvoid should be given to a pregnant woman only if clearly needed.
Nursing Mothers: It is not known whether this drug is excreted in human milk. Because many drugs are excreted in human milk, caution should be exercised when Duvoid is administered to a nursing woman.
Pediatric Use: Safety and effectiveness in children below the age of 8 years have not been established.

ADVERSE REACTIONS
Adverse reactions are infrequent with Duvoid. The following may occur:
Cardiovascular: Fall in blood pressure. (See **Warnings.**)
Gastrointestinal: Involuntary defecation, vomiting, colicky pain, abdominal cramps, diarrhea, nausea and belching, salivation, and borborygmi.
Respiratory: Asthmatic attacks and dyspnea.
Neurologic: Headache, facial flushing.
Urogenital: Urinary urgency.
Miscellaneous: Substernal pressure or pain (see **Warnings**), malaise.

OVERDOSAGE
Maintain artificial respiration until antidote can be given. Atropine sulfate is a specific antidote and may be given in doses of 0.6 mg–1.2 mg intravenously (slowly), intramuscularly, or subcutaneously to counteract severe toxic cardiovascular or bronchoconstrictor responses to bethanechol chloride.

DOSAGE AND ADMINISTRATION
Dosage must be individualized, depending on type and severity of the condition to be treated.
Preferably give the drug on an empty stomach to minimize the possibility of nausea and vomiting.
The usual adult oral dose ranges from 10 to 50 mg three or four times a day. The minimum effective dose is determined by giving 5 or 10 mg initially, and repeating the same amount at hourly intervals until satisfactory response occurs, or until a maximum of 50 mg has been given. The effects of the drug sometimes appear within 30 minutes, and are usually maximal within 90 minutes. The drug's effects persist for about one hour.

HOW SUPPLIED
Duvoid is available as follows:
10 mg: pale orange, scored tablets coded "Eaton 045"
NDC 0149-0045-05 bottle of 100
NDC 0149-0045-77 hospital unit-dose strips in box of 100.
25 mg: white, scored tablets coded "Eaton 046"
NDC 0149-0046-05 bottle of 100
NDC 0149-0046-77 hospital unit-dose strips in box of 100.
50 mg: tan, scored tablets coded "Eaton 047"
NDC 0149-0047-05 bottle of 100
NDC 0149-0047-77 hospital unit-dose strips in box of 100.

CAUTION
Federal law prohibits dispensing without prescription.
Keep container tightly closed. Avoid excessive heat (over 104°F or 40°C).
REVISED FEBRUARY 1985 DUV-P7

ENTEX® ℞
[*n* '*tex*]
(phenylephrine hydrochloride/phenylpropanolamine hydrochloride/guaifenesin)

DESCRIPTION
Each ENTEX orange and white capsule for oral administration contains:
phenylephrine hydrochloride .... 5 mg
phenylpropanolamine hydrochloride .... 45 mg
guaifenesin .... 200 mg
This product contains ingredients of the following therapeutic classes: decongestant and expectorant.
Phenylephrine hydrochloride is a decongestant having the chemical name, 3-hydroxy-α-[(methylamino)methyl]benzenemethanol hydrochloride, with the following structure:
[See Chemical Formula at top of next column].

OH, C—CH₂NHCH₃ · HCl, OH

Phenylpropanolamine hydrochloride is a decongestant having the chemical name, benzenemethanol, α-(1-aminoethyl)-, hydrochloride (R*, S*), (±), with the following structure:

CH—CH—CH₃ · HCl, OH NH₂

Guaifenesin is an expectorant having the chemical name, 1,2-propanediol,3-(2-methoxyphenoxy)-, with the following structure:

OH, OCH CHCH₂OH, OCH₃

INACTIVE INGREDIENTS
Each capsule contains edible black ink, gelatin, FD&C Red #3, silica gel, starch, titanium dioxide, FD&C Yellow #6, and may contain zinc stearate.

CLINICAL PHARMACOLOGY
Phenylephrine hydrochloride and phenylpropanolamine hydrochloride are α-adrenergic receptor agonists (sympathomimetics) which produce vasoconstriction by stimulating α-receptors within the mucosa of the respiratory tract. Clinically, phenylephrine and phenylpropanolamine shrink swollen mucous membranes, reduce tissue hyperemia, edema, and nasal congestion, and increase nasal airway patency. Guaifenesin promotes lower respiratory tract drainage by thinning bronchial secretions, lubricates irritated respiratory tract membranes through increased mucous flow, and facilitates removal of viscous, inspissated mucus. As a result, sinus and bronchial drainage is improved, and dry, nonproductive coughs become more productive and less frequent.

INDICATIONS AND USAGE
ENTEX is indicated for the symptomatic relief of sinusitis, bronchitis, pharyngitis, and coryza when these conditions are associated with nasal congestion and viscous mucus in the lower respiratory tract.

CONTRAINDICATIONS
ENTEX is contraindicated in individuals with known hypersensitivity to sympathomimetics, severe hypertension, or in patients receiving monoamine oxidase inhibitors.

WARNINGS
Sympathomimetic amines should be used with caution in patients with hypertension, diabetes mellitus, heart disease, peripheral vascular disease, increased intraocular pressure, hyperthyroidism, or prostatic hypertrophy.

PRECAUTIONS
Drug Interactions: ENTEX should not be used in patients taking monoamine oxidase inhibitors or other sympathomimetics.
Drug/Laboratory Test Interactions: Guaifenesin has been reported to interfere with clinical laboratory determinations of urinary 5-hydroxyindoleacetic acid (5-HIAA) and urinary vanilmandelic acid (VMA).
Pregnancy: Pregnancy Category C. Animal reproduction studies have not been conducted with ENTEX. It is also not known whether ENTEX can cause fetal harm when administered to a pregnant woman or can affect reproduction capacity. ENTEX should be given to a pregnant woman only if clearly needed.
Nursing Mothers: It is not known whether the drugs in ENTEX are excreted in human milk. Because many drugs are excreted in human milk and because of the potential for serious adverse reactions in nursing infants, a decision should be made whether to discontinue nursing or to discontinue the product, taking into account the importance of the drug to the mother.
Pediatric Use: Safety and effectiveness of ENTEX capsules in children below the age of 12 have not been established.

ADVERSE REACTIONS
Possible adverse reactions include nervousness, insomnia, restlessness, headache, nausea, or gastric irritation. These reactions seldom, if ever, require discontinuation of therapy. Urinary retention may occur in patients with prostatic hypertrophy.

OVERDOSAGE
The treatment of overdosage should provide symptomatic and supportive care. If the amount ingested is considered dangerous or excessive, induce vomiting with ipecac syrup unless the patient is convulsing, comatose, or has lost the gag reflex, in which case perform gastric lavage using a large-bore tube. If indicated, follow with activated charcoal and a saline cathartic.

DOSAGE AND ADMINISTRATION
Adults and children 12 years of age and older—one capsule four times daily (every 6 hours) with food or fluid. ENTEX is not recommended for children under 12 years of age.

HOW SUPPLIED
ENTEX orange and white capsules are imprinted with "ENTEX" and "0149 0412".
NDC 0149-0412-01 Bottle of 100
NDC 0149-0412-05 Bottle of 500

CAUTION
Federal law prohibits dispensing without prescription.
REVISED SEPTEMBER 1985 ENXCP-P6

ENTEX® LIQUID ℞
[*n* '*tex*]
(phenylephrine hydrochloride/phenylpropanolamine hydrochloride/guaifenesin)

DESCRIPTION
Each 5 ml (one teaspoonful) for oral administration contains:
phenylephrine hydrochloride .... 5 mg
phenylpropanolamine hydrochloride .... 20 mg
guaifenesin .... 100 mg
alcohol 5%
This product contains ingredients of the following therapeutic classes: decongestant and expectorant.
Phenylephrine hydrochloride is a decongestant having the chemical name, 3-hydroxy-α-[(methylamino)methyl]benzenemethanol hydrochloride, with the following structure:

OH, C—CH₂NHCH₃ · HCl, H, OH

Phenylpropanolamine hydrochloride is a decongestant having the chemical name, benzenemethanol, α-(1-aminoethyl)-, hydrochloride (R*, S*), (±), with the following structure:

CH—CH—CH₃ · HCl, OH NH₂

Guaifenesin is an expectorant having the chemical name, 1,2-propanediol, 3-(2-methoxyphenoxy)-, with the following structure:

OH, OCH₂CHCH₂OH, OCH₃

INACTIVE INGREDIENTS
Entex liquid contains citric acid, flavoring, glycerin, purified water, saccharin sodium, sodium benzoate, sodium chloride, sorbitol solution, sucrose, and FD&C Yellow #6.

CLINICAL PHARMACOLOGY
Phenylephrine hydrochloride and phenylpropanolamine hydrochloride are α-adrenergic receptor agonists (sympathomimetics) which produce vasoconstriction by stimulating α-receptors within the mucosa of the respiratory tract. Clinically, phenylephrine and phenylpropanolamine shrink swollen mucous membranes, reduce tissue hyperemia, edema, and nasal congestion, and increase nasal airway patency. Guaifenesin promotes lower respiratory tract drainage by thinning bronchial secretions, lubricates irritated respiratory tract membranes through increased mucous flow, and facilitates removal of viscous, inspissated mucus. As a result, sinus and bronchial drainage is improved, and dry, nonproductive coughs become more productive and less frequent.

INDICATIONS AND USAGE
ENTEX LIQUID is indicated for the symptomatic relief of sinusitis, bronchitis, pharyngitis, and coryza when these conditions are associated with nasal congestion and inspissated mucus in the lower respiratory tract.

CONTRAINDICATIONS
ENTEX LIQUID is contraindicated in individuals with hypersensitivity to sympathomimetics, severe hypertension, or in patients receiving monoamine oxidase inhibitors.

WARNINGS

Sympathomimetic amines should be used with caution in patients with hypertension, diabetes mellitus, heart disease, peripheral vascular disease, increased intraocular pressure, hyperthyroidism, or prostatic hypertrophy.

PRECAUTIONS

Drug Interactions: ENTEX LIQUID should not be used in patients taking monoamine oxidase inhibitors or other sympathomimetics.

Drug/Laboratory Test Interactions: Guaifenesin has been reported to interfere with clinical laboratory determinations of urinary 5-hydroxyindoleacetic acid (5-HIAA) and urinary vanilmandelic acid (VMA).

Pregnancy: Pregnancy Category C. Animal reproduction studies have not been conducted with ENTEX LIQUID. It is also not known whether ENTEX LIQUID can cause fetal harm when administered to a pregnant woman or can affect reproduction capacity. ENTEX LIQUID should be given to a pregnant woman only if clearly needed.

Nursing Mothers: It is not known whether the drugs in EXTEX LIQUID are excreted in human milk. Because many drugs are excreted in human milk and because of the potential for serious adverse reactions in nursing infants, a decision should be made whether to discontinue nursing or to discontinue the product, taking into account the importance of the drug to the mother.

Pediatric Use: Safety and effectiveness of ENTEX LIQUID in children below the age of 2 have not been established.

ADVERSE REACTIONS

Possible adverse reactions include nervousness, insomnia, restlessness, headache, nausea, or gastric irritation. These reactions seldom, if ever, require discontinuation of therapy. Urinary retention may occur in patients with prostatic hypertrophy.

OVERDOSAGE

The treatment of overdosage should provide symptomatic and supportive care. If the amount ingested is considered dangerous or excessive, induce vomiting with ipecac syrup unless the patient is convulsing, comatose, or has lost the gag reflex, in which case perform gastric lavage using a large-bore tube. If indicated, follow with activated charcoal and a saline cathartic.

DOSAGE AND ADMINISTRATION

All dosage should be administered four times daily (every 6 hours).

Children:
2 to under 4 years .... ½ teaspoonful (2.5 ml)
4 to under 6 years .... 1 teaspoonful (5.0 ml)
6 to under 12 years .... 1½ teaspoonfuls (7.5 ml)
Adults and children 12 years
of age and older .... 2 teaspoonfuls (10.0 ml)

HOW SUPPLIED

ENTEX LIQUID is available as an orange-colored, pleasant-tasting liquid.

NDC 0149-0414-16 16 FL. OZ. (1 Pint) bottle

CAUTION

Federal law prohibits dispensing without prescription.
REVISED SEPTEMBER 1985 ENXLQ-P4

ENTEX® LA ℞

[n'tex]

(phenylpropanolamine hydrochloride/guaifenesin)

DESCRIPTION

Each ENTEX LA blue, scored, long-acting tablet for oral administration contains:
phenylpropanolamine hydrochloride .... 75 mg
guaifenesin .... 400 mg
in a special base to provide a prolonged therapeutic effect.
This product contains ingredients of the following therapeutic classes: decongestant and expectorant.

Phenylpropanolamine hydrochloride is a decongestant having the chemical name, benzenemethanol, α-(1-aminoethyl)-, hydrochloride (R*, S*), (±), with the following structure:

CH—CH—CH₃ · HCl
OH NH₂

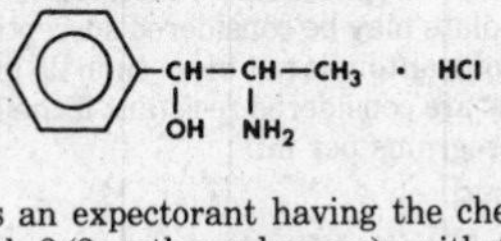

Guaifenesin is an expectorant having the chemical name, 1,2-propanediol, 3-(2-methoxyphenoxy)-, with the following structure:

OH
OCH₂CHCH₂OH
OCH₃

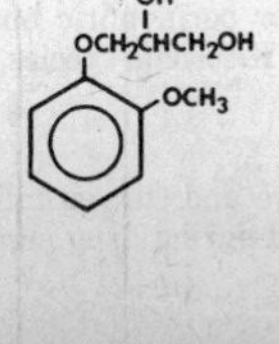

INACTIVE INGREDIENTS

Each tablet contains FD&C Blue #1, carbomer 934P, compressible sugar, stearic acid, and zinc stearate.

CLINICAL PHARMACOLOGY

Phenylpropanolamine hydrochloride is an α-adrenergic receptor agonist (sympathomimetic) which produces vasoconstriction by stimulating α-receptors within the mucosa of the respiratory tract. Clinically, phenylpropanolamine shrinks swollen mucous membranes, reduces tissue hyperemia, edema, and nasal congestion, and increases nasal airway patency. Guaifenesin promotes lower respiratory tract drainage by thinning bronchial secretions, lubricates irritated respiratory tract membranes through increased mucous flow, and facilitates removal of viscous, inspissated mucous. As a result, sinus and bronchial drainage is improved, and dry, nonproductive coughs become more productive and less frequent.

INDICATIONS AND USAGE

ENTEX LA is indicated for the symptomatic relief of sinusitis, bronchitis, pharyngitis, and coryza when these conditions are associated with nasal congestion and viscous mucous in the lower respiratory tract.

CONTRAINDICATIONS

ENTEX LA is contraindicated in individuals with known hypersensitivity to sympathomimetics, severe hypertension, or in patients receiving monoamine oxidase inhibitors.

WARNINGS

Sympathomimetic amines should be used with caution in patients with hypertension, diabetes mellitus, heart disease, peripheral vascular disease, increased intraocular pressure, hyperthyroidism, or prostatic hypertrophy.

PRECAUTIONS

Information for Patients: Do not crush or chew ENTEX LA tablets prior to swallowing.

Drug Interactions: ENTEX LA should not be used in patients taking monoamine oxidase inhibitors or other sympathomimetics.

Drug/Laboratory Test Interactions: Guaifenesin has been reported to interfere with clinical laboratory determinations of urinary 5-hydroxyindoleacetic acid (5-HIAA) and urinary vanilmandelic acid (VMA).

Pregnancy: Pregnancy Category C. Animal reproduction studies have not been conducted with ENTEX LA. It is also not known whether ENTEX LA can cause fetal harm when administered to a pregnant woman or can affect reproduction capacity. ENTEX LA should be given to a pregnant woman only if clearly needed.

Nursing Mothers: It is not known whether the drugs in ENTEX LA are excreted in human milk. Because many drugs are excreted in human milk and because of the potential for serious adverse reactions in nursing infants, a decision should be made whether to discontinue nursing or to discontinue the product, taking into account the importance of the drug to the mother.

Pediatric Use: Safety and effectiveness of ENTEX LA tablets in children below the age of 6 have not been established.

ADVERSE REACTIONS

Possible adverse reactions include nervousness, insomnia, restlessness, headache, nausea, or gastric irritation. These reactions seldom, if ever, require discontinuation of therapy. Urinary retention may occur in patients with prostatic hypertrophy.

OVERDOSAGE

The treatment of overdosage should provide symptomatic and supportive care. If the amount ingested is considered dangerous or excessive, induce vomiting with ipecac syrup unless the patient is convulsing, comatose, or has lost the gag reflex, in which case perform gastric lavage using a large-bore tube. If indicated, follow with activated charcoal and a saline cathartic. Since the effects of ENTEX LA may last up to 12 hours, treatment should be continued for at least that length of time.

DOSAGE AND ADMINISTRATION

Adults and children 12 years of age and older—one tablet twice daily (every 12 hours); children 6 to under 12 years—one-half (½) tablet twice daily (every 12 hours). ENTEX LA is not recommended for children under 6 years of age. Tablets may be broken in half for ease of administration without affecting release of medication but should not be crushed or chewed prior to swallowing.

HOW SUPPLIED

ENTEX LA is available as a blue, scored tablet imprinted with "ENTEX LA" on the smooth side.

NDC 0149-0436-01 bottle of 100

CAUTION

Federal law prohibits dispensing without prescription.

Shown in Product Identification Section, page 419

REVISED JULY 1985 ENXLATB-P7

FURACIN® ℞

[fewr'a-sin]

(nitrofurazone) SOLUBLE DRESSING

DESCRIPTION

Chemically, Furacin is nitrofurazone, 2-[(5-nitro-2-furanyl)methylene]hydrazinecarboxamide, with the following structure:

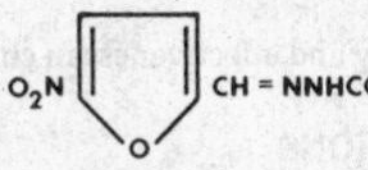

O₂N CH = NNHCONH₂
O

Furacin Soluble Dressing is a preparation containing 0.2% nitrofurazone in Solubase® (a water-soluble base of polyethylene glycols 3350, 900, and 300).

Furacin Soluble Dressing is an antibacterial agent for topical use.

CLINICAL PHARMACOLOGY

Furacin Soluble Dressing (nitrofurazone) is a nitrofuran that is bactericidal for most pathogens commonly causing surface infections, including *Staphylococcus aureus, Streptococcus, Escherichia coli, Clostridium perfringens, Aerobacter aerogenes,* and *Proteus.*

Furacin Soluble Dressing inhibits a number of bacterial enzymes, especially those involved in the aerobic and anaerobic degradation of glucose and pyruvate. The activity appears to involve the pyruvate dehydrogenase system as well as citrate synthetase, malate dehydrogenase, glutathione reductase, and pyruvate decarboxylase. Glutathione reductase inhibition may be caused by control of pentose phosphate metabolism. Although Furacin Soluble Dressing inhibits a variety of enzymes, it is not considered to be a general enzyme inactivator since many enzymes are not inhibited by this compound.

INDICATIONS AND USAGE

Furacin Soluble Dressing is a topical antibacterial agent indicated for adjunctive therapy of patients with second- and third-degree burns when bacterial resistance to other agents is a real or potential problem.

It is also indicated in skin grafting where bacterial contamination may cause graft rejection and/or donor site infection particularly in hospitals with historical resistant-bacteria epidemics.

There is no known evidence of effectiveness of this product in the treatment of minor burns or surface bacterial infections involving wounds, cutaneous ulcers, or the various pyodermas.

CONTRAINDICATIONS

Known sensitization to any of the components of this preparation is a contraindication for use.

WARNINGS

Nitrofurazone has been shown to produce mammary tumors when fed at high doses to female Sprague-Dawley rats. The relevance of this to topical use in humans is unknown.

Furacin Soluble Dressing should be used with caution in patients with known or suspected renal impairment. The polyethylene glycols in the base can be absorbed through denuded skin and may not be excreted normally by the compromised kidney. This may lead to symptoms of progressive renal impairment such as increased BUN, anion gap, and metabolic acidosis. (NOTE: Furacin (nitrofurazone) Topical Cream does not contain polyethylene glycols.)

PRECAUTIONS

General: Use of topical antimicrobials occasionally allows overgrowth of nonsusceptible organisms including fungi. If this occurs, or if irritation, sensitization or superinfection develops, treatment with Furacin Soluble Dressing should be discontinued and appropriate therapy instituted.

Carcinogenesis, mutagenesis, and impairment of fertility: Nitrofurazone has been shown to produce mammary tumors when fed at high doses to female Sprague-Dawley rats. The relevance of this to topical use in humans is unknown. Dietary dosage levels of 60 and 30 mg/kg/day shortened the onset time of the typical mammary gland tumors associated with older female rats. These tumors exhibited the same histological characteristics seen in the spontaneously occurring tumors, and were seen only in the female animals. No mammary tumors were seen in rats treated with nitrofurazone orally in the diet for 1 year at levels of approximately 11 mg/kg/day. Spermatogenic arrest was noted in the male rats in dietary dosage levels of 30 mg/kg/day and above, after one year on test.

Usage in Pregnancy: Pregnancy Category C: Nitrofurazone has been shown to have an embryocidal effect in rabbits when given in oral doses thirty times the human dose. There are no adequate and well controlled studies in pregnant women.

Furacin Soluble Dressing should be used during pregnancy only if the potential benefit justifies the potential risk to the fetus.

Continued on next page

Norwich Eaton—Cont.

Nursing mothers: It is not known whether this drug is excreted in human milk. Because many drugs are excreted in human milk and because of the potential for tumorigenicity shown for nitrofurazone in animal studies, a decision should be made whether to discontinue nursing or to discontinue the drug, taking into account the importance of the drug to the mother.
Pediatric use: Safety and effectiveness in children have not been established.

ADVERSE REACTIONS
In quantitative studies published during the period 1945-70, 206 instances of clinical skin reaction were reported out of 18,249 patients (an incidence of 1.1%) treated with Furacin formulations. Symptoms appeared as varying degrees of contact dermatitides such as rash, pruritus, and local edema. Allergic reactions to Furacin Soluble Dressing should be treated symptomatically.

DOSAGE AND ADMINISTRATION
Burns: Apply directly to the lesion with a spatula, or first place on gauze. Impregnated gauze may be used. Reapply depending on the preferred dressing technique. Flushing the dressing with sterile saline facilitates its removal.
Preparation of Impregnated Gauze: Sterile gauze strips are placed in a tray and covered with Furacin Soluble Dressing. Repeat the procedure, adding several layers of gauze for each layer of Furacin Soluble Dressing. Sprinkling a little sterile water on each layer of dressing will minimize any color change from autoclaving. Cover the tray very loosely and autoclave at 121°C for 30 minutes at 15 to 20 pounds pressure.
To impregnate bandage rolls, place some Furacin Soluble Dressing in the bottom of a glass jar. Stand rolls on end. Place more Furacin Soluble Dressing on top. Cover top of jar with aluminum foil. Autoclave at 121°C for 45 minutes at 15 to 20 pounds pressure. Do not store impregnated bandage rolls for more than 24 hours.
Autoclaving more than once is not recommended.

HOW SUPPLIED
Furacin Soluble Dressing is available in:
NDC 0149-0704-12 tube of 28 grams
NDC 0149-0704-11 tube of 56 grams
NDC 0149-0704-51 jar of 135 grams
NDC 0149-0704-61 jar of 454 grams

ANIMAL TOXICOLOGY
The oral administration of nitrofurazone for 7 days to rats at extremely high dosage levels of 240 mg/kg/day produced severe hepatorenal lesions whereas only renal changes were seen when the dosage level was reduced to 60 mg/kg/day for 60 days.
Dogs treated orally with nitrofurazone for 400 days at levels of 11 mg/kg/day showed no toxic effects related to drug treatment. The single intravenous administration in dogs of 20, 35, or 75 mg/kg nitrofurazone produced clinical signs of lacrimation, salivation, emesis, diarrhea, excitation, weakness, ataxia, and weight loss, whereas 100 mg/kg produced convulsions and death.
There was no evidence of toxicosis in rhesus monkeys treated with doses of nitrofurazone as high as 58 mg/kg/day for 10 weeks and 23 mg/kg/day for 63 weeks.
The peroral LD_{50} of nitrofurazone in mice and rats is 747 and 590 mg/kg respectively.
For bacterial sensitivity tests: Furacin Sensi-Discs are available from BBL, Division of BioQuest.
REVISED JUNE 1984 FSD-P7

FURACIN® TOPICAL CREAM ℞
[fewr 'a-sin]
(nitrofurazone)

DESCRIPTION
Chemically, Furacin is nitrofurazone, 2-[(5-nitro-2-furanyl)methylene]hydrazinecarboxamide, with the following structure:

O_2N … CH = $NNHCONH_2$

Furacin Topical Cream is a preparation containing 0.2% Furacin in a water-miscible base consisting of glycerin, cetyl alcohol, mineral oil, an ethoxylated fatty alcohol, methylparaben, propylparaben, and purified water.
Furacin Topical Cream is an antibacterial agent for topical use.

CLINICAL PHARMACOLOGY
Furacin Topical Cream is a nitrofuran that is bactericidal for most pathogens commonly causing surface infections, including *Staphylococcus aureus, Streptococcus, Escherichia coli, Clostridium perfringens, Aerobacter aerogenes,* and *Proteus.*
Furacin Topical Cream inhibits a number of bacterial enzymes, especially those involved in the aerobic and anaerobic degradation of glucose and pyruvate. The activity appears to involve the pyruvate dehydrogenase system as well as citrate synthetase, malate dehydrogenase, glutathione reductase, and pyruvate decarboxylase. Glutathione reductase inhibition may be caused by control of pentose phosphate metabolism. Although Furacin Topical Cream inhibits a variety of enzymes, it is not considered to be a general enzyme inactivator since many enzymes are not inhibited by this compound.

INDICATIONS AND USAGE
Furacin Topical Cream is a topical antibacterial agent indicated for adjunctive therapy of patients with second- and third-degree burns when bacterial resistance to other agents is a real or potential problem.
It is also indicated in skin grafting where bacterial contamination may cause graft rejection and/or donor site infection particularly in hospitals with historical resistant-bacteria epidemics.
There is no known evidence of effectiveness of this product in the treatment of minor burns or surface bacterial infections involving wounds, cutaneous ulcers or the various pyodermas.

CONTRAINDICATIONS
Known sensitization to any of the components of this preparation is a contraindication for use.

WARNINGS
None.

PRECAUTIONS
General: Use of Furacin Topical Cream occasionally allows overgrowth of nonsusceptible organisms including fungi and *Pseudomonas.* If this occurs, or if irritation, sensitization or superinfection develops, treatment with Furacin Topical Cream should be discontinued and appropriate therapy instituted.
Information for Patients: Patients should be told to use Furacin Topical Cream only as directed by a physician. Patients should be advised to discontinue the drug and contact a physician should rash or irritation occur.
Carcinogenesis, Mutagenesis, and Impairment of Fertility: Nitrofurazone has been shown to produce mammary tumors when fed at high doses to female Sprague-Dawley rats. The relevance of this to topical use in humans is unknown.
Dietary dosage levels of 60 and 30 mg/kg/day shortened the onset time of the typical mammary gland tumors associated with older female rats. These tumors exhibited the same histological characteristics seen in the spontaneously occurring tumors, and were seen only in the female animals. No mammary tumors were seen in rats treated with nitrofurazone orally in the diet for 1 year at levels approximately 11 mg/kg/day. Spermatogenic arrest was noted in the male rats in dietary dosage levels of 30 mg/kg/day and above, after one year on test.
Usage in Pregnancy: Pregnancy Category C: Nitrofurazone, when administered orally to pregnant rabbits, caused a slight increase in the frequency of stillbirths when given in doses thirty times the human dose. There are no adequate and well controlled studies in pregnant women. Furacin Topical Cream should be used during pregnancy only if the potential benefit justifies the potential risk to the fetus.
Nursing Mothers: It is not known whether this drug is excreted in human milk. Because many drugs are excreted in human milk and because of the potential for tumorigenicity shown for nitrofurazone in animal studies, a decision should be made whether to discontinue nursing or to discontinue the drug, taking into account the importance of the drug to the mother.

ADVERSE REACTIONS
In quantitative studies published during the period 1945–70, 206 instances of clinical skin reaction were reported out of 18,249 patients (an incidence of 1.1%) treated with Furacin formulations. Symptoms appeared as varying degrees of contact dermatitides such as rash, pruritus, and local edema. Allergic reactions to Furacin Topical Cream should be treated symptomatically.

DOSAGE AND ADMINISTRATION
Apply Furacin Topical Cream directly to the lesion, or first place on gauze. Reapply once daily or every few days, depending on the usual dressing technique.

HOW SUPPLIED
Furacin Topical Cream is available in:
NDC 0149-0777-15 tube of 14 grams
NDC 0149-0777-12 tube of 28 grams
NDC 0149-0777-61 jar of 368 grams

STORAGE
Avoid exposure to direct sunlight, strong fluorescent lighting, alkaline materials, and excessive heat (over 104°F or 40°C).

ANIMAL TOXICOLOGY
The oral administration of nitrofurazone for 7 days to rats at extremely high dosage levels of 240 mg/kg/day produced severe hepatorenal lesions whereas only renal changes were seen when the dosage level was reduced to 60 mg/kg/day for 60 days.
Dogs treated orally with nitrofurazone for 400 days at levels of 11 mg/kg/day showed no toxic effects related to drug treatment.
There was no evidence of toxicosis in rhesus monkeys treated with doses of nitrofurazone as high as 58 mg/kg/day for 10 weeks and 23 mg/kg/day for 63 weeks.
The peroral LD_{50} of nitrofurazone in mice and rats is 747 and 590 mg/kg respectively.
For bacterial sensitivity tests: Furacin Sensi-Discs are available from BBL, Division of BioQuest.

CAUTION
Federal law prohibits dispensing without prescription.
REVISED OCTOBER 1983 FTOPCR-P2

FURADANTIN® ℞
[fewr-a-dan 'tin]
(nitrofurantoin)

DESCRIPTION
Furadantin is 1-[[(5-nitro-2-furanyl) methylene]amino]-2, 4-imidazolidinedione, a synthetic antimicrobial agent. It is a yellow, stable crystalline compound:

O_2N—…—CH=N—N—C=O, NH, CH_2—C=O

INACTIVE INGREDIENTS
Furadantin tablets contain calcium pyrophosphate, magnesium stearate, starch, and sucrose. Furadantin Oral Suspension contains carboxymethylcellulose sodium, citric acid, flavors, glycerin, magnesium aluminum silicate, methylparaben, propylparaben, purified water, saccharin, sodium citrate, and sorbitol.

ACTIONS
Clinical Pharmacology: Orally administered Furadantin is readily absorbed and rapidly excreted in urine. Blood concentrations at therapeutic dosage are usually low. It is highly soluble in urine, to which it may impart a brown color. Following a therapeutic dose regimen (100 mg q.i.d. for 7 days) average urinary drug recoveries (0–24 hours) on day 1 and day 7 were 42.7% and 43.6%, respectively, for Furadantin.
Microbiology: Furadantin, *in vitro,* is bacteriostatic in low concentrations (10 mcg/ml to 5 mcg/ml) and is considered to be bactericidal in higher concentrations. Its presumed mode of action is based upon its interference with several bacterial enzyme systems. Bacteria develop only a limited resistance to furan derivatives clinically. Furadantin is usually active against the following organisms *in vitro: Escherichia coli,* enterococci (e.g. *Streptococcus faecalis) Staphylococcus aureus.*
Note: Some strains of *Enterobacter* species and *Klebsiella* species are resistant to Furadantin. It is not active against most strains of *Proteus* species, and *Serratia* species. It has no activity against *Pseudomonas* species.
Susceptibility Tests—Quantitative methods that require measurement of zone diameters give the most precise estimates of antimicrobial susceptibility. One recommended procedure, (NCCLS, ASM-2)*, uses a disc containing 300 micrograms for testing susceptibility; interpretations correlate zone diameters of this disc test with MIC values for nitrofurantoin. Reports from the laboratory should be interpreted according to the following criteria:
Susceptible organisms produce zones of 17 mm or greater, indicating that the tested organism is likely to respond to therapy.
Organisms of intermediate susceptibility produce zones of 15 to 16 mm, indicating that the tested organism would be susceptible if high dosage is used.
Resistant organisms produce zones of 14 mm or less, indicating that other therapy should be selected.
A bacterial isolate may be considered susceptible if the MIC value for nitrofurantoin is not more than 25 micrograms per ml. Organisms are considered resistant if the MIC is not less than 100 micrograms per ml.

INDICATIONS
Furadantin is indicated for the treatment of urinary tract infections when due to susceptible strains of *E. coli,* enterococci, *S. aureus* (it is not indicated for the treatment of associated renal cortical or perinephric abscesses), and certain susceptible strains of *Klebsiella* species, *Enterobacter* species, and *Proteus* species.

NOTE
Specimens for culture and susceptibility testing should be obtained prior to and during drug administration.

CONTRAINDICATIONS

Anuria, oliguria, or significant impairment of renal function (creatinine clearance under 40 ml per minute) are contraindications to therapy with this drug. Treatment of this type of patient carries an increased risk of toxicity because of impaired excretion of the drug. For the same reason, this drug is much less effective under these circumstances.

The drug is contraindicated in pregnant patients at term as well as in infants under one month of age because of the possibility of hemolytic anemia due to immature enzyme systems (glutathione instability).

The drug is also contraindicated in those patients with known hypersensitivity to Furadantin, Macrodantin® (nitrofurantoin macrocrystals), and other nitrofurantoin preparations.

WARNINGS

Acute, subacute and chronic pulmonary reactions have been observed in patients treated with nitrofurantoin products. If these reactions occur, the drug should be withdrawn and appropriate measures should be taken.

An insidious onset of pulmonary reactions (diffuse interstitial pneumonitis or pulmonary fibrosis, or both) in patients on long-term therapy warrants close monitoring of these patients.

There have been isolated reports giving pulmonary reactions as a contributing cause of death. (See Hypersensitivity reactions.)

Cases of hemolytic anemia of the primaquine sensitivity type have been induced by Furadantin. The hemolysis appears to be linked to a glucose-6-phosphate dehydrogenase deficiency in the red blood cells of the affected patients. This deficiency is found in 10 percent of Negroes and a small percentage of ethnic groups of Mediterranean and Near-Eastern origin. Any sign of hemolysis is an indication to discontinue the drug. Hemolysis ceases when the drug is withdrawn.

Hepatitis, including chronic active hepatitis, occurs rarely. Fatalities have been reported. The onset of chronic active hepatitis may be insidious, and patients receiving long-term therapy should be monitored periodically for changes in liver function. If hepatitis occurs, the drug should be withdrawn immediately and appropriate measures should be taken.

PRECAUTIONS

Peripheral neuropathy may occur with Furandantin therapy; this may become severe or irreversible. Fatalities have been reported. Predisposing conditions such as renal impairment (creatinine clearance under 40 ml per minute), anemia, diabetes, electrolyte imbalance, vitamin B deficiency, and debilitating disease may enhance such occurrence.

Usage in Pregnancy: The safety of Furadantin during pregnancy and lactation has not been established. Use of this drug in women of childbearing potential requires that the anticipated benefit be weighed against the possible risks.

ADVERSE REACTIONS

Gastrointestinal reactions: Anorexia, nausea and emesis are the most frequent reactions; abdominal pain and diarrhea occur less frequently. These dose-related toxicity reactions can be minimized by reduction of dosage, especially in the female patient. Hepatitis, including chronic active hepatitis, has been observed rarely. The mechanism appears to be of an idiosyncratic hypersensitive type.

Hypersensitivity reactions: Pulmonary sensitivity reactions may occur, which can be acute, subacute, or chronic. Acute reactions are commonly manifested by fever, chills, cough, chest pain, dyspnea, pulmonary infiltration with consolidation or pleural effusion on x-ray, and eosinophilia. The acute reactions usually occur within the first week of treatment and are reversible with cessation of therapy. Resolution may be dramatic.

In subacute reactions, fever and eosinophilia are observed less often. Recovery is somewhat slower, perhaps as long as several months. If the symptoms are not recognized as being drug related and nitrofurantoin is not withdrawn, symptoms may become more severe.

Chronic pulmonary reactions are more likely to occur in patients who have been on continuous nitrofurantoin therapy for six months or longer. The insidious onset of malaise, dyspnea on exertion, cough, and altered pulmonary function are common manifestations. Roentgenographic and histologic findings of diffuse interstitial pneumonitis or fibrosis, or both, are also common manifestations. Fever is rarely prominent.

The severity of these chronic pulmonary reactions and the degree of their resolution appear to be related to the duration of therapy after the first clinical signs appear. Pulmonary function may be permanently impaired even after cessation of nitrofurantoin therapy. This risk is greater when pulmonary reactions are not recognized early.

Dermatologic reactions: Exfoliative dermatitis and erythema multiforme (including Stevens-Johnson Syndrome) have been reported rarely. Maculopapular, erythematous or eczematous eruption, pruritus, urticaria, and angioedema.

Other hypersensitivity reactions: Anaphylaxis, asthmatic attack in patients with history of asthma, cholestatic jaundice, hepatitis, drug fever, arthralgia, sialadenitis, and pancreatitis.

Hematologic reactions: Hemolytic anemia, granulocytopenia, agranulocytosis, leukopenia, thrombocytopenia, eosinophilia, and megaloblastic anemia. Return of the blood picture to normal has followed cessation of therapy. Aplastic anemia has been reported rarely.

Neurological reactions: Peripheral neuropathy, headache, dizziness, nystagmus, and drowsiness.

Miscellaneous reactions: Transient alopecia. As with other antimicrobial agents, superinfections by resistant organisms, e.g., *Pseudomonas*, may occur. With Furadantin, however, these are limited to the genitourinary tract because suppression of normal bacterial flora elsewhere in the body does not occur.

DOSAGE AND ADMINISTRATION

Furadantin should be given with food to improve drug absorption and, in some patients, tolerance.

Adults: 50–100 mg four times a day—the lower dosage level is recommended for uncomplicated urinary tract infections.

Children: 5-7 mg/kg of body weight per 24 hours, to be given in four divided doses (contraindicated under one month of age). The following table can be used to calculate an average dose of Furadantin Oral Suspension (5 mg/ml) for children (one 5 ml teaspoon of Furadantin Oral Suspension contains 25 mg of Furadantin):

Body Weight		No. Teaspoonfuls
Pounds	**Kilograms**	**4 Times Daily**
15 to 26	7 to 11	½ (2.5 ml)
27 to 46	12 to 21	1 (5 ml)
47 to 68	22 to 30	1½ (7.5 ml)
69 to 91	31 to 41	2 (10 ml)

Therapy should be continued for at least one week and for at least 3 days after sterility of the urine is obtained. Continued infection indicates the need for reevaluation.

For long-term suppressive therapy in adults, a reduction of dosage to 50-100 mg at bedtime may be adequate. See WARNINGS section regarding risks associated with long-term therapy. For long-term suppressive therapy in children, doses as low as 1 mg/kg per 24 hours, given in a single or in two divided doses, may be adequate.

HOW SUPPLIED

Furadantin is available in:

50-mg scored, yellow tablets coded "Eaton 036"

NDC 0149-0036-05 bottle of 100
NDC 0149-0036-66 bottle of 500
NDC 0149-0036-06 hospital unit-dose strips in box of 100

100-mg scored, yellow tablets coded "Eaton 037"

NDC 0149-0037-05 bottle of 100
NDC 0149-0037-66 bottle of 500
NDC 0149-0037-07 hospital unit-dose strips in box of 100

It should be dispensed in amber bottles.

Furadantin (nitrofurantoin) Oral Suspension is available in:

NDC 0149-0735-15 amber bottle of 60 ml
NDC 0149-0735-61 amber bottle of 470 ml

Avoid exposure to strong light which may darken the drug. It is stable in storage. It should be dispensed in amber bottles.

Furadantin 300 mcg Sensi-Discs for the laboratory determination of bacterial sensitivity are available from BBL, division of BioQuest. For information on simple Furadantin assays in blood, serum, and urine, write or call the Medical Department. Literature sent to physicians on request.

Address medical inquiries to Norwich Eaton Pharmaceuticals, Inc., Medical Department, Norwich, NY 13815.

* National Committee for Clinical Laboratory Standards. Approved Standard: ASM-2, Performance Standards for Antimicrobial Disc Susceptibility Tests, July, 1975.

Manufactured by
Eaton Laboratories, Inc.
Manati, Puerto Rico 00701
Distributed by
Norwich Eaton Pharmaceuticals, Inc.
Norwich, New York 13815
A Procter & Gamble Company
REVISED APRIL 1985 FDN-P6

FUROXONE® ℞

[fewr-ox 'ōne]
(furazolidone)
Available both in Tablet Form and as a Liquid Suspension

DESCRIPTION

Furoxone (furazolidone) is one of the synthetic antimicrobial nitrofurans. It is a stable, yellow, crystalline compound with the following structure:

3-(5-nitrofurfurylideneamino)-2-oxazolidinone

INACTIVE INGREDIENTS

Furoxone tablets contain calcium pyrophosphate, FD&C Blue #2, FD&C Red #3, magnesium stearate, starch, and sucrose. Furoxone liquid contains carboxymethylcellulose sodium, flavors, glycerin, magnesium aluminum silicate, methylparaben, propylparaben, purified water, and saccharin sodium.

ACTION

Furoxone has a broad antibacterial spectrum covering the majority of gastrointestinal tract pathogens including *E. coli*, staphylococci, *Salmonella, Shigella, Proteus, Aerobacter aerogenes, Vibrio cholerae*[9,10,11] *and Giardia lamblia.*[5,6] Its bactericidal activity is based upon its interference with several bacterial enzyme systems; this antimicrobial action minimizes the development of resistant organisms. It neither significantly alters the normal bowel flora nor results in fungal overgrowth. The brown color found in the urine with adequate dosage is of no clinical significance.

INDICATIONS

Indicated in the specific and symptomatic treatment of bacterial or protozoal diarrhea and enteritis caused by susceptible organisms. Furoxone products are well tolerated, have a very low incidence of adverse reactions.

CONTRAINDICATIONS

1. To obviate an Antabuse® (disulfiram)-like reaction which may occur in some patients, the ingestion of alcohol should be avoided during or within four days after Furoxone therapy. (See ADVERSE REACTIONS)
2. IN GENERAL, MAOI DRUGS, TYRAMINE CONTAINING FOODS AND INDIRECTLY ACTING SYMPATHOMIMETIC AMINES ARE CONTRAINDICATED OR SHOULD BE USED WITH CAUTION IN PATIENTS RECEIVING FUROXONE (SEE PRECAUTIONS.)
3. INFANTS UNDER 1 MONTH SHOULD NOT RECEIVE FUROXONE (SEE ADVERSE REACTIONS AND DOSAGE FOR CHILDREN).[4] THE FUROXONE CONCENTRATION IN THE BREAST MILK OF LACTATING WOMEN HAS NOT BEEN DETERMINED, THEREFORE THE SAFETY IN THIS CIRCUMSTANCE HAS NOT BEEN ESTABLISHED.
4. Prior sensitivity to Furoxone is a contraindication.

WARNINGS

(See CONTRAINDICATIONS listed above.)

Use in Pregnancy: The safety of Furoxone during the childbearing age has not been established; as with any potent antibacterial, Furoxone must be administered with caution during the childbearing age. However, animal breeding studies have revealed no evidence of teratogenicity following the administration of Furoxone for long periods of time and at doses far in excess of those recommended for the human. There have been no clinical reports regarding this possible adverse effect on the fetus or the newborn infant.

PRECAUTIONS

Monoamine Oxidase Inhibition:[7] Effective inhibition of monoamine oxidase by furazolidone has been demonstrated experimentally in man by the enhancement of tyramine and amphetamine sensitivity and by the directly measured monamine oxidase inhibition.

A period of five days of furazolidone administration in the recommended doses in these patients was required to give an enhancement of the tyramine and amphetamine sensitivities by two to threefold. Administration of furazolidone in the recommended dose of 400 mg/day for a period of five days should not subject the adult patient to an undue hazard of hypertensive crisis due to monoamine oxidase inhibition. Hypertensive crises have never been reported even after the peroral administration of larger doses and/or for longer periods of time. Controlled studies reveal no signs or symptoms of hypertensive crisis even after the peroral administration of Furoxone in doses of 400 mg/day in excess of 48 consecutive months.[8]

Continued on next page

Norwich Eaton—Cont.

If administered in doses larger than recommended or in excess of five days, the indications must be weighed against the possible hazards of hypertensive crisis related to the accumulation of monoamine oxidase inhibition. If indications are sufficient, the patients should be informed of drugs and foods which predispose to hypertensive crises:

(A) Other known MAOI drugs; however, when indicated they should be prescribed with caution and at a reduced dosage.
(B) Tyramine-containing foods such as broad beans, yeast extracts, strong unpasteurized cheeses, beer, wine, pickled herring, chicken livers and fermented products are contraindicated.
(C) Indirectly-acting sympathomimetic amines such as those found in nasal decongestants (phenylephrine, ephedrine) and anorectics (amphetamines) are contraindicated.
(D) Likewise, sedatives, antihistamines, tranquilizers and narcotics should be used in reduced dosages and with caution.

Orthostatic hypotension and hypoglycemia may occur.

Carcinogenesis, Mutagenesis, Impairment of Fertility: Furazolidone has shown evidence of tumorigenic activity in several studies involving chronic, high-dose oral administration to rodents. Promotion of the development of mammary neoplasia has been demonstrated in rats of two strains. Prominent among the findings in mice was that furazolidone caused significant increases in malignant lung tumors. The relevance of these animals findings, particularly in relationship to short-term therapy in humans, is not established.

ADVERSE REACTIONS

A few hypersensitivity reactions to Furoxone have been reported including a fall in blood pressure, urticaria, fever, arthralgia and a vesicular morbilliform rash. These reactions subsided following withdrawal of the drug.

Nausea, emesis, headache or malaise occur occasionally and may be minimized or eliminated by reduction in dosage or withdrawal of the drug.

Rarely, individuals receiving Furoxone have exhibited an Antabuse® (disulfiram)-like reaction to alcohol characterized by flushing, slight temperature elevation, dyspnea, and in some instances, a sense of constriction within the chest. All symptomatology disappeared within 24 hours with no lasting ill effects. During nine years of clinical use and approximately 3.5 million courses of therapy (in the U.S.A. alone) in the published literature and documented case reports 43 cases have been reported—of which 14 were produced under experimental conditions with planned doses of the compound in excess of those recommended.

Three of these experienced a fall in blood pressure necessitating active therapy. Indications are that levarterenol (Levophed®) may be used to combat such hypotensive episodes since human studies show that this drug is not potentiated in patients treated with Furoxone. (Indirectly acting pressor agents should be avoided.) The ingestion of alcohol in any form should be avoided during Furoxone therapy and for four days thereafter to prevent this reaction.

Furoxone may cause mild reversible intravascular hemolysis in certain ethnic groups of Mediterranean and Near-Eastern origin, and Negroes.[1,3] This is due to an intrinsic defect of red blood cell metabolism in a small percentage of these ethnic groups, making them unusually susceptible to hemolysis by numerous compounds.[2] It is necessary to observe such patients closely while receiving Furoxone and to discontinue its use if there is any indication of hemolysis.

Should not be administered to infants under 1 month of age because of the possibility of producing a hemolytic anemia due to immature enzyme systems (glutathione instability) in the early neonatal period.[4]

Colitis, proctitis, anal pruritus, staphylococcic enteritis, renal or hepatic toxicity have not been a significant problem with Furoxone.

DOSAGE AND ADMINISTRATION

FUROXONE TABLETS, 100 mg each, are brown and scored to facilitate adjustment of dosage.

Average Adult Dosage: One 100 mg tablet four times daily.

Average Dosage for Children: Those 5 years of age or older should receive 25 to 50 mg (¼ to ½ tablet) four times daily. The tablet dosage may be crushed and given in a spoonful of corn syrup.

FUROXONE LIQUID composition: each 15 ml tablespoonful contains Furoxone 50 mg per 15 ml (3.33 mg per ml) in a light-yellow aqueous vehicle. Suitable flavoring, suspending and preservative agents complete the formulation. It is stable in storage. Prior to administering Furoxone Liquid shake the bottle vigorously. It should be dispensed in amber bottles.

Average Adult Dosage: Two tablespoonfuls four times daily.

Average Dosage for Children:

5 years or older—½ to 1 tablespoonful four times daily (7.5–15.0 ml)

1 to 4 years old—1 to 1½ teaspoonfuls four times daily (5.0–7.5 ml)

1 month to 1 year—½ to 1 teaspoonful four times daily (2.5–5.0 ml)

This dosage is based on an average dose of 5 mg of Furoxone per Kg (2.3 mg per lb) of body weight given in four equally divided doses during 24 hours. The maximal dose of 8.8 mg of Furoxone per Kg (4 mg per lb) of body weight per 24 hours should probably not be exceeded because of the possibility of producing nausea or emesis. If these are severe, the dosage should be reduced.

The average case of diarrhea treated with Furoxone will respond within 2 to 5 days of therapy. Occasional patients may require a longer term of therapy. If satisfactory clinical response is not obtained within 7 days it indicates that the pathogen is refractory to Furoxone and the drug should be discontinued. Adjunctive therapy with other antibacterial agents or bismuth salts is not contraindicated. (N.B. Refer to Warnings.)

In order to administer furazolidone in doses larger than recommended or in excess of five days the indications must be weighed against the possible hazards of hypertensive crisis related to the accumulation of monoamine oxidase inhibition. If indications are sufficient, the patient should be informed of drugs and foods which predispose to hypertensive crisis. (See PRECAUTIONS.)

HOW SUPPLIED

Furoxone Tablets, 100 mg each, coded "Eaton 072", are supplied in amber bottles containing 20 and 100 tablets. (Should be dispensed in amber bottles.)

Furoxone Liquid is supplied in amber bottles containing 60 ml and 473 ml. (Should be dispensed in amber bottles.)

REFERENCES

(1) Kellermeyer, R.S.; Tarlov, A.R.; Schrier, S.L., and Alving, A.S.: J. Lab. Clin. Med. 52:827–828 (Nov.) 1958.
(2) Tarlov et al.: Arch. Int. Med. 109:209–234, 1962.
(3) Kellermeyer et al.: J.A.M.A. 180: No. 5, 388–394, 1962.
(4) Zinkham, Pediatrics, 23:18–32, 1959; Gross & Hurwitz, Pediatrics 22:453, 1958.
(5) Fallas Vargas, M. Un Nuevo Tratamiento para la Giardiasis (A New Treatment for Giardiasis). Rev. Med. Costa Rica 19:269–284 (July 1962).
(6) Webster, B.H. Furazolidone in the Treatment of Giardiasis. Amer. J. Dig. Diseases 5:618–622 (July) 1960.
(7) Oates, J.A.; Pettinger, W.A. Inhibition of Monoamine Oxidase by Furazolidone in Man. Data on file: Office of the Medical Director, Norwich Eaton Pharmaceuticals, Inc. Available upon request.
(8) Kirsner, Joseph B., M.D., Ph.D. Data on file: Office of the Medical Director, Norwich Eaton Pharmaceuticals, Inc. Available upon request.
(9) Neogy, K.N., et al. Furazolidone in Cholera, Journ. Indian Med. Assoc. 48:137, 1967.
(10) Chaudhuri, R.N. et al. Furazolidone in Cholera. Lancet 2:909 (Oct. 30) 1965.
(11) Curlin, G. Comparison of Antibiotic Regimens in Cholera. Abstracts of papers, Epidemiological Intelligence Service Conference, Atlanta, Ga., April 11–14, 1967, p. 11.

FUROXONE (FURAZOLIDONE) SENSI-DISCS for laboratory determination of bacterial sensitivity are available from BBL, division of BioQuest.

CAUTION

Federal law prohibits dispensing without prescription.

Literature available to physicians on request.

Shown in Product Identification Section, page 419

REVISED APRIL 1985 FUROX-P4

MACRODANTIN® ℞

[mak"rō-dan'tin]

(nitrofurantoin macrocrystals)

DESCRIPTION

Macrodantin is a synthetic chemical of controlled crystal size. It is a stable, yellow crystalline compound. It is supplied in capsules containing 25 mg, 50 mg, and 100 mg.

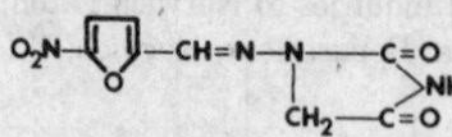

1-[[(5-nitro-2-furanyl)methylene] amino]-2, 4-imidazolidinedione

INACTIVE INGREDIENTS

Each capsule contains edible black ink, gelatin, lactose, starch, talc, titanium dioxide, and may contain FD&C Yellow #6 and D&C Yellow #10.

ACTIONS

Clinical Pharmacology: Macrodantin is a larger crystal form of Furadantin® (nitrofurantoin). The absorption of Macrodantin is slower and its excretion somewhat less when compared to Furandantin. Blood concentrations at therapeutic dosage are usually low. A number of patients who cannot tolerate Furadantin (nitrofurantoin) Tablets are able to take Macrodantin Capsules without nausea. It is highly soluble in urine, to which it may impart a brown color. Following a therapeutic dose regimen (100 mg q.i.d. for 7 days) average urinary drug recoveries (0-24 hours) on day 1 and 7 were 37.9% and 35.0%, respectively, for Macrodantin.

Microbiology: Macrodantin, *in vitro*, is bacteriostatic in low concentrations (10 mcg/ml to 5 mcg/ml) and is considered to be bactericidal in higher concentrations. Its presumed mode of action is based upon its interference with several bacterial enzyme systems. Bacteria develop only a limited resistance to furan derivatives clinically.

Macrodantin is usually active against the following organisms *in vitro: Escherichia coli*, enterococci (e.g. *Streptococcus faecalis*), *Staphylococcus aureus.*

Note: Some strains of *Enterobacter* species and *Klebsiella* species are resistant to Macrodantin. It is not active against most strains of *Proteus* species, and *Serratia* species. It has no activity against *Pseudomonas* species.

Susceptibility Tests—Quantitative methods that require measurement of zone diameters give the most precise estimates of antimicrobial susceptibility. One recommended procedure, (NCCLS, ASM-2)*, uses a disc containing 300 micrograms for testing susceptibility; interpretations correlate zone diameters of this disc test with MIC values for nitrofurantoin.

Reports from the laboratory should be interpreted according to the following criteria:

Susceptible organisms produce zones of 17 mm or greater, indicating that the tested organism is likely to respond to therapy.

Organisms of intermediate susceptibility produce zones of 15 to 16 mm, indicating that the tested organism would be susceptible if high dosage is used.

Resistant organisms produce zones of 14 mm or less, indicating that other therapy should be selected.

A bacterial isolate may be considered susceptible if the MIC value for nitrofurantoin is not more than 25 micrograms per ml. Organisms are considered resistant if the MIC is not less than 100 micrograms per ml.

INDICATIONS

Macrodantin is indicated for the treatment of urinary tract infections when due to susceptible strains of *E. coli*, enterococci, *S. aureus* (it is not indicated for the treatment of associated renal cortical or perinephric abscesses), and certain susceptible strains of *Klebsiella* species, *Enterobacter* species and *Proteus* species.

Note: Specimens for culture and susceptibility testing should be obtained prior to and during drug administration.

CONTRAINDICATIONS

Anuria, oliguria, or significant impairment of renal function (creatinine clearance under 40 ml per minute) are contraindications to therapy with this drug. Treatment of this type of patient carries an increased risk of toxicity because of impaired excretion of the drug. For the same reason, this drug is much less effective under these circumstances.

The drug is contraindicated in pregnant patients at term as well as in infants under one month of age because of the possibility of hemolytic anemia due to immature enzyme systems (glutathione instability).

The drug is also contraindicated in those patients with known hypersensitivity to Macrodantin, Furadantin (nitrofurantoin), and other nitrofurantoin preparations.

WARNINGS

Acute, subacute and chronic pulmonary reactions have been observed in patients treated with nitrofurantoin products. If these reactions occur, the drug should be withdrawn and appropriate measures should be taken.

An insidious onset of pulmonary reactions (diffuse interstitial pneumonitis or pulmonary fibrosis, or both) in patients on long-term therapy warrants close monitoring of these patients.

There have been isolated reports giving pulmonary reactions as a contributing cause of death. (See Hypersensitivity reactions.)

Cases of hemolytic anemia of the primaquine sensitivity type have been induced by Macrodantin. The hemolysis appears to be linked to a glucose-6-phosphate dehydrogenase deficiency in the red blood cells of the affected patients. This deficiency is found in 10 percent of Negroes and a small percentage of ethnic groups of Mediterranean and Near-Eastern origin. Any sign of hemolysis is an indication to discontinue the drug. Hemolysis ceases when the drug is withdrawn.

Hepatitis, including chronic active hepatitis, occurs rarely. Fatalities have been reported. The onset of chronic active hepatitis may be insidious, and patients receiving long-term therapy should be monitored periodically for changes in liver function. If hepatitis occurs, the drug should be withdrawn immediately and appropriate measures should be taken.

PRECAUTIONS

Peripheral neuropathy may occur with Macrodantin therapy; this may become severe or irreversible. Fatalities have been reported. Predisposing conditions such as renal impairment (creatinine clearance under 40 ml per minute), anemia, diabetes, electrolyte imbalance, vitamin B deficiency, and debilitating disease may enhance such occurrence.

Usage in Pregnancy: The safety of Macrodantin during pregnancy and lactation has not been established. Use of this drug in women of childbearing potential requires that the anticipated benefit be weighed against the possible risks.

ADVERSE REACTIONS

Gastrointestinal reactions: Anorexia, nausea and emesis are the most frequent reactions; abdominal pain and diarrhea occur less frequently. These dose-related toxicity reactions can be minimized by reduction of dosage, especially in the female patient.

Hepatitis, including chronic active hepatitis, has been observed rarely. The mechanism appears to be of an idiosyncratic hypersensitive type.

Hypersensitivity reactions: Pulmonary sensitivity reactions may occur, which can be acute, subacute, or chronic. Acute reactions are commonly manifested by fever, chills, cough, chest pain, dyspnea, pulmonary infiltration with consolidation or pleural effusion on x-ray, and eosinophilia. The acute reactions usually occur within the first week of treatment and are reversible with cessation of therapy. Resolution may be dramatic.

In subacute reactions, fever and eosinophilia are observed less often. Recovery is somewhat slower, perhaps as long as several months. If the symptoms are not recognized as being drug related and nitrofurantoin is not withdrawn, symptoms may become more severe.

Chronic pulmonary reactions are more likely to occur in patients who have been on continuous nitrofurantoin therapy for six months or longer. The insidious onset of malaise, dyspnea on exertion, cough, and altered pulmonary function are common manifestations. Roentgenographic and histologic findings of diffuse interstitial pneumonitis or fibrosis, or both, are also common manifestations. Fever is rarely prominent. The severity of these chronic pulmonary reactions and the degree of their resolution appear to be related to the duration of therapy after the first clinical signs appear. Pulmonary function may be permanently impaired even after cessation of nitrofurantoin therapy. This risk is greater when pulmonary reactions are not recognized early.

Dermatologic reactions: Exfoliative dermatitis and erythema multiforme (including Stevens-Johnson Syndrome) has been reported rarely. Maculopapular, erythematous, or eczematous eruption, pruritus, urticaria and angioedema.

Other hypersensitivity reactions: Anaphylaxis, asthmatic attack in patients with history of asthma, cholestatic jaundice, hepatitis, drug fever, arthralgia, sialadenitis, and pancreatitis.

Hematologic reactions: Hemolytic anemia, granulocytopenia, agranulocytosis, leukopenia, thrombocytopenia, eosinophilia, and megaloblastic anemia. Return of the blood picture to normal has followed cessation of therapy. Aplastic anemia has been reported rarely.

Neurological reactions: Peripheral neuropathy, headache, dizziness, nystagmus, and drowsiness.

Miscellaneous reactions: Transient alopecia. As with other antimicrobial agents, superinfections by resistant organisms, e.g., *Pseudomonas*, may occur. With Macrodantin, however, these are limited to the genitourinary tract because suppression of normal bacterial flora elsewhere in the body does not occur.

DOSAGE AND ADMINISTRATION

Macrodantin should be given with food to improve drug absorption and, in some patients, tolerance.

Adults: 50–100 mg four times a day—the lower dosage level is recommended for uncomplicated urinary tract infections.

Children: 5–7 mg/kg of body weight per 24 hours given in four divided doses (contraindicated under one month of age).

Therapy should be continued for at least one week and for at least 3 days after sterility of the urine is obtained. Continued infection indicates the need for reevaluation.

For long-term suppressive therapy in adults, a reduction of dosage to 50–100 mg at bedtime may be adequate. See WARNINGS section regarding risks associated with long-term therapy. For long-term suppressive therapy in children, doses as low as 1 mg/kg per 24 hours, given in a single or in two divided doses, may be adequate.

HOW SUPPLIED

Macrodantin is available as follows:

100 mg: opaque, yellow capsule imprinted with three black lines encircling the capsule and coded "Macrodantin 100 mg" and "0149 0009".*

NDC 0149-0009-05 bottle of 100
NDC 0149-0009-66 bottle of 500
NDC 0149-0009-67 bottle of 1000
NDC 0149-0009-77 hospital unit-dose strips in box of 100

50 mg: opaque, yellow and white capsule imprinted with two black lines encircling the capsule and coded "Macrodantin 50 mg" and "0149 0008".*

NDC 0149-0008-05 bottle of 100
NDC 0149-0008-66 bottle of 500
NDC 0149-0008-67 bottle of 1000
NDC 0149-0008-77 hospital unit-dose strips in box of 100

25 mg: opaque, white capsule imprinted with one black line encircling the capsule and coded "Macrodantin 25 mg" and "0149 0007".

NDC 0149-0007-05 bottle of 100

* capsule design, registered trademark of Eaton Laboratories, Inc.

Furadantin (nitrofurantoin)/Macrodantin Sensi-Discs for the laboratory determination of bacterial sensitivity are available from BBL, Division of BioQuest. For information on simple nitrofurantoin assays in blood, serum, and urine, write or call the Medical Department. Literature sent to physicians on request.

Address medical inquires to Norwich Eaton Pharmaceuticals, Inc. Medical Department, Norwich, NY 13815.

Manufactured by
Eaton Laboratories, Inc.
Manati, Puerto Rico 00701
Distributed by
Norwich Eaton Pharmaceuticals, Inc.
Norwich, New York 13815
A Procter & Gamble Company

Shown in Product Identification Section, page 419

REVISED APRIL 1985 MACRO-P7

TOPICYCLINE® ℞

[*top'i-sī-klēn"*]
(tetracycline hydrochloride for Topical Solution)

DESCRIPTION

TOPICYCLINE is a topical antibiotic preparation containing 2.2 mg of tetracycline hydrochloride per ml as the active ingredient, as well as 4-epitetracycline hydrochloride and sodium bisulfite in an aqueous base of 40% ethanol, citric acid and n-decyl methyl sulfoxide.

Tetracycline is 4-(dimethylamino)-1,4,4a,5,5a, 6, 11, 12a-octahydro-3, 6, 10, 12, 12a-pentahydroxy-6-methyl-1, 11-dioxo-2-naphthacenecarboxamide, the structural formula of which is:

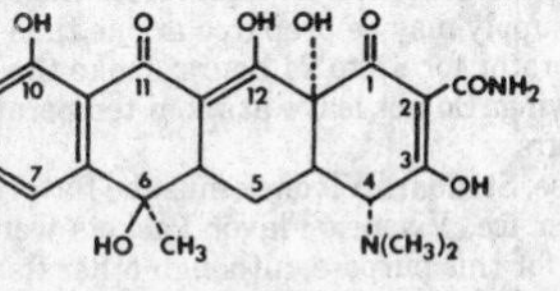

OH O OH OH O; CONH₂ → $CONH_2$; OH; HO CH₃; N(CH₃)₂ → $N(CH_3)_2$; ring positions 1–12

CLINICAL PHARMACOLOGY

TOPICYCLINE delivers tetracycline to the pilosebaceous apparatus and the adjacent tissues. TOPICYCLINE reduces inflammatory acne lesions, but its mode of action is not fully understood.

In clinical studies, use of TOPICYCLINE on the face and neck twice daily delivered to the skin an average dose of 2.9 mg of tetracycline hydrochloride per day. Patients who used the medication twice daily on other acne-involved areas in addition to the face and neck applied an average dose of 4.8 mg of tetracycline hydrochloride per day.

TOPICYCLINE has been formulated such that the recrystallization properties of the tetracyclines on the skin greatly reduce or eliminate the yellow color often associated with topical tetracycline.

INDICATIONS AND USAGE

TOPICYCLINE is indicated in the treatment of acne vulgaris.

CONTRAINDICATIONS

TOPICYCLINE is contraindicated in persons who have shown hypersensitivity to any of its ingredients or to any of the other tetracyclines.

WARNINGS

Contains sodium bisulfite, a sulfite that may cause allergic-type reactions (e.g., hives, itching, wheezing, anaphylaxis) in certain susceptible persons. Although the overall prevalence of sulfite sensitivity in the general population is probably low, it is seen more frequently in asthmatics or in atopic nonasthmatic persons.

PRECAUTIONS

General: This drug is for external use only and care should be taken to keep it out of the eyes, nose, and mouth.

Carcinogenesis, Mutagenesis, and Impairment of Fertility: A two-year dermal study in mice has been performed with TOPICYCLINE and indicates there is no carcinogenic potential with this drug.

Pregnancy: Pregnancy Category B. Reproduction studies have been performed in rats and rabbits at doses of up to 246 times the human dose (assuming the human dose to be 1.3 ml/40kg/day) and have revealed no evidence of impaired fertility or harm to the fetus from TOPICYCLINE. There are, however, no adequate and well-controlled studies in pregnant women. Because animal reproduction studies are not always predictive of human response, this drug should be used during pregnancy only if clearly needed.

Nursing Mothers: It is not known whether tetracycline or any other component of TOPICYCLINE administered in this topical form is excreted in human milk. Because many drugs are excreted in human milk, caution should be exercised when TOPICYCLINE is administered to a nursing woman.

Pediatric Use: Safety and effectiveness in children below the age of eleven have not been established.

ADVERSE REACTIONS

Among the 838 patients treated with TOPICYCLINE under normal usage conditions during clinical evaluation, there was one instance of severe dermatitis requiring systemic steroid therapy.

About one-third of patients are likely to experience a stinging or burning sensation upon application of TOPICYCLINE. The sensation ordinarily lasts no more than a few minutes, and does not occur at every application. There has been no indication that patients experience sufficient discomfort to reduce the frequency of use or to discontinue use of the product.

The kinds of side effects often associated with oral or parenteral administration of tetracyclines (e.g., various gastrointestinal complaints, vaginitis, hematologic abnormalities, manifestations of systemic hypersensitivity reactions, and dental and skeletal disorders) have not been observed with TOPICYCLINE. Because of TOPICYCLINE's topical form of administration, it is highly unlikely that such side effects will occur from its use.

DOSAGE AND ADMINISTRATION

It is recommended that TOPICYCLINE be applied generously twice-daily to the entire affected area (not just to individual lesions) until the skin is thoroughly wet. Instructions to the patients for proper application are provided on the TOPICYCLINE bottle label. Patients may continue their normal use of cosmetics.

Concomitant use with benzoyl peroxide or oral tetracycline has been reported without observed problems.

HOW SUPPLIED

TOPICYCLINE is supplied in a single carton containing a powder and a liquid which must be combined prior to using. Complete instructions for mixing are provided on the carton. Once combined, the TOPICYCLINE bottle contains 70 ml of medication. This constitutes about an eight-week supply for treating the face and neck, or about a four-week supply for treating the face, neck and additional acne-involved areas. Differences in individual usage habits will result in variation from these averages.

NDC 0149-0401-03 70 ml as dispensed.

TOPICYCLINE should be kept at controlled room temperature 59°F–86°F (15°C–30°C) or below.

CAUTION

Federal law prohibits dispensing without prescription.

Manufactured for
Norwich Eaton Pharmaceuticals, Inc.
A Procter & Gamble Company
Norwich, New York 13815
by **Taylor Pharmacal**
Decatur, Illinois 62525

REVISED JANUARY 1986 TOPI-P3

STANDARD VIVONEX®

[*vī'vō-nex"*]

NUTRITIONAL INFORMATION AND USE INSTRUCTIONS

Standard Vivonex® is a patented, nutritionally complete elemental diet formulated for the nutritional management of patients with impaired digestion and/or malabsorption.

COMPOSITION

Standard Vivonex is a chemically defined diet composed of all essential nutrients in simple, readily absorbable form: free amino acids, predigested carbohydrates, safflower oil, vitamins, minerals, electrolytes and trace elements. One 80-gram packet provides 300 Calories and 0.98 grams of available nitrogen with a caloric density of 1 Calorie per ml when diluted with 255 ml water to a total standard dilution volume of 300 ml:

[See table on bottom next page].

Six 80-g packets of Standard Vivonex supply 5.88 grams of available nitrogen, 2.61 grams fat, 407 grams carbohydrate,

Continued on next page

Norwich Eaton—Cont.

and the following vitamins, minerals, electrolytes and amino acid profile:
[See table right].

Electrolytes	mEq per 1000 ml (Standard dilution)	Wt per 1000 ml (Standard dilution)
CATIONS		
Sodium	20.4	468 mg
Potassium	30.0	1172 mg
Calcium	27.7	556 mg
Magnesium	18.3	222 mg
Manganese	0.057	1.56 mg
Iron	0.358	10 mg
Copper	0.035	1.11 mg
Zinc	0.255	8.33 mg
Selenium+	0.002*	83.3 mcg
Molybdenum+	0.002**	83.3 mcg
Chromium+	0.002	27.8 mcg
ANIONS		
Chloride	20.4	722 mg
Phosphorus	54.0‡	556 mg
Acetate	18.7	1106 mg
Iodide	0.0007	83.3 mcg

\+ Represents amounts of these elements added.
* Calculated as Selenite SeO_3^{-2}
** Calculated as Molybdate MoO_4^{-2}
‡ Calculated as Phosphate PO_4^{-3}

Amino Acid Profile	% Total Amino Acids
ESSENTIALS	
L-Isoleucine	4.55
L-Leucine	7.20
L-Valine	5.02
L-Lysine	5.41
L-Methionine	4.66
L-Phenylalanine	5.18
L-Threonine	4.55
L-Tryptophan	1.41
Total essential amino acids	37.98
NON-ESSENTIAL	
L-Alanine	4.85
L-Arginine	8.87
L-Aspartic Acid	10.35
L-Glutamine	17.07
Glycine	7.91
L-Histidine	2.21
L-Proline	6.48
L-Serine	3.34
L-Tyrosine	0.94
Total non-essential amino acids	62.02

In the standard solution of 1 Calorie/ml, Standard Vivonex has a pH of approximately 5.5 and an average osmolality of 550 mOsm/kg.

ACTIONS AND USES

Standard Vivonex is a nutritionally complete, elemental diet that is rapidly utilized, since digestion is virtually obviated, and absorption can take place without the aid of peptidases. Standard Vivonex is absorbed within the first 100 cm of functional small intestine. It is essentially a non-residue diet. There is minimal stimulation of biliary, pancreatic, and intestinal secretions, because of its free L-amino acid nitrogen (protein) source, glucose oligosaccharide primary energy source, and low fat content. The low fat content also permits rapid gastric emptying and eliminates gastric residuals, thus minimizing the possibility of aspiration.
The balanced amino acid profile of Standard Vivonex insures optimum utilization and retention of its readily absorbed, elemental nitrogen source.
Standard Vivonex is useful in the dietary management of patients with impaired digestion and absorption which are secondary to a variety of diseases and disorders such as gastrointestinal disease, e.g. inflammatory bowel disease, cancer, intestinal atresia; conditions leading to partial function of the gastrointestinal tract, e.g. pancreatitis, fistula, partial obstruction, short-gut syndrome. Standard Vivonex is also useful in the dietary management of neonates and infants suffering from intractable diarrhea, as an aid in preparing the bowel for diagnostic and surgical procedures, and as a transition diet between parenteral and normal oral feeding.
It is synthetically derived and contains no whole foodstuffs and therefore is hypoallergenic and well tolerated by patients with known food sensitivites. Standard Vivonex has been proven useful as an elimination diet for patients undergoing diagnosis of specific food allergens.
One packet diluted with 255 ml (8½ oz.) of water makes a single serving. Six packets of Standard Vivonex mixed thoroughly with 1530 ml of water provide a full day's supply for the average adult with 1800 Calories, 5.88 grams available nitrogen, 2.61 grams fat, and 415 grams carbohydrate. Standard Vivonex is a perishable liquid food when in solution. A full day's supply may be prepared at one time and stored in the refrigerator for up to 24 hours; shake the liquid briefly before serving. Do not leave at room temperature for more than 8 hours.
For oral use, Standard Vivonex must be flavored and served chilled over ice. Vivonex Flavor Packets were specifically developed for this purpose, although other flavoring agents may be used if their contribution to the elemental and nutritional qualities of the diet are kept in mind. Standard Vivonex should be sipped slowly, preferably with a straw, when served as a beverage. Initiate oral feeding with dilute solution, e.g. one packet diluted with 555 ml (18½ oz.), and gradually increase volume and concentration.
Oral feedings of elemental diets are sometimes met by poor patient acceptance because of taste and the lack of the usual appetite cues of normal meals. Varying the available flavors, serving chilled over ice and sipping through a straw, and educating and motivating the patient as to the therapeutic importance of this form of diet, are reportedly effective in improving patient acceptability.
Standard Vivonex may also be administered via feeding tube placed nasogastrically or into an esophagostomy, gastrostomy, or jejunostomy. Because of its homogeneity and low viscosity, as small as a 16 gauge catheter or #5 French feeding tube may be used to optimize patient tolerance. It is suggested that the diet be given at room temperature by continuous drip technique using the Vivonex® Acutrol® Enteral Feeding System, the Vivonex® Delivery System, or a suitable infusion pump. At the 1 Calorie per ml dilution, Standard Vivonex supplies most of the daily fluid requirements. Additional fluids should be given when necessary to maintain adequate urine output.
During the first two days of use, Standard Vivonex may need to be over-diluted for the osmotically sensitive patient, gradually titrating up to full strength. The following administration schedule will facilitate GI adaptation, in most patients, within three days:
[See table on top next page].
If diarrhea is encountered, revert one step to a more dilute solution, maintaining the patient at the last tolerated rate until free of symptoms for 8 hours. Then continue with progressive schedule until desired caloric/nitrogen intake is achieved.

PRECAUTIONS

DO NOT ADMINISTER STANDARD VIVONEX PARENTERALLY.

For use only under medical supervision.
Nausea, vomiting, abdominal cramps and distention, and diarrhea have been reported. Nausea is usually due to feeding rate, while diarrhea may also be caused by the diet concentration. If encountered, revert one step in the above administration schedule, and then continue slowly with a progressive schedule until desired caloric/nitrogen intake is achieved. Local water conditions have also been implicated in instances of diarrhea. Using deionized or distilled water in diet preparation, until patient tolerance with full strength diet is achieved, has been reported to be effective in this circumstance.
Aspiration is an uncommon complication with Standard Vivonex because of its low fat content. However, in patients suspected at risk, radiologically confirm the anatomic position of the feeding tube, elevate the head of the bed 30° while the patient is receiving diet intragastrically, and control the administration to 150 ml/hour or less, depending upon patient tolerance. Jejunal administration should also be considered.
Additional professional and technical information on all Vivonex products is available through your local Norwich Eaton Pharmaceuticals representative.

SUPPLY INFORMATION

Standard Vivonex (NDC 0149-0052-01) is available in cartons of six 80-g sealed packets for individual servings. Each packet provides 300 Calories in a total volume of 300 ml when mixed with 255 ml water.
Vivonex Flavor Packets are available in Vanilla (NDC 0149-0054-02), Strawberry (NDC 0149-0056-02), Orange-Pineapple (NDC 0149-0058-02), and Lemon-Lime (NDC 0149-0057-02) flavors.
The Vivonex Acutrol Enteral Feeding System (NDC 0149-0065-06) is a one-liter, universal, gravity feeding system offering a unique rapid-fill funnel cap, easy-to-read fluid level graduations, macro-drip sight chamber, precise control roller clamp, universal luer adapter, and a built-in burette.
The Vivonex Delivery System (NDC 0149-0050-10) is a disposable, gravity-drip tube feeding system with one liter capacity, complete with micro-drop cannula and connecting tubing.
Patent No. 3,697,287
REVISED FEBRUARY 1984 STDVIV-P6

Vitamins, Minerals and Trace Elements	Per 1000 ml (Standard dilution)	Per 6 Packets (480 Grams)	% U.S. RDA Per 6 Packets
Vitamin A	2778 IU	5000 IU	100
Vitamin D_3	222 IU	400 IU	100
Vitamin E	16.7 IU	30 IU	100
Vitamin C	33.3 mg	60 mg	100
Folic Acid	0.22 mg	0.4 mg	100
Thiamine	0.83 mg	1.5 mg	100
Riboflavin	0.94 mg	1.7 mg	100
Niacin	11.1 mg	20 mg	100
Vitamin B_6	1.11 mg	2 mg	100
Vitamin B_{12}	3.33 mcg	6 mcg	100
Biotin	0.17 mg	0.3 mg	100
Pantothenic Acid	5.55 mg	10 mg	100
Vitamin K_1	37.2 mcg	67 mcg	•
Choline	40.9 mg	73.7 mg	•
Calcium	0.55 g	1 g	100
Phosphorus	0.55 g	1 g	100
Iodine	83.3 mcg	150 mcg	100
Iron	10 mg	18 mg	100
Magnesium	222 mg	400 mg	100
Copper	1.11 mg	2 mg	100
Zinc	8.33 mg	15 mg	100
Manganese	1.56 mg	2.81 mg	•
Selenium+	83.3 mcg	150 mcg	•
Molybdenum+	83.3 mcg	150 mcg	•
Chromium+	27.8 mcg	50 mcg	•

• No U.S. RDA established
\+ Represents amounts of these elements added.

	Amount per 80 g	Amount per 1000 ml (Standard dilution)	Energy Distribution
Total energy (Calories)	300	1000	
Amino acids (free base equivalent)	6.18 g	20.6 g	8.2%
Carbohydrate (dry basis)	67.9 g	226.3 g	90.5%
Fat	0.435 g	1.45 g	1.3%
Linoleic acid	0.348 g	1.16 g	1.0%

Day	Strength	Approx. Rate (ml/hour)	Standard Vivonex (No. of Packets)	+	Total Water (ml)	=	Volume (ml)	Calories (Cal.)	Nitrogen (g)
1	½	75	3	+	1,665	=	1,800	900	3
2	⅔	75	4	+	1,620	=	1,800	1,200	4
3	Full	75	6	+	1,530	=	1,800	1,800	6

VIVONEX®
[*vī 'vō-nex "*]
FLAVOR PACKETS—Lemon-Lime, Orange-Pineapple, Strawberry or Vanilla
NONNUTRITIVE

Exclusively for use with Vivonex T.E.N., High Nitrogen Vivonex or Standard Vivonex.

VIVONEX® ACUTROL® ℞
[*vī 'vō-nex " ak 'ū-trawl*]
Enteral Feeding System

VIVONEX® Delivery System
[*vī 'vō-nex "*]
Tube Feeding System

VIVONEX® JEJUNOSTOMY KIT
[*vī 'vō-nex " jā-jū-nos 'tō-me*]
Needle catheter jejunostomy kit

VIVONEX® TUNGSTEN TIP TUBE
[*vī-vō-nex "*]

Nasogastric/Nasointestinal Feeding Tube

VIVONEX® T.E.N.
[*vī 'vō-nex*]
Elemental Diet For TOTAL ENTERAL NUTRITION an effective substitute for intravenous feeding (TPN)

Vivonex® T.E.N. is a high nitrogen, elemental diet for total enteral nutrition. Vivonex T.E.N. is an effective substitute for intravenous feeding (TPN), except in patients where enteral feeding may be contraindicated (i.e., less than 60 cm of functioning small intestine). Its high essential to nonessential amino acid ratio (52:48), enhanced branched-chain amino acid content (33% of total amino acids), and optimal quantity of protein-sparing carbohydrate in a 175:1 Calorie to nitrogen ratio, make it especially useful in stressed, catabolic patients. Vivonex T.E.N. will further benefit those patients requiring a low residue feeding that permits maximal absorption with minimal digestion.

INDICATIONS

Vivonex T.E.N. is recommended in the dietary management of the following conditions:

- Stress
  - multiple trauma
  - burns
  - immediate postoperative malnutrition
  - sepsis
- Impaired digestion and absorption
  - inflammatory bowel disease
  - cancer
  - intestinal atresia
  - pancreatitis
  - fistula
  - partial obstruction
  - short-gut syndrome
- Malnutrition and cachexia
- Bowel preparation prior to diagnostic and surgical procedures
- Transition diet between parenteral and normal oral feeding
- Food sensitivities

COMPOSITION

Vivonex T.E.N. is a chemically defined diet composed of all essential nutrients in simple, readily absorbable form: free amino acids, predigested carbohydrates, safflower oil, vitamins, minerals, electrolytes, and trace elements. One 80.4-gram packet provides 300 Calories and 1.71 grams of available nitrogen with a caloric density of 1 Calorie per ml when diluted with 250 ml water to a total standard dilution volume of 300 ml:

[See table below].

Ten 80.4-gram packets of Vivonex T.E.N. meet or exceed the quantity of nutrients and energy required by the average catabolic adult: 17.1 grams of available nitrogen, 115 grams amino acids, 8.33 grams fat, 617 grams carbohydrate, and the following vitamins, minerals, electrolytes, and amino acid profile:

[See table on bottom next page].

Electrolytes	mEq per 1000 ml (standard dilution)	Wt. Per 1000 ml (standard dilution)
Cations		
Sodium	20	460 mg
Potassium	20	782 mg
Calcium	25	500 mg
Magnesium	16.5	200 mg
Manganese	0.034	937 mcg
Iron	0.322	9 mg
Copper	0.032	1 mg
Zinc	0.306	10 mg
Selenium†	0.001*	50 mcg
Molybdenum†	0.001**	50 mcg
Chromium†	0.001	17 mcg
Anions		
Chloride	23.1	819 mg
Phosphorus	48.5‡	500 mg
Acetate	31.0	1830 mg
Iodide	0.0006	75 mcg

† Represents amounts of these elements added
* Calculated as Selenite, SeO_3^{-2}
** Calculated as Molybdate, MoO_4^{-2}
‡ Calculated as Phosphate, PO_4^{-3}

Amino Acid Profile	% Total Amino Acids
Essential	
L-Isoleucine	8.27
L-Leucine	16.56
L-Valine	8.27
L-Lysine	5.10
L-Methionine	3.66
L-Phenylalanine	5.16
L-Threonine	4.00
L-Tryptophan	1.28
Total essential amino acids	52.30
Non-essential	
L-Alanine	5.18
L-Arginine	7.64
L-Aspartic Acid	7.01
L-Glutamine	12.85
Glycine	4.01
L-Histidine	2.36
L-Proline	4.88
L-Serine	2.93
L-Tryosine	0.84
Total nonessential amino acids	47.70
Branched-chain amino acids (Isoleucine, Leucine, Valine)	33.10
Aromatic amino acids (Phenylalanine, Tyrosine)	6.00
Branched-chain: Aromatic amino acid molar ratio	7.4 : 1

In the standard dilution of 1 Calorie/ml, Vivonex T.E.N. has a pH of approximately 5.0 and an average osmolality of 630 mOsm/kg.

MIXING AND STORAGE

To prepare 300 ml of full strength diet (1 packet):

1. Add 1 packet of diet to 250 ml of warm water in a 1 pint container.
2. Cover and shake for 20 seconds.

Any remaining undissolved particles will dissolve spontaneously after standing 5–10 minutes.

NOTE: For larger quantities the container should be no more than ¾ full after diet is added to water, and more time may be required to shake product into solution. Vivonex T.E.N. can also be blenderized if desired.

Vivonex T.E.N. is a perishable liquid food when in solution. A full day's supply may be prepared at one time and stored in the refrigerator for up to 48 hours; shake the liquid briefly before serving. Do not leave at room temperature for more than 8 hours.

Feeding Tube Administration: VIVONEX T.E.N. may be administered via a nasogastric, nasointestinal, esophagostomy, gastrostomy, or jejunostomy feeding tube. Because of its homogeneity and low viscosity, small bore feeding tubes (16 gauge catheter or #5 French tube) may be used to optimize patient tolerance. The diet should be given at room temperature by continuous drip technique, using the Vivonex® Acutrol® Enteral Feeding System, the Vivonex® Delivery System, or a suitable infusion pump. At the 1 Calorie per ml dilution, Vivonex T.E.N. supplies most of the daily fluid requirements. Additional fluids should be given when necessary to maintain hydration and adequate urine output.

Generally, patient tolerance is optimized with any enteral diet by beginning with a dilute solution, titrating up to the desired calorie and nitrogen input. Although a more aggressive administration schedule may be considered, especially for gastric feeding or patients with a serum albumin level greater than 3.5 g/dl, the following schedule has been found to facilitate adaptation in most patients:

[See table on top next page].

Once full strength T.E.N. is being administered, nutrient intake can be increased by raising the continuous flow rate in 25 ml increments and/or raising the concentration, e.g., one packet + 150 ml water = 200 ml of 1.5 Cal/ml diet.

Diarrhea is the most common side effect with any liquid diet. Concomitant use of an antidiarrheal will often allow uninterrupted titration of the diet. However, in some instances, it may be necessary to revert one step to a more dilute solution, maintaining the patient at the last tolerated rate until free of symptoms for eight hours. Then, continue with progressive schedule until desired calorie and nitrogen intake is achieved.

ORAL ADMINISTRATION

For oral use, Vivonex T.E.N. should be flavored and served chilled over ice. Vivonex Flavor Packets were specifically developed for this purpose, although other flavoring agents may be used if their contribution to the elemental and nutritional qualities of the diet are kept in mind. Vivonex T.E.N. should be sipped slowly, preferably through a straw, when served as a beverage. Initiate oral feeding with dilute solution, e.g., one packet diluted with 550 ml (18⅓ oz.), and gradually increase volume and concentration.

Oral feedings of elemental diets are sometimes met with poor patient acceptance because of taste and the lack of the usual appetite cues of normal meals. Varying the available flavors, serving chilled over ice and sipping through a straw, and educating and motivating the patient as to the therapeutic importance of this form of diet, are reportedly effective in improving patient acceptability.

PRECAUTIONS

DO NOT ADMINISTER VIVONEX T.E.N. PARENTERALLY. For use only under medical supervision. Nausea, vomiting, abdominal cramps, distention, and diarrhea are possible. Nausea and diarrhea are usually due to feeding rate or diet concentration. Local water conditions may be implicated in instances of diarrhea. Preparing diet with deionized or distilled water may be effective in this circumstance.

Aspiration is an uncommon complication with Vivonex T.E.N. because of its low fat content. However, radiologically confirm the anatomic position of the feeding tube, elevate the head of the bed 30° while the patient is receiving diet intragastrically, and control the administration to 150 ml/hour or less, depending upon patient tolerance. Jejunal administration should also be considered.

Diabetics and patients with renal insufficiency receiving this diet should be closely monitored. Use in children may require adjusting the daily consumption to meet the Recommended Daily Allowance for the age group involved.

	Amount per 80.4 g	Amount per 1000 ml (standard dilution)	Energy Distribution
Total energy (Calories)	300	1000	
Amino acids (free base equivalent)	11.46 g	38.20 g	15.3%
Carbohydrate (dry basis)	61.67 g	205.57 g	82.2%
Fat	0.83 g	2.77 g	2.5%
Linoleic acid	0.65 g	2.17 g	2.0%

Continued on next page

Norwich Eaton—Cont.

SUPPLY INFORMATION

Vivonex T.E.N. (NDC 0149-0067-01) is available in cartons of ten 80.4-gram sealed packets, each providing 300 Calories. Vivonex Flavor Packets are available in Vanilla (NDC 0149-0054-02), Strawberry (NDC 0149-0056-02), Orange-Pineapple (NDC 0149-0058-02), and Lemon-Lime (NDC 0149-0057-02) flavors.

The Vivonex Acutrol Enteral Feeding System (NDC 0149-0065-06) is a one-liter, universal, gravity feeding system offering a unique rapid-fill funnel cap, easy-to-read fluid level graduations, macro-drip sight chamber, precise control roller clamp, universal luer adapter, and a built-in burette. The Vivonex Delivery System (NDC 0149-0050-10) is a disposable, gravity-drip tube feeding system with one liter capacity, complete with micro-drop cannula and connecting tubing.

Additional professional and technical information on all Vivonex products is available through local Norwich Eaton Pharmaceuticals representatives.

REVISED MAY 1986 VIVTEN-P4

EDUCATIONAL MATERIAL

Norwich Eaton offers a wide range of Professional Services to the medical profession free of charge. Please write to the Director of Professional Services, Norwich Eaton Pharmaceuticals, Inc., Norwich, NY 13815-0231, for further information.

- ***The Norwich Eaton Audio-Visual Library***—nearly 300 film, slide and videotape programs are available on free-loan (Directory available upon request)
- ***Professional Speaker Bureaus*** (UTI, Nutrition, Clinical Management of Pain, and Clinical Disorders of Bone)
- ***Calendars of CME Events*** (Ob/Gyn, Urology, Allergy)
- ***Patient Education Brochures and Films*** (Urology)
- ***ACOG Physician Placement Service***
- ***AUA Physician Placement Service***

Important Notice
Before prescribing or administering any product described in PHYSICIANS' DESK REFERENCE always consult the PDR Supplement for possible new or revised information

Day	Strength	Approx. Rate (ml/hour)	Vivonex T.E.N. (no. of packets)	+	Water (ml)	=	Total Volume (ml)	Calories (Cal.)	Nitrogen (g)
1	½	50	2	+	1100	=	1200	600	3.42
2	½	100	4	+	2200	=	2400	1200	6.84
3	¾	100	6	+	2100	=	2400	1800	10.26
4	Full	100	8	+	2000	=	2400	2400	13.68

NTRON International Sales Co.

3833 REDWOOD HWY.
P.O. BOX 7000
SAN RAFAEL, CA 94912

NTRON TENS ℞

[*ĕn 'trŏn*]

Transcutaneous Electrical Nerve Stimulator

DESCRIPTION

The NTRON TENS is a portable, battery-powered electrical generator. It produces small amounts of pulsatile alternating current which is transported through the patient's skin by non-invasive surface electrodes. The effects are comfortable for most patients.

ACTIONS

The physiological means by which TENS produces analgesia is as yet incompletely understood. Current theory suggests that electrical stimulation of the large, faster-conducting non-nociceptive A-beta nerve fibers may block impulses from the smaller, slower-conducting nociceptive A-delta and C fibers at the substantia gelatinosa. It is also suggested that TENS may increase the body's production of endogenous opiates.

INDICATIONS

TENS may be indicated for the treatment of chronic intractable pain as a conservative alternative to pharmaceutical or surgical analgesic treatments. It has been shown to be effective in reducing or eliminating pain associated with a wide variety of syndromes, including low back pain, sciatica, causalgia, phantom limb, osteoarthritis, post herpetic neuralgias, bursitis, and tension and migraine headaches.

TENS therapy may also be effective in relieving acute pain due to trauma, and to relieve incisional pain following surgery, while reducing ileus and atelectasis.

CONTRAINDICATIONS

There are no known short or long term complications. The possibility that TENS may effect the nervous system in some presently unknown way should not be overlooked.

WARNINGS

The stimulation of the NTRON TENS is not enough to effect the function of the heart in normal individuals. Adequate precautions should be taken with suspected heart patients. Electrical stimulation may interfere with the proper functioning of demand-type pacemakers. Care should be exercised in avoiding stimulation in paths that include the pacemaker and pacemaker cables. Electrodes should not be placed directly over the eye, in the mouth, or over the carotid sinus. Power should be increased slowly so as not to startle the patient or cause a secondary accident. The conductive gel under the electrodes should not be allowed to dry, as this may result in skin burn or irritation.

PRECAUTIONS

Though no adverse effects have been reported, the safety of TENS during pregnancy, labor and delivery has not been established. As with all analgesics, TENS should be used only to relieve pain and not replace proper medical procedure for a correctable condition.

ADVERSE REACTIONS

Cases of skin irritation under the electrodes may be avoided by periodic relocation of the electrodes after extended wear or by selection of a compatible electrode gel, adhesive and/or use of a skin barrier preparation.

DOSAGE AND ADMINISTRATION

The efficacy of TENS therapy is quite patient-specific. The most effective electrode placements, number of electrodes, device settings, and length of treatment time for optimum results may vary from patient to patient. One or more clinical training sessions will be necessary to establish the most effective regimen and to train the patient in the proper use of the instrument. After clinical training, unsupervised self-administration by the patient can be considered. Treatment time should be determined by patient comfort and clinical effect. Treatments may vary from a few minutes up to 24 hours per day. Once a trial period of self-administered patient use has been evaluated, TENS may be considered for long term use.

OVERDOSAGE

Within the strictures of the aforementioned warnings and precautions, treatment with the TENS has been used indefinitely with no reported ill effects. It is a non-addictive and completely reversible form of analgesia with no known combinatory disadvantages.

HOW SUPPLIED

NTRON Transcutaneous Electrical Nerve Stimulator. The device is housed in an attractive 3 × 2 × 1″ plastic case. Electrodes and cables, 9 Volt alkaline battery, electrode gel, adhesives, and Patient Instruction Booklet are supplied. Accessories are available for special requirements. Clinical training materials are available.

CAUTION

Federal law prohibits dispensing without prescription.

Organon Inc.

375 MT. PLEASANT AVE.
WEST ORANGE, NJ 07052

Below are listed the currently available products. For a complete catalog and price list direct inquiries to Customer Service. For specific product information, direct inquiries to the Professional Services Department.

CALDEROL® ℞

[*kal-dah 'rol*]

(calcifediol capsules, USP)

DESCRIPTION

Calderol Capsules contain calcifediol, USP, which is the colorless, crystalline monohydrate of 25-hydroxycholecalciferol prepared by chemical synthesis and is identical to the natural vitamin metabolite. Calcifediol has a calculated molecular weight of 418.67 and is soluble in organic solvents but relatively insoluble in water. Chemically, calcifediol is (5Z,7E)-9,10-secocholesta-5,7,10(19)-triene-3β, 25-diol monohydrate. The structural formula is represented below:

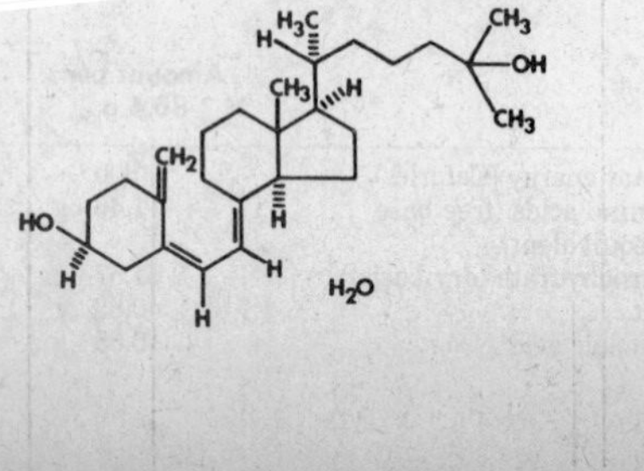

Vitamins, Minerals and Trace Elements	Per 1000 ml (standard dilution)		Per 10 Packets (804 Grams)		% U.S. RDA Per 10 Packets
Vitamin A	2500	IU	7500	IU	150
Vitamin D_3	200	IU	600	IU	150
Vitamin E	15	IU	45	IU	150
Vitamin C	60	mg	180	mg	300
Folic Acid	0.4	mg	1.2	mg	300
Thiamine	1.5	mg	4.5	mg	300
Riboflavin	1.7	mg	5.1	mg	300
Niacin	20	mg	60	mg	300
Vitamin B_6	2	mg	6	mg	300
Vitamin B_{12}	6	mcg	18	mcg	300
Biotin	0.3	mg	0.9	mg	300
Pantothenic Acid	10	mg	30	mg	300
Vitamin K_1	22.3	mcg	67	mcg	*
Choline	73.7	mg	221	mg	*
Calcium	0.5	g	1.5	g	150
Phosphorus	0.5	g	1.5	g	150
Iodine	75	mcg	225	mcg	150
Iron	9	mg	27	mg	150
Magnesium	200	mg	600	mg	150
Copper	1	mg	3	mg	150
Zinc	10	mg	30	mg	200
Manganese	0.94	mg	2.81	mg	*
Selenium†	50	mcg	150	mcg	*
Molybdenum†	50	mcg	150	mcg	*
Chromium†	16.67	mcg	50	mcg	*

* No U.S. RDA established.
† Represents amounts of these elements added.

The other names frequently used for 25-hydroxycholecalciferol are 25-hydroxyvitamin D_3, 25-HCC, 25-OHCC, and 25-OHD_3.
Calderol for oral administration is available in two strengths: a white capsule containing 20 mcg calcifediol and an orange capsule containing 50 mcg calcifediol.

CLINICAL PHARMACOLOGY

The natural supply of vitamin D in man mainly depends on the ultraviolet rays of the sun for conversion of 7-dehydrocholesterol to vitamin D_3 (cholecalciferol). It is now known that vitamin D_3 must first be converted to 25-OHD_3 (25-hydroxycholecalciferol) by a vitamin D_3-25-hydroxylase enzyme (25-OHase) present in the liver. 25-Hydroxycholecalciferol is the major transport form of vitamin D_3 and can be readily monitored in the serum. It is further converted to 1,25-dihydroxycholecalciferol (1,25-$(OH)_2D_3$) and 24,25-dihydroxycholecalciferol (24,25-$(OH)_2D_3$) in the kidney. 1,25-$(OH)_2D_3$ stimulates resorption of calcium from bone and increases intestinal calcium absorption. The physiologic role of 24,25-$(OH)_2D_3$ has not been clearly established. The metabolic activity of calcifediol in clinical use appears to be related not only to its conversion to other metabolites but also due to its intrinsic activity.
When administered orally, calcifediol is rapidly absorbed from the intestine, with peak 25-OHD_3 concentrations in the serum reported after about 4 hours. 25-Hydroxycholecalciferol is known to be transported in blood, bound to a specific plasma protein. The terminal half-life of orally administered calcifediol in the serum is about 16 days.

INDICATIONS AND USAGE

Calderol (calcifediol) is indicated in the treatment and management of metabolic bone disease or hypocalcemia associated with chronic renal failure in patients undergoing renal dialysis.
In studies to date it has been shown to increase serum calcium levels, to decrease alkaline phosphatase and parathyroid hormone levels in some patients, to decrease subperiosteal bone resorption in some patients, and to decrease histological signs of hyperparathyroid bone disease and mineralization defects in some patients.

CONTRAINDICATIONS

Calderol (calcifediol) should not be given to patients with hypercalcemia or evidence of vitamin D toxicity.

WARNINGS

Since calcifediol is a metabolite of vitamin D, vitamin D and its derivatives should be withheld during treatment.
Aluminum carbonate or hydroxide gels should be used to control serum phosphorus levels in patients undergoing dialysis.
Overdosage of any form of vitamin D is dangerous (see also **Overdosage**). Progressive hypercalcemia may be so severe as to require emergency attention. Chronic hypercalcemia can lead to generalized vascular calcification, nephrocalcinosis, and other soft-tissue calcification. The serum calcium times phosphorus (Ca × P) product should not be allowed to exceed 70. Radiographic and/or slit lamp evaluation of suspect anatomical regions may be useful in the early detection of this condition.

PRECAUTIONS

i) ***General:*** Excessive dosage of Calderol (calcifediol) induces hypercalcemia and in some instances hypercalciuria; therefore, early in treatment during dosage adjustment, serum calcium should be determined frequently (at least weekly). Should hypercalcemia develop, the drug should be discontinued immediately. After achieving normocalcemia, the drug may be readministered at a lower dosage. Calderol should be given cautiously to patients receiving digitalis, because hypercalcemia in such patients may precipitate cardiac arrhythmias.
ii) ***Information for the Patient:*** The patient and his or her parents or spouse should be informed about compliance with dosage instructions, adherence to instructions about diet, calcium supplementation, phosphate binder usage, and avoidance of non approved prescription drugs. Patients should also be informed about the symptoms of hypercalcemia (see **Adverse Reactions**).
iii) ***Essential Laboratory Tests:*** Serum calcium, phosphorus and alkaline phosphatase and 24-hour urinary calcium and phosphorus should be determined periodically. During the initial phase of the medication, serum calcium should be determined more frequently (at least weekly).
iv) ***Drug Interactions:*** Cholestyramine has been reported to reduce absorption of fat-soluble vitamins; as such, it may impair intestinal absorption of calcifediol. The administration of anticonvulsants has been shown to affect the calcifediol requirements in some patients.
v) ***Carcinogenesis, Mutagenesis, Impairment of Fertility:*** - Long-term studies in animals have not been completed to evaluate the carcinogenic potential of Calderol. No significant effects of calcifediol on fertility and/or general reproductive performances were reported.
vi) ***Use in Pregnancy:*** Teratogenic effects:
Pregnancy Category C: Calcifediol has been shown to be teratogenic in rabbits when given in doses of 6 to 12 times the human dose. There are no adequate and well-controlled studies in pregnant women. Calderol should be used during pregnancy only if the potential benefit justifies potential risk to the fetus.
When calcifediol was given orally to bred rabbits on the 6th through the 18th day of gestation, gross visceral and skeletal examination of pups indicated that the compound was teratogenic at doses of 25 and 50 mcg/kg/day. A dose of 5 mcg/kg/day was not teratogenic. In a similar study in rats, calcifediol was not teratogenic at doses up to and including 60 mcg/kg/day.
vii) ***Labor and Delivery:*** The effect of this drug on the mother and the fetus during labor and delivery is not known.
viii) ***Nursing Mothers:*** It is not known whether this drug is excreted in human milk. Because many drugs are excreted in human milk, caution should be exercised when Calderol is administered to a nursing woman.
ix) ***Pediatric Use:*** The safety and effectiveness of Calderol in children have not been established.

ADVERSE REACTIONS

Since calcifediol is an active metabolite of vitamin D, adverse effects are, in general, similar to those encountered with excessive vitamin D intake. The early and late signs and symptoms of vitamin D intoxication associated with hypercalcemia include:
a. ***Early:*** Weakness, headache, somnolence, nausea, vomiting, dry mouth, constipation, muscle pain, bone pain, and metallic taste.
b. ***Late:*** Polyuria, polydipsia, anorexia, irritability, weight loss, nocturia, conjunctivitis (calcific), pancreatitis, photophobia, rhinorrhea, pruritus, hyperthermia, decreased libido, elevated BUN, albuminuria, hypercholesterolemia, elevated SGOT and SGPT, ectopic calcification, hypertension, cardiac arrhythmias, and, rarely, overt psychosis.

OVERDOSAGE

Administration of Calderol (calcifediol) to patients in excess of their daily requirements can cause hypercalcemia, hypercalciuria, and hyperphosphatemia. High intake of calcium and phosphate concomitant with Calderol may lead to similar abnormalities.
Treatment of Hypercalcemia and Overdosages: General treatment of hypercalcemia (greater than 1 mg/dl above the upper limit of the normal range) consists of discontinuation of therapy with Calderol. Serum calcium measurements should be performed regularly until normocalcemia ensues. Hypercalcemia usually resolves in two to four weeks. When serum calcium levels have returned to within normal limits, therapy with Calderol may be reinstituted at a dosage lower than prior therapy. Serum calcium levels should be obtained at least weekly after all dosage changes and subsequent dosage titration. Persistent or markedly elevated calcium levels in dialysis patients may be corrected by dialysis against a calcium-free dialysate.
Treatment of Accidental Overdosage: The treatment of acute accidental overdosage of Calderol should consist of general supportive measures. If drug ingestion is discovered within a relatively short time, induction of emesis or gastric lavage may be of benefit in preventing further absorption. If the drug has passed through the stomach, the administration of mineral oil may promote fecal elimination. Serial serum calcium determination, rate of urinary calcium excretion, and an assessment of electrocardiographic abnormalities due to hypercalcemia should be obtained. Such monitoring is critical in patients receiving digitalis. Discontinuation of supplemental calcium and a low calcium diet are also indicated in accidental overdosage. Because the conversion of calcifediol to 1.25-$(OH)_2D_3$ is tightly regulated by the body's needs, further measures are probably unnecessary. Should persistent and marked hypercalcemia occur, however, there are a variety of therapeutic measures that may be considered, depending on the patient's underlying condition. These include the use of drugs such as phosphates and corticosteroids as well as measures to induce an appropriate forced diuresis. The use of peritoneal dialysis against a calcium-free dialysate may also be considered.
The Oral LD_{50} in the rat is >320 mg/kg.

DOSAGE AND ADMINISTRATION

The optimal daily dose of Calderol (calcifediol) must be carefully determined for each patient. The recommended initial dosage of Calderol is based on the assumption that each patient is receiving an adequate daily intake of calcium from dietary sources or from the addition of calcium supplements. The RDA for calcium in adults is 1000 mg. To ensure that each patient receives an adequate daily intake of calcium, the physician should either prescribe a calcium supplement or instruct the patients in proper dietary measures.
Chronic Renal Failure—Dialysis Patients: The recommended initial dose of Calderol is 300 to 350 mcg of calcifediol weekly, administered on a daily or alternate-day schedule. If a satisfactory response in the biochemical parameters and clinical manifestations of the disease state is not observed, dosage may be increased at four-week intervals. During this titration period, serum calcium levels should be obtained at least weekly, and if hypercalcemia is noted, the drug should be discontinued until normocalcemia ensues.
Some patients with normal serum calcium levels may respond to doses of 20 mcg of calcifediol every other day. Most patients respond to doses between 50 and 100 mcg daily or between 100 and 200 mcg on alternate days.

HOW SUPPLIED

Calderol (calcifediol capsules, USP) are available in the following strengths and package sizes:

Strength	Packaged	NDC Number
20 mcg	Bottle of 60 (white, soft elastic capsules)	0052-0472-60
50 mcg	Bottle of 60 (orange, soft elastic capsules)	0052-0474-60

Caution: Federal law prohibits dispensing without prescription.

Distributed by: **Organon Inc., W. Orange, NJ 07052**
Manufactured by: The Upjohn Co., Kalamazoo, MI 49001
Revised 4/85
Shown in Product Identification Section, page 419

CORTROPHIN®—Zinc ACTH ℞

(Sterile Corticotropin Zinc Hydroxide Suspension, USP)

HOW SUPPLIED

Vials, 5 ml (40 USP Units/ml).

CORTROSYN® ℞

Cosyntropin is α 1–24 corticotropin, a synthetic subunit of ACTH.

HOW SUPPLIED

Available as a lyophilized powder in vials containing 0.25 mg of Cosyntropin and 10 mg of mannitol, (Boxes of 10 × 1 ml vials of powder and 10 × 1 ml amps diluent).

COTAZYM® ℞

[*kōt 'a zīm*]
(Pancrelipase Capsules, USP)

DESCRIPTION

Cotazym (Pancrelipase, USP) is a powder containing enzymes obtained from the pancreas of the hog. These include amylase and protease but principally lipase. Each capsule (regular or cherrry flavored) contains:
Lipase—8,000 USP Units
Protease—30,000 USP Units
Amylase—30,000 USP Units
Precipitated calcium carbonate 25 mg.

INDICATIONS AND USAGE

It is indicated in conditions where pancreatic enzymes are either absent or deficient with resultant inadequate fat digestion. Such conditions include but are not limited to chronic pancreatitis, pancreatectomy, cystic fibrosis and steatorrhea of diverse etiologies.

CONTRAINDICATIONS

Known hypersensitivity to pork protein.

PRECAUTIONS

In the event that capsules are opened for any reason care should be taken so that powder is not inhaled or spilled on hands since it may prove irritating to the skin or mucous membranes.

ADVERSE REACTIONS

No adverse reactions have been reported. It should be noted, however, that extremely high doses of exogenous pancreatic enzymes have been associated with hyperuricosuria and hyperuricemia.

DOSAGE AND ADMINISTRATION

One to three capsules just prior to each meal or snack or as directed by physician. Severe cases may require higher dosage and dietary adjustment.

STORAGE

Not to exceed 25°C (77°F). Dry place when opened.

DISPENSE

In tight container as defined in the USP.

SUPPLIED

Cotazym capsules (regular) bottles of 100 and 500. NDC # 0052-0381-91, NDC # 0052-0381-95.
Cotazym capsules (cherry flavored) bottles of 100. NDC # 0052-0386-91.
Shown in Product Identification Section, page 419

Continued on next page

Organon—Cont.

COTAZYM-S™ ℞
[kōt'a zīm-s]
Enteric coated spheres
(Pancrelipase, USP)

DESCRIPTION
Cotazym-S contains enteric coated spheres of pancrelipase, a substance containing enzymes, principally lipase, with amylase and protease, obtained from the pancreas of the hog.
Each capsule contains:
Lipase—5,000 USP Units
Protease—20,000 USP Units
Amylase—20,000 USP Units
COTAZYM-S™

CLINICAL PHARMACOLOGY
Cotazym-S is protected against inactivation by gastric acidity, and active enzymes are released in the duodenum. The enzymes promote hydrolysis of fats into glycerol and fatty acids, protein into proteases and derived substances, and starch into dextrans and sugars.

INDICATIONS AND USAGE
Cotazym-S is indicated in conditions where pancreatic enzymes are either absent or deficient with resultant inadequate fat digestion. Such conditions include but are not limited to chronic pancreatitis, pancreatectomy, cystic fibrosis and steatorrhea of diverse etiologies.

CONTRAINDICATIONS
Known hypersensitivity to pork protein.

PRECAUTIONS
To maintain enteric coating integrity, do not chew or crush spheres.

ADVERSE REACTIONS
No adverse reactions have been reported. It should be noted, however, that extremely high doses of exogenous pancreatic enzymes have been associated with hyperuricosuria and hyperuricemia.

DOSAGE AND ADMINISTRATION
One to two capsules with each meal or snack or as directed by physician. Severe cases may require higher dosage and dietary adjustment. Cotazym-S capsules are usually easy to swallow, but in case of any difficulty, capsules may be opened and the spheres taken with liquids or soft foods which do not require chewing.

STORAGE
Not to exceed 25°C (77°F). Dry place when opened.

DISPENSE
In tight container as defined in the USP.

SUPPLIED
Cotazym-S bottles of 100. NDC #0052-0388-91. Bottles of 500. NDC #0052-0388-95.
Shown in Product Identification Section, page 419

DECA-DURABOLIN® ℞
(Nandrolone Decanoate Injection, USP)

HOW SUPPLIED
50 mg/ml—1 ml ampuls, 2 ml vials, 1 ml prefilled syringe.
100 mg/ml—2 ml vials, 1 ml prefilled syringe.
200 mg/ml—1 ml vials, 1 ml prefilled syringe.

DURABOLIN® ℞
(Nandrolone Phenpropionate Injection, USP)

HOW SUPPLIED
25 mg/ml—5 ml vials.
50 mg/ml—2 ml vials.

HEPARIN SODIUM ℞
Injection, USP
(From Beef Lung)

HOW SUPPLIED
1,000 USP Units/ml (aqueous) Vials, 10 ml and 30 ml
5,000 USP Units/ml (aqueous) Vials, 1 ml and 10 ml
10,000 USP Units/ml (aqueous) Vials, 1 ml and 4 ml

HEXADROL® Elixir ℞
(Dexamethasone Elixir, USP)

Each 5 ml contains: 0.5 mg dexamethasone with 5% alcohol.

HOW SUPPLIED
Elixir (0.5 mg/5 ml)—Bottle of 120 ml

HEXADROL® ℞
(Dexamethasone Tablets, USP)

HOW SUPPLIED
Tablets (0.5 mg yellow, scored)—bottle of 100
Tablets (0.75 mg white, scored)—bottle of 100
Tablets (1.5 mg peach, scored)—bottle of 100
Tablets (4 mg green, scored)—bottle of 100
Shown in Product Identification Section, page 419

HEXADROL® STRIP PACKS ℞
(Dexamethasone Tablets, USP)

HOW SUPPLIED
Box of 100 (10 strips–10 per strip) in the following strengths:
0.5 mg yellow, scored
0.75 mg white, scored
1.5 mg peach, scored
4 mg green, scored

HEXADROL® ℞
Therapeutic Pack
(Dexamethasone Tablets, USP)

HOW SUPPLIED
Each pack contains: 6 × 1.5 mg tablets, (peach scored); 8 × 0.75 mg tablets, (white, scored).
Shown in Product Identification Section, page 419

HEXADROL® ℞
Phosphate Injection
(Dexamethasone Sodium Phosphate Injection, USP)

HOW SUPPLIED
Available in three potencies:
4 mg/ml—1 ml vials, 5 ml vials, 1 ml prefilled syringe.
10 mg/ml—10 ml vials, 1 ml prefilled syringe.
20 mg/ml—5 ml vial, 5 ml prefilled syringe.

HYDROCORTISONE, USP ℞
Micronized Powder
Non-Sterile: For Prescription Compounding Only

HOW SUPPLIED
Available in 10, 25 and 100 gram containers.

LIQUAEMIN® Sodium ℞
(Heparin Sodium Injection, USP)
from porcine intestinal mucosa

HOW SUPPLIED
1,000 USP Units/ml Vials, 10 ml & 30 ml
5,000 USP Units ml Ampuls, 1 ml Vials, 1 ml & 10 ml
10,000 USP Units/ml Ampuls, 1 ml Vials, 1 ml & 4 ml
20,000 USP Units/ml Vials, 1 ml, 2 ml & 5 ml
40,000 USP Units/ml Vials, 1 ml
Preservative Free
1,000 USP Units/ml, Ampuls, 1 ml
5,000 USP Units/ml, Ampuls, 1 ml

MAXIBOLIN® ℞
(ethylestrenol)

HOW SUPPLIED
Tablets, 2 mg—bottle of 100.
Elixir, 2 mg/5 ml—120 ml bottle.

NORCURON® ℞
(vecuronium bromide for injection)

THIS DRUG SHOULD BE ADMINISTERED BY ADEQUATELY TRAINED INDIVIDUALS FAMILIAR WITH ITS ACTIONS, CHARACTERISTICS, AND HAZARDS.

DESCRIPTION
NORCURON® (vecuronium bromide) injection is a nondepolarizing neuromuscular blocking agent of intermediate duration, chemically designated as piperidinium, 1-[(2β, 3α, 5α, 16β, 17β)-3, 17-bis(acetyloxy)-2-(1-piperidinyl)androstan-16-yl]-1-methyl-, bromide. The structural formula is:

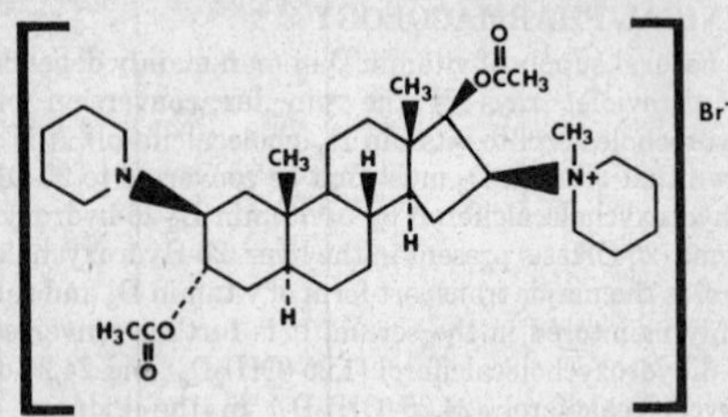

Norcuron® is supplied as a sterile nonpyrogenic freeze-dried buttered cake of very fine microscopic crystalline particles for intravenous injection only. Following reconstitution with solvent (water for injection) the resultant solution is isotonic and has a pH of 4. Each 5 ml vial contains 10 mg vecuronium bromide. Each vial also contains citric acid, dibasic sodium phosphate, sodium hydroxide, and/or phosphoric acid to buffer and adjust pH and mannitol to make isotonic.

CLINICAL PHARMACOLOGY
Norcuron® (vecuronium bromide) injection is a nondepolarizing neuromuscular blocking agent possessing all of the characteristic pharmacological actions of this class of drugs (curariform). It acts by competing for cholinergic receptors at the motor end-plate. The antagonist to acetycholine is inhibited and neuromuscular block is reversed by acetylcholinesterase inhibitors such as neostigmine, edrophonium, and pyridostigmine. Norcuron® is about ⅓ more potent than pancuronium; the duration of neuromuscular blockade produced by Norcuron® is shorter than that of pancuronium at initially equipotent doses. The time to onset of paralysis decreases and the duration of maximum effect increases with increasing Norcuron® doses. The use of a peripheral nerve stimulator is of benefit in assessing the degree of muscular relaxation.
The ED_{90} (dose required to produce 90% suppression of the muscle twitch reponse with balanced anesthesia) has averaged 0.057 mg/kg (0.049 to 0.062 mg/kg in various studies). An initial Norcuron® dose of 0.08 to 0.10 mg/kg generally produces first depression of twitch in approximately 1 minute, good or excellent intubation conditions within 2.5 to 3.0 minutes, and maximum neuromuscular blockade within 3 to 5 minutes of injection in most patients. Under balanced anesthesia, the time to recovery to 25% of control (clinical duration) is approximately 25 to 40 minutes after injection and recovery is usually 95% complete approximately 45–65 minutes after injection of intubating dose. The neuromuscular blocking action of Norcuron® is slightly enhanced in the presence of potent inhalation anesthetics. If Norcuron® is first administered more than 5 minutes after the start of the inhalation of enflurane, isoflurane, or halthane, or when steady state has been achieved, the intubating dose of Norcuron® may be decreased by approximately 15% (see DOSAGE AND ADMINISTRATION section). Prior administration of succinylcholine may enhance the neuromuscular blocking effect of Norcuron® and its duration of action. With succinylcholine as the intubating agent, initial doses of 0.04–0.06 mg/kg of Norcuron® will produce complete neuromuscular block with clinical duration of action of 25–30 minutes. If succinylcholine is used prior to Norcuron®, the administration of Norcuron® should be delayed until the patient starts recovering from succinylcholine-induced neuromuscular blockade. The effect of prior use of other nondepolarizing neuromuscular blocking agents on the activity of Norcuron® has not been studied (see Drug Interactions).
Repeated administration of maintenance doses of Norcuron® has little or no cumulative effect on the duration of neuromuscular blockade. Therefore, repeat doses can be administered at relatively regular intervals with predictable results. After an initial dose of 0.08 to 0.10 mg/kg under balanced anesthesia, the first maintenance dose (suggested maintenance dose is 0.010 to 0.015 mg/kg) is generally required within 25 to 40 minutes; subsequent maintenance doses, if required, may be administered at approximately 12 to 15 minute intervals. Halothane anesthesia increases the clinical duration of the maintenance dose only slightly. Under enflurane a maintenance dose of 0.010 mg/kg is approximately equal to 0.015 mg/kg dose under balanced anesthesia.
The recovery index (time from 25% to 75% recovery) is approximately 15–25 minutes under balanced or halothane anesthesia. When recovery from Norcuron® neuromuscular blocking effect begins, it proceeds more rapidly than recovery from pancuronium. Once spontaneous recovery has started, the neuromuscular block produced by Norcuron® is readily reversed with various anticholinesterase agents, e.g.

pyridostigmine, neostigmine, or edrophonium in conjunction with an anti-cholinergic agent such as atropine or glycopyrrolate. There have been no reports of recurarization following satisfactory reversal of Norcuron® induced neuromuscular blockade; rapid recovery is a finding consistent with its short elimination half-life.

Pharmacokinetics: At clinical doses of 0.04–0.10 mg/kg, 60–80% of Norcuron® is usually bound to plasma protein. The distribution half-life following a single intravenous dose (range 0.025–0.280 mg/kg) is approximately 4 minutes. Elimination half-life over this same dosage range is approximately 65–75 minutes in healthy surgical patients and in renal failure patients undergoing transplant surgery. In late pregnancy, elimination half-life may be shortened to approximately 35–40 minutes. The volume of distribution at steady state is approximately 300–400 ml/kg; systemic rate of clearance is approximately 3–4.5 ml/minute/kg. In man, urine recovery of Norcuron® varies from 3–35% within 24 hours. Data derived from patients requiring insertion of a T-tube in the common bile duct suggests that 25–50% of a total intravenous dose of vecuronium may be excreted in bile within 42 hours. Only unchanged Norcuron® (vercuronium bromide) injection has been detected in human plasma following clinical use. One metabolite, 3-deacetyl vecuronium, has been recovered in the urine of some patients in quantities that account for up to 10% of injected dose; 3-deacetyl vecuronium has also been recovered by T-tube in some patients accounting for up to 25% of the injected dose.

This metabolite has been judged by animal screening (dogs and cats) to have 50% or more of the potency of Norcuron®; equipotent doses are of approximately the same duration as Norcuron® in dogs and cats. Biliary excretion accounts for about half the dose of Norcuron® within 7 hours in the anesthetized rat. Circulatory bypass of the liver (cat preparation) prolongs recovery from Norcuron®. Limited data derived from patients with cirrhosis or cholestasis suggests that some measurements of recovery may be doubled in such patients. In patients with renal failure, measurements of recovery do not differ significantly from similar measurements in healthy patients.

Studies involving routine hemodynamic monitoring in good risk surgical patients reveal that the administration of Norcuron® in doses up to three times that needed to produce clinical relaxation (0.15 mg/kg) did not produce clinically significant changes in systolic, diastolic or mean arterial pressure. The heart rate, under similar monitoring, remained unchanged in some studies and was lowered by a mean of up to 8% in other studies. A large dose of 0.28 mg/kg administered during a period of no stimulation, while patients were being prepared for coronary artery bypass grafting, was not associated with alterations in rate-pressure-product or pulmonary capillary wedge pressure. Systemic vascular resistance was lowered slightly and cardiac output was increased insignficantly. (The drug has not been studied in patients with hemodynamic dysfunction secondary to cardiac valvular disease). Limited clinical experience (3 patients) with use of Norcuron® during surgery for pheochromocytoma has shown that administration of this drug is not associated with changes in blood pressure or heart rate.

Unlike other nondepolarizing skeletal muscle relaxants, Norcuron® has no clinically significant effects on hemodynamic parameters and will not counteract those hemodynamic changes or known side effects produced by or associated with anesthetic agents.

Preliminary data on histamine assay in 16 patients and available clinical experience in more than 600 patients indicate that hypersensitivity reactions such as bronchospasm, flushing, redness, hypotension, tachycardia, and other reactions commonly associated with histamine release are unlikely to occur.

INDICATIONS AND USAGE

Norcuron® is indicated as an adjunct to general anesthesia, to facilitate endotracheal intubation and to provide skeletal muscle relaxation during surgery or mechanical ventilation.

CONTRAINDICATIONS

None known.

WARNINGS

NORCURON® SHOULD BE ADMINISTERED IN CAREFULLY ADJUSTED DOSAGE BY OR UNDER THE SUPERVISION OF EXPERIENCED CLINICIANS WHO ARE FAMILIAR WITH ITS ACTIONS AND THE POSSIBLE COMPLICATIONS THAT MIGHT OCCUR FOLLOWING ITS USE. THE DRUG SHOULD NOT BE ADMINISTERED UNLESS FACILITIES FOR INTUBATION, ARTIFICIAL RESPIRATION, OXYGEN THERAPY, AND REVERSAL AGENTS ARE IMMEDIATELY AVAILABLE. THE CLINICIAN MUST BE PREPARED TO ASSIST OR CONTROL RESPIRATION. In patients who are known to have myasthenia gravis or the myasthenic (Eaton-Lambert) syndrome, small doses of Norcuron® may have profound effects. In such patients, a peripheral nerve stimulator and use of a small test dose may be of value in monitoring the response to administration of muscle relaxants.

PRECAUTIONS

Renal Failure: Norcuron® is well-tolerated without clinically significant prolongation of neuromuscular blocking effect in patients with renal failure who have been optimally prepared for surgery by dialysis. Under emergency conditions in anephric patients some prolongation of neuromuscular blockade may occur; therefore, if anephric patients cannot be prepared for non-elective surgery, a lower initial dose of Norcuron® should be considered.

Altered Circulation Time: Conditions associated with slower circulation time in cardiovascular disease, old age, edematous states resulting in increased volume of distribution may contribute to a delay in onset time; therefore dosage should not be increased.

Hepatic Disease: Limited experience in patients with cirrhosis or cholestasis has revealed prolonged recovery time in keeping with the role the liver plays in Norcuron® metabolism and excretion (see Pharmocokinetics). Data currently available do not permit dosage recommendations in patients with impaired liver function.

UNDER THE ABOVE CONDITIONS, USE OF A PERIPHERAL NERVE STIMULATOR FOR ADEQUATE MONITORING OF NEUROMUSCULAR BLOCKING EFFECT WILL PRECLUDE INADVERTANT EXCESS DOSING.

Severe Obesity or Neuromuscular Disease: Patients with severe obesity or neuromuscular disease may pose airway and/or ventilatory problems requiring special care before, during and after the use of neuromuscular blocking agents such as Norcuron®.

Malignant Hyperthermia: Many drugs used in anesthetic practice are suspected of being capable of triggering a potentially fatal hypermetabolism of skeletal muscle known as malignant hyperthermia. There are insufficient data derived from screening in susceptible animals (swine) to establish whether or not Norcuron® is capable of triggering malignant hyperthermia.

Norcuron® has no known effect on consciousness, the pain threshold or cerebration. Administration must be accompanied by adequate anesthesia.

Drug Interactions: Prior administration of succinylcholine may enhance the neuromuscular blocking effect of Norcuron® (vecuronium bromide) injection and its duration of action. If succinylcholine is used before Norcuron®, the administration of Norcuron® should be delayed until the succinylcholine effect shows signs of wearing off. With succinylcholine as the intubating agent, initial doses of 0.04–0.06 mg/kg of Norcuron® may be administered to produce complete neuromuscular block with clinical duration of action of 25–30 minutes (see CLINICAL PHARMACOLOGY). The use of Norcuron® before succinylcholine, in order to attenuate some of the side effects of succinylcholine, has not been sufficiently studied.

Other nondepolarizing neuromuscular blocking agents (pancuronium, d-tubocurarine, metocurine, and gallamine) act in the same fashion as does Norcuron®; therefore these drugs and Norcuron® may manifest an additive effect when used together. There are insufficient data to support concomitant use of Norcuron® and other competitive muscle relaxants in the same patient.

Inhalational Anesthetics: Use of volatile inhalational anesthetics such as enflurane, isoflurane, and halothane with Norcuron® will enhance neuromuscular blockade. Potentiation is most prominent with use of enflurane and isoflurane. With the above agents the initial dose of Norcuron® may be the same as with balanced anesthesia unless the inhalational anesthetic has been administered for a sufficient time at a sufficient dose to have reached clinical equilibrium (see CLINICAL PHARMACOLOGY).

Antibiotics: Parenteral/intraperitoneal administration of high doses of certain antibiotics may intensify or produce neuromuscular block on their own. The following antibiotics have been associated with various degrees of paralysis: aminoglycosides (such as neomycin, streptomycin, kanamycin, gentamicin, and dihydrostreptomycin); tetracyclines; bacitracin; polymyxin B; colistin; and sodium colistimethate. If these or other newly introduced antibiotics are used in conjunction with Norcuron® during surgery. unexpected prolongation of neuromuscular block should be considered a possibility.

Other: Experience concerning injection of quinidine during recovery from use of other muscle relaxants suggests that recurrent paralysis may occur. This possibility must also be considered for Norcuron®. Norcuron® induced neuromuscular blockade has been counteracted by alkalosis and enhanced by acidosis in experimental animals (cat). Electrolyte imbalance and diseases which lead to electrolyte imbalance, such as adrenal cortical insufficiency, have been shown to alter neuromuscular blockade. Depending on the nature of the imbalance, either enhancement or inhibition may be expected. Magnesium salts, administered for the management of toxemia of pregnancy, may enhance the neuromuscular blockade.

Drug/laboratory test interactions: None known.

Carcinogenesis, Mutagenesis, Impairment of Fertility: Long-term studies in animals have not been peformed to evaluate carcinogenic or mutagenic potential or impairment of fertility.

Pregnancy: Pregnancy Category C: Animal reproduction studies have not been conducted with Norcuron®. It is also not known whether Norcuron® can cause fetal harm when administered to a pregnant woman or can affect reproduction capacity. Norcuron® should be given to a pregnant woman only if clearly needed.

Pediatric Use: Infants under 1 year of age but older than 7 weeks, also tested under halothane anesthesia, are moderately more sensitive to Norcuron® on a mg/kg basis than adults and take about 1½ times as long to recover. Information presently available does not permit recommendations for usage in neonates.

ADVERSE REACTIONS

Norcuron® was well-tolerated and produced no adverse reactions during extensive clinical trials. The most frequent adverse reaction to nondepolarizing blocking agents as a class consists of an extension of the drug's pharmacological action beyond the time period needed for surgery and anesthesia. This may vary from skeletal muscle weakness to profound and prolonged skeletal muscle paralysis resulting in respiratory insufficiency or apnea.

Inadequate reversal of the neuromuscular blockade, although not yet reported, is possible with Norcuron® as with all curariform drugs. These adverse reactions are managed by manual or mechanical ventilation until recovery is judged adequate. Little or no increase in intensity of blockade or duration of action of Norcuron® is noted from the use of thiobarbiturates, narcotic analgesics, nitrous oxide, or droperidol. See OVERDOSAGE for discussion of other drugs used in anesthetic practice which also cause respiratory depression.

OVERDOSAGE

There has been no experience with Norcuron® overdosage. The possibility of iatrogenic overdosage can be minimized by carefully monitoring muscle twitch response to peripheral nerve stimulation.

Excessive doses of Norcuron® can be expected to produce enhanced pharmacological effects. Residual neuromuscular blockade beyond the time period needed for surgery and anesthesia may occur with Norcuron® as with other neuromuscular blockers. This may be manifested by skeletal muscle weakness, decreased respiratory reserve, low tidal volume, or apnea. A peripheral nerve stimulator may be used to assess the degree of residual neuromuscular blockade and help to differentiate residual neuromuscular blockade from other causes of decreased respiratory reserve.

Respiratory depression may be due either wholly or in part to other drugs used during the conduct of general anesthesia such as narcotics, thiobarbiturates and other central nervous system depressants. Under such circumstances the primary treatment is maintenance of a patent airway and manual or mechanical ventilation until complete recovery of normal respiration is assured. Regonol® (pyridostigmine bromide injection), neostigmine, or edrophonium, in conjunction with atropine or glycopyrrolate will usually antagonize the skeletal muscle relaxant action of Norcuron®. Satisfactory reversal can be judged by adequacy of skeletal muscle tone and by adequacy of respiration. A peripheral nerve stimulator may also be used to monitor restoration of twitch height. Failure of prompt reversal (within 30 minutes) may occur in the presence of extreme debilitation, carcinomatosis, and with concomitant use of certain broad spectrum antibiotics, or anesthetic agents and other drugs which enhance neuromuscular blockade or cause respiratory depression of their own. Under such circumstances the management is the same as that of prolonged neuromuscular blockade. Ventilation must be supported by artificial means until the patient has resumed control of his respiration. Prior to the use of reversal agents, reference should be made to the specific package insert of the reversal agent.

DOSAGE AND ADMINISTRATION

Norcuron® (vecuronium bromide) injection is for intravenous use only. This drug should be administered by or under the supervision of experienced clinicians familiar with the use of neuromuscular blocking agents. Dosage must be individualized in each case. The dosage information which follows is derived from studies based upon units of drug per unit of body weight and is intended to serve as a guide only, especially regarding enhancement of neuromuscular blockade of Norcuron® by volatile anesthetics and by prior use of succinylcholine (see PRECAUTIONS/Drug Interactions). Parenteral drug products should be inspected visually for particulate matter and discoloration prior to administration, whenever solution and container permit.

To obtain maximum clinical benefits of Norcuron® and to minimize the possibility of overdosage, the monitoring of muscle twitch response to peripheral nerve stimulation is advised.

The recommended initial dose of Norcuron® is 0.08 to 0.10 mg/kg (1.4 to 1.75 times the ED_{90}) given as an intravenous

Continued on next page

Organon—Cont.

bolus injection. This dose can be expected to produce good or excellent non-emergency intubation conditions in 2.5 to 3.0 minutes after injection. Under balanced anesthesia, clinically required neuromuscular blockade lasts approximately 25–30 minutes, with recovery to 25% of control achieved approximately 25 to 40 minute after injection and recovery to 95% of control achieved approximately 25 to 40 minutes after injection. In the presence of potent inhalation anesthetics, the neuromuscular blocking effect of Norcuron® is enhanced. If Norcuron® is first administered more than 5 minutes after the start of inhalation agent or when steady state has been achieved, the initial Norcuron® dose may be reduced by approximately 15%, i.e., 0.060 to 0.085 mg/kg.
Prior administration of succinylcholine may enhance the neuromuscular blocking effect and duration of action of Norcuron®. If intubation is performed using succinylcholine, a reduction of initial dose of Norcuron® to 0.04–0.06 mg/kg with inhalation anesthesia and 0.05–0.06 mg/kg with balanced anesthesia may be required.
During prolonged surgical procedures, maintenance doses of 0.010 to 0.015 mg/kg of Norcuron® are recommended; after the initial Norcuron® injection, the first maintenance dose will generally be required within 25 to 40 minutes. However, clinical criteria should be used to determine the need for maintenance doses. Since Norcuron® lacks clinically important cumulative effects, subsequent maintenance doses, if required, may be administered at relatively regular intervals for each patient, ranging approximately from 12 to 15 minutes under balanced anesthesia, slightly longer under inhalation agents. (If less frequent administration is desired, higher maintenance doses may be administered.)
Should there be reason for the selection of larger doses in individual patients, initial doses ranging from 0.15 mg/kg up to 0.28 mg/kg have been administered during surgery under halothane anesthesia without ill effects to the cardiovascular system being noted as long as ventilation is properly maintained (see CLINICAL PHARMACOLOGY).
Dosage in Children: Older children (10 to 17 years of age) have approximately the same dosage requirements (mg/kg) as adults and may be managed the same way. Younger children (1 to 10 years of age) may require a slightly higher initial dose and may also require supplementation slightly more often than adults. Infants under one year of age but older than 7 weeks are moderately more sensitive to Norcuron® on a mg/kg basis than adults and take about 1½ times as long to recover. See also subsection of PRECAUTIONS titled Pediatric Use. Information presently available does not permit recommendation on usage in neonates (see PRECAUTIONS).

COMPATIBILITY

Norcuron® is compatible in solution with:

0.9% NaCl solution	5% glucose in saline
5% glucose in water	Lactated Ringers

HOW SUPPLIED

5 ml vials (contains 10 mg of active ingredient) and 5 ml ampuls of sterile water for injection, U.S.P. as diluent.
Boxes of 10 NDC#0052-0442-17
5 ml vials (contains 10 mg of active ingredient) only. **DILUENT,** sterile water for injection U.S.P., **NOT SUPPLIED.**
Boxes of 10 NDC#0052-0442-57

STORAGE

PROTECT FROM LIGHT. Store at 15°-30°C (59°-86°F)

AFTER RECONSTITUTION

Solution may be stored in refrigerator or kept at room temperature not to exceed 30°C (86°F) DISCARD SOLUTION AFTER 24 HOURS.
DISCARD UNUSED PORTION. SINGLE USE VIALS
Manufactured for ORGANON INC.
By BEN VENUE LABORATORIES, INC. Bedford, Ohio 44146

PAVULON® ℞
[*pāv-u-lon*]
(pancuronium bromide injection)

THIS DRUG SHOULD BE ADMINISTERED BY ADEQUATELY TRAINED INDIVIDUALS FAMILIAR WITH ITS ACTIONS, CHARACTERISTICS, AND HAZARDS.

DESCRIPTION

Pavulon® (pancuronium bromide injection) is a nondepolarizing neuromuscular blocking agent chemically designated as the aminosteroid 2 β, 16β-dipiperidino-5α-androstane-3 α, 17-βdiol diacetate dimethobromide. The structural formula is:
[See Chemical Formula at top of next column].

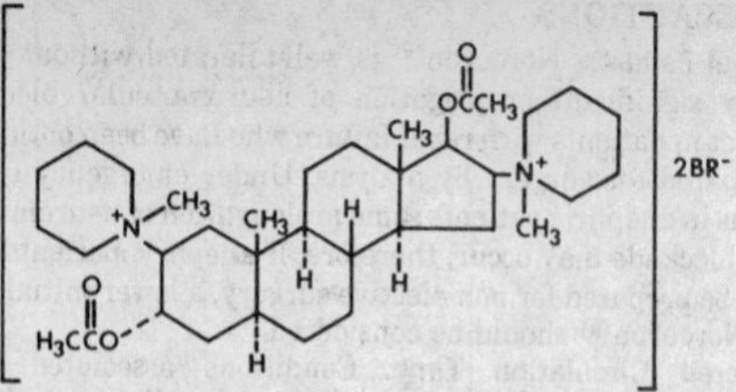

Pavulon® is supplied as a sterile, isotonic, nonpyrogenic solution for injection. Each ml contains 1 mg or 2 mg pancuronium bromide, 2 mg sodium acetate and 1% benzyl alcohol as preservative. The solution is adjusted to isotonicity with sodium chloride and to a pH of 4 with acetic acid and/or sodium hydroxide; water is used as the solvent.

CLINICAL PHARMACOLOGY

Pavulon® is a nondepolarizing neuromuscular blocking agent possessing all the characteristic pharmacological actions of this class of drugs (curariform). It acts by competing for cholinergic receptors at the motor end-plate. The antagonism to acetylcholine is inhibited and neuromuscular block is reversed by anticholinesterase agents such as pyridostigmine, neostigmine, and edrophonium. Pavulon® is approximately ⅓ less potent than vecuronium and approximately 5 times as potent as d-tubocurarine; the duration of neuromuscular blockade produced by Pavulon® is longer, than that of vecuronium at initially equipotent doses.
The ED_{95} (dose required to produce 95% suppression of muscle twitch response) is approximately 0.05 mg/kg under balanced anesthesia and 0.03 mg/kg under halothane anesthesia. These doses produce effective skeletal muscle relaxation (as judged by time from maximum effect to 25% recovery of control twitch height) for approximately 22 minutes; the duration from injection to 90% recovery of control twitch height is approximately 65 minutes. The intubating dose of 0.1 mg/kg (balanced anesthesia) will effectively abolish twitch response within approximately 4 minutes; time from injection to 25% recovery from this dose is approximately 100 minutes.
Supplemental doses to maintain muscle relaxation slightly increase the magnitude of block and significantly increase the duration of block. The use of a peripheral nerve stimulator is of benefit in assessing the degree of neuromuscular blockade.
The most characteristic circulatory effects of pancuronium, studied under halothane anesthesia, are a moderate rise in heart rate, mean arterial pressure and cardiac output; systemic vascular resistance is not changed significantly and central venous pressure may fall slightly. The heart rate rise is inversely related to the rate immediately before administration of pancuronium, is blocked by prior administration of atropine, and appears unrelated to the concentration of halothane or dose of pancuronium.
Data on histamine assays and available clinical experience indicate that hypersensitivity reactions such as bronchospasm, flushing, redness, hypotension, tachycardia, and other reactions commonly associated with histamine release are rare. (See **ADVERSE REACTIONS**).
Pharmacokinetics: The elimination half-life of pancuronium has been reported to range between 89-161 minutes. The volume of distribution ranges from 241-280 ml/kg and plasma clearance is approximately 1.1-1.9 ml/minute/kg. Approximately 40% of the total dose of pancuronium has been recovered in urine as unchanged pancuronium and its metabolites while approximately 11% has been recovered in bile. As much as 25% of an injected dose may be recovered as 3-hydroxy metabolite, which is half as potent a blocking agent as pancuronium. Less than 5% of the injected dose is recovered as 17-hydroxy metabolite and 3.17-dihydroxy metabolite, which have been judged to be approximately 50 times less potent than pancuronium. Pancuronium exhibits strong binding to gamma globulin and moderate binding to albumin. Approximately 13% is unbound to plasma protein. In patients with cirrhosis the volume of distribution is increased by approximaty 50%, the plasma clearance is decreased by approximately 22% and the elimination half-life is doubled. Similar results were noted in patients with biliary obstruction, except that plasma clearance was less than half the normal rate. The initial total dose to achieve adequate relaxation may thus be high in patients with hepatic and/or biliary tract dysfunction, while the duration of action is greater than usual.
The elimination half-life is doubled and the plasma clearance is reduced by approximately 50% in patients with renal failure. The volume of distribution is variable, and in some cases elevated. The rate of recovery of neuromuscular blockade, as determined by peripheral nerve stimulation, is variable and sometimes very much slower than normal.

INDICATIONS AND USAGE

Pavulon® (pancuronium bromide injection) is indicated as an adjunct to general anesthesia, to facilitate tracheal intubation and to provide skeletal muscle relaxation during surgery or mechanical ventilation.

CONTRAINDICATIONS

Pavulon® is contraindicated in patients known to be hypersensitive to the drug.

WARNINGS

PAVULON® SHOULD BE ADMINISTERED IN CAREFULLY ADJUSTED DOSES BY OR UNDER THE SUPERVISION OF EXPERIENCED CLINICIANS WHO ARE FAMILIAR WITH ITIS ACTIONS AND THE POSSIBLE COMPLICATIONS THAT MIGHT OCCUR FOLLOWING ITS USE. THE DRUG SHOULD NOT BE ADMINISTERED UNLESS FACILITIES FOR INTUBATION, ARTIFICIAL RESPIRATION, OXYGEN THERAPY, AND REVERSAL AGENTS ARE IMMEDIATELY AVAILABLE. THE CLINICIAN MUST BE PREPARED TO ASSIST OR CONTROL RESPIRATION.
In patients who are known to have myasthenia gravis or the myasthenic (Eaton-Limbert) syndrome, small doses of Pavulon® may have profound effects. In such patients, a peripheral nerve stimulator and use of a small test dose may be of value in monitoring the response to administration of muscle relaxants.

PRECAUTIONS

USE OF A PERIPHERAL NERVE STIMULATOR WILL USUALLY BE OF VALUE FOR MONITORING OF NEUROMUSCULAR BLOCKING EFFECT, AVOIDING OVERDOSAGE AND ASSISTING IN EVALUATION OF RECOVERY.
General: Although Pavulon® has been used successfully in many patients with pre-existing pulmonary, hepatic, or renal disease, caution should be exercised in these situations.
Renal Failure: A major portion of pancuronium, as well as an active metabolite, are recovered in urine. The elimination half-life is doubled and the plasma clearance is reduced in patients with renal failure; at the same time, the rate of recovery of neuromuscular blockade is variable and sometimes very much slower than normal (see Pharmocokinetics). This information should be taken into consideration if pancuronium is selected for other reasons to be used in a patient with renal failure.
Altered Circulation Time: Conditions associated with slower circulation time in cardiovascular disease, old age, edematous states resulting in increased volume of distribution may contribute to a delay in onset time; therefore dosage should not be increased.
Hepatic and/or Biliary Tract Disease: The doubled elimination half-life and reduced plasma clearance determined in patients with hepatic and/or biliary tract disease, as well as limited data showing that recovery time is prolonged an average of 65% in patients with biliary tract obstruction, suggests that prolongation of neuromuscular blockade may occur. At the same time, these conditions are characterized by an approximately 50% increase in volume of distribution of pancuronium, suggesting that the total initial dose to achieve adequate relaxation may in some cases be high. The possibility of slower onset, higher total dosage and prolongation of neuromuscular blockade must be taken into consideration when pancuronium is used in these patients. (See also **Pharmacokinetics**).
Severe Obesity or Neuromuscular Disease: Patients with severe obesity or neuromuscular disease may pose airway and/or ventilatory problems requiring special care before, during and after the use of neuromuscular blocking agents such as Pavulon®.
Pavulon® has no known effect on consciousness, the pain threshold or cerebration. Administration should be accompanied by adequate anesthesia.
Drug Interactions: Prior Administration of succinylcholine may enhance the neuromuscular blocking effect of Pavulon® and increase its duration of action. If succinylcholine is used before Pavulon® the administration of Pavulon® should be delayed until the patient starts recovering from succinylcholine-induced neuromuscular blockade.
If a small dose of Pavulon® is given at least 3 minutes prior to the administration of succinylcholine, in order to reduce the incidence and intensity of succinylcholine-induced fasiculations, this dose may induce a degree of neuromuscular block sufficient to cause respiratory depression in some patients.
Other nondepolarizing neuromuscular blocking agents (vecuronium, atracurium, d-tubocurarine, metocurine, and gallamine) behave in a clinically similar fashion to Pavulon® The combinations of Pavulon®-metocurine and Pavulon®-d-tubocurarine are significantly more potent than the additive effects of each of the individual drugs given alone, however, the duration of blockade of these combinations is not prolonged. There are insufficient data to support concomitant use of pancuronium and the other three above mentioned muscle relaxants in the same patient.
Inhalational Anesthetics: Use of volatile inhalational anesthetics such as enflurane, isoflurane, and halothane with Pavulon® will enhance neuromuscular blockade.

Potentiation is most prominent with use of enflurane and isoflurane.

With the above agents, the intubating dose of Pavulon® may be the same as with balanced anesthesia unless the inhalational anesthetic has been administered for a sufficient time at a sufficient dose to have reached clinical equilibrium. The relatively long duration of action of pancuronium should be taken into consideration when the drug is selected for intubation in these circumstances.

Clinical experience and animal experiments suggest that pancuronium should be given with caution to patients receiving chronic tricyclic antidepressant therapy who are anesthetized with halothane because severe ventricular arrythmias may result from the combintion. The severity of the arrhythmias appear in part related to the dose of pancuronium.

Antibiotics: Parenteral/intraperitoneal administration of high doses of certain antibiotics may intensify, or produce neuromuscular block on their own. The following antibiotics have been associated with various degrees of paralysis: aminoglycosides (such as neomycin, streptomycin, kanamycin, gentamicin, and dihydrostreptomycin); tetracyclines; bacitracin; polymyxin B; colistin; and sodium colistimethate. If these or other newly introduced antibiotics are used preoperatively or in conjunction with Pavulon® during surgery, unexpected prolongation of neuromuscular block should be considered a possibility.

Other: Experience concerning injection of quinidine during recovery from use of other muscle relaxants suggests that recurrent paralysis may occur. This possibility must also be considered for Pavulon® (pancuronium bromide injection). Electrolyte imbalance and diseases which lead to electrolyte imbalance, such as adrenal cortical insufficiency, have been shown to alter neuromuscular blockade. Depending on the nature of the imbalance, either enhancement or inhibition may be expected. Magnesium salts, administered for the management of toxemia of pregnancy, may enhance the neuromuscular blockade.

Drug/laboratory test interactions: None known.

Carcinogenesis, Mutagenesis, Impairment of Fertility: Long-term studies in animals have not been performed to evaluate carcinogenic or mutagenic potential or impairment of fertility.

Pregnancy: Pregnancy Category C: Animal reproduction studies have not been performed. It is ot known whether Pavulon® can cause fetal harm when administered to a pregnant woman or can affect reproduction capacity. Pavulon® should be given to a pregnant woman only if the administering clinician decides that the benefits outweigh the risks.

Pavulon® may be used in operative obstetrics (Cesarean section), but reversal of pancuronium may be unsatisfactory in patients receiving magnesium sulfate for toxemia of pregnancy, because magnesium salts enhance neuromuscular blockade. Dosage should usually be reduced, as indicated, in such cases. It is also recommended that the interval between use of pancuronium and delivery be reasonably short to avoid clinically significant placental transfer.

Pediatric Use: Dose response studies in children indicate that, with the exception of neonates, dosage requirements are the same as for adults. Neonates are especially sensitive to nondepolarizing neuromuscular blocking agents, such as Pavulon®, during the first month of life. It is recommended that a test dose of 0.02 mg/kg be given first in this group to measure responsiveness.

The prolonged use of Pavulon® is for the management of neonates undergong mechanical ventilation has been associated in rare cases with severe skeletal muscle weakness that may first be noted during attempts to wean such patients from the ventilator; such patients usually receive other drugs such as antibiotics which may enhance neuromuscular blockade. Microscopic changes consistent with disuse atrophy have been noted at autopsy. Although a cause-and-effect relationship has not been established, the benefits-to-risk ratio must be considered when there is a need for neuromuscular blockade to facilitate long term mechanical ventilation of neonates.

Rare cases of unexplained, clinically significant methemoglobinemia have been reported in premature neonates, undergoing emergency anesthesia and surgery which included combined use of pancuronium fentanyl and atropine. A direct cause-and-effect relationship between the combined use of these drugs and the reported cases of methemoglobinemia has not been established.

ADVERSE REACTIONS

Neuromuscular: The most frequent adverse reaction to nondepolarizing blocking agents as a class consists of an extension of the drug's pharmacological action beyond the time period needed for surgery and anesthesia. This may vary from skeletal muscle weakness to profound and prolonged skeletal muscle paralysis resulting in respiratory insufficiency or apnea. (See **PRECAUTIONS: Pediatric Use**).

Inadequate reversal of the neuromuscular blockade is possible with Pavulon® as with all curariform drugs. These adverse experiences are managed by manual or mechanical ventilation until recovery is judged adequate.

Cardiovascular: See discussion of circulatory effects in **CLINICAL PHARMACOLOGY.**

Gastrointestinal: Salivation is sometimes noted during very light anesthesia, especially if no anticholinergic premedication is used.

Skin: An occasional transient rash is noted accompanying the use of Pavulon®.

Other: Although histamine release is not a characteristic action of Pavulon®, rare hypersensitivity reactions such as bronchospasm, flushing, redness, hypotension, tachycardia and other reactions possibly mediated by histamine release have been reported.

OVERDOSAGE

The possibility of iatrogenic overdosage can be minimized by carefully monitored the muscle twitch to peripheral nerve stimulation.

Excessive doses of Pavulon® can be expected to produce enhanced pharmacological effects. Residual neuromuscular blockade beyond the time period needed for surgery and anesthesia may occur with Pavulon® as with other neuromuscular blockers. This may be manifested by skeletal muscle weakness, decreased respiratory reserve, low tidal volume, or apnea. A peripheral nerve stimulator may be used to assess the degree of residual neuromuscular blockade and help to differentiate residual or neuromuscular blockade from other causes of decreased respiratory reserve.

Respiratory depression may be due either wholly or in part to other drugs used during the conduct of general anesthesia, such as narcotics, thiobarbiturates and other central nervous system depressants. Under such circumstances, the primary treatment is maintenance of a patent airway and manual or mechanical ventilation until complete recovery of normal respiration is assured.

Regonol® (pyridostigmine bromide injection), neostigmine, or edrophonium, in conjunction with atropine or glycopyrrolate, will usually antagonize the skeletal muscle relaxant action of Pavulon®. Satisfactory reversal can be judged by adequacy of skeletal muscle tone and by adequacy of respiration. A peripheral nerve stimulator may also be used to monitor restoration of twitch response.

Failure of prompt reversal (within 30 minutes) may occur in the presence of extreme debilitation, carcinomatosis, and with concomitant use of certain broad spectrum antibiotics, or anesthetic agents and other drugs which enhance neuromuscular blockade or cause respiratory depression of their own. Under such circumstances, the management is the same as that of prolonged neuromuscular blockade. Ventilation must be supported by artificial means until the patient has resumed control of his respiration. Prior to the use of reversal agents, reference should be made to the specific package insert of the reversal agent.

DOSAGE AND ADMINISTRATION

Pavulon® (pancuronium bromide injection) is for intravenous use only. This drug should be administered by or under the supevision of experienced clinicians familiar with the use of neuromuscular blocking agents. DOSAGE MUST BE INDIVDUALIZED IN EACH CASE. The dosage information which follows is derived from studies based upon units of drug per unit of body weight and is intended to serve as a guide only. Since potent inhalational anesthetics or prior use of succinylcholine may enhance the intensity and duration of Pavulon® (See **PRECAUTIONS: Drug Interactions**), the lower end of the recommended initial dosage range may suffice when Pavulon® is first used after intubation with succinylcholine and/or after maintenance doses of volatile liquid inhalational anesthetics are started. To obtain maximum clinical benefits of Pavulon® and to minimize the possibility of overdosage, the monitoring of muscle twitch reponse to a peripheral nerve stimulator is advised.

In adults under balanced anesthesia the initial intravenous dosage range is 0.04 to 0.1 mg/kg. Later incremental doses starting at 0.01 mg/kg may be used. These increments slightly increase the magnitude of the blockade and significantly increase the duration of blockade, because a significant number of myoneural junctions are still blocked when there is a clinical need for more drug.

If Pavulon® is used to provide skeletal muscle relaxation for endotracheal intubation, a bolus dosage of 0.06 to 0.1 mg/kg are recommended. Conditions satisfactory for intubation are usually present within 2 to 3 minutes.

Dosage in Children: Dose response studies in children indicate that, with the exception of neonates, dosage requirements are the same as for adults. Neonates are especially sensitive to nondepolarizing neuromuscular blocking agents, such as Pavulon® (pancuronium bromide injection) during the first month of life. It is recommended that a test dose of 0.02 mg/kg be given first in this group to measure responsiveness.

Cesarean Section: The dosage to provide relaxation for intubation and operation is the same as for general surgical procedures. The dosage to provide relaxation, following usage of succinylcholine for intubation (see **PRECAUTIONS: Drug Interactions**), is the same as for general surgical procedures.

Compatibility: Pavulon® is compatible in solution with:

0.9% sodium chloride injection	5% dextrose and sodium chloride injection
5% dextrose injection	Lactate Ringer's injection

Parenteral drug products should be inspected visually for particulate matter and discoloration prior to administration, whenever solution and container permit.

When mixed with the above solutions in glass or plastic containers, Pavulon® will remain stable in solution for 48 hours with no alteration in potency or pH; no decomposition is observed and there is no absorption to either the glass or plastic container.

HOW SUPPLIED

Pavulon® is packaged in the following forms:
2 ml ampuls—2 mg/ml—boxes of 25, NDC#0052-0444-26;
5 ml ampuls—2 mg/ml—boxes of 25, NDC#0052-0444-25;
10 ml vials—1 mg/ml—boxes of 25, NDC#0052-0443-25.

STORAGE

Both concentrations of Pavulon® will maintain full clinical potency for six months if kept at room temperature of 18°to 22°(65°to 72°F.); or for 2 years when refrigerated at 2°to 8°C. (36°to 46°F).

PREGNYL® ℞

(Chorionic Gonadotropin For Injection, U.S.P.)

DESCRIPTION

Human chorionic gonadotropin (HCG), a polypeptide hormone produced by the human placenta, is composed of an alpha and a beta sub-unit. The alpha sub-unit is essentially identical to the alpha sub-units of the human pituitary gonadotropins, luteinizing hormone (LH) and follicle-stimulating hormone (FSH), as well as to the alpha sub-unit of human thyroid-stimulating hormone (TSH). The beta sub-units of these hormones differ in amino acid sequence. Chorionic Gonadotropin is derived from the urine of pregnant women. It is standardized by a biological assay procedure.

CLINICAL PHARMACOLOGY

The action of HCG is virtually identical to that of pituitary LH although HCG appears to have a small degree of FSH activity as well. It stimulates production of gonadal steroid hormones by stimulating the interstitial cells, (Leydig cells) of the test is to produce androgens and the corpus luteum of the ovary to produce progesterone. Androgen stimulations in the male leads to the development of secondary sex characteristics and may stimulate testicular descent when no anatomical impediment to descent is present. This descent is usually reversible when HCG is discontinued. During the normal menstrual cycle, LH participates with FSH in the development and maturation of the normal ovarian follicle and the mid-cycle LH surge triggers ovulation. HCG can substitute for LH in this function. During a normal pregnancy, HCG secreted by the placenta maintains the corpus luteum after LH secretion decreases, supporting continued secretion of estrogen and progesterone and preventing menstruation. HCG HAS NO KNOWN EFFECT ON FAT MOBILIZATION, APPETITE OR SENSE OF HUNGER, OR BODY FAT DISTRIBUTION.

INDICATIONS

HCG HAS NOT BEEN DEMONSTRATED TO BE EFFECTIVE ADJUNCTIVE THERAPY IN THE TREATMENT OF OBESITY THERE IS NO SUBSTANTIAL EVIDENCE THAT IT INCREASES WEIGHT LOSS BEYOND THAT RESULTING FROM CALORIC RESTRICTION THAT IT CAUSES A MORE ATTRACTIVE OR "NORMAL" DISTRIBUTION OF FAT, OR THAT IT DECREASES THE HUNGER AND DISCOMFORT ASSOCIATED WITH CALORIE-RESTRICTED DIETS.

1. Prepubertal cryptorchidism not due to anatomical obstruction. In general, HCG is thought to induce testicular descent in situations when descent would have occurred at puberty. HCG thus may help predict whether or not orchiopexy will be needed in the future. Although in some cases, descent following HCG administration is permanent in most cases, the response is temporary. Therapy is usually instituted between the ages 4 and 9.
2. Selected cases of hypogonadotropic hypogonadism (hypogonadism secondary to a pituitary deficiency) in males.
3. Induction of ovulation and pregnancy in the anovulatory, infertile woman in whom the cause of anovulation is secondary and not due to primary ovarian failure and who has been appropiately pretreated with human menotropins.

CONTRAINDICATIONS

Precocious puberty, prostatic carcinoma or other androgen-dependent neoplasm, prior allergic reaction to HCG.

Continued on next page

Organon—Cont.

WARNINGS

HCG should be used in conjunction with human menopausal gonadotropins only by physicians experienced with infertility problems who are familiar with the criteria for patient selection, contraindications, warnings, precautions and adverse reactions described in the package insert for menotropins. The principal serious adverse reactions during this use are: (1) Ovarian hyperstimulation a syndrome of sudden ovarian enlargement ascites with or without pain, and/or pleural effusion, (2) Rupture of ovarian cysts with resultant hemoperitoneum, (3) Multiple births, and (4) Arterial thromboembolism.

PRECAUTIONS

Induction of androgen secretion by HCG may induce precocious puberty in patients treated for cryptorchidism. Therapy should be discontinued if signs of precocious puberty occur.
Since androgens may cause fluid retention, HCG should be used with caution in patients with cardiac or renal disease, epilepsy, migraine, or asthma.

ADVERSE REACTIONS

Headache, irritability, restlessness, depression, fatigue, edema, precocious puberty, gynecomastia, pain at the site of injection.

DOSAGE AND ADMINISTRATION

(Intramuscular Use Only): The dosage regimen employed in any particular case will depend upon the indication for use, the age and weight of the patient, and the physician's preference. The following regimens have been advocated by various authorities.

Prepubertal cryptochidism not due to anatomical obstruction.

1 4,000 U.S.P. Units three times weekly for three weeks.
2 5,000 U.S.P. Units every second day for four injections.
3 15 injections of 500 to 1,000 U.S.P. Units over a period of six weeks.
4 500 U.S.P. Units three times weekly for four to six weeks. If this course of treatment is not successful, another is begun one month later giving 1,000 U.S.P. Units per injection.

Selected cases of hypogonadotropic hypogonadism in males

1 500 to 1,000 U.S.P. Units three times a week for three weeks, followed by the same dose twice a week for three weeks.
2 4,000 U.S.P. Units three times weekly for six to nine months, following which the dosage may be reduced to 2,000 U.S.P. Units three times weekly for an additional three months.

Induction of ovulation and pregnancy in the anovulatory infertile woman in whom the cause of anovulation is secondary and not due to primary ovarian failure and who has been appropriately pre-treated with human menotropins. (See prescribing information for menotropins for dosage and administration for that drug product). 5,000 to 10,000 U.S.P. Units one day following the last dose of menotropins. (A dosage of 10,000 U.S.P. Units is recommended in the labeling for menotropins).
IMPORTANT: USE COMPLETELY WITHIN 60 DAYS AFTER RECONSTITUTION REFRIGERATE AFTER RECONSTITUTION.

HOW SUPPLIED

The freeze-dried stabilized active principle is supplied in a two vial package including Bacteriostatic Water for Injection as diluent
When reconstituted, each vial contains in U.S.P. Units:

VIAL SIZE	10 ml
Chorionic Gonadotropin	10,000 U.
Mannitol, U.S.P.	100 mg.
Benzyl Alcohol, N F	0.9%

with Sodium Phosphate Dibasic and Sodium Phosphate Monobasic to adjust pH.
The product is assayed in accord with the U.S.P. method and potencies refer to U.S.P. Units (International Units) defined in terms of the U.S.P. Chorionic Gonadotropin Reference Standard.

CAUTION

Federal (USA) law prohibits dispensing without prescription.

DIRECTIONS FOR RECONSTITUTION

TWO-VIAL PACKAGE: Withdraw sterile air from lyophilized vial and inject into diluent vial. Remove 10 ml from diluent and add to lyophilized vial, agitate gently until solution is complete.
Refrigerate after reconstitution and use within 60 days.

REGONOL® ℞

[re-gō-nol]
(pyridostigmine bromide) injection, USP

DESCRIPTION

Regonol (pyridostigmine bromide injection, USP) is an active cholinesterase inhibitor. Chemically, pyridostigmine bromide is 3-hydroxy-1-methylpyridinium bromide dimethylcarbamate. Its structural formula is:

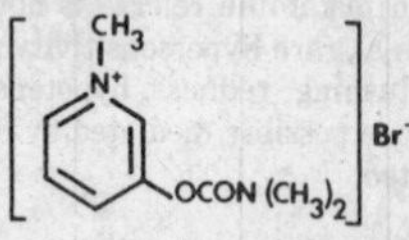

Each ml. contains 5 mg. of pyridostigmine bromide compounded with 1% benzyl alcohol as the preservative. The pH is buffered with sodium citrate and citric acid and adjusted with sodium hydroxide if necessary.

ACTIONS

Pyridostigmine bromide facilitates the transmission of impulses across the myoneural junction by inhibiting the destruction of acetylcholine by cholinesterase. Pyridostigmine is an analog of neostigmine but differs from it clinically by having fewer side effects. Currently available data indicate that pyridostigmine may have a significantly lower degree and incidence of bradycardia, salivation and gastrointestinal stimulation. Animal studies using the injectable form of pyridostigmine and human studies using the oral preparation have indicated that pyridostigmine has a longer duration of action than does neostigmine measured under similar circumstances.

INDICATIONS

Pyridostigmine bromide is useful as a reversal agent or antagonist to nondepolarizing muscle relaxants.

CONTRAINDICATIONS

Known hypersensitivity to anticholinesterase agents; intestinal and urinary obstructions of mechanical type.

WARNINGS

Pyridostigmine bromide should be used with particular caution in patients with bronchial asthma or cardiac dysrhythmias. Transient bradycardia may occur and be relieved by atropine sulfate. Atropine should also be used with caution in patients with cardiac dysrhythmias. When large doses of pyridostigmine bromide are administered, as during reversal of muscle relaxants, prior or simultaneous injection of atropine sulfate is advisable. Because of the possibility of hypersensitivity in an occasional patient, atropine and antishock medication should always be readily available.
When used as an antagonist to nondepolarizing muscle relaxants, adequate recovery of voluntary respiration and neuromuscular transmission must be obtained prior to discontinuation of respiratory assistance and there should be continuous patient observation. Satisfactory recovery may be defined by a combination of clinical judgement, respiratory measurements and observation of the effects of peripheral nerve stimulation. If there is any doubt concerning the adequacy of recovery from the effects of the nondepolarizing muscle relaxant, artificial ventilation should be continued until all doubt has been removed.
Use in Pregnancy—The safety of pyridostigmine bromide during pregnancy or lactation in humans has not been established. Therefore its use in women who are pregnant requires weighing the drug's potential benefits against its possible hazards to mother and child.

ADVERSE REACTIONS

The side effects of pyridostigmine bromide are most commonly related to overdosage and generally are of two varieties, muscarinic and nicotinic. Among those in the former group are nausea, vomiting, diarrhea, abdominal cramps, increased peristalsis, increased salivation, increased bronchial secretions, miosis and diaphoresis. Nicotinic side effects are comprised chiefly of muscle cramps, fasciculation and weakness. Muscarinic side effects can usually be counteracted by atropine. As with any compound containing the bromide radical, a skin rash may be seen in an occasional patient. Such reactions usually subside promptly upon discontinuance of the medication. Thrombophlebitis has been reported subsequent to intravenous administration.

DOSAGE AND ADMINISTRATION

When pyridostigmine bromide is given intravenously to reverse the action of muscle relaxant drugs, it is recommended that atropine sulfate (0.6 to 1.2 mg.) or glycopyrrolate in equipotent doses be given intravenously immediately prior to or simultaneous with its administration. Side effects, notably excessive secretions and bradycardia are thereby minimized. Reversal dosages range from 0.1 - 0.25 mg/kg. Usually 10 or 20 mg. of pyridostigmine bromide will be sufficient for antagonism of the effects of the nondepolarizing muscle relaxants. Although full recovery may occur within 15 minutes in most patients, others may require a half hour or more. Satisfactory reversal can be evident by adequate voluntary respiration, respiratory measurements and use of a peripheral nerve stimulator device. It is recommended that the patient be well ventilated and a patent airway maintained until complete recovery of normal respiration is assured. Once satisfactory reversal has been attained, recurarization has not been reported.
Failure of pyridostigmine bromide to provide prompt (within 30 minutes) reversal may occur, e.g. in the presence of extreme debilitation, carcinomatosis, or with concomitant use of certain broad spectrum antibiotics or anesthetic agents, notably ether. Under these circumstances ventilation must be supported by artificial means until the patient has resumed control of his respiration.

HOW SUPPLIED

Regonol is available in:
5 mg./ml.: 2 ml. ampuls—boxes of 25—NDC-0052-0460-02
5 ml. vials—boxes of 25—NDC-0052-0460-05
Protect from light.

SUCCINYLCHOLINE CHLORIDE INJECTION USP ℞

HOW SUPPLIED

20 mg/ml-10 ml vials, boxes of 25.

WIGRAINE® ℞

DESCRIPTION

Wigraine Tablet: Each tablet contains the following:

Ergotamine tartrate, USP	1 mg
Caffeine, USP	100 mg

Wigraine tablets are uncoated and prepared to insure rapid disintegration (by an exclusive manufacturing process) and facilitate quick absorption. Rapid onset of effect is important for the satisfactory treatment of acute attacks of vascular headaches.
Wigraine Suppository: Each suppository contains the following:

Ergotamine tartrate, USP	2 mg
Caffeine, USP	100 mg
Tartaric Acid	21.5 mg

Wigraine suppositories contain the active ingredients in a synthetic cocoa butter base which melts rapidly at room temperature.

CLINICAL PHARMACOLOGY

Ergotamine is an alpha adrenergic blocking agent with a direct stimulating effect on the smooth muscle of peripheral and cranial blood vessels and produces depression of central vasomotor centers. The compound also has the properties of serotonin antagonism. In comparison to hydrogenated ergotamine, the adrenergic blocking actions are less pronounced and vasoconstrictive actions are greater. Caffeine, also a cranial vasoconstrictor is added to further enhance the vasoconstrictive effect without the necessity of increasing ergotamine dosage.

INDICATIONS AND USAGE

Wigraine is indicated as therapy to abort or prevent vascular headaches such as migraine, migraine variants, or so-called histamine cephalalgia.

CONTRAINDICATIONS

Wigraine can cause fetal harm when administered to a pregnant women. It can produce prolonged uterine contractions which can result in abortion. Wigraine is contraindicated in women who are or may become pregnant. If this drug is used during pregnancy, or if the patient becomes pregnant while taking this drug, the patient should be advised of the potential hazard to the fetus.
Peripheral vascular disease, coronary heart disease, hypertension, impaired hepatic or renal function, sepsis, and hypersensitivity to any of the components.

PRECAUTIONS

Although signs and symptoms of ergotism rarely develop even after long term intermittent use of the orally or rectally administered drugs, care should be exercised to remain within the limits of recommended dosage.
Pregnancy Category X. See Contraindications section.
Nursing Mothers. It is not known whether the ergotamine tartrate in Wigraine is excreted in human milk. Because some ergot alkaloids have been found in the milk of nursing mothers resulting in symptoms of ergotism in their children, a decision should be made whether to discontinue nursing or to discontinue the drug, taking into account the importance of the drug to the mother.
Pediatric Usage. Safety and effectiveness in children have not been established.

ADVERSE REACTIONS

In order of decreasing severity; precordial distress and pain, muscle pains in the extremities, numbness and tingling in fingers and toes, transient tachycardia or bradycardia, vomiting, nausea, weakness in the legs, diarrhea, localized edema and itching.

DOSAGE AND ADMINISTRATION

Best results are obtained if the tablets or suppositories are administered at the first sign of an attack. Wigraine Tablet: the average oral adult dose is 2 tablets at the start of a vascular headache (migraine) attack; followed by one additional tablet every ½ hour if needed, up to 6 tablets per attack. Total weekly dosage should not exceed 10 tablets. Wigraine Suppository: the maximum adult dose is 2 suppositories for an individual attack. In carefully selected patients, with due consideration of maximum dosage recommendations, administration of the drug at bedtime may be an appropriate short-term preventive measure.

OVERDOSAGE

The toxic effects of an acute overdosage of Wigraine are due primarily to the ergotamine component. The amount of caffeine is such that its toxic effects will be overshadowed by those of ergotamine. Symptoms include vomiting, numbness, tingling, pain and cyanosis of the extremities associated with diminished or absent peripheral pulses, hypertension or hypotension, drowsiness, stupor, coma, convulsions, and shock. Treatment consists of removal of the offending drug by induction of emesis, gastric lavage and catharsis. Maintenance of adequate pulmonary ventilation, correction of hypotension and control of convulsions are important considerations. Treatment of peripheral vasospasm should consist of warmth, but not heat, and protection of the ischemic limbs. Vasodilators may be used with benefit but caution must be exercised to avoid aggravating an already existing hypotension.

The LD_{50} limits of the various components as outlined in NIOSH 1981-82 Registry of Toxic Effects of Chemical Substances, published by U.S. Department of Health and Human Services are as follows: Ergotamine Tartrate IV LD_{50} in rats = 80mg/kg, Caffeine IV LD_{50} in rats = 105mg/kg.

HOW SUPPLIED

Wigraine tablets are white tablets embossed with "ORGANON 542" on one side. They are individually foil stripped and packaged in boxes of 20 NDC #0052-0542-20 and 100's NDC #0052-0542-91. Wigraine suppositories are individuallly foil wrapped and packaged in boxes of 12. NDC #0052-0548-12 Wigraine tablets should be stored at a maximum of 30°C (86°F) and the suppositories should be refrigerated at 2°-8°C (36°-46°F).

Shown in Product Identification Section, page 419

Ortho Diagnostic Systems Inc.

ROUTE 202
RARITAN, NEW JERSEY 08869

MICRhoGAM™ ℞

[mike'ro-gam]

Rh_o (D) Immune Globulin (Human)
For Intramuscular Use Only

Micro-Dose for use *only* after spontaneous or induced abortion or termination of ectopic pregnancy up to and including 12 weeks' gestation.

DESCRIPTION

MICRhoGAM Rh_o(D) Immune Globulin (Human) is a sterile solution containing IgG anti-Rh_o(D) for use in preventing Rh immunization in Rh negative individuals exposed to Rh positive red blood cells. It may include globulin derived from fractionated plasma prepared by other licensed manufacturers which does not contain anti-Rh_o(D). A single dose of MICRhoGAM contains sufficient anti-Rh_o(D) (approximately 50 μg)† to suppress the immune response to 2.5 ml (or less) of Rh positive red blood cells.

All plasma used in the preparation of MICRhoGAM was tested for hepatitis B surface antigen (HBsAg) by a licensed third generation test and found to be nonreactive. All donors are carefully screened to eliminate those in high risk groups for disease transmission. Fractionation of the plasma is done by a modification of the cold alcohol procedure. Human immune globulins prepared by cold alcohol fractionation have not been reported to transmit hepatitis or other infectious diseases. Glycine (15 mg/ml) is included in the final product as a stabilizer. The final product contains 15% ± 1.5% globulin, 2.9 mg/ml sodium chloride and 0.01% thimerosal (mercury derivative).

This product is for intramuscular injection only.

† A full dose of Rh_o(D) Immune Globulin (Human) has traditionally been referred to as a "300 μg" dose and this usage is employed here for convenience in terminology. *It should not be construed as the actual anti-D content.* Each full dose of Rh_o(D) Immune Globulin (Human) must contain at least as much anti-D as 1 milliliter of the U.S. Reference Rh_o(D) Immune Globulin (Human). Studies performed at the Food and Drug Administration have shown that the U.S. Reference contains 820 international units (IU) of anti-D per milliliter. When the conversion factor determined for the International (WHO) Reference Preparation is used, 820 IU per milliliter is equivalent to 164 μg per milliliter of anti-D.

MICRhoGAM contains approximately one-sixth the amount of anti-D contained in the full dose.

CLINICAL PHARMACOLOGY

MICRhoGAM acts by suppressing the immune response of Rh negative women to Rh positive red blood cells. The risk of immunization is related to the number of Rh positive red cells received. The risk was found to be 3% when 0.1 ml of fetal red blood cells is present in the mother and 65% when 5 ml is present. In the first 12 weeks of gestation the total volume of red blood cells in the fetus is estimated at less than 2.5 ml.

Clinical studies demonstrated that administration of MICRhoGAM within three (3) hours following abortion was 100% effective in preventing Rh immunization. Studies in male volunteers showed MICRhoGAM to be effective when given as long as 72 hours after the infusion of Rh positive red cells. A lesser degree of protection is afforded if the antibody is administered beyond this time period.

INDICATIONS AND USAGE

MICRhoGAM is indicated for an Rh negative woman following spontaneous or induced abortion or termination of ectopic pregnancy up to and including 12 weeks' gestation, unless the father is conclusively shown to be Rh negative.

CONTRAINDICATIONS

MICRhoGAM must not be used for genetic amniocentesis at 15 to 18 weeks' gestation or antepartum prophylaxis at 28 weeks' gestation. RhoGAM™ Rh_o(D) Immune Globulin (Human) is recommended for any indication beyond 12 weeks' gestation.

Individuals known to have had an anaphylactic or severe systemic reaction to human globulin should not receive MICRhoGAM or any other Rh_o(D) Immune Globulin (Human).

WARNINGS

Do not inject intravenously.

PRECAUTIONS

Pregnancy Category C—Animal reproduction studies have not been conducted with MICRhoGAM. It is also not known whether Rh_o(D) Immune Globulin (Human) can cause fetal harm when administered to a pregnant woman or can affect reproduction capacity. Rh_o(D) Immune Globulin (Human) should be given to a pregnant woman only if clearly needed.

ADVERSE REACTIONS

Systemic reactions associated with administration of MICRhoGAM are extremely rare. Discomfort at the site of injection has been reported and a small number of women have noted a slight elevation in temperature.

DOSAGE AND ADMINISTRATION

Parenteral drug products should be inspected visually for particulate matter and discoloration prior to administration, whenever solution and container permit.

A single dose (approximately 50 μg)† of MICRhoGAM will completely suppress the immune response to 2.5 ml of Rh positive red blood cells (packed cells, not whole blood).

Administer a single dose of MICRhoGAM intramuscularly as soon as possible after termination of a pregnancy up to and including 12 weeks' gestation. At or beyond 13 weeks' gestation it is recommended that a single dose of RhoGAM Rh_o(D) Immune Globulin (Human) (approximately 300 μg)† be given instead of MICRhoGAM.

Since there is no lot number and expiration date on the prefilled syringes, they should not be removed from the protective pouch until immediately before use.

† See footnote under Description.

HOW SUPPLIED

- 5 prefilled single-dose syringes of MICRhoGAM (Product code 8040) NDC 0562-8010-40
- package insert
- 5 control forms
- 5 patient identification cards

and

- 25 prefilled single-dose syringes of MICRhoGAM (Product code 8045) NDC 0562-8010-45
- package insert
- 25 control forms
- 25 patient identification cards

STORAGE

Store at 2° to 8°C. DO NOT FREEZE.

RhoGAM™ ℞

[ro'gam]

Rh_o (D) Immune Globulin (Human)
For Intramuscular Use Only

DESCRIPTION

RhoGAM Rh_o(D) Immune Globulin (Human) is a sterile solution containing IgG anti-Rh_o(D) for use in preventing Rh immunization in Rh negative individuals exposed to Rh positive red blood cells. It may include globulin derived from fractionated plasma prepared by other licensed manufacturers which does not contain anti-Rh_o(D). Each single dose of RhoGAM contains sufficient anti-Rh_o(D) (approximately 300 μg)† to suppress the immune response to 15 ml (or less) of Rh positive red blood cells.

All plasma used in the preparation of RhoGAM was tested for hepatitis B surface antigen (HBsAg) by a licensed third generation test and found to be nonreactive. All donors are carefully screened to eliminate those in high risk groups for disease transmission. Fractionation of the plasma is done by a modification of the cold alcohol procedure. Human immune globulins prepared by cold alcohol fractionation have not been reported to transmit hepatitis or other infectious diseases. Glycine (15 mg/ml) is included in the final product as a stabilizer. The final product contains 15% ± 1.5% globulin, 2.9 mg/ml sodium chloride and 0.01% thimerosal (mercury derivative).

This product is for intramuscular injection only.

† A full dose of Rh_o(D) Immune Globulin (Human) has traditionally been referred to as a "300 μg" dose and this usage is employed here for convenience in terminology. *It should not be construed as the actual anti-D content.* Each full dose of Rh_o(D) Immune Globulin (Human) must contain at least as much anti-D as 1 milliliter of the U.S. Reference Rh_o(D) Immune Globulin (Human). Studies performed at the Food and Drug Administration have shown that the U.S. Reference contains 820 international units (IU) of anti-D per milliliter. When the conversion factor determined for the International (WHO) Reference Preparation is used, 820 IU per milliliter is equivalent to 164 μg per milliliter of anti-D.

CLINICAL PHARMACOLOGY

RhoGAM acts by suppressing the immune response of Rh negative individuals to Rh positive red blood cells. The risk of immunization is related to the number of Rh positive red blood cells received and the route of introduction.

The obstetrical patient may be exposed to red blood cells from her Rh positive fetus during the normal course of pregnancy as a consequence of abdominal trauma, amniocentesis, abortion, or full-term delivery. Clinical studies proved that the incidence of Rh immunization as a result of pregnancy was reduced to 1% to 2% when RhoGAM was given within 72 hours following delivery, compared with 12% to 13% incidence in untreated women. Further studies in which patients received two doses of Rh immune globulin, one at 28 to 32 weeks of gestation and another after delivery if the baby was Rh positive, showed this regimen reduced the risk of immunization to less than 0.1%.

An Rh negative individual who receives a transfusion of one unit of Rh positive whole blood or Rh positive red blood cells has about an 80% likelihood of producing anti-Rh_o(D).

Protection from Rh immunization has been accomplished by administering the appropriate number of single doses of RhoGAM as described under Dosage and Administration.

INDICATIONS AND USAGE

Pregnancy and Other Obstetric Conditions—RhoGAM is indicated whenever it is known or suspected that fetal red cells have entered the circulation of an Rh negative mother unless the fetus or the father can be shown conclusively to be Rh negative. Small fetal-maternal hemorrhages that could cause the mother to produce anti-Rh_o(D) have been reported in association with abortion, amniocentesis, full-term delivery and in the normal course of pregnancy.

Transfusion—RhoGAM is indicated for any Rh negative female of childbearing age who receives Rh positive red blood cells or whole blood, or components such as platelets or granulocytes prepared from Rh positive blood.

CONTRAINDICATIONS

Individuals known to have had an anaphylactic or severe systemic reaction to human globulin should not receive RhoGAM or any other Rh_o(D) Immune Globulin (Human).

WARNINGS

Do not inject intravenously.
Do not inject infant.

PRECAUTIONS

The presence of passively acquired anti-Rh_o(D) in the maternal serum may cause a positive antibody screening test subsequent to administration of Rh_o(D) Immune Globulin (Human). This does not preclude further antepartum or postpartum prophylaxis.

Continued on next page

Ortho Diagnostic—Cont.

Some babies born of women given $Rh_o(D)$ Immune Globulin (Human) antepartum have weakly positive direct antiglobulin tests at birth.

Late in pregnancy or following delivery there may be sufficient fetal red blood cells in the maternal circulation to cause a positive result if one tests for the $Rh_o(D)$ variant known as D^u. When there is any doubt as to the patient's Rh type, RhoGAM should be administered.

Pregnancy Category C—Animal reproduction studies have not been conducted with RhoGAM. It is also not known whether $Rh_o(D)$ Immune Globulin (Human) can cause fetal harm when administered to a pregnant woman or can affect reproduction capacity. $Rh_o(D)$ Immune Globulin (Human) should be given to a pregnant woman only if clearly needed. However, use of Rh antibody during the third trimester in full doses of antibody has been reported to produce no evidence of hemolysis in the infant.

ADVERSE REACTIONS

Systemic reactions associated with administration of RhoGAM are extremely rare. Discomfort at the site of injection has been reported and a small number of women have noted a slight elevation in temperature.

About one-quarter of a group of 22 individuals who were given multiple doses of RhoGAM to treat mismatched transfusions noted fever, myalgia and lethargy. Bilirubin levels of 0.4 to 6.8 mg/dl were observed in some of the treated individuals and one had splenomegaly.

DOSAGE AND ADMINISTRATION

Parenteral drug products should be inspected visually for particulate matter and discoloration prior to administration, whenever solution and container permit.

A single dose (approximately 300 μg)† is contained in each vial or prefilled syringe of RhoGAM. This is the usual dose for the indications associated with pregnancy unless there is clinical or laboratory evidence of a fetal-maternal hemorrhage in excess of 15 ml of Rh positive red blood cells. The indications and recommended dosage for RhoGAM are summarized in the following table.

Indications and Recommended Dosage

Indication	Dose (approximately)
Threatened abortion at any stage of gestation with continuation of pregnancy	300 μg†
Abortion or termination of ectopic pregnancy at or beyond 13 weeks' gestation**	300 μg
Genetic amniocentesis at 15 to 18 weeks' gestation	300 μg
Abdominal trauma in second or third trimester	300 μg
Third trimester amniocentesis	300 μg
Antepartum prophylaxis at 26 to 28 weeks' gestation††	300 μg
Postpartum (if newborn Rh positive)	300 μg

†See footnote under Description

**If abortion or termination of ectopic pregnancy occurs up to and including 12 weeks' gestation, a single dose of MICRhoGAM™ $Rh_o(D)$ Immune Globulin (Human) (approximately 50 μg)† may be used instead of RhoGAM.

††If antepartum prophylaxis is indicated, it is essential that the mother receive a postpartum dose if the infant is Rh positive.

If abdominal trauma, amniocentesis, abortion, or other adverse event requires the administration of RhoGAM at 13 to 18 weeks of gestation, another dose should be given at 26 to 28 weeks. To maintain protection throughout pregnancy, the level of passively acquired anti-$Rh_o(D)$ should not be allowed to fall below the level required to prevent an immune response to Rh positive red cells. The half-life of IgG is 23 to 26 days. In any case, a dose of RhoGAM should be given within 72 hours after delivery if the baby is Rh positive. If delivery occurs within three weeks after the last dose, the postpartum dose may be withheld unless there is a fetal-maternal hemorrhage in excess of 15 ml of Rh positive red blood cells.

Whenever there is a fetal-maternal hemorrhage in excess of 15 ml of Rh positive red blood cells, multiple doses of RhoGAM are required. Based on the blood volume of the fetus at different stages of gestation, a fetal-maternal hemorrhage of this magnitude is unlikely prior to the last trimester of pregnancy. Patients who may need multiple doses of RhoGAM can be identified by a screening test based on rosetting. If the test is positive, the volume of the fetal-maternal hemorrhage should be determined by using an approved laboratory assay and a single dose of RhoGAM administered for every 15 ml of fetal red blood cells. If the dose calculation results in a fraction, administer the next number of whole vials or prefilled syringes of RhoGAM.

Multiple doses of RhoGAM are usual for indications associated with transfusion. For every 15 ml of Rh positive red blood cells transfused, whether as red blood cells, in whole blood or in components such as platelets or granulocytes prepared from Rh positive blood, the patient should receive a single dose of RhoGAM.

Administer RhoGAM intramuscularly. Do not inject intravenously. The contents of multiple vials or prefilled syringes may be given at one time into different sites, or at different times, as long as the total dose is administered within three days after delivery or receipt of Rh positive red cells.

Since there is no lot number and expiration date on the prefilled syringes, they should not be removed from the protective pouch until immediately before use.

HOW SUPPLIED

RhoGAM is supplied in packages containing:

- 1 single-dose vial of RhoGAM (Product code 8020) NDC 0562-8000-71
- package insert
- control form
- patient identification card

and

- 25 single-dose vials of RhoGAM (Product code 8003) NDC 0562-8000-72
- package insert
- 25 control forms
- 25 patient identification cards

and

- 5 prefilled single-dose syringes of RhoGAM (Product code 8030) NDC 0562-8000-30
- package insert
- 5 control forms
- 5 patient identification cards

and

- 5 prefilled single-dose syringes of RhoGAM (Product code 8033) NDC 0562-8000-33
- package insert
- suggested office protocol
- 5 injection records
- 5 patient information booklets
- 5 patient identification cards
- 5 labels for patients' charts

and

- 25 prefilled single-dose syringes of RhoGAM (Product code 8032) NDC 0562-8000-32
- package insert
- 25 control forms
- 25 patient identification cards

STORAGE

Store at 2° to 8°C. DO NOT FREEZE.

Ortho Pharmaceutical Corporation
RARITAN, NJ 08869

ACI-JEL® Therapeutic Vaginal Jelly ℞

DESCRIPTION

ACI-JEL Vaginal Jelly is a bland, non-irritating, water-dispersible, buffered acid jelly for intravaginal use. ACI-JEL is classified as a Vaginal Therapeutic Jelly. ACI-JEL contains 0.921% glacial acetic acid ($C_2H_4O_2$), 0.025% oxyquinoline sulfate ($C_{18}H_{16}N_2O_6S$), 0.7% ricinoleic acid ($C_{18}H_{34}O_3$), and 5% glycerin ($C_3H_8O_3$) compounded with tragacanth, acacia, propylparaben, potassium hydroxide, stannous chloride, egg albumen, potassium bitartrate, perfume and purified water. ACI-JEL is formulated to pH 3.9–4.1.

CLINICAL PHARMACOLOGY

ACI-JEL acts to restore and maintain normal vaginal acidity through its buffer action.

INDICATIONS AND USAGE

ACI-JEL is indicated as adjunctive therapy in those cases where restoration and maintenance of vaginal acidity are desirable.

CONTRAINDICATIONS

None known.

WARNINGS

No serious adverse reactions or potential safety hazards have been reported with the use of ACI-JEL.

PRECAUTIONS

General: No special care is required for the safe and effective use of ACI-JEL. *Drug Interactions:* No incidence of drug interactions have been reported with concomitant use of ACI-JEL and any other medications. *Laboratory Tests:* The monitoring of vaginal acidity (pH) may be helpful in following the patient's response. (The normal vaginal pH has been shown to be in the range of 4.0 to 5.0.) *Carcinogenesis:* No long-term studies in animals have been performed to evaluate carcinogenic potential. *Pregnancy:* Pregnancy Category C. Animal reproduction studies have not been conducted with ACI-JEL. It is also not known whether ACI-JEL can cause fetal harm when administered to a pregnant woman or can affect reproduction capacity. ACI-JEL should be given to a pregnant woman only if clearly needed. *Nursing Mothers:* It is not known whether this drug is excreted in human milk. Because many drugs are excreted in human milk, caution should be exercised when ACI-JEL is administered to a nursing woman.

ADVERSE REACTIONS

Occasional cases of local stinging and burning have been reported.

DOSAGE AND ADMINISTRATION

The usual dose is one applicatorful, administered intravaginally, morning and evening. Duration of treatment may be determined by the patient's response to therapy.

HOW SUPPLIED

85g Tube with ORTHO® Measured-Dose Applicator.
NDC 0062-5421-01

CONCEPTROL® Birth Control Cream

(See PDR For Nonprescription Drugs)

CONCEPTROL® Contraceptive Gel Disposable

(See PDR For Nonprescription Drugs)

DELFEN® Contraceptive Foam

(See PDR For Nonprescription Drugs)

DIENESTROL Cream ℞

(See ORTHO® Dienestrol Cream)

GYNOL II® Contraceptive Jelly

(See PDR For Nonprescription Drugs)

LIPPES LOOP™ Intrauterine Device ℞

DESCRIPTION

The LIPPES LOOP is made of polyethylene in the shape of a double S. Four different sizes are manufactured to allow for the variability in the size of the uterus. (See below.) A fine, double thread or "tail" made of polyethylene suture (monofilament) is attached to the lower end to facilitate removal. In addition, palpation of the tail through the cervix by the patient, or visualization by the physician, can assist in determining whether or not an undetected expulsion has occurred. A LIPPES LOOP comes prepackaged and sterilized with an introducer, together with an insertion tube in a polyethylene pouch. The insertion tube is equipped with a flange to aid in gauging the depth to which the insertion tube should be inserted through the cervical canal and into the uterine cavity. The four available sizes are as follows:

Loop A—22.2 mm. Blue thread. For those women who cannot tolerate a larger size device.

Loop B—27.5 mm. WITH REDUCED RADII. Black thread. Suggested for women who have had premature pregnancy losses and multiparous females whose uteri sound out less than 6 cm.

Loop C—30 mm. WITH REDUCED RADII. Yellow thread. Suggested for use when Loop D is removed for bleeding or pain. The physician is advised to wait two to four weeks between removing a loop for bleeding and reinserting a second loop.

Loop D—30 mm. White thread. Suggested for use in women with one or more children.

Mode of Action or Principles of IUD Design:
The exact mechanism of action of the LIPPES LOOP is not known. However, it is believed to interfere in some manner with nidation in the endometrium, probably through foreign body reaction in the uterus.

INDICATIONS AND USAGE

LIPPES LOOP is indicated for contraception.

CONTRAINDICATIONS

IUD's should not be inserted when the following conditions exist:

1. Pregnancy or suspicion of pregnancy.
2. Abnormalities of the uterus resulting in distortion of the uterine cavity.
3. Pelvic inflammatory disease or a history of repeated pelvic inflammatory disease.
4. Postpartum endometritis or infected abortion in the past three months.
5. Known or suspected uterine or cervical malignancy including unresolved, abnormal "Pap" smear.
6. Genital bleeding of unknown etiology.
7. Cervicitis until infection is controlled.

WARNINGS

1. **Pregnancy. a. Long-term effects.** Long-term effects on the offspring when pregnancy occurs with LIPPES LOOP in place are unknown.

b. Septic abortion. Reports have indicated an increased incidence of septic abortion associated in some instances with septicemia, septic shock, and death in patients becoming pregnant with an IUD in place. Most of these reports have been associated with the mid-trimester of pregnancy. In some cases, the initial symptoms have been insidious and not easily recognized. If pregnancy should occur with an IUD in place, the IUD should be removed if the string is visible or, if removal proves to be or would be difficult, termination of the pregnancy should be considered and offered the patient as an option, bearing in mind that the risks associated with an elective abortion increase with gestational age.

c. Continuation of pregnancy. If the patient chooses to continue the pregnancy, she must be warned of the increased risk of spontaneous abortion and of the increased risk of sepsis, including death, if the pregnancy continues with the IUD in place. The patient must be closely observed and she must be advised to report all abnormal symptoms, such as flu-like syndrome, fever, abdominal cramping and pain, bleeding, or vaginal discharge, immediately because generalized symptoms of septicemia may be insidious.

2. **Ectopic pregnancy. a.** A pregnancy that occurs with an IUD in place is more likely to be ectopic than a pregnancy occurring without an IUD in place. Accordingly, patients who become pregnant while using the IUD should be carefully evaluated for the possibility of an ectopic pregnancy.

b. Special attention should be directed to patients with delayed menses, slight metrorrhagia and/or unilateral pelvic pain, and to those patients who wish to terminate a pregnancy because of IUD failure, to determine whether ectopic pregnancy has occurred.

3. **Pelvic infection.** An increased risk of pelvic infection has been reported with the IUD in place. Although the etiology of this risk is not understood, it has been suggested that the tail may act as a mechanism for the passage of vaginal bacteria into the uterus. This, at times, may result in the development of bilateral or unilateral tubo-ovarian abscesses or general peritonitis. Pelvic infection may lead to hospitalization or surgery and infertility. Appropriate aerobic and anaerobic bacteriological studies should be done and antibiotic therapy initiated. The IUD should be removed and the continuing treatment reassessed based upon the results of culture and sensitivity tests.

Because of the increased risk of pelvic infection, the physician may wish each woman who has an IUD in place to have a periodic cervical vaginal "Pap" smear and pelvic exam. All "Pap" smears should include specific evaluation for actinomycosis.

4. **Effect on future fertility.** An increased risk of tubal infertility, with or without prior symptoms of pelvic infection, has been associated with the use of IUD's, particularly inert IUD's, including the LIPPES LOOP. This risk appears to be greatest for nulliparous women and those exposed to multiple sexual partners. The decision to use an IUD must be made by the physician and patient with appropriate regard for the possibility of future infertility. This consideration is especially important for women, particularly nulliparous women, who may wish to have children at a later date.

5. **Embedment.** Partial penetration or lodging of the IUD in the endometrium can result in difficult removals.

6. **Perforation.** Partial or total perforation of the uterine wall or cervix may occur with the use of IUDs. The possibility of perforation must be kept in mind during insertion and at the time of any subsequent examination. If perforation occurs, the IUD should be removed. Adhesions, foreign body reactions, and intestinal obstruction may result if an IUD is left in the peritoneal cavity. There are a few reports that there has been migration after insertion apparently in the absence of perforation at insertion. In any event, it is possible for the IUD to perforate outside the uterus.

PRECAUTIONS

1. **Patient counseling.** Prior to insertion, the physician, nurse or other trained health professional must provide the patient with the Patient Brochure. The patient should be given the opportunity to read the brochure and discuss fully any questions she may have concerning the IUD as well as other methods of contraception.

2. **Patient evaluation and clinical considerations. a.** A complete medical history should be obtained to determine conditions that might influence the selection of an IUD. Physical examination should include a pelvic examination, "Pap" smear, gonorrhea culture and, if indicated, appropriate tests for other forms of venereal disease. Papanicolaou smears should include specific evaluation for actinomycosis.

b. The uterus should be carefully sounded prior to insertion to determine the degree of patency of the endocervical canal and the internal os, and the direction and depth of the uterine cavity. In occasional cases, severe cervical stenosis may be encountered. Do not use excessive force to overcome this resistance.

c. The uterus should sound to a depth of 6 to 8 centimeters (cm). Insertion of an IUD into a uterine cavity measuring less than 6.5 cm by sounding may increase the incidence of expulsion, bleeding, pain and perforation.

d. The possibility of insertion in the presence of an existing undetermined pregnancy is reduced if insertion is performed during or shortly following a menstrual period. The IUD should not be inserted postpartum or postabortion until involution of the uterus is completed. The incidence of perforation and expulsion is greater if involution is not completed.

e. IUD's should be used with caution in those patients who have anemia or a history of menorrhagia or hypermenorrhea. Patients experiencing menorrhagia and/or metrorrhagia following IUD insertion may be at risk for the development of hypochromic microcytic anemia. Also, IUD's should be used with caution in patients receiving anticoagulants or having a coagulopathy.

f. Syncope, bradycardia, or other neurovascular episodes may occur during insertion or removal of IUD's especially in patients with a previous disposition to these conditions.

g. Patients with valvular or congenital heart disease are more prone to develop subacute bacterial endocarditis than patients who do not have valvular or congenital heart disease. Use of an IUD in these patients may represent a potential source of septic emboli.

h. Use of an IUD in those patients with cervicitis should be postponed until treatment has cured the infection (see CONTRAINDICATIONS Section).

i. Since an IUD may be expelled or displaced, patients should be reexamined and evaluated shortly after the first postinsertion menses, but definitely within three months after insertion. Thereafter, annual examination with appropriate medical and laboratory examination should be carried out.

j. The patient should be told that some bleeding and cramps may occur during the first few weeks after insertion, but if these symptoms continue or are severe, she should report them to her physician. The patient should be instructed on how to check to make certain that the thread still protrudes from the cervix, and she should be cautioned that there is no contraceptive protection if the IUD is expelled. She should be instructed to check the tail as often as possible, but at least after each menstrual period. The patient should be cautioned not to pull on the thread and displace the IUD. If partial expulsion occurs, removal is indicated and a new IUD may be inserted.

k. The use of medical diathermy (shortwave and microwave) in patients with metal-containing IUD's may cause heat injury to the surrounding tissue. Therefore, medical diathermy to the abdominal and sacral areas should not be used.

[LIPPES LOOP contains no metals. This section does not apply to LIPPES LOOP].

ADVERSE REACTIONS

These adverse reactions are not listed in any order of frequency or severity.

Reported adverse reactions include: endometritis, spontaneous abortion, septic abortion, septicemia, perforation of the uterus and cervix, embedment, migration resulting in partial or complete perforation, fragmentation of the IUD, pelvic infection (pelvic inflammatory disease), future infertility, vaginitis, leukorrhea, cervical erosion, pregnancy, ectopic pregnancy, difficult removal, complete or partial expulsion of the IUD, intermenstrual spotting, prolongation of menstrual flow, anemia, pain and cramping, dysmenorrhea, backaches, dyspareunia, neurovascular episodes, including bradycardia and syncope secondary to insertion. Perforation into the abdomen has been followed by abdominal adhesions, intestinal penetration, intestinal obstruction, and cystic masses in the pelvis.

DIRECTIONS FOR USE

Preinsertion

1. It is imperative that sterile technique be maintained throughout the insertion procedure.

2. Perform a through pelvic examination to determine freedom from overt disease and to determine position and shape of the uterus. RULE OUT PREGNANCY AND OTHER CONTRAINDICATIONS.

3. With a speculum in place, gently insert a sterile sound to determine the depth and direction of the uterine canal. Be sure to determine the position of the uterus before insertion. Occasionally a tenaculum is required if the uterine canal needs to be straightened. If a stenotic cervix must be dilated, use a sterile Hank's dilator rather than a Hegar's; dilation to a Hank's 16 to 18 should be sufficient.

Insertion

Caution: It is generally felt that perforations are caused at the time of insertion, although the perforation may not be detected until some time later. The position of the uterus should be determined during the preinsertion examination. Great care must be exercised during the preinsertion sounding and subsequent insertion. No attempt should be made to force the insertion. There are a few reports, however, that there has been migration after insertion apparently in the absence of perforation at insertion. In any event, it is possible for the IUD to perforate outside the uterus.

1. How to prepare the LIPPES LOOP Intrauterine Double-S inserter.

Using sterile gloves, hold tube in one hand and with the other draw LOOP into inserter by pulling the push rod. As the LOOP is drawn into the inserter you will encounter some resistance. It is important to use a slow steady pulling action until all but the bulbous tip of the LOOP is entirely within the inserter. At this point, insure that both the flat surface of the bulbous tip and the inserter flange are in a horizontal plane.

Do this not more than one minute before insertion.

2. How to insert LIPPES LOOP Intrauterine Double-S.

Insert the loaded inserter gently through the endocervical canal, with the flange in a horizontal plane. DO NOT FORCE THE INSERTION. If resistance is encountered, do not proceed; perforation of the uterus may occur. If the flange makes contact with the cervix WITHOUT the inserter touching the fundal wall, withdraw ¼ inch before pressing the push rod to release the device in utero. Should the inserter touch the fundal wall BEFORE the flange makes contact, withdraw ½ inch prior to pressing the push rod to release the device in utero. With the inserter now in place, proceed, and WITHOUT UNDUE PRESSURE, push the rod slowly as far as it will go. LIPPES LOOP Intrauterine Double-S should now be in place. Withdraw the inserter tube and push rod from the cervical os until the tail is visible. Cut the tail leaving it as long as possible.

Time of Insertion

LIPPES LOOP Intrauterine Double-S should be inserted preferably the last one or two days of a normal menstrual period or the two days following the last day.

The expulsion and perforation rate may be increased when insertions are made before normal uterine involution occurs (usually four to six weeks postpartum or postabortion).

To Remove

To remove LIPPES LOOP Intrauterine Double-S, pull gently on the exposed tail. On those rare occasions that the tail is not available, the device should be carefully removed.

CLINICAL STUDIES

Different event rates have been recorded with the use of different IUD's. Inasmuch as these rates are usually derived from separate studies conducted by different investigators in several population groups, they cannot be compared with precision. Furthermore, event rates tend to be lower as clinical experience is expanded, possibly due to retention in the clinical study of those patients who accept the treatment regimen and do not discontinue due to adverse reactions or pregnancy. In clinical trials conducted by the Population Council with the LIPPES LOOP, use effectiveness was determined as follows for women, as tabulated by the life table method. (Rates are expressed as events per 100 women through 12 and 24 months of use). This experience is based on 198,257 woman/months of use, including 121,489 woman/months of use in first year after insertion, and 76,768 woman/months of use in second year after insertion. LIPPES LOOP Intrauterine Double-S devices are manufactured in four different sizes, and the figures given above represent the totals for the four sizes. The following table presents these figures individually for each size LOOP:

[See table above].

TABLE I

LIPPES LOOP Size	Number Woman/Months	Woman/Months of Use 1st Year After Insertion	Woman/Months of Use 2nd Year After Insertion
A	13,453	8,751	4,702
B	12,463	9,660	2,803
C	50,775	31,032	19,743
D	121,566	72,046	49,520

Tables II–V below give the pregnancy expulsion, medical removal and continuation rates for each individual size LOOP:

Continued on next page

Ortho Pharm.—Cont.

TABLE II
LOOP A
(Annual Rates Per 100 Users)

	12 Months	24 Months (cumulative)
Pregnancy	5.3	9.7
Expulsion	23.9	27.7
Medical Removal	12.2	20.0
Continuation Rate	75.2	63.6

TABLE III
LOOP B
(Annual Rates Per 100 Users)

	12 Months	24 Months (cumulative)
Pregnancy	3.4	6.3
Expulsion	18.9	24.9
Medical Removal	15.1	23.8
Continuation Rate	74.6	59.2

TABLE IV
LOOP C
(Annual Rates Per 100 Users)

	12 Months	24 Months (cumulative)
Pregnancy	3.0	4.8
Expulsion	19.1	24.6
Medical Removal	14.3	22.1
Continuation Rate	76.5	62.8

TABLE V
LOOP D
(Annual Rates Per 100 Users)

	12 Months	24 Months (cumulative)
Pregnancy	2.7	4.2
Expulsion	12.7	16.0
Medical Removal	15.2	23.3
Continuation Rate	77.4	65.6

MASSE' ® Breast Cream

(See PDR For Nonprescription Drugs)

MONISTAT® 7 Vaginal Cream ℞
(miconazole nitrate 2%)

DESCRIPTION
MONISTAT 7 Vaginal Cream (miconazole nitrate 2%) is a water-miscible, white cream containing as the active ingredient, 2% miconazole nitrate, 1-[2,4-dichloro-β-(2,4-dichlorobenzyloxy) phenethyl] imidazole nitrate.

ACTIONS
MONISTAT 7 Vaginal Cream exhibits fungicidal activity *in vitro* against species of the genus *Candida*. The pharmacologic mode of action is unknown.

INDICATIONS
MONISTAT 7 Vaginal Cream is indicated for the local treatment of vulvovaginal candidiasis (moniliasis). As MONISTAT 7 Vaginal Cream is effective only for candidal vulvovaginitis, the diagnosis should be confirmed by KOH smears and/or cultures. Other pathogens commonly associated with vulvovaginitis (*Trichomonas* and *Haemophilus vaginalis* [*Gardnerella*]) should be ruled out by appropriate laboratory methods.
MONISTAT 7 is effective in both pregnant and non-pregnant women, as well as in women taking oral contraceptives. (See PRECAUTIONS.)

CONTRAINDICATIONS
Patients known to be hypersensitive to this drug.

PRECAUTIONS
General: Discontinue drug if sensitization or irritation is reported during use. Laboratory Tests: If there is a lack of response to MONISTAT 7, appropriate microbiological studies should be repeated to confirm the diagnosis and rule out other pathogens.
Pregnancy: Since MONISTAT is absorbed in small amounts from the human vagina, it should be used in the first trimester of pregnancy only when the physician considers it essential to the welfare of the patient.
Clinical studies, during which MONISTAT was used for 14 days, included 209 pregnant patients. Follow-up reports now available in 117 of these patients reveal no adverse effects or complications attributable to MONISTAT therapy in infants born to these women.

ADVERSE REACTIONS
During clinical studies with MONISTAT for a 14-day regimen, 39 of the 528 patients (7.4%) treated with MONISTAT reported complaints during therapy that were possibly drug-related. Most complaints were reported during the first week of therapy. Vulvovaginal burning, itching or irritation occurred in 6.6%, while other complaints such as vaginal burning, pelvic cramps, hives, skin rash and headache occurred rarely (each less than 0.2% patient incidence). The therapy-related dropout rate was 0.9%.

CLINICAL
Statistical analysis of randomized clinical trials, conducted to determine the shortest effective course of therapy with MONISTAT, demonstrates that a regimen of seven or more days has a cure rate equivalent to the 14-day regimen.
The graphic representation of this conclusion plots Days of Therapy versus Cure Rates. The solid line represents the mean therapeutic cure rate and the shaded area represents the 95% confidence interval.

DOSE RESPONSE CURVE

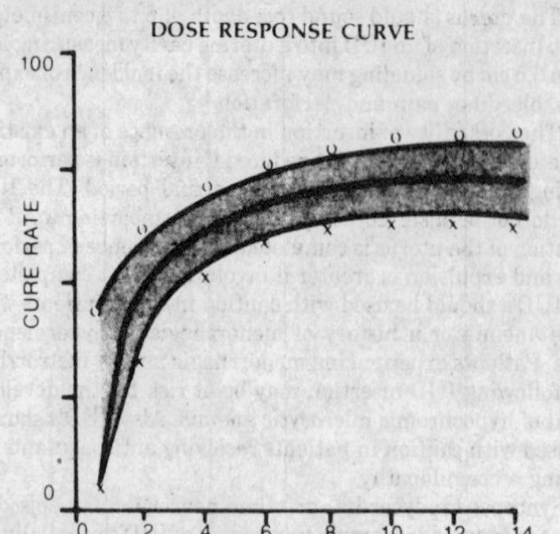

DOSAGE AND ADMINISTRATION
One applicatorful is administered intravaginally once daily at bedtime for seven days. Course of therapy may be repeated after other pathogens have been ruled out by appropriate smears and cultures.

HOW SUPPLIED
MONISTAT 7 Vaginal Cream is available in 1.59 oz. (45 g) tubes (NDC 0062-5431-07) with ORTHO® Measured-Dose Applicator.

Shown in Product Identification Section, page 419

MONISTAT® 3 ℞
(miconazole nitrate, 200 mg)
Vaginal Suppositories

DESCRIPTION
MONISTAT 3 Vaginal Suppositories are white to off-white suppositories, each containing the antifungal agent, miconazole nitrate, 1-[2,4-dichloro-β(2,4-dichlorobenzyloxy) phenethyl] imidazole nitrate, 200 mg, in a hydrogenated vegetable oil base. Miconazole nitrate for vaginal use is also available as MONISTAT 7 Vaginal Cream and MONISTAT 7 Vaginal Suppositories.

MICONAZOLE NITRATE

N
N
Cl
CH_2—CH—O—CH_2
Cl
Cl
Cl
$\cdot HNO_3$

CLINICAL PHARMACOLOGY
Miconazole nitrate exhibits fungicidal activity *in vitro* against species of the genus *Candida*. The pharmacologic mode of action is unknown. Following intravaginal administration of miconazole nitrate, small amounts are absorbed. Administration of a single dose of miconazole nitrate suppositories (100mg) to healthy subjects resulted in a total recovery from the urine and feces of 0.85% (±0.43%) of the administered dose.
Animal studies indicate that the drug crossed the placenta and doses above those used in humans result in embryo and feto-toxicity (80 mg/kg, orally), although this has not been reported in human subjects (See PRECAUTIONS).
In multi-center clinical trials in 440 women with vulvovaginal candidiasis, the efficacy of treatment with the MONISTAT 3 Vaginal Suppository for 3 days was compared with treatment for 7 days with MONISTAT 7 Vaginal Cream. The clinical cure rates (free of microbiological evidence and clinical signs and symptoms of candidiasis at 8–10 days and 30–35 days post-therapy) were numerically lower, although not statistically different, with the 3-Day Suppository when compared with the 7-Day Cream.

INDICATIONS AND USAGE
MONISTAT 3 Vaginal Suppositories are indicated for the local treatment of vulvovaginal candidiasis (moniliasis). Effectiveness in pregnancy and in diabetic patients has not been established. As MONISTAT is effective only for candidal vulvovaginitis, the diagnosis should be confirmed by KOH smear and/or cultures. Other pathogens commonly associated with vulvovaginitis (*Trichomonas* and *Haemophilus vaginalis* [*Gardnerella*]) should be ruled out by appropriate laboratory methods.

CONTRAINDICATIONS
Patients known to be hypersensitive to this drug.

PRECAUTIONS
General: Discontinue drug if sensitization or irritation is reported during use. The base contained in the suppository formulation may interact with certain latex products, such as that used in vaginal contraceptive diaphragms. Concurrent use is not recommended. MONISTAT 7 Vaginal Cream may be considered for use under these conditions.
Laboratory Tests: If there is a lack of response to MONISTAT 3 Vaginal Suppositories, appropriate microbiological studies (standard KOH smear and/or cultures) should be repeated to confirm the diagnosis and rule out other pathogens.
Carcinogenesis, Mutagenesis, Impairment of Fertility: Long-term animal studies to determine carcinogenic potential have not been performed.
Fertility (Reproduction): Oral administration of miconazole nitrate in rats has been reported to produce prolonged gestation. However, this effect was not observed in oral rabbit studies. In addition, signs of fetal and embryo toxicity were reported in rat and rabbit studies, and dystocia was reported in rat studies after oral doses at and above 80 mg per kg. Intravaginal administration did not produce these effects in rats.
Pregnancy: Since imidazoles are absorbed in small amounts from the human vagina, they should not be used in the first trimester of pregnancy unless the physician considers it essential to the welfare of the patient.
Clinical studies, during which miconazole nitrate vaginal cream and suppositories were used for up to 14 days, were reported to include 514 pregnant patients. Follow-up reports available in 471 of these patients reveal no adverse effects or complications attributable to miconazole nitrate therapy in infants born to these women.
Nursing Mothers: It is not known whether miconazole nitrate is excreted in human milk. Because many drugs are excreted in human milk, caution should be exercised when miconazole nitrate is administered to a nursing woman.

ADVERSE REACTIONS
During clinical studies with the MONISTAT 3 Vaginal Suppository (miconazole nitrate, 200 mg) 301 patients were treated. The incidence of vulvovaginal burning, itching or irritation was 2%. Complaints of cramping (2%) and headaches (1.3%) were also reported. Other complaints (hives, skin rash) occurred with less than a 0.5% incidence. The therapy-related dropout rate was 0.3%.

OVERDOSE
Overdose of miconazole nitrate in humans has not been reported to date. In mice, rats, guinea pigs and dogs, the oral LD 50 values were found to be 578.1, >640, 275.9 and >160 mg/kg, respectively.

DOSAGE AND ADMINISTRATION
MONISTAT 3 Vaginal Suppositories: One suppository (miconazole nitrate, 200 mg) is inserted intravaginally once daily at bedtime for three consecutive days. Before prescribing another course of therapy, the diagnosis should be reconfirmed by smears and/or cultures to rule out other pathogens.

HOW SUPPLIED
MONISTAT 3 Suppositories (miconazole nitrate, 200 mg) are available as 2.5 gm, elliptically shaped white to off-white suppositories in packages of three (NDC 0062-5437-01) with a vaginal applicator. Store at 59°–86° F (13–30° C).

Shown in Product Identification Section, page 419

MONISTAT® 7 Vaginal Suppositories ℞
(100 mg miconazole nitrate)

DESCRIPTION
MONISTAT 7 Vaginal Suppositories are white to off-white suppositories, each containing the antifungal agent, miconazole nitrate, 1-[2,4-dichloro-β-(2,4-dichloro-benzyloxy) phenethyl] imidazole nitrate, 100 mg, in a hydrogenated vegetable oil base. Miconazole nitrate for vaginal use is also available as MONISTAT 7 Vaginal Cream.
[See Chemical Formula at top of next page].

CLINICAL PHARMACOLOGY
Miconazole nitrate exhibits fungicidal activity *in vitro* against species of the genus *Candida*. The pharmacologic

mode of action is unknown. Following intravaginal administration of MONISTAT 7 Vaginal Suppositories or MONISTAT 7 Vaginal Cream, small amounts are absorbed. Administration of a single dose of MONISTAT 7 Vaginal Suppositories to healthy subjects resulted in a total recovery from the urine and feces of 0.85% (±0.43%) of the administered dose. For MONISTAT 7 Vaginal Cream the corresponding figure was 1.03% (±0.51%) of the administered dose.

Animal studies indicate that the drug crossed the placenta and doses above those used in humans result in embryo and feto-toxicity (80 mg/kg-orally) although this has not been reported in human subjects (see Precautions).

INDICATIONS AND USAGE

MONISTAT 7 Vaginal Suppositories are indicated for the local treatment of vulvovaginal candidiasis (moniliasis). Effectiveness in pregnancy has not been established. As MONISTAT 7 is effective only for candidal vulvovaginitis, the diagnosis should be confirmed by KOH smear and/or cultures. Other pathogens commonly associated with vulvovaginitis (*Trichomonas* and *Haemophilus vaginalis* [*Gardnerella*]) should be ruled out by appropriate laboratory methods.

Clinical: Statistical analyses of randomized clinical trials, conducted to determine the shortest effective course of therapy with miconazole nitrate vaginal cream and suppositories, demonstrate that a regimen of seven or more days had a cure rate equivalent to a 14-day regimen.

The graphic representation of this conclusion plots Days of Therapy versus Cure Rate for miconazole nitrate vaginal cream. (Results were similar with suppositories.) The solid line represents the mean therapeutic cure rate and the shaded area represents the 95% confidence interval.

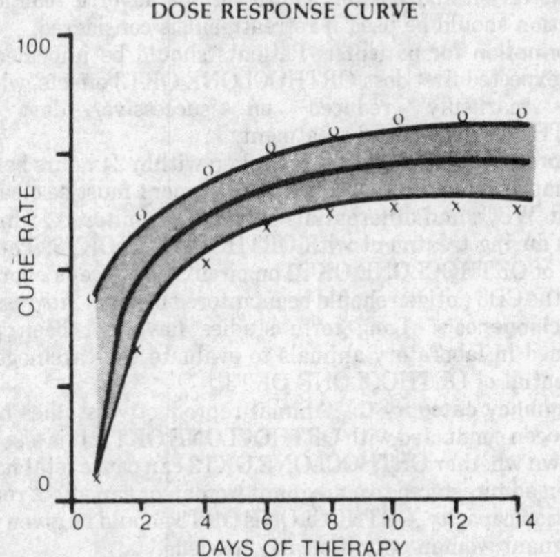

CONTRAINDICATIONS

Patients known to be hypersensitive to this drug.

PRECAUTIONS

General: Discontinue drug if sensitization or irritation is reported during use. The base contained in the suppository formulation may interact with certain latex products, such as that used in vaginal contraceptive diaphragms. Concurrent use is not recommended. MONISTAT 7 Vaginal Cream may be considered for use under these conditions.

Laboratory Tests: If there is a lack of response to MONISTAT 7, appropriate microbiological studies (standard KOH smear and/or cultures) should be repeated to confirm the diagnosis and rule out other pathogens.

Carcinogenesis, Mutagenesis, Impairment of Fertility: Long-term animal studies to determine carcinogenic potential have not been performed.

Fertility (reproduction): Oral administration of miconazole nitrate in rats has been reported to produce prolonged gestation. However, this effect was not observed in oral rabbit studies. In addition, signs of fetal and embryotoxicity were reported in rat and rabbit studies and dystocia in rat studies after oral doses at and above 80 mg per kg. Intravaginal administration did not produce these effects in rats.

Pregnancy: Since imidazoles are absorbed in small amounts from the human vagina, they should not be used in the first trimester of pregnancy unless the physician considers it essential to the welfare of the patient.

Clinical studies, during which miconazole nitrate vaginal cream and suppositories were used for up to 14 days, were reported to include 487 pregnant patients. Follow-up reports available on 446 of these patients reveal no adverse effects or complications attributable to miconazole nitrate therapy in infants born to these women.

Nursing Mothers: It is not known whether miconazole nitrate is excreted in human milk. Because many drugs are excreted in human milk, caution should be exercised when miconazole nitrate is administered to a nursing woman.

ADVERSE REACTIONS

During clinical studies with miconazole nitrate cream for a 14-day regimen, 39 of the 528 patients (7.4%) treated with miconazole nitrate cream reported complaints during therapy that were possibly drug-related. Most complaints were reported during the first week of therapy. Vulvovaginal burning, itching or irritation occurred in 6.6%, while other complaints such as vaginal burning, pelvic cramps, hives, skin rash and headache occurred rarely (each less than 0.2% patient incidence). The therapy-related dropout rate was 0.9%.

During clinical studies with regimens which varied from 1 to 14 days, 1,057 patients were treated with miconazole nitrate suppositories. The incidence of vulvovaginal burning, itching or irritation was 0.5%, while complaints of skin rash occurred at only a 0.2% incidence.

OVERDOSE

Overdosage of miconazole nitrate in humans has not been reported to date. In mice, rats, guinea pigs and dogs, the oral LD_{50} values were found to be 578.1, >640, 275.9 and >160 mg/kg, respectively.

DOSAGE AND ADMINISTRATION

MONISTAT 7 Vaginal Suppositories: One suppository (100 mg miconazole nitrate) is inserted intravaginally once daily at bedtime for seven days. Before prescribing another course of therapy, the diagnosis should be reconfirmed by smears and/or cultures to rule out other pathogens.

HOW SUPPLIED

MONISTAT 7 Vaginal Suppositories are available as 2.5g (100 mg miconazole nitrate) elliptically shaped white to off-white suppositories in packages of seven (NDC 0062-5432-01) with a vaginal applicator. Store at 59°-86°F (13°-30°C).

Shown in Product Identification Section, page 419

MONISTAT® Ɍ
(miconazole nitrate)
DUAL-PAK®

3 DAY SUPPOSITORY THERAPY
MONISTAT® 3
(miconazole nitrate, 200 mg)
Vaginal Suppositories

DESCRIPTION

MONISTAT 3 Vaginal Suppositories are water-miscible, white to off-white suppositories, each containing the antifungal agent, micronazole nitrate, 1-[2,4-dichloro-β(2,4-dichlorobenzyloxy) phenethyl] imidazole nitrate, 200 mg., in a hydrogenated vegetable oil base. Miconazole nitrate for vaginal use is also available as MONISTAT 7 Vaginal Cream and MONISTAT 7 Vaginal Suppositories.

MICONAZOLE NITRATE

CLINICAL PHARMACOLOGY

Miconazole nitrate exhibits fungicidal activity *in vitro* against species of the genus *Candida*. The pharmacologic mode of action is unknown. Following intravaginal administration of miconazole nitrate, small amounts are absorbed. Administration of a single dose of miconazole nitrate suppositories (100 mg) to healthy subjects resulted in a total recovery from the urine and feces of 0.85% (±0.43%) of the administered dose.

Animal studies indicate that the drug crossed the placenta and doses above those used in humans result in embryo and feto-toxicity (80 mg/kg, orally), although this has not been reported in human subjects (See PRECAUTIONS).

In multi-center clinical trials in 440 women with vulvovaginal candidiasis, the efficacy of treatment with the MONISTAT 3 Vaginal Suppository for 3 days was compared with treatment for 7 days with MONISTAT 7 Vaginal Cream. The clinical cure rates (free of microbiological evidence and clinical signs and symptoms of candidiasis at 8–10 days and 30–35 days post-therapy) were numerically lower, although not statistically different, with the 3-Day Suppository when compared with the 7-Day Cream.

INDICATIONS AND USAGE

MONISTAT 3 Vaginal Suppositories are indicated for the local treatment of vulvovaginal candidiasis (moniliasis). Effectiveness in pregnancy and in diabetic patients has not been established. As MONISTAT is effective only for candidal vulvovaginitis, the diagnosis should be confirmed by KOH smear and/or cultures. Other pathogens commonly associated with vulvovaginitis (*Trichomonas* and *Haemophilus vaginalis* [*Gardnerella*]) should be ruled out by appropriate laboratory methods.

CONTRAINDICATIONS

Patients known to be hypersensitive to this drug.

PRECAUTIONS

General: Discontinue drug if sensitization or irritation is reported during use. The base contained in the suppository formulation may interact with certain latex products, such as that used in vaginal contraceptive diaphragms. Concurrent use is not recommended. MONISTAT 7 Vaginal Cream may be considered for use under these conditions.

Laboratory Tests: If there is a lack of response to MONISTAT 3 Vaginal Suppositories, appropriate microbiological studies (standard KOH smear and/or cultures) should be repeated to confirm the diagnosis and rule out other pathogens.

Carcinogenesis, Mutagenesis, Impairment of Fertility: Long-term animal studies to determine carcinogenic potential have not been performed.

Fertility (Reproduction): Oral administration of miconazole nitrate in rats has been reported to produce prolonged gestation. However, this effect was not observed in oral rabbit studies. In addition, signs of fetal and embryo toxicity were reported in rat and rabbit studies, and dystocia was reported in rat studies after oral doses at and above 80 mg per kg. Intravaginal administration did not produce these effects in rats.

Pregnancy: Since imidazoles are absorbed in small amounts from the human vagina, they should not be used in the first trimester of pregnancy unless the physician considers it essential to the welfare of the patient.

Clinical studies, during which miconazole nitrate vaginal cream and suppositories were used for up to 14 days, were reported to include 514 pregnant patients. Follow-up reports available in 471 of these patients reveal no adverse effects or complications attributable to miconazole nitrate therapy in infants born to these women.

Nursing Mothers: It is not known whether miconazole nitrate is excreted in human milk. Because many drugs are excreted in human milk, caution should be exercised when miconazole nitrate is administered to a nursing woman.

ADVERSE REACTIONS

During clinical studies with the MONISTAT 3 Vaginal Suppository (miconazole nitrate, 200 mg) 301 patients were treated. The incidence of vulvo-vaginal burning, itching or irritation was 2%. Complaints of cramping (2%) and headaches (1.3%) were also reported. Other complaints (hives, skin rash) occurred with less than a 0.5% incidence. The therapy-related dropout rate was 0.3%.

OVERDOSE

Overdose of miconazole nitrate in humans has not been reported to date. In mice, rats, guinea pigs and dogs, the oral LD 50 values were found to be 578.1, >640, 275.9 and >160 mg/kg, respectively.

DOSAGE AND ADMINISTRATION

MONISTAT 3 Vaginal Suppositories: One suppository (miconazole nitrate, 200 mg) is inserted intravaginally once daily at bedtime for three consecutive days. Before prescribing another course of therapy, the diagnosis should be reconfirmed by smears and/or cultures to rule out other pathogens.

HOW SUPPLIED

MONISTAT 3 Suppositories (miconazole nitrate, 200 mg) are available as 2.5 gm, elliptically shaped white to off-white suppositories in packages of three (NDC 0062-5437-01) with a vaginal applicator. Store at 59–86°F (13–30°C).

14 DAY CREAM THERAPY
MONISTAT-DERM®
(miconazole nitrate 2%)
Cream and Lotion
For Topical Use Only

DESCRIPTION

MONISTAT-DERM (miconazole nitrate 2%) Cream and Lotion each contain miconazole nitrate* 2%, formulated into a water-miscible base consisting of pegoxol 7 stearate, peglicol 5 oleate, mineral oil, benzoic acid, butylated hydroxynisole and purified water.

Continued on next page

Ortho Pharm.—Cont.

ACTIONS

Miconazole nitrate is a synthetic antifungal agent which inhibits the growth of the common dermatophytes, *Trichophyton rubrum, Trichophyton mentagrophytes,* and *Epidermophyton floccosum,* the yeast-like fungus, *Candida albicans,* and the organism responsible for tinea versicolor *(Malessezia furfur).*

INDICATIONS

For topical application in the treatment of tinea pedis (athlete's foot), tinea cruris, and tinea corporis caused by *Trichophyton rubrum, Tichophyton mentagrophytes,* and *Epidermophyton floccosum,* in the treatment of cutaneous candidiasis (moniliasis), and in the treatment of tinea versicolor.

CONTRAINDICATIONS

MONISTAT-DERM (miconazole nitrate 2%) Cream and Lotion have no known contraindications.

PRECAUTIONS

If a reaction suggesting sensitivity or chemical irritation should occur, use of the medication should be discontinued. For external use only. Avoid introduction of MONISTAT-DERM Cream and Lotion into the eyes.

ADVERSE REACTIONS

There have been isolated reports of irritation, burning, maceration, and allergic contact dermatitis associated with the application of MONISTAT-DERM.

DOSAGE AND ADMINISTRATION

Sufficient MONISTAT-DERM Cream should be applied to cover affected areas twice daily (morning and evening) in patients with tinea pedis, tinea cruris, tinea corporis, and cutaneous candidiasis, and once daily in patients with tinea versicolor. It is preferable to use MONISTAT-DERM Lotion in intertriginous areas; if the cream is used, it should be applied sparingly and smoothed in well to avoid maceration effects.

Early relief of symptoms (2 to 3 days) is experienced by the majority of patients and clinical improvement may be seen fairly soon after treatment is begun; however, *Candida* infections and tinea cruris and corporis should be treated for two weeks and tinea pedis for one month in order to reduce the possibility of recurrence. If a patient shows no clinical improvement after a month of treatment, the diagnosis should be redetermined. Patients with tinea versicolor usually exhibit clinical and mycological clearing after two weeks of treatment.

HOW SUPPLIED

MONISTAT-DERM (miconazole nitrate 2%) Cream containing miconazole nitrate at 2% strength is supplied in 15 g., 1 oz. and 3 oz. tubes. MONISTAT-DERM (miconazole nitrate 2%) Lotion containing miconazole nitrate at 2% w/w strength is supplied in polyethylene squeeze bottles in quantities of 30 ml. and 60 ml.

*Chemical name: 1-[2,4-dichloro-β-{(2,4- dichlorobenzyl) oxy}phenethyl] imidazole mononitrate.

Shown in Product Identification Section, page 419

ORTHOCLONE OKT®3 Sterile Solution ℞

(muromonab-CD3)
For Intravenous Use Only

> **WARNING**
>
> Only physicians experienced in immunosuppressive therapy and management of renal transplant patients should use ORTHOCLONE OKT3 (muromonab-CD3).
> Patients receiving ORTHOCLONE OKT3 should be managed in facilities equipped and staffed for cardiopulmonary resuscitation.
> Severe pulmonary edema has occurred in patients with fluid overload prior to treatment with ORTHOCLONE OKT3.

DESCRIPTION

ORTHOCLONE OKT3 (muromonab-CD3) Sterile Solution is a murine nonoclonal antibody to the T3 (CD3) antigen of human T cells which functions as an immunosuppressant. It is for intravenous use only. The antibody is a biochemically purified IgG_{2a} immunoglobulin with a heavy chain of approximately 50,000 daltons and a light chain of approximately 25,000 daltons. It is directed to a glycoprotein with a molecular weight of 20,000 in the human T cell surface which is essential for T cell functions. Because it is a monoclonal antibody preparation, ORTHOCLONE OKT3 Sterile Solution is a homogeneous, reproducible antibody product with consistent, measurable reactivity to human T cells.

Each 5 ml ampule of ORTHOCLONE OKT3 Sterile Solution contains 5 mg (1 mg/ml) of muromonab-CD3 in a clear colorless solution which may contain a few fine translucent protein particles. Each ampule contains a buffered solution (pH 7.0 ±0.5) of monobasic sodium phosphate (2.25 mg), dibasic sodium phosphate (9.0 mg), sodium chloride (43 mg) and polysorbate 80 (1.0 mg) in water for injection.

The proper name, muromonab-CD3, is derived from the descriptive term murine monoclonal antibody. The CD3 designation identifies the specificity of the antibody as the Cell Differentiation (CD) cluster 3 defined by the First International Workshop on Human Leukocyte Differentiation Antigens.

CLINICAL PHARMACOLOGY

ORTHOCLONE OKT3 reverses graft rejection, most probably by blocking the function of all T cells which play a major role in acute renal rejection.

ORTHOCLONE OKT3 reacts with and blocks the function of a 20,000 dalton molecule (CD3) in the membrane of human T cells that has been associated *in vitro* with the antigen recognition structure of T cells and is essential for signal transduction. In *in vitro* cytolytic assays, ORTHOCLONE OKT3 blocks both the generation and function of effector cells. It is a potent mitogen *in vitro* in calf serum, but this mitogenicity is markedly reduced in human serum. ORTHOCLONE OKT3 thus blocks all known T cell functions.

In vivo, ORTHOCLONE OKT3 reacts with most peripheral blood T cells and T cells in body tissues, but has not been found to react with other hematopoietic elements or other tissues of the body.

In all patients studied, a rapid and concomitant decrease in the number of circulating CD3 positive, CD4 positive and CD8 positive T cells was observed within minutes after the administration of ORTHOCLONE OKT3. Between days two and seven increasing numbers of circulating CD4 positive and CD8 positive cells have been observed in patients although CD3 positive cells are not detectable. The presence of these CD4 and CD8 positive cells has not been found to affect the clinical course of the patient. CD3 positive cells reappear rapidly and reach pre-treatment levels within a week after termination of ORTHOCLONE OKT3 therapy. Increasing numbers of CD3 positive cells have been observed in some patients during the second week of ORTHOCLONE OKT3 therapy, possibly as a result of the development of neutralizing antibodies to ORTHOCLONE OKT3.

Antibodies to ORTHOCLONE OKT3 have been observed, occurring with an incidence of 21% (n=43) for IgM, 86% (n=43) for IgG and 29% (n=35) for IgE. The mean time of appearance of IgG antibodies was 20±2 (mean ±SD) days. Early IgG antibodies appeared towards the end of the second week of treatment in 3% (n=86) of the patients.

Serum levels of ORTHOCLONE OKT3 are measurable using an enzyme-linked immunosorbent assay (ELISA). During treatment with 5 mg per day for 14 days, mean serum trough levels of the drug rose over the first three days and then averaged 0.9 μg/ml on days 3 to 14. The levels obtained during therapy have been shown to block T cell effector functions *in vitro.*

INDICATIONS AND USAGE

ORTHOCLONE OKT3 is indicated for the treatment of acute allograft rejection in renal transplant patients.

In a controlled randomized clinical trial, ORTHOCLONE OKT3 was significantly more effective than conventional high dose steroid therapy in reversing acute renal allograft rejection. In this trial, 122 evaluable patients undergoing acute rejection of cadaveric renal transplants were treated either with ORTHOCLONE OKT3 daily for a mean of 14 days, with concomitant lowering of the dosage of azathioprine and maintenance steroids (62 patients), or with conventional high dose steroids (60 patients). ORTHOCLONE OKT3 reversed 94% of the rejections compared to a 75% reversal rate obtained with conventional high dose steroid treatment (p=0.006). The one year Kaplan-Meier (actuarial) estimates of graft survival rates for these patients who had acute rejection were 62% and 45% for ORTHOCLONE OKT3 and steroid treated patients, respectively (p=0.04). At two years the rates were 56% and 42%, respectively (p=0.06).

One- and two-year patient survivals were not significantly different between the two groups, being 85% and 75% for ORTHOCLONE OKT3 treated patients and 90% and 85% for steroid treated patients.

In additional open clinical trials, the observed rate of reversal of acute renal allograft rejection was 92% (n=126) for ORTHOCLONE OKT3 therapy. ORTHOCLONE OKT3 also was effective in reversing acute renal allograft rejections in 65% (n=225) of cases where steroids and lymphocyte immune globulin preparations were contraindicated or were not successful (rescue).

The dosage of other immunosuppressive agents used in conjunction with ORTHOCLONE OKT3 should be lowered to minimal levels (See DOSAGE AND ADMINISTRATION Section).

CONTRAINDICATIONS

ORTHOCLONE OKT3 should not be used in patients who are hypersensitive to this or any other product of murine origin nor in patients who are in fluid overload, as evidenced by chest x-ray or a greater than 3 percent weight gain within the week prior to planned ORTHOCLONE OKT3 administration.

WARNINGS

SEE BOXED WARNINGS

Immunosuppressive therapy can lead to increased susceptibility to infection. Further, lymphomas have been reported following immunosuppressive therapy, and data suggest that their occurrence is related to the intensity and duration of immunosuppression rather than the use of specific agents.

Significant fever, chills, dyspnea and malaise may occur ½ to 6 hours after the first dose of ORTHOCLONE OKT3. Therefore, the injection of the first dose should be performed in a facility where the patient can be closely monitored and which is equipped and staffed for cardio-pulmonary resuscitation. The most serious first-dose reaction—potentially fatal severe pulmonary edema—has occurred infrequently (4.7% of the initial 107 patients and 0.0% in the subsequent 311 patients treated with first-dose restrictions). In each case of severe pulmonary edema, fluid overload was present before treatment. Therefore, patients should be evaluated for fluid overload by chest x-ray or weight gain of greater than 3%. Weight should be brought to a value less than or equal to 3% above the minimum weight in the prior week before ORTHOCLONE OKT3 treatment is initiated. Reactions to the first dose may be minimized by using the recommended steroid regimen (See DOSAGE AND ADMINISTRATION Section).

This formulation of ORTHOCLONE OKT3 contains polysorbate 80 and must not be used for the *in vitro* treatment of bone marrow.

PRECAUTIONS

General

If the patient temperature exceeds 37.8°C (100°F), it should be lowered by antipyretics before ORTHOCLONE OKT3 administration.

Use a low protein-binding 0.2 or 0.22 micrometer (μm) filter to prepare the injections (See ADMINISTRATION INSTRUCTIONS).

ORTHOCLONE OKT3 is a heterologous protein and induces detectable antibodies in most patients. Only limited data are available regarding retreatment with ORTHOCLONE OKT3. The presence of antibodies to ORTHOCLONE OKT3 could limit its efficacy following readministration and possibly cause serious adverse reactions. Caution should be used if retreatment is considered.

Information for patients: Patients should be informed of the expected first dose ORTHOCLONE OKT3 effects, which are markedly reduced on successive days of ORTHOCLONE OKT3 treatment.

Laboratory tests: Chest x-ray taken within 24 hours before initiating ORTHOCLONE OKT3 treatment must be clear of fluid. WBCs and differentials should be monitored at intervals during treatment with ORTHOCLONE OKT3. The effect of ORTHOCLONE OKT3 on circulating T cells expressing the CD3 antigen should be monitored by an *in vitro* assay.

Carcinogenesis: Long term studies have not been performed in laboratory animals to evaluate the carcinogenic potential of ORTHOCLONE OKT3.

Pregnancy category C: Animal reproductive studies have not been conducted with ORTHOCLONE OKT3. It is also not known whether ORTHOCLONE OKT3 can cause fetal harm when administered to a pregnant woman or can affect reproduction capacity. ORTHOCLONE OKT3 should be given to a pregnant woman only if clearly needed.

Pediatric use: Safety and effectiveness in children have not been established. Although no adequate controlled studies have been conducted in children, patients as young as two years of age have received ORTHOCLONE OKT3 with no unexpected adverse effects.

ADVERSE REACTIONS

Determinations of adverse experiences with ORTHOCLONE OKT3 have been primarily documented in clinical trials of renal rejection following cadaveric transplantation. These patients were simultaneously receiving low-dose immunosuppressive therapy, primarily azathioprine and corticosteroids.

Compared to conventional treatment, patients treated with ORTHOCLONE OKT3 experienced increased adverse reactions during the first two days of treatment. During this period the majority of patients experienced pyrexia (73%) of which 2% were 40.0°C (104°F) or above, and chills (57%). In addition, other adverse experiences occurring in more than 8% of the patients during the first two days of ORTHOCLONE OKT3 therapy included dyspnea (21%), chest pain (14%), vomiting (13%, wheezing (11%), nausea (11%), diarrhea (10%), and tremor (10%). Similar adverse effects were observed in the additional open clinical studies.

Potentially fatal severe pulmonary edema was reported following the first dose in less than 2% of the cases and was always associated with fluid overload. It is therefore essential that patients receiving ORTHOCLONE OKT3 not be in fluid overload and remain under close medical supervision

for 48 hours after the first dose administration. The first dose should be administered as detailed in the DOSAGE AND ADMINISTRATION Section.
In the ORTHOCLONE OKT3 treated patients in the randomized controlled trial, the most common infections observed in the first 45 days following start of ORTHOCLONE OKT3 therapy were due to cytomegalovirus (19%) and Herpes simplex (27%). Other severe and life-threatening infections seen in these patients during this period were *Staphylococcus epidermidis* (4.8%), *Pneumocystis carinii* (3.1%), Legionella (1.6%), Cryptococcus (1.6%), Serratia (1.6%) and gram-negative bacteria (1.6%). The incidence of infections was not statistically different with ORTHOCLONE OKT3 than with high dose steroids.
Additional clinically significant adverse reactions were observed whose causal relationship to ORTHOCLONE OKT3 therapy is unclear. They were anaphylaxis (1 patient), serum sickness (2 patients) and lymphoma (2 patients).
A monoclonal B-lymphoproliferative disorder, similar to Epstein-Barr virus (EBV) associated B-lymphoproliferation, occurred in one of 22 bone marrow transplantation patients treated for graft-versus-host disease with ORTHOCLONE OKT3. This patient also received treatment with corticosteroids, cyclosporine, methotrexate and anti-thymocyte globulin. One patient with acute renal rejection was diagnosed as having generalized lymphoma three weeks after receiving three days of ORTHOCLONE OKT3. This patient also received treatment with high dose steroids, cyclosporine, antithymocyte globulin and azathioprine. Long term risk for increased incidence of lymphoma or other malignancies has not been determined.

OVERDOSAGE
The maximum amount of ORTHOCLONE OKT3 that can safely be administered in single or multiple doses has not been determined.

DOSAGE AND ADMINISTRATION
The recommended dose of ORTHOCLONE OKT3 for the treatment of acute renal allograft rejection is 5 mg per day for 10 to 14 days. Treatment should begin once acute renal rejection is diagnosed.
Patients should be monitored closely for 48 hours after the first dose is administered. Intravenous methylprednisolone sodium succinate 1.0 mg/kg given prior to ORTHOCLONE OKT3 administration and intravenous hydrocortisone sodium succinate 100 mg given 30 minutes after ORTHOCLONE OKT3 administration is strongly recommended to decrease the incidence of reactions to the first dose. Acetaminophen and antihistamines can be given concomitantly with ORTHOCLONE OKT3 to reduce early reactions. Patient temperature should not exceed 37.8°C (100°F) at the time of first ORTHOCLONE OKT3 administration (See TABLE I).
Conventional concomitant immunosuppressive therapy should be lowered during ORTHOCLONE OKT3 administration to a daily dose of prednisone 0.5 mg/kg and azathioprine 25 mg. Preliminary studies suggest that during ORTHOCLONE OKT3 treatment the use of cyclosporine should be reduced or discontinued. Maintenance immunosuppression should be resumed approximately three days prior to cessation of ORTHOCLONE OKT3 therapy.

TABLE I
Suggested Prevention And Treatment Of ORTHOCLONE OKT3 First Dose Effects

Adverse Reaction	Effective Prevention or Palliation	Supportive Treatment
1. Severe pulmonary edema	• Clear chest x-ray within 24 hrs. preinjection	• Prompt intubation and oxygenation
	• Weight restriction to ≤3% gain over 7 days pre-injection	• 24 hr. close observation
2. Fever, chills	• 1.0 mg/kg methyl-prednisolone sodium succinate preinjection	• Cooling blanket
	• Fever reduction below 37.8°C (100°F) preinjection	• Acetaminophen p.r.n.
3. Respiratory Effects	• 100 mg hydrocortisone sodium succinate 30 min. post-injection	• Additional 100 mg hydrocortisone sodium succinate p.r.n.

ADMINISTRATION INSTRUCTIONS
1. Parenteral drug products should be inspected visually for particulate matter and discoloration prior to administration. Because ORTHOCLONE OKT3 is a protein solution, it may develop a few fine translucent particles which have been shown not to affect its potency.
2. Prepare ORTHOCLONE OKT3 for injection by drawing solution into a syringe through a low protein-binding 0.2 or 0.22 micrometer (μm) filter. Discard filter and attach needle for IV bolus injection.
3. Administer ORTHOCLONE OKT3 as an IV bolus in less than one minute. Do not administer by intravenous infusion or in conjunction with other drug solutions.

HOW SUPPLIED
ORTHOCLONE OKT3 is supplied as a sterile solution in packages of 5 ampules (NDC 0062-7102-01). Each 5 ml ampule contains 5 mg of muromonab-CD3.
Storage: Store in a refrigerator at 2 to 8°C (36 to 46°F).
DO NOT FREEZE OR SHAKE.

REFERENCES

1. Kung, P.C., Goldstein, G., Reinherz, E.L. and Schlossman, S.F. (1979), "Monoclonal Antibodies Defining Distinctive Human T Cell Surface Antigens". Science *206*: 347–349.
2. ORTHO Multicenter Transplant Study Group (1985), "A Randomized Clinical Trial of OKT3 Monoclonal Antibody for Acute Rejection of Cadaveric Renal Transplants". New England Journal of Medicine. *313*: 337–342.
3. Nomenclature Subcommittee, (1984), "Differentiation Human Leukocyte Antigens: A Proposed Nomenclature". Immunology Today *5*, No. 6.: 158–159.

ORTHO PHARMACEUTICAL CORPORATION
Immunobiology Division
Raritan, New Jersey 08869, USA
 Issued June 1986

ORTHO-CREME® Contraceptive Cream

(See PDR For Nonprescription Drugs)

ORTHO™ DIAPHRAGM KITS

DESCRIPTION
ORTHO Diaphragm Kits include three different types in a variety of sizes.
1. The ALL-FLEX* Arcing Spring Diaphragm is a molded, buff-colored, latex vaginal diaphragm containing a distortion-free, dual spring-within-a-spring which provides unique arcing action no matter where the rim is compressed. It is ideal not only where ordinary diaphragms are indicated, but also in patients with mild cystocele, rectocele or retroversion.
2. The ORTHO* Coil Spring Diaphragm is a molded latex vaginal diaphragm. The rim encases a tension-adjusted, cadmium-plated coil spring.
3. The ORTHO-WHITE* Flat Spring Diaphragm is a molded, pure white, latex vaginal diaphragm containing a flat, watch-type spring which allows compressibility in one plane only, thus facilitating insertion.

ORTHO Diaphragms are used in conjunction with spermicides, e.g., GYNOL II* Contraceptive Jelly, ORTHO-GYNOL* Contraceptive Jelly or ORTHO-CREME* Contraceptive Cream in conception control.

ACTION
These diaphragms when properly fitted serve two purposes:
a. To stop the sperm from entering the cervical canal;
b. To hold the spermicide.

INDICATIONS
ORTHO Diaphragms, in conjunction with an appropriate spermicide, are indicated for the prevention of pregnancy in women who elect to use diaphragms as a method of contraception.

PRECAUTIONS
Although an association has not been established between diaphragm use and toxic shock syndrome (TSS), symptoms of this condition have been reported in a few women using diaphragms. In most of these cases, the women wore a diaphragm continuously for more than 24 hours. Therefore, continuous wearing of the diaphragm for more than 24 hours is not recommended.
Primary symptoms of TSS are sudden high fever (usually 102°F or more) and vomiting, diarrhea, fainting or near fainting when standing up, dizziness or a rash that looks like a sunburn. There may also be other signs of TSS, such as aching of muscles and joints, redness of the eyes, sore throat and weakness. The patient should be instructed that if she has sudden high fever and one or more of the other symptoms, she should remove her diaphragm and consult her physician immediately.

INSTRUCTIONS
1. Proper placement of the diaphragm is vital for effectiveness.
2. To be fully effective the diaphragm should never be used without contraceptive cream or jelly. This contraceptive cream or jelly must be spread around the inner surface of the diaphragm as well as around the rim.
3. The diaphragm may be inserted up to six hours before intercourse. If more than six hours has elapsed between insertion of the diaphragm and intercourse, additional contraceptive jelly or cream must be applied. The diaphragm should not be removed to apply this additional cream or jelly.
4. The diaphragm should not be removed nor should the patient douche for six to eight hours after intercourse. The diaphragm should not remain in position for more than 24 hours.

HOW SUPPLIED
All ORTHO Diaphragm Kits are available individually and contain a sample tube of GYNOL II Contraceptive Jelly. Each diaphragm is contained in an attractive plastic compact.
1. The ALL-FLEX Arcing Spring Diaphragm is available in sizes 55mm through 95mm in 5mm increments.
2. The ORTHO Coil Spring Diaphragm is available in sizes 50mm through 105mm in 5mm increments.
3. The ORTHO-WHITE Flat Spring Diaphragm is available in sizes 55mm through 95mm in 5mm increments.

*Trademark

ORTHO® Dienestrol Cream ℞

1. ESTROGENS HAVE BEEN REPORTED TO INCREASE THE RISK OF ENDOMETRIAL CARCINOMA.
Three independent case control studies have shown an increased risk of endometrial cancer in postmenopausal women exposed to exogenous estrogens for prolonged periods.[1–3] This risk was independent of the other known risk factors for endometrial cancer. These studies are further supported by the finding that incidence rates of endometrial cancer have increased sharply since 1969 in eight different areas of the United States with population-based cancer reporting systems, an increase which may be related to the rapidly expanding use of estrogens during the last decade.[4]
The three case control studies reported that the risk of endometrial cancer in estrogen users was about 4.5 to 13.9 times greater than in nonusers. The risk appears to depend on both duration of treatment[1] and on estrogen dose.[3] In view of these findings, when estrogens are used for the treatment of menopausal symptoms, the lowest dose that will control symptoms should be utilized and medication should be discontinued as soon as possible. When prolonged treatment is medically indicated, the patient should be reassessed on at least a semiannual basis to determine the need for continued therapy. Although the evidence must be considered preliminary, one study suggests that cyclic administration of low doses of estrogen may carry less risk than continuous administration;[3] it therefore appears prudent to utilize such a regimen.
Close clinical surveillance of all women taking estrogens is important. In all cases of undiagnosed persistent or recurring abnormal vaginal bleeding, adequate diagnostic measures should be undertaken to rule out malignancy.
There is no evidence at present that "natural" estrogens are more or less hazardous than "synthetic" estrogens at equiestrogenic doses.
2. ESTROGENS SHOULD NOT BE USED DURING PREGNANCY
The use of female sex hormones, both estrogens and progestogens, during early pregnancy may seriously damage the offspring. It has been shown that females exposed *in utero* to diethylstilbestrol, a non-steroidal estrogen, have an increased risk of developing in later life a form of vaginal or cervical cancer that ordinarily is extremely rare.[5,6] This risk has been estimated as not greater than 4 per 1000 exposures.[7] Furthermore, a high percentage of such exposed women (from 30 to 90 percent) have been found to have vaginal adenosis,[8,13] epithelial changes of the vagina and cervix. Although these changes are histologically benign, it is not known whether they are precursors of malignancy. Although similar data are not available with the use of other estrogens, it cannot be presumed they would not induce similar changes.
Several reports suggest an association between intrauterine exposure to female sex hormones and congenital anomalies, including congenital heart defects and limb reduction defects.[13–16] One case control study[16] estimated a 4.7 fold increased risk of limb reduction defects in infants exposed in utero to sex hormones (oral contraceptives, hormone withdrawal tests for pregnancy, or attempted treatment for threatened abortion). Some of these exposures were very short and involved only a few days of treatment. The data suggest

Continued on next page

Ortho Pharm.—Cont.

that the risk of limb reduction defects in exposed fetuses is somewhat less than 1 per 1000.
In the past, female sex hormones have been used during pregnancy in an attempt to treat threatened or habitual abortion. There is considerable evidence that estrogens are ineffective for these indications, and there is no evidence from well controlled studies that progestogens are effective for these uses.
If ORTHO Dienestrol Cream is used during pregnancy, or if the patient becomes pregnant while using this drug, she should be apprised of the potential risks to the fetus, and the advisability of pregnancy continuation.

DESCRIPTION

ORTHO Dienestrol Cream
Cream for Intravaginal use only
Active ingredient: Dienestrol 0.01%.
Dienestrol is a synthetic, non-steroidal estrogen. It is compounded in a cream base suitable for intravaginal use only. The cream base is composed of glyceryl monostearate, peanut oil, glycerin, benzoic acid, glutamic acid, butylated hydroxyanisole, citric acid, sodium hydroxide and water. The pH is approximately 4.3.

CLINICAL PHARMACOLOGY

Systemic absorption and mode of action are undetermined.

INDICATIONS AND USAGE

ORTHO Dienestrol Cream is indicated in the treatment of atrophic vaginitis and kraurosis vulvae.
ORTHO DIENESTROL CREAM HAS NOT BEEN SHOWN TO BE EFFECTIVE FOR ANY PURPOSE DURING PREGNANCY AND ITS USE MAY CAUSE SEVERE HARM TO THE FETUS (*SEE* BOXED WARNING).
The lowest effective dose appropriate for the specific indication should be utilized. Studies of the addition of a progestin for seven or more days of a cycle of estrogen administration have reported a lowered incidence of endometrial hyperplasia. Morphological and biochemical studies of endometrium suggest that 10 to 13 days of progestin are needed to provide maximal maturation of the endometrium and to eliminate any hyperplastic changes. Whether this will provide protection from endometrial carcinoma has not been clearly established. There are possible additional risks which may be associated with the inclusion of progestin in estrogen replacement regimens. The potential risks include adverse effects on carbohydrate and lipid metabolism. The choice of progestin and dosage may be important in minimizing these adverse effects.

CONTRAINDICATIONS

Estrogens may cause fetal harm when administered to a pregnant woman (see Boxed Warning). Estrogens are contraindicated in women who are or may become pregnant. If this drug is used during pregnancy, or if the patient becomes pregnant while using this drug, the patient should be apprised of the potential hazard to the fetus.
Estrogens should also not be used in women with any of the following conditions:
1. Known or suspected cancer of the breast.
2. Known or suspected estrogen-dependent neoplasia.
3. Undiagnosed abnormal genital bleeding.
4. Active thrombophlebitis or thromboembolic disorders.
5. A past history of thrombophlebitis, thrombosis, or thromboembolic disorders associated with previous estrogen use.

WARNINGS

1. *Induction of malignant neoplasms.* Long-term continuous administration of natural and synthetic estrogens in certain animal species increases the frequency of carcinomas of the breast, cervix, vagina, and liver. There is now evidence that estrogens increase the risk of carcinoma of the endometrium in humans. (*See* Boxed Warning.)
At the present time there is no satisfactory evidence that estrogens given to postmenopausal women increase the risk of cancer of the breast,[18] although a recent long-term followup of a single physician's practice has raised this possibility.[18a] Because of the animal data, there is a need for caution in prescribing estrogens for women with a strong family history of breast cancer or who have breast nodules, fibrocystic disease, or abnormal mammograms.
2. *Gall bladder disease.* A recent study has reported a 2 to 3-fold increase in the risk of surgically confirmed gall bladder disease in women receiving postmenopausal estrogens,[18] similar to the 2-fold increase previously noted in users of oral contraceptives.[19,24] In the case of oral contraceptives the increased risk appeared after two years of use.[24]
3. *Effects similar to those caused by estrogen-progestogen oral contraceptives.* There are several serious adverse effects of oral contraceptives, most of which have not, up to now, been documented as consequences of postmenopausal estrogen therapy. This may reflect the comparatively low doses of estrogen used in postmenopausal women. It would be expected that the larger doses of estrogen used to treat prostatic or breast cancer or postpartum breast engorgement are more likely to result in these adverse effects, and, in fact, it has been shown that there is an increased risk of thrombosis in men receiving estrogens for prostatic cancer and women for postpartum breast engorgement.[20-23]
a. *Thromboembolic disease.* It is now well established that users of oral contraceptives have an increased risk of various thromboembolic and thrombotic vascular diseases, such as thrombophlebitis, pulmonary embolism, stroke, and myocardial infarction.[24-31] Cases of retinal thrombosis, mesenteric thrombosis, and optic neuritis have been reported in oral contraceptive users. There is evidence that the risk of several of these adverse reactions is related to the dose of the drug.[32,33] An increased risk of postsurgery thromboembolic complications has also been reported in users of oral contraceptives.[34,35] If feasible, estrogen should be discontinued at least 4 weeks before surgery of the type associated with an increased risk of thromboembolism, or during periods of prolonged immobilization.
While an increased risk of thromboembolic and thrombotic disease in postmenopausal users of estrogens has not been found,[18,36] this does not rule out the possibility that such an increase may be present or that subgroups of women who have underlying risk factors or who are receiving relatively large doses of estrogens may have increased risk. Therefore estrogens should not be used in persons with active thrombophlebitis or thromboembolic disorders, and they should not be used (except in treatment of malignancy) in persons with a history of such disorders in association with estrogen use. They should be used with caution in patients with cerebral vascular or coronary artery disease and only for those in whom estrogens are clearly needed.
Large doses of estrogen (5 mg conjugated estrogens per day), comparable to those used to treat cancer of the prostate and breast, have been shown in a large prospective clinical trial in men to increase the risk of nonfatal myocardial infarction, pulmonary embolism and thrombophlebitis. When estrogen doses of this size are used, any of the thromboembolic and thrombotic adverse effects associated with oral contraceptive use should be considered a clear risk.
b. *Hepatic adenoma.* Benign hepatic adenomas appear to be associated with the use of oral contraceptives.[38-40] Although benign, and rare, these may rupture and may cause death through intra-abdominal hemorrhage. Such lesions have not yet been reported in association with other estrogen or progestogen preparations but should be considered in estrogen users having abdominal pain and tenderness, abdominal mass, or hypovolemic shock. Hepatocellular carcinoma has also been reported in women taking estrogen-containing oral contraceptives.[39] The relationship of this malignancy to these drugs is not known at this time.
c. *Elevated blood pressure.* Increased blood pressure is not uncommon in women using oral contraceptives. There is now a report that this may occur with use of estrogens during menopause.[41] Blood pressure should be monitored with estrogen use, especially if high doses are used.
d. *Glucose tolerance.* A worsening of glucose tolerance has been observed in a significant percentage of patients on estrogen-containing oral contraceptives. For this reason, diabetic patients should be carefully observed while receiving estrogen.
4. *Hypercalcemia.* Administration of estrogens may lead to severe hypercalcemia in patients with breast cancer and bone metastases. If this occurs, the drug should be stopped and appropriate measures taken to reduce the serum calcium level.

PRECAUTIONS

A. General
1. A complete medical and family history should be taken prior to the initiation of any estrogen therapy. The pretreatment and periodic physical examinations should include special reference to blood pressure, breasts, abdomen, and pelvic organs, and should include a Papanicolaou smear. As a general rule, estrogen should not be prescribed for longer than one year without another physical examination being performed.
2. Fluid retention—Because estrogens may cause some degree of fluid retention, conditions which might be influenced by this factor such as epilepsy, migraine, and cardiac or renal dysfunction, require careful observation.
3. Certain patients may develop undesirable manifestations of excessive estrogenic stimulation, such as abnormal or excessive uterine bleeding, mastodynia, etc.
4. Oral contraceptives appear to be associated with an increased incidence of mental depression.[24] Although it is not clear whether this is due to the estrogenic or progestogenic component of the contraceptive, patients with a history of depression should be carefully observed.
5. Preexisting uterine leiomyomata may increase in size during estrogen use.
6. The pathologist should be advised of estrogen therapy when relevant specimens are submitted.
7. Patients with a past history of jaundice during pregnancy have an increased risk of recurrence of jaundice while receiving estrogen-containing oral contraceptive therapy. If jaundice develops in any patient receiving estrogen, the medication should be discontinued while the cause is investigated.
8. Estrogens may be poorly metabolized in patients with impaired liver function and they should be administered with caution in such patients.
9. Because estrogens influence the metabolism of calcium and phosphorus, they should be used with caution in patients with metabolic bone diseases that are associated with hypercalcemia or in patients with renal insufficiency.
10. Because of the effects of estrogens on epiphyseal closure, they should be used judiciously in young patients in whom bone growth is not complete.
B. Information for Patients: See text of Patient Package Information which is reproduced below.
C. Drug/Laboratory Test Interactions
Certain endocrine and liver function tests may be affected by estrogen-containing oral contraceptives. The following similar changes may be expected with larger doses of estrogen:
1. Increased sulfobromophthalein retention.
2. Increased prothrombin and factors VII, VIII, IX and X; decreased antithrombin 3; increased norepinephrine-induced platelet aggregability.
3. Increased thyroid-binding globulin (TBG) leading to increased circulating total thyroid hormone, as measured by PBI, T4 by column, or T4 by radioimmunoassay. Free T3 resin uptake is decreased, reflecting the elevated TBG; free T4 concentration is unaltered.
4. Impaired glucose tolerance.
5. Decreased pregnanediol excretion.
6. Reduced response to metyrapone test.
7. Reduced serum folate concentration.
8. Increased serum triglyceride and phospholipid concentration.
D. Carcinogenesis, Mutagenesis, Impairment of Fertility: See "Warnings" section for information on carcinogenesis, mutagenesis and impairment of fertility.
E. Pregnancy:
Teratogenic Effects.
Pregnancy Category X.
See "Contraindications" section.
F. Nursing Mothers: It is not known whether this drug is excreted in human milk. Because many drugs are excreted in human milk, caution should be exercised when estrogens are administered to a nursing woman.

ADVERSE REACTIONS

(*See* Warnings regarding induction of neoplasia, adverse effects on the fetus, increased incidence of gall bladder disease, and adverse effects similar to those of oral contraceptives, including thromboembolism.) The following additional adverse reactions have been reported with estrogenic therapy, including oral contraceptives:
1. *Genitourinary system.*
Increase in size of uterine fibromyomata.
Vaginal candidiasis.
Breakthrough bleeding, spotting, change in menstrual flow.
Dysmenorrhea.
Premenstrual-like syndrome.
Amenorrhea during and after treatment.
Change in cervical eversion and in degree of cervical secretion.
Cystitis-like syndrome.
2. *Breasts.*
Tenderness, enlargement, secretion.
3. *Gastrointestinal.*
Cholestatic jaundice.
Nausea, vomiting.
Abdominal cramps, bloating.
4. *Skin.*
Erythema multiforme.
Erythema nodosum.
Hemorrhagic eruption.
Loss of scalp hair.
Hirsutism.
Chloasma or melasma which may persist when drug is discontinued.
5. *Eyes.*
Steepening of corneal curvature.
Intolerance to contact lenses.
6. *CNS.*
Mental depression.
Headache, migraine, dizziness.
Chorea.
7. *Miscellaneous.*
Reduced carbohydrate tolerance.
Aggravation of porphyria.
Edema.
Changes in libido.
Increase or decrease in weight.

OVERDOSAGE

Numerous reports of ingestion of large doses of estrogen-containing oral contraceptives by young children indicate that serious ill effects do not occur. Overdosage of estrogen may cause nausea, and withdrawal bleeding may occur in females.

DOSAGE AND ADMINISTRATION

Given cyclically for short term use only:

For treatment of atrophic vaginitis, or kraurosis vulvae associated with the menopause.

The lowest dose that will control symptoms should be chosen and medication should be discontinued as promptly as possible.

Attempts to discontinue or taper medication should be made at 3 to 6 month intervals.

The usual dosage range is one or two applicatorsful per day for one or two weeks, then gradually reduced to one half initial dosage for a similar period. A maintenance dosage of one applicatorful, one to three times a week, may be used after restoration of the vaginal mucosa has been achieved.

Treated patients with an intact uterus should be monitored closely for signs of endometrial cancer and appropriate diagnostic measures should be taken to rule out malignancy in the event of persistent or recurring abnormal vaginal bleeding.

SUPPLIED

Available in 2.75 oz. (78g) tubes with or without ORTHO® Measured-Dose Applicator.

With applicator: NDC 0062-5450-77

Without applicator: NDC 0062-5450-00

Store at controlled room temperature.

1. Ziel, H.K. and W.D. Finkle, "Increased Risk of Endometrial Carcinoma Among Users of Conjugated Estrogens," *New England Journal of Medicine,* 293:1167–1170, 1975.

2. Smith, D.C., R. Prentic, D.J. Thompson, and W.L. Hermann, "Association of Exogenous Estrogen and Endometrial Carcinoma," *New England Journal of Medicine,* 293:1164–1167, 1975.

3. Mack, T.M., M.C. Pike, B.E. Henderson, R.I. Pfeffer, V.R. Gerkins, M. Arthur, and S.E. Brown, "Estrogens and Endometrial Cancer in a Retirement Community," *New England Journal of Medicine,* 294:1267–1287, 1976.

4. Weiss, N.S., D.R. Szekely and D.F. Austin, "Increasing Incidence of Endometrial Cancer in the United States," *New England Journal of Medicine,* 294:1259–1262, 1976.

5. Herbst, A.L., H. Ulfelder and D.C. Poskanzer, "Adenocarcinoma of Vagina," *New England Journal of Medicine,* 284:878–881, 1971.

6. Greenwald, P., J. Barlow, P. Nasca, and W. Burnett, "Vaginal Cancer after Maternal Treatment with Synthetic Estrogens," *New England Journal of Medicine,* 285:390–392, 1971.

7. Lanier, A., K. Noller, D. Decker, L. Elveback, and L. Kurland, "Cancer and Stilbestrol. A Follow-up of 1719 Persons Exposed to Estrogens in Utero and Born 1943–1959," *Mayo Clinic Proceedings,* 48:793–799, 1973.

8. Herbst, A., R. Kurman, and R. Scully, "Vaginal and Cervical Abnormalities After Exposure to Stilbestrol In Utero," *Obstetrics and Gynecology,* 40:287–298, 1972.

9. Herbst, A., S. Robboy, G. Macdonald, and R. Scully, "The Effects of Local Progesterone on Stilbestrol-Associated Vaginal Adenosis," *American Journal of Obstetrics and Gynecology* 118:607–615, 1974.

10. Herbst, A., D. Poskanzer, S. Robboy, L. Friedlander, and R. Scully, "Prenatal Exposure to Stilbestrol, A Prospective Comparison of Exposed Female Offspring with Unexposed Controls," *New England Journal of Medicine,* 292:334–339, 1975.

11. Staffi, A., R. Mattingly, D. Foley, and W. Fetherston, "Clinical Diagnosis of Vaginal Adenosis," *Obstetrics and Gynecology,* 43:118–128, 1974.

12. Sherman, A.I., M. Goldrath, A. Berlin, V. Vakhariya, F. Banooni, W. Michaels, P. Goodman, S. Brown, "Cervical-Vaginal Adenosis After *In Utero* Exposure to Synthetic Estrogens," *Obstetrics and Gynecology,* 44:531–545, 1974.

13. Gal, I., B. Kirman, and J. Stern, "Hormone Pregnancy Tests and Congenital Malformation," *Nature,* 216:83, 1967.

14. Levy, E.P., A. Cohen, and F.C. Fraser, "Hormone Treatment During Pregnancy and Congenital Heart Defects," *Lancet,* 1:611, 1973.

15. Nora, J. and A. Nora, "Birth Defects and Oral Contraceptives," *Lancet,* 1:941–942, 1973.

16. Janerich, D.T., J.M. Piper, and D.M. Glebatis, "Oral Contraceptives and Congenital Limb-Reduction Defects," *New England Journal of Medicine,* 291:697–700, 1974.

17. "Estrogens for Oral or Parenteral Use," *Federal Register,* 40:8212, 1975.

18. Boston Collaborative Drug Surveillance Program, "Surgically Confirmed Gall Bladder Disease, Venous Thromboembolism and Breast Tumors in Relation to Post-Menopausal Estrogen Therapy," *New England Journal of Medicine,* 290:15–19, 1974.

18a. Hoover, R., L.A. Gray, Sr., P. Cole, and B. MacMahon, "Menopausal Estrogens and Breast Cancer," *New England Journal of Medicine,* 295:401–405, 1976.

19. Boston Collaborative Drug Surveillance Program, "Oral Contraceptives and Venous Thromboembolic Disease, Surgically Confirmed Gall Bladder Disease, and Breast Tumors," *Lancet* 1:1399–1404, 1973.

20. Daniel, D.G., H. Campbell, and A.C. Turnbull, "Puerperal Thromboembolism and Suppression of Lactation," *Lancet,* 2:287–289, 1967.

21. The Veterans Administration Cooperative Urological Research Group, "Carcinoma of the Prostate: Treatment Comparisons," *Journal of Urology,* 98:516–522, 1967.

22. Bailer, J.C., "Thromboembolism and Oestrogen Therapy," *Lancet,* 2:560, 1967.

23. Blackard, C., R. Doe, G. Mellinger, and D. Byar, "Incidence of Cardiovascular Disease and Death In Patients Receiving Diethylstilbestrol for Carcinoma of the Prostate," *Cancer,* 26:249–256, 1970.

24. Royal College of General Practitioners, "Oral Contraception and Thromboembolic Disease," *Journal of the Royal College of General Practitioners,* 13:267–279, 1967.

25. Inman, W.H.W. and M.P. Vessey, "Investigation of Deaths from Pulmonary, Coronary, and Cerebral Thrombosis and Embolism in Women of Child-Bearing Age," *British Medical Journal,* 2:193–199, 1968.

26. Vessey, M.P. and R. Doll, "Investigation of Relation Between Use of Oral Contraceptives and Thromboembolic Disease, A Further Report," *British Medical Journal,* 2:651–657, 1969.

27. Sartwell, P.E., A.T. Masi, F.G. Arthes, G.R. Greene, and H.E. Smith, "Thromboembolism and Oral Contraceptives: An Epidemiological Case Control Study," *American Journal of Epidemiology,* 90:365–380, 1969.

28. Collaborative Group for the Study of Stroke In Young Women, "Oral Contraception and Increased Risk of Cerebral Ischemia or Thrombosis," *New England Journal of Medicine,* 288:871–878, 1973.

29. Collaborative Group for the Study of Stroke in Young Women, "Oral Contraceptives and Stroke in Young Women: Associated Risk Factors," *Journal of the American Medical Association,* 231:718–722, 1975.

30. Mann, J.I. and W.H.W. Inman, "Oral Contraceptives and Death from Myocardial Infarction," *British Medical Journal,* 2:245–248, 1975.

31. Mann, J.I., M.P. Vessey, M. Thorogood, and R. Doll., "Myocardial Infarction in Young Women with Special Reference to Oral Contraceptive Practice," *British Medical Journal,* 2:241–245, 1975.

32. Inman, W.H.W., V.P. Vessey, B. Westerholm, and A. Engelund, "Thromboembolic Disease and the Steroidal Content of Oral Contraceptives," *British Medical Journal,* 2:203–209, 1970.

33. Stolley, P.D., J.A. Tonascia, M.S. Tockman, P.E. Sartwell, A.H. Rutledge, and M.P. Jacobs, "Thrombosis with Low-Estrogen Oral Contraceptives," *American Journal of Epidemiology,* 102:197–208, 1975.

34. Vessey, M.P., R. Doll, A.S. Fairbairn, and G. Glober, "Post-Operative Thromboembolism and the Use of the Oral Contraceptives," *British Medical Journal,* 3:123–126, 1970.

35. Greene, G.R. and P.E. Sartwell, "Oral Contraceptive Use in Patients with Thromboembolism Following Surgery, Trauma or Infection," *American Journal of Public Health,* 62:680–685, 1972.

36. Rosenberg, L., M.B. Armstrong and H. Jick, "Myocardial Infarction and Estrogen Therapy in Postmenopausal Women," *New England Journal of Medicine,* 294:1256–1259, 1976.

37. Coronary Drug Project Research Group, "The Coronary Drug Project: Initial Findings Leading to Modifications of Its Research Protocol," *Journal of the American Medical Association,* 214:1303–1313, 1970.

38. Baum, J., F. Holtz, J.J. Bookstein, and E.W. Klein, "Possible Association between Benign Hepatomas and Oral Contraceptives," *Lancet,* 2:926–928, 1973.

39. Mays, E.T., W.M. Christopherson, M.M. Mahr, and H.C. Williams, "Hepatic Changes in Young Women Ingesting Contraceptive Steroids, Hepatic Hemorrhage and Primary Hepatic Tumors." *Journal of the American Medical Association,* 235:730–782, 1976.

40. Edmondson, H.A., B. Henderson, and B. Benton, "Liver Cell Adenomas Associated with the Use of Oral Contraceptives," *New England Journal of Medicine,* 294:470–472, 1976.

41. Pfeffer, R.I. and S. Van Den Noore, "Estrogen Use and Stroke Risk in Postmenopausal Women," *American Journal of Epidemiology,* 103:445–456, 1976.

PATIENT INFORMATION ABOUT ESTROGENS

Estrogens are female hormones produced by the ovaries. The ovaries make several different kinds of estrogens. In addition, scientists have been able to make a variety of synthetic estrogens. As far as we know, all these synthetic estrogens have similar properties and therefore much the same usefulness, side effects, and risks. This leaflet is intended to help you understand what estrogens are used for, some of the risks involved in their use, and to help minimize these risks.

This leaflet includes important information about estrogens, but not all the information. If you want to know more, you can ask your doctor or pharmacist to let you read the package insert prepared for the doctor.

USES OF ESTROGEN

THERE IS NO PROPER USE OF ESTROGENS IN A PREGNANT WOMAN

Estrogens are prescribed by doctors for a number of purposes, including:

1. To provide estrogen during a period of adjustment when a woman's ovaries no longer produce it, in order to prevent certain uncomfortable symptoms of estrogen deficiency. (All women normally decrease the production of estrogens, generally between the ages of 45 and 55; this is called the menopause.)
2. To prevent symptoms of estrogen deficiency when a woman's ovaries have been removed surgically before the natural menopause.
3. To prevent pregnancy. (Estrogens are given along with a progestogen, another female hormone; these combinations are called oral contraceptives or birth control pills. Patient labeling is available to women taking oral contraceptives and they will not be discussed in this leaflet.)
4. To treat certain cancers in women and men.
5. To prevent painful swelling of the breasts after pregnancy in women who choose not to nurse their babies.

ESTROGENS IN THE MENOPAUSE

In the natural course of their lives, all women eventually experience a decrease in estrogen production. This usually occurs between ages 45 and 55 but may occur earlier or later. Sometimes the ovaries may need to be removed by an operation before natural menopause, producing a "surgical menopause."

When the amount of estrogen in the blood begins to decrease, many women may develop typical symptoms: Feelings of warmth in the face, neck, and chest or sudden intense episodes of heat and sweating throughout the body (called "hot flashes" or "hot flushes"). These symptoms are sometimes very uncomfortable. A few women eventually develop changes in the vagina (called "atrophic vaginitis") which cause discomfort, especially during and after intercourse.

Estrogens can be prescribed to treat these symptoms of the menopause. It is estimated that considerably more than half of all women undergoing the menopause have only mild symptoms or no symptoms at all and therefore do not need estrogens. Other women may need estrogens for a few months, while their bodies adjust to lower estrogen levels. Sometimes the need will be for periods longer than six months. In an attempt to avoid over-stimulation of the uterus (womb), estrogens are usually given cyclically during each month of use, that is three weeks of pills followed by one week without pills.

Sometimes women experience nervous symptoms or depression during menopause. There is no evidence that estrogens are effective for such symptoms and they should not be used to treat them, although other treatment may be needed.

You may have heard that taking estrogens for long periods (years) after the menopause will keep your skin soft and supple and keep you feeling young. There is no evidence that this is so, however, and such long-term treatment carries important risks.

Estrogens to Prevent Swelling of the Breasts After Pregnancy: If you do not breast-feed your baby after delivery, your breasts may fill up with milk and become painful and engorged. This usually begins about three to four days after delivery and may last for a few days to up to a week or more. Sometimes the discomfort is severe, but usually it is not and can be controlled by pain-relieving drugs such as aspirin and by binding the breasts up tightly. Estrogens can be used to try to prevent the breasts from filling up. While this treatment is sometimes successful, in many cases the breasts fill up to some degree in spite of treatment. The dose of estrogens needed to prevent pain and swelling of the breasts is much larger than the dose needed to treat symptoms of the menopause and this may increase your chances of developing blood clots in the legs or lungs (see below). Therefore, it is important that you discuss the benefits and the risks of estrogen use with your doctor if you have decided not to breast-feed your baby.

Some of the Dangers of Estrogen:

1. *Cancer of the uterus.* If estrogens are used in the postmenopausal period for more than a year, there is an increased risk of *endometrial cancer* (cancer of the uterus). Women taking estrogens have roughly five to ten times as great a chance of getting this cancer as women who take no estrogens. To put this another way, while a postmenopausal woman not taking estrogens has one chance in 1,000 each year of getting cancer of the uterus, a woman taking estrogens has five to ten chances in 1,000 each year. For this reason *it is important to take estrogens only when you really need them.*

Continued on next page

Ortho Pharm.—Cont.

The risk of this cancer is greater the longer estrogens are used and also seems to be greater when larger doses are taken. For this reason *it is important to take the lowest dose of estrogen that will control symptoms and to take it only as long as it is needed.* If estrogens are needed for longer periods of time, your doctor will want to reevaluate your need for estrogens at least every six months.

Women using estrogens should report any irregular vaginal bleeding to their doctors; such bleeding may be of no importance, but it can be an early warning of cancer of the uterus. If you have undiagnosed vaginal bleeding, you should not use estrogens until a diagnosis is made and you are certain there is no cancer of the uterus.

If you have had your uterus completely removed (total hysterectomy), there is no danger of developing cancer of the uterus.

2. *Other possible cancers.* Estrogens can cause development of other tumors in animals, such as tumors of the breast, cervix, vagina, or liver, when given for a long time. At present there is no good evidence that women using estrogen in the menopause have an increased risk of such tumors, but there is no way yet to be sure they do not; and one study raises the possibility that use of estrogens in the menopause may increase the risk of breast cancer many years later. This is a further reason to use estrogens only when clearly needed. While you are taking estrogens, it is important that you go to your doctor at least once a year for a physical examination. Also, if members of your family have had breast cancer or if you have breast nodules or abnormal mammograms (breast x-rays), your doctor may wish to carry out more frequent examinations of your breasts.

3. *Gall bladder disease.* Women who use estrogens after menopause are more likely to develop gall bladder disease needing surgery than women who do not use estrogens. Birth control pills have a similar effect.

4. *Abnormal blood clotting.* Oral contraceptives, some of which contain estrogens, increase the risk of blood clotting in various parts of the body. This can result in a stroke (if the clot is in the brain), a heart attack (clot in a blood vessel of the heart), or a pulmonary embolus (a clot which forms in the legs or pelvis, then breaks off and travels to the lungs). Any of these can be fatal. Blood clots may result in the loss of a limb, paralysis or loss of sight, depending on where the blood clot is formed or lodges if it breaks loose.

The larger doses of estrogen used to prevent swelling of the breasts after pregnancy have been reported to cause clotting in the legs and lungs.

It is recommended that if you have had any blood clotting disorders including clotting in the legs or lungs, or a heart attack or stroke, you should not use estrogens.

Special Warning About Pregnancy: You should not receive estrogen if you are pregnant. If this should occur, there is a greater than usual chance that the developing child will be born with a birth defect, although the possibility remains fairly small. A female child may have an increased risk of developing cancer of the vagina or cervix later in life (in the teens or twenties). Every possible effort should be made to avoid exposure to estrogens during pregnancy. If exposure occurs, see your doctor.

Some Other Effects of Estrogens: In addition to the serious known risks of estrogens described above, estrogens have the following side effects and potential risks:

1. *Nausea and vomiting.* The most common side effect of estrogen therapy is nausea. Vomiting is less common.
2. *Effects on breasts.* Estrogens may cause breast tenderness or enlargement and may cause the breasts to secrete a liquid.
3. *Effects on the uterus.* Estrogens may cause benign fibroid tumors of the uterus to get larger.

Some women will have menstrual bleeding when estrogens are stopped. But if the bleeding occurs on days you are still taking estrogens you should report this to your doctor.

4. *Effects on liver.* Women taking estrogens develop on rare occasions a tumor of the liver which can rupture and bleed into the abdomen. You should report any swelling or unusual pain or tenderness in the abdomen to your doctor immediately.

Women with a past history of jaundice (yellowing of the skin and white parts of the eyes) may get jaundice again during estrogen use.

5. *Other effects.* Estrogens may cause excess fluid to be retained in the body. This may make some conditions worse, such as epilepsy, migraine, heart disease, or kidney disease.

If any of the above occur, stop taking estrogens and call your doctor.

SUMMARY

Estrogens have important uses, but they have serious risks as well. You must decide, with your doctor, whether the risks are acceptable to you in view of the benefits of treatment. Except where your doctor has prescribed estrogens for use in special cases of cancer of the breast or prostate, you should not use estrogens if you have cancer of the breast or uterus, are pregnant, have undiagnosed abnormal vaginal bleeding, blood clotting disorders including clotting in the legs or lungs, or have had a stroke, heart attack or angina.

You must understand that your doctor will require regular physical examinations while you are taking them and will try to discontinue the drug as soon as possible and use the smallest dose possible. You can help minimize the risk by being alert for signs of trouble including:

1. Abnormal bleeding from the vagina.
2. Pains in the calves or chest or sudden shortness of breath, or coughing blood (indicating possible clots in the legs, heart or lungs).
3. Severe headache, dizziness, faintness, or changes in vision (indicating possible developing clots in the brain or eye).
4. Breast lumps (you should ask your doctor how to examine your own breasts).
5. Jaundice (yellowing of the skin).
6. Mental depression.
7. <u>Any</u> other unusual condition or problem.

Based on his or her assessment of your medical needs, your doctor has prescribed this drug for you. Do not give the drug to anyone else.

HOW SUPPLIED

Available in 2.75 oz. (78g) tubes with or without ORTHO® Measured-Dose Applicator.
With applicator: NDC 0062-5450-77
Without applicator: NDC 0062-5450-00
Store at controlled room temperature.

ORTHO® Disposable Applicator

(See PDR For Nonprescription Drugs)

ORTHO® Personal Lubricant

(See PDR For Nonprescription Drugs)

ORTHO-GYNOL® Contraceptive Jelly

(See PDR For Nonprescription Drugs)

ORTHO-NOVUM® Tablets ℞
(norethindrone/mestranol) or (norethindrone/ethinyl estradiol) and

MODICON® Tablets ℞
(norethindrone/ethinyl estradiol) and

MICRONOR® Tablets ℞
(norethindrone)

DESCRIPTION

ORTHO-NOVUM 7/7/7□21 Tablets are a combination oral contraceptive. Each white ORTHO-NOVUM 7/7/7□21 Tablet contains 0.5 mg of the progestational compound, norethindrone (17-hydroxy-19-nor-17α-pregn-4-en-20-yn-3-one), together with 0.035 mg of the estrogenic compound ethinyl estradiol (19-nor-17α-pregna-1,3,5(10)-trien-20-yne-3,17-diol). Inactive ingredients include FD&C Yellow No. 6, lactose, magnesium stearate, and pregelatinized starch. Each light peach ORTHO-NOVUM 7/7/7□21 Tablet contains 0.75 mg of the progestational compound, norethindrone (17-hydroxy-19-nor-17α-pregn-4-en-20-yn-3-one), together with 0.035 mg of the estrogenic compound, ethinyl estradiol (19-nor-17α-pregna-1,3,5(10)-trien-20-yne-3,17-diol). Inactive ingredients include FD&C Yellow No. 6, lactose, magnesium stearate, and pregelatinized starch. Each peach ORTHO-NOVUM 7/7/7□21 Tablet contains 1 mg of the progestational compound, norethindrone (17-hydroxy-19-nor-17α-pregn-4-en-20-yn-3-one), together with 0.035 mg of the estrogenic compound, ethinyl estradiol (19-nor-17α-pregna-1,3,5(10)-trien-20-yne-3,17-diol). Inactive ingredients include FD&C Yellow No. 6, lactose, magnesium stearate, and pregelatinized starch.

ORTHO-NOVUM 7/7/7□28 Tablets are a combination oral contraceptive. Each white ORTHO-NOVUM 7/7/7□28 Tablet contains 0.5 mg of the progestational compound, norethindrone (17-hydroxy-19-nor-17α-pregn-4-en-20-yn-3-one), together with 0.035 mg of the estrogenic compound, ethinyl estradiol (19-nor-17α-pregna-1,3,5(10)-trien-20-yne-3,17-diol). Inactive ingredients include lactose, magnesium stearate, and pregelatinized starch. Each light peach ORTHO-NOVUM 7/7/7□28 Tablet contains 0.75 mg of the progestational compound, norethindrone (17-hydroxy-19-nor-17α-pregn-4-en-20-yn-3-one), together with 0.035 mg of the estrogenic compound, ethinyl estradiol (19-nor-17α-pregna-1,3,5(10)-trien-20-yne-3,17-diol). Inactive ingredients include lactose, magnesium stearate, and pregelatinized starch. Each peach ORTHO-NOVUM 7/7/7□28 Tablet contains 1 mg of the progestational compound norethindrone (17-hydroxy-19-nor-17α-pregn-4-en-20-yn-3-one), together with 0.035 mg of the estrogenic compound, ethinyl estradiol (19-nor-17α-pregna-1,3,5(10)-trien-20-yne-3,17-diol). Inactive ingredients include FD&C Yellow No. 6, lactose, magnesium stearate, and pregelatinized starch. Each green tablet contains the following inert ingredients: D&C Yellow No. 10 Aluminum Lake, FD&C Blue No. 2 Aluminum Lake, lactose, magnesium stearate, microcrystalline cellulose, and pregelatinized starch.

ORTHO-NOVUM 10/11□21 Tablets are a combination oral contraceptive. Each white ORTHO-NOVUM 10/11□21 Tablet contains 0.5 mg of the progestational compound, norethindrone (17-hydroxy-19-nor-17α-pregn-4-en-20-yn-3-one), together with 0.035 mg of the estrogenic compound, ethinyl estradiol (19-nor-17α-pregna-1,3,5(10)-trien-20-yne-3,17-diol). Inactive ingredients include lactose, magnesium stearate, and pregelatinized starch. Each peach ORTHO-NOVUM 10/11□21 Tablet contains 1 mg of the progestational compound, norethindrone (17-hydroxy-19-nor-17α-pregn-4-en-20-yn-3-one), together with 0.035 mg of the estrogenic compound, ethinyl estradiol (19-nor-17α-pregna-1,3,5(10)-trien-20-yne-3,17-diol). Inactive ingredients include FD&C Yellow No. 6, lactose, magnesium stearate, and pregelatinized starch.

ORTHO-NOVUM 10/11□28 Tablets are a combination oral contraceptive. Each white ORTHO-NOVUM 10/11□28 Tablet contains 0.5 mg of the progestational compound, norethindrone (17-hydroxy-19-nor-17α-pregn-4-en-20-yn-3-one), together with 0.035 mg of the estrogenic compound, ethinyl estradiol (19-nor-17α-pregna-1,3,5(10)-trien-20-yne-3,17-diol). Inactive ingredients include lactose, magnesium stearate, and pregelatinized starch. Each peach ORTHO-NOVUM 10/11□28 Tablet contains 1 mg of the progestational compound, norethindrone (17-hydroxy-19-nor-17α-pregn-4-en-20-yn-3-one), together with 0.035 mg of the estrogenic compound, ethinyl estradiol (19-nor-17α-pregna-1,3,5(10)-trien-20-yne-3,17-diol). Inactive ingredients include FD&C Yellow No. 6, lactose, magnesium stearate, and pregelatinized starch. Each green tablet contains inert ingredients. (See inactive ingredient listing for inert green tablets in ORTHO-NOVUM 7/7/7□28).

ORTHO-NOVUM 1/35□21 Tablets are a combination oral contraceptive. Each ORTHO-NOVUM 1/35□21 Tablet contains 1 mg of the progestational compound, norethindrone (17- hydroxy-19-nor-17α -pregn- 4 -en- 20-yn-3- one), together with 0.035 mg of the estrogenic compound, ethinyl estradiol (19-nor-17α-pregna-1,3,5(10)-trien-20-yne-3,17-diol). Inactive ingredients include FD&C Yellow No. 6, lactose, magnesium stearate, and pregelatinized starch.

ORTHO-NOVUM 1/35□28 Tablets are a combination oral contraceptive. Each peach ORTHO-NOVUM 1/35□28 Tablet contains 1 mg of the progestational compound, norethindrone (17-hydroxy-19-nor-17α-pregn-4-en-20-yn-3-one), together with 0.035 mg of the estrogenic compound ethinyl estradiol (19-nor-17α-pregna-1,3,5(10)-trien-20-yne-3, 17-diol). Inactive ingredients include FD&C Yellow No. 6, lactose, magnesium stearate, and pregelatinized starch. Each green tablet contains inert ingredients. (See inactive ingredient listing for inert green tablets in ORTHO-NOVUM 7/7/7□28).

MODICON 21 Tablets are a combination oral contraceptive. Each MODICON 21 Tablet contains 0.5 mg of the progestational compound, norethindrone (17-hydroxy-19-nor-17α-pregn-4-en-20-yn-3-one), together with 0.035 mg of the estrogenic compound, ethinyl estradiol (19-nor-17α-pregna-1,3,5(10)-trien-20-yne-3,17-diol). Inactive ingredients include lactose, magnesium stearate, and pregelatinized starch.

MODICON 28 Tablets are a combination oral contraceptive. Each white MODICON 28 Tablet contains 0.5 mg of the progestational compound, norethindrone (17-hydroxy-19-nor-17α-pregn-4-en-20-yn-3-one), together with 0.035 mg of the estrogenic compound, ethinyl estradiol (19-nor-17α-pregna-1,3,5(10)-trien-20-yne-3,17-diol). Inactive ingredients include lactose, magnesium stearate, and pregelatinized starch. Each green tablet contains inert ingredients. (See inactive ingredient listing for inert green tablets in ORTHO-NOVUM 7/7/7□28).

ORTHO-NOVUM 1/50□21 Tablets are a combination oral contraceptive. Each ORTHO-NOVUM 1/50□21 Tablet contains 1 mg of the progestational compound, norethindrone (17-hydroxy-19-nor- 17α -pregn-4-en-20-yn-3-one), together with 0.05 mg of the estrogenic compound, mestranol (3-methoxy-19-nor-17α-pregna-1,3,5(10)-trien-20-yn-17-ol). Inactive ingredients include D&C Yellow No. 10, lactose, magnesium stearate, and pregelatinized starch.

ORTHO-NOVUM 1/50□28 Tablets are a combination oral contraceptive. Each yellow ORTHO-NOVUM 1/50□28 Tablet contains 1 mg of the progestational compound, norethindrone (17-hydroxy-19-nor-17α-pregn-4-en-20-yn-3-one), together with 0.05 mg of the estrogenic compound, mestranol (3-methoxy-19-nor-17α-pregna-1,3,5 (10)-trien-20-yn-17-ol). Inactive ingredients include D&C Yellow No. 10, lactose, magnesium stearate, and pregelatinized starch. Each green tablet contains inert ingredients. (See inactive ingredient listing for inert green tablets in ORTHO-NOVUM 7/7/7□28).

ORTHO-NOVUM 1/80□21 Tablets are a combination oral contraceptive. Each ORTHO-NOVUM 1/80□21 Tablet contains 1 mg of the progestational compound, norethindrone (17-hydroxy-19-nor- 17α -pregn-4-en-20-yn-3-one), together with 0.08 mg of the estrogenic compound, mestranol (3-methoxy-19-nor-17α-pregna-1,3,5(10)-trien-20-yn-17-ol). Inactive ingredients include lactose, magnesium stearate, and pregelatinized starch.

ORTHO-NOVUM 1/80□28 Tablets are a combination oral contraceptive. Each white ORTHO-NOVUM 1/80□28 Tablet contains 1 mg of the progestational compound, norethindrone (17-hydroxy-19-nor-17α-pregn-4-en-20-yn-3-one), together with 0.08 mg of the estrogenic compound, mestranol (3-methoxy-19-nor-17α-pregna-1,3,5 (10)-trien-20-yn-17-ol). Inactive ingredients include lactose, magnesium stearate, and pregelatinized starch. Each green tablet contains inert ingredients. (See inactive ingredient listing for inert green tablets in ORTHO-NOVUM 7/7/7□28).

ORTHO-NOVUM 2 mg□21 Tablets are a combination oral contraceptive. Each ORTHO-NOVUM 2 mg□21 Tablet contains 2 mg of the progestational compound, norethindrone (17-hydroxy-19-nor-17α-pregn-4-en-20-yn-3- one), together with 0.10 mg of the estrogenic compound, mestranol (3-methoxy-19-nor-17α-pregna-1,3,5(10)-trien-20-yn-17-ol). Inactive ingredients include lactose, magnesium stearate, and pregelatinized starch.

MICRONOR Tablets are a progestogen-only oral contraceptive. Each MICRONOR Tablet contains 0.35 mg of the progestational compound, norethindrone (17-hydroxy-19-nor-17α-pregn-4-en-20-yn-3-one), a synthetic progestogen. Inactive ingredients include D&C Green No. 5, D&C Yellow No. 10, lactose, magnesium stearate, povidone, and starch.

Clinical Pharmacology Combination Oral Contraceptives Only: Combination oral contraceptives act primarily through the mechanism of gonadotropin suppression due to the estrogenic and progestational activity of the ingredients. Although the primary mechanism of action is inhibition of ovulation, alterations in the genital tract including changes in the cervical mucus (which increase the difficulty of sperm penetration) and the endometrium (which reduce the likelihood of implantation) may also contribute to contraceptive effectiveness.

Clinical Pharmacology Progestogen Oral Contraceptives: The primary mechanism through which MICRONOR prevents conception is not known, but progestogen-only contraceptives are known to alter the cervical mucus, exert a progestational effect on the endometrium, interfering with implantation, and, in some patients, suppress ovulation.

INDICATIONS AND USAGE

ORTHO-NOVUM 7/7/7□21, ORTHO-NOVUM 7/7/7□28, ORTHO-NOVUM 10/11□21, ORTHO-NOVUM 10/11□28, ORTHO-NOVUM 1/35□21, ORTHO-NOVUM 1/35□28, MODICON 21, MODICON 28, ORTHO-NOVUM 1/50□21, ORTHO-NOVUM 1/50□28, ORTHO-NOVUM 1/80□21, ORTHO-NOVUM 1/80□28, and MICRONOR are indicated for the prevention of pregnancy in women who elect to use oral contraceptives as a method of contraception.

ORTHO-NOVUM 2 mg□21 is indicated for the treatment of hypermenorrhea. ORTHO-NOVUM 2 mg□21 is indicated for the prevention of pregnancy in women who elect to use oral contraceptives as a method of contraception. (See first paragraph immediately following the opening WARNINGS statement.)

Oral contraceptives are highly effective. The pregnancy rate in women using conventional combination oral contraceptives (containing 35 mcg or more of ethinyl estradiol or 50 mcg or more of mestranol) is generally reported as less than one pregnancy per 100 woman-years of use. Slightly higher rates (somewhat more than one pregnancy per 100 woman-years of use) are reported for some combination products containing 35 mcg or less of ethinyl estradiol, and rates on the order of three pregnancies per 100 woman-years are reported for the progestogen-only oral contraceptives.

These rates are derived from separate studies conducted by different investigators in several population groups and cannot be compared precisely. Furthermore, pregnancy rates tend to be lower as clinical studies are continued, possibly due to selective retention in the longer studies of those patients who accept the treatment regimen and do not discontinue as a result of adverse reactions, pregnancy or other reasons.

The ORTHO-NOVUM 7/7/7□21 Tablet regimen consists of 7 white tablets containing 0.5 mg norethindrone together with 0.035 mg ethinyl estradiol, followed by 7 light peach tablets containing 0.75 mg norethindrone together with 0.035 mg ethinyl estradiol, followed by 7 peach tablets containing 1 mg norethindrone together with 0.035 mg ethinyl estradiol.

The ORTHO-NOVUM 7/7/7□28 Tablet regimen consists of 7 white tablets containing 0.5 mg norethindrone together with 0.035 mg ethinyl estradiol, followed by 7 light peach tablets containing 0.75 mg norethindrone together with 0.035 mg ethinyl estradiol, followed by 7 peach tablets containing 1 mg norethindrone together with 0.035 mg ethinyl estradiol and 7 green placebo tablets.

7 WHITE TABLETS

In clinical trials with a formulation containing 0.5 mg of norethindrone and 0.035 mg of ethinyl estradiol, 1,168 patients completed 16,345 cycles of use and a total of three pregnancies was reported. This represents a pregnancy rate of 0.22 per 100 woman-years.

7 PEACH TABLETS

In clinical trials with a formulation containing 1 mg of norethindrone and 0.035 mg of ethinyl estradiol, 940 subjects completed 14,366 cycles of use. Two pregnancies were reported for a pregnancy rate of 0.17 per 100 woman-years.

Table 1 gives ranges of pregnancy rates reported in the literature for other means of contraception. The efficacy of these means of contraception (except the IUD) depends upon the degree of adherence to the method.

The ORTHO-NOVUM 10/11□21 Tablet regimen consists of 10 white tablets followed by 11 peach tablets.

The ORTHO-NOVUM 10/11□28 Tablet regimen consists of 10 white tablets followed by 11 peach tablets and 7 green placebo tablets.

10 WHITE TABLETS

In clinical trials with a formulation containing 0.5 mg of norethindrone and 0.035 mg of ethinyl estradiol, 1,168 patients completed 16,345 cycles of use and a total of three pregnancies was reported. This represents a pregnancy rate of 0.22 per 100 woman-years.

11 PEACH TABLETS

In clinical trials with a formulation containing 1 mg norethindrone and 0.035 mg of ethinyl estradiol, 940 subjects completed 14,366 cycles of use. Two pregnancies were reported for a pregnancy rate of 0.17 per 100 woman-years.

The dropout rate for medical reasons, as observed in the clinical trials conducted with ORTHO-NOVUM 1/35 and MODICON, appears to be somewhat higher than observed with higher dose combination products. The dropout rate due to menstrual disorders and irregularities was also somewhat higher, dropouts being equally split between menstrual disorders and irregularities and other medical reasons attributable to the drug.

In clinical trials with ORTHO-NOVUM 1/35□21 and ORTHO-NOVUM 1/35□28, 940 subjects completed 14,366 cycles of use. Two pregnancies were reported for a pregnancy rate of 0.17 per 100 woman-years.

In clinical trials with MODICON and MODICON 28, 1,168 patients completed 16,345 cycles of use, and a total of three pregnancies was reported. This represents a pregnancy rate of 0.22 per 100 woman-years.

In clinical trials with ORTHO-NOVUM 1/50□21, 3,852 patients completed 45,937 cycles, and a total of 10 pregnancies was reported. This represents a pregnancy rate of 0.26 per 100 woman-years.

In clinical trials with ORTHO-NOVUM 1/50□28, 1,590 patients completed 7,330 cycles, and a total of three pregnancies was reported. This represents a pregnancy rate of 0.5 per 100 woman-years.

In clinical trials with ORTHO-NOVUM 1/80□21, and ORTHO-NOVUM 1/80□28, 3,464 patients completed 34,068 cycles, and a total of five pregnancies was reported. This represents a pregnancy rate of 0.18 per 100 woman-years.

In clinical trials with ORTHO-NOVUM 2 mg□20, 6,097 patients completed 121,233 cycles, and a total of 13 pregnancies was reported. This represents a pregnancy rate of 0.13 per 100 woman-years. In clinical trials with ORTHO-NOVUM 2 mg□21, 965 patients completed 3,743 cycles, and no pregnancies were reported. This represents a pregnancy rate of 0.0 per 100 woman-years.

In clinical trials with MICRONOR, 2,963 patients completed 25,901 cycles of therapy, and a total of 55 pregnancies was reported. This represents an average pregnancy rate of 2.54 per 100 woman-years.

A higher pregnancy rate of 3.72 was recorded in "fresh" patients (those who had never taken oral contraceptives prior to starting MICRONOR therapy) to a large extent because of incorrect tablet intake. This compares to the lower pregnancy rate of 1.95 recorded in "changeover" patients (those switched from other oral contraceptives).

This difference was found to be statistically significant. Furthermore, an even greater statistically significant difference in pregnancy rates between these two groups was found during the first six months of MICRONOR therapy. Therefore, it is especially important for "fresh" patients to strictly adhere to the regimen.

Table 1 gives ranges of pregnancy rates reported in the literature[1] for other means of contraception. The efficacy of these means of contraception (except the IUD) depends upon the degree of adherence to the method.

Table 1
Pregnancies Per 100 Woman-Years

IUD, less than 1–6;

Diaphragm with spermicidal product (creams or jellies), 2–20; Condom, 3–36; Aerosol foams, 2–29; Jellies and creams, 4–36; Periodic abstinence (rhythm) all types, less than 1–47;

1. Calendar method, 14–47;
2. Temperature method, 1–20;
3. Temperature method—intercourse only in postovulatory phase, less than 1–7;
4. Mucus method, 1–25;

No contraception, 60–80.

Dose-Related Risk of Thromboembolism From Oral Contraceptives: Two studies have shown a positive association between the dose of estrogens in oral contraceptives and the risk of thromboembolism.[2,3] For this reason, it is prudent and in keeping with good principles of therapeutics to minimize exposure to estrogen. The oral contraceptive product prescribed for any given patient should be that product which contains the least amount of estrogen that is compatible with an acceptable pregnancy rate and patient acceptance. It is recommended that new acceptors of oral contraceptives be started on preparations containing .05 mg or less of estrogen.

CONTRAINDICATIONS

Oral contraceptives should not be used in women with any of the following conditions:

1. Thrombophlebitis or thromboembolic disorders.
2. A past history of deep vein thrombophlebitis or thromboembolic disorders.
3. Cerebral vascular or coronary artery disease.
4. Known or suspected carcinoma of the breast.
5. Known or suspected estrogen-dependent neoplasia.
6. Undiagnosed, abnormal genital bleeding.
7. Oral contraceptive tablets may cause fetal harm when administered to a pregnant woman. Oral contraceptive tablets are contraindicated in women who are pregnant. If the patient becomes pregnant while taking this drug, the patient should be apprised of the potential hazard to the fetus (see WARNINGS, No. 5).
8. Benign or malignant liver tumor which developed during the use of oral contraceptives or other estrogen-containing products.

WARNINGS

Cigarette smoking increases the risk of serious cardiovascular side effects from oral contraceptive use. This risk increases with age and with heavy smoking (15 or more cigarettes per day) and is quite marked in women over 35 years of age. Women who use oral contraceptives should be strongly advised not to smoke.

The use of oral contraceptives is associated with increased risk of several serious conditions including thromboembolism, stroke, myocardial infarction, hepatic adenoma, gallbladder disease, hypertension. Practitioners prescribing oral contraceptives should be familiar with the following information relating to these risks.

ORTHO-NOVUM 2 mg□21 should only be used for contraception when lower dose formulations prove unacceptable.

1. THROMBOEMBOLIC DISORDERS AND OTHER VASCULAR PROBLEMS. An increased risk of thromboembolic and thrombotic disease associated with the use of oral contraceptives is well-established. Four principal studies in Great Britain[4,5,6,26] and three in the United States[7–10] have demonstrated an increased risk of fatal and nonfatal venous thromboembolism and stroke, both hemorrhagic and thrombotic. These studies estimate that users of oral contraceptives are 4 to 11 times more likely than nonusers to develop these diseases without evident cause (Tables 2,4). Overall excess mortality due to pulmonary embolism or stroke is on the order of 1.0 to 3.5 deaths annually per 100,000 users and increases with age (Table 3).

Table 2
Hospitalization Rates Due to Venous Thromboembolic Disease[6]

	Admissions annually per 100,000 women, age 20–44
Users of oral contraceptives	45
Nonusers	5

Table 3
Death Rates Due to Pulmonary Embolism or Cerebral Thrombosis[5]—Deaths Annually Per 100,000 Nonpregnant Women

	Age 20 to 34	Age 35 to 44
Users of oral contraceptives	1.5	3.9
Nonusers	.2	.5

Cerebrovascular Disorders: In a collaborative American study[9,10] of cerebrovascular disorders in women with and without predisposing causes, it was estimated that the risk of hemorrhagic stroke was 2.0 times greater in users than in nonusers and the risk of thrombotic stroke was 4.0 to 9.5 times greater in users than in nonusers (Table 4).

Continued on next page

Ortho Pharm.—Cont.

Table 4

Summary of Relative Risk of Thromboembolic Disorders and Other Vascular Problems in Oral Contraceptive Users Compared to Nonusers

	Relative risk, times greater
Idiopathic thromboembolic disease	4–11
Post surgery thromboembolic complications	4–6
Thrombotic stroke	4–9.5
Hemorrhagic stroke	2
Myocardial infarction	2–12

A prospective study conducted in Great Britain[57] estimated that former users have a risk for all cerebrovascular disease 2.6 times greater than that of non-users. This risk remained elevated for at least six years after last oral contraceptive use. A prospective study conducted in the United States[55] found that past use of oral contraceptives was associated with increased risk of subarachnoid hemorrhage, the relative risk being 5.3. There was also some evidence from this study that the degree of risk may be related to duration of oral contraceptive use.

Myocardial Infarction: An increased risk of myocardial infarction associated with the use of oral contraceptives has been reported[11,12,13] confirming a previously suspected association (Tables 5 & 6). These studies, conducted in the United Kingdom, found, as expected, that the greater the number of underlying risk factors for coronary artery disease (cigarette smoking, hypertension, hypercholesterolemia, obesity, diabetes, history of preeclamptic toxemia), the higher the risk of developing myocardial infarction, regardless of whether the patient was an oral contraceptive user or not. Oral contraceptives, however, were found to be a clear additional risk factor.

The annual excess case rate (increased risk) of myocardial infarction (fatal and nonfatal) in oral contraceptive users was estimated to be approximately 7 cases per 100,000 women users in the 30–39 age group and 67 cases per 100,000 women users in the 40–44 age group.

In terms of relative risk, it has been estimated[52] that oral contraceptive users who do not smoke (smoking is considered a major predisposing condition to myocardial infarction) are about twice as likely to have a fatal myocardial infarction as nonusers who do not smoke. Oral contraceptive users who are also smokers have about a 5-fold increased risk of fatal infarction compared to users who do not smoke, but about a 10- to 12-fold increased risk compared to nonusers who do not smoke. Furthermore, the amount of smoking is also an important factor. In determining the importance of these relative risks, however, the baseline rates for various age groups, as shown in Table 5, must be given serious consideration. The importance of other predisposing conditions mentioned above in determining relative and absolute risks has not as yet been quantified; it is quite likely that the same synergistic action exists, but perhaps to a lesser extent.

A study[56] suggests that some increased risk of myocardial infarction in oral contraceptive users persists following discontinuation of oral contraceptives and that the degree of the residual risk is related to the duration of past use.

Table 5

Estimated Annual Mortality Rate Per 100,000 Women From Myocardial Infarction By Use Of Oral Contraceptives, Smoking Habits, And Age (in years)

	Myocardial Infarction			
	Women aged 30–39		Women aged 40–44	
Smoking habits	Users	Non-users	Users	Non-users
All smokers	10.2	2.6	62.0	15.9
Heavy[1]	13.0	5.1	78.7	31.3
Light	4.7	.9	28.6	5.7
Nonsmokers	1.8	1.2	10.7	7.4
Smokers and nonsmokers	5.4	1.9	32.8	11.7

[1]Heavy smoker: 15 or more cigarettes per day. From Jain, A.K., Studies in Family Planning. 8:50, 1977.

[See table below].

Risk of dose: In an analysis of data derived from several national adverse reaction reporting systems,[2] British investigators concluded that the risk of thromboembolism including coronary thrombosis is directly related to the dose of estrogen used in oral contraceptives. Preparations containing 100 mcg or more of estrogen were associated with a higher risk of thromboembolism than those containing 50–80 mcg of estrogen. Their analysis did suggest, however, that the quantity of estrogen may not be the sole factor involved. This finding has been confirmed in the United States.[3] Careful epidemiological studies to determine the degree of thromboembolic risk associated with progestogen-only oral contraceptives have not been performed. Cases of thromboembolic disease have been reported in women using these products, and they should not be presumed to be free of excess risk.

The risk of thromboembolic and thrombotic disorders, in both users and nonusers of oral contraceptives, increases with age. Oral contraceptives are, however, an independent risk factor for these events.

Estimate of Excess Mortality From Circulatory Diseases: A large prospective study[53] carried out in the United Kingdom estimated the mortality rate per 100,000 women per year from diseases of the circulatory system for users and nonusers of oral contraceptives according to age, smoking habits, and duration of use. The overall excess death rate annually from circulatory diseases for oral contraceptive users was estimated to be 20 per 100,000 (ages 15–34—5/100,000; ages 35–44—33/100,000; ages 45–49—140/100,000), the risk being concentrated in older women, in those with a long duration of use and in cigarette smokers. It was not possible, however, to examine the interrelationships of age, smoking, and duration of use, nor to compare the effects of continuous versus intermittent use. Although the study showed a 10-fold increase in death due to circulatory diseases in users for five or more years, all of these deaths occurred in women 35 or older. Until larger numbers of women under 35 with continuous use for five or more years are available, it is not possible to assess the magnitude of the relative risk for this younger age group.

This study reports that the increased risk of circulatory disease mortatilty[57] may persist after the pill is discontinued. Another study published at the same time confirms a previously reported increase of mortality in pill users from cardiovascular disease.[54]

The available data from a variety of sources have been analyzed[14] to estimate the risk of death associated with various methods of contraception. The estimates of risk of death for each method include the combined risk of the contraceptive method (e.g., thromboembolic and thrombotic disease in the case of oral contraceptives) plus the risk attributable to pregnancy or abortion in the event of method failure. This latter risk varies with the effectiveness of the contraceptive method. The findings of this analysis are shown in Figure 1 below.[14] The study concluded that the mortality associated with all methods of birth control is low and below that associated with childbirth, with the exception of oral contraceptives in women over 40 who smoke. (The rates given for pill only/smokers for each age group are for smokers as a class. For "heavy" smokers [more than 15 cigarettes a day], the rates given would be about double; for "light" smokers [less than 15 cigarettes a day], about 50 percent.)

The mortality associated with oral contraceptive use in nonsmokers over 40 is higher than with any other method of contraception in that age group.

The lowest mortality is associated with the condom or diaphragm backed up by early abortion.

The risk of thromboembolic and thrombotic disease associated with oral contraceptives increases with age after approximately age 30 and, for myocardial infarction, is further increased by hypertension, hypercholesterolemia, obesity, diabetes, or history of preeclamptic toxemia and especially by cigarette smoking. The risk of myocardial infarction in oral contraceptive users is substantially increased in women age 40 and over, especially those with other risk factors.

Based on the data currently available, the following chart gives a gross estimate of the risk of death from circulatory disorders associated with the use of oral contraceptives:

Smoking Habits and Other Predisposing Conditions—Risk Associated With Use Of Oral Contraceptives

Age	Below 30	30–39	40+
Heavy smokers	C	B	A
Light smokers	D	C	B
Nonsmokers (no predisposing conditions)	D	C,D	C
Nonsmokers (other predisposing conditions)	C	C,B	B,A

A—Use associated with very high risk.
B—Use associated with high risk.
C—Use associated with moderate risk.
D—Use associated with low risk.

The physician and the patient should be alert to the earliest manifestations of thromboembolic and thrombotic disorders (e.g., thrombophlebitis, pulmonary embolism, cerebrovascular insufficiency, coronary occlusion, retinal thrombosis, and mesenteric thrombosis). Should any of these occur or be suspected, the drug should be discontinued immediately.

A four- to six-fold increased risk of post surgery thromboembolic complications has been reported in oral contraceptives users.[15,16] If feasible, oral contraceptives should be discontinued at least four weeks before surgery of a type associated with an increased risk of thromboembolism or prolonged immobilization.

2. OCULAR LESIONS. There have been reports of neuro-ocular lesions such as optic neuritis or retinal thrombosis associated with the use of oral contraceptives. Discontinue oral contraceptive medication if there is unexplained, sudden or gradual, partial or complete loss of vision; onset of proptosis or diplopia; papilledema; or retinal vascular lesions and institute appropriate diagnostic and therapeutic measures.

3. CARCINOMA. Long-term continuous administration of either natural or synthetic estrogen in certain animal species increases the frequency of carcinoma of the breast, cervix, vagina, and liver. Certain synthetic progestogens, none currently contained in oral contraceptives, have been noted to increase the incidence of mammary nodules, benign and malignant, in dogs.

In humans, three case control studies have reported an increased risk of endometrial carcinoma associated with the prolonged use of exogenous estrogen in postmenopausal women.[17,18,19] One publication[20] reported on the first 21 cases submitted by physicians to a registry of cases of adenocarcinoma of the endometrium in women under 40 on oral contraceptives. Of the cases found in women without predisposing risk factors for adenocarcinoma of the endometrium (e.g., irregular bleeding at the time oral contraceptives were first given, polycystic ovaries), nearly all occurred in women who had used a sequential oral contraceptive. These products are no longer marketed. No evidence has been reported suggesting an increased risk of endometrial cancer in users of conventional combination or progestogen-only oral contraceptives.

Several studies[8,21–24] have found no increases in breast cancer in women taking oral contraceptives or estrogens. One study[25], however, while also noting no overall increased risk of breast cancer in women treated with oral contraceptives, found an excess risk in the subgroups of oral contraceptive users with documented benign breast disease. A reduced occurrence of benign breast tumors in users of oral contraceptives has been well- documented.[8,21,25,26,27] In summary, there is at present no confirmed evidence from human studies of an increased risk of cancer associated with oral contraceptives. Close clinical surveillance of all women taking oral contraceptives is, nevertheless, essential. In all cases of undiagnosed persistent or recurrent abnormal vaginal bleeding, appropriate diagnostic measures should be taken to rule out malignancy. Women with a strong family history of breast cancer or who have breast nodules, fibrocystic disease or abnormal mammograms should be monitored with particular care if they elect to use oral contraceptives instead of other methods of contraception.

4. HEPATIC TUMORS. Benign hepatic adenomas have been found to be associated with the use of oral contraceptives.[28,29,30,46] One study[46] showed that oral contraceptive formulations with high hormonal potency were associated with a higher risk than lower potency formulations and use of oral contraceptives with high hormonal potency and age over 30 years may further increase the woman's risk of hepatocellular adenoma. Although benign, hepatic adenomas may rupture and may cause death through intra-abdominal hemorrhage. This has been reported in short-term as well as long-term users of oral contraceptives. Two studies relate risk with duration of use of the contraceptive, the risk being much greater after four or more years of oral contraceptive use.[30,46] While hepatic adenoma is a rare lesion, it should be considered in women presenting abdominal pain and tenderness, abdominal mass or shock.

Table 6

Myocardial Infarction Rates in Users And Nonusers Of Oral Contraceptives in Britain[11,12,13]—Cases Annually Per 100,000 Women

	Nonfatal		Fatal	
	Age 30 to 39	Age 40 to 44	Age 30 to 39	Age 40 to 44
Users of oral contraceptives	5.6	56.9	5.4	32.0
Nonusers of oral contraceptives	2.1	9.9	1.9	12.0
Relative risk	2.7	5.7	2.8	2.8

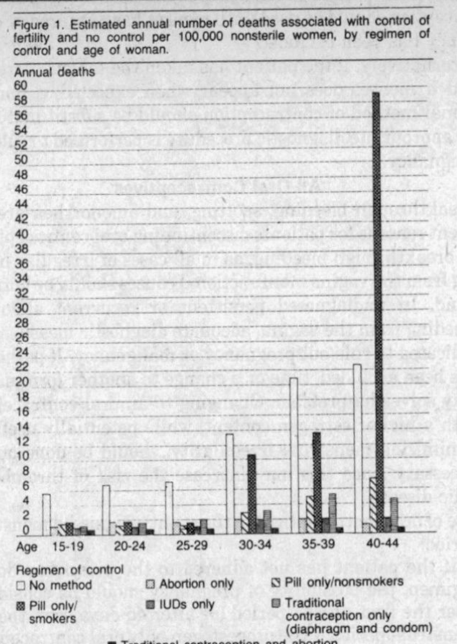

Figure 1. Estimated annual number of deaths associated with control of fertility and no control per 100,000 nonsterile women, by regimen of control and age of woman.

Cases of hepatocellular carcinoma, although rare, have been reported in women taking oral contraceptives. Retrospective studies conducted in the United States[58] and Britain[59,60] report an increased risk of hepatocellular carcinoma in oral contraceptive users, particularly with increased duration of use.

5. USE IN OR IMMEDIATELY PRECEDING PREGNANCY, BIRTH DEFECTS IN OFFSPRING, AND MALIGNANCY IN FEMALE OFFSPRING. The use of female sex hormones— both estrogenic and progestational agents—during early pregnancy may seriously damage the offspring. It has been shown that females exposed in utero to diethylstilbestrol, a nonsteroidal estrogen, have an increased risk of developing in later life a form of vaginal or cervical cancer that is ordinarily extremely rare.[31,32] This risk has been estimated to be of the order of 1 to 4 in 1000 exposures.[33,47] Although there is no evidence at the present time that oral contraceptives further enhance the risk of developing this type of malignancy, such patients should be monitored with particular care if they elect to use oral contraceptives instead of other methods of contraception. Furthermore, a high percentage of such exposed women (from 30 to 90%) have been found to have epithelial changes of the vagina and cervix.[34–38] Although these changes are histologically benign, it is not known whether this condition is a precursor of vaginal malignancy. Male children so exposed may develop abnormalities of the urogenital tract.[48,49,50] Although similar data are not available with the use of other estrogens, it cannot be presumed that they would not induce similar changes.

An increased risk of congenital anomalies, including heart defects and limb defects, has been reported with the use of sex hormones, including oral contraceptives, in pregnancy.[39–42,51] One case control study[42] has estimated a 4.7-fold increase in risk of limb-reduction defects in infants exposed in utero to sex hormones (oral contraceptives, hormonal withdrawal tests for pregnancy or attempted treatment for threatened abortion). Some of these exposures were very short and involved only a few days of treatment. The data suggest that the risk of limb-reduction defects in exposed fetuses is somewhat less than one in 1,000 live births.

In the past, female sex hormones have been used during pregnancy in an attempt to treat threatened or habitual abortion. There is considerable evidence that estrogens are ineffective for these indications, and there is no evidence from well-controlled studies that progestogens are effective for these uses.

There is some evidence that triploidy and possibly other types of polyploidy are increased among abortuses from women who become pregnant soon after ceasing oral contraceptives.[43] Embryos with these anomalies are virtually always aborted spontaneously. Whether there is an overall increase in spontaneous abortion of pregnancies conceived soon after stopping oral contraceptives is unknown. It is recommended that for any patient who has missed two consecutive periods, pregnancy should be ruled out before continuing the contraceptive regimen. If the patient has not adhered to the prescribed schedule, the possibility of pregnancy should be considered at the time of the first missed period (or after 45 days from the last menstrual period if the progestogen-only oral contraceptives are used), and further use of oral contraceptives should be withheld until pregnancy has been ruled out. If pregnancy is confirmed, the patient should be apprised of the potential risks to the fetus and the advisability of continuation of the pregnancy should be discussed in the light of these risks.

It is also recommended that women who discontinue oral contraceptives with the intent of becoming pregnant use an alternate form of contraception for a period of time before attempting to conceive. Many clinicians recommend three months although no precise information is available on which to base this recommendation.

The administration of progestogen-only or progestogen-estrogen combinations to induce withdrawal bleeding should not be used as a test of pregnancy.

6. GALLBLADDER DISEASE. Studies[8,23,26] report an increased risk of surgically confirmed gallbladder disease in users of oral contraceptives and estrogens. In one study, an increased risk appeared after two years of use and doubled after four or five years of use. In one of the other studies, an increased risk was apparent between six and twelve months of use.

7. CARBOHYDRATE AND LIPID METABOLIC EFFECTS. A decrease in glucose tolerance has been observed in a significant percentage of patients on oral contraceptives. For this reason, prediabetic and diabetic patients should be carefully observed while receiving oral contraceptives.

An increase in triglycerides and total phospholipids has been observed in patients receiving oral contraceptives.[44] The clinical significance of this finding remains to be defined.

8. ELEVATED BLOOD PRESSURE. An increase in blood pressure has been reported in patients receiving oral contraceptives.[26] In some women hypertension may occur within a few months of beginning oral contraceptive use. In the first year of use, the prevalence of women with hypertension is low in users and may be no higher than that of a comparable group of nonusers. The prevalence in users increases, however, with longer exposure, and in the fifth year of use is two and a half to three times the reported prevalence in the first year. Age is also strongly correlated with the development of hypertension in oral contraceptive users. Women who previously have had hypertension during pregnancy may be more likely to develop elevation of blood pressure when given oral contraceptives. Hypertension that develops as a result of taking oral contraceptives usually returns to normal after discontinuing the drug.

9. HEADACHE. The onset or exacerbation of migraine or development of headache of a new pattern which is recurrent, persistent, or severe, requires discontinuation of oral contraceptives and evaluation of the cause.

10. BLEEDING IRREGULARITIES. Breakthrough bleeding, spotting, and amenorrhea are frequent reasons for patients discontinuing oral contraceptives. In breakthrough bleeding, as in all cases of irregular bleeding from the vagina, nonfunctional causes should be borne in mind. In undiagnosed persistent or recurrent abnormal bleeding from the vagina, adequate diagnostic measures are indicated to rule out pregnancy or malignancy. If pathology has been excluded, time or a change to another formulation may solve the problem. Changing to an oral contraceptive with a higher estrogen content, while potentially useful in minimizing menstrual irregularity, should be done only if necessary since this may increase the risk of thromboembolic disease.

An alteration in menstrual patterns is likely to occur in women using progestogen-only oral contraceptives. The amount and duration of flow, cycle length, breakthrough bleeding, spotting and amenorrhea will probably be quite variable. Bleeding irregularities occur more frequently with the use of progestogen-only oral contraceptives than with the combinations and the dropout rate due to such conditions is higher.

Women with a past history of oligomenorrhea or secondary amenorrhea or young women without regular cycles may have a tendency to remain anovulatory or to become amenorrheic after discontinuation of oral contraceptives. Women with these preexisting problems should be advised of this possibility and encouraged to use other contraceptive methods. Postuse anovulation, possibly prolonged, may also occur in women without previous irregularities.

11. ECTOPIC PREGNANCY. Ectopic as well as intrauterine pregnancy may occur in contraceptive failures. However, in progestogen-only oral contraceptive failures, the ratio of ectopic to intrauterine pregnancies is higher than in women who are not receiving oral contraceptives, since the drugs are more effective in preventing intrauterine than ectopic pregnancies.

12. BREAST FEEDING. Oral contraceptives given in the postpartum period may interfere with lactation. There may be a decrease in the quantity and quality of the breast milk. Furthermore, a small fraction of the hormonal agents in oral contraceptives has been identified in the milk of mothers receiving these drugs.[45] The effects, if any, on the breast-fed child have not been determined. If feasible, the use of oral contraceptives should be deferred until the infant has been weaned.

PRECAUTIONS

General

1. A complete medical and family history should be taken prior to the initiation of oral contraceptives. The pretreatment and periodic physical examinations should include special reference to blood pressure, breasts, abdomen and pelvic organs, including Papanicolaou smear and relevant laboratory tests. As a general rule, oral contraceptives should not be prescribed for longer than one year without another physical examination being performed.

2. Under the influence of estrogen-progestogen preparations, preexisting uterine leiomyomata may increase in size.

3. Patients with a history of psychic depression should be carefully observed and the drug discontinued if depression recurs to a serious degree. Patients becoming significantly depressed while taking oral contraceptives should stop the medication and use an alternate method of contraception in an attempt to determine whether the symptom is drug-related.

4. Oral contraceptives may cause some degree of fluid retention. They should be prescribed with caution, and only with careful monitoring, in patients with conditions which might be aggravated by fluid retention, such as convulsive disorders, migraine syndrome, asthma, or cardiac or renal insufficiency.

5. Patients with a past history of jaundice during pregnancy have an increased risk of recurrence of jaundice while receiving oral contraceptive therapy. If jaundice develops in any patient receiving such drugs, the medication should be discontinued.

6. Steroid hormones may be poorly metabolized in patients with impaired liver function and should be administered with caution in such patients.

7. Oral contraceptive users may have disturbances in normal tryptophan metabolism which may result in a relative pyridoxine deficiency. The clinical significance of this is yet to be determined.

8. Serum folate levels may be depressed by oral contraceptive therapy. Since the pregnant woman is predisposed to the development of folate deficiency and the incidence of folate deficiency increases with increasing gestation, it is possible that if a woman becomes pregnant shortly after stopping oral contraceptives, she may have a greater chance of developing folate deficiency and complications attributed to this deficiency.

INFORMATION FOR THE PATIENT

(See Patient Labeling printed below.)

DRUG INTERACTIONS

Reduced efficacy and increased incidence of breakthrough bleeding have been associated with concomitant use of rifampin. A similar association has been suggested with barbiturates, phenylbutazone, phenytoin sodium, ampicillin, griseofulvin, and tetracycline.

Drug/Laboratory Test Interactions: The pathologist should be advised of oral contraceptive therapy when relevant specimens are submitted.

Certain endocrine and liver function tests and blood components may be affected by estrogen-containing oral contraceptives:

a. Increased sulfobromophthalein retention.

b. Increased prothrombin and factors VII, VIII, IX, and X; decreased antithrombin 3; increased norepinephrine-induced platelet aggregability.

c. Increased thyroid-binding globulin (TBG) leading to increased circulating total thyroid hormone, as measured by protein-bound iodine (PBI), T4 by column, or T4 by radioimmunoassay. Free T3 resin uptake is decreased, reflecting the elevated TBG, free T4 concentration is unaltered.

d. Decreased pregnanediol excretion.

e. Reduced response to metyrapone test.

Carcinogenesis, Mutagenesis, Impairment of Fertility: See WARNINGS section for information on carcinogenesis, mutagenesis and impairment of fertility.

Pregnancy: Pregnancy category X. See CONTRAINDICATIONS and WARNINGS.

Nursing Mothers: Because of the potential for tumorigenicity shown for oral contraceptives in animal and human studies, a decision should be made whether to discontinue the drug, taking into account the importance of the drug to the mother (see WARNINGS).

ADVERSE REACTIONS

An increased risk of the following serious adverse reactions has been associated with the use of oral contraceptives (see WARNINGS):

Thrombophlebitis	Hypertension.
Pulmonary embolism.	Gallbladder disease.
Coronary thrombosis.	Liver tumors.
Cerebral thrombosis.	Congenital anomalies.
Cerebral hemorrhage.	

There is evidence of an association between the following conditions and the use of oral contraceptives, although additional confirmatory studies are needed.

Mesenteric thrombosis.

Neuro-ocular lesion, e.g., retinal thrombosis and optic neuritis.

The following adverse reactions have been reported in patients receiving oral contraceptives and are believed to be drug-related:

Continued on next page

Ortho Pharm.—Cont.

Nausea and/or vomiting, usually the most common adverse reactions, occur in approximately 10 percent or less of patients during the first cycle. Other reactions, as a general rule, are seen much less frequently or only occasionally.

Gastrointestinal symptoms (such as abdominal cramps and bloating).

Breakthrough bleeding.
Spotting.
Change in menstrual flow.
Dysmenorrhea.
Amenorrhea during and after treatment.
Temporary infertility after discontinuance of treatment.
Edema.
Chloasma or melasma which may persist.
Breast changes: tenderness, enlargement, and secretion.
Change in weight (increase or decrease).
Change in cervical erosion and cervical secretion.
Possible diminution in lactation when given immediately postpartum.
Cholestatic jaundice.
Migraine.
Increase in size of uterine leiomyomata.
Rash (allergic).
Mental depression.
Reduced tolerance to carbohydrates.
Vaginal candidiasis.
Change in corneal curvature (steepening).
Intolerance to contact lenses.

The following adverse reactions have been reported in users of oral contraceptives, and the association has been neither confirmed nor refuted:

Premenstrual-like syndrome.
Cataracts.
Changes in libido.
Chorea.
Changes in appetite.
Cystitis-like syndrome.
Headache.
Nervousness.
Dizziness.
Hirsutism.
Loss of scalp hair.
Erythema multiforme.
Erythema nodosum.
Hemorrhagic eruption.
Vaginitis.
Porphyria.
Impaired renal function.
Hemolytic uremic syndrome.

OVERDOSAGE

Serious ill effects have not been reported following acute ingestion of large doses of oral contraceptives by young children. Overdosage may cause nausea, and withdrawal bleeding may occur in females.

DOSAGE AND ADMINISTRATION

To achieve maximum contraceptive effectiveness, ORTHO-NOVUM Tablets, MODICON Tablets and MICRONOR must be taken exactly as directed and at intervals not exceeding 24 hours.

21-DAY REGIMEN (Sunday Start)

When taking ORTHO-NOVUM 7/7/7□21, the first white tablet should be taken on the first Sunday after menstruation begins. If period begins on Sunday, the first white tablet is taken on that day. Tablets are taken as follows: One white tablet daily for 7 days, then one light peach tablet daily for 7 days, then one peach tablet for 7 days. For subsequent cycles, no tablets are taken for seven days, then a white tablet is taken the next day (Sunday), etc.

When taking ORTHO-NOVUM 10/11□21, the first white tablet should be taken on the first Sunday after menstruation begins. If period begins on Sunday, the first white tablet is taken on that day. Tablets are taken as follows: One white tablet daily for 10 days, then one peach tablet daily for 11 days. For subsequent cycles, no tablets are taken for 7 days, then a white tablet is taken the next day (Sunday) etc. Contraceptives reliance should not be placed on these products until after the first 7 consecutive days of administration.

The use of ORTHO-NOVUM 7/7/7□21 and ORTHO-NOVUM 10/11□21 for contraception may be initiated postpartum. When the tablets are administered during the postpartum period, the increased risk of thromboembolic disease associated with the postpartum period must be considered. (See CONTRAINDICATIONS, WARNINGS, and PRECAUTIONS concerning thromboembolic disease.) The possibility of ovulation and conception prior to initiation of medication should be considered. If the patient misses more than one tablet, the patient should begin taking tablets again as soon as remembered and another method of contraception used for the balance of that tablet cycle.

21-DAY REGIMEN (21 days on, 7 days off)

The dosage of ORTHO-NOVUM 1/35□21, MODICON 21, ORTHO-NOVUM 1/50□21, ORTHO-NOVUM 1/80□21 and ORTHO-NOVUM 2 mg□21 for the initial cycle of therapy is one tablet administered daily from the 5th day through the 25th day of the menstrual cycle, counting the first day of menstrual flow as "Day 1." The use of these products for contraception may be initiated postpartum. When the tablets are administered during the postpartum period, the increased risk of thromboembolic disease associated with the postpartum period must be considered. (See CONTRAINDICATIONS, WARNINGS, and PRECAUTIONS concerning thromboembolic disease.) If ORTHO-NOVUM 1/35□21, MODICON 21, ORTHO-NOVUM 1/50□21, ORTHO-NOVUM 1/80□21, and ORTHO-NOVUM 2 mg□21 are first taken later than the fifth day of the first menstrual cycle of medication or postpartum, contraceptive reliance should not be placed on these products until after the first seven consecutive days of administration. For subsequent cycles, no tablets are taken for 7 days, then a new course is started of one tablet a day for 21 days. The dosage regimen then continues with 7 days of no medication, followed by 21 days of medication, instituting a three-weeks-on, one-week-off dosage regimen. The possibility of ovulation and conception prior to initiation of medication should be considered. If the patient misses more than one tablet, the patient should begin taking tablets again as soon as remembered and another method of contraception used for the balance of that tablet cycle.

ORTHO-NOVUM 2 mg□21: Following three months of treatment of hypermenorrhea, medication may be discontinued to determine the need for further therapy.

(See discussion of Dose-Related Risk of Thromboembolism from Oral Contraceptives.)

28-DAY REGIMEN (Sunday Start)

When taking ORTHO-NOVUM 7/7/7□28, the first white tablet should be taken on the first Sunday after menstruation begins. If period begins on Sunday, the first white tablet is taken on that day. Tablets are taken without interruption as follows: One white tablet daily for 7 days, one light peach tablet daily for 7 days, one peach tablet daily for 7 days, then one green tablet daily for 7 days. After 28 tablets have been taken, a white tablet is then taken the next day (Sunday), etc.

When taking ORTHO-NOVUM 10/11□28, the first white tablet should be taken on the first Sunday after menstruation begins. If period begins on Sunday, the first white tablet is taken on that day. Tablets are taken without interruption as follows: one white tablet daily for 10 days, one peach tablet daily for 11 days, then one green tablet daily for 7 days. After 28 tablets have been taken, a white tablet is then taken the next day (Sunday) etc.

When taking ORTHO-NOVUM 1/35□28, the first peach tablet should be taken on the first Sunday after mestruation begins. When taking MODICON 28 or ORTHO-NOVUM 1/80□28, the first white tablet should be taken on the first Sunday after menstruation begins. When taking ORTHO-NOVUM 1/50□28, the first yellow tablet should be taken on the first Sunday after menstruation begins. If period begins on Sunday, the first peach tablet, white tablet or yellow tablet is taken on that day. Tablets are taken without interruption as follows: One peach, white or yellow tablet daily for 21 days, then one green tablet daily for 7 days. After 28 tablets have been taken, a peach, white or yellow tablet is then taken the next day (Sunday) etc. Contraceptive reliance should not be placed on these products until after the first 7 consecutive days of administration.

The use of ORTHO-NOVUM 7/7/7□28, ORTHO-NOVUM 10/11□ 28, ORTHO-NOVUM 1/35□28, MODICON 28, ORTHO-NOVUM 1/50□28, and ORTHO-NOVUM 1/80□28 for contraception may be initiated postpartum. When the tablets are administered during the postpartum period, the increased risk of thromboembolic disease associated with the postpartum period must be considered. (See CONTRAINDICATIONS, WARNINGS, and PRECAUTIONS concerning thromboembolic disease.) The possibility of ovulation and conception prior to initiation of medication should be considered. If the patient misses more than one tablet, the patient should begin taking tablets again as soon as remembered and another method of contraception used for the balance of that tablet cycle.

MICRONOR (Continuous Regimen)

MICRONOR (norethindrone) is administered on a continuous daily dosage regimen starting on the first day of menstruation, i.e., one tablet each day, every day of the year. Tablets should be taken at the same time each day and continued daily. The patient should be advised that if prolonged bleeding occurs, she should consult her physician.

The use of MICRONOR for contraception may be initiated postpartum (see WARNINGS section). When MICRONOR is administered during the postpartum period, the increased risk of thromboembolic disease associated with the postpartum period must be considered. (See CONTRAINDICATIONS, WARNINGS, and PRECAUTIONS concerning thromboembolic disease.)

If the patient misses one tablet, MICRONOR should be discontinued immediately and a method of nonhormonal contraception should be used until menses has appeared or pregnancy has been excluded.

Alternatively, if the patient has taken the tablets correctly, and if menses does not appear when expected, a nonhormonal method of contraception should be substituted until an appropriate diagnostic procedure is performed to rule out pregnancy.

All Oral Contraceptives

Breakthrough bleeding, spotting, and amenorrhea are frequent reasons for patients discontinuing oral contraceptives. In breakthrough bleeding, as in all cases of irregular bleeding from the vagina, nonfunctional causes should be borne in mind. In undiagnosed persistent or recurrent abnormal bleeding from the vagina, adequate diagnostic measures are indicated to rule out pregnancy or malignancy. If pathology has been excluded, time or a change to another formulation may solve the problem. Changing to an oral contraceptive with a higher estrogen content, while potentially useful in minimizing menstrual irregularity, should be done only if necessary since this may increase the risk of thromboembolic disease.

Use of oral contraceptives in the event of a missed menstrual period:

1. If the patient has not adhered to the prescribed dosage regimen, the possibility of pregnancy should be considered after the first missed period (or after 45 days from the last menstrual period if the progestogen-only oral contraceptives are used) and oral contraceptives should be withheld until pregnancy has been ruled out.
2. If the patient has adhered to the prescribed regimen and misses two consecutive periods, pregnancy should be ruled out before continuing the contraceptive regimen.

HOW SUPPLIED

ORTHO-NOVUM 7/7/7□21 Tablets are available in a DIALPAK* Tablet Dispenser (NDC 0062-1780-15) containing 21 tablets. Each white tablet contains 0.5 mg of the progestational compound, norethindrone, together with 0.035 mg of the estrogenic compound, ethinyl estradiol. Each light peach tablet contains 0.75 mg of the progestational compound, norethindrone, together with 0.035 mg of the estrogenic compound, ethinyl estradiol. Each peach tablet contains 1 mg of the progestational compound, norethindrone, together with 0.035 mg of the estrogenic compound, ethinyl estradiol. The white tablets are unscored with "Ortho" and "535" debossed on each side; the light peach tablets are unscored with "Ortho" and "75" debossed on each side; the peach tablets are unscored with "Ortho" and "135" debossed on each side.

ORTHO-NOVUM 7/7/7□21 is available for clinic usage in a VERIDATE* Tablet Dispenser (unfilled) and VERIDATE Refills (NDC 0062-1780-20).

ORTHO-NOVUM 7/7/7□28 Tablets are available in a DIALPAK Tablet Dispenser (NDC 0062-1781-15) containing 28 tablets. Each white tablet contains 0.5 mg of the progestational compound, norethindrone, together with 0.035 mg of the estrogenic compound, ethinyl estradiol. Each light peach tablet contains 0.75 mg of the progestational compound, norethindrone, together with 0.035 mg of the estrogenic compound, ethinyl estradiol. Each peach tablet contains 1 mg of the progestational compound, norethindrone, together with 0.035 mg of the estrogenic compound, norethindrone, together with 0.035 mg of the estrogenic compound, ethinyl estradiol. Each green tablet contains inert ingredients. The white tablets are unscored with "Ortho" and "535" debossed on each side; the light peach tablets are unscored with "Ortho" and "75" debossed on each side; the peach tablets are unscored with "Ortho" and "135" debossed on each side.

ORTHO-NOVUM 7/7/7□28 is available for clinic usage in a VERIDATE Tablet Dispenser (unfilled) and VERIDATE Refills (NDC 0062-1781-20).

ORTHO-NOVUM 10/11□21 Tablets are available in a DIALPAK* Tablet Dispenser (NDC 0062-1770-15) containing 21 tablets. Each white tablet contains 0.5 mg of the progestational compound, norethindrone, together with a 0.035 mg of the estrogenic compound, ethinyl estradiol. Each peach tablet contains 1 mg of the progestational compound, norethindrone, together with 0.035 mg of the estrogenic compound, ethinyl estradiol. The white tablets are unscored with "Ortho" and "535" debossed on each side; the peach tablets are unscored with "Ortho" and "135" debossed on each side.

ORTHO-NOVUM 10/11□21 is available for clinic usage in a VERIDATE* Tablet Dispenser (unfilled) and VERIDATE Refills. (NDC 0062-1770-20).

ORTHO-NOVUM 10/11□28 Tablets are available in a DIALPAK Tablet Dispenser (NDC 0062-1771-15) containing 28 tablets. Each white tablet contains 0.5 mg of the progestational compound, norethindrone, together with 0.035 mg of the estrogenic compound, ethinyl estradiol. Each peach tablet contains 1 mg of the progestational compound, norethindrone, together with 0.035 mg of the estrogenic compound, ethinyl estradiol. Each green tablet contains inert ingredients. The white tablets are unscored with "Ortho" and "535" debossed on each side; the peach tablets are unscored with "Ortho" and "135" debossed on each side.

ORTHO-NOVUM 10/11□28 is available for clinic usage in VERIDATE Tablet Dispenser (unfilled) and VERIDATE Refills. (NDC 0062-1771-20).

ORTHO-NOVUM 1/35□21 Tablets (as peach unscored tablets with "Ortho" and "135" debossed on each side) are available in a DIALPAK Tablet Dispenser (NDC 0062-1760-15) containing 21 tablets. Each peach tablet contains 1 mg of the progestational compound, norethindrone, together with 0.035 mg of the estrogenic compound, ethinyl estradiol.

ORTHO-NOVUM 1/35□21 is available for clinic usage in a VERIDATE Tablet Dispenser (unfilled) and VERIDATE Refills. (NDC 0062-1760-20).

ORTHO-NOVUM 1/35□28 Tablets (as peach unscored tablets with "Ortho" and "135" debossed on each side) are available in a DIALPAK Tablet Dispenser (NDC 0062-1761-15) containing 28 tablets, 21 peach norethindrone with ethinyl estradiol tablets, and 7 green tablets containing inert ingredients. Each peach ORTHO-NOVUM 1/35□28 Tablet contains 1 mg of the progestational compound, norethindrone, together with 0.035 mg of the estrogenic compound, ethinyl estradiol.

ORTHO-NOVUM 1/35□28 is available for clinic usage in a VERIDATE Tablet Dispenser (unfilled) and VERIDATE Refills (NDC 0062-1761-20).

MODICON 21 Tablets (as white unscored tablets with "Ortho" and "535" debossed on each side) are available in a DIALPAK Tablet Dispenser (NDC 0062-1712-15) containing 21 tablets. Each white tablet contains 0.5 mg of the progestational compound, norethindrone, together with 0.035 mg of the estrogenic compound, ethinyl estradiol.

MODICON 21 is available for clinic usage in a VERIDATE Tablet Dispenser (unfilled) and VERIDATE Refills (NDC 0062-1712-20).

MODICON 28 Tablets (as white unscored tablets with "Ortho" and "535" debossed on each side) are available in a DIALPAK Tablet Dispenser (NDC 0062-1714-15) containing 28 tablets, 21 white norethindrone with ethinyl estradiol tablets and 7 green tablets containing inert ingredients. Each white MODICON 28 Tablet contains 0.5 mg of the progestational compound, norethindrone, together with 0.035 mg of the estrogenic compound, ethinyl estradiol.

MODICON 28 is available for clinic usage in a VERIDATE Tablet Dispenser (unfilled) and VERIDATE Refills (NDC 0062-1714-20).

ORTHO-NOVUM 1/50□21 Tablets (as yellow unscored tablets with "Ortho" and "150" debossed on each side) are available in a DIALPAK Tablet Dispenser (NDC 0062-1331-15) containing 21 tablets and a dispensing unit which contains one DIALPAK and two refills of 21 tablets each. Each yellow ORTHO-NOVUM 1/50□21 Tablet contains 1 mg of the progestational compound, norethindrone, together with 0.05 mg of the estrogenic compound, mestranol.

ORTHO-NOVUM 1/50□21 is available for clinic usage in a VERIDATE Tablet Dispenser (unfilled) and VERIDATE Refills (NDC 0062-1331-20).

ORTHO-NOVUM 1/50□28 Tablets (as yellow unscored tablets with "Ortho" and "150" debossed on each side) are available in a DIALPAK Tablet Dispenser (NDC 0062-1332-15) containing 28 tablets, 21 yellow norethindrone with mestranol tablets and 7 green tablets containing inert ingredients. Each yellow ORTHO-NOVUM 1/50□28 Tablet contains 1 mg of the progestational compound, norethindrone, together with 0.05 mg of the estrogenic compound, mestranol.

ORTHO-NOVUM 1/50□28 is available for clinic usage in a VERIDATE Tablet Dispenser (unfilled) and VERIDATE Refills (NDC 0062-1332-20).

ORTHO-NOVUM 1/80□21 Tablets (as white unscored tablets with "Ortho" and "1" debossed on each side) are available in a DIALPAK Tablet Dispenser (NDC 0062-1390-15) containing 21 tablets and a dispensing unit which contains one DIALPAK and two refills of 21 tablets each. Each white ORTHO-NOVUM 1/80□21 Tablet contains 1 mg of the progestational compound, norethindrone, together with 0.08 mg of the estrogenic compound, mestranol.

ORTHO-NOVUM 1/80□28 Tablets (as white unscored tablets with "Ortho" and "1" debossed on each side) are available in a DIALPAK Tablet Dispenser (NDC 0062-1391-15) containing 28 tablets, 21 white norethindrone with mestranol tablets and 7 green tablets containing inert ingredients. Each white ORTHO-NOVUM 1/80□28 Tablet contains 1 mg of the progestational compound, norethindrone, together with 0.08 mg of the estrogenic compound, mestranol.

ORTHO-NOVUM 1/80□28 is available for clinic usage in a VERIDATE Tablet Dispenser (unfilled) and VERIDATE Refills (NDC 0062-1391-20).

ORTHO-NOVUM 2 mg□21 Tablets (as white unscored tablets with "Ortho" and "2" debossed on each side) are available in a DIALPAK Tablet Dispenser (NDC 0062-1351-08) containing 21 tablets. Each white ORTHO-NOVUM 2 mg□21 Tablet contains 2 mg of the progestational compound, norethindrone, together with 0.10 mg of the estrogenic compound, mestranol.

MICRONOR Tablets (as lime unscored tablets with "Ortho" and "0.35" debossed on each side) are available in a DIALPAK Tablet Dispenser (NDC 0062-1411-01) containing 28 tablets. Each lime MICRONOR Tablet contains 0.35 mg of the progestational compound norethindrone.

MICRONOR is available for clinic usage in a VERIDATE Tablet Dispenser (unfilled) and VERIDATE Refills (NDC 0062-1411-23).

REFERENCES

1. "Population Reports," Series H, Number 2, May 1974; Series I, Number 1, June 1974; Series B, Number 2, January 1975; Series H, Number 3, 1975; Series H, Number 4, January 1976 (published by the Population Information Program, The George Washington University Medical Center, 2001 S. St. NW, Washington, D.C.). **2.** Inman, W.H.W., M.P. Vessey, B. Westerholm, and A. Engelund, "Thromboembolic disease and the steroidal content of oral contraceptives. A report to the Committee on Safety of Drugs," Brit Med J *2:* 203–209, 1970. **3.** Stolley, P.D., J.A. Tonascia, M.S. Tockman, P.E. Sartwell, A.H. Rutledge, and M.P. Jacobs, "Thrombosis with low-estrogen oral contraceptives," Am J Epidemiol *102:* 197–208, 1975. **4.** Royal College of General Practitioners, "Oral contraception and thromboembolic disease," J Coll Gen Pract *13:* 267–279, 1967. **5.** Inman, W.H.W. and M.P. Vessey, "Investigation of deaths from pulmonary, coronary, and cerebral thrombosis and embolism in women of childbearing age," Brit Med J *2:* 193–199, 1968. **6.** Vessey, M.P. and R. Doll, "Investigation of relation between use of oral contraceptives and thromboembolic disease. A further report," Brit Med J *2:* 651–657, 1969. **7.** Sartwell, P.E., A.T. Masi, F.G. Arthes, G.R. Greene and H.E. Smith, "Thromboembolism and oral contraceptives: an epidemiological case control study," Am J Epidemiol *90:* 365–380, 1969. **8.** Boston Collaborative Drug Surveillance Program, "Oral contraceptives and venous thromboembolic disease, surgically confirmed gall bladder disease and breast tumors," Lancet *1:* 1399–1404, 1973. **9.** Collaborative Group for the Study of Stroke in Young Women, "Oral contraception and increased risk of cerebral ischemia or thrombosis," N Engl J Med *288:* 871–878, 1973. **10.** Collaborative Group for the Study of Stroke in Young Women, "Oral contraceptives and strokes in young women: associated risk factors," JAMA *231:* 718–722, 1975. **11.** Mann, J.I. and W.H.W. Inman, "Oral contraceptives and death from myocardial infarction," Brit Med J *2:* 245–248, 1975. **12.** Mann, J.I., W.H.W. Inman, and M. Thorogood, "Oral contraceptive use in older women and fatal myocardial infarction," Brit Med J *2:* 445–447, 1976. **13.** Mann. J.I., M.P. Vessey, M. Thorogood, and R. Doll, "Myocardial infarction in young women with special reference to oral contraceptive practice," Brit Med J *2:* 241–245, 1975. **14.** Tietze, C., "New Estimate of Mortality Associated with Fertility Control," Family Planning Perspectives Vol. 9, No. 2, 74–76, 1977. **15.** Vessey, M.P., R. Doll, A.S. Fairbairn, and G. Glober, "Post-operative thromboembolism and the use of oral contraceptives," Brit Med J *3:* 123–126, 1970. **16.** Greene, G.R., and P.E. Sartwell, "Oral contraceptive use in patients with thromboembolism following surgery, trauma, or infection," Am J Pub Health *62:* 680–685, 1972. **17.** Smith, D.C., R. Prentice, D.J. Thompson, and W.L. Herrmann, "Association of exogenous estrogen and endometrial carcinoma," N Engl J Med *293:* 1164–1167, 1975. **18.** Ziel, H.K. and W.D. Finkle, "Increased risk of endometrial carcinoma among users of conjugated estrogens," N Engl J Med *293:* 1167–1170, 1975. **19.** Mack, T.N., M.C. Pike, B.E. Henderson, R.I. Pfeffer, V.R. Gerkins, M. Arthur, and S.E. Brown, "Estrogens and endometrial cancer in a retirement community," N Engl J Med *294:* 1262–1267, 1976. **20.** Silverberg, S.G., and E.L. Makowski, "Endometrial carcinoma in young women taking oral contraceptive agents," Obstet Gynecol *46:* 503–506, 1975. **21.** Vessey, M.P., R. Doll, and P.M. Sutton, "Oral contraceptives and breast neoplasia: a retrospective study," Brit Med J *3:* 719–724, 1972. **22.** Vessey, M.P., R. Doll, and K. Jones, "Oral contraceptives and breast cancer. Progress report of an epidemiological study," Lancet *1:* 941–943, 1975. **23.** Boston Collaborative Drug Surveillance Program, "Surgically confirmed gall bladder disease, venous thromboembolism and breast tumors in relation to postmenopausal estrogen therapy," N Engl J Med *290:* 15–19, 1974. **24.** Arthes, F.G., P.E. Sartwell, and E.F. Lewison, "The Pill, estrogens, and the breast. Epidemiological aspects," Cancer *28:* 1391–1394, 1971. **25.** Fasal, E., and R.S. Paffenbarger, "Oral contraceptives as related to cancer and benign lesions of the breast," J Natl Cancer Inst *55:* 767–773, 1975. **26.** Royal College of General Practitioners, "Oral Contraceptives and Health," London, Pitman, 1974. **27.** Ory, H., P. Cole, B. MacMahon and R. Hoover, "Oral contraceptives and reduced risk of benign breast diseases," N Engl J Med *294:* 419–422, 1976. **28.** Baum, J., F. Holtz, J.J. Bookstein, and E.W. Klein, "Possible association between benign hepatomas and oral contraceptives," Lancet *2:* 926–928, 1973. **29.** Mays, E.T., W.M. Christopherson, M.M. Mahr, and H.C. Williams, "Hepatic changes in young women ingesting contraceptive steroids. Hepatic hemorrhage and primary hepatic tumors," JAMA *235:* 730–732, 1976. **30.** Edmonsen, H.A., B. Henderson, and B. Benton, "Liver-cell adenomas associated with the use of oral contraceptives," N Engl J Med *294:* 470–472, 1976. **31.** Herbst, A.L., H. Ulfedler, and D.C. Poskanzer, "Adenocarcinoma of the vagina," N Engl J Med *284:* 878-881, 1971. **32.** Greenwald, P., J.J. Barlow, P.C. Nasca, and W. Burnett, "Vaginal cancer after maternal treatment with synthetic estrogens," N Engl J Med *285:* 390–392, 1971. **33.** Lanier, A.P., K.L. Noller, D.G. Decker, L. Elveback, and L.T. Kurland, "Cancer and stilbestrol. A follow-up of 1719 persons exposed to estrogen in utero and born 1943–1959," Mayo Clinic Pro *48:* 793–799, 1973. **34.** Herbst, A.L., R.J. Kurman, and R.E. Scully, "Vaginal and cervical abnormalities after exposure to stilbestrol in utero," Obstet Gynecol *40:* 287–298, 1972. **35.** Herbst, A.L., S.J. Robboy, G.J. Macdonald, and R.E. Scully, "The effects of local progesterone on stilbestrol-associated vaginal adenosis," Am J Obstet Gynecol *118:* 607–615, 1974. **36.** Herbst, A.L., D.C. Poskanzer, S.J. Robboy, L. Friedlander, and R.E. Scully, "Prenatal exposure to stilbestrol: a prospective comparison of exposed female offspring with unexposed controls," N Engl J Med *292:* 334–339, 1975. **37.** Stafi, A., R.F. Mattingly, D.V. Foley, W. Fetherston, "Clinical diagnosis of vaginal adenosis," Obstet Gynecol *43:* 118–128, 1974. **38.** Sherman, A.I., M. Goldrath, A. Berlin, V. Vakhariya, F. Banooni, W. Michaels, P. Goodman, and S. Brown, "Cervical-vaginal adenosis after in utero exposure to synthetic estrogens," Obstet Gynecol *44:* 531–545, 1974. **39.** Gal, I., B. Kirman, and J. Stern, "Hormone pregnancy tests and congenital malformation," Nature *216:* 83, 1967. **40.** Levy, E.P., A. Cohen, and F.C. Fraser, "Hormone treatment during pregnancy and congenital heart defects," Lancet *1:* 611, 1973. **41.** Nora, J.J. and A.H. Nora, "Birth defects and oral contraceptives," Lancet *1:* 941–942, 1973. **42.** Janerich, D.T., J.M. Piper, and D.M. Glebatis, "Oral contraceptives and congenital limb-reduction defects," N Engl J Med *291:* 697–700, 1974. **43.** Carr, D.H., "Chromosome studies in selected spontaneous abortions: I. Conception after oral contraceptives," Canad Med Assoc J *103:* 343–348, 1970. **44.** Wynn, V., J.W.H. Doar, and G.L. Mills, "Some effects of oral contraceptives on serum-lipid and lipoprotein levels," Lancet *2:* 720–723, 1966. **45.** Laumas, K.R., P.K. Malkani, S. Bhatnagar, and V. Laumas, "Radioactivity in the breast milk of lactating women after oral administration of 3 H-norethynodrel," Amer J Obstet Gynecol *98:* 411–413, 1967. **46.** Rooks, et al., "Epidemiology of Hepatocellular Ademona, the Role of Oral Contraceptive Use," JAMA *242:* 644, 1979. **47.** Herbst, A.L., P. Cole, T. Colton, S.J. Robboy, R. E. Scully, "Age-incidence and Risk of Diethylstilbestrol-related Clear Cell Adenocarcinoma of the Vagina and Cervix," Am J Obstet Gynecol, *128:* 43–50, 1977. **48.** Bibbo, M., M. Al-Naqeeb, I. Baccarini, W. Gill, M. Newton, K.M. Sleeper, M. Sonek, G.L. Wied, "Follow-up Study of Male and Female Offspring of DES-treated Mothers. A Preliminary Report," Jour of Repro Med, *15:* 29–32, 1975. **49.** Gill, W.B., G.F.B. Schumacher, M. Bibbo, "Structural and Functional Abnormalities in the Sex Organs of Male Offspring of Mothers Treated with Diethylstilbestrol (DES)," Jour of Repro Med, *16:* 147–153, 1976. **50.** Henderson, B.E., B. Senton, M. Cosgrove, J. Baptista, J. Aldrich, D. Townsend, W. Hart, T. Mack, "Urogenital Tract Abnormalities in Sons of Women Treated with Diethylstilbestrol," Pediatrics, *58:* 505–507, 1976. **51.** Heinonen, O.P., D. Slone, R.R. Nonson, E.B. Hook, S. Shapiro, "Cardiovascular Birth Defects and Antenatal Exposure to Female Sex Hormones," N Engl J Med, *296:* 67–70, 1977. **52.** Jain, A.K., "Mortality Risk Associated with the Use of Oral Contraceptives," Studies in Family Planning, *8:* 50–54, 1977. **53.** Beral, V., "Mortality Among Oral Contraceptive Users," Lancet, *2:* 727–731, 1977. **54.** Vessey, M.P., McPherson, K., and Johnson, B., "Mortality Among Women Participating in the Oxford/Family Planning Association Contraceptive Study," Lancet *2:* 731–733, 1977. **55.** Petitti, D.B., Wingerd, J., "Use of Oral Contraceptives, Cigarette Smoking, and Risk of Subarachnoid Haemorrhage," Lancet, 2:234–6, 1978. **56.** Slone, D., et al, "Risk of Myocardial Infarction in Relation to Current and Discontinued Use of Oral Contraceptives," N Engl J Med, 305:420–424, 1981. **57.** Royal College of General Practitioners, "Incidence of Arterial Disease Among Oral Contraceptive Users." J Coll Gen Pract 33:75–82, 1983. **58.** Henderson, B.E., S. Preston-Martin, H.A. Edmondson, R.L. Peters and M.C. Pike, "Hepatocellular carcinoma and oral contraceptives," Br. J. Cancer 48:437–440, 1983. **59.** Neuberger, J., D. Forman, R. Doll and R. Williams, "Oral Contraceptives and hepatocellular carcinoma," Brit Med J, 292:1355–1357, 1986. **60.** Forman, D., T.J. Vincent and R. Doll, "Cancer of the liver and the use of oral contraceptives," Brit Med J, 292:1357–1361, 1986.

Brief Summary Patient Package Insert

Cigarette smoking increases the risk of serious adverse effects on the heart and blood vessels from oral contraceptive use. This risk increases with age and with heavy smoking (15 or more cigarettes per day) and is quite marked in women over 35 years of age. Women who use oral contraceptives should not smoke.

Continued on next page

Ortho Pharm.—Cont.

Oral contraceptives taken as directed are about 99% effective in preventing pregnancy. (The mini-pill, however, is somewhat less effective.) Forgetting to take your pills increases the chance of pregnancy. Various drugs, such as antibiotics, may also decrease the effectiveness of oral contraceptives.
Women who have or have had clotting disorders, cancer of the breast or sex organs, unexplained vaginal bleeding, a stroke, heart attack, angina pectoris, or who suspect they may be pregnant should not use oral contraceptives.

Most side effects of the pill are not serious. The most common side effects are nausea, vomiting, bleeding between menstrual periods, weight gain, and breast tenderness. However, proper use of oral contraceptives requires that they be taken under your doctor's continuous supervision, because they can be associated with serious side effects which may be fatal. Fortunately, these occur very infrequently. The serious side effects are:

1. Blood clots in the legs, lungs, brain, heart or other organs and hemorrhage into the brain due to bursting of a blood vessel. There is evidence that these risks may continue for a number of years after stopping oral contraceptive use.
2. Liver tumors, which may rupture and cause severe bleeding.
3. Birth defects if the pill is taken while you are pregnant.
4. High blood pressure.
5. Gallbladder disease.

Some of the symptoms associated with these serious side effects are discussed in the detailed leaflet given you with your supply of pills. Notify your doctor if you notice any unusual physical disturbance while taking the pill.
The estrogen in oral contraceptives has been found to cause breast cancer and other cancers in certain animals. These findings suggest that oral contraceptives may also cause cancer in humans. However, studies to date in women taking currently marketed oral contraceptives have not confirmed that oral contraceptives cause cancer in humans.
The detailed leaflet describes more completely the benefits and risks of oral contraceptives. It also provides information on other forms of contraception. Read it carefully. If you have any questions, consult your doctor.
Caution: Oral contraceptives are of no value in the prevention or treatment of venereal disease.

Detailed Patient Labeling

PLEASE NOTE: **This labeling is revised from time to time as important new medical information becomes available. Therefore, please review this labeling carefully.**

What You Should Know About Oral Contraceptives: Oral contraceptives ("the pill") are the most effective way (except for sterilization) to prevent pregnancy. They are also convenient and, for most women, free of serious or unpleasant side effects. Oral contraceptives must always be taken under the continuous supervision of a physician.
The information in this leaflet under the headings "Who Should Not Use Oral Contraceptives," "The Dangers of Oral Contraceptives," and "How to Use Oral Contraceptives As Effectively As Possible, Once You Have Decided to Use Them" is also applicable when these drugs are used for other indications.
ORTHO-NOVUM 2 mg□21 may be prescribed for the treatment of hypermenorrhea.
It is important that any woman who considers using an oral contraceptive understand the risks involved. Although the oral contraceptives have important advantages over other methods of contraception, they have certain risks that no other method has. Only you can decide whether the advantages are worth these risks. This leaflet will tell you about the most important risks. It will explain how you can help your doctor prescribe the pill as safely as possible by telling him about yourself and being alert for the earliest signs of trouble. And it will tell you how to use the pill properly, so that it will be as effective as possible. There is more detailed information available in the leaflet prepared for doctors. Your pharmacist can show you a copy; you may need your doctor's help in understanding parts of it.

Who Should Not Use Oral Contraceptives:

A. If you have now, or have had in the past, any of the following conditions you should not use the pill:
1. Heart attack or stroke.
2. Clots in the legs or lungs.
3. Angina pectoris.
4. Known or suspected cancer of the breast or sex organs.
5. Unusual vaginal bleeding that has not yet been diagnosed.

B. If you are pregnant or suspect that you are pregnant, do not use the pill.

C. Cigarette smoking increases the risk of serious adverse effects on the heart and blood vessels from oral contraceptive use. This risk increases with age and with heavy smoking (15 or more cigarettes per day) and is quite marked in women over 35 years of age. Women who use oral contraceptives should not smoke.

D. If you have scanty or irregular periods or are a young woman without a regular cycle, you should use another method of contraception because, if you use the pill, you may have difficulty becoming pregnant or may fail to have menstrual periods after discontinuing the pill.

Deciding To Use Oral Contraceptives: If you do not have any of the conditions listed above and are thinking about using oral contraceptives, to help you decide, you need information about the advantages and risks of oral contraceptives and of other contraceptive methods as well. This leaflet describes the advantages and risks of oral contraceptives. Except for sterilization, the IUD and abortion, which have their own exclusive risks, the only risks of other methods of contraception are those due to pregnancy should the method fail. Your doctor can answer questions you may have with respect to other methods of contraception. He can also answer any questions you may have after reading this leaflet on oral contraceptives.

1. What Oral Contraceptives Are and How They Work. Oral contraceptives are of two types. The most common, often simply called "the pill," is a combination of an estrogen and a progestogen, the two kinds of female hormones. The amount of estrogen and progestogen can vary, but the amount of estrogen is most important because both the effectiveness and some of the dangers of oral contraceptives are related to the amount of estrogen. This kind of oral contraceptive works principally by preventing release of an egg from the ovary. When the amount of estrogen is 50 micrograms or more, and the pill is taken as directed, oral contraceptives are more than 99% effective (i.e., there would be less than one pregnancy if 100 women used the pill for one year). Pills that contain 20 to 35 micrograms of estrogen vary slightly in effectiveness, ranging from 98% to more than 99% effective.
The second type of oral contraceptive, often called the "mini-pill," contains only a progestogen. It works in part by preventing release of an egg from the ovary but also by keeping sperm from reaching the egg and by making the uterus (womb) less receptive to any fertilized egg that reaches it. The mini-pill is less effective than the combination oral contraceptive, about 97% effective. In addition, the progestogen-only pill has a tendency to cause irregular bleeding which may be quite inconvenient, or cessation of bleeding entirely. The progestogen-only pill is used despite its lower effectiveness in the hope that it will prove not to have some of the serious side effects of the estrogen-containing pill (see below) but it is not yet certain that the mini-pill does in fact have fewer serious side effects. The discussion below, while based mainly on information about the combination pills, should be considered to apply as well to the mini-pill.

2. Other Nonsurgical Ways to Prevent Pregnancy. As this leaflet will explain, oral contraceptives have several serious risks. Other methods of contraception have lesser risks or none at all. They are also less effective than oral contraceptives, but, used properly, may be effective enough for many women. The following table gives reported pregnancy rates (the number of women out of 100 who would become pregnant in one year) for these methods:

Pregnancies Per 100 Women Per Year

Intrauterine device (IUD), less than 1–6;
Diaphragm with spermicidal products (creams or jellies), 2–20;
Condom (rubber), 3–36; Aerosol foams, 2–29; Jellies and creams, 4–36;
Periodic abstinence (rhythm) all types, less than 1–47;
1. Calendar method, 14–47;
2. Temperature method, 1–20;
3. Temperature method—intercourse only in postovulatory phase, less than 1–7;
4. Mucus method, 1–25;

No contraception, 60–80.
The figures (except for the IUD) vary widely because people differ in how well they use each method. Very faithful users of the various methods obtain very good results, except for users of the calendar method of periodic abstinence (rhythm). Except for the IUD, effective use of these methods requires somewhat more effort than simply taking a single pill every morning, but it is an effort that many couples undertake successfully. Your doctor can tell you a great deal more about these methods of contraception.

3. The Dangers of Oral Contraceptives.

a. *Circulatory disorders (abnormal blood clotting, heart attack, and stroke due to hemorrhage).* Blood clots (in various blood vessels of the body) are the most common of the serious side effects of oral contraceptives. A clot can result in a stroke (if the clot is in the brain), a heart attack (if the clot is in a blood vessel of the heart), or a pulmonary embolus (a clot which forms in the legs or pelvis, then breaks off and travels to the lungs). Any of these can be fatal. Clots also occur rarely in the blood vessels of the eye, resulting in blindness or impairment of vision in that eye. There is evidence that the risk of clotting increases with higher estrogen doses. It is therefore important to keep the dose of estrogen as low as possible, so long as the oral contraceptive used has an acceptable pregnancy rate and doesn't cause unacceptable changes in the menstrual pattern. Furthermore, cigarette smoking by oral contraceptive users increases the risk of serious adverse effects on the heart and blood vessels. This risk increases with age and with heavy smoking (15 or more cigarettes per day) and begins to become quite marked in women over 35 years of age. For this reason, women who use oral contraceptives should not smoke.

The risk of abnormal blood clotting increases with age in both users and nonusers of oral contraceptives, but the increased risk from the oral contraceptive appears to be present at all ages. For women aged 20 to 44 it is estimated that about 1 in 2,000 using oral contraceptives will be hospitalized each year because of abnormal clotting. Among nonusers in the same age group, about 1 in 20,000 would be hospitalized each year. For oral contraceptive users in general, it has been estimated that in women between the ages of 15 and 34 the risk of death due to a circulatory disorder is about 1 in 12,000 per year, whereas for nonusers the rate is about 1 in 50,000 per year. In the age group 35 to 44, the risk is estimated to be about 1 in 2,500 per year for oral contraceptive users and about 1 in 10,000 per year for nonusers.
Even without the pill the risk of having a heart attack increases with age and is also increased by such heart attack risk factors as high blood pressure, high cholesterol, obesity, diabetes, and cigarette smoking. Without any risk factors present, the use of oral contraceptives alone may double the risk of heart attack. However, the combination of cigarette smoking, especially heavy smoking, and oral contraceptive use greatly increases the risk of heart attack. Oral contraceptive users who smoke are about five times more likely to have a heart attack than users who do not smoke and about ten times more likely to have a heart attack than nonusers who do not smoke. It has been estimated that users between the ages of 30 and 39 who smoke have about a 1-in-10,000 chance each year of having a fatal heart attack compared to about a 1-in-50,000 chance in users who do not smoke, and about a 1-in-100,000 chance in nonusers who do not smoke. In the age group 40 to 44, the risk is about 1 in 1,700 per year for users who smoke compared to about 1 in 10,000 for users who do not smoke and to about one in 14,000 per year for nonusers who do not smoke. Heavy smoking (about 15 cigarettes or more a day) further increases the risk. If you do not smoke and have none of the other heart attack risk factors described above, you will have a smaller risk than listed. If you have several heart attack risk factors, the risk may be considerably greater than listed.
In addition to blood clotting disorders, it has been estimated that women taking oral contraceptives are twice as likely as nonusers to have a stroke due to rupture of a blood vessel in the brain.
One report suggests that the risk of circulatory diseases appears to increase the longer you are on the pill.
Several reports suggest that an increased risk of heart attack, stroke and other blood clotting disorders may continue for a number of years after stopping oral contraceptives. There is also some evidence that the size of this continuing risk may be greater with longer duration of oral contraceptive use.

b. *Formation of tumors.* Studies have found that when certain animals are given the female sex hormone estrogen, which is an ingredient of oral contraceptives, continuously for long periods, cancers may develop in the breast, cervix, vagina, and liver.
These findings suggest that oral contraceptives may cause cancer in humans. However, studies to date in women taking currently marketed oral contraceptives have not confirmed that oral contraceptives cause cancer in humans. Several studies have found no increase in breast cancer in users, although one study suggested oral contraceptives might cause an increase in breast cancer in women who already have benign breast disease (e.g., cysts).
Women with a strong family history of breast cancer or who have breast nodules, fibrocystic disease, or abnormal mammograms or who were exposed to DES (diethylstilbestrol), an estrogen, during their mother's pregnancy must be followed very closely by their doctors if they choose to use oral contraceptives instead of another method of contraception.
Many studies have shown that women taking oral contraceptives have less risk of getting benign breast disease than those who have not used oral contraceptives. Recently, strong evidence has emerged that estrogens (one component of oral contraceptives), when given for periods of more than one year to women after the menopause, increase the risk of cancer of the uterus (womb). There is also some evidence that a kind of oral contraceptive which is no longer marketed, the sequential oral contraceptive, may increase the risk of cancer of the uterus. There remains no evidence, however, that the oral contraceptives now available increase the risk of this cancer.
Oral contraceptives do cause, although rarely, a benign (nonmalignant) tumor of the liver. These tumors do not spread, but they may rupture and cause internal bleeding, which

may be fatal. A few studies have reported an increased risk of rare malignant liver tumors in women taking oral contraceptives, particularly in users of long duration.

c. *Dangers to a developing child if oral contraceptives are used in or immediately preceding pregnancy.* Oral contraceptives should not be taken by pregnant women because they may damage the developing child. An increased risk of birth defects, including heart defects and limb defects, has been associated with the use of sex hormones, including oral contraceptives, in pregnancy. In addition, the developing female child whose mother has received DES (diethylstilbestrol), an estrogen, during pregnancy has a risk of getting cancer of the vagina or cervix in her teens or young adulthood. This risk is estimated to be about 1 to 4 in 1000 exposures. Abnormalities of the urinary and sex organs have been reported in male offspring so exposed. It is possible that other estrogens, such as the estrogens in oral contraceptives, could have the same effect in the child if the mother takes them during pregnancy.

If you stop taking oral contraceptives to become pregnant, your doctor may recommend that you use another method of contraception for a short while, for example three months. The reason for this is that there is evidence from studies in women who have had "miscarriages" soon after stopping the pill, that the lost fetuses are more likely to be abnormal. Whether there is an overall increase in "miscarriage" in women who become pregnant soon after stopping the pill as compared with women who do not use the pill is not known, but it is possible that there may be. If, however, you do become pregnant soon after stopping oral contraceptives, and do not have a miscarriage, there does not appear to be evidence that the baby has an increased risk of being abnormal.

d. *Gallbladder disease.* Women who use oral contraceptives have a greater risk than nonusers of having gallbladder disease requiring surgery. The increased risk may first appear within one year of use and may double after four or five years of use.

e. *Other side effects of oral contraceptives.* Some women using oral contraceptives experience unpleasant side effects. Some of these may be temporary. Your breasts may feel tender, nausea and vomiting may occur, you may gain or lose weight, and your ankles may swell. A spotty darkening of the skin, particularly of the face, is possible and may persist. You may notice unexpected vaginal bleeding or changes in your menstrual period. Irregular bleeding is frequently seen when using the mini-pill or combination oral contraceptives containing less than 50 micrograms of estrogen.

More serious side effects include worsening of migraine, asthma, epilepsy, and kidney or heart disease because of a tendency for water to be retained in the body when oral contraceptives are used. Other side effects are growth of preexisting fibroid tumors of the uterus; mental depression; and liver problems with jaundice (yellowing of the skin). Your doctor may find that levels of sugar and fatty substances in your blood are elevated; the long-term effects of these changes are not known. Some women develop high blood pressure while taking oral contraceptives, which ordinarily returns to the original levels when the oral contraceptive is stopped.

Other reactions, although not proved to be caused by oral contraceptives, are occasionally reported. These include more frequent urination and some discomfort when urinating, kidney disease including blood cell breakdown with kidney failure, nervousness, dizziness, some loss of scalp hair, an increase in body hair, an increase or decrease in sex drive, appetite changes, cataracts, and a need for a change in contact lens prescription or inability to use contact lenses.

After you stop using oral contraceptives there may be a delay before you are able to become pregnant or before you resume having menstrual periods. This is especially true of women who had irregular menstrual cycles prior to the use of oral contraceptives. As discussed previously, your doctor may recommend that you wait a short while after stopping the pill before you try to become pregnant. During this time, use another form of contraception. You should consult your physician before resuming use of oral contraceptives after childbirth, especially if you plan to nurse your baby. Drugs in oral contraceptives are known to appear in the milk, and the long-range effect on infants is not known at this time. Furthermore, oral contraceptives may cause a decrease in your milk supply as well as in the quality of the milk.

4. Comparison of the Risks of Oral Contraceptives and Other Contraceptive Methods. The many studies on the risks and effectiveness of oral contraceptives and other methods of contraception have been analyzed to estimate the risk of death associated with various methods of contraception. This risk has two parts: (a) the risk of the method itself (e.g., the risk that oral contraceptives will cause death due to abnormal clotting), and (b) the risk of death due to pregnancy or abortion in the event the method fails. The results of this analysis are shown in the bar graph (Figure 1). The height of the bars is the number of deaths per 100,000 women each year. There are six sets of bars, each set referring to a specific age group of women. Within each set of bars there is a single bar for each of the different contraceptive methods. For oral contraceptives, there are two bars—one for smokers and the other for nonsmokers. The analysis is based on present knowledge and new information could, of course, alter it. The analysis shows that the risk of death from all methods of birth control is low and below that associated with childbirth, except for oral contraceptives in women over 40 who smoke. It shows that the lowest risk of death is associated with the condom or diaphragm (traditional contraception) backed up by early abortion in case of failure of the condom or diaphragm to prevent pregnancy. Also, at any age the risk of death (due to unexpected pregnancy) from the use of traditional contraception, even without a backup of abortion, is generally the same as or less than that from use of oral contraceptives.

How To Use Oral Contraceptives As Effectively As Possible, Once You Have Decided To Use Them:

1. What to Tell your Doctor.

You can make use of the pill as effectively as possible by telling your doctor if you have any of the following:

a. Conditions that mean you should not use oral contraceptives:

Clots in the legs or lungs.
Clots in the legs or lungs in the past.
A stroke, heart attack, or angina pectoris.
Known or suspected cancer of the breast or sex organs.
Unusual vaginal bleeding that has not yet been diagnosed.
Known or suspected pregnancy.

b. Conditions that your doctor will want to watch closely or which might cause him to suggest another method of contraception:

A family history of breast cancer.
Breast nodules, fibrocystic disease of the breast, or an abnormal mammogram.

Diabetes.	Heart or kidney disease.
High blood pressure.	Epilepsy.
High cholesterol.	Mental depression.
Cigarette smoking.	Fibroid tumors of the uterus.
Migraine headaches.	Gallbladder disease.

c. Once you are using oral contraceptives, you should be alert for signs of a serious adverse effect and call your doctor if they occur:

Sharp pain in the chest, coughing blood, or sudden shortness of breath (indicating possible clots in the lungs).
Pain in the calf (possible clot in the leg).
Crushing chest pain or heaviness (indicating possible heart attack).
Sudden severe headache or vomiting, dizziness or fainting, disturbance of vision or speech or weakness or numbness in an arm or leg (indicating a possible stroke).
Sudden partial or complete loss of vision (indicating a possible clot in the eye).
Breast lumps (you should ask your doctor to show you how to examine your own breasts).
Severe pain in the abdomen (indicating a possible ruptured tumor of the liver).
Severe depression.
Yellowing of the skin (jaundice).

2. How to Take the Pill So That it is Most Effective.

Reduced effectiveness and an increased incidence of breakthrough bleeding have been associated with the use of oral contraceptives with antibiotics such as rifampicin, ampicillin, griseofulvin, and tetracycline or with certain other drugs, such as barbiturates, phenylbutazone or phenytoin sodium. You should use an additional means of contraception during any cycle in which any of these drugs are taken. To achieve maximum contraceptive effectiveness, ORTHO-NOVUM, MODICON, and MICRONOR must be taken exactly as directed and at intervals not exceeding 24 hours.

ORTHO-NOVUM 7/7/7 Sunday-Start Package:

21-Day Regimen: The first white tablet should be taken on the first Sunday after the menstrual period begins. If period begins on Sunday, the first white tablet is taken on that day. Take one white tablet at the same time each day for 7 consecutive days, take one light peach tablet daily for 7 days, then take one peach tablet daily for 7 days. During the FIRST cycle, it is important that you use another method of birth control until you have taken a white tablet daily for seven consecutive days. After taking your last peach tablet, wait for seven days during which time a menstrual period usually occurs. After the seven-day waiting period, on Sunday, start taking a white tablet each day for the next 7 days; a light peach tablet for the next 7 days; then a peach tablet for the next 7 days, thus using a three-week-on, one-week-off regimen.

28-Day Regimen: The first white tablet should be taken on the first Sunday after the menstrual period begins. If period begins on Sunday, begin taking tablets that day. Take one white tablet at the same time each day for 7 consecutive days; take one light peach tablet daily for 7 days; take one peach tablet daily for 7 days, then take one green tablet daily for 7 days, during which time your period usually occurs. During the FIRST cycle, it is important that you use another method of birth control until you have taken a white tablet daily for seven consecutive days. After 28 tablets have been taken, (last green tablet will always be taken on Saturday) take the first tablet (white) from your next package the following day (Sunday) whether or not you are still menstruating. With the 28-day regimen, tablets are taken every day of the year.

ORTHO-NOVUM 10/11 — Sunday-Start Package

21-Day Regimen: The first white tablet should be taken on the first Sunday after the menstrual period begins. If period begins on Sunday, begin taking tablets that day. Take one white tablet at the same time each day for 10 consecutive days, then take one peach tablet daily for 11 days. During the FIRST cycle, it is important that you use another method of birth control until you have taken a white tablet daily for seven consecutive days. After taking your last peach tablet, wait for seven days during which time a menstrual period usually occurs. After the seven-day waiting period, on Sunday, start taking a white tablet each day for the next 10 days, then a peach tablet for the next 11 days, thus using a three-week-on, one-week-off regimen.

28-Day Regimen: The first white tablet should be taken on the first Sunday after the menstrual period begins. If period begins on Sunday, begin taking tablets that day. Take one white tablet at the same time each day for 10 consecutive days, take one peach tablet daily for 11 days, then take one green tablet daily for 7 days, during which time your period usually occurs. During the FIRST cycle, it is important that you use another method of birth control until you have taken a white tablet daily for seven consecutive days. After 28 tablets have been taken, (last green tablet will always be taken on a Saturday) take the first tablet (white) from your next package the following day (Sunday) whether or not you are still menstruating. With the 28-day regimen, pills are taken every day of the year.

ORTHO-NOVUM 1/35, MODICON, ORTHO-NOVUM 1/50, ORTHO-NOVUM 1/80 and ORTHO-NOVUM 2 mg

21-day Regimen: Counting the first day of menstrual flow as "Day 1," take one tablet daily from the 5th through the 25th day of the menstrual cycle. If the first tablet is taken later than the 5th day of the menstrual cycle or postpartum, contraceptive reliance should not be placed on ORTHO-NOVUM or MODICON until after the first seven consecutive days of administration. Take a tablet the same time each day, preferably at bedtime, for 21 days, then wait for 7 days during which time a menstrual period usually occurs. Following this 7-day waiting period, start taking a tablet each day for the next 21 days, thus using a three-weeks-on, one-week-off dosage regimen.

When ORTHO-NOVUM 2 mg□21 Tablets are used for the treatment of hypermenorrhea, your physician will discuss the regimen with you.

ORTHO-NOVUM 1/35, MODICON, ORTHO-NOVUM 1/50 and ORTHO-NOVUM 1/80.

28-Day Regimen: The first white, yellow or peach tablet should be taken on the first Sunday after the menstrual period begins. If period begins on Sunday, begin taking tablets that day. Take one white, yellow or peach tablet at the same time each day for 21 consecutive days, then take one green tablet daily for 7 days during which time your menstrual period usually occurs. During the FIRST cycle, it is important that you use another method of birth control until you have taken a white, yellow or peach tablet daily for seven consecutive days. After 28 tablets have been taken, (last green tablet will always be taken on a Saturday) take the first tablet (white, yellow or peach) from your next package the following day (Sunday) whether or not you are still menstruating. With the 28-day regimen, pills are taken every day of the year.

Continuous Regimen (MICRONOR): The first MICRONOR Tablet should be taken on the first day of the menstrual period.

Take one tablet at the same time each day without interruption for as long as contraceptive protection is desired. The effectiveness of progestogen-only oral contraceptives, such as MICRONOR, is lower than that of the combination oral contraceptives containing both estrogen and progestogen. If 100 women utilized an estrogen-containing oral contraceptive for a period of one year, generally less than one pregnancy would be expected to occur; however, if MICRONOR had been utilized, approximately three pregnancies might occur.

Women who participated in the clinical studies with MICRONOR and who had not taken other oral contraceptives before starting MICRONOR had a higher pregnancy rate (four women out of 100), particularly during the first six months of therapy, and to a large extent because they did not take their tablets correctly.

Of course, if you don't take your tablets as directed, or forget to take them every day, the chance you may become pregnant is naturally greater.

MICRONOR (norethindrone) will probably cause some changes in your menstrual pattern. Your cycle, that is the time between menstrual periods, will vary. For example, you might have a 28-day cycle, followed by a 17-day cycle, followed by a 35-day cycle, etc. This is common with MICRONOR.

Continued on next page

Ortho Pharm.—Cont.

While using MICRONOR, your period may be longer or shorter than before. If bleeding lasts more than eight days, be sure to let your doctor know.

At times there may be no menstrual period after a cycle of pills. Therefore, if you miss one menstrual period but have taken the pills *exactly as you were supposed to,* continue as usual into the next cycle. If you have not taken them correctly and miss a menstrual period, or if you are taking minipills and it is 45 days or more from the start of your last menstrual period, you may be pregnant and should stop taking oral contraceptives until your doctor determines whether or not you are pregnant. Until you can get to your doctor, use another form of contraception. If two consecutive menstrual periods are missed, you should stop taking pills until it is determined whether you are pregnant. If you do become pregnant while using oral contraceptives, you should discuss the risks to the developing child with your doctor.

3. Periodic Examination.

Your doctor will take a complete medical and family history before prescribing oral contraceptives. At that time and about once a year thereafter, he will generally examine your blood pessure, breasts, abdomen, and pelvic organs (including a Papanicolaou smear, i.e., test for cancer).

SUMMARY

Oral contraceptives are the most effective method, except sterilization, for preventing pregnancy. Other methods, when used conscientiously, are also very effective and have fewer risks.

Women who use oral contraceptives should not smoke.

In addition, if you have certain conditions or have had these conditions in the past, you should not use oral contraceptives because the risk is too great. These conditions are listed in the booklet. If you do not have these conditions and decide to use the "pill," please read the booklet carefully so that you can use the "pill."

Based on his or her assessment of your medical needs, your doctor has prescribed this drug for you. Do not give the drug to anyone else.

Revised August 1985

Shown in Product Identification Section, page 419

PROTOSTAT® ℞
(metronidazole) Tablets

> **WARNING**
> Metronidazole has been shown to be carcinogenic in mice and rats. *(See Warnings.)* Unnecessary use of this drug should be avoided. Its use should be reserved for the conditions described in the *Indications And Usage* section below.

DESCRIPTION

PROTOSTAT (metronidazole) is a 1-(β-hydroxyethyl)-2-methyl-5-nitroimidazole. Both the 250 mg and 500 mg tablets include the following inactive ingredients: Lactose, magnesium stearate, microcrystalline cellulose, povidone, sodium starch glycolate, and stearic acid. Metronidazole is classified therapeutically as an antiprotozoal *(Trichomonas),* and antibacterial (antianaerobic) agent. It occurs as pale yellow crystals that are slightly soluble in water and alcohol. Metronidazole has the following structural formula:

CLINICAL PHARMACOLOGY

Metronidazole is usually well absorbed after oral administration, with peak plasma concentrations occurring between one and two hours. An average elimination half-life is 8 hours in healthy humans. Plasma concentrations of metronidazole are proportional to the administered dose. Oral administration of 250 mg., 500 mg., or 2,000 mg. produced peak plasma concentrations of 6 mcg/ml, 12 mcg/ml, and 40 mcg/ml, respectively. Studies reveal no significant bioavailability differences between males and females; however, because of weight differences, the resulting plasma levels in males are generally lower.

Metronidazole is the major component appearing in the plasma, with lesser quantities of the 2-hydroxymethyl metabolite also being present. Less than 20% of the circulating metronidazole is bound to plasma proteins. Both the parent compound and the metabolite possess *in vitro* trichomonacidal activity and *in vitro* bactericidal activity against most strains of anaerobic bacteria.

The major route of elimination of metronidazole and its metabolites is via the urine (60-80% of the dose), with fecal excretion accounting for 6-15% of the dose. The metabolites that appear in the urine result primarily from side-chain oxidation [1-(β-hydroxyethyl)-2-hydroxymethyl-5-nitroimidazole and 2-methyl-5-nitroimidazole-1-yl-acetic acid] and glucuronide conjugation, with unchanged metronidazole accounting for approximately 20% of the total. Renal clearance of metronidazole is approximately 10 ml/min/1.73m^2.

Decreased renal function does not alter the single-dose pharmacokinetics of metronidazole. However, plasma clearance of metronidazole is decreased in patients with decreased liver function.

Metronidazole appears in cerebrospinal fluid, saliva, and breast milk in concentrations similar to those found in plasma. Bactericidal concentrations of metronidazole have also been detected in pus from hepatic abscesses.

Microbiology: Metronidazole possesses direct trichomonacidal and amoebicidal activity against *Trichomonas Vaginalis* and *Entamoeba histolytica.* The *in vitro* minimal inhibitory concentration (MIC) for most strains of these organisms is 1 mcg/ml or less. Metronidazole's mechanism of antiprotozoal action is unknown.

Anaerobic Bacteria: Metronidazole is active *in vitro* against obligate anaerobes, but does not appear to possess any clinically relevant activity against facultative anaerobes or obligate aerobes. Against susceptible organisms, metronidazole is generally bactericidal at concentrations equal to or slightly higher than the minimal inhibitory concentrations (MIC). Metronidazole has been shown to have *in vitro* and clinical activity against the following organisms:

Anaerobic gram-negative bacilli, including:
Bacteroides species, including the *Bacteroides fragilis* group *(B. fragilis, B. distasonis, B. ovatus, B. thetaiotaomicron, B. vulgatus)*
Fusobacterium species
Anaerobic gram-positive bacilli, including:
Clostridium species and susceptible strains of *Eubacterium*
Anaerobic gram-positive cocci, including:
Peptococcus species
Peptostreptococcus species

Susceptibility tests: Bacteriologic studies should be performed to determine the causative organisms and their susceptibility to metronidazole; however, the rapid, routine susceptibility testing of individual isolates of anaerobic bacteria is not always practical, and therapy may be started while awaiting these results.

Quantitative methods give the most precise estimates of susceptibility to antibacterial drugs. A standardized agar dilution method and a broth microdilution method are recommended.[1]

Control strains are recommended for standardized susceptibility testing. Each time the test is performed, one or more of the following strains should be included: *Clostridium perfringens* ATCC 13124, *Bacteroides fragilis* ATCC 25285, and *Bacteroides thetaiotaomicron* ATCC 29741. The mode metronidazole MIC's for those three strains are reported to be 0.25, 0.25, and 0.5 mcg/ml, respectively.

A clinical laboratory is considered under acceptable control if the results of the control strains are within one doubling dilution of the mode MIC's reported for metronidazole.

A bacterial isolate may be considered susceptible if the MIC value for metronidazole is not more than 16 mcg/ml. An organism is considered resistant if the MIC is greater than 16 mcg/ml. A report of "resistant" from the laboratory indicates that the infecting organism is not likely to respond to therapy.

INDICATIONS AND USAGE

Symptomatic Trichomoniasis: PROTOSTAT is indicated for the treatment of symptomatic trichomoniasis in females and males when the presence of trichomonad has been confirmed by appropriate laboratory procedures (wet smears and/or cultures).

Asymptomatic Trichomoniasis: PROTOSTAT is indicated in the treatment of asymptomatic females when the organism is associated with endocervicitis, cervicitis, or cervical erosion. Since there is evidence that presence of the trichomonad can interfere with accurate assessment of abnormal cytological smears, additional smears should be performed after eradication of the parasite.

Treatment of Asymptomatic Consorts: T. vaginalis infection is a venereal disease. Therefore, asymptomatic sexual partners of treated patients should be treated simultaneously if the organism has been found to be present in order to prevent reinfection of the partner. The decision as to whether to treat an asymptomatic male partner with a negative culture or one in whom no culture has been attempted is an individual one. In making this decision, it should be noted that there is evidence that women may become reinfected if the consort is not treated. Also, since there can be considerable difficulty in isolating the organism from the asymptomatic male carrier, negative smears and cultures cannot be relied upon in this regard. In any event, the consort should be treated with PROTOSTAT in cases of reinfection.

Amoebiasis: PROTOSTAT is indicated in the treatment of acute intestinal amoebiasis (amoebic dysentery) and amoebic liver abscess.

In amoebic liver abscess, PROTOSTAT therapy does not obviate the need for aspiration or drainage of pus.

Anaerobic Bacterial Infections: PROTOSTAT is indicated in the treatment of serious infections caused by susceptible anaerobic bacteria. Indicated surgical procedures should be performed in conjunction with PROTOSTAT therapy. In a mixed aerobic and anaerobic infection, antibiotics appropriate for the treatment of aerobic infection should be used in addition to PROTOSTAT. In the treatment of most serious anaerobic infections the intravenous form of metronidazole is usually administered initially. This may be followed by oral therapy with PROTOSTAT at the discretion of the physician.

INTRA-ABDOMINAL INFECTION, including peritonitis, intra-abdominal abscess, and liver abscess, caused by *Bacteroides* species including the *B. fragilis* group *(B. fragilis, B. distasonis, B. ovatus, B. thetaiotaomicron, B. vulgatus), Clostridium* species, *Eubacterium* species, *Peptococcus* species, and *Peptostreptococcus* species.

SKIN AND SKIN STRUCTURE INFECTIONS caused by *Bacteroides* species including the *B. fragilis* group, *Clostridium* species, *Peptococcus* species, *Peptostreptococcus* species, and *Fusobacterium* species.

GYNECOLOGIC INFECTIONS, including endometritis, endomyometritis, tubo-ovarian abscess, and post-surgical vaginal cuff infection, caused by *Bacteroides* species including the *B. fragilis* group, *Clostridium* species, *Peptococcus* species, and *Peptostreptococcus* species.

BACTERIAL SEPTICEMIA caused by *Bacteroides* species including the *B. fragilis* group, and *Clostridium* species.

BONE AND JOINT INFECTIONS, as adjunctive therapy, caused by *Bacteroides* species including the *B. fragilis* group.

CENTRAL NERVOUS SYSTEM (CNS) INFECTIONS, including meningitis and brain abscess, caused by *Bacteroides* species including the *B. fragilis* group.

LOWER RESPIRATORY TRACT INFECTIONS, including pneumonia, empyema, and lung abscess, caused by *Bacteroides* species including the *B. fragilis* group.

ENDOCARDITIS caused by *Bacteroides* species including the *B. fragilis* group.

CONTRAINDICATIONS

PROTOSTAT is contraindicated in patients with a prior history of hypersensitivity to metronidazole or other nitroimidazole derivatives. In patients with trichomoniasis, PROTOSTAT is contraindicated during the first trimester of pregnancy. *(See Warnings.)*

WARNINGS

Convulsive Seizures and Peripheral Neuropathy: Convulsive seizures and peripheral neuropathy, the latter characterized mainly by numbness or paresthesia of an extremity, have been reported in patients treated with metronidazole. The appearance of abnormal neurologic signs demands the prompt discontinuation of PROTOSTAT therapy. PROTOSTAT should be administered with caution to patients with central nervous system diseases.

Tumorigenicity Studies in Rodents: Metronidazole has shown evidence of carcinogenic activity in a number of studies involving chronic, oral administration in mice and rats. Prominent among the effects in the mouse was the promotion of pulmonary tumorigenesis. This has been observed in all six reported studies in that species, including one study in which the animals were dosed on an intermittent schedule (administration during every fourth week only). At very high dose levels (approx. 500mg/kg/day) there was a statistically significant increase in the incidence of malignant liver tumors in males. Also, the published results of one of the mouse studies indicated an increase in the incidence of malignant lymphomas as well as pulmonary neoplasms associated with lifetime feeding of the drug. All these effects are statistically significant.

Several long-term oral dosing studies in the rats have been completed. There was a statistically significant increase in the incidence of various neoplasms, particularly in mammary and hepatic tumors, among female rats administered metronidazole over those noted in the concurrent female control groups.

Two lifetime tumorigenicity studies in hamsters have been performed and reported to be negative.

Mutagenicity Studies: Although metronidazole has shown mutagenic activity in a number of *in vitro* assay systems, studies in mammals (*in vivo*) have failed to demonstrate a potential for genetic damage.

PRECAUTIONS

General: Patients with severe hepatic disease metabolize metronidazole slowly, with resultant accumulation of metronidazole and its metabolites in the plasma. Accordingly, for such patients, doses below those usually recommended should be administered cautiously.

Known or previously unrecognized candidiasis may present more prominent symptoms during therapy with

PROTOSTAT and requires treatment with a candicidal agent.

Laboratory Tests: PROTOSTAT (metronidazole) is a nitroimidazole and should be used with care in patients with evidence of, or history of, blood dyscrasia. A mild leukopenia has been observed during its administration; however, no persistent hematologic abnormalities attributable to metronidazole have been observed in clinical studies. Total and differential leukocyte counts are recommended before and after therapy for trichomoniasis and amoebiasis, especially if a second course of therapy is necessary, and before and after therapy for anaerobic infection.

Drug Interactions: Metronidazole has been reported to potentiate the anticoagulant effect of coumarin and warfarin resulting in a prolongation of prothrombin time. This possible drug interaction should be considered when PROTOSTAT is prescribed for patients on this type of anticoagulant therapy.

Alcoholic beverages should not be consumed during PROTOSTAT therapy because abdominal cramps, nausea, vomiting, headache, and flushing may occur.

The simultaneous administration of drugs that induce microsomal liver enzymes, such as phenytoin or phenobarbital, may accelerate the elimination of metronidazole, resulting in reduced plasma levels.

Drug/Laboratory Test Interactions: Metronidazole may interfere with certain chemical analyses for serum glutamic oxalacetic transaminase, resulting in decreased values. Values of zero may be observed.

Carcinogenesis: (See Warnings.)

Pregnancy: Teratogenic Effects—Pregnancy Category B: Metronidazole crosses the placental barrier and enters the fetal circulation rapidly. Reproduction studies have been performed in rabbits and rats at doses up to five times the human dose and have revealed no evidence of impaired fertility or harm to the fetus due to metronidazole. There are, however, no adequate and well-controlled studies in pregnant women. Because animal reproduction studies are not always predictive of human response, and because metronidazole is a carcinogen in rodents, this drug should be used during pregnancy only if clearly needed. *(See Contraindications.)*

Use of PROTOSTAT for trichomoniasis in the second and third trimesters should be restricted to those in whom local palliative treatment has been inadequate to control symptoms.

Nursing Mothers: Because of the potential for tumorigenicity shown for metronidazole in mouse and rat studies, a decision should be made whether to discontinue nursing or to discontinue the drug, taking into account the importance of the drug to the mother. Metronidazole is secreted in breast milk in concentrations similar to those found in plasma.

Pediatric Use: Safety and effectiveness in children have not been established, except for the treatment of amoebiasis.

ADVERSE REACTIONS

The two most serious adverse reactions reported in patients treated with PROTOSTAT (metronidazole) have been convulsive seizures and peripheral neuropathy, the latter characterized mainly by numbness or paresthesia of an extremity. Since persistent peripheral neuropathy has been reported in some patients receiving prolonged administration of PROTOSTAT, patients should be specifically warned about these reactions and should be told to stop the drug and report immediately to their physicians if any neurologic symptoms occur.

The most common adverse reactions reported have been referable to the gastrointestinal tract, particularly nausea, sometimes accompanied by headache, anorexia, and occasionally vomiting; diarrhea; epigastric distress; and abdominal cramping. Constipation has also been reported.

The following reactions have also been reported during treatment with PROTOSTAT (metronidazole):

Mouth: A sharp, unpleasant metallic taste is not unusual. Furry tongue, glossitis, and stomatitis have occurred; these may be associated with a sudden overgrowth of *Candida* which may occur during effective therapy.

Hematopoietic: Reversible neutropenia (leukopenia).

Cardiovascular: Flattening of the T-wave may be seen in electrocardiographic tracings.

Central Nervous System: Convulsive seizures, peripheral neuropathy, dizziness, vertigo, incoordination, ataxia, confusion, irritability, depression, weakness, and insomnia.

Hypersensitivity: Urticaria, erythematous rash, flushing, nasal congestion, dryness of mouth (or vagina or vulva), and fever.

Renal: Dysuria, cystitis, polyuria, incontinence, and a sense of pelvic pressure. Instances of darkened urine have been reported, and this manifestation has been the subject of a special investigation. Although the pigment which is probably responsible for this phenomenon has not been positively identified, it is almost certainly a metabolite of metronidazole and seems to have no clinical significance.

Other: Proliferation of *Candida* in the vagina, dyspareunia, decrease of libido, proctitis, and fleeting joint pains sometimes resembling "serum sickness." If patients receiving PROTOSTAT drink alcoholic beverages, they may experience abdominal distress, nausea, vomiting, flushing, or headache. A modification of the taste of alcoholic beverages has also been reported.

OVERDOSAGE

Single oral doses of metronidazole, up to 15 g, have been reported in suicide attempts and accidental overdoses. Symptoms reported include nausea, vomiting, and ataxia. Oral metronidazole has been studied as a radiation sensitizer in the treating of malignant tumors. Neurotoxic effects, including seizures and peripheral neuropathy, have been reported after 5 to 7 days of doses of 6 to 10.4 g every other day.

Treatment: There is no specific antidote for PROTOSTAT overdose; therefore, management of the patient should consist of symptomatic and supportive therapy.

DOSAGE AND ADMINISTRATION

Trichomoniasis:

In The Female: One-day treatment—two grams of PROTOSTAT given either as a single dose or in two divided doses of one gram each given in the same day.

Seven-day course of treatment—250 mg three times daily for seven consecutive days. There is some indication from controlled comparative studies that cure rates as determined by vaginal smears, signs and symptoms, may be higher after a seven-day course of treatment than after a one-day treatment regimen.

The dosage regimen should be individualized. Single-dose treatment can assure compliance, especially if administered under supervision, in those patients who cannot be relied on to continue the seven-day regimen.

A seven-day course of treatment may minimize reinfection of the female long enough to treat sexual contacts. Further, some patients may tolerate one course of therapy better than the other.

Pregnant patients should not be treated during the first trimester with either regimen. If treated during the second or third trimester, the one-day course of therapy should not be used, as it results in higher serum levels which reach the fetal circulation. *(See Contraindications and Precautions.)*

When repeated courses of the drug are required, it is recommended that an interval of four to six weeks elapse between courses and that the presence of the trichomonad be reconfirmed by appropriate laboratory measures. Total and differential leukocyte counts should be made before and after treatment.

In The Male: Treatment should be individualized as for the female.

Amoebiasis: Adults: For Acute Intestinal Amoebiasis (Acute Amoebic Dysentery):

750 mg. orally 3 times daily for 5 to 10 days.

For Amoebic Liver Abscess: 500 mg or 750 mg orally 3 times daily for 5 to 10 days.

Children: 35 to 50 mg/kg of body weight/24 hours divided into 3 doses, orally for 10 days.

Anaerobic Bacterial Infections: In the treatment of most serious anaerobic infections the intravenous form of metronidazole is usually administered initially.

Following intravenous therapy, oral metronidazole may be used when conditions warrant based upon the severity of the disease and the response of the patient to intravenous treatment.

The usual adult *oral* dosage is 7.5 mg/kg every six hours (approximately 500 mg for a 70 kg adult). A maximum of 4.0 g should not be exceeded during a 24-hour period.

The usual duration of therapy is 7 to 10 days; however, infections of the bone and joint, lower respiratory tract, and endocardium may require longer treatment.

Patients with severe hepatic disease metabolize metronidazole slowly, with resultant accumulation of metronidazole and its metabolites in the plasma. Accordingly, for such patients, doses below those usually recommended should be administered cautiously. Close monitoring of plasma metronidazole levels[2] and toxicity is recommended.

The dose of PROTOSTAT should not be specifically reduced in anuric patients since accumulated metabolites may be rapidly removed by dialysis.

HOW SUPPLIED

Available in tablets containing 250 mg. and 500 mg. of metronidazole, USP. PROTOSTAT 250 mg. is a white to off-white capsule-shaped, convex tablet. Each 250 mg. PROTOSTAT Tablet is scored on one side and imprinted with ORTHO 1570 on the other side, packaged in a bottle of 100 tablets (NDC 0062-1570-01). PROTOSTAT 500 mg. is a white to off-white capsule-shaped, convex tablet. Each 500 mg. PROTOSTAT tablet is scored on one side and imprinted with ORTHO 1571 on the other side, packaged in a bottle of 50 tablets (NDC 0062-1571-01).

Dispense in well-closed, light-resistant containers as defined in the USP.

Store below 86°F (30°C).

1. Proposed standard: PSM-11—Proposed Reference Dilution Procedure for Antimicrobic Susceptibility Testing of Anaerobic Bacteria, National Committee for Clinical Laboratory Standards, and Sutter, et al: Collaborative Evaluation of a Proposed Reference Dilution Method of Susceptibility Testing of Anaerobic Bacteria, Antimicrob. Agents Chemother. *16*:495-502 (Oct.) 1979; and Talley, et al: *In Vitro* Activity of Thienamycin Antimicrob. Agents Chemother. *14*:436–438 (Sept.) 1978.

2. Ralph, E.D., and Kirby, W.M.M.: Bioassay of Metronidazole With Either Anaerobic or Aerobic Incubation, J. Infect. Dis. *132*:587–591 (Nov.) 1975; or Gulaid, et al: Determination of Metronidazole and Its Major Metabolites in Biological Fluids by High Pressure Liquid Chromatography, Br. J. Clin. Pharmacol. *6*:430–432, 1978.

Shown in Product Identification Section, page 419

SULTRIN® Triple Sulfa Cream and Vaginal Tablets ℞

COMPOSITION

SULTRIN Cream contains sulfathiazole 3.42%, sulfacetamide 2.86%, sulfabenzamide 3.7% and urea 0.64%, compounded with glyceryl monostearate, cetyl alcohol, stearic acid, cholesterol, lanolin, lecithin, peanut oil, propylparaben, propylene glycol, diethylaminoethyl stearamide, phosphoric acid, methylparaben and purified water.

COMPOSITION

Each SULTRIN Tablet contains sulfathiazole 172.5 mg, sulfacetamide 143.75 mg, and sulfabenzamide 184.0 mg, compounded with urea, lactose, guar gum, starch and magnesium stearate.

INDICATIONS

SULTRIN Cream and SULTRIN Tablets are indicated for treatment of *Haemophilus vaginalis* (*Gardnerella*) vaginitis.

Contraindications: Sulfonamide sensitivity and kidney disease.

Dosage: SULTRIN Cream. One applicatorful intravaginally twice daily for 4 to 6 days. The dosage may then be reduced one-half to one-quarter.

SULTRIN Vaginal Tablets. 1 tablet intravaginally before retiring and again in the morning for 10 days. This course may be repeated if necessary.

PACKAGING

Cream—78 g tubes with the ORTHO® Measured-Dose Applicator.

Vaginal Tablets—Package of 20 foil-wrapped tablets with vaginal applicator.

EDUCATIONAL MATERIAL

THE ORTHO FILM LIBRARY

Ortho Pharmaceutical Corporation can provide a number of educational films on a free-loan basis to hospitals, medical schools and health care professionals for use in training and educational programs.

These films, which are available directly from the distributor, KAROL MEDIA, 22 Riverview Drive, Wayne, New Jersey 07470, or by calling (201) 628-9111 are:

Modern Obstetrics: Cesarean Section
Modern Obstetrics: Diabetes in Pregnancy
Modern Obstetrics: Fetal Evaluation
Modern Obstetrics: Normal Labor and Delivery—no printed narration available
Modern Obstetrics: Postpartum Hemorrhage
Modern Obstetrics: Pre-Eclampsia—Eclampsia
Chorionic Villi Sampling—no printed narration available

Printed narrations of these Modern Obstetrics films are available upon written request from: Professional Affairs Department, Ortho Pharmaceutical Corporation, Route 202, P.O. Box 300, Raritan, New Jersey 08869-0602.

Ortho Pharmaceutical Corporation

DERMATOLOGICAL DIVISION
P.O. BOX 300
ROUTE 202
RARITAN, NJ 08869-0602

ERYCETTE™ ℞
(erythromycin 2%)
TOPICAL SOLUTION

DESCRIPTION

Erythromycin is an antibiotic produced from a strain of Streptomyces erythraeus. It is basic and readily forms salts with acids. Each ml of ERYCETTE (erythromycin 2%) Topical Solution contains 20 mg of erythromycin base in a vehicle consisting of alcohol (66%) and propylene glycol. It may contain citric acid to adjust pH.

ACTIONS

Although the mechanism by which ERYCETTE Solution acts in reducing inflammatory lesions of acne vulgaris is unknown, it is presumably due to its antibiotic action.

INDICATIONS

ERYCETTE Solution is indicated for the topical control of acne vulgaris.

CONTRAINDICATIONS

ERYCETTE Solution is contraindicated in persons who have shown hypersensitivity to any of its ingredients.

WARNINGS

The safe use of ERYCETTE (erythromycin 2%) Solution during pregnancy or lactation has not been established.

PRECAUTIONS

ERYCETTE Solution is for external use only and should be kept away from the eyes, nose, mouth and other mucous membranes. Concomitant topical acne therapy should be used with caution because a cumulative irritant effect may occur, especially with the use of peeling, desquamating, or abrasive agents.
The use of antimicrobial agents may be associated with the overgrowth of antibiotic-resistant organisms; in such a case, antibiotic administration should be stopped and appropriate measures taken.

ADVERSE REACTIONS

Adverse conditions reported include dryness, tenderness, pruritis, desquamation, erythema, oiliness, and burning sensation. Irritation of the eyes has also been reported. A case of generalized urticarial reaction, possibly related to the drug, which required the use of systemic steroid therapy has been reported.

DOSAGE AND ADMINISTRATION

The ERYCETTE pledget should be rubbed over the affected area twice a day after the skin is thoroughly washed with warm water and soap and patted dry. Acne lesions on the face, neck, shoulders, chest and back may be treated in this manner. Additional pledgets may be used, if needed.

HOW SUPPLIED

ERYCETTE (erythromycin 2%) Topical Solution is supplied as foil-covered saturated pledgets (swabs) in boxes of 60 (NDC 0062-1185-01).
Store at controlled room temperature (59°-86°F).

GRIFULVIN V® ℞
(griseofulvin microsize)
Tablets/Suspension

DESCRIPTION

Griseofulvin is an antibiotic derived from a species of *Penicillium.* Each GRIFULVIN V Tablet contains either 250 mg or 500 mg of griseofulvin microsize, and also contains calcium stearate, colloidal silicon dioxide, starch, and wheat gluten. Additionally, the 250 mg tablet also contains dibasic calcium phosphate. Each 5 ml of GRIFULVIN V Suspension contains 125 mg of griseofluvin microsize and also contains alcohol 0.008%, docusate sodium, FD&C Red No. 40, FD&C Yellow No. 6, flavors, magnesium aluminium silicate, menthol, methylparaben, propylene glycol, propylparaben, saccharin sodium, simethicone emulsion, sodium alginate, sucrose, and purified water.

CLINICAL PHARMACOLOGY

GRIFULVIN V (griseofulvin microsize) acts systemically to inhibit the growth of Trichophyton, Microsporum and Epidermophyton genera of fungi. Fungistatic amounts are deposited in the keratin, which is gradually exfoliated and replaced by noninfected tissue.
Griseofulvin absorption from the gastrointestinal tract varies considerably among individuals, mainly because of insolubility of the drug in aqueous media of the upper G.I. tract. The peak serum level found in fasting adults given 0.5 gm. occurs at about four hours and ranges between 0.5 and 2.0 mcg./ml.
It should be noted that some individuals are consistently "poor absorbers" and tend to attain lower blood levels at all times. This may explain unsatisfactory therapeutic results in some patients. Better blood levels can probably be attained in most patients if the tablets are administered after a meal with a high fat content.

INDICATIONS AND USAGE

Major indications for GRIFULVIN V griseofulvin microsize are:

Tinea capitis (ringworm of the scalp)
Tinea corporis (ringworm of the body)
Tinea pedis (athlete's foot)
Tinea unguium (onychomycosis; ringworm of the nails)
Tinea cruris (ringworm of the thigh)
Tinea barbae (barber's itch)

GRIFULVIN V (griseofulvin microsize) inhibits the growth of those genera of fungi that commonly cause ringworm infections of the hair, skin, and nails, such as:

Trichophyton rubrum
Trichophyton tonsurans
Trichophyton mentagrophytes
Trichophyton interdigitalis
Trichophyton verrucosum
Trichophyton sulphureum
Trichophyton schoenleini
Microsporum audouini
Microsporum canis
Microsporum gypseum
Epidermophyton floccosum
Trichophyton megnini
Trichophyton gallinae
Trichophyton crateriform

Note: Prior to therapy, the type of fungi responsible for the infection should be indentified. The use of the drug is not justified in minor or trivial infections which will respond to topical antifungal agents alone.
It is *not* effective in:

Bacterial infections
Candidiasis (Moniliasis)
Histoplasmosis
Actinomycosis
Sporotrichosis
Chromoblastomycosis
Coccidioidomycosis
North American Blastomycosis
Cryptococcosis (Torulosis)
Tinea versicolor
Nocardiosis

CONTRAINDICATIONS

This drug is contraindicated in patients with porphyria, hepatocellular failure, and in individuals with a history of hypersensitivity to griseofulvin.

WARNINGS

Usage in Pregnancy: Safe use of GRIFULVIN V (griseofulvin microsize) in pregnancy has not been established.
Prophylactic Usage: Safety and efficacy of prophylactic use of this drug has not been established.
Chronic feeding of griseofulvin, at levels ranging from 0.5-2.5% of the diet, resulted in the development of liver tumors in several strains of mice, particularly in males. Smaller particle sizes result in an enhanced effect. Lower oral dosage levels have not been tested. Subcutaneous administration of relatively small doses of griseofulvin once a week during the first three weeks of life has also been reported to induce hepatomata in mice. Although studies in other animal species have not yielded evidence of tumorigenicity, these studies were not of adequate design to form a basis for conclusions in this regard.
In subacute toxicity studies, orally administered griseofulvin produced hepatocellular necrosis in mice, but this has not been seen in other species. Disturbances in porphyrin metabolism have been reported in griseofulvin-treated laboratory animals. Griseofulvin has been reported to have a colchicine-like effect on mitosis and cocarcinogenicity with methylcholanthrene in cutaneous tumor induction in laboratory animals.
Reports of animal studies in the Soviet literature state that a griseofulvin preparation was found to be embryotoxic and teratogenic on oral administration to pregnant Wistar rats. Rat reproduction studies done thus far in the United States and Great Britain have been inconclusive in this regard, and additional animal reproduction studies are underway. Pups with abnormalities have been reported in the litters of a few bitches treated with griseofulvin.
Suppression of spermatogenesis has been reported to occur in rats but investigation in man failed to confirm this.

PRECAUTIONS

Patients on prolonged therapy with any potent medication should be under close observation. Periodic monitoring of organ system function, including renal, hepatic and hemopoietic, should be done.
Since griseofulvin is derived from species of penicillin, the possibility of cross sensitivity with penicillin exists; however, known penicillin-sensitive patients have been treated without difficulty.
Since a photosensitivity reaction is occasionally associated with griseofulvin therapy, patients should be warned to avoid exposure to intense natural or artificial sunlight. Should a photosensitivity reaction occur, lupus erythematosus may be aggravated.
Drug Interactions: Patients on warfarin-type anticoagulant therapy may require dosage adjustment of the anticoagulant during and after griseofulvin therapy. Concomitant use of barbiturates usually depresses griseofulvin activity and may necessitate raising the dosage.
The concomitant administration of griseofulvin has been reported to reduce the efficacy of oral contraceptives and to increase the incidence of breakthrough bleeding.

ADVERSE REACTIONS

When adverse reactions occur, they are most commonly of the hypersensitivity type such as skin rashes, urticaria and rarely, angioneurotic edema, and may necessitate withdrawal of therapy and appropriate countermeasures. Paresthesias of the hands and feet have been reported rarely after extended therapy. Other side effects reported occasionally are oral thrush, nausea, vomiting, epigastric distress, diarrhea; headache, fatigue, dizziness, insomnia, mental confusion and impairment of performance of routine activities.
Proteinuria and leukopenia have been reported rarely. Administration of the drug should be discontinued if granulocytopenia occurs.
When rare, serious reactions occur with griseofulvin, they are usually associated with high dosages, long periods of therapy, or both.

DOSAGE AND ADMINISTRATION

Accurate diagnosis of the infecting organism is essential. Identification should be made either by direct microscopic examination of a mounting of infected tissue in a solution of potassium hydroxide or by culture on an appropriate medium.
Medication must be continued until the infecting organism is completely eradicated as indicated by appropriate clinical or laboratory examination. Representative treatment periods are tinea capitis, 4 to 6 weeks; tinea corporis, 2 to 4 weeks; tinea pedis, 4 to 8 weeks; tinea unguium—depending on rate of growth —fingernails, at least 4 months; toenails, at least 6 months.
General measures in regard to hygiene should be observed to control sources of infection or reinfection. Concommitant use of appropriate topical agents is usually required, particularly in treatment of tinea pedis since in some forms of athlete's foot, yeasts and bacteria may be involved. Griseofulvin will not eradicate the bacterial or monilial infection.
Adults: A daily dose of 500 mg. will give a satisfactory response in most patients with tinea corporis, tinea cruris, and tinea capitis.
For those fungus infections more difficult to eradicate such as tinea pedis and tinea unguium, a daily dose of 1.0 gram is recommended.
Children: Approximately 5 mg. per pound of body weight per day is an effective dose for most children. On this basis the following dosage schedule for children is suggested:

Children weighing 30 to 50 pounds—125 mg. to 250 mg. daily.
Children weighing over 50 pounds—250 mg. to 500 mg. daily.

HOW SUPPLIED

GRIFULVIN V (griseofulvin microsize) 250 mg. Tablets in bottles of 100 (NDC 0062-0211-60) (white, scored, imprinted "ORTHO 211").
GRIFULVIN V (griseofulvin microsize) 500 mg. Tablets in bottles of 100 (NDC 0062-0214-60) and 500 (NDC 0062-0214-70) (white, scored, imprinted "ORTHO 214").
Dispense GRIFULVIN V tablets in well-closed container as defined in the official compendia.
GRIFULVIN V (griseofulvin microsize) Suspension 125 mg. per 5 cc. in bottles of 4 fl. oz. (NDC 0062-0206-04).
Dispense GRIFULVIN V suspension in tight, light-resistant container as defined in the official compendia.
STORE AT ROOM TEMPERATURE

MECLAN® ℞
(meclocycline sulfosalicylate)
Cream 1%
For Topical Use Only

DESCRIPTION

MECLAN (meclocycline sulfosalicylate) Cream 1% is a homogeneous smooth yellow cream, each gram of which contains meclocycline sulfosalicylate equivalent to 10 mg. of meclocycline activity in an aqueous cream vehicle consisting of glyceryl stearate, propylene glycol stearate, caprylic/cap-

ric triglyceride, paraffin, trihydroxystearin, polysorbate 40, sorbitol solution, propyl gallate, sorbic acid, sodium formaldehyde sulfoxylate, perfume, and water. The vehicle is pharmaceutically compatible with both oil- and water-based systems.
Chemically meclocycline sulfosalicylate is [4S-(4α, 4aα, 5α, 5aα, 12aα)]-7-chloro-4-(dimethyl- amino) - 1, 4,4a,5,5a,6,11,-12a-octahydro-3,5,10, 12,12a-pentahydroxy-6-methylene-1, 11- dioxo- 2-naphthacenecarboxamide 5-sulfosalicylate.

ACTIONS (CLINICAL PHARMACOLOGY)

The mode of action of MECLAN Cream in the treatment of acne is not fully understood. However, it appears that meclocycline possesses a localized effect, since it is not absorbed through the skin in sufficient quantities to be detected systemically. In subtotal body inunction studies, up to 40 times the average treatment dose was applied to 20 human subjects daily for 28 days. No measurable amounts of meclocycline appeared in the blood (0.1 microgram/ml. level of detectability) or urine (0.02 microgram/ml. level of detectability).

INDICATION

MECLAN Cream (meclocycline sulfosalicylate) is indicated for topical application in the treatment of acne vulgaris.

CONTRAINDICATIONS

MECLAN is contraindicated in persons who have shown hypersensitivity to any of its ingredients or to any of the other tetracyclines.

WARNINGS

Although no absorption has been demonstrated by 28-day inunction studies in humans, the possibility exists that significant percutaneous absorption may result from prolonged use. Therefore, caution is advised in administering MECLAN (meclocycline sulfosalicylate) to persons with hepatic or renal dysfunction.

PRECAUTIONS

This drug is for external use only and should be kept out of the eyes, nose, and mouth. It should be used with caution by patients who are sensitive to formaldehyde.
Pregnancy: Pregnancy Category B. Reproduction studies have been performed in rats and rabbits at oral doses up to 1000 times the human dose (assuming the human dose to be one gram of cream per day) and have revealed no evidence of impaired fertility or harm to the fetus due to meclocycline sulfosalicylate. There was, however, a slight delay in ossification in rabbits when meclocycline was applied topically. There are no adequate and well-controlled studies in pregnant women. Because animal reproduction studies are not always predictive of human response, this drug should be used during pregnancy only if clearly needed.
Nursing Mothers: It is not known whether this drug is excreted in human milk. Because many drugs are excreted in human milk, caution should be exercised when meclocycline sulfosalicylate is administered to a nursing woman.

ADVERSE REACTIONS

MECLAN is well tolerated by the skin. In the clinical trials there was one report of acute contact dermatitis. There were isolated reports of skin irritation. Temporary follicular staining may occur with excessive application. Patch testing has demonstrated no photosensitivity or contact allergy potential.

DOSAGE AND ADMINISTRATION

It is recommended that MECLAN be applied to the affected area twice daily, morning and evening. Less frequent application may be used depending on patient response. Excessive use of MECLAN Cream may cause staining of some fabrics.

HOW SUPPLIED

MECLAN (meclocycline sulfosalicylate) Cream 1% is supplied in 20 gram and 45 gram sealed tubes.

MONISTAT-DERM™ ℞

(miconazole nitrate 2%)
Cream and Lotion
For Topical Use Only

DESCRIPTION

MONISTAT-DERM (miconazole nitrate 2%) Cream and Lotion each contain miconazole nitrate* 2%, formulated into a water-miscible base consisting of pegoxol 7 stearate, peglicol 5 oleate, mineral oil, benzoic acid, and butylated hydroxyanisole and purified water.
*Chemical name: 1-[2,4-dichloro-β-{(2,4-dichlorobenzyl)oxy} phenethyl] imidazole mononitrate.

ACTIONS

Miconazole nitrate is a synthetic antifungal agent which inhibits the growth of the common dermatophytes, *Trichophyton rubrum, Trichophyton mentagrophytes,* and *Epidermophyton floccosum,* the yeast-like fungus. *Candida albicans,* and the organism responsible for tinea versicolor *(Malassezia furfur).*

INDICATIONS

For topical application in the treatment of tinea pedis (athlete's foot), tinea cruris, and tinea corporis caused by *Trichophyton rubrum, Trichophyton mentagrophytes,* and *Epidermophyton floccosum,* in the treatment of cutaneous candidiasis (moniliasis), and in the treatment of tinea versicolor.

CONTRAINDICATIONS

MONISTAT-DERM (miconazole nitrate 2%) Cream and Lotion have no known contraindications.

PRECAUTIONS

If a reaction suggesting sensitivity or chemical irritation should occur, use of the medication should be discontinued. For external use only. Avoid introduction of MONISTAT-DERM Cream and Lotion into the eyes.

ADVERSE REACTIONS

There have been isolated reports of irritation, burning, maceration, and allergic contact dermatitis associated with application of MONISTAT-DERM.

DOSAGE AND ADMINISTRATION

Sufficient MONISTAT-DERM Cream should be applied to cover affected areas twice daily (morning and evening) in patients with tinea pedis, tinea cruris, tinea corporis, and cutaneous candidiasis, and once daily in patients with tinea versicolor. It is preferable to use MONISTAT-DERM Lotion in intertriginous areas; if the cream is used, it should be applied sparingly and smoothed in well to avoid maceration effects.
Early relief of symptoms (2 to 3 days) is experienced by the majority of patients and clinical improvement may be seen fairly soon after treatment is begun; however, *Candida* infections and tinea cruris and corporis should be treated for two weeks and tinea pedis for one month in order to reduce the possibility of recurrence. If a patient shows no clinical improvement after a month of treatment, the diagnosis should be redetermined. Patients with tinea versicolor usually exhibit clinical and mycological clearing after two weeks of treatment.

HOW SUPPLIED

MONISTAT-DERM (miconazole nitrate 2%) Cream containing miconazole nitrate at 2% strength is supplied in 15 g., 1 oz. and 3 oz. tubes. MONISTAT-DERM (miconazole nitrate 2%) Lotion containing miconazole nitrate at 2% w/w strength is supplied in polyethylene squeeze bottles in quantities of 30 ml. and 60 ml.

PERSA–GEL® 5% & 10% ℞

(benzoyl peroxide)
acetone-base gel

PERSA-GEL W 5% & 10%

(benzoyl peroxide)
water-base gel

DESCRIPTION

PERSA-GEL and PERSA-GEL W 5% and 10% (benzoyl peroxide 5% and 10%) are topical gel preparations for use in the treatment of acne vulgaris. Benzoyl peroxide is an oxidizing agent which possesses antibacterial properties and is classified as a keratolytic.
PERSA-GEL contains benzoyl peroxide 5% or 10% as the active ingredient in a gel base containing acetone, carbomer 940, trolamine, sodium lauryl sulfate, propylene glycol and purified water.
PERSA-GEL W contains benzoyl peroxide 5% or 10% as the active ingredient containing purified water, carbomer, sodium hydroxide, hydroxypropyl methylcellulose 2906, and laureth 4.

CLINICAL PHARMACOLOGY

The mechanism of action of benzoyl peroxide has not been determined but may be related to its antibacterial activity against **Propionibacterium acnes** and its ability to cause drying and peeling. Benzoyl peroxide reduces the concentration of free fatty acids in the sebum. Little is known about the percutaneous penetration, metabolism, and excretion of benzoyl peroxide, although it is likely that benzoic acid is a major metabolite. There is no evidence of systemic toxicity caused by benzoyl peroxide in humans.

INDICATIONS AND USAGE

These products are indicated for the topical treatment of acne vulgaris.

CONTRAINDICATIONS

These products are contraindicated in patients with a history of hypersensitivity to any of the components of the preparations.

PRECAUTIONS

General: For external use only. If severe irritation develops, discontinue use and institute appropriate therapy. After the reaction clears, treatment may often be resumed with less frequent application. This preparation should not be used in or near the eyes or on mucous membranes.

Information for Patients: Avoid contact with eyes, eyelids, lips and mucous membranes. If accidental contact occurs, rinse with water. May bleach hair and colored fabrics. If excessive irritation develops, discontinue use and consult your physician.
Carcinogenesis, Mutagenesis, Impairment of Fertility: There is no evidence in the published literature that benzoyl peroxide is carcinogenic, mutagenic or that it impairs fertility.
Pregnancy: Pregnancy Category C: Animal reproduction studies have not been conducted with benzoyl peroxide. It is also not known whether benzoyl peroxide can cause fetal harm when administered to a pregnant woman or can affect reproduction capacity. Benzoyl peroxide should be used by a pregnant woman only if clearly needed. There are no data available on the effect of benzoyl peroxide on the growth, development and functional maturation of the unborn child.
Nursing Mothers: It is not known whether this drug is excreted in human milk. Because many drugs are excreted in human milk, caution should be exercised when benzoyl peroxide is administered to a nursing woman.
Pediatric Use: Safety and effectiveness in children have not been established.

ADVERSE REACTIONS

Allergic contact dermatitis has been reported with topical benzoyl peroxide therapy.

DOSAGE AND ADMINISTRATION

PERSA-GEL or PERSA-GEL W 5% or 10% should be applied once or twice daily to affected areas after washing with a mild cleanser and water. The degree of drying and peeling can be adjusted by modification of the dosage schedule.

HOW SUPPLIED

PERSA-GEL 5%, 1.5 oz. tubes
(NDC 0062-8610-31)
PERSA-GEL 5%, 3 oz. tubes
(NDC 0062-8610-03)
PERSA-GEL 10%, 1.5 oz. tubes
(NDC 0062-8600-31)
PERSA-GEL 10%, 3 oz. tubes
(NDC 0062-8600-03)
PERSA-GEL W 5% 1.5 oz. tubes
(NDC 0062-8630-31)
PERSA-GEL W 5% 3.0 oz. tubes
(NDC 0062-8630-03)
PERSA-GEL W 10% 1.5 oz. tubes
(NDC 0062-8620-31)
PERSA-GEL W 10% 3.0 oz. tubes
(NDC 0062-8620-03)
Store at controlled room temperature (59°– 86°F).

PURPOSE® Dry Skin Cream

(See PDR For Nonprescription Drugs)

PURPOSE® Shampoo

(See PDR For Nonprescription Drugs)

PURPOSE® Soap

(See PDR For Nonprescription Drugs)

RETIN–A™ ℞

(tretinoin)
Cream•Gel•Liquid
For Topical Use Only

DESCRIPTION

RETIN-A Gel, Cream and Liquid, containing tretinoin, are used for the topical treatment of acne vulgaris. RETIN-A Gel contains tretinoin (retinoic acid; vitamin A acid) in either of two strengths, 0.025% of 0.01% by weight, in a gel vehicle of butylated hydroxytoluene, hydroxypropyl cellulose, and alcohol 90% w/w. RETIN-A (tretinoin) Cream contains tretinoin in either of two strengths, 0.1% or 0.05% by weight, in a hydrophilic cream vehicle of stearic acid, isopropyl myristate, polyoxyl 40 stearate, stearyl alcohol, xanthan gum, sorbic acid, butylated hydroxytoluene, and purified water. RETIN-A Liquid contains tretinoin 0.05% by weight, polyethylene glycol 400, butylated hydroxytoluene, and alcohol 55%.

CLINICAL PHARMACOLOGY

Although the exact mode of action of tretinoin is unknown, current evidence suggests that topical tretinoin decreases cohesiveness of follicular epithelial cells with decreased microcomedo formation. Additionally, tretinoin stimulates mitotic activity and increased turnover of follicular epithelial cells, causing extrusion of the comedones.

Continued on next page

Ortho Derm.—Cont.

INDICATIONS AND USAGE
RETIN-A is indicated for topical application in the treatment of acne vulgaris.

CONTRAINDICATIONS
Use of the product should be discontinued if hypersensitivity to any of the ingredients is noted.

PRECAUTIONS
General: If a reaction suggesting sensitivity or chemical irritation occurs, use of the medication should be discontinued. Exposure to sunlight, including sunlamps, should be minimized during the use of RETIN-A, and patients with sunburn should be advised not to use the product until fully recovered because of heightened susceptibility to sunlight as a result of the use of tretinoin. Patients who may be required to have considerable sun exposure due to occupation and those with inherent sensitivity to the sun should exercise particular caution. Use of sunscreen products and protective clothing over treated areas may be prudent when exposure cannot be avoided. Weather extremes, such as wind or cold, also may be irritating to patients under treatment with tretinoin.

RETIN-A (tretinoin) acne treatment should be kept away from the eyes, the mouth, angles of the nose, and mucous membranes. Topical use may induce severe local erythema and peeling at the site of application. If the degree of local irritation warrants, patients should be directed to use the medication less frequently, discontinue use temporarily, or discontinue use altogether. Tretinoin has been reported to cause severe irritation on eczematous skin and should be used with utmost caution in patients with this condition.

Drug Interactions: Concomitant topical medication, medicated or abrasive soaps and cleansers, soaps and cosmetics that have a strong drying effect, and products with high concentrations of alcohol, astringents, spices or lime should be used with caution because of possible interaction with tretinoin. Particular caution should be exercised in using preparations containing sulfur, resorcinol, or salicylic acid with RETIN-A. It is also advisable to "rest" a patient's skin until the effects of such preparations subside before use of RETIN-A is begun.

Carcinogenesis: Long-term animal studies to determine the carcinogenic potential of tretinoin have not been performed. Studies in hairless albino mice suggest that tretinoin may accelerate the tumorigenic potential of ultraviolet radiation. Although the significance to man is not clear, patients should avoid or minimize exposure to sun.

Pregnancy: Pregnancy Category B. Reproduction studies performed in rats and rabbits at dermal doses up to 50 times the human dose (assuming the human dose to be 500 mg of gel per day) have revealed no evidence of impaired fertility or harm to the fetus due to tretinoin (retinoic acid). There was, however, a slightly higher incidence of irregularly contoured or partially ossified skull bones in some rat and rabbit fetuses. There are no adequate and well-controlled studies in pregnant women. Because animal reproduction studies are not always predictive of human response, this drug should be used during pregnancy only if clearly needed.

Nursing Mothers: It is not known whether this drug is excreted in human milk. Because many drugs are excreted in human milk, caution should be exercised when tretinoin is administered to a nursing woman.

ADVERSE REACTIONS
The skin of certain sensitive individuals may become excessively red, edematous, blistered, or crusted. If these effects occur, the medication should either be discontinued until the integrity of the skin is restored, or the medication should be adjusted to a level the patient can tolerate. True contact allergy to topical tretinoin is rarely encountered. Temporary hyper- or hypopigmentation has been reported with repeated application of RETIN-A. Some individuals have been reported to have heightened susceptibility to sunlight while under treatment with RETIN-A. To date, all adverse effects of RETIN-A have been reversible upon discontinuation of therapy (see Dosage and Administration Section).

OVERDOSAGE
If medication is applied excessively, no more rapid or better results will be obtained and marked redness, peeling, or discomfort may occur.

Oral LD_{50} values for the various dosage forms of RETIN-A were found to be:

	0.05% Solution	0.1% Cream	0.05% Gel*
Mice	19.0 ml/Kg	Sublethal	11.83 ml/Kg
Rats	20.9 ml/Kg	Sublethal	20.21 ml/Kg

The intravenous LD_{50} values of the 0.05% solution in mice and rats were found to be 5.2 ml/Kg and 8.7 ml/Kg respectively.

DOSAGE AND ADMINISTRATION
RETIN-A Gel, Cream or Liquid should be applied once a day, before retiring, to the skin where acne lesions appear, using enough to cover the entire affected area lightly. Liquid: The liquid may be applied using a fingertip, gauze pad, or cotton swab. If gauze or cotton is employed, care should be taken not to oversaturate it to the extent that the liquid would run into areas where treatment is not intended. Gel: Excessive application results in "pilling" of the gel, which minimizes the likelihood of overapplication by the patient.

Application may cause a transitory feeling of warmth or slight stinging. In cases where it has been necessary to temporarily discontinue therapy or to reduce the frequency of application, therapy may be resumed or frequency of application increased when the patients become able to tolerate the treatment.

It should be noted that just as some patients require less frequent applications or other dosage forms, others may respond better to more frequent application of tretinoin. Alterations of vehicle, drug concentration, or dose frequency should be closely monitored by careful observation of the clinical therapeutic response and skin tolerance.

During the early weeks of therapy, an *apparent* exacerbation of inflammatory lesions may occur. This is due to the action of the medication on deep, previously unseen lesions and should not be considered a reason to discontinue therapy.

Therapeutic results should be noticed after two to three weeks but more than six weeks of therapy may be required before definite beneficial effects are seen.

Once the acne lesions have responded satisfactorily, it may be possible to maintain the improvement with less frequent applications or other dosage forms.

Patients treated with RETIN-A (tretinoin) acne treatment may use cosmetics, but the areas to be treated should be cleansed thoroughly before the medication is applied.

HOW SUPPLIED
RETIN-A (tretinoin) is supplied as:

1. A 0.025% Gel in tubes of 15 grams (NDC 0062-0475-42) and 45 grams (NDC 0062-0475-45) and a 0.01% Gel in tubes of 15 grams (NDC 0062-0575-44) and 45 grams (NDC 0062-0575-46).
2. A 0.1% Cream in tubes of 20 grams (NDC 0062-0275-23) and a 0.05% Cream in tubes of 20 grams (NDC 0062-0175-12) and 45 grams (NDC 0062-0175-13).
3. A 0.05% Liquid in amber bottles containing 28 ml (NDC 0062-0075-07).

Storage Conditions: RETIN-A Liquid 0.05%, and RETIN-A Gel 0.025% and 0.01%; store below 86°F.

RETIN-A Cream 0.1% and 0.05% store below 80°F.

**The 0.05% Gel was never marketed.*

SPECTAZOLE™ ℞
(econazole nitrate 1%)
Cream
For Topical Use Only

DESCRIPTION
SPECTAZOLE Cream contains the antifungal agent, econazole nitrate 1%, in a water-miscible base consisting of pegoxol 7 stearate, peglicol 5 oleate, mineral oil, benzoic acid, butylated hydroxyanisole, and purified water. The white to off-white soft cream is for topical use only.

Chemically, econazole nitrate is 1-[2-{(4-chlorophenyl)methoxy}-2-(2,4-dichlorophenyl)ethyl]-1H-imidazole mononitrate. Its structure is as follows:

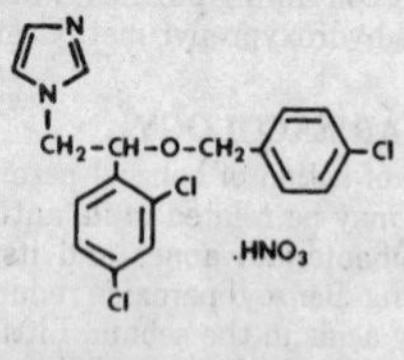

CLINICAL PHARMACOLOGY
After topical application to the skin of normal subjects, systemic absorption of econazole nitrate is extremely low. Although most of the applied drug remains on the skin surface, drug concentrations were found in the stratum corneum which, by far, exceeded the minimum inhibitory concentration for dermatophytes. Inhibitory concentrations were achieved in the epidermis and as deep as the middle region of the dermis. Less than 1% of the applied dose was recovered in the urine and feces.

Microbiology: In *in-vitro* studies, econazole nitrate exhibits broad-spectrum antifungal activity against the dermatophytes, *Trichophyton rubrum, Trichophyton mentagrophytes, Trichophyton tonsurans, Microsporum canis, Microsporum audouini, Microsporum gypseum,* and *Epidermophyton floccosum,* the yeasts, *Candida albicans* and *Pityrosporum orbiculare* (the organism responsible for tinea versicolor), and certain gram positive bacteria.

INDICATIONS AND USAGE
SPECTAZOLE Cream is indicated for topical application in the treatment of tinea pedis, tinea cruris, and tinea corporis caused by *Trichophyton rubrum, Trichophyton mentagrophytes, Trichophyton tonsurans, Microsporum canis, Microsporum audouini, Microsporum gypseum,* and *Epidermophyton floccosum,* in the treatment of cutaneous candidiasis, and in the treatment of tinea versicolor.

CONTRAINDICATIONS
SPECTAZOLE Cream is contraindicated in individuals who have shown hypersensitivity to any of its ingredients.

WARNINGS
SPECTAZOLE is not for ophthalmic use.

PRECAUTIONS
General: If a reaction suggesting sensitivity or chemical irritation should occur, use of the medication should be discontinued.

For external use only. Avoid introduction of SPECTAZOLE Cream into the eyes.

Carcinogenicity Studies: Long-term animal studies to determine carcinogenic potential have not been performed.

Fertility (Reproduction): Oral administration of econazole nitrate in rats has been reported to produce prolonged gestation. Intravaginal administration in humans has not shown prolonged gestation or other adverse reproductive effects attributable to econazole nitrate therapy.

Pregnancy: Pregnancy Category C. Econazole nitrate has not been shown to be teratogenic when administered orally to mice, rabbits or rats. Fetotoxic or embryotoxic effects were observed in Segment I oral studies with rats receiving 10 to 40 times the human dermal dose. Similar effects were observed in Segment II or Segment III studies with mice, rabbits and/or rats receiving oral doses 80 or 40 times the human dermal dose.

Econazole should be used in the first trimester of pregnancy only when the physician considers it essential to the welfare of the patient. The drug should be used during the second and third trimesters of pregnancy only if clearly needed.

Nursing Mothers: It is not known whether econazole nitrate is excreted in human milk. Following oral administration of econazole nitrate to lactating rats, econazole and/or metabolites were excreted in milk and were found in nursing pups. Also, in lactating rats receiving large oral doses (40 or 80 times the human dermal dose), there was a reduction in post partum viability of pups and survival to weaning; however, at these high doses, maternal toxicity was present and may have been a contributing factor. Caution should be exercised when econazole nitrate is administered to a nursing woman.

ADVERSE REACTIONS
During clinical trials, 12 (3.3%) of 366 patients treated with econazole nitrate 1% cream reported side effects, consisting mainly of burning, itching, stinging and erythema.

OVERDOSE
Overdosage of econazole nitrate in humans has not been reported to date. In mice, rats, guinea pigs and dogs, the oral LD 50 values were found to be 462, 668, 272, and > 160 mg/kg, respectively.

DOSAGE AND ADMINISTRATION
Sufficient SPECTAZOLE Cream should be applied to cover affected areas twice daily (morning and evening) in patients with tinea pedis, tinea cruris, tinea corporis, and cutaneous candidiasis, and once daily in patients with tinea versicolor.

Early relief of symptoms is experienced by the majority of patients and clinical improvement may be seen fairly soon after treatment is begun; however, candidal infections and tinea cruris and corporis should be treated for two weeks and tinea pedis for one month in order to reduce the possibility of recurrence. If a patient shows no clinical improvement after the treatment period, the diagnosis should be redetermined. Patients with tinea versicolor usually exhibit clinical and mycological clearing after two weeks of treatment.

HOW SUPPLIED
SPECTAZOLE (econazole nitrate 1%) Cream is supplied in tubes of 15 grams (NDC 0062-5460-02), 30 grams (NDC 0062-5460-01), and 85 grams (NDC 0062-5460-03).

Store SPECTAZOLE Cream below 86°F.

Products are cross-indexed by generic and chemical names in the **YELLOW SECTION**

Owen Laboratories

Division of Dermatological Products of Texas, Inc.
SAN ANTONIO, TX 78296
An Affiliate of Alcon Laboratories, Inc.
FORT WORTH, TX 76134

CETAPHIL® Lotion
Skin Cleanser—Soap Substitute

COMPOSITION
Contains water, cetyl alcohol, propylene glycol, sodium lauryl sulfate, stearyl alcohol, methylparaben, propylparaben and butylparaben.

ACTION AND USES
CETAPHIL® Lotion is an alternative for soap intolerant skin. It allows gentle, thorough cleansing without the irritancy of harsh soaps. The unique oil-free formula is particularly well-suited for atopic dermatitis, diaper dermatitis and other eczematous skin conditions. Its emollient quality helps soften as it cleanses, providing comfort for sensitive, irritated skin. CETAPHIL Lotion is free of animal, vegetable and mineral fats.

ADMINISTRATION AND DOSAGE
Apply liberal amount to skin and rub gently to produce lather. Remove excess with soft cloth or tissue.

HOW SUPPLIED
CETAPHIL Lotion 8 oz. (NDC 0299-3921-08); CETAPHIL Lotion 16 oz. (NDC 0299-3921-16).

DESOWEN™ ℞
(desonide)
Cream 0.05%

DESCRIPTION
DESOWEN™ Cream contains the topical corticosteroid, desonide, nonfluorinated corticosteroid. It has the chemical name: Pregna-1,4-diene-3,20-dione,11,21-dihydroxy-16,17-[(1-methylethylidene)bis(oxy)]-, (11β, 16α)-; the empirical formula: $C_{24}H_{32}O_6$; molecular weight: 416.5.
Each gram of DESOWEN Cream contains 0.5 mg of desonide microdispersed in a compatible vehicle buffered to the pH range of normal skin. It contains propylene glycol, polysorbate 60, emulsifying wax, isopropylpalmitate, stearic acid, synthetic beeswax, citric acid, sodium hydroxide and purified water. It is preserved with sorbic acid and potassium sorbate.

CLINICAL PHARMACOLOGY
Topical corticosteroids share anti-inflammatory, antipurtic and vasoconstrictive actions.
The mechanism of anti-inflammatory activity of the topical corticosteroids is unclear. Various laboratory methods, including vasoconstrictor assays, are used to compare and predict potencies and/or clinical efficacies of the topical corticosteroids. There is some evidence to suggest that a recognizable correlation exists between vasoconstrictor potency and therapeutic efficacy in man.
Pharmacokinetics: The extent of percutaneous absorption of topical corticosteroids is determined by many factors including the vehicle, the integrity of the epidermal barrier, and the use of occlusive dressings.
Topical corticosteroids can be absorbed from normal intact skin. Inflammation and/or other disease processes in the skin increase percutaneous absorption. Occlusive dressings substantially increase the percutaneous absorption of topical corticosteroids.
Thus, occlusive dressings may be a valuable therapeutic adjunct for treatment of resistant dermatoses. (See DOSAGE AND ADMINISTRATION.)
Once absorbed through the skin, topical corticosteroids are handled through pharmacokinetic pathways similar to systemically administered corticosteroids. Corticosteroids are bound to plasma proteins in varying degrees. Corticosteroids are metabolized primarily in the liver and are then excreted by the kidneys. Some of the topical corticosteroids and their metabolites are also excreted into the bile.

INDICATIONS AND USAGE
DESOWEN Cream 0.05% (desponide) is indicated for the relief of the inflammatory and pruritic manifestations of corticosteroid-responsive dermatoses.

CONTRAINDICATIONS
Topical corticosteroids are contraindicated in those patients with a history of hypersensitivity to any of the components of the preparation.

PRECAUTIONS
General: Systemic absorption of topical corticosteroids has produced reversible hypothalamic-pituitary-adrenal (HPA) axis suppression, manifestations of Cushings syndrome, hyperglycemia, and glucosuria in some patients.
Conditions which augment systemic absorption include the application of the more potent steroids, use over large surface areas, prolonged use, and the addition of occlusive dressings.
Therefore, patients receiving a large dose of a potent topical steroid applied to a large surface area or under an occlusive dressing should be evaluated periodically for evidence of HPA axis supression by using the urinary free cortisol and ACTH stimulation tests. If HPA axis suppression is noted, an attempt should be made to withdraw the drug, to reduce the frequency of application, or to substitute a less potent steroid.
Recovery of HPA axis function is generally prompt and complete upon discontinuation of the drug. Infrequently, signs and symptoms of steroid withdrawal may occur, requiring supplemental systemic corticosteroids.
Children may absorb proportionally larger amounts of topical corticosteroids and thus be more susceptible to systemic toxicity. (See PRECAUTIONS—PEDIATRIC USE).
If irritation develops, topical corticosteroids should be discontinued and appropriate therapy instituted.
In the presence of dematological infections, the use of an appropriate antifungal or antibacterial agent should be instituted. If a favorable response does not occur promptly, the corticosteroid should be discontinued until the infection has been adquately controlled.
Information for the Patient: Patients using topical corticosteroids should receive the following information and instructions:

1. This medication is to be used as directed by the physician. It is for external use only. Avoid contact with the eyes.
2. Patients should be advised not to use this medication for any disorder other than for which it was prescribed.
3. The treated skin area should not be bandaged or otherwise covered or wrapped as to be occlusive unless directed by the physician.
4. Patients should report any signs of local adverse reactions especially under occlusive dressing.
5. Parents of pediatric patients should be advised not to use tight-fitting diapers or plastic pants on a child being treated in the diaper area, as these garments may constitute occlusive dressings.

Laboratory Tests: The following tests may be helpful in evaluating the HPA axis suppression.
Unirary free cortisol test
ACTH stimulation test
Carcinogenesis, Mutagenesis, and Impairment of Fertility: - Long-term animal studies have not been performed to evaluate the carcinogenic potential or the effect on fertility of topical corticosteroids.
Studies to determine mutagenicity with prednisolone and hydrocortisone have revealed negative results.
Pregnancy Category C: Corticosteroids are generally teratogenic in laboratory animals when administered systemically at relatively low dosage levels. The more potent corticosteroids have been shown to be teratogenic after dermal application in laboratory animals. There are no adequate and well-controlled studies in pregnant women on teratogenic effects from topically applied corticosteroids. Therefore, topical corticosteroids should be used during pregnancy only if the potential benefit justifies the potential risk to the fetus. Drugs of this class should not be used extensively on pregnant patients, in large amounts, or for prolonged periods of time.
Nursing Mothers: It is not known whether topical administration of corticosteroids could result in sufficient systemic absorption to produce detectable quantities in breast milk. Systemically administered corticosteroids are secreted into breast milk, in quantities not likely to have deleterious effect on the infant. Nevertheless, caution should be exercised when topical corticosteroids are administered to a nursing woman.
Pediatric Use: *Pediatric patients may demonstrate greater susceptibility to topical corticosteroid-induced HPA axis suppression and Cushing's syndrome than mature patients because of a larger skin surface area to body weight ratio.*
Hypothalamic-pituitary-adrenal (HPA) axis suppression, Cushing's syndrome, and intracranial hypertension have been reported in children receiving topical corticosteroids. Manifestations of adrenal suppression in children include linear growth retardation, delayed weight gain, low plasma cortisol levels, and absence of response to ACTH stimulation. Manifestations of intracranial hypertension include bulging fontanelles, headaches, and bilateral papilledema. Administration of topical corticosteroids to children should be limited to the least amount compatible with an effective therapeutic regimen. Chronic corticosteroid therapy may interfere with the growth and development of children.

ADVERSE REACTIONS
The following local adverse reactions are reported infrequently with topical corticosteroids, but may occur more frequently with the use of occlusive dressings. These reactions are listed in an aproximately decreasing order of occurrence: burning, itching, irritation, dryness, folliculitis, hypertrichosis, acneiform eruptions, hypopigmentation, perioral dermatitis, allergic contact dermatitis, maceration of the skin, secondary infection, skin atrophy, striae, miliaria.

OVERDOSAGE
Topically applied corticosteroids can be absorbed in sufficient amounts to produce systemic effects (See PRECAUTIONS).

DOSAGE AND ADMINISTRATION
DESOWEN Cream 0.05% (desonide) should be applied to the affected area as a thin film from two to three times daily depending on the severity of the condition. Occlusive dressings may be used for the management of psoriasis or recalcitrant conditions.
If an infection develops, the use of occlusive dressings should be discontinued and approrpiate antimicrobial therapy instituted.

CAUTION
Federal law prohibits dispensing without prescription.

HOW SUPPLIED
DESOWEN Cream 0.05% (desonide) is supplied in tubes containing:
15 gram—**NDC** 0299-5770-15
60 gram—**NDC** 0299-5770-60
Storage Conditions: Store below 86°F (30°C), avoid freezing.

IONIL® Shampoo
Antiseborrheic Treatment Shampoo

COMPOSITION
OWENETHER® (special blend of polyoxyethylene ethers), alcohol 12%, salicylic acid and benzalkonium chloride.

ACTION AND USES
IONIL relieves the itching, irritation, and flaking associated with dandruff, seborrheic dermatitis, and psoriasis of the scalp. IONIL contains no anionic detergents or soaps making it gentle enough for daily use.

ADMINISTRATION AND DOSAGE
Wet hair, apply IONIL, and massage into scalp. Don't expect as much initial sudsing as the anionic non-medicated shampoos. Rinse, then apply IONIL again and massage into a lather. Allow to remain in hair for about five minutes before rinsing.

CAUTION
For external use only. Rinse eyes with water if contact is made. Keep this and all drugs out of the reach of children.

HOW SUPPLIED
4 oz. (NDC 0299-3730-02), 8 oz. (NDC 0299-3730-04), 16 oz. (NDC 0299-3730-05), and 32 oz. (NDC 0299-3730-06) bottles.

IONIL® PLUS Shampoo
Antiseborrheic Treatment Shampoo

COMPOSITION
Salicylic Acid 2%. Also contains: Water, Sodium Laureth Sulfate, Lauramide Dea, Quaternium-22, Talloweth-60 Myristyl Glycol, Laureth-23, Tea Lauryl Sulfate, Glycol Distearate, Laureth-4, Tea-Abietoyl Hydrolyzed Collagen, DMDM Hydantoin, Tetrasodium EDTA, Sodium Hydroxide, Fragrance, FD&C Blue No. 1.

ACTION AND USES
IONIL PLUS Shampoo relieves the itching, irritation and flaking associated with dandruff, seborrheic dermatitis, and psoriasis of the scalp. IONIL PLUS shampoo is gentle enough for daily use and leaves hair manageable.

ADMINISTRATION AND DOSAGE
Wet hair, apply IONIL PLUS and massage into scalp. Let lather stand one minute, then rinse. Repeat application, if needed. May be used daily.

CAUTION
For external use only. Rinse eyes with water if contact is made. Keep this and all drugs out of the reach of children.

HOW SUPPLIED
4 oz. (NDC 0299-3731-04) and 8 oz. (NDC 0299-3731-08) bottles.

IONIL® T Shampoo
Antiseborrheic Tar Shampoo

COMPOSITION
OWENTAR® (coal tar solution), salicylic acid, benzalkonium chloride, OWENETHERS® (special blend of polyoxyethylene ethers), alcohol 12%, isopropyl alcohol 4%.

Continued on next page

Owen—Cont.

ACTION AND USES

IONIL T relieves the itching, irritation, and flaking associated with dandruff, seborrheic dermatitis, and psoriasis of the scalp. IONIL T contains no anionic detergents or soaps making it gentle enough for daily use.

ADMINISTRATION AND DOSAGE

Wet hair, apply IONIL T, and massage into scalp. Don't expect as much initial sudsing as the anionic non-medicated shampoos. Rinse, then apply IONIL T again and massage into a lather. Allow to remain in hair for about five minutes before rinsing.

CAUTION

For external use only. Rinse eyes with water if contact is made. Keep this and all drugs out of the reach of children.

HOW SUPPLIED

4 oz. (NDC 0299-3750-02), 8 oz. (NDC 0299-3750-04), 16 oz. (NDC 0299-3750-05), and 32 oz. (NDC 0299-3750-06) bottles.

IONIL T® PLUS Shampoo

Antiseborrheic Tar Shampoo

COMPOSITION

OWENTAR® II (coal tar distillate equivalent to 2% crude coal tar). Also contains: Water, Sodium Laureth Sulfate, Lauramide Dea, Quaternium-22, Laureth-23, Talloweth-60 Myristyl Glycol, Tea Lauryl Sulfate, Glycol Distearate, Laureth-4, Tea-Abietoyl Hydrolyzed Collagen, DMDM Hydantoin, Disodium EDTA, Fragrance, FD&C Blue No. 1, Ext. D&C Yellow No. 7.

ACTION AND USES

IONIL T PLUS Shampoo relieves the itching, irritation and flaking associated with dandruff, seborrheic dermatitis, and psoriasis of the scalp. Will not discolor white or light colored hair. IONIL T PLUS is gentle enough for daily use and leaves hair manageable.

ADMINISTRATION AND DOSAGE

Wet hair, apply IONIL T PLUS, and massage into scalp. Let lather stand one minute and then rinse. Repeat application, if needed. May be used daily.

CAUTION

For external use only. Rinse eyes with water if contact is made. Keep this and all drugs out of the reach of children.

HOW SUPPLIED

4 oz. (NDC 0299-3752-04) and 8 oz. (NDC 0299-3752-08) bottles.

LOCOID® ℞

(hydrocortisone butyrate)
Cream 0.1%
Ointment 0.1%

CAUTION: Federal law prohibits dispensing without prescription.

DESCRIPTION

LOCOID cream and ointment contain the topical corticosteroid, hydrocortisone butyrate, a non-fluorinated ester of hydrocortisone. It has the chemical name: pregn-4-ene-3,20-dione, 11,21-dihydroxy-17-[(1-oxobutyl)oxy]-, (11_{β})-; the empirical formula: $C_{25}H_{36}O_6$; the molecular weight: 432.54 and the CAS registry number: 13609-67-1.

LOCOID® Cream 0.1%

Each gram of LOCOID cream contains 1 mg of hydrocortisone butyrate in a hydrophilic base consisting of cetostearyl alcohol, ceteth-20, mineral oil, white petrolatum, citric acid, sodium citrate, methylparaben (preservative) and purified water.

LOCOID® Ointment 0.1%

Each gram of LOCOID ointment contains 1 mg of hydrocortisone butyrate in a base consisting of mineral oil and polyethylene.

CLINICAL PHARMACOLOGY

Topical corticosteroids share anti-inflammatory, anti-pruritic and vasoconstrictive actions.

The mechanism of anti-inflammatory activity of the topical corticosteroids is unclear. Various laboratory methods, including vasoconstrictor assays, are used to compare and predict potencies and/or clinical efficacies of the topical corticosteroids. There is some evidence to suggest that a recognizable correlation exists between vasoconstrictor potency and therapeutic efficacy in man.

Pharmacokinetics

The extent of percutaneous absorption of topical corticosteroids is determined by many factors including the vehicle, the integrity of the epidermal barrier, and the use of occlusive dressings.

Topical corticosteroids can be absorbed from normal intact skin. Inflammation and/or other disease processes in the skin increase percutaneous absorption. Occlusive dressings substantially increase the percutaneous absorption of topical corticosteroids.

Thus, occlusive dressings may be a valuable therapeutic adjunct for treatment of resistant dermatoses. (See DOSAGE AND ADMINISTRATION.)

Once absorbed through the skin, topical corticosteroids are handled through pharmacokinetic pathways similar to systemically administered corticosteroids. Corticosteroids are bound to plasma proteins in varying degrees. Corticosteroids are metabolized primarily in the liver and are then excreted by the kidneys. Some of the topical corticosteroids and their metabolites are also excreted into the bile.

INDICATIONS AND USAGE

LOCOID cream 0.1% and ointment 0.1% (hydrocortisone butyrate) are indicated for the relief of the inflammatory and pruritic manifestations of corticosteroid-responsive dermatoses.

CONTRAINDICATIONS

Topical corticosteroids are contraindicated in those patients with a history of hypersensitivity to any of the components of the preparation.

PRECAUTIONS

General: Systemic absorption of topical corticosteroids has produced reversible hypothalamic-pituitary-adrenal (HPA) axis suppression, manifestations of Cushing's syndrome, hyperglycemia, and glucosuria in some patients.

Conditions which augment systemic absorption include the application of the more potent steroids, use over large surface areas, prolonged use, and the addition of occlusive dressings.

Therefore, patients receiving a large dose of a potent topical steroid applied to a large surface area or under an occlusive dressing should be evaluated periodically for evidence of HPA axis suppression by using the urinary free cortisol and ACTH stimulation tests. If HPA axis suppression is noted, an attempt should be made to withdraw the drug, to reduce the frequency of application, or to substitute a less potent steroid.

Recovery of HPA axis function is generally prompt and complete upon discontinuation of the drug. Infrequently, signs and symptoms of steroid withdrawal may occur, requiring supplemental systemic corticosteroids.

Children may absorb proportionally larger amounts of topical corticosteroids and thus be more susceptible to systemic toxicity (See PRECAUTIONS—PEDIATRIC USE).

If irritation develops, topical corticosteroids should be discontinued and appropriate therapy instituted.

In the presence of dermatological infections, the use of an appropriate antifungal or antibacterial agent should be instituted. If a favorable response does not occur promptly, the corticosteroid should be discontinued until the infection has been adequately controlled.

Information for the patient

Patients using topical corticosteroids should receive the following information and instructions:

1. This medication is to be used as directed by the physician. It is for external use only. Avoid contact with the eyes.
2. Patients should be advised not to use this medication for any disorder other than for which it was prescribed.
3. The treated skin area should not be bandaged or otherwise covered or wrapped as to be occlusive unless directed by the physician.
4. Patients should report any signs of local adverse reactions especially under occlusive dressing.
5. Parents of pediatric patients should be advised not to use tight-fitting diapers or plastic pants on a child being treated in the diaper area, as these garments may constitute occlusive dressings.

Laboratory tests

The following tests may be helpful in evaluating the HPA axis suppression:
Urinary free cortisol test
ACTH stimulation test

Carcinogenesis, mutagenesis, and impairment of fertility

Long-term animal studies have not been performed to evaluate the carcinogenic potential or the effect on fertility of topical corticosteroids.

Studies to determine mutagenicity with prednisolone and hydrocortisone have revealed negative results.

Pregnancy category C

Corticosteroids are generally teratogenic in laboratory animals when administered systemically at relatively low dosage levels. The more potent corticosteroids have been shown to be teratogenic after dermal application in laboratory animals. There are no adequate and well-controlled studies in pregnant women on teratogenic effects from topically applied corticosteroids. Therefore, topical corticosteroids should be used during pregnancy only if the potential benefit justifies the potential risk to the fetus. Drugs of this class should not be used extensively on pregnant patients, in large amounts, or for prolonged periods of time.

Nursing mothers

It is not known whether topical administration of corticosteroids could result in sufficient systemic absorption to produce detectable quantities in breast milk. Systemically administered corticosteroids are secreted into breast milk, in quantities not likely to have a deleterious effect on the infant. Nevertheless, caution should be exercised when topical corticosteroids are administered to a nursing woman.

Pediatric use

Pediatric patients may demonstrate greater susceptibility to topical corticosteroid-induced HPA axis suppression and Cushing's syndrome than mature patients because of a larger skin surface area to body weight ratio.

Hypothalamic-pituitary-adrenal (HPA) axis suppression, Cushing's syndrome, and intracranial hypertension have been reported in children receiving topical corticosteroids. Manifestations of adrenal suppression in children include linear growth retardation, delayed weight gain, low plasma cortisol levels, and absence of response to ACTH stimulation. Manifestations of intracranial hypertension include bulging fontanelles, headaches, and bilateral papilledema.

Administration of topical corticosteroids to chldren should be limited to the least amount compatible with an effective therapeutic regimen. Chronic corticosteroid therapy may interfere with the growth and development of children.

ADVERSE REACTIONS

The following local adverse reactions are reported infrequently with topical corticosteroids, but may occur more frequently with the use of occlusive dressings. These reactions are listed in an approximately decreasing order of occurrence: burning, itching, irritation, dryness, foliculitis, hypertrichosis, acneiform eruptions, hypopigmentation, perioral dermatitis, allergic contact dermatitis, maceration of the skin, secondary infection, skin atrophy, striae, milaria.

OVERDOSAGE

Topically applied corticosteroids can be absorbed in sufficient amounts to produce systemic effects (See PRECAUTIONS).

DOSAGE AND ADMINISTRATION

LOCOID cream 0.1% or LOCOID ointment 0.1% (hydrocortisone butyrate) should be applied to the affected area as a thin film from two to three times daily depending on the severity of the condition.

Occlusive dressings may be used for the management of psoriasis or recalcitrant conditions.

If an infection develops, the use of occlusive dressings should be discontinued and appropriate antimicrobial therapy instituted.

HOW SUPPLIED

LOCOID cream 0.1% (hydrocortisone butyrate) is supplied in tubes containing:
15 g NDC 0299-2000-15
45 g NDC 0299-2000-45
LOCOID ointment 0.1% (hydrocortisone butyrate) is supplied in tubes containing:
15 g NDC 0299-2010-15
45 g NDC 0299-2010-45

STORAGE CONDITIONS

LOCOID cream 0.1%: Store between 46° and 77°F (8° and 25°C).

LOCOID ointment 0.1%: Store below 86°F (30°C). Avoid freezing.

Manufactured under
license from Gist-Brocades, N.V.
Delft-Netherlands

NUTRACORT® ℞

(hydrocortisone)
Cream 1%
Lotion 1%

DESCRIPTION

NUTRACORT® cream and lotion are topical hydrocortisone preparations. Hydrocortisone is therapeutically classed as an anti-inflammatory and anti-pruritic agent. Hydrocortisone is a white crystalline powder that is very slightly soluble in water and ether and sparingly soluble in acetone and in alcohol.

Chemical Name: Pregn-4-ene-3,20-dione, 11, 17, 21-trihydroxy-,(11β)-.
Empirical Formula: $C_{21}H_{30}O_5$
Molecular Weight: 362.47

NUTRACORT® Cream 1% contains: Hydrocortisone 1.0% (10 mg/g) in a cream base containing propylene glycol, polysorbate 60, emulsifying wax, synthetic beeswax, stearic acid, isopropyl palmitate, sorbic acid, potassium sorbate, propyl gallate, citric acid and/or sodium hydroxide (to adjust pH), purified water and certified color.

NUTRACORT® Lotion 1% contains: Hydrocortisone 1.0% (10 mg/ml) in a lotion base containing sodium lauryl sulfate, light mineral oil, cetyl alcohol, stearyl alcohol, methylparaben, propylparaben, sorbitan monostearate, glyceryl monostearate, edetate sodium, purified water and certified color. May contain citric acid and/or sodium hydroxide for pH adjustment.

CLINICAL PHARMACOLOGY

Topical corticosteroids share anti-inflammatory, anti-pruritic and vasoconstrictive actions.

The mechanism of anti-inflammatory activity of the topical corticosteroids is unclear. Various laboratory methods, including vasoconstrictor assays, are used to compare and predict potencies and/or clinical efficacies of the topical corticosteroids. There is some evidence to suggest that a recognizable correlation exists between vasoconstrictor potency and therapeutic efficacy in man.

Pharmacokinetics: The extent of percutaneous absorption of topical corticosteroids is determined by many factors including the vehicle, the integrity of the epidermal barrier, and the use of occlusive dressings.

Topical corticosteroids can be absorbed from normal intact skin. Inflammation and/or other disease processes in the skin increase percutaneous absorption. Occlusive dressings substantially increase the percutaneous absorption of topical corticosteroids. Thus, occlusive dressings may be a valuable therapeutic adjunct for treatment of resistant dermatoses. (See DOSAGE AND ADMINISTRATION.)

Once absorbed through the skin, topical corticosteroids are handled through pharmacokinetic pathways similar to systemically administered corticosteroids. Corticosteroids are bound to plasma proteins in varying degrees. Corticosteroids are metabolized primarily in the liver and are then excreted by the kidneys. Some of the topical corticosteroids and their metabolites are also excreted into the bile.

INDICATIONS AND USAGE

Topical corticosteroids are indicated for the relief of the inflammatory and pruritic manifestations of corticosteroid-responsive dermatoses.

CONTRAINDICATIONS

Topical corticosteroids are contraindicated in those patients with a history of hypersensitivity to any of the components of the preparation.

PRECAUTIONS

General: Systemic absorption of topical corticosteroids has produced reversible hypothalamic-pituitary-adrenal (HPA) axis suppression, manifestations of Cushing's syndrome, hyperglycemia, and glucosuria in some patients.

Conditions which augment systemic absorption include the application of the more potent steroids, use over large surface areas, prolonged use, and the addition of occlusive dressings.

Therefore, patients receiving a large dose of a potent topical steroid applied to a large surface area or under an occlusive dressing should be evaluated periodically for evidence of HPA axis suppression by using the urinary free cortisol and ACTH stimulation tests. If HPA axis suppression is noted, an attempt should be made to withdraw the drug, to reduce the frequency of application, or to substitute a less potent steroid. Recovery of HPA axis function is generally prompt and complete upon discontinuation of the drug. Infrequently, signs and symptoms of steroid withdrawal may occur, requiring supplemental systemic corticosteroids.

Children may absorb proportionally larger amounts of topical corticosteroids and thus be more susceptible to systemic toxicity. (See PRECAUTIONS—Pediatric Use.)

If irritation develops, topical corticosteroids should be discontinued and appropriate therapy instituted.

In the presence of dermatological infections, the use of an appropriate antifungal or antibacterial agent sould be instituted. If a favorable response does not occur promptly, the corticosteroid should be discontinued until the infection has been adequately controlled.

Information for the Patient: Patients using topical corticosteroids should receive the following information and instructions:

1. This medication is to be used as directed by the physician. It is for external use only. Avoid contact with the eyes.
2. Patients should be advised not to use this medication for any disorder other than for which it was prescribed.
3. The treated skin area should not be bandaged or otherwise covered or wrapped as to be occlusive unless directed by the physician.
4. Patients should report any signs of local adverse reactions especially under occlusive dressing.
5. Parents of pediatric patients should be advised not to use tight-fitting diapers or plastic pants on a child being treated in the diaper area, as these garments may constitute occlusive dressings.

Laboratory Tests: The following tests may be helpful in evaluating the HPA axis suppression:

Urinary free cortisol test
ACTH stimulation test

Carcinogenesis, Mutagenesis, and Impairment of Fertility: Long-term animal studies have not been performed to evaluate the carcinogenic potential or the effect on fertility of topical corticosteroids.

Studies to determine mutagencity with prednisolone and hydrocortisone have revealed negative results.

Pregnancy Category C: Corticosteroids are generally teratogenic in laboratory animals when administered systemically at relatively low dosage levels. The more potent corticosteroids have been shown to be teratogenic after dermal application in laboratory animals. There are no adequate and well-controlled studies in pregnant women on teratogenic effects from topically applied corticosteroids. Therefore, topical corticosteroids should be used during pregnancy only if the potential benefit justifies the potential risk to the fetus. Drugs of this class should not be used extensively on pregnant patients, in large amounts, or for prolonged periods of time.

Nursing Mothers: It is not known whether topical administration of corticosteroids could result in sufficient systemic absorption to produce detectable quantities in breast milk. Systemically administered corticosteroids are secreted into breast milk in quantities *not* likely to have a deleterious effect on the infant. Nevertheless, caution should be exercised when topical corticosteroids are administered to a nursing woman.

Pediatric Use: *Pediatric patients may demonstrate greater susceptibility to topical corticosteroid-induced HPA axis suppression and Cushing's syndrome than mature patients because of a larger skin surface area to body weight ratio.*

Hypothalamic-pituitary-adrenal (HPA) axis suppression, Cushing's syndrome, and intracranial hypertension have been reported in children receiving topical corticosteroids. Manifestations of adrenal suppression in children include linear growth retardation, delayed weight gain, low plasma cortisol levels, and absence of response to ACTH stimulation. Manifestations of intracranial hypertension include bulging fontanelles, headaches, and bilateral papilledema.

Administration of topical corticosteroids to children should be limited to the least amount compatible with an effective therapeutic regimen. Chronic corticosteroid therapy may interfere with the growth and development of children.

ADVERSE REACTIONS

The following local adverse reactions are reported infrequently with topical corticosteroids, but may occur more frequently with the use of occlusive dressings. These reactions are listed in an approximate decreasing order of occurrence:

Burning, Itching, Irritation, Dryness, Folliculitis, Hypertrichosis, Acneiform eruptions, Hypopigmentation, Perioral dermatitis, Allergi contact dermatitis, Maceration of the skin, Secondary infection, Skin Atrophy, Straie, Miliaria.

OVERDOSAGE

Topically applied corticosteroids can be absorbed in sufficient amounts to produce systemic effects (See PRECAUTIONS).

DOSAGE AND ADMINISTRATION

Topical corticosteroids are generally applied to the affected area as a thin film from three to four times daily depending on the severity of the condition.

Occlusive dressings may be used for the management of psoriasis or recalcitrant conditions.

If an infection develops, the use of occlusive dressings should be discontinued and appropriate antimicrobial therapy instituted.

HOW SUPPLIED

NUTRACORT® Cream 1% is supplied in high density polyethylene (HDPE) tubes:
30g—**NDC** 0299-5821-30
60g—**NDC** 0299-5821-60
and in polypropylene jars:
4 oz—**NDC** 0299-5821-04
NUTRACORT® Lotion 1% is supplied in HDPE bottles:
2 fl. oz.—NDC 0299-5830-01
4 fl. oz.—NDC 0299-5830-02
Store at room temperature.

NUTRADERM® Lotion
Skin-Lubricant—Moisturizer

NUTRADERM® Cream
Moisturizer—Emollient

COMPOSITION

Lotion contains mineral oil in water, sorbitan stearate, stearyl alcohol, sodium lauryl sulfate, cetyl alcohol, carbomer-940, methylparaben triethanolamine, propylparaben and fragrance.

Cream contains mineral oil in water, sorbitan stearate, stearyl alcohol, cetyl alcohol, sorbitol, isopropyl palmitate, cetyl esters wax, sodium lauryl sulfate, dimethicone, methylparabens, propylparabens, citric acid and fragrance.

ACTIONS AND USES

NUTRADERM Lotion lubricates and moisturizes the skin through hydration. It helps retain the normal moisture balance of the skin and helps the protective action of skin lipids. Indicated for the generalized dryness and itching associated with chapped or chafed skin, sunburn, winter-itch, aging, heat rash, diaper rash and detergent hands.

ADMINISTRATION AND DOSAGE

Apply freely to dry skin areas as necessary, or as directed by your dermatologist.

HOW SUPPLIED

NUTRADERM Lotion 8 oz. (NDC 0299-5880-04), NUTRADERM Lotion 16 oz. (NDC 0299-5880-05) plastic bottles; also available as NUTRADERM Cream 1.5 oz. (NDC 0299-5850-01), NUTRADERM Cream 3 oz. (NDC 0299-5850-30) plastic tubes; NUTRADERM Cream 1 lb. (NDC 0299-5850-05) plastic jar.

Paddock Laboratories, Inc.

3101 LOUISIANA AVENUE NORTH
MINNEAPOLIS, MN 55427

ACTIDOSE™ **OTC**
[act 'ĭ -dose]
(Activated Charcoal Suspension)

Actidose (Activated charcoal) is supplied in bottles containing 25 grams and 50 grams activated charcoal suspension. Each milliliter contains 208 mg (0.208 grams) activated charcoal and 400 mg (0.4 grams) sorbitol.

ACTIDOSE–AQUA **OTC**
[act 'ĭ 'dose a-qua]
(Activated Charcoal Suspension)

Actidose-Aqua (Activated Charcoal) is supplied in bottles containing 25 grams and 50 grams activated charcoal suspension. Each milliliter contains 208 mg (0.208 grams) activated charcoal in aqueous suspension.

ETS–2%™ ℞
(Erythromycin Topical Solution)

DESCRIPTION

Erythromycin is an antibiotic produced from a strain of Streptomyces erythraeus. It is basic and readily forms salts with acids. Erythromycin 2 percent Topical Solution containing 20 mg/ml erythromycin base in a clear solution vehicle of 66 percent alcohol, propylene glycol and citric acid.

CLINICAL PHARMACOLOGY

Although the mechanism by which Erythromycin Solution acts in reducing inflammatory lesions of acne vulgaris is unknown, it is presumably due to its antibiotic action.

INDICATIONS AND USAGE

Erythromycin Solution is indicated for the topical control of acne vulgaris.

CONTRAINDICATIONS

Erythromycin Solution is contraindicated in persons who have shown hypersensitivity to erythromycin or any of the other listed ingredients.

WARNING

The safe use of Erythromycin Solution during pregnancy or lactation has not been established.

PRECAUTIONS

Erythromycin Solution is recommended for external use only and should be kept away from the eyes, nose, mouth and other mucous membranes. Concomitant topical acne therapy should be used with caution because a cumulative irritancy effect may occur, especially with the use of peeling, desquamating or abrasive agents.

The use of antibiotic agents may be associated with the overgrowth of antibiotic-resistant organisms. If this occurs, administration of this drug should be discontinued and appropriate measures taken.

ADVERSE REACTIONS

Adverse conditions reported include dryness, tenderness, pruritus, desquamation, erythema, oiliness, and burning sensation. Irritation of the eyes has also been reported. A case of generalized urticarial reaction, possibly related to the drug, which required the use of systemic steroid therapy has been reported.

DOSAGE AND ADMINISTRATION

Erythromycin Solution should be applied to the affected area each morning and evening after the skin is thoroughly washed with warm water and soap and patted dry. Apply contents by tilting bottle and rubbing applicator over affected area until skin is thoroughly wet. Close tightly after each use.

Continued on next page

Paddock—Cont.

HOW SUPPLIED
Bottles of 2 fl. oz. (59 ml). Store at controlled room temperature (59°F–86°F). NDC 0574-0014-02

CAUTION
Federal law prohibits dispensing without prescription.

EMULSOIL®
(Self-Emulsifying Castor Oil)

(See PDR For Nonprescription Drugs)

GLUTOSE®
(Dextrose Gel)
For Insulin Reactions

(See PDR For Nonprescription Drugs)

IPECAC SYRUP

(See PDR For Nonprescription Drugs)

NYSTATIN, USP ℞
For Extemporaneous Preparation of Oral Suspension

DESCRIPTION
Nystatin, USP is an antifungal antibiotic which is both fungistatic and fungicidal *in vitro* against a wide variety of yeasts and yeast-like fungi. It is a polyene antibiotic of undetermined structural formula that is obtained from *Streptomyces noursei.* Nystatin, USP, which contains no excipients or preservatives, is a ready-to-use non-sterile powder for oral administration available in bottles of 50-million, 150-million, 500-million and 5-billion units.

CLINICAL PHARMACOLOGY
Nystatin probably acts by binding to sterols in the cell membrane of the fungus with a resultant change in membrane permeability allowing leakage of intracellular components. It is absorbed very sparingly following oral administration, with no detectable blood levels when given in the recommended doses. Most of the orally administered nystatin is passed unchanged in the stool.

INDICATIONS AND USAGE
For the treatment of infections of the oral cavity caused by *Candida albicans* (monilia).

CONTRAINDICATIONS
Hypersensitivity to the drug.

ADVERSE REACTIONS
Large oral doses of nystatin have occasionally produced diarrhea, gastrointestinal distress, nausea and vomiting.

DOSAGE AND ADMINISTRATION
Adults and older children: Add ⅛ tsp. (500,000 units) of nystatin, USP to approximately ½ to 1 cup (120 to 240 ml, or 4 to 8 oz.) of water and stir well. The entire dose should then be used to thoroughly rinse the mouth and the dose should be retained in the mouth as long as possible before swallowing. This dose should be given orally four times daily, and should be continued for at least 48 hours after perioral symptoms have disappeared and cultures have returned to normal. One-eighth tsp. of nystatin, USP is equivalent to the recommended dose for adults and children of Nystatin Oral Suspension (4 to 6 ml, or 400,000 to 600,000 units). This product contains no preservative and therefore should be used immediately after mixing and should not be stored.

HOW SUPPLIED
Bottles containing 50-million units, 150-million units, 500-million units and 5-billion units—(1 billion units is approximately 170 to 200 g depending on potency of the powder).
NDC 0574-0403-05—50-Million Units
NDC 0574-0403-15—150-Million Units
NDC 0574-0403-50—500 Million Units
NDC 0574-0403-01—5-Billion Units
Store under refrigeration 2–8°C (36–46°F) in tight light-resistant containers.
Note: The potency of this product cannot be assured for longer than 90 days after the container is first opened.
6/85

Products are cross-indexed by generic and chemical names in the **YELLOW SECTION**

Palisades Pharmaceuticals, Inc.
219 COUNTY ROAD
TENAFLY, NEW JERSEY 07670

SCLEROMATE™ ℞
[*skle″ro-māt*]
MORRHUATE SODIUM INJECTION U.S.P.

DESCRIPTION
Morrhuate Sodium Injection, U.S.P. is a mixture of the sodium salts of the saturated and unsaturated fatty acids of Cod Liver Oil. SCLEROMATE Morrhuate Sodium Injection, U.S.P. is prepared by the saponification of selected Cod Liver Oils, it is overlaid with filtered Nitrogen to prevent discoloration that occurs on exposure to oxygen. Morrhuate Sodium occurs as a pale-yellowish, granular powder with a slight fishy odor and is soluable in water and in alcohol.
NOTE: Solid matter may develop a hazy appearance on standing and the injection should not be used if the solid matter does not dissolve completely on warming. The pH of the injection is adjusted to approximately 9.5.

CLINICAL PHARMACOLOGY
Morrhuate Sodium, when injected into the vein, causes inflamation of the intima and formation of a thrombus. This blood clot occludes the injected vein and fibrous tissue develops, resulting in the obliteration of the vein.

INDICATIONS AND USAGE
Morrhuate Sodium Injection is used for the obliteration of primary varicosed veins that consist of simple dilation with competent valves.
Sclerotherapy should not be used in patients with significant valvular or deep vein incompetence. (See Precautions)
Although a Morrhuate Sodium has been used as a sclerosing agent for the treatment of internal hemorrhoids, there is no substantial evidence that the drug is useful for this purpose.
Most patients with symptomatic primary varicosed veins should be treated initially with compression stockings. If this treatment is inadequate, surgery may be required. Sclerosing agents may be useful as a supplement to venous ligation to obliterate residual varicosed veins or in patients who have conditions which increase the risk of surgery. However, many clinicians consider sclerotherapy if not effective may decrease the potential success of later surgery, should this be required.

CONTRAINDICATIONS
Morrhuate Sodium is contraindicated in patients who have shown a previous hypersensitivity reaction to the drug or to the fatty acids of cod liver oil. Continued administration of the drug is contraindicated when an unusual local reaction at the injection site or a systemic reaction occurs.
Thrombosis induced by Morrhuate Sodium may extend into the deep venous system in patients with significant valvular incompetence, therefore, valvular competency, deep vein patency, and deep vein competency should be determined by angiography and/or by tests such as the Trendelenberg and Perthes before injection of sclerosing agents. The drug is contraindicated for obliterations of superficial veins in patients with persistent occlusion of the deep veins. Morrhuate Sodium is also contraindicated in patients with acute superficial thrombophlebitis; underlying arterial disease; varicosities caused by abdominal and pelvic tumors, uncontrolled diabetes melitus, thyrotoxicosis, tuberculosis, neoplasms, asthma, sepsis, blood dyscrasias, acute respiratory or skin disease; and in bedridden patients. Treatment with Morrhuate Sodium should be delayed in patients with acute local or systemic infections (including infected ulcers). Extensive therapy with the drug is inadvisable in patients who are severely debilitated or senile.

PRECAUTIONS
Burning or cramping sensations indicate local reactions. Urticaria may result. Sloughing and necrosis of tissue may occur with extravasation of the drug. Technique development is essential for optimal success in sclerotherapy, therefore the drug should be administered only by a physician familiar with proper injection technique. Drowsiness and headache may occur rarely. Pulmonary embolism has been reported.
Rarely, patients may have, or may develop hypersensitivity to Morrhuate Sodium, characterized by dizziness, weakness, vascular collapse, asthma, respiratory depression, gastrointestinal disturbances (i.e., Nausea, vomiting), and urticaria. Anaphylactic reactions may occur within a few minutes after injection of the drug and are most likely to occur when therapy is reinstituted after an interval of several weeks. Morrhuate Sodium should only be administered when adequate facilities, drugs (i.e., epinephrine, antihistamines, corticosteroids), and personnel are available for the treatment of anaphylactic reactions.

PREGNANCY
Safety in use of Morrhuate Sodium during pregnancy has not been established.

DOSAGE
Morrhuate Sodium is administered only by INTRAVENOUS Injection. Care must be taken to avoid extravasation. (see Precautions.) Specialized references should be consulted for specific procedures and techniques of administration. When small veins are injected, or the injection solution is cold, or if solid matter has separated in the solution, the ampul or vial should be warmed by immersing in hot water. The solution should become clear on warming; only a clear solution should be used. Because the solution froths easily, a large bore needle should be used to fill the syringe, however, a small bore needle should be used for the injection.
To determine possible sensitivity to the drug, some clinicians recommend injection of 0.25–1 ml of 5% Morrhuate Sodium injection into a varicosity 24 hours before administration of a large dose.
Dosage of Morrhuate Sodium depends on the size and degree of varicosity. The usual adult dose for obliteration of small or medium veins is 50–100mg (1–2ml of the 5% injection). For large veins, 150–250 (3–5ml of the injection) is used. The drug may be given as multiple injections at one time or in single doses. Therapy may be repeated at 5–7 day intervals, according to the patient's response. Following injection of Morrhuate Sodium, the vein promptly becomes hard and swollen for 2–4 inches, depending on the size and response of the vein. After 24 hours, the vein is hard and slightly tender to the touch (with little or no periphlebitis). The skin around the injection becomes light-bronze; this color usually disappears shortly. An aching sensation and feeling of stiffness usually occur and last approximately 48 hours.

HOW SUPPLIED

MORRHUATE SODIUM INJECTION 5%

NDC-53159-003-25	5ml Ampuls in boxes of 25's
NDC-53159-003-01	30ml Multiple use Vials
NDC-53159-003-10	10ml fill in 20ml Multiple use Vials

STORAGE
Store below 40 degrees C. (104 degrees F.) preferably in a refrigerator, or between 15–30 degrees C. (59–86 degrees F.)
Rev. July 1985

YOCON® ℞
[*yō′kon*]
(brand of yohimbine hydrochloride)

DESCRIPTION
Yohimbine is a 3α-15α-20β-17α-hydroxy Yohimbine-16α-carboxylic acid methyl ester. The alkaloid is found in Rubaceae and related trees. Also in Rauwolfia Serpentina (L) Benth.
Yohimbine is an indolalkylamine alkaloid with chemical similarity to reserpine. It is a crystalline powder, odorless. Each compressed tablet contains (1/12 gr.) 5.4 mg of Yohimbine Hydrochloride.

ACTION
Yohimbine blocks presynaptic alpha-2 adrenergic receptors. Its action on peripheral blood vessels resembles that of reserpine, though it is weaker and of short duration. Yohimbine's peripheral autonomic nervous system effect is to increase parasympathetic (cholinergic) and decrease sympathetic (adrenergic) activity. It is to be noted that in male sexual performance, erection is linked to cholinergic activity and to alpha-2 adrenergic blockade which may theoretically result in increased penile inflow, decreased penile outflow or both.
Yohimbine exerts a stimulating action on the mood and may increase anxiety. Such actions have not been adequately studied or related to dosage although they appear to require high doses of the drug. Yohimbine has a mild anti-diuretic action, probably via stimulation of hypothalmic centers and release of posterior pituitary hormone.
Reportedly, Yohimbine exerts no significant influence on cardiac stimulation and other effects mediated by β-adrenergic receptors, its effect on blood pressure, if any, would be to lower it; however, no adequate studies are at hand to quantitate this effect in terms of Yohimbine dosage.

INDICATIONS
YOCON is indicated as a sympathicolytic and mydriatic. It may have activity as an aphrodisiac.

CONTRAINDICATIONS
Renal diseases, and patient's sensitive to the drug. In view of the limited and inadequate information at hand, no precise tabulation can be offered of additional contra-indications.

WARNING
Generally, this drug is not proposed for use in females and certainly must not be used during pregnancy. Neither is this drug proposed for use in pediatric, geriatric or cardio-renal patients with gastric or duodenal ulcer history. Nor should it be used in conjunction with mood-modifying drugs such as antidepressants, or in psychiatric patients in general.

ADVERSE REACTIONS

Yohimbine readily penetrates the (CNS) and produces a complex pattern of responses in lower doses than required to produce peripheral α-adrenergic blockade. These include, anti-diuresis, a general picture of central excitation including elevation of blood pressure and heart rate increased motor activity, irritability and tremor. Sweating, nausea and vomiting are common after parenteral administration of the drug.[1,2] Also dizziness, headache, skin flushing reported when used orally[1,3].

DOSAGE AND ADMINISTRATION

Experimental dosage reported in treatment of erectile impotence:[1,3,4] 1 tablet (5.4 mg) 3 times a day, to adult males taken orally. Occasional side effects reported with this dosage are nausea, dizziness or nervousness. In the event of side effects dosage is to be reduced to ½ tablet 3 times a day, followed by gradual increases to 1 tablet 3 times a day. Reported therapy not more than 10 weeks[3].

HOW SUPPLIED

Oral tablets of Yocon® 1/12 gr 5.4 mg in bottles of 100's **NDC** 53159-001-01 and 1000's **NDC** 53159-001-10.

REFERENCES

1. A. Morales et al., New England Journal of Medicine: 1221. November 12, 1981.
2. Goodman, Gilman —The Pharmacological basis of Therapeutics 6th ed., p. 176-188, McMillan
3. Weekly Urological Clinical letter, 27:2, July 4, 1983.
4. A. Morales et al., The Journal of Urology *128*: 45-47, 1982.

Rev. January 1985

Parke-Davis

Division of Warner-Lambert Company
201 TABOR ROAD
MORRIS PLAINS, NEW JERSEY 07950

PARCODE®
(Parke-Davis Accurate Recognition Code)

Code Number — Product Name

001 Peritrate® Tablets
Each tablet contains 20 mg pentaerythritol tetranitrate.

002-003 *Unassigned*

004 Peritrate® SA Sustained Action Tablets
Each tablet contains 80 mg pentaerythritol tetranitrate (20 mg in the immediate release layer and 60 mg in the sustained release base).

005-006 *Unassigned*

007 Dilantin® Infatabs®
Each tablet contains 50 mg phenytoin sodium, USP.

008 Peritrate® Tablets
Each tablet contains 40 mg pentaerythritol tetranitrate.

009 *Unassigned*

010 Chlorpromazine Hydrochloride Tablets, USP (Promapar®)
Each tablet contains 10 mg chlorpromazine hydrochloride, USP.

011-012 *Unassigned*

013 Peritrate® Tablets
Each tablet contains 10 mg pentaerythritol tetranitrate.

014-024 *Unassigned*

025 Chlorpromazine Hydrochloride Tablets, USP (Promapar®)
Each tablet contains 25 mg chlorpromazine hydrochloride, USP.

026-036 *Unassigned*

037 Ferrous Sulfate Filmseals®, USP (325 mg)

038-049 *Unassigned*

050 Chlorpromazine Hydrochloride Tablets, USP (Promapar®)
Each tablet contains 50 mg chlorpromazine hydrochloride, USP.

051-099 *Unassigned*

100 Chlorpromazine Hydrochloride Tablets, USP (Promapar®)
Each tablet contains 100 mg chlorpromazine hydrochloride, USP.

101-110 *Unassigned*

111 Ergostat® Sublingual Tablets
Each tablet contains 2 mg ergotamine tartrate.

112-116 *Unassigned*

117 Diphenoxylate Hydrochloride and Atropine Sulfate Tablets, USP
Each tablet contains 2.5 mg diphenoxylate hydrochloride and 0.025 mg atropine sulfate, USP.

118-120 *Unassigned*

121 Chlorthalidone Tablets, USP
Each tablet contains 50 mg chlorthalidone, USP.

122 *Unassigned*

123 Chlorthalidone Tablets, USP
Each tablet contains 25 mg chlorthalidone, USP.

124-140 *Unassigned*

141 Diazepam Tablets, USP
Each tablet contains 2 mg diazepam, USP.

142 Diazepam Tablets, USP
Each tablet contains 5 mg diazepam, USP.

143 Diazepam Tablets, USP
Each tablet contains 10 mg diazepam, USP.

144-165 *Unassigned*

166 Mandelamine® Tablets
Each tablet contains 0.5 gram methenamine mandelate, USP.

167 Mandelamine® Tablets
Each tablet contains 1.0 gram methenamine mandelate, USP.

168-176 *Unassigned*

177 Sinubid ® Tablets
Each tablet contains 300 mg acetaminophen, 100 mg phenylpropanolamine hydrochloride, and 66 mg phenyltoloxamine citrate.

178-179 *Unassigned*

180 Pyridium® Tablets
Each tablet contains 100 mg phenazopyridine hydrochloride, USP.

181 Pyridium® Tablets
Each tablet contains 200 mg phenazopyridine hydrochloride, USP.

182 Pyridium® Plus Tablets
Each tablet contains 150 mg phenazopyridine hydrochloride (Pyridium®), 0.3 mg hyoscyamine hydrobromide, and 15 mg butabarbital.

183-199 *Unassigned*

200 Brondecon® Tablets
Each tablet contains 200 mg oxtriphylline and 100 mg guaifenesin.

201 Chlorpromazine Hydrochloride Tablets, USP (Promapar®)
Each tablet contains 200 mg chlorpromazine hydrochloride, USP.

202 Procan® SR Tablets, 250 mg
Each sustained-release tablet contains 250 mg procainamide hydrochloride.

203 *Unassigned*

204 Procan® SR Tablets, 500 mg
Each sustained-release tablet contains 500 mg procainamide hydrochloride.

205 Procan® SR Tablets, 750 mg
Each sustained-release tablet contains 750 mg procainamide hydrochloride.

206 *Unassigned*

207 Procan® SR Tablets, 1000 mg
Each sustained-release tablet contains 1000 mg procainamide hydrochloride.

208-209 *Unassigned*

210 Choledyl® Tablets
Each tablet contains 100 mg oxtriphylline, USP.

211 Choledyl® Tablets
Each tablet contains 200 mg oxtriphylline, USP.

212-213 *Unassigned*

214 Choledyl® SA Tablets
Each sustained-action tablet contains 400 mg oxtriphylline, USP.

215-220 *Unassigned*

221 Choledyl® SA Tablets
Each sustained-action tablet contains 600 mg oxtriphylline, USP.

222-229 *Unassigned*

230 Tedral® Tablets
Each tablet contains 130 mg theophylline, 24 mg ephedrine hydrochloride, and 8 mg phenobarbital.

231 Tedral® SA Tablets
Each sustained-action tablet contains 180 mg anhydrous theophylline (90 mg in the immediate release layer and 90 mg in the sustained-release layer); 48 mg ephedrine hydrochloride (16 mg in the immediate release layer and 32 mg in the sustained-release layer); 25 mg phenobarbital in the immediate release layer.

232-236 *Unassigned*

237 Zarontin® Capsules
Each capsule contains 250 mg ethosuximide, USP.

238-246 *Unassigned*

247 D-S-S Capsules
Each capsule contains 100 mg docusate sodium.

248 D-S-S Plus Capsules
Each capsule contains 100 mg docusate sodium and 30 mg casanthranol.

249-250 *Unassigned*

251 Proloid® Tablets
Each tablet contains ½ grain thyroglobulin, USP.

252 Proloid® Tablets
Each tablet contains 1 grain thyroglobulin, USP.

253 Proloid® Tablets
Each tablet contains 1½ grains thyroglobulin, USP.

254 Proloid® Tablets
Each tablet contains 3 grains thyroglobulin, USP.

255-256 *Unassigned*

257 Proloid® Tablets
Each tablet contains 2 grains thyroglobulin, USP.

258-259 *Unassigned*

260 Euthroid®-½ Tablets
Each tablet contains 30 mcg levothyroxine sodium (T_4), 7.5 mcg liothyronine sodium (T_3).

261 Euthroid®-1 Tablets
Each tablet contains 60 mcg levothyroxine sodium (T_4), 15 mcg liothyronine sodium (T_3).

262 Euthroid®-2 Tablets
Each tablet contains 120 mcg levothyroxine sodium (T_4), 30 mcg liothyronine sodium (T_3).

263 Euthroid®-3 Tablets
Each tablet contains 180 mcg levothyroxine sodium (T_4), 45 mcg liothyronine sodium (T_3).

264-267 *Unassigned*

268 Meclomen® Capsules
Each capsule contains 50 mg meclofenamate sodium.

269 Meclomen® Capsules
Each capsule contains 100 mg meclofenamate sodium.

270 Nardil® Tablets
Each tablet contains 15 mg phenelzine sulfate, USP.

271 Amitriptyline Hydrochloride Tablets
Each tablet contains 100 mg amitriptyline hydrochloride, USP.

272 Amitriptyline Hydrochloride Tablets
Each tablet contains 10 mg amitriptyline hydrochloride, USP.

273 Amitriptyline Hydrochloride Tablets
Each tablet contains 25 mg amitriptyline hydrochloride, USP.

274 Amitriptyline Hydrochloride Tablets
Each tablet contains 50 mg amitriptyline hydrochloride, USP.

275 Amitriptyline Hydrochloride Tablets
Each tablet contains 75 mg amitriptyline hydrochloride, USP.

276 Ⓒ Centrax® Tablets
Each tablet contains 10 mg prazepam.

277 *Unassigned*

278 Amitriptyline Hydrochloride Tablets
Each tablet contains 150 mg amitriptyline hydrochloride, USP.

Continued on next page

This product information was prepared in August, 1986. On these and other Parke-Davis Products, information may be obtained by addressing PARKE-DAVIS, Division of Warner-Lambert Company, Morris Plains, New Jersey 07950.

Parke-Davis—Cont.

279-
281 *Unassigned*

282 **Natafort® Filmseal®**
Each tablet represents vitamin A (acetate), 6,000 IU; vitamin D 400 IU; folic acid, 1 mg; vitamin B_1 (thiamine mononitrate), 3 mg; vitamin B_2 (riboflavin), 2 mg; vitamin B_6 (pyridoxine hydrochloride), 15 mg; vitamin B_{12} (cyanocobalamin), crystalline, 6 mcg; vitamin C (ascorbic acid), 120 mg; nicotinamide (niacinamide), 20 mg; vitamin E (*dl*-alpha tocopheryl acetate), 30 IU; calcium (as calcium carbonate), 350 mg; magnesium (as magnesium oxide), 100 mg; iodine (as potassium iodide), 0.15 mg; iron (as ferrous fumarate), 65 mg; zinc (as zinc oxide), 25 mg.

283-
319 *Unassigned*

320 **Parsidol® Tablets**
Each tablet contains 10 mg ethopropazine hydrochloride, USP.

321 **Parsidol® Tablets**
Each tablet contains 50 mg ethopropazine hydrochloride, USP.

322-
336 *Unassigned*

337 **Eldec® Kapseals®**
Each capsule represents vitamin A (acetate), (0.5 mg) 1,667 IU; vitamin C (ascorbic acid), 66.7 mg; vitamin B_1 (thiamine mononitrate), 10 mg; vitamin B_2 (riboflavin), 0.87 mg; vitamin B_6 (pyridoxine hydrochloride), 0.67 mg; nicotinamide (niacinamide), 16.7 mg; *dl*-panthenol, 10 mg; ferrous sulfate, dried, 16.7 mg; iodine (as potassium iodide), 0.05 mg; calcium carbonate, 66.7 mg; vitamin E (*dl*-alpha tocopheryl acetate), (10 mg) 10 IU; vitamin B_{12} (cyanocobalamin), 2 mcg; folic acid, 0.33 mg. The Kapseal is a Dark Blue No. 1 capsule with Light Blue opaque band.

338-
361 *Unassigned*

362 **Dilantin® Kapseals®**
Each Kapseal contains 100 mg extended phenytoin sodium, USP. The Kapseal is a No. 3 capsule with Orange band. (The Orange band on White capsule is a trademark registered in the US Patent Office.)

363-
364 *Unassigned*

365 **Dilantin® Kapseals®**
Each Kapseal contains 30 mg extended phenytoin sodium, USP. The Kapseal is a No. 4 capsule with Pink opaque band.

366-
372 *Unassigned*

373 **Benadryl® Kapseals®**
Each Kapseal contains 50 mg diphenhydramine hydrochloride. The Kapseal is a Pink No. 4 capsule with White opaque band. (The White band on Pink capsule is a trademark registered in the US Patent Office.)

374 *Unassigned*

375 **Dilantin® with Phenobarbital (1/4 grain) Kapseals®**
Each Kapseal contains Dilantin (phenytoin sodium), 100 mg; phenobarbital, 16 mg (1/4 grain). The Kapseal is a No. 3 capsule with Garnet band.

376-
378 *Unassigned*

379 **Chloromycetin® Kapseals®**
Each Kapseal contains 250 mg chloramphenicol. The Kapseal is a White opaque No. 2 capsule with Gray opaque band. (The Gray band on White capsule is a trademark registered in the US Patent Office.)

380-
389 *Unassigned*

390 **Natabec® Kapseals®**
Each Kapseal represents vitamin A (acetate), (1.2 mg), 4,000 IU*; vitamin D, 400 IU; vitamin C (ascorbic acid), 50 mg; vitamin B_1 (thiamine mononitrate), 3 mg; vitamin B_2 (riboflavin), 2 mg; nicotinamide +, 10 mg; vitamin B_6 (pyridoxine HCl), 3 mg; vitamin B_{12} crystalline (cyanocobalamin), 5 mcg; precipitated calcium carbonate, 600 mg; iron (as dried ferrous sulfate), 30 mg.

---
*IU = International Units
+Supplied as niacinamide

391-
392 *Unassigned*

393 **Milontin® Kapseals®**
Each Kapseal contains 500 mg phensuximide, USP. The Kapseal is a Light Orange No. 0 capsule with Orange band.

394-
401 *Unassigned*

402 **Amcill® Capsules, 250 mg**
Each capsule contains ampicillin trihydrate equivalent to 250 mg ampicillin.

403 *Unassigned*

404 **Amcill® Capsules, 500 mg**
Each capsule contains ampicillin trihydrate equivalent to 500 mg ampicillin.

405-
406 *Unassigned*

407 **Tetracycline Hydrochloride Capsules, USP, 250 mg (Cyclopar®)**
Each capsule contains 250 mg tetracycline hydrochloride, USP.

408-
419 *Unassigned*

420 **Quinine Sulfate Capsules, USP**
Each capsule contains 0.325 g (5 grains) quinine sulfate.

421-
436 *Unassigned*

437 **Estrovis® Tablets**
Each tablet contains 100 mcg quinestrol.

438-
439 *Unassigned*

440 **Furosemide Tablets, USP, 20 mg**
Each tablet contains 20 mg furosemide, USP.

441 **Furosemide Tablets, USP, 40 mg**
Each tablet contains 40 mg furosemide, USP.

442 **Furosemide Tablets, USP, 80 mg**
Each tablet contains 80 mg furosemide, USP.

443-
470 *Unassigned*

471 **Benadryl® Capsules**
Each capsule contains 25 mg diphenhydramine hydrochloride.

472-
489 *Unassigned*

490 **Easprin® Enteric Coated Tablets**
Each tablet contains 15 grains (975 mg) aspirin, USP.

491-
524 *Unassigned*

525 **Celontin® Kapseals®**
Each Kapseal contains 300 mg methsuximide, USP. The Kapseal is a Yellow Tint No. 2 capsule with Orange band.

526-
528 *Unassigned*

529 **Humatin® Capsules**
Each capsule contains paromomycin sulfate, USP, equivalent to 250 mg paromomycin.

530 *Unassigned*

531 **Dilantin® with Phenobarbital (1/2 grain) Kapseals®**
Each Kapseal contains Dilantin (phenytoin sodium), 100 mg; phenobarbital, 32 mg (1/2 grain). The Kapseal is a No. 3 capsule with Black band.

532 *Unassigned*

533 **Calcium Lactate Tablets, USP**
Each tablet contains 325 mg calcium lactate.

534 **Natabec® with Fluoride Kapseals®**
Each Kapseal represents vitamin A (acetate) (1.2 mg), 4,000 IU*; vitamin D (ergocalciferol) (10 mcg), 400 IU; vitamin C (ascorbic acid), 50 mg; thiamine mononitrate (vitamin B_1), 3 mg; riboflavin (vitamin B_2), 2.0 mg; nicotinamide (niacinamide), 20 mg; vitamin B_6 (pyridoxine hydrochloride), 3 mg; vitamin B_{12}, crystalline (cyanocobalamin), 5 mcg; ferrous sulfate, 150 mg; calcium carbonate, 600 mg; sodium fluoride, 2.2 mg.

*International Units
The Kapseal is a Pastel Pink No. 0 capsule with Ruby Red opaque band.

535-
536 *Unassigned*

537 **Celontin® (Half Strength) Kapseals®**
Each Kapseal contains 150 mg methsuximide, USP. The Kapseal is a Yellow Tint No. 4 capsule with Brown opaque band.

538-
539 *Unassigned*

540 **Ponstel® Kapseals®**
Each Kapseal contains 250 mg mefenamic acid. The Kapseal is an Ivory opaque No. 1 capsule with Light Blue opaque band. The blue band on ivory capsule combination is a Parke-Davis trademark.

541 **Natabec-FA® Kapseals®**
Each Kapseal represents vitamin A (acetate), (1.2 mg) 4,000 IU; ergocalciferol (10 mcg), 400 IU; ascorbic acid, 50 mg; thiamine mononitrate, 3 mg; riboflavin, 2 mg; pyridoxine hydrochloride, 3 mg; cyanocobalamin, 5 mcg; folic acid, 0.1 mg; niacinamide, 20 mg; calcium carbonate, 600 mg; ferrous sulfate,* 150 mg.

---
*Supplied as dried ferrous sulfate equivalent to the labeled amount of ferrous sulfate.
The Kapseal is a Pink Tint opaque No. 0 capsule with White opaque band.

542-
543 *Unassigned*

544 **Geriplex-FS® Kapseals®**
Each capsule represents vitamin A (acetate) (1.5 mg), 5,000 IU; ascorbic acid,* 50 mg; thiamine mononitrate, 5 mg; riboflavin, 5 mg; cyanocobalamin, 2 mcg; choline dihydrogen citrate, 20 mg; niacinamide, 15 mg; *dl*-alpha tocopheryl acetate (5 mg), 5 IU; iron,† 6 mg; copper sulfate, 4 mg; manganese sulfate (monohydrate), 4 mg; zinc sulfate, 2 mg; calcium phosphate, dibasic (anhydrous), 200 mg; Taka-Diastase® (*aspergillus oryzae enzymes*); 2 1/2 gr; docusate sodium, 100 mg.

*Supplied as sodium ascorbate.
†Supplied as dried ferrous sulfate.
The Kapseal is a Blue No. 0 capsule with White opaque band.

545-
546 *Unassigned*

547 **Natabec ℞® Kapseals®**
Each Kapseal represents vitamin A (acetate) (1.2 mg), 4,000 IU; Vitamin D (10 mcg) 400 IU; ascorbic acid, 50 mg; thiamine mononitrate, 3 mg; riboflavin, 2 mg; pyridoxine hydrochloride, 3 mg; cyanocobalamin, 5 mcg; niacinamide, 10 mg; folic acid, 1 mg; calcium carbonate, precipitated, 600 mg; iron* 30 mg.

---
*Supplied as dried ferrous sulfate.
The Kapseal is a Blue opaque No. 0 capsule with Pink opaque band. The banded capsule is a Warner-Lambert trademark registered in the US Patent Office.

548-
551 *Unassigned*

552 **CIV Centrax® Capsules**
Each capsule contains 5 mg prazepam.

553 **CIV Centrax® Capsules**
Each capsule contains 10 mg prazepam.

554 **CIV Centrax® Capsules**
Each capsule contains 20 mg prazepam.

555-
603 *Unassigned*

604 **Calcium Lactate Tablets, USP**
Each tablet contains 650 mg (10 grains) calcium lactate.

605 *Unassigned*

606 **Aspirin Tablets, USP (White)**
Each tablet contains 325 mg (5 grains) aspirin.

607 **CIV Phenobarbital Tablets, USP**
Each tablet contains 60 mg (1 grain) phenobarbital.

608-
617 *Unassigned*

618 **Placebo tablet in Norlestrin 28 1/50.**

619-
621 *Unassigned*

622 **Ferrous Fumarate Tablets**
Each tablet contains 75 mg ferrous fumarate, USP.

623-
633 *Unassigned*

634 **CIII Acetaminophen with Codeine Phosphate Tablets, No. 2**
Each tablet contains 300 mg acetaminophen and 15 mg (1/4 grain) codeine phosphate.

635 **CIII Acetaminophen with Codeine Phosphate Tablets, No. 3**
Each tablet contains 300 mg acetaminophen and 30 mg (1/2 grain) codeine phosphate.

636 *Unassigned*

637 **CIII Acetaminophen with Codeine Phosphate Tablets, No. 4**
Each tablet contains 300 mg acetaminophen and 60 mg (1 grain) codeine phosphate.

638 **Tabron® Filmseal®**
Each tablet represents ferrous fumarate, 304.2 mg (represents 100 mg of elemental iron); vitamin C (ascorbic acid), 500 mg; vitamin B_1 (thiamine mononitrate), 6 mg; vitamin B_2 (riboflavin), 6 mg; vitamin B_6 (pyridoxine hydrochloride), 5 mg; vitamin B_{12} (cyanocobalamin), crystalline, 25 mcg; folic acid, 1

mg; nicotinamide (niacinamide), 30 mg; calcium pantothenate, 10 mg; vitamin E (*dl*-alpha tocopheryl acetate), (30 mg), 30 IU; docusate sodium, 50 mg.

639 *Unassigned*

640 **Acetaminophen Tablets, USP (Tapar®)**
Each tablet contains 325 mg (5 grains) acetaminophen, USP.

641-
647 *Unassigned*

648 **Penicillin V Potassium Tablets, USP, 250 mg (Penapar VK®)**
Each tablet contains penicillin V potassium equivalent to 250 mg (400,000 units) penicillin V.

649-
668 *Unassigned*

669 **Lopid® Capsules**
Each capsule contains 300 mg gemfibrozil.

670-
671 *Unassigned*

672 **Erythromycin Stearate Filmseals (Erypar®)**
Each Filmseal® contains 250 mg erythromycin as erythromycin stearate.

673 **Penicillin V Potassium Tablets, USP, 500 mg (Penapar VK®)**
Each tablet contains penicillin V potassium equivalent to 500 mg (800,000 units) penicillin V.

674-
691 *Unassigned*

692 **ⒸIV Propoxyphene Hydrochloride Capsules, USP**
Each capsule contains 65 mg propoxyphene hydrochloride.

693-
695 *Unassigned*

696 **ERYC® Capsules**
Each capsule contains 250 mg erythromycin, USP.

697 **Tetracycline Hydrochloride Capsules, USP, 500 mg (Cyclopar® 500)**
Each capsule contains 500 mg tetracycline hydrochloride, USP.

698 **ⒸIV Phenobarbital Tablets, USP**
Each tablet contains 100 mg ($1\frac{1}{2}$ grains) phenobarbital.

699 **ⒸIV Phenobarbital Tablets, USP**
Each tablet contains 15 mg ($\frac{1}{4}$ grain) phenobarbital.

700 **ⒸIV Phenobarbital Tablets, USP**
Each tablet contains 30 mg ($\frac{1}{2}$ grain) phenobarbital.

701 *Unassigned*

702 **Hydrochlorothiazide Tablets, USP (Thiuretic®)**
Each tablet contains 25 mg hydrochlorothiazide.

703-
709 *Unassigned*

710 **Hydrochlorothiazide Tablets, USP (Thiuretic®)**
Each tablet contains 50 mg hydrochlorothiazide.

711- *Unassigned*

712 **Spironolactone with Hydrochlorothiazide Tablets**
Each tablet contains 25 mg spironolactone and 25 mg hydrochlorothiazide.

713 **Spironolactone Tablets, USP**
Each tablet contains 25 mg spironolactone, USP.

714-
724 *Unassigned*

725 **ⒸIII Aspirin with Codeine Phosphate Tablets, No. 2**
Each tablet contains codeine phosphate, $\frac{1}{4}$ grain; aspirin, 325 mg.

726 **ⒸIII Aspirin with Codeine Phosphate Tablets, No. 3**
Each tablet contains codeine phosphate, $\frac{1}{2}$ grain; aspirin, 325 mg.

727 **ⒸIII Aspirin with Codeine Phosphate Tablets, No. 4**
Each tablet contains codeine phosphate, 1 grain; aspirin, 325 mg.

728-
729 *Unassigned*

730 **Amoxicillin Capsules (Utimox®), USP, 250 mg**
Each capsule contains 250 mg amoxicillin.

731 **Amoxicillin Capsules (Utimox®), USP, 500 mg**
Each capsule contains 500 mg amoxicillin.

732 -
799 *Unassigned*

800 **ⒸIV Chlordiazepoxide Hydrochloride Capsules, USP**
Each capsule contains 5 mg chlordiazepoxide hydrochloride.

801 **ⒸIV Chlordiazepoxide Hydrochloride Capsules, USP**
Each capsule contains 10 mg chlordiazepoxide hydrochloride.

802 **ⒸIV Chlordiazepoxide Hydrochloride Capsules, USP**
Each capsule contains 25 mg chlordiazepoxide hydrochloride.

803-
812 *Unassigned*

813 **Doxycycline Hyclate Tablets, USP**
Each tablet contains 100 mg doxycycline hyclate, USP.

814-
828 *Unassigned*

829 **Doxycycline Hyclate Capsules, USP**
Each capsule contains 50 mg doxycycline hyclate, USP.

830 **Doxycycline Hyclate Capsules, USP**
Each capsule contains 100 mg doxycycline hyclate, USP.

831-
848 *Unassigned*

849 **Quinidine Sulfate Tablets, USP**
Each tablet contains 3 grains (200 mg) quinidine sulfate.

850 **Duraquin® (quinidine gluconate) Tablets, 330 mg**
Each scored, white, sustained-release tablet contains 330 mg quinidine gluconate.

851-
864 *Unassigned*

865 **Methyldopa Tablets, USP**
Each tablet contains 250 mg methyldopa, USP.

866 **Methyldopa Tablets, USP**
Each tablet contains 500 mg methyldopa, USP.

867-
881 *Unassigned*

882 **Norlutin® Tablets**
Each tablet contains 5 mg norethindrone, USP.

883-
886 *Unassigned*

887 **Indomethacin Capsules, USP**
Each capsule contains 25 mg indomethacin, USP.

888 **Indomethacin Capsules, USP**
Each capsule contains 50 mg indomethacin, USP.

889-
900 *Unassigned*

901 **Norlestrin® 2.5/50 Tablets**
Each tablet contains norethindrone acetate, 2.5 mg; ethinyl estradiol, 50 mcg.

902-
903 *Unassigned*

904 **Norlestrin® 1/50 Tablets**
Each tablet contains norethindrone acetate, 1 mg; ethinyl estradiol, 50 mcg.

905-
914 *Unassigned*

915 **Loestrin® 1/20 Tablets**
Each tablet contains norethindrone acetate, 1 mg; ethinyl estradiol, 20 mcg.

916 **Loestrin® 1.5/30 Tablets**
Each tablet contains norethindrone acetate, 1.5 mg; ethinyl estradiol, 30 mcg.

917 *Unassigned*

918 **Norlutate® Tablets**
Each tablet contains 5 mg norethindrone acetate.

919 **Erythromycin Stearate Filmseals (Erypar®)**
Each Filmseal® contains 500 mg erythromycin as erythromycin stearate.

920-
999 *Unassigned*

ADRENALIN® CHLORIDE SOLUTION ℞

[*ă-drĕn 'ă-lĭn" chlō 'rīde*]

(Epinephrine Injection, USP), 1:1000

DESCRIPTION

A sterile solution intended for subcutaneous or intramuscular injection. When diluted, it may also be administered intracardially or intravenously. Each milliliter contains 1 mg Adrenalin (epinephrine) as the hydrochloride dissolved in Water for Injection, USP, with sodium chloride added for isotonicity. The ampoules contain not more than 0.1% sodium bisulfite as an antioxidant, and the air in the ampoule has been displaced by nitrogen. The Steri-Vials® contain 0.5% Chloretone® (chlorobutanol) (chloroform derivative) as a preservative and not more than 0.15% sodium bisulfite as an antioxidant. Epinephrine is the active principle of the adrenal medulla, chemically described as (−)-3,4-Dihydroxy-α-[(methylamino) methyl] benzyl alcohol.

CLINICAL PHARMACOLOGY

Adrenalin (epinephrine) is a sympathomimetic drug. It activates an adrenergic receptive mechanism on effector cells and imitates all actions of the sympathetic nervous system except those on the arteries of the face and sweat glands. Epinephrine acts on both alpha and beta receptors and is the most potent alpha receptor activator.

INDICATIONS AND USAGE

In general, the most common uses of epinephrine are to relieve respiratory distress due to bronchospasm, to provide rapid relief of hypersensitivity reactions to drugs and other allergens, and to prolong the action of infiltration anesthetics. Its cardiac effects may be of use in restoring cardiac rhythm in cardiac arrest due to various causes, but it is not used in cardiac failure or in hemorrhagic, traumatic, or cardiogenic shock.

Epinephrine is used as a hemostatic agent. It is also used in treating mucosal congestion of hay fever, rhinitis, and acute sinusitis; to relieve bronchial asthmatic paroxysms; in syncope due to complete heart block or carotid sinus hypersensitivity; for symptomatic relief of serum sickness, urticaria, angioneurotic edema; for resuscitation in cardiac arrest following anesthetic accidents; in simple (open angle) glaucoma; for relaxation of uterine musculature and to inhibit uterine contractions. Epinephrine Injection can be utilized to prolong the action of intraspinal and local anesthetics (see Contraindications).

CONTRAINDICATIONS

Epinephrine is contraindicated in narrow angle (congestive) glaucoma, shock, during general anesthesia with halogenated hydrocarbons or cyclopropane and in individuals with organic brain damage. Epinephrine is also contraindicated with local anesthesia of certain areas, eg, fingers, toes, because of the danger of vasoconstriction producing sloughing of tissue; in labor because it may delay the second stage; in cardiac dilatation and coronary insufficiency.

WARNINGS

Administer with caution to elderly people; to those with cardiovascular disease, hypertension, diabetes or hyperthyroidism; in psychoneurotic individuals, and in pregnancy.

Patients with long-standing bronchial asthma and emphysema who have developed degenerative heart disease should be administered the drug with extreme caution.

Overdosage or inadvertent intravenous injection of epinephrine may cause cerebrovascular hemorrhage resulting from the sharp rise in blood pressure.

Fatalities may also result from pulmonary edema because of the peripheral constriction and cardiac stimulation produced. Rapidly acting vasodilators such as nitrites, or alpha blocking agents may counteract the marked pressor effects of epinephrine.

PRECAUTIONS

General: Adrenalin (epinephrine injection) should be protected from exposure to light. Do not remove ampoules or syringes from carton until ready to use. The solution should not be used if it is brown in color or contains a precipitate.

Epinephrine is readily destroyed by alkalies and oxidizing agents. In the latter category are oxygen, chlorine, bromine, iodine, permanganates, chromates, nitrites and salts of easily reducible metals, especially iron.

Drug Interactions: Use of epinephrine with excessive doses of digitalis, mercurial diuretics, or other drugs that sensitize the heart to arrhythmias is not recommended. Anginal pain may be induced when coronary insufficiency is present.

The effects of epinephrine may be potentiated by tricyclic antidepressants; certain antihistamines, eg, diphenhydramine, tripelennamine, d-chlorpheniramine; and sodium l-thyroxine.

Usage in Pregnancy: Pregnancy Category C. Adrenalin (epinephrine) has been shown to be teratogenic in rats when given in doses about 25 times the human dose. There are no adequate and well controlled studies in pregnant women. Adrenalin should be used during pregnancy only if the potential benefit justifies the potential risk to the fetus.

ADVERSE REACTIONS

Transient and minor side effects of anxiety, headache, fear and palpitations often occur with therapeutic doses, especially in hyperthyroid individuals. Repeated local injections can result in necrosis at sites of injection from vascular constriction. "Epinephrine-fastness" can occur with prolonged use.

DOSAGE AND ADMINISTRATION

Subcutaneously or intramuscularly—0.2 to 1 ml (mg). Start with a small dose and increase if required.

Note: The subcutaneous is the preferred route of administration. If given intramuscularly, injection into the buttocks should be avoided.

Continued on next page

This product information was prepared in August, 1986. On these and other Parke-Davis Products, information may be obtained by addressing PARKE-DAVIS, Division of Warner-Lambert Company, Morris Plains, New Jersey 07950.

Parke-Davis—Cont.

For bronchial asthma and certain allergic manifestations, eg, angioedema, urticaria, serum sickness, anaphylactic shock, use epinephrine subcutaneously. For bronchial asthma in pediatric patients, administer 0.01 mg/kg or 0.3 mg/m^2 to a maximum of 0.5 mg subcutaneously, repeated every four hours if required.
For cardiac resuscitation—A dose of 0.5 ml (0.5 mg) diluted to 10 ml with sodium chloride injection can be administered intravenously or intracardially to restore myocardial contractility. External cardiac massage should follow intracardial administration to permit the drug to enter coronary circulation. The drug should be used secondarily to unsuccessful attempts with physical or electromechanical methods.
Ophthalmologic use (for producing conjunctival decongestion, to control hemorrhage, produce mydriasis and reduce intraocular pressure)—use a concentration of 1:10,000 (0.1 mg/ml) to 1:1,000 (1 mg/ml).
Intraspinal use (Amp 88)—Usual dose is 0.2 to 0.4 ml (0.2 to 0.4 mg) added to anesthetic spinal fluid mixture (may prolong anesthetic action by limiting absorption). For use with local anesthetic—Epinephrine 1:100,000 (0.01 mg /ml) to 1:20,000 (0.05 mg/ml) is the usual concentration employed with local anesthetics.

HOW SUPPLIED

N 0071-4188-03 (Amp 88) Sterile solution containing 1 mg Adrenalin (epinephrine) as the hydrochloride in each 1-ml ampoule (1:1000). For intramuscular or subcutaneous use. When diluted, it may also be administered intracardially, intravenously, or intraspinally. Supplied in packages of ten.
N 0071-4011-13 (S.V. 11) Sterile solution containing 1 mg Adrenalin (epinephrine) as the hydrochloride (1:1000). For intramuscular or subcutaneous use. When diluted, it may also be administered intracardially or intravenously. Supplied in a 30 ml Steri-Vial® (rubber-diaphragm-capped vial.)
4188G040

AMCILL® ℞

[ăm 'cĭll ″]
(ampicillin, USP) as the trihydrate
Ampicillin Capsules, USP—250 mg and 500 mg
Ampicillin for Oral Suspension, USP 125 mg/5 ml and 250 mg/5 ml

DESCRIPTION

Ampicillin is a semisynthetic penicillin derived from the basic penicillin nucleus, 6-aminopenicillanic acid.
Ampicillin Capsules also contain magnesium stearate, NF. The capsule shell contains black iron oxide, D&C red No. 28; FD&C blue No. 1; gelatin, NF; sodium bisulfite; titanium dioxide, USP.
Ampicillin for Oral Suspension also contains flavors: microcrystalline cellulose, NF; povidone, USP; saccharine sodium, USP; silicon dioxide, NF; sodium benzoate, NF; sodium citrate, USP; sodium propionate, NF; sucrose, NF.

ACTIONS

Microbiology: *In vitro* studies have shown sensitivity of the following microorganisms to ampicillin:
Gram Positive: Alpha- and beta-hemolytic streptococci, *Diplococcus pneumoniae,* staphylococci (nonpenicillinase-producing), *Bacillus anthracis, Clostridia* spp, *Corynebacterium xerose,* and most strains of enterococci.
The drug does not resist destruction by penicillinase, hence is not effective against penicillin G-resistant staphylococci.
Gram Negative: *Haemophilus influenzae, Neisseria gonorrhoeae, N meningitidis, Proteus mirabilis,* and many strains of *Salmonella* (including *S typhosa), Shigella* spp, and *Escherichia coli.*
Testing for Susceptibility: The invading organism should be cultured and its sensitivity demonstrated as a guide to therapy. If the Kirby-Bauer method of disc sensitivity is used, a 10-mcg ampicillin disc should be used to determine the relative *in vitro* susceptibility.
Human Pharmacology: Ampicillin is stable in the presence of gastric acid and is well-absorbed from the gastrointestinal tract. It diffuses readily into most body tissues and fluids. However, penetration into the cerebrospinal fluid and brain occurs only with meningeal inflammation. Ampicillin is excreted largely unchanged in the urine. Its excretion can be delayed by concurrent administration of probenecid. Ampicillin is the least serum bound of all the penicillins, averaging 20% compared to 60% to 90% for other penicillins. Average peak blood serum levels of approximately 3 mcg/ml are attained in approximately two hours following a 500-mg dose of ampicillin in the capsule form. A dose of 250 mg ampicillin, as the oral suspension, produces average blood serum levels of approximately 2 mcg/ml within one and one-half hours.

Indications: Ampicillin is indicated primarily in the treatment of infections caused by susceptible strains of the following microorganisms: *Shigella, Salmonella* (including *S typhosa), E coli, H influenzae, P mirabilis,* and *N gonorrhoeae.* Ampicillin may also be indicated in certain infections caused by susceptible gram positive organisms: penicillin G-sensitive staphylococci, streptococci, pneumococci, and enterococci.
Bacteriology studies to determine the causative organisms and their sensitivity to ampicillin should be performed. Therapy may be instituted prior to the results of sensitivity testing.

CONTRAINDICATION

Ampicillin is contraindicated in patients with a history of a hypersensitivity reaction to the penicillins.

WARNING

Serious and occasionally fatal hypersensitivity (anaphylactic) reactions have been reported in patients on penicillin therapy. Although anaphylaxis is more frequent following parenteral therapy, it has occurred in patients on oral penicillins. These reactions are more apt to occur in individuals with a history of sensitivity to multiple allergens.
There have been reports of individuals with a history of penicillin hypersensitivity who experienced severe reactions when treated with cephalosporins. Before therapy with any penicillin, careful inquiry should be made concerning previous hypersensitivity reactions to penicillins, cephalosporins, or other allergens. Serious anaphylactoid reactions require immediate emergency treatment with epinephrine. Oxygen, intravenous steroids, and airway management, including intubation, should also be administered as indicated.
Usage in Pregnancy: Safety for use in pregnancy has not been established.

PRECAUTIONS

As with any potent drug, periodic assessment of renal, hepatic, and hematopoietic functions should be made during prolonged therapy.
The possibility of superinfections with mycotic or bacterial pathogens should be kept in mind during therapy. If superinfections occur, appropriate therapy should be instituted.

ADVERSE REACTIONS

As with other penicillins, it may be expected that untoward reactions will be essentially limited to sensitivity phenomena. They are more likely to occur in individuals who have previously demonstrated hypersensitivity to penicillins and in those with a history of allergy, asthma, hay fever, or urticaria.
The following adverse reactions have been reported as associated with the use of ampicillin.
Gastrointestinal—Glossitis, stomatitis, black "hairy" tongue, nausea, vomiting, enterocolitis, pseudomembranous colitis, and diarrhea have been reported. (These reactions are usually associated with oral dosage forms.)
Hypersensitivity Reactions—Erythematous maculopapular rashes have been reported fairly frequently. Urticaria, erythema multiforme, and an occasional case of exfoliative dermatitis have been reported. Anaphylaxis is the most serious reaction experienced and has usually been associated with the parenteral dosage form.
NOTE: Urticaria, other skin rashes, and serum sickness-like reactions may be controlled with antihistamines and, if necessary, systemic corticosteroids. Whenever such reactions occur, ampicillin should be discontinued unless, in the opinion of the physician, the condition being treated is life-threatening and amenable only to ampicillin therapy. Serious anaphylactic reactions require the immediate use of epinephrine, oxygen, and intravenous steroids.
Liver—A moderate rise in serum glutamic oxaloacetic transaminase (SGOT) has been noted, particularly in infants, but the significance of this finding is unknown.
Hemic and Lymphatic Systems—Anemia, thrombocytopenia, thrombocytopenic purpura, eosinophilia, leukopenia, and agranulocytosis have been reported during therapy with the penicillins. These reactions are usually reversible on discontinuation of therapy and are believed to be hypersensitivity phenomena.
Other—Since infectious mononucleosis is viral in origin, ampicillin should not be used in the treatment. A high percentage of patients with mononucleosis who received ampicillin developed a skin rash.

DOSAGE AND ADMINISTRATION

Infections of the respiratory tract and soft tissues
Patients weighing 20 kg (44 lb) or more: 250 mg every six hours
Patients weighing less than 20 kg (44 lb): 50 mg/kg/day in equally divided doses at 6- or 8-hour intervals
Infections of the gastrointestinal and genitourinary tracts
Patients weighing 20 kg (44 lb) or more: 500 mg every six hours
Patients weighing less than 20 kg (44 lb): 100 mg/kg/day in equally divided doses at 6- or 8-hour intervals
In the treatment of chronic urinary tract and intestinal infections, frequent bacteriologic and clinical appraisal is necessary. Smaller doses than those recommended above should not be used. Higher doses should be used for stubborn or severe infections. In stubborn infections, therapy may be required for several weeks. It may be necessary to continue clinical and/or bacteriologic follow-up for several months after cessation of therapy.
Urethritis in males or females due to *N gonorrhoeae:*
3.5 grams with 1 gram probenecid, administered simultaneously.
In the treatment of complications of gonorrheal urethritis, such as prostatitis and epididymitis, prolonged and intensive therapy is recommended. Cases of gonorrhea with a suspected primary lesion of syphilis should have darkfield examinations before receiving treatment. In all other cases where concomitant syphilis is suspected, monthly serologic tests should be made for a minimum of four months.
Treatment of all infections should be continued for a minimum of 48 to 72 hours beyond the time that the patient becomes asymptomatic or evidence of bacterial eradication has been obtained. A minimum of ten days treatment is recommended for any infection caused by Group A beta-hemolytic streptococci to help prevent the occurrence of acute rheumatic fever or acute glomerulonephritis.
Directions For Dispensing Oral Suspensions
Prepare suspension at time of dispensing. For ease in preparation, add water to the bottle in two portions, and shake well after each addition.
125 MG/5 ML
Add a total of 88 ml to the 100-ml package and 173 ml to the 200-ml package. This will provide 100 and 200 ml of suspension. Each 5 ml (teaspoonful) will contain ampicillin trihydrate equivalent to 125 mg ampicillin. The reconstituted suspension is stable for 14 days under refrigeration.
250 MG/5 ML
Add a total of 70 ml to the 100-ml package and 140 ml to the 200-ml package. This will provide 100 and 200 ml of suspension. Each 5 ml (teaspoonful) will contain ampicillin trihydrate equivalent to 250 mg ampicillin. The reconstituted suspension is stable for 14 days under refrigeration.

HOW SUPPLIED

N 0071-0402 (Capsule 402)—Amcill Capsules, 250 mg. Each capsule contains ampicillin trihydrate equivalent to 250 mg ampicillin. Bottles of 100 and 500, and unit-dose packages of 100 (10 strips of 10 capsules each).
N 0071-0404 (Capsule 404)—Amcill Capsules, 500 mg. Each capsule contains ampicillin trihydrate equivalent to 500 mg ampicillin. Bottles of 100 and 500, and unit-dose packages of 100 (10 strips of 10 capsules each).
Shown in Product Identification Section, page 419
N 0071-2301—Amcill for Oral Suspension 125 mg/5 ml. Each 5 ml of reconstituted suspension contains ampicillin trihydrate equivalent to 125 mg ampicillin. Available in 100-ml and 200-ml individual bottles and packs of six.
N 0071-2302—Amcill for Oral Suspension 250 mg/5 ml. Each 5 ml of reconstituted suspension contains ampicillin trihydrate equivalent to 250 mg ampicillin. Available in 100-ml and 200-ml individual bottles and packs of six.
AHFS 8:12.16 **7000G093**
Amcill products are manufactured by John D. Copanos Inc., Baltimore, MD 21225 and distributed by Parke-Davis, Morris Plains, NJ 07950.

AMITRIPTYLINE HYDROCHLORIDE ℞

[ă ″mĭ-trip ′ty-lēne]
Tablets USP
(Amitril®)

DESCRIPTION

Amitriptyline HCl, a dibenzocycloheptadiene derivative, is a white, crystalline compound that is readily soluble in water. It is designated chemically as 5-(3-dimethylamino-propylidene)-dibenzo [a,d] [1,4] cycloheptadiene hydrochloride. The molecular weight is 313.87. The empirical formula is $C_{20}H_{23}N \cdot HCl$.
AmitriptylineHCl is available as 10 mg, 25 mg, 50 mg, 75 mg, 100 mg, and 150 mg tablets for oral administration. Each tablet also contains candelilla wax; cellulose, NF; hydroxypropyl cellulose; hydroxypropylmethylcellulose; lactose, NF; magnesium stearate, NF; polyethylene glycol 3350, NF; povidone, USP; propylene glycol, USP; starch, NF; and talc, USP. Also contains Opaspray tan (10 mg), Opaspray coral pink (25 mg), Opaspray purple (50mg), Opaspray light green (75 mg), Opaspray light brown (100 mg), and Opaspray orange (150 mg).

CLINICAL PHARMACOLOGY

Amitriptyline HCl is an antidepressant with sedative effects. Its mechanism of action in man is not known. It is not a monoamine oxidase inhibitor and it does not act primarily by stimulation of the central nervous system.
Amitriptyline inhibits the membrane pump mechanism responsible for reuptake of norepinephrine and serotonin into adrenergic and serotonergic neurons. Pharmacologically this action may potentiate or prolong neuronal activity

since reuptake of these biogenic amines is important physiologically in terminating its transmitting activity. This interference with reuptake of norepinephrine and/or serotonin is believed by some to underlie the antidepressant activity of amitriptyline.

INDICATIONS AND USAGE

For the relief of symptoms of depression. Endogenous depression is more likely to be alleviated than are other depressive states.

CONTRAINDICATIONS

Amitriptyline HCl is contraindicated in patients who have shown prior hypersensitivity to it. It should not be given concomitantly with a monoamine oxidase inhibitor. Hyperpyretic crises, severe convulsions, and deaths have occurred in patients receiving tricyclic antidepressant and monoamine oxidase inhibiting drugs simultaneously. When it is desired to replace a monoamine oxidase inhibitor with amitriptyline, a minimum of 14 days should be allowed to elapse after the former is discontinued. Amitriptyline HCl should then be initiated cautiously with gradual increase in dosage until optimum response is achieved.

This drug is not recommended for use during the acute recovery phase following myocardial infarction.

WARNINGS

Amitriptyline HCl may block the antihypertensive action of guanethidine or similarly acting compounds.

It should be used with caution in patients with a history of seizures and because of its atropine-like action, in patients with a history of urinary retention, angle-closure glaucoma, or increased intraocular pressure. In patients with angle-closure glaucoma, even average doses may precipitate an attack.

Patients with cardiovascular disorders should be watched closely. Tricyclic antidepressant drugs, including amitriptyline, particularly when given in high doses, have been reported to produce arrhythmias, sinus tachycardia, and prolongation of the conduction time. Myocardial infarction and stroke have been reported with drugs of this class.

Close supervision is required when amitriptyline is given to hyperthyroid patients or those receiving thyroid medication.

This drug may impair mental and/or physical abilities required for performance of hazardous tasks, such as operating machinery or driving a motor vehicle.

Amitriptyline may enhance the response to alcohol and the effects of barbiturates and other CNS depressants. In patients who may use alcohol excessively, it should be borne in mind that the potentiation may increase the danger inherent in any suicide attempt or overdosage.

Usage in Pregnancy—Safe use of amitriptyline during pregnancy and lactation has not been established; therefore, in administering the drug to pregnant patients, nursing mothers, or women who may become pregnant, the possible benefits must be weighed against the possible hazards to mother and child.

Animal reproduction studies have been inconclusive and clinical experience has been limited.

Usage in Children—In view of the lack of experience in children, the drug is not recommended at the present time for patients under 12 years of age.

PRECAUTIONS

Schizophrenic patients may develop increased symptoms of psychosis; patients with paranoid symptomatology may have an exaggeration of such symptoms; manic depressive patients may experience a shift to the manic phase.

In these circumstances the dose of amitriptyline may be reduced or a major tranquilizer such as perphenazine may be administered concurrently.

When this drug is given with anticholinergic agents or sympathomimetic drugs, including epinephrine combined with local anesthetics, close supervision and careful adjustment of dosages are required.

Paralytic ileus may occur in patients taking tricyclic antidepressants in combination with anticholinergic-type drugs.

Caution is advised if patients receive large doses of ethchlorvynol concurrently. Transient delirium has been reported in patients who were treated with one gram of ethchlorvynol and 75 to 150 mg of amitriptyline.

The possibility of suicide in depressed patients remains until significant remission occurs. Potentially suicidal patients should not have access to large quantities of this drug. Prescriptions should be written for the smallest amount feasible.

Concurrent administration of amitriptyline and electroshock therapy may increase the hazards associated with such therapy. Such treatment should be limited to patients for whom it is essential.

Discontinue the drug several days before elective surgery if possible.

Both elevation and lowering of blood sugar levels have been reported.

Amitriptyline should be used with caution in patients with impaired liver function.

ADVERSE REACTIONS

Note: Included in the listing which follows are a few adverse reactions which have not been reported with this specific drug. However, pharmacological similarities among the tricyclic antidepressant drugs require that each of the reactions be considered when amitriptyline is administered.

Cardiovascular: Hypotension, hypertension, tachycardia, palpitation, myocardial infarction, arrhythmias, heart block, stroke.

CNS and Neuromuscular: Confusional states, disturbed concentration; disorientation; delusions; hallucinations; excitement; anxiety; restlessness; insomnia; nightmares; numbness, tingling, and paresthesias of the extremities; peripheral neuropathy; incoordination; ataxia; tremors; seizures; alteration in EEG patterns; extrapyramidal symptoms; tinnitus.

Anticholinergic: Dry mouth, blurred vision, disturbance of accommodation, constipation, paralytic ileus, urinary retention, dilatation of urinary tract.

Allergic: Skin rash, urticaria, photosensitization, edema of face and tongue.

Hematologic: Bone marrow depression including agranulocytosis, leukopenia, eosinophilia, purpura, thrombocytopenia.

Gastrointestinal: Nausea, epigastric distress, vomiting, anorexia, stomatitis, peculiar taste, diarrhea, parotid swelling, black tongue. Rarely hepatitis (including altered liver function and jaundice).

Endocrine: Testicular swelling and gynecomastia in the male, breast enlargement and galactorrhea in the female, increased or decreased libido, elevation and lowering of blood sugar levels.

Other: Dizziness, weakness, fatigue, headache, weight gain or loss, increased perspiration, urinary frequency, mydriasis, drowsiness, alopecia.

Withdrawal Symptoms: Abrupt cessation of treatment after prolonged administration may produce nausea, headache, and malaise. These are not indicative of addiction.

OVERDOSAGE

Manifestations—High doses may cause temporary confusion, disturbed concentration, or transient visual hallucinations. Overdosage may cause drowsiness; hypothermia; tachycardia and other arrhythmic abnormalities, such as bundle branch block; ECG evidence of impaired conduction; congestive heart failure; dilated pupils; convulsions; severe hypotension; stupor; and coma. Other symptoms may be agitation, hyperactive reflexes, muscle rigidity, vomiting, hyperpyrexia, or any of those listed under ADVERSE REACTIONS.

All patients suspected of having taken an overdosage should be admitted to a hospital as soon as possible.

Treatment is symptomatic and supportive. Empty the stomach as quickly as possible by emesis followed by gastric lavage upon arrival at the hospital. Following gastric lavage, activated charcoal may be administered. Twenty to 30 g of activated charcoal may be given every four to six hours during the first 24 to 48 hours after ingestion. An ECG should be taken and close monitoring of cardiac function instituted if there is any sign of abnormality. Maintain an open airway and adequate fluid intake; regulate body temperature.

The intravenous administration of 1–3 mg of physostigmine salicylate has been reported to reverse the symptoms of tricyclic antidepressant poisoning. Because physostigmine is rapidly metabolized, the dosage of physostigmine should be repeated as required particularly if life threatening signs such as arrhythmias, convulsions, and deep coma recur or persist after the initial dosage of physostigmine. Because physostigmine itself may be toxic, it is not recommended for routine use.

Standard measures should be used to manage circulatory shock and metabolic acidosis. Cardiac arrhythmias may be treated with neostigmine, pyridostigmine, or propranolol. Should cardiac failure occur, the use of digitalis should be considered. Close monitoring of cardiac function for not less than five days is advisable.

Anticonvulsants may be given to control convulsions. Amitriptyline increases the CNS depressant action, but not the anticonvulsant action of barbiturates; therefore, an inhalation anesthetic, diazepam, or paraldehyde is recommended for control of convulsions.

Dialysis is of no value because of low plasma concentrations of the drug.

Since overdosage is often deliberate, patients may attempt suicide by other means during the recovery phase.

Deaths by deliberate or accidental overdosage have occurred with this class of drugs.

DOSAGE AND ADMINISTRATION

Oral Dosage—Dosage should be initiated at a low level and increased gradually, noting carefully the clinical response and any evidence of intolerance.

Initial Dosage for Adults—Twenty-five mg three times a day usually is satisfactory for outpatients. If necessary this may be increased to a total of 150 mg a day. Increases are made preferably in the late afternoon and/or bedtime doses. A sedative effect may be apparent before the antidepressant effect is noted, but an adequate therapeutic effect may take as long as 30 days to develop.

An alternative method of initiating therapy in outpatients is to begin with 50 to 100 mg amitriptyline HCl at bedtime. This may be increased by 25 to 50 mg as necessary in the bedtime dose to a total of 150 mg per day.

Hospitalized patients may require 100 mg a day initially. This can be increased gradually to 200 mg a day if necessary. A small number of hospitalized patients may need as much as 300 mg a day.

Adolescent and Elderly Patients—In general, lower dosages are recommended for these patients. Ten mg three times a day with 20 mg at bedtime may be satisfactory in adolescent and elderly patients who do not tolerate higher dosages.

Maintenance—The usual maintenance dose is 25 mg two to four times a day. In some patients 10 mg four times a day is sufficient. When satisfactory improvement has been reached, dosage should be reduced to the lowest amount that will maintain relief of symptoms. It is appropriate to continue maintenance therapy three months or longer to lessen the possibility of relapse.

Usage in Children—In view of the lack of experience in children, this drug is not recommended at the present time for patients under 12 years of age.

HOW SUPPLIED

Amitriptyline HCl tablets are supplied as film-coated tablets as follows:

N 0071-0272 10 mg (tan, P-D 272), in bottles of 100 and unit-dose packages of 100 (10 strips of 10 tablets each).

N 0071-0273 25 mg (coral, P-D 273), in bottles of 100 and 1000 and unit-dose packages of 100 (10 strips of 10 tablets each).

N 0071-0274 50 mg (blue/purple, P-D 274), in bottles of 100 and 1000 and unit-dose packages of 100 (10 strips of 10 tablets each).

N 0071-0275 75 mg (green, P-D 275), in bottles of 100.

N 0071-0271 100 mg (brown/mustard, P-D 271), in bottles of 100 and unit-dose packages of 100 (10 strips of 10 tablets each).

N 0071-0278 150 mg (orange, P-D 278), in bottles of 100.

Store at controlled room temperature between 15°–30°C (59°–86°F).

6000G035

Shown in Product Identification Section, page 420

AMOXICILLIN ℞

[ă-mŏx 'ă-cĭll "ĭn]

(Utimox®)

Amoxicillin Capsules, USP—250 and 500 mg

Amoxicillin for Oral Suspension, USP—125 mg/5 ml and 250 mg/5 ml

DESCRIPTION

Amoxicillin is a semisynthetic penicillin, an analogue of ampicillin, with a broad spectrum of bactericidal activity against many gram-positive and gram-negative microorganisms. Chemically, it is D-(-)-α-amino-*p*-hydroxybenzyl penicillin trihydrate.

Amoxicillin Capsules also contain magnesium stearate, NF; sodium laurel sulfate, NF. The capsule shell contains D&C red No. 33; FD&C blue No. 1; FD&C red No. 40; FD&C yellow No. 6; gelatin, NF; titanium dioxide, USP.

Amoxicillin for Oral Suspension also contains flavors, Hercules casting color 27-75; microcrystalline cellulose, NF; saccharin sodium, USP; silicon dioxide, NF; sodium citrate, USP; sodium propionate, NF; sucrose, NF.

ACTIONS

Pharmacology

Amoxicillin is stable in the presence of gastric acid and may be given with no regard for food. It is rapidly absorbed after oral administration. It diffuses readily into most body tissues and fluids, with the exception of brain and spinal fluid, except when meninges are inflamed. The half-life of amoxicillin is 1 hour. Most of the amoxicillin is excreted unchanged in the urine; its excretion can be delayed by concurrent administration of probenecid. Amoxicillin is not highly protein-bound. In blood serum, amoxicillin is approximately 20% protein-bound as compared to 60% for penicillin G.

Orally administered doses of 250 mg and 500 mg amoxicillin capsules result in average peak blood levels, one to two hours after administration, in the range of 3.5 mcg/ml to 5.0 mcg/ml, and 5.5 mcg/ml to 7.5 mcg/ml, respectively.

Continued on next page

This product information was prepared in August, 1986. On these and other Parke-Davis Products, information may be obtained by addressing PARKE-DAVIS, Division of Warner-Lambert Company, Morris Plains, New Jersey 07950.

Parke-Davis—Cont.

Orally administered doses of amoxicillin suspension 125 mg/5 ml and 250 mg/5 ml result in average peak blood levels, one to two hours after administration, in the range of 1.5 mcg/ml to 3.0 mcg/ml, and 3.5 mcg/ml to 5.0 mcg/ml, respectively.

Detectable serum levels are observed up to 8 hours after an orally administered dose of amoxicillin. Approximately 60% of an orally administered dose of amoxicillin is excreted in the urine within six to eight hours.

Microbiology

Amoxicillin is similar to ampicillin in its bactericidal action against susceptible organisms during the stage of active multiplication. It acts through the inhibition of biosynthesis of cell wall mucopeptide. *In vitro* studies have demonstrated the susceptibility of most strains of the following gram-positive bacteria: alpha- and beta-hemolytic streptococci, *Diplococcus pneumoniae,* nonpenicillinase-producing staphylococci, and *Streptococcus faecalis.* Amoxicillin is active *in vitro* against many strains of *Haemophilus influenzae, Neisseria gonorrhoeae, Escherichia coli,* and *Proteus mirabilis.* Because it does not resist destruction by penicillinase, the drug is not effective against penicillinase-producing bacteria, particularly resistant staphylococci. All strains of *Pseudomonas* and most strains of *Klebsiella* and *Enterobacter* are resistant.

Disc Susceptibility Tests

Quantitative methods that require measurement of zone diameters give the most precise estimates of antibiotic susceptibility. One such procedure* has been recommended for use with discs for testing susceptibility to ampicillin class antibiotics. Interpretations correlate diameters of the disc test with MIC values for amoxicillin. With this procedure, a report from the laboratory of "susceptible" indicates that the infecting organism is likely to respond to therapy. A report of "resistant" indicates that the infecting organism is not likely to respond to therapy. A report of "intermediate susceptibility" suggests that the organism would be susceptible if high dosage is used, or if the infection is confined to tissues and fluids (eg, urine), in which high antibiotic levels are attained.

INDICATIONS

Amoxicillin is indicated in the treatment of infections due to susceptible strains of the following.

Gram-negative organisms—*H influenzae, E coli, P mirabilis,* and *N gonorrhoeae*

Gram-positive organisms—Streptococci (including *Str faecalis), D pneumoniae,* and nonpenicillinase-producing staphylococci

Therapy may be instituted prior to obtaining results from bacteriological and susceptibility studies to determine the causative organisms and their susceptibility to amoxicillin. Indicated surgical procedures should be performed.

CONTRAINDICATION

The use of this drug is contraindicated in individuals with a history of an allergic reaction to the penicillins.

WARNINGS

SERIOUS AND OCCASIONALLY FATAL HYPERSENSITIVITY (ANAPHYLACTOID) REACTIONS HAVE BEEN REPORTED IN PATIENTS ON PENICILLIN THERAPY. ALTHOUGH ANAPHYLAXIS IS MORE FREQUENT FOLLOWING PARENTERAL THERAPY, IT HAS OCCURRED IN PATIENTS ON ORAL PENICILLINS. THESE REACTIONS ARE MORE APT TO OCCUR IN INDIVIDUALS WITH A HISTORY OF SENSITIVITY TO MULTIPLE ALLERGENS.

THERE HAVE BEEN REPORTS OF INDIVIDUALS WITH A HISTORY OF PENICILLIN HYPERSENSITIVITY WHO HAVE EXPERIENCED SEVERE REACTIONS WHEN TREATED WITH CEPHALOSPORINS. BEFORE THERAPY WITH ANY PENICILLIN, CAREFUL INQUIRY SHOULD BE MADE CONCERNING PREVIOUS HYPERSENSITIVITY REACTIONS TO PENICILLINS, CEPHALOSPORINS, AND OTHER ALLERGENS. IF AN ALLERGIC REACTION OCCURS, APPROPRIATE THERAPY SHOULD BE INSTITUTED AND DISCONTINUANCE OF AMOXICILLIN THERAPY CONSIDERED.

SERIOUS ANAPHYLACTOID REACTIONS REQUIRE IMMEDIATE EMERGENCY TREATMENT WITH EPINEPHRINE. OXYGEN, INTRAVENOUS STEROIDS, AND AIRWAY MANAGEMENT, INCLUDING INTUBATION, SHOULD ALSO BE ADMINISTERED AS INDICATED.

Usage in Pregnancy—Safety for use in pregnancy has not been established.

PRECAUTIONS

As with any potent drug, periodic assessment of renal, hepatic, and hematopoietic functions should be made during prolonged therapy.

The possibility of superinfections with mycotic or bacterial pathogens should be kept in mind during therapy. If superinfections occur (usually involving *Enterobacter, Pseudomonas,* or *Candida),* the drug should be discontinued and/or appropriate therapy instituted.

ADVERSE REACTIONS

As with other penicillins, it may be expected that untoward reactions will be essentially limited to sensitivity phenomena. They are more likely to occur in individuals who have previously demonstrated hypersensitivity to penicillins and in those with a history of allergy, asthma, hay fever, or urticaria.

The following adverse reactions have been reported as associated with the use of penicillins.

Gastrointestinal—Nausea, vomiting, and diarrhea

Hypersensitivity Reactions—Erythematous maculopapular rashes and urticaria have been reported.

Note—Urticaria, other skin rashes, and serum sickness-like reactions may be controlled with antihistamines and, if necessary, systemic corticosteroids. Whenever such reactions occur, amoxicillin should be discontinued unless, in the opinion of the physician, the condition being treated is life-threatening and amenable only to amoxicillin therapy.

Liver—A moderate rise in serum glutamic oxaloacetic transaminase (SGOT) has been noted, but the significance of this finding is unknown.

Hemic and Lymphatic Systems—Anemia, thrombocytopenia, thrombocytopenic purpura, eosinophilia, leukopenia, and agranulocytosis have been reported during therapy with the penicillins. These reactions are usually reversible on discontinuation of therapy and are believed to be hypersensitivity phenomena.

DOSAGE AND ADMINISTRATION

Infections of the ear, nose, and throat due to streptococci, pneumococci, nonpenicillinase-producing staphylococci, and *H influenzae:*

Infections of the genitourinary tract due to *E coli, P mirabilis,* and *Str faecalis:*

Infections of the skin and soft tissues due to streptococci, susceptible staphylococci, and *E coli:*

Usual Dosage:

Adults: 250 mg every 8 hours

Children: 20 mg/kg/day in divided doses every 8 hours.

Children weighing 20 kg or more should be dosed according to the adult recommendations.

In severe infections or those caused by less susceptible organisms: 500 mg every 8 hours for adults, and 40 mg/kg/day in divided doses every 8 hours for children may be needed.

Infections of the lower respiratory tract due to streptococci, pneumococci, nonpenicillinase-producing staphylococci, and *H influenzae:*

Usual Dosage:

Adults: 500 mg every 8 hours

Children: 40/kg/day in divided doses every 8 hours

Children weighing 20 kg or more should be dosed according to the adult recommendations.

Gonorrhea, acute, uncomplicated anogenital and urethral infections due to *N gonorrhoeae:* (males and females) 3 grams as a single dose.

Cases of gonorrhea with a suspected lesion of syphilis should have darkfield examinations before receiving amoxicillin and monthly serological tests for a minimum of four months.

Larger doses may be required for stubborn or severe infections.

The children's dosage is intended for individuals whose weight will not cause a dosage to be calculated greater than that recommended for adults.

It should be recognized that in the treatment of chronic urinary tract infections, frequent bacteriological and clinical appraisals are necessary. Smaller doses than those recommended above should not be used. Even higher doses may be needed at times. In stubborn infections, therapy may be required for several weeks. It may be necessary to continue clinical and/or bacteriological follow-up for several months after cessation of therapy. Except for gonorrhea, treatment should be continued for a minimum of 48 to 72 hours beyond the time that the patient becomes asymptomatic or evidence of bacterial eradication has been obtained.

It is recommended that there be at least 10 days' treatment for any infection caused by hemolytic streptococci to prevent the occurrence of acute rheumatic fever or glomerulonephritis.

After reconstitution, the required amount of suspension should be placed directly on the child's tongue for swallowing. Alternate means of administration are to add the required amount of suspension to formula, milk, fruit juice, water, ginger ale, or cold drinks. These preparations should then be taken immediately. To be certain the child is receiving full dosage, such preparations should be consumed in entirety.

Directions for Preparing Oral Suspension: Prepare suspension at the time of dispensing. Shake bottle to loosen powder or break up the cake that may have formed. For ease of preparation, add water to the bottle in two portions and shake well after each addition. Each teaspoonful (5 ml) will contain 125 mg or 250 mg amoxicillin.

Product	Bottle Size	Amount of Water Required for Reconstitution
125 mg/5 ml	80 ml	70 ml
	100 ml	87 ml
	150 ml	130 ml
	200 ml	170 ml
250 mg/5 ml	80 ml	56 ml
	100 ml	70 ml
	150 ml	105 ml
	200 ml	140 ml

NOTE

SHAKE THE ORAL SUSPENSION WELL BEFORE USING.

Keep bottle tightly closed. The reconstituted suspension is stable for 14 days. Refrigeration is preferable but not required.

HOW SUPPLIED

Amoxicillin Capsules are supplied as:

N 0071-0730-24 250 mg—Bottles of 100
N 0071-0730-30 250 mg—Bottles of 500
N 0071-0730-40 250 mg—Unit dose packages of 100 (10 strips of 10)

Each capsule contains amoxicillin trihydrate equivalent to 250 mg amoxicillin.

N 0071-0731-24 500 mg—Bottles of 100
N 0071-0731-40 500 mg—Unit dose packages of 100 (10 strips of 10)

Each capsule contains amoxicillin trihydrate equivalent to 500 mg amoxicillin.

Shown in Product Identification Section, page 419

Amoxicillin for Oral Suspension is supplied as:

N 0071-2500-16 125 mg/5 ml—80 ml individual bottles and packs of six.
N 0071-2500-17 125 mg/5 ml—100 ml individual bottles and packs of six.
N 0071-2500-18 125 mg/5 ml—150 ml individual bottles and packs of six.
N 0071-2500-20 125 mg/5 ml—200 ml individual bottles and packs of six.

When reconstituted according to directions, each 5 ml of reconstituted suspension contains amoxicillin trihydrate equivalent to 125 mg amoxicillin.

N 0071-2501-16 250 mg/5 ml—80 ml individual bottles and packs of six.
N 0071-2501-17 250 mg/5 ml—100 ml individual bottles and packs of six.
N 0071-2501-18 250 mg/5 ml—150 ml individual bottles and packs of six.
N 0071-2501-20 250 mg/5 ml—200 ml individual bottles and packs of six.

When reconstituted according to directions, each 5 ml of reconstituted suspension contains amoxicillin trihydrate equivalent to 250 mg amoxicillin.

* Bauer, A.W., Kirby, W.M.M., Sherris, J.C., and Turck, M.: Antibiotic Testing by a Standardized Single Disc Method, *Am. J. Clin. Pathol.,* 45:493, 1966; Standardized Disc Susceptibility Test, *FEDERAL REGISTER* 37:20527-29, 1972.

Manufactured by John D. Copanos Inc., Baltimore, MD 21225 and distributed by Parke-Davis, Morris Plains, NJ 07950.

AHFS: 8:12.16 **7000G085**

ANUSOL-HC® SUPPOSITORIES ℞

[ăn ′ū-sōl″]

Hemorrhoidal Suppositories

ANUSOL-HC® CREAM ℞

Rectal Cream

with Hydrocortisone Acetate

DESCRIPTION

	Anusol-HC Suppositories each contains	Anusol-HC Cream each gram
Hydrocortisone Acetate	10.0 mg	5.0 mg
Bismuth Subgallate	2.25%	22.5 mg
Bismuth Resorcin Compound	1.75%	17.5 mg
Benzyl Benzoate	1.2 %	12.0 mg
Peruvian Balsam	1.8 %	18.0 mg
Zinc Oxide	11.0 %	110.0 mg
	Also contains the following inactive ingredients: dibasic calcium phosphate and certified coloring in a hydrogenated vegetable oil base.	Also contains the following inactive ingredients: propylene glycol, propylparaben, methylparaben, polysorbate 60 and sorbitan monostearate in a water-miscible base of mineral oil, glyceryl monostearate and water.

ACTIONS

Anusol-HC Suppositories and Anusol-HC Cream help to relieve pain, itching and discomfort arising from irritated anorectal tissues. These preparations have a soothing, lubricant action on mucous membranes, and the antiinflammatory action of hydrocortisone acetate in Anusol-HC helps to reduce hyperemia and swelling.
The hydrocortisone acetate in Anusol-HC is primarily effective because of its antiinflammatory, antipruritic and vasoconstrictive actions.

INDICATIONS

Anusol-HC Suppositories and Anusol-HC Cream are adjunctive therapy for the symptomatic relief of pain and discomfort in: external and internal hemorrhoids, proctitis, papillitis, cryptitis, anal fissures, incomplete fistulas and relief of local pain and discomfort following anorectal surgery.
Anusol-HC Cream is also indicated for pruritus ani.
Anusol-HC is especially indicated when inflammation is present. After acute symptoms subside, most patients can be maintained on regular Anusol® Suppositories or Ointment.

CONTRAINDICATIONS

Anusol-HC Suppositories and Anusol-HC Cream are contraindicated in those patients with a history of hypersensitivity to any of the components of the preparations.

WARNINGS

The safe use of topical steroids during pregnancy has not been fully established. Therefore, during pregnancy, they should not be used unnecessarily on extensive areas, in large amounts, or for prolonged periods of time.

PRECAUTIONS

Symptomatic relief should not delay definitive diagnoses or treatment.
If irritation develops, Anusol-HC Suppositories and Anusol-HC Cream should be discontinued and appropriate therapy instituted.
In the presence of an infection the use of an appropriate antifungal or antibacterial agent should be instituted. If a favorable response does not occur promptly, the corticosteroid should be discontinued until the infection has been adequately controlled.
Care should be taken when using the corticosteroid hydrocortisone acetate in children and infants.
Anusol-HC is not for ophthalmic use.

DOSAGE AND ADMINISTRATION

Anusol-HC Suppositories—Adults: Remove foil wrapper and insert suppository into the anus. Insert one suppository in the morning and one at bedtime, for 3 to 6 days or until inflammation subsides. Then maintain patient comfort with regular Anusol Suppositories.
Anusol-HC Cream—Adults: After gentle bathing and drying of the anal area, remove tube cap and apply to the exterior surface and gently rub in. For internal use, attach the plastic applicator and insert into the anus by applying gentle continuous pressure. Then squeeze the tube to deliver medication. Cream should be applied 3 or 4 times a day for 3 to 6 days until inflammation subsides. Then maintain patient comfort with regular Anusol Ointment.
NOTE: If staining from either of the above products occurs, the stain may be removed from fabric by hand or machine washing with household detergent.

HOW SUPPLIED

Anusol-HC Suppositories— boxes of 12 (N 0071-1089-07) and boxes of 24 (N 0071-1089-13); in silver foil strips.
Shown in Product Identification Section, page 420
Anusol-HC Cream—one-ounce tube (N 0071-3090-13); with plastic applicator.
Store between 15°-30° C (59°-86° F).
Shown in Product Identification Section, page 420

1089 G 010

APLISOL® ℞

[*ă'plĭ-sŏl"*]
(tuberculin purified protein derivative, diluted [Stabilized Solution])

For complete product information, consult Diagnostic Products Information Section.

APLITEST® ℞

[*ă'plĭ-tĕst"*]
(tuberculin purified protein derivative)
Multiple-Puncture Device

For complete product information, consult Diagnostic Products Information Section.

BENADRYL® ℞

[*bĕ'nă-dril*]
(Diphenhydramine Hydrochloride Capsules, USP)

DESCRIPTION

Benadryl (diphenhydramine hydrochloride) is an antihistamine drug having the chemical name 2-(Diphenylmethoxy)-N, N-dimethylethylamine hydrochloride and has the empirical formula $C_{17}H_{21}NO \cdot HCl$ (molecular weight 291.82). It occurs as a white, crystalline powder and is freely soluble in water and alcohol.
Each Benadryl capsule contains 25 mg or 50 mg diphenhydramine hydrochloride for oral administration.
The 25-mg capsule also contains lactose, NF and magnesium stearate, NF. The capsule shell and/or band contains D&C red No. 28; FD&C blue No. 1; FD&C red No. 3; FD&C red No. 40; gelatin, NF; colloidal silicon dioxide, NF; sodium bisulfite, NF; and sodium lauryl sulfate, NF.
The 50-mg capsule also contains confectioner's sugar, NF and talc, USP. The capsule shell and/or band contains FD&C blue No. 1; FD&C red No. 3; gelatin, NF; glyceryl monooleate; colloidal silicon dioxide, NF; sodium bisulfite, NF; sodium lauryl sulfate, NF; and titanium dioxide, USP.

CLINICAL PHARMACOLOGY

Diphenhydramine hydrochloride is an antihistamine with anticholinergic (drying) and sedative effects. Antihistamines appear to compete with histamine for cell receptor sites on effector cells.
A single oral dose of diphenhydramine hydrochloride is quickly absorbed with maximum activity occurring in approximately one hour. The duration of activity following an average dose of Benadryl is from four to six hours. Diphenhydramine is widely distributed throughout the body, including the CNS. Little, if any, is excreted unchanged in the urine; most appears as the degradation products of metabolic transformation in the liver, which are almost completely excreted within 24 hours.

INDICATIONS AND USAGE

Benadryl in the oral form is effective for the following indications:
Antihistaminic: For allergic conjunctivitis due to foods; mild, uncomplicated allergic skin manifestations of urticaria and angioedema; amelioration of allergic reactions to blood or plasma; dermatographism; as therapy for anaphylactic reactions *adjunctive* to epinephrine and other standard measures after the acute manifestations have been controlled.
Motion sickness: For active and prophylactic treatment of motion sickness.
Antiparkinsonism: For parkinsonism (including drug-induced) in the elderly unable to tolerate more potent agents; mild cases of parkinsonism (including drug-induced) in other age groups; in other cases of parkinsonism (including drug-induced) in combination with centrally acting anticholinergic agents.
Nighttime sleep-aid.

CONTRAINDICATIONS

Use in Newborn or Premature Infants
This drug should *not* be used in newborn or premature infants.
Use in Nursing Mothers
Because of the higher risk of antihistamines for infants generally, and for newborns and prematures in particular, antihistamine therapy is contraindicated in nursing mothers.
Antihistamines are also contraindicated in the following conditions:
Hypersensitivity to diphenhydramine hydrochloride and other antihistamines of similar chemical structure.

WARNINGS

Antihistamines should be used with considerable caution in patients with narrow-angle glaucoma, stenosing peptic ulcer, pyloroduodenal obstruction, symptomatic prostatic hypertrophy, or bladder-neck obstruction.
Use in Children
In infants and children, especially, antihistamines in *overdosage* may cause hallucinations, convulsions, or death.
As in adults, antihistamines may diminish mental alertness in children. In the young child, particularly, they may produce excitation.
Use in the Elderly (approximately 60 years or older).
Antihistamines are more likely to cause dizziness, sedation, and hypotension in elderly patients.

PRECAUTIONS

General: Diphenhydramine hydrochloride has an atropine-like action and therefore should be used with caution in patients with a history of bronchial asthma, increased intraocular pressure, hyperthyroidism, cardiovascular disease or hypertension.
Information for Patients: Patients taking diphenhydramine hydrochloride should be advised that this drug may cause drowsiness and has an additive effect with alcohol.
Patients should be warned about engaging in activities requiring mental alertness such as driving a car or operating appliances, machinery, etc.
Drug Interactions: Diphenhydramine hydrochloride has additive effects with alcohol and other CNS depressants (hypnotics, sedatives, tranquilizers, etc).
CAUTION—Patients taking monoamine oxidase inhibitors should not receive antihistamine therapy concurrently.
MAO inhibitors prolong and intensify the anticholinergic (drying) effects of antihistamines.
Carcinogenesis, Mutagenesis, Impairment of Fertility: Long-term studies in animals to determine mutagenic and carcinogenic potential have not been performed.
Pregnancy: Pregnancy Category B. Reproduction studies have been performed in rats and rabbits at doses up to 5 times the human dose and have revealed no evidence of impaired fertility or harm to the fetus due to diphenhydramine hydrochloride. There are, however, no adequate and well-controlled studies in pregnant women. Because animal reproduction studies are not always predictive of human response, this drug should be used during pregnancy only if clearly needed.

ADVERSE REACTIONS

The most frequent adverse reactions are underscored.

1. *General:* Urticaria, drug rash, anaphylactic shock, photosensitivity, excessive perspiration, chills, dryness of mouth, nose, and throat.
2. *Cardiovascular System:* Hypotension, headache, palpitations, tachycardia, extrasystoles.
3. *Hematologic System:* Hemolytic anemia, thrombocytopenia, agranulocytosis.
4. *Nervous System:* <u>Sedation</u>, <u>sleepiness</u>, <u>dizziness</u>, <u>disturbed coordination</u>, fatigue, confusion, restlessness, excitation, nervousness, tremor, irritability, insomnia, euphoria, paresthesia, blurred vision, diplopia, vertigo, tinnitus, acute labyrinthitis, neuritis, convulsions.
5. *GI System:* <u>Epigastric distress</u>, anorexia, nausea, vomiting, diarrhea, constipation.
6. *GU System:* Urinary frequency, difficult urination, urinary retention, early menses.
7. *Respiratory System:* <u>Thickening of bronchial secretions</u>, tightness of chest and wheezing, nasal stuffiness.

OVERDOSAGE

Antihistamine overdosage reactions may vary from central nervous system depression to stimulation. Stimulation is particularly likely in children. Atropine-like signs and symptoms, dry mouth; fixed, dilated pupils; flushing, and gastrointestinal symptoms may also occur.
If vomiting has not occurred spontaneously the patient should be induced to vomit. This is best done by having him drink a glass of water or milk after which he should be made to gag. Precautions against aspiration must be taken, especially in infants and children.
If vomiting is unsuccessful gastric lavage is indicated within 3 hours after ingestion and even later if large amounts of milk or cream were given beforehand. Isotonic or ½ isotonic saline is the lavage solution of choice.
Saline cathartics, as milk of magnesia, by osmosis draw water into the bowel and therefore are valuable for their action in rapid dilution of food content.
Stimulants should not be used.
Vasopressors may be used to treat hypotension.

DOSAGE AND ADMINISTRATION

DOSAGE SHOULD BE INDIVIDUALIZED ACCORDING TO THE NEEDS AND THE RESPONSE OF THE PATIENT.
A single oral dose of diphenhydramine hydrochloride is quickly absorbed with maximum activity occurring in approximately one hour. The duration of activity following an average dose of Benadryl is from four to six hours.
ADULTS: 25 to 50 mg three or four times daily. The nighttime sleep-aid dosage is 50 mg at bedtime.
CHILDREN: (over 20 lb): 12.5 to 25 mg three to four times daily. Maximum daily dosage not to exceed 300 mg. For physicians who wish to calculate the dose on the basis of body weight or surface area, the recommended dosage is 5 mg/kg/24 hours or 150 mg/m^2/24 hours.
Data are not available on the use of diphenhydramine hydrochloride as a nighttime sleep-aid in children under 12 years.
The basis for determining the most effective dosage regimen will be the response of the patient to medication and the condition under treatment.
In motion sickness, full dosage is recommended for prophylactic use, the first dose to be given 30 minutes before exposure to motion and similar doses before meals and upon retiring for the duration of exposure.

Continued on next page

This product information was prepared in August, 1986. On these and other Parke-Davis Products, information may be obtained by addressing PARKE-DAVIS, Division of Warner-Lambert Company, Morris Plains, New Jersey 07950.

Parke-Davis—Cont.

HOW SUPPLIED

Benadryl 50 mg (P-D 373)—each banded capsule (Kapseals®) contains 50 mg diphenhydramine hydrochloride. Available as a pink capsule with white band in bottles of 100 (N 0071-0373-24), 1000 (N 0071-0373-32), and unit dose 100 (N 0071-0373-40).

Benadryl 25 mg (P-D 471)—each capsule contains 25 mg diphenhydramine hydrochloride. Available as a pink/white capsule in bottles of 100 (N 0071-0471-24), 1000 (N 0071-0471-32), and unit dose 100 (N 0071-0471-40).

Storage Conditions:

Store at controlled room temperature 15°–30°C (59°–86°F). Protect from moisture.

Caution—Federal law prohibits dispensing without prescription.

Shown in Product Identification Section, page 420

0373G212

ELIXIR

BENADRYL®

[*bē'nă-dril*]

(Diphenhydramine Hydrochloride Elixir, USP)

DESCRIPTION

Benadryl (diphenhydramine hydrochloride) is an antihistamine drug having the chemical name 2-(Diphenylmethoxy)-N, N-dimethylethylamine hydrochloride and has the empirical formula $C_{17}H_{21}NO \cdot HCl$ (molecular weight 291.82). It occurs as a white, crystalline powder and is freely soluble in water and alcohol.

Each 5 mL of Benadryl Elixir contains 12.5 mg diphenhydramine hydrochloride with 14% alcohol for oral administration. Benadryl Elixir has an apparent pH of about 5.0 to 8.0. Also contains: anethole, NF; cinnamon oil, NF; clove oil, NF; coriander oil, NF; D&C red No 33; FD&C red No. 40; orange oil, NF; sucrose, NF; and purified water, USP.

CLINICAL PHARMACOLOGY

Diphenhydramine hydrochloride is an antihistamine with anticholinergic (drying) and sedative effects. Antihistamines appear to compete with histamine for cell receptor sites on effector cells.

A single oral dose of diphenhydramine hydrochloride is quickly absorbed with maximum activity occurring in approximately one hour. The duration of activity following an average dose of Benadryl is from four to six hours. Diphenhydramine is widely distributed throughout the body, including the CNS. Little, if any, is excreted unchanged in the urine; most appears as the degradation products of metabolic transformation in the liver, which are almost completely excreted within 24 hours.

INDICATIONS AND USAGE

Benadryl in the oral form is effective for the following indications:

Antihistaminic: For perennial and seasonal (hay fever) allergic rhinitis; vasomotor rhinitis; allergic conjunctivitis due to inhalant allergens and foods; mild, uncomplicated allergic skin manifestations of urticaria and angioedema; amelioration of allergic reactions to blood or plasma; dermatographism; as therapy for anaphylactic reactions *adjunctive* to epinephrine and other standard measures after the acute manifestations have been controlled.

Motion sickness: For active and prophylactic treatment of motion sickness.

Antiparkinsonism: For parkinsonism (including drug-induced) in the elderly unable to tolerate more potent agents; mild cases of parkinsonism (including drug-induced) in other age groups; in other cases of parkinsonism (including drug-induced) in combination with centrally acting anticholinergic agents.

Nighttime sleep-aid.

CONTRAINDICATIONS

Use in Newborn or Premature Infants

This drug should *not* be used in newborn or premature infants.

Use in Nursing Mothers

Because of the higher risk of antihistamines for infants generally, and for newborns and prematures in particular, antihistamine therapy is contraindicated in nursing mothers.

Antihistamines are also contraindicated in the following conditions:

Hypersensitivity to diphenhydramine hydrochloride and other antihistamines of similar chemical structure.

WARNINGS

Antihistamines should be used with considerable caution in patients with narrow-angle glaucoma, stenosing peptic ulcer, pyloroduodenal obstruction, symptomatic prostatic hypertrophy, or bladder-neck obstruction.

Use in Children

In infants and children, especially, antihistamines in *overdosage* may cause hallucinations, convulsions, or death.

As in adults, antihistamines may diminish mental alertness in children. In the young child, particularly, they may produce excitation.

Use in the Elderly (approximately 60 years or older).

Antihistamines are more likely to cause dizziness, sedation, and hypotension in elderly patients.

PRECAUTIONS

General: Diphenhydramine hydrochloride has an atropine-like action and therefore should be used with caution in patients with a history of lower respiratory disease, including asthma, increased intraocular pressure, hyperthyroidism, cardiovascular disease or hypertension.

Information for patients: Patients taking diphenhydramine hydrochloride should be advised that this drug may cause drowsiness and has an additive effect with alcohol.

Patients should be warned about engaging in activities requiring mental alertness such as driving a car or operating appliances, machinery, etc.

Drug Interactions: Diphenhydramine hydrochloride has additive effects with alcohol and other CNS depressants (hypnotics, sedatives, tranquilizers, etc.).

MAO inhibitors prolong and intensify the anticholinergic (drying) effects of antihistamines.

Carcinogenesis, Mutagenesis, Impairment of Fertility: Long-term studies in animals to determine mutagenic and carcinogenic potential have not been performed.

Pregnancy: Pregnancy Category B. Reproduction studies have been performed in rats and rabbits at doses up to 5 times the human dose and have revealed no evidence of impaired fertility or harm to the fetus due to diphenhydramine hydrochloride. There are, however, no adequate and well-controlled studies in pregnant women. Because animal reproduction studies are not always predictive of human response, this drug should be used during pregnancy only if clearly needed.

ADVERSE REACTIONS

The most frequent adverse reactions are underscored.

1. *General:* Urticaria, drug rash, anaphylactic shock, photosensitivity, excessive perspiration, chills, dryness of mouth, nose, and throat
2. *Cardiovascular System:* Hypotension, headache, palpitations, tachycardia, extrasystoles
3. *Hematologic System:* Hemolytic anemia, thrombocytopenia, agranulocytosis
4. *Nervous System:* <u>Sedation, sleepiness, dizziness, disturbed coordination,</u> fatigue, confusion, restlessness, excitation, nervousness, tremor, irritability, insomnia, euphoria, paresthesia, blurred vision, diplopia, vertigo, tinnitus, acute labyrinthitis, neuritis, convulsions
5. *GI System:* <u>Epigastric distress,</u> anorexia, nausea, vomiting, diarrhea, constipation
6. *GU System:* Urinary frequency, difficult urination, urinary retention, early menses
7. *Respiratory System:* <u>Thickening of bronchial secretions,</u> tightness of chest and wheezing, nasal stuffiness

OVERDOSAGE

Antihistamine overdosage reactions may vary from central nervous system depression to stimulation. Stimulation is particularly likely in children. Atropine-like signs and symptoms, dry mouth; fixed, dilated pupils; flushing, and gastrointestinal symptoms may also occur.

If vomiting has not occurred spontaneously the patient should be induced to vomit. This is best done by having him drink a glass of water or milk after which he should be made to gag. Precautions against aspiration must be taken, especially in infants and children.

If vomiting is unsuccessful gastric lavage is indicated within 3 hours after ingestion and even later if large amounts of milk or cream were given beforehand. Isotonic or ½ isotonic saline is the lavage solution of choice.

Saline cathartics, as milk of magnesia, by osmosis draw water into the bowel and therefore are valuable for their action in rapid dilution of bowel content.

Stimulants should not be used.

Vasopressors may be used to treat hypotension.

DOSAGE AND ADMINISTRATION

DOSAGE SHOULD BE INDIVIDUALIZED ACCORDING TO THE NEEDS AND THE RESPONSE OF THE PATIENT.

A single oral dose of diphenhydramine hydrochloride is quickly absorbed with maximum activity occurring in approximately one hour. The duration of activity following an average dose of Benadryl is from four to six hours.

CHILDREN: (over 20 lb): one to two teaspoonfuls three to four times daily. Maximum daily dosage not to exceed 300 mg.

For physicians who wish to calculate the dose on the basis of body weight or surface area, the recommended dosage is 5 mg/kg/24 hours or 150 mg/m^2/24 hours. Data are not available on the use of diphenhydramine hydrochloride as a nighttime sleep-aid in children under 12 years.

ADULTS: Two to four teaspoonfuls three to four times daily. The nighttime sleep-aid dosage is four teaspoonfuls at bedtime.

The basis of determining the most effective dosage regimen will be the response of the patient to medication and the condition under treatment.

In motion sickness, full dosage is recommended for prophylactic use, the first dose to be given 30 minutes before exposure to motion and similar doses before meals and upon retiring for the duration of exposure.

HOW SUPPLIED

Benadryl Elixir—each 5 mL contains 12.5 mg diphenhydramine hydrochloride with 14% alcohol. Available in 4-oz bottles (N 0071-2220-17),
pint bottles (N 0071-2220-23),
gallon bottles (N 0071-2220-32) and
unit-dose (5 mL × 100) (N 0071-2220-40).

Storage Conditions:

Store at controlled room temperature 15°–30°C (59°–86°F). Protect from moisture.

2220G304

BENADRYL® ℞

[*bē'nă-dril*]

(Diphenhydramine Hydrochloride Injection, USP)

DESCRIPTION

Benadryl (diphenhydramine hydrochloride) is 2-(Diphenylmethoxy)-N,N-dimethylethylamine hydrochloride and occurs as a white, crystalline powder and is freely soluble in water and alcohol.

ACTIONS

Diphenhydramine hydrochloride is an antihistamine with anticholinergic (drying), and sedative side effects. Antihistamines appear to compete with histamine for cell receptor sites on effector cells.

INDICATIONS

Benadryl in the injectable form is effective for the following conditions when Benadryl in the oral form is impractical.

Antihistaminic: For amelioration of allergic reactions to blood or plasma, in anaphylaxis as an adjunct to epinephrine and other standard measures after the acute symptoms have been controlled; and for other uncomplicated allergic conditions of the immediate type when oral therapy is impossible or contraindicated.

Motion Sickness: For active treatment of motion sickness.

Antiparkinsonism: For use in parkinsonism, when oral therapy is impossible or contraindicated, as follows: parkinsonism in the elderly who are unable to tolerate more potent agents, mild cases of parkinsonism in other age groups, and in other cases of parkinsonism in combination with centrally acting anticholinergic agents.

CONTRAINDICATIONS

Use in Newborn or Premature Infants

This drug should *not* be used in newborn or premature infants.

Use in Nursing Mothers

Because of the higher risk of antihistamines for infants generally, and for newborns and prematures in particular, antihistamine therapy is contraindicated in nursing mothers.

Antihistamines are also contraindicated in the following conditions.

Hypersensitivity to diphenhydramine hydrochloride and other antihistamines of similar chemical structure.

WARNINGS

Antihistamines should be used with considerable caution in patients with narrow-angle glaucoma, stenosing peptic ulcer, pyloroduodenal obstruction, symptomatic prostatic hypertrophy, bladder-neck obstruction.

Use in Children

In infants and children, especially, antihistamines in *overdosage* may cause hallucinations, convulsions, or death.

As in adults, antihistamines may diminish mental alertness in children. In the young child, particularly, they may produce excitation.

Use in Pregnancy

Experience with this drug in pregnant women is inadequate to determine whether there exists a potential for harm to the developing fetus.

Use With CNS Depressants

Diphenhydramine hydrochloride has additive effects with alcohol and other CNS depressants (hypnotics, sedatives, tranquilizers, etc).

Use in Activities Requiring Mental Alertness

Patients should be warned about engaging in activities requiring mental alertness such as driving a car or operating appliances, machinery, etc.

Use in the Elderly (approximately 60 years or older)

Antihistamines are more likely to cause dizziness, sedation, and hypotension in elderly patients.

PRECAUTIONS

Diphenhydramine hydrochloride has an atropine-like action and, therefore, should be used with caution in patients with a history of bronchial asthma, increased intraocular pressure, hyperthyroidism, cardiovascular disease, hypertension. Use with caution in patients with lower respiratory disease, including asthma.

DRUG INTERACTIONS

MAO inhibitors prolong and intensify the anticholinergic (drying) effects of antihistamines.

ADVERSE REACTIONS

The most frequent adverse reactions are underscored.

1. *General:* Urticaria, drug rash, anaphylactic shock, photosensitivity, excessive perspiration, chills, dryness of mouth, nose, and throat
2. *Cardiovascular System:* Hypotension, headache, palpitations, tachycardia, extrasystoles.
3. *Hematologic System:* Hemolytic anemia, thrombocytopenia, agranulocytosis
4. *Nervous System:* Sedation, sleepiness, dizziness, disturbed coordination, fatigue, confusion, restlessness, excitation, nervousness, tremor, irritability, insomnia, euphoria, paresthesia, blurred vision, diplopia, vertigo, tinnitus, acute labyrinthitis, hysteria, neuritis, convulsions.
5. *GI System:* Epigastric distress, anorexia, nausea, vomiting, diarrhea, constipation
6. *GU System:* Urinary frequency, difficult urination, urinary retention, early menses
7. *Respiratory System:* Thickening of bronchial secretions, tightness of chest and wheezing, nasal stuffiness

OVERDOSAGE

Antihistamine overdosage reactions may vary from central nervous system depression to stimulation. Stimulation is particularly likely in children. Atropine-like signs and symptoms—dry mouth; fixed, dilated pupils; flushing, and gastrointestinal symptoms may also occur.

Stimulants should *not* be used.

Vasopressors may be used to treat hypotension.

DOSAGE AND ADMINISTRATION

Benadryl in the injectable form is indicated when the oral form is impractical. DOSAGE SHOULD BE INDIVIDUALIZED ACCORDING TO THE NEEDS AND THE RESPONSE OF THE PATIENT.

CHILDREN: 5 mg/kg/24 hr or 150 mg/m^2/24 hr. Maximum daily dosage is 300 mg. Divide into four doses, administered intravenously or deeply intramuscularly.

ADULTS: 10 to 50 mg intravenously or deeply intramuscularly; 100 mg if required; maximum daily dosage is 400 mg.

HOW SUPPLIED

Benadryl in parenteral form is supplied as:

N 0071-4015-10 (Steri-Vial®15)

N 0071-4015-13 (Steri-Vial 108)

Sterile solution containing 10 mg diphenhydramine hydrochloride in each milliliter of solution with 0.1 mg/ml benzethonium chloride as a germicidal agent. Supplied in 10-ml and 30-ml Steri-Vials (rubber-diaphragm-capped vials).

N 0071-4402-10 (Steri-Vial 1402)

Sterile solution containing 50 mg diphenhydramine hydrochloride in each milliliter of solution with 0.1 mg/ml benzethonium chloride as a germicidal agent. Supplied in 10-ml Steri-Vials.

N 0071-4259-03 (Amp. 259)

Sterile solution containing 50 mg diphenhydramine hydrochloride in a 1-ml ampoule. Supplied in packages of ten.

N 0071-4259-40 (Steri-Dose® 1406)

N 0071-4259-41 (Steri-Dose 1406)

Sterile solution containing 50 mg diphenhydramine hydrochloride in a 1-ml disposable syringe. Supplied in packages of ten (individually cartoned, and in packages of two trays of 5 syringes each).

The pH of the solutions for parenteral use may have been adjusted with either sodium hydroxide or hydrochloric acid.

4259G012

BRONDECON® ℞

[*brŏn 'dĕ-cŏn "*]

oxtriphylline and guaifenesin

DESCRIPTION

Each tablet contains 200 mg oxtriphylline, USP and 100 mg guaifenesin, USP. Also contains: acacia, NF; colloidal silicon dioxide, NF; corn starch, NF; ethylcellulose, NF; FD&C red No. 40; FD&C yellow No. 6; hydrogenated vegetable oil, NF; lactose, NF; magnesium stearate, NF; methylcellulose, USP; pregelatinized starch, NF; saccharin sodium, USP; sucrose, NF.

Each 5 mL teaspoonful of elixir contains 100 mg oxtriphylline, USP and 50 mg guaifenesin, USP; alcohol 20%. Also contains: citric acid, USP; D&C red No. 33; FD&C red No. 40; flavors; glycerin, USP; purified water, USP; saccharin sodium, USP; sodium citrate, USP; sucrose, NF.

NOTE: 100 mg oxtriphylline is equivalent to 64 mg anhydrous theophylline.

ACTIONS

Brondecon, a bronchodilator and expectorant, helps to relieve symptoms of bronchospasm as well as obstruction caused by viscid mucus in the bronchioles.

Oxtriphylline, the choline salt of theophylline, is a xanthine bronchodilating agent. Compared to aminophylline, oxtriphylline is less irritating to the gastric mucosa, better absorbed from the gastrointestinal tract, more stable and more soluble. The expectorant component of Brondecon is guaifenesin, which tends to increase the secretion and decrease the viscosity of fluids of the respiratory tract. These physiologic fluids help to lubricate the inflamed mucous membranes of the bronchi and also help the patient to expel viscid mucus thus making cough more productive.

INDICATIONS

Brondecon is an adjunct in the management of bronchitis, bronchial asthma, asthmatic bronchitis, pulmonary emphysema, and similar chronic obstructive lung disease. It is indicated when both relaxation of bronchospasm and expectorant action are desirable.

PRECAUTIONS

Concurrent use of other xanthine preparations may lead to adverse reactions, particularly CNS stimulation in children.

ADVERSE REACTIONS

Gastric distress and, occasionally, palpitation and CNS stimulation have been reported.

DOSAGE

Tablets—over 12 years of age: one tablet, 4 times a day.

Elixir—over 12 years of age: two teaspoonfuls, 4 times a day; from 2 to 12 years: one teaspoonful per 60 lb body weight, 4 times a day.

Above recommendations are averages. Dosage should be individualized.

SUPPLIED

Salmon-pink tablets in bottles of 100 (N 0071-0200-24).

Elixir, dark red, cherry-flavored in 237 ml (8 fl oz) (N 0071-2201-20) and 474 ml (16 fl oz) (N 0071-2201-23) bottles.

Store between 15° and 30°C (59° and 86°F).

Shown in Product Identification Section, page 420

0200G011

CELONTIN® KAPSEALS® ℞

[*cĕ "lŏn 'tĭn*]

(methsuximide capsules, USP)

DESCRIPTION

Celontin (methsuximide) is an anticonvulsant succinimide, chemically designated as N,2-Dimethyl-2-phenylsuccinimide.

Each Celontin capsule contains 150 mg or 300 mg methsuximide, USP. Also contains starch, NF. The capsule and band contain citric acid, USP; colloidal silicon dioxide, NF; D&C yellow No. 10; FD&C red No. 3; FD&C yellow No. 6, gelatin, NF; glycerylmonooleate; sodium benzoate, NF; sodium lauryl sulfate NF. The 150-mg capsule and band also contain FD&C blue No. 1; titanium dioxide, USP. The 300-mg capsule and band also contain polyethylene glycol 200.

ACTION

Methsuximide suppresses the paroxysmal three-cycle-per-second spike and wave activity associated with lapses of consciousness which is common in absence (petit mal) seizures. The frequency of epileptiform attacks is reduced, apparently by depression of the motor cortex and elevation of the threshold of the central nervous system to convulsive stimuli.

INDICATION

Celontin is indicated for the control of absence (petit mal) seizures that are refractory to other drugs.

CONTRAINDICATION

Methsuximide should not be used in patients with a history of hypersensitivity to succinimides.

WARNINGS

Blood dyscrasias, including some with fatal outcome, have been reported to be associated with the use of succinimides; therefore, periodic blood counts should be performed.

It has been reported that succinimides have produced morphological and functional changes in animal liver. For this reason, methsuximide should be administered with extreme caution to patients with known liver or renal disease. Periodic urinalysis and liver function studies are advised for all patients receiving the drug.

Cases of systemic lupus erythematosus have been reported with the use of succinimides. The physician should be alert to this possibility.

USAGE IN PREGNANCY

The effects of Celontin in human pregnancy and nursing infants are unknown.

Recent reports suggest an association between the use of anticonvulsant drugs by women with epilepsy and an elevated incidence of birth defects in children born to these women. Data are more extensive with respect to phenytoin and phenobarbital, but these are also the most commonly prescribed anticonvulsants; less systematic or anecdotal reports suggest a possible similar association with the use of all known anticonvulsant drugs.

The reports suggesting an elevated incidence of birth defects in children of drug-treated epileptic women cannot be regarded as adequate to prove a definite cause-and-effect relationship. There are intrinsic methodologic problems in obtaining adequate data on drug teratogenicity in humans; the possibility also exists that other factors, eg, genetic factors or the epileptic condition itself, may be more important than drug therapy in leading to birth defects. The great majority of mothers on anticonvulsant medication deliver normal infants. It is important to note that anticonvulsant drugs should not be discontinued in patients in whom the drug is administered to prevent major seizures because of the strong possibility of precipitating status epilepticus with attendant hypoxia and threat to life. In individual cases where the severity and frequency of the seizure disorder are such that the removal of medication does not pose a serious threat to the patient, discontinuation of the drug may be considered prior to and during pregnancy, although it cannot be said with any confidence that even minor seizures do not pose some hazard to the developing embryo or fetus.

The prescribing physician will wish to weigh these considerations in treating or counseling epileptic women of childbearing potential.

Hazardous Activities: Methsuximide may impair the mental and/or physical abilities required for the performance of potentially hazardous tasks, such as driving a motor vehicle or other such activity requiring alertness; therefore, the patient should be cautioned accordingly.

PRECAUTIONS

It is recommended that the physician withdraw the drug slowly on the appearance of unusual depression, aggressiveness, or other behavioral alterations.

As with other anticonvulsants, it is important to proceed slowly when increasing or decreasing dosage, as well as when adding or eliminating other medication. Abrupt withdrawal of anticonvulsant medication may precipitate absence (petit mal) status.

Methsuximide, when used alone in mixed types of epilepsy, may increase the frequency of grand mal seizures in some patients.

ADVICE TO THE PHARMACIST AND PATIENT: Since methsuximide has a relatively low melting temperature (124°F), storage conditions which may promote high temperatures (closed cars, delivery vans, or storage near steam pipes) should be avoided. Do not dispense or use capsules that are not full or in which contents have melted. Effectiveness may be reduced. Protect from excessive heat (104°F).

ADVERSE REACTIONS

Gastrointestinal System: Gastrointestinal symptoms occur frequently and have included nausea or vomiting, anorexia, diarrhea, weight loss, epigastric and abdominal pain, and constipation.

Hemopoietic System: Hemopoietic complications associated with the administration of methsuximide have included eosinophilia, leukopenia, monocytosis, and pancytopenia.

Nervous System: Neurologic and sensory reactions reported during therapy with methsuximide have included drowsiness, ataxia or dizziness, irritability and nervousness, headache, blurred vision, photophobia, hiccups, and insomnia. Drowsiness, ataxia, and dizziness have been the most frequent side effects noted. Psychologic abnormalities have included confusion, instability, mental slowness, depression, hypochondriacal behavior, and aggressiveness. There have been rare reports of psychosis, suicidal behavior, and auditory hallucinations.

Integumentary System: Dermatologic manifestations which have occurred with the administration of methsuximide have included urticaria, Stevens-Johnson syndrome, and pruritic erythematous rashes.

Other: Miscellaneous reactions reported include periorbital edema and hyperemia.

DOSAGE AND ADMINISTRATION

Optimum dosage of Celontin must be determined by trial. A suggested dosage schedule is 300 mg per day for the first week. If required, dosage may be increased thereafter at weekly intervals by 300 mg per day for the three weeks following to a daily dosage of 1.2 g. Because therapeutic effect

Continued on next page

This product information was prepared in August, 1986. On these and other Parke-Davis Products, information may be obtained by addressing PARKE-DAVIS, Division of Warner-Lambert Company, Morris Plains, New Jersey 07950.

Parke-Davis—Cont.

and tolerance vary among patients, therapy with Celontin must be individualized according to the response of each patient. Optimal dosage is that amount of Celontin which is barely sufficient to control seizures so that side effects may be kept to a minimum. The smaller capsule (150 mg) facilitates administration to small children.
Celontin may be administered in combination with other anticonvulsants when other forms of epilepsy coexist with absence (petit mal.)

HOW SUPPLIED
N 0071-0525-24 (P-D 525)—Celontin Kapseals, each containing 300 mg methsuximide; bottles of 100.
N 0071-0537-24 (P-D 537)—Celontin Kapseals, Half Strength, each containing 150 mg methsuximide, bottles of 100.
Store at controlled room temperature 15°-30°C (59°-86°F). Protect from light and moisture.

0537G012

Shown in Product Identification Section, page 420

CENTRAX® ℂ ℞
[*cĕn'trăx*]
(prazepam capsules and tablets, USP)

DESCRIPTION
Centrax (prazepam) is a benzodiazepine derivative. Chemically, prazepam is 7-chloro-1-(cyclopropylmethyl)-1, 3-dihydro-5-phenyl-2H-1, 4-benzodiazepin-2- one, and has a molecular weight of 324.8.

CLINICAL PHARMACOLOGY
Studies in normal subjects have shown that Centrax (prazepam) has depressant effects on the central nervous system. Oral administration of single doses as high as 60 mg and of divided doses up to 100 mg three times a day (300 mg total daily dosage) were without toxic effects.
Single, oral doses of Centrax (prazepam) in normal subjects produced average peak blood levels of the major metabolite norprazepam at 6 hours postadministration, with significant amounts still present after 48 hours. Prazepam was slowly absorbed over a prolonged period; rather constant blood levels were maintained on multiple-dose schedules; and excretion was prolonged. The mean half-life of norprazepam measured in subjects given 10 mg prazepam three times a day for one week was 63 (± 15 SD) hours before and 70 (± 10 SD) hours after multiple dosing—a nonsignificant difference. Human metabolism studies showed that prior to elimination from the body, prazepam is metabolized in large part to 3-hydroxyprazepam and oxazepam.

INDICATIONS
Centrax is indicated for the management of anxiety disorders or for the short-term relief of the symptoms of anxiety. Anxiety or tension associated with the stress of everyday life usually does not require treatment with an anxiolytic.
The effectiveness of Centrax in long-term use, that is, more than 4 months, has not been assessed by systematic clinical studies. The physician should periodically reassess the usefulness of the drug for the individual patient.

CONTRAINDICATIONS
Centrax (prazepam) is contraindicated in patients with a known hypersensitivity to the drug and in those with acute narrow-angle glaucoma.

WARNINGS
Centrax (prazepam) is not recommended in psychotic states and in those psychiatric disorders in which anxiety is not a prominent feature.
Patients taking Centrax should be cautioned against engaging in hazardous occupations requiring mental alertness, such as operating dangerous machinery including motor vehicles.
Since Centrax has a central nervous system depressant effect, patients should be advised against the simultaneous ingestion of alcohol and other CNS-depressant drugs during Centrax therapy.
Physical and Psychological Dependence: Withdrawal symptoms similar in character to those noted with barbiturates and alcohol have occurred following abrupt discontinuance of benzodiazepine drugs. These symptoms include convulsions, tremor, abdominal and muscle cramps, vomiting and sweating. Addiction-prone individuals, such as drug addicts and alcoholics, should be under careful surveillance when receiving benzodiazepines because of the predisposition of such patients to habituation and dependence.
Withdrawal symptoms have also been reported following abrupt discontinuance of benzodiazepines taken continuously at therapeutic levels for several months.

PRECAUTIONS
Usage in Pregnancy and Lactation: An increased risk of congenital malformations associated with the use of minor tranquilizers (chlordiazepoxide, diazepam, and meprobamate) during the first trimester of pregnancy has been suggested in several studies. Prazepam, a benzodiazepine derivative, has not been studied adequately to determine whether it, too, may be associated with an increased risk of fetal abnormality. Because use of these drugs is rarely a matter of urgency, their use during this period should almost always be avoided. The possibility that a woman of childbearing potential may be pregnant at the time of institution of therapy should be considered. Patients should be advised that if they become pregnant during therapy or intend to become pregnant, they should communicate with their physicians about the desirability of discontinuing the drug. In view of their molecular size, prazepam and its metabolites are probably excreted in human milk. Therefore, this drug should not be given to nursing mothers.
In those patients in whom a degree of depression accompanies the anxiety, suicidal tendencies may be present and protective measures may be required. The least amount of drug that is feasible should be available to the patient at any one time.
Patients taking Centrax (prazepam) for prolonged periods should have blood counts and liver function tests periodically. The usual precautions in treating patients with impaired renal or hepatic functions should also be observed. Hepatomegaly and cholestasis were observed in chronic toxicity studies in rats and dogs.
In elderly or debilitated patients, the initial dose should be small, and increments should be made gradually, in accordance with the response of the patient, to preclude ataxia or excessive sedation.
If Centrax is to be combined with other psychotropic agents or anticonvulsant drugs, careful consideration should be given to the pharmacology of the agents to be employed—particularly with known compounds which may potentiate the action of Centrax, such as phenothiazines, narcotics, barbiturates, MAO inhibitors and other antidepressants.
Pediatric Use: Safety and effectiveness in patients below the age of 18 have not been established.

ADVERSE REACTIONS
The side effects most frequently reported during double-blind, placebo-controlled trials employing a typical 30-mg divided total daily dosage and the percent incidence in the prazepam group were fatigue (11.6%), dizziness (8.7%), weakness (7.7%), drowsiness (6.8%), lightheadedness (6.8%), and ataxia (5.0%). Less frequently reported were headache, confusion, tremor, vivid dreams, slurred speech, palpitation, stimulation, dry mouth, diaphoresis, and various gastrointestinal complaints. Other side effects included pruritus, transient skin rashes, swelling of feet, joint pains, various genitourinary complaints, blurred vision, and syncope. Single, nightly dose, controlled trials of variable dosages showed a dose-related incidence of these same side effects. Transient and reversible aberrations of liver function tests have been reported, as have been slight decreases in blood pressure and increases in body weight.
These findings are characteristic of benzodiazepine drugs.

OVERDOSAGE
As in the management of overdosage with any drug, it should be borne in mind that multiple agents may have been taken. Vomiting should be induced if it has not occurred spontaneously. Immediate gastric lavage is also recommended. General supportive care, including frequent monitoring of vital signs and close observation of the patient, is indicated. Hypotension, though unlikely, may be controlled with Levophed® (levarterenol bitartrate), or Aramine® (metaraminol bitartrate).

DOSAGE AND ADMINISTRATION
Centrax (prazepam) is administered orally in divided doses. The usual daily dose is 30 mg. The dose should be adjusted gradually within the range of 20 mg to 60 mg daily in accordance with the response of the patient. In elderly or debilitated patients it is advisable to initiate treatment at a divided daily dose of 10 mg to 15 mg (see Precautions).
Centrax may also be administered as a single, daily dose at bedtime. The recommended starting nightly dose is 20 mg. The response of the patient to several days' treatment will permit the physician to adjust the dose upwards or, occasionally, downwards to maximize antianxiety effect with a minimum of daytime drowsiness. The optimum dosage will usually range from 20 mg to 40 mg.

DRUG INTERACTIONS
If Centrax (prazepam) is to be combined with other drugs acting on the central nervous system, careful consideration should be given to the pharmacology of the agents to be employed. The actions of the benzodiazepines may be potentiated by barbiturates, narcotics, phenothiazines, monoamine oxidase inhibitors, or other antidepressants.
If Centrax (prazepam) is used to treat anxiety associated with somatic disease states, careful attention must be paid to possible drug interaction with concomitant medication.

HOW SUPPLIED
Centrax 5 mg—Each capsule contains 5 mg prazepam. Available in bottles of 100 (N 0710-0552-24), and 500 (N 0710-0552-30). Centrax 10 mg—Each capsule contains 10 mg prazepam. Available in bottles of 100 (N 0710-0553-24), and 500 (N 0710-0553-30). Centrax 20 mg—Each capsule contains 20 mg prazepam. Available in bottles of 100 (N 0710-0554-24).
Also supplied as Centrax Tablets (prazepam tablets, USP) 10 mg light blue, scored tablets in bottles of 100 (N 0710-0276-24) and unit dose (N 0710-0276-40).

Direct Medical Inquiries to:
Parke-Davis, Div Warner-Lambert Inc
c/o Warner-Lambert Co
201 Tabor Road, Morris Plains, NJ 07950.
Attn: Medical Affairs Dept

0552G122

Shown in Product Identification Section, page 420

CHLOROMYCETIN® CREAM, 1% ℞
[*chlō"rō-my-cē'tĭn*]
(chloramphenicol cream, USP) 1%

DESCRIPTION
Each gram of Chloromycetin Cream, 1%, contains 10 mg chloramphenicol with 0.1% propylparaben in a water-miscible ointment base of liquid petrolatum, cetyl alcohol, sodium lauryl sulfate, sodium phosphate buffer, and water.

CLINICAL PHARMACOLOGY
Chloramphenicol is a broad-spectrum antibiotic originally isolated from *Streptomyces venezuelae.* It is primarily bacteriostatic and acts by inhibition of protein synthesis by interfering with the transfer of activated amino acids from soluble RNA to ribosomes. Development of resistance to chloramphenicol can be regarded as minimal for staphylococci and many other species of bacteria.

INDICATIONS AND USAGE
Chloromycetin (chloramphenicol) Cream, 1%, is indicated for the treatment of surface skin infections caused by bacteria susceptible to chloramphenicol. Deeper cutaneous infections should be treated with appropriate systemic antibiotics.

CONTRAINDICATION
This product is contraindicated in persons sensitive to any of its components.

WARNINGS
Bone marrow hypoplasia, including aplastic anemia and death, has been reported following the local application of chloramphenicol.

PRECAUTIONS
The prolonged use of antibiotics may occasionally result in overgrowth of nonsusceptible organisms, including fungi. If new infections appear during medication, the drug should be discontinued and appropriate measures should be taken.
In all except very superficial infections, the topical use of chloramphenicol should be supplemented by appropriate systemic medication.

ADVERSE REACTIONS
Signs of local irritation with subjective symptoms of itching or burning, angioneurotic edema, urticaria, vesicular and maculopapular dermatitis have been reported in patients sensitive to chloramphenicol and are causes for discontinuing the medication. Similar sensitivity reactions to other materials in topical preparations may also occur. Blood dyscrasias have been reported in association with the use of chloramphenicol (See WARNINGS).

DOSAGE AND ADMINISTRATION
Apply to the infected area three or four times daily after cleansing.

HOW SUPPLIED
N 0071-3166-13 (Ointment 66)
Chloromycetin Cream (chloramphenicol cream), 1%, is supplied in 1-oz tubes.
AHFS 84:04.04 3166G012

CHLOROMYCETIN® ℞
[*chlō"rō-my-cē'tĭn*]
HYDROCORTISONE OPHTHALMIC
(Chloramphenicol and Hydrocortisone Acetate for Suspension, USP)

WARNING
Bone marrow hypoplasia including aplastic anemia and death has been reported following local application of chloramphenicol. Chloramphenicol should not be used

when less potentially dangerous agents would be expected to provide effective treatment.

DESCRIPTION

Chloromycetin® Hydrocortisone Ophthalmic (Chloramphenicol and Hydrocortisone Acetate for Suspension, USP) is a sterile, buffered antibiotic/antiinflammatory dry mixture for suspension for ophthalmic administration. Each vial of Chloromycetin Hydrocortisone Ophthalmic contains 12.5 mg chloramphenicol and 25 mg hydrocortisone acetate with boric acid-sodium borate buffer, cholesterol, methylcellulose, sodium chloride, and Phemerol® (benzethonium chloride), 0.1 mg per ml, in the suspension when prepared as directed. A 5 ml vial of Sterile Distilled Water is included in each package for use as a diluent in the preparation of a suspension of Chloromycetin Hydrocortisone suitable for ophthalmic use.

The chemical names for chloramphenicol are:

(1) Acetamide,2,2-dichloro-N-[2-hydroxy-1-(hydroxymethyl)-2-(4-nitrophenyl) ethyl]-, and

(2) D-*threo* -(–)-2,2-Dichloro-N-[β-hydroxy-α-(hydroxymethyl)-*p* -nitrophenethyl] acetamide

The chemical names for hydrocortisone acetate are:

(1) Pregn-4-ene-3,20-dione,21-(acetyloxy)-11,17-dihydroxy-,(11β)-, and

(2) 17-Hydroxycorticosterone 21-acetate

CLINICAL PHARMACOLOGY

Corticoids suppress the inflammatory response to a variety of agents and they probably delay or slow healing. Since corticoids may inhibit the body's defense mechanism against infection, a concomitant antimicrobial drug may be used when this inhibition is considered to be clinically significant in a particular case.

The antiinfective component in this combination is included to provide action against specific organisms susceptible to it. Chloramphenicol is considered active against a wide spectrum of gram-negative and gram-positive organisms such as *Escherichia coli, Hemophilus influenzae, Staphylococcus aureus, Streptococcus hemolyticus,* and *Moraxella lacunata* (Morax-Axenfeld bacillus). Development of resistance to chloramphenicol can be regarded as minimal for staphylococci and many other species of bacteria. Chloramphenicol is primarily bacteriostatic and acts by inhibition of protein synthesis by interfering with the transfer of activated amino acids from soluble RNA to ribosomes. It has been noted that chloramphenicol is found in measurable amounts in the aqueous humor following local application to the eye.

When a decision to administer both a corticoid and an antimicrobial is made, the administration of such drugs in combination has the advantage of greater patient compliance and convenience, with the added assurance that the appropriate dosage of both drugs is administered, plus assured compatibility of ingredients when both types of drug are in the same formulation and, particularly, that the correct volume of drug is delivered and retained.

The relative potency of corticosteroids depends on the molecular structure, concentration, and release from the vehicle.

INDICATIONS AND USAGE

Chloramphenicol should be used only in those serious infections for which less potentially dangerous drugs are ineffective or contraindicated. Bacteriological studies should be performed to determine the causative organisms and their sensitivity to chloramphenicol (See Box Warning).

For steroid-responsive inflammatory ocular conditions for which a corticosteroid is indicated and where bacterial infection or a risk of bacterial ocular infection exists.

Ocular steroids are indicated in inflammatory conditions of the palpebral and bulbar conjunctiva, cornea, and anterior segment of the globe where the inherent risk of steroid use in certain infective conjunctivitides is accepted to obtain a diminution in edema and inflammation. They are also indicated in chronic anterior uveitis and corneal injury from chemical radiation, thermal burns, or penetration of foreign bodies.

The use of a combination drug with an antiinfective component is indicated where the risk of infection is high or where there is an expectation that potentially dangerous numbers of bacteria will be present in the eye.

The particular antiinfective drug in this product is active against the following common bacterial eye pathogens:

Staphylococcus aureus
Streptococci, including *Streptococcus pneumoniae*
Escherichia coli
Hemophilus influenzae
Klebsiella/Enterobacter species
Moraxella lacunata (Morax-Axenfeld bacillus)
Neisseria species

The product does not provide adequate coverage against:

Pseudomonas aeruginosa
Serratia marcescens

CONTRAINDICATIONS

Epithelial herpes simplex keratitis (dendritic keratitis), vaccinia, varicella, and many other viral diseases of the cornea and conjunctiva. Mycobacterial infection of the eye. Fungal diseases of ocular structures. Hypersensitivity to a component of the medication. (Hypersensitivity to the antibiotic component occurs at a higher rate than for other components).

The use of these combinations is always contraindicated after uncomplicated removal of a corneal foreign body.

WARNINGS

SEE BOX WARNING

Prolonged use of steroids may result in glaucoma, with damage to the optic nerve, defects in visual acuity and fields of vision, and posterior subcapsular cataract formation. Prolonged use may suppress the host response and thus increase the hazard of secondary ocular infections. In those diseases causing thinning of the cornea or sclera, perforations have been known to occur with the use of topical steroids. In acute purulent conditions of the eye, steroids may mask infection or enhance existing infection. If these products are used for 10 days or longer, intraocular pressure should be routinely monitored even though it may be difficult in children and uncooperative patients.

Employment of steroid medication in the treatment of herpes simplex requires great caution.

PRECAUTIONS

The initial prescription and renewal of the medication order beyond 20 milliliters should be made by a physician only after examination of the patient with the aid of magnification, such as slit lamp biomicroscopy and, where appropriate, fluorescein staining.

The possibility of persistent fungal infections of the cornea should be considered after prolonged steroid dosing.

The prolonged use of antibiotics may occasionally result in overgrowth of nonsusceptible organisms, including fungi. If new infections appear during medication, the drug should be discontinued and appropriate measures should be taken.

In all serious infections the topical use of chloramphenicol should be supplemented by appropriate systemic medication.

ADVERSE REACTIONS

Blood dyscrasias have been reported in association with the use of chloramphenicol. (See **Warnings**).

Adverse reactions have occurred with steroid /antiinfective combination drugs which can be attributed to the steroid component, the antiinfective component, or the combination. Exact incidence figures are not available since no denominator of treated patients is available.

Reactions occurring most often from the presence of the antiinfective ingredient are allergic sensitizations. The reactions due to the steroid component in decreasing order of frequency are: elevation of intraocular pressure (IOP) with possible development of glaucoma, and infrequent optic nerve damage; posterior subcapsular cataract formation; and delayed wound healing.

Secondary Infection: The development of secondary infection has occurred after use of combinations containing steroids and antimicrobials. Fungal infections of the cornea are particularly prone to develop coincidentally with long-term applications of steroid. The possibility of fungal invasion must be considered in any persistent corneal ulceration where steroid treatment has been used.

Secondary bacterial ocular infection following suppression of host responses also occurs.

DOSAGE AND ADMINISTRATION

Two drops applied to the affected eye every three hours, or more frequently if deemed advisable by the prescribing physician. Administration should be continued day and night for the first 48 hours, after which the interval between applications may be increased. Treatment should be continued for at least 48 hours after the eye appears normal.

Directions for dispensing—Add 5 ml sterile distilled water to contents of vial under aseptic conditions. Shake to make uniform suspension. Place sterile dropper in vial. Each ml of suspension prepared as directed contains 2.5 mg Chloromycetin (chloramphenicol) and 5 mg Hydrocortisone Acetate.

Not more than 20 milliliters should be prescribed initially and the prescription should not be refilled without further evaluation as outlined in Precautions above.

HOW SUPPLIED

N 0071-3228-36 Chloromycetin Hydrocortisone Ophthalmic (Chloramphenicol and Hydrocortisone Acetate for Suspension, USP) is supplied in a package containing dry ingredients in a 5 ml vial and also a vial containing 5 ml of Sterile Distilled Water for use as a diluent in preparation of the ophthalmic suspension. After dispensing, the product may be stored at room temperature for a period of not more than 10 days. A sterilized dropper-cap assembly for use with the vial is included in the package.

Chloromycetin, brand of chloramphenicol, Reg US Pat Off.

3228G014

KAPSEALS®/CAPSULES CHLOROMYCETIN® ℞

[*chlō″rō-my-cē′tĭn*]

(chloramphenicol capsules, USP)

WARNING

Serious and fatal blood dyscrasias (aplastic anemia, hypoplastic anemia, thrombocytopenia, and granulocytopenia) are known to occur after the administration of chloramphenicol. In addition, there have been reports of aplastic anemia attributed to chloramphenicol which later terminated in leukemia. Blood dyscrasias have occurred after both short-term and prolonged therapy with this drug. Chloramphenicol must not be used when less potentially dangerous agents will be effective, as described in the Indications section. *It must not be used in the treatment of trivial infections or where it is not indicated, as in colds, influenza, infections of the throat; or as a prophylactic agent to prevent bacterial infections.*

Precautions: It is essential that adequate blood studies be made during treatment with the drug. While blood studies may detect early peripheral blood changes, such as leukopenia, reticulocytopenia, or granulocytopenia, before they become irreversible, such studies cannot be relied on to detect bone marrow depression prior to development of aplastic anemia. To facilitate appropriate studies and observation during therapy, it is desirable that patients be hospitalized.

DESCRIPTION

Chloramphenicol is an antibiotic that is clinically useful for, *and should be reserved for,* serious infections caused by organisms susceptible to its antimicrobial effects when less potentially hazardous therapeutic agents are ineffective or contraindicated. Sensitivity testing is essential to determine its indicated use, but may be performed concurrently with therapy initiated on clinical impression that one of the indicated conditions exists (see Indications and Usage section).

Each capsule contains 250 mg chloramphenicol. Also contains lactose, NF. The capsule shell and/or band contains gelatin, NF; colloidal silicon dioxide, NF; glyceryl monooleate; gray Opatint OD-7502; sodium lauryl sulfate, NF; titanium dioxide USP.

CLINICAL PHARMACOLOGY

In vitro chloramphenicol exerts mainly a bacteriostatic effect on a wide range of gram-negative and gram-positive bacteria and is active *in vitro* against rickettsiae, the lymphogranuloma psittacosis group, and *Vibrio cholerae.* It is particularly active against *Salmonella typhi* and *Hemophilus influenzae.* The mode of action is through interference or inhibition of protein synthesis in intact cells and in cell-free systems.

Chloramphenicol administered orally is absorbed rapidly from the intestinal tract. In controlled studies in adult volunteers using the recommended dosage of 50 mg/kg/day, a dosage of 1 g every 6 hours for 8 doses was given. Using the microbiological assay method, the average peak serum level was 11.2 mcg/ml one hour after the first dose. A cumulative effect gave a peak rise to 18.4 mcg/ml after the fifth dose of 1 g. Mean serum levels ranged from 8 to 14 mcg/ml over the 48-hour period. Total urinary excretion of chloramphenicol in these studies ranged from a low of 68% to a high of 99% over a three-day period. From 8 to 12% of the antibiotic excreted is in the form of free chloramphenicol; the remainder consists of microbiologically inactive metabolites, principally the conjugate with glucuronic acid. Since the glucuronide is excreted rapidly, most chloramphenicol detected in the blood is in the microbiologically active free form. Despite the small proportion of unchanged drug excreted in the urine, the concentration of free chloramphenicol is relatively high, amounting to several hundred mcg/ml in patients receiving divided doses of 50 mg/kg/day. Small amounts of active drug are found in bile and feces. Chloramphenicol diffuses rapidly, but its distribution is not uniform. Highest concentrations are found in liver and kidney, and lowest concentrations are found in brain and cerebrospinal fluid. Chloramphenicol enters cerebrospinal fluid even in the absence of meningeal inflammation, appearing in concentrations about half of those found in the blood. Measurable levels are also detected in pleural and in ascitic fluids, saliva, milk, and in the aqueous and vitreous humors. Transport across the placental barrier occurs with somewhat

Continued on next page

This product information was prepared in August, 1986. On these and other Parke-Davis Products, information may be obtained by addressing PARKE-DAVIS, Division of Warner-Lambert Company, Morris Plains, New Jersey 07950.

Parke-Davis—Cont.

lower concentration in cord blood of newborn infants than in maternal blood.

INDICATIONS AND USAGE

In accord with the concepts in the warning box and this indications section, chloramphenicol must be used only in those serious infections for which less potentially dangerous drugs are ineffective or contraindicated. However, chloramphenicol may be chosen to initiate antibiotic therapy on the clinical impression that one of the conditions below is believed to be present; *in vitro* sensitivity tests should be performed concurrently so that the drug may be discontinued as soon as possible if less potentially dangerous agents are indicated by such tests. The decision to continue use of chloramphenicol rather than another antibiotic when both are suggested by *in vitro* studies to be effective against a specific pathogen should be based upon severity of the infection, susceptibility of the pathogen to the various antimicrobial drugs, efficacy of the various drugs in the infection, and the important additional concepts contained in the Warning Box above:

1. Acute infections caused by *Salmonella typhi*
Chloramphenicol is a drug of choice.* It is not recommended for the routine treatment of the typhoid carrier state.

2. Serious infections caused by susceptible strains in accordance with the concepts expressed above:

a. *Salmonella* species
b. *H influenzae*, specifically meningeal infections
c. Rickettsia
d. Lymphogranuloma-psittacosis group
e. Various gram-negative bacteria causing bacteremia, meningitis, or other serious gram-negative infections
f. Other susceptible organisms which have been demonstrated to be resistant to all other appropriate antimicrobial agents.

3. Cystic fibrosis regimens

CONTRAINDICATIONS

Chloramphenicol is con- traindicated in individuals with a history of previous hypersensitivity and/or toxic reaction to it. *It must not be used in the treatment of trivial infections or where it is not indicated, as in colds, influenza, infections of the throat; or as a prophylactic agent to prevent bacterial infections.*

---

* In the treatment of typhoid fever, some authorities recommend that chloramphenicol be administered at therapeutic levels for 8 to 10 days after the patient has become afebrile to lessen the possibility of relapse.

PRECAUTIONS

1. Baseline blood studies should be followed by periodic blood studies approximately every two days during therapy. The drug should be discontinued upon appearance of reticulocytopenia, leukopenia, thrombocytopenia, anemia, or any other blood study findings attributable to chloramphenicol. However, it should be noted that such studies do not exclude the possible later appearance of the irreversible type of bone marrow depression.

2. Repeated courses of the drug should be avoided if at all possible. Treatment should not be continued longer than required to produce a cure with little or no risk of relapse of the disease.

3. Concurrent therapy with other drugs that may cause bone marrow depression should be avoided.

4. Excessive blood levels may result from administration of the recommended dose to patients with impaired liver or kidney function, including that due to immature metabolic processes in the infant. The dosage should be adjusted accordingly or, preferably, the blood concentration should be determined at appropriate intervals.

5. There are no studies to establish the safety of this drug in pregnancy.

6. Since chloramphenicol readily crosses the placental barrier, caution in use of the drug is particularly important during pregnancy at term or during labor because of potential toxic effects on the fetus ("gray syndrome").

7. Precaution should be used in therapy of premature and full-term infants to avoid "gray syndrome" toxicity. (See Adverse Reactions.) Serum drug levels should be carefully followed during therapy of the newborn infant.

8. Precaution should be used in therapy during lactation because of the possibility of toxic effects on the nursing infant.

9. The use of this antibiotic, as with other antibiotics, may result in an overgrowth of nonsusceptible organisms, including fungi. If infections caused by nonsusceptible organisms appear during therapy, appropriate measures should be taken.

ADVERSE REACTIONS

1. Blood Dyscrasias
The most serious adverse effect of chloramphenicol is bone marrow depression. Serious and fatal blood dyscrasias (aplastic anemia, hypoplastic anemia, thrombocytopenia, and granulocytopenia) are known to occur after the administration of chloramphenicol. An irreversible type of marrow depression leading to aplastic anemia with a high rate of mortality is characterized by the appearance weeks or months after therapy of bone marrow aplasia or hypoplasia. Peripherally, pancytopenia is most often observed, but in a small number of cases only one or two of the three major cell types (erythrocytes, leukocytes, platelets) may be depressed.
A reversible type of bone marrow depression, which is dose-related, may occur. This type of marrow depression is characterized by vacuolization of the erythroid cells, reduction of reticulocytes, and leukopenia, and responds promptly to the withdrawal of chloramphenicol.
An exact determination of the risk of serious and fatal blood dyscrasias is not possible because of lack of accurate information regarding (1) the size of the population at risk, (2) the total number of drug-associated dyscrasias, and (3) the total number of nondrug-associated dyscrasias.
In a report to the California State Assembly by the California Medical Association and the State Department of Public Health in January 1967, the risk of fatal aplastic anemia was estimated at 1:24,200 to 1:40,500 based on two dosage levels.
There have been reports of aplastic anemia attributed to chloramphenicol which later terminated in leukemia.
Paroxysmal nocturnal hemoglobinuria has also been reported.

2. Gastrointestinal Reactions
Nausea, vomiting, glossitis and stomatitis, diarrhea, and enterocolitis may occur in low incidence.

3. Neurotoxic Reactions
Headache, mild depression, mental confusion, and delirium have been described in patients receiving chloramphenicol. Optic and peripheral neuritis have been reported, usually following long-term therapy. If this occurs, the drug should be promptly withdrawn.

4. Hypersensitivity Reactions
Fever, macular and vesicular rashes, angioedema, urticaria, and anaphylaxis may occur. Herxheimer reactions have occurred during therapy for typhoid fever.

5. "Gray Syndrome"
Toxic reactions including fatalities have occurred in the premature and newborn; the signs and symptoms associated with these reactions have been referred to as the "gray syndrome". One case of "gray syndrome" has been reported in an infant born to a mother having received chloramphenicol during labor. One case has been reported in a 3-month-old infant. The following summarizes the clinical and laboratory studies that have been made on these patients:

(a) In most cases, therapy with chloramphenicol had been instituted within the first 48 hours of life.
(b) Symptoms first appeared after 3 to 4 days of continued treatment with high doses of chloramphenicol.
(c) The symptoms appeared in the following order:
  (1) abdominal distention with or without emesis;
  (2) progressive pallid cyanosis;
  (3) vasomotor collapse, frequently accompanied by irregular respiration;
  (4) death within a few hours of onset of these symptoms.
(d) The progression of symptoms from onset to exitus was accelerated with higher dose schedules.
(e) Preliminary blood serum level studies revealed unusually high concentrations of chloramphenicol (over 90 mcg/ml after repeated doses).
(f) Termination of therapy upon early evidence of the associated symptomatology frequently reversed the process with complete recovery.

DOSAGE AND ADMINISTRATION

Dosage Recommendations For Oral Chloramphenicol Preparations

The majority of microorganisms susceptible to chloramphenicol will respond to a concentration between 5 and 20 mcg/ml. The desired concentration of active drug in blood should fall within this range over most of the treatment period. Dosage of 50 mg/kg/day divided into 4 doses at intervals of 6 hours will usually achieve and sustain levels of this magnitude.
Except in certain circumstances (eg, premature and newborn infants and individuals with impairment of hepatic or renal function), lower doses may not achieve these concentrations. Chloramphenicol, like other potent drugs, should be prescribed at recommended doses known to have therapeutic activity. Close observation of the patient should be maintained and in the event of any adverse reactions, dosage should be reduced or the drug discontinued, if other factors in the clinical situation permit.

Adults
Adults should receive 50 mg/kg/day (approximately one 250-mg capsule per each 10 lbs body weight) in divided doses at 6-hour intervals. In exceptional cases, patients with infections due to moderately resistant organisms may require increased dosage up to 100 mg/kg/day to achieve blood levels inhibiting the pathogen, but these high doses should be decreased as soon as possible. Adults with impairment of hepatic or renal function or both may have reduced ability to metabolize and excrete the drug. In instances of impaired metabolic processes, dosages should be adjusted accordingly. (See discussion under Newborn Infants.) Precise control of concentration of the drug in the blood should be carefully followed in patients with impaired metabolic processes by the available microtechniques (information available on request).

Children
Dosage of 50 mg/kg/day divided into 4 doses at 6-hour intervals yields blood levels in the range effective against most susceptible organisms. Severe infections (eg, bacteremia or meningitis), especially when adequate cerebrospinal fluid concentrations are desired, may require dosage up to 100 mg/kg/day; however, it is recommended that dosage be reduced to 50 mg/kg/day as soon as possible. Children with impaired liver or kidney function may retain excessive amounts of the drug.

Newborn Infants
(See section titled "Gray Syndrome" under Adverse Reactions.)
A total of 25 mg/kg/day in 4 equal doses at 6-hour intervals usually produces and maintains concentrations in blood and tissues adequate to control most infections for which the drug is indicated. Increased dosage in these individuals, demanded by severe infections, should be given only to maintain the blood concentration within a therapeutically effective range. After the first two weeks of life, full-term infants ordinarily may receive up to a total of 50 mg/kg/day equally divided into 4 doses at 6-hour intervals. **These dosage recommendations are extremely important because blood concentration in all premature infants and full-term infants under two weeks of age differs from that of other infants.** This difference is due to variations in the maturity of the metabolic functions of the liver and the kidneys.
When these functions are immature (or seriously impaired in adults), high concentrations of the drug are found which tend to increase with succeeding doses.

Infants and Children with Immature Metabolic Processes
In young infants and other children in whom immature metabolic functions are suspected, a dose of 25 mg/kg/day will usually produce therapeutic concentrations of the drug in the blood. In this group particularly, the concentration of the drug in the blood should be carefully following by microtechniques. (Information available on request.)

HOW SUPPLIED

Kapseals No. 379, Chloromycetin (Chloramphenicol Capsules), each contain 250 mg chloramphenicol.
N 0071-0379-09 Bottles of 16.
N 0071-0379-24 Bottles of 100.
N 0071-0379-40 Unit dose packages of 100 (10/10's).
Shown in Product Identification Section, page 420
AHFS 8:12.08 **0379G101**

Chloromycetin, brand of chloramphenicol.
Reg. US Pat Off

STORAGE

Store at a room temperature below 86°F(30°C). Protect from moisture and excessive heat.
Caution—Federal law prohibits dispensing without prescription.

CHLOROMYCETIN® OPHTHALMIC ℞

[*chlō"rō-my-cē'tĭn*]
(Chloramphenical for Ophthalmic Solution, USP)

> **WARNING**
> Bone marrow hypoplasia including aplastic anemia and death has been reported following local application of chloramphenicol. Chloramphenicol should not be used when less potentially dangerous agents would be expected to provide effective treatment.

DESCRIPTION

Each vial of Chloromycetin Ophthalmic contains 25 mg of Chloromycetin (chloramphenicol) with boric acid-sodium borate buffer. Sodium hydroxide may have been added for adjustment of pH. A 15 ml bottle of Sterile Distilled Water is included in each package for use as a diluent in the preparation of a solution of Chloromycetin suitable for ophthalmic use. By varying the quantity of diluent used solutions ranging in strength from 0.16% to 0.5% may be prepared. Both the powder for solution and the diluent contain no preservatives. Sterile powder.
The chemical names for chloramphenicol are:

(1) Acetamide,2,2-dichloro-*N*-[2-hydroxy-1-(hydroxymethyl)-2-(4-nitrophenyl) ethyl]-, and
(2) D-*threo* -(–)-2,2-Dichloro-*N*-[β-hydroxy-α-(hydroxymethyl)-*p*-nitrophenethyl] acetamide

CLINICAL PHARMACOLOGY

Chloramphenicol is a broad-spectrum antibiotic originally isolated from *Streptomyces venezuelae.* It is primarily bacteriostatic and acts by inhibition of protein synthesis by interfering with the transfer of activated amino acids from soluble RNA to ribosomes. It has been noted that chloramphenicol is found in measurable amounts in the aqueous humor following local application to the eye. Development of resistance to chloramphenicol can be regarded as minimal for staphylococci and many other species of bacteria.

INDICATIONS AND USAGE

Chloramphenicol should be used only in those serious infections for which less potentially dangerous drugs are ineffective or contraindicated. Bacteriological studies should be performed to determine the causative organisms and their sensitivity to chloramphenicol (See Box Warning).

Chloromycetin (chloramphenicol) Ophthalmic is indicated for the treatment of surface ocular infections involving the conjunctiva and/or cornea caused by chloramphenicol-susceptible organisms.

The particular antiinfective drug in this product is active against the following common bacterial eye pathogens:

Staphylococcus aureus
Streptococci, including *Streptococcus pneumoniae*
Escherichia coli
Haemophilus influenzae
Klebsiella/Enterobacter species
Moraxella lacunata (Morax-Axenfeld bacillus)
Neisseria species

The product does not provide adequate coverage against:

Pseudomonas aeruginosa
Serratia marcescens

CONTRAINDICATIONS

This product is contraindicated in persons sensitive to any of its components.

WARNINGS

SEE BOX WARNING

PRECAUTIONS

The prolonged use of antibiotics may occasionally result in overgrowth of nonsusceptible organisms, including fungi. If new infections appear during medication, the drug should be discontinued and appropriate measures should be taken.

In all serious infections the topical use of chloramphenicol should be supplemented by appropriate systemic medication.

ADVERSE REACTIONS

Blood dyscrasias have been reported in association with the use of chloramphenicol (See WARNINGS).

DOSAGE AND ADMINISTRATION

Two drops applied to the affected eye every three hours, or more frequently if deemed advisable by the prescribing physician. Administration should be continued day and night for the first 48 hours, after which the interval between applications may be increased. Treatment should be continued for at least 48 hours after the eye appears normal.

Directions for dispensing—Prepare solution by adding sterile distilled water to the vial as follows:

Strength of solution desired	Add sterile distilled water
0.5%	5 ml
0.25%	10 ml
0.16%	15 ml

Solutions remain stable at room temperature for ten days.

HOW SUPPLIED

N 0071-3213-35 Chloromycetin (chloramphenicol) Ophthalmic is supplied in a package containing dry ingredients in a 15 ml vial and also a vial containing 15 ml of Sterile Distilled Water for use as a diluent in preparing the solution for ophthalmic use. A sterilized dropper-cap assembly for use on the vial of solution is included in the package.

Store below 30°C (86°F).

Chloromycetin, brand of chloramphenicol. Reg US Pat Off

3213G011

CHLOROMYCETIN® ℞

[*chlō"rō-my-cē'tĭn*]

OPHTHALMIC OINTMENT, 1%
(chloramphenicol ophthalmic ointment, USP)

> **WARNING**
> Bone marrow hypoplasia including aplastic anemia and death has been reported following local application of chloramphenicol. Chloramphenicol should not be used when less potentially dangerous agents would be expected to provide effective treatment.

DESCRIPTION

Each gram of Chloromycetin Ophthalmic Ointment, 1% contains 10 mg chloramphenicol in a special base of liquid petrolatum and polyethylene. It contains no preservatives. Sterile ointment.

The chemical names for chloramphenicol are:

(1) Acetamide,2,2-dichloro-*N*-[2-hydroxy-1- (hydroxymethyl)-2-(4-nitrophenyl) ethyl]-, and
(2) D-*threo*-(–)-2,2-Dichloro-*N*-[β-hydroxy-α-(hydroxymethyl)-*p*-nitrophenethyl] acetamide

CLINICAL PHARMACOLOGY

Chloramphenicol is a broad-spectrum antibiotic originally isolated from *Streptomyces venezuelae.* It is primarily bacteriostatic and acts by inhibition of protein synthesis by interfering with the transfer of activated amino acids from soluble RNA to ribosomes. It has been noted that chloramphenicol is found in measurable amounts in the aqueous humor following local application to the eye. Development of resistance to chloramphenicol can be regarded as minimal for staphylococci and many other species of bacteria.

INDICATIONS AND USAGE

Chloramphenicol should be used only in those serious infections for which less potentially dangerous drugs are ineffective or contraindicated. Bacteriological studies should be performed to determine the causative organisms and their sensitivity to chloramphenicol (See Box Warning).

Chloromycetin (chloramphenicol) Ophthalmic Ointment, 1% is indicated for the treatment of surface ocular infections involving the conjunctiva and/or cornea caused by chloramphenicol-susceptible organisms.

The particular antiinfective drug in this product is active against the following common bacterial eye pathogens:

Staphylococcus aureus
Streptococci, including *Streptococcus pneumoniae*
Escherichia coli
Haemophilus influenzae
Klebsiella/Enterobacter species
Moraxella lacunata (Morax-Axenfeld bacillus)
Neisseria species

The product does not provide adequate coverage against:

Pseudomonas aeruginosa
Serratia marcescens

CONTRAINDICATIONS

This product is contraindicated in persons sensitive to any of its components.

WARNINGS

SEE BOX WARNING
Ophthalmic ointments may retard corneal wound healing.

PRECAUTIONS

The prolonged use of antibiotics may occasionally result in overgrowth of nonsusceptible organisms, including fungi. If new infections appear during medication, the drug should be discontinued and appropriate measures should be taken.

In all serious infections the topical use of chloramphenicol should be supplemented by appropriate systemic medication.

ADVERSE REACTIONS

Blood dyscrasias have been reported in association with the use of chloramphenicol (See WARNINGS).

DOSAGE AND ADMINISTRATION

A small amount of ointment placed in the lower conjunctival sac every three hours, or more frequently if deemed advisable by the prescribing physician. Administration should be continued day and night for the first 48 hours, after which the interval between applications may be increased. Treatment should be continued for at least 48 hours after the eye appears normal.

HOW SUPPLIED

N 0071-3070-07

Chloromycetin Ophthalmic Ointment, 1% (Chloramphenicol Ophthalmic Ointment, USP) is supplied, sterile, in ophthalmic ointment tubes of 3.5 grams.

Chloromycetin, brand of chloramphenicol. Reg US Pat Off

AHFS Category 52:04.04 **3070G021**

CHLOROMYCETIN® OTIC ℞

[*chlō"rō-my-cē'tĭn ō'-tĭc*]

(chloramphenicol otic)

> **WARNING**
> Bone marrow hypoplasia including aplastic anemia and death has been reported following local application of chloramphenicol. Chloramphenicol should not be used when less potentially dangerous agents would be expected to provide effective treatment.

DESCRIPTION

Each milliliter of Chloromycetin Otic contains 5 mg (0.5%) chloramphenicol in propylene glycol. Sterile.

The chemical names for chloramphenicol are:

(1) Acetamide,2,2-dichloro -*N*- [2-hydroxy-1-(hydroxymethyl) -2- (4-nitro-phenyl) ethyl]-, and
(2) D- *threo* - (—) -2,2 -Dichloro -*N*- [β-hydroxy-α(hydroxymethyl)-*p* -nitrophenethyl]acetamide

CLINICAL PHARMACOLOGY

Chloramphenicol is a broad-spectrum antibiotic originally isolated from *Streptomyces venezuelae.* It is primarily bacteriostatic and acts by inhibition of protein synthesis by interfering with the transfer of activated amino acids from soluble RNA to ribosomes. Development of resistance to chloramphenicol can be regarded as minimal for staphylococci and many other species of bacteria.

INDICATIONS AND USAGE

Chloromycetin (chloramphenicol) Otic is indicated for the treatment of surface infections of the external auditory canal caused by susceptible strains of various gram-positive and gram-negative organisms including:

Staphylococcus aureus, Escherichia coli, Hemophilus influenzae, Pseudomonas aeruginosa, Aerobacter aerogenes, Klebsiella pneumoniae and *Proteus* species.

Deeper infections should be treated with appropriate systemic antibiotics.

CONTRAINDICATIONS

This product is contraindicated in persons sensitive to any of its components.

WARNINGS

SEE BOX WARNING.

PRECAUTIONS

The prolonged use of antibiotics may occasionally result in overgrowth of nonsusceptible organisms, including fungi. If new infections appear during medication, the drug should be discontinued and appropriate measures should be taken.

In all serious infections, the topical use of chloramphenicol should be supplemented by appropriate systemic medication.

The possibility of the occurrence of ototoxicity must be considered if this product is allowed to enter the middle ear.

ADVERSE REACTION

Signs of local irritation with subjective symptoms of itching or burning, angioneurotic edema, urticaria, vesicular and maculopapular dermatitis have been reported in patients sensitive to chloramphenicol and are causes for discontinuing the medication. Similar sensitivity reactions to other materials in topical preparations may also occur. Blood dyscrasias have been reported in association with the use of chloramphenicol (See WARNINGS).

DOSAGE AND ADMINISTRATION

Instill 2 or 3 drops into the affected ear three times daily.

HOW SUPPLIED

N0071-3313-35 Chloromycetin (chloramphenicol) Otic is supplied in 15 mL vials with droppers.

Store below 30°C (86°F).

Chloromycetin, brand of chloramphenicol, Reg US Pat Off.

Caution—Federal law prohibits dispensing without prescription.

3313G022

ORAL SUSPENSION

CHLOROMYCETIN® PALMITATE ℞

[*chlō"rō-my-ce'tĭn păl'mĭ-tāte"*]

(chloramphenicol palmitate oral suspension, USP)

> **WARNING**
> **Serious and fatal blood dyscrasias (aplastic anemia, hypoplastic anemia, thrombocytopenia, and granulocytopenia) are known to occur after the administration of chloramphenicol. In addition, there have been reports of aplastic anemia attributed to chloramphenicol which later terminated in leukemia. Blood dyscrasias have occurred after both short-term and prolonged therapy with this drug. Chloramphenicol must not be used**

Continued on next page

This product information was prepared in August, 1986. On these and other Parke-Davis Products, information may be obtained by addressing PARKE-DAVIS, Division of Warner-Lambert Company, Morris Plains, New Jersey 07950.

Parke-Davis—Cont.

when less potentially dangerous agents will be effective, as described in the Indications section. *It must not be used in the treatment of trivial infections or where it is not indicated, as in colds, influenza, infections of the throat; or as a prophylactic agent to prevent bacterial infections.*
Precautions: It is essential that adequate blood studies be made during treatment with the drug. While blood studies may detect early peripheral blood changes, such as leukopenia, reticulocytopenia, or granulocytopenia, before they become irreversible, such studies cannot be relied on to detect bone marrow depression prior to development of aplastic anemia. To facilitate appropriate studies and observation during therapy, it is desirable that patients be hospitalized.

DESCRIPTION

Chloromycetin Palmitate Oral Suspension contains chloramphenicol palmitate equivalent to 150 mg chloramphenicol per 5 mL. Also contains alcohol, USP; carboxymethylcellulose sodium, USP; citric acid, USP; custard flavor, imitation; glycerin, USP; povidone, USP; propylene glycol, USP; sodium benzoate, NF; sorbitan monolaurate, NF; sucrose, NF; veegum, HV; purified water, USP.
Chloramphenicol is an antibiotic that is clinically useful for, *and should be reserved for,* serious infections caused by organisms susceptible to its antimicrobial effects when less potentially hazardous therapeutic agents are ineffective or contraindicated. Sensitivity testing is essential to determine its indicated use, but may be performed concurrently with therapy initiated on clinical impression that one of the indicated conditions exists (see Indications section).

CLINICAL PHARMACOLOGY

In vitro chloramphenicol exerts mainly a bacteriostatic effect on a wide range of gram-negative and gram-positive bacteria and is active *in vitro* against rickettsiae, the lymphogranuloma-psittacosis group and *Vibrio cholerae.* It is particularly active against *Salmonella typhi* and *Hemophilus influenzae.* The mode of action is through interference or inhibition of protein synthesis in intact cells and in cell-free systems.
Chloramphenicol administered orally is absorbed rapidly from the intestinal tract. In controlled studies in adult volunteers using the recommended dosage of 50 mg/kg/day, a dosage of 1 g every 6 hours for 8 doses was given. Using the microbiological assay method, the average peak serum level was 11.2 mcg/ml one hour after the first dose.
A cumulative effect gave a peak rise to 18.4 mcg/ml after the fifth dose of 1 g. Mean serum levels ranged from 8 to 14 mcg/ml over the 48-hour period. Total urinary excretion of chloramphenicol in these studies ranged from a low of 68% to a high of 99% over a three-day period. From 8% to 12% of the antibiotic excreted is in the form of free chloramphenicol; the remainder consists of microbiologically inactive metabolites, principally the conjugate with glucuronic acid. Since the glucuronide is excreted rapidly, most chloramphenicol detected in the blood is in the microbiologically active free form. Despite the small proportion of unchanged drug excreted in the urine, the concentration of free chloramphenicol is relatively high, amounting to several hundred mcg/ml in patients receiving divided doses of 50 mg/kg/day. Small amounts of active drug are found in bile and feces. Chloramphenicol diffuses rapidly, but its distribution is not uniform. Highest concentrations are found in liver and kidney, and lowest concentrations are found in brain and cerebrospinal fluid. Chloramphenicol enters cerebrospinal fluid even in the absence of meningeal inflammation, appearing in concentrations about half of those found in the blood. Measurable levels are also detected in pleural and in ascitic fluids, saliva, milk and in the aqueous and vitreous humors. Transport across the placental barrier occurs with somewhat lower concentration in cord blood of newborn infants than in maternal blood.

INDICATIONS AND USAGE

In accord with the concepts in the Warning Box and this Indications section, chloramphenicol must be used only in those serious infections for which less potentially dangerous drugs are ineffective or contraindicated. However, chloramphenicol may be chosen to initiate antibiotic therapy on the clinical impression that one of the conditions below is believed to be present; *in vitro* sensitivity tests should be performed concurrently so that the drug may be discontinued as soon as possible if less potentially dangerous agents are indicated by such tests. The decision to continue use of chloramphenicol rather than another antibiotic when both are suggested by *in vitro* studies to be effective against a specific pathogen should be based upon severity of the infection, susceptibility of the pathogen to the various antimicrobial drugs, efficacy of the various drugs in the infection, and the important additional concepts contained in the Warning Box above.

1. Acute infections caused by *Salmonella typhi*
Chloramphenicol is a drug of choice.* It is not recommended for the routine treatment of the typhoid carrier state.
2. Serious infections caused by susceptible strains in accordance with the concepts expressed above:
a. Salmonella species
b. *H influenzae,* specifically meningeal infections
c. Rickettsia
d. Lymphogranuloma-psittacosis group
e. Various gram-negative bacteria causing bacteremia, meningitis or other serious gram-negative infections
f. Other susceptible organisms which have been demonstrated to be resistant to all other appropriate antimicrobial agents.
3. Cystic fibrosis regimens

* In the treatment of typhoid fever some authorities recommend that chloramphenicol be administered at therapeutic levels for 8 to 10 days after the patient has become afebrile to lessen the possibility of relapse.

CONTRAINDICATIONS

Chloramphenicol is contraindicated in individuals with a history of previous hypersensitivity and/or toxic reaction to it. *It must not be used in the treatment of trivial infections or where it is not indicated, as in colds, influenza, infections of the throat; or as a prophylactic agent to prevent bacterial infections.*

PRECAUTIONS

1. Baseline blood studies should be followed by periodic blood studies approximately every two days during therapy. The drug should be discontinued upon appearance of reticulocytopenia, leukopenia, thrombocytopenia, anemia, or any other blood study findings attributable to chloramphenicol. However, it should be noted that such studies do not exclude the possible later appearance of the irreversible type of bone marrow depression.
2. Repeated courses of the drug should be avoided if at all possible. Treatment should not be continued longer than required to produce a cure with little or no risk of relapse of the disease.
3. Concurrent therapy with other drugs that may cause bone marrow depression should be avoided.
4. Excessive blood levels may result from administration of the recommended dose to patients with impaired liver or kidney function, including that due to immature metabolic processes in the infant. The dosage should be adjusted accordingly or, preferably, the blood concentration should be determined at appropriate intervals.
5. There are no studies to establish the safety of this drug in pregnancy.
6. Since chloramphenicol readily crosses the placental barrier, caution in use of the drug is particularly important during pregnancy at term or during labor because of potential toxic effects on the fetus (gray syndrome).
7. Precaution should be used in therapy of premature and full-term infants to avoid "gray syndrome" toxicity. (See "Adverse Reactions.") Serum drug levels should be carefully followed during therapy of the newborn infant.
8. Precaution should be used in therapy during lactation because of the possibility of toxic effects on the nursing infant.
9. The use of this antibiotic, as with other antibiotics, may result in an overgrowth of nonsusceptible organisms, including fungi. If infections caused by nonsusceptible organisms appear during therapy, appropriate measures should be taken.

ADVERSE REACTIONS

1. Blood Dyscrasias
The most serious adverse effect of chloramphenicol is bone marrow depression. Serious and fatal blood dyscrasias (aplastic anemia, hypoplastic anemia, thrombocytopenia, and granulocytopenia) are known to occur after the administration of chloramphenicol. An irreversible type of marrow depression leading to aplastic anemia with a high rate of mortality is characterized by the appearance weeks or months after therapy of bone marrow aplasia or hypoplasia. Peripherally, pancytopenia is most often observed, but in a small number of cases only one or two of the three major cell types (erythrocytes, leukocytes, platelets) may be depressed.
A reversible type of bone marrow depression, which is dose related, may occur. This type of marrow depression is characterized by vacuolization of the erythroid cells, reduction of reticulocytes and leukopenia, and responds promptly to the withdrawal of chloramphenicol.
An exact determination of the risk of serious and fatal blood dyscrasias is not possible because of lack of accurate information regarding 1) the size of the population at risk, 2) the total number of drug-associated dyscrasias, and 3) the total number of nondrug associated dyscrasias.
In a report to the California State Assembly by the California Medical Association and the State Department of Public Health in January 1967, the risk of fatal aplastic anemia was estimated at 1:24,200 to 1:40,500 based on two dosage levels.
There have been reports of aplastic anemia attributed to chloramphenicol which later terminated in leukemia.
Paroxysmal nocturnal hemoglobinuria has also been reported.
2. Gastrointestinal Reactions
Nausea, vomiting, glossitis and stomatitis, diarrhea and enterocolitis may occur in low incidence.
3. Neurotoxic Reactions
Headache, mild depression, mental confusion and delirium have been described in patients receiving chloramphenicol. Optic and peripheral neuritis have been reported, usually following long-term therapy. If this occurs, the drug should be promptly withdrawn.
4. Hypersensitivity Reactions
Fever, macular and vesicular rashes, angioedema, urticaria and anaphylaxis may occur. Herxheimer reactions have occurred during therapy for typhoid fever.
5. "Gray Syndrome"
Toxic reactions including fatalities have occurred in the premature and newborn, the signs and symptoms associated with these reactions have been referred to as the gray syndrome. One case of gray syndrome has been reported in an infant born to a mother having received chloramphenicol during labor. One case has been reported in a 3-month-old infant. The following summarizes the clinical and laboratory studies that have been made on these patients.
(a) In most cases therapy with chloramphenicol had been instituted within the first 48 hours of life.
(b) Symptoms first appeared after 3 to 4 days of continued treatment with high doses of chloramphenicol
(c) The symptoms appeared in the following order:
1) abdominal distention with or without emesis;
2) progressive pallid cyanosis;
3) vasomotor collapse, frequently accompanied by irregular respiration;
4) death within a few hours of onset of these symptoms.
(d) The progression of symptoms from onset to exitus was accelerated with higher dose schedules.
(e) Preliminary blood serum level studies revealed unusually high concentrations of chloramphenicol (over 90 mcg/ml after repeated doses).
(f) Termination of therapy upon early evidence of the associated symptomatology frequently reversed the process with complete recovery.

DOSAGE AND ADMINISTRATION

Dosage Recommendations
The majority of microorganisms susceptible to chloramphenicol will respond to a concentration between 5 and 20 mcg/ml. The desired concentration of active drug in blood should fall within this range over most of the treatment period. Dosage of 50 mg/kg/day divided into 4 doses at intervals of 6 hours will usually achieve and sustain levels of this magnitude.
Except in certain circumstances (eg. premature and newborn infants and individuals with impairment of hepatic or renal function) lower doses may not achieve these concentrations. Chloramphenicol, like other potent drugs, should be prescribed at recommended doses known to have therapeutic activity. Close observation of the patient should be maintained and in the event of any adverse reactions, dosage should be reduced or the drug discontinued, if other factors in the clinical situation permit.
Adults
Adults should receive 50 mg/kg/day in divided doses at 6-hour intervals. In exceptional cases patients with infections due to moderately resistant organisms may require increased dosage up to 100 mg/kg/day to achieve blood levels inhibiting the pathogen, but these high doses should be decreased as soon as possible. Adults with impairment of hepatic or renal function or both may have reduced ability to metabolize and excrete the drug. In instances of impaired metabolic processes, dosages should be adjusted accordingly. (See discussion under Newborn Infants.) Precise control of concentration of the drug in the blood should be carefully followed in patients with impaired metabolic processes by the available microtechniques (information available on request).
Children
Dosage of 50 mg/kg/day divided into 4 doses at 6-hour intervals yields blood levels in the range effective against most susceptible organisms. Severe infections (eg. bacteremia or meningitis), especially when adequate cerebrospinal fluid concentrations are desired, may require dosage up to 100 mg/kg/day; however, it is recommended that dosage be reduced to 50 mg/kg/day as soon as possible. Children with impaired liver or kidney function may retain excessive amounts of the drug.
Newborn Infants
(See section titled "Gray Syndrome" under Adverse Reactions.)
A total of 25 mg/kg/day in 4 equal doses at 6-hour intervals usually produces and maintains concentrations in blood and tissues adequate to control most infections for which the drug is indicated. Increased dosage in these individuals, demanded by severe infections, should be given only to main-

tain the blood concentration within a therapeutically effective range. After the first two weeks of life, full-term infants ordinarily may receive up to a total of 50 mg/kg/day equally divided into 4 doses at 6-hour intervals. *These dosage recommendations are extremely important because blood concentration in all premature infants and full-term infants under two weeks of age differs from that of other infants.* This difference is due to variations in the maturity of the metabolic functions of the liver and the kidneys.

When these functions are immature (or seriously impaired in adults), high concentrations of the drug are found which tend to increase with succeeding doses.

Infants and Children with Immature Metabolic Processes

In young infants and other children in whom immature metabolic functions are suspected, a dose of 25 mg/kg/day will usually produce therapeutic concentrations of the drug in the blood. In this group particularly, the concentration of the drug in the blood should be carefully followed by microtechniques. (Information available on request.)

HOW SUPPLIED

N 0071-2310-15

Oral Suspension Chloromycetin Palmitate (Chloramphenicol Palmitate Oral Suspension, USP), each 5 ml contains chloramphenicol palmitate equivalent to 150 mg chloramphenicol with 0.5% sodium benzoate as preservative, in bottles of 60 ml.

Chloramphenicol Palmitate is hydrolyzed to chloramphenicol before absorption. Resulting blood concentration is similar to that produced by the oral administration of chloramphenicol.

Chloromycetin, brand of chloramphenicol. Reg. US Pat Off

2310G042

Caution—Federal law prohibits dispensing without prescription.

CHLOROMYCETIN® ℞

[*chlō"rō-my-cē'tĭn sŭc'cĭ-nāte"*]

SODIUM SUCCINATE

(sterile chloramphenicol sodium succinate, USP)

FOR INTRAVENOUS ADMINISTRATION

WARNING

Serious and fatal blood dyscrasias (aplastic anemia, hypoplastic anemia, thrombocytopenia, and granulocytopenia) are known to occur after the administration of chloramphenicol. In addition, there have been reports of aplastic anemia attributed to chloramphenicol which later terminated in leukemia. Blood dyscrasias have occurred after both short-term and prolonged therapy with this drug. Chloramphenicol must not be used when less potentially dangerous agents will be effective, as described in the Indications section. *It must not be used in the treatment of trivial infections or where it is not indicated, as in colds, influenza, infections of the throat; or as a prophylactic agent to prevent bacterial infections.*

Precautions: It is essential that adequate blood studies be made during treatment with the drug. While blood studies may detect early peripheral blood changes, such as leukopenia, reticulocytopenia, or granulocytopenia, before they become irreversible, such studies cannot be relied on to detect bone marrow depression prior to development of aplastic anemia. To facilitate appropriate studies and observation during therapy, it is desirable that patients be hospitalized.

IMPORTANT CONSIDERATIONS IN PRESCRIBING INJECTABLE CHLORAMPHENICOL SODIUM SUCCINATE CHLORAMPHENICOL SODIUM SUCCINATE IS INTENDED FOR INTRAVENOUS USE ONLY. IT HAS BEEN DEMONSTRATED TO BE INEFFECTIVE WHEN GIVEN INTRAMUSCULARLY.

1. Chloramphenicol sodium succinate must be hydrolyzed to its microbiologically active form and there is a lag in achieving adequate blood levels compared with the base given intravenously.
2. The oral form of chloramphenicol is readily absorbed and adequate blood levels are achieved and maintained on the recommended dosage.
3. Patients started on intravenous chloramphenicol sodium succinate should be changed to the oral form as soon as practicable.

DESCRIPTION

Chloramphenicol is an antibiotic that is clinically useful for, *and should be reserved for,* serious infections caused by organisms susceptible to its antimicrobial effects when less potentially hazardous therapeutic agents are ineffective or contraindicated. Sensitivity testing is essential to determine its indicated use, but may be performed concurrently with therapy initiated on clinical impression that one of the indicated conditions exists (see Indications section).

Each gram (10 ml of a 10% solution) of chloramphenicol sodium succinate contains approximately 52 mg (2.25 mEq) of sodium.

ACTIONS AND PHARMACOLOGY

In vitro chloramphenicol exerts mainly a bacteriostatic effect on a wide range of gram-negative and gram-positive bacteria and is active *in vitro* against rickettsiae, the lymphogranuloma-psittacosis group, and *Vibrio cholerae.* It is particularly active against *Salmonella typhi* and *Hemophilus influenzae.* The mode of action is through interference or inhibition of protein synthesis in intact cells and in cell-free systems.

Chloramphenicol administered orally is absorbed rapidly from the intestinal tract. In controlled studies in adult volunteers using the recommended dosage of 50 mg/kg/day, a dosage of 1 g every 6 hours for 8 doses was given. Using the microbiological assay method, the average peak serum level was 11.2 mcg/ml one hour after the first dose. A cumulative effect gave a peak rise to 18.4 mcg/ml after the fifth dose of 1 g. Mean serum levels ranged from 8 to 14 mcg/ml over the 48-hour period. Total urinary excretion of chloramphenicol in these studies ranged from a low of 68% to a high of 99% over a three-day period. From 8 to 12% of the antibiotic excreted is in the form of free chloramphenicol; the remainder consists of microbiologically inactive metabolites, principally the conjugate with glucuronic acid. Since the glucuronide is excreted rapidly, most chloramphenicol detected in the blood is in the microbiologically active free form. Despite the small proportion of unchanged drug excreted in the urine, the concentration of free chloramphenicol is relatively high, amounting to several hundred mcg/ml in patients receiving divided doses of 50 mg/kg/day. Small amounts of active drug are found in bile and feces. Chloramphenicol diffuses rapidly, but its distribution is not uniform. Highest concentrations are found in liver and kidney, and lowest concentrations are found in brain and cerebrospinal fluid. Chloramphenicol enters cerebrospinal fluid even in the absence of meningeal inflammation, appearing in concentrations about half of those found in the blood. Measurable levels are also detected in pleural and in ascitic fluids, saliva, milk, and in the aqueous and vitreous humors. Transport across the placental barrier occurs with somewhat lower concentration in cord blood of newborn infants than in maternal blood.

INDICATIONS

In accord with the concepts in the warning box and this Indications section, chloramphenicol must be used only in those serious infections for which less potentially dangerous drugs are ineffective or contraindicated. However, chloramphenicol may be chosen to initiate antibiotic therapy on the clinical impression that one of the conditions below is believed to be present; *in vitro* sensitivity tests should be performed concurrently so that the drug may be discontinued as soon as possible if less potentially dangerous agents are indicated by such tests. The decision to continue use of chloramphenicol rather than another antibiotic when both are suggested by *in vitro* studies to be effective against a specific pathogen should be based upon severity of the infection, susceptibility of the pathogen to the various antimicrobial drugs, efficacy of the various drugs in the infection, and the important additional concepts contained in the Warning Box above:

1. Acute infections caused by *S typhi**

It is not recommended for the routine treatment of the typhoid carrier state.

2. Serious infections caused by susceptible strains in accordance with the concepts expressed above:

a. *Salmonella* species
b. *H influenzae,* specifically meningeal infections
c. Rickettsia
d. Lymphogranuloma-psittacosis group
e. Various gram-negative bacteria causing bacteremia, meningitis, or other serious gram-negative infections
f. Other susceptible organisms which have been demonstrated to be resistant to all other appropriate antimicrobial agents.

3. Cystic fibrosis regimens

*In the treatment of typhoid fever, some authorities recommend that chloramphenicol be administered at therapeutic levels for 8 to 10 days after the patient has become afebrile to lessen the possibility of relapse.

CONTRAINDICATIONS

Chloramphenicol is contraindicated in individuals with a history of previous hypersensitivity and/or toxic reaction to it. *It must not be used in the treatment of trivial infections or where it is not indicated, as in colds, influenza, infections of the throat; or as a prophylactic agent to prevent bacterial infection.*

PRECAUTIONS

1. Baseline blood studies should be followed by periodic blood studies approximately every two days during therapy. The drug should be discontinued upon appearance of reticulocytopenia, leukopenia, thrombocytopenia, anemia, or any other blood study findings attributable to chloramphenicol. However, it should be noted that such studies do not exclude the possible later appearance of the irreversible type of bone marrow depression.
2. Repeated courses of the drug should be avoided if at all possible. Treatment should not be continued longer than required to produce a cure with little or no risk of relapse of the disease.
3. Concurrent therapy with other drugs that may cause bone marrow depression should be avoided.
4. Excessive blood levels may result from administration of the recommended dosage to patients with impaired liver or kidney function, including that due to immature metabolic processes in the infant. The dosage should be adjusted accordingly or, preferably, the blood concentration should be determined at appropriate intervals.
5. There are no studies to establish the safety of this drug in pregnancy.
6. Since chloramphenicol readily crosses the placental barrier, caution in use of the drug is particularly important during pregnancy at term or during labor because of potential toxic effects on the fetus (gray syndrome).
7. Precaution should be used in therapy of premature and full-term infants to avoid gray syndrome toxicity (see Adverse Reactions). Serum drug levels should be carefully followed during therapy of the newborn infant.
8. Precaution should be used in therapy during lactation because of the possibility of toxic effects on the nursing infant.
9. The use of this antibiotic, as with other antibiotics, may result in an overgrowth of nonsusceptible organisms, including fungi. If infections caused by nonsusceptible organisms appear during therapy, appropriate measures should be taken.

ADVERSE REACTIONS

1. Blood Dyscrasias

The most serious adverse effect of chloramphenicol is bone marrow depression. Serious and fatal blood dyscrasias (aplastic anemia, hypoplastic anemia, thrombocytopenia, and granulocytopenia) are known to occur after the administration of chloramphenicol. An irreversible type of marrow depression leading to aplastic anemia with a high rate of mortality is characterized by the appearance weeks or months after therapy of bone marrow aplasia or hypoplasia. Peripherally, pancytopenia is most often observed, but in a small number of cases only one or two of the three major cell types (erythrocytes, leukocytes, platelets) may be depressed.

A reversible type of bone marrow depression, which is dose-related, may occur. This type of marrow depression is characterized by vacuolization of the erythroid cells, reduction of reticulocytes, and leukopenia, and responds promptly to the withdrawal of chloramphenicol.

An exact determination of the risk of serious and fatal blood dyscrasias is not possible because of lack of accurate information regarding (1) the size of the population at risk, (2) the total number of drug-associated dyscrasias, and (3) the total number of nondrug-associated dyscrasias.

In a report to the California State Assembly by the California Medical Association and the State Department of Public Health in January 1967, the risk of fatal aplastic anemia was estimated at 1:24,200 to 1:40,500 based on two dosage levels.

There have been reports of aplastic anemia attributed to chloramphenicol which later terminated in leukemia.

Paroxysmal nocturnal hemoglobinuria has also been reported.

2. Gastrointestinal Reactions

Nausea, vomiting, glossitis and stomatitis, diarrhea, and enterocolitis may occur in low incidence.

3. Neurotoxic Reactions

Headache, mild depression, mental confusion, and delirium have been described in patients receiving chloramphenicol. Optic and peripheral neuritis have been reported, usually following long-term therapy. If this occurs, the drug should be promptly withdrawn.

4. Hypersensitivity Reactions

Fever, macular and vesicular rashes, angio- edema, urticaria, and anaphylaxis may occur. Herxheimer reactions have occurred during therapy for typhoid fever.

Continued on next page

This product information was prepared in August, 1986. On these and other Parke-Davis Products, information may be obtained by addressing PARKE-DAVIS, Division of Warner-Lambert Company, Morris Plains, New Jersey 07950.

Parke-Davis—Cont.

5. "Gray Syndrome"
Toxic reactions including fatalities have occurred in the premature and newborn; the signs and symptoms associated with these reactions have been referred to as the gray syndrome. One case of gray syndrome has been reported in an infant born to a mother having received chloramphenicol during labor. One case has been reported in a 3-month-old infant. The following summarizes the clinical and laboratory studies that have been made on these patients:

a) In most cases, therapy with chloramphenicol had been instituted within the first 48 hours of life.
b) Symptoms first appeared after 3 to 4 days of continued treatment with high doses of chloramphenicol.
c) The symptoms appeared in the following order:
   (1) abdominal distention with or without emesis;
   (2) progressive pallid cyanosis;
   (3) vasomotor collapse, frequently accompanied by irregular respiration;
   (4) death within a few hours of onset of these symptoms.
d) The progression of symptoms from onset to exitus was accelerated with higher dose schedules.
e) Preliminary blood serum level studies revealed unusually high concentrations of chloramphenicol (over 90 mcg/ml after repeated doses).
f) Termination of therapy upon early evidence of the associated symptomatology frequently reversed the process with complete recovery.

ADMINISTRATION
Chloramphenicol, like other potent drugs, should be prescribed at recommended doses known to have therapeutic activity. Administration of 50 mg/kg/day in divided doses will produce blood levels of the magnitude to which the majority of susceptible microorganisms will respond.

As soon as feasible, an oral dosage form of chloramphenicol should be substituted for the intravenous form because adequate blood levels are achieved with chloramphenicol by mouth.

The following method of administration is recommended:
Intravenously as a 10% (100 mg/ml) solution to be injected over at least a one-minute interval. This is prepared by the addition of 10 ml of an aqueous diluent, such as water for injection or 5% dextrose injection.

DOSAGE
Adults
Adults should receive 50 mg/kg/day in divided doses at 6-hour intervals. In exceptional cases, patients with infections due to moderately resistant organisms may require increased dosage up to 100 mg/kg/day to achieve blood levels inhibiting the pathogen, but these high doses should be decreased as soon as possible. Adults with impairment of hepatic or renal function or both may have reduced ability to metabolize and excrete the drug. In instances of impaired metabolic processes, dosages should be adjusted accordingly. (See discussion under Newborn Infants.) Precise control of concentration of the drug in the blood should be carefully followed in patients with impaired metabolic processes by the available microtechniques (information available on request).

Children
Dosage of 50 mg/kg/day divided into 4 doses at 6-hour intervals yields blood levels in the range effective against most susceptible organisms. Severe infections (eg, bacteremia or meningitis), especially when adequate cerebrospinal fluid concentrations are desired, may require dosage up to 100 mg/kg/day; however, it is recommended that dosage be reduced to 50 mg/kg/day as soon as possible. Children with impaired liver or kidney function may retain excessive amounts of the drug.

Newborn Infants
(See section titled Gray Syndrome under Adverse Reactions.)
A total of 25 mg/kg/day in 4 equal doses at 6-hour intervals usually produces and maintains concentrations in blood and tissues adequate to control most infections for which the drug is indicated. Increased dosage in these individuals, demanded by severe infections, should be given only to maintain the blood concentration within a therapeutically effective range. After the first two weeks of life, full-term infants ordinarily may receive up to a total of 50 mg/kg/day equally divided into 4 doses at 6-hour intervals. *These dosage recommendations are extremely important because blood concentration in all premature infants and full-term infants under two weeks of age differs from that of other infants.* This difference is due to variations in the maturity of the metabolic functions of the liver and the kidneys.

When these functions are immature (or seriously impaired in adults), high concentrations of the drug are found which tend to increase with succeeding doses.

Infants and Children with Immature Metabolic Processes
In young infants and other children in whom immature metabolic functions are suspected, a dose of 25 mg/kg/day will usually produce therapeutic concentrations of the drug in the blood. In this group particularly, the concentration of the drug in the blood should be carefully followed by microtechniques. (Information available on request.)

HOW SUPPLIED
N 0071-4057-03—(Steri-Vial® No. 57) Chloromycetin Sodium Succinate (Chloramphenicol Sodium Succinate for Injection, USP) is freeze-dried in the vial and supplied in Steri-Vials (rubber diaphragm-capped vials). When reconstituted as directed, each vial contains a sterile solution equivalent to 100 mg of chloramphenicol per milliliter (1 g/10 ml). Available in packages of 10 vials.
Chloromycetin, brand of chloramphenicol, Reg US Pat Off
AHFS 8:12.08 **4057G020**

CHLORTHALIDONE ℞
[*chlōr-thă 'lĭ-dōne* "]
Tablets, USP

DESCRIPTION
Chlorthalidone is a monosulfamyl diuretic that differs chemically from thiazide diuretics in that a double-ring system is incorporated in its structure. Chemically it is designated 2-chloro-5-(1-hydroxy-3-oxo-1-isoindo-linyl) benzenesulfonamide. Its empirical formula is $C_{14}H_{11}ClN_2O_4S$.
Chlorthalidone Tablets, USP are available in strengths of 25 mg and 50 mg for oral administration.

CLINICAL PHARMACOLOGY
Chlorthalidone is an oral diuretic with prolonged action (48 to 72 hours) and low toxicity. The diuretic effect of the drug occurs within two hours of an oral dose and continues for up to 72 hours. It produces copious diuresis with greatly increased excretion of sodium and chloride. At maximal therapeutic dosage, chlorthalidone is approximately equal in its diuretic effect to comparable maximal therapeutic doses of benzothiadiazine diuretics. The site of action appears to be the cortical diluting segment of the ascending limb of Henle's loop of the nephron.

INDICATIONS AND USAGE
Diuretics such as chlorthalidone are indicated in the management of hypertension either as the sole therapeutic agent or to enhance the effect of other antihypertensive drugs in the more severe forms of hypertension.
Chlorthalidone is indicated as adjunctive therapy in edema associated with congestive heart failure, hepatic cirrhosis, and corticosteroid and estrogen therapy.
Chlorthalidone has also been found useful in edema due to various forms of renal dysfunction such as nephrotic syndrome, acute glomerulonephritis, and chronic renal failure.
Usage in Pregnancy: The routine use of diuretics in an otherwise healthy woman is inappropriate and exposes mother and fetus to unnecessary hazard. Diuretics do not prevent development of toxemia of pregnancy, and there is no satisfactory evidence that they are useful in the treatment of developed toxemia.
Edema during pregnancy may arise from pathological causes or from the physiologic and mechanical consequences of pregnancy. Chlorthalidone is indicated in pregnancy when edema is due to pathologic causes, just as it is in the absence of pregnancy (however, see PRECAUTIONS, below). Dependent edema in pregnancy, resulting from restriction of venous return by the expanded uterus, is properly treated through elevation of the lower extremities and use of support hose; use of diuretics to lower intravascular volume in this case is illogical and unnecessary. There is hypervolemia during normal pregnancy which is harmful to neither the fetus nor the mother (in the absence of cardiovascular disease), but which is associated with edema, including generalized edema, in the majority of pregnant women. If this edema produces discomfort, increased recumbency will often provide relief. In rare instances, this edema may cause extreme discomfort that is not relieved by rest. In these cases, a short course of diuretics may provide relief and may be appropriate.

CONTRAINDICATIONS
Anuria.
Hypersensitivity to chlorthalidone or other sulfonamide-derived drugs.

WARNINGS
Should be used with caution in severe renal disease. In patients with renal disease, chlorthalidone or related drugs may precipitate azotemia. Cumulative effects of the drug may develop in patients with impaired renal function.
Chlorthalidone should be used with caution in patients with impaired hepatic function or progressive liver disease, since minor alterations of fluid and electrolyte balance may precipitate hepatic coma.
Chlorthalidone may add to or potentiate the action of the other antihypertensive drugs. Potentiation occurs with ganglionic or peripheral adrenergic blocking drugs.
Sensitivity reactions may occur in patients with a history of allergy or bronchial asthma.
The possibility of exacerbation or activation of systemic lupus erythematosus has been reported with thiazide diuretics, which are structurally related to chlorthalidone. However, systemic lupus erythematosus has not been reported following chlorthalidone administration.

PRECAUTIONS
Periodic determination of serum electrolytes to detect possible electrolyte imbalance should be performed at appropriate intervals.
All patients receiving chlorthalidone should be observed for clinical signs of fluid or electrolyte imbalance; namely, hyponatremia, hypochloremic alkalosis, and hypokalemia. Serum and urine electrolyte determinations are particularly important when the patient is vomiting excessively or receiving parenteral fluids. Medication such as digitalis may also influence serum electrolytes. Warning signs, irrespective of cause are: dryness of mouth, thirst, weakness, lethargy, drowsiness, restlessness, muscle pains or cramps, muscular fatigue, hypotension, oliguria, tachycardia, and gastrointestinal disturbances such as nausea and vomiting.
Hypokalemia may develop with chlorthalidone as with any other potent diuretic, especially with brisk diuresis, when severe cirrhosis is present, or during concomitant use of corticosteroids or ACTH.
Interference with adequate oral electrolyte intake will also contribute to hypokalemia. Digitalis therapy may exaggerate metabolic effects of hypokalemia especially with reference to myocardial activity.
Any chloride deficit is generally mild and usually does not require specific treatment except under extraordinary circumstances (as in liver disease or renal disease). Dilutional hyponatremia may occur in edematous patients in hot weather; appropriate therapy is water restriction rather than administration of salt except in rare instances when the hyponatremia is life-threatening. In actual salt depletion, appropriate replacement is the therapy of choice.
Hyperuricemia may occur or frank gout may be precipitated in certain patients receiving chlorthalidone.
Insulin requirements in diabetic patients may be increased, decreased, or unchanged. Latent diabetes mellitus may become manifest during chlorthalidone administration.
Chlorthalidone and related drugs may increase the responsiveness to tubocurarine.
The antihypertensive effects of the drug may be enhanced in the postsympathectomy patient.
Chlorthalidone and related drugs may decrease arterial responsiveness to norepinephrine. This diminution is not sufficient to preclude effectiveness of the pressor agent for therapeutic use.
If progressive renal impairment becomes evident, as indicated by a rising nonprotein nitrogen or blood urea nitrogen, a careful reappraisal of therapy is necessary with consideration given to withholding or discontinuing diuretic therapy.
Chlorthalidone and related drugs may decrease serum PBI levels without signs of thyroid disturbance.
Usage in Pregnancy: Reproduction studies in various animal species at multiples of the human dose showed no significant level of teratogenicity; no fetal or congenital abnormalities were observed. Animal data should not be extrapolated for clinical application.
Thiazides cross the placental barrier and appear in cord blood. The use of chlorthalidone and related drugs in pregnant women requires that the anticipated benefits of the drug be weighed against possible hazards to the fetus. These hazards include fetal or neonatal jaundice, thrombocytopenia, and possibly other adverse reactions which have occurred in the adult.
Nursing Mothers: Thiazides cross the placental barrier and appear in breast milk. If use of the drug is deemed essential, the patient should stop nursing.

ADVERSE REACTIONS
Gastrointestinal System Reactions:
anorexia
gastric irritation
nausea
vomiting
cramping
diarrhea
constipation
jaundice (intrahepatic cholestatic jaundice)
pancreatitis
Central Nervous System Reactions:
dizziness
vertigo
paresthesias
headache
xanthopsia
Hematologic Reactions:
leukopenia
agranulocytosis
thrombocytopenia
aplastic anemia
Dermatologic-Hypersensitivity Reactions:
purpura

photosensitivity
rash
urticaria
necrotizing angiitis (vasculitis) (cutaneous vasculitis)
Lyell's syndrome (toxic epidermal necrolysis)

Cardiovascular Reaction: Orthostatic hypotension may occur and may be aggravated by alcohol, barbiturates or narcotics.

Other Adverse Reactions:
hyperglycemia
glycosuria
hyperuricemia
muscle spasm
weakness
restlessness
impotence

Whenever adverse reactions are moderate or severe, chlorthalidone dosage should be reduced or therapy withdrawn.

OVERDOSAGE

Symptoms of overdosage include nausea, weakness, dizziness and disturbances of electrolyte balance. There is no specific antidote, but gastric lavage is recommended, followed by supportive treatment. Where necessary, this may include intravenous dextrose-saline with potassium, administered with caution.

DOSAGE AND ADMINISTRATION

Therapy should be individualized according to patient response. This therapy should be titrated to gain maximal therapeutic response as well as the minimal dose possible to maintain that therapeutic response. A single dose given in the morning with food is recommended; divided doses are unnecessary.

Hypertension. *Initiation:* Therapy should be initiated with a dose of 25 mg or 50 mg as a single daily dose. In some patients a 100-mg dose may lower the blood pressure further, but dosage above this level usually does not increase effectiveness. Increases in serum uric acid and decreases in serum potassium are dose-related over the 25–100 mg/day range.

Maintenance: Maintenance doses may often be lower than initial doses and should be adjusted according to the individual patient. Effectiveness is well sustained during continued use.

Edema. *Initiation:* Adults, initially 50 to 100 mg daily, or 100 mg on alternate days. Some patients may require 150 to 200 mg at these intervals, or up to 200 mg daily. Dosages above this level, however, do not usually produce a greater response.

Maintenance: Maintenance doses may often be lower than initial doses and should be adjusted according to the individual patient. Effectiveness is well sustained during continued use.

HOW SUPPLIED

Chlorthalidone Tablets, USP 25 mg (orange, P-D 123) are supplied as:
N 0071-0123-24 Bottle of 100
N 0071-0123-32 Bottle of 1000
N 0071-0123-40 Unit-Dose packages of 100
(10 strips of 10 tablets each).

Chlorthalidone Tablets, USP 50 mg (light blue, P-D 121) are supplied as:
N 0071-0121-24 Bottle of 100
N 0071-0121-32 Bottle of 1000
N 0071-0121-40 Unit-Dose packages of 100
(10 strips of 10 tablets each).

ANIMAL PHARMACOLOGY

Biochemical studies in animals have suggested reasons for the prolonged effect of chlorthalidone. Absorption from the gastrointestinal tract is slow because of low solubility. After passage to the liver, some of the drug enters the general circulation, while some is excreted in the bile to be reabsorbed later. In the general circulation, it is distributed widely to the tissues, but is taken up in highest concentrations by the kidneys, where amounts have been found 72 hours after ingestion, long after it has disappeared from other tissues. The drug is excreted unchanged in the urine.

0121G011

Caution—Federal law prohibits dispensing without prescription.

CHOLEDYL® ℞

[*clō'lĕ-dyl"*]
Tablets/Elixir
(oxtriphylline, USP)

DESCRIPTION

Each enteric-coated tablet contains 200 mg or 100 mg oxtriphylline. Each tablet also contains acacia, NF; precipitated calcium carbonate, USP; tribasic calcium phosphate, NF; carnauba wax; confectioner's sugar, NF; gelatin, NF; kaolin, USP; magnesium stearate, NF; pharmaceutical glaze; starch, NF; sucrose, NF; talc, USP; titanium dioxide, USP; tragacauth, NF; and white wax, NF. The 100-mg tablet also contains D&C red No. 7 Lake and FD&C yellow No. 6 Lake. The 200-mg tablet also contains D&C yellow No. 10. Each 5-ml teaspoonful of elixir contains 100 mg oxtriphylline; alcohol 20%. Also contains citric acid, USP; D&C green No. 5; D&C yellow No. 10; FD&C red No. 40; flavor; glycerin, USP; saccharin sodium, USP; sodium chloride, USP; sodium citrate, USP; sorbitol solution, USP; sucrose, NF; and purified water, USP. Note: 100 mg oxtriphylline is equivalent to 64 mg anhydrous theophylline.

ACTIONS

Choledyl (oxtriphylline) is a xanthine bronchodilator—the choline salt of theophylline. Choledyl, compared to aminophylline, is less irritating to the gastric mucosa, more readily absorbed from the gastrointestinal tract, more stable and more soluble.

Like other xanthines, oxtriphylline is known to increase vital capacity which has been impaired by bronchospasm and air-trapping. Development of tolerance has been reported infrequently, and therefore Choledyl is useful for long-term therapy of bronchospasm.

INDICATIONS

Choledyl (oxtriphylline) is indicated for relief of acute bronchial asthma and for reversible bronchospasm associated with chronic bronchitis and emphysema.

WARNING

Use in pregnancy—animal studies revealed no evidence of teratogenic potential. Safety in human pregnancy has not been established; use during lactation or in patients who are or who may become pregnant requires that the potential benefits of the drug be weighed against its possible hazards to the mother and child.

PRECAUTIONS

Concurrent use of other xanthine-containing preparations may lead to adverse reactions, particularly CNS stimulation in children.

ADVERSE REACTIONS

Gastric distress and, occasionally, palpitation and CNS stimulation have been reported.

DOSAGE

Tablets—Adults: 200 mg, 4 times a day.
Elixir—Adults: 200 mg (two teaspoonfuls or 10 ml), 4 times a day; Children (2 to 12): 100 mg (one teaspoonful or 5 ml) per 60 lb body weight, 4 times a day.

Above recommendations are averages. Dosage should be individualized.

SUPPLIED

N 0071-0211—Choledyl 200 mg, yellow, partially enteric coated tablets in bottles of 100, 1000, and unit dose packages (10 x 10 strips);
N 0071-0210-24 Choledyl 100 mg, red partially enteric coated tablets in bottles of 100;
N 0071-2215-23 Choledyl elixir, sherry-flavored in bottles of 16 fl oz (1 pint) 474 ml.
Store between 59° and 86°F (15° and 30°C).

Toxicity:
Oxtriphylline, aminophylline and caffeine appear to be more toxic to newborn than to adult rats. No teratogenic effects have been seen.

Shown in Product Identification Section, page 420

0210 G052

CHOLEDYL® PEDIATRIC SYRUP ℞

[*chō'lĕ-dyl"*]
(oxtriphylline)

DESCRIPTION

Choledyl (oxtriphylline) is a xanthine bronchodilator—the choline salt of theophylline.

Each 5 ml of Choledyl Pediatric Syrup contains 50 mg oxtriphylline (equivalent to 32 mg of anhydrous theophylline). Also contains: caramel acid proof; citric acid, USP; FD&C red No. 40; flavors; glycerin, USP; invert sugar; menthol, USP; saccharin sodium, USP; sodium citrate, USP; sodium hydroxide; sorbitol solution, USP and purified water, USP.

CLINICAL PHARMACOLOGY

Theophylline directly relaxes the smooth muscle of the bronchial airways and pulmonary blood vessels, thus acting mainly as a bronchodilator, pulmonary vasodilator and smooth muscle relaxant. The drug also possesses other actions typical of the xanthine derivatives: coronary vasodilator, diuretic, cardiac stimulant, cerebral stimulant and skeletal muscle stimulant. The actions of theophylline may be mediated through inhibition of phosphodiesterase and a resultant increase in intracellular cyclic AMP which could mediate smooth muscle relaxation. At concentrations higher than attained *in vivo*, theophylline also inhibits the release of histamine by mast cells.

Theophylline has been shown to react additively with beta agonists that increase intracellular cyclic AMP through the stimulation of adenyl cyclase (isoproterenol).

Apparently, the development of tolerance does not occur with chronic use of theophylline.

The half-life is shortened with cigarette smoking. The half-life is prolonged in alcoholism, reduced hepatic or renal function, congestive heart failure, and in patients receiving antibiotics such as TAO (troleandomycin), erythromycin and clindamycin. High fever for prolonged periods may decrease theophylline elimination.

Theophylline Elimination Characteristics

	Theophylline Clearance Rates (mean ± S.D.)	Half-life Average (mean ± S.D.)
Children (over 6 months of age)	1.45 ± .58 ml/kg/min	3.7 ± 1.1 hours
Adult non-smokers with uncomplicated asthma	.65 ± .19 ml/kg/min	8.7 ± 2.2 hours

Newborn infants have extremely slow clearances and half-lives exceeding 24 hours, which approach those seen for older children after about 3–6 months.

The half-life of theophylline is prolonged in patients with congestive heart failure, in those with reduced hepatic or renal function, and in alcoholism. The half-life of theophylline may also be prolonged by concurrent use of various drugs such as phenobarbital, and certain antibiotics, including troleandomycin, erythromycin, and lincomycin.

Theophylline half-life is shortened in cigarette smokers (1 to 2 packs/day) as compared to nonsmokers. The increase in theophylline clearance caused by smoking is probably the result of induction of drug metabolizing enzymes that do not readily normalize after cessation of smoking. It appears that between 3 months and 2 years may be necessary for normalization of the effect of smoking on theophylline pharmacokinetics.

ACTIONS

Choledyl (oxtriphylline), the choline salt of theophylline, effects significant improvement in pulmonary function parameters which have been impaired by bronchospasm. It is more soluble than either aminophylline or theophylline.

INDICATIONS

Choledyl (oxtriphylline) is indicated for relief of acute and chronic bronchial asthma and for reversible bronchospasm associated with chronic bronchitis and emphysema.

CONTRAINDICATIONS

Choledyl is contraindicated in individuals who have shown hypersensitivity to theophylline or to Choledyl (oxtriphylline) or any of its components.

WARNINGS

Status asthmaticus is a medical emergency. Optimal therapy frequently requires additional medication including corticosteroids when the patient is not rapidly responsive to bronchodilators.

Excessive theophylline doses may be associated with toxicity, and serum theophylline levels are recommended to assure maximal benefit without excessive risk; incidence of toxicity increases at levels greater than 20 mcg theophylline/ml. Morphine, curare, and stilbamidine should be used with caution in patients with airflow obstruction since they stimulate histamine release and can induce asthmatic attacks. These drugs may also suppress respiration leading to respiratory failure. Alternative drugs should be chosen whenever possible.

There is excellent correlation between high blood levels of theophylline resulting from conventional doses and associated clinical manifestations of toxicity in patients with liver dysfunction or chronic obstructive lung disease.

There is excellent correlation between high serum levels of theophylline (over 20 mcg/ml) and the clinical manifestations of toxicity. Careful reduction of dosage and monitoring of serum levels are especially important in patients manifesting a decrease in total body theophylline clearance rate, including those with generalized debility, acute hypoxia, cardiac decompensation, hepatic dysfunction, or renal failure. Dosage reduction may also be necessary in patients who are older than 55 years of age, particularly males.

Serious toxic effects may occur suddenly and are not invariably preceded by minor adverse effects such as nausea, vom-

Continued on next page

This product information was prepared in August, 1986. On these and other Parke-Davis Products, information may be obtained by addressing PARKE-DAVIS, Division of Warner-Lambert Company, Morris Plains, New Jersey 07950.

Parke-Davis—Cont.

iting, and restlessness. Convulsions, tachycardia, or ventricular arrhythmias may be the first sign of toxicity.
Children have a marked sensitivity to the CNS stimulant action of theophylline. Serious toxic effects, including fatalities have been reported in children as well as adults.
Theophylline products may worsen pre-existing arrhythmias.

PRECAUTIONS

General: Mean half-life in smokers is shorter than nonsmokers. Therefore, smokers may require larger doses of theophylline. Theophylline should not be administered concurrently with other xanthine medications or with xanthine-containing beverages or foods. Use with caution in patients with severe cardiac disease, severe hypoxemia, hypertension, hyperthyroidism, acute myocardial injury, cor pulmonale, congestive heart failure, or liver disease, and in the elderly (especially males) and in neonates. Great caution should especially be used in giving theophylline to patients in congestive heart failure. Such patients have shown markedly prolonged theophylline blood level curves with theophylline persisting in serum for long periods following discontinuation of the drug.
Use theophylline cautiously in patients with a history of peptic ulcer. Theophylline may occasionally act as a local irritant to the G.I. tract although gastrointestinal symptoms are more commonly central and associated with serum theophylline concentrations over 20 mcg/ml.

DRUG INTERACTIONS

Theophylline-containing preparations have exhibited interaction with the following drugs:

Drug	Effect
Lithium carbonate	Increased excretion of lithium carbonate.
Propranolol	Antagonism of propranolol effect.
Furosemide	Increased furosemide diuresis.
Hexamethonium	Decreased hexamethonium-induced chronotropic effect.
Reserpine	Reserpine-induced tachycardia.
Chlordiazepoxide	Chlordiazepoxide-induced fatty acid mobilization.
Troleandomycin erythromycin or lincomycin	Increased theophylline plasma levels.

USAGE IN PREGNANCY

Safe use of Choledyl (oxtriphylline) in pregnancy and lactation has not been established relative to possible adverse effects on fetal or neonatal development. Therefore Choledyl (oxtriphylline) should not be used in patients who are pregnant or who may become pregnant, or during lactation unless, in the judgment of the physician, the potential benefits outweigh the possible hazards.

ADVERSE REACTIONS

The most consistent adverse reactions are usually due to overdose and are:

1. Gastrointestinal: nausea, vomiting, epigastric pain, hematemesis, diarrhea.
2. Central nervous system: headaches, irritability, restlessness, insomnia, reflex hyperexcitability, muscle twitching, clonic and tonic generalized convulsions.
3. Cardiovascular: palpitation, tachycardia, extrasystoles, flushing, hypotension, circulatory failure, life-threatening ventricular arrhythmias.
4. Respiratory: tachypnea.
5. Renal: albuminuria, increased excretion of renal tubular cells and red blood cells, diuresis.
6. Others: hyperglycemia and inappropriate antidiuretic hormone (ADH) syndrome.

Approximate Choledyl Pediatric Syrup Dosage (administered every 6 hours)

Body Weight		<9 years		9–12 years		12–16 years		>16 years	
		Initial Dose	Max. Dose	Initial Dose	Max. Dose	Initial Dose	Max. Dose	Initial Dose	Max. Dose
lbs.	Kg.	6.2 mg/kg	9.4 mg/kg	6.2 mg/kg	7.8 mg/kg	6.2 mg/kg	7 mg/kg	6.2 mg/kg	5
18	8	1 tsp	$1\frac{1}{2}$ tsp	—	—	—	—	—	—
36	16	2 tsp	3 tsp	2 tsp	$2\frac{1}{2}$ tsp	—	—	—	—
54	24	3 tsp*	$4\frac{1}{2}$ tsp	3 tsp*	$3\frac{1}{2}$ tsp	3 tsp*	$3\frac{1}{2}$ tsp	—	—
72	32	3 tsp*	6 tsp	3 tsp*	5 tsp	3 tsp*	$4\frac{1}{2}$ tsp	3 tsp*	3 tsp
90	40	3 tsp*	7 tsp**	3 tsp*	6 tsp	3 tsp*	$5\frac{1}{2}$ tsp	3 tsp*	4 tsp
108	48	3 tsp*	7 tsp**	3 tsp*	7 tsp**	3 tsp*	$6\frac{1}{2}$ tsp	3 tsp*	5 tsp

NOTE: The initial dosage may be increased in approximately 25 percent increments at 2 to 3 day intervals as clinically indicated and tolerated until the maximum dosage is reached.
1 mg Choledyl (oxtriphylline) = 0.64 mg anhydrous theophylline
*Initial Dosage should not exceed 625 mg/day Choledyl (400 mg/day theophylline)
**Maximum Dosage should not exceed 1400 mg/day Choledyl (900 mg/day theophylline)

DOSAGE AND ADMINISTRATION

Therapeutic serum levels associated with optimal likelihood of benefit and minimal risk of toxicity are considered to be between 10 mcg/ml and 20 mcg/ml. Levels above 20 mcg/ml may produce toxic effects. There is great variation from patient to patient in dosage needed in order to achieve a therapeutic blood level because of variable rates of elimination. Because of this wide variation from patient to patient and the relatively narrow therapeutic blood level range, dosage must be individualized; monitoring of theophylline serum levels is highly recommended.
Dosage should be calculated on the basis of lean (ideal) body weight—mg/kg. Theophylline does not distribute into fatty tissue.
Giving theophylline with food may prevent the rare case of stomach irritation, and although absorption may be slower, it is still complete.
When rapidly absorbed products such as solutions are used, dosing to maintain "around the clock" blood levels generally requires administration every 6 hours to obtain the greatest efficacy for use in children; dosing intervals up to 8 hours may be satisfactory for adults because of their slower elimination. Children and adults requiring higher than average doses may benefit from products with slower absorption. This may allow longer dosing intervals and/or less fluctuation in serum concentration over a dosing interval during chronic therapy. In patients receiving concurrent bronchodilator therapy, eg, beta agonists, downward adjustment of Choledyl (oxtriphylline) dosage is necessary.
[See table below].
II. *Those currently receiving theophylline products:*
Determine where possible, the time, amount, route of administration and form of the patient's last dose.
The loading dose for theophylline will be based on the principle that each 0.8 mg/kg of Choledyl (oxtriphylline) (0.5 mg/kg of theophylline) administered as a loading dose will result in a 1 mcg/ml increase in serum theophylline concentration. Ideally, then, the loading dose should be deferred if a serum theophylline concentration can be rapidly obtained. If this is not possible, the clinician must exercise his judgment in selecting a dose based on the potential for benefit and risk. When there is sufficient respiratory distress to warrant a small risk, 4 mg/kg Choledyl (oxtriphylline) (2.5 mg/kg of theophylline) is likely to increase the serum concentration when administered as a loading dose in rapidly absorbed form by only about 5 mcg/ml. If the patient is not already experiencing theophylline toxicity, this is unlikely to result in dangerous adverse effects.
Following the decision regarding loading dose in this group of patients, the subsequent maintenance dosage recommendations are the same as those described above.
To achieve optimal therapeutic theophylline dosage, monitoring of serum theophylline concentrations is recommended. However, it is not always possible or practical to obtain a serum theophylline level.
Patients should be closely monitored for signs of toxicity. The present data suggest that the above dosage recommendations will achieve therapeutic serum concentrations with minimal risk of toxicity for most patients. However, some risk of toxic serum concentration is still present.
Adverse reactions to theophylline often occur when serum theophylline levels exceed 20 mcg/ml.

CHOLEDYL (OXTRIPHYLLINE) DOSAGE FOR PATIENT POPULATION

Acute Symptoms of Asthma Requiring Rapid Theophyllinization:
I. *Not currently receiving theophylline products:*

GROUP	ORAL LOADING DOSE CHOLEDYL	MAINTENANCE DOSE FOR NEXT 12 HOURS CHOLEDYL	MAINTENANCE DOSE BEYOND 12 HOURS CHOLEDYL
1. Children 6 months to 9 years	9.4 mg/kg *(6 mg/kg)	6.2 mg/kg q4 hrs *(4 mg/kg q4 hrs)	6.2 mg/kg q6 hrs *(4 mg/kg q6 hrs)
2. Children age 9–16 and young adult smokers	9.4 mg/kg *(6 mg/kg)	4.7 mg/kg q4 hrs *(3 mg/kg q4 hrs)	4.7 mg/kg q6 hrs *(3 mg/kg q6 hrs)
3. Otherwise healthy nonsmoking adults	9.4 mg/kg *(6 mg/kg)	4.7 mg/kg q6 hrs *(3 mg/kg q6 hrs)	4.7 mg/kg q8 hrs *(3 mg/kg q8 hrs)
4. Older patients and patients with cor pulmonale	9.4 mg/kg *(6 mg/kg)	3.1 mg/kg q6 hrs *(2 mg/kg q6 hrs)	3.1 mg/kg q8 hrs *(2 mg/kg q8 hrs)
5. Patients with congestive heart failure, liver failure	9.4 mg/kg *(6 mg/kg)	3.1 mg/kg q8 hrs *(2 mg/kg q8 hrs)	1.6–3.1 mg/kg q12 hrs *(1–2 mg/kg q12 hrs)

*Anhydrous theophylline indicated in ()

Chronic Asthma

Theophyllinization is a treatment of first choice for the management of chronic asthma (to prevent symptoms and maintain patent airways). Slow clinical titration is generally preferred to assure acceptance and safety of the medication.

Choledyl (oxtriphylline)

Initial dose:	25 mg*/kg/day or 625 mg/day (whichever is lower) in 3 to 4 divided doses at 6–8 hour intervals.
Increased dose:	The above dosage may be increased in approximately 25 percent increments at 2 to 3 day intervals so long as no intolerance is observed until the maximum, indicated below, is reached.

*25 mg Choledyl = 16 mg anhydrous theophylline

Maximum dose of Choledyl Pediatric Syrup without measurement of serum theophylline concentration:
Not to exceed the following: (WARNING: DO NOT ATTEMPT TO MAINTAIN ANY DOSE THAT IS NOT TOLERATED)

Age <9 years	—37.5 mg/kg/day **(24 mg/kg/day)
Age 9–12 years	—31 mg/kg/day **(20 mg/kg/day)
Age 12–16 years	—28 mg/kg/day **(18 mg/kg/day)
Age >16 years	—20 mg/kg/day or 1400 mg/day (WHICHEVER IS LESS) **(13 mg/kg/day or 900 mg/day) (WHICHEVER IS LESS)

NOTE: Use ideal body weight for obese patients.
**anhydrous theophylline indicated in ()
To assist in determining dosage of Choledyl Pediatric Syrup in chronic asthma the above information has been summarized in the Approximate Choledyl Pediatric Syrup Dosage table.
[See table above].

Measurement of serum theophylline concentration during chronic therapy

If the above maximum dosages are to be maintained or exceeded, serum theophylline measurement is recommended. This should be obtained at the approximate time of peak absorption (1 to $1\frac{1}{2}$ hours after dosing) during chronic therapy. It is important that the patient will have missed *no* doses during the previous 48 hours and that dosing intervals will have been reasonably typical, with no added doses during that period of time.
DOSAGE ADJUSTMENT BASED ON SERUM THEOPHYLLINE MEASUREMENTS IF THE ABOVE INSTRUCTIONS HAVE NOT BEEN FOLLOWED MAY RESULT IN RISK OF TOXICITY TO THE PATIENT.
Caution should be exercised for younger children who cannot complain of minor side effects. Older adults, those with cor pulmonale, congestive heart failure, and/or liver disease, may have unusually low dosage requirements and thus may

experience toxicity at the maximal dosage recommended above.
It is important that no patient be maintained on any dosage that he is not tolerating. In instructing patients to increase dosage according to the schedule above, they should be instructed to not take a subsequent dose if apparent side effects occur and to resume therapy at a lower dose once adverse effects have disappeared.

OVERDOSAGE

Serious toxic effects due to overdosage may occur suddenly and are not invariably preceded by minor adverse effects. Therefore, careful observation of the patient and prompt institution of appropriate therapeutic measures are essential in all cases of overdosage. All patients suspected of overdosage should be hospitalized.
Signs and symptoms of overdosage are related primarily to the cardiovascular, gastrointestinal, and central nervous systems.
Cardiovascular symptoms include precordial pain, tachycardia, ventricular and other arrhythmias; also varying degrees of hypotension including in extreme cases, severe shock, cardiovascular collapse and death.
Gastrointestinal symptoms include abdominal pain, nausea, persistent vomiting, and hematemesis.
Central nervous system symptoms include headache, dizziness, restlessness, irritability, tremors, hyperactivity, and agitation followed, in severe cases, by convulsions, drowsiness, coma and death.
Treatment of overdosage should be directed toward minimizing absorption and supporting vital functions.
In the alert patient emesis should be induced, followed by appropriate additional measures, as listed below. In the obtunded patient, the airway should be secured immediately by means of an endotracheal tube with cuff inflated. After the airway has been secured, lavage should be carried out, and activated charcoal slurry and a cathartic should be administered.
CNS stimulation may be controlled with diazepam, 0.1–0.3 mg/kg intravenously in children, and 10 mg intravenously in adults. Respiration should be supported by appropriate means. Hypotension and shock should be treated with appropriate fluid replacement, avoiding the use of vasopressors, if possible. Additional supportive measures should be carried out as required.
Serial serum theophylline levels are of value in following the patient's course and in guiding further management.
Forced diuresis is of no value because of the small amount of theophylline excreted unchanged by the kidney. There has been a single report of survival with the use of an activated charcoal column (hemoperfusion) in massive theophylline overdosage.

HOW SUPPLIED

N 0071-2217-23—Choledyl Pediatric Syrup, 50 mg oxtriphylline/5 ml (equivalent to 32 mg anhydrous theophylline), is supplied as a vanilla-mint flavored syrup in bottles of 16 fl oz (474 ml).

2217G052

CHOLEDYL® SA ℞

[chō'lĕ-dyl"]
(Oxtriphylline)
Sustained Action

DESCRIPTION

Choledyl (oxtriphylline) is a xanthine bronchodilator—the choline salt of theophylline.
Each film-coated Choledyl SA tablet contains 400 mg or 600 mg oxtriphylline (equivalent to 254 mg or 382 mg anhydrous theophylline, respectively). Each tablet also contains, candelilla wax, confectioner's sugar, NF; magnesium stearate, NF; Opaseal pharmaceutical sealant; talc, USP and other ingredients. The 400-mg tablet also contains Opaspray pink and triethyl citrate. The 600-mg tablet also contains Opaspray tan.
Each tablet of Choledyl SA contains oxtriphylline in a tablet matrix specially designed for the prolonged release of the drug in the gastrointestinal tract. Following release of the drug, the expended wax tablet matrix, which is not absorbed, may be detected in the stool.

CLINICAL PHARMACOLOGY

Choledyl (oxtriphylline), the choline salt of theophylline, effects significant improvement in pulmonary function parameters which have been impaired by bronchospasm. It is more soluble than either aminophylline or theophylline. Film-coated Choledyl SA tablets are less irritating to the gastric mucosa than aminophylline.
Choledyl SA tablets have been formulated to provide therapeutic serum levels when administered every 12 hours and minimize the peaks and valleys of serum levels commonly found with shorter acting theophylline products.
The sustained action characteristic of Choledyl SA tablets has been demonstrated in studies in human subjects. Single and multiple dose studies have shown equivalent steady-state theophylline plasma levels of Choledyl SA tablets given every 12 hours when compared with an equal total daily dose of (the nonsustained action) Choledyl Elixir given every six hours.
Theophylline directly relaxes the smooth muscle of the bronchial airways and pulmonary blood vessels, thus acting mainly as a bronchodilator, pulmonary vasodilator and smooth muscle relaxant. The drug also possesses other actions typical of the xanthine derivatives: coronary vasodilator, diuretic, cardiac stimulant, cerebral stimulant and skeletal muscle stimulant. The actions of theophylline may be mediated through inhibition of phosphodiesterase and a resultant increase in intracellular cyclic AMP which could mediate smooth muscle relaxation. At concentrations higher than attained *in vivo*, theophylline also inhibits the release of histamine by mast cells.
Theophylline has been shown to react synergistically with beta agonists that increase intracellular cyclic AMP through the stimulation of adenyl cyclase (isoproterenol).
Apparently, the development of tolerance does not occur with chronic use of theophylline.
The half-life is shortened with cigarette smoking. The half-life is prolonged in alcoholism, reduced hepatic or renal function, congestive heart failure, and in patients receiving antibiotics such as TAO (troleandomycin), erythromycin and clindamycin. High fever for prolonged periods may decrease theophylline elimination.

Theophylline Elimination Characteristics

	Theophylline Clearance Rates (mean ± S.D.)	Half-Life Average (mean ± S.D.)
Children (over 6 months of age)	1.45 ± .58 ml/kg/min	3.7 ± 1.1 hours
Adult non-smokers with uncomplicated asthma	.65 ± .19 ml/kg/min	8.7 ±2.2 hours

Newborn infants have extremely slow clearance and half-lives exceeding 24 hours, which approach those seen for older children after about 3–6 months.
Older adults with chronic obstructive pulmonary disease, and patients with cor pulmonale or other causes of heart failure, and patients with liver pathology may have much lower clearances with half-lives that may exceed 24 hours.
The half-life of theophylline is prolonged in patients with congestive heart failure, in those with reduced hepatic or renal function, and in alcoholism. The half-life of theophylline may also be prolonged by concurrent use of various drugs such as phenobarbital, and certain antibiotics, including troleandomycin, erythromycin, and lincomycin.
Theophylline half-life is shortened in cigarette smokers (1 to 2 packs/day) as compared to nonsmokers. The increase in theophylline clearance caused by smoking is probably the result of induction of drug metabolizing enzymes that do not readily normalize after cessation of smoking. It appears that between 3 months and 2 years may be necessary for normalization of the effect of smoking on theophylline pharmacokinetics.

INDICATIONS

Choledyl (oxtriphylline) is indicated for relief of acute and chronic bronchial asthma and for reversible bronchospasm associated with chronic bronchitis and emphysema.

CONTRAINDICATIONS

Choledyl is contraindicated in individuals who have shown hypersensitivity to theophylline or to Choledyl (oxtriphylline) or any of its components.

WARNINGS

Status asthmaticus is a medical emergency. Optimal therapy frequently requires additional medication including corticosteroids when the patient is not rapidly responsive to bronchodilators.
Excessive theophylline doses may be associated with toxicity, and serum theophylline levels are recommended to assure maximal benefit without excessive risk; incidence of toxicity increases at levels greater than 20 mcg theophylline/ml. Morphine, curare, and stilbamidine should be used with caution in patients with airflow obstruction since they stimulate histamine release and can induce asthmatic attacks. These drugs may also suppress respiration leading to respiratory failure. Alternative drugs should be chosen whenever possible.
There is an excellent correlation between high blood levels of theophylline resulting from conventional doses and associated clinical manifestations of toxicity in patients with liver dysfunction or chronic obstructive lung disease.
There is excellent correlation between high serum levels of theophylline (over 20 mcg/ml) and the clinical manifestations of toxicity. Careful reduction of dosage and monitoring of serum levels are especially important in patients manifesting a decrease in total body theophylline clearance rate, including those with generalized debility, acute hypoxia, cardiac decompensation, hepatic dysfunction, or renal failure. Dosage reduction may also be necessary in patients who are older than 55 years of age, particularly males.
Serious toxic effects may occur suddenly and are not invariably preceded by minor adverse effects such as nausea, vomiting, and restlessness. Convulsions, tachycardia, or ventricular arrhythmias may be the first sign of toxicity.
Children have a marked sensitivity to the CNS stimulant action of theophylline. Serious toxic effects, including fatalities have been reported in children as well as adults.
Theophylline products may worsen pre-existing arrhythmias.

USAGE IN PREGNANCY

Safe use of Choledyl (oxtriphylline) in pregnancy and lactation has not been established relative to possible adverse effects on fetal or neonatal development. Therefore Choledyl (oxtriphylline) should not be used in patients who are pregnant or who may become pregnant, or during lactation unless, in the judgment of the physician, the potential benefits outweigh the possible hazards.

PRECAUTIONS

Mean half-life in smokers is shorter than nonsmokers, therefore, smokers may require larger doses of theophylline. Theophylline should not be administered concurrently with other xanthine medications or with xanthine-containing beverages or foods. Use with caution in patients with severe cardiac disease, severe hypoxemia, hypertension, hyperthyroidism, acute myocardial injury, cor pulmonale, congestive heart failure, or liver disease, and in the elderly (especially males) and in neonates. Great caution should especially be used in giving theophylline to patients in congestive heart failure. Such patients have shown markedly prolonged theophylline blood level curves with theophylline persisting in serum for long periods following discontinuation of the drug.
Use theophylline cautiously in patients with a history of peptic ulcer. Theophylline may occasionally act as a local irritant to the GI tract although gastrointestinal symptoms are more commonly central and associated with serum theophylline concentrations over 20 mcg/ml.

ADVERSE REACTIONS

The most consistent adverse reactions are usually due to overdose and are:
1. Gastrointestinal: nausea, vomiting, epigastric pain, hematemesis, diarrhea.
2. Central nervous system: headaches, irritability, restlessness, insomnia, reflex hyperexcitability, muscle twitching, clonic and tonic generalized convulsions.
3. Cardiovascular: palpitation, tachycardia, extrasystoles, flushing, hypotension, circulatory failure, life-threatening ventricular arrhythmias.
4. Respiratory: tachypnea.
5. Renal: albuminuria, increased excretion of renal tubular cells and red blood cells, diuresis.
6. Others: hyperglycemia and inappropriate antidiuretic hormone (ADH) syndrome.

Drug Interactions: Theophylline-containing preparations have exhibited interaction with the following drugs:

Drug	Effect
Lithium carbonate	Increased excretion of lithium carbonate.
Propranolol	Antagonism of propranolol effect.
Furosemide	Increased furosemide diuresis.
Hexamethonium	Decreased hexamethonium-induced chronotropic effect
Reserpine	Reserpine-induced tachycardia.
Chlordiazepoxide	Chlordiazepoxide-induced fatty acid mobilization.
Troleandomycin, erythromycin or lincomycin	Increased theophylline plasma levels.

Continued on next page

This product information was prepared in August, 1986. On these and other Parke-Davis Products, information may be obtained by addressing PARKE-DAVIS, Division of Warner-Lambert Company, Morris Plains, New Jersey 07950.

Parke-Davis—Cont.

DOSAGE AND ADMINISTRATION

Therapy should be initiated and daily dosage requirements established utilizing a nonsustained-action form of Choledyl (oxtriphylline) (eg, Choledyl Tablets, Elixir).

If the total daily maintenance dosage requirement of the Choledyl (oxtriphylline) nonsustained preparation is established at approximately 1200 mg, Choledyl SA 600 mg Sustained Action Tablets, one every 12 hours, may be substituted to provide smoother steady-state theophylline levels and the convenience of bid dosage. Similarly, if the total daily maintenance dosage is established at approximately 800 mg, Choledyl SA 400 mg Sustained Action Tablets, one every 12 hours, may be substituted.

Therapeutic serum levels associated with optimal likelihood of benefit and minimal risk of toxicity are considered to be between 10 mcg/ml and 20 mcg/ml. Levels above 20 mcg/ml may produce toxic effects.

There is great variation from patient to patient in dosage needed in order to achieve a therapeutic blood level because of variable rates of elimination. Because of this wide variation from patient to patient and the relatively narrow therapeutic blood level range, dosage must be individualized; monitoring of theophylline serum levels is highly recommended.

Dosage should be calculated on the basis of lean (ideal) body weight—mg/kg. Theophylline does not distribute into fatty tissue.

Giving Choledyl (oxtriphylline) with food may prevent the rare case of stomach irritation, and although absorption may be slower, it is still complete.

When rapidly absorbed products such as solutions are used, dosing to maintain "around the clock" blood levels generally requires administration every 6 hours to obtain the greatest efficacy for use in children, dosing intervals up to 8 hours may be satisfactory for adults because of their slower elimination. Children and adults requiring higher than average doses may benefit from products with slower absorption. This may allow longer dosing intervals and/or less fluctuation in serum concentration over a dosing interval during chronic therapy. In patients receiving concurrent bronchodilator therapy, eg, beta agonists, downward adjustment of Choledyl (oxtriphylline) dosage is necessary.

The following dosage information relates to initiation and titration of daily dosage requirements utilizing a nonsustained action form of Choledyl (eg Choledyl Tabs, Elixir).
[See table below].

II. *Those currently receiving theophylline products:*
Determine where possible, the time, amount, route of administration and form of the patient's last dose.

The loading dose for theophylline will be based on the principle that each 0.8 mg/kg of Choledyl (oxtriphylline) (0.5 mg/kg of theophylline) administered as a loading dose will result in a 1 mcg/ml increase in serum theophylline concentration. Ideally, then, the loading dose should be deferred if a serum theophylline concentration can be rapidly obtained. If this is not possible, the clinician must exercise his judgment in selecting a dose based on the potential for benefit and risk. When there is sufficient respiratory distress to warrant a small risk, 4 mg/kg Choledyl (oxtriphylline) (2.5 mg/kg of theophylline) is likely to increase the serum concentration when administered as a loading dose in rapidly absorbed form by only about 5 mcg/ml. If the patient is not already experiencing theophylline toxicity, this is unlikely to result in dangerous adverse effect.

	Choledyl (oxtriphylline)
Initial dose:	25 mg*/kg/day or 625 mg/day (whichever is lower) in 3 to 4 divided doses at 6–8 hour intervals.
Increased dose:	The above dosage may be increased in approximately 25 percent increments at 2 to 3 day intervals so long as no intolerance is observed until the maximum indicated below is reached.

*25 mg Choledyl = 16 mg anhydrous theophylline

Following the decision regarding loading dose in this group of patients, the subsequent maintenance dosage recommendations are the same as those described above.

To achieve optimal therapeutic theophylline dosage, monitoring of serum theophylline concentrations is recommended. However, it is not always possible or practical to obtain a serum theophylline level.

Patients should be closely monitored for signs of toxicity. The present data suggests that the above dosage recommendations will achieve therapeutic serum concentrations with minimal risk of toxicity for most patients. However, some risk of toxic serum concentrations is still present.

Adverse reactions to theophylline often occur when serum theophylline levels exceed 20 mcg/ml.

Chronic Asthma
Theophyllinization is a treatment of first choice for the management of chronic asthma (to prevent symptoms and maintain patent airways). Slow clinical titration is generally preferred to assure acceptance and safety of the medication. [See table above].

Maximum dose of Choledyl (oxtriphylline) without measurement of serum theophylline concentration:
Not to exceed the following: (WARNING: DO NOT ATTEMPT TO MAINTAIN ANY DOSE THAT IS NOT TOLERATED)

Age <9 years	—37.5 mg/kg/day **(24 mg/kg/day)
Age 9–12 years	—31 mg/kg/day **(20 mg/kg/day)
Age 12–16 years	—28 mg/kg/day **(18 mg/kg/day)
Age >16 years	—20 mg/kg/day or 1400 mg/day (WHICHEVER IS LESS) **(13 mg/kg/day or 900 mg/day) (WHICHEVER IS LESS)

Note: Use ideal body weight for obese patients.
**anhydrous theophylline indicated in ( )

If the total daily maintenance dosage requirement of the Choledyl (oxtriphylline) nonsustained preparation is established at approximately 1200 mg, Choledyl SA 600 mg Sustained Action Tablets, one every 12 hours, may be substituted to provide smoother steady-state theophylline levels and the convenience of bid dosage. Similarly, if the total daily maintenance dosage is established at approximately 800 mg, Choledyl SA 400 mg Sustained Action Tablets, one every 12 hours, may be substituted.

Measurement of serum theophylline concentration during chronic therapy
If the above maximum dosages are to be maintained or exceeded, serum theophylline measurement is recommended. This should be obtained at the approximate time of peak absorption (1 to 2 hours after dosing) during chronic therapy. It is important that the patient will have missed *no* doses during the previous 48 hours and that dosing intervals will have been reasonably typical, with no added doses during that period of time.

CHOLEDYL (OXTRIPHYLLINE) DOSAGE FOR PATIENT POPULATION

Acute Symptoms of Asthma Requiring Rapid Theophyllinization:
1. *Not currently receiving theophylline products:*

GROUP	ORAL LOADING DOSE CHOLEDYL	MAINTENANCE DOSE FOR NEXT 12 HOURS CHOLEDYL	MAINTENANCE DOSE BEYOND 12 HOURS CHOLEDYL
1. Children 6 months to 9 years	9.4 mg/kg *(6 mg/kg)	6.2 mg/kg q4 hrs *(4 mg/kg q4 hrs)	6.2 mg/kg q6 hrs *(4 mg/kg q6 hrs)
2. Children age 9–16 and young adult smokers	9.4 mg/kg *(6 mg/kg)	4.7 mg/kg q4 hrs *(3 mg/kg q4 hrs)	4.7 mg/kg q6 hrs *(3 mg/kg q6 hrs)
3. Otherwise healthy nonsmoking adults	9.4 mg/kg *(6 mg/kg)	4.7 mg/kg q6 hrs *(3 mg/kg q6 hrs)	4.7 mg/kg q8 hrs *3 mg/kg q8 hrs)
4. Older patients and patients with cor pulmonale	9.4 mg/kg *(6 mg/kg)	3.1 mg/kg q6 hrs *(2 mg/kg q6 hrs)	3.1 mg/kg q8 hrs *(2 mg/kg q8 hrs)
5. Patients with congestive heart failure, liver failure	9.4 mg/kg *(6 mg/kg)	3.1 mg/kg q8 hrs *(2 mg/kg q8 hrs)	1.6–3.1 mg/kg q12 hrs *(1–2 mg/kg q12 hrs)

*Anhydrous theophylline indicated in ( )

DOSAGE ADJUSTMENT BASED ON SERUM THEOPHYLLINE MEASUREMENTS IF THE ABOVE INSTRUCTIONS HAVE NOT BEEN FOLLOWED MAY RESULT IN RISK OF TOXICITY TO THE PATIENT.

Caution should be exercised for younger children who cannot complain of minor side effects. Older adults, those with cor pulmonale, congestive heart failure, and/or liver disease, may have unusually low dosage requirements and thus may experience toxicity at the maximal dosage recommended above.

It is important that no patient be maintained on any dosage that he is not tolerating. In instructing patients to increase dosage according to the schedule above, they should be instructed to not take a subsequent dose if apparent side effects occur and to resume therapy at a lower dose once adverse effects have disappeared.

OVERDOSAGE

Serious toxic effects due to overdosage may occur suddenly and are not invariably preceded by minor adverse effects. Therefore, careful observation of the patient and prompt institution of appropriate therapeutic measures are essential in all cases of overdosage. All patients suspected of overdosage should be hospitalized.

Signs and symptoms of overdosage are related primarily to the cardiovascular, gastrointestinal, and central nervous systems.

Cardiovascular symptoms include precordial pain, tachycardia, ventricular and other arrhythmias; also varying degrees of hypotension including, in extreme cases, severe shock, cardiovascular collapse and death.

Gastrointestinal symptoms include abdominal pain, nausea, persistent vomiting, and hematemesis.

Central nervous system symptoms include headache, dizziness, restlessness, irritability, tremors, hyperactivity, and agitation followed, in severe cases, by convulsions, drowsiness, coma and death.

Treatment of overdosage should be directed toward minimizing absorption and supporting vital functions.

In the alert patient emesis should be induced, followed by appropriate additional measures, as listed below.

In the obtunded patient, the airway should be secured immediately by means of an endotracheal tube with cuff inflated. After the airway has been secured, lavage should be carried out, and activated charcoal slurry and a cathartic should be administered.

CNS stimulation may be controlled with diazepam, 0.1–0.3 mg/kg intravenously in children, and 10 mg intravenously in adults. Respiration should be supported by appropriate means. Hypotension and shock should be treated with appropriate fluid replacement, avoiding the use of vasopressors, if possible. Additional supportive measures should be carried out as required.

Serial serum theophylline levels are of value in following the patient's course and in guiding further management.

Forced diuresis is of no value because of the small amount of theophylline excreted unchanged by the kidney. There has been a single report of survival with the use of an activated charcoal column (hemoperfusion) in massive theophylline overdosage.

HOW SUPPLIED

Choledyl SA 400 mg—each sustained action tablet contains 400 mg oxtriphylline. Available as pink film-coated tablets in bottles of 100 (N 0071-0214-24), and unit-dose 100's (N 0071-0214-40).

Choledyl SA 600 mg—each sustained action tablet contains 600 mg oxtriphylline. Available as tan film-coated tablets in bottles of 100 (N 0071-0221-24), and unit-dose 100's (N 0071-0221-40).

0214G092

Shown in Product Identification Section, page 420

COLY-MYCIN® M PARENTERAL ℞

[*cō″ly-my′cĭn pă″rĕn′tĕr-ăl*]
(sterile colistimethate sodium, USP)
for intramuscular and intravenous use

DESCRIPTION

Coly-Mycin M Parenteral (sterile colistimethate sodium) contains the sodium salt of colistimethate. Colistimethate sodium is a polypeptide antibiotic with an approximate molecular weight of 1750; the empirical formula is $C_{58}H_{105}N_{16}Na_5O_{28}S_5$.

CLINICAL PHARMACOLOGY

Microbiology

Coly-Mycin M Parenteral has bactericidal activity against the following gram-negative bacilli: *Enterobacter aerogenes, Escherichia coli, Klebsiella pneumoniae,* and *Pseudomonas aeruginosa.*

Human Pharmacology

Typical serum and urine levels following a single 150 mg dose of Coly-Mycin M Parenteral IM or IV in normal adult subjects are shown in Figure 1.

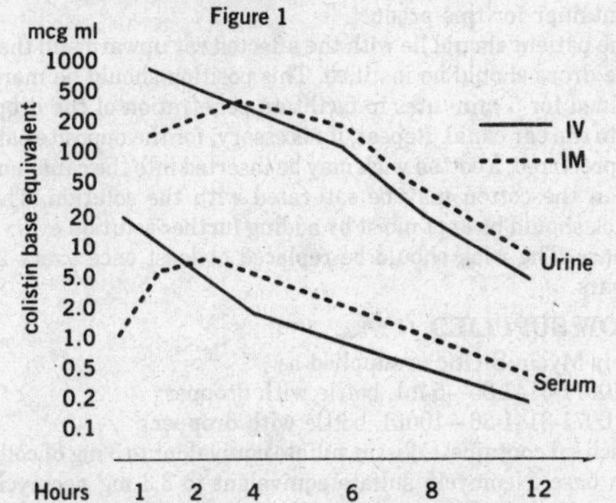

Figure 1. Urine and serum values in adults following parenteral (IM or IV) administration of Coly-Mycin M Parenteral Higher serum levels were obtained at 10 min- utes following IV administration. Serum concentration declined with a half-life of 2-3 hours following either intravenous or intramuscular administration in adults and children, including premature infants.

Colistimethate sodium is transferred across the placental barrier, and blood levels of about 1 mcg/ml are obtained in the fetus following intravenous administration to the mother.

Average urine levels ranged from about 270 mcg/ml at 2 hours to about 15 mcg/ml at 8 hours after intravenous administration and from about 200 to about 25 mcg/ml during a similar period following intramuscular administration.

INDICATIONS AND USAGE

Coly-Mycin M Parenteral (sterile colistimethate sodium) is indicated for the treatment of acute or chronic infections due to sensitive strains of certain gram-negative bacilli. It is particularly indicated when the infection is caused by sensitive strains of ***Pseudomonas aeruginosa.*** This antibiotic is not indicated for infections due to *Proteus* or *Neisseria.* Coly-Mycin M Parenteral has proven clinically effective in treatment of infections due to the following gram-negative organisms: ***Enterobacter aerogenes, Escherichia coli, Klebsiella pneumoniae,*** and ***Pseudomonas aeruginosa.***

Pending results of appropriate bacteriologic cultures and sensitivity tests, Coly-Mycin M Parenteral may be used to initiate therapy in serious infections that are suspected to be due to gram-negative organisms.

CONTRAINDICATIONS

The use of Coly-Mycin M Parenteral is contraindicated for patients with a history of sensitivity to the drug.

WARNING

Maximum daily dose should not exceed 5 mg/kg/day (2.3 mg/lb) with normal renal function.

Transient neurological disturbances may occur. These include circumoral paresthesias or numbness, tingling or formication of the extremities, generalized pruritus, vertigo, dizziness, and slurring of speech. For these reasons, patients should be warned not to drive vehicles or use hazardous machinery while on therapy. Reduction of dosage may alleviate symptoms. Therapy need not be discontinued, but such patients should be observed with particular care. Overdosage can result in renal insufficiency, muscle weakness and apnea. See PRECAUTIONS for use concomitantly with curariform drugs, and DOSAGE and ADMINISTRATION Section for use in renal impairment.

PRECAUTIONS

Since Coly-Mycin M Parenteral (sterile colistimethate sodium) is eliminated mainly by renal excretion, it should be used with caution when the possibility of impaired renal function exists. The decline in renal function with advanced age should be considered.

When actual renal impairment is present, Coly-Mycin M Parenteral may be used, but the greatest caution should be exercised and the dosage should be reduced in proportion to the extent of the impairment. Administration of amounts of Coly-Mycin M Parenteral in excess of renal excretory capacity will lead to high serum levels and can result in further impairment of renal function, initiating a cycle which, if not recognized, can lead to acute renal insufficiency, renal shutdown and further concentration of the antibiotic to toxic levels in the body. At this point, interference of nerve transmission at neuromuscular junctions may occur and result in muscle weakness and apnea.

Table 1

SUGGESTED MODIFICATION OF DOSAGE SCHEDULES OF COLY-MYCIN M PARENTERAL (STERILE COLISTIMETHATE SODIUM) FOR ADULTS WITH IMPAIRED RENAL FUNCTION

RENAL FUNCTION		DEGREE OF IMPAIRMENT		
	Normal	Mild	Moderate	Considerable
Plasma creatinine, (mg/100 ml)	0.7–1.2	1.3–1.5	1.6–2.5	2.6–4.0
Urea clearance, % of normal	80–100	40–70	25–40	10–25
DOSAGE				
Unit dose of Coly-Mycin M, mg	100–150	75–115	66–150	100–150
Frequency, times/day	4 to 2	2	2 or 1	every 36 hr
Total daily dose, mg	300	150–230	133–150	100
Approximate daily dose, mg/kg/day	5.0	2.5–3.8	2.5	1.5

NOTE

The suggested unit dose is 2.5–5 mg/kg; however, the time INTERVAL between injections should be increased in the presence of impaired renal function.

Easily recognized signs indicating the development of impaired renal function are diminishing urine output, rising BUN and serum creatinine. If present, therapy with Coly-Mycin M Parenteral (sterile colistimethate sodium) should be discontinued immediately.

If a life-threatening situation exists, therapy may be reinstated at a lower dosage after blood levels have fallen.

Certain other antibiotics (kanamycin, streptomycin, dihydrostreptomycin, polymyxin, neomycin) have also been reported to interfere with the nerve transmission at the neuromuscular junction. Based on this reported activity, they should not be given concomitantly with Coly-Mycin M Parenteral except with the greatest caution. The antibiotics with a gram-positive antimicrobial spectrum, e.g., penicillin, tetracycline, sodium cephalothin, have not been reported to interfere with nerve transmission and, accordingly, would not be expected to potentiate this activity of Coly-Mycin M Parenteral.

Other drugs, including curariform muscle relaxants (ether, tubocurarine, succinylcholine, gallamine, decamethonium and sodium citrate), potentiate the neuromuscular blocking effect and should be used with extreme caution in patients being treated with Coly-Mycin M Parenteral.

If apnea occurs, it may be treated with assisted respiration, oxygen, and calcium chloride injections.

USE IN PREGNANCY

The safety of colistimethate sodium during human pregnancy has not been established.

ADVERSE REACTIONS

Respiratory arrest has been reported following intramuscular administration of colistimethate sodium. Impaired renal function increases the possibility of apnea and neuromuscular blockade following administration of colistimethate sodium. This has been generally due to failure to follow recommended guidelines, usually overdosage, failure to reduce dose commensurate with degree of renal impairment, and/or concomitant use of other antibiotics or drugs with neuromuscular blocking potential.

A decrease in urine output or increase in blood urea nitrogen or serum creatinine can be interpreted as signs of nephrotoxicity, which is probably a dose-dependent effect of colistimethate sodium. These manifestations of nephrotoxicity are reversible following discontinuation of the antibiotic.

Increases of blood urea nitrogen have been reported for patients receiving Coly-Mycin M Parenteral (sterile colistimethate sodium) at dose levels of 1.6-5 mg/kg per day. The BUN values returned to normal following cessation of Coly-Mycin M Parenteral administration.

Paresthesia, tingling of the extremities or tingling of the tongue and generalized itching or urticaria have been reported by patients who received Coly-Mycin M Parenteral by intravenous or intramuscular injection. In addition, the following adverse reactions have been reported for colistimethate sodium: drug fever and gastrointestinal upset, vertigo, and slurring of speech. The subjective symptoms reported by the adult may not be manifest in infants or young children, thus requiring close attention to renal function.

DOSAGE AND ADMINISTRATION

Important: Coly-Mycin M Parenteral (sterile colistimethate sodium) is supplied in vials containing colistimethate sodium equivalent to 150 mg colistin base activity per vial.

Reconstitution: The *150-mg* vial should be reconstituted with *2.0 ml* Sterile Water for Injection USP. The reconstituted solution provides colistimethate sodium at a concentration of 75 mg/ml.

During reconstitution swirl *gently* to avoid frothing.

DOSAGE

Adults and children—intravenous or intramuscular administration—Coly-Mycin M Parenteral should be given in 2 to 4 divided doses at dose levels of 2.5 to 5 mg/kg per day for patients with normal renal function, depending on the severity of the infection.

The daily dose should be reduced in the presence of any renal impairment, which can often be anticipated from the history.

Modifications of dosage in the presence of renal impairment are presented in Table 1.

[See table above].

INTRAVENOUS ADMINISTRATION

1. Direct Intermittent Administration — slowly inject one-half of the total daily dose over a period of 3 to 5 minutes every 12 hours.
2. Continuous Infusion — slowly inject one-half the total daily dose over 3 to 5 minutes. Add the remaining half of the total daily dose of Coly-Mycin M Parenteral to one of the following: 0.9% NaCl; 5% dextrose in 0.9% NaCl; 5% dextrose in water; 5% dextrose in 0.45% NaCl; 5% dextrose in 0.225% NaCl; lactated Ringer's solution, or 10% invert sugar solution. There are not sufficient data to recommend usage of Coly-Mycin M Parenteral with other drugs or with other than the above listed infusion solutions.

Administer by slow intravenous infusion starting 1 to 2 hours after the initial dose at a rate of 5-6 mg/hr in the presence of normal renal function. In the presence of impaired renal function, reduce the infusion rate depending on the degree of renal impairment.

The choice of intravenous solution and the volume to be employed are dictated by the requirements of fluid and electrolyte management.

Any infusion solution containing colistimethate sodium should be freshly prepared and used for no longer than 24 hours.

HOW SUPPLIED

Coly-Mycin M Parenteral (sterile colistimethate sodium) is supplied in vials containing colistimethate sodium (150 mg colistin base equivalent per vial) as a white to slightly yellow lyophilized cake and is available as one vial per carton (N 0071-4145-01) or as 50 vials per carton (N 0071-4145-47).

STORE AT CONTROLLED ROOM TEMPERATURE (15° to 30°C) (59° to 86°F).

STORE RECONSTITUTED SOLUTION IN REFRIGERATOR (2° to 8°C) (36° to 46°F) OR AT CONTROLLED ROOM TEMPERATURE (15° to 30°C) (59° to 86°F), and use within 7 days.

Continued on next page

This product information was prepared in August, 1986. On these and other Parke-Davis Products, information may be obtained by addressing PARKE-DAVIS, Division of Warner-Lambert Company, Morris Plains, New Jersey 07950.

Parke-Davis—Cont.

Toxicology and Animal Pharmacology:

Acute Toxicity: The intravenous LD_{50} was 41.5 mg/kg in the dog and 739 mg/kg in the mouse; intramuscular toxicity was 42 mg/kg in the dog and 267 mg/kg in the mouse.

Subacute Toxicity: In albino rabbits and beagle dogs, IV doses of 5, 10 and 20 mg/kg/day for 28 days resulted in elevated blood urea nitrogen in the dog (10 mg/kg/day dose group) and in both 20 mg/kg dose groups.

Clinical Studies: Clinically, Coly-Mycin M Parenteral (sterile colistimethate sodium) has been of particular therapeutic value in acute and chronic urinary tract infections caused by sensitive strains of *Pseudomonas aeruginosa.* Colistimethate sodium is clinically effective in the treatment of infections due to other sensitive gram-negative pathogenic bacilli that have become resistant to broad-spectrum antibiotics.

Colistimethate sodium has been used to treat bacteriuria and overt urinary infections in pregnant women during the third trimester. However, in view of the evidence of possible embryotoxic and teratogenic effects of colistimethate sodium in pregnant rabbits, caution should be exercised in use of this drug in women of childbearing potential.

4145G013

COLY-MYCIN® S FOR ORAL SUSPENSION ℞

[*cō "ly-my 'cĭn*]

(colistin sulfate for oral suspension, USP)

FOR ORAL USE ONLY

DESCRIPTION

Coly-Mycin S For Oral Suspension (colistin sulfate for oral suspension) contains the sulfate salt of colistin, a polypeptide antibiotic with a molecular weight of approximately 1170. The empirical formula of colistin is $C_{53}H_{100}N_{16}O_{13}$.

Each 5 mL of Coly-Mycin S Suspension contains the equivalent of 25 mg colistin base. Also contains citric acid, USP; cocoa, NF; dried low fat milk solids; guar gum, NF; imitation chocolate flavor; imitation vanilla bean flavor; magnesium stearate, NF; menthol, USP; methylparaben, NF; propylparaben, NF; saccharin sodium, USP; sodium chloride, USP; sorbitol, NF; sucrose, NF.

CLINICAL PHARMACOLOGY

Colistin sulfate has *in vitro* bactericidal activity against most gram-negative enteric pathogens, especially enteropathogenic *E. coli* and *Shigella* (but not *Proteus*). In infants and children, it has effectively controlled acute infections of the intestinal tract due to these pathogens. Susceptible strains of *E. coli* and *Shigella in vitro* or *in vivo* rarely develop resistance to colistin sulfate. Cross resistance to polymyxin B sulfate does exist, but cross resistance to broad spectrum antibiotics has not been encountered.

INDICATIONS AND USAGE

Diarrhea in infants and children, caused by susceptible strains of enteropathogenic *E. coli.*

Gastroenteritis due to *Shigella* organisms. Clinical response may vary due to the absence of tissue levels in the bowel wall.

CONTRAINDICATIONS

Known hypersensitivity to the drug.

WARNINGS

Although colistin sulfate is not absorbed systemically in measurable amounts, it is assumed that slight absorption may occur. Therefore, in the presence of azotemia or, if dosages above the recommended range are used, a potential for possible renal toxicity exists.

With prolonged usage, suppression of intestinal bacterial flora may occur. There may be a resultant overgrowth of organisms (such as *Proteus*); appropriate therapy should be initiated immediately.

PRECAUTIONS

Renal function should be assessed prior to initiation of therapy.

ADVERSE REACTIONS

Within the recommended dosage range, none reported.

DOSAGE AND ADMINISTRATION

The usual dosage of colistin base (supplied as the sulfate) is 5–15 mg/kg/day (2.3–6.8 mg/pound/day) given in three divided doses. Higher doses may be necessary. Each 5 ml of suspension contains the equivalent of 25 mg colistin base. A 10-pound infant would require a total daily dose of 23–68 mg colistin base, given in divided doses (approximately ⅓ to 1 teaspoonful three times a day). A 50-pound patient would require a total daily dose of 115–340 mg colistin base, given in divided doses (approximately 1½–4½ teaspoonfuls three times a day).

PREPARATION

Coly-Mycin S For Oral Suspension (colistin sulfate for oral suspension) is a dry powder which is reconstituted with 37 ml of distilled water. To reconstitute, slowly add one half of the diluent, replace the cap and shake well. Add the remaining diluent and repeat shaking. Volume after reconstitution is 60 ml. When reconstituted, Coly-Mycin S Oral Suspension is a chocolate-flavored mixture, each 5 ml teaspoonful containing the equivalent of 25 mg of colistin base. Reconstituted Coly-Mycin S Oral Suspension is stable for two weeks when kept below 15°C (59°F).

SUPPLIED

Bottles containing colistin sulfate equivalent to 300 mg colistin base (N 0071-2142-15).

Before reconstitution store between 15° and 30°C.

2142G012

Caution—Federal law prohibits dispensing without prescription.

COLY-MYCIN® S OTIC ℞

[*cō "ly-my 'cĭn s ō 'tĭc*]

with Neomycin and Hydrocortisone

(colistin sulfate—neomycin sulfate—thonzonium bromide—hydrocortisone acetate otic suspension)

DESCRIPTION

Coly-Mycin S Otic with Neomycin and Hydrocortisone (colistin sulfate-neomycin sulfate-thonzonium bromide-hydrocortisone acetate otic suspension) is a sterile aqueous suspension containing in each ml: Colistin base activity, 3 mg (as the sulfate); Neomycin base activity, 3.3 mg (as the sulfate); Hydrocortisone acetate, 10 mg (1%); Thonzonium bromide, 0.5 mg (0.05%); Polysorbate 80, acetic acid, and sodium acetate in a buffered aqueous vehicle. Thimerosal (mercury derivative), 0.002%, added as a preservative. It is a nonviscous liquid, buffered at pH 5, for instillation into the canal of the external ear or direct application to the affected aural skin.

CLINICAL PHARMACOLOGY

1. Colistin sulfate—an antibiotic with bactericidal action against most gram-negative organisms, notably *Pseudomonas aeruginosa, E. coli.,* and *Klebsiella-Aerobacter.*
2. Neomycin sulfate—a broad-spectrum antibiotic, bactericidal to many pathogens, notably *Staph aureus* and *Proteus* sp.
3. Hydrocortisone acetate—a corticosteroid that controls inflammation, edema, pruritus and other dermal reactions.
4. Thonzonium bromide—a surface-active agent that promotes tissue contact by dispersion and penetration of the cellular debris and exudate.

INDICATIONS AND USAGE

For the treatment of superficial bacterial infections of the external auditory canal, caused by organisms susceptible to the action of the antibiotics; and for the treatment of infections of mastoidectomy and fenestration cavities, caused by organisms susceptible to the antibiotics.

CONTRAINDICATIONS

This product is contraindicated in those individuals who have shown hypersensitivity to any of its components, and in herpes simplex, vaccinia and varicella.

WARNINGS

As with other antibiotic preparations, prolonged treatment may result in overgrowth of nonsusceptible organisms and fungi.

If the infection is not improved after one week, cultures and susceptibility tests should be repeated to verify the identity of the organism and to determine whether therapy should be changed.

Patients who prefer to warm the medication before using should be cautioned against heating the solution above body temperature, in order to avoid loss of potency.

PRECAUTIONS

General: If sensitization or irritation occurs, medication should be discontinued promptly.

This drug should be used with care in cases of perforated eardrum and in longstanding cases of chronic otitis media because of the possibility of ototoxicity caused by neomycin. Treatment should not be continued for longer than ten days.

Allergic cross-reactions may occur which could prevent the use of any or all of the following antibiotics for the treatment of future infections: kanamycin, paromomycin, streptomycin, and possibly gentamicin.

ADVERSE REACTIONS

Neomycin is a not uncommon cutaneous sensitizer. There are articles in the current literature that indicate an increase in the prevalence of persons sensitive to neomycin.

DOSAGE AND ADMINISTRATION

The external auditory canal should be thoroughly cleansed and dried with a sterile cotton applicator.

When using the calibrated dropper:

For adults, 5 drops of the suspension should be instilled into the affected ear 3 or 4 times daily. For infants and children, 4 drops are suggested because of the smaller capacity of the ear canal.

This dosage correlates to the 4 drops (for adults) and 3 drops (for children) recommended when using the dropper-bottle container for this product.

The patient should lie with the affected ear upward and then the drops should be instilled. This position should be maintained for 5 min- utes to facilitate penetration of the drops into the ear canal. Repeat, if necessary, for the opposite ear.

If preferred, a cotton wick may be inserted into the canal and then the cotton may be saturated with the solution. This wick should be kept moist by adding further solution every 4 hours. The wick should be replaced at least once every 24 hours.

HOW SUPPLIED

Coly-Mycin S Otic is supplied as:

N 0071-3141-35—5-mL bottle with dropper

N 0071-3141-36—10-mL bottle with dropper

Each ml contains: Colistin sulfate equivalent to 3 mg of colistin base, Neomycin sulfate equivalent to 3.3 mg neomycin base, Hydrocortisone acetate 10 mg (1%), Thonzonium bromide 0.5 mg (0.05%), and Polysorbate 80 in an aqueous vehicle buffered with acetic acid and sodium acetate. Thimerosal (mercury derivative) 0.002% added as a preservative.

Shake well before using.

Store at controlled room temperature 15°–30°C (59°–86°F). Stable for 18 months at room temperature; prolonged exposure to higher temperatures should be avoided.

3141G033

Caution—Federal law prohibits dispensing without prescription.

DIAZEPAM Ⓒ ℞

[*dī-ā 'zĭ-păm*]

Tablets, USP

DESCRIPTION

Diazepam, a benzodiazepine derivative, occurs as an off-white to yellow, practically odorless, crystalline powder that is stable in air and sensitive to light. It is insoluble in water, soluble in alcohol, and sparingly soluble in propylene glycol. Chemically, diazepam is 7-chloro-1,3-dihydro-1-methyl-5-phenyl-2H-1,4-benzodiazepin-2-one.

Diazepam is subject to control as a Schedule IV substance under the Federal Controlled Substances Act of 1970. It is available as tablets for oral administration in strengths of 2 mg, 5 mg and 10 mg. Also contains calcium stearate, NF; lactose, NF; microcrystalline cellulose, NF; povidone, USP; starch, NF.

CLINICAL PHARMACOLOGY

In animals diazepam appears to act on parts of the limbic system, the thalamus and hypothalamus, and induces calming effects. Diazepam, unlike chlorpromazine and reserpine, has no demonstrable peripheral autonomic blocking action, nor does it produce extrapyramidal side effects; however, animals treated with diazepam do have a transient ataxia at higher doses. Diazepam has transient cardiovascular depressor effects in dogs. Long-term experiments in rats reveal no disturbances of endocrine function.

Oral LD_{50} of diazepam is 720 mg/kg in mice and 1240 mg/kg in rats. Intraperitoneal administration of 400 mg/kg to a monkey was reported to have resulted in death on the sixth day.

Reproduction Studies: A series of rat reproduction studies performed with diazepam in oral doses of 1, 10, 80 and 100 mg/kg were reported. At 100 mg/kg there was a decrease in the number of pregnancies and surviving offspring in these rats. Neonatal survival of rats at doses lower than 100 mg/kg was within normal limits. Several neonates in these rat reproduction studies showed skeletal or other defects. Further studies in rats at doses up to and including 80 mg/kg/day did not reveal teratological effects on the offspring.

In humans, measurable blood levels of diazepam are obtained in maternal and cord blood, indicating placental transfer of the drug.

INDICATIONS AND USAGE

For management of anxiety disorders or for short-term relief of the symptoms of anxiety. The effectiveness of diazepam in long-term use (more than 4 months) has not been assessed by systematic clinical studies. The physician should periodically reassess the usefulness of the drug for the individual patient. Anxiety or tension associated with the stress of everyday life usually does not require treatment with an anxiolytic.

In acute alcohol withdrawal, for the symptomatic relief of acute agitation, tremor, impending or acute delirium tremens, and hallucinosis.

As an adjunct for relief of:

—skeletal muscle spasm due to reflex spasm to local pathology (such as inflammation of the muscles or joints, or secondary to trauma).
—spasticity caused by upper motor neuron disorders (such as cerebral palsy and paraplegia)
—athetosis
—stiff-man syndrome

Oral diazepam may be used adjunctively in disorders, although it has not proved useful as the sole therapy.

CONTRAINDICATIONS

In patients with known hypersensitivity to diazepam.
In patients with acute narrow angle glaucoma (but may be used in patients with open angle glaucoma who are receiving appropriate therapy).
In children under 6 months of age (because of lack of sufficient clinical experience).

WARNINGS

Diazepam is not of value in the treatment of psychotic patients and should not be employed in lieu of appropriate treatment. As is true of most preparations containing CNS-acting drugs, patients receiving diazepam should be cautioned against engaging in hazardous occupations requiring complete mental alertness such as operating machinery or driving a motor vehicle.

As with other agents which have anticonvulsant activity, when diazepam is used as an adjunct in treating convulsive disorders, the possibility of an increase in the frequency and /or severity of grand mal seizures may require an increase in the dosage of standard anticonvulsant medication. Abrupt withdrawal of diazepam in such cases may also be associated with a temporary increase in the frequency and/or severity of seizures.

Since diazepam has a central nervous system depressant effect, patients should be advised against the simultaneous ingestion of alcohol and other CNS-depressant drugs during diazepam therapy.

Physical and Psychological Dependence: Withdrawal symptoms (similar in character to those noted with barbiturates and alcohol) have occurred following abrupt discontinuance of diazepam (convulsions, tremor, abdominal and muscle cramps, vomiting and sweating). These were usually limited to those patients who had received excessive doses over an extended period of time.

Although infrequently seen, milder withdrawal symptoms have also been reported following abrupt discontinuance of benzodiazepines taken continuously, generally at higher therapeutic levels, for at least several months. Consequently, after extended therapy, abrupt discontinuation should generally be avoided and a gradual tapering in dosage followed. Particularly addiction-prone individuals (such as drug addicts or alcoholics) should be under careful surveillance when receiving diazepam or other psychotropic agents because of the predisposition of such patients to habituation and dependence.

Usage in Pregnancy: An increased risk of congenital malformations associated with the use of minor tranquilizers (diazepam, meprobamate and chlordiazepoxide) during the first trimester of pregnancy has been suggested in several studies. Because use of these drugs is rarely a matter of urgency, their use during this period should almost always be avoided. The possibility that a woman of childbearing potential may be pregnant at the time of institution of therapy should be considered. Patients should be advised that if they become pregnant during therapy or intend to become pregnant they should communicate with their physicians about the desirability of discontinuing the drug.

Management of Overdosage: Manifestations of diazepam overdosage include somnolence, confusion, coma and diminished reflexes. Respiration, pulse and blood pressure should be monitored, as in all cases of drug overdosage, although, in general, these effects have been minimal following overdosage. General supportive measures should be employed along with immediate gastric lavage. Intravenous fluids should be administered and an adequate airway maintained. Hypotension may be combated by the use of norepinephrine or metaraminol. Dialysis is of limited value. As with the management of intentional overdosage with any drug, it should be borne in mind that multiple agents may have been ingested.

PRECAUTIONS

If diazepam is to be combined with other psychotropic agents or anticonvulsant drugs, careful consideration should be given to the pharmacology of the agents to be employed—particularly with known compounds which may potentiate the action of diazepam, such as phenothiazines, narcotics, barbiturates, MAO inhibitors and other antidepressants. The usual precautions are indicated for severely depressed patients or those in whom there is any evidence of latent depression; particularly the recognition that suicidal tendencies may be present and protective measures may be necessary. The usual precautions in treating patients with impaired renal or hepatic function should be observed.

In elderly and debilitated patients, it is recommended that the dosage be limited to the smallest effective amount to preclude the development of ataxia or oversedation (2 mg to 2 ½ mg once or twice daily, initially, to be increased gradually as needed and tolerated.)

The clearance of diazepam and certain other benzodiazepines can be delayed in association with Tagamet* (cimetidine) administration. The clinical significance of this is unclear.

ADVERSE REACTIONS

Side effects most commonly reported were drowsiness, fatigue and ataxia. Infrequently encountered were confusion, constipation, depression, diplopia, dysarthria, headache, hypotension, incontinence, jaundice, changes in libido, nausea, changes in salivation, skin rash, slurred speech, tremor, urinary retention, vertigo and blurred vision. Paradoxical reactions such as acute hyperexcited states, anxiety, hallucinations, increased muscle spasticity, insomnia, rage, sleep disturbances and stimulation have been reported; should these occur, use of the drug should be discontinued.

Because of isolated reports of neutropenia and jaundice, periodic blood counts and liver function tests are advisable during long-term therapy. Minor changes in EEG patterns, usually low-voltage fast activity, have been observed in patients during and after diazepam therapy and are of no known signficance.

DOSAGE AND ADMINISTRATION

Dosage should be individualized for maximum beneficial effect. While the usual daily dosages given below will meet the needs of most patients, there will be some who may require higher dosages. In such cases dosage should be increased cautiously to avoid adverse effects.

Since diazepam and its metabolites have long elimination half-lives, time to reach steady-state plasma levels should be considered when dosage adjustments are made.

Adults	**Usual Daily Dose**
Management of anxiety disorders and relief of symptoms of anxiety	Depending upon severity of symptoms—2 mg to 10 mg. bid to qid
Symptomatic relief in acute alcohol withdrawal	10 mg. 3 to 4 times during the first 24 hours reducing to 5 mg tid or qid as needed.
Adjunctively in convulsive disorders	2 mg to 10 mg bid to qid
Adjunctively for relief of skeletal muscle spasm	2 mg to 10 mg bid to qid
Geriatric patients or in the presence of debilitating disease.	2 mg to 2 ½ mg daily or bid initially increase gradually as needed and tolerated.
Children	
Because of the varied response of children to CNS-acting drugs, initiate therapy with lowest dose and increase as required	1 mg to 2 ½ mg tid or qid initially increase gradually as needed and tolerated.

Not for use in children younger than 6 months of age.

HOW SUPPLIED

Diazepam Tablets USP, 2 mg (flat, oval, white scored tablets coded P-D 141) are supplied as follows.

N 0071-0141-24	Bottles of 100
N 0071-0141-30	Bottles of 500
N 0071-0141-40	Unit-dose packages of 100 (10 strips of 10 tablets each)
N 0071-0141-41	Hospital Pack of 100 (4 cards of 25 tablets each)

Diazepam Tablets USP, 5 mg (flat, triangular, white scored tablets coded P-D 142) are supplied as follows.

N 0071-0142-24	Bottles of 100
N 0071-0142-30	Bottles of 500
N 0071-0142-40	Unit-dose packages of 100 (10 strips of 10 tablets each)
N 0071-0142-41	Hospital Pack of 100 (4 cards of 25 tablets each)

Diazepam Tablets USP, 10 mg (flat, round, white, scored tablets coded P-D 143) are supplied as follows.

N 0071-0143-24	Bottles of 100
N 0071-0143-30	Bottles of 500
N 0071-0143-40	Unit-dose packages of 100 (10 strips of 10 tablets each) Hospital Pack of 100
N 0071-0143-41	Hospital Pack of 100 (4 cards of 25 tablets each)

Special Handling and Storage Conditions
Protect from light and moisture.
Store at controlled room temperature, 15–30 C (59–86 F).

Caution: Diazepam is subject to control as a Schedule IV substance under the Federal Controlled Substances Act of 1970. Federal law prohibits dispensing without prescription.

0141G013

Shown in Product Identification Section, page 420

KAPSEALS®
DILANTIN® ℞
[*dī-lăn ′tĭn ″*]
(Extended Phenytoin Sodium Capsules, USP)

DESCRIPTION

Phenytoin Sodium is an antiepileptic drug. Phenytoin sodium is related to the barbiturates in chemical structure, but has a five-membered ring. The chemical name is sodium 5,5-diphenyl-2,4-imidazolidinedione.

Each Dilantin—*Extended Phenytoin Sodium Capsule* USP contains 30 mg or 100 mg phenytoin sodium. Product *in vivo* performance is characterized by a slow and extended rate of absorption with peak blood concentrations expected in 4 to 12 hours as contrasted to *Prompt Phenytoin Sodium Capsules* USP with a rapid rate of absorption with peak blood concentration expected in 1½ to 3 hours.

CLINICAL PHARMACOLOGY

Phenytoin is an antiepileptic drug which can be useful in the treatment of epilepsy. The primary site of action appears to be *the motor cortex* where spread of seizure activity is inhibited. Possibly by promoting sodium efflux from neurons, phenytoin tends to *stabilize* the threshold against hyperexcitability caused by excessive stimulation or environmental changes capable of reducing membrane sodium gradient. This includes the reduction of posttetanic potentiation at synapses. Loss of posttetanic potentiation prevents cortical seizure foci from detonating adjacent cortical areas. Phenytoin reduces the maximal activity of brain stem centers responsible for the tonic phase of tonic-clonic (grand mal) seizures.

The plasma half-life in man after oral administration of phenytoin averages 22 hours, with a range of 7 to 42 hours. Steady-state therapeutic levels are achieved 7 to 10 days after initiation of therapy with recommended doses of 300 mg/day.

When serum level determinations are necessary, they should be obtained at least 5-7 half-lives after treatment initiation, dosage change, or addition or subtraction of another drug to the regimen so that equilibrium or steady-state will have been achieved. Trough levels provide information about clinically effective serum level range and confirm patient compliance and are obtained just prior to the patient's next scheduled dose. Peak levels indicate an individual's threshold for emergence of dose-related side effects and are obtained at the time of expected peak concentration. For Dilantin Kapseals peak serum levels occur 4-12 hours after administration.

Optimum control without clinical signs of toxicity occurs more often with serum levels between 10 and 20 mcg/ml, although some mild cases of tonic-clonic (grand mal) epilepsy may be controlled with lower-serum levels of phenytoin.

In most patients maintained at a steady dosage, stable phenytoin serum levels are achieved. There may be wide interpatient variability in phenytoin serum levels with equivalent dosages. Patients with unusually low levels may be noncompliant or hypermetabolizers of phenytoin. Unusually high levels result from liver disease, congenital enzyme deficiency or drug interactions which result in metabolic interference. The patient with large variations in phenytoin plasma levels, despite standard doses, presents a difficult clinical problem. Serum level determinations in such patients may be particularly helpful.

Most of the drug is excreted in the bile as inactive metabolites which are then reabsorbed from the intestinal tract and excreted in the urine. Urinary excretion of phenytoin and its metabolites occurs partly with glomerular filtration but more importantly, by tubular secretion. Because phenytoin is hydroxylated in the liver by an enzyme system which is saturable, small incremental doses may produce very substantial increases in serum levels, when these are in the upper range. The steady-state level may be disproportionately increased, with resultant intoxication, from an increase in dosage of 10% or more.

INDICATIONS AND USAGE

Dilantin is indicated for the control of tonic-clonic and psychomotor (grand mal and temporal lobe) seizures and prevention and treatment of seizures occurring during or following neurosurgery.

Phenytoin serum level determinations may be necessary for optimal dosage adjustments (see Dosage and Administration).

Continued on next page

This product information was prepared in August, 1986. On these and other Parke-Davis Products, information may be obtained by addressing PARKE-DAVIS, Division of Warner-Lambert Company, Morris Plains, New Jersey 07950.

Parke-Davis—Cont.

CONTRAINDICATIONS

Phenytoin is contraindicated in those patients who are hypersensitive to phenytoin or other hydantoins.

WARNINGS

Abrupt withdrawal of phenytoin in epileptic patients may precipitate status epilepticus. When, in the judgment of the clinician, the need for dosage reduction, discontinuation, or substitution of alternative antiepileptic medication arises, this should be done gradually. However, in the event of an allergic or hypersensitivity reaction, rapid substitution of alternative therapy may be necessary. In this case, alternative therapy should be an antiepileptic drug not belonging to the hydantoin chemical class.

There have been a number of reports suggesting a relationship between phenytoin and the development of lymphadenopathy (local or generalized) including benign lymph node hyperplasia, pseudolymphoma, lymphoma, and Hodgkin's Disease.

Although a cause and effect relationship has not been established, the occurrence of lymphadenopathy indicates the need to differentiate such a condition from other types of lymph node pathology. Lymph node involvement may occur with or without symptoms and signs resembling serum sickness eg, fever, rash and liver involvement.

In all cases of lymphadenopathy, follow-up observation for an extended period is indicated and every effort should be made to achieve seizure control using alternative antiepileptic drugs.

Acute alcoholic intake may increase phenytoin serum levels while chronic alcoholic use may decrease serum levels.

Usage in Pregnancy:

A number of reports suggests an association between the use of antiepileptic drugs by women with epilepsy and a higher incidence of birth defects in children born to these women. Data are more extensive with respect to phenytoin and phenobarbital, but these are also the most commonly prescribed antiepileptic drugs; less systematic or anecdotal reports suggest a possible similar association with the use of all known antiepileptic drugs.

The reports suggesting a higher incidence of birth defects in children of drug-treated epileptic women cannot be regarded as adequate to prove a definite cause and effect relationship. There are intrinsic methodologic problems in obtaining adequate data on drug teratogenicity in humans; genetic factors or the epileptic condition itself may be more important than drug therapy in leading to birth defects. The great majority of the mothers on antiepileptic medication deliver normal infants. It is important to note that antiepileptic drugs should not be discontinued in patients in whom the drug is administered to prevent major seizures, because of the strong possibility of precipitating status epilepticus with attendant hypoxia and threat to life. In individual cases where the severity and frequency of the seizure disorder are such that the removal of medication does not pose a serious threat to the patient, discontinuation of the drug may be considered prior to and during pregnancy, although it cannot be said with any confidence that even minor seizures do not pose some hazards to the developing embryo or fetus. The prescribing physician will wish to weigh these considerations in treating and counseling epileptic women of childbearing potential.

In addition to the reports of increased incidence of congenital malformation, such as cleft lip/palate and heart malformations in children of women receiving phenytoin and other antiepileptic drugs, there have more recently been reports of a fetal hydantoin syndrome. This consists of prenatal growth deficiency, microcephaly and mental deficiency in children born to mothers who have received phenytoin, barbiturates, alcohol, or trimethadione. However, these features are all interrelated and are frequently associated with intrauterine growth retardation from other causes.

There have been isolated reports of malignancies, including neuroblastoma, in children whose mothers received phenytoin during pregnancy.

An increase in seizure frequency during pregnancy occurs in a high proportion of patients, because of altered phenytoin absorption or metabolism. Periodic measurement of serum phenytoin levels is particularly valuable in the management of a pregnant epileptic patient as a guide to an appropriate adjustment of dosage. However, postpartum restoration of the original dosage will probably be indicated.

Neonatal coagulation defects have been reported within the first 24 hours in babies born to epileptic mothers receiving phenobarbital and/or phenytoin. Vitamin K_1 has been shown to prevent or correct this defect and has been recommended to be given to the mother before delivery and the neonate after birth.

PRECAUTIONS

General:

The liver is the chief site of biotransformation of phenytoin; patients with impaired liver function, elderly patients, or those who are gravely ill may show early signs of toxicity.

A small percentage of individuals who have been treated with phenytoin have been shown to metabolize the drug slowly. Slow metabolism may be due to limited enzyme availability and lack of induction; it appears to be genetically determined.

Phenytoin should be discontinued if a skin rash appears (see "Warnings" section regarding drug discontinuation). If the rash is exfoliative, purpuric, or bullous or if lupus erythematosus or Stevens-Johnson syndrome is suspected, use of the drug should not be resumed. (See Adverse Reactions.) If the rash is of a milder type (measles-like or scarlatiniform), therapy may be resumed after the rash has completely disappeared. If the rash recurs upon reinstitution of therapy, further phenytoin medication is contraindicated.

Hyperglycemia, resulting from the drug's inhibitory effects on insulin release, has been reported. Phenytoin may also raise the serum glucose level in diabetic patients.

Osteomalacia has been associated with phenytoin therapy and is considered to be due to phenytoin's interference with Vitamin D metabolism.

Phenytoin is not indicated for seizures due to hypoglycemic or other causes. Appropriate diagnostic procedures should be performed as indicated.

Phenytoin is not effective for absence (petit mal) seizures. If tonic-clonic (grand-mal) and absence (petit mal) seizures are present, combined drug therapy is needed.

Serum levels of phenytoin sustained above the optimal range may produce confusional states referred to as "delirium," "psychosis," or "encephalopathy," or rarely irreversible cerebellar dysfunction. Accordingly, at the first sign of acute toxicity, plasma levels are recommended. Dose reduction of phenytoin therapy is indicated if plasma levels are excessive; if symptoms persist, termination is recommended. (See Warnings.)

Information for Patients:

Patients taking phenytoin should be advised of the importance of adhering strictly to the prescribed dosage regimen, and of informing the physician of any clinical condition in which it is not possible to take the drug orally as prescribed, eg, surgery, etc.

Patients should also be cautioned on the use of other drugs or alcoholic beverages without first seeking the physician's advice.

Patients should be instructed to call their physician if skin rash develops.

The importance of good dental hygiene should be stressed in order to minimize the development of gingival hyperplasia and its complications.

Laboratory Tests:

Phenytoin serum level determinations may be necessary to achieve optimal dosage adjustments.

Drug Interactions:

There are many drugs which may increase or decrease phenytoin levels or which phenytoin may affect. The most commonly occurring drug interactions are listed below:

1. Drugs which may increase phenytoin serum levels include: chloramphenicol, dicumarol, disulfiram, tolbutamide, isoniazid, phenylbutazone, acute alcohol intake, salicylates, chlordiazepoxide, phenothiazines, diazepam, estrogens, ethosuximide, halothane, methylphenidate, sulfonamides, cimetidine, trazodone.
2. Drugs which may decrease phenytoin levels include: carbamazepine, chronic alcohol abuse, reserpine. Moban® brand of Molindone Hydrochloride contains calcium ions which interfere with the absorption of phenytoin. Ingestion times of phenytoin and antacid preparations containing calcium should be staggered in patients with low serum phenytoin levels to prevent absorption problems.
3. Drugs which may either increase or decrease phenytoin serum levels include: phenobarbital, valproic acid, and sodium valproate. Similarly, the effect of phenytoin on phenobarbital, valproic acid and sodium valproate serum levels is unpredictable.
4. Although not a true drug interaction, tricyclic antidepressants may precipitate seizures in susceptible patients and phenytoin dosage may need to be adjusted.
5. Drugs whose efficacy is impaired by phenytoin include: corticosteroids, coumarin anticoagulants, oral contraceptives, quinidine, vitamin D, digitoxin, rifampin, doxycycline, estrogens, furosemide.

Serum level determinations are especially helpful when possible drug interactions are suspected.

Drug/Laboratory Test Interactions:

Phenytoin may cause decreased serum levels of protein-bound iodine (PBI). It may also produce lower than normal values for dexamethasone or metyrapone tests. Phenytoin may cause raised serum levels of glucose, alkaline phosphatase, and gamma glutamyl transpeptidase (GGT).

Carcinogenesis:

See 'Warnings' section for information on carcinogenesis.

Pregnancy:

See Warnings

Nursing Mothers:

Infant breast feeding is not recommended for women taking this drug because phenytoin appears to be secreted in low concentrations in human milk.

ADVERSE REACTIONS

Central Nervous System: The most common manifestations encountered with phenytoin therapy are referable to this system and are usually dose-related. These include nystagmus, ataxia, slurred speech, and mental confusion. Dizziness, insomnia, transient nervousness, motor twitchings, and headaches have also been observed. There have also been rare reports of phenytoin induced dyskinesias, including chorea, dystonia, tremor and asterixis, similar to those induced by phenothiazine and other neuroleptic drugs.

A predominantly sensory peripheral polyneuropathy has been observed in patients receiving long-term phenytoin therapy.

Gastrointestinal System: Nausea, vomiting and constipation.

Integumentary System: Dermatological manifestations sometimes accompanied by fever have included scarlatiniform or morbilliform rashes. A morbilliform rash (measles-like) is the most common; other types of dermatitis are seen more rarely. Other more serious forms which may be fatal have included bullous, exfoliative or purpuric dermatitis, lupus erythematosus, and Stevens-Johnson syndrome (see Precautions).

Hemopoietic System: Hemopoietic complications, some fatal, have occasionally been reported in association with administration of phenytoin. These have included thrombocytopenia, leukopenia, granulocytopenia, agranulocytosis, and pancytopenia. While macrocytosis and megaloblastic anemia have occurred, these conditions usually respond to folic acid therapy. Lymphadenopathy including benign lymph node hyperplasia, pseudolymphoma, lymphoma, and Hodgkin's Disease have been reported (see Warnings).

Connective Tissue System: Coarsening of the facial features, enlargement of the lips, gingival hyperplasia, hirsutism, and Peyronie's Disease.

Other: Systemic lupus erythematosus, periarteritis nodosa, toxic hepatitis, liver damage, and immunoglobulin abnormalities may occur.

OVERDOSAGE

The lethal dose in children is not known. The lethal dose in adults is estimated to be 2 to 5 grams. The initial symptoms are nystagmus, ataxia, and dysarthria. Other signs are tremor, hyperflexia, lethargy, slurred speech, nausea, vomiting. The patient may become comatose and hypertensive. Death is due to respiratory and circulatory depression.

There are marked variations among individuals with respect to phenytoin plasma levels where toxicity may occur. Nystagmus, on lateral gaze, usually appears at 20 mcg/ml, ataxia at 30 mcg/ml, dysarthria and lethargy appear when the plasma concentration is over 40 mcg/ml, but as high a concentration as 50 mcg/ml has been reported without evidence of toxicity. As much as 25 times the therapeutic dose has been taken to result in a serum concentration over 100 mcg/ml with complete recovery.

Treatment:

Treatment is nonspecific since there is no known antidote. The adequacy of the respiratory and circulatory systems should be carefully observed and appropriate supportive measures employed. Hemodialysis can be considered since phenytoin is not completely bound to plasma proteins. Total exchange transfusion has been used in the treatment of severe intoxication in children.

In acute overdosage the possibility of other CNS depressants, including alcohol, should be borne in mind.

DOSAGE AND ADMINISTRATION

Serum concentrations should be monitored in changing from extended Phenytoin Sodium Capsules USP (Dilantin) to Prompt Phenytoin sodium capsules USP, and from the sodium salt to the free acid form.

Dilantin® Kapseals,® Dilantin Parenteral, and Dilantin with Phenobarbital are formulated with the sodium salt of phenytoin. The free acid form of phenytoin is used in Dilantin-30 Pediatric and Dilantin-125 Suspensions and Dilantin Infatabs. Because there is approximately an 8% increase in drug content with the free acid form than the sodium salt, dosage adjustments and serum level monitoring may be necessary when switching from a product formulated with the free acid to a product formulated with the sodium salt and vice versa.

General:

Dosage should be individualized to provide maximum benefit. In some cases serum blood level determinations may be necessary for optimal dosage adjustments—the clinically effective serum level is usually 10-20 mcg/ml. With recommended dosage, a period of seven to ten days may be required to achieve steady-state blood levels with phenytoin and changes in dosage (increase or decrease) should not be carried out at intervals shorter than seven to ten days.

Adult Dosage:

Divided Daily Dosage

Patients who have received no previous treatment may be started on one 100 mg Dilantin (Extended Phenytoin Sodium Capsule) three times daily and the dosage then adjusted to suit individual requirements. For most adults, the satisfactory maintenance dosage will be one capsule three to four times a day. An increase up to two capsules three times a day may be made, if necessary.

Once-a-Day Dosage:

In adults, if seizure control is established with divided doses of three 100 mg Dilantin capsules daily, once-a-day dosage with 300 mg of extended phenytoin sodium capsules may be considered. Studies comparing divided doses of 300 mg with a single daily dose of this quantity indicated absorption, peak plasma levels, biologic half-life, difference between peak and minimum values, and urinary recovery were equivalent. Once-a-day dosage offers a convenience to the individual patient or to nursing personnel for institutionalized patients and is intended to be used only for patients requiring this amount of drug daily. A major problem in motivating noncompliant patients may also be lessened when the patient can take this drug once a day. However, patients should be cautioned not to miss a dose, inadvertently.

Only extended phenytoin sodium capsules are recommended for once-a-day dosing. Inherent differences in dissolution characteristics and resultant absorption rates of phenytoin due to different manufacturing procedures and/or dosage forms preclude such recommendation for other phenytoin products. When a change in the dosage form or brand is prescribed, careful monitoring of phenytoin serum levels should be carried out.

Loading Dose:

Some authorities have advocated use of an oral loading dose of phenytoin in adults who require rapid steady-state serum levels and where intravenous administration is not desirable. This dosing regimen should be reserved for patients in a clinic or hospital setting where phenytoin serum levels can be closely monitored. Patients with a history of renal or liver disease should not receive the oral loading regimen.

Initially, one gram of phenytoin capsules is divided into 3 doses (400 mg, 300 mg, 300 mg) and administered at two-hourly intervals. Normal maintenance dosage is then instituted 24 hours after the loading dose, with frequent serum level determinations.

Pediatric Dosage:

Initially, 5 mg/kg/day in two or three equally divided doses, with subsequent dosage individualized to a maximum of 300 mg daily. A recommended daily maintenance dosage is usually 4 to 8 mg/kg. Children over 6 years old may require the minimum adult dose (300 mg/day).

HOW SUPPLIED

N 0071-0362 (Kapseal 362)—Dilantin 100 mg; in 100's, 1,000's, and unit dose 100's and in a Memo Pack containing 84 unit dose capsules (28 days dosage regimen).

N 0071-0365 (Kapseal 365)—Dilantin 30 mg; in 100's, 1,000's and unit dose 100's.

Shown in Product Identification Section, page 420

Also available as:

N 0071-2214—Dilantin-125® Suspension 125 mg phenytoin/5 ml with a maximum alcohol content not greater than 0.6 percent, available in 8-oz bottles and individual unit dose foil pouches which deliver 5 ml (125 mg phenytoin). The minimum sales unit is 100 pouches.

N 0071-2315—Dilantin-30® Pediatric Suspension 30 mg phenytoin/5 ml with a maximum alcohol content not greater than 0.6 percent; available in 8-oz bottles and individual unit dose foil pouches which deliver 5 ml (30 mg phenytoin). The minimum sales unit is 100 pouches.

N 0071-0375 (Kapseal 375)—Dilantin with Phenobarbital each contain 100 mg phenytoin sodium with 16 mg (¼ gr) phenobarbital; in 100's and 1,000's.

N 0071-0531 (Kapseal 531)—Dilantin with Phenobarbital each contain 100 mg phenytoin sodium with 32 mg (½ gr) phenobarbital; in 100's, 1,000's and unit dose 100's.

N 0071-0007 (Tablet 7)—Dilantin Infatabs® each contain 50 mg phenytoin, 100's and unit dose 100's.

For Parenteral Use:

N 0071-4488-05 (Ampoule 1488)—Dilantin ready-mixed solution containing 50 mg phenytoin sodium per milliliter is supplied in 2-ml ampoules. Packages of ten.

N 0071-4488-41 (Steri-Dose® 4488)—Dilantin ready-mixed solution containing 50 mg phenytoin sodium per milliliter is supplied in a 2-ml sterile disposable syringe (22 gauge × 1¼ inch needle). Packages of ten individually cartoned syringes.

N 0071-4475-35 (Ampoule 1475)—Dilantin ready-mixed solution containing 50 mg phenytoin sodium per milliliter is supplied in 5-ml ampoules with one 6-ml sterile disposable syringe (22 gauge × 1¼ inch needle). Packages of ten.

N 0071-4475-08 (Ampoule 1475)—Dilantin ready-mixed solution containing 50 mg phenytoin sodium per milliliter is supplied in packages of ten 5-ml ampoules without syringes.

Store below 30°C (86°F). Protect from light and moisture.

0362G023

INFATABS®
DILANTIN® ℞
[*dī-lăn'tĭn" ĭn'fă-tăbs"*]
(Phenytoin Tablets, USP)

NOT FOR ONCE A DAY DOSING

DESCRIPTION

Dilantin is an antiepileptic drug.

Dilantin (phenytoin) is related to the barbiturates in chemical structure, but has a five-membered ring. The chemical name is 5,5-diphenyl-2,4-imidazolidinedione.

Each Dilantin Infatab, for oral administration, contains 50 mg phenytoin, USP. Also contains: D&C yellow No. 10, Al lake; FD&C yellow No. 6, Al lake flavor; saccharin sodium, USP; sucrose, NF; talc, USP; and other ingredients.

CLINICAL PHARMACOLOGY

Phenytoin is an antiepileptic drug which can be useful in the treatment of epilepsy. The primary site of action appears to be the motor cortex where spread of seizure activity is inhibited. Possibly by promoting sodium efflux from neurons, phenytoin tends to stabilize the threshold against hyperexcitability caused by excessive stimulation or environmental changes capable of reducing membrane sodium gradient. This includes the reduction of posttetanic potentiation at synapses. Loss of posttetanic potentiation prevents cortical seizure foci from detonating adjacent cortical areas. Phenytoin reduces the maximal activity of brain stem centers responsible for the tonic phase of tonic-clonic (grand mal) seizures.

Clinical studies using Dilantin Infatabs have shown an average plasma half-life of 14 hours with a range of 7 to 29 hours. Steady-state therapeutic levels are achieved at least 7 to 10 days (5-7 half-lives) after initiation of therapy with recommended doses of 300 mg/day.

When serum level determinations are necessary, they should be obtained at least 5-7 half-lives after treatment initiation, dosage change, or addition or subtraction of another drug to the regimen so that equilibrium or steady-state will have been achieved. Trough levels provide information about clinically effective serum level range and confirm patient compliance and are obtained just prior to the patient's next scheduled dose. Peak levels indicate an individual's threshold for emergence of dose-related side effects and are obtained at the time of expected peak concentration. For Dilantin Infatabs peak levels occur 1½-3 hours after administration.

Optimum control without clinical signs of toxicity occurs more often with serum levels between 10 and 20 mcg/ml, although some mild cases of tonic-clonic (grand mal) epilepsy may be controlled with lower-serum levels of phenytoin.

In most patients maintained at a steady dosage, stable phenytoin serum levels are achieved. There may be wide interpatient variability in phenytoin serum levels with equivalent dosages. Patients with unusually low levels may be noncompliant or hypermetabolizers of phenytoin. Unusually high levels result from liver disease, congenital enzyme deficiency or drug interactions which result in metabolic interference. The patient with large variations in phenytoin plasma levels, despite standard doses, presents a difficult clinical problem. Serum level determinations in such patients may be particularly helpful.

Most of the drug is excreted in the bile as inactive metabolites which are then reabsorbed from the intestinal tract and excreted in the urine. Urinary excretion of phenytoin and its metabolites occurs partly with glomerular filtration but more importantly, by tubular secretion. Because phenytoin is hydroxylated in the liver by an enzyme system which is saturable at high plasma levels small incremental doses may increase the half-life and produce very substantial increases in serum levels, when these are in the upper range. The steady-state level may be disproportionately increased, with resultant intoxication, from an increase in dosage of 10% or more.

Clinical studies show that chewed and unchewed Dilantin Infatabs are bioequivalent, yield approximately equivalent plasma levels, and are more rapidly absorbed than 100-mg Dilantin Kapseals.®

INDICATIONS AND USAGE

Dilantin Infatabs (Phenytoin Tablets, USP) are indicated for the control of generalized tonic-clonic (grand mal) and complex partial (psychomotor, temporal lobe) seizures and prevention and treatment of seizures occurring during or following neurosurgery. Phenytoin serum level determinations may be necessary for optimal dosage adjustments (see Dosage and Administration and Clinical Pharmacology).

CONTRAINDICATIONS

Phenytoin is contraindicated in those patients who are hypersensitive to phenytoin or other hydantoins.

WARNINGS

Abrupt withdrawal of phenytoin in epileptic patients may precipitate status epilepticus. When, in the judgment of the clinician, the need for dosage reduction, discontinuation, or substitution of alternative antiepileptic medication arises, this should be done gradually. However, in the event of an allergic or hypersensitivity reaction, rapid substitution of alternative therapy may be necessary. In this case, alternative therapy should be an antiepileptic drug not belonging to the hydantoin chemical class.

There have been a number of reports suggesting a relationship between phenytoin and the development of lymphadenopathy (local or generalized) including benign lymph node hyperplasia, pseudolymphoma, lymphoma, and Hodgkin's Disease. Although a cause and effect relationship has not been established, the occurrence of lymphadenopathy indicates the need to differentiate such a condition from other types of lymph node pathology. Lymph node involvement may occur with or without symptoms and signs resembling serum sickness eg, fever, rash and liver involvement. In all cases of lymphadenopathy, follow-up observation for an extended period is indicated and every effort should be made to achieve seizure control using alternative antiepileptic drugs. Acute alcoholic intake may increase phenytoin serum levels while chronic alcoholic use may decrease serum levels.

Usage in Pregnancy

A number of reports suggest an association between the use of antiepileptic drugs by women with epilepsy and a higher incidence of birth defects in children born to these women. Data are more extensive with respect to phenytoin and phenobarbital, but these are also the most commonly prescribed antiepileptic drugs; less systematic or anecdotal reports suggest a possible similar association with the use of all known antiepileptic drugs.

The reports suggesting a higher incidence of birth defects in children of drug-treated epileptic women cannot be regarded as adequate to prove a definite cause and effect relationship. There are intrinsic methodologic problems in obtaining adequate data on drug teratogenicity in humans: genetic factors or the epileptic condition itself, may be more important than drug therapy in leading to birth defects. The great majority of mothers on antiepileptic medication deliver normal infants. It is important to note that antiepileptic drugs should not be discontinued in patients in whom the drug is administered to prevent major seizures, because of the strong possibility of precipitating status epilepticus with attendant hypoxia and threat to life. In individual cases where the severity and frequency of the seizure disorder are such that the removal of medication does not pose a serious threat to the patient, discontinuation of the drug may be considered prior to and during pregnancy, although it cannot be said with any confidence that even minor seizures do not pose some hazard to the developing embryo or fetus. The prescribing physician will wish to weigh these considerations in treating or counseling epileptic women of childbearing potential.

In addition to the reports of increased incidence of congenital malformations, such as cleft lip/palate and heart malformations in children of women receiving phenytoin and other antiepileptic drugs, there have more recently been reports of a fetal hydantoin syndrome. This consists of prenatal growth deficiency, microcephaly and mental deficiency in children born to mothers who have received phenytoin, barbiturates, alcohol, or trimethadione. However, these features are all interrelated and are frequently associated with intrauterine growth retardation from other causes.

There have been isolated reports of malignancies, including neuroblastoma, in children whose mothers received phenytoin during pregnancy.

An increase in seizure frequency during pregnancy occurs in a high proportion of patients, because of altered phenytoin absorption or metabolism. Periodic measurement of serum phenytoin levels is particularly valuable in the management of a pregnant epileptic patient as a guide to an appropriate adjustment of dosage. However, postpartum restoration of the original dosage will probably be indicated.

Neonatal coagulation defects have been reported within the first 24 hours in babies born to epileptic mothers receiving phenobarbital and/or phenytoin. Vitamin K has been shown to prevent or correct this defect and has been recommended to be given to the mother before delivery and to the neonate after birth.

Continued on next page

This product information was prepared in August, 1986. On these and other Parke-Davis Products, information may be obtained by addressing PARKE-DAVIS, Division of Warner-Lambert Company, Morris Plains, New Jersey 07950.

Parke-Davis—Cont.

PRECAUTIONS

General

The liver is the chief site of biotransformation of phenytoin; patients with impaired liver function, elderly patients, or those who are gravely ill may show early signs of toxicity.

A small percentage of individuals who have been treated with phenytoin have been shown to metabolize the drug slowly. Slow metabolism may be due to limited enzyme availability and lack of induction; it appears to be genetically determined.

Phenytoin should be discontinued if a skin rash appears (see "Warnings" section regarding drug discontinuation). If the rash is exfoliative, purpuric, or bullous or if lupus erythematosus or Stevens-Johnson syndrome is suspected, use of the drug should not be resumed, and alternative therapy should be considered (see Adverse Reactions). If the rash is of a milder type (measles-like or scarlatiniform), therapy may be resumed after the rash has completely disappeared. If the rash recurs upon reinstitution of therapy, further phenytoin medication is contraindicated.

Hyperglycemia, resulting from the drug's inhibitory effects on insulin release, has been reported. Phenytoin may also raise the serum glucose level in diabetic patients.

Osteomalacia has been associated with phenytoin therapy and is considered to be due to phenytoin's interference with Vitamin D metabolism.

Phenytoin is not indicated for seizures due to hypoglycemic or other metabolic causes. Appropriate diagnostic procedures should be performed as indicated.

Phenytoin is not effective for absence (petit mal) seizures. If tonic-clonic (grand-mal) and absence (petit mal) seizures are present, combined drug therapy is needed.

Serum levels of phenytoin sustained above the optimal range may produce confusional states referred to as "delirium," "psychosis," or "encephalopathy," or rarely irreversible cerebellar dysfunction. Accordingly, at the first sign of acute toxicity, plasma levels are recommended. Dose reduction of phenytoin therapy is indicated if plasma levels are excessive, if symptoms persist, termination is recommended. (See Warnings).

Information for Patients

Patients taking phenytoin should be advised of the importance of adhering strictly to the prescribed dosage regimen, and of informing the physician of any clinical condition in which it is not possible to take the drug orally as prescribed, eg, surgery, etc.

Patients should also be cautioned on the use of other drugs or alcoholic beverages without first seeking the physician's advice.

Patients should be instructed to call their physician if skin rash develops.

The importance of good dental hygiene should be stressed in order to minimize the development of gingival hyperplasia and its complications.

Laboratory Tests

Phenytoin serum level determinations may be necessary to achieve optimal dosage adjustments.

Drug Interactions

There are many drugs which may increase or decrease phenytoin levels or which phenytoin may affect. The most commonly occurring drug interactions are listed below:

1. Drugs which may increase phenytoin serum levels include: chloramphenicol, dicumarol, disulfiram, tolbutamide, isoniazid, phenylbutazone, acute alcohol intake, salicylates, chlordiazepoxide, phenothiazines, diazepam, estrogens, ethosuximide, halothane, methylphenidate, sulfonamides, cimetidine, trazodone.
2. Drugs which may decrease phenytoin serum levels include: carbamazepine, chronic alcohol abuse, reserpine. Moban® brand of Molindone Hydrochloride contains calcium ions which interfere with the absorption of phenytoin. Ingestion times of phenytoin and antacid preparations containing calcium should be staggered in patients with low serum phenytoin levels to prevent absorption problems.
3. Drugs which may either increase or decrease phenytoin serum levels include: Phenobarbital, valproic acid, and sodium valproate. Similarly, the effect of phenytoin on phenobarbital, valproic acid and sodium valproate serum levels is unpredictable.
4. Although not a true drug interaction, tricyclic antidepressants may precipitate seizures in susceptible patients and phenytoin dosage may need to be adjusted.
5. Drugs whose efficacy is impaired by phenytoin include: corticosteroids, coumarin anticoagulants, oral contraceptives, quinidine, vitamin D, digitoxin, rifampin, doxycycline, estrogens, furosemide.

Serum level determinations are especially helpful when possible drug interactions are suspected.

Drug/Laboratory Test Interactions

Phenytoin may cause decreased serum levels of protein-bound iodine (PBI). It may also produce lower than normal values for dexamethasone or metyrapone tests. Phenytoin may cause increased serum levels of glucose, alkaline phosphatase, and gamma glutamyl transpeptidase (GGT).

Carcinogenesis

See 'Warnings' section for information on carcinogenesis.

Pregnancy

See Warnings

Nursing Mothers

Infant breast-feeding is not recommended for women taking this drug because phenytoin appears to be secreted in low concentrations in human milk.

ADVERSE REACTIONS

Central Nervous System: The most common manifestations encountered with phenytoin therapy are referable to this system and are usually dose-related. These include nystagmus, ataxia, slurred speech, decreased coordination and mental confusion. Dizziness, insomnia, transient nervousness, motor twitchings, and headache have also been observed.

There have also been rare reports of phenytoin induced dyskinesias, including chorea, dystonia, tremor and asterixis, similar to those induced by phenothiazine and other neuroleptic drugs.

A predominantly sensory peripheral polyneuropathy has been observed in patients receiving long-term phenytoin therapy.

Gastrointestinal System: Nausea, vomiting, and constipation.

Integumentary System: Dermatological manifestations sometimes accompanied by fever have included scarlatiniform or morbilliform rashes. A morbilliform rash (measles-like) is the most common; other types of dermatitis are seen more rarely. Other more serious forms which may be fatal have included bullous, exfoliative or purpuric dermatitis, lupus erythematosus, and Stevens-Johnson syndrome (see Precautions).

Hemopoietic System: Hemopoietic complications, some fatal, have occasionally been reported in association with administration of phenytoin. These have included thrombocytopenia, leukopenia, granulocytopenia, agranulocytosis, and pancytopenia with or without bone marrow suppression. While macrocytosis and megaloblastic anemia have occurred, these conditions usually respond to folic acid therapy. Lymphadenopathy including benign lymph node hyperplasia, pseudolymphoma, lymphoma, and Hodgkin's Disease have been reported (see Warnings).

Connective Tissue System: Coarsening of the facial features, enlargement of the lips, gingival hyperplasia, hypertrichosis, and Peyronie's Disease.

Other: Systemic lupus erythematosus, periarteritis nodosa, toxic hepatitis, liver damage, and immunoglobulin abnormalities may occur.

OVERDOSAGE

The lethal dose in children is not known. The lethal dose in adults is estimated to be 2 to 5 grams. The initial symptoms are nystagmus, ataxia, and dysarthria. Other signs are tremor, hyperflexia, lethargy, slurred speech, nausea, vomiting. The patient may become comatose and hypertensive. Death is due to respiratory and circulatory depression.

There are marked variations among individuals with respect to phenytoin plasma levels where toxicity may occur. Nystagmus on lateral gaze usually appears at 20 mcg/ml, ataxia at 30 mcg/ml, dysarthria and lethargy appear when the plasma concentration is over 40 mcg/ml, but as high a concentration as 50 mcg/ml has been reported without evidence of toxicity. As much as 25 times the therapeutic dose has been taken to result in a serum concentration over 100 mcg/ml with complete recovery.

Treatment

Treatment is nonspecific since there is no known antidote. The adequacy of the respiratory and circulatory systems should be carefully observed and appropriate supportive measures employed. Hemodialysis can be considered since phenytoin is not completely bound to plasma proteins. Total exchange transfusion has been used in the treatment of severe intoxication in children.

In acute overdosage the possibility of other CNS depressants, including alcohol, should be borne in mind.

DOSAGE AND ADMINISTRATION

When given in equal doses, Dilantin Infatabs yield higher plasma levels than Dilantin Kapseals.® For this reason serum concentrations should be monitored and care should be taken when switching a patient from the sodium salt to the free acid form.

Dilantin® Kapseals,® Dilantin Parenteral, and Dilantin with Phenobarbital are formulated with the sodium salt of phenytoin. The free acid form of phenytoin is used in Dilantin-30 Pediatric and Dilantin-125 Suspensions and Dilantin Infatabs. Because there is approximately an 8% increase in drug content with the free acid form over that of the sodium salt, dosage adjustments and serum level monitoring may be necessary when switching from a product formulated with the free acid to a product formulated with the sodium salt and vice versa.

General

Not for once a day dosing.

Dosage should be individualized to provide maximum benefit. In some cases, serum blood level determinations may be necessary for optimal dosage adjustments—the clinically effective serum level is usually 10–20 mcg/ml. With recommended dosage, a period of seven to ten days may be required to achieve steady-state blood levels with phenytoin and changes in dosage (increase or decrease) should not be carried out at intervals shorter than seven to ten days.

Dilantin Infatabs can be either chewed thoroughly before being swallowed or swallowed whole.

Adult Dosage

Patients who have received no previous treatment may be started on two Infatabs three times daily, and the dose is then adjusted to suit individual requirements. For most adults, the satisfactory maintenance dosage will be six to eight Infatabs daily; an increase to twelve Infatabs daily may be made, if necessary.

Pediatric Dosage

Initially, 5 mg/kg/day in two or three equally divided doses, with subsequent dosage individualized to a maximum of 300 mg daily. A recommended daily maintenance dosage is usually 4 to 8 mg/kg. Children over 6 years old may require the minimum adult dose (300 mg/day). If the daily dosage cannot be divided equally, the larger dose should be given before retiring.

HOW SUPPLIED

Dilantin Infatabs are supplied as:
N 0071-0007-24—Bottle of 100.
N 0071-0007-40—Unit dose (10/10's).
Each tablet contains 50 mg phenytoin.

Shown in Product Identification Section, page 420

Store at controlled room temperature (59°–86°F).
Protect from moisture.
Dilantin is also supplied in the following forms:
N 0071-0362-24—Bottle of 100.
N 0071-0362-32—Bottle of 1000.
N 0071-0362-40—Unit dose (10/10's).
Each capsule contains 100 mg phenytoin sodium.
N 0071-0365-24—Bottle of 100.
N 0071-0365-32—Bottle of 1000.
N 0071-0365-40—Unit dose (10/10's).
Each capsule contains 30 mg phenytoin sodium.
N 0071-2214-20—8 oz bottle.
N 0071-2214-40—Unit dose pouches (5 ml × 100).
Each 5 ml of suspension contains 125 mg phenytoin with a maximum alcohol content not greater than 0.6 percent.
N 0071-2315-20—8 oz bottle.
N 0071-2315-40—Unit dose pouches (5 ml × 100).
Each 5 ml of suspension contains 30 mg phenytoin with a maximum alcohol content not greater than 0.6 percent.
N 0071-0375-24—Bottle of 100.
N 0071-0375-32—Bottle of 1000.
Each capsule contains phenytoin sodium 100 mg and phenobarbital 16 mg (1/4 gr).
N 0071-0531-24—Bottle of 100.
N 0071-0531-32—Bottle of 1000.
N 0071-0531-40—Unit dose (10/10's).
Each capsule contains phenytoin sodium 100 mg and phenobarbital 32 mg (1/2 gr).
N 0071-4488-05—2-ml ampoules.
A sterile solution for parenteral use containing 50 mg phenytoin sodium per ml. Supplied in packages of ten.
N 0071-4488-41—2-ml prefilled syringes.
A sterile solution for parenteral use containing 50 mg phenytoin sodium per ml in an individually cartoned disposable syringe (22 gauge × 1 1/4 inch needle). Supplied in packages of ten.
N 0071-4475-35—5-ml ampoules with syringes.
A sterile solution for parenteral use containing 50 mg phenytoin sodium per ml. One 6-ml sterile disposable syringe (22 gauge ×1 1/4 inch needle). Supplied in packages of ten.
N 0071-4475-08—5-ml ampoules.
A sterile solution for parenteral use containing 50 mg phenytoin sodium per ml. Supplied in packages of ten.

0007G043

Parenteral
DILANTIN® ℞
[dī-lăn′ tĭn″]
(Phenytoin Sodium Injection, USP)

IMPORTANT NOTE
This drug must be administered slowly. In adults do not exceed 50 mg per minute intravenously. In neonates, the drug should be administered at a rate not exceeding 1–3 mg/kg/min.

DESCRIPTION

Dilantin (phenytoin sodium injection, USP) is a ready-mixed solution of phenytoin sodium in a vehicle containing 40%

propylene glycol and 10% alcohol in water for injection, adjusted to pH 12 with sodium hydroxide. Phenytoin sodium is related to the barbiturates in chemical structure, but has a five-membered ring. The chemical name is sodium 5,5-diphenyl-2,4-imidazolidinedione.

CLINICAL PHARMACOLOGY

Phenytoin is an anticonvulsant which may be useful in the treatment of status epilepticus of the grand mal type. The primary site of action appears to be the motor cortex where spread of seizure activity is inhibited. Possibly by promoting sodium efflux from neurons, phenytoin tends to stabilize the threshold against hyperexcitability caused by excessive stimulation or environmental changes capable of reducing membrane sodium gradient. This includes the reduction of posttetanic potentiation at synapses. Loss of posttetanic potentiation prevents cortical seizure foci from detonating adjacent cortical areas. Phenytoin reduces the maximal activity of brain stem centers responsible for the tonic phase of grand mal seizures.

The plasma half-life in man after intravenous administration ranges from 10 to 15 hours. Optimum control without clinical signs of toxicity occurs most often with serum levels between 10 and 20 mcg/mL.

A fall in plasma levels may occur when patients are changed from oral to intramuscular administration. The drop is caused by slower absorption, as compared to oral administration, due to the poor water solubility of phenytoin. Intravenous administration is the preferred route for producing rapid therapeutic serum levels.

There are occasions when intramuscular administration may be required, ie, postoperatively, in comatose patients, for GI upsets. During these periods, a sufficient dose must be administered intramuscularly to maintain the plasma level within the therapeutic range. Where oral dosage is resumed following intramuscular usage, the oral dose should be properly adjusted to compensate for the slow, continuing IM absorption to avoid toxic symptoms.

Patients stabilized on a daily oral regimen of Dilantin experience a drop in peak blood levels to 50–60 percent of stable levels if crossed over to an equal dose administered intramuscularly. However, the intramuscular depot of poorly soluble material is eventually absorbed, as determined by urinary excretion of 5-(p-hydroxyphenyl)-5-phenylhydantoin (HPPH), the principal metabolite, as well as the total amount of drug eventually appearing in the blood.

A short-term (one week) study indicates that patients do not experience the expected drop in blood levels when crossed over to the intramuscular route if the Dilantin IM dose is increased by 50 percent over the previously established oral dose. To avoid drug cumulation due to absorption from the muscle depots, it is recommended that for the first week back on oral Dilantin, the dose be reduced to half of the original oral dose (one third of the IM dose). Experience for periods greater than one week is lacking and blood level monitoring is recommended. For administration of Dilantin in patients who cannot take oral medication for periods greater than a week, gastric intubation may be considered.

INDICATIONS

Parenteral Dilantin is indicated for the control of status epilepticus of the grand mal type, and prevention and treatment of seizures occurring during neurosurgery.

CONTRAINDICATIONS

Phenytoin is contraindicated in patients with a history of hypersensitivity to hydantoin products.

Because of its effect on ventricular automaticity, phenytoin is contraindicated in sinus bradycardia, sino-atrial block, second and third degree A-V block, and patients with Adams-Stokes syndrome.

WARNINGS

Intravenous administration should not exceed 50 mg per minute in adults. In neonates, the drug should be administered at a rate not exceeding 1–3mg/kg/min.

Severe cardiotoxic reactions and fatalities have been reported with atrial and ventricular conduction depression and ventricular fibrillation. Severe complications are most commonly encountered in elderly or gravely ill patients.

Phenytoin should be used with caution in patients with hypotension and severe myocardial insufficiency.

Hypotension usually occurs when the drug is administered rapidly by the intravenous route.

The intramuscular route is not recommended for the treatment of status epilepticus since blood levels of phenytoin in the therapeutic range cannot be readily achieved with doses and methods of administration ordinarily employed.

There have been a number of reports suggesting a relationship between phenytoin and the development of lymphadenopathy (local or generalized) including benign lymph node hyperplasia, pseudolymphoma, lymphoma, and Hodgkin's Disease. Although a cause and effect relationship has not been established, the occurrence of lymphadenopathy indicates the need to differentiate such a condition from other types of lymph node pathology. Lymph node involvement may occur with or without symptoms and signs resembling serum sickness eg, fever, rash and liver involvement.

In all cases of lymphadenopathy, follow-up observation for an extended period is indicated and every effort should be made to achieve seizure control using alternative antiepileptic drugs.

Acute alcoholic intake may increase phenytoin serum levels while chronic alcoholic use may decrease serum levels.

Usage in Pregnancy: A number of reports suggests an association between the use of antiepileptic drugs by women with epilepsy and a higher incidence of birth defects in children born to these women. Data are more extensive with respect to phenytoin and phenobarbital, but these are also the most commonly prescribed antiepileptic drugs; less systematic or anecdotal reports suggest a possible similar association with the use of all known antiepileptic drugs.

The reports suggesting a higher incidence of birth defects in children of drug-treated epileptic women cannot be regarded as adequate to prove a definite cause and effect relationship. There are intrinsic methodologic problems in obtaining adequate data on drug teratogenicity in humans; genetic factors or the epileptic condition itself may be more important than drug therapy in leading to birth defects. The great majority of mothers on antiepileptic medication deliver normal infants. It is important to note that antiepileptic drugs should not be discontinued in patients in whom the drug is administered to prevent major seizures, because of the strong possibility of precipitating status epilepticus with attendant hypoxia and threat to life. In individual cases where the severity and frequency of the seizure disorder are such that the removal of medication does not pose a serious threat to the patient, discontinuation of the drug may be considered prior to and during pregnancy, although it cannot be said with any confidence that even minor seizures do not pose some hazard to the developing embryo or fetus. The prescribing physician will wish to weigh these considerations in treating or counseling epileptic women of childbearing potential.

In addition to the reports of increased incidence of congenital malformation, such as cleft lip/palate and heart malformations in children of women receiving phenytoin and other antiepileptic drugs, there have more recently been reports of a fetal hydantoin syndrome. This consists of prenatal growth deficiency, microcephaly and mental deficiency in children born to mothers who have received phenytoin, barbiturates, alcohol, or trimethadione. However, these features are all interrelated and are frequently associated with intrauterine growth retardation from other causes.

There have been isolated reports of malignancies, including neuroblastoma, in children whose mothers received phenytoin during pregnancy.

An increase in seizure frequency during pregnancy occurs in a high proportion of patients, because of altered phenytoin absorption or metabolism. Periodic measurement of serum phenytoin levels is particularly valuable in the management of a pregnant epileptic patient as a guide to an appropriate adjustment of dosage. However, postpartum restoration of the original dosage will probably be indicated.

Neonatal coagulation defects have been reported within the first 24 hours in babies born to epileptic mothers receiving phenobarbital and/or phenytoin. Vitamin K has been shown to prevent or correct this defect and has been recommended to be given to the mother before delivery and the neonate after birth.

PRECAUTIONS

General: The addition of Dilantin solution to intravenous infusion is not recommended due to lack of solubility and resultant precipitation.

The liver is the site of biotransformation. Patients with impaired liver function, elderly patients, or those who are gravely ill may show early toxicity.

A small percentage of individuals who have been treated with phenytoin have been shown to metabolize the drug slowly. Slow metabolism may be due to limited enzyme availability and lack of induction; it appears to be genetically determined.

Phenytoin should be discontinued if a skin rash appears (see "Warnings" section regarding drug discontinuation). If the rash is exfoliative, purpuric, or bullous or if lupus erythematosus or Stevens-Johnson syndrome is suspected, use of this drug should not be resumed and alternative therapy should be considered. (See Adverse Reactions.) If the rash is of a milder type (measles-like or scarlatiniform), therapy may be resumed after the rash has completely disappeared. If the rash recurs upon reinstitution of therapy, further phenytoin medication is contraindicated.

Hyperglycemia, resulting from the drug's inhibitory effects on insulin release, has been reported. Phenytoin may also raise the serum glucose level in diabetic patients.

Phenytoin is not indicated for seizures due to hypoglycemic or other metabolic causes. Appropriate diagnostic procedures should be performed as indicated.

Each injection of intravenous Dilantin should be followed by an injection of sterile saline through the same needle or intravenous catheter to avoid local venous irritation due to the alkalinity of the solution. Continuous infusion should be avoided.

Soft tissue irritation and inflammation has occurred at the site of injection with and without extravasation of intravenous phenytoin. Soft tissue irritation varying from slight tenderness to extensive necrosis and sloughing has been noted. Subcutaneous or perivascular injection should be avoided.

Phenytoin is not effective for absence (petit mal) seizures. If tonic-clonic (grand-mal) and absence (petit mal) seizures are present, combined drug therapy is needed.

Serum levels of phenytoin sustained above the optimal range may produce confusional states referred to as "delirium," "psychosis," or "encephalopathy," or rarely irreversible cerebellar dysfunction. Accordingly, at the first sign of acute toxicity, plasma levels are recommended. Dose reduction of phenytoin therapy is indicated if plasma levels are excessive; if symptoms persist, termination is recommended. (See Warnings)

Laboratory Tests: Phenytoin serum level determinations may be necessary to achieve optimal dosage adjustments.

Drug Interactions: There are many drugs which may increase or decrease phenytoin levels or which phenytoin may affect. The most commonly occurring drug interactions are listed below:

1. Drugs which may increase phenytoin serum levels include: chloramphenicol, dicumarol, disulfiram, tolbutamide, isoniazid, phenylbutazone, acute alcohol intake, salicylates, chlordiazepoxide, phenothiazines, diazepam, estrogens, ethosuximide, halothane, methylphenidate, sulfonamides, cimetidine, trazodone.
2. Drugs which may decrease phenytoin levels include: carbamazepine, chronic alcohol abuse, reserpine. Moban* brand of Molindone Hydrochloride contains calcium ions which interfere with the absorption of phenytoin. Ingestion times of phenytoin and antacid preparations containing calcium should be staggered in patients with low serum phenytoin levels to prevent absorption problems.
3. Drugs which may either increase or decrease phenytoin serum levels include: phenobarbital, valproic acid, and sodium valproate. Similarly, the effect of phenytoin on phenobarbital, valproic acid and sodium valproate serum levels is unpredictable.
4. Although not a true drug interaction, tricyclic antidepressants may precipitate seizures in susceptible patients and phenytoin dosage may need to be adjusted.
5. Drugs whose efficacy is impaired by phenytoin include: corticosteroids, coumarin anticoagulants, oral contraceptives, quinidine, vitamin D, digitoxin, rifampin, doxycycline, estrogens, furosemide.

Serum level determinations are especially helpful when possible drug interactions are suspected.

Drug/Laboratory Test Interactions: Phenytoin may cause decreased serum levels of protein-bound iodine (PBI). It may also produce lower than normal values for dexamethasone or metyrapone tests. Phenytoin may cause increased serum levels of glucose, alkaline phosphatase, and gamma glutamyl transpeptidase (GGT).

Carcinogenesis: See 'Warnings' section for information on carcinogenesis.

Pregnancy: See Warnings

Nursing Mothers: Infant breast feeding is not recommended for women taking this drug because phenytoin appears to be secreted in low concentrations in human milk.

ADVERSE REACTIONS

The most notable signs of toxicity associated with the intravenous use of this drug are cardiovascular collapse and/or central nervous system depression. Hypotension does occur when the drug is administered rapidly by the intravenous route. The *rate* of administration is very important; it should not exceed 50 mg per minute in adults, and 1–3 mg/kg/min in neonates. At this rate, toxicity should be minimized.

Cardiovascular: Severe cardiotoxic reactions and fatalities have been reported with atrial and ventricular conduction depression and ventricular fibrillation. Severe complications are most commonly encountered in elderly or gravely ill patients.

Central Nervous System: The most common manifestations encountered with phenytoin therapy are referable to this system and are usually dose-related. These include nystagmus, ataxia, slurred speech, decreased coordination and mental confusion. Dizziness, insomnia, transient nervousness, motor twitchings, and headaches have also been observed. There have also been rare reports of phenytoin induced dyskinesias, including chorea, dystonia, tremor and

Continued on next page

This product information was prepared in August, 1986. On these and other Parke-Davis Products, information may be obtained by addressing PARKE-DAVIS, Division of Warner-Lambert Company, Morris Plains, New Jersey 07950.

Parke-Davis—Cont.

asterixis, similar to those induced by phenothiazine and other neuroleptic drugs.
A predominantly sensory peripheral polyneuropathy has been observed in patients receiving long-term phenytoin therapy.
Gastrointestinal System: Nausea, vomiting, and constipation.
Integumentary System: Dermatological manifestations sometimes accompanied by fever have included scarlatiniform or morbilliform rashes. A morbilliform rash (measles-like) is the most common; other types of dermatitis are seen more rarely. Other more serious forms which may be fatal have included bullous, exfoliative or purpuric dermatitis, lupus erythematosus, and Stevens-Johnson syndrome (see Precautions).
Hemopoietic System: Hemopoietic complications, some fatal, have occasionally been reported in association with administration of phenytoin. These have included thrombocytopenia, leukopenia, granulocytopenia, agranulocytosis, and pancytopenia with or without bone marrow suppression. While macrocytosis and megaloblastic anemia have occurred, these conditions usually respond to folic acid therapy. Lymphadenopathy including benign lymph node hyperplasia, pseudolymphoma, lymphoma, and Hodgkin's Disease have been reported (see Warnings).
Connective Tissue System: Coarsening of the facial features, enlargement of the lips, gingival hyperplasia, hypertrichosis, and Peyronie's Disease.
Injection Site: Local irritation, inflammation, tenderness, necrosis, and sloughing have been reported with or without extravasation of intravenous phenytoin.
Other: Systemic lupus erythematosus, periarteritis nodosa, toxic hepatitis, liver damage, and immunoglobulin abnormalities may occur.

OVERDOSAGE

The lethal dose in children is not known. The lethal dose in adults is estimated to be 2 to 5 grams. The initial symptoms are nystagmus, ataxia and dysarthria. Other signs are tremor, hyperflexia, lethargy, slurred speech, nausea, vomiting. The patient may become comatose and hypertensive. Death is due to respiratory and circulatory depression.
There are marked variations among individuals with respect to phenytoin plasma levels where toxicity may occur. Nystagmus, on lateral gaze, usually appears at 20 mcg/mL, ataxia at 30 mcg/mL, dysarthria and lethargy appear when the plasma concentration is over 40 mcg/mL, but as high a concentration as 50 mcg/mL has been reported without evidence of toxicity. As much as 25 times the therapeutic dose has been taken to result in a serum concentration over 100 mcg/mL with complete recovery.
Treatment: Treatment is nonspecific since there is no known antidote.
The adequacy of the respiratory and circulatory systems should be carefully observed and appropriate supportive measures employed. Hemodialysis can be considered since phenytoin is not completely bound to plasma proteins. Total exchange transfusion has been used in the treatment of severe intoxication in children.
In acute overdosage the possibility of other CNS depressants, including alcohol, should be borne in mind.

DOSAGE AND ADMINISTRATION

The addition of Dilantin solution to intravenous infusion is not recommended due to lack of solubility and resultant precipitation.
Not to exceed 50 mg per minute, intravenously in adults, and not exceeding 1–3 mg/kg/min in neonates There is a relatively small margin between full therapeutic effect and minimally toxic doses of this drug.
The solution is suitable for use as long as it remains free of haziness and precipitate. Upon refrigeration or freezing, a precipitate might form; this will dissolve again after the solution is allowed to stand at room temperature. The product is still suitable for use. Only a clear solution should be used. A faint yellow coloration may develop; however, this has no effect on the potency of the solution.
In the treatment of status epilepticus, the intravenous route is preferred because of the delay in absorption of phenytoin when administered intramuscularly.
Serum concentrations should be monitored and care should be taken when switching a patient from the sodium salt to the free acid form.
Dilantin® Kapseals®, Dilantin Parenteral, and Dilantin with Phenobarbital are formulated with the sodium salt of phenytoin. The free acid form of phenytoin is used in Dilantin-30 Pediatric and Dilantin-125 Suspensions and Dilantin Infatabs. Because there is approximately an 8% increase in drug content with the free acid form over that of the sodium salt, dosage adjustments and serum level monitoring may be necessary when switching from a product formulated with the free acid to a product formulated with the sodium salt and vice versa.
Status Epilepticus: In adults, a loading dose of 10 to 15 mg/kg should be administered slowly intravenously, at a rate not exceeding 50 mg per minute (this will require approximately 20 minutes in a 70-kg patient). The loading dose should be followed by maintenance doses of 100 mg orally or intravenously every 6–8 hours.
Recent work in neonates and children has shown that absorption of phenytoin is unreliable after oral administration, but a loading dose of 15–20 mg/kg of Dilantin intravenously will usually produce plasma concentrations of phenytoin within the generally accepted therapeutic range (10–20 mcg/mL). The drug should be injected slowly intravenously at a rate not exceeding 1–3 mg/kg/min.
Parenteral Dilantin should be injected *slowly* and directly into a large vein through a large-gauge needle or intravenous catheter. Each injection of intravenous Dilantin should be followed by an injection of sterile saline through the same needle or catheter to avoid local venous irritation due to alkalinity of the solution. Continuous infusion should be avoided; the addition of Parenteral Dilantin to intravenous infusion fluids is not recommended because of the likelihood of precipitation.
Continuous monitoring of the electrocardiogram and blood pressure is essential. The patient should be observed for signs of respiratory depression. Determination of phenytoin plasma levels is advised when using Dilantin in the management of status epilepticus and in the subsequent establishment of maintenance dosage.
Other measures, including concomitant administration of an intravenous benzodiazepine such as diazepam, or an intravenous short-acting barbiturate, will usually be necessary for rapid control of seizures because of the required slow rate of administration of Dilantin.
If administration of Parenteral Dilantin does not terminate seizures, the use of other anticonvulsants, intravenous barbiturates, general anesthesia, and other appropriate measures should be considered.
Intramuscular administration should not be used in the treatment of status epilepticus because the attainment of peak plasma levels may require up to 24 hours.
Neurosurgery: Prophylactic dosage—100 to 200 mg (2 to 4 mL) intramuscularly at approximately 4-hour intervals during surgery and continued during the postoperative period.
When intramuscular administration is required for a patient previously stabilized orally, compensating dosage adjustments are necessary to maintain therapeutic plasma levels. An intramuscular dose 50% greater than the oral dose is necessary to maintain these levels. When returned to oral administration, the dose should be reduced by 50% of the original oral dose for one week to prevent excessive plasma levels due to sustained release from intramuscular tissue sites.
If the patient requires more than a week of IM Dilantin, alternative routes should be explored, such as gastric intubation. For time periods less than one week, the patient shifted back from IM administration should receive one half the original oral dose for the same period of time the patient received IM Dilantin. Monitoring plasma levels would help prevent a fall into the subtherapeutic range. Serum blood level determinations are especially helpful when possible drug interactions are suspected.

HOW SUPPLIED

N 0071-4488-05 (Ampoule 1488) Dilantin ready-mixed solution containing 50 mg phenytoin sodium per milliliter is supplied in 2-mL ampoules. Packages of ten.
N 0071-4488-41 (Steri-Dose® 4488) Dilantin ready-mixed solution containing 50 mg phenytoin sodium per milliliter is supplied in a 2-mL sterile disposable syringe (22 gauge × 1¼ inch needle). Packages of ten individually cartoned syringes.
N 0071-4475-35 (Ampoule 1475) Dilantin ready-mixed solution containing 50 mg phenytoin sodium per milliliter is supplied in 5-mL ampoules with one 6-mL sterile disposable syringe (22 gauge × 1¼ inch needle). Packages of ten.
N 0071-4475-08 (Ampoule 1475) Dilantin ready-mixed solution contaning 50 mg phenytoin sodium per milliliter is supplied in packages of ten 5-mL ampoules without syringes.
Caution—Federal law prohibits dispensing without prescription.

4475G023

DILANTIN-30® PEDIATRIC/ DILANTIN-125® ℞

[*dī-lăn 'tĭn*]
(Phenytoin Oral Suspension, USP)

DESCRIPTION

Dilantin (phenytoin) is related to the barbiturates in chemical structure, but has a five-membered ring. The chemical name is 5.5-diphenyl-2,4 imidazolidinedione.
Each teaspoonful of suspension contains 30 mg or 125 mg of phenytoin, USP with a maximum alcohol content not greater than 0.6 percent. Also contains carboxymethylcellulose sodium, USP; citric acid; anhydrous, USP; flavors; glycerin, USP; magnesium aluminum silicate, NF; polysorbate 40, NF; purified water, USP; sodium benzoate, NF; sucrose, NF; vanillin NF. The 30 mg per teaspoonful suspension also contains D&C red No. 33; FD&C red No. 40. The 125 mg per teaspoonful suspension also contains FD&C yellow No. 6.

CLINICAL PHARMACOLOGY

Phenytoin is an antiepileptic drug which can be useful in the treatment of epilepsy. The primary site of action appears to be *the motor cortex* where spread of seizure activity is inhibited. Possibly by promoting sodium efflux from neurons, phenytoin tends to *stabilize* the threshold against hyperexcitability caused by excessive stimulation or environmental changes capable of reducing membrane sodium gradient. This includes the reduction of posttetanic potentiation at synapses. Loss of posttetanic potentiation prevents cortical seizure foci from detonating adjacent cortical areas. Phenytoin reduces the maximal activity of brain stem centers responsible for the tonic phase of tonic-clonic (grand mal) seizures.
The plasma half-life in man after oral administration of phenytoin averages 22 hours, with a range of 7 to 42 hours. Steady-state therapeutic levels are achieved at least 7 to 10 days (5–7 half-lives) after initiation of therapy with recommended doses of 300 mg/day.
When serum level determinations are necessary, they should be obtained at least 5–7 half-lives after treatment initiation, dosage change, or addition or subtraction of another drug to the regimen so that equilibrium or steady-state will have been achieved. Trough levels provide information about clinically effective serum level range and confirm patient compliance and are obtained just prior to the patient's next scheduled dose. Peak levels indicate an individual's threshold for emergence of dose-related side effects and are obtained at the time of expected peak concentration. For Dilantin-30 Pediatric and Dilantin-125 Suspensions peak levels occur 1½–3 hours after administration.
Optimum control without clinical signs of toxicity occurs more often with serum levels between 10 and 20 mcg/mL, although some mild cases of tonic-clonic (grand mal) epilepsy may be controlled with lower serum levels of phenytoin.
In most patients maintained at a steady dosage, stable phenytoin serum levels are achieved. There may be wide interpatient variability in phenytoin serum levels with equivalent dosages. Patients with unusually low levels may be noncompliant or hypermetabolizers of phenytoin. Unusally high levels result from liver disease, congenital enzyme deficiency or drug interactions which result in metabolic interference. The patient with large variations in phenytoin plasma levels, despite standard doses, presents a difficult clinical problem. Serum level determinations in such patients may be particularly helpful.
Most of the drug is excreted in the bile as inactive metabolites which are then reabsorbed from the intestinal tract and excreted in the urine. Urinary excretion of phenytoin and its metabolites occurs partly with glomerular filtration but more importantly, by tubular secretion. Because phenytoin is hydroxylated in the liver by an enzyme system which is saturable at high plasma levels small incremental doses may increase the half-life and produce very substantial increases in serum levels, when these are in the upper range. The steady-state level may be disproportionately increased, with resultant intoxication, from an increase in dosage of 10% or more.

INDICATIONS

Dilantin (phenytoin) is indicated for the control of tonic-clonic (grand mal) and psychomotor (temporal lobe) seizures. Phenytoin serum level determinations may be necessary for optimal dosage adjustments (see Dosage and Administration and Clinical Pharmacology).

CONTRAINDICATION

Dilantin is contraindicated in those patients with a history of hypersensitivity to hydantoin products.

WARNINGS

Abrupt withdrawal of phenytoin in epileptic patients may precipitate status epilepticus. When in the judgment of the clinician the need for dosage reduction, discontinuation, or substitution of alternative anticonvulsant medication arises, this should be done gradually. In the event of an allergic or hypersensitivity reaction, more rapid substitution of alternative therapy may be necessary. In this case, alternative therapy should be an anticonvulsant not belonging to the hydantion chemical class.
There have been a number of reports suggesting a relationship between phenytoin and the development of lymphadenopathy (local or generalized) including benign lymph node hyperplasia, pseudolymphoma, lymphoma, and Hodgkin's Disease. Although a cause and effect relationship has not been established, the occurrence of lymphadenopathy indicates the need to differentiate such a condition from other types of lymph node pathology. Lymph node involvement may occur with or without symptoms and signs resembling serum sickness eg, fever, rash and liver involvement.

In all cases of lymphadenopathy, follow-up observation for an extended period is indicated and every effort should be made to achieve seizure control using alternative antiepileptic drugs. Acute alcoholic intake may increase phenytoin serum levels while chronic alcoholic use may decrease serum levels.

Usage in Pregnancy: A number of reports suggests an association between the use of antiepileptic drugs by women with epilepsy and a higher incidence of birth defects in children born to these women. Data are more extensive with respect to phenytoin and phenobarbital, but these are also the most commonly prescribed antiepileptic drugs; less systematic or anecdotal reports suggest a possible similar association with the use of all known antiepileptic drugs.

The reports suggesting a higher incidence of birth defects in children of drug-treated epileptic women cannot be regarded as adequate to prove a definite cause and effect relationship. There are intrinsic methodologic problems in obtaining adequate data on drug teratogenicity in humans; genetic factors or the epileptic condition itself may be more important than drug therapy in leading to birth defects. The great majority of mothers on antiepileptic medication deliver normal infants. It is important to note that antiepileptic drugs should not be discontinued in patients in whom the drug is administered to prevent major seizures, because of the strong possibility of precipitating status epilepticus with attendant hypoxia and threat to life. In individual cases where the severity and frequency of the seizure disorder are such that the removal of medication does not pose a serious threat to the patient, discontinuation of the drug may be considered prior to and during pregnancy, although it cannot be said with any confidence that even minor seizures do not pose some hazards to the developing embryo or fetus. The prescribing physician will wish to weigh these considerations in treating and counseling epileptic women of childbearing potential.

In addition to the reports of increased incidence of congenital malformation, such as cleft lip/palate and heart malformations in children of women receiving phenytoin and other antiepileptic drugs, there have more recently been reports of a fetal hydantoin syndrome. This consists of prenatal growth deficiency, microcephaly and mental deficiency in children born to mothers who have received phenytoin, barbiturates, alcohol, or trimethadione. However, these features are all interrelated and are frequently associated with intrauterine growth retardation from other causes.

There have been isolated reports of malignancies, including neuroblastoma, in children whose mothers received phenytoin during pregnancy.

An increase in seizure frequency during pregnancy occurs in a high proportion of patients, because of altered phenytoin absorption or metabolism. Periodic measurement of serum phenytoin levels is particularly valuable in the management of a pregnant epileptic patient as a guide to an appropriate adjustment of dosage. However, postpartum restoration of the original dosage will probably be indicated.

Neonatal coagulation defects have been reported within the first 24 hours in babies born to epileptic mothers receiving phenobarbital and/or phenytoin. Vitamin K has been shown to prevent or correct this defect and has been recommended to be given to the mother before delivery and the neonate after birth.

PRECAUTIONS

General: The liver is the chief site of biotransformation of phenytoin; patients wth impaired liver function, elderly patients, or those who are gravely ill may show early signs of toxicity.

A small percentage of individuals who have been treated with phenytoin have been shown to metabolize the drug slowly. Slow metabolism may be due to limited enzyme availability and lack of induction; it appears to be genetically determined.

Phenytoin should be discontinued if a skin rash appears (see "Warnings" section regarding drug discontinuation). If the rash is exfoliative, purpuric, or bullous or if lupus erythematosus or Stevens-Johnson syndrome is suspected, use of this drug should not be resumed and alternative therapy should be considered. (See Adverse Reactions). If the rash is of a milder type (measles-like or scarlatiniform), therapy may be resumed after the rash has completely disappeared. If the rash recurs upon reinstitution of therapy, further phenytoin medication is contraindicated. Hyperglycemia, resulting from the drug's inhibitory effects on insulin release, has been reported. Phenytoin may also raise the serum glucose level in diabetic patients.

Osteomalacia has been associated with phenytoin therapy and is considered to be due to phenytoin's interference with Vitamin D metabolism.

Phenytoin is not indicated for seizures due to hypoglycemic or other metabolic causes. Appropriate diagnostic procedures should be performed as indicated.

Phenytoin is not effective for absence (petit mal) seizures. If tonic-clonic (grand mal) and absence (petit mal) seizures are present, combined drug therapy is needed.

Serum levels of phenytoin sustained above the optimal range may produce confusional states referred to as "delirium," "psychosis" or "encephalopathy," or rarely irreversible cerebellar dysfunction. Accordingly, at the first sign of acute toxicity, plasma levels are recommended. Dose reduction of phenytoin therapy is indicated if plasma levels are excessive; if symptoms persist, termination is recommended. (See Warnings).

Information for Patients: Patients taking phenytoin should be advised of the importance of adhering strictly to the prescribed dosage regimen, and of informing the physician of any clinical condition in which it is not possible to take the drug orally as prescribed, eg, surgery, etc.

Patients should also be cautioned on the use of other drugs or alcoholic beverages without first seeking the physician's advice.

Patients should be instructed to call their physician if skin rash develops.

The importance of good dental hygiene should be stressed in order to minimize the development of gingival hyperplasia and its complications.

Laboratory Tests: Phenytoin serum level determinations may be necessary to achieve optimal dosage adjustments.

Drug Interactions: There are many drugs which may increase or decrease phenytoin levels or which phenytoin may affect. The most commonly occurring drug interactions are listed below:

1. Drugs which may increase phenytoin serum levels include: chloramphenicol, dicumarol, disulfiram, tolbutamide, isoniazid, phenylbutazone, acute alcohol intake, salicylates, chlordiazepoxide, phenothiazines, diazepam, estrogens, ethosuximide, halothane, methylphenidate, sulfonamides, cimetidine, trazodone.
2. Drugs which may decrease phenytoin levels include: carbamazepine, chronic alcohol abuse, reserpine. Moban® brand of Molindone Hydrochloride contains calcium ions which interfere with the absorption of phenytoin. Ingestion times of phenytoin and antacid preparations containing calcium should be staggered in patients with low serum phenytoin levels to prevent absorption problems.
3. Drugs which may either increase or decrease phenytoin serum levels include; phenobarbital, valproic acid, and sodium valproate. Similarly, the effect of phenytoin on phenobarbital, valproic acid, and sodium valproate serum levels is unpredictable.
4. Although not a true drug interaction, tricyclic antidepressants may precipitate seizures in susceptible patients and phenytoin dosage may need to be adjusted.
5. Drugs whose efficacy is impaired by phenytoin include: corticosteroids, coumarin anticoagulants, oral contraceptives, quinidine, vitamin D, digitoxin, rifampin, doxycycline, estrogens, furosemide.

Serum level determinations are especially helpful when possible drug interactions are suspected.

Drug/Laboratory Test Interactions: Phenytoin may cause decreased serum levels of protein-bound iodine (PBI). It may also produce lower than normal values for dexamethasone or metyrapone tests. Phenytoin may cause increased serum levels of glucose, alkaline phosphatase, and gamma glutamyl transpeptidase (GGT).

Carcinogenesis: See 'Warnings' section for information on carcinogenesis.

Pregnancy: See Warnings

Nursing Mothers: Infant breast feeding is not recommended for women taking this drug because phenytoin appears to be secreted in low concentrations in human milk.

ADVERSE REACTIONS

Central Nervous System: The most common manifestations encountered with phenytoin therapy are referable to this system and are usually dose-related. These include nystagmus, ataxia, slurred speech, decreased coordination, and mental confusion. Dizziness, insomnia, transient nervousness, motor twitchings, and headaches have also been observed. There have also been rare reports of phenytoin induced dyskinesias, including chorea, dystonia, tremor and asterixis, similar to those induced by phenothiazine and other neuroleptic drugs.

A predominantly sensory peripheral polyneuropathy has been observed in patients receiving long-term phenytoin therapy.

Gastrointestinal System: Nausea, vomiting, and constipation.

Integumentary System: Dermatological manifestations sometimes accompanied by fever have included scarlatiniform or morbilliform rashes. A morbilliform rash (measles-like) is the most common; other types of dermatitis are seen more rarely. Other more serious forms which may be fatal have included bullous, exfoliative or purpuric dermatitis, lupus erythematosus, and Stevens-Johnson syndrome (see Precautions).

Hemopoietic System: Hemopoietic complications, some fatal, have occasionally been reported in association with administration of phenytoin. These have included thrombocytopenia, leukopenia, granulocytopenia, agranulocytosis, and pancytopenia with or without bone marrow suppression. While macrocytosis and megaloblastic anemia have occurred, these conditions usually respond to folic acid therapy. Lymphadenopathy including benign lymph node hyperplasia, pseudolymphoma, lymphoma, and Hodgkin's Disease have been reported (see Warnings).

Connective Tissue System: Coarsening of the facial features, enlargement of the lips, gingival hyperplasia, hypertrichosis, and Peyronie's Disease.

Other: Systemic lupus erythematosus, periarteritis nodosa, toxic hepatitis, liver damage, and immunoglobulin abnormalities may occur.

OVERDOSAGE

The lethal dose in children is not known. The lethal dose in adults is estimated to be 2 to 5 grams. The initial symptoms are nystagmus, ataxia, and dysarthria. Other signs are tremor, hyperflexia, lethargy, slurred speech, nausea, vomiting. The patient may become comatose and hypertensive. Death is due to respiratory and circulatory depression.

There are marked variations among individuals with respect to phenytoin plasma levels where toxicity may occur. Nystagmus, on lateral gaze, usually appears at 20 mcg/mL, ataxia at 30 mcg/mL, dysarthria and lethargy appear when the plasma concentration is over 40 mcg/mL, but as high a concentration as 50 mcg/mL has been reported without evidence of toxicity. As much as 25 times the therapeutic dose has been taken to result in a serum concentration over 100 mcg/mL with complete recovery.

Treatment: Treatment is nonspecific since there is no known antidote.

The adequacy of the respiratory and circulatory systems should be carefully observed and appropriate supportive measures employed. Hemodialysis can be considered since phenytoin is not completely bound to plasma proteins. Total exchange transfusion has been used in the treatment of severe intoxication in children.

In acute overdosage the possibility of other CNS depressants, including alcohol, should be borne in mind.

DOSAGE AND ADMINISTRATION

Serum concentrations should be monitored and care should be taken when switching a patient from the sodium salt to the free acid form.

Dilantin® Kapseals®, Dilantin Parenteral, and Dilantin with Phenobarbital are formulated with the sodium salt of phenytoin. The free acid form of phenytoin is used in Dilantin-30 Pediatric and Dilantin-125 Suspensions and Dilantin Infatabs. Because there is approximately an 8% increase in drug content with the free acid form over that of the sodium salt, dosage adjustments and serum level monitoring may be necessary when switching from a product formulated with the free acid to a product formulated with the sodium salt and vice versa.

General: Dosage should be individualized to provide maximum benefit. In some cases serum blood level determinations may be necessary for optimal dosage adjustments—the clinically effective serum level is usually 10–20 mcg/mL. With recommended dosage, a period of seven to ten days may be required to achieve steady-state blood levels with phenytoin and changes in dosage (increase or decrease) should not be carried out at intervals shorter than seven to ten days.

Adult Dose: Patients who have received no previous treatment may be started on one teaspoonful (5 mL) of Dilantin-125 Suspension three times daily, and the dose is then adjusted to suit individual requirements. An increase to five teaspoonfuls daily may be made, if necessary.

Pediatric Dose: Initially, 5 mg/kg/day in two or three equally divided doses, with subsequent dosage individualized to a maximum of 300 mg daily. A recommended daily maintenance dosage is usually 4 to 8 mg/kg. Children over 6 years may require the minimum adult dose (300 mg/day).

HOW SUPPLIED

N 0071-2214—Dilantin-125® Suspension (phenytoin oral suspension, USP), 125 mg phenytoin/5 mL with a maximum alcohol content not greater than 0.6 percent; available in 8-oz bottles and individual unit dose foil pouches which deliver 5 mL (125 mg phenytoin). The minimum sales unit is 100 pouches.

N 0071-2315—Dilantin-30® Pediatric Suspension (phenytoin oral suspension, USP), 30 mg phenytoin/5 mL with a maximum alcohol content not greater than 0.6 percent; available in 8-oz bottles and individual unit dose foil pouches which deliver 5 mL (30 mg phenytoin). The minimum sales unit is 100 pouches.

Also available as:

N 0071-0362 (Kapseal® 362)—Dilantin (extended phenytoin sodium capsules, USP) 100 mg; in 100's, 1000's, unit dose 100's and in a Memo Pack containing 84 unit-dose capsules (28 days dosage regimen).

Continued on next page

This product information was prepared in August, 1986. On these and other Parke-Davis Products, information may be obtained by addressing PARKE-DAVIS, Division of Warner-Lambert Company, Morris Plains, New Jersey 07950.

Parke-Davis—Cont.

N 0071-0365 (Kapseal 365)—Dilantin (extended phenytoin sodium capsules, USP) 30 mg; in 100's, 1000's and unit dose 100's .
N 0071-0375 (Kapseal 375)—Dilantin with Phenobarbital each contain 100 mg phenytoin sodium with 16 mg (¼ gr) phenobarbital; in 100's and 1000's .
N 0071-0531 (Kapseal 531)—Dilantin with Phenobarbital each contain 100 mg phenytoin sodium with 32 mg (½ gr) phenobarbital; in 100's, 1000's and unit dose 100's.
N 0071-0007 (Tablet 7)—Dilantin Infatabs® (phenytoin tablets, USP) each contain 50 mg phenytoin; 100's and unit dose 100's.
For Parenteral Use:
N 0071-4488-05 (Ampoule 1488)—Dilantin ready-mixed solution containing 50 mg phenytoin sodium per milliliter is supplied in 2-mL ampoules. Packages of ten.
N 0071-4475-35 (Ampoule 1475)—Dilantin (phenytoin sodium injection) ready-mixed solution containing 50 mg phenytoin sodium per milliliter is supplied in 5-mL ampoules with one 6-mL sterile disposable syringe (22 gauge × 1¼ inch needle). Packages of ten.
N 0071-4475-08 (Ampoule 1475)—Dilantin ready-mixed solution containing 50 mg phenytoin sodium per milliliter is supplied in packages of ten 5-mL ampoules without syringes.
N 0071-4488-41 (Steri-Dose® 4488)—Dilantin ready-mixed solution containing 50 mg phenytoin sodium per milliliter is supplied in a 2-mL sterile disposable syringe (22 gauge × 1¼ inch needle). Packages of ten individually cartoned syringes.
Caution—Federal law prohibits dispensing without prescription.

2214G104

KAPSEALS®
DILANTIN® ℞
[di-lăn'tĭn]
(Phenytoin Sodium) with Phenobarbital

Each Dilantin® with ¼ gr Phenobarbital Kapseal® contains:
Dilantin (phenytoin sodium) .... 100 mg
Phenobarbital .... 16 mg (¼ gr)
(Warning—May be habit forming)
Each Dilantin with ½ gr Phenobarbital Kapseal contains:
Dilantin (phenytoin sodium) .... 100 mg
Phenobarbital .... 32 mg (½ gr)
(Warning—May be habit forming)

DESCRIPTION

Dilantin (phenytoin sodium) is related to the barbiturates in chemical structure, but has a five-membered ring. The chemical name is sodium 5,5-diphenyl-2,4-imidazolidinedione.
Phenobarbital is a derivative of barbituric acid and is chemically described as 5-ethyl-5-phenylbarbituric acid.
Also contains confectioner's sugar NF, magnesium stearate, NF; talc, USP. The capsule shell and band contain citric acid, USP; colloidal silicon dioxide, NF; FD&C blue No. 1; FD&C red No. 40; gelatin NF; glyceryl monooleate; polyethylene glycol 200; sodium benzoate, NF; sodium bisulfite; sodium lauryl sulfate, NF. The Dilantin with Phenobarbital ¼ gr capsule shell and band also contain FD&C red No. 3; hydrogen peroxide 3%. The Dilantin with Phenobarbital ½ gr capsule shell and band also contain FD&C yellow No. 6.

CLINICAL PHARMACOLOGY

Phenytoin—Phenytoin is an antiepileptic drug which can be useful in the treatment of epilepsy. The primary site of action appears to be the *motor cortex* where spread of seizure activity is inhibited. Possibly by promoting sodium efflux from neurons, phenytoin tends to *stabilize* the threshold against hyperexcitability caused by excessive stimulation or environmental changes capable of reducing membrane sodium gradient. This includes the reduction of posttetanic potentiation at synapses. Loss of posttetanic potentiation prevents cortical seizure foci from detonating adjacent cortical areas. Phenytoin reduces the maximal activity of brain stem centers responsible for the tonic phase of tonic-clonic (grand mal) seizures.
The plasma half-life in man after oral administration of phenytoin averages 22 hours, with a range of 7 to 42 hours. Steady-state therapeutic levels are achieved at least 7 to 10 days (5–7 half-lives) after initiation of therapy with recommended doses of 300 mg/day.
When serum level determinations are necessary, they should be obtained at least 5–7 half-lives after treatment initiation, dosage change, or addition or subtraction of another drug to the regimen so that equilibrium or steady-state will have been achieved. Trough levels provide information about clinically effective serum level range and confirm patient compliance and are obtained just prior to the patient's next scheduled dose. Peak levels indicate an individual's threshold for emergence of dose-related side effects and are obtained at the time of expected peak concentration. For Dilantin with Phenobarbital Kapseals peak serum levels occur 1½–3 hours after administration.
Optimum control without clinical signs of toxicity occurs more often with serum levels between 10 and 20 mcg/mL, although some mild cases of tonic-clonic (grand mal) epilepsy may be controlled with lower serum levels of phenytoin.
In most patients maintained at a steady dosage, stable phenytoin serum levels are achieved. There may be wide interpatient variability in phenytoin serum levels with equivalent dosages. Patients with unusually low levels may be noncompliant or hypermetabolizers of phenytoin. Unusually high levels result from liver disease, congenital enzyme deficiency or drug interactions which result in metabolic interference. The patient with large variations in phenytoin plasma levels, despite standard doses, presents a difficult clinical problem. Serum level determinations in such patients may be particularly helpful.
Most of the drug is excreted in the bile as inactive metabolites which are then reabsorbed from the intestinal tract and excreted in the urine. Urinary excretion of phenytoin and its metabolites occurs partly with glomerular filtration, but more importantly, by tubular secretion. Because phenytoin is hydroxylated in the liver by an enzyme system which is saturable at high plasma levels small incremental doses may increase the half-life and produce very substantial increases in serum levels, when these are in the upper range. The steady-state level may be disproportionately increased, with resultant intoxication, from an increase in dosage of 10% or more.
Phenobarbital—Phenobarbital produces its anticonvulsant effect by depressing the motor cortex and raising the seizure threshold.
Phenobarbital is absorbed completely, although slowly, following oral administration and undergoes partial biotransformation in the liver by hydroxylation. Phenobarbital is excreted via the kidneys, 10% to 25% as free drug and the reminder primarily as the inactive para-hydroxyphenyl metabolite. The plasma half-life is long, approximately two to six days in adults, and shorter and more variable in children.
In adults, the oral anticonvulsant dose of 1 to 3 mg/kg will produce therapeutic concentrations of 10 to 30 mcg/mL in the serum, the levels usually necessary for seizure control. At this dose, approximately three weeks may be required for the serum levels to achieve steady-state.
High serum levels occur when liver disease, diminished urinary flow, acidosis, or obesity is present. Low serum levels in adults may be due to poor patient compliance.
When used as an anticonvulsant, the clinical phenomenon of breakthrough seizures has been seen. Whether this is a case of true pharmacologic tolerance or some form of spontaneous variation is not known. Physical dependence does develop and may produce accentuation of seizures in epileptics when the drug is abruptly withdrawn.

INDICATIONS AND USAGE

Dilantin with Phenobarbital is indicated for the control of generalized tonic-clonic (grand mal) and complex partial (psychomotor, temporal lobe) seizures, only in those patients who require both drugs for seizure control and who previously have had their daily anticonvulsant requirements determined by the administration of the two drugs separately. Combinations should not be used to initiate anticonvulsant therapy and are provided as a convenience for epileptic patients.
Phenytoin serum level determinations may be necessary for optimal dosage adjustments (see Dosage and Administration and Clinical Pharmacology).

CONTRAINDICATIONS

Phenytoin is contraindicated in those patients with a history of hypersensitivity to hydantoin products.
Phenobarbital is contraindicated in the following conditions: latent or manifest porphyria or familial history of intermittent porphyria, history of confusion or restlessness from hypnotics, history of abnormal reaction or known hypersensitivity to barbital and its derivatives, including phenobarbital, or a known previous addiction to sedative-hypnotics. Other contraindications include renal and hepatic impairment and severe pulmonary insufficiency.

WARNINGS

Warning—Phenobarbital may be habit forming. Abrupt withdrawal of phenytoin in epileptic patients may precipitate status epilepticus. When, in the judgment of the clinician, the need for dosage reduction, discontinuation, or substitution of alternative anticonvulsant medication arises, this should be done gradually. In the event of an allergic or hypersensitivity reaction, more rapid substitution of alternative therapy may be necessary. In this case, alternative therapy should be an anticonvulsant not belonging to the hydantoin chemical class.
There have been a number of reports suggesting a relationship between phenytoin and the development of lymphadenopathy (local or generalized) including benign lymph node hyperplasia, pseudolymphoma, lymphoma, and Hodgkin's Disease. Although a cause and effect relationship has not been established, the occurrence of lymphadenopathy indicates the need to differentiate such a condition from other types of lymph node pathology. Lymph node involvement may occur with or without symptoms and signs resembling serum sickness eg, fever, rash and liver involvement.
In all cases of lymphadenopathy, follow-up observation for an extended period is indicated and every effort should be made to achieve seizure control using alternative antiepileptic drugs.
Acute alcoholic intake may increase phenytoin serum levels while chronic alcoholic use may decrease serum levels.
Usage in Pregnancy: A number of reports suggests an association between the use of antiepileptic drugs by women with epilepsy and a higher incidence of birth defects in children born to these women. Data are more extensive with respect to phenytoin and phenobarbital, but these are also the most commonly prescribed antiepileptic drugs; less systematic or anecdotal reports suggest a possible similar association with the use of all known antiepileptic drugs.
The reports suggesting a higher incidence of birth defects in children of drug-treated epileptic women cannot be regarded as adequate to prove a definite cause and effect relationship. There are intrinsic methodologic problems in obtaining adequate data on drug teratogenicity in humans; genetic factors or the epileptic condition itself may be more important than drug therapy in leading to birth defects. The great majority of mothers on antiepileptic medication deliver normal infants. It is important to note that antiepileptic drugs should not be discontinued in patients in whom the drug is administered to prevent major seizures, because of the strong possibility of precipitating status epilepticus with attendant hypoxia and threat to life. In individual cases where the severity and frequency of the seizure disorder are such that the removal of medication does not pose a serious threat to the patient, discontinuation of the drug may be considered prior to and during pregnancy, although it cannot be said with any confidence that even minor seizures do not pose some hazards to the developing embryo or fetus. The prescribing physician will wish to weigh these considerations in treating and counseling epileptic women of childbearing potential.
In addition to the reports of increased incidence of congenital malformation, such as cleft lip/palate and heart malformations in children of women receiving phenytoin and other antiepileptic drugs, there have more recently been reports of a fetal hydantoin syndrome. This consists of prenatal growth deficiency, microcephaly and mental deficiency in children born to mothers who have received phenytoin, barbiturates, alcohol, or trimethadione. However, these features are all interrelated and are frequently associated with intrauterine growth retardation from other causes.
There have been isolated reports of malignancies, including neuroblastoma, in children whose mothers received phenytoin during pregnancy.
An increase in seizure frequency during pregnancy occurs in a high proportion of patients, because of altered phenytoin absorption or metabolism. Periodic measurement of serum phenytoin levels is particularly valuable in the management of a pregnant epileptic patient as a guide to an appropriate adjustment of dosage. However, postpartum restoration of the original dosage will probably be indicated.
Neonatal coagulation defects have been reported within the first 24 hours in babies born to epileptic mothers receiving phenobarbital and/or phenytoin. Vitamin K has been shown to prevent or correct this defect and has been recommended to be given to the mother before delivery and the neonate after birth.

PRECAUTIONS

Phenytoin
General: The liver is the chief site of biotransformation of phenytoin; patients with impaired liver function may show early signs of toxicity. Elderly patients or those who are gravely ill may show early signs of toxicity.
A small percentage of indiviauals who have been treated with phenytoin have been shown to metabolize the drug slowly. Slow metabolism may be due to limited enzyme availability and lack of induction; it appears to be genetically determined.
Phenytoin should be discontinued if a skin rash appears (see "Warnings" section regarding drug discontinuation). If the rash is exfoliative, purpuric, or bullous or if lupus erythematosus or Stevens-Johnson syndrome is suspected, use of this drug should not be resumed and alternative therapy should be considered. (See Adverse Reactions.) If the rash is of a milder type (measles-like or scarlatiniform), therapy may be resumed after the rash has completely disappeared. If the rash recurs upon reinstitution of therapy, further phenytoin medication is contraindicated.
Hyperglycemia, resulting from the drug's inhibitory effects on insulin release, has been reported. Phenytoin may also raise the serum glucose level in diabetic patients.
Osteomalacia has been associated with phenytoin therapy and is considered to be due to phenytoin's interference with Vitamin D metabolism.

Phenytoin is not indicated for seizures due to hypoglycemic or other metabolic causes. Appropriate diagnostic procedures should be performed as indicated.
Phenytoin is not effective for absence (petit mal) seizures. If tonic-clonic (grand mal) and absence (petit mal) seizures are present, combined drug therapy is needed.
Serum levels of phenytoin sustained above the optimal range may produce confusional states referred to as "delirium," "psychosis," or "encephalopathy," or rarely irreversible cerebellar dysfunction. Accordingly, at the first sign of acute toxicity, plasma levels are recommended. Dose reduction of phenytoin therapy is indicated if plasma levels are excessive; if symptoms persist termination is recommended. (See Warnings)
Information for Patients: Patients taking phenytoin should be advised of the importance of adhering strictly to the prescribed dosage regimen, and of informing the physician of any clinical condition in which it is not possible to take the drug orally as prescribed, eg, surgery, etc.
Patients should also be cautioned on the use of other drugs or alcoholic beverages without first seeking the physician's advice.
Patients should be instructed to call their physician if skin rash develops.
The importance of good dental hygiene should be stressed in order to minimize the development of gingival hyperplasia and its complications.
Laboratory Tests: Phenytoin serum level determinations may be necessary to achieve optimal dosage adjustments.
Drug Interactions: There are many drugs which may increase or decrease phenytoin levels or which phenytoin may affect. The most commonly occurring drug interactions are listed below:

1. Drugs which may increase phenytoin serum levels include: chloramphenicol, dicumarol, disulfiram, tolbutamide, isoniazid, phenylbutazone, acute alcohol intake, salicylates, chlordiazepoxide, phenothiazines, diazepam, estrogens, ethosuximide, halothane, methylphenidate, sulfonamides, cimetidine, trazodone.
2. Drugs which may decrease phenytoin levels include: carbamazepine, chronic alcohol abuse, reserpine. Moban® brand of Molindone Hydrochloride contains calcium ions which interfere with the absorption of phenytoin. Ingestion times of phenytoin and antacid preparations containing calcium should be staggered in patients with low serum phenytoin levels to prevent absorption problems.
3. Drugs which may either increase or decrease phenytoin serum levels include: phenobarbital, valproic acid, and sodium valproate. Similarly, the effect of phenytoin on phenobarbital, valproic acid and sodium valproate serum levels is unpredictable.
4. Although not a true drug interaction, tricyclic antidepressants may precipitate seizures in susceptible patients and phenytoin dosage may need to be adjusted.
5. Drugs whose efficacy is impaired by phenytoin include: corticosteroids, coumarin anticoagulants, oral contraceptives, quinidine, vitamin D, digitoxin, rifampin, doxycycline, estrogens, furosemide. Serum level determinations are especially helpful when possible drug interactions are suspected.

Drug/Laboratory Test Interactions: Phenytoin may cause decreased serum levels of protein-bound iodine (PBI). It may also produce lower than normal values for dexamethasone or metyrapone tests. Phenytoin may cause increased serum levels of glucose, alkaline phosphatase, and gamma glutamyl transpeptidase (GGT).
Carcinogenesis: See 'Warnings' section for information on carcinogenesis.
Pregnancy: See Warnings.
Nursing Mothers: Infant breast-feeding is not recommended for women taking this drug because phenytoin appears to be secreted in low concentrations in human milk.
Phenobarbital
Withdrawal symptoms, including convulsions and delirium, may occur upon discontinuance of phenobarbital in patients with chronic intoxication. Analgesics, if used with phenobarbital, should be prescribed with caution because of possible additive effects. Caution should be exercised in prescribing this drug to patients with suicidal tendencies or with a predilection to abusive use of barbiturates.
Phenobarbital should be used with caution in debilitating and pulmonary diseases.
Phenobarbital should be used with caution in patients with severely impaired liver function, severe anemia, congestive heart failure, fever, neuroses, hyperthyroidism, diabetes mellitus, and any conditions in which respiratory depression may be characteristic. Marked excitement rather than depression may occur in aged or debilitated patients, particularly those with cerebral arteriosclerosis.
Confusion or euphoria may result from use of this drug. Symptoms in mentally ill, phobic, and emotionally disturbed patients may be accentuated. Prolonged usage may produce psychological habituation. Sudden discontinuation or radical reduction of dosage may precipitate withdrawal symptoms in patients who have taken the drug for prolonged periods; dosage should be gradually reduced to the point of complete discontinuation.
Barbiturates should be prescribed with extreme caution for persons known or suspected of routinely or periodically consuming large quantities of alcoholic beverages. Potentiation of effect, even to the extent of causing death, may result from consumption of barbiturates by patients with a high serum alcohol level.
Information for Patients: Phenobarbital may impair the mental and/or physical abilities required for the performance of potentially hazardous tasks, such as driving a motor vehicle or other such activity requiring alertness; therefore, the patient should be cautioned accordingly.
Drug Interactions: The effects of phenobarbital may be increased by many drugs, including antihistamines, tranquilizers, corticosteroids, monoamine oxidase inhibitors, narcotic analgesics, amitriptyline, imipramine, and rauwolfia alkaloids.
Pregnancy
See WARNINGS
Nursing Mothers: Evidence that phenobarbital is secreted in human milk is inadequate. The drug appears to be secreted in low concentrations which are unlikely to affect the infant. If the mother is receiving large doses of phenobarbital, however, the drug concentration in milk might increase. For this reason, artificial feeding of the infant is recommended for women taking this drug.
Labor and Delivery: Barbiturates readily cross the placental barrier and, if administered during labor, may have a depressant effect on the fetus; infants born of mothers receiving barbiturates may have difficulty breathing spontaneously.

ADVERSE REACTIONS

Phenytoin
Central Nervous System: The most common manifestations encountered with phenytoin therapy are referable to this system and are usually dose-related. These include nystagmus, ataxia, slurred speech, decreased coordination and mental confusion. Dizziness, insomnia, transient nervousness, motor twitchings, and headaches have also been observed. There have also been rare reports of phenytoin induced dyskinesias, including chorea, dystonia, tremor and asterixis, similar to those induced by phenothiazine and other neuroleptic drugs.
A predominantly sensory peripheral polyneuropathy has been observed in patients receiving long-term phenytoin therapy.
Gastrointestinal System: Nausea, vomiting, and constipation.
Integumentary System: Dermatological manifestations sometimes accompanied by fever have included scarlatiniform or morbilliform rashes. A morbilliform rash (measles-like) is the most common; other types of dermatitis are seen more rarely. Other more serious forms which may be fatal have included bullous, exfoliative, or purpuric dermatitis, lupus erythematosus, and Stevens-Johnson syndrome (see Precautions).
Hemopoietic System: Hemopoietic complications, some fatal, have occasionally been reported in association with administration of phenytoin. These have included thrombocytopenia, leukopenia, granulocytopenia, agranulocytosis, and pancytopenia with or without bone marrow suppression. While macrocytosis and megaloblastic anemia have occurred, these conditions usually respond to folic acid therapy. Lymphadenopathy including benign lymph node hyperplasia, pseudolymphoma, lymphoma, and Hodgkin's Disease have been reported (see Warnings).
Connective Tissue System: Coarsening of the facial features, enlargement of the lips, gingival hyperplasia, hypertrichosis, and Peyronie's Disease.
Other: Systemic lupus erythematosus, periarteritis nodosa, toxic hepatitis, liver damage, and immunoglobulin abnormalities may occur.
Phenobarbital
Central Nervous System: With larger doses, the most common manifestations relate to this system. These include drowsiness, vertigo, ataxia, hebetude, headache, delirium and stupor.
Gastrointestinal System: Phenobarbital may cause gastrointestinal discomfort and nausea.
Integumentary System: Hypersensitivity reactions are rare. Cutaneous eruptions are principally due to idiosyncrasy. Fatalities from exfoliative dermatitis and cutaneous eruptions have been reported. There are two syndromes associated with phenobarbital administration: Stevens-Johnson and a phenobarbital sensitivity syndrome. The phenobarbital sensitivity syndrome, which has resulted in fatalities, is characterized by an erythematous rash, high fever, jaundice, mental confusion, and toxic damage of "parenchymatous organs."
Hemopoietic System: Megaloblastic anemia has been reported; this condition usually responds to folic acid therapy.

OVERDOSAGE

The therapeutic ranges for phenytoin and phenobarbital in adults are 10 to 20 mcg/mL and 10 to 30 mcg/mL, respectively. Following acute overdosage of this combination, the patient at steady-state may experience evidence of phenytoin toxicity ahead of phenobarbital toxicity because phenytoin plasma levels rise more rapidly than phenobarbital levels. Phenytoin also has a narrower margin between therapeutic and toxic levels than does phenobarbital.
Phenytoin
The lethal dose in children is not known. The lethal dose in adults is estimated to be 2 to 5 grams. The initial symptoms are nystagmus, ataxia, and dysarthria. Other signs are tremor, hyperflexia, lethargy, slurred speech, nausea, vomiting. The patient may become comatose and hypertensive. Death is due to respiratory and circulatory depression.
There are marked variations among individuals with respect to phenytoin plasma levels where toxicity may occur. Nystagmus, on lateral gaze, usually appears at 20 mcg/mL, ataxia at 30 mcg/mL, dysarthria and lethargy appear when the plasma concentration is over 40 mcg/mL, but as high a concentration as 50 mcg/mL has been reported without evidence of toxicity. As much as 25 times the therapeutic dose has been taken to result in a serum concentration over 100 mcg/mL with complete recovery.
Treatment is nonspecific since there is no known antidote. The adequacy of the respiratory and circulatory systems should be carefully observed and appropriate supportive measures employed. Hemodialysis can be considered since phenytoin is not completely bound to plasma proteins. Total exchange transfusion has been used in the treatment of severe intoxication in children.
In acute overdosage the possibility of other CNS depressants, including alcohol, should be borne in mind.
Phenobarbital
The lethal dose of phenobarbital is believed to be 5 grams. The highest known blood level from which a patient recovered was 580 mcg/mL. An overdose of phenobarbital will include the classical picture of progressive central nervous system depression. In its severest form this syndrome leads to respiratory arrest as a result of general reflex paralysis. The milder forms of this syndrome may mimic any stage of clinical anesthesia. Except for a rapid (and weak) pulse, vital signs are characteristically reduced. In addition to direct inhibition of the cardiac contractile mechanism with consequent hypotension, circulatory insufficiency may be aggravated by hypoxia from inadequate pulmonary ventilation. Early deaths are usually due to respiratory arrest, but delayed fatalities may arise from one or any combination of the following complications: hypostatic pneumonia, bronchopneumonia, lung abscess, pulmonary edema, cerebral edema, circulatory collapse, and irreversible renal shutdown. The treatment of barbiturate poisoning consists in removing any unabsorbed drug from the stomach, supporting the respiration and circulation, and expediting elimination of the drug which has been absorbed.

DOSAGE AND ADMINISTRATION

Serum concentrations should be monitored and care should be taken when switching a patient from the sodium salt to the free acid form.
Dilantin® Kapseals®, Dilantin Parenteral, and Dilantin with Phenobarbital are formulated with the sodium salt of phenytoin. The free acid form of phenytoin is used in Dilantin-30 Pediatric and Dilantin-125 Suspensions and Dilantin Infatabs. Because there is approximately an 8% increase in drug content with the free acid form over that of the sodium salt, dosage adjustments and serum level monitoring may be necessary when switching from a product formulated with the free acid to a product formulated with the sodium salt and vice versa.
The combination of Dilantin with Phenobarbital Kapseals is provided as a convenience for epileptic patients who require both drugs for seizure control. Anticonvulsant therapy should be initiated with either phenytoin or phenobarbital and, if indicated, the other drug can then be added. If the total daily doses of the two drugs used separately are within those given below, the combination of Dilantin with Phenobarbital Kapseals can then be substituted in equivalent amounts. When plasma level determinations are necessary for optimal dosage adjustments, the clinically effective level of Dilantin is usually 10 to 20 mcg/mL and for phenobarbital 10 to 30 mcg/mL in adults. Serum blood level determinations are especially helpful when possible drug interactions are suspected.

Continued on next page

This product information was prepared in August, 1986. On these and other Parke-Davis Products, information may be obtained by addressing PARKE-DAVIS, Division of Warner-Lambert Company, Morris Plains, New Jersey 07950.

Parke-Davis—Cont.

If either the phenytoin or phenobarbital dosage requires adjustment, this should be done by switching the patient to separate phenytoin and phenobarbital dosage forms in order to enable subsequent dosage adjustment of either or both drugs.
The recommended starting phenobarbital dose for children is 2 to 3 mg/kg/day in two or three equally divided doses.
The recommended starting Dilantin dose for children is 5 mg/kg/day in two or three equally divided doses.
Adult Dosage: For maintenance (see above)—usually three or four capsules daily. An increase to six capsules daily may be made, if necessary.
Pediatric Dosage: For maintenance (see above)—individualized to a maximum of 300 mg Dilantin daily.

HOW SUPPLIED

N 0071-0375 (Kapseal 375)—Dilantin with Phenobarbital each contain 100 mg phenytoin sodium with 16 mg (1/4 gr) phenobarbital; in 100's and 1000's.
N 0071-0531 (Kapseal 531)—Dilantin with Phenobarbital each contain 100 mg phenytoin sodium with 32 mg (1/2 gr) phenobarbital in 100's, 1000's and unit dose 100's.
Store at room temperature below 30°C (86°F).
Protect from moisture and light.
Also Available As:
N 0071-0362 (Kapseal 362)—Dilantin (phenytoin sodium) 100 mg; in 100's, 1000's, unit dose 100's and in a Memo Pack containing 84 unit-dose capsules (28 day dosage regimen).
N 0071-0365 (Kapseal 365)—Dilantin (phenytoin sodium) 30 mg in 100's, 1000's, and unit dose 100's.
N 0071-0007 (Tablet 7)—Dilantin Infatabs® each contain 50 mg phenytoin; 100's, and unit dose 100's.
N 0071-2214—Dilantin-125® Suspension (phenytoin oral suspension USP.) 125 mg phenytoin/5 mL with a maximum alcohol content not greater than 0.6 percent; available in 8-oz bottles and individual dose foil pouches which deliver 5 mL (125 mg phenytoin). The minimum sales unit is 100 pouches.
N 0071-2315—Dilantin-30® Pediatric Suspension (phenytoin oral suspension, USP.) 30 mg phenytoin/5 mL with a maximum alcohol content not greater than 0.6 percent; available in 8-oz bottles and individual unit dose foil pouches which deliver 5 mL (30 mg phenytoin). The minimum sales unit is 100 pouches.
For Parenteral Use:
N 0071-4488-05 (Ampoule 1488)—Dilantin ready-mixed solution containing 50 mg phenytoin sodium per milliliter is supplied in 2-mL ampoules. Packages of ten.
N 0071-4488-41 (Steri-Dose® 4488)—Dilantin ready-mixed solution containing 50 mg phenytoin sodium per milliliter is supplied in a 2-mL sterile disposable syringe (22 gauge × 1 1/4 inch needle).
Packages of ten individually cartoned syringes.
N 0071-4475-35 (Ampoule 1475)—Dilantin ready-mixed solution containing 50 mg phenytoin sodium per milliliter is supplied in 5-mL ampoules with one 6-mL sterile disposable syringe (22 gauge × 1 1/4 inch needle). Packages of ten.
N 0071-4475-08 (Ampoule 1475)—Dilantin ready-mixed solution containing 50 mg phenytoin sodium per milliliter is supplied in packages of ten 5-mL ampoules without syringes.

REFERENCES

1. Woodbury, DM and Fingl, E. "Drugs Effective in the Therapy of the Epilepsies," in Goodman, LS and Gilman, A(eds): The Pharmacological Basis of Therapeutics ed 5. New York, Macmillan Publishing Co, Inc, 1975, pp 201–226.
2. Henn, K. "Diphenylhydantoin: Relation of Plasma Levels to Clinical Control," in Woodbury, DM, Penry, JK, and Schmidt, RP, (eds): Antiepileptic Drugs, New York, Raven Press, Publishers, 1972, pp 211–218.

Caution—Federal law prohibits dispensing without prescription.

0375G013

Shown in Product Identification Section, page 420

DOPAMINE HYDROCHLORIDE INJECTION, USP DOPASTAT® ℞

DESCRIPTION

Dopamine, a sympathomimetic amine vasopressor, is the naturally occurring immediate precursor of norepinephrine. Dopamine HCl is a white, odorless, crystalline powder that is freely soluble in water and soluble in alcohol. It is sensitive to light, alkalis, iron salts, and oxidizing agents. Chemically it is designated as 4-(2-Aminoethyl) pyrocatechol hydrochloride.
Dopastat is a clear, practically colorless, sterile, pyrogen-free, aqueous solution of dopamine HCl for intravenous infusion after dilution. Each mL contains dopamine HCl (either 40 mg, equivalent to 32.31 mg dopamine base, or 80 mg, equivalent to 64.62 mg dopamine base) in Water for Injection, USP, and 1% sodium metabisulfite as an antioxidant. Hydrochloric acid may have been added for pH adjustment. Dopastat must be diluted in an appropriate, sterile parenteral solution before intravenous administration. (See DOSAGE AND ADMINISTRATION.)

CLINICAL PHARMACOLOGY

Dopamine is a natural catecholamine formed by the decarboxylation of 3,4-dihydroxyphenyl-alanine (DOPA). It is a precursor to norepinephrine in noradrenergic nerves and is also a neurotransmitter in certain areas of the central nervous system, especially in the nigrostriatal tract, and in a few peripheral sympathetic nerves.
Dopamine produces positive chronotropic and inotropic effects on the myocardium, resulting in increased heart rate and cardiac contractility. This is accomplished directly by exerting an agonist action on beta-adrenoceptors and indirectly by causing release of norepinephrine from storage sites in sympathetic nerve endings.
Dopamine's onset of action occurs within 5 minutes of intravenous administration, and with dopamine's plasma half-life of about two minutes, the duration of action is less than ten minutes. However, if monoamine oxidase (MAO) inhibitors are present, the duration may increase to one hour. The drug is widely distributed in the body but does not cross the blood-brain barrier to a significant extent. Dopamine is metabolized in the liver, kidney, and plasma by MAO and catechol-O-methyltransferase to the inactive compounds homovanillic acid (HVA) and 3,4- dihydroxyphenylacetic acid. About 25% of the dose is taken up into specialized neurosecretory vesicles (the adrenergic nerve terminals), where it is hydroxylated to form norepinephrine. It has been reported that about 80% of the drug is excreted in the urine within 24 hours, primarily as HVA and its sulfate and glucoronide conjugates and as 3,4-dihydroxy-phenylacetic acid. A very small portion is excreted unchanged.
The predominant effects of dopamine are dose-related, although it should be noted that actual reponse of an individual patient will largely depend on the clinical status of the patient at the time the drug is administered. At low rates of infusion (0.5-2 mcg/kg/min) dopamine causes vasodilation that is presumed to be due to a specific agonist action on dopamine receptors (distinct from alpha- and beta-adrenoceptors) in the renal, mesenteric, coronary, and intracerebral vascular beds. At these dopamine receptors, haloperidol is an antagonist. The vasodilation in these vascular beds is accompanied by increased glomerular filtration rate, renal blood flow, sodium excretion, and urine flow. Hypotension sometimes occurs. An increase in urinary output produced by dopamine is usually not associated with a decrease in osmolality of the urine.
At intermediate rates of infusion (2–10 mcg/kg/min) dopamine acts to stimulate the $beta_1$-adrenoceptors, resulting in improved myocardial contractility, increased SA rate and enhanced impulse conduction in the heart. There is little, if any, stimulation of the $beta_2$-adrenoceptors (peripheral vasodilation). Dopamine causes less increase in myocardial oxygen consumption that isoproterenol, and its use is not usually associated with a tachyarrhythmia. Clinical studies indicate that it usually increases systolic and pulse pressure with either no effect or a slight increase in diastolic pressure. Blood flow to the peripheral vascular beds may decrease while mesenteric flow increases due to increased cardiac output. Total peripheral resistance (alpha effects) at low and intermediate doses is usually unchanged.
At higher rates of infusion (10–20 mcg/kg/min) there is some effect on alpha-adrenoceptors, with consequent vasoconstrictor effects and a rise in blood pressure. The vasoconstrictor effects are first seen in the skeletal muscle vascular beds, but with increasing doses, they are also evident in the renal and mesenteric vessels. At very high rates of infusion (above 20 mcg/kg/min), stimulation of alpha- adrenoceptors predominates and vasoconstriction may compromise the circulation of the limbs and override the dopaminergic effects of dopamine, reversing renal dilation and naturesis.

INDICATIONS AND USAGE

Dopamine HCl is indicated for the correction of hemodynamic imbalances present in the shock syndrome due to myocardial infarction, trauma, endotoxic septicemia, open-heart surgery, renal failure, and chronic cardiac decompensation as in congestive failure.
Patients most likely to respond adequately to dopamine HCl are those in whom physiological parameters, such as urine flow, myocardial function, and blood pressure, have not undergone profound deterioration. Multiclinic trials indicate that the shorter the time interval between onset of signs and symptoms and initiation of therapy with blood volume correction and dopamine HCl, the better the prognosis. Where appropriate, blood volume restoration with a suitable plasma expander or whole blood should be accomplished prior to administration of dopamine HCl.
Poor Perfusion of Vital Organs—Urine flow appears to be one of the better diagnostic signs by which adequacy of vital organ perfusion can be monitored. Nevertheless, the physician should also observe the patient for signs of reversal of confusion or reversal of comatose condition. Loss of pallor, increase in toe temperature, and/or adequacy of nail bed capillary filling may also be used as indices of adequate dosage. Clinical studies have shown that when dopamine HCl is administered before urine flow has diminished to levels approximately 0.3 mL/minute, prognosis is more favorable. Nevertheless, in a number of oliguric or anuric patients, administration of dopamine HCl has resulted in an increase in urine flow in patients whose output is within normal limits and thus may be of value in reducing the degree of preexisting fluid accumulation. It should be noted that at doses above those optimal for the individual patient, urine flow may decrease, necessitating reduction of dosage.
Low Cardiac Output—Increased cardiac output is related to dopamine's direct inotropic effect on the myocardium. Increased cardiac output at low or moderate doses appears to be related to a favorable prognosis. Increase in cardiac output has been associated with either static or decreased systemic vascular resistance (SVR). Static or decreased SVR associated with low or moderate movements in cardiac output is believed to be a reflection of differential effects on specific vascular beds with increased resistance in peripheral beds (e.g., femoral) and concomitant decreases in mesenteric and renal vascular beds.
Redistribution of blood flow parallels these changes so that an increase in cardiac output is accompanied by an increase in mesenteric and renal blood flow. In many instances the renal fraction of the total cardiac output has been found to increase. Increase in cardiac output produced by dopamine is not associated with substantial decreases in systemic vascular resistance as may occur with isoproterenol.
Hypotension—Hypotension due to inadequate cardiac output can be managed by administration of low to moderate doses of dopamine HCl which have little effect on SVR. At high therapeutic doses, dopamine's alpha-adrenergic activity becomes more prominent and thus may correct hypotension due to diminished SVR. As in the case of other circulatory decompensation states, prognosis is better in patients whose blood pressure and urine flow have not undergone profound deterioration. Therefore, it is suggested that the physician administer dopamine HCl as soon as a definite trend toward decreased systolic and diastolic pressure becomes evident.

CONTRAINDICATIONS

Dopamine HCl should not be used in patients with pheochromocytoma.
Dopamine HCl should not be administered to patients with uncorrected tachyarrhythmias or ventricular fibrillation.

WARNINGS

Do NOT add dopamine HCl to any alkaline diluent solution since the drug is inactivated in alkaline solution.
Patients who have been receiving MAO inhibitors prior to the administration of dopamine HCl will require substantially reduced dosage. See Drug Interactions below.

PRECAUTIONS

General

1. **Monitoring**—Careful monitoring of the following indices is necessary during dopamine HCl infusion, as with any adrenergic agent: blood pressure, urine flow, and, when possible, cardiac output and pulmonary wedge pressure.
2. **Hypovolemia**—Prior to treatment with dopamine HCl, hypovolemia should be fully corrected, if possible, with either whole blood or plasma as indicated. Monitoring of central venous pressure or left ventricular filling pressure may be helpful in detecting and treating hypovolemia.
3. **Hypoxia, Hypercapnia, Acidosis**—These conditions, which may also reduce the effectiveness and/or increase the incidence of adverse effects of dopamine, must be identified and corrected prior to, or concurrently with, administration of dopamine HCl.
4. **Decreased Pulse Pressure**—If a disproportionate increase in diastolic blood pressure and a marked decrease in pulse pressure are observed in patients receiving dopamine HCl, the rate of infusion should be decreased and the patient observed carefully for further evidence of predominant vasoconstrictor activity, unless such effect is desired.
5. **Ventricular Arrhythmias**—If an increased number of ectopic beats are observed, the dose should be reduced if possible.
6. **Hypotension**—At lower infusion rates, if hypotension occurs, the infusion rate should be rapidly increased until adequate blood pressure is obtained. If hypotension persists, dopamine HCl should be discontinued and a more potent vasoconstrictor agent such as norepinephrine should be administered.
7. **Extravasation**—Dopamine HCl should be infused into a large vein whenever possible to prevent the possibility of extravasation into tissue adjacent to the infusion site. Extravasation may cause necrosis and sloughing of surrounding tissue. Large veins of the antecubital fossa are preferred to veins in the dorsum of the hand or ankle. Less suitable infusion sites should be used only if the patient's condition requires immediate attention. The physician

should switch to more suitable sites as rapidly as possible. The infusion site should be continuously monitored for free flow.

8. **Occlusive Vascular Disease**—Patients with a history of occlusive vascular disease (for example, atherosclerosis, arterial embolism, Raynaud's disease, cold injury, diabetic endarteritis, and Buerger's disease) should be closely monitored for any changes in color or temperature of the skin in the extremities. If a change in skin color or temperature occurs and is thought to be the result of compromised circulation in the extremities, the benefits of continued dopamine HCl infusion should be weighed against the risk of possible necrosis. This condition may be reversed by either decreasing the rate or discontinuing the infusion.

IMPORTANT

Antidote for Peripheral Ischemia: To prevent sloughing and necrosis in ischemic areas, the area should be infiltrated as soon as possible with 10 to 15 mL of saline solution containing from 5 to 10 mg of Regitine® (brand of phentolamine), an adrenergic blocking agent. A syringe with a fine hypodermic needle should be used, and the solution liberally infiltrated throughout the ischemic area. Sympathetic blockade with phentolamine causes immediate and conspicuous local hyperemic changes if the area is infiltrated within 12 hours. Therefore, *phentolamine should be given as soon as possible* after the extravasation is noted.

9. **Weaning**—When discontinuing the infusion, it may be necessary to gradually decrease the dose of dopamine HCl while expanding blood volume with IV fluids, since sudden cessation may result in marked hypotension.

Drug Interactions

1. Because dopamine is metabolized by monoamine oxidase (MAO), inhibition of this enzyme prolongs and potentiates the effect of dopamine. Patients who have been treated with **MAO inhibitors** within two to three weeks prior to the administration of dopamine HCl should receive initial doses of dopamine HCl no greater than one tenth (1/10) of the usual dose.
2. Concurrent administration of dopamine HCl and **diuretic agents** may produce an additive or potentiating effect on urine flow.
3. **Tricyclic antidepressants** may potentiate the pressor response to adrenergic agents.
4. Cardiac effects of dopamine are antagonized by **beta-adrenergic blocking agents,** such as propranolol and metoprolol. The peripheral vasoconstriction caused by high doses of dopamine HCl is antagonized by **alpha-adrenergic blocking agents.** Dopamine-induced renal and mesenteric vasodilation is not antagonized by either alpha- or beta-adrenergic blocking agents.
5. **Haloperidol** appears to have strong central antidopaminergic properties. Haloperidol and haloperidol-like drugs suppress the dopaminergic renal and mesenteric vasodilation induced at low rates of dopamine infusion.
6. **Cyclopropane or halogenated hydrocarbon anesthetics** increase cardiac autonomic irritability and may sensitize the myocardium to the action of certain intravenously administered catecholamines, such as dopamine. This interaction appears to be related both to pressor activity and to beta-adrenergic stimulating properties of these catecholamines and may produce ventricular arrhythmias and hypertension. Therefore, EXTREME CAUTION should be exercised when administering dopamine HCl to patients receiving cyclopropane or halogenated hydrocarbon anesthetics. It has been reported that results of studies in animals indicate that dopamine-induced ventricular arrhythmias during anesthesia can be reversed by propranolol.
7. The concomitant use of vasopressors and some **oxytocic drugs** may result in severe persistent hypertension. See Labor and Delivery below.
8. Administration of **phenytoin** to patients receiving dopamine HCl has been reported to lead to hypotension and bradycardia. It is suggested that in patients receiving dopamine HCl, alternatives to phenytoin should be used if anticonvulsant therapy is needed.

Pregnancy

Pregnancy Category C. Animal studies have revealed no evidence of teratogenic effects due to dopamine. However, in one study, administration of dopamine HCl to pregnant rats resulted in a decreased survival rate of the newborn and a potential for cataract formation in the survivors. There are no adequate and well-controlled studies in pregnant women and it is not known if dopamine crosses the placental barrier. Because animal reproduction studies are not always predictive of human response, this drug should be used during pregnancy only if, in the judgment of the physician, the potential benefit justifies the potential risk to the fetus.

Labor and Delivery

In obstetrics, if vasopressor drugs are used to correct hypotension or are added to a local anesthetic solution, some oxytocic drugs may cause severe persistent hypertension and may even cause rupture of a cerebral blood vessel to occur during the postpartum period.

Nursing Mothers

It is not known whether this drug is excreted in human milk. Because many drugs are excreted in human milk, caution should be exercised when dopamine HCl is administered to a nursing woman.

Pediatric Use

Safety and effectiveness in children have not been established. Dopamine HCl has been used in a limited number of pediatric patients. but such use has been inadequate to fully define proper dosage and limitations for use.

ADVERSE REACTIONS

The following adverse reactions have been observed, but there are not enough data to support an estimate of their frequency.

Cardiovascular System

ventricular arrhythmia (at very high doses)
ectopic beats
tachycardia
anginal pain
palpitation
cardiac conduction abnormalities
widened QRS complex
bradycardia
hypotension
hypertension
vasoconstriction

Respiratory System

dyspnea

Gastrointestinal System

nausea
vomiting

Metabolic/Nutritional System

azotemia

Central Nervous System

headache
anxiety

Dermatological System

piloerection

Other

Gangrene of the extremities has occurred when high doses were administered for prolonged periods or in patients with occlusive vascular disease receiving low doses of dopamine HCl.

OVERDOSAGE

In case of accidental overdosage, as evidenced by excessive elevation of blood pressure, reduce rate of administration or temporarily discontinue dopamine HCl until patient's condition stabilizes. Since dopamine's duration of action is quite short, no additional remedial measures are usually necessary. If these measures fail to stabilize the patient's condition, use of the short-acting alpha-adrenergic blocking agent phentolamine should be considered.

DOSAGE AND ADMINISTRATION

WARNING: This is a potent drug. It must be diluted before administration to patient.

Parenteral drug products should be inspected visually for particulate matter and discoloration prior to administration, whenever solution and container permit. Dopastat is a clear, practically colorless solution. Do not use if solution is darker than slightly yellow or discolored in any other way.

Suggested Dilution

Transfer contents of one or more ampoules or vials (each containing 200 mg or 400 mg dopamine HCl) by aseptic technique to either a 250-mL or 500-mL bottle of one of the following sterile intravenous solutions.

1. Sodium Chloride Injection, USP
2. Dextrose 5% Injection, USP
3. Dextrose (5%) and Sodium Chloride (0.9%) Injection, USP
4. Dextrose (5%) and Sodium Chloride (0.45%) Injection, USP
5. Dextrose (5%) and Lactated Ringer's Injection
6. Sodium Lactate (1/6 Molar) Injection, USP
7. Lactated Ringer's Injection, USP

Dopamine HCl has been found to be stable for a minimum of 24 hours after dilution in the sterile intravenous solutions listed above. However, as with all intravenous admixtures, dilution should be made just prior to administration.

Do NOT add dopamine HCl parenteral solution to 5% Sodium Bicarbonate or other alkaline intravenous solutions, since the drug is inactivated in alkaline solution.

Rate of Administration

Dopamine HCl, after dilution, is administered intravenously through a suitable intravenous catheter or needle. An IV drip chamber or other suitable metering device is essential for controlling the rate of flow in drops/minute. Each patient must be individually titrated to the desired hemodynamic and/or renal response with dopamine HCl. In titrating to the desired increase in systolic blood pressure, the optimum dosage rate for renal response may be exceeded, thus necessitating a reduction in rate after the hemodynamic condition is stabilized.

Administration at rates greater than 50 mcg/kg/minute have safely been used in advanced circulatory decompensation states. If unnecessary fluid expansion is of concern, adjustment of drug concentration may be preferred over increasing the flow rate of a less concentrated dilution.

Suggested Regimen

1. When appropriate, increase blood volume with whole blood or plasma until central venous pressure is 10 to 15 cm H_2O or pulmonary wedge pressure is 14 to 18 mm Hg.
2. Begin administration of diluted solution at doses of 2–5 mcg/kg/minute dopamine HCl in patients who are likely to respond to modest increments of heart force and renal perfusion.

In more seriously ill patients, begin administration of diluted solution at doses of 5 mcg/kg/minute dopamine HCl and increase gradually using 5–10 mcg/kg/minute increments up to 20–50 mcg/kg/minute as needed. If doses of dopamine HCl in excess of 50 mcg/kg/minute are required, it is suggested that urine output be checked frequently. Should urine flow begin to decrease in the absence of hypotension, reduction of dopamine HCl dosage should be considered. Multiclinic trials have shown that more than 50% of the patients were satisfactorily maintained on doses of dopamine HCl of less than 20 mcg/kg/minute. In patients who do not respond to these doses with adequate arterial pressures or urine flow, additional increments of dopamine HCl may be employed in an effort to produce an appropriate arterial pressure and central perfusion.

3. Treatment of all patients requires constant evaluation of therapy in terms of the blood volume, augmentation of myocardial contractility, and distribution of peripheral perfusion. Dosage of dopamine HCl should be adjusted according to the patient's response, with particular attention to diminution of established urine flow rate, increasing tachycardia or development of new dysrhythmias as indices for decreasing or temporarily suspending the dosage.
4. As with all potent intravenously administered drugs, care should be taken to control the rate of administration to avoid inadvertent administration of a bolus of drug.

HOW SUPPLIED

Dopastat® is a parenteral solution of dopamine HCl for infusion after dilution. It is supplied as follows:

N 0071-4210-08 Packages of ten individually cartoned 5-mL ampoules, (color coded white) containing 200 mg dopamine HCl (40 mg/mL dopamine HCl, equivalent to 32.31 mg/mL dopamine base).

N 0071-4210-45 Packages of ten individually cartoned 5-mL vials, (color coded white) containing 200 mg dopamine HCl (40 mg/mL dopamine HCl, equivalent to 32.31 mg/mL dopamine base).

N 0071-4220-08 Packages of ten individually cartoned 5- mL vials, (color coded green) containing 400 mg dopamine HCl (80 mg/mL dopamine HCl, equivalent to 64.62 mg/mL dopamine base).

SPECIAL HANDLING AND STORAGE CONDITIONS

Store at controlled room temperature, 15°–30°C (59°–86°F). Protect from light.

Avoid contact with alkalies (including sodium bicarbonate), oxidizing agents, or iron salts.

Caution—Federal law prohibits dispensing without prescription.

4210G045

DORYX® ℞

(Coated Doxycycline Hyclate Pellets)

DESCRIPTION

DORYX® Capsules contain specially coated pellets of doxycycline hyclate for oral administration. Also contains lactose, NF; microcrystalline cellulose, NF; povidone, USP. The capsule shell and/or band contains FD and C blue No. 1; FD and C yellow No. 6; D and C yellow No. 10; gelatin, NF; silicon dioxide; sodium lauryl sulfate, NF; titanium dioxide, USP. Doxycycline is a broad-spectrum antibiotic synthetically derived from oxytetracycline and available as doxycycline hyclate. The chemical designation of this light-yellow crystalline powder is alpha-6-desoxy-5-oxytetracycline. Doxycycline has a high degree of lipoid solubility and a low affinity for calcium binding. It is highly stable in normal human serum. Doxycycline will not degrade into an epianhydro form.

Continued on next page

This product information was prepared in August, 1986. On these and other Parke-Davis Products, information may be obtained by addressing PARKE-DAVIS, Division of Warner-Lambert Company, Morris Plains, New Jersey 07950.

Parke-Davis—Cont.

CLINICAL PHARMACOLOGY

Tetracyclines are readily absorbed and are bound to plasma proteins in varying degree. They are concentrated by the liver in the bile, and excreted in the urine and feces at high concentrations and in a biologically active form.

Doxycycline is virtually completely absorbed after oral administration. Following a 200 mg dose, normal adult volunteers averaged peak serum levels of 2.6 mcg/mL of doxycycline at 2 hours decreasing to 145 mcg/mL at 24 hours. Excretion of doxycycline by the kidney is about 40%/72 hours in individuals with normal function (creatinine clearance about 75 mL/min). This percentage excretion may fall as low as 1–5%/72 hours in individuals with severe renal insufficiency (creatinine clearance below 10 mL/min). Studies have shown no significant difference in serum half-life of doxycycline (range 18–22 hours) in individuals with normal and severely impaired renal function.

Hemodialysis does not alter serum half-life.

Microbiology: Doxycycline is primarily bacteriostatic and is thought to exert its antimicrobial effect by the inhibition of protein synthesis. Doxycycline is active against a wide range of gram-positive and gram-negative organisms. The drugs in the tetracycline class have closely similar antimicrobial spectra and cross resistance among them is common.

Susceptibility Tests: Diffusion Techniques: The use of antibiotic disc susceptibility test methods which measure zone diameter gives an accurate estimation of susceptibility of organisms to DORYX: One such standard procedure[1] has been recommended for use with discs for testing antimicrobials. Doxycycline 30 mcg discs should be used for the determination of the susceptibility of organisms to doxycycline.

With this type of procedure, a report of "susceptible" from the laboratory indicates that the infecting organism is likely to respond to therapy. A report of "intermediate susceptibility" suggests that the organism would be susceptible if high dosage is used or if the infection is confined to tissue and fluids (e.g., urine) in which high antibiotic levels are obtained. A report of "resistant" indicates that the infecting organism is not likely to respond to therapy. With the doxycycline disc, a zone of 16 mm or greater indicates susceptibility, zone sizes of 12 mm or less indicate resistance, and zone sizes of 13 to 15 mm indicate intermediate susceptibility.

Standardized procedures require the use of laboratory control organisms. The 30 mcg tetracycline disc should give zone diameters between 19 and 28 mm for *S.aureus* ATCC 25923 and between 18 and 25 mm for *E.coli* ATCC 25922. The 30 mcg doxycycline disc should give zone diameters between 23 and 29 mm for *S.aureus* ATCC 25923, and between 18 and 24 mm for *E.coli* ATCC 25922.

Dilution Techniques: A bacterial isolate may be considered susceptible if the MIC (minimal inhibitory concentration) value for doxycycline is less than 4 mcg/mL. Organisms are considered resistant if the MIC is greater than 12.5 mcg/mL. MICs greater than 4.0 mcg/mL and less than 12.5 mcg/mL indicate intermediate susceptibility.

As with standard diffusion methods, dilution procedures require the use of laboratory control mechanisms. Standard doxycycline powder should give MIC values in the range of 0.25 mcg/mL and 1.0 mcg/mL for *S.aureus* ATCC 25923. For *E.coli* ATCC 25922 the MIC range should be between 1.0 mcg/mL and 4.0 mcg/mL.

INDICATIONS AND USAGE

Doxycycline is indicated in infections caused by the following microorganisms:

Rickettsiae (Rocky Mountain spotted fever, typhus fever and the typhus group, Q fever, rickettsialpox and tick fevers).

Mycoplasma pneumoniae (PPLO, Eaton's agent).

Agents of psittacosis and ornithosis.

Agents of lymphogranuloma venereum and granuloma inguinale.

The following gram-negative microorganisms:

Haemophilus ducreyi (chancroid)
Yersinia pestis (formerly *Pasteurella pestis*)
Francisella tularensis (formerly *Pasteurella tularensis*)
Bartonella bacilliformis
Bacteroides species
Vibrio cholerae (formerly *Vibrio comma*)
Campylobacter fetus (formerly *Vibrio fetus*)
Brucella species (in conjunction with streptomycin)

Because many strains of the following groups of microorganisms have been shown to be resistant to tetracyclines, culture and susceptibility testing are recommended.

Doxycycline is indicated for treatment of infections caused by the following gram-negative microorganisms, when bacteriological testing indicates appropriate susceptibility to the drug:

Escherichia coli
Enterobacter aerogenes (formerly *Aerobacter aerogenes*)
Shigella species
Mima species and *Herellea* species
Haemophilus influenzae (respiratory infections)
Klebsiella species (respiratory and urinary infections)

Doxycycline is indicated for treatment of infections caused by the following gram-positive microorganisms when bacteriological testing indicates appropriate susceptibility to the drug:

Streptococcus species:

Up to 44 percent of strains of *Streptococcus pyogenes* and 74 percent of *Streptococcus faecalis* have been found to be resistant to tetracycline drugs. Therefore, tetracyclines should not be used for streptococcal disease unless the organism has been demonstrated to be susceptible.

For upper respiratory infections due to group A beta-hemolytic streptococci, penicillin is the usual drug of choice, including prophylaxis of rheumatic fever.

Diplococcus pneumoniae.

Staphylococcus aureus, (respiratory, skin and soft-tissue infections). Tetracyclines are not the drug of choice in the treatment of any type of staphylococcal infection.

When penicillin is contraindicated, doxycycline is an alternative drug in the treatment of infections due to:

Treponema pallidum and *Treponema pertenue* (syphilis and yaws)
Listeria monocytogenes
Clostridium species
Bacillus anthracis
Fusobacterium fusiforme (Vincent's infection)
Actinomyces species

In acute intestinal amebiasis doxycycline may be a useful adjunct to amebicides.

In severe acne doxycycline may be useful adjunctive therapy.

Doxycycline is indicated in the treatment of trachoma, although the infectious agent is not always eliminated, as judged by immunofluorescence.

Inclusion conjunctivitis may be treated with oral doxycycline alone, or with a combination of topical agents.

Doxycycline is indicated for the treatment of uncomplicated urethral, endocervical or rectal infections in adults caused by *Chlamydia trachomatis.*[2]

Doxycycline is indicated for the treatment of nongonococcal urethritis caused by *Chlamydia trachomatis* and *Ureaplasma urealyticum* and for the treatment of acute epididymo-orchitis caused by *Chlamydia trachomatis.*[2]

Doxycycline is indicated for the treatment of uncomplicated gonococcal infections in adults (except for anorectal infections in men), the gonococcal arthritis-dermatitis syndrome and acute epididymo-orchitis caused by *N. gonorrhoeae.*[2]

CONTRAINDICATIONS

The drug is contraindicated in persons who have shown hypersensitivity to any of the tetracyclines.

WARNINGS

THE USE OF DRUGS OF THE TETRACYCLINE CLASS DURING TOOTH DEVELOPMENT (LAST HALF OF PREGNANCY, INFANCY AND CHILDHOOD TO THE AGE OF 8 YEARS) MAY CAUSE PERMANENT DISCOLORATION OF THE TEETH (YELLOW-GRAY-BROWN). This adverse reaction is more common during long term use of the drugs but has been observed following repeated short term courses. Enamel hypoplasia has also been reported. TETRACYCLINE DRUGS, THEREFORE, SHOULD NOT BE USED IN THIS AGE GROUP UNLESS OTHER DRUGS ARE NOT LIKELY TO BE EFFECTIVE OR ARE CONTRAINDICATED.

Results of animal studies indicate that tetracyclines cross the placenta, are found in fetal tissues and can have toxic effects on the developing fetus (often related to retardation of skeletal development). Evidence of embryotoxicity has been noted in animals treated early in pregnancy. If any tetracycline is used during pregnancy or if the patient becomes pregnant while taking these drugs, the patient should be apprised of potential hazard to the fetus.

As with other tetracyclines, doxycycline forms a stable calcium complex in any bone-forming tissue. A decrease in the fibula growth rate has been observed in prematures given oral tetracycline in doses of 25 mg/kg every six hours. This reaction was shown to be reversible when the drug was discontinued.

Photosensitivity manifested by an exaggerated sunburn reaction has been observed in some individuals taking tetracyclines. Patients apt to be exposed to direct sunlight or ultraviolet light should be advised that this reaction can occur with tetracycline drugs, and treatment should be discontinued at the first evidence of skin erythema.

The antianabolic action of the tetracyclines may cause an increase in BUN. Studies to date indicate that this does not occur with the use of doxycycline in patients with impaired renal function.

PRECAUTIONS

As with other antibiotic preparations, use of this drug may result in overgrowth of nonsusceptible organisms, including fungi. If superinfection occurs, the antibiotic should be discontinued and appropriate therapy instituted.

All infections due to group A beta-hemolytic streptococci should be treated for at least 10 days.

Laboratory tests: In venereal disease when coexistent syphilis is suspected, dark-field examination should be done before treatment is started and the blood serology repeated monthly for at least 4 months.

In long term therapy, periodic laboratory evaluation of organ systems, including hematopoietic, renal and hepatic studies should be performed.

Drug interactions: Because tetracyclines have been shown to depress plasma prothrombin activity, patients who are on anticoagulant therapy may require downward adjustment of their anticoagulant dosage.

Since bacteriostatic drugs may interfere with the bactericidal action of penicillin, it is advisable to avoid giving tetracyclines in conjunction with penicillin.

For concomitant therapy with antacids or iron-containing preparations and food see "Dosage and Administration" section.

Carcinogenesis, mutagenesis, impairment of fertility: Long term studies are currently being conducted to determine whether tetracyclines have carcinogenic potential. Animal studies conducted in rats and mice have not provided conclusive evidence that tetracyclines may be carcinogenic or that they impair fertility. In two mammalian cell assays (L51784 mouse lymphoma and Chinese hamster lung cells *in vitro*) positive responses for mutagenicity occurred at concentrations of 60 and 10 mcg/mL respectively. In humans no association between tetracyclines and these effects have been made.

Pregnancy: Pregnancy Category D (See Warnings section).

Nursing mothers: Tetracyclines are present in the milk of lactating women who are taking a drug in this class. Because of the potential for serious adverse reactions in nursing infants from the tetracyclines, a decision should be made whether to discontinue nursing or discontinue the drug, taking into account the importance of the drug to the mother (see Warnings section).

Pediatric use: See Warnings and Dosage and Administration sections.

ADVERSE REACTIONS

Due to oral doxycycline's virtually complete absorption, side effects to the lower bowel, particularly diarrhea, have been infrequent. The following adverse reactions have been observed in patients receiving tetracyclines:

Gastrointestinal: Anorexia, nausea, vomiting, diarrhea, glossitis, dysphagia, enterocolitis, and inflammatory lesions (with monilial overgrowth) in the anogenital region. These reactions have been caused by both the oral and parenteral administration of tetracyclines. Rare instances of esophagitis and esophageal ulcerations have been reported in patients receiving capsule and tablet forms of drugs in the tetracycline class. Most of these patients took medications immediately before going to bed. (See Dosage and Administration).

Skin: Maculopapular and erythematous rashes. Exfoliative dermatitis has been reported but is uncommon. Photosensitivity is discussed above (see Warnings).

Renal toxicity: Rise in BUN has been reported and is apparently dose related. (See Warnings).

Hypersensitivity reactions: Urticaria, angioneurotic edema, anaphylaxis, anaphylactoid purpura, pericarditis, and exacerbation of systemic lupus erythematosus.

Bulging fontanels in infants and benign intracranial hypertension in adults have been reported in individuals receiving tetracyclines. These conditions disappeared when the drug was discontinued.

Blood: Hemolytic anemia, thrombocytopenia, neutropenia, and eosinophilis have been reported with tetracyclines.

When given over prolonged periods, tetracyclines have been reported to produce brown-black microscopic discoloration of thyroid glands. No abnormalities of thyroid function are known to occur.

DOSAGE AND ADMINISTRATION

THE USUAL DOSAGE AND FREQUENCY OF ADMINISTRATION OF DOXYCYCLINE DIFFERS FROM THAT OF THE OTHER TETRACYCLINES. EXCEEDING THE RECOMMENDED DOSAGE MAY RESULT IN AN INCREASED INCIDENCE OF SIDE EFFECTS.

Adults: The usual dose of oral doxycycline is 200 mg on the first day of treatment (administered 100 mg every 12 hours) followed by a maintenance dose of 100 mg/day. The maintenance dose may be administered as a single dose or as 50 mg every 12 hours. In the management of more severe infections (particularly chronic infections of the urinary tract), 100 mg every 12 hours is recommended.

For children above eight years of age: The recommended dosage schedule for children weighing 100 pounds or less is 2 mg/lb of body weight divided into two doses on the first day of treatment, followed by 1 mg/lb of body weight given as a single daily dose or divided into two doses on subsequent days. For more severe infections up to 2 mg/lb of body weight may be used. For children over 100 pounds, the usual adult dose should be used.

Uncomplicated gonococcal infections in adults (except anorectal infections in men): 100 mg, by mouth, twice-a-day for 7 days.[2] As an alternate single visit dose, administer 300 mg stat followed in one hour by a second 300 mg dose. The dose may be administered with food, including milk or carbonated beverage, as required.
Acute epididymo-orchitis caused by *N. gonorrhoeae:* 100 mg, by mouth, twice-a-day for at least 10 days.[2]
Primary and secondary syphilis: 300 mg a day in divided doses for at least 10 days.
Uncomplicated urethral, endocervical, or rectal infection in adults caused by *Chlamydia trachomatis:* 100 mg by mouth, twice-a-day for at least 7 days.[2]
Nongonococcal urethritis caused by *C. trachomatis* and *U. urealyticum:* 100 mg, by mouth, twice-a-day for at least 7 days.[2]
Acute epididymo-orchitis caused by *C. trachomatis:* 100 mg, by mouth, twice-a-day for at least 10 days.[2]
The therapeutic antibacterial serum activity will usually persist for 24 hours following recommended dosage.
When used in streptococcal infections, therapy should be continued for 10 days.
Administration of adequate amounts of fluid along with capsule and tablet forms of drugs in the tetracycline class is recommended to wash down the drugs and reduce the risk of esophageal irritation and ulceration (see Adverse Reactions).
If gastric irritation occurs, it is recommended that doxycycline be given with food or milk. The absorption of doxycycline is not markedly influenced by simultaneous ingestion of food or milk.
Concomitant therapy: Antacids containing aluminum, calcium or magnesium, sodium bicarbonate, and iron-containing preparations should not be given to patients taking oral tetracyclines.
Studies to date have indicated that administration of doxycycline at the usual recommended doses does not lead to excessive accumulation of the antibiotic in patients with renal impairment.

HOW SUPPLIED

DORYX® Capsules have a yellow transparent body with light blue opaque cap; the capsule bearing the inscription "DORYX" in white. Pellets are colored yellow. Each capsule contains specially coated pellets of doxycycline hyclate equivalent to 100 mg of doxycycline, supplied in:
Bottles of 50 capsules ....N 0071-0838-19

STORAGE CONDITIONS

Store at controlled room temperature below 25° C (77° F).

References:

1. NCCLS Approved Standard:
M2-A3, Vol. 4, Performance Standards for Antimicrobial Disk Susceptibility Tests, Third Edition: available from the National Committee for Clinical Laboratory Standards, 771 East Lancaster Avenue, Villanova, Pa. 19085
2. CDC Sexually Transmitted Diseases Treatment Guidelines 1982

Caution—Federal law prohibits dispensing without prescription.
Manufactured by
Faulding International
129 Dew Street,
Thebarton, South Australia, 5031
Distributed by
PARKE-DAVIS
Div of Warner-Lambert Co
Morris Plains, NJ 07950 USA

0838G021

Shown in Product Identification Section, page 420

DOXYCYCLINE HYCLATE ℞
Capsules, USP
50 mg and 100 mg
DOXYCYCLINE HYCLATE ℞
Tablets, USP
100 mg

DESCRIPTION

Doxycycline is a broad-spectrum antibiotic synthetically derived from oxytetracycline. Each 100 mg tablet also contains croscarmellose sodium type A, NF; magnesium stearate, NF; methylcellulose, USP; microcrystalline cellulose, NF; Opadry clear; Opadry orange; stearic acid, NF. Each 50 mg and 100 mg capsule also contains lactose, NF; magnesium stearate, NF. The capsule shell and/or band contains FD and C blue No. 1; FD and C green No. 3; gelatin, NF; silicon dioxide; sodium lauryl sulfate, NF; titanium dioxide, USP. The chemical designation of this light-yellow crystalline powder is alpha-6-deoxy-5-oxytetracycline. Doxycycline has a high degree of lipoid solubility and a low affinity for calcium binding. It is highly stable in normal human serum. Doxycycline will not degrade into an epianhydro form.

CLINICAL PHARMACOLOGY

Doxycycline is primarily bacteriostatic and is thought to exert its antimicrobial effect by the inhibition of protein synthesis. Doxycycline is active against a wide range of gram-positive and gram-negative organisms.
The drugs in the tetracycline class have closely similar antimicrobial spectra, and cross resistance among them is common. Microorganisms may be considered susceptible if the M.I.C. (minimum inhibitory concentration) is less than 4.0 mcg/mL and intermediate if the M.I.C. is 4.0 to 12.5 mcg/mL.
Susceptibility plate testing: If the Kirby-Bauer method of disc susceptibility testing is used, a 30 mcg doxycycline disc should give a zone of at least 16 mm when tested against a doxycycline-susceptible bacterial strain. A tetracycline disc may be used to determine microbial susceptibility. If the Kirby-Bauer method of disc susceptibility testing is used, a 30 mcg tetracycline disc should give a zone of at least 19 mm when tested against a tetracycline-susceptible bacterial strain.
Tetracyclines are readily absorbed and are bound to plasma proteins in varying degree. They are concentrated by the liver in the bile, and excreted in the urine and feces at high concentrations and in a biologically active form. Doxycycline is virtually completely absorbed after oral administration.
Following a 200 mg dose, normal adult volunteers averaged peak serum levels of 2.6 mcg/mL of doxycycline at 2 hours decreasing to 1.45 mcg/mL at 24 hours. Excretion of doxycycline by the kidney is about 40%/72 hours in individuals with normal function (creatinine clearance about 75 mL/min). This percentage excretion may fall as low as 1–5%/72 hours in individuals with severe renal insufficiency (creatinine clearance below 10 mL/min). Studies have shown no significant difference in serum half-life of doxycycline (range 18–22 hours) in individuals with normal and severely impaired renal function.
Hemodialysis does not alter serum half-life.

INDICATIONS AND USAGE

Doxycycline is indicated in infections caused by the following microorganisms:
Rickettsiae: Rocky Mountain spotted fever, typhus fever and the typhus group, Q fever, rickettsialpox, and tick fevers.
Mycoplasma pneumoniae (PPLO, Eaton agent).
Agents of psittacosis and ornithosis.
Agents of lymphogranuloma venereum and granuloma inguinale.
The spirochetal agent of relapsing fever *(Borrelia recurrentis).*
The following gram-negative microorganisms:
Haemophilus ducreyi (chancroid).
Pasteurella pestis, and *Pasteurella tularensis.*
Bartonella bacilliformis.
Bacteroides species.
Vibrio comma and *Vibrio fetus.*
Brucella species (in conjunction with streptomycin).
Because many strains of the following groups of microorganisms have been shown to be resistant to tetracyclines, culture and susceptibility testing are recommended.
Doxycycline is indicated for treatment of infections caused by the following gram-negative microorganisms, when bacteriologic testing indicates appropriate susceptibility to the drug:
Escherichia coli,
Enterobacter aerogenes (formerly *Aerobacter aerogenes),*
Shigella species,
Mima species and *Herellea* species,
Haemophilus influenzae (respiratory infections),
Klebsiella species (respiratory and urinary infections),
Doxycycline is indicated for treatment of infections caused by the following gram-positive microorganisms when bacteriologic testing indicates appropriate susceptibility to the drug:
***Streptococcus* species:**
Up to 44 percent of strains of *Streptococcus pyogenes* and 74 percent of *Streptococcus faecalis* have been found to be resistant to tetracycline drugs. Therefore, tetracyclines should not be used for streptococcal disease unless the organism has been demonstrated to be sensitive.
For upper respiratory infections due to group A beta hemolytic streptococci, penicillin is the usual drug of choice, including prophylaxis of rheumatic fever.
Diplococcus pneumoniae.
Staphylococcus aureus, respiratory, skin and soft-tissue infections. Tetracyclines are not the drug of choice in the treatment of any type of staphylococcal infection.
When penicillin is contraindicated, doxycycline is an alternative drug in the treatment of infections due to:
Treponema pallidum and *Treponema pertenue* (syphilis and yaws),
Listeria monocytogenes,
Clostridium species,
Bacillus anthracis,
Fusobacterium fusiforme (Vincent's infection),
Actinomyces species.
In acute intestinal amebiasis doxycycline may be a useful adjunct to amebicides.
In severe acne doxycycline may be useful adjunctive therapy.
Doxycycline is indicated in the treatment of trachoma, although the infectious agent is not always eliminated, as judged by immunofluorescence.
Inclusion conjunctivitis may be treated with oral doxycycline alone, or with a combination of topical agents.
Doxycycline is indicated for the treatment of uncomplicated urethral, endocervical, or rectal infections in adults caused by *Chlamydia trachomatis.*[1]
Doxycycline is indicated for treatment of nongonococcal urethritis caused by *Chlamydia trachomatis* and *Ureaplasma urealyticum* and for the treatment of acute epididymo-orchitis caused by *Chlamydia trachomatis.*[1]
Doxycycline is indicated for the treatment of uncomplicated gonococcal infections in adults (except for anorectal infections in men) and acute epididymo-orchitis caused by *N gonorrhoeae.*[1]

CONTRAINDICATIONS

This drug is contraindicated in persons who have shown hypersensitivity to any of the tetracyclines.

WARNINGS

THE USE OF DRUGS OF THE TETRACYCLINE CLASS DURING TOOTH DEVELOPMENT (LAST HALF OF PREGNANCY, INFANCY AND CHILDHOOD TO THE AGE OF 8 YEARS) MAY CAUSE PERMANENT DISCOLORATION OF THE TEETH (YELLOW-GRAY-BROWN). This adverse reaction is more common during long term use of the drugs but has been observed following repeated short term courses. Enamel hypoplasia has also been reported. *TETRACYCLINE DRUGS, THEREFORE, SHOULD NOT BE USED IN THIS AGE GROUP UNLESS OTHER DRUGS ARE NOT LIKELY TO BE EFFECTIVE OR ARE CONTRAINDICATED.*
Photosensitivity manifested by an exaggerated sunburn reaction has been observed in some individuals taking tetracyclines. Patients apt to be exposed to direct sunlight or ultraviolet light should be advised that this reaction can occur with tetracycline drugs, and treatment should be discontinued at the first evidence of skin erythema.
The antianabolic action of the tetracyclines may cause an increase in BUN. Studies to date indicate that this does not occur with the use of doxycycline in patients with impaired renal function.
Usage in Pregnancy: (See above "WARNINGS" about use during tooth development.) Results of animal studies indicate that tetracyclines cross the placenta, are found in fetal tissues, and can have toxic effects on the developing fetus (often related to retardation of skeletal development). Evidence of embryotoxicity has also been noted in animals treated early in pregnancy.
Usage in Newborns, Infants, and Children: (See above "WARNINGS" about use during tooth development.) As with other tetracyclines, doxycycline forms a stable calcium complex in any bone-forming tissue. A decrease in the fibula growth rate has been observed in prematures given oral tetracycline in doses of 25 mg/kg every six hours. This reaction was shown to be reversible when the drug was discontinued.
Tetracyclines are present in the milk of lactating women who are taking a drug in this class.

PRECAUTIONS

As with other antibiotic preparations, use of this drug may result in overgrowth of nonsusceptible organisms, including fungi. If superinfection occurs, the antibiotic should be discontinued and appropriate therapy should be instituted.
In venereal disease when coexistent syphilis is suspected, a dark field examination should be done before treatment is started and the blood serology repeated monthly for at least four months.
Because the tetracyclines have been shown to depress plasma prothrombin activity, patients who are on anticoagulant therapy may require downward adjustment of their anticoagulant dosage.
In long term therapy, periodic laboratory evaluation of organ systems, including hematopoietic, renal, and hepatic studies should be performed.
All infections due to group A beta-hemolytic streptococci should be treated for at least 10 days.
Since bacteriostatic drugs may interfere with the bactericidal action of penicillin, it is advisable to avoid giving tetracycline in conjunction with penicillin.

ADVERSE REACTIONS

Due to oral doxycycline's virtually complete absorption, side effects of the lower bowel, particularly diarrhea, have been infrequent. The following adverse reactions have been observed in patients receiving tetracyclines:

Continued on next page

This product information was prepared in August, 1986. On these and other Parke-Davis Products, information may be obtained by addressing PARKE-DAVIS, Division of Warner-Lambert Company, Morris Plains, New Jersey 07950.

Parke-Davis—Cont.

Gastrointestinal: anorexia, nausea, vomiting, diarrhea, glossitis, dysphagia, enterocolitis, and inflammatory lesions (with monolial overgrowth) in the anogenital region. These reactions have been caused by both the oral and parenteral administration of tetracyclines. Rare instances of esophagitis and esophageal ulcerations have been reported in patients receiving capsule and tablet forms of drugs in the tetracycline class. Most of these patients took medications immediately before going to bed. (See Dosage and Administration.)
Skin: maculopapular and erythematous rashes. Exfoliative dermatitis has been reported but is uncommon. Photosensitivity is discussed above (see "WARNINGS").
Renal toxicity: Rise in BUN has been reported and is apparently dose related. (See "WARNINGS".)
Hypersensitivity reactions: Urticaria, angioneurotic edema, anaphylaxis, anaphylactoid purpura, pericarditis, and exacerbation of systemic lupus erythematosus.
Bulging fontanels in infants and benign intracranial hypertension in adults have been reported in individuals receiving full therapeutic dosages. These conditions disappeared rapidly when the drug was discontinued.
Blood: Hemolytic anemia, thrombocytopenia, neutropenia, and eosinophilia have been reported with tetracyclines.
When given over prolonged periods, tetracyclines have been reported to produce brown-black microscopic discoloration of thyroid glands. No abnormalities of thyroid function studies are known to occur.

DOSAGE AND ADMINISTRATION

THE USUAL DOSAGE AND FREQUENCY OF ADMINISTRATION OF DOXYCYCLINE DIFFERS FROM THAT OF THE OTHER TETRACYCLINES. EXCEEDING THE RECOMMENDED DOSAGE MAY RESULT IN AN INCREASED INCIDENCE OF SIDE EFFECTS.
Adults: The usual dose of oral doxycycline is 200 mg on the first day of treatment (administered 100 mg every 12 hours) followed by a maintenance dose of 100 mg/day. The maintenance dose may be administered as a single dose or as 50 mg every 12 hours. In the management of more severe infections (particularly chronic infections of the urinary tract), 100 mg every 12 hours is recommended.
For children above eight years of age: The recommended dosage schedule for children weighing 100 pounds or less is 2 mg/lb of body weight divided into two doses on the first day of treatment, followed by 10 mg/lb of body weight given as a single daily dose or divided into two doses, on subsequent days. For more severe infections up to 2 mg/lb of body weight may be used. For children over 100 lbs the usual adult dose should be used.
Uncomplicated gonococcal infections in adults (except anorectal infections in men): 100 mg, by mouth, twice a day for 7 days.[1]
As an alternate single visit dose, administer 300 mg stat followed in one hour by a second 300 mg dose. The dose may be administered with food, including milk or carbonated beverage as required.
Acute epididymo-orchitis caused by N gonorrhoeae: 100 mg, by mouth, twice a day for at least 10 days.[1]
Primary and secondary syphilis: 300 mg a day in divided doses for at least 10 days.
The therapeutic antibacterial serum activity will usually persist for 24 hours following recommended dosage.
When used in streptococcal infections, therapy should be continued for 10 days.
Administration of adequate amounts of fluid along with capsule and tablet forms of drugs in the tetracycline class is recommended to wash down the drugs and reduce the risk of esophageal irritation and ulceration. (See Adverse Reactions.)
If gastric irritation occurs, it is recommended that doxycycline be given with food or milk. The absorption of doxycycline is not markedly influenced by simultaneous ingestion of food or milk.
Uncomplicated urethral, endocervical, or rectal infection in adults caused by *Chlamydia trachomatis:* 100 mg. by mouth, twice a day for at least 7 days.[1]
Nongonococcal urethritis caused by *C trachomatis* and *U urealyticum:* 100 mg. by mouth, twice a day for at least 10 days.[1]
Acute epididymo-orchitis caused by *C trachomatis:* 100 mg. by mouth, twice a day for at least 10 days.[1]
Concomitant therapy: Antacids containing aluminum, calcium, or magnesium impair absorption and should not be given to patients taking oral doxycycline.
Studies to date have indicated that administration of doxycycline at the usual recommended doses does not lead to excessive accumulation of the antibiotic in patients with renal impairment.

HOW SUPPLIED

Doxycycline hyclate capsules:
N 0071-0829-19 50 mg Bottles of 50
Each capsule contains doxycycline hyclate equivalent to 50 mg doxycycline.
N 0071-0830-19 100 mg Bottles of 50
Each capsule contains doxycycline hyclate equivalent to 100 mg doxycycline.
Doxycycline hyclate tablets:
N 0071-0813-19 100 mg Bottles of 50
Each tablet contains doxycycline hyclate equivalent to 100 mg doxycycline.

REFERENCE

[1] CDC Sexually Transmitted Diseases Treatment Guidelines 1982.

Store at controlled room temperature 15°-30°C (59°-86°F). Protect from moisture.
Caution—Federal law prohibits dispensing without prescription.

0829G021

DURAQUIN® ℞

[dŭ'ră-quĭn]
(quinidine gluconate tablets)
SUSTAINED RELEASE

DESCRIPTION

Quinidine gluconate is the gluconate of an alkaloid which may be obtained from various species of Cinchona and their hybrids, from *Remijia pedunculata* Fluckiger (Fam. Rubiaceae), or prepared from quinine. Quinidine gluconate contains, on the dry basis, not less than 99% of $C_{20}H_{24}N_2O_2 \cdot C_6H_{12}O_7$ (520.58). Quinidine is chemically described as 6-methoxy-alpha-(5-vinyl-2 quinuclidinyl)-4 quinolinemethanol and is the dextrorotatory isomer of quinine. Each 330-mg sustained-release tablet, representing 206 mg of quinidine base, is equivalent to 248 mg of quinidine sulfate.
Each tablet also contains magnesium stearate, NF; povidone, USP; and other ingredients.

ACTIONS

The antiarrhythmic activity consists of two actions: (a) prolongation of effective refractory period of the atrial or ventricular muscle which leads to termination of arrhythymia; (b) decrease in excitability of ectopic foci of the heart. In addition, quinidine blocks vagal innervation and facilitates conduction in the atrial-ventricular junction.

CLINICAL PHARMACOLOGY

In clinical studies, single doses of Duraquin produced a mean maximum plasma level at 2 hours which was maintained for 12 hours. This broad plateau indicates slow, continuous absorption from the gastrointestinal tract.
In multiple-dose studies, administration of Duraquin tablets, 660 mg every 12 hours, produced steady state (equilibrium) plasma levels shortly after 24 hours. The average quinidine plasma levels (Cramer and Isaksson assay[1]) were 0.81 mcg/ml and the mean peak levels were 1.16 mcg/ml in a group of normal male subjects weighing 75 kg. Following the last dose at steady state, quinidine plasma levels decreased at an approximate rate of 50% in 10 hours. This compares to the expected plasma half-life of 6.3 hours for quinidine sulfate tablets, USP.
Therapeutic and toxic effects coordinate better with plasma levels than with dosage. While therapeutic levels of 3 to 6 mcg/ml with a range of 1.5 to 9 mcg/ml have been reported, these values are based on peak plasma levels determined by the less specific Edgar and Sokolow assay.[2] This procedure yields quinidine levels averaging 22% higher than the Cramer and Isaksson assay. Plasma levels vary considerably in patients receiving identical doses. Therefore, it is advisable to adjust the dosage by monitoring plasma quinidine levels.

INDICATIONS

Duraquin tablets are indicated for the prevention of premature atrial, nodal, or ventricular contractions. They are also indicated for the maintenance of normal sinus rhythm following spontaneous reversion or electrical conversion of atrial, nodal, or ventricular tachycardia, atrial flutter and fibrillation (either paroxysmal or chronic).

CONTRAINDICATIONS

1. History of hypersensitivity to quinidine manifested by thrombocytopenia, skin eruption, febrile reactions, etc.
2. Complete A-V block
3. Complete bundle branch block or other severe intraventricular conduction defects exhibiting marked QRS widening or bizarre complexes
4. Myasthenia gravis
5. Arrhythmias associated with digitalis toxicity

WARNINGS

1. (a) In the treatment of atrial fibrillation with rapid ventricular response, ventricular rate should be controlled with digitalis glycosides *prior* to administration of quinidine.
   (b) In the treatment of atrial flutter with quinidine, reversion to sinus rhythm may be preceded by progressive reduction in the degree of A-V block to a 1:1 ratio resulting in an extremely high ventricular rate. This potential hazard may be reduced by digitalization prior to administration of quinidine.

Recent reports have described increased, potentially toxic, digoxin plasma levels when quinidine is administered concurrently. When concurrent use is necessary, digoxin dosage should be reduced and plasma concentration should be monitored and patients observed closely for digitalis intoxication.

2. Quinidine cardiotoxicity may be manifested by increased PR and QT intervals, 50% widening of QRS, and/or ventricular ectopic beats or tachycardia. Appearance of these toxic signs during quinidine administration mandates immediate discontinuation of the drug, and/or close clinical and electrocardiographic monitoring. Note: Quinidine effect is enhanced by potassium and reduced in the presence of hypokalemia.
3. "Quinidine Syncope" may occur as a complication of long-term therapy. It is manifested by sudden loss of consciousness and ventricular arrhythmias with bizarre QRS complexes. This syndrome does not appear to be related to dose or plasma levels but occurs more often with prolonged QT intervals.
4. Because quinidine antagonizes the effect of vagal excitation upon the atrium and the A-V node, the administration of parasympathomimetic drugs (choline esters) or the use of any other procedure to enhance vagal activity may fail to terminate paroxysmal supraventricular tachycardia in patients receiving quinidine.
5. Quinidine should be used with extreme caution in: a) the presence of incomplete A-V block, since a complete block and asystole may result. Quinidine may cause unpredictable abnormalities of rhythm in digitalized hearts. Therefore, it should be used with caution in the presence of digitalis intoxication. (See 1.(b) above).
   b) Partial bundle branch block.
   c) Severe congestive heart failure and hypotensive states due to the depressant effects of quinidine on myocardial contractility and arterial pressure.
   d) Poor renal function, especially renal tubular acidosis, because of the potential accumulation of quinidine in plasma leading to toxic concentrations.

PRECAUTIONS

1. Test Dose
A preliminary test dose of a single tablet of quinidine *sulfate* should be administered prior to the initiation of the sustained release gluconate to determine whether the patient has an idiosyncrasy to the quinidine molecule.
2. Hypersensitivity
During the first weeks of therapy; hypersensitivity to quinidine, although rare, should be considered (eg, angioedema, purpura, acute asthmatic episode, vascular collapse).
3. Long-Term Therapy
Periodic blood counts and liver and kidney function tests should be performed during long-term therapy and the drug should be discontinued if blood dyscrasias or signs of hepatic or renal disorders occur.
4. Large Doses
ECG monitoring and determination of plasma quinidine levels are recommended when doses greater than 2.5 g/day are administered.
5. Usage in Pregnancy
The use of quinidine, in pregnancy, should be reserved only for those cases where the benefits outweigh the possible hazards to the patient and fetus.
6. Nursing Mothers
The drug should be used with extreme caution in nursing mothers because the drug is excreted in breast milk.
7. General
In patients exhibiting asthma, muscle weakness, and infection with fever *prior* to quinidine administration, hypersensitivity reactions to the drug may be masked.

DRUG INTERACTIONS

1. Caution should be used when quinidine and its analogs are administered concurrently with coumarin anticoagulants. This combination may reduce prothrombin levels and cause bleeding.
2. Quinidine, a weak base, may have its half-life prolonged in patients who are concurrently taking drugs that can alkalize the urine, such as thiazide diuretics, sodium bicarbonate, and carbonic anhydrase inhibitors. Quinidine and drugs which alkalize the urine should be used together cautiously.
3. Quinidine exhibits a distinct anticholinergic activity in the myocardial tissues. An additive vagolytic effect may be seen when quinidine and drugs having anticholinergic blocking activity are used together. Drugs having cholinergic activity may be antagonized by quinidine.
4. Quinidine and other antiarrhythmic agents may produce additive cardiac depressant effects when administered together.

5. Quinidine interaction with cardiac glycosides (digoxin); See Warnings.
6. Antacids may delay absorption of quinidine but appear unlikely to cause incomplete absorption.
7. Phenobarbital and phenytoin may reduce plasma half-life of quinidine by 50%.
8. Quinidine may potentiate the neuromuscular blocking effect in ventilatory depression of patients receiving decamethonium, tubocurare, or succinylcholine.

ADVERSE REACTIONS

Symptoms of cinchonism (ringing in the ears, headache, disturbed vision) may appear in sensitive patients after a single dose of the drug.

Gastrointestinal: The most common side effects encountered with quinidine are referable to this system. Diarrhea frequently occurs, but it rarely necessitates withdrawal of the drug. Nausea, vomiting, and abdominal pain also occur. Some of these effects may be minimized by administering the drug with meals.

Cardiovascular: Widening of QRS complex, cardiac asystole, ventricular ectopic beats, idioventricular rhythms including ventricular tachycardias and fibrillation; paradoxical tachycardia, arterial embolism and hypotension.

Hematologic: acute hemolytic anemia, hypoprothrombinemia, thrombocytopenic purpura, agranulocytosis.

CNS: headache, fever, vertigo, apprehension, excitement, confusion, delirium and syncope, disturbed hearing (tinnitus, decreased auditory acuity), disturbed vision (mydriasis, blurred vision, disturbed color perception, photophobia, diplopia, night blindness, scotomata); optic neuritis.

Dermatologic: cutaneous flushing with intense pruritus.

Hypersensitivity reactions: angioedema, acute asthmatic episode, vascular collapse, respiratory arrest.

DOSAGE AND ADMINISTRATION

Dosage should be titrated to give the desired clinical effect, e.g., elimination of paroxysmal rhythm or reduction in premature contractions (See Clinical Pharmacology). This will often require prolonged ambulatory ECG monitoring, as hour-to-hour variability renders brief ECG recordings unreliable. When doses larger than 2.5g/day are used, quinidine blood levels should be monitored, if possible, and serial ECGs should be followed (See Warnings and Precautions).

For prevention of premature contractions and maintenance of normal sinus rhythm following spontaneous reversion or electrical conversion, the usual dosage is from 330 mg to 660 mg every eight hours, most patients requiring the higher dosage.

In elderly patients, and in patients in the lower end of the normal weight range, plasma quinidine determinations should be considered. Dosage adjustments may be required.

OVERDOSAGE

Cardiotoxic effects of quinidine may be reversed in part by molar sodium lactate; the hypotension may be reversed by vasoconstrictors and by catecholamines (since the vasodilation is partly due to alpha-adrenergic blockade).

HOW SUPPLIED

N 0071-0850 (P-D 850) Duraquin (quinidine gluconate tablets) 330-mg tablets are supplied in bottles of 100 and in unit-dose packages of 100 (10 strips of 10 tablets each).

0850G011

[1] Cramer, G. and Isaksson, B. Quantitative Determination of Quinidine in Plasma, Scandinavian J. Clin. & Lab Investigation 15, 553, 1963.

[2] Edgar, A.L. and Sokolow, M. Experiences with the Photofluorometric Determination of Quinidine in Blood J. Lab Clin. Med. 36, 478, 1950.

Shown in Product Identification Section, page 420

EASPRIN® ℞

[ēas'prĭn"]
(Aspirin Tablets, USP)
Enteric Coated Tablets

Caution—Federal law prohibits dispensing without prescription.

DESCRIPTION

Easprin (Aspirin Tablets, USP) enteric coated tablets contain 15 grains (975 mg) aspirin for oral administration. Also contains: candelilla wax; colloidal silicon dioxide, NF; corn starch 1500; dusty rose Opaspray; hydroxypropyl methylcellulose, USP (15 cps); methylparaben, NF; microcrystalline cellulose, NF; mistron spray talc; polyethylene glycol 3350, NF; propylparaben, NF; stearic acid powder; vanillin, NF; zinc stearate, USP. The enteric coating is designed to prevent the release of aspirin in the stomach and thereby reduce gastric irritation and total occult blood loss. The pharmacologic effects of aspirin include analgesia, antipyresis, antiinflammatory activity, and antirheumatic activity.

CLINICAL PHARMACOLOGY

Aspirin is a salicylate that has demonstrated antiinflammatory, analgesic, antipyretic, and antirheumatic activity.

Aspirin's mode of action as an antiinflammatory and antirheumatic agent may be due to inhibition of synthesis and release of prostaglandins.

Aspirin appears to produce analgesia by virtue of both a peripheral and CNS effect. Peripherally, aspirin acts by inhibiting the synthesis and release of prostaglandins. Acting centrally, it would appear to produce analgesia at a hypothalamic site in the brain, although the mode of action is not known.

Aspirin also acts on the hypothalamus to produce antipyresis; heat dissipation is increased as a result of vasodilation and increased peripheral blood flow. Aspirin's antipyretic activity may also be related to inhibition of synthesis and release of prostaglandins.

In a crossover study, Easprin at a dose of one tablet (15 grains) three times a day produced an average fecal blood loss of 1.54 ml per day. Uncoated aspirin at a dosage of three 5 grain tablets given three times a day caused an average fecal blood loss of 4.33 ml per day.

Easprin Tablets are enteric coated. This coating acts to prevent the release of aspirin in the stomach but permits the tablet to dissolve with resultant absorption in the upper portion of the small intestine. This reduces any gastric irritation that may occur with uncoated aspirin but does delay the onset of action. Aspirin is rapidly hydrolyzed primarily in the liver to salicylic acid, which is conjugated with glycine (forming salicyluric acid) and glucuronic acid and excreted largely in the urine. As a result of the rapid hydrolysis, plasma concentrations of aspirin are always low and rarely exceed 20 mcg/ml at ordinary therapeutic doses. The peak salicylate level for uncoated aspirin occurs in about 2 hours; however with enteric coated aspirin tablets this is delayed. A direct correlation between salicylate plasma levels and clinical analgesic effectiveness has not been definitely established, but effective analgesia is usually achieved at plasma levels of 15 to 30 mg per 100 ml. Effective antiinflammatory activity is usually achieved at salicylate plasma levels of 20 to 30 mg per 100 ml. There is also poor correlation between toxic symptoms and plasma salicylate concentrations, but most patients exhibit symptoms of salicylism at plasma salicylate levels of 35 mg per 100 ml. The plasma half-life for aspirin is approximately 15 minutes; that for salicylate lengthens as the dose increases: Doses of 300 to 650 mg have a half-life of 3.1 to 3.2 hours; with doses of 1 gram, the half-life is increased to 5 hours and with 2 grams it is increased to about 9 hours.

Salicylates are excreted mainly by the kidney. Studies in man indicate that salicylate is excreted in the urine as free salicylic acid (10%), salicyluric acid (75%), salicylic phenolic (10%), and acyl (5%) glucuronides and gentisic acid.

INDICATIONS AND USAGE

Easprin is indicated in patients who need the higher 15 grain dose of aspirin in the long-term palliative treatment of mild to moderate pain and inflammation of arthritic and other inflammatory conditions.

CONTRAINDICATIONS

Easprin should not be used in patients who have previously exhibited hypersensitivity to aspirin and/or nonsteroidal antiinflammatory agents.

Easprin should not be given to patients with a recent history of gastrointestinal bleeding or in patients with bleeding disorders (eg, hemophilia).

WARNINGS

Easprin Tablets should be used with caution when anticoagulants are prescribed concurrently, for aspirin may depress the concentration of prothrombin in plasma and thereby increase bleeding time. Large doses of salicylates have a hypoglycemic action and may enhance the effect of the oral hypoglycemics. Consequently, they should not be given concomitantly; if however, this is necessary, the dosage of the hypoglycemic agent must be reduced while the salicylate is given. This hypoglycemic action may also affect the insulin requirements of diabetics.

Although salicylates in large doses are uricosuric agents, smaller amounts may decrease the uricosuric effects of probenecid, sulfinpyrazone, and phenylbutazone.

PRECAUTIONS

General: Easprin Tablets should be administered with caution to patients with asthma, nasal polyps, or nasal allergies. In patients receiving large doses of aspirin and/or prolonged therapy, mild salicylate intoxication (salicylism) may develop that may be reversed by reduction in dosage.

Although the fecal blood loss with Easprin is less than that with uncoated aspirin tablets, Easprin Tablets should be administered with caution to patients with a history of gastric distress, ulcer, or bleeding problems. Occult gastrointestinal bleeding occurs in many patients but is not correlated with gastric distress. The amount of blood lost is usually insignificant clinically, but with prolonged administration, it may result in iron deficiency anemia.

Sodium excretion produced by spironolactone may be decreased in the presence of salicylates.

Salicylates can produce changes in thyroid function tests.

Salicylates should be used with caution in patients with severe hepatic damage, preexisting hypoprothrombinemia, or Vitamin K deficiency, and in those undergoing surgery.

DRUG INTERACTIONS

Anticoagulants: See Warnings.

Hypoglycemic Agents: See Warnings.

Uricosuric Agents: Aspirin may decrease the effects of probenecid, sulfinpyrazone, and phenylbutazone.

Spironolactone: See general precautions above.

Alcohol: Has a synergistic effect with aspirin in causing gastrointestinal bleeding.

Corticosteroids: Concomitant administration with aspirin may increase the risk of gastrointestinal ulceration.

Pyrazolone Derivatives (phenylbutazone, oxyphenbutazone, and possibly dipyrone): Concomitant administration with aspirin may increase the risk of gastrointestinal ulceration.

Nonsteroidal Antiinflammatory Agents: Aspirin is contraindicated in patients who are hypersensitive to nonsteroidal antiinflammatory agents.

Urinary Alkalinizers: Decrease aspirin effectiveness by increasing the rate of salicylate renal excretion.

Phenobarbital: Decreases aspirin effectiveness by enzyme induction.

Propranolol: May decrease aspirin's antiinflammatory action by competing for the same receptors.

Antacids: Easprin should not be given concurrently with antacids, since an increase in the pH of the stomach may affect the enteric coating of the tablets.

Usage in Pregnancy: Aspirin does not appear to have any teratogenic effects. However, it has been reported that adverse effects were increased in the mother and fetus following chronic ingestion of aspirin. Prolonged pregnancy and labor with increased bleeding before and after delivery, as well as decreased birth weight and increased rate of stillbirth were correlated with high blood salicylate levels. Because of possible adverse effects on the neonate and the potential for increased maternal blood loss, aspirin should be avoided during the last three months of pregnancy.

ADVERSE REACTIONS

Gastrointestinal: Dyspepsia, nausea, vomiting, diarrhea, gastrointestinal bleeding, and/or ulceration.

Ear: Tinnitus, vertigo, reversible hearing loss.

Hematologic: Prolongation of bleeding time, leukopenia, thrombocytopenia, purpura, decreased plasma iron concentration and shortened erythrocyte survival time.

Dermatologic and Hypersensitivity: Urticaria, angioedema, pruritus, various skin eruptions, asthma, and anaphylaxis.

Miscellaneous: Acute reversible hepatotoxicity, mental confusion, drowsiness, sweating, dizziness, headache, fever, thirst, and dimness of vision.

OVERDOSAGE

Overdosage of 200 to 500 mg/kg is in the fatal range. Early symptoms are CNS stimulation with vomiting, hyperpnea, hyperactivity, and possibly convulsions. This progresses quickly to depression, coma, respiratory failure, and collapse. These symptoms are accompanied by severe electrolyte disturbances.

In the treatment of salicylate overdosage, intensive supportive therapy should be instituted immediately. Plasma salicylate levels should be measured in order to determine the severity of the poisoning and to provide a guide for therapy. Emptying of the stomach should be accomplished as soon as possible with ipecac syrup unless the patient is depressed. In depressed patients use airway protected gastric lavage. Delay absorption with activated charcoal and give a saline cathartic. Proceed according to Standard Reference Procedures for Salicylate Intoxication.

DOSAGE AND ADMINISTRATION

Usual Adult Dosage: One tablet 3 to 4 times daily.

Patients who have displayed no significant adverse effects on a long term qid regimen and who receive a total daily dosage of aspirin no greater than 3.9 grams may be considered for a bid regimen (2 tablets of Easprin twice daily). Patients on the bid Easprin regimen should be closely monitored for serum salicylate levels, increased incidence of CNS-related adverse effects, increased fecal blood loss, or any other signs or symptoms suggestive of significant blood loss.

If necessary, dosage may be increased until relief is obtained, but dosage should be maintained slightly below that which produces tinnitus. Plasma salicylate levels may also be help-

Continued on next page

This product information was prepared in August, 1986. On these and other Parke-Davis Products, information may be obtained by addressing PARKE-DAVIS, Division of Warner-Lambert Company, Morris Plains, New Jersey 07950.

Parke-Davis—Cont.

ful in determining proper dosage (see Clinical Pharmacology section).

HOW SUPPLIED

Easprin enteric coated tablets each containing 15 grains (975 mg) aspirin are available:
N 0071-0490-24—Bottles of 100

Storage: Store at controlled room temperature 15° to 30°C (59° to 86°F).

AHFS Category 28:08 **0490G014**

Shown in Product Identification Section, page 420

ELASE® ℞
[ē'lāse"]
(fibrinolysin and desoxyribonuclease, combined [bovine])

ELASE OINTMENT ℞
(fibrinolysin and desoxyribonuclease, combined [bovine], ointment)

ELASE–CHLOROMYCETIN® OINTMENT ℞
(fibrinolysin and desoxyribonuclease, combined [bovine], with chloramphenicol ointment)

DESCRIPTION

Elase is a combination of two lytic enzymes, fibrinolysin and desoxyribonuclease, supplied as a lyophilized powder and in an ointment base of liquid petrolatum and polyethylene. The fibrinolysin component is derived from bovine plasma and the desoxyribonuclease is isolated in a purified form from bovine pancreas. The fibrinolysin used in the combination is activated by chloroform.

Elase-Chloromycetin Ointment: Elase-Chloromycetin Ointment contains two lytic enzymes, fibrinolysin and desoxyribonuclease, combined with chloramphenicol in an ointment base.

Chloramphenicol is a broad-spectrum antibiotic originally isolated from *Streptomyces venezuelae.* It is therapeutically active against a wide variety of susceptible organisms, both gram-positive and gram-negative. Chemically, chloramphenicol may be identified as D(-)- *threo*-1-*p*- nitrophenyl -2 - dichloroacetamido- 1, 3-propanediol.

ACTION

Combination of these two enzymes is based on the observation that purulent exudates consist largely of fibrinous material and nucleoprotein. Desoxyribonuclease attacks the desoxyribonucleic acid (DNA) and fibrinolysin attacks principally fibrin of blood clots and fibrinous exudates.

The activity of desoxyribonuclease is limited principally to the production of large polynucleotides, which are less likely to be absorbed than the more diffusible protein fractions liberated by certain enzyme preparations obtained from bacteria. The fibrinolytic action of Elase and of the enzymes in Elase Ointment and Elase-Chloromycetin Ointment is directed mainly against denatured proteins, such as those found in devitalized tissue, while protein elements of living cells remain relatively unaffected.

Elase, Elase Ointment, and Elase-Chloromycetin Ointment are combinations of active enzymes. This is an important consideration in treating patients suffering from lesions resulting from impaired circulation.

The enzymatic action of Elase helps to produce clean surfaces and thus supports healing in a variety of exudative lesions.

Elase-Chloromycetin Ointment:

Chloramphenicol is a broad-spectrum antibiotic that is primarily bacteriostatic and acts by inhibition of protein synthesis by interfering with the transfer of activated amino acids from soluble RNA to ribosomes. Development of resistance to chloramphenicol can be regarded as minimal for staphylococci and many other species of bacteria.

The action of Elase-Chloromycetin helps to produce clean surfaces and thus supports healing in a variety of exudative lesions.

INDICATIONS

Elase and Elase Ointment are indicated for topical use as debriding agents in a variety of inflammatory and infected lesions. These include: (1) general surgical wounds; (2) ulcerative lesions—trophic, decubitus, stasis, arteriosclerotic; (3) second- and third-degree burns; (4) circumcision and episiotomy. Elase and Elase Ointment are used intravaginally in: (1) cervicitis—benign, postpartum, and postconization, and (2) vaginitis. Elase is used as an irrigating agent in the following conditions: (1) infected wounds—abscesses, fistulae, and sinus tracts; (2) otorhinolaryngologic wounds; (3) superficial hematomas (except when the hematoma is adjacent to or within adipose tissue).

Elase-Chloromycetin Ointment:

Elase-Chloromycetin Ointment is indicated for use in the treatment of infected lesions, such as burns, ulcers, and wounds where the actions of both a debriding agent and a topical antibiotic are desired. This dual-purpose approach is especially useful in the treatment of infections caused by organisms that utilize a process of fibrin deposition as protective device (ie, coagulase and the staphylococcus). Appropriate measures should be taken to determine the susceptibility of the pathogen to chloramphenicol.

CONTRAINDICATIONS

These products (Elase, Elase Ointment, Elase-Chloromycetin Ointment) are contraindicated in individuals with a history of hypersensitivity reactions to any of their components. Elase is not recommended for parenteral use because the bovine fibrinolysin may be antigenic.

WARNINGS

Elase-Chloromycetin Ointment:

Bone marrow hypoplasia, including aplastic anemia and death, has been reported following the local application of chloramphenicol.

PRECAUTIONS

Elase-Chloromycetin Ointment: The prolonged use of antibiotics may occasionally result in overgrowth of nonsusceptible organisms, including fungi. If new infections appear during medication, the drug should be discontinued and appropriate measures should be taken.

In all except very superficial infections, the topical use of chloramphenicol should be supplemented by appropriate systemic medication.

Elase, Elase Ointment, Elase-Chloromycetin Ointment: The usual precautions against allergic reactions should be observed, particularly in persons with a history of sensitivity to materials of bovine origin or to mercury compounds.

Elase: To be maximally effective, Elase solutions must be freshly prepared before use. The loss in activity is reduced by refrigeration; however, even when stored in a refrigerator, the solution should not be used 24 hours or more after reconstitution.

ADVERSE REACTIONS

Side effects attributable to the enzymes have not been a problem at the dose and for the indications recommended herein. With higher concentrations, side effects have been minimal, consisting of local hyperemia.

Chills and fever attributable to antigenic action of profibrinolysin activators of bacterial origin are not a problem with Elase, Elase Ointment, or Elase-Chloromycetin Ointment.

Elase-Chloromycetin Ointment: Signs of local irritation, with subjective symptoms of itching or burning, angioneurotic edema, urticaria, vesicular and maculopapular dermatitis have been reported in patients sensitive to chloramphenicol and are causes for discontinuing the medication. Similar sensitivity reactions to other materials in topical preparations may also occur. Blood dyscrasias have been associated with the use of chloramphenicol.

Preparation of Elase Solution: The contents of each vial may be reconstituted with 10 ml of isotonic sodium chloride solution. Higher or lower concentrations can be prepared if desired by varying the amount of the diluent.

DOSAGE AND ADMINISTRATION

Since the conditions for which Elase and Elase Ointment and Elase-Chloromycetin Ointment are helpful vary considerably in severity, dosage must be adjusted to the individual case; however, the following general recommendations can be made.

Successful use of enzymatic debridement depends on several factors: (1) dense, dry eschar, if present, should be removed surgically before enzymatic debridement is attempted; (2) the enzyme must be in constant contact with the substrate; (3) accumulated necrotic debris must be periodically removed; (4) the enzyme must be replenished at least once daily; and (5) secondary closure or skin grafting must be employed as soon as possible after optimal debridement has been attained. It is further essential that wound-dressing techniques be performed carefully under aseptic conditions and that appropriate systemically acting antibiotics be administered concomitantly if, in the opinion of the physician, they are indicated.

General Topical Uses: ***Elase Ointment:*** Local application should be repeated at intervals for as long as enzyme action is desired. After application Elase Ointment becomes rapidly and progressively less active and is probably exhausted for practical purposes at the end of 24 hours. A recommended procedure for application of Elase Ointment follows.

1. Clean the wound with water, peroxide, or normal saline and dry area gently. If there is a dense, dry eschar present, it should be removed surgically before applying Elase.
2. Apply a *thin* layer of Elase Ointment.
3. Cover with petrolatum gauze or another type of nonadhering dressing.
4. Change the dressing at least ONCE a day, preferably two or three times daily. Frequency of application is more important than the amount of Elase used. Flush away the necrotic debris and fibrinous exudates with saline, peroxide, or warm water so that newly applied ointment can be in direct contact with the substrate.

Elase: Local application should be repeated at intervals for as long as enzyme action is desired. Elase solution may be applied topically as a liquid, spray, or wet dressing. Application of a gentle spray of the solution can be accomplished by using a conventional atomizer. After application, Elase, especially in solution, becomes rapidly and progressively less active and is probably exhausted for practical purposes at the end of 24 hours. The dry material for solution is stable at room temperature through the expiration date printed on the package. A recommended procedure for application of a solution of Elase using a Wet-to-Dry method follows.

1. Mix one vial of Elase powder with 10 to 50 ml of saline and saturate strips of fine-mesh gauze or an unfolded sterile gauze sponge with the Elase solution.
2. Pack ulcerated area with the Elase-saturated gauze, making sure the gauze remains in contact with the necrotic substrate (if the lesion is covered with a heavy eschar, it must be removed surgically before wet-to-dry debridement is begun).
3. ALLOW GAUZE TO DRY IN CONTACT WITH THE ULCERATED LESION (approximately six to eight hours). As the gauze dries, the necrotic tissues slough and become enmeshed in the gauze.
4. Remove dried gauze. This mechanically debrides the area. Repeat wet-to-dry procedure three or four times daily, since frequent dressing changes greatly enhance results. After two, three, or four days, the area becomes clean and starts to fill in with granulation tissue.

Intravaginal use: ***Elase Ointment:*** In mild to moderate vaginitis and cervicitis, 5 ml of Elase Ointment should be deposited deep in the vagina once nightly at bedtime for approximately five applications, or until the entire contents of one 30-g tube has been used. The patient should be checked by her physician to determine possible need for further therapy. In more severe cervicitis and vaginitis, some physicians prefer to initiate therapy with an application of Elase (fibrinolysin and desoxyribonuclease, combined, [bovine]) in solution. See Elase package insert.

Elase: In severe cervicitis and vaginitis, the physician may instill 10 ml of the solution intravaginally, wait one or two minutes for the enzyme to disperse and then insert a cotton tampon in the vaginal canal. The tampon should be removed the next day. Continuing therapy should then be instituted with Elase Ointment (fibrinolysin and desoxyribonuclease, combined [bovine] ointment). See Elase Ointment package insert.

Abscesses, empyema cavities, fistulae, sinus tracts or subcutaneous hematomas: Despite the contraindication against parenteral use, Elase has been used in irrigating these specific conditions. The Elase solution should be drained and replaced at intervals of six to ten hours to reduce the amount of by-product accumulation and minimize loss of enzyme activity. Traces of blood in the discharge usually indicate active filling in of the cavity.

HOW SUPPLIED

ELASE (fibrinolysin and desoxyribonuclease, combined [bovine])
N 0071-4256-01 Elase—lyophilized powder for solution
Elase is supplied in rubber diaphragm-capped vials of 30-ml capacity containing 25 units (Loomis) of fibrinolysin and 15,000 units (modified Christensen method) of desoxyribonuclease with 0.1 mg thimerosal (mercury derivative).
This product also contains sodium chloride and sucrose as incidental ingredients.

Shown in Product Identification Section, page 420

121 876350/ZF

ELASE OINTMENT (fibrinolysin and desoxyribonuclease, combined [bovine], ointment)
N 0071-4279-10 Elase Ointment, 10 g.
The 10-g tube contains 10 units of fibrinolysin and 6,666 units of desoxyribonuclease with 0.04 mg thimerosal (mercury derivative) in a special ointment base of liquid petrolatum and polyethylene.
N 0071-4279-13 Elase Ointment, 30 g.
The 30-g tube contains 30 units of fibrinolysin and 20,000 units of desoxyribonuclease with 0.12 mg thimerosal (mercury derivative) in a special ointment base of liquid petrolatum and polyethylene. For gynecologic use, six disposable vaginal applicators (V-Applicator*) as a separate package are available for this tube when required to facilitate administration of the proper dose.
These products also contain sodium chloride and sucrose as incidental ingredients.

Shown in Product Identification Section, page 420

4279G020

ELASE-CHLOROMYCETIN OINTMENT (fibrinolysin and desoxyribonuclease, combined [bovine], with chloramphenicol ointment)
Elase-Chloromycetin (fibrinolysin-desoxyribonuclease-chloramphenicol) is supplied in 30-g and 10-g ointment tubes. The 10-g tubes have an elongated nozzle to facilitate the application to surface lesions.
The 30-g tubes contain 30 units (Loomis) of fibrinolysin (bovine) and 20,000 units** of desoxyribonuclease with 0.12 mg thimerosal (mercury derivative) (as a preservative) and 0.3

g† chloramphenicol in a special ointment base of liquid petrolatum and polyethylene.
The 10-g tubes contain 10 units (Loomis) of fibrinolysin (bovine) and 6,666 units** of desoxyribonuclease with 0.04 mg thimerosal (mercury derivative) (as a preservative) and 0.1 g† chloramphenicol in a special ointment base of liquid petrolatum and polyethylene.
The ointment contains sodium chloride and sucrose used in its manufacture.

*Trademark
**Modified Christensen method.
†10 mg chloramphenicol per gram, or 1%.

Shown in Product Identification Section, page 420

4281G020

ELDEC® KAPSEALS® ℞

[*ĕl 'dĕc"*]

COMPOSITION

Each capsule contains vitamin A (acetate), 1,667 IU; vitamin C (ascorbic acid), 66.7 mg; vitamin B_1 (thiamine mononitrate), 10 mg; vitamin B_2 (riboflavin), 0.87 mg; vitamin B_6 (pyridoxine hydrochloride), 0.67 mg; nicotinamide (niacinamide), 16.7 mg; *dl*-panthenol, 10 mg; ferrous sulfate, dried, 16.7 mg; iodine (as potassium iodide), 0.05 mg; calcium carbonate, precipitated, 66.7 mg; vitamin E (*dl*-alpha tocopheryl acetate), (10 mg) 10 IU; vitamin B_{12} (cyanocobalamin), 2 mcg; folic acid, 0.33 mg.

ACTION AND USES

For certain vitamin and mineral deficiencies.
Caution—Folic acid in doses above 0.1 mg daily may obscure pernicious anemia in that hematologic remission can occur while neurological manifestations remain progressive.

DOSAGE

The usual dosage of Eldec is one capsule three times a day.

HOW SUPPLIED

N 0071-0337-24 Eldec (Kapseal 398), bottles of 100. Parcode® No. 337; new ID code imprint, formerly 398—no formula change.

Shown in Product Identification Section, page 420

ERGOSTAT® ℞

(Ergotamine Tartrate Tablets) sublingual

DESCRIPTION

Each sublingual tablet contains 2 mg ergotamine tartrate. Also contains hydroxypropyl cellulose, NF; FD&C yellow No. 6 Al lake; lactose, NF; magnesium stearate, NF; mannitol, USP; artificial peppermint flavor; saccharin, NF; saccharin sodium, USP; and corn starch, NF.
Pharmacological Category: Vasoconstrictor, uterine stimulant, alpha adrenoreceptor antagonist.
Therapeutic Class: Antimigraine.
Chemical Name: Ergotaman-3′,6′,18-trione,12′-hydroxy-2′-methyl-5′-(phenylmethyl)-,(5′α)-,[R-(R*,R*)]-2,3-dihydroxybutanedioate (2:1) salt.

CLINICAL PHARMACOLOGY

The pharmacological properties of ergotamine are extremely complex; some of its actions are unrelated to each other, and even mutually antagonistic. The drug has partial agonist and/or antagonist activity against tryptaminergic, dopaminergic and alpha adrenergic receptors depending upon their site, and it is a highly active uterine stimulant. It causes constriction of peripheral and cranial blood vessels and produces depression of central vasomotor centers. The pain of a migraine attack is believed to be due to greatly increased amplitude of pulsations in the cranial arteries, especially the meningeal branches of the external carotid artery. Ergotamine reduces extracranial blood flow, causes a decline in the amplitude of pulsation in the cranial arteries, and decreases hyperperfusion of the territory of the basilar artery. It does not reduce cerebral hemispheric blood flow. Long-term usage has established the fact that ergotamine tartrate is effective in controlling up to 70% of acute migraine attacks, so that it is now considered specific for the treatment of this headache syndrome. Ergotamine produces constriction of both arteries and veins. In doses used in the treatment of vascular headaches, ergotamine usually produces only small increases in blood pressure, but it does increase peripheral resistance and decrease blood flow in various organs. Small doses of the drug increase the force and frequency of uterine contraction; larger doses increase the resting tone of the uterus also. The gravid uterus is particularly sensitive to these effects of ergotamine. Although specific teratogenic effects attributable to ergotamine have not been found, the fetus suffers if ergotamine is given to the mother. Retarded fetal growth and an increase in intrauterine death and resorption have been seen in animals. These are thought to result from ergotamine-induced increases in uterine motility and vasoconstriction in the placental vascular bed.
The bioavailability of sublingually administered ergotamine has not been determined.
Ergotamine is metabolized in the liver by largely undefined pathways, and 90% of the metabolites are excreted in the bile. The unmetabolized drug is erratically secreted in the saliva, and only traces of unmetabolized drug appear in the urine and feces. Ergotamine is secreted into breast milk. The elimination half-life of ergotamine from plasma is about 2 hours, but the drug may be stored in some tissues, which would account for its long-lasting therapeutic and toxic actions.

INDICATIONS AND USAGE

Ergotamine tartrate is indicated as therapy to abort or prevent vascular headache, e.g., migraine, migraine variants, or so called "histaminic cephalalgia".

CONTRAINDICATIONS

Ergotamine is contraindicated in peripheral vascular disease (thromboangiitis obliterans, luetic arteritis, severe arteriosclerosis, thrombophlebitis, Raynaud's disease), coronary heart disease, hypertension, impaired hepatic or renal function, severe pruritus, and sepsis. It is also contraindicated in patients who are hypersensitive to any of its components. Ergotamine may cause fetal harm when administered to a pregnant woman by virtue of its powerful uterine stimulant actions. It is contraindicated in women who are, or may become, pregnant.

PRECAUTIONS

General: Although signs and symptoms of ergotism rarely develop even after long-term intermittent use of ergotamine, care should be exercised to remain within the limits of recommended dosage.
Drug Interactions: The effects of ergotamine tartrate may be potentiated by triacetyloleandomycin which inhibits the metabolism of ergotamine. The pressor effects of ergotamine and other vasoconstrictor drugs can combine to cause dangerous hypertension.
Carcinogenesis: No studies have been performed to investigate ergotamine tartrate for carcinogenic effects.
Pregnancy: Pregnancy Category X—See CONTRAINDICATIONS.
Nursing Mothers: Ergotamine is secreted into human milk. It can reach the breast-fed infant by this route and exert pharmacologic effects in it. Caution should be exercised when ergotamine is administered to a nursing woman. Excessive dosing or prolonged administration of ergotamine may inhibit lactation.

ADVERSE REACTIONS

Nausea and vomiting occur in up to 10% of patients after ingestion of therapeutic doses of ergotamine. Weakness of the legs and pain in limb muscles are also frequent complaints. Numbness and tingling of the fingers and toes, precordial pain, transient changes in heart rate and localized edema and itching may also occur, particularly in patients who are sensitive to the drug.

DRUG ABUSE AND DEPENDENCE

Patients who take ergotamine for extended periods of time may become dependent upon it and require progressively increasing doses for relief of vascular headaches, and for prevention of dysphoric effects which follow withdrawal of the drug.

OVERDOSAGE

Overdosage with ergotamine causes nausea, vomiting, weakness of the legs, pain in limb muscles, numbness and tingling of the fingers and toes, precordial pain, tachycardia or bradycardia, hypertension or hypotension and localized edema and itching together with signs and symptoms of ischemia due to vasconstriction of peripheral arteries and arterioles. The feet and hands become cold, pale and numb. Muscle pain occurs while walking and later at rest also. Gangrene may ensue. Confusion, depression, drowsiness, and convulsions are occasional signs of ergotamine toxicity. Overdosage is particularly likely to occur in patients with sepsis or impaired renal or hepatic function. Patients with peripheral vascular disease are especially at risk of developing peripheral ischemia following treatment with ergotamine. Some cases of ergotamine poisoning have been reported in patients who have taken less than 5 mg of the drug. Usually, however, toxicity is seen at doses of ergotamine tartrate in excess of about 15 mg in 24 hours or 40 mg in a few days.
Treatment of ergotamine overdosage consists of the withdrawal of the drug followed by symptomatic measures including attempts to maintain an adequate circulation in the affected parts. Anticoagulant drugs, low molecular weight dextran and potent vasodilator drugs may all be beneficial. Intravenous infusion of sodium nitroprusside has also been reported to be successful. Vasodilators must be used with special care in the presence of hypotension.
Nausea and vomiting may be relieved by atropine or antiemetic compounds of the phenothiazine group. Ergotamine is dialyzable.

DOSAGE AND ADMINISTRATION

All efforts should be made to initiate therapy as soon as possible after the first symptoms of the attack are noted, because success is proportional to rapidity of treatment, and lower dosages will be effective. At the first sign of an attack or to relieve the symptoms of the full-blown attack, one sublingual tablet (2 mg) is placed under the tongue. Another sublingual tablet (2 mg) should be placed under the tongue at half-hourly intervals thereafter, if necessary, for a total of three tablets (6 mg). Dosage must not exceed three tablets (6 mg) in any 24-hour period. Limit dosage to not more than five tablets (10 mg) in any one week.

HOW SUPPLIED

Ergostat (Ergotamine Tartrate Tablets) sublingual, 2 mg (round, orange, coded P-D 111), is supplied as follows:
N 0071-0111-13 Vial containing 24 individually packaged tablets.
Store at controlled room temperature 15°–30°C (59°–86°F).
AHFS Category 12:16 **0111G013**

Shown in Product Identification Section, page 420

ERYC® ℞

[*ĕ 'ryc*]
(Erythromycin Capsules, USP)

DESCRIPTION

ERYC Capsules contain enteric-coated pellets of erythromycin base for oral administration. Erythromycin is produced by a strain of *Streptomyces erythraeus* and belongs to the macrolide group of antibiotics. It is basic and readily forms salts with acids, but it is the base which is microbiologically active. Each ERYC Capsule contains 250 milligrams of erythromycin base. Also contains: lactose NF; povidone USP; FD&C Yellow #6. The capsule shell contains gelatin NF; titanium dioxide USP; FD&C Yellow #6. Erythromycin base is (3*R**, 4*S**, 5*S**, 6*R**, 7*R**, 9*R**, 11*R**, 12*R**, 13*S**, 14*R**)-4-[(2,6-Dideoxy-3-*C*-methyl-3-*O*-methyl-α-L-*ribo*-hexopyranosyl)-oxy]-14-ethyl-7, 12, 13-trihydroxy-3, 5, 7, 9, 11, 13-hexamethyl-6-[[3, 4, 6-trideoxy-3-(dimethylamino)-β-D-*xylo*-hexopyranosyl]oxy]oxacyclotetradecane-2, 10-dione.

CLINICAL PHARMACOLOGY

Orally administered erythromycin base and its salts are readily absorbed in the microbiologically active form. Interindividual variations in the absorption of erythromycin are, however, observed, and some patients do not achieve acceptable serum levels. Erythromycin is largely bound to plasma proteins, and the freely dissociating bound fraction after administration of erythromycin base represents 90% of the total erythromycin absorbed. After absorption erythromycin diffuses readily into most body fluids. In the absence of meningeal inflammation, low concentrations are normally achieved in the spinal fluid but the passage of the drug across the blood-brain barrier increases in meningitis. Erythromycin is excreted in breast milk. The drug crosses the placental barrier but fetal plasma levels are low.
In the presence of normal hepatic function erythromycin is concentrated in the liver and is excreted in the bile; the effect of hepatic dysfunction on biliary excretion of erythromycin is not known. After oral administration less than 5% of the administered dose can be recovered in the active form in the urine.
The enteric coating of pellets in ERYC Capsules protects the erythromycin base from inactivation by gastric acidity. Because of their small size and enteric coating, the pellets readily pass intact from the stomach to the small intestine and dissolve efficiently to allow absorption of erythromycin in a uniform manner. After administration of a single dose of a 250 mg ERYC capsule, peak serum levels in the range of 1.13 to 1.68 mcg/ml are attained in approximately 3 hours and decline to 0.30-0.42 mcg/ml in 6 hours. Optimal conditions for stability in the presence of gastric secretion and for complete absorption are attained when ERYC is taken on an empty stomach.
Microbiology Erythromycin acts by inhibition of protein synthesis by binding 50 S ribosomal subunits of susceptible organisms. It does not affect nucleic acid synthesis. Antagonism has been demonstrated between clindamycin and erythromycin. Resistance to erythromycin by some strains of *Haemophilus influenzae* and staphylococci has been demonstrated. Specimens should be obtained for culture and susceptibility testing.
Erythromycin is usually active against the following organisms in *vitro* and in clinical infections:

Streptococcus pyogenes
Alpha hemolytic streptococci (viridans group)

Continued on next page

This product information was prepared in August, 1986. On these and other Parke-Davis Products, information may be obtained by addressing PARKE-DAVIS, Division of Warner-Lambert Company, Morris Plains, New Jersey 07950.

Parke-Davis—Cont.

Staphylococcus aureus (Resistant organisms may emerge during treatment.)
Streptococcus pneumoniae
Mycoplasma pneumoniae (Eaton's Agent)
Haemophilus influenzae (Many strains are resistant to erythromycin alone, but are susceptible to erythromycin and sulfonamides together.)
Treponema pallidum
Corynebacterium diphtheriae
Corynebacterium minutissimum
Entamoeba histolytica
Listeria monocytogenes
Neisseria gonorrhoeae
Bordetella pertussis
Legionella pneumophila (agent of Legionnaires' Disease)

Susceptibility Testing Quantitative methods that require measurement of zone diameters give the most precise estimates of antibiotic susceptibility. One such standardized single disc procedure has been recommended for use with discs to test susceptibility to erythromycin.[1] Interpretation involves correlation of the zone diameters obtained in the disc test with minimum inhibitory concentration (MIC) values for erythromycin.

Reports from the laboratory giving results of the standardized single-disc susceptibility test using a 15 mcg erythromycin disc should be interpreted according to the following criteria:

Susceptible organisms produce zones of 18 mm or greater indicating that the tested organism is likely to respond to therapy.

Resistant organisms produce zones of 13 mm or less, indicating that other therapy should be selected.

Organisms of intermediate susceptibility produce zones of 14 to 17 mm. The "intermediate" category provides a "buffer zone" which should prevent small uncontrolled technical factors from causing major discrepancies in interpretations, thus when a zone diameter falls within the "intermediate" range, the results may be considered equivocal. If alternate drugs are not available, confirmation by dilution tests may be indicated.

A bacterial isolate may be considered susceptible if the MIC value[2] (minimal inhibitory concentration) for erythromycin is not more than 2 mcg/ml. Organisms are considered resistant if the MIC is 8 mcg/ml or higher.

INDICATIONS AND USAGE

ERYC is indicated in children and adults for the treatment of the following conditions:

Upper respiratory tract infections of mild to moderate degree caused by *Streptococcus pyogenes* (group A beta hemolytic streptococci); *Streptococcus pneumoniae (Diplococcus pneumoniae); Haemophilus influenzae* (when used concomitantly with adequate doses of sulfonamides, since not all strains of *H influenzae* are susceptible at the erythromycin concentrations ordinarily achieved). (See appropriate sulfonamide labeling for prescribing information.)

Lower respiratory tract infections of mild to moderate severity caused by *Streptococcus pyogenes* (group A beta hemolytic streptococci): *Streptococcus pneumoniae (Diplococcus pneumoniae).*

Respiratory tract infections due to *Mycoplasma pneumoniae (Eaton's agent).*

Pertussis (whooping cough) caused by *Bordetella pertussis.* Erythromycin is effective in eliminating the organism from the nasopharynx of infected individuals, rendering them noninfectious. Some clinical studies suggest that erythromycin may be helpful in the prophylaxis of pertussis in exposed susceptible individuals.

Diphtheria—As an adjunct to antitoxin in infections due to *Corynebacterium diphtheriae,* to prevent establishment of carriers and to eradicate the organism in carriers.

Erythrasma—In the treatment of infections due to *Corynebacterium minutissimum.*

Intestinal amebiasis caused by *Entamoeba histolytica* (oral erythromycins only). Extraenteric amebiasis requires treatment with other agents.

Infections due to *Listeria monocytogenes.*

Skin and soft tissue infections of mild to moderate severity caused by *Streptococcus pyogenes* and *Staphylococcus aureus* (Resistant staphylococci may emerge during treatment.)

Primary syphilis caused by *Treponema pallidum.* Erythromycin (oral forms only) is an alternate choice of treatment for primary syphilis in patients allergic to the penicillins. In treatment of primary syphilis, spinal fluid should be examined before treatment and as part of the follow-up after therapy. The use of erythromycin for the treatment of *in utero* syphilis is not recommended (See CLINICAL PHARMACOLOGY).

Erythromycins are indicated for treatment of the following infections caused by *Chlamydia trachomatis:* conjunctivitis of the newborn, pneumonia of infancy, urogenital infections during pregnancy. When tetracyclines are contraindicated or not tolerated, erythromycin is indicated for the treatment of uncomplicated urethral, endocervical, or rectal infections in adults due to *Chlamydia trachomatis*[4].

Legionnaires' disease caused by *Legionella pneumophila.* Although no controlled clinical efficacy studies have been conducted, *in vitro* and limited preliminary clinical data suggest that erythromycin may be effective in treating Legionnaires' disease.

Therapy with erythromycin should be monitored by bacteriological studies and by clinical response (See CLINICAL PHARMACOLOGY—Microbiology).

Injectable benzathine penicillin G is considered by the American Heart Association to be the drug of choice in the treatment and prevention of streptococcal pharyngitis and in long-term prophylaxis of rheumatic fever. When oral medication is preferred for treatment of the above conditions, penicillin G, V, or erythromycin are alternate drugs of choice.

Although no controlled clinical efficacy trials have been conducted, erythromycin has been suggested by the American Heart Association and the American Dental Association for use in a regimen for prophylaxis against bacterial endocarditis in patients allergic to penicillin who have congenital and/or rheumatic or other acquired valvular heart disease when they undergo dental procedures and surgical procedures of the upper respiratory tract.[3] (Erythromycin is not suitable prior to genitourinary surgery where the organisms likely to lead to bacteremia are gram-negative bacilli or the enterococcal group of streptococci).

NOTE: When selecting antibiotics for the prevention of bacterial endocarditis the physician or dentist should read the full joint 1984 statement of the American Heart Association and the American Dental Association.[3]

CONTRAINDICATION

ERYC is contraindicated in patients with known hypersensitivity to this antibiotic.

WARNING

There have been a few reports of hepatic dysfunction, with or without jaundice, occurring in patients receiving erythromycin ethylsuccinate, base, and stearate products.

PRECAUTIONS

Caution should be exercised when erythromycin is administered to patients with impaired hepatic function (see CLINICAL PHARMACOLOGY and WARNING).

Erythromycin use in patients who are receiving high doses of theophylline may be associated with an increase in serum theophylline levels and potential theophylline toxicity. In case of theophylline toxicity and/or elevated serum theophylline levels, the dose of theophylline should be reduced while the patient is receiving concomitant erythromycin therapy.

Erythromycin interferes with the fluorometric determination of urinary catecholamines.

Prolonged or repeated use of erythromycin may result in an overgrowth of nonsusceptible bacteria or fungi. If superinfection occurs, erythromycin should be discontinued and appropriate therapy instituted.

When indicated, incision and drainage or other surgical procedures should be performed in conjunction with antibiotic therapy.

Pregnancy Category B—Reproduction studies have been performed in rats, mice and rabbits using erythromycin and its various salts and esters, at doses which were several times multiples of the usual human dose. No evidence of impaired fertility or harm to the fetus that appeared related to erythromycin was reported in these studies. There are, however, no adequate and well-controlled studies in pregnant women. Because animal reproduction studies are not always predictive of human response, this drug should be used during pregnancy only if clearly needed.

Labor and Delivery—The effect of ERYC on labor and delivery is unknown.

Nursing Mothers—Erythromycin is excreted in milk (see CLINICAL PHARMACOLOGY).

Pediatric Use—See INDICATIONS AND USAGE and DOSAGE AND ADMINISTRATION.

ADVERSE REACTIONS

The most frequent side effects of oral erythromycin preparations are gastrointestinal and are dose-related. They include nausea, vomiting, abdominal pain, diarrhea and anorexia. Symptoms of hepatic dysfunction and/or abnormal liver function test results may occur (see WARNING).

Mild allergic reactions such as rashes with or without pruritus, urticaria, bullous fixed eruptions, and eczema have been reported with erythromycin. Serious allergic reactions, including anaphylaxis have been reported.

A few cases of transient deafness have been reported with high doses of erythromycin.

DOSAGE AND ADMINISTRATION

Administration of a dose of ERYC in the presence of food lowers the blood levels of systemically available erythromycin. Although the blood levels obtained upon administration of enteric-coated erythromycin products in the presence of food are still above minimum inhibitory concentrations (MICs) of most organisms for which erythromycin is indicated, optimum blood levels are obtained on a fasting stomach (administration of at least ½ hour and preferably two hours before or after a meal).

ADULTS: The usual dose is 250 mg every 6 hours taken one hour before meals. If twice-a-day dosage is desired, the recommended dose is 500 mg every 12 hours. Dosage may be increased up to 4 grams per day, according to the severity of infection. Twice-a-day dosing is not recommended when doses larger than 1 gram daily are administered.

CHILDREN: Age, weight, and severity of the infection are important factors in determining the proper dosage. The usual dosage is 30 to 50 mg/kg/day in divided doses. For the treatment of more severe infections, this dose may be doubled.

Streptococcal infections: A therapeutic dosage of oral erythromycin should be administered for at least 10 days. For continuous prophylaxis against recurrences of streptococcal infections in persons with a history of rheumatic heart disease, the dose is 250 mg twice a day.

For the prevention of bacterial endocarditis in penicillin-allergic patients with valvular heart disease who are to undergo dental procedures or surgical procedures of the upper respiratory tract, the adult dose is 1.0 grams orally (20 mg/kg for children) one and one-half to 2 hours prior to the procedure and then 500 mg (10 mg/kg for children) orally every 6 hours for 8 doses.[3] (See INDICATIONS AND USAGE).

Primary syphilis: 30-40 grams given in divided doses over a period of 10-15 days.

Intestinal amebiasis: 250 mg four times daily for 10 to 14 days for adults; 30 to 50 mg/kg/day in divided doses for 10 to 14 days for children.

Legionnaires' Disease: Although optimal doses have not been established, doses utilized in reported clinical data were those recommended above (1 to 4 grams daily in divided doses).

Urogenital infections during pregnancy due to *Chlamydia trachomatis:* Although the optimal dose and duration of therapy have not been established, the suggested treatment is erythromycin 500 mg, by mouth, 4 times a day on an empty stomach for at least 7 days. For women who cannot tolerate this regimen, a decreased dose of 250 mg, by mouth, 4 times a day should be used for at least 14 days[4].

For adults with uncomplicated urethral, endocervical, or rectal infections caused by *Chlamydia trachomatis* in whom tetracyclines are contraindicated or not tolerated: 500 mg. by mouth, 4 times a day for at least 7 days[4].

Pertussis: Although optimum dosage and duration of therapy have not been established, doses of erythromycin utilized in reported clinical studies were 40-50 mg/kg/day, given in divided doses for 5 to 14 days.

HOW SUPPLIED

ERYC (Capsule 696), clear and orange opaque capsules, each containing 250 mg erythromycin as enteric coated pellets, are available as follows:

N 0071-0696-16 Bottles of 40
N 0071-0696-24 Bottles of 100
N 0071-0696-30 Bottles of 500
N 0071-0696-40 Unit dose package of 100 (10 strips of 10 capsules each).

Storage Conditions: Store at a room temperature below 30°C (86°F). Protect from moisture and light.

REFERENCES

1. Approved Standard ASM-2 "Performance Standards for Anti-microbial Disc Susceptibility Test." National Committee for Clinical Laboratory Standards. 771 East Lancaster Avenue, Villanova. PA 19085.
2. Ericson, H.M. and Sherris, J.C.: "Antibiotic Sensitivity Testing Report of an International Collaborative Study." *Acta Pathologica et Microbiologica Scandinavica.* Section B. Supp. 217, 1971, pp. 1-90.
3. Am. Heart Assoc. and Am. Dental Assoc. "Prevention of Bacterial Endocarditis." *Circulation:*" Vol. 56, No. 1, July, 1977. 139A-143A.
4. CDC Sexually Transmitted Diseases Treatment Guidelines 1982.

Shown in Product Identification Section, page 420

0696G015

ERYC® 125 ℞

(Erythromycin Capsules, USP)
Pediatric Pellets 125 mg

DESCRIPTION

ERYC 125 (erythromycin capsules, USP) contain enteric-coated pellets of erythromycin base for oral administration.

The pellet form makes ERYC 125 ideal for children and other patients who are unable to swallow a tablet or capsule. The enteric coating on the pellets covers the bitter tasting erythromycin as well as protects the erythromycin from gastric acid destruction during the passage through the stomach. Each capsule is size #0 (oversized) for ease of opening.

Erythromycin is produced by a strain of *Streptomyces erythraeus* and belongs to the macrolide group of antibiotics. It is basic and readily forms salts with acids, but it is the base which is microbiologically active. Each ERYC 125 capsule contains 125 mg of erythromycin base. Also contains lactose, NF; povidone, USP. The capsule shell contains gelatin, NF; colloidal silicon dioxide, NF; sodium lauryl sulfate, NF; titanium dioxide, USP; D&C Yellow No. 10; FD&C Red No. 40. Erythromycin bases is (3*R* *, 4*S* *, 5*S* *, 6*R* *, 7*R* *, 9*R* *, 11*R* *, 12*R* *, 13*S* *, 14*R* *)-4-[(2,6-Dideoxy-3-*C*-methyl-3-*O*-methyl-α-L-*ribo*-hexopyranosyl) oxy]-14-ethyl-7,12,13-trihydroxy-3,5,7,9,11,13-hexamethyl-6-[[3,4,6-trideoxy-3-(dimethyl-amino)-β-D-*xylo*-hexopyranosyl]oxy]oxacyclotetradecane-2,10-dione.

CLINICAL PHARMACOLOGY

Orally administered erythromycin base and its salts are readily absorbed in the microbiologically active form. Interindividual variations in the absorption of erythromycin are, however, observed, and some patients do not achieve acceptable serum levels. Erythromycin is largely bound to plasma proteins, and the freely dissociating bound fraction after administration of erythromycin base represents 90% of the total erythromycin absorbed. After absorption erythromycin diffuses readily into most body fluids. In the absence of meningeal inflammation, low concentrations are normally achieved in the spinal fluid but the passage of the drug across the blood-brain barrier increases in meningitis. Erythromycin is excreted in breast milk. The drug crosses the placental barrier but fetal plasma levels are low.

In the presence of normal hepatic function erythromycin is concentrated in the liver and is excreted in the bile; the effect of hepatic dysfunction on biliary excretion of erythromycin is not known. After oral administration less than 5% of the administered dose can be recovered in the active form in the urine.

The enteric coating of pellets in ERYC 125 Capsules protects the erythromycin base from inactivation by gastric acidity. Because of their small size, the pellets readily pass intact from the stomach to the small intestine and dissolve efficiently to allow absorption of erythromycin in a uniform manner. After administration of a single dose of 125 mg ERYC 125 Capsules to adults, a mean peak serum level of 0.84 mcg/mL was attained in approximately 3 hours, and the levels declined to a mean of 0.25 mcg/mL in 6 hours. Optimal conditions for stability in the presence of gastric secretion and for complete absorption are attained when ERYC 125 is taken on an empty stomach.

Microbiology: Erythromycin acts by inhibition of protein synthesis by binding 50 S ribosomal subunits of susceptible organisms. It does not affect nucleic acid synthesis. Antagonism has been demonstrated between clindamycin and erythromycin. Resistance to erythromycin by some strains of *Haemophilus influenzae* and staphylococci has been demonstrated. Specimens should be obtained for culture and susceptibility testing.

Erythromycin is usually active against the following organisms in vitro and in clinical infections:

Streptococcus pyogenes
Alpha hemolytic streptococci (viridans group)
Staphylococcus aureus (Resistant organisms may emerge during treatment)
Streptococcus pneumoniae
Mycoplasma pneumoniae (Eaton's agent)
Haemophilus influenzae (Many strains are resistant to erythromycin alone, but are susceptible to erythromycin and sulfonamides together)
Treponema pallidum
Corynebacterium diphtheriae
Corynebacterium minutissimum
Entamoeba histolytica
Listeria monocytogenes
Neisseria gonorrhoeae
Bordetella pertussis
Legionella pneumophila (agent of Legionnaires' Disease)
Chlamydia trachomatis
Ureaplasma urealyticum

Susceptibility Testing: Quantitative methods that require measurement of zone diameters give the most precise estimates of antibiotic susceptibility. One such standardized single disc procedure has been recommended for use with discs to test susceptiblity to erythromycin.[1] Interpretation involves correlation of the zone diameters obtained in the disc test with minimal inhibitory concentration (MIC) values for erythromycin.

Reports from the laboratory giving results of the standardized single-disc susceptibility test using a 15 mcg erythromycin disc should be interpreted according to the following criteria:

Susceptible organisms produce zones of 18 mm or greater indicating that the tested organism is likely to repond to therapy.

Resistant organisms produce zones of 13 mm or less, indicating that other therapy should be selected.

Organisms of intermediate susceptibility produce zones of 14 to 17 mm. The "intermediate" category provides a "buffer zone" which should prevent small uncontrolled technical factors from causing major discrepancies in interpretations, thus when a zone diameter falls within the "intermediate" range, the results may be considered equivocal. If alternative drugs are not available, confirmation by dilution tests may be indicated.

Standardized procedures require the use of control organisms. The 15 mcg erythromycin disc should give zone diameters between 22 and 30 millimeters for the *S. aureus* ATCC 25923 control strain.

A bacterial isolate may be considered susceptible if the MIC value[2] for erythromycin is not more than 2 mcg/mL. Organisms are considered resistant if the MIC is 8 mcg/mL or higher. The MIC of erythromycin for *S. aureus* ATCC 29213 control strain should be between 0.12 and 0.5 mcg/mL.

INDICATIONS AND USAGE

ERYC 125 is indicated in children and adults for the treatment of the following conditions:

Upper respiratory tract infections of mild to moderate degree caused by *Streptococcus pyogenes* (group A beta hemolytic streptococci); *Streptococcus pneumoniae (Diplococcus pneumoniae); Haemophilus influenzae* (when used concomitantly with adequate doses of sulfonamides, since not all strains of *H influenzae* are susceptible at the erythromycin concentrations ordinarily achieved). (See appropriate sulfonamide labeling for prescribing information.)

Lower respiratory tract infections of mild to moderate severity caused by *Streptococcus pyogenes* (group A beta hemolytic streptococci); *Streptococcus pneumoniae (Diplococcus pneumoniae).*

Respiratory tract infections due to *Mycoplasma pneumoniae* (Eaton's agent).

Skin and skin structures infections of mild to moderate severity caused by *Streptococcus pyogenes* and *Staphylococcus aureus* (resistant staphylococci may emerge during treatment).

Pertussis (whooping cough) caused by *Bordetella pertussis.* Erythromycin is effective in eliminating the organism from the nasopharynx of infected individuals, rendering them noninfectious. Some clinical studies suggest that erythromycin may be helpful in the prophylaxis of pertussis in exposed susceptible individuals.

Diphtheria—As an adjunct to antitoxin infections due to *Corynebacterium diphtheriae,* to prevent establishment of carriers and to eradicate the organism in carriers.

Erythrasma—In the treatment of infections due to *Corynebacterium minutissimum.*

Intestinal amebiasis caused by *Entamoeba histolytica* (oral erythromycins only). Extraenteric amebiasis requires treatment with other agents.

Infections due to *Listeria monocytogenes.*

Erythromycin is indicated for treatment of the following infections caused by *Chlamydia trachomatis:* conjunctivitis of the newborn, pneumonia of infancy and urogenital infections during pregnancy. When tetracyclines are contraindicated or not tolerated, erythromycin is indicated for the treatment of uncomplicated urethral, endocervical, or rectal infections in adults due to *Chlamydia trachomatis.*[4]

When tetracyclines are contraindicated or not tolerated erythromycin is indicated for the treatment of nongonococcal urethritis caused by *Ureaplasma urealyticum.*[4]

Primary syphilis caused by *Treponema pallidum.* Erythromycin (oral forms only) is an alternative choice of treatment for primary syphilis in patients allergic to the penicillins. In treatment of primary syphilis, spinal fluid should be examined before treatment and as part of the follow-up after therapy.

Legionnaires' Disease caused by *Legionella pneumophila.* Although no controlled clinical efficacy studies have been conducted, in vitro and limited preliminary clinical data suggest that erythromycin may be effective in treating Legionnaires' Disease.

Prevention of Initial Attacks of Rheumatic Fever—Penicillin is considered by the American Heart Association to be the drug of choice in the prevention of initial attacks of rheumatic fever (treatment of group A beta-hemolytic streptococcal infections of the upper respiratory tract, e.g. tonsillitis or pharyngitis).[3]

Erythromycin is indicated for the treatment of penicillin-allergic patients. A therapeutic dose should be administered for ten days.

Prevention of Recurrent Attacks of Rheumatic Fever—Penicillin or sulfonamides are considered by the American Heart Association to be the drugs of choice in the prevention of recurrent attacks of rheumatic fever.

In patients who are allergic to penicillin and sulfonamides, oral erythromycin is recommended by the American Heart Association in the long-term prophylaxis of streptococcal pharyngitis (for the prevention of recurrent attacks of rheumatic fever).[3]

Prevention of Bacterial Endocarditis—Although no controlled clinical efficacy trials have been conducted, oral erythromycin has been recommended by the American Heart Association for prevention of bacterial endocarditis in penicillin-allergic patients with prosthetic cardiac valves, most congenital cardiac malformations, surgically constructed systemic-pulmonary shunts, rheumatic or other acquired valvular dysfunction, idiopathic hypertrophic subaortic stenosis (IHSS), previous history of bacterial endocarditis and mitral valve prolapse with insufficiency when they undergo dental procedures and surgical procedures of the upper respiratory tract.[5]

CONTRAINDICATION

ERYC 125 is contraindicated in patients with known hypersensitivity to this antibiotic.

WARNING

There have been a few reports of hepatic dysfunction, with or without jaundice, occurring in patients receiving erythromycin ethylsuccinate, base, estolate and stearate products.

PRECAUTIONS

Caution should be exercised when erythromycin is administered to patients with impaired hepatic function (see CLINICAL PHARMACOLOGY and WARNING section).

Prolonged or repeated use of erythromycin may result in an overgrowth of non-susceptible bacteria or fungi. If superinfection occurs, erythromycin should be discontinued and appropriate therapy instituted. When indicated, incision and drainage or other surgical procedures should be performed in conjunction with antibiotic therapy.

Laboratory Tests: Erythromycin interferes with the fluorometric determination of urinary catecholamines.

Drug Interactions: Erythromycin use in patients who are receiving high doses of theophylline may be associated with an increase in serum theophylline levels and potential theophylline toxicity. In case of theophylline toxicity and/or elevated serum theophylline levels, the dose of theophylline should be reduced while the patient is receiving concomitant erythromycin therapy.

Erythromycin administration in patients receiving carbamazepine has been reported to cause increased blood levels of carbamazepine toxicity.

Pregnancy Category B—Reproduction studies have been performed in rats, mice and rabbits using erythromycin and its various salts and esters, at doses which were several times the usual human dose. No evidence of impaired fertility or harm to the fetus that appeared related to erythromycin was reported in these studies. There are, however, no adequate well-controlled studies in pregnant women. Because animal reproduction studies are not always predictive of human response, this drug should be used during pregnancy only if clearly needed.

Labor and Delivery—The effect of ERYC 125 on labor and delivery is unknown.

Nursing Mothers—Erythromycin is excreted in milk (see CLINICAL PHARMACOLOGY).

Pediatric Use—See INDICATIONS AND USAGE and DOSAGE AND ADMINISTRATION.

ADVERSE REACTIONS

The most frequent side effects of oral erythromycin preparations are gastrointestinal and are dose-related. They include nausea, vomiting, abdominal pain, diarrhea and anorexia. Symptoms of hepatic dysfunction and/or abnormal liver function test results may occur (see WARNING).

Mild allergic reactions such as rashes with or without pruritus, urticaria, bullous fixed eruptions, and eczema have been reported with erythromycin. Serious allergic reactions, including anaphylaxis, have been reported.

There have been isolated reports of reversible hearing loss occurring chiefly in patients with renal insufficiency and in patients receiving high doses of erythromycin.

DOSAGE AND ADMINISTRATION

The entire contents of an ERYC 125 Capsule should be sprinkled on a small amount of apple sauce prior to ingestion. SUBDIVIDING THE CONTENTS OF A CAPSULE IS NOT RECOMMENDED. If desired ERYC 125 Capsule may be swallowed whole.

Optimum and uniform serum levels of erythromycin are obtained when ERYC 125 is administered in the fasting state, (at least 1 hour before meals).

ADULTS: The usual dose is 250 mg every 6 hours. If twice-a-day dosage is desired, the recommended dose is 500 mg every 12 hours. Dosage may be increased up to 4 grams per day,

Continued on next page

This product information was prepared in August, 1986. On these and other Parke-Davis Products, information may be obtained by addressing PARKE-DAVIS, Division of Warner-Lambert Company, Morris Plains, New Jersey 07950.

Parke-Davis—Cont.

according to the severity of infection. Twice-a-day dosing is not recommended when doses larger than 1 gram daily are administered.
CHILDREN: Age, weight, and severity of the infection are important factors in determining the proper dosage. The usual dosage is 30–50 mg/kg/day in equally divided doses. For the treatment of more severe infections this dosage may be doubled.
In the treatment of group A beta-hemolytic streptococcal infections of the upper respiratory tract (e.g., tonsillitis or pharyngitis) a therapeutic dosage of erythromycin should be administered for ten days.
The American Heart Association suggests a dosage of 250 mg of erythromycin orally twice a day in long-term prophylaxis of streptococcal upper respiratory tract infections for the prevention of recurrent attacks of rheumatic fever in patients allergic to penicillin and sulfonamide.[3]
In prophylaxis against bacterial endocarditis (see Indications), the oral regimen for penicillin-allergic patients is erythromycin 1.0 g one hour before the procedure followed by 500 mg six hours later.[5]
Conjunctivitis of the newborn caused by *Chlamydia trachomatis:* Oral erythromycin syrup 50 mg/kg/day in four divided doses for at least two weeks.[4]
Pneumonia of infancy caused by *Chlamydia trachomatis:* Although the optimal duration of therapy has not been established, the recommended therapy is oral erythromycin syrup 50 mg/kg/day in four divided doses for at least three weeks.[4]
Urogenital infections during pregnancy due to *Chlamydia trachomatis:* Although the optimal dose and duration of the therapy have not been established, the suggested treatment is erythromycin 500 mg. by mouth, four times a day on an empty stomach for at least seven days. For women who cannot tolerate this regimen, a decreased dose of 250 mg. by mouth, four times a day should be used for at least fourteen days.[4]
For adults with uncomplicated urethral, endocervical, or rectal infections caused by *Chlamydia trachomatis* in whom tetracyclines are contraindicated or not tolerated: 500 mg. by mouth, four times a day for at least seven days.[4]
For patients with nongonococcal urethritis caused by *Ureaplasma urealyticum* in whom tetracyclines are contraindicated or not tolerated: 500 mg. by mouth, four times a day for at least seven days.[4]
Primary syphilis: 30–40 grams given in divided doses over a period of ten to fifteen days.
Intestinal amebiasis: 250 mg. four times daily, for ten to fourteen days for adults 30 to 50 mg/kg/day in divided doses for ten to fourteen days for children.
Legionnaires' Disease: Although optimal doses have not been established, doses utilized in reported clinical data were those recommended above (1 to 4 grams daily in divided doses).
Pertussis: Although optimum dosage and duration of therapy have not been established, doses of erythromycin utilized in reported clinical studies were 40–50 mg/kg/day, given in divided doses for five to fourteen days.

HOW SUPPLIED

Capsules containing enteric-coated pellets. The capsules have an opaque orange cap and a clear body. They bear the inscription 'This end up' and 'PD' on the cap and 'Eryc 125' on the body. The pellets are colored white.
ERYC 125 (Capsule 663) each containing 125 mg erythromycin base as enteric-coated pellets, is available as follows:
N 0071-0663-24 Bottles of 100
Storage Condition: Maintain at a temperature not exceeding 30°C.

REFERENCES

1. Approved Standard ASM-2 "Performance Standards for Anti-microbial Disc Susceptibility Test." National Committee for Clinical Laboratory Standards, 771 East Lancaster Avenue, Villanova, PA 19085.
2. Ericson, H.M. and Sherris, J.C. "Antibiotic Sensitivity Testing Report of an International Collaborative Study." *Acta Pathologica et Microbiologica Scandinavica,* Section B, Supp. 217, 1971, pp. 1–90.
3. Committee on Rheumatic Fever and Infective Endocarditis of the Council on Cardiovascular Disease in the Young: Prevention of Rheumatic Fever, *Circulation* 70: 1118A, 1984.
4. CDC Sexually Transmitted Diseases Treatment Guidelines 1982.
5. Committee on Rheumatic Fever and Infective Endocarditis of the Council on Cardiovascular Disease in the Young: Prevention of Bacterial Endocarditis, *Circulation* 70: 1123A, 1984.

Caution—Federal law prohibits dispensing without prescription.

Manufactured by
Faulding International
129 Dew Street
Thebarton, South Australia 5031
Distributed by
PARKE-DAVIS
Div of Warner-Lambert Co
Morris Plains, NJ 07950 USA

0663G111

Shown in Product Identification Section, page 420

ERYTHROMYCIN STEARATE ℞
[*ĕ-ry 'thrō-my "cĭn stēa 'rāte "*]
TABLETS, USP
(Erypar®)

DESCRIPTION

Erythromycin is produced by a strain of *Streptomyces erythraeus* and belongs to the macrolide group of antibiotics. It is basic and readily forms salts with acids. The base, the stearate salt, and the esters are poorly soluble in water, and are suitable for oral administration.
The film-coated tablets contain 250 mg or 500 mg of erythromycin as erythromycin stearate, USP.
Erythromycin Stearate 250 mg also contains: hydroxypropyl cellulose, NF; magnesium stearate, NF; Opaseal pharmaceutical sealant; Opaspray yellow K-1-2227; polysorbate 80, NF; povidone, USP; N-vinyl-2-pyrrolidone polyvinylpoly-pyrrolidone; sodium citrate, USP; carboxymethyl starch; Mistron spray talc.
Erythromycin Stearate 500 mg also contains: croscarmellous sodium, NF; hydroxypropyl cellulose, NF; hydroxypropyl methylcellulose 2910, USP; magnesium stearate, NF; methylparaben, NF; Opaspray yellow K-1-2227; polyethylene glycol, NF; dibasic potassium phosphate; monobasic potassium phosphate, NF; polyvinyl acetate phthalate; propylparaben, NF; silica gel, NF; sodium citrate, USP; starch, NF; pregelatinized starch, NF; Mistron spray talc; triethyl citrate.

CLINICAL PHARMACOLOGY

The mode of action of erythromycin is by inhibition of protein synthesis without affecting nucleic acid synthesis. Resistance to erythromycin of some strains of *Hemophilus influenzae* and staphylococci has been demonstrated. Culture and susceptibility testing should be done. If the Kirby-Bauer method of disc susceptibility is used, a 15-mcg erythromycin disc should give a zone diameter of at least 18 mm when tested against an erythromycin-susceptible organism.
Orally administered erythromycin is readily absorbed by most patients, especially on an empty stomach, but patient variation is observed.
After absorption, erythromycin diffuses readily into most body fluids. In the absence of meningeal inflammation, low concentrations are normally achieved in the spinal fluid, but passage of the drug across the blood-brain barrier increases in meningitis. In the presence of normal hepatic function, erythromycin is concentrated in the liver and excreted in the bile; the effect of hepatic dysfunction on excretion of erythromycin by the liver into the bile is not known. After oral administration, less than 5 percent of the activity of the administered dose can be recovered in the urine.
Erythromycin crosses the placental barrier but fetal plasma levels are generally low.

INDICATIONS AND USAGE

Streptococcus pyogenes (Group A beta-hemolytic *Streptococcus*): Upper and lower respiratory tract, skin, and soft-tissue infections of mild to moderate severity
Injectable benzathine penicillin G is considered by the American Heart Association to be the drug of choice in the treatment and prevention of streptococcal pharyngitis and in the long-term prophylaxis of rheumatic fever.
When oral medication is preferred for treatment of streptococcal pharyngitis, penicillin G, V, or erythromycin are alternate drugs of choice.
When oral medication is given, the importance of strict adherence by the patient to the prescribed dosage regimen must be stressed. A therapeutic dose should be administered for at least 10 days.
Although no controlled clinical efficacy trials have been conducted, oral erythromycin has been suggested by the American Heart Association and American Dental Association for use in a regimen for prophylaxis against bacterial endocarditis in patients allergic to penicillin who have congenital heart disease or rheumatic or other acquired valvular heart disease when they undergo dental procedures and surgical procedures of the upper respiratory tract.[1] Erythromycin is not suitable prior to genitourinary or gastrointestinal tract surgery.
Note: When selecting antibiotics for the prevention of bacterial endocarditis, the physician or dentist should read the full joint statement of the American Heart Association and the American Dental Association.[1]
Staphylococcus aureus: Acute infections of skin and soft tissue of mild to moderate severity. Resistant organisms may emerge during treatment.
Diplococcus pneumoniae: Upper respiratory tract infections (eg, otitis media, pharyngitis) and lower respiratory tract infections (eg, pneumonia) of mild to moderate degree
Mycoplasma pneumoniae (Eaton agent, PPLO): In the treatment of primary atypical pneumonia, when due to this organism
Treponema pallidum: Erythromycin is an alternate choice of treatment for primary syphilis in patients allergic to the penicillins. In treatment of primary syphilis, spinal fluid examinations should be done before treatment and as part of follow-up after therapy.
Erythromycins are indicated for treatment of the following infections caused by *Chlamydia trachomatis:* conjunctivitis of the newborn, pneumonia of infancy, urogenital infections during pregnancy. When tetracyclines are contraindicated or not tolerated, erythromycin is indicated for the treatment of uncomplicated urethral, endocervical, or rectal infections in adults due to *Chlamydia trachomatis.*[2]
Corynebacterium diphtheriae and *C minutissimum:* As an adjunct to antitoxin, to prevent establishment of carriers, and to eradicate the organism in carriers
In the treatment of erythrasma
Entamoeba histolytica: In the treatment of intestinal amebiasis only. Extra-enteric amebiasis requires treatment with other agents.
Listeria monocytogenes: Infections due to this organism
Legionnaires' Disease: Although no controlled clinical efficacy studies have been conducted, *in vitro* and limited preliminary clinical data suggest that erythromycin may be effective in treating Legionnaires' Disease.

CONTRAINDICATION

Erythromycin is contraindicated in patients with known hypersensitivity to this antibiotic.

PRECAUTIONS

Erythromycin is principally excreted by the liver. Caution should be exercised in administering the antibiotic to patients with impaired hepatic function. There have been reports of hepatic dysfunction, with or without jaundice, occurring in patients receiving oral erythromycin products.
Recent data from studies of erythromycin reveal that its use in patients who are receiving high doses of theophylline may be associated with an increase of serum theophylline levels and potential theophylline toxicity. In case of theophylline toxicity and/or elevated serum theophylline levels, the dose of theophylline should be reduced while the patient is receiving concomitant erythromycin therapy.
Surgical procedures should be performed when indicated.
Usage during pregnancy and lactation: The safety of erythromycin for use during pregnancy has not been established. Erythromycin crosses the placental barrier. Erythromycin also appears in breast milk.

ADVERSE REACTIONS

The most frequent side effects of oral erythromycin preparations are gastrointestinal, such as abdominal cramping and discomfort, and are dose-related. Nausea, vomiting, and diarrhea occur infrequently with usual oral doses.
During prolonged or repeated therapy, there is a possibility of overgrowth of nonsusceptible bacteria or fungi. If such infections occur, the drug should be discontinued and appropriate therapy instituted.
Mild allergic reactions, such as urticaria and other skin rashes, have occurred. Serious allergic reactions, including anaphylaxis, have been reported.

DOSAGE AND ADMINISTRATION

Optimum blood levels are obtained when doses are given on an empty stomach.
Adults: 250 mg every six hours is the usual dose; or 500 mg every 12 hours, one hour before meals. Dosage may be increased up to 4 grams per day according to the severity of the infection.
Children: Age, weight, and severity of the infection are important factors in determining the proper dosage: 30 to 50 mg/kg/day, in divided doses, is the usual dose. For more severe infections, this dosage may be doubled.
If dosage is desired on a twice-a-day schedule in either adults or children, one half of the total daily dose may be given every 12 hours, one hour before meals.
In the treatment of streptococcal infections, a therapeutic dosage of erythromycin should be administered for at least 10 days. In continuous *prophylaxis* of streptococcal infections in persons with a history of rheumatic heart disease, the dose is 250 mg twice a day.
For prophylaxis against bacterial endocarditis[1] in patients with congenital heart disease or rheumatic or other acquired valvular heart disease when undergoing dental procedures or surgical procedures of the upper respiratory tract, give 1.0 gm (20 mg/kg for children) orally 1½-2 hours before the procedure, and then 500 mg (10 mg/kg for children) orally every 6 hours for 8 doses.

For treatment of primary syphilis: 30 to 40 grams given in divided doses over a period of 10 to 15 days.
For dysenteric amebiasis: Adults: 250 mg four times daily for 10 to 14 days. Children: 30 to 50 mg/kg/day in divided doses for 10 to 14 days.
For treatment of Legionnaires' Disease: Although optimal doses have not been established, doses utilized in reported clinical data were those recommended above (1 to 4 grams erythromycin stearate daily in divided doses).

HOW SUPPLIED

Erythromycin Stearate Tablets, USP are supplied as:
N 0071-0672-24—bottle of 100
N 0071-0672-30—bottle of 500
N 0071-0672-40—unit dose (10/10's)
Each film-coated tablet contains 250 mg erythromycin as erythromycin stearate.
N 0071-0919-24—bottle of 100
Each film-coated tablet contains 500 mg erythromycin as erythromycin stearate.
AHFS 8:12.12 **0672G013**

Shown in Product Identification Section, page 420

REFERENCE

1. American Heart Association. Prevention of bacterial endocarditis. *Circulation.* 70:1123A-1127A, 1984.
2. CDC Sexually Transmitted Diseases Treatment Guidelines 1982.

ESTROVIS® ℞
[ĕs-trō'vĭs"]
(Quinestrol tablets, USP)*

*Product of Warner-Lambert Inc

WARNING

1. Estrogens Have Been Reported to Increase the Risk of Endometrial Carcinoma.

Three independent case control studies have shown an increased risk of endometrial cancer in postmenopausal women exposed to exogenous estrogens for prolonged periods.[1–3] This risk was independent of the other known risk factors for endometrial cancer. These studies are further supported by the finding that incidence rates of endometrial cancer have increased sharply since 1969 in eight different areas of the United States with population-based cancer reporting systems, an increase which may be related to the rapidly expanding use of estrogens during the last decade.[4]

The three case control studies reported that the risk of endometrial cancer in estrogen users was about 4.5 to 13.9 times greater than in nonusers. The risk appears to depend on both duration of treatment[1] and on estrogen dose.[3] In view of these findings, when estrogens are used for the treatment of menopausal symptoms, the lowest dose that will control symptoms should be utilized and medication should be discontinued as soon as possible. When prolonged treatment is medically indicated, the patient should be reassessed on at least a semiannual basis to determine the need for continued therapy. Although the evidence must be considered preliminary, one study suggests that cyclic administration of low doses of estrogen may carry less risk than continuous administration.[3] Therefore, while it appears prudent to utilize such a regimen with other orally administered estrogens, Estrovis may be administered, following a seven-day priming schedule, on a once weekly maintenance dosage beginning two weeks after the start of treatment.

Close clinical surveillance of all women taking estrogens is important. In all cases of undiagnosed persistent or recurring abnormal vaginal bleeding, adequate diagnostic measures should be undertaken to rule out malignancy.

There is no evidence at present that "natural" estrogens are more or less hazardous than "synthetic" estrogens at equiestrogenic doses.

2. Estrogens Should not be Used During Pregnancy.

The use of female sex hormones, both estrogens and progestogens, during early pregnancy may seriously damage the offspring. It has been shown that females exposed *in utero* to diethylstilbestrol, a nonsteroidal estrogen, have an increased risk of developing in later life a form of vaginal or cervical cancer that is ordinarily extremely rare.[5–6] This risk has been estimated as not greater than 4 per 1,000 exposures.[7] Furthermore, a high percentage of such exposed women (from 30 to 90%) have been found to have vaginal adenosis,[8–12] epithelial changes of the vagina and cervix. Although these changes are histologically benign, it is not known whether they are precursors of malignancy. Although similar data are not available with the use of other estrogens, it cannot be presumed they would not induce similar changes.

Several reports suggest an association between intrauterine exposure to female sex hormones and congenital anomalies, including congenital heart defects and limb- reduction defects.[13–16] One case control study[16] estimated a 4.7-fold increased risk of limb-reduction defects in infants exposed *in utero* to sex hormones (oral contraceptives, hormone withdrawal tests for pregnancy, or attempted treatment for threatened abortion). Some of these exposures were very short and involved only a few days of treatment. The data suggest that the risk of limb-reduction defects in exposed fetuses is somewhat less than 1 per 1,000.

In the past, female sex hormones have been used during pregnancy in an attempt to treat threatened or habitual abortion. There is considerable evidence that estrogens are ineffective for these indications, and there is no evidence from well-controlled studies that progestogens are effective for these uses.

If Estrovis (quinestrol) is used during pregnancy, or if the patient becomes pregnant while taking this drug, she should be apprised of the potential risks to the fetus and the advisability of pregnancy continuation.

DESCRIPTION

Estrovis is the 3-cyclopentylether of ethinyl estradiol. It is an estrogenic agent for oral administration. Each tablet contains 100 mcg quinestrol, USP. Estrovis also contains: FD&C blue No. 1 Al lake; lactose, NF; and magnesium stearate, NF. The chemical name is 3-cyclopentyloxy-17α-ethynylestra-1,3,5(10)-trien-17β-ol.

It is a white, essentially odorless powder, insoluble in water and soluble in alcohol, chloroform, and ether.

CLINICAL PHARMACOLOGY

Estrovis (quinestrol) is an orally effective estrogen as judged by conventional assay procedures employing vagina and uterine end-points in mice, rats and rabbits.

The estrogenic effects of Estrovis have been demonstrated in clinical studies by its effects on the endometrium, maturation of the vaginal epithelium, thinning of cervical mucus, suppression of pituitary gonadotropin, inhibition of ovulation, and prevention of postpartum breast discomfort.

INDICATIONS

Estrovis (quinestrol) is indicated in the treatment of:

1. Moderate to severe vasomotor symptoms associated with the menopause. (There is no evidence that estrogens are effective for nervous symptoms or depression which might occur during menopause, and they should not be used to treat these conditions.)
2. Atrophic vaginitis
3. Kraurosis vulvae
4. Female hypogonadism
5. Female castration
6. Primary ovarian failure

Estrovis (Quinestrol) Has Not Been Shown to be Effective for any Purpose during Pregnancy and Its Use May Cause Severe Harm to the Fetus (See Boxed Warning).

CONTRAINDICATIONS

Estrogens should not be used in women (or men) with any of the following conditions:

1. Known or suspected cancer of the breast except in appropriately selected patients being treated for metastatic disease
2. Known or suspected estrogen-dependent neoplasia
3. Known or suspected pregnancy (See Boxed Warning)
4. Undiagnosed abnormal genital bleeding
5. Active thrombophlebitis or thromboembolic disorders
6. A past history of thrombophlebitis, thrombosis, or thromboembolic disorders associated with previous estrogen use (except when used in treatment of breast or prostatic malignancy)

WARNINGS

1. *Induction of malignant neoplasms.* Long-term continuous administration of natural and synthetic estrogens in certain animal species increases the frequency of carcinomas of the breast, cervix, vagina, and liver. There is now evidence that estrogens increase the risk of carcinoma of the endometrium in humans. (See Boxed Warning.)

At the present time, there is no satisfactory evidence that estrogens given to postmenopausal women increase the risk of cancer of the breast,[18] although a recent long-term follow up of a single physician's practice has raised this possibility.[18a] Because of the animal data, there is a need for caution in prescribing estrogens for women with a strong family history of breast cancer or who have breast nodules, fibrocystic disease, or abnormal mammograms.

2. *Gallbladder disease.* A recent study has reported a 2- to 3-fold increase in the risk of surgically confirmed gallbladder disease in women receiving postmenopausal estrogens,[18] similar to the 2-fold increase previously noted in users of oral contraceptives.[19–24] In the case of oral contraceptives, the increased risk appeared after two years of use.[24]

3. *Effects similar to those caused by estrogen-progestogen oral contraceptives.* There are several serious adverse effects of oral contraceptives, most of which have not, up to now, been documented as consequences of postmenopausal estrogen therapy. This may reflect the comparatively low doses of estrogen used in postmenopausal women. It would be expected that the larger doses of estrogen used to treat prostatic or breast cancer or postpartum breast engorgement are more likely to result in these adverse effects, and, in fact, it has been shown that there is an increased risk of thrombosis in men receiving estrogens for prostatic cancer and women for postpartum breast engorgement.[20-23]

a. *Thromboembolic disease.* It is now well established that users of oral contraceptives have an increased risk of various thromboembolic and thrombotic vascular diseases, such as thrombophlebitis, pulmonary embolism, stroke, and myocardial infarction.[24–31] Cases of retinal thrombosis, mesenteric thrombosis, and optic neuritis have been reported in oral contraceptive users. There is evidence that the risk of several of these adverse reactions is related to the dose of the drug.[32,33] An increased risk of postsurgery thromboembolic complications has also been reported in users of oral contraceptives.[34,35] If feasible, estrogen should be discontinued at least 4 weeks before surgery of the type associated with an increased risk of thromboembolism, or during periods of prolonged immobilization.

While an increased rate of thromboembolic and thrombotic disease in postmenopausal users of estrogens has not been found,[18,36] this does not rule out the possibility that such an increase may be present or that subgroups of women who have underlying risk factors or who are receiving relatively large doses of estrogens may have increased risk. Therefore, estrogens should not be used in persons with active thrombophlebitis or thromboembolic disorders, and they should not be used (except in treatment of malignancy) in persons with a history of such disorders in association with estrogen use. They should be used with caution in patients with cerebral vascular or coronary artery disease and only for those in whom estrogens are clearly needed.

Large doses of estrogen (5 mg conjugated estrogens per day), comparable to those used to treat cancer of the prostate and breast, have been shown in a large prospective clinical trial in men[37] to increase the risk of nonfatal myocardial infarction, pulmonary embolism, and thrombophlebitis. When estrogen doses of this size are used, any of the thromboembolic and thrombotic adverse effects associated with oral contraceptive use should be considered a clear risk.

b. *Hepatic adenoma.* Benign hepatic adenomas appear to be associated with the use of oral contraceptives.[38–40] Although benign, and rare, these may rupture and may cause death through intra-abdominal hemorrhage. Such lesions have not yet been reported in association with other estrogen or progestogen preparations but should be considered in estrogen users having abdominal pain and tenderness, abdominal mass, or hypovolemic shock. Hepatocellular carcinoma has also been reported in women taking estrogen-containing oral contraceptives.[39] The relationship of this malignancy to these drugs is not known at this time.

c. *Elevated blood pressure.* Increased blood pressure is not uncommon in women using oral contraceptives. There is now a report that this may occur with use of estrogens in the menopause[11] and blood pressure should be monitored with estrogen use, especially if high doses are used.

d. *Glucose tolerance.* A worsening of glucose tolerance has been observed in a significant percentage of patients on estrogen-containing oral contraceptives. For this reason, diabetic patients should be carefully observed while receiving estrogen.

4. *Hypercalcemia.* Administration of estrogens may lead to severe hypercalcemia in patients with breast cancer and bone metastases. If this occurs, the drug should be stopped and appropriate measures taken to reduce the serum calcium level.

PRECAUTIONS

A. General Precautions

1. A complete medical and family history should be taken prior to the initiation of any estrogen therapy. The pretreatment and periodic physical examinations should include special reference to blood pressure, abdomen, and pelvic organs, and should include a Papanicolaou smear. As a general rule, estrogen should not be prescribed for longer than one year without another physical examination being performed.
2. Fluid retention—Because estrogens may cause some degree of fluid retention, conditions which might be influenced by this factor, such as epilepsy, migraine, and cardiac or renal dysfunction, require careful observation.

Continued on next page

This product information was prepared in August, 1986. On these and other Parke-Davis Products, information may be obtained by addressing PARKE-DAVIS, Division of Warner-Lambert Company, Morris Plains, New Jersey 07950.

Parke-Davis—Cont.

3. Certain patients may develop undesirable manifestations of excessive estrogenic stimulation, such as abnormal or excessive uterine bleeding, mastodynia, etc.
4. Oral contraceptives appear to be associated with an increased incidence of mental depression.[24] Although it is not clear whether this is due to the estrogenic or progestogenic component of the contraceptive, patients with a history of depression should be carefully observed.
5. Preexisting uterine leiomyomata may increase in size during estrogen use.
6. The pathologist should be advised of estrogen therapy when relevant specimens are submitted.
7. Patients with a past history of jaundice during pregnancy have an increased risk of recurrence of jaundice while receiving estrogen-containing oral contraceptive therapy. If jaundice develops in any patient receiving estrogen, the medication should be discontinued while the cause is investigated.
8. Estrogens may be poorly metabolized in patients with impaired liver function and they should be administered with caution in such patients.
9. Because estrogens influence the metabolism of calcium and phosphorus, they should be used with caution in patients with metabolic bone diseases that are associated with hypercalcemia or in patients with renal insufficiency.
10. Because of the effects of estrogens on epiphyseal closure, they should be used judiciously in young patients in whom bone growth is not complete.
11. Certain endocrine and liver function tests may be affected by estrogen-containing oral contraceptives. The following similar changes may be expected with larger doses of estrogen:
a. Increased sulfobromophthalein retention.
b. Increased prothrombin and factors VII, VIII, IX, and X; decreased antithrombin 3; increased norepinephrine-induced platelet aggregability.
c. Increased thyroid binding globulin (TBG) leading to increased circulating total thyroid hormone, as measured by PHI, T4 by column, or T4 by radioimmunoassay. Free T3 resin uptake is decreased, reflecting the elevated TBG; free T4 concentration is unaltered.
d. Impaired glucose tolerance.
e. Decreased pregnanediol excretion.
f. Reduced response to metyrapone test.
g. Reduced serum folate concentration.
h. Increased serum triglyceride and phospholipid concentration.
B. Information for the patient. See text of Patient Package Insert.
C. Pregnancy. See Contraindications and Boxed Warning.
D. Nursing Mothers. As a general principle, the administration of any drug to nursing mothers should be done only when clearly necessary because many drugs are excreted in human milk.

ADVERSE REACTIONS

(See Warnings regarding induction of neoplasia, adverse effects on the fetus, increased incidence of gallbladder disease, and adverse effects similar to those of oral contraceptives, including thromboembolism.) The following additional adverse reactions have been reported with estrogenic therapy, including oral contraceptives:
1. *Genitourinary system.*
Breakthrough bleeding, spotting, change in menstrual flow
Dysmenorrhea
Premenstrual-like syndrome
Amenorrhea during and after treatment
Increase in size of uterine fibromyomata
Vaginal candidiasis
Change in cervical eversion and in degree of cervical secretion
Cystitis-like syndrome
2. *Breasts.*
Tenderness, enlargement, secretion
3. *Gastrointestinal.*
Nausea, vomiting
Abdominal cramps, bloating
Cholestatic jaundice
4. *Skin.*
Chloasma or melasma which may persist when drug is discontinued
Erythema multiforme
Erythema nodosum
Hemorrhagic eruption
Loss of scalp hair
Hirsutism
5. *Eyes.*
Steepening of corneal curvature
Intolerance to contact lenses
6. *CNS.*
Headache, migraine, dizziness
Mental depression
Chorea
7. *Miscellaneous.*
Increase or decrease in weight
Reduced carbohydrate tolerance
Aggravation of porphyria
Edema
Changes in libido

ACUTE OVERDOSAGE

Numerous reports of ingestion of large doses of estrogen-containing oral contraceptives by young children indicate that serious ill effects do not occur. Overdosage of estrogen may cause nausea, and withdrawal bleeding may occur in females.

DOSAGE AND ADMINISTRATION

For treatment of moderate to severe vasomotor symptoms associated with the menopause, and for atrophic vaginitis, kraurosis vulvae, female hypogonadism, female castration, and primary ovarian failure.
One Estrovis (quinestrol) 100-mcg tablet once daily for seven days, followed by one 100-mcg tablet weekly as a maintenance schedule, commencing two weeks after inception of treatment. The dosage may be increased to 200 mcg weekly if the therapeutic response is not that which may be desirable or considered optimal.
The lowest maintenance dose that will control symptoms should be chosen and medication should be discontinued as promptly as possible.
Attempts to discontinue or taper medication should be made at three- to six-month intervals.
Treated patients with an intact uterus should be monitored closely for signs of endometrial cancer and appropriate diagnostic measures should be taken to rule out malignancy in the event of persistent or recurring abnormal vaginal bleeding.

HOW SUPPLIED

N 0071-0437-24 (P-D 437) Estrovis (quinestrol) 100-mcg tablets are supplied in bottles of 100.

0437G024

PHYSICIAN REFERENCES

1. Ziel, H.K. and W.D. Finkle, "Increased Risk of Endometrial Carcinoma Among Users of Conjugated Estrogens." *New England Journal of Medicine,* 293:1167–1170, 1975.
2. Smith, D.C., R. Prentic, D.J. Thompson, and W.L. Hermann, "Association of Exogenous Estrogen and Endometrial Carcinoma." *New England Journal of Medicine,* 293:1164–1167, 1975.
3. Mack, T.M., M.C. Pike, B.E. Henderson, R.I. Pfeffer, V.R. Gerkins, M. Arthur, and S.E. Brown, "Estrogens and Endometrial Cancer in a Retirement Community." *New England Journal of Medicine,* 294:1262–1267, 1976.
4. Weiss, N.D., D.R. Szekely and D.F. Austin, "Increasing Incidence of Endometrial Cancer in the United States." *New England Journal of Medicine,* 294:1259–1262, 1976.
5. Herbst, A.L., H. Ulfelder and D.C. Poskanzer, "Adenocarcinoma of Vagina." *New England Journal of Medicine,* 284:878–881, 1971.
6. Greenwald, P., J. Barlow, P. Nasca, and W. Burnett, "Vaginal Cancer after Maternal Treatment with Synthetic Estrogens." *New England Journal of Medicine,* 285:390–392, 1971.
7. Lanier, A., K. Noller, D. Decker, L. Elveback, and L. Kurland, "Cancer and Stilbestrol, A Follow-Up of 1719 Persons Exposed to Estrogens in Utero and Born 1943–1959." *Mayo Clinic Proceedings,* 48:793–799, 1973.
8. Herbst, A., R. Kurman, and R. Scully, "Vaginal and Cervical Abnormalities After Exposure to Stilbestrol in Utero." *Obstetrics and Gynecology,* 40:287–298, 1972.
9. Herbst, A., S. Robboy, G. Macdonald, and R. Scully, "The Effects of Local Progesterone on Stilbestrol-Associated Vaginal Adenosis." *American Journal of Obstetrics and Gynecology,* 118:607–615, 1974.
10. Herbst, A., D. Poskanzer, S. Robboy, L. Friedlander, and R. Scully, "Prenatal Exposure to Stilbestrol, A Prospective Comparison of Exposed Female Offspring with Unexpected Controls." *New England Journal of Medicine,* 292:334–339, 1975.
11. Stafl, A., R. Mattingly, D. Foley, and W. Fetherston, "Clinical Diagnosis of Vaginal Adenosis." *Obstetrics and Gynecology,* 43:118–128, 1974.
12. Sherman, A.I., M. Goldrath, A. Berlin, V. Vakhariya, F. Banooni, W. Michaels, P. Goodman, S. Brown, "Cervical-Vaginal Adenosis After *In Utero* Exposure to Synthetic Estrogens," *Obstetrics and Gynecology,* 44:531–545, 1974.
13. Gal, I., B. Kirman, and J. Stern, "Hormone Pregnancy Tests and Congenital Malformation," *Nature,* 216:83, 1967.
14. Levy, E.P., A. Cohen, and F.C. Fraser, "Hormone Treatment During Pregnancy and Congenital Heart Defects," *Lancet,* 1:611, 1973.
15. Nora, J. and A. Nora, "Birth Defects and Oral Contraceptives," *Lancet,* 1:941–942, 1973.
16. Janerich, D.T., J.M. Piper, and D.M. Glebatis, "Oral Contraceptives and Congenital Limb-Reduction Defects," *New England Journal of Medicine,* 291:697–700, 1974.
17. "Estrogens for Oral or Parenteral Use," *Federal Register,* 40:8212, 1975.
18. Boston Collaborative Drug Surveillance Program "Surgically Confirmed Gallbladder Disease, Venous Thromboembolism and Breast Tumors in Relation to Post-Menopausal Estrogen Therapy," *New England Journal of Medicine,* 210:15–19, 1974.
18a. Hoover, R., L.A. Gray, Sr., P. Cole, and B. MacMahon, "Menopausal Estrogens and Breast Cancer." *New England Journal of Medicine,* 295:401–405, 1976.
19. Boston Collaborative Drug Surveillance Program, "Oral Contraceptives and Venous Thromboembolic Disease, Surgically Confirmed Gallbladder Disease, and Breast Tumors," *Lancet,* 1:1399–1404, 1973.
20. Daniel, D.G., H. Campbell, and A.C. Turnbull, "Puerperal Thromboembolism and Suppression of Lactation." *Lancet,* 2:287–289, 1967.
21. The Veterans Administration Cooperative Urological Research Group, "Carcinoma of the Prostate: Treatment Comparisons," *Journal of Urology,* 98:516–522, 1967.
22. Ballar, J.C., "Thromboembolism and Oestrogen Therapy," *Lancet,* 2, 560. 1967.
23. Blackard, C., R. Doe, G. Mellinger, and D. Byar, "Incidence of Cardiovascular Disease and Death in Patients Receiving Diethylstilbestrol for Carcinoma of the Prostate," *Cancer,* 26:249–256, 1970.
24. Royal College of General Practitioners, "Oral Contraception and Thromboembolic Disease," *Journal of the Royal College of General Practitioners,* 13, 267–279, 1967.
25. Inman, W.H.W. and M.P. Vessey, "Investigation of Deaths from Pulmonary, Coronary, and Cerebral Thrombosis and Embolism in Women of Child-Bearing Age." *British Medical Journal,* 2:193–199, 1968.
26. Vessey, M.P. and R. Doll, "Investigation of Relation Between Use of Oral Contraceptives and Thromboembolic Disease, A Further Report," *British Medical Journal,* 2:651–657, 1969.
27. Sartwell, P.E., A.T. Masi, F.G. Arthes, G.R. Greene and H.E. Smith, "Thromboembolism and Oral Contraceptives: An Epidemiological Case Control Study." *American Journal of Epidemiology,* 90:365–380, 1969.
28. Collaborative Group for the Study of Stroke in Young Women, "Oral Contraception and Increased Risk of Cerebral Ischemia or Thrombosis," *New England Journal of Medicine,* 288:871–878, 1973.
29. Collaborative Group for the Study of Stroke in Young Women: "Oral Contraceptives and Stroke in Young Women: Associated Risk Factors," 231:718–722, 1975. *Journal of the American Medical Assoc.* 231:718–722, 1975.
30. Mann, J.I. and W.H.W. Inman, "Oral Contraceptives and Death from Myocardial Infarction," *British Medical Journal,* 2:245–248, 1975.
31. Mann, J.I., M.P. Vessey, M. Thorogood, and R. Doll, "Myocardial Infarction in Young Women with Special Reference to Oral Contraceptive Practice," *British Medical Journal,* 2:241–245, 1975.
32. Inman, W.H.W., M.P. Vessey, B. Westerholm, and A. Engelund. "Thromboembolic Disease and the Steroidal Content of Oral Contraceptives," *British Medical Journal,* 2:203–209, 1970.
33. Stolley, P.D., J.A. Tonascia, M.S. Tockman, P.E. Sartwell, A.H. Rutledge, and M.P. Jacobs, "Thrombosis with Low-Estrogen Oral Contraceptives," *American Journal of Epidemiology,* 102:197–208, 1975.
34. Vessey, M.P., R. Doll, A.S. Fairbairn, and G. Glober, "Post-Operative Thromboembolism and the use of the Oral Contraceptives," *British Medical Journal,* 3:123–126, 1970.
35. Greene, G.R. and P.E. Sartwell, "Oral Contraceptive Use in Patients with Thromboembolism Following Surgery, Trauma or Infection," *American Journal of Public Health,* 62:680–685, 1972.
36. Rosenberg, L., M.B. Armstrong and H. Jick "Myocardial Infarction and Estrogen Therapy in Post-menopausal Women," *New England Journal of Medicine,* 294:1256–1259, 1976.
37. Coronary Drug Project Research Group, "The Coronary Drug Project: Initial Findings Leading to Modifications of Its Research Protocol," *Journal of the American Medical Association,* 214:1303–1313, 1970.
38. Baum, J., F. Holtz, J.J. Bookstein, and E.W. Klein, "Possible Association between Benign Hepatomas and Oral Contraceptives," *Lancet,* 2:926–928, 1973.
39. Mays, E.T., W.M. Christopherson, M.M. Mahr, and H.C. Williams, "Hepatic Changes in Young Women Ingesting Contraceptive Steroids, Hepatic Hemorrhage and Primary Hepatic Tumors," *Journal of the American Medical Association,* 235:780–782, 1976.
40. Edmondson, H.A., B. Henderson, and B. Benton, "Liver Cell Adenomas Association with the Use of Oral Contraceptives," *New England Journal of Medicine,* 294:470–472, 1976.
41. Pfeffer, A.I. and S. Van Den Noore, "Estrogen use and Stroke Risk in Post-menopausal Women," *American Journal of Epidemiology,* 103:545–546, 1976.

Shown in Product Identification Section, page 420

EUTHROID® ℞

[ūth ′roid]

(Liotrix Tablets, USP)

DESCRIPTION

Euthroid is synthetic microcrystalline levothyroxine sodium (T_4) USP and synthetic microcrystalline liothyronine sodium (T_3) USP combined in a constant 4:1 ratio.

CLINICAL PHARMACOLOGY

Euthroid provides replacement therapy for the thyroactive material normally supplied by the human thyroid. The normal thyroid gland produces and stores thyroglobulin, the active components of which are two metabolically active hormones: levothyroxine and liothyronine. Euthroid (liotrix) provides a combination of these hormones in purified, synthetic form, supplied in a constant 4:1 ratio in order to simulate as closely as possible the physiologic and metabolic effects of normal endogenous thyroid secretions.

In contrast with the individual synthetic, metabolically active hormones, Euthroid will usually produce normal results for PBI, T_3, and other thyroid function tests—consistent with clinical progress—when persons with endogenous thyroid deficiencies are made euthyroid. Liothyronine sodium (T_3) acts more rapidly and for a shorter period of time than preparations of biological origin. Customarily, its use as a single agent produces inappropriately decreased PBI values. Levothyroxine sodium (T_4), on the other hand, is more tightly bound by plasma protein fractions and is somewhat slower acting than liothyronine sodium (T_3); its use as a single agent tends to produce inappropriately elevated PBI values. Euthroid, with its unvarying 4:1 ratio of T_4/T_3, permits interpretation of appropriate laboratory tests consistent with the total clinical status of the patient.

INDICATIONS AND USAGE

Euthroid provides thyroid replacement therapy in all conditions of inadequate production of thyroid hormones, namely:

1) Hypothyroidism, including cretinism and myxedema.
2) Simple (nontoxic) goiter.
3) Subacute or chronic thyroiditis including Hashimoto's disease.
4) Prevention of goiter in hyperthyroid patients undergoing treatment with thiouracil derivatives.
5) Usage in patients who may manifest intolerance to thyroid products of animal origin.

CONTRAINDICATIONS

Acute myocardial infarction, adrenal insufficiency, hypersensitivity to any component of this drug.

WARNINGS

> Drugs with thyroid hormone activity, alone or together with other therapeutic agents, have been used for the treatment of obesity. In euthyroid patients, doses within the range of daily hormonal requirements are ineffective for weight reduction. Larger doses may produce serious or even life-threatening manifestations of toxicity, particularly when given in association with sympathomimetic amines such as those used for their anorectic effects.

Liotrix should not be used in the presence of cardiovascular disease unless thyroid replacement therapy is clearly indicated. If the latter exists, low doses should be instituted (Euthroid-½ or Euthroid-1) and increased by the same amount in increments at 2-week intervals. This demands careful clinical judgment.

Morphologic hypogonadism and nephroses should be ruled out and adrenal deficiency due to hypopituitarism corrected before liotrix therapy is started.

If hypothyroidism and adrenal insufficiency exist concomitantly, cortisone or similar steroids should be given at dose levels sufficient to correct the adrenal insufficiency before attempting replacement therapy with thyroid hormones.

Likewise, the possibility of alterations in the prothrombin time must be considered and closely monitored in patients on anticoagulant therapy.

Myxedematous patients are very sensitive to thyroid hormones, and dosage should be started at a very low level and increased gradually.

Surgery: Euthroid-treated patients with coronary artery disease should be carefully observed during surgery, since the possibility of precipitating cardiac arrhythmias may be greater in patients treated with thyroid hormones.

PRECAUTIONS

Hypothyroid patients are especially sensitive to thyroid preparations, and those with severe hypothyroidism may be unusually so.

Initiation of thyroid replacement therapy in patients with diabetes must be carefully monitored because of potential fluctuation in daily insulin or oral hypoglycemic requirements.

Euthroid (liotrix tablets, USP)			Approximate Equivalents		
			Natural	Synthetic	
Tablet	T_4*/T_3** mcg	Color	Thyroid USP	T_4*	T_3**
Euthroid-½	(30/7.5)	pale orange	½ grain	.05 mg	12.5 mcg
Euthroid-1	(60/15)	light brown	1 grain	.1 mg	25.0 mcg
Euthroid-2	(120/30)	violet	2 grains	.2 mg	50.0 mcg
Euthroid-3	(180/45)	gray	3 grains	.3 mg	75.0 mcg

*T_4= levothyroxine sodium (*l*-thyroxine)

**T_3= liothyronine sodium (*l*-triiodothyronine)

As with all thyroid preparations, this drug will alter the results of thyroid function tests.

Euthroid-½, -1, -3 contains FD&C Yellow No. 5 (tartrazine) which may cause allergic-type reactions (including bronchial asthma) in certain susceptible individuals. Although the overall incidence of FD&C Yellow No. 5 (tartrazine) sensitivity in the population is low, it is frequently seen in patients who also have aspirin hypersensitivity.

Drug Interactions

The possibility of alterations in the prothrombin time must be considered and closely monitored in patients on anticoagulant therapy.

ADVERSE REACTIONS

Overdosage or too rapid increase in dosage of thyroid preparations can produce signs and symptoms of hyperthyroidism, such as menstrual irregularities, nervousness, cardiac arrhythmias, and angina pectoris.

OVERDOSAGE

Symptoms: Headache, instability, nervousness, sweating, tachycardia, and unusual bowel motility. Angina pectoris or congestive heart failure may be induced or aggravated. Shock may develop. Massive overdosage may result in symptoms resembling thyroid storm; chronic excessive dosage will produce the signs and symptoms of hyperthyroidism.

Treatment: Shock—supportive measures should be utilized. Treatment of unrecognized adrenal insufficiency should be considered.

DOSAGE AND ADMINISTRATION

Initial dosage should be low and gradually increased at 2-week intervals until the desired clinical response is obtained. Laboratory criteria of euthyroidism include a PBI of 3.5 to 8 mcg; T_3, T_4 and BEI tests are useful.

For most patients, a single daily dose of Euthroid-1, -2. -3 will maintain euthyroidism. Transfer of a patient from a maintenance dose of another thyroid preparation to Euthroid can usually be effected smoothly. See table for initiating therapy or converting from other thyroid preparations.

[See table above].

Dosage for cretinism or severe hypothyroidism in children is the same as for adults with myxedema. Eventual maintenance dosage in the growing child may be higher than in the adult.

HOW SUPPLIED

Square monogrammed tablets of four potencies, each identified by a different color (see table).

Euthroid-½ is supplied as: N 0710-0260-24—Bottles of 100.
Euthroid-1 is supplied as: N 0710-0261-24—Bottles of 100.
N 0710-0261-32—Bottles of 1000.
Euthroid-2 is supplied as: N 0710-0262-24—Bottles of 100.
Euthroid-3 is supplied as: N 0710-0263-24—Bottles of 100.

Store between 59°-86°F (15°–30°C).

0260G021

Shown in Product Identification Section, page 420

FLUOGEN® ℞

[*flŭ ′ō-jĕn″*]

(influenza virus vaccine)

The formulation of influenza virus vaccine for use during each season is established by the Office of Biologics, Food and Drug Administration, Public Health Service. For information regarding the current formulation, please refer to the product package insert, contact your Parke-Davis representative, or call (201) 540-2000.

FUROSEMIDE INJECTION, USP ℞

[*fū-rō ′sĕ-mīde″*]

(10 mg/ml)

WARNING

Furosemide is a potent diuretic which, if given in excessive amounts, can lead to a profound diuresis with water and electrolyte depletion. Therefore, careful medical supervision is required and dose and dose schedule have to be adjusted to the individual patient's needs. (See under "DOSAGE AND ADMINISTRATION.")

DESCRIPTION

Furosemide is an anthranilic acid derivative. It is a white to slightly yellow, odorless, crystalline powder. It is practically insoluble in water; freely soluble in acetone, in dimethylformamide, and in solutions of alkali hydroxides; soluble in methanol; sparingly soluble in alcohol; slightly soluble in ether; very slightly soluble in chloroform. Chemically it is 4-chloro-N-furfuryl-5-sulfamoyl-anthranilic acid.

CLINICAL PHARMACOLOGY

Investigations into the mode of action of furosemide have utilized micropuncture studies in rats, stop flow experiments in dogs and various clearance studies in both humans and experimental animals. It has been demonstrated that furosemide inhibits primarily the reabsorption of sodium and chloride not only in the proximal and distal tubules but also in the loop of Henle. The high degree of efficacy is largely due to this unique site of action. The action of the distal tubule is independent of any inhibitory effect on carbonic anhydrase and aldosterone.

The onset of diuresis following intravenous administration is within 5 minutes and somewhat later after intramuscular administration. The peak effect occurs within the first half hour. The duration of diuretic effect is approximately 2 hours.

INDICATIONS AND USAGE

Parenteral therapy should be reserved for patients unable to take oral medication or for patients in emergency clinical situations.

If gastrointestinal absorption is impaired or oral medication is not practical for any reason, furosemide is indicated by the intravenous or intramuscular route. Parenteral use should be replaced with oral furosemide as soon as practical.

Edema Furosemide is indicated for the treatment of edema associated with congestive heart failure, cirrhosis of the liver, and renal disease, including the nephrotic syndrome. Furosemide is particularly useful when an agent with greater diuretic potential than that of those commonly employed is desired.

Acute Pulmonary Edema Furosemide is indicated as adjunctive therapy in acute pulmonary edema. The intravenous administration of furosemide is indicated when a rapid onset of diuresis is desired, eg, in acute pulmonary edema.

CONTRAINDICATIONS

Furosemide is contraindicated in anuria. It is contraindicated in patients with a history of hypersensitivity to this compound.

WARNINGS

Excessive diuresis may result in dehydration and reduction in blood volume with circulatory collapse and with the possibility of vascular thrombosis and embolism, particularly in elderly patients. Excessive loss of potassium in patients receiving digitalis glycosides may precipitate digitalis toxicity. Care should also be exercised in patients receiving potassium-depleting steroids.

Frequent serum electrolyte, CO_2 and BUN determinations should be performed during the first few months of therapy and periodically thereafter, and abnormalities corrected or the drug temporarily withdrawn.

In patients with hepatic cirrhosis and ascites, initiation of therapy with furosemide is best carried out in the hospital. In hepatic coma and in states of electrolyte depletion, therapy should not be instituted until the basic condition is improved. Sudden alterations of fluid and electrolyte balance in patients with cirrhosis may precipitate hepatic coma; therefore, strict observation is necessary during the period of diuresis. Supplemental potassium chloride and, if required, an aldosterone antagonist are helpful in preventing hypokalemia and metabolic alkalosis.

Continued on next page

This product information was prepared in August, 1986. On these and other Parke-Davis Products, information may be obtained by addressing PARKE-DAVIS, Division of Warner-Lambert Company, Morris Plains, New Jersey 07950.

Parke-Davis—Cont.

If increasing azotemia and oliguria occur during treatment of severe progressive renal disease, the drug should be discontinued.
As with many other drugs, patients should be observed regularly for the possible occurrence of blood dyscrasias, liver damage, or other idiosyncratic reactions.
Patients with known sulfonamide sensitivity may show allergic reactions to furosemide.
Furosemide may add to or potentiate the therapeutic effect of other antihypertensive drugs. Potentiation occurs with ganglionic or peripheral adrenergic blocking drugs.
The possibility exists of exacerbation or activation of systemic lupus erythematosus.
Furosemide appears in breast milk. If use of the drug is deemed essential, the patient should stop nursing.
Parenterally administered furosemide may increase the ototoxic potential of aminoglycoside antibiotics. Especially in the presence of impaired renal function, the use of parenterally administered furosemide in patients to whom aminoglycoside antibiotics are also being given should be avoided, except in life-threatening situations.
Cases of tinnitus and reversible hearing impairments have been reported. There have also been some reports of cases in which irreversible hearing impairment occurred. Usually, ototoxicity has been reported when furosemide was injected rapidly in patients with severe impairment of renal function at doses exceeding several times the usual recommended dose and in whom other drugs known to be ototoxic were given. If the physician elects to use high dose parenteral therapy in patients with severely impaired renal function, controlled intravenous infusion is advisable [for adults, an infusion rate not exceeding 4 mg furosemide per minute has been used].

PRECAUTIONS

As with any effective diuretic, electrolyte depletion may occur during therapy with furosemide, especially in patients receiving higher doses and a restricted salt intake. Periodic determinations of serum electrolytes to detect possible imbalance should be performed at appropriate intervals.
All patients receiving furosemide therapy should be observed for signs of fluid or electrolyte imbalance: namely, hyponatremia, hypochloremic alkalosis and hypokalemia. Serum and urine electrolyte determinations are particularly important when the patient is vomiting excessively or receiving parenteral fluids. Medication such as digitalis may also influence serum electrolytes. Warning signs, irrespective of cause, are dryness of mouth, thirst, weakness, lethargy, drowsiness, restlessness, muscle pains or cramps, muscular fatigue, hypotension, oliguria, tachycardia, arrhythmia and gastrointestinal disturbances such as nausea and vomiting.
Hypokalemia may develop with furosemide as with any other potent diuretic, especially with brisk diuresis, when cirrhosis is present, or during concomitant use of corticosteroids or ACTH.
Interference with adequate oral electrolyte intake will also contribute to hypokalemia. Digitalis therapy may exaggerate metabolic effects of hypokalemia, especially with reference to myocardial activity.
Asymptomatic hyperuricemia can occur and gout may rarely be precipitated.
Periodic checks on urine and blood glucose should be made in diabetics and even those suspected of latent diabetes when receiving furosemide. Increases in blood glucose and alterations in glucose tolerance tests with abnormalities of the fasting and 2-hour postprandial sugar have been observed, and rare cases of precipitation of diabetes mellitus have been reported.
Furosemide may lower serum calcium levels, and rare cases of tetany have been reported. Accordingly, periodic serum calcium levels should be obtained.
Reversible elevations of BUN may be seen. These have been observed in association with dehydration, which should be avoided, particularly in patients with renal insufficiency.
Patients receiving high doses of salicylates, as in rheumatic disease, in conjunction with furosemide may experience salicylate toxicity at lower doses because of competitive renal excretory sites.
Furosemide has a tendency to antagonize the skeletal muscle relaxing effect of tubocurarine and may potentiate the action of succinylcholine.
Lithium generally should not be given with diuretics because they reduce its renal clearance and add a high risk of lithium toxicity.
It has been reported in the literature that diuretics such as furosemide may enhance the nephrotoxicity of cephaloridine. Therefore, furosemide and cephaloridine should not be administered simultaneously.
Furosemide may decrease arterial responsiveness to norepinephrine. This diminution is not sufficient to preclude effectiveness of the pressor agent for therapeutic use.
It has been reported in the literature that coadministration of indomethacin may reduce the natriuretic and antihypertensive effects of furosemide in some patients. This effect has been attributed to inhibition of prostaglandin synthesis by indomethacin. Indomethacin may also affect plasma renin levels and aldosterone excretion; this should be borne in mind when a renin profile is evaluated in hypertensive patients. Patients receiving both indomethacin and furosemide should be observed closely to determine if the desired diuretic and/or antihypertensive effect of furosemide is achieved.
Renal calcifications (from barely visible on x-ray to staghorn) have occurred in some severely premature infants treated with intravenous furosemide for edema due to patent ductus arteriosus and hyaline membrane disease. The concurrent use of chlorothiazide has been reported to decrease hypercalciuria and to dissolve some calculi.

PREGNANCY

Pregnancy Category C. Furosemide has been shown to cause unexplained maternal deaths and abortions in rabbits at 2, 4 and 8 times the human dose. There are no adequate and well-controlled studies in pregnant women. Furosemide should be used during pregnancy only if the potential benefit justifies the potential risk to the fetus.
The effects of furosemide on embryonic and fetal development and on pregnant dams were studied in mice, rats and rabbits.
Furosemide caused unexplained maternal deaths and abortions in the rabbit when 50 mg/kg (4 times the maximal recommended human dose of 600 mg per day) was administered between days 12 and 17 of gestation. In a previous study the lowest dose of only 25 mg/kg (2 times the maximal recommended human dose of 600 mg per day) caused maternal deaths and abortions. In a third study, none of the pregnant rabbits survived a dose of 100 mg/kg. Data from the above studies indicate fetal lethality that can precede maternal deaths.
The results of the mouse study and one of the three rabbit studies also showed an increased incidence of hydronephrosis (distention of the renal pelvis and, in some cases, of the ureters) in fetuses derived from treated dams as compared to the incidence in fetuses from the control group.

ADVERSE REACTIONS

Gastrointestinal System Reactions
1. anorexia
2. oral and gastric irritation
3. nausea
4. vomiting
5. cramping
6. diarrhea
7. constipation
8. jaundice (intrahepatic cholestatic jaundice)
9. pancreatitis

Central Nervous System Reactions
1. dizziness
2. vertigo
3. paresthesias
4. headache
5. xanthopsia
6. blurred vision
7. tinnitus and hearing loss

Hematologic Reactions
1. anemia
2. leukopenia
3. agranulocytosis (rare)
4. thrombocytopenia
5. aplastic anemia (rare)

Dermatologic-Hypersensitivity Reactions
1. purpura
2. photosensitivity
3. rash
4. uticaria
5. necrotizing angiitis (vasculitis, cutaneous vasculitis)
6. exfoliative dermatitis
7. erythema multiforme
8. pruritus

Cardiovascular Reactions
Orthostatic hypotension may occur and be aggravated by alcohol, barbiturates or narcotics.

Other
1. hyperglycemia
2. glycosuria
3. hyperuricemia
4. muscle spasm
5. weakness
6. restlessness
7. urinary bladder spasm
8. thrombophlebitis
9. transient pain at the injection site following intramuscular injection

Whenever adverse reactions are moderate or severe, furosemide dosage should be reduced or therapy withdrawn.

DOSAGE AND ADMINISTRATION

Parenteral drug products should be inspected visually for particulate matter and discoloration prior to administration, whenever solution and container permit.
Do not use if solution is discolored.
Adults—Parenteral therapy should be reserved for patients for whom oral medication is not practical or in emergency situations where prompt diuresis is desired. Parenteral therapy should be replaced by oral therapy as soon as this is practical for continued mobilization of edema.
Edema The usual initial dose of furosemide is 20 to 40 mg given as a single dose, injected intramuscularly or intravenously. The intravenous injection should be given slowly (1 to 2 minutes). Ordinarily, a prompt diuresis ensues. Depending on the patient's response, a second dose can be administered 2 hours after the first dose or later.
If the diuretic response with a single dose of 20 to 40 mg is not satisfactory, increase this dose by increments of 20 mg not sooner than 2 hours after the previous dose until the desired diuretic effect has been obtained. This individually determined single dose should then be given once or twice daily.
If the physician elects to use high dose parenteral therapy it should be administered as a controlled infusion at a rate not exceeding 4 mg/min. Furosemide Injection, USP is a mildly buffered alkaline solution which should not be mixed with acidic solutions of pH below 5.5. To prepare infusion solutions, isotonic saline and lactated Ringer's injection and 5% dextrose injection have been used after pH has been adjusted when necessary.
Therapy should be individualized according to patient response. This therapy should be titrated to gain maximal therapeutic response as well as the minimal dose possible to maintain that therapeutic response. Close medical supervision is necessary.
Acute Pulmonary Edema The usual initial dose of furosemide is 40 mg injected intravenously. The injection should be given slowly (1 to 2 minutes). If 40 mg furosemide does not produce a satisfactory response within 1 hour, the dose may be increased to 80 mg given intravenously (over 1 to 2 minutes).
If deemed necessary, additional therapy (eg, digitalis, oxygen) can be administered concomitantly.
Infants and Children—Parenteral therapy should be reserved for patients for whom oral medication is not practical or in emergency situations where prompt diuresis is desired. Parenteral therapy should be replaced by oral therapy as soon as this is practical for continued mobilization of edema.
The usual initial dose of furosemide, injected intravenously or intramuscularly, in infants and children is 1 mg/kg body weight and should be given slowly under close medical supervision. If the diuretic response after the initial dose is not satisfactory, dosage may be increased by 1 mg/kg not sooner than 2 hours after the previous dose, until the desired diuretic effect has been obtained. Doses greater than 6 mg/kg body weight are not recommended.

HOW SUPPLIED

Furosemide Injection, USP is supplied as a sterile solution for parenteral use as follows:
N 0071-4143-05 2 ml amber ampoule, carton of 10 ampoules
N 0071-4143-08 4 ml amber ampoule, carton of 10 ampoules
N 0071-4143-10 10 ml amber ampoule, carton of 10 ampoules
Each milliliter of solution contains 10 mg furosemide, with sodium chloride for isotonicity and sodium hydroxide to make the solution slightly alkaline.
Store at controlled room temperature, 15°-30°C (59°-86°F). Do not use if solution is discolored.
Protect from light.
Caution: Federal law prohibits dispensing without a prescription.

4143G011

FUROSEMIDE Tablets, USP ℞

[*fū "rō 'sĕ-mīde*]

> **WARNING**
> Furosemide is a potent diuretic which, if given in excessive amounts, can lead to a profound diuresis with water and electrolyte depletion. Therefore, careful medical supervision is required and dose and dose schedule have to be adjusted to the individual patient's needs. (See under "DOSAGE AND ADMINISTRATION.")

DESCRIPTION

Furosemide is an anthranilic acid derivative. It is a white to slightly yellow, odorless, crystalline powder. It is practically insoluble in water; freely soluble in acetone, in dimethylformamide, and in solutions of alkali hydroxides; soluble in methanol; sparingly soluble in alcohol; slightly soluble in ether; very slightly soluble in chloroform. Chemically it is 4-chloro-N-furfuryl-5-sulfamoyl-anthranilic acid.

Furosemide Tablets, USP are available in strengths of 20 mg, 40 mg and 80 mg for oral administration. Each tablet also contains microcrystalline cellulose. NF; hydroxypropyl cellulose, lactose, NF; magnesium stearate. NF; sodium bisulfite; starch, NF; and stearic acid. NF.

CLINICAL PHARMACOLOGY

Investigations into the mode of action of furosemide have utilized micropuncture studies in rats, stop flow experiments in dogs and various clearance studies in both humans and experimental animals. It has been demonstrated that furosemide inhibits primarily the reabsorption of sodium and chloride not only in the proximal and distal tubules but also in the loop of Henle. The high degree of efficacy is largely due to this unique site of action. The action on the distal tubule is independent of any inhibitory effect on carbonic anhydrase and aldosterone.

The onset of diuresis following oral administration is within 1 hour. The peak effect occurs within the first or second hour. The duration of diuretic effect is 6 to 8 hours.

INDICATIONS

Edema: Furosemide is indicated for the treatment of edema associated with congestive heart failure, cirrhosis of the liver, and renal disease, including the nephrotic syndrome. Furosemide is particularly useful when an agent with greater diuretic potential than that of those commonly employed is desired.

If gastrointestinal absorption is impaired or oral medication is not practical for any reason, furosemide is indicated by the intravenous or intramuscular route. Parenteral use should be replaced with oral furosemide as soon as practical.

Hypertension: Furosemide may be used for the treatment of hypertension alone or in combination with other antihypertensive agents. Hypertensive patients who cannot be adequately controlled with thiazides will probably also not be adequately controlled with furosemide alone.

CONTRAINDICATIONS

Furosemide is contraindicated in anuria. It is contraindicated in patients with a history of hypersensitivity to this compound.

WARNINGS

Excessive diuresis may result in dehydration and reduction in blood volume with circulatory collapse and with the possibility of vascular thrombosis and embolism, particularly in elderly patients. Excessive loss of potassium in patients receiving digitalis glycosides may precipitate digitalis toxicity. Care should also be exercised in patients receiving potassium-depleting steroids.

Frequent serum electrolyte, CO_2 and BUN determinations should be performed during the first few months of therapy and periodically thereafter, and abnormalities corrected or the drug temporarily withdrawn.

In patients with hepatic cirrhosis and ascites, initiation of therapy with furosemide is best carried out in the hospital. In hepatic coma and in states of electrolyte depletion, therapy should not be instituted until the basic condition is improved. Sudden alterations of fluid and electrolyte balance in patients with cirrhosis may precipitate hepatic coma; therefore, strict observation is necessary during the period of diuresis. Supplemental potassium chloride and, if required, an aldosterone antagonist are helpful in preventing hypokalemia and metabolic alkalosis.

If increasing azotemia and oliguria occur during treatment of severe progressive renal disease, the drug should be discontinued.

As with many other drugs, patients should be observed regularly for the possible occurrence of blood dyscrasias, liver damage, or other idiosyncratic reactions.

Patients with known sulfonamide sensitivity may show allergic reactions to furosemide.

Furosemide may add to or potentiate the therapeutic effect of other antihypertensive drugs. Potentiation occurs with ganglionic or peripheral adrenergic blocking drugs.

The possibility exists of exacerbation or activation of systemic lupus erythematosus.

Furosemide appears in breast milk. If use of the drug is deemed essential, the patient should stop nursing.

When parenteral use of furosemide precedes its oral use, it should be kept in mind that cases of tinnitus and reversible hearing impairments have been reported. There have also been some reports of cases in which irreversible hearing impairment occurred. Usually ototoxicity has been reported when furosemide was injected rapidly in patients with severe impairment of renal function at doses exceeding several times the usual recommended dose and in whom other drugs known to be ototoxic were given. If the physician elects to use high dose parenteral therapy in patients with severely impaired renal function, controlled intravenous infusion is advisable [for adults, an infusion rate not exceeding 4 mg furosemide per minute has been used].

PRECAUTIONS

As with any effective diuretic, electrolyte depletion may occur during therapy with furosemide, especially in patients receiving higher doses and a restricted salt intake. Periodic determinations of serum electrolytes to detect possible imbalance should be performed at appropriate intervals.

All patients receiving furosemide therapy should be observed for signs of fluid or electrolyte imbalance: namely, hyponatremia, hypochloremic alkalosis and hypokalemia. Serum and urine electrolyte determinations are particularly important when the patient is vomiting excessively or receiving parenteral fluids. Medication such as digitalis may also influence serum electrolytes. Warning signs, irrespective of cause are dryness of mouth, thirst, weakness, lethargy, drowsiness, restlessness, muscle pains or cramps, muscular fatigue, hypotension, oliguria, tachycardia, arrhythmia and gastrointestinal disturbances such as nausea and vomiting.

Hypokalemia may develop with furosemide as with any other potent diuretic, especially with brisk diuresis, when cirrhosis is present, or during concomitant use of corticosteroids or ACTH.

Interference with adequate oral electrolyte intake will also contribute to hypokalemia. Digitalis therapy may exaggerate metabolic effects of hypokalemia, especially with reference to myocardial activity.

Asymptomatic hyperuricemia can occur and gout may rarely be precipitated.

Periodic checks on urine and blood glucose should be made in diabetics and even those suspected of latent diabetes when receiving furosemide. Increases in blood glucose and alterations in glucose tolerance tests with abnormalities of the fasting and 2-hour postprandial sugar have been observed, and rare cases of precipitation of diabetes mellitus have been reported.

Furosemide may lower serum calcium levels, and rare cases of tetany have been reported. Accordingly, periodic serum calcium levels should be obtained.

Reversible elevations of BUN may be seen. These have been observed in association with dehydration, which should be avoided, particularly in patients with renal insufficiency.

Patients receiving high doses of salicylates, as in rheumatic disease, in conjunction with furosemide may experience salicylate toxicity at lower doses because of competitive renal excretory sites.

Furosemide has a tendency to antagonize the skeletal muscle relaxing effect of tubocurarine and may potentiate the action of succinylcholine.

Lithium generally should not be given with diuretics because they reduce its renal clearance and add a high risk of lithium toxicity.

It has been reported in the literature that diuretics such as furosemide may enhance the nephrotoxicity of cephaloridine. Therefore, furosemide and cephaloridine should not be administered simultaneously.

Furosemide may decrease arterial responsiveness to norepinephrine. This diminution is not sufficient to preclude effectiveness of the pressor agent for therapeutic use.

It has been reported in the literature that coadministration of indomethacin may reduce the natriuretic and antihypertensive effects of furosemide in some patients. This effect has been attributed to inhibition of prostaglandin synthesis by indomethacin. Indomethacin may also affect plasma renin levels and aldosterone excretion; this should be borne in mind when a renin profile is evaluated in hypertensive patients. Patients receiving both indomethacin and furosemide should be observed closely to determine if the desired diuretic and/or antihypertensive effect of furosemide is achieved.

PREGNANCY

Pregnancy Category C. Furosemide has been shown to cause unexplained maternal deaths and abortions in rabbits at 2, 4 and 8 times the human dose. There are no adequate and well-controlled studies in pregnant women. Furosemide should be used during pregnancy only if the potential benefit justifies the potential risk to the fetus.

The effects of furosemide on embryonic and fetal development and on pregnant dams were studied in mice, rats and rabbits.

Furosemide caused unexplained maternal deaths and abortions in the rabbit when 50 mg/kg (4 times the maximal recommended human dose of 600 mg per day) was administered between days 12 and 17 of gestation. In a previous study the lowest dose of only 25 mg/kg (2 times the maximal recommended human dose of 600 mg per day) caused maternal deaths and abortions. In a third study, none of the pregnant rabbits survived a dose of 100 mg/kg. Data from the above studies indicate fetal lethality that can precede maternal deaths.

The results of the mouse study and one of the three rabbit studies also showed an increased incidence of hydronephrosis (distention of the renal pelvis and, in some cases, of the ureters) in fetuses derived from treated dams as compared to the incidence in fetuses from the control group.

ADVERSE REACTIONS

Gastrointestinal System Reactions

1. anorexia
2. oral and gastric irritation
3. nausea
4. vomiting
5. cramping
6. diarrhea
7. constipation
8. jaundice (intrahepatic cholestatic jaundice)
9. pancreatitis

Central Nervous System Reactions

1. dizziness
2. vertigo
3. paresthesias
4. headache
5. xanthopsia
6. blurred vision
7. tinnitus and hearing loss

Hematologic Reactions

1. anemia
2. leukopenia
3. agranulocytosis (rare)
4. thrombocytopenia
5. aplastic anemia (rare)

Dermatologic-Hypersensitivity Reactions

1. purpura
2. photosensitivity
3. rash
4. urticaria
5. necrotizing angiitis (vasculitis, cutaneous vasculitis)
6. exfoliative dermatitis
7. erythema multiforme
8. pruritus

Cardiovascular Reactions

Orthostatic hypotension may occur and be aggravated by alcohol, barbiturates or narcotics.

Other

1. hyperglycemia
2. glycosuria
3. hyperuricemia
4. muscle spasm
5. weakness
6. restlessness
7. urinary bladder spasm
8. thrombophlebitis

Whenever adverse reactions are moderate or severe, furosemide dosage should be reduced or therapy withdrawn.

DOSAGE AND ADMINISTRATION

Edema

Therapy should be individualized according to patient response. This therapy should be titrated to gain maximal therapeutic response as well as the minimal dose possible to maintain that therapeutic response.

Parenteral therapy should be reserved for patients unable to take oral medication or in emergency situations.

Adults: The usual daily dose of furosemide is 20 to 80 mg given as a single dose. Ordinarily a prompt diuresis ensues. Depending on the patient's response, a second dose can be administered 6 to 8 hours later.

If the diuretic response to a single dose of 20 to 80 mg is not satisfactory, increase this dose by increments of 20 or 40 mg not sooner than 6 to 8 hours after the previous dose until the desired diuretic effect has been obtained. This individually determined single dose should then be given once or twice daily (eg, at 8:00 a.m. and 2:00 p.m.). The dose of furosemide may be carefully titrated up to 600 mg/day in those patients with severe clinical edematous states.

The mobilization of edema may be most efficiently and safely accomplished by utilizing an intermittent dosage schedule in which the diuretic is given for 2 to 4 consecutive days each week.

When doses exceeding 80 mg/day are given for prolonged periods, careful clinical and laboratory observations are particularly advisable.

Infants and Children: The usual initial dose of furosemide in infants and children is 2 mg/kg body weight, given as a single dose. If the diuretic response is not satisfactory after the initial dose, dose may be increased by 1 or 2 mg/kg no sooner than 6 to 8 hours after the previous dose. Doses greater than 6 mg/kg body weight are not recommended. For maintenance therapy in infants and children, the dose should be adjusted to the minimum effective level.

Hypertension

Therapy should be individualized according to patient response. This therapy should be titrated to gain maximal therapeutic response as well as the minimal dose possible to maintain that therapeutic response.

Adults: The usual initial daily dose of furosemide for antihypertensive therapy is 80 mg, usually divided into 40 mg twice a day. Dosage should then be adjusted according to response. If the patient does not respond, add other antihypertensive agents.

Careful observations for changes in blood pressure must be made when this compound is used with other antihypertensive drugs, especially during initial therapy. The dosage of other agents must be reduced by at least 50 percent as soon as furosemide is added to the regimen, to prevent excessive drop in blood pressure. As the blood pressure falls under the potentiating effect of furosemide, a further reduction in dos-

Continued on next page

This product information was prepared in August, 1986. On these and other Parke-Davis Products, information may be obtained by addressing PARKE-DAVIS, Division of Warner-Lambert Company, Morris Plains, New Jersey 07950.

Parke-Davis—Cont.

age or even discontinuation of other antihypertensive drugs may be necessary.

HOW SUPPLIED

Furosemide Tablets, USP, 20 mg are supplied as white, oval tablets (P-D 440).
N 0071-0440-24 Bottles of 100
Furosemide Tablets, USP, 40 mg are supplied as white, round scored tablets (P-D 441).
N 0071-0441-24 Bottles of 100
N 0071-0441-30 Bottles of 500
N 0071-0441-40 Unit-dose packages of 100 (10 strips of 10 tablets each)
Furosemide Tablets, USP, 80 mg are supplied as white, round tablets (P-D 442).
N 0071-0442-24 Bottles of 100

Note: Dispense in tight, light resistant containers. Discolored tablets should not be dispensed.

Store bottles at room temperature below 30°C (86°F) and unit-dose packages at controlled room temperature 15°-30°C (59°-86°F).

Protect from light and moisture.

0440G015

Caution—Federal law prohibits dispensing without prescription.

GENERICS

The following is a list of the generic names of all Parke-Davis solid-oral product forms which are marketed under the generic name or a trade name.

0634- C-III **Acetaminophen with Codeine Phosphate Tablets, No. 2**
0635- C-III **Acetaminophen with Codeine Phosphate Tablets, No. 3**
0637- C-III **Acetaminophen with Codeine Phosphate Tablets, No. 4**
0640- **Acetaminophen Tablets, USP (Tapar®), 325 mg**
0272- **Amitriptyline Hydrochloride Tablets, USP (Amitril®), 10 mg**
0273- **Amitriptyline Hydrochloride Tablets, USP (Amitril®), 25 mg**
0274- **Amitriptyline Hydrochloride Tablets, USP (Amitril®), 50 mg**
0275- **Amitriptyline Hydrochloride Tablets, USP (Amitril®), 75 mg**
0271- **Amitriptyline Hydrochloride Tablets, USP (Amitril®), 100 mg**
0278- **Amitriptyline Hydrochloride Tablets, USP (Amitril®), 150 mg**
0730- **Amoxicillin (Utimox®) Capsules, 250 mg**
0731- **Amoxicillin (Utimox®) Capsules, 500 mg**
0402- **Ampicillin Capsules, USP (Amcill® Capsules), 250 mg**
0404- **Ampicillin Capsules, USP (Amcill® Capsules), 500 mg**
0606- **Aspirin Tablets, USP, 325 mg**
0533- **Calcium Lactate Tablets, USP, 325 mg**
0604- **Calcium Lactate Tablets, USP, 650 mg**
0379- **Chloramphenicol Capsules, USP (Chloromycetin® Kapseals), 250 mg**
0800- C-IV **Chlordiazepoxide Hydrochloride Capsules, USP, 5 mg**
0801- C-IV **Chlordiazepoxide Hydrochloride Capsules, USP, 10 mg**
0802- C-IV **Chlordiazepoxide Hydrochloride Capsules, USP, 25 mg**
0010- **Chlorpromazine Hydrochloride Tablets, USP (Promapar®), 10 mg**
0025 **Chlorpromazine Hydrochloride Tablets, USP, 25 mg**
0050- **Chlorpromazine Hydrochloride Tablets, USP, 50 mg**
0100- **Chlorpromazine Hydrochloride Tablets, USP, 100 mg**
0201- **Chlorpromazine Hydrochloride Tablets, USP, 200 mg**
0123- **Chlorthalidone Tablets, USP, 25 mg**
0121- **Chlorthalidone Tablets, USP, 50 mg**
0141- **Diazepam Tablets, USP, 2 mg**
0142- **Diazepam Tablets, USP, 5 mg**
0143- **Diazepam Tablets, USP, 10 mg**
0471- **Diphenhydramine Hydrochloride Capsules, USP (Benadryl®), 25 mg**
0373- **Diphenhydramine Hydrochloride Capsules, USP (Benadryl® Kapseals), 50 mg**
0247- **Docusate Sodium Capsules, USP (DSS Capsules), 100 mg**
0248- **Docusate Sodium with Casanthranol Capsules (DSS Plus Capsules)**
0813- **Doxycycline Hyclate Tablets, USP, 100 mg**
0829- **Doxycycline Hyclate Capsules, USP, 50 mg**
0830- **Doxycycline Hyclate Capsules, USP, 100 mg**
0111- **Ergotamine Tartrate Tablets (Ergostat® Sublingual Tablets), 2 mg**
0672- **Erythromycin Stearate Tablets, USP (Erypar® Filmseal), 250 mg**
0919- **Erythromycin Stearate Tablets, USP (Erypar® Filmseal), 500 mg**
0237- **Ethosuximide Capsules, USP (Zarontin® Capsules), 250 mg**
0037- **Ferrous Sulfate Filmseal, 325 mg**
0440- **Furosemide Tablets, USP, 20 mg**
0441- **Furosemide Tablets, USP, 40 mg**
0442- **Furosemide Tablets, USP, 80 mg**
0702- **Hydrochlorothiazide Tablets, USP (Thiuretic®), 25 mg**
0710- **Hydrochlorothiazide Tablets, USP (Thiuretic®), 50 mg**
0887- **Indomethacin Capsules, USP, 25 mg**
0888- **Indomethacin Capsules, USP, 50 mg**
0268- **Meclofenamate Sodium (Meclomen®) Capsules, 50 mg**
0269- **Meclofenamate Sodium (Meclomen) Capsules, 100 mg**
0540- **Mefenamic Acid (Ponstel® Kapseals), 250 mg**
0525- **Methsuximide Capsules, USP (Celontin® Kapseals), 300 mg**
0537- **Methsuximide Capsules, USP (Celontin® Kapseals), 150 mg**
0865- **Methyldopa Tablets, USP, 250 mg**
0866- **Methyldopa Tablets, USP, 500 mg**
1460- **Nitroglycerin Tablets, USP (Nitrostat® Sublingual Tablets), 0.15 mg**
1469- **Nitroglycerin Tablets, USP (Nitrostat® Sublingual Tablets), 0.3 mg**
1470- **Nitroglycerin Tablets, USP (Nitrostat® Sublingual Tablets), 0.4 mg**
1471- **Nitroglycerin Tablets, USP (Nitrostat® Sublingual Tablets), 0.6 mg**
0882- **Norethindrone Tablets, USP (Norlutin® Tablets), 5 mg**
0918- **Norethindrone Acetate Tablets, USP (Norlutate® Tablets), 5 mg**
0210- **Oxtriphylline (Choledyl) Tablets, USP, 100 mg**
0211- **Oxtriphylline (Choledyl) Tablets, USP, 200 mg**
0529- **Paromomycin Sulfate Capsules, USP (Humatin® Capsules), 250 mg**
0648- **Penicillin V Potassium Tablets, USP (Penapar VK®), 250 mg**
0673- **Penicillin V Potassium Tablets, USP (Penapar VK®), 500 mg**
0699- C-IV **Phenobarbital Tablets, USP, 15 mg**
0700- C-IV **Phenobarbital Tablets, USP, 30 mg**
0607- C-IV **Phenobarbital Tablets, USP, 60 mg**
0698- C-IV **Phenobarbital Tablets, USP, 100 mg**
0393- **Phensuximide Capsules, USP (Milontin® Kapseals), 500 mg**
0007- **Phenytoin Tablets, USP (Dilantin® Infatabs®), 50 mg**
0362- **Phenytoin Sodium, Extended, Capsules, USP (Dilantin® Kapseals), 100 mg**
0365- **Phenytoin Sodium, Extended, Capsules, USP (Dilantin® Kapseals), 30 mg**
0552- C-IV **Prazepam (Centrax®) Capsules, 5 mg**
0553- C-IV **Prazepam (Centrax®) Capsules, 10 mg**
0554 C-IV **Prazepam (Centrax®) Capsules, 20 mg**
0276- C-IV **Prazepam (Centrax®) Tablets, 10 mg**
0202 **Procainamide Hydrochloride Tablets, Sustained Release (Procan® SR), 250 mg**
0204 **Procainamide Hydrochloride Tablets, Sustained Release (Procan® SR), 500 mg**
0205 **Procainamide Hydrochloride Tablets, Sustained Release (Procan® SR), 750 mg**
0692- C-IV **Propoxyphene Hydrochloride Capsules, USP, 65 mg**
0437- **Quinestrol Tablets (Estrovis® Tablets), 100 mcg**
0850- **Quinidine Gluconate Tablets, Sustained Release, (Duraquin® Tablets), 330 mg**
0849- **Quinidine Sulfate Tablets, USP, 200 mg**
0420- **Quinine Sulfate Capsules, USP, 325 mg**
0713- **Spironolactone Tablets, USP**
0712- **Spironolactone with Hydrochlorothiazide Tablets**
0407- **Tetracycline Hydrochloride Capsules, USP (Cyclopar®), 250 mg**
0697- **Tetracycline Hydrochloride Capsules, USP (Cyclopar® 500), 500 mg**
0251- **Thyroglobulin Tablets (Proloid®), ½ grain**
0252- **Thyroglobulin Tablets (Proloid®), 1 grain**
0253- **Thyroglobulin Tablets (Proloid®), 1½ grains**
0257- **Thyroglobulin Tablets (Proloid®), 2 grains**
0254- **Thyroglobulin Tablets (Proloid®), 3 grains**

GERIPLEX-FS® KAPSEALS® OTC

[jĕ′-rĭ-plĕx″]

COMPOSITION

Each capsule represents:
Vitamin A .... (1.5 mg) 5,000 IU*
(acetate)
Vitamin C .... 50 mg
(ascorbic acid)†
Vitamin B_1 .... 5 mg
(thiamine mononitrate)
Vitamin B_2 .... 5 mg
(riboflavin)
Vitamin B_{12}, crystalline
(cyanocobalamin) .... 2 mcg
Choline dihydrogen
citrate .... 20 mg
Nicotinamide .... 15 mg
(niacinamide)
Vitamin E (*dl*-alpha tocopheryl acetate, 5 mg) .... 5 IU*
Iron‡ .... 6 mg
Copper sulfate .... 4 mg
Manganese sulfate
(monohydrate) .... 4 mg
Zinc sulfate .... 2 mg
Calcium phosphate, dibasic
(anhydrous) .... 200 mg
Taka-Diastase® (aspergillus
oryzae enzymes) .... 2½ gr
Docusate sodium .... 100 mg

* International Units
†Supplied as sodium ascorbate
‡Supplied as dried ferrous sulfate

Action and Uses: A preparation containing vitamins, minerals, and a fecal softener for middle-aged and older individuals. The fecal softening agent, docusate sodium, acts to soften stools and make bowel movements easier.

Administration and Dosage: USUAL DOSAGE—One capsule daily, with or immediately after a meal.

How Supplied: N 0071-0544-24—Bottles of 100. Parcode® No. 544.

0544G031

Shown in Product Identification Section, page 420

GERIPLEX-FS® OTC

[jĕ′rĭ-plĕx″]

LIQUID

Geriatric Vitamin Formula with Iron and a Fecal Softener

COMPOSITION

Each 30 ml represents vitamin B_1 (thiamine hydrochloride), 1.2 mg; vitamin B_2 (as riboflavin-5′-phosphate sodium), 1.7 mg; vitamin B_6 (pyridoxine hydrochloride), 1 mg; vitamin B_{12} (cyanocobalamin) crystalline, 5 mcg; niacinamide, 15 mg; iron (as ferric ammonium citrate, green), 15 mg; Pluronic® F-68,* 200 mg; alcohol, 18%.

Also contains: brandy, caramel NF; citric acid anhydrous NF; D&C red no. 33; flavors; FD&C red no. 40, glucono delta lactone; glucose liquid, USP; glycerin USP; sodium citrate USP; sodium saccharin NF; sorbitol solution USP; sugar, water purified.

ADMINISTRATION AND DOSAGE

USUAL ADULT DOSAGE—Two tablespoonfuls (30 ml) daily or as recommended by the physician.

HOW SUPPLIED

N 0071-2454-23—16-oz bottles.

2454G012

*Pluronic is a registered trademark of BASF Wyandotte Corporation for polymers of ethylene oxide and propylene oxide.

HUMATIN® ℞

[hu'mah-tin]
(Paromomycin Sulfate, USP)

DESCRIPTION

Humatin is a broad spectrum antibiotic produced by *Streptomyces rimosus* var. *paromomycinus*. It is a white, amorphous, stable, water-soluble product supplied as capsules containing the equivalent of 250 mg paromomycin. The capsule contains D&C yellow No. 10; FD&C blue No. 1; FD&C red No. 3; FD&C yellow No. 6; gelatin, NF; and titanium dioxide, USP.

ACTION

The *in vitro* and *in vivo* antibacterial action of paromomycin closely parallels that of neomycin. It is poorly absorbed after oral administration, with almost 100% of the drug recoverable in the stool.

INDICATIONS

Humatin is indicated for intestinal amebiasis—acute and chronic (NOTE—It is not effective in extra-intestinal amebiasis); management of hepatic coma—as adjunctive therapy.

CONTRAINDICATIONS

Paromomycin sulfate is contraindicated in individuals with a history of previous hypersensitivity reactions to it. It is also contraindicated in intestinal obstruction.

PRECAUTIONS

The use of this antibiotic, as with other antibiotics, may result in an overgrowth of nonsusceptible organisms, including fungi. Constant observation of the patient is essential. If new infections caused by nonsusceptible organisms appear during therapy, appropriate measures should be taken.
The drug should be used with caution in individuals with ulcerative lesions of the bowel to avoid renal toxicity through inadvertent absorption.

ADVERSE REACTIONS

Nausea, abdominal cramps, and diarrhea have been reported in patients on doses over 3 g daily.

DOSAGE AND ADMINISTRATION

Intestinal amebiasis: Adults and Children: Usual dose—25 to 35 mg/kg body weight daily, administered in three doses with meals, for five to ten days.
Management of hepatic coma: Adults: Usual dose—4 g daily in divided doses, given at regular intervals for five to six days.

HOW SUPPLIED

N0071-0529-09 Humatin Capsules, each containing paromomycin sulfate equivalent to 250 mg paromomycin, are supplied in bottles of 16.
Shown in Product Identification Section, page 420
0529G031

HYDROCHLOROTHIAZIDE TABLETS, USP ℞

[hy"drō-chlō"rō-thī'ă-zīde]
(Thiuretic®)

DESCRIPTION

Hydrochlorothiazide is a member of the benzothiadiazine (thiazide) family of drugs, closely related to chlorothiazide. Its chemical name is 6-chloro-3,4-dihydro-2*H*-1,2, 4-benzothiadiazine-7-sulfonamide 1,1-dioxide.
Hydrochlorothiazide is a white, or practically white, crystalline compound which is slightly soluble in water and soluble in alcohol.
Clinically, hydrochlorothiazide is a diuretic-antihypertensive agent, available in 25 mg and 50 mg strength tablets for oral administration.

CLINICAL PHARMACOLOGY

The diuretic and saluretic effects of hydrochlorothiazide result from a drug-induced inhibition of the renal tubular reabsorption of electrolytes. The excretion of sodium and chloride is greatly enhanced. Potassium excretion is also enhanced to a variable degree, as it is with the other thiazides. Although urinary excretion of bicarbonate is increased slightly, there is usually no significant change in urinary pH. Hydrochlorothiazide has a per mg natriuretic activity approximately 10 times that of the prototype thiazide, chlorothiazide. At maximal therapeutic dosages, all thiazides are approximately equal in their diuretic/natriuretic effects.
There is significant natriuresis and diuresis within two hours after administration of a single oral dose of hydrochlorothiazide. These effects reach a peak in about six hours and persist for about 12 hours following oral administration of a single dose.
Like other benzothiadiazines, hydrochlorothiazide also has antihypertensive properties, and may be used for this purpose either alone or to enhance the antihypertensive action of other drugs. The mechanism by which the benzothiadiazines, including hydrochlorothiazide, produce a reduction of elevated blood pressure is not known. However, sodium depletion appears to be involved.
Hydrochlorothiazide is readily absorbed from the gastrointestinal tract and is excreted unchanged by the kidneys. Excretion of the drug is essentially complete within 24 hours.

INDICATIONS AND USAGE

Hydrochlorothiazide is indicated in the management of hypertension either as the sole therapeutic agent or to enhance the effectiveness of other antihypertensive drugs in the more severe forms of hypertension.
Hydrochlorothiazide is indicated as adjunctive therapy in edema associated with congestive heart failure, hepatic cirrhosis, and corticosteroid and estrogen therapy.
Hydrochlorothiazide has also been found useful in edema due to various forms of renal dysfunction such as the nephrotic syndrome, acute glomerulonephritis, and chronic renal failure.
Usage in Pregnancy: The routine use of diuretics in an otherwise healthy pregnant woman is inappropriate and exposes mother and fetus to unnecessary hazard. Diuretics do not prevent development of toxemia of pregnancy, and there is no satisfactory evidence that they are useful in the treatment of developed toxemia.
Edema during pregnancy may arise from pathological causes or from the physiological and mechanical consequences of pregnancy. Thiazides are indicated in pregnancy when edema is due to pathological causes, just as they are in the absence of pregnancy (however, see PRECAUTIONS below). Dependent edema in pregnancy, resulting from restriction of venous return by the expanded uterus, is properly treated through elevation of the lower extremities and use of support hose; use of diuretics to lower intravascular volume in this case is illogical and unnecessary. There is hypervolemia during normal pregnancy which is harmful to neither the fetus nor the mother (in the absence of cardiovascular disease), but which is associated with edema, including generalized edema, in the majority of pregnant women. If this edema produces discomfort, increased recumbency will often provide relief. In rare instances, this edema may cause extreme discomfort which is not relieved by rest. In these cases, a short course of diuretics may provide relief and may be appropriate.

CONTRAINDICATIONS

Anuria.
Hypersensitivity to this or other sulfonamide-derived drugs.

WARNINGS

Thiazides should be used with caution in patients with renal disease or significant impairment of renal function. In patients with renal disease, thiazides may precipitate azotemia. Cumulative effects of the drug may develop in patients with impaired renal function.
Thiazides should be used with caution in patients with impaired hepatic function or progressive liver disease, since minor alterations of fluid and electrolyte balance may precipitate hepatic coma.
Thiazides may add to or potentiate the action of other antihypertensive drugs. Potentiation occurs with ganglionic or peripheral adrenergic blocking drugs.
Sensitivity reactions may occur in patients with a history of allergy or bronchial asthma.
The possibility of exacerbation or activation of systemic lupus erythematosus has been reported.

PRECAUTIONS

Periodic determinations of serum electrolytes should be performed at appropriate intervals for the purpose of detecting possible electrolyte imbalances. All patients receiving thiazide therapy should be observed for clinical signs of fluid or electrolyte imbalance, namely, hyponatremia, hypochloremic alkalosis, and hypokalemia. Serum and urine electrolyte determinations are particularly important when a patient is vomiting excessively or receiving parenteral fluids. Warning signs of electrolyte imbalance include dryness of mouth, thirst, weakness, lethargy, drowsiness, restlessness, muscle pains or cramps, muscular fatigue, hypotension, oliguria, tachycardia, and gastrointestinal disturbances such as nausea and vomiting.
Hypokalemia may develop with thiazides as with any other potent diuretic, especially when brisk diuresis occurs, severe cirrhosis is present, or when corticosteroids or ACTH are given concomitantly. Interference with the adequate oral intake of electrolytes will also contribute to the possible development of hypokalemia. Potassium depletion, even of a mild degree, resulting from thiazide use may sensitize a patient to the effects of cardiac glycosides such as digitalis.
Any chloride deficit is generally mild and usually does not require specific treatment except under extraordinary circumstances (as in liver disease or renal disease). Dilutional hyponatremia may occur in edematous patients in hot weather; appropriate therapy is water restriction rather than administration of salt except in rare instances where the hyponatremia is life threatening.
In actual salt depletion, appropriate replacement is the therapy of choice.
Hyperuricemia may occur or frank gout may be precipitated in certain patients receiving thiazide therapy.
Insulin requirements in diabetic patients may be increased, decreased or unchanged. Latent diabetes mellitus may become manifest during thiazide administration.
Thiazide drugs may increase the responsiveness to tubocurarine.
The antihypertensive effects of the drug may be enhanced in the postsympathectomy patient.
Thiazides may decrease arterial responsiveness to norepinephrine. This diminution is not sufficient to preclude effectiveness of the pressor agent for therapeutic use.
If progressive renal impairment becomes evident as indicated by a rising nonprotein nitrogen or blood urea nitrogen, a careful reappraisal of therapy is necessary with consideration given to withholding or discontinuing diuretic therapy.
Thiazides may decrease serum PBI levels without signs of thyroid disturbance.
Thiazides have been reported, on rare occasions, to have elevated serum calcium to hypercalcemic levels. The serum calcium levels have returned to normal when the medication has been stopped. This phenomenon may be related to the ability of the thiazide diuretics to lower the amount of calcium excreted in the urine.
Usage in Pregnancy: Thiazides cross the placental barrier and appear in cord blood. The use of thiazides in pregnant women requires that the anticipated benefit be weighed against possible hazards to the fetus. These hazards include fetal or neonatal jaundice, thrombocytopenia, and possible other adverse reactions that have occurred in the adults. (Also see INDICATIONS AND USAGE, above.)
Nursing Mothers: Thiazides appear in breast milk. If use of the drug is deemed essential, the patient should stop nursing.

ADVERSE REACTIONS

A. *Gastrointestinal System*
1. anorexia
2. gastric irritation
3. nausea
4. vomiting
5. cramping
6. diarrhea
7. constipation
8. jaundice (intrahepatic cholestatic jaundice)
9. pancreatitis

B. *Central Nervous System*
1. dizziness
2. vertigo
3. paresthesias
4. headache
5. xanthopsia

C. *Hematologic*
1. leukopenia
2. agranulocytosis
3. thrombocytopenia
4. aplastic anemia

D. *Dermatologic-Hypersensitivity*
1. purpura
2. photosensitivity
3. rash
4. urticaria
5. necrotizing angiitis (vasculitis) (cutaneous vasculitis)

E. *Cardiovascular*
Orthostatic hypotension may occur and may be aggravated by alcohol, barbiturates, or narcotics.

F. *Other*
1. hyperglycemia
2. glycosuria
3. hypercalcemia
4. hyperuricemia
5. muscle spasm
6. weakness
7. restlessness
8. severe fluid and electrolyte derangements (rarely)

Whenever adverse reactions are moderate or severe, thiazide dosage should be reduced or therapy withdrawn.

OVERDOSAGE

Symptoms of overdosage include electrolyte imbalance and signs of potassium deficiency such as confusion, dizziness, muscular weakness and gastrointestinal disturbances. General supportive measures including replacement of fluids and electrolytes may be indicated in treatment of overdosage.

Continued on next page

This product information was prepared in August, 1986. On these and other Parke-Davis Products, information may be obtained by addressing PARKE-DAVIS, Division of Warner-Lambert Company, Morris Plains, New Jersey 07950.

Parke-Davis—Cont.

DOSAGE AND ADMINISTRATION

Hydrochlorothiazide is administered orally. Therapy should be individualized according to the patient's requirements and response. The response of the patient depends on factors such as the nature and degree of the disease, state of hydration, cardiac output, physical activity, diet, and concurrent administration of other drugs. Therapy should be titrated to attain the maximum therapeutic effect at minimum dosage.

Adult Dose: For the management of edema, the usual initial adult dosage is 25 to 200 mg daily given in 1 to 3 doses. When nonedematous weight is attained, a maintenance dosage of 25 to 100 mg daily or intermittently may be instituted. Occasionally, up to 200 mg daily is required in refractory patients.

For the management of hypertension, the usual initial adult dosage is 50 to 100 mg daily, given in 2 divided doses. The dosage may be increased if necessary to a maximum of 200 mg daily, given in 2 divided doses. Maintenance dosage is determined by the patient's blood pressure and usually ranges from 25 to 100 mg daily in a single dose.

When therapy is prolonged or large doses are used, particular attention should be given to the patient's electrolyte status. Supplemental potassium may be required.

In the treatment of hypertension, hydrochlorothiazide may be employed either alone or concurrently with other antihypertensive drugs. Combined therapy may provide adequate control of hypertension with lower dosage of the component drugs and fewer or less severe side effects.

For treatment of moderate to severe hypertension, supplemental use of other more potent antihypertensive agents may be indicated.

When other antihypertensive agents are to be added to the regimen, this should be accomplished gradually. Additional potent antihypertensive agents should be given at only half the usual dose since their effect is potentiated by pretreatment with hydrochlorothiazide.

Pediatric Dose: The usual pediatric dosage is 1 mg hydrochlorothiazide per pound of body weight per day, given in 2 divided doses. Infants younger than 6 months of age may require up to 1.5 mg per pound per day in 2 divided doses.

HOW SUPPLIED

Hydrochlorothiazide Tablets, USP, 25 mg (white, round, scored, coded P-D 702) are available in bottles of 100 (N 0071-0702-24).

Hydrochlorothiazide Tablets, USP, 50 mg (white, round, scored, coded P-D 710) are available in bottles of 100 (N 0071-0710-24), bottles of 1000 (N 0071-0710-32), and unit dose packages of 100 (N 0071-0710-40).

0702G011

INDOMETHACIN Capsules, USP ℞

DESCRIPTION

Indomethacin cannot be considered a simple analgesic and should not be used in conditions other than those recommended under INDICATIONS AND USAGE.

Indomethacin is supplied as capsules for oral administration containing 25 mg or 50 mg of indomethacin. Also contains colloidal silicon dioxide, NF; corn starch, NF; hydrogenated vegetable oil, NF; lactose, NF; polysorbate 80, NF; povidone, USP. The capsule contains colloidal silicon dioxide, NF; D&C red No. 28, FD&C blue No. 1; FD&C green No. 3; FD&C red No. 40; gelatin, NF; sodium lauryl sulfate, NF; titanium dioxide, USP. Indomethacin is a nonsteroidal antiinflammatory indole derivative designated chemically as 1-(4-chlorobenzoyl)-5-methoxy-2-methyl-1 H-indole-3-acetic acid. Its empirical formula is $C_{19}H_{16}ClNO_4$.

CLINICAL PHARMACOLOGY

Indomethacin is a nonsteroidal drug with antiinflammatory, antipyretic and analgesic properties. Its mode of action, like that of other antiinflammatory drugs, is not known. However, its therapeutic action is not due to pituitary-adrenal stimulation.

Indomethacin is a potent inhibitor of prostaglandin synthesis *in vitro*. Concentrations are reached during therapy which have been demonstrated to have an effect *in vivo* as well. Prostaglandins sensitize afferent nerves and potentiate the action of bradykinin in inducing pain in animal models. Moreover, prostaglandins are known to be among the mediators of inflammation. Since indomethacin is an inhibitor of prostaglandin synthesis, its mode of action may be due to a decrease of prostaglandins in peripheral tissues.

Indomethacin has been shown to be an effective antiinflammatory agent, appropriate for long-term use in rheumatoid arthritis, ankylosing spondylitis, and osteoarthritis.

Indomethacin affords relief of symptoms; it does not alter the progressive course of the underlying disease.

Indomethacin suppresses inflammation in rheumatoid arthritis as demonstrated by relief of pain, and reduction of fever, swelling and tenderness. Improvement in patients treated with indomethacin for rheumatoid arthritis has been demonstrated by a reduction in joint swelling, average number of joints involved, and morning stiffness; by increased mobility as demonstrated by a decrease in walking time; and by improved functional capability as demonstrated by an increase in grip strength.

Indomethacin has been found effective in relieving the pain, reducing the fever, swelling, redness, and tenderness of acute gouty arthritis.

Following single oral doses of indomethacin 25 mg or 50 mg, indomethacin is readily absorbed, attaining peak plasma concentrations of about 1 and 2 mcg/mL, respectively, at about 2 hours. Orally administered Indomethacin Capsules, USP are virtually 100% bioavailable, with 90% of the dose absorbed within 4 hours.

Indomethacin is eliminated via renal excretion, metabolism, and biliary excretion. Indomethacin undergoes appreciable enterohepatic circulation. The mean half-life of indomethacin is estimated to be about 4.5 hours. With a typical therapeutic regimen of 25 or 50 mg t.i.d., the steady-state plasma concentrations of indomethacin are an average 1.4 times those following the first dose.

Indomethacin exists in the plasma as the parent drug and its desmethyl, desbenzoyl, and desmethyl-desbenzoyl metabolites, all in the unconjugated form. About 60 percent of an oral dosage is recovered in urine as drug and metabolites (26 percent as indomethacin and its glucuronide), and 33 percent is recovered in feces (1.5 percent as indomethacin).

About 90% of indomethacin is bound to protein in plasma over the expected range of therapeutic plasma concentrations.

INDICATIONS AND USAGE

Because of its potential to cause adverse reactions, particularly at high dose levels, the use of indomethacin in rheumatoid arthritis and osteoarthritis in adults should be carefully considered for active disease unresponsive to adequate trial with salicylates and other measures of established value, such as appropriate rest.

In accord with this important concept indomethacin has been found effective in active stages of the following:

1. Moderate to severe rheumatoid arthritis including acute flares of chronic disease.
2. Moderate to severe ankylosing spondylitis.
3. Moderate to severe osteoarthritis.
4. Acute painful shoulder (bursitis and/or tendinitis).
5. Acute gouty arthritis.

Indomethacin may enable the reduction of steroid dosage in patients receiving steroids for the more severe forms of rheumatoid arthritis. In such instances the steroid dosage should be reduced slowly and the patients followed very closely for any possible adverse effects.

The use of indomethacin in conjunction with aspirin or other salicylates is not recommended. Controlled clinical studies have shown that the combined use of indomethacin and aspirin does not produce any greater therapeutic effect than the use of indomethacin alone. Furthermore, in one of these clinical studies, the incidence of gastrointestinal side effects was significantly increased with combined therapy. (See DRUG INTERACTIONS).

CONTRAINDICATIONS

Indomethacin is contraindicated in patients who are allergic to indomethacin or who have nasal polyps associated with angioedema or a bronchospastic reaction to aspirin or other nonsteroidal antiinflammatory drugs.

WARNINGS

General

Because of the variability of the potential of indomethacin to cause adverse reactions in the individual patient, the following are strongly recommended:

1. The lowest possible effective dose for the individual patient should be prescribed. Increased dosage tends to increase adverse effects, particularly in doses over 150–200 mg/day, without corresponding increase in clinical benefits.
2. Careful instructions to, and observations of, the individual patient are essential to the prevention of serious adverse reactions. As advancing years appear to increase the possibility of adverse reactions, indomethacin should be used with greater care in the aged.
3. Safe conditions for use in children have not been established; therefore, indomethacin should not be prescribed for children 14 years of age and under except under circumstances where lack of efficacy or toxicity associated with other drugs warrants the risk. Such patients should be monitored closely.

Gastrointestinal Effects

Single or multiple ulcerations, including perforation and hemorrhage of the esophagus, stomach, duodenum or small intestine, have been reported to occur with indomethacin. Fatalities have been reported in some instances. Rarely, intestinal ulceration has been associated with stenosis and obstruction.

Gastrointestinal bleeding without obvious ulcer formation and perforation of preexisting sigmoid lesions (diverticulum, carcinoma, etc.) have occurred. Increased abdominal pain in ulcerative colitis patients or the development of ulcerative colitis and regional ileitis have been reported to occur rarely.

Because of the occurrence, and at times severity, of gastrointestinal reactions to indomethacin, the prescribing physician must be continuously alert for any sign or symptom signaling a possible gastrointestinal reaction. The risks of continuing therapy with indomethacin in the face of such symptoms must be weighed against the possible benefits to the individual patient.

Indomethacin should not be given to patients with active gastrointestinal lesions or with a history of recurrent gastrointestinal lesions except under circumstances which warrant the very high risk and where patients can be monitored very closely. The gastrointestinal effects may be reduced by giving indomethacin immediately after meals, with food, or with antacids.

Renal Effects

Because adequate renal function can depend upon renal prostaglandin synthesis, indomethacin can precipitate renal insufficiency, including acute renal failure. The risk is greater in patients with any of a number of underlying conditions, e.g., those with renal or hepatic dysfunction, complications associated with advanced age, extracellular volume depletion from any cause, congestive heart failure, sepsis, or concomitant use of any nephrotoxic drug. However, the drug should be given with caution and renal function should be monitored in any patient who may have reduced renal reserve. Most of the renal abnormalities have been reversible upon discontinuation of the drug.

Ocular Effects

Corneal deposits and retinal disturbances, including those of the macula, have been observed in some patients who had received prolonged therapy with indomethacin. The prescribing physician should be alert to the possible association between the changes noted and indomethacin. It is advisable to discontinue therapy if such changes are observed. Blurred vision may be a significant symptom and warrants a thorough ophthalmological examination. Since these changes may be asymptomatic, ophthalmologic examination at periodic intervals is desirable in patients where therapy is prolonged.

Central Nervous System Effects

Indomethacin may aggravate depression or other psychiatric disturbances, epilepsy, and parkinsonism, and should be used with considerable caution in patients with these conditions. If severe CNS adverse reactions develop, indomethacin should be discontinued.

Indomethacin may cause drowsiness; therefore, patients should be cautioned about engaging in activities requiring mental alertness and motor coordination, such as driving a car. Indomethacin may also cause headache. Headache which persists despite dosage reduction requires cessation of therapy with indomethacin.

Use in Pregnancy and the Neonatal Period

Indomethacin is not recommended for use in pregnant women, since safety for use has not been established, and because of the known effect of drugs of this class on the human fetal cardiovascular system (closure of the ductus arteriosus) during the third trimester of pregnancy.

Teratogenic studies were conducted in mice and rats at dosages of 0.5, 1.0, 2.0, and 4.0 mg/kg/day. Except for retarded fetal ossification at 4 mg/kg/day considered secondary to the decreased average fetal weights, no increase in fetal malformations was observed as compared with control groups. Other studies in mice reported in the literature using higher doses (5 to 15 mg/kg/day) have described maternal toxicity and death, increased fetal resorptions, and fetal malformations. Comparable studies in rodents using high doses of aspirin have shown similar maternal and fetal effects.

As with other nonsteroidal antiinflammatory agents which inhibit prostaglandin synthesis, indomethacin has been found to delay parturition in rats.

In rats and mice, 4.0 mg/kg/day given during the last three days of gestation caused a decrease in maternal weight gain and some maternal and fetal deaths. An increased incidence of neuronal necrosis in the diencephalon in the live-born fetuses was observed. At 2.0 mg/kg/day, no increase in neuronal necrosis was observed as compared to the control groups. Administration of 0.5 and 4.0 mg/kg/day during the first three days of life did not cause an increase in neuronal necrosis at either dose level.

Use in Nursing Mothers

Indomethacin is excreted in the milk of lactating mothers. Indomethacin is not recommended for use in nursing mothers.

PRECAUTIONS

Indomethacin may mask the usual signs and symptoms of infection. Therefore, the physician must be continually on the alert for this and should use the drug with extra care in the presence of existing controlled infection.

Indomethacin, like other nonsteroidal antiinflammatory agents, can inhibit platelet aggregation. This effect is of shorter duration than that seen with aspirin and usually disappears within 24 hours after discontinuation of indomethacin. Indomethacin has been shown to prolong bleeding time (but within the normal range) in normal subjects. Because this effect may be exaggerated in patients with underlying hemostatic defects, indomethacin should be used with caution in persons with coagulation defects.

As with other nonsteroidal antiinflammatory drugs, borderline elevations of one or more liver tests may occur in up to 15% of patients. These abnormalities may progress, may remain essentially unchanged, or may be transient with continued therapy. The SGPT (ALT) test is probably the most sensitive indicator of liver dysfunction. Meaningful (3 times the upper limit of normal) elevations of SGPT or SGOT (AST) occurred in controlled clinical trials in less than 1% of patients. A patient with symptoms and/or signs suggesting liver dysfunction, or in whom an abnormal liver test has occurred, should be evaluated for evidence of the development of more severe hepatic reaction while on therapy with indomethacin. Severe hepatic reactions, including jaundice and cases of fatal hepatitis, have been reported with indomethacin as with other nonsteroidal antiinflammatory drugs. Although such reactions are rare, if abnormal liver tests persist or worsen, if clinical signs and symptoms consistent with liver disease develop, or if systemic manifestations occur (e.g. eosinophilia, rash, etc), indomethacin should be discontinued.

Drug Interactions

In normal volunteers receiving indomethacin, the administration of diflunisal decreased the renal clearance and significantly increased the plasma levels of indomethacin. In some patients, combined use of indomethacin and diflunisal has been associated with fatal gastrointestinal hemorrhage. Therefore, diflunisal and indomethacin should not be used concomitantly.

In a study in normal volunteers, it was found that chronic concurrent administration of 3.6 g of aspirin per day decreases indomethacin blood levels approximately 20%.

Clinical studies have shown that indomethacin does not influence the hypoprothrombinemia produced by anticoagulants. However, when any additional drug, including indomethacin, is added to the treatment of patients on anticoagulant therapy, the patient should be observed for alterations of the prothrombin time.

When indomethacin is given to patients receiving probenecid, the plasma levels of indomethacin are likely to be increased. Therefore, a lower total daily dosage of indomethacin may produce a satisfactory therapeutic effect. When increases in the dose of indomethacin are made, they should be made carefully and in small increments.

Indomethacin Capsules, USP, 50 mg t.i.d. produced a clinically relevant elevation of plasma lithium and reduction in renal lithium clearance in psychiatric patients and normal subjects with steady state plasma lithium concentrations. This effect has been attributed to inhibition of prostaglandin synthesis. As a consequence, when indomethacin and lithium are given concomitantly, the patient should be carefully observed for signs of lithium toxicity. (Read circulars for lithium preparations before use of such concomitant therapy). In addition, the frequency of monitoring serum lithium concentration should be increased at the outset of such combination drug treatment.

Clinical studies have shown that the administration of indomethacin can reduce the natriuretic and antihypertensive effect of furosemide and thiazides in some patients. This response has been attributed to inhibition of renal prostaglandin synthesis by nonsteroidal antiinflammatory drugs. Therefore, when indomethacin is added to the treatment of a patient receiving furosemide or thiazides, or furosemide or thiazides are added to the treatment of a patient receiving indomethacin, the patient should be observed closely to determine if the desired effect of furosemide or thiazides is obtained.

Indomethacin blocks the furosemide-induced increase in plasma renin activity. This fact should be kept in mind when evaluating plasma renin activity in hypertensive patients.

There is a report of a clinical pharmacology study in which triamterene was added to a maintenance schedule of indomethacin for four healthy volunteers. Two of the subjects developed azotemia and reduced creatinine clearance after several days of combined drug administration. This effect was reversible and may be mediated by prostaglandin inhibition. Nonetheless, indomethacin and triamterene should not be used together.

Blunting of the antihypertensive effect of beta-adrenoceptor blocking agents by nonsteroidal antiinflammatory drugs including indomethacin has been reported. Therefore, when using these blocking agents to treat hypertension, patients should be observed carefully in order to confirm that the desired therapeutic effect has been obtained. There are reports that indomethacin can reduce the antihypertensive effect of captopril in some patients.

ADVERSE REACTIONS

The adverse reactions listed below have been arranged into two groups:
(1) incidence greater than 1%; and (2) incidence less than 1%. The incidence for group (1) was obtained from 33 double-blind controlled clinical trials reported in the literature (1,092 patients). The incidence for group (2) was based on reports in clinical trials, in the literature, and on voluntary reports since marketing. The probability of a causal relationship exists between indomethacin and these adverse reactions, some of which have been reported only rarely.

A. GASTROINTESTINAL

1. Incidence greater than 1%

a) nausea, with or without vomiting (3% to 9%)
b) dyspepsia, including indigestion, heartburn, and epigastric pain (3% to 9%)
c) diarrhea (1% to 3%)
d) abdominal distress or pain (1% to 3%)
e) constipation (1% to 3%)

2. Incidence less than 1%

a) anorexia
b) bloating (includes distension)
c) flatulence
d) peptic ulcer
e) gastroenteritis
f) rectal bleeding
g) proctitis
h) perforation and hemorrhage of the esophagus, stomach, duodenum, or small intestine
i) intestinal ulceration associated with stenosis and obstruction
j) gastrointestinal bleeding without obvious ulcer formation and perforation of preexisting sigmoid lesions (diverticulum, carcinoma, etc)
k) development of ulcerative colitis and regional ileitis
l) ulcerative stomatitis
m) toxic hepatitis and jaundice (some fatal cases have been reported)

B. CENTRAL NERVOUS SYSTEM

1. Incidence greater than 1%

a) headache (over 10%)
b) dizziness (3% to 9%)
c) vertigo (1% to 3%)
d) somnolence (1% to 3%)
e) depression and fatigue (including malaise and listlessness) (1% to 3%)

2. Incidence less than 1%

a) anxiety (includes nervousness)
b) muscle weakness
c) involuntary muscle movements
d) insomnia
e) muzziness
f) psychic disturbances including psychotic episodes
g) mental confusion
h) drowsiness
i) lightheadedness
j) syncope
k) paresthesia
l) aggravation of epilepsy and parkinsonism
m) depersonalization
n) coma
o) peripheral neuropathy
p) convulsions

C. SPECIAL SENSES

1. Incidence greater than 1%

a) tinnitus (1% to 3%)

2. Incidence less than 1%

a) corneal deposits and retinal disturbances, including those of the macula, have been reported with prolonged therapy
b) blurred vision
c) hearing disturbances
d) deafness

D. CARDIOVASCULAR

1. Incidence less than 1%

a) hypertension
b) tachycardia
c) chest pain
d) congestive heart failure
e) arrhythmia
f) palpitations

E. METABOLIC

1. Incidence less than 1%

a) edema
b) weight gain
c) flushing or sweating
d) hyperglycemia
e) glycosuria
f) hyperkalemia

F. INTEGUMENTARY

1. Incidence less than 1%

a) pruritus
b) rash
c) urticaria
d) petechiae or ecchymosis
e) exfoliative dermatitis
f) erythema nodosum
g) loss of hair
h) Stevens-Johnson Syndrome
i) erythema multiforme
j) toxic epidermal necrolysis

G. HEMATOLOGIC

1. Incidence less than 1%

a) leukopenia
b) bone marrow depression
c) anemia secondary to obvious or occult gastrointestinal bleeding
d) aplastic anemia
e) hemolytic anemia
f) agranulocytosis
g) thrombocytopenic purpura

H. HYPERSENSITIVITY

1. Incidence less than 1%

a) acute respiratory distress
b) rapid fall in blood pressure resembling a shock-like state
c) angioedema
d) dyspnea
e) asthma
f) purpura
g) angiitis
h) pulmonary edema

I. GENITOURINARY

1. Incidence less than 1%

a) hematuria
b) vaginal bleeding
c) BUN elevation
d) renal insufficiency, including renal failure

J. MISCELLANEOUS

1. Incidence less than 1%

a) epistaxis
b) breast changes including enlargement, tenderness, or gynecomastia

Causal relationship unknown: Other reactions have been reported but occurred under circumstances where a causal relationship could not be established. However, in these rarely reported events the possibility cannot be excluded. Therefore, these observations are being listed to serve as alerting information to physicians.

A. HEMATOLOGIC: although there have been several reports of leukemia, the supporting information is weak.

B. GENITOURINARY: urinary frequency.

DOSAGE AND ADMINISTRATION

Indomethacin is available as 25 and 50 mg capsules for oral use.

Adverse reactions appear to correlate with the size of the dose of indomethacin in most patients but not all. Therefore, every effort should be made to determine the smallest effective dosage for the individual patient.

Always give indomethacin with food, immediately after meals, or with antacids to reduce gastric irritation.

Indomethacin should not ordinarily be prescribed for children 14 years of age and under because safe conditions for use have not been established. (See WARNINGS)

Dosage Recommendations for Active Stages of the Following:

1. Moderate to severe rheumatoid arthritis including acute flares of chronic disease; moderate to severe ankylosing spondylitis, and moderate to severe osteoarthritis.

Suggested Dosage:

25 mg b.i.d. or t.i.d. If this is well tolerated, increase the daily dosage by 25 or by 50 mg, if required by continuing symptoms, at weekly intervals until a satisfactory response is obtained or until a total daily dose of 150–200 mg is reached. DOSES ABOVE THIS AMOUNT GENERALLY DO NOT INCREASE THE EFFECTIVENESS OF THE DRUG.

In patients who have persistent night pain and/or morning stiffness, the giving of a large portion, up to a maximum of 100 mg, of the total daily dose at bedtime may be helpful in affording relief. The total daily dose should not exceed 200 mg. In acute flares of chronic rheumatoid arthritis, it may be necessary to increase the dosage by 25 mg or, if required, by 50 mg daily.

If minor adverse effects develop as the dosage is increased, reduce the dosage rapidly to a tolerated dose and OBSERVE THE PATIENT CLOSELY. If severe adverse reactions occur, STOP THE DRUG. After the acute phase of the disease is under control, an attempt to reduce the daily dose should be made repeatedly until the patient is receiving the smallest effective dose or the drug is discontinued.

Careful instructions to, and observations of, the individual patient are essential to the prevention of serious, irreversible, including fatal, adverse reactions.

As advancing years appear to increase the possibility of adverse reactions, indomethacin should be used with greater care in the aged.

Continued on next page

This product information was prepared in August, 1986. On these and other Parke-Davis Products, information may be obtained by addressing PARKE-DAVIS, Division of Warner-Lambert Company, Morris Plains, New Jersey 07950.

Parke-Davis—Cont.

2. Acute painful shoulder (bursitis and/or tendinitis)
Initial Dose:
75–150 mg daily in 3 or 4 divided doses.
The drug should be discontinued after the signs and symptoms of inflammation have been controlled for several days. The usual course of therapy is 7–14 days.
3. Acute gouty arthritis.
Suggested Dosage:
50 mg t.i.d. until pain is tolerable. The dose should then be rapidly reduced to complete cessation of the drug. Definite relief of pain has been reported within 2 to 4 hours. Tenderness and heat usually subside in 24 to 36 hours, and swelling gradually disappears in 3 to 5 days.

HOW SUPPLIED

Indomethacin Capsules, USP, 25 mg (#3 capsule with dark blue opaque cap and light aqua opaque body, coded P-D 887) are supplied as follows:
N 0071-0887-24 Bottles of 100
N 0071-0887-32 Bottles of 1000
Indomethacin Capsules, USP, 50 mg (#1 capsule with dark blue opaque cap and light aqua opaque body, coded P-D 888) are supplied as follows:
N 0071-0888-24 Bottles of 100

Special Handling and Storage Conditions:
Store bottles at room temperature below 30°C (86°F).
Store unit dose packages at controlled room temperature, 15°–30°C (59°–86°F)
Protect from light and moisture.
Caution: Federal law prohibits dispensing without a prescription.

0887G011

Shown in Product Identification Section, page 420

KETALAR® ℞

[*kē'tă-lăr"*]
(Ketamine Hydrochloride Injection, USP)

SPECIAL NOTE

EMERGENCE REACTIONS HAVE OCCURRED IN APPROXIMATELY 12 PERCENT OF PATIENTS.
THE PSYCHOLOGICAL MANIFESTATIONS VARY IN SEVERITY BETWEEN PLEASANT DREAM-LIKE STATES, VIVID IMAGERY, HALLUCINATIONS, AND EMERGENCE DELIRIUM. IN SOME CASES THESE STATES HAVE BEEN ACCOMPANIED BY CONFUSION, EXCITEMENT, AND IRRATIONAL BEHAVIOR WHICH A FEW PATIENTS RECALL AS AN UNPLEASANT EXPERIENCE. THE DURATION ORDINARILY IS NO MORE THAN A FEW HOURS; IN A FEW CASES, HOWEVER, RECURRENCES HAVE TAKEN PLACE UP TO 24 HOURS POSTOPERATIVELY. NO RESIDUAL PSYCHOLOGICAL EFFECTS ARE KNOWN TO HAVE RESULTED FROM USE OF KETALAR.
THE INCIDENCE OF THESE EMERGENCE PHENOMENA IS LEAST IN THE YOUNG (15 YEARS OF AGE OR LESS) AND ELDERLY (OVER 65 YEARS OF AGE) PATIENT. ALSO, THEY ARE LESS FREQUENT WHEN THE DRUG IS GIVEN INTRAMUSCULARLY AND THE INCIDENCE IS REDUCED AS EXPERIENCE WITH THE DRUG IS GAINED.
THE INCIDENCE OF PSYCHOLOGICAL MANIFESTATIONS DURING EMERGENCE, PARTICULARLY DREAM-LIKE OBSERVATIONS AND EMERGENCE DELIRIUM, MAY BE REDUCED BY USING LOWER RECOMMENDED DOSAGES OF KETALAR IN CONJUNCTION WITH INTRAVENOUS DIAZEPAM DURING INDUCTION AND MAINTENANCE OF ANESTHESIA. (See Dosage and Administration.) ALSO, THESE REACTIONS MAY BE REDUCED IF VERBAL, TACTILE AND VISUAL STIMULATION OF THE PATIENT IS MINIMIZED DURING THE RECOVERY PERIOD. THIS DOES NOT PRECLUDE THE MONITORING OF VITAL SIGNS.
IN ORDER TO TERMINATE A SEVERE EMERGENCE REACTION THE USE OF A SMALL HYPNOTIC DOSE OF A SHORT-ACTING OR ULTRASHORT-ACTING BARBITURATE MAY BE REQUIRED.
WHEN KETALAR IS USED ON AN OUTPATIENT BASIS, THE PATIENT SHOULD NOT BE RELEASED UNTIL RECOVERY FROM ANESTHESIA IS COMPLETE AND THEN SHOULD BE ACCOMPANIED BY A RESPONSIBLE ADULT.

DESCRIPTION

Ketalar is a nonbarbiturate anesthetic, chemically designated *dl* 2-(o-chlorophenyl)-2-(methylamino) cyclohexanone hy- drochloride. It is formulated as a slightly acid (pH 3.5-5.5) sterile solution for intravenous or intramuscular injection in concentrations containing the equivalent of either 10, 50 or 100 mg ketamine base per milliliter and contains not more than 0.1 mg/ml Phemerol® (benzethonium chloride) added as a preservative. The 10 mg/ml solution has been made isotonic with sodium chloride.

CLINICAL PHARMACOLOGY

Ketalar is a rapid-acting general anesthetic producing an anesthetic state characterized by profound analgesia, normal pharyngeal-laryngeal reflexes, normal or slightly enhanced skeletal muscle tone, cardiovascular and respiratory stimulation, and occasionally a transient and minimal respiratory depression.
A patent airway is maintained partly by virtue of unimpaired pharyngeal and laryngeal reflexes. (See Warnings and Precautions.)
The biotransformation of Ketalar includes N-dealkylation (metabolite I), hydroxylation of the cyclohexone ring (metabolites III and IV), conjugation with glucuronic acid and dehydration of the hydroxylated metabolites to form the cyclohexene derivative (metabolite II).
Following intravenous administration, the ketamine concentration has an initial slope (alpha phase) lasting about 45 minutes with a half-life of 10 to 15 minutes. This first phase corresponds clinically to the anesthetic effect of the drug. The anesthetic action is terminated by a combination of redistribution from the CNS to slower equilibrating peripheral tissues and by hepatic biotransformation to metabolite I. This metabolite is about 1/3 as active as ketamine in reducing halothane requirements (MAC) of the rat. The later half-life of ketamine (beta phase) is 2.5 hours.
The anesthetic state produced by Ketalar has been termed "dissociative anesthesia" in that it appears to selectively interrupt association pathways of the brain before producing somesthetic sensory blockade. It may selectively depress the thalamoneocortical system before significantly obtunding the more ancient cerebral centers and pathways (reticular-activating and limbic systems).
Elevation of blood pressure begins shortly after injection, reaches a maximum within a few minutes and usually returns to preanesthetic values within 15 minutes after injection. In the majority of cases, the systolic and diastolic blood pressure peaks from 10% to 50% above preanesthetic levels shortly after induction of anesthesia, but the elevation can be higher or longer in individual cases (see Contraindications).
Ketamine has a wide margin of safety; several instances of unintentional administration of overdoses of Ketalar (up to ten times that usually required) have been followed by prolonged but complete recovery.
Ketalar has been studied in over 12,000 operative and diagnostic procedures, involving over 10,000 patients from 105 separate studies. During the course of these studies Ketalar was administered as the sole agent, as induction for other general agents, or to supplement low-potency agents.
Specific areas of application have included the following:
1. debridement, painful dressings, and skin grafting in burn patients, as well as other superficial surgical procedures.
2. neurodiagnostic procedures such as pneumoencephalograms, ventriculograms, myelograms, and lumbar punctures. See also Precaution concerning increased intracranial pressure.
3. diagnostic and operative procedures of the eye, ear, nose, and mouth, including dental extractions.
4. diagnostic and operative procedures of the pharynx, larynx, or bronchial tree. NOTE: Muscle relaxants, with proper attention to respiration, may be required (see Precautions).
5. sigmoidoscopy and minor surgery of the anus and rectum, and circumcision.
6. extraperitoneal procedures used in gynecology such as dilatation and curettage.
7. orthopedic procedures such as closed reductions, manipulations, femoral pinning, amputations, and biopsies.
8. as an anesthetic in poor-risk patients with depression of vital functions.
9. in procedures where the intramuscular route of administration is preferred.
10. in cardiac catheterization procedures.

In these studies, the anesthesia was rated either "excellent" or "good" by the anesthesiologist and the surgeon at 90% and 93%, respectively; rated "fair" at 6% and 4%, respectively; and rated "poor" at 4% and 3%, respectively. In a second method of evaluation, the anesthesia was rated "adequate" in at least 90%, and "inadequate" in 10% or less of the procedures.

INDICATIONS AND USAGE

Ketalar is indicated as the sole anesthetic agent for diagnostic and surgical procedures that do not require skeletal muscle relaxation. Ketalar is best suited for short procedures but it can be used, with additional doses, for longer procedures.
Ketalar is indicated for the induction of anesthesia prior to the administration of other general anesthetic agents.
Ketalar is indicated to supplement low-potency agents, such as nitrous oxide.
Specific areas of application are described in the Clinical Pharmacology section.

CONTRAINDICATIONS

Ketamine hydrochloride is contraindicated in those in whom a significant elevation of blood pressure would constitute a serious hazard and in those who have shown hypersensitivity to the drug.

WARNINGS

Cardiac function should be continually monitored during the procedure in patients found to have hypertension or cardiac decompensation.
Postoperative confusional states may occur during the recovery period. (See Special Note.)
Respiratory depression may occur with overdosage or too rapid a rate of administration of Ketalar, in which case supportive ventilation should be employed. Mechanical support of respiration is preferred to administration of analeptics.

PRECAUTIONS

General
Ketalar should be used by or under the direction of physicians experienced in administering general anesthetics and in maintenance of an airway and in the control of respiration.
Because pharyngeal and laryngeal reflexes are usually active, Ketalar should not be used alone in surgery or diagnostic procedures of the pharynx, larynx, or bronchial tree. Mechanical stimulation of the pharynx should be avoided, whenever possible, if Ketalar is used alone. Muscle relaxants, with proper attention to respiration, may be required in both of these instances.
Resuscitative equipment should be ready for use.
The incidence of emergence reactions may be reduced if verbal and tactile stimulation of the patient is minimized during the recovery period. This does not preclude the monitoring of vital signs (see Special Note).
The intravenous dose should be administered over a period of 60 seconds. More rapid administration may result in respiratory depression or apnea and enhanced pressor response.
In surgical procedures involving visceral pain pathways, Ketalar should be supplemented with an agent which obtunds visceral pain.
Use with caution in the chronic alcoholic and the acutely alcohol-intoxicated patient.
An increase in cerebrospinal fluid pressure has been reported following administration of ketamine hydrochloride. Use with extreme caution in patients with preanesthetic elevated cerebrospinal fluid pressure.

Information for Patients
As appropriate, especially in cases where early discharge is possible, the duration of Ketalar and other drugs employed during the conduct of anesthesia should be considered. The patients should be cautioned that driving an automobile, operating hazardous machinery or engaging in hazardous activities should not be undertaken for 24 hours or more (depending upon the dosage of Ketalar and consideration of other drugs employed) after anesthesia.

Drug Interactions
Prolonged recovery time may occur if barbiturates and/or narcotics are used concurrently with Ketalar.
Ketalar is clinically compatible with the commonly used general and local anesthetic agents when an adequate respiratory exchange is maintained.

Usage in Pregnancy
Since the safe use in pregnancy, including obstetrics (either vaginal or abdominal delivery), has not been established, such use is not recommended (see Animal Reproduction).

ADVERSE REACTIONS

Cardiovascular: Blood pressure and pulse rate are frequently elevated following administration of Ketalar alone. However, hypotension and bradycardia have been observed. Arrhythmia has also occurred.
Respiration: Although respiration is frequently stimulated, severe depression of respiration or apnea may occur following rapid intravenous administration of high doses of Ketalar. Laryngospasms and other forms of airway obstruction have occurred during Ketalar anesthesia.
Eye: Diplopia and nystagmus have been noted following Ketalar administration.
It also may cause a slight elevation in intraocular pressure measurement.
Psychological: (See Special Note).
Neurological: In some patients, enhanced skeletal muscle tone may be manifested by tonic and clonic movements sometimes resembling seizures (see Dosage and Administration).
Gastrointestinal: Anorexia, nausea and vomiting have been observed; however this is not usually severe and allows the great majority of patients to take liquids by mouth shortly after regaining consciousness (see Dosage and Administration).
General: Local pain and exanthema at the injection site have infrequently been reported. Transient erythema and/or morbilliform rash have also been reported.

OVERDOSAGE

Respiratory depression may occur with overdosage or too rapid a rate of administration of Ketalar, in which case supportive ventilation should be employed. Mechanical support of respiration is preferred to administration of analeptics.

DOSAGE AND ADMINISTRATION

Note: Barbiturates and Ketalar, being chemically incompatible because of precipitate formation, *should not* be injected from the same syringe.

If the Ketalar dose is augmented with diazepam, the two drugs must be given separately. Do not mix Ketalar and diazepam in syringe or infusion flask. For additional information on the use of diazepam, refer to the Warnings and Dosage and Administration Sections of the diazepam insert.

Preoperative Preparations:

1. While vomiting has been reported following Ketalar administration, some airway protection may be afforded because of active laryngeal-pharyngeal reflexes. However, since aspiration may occur with Ketalar and since protective reflexes may also be diminished by supplementary anesthetics and muscle relaxants, the possibility of aspiration must be considered. Ketalar is recommended for use in the patient whose stomach is not empty when, in the judgment of the practitioner, the benefits of the drug outweigh the possible risks.
2. Atropine, scopolamine, or another drying agent should be given at an appropriate interval prior to induction.

Onset and Duration:

Because of rapid induction following the initial intravenous injection, the patient should be in a supported position during administration.

The onset of action of Ketalar is rapid; an intravenous dose of 2 mg/kg (1 mg/lb) of body weight usually produces surgical anesthesia within 30 seconds after injection, with the anesthetic effect usually lasting five to ten minutes. If a longer effect is desired, additional increments can be administered intravenously or intramuscularly to maintain anesthesia without producing significant cumulative effects.

Intramuscular doses, from experience primarily in children, in a range of 9 to 13 mg/kg (4 to 6 mg/lb) usually produce surgical anesthesia within 3 to 4 minutes following injection, with the anesthetic effect usually lasting 12 to 25 minutes.

Dosage:

As with other general anesthetic agents, the individual response to Ketalar is somewhat varied depending on the dose, route of administration, and age of patient, so that dosage recommendation cannot be absolutely fixed. The drug should be titrated against the patient's requirements.

Induction:

Intravenous Route: The initial dose of Ketalar administered intravenously may range from 1 mg/kg to 4.5 mg/kg (0.5 to 2 mg/lb). The average amount required to produce five to ten minutes of surgical anesthesia has been 2 mg/kg (1 mg/lb).

Alternatively, in adult patients an induction dose of 1.0 mg to 2.0 mg/kg intravenous ketamine at a rate of 0.5 mg/kg/min may be used for induction of anesthesia. In addition, diazepam in 2 mg to 5 mg doses, administered in a separate syringe over 60 seconds, may be used. In most cases, 15.0 mg of intravenous diazepam *or less* will suffice. The incidence of psychological manifestations during emergence, particularly dream-like observations and emergence delirium, may be reduced by this induction dosage program.

Note: The 100 mg/ml concentration of Ketalar *should not* be injected intravenously without proper dilution. It is recommended the drug be diluted with an equal volume of either Sterile Water for Injection, USP, Normal Saline, or 5% Dextrose in Water.

Rate of Administration: It is recommended that Ketalar be administered slowly (over a period of 60 seconds). More rapid administration may result in respiratory depression and enhanced pressor response.

Intramuscular Route: The initial dose of Ketalar administered intramuscularly may range from 6.5 to 13 mg/kg (3 to 6 mg/lb). A dose of 10 mg/kg (5 mg/lb) will usually produce 12 to 25 minutes of surgical anesthesia.

Maintenance of Anesthesia:

The maintenance dose should be adjusted according to the patient's anesthetic needs and whether an additional anesthetic agent is employed.

Increments of one-half to the full induction dose may be repeated as needed for maintenance of anesthesia. However, it should be noted that purposeless and tonic-clonic movements of extremities may occur during the course of anesthesia. These movements do not imply a light plane and are not indicative of the need for additional doses of the anesthetic. It should be recognized that the larger the total dose of Ketalar administered, the longer will be the time to complete recovery.

Adult patients induced with Ketalar augmented with intravenous diazepam may be maintained on Ketalar given by slow microdrip infusion technique at a dose of 0.1 to 0.5 mg/minute, augmented with diazepam 2 to 5 mg administered intravenously as needed. In many cases 20 mg *or less* of intravenous diazepam total for combined induction and maintenance will suffice. However, slightly more diazepam may be required depending on the nature and duration of the operation, physical status of the patient, and other factors. The incidence of psychological manifestations during emergence, particularly dream-like observations and emergence delirium, may be reduced by this maintenance dosage program.

Dilution: To prepare a dilute solution containing 1 mg of ketamine per ml, aseptically transfer 10 ml (50 mg per ml Steri-Vial) or 5 ml (100 mg per ml Steri-Vial) to 500 ml of 5% Dextrose Injection, USP or Sodium Chloride (0.9%) Injection, USP (Normal Saline) and mix well. The resultant solution will contain 1 mg of ketamine per ml.

The fluid requirements of the patient and duration of anesthesia must be considered when selecting the appropriate dilution of Ketalar. If fluid restriction is required, Ketalar can be added to a 250 ml infusion as described above to provide a Ketalar concentration of 2 mg/ml.

Ketalar Steri-Vials, 10 mg/ml are not recommended for dilution.

Supplementary Agents:

Ketalar is clinically compatible with the commonly used general and local anesthetic agents when an adequate respiratory exchange is maintained.

The regimen of a reduced dose of Ketalar supplemented with diazepam can be used to produce balanced anesthesia by combination with other agents such as nitrous oxide and oxygen.

HOW SUPPLIED

Ketalar is supplied as the hydrochloride in concentrations equivalent to ketamine base.

N 0071-4581-15—Each 50-ml vial contains 10 mg/ml. Supplied in cartons of 10.

N 0071-4581-13—Each 25-ml vial contains 10 mg/ml. Supplied in cartons of 10.

N 0071-4581-12—Each 20-ml vial contains 10 mg/ml. Supplied in cartons of 10.

N 0071-4582-10—Each 10-ml vial contains 50 mg/ml. Supplied in cartons of 10.

N 0071-4585-08—Each 5-ml vial contains 100 mg/ml. Supplied in cartons of 10.

Animal Pharmacology and Toxicology:

Toxicity: The acute toxicity of Ketalar has been studied in several species. In mature mice and rats, the intraperitoneal LD_{50} values are approximately 100 times the average human intravenous dose and approximately 20 times the average human intramuscular dose. A slightly higher acute toxicity observed in neonatal rats was not sufficiently elevated to suggest an increased hazard when used in children. Daily intravenous injections in rats of five times the average human intravenous dose and intramuscular injections in dogs at four times the average human intramuscular dose demonstrated excellent tolerance for as long as 6 weeks. Similarly, twice weekly anesthetic sessions of one, three, or six hours' duration in monkeys over a four-to six-week period were well tolerated.

Interaction With Other Drugs Commonly Used For Preanesthetic Medication: Large doses (three or more times the equivalent effective human dose) of morphine, meperidine, and atropine increased the depth and prolonged the duration of anesthesia produced by a standard anesthetizing dose of Ketalar in Rhesus monkeys. The prolonged duration was not of sufficient magnitude to contraindicate the use of these drugs for preanesthetic medication in human clinical trials.

Blood Pressure: Blood pressure responses to Ketalar vary with the laboratory species and experimental conditions. Blood pressure is increased in normotensive and renal hypertensive rats with and without adrenalectomy and under pentobarbital anesthesia.

Intravenous Ketalar produces a fall in arterial blood pressure in the Rhesus monkey and a rise in arterial blood pressure in the dog. In this respect the dog mimics the cardiovascular effect observed in man. The pressor response to Ketalar injected into intact, unanesthetized dogs is accompanied by a tachycardia, rise in cardiac output and a fall in total peripheral resistance. It causes a fall in perfusion pressure following a large dose injected into an artificially perfused vascular bed (dog hindquarters), and it has little or no potentiating effect upon vasoconstriction responses of epinephrine or norepinephrine. The pressor response to Ketalar is reduced or blocked by chlorpromazine (central depressant and peripheral α-adrenergic blockade), by β-adrenergic blockade, and by ganglionic blockade. The tachycardia and increase in myocardial contractile force seen in intact animals does not appear in isolated hearts (Langendorff) at a concentration of 0.1 mg of Ketalar nor in Starling dog heart-lung preparations at a Ketalar concentration of 50 mg/kg of HLP. These observations support the hypothesis that the hypertension produced by Ketalar is due to selective activation of central cardiac stimulating mechanisms leading to an increase in cardiac output. The dog myocardium is not sensitized to epinephrine and Ketalar appears to have a weak antiarrhythmic activity.

Metabolic Disposition: Ketalar is rapidly absorbed following parenteral administration. Animal experiments indicated that Ketalar was rapidly distributed into body tissues, with relatively high concentrations appearing in body fat, liver, lung, and brain; lower concentrations were found in the heart, skeletal muscle, and blood plasma. Placental transfer of the drug was found to occur in pregnant dogs and monkeys. No significant degree of binding to serum albumin was found with Ketalar.

Balance studies in rats, dogs, and monkeys resulted in the recovery of 85% to 95% of the dose in the urine, mainly in the form of degradation products. Small amounts of drug were also excreted in the bile and feces. Balance studies with tritium-labeled Ketalar in human subjects (1 mg/lb given intravenously) resulted in the mean recovery of 91% of the dose in the urine and 3% in the feces. Peak plasma levels averaged about 0.75 μg/ml, and CSF levels were about 0.2 μg/ml, 1 hour after dosing.

Ketalar undergoes N-demethylation and hydroxylation of the cyclohexanone ring, with the formation of water-soluble conjugates which are excreted in the urine. Further oxidation also occurs with the formation of a cyclohexanone derivative. The unconjugated N-demethylated metabolite was found to be less than one-sixth as potent as Ketalar. The unconjugated demethyl cyclohexanone derivative was found to be less than one-tenth as potent as Ketalar. Repeated doses of Ketalar administered to animals did not produce any detectable increase in microsomal enzyme activity.

Reproduction: Male and female rats, when given five times the average human intravenous dose of Ketalar for three consecutive days about one week before mating, had a reproductive performance equivalent to that of saline-injected controls. When given to pregnant rats and rabbits intramuscularly at twice the average human intramuscular dose during the respective periods of organogenesis, the litter characteristics were equivalent to those of saline-injected controls. A small group of rabbits was given a single large dose (six times the average human dose) of Ketalar on Day 6 of pregnancy to simulate the effect of an excessive clinical dose around the period of nidation. The outcome of pregnancy was equivalent in control and treated groups.

To determine the effect of Ketalar on the perinatal and postnatal period, pregnant rats were given twice the average human intramuscular dose during Days 18 to 21 of pregnancy. Litter characteristics at birth and through the weaning period were equivalent to those of the control animals. There was a slight increase in incidence of delayed parturition by one day in treated dams of this group. Three groups each of mated beagle bitches were given 2.5 times the average human intramuscular dose twice weekly for the three weeks of the first, second, and third trimesters of pregnancy, respectively, without the development of adverse effects in the pups.

4581G030

LOESTRIN® 21 1/20 ℞

[lō″ĕs′trĭn]

(Each white tablet contains 1 mg norethindrone acetate and 20 mcg ethinyl estradiol.)

LOESTRIN® 21 1.5/30 ℞

(Each green tablet contains 1.5 mg norethindrone acetate and 30 mcg ethinyl estradiol.)

LOESTRIN® Fe 1/20 ℞

(Each white tablet contains 1 mg norethindrone acetate and 20 mcg ethinyl estradiol. Each brown tablet contains 75 mg ferrous fumarate, USP.)

LOESTRIN® Fe 1.5/30 ℞

(Each green tablet contains 1.5 mg norethindrone acetate and 30 mcg ethinyl estradiol. Each brown tablet contains 75 mg ferrous fumarate, USP)

Each white tablet contains: norethindrone acetate (17 alpha-ethinyl-19-nortestosterone acetate), 1 mg; ethinyl estradiol (17 alpha-ethinyl-1,3,5(10)-estratriene-3,17 beta-diol), 20 mcg.

Each green tablet contains: norethindrone acetate (17 alpha-ethinyl-19-nortestosterone acetate). 1.5 mg; ethinyl estradiol (17 alpha-ethinyl-1,3,5(10)-estratriene-3, 17 beta-diol), 30 mcg.

Each brown tablet contains 75 mg ferrous fumarate, USP.

DESCRIPTION

Loestrin is a progestogen-estrogen combination.

Loestrin Fe 1/20 and 1.5/30 provides a continuous dosage regimen consisting of 21 oral contraceptive tablets and seven ferrous fumarate tablets. The ferrous fumarate tablets are present to facilitate ease of drug administration via a 28-day

Continued on next page

This product information was prepared in August, 1986. On these and other Parke-Davis Products, information may be obtained by addressing PARKE-DAVIS, Division of Warner-Lambert Company, Morris Plains, New Jersey 07950.

Parke-Davis—Cont.

regimen and are not intended to serve any therapeutic purpose.

CLINICAL PHARMACOLOGY

Combination oral contraceptives act primarily through the mechanism of gonadotropin suppression due to the estrogenic and progestational activity of the ingredients. Although the primary mechanism of action is inhibition of ovulation, alterations in the genital tract, including changes in the cervical mucus (which increase the difficulty of sperm penetration) and the endometrium (which reduce the likelihood of implantation) may also contribute to contraceptive effectiveness.

INDICATIONS AND USAGE

Loestrin is indicated for the prevention of pregnancy in women who elect to use oral contraceptives as a method of contraception.

Oral contraceptives are highly effective. The pregnancy rate in women using conventional combination oral contraceptives (containing 35 mcg or more of ethinyl estradiol or 50 mcg or more of mestranol) is generally reported as less than one pregnancy per 100 women-years of use. Slightly higher rates (somewhat more than one pregnancy per 100 woman-years of use) are reported for some combination products containing 35 mcg or less of ethinyl estradiol, and rates on the order of three pregnancies per 100 woman-years are reported for the progestogen-only oral contraceptives.

These rates are derived from separate studies conducted by different investigators in several population groups and cannot be compared precisely. Furthermore, pregnancy rates tend to be lower as clinical studies are continued, possibly due to selective retention in the longer studies of those patients who accept the treatment regimen and do not discontinue as a result of adverse reactions, pregnancy, or other reasons.

In clinical trials with Loestrin 1/20, 1,431 patients completed 15,899 cycles and a total of 10 pregnancies were reported. This represents a pregnancy rate of 0.75 per 100 woman-years based upon data that include the cases where patients failed to comply with the dosage regimen. The pregnancy rate in patients who adhered to the dosage regimen was 0.30 per 100 woman-years (four pregnancies in these trials).

In clinical trials with Loestrin 1.5/30, 1,289 patients completed 17,139 cycles and a total of 7 pregnancies were reported. This represents a pregnancy rate of 0.49 per 100 woman-years based upon data that include the cases where patients failed to comply with the dosage regimen. The pregnancy rate in patients who adhered to the dosage regimen was 0.07 per 100 woman-years (one pregnancy in these trials).

Table 1 gives ranges of pregnancy rates reported in the literature[1] for other means of contraception. The efficacy of these means of contraception (except the IUD) depends upon the degree of adherence to the method.

Table 1 Pregnancies per 100 Woman-Years

IUD, less than 1–6; Diaphragm with spermicidal products (creams or jellies), 2–20; Condom, 3–36; Aerosol foams, 2–29; Jellies and creams, 4–36; Periodic abstinence (rhythm) all types less than 1–47; *1. Calendar method, 14–47; 2. Temperature method, 1–20; 3. Temperature method—intercourse only in post-ovulatory phase, less than 1–7; 4. Mucus method, 1–25;* No contraception, 60–80.

Dose-Related Risk of Thromboembolism from Oral Contraceptives

Two studies have shown a positive association between the dose of estrogens in oral contraceptives and the risk of thromboembolism.[2,3] For this reason, it is prudent and in keeping with good principles of therapeutics to minimize exposure to estrogen. The oral contraceptive product prescribed for any given patient should be that product which contains the least amount of estrogen that is compatible with an acceptable pregnancy rate and patient acceptance. It is recommended that new acceptors of oral contraceptives be started on preparations containing 0.05 mg or less of estrogen.

CONTRAINDICATIONS

Oral contraceptives should not be used in women with any of the following conditions.

1. Thrombophlebitis or thromboembolic disorders
2. A past history of deep vein thrombophlebitis or thromboembolic disorders.
3. Cerebral vascular or coronary artery disease
4. Known or suspected carcinoma of the breast
5. Known or suspected estrogen-dependent neoplasia
6. Undiagnosed abnormal genital bleeding
7. Known or suspected pregnancy (see Warning No. 5)
8. Benign or malignant liver tumor which developed during the use of oral contraceptives or other estrogen-containing products.

WARNINGS

Cigarette smoking increases the risk of serious cardiovascular side effects from oral contraceptive use. This risk increases with age and with heavy smoking (15 or more cigarettes per day) and is quite marked in women over 35 years of age. Women who use oral contraceptives should be strongly advised not to smoke.

The use of oral contraceptives is associated with increased risk of several serious conditions including thromboembolism, stroke, myocardial infarction, hepatic adenoma, gallbladder disease, and hypertension. Practitioners prescribing oral contraceptives should be familiar with the following information relating to these risks.

1. *Thromboembolic Disorders and Other Vascular Problems.* An increased risk of thromboembolic and thrombotic disease associated with the use of oral contraceptives is well established. Three principal studies in Great Britain[4–6] and three in the United States[7–10] have demonstrated an increased risk of fatal and nonfatal venous thromboembolism and stroke, both hemorrhagic and thrombotic. These studies estimate that users of oral contraceptives are 4 to 11 times more likely than nonusers to develop these diseases without evident cause (Table 2).

Cerebrovascular Disorders

In a collaborative American study[9,10] of cerebrovascular disorders in women with and without predisposing causes, it was estimated that the risk of hemorrhagic stroke was 2.0 times greater in users than nonusers and the risk of thrombotic stroke was 4 to 9.5 times greater in users than in nonusers (Table 2).

Table 2

Summary of relative risk of thromboembolic disorders and other vascular problems in oral contraceptive users compared to nonusers

	Relative risk, times greater
Idiopathic thromboembolic disease	4–11
Postsurgery thromboembolic complications	4–6
Thrombotic stroke	4–9.5
Hemorrhagic stroke	2
Myocardial infarction	2–12

Myocardial Infarction

An increased risk of myocardial infarction associated with the use of oral contraceptives has been reported[11–13] confirming a previously suspected association. These studies, conducted in the United Kingdom, found, as expected, that the greater the number of underlying risk factors for coronary artery disease (cigarette smoking, hypertension, hypercholesterolemia, obesity, diabetes, history of preeclamptic toxemia) the higher the risk of developing myocardial infarction, regardless of whether the patient was an oral contraceptive user or not. Oral contraceptives, however, were found to be a clear additional risk factor.

In terms of relative risk, it has been estimated[52] that oral contraceptive users who do not smoke (smoking is considered a major predisposing condition to myocardial infarction) are about twice as likely to have a fatal myocardial infarction as nonusers who do not smoke. Oral contraceptive users who are also smokers have about a 5-fold increased risk of fatal infarction compared to users who do not smoke, but about a 10- to 12-fold increased risk compared to nonusers who do not smoke. Furthermore, the amount of smoking is also an important factor. In determining the importance of these relative risks, however, the baseline rates for various age groups, as shown in Table 3, must be given serious consideration. The importance of other predisposing conditions mentioned above in determining relative and absolute risks has not as yet been quantified; it is quite likely that the same synergistic action exists, but perhaps to a lesser extent.

Table 3

Estimated annual mortality rate per 100,000 women from myocardial infarction by use of oral contraceptives, smoking habits, and age (in years)

[See table below].

Risk of Dose

Persistence of Risk

In confirmation of earlier reports,[53,54] two studies have suggested that an increased risk may persist for as long as 6 years after discontinuation of oral contraceptive use for cerebrovascular disease[55] and 9 years for myocardial infarction[56]. In addition, a prospective study suggested the persistence of risk for subarachnoid hemorrhage.[57]

In an analysis of data derived from several national adverse reaction reporting systems,[2] British investigators concluded that the risk of thromboembolism, including coronary thrombosis, is directly related to the dose of estrogen used in oral contraceptives. Preparations containing 100 mcg or more of estrogen were associated with a higher risk of thromboembolism than those containing 50 to 80 mcg of estrogen. Their analysis did suggest, however, that the quantity of estrogen may not be the sole factor involved. This finding has been confirmed in the United States. Careful epidemiological studies to determine the degree of thromboembolic risk associated with progestogen-only oral contraceptives have not been performed. Cases of thromboembolic disease have been reported in women using these products, and they should not be presumed to be free of excess risk.

Estimate of Excess Mortality from Circulatory Diseases

A large prospective study [53] carried out in the U.K. estimated the mortality rate per 100,000 women per year from diseases of the circulatory system for users and nonusers of oral contraceptives according to age, smoking habits, and duration of use. The overall excess death rate annually from circulatory diseases for oral contraceptive users was estimated to be 20 per 100,000 (ages 15 to 34—5/100,000; ages 35 to 44— 33/100,000; ages 45 to 49—140/100,000), the risk being concentrated in older women, in those with a long duration of use, and in cigarette smokers. It was not possible, however, to examine the interrelationships of age, smoking, and duration of use, nor to compare the effects of continuous versus intermittent use. Although the study showed a 10-fold increase in death due to circulatory diseases in users for 5 or more years, all of these deaths occurred in women 35 or older. Until larger numbers of women under 35 with continuous use for 5 or more years are available, it is not possible to assess the magnitude of the relative risk for this younger age group.

The available data from a variety of sources have been analyzed[14] to estimate the risk of death associated with various methods of contraception. The estimates of risk of death for each method include the combined risk of the contraceptive method (eg, thromboembolic and thrombotic disease in the case of oral contraceptives) plus the risk attributable to pregnancy or abortion in the event of method failure. This latter risk varies with the effectiveness of the contraceptive method. The findings of this analysis are shown in Figure 1 which follows.[14] The study concluded that the mortality associated with all methods of birth control is low and below that associated with childbirth, with the exception of oral contraceptives in women over 40 who smoke. (The rates given for pill only/smokers for each age group are for smokers as a class. For "heavy" smokers [more than 15 cigarettes a day] the rates given would be about double, for "light" smokers [less than 15 cigarettes a day] about 50 percent.) The lowest mortality is associated with the condom or diaphragm backed up by early abortion.

[See Figure 1 on next page].

The risk of thromboembolic and thrombotic disease associated with oral contraceptives increases with age after approximately age 30 and, for myocardial infarction, is further increased by hypertension, hypercholesterolemia, obesity, diabetes, or history of preeclamptic toxemia and especially by cigarette smoking.

Based on the data currently available, the following chart gives a gross estimate of the risk of death from circulatory disorders associated with the use of oral contraceptives.

[See chart next page]

The physician and the patient should be alert to the earliest manifestations of thromboembolic and thrombotic disorders (eg, thrombophlebitis, pulmonary embolism, cerebrovascular insufficiency, coronary occlusion, retinal thrombosis, and mesenteric thrombosis). Should any of these occur or be suspected, the drug should be discontinued immediately.

A four- to six-fold increased risk of postsurgery thromboembolic complications has been reported in oral contraceptive

Loestrin

	Myocardial infarction			
	Women aged 30–39		Women aged 40–44	
Smoking habits	Users	Nonusers	Users	Nonusers
All smokers	10.2	2.6	62.0	15.9
Heavy*	13.0	5.1	78.7	31.3
Light	4.7	0.9	28.6	5.7
Nonsmokers	1.8	1.2	10.7	7.4
Smokers and nonsmokers	5.4	1.9	32.8	11.7

*Heavy smoker: 15 or more cigarettes per day. From Jain, A.K., Studies in Family Planning 8:50, 1977.

Smoking Habits and Other Predisposing Conditions—Risk Associated with Use of Oral Contraceptives

Age	Below 30	30–39	40+
Heavy smokers	C	B	A
Light smokers	D	C	B
Nonsmokers (no predisposing conditions)	D	C,D	C
Nonsmokers (other predisposing conditions)	C	C,B	B,A

A—Use associated with very high risk
B—Use associated with high risk
C—Use associated with moderate risk
D—Use associated with low risk

users.[15,16] If feasible, oral contraceptives should be discontinued at least 4 weeks before surgery of a type associated with an increased risk of thromboembolism or prolonged immobilization.

2. *Ocular Lesions.* There have been reports of neuro-ocular lesions, such as optic neuritis or retinal thrombosis, associated with the use of oral contraceptives. Discontinue oral contraceptive medication if there is unexplained, sudden or gradual, partial or complete loss of vision; onset of proptosis or diplopia; papilledema; or retinal vascular lesions and institute appropriate diagnostic and therapeutic measures.

3. *Carcinoma.* Long-term continuous administration of either natural or synthetic estrogen in certain animal species increases the frequency of carcinoma of the breast, cervix, vagina, and liver. Certain synthetic progestogens, none currently contained in oral contraceptives, have been noted to increase the incidence of mammary nodules, benign and malignant, in dogs.

In humans, three case control studies have reported an increased risk of endometrial carcinoma associated with the prolonged use of exogenous estrogen in post-menopausal women.[17–19] One publication[20] reported on the first 21 cases submitted by physicians to a registry of cases of adenocarcinoma of the endometrium in women under 40 on oral contraceptives. Of the cases found in women without predisposing risk factors for adenocarcinoma of the endometrium (eg, irregular bleeding at the time oral contraceptives were first given, polycystic ovaries), nearly all occurred in women who had used a sequential oral contraceptive. These products are no longer marketed. No evidence has been reported suggesting an increased risk of endometrial cancer in users of conventional-combination or progestogen-only oral contraceptives.

Several studies[8,21–24] have found no increase in breast cancer in women taking oral contraceptives or estrogens. One study,[25] however, while also noting no overall increased risk of breast cancer in women treated with oral contraceptives, found an excess risk in the subgroups of oral contraceptive users with documented benign breast disease. A reduced occurrence of benign breast tumors in users of oral contraceptives has been well-documented.[8,21,25–27]

In summary, there is at present no confirmed evidence from human studies of an increased risk of cancer associated with oral contraceptives. Close clinical surveillance of all women taking oral contraceptives is, nevertheless, essential. In all cases of undiagnosed persistent or recurrent abnormal vaginal bleeding, appropriate diagnostic measures should be taken to rule out malignancy. Women with a strong family history of breast cancer or who have breast nodules, fibrocystic disease, or abnormal mammograms, should be monitored with particular care if they elect to use oral contraceptives instead of other methods of contraception.

4. *Hepatic Tumors.* Benign hepatic adenomas have been found to be associated with the use of oral contraceptives.[28–30,46] One study[46] showed that oral contraceptive formulations with high hormonal potency were associated with a higher risk than lower potency formulations. Although benign, hepatic adenomas may rupture and may cause death through intra-abdominal hemorrhage. This has been reported in short-term as well as long-term users of oral contraceptives. Two studies relate risk with duration of use of the contraceptive, the risk being much greater after 4 or more years of oral contraceptive use.[30,46] While hepatic adenoma is a rare lesion, it should be considered in women presenting abdominal pain and tenderness, abdominal mass or shock.

A few cases of hepatocellular carcinoma have been reported in women taking oral contraceptives. The relationship of these drugs to this type of malignancy is not known at this time.

5. *Use in or Immediately Preceding Pregnancy, Birth Defects in Offspring, and Malignancy in Female Offspring.* The use of female sex hormones— both estrogenic and progestational agents—during early pregnancy may seriously damage the offspring. It has been shown that females exposed *in utero* to diethylstilbestrol, a nonsteroidal estrogen, have an increased risk of developing in later life a form of vaginal or

Figure 1. Estimated annual number of deaths associated with control of fertility and no control per 100,000 nonsterile women, by regimen of control and age of woman.

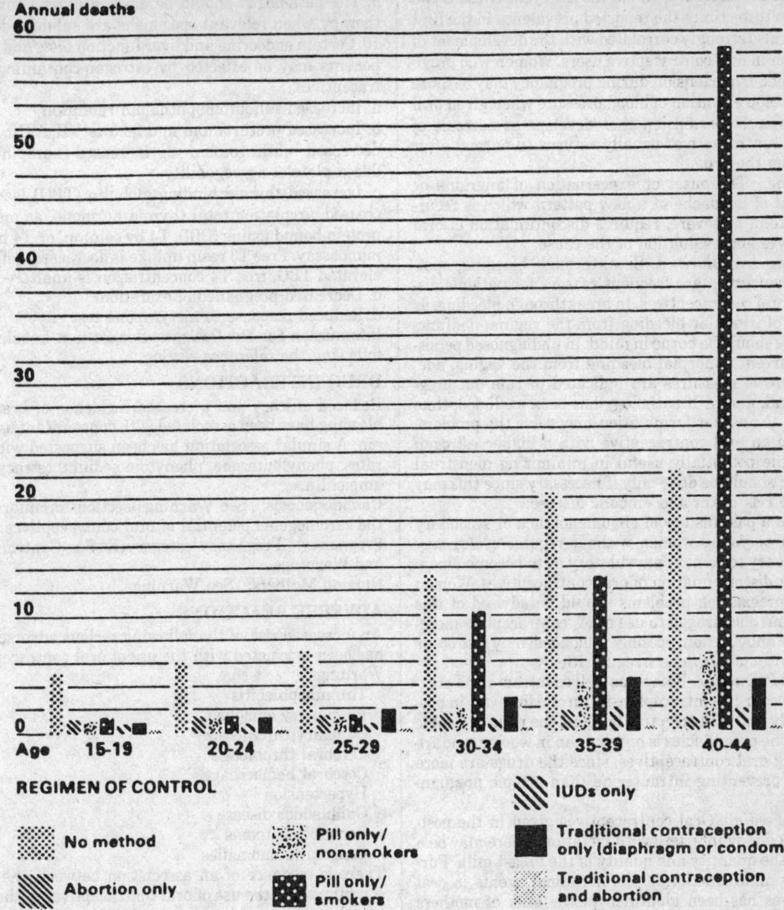

cervical cancer that is ordinarily extremely rare.[31,32] This risk has been estimated to be of the order of 1 in 1,000 exposures or less.[33,47] Although there is no evidence at the present time that oral contraceptives further enhance the risk of developing this type of malignancy, such patients should be monitored with particular care if they elect to use oral contraceptives instead of other methods of contraception. Furthermore, a high percentage of such exposed women (from 30% to 90%) have been found to have epithelial changes of the vagina and cervix.[34–38] Although these changes are histologically benign, it is not known whether this condition is a precursor of vaginal malignancy. Male children so exposed may develop abnormalities of the urogenital tract.[48–50] Although similar data are not available with the use of other estrogens, it cannot be presumed that they would not induce similar changes.

An increased risk of congenital anomalies, including heart defects and limb defects, has been reported with the use of sex hormones, including oral contraceptives, in pregnancy.[39–42,51] One case control study[42] has estimated a 4.7-fold increase in risk of limb-reduction defectes in infants exposed *in utero* to sex hormones (oral contraceptives, hormonal withdrawal tests for pregnancy or attempted treatment for threatened abortion). Some of these exposures were very short and involved only a few days of treatment. The data suggest that the risk of limb-reduction defects in exposed fetuses is somewhat less than 1 in 1,000 live births.

In the past, female sex hormones have been used during pregnancy in an attempt to treat threatened or habitual abortion. There is considerable evidence that estrogens are ineffective for these indications, and there is no evidence from well-controlled studies that progestogens are effective for these uses.

There is some evidence that triploidy and possibly other types of polyploidy are increased among abortuses from women who become pregnant soon after ceasing oral contraceptives.[43] Embryos with these anomalies are virtually always aborted spontaneously. Whether there is an overall increase in spontaneous abortion of pregnancies conceived soon after stopping oral contraceptives is unknown.

It is recommended that for any patient who has missed two consecutive periods, pregnancy should be ruled out before continuing the contraceptive regimen. If the patient has not adhered to the prescribed schedule, the possibility of pregnancy should be considered at the time of the first missed period, and further use of oral contraceptives should be withheld until pregnancy has been ruled out. If pregnancy is confirmed, the patient should be apprised of the potential risks to the fetus and the advisability of continuation of the pregnancy should be discussed in the light of these risks.

It is also recommended that women who discontinue oral contraceptives with the intent of becoming pregnant use an alternate form of contraception for a period of time before attempting to conceive. Many clinicians recommend 3 months although no precise information is available on which to base this recommendation.

The administration of progestogen-only or progestogen-estrogen combinations to induce withdrawal bleeding should not be used as a test of pregnancy.

6. *Gallbladder Disease.* Studies[8,23,26] report an increased risk of surgically confirmed gallbladder disease in users of oral contraceptives and estrogens. In one study, an increased risk appeared after 2 years of use and doubled after 4 or 5 years of use. In one of the other studies, an increased risk was apparent between 6 and 12 months of use.

7. *Carbohydrate and Lipid Metabolic Effects.* A decrease in glucose tolerance has been observed in a significant percentage of patients on oral contraceptives. For this reason, prediabetic and diabetic patients should be carefully observed while receiving oral contraceptives.

An increase in triglycerides and total phospholipids has been observed in patients receiving oral contraceptives.[44] The clinical significance of this finding remains to be defined.

8. *Elevated Blood Pressure.* An increase in blood pressure has been reported in patients receiving oral contraceptives.[26] In some women, hypertension may occur within a few months of beginning oral contraceptive use. In the first year of use, the prevalence of women with hypertension is low in users and may be no higher than that of a comparable group of nonusers. The prevalance in users increases, how-

Continued on next page

This product information was prepared in August, 1986. On these and other Parke-Davis Products, information may be obtained by addressing PARKE-DAVIS, Division of Warner-Lambert Company, Morris Plains, New Jersey 07950.

Parke-Davis—Cont.

ever, with longer exposure, and in the fifth year of use is two and a half to three times the reported prevalence in the first year. Age is also strongly correlated with the development of hypertension in oral contraceptive users. Women who previously have had hypertension during pregnancy may be more likely to develop elevation of blood pressure when given oral contraceptives. Hypertension that develops as a result of taking oral contraceptives usually returns to normal after discontinuing the drug.

9. *Headache.* The onset or exacerbation of migraine or development of headache of a new pattern which is recurrent, persistent, or severe, requires discontinuation of oral contraceptives and evaluation of the cause.

10. *Bleeding Irregularities.* Breakthrough bleeding, spotting and amenorrhea are frequent reasons for patients discontinuing oral contraceptives. In breakthrough bleeding, as in all cases of irregular bleeding from the vagina, nonfunctional causes should be borne in mind. In undiagnosed persistent or recurrent abnormal bleeding from the vagina, adequate diagnostic measures are indicated to rule out pregnancy or malignancy. If pathology has been excluded, time or a change to another formulation may solve the problem. Changing to an oral contraceptive with a higher estrogen content, while potentially useful in minimizing menstrual irregularity, should be done only if necessary since this may increase the risk of thromboembolic disease.

Women with a past history of oligomenorrhea or secondary amenorrhea or young women without regular cycles may have a tendency to remain anovulatory or to become amenorrheic after discontinuation of oral contraceptives. Women with these preexisting problems should be advised of this possibility and encouraged to use other contraceptive methods. Post-use anovulation, possibly prolonged, may also occur in women without previous irregularities.

11. *Ectopic Pregnancy.* Ectopic as well as intrauterine pregnancy may occur in contraceptive failures. However, in progestogen-only oral contraceptive failures, the ratio of ectopic to intrauterine pregnancies is higher than in women who are not receiving oral contraceptives, since the drugs are more effective in preventing intrauterine than ectopic pregnancies.

12. *Breast-Feeding.* Oral contraceptives given in the postpartum period may interfere with lactation. There may be a decrease in the quantity and quality of the breast milk. Furthermore, a small fraction of the hormonal agents in oral contraceptives has been identified in the milk of mothers receiving these drugs.[45] The effects, if any, on the breast-fed child have not been determined. If feasible, the use of oral contraceptives should be deferred until the infant has been weaned.

PRECAUTIONS

General

1. A complete medical and family history should be taken prior to the initiation of oral contraceptives. The pretreatment and periodic physical examinations should include special reference to blood pressure, breasts, abdomen and pelvic organs, including Papanicolaou smear and relevant laboratory tests. As a general rule, oral contraceptives should not be prescribed for longer than 1 year without another physical examination being performed.
2. Under the influence of estrogen-progestogen preparations preexisting uterine leiomyomata may increase in size.
3. Patients with a history of psychic depression should be carefully observed and the drug discontinued if depression recurs to a serious degree. Patients becoming significantly depressed while taking oral contraceptives should stop the medication and use an alternate method of contraception in an attempt to determine whether the symptom is drug related.
4. Oral contraceptives may cause some degree of fluid retention. They should be prescribed with caution, and only with careful monitoring, in patients with conditions which might be aggravated by fluid retention, such as convulsive disorders, migraine syndrome, asthma, or cardiac or renal insufficiency.
5. Patients with a past history of jaundice during pregnancy have an increased risk of recurrence of jaundice while receiving oral contraceptive therapy. If jaundice develops in any patient receiving such drugs, the medication should be discontinued.
6. Steroid hormones may be poorly metabolized in patients with impaired liver function and should be administered with caution in such patients.
7. Oral contraceptive users may have disturbances in normal tryptophan metabolism which may result in a relative pyridoxine deficiency. The clinical significance of this is yet to be determined.
8. Serum folate levels may be depressed by oral contraceptive therapy. Since the pregnant woman is predisposed to the development of folate deficiency and the incidence of folate deficiency increases with increasing gestation, it is possible that if a woman becomes pregnant shortly after stopping oral contraceptives, she may have a greater chance of developing folate deficiency and complications attributed to this deficiency.
9. The pathologist should be advised of oral contraceptive therapy when relevant specimens are submitted.
10. Certain endocrine and liver function tests and blood components may be affected by estrogen-containing oral contraceptives:

a. Increased sulfobromophthalein retention
b. Increased prothrombin and factors VII, VIII, IX, and X; decreased antithrombin 3; increased norepinephrine-induced platelet aggregability
c. Increased thyroid binding globulin (TBG) leading to increased circulating total thyroid hormone, as measured by protein-bound iodine (PBI), T4 by column, or T4 by radioimmunoassay. Free T3 resin uptake is decreased, reflecting the elevated TBG, free T4 concentration is unaltered
d. Decreased pregnanediol excretion
e. Reduced response to metyrapone test

Information For The Patient: See Patient Labeling printed following the reference section.

DRUG INTERACTIONS

Reduced efficacy and increased incidence of breakthrough bleeding have been associated with concomitant use of rifampin. A similar association has been suggested with barbiturates, phenylbutazone, phenytoin sodium, tetracycline, and ampicillin.

Carcinogenesis: See Warnings section for information on the carcinogenic potential of oral contraceptives.

Pregnancy: Pregnancy category X. See Contraindications and Warnings.

Nursing Mothers: See Warnings.

ADVERSE REACTIONS

An increased risk of the following serious adverse reactions has been associated with the use of oral contraceptives (see Warnings):

- Thrombophlebitis
- Pulmonary embolism
- Coronary thrombosis
- Cerebral thrombosis
- Cerebral hemorrhage
- Hypertension
- Gallbladder disease
- Benign hepatomas
- Congenital anomalies

There is evidence of an association between the following conditions and the use of oral contraceptives, although additional confirmatory studies are needed:

- Mesenteric thrombosis
- Neuro-ocular lesions, eg, retinal thrombosis and optic neuritis

The following adverse reactions have been reported in patients receivng oral contraceptives and are believed to be drug related:

Nausea and/or vomiting, usually the most common adverse reactions, occur in approximately 10 percent or less of patients during the first cycle. Other reactions, as a general rule, are seen much less frequently or only occasionally:

- Gastrointestinal symptoms (such as abdominal cramps and bloating)
- Breakthrough bleeding
- Spotting
- Change in menstrual flow
- Dysmenorrhea
- Amenorrhea during and after treatment
- Temporary infertility after discontinuance of treatment
- Edema
- Chloasma or melasma which may persist
- Breast changes: tenderness, enlargement and secretion
- Change in weight (increase or decrease)
- Change in cervical erosion and cervical secretion
- Possible diminution in lactation when given immediately postpartum
- Cholestatic jaundice
- Migraine
- Increase in size of uterine leiomyomata
- Rash (allergic)
- Mental depression
- Reduced tolerance to carbohydrates
- Vaginal candidiasis
- Change in corneal curvature (steepening)
- Intolerance to contact lenses

The following adverse reactions have been reported in users of oral contraceptives, and the association has been neither confirmed nor refuted:

- Premenstrual-like syndrome
- Cataracts
- Changes in libido
- Chorea
- Changes in appetite
- Cystitis-like syndrome
- Headache
- Nervousness
- Dizziness
- Hirsutism
- Loss of scalp hair
- Erythema multiforme
- Erythema nodosum
- Hemorrhagic eruption
- Vaginitis
- Porphyria

ACUTE OVERDOSE

Serious ill effects have not been reported following acute ingestion of large doses of oral contraceptives by young children. Overdosage may cause nausea, and withdrawal bleeding may occur in females.

Dosage and Administration For 21-Day Dosage Regimen: To achieve maximum contraceptive effectiveness, Loestrin must be taken exactly as directed and at intervals not exceeding 24 hours. Loestrin **21** provides the patient with a convenient tablet schedule of "3 weeks on—1 week off."

The first day of menstrual flow is considered Day 1. Initially, the patient begins taking tablets on Day 5 and takes one tablet daily for 21 days. She then takes no tablets for seven days. After the seven days during which no tablets are taken, the patient begins a new course of one tablet daily for 21 days. Each course of tablets will begin on the same day of the week as the first course. Likewise, the interval of no tablets will always start on the same day of the week.

Tablets should be taken regularly with a meal or at bedtime. It should be stressed that efficacy of medication depends on strict adherence to the dosage schedule.

Special Notes on Administration

Menstruation usually begins two or three days, but may begin as late as the fourth or fifth day after discontinuing medication. Because of the relatively low estrogenic content, Loestrin is not a good cyclic regulator. There are patients whose inherent hormone balance will require larger amounts of estrogen to achieve cyclic regularity than that contained in Loestrin. These patients experience altered bleeding patterns, which do not conform to treatment schedules, while taking Loestrin tablets. However, it is important that patients adhere to the dosage schedule regardless of when bleeding occurs.

The occurrence of altered bleeding is highest in Cycle 1. The majority of patients will have seven days or less of total bleeding during the 28-day cycle (including both withdrawal bleeding and breakthrough bleeding and spotting). Should irregular bleeding occur, patients should be reassured and instructed to continue taking the tablets as directed. If by the third cycle the irregular patterns are unacceptable, consideration should be given to changing the medication to a product with a higher estrogen content (Norlestrin® *1/50 or Norlestrin 2.5/50). The physician should be alert to the fact that the irregular bleeding patterns could mask bleeding from organic causes, and appropriate diagnostic measures should be taken if the bleeding persists or continues after changing to a higher estrogen-content product.

If a patient forgets to take one or more tablets, the following is suggested. If one tablet is missed, take it as soon as remembered, or take two tablets the next day. If two consecutive tablets are missed, take two tablets daily for the next two days, then resume the regular schedule. While there is little likelihood of pregnancy occurring if the patient misses only one or two tablets, the possibility of pregnancy increases with each successive day that tablets are missed. *However if the patient is taking* Loestrin **21** 1/20, *in addition to taking two white tablets a day for two days the patient should use an additional means of contraception for seven consecutive days.* If three consecutive tablets are missed, begin a new compact of tablets starting seven days after the last tablet was taken. The patient should use an alternate means of contraception, other than oral tablets, until the start of the next menstrual period.

The possibility of ovulation occurring increases with each successive day that scheduled tablets are missed. While there is little likelihood of ovulation occurring if only one tablet is missed, the possibility of spotting or bleeding is increased. This is particularly likely to occur if two or more consecutive tablets are missed.

*Norlestrin (Norethindrone Acetate and Ethinyl Estradiol Tablets, USP)

Dosage and Administration For 28-Day Dosage Regimen: To achieve maximum contraceptive effectiveness, Loestrin must be taken exactly as directed and at intervals not exceeding 24 hours.

Loestrin **Fe** provides a continuous administration regimen consisting of 21 *light-colored* tablets of Loestrin and 7 brown tablets of ferrous fumarate. There is no need for the patient to count days between cycles because there are no "off-tablet days."

The dosage schedule is one *light-colored* tablet daily for 21 days, starting initially on Day 5 of the menstrual cycle, followed without interruption by one brown tablet daily for 7 days. The first day of menstrual flow is considered Day 1. Upon completion of this first course of tablets, a second course of tablets is started without interruption. All subsequent courses also are taken without interruption.

Tablets should be taken regularly with a meal or at bedtime. It should be stressed that efficacy of medication depends on strict adherence to the dosage schedule.

Special Notes on Administration

Menstruation usually begins two or three days, but may begin as late as the fourth or fifth day, after the brown tablets have been started. Because of the relatively low estrogenic content, Loestrin is not a good cyclic regulator. There are patients whose inherent hormone balance will require larger amounts of estrogen to achieve cyclic regularity than that contained in Loestrin. These patients experience altered bleeding patterns, which do not conform to treatment schedules, while taking the *light-colored* Loestrin tablets. However, it is important that patients adhere to the dosage schedule regardless of when bleeding occurs.

The occurrence of altered bleeding is highest in Cycle 1. The majority of patients will have seven days or less of total bleeding during the 28-day cycle (including both withdrawal bleeding and breakthrough bleeding and spotting). Should irregular bleeding occur, patients should be reassured and instructed to continue taking the tablets as directed. If by the third cycle the irregular patterns are unacceptable, consideration should be given to changing the medication to a product with a higher estrogen content (Norlestrin *1/50 or Norlestrin 2.5/50). The physician should be alert to the fact that the irregular bleeding patterns could mask bleeding from organic causes, and appropriate diagnostic measures should be taken if the bleeding persists or continues after changing to a higher estrogen-content product.

If a patient forgets to take one or more *light-colored* tablets, the following is suggested. If one *light-colored* tablet is missed, take it as soon as remembered, or take two *light-colored* tablets the next day. If two consecutive *light-colored* tablets are missed, take two *light-colored* tablets daily for the next two days, then resume the regular schedule. While there is little likelihood of pregnancy occurring if the patient misses only one or two *light-colored* tablets, the possibility of pregnancy increases with each successive day that *light-colored* tablets are missed. *However, if the patient is taking* Loestrin **Fe** 1/20, *in addition to taking two white tablets a day for two days, the patient should use an additional means of contraception for seven consecutive days.* If three consecutive *light-colored* tablets are missed, begin a new compact of tablets, starting seven days after the last *light-colored* tablet was taken. The patient should use an alternate means of contraception, other than oral tablets, until the start of the next menstrual period.

The possibility of ovulation occurring increases with each successive day that scheduled *light-colored* tablets are missed. While there is little likelihood of ovulation occurring if only one *light-colored* tablet is missed, the possibility of spotting or bleeding is increased. This is particularly likely to occur if two or more consecutive *light-colored* tablets are missed.

If one or more brown tablets are missed, the *light-colored* tablets should be started no later than the eighth day after the last *light-colored* tablet was taken. The possibility of conception occurring is not increased if brown tablets are missed.

*Norlestrin (Norethindrone Acetate and Ethinyl Estradiol Tablets, USP)

Use of oral contraceptives in the event of a missed menstrual period:

1. If the patient has not adhered to the prescribed dosage regimen, the possibility of pregnancy should be considered after the first missed period and oral contraceptives should be withheld until pregnancy has been ruled out.
2. If the patient has adhered to the prescribed regimen and misses two consecutive periods, pregnancy should be ruled out before continuing the contraceptive regimen.

After several months on treatment, bleeding may be reduced to a point of virtual absence. This reduced flow may occur as a result of medication, in which event it is not indicative of pregnancy.

HOW SUPPLIED

Loestrin **21** 1/20 is available in compacts each containing 21 tablets. Each tablet contains 1 mg of norethindrone acetate and 20 mcg of ethinyl estradiol. Available in packages of five compacts and packages of five refills.

Loestrin **Fe** 1/20 is available in compacts each containing 21 white tablets and 7 brown tablets. Each white tablet contains 1 mg of norethindrone acetate and 20 mcg of ethinyl estradiol. Each brown tablet contains 75 mg ferrous fumarate, USP. Available in packages of five compacts and packages of five refills.

Loestrin **21** 1.5/30 is available in compacts each containing 21 tablets. Each tablet contains 1.5 mg of norethindrone acetate and 30 mcg of ethinyl estradiol. Available in packages of five compacts and packages of five refills.

Loestrin **Fe** 1.5/30 is available in compacts each containing 21 green tablets and 7 brown tablets. Each green tablet contains 1.5 mg of norethindrone acetate and 30 mcg of ethinyl estradiol. Each brown tablet contains 75 mg ferrous fumarate, USP. Available in packages of five compacts and packages of five refills.

References:

1. "*Population Reports,*" Series H, Number 2, May 1974; Series 1, Number 1, June 1974; Series B, Number 2, January 1975; Series H, Number 3, 1975; Series H, Number 4, January 1976 (published by the Population Information Program, The George Washington University Medical Center, 2001 S. St. NW., Washington, D.C.)
2. Inman, W. H. W., M. P. Vessey, B. Westerholm, and A. Engelund. "Thromboembolic disease and the steroidal content of oral contraceptives. A report to the Committee on Safety of Drugs," *Brit Med J* 2:203–209, 1970.
3. Stolley, P.D., J. A. Tonascia, M. S. Tockman, P. E. Sartwell, A. H. Rutledge, and M. P. Jacobs, "Thrombosis with low-estrogen oral contraceptives," *Am J Epidemiol* 102: 197–208, 1975.
4. Royal College of General Practitioners, "Oral contraception and thromboembolic disease," *J Coll Gen Pract* 13:267–279, 1967.
5. Inman, W. H. W. and M. P. Vessey, "Investigation of deaths from pulmonary, coronary and cerebral thrombosis and embolism in women of childbearing age," *Brit Med. J* 2-193–199, 1968.
6. Vessey, M. P. and R. Doll, "Investigation of relation between use of oral contraceptives and thromboembolic disease. A further report," *Brit Med J* 2:651–657, 1969.
7. Sartwell, P. E., A. T. Masi, F. G. Arthes, G. R. Greene, and H. E. Smith, "Thromboembolism and oral contraceptives an epidemiological case control study," *Am J Epidemiol* 90:365–380, 1969.
8. Boston Collaborative Drug Surveillance Program. "Oral contraceptives and venous thromboembolic disease, surgically confirmed gallbladder disease and breast tumors," *Lancet* 1:1399–1404, 1973.
9. Collaborative Group for the Study of Stroke in Young Women, "Oral contraception and increased risk of cerebral ischemia or thrombosis," *N Engl J Med* 288:871–878, 1973.
10. Collaborative Group for the Study of Stroke in Young Women, "Oral contraceptives and stroke in young women: associated risk factors," *JAMA* 231:718–722, 1975.
11. Mann, J. I., and W. H. W. Inman, "Oral contraceptives and death from myocardial infarction," *Brit Med J* 2:245–248, 1975.
12. Mann, J. I., W. H. W. Inman, and M. Thorogood, "Oral contraceptive use in older women and fatal myocardial infarction," *Brit Med J* 2:445–447, 1976.
13. Mann, J. I., M. P. Vessey, M. Thorogood and R. Doll, "Myocardial infarction in young women with special reference to oral contraceptive practice," *Brit Med J* 2:241–245, 1975.
14. Tietze, C., "New Estimates of Mortality Associated with Fertility Control," *Family Planning Perspectives,* 9:74–76, 1977.
15. Vessey, M. P., R. Doll, A. S. Fairbairn, and G. Glober, "Post-operative thromboembolism and the use of oral contraceptives," *Brit Med J* 3:123–126, 1970.
16. Greene, G. R., P. E. Sartwell, "Oral contraceptive use in patients with thromboembolism following surgery, trauma or infection," *Am J Pub Health* 62:680–685, 1972.
17. Smith, D. C., R. Prentice, D. J. Thompson and W. L. Herrmann, "Association of exogenous estrogen and endometrial carcinoma," *N Engl J Med* 293:1164–1167, 1975.
18. Ziel, H. K., and W. D. Finkle, "Increased risk of endometrial carcinoma among users of conjugated estrogens," *N Engl J Med* 293: 1167–1170, 1975.
19. Mack, T. N., M. C. Pike, B. E. Henderson, R. I. Pfeffer, V. R. Gerkins, M. Arthur and S. E. Brown, "Estrogens and endometrial cancer in a retirement community," *N Engl J Med* 294: 1262–1267, 1976.
20. Silverberg, S. G., and E. L. Makowski, "Endometrial carcinoma in young women taking oral contraceptive agents," *Obstet Gynecol* 46:503–506, 1975.
21. Vessey, M. P., R. Doll, and P. M. Sutton, "Oral contraceptives and breast neoplasia: a retrospective study," *Brit Med J* 3:719–724, 1972.
22. Vessey, M. P., R. Doll, and K. Jones, "Oral contraceptives and breast cancer. Progress report of an epidemiological study," *Lancet* 1:941–943, 1975.
23. Boston Collaborative Drug Surveillance Program, "Surgically confirmed gallbladder disease, venous thromboembolism and breast tumors in relation to postmenopausal estrogen therapy," *N Engl J Med* 290:14–19, 1974.
24. Arthes, F. G., P. E. Sartwell, and E. F. Lewison, "The pill, estrogens, and the breast, Epidemiologic aspects," *Cancer* 28:1391–1394, 1971.
25. Fasal, E., and R. S. Paffenbarger, "Oral contraceptives as related to cancer and benign lesions of the breast." *J Natl Cancer Inst* 55:767–773, 1975.
26. Royal College of General Practitioners, "Oral Contraceptives and Health," London, Pitman, 1974.
27. Ory, H., P. Cole, B. MacMahon, and R. Hoover, "Oral contraceptives and reduced risk of benign breast diseases," *N Engl J Med* 294:419–422, 1976.
28. Baum, J., F. Holtz, J. J. Bookstein, and E. W. Klein, "Possible association between benign hepatomas and oral contraceptives," *Lancet* 2:926–928, 1973.
29. Mays, E. T., W. M. Christopherson, M. M. Mahr, and H. C. Williams, "Hepatic changes in young women ingesting contraceptive steroids. Hepatic hemorrhage and primary hepatic tumors," *JAMA* 235:730–732, 1976.
30. Edmondson, H. A., B. Henderson, and B. Benton, "Liver-cell adenomas associated with use of oral contraceptives," *N Engl J Med* 294:470–472, 1976.
31. Herbst, A. L., H. Ulfelder, and D. C. Poskanzer, "Adenocarcinoma of the vagina," *N Engl J Med* 284:878–881, 1971.
32. Greenwald, P., J. J. Barlow, P. C. Nasca and W. Burnett, "Vaginal cancer after maternal treatment with synthetic estrogens," *N Engl J Med* 285:390–392, 1971.
33. Lanier, A. P., K. L. Noller, D. G. Decker, L. Elveback, and L. T. Kurland, "Cancer and stilbestrol. A follow-up of 1719 persons exposed to estrogens in utero and born 1943–1959," *Mayo Clin Pro* 48:793–799, 1973.
34. Herbst, A. L., R. J. Kurman, and R. E. Scully, "Vaginal and cervical abnormalities after exposure to stilbestrol in utero," *Obstet Gynecol* 40:287–298, 1972.
35. Herbst, A. L., S. J. Robboy, G. J. Macdonald, and R. E. Scully, "The effects of local progesterone on stilbestrol-associated vaginal adenosis," *Am J. Obstet Gynecol* 118:607–615, 1974.
36. Herbst, A. L., D. C. Poskanzer, S. J. Robboy, L. Friedlander, and R. E. Scully, "Prenatal exposure to stilbestrol: a prospective comparison of exposed female offspring with unexposed controls," *N Engl J Med* 292:334–339, 1975.
37. Stafl, A., R. F. Mattingly, D. V. Foley, W. Fetherston, "Clinical diagnosis of vaginal adenosis," *Obstet Gynecol* 43:118–128, 1974.
38. Sherman, A. I., M. Goldrath, A. Berlin, V. Vakhariya, F. Banooni, W. Michaels, P. Goodman, and S. Brown, "Cervical-vaginal adenosis after in utero exposure to synthetic estrogens," *Obstet Gynecol* 44:531–545, 1974.
39. Gal, I., B. Kirman, and J. Stern, "Hormone pregnancy tests and congenital malformation," *Nature* 216:83, 1967.
40. Levy, E. P., A. Cohen, and F. C. Fraser, "Hormone treatment during pregnancy and congenital heart defects," *Lancet* 1:611, 1973.
41. Nora, J. J., and A. H. Nora, "Birth defects and oral contraceptives," *Lancet* 1:941–942, 1973.
42. Janerich, D. T., J. M. Piper, and D. M. Glebatis, "Oral contraceptives and congenital limb-reduction defects," *N Engl J Med* 291:697–700, 1974.
43. Carr, D. H., "Chromosome studies in selected spontaneous abortions: I. Conception after oral contraceptives," *Canad Med Assoc J* 103:343–348, 1970.
44. Wynn, V., J. W. H. Doar, and G. L. Mills, "Some effects of oral contraceptives on serum-lipid and lipoprotein levels," *Lancet* 2:720–723, 1966.
45. Laumas, K. R., P. K. Malkani, S. Bhatnagar, and V. Laumas, "Radioactivity in the breast milk of lactating women after oral administration of 3 H-norethynodrel," *Amer J Obstet Gynecol* 98:411–413, 1967.
46. Center for Disease Control, "Increased Risk of Hepatocellular Adenoma in Women with Long-term use of Oral Contraceptives," *Morbidity and Mortality Weekly Report* 26:293–294, 1977.
47. Herbst, A. L., P. Cole, T. Colton, S. J. Robboy, R. E. Scully, "Age-incidence and Risk of Diethylstilbestrol-related Clear Cell Adenocarcinoma of the Vagina and Cervix," *Am J. Obstet Gynecol* 128:43–50, 1977.
48. Bibbo, M., M. Al-Naqeeb, I. Baccarini, W. Gill, M. Newton, K. M. Sleeper, M. Sonek, G. L. Wied, "Follow-Up Study of Male and Female Offspring of DES-treated Mothers. A Preliminary Report," *Jour of Repro Med* 15:29–32, 1975.
49. Gill, W. B., G. F. B. Schumacher, M. Bibbo, "Structural and Functional Abnormalities in the Sex Organs of Male Offpsring of Mothers Treated with Diethylstilbestrol (DES)," *Jour of Repro Med* 16:147–153, 1976.
50. Henderson, B. E., B. Benton, M. Cosgrove, J. Baptista, J. Aldrich, D. Townsend, W. Hart, T. Mack, "Urogenital Tract Abnormalities in Sons of Women Treated with Diethylstilbestrol," *Pediatrics* 58:505–507, 1976.
51. Heinonen, O. P., D. Slone, R. R. Nonson, E. B. Hook, S. Shapiro, "Cardiovascular Birth Defects and Antenatal Exposure to Female Sex Hormones," *N Engl J Med* 296:67–70, 1977.
52. Jain, A. K., "Mortality Risk Associated with the Use of Oral Contraceptives," *Studies in Family Planning* 8:50–54, 1977.
53. Beral, V., "Mortality Among Oral Contraceptive Users," *Lancet* 2:727–731, 1977.
54. Layde, P.M., et al.: *Lancet* 1:541–546, 1981.
55. Royal College of General Practitioners: *J Coll Gen Pract* 33:75, 19.

Continued on next page

This product information was prepared in August, 1986. On these and other Parke-Davis Products, information may be obtained by addressing PARKE-DAVIS, Division of Warner-Lambert Company, Morris Plains, New Jersey 07950.

Parke-Davis—Cont.

56. Slone D., et al.: *NEJM* 305:4 1981.
57. Petitti, D.B., et al.: *Lancet* 2:234, 1978.

The patient labeling for oral contraceptive drug products is set forth below:

Brief Summary Patient Package Insert

> Cigarette smoking increases the risk of serious adverse effects on the heart and blood vessels from oral contraceptive use. This risk increases with age and with heavy smoking (15 or more cigarettes per day) and is quite marked in women over 35 years of age. Women who use oral contraceptives should not smoke.

Oral contraceptives taken as directed are about 99% effective in preventing pregnancy. (The mini-pill, however is somewhat less effective.) Forgetting to take your pills increases the chance of pregnancy. Various drugs, such as antibiotics, may also decrease the effectiveness of oral contraceptives.

Women who have or have had clotting disorders, cancer of the breast or sex organs, unexplained vaginal bleeding, a stroke, heart attack, angina pectoris, or who suspect they may be pregnant should not use oral contraceptives.

Most side effects of the pill are not serious. The most common side effects are nausea, vomiting, bleeding between menstrual periods, weight gain, and breast tenderness. However, proper use of oral contraceptives requires that they be taken under your doctor's continuous supervision, because they can be associated with serious side effects which may be fatal. Fortunately, these occur very infrequently.

The serious side effects are:

1. Blood clots in the legs, lungs, brain, heart or other organs and hemorrhage into the brain due to bursting of a blood vessel. Certain of these effects may occur after pill use has been stopped
2. Liver tumors, which may rupture and cause severe bleeding
3. Birth defects if the pill is taken while you are pregnant
4. High blood pressure
5. Gallbladder disease

The symptoms associated with these serious side effects are discussed in the detailed leaflet given you with your supply of pills. Notify your doctor if you notice any unusual physical disturbance while taking the pill.

The estrogen in oral contraceptives has been found to cause breast cancer and other cancers in certain animals. These findings suggest that oral contraceptives may also cause cancer in humans. However, studies to date in women taking currently marketed oral contraceptives have not confirmed that oral contraceptives cause cancer in humans.

The detailed leaflet describes more completely the benefits and risks of oral contraceptives. It also provides information on other forms of contraception. Read it carefully. If you have any questions, consult your doctor.

Caution: Oral contraceptives are of no value in the prevention or treatment of venereal disease.

Detailed Patient Labeling

What You Should Know About Oral Contraceptives

Oral contraceptives ("the pill") are the most effective way (except for sterilization) to prevent pregnancy. They are also convenient and, for most women, free of serious or unpleasant side effects. Oral contraceptives must always be taken under the continuous supervision of a physician.

It is important that any woman who considers using an oral contraceptive understand the risks involved. Although the oral contraceptives have important advantages over other methods of contraception, they have certain risks that no other method has, and some of these risks may continue after you have stopped using the pill. Only you can decide whether the advantages are worth these risks. This leaflet will tell you about the most important risks. It will explain how you can help your doctor prescribe the pill as safely as possible by telling him about yourself and being alert for the earliest signs of trouble. And it will tell you how to use the pill properly, so that it will be as effective as possible. There is more detailed information available in the leaflet prepared for doctors. Your pharmacist can show you a copy; you may need your doctor's help in understanding parts of it.

Who Should Not Use Oral Contraceptives

A. If you have any of the following conditions you should not use the pill:

1. Clots in the legs or lungs
2. Angina pectoris
3. Known or suspected cancer of the breast or sex organs
4. Unusual vaginal bleeding that has not yet been diagnosed
5. Known or suspected pregnancy

B. If you have had any of the following conditions you should not use the pill:

1. Heart attack or stroke
2. Clots in the legs or lungs

> C. Cigarette smoking increases the risk of serious adverse effects on the heart and blood vessels from oral contraceptive use. This risk increases with age and with heavy smoking (15 or more cigarettes per day) and is quite marked in women over 35 years of age. Women who use oral contraceptives should not smoke.

D. If you have scanty or irregular periods or are a young woman without a regular cycle, you should use another method of contraception because, if you use the pill, you may have difficulty becoming pregnant or may fail to have menstrual periods after discontinuing the pill.

Deciding To Use Oral Contraceptives

If you do not have any of the conditions listed above and are thinking about using oral contraceptives, to help you decide, you need information about the advantages and risks of oral contraceptives and of other contraceptive methods as well. This leaflet describes the advantages and risks of oral contraceptives. Except for sterilization, the IUD and abortion, which have their own exclusive risks, the only risks of other methods of contraception are those due to pregnancy should the method fail. Your doctor can answer questions you may have with respect to other methods of contraception. He can also answer any questions you may have after reading this leaflet on oral contraceptives.

1. What Oral Contraceptives Are and How They Work. Oral contraceptives are of two types. The most common, often simply called "the pill," is a combination of an estrogen and a progestogen, the two kinds of female hormones. The amount of estrogen and progestogen can vary, but the amount of estrogen is most important because both the effectiveness and some of the dangers of oral contraceptives are related to the amount of estrogen. This kind of oral contraceptive works principally by preventing release of an egg from the ovary. When the amount of estrogen is 50 micrograms or more, and the pill is taken as directed, oral contraceptives are more than 99% effective (ie, there would be less than one pregnancy if 100 women used the pill for 1 year). Pills that contain 20 to 35 micrograms of estrogen vary slightly in effectiveness, ranging from 98% to more than 99% effective. Norlestrin was shown in clinical trials to be more than 99% effective.

The second type of oral contraceptive, often called the "mini-pill," contains only a progestogen. It works in part by preventing release of an egg from the ovary but also by keeping sperm from reaching the egg and by making the uterus (womb) less receptive to any fertilized egg that reaches it. The mini-pill is less effective than the combination oral contraceptive, about 97% effective.

In addition, the progestogen-only pill has a tendency to cause irregular bleeding which may be quite inconvenient, or cessation of bleeding entirely. The progestogen-only pill is used despite its lower effectiveness in the hope that it will prove not to have some of the serious side effects of the estrogen-containing pill (which follows) but it is not yet certain that the mini-pill does in fact have fewer serious side effects. The discussion which follows, while based mainly on information about the combination pills, should be considered to apply, as well, to the mini-pill.

2. Other Nonsurgical Ways to Prevent Pregnancy. As this leaflet will explain, oral contraceptives have several serious risks. Other methods of contraception have lesser risks or none at all. They are also less effective than oral contraceptives but, used properly, may be effective enough for many women. The following gives reported pregnancy rates (the number of women out of 100 who would become pregnant in 1 year) for these methods:

Pregnancies Per 100 Women Per Year

Intrauterine device (IUD), less than 1-6; Diaphragm with spermicidal products (creams or jellies), 2-20; Condom (rubber), 3-36; Aerosol foams, 2-29; Jellies and creams, 4-36; Periodic abstinence (rhythm) all types, less than 1-47; *1. Calendar method, 14-47; 2. Temperature method, 1-20; 3. Temperature method—intercourse only in post-ovulatory phase, less than 1-7; 4. Mucus method, 1-25;* No contraception, 60-80.

The figures (except for the IUD) vary widely because people differ in how well they use each method. Very faithful users of the various methods obtain very good results except for users of the calendar method of periodic abstinence (rhythm). Except for the IUD, effective use of these methods requires somewhat more effort than simply taking a single pill every morning, but it is an effort that many couples undertake successfully. Your doctor can tell you a great deal more about these methods of contraception.

3. The Dangers of Oral Contraceptives.

a. *Circulatory disorders (abnormal blood clotting and stroke due to hemorrhage).* Blood clots (in various blood vessels of the body) are the most common of the serious side effects of oral contraceptives. A clot can result in a stroke (if the clot is in the brain), a heart attack (if the clot is in a blood vessel of the heart), or a pulmonary embolus (a clot which forms in the legs or pelvis, then breaks off and travels to the lungs). Any of these can be fatal. Clots also occur rarely in the blood vessels of the eye, resulting in blindness or impairment of vision in that eye. There is evidence that the risk of clotting increases with higher estrogen doses. It is, therefore, important to keep the dose of estrogen as low as possible, so long as the oral contraceptive used has an acceptable pregnancy rate and doesn't cause unacceptable changes in the menstrual pattern. Furthermore, cigarette smoking by oral contraceptive users increases the risk of serious adverse effects on the heart and blood vessels. This risk increases with age and with heavy smoking (15 or more cigarettes per day) and begins to become quite marked in women over 35 years of age. For this reason, women who use oral contraceptives should not smoke.

The risk of abnormal clotting increases with age in both users and nonusers of oral contraceptives, but the increased risk from the contraceptives appears to be present at all ages. For oral contraceptive users in general, it has been estimated that in women between the ages of 15 and 34 the risk of death due to a circulatory disorder is about 1 in 12,000 per year, whereas for nonusers the rate is about 1 in 50,000 per year. In the age group 35 to 44, the risk is estimated to be about 1 in 2,500 per year for oral contraceptive users and about 1 in 10,000 per year for nonusers.

Even without the pill the risk of having a heart attack increases with age and is also increased by such heart attack risk factors as high blood pressure, high cholesterol, obesity, diabetes, and cigarette smoking. Without any risk factors present, the use of oral contraceptives alone may double the risk of heart attack. However, the combination of cigarette smoking, especially heavy smoking, and oral contraceptive use greatly increases the risk of heart attack. Oral contraceptive users who smoke are about 5 times more likely to have a heart attack than users who do not smoke and about 10 times more likely to have a heart attack than nonusers who do not smoke. It has been estimated that users between the ages of 30 and 39 who smoke have about a 1 in 10,000 chance each year of having a fatal heart attack compared to about a 1 in 50,000 chance in users who do not smoke, and about a 1 in 100,000 chance in nonusers who do not smoke. In the age group 40 to 44, the risk is about 1 in 1,700 per year for users who smoke compared to about 1 in 10,000 for users who do not smoke and to about 1 in 14,000 per year for nonusers who do not smoke. Heavy smoking (about 15 cigarettes or more a day) further increases the risk. If you do not smoke and have none of the other heart attack risk factors described above, you will have a smaller risk than listed. If you have several heart attack risk factors, the risk may be considerably greater than listed.

In addition to blood-clotting disorders, it has been estimated that women taking oral contraceptives are twice as likely as nonusers to have a stroke due to rupture of a blood vessel in the brain.

b. *Formation of tumors.* Studies have found that when certain animals are given the female sex hormone estrogen, which is an ingredient of oral contraceptives, continuously for long periods, cancers may develop in the breast, cervix, vagina, and liver.

These findings suggest that oral contraceptives may cause cancer in humans. However, studies to date in women taking currently marketed oral contraceptives have not confirmed that oral contraceptives cause cancer in humans. Several studies have found no increase in breast cancer in users, although one study suggested oral contraceptives might cause an increase in breast cancer in women who already have benign breast disease (eg, cysts).

Women with a strong family history of breast cancer or who have breast nodules, fibrocystic disease, or abnormal mammograms or who were exposed to DES (diethylstilbestrol), an estrogen, during their mother's pregnancy must be followed very closely by their doctors if they choose to use oral contraceptives instead of another method of contraception. Many studies have shown that women taking oral contraceptives have less risk of getting benign breast disease than those who have not used oral contraceptives. Recently, strong evidence has emerged that estrogens (one component of oral contraceptives), when given for periods of more than one year to women after the menopause, increase the risk of cancer of the uterus (womb). There is also some evidence that a kind of oral contraceptive which is no longer marketed, the sequential oral contraceptive, may increase the risk of cancer of the uterus. There remains no evidence, however, that the oral contraceptives now available increase the risk of this cancer.

Oral contraceptives do cause, although rarely, a benign (nonmalignant) tumor of the liver. These tumors do not spread, but they may rupture and cause internal bleeding, which may be fatal. A few cases of cancer of the liver have been reported in women using oral contraceptives, but it is not yet known whether the drug caused them.

c. *Dangers to a developing child if oral contraceptives are used in or immediately preceding pregnancy.* Oral contraceptives should not be taken by pregnant women because they may damage the developing child. An increased risk of birth defects, including heart defects and limb defects, has been associated with the use of sex hormones, including oral contraceptives, in pregnancy. In addition, the developing female child whose mother has received DES (diethylstilbestrol), an estrogen, during pregnancy has a risk of getting cancer of the vagina or cervix in her teens or young adulthood. This risk is estimated to be about 1 in 1,000 exposures or less. Abnormalities of the urinary and sex organs have been reported in male offspring so exposed. It is possible that other estrogens, such as the estrogens in oral contraceptives, could have the same effect in the child if the mother takes them during pregnancy.

If you stop taking oral contraceptives to become pregnant, your doctor may recommend that you use another method of contraception for a short while. The reason for this is that there is evidence from studies in women who have had "miscarriages" soon after stopping the pill, that the lost fetuses are more likely to be abnormal. Whether there is an overall increase in "miscarriage" in women who become pregnant soon after stopping the pill, as compared with women who do not use the pill, is not known, but it is possible that there may be. If, however, you do become pregnant soon after stopping oral contraceptives, and do not have a miscarriage, there is no evidence that the baby has an increased risk of being abnormal.

d. *Gallbladder disease.* Women who use oral contraceptives have a greater risk than nonusers of having gallbladder disease requiring surgery. The increased risk may first appear within 1 year of use and may double after 4 or 5 years of use.

e. *Other side effects of oral contraceptives.* Some women using oral contraceptives experience unpleasant side effects that are not dangerous and are not likely to damage their health. Some of these may be temporary. Your breasts may feel tender, nausea and vomiting may occur, you may gain or lose weight, and your ankles may swell. A spotty darkening of the skin, particularly of the face, is possible and may persist. You may notice unexpected vaginal bleeding or changes in your menstrual period. Irregular bleeding is frequently seen when using the mini-pill or combination oral contraceptives containing less than 50 micrograms of estrogen.

More serious side effects include worsening of migraine, asthma, epilepsy, and kidney or heart disease because of a tendency for water to be retained in the body when oral contraceptives are used. Other side effects are growth of preexisting fibroid tumors of the uterus, mental depression, and liver problems with jaundice (yellowing of the skin). Your doctor may find that levels of sugar and fatty substances in your blood are elevated; the long-term effects of these changes are not known. Some women develop high blood pressure while taking oral contraceptives, which ordinarily returns to the original levels when the oral contraceptive is stopped.

Other reactions, although not proved to be caused by oral contraceptives, are occasionally reported. These include more frequent urination and some discomfort when urinating, nervousness, dizziness, some loss of scalp hair, an increase in body hair, an increase or decrease in sex drive, appetite changes, cataracts, and a need for a change in contact lens prescription or inability to use contact lenses.

After you stop using oral contraceptives there may be a delay before you are able to become pregnant or before you resume having menstrual periods. This is especially true of women who had irregular menstrual cycles prior to the use of oral contraceptives. As discussed previously, your doctor may recommend that you wait a short while after stopping the pill before you try to become pregnant. During this time, use another form of contraception. You should consult your physican before resuming use of oral contraceptives after childbirth, especially if you plan to nurse your baby. Drugs in oral contraceptives are known to appear in the milk, and the long-range effect on infants is not known at this time. Furthermore, oral contraceptives may cause a decrease in your milk supply as well as in the quality of the milk.

4. Comparison of the Risks of Oral Contraceptives and Other Contraceptive Methods. The many studies on the risks and effectiveness of oral contraceptives and other methods of contraception have been analyzed to estimate the risk of death associated with various methods of contraception. This risk has two parts: (a) the risk of the method itself (eg, the risk that oral contraceptives will cause death due to abnormal clotting); and (b) the risk of death due to pregnancy or abortion in the event the method fails. The results of this analysis are shown in the following bar graph. The height of the bars is the number of deaths per 100,000 women each year. There are six sets of bars, each set referring to a specific age group of women. Within each set of bars, there is a single bar for each of the different contraceptive methods. For oral contraceptives, there are two bars—one for smokers and the other for nonsmokers. The analysis is based on present knowledge and new information could, of course, alter it. The analysis shows that the risk of death from all methods of birth control is low and below that associated with childbirth, except for oral contraceptives in women over 40 who smoke. It shows that the lowest risk of death is associated with the condom or diaphragm (traditional contraception) backed up by early abortion in case of failure of the condom or diaphragm to prevent pregnancy. Also, at any age the

Figure 1. Estimated annual number of deaths associated with control of fertility and no control per 100,000 nonsterile women, by regimen of control and age of woman.

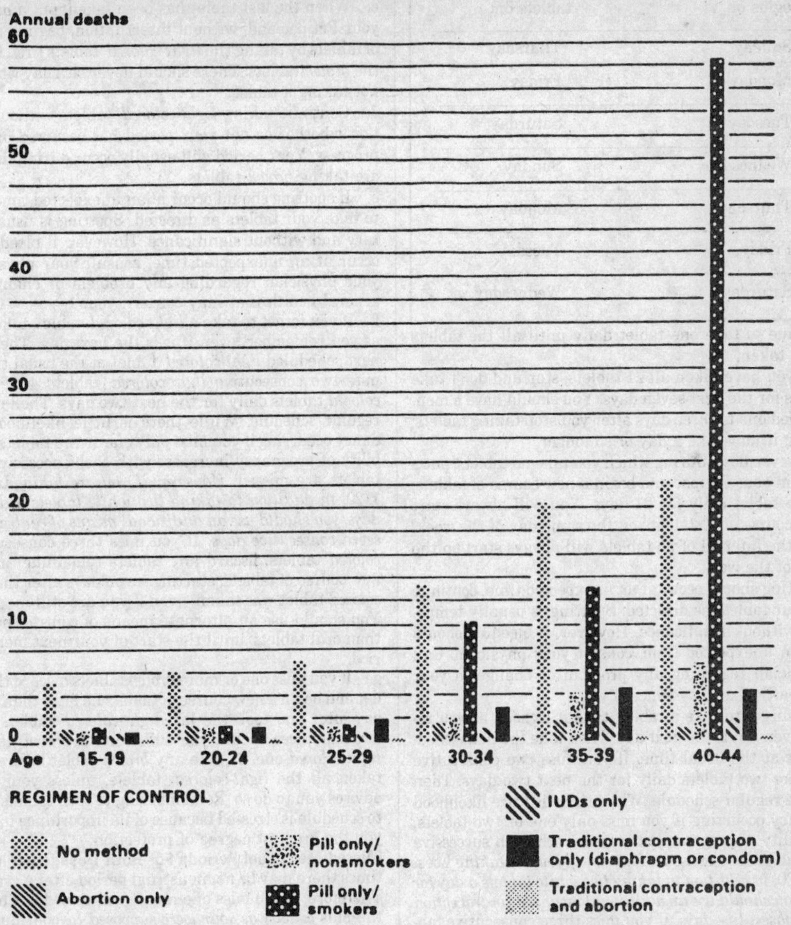

risk of death (due to unexpected pregnancy) from the use of traditional contraception, even without a backup of abortion, is generally the same as or less than that from use of oral contraceptives.

[See Figure 1 above].

How to Use Oral Contraceptives As Safely and Effectively As Possible, Once You Have Decided to Use Them

1. What to Tell your Doctor.

You can make use of the pill as safely as possible, by telling your doctor if you have any of the following:

a. Conditions that mean you should not use oral contraceptives:

Clots in the legs or lungs
Clots in the legs or lungs in the past
A stroke, heart attack, or angina pectoris
Known or suspected cancer of the breast or sex organs
Unusual vaginal bleeding that has not yet been diagnosed
Known or suspected pregnancy

b. Conditions that your doctor will want to watch closely or which might cause him to suggest another method of contraception:

A family history of breast cancer
Breast nodules, fibrocystic disease of the breast, or an abnormal mammogram
Diabetes
High blood pressure
High cholesterol
Cigarette smoking
Migraine headaches
Heart or kidney disease
Epilepsy
Mental depression
Fibroid tumors of the uterus
Gallbladder disease

c. Once you are using oral contraceptives, you should be alert for signs of a serious adverse effect and call your doctor if they occur:

Sharp pain in the chest, coughing blood, or sudden shortness of breath (indicating possible clots in the lungs)
Pain in the calf (possible clot in the leg)
Crushing chest pain or heaviness (indicating possible heart attack)

Sudden severe headache or vomiting, dizziness or fainting, disturbance of vision or speech, or weakness or numbness in an arm or leg (indicating a possible stroke)

Sudden partial or complete loss of vision (indicating a possible clot in the eye)

Breast lumps (you should ask your doctor to show you how to examine your own breasts)

Severe pain in the abdomen (indicating a possible ruptured tumor of the liver)

Severe depression

Yellowing of the skin (jaundice)

2. How to Take the Pill So That It Is Most Effective.

Reduced effectiveness and an increased incidence of breakthrough bleeding have been associated with the use of oral contraceptives with antibiotics such as rifampin, ampicillin, and tetracycline or with certain other drugs, such as barbiturates, phenylbutazone or phenytoin sodium. You should use an additional means of contraception during any cycle in which any of these drugs are taken.

Directions For 21-Day Dosage Regimen

a. The first day of your period is Day 1. On the fifth day (Day 5), start taking one tablet daily, beginning with the tablet in the upper left corner of the Petipac. In the space provided, write the day you start. To remove a tablet, press down on it with your thumb or finger. The tablet will drop through a hole in the bottom of the Petipac. Do not press on the tablet with your thumbnail or fingernail, or any other sharp object.

Continued on next page

This product information was prepared in August, 1986. On these and other Parke-Davis Products, information may be obtained by addressing PARKE-DAVIS, Division of Warner-Lambert Company, Morris Plains, New Jersey 07950.

Parke-Davis—Cont.

If your period begins on:	Start taking tablets on:
Sunday	Thursday
Monday	Friday
Tuesday	Saturday
Wednesday	Sunday
Thursday	Monday
Friday	Tuesday
Saturday	Wednesday

b. Continue to take one tablet daily until all the tablets have been taken.
c. After you have taken all 21 tablets, stop and don't take any tablets for the next seven days. You should have a menstrual period one to three days after you stop taking tablets; sometimes, it may take a day or so longer.
d. After seven days, during which you take no tablets, put a new refill in your Petipac and begin a new course of tablets, taking one tablet daily for 21 days. You will always start each new course of 21 tablets on the same day of the week. Likewise, the interval of no tablets will always start on the same day of the week.
e. If spotting should occur at an unexpected time, continue to take your tablets as directed. Spotting is usually temporary and without significance. However, if bleeding should occur at an unexpected time, consult your physician. Call your physician regarding any problem or change in your general health that may concern you.
f. If you forget to take a tablet, take it as soon as you remember, even if it is the next day. Then take the next scheduled tablet at the usual time. If you miss two consecutive tablets, take two tablets daily for the next two days. Then resume the regular schedule. While there is little likelihood of pregnancy occurring if you miss only one or two tablets, the possibility of pregnancy increases with each successive day that tablets are missed. *However, if you are taking* Loestrin **21** 1/20, *in addition to taking two white tablets a day for two days, you should use an additional means of contraception for seven consecutive days.* If you miss three consecutive tablets, discard any tablets remaining and begin a new course of tablets, starting seven days after the last tablet was taken, even if you are still menstruating. You should use an alternate means of contraception, other than oral tablets, until the start of your next menstrual period.
Remembering to take tablets according to schedule is stressed because of its importance in providing you the greatest degree of protection.

Directions For 28-Day Dosage Regimen
a. The first day of your period is Day 1. On the fifth day (Day 5), start taking one *light-colored* tablet daily, beginning with the tablet in the upper left corner of the Petipac. In the space provided, write the day you start. Take all the tablets in the top row first, followed by the second row, and so on. To remove a tablet, press down on it with your thumb or finger. The tablet will drop through a hole in the bottom of the Petipac. Do not press on the tablet with your thumbnail or fingernail, or any other sharp object.

If your period begins on:	Start taking tablets on:
Sunday	Thursday
Monday	Friday
Tuesday	Saturday
Wednesday	Sunday
Thursday	Monday
Friday	Tuesday
Saturday	Wednesday

b. On the day after taking the last *light-colored* tablet, begin taking one *brown* tablet daily until all the tablets have been taken.
c. When the last tablet has been taken, put a new refill in your Petipac and, without interruption, begin a new course of tablets by taking the *light-colored* tablets first, followed by the *brown* tablets. There should never be a day when you are not taking a tablet.
d. Continue taking *light-colored* tablets without interruption whether or not your period has occurred or is still in progress. Your period will usually occur during the time you are taking *brown* tablets.
e. If spotting should occur at an unexpected time, continue to take your tablets as directed. Spotting is usually temporary and without significance. However, if bleeding should occur at an unexpected time, consult your physician. Call your physician regarding any problem or change in your general health that may concern you.
f. If you forget to take a *light-colored* tablet, take it as soon as you remember, even if it is the next day. Then take the next scheduled *light-colored* tablet at the usual time. If you miss two consecutive *light-colored* tablets, take two *light-colored* tablets daily for the next two days. Then resume the regular schedule. While there is little likelihood of pregnancy occurring if you miss only one or two tablets, the possibility of pregnancy increases with each successive day that tablets are missed. *However, if you are taking* Loestrin **Fe** 1/20, *in addition to taking two white tablets a day for two days, you should use an additional means of contraception for seven consecutive days.* If you miss three consecutive *light-colored* tablets discard any tablets remaining and begin a new course of tablets, starting seven days after the last *light-colored* tablet was taken, even if you are still menstruating. You should use an alternate means of contraception, other than oral tablets, until the start of your next menstrual period.
g. If you miss one or more *brown* tablets discard the remainder and begin a new course of tablets no later than the eighth day after you took the last *light-colored* tablet. Under no circumstances should you substitute a *brown* tablet for a *light-colored* one, or take any *brown* tablet before you have taken all the *light-colored* tablets, unless your physician advises you to do so. Remembering to take tablets according to schedule is stressed because of its importance in providing you the greatest degree of protection.

Missed Menstrual Periods For Both Dosage Regimens: At times there may be no menstrual period after a cycle of pills. Therefore, if you miss one menstrual period but have taken the pills *exactly as your were supposed to,* continue as usual into the next cycle. If you have not taken the pills correctly and miss a menstrual period, *you may be pregnant* and should stop taking oral contraceptives until your doctor determines whether or not you are pregnant. Until you can get to your doctor, use another form of contraception. If two consecutive menstrual periods are missed, you should stop taking pills until it is determined whether you are pregnant. If you do become pregnant while using oral contraceptives, you should discuss the risks to the developing child with your doctor.
Periodic Examination
Your doctor will take a complete medical and family history before prescribing oral contraceptives. At that time and about once a year thereafter, he will generally examine your blood pressure, breasts, abdomen, and pelvic organs (including a Papanicolaou smear, ie, test for cancer).

SUMMARY

Oral contraceptives are the most effective method, except sterilization, for preventing pregnancy. Other methods, when used conscientiously, are also very effective and have fewer risks. Although the serious risks of oral contraceptives are uncommon, some of the risks may persist after you stop using the pill. On the other hand, the "pill" is a very convenient method of preventing pregnancy.
If you have certain conditions or have had these conditions in the past, you should not use oral contraceptives because the risk is too great. These conditions are listed in this leaflet. If you do not have these conditions, and decide to use the "pill," please read this leaflet carefully so that you can use the "pill" most safely and effectively.
Based on his or her assessment of your medical needs, your doctor has prescribed this drug for you. Do not give this drug to anyone else.

0913G151

Shown in Product Identification Section, page 420

Lopid

HLP Type	TRIGLYCERIDE	CHOLESTEROL				RATIO:
		Total	VLDL	LDL	HDL	HDL Cholesterol / Total Cholesterol
IIa	−44%	−4.2%	−44.3%	−5.8%	+24.6%	+33%
IIb	−45%	−8.6%	−45.0%	−6.4%	+19.5%	+34%
IV	−40%	−1.8%	−40.8%	+14.6%	+17.4%	+23%

LOPID® ℞

[lō′pĭd]
(gemfibrozil capsules, USP)

DESCRIPTION

LOPID (gemfibrozil) is a lipid regulating agent. It is available as capsules for oral administration. Each capsule contains 300 mg gemfibrozil. The chemical name is 5-(2,5-dimethylphenoxy)-2,2-dimethylpentanoic acid.
The empirical formula is $C_{15}H_{22}O_3$ and the molecular weight is 250.35; the solubility in water and acid is 0.0019% and in dilute base it is greater than 1%. The melting point is 58°-61°C. Gemfibrozil is a white solid which is stable under ordinary conditions.

CLINICAL PHARMACOLOGY

LOPID is a lipid regulating agent which lowers elevated serum lipids primarily by decreasing serum triglyceride with a variable reduction in total serum cholesterol. These decreases occur primarily in the very low density lipoprotein (VLDL) fraction and less frequently in the low density lipoprotein (LDL) fraction. It has been reported that Lopid may increase levels of high density lipoprotein (HDL) subfractions, HDL_2 and HDL_3 as well as apolipoproteins AI and AII. Epidemiological studies have shown that both low HDL-cholesterol and high LDL-cholesterol are independent risk factors for coronary heart disease. It is not yet known whether pharmacological interventions designed to raise HDL-cholesterol alter morbidity or mortality due to coronary heart disease. The mechanism of action has not been definitively established. In man, LOPID has been shown to inhibit peripheral lipolysis and to decrease the hepatic extraction of free fatty acids, thus reducing hepatic triglyceride production. LOPID inhibits synthesis and increases clearance of VLDL carrier apolipoprotein B, leading to a decrease in VLDL production.
Animal studies suggest that LOPID may, in addition to elevating HDL cholesterol, reduce incorporation of long-chain fatty acids into newly formed triglycerides, accelerate turnover and removal of cholesterol from the liver, and increase excretion of cholesterol in the feces.
LOPID is well absorbed from the gastrointestinal tract after oral administration. Peak plasma levels occur in one to two hours with a plasma half-life of 1.5 hours following single doses and 1.3 hours following multiple doses. Plasma levels appear proportional to dose and do not demonstrate accumulation across time following multiple doses.
LOPID mainly undergoes oxidation of a ring methyl group to successively form a hydroxymethyl and a carboxyl metabolite. Approximately seventy percent of the administered human dose is excreted in the urine, primarily as unchanged gemfibrozil. Six percent of the dose is accounted for in the feces. In a large, controlled multicenter trial of 427 patients, lipid and lipoprotein changes from average baseline (%) by hyperlipoproteinemic (HLP) type are summarized below for those patients receiving gemfibrozil, 1200 mg/day, at the end of 12 weeks.
[See table left].

INDICATIONS AND USAGE

Drug therapy should not be used for the routine treatment of elevated blood lipids for the prevention of coronary heart disease. Dietary therapy specific for the type of hyperlipidemia is the initial treatment of choice. Excess body weight and excess alcoholic intake may be important factors in hypertriglyceridemia and should be addressed prior to any drug therapy. Physical exercise can be an important ancillary measure.
Contributory diseases such as hypothyroidism or diabetes mellitus should be looked for and adequately treated. The use of drugs should be considered only when reasonable attempts have been made to obtain satisfactory results with nondrug methods. If the decision is to use drugs, the patient should be instructed that this does not reduce the importance of adhering to diet.
Because of chemical, pharmacological, and clinical similarities between gemfibrozil and clofibrate, and the adverse findings with clofibrate in two large clinical studies (see Warnings), use of gemfibrozil should be restricted to the following indications. LOPID may be considered for the treatment of adult patients with very high serum triglyceride levels (type IV or type V hyperlipoproteinemia) who present a risk of abdominal pain and pancreatitis and who do not respond adequately to a determined dietary effort to control them. Patients with triglyceride levels in excess of 750 mg per deciliter are likely to present such risk. LOPID (gemfibrozil) has little effect on elevated cholesterol levels in most subjects. A minority of subjects show a more pronounced response. Therefore, the physician should be very selective and confine gemfibrozil treatment to patients with clearly defined risk due to severe hypercholesterolemia (eg, individuals with familial hypercholesterolemia starting in childhood) who inadequately respond to appropriate diet and more effective cholesterol-lowering drugs.
LOPID is not useful for the hypertriglyceridemia of Type I hyperlipidemia.

The biochemical response to gemfibrozil is variable, and it is not always possible to predict from the lipoprotein type or other factors which patients will obtain favorable results. It is essential that lipid levels be assessed and that the drug be discontinued after three months in any patient in whom lipids do not show significant improvement.
The effect of drug-induced reduction of serum cholesterol or triglyceride levels or elevation of HDL cholesterol levels on morbidity or mortality due to coronary heart disease has not been established. Several years may be required before ongoing long-term investigations will resolve this question.

CONTRAINDICATIONS

1. Hepatic or severe renal dysfunction, including primary biliary cirrhosis.
2. Preexisting gallbladder disease. (See Warnings).
3. Hypersensitivity to gemfibrozil.

WARNINGS

1. Because of chemical, pharmacological, and clinical similarities between gemfibrozil and clofibrate, the adverse findings with clofibrate in two large clinical studies may also apply to gemfibrozil. In the first of those studies, the Coronary Drug Project, 1000 subjects with previous myocardial infarction were treated for five years with clofibrate. There was no difference in mortality between the clofibrate-treated subjects and 3000 placebo-treated subjects, but twice as many clofibrate-treated subjects developed cholelithiasis and cholecystitis requiring surgery. In the other study, conducted by the World Health Organization, 5000 subjects without known coronary heart disease were treated with clofibrate for five years and followed one year beyond. There was a statistically significant 36% higher total mortality in the clofibrate-treated than in a comparable placebo-treated control group. The excess mortality was due to noncardiovascular causes, including malignancy, postcholecystectomy complications, and pancreatitis. The higher risk of clofibrate-treated subjects for gallbladder disease was confirmed.
2. Long-Term Toxicity and Animal Tumorigenicity Studies: Long-term studies have been conducted in rats and mice at one and ten times the human dose. The incidence of benign liver nodules and liver carcinomas was significantly increased in high dose male rats. The incidence of liver carcinomas increased also in low dose males, but this increase was not statistically significant (p greater than 0.05). There were no statistically significant differences from controls in the incidence of liver tumors in female rats, and in male and female mice.
Electron microscopy studies have demonstrated a florid hepatic peroxisome proliferation following LOPID administration to the male rat. Similar changes have not been found in the human liver.
Male rats had a dose-related increase of benign Leydig cell tumors. Subcapsular bilateral cataracts occurred in 10%, and unilateral in 6.3% of the high dose males.
3. Since a reduction of mortality from coronary artery disease has not been demonstrated and liver and interstitial cell testicular tumors were increased in male rats, LOPID should be administered only to those patients described in the Indications and Usage Section. If a significant serum lipid response is not obtained, LOPID should be discontinued.
4. Cholelithiasis—LOPID may increase cholesterol excretion into the bile leading to cholelithiasis. If cholelithiasis is suspected gallbladder studies are indicated. LOPID therapy should be discontinued if gallstones are found.
5. Concomitant Anticoagulants—Caution should be exercised when anticoagulants are given in conjunction with LOPID. The dosage of the anticoagulant should be reduced to maintain the prothrombin time at the desired level to prevent bleeding complications. Frequent prothrombin determinations are advisable until it has been definitely determined that the prothrombin level has stabilized.

PRECAUTIONS

1. **Initial Therapy**—Before instituting LOPID (gemfibrozil) therapy, every attempt should be made to control serum lipids with appropriate diet, exercise, weight loss in obese patients, and other medical problems such as diabetes mellitus and hypothyroidism.
2. **Continued Therapy**—Pretreatment laboratory studies should be performed to ensure that patients have abnormal levels of serum lipids. Periodic determinations of serum lipids should be obtained during LOPID administration. The drug should be withdrawn after three months if the lipid response is inadequate.
3. **Impairment of Fertility**—Administration of approximately three and ten times the human dose to male rats for 10 weeks resulted in a dose-related decrease of fertility. Subsequent studies demonstrated that this effect was reversed after a drug-free period of about eight weeks, and it was not transmitted to their offspring.
4. **Pregnancy Category B**—Reproduction studies have been performed in the rat at doses 3 and 9 times the human dose, and in the rabbit at 2 and 6.7 times the human dose. These studies have revealed no evidence of impaired fertility in females or harm to the fetus due to LOPID. Minor fetotoxicity was manifested by reduced birth rates observed at the high dose levels. No significant malformations were found among almost 400 offspring from 36 litters of rats and 100 fetuses from 22 litters of rabbits.
There are no studies in pregnant women. In view of the fact that LOPID is tumorigenic in male rats, the use of LOPID in pregnancy should be reserved for those patients where the benefit clearly outweighs the possible risk to the patient or fetus.
5. **Nursing Mothers**—Because of the potential for tumorigenicity shown for gemfibrozil in male rats, a decision should be made whether to discontinue nursing or discontinue the drug, taking into account the importance of the drug to the mother.
6. **Hematologic Changes**—Mild hemoglobin, hematocrit and white blood cell decreases have been observed in occasional patients following initiation of LOPID therapy. However, these levels stabilize during long-term administration. Therefore, periodic blood counts are recommended during the first 12 months of LOPID administration.
7. **Liver Function**—Abnormal liver function tests have been observed occasionally during LOPID administration, including elevations of SGOT, SGPT, LDH, and alkaline phosphatase. These are usually reversible when LOPID is discontinued. Therefore periodic liver function studies are recommended and LOPID therapy should be terminated if abnormalities persist.
8. **Use in Children**—Safety and efficacy in children have not been established.

ADVERSE REACTIONS

In controlled clinical trials of 805 patients, including 245 who received LOPID for at least one year, the most frequently reported adverse reactions associated with LOPID involved the gastrointestinal system. In decreasing order of frequency, these were abdominal pain (6.0%), epigastric pain (4.9%), diarrhea (4.8%), nausea (4.0%), vomiting (1.6%), and flatulence (1.1%). Other adverse reactions where the probability of a causal relationship to LOPID therapy exists are listed by system.

Integumentary: rash, dermatitis, pruritus, urticaria
Central Nervous System: headache, dizziness, blurred vision
Musculoskeletal: painful extremities
Hematopoietic: anemia, eosinophilia, leukopenia

Other reactions have been reported under conditions where a causal relationship is difficult to establish, thus the physician should be alert to these occurrences. Reports of viral and bacterial infections (common cold, cough, and urinary tract infections) were more common in gemfibrozil than in placebo-treated patients.

Other reactions were:
Gastrointestinal: dry mouth, constipation, anorexia, gas pain, dyspepsia
Musculoskeletal: back pain, arthralgia, muscle cramps, myalgia, swollen joints
Central Nervous System: vertigo, insomnia, paresthesia, tinnitus
Clinical Laboratory: hypokalemia, liver function abnormalities (increased SGOT, SGPT, LDH, CPK, alkaline phosphatase)
Miscellaneous: fatigue, malaise, syncope, alopecia

DOSAGE AND ADMINISTRATION

The recommended dose for adults is 1200 mg administered in two divided doses 30 minutes before the morning and evening meal. Some patients will experience therapeutic effects on 900 mg/day; a few may require 1500 mg/day for satisfactory results.

DRUG INTERACTIONS

CAUTION SHOULD BE EXERCISED WHEN ANTICOAGULANTS ARE GIVEN IN CONJUNCTION WITH LOPID (GEMFIBROZIL). THE DOSAGE OF THE ANTICOAGULANT SHOULD BE REDUCED TO MAINTAIN THE PROTHROMBIN TIME AT THE DESIRED LEVEL TO PREVENT BLEEDING COMPLICATIONS. FREQUENT PROTHROMBIN DETERMINATIONS ARE ADVISABLE UNTIL IT HAS BEEN DEFINITELY DETERMINED THAT THE PROTHROMBIN LEVEL HAS STABILIZED.

MANAGEMENT OF OVERDOSAGE

While there has been no reported case of overdosage, symptomatic supportive measures should be taken should it occur.

HOW SUPPLIED

LOPID (Capsule 669), white and maroon opaque capsules, each containing 300 mg gemfibrozil, are available as follows:
N 0071-0669-24 Bottles of 100
N 0071-0669-30 Bottles of 500
Parcode® No. 669.
Storage: Store below 30°C (86°F).

0669G016

Shown in Product Identification Section, page 420

MANDELAMINE® TABLETS ℞
[*măn "dĕ 'lă-mīne*]
(methenamine mandelate tablets, USP)

MANDELAMINE SUSPENSION FORTE, 500 mg/5ml ℞

MANDELAMINE SUSPENSION, 250 mg/5ml ℞
(methenamine mandelate oral suspension, USP)

MANDELAMINE GRANULES ℞
(methenamine mandelate)

DESCRIPTION

Mandelamine (methenamine mandelate, USP), a urinary antibacterial agent, is the chemical combination of mandelic acid with methenamine. Mandelamine is available for oral use as film-coated tablets, suspension, and granules.
Each tablet contains 0.5 g or 1.0 g of methenamine mandelate, USP; and also contains calcium stearate, NF; candelilla wax; colloidal silicon dioxide, NF; croscarmellose sodium, NF; hydroxypropylmethylcellulose; Opaspray brown (0.5 g tablet) or Opaspray purple (1.0 g tablet); povidone, USP; propylene glycol, USP; and silica gel.
Each teaspoonful of suspension contains 250 mg or 500 mg of methenamine mandelate, USP; and also contains flavors; propylparaben, NF; saccharin sodium, USP; sesame oil, NF and thixcin. The 500 mg per teaspoonful suspension also contains FD&C red No. 3 Lake.
Each packet of granules contains 0.5 g or 1.0 g of methenamine mandelate, USP; and also contains colloidal silicon dioxide, NF; D&C yellow No. 10; FD&C yellow No. 6; flavors; povidone, USP; saccharin sodium, USP; and sucrose, NF.

CLINICAL PHARMACOLOGY

Mandelamine is readily absorbed but remains essentially inactive until it is excreted by the kidney and concentrated in the urine. An acid urine is essential for antibacterial action, with maximum efficacy occurring at pH 5.5 or less. In an acid urine, mandelic acid exerts its antibacterial action and also contributes to the acidification of the urine. Mandelic acid is excreted by both glomerular filtration and tubular excretion. The methenamine component, in an acid urine, is hydrolyzed to ammonia and to the bactericidal agent formaldehyde. There is equally effective antibacterial activity against both gram-positive and gram-negative organisms, since the antibacterial action of mandelic acid and formaldehyde is nonspecific. There are reports that Mandelamine is ineffective in some infections with *Proteus vulgaris* and urea-splitting strains of *Pseudomonas aeruginosa* and *A aerogenes.* Since urea-splitting strains may raise the pH of the urine, particular attention to supplementary acidification is required. However, results in any single case will depend to a large extent on the underlying pathology and the overall management.

INDICATIONS AND USAGE

Mandelamine is indicated for the suppression or elimination of bacteriuria associated with pyelonephritis, cystitis, and other chronic urinary tract infections; also for infected residual urine sometimes accompanying neurologic diseases. When used as recommended, Mandelamine is particularly suitable for long-term therapy because of its safety and because resistance to the nonspecific bactericidal action of formaldehyde does not develop. Pathogens resistant to other antibacterial agents may respond to Mandelamine because of the non-specific effect of formaldehyde formed in an acid urine.
Prophylactic use rationale: Urine is a good culture medium for many urinary pathogens. Inoculation by a few organisms (relapse or reinfection) may lead to bacteriuria in susceptible individuals. Thus, the rationale of management in recurring urinary tract infection (bacteriuria) is to change the urine from a growth-supporting to a growth-inhibiting medium. There is a growing body of evidence that long-term administration of Mandelamine can prevent the recurrence of bacteriuria in patients with chronic pyelonephritis.
Therapeutic use rationale: Mandelamine helps to sterilize the urine, and in some situations in which underlying pathologic conditions prevent sterilization by any means, it can help to suppress the bacteriuria. Mandelamine should not be used alone for acute infections with parenchymal involvement causing systemic symptoms such as chills and fever. A thorough diagnostic investigation as a part of the overall management of the urinary tract infection should accompany the use of Mandelamine.

Continued on next page

This product information was prepared in August, 1986. On these and other Parke-Davis Products, information may be obtained by addressing PARKE-DAVIS, Division of Warner-Lambert Company, Morris Plains, New Jersey 07950.

Parke-Davis—Cont.

CONTRAINDICATIONS

Contraindicated in renal insufficiency.
Mandelamine should not be used in patients who have previously exhibited hypersensitivity to it.

PRECAUTIONS

General: Dysuria may occur (usually at higher than recommended dosage). This can be controlled by reducing the dosage and the acidification. When urine acidification is contraindicated or unattainable (as with some urea-splitting bacteria), the drug is not recommended.
To avoid inducing lipid pneumonia, administer Mandelamine Suspension Forte and Mandelamine Suspension with care to elderly, debilitated or otherwise susceptible patients.
Drug Interactions: Formaldehyde and sulfamethizole form an insoluble precipitate in acid urine; therefore, Mandelamine should not be administered concurrently with sulfamethizole.
Drug/Laboratory Test Interactions: Formaldehyde interferes with fluorometric procedures for determination of urinary catecholamines and vanilmandelic acid (VMA) causing erroneously high results. Formaldehyde also causes falsely decreased urine estriol levels by reacting with estriol when acid hydrolysis techniques are used; estriol determinations which use enzymatic hydrolysis are unaffected by formaldehyde. Formaldehyde causes falsely elevated 17-hydroxycorticosteroid levels when the Porter-Silber method is used and falsely decreased 5-hydroxy-indoleacetic acid (5HIAA) levels by inhibiting color development when nitrosonaphthol methods are used.
Pregnancy Category C. Animal reproduction studies have not been conducted with Mandelamine. It is also not known whether Mandelamine can cause fetal harm when administered to a pregnant woman or can affect reproduction capacity. Mandelamine should be given to a pregnant woman only if clearly needed.
Since introduction, published reports on the use of Mandelamine in pregnant women have not shown an increased risk of fetal abnormalities from use during pregnancy.

ADVERSE REACTIONS

An occasional patient may experience gastrointestinal disturbance or a generalized skin rash. Microscopic and rarely gross hematuria have been described.

DOSAGE AND ADMINISTRATION

Directions for using Granules: dissolve contents of packet in 2–4 oz of water immediately before using. Solution formed may remain turbid.
Suspensions: Shake well before using.
The average adult dosage is 4 grams daily given as 1.0 gram after each meal and at bedtime. Children 6 to 12 should receive half the adult dose and children under 6 years of age should receive 250 mg per 30 lb body weight, four times daily. (See chart.) Since an acid urine is essential for antibacterial activity, with maximum efficacy occurring at pH 5.5 or below, restriction of alkalinizing foods and medication is thus desirable. If testing of urine pH reveals the need, supplemental acidification should be given.

DOSAGES

Dosage	Adults	Children
Tablets and Granules		
1.0 gram	1 tablet qid	—
	1 packet qid	—
0.5 gram	2 tablets qid	(Ages 6–12) 1 tablet qid
	—	(Ages 6–12) 1 packet qid
Suspension Forte		
500 mg/ 5 ml teasp.	2 teaspoonfuls (10 ml) qid	(Ages 6–12) 1 teaspoonful (5 ml) qid
Suspension		
250 mg/5 ml teasp.	—	(Age under 6) 1 teaspoonful (5 ml) per 30 lb body weight qid

HOW SUPPLIED

Mandelamine Tablets are supplied as:
N 0071-0166-24 0.5 g—Bottles of 100
N 0071-0166-32 0.5 g—Bottles of 1000
N 0071-0166-40 0.5 g—Unit dose packages of 100 (10 × 10 strips)
Each tablet is film coated, brown, and bears the P-D 166 monogram.
N 0071-0167-24 1.0 g—Bottles of 100
N 0071-0167-30 1.0 g—Bottles of 500
N 0071-0167-40 1.0 g—Unit dose packages of 100 (10 × 10 strips)
Each tablet is film coated, and bears the P-D 167 monogram.
Mandelamine Granules are supplied as:
N 0071-2177-02 0.5 g—Cartons of 56 individual packets.
N 0071-2176-03 1.0 g—Cartons of 56 individual packets.
Granules are orange flavored.
Mandelamine Suspension is supplied as:
N 0071-2173-23 250 mg/5 ml—Bottles of 16 fl oz
Suspension is cream colored, coconut flavored, and in vegetable oil.
Mandelamine Suspension Forte is supplied as:
N 0071-2174-20 500 mg/5 ml—Bottles of 8 fl oz
N 0071-2174-23 500 mg/5 ml—Bottles of 16 fl oz
Suspension is rosy pink, cherry flavored, and in vegetable oil.
Store between 15°–30°C (59°–86°F).

0166G035

Shown in Product Identification Section, page 420

MECLOMEN® ℞

[mĕʹclō″mĕn]
(Meclofenamate Sodium Capsules, USP)

DESCRIPTION

Meclomen (meclofenamate sodium) is N-(2, 6-dichloro-m-tolyl) anthranilic acid, sodium salt, monohydrate. It is an antiinflammatory drug for oral administration. Meclomen capsules contain 50 mg or 100 mg meclofenamic acid as the sodium salt. Also contain lactose, NF, magnesium stearate, NF; silica gel, NF; sodium lauryl sulfate, NF. The capsule shell contains colloidal silicon dioxide, NF, FD&C yellow No. 6, gelatin, NF, sodium lauryl sulfate, NF, titanium dioxide, USP.
It is a white powder with melting point 287° to 291°C, molecular weight 336.15, and water solubility greater than 250 mg/ml.

CLINICAL PHARMACOLOGY

Meclomen is a nonsteroidal agent which has demonstrated antiinflammatory, analgesic, and antipyretic activity in laboratory animals. The mode of action, like that of other nonsteroidal antiinflammatory agents, is not known. Therapeutic action does not result from pituitary-adrenal stimulation. In animal studies, Meclomen was found to inhibit prostaglandin synthesis and to compete for binding at the prostaglandin receptor site. These properties may be responsible for the antiinflammatory action of Meclomen. There is no evidence that Meclomen alters the course of the underlying disease.
Following a single oral dose to normal human volunteers, peak plasma levels occurred in 0.5 to 1 hr, with a half-life of 2 hr (3.3 hr following multiple doses). Plasma levels are proportional to dose. There is no evidence of accumulation of drug. Urinary and fecel excretion of tritium-labeled Meclomen account for 80% to 102% of the total dose, with about two thirds appearing in urine and one third in feces. Most of the urinary excretion occurs as the glucuronide conjugates of the metabolites, with only small amounts of free drug recovered.
In several human isotope studies, Meclomen, at a dosage of 300 mg/day, produced a fecal blood loss of 1 to 2 ml per day, and 2 to 3 ml per day at 400 mg/day. Aspirin, at a dosage of 3.6 g/day, caused a fecal blood loss of 6 ml per day.
In a multiple-dose, one-week study in normal human volunteers, Meclomen had little or no effect on collagen-induced platelet aggregation, platelet count, or bleeding time. In comparison, aspirin suppressed collagen-induced platelet aggregation and increased bleeding time. The concomitant administration of antacids (aluminum and magnesium hydroxides) does not interfere with absorption of Meclomen.
Controlled clinical trials comparing Meclomen with aspirin demonstrated comparable efficacy in rheumatoid arthritis. The Meclomen-treated patients had fewer reactions involving the special senses, specifically tinnitus, but more gastrointestinal reactions, specifically diarrhea.
The incidence of patients who discontinued therapy due to adverse reactions was similar for both the Meclomen and aspirin-treated groups.
The improvement with Meclomen reported by patients and the reduction of the disease activity as evaluated by both physicians and patients with rheumatoid arthritis are associated with a significant reduction in number of tender joints, severity of tenderness, and duration of morning stiffness.
The improvement reported by patients and as evaluated by physicians in patients treated with Meclomen for osteoarthritis is associated with a significant reduction in night pain, pain on walking, degree of starting pain, and pain on passive motion. The function of knee joints also improved significantly.
Meclomen has been used in combination with gold salts or corticosteroids in patients with rheumatoid arthritis. Studies have demonstrated that Meclomen contributes to the improvement of patients' conditions while maintained on gold salts or corticosteroids. Data are inadequate to demonstrate that Meclomen in combination with salicylates produces greater improvement than that achieved with Meclomen alone.

INDICATIONS AND USAGE

Meclomen is indicated for relief of the signs and symptoms of acute and chronic rheumatoid arthritis and osteoarthritis.
As with all nonsteroidal antiinflammatory drugs, selection of Meclomen requires a careful assessment of the benefit/risk ratio. (See Warnings, Precautions and Adverse Reactions sections.)
The safety and effectiveness of Meclomen have not been established in those patients with rheumatoid arthritis who are designated by the American Rheumatism Association as Functional Class IV (incapacitated, largely or wholly bedridden, or confined to a wheelchair, little or no self-care).
Meclomen is not recommended in children because adequate studies to demonstrate safety and efficacy have not been carried out.

CONTRAINDICATIONS

Meclomen should not be used in patients who have previously exhibited hypersensitivity to it.
Because the potential exists for cross sensitivity to aspirin or other nonsteroidal antiinflammatory drugs, Meclomen should not be given to patients in whom these drugs induce symptoms of bronchospasm, allergic rhinitis, or urticaria.

WARNINGS

In patients with a history of upper gastrointestinal tract disease, Meclomen should be given under close supervision and only after consulting the Adverse Reactions section.
Peptic ulceration and gastrointestinal bleeding, sometimes severe, including one fatality, have been reported in patients receiving Meclomen.
Diarrhea, gastrointestinal irritation, and abdominal pain may be associated with Meclomen therapy. Dosage reduction or temporarily stopping the drug have generally controlled these symptoms. (See Adverse Reactions and Dosage and Administration sections.)

PRECAUTIONS

General: Patients receiving nonsteroidal antiinflammatory agents, such as Meclomen, should be evaluated periodically to insure that the drug is still necessary and well tolerated. (See other Precautions, Warnings, and Adverse Reactions.)
Diarrhea, gastrointestinal irritation and abdominal pain may be associated with Meclomen therapy. Dosage reduction or temporarily stopping the drug have generally controlled these symptoms. (See Adverse Reactions and Dosage and Administration sections).
Decreases in hemoglobin and/or hematocrit levels have occurred in approximately 1 of 6 patients, but rarely required discontinuation of Meclomen therapy. The clinical data revealed no evidence of increased chronic blood loss, bone-marrow suppression, or hemolysis to account for the decreases in hemoglobin or hematocrit levels. Patients who are receiving long-term Meclomen therapy should have hemoglobin and hematocrit values determined if anemia is suspected on clinical grounds.
If a patient develops visual symptoms (see Adverse Reactions) during Meclomen therapy, the drug should be discontinued and the patient should have a complete ophthalmologic examination.
When Meclomen is used in combination with steroid therapy, any reduction in steroid dosage should be gradual to avoid the possible complications of sudden steroid withdrawal.
Adverse effects are seen more commonly in the elderly, therefore a lower starting dose and careful follow-up are advised.
As with other nonsteroidal antiinflammatory drugs, borderline evalutions of one or more liver tests may occur in some patients. These abnormalities may progress, may remain essentially unchanged, or may be transient with continued therapy. The SGPT (ALT) test is probably the most sensitive indicator of liver dysfunction. Meaningful (3 times the upper limit of normal) elevations of SGPT or SGOT (AST) occurred in controlled clinical trials in less than 1% of patients. A patient with symptoms and/or signs suggesting liver dysfunction, or in whom an abnormal liver test has occurred, should be evaluated for evidence of the development of more severe hepatic reaction while on therapy with Meclomen. Severe hepatic reactions, including jaundice and cases of fatal hepatitis, have been reported with other nonsteroidal antiinflammatory drugs. Although such reactions are rare, if abnormal liver tests persist or worsen, if clinical signs and symptoms consistent with liver disease develop, or if sys-

temic manifestations occur (eg, eosinophilia, rash), Meclomen should be discontinued.

Renal Effects: As with other nonsteroidal antiinflammatory drugs, long-term administration of meclofenamate sodium to animals has resulted in renal papillary necrosis and other abnormal renal pathology. In humans, there have been reports of acute interstitial nephritis with hematuria, proteinuria, and occasionally nephrotic syndrome.

A second form of renal toxicity has been seen in patients with prerenal conditions leading to a reduction in renal blood flow or blood volume, where the renal prostaglandins have a supportive role in the maintenance of renal perfusion. In these patients administration of an NSAID may cause a dose-dependent reduction in prostaglandin formation and may precipitate overt renal decompensation. Patients at greatest risk of this reaction are those with impaired renal function, heart failure, liver dysfunction, those taking diuretics, and the elderly. Discontinuation of NSAID therapy is typically followed by recovery to the pretreatment state.

Since Meclomen is eliminated primarily by the kidneys, patients with significantly impaired renal function should be closely monitored; a lower daily dosage should be anticipated to avoid excessive drug accumulation.

Information for Patients: Patients should be advised that nausea, vomiting, diarrhea, and abdominal pain have been associated with the use of Meclomen. The patient should be made aware of a possible drug connection and accordingly should consider discontinuing the drug and contacting his or her physician if any of these conditions are severe.

Meclomen may be taken with meals or milk to control gastrointestinal complaints. Concomitant administration of an antacid (specifically, aluminum and magnesium hydroxides) does not interfere with the absorption of the drug.

Laboratory Tests: Patients receiving long-term Meclomen therapy should have hemoglobin and hematocrit values determined if signs or symptoms of anemia occur.

Low white blood cell counts were rarely observed in clinical trials. These low counts were transient and usually returned to normal while the patient continued on Meclomen therapy. Persistent leukopenia, granulocytopenia, or thrombocytopenia warrant further clinical evaluation and may require discontinuation of the drug.

When abnormal blood chemistry values are obtained, follow-up studies are indicated.

Elevations of serum transaminase levels and of alkaline phosphatase levels occurred in approximately 4% of patients. An occasional patient had elevations of serum creatinine or BUN levels.

DRUG INTERACTIONS

1. **Warfarin:** Meclomen enhances the effect of warfarin. Therefore, when Meclomen is given to a patient receiving warfarin, the dosage of warfarin should be reduced to prevent excessive prolongation of the prothrombin time.
2. **Aspirin:** Concurrent administration of aspirin may lower Meclomen plasma levels, possibly by competing for protein-binding sites. The urinary excretion of Meclomen is unaffected by aspirin, indicating no change in Meclomen absorption. Meclomen does not affect serum salicylate levels. Greater fecal blood loss results from concomitant administration of both drugs than from either drug alone.
3. **Propoxyphene:** The concurrent administration of propoxyphene hydrochloride does not affect the bioavailability of Meclomen.
4. **Antacids:** Concomitant administration of aluminum and magnesium hydroxides does not interfere with absorption of Meclomen.

Carcinogenesis: An 18-month study in rats revealed no evidence of carcinogenicity.

Usage in Pregnancy: Meclomen like aspirin and other nonsteroidal antiinflammatory drugs causes fetotoxicity, minor skeletal malformations, eg, supernumerary ribs, and delayed ossification in rodent reproduction trials, but no major teratogenicity. Similarly, it prolongs gestation and interferes with parturition and with normal development of young before weaning. Meclomen is not recommended for use during pregnancy, particularly in the 1st and 3rd trimesters based on these animal findings. There are, however, no adequate and well-controlled studies in pregnant women.

Usage in Nursing Mothers: It is not known whether Meclomen is excreted in human milk. Because of the effects on suckling rodents and the fact that many drugs are excreted in human milk, Meclomen is not recommended for nursing women.

Pediatric Use: Safety and effectiveness in children below the age of 14 have not been established.

ADVERSE REACTIONS

Incidence Greater than 1%

The following adverse reactions were observed in clinical trials and included observations from more than 2,700 patients, 594 of whom were treated for one year and 248 for at least two years.

Gastrointestinal: The most frequently reported adverse reactions associated with Meclomen involve the gastrointestinal system. In controlled studies of up to six months duration, these disturbances occurred in the following decreasing order of frequency with the approximate incidences in parentheses: diarrhea (10–33%), nausea with or without vomiting (11%), other gastrointestinal disorders (10%), and abdominal pain.* In long-term uncontrolled studies of up to four years duration, one third of the patients had at least one episode of diarrhea some time during Meclomen therapy.

In approximately 4% of the patients in controlled studies, diarrhea was severe enough to require discontinuation of Meclomen. The occurrence of diarrhea is dose related, generally subsides with dose reduction, and clears with termination of therapy. The incidence of diarrhea in patients with osteoarthritis is generally lower than that reported in patients with rheumatoid arthritis.

Other reactions less frequently reported were pyrosis,* flatulence,* anorexia, constipation, stomatitis, and peptic ulcer. The majority of the patients with peptic ulcer had either a history of ulcer disease or were receiving concomitant antiinflammatory drugs, including corticosteroids which are known to produce peptic ulceration.

Cardiovascular: edema

Dermatologic: rash,* urticaria, pruritus

Central Nervous System: headache,* dizziness*

Special Senses: tinnitus

*Incidence between 3% and 9%. Those reactions occurring in 1% to 3% of patients are not marked with an asterisk.

Incidence Less than 1%.
Probably Causally Related

The following adverse reactions were reported less frequently than 1% during controlled clinical trials and through voluntary reports since marketing. The probability of a causal relationship exists between the drug and these adverse reactions.

Gastrointestinal: Bleeding and/or perforation with or without obvious ulcer formation, colitis, cholestatic jaundice

Renal: Renal failure.

Hematologic: Neutropenia, thrombocytopenic purpura, leukopenia, agranulocytosis, hemolytic anemia, eosinophilia, decrease in hemoglobin and/or hematocrit

Dermatologic: Erythema multiforme, Stevens-Johnson syndrome, exfoliative dermatitis

Hepatic: Alteration of liver function tests

Allergic: Lupus and serum sickness-like symptoms

Incidence Less than 1%
Causal Relationship Unknown

Other reactions have been reported but under conditions where a causal relationship could not be established. However, in these rarely reported events, that possibility cannot be excluded. Therefore, these observations are listed to alert physicians.

Cardiovascular: palpitations

Central Nervous System: malaise, fatigue, paresthesia, insomnia, depression

Special Senses: blurred vision, taste disturbances, decreased visual acuity, temporary loss of vision, reversible loss of color vision, retinal changes including macular fibrosis, macular and perimacular edema, conjunctivitis, iritis

Renal: nocturia

Gastrointestinal: paralytic ileus

Dermatologic: erythema nodosum, hair loss

OVERDOSAGE

The following is based on the little information available concerning overdosage with Melcomen and related compounds. After a massive overdose, CNS stimulation may be manifested by irrational behavior, marked agitation and generalized seizures. Following this phase, renal toxicity (falling urine output, rising creatinine, abnormal urinary cellular elements) may be noted with possible oliguria or anuria and azotemia. One patient was anuric for about a week before diuresis and recovery occurred.

Management consists of emptying the stomach by emesis or lavage and instilling an ample dose of activated charcoal into the stomach. There is some evidence that charcoal will actively absorb Meclomen, but dialysis or hemoperfusion may be less effective because of plasma protein binding. The seizures should be controlled by an appropriate anticonvulsant regimen. Attention should be directed throughout, by careful monitoring, to the preservation of vital functions and fluid-electrolyte balance. Dialysis may be required to correct serious azotemia or electrolyte imbalance.

DOSAGE AND ADMINISTRATION

Usual Dosage: For rheumatoid arthritis and osteoarthritis, including acute exacerbations of chronic disease, the dosage is 200 to 400 mg per day, administered in three or four equal doses.

Therapy should be initiated at the lower dosage, then increased as necessary to improve clinical response. The dosage should be individually adjusted for each patient depending on the severity of the symptoms and the clinical response. The daily dosage should not exceed 400 mg per day. The smallest dosage of Meclomen that yields clinical control should be employed.

Although improvement may be seen in some patients in a few days, two to three weeks of treatment may be required to obtain the optimum therapeutic benefit.

After a satisfactory response has been achieved, the dosage should be adjusted as required. A lower dosage may suffice for long-term administration.

If gastrointestinal complaints occur, see Warnings and Precautions. Meclomen may be administered with meals or with milk. If intolerance occurs, the dosage may need to be reduced. Therapy should be terminated if any severe adverse reactions occur.

HOW SUPPLIED

(Capsule 268) Meclomen Capsules, each containing meclofenamate sodium monohydrate equivalent to 50 mg meclofenamic acid, are available:

N 0710-0268-24—bottles of 100
N 0710-0268-40—Uni/Use® 100's (10×10)

(Capsule 269) Meclomen Capsules, each containing meclofenamate sodium monohydrate equivalent to 100 mg meclofenamic acid, are available:

N 0710-0269-24—bottles of 100
N 0710-0269-30—bottles of 500
N 0710-0269-40—Uni/Use 100's (10×10)

Storage: Store at room temperature below 30°C (86°F). Protect from moisture and light.

0268G133

Shown in Product Identification Section, page 420

METHYLDOPA ℞

[*mĕ-thĕl-dō ′pă*]
Tablets, USP

DESCRIPTION

Methyldopa is the *L*-isomer of alpha-methyldopa. Its chemical name is levo-3-(3,4-dihydroxyphenyl)-2-methylalanine. Methyldopa Tablets, USP, is supplied as 250-mg and 500-mg tablets and contains no sulfites. Also contains: blue Opaspray; candelilla wax; colloidal silicon dioxide, NF; edetate disodium, USP; hydoxypropyl cellulose, NF; hydroxypropyl methylcellulose 2910, USP; methylparaben, NF; microcrystalline cellulose, NF; polyethylene glycol 3350, NF; pregelatinized starch, NF; propylparaben, NF; stearic acid, NF.

ACTIONS

Methyldopa Tablets, USP, a unique antihypertensive, is an aromatic-amino-acid decarboxylase inhibitor in animals and in man. Although the mechanism of action has yet to be conclusively demonstrated, the antihypertensive effect of methyldopa probably is due to its metabolism to alpha-methylnorepinephrine, which then lowers arterial pressure by stimulation of central inhibitory alpha-adrenergic receptors, false neurotransmission, and/or reduction of plasma renin activity. Methyldopa has been shown to cause a net reduction in the tissue concentration of serotonin, dopamine, norepinephrine, and epinephrine.

Only methyldopa, the *L*-isomer of alpha-methyldopa, has the ability to inhibit dopa decarboxylase and to deplete animal tissues of norepinephrine. In man the antihypertensive activity appears to be due solely to the *L*-isomer. About twice the dose of the racemate (*DL*-alpha-methyldopa) is required for equal antihypertensive effect.

Methyldopa has no direct effect on cardiac function and usually does not reduce glomerular filtration rate, renal blood flow, or filtration fraction. Cardiac output usually is maintained without cardiac acceleration. In some patients the heart rate is slowed.

Normal or elevated plasma renin activity may decrease in the course of methyldopa therapy.

Methyldopa Tablets, USP, reduces both supine and standing blood pressure. Methyldopa usually produces highly effective lowering of the supine pressure with infrequent symptomatic postural hypotension. Exercise hypotension and diurnal blood pressure variations rarely occur.

INDICATION

Hypertension.

CONTRAINDICATIONS

Active hepatic disease, such as acute hepatitis and active cirrhosis.

If previous methyldopa therapy has been associated with liver disorders (see WARNINGS).

Continued on next page

This product information was prepared in August, 1986. On these and other Parke-Davis Products, information may be obtained by addressing PARKE-DAVIS, Division of Warner-Lambert Company, Morris Plains, New Jersey 07950.

Parke-Davis—Cont.

Hypersensitivity.

WARNINGS

It is important to recognize that a positive Coombs test, hemolytic anemia, and liver disorders may occur with methyldopa therapy. The rare occurrences of hemolytic anemia or liver disorders could lead to potentially fatal complications unless properly recognized and managed. Read this section carefully to understand these reactions.

With prolonged methyldopa therapy, 10 to 20 percent of patients develop a positive direct Coombs test which usually occurs between 6 and 12 months of methyldopa therapy. Lowest incidence is at daily dosage of 1 g or less. This on rare occasions may be associated with hemolytic anemia, which could lead to potentially fatal complications. One cannot predict which patients with a positive direct Coombs test may develop hemolytic anemia.

Prior existence or development of a positive direct Coombs test is not in itself a contraindication to use of methyldopa. If a positive Coombs test develops during methyldopa therapy, the physician should determine whether hemolytic anemia exists and whether the positive Coombs test may be a problem. For example, in addition to a positive direct Coombs test there is less often a positive indirect Coombs test which may interfere with cross matching of blood.

At the start of methyldopa therapy, it is desirable to do a blood count (hematocrit, hemoglobin, or red cell count) for a baseline or to establish whether there is anemia. Periodic blood counts should be done during therapy to detect hemolytic anemia. It may be useful to do a direct Coombs test before therapy and at 6 and 12 months after the start of therapy.

If Coombs-positive hemolytic anemia occurs, the cause may be methyldopa and the drug should be discontinued. Usually the anemia remits promptly. If not, corticosteroids may be given and other causes of anemia should be considered. If the hemolytic anemia is related to methyldopa, the drug should not be reinstituted. When methyldopa causes Coombs positivity alone or with hemolytic anemia, the red cell is usually coated with gamma globulin of the IgG (gamma G) class only. The positive Coombs test may not revert to normal until weeks to months after methyldopa is stopped.

Should the need for transfusion arise in a patient receiving methyldopa, both a direct and an indirect Coombs test should be performed on his or her blood. In the absence of hemolytic anemia, usually only the direct Coombs test will be positive. A positive direct Coombs test alone will not interfere with typing or cross matching. If the indirect Coombs test is also positive, problems may arise in the major cross match and the assistance of a hematologist or transfusion expert will be needed.

Occasionally, fever has occurred within the first 3 weeks of methyldopa therapy, associated in some cases with eosinophilia or abnormalities in one or more liver function tests, such as serum alkaline phosphatase, serum transaminases (SGOT, SGPT), bilirubin, cephalin cholesterol flocculation, prothrombin time, and bromsulphalein retention. Jaundice, with or without fever, may occur with onset usually within the first 2 to 3 months of therapy. In some patients the findings are consistent with those of cholestasis.

Rarely fatal hepatic necrosis has been reported after use of methyldopa. These hepatic changes may represent hypersensitivity reactions. Periodic determinations of hepatic function should be done particularly during the first 6 to 12 weeks of therapy or whenever an unexplained fever occurs. If fever, abnormalities in liver function tests, or jaundice appear, stop therapy with methyldopa. If caused by methyldopa, the temperature and abnormalities in liver function characteristically have reverted to normal when the drug was discontinued. Methyldopa should not be reinstituted in such patients.

Rarely, a reversible reduction of the white blood cell count with a primary effect on the granulocytes has been seen. The granulocyte count returned promptly to normal on discontinuance of the durg. Rare cases of granulocytopenia have been reported. In each instance, upon stopping the drug, the white cell count returned to normal. Reversible thrombocytopenia has occurred rarely. When methyldopa is used with other antihypertensive drugs, potentiation of antihypertensive effect may occur. Patients should be followed carefully to detect side reactions or unusual manifestations of drug idiosyncrasy.

Pregnancy and Nursing

Use of any drug in women who are or may become pregnant or intend to nurse requires that anticipated benefits be weighed against possible risks. Methyldopa crosses the placental barrier, appears in cord blood, and appears in breast milk.

No unusual adverse reactions have been reported in association with the use of methyldopa during pregnancy. Though no obvious teratogenic effects have been reported, the possibility of fetal injury cannot be excluded. Also, the possibility of injury to a nursing infant cannot be excluded.

PRECAUTIONS

Methyldopa should be used with caution in patients with a history of previous liver disease or dysfunction (see WARNINGS).

Methyldopa may interfere with measurement of: urinary uric acid by the phosphotungstate method, serum creatinine by the alkaline picrate method, and SGOT by colorimetric methods. Interference with spectrophotometric methods for SGOT analysis has not been reported.

Since methyldopa causes fluorescence in urine samples at the same wave lengths as catecholamines, falsely high levels of urinary catecholamines may be reported. This will interfere with the diagnosis of pheochromocytoma. It is important to recognize this phenomenon before a patient with a possible pheochromocytoma is subjected to surgery. Methyldopa does not interfere with measurement of VMA (vanillylmandelic acid), a test for pheochromocytoma, by those methods which convert VMA to vanillin. Methyldopa is not recommended for the treatment of patients with pheochromocytoma. Rarely, when urine is exposed to air after voiding, it may darken because of breakdown of methyldopa or its metabolites.

Rarely involuntary choreoathetotic movements have been observed during therapy with methyldopa in patients with severe bilateral cerebrovascular disease. Should these movements occur, stop therapy.

Patients may require reduced doses of anesthetics when on methyldopa. If hypotension does occur during anesthesia, it usually can be controlled by vasopressors. The adrenergic receptors remain sensitive during treatment with methyldopa.

Hypertension has recurred occasionally after dialysis in patients given methyldopa because the drug is removed by this procedure.

ADVERSE REACTIONS

Sedation, usually transient, may occur during the initial period of therapy or whenever the dose is increased. Headache, asthenia, or weakness may be noted as early and transient symptoms. However, significant adverse effects due to Methyldopa Tablets, USP, have been infrequent and this agent usually is well tolerated.

Nervous System/Psychiatric: Sedation, headache, asthenia or weakness, dizziness, lightheadedness, symptoms of cerebrovascular insufficiency, paresthesias, parkinsonism, Bell's palsy, decreased mental acuity, involuntary choreoathetotic movements. Psychic disturbances including nightmares and reversible mild psychoses or depression.

Cardiovascular: Bradycardia, prolonged carotid sinus hypersensitivity, aggravation of angina pectoris. Orthostatic hypotension (decrease daily dosage). Edema (and weight gain) usually relieved by use of a diuretic. (Discontinue methyldopa if edema progresses or signs of heart failure appear.)

Digestive: Nausea, vomiting, distention, constipation, flatus, diarrhea, colitis, mild dryness of mouth, sore or "black" tongue, pancreatitis, sialadenitis.

Hepatic: Abnormal liver function tests, jaundice, liver disorders.

Hematologic: Positive Coombs test, hemolytic anemia. Bone marrow depression, leukopenia, granulocytopenia, thrombocytopenia. Positive tests for antinuclear antibody, LE cells, and rheumatoid factor.

Allergic: Drug-related fever, lupus-like syndrome, myocarditis, pericarditis.

Skin: Rash as in eczema or lichenoid eruption; toxic epidermal necrolysis.

Respiratory: Nasal stuffiness.

Metabolic: Rise in BUN.

Urogenital: Breast enlargement, gynecomastia, lactation, amenorrhea, impotence, decreased libido.

Endocrine: Hyperprolactinemia.

Musculoskeletal: Mild arthralgia, with or without joint swelling; myalgia.

DOSAGE AND ADMINISTRATION

ADULTS

Initiation of Therapy

The usual starting dosage of Methyldopa Tablets is 250 mg two or three times a day in the first 48 hours. The daily dosage then may be increased or decreased, preferably at intervals of not less than two days, until an adequate response is achieved. To minimize the sedation, start dosage increases in the evening. By adjustment of dosage, morning hypotension may be prevented without sacrificing control of afternoon blood pressure.

When methyldopa is given to patients on other antihypertensives, the doses of these agents may need to be adjusted to effect a smooth transition. When Methyldopa Tablets are given with antihypertensives other than thiazides, the initial dosage of Methyldopa Tablets should be limited to 500 mg daily in divided doses, when Methyldopa Tablets are added to a thiazide, the dosage of thiazide need not be changed.

Maintenance Therapy

The usual daily dosage is 500 mg to 2.0 g in two to four doses. Although occasional patients have responded to higher doses, the maximum recommended daily dosage is 3.0 g. Once an effective dosage range is attained, a smooth blood pressure response occurs in most patients in 12 to 24 hours. Since methyldopa has a relatively short duration of action, withdrawal is followed by return of hypertension usually within 48 hours. This is not complicated by an overshoot of blood pressure.

Occasionally tolerance may occur, usually between the second and third month of therapy. Adding a diuretic or increasing the dosage of methyldopa frequently will restore effective control of blood pressure. A thiazide may be added at any time during methyldopa therapy and is recommended if therapy has not been started with a thiazide or if effective control of blood pressure cannot be maintained on 2.0 g of methyldopa daily. Methyldopa is largely excreted by the kidney and patients with impaired renal function may respond to smaller doses. Syncope in older patients may be related to an increased sensitivity and advanced arteriosclerotic vascular disease. This may be avoided by lower doses.

CHILDREN

Initial dosage is based on 10 mg/kg of body weight daily in two to four doses. The daily dosage then is increased or decreased until an adequate response is achieved. The maximum dosage is 65 mg/kg or 3.0 g daily, whichever is less.

HOW SUPPLIED

Methyldopa Tablets, USP, 250 mg (round, medium blue, film-coated tablet, $^{13}/_{32}$ inch in diameter, coded P-D 865) are supplied as follows:
N0071-0865-24 bottles of 100
N0071-0865-32 bottles of 1000

Methyldopa Tablets, USP, 500 mg (round, medium blue, film-coated tablet, ½ inch in diameter, coded P-D 866) are supplied as follows:
N0071-0866-24 bottles of 100
N0071-0866-30 bottles of 500

STORAGE CONDITIONS

Store at room temperature below 30°C (86°F).
Protect from moisture.

Caution—Federal law prohibits dispensing without prescription.

0865G021

Shown in Product Identification Section, page 420

MILONTIN® ℞

[*mĭ″lŏn′tĭn*]
(phensuximide, USP)

DESCRIPTION

Milontin (phensuximide) is an anticonvulsant succinimide, chemically designated as N-methyl-2-phenylsuccinimide.

Each Milontin capsule contains 500 mg phensuximide USP. The capsule and band contain citric acid, USP; colloidal silicon dioxide, NF; D&C yellow No. 10, FD&C red No. 3, FD&C yellow No. 6, gelatin, NF; glyceryl monooleate, polyethylene glycol 200, sodium benzoate, NF; sodium lauryl sulfate, NF.

ACTION

Phensuximide suppresses the paroxysmal three-cycle-per-second spike and wave activity associated with lapses of consciousness which is common in absence (petit mal) seizures. The frequency of epileptiform attacks is reduced, apparently by depression of the motor cortex and elevation of the threshold of the central nervous system to convulsive stimuli.

INDICATION

Milontin is indicated for the control of absence (petit mal) seizures.

CONTRAINDICATION

Phensuximide should not be used in patients with a history of hypersensitivity to succinimides.

WARNINGS

Blood dyscrasias, including some with fatal outcome, have been reported to be associated with the use of succinimides; therefore, periodic blood counts should be performed.

It has been reported that succinimides have produced morphological and functional changes in animal liver. For this reason, phensuximide should be administered with extreme caution to patients with known liver or renal diseases. Periodic urinalysis and liver function studies are advised for all patients receiving the drug.

Cases of systemic lupus erythematosus have been reported with the use of succinimides. The physician should be alert to this possibility.

Usage in pregnancy: The effects of Milontin in human pregnancy and nursing infants are unknown.

Recent reports suggest an association between the use of anticonvulsant drugs by women with epilepsy and an elevated incidence of birth defects in children born to these women. Data is more extensive with respect to phenytoin and phenobarbital, but these are also the most commonly prescribed anticonvulsants; less systematic or anecdotal reports suggest a possible similar association with the use of all known anticonvulsant drugs.

The reports suggesting an elevated incidence of birth defects in children of drug-treated epileptic women cannot be regarded as adequate to prove a definite cause-and-effect relationship. There are intrinsic methodologic problems in obtaining adequate data on drug teratogenicity in humans; the possibility also exists that other factors, eg, genetic factors or the epileptic condition itself, may be more important than drug therapy in leading to birth defects. The great majority of mothers on anticonvulsant medication deliver normal infants. It is important to note that anticonvulsant drugs should not be discontinued in patients in whom the drug is administered to prevent major seizures because of the strong possibility of precipitating status epilepticus with attendant hypoxia and threat to life. In individual cases where the severity and frequency of the seizure disorder are such that the removal of medication does not pose a serious threat to the patient, discontinuation of the drug may be considered prior to and during pregnancy, although it cannot be said with any confidence that even minor seizures do not pose some hazard to the developing embryo or fetus.

The prescribing physician will wish to weigh these considerations in treating or counseling epileptic women of childbearing potential.

Hazardous activities: Phensuximide may impair the mental and/or physical abilities required for the performance of potentially hazardous tasks, such as driving a motor vehicle or other such activity requiring alertness; therefore, the patient should be cautioned accordingly.

PRECAUTIONS

Phensuximide, when used alone in mixed types of epilepsy, may increase the frequency of grand mal seizures in some patients.

As with other anticonvulsants, it is important to proceed slowly when increasing or decreasing dosage, as well as when adding or eliminating other medication. Abrupt withdrawal of anticonvulsant medication may precipitate absence (petit mal) status.

ADVERSE REACTIONS

Gastrointestinal System: Gastrointestinal symptoms, such as nausea, vomiting, and anorexia, occur frequently, but may be the result of overdosage.

Nervous System: Neurologic and sensory reactions reported during therapy with phensuximide have included drowsiness, dizziness, ataxia, headache, dreamlike state, and lethargy. Side effects, such as drowsiness and dizziness, may be relieved by a reduction in total dosage.

Integumentary System: Dermatologic manifestations reported to be associated with the administration of phensuximide have included pruritus, skin eruptions, erythema multiforme, and erythematous rashes.

Genitourinary System: Genitourinary complications which have been reported include urinary frequency, renal damage, and hematuria.

Hemopoietic System: Hemopoietic complications associated with the administration of phensuximide include granulocytopenia, transient leukopenia, and pancytopenia.

Other: Miscellaneous reactions reported have been alopecia and muscular weakness.

DOSAGE AND ADMINISTRATION

Milontin (phensuximide capsules, USP) is administered by the oral route in doses of 500 mg to 1 g two or three times daily. As with other anticonvulsant medication, the dosage should be adjusted to suit individual requirements. The total dosage, irrespective of age, may, therefore, vary between 1 and 3 g per day, the average being 1.5 g.

Milontin may be administered in combination with other anticonvulsants when other forms of epilepsy coexist with absence (petit mal).

HOW SUPPLIED

N 0071-0393-24 (Kapseal® 393)—Milontin Kapseals, each containing 0.5 g phensuximide; bottles of 100.

0393G012

Shown in Product Identification Section, page 421

NARDIL® ℞

[*när'dĭl"*]

(Phenelzine Sulfate Tablets, USP)

DESCRIPTION

Nardil (phenelzine sulfate) is a potent inhibitor of monoamine oxidase (MAO). Chemically, it is a hydrazine derivative. Each tablet contains phenelzine sulfate equivalent to 15 mg of phenelzine base. Also contains acacia, NF; calcium carbonate, carnauba wax, NF; corn starch, NF; FD and C yellow No. 6; gelatin, NF; kaolin, USP; magnesium stearate, NF; mannitol, USP; pharmaceutical glaze, NF; povidone, USP; sucrose, NF; talc, USP; white wax, NF; white wheat flour.

ACTIONS

Monoamine oxidase is a complex enzyme system, widely distributed throughout the body. Drugs that inhibit monoamine oxidase in the laboratory are associated with a number of clinical effects. Thus, it is unknown whether MAO inhibition *per se*, other pharmacologic actions, or an interaction of both is responsible for the clinical effects observed. Therefore, the physician should become familiar with all the effects produced by drugs of this class.

INDICATIONS

Nardil has been found to be effective in depressed patients clinically characterized as "atypical," "nonendogenous," or "neurotic." These patients often have mixed anxiety and depression and phobic or hypochondriacal features. There is less conclusive evidence of its usefulness with severely depressed patients with endogenous features.

Nardil should rarely be the first antidepressant drug used. Rather, it is more suitable for use with patients who have failed to respond to the drugs more commonly used for these conditions.

CONTRAINDICATIONS

Nardil is contraindicated in patients with known sensitivity to the drug, pheochromocytoma, congestive heart failure, a history of liver disease, or abnormal liver function tests.

The potentiation of sympathomimetic substances and related compounds by MAO inhibitors may result in hypertensive crises (See WARNINGS). Therefore, patients being treated with Nardil should not take sympathomimetic drugs (including amphetamines, cocaine, methylphenidate, dopamine, epinephrine and norepinephrine) or related compounds (including methyldopa, L-dopa, L-tryptophan, L-tyrosine, and phenylalanine). Hypertensive crises during Nardil therapy may also be caused by the ingestion of foods with a high concentration of tyramine or dopamine. Therefore, patients being treated with Nardil should avoid high protein food that has undergone protein breakdown by aging, fermentation, pickling, smoking, or bacterial contamination; patients should also avoid cheeses (especially aged varieties), pickled herring, beer, wine, liver, yeast extract (including brewer's yeast in large quantities), dry sausage (including Genoa salami, hard salami, pepperoni, and Lebanon bologna), pods of broad beans (Fava beans), and yogurt. Excessive amounts of caffeine and chocolate may also cause hypertensive reactions.

Nardil should not be used in combination with CNS depressants such as alcohol and certain narcotics. Excitation, seizures, delirium, hyperpyrexia, circulatory collapse, coma, and death have been reported in patients receiving MAOI therapy who have been given a single dose of meperidine. Nardil should not be administered together with or in rapid succession to other MAO inhibitors because HYPERTENSIVE CRISES and convulsive seizures, fever, marked sweating, excitation, delirium, tremor, coma, and circulatory collapse may occur.

List of MAO Inhibitors

Generic Name	*Trademark*
pargyline hydrochloride	Eutonyl® (Abbott Laboratories)
pargyline hydrochloride and methyclothiazide	Eutron® (Abbott Laboratories)
furazolidone	Furoxone® (Eaton Laboratories)
isocarboxazid	Marplan® (Roche)
procarbazine	Matulane® (Roche)
tranylcypromine	Parnate® (Smith Kline & French Laboratories)

Patients taking Nardil should not undergo elective surgery requiring general anesthesia. Also, they should not be given cocaine or local anesthesia containing sympathomimetic vasoconstrictors. The possible combined hypotensive effects of Nardil and spinal anesthesia should be kept in mind. Nardil should be discontinued at least 10 days prior to elective surgery.

IMPORTANT

Warnings: The most serious reactions to Nardil involve changes in blood pressure.

Hypertensive Crises: The most important reaction associated with Nardil administration is the occurrence of hypertensive crises, which have sometimes been fatal.

These crises are characterized by some or all of the following symptoms: occipital headache which may radiate frontally, palpitation, neck stiffness or soreness, nausea, vomiting, sweating (sometimes with fever and sometimes with cold, clammy skin), dilated pupils, and photophobia. Either tachycardia or bradycardia may be present and can be associated with constricting chest pain.

NOTE: Intracranial bleeding has been reported in association with the increase in blood pressure.

Blood pressure should be observed frequently to detect evidence of any pressor response in all patients receiving Nardil. Therapy should be discontinued immediately upon the occurrence of palpitation or frequent headaches during therapy.

Recommended treatment in hypertensive crisis: If a hypertensive crisis occurs, Nardil should be discontinued immediately and therapy to lower blood pressure should be instituted immediately. On the basis of present evidence, phentolamine is recommended. (The dosage reported for phentolamine is 5 mg intravenously.) Care should be taken to administer this drug slowly in order to avoid producing an excessive hypotensive effect. Fever should be managed by means of external cooling.

Warning to the patient: All patients should be warned that the following foods, beverages and medications must be avoided while taking Nardil, and for two weeks after discontinuing use.

Foods and Beverages To Avoid

Meat and Fish
Pickled herring
Liver
Dry sausage (including Genoa salami, hard salami, pepperoni, and Lebanon bologna)

Vegetables
Broad bean pods (fava bean pods)

Dairy Products
Cheese (cottage cheese and cream cheese are allowed)
Yogurt

Beverages
Beer and wine

Miscellaneous
Yeast extract (including brewer's yeast in large quantities)
Excessive amounts of chocolate and caffeine

Also, any spoiled or improperly refrigerated, handled or stored protein-rich foods such as meats, fish, and dairy products, including foods that may have undergone protein changes by aging, pickling, fermentation, or smoking to improve flavor should be avoided.

OTC Medications To Avoid
Cold tablets or liquids
Nasal decongestants (tablets, drops or spray)
Hay-fever medications
Sinus medications
Asthma inhalant medications
Antiappetite medicines
Weight-reducing preparations
"Pep" pills
L-tryptophan containing preparations

Also, certain prescription drugs should be avoided. Therefore, patients under the care of another physician or dentist, should inform him/her they are taking Nardil.

Patients should be warned that the use of the above foods, beverages or medications may cause a reaction characterized by headache and other serious symptoms due to a rise in blood pressure.

Patients should be instructed to report promptly the occurrence of headache or other unusual symptoms.

Concomitant Use with Dibenzazepine Derivative Drugs

If the decision is made to administer Nardil concurrently with other antidepressant drugs, or within less than 10 days after discontinuation of antidepressant therapy, the patient should be cautioned by the physician regarding the possibility of adverse drug interaction.

List of Dibenzazepine Derivative Drugs

Generic Name	*Trademark*
nortriptyline hydrochloride	Aventyl® (Eli Lilly & Co.)
amitriptyline hydrochloride	Amitril® (Parke-Davis)
amitriptyline hydrochloride	Elavil® (Merck Sharp & Dohme)
amitriptyline hydrochloride	Endep® (Roche)
perphenazine and amitriptyline hydrochloride	Etrafon® (Schering Corporation)
perphenazine and amitriptyline hydrochloride	Triavil® (Merck Sharp & Dohme)
desipramine hydrochloride	Norpramin® (Merrell-National)
desipramine hydrochloride	Pertofrane® (USV)
imipramine hydrochloride	Tofranil® (Geigy)
doxepin	Adapin® (Pennwalt)
doxepin	Sinequan® (Pfizer)

Continued on next page

This product information was prepared in August, 1986. On these and other Parke-Davis Products, information may be obtained by addressing PARKE-DAVIS, Division of Warner-Lambert Company, Morris Plains, New Jersey 07950.

Parke-Davis—Cont.

carbamazepine	Tegretol® (Geigy)
cyclobenzaprine HCl	Flexeril® (Merck Sharp & Dohme)
amoxapine	Asendin® (Lederle)
maprotiline HCl	Ludiomil® (CIBA)
trimipramine maleate	Surmontil® (Ives)

Nardil should be used with caution in combination with antihypertensive drugs, including thiazide diuretics and β-blockers, since exaggerated hypotensive effects may result. MAO inhibitors including Nardil are contraindicated in patients receiving guanethidine.

Use in Pregnancy: The safe use of Nardil during pregnancy or lactation has not been established. The potential benefit of this drug, if used during pregnancy, lactation, or in women of childbearing age, should be weighed against the possible hazard to the mother or fetus.

Doses of Nardil in pregnant mice well exceeding the maximum recommended human dose have caused a significant decrease in the number of viable offspring per mouse. In addition, the growth of young dogs and rats has been retarded by doses exceeding the maximum human dose.

Use in Children: Nardil is not recommended for patients under 16 years of age since there are no controlled studies of safety in this age group.

Nardil, as with other hydrazine derivatives, has been reported to induce pulmonary and vascular tumors in an uncontrolled lifetime study in mice.

PRECAUTIONS

In depressed patients, the possibility of suicide should always be considered and adequate precautions taken. It is recommended that careful observations of patients undergoing Nardil treatment be maintained until control of depression is achieved. If necessary, additional measures (ECT, hospitalization, etc.) should be instituted.

All patients undergoing treatment with Nardil should be closely followed for symptoms of postural hypotension. Hypotensive side effects have occurred in hypertensive as well as normal and hypotensive patients. Blood pressure usually returns to pretreatment levels rapidly when the drug is discontinued or the dosage is reduced.

Because the effect of Nardil on the convulsive threshold may be variable, adequate precautions should be taken when treating epileptic patients.

Of the more severe side effects that have been reported with any consistency, hypomania has been the most common. This reaction has been largely limited to patients in whom disorders characterized by hyperkinetic symptoms coexist with, but are obscured by, depressive affect; hypomania usually appeared as depression improved. If agitation is present, it may be increased with Nardil. Hypomania and agitation have also been reported at higher than recommended doses, or following long-term therapy.

Nardil may cause excessive stimulation in schizophrenic patients; in manic-depressive states it may result in a swing from a depressive to a manic phase.

MAO inhibitors, including Nardil potentiate hexobarbital hypnosis in animals. Therefore, barbiturates should be given at a reduced dose with Nardil.

MAO inhibitors inhibit the destruction of serotonin and norepinephrine, which are believed to be released from tissue stores by rauwolfia alkaloids. Accordingly, caution should be exercised when rauwolfia is used concomitantly with an MAO inhibitor, including Nardil.

There is conflicting evidence as to whether or not MAO inhibitors affect glucose metabolism or potentiate hypoglycemic agents. This should be kept in mind if Nardil is administered to diabetics.

ADVERSE REACTIONS

Nardil is a potent inhibitor of monoamine oxidase. Because this enzyme is widely distributed throughout the body, diverse pharmacologic effects can be expected to occur. When they occur, such effects tend to be mild or moderate in severity (see below), often subside as treatment continues, and can be minimized by adjusting dosage; rarely is it necessary to institute counteracting measures or to discontinue Nardil.

Common side effects include dizziness, constipation, dry mouth, postural hypotension, drowsiness, weakness and fatigue, edema, gastrointestinal disturbances, tremors, twitching, hyperreflexia, and sexual disturbances, ie, anorgasmia and ejaculatory disturbances.

Less common mild to moderate side effects, some of which have been reported in a single patient or by a single physician, include blurred vision, glaucoma, sweating, skin rash, jitteriness, palilalia, urinary retention, weight gain, euphoria, nystagmus, sexual disturbances and hypernatremia.

Although reported less frequently, and sometimes only once, additional severe side effects have included ataxia, shock-like coma, edema of the glottis, transient respiratory and cardiovascular depression following ECT, leukopenia, toxic delirium, reversible jaundice, manic reaction, convulsions, acute anxiety reaction and precipitation of schizophrenia. To date, fatal progressive necrotizing hepatocellular damage has been reported in a very few patients.

An uncommon withdrawal syndrome following abrupt withdrawal of Nardil has been infrequently reported. Signs and symptoms of this syndrome generally commence 24 to 72 hours after drug discontinuation and may range from vivid nightmares with agitation to frank psychosis. This syndrome generally responds to reinstitution of low-dose Nardil therapy followed by cautious downward titration and discontinuation.

DOSAGE AND ADMINISTRATION

Initial dose: the usual starting dose of Nardil is one tablet (15 mg) three times a day.

Early phase treatment: dosage should be increased to at least 60 mg per day at a fairly rapid pace consistent with patient tolerance. It may be necessary to increase dosage up to 90 mg per day to obtain sufficient MAO inhibition. Many patients do not show a clinical response until treatment at 60 mg has been continued for at least 4 weeks.

Maintenance dose: after maximum benefit from Nardil is achieved, dosage should be reduced slowly over several weeks. Maintenance dose may be as low as 1 tablet, 15 mg, a day or every other day, and should be continued for as long as is required.

OVERDOSAGE

Note—For management of *hypertensive crises* see Warnings.

Accidental or intentional overdosage may be more common in patients who are depressed. It should be remembered that multiple drugs and/or alcohol may have been ingested.

Depending on the amount of overdosage with Nardil, a varying and mixed clinical picture may develop, involving signs and symptoms of central nervous system and cardiovascular stimulation and/or depression. Signs and symptoms may be absent or minimal during the initial 12-hour period following ingestion and may develop slowly thereafter, reaching a maximum in 24–48 hours. Death has been reported following overdosage. Therefore, immediate hospitalization, with continuous patient observation and monitoring throughout this period, is essential.

Signs and symptoms of overdosage may include, alone or in combination, any of the following: drowsiness, dizziness, faintness, irritability, hyperactivity, agitation, severe headache, hallucinations, trismus, opisthotonus, convulsions and coma; rapid and irregular pulse, hypertension, hypotension and vascular collapse; precordial pain, respiratory depression and failure, hyperpyrexia, diaphoresis, and cool, clammy skin.

Intensive symptomatic and supportive treatment may be required. Induction of emesis or gastric lavage with instillation of charcoal slurry may be helpful in early poisoning, provided the airway has been protected against aspiration. Signs and symptoms of central nervous system stimulation, including convulsions, should be treated with diazepam, given slowly intravenously. Phenothiazine derivatives and central nervous system stimulants should be avoided. Hypotension and vascular collapse should be treated with intravenous fluids and, if necessary, blood pressure titration with an intravenous infusion of dilute pressor agent. It should be noted that adrenergic agents may produce a markedly increased pressor response.

Respiration should be supported by appropriate measures, including management of the airway, use of supplemental oxygen, and mechanical ventilatory assistance, as required.

Body temperature should be monitored closely. Intensive management of hyperpyrexia may be required. Maintenance of fluid and electrolyte balance is essential.

There are no data on the lethal dose in man. The pathophysiologic effects of massive overdosage may persist for several days, since the drug acts by inhibiting physiologic enzyme systems. With symptomatic and supportive measures, recovery from *mild* overdosage may be expected within 3 to 4 days. Hemodialysis, peritoneal dialysis, and charcoal hemoperfusion may be of value in massive overdosage, but sufficient data are not available to recommend their routine use in these cases.

Toxic blood levels of phenelzine have not been established, and assay methods are not practical for clinical or toxicological use.

HOW SUPPLIED

Tablets—each orange-coated tablet bears the P-D 270 monogram and contains phenelzine sulfate equivalent to 15 mg of phenelzine base; bottles of 100 (N 0071-0270-24). Store between 15°–30°C (59°–86°F).

US Patent 3,314,855

Shown in Product Identification Section, page 421

0270G025

NATABEC® KAPSEALS®

[*nā 'tă-bĕc*]

Each capsule represents:

Vitamins	
Vitamin A (acetate)	(1.2 mg) 4,000 IU*
Vitamin D	400 IU
Vitamin C (ascorbic acid)	50 mg
Vitamin B_1 (thiamine mononitrate)	3 mg
Vitamin B_2 (riboflavin)	2.0 mg
Nicotinamide +	10 mg
Vitamin B_6 (pyridoxine HCl)	3 mg
Vitamin B_{12} crystalline (cyanocobalamin)	5 mcg
Minerals	
Precipitated Calcium Carbonate	600 mg
Iron (as dried ferrous sulfate)	30 mg

*IU = International Units

+Supplied as niacinamide

ACTION AND USES

A multivitamin and mineral supplement for use during pregnancy and lactation

DOSAGE

One capsule daily, or as directed by physician

HOW SUPPLIED

N 0071-0390-24. In bottles of 100, Parcode® 390

The color combination of the banded capsule is a Warner-Lambert trademark.

Shown in Product Identification Section, page 421

NATABEC Rx® KAPSEALS® ℞

[*nā 'tă-bĕc"*]

Vitamin and Mineral Formula Containing Folic Acid

Each Kapseal Represents:

Vitamin A (acetate)	4,000 units
Vitamin D	400 units
Vitamin C (ascorbic acid)	50 mg
Vitamin B_1 (thiamine mononitrate)	3 mg
Vitamin B_2 (riboflavin)	2 mg
Vitamin B_6 (pyridoxine hydrochloride)	3 mg
Vitamin B_{12} (cyanocobalamin) crystalline	5 mcg
Nicotinamide (niacinamide)	10 mg
Folic acid	1 mg
Calcium carbonate, precipitated	600 mg
Iron*	30 mg

* Supplied as dried ferrous sulfate.

ACTION AND USES

Vitamin and mineral formula containing 1 mg folic acid for use during pregnancy and lactation

Caution—Folic acid in doses above 0.1 mg daily may obscure pernicious anemia in that hematologic remission can occur while neurological manifestations remain progressive.

DOSAGE

One capsule daily or as directed by the physician.

HOW SUPPLIED

N 0071-0547-24—bottles of 100.

The pink band on blue capsule is a Warner-Lambert trademark registered in the US Patent Office.

Shown in Product Identification Section, page 421

NATAFORT® FILMSEAL® ℞

[*nā 'tă-fōrt"*]

Each tablet represents:

Vitamin A (acetate)	6,000 IU*
Vitamin D	400 IU
Vitamin C (ascorbic acid)	120 mg
Thiamine (vitamin B_1) (thiamine mononitrate)	3 mg
Riboflavin (vitamin B_2)(riboflavin)	2 mg
Vitamin B_6 (pyridoxine HCl)	15 mg
Vitamin B_{12} (cyanocobalamin) crystalline	6 mcg
Folic acid	1 mg
Nicotinamide (niacinamide)	20 mg
Vitamin E (*dl* alpha tocopheryl acetate)	30 IU
Calcium†	350 mg
Iodine†	0.15 mg
Iron†	65 mg
Magnesium†	100 mg
Zinc†	25 mg

* IU = International Units

† The minerals are supplied as calcium carbonate, magnesium oxide, potassium iodide, ferrous fumarate, and zinc oxide.

INDICATIONS

Comprehensive prenatal vitamin and mineral formula including 1 mg of folic acid to prevent megaloblastic anemia of pregnancy.
Caution—Folic acid in doses above 0.1 mg daily may obscure pernicious anemia in that hematologic remission can occur while neurological manifestations remain progessive.

USUAL DOSAGE

One tablet daily.

HOW SUPPLIED

N 0071-0282-24 bottles of 100.

Shown in Product Identification Section, page 421

NITROSTAT® Ointment 2% ℞

[nī'trō"stăt]
(Nitroglycerin)

DESCRIPTION

Nitrostat® ointment contains 2% nitroglycerin in an ointment base composed of lanolin, lactose, and white petrolatum, formulated to provide a controlled release of the active ingredient. Each inch, as squeezed from the tube, contains 15 mg nitroglycerin.

ACTIONS

When the ointment is spread on the skin, nitroglycerin is absorbed continuously into the systemic circulation. Nitrostat ointment reduces the work load of the heart by virtue of its smooth muscle relaxation. This results predominantly in peripheral venous dilatation, which reduces preload, but also to a lesser degree in peripheral arteriolar dilatation, which reduces afterload. These hemodynamic effects have been advanced as explanations for the beneficial actions of nitroglycerin ointment in angina pectoris.
Computerized digital plethysmographic studies have shown the duration of action of nitroglycerin ointment (2 inches applied to the chest) to be eight hours in comparison to placebo; the onset of action occurred within thirty minutes of administration. Controlled clinical studies have demonstrated that nitrocylcerin ointment increased measured exercise tolerance in patients with angina pectoris up to three hours after application (the maximal time interval studied).

INDICATIONS

This drug product has been conditionally approved by the FDA for the prevention and treatment of angina pectoris due to coronary artery disease. The conditional approval reflects a determination that the drug may be marketed while further investigation of its effectiveness is undertaken. A final evaluation of the effectiveness of the product will be announced by the FDA.

CONTRAINDICATIONS

In patients known to be intolerant of the organic nitrate drugs.

WARNINGS

In acute myocardial infarction or congestive heart failure, Nitrostat ointment should be used under careful clinical and/or hemodynamic monitoring.

PRECAUTIONS

Nitrostat ointment should not be used for treatment of acute anginal attacks. Symptoms of hypotension, particularly during sudden arising from the recumbent position, are signs of overdosage. When they occur, the dosage should be reduced.

ADVERSE REACTIONS

Transient headaches are the most common side effect, especially at higher dosages. Headaches should be treated with mild analgesics, and nitroglycerin ointment continued. Only with untreatable headaches should the dosage be reduced.
Although uncommon, hypotension, an increase in heart rate, faintness, flushing, dizziness, and nausea may occur. These are all attributable to the pharmacologic effects of nitroglycerin on the cardiovascular system but are symptoms of overdosage. When they occur and persist, the dosage should be reduced.

DOSAGE AND ADMINISTRATION

When applying the ointment, place the specially designed dose-measuring applicator supplied with the package on a flat surface with the printed side down and squeeze the necessary amount of ointment from the tube onto the applicator. Then place the applicator with the ointment side down onto the desired area of skin, usually the chest (although other areas can be used).
Using the applicator, spread the ointment in a thin, uniform layer over an area approximately the size of the applicator or larger. Cover the area, including the applicator, with plastic wrap, which can be held in place by adhesive tape. The applicator allows the patient to measure the necessary amount of ointment and to spread it without its being absorbed through the fingers during application to the skin surface.
The usual therapeutic dose is 2 inches (50 mm) applied every eight hours, although some patients may require as much as 4 to 5 inches (100 to 125 mm) and/or application every four hours.
Start at ½ inch (12.5 mm) every eight hours and increase the dose by ½ inch (12.5 mm) with each successive application to achieve the desired clinical effects. The optimal dosage should be selected based upon the clinical response, side effects, and the effects of therapy upon blood pressure. The greatest attainable decrease in resting blood pressure that is not associated with clinical symptoms of hypotension, especially during orthostasis, indicates the optimal dosage. To decrease adverse reactions, the dose and frequency of application should be tailored to the individual patient's needs.
Keep the tube tightly closed and store at controlled room temperature 15° to 30°C (59° to 86°F). Avoid excessive heat.
Patient Instructions For Application: Information furnished with dose-measuring applicators.

HOW SUPPLIED

Nitrostat ointment 2% is supplied as:
N 0071-3001-13—30-gram tube
N 0071-3001-15—60-gram tube
Each gram of ointment contains 20 mg of nitroglycerin.

3001G032

Shown in Product Identification Section, page 421

NITROSTAT® ℞

[nī'trō"stăt]
(nitroglycerin tablets, USP)

DESCRIPTION

Nitrostat is a stabilized sublingual nitroglycerin tablet manufactured by a patented process* which prevents the migration of nitroglycerin by adding the nonvolatile fixing agent polyethylene glycol 3350. This stabilized formulation has been shown to be more stable and more uniform than conventional molded tablets. Nitrostat tablets contain 0.15 mg (1/400 grain), 0.3 mg (1/200 grain), 0.4 mg (1/150 grain) and 0.6 mg (1/100 grain) nitroglycerin. Also contains lactose, NF; polyethylene glycol 3350, NF; sucrose, NF.
Nitroglycerin, an organic nitrate, is a vasodilating agent. The chemical name for nitroglycerin is 1,2,3 propanetriol trinitrate.

CLINICAL PHARMACOLOGY

Relaxation of vascular smooth muscle is the principal pharmacologic action of nitroglycerin. The mechanism by which nitroglycerin produces relaxation of smooth muscle is unknown. Although venous effects predominate, nitroglycerin produces, in a dose-related manner, dilation of both arterial and venous beds. Dilation of the postcapillary vessels, including large veins, promotes peripheral pooling of blood and decreases venous return to the heart, reducing left ventricular end-diastolic pressure (preload). Arteriolar relaxation reduces systemic vascular resistance and arterial pressure (afterload). Myocardial oxygen consumption or demand (as measured by the pressure-rate product, tension-time index and stroke-work index) is decreased by both the arterial and venous effects of nitroglycerin, and a more favorable supply-demand ratio can be achieved.
Therapeutic doses of nitroglycerin may reduce systolic, diastolic and mean arterial blood pressure. Effective coronary perfusion pressure is usually maintained, but can be compromised if blood pressure falls excessively or increased heart rate decreases diastolic filling time.
Elevated central venous and pulmonary capillary wedge pressures, pulmonary vascular resistance and systemic vascular resistance are also reduced by nitroglycerin therapy. Heart rate is usually slightly increased, presumably a reflex response to the fall in blood pressure. Cardiac index may be increased, decreased, or unchanged. Patients with elevated left ventricular filling pressure and systemic vascular resistance values in conjunction with a depressed cardiac index are likely to experience an improvement in cardiac index. On the other hand, when filling pressures and cardiac index are normal, cardiac index may be slightly reduced by intravenous nitroglycerin.
Nitroglycerin is rapidly absorbed following sublingual administration. Its onset of action is approximately one to three minutes. Significant pharmacologic effects are present for 30 to 60 minutes following administration by the above route.
Nitroglycerin is rapidly metabolized to dinitrates and mononitrates, with a short half-life, estimated at 1 to 4 minutes. At plasma concentrations of between 50 and 500 ng/ml, the binding of nitroglycerin to plasma proteins is approximately 60%, while that of 1,2 dinitroglycerin and 1,3 dinitroglycerin is 60% and 30% respectively. The activity and half-life of 1,2 dinitroglycerin and 1,3 dinitroglycerin are not well characterized. The mononitrate is not active.

INDICATIONS AND USAGE

Nitroglycerin is indicated for the prophylaxis, treatment and management of patients with angina pectoris.

CONTRAINDICATIONS

Sublingual nitroglycerin therapy is contraindicated in patients with early myocardial infarction, severe anemia, increased intracranial pressure, and those with a known hypersensitivity to nitroglycerin.

PRECAUTIONS

General: Only the smallest dose required for effective relief of the acute anginal attack should be used. Excessive use may lead to the development of tolerance. Nitrostat tablets are intended for sublingual or buccal administration and should not be swallowed. The drug should be discontinued if blurring of vision or drying of the mouth occurs. Excessive dosage of nitroglycerin may produce severe headaches.
Information for Patients: If possible, patients should sit down when taking Nitrostat tablets. This eliminates the possibility of falling due to lightheadedness or dizziness.
Drug Interactions: Concomitant use of nitrates and alcohol may cause hypotension. Patients receiving antihypertensive drugs, beta-adrenergic blockers, or phenothiazines and nitrates should be observed for possible additive hypotensive effects.
Drug/Laboratory Test Interactions: Nitrates may interfere with the Zlatkis-Zak color reaction causing a false report of decreased serum cholesterol.
Carcinogenesis, Mutagenesis, Impairment of Fertility: No long-term studies in animals were performed to evaluate the carcinogenic potential of nitroglycerin.
Pregnancy Category C: Animal reproduction studies have not been conducted with nitroglycerin. It is also not known whether nitroglycerin can cause fetal harm when administered to a pregnant woman or can affect reproduction capacity. Nitroglycerin should be given to a pregnant woman only if clearly needed.
Nursing Mother: It is not known whether nitroglycerin is excreted in human milk. Because many drugs are excreted in human milk, caution should be exercised when intravenous nitroglycerin is administered to a nursing woman.
Pediatric Use: The safety and effectiveness of nitroglycerin in children have not been established.

ADVERSE REACTIONS

Transient headache may occur immediately after use. Vertigo, weakness, palpitation, and other manifestations of postural hypotension may develop occasionally, particularly in erect, immobile patients. Syncope due to nitrate vasodilation has been reported.

DOSAGE AND ADMINISTRATION

One tablet should be dissolved under the tongue or in the buccal pouch at the first sign of an acute anginal attack. The dose may be repeated approximately every five minutes until relief is obtained. If the pain persists after a total of 3 tablets in a 15-minute period, the physician should be notified. Nitrostat may be used prophylactically five to ten minutes prior to engaging in activities which might precipitate an acute attack.

HOW SUPPLIED

Nitrostat is supplied in four strengths in bottles containing 100 tablets each, with color-coded labels, and in color-coded Patient Convenience Packages of four bottles of 25 tablets each.
0.15 mg (1/400 grain):
N 0071-0568-24—Bottle of 100 tablets
N 0071-0568-13—Convenience Package
0.3 mg (1/200 grain):
N 0071-0569-24—Bottle of 100 tablets
N 0071-0569-13—Convenience Package
0.4 mg (1/150 grain):
N 0071-0570-24—Bottle of 100 tablets
N 0071-0570-13—Convenience Package
0.6 mg (1/100 grain):
N 0071-0571-24—Bottle of 100 tablets
N 0071-0571-13—Convenience Package
Store at controlled room temperature 15°–30°C (59°–86°F). Protect from moisture.
*US Patent No. 3,789,119

0568G063

Shown in Product Identification Section, page 421

Continued on next page

This product information was prepared in August, 1986. On these and other Parke-Davis Products, information may be obtained by addressing PARKE-DAVIS, Division of Warner-Lambert Company, Morris Plains, New Jersey 07950.

Parke-Davis—Cont.

NITROSTAT® IV ℞
[nī'trō"stăt]
(Nitroglycerin for Infusion)
FOR INTRAVENOUS USE ONLY

NOT FOR DIRECT INTRAVENOUS INJECTION. NITROSTAT IV IS A CONCENTRATED, POTENT DRUG WHICH MUST BE DILUTED IN DEXTROSE (5%) INJECTION, USP OR SODIUM CHLORIDE (0.9%) INJECTION, USP PRIOR TO ITS INFUSION. THE CONTAINER AND ADMINISTRATION SET USED FOR INFUSION MAY AFFECT THE AMOUNT OF INTRAVENOUS NITROGLYCERIN DELIVERED TO THE PATIENT. (SEE WARNINGS AND DOSAGE AND ADMINISTRATION SECTIONS.)
CAUTION: SEVERAL PREPARATIONS OF NITROGLYCERIN FOR INJECTION ARE AVAILABLE. THEY DIFFER IN CONCENTRATION AND/OR VOLUME PER VIAL. WHEN SWITCHING FROM ONE PRODUCT TO ANOTHER, ATTENTION MUST BE PAID TO THE DILUTION AND DOSAGE AND ADMINISTRATION INSTRUCTIONS.

DESCRIPTION

Nitrostat IV is a clear, practically colorless additive solution for intravenous infusion after dilution. Each milliliter contains 0.8 mg nitroglycerin, with citric acid and sodium citrate as buffers, and 5% alcohol in Water for Injection, USP. The solution is sterile, nonpyrogenic, and nonexplosive. Intravenous nitroglycerin, an organic nitrate, is a vasodilator. The chemical name for nitroglycerin is 1,2,3 propanetriol trinitrate and its chemical structure is:

$H_2C-O-NO_2$
|
$HC-O-NO_2$
|
$H_2C-O-NO_2$

CLINICAL PHARMACOLOGY

Relaxation of vascular smooth muscle is the principal pharmacologic action of intravenous nitroglycerin. Although venous effects predominate, nitroglycerin produces, in a dose-related manner, dilation of both arterial and venous beds. Dilation of the postcapillary vessels, including large veins, promotes peripheral pooling of blood and decreases venous return to the heart, reducing left ventricular end-diastolic pressure (preload). Arteriolar relaxation reduces systemic vascular resistance and arterial pressure (afterload). Myocardial oxygen consumption or demand (as measured by the pressure-rate product, tension-time index and stroke-work index) is decreased by both the arterial and venous effects of nitroglycerin, and a more favorable supply-demand ratio can be achieved.
Therapeutic doses of intravenous nitroglycerin reduce systolic, diastolic and mean arterial blood pressure. Effective coronary perfusion pressure is usually maintained, but can be compromised if blood pressure falls excessively or increased heart rate decreases diastolic filling time.
Elevated central venous and pulmonary capillary wedge pressures, pulmonary vascular resistance and systemic vascular resistance are also reduced by nitroglycerin therapy. Heart rate is usually slightly increased, presumably a reflex response to the fall in blood pressure. Cardiac index may be increased, decreased, or unchanged. Patients with elevated left ventricular filling pressure and systemic vascular resistance values in conjunction with a depressed cardiac index are likely to experience an improvement in cardiac index. On the other hand, when filling pressures and cardiac index are normal, cardiac index may be slightly reduced by intravenous nitroglycerin.
Nitroglycerin is widely distributed in the body with an apparent volume of distribution of approximately 200 liters in adult male subjects, and is rapidly metabolized to dinitrates and mononitrates, with a short half-life, estimated at 1 to 4 minutes. This results in a low plasma concentration after intravenous infusion. At plasma concentrations of between 50 and 500 ng/ml, the binding of nitroglycerin to plasma proteins is approximately 60%, while that of 1,2 dinitroglycerin and 1,3 dinitroglycerin is 60% and 30% respectively. The activity and half-life of 1,2 dinitroglycerin and 1,3 dinitroglycerin are not well characterized. The mononitrate is not active.

INDICATIONS AND USAGE

Nitrostat IV is indicated for:
1. *Control of blood pressure in perioperative hypertension*, ie, hypertension associated with surgical procedures, especially cardiovascular procedures, such as the hypertension seen during intratracheal intubation, anesthesia, skin incision, sternotomy, cardiac bypass, and in the immediate postsurgical period.
2. *Congestive Heart Failure Associated with Acute Myocardial Infarction.*
3. *Treatment of Angina Pectoris* in patients who have not responded to recommended doses of organic nitrates and/or a beta blocker.
4. *Production of controlled hypotension during surgical procedures.*

CONTRAINDICATIONS

Nitrostat IV should not be administered to individuals with:
1. A known hypersensitivity to nitroglycerin or a known idiosyncratic reaction to organic nitrates.
2. Hypotension or uncorrected hypovolemia, as the use of Nitrostat IV in such states could produce severe hypotension or shock.
3. Increased intracranial pressure (eg, head trauma or cerebral hemorrhage).
4. Constrictive pericarditis and pericardial tamponade.

WARNINGS

1. Nitroglycerin readily migrates into many plastics. To avoid absorption of nitroglycerin into plastic parenteral solution containers, the dilution and storage of nitroglycerin for intravenous infusion should be made only in glass parenteral solution bottles.
2. Some filters also absorb nitroglycerin; they should be avoided if possible.
3. Forty to 80% of the total amount of nitroglycerin in the final diluted solution for infusion is absorbed by the polyvinyl chloride (PVC) tubing of the intravenous administration sets currently in general use. The higher rates of absorption occur when flow rates are low, nitroglycerin concentrations are high, and tubing is long. Although the rate of loss is highest during the early phase of administration (when flow rates are lowest), the loss is neither constant nor self-limiting; consequently no simple calculation or correction can be performed to convert the theoretical infusion rate (based on the concentration of the infusion solution) to the actual delivery rate.

Because of this problem, Parke-Davis, Division of Warner-Lambert Company has developed a nonabsorbing infusion set, Nitrostat IV intravenous infusion set, in which the loss of nitroglycerin is minimal (less than 5%). The Nitrostat IV intravenous infusion set or a similar infusion set is recommended for infusions of intravenous nitroglycerin.
Dosage instructions must be followed with care. It should be noted that when these infusion sets are used, the calculated dose will be delivered to the patient because the loss of nitroglycerin due to absorption in standard PVC tubing will be kept to a minimum. Note that the dosages commonly used in published studies utilized general-use PVC infusion sets and recommended doses based on this experience are too high if the new infusion sets are used.

PRECAUTIONS

Nitrostat IV should be used with caution in patients who have severe hepatic or renal disease.
Excessive hypotension, especially for prolonged periods of time, must be avoided because of possible deleterious effects on the brain, heart, liver, and kidney from poor perfusion and the attendant risk of ischemia, thrombosis, and altered function of these organs. Paradoxical bradycardia and increased angina pectoris may accompany nitroglycerin-induced hypotension. Patients with normal or low pulmonary capillary wedge pressure are especially sensitive to the hypotensive effects of intravenous nitroglycerin. If pulmonary capillary wedge pressure is being monitored, it will be noted that a fall in wedge pressure precedes the onset of arterial hypotension, and the pulmonary capillary wedge pressure is thus a useful guide to safe titration of the drug.
NITROSTAT IV CONTAINS ALCOHOL. SAFETY FOR INTRACORONARY INJECTION HAS NOT BEEN SHOWN.

Carcinogenesis, Mutagenesis, Impairment of Fertility:
No long-term studies in animals were performed to evaluate the carcinogenic potential of nitroglycerin.

Pregnancy:
Category C: Animal reproduction studies have not been conducted with nitroglycerin. It is also not known whether nitroglycerin can cause fetal harm when administered to a pregnant woman or can affect reproduction capacity. Nitroglycerin should be given to a pregnant woman only if clearly needed.

Nursing Mother:
It is not known whether nitroglycerin is excreted in human milk. Because many drugs are excreted in human milk, caution should be exercised when intravenous nitroglycerin is administered to a nursing woman.

Pediatric Use:
The safety and effectiveness of nitroglycerin in children have not been established.

ADVERSE REACTIONS

The most frequent adverse reaction in patients treated with nitroglycerin is headache, which occurs in approximately 2% of patients. Other adverse reactions occurring in less than 1% of patients are the following: tachycardia, nausea, vomiting, apprehension, restlessness, muscle twitching, retrosternal discomfort, palpitations, dizziness and abdominal pain.
The following additional adverse reactions have been reported with the oral and/or topical use of nitroglycerin: cutaneous flushing, weakness, and occasionally drug rash or exfoliative dermatitis.

OVERDOSAGE

Accidental overdosage of nitroglycerin may result in severe hypotension and reflex tachycardia which can be treated by elevating the legs and decreasing or temporarily terminating the infusion until the patient's condition stabilizes. Since the duration of the hemodynamic effects following nitroglycerin administration is quite short, additional corrective measures are usually not required. However, if further therapy is indicated, administration of an intravenous alpha adrenergic agonist (eg, methoxamine or phenylephrine) should be considered.

DOSAGE AND ADMINISTRATION

NOT FOR DIRECT INTRAVENOUS INJECTION
NITROSTAT IV IS A CONCENTRATED, POTENT DRUG WHICH MUST BE DILUTED IN DEXTROSE (5%) INJECTION, USP OR SODIUM CHLORIDE (0.9%) INJECTION, USP PRIOR TO ITS INFUSION.
NITROSTAT IV SHOULD NOT BE ADMIXED WITH OTHER DRUGS.
Dilution: It is important to consider the fluid requirements of the patient as well as the expected duration of infusion in selecting the appropriate dilution of nitroglycerin.
Solution Preparation for an Infusion Pump (60 microdrops = 1 ml)
Aseptically transfer 10 ml (8 mg nitroglycerin) of Nitrostat IV into a *glass*, IV bottle containing 250 ml of 5% Dextrose Injection, USP or 0.9% Sodium Chloride Injection, USP and mix well. The resultant solution will contain approximately 30 mcg/ml of nitroglycerin and is stable for at least 96 hours at controlled room temperature (15° to 30° C) or under refrigeration.

RATE OF ADMINISTRATION
(microdrops per minute or milliliters per hour)

Desired Dose (mcg/min)	10 ml in 250 ml = 30 mcg/ml (approx) Microdrops Per Minute	ml/hour
5	10	10
10	20	20
15	30	30
20	40	40
30	60	60
40	80	80
50	100	100

The tables below contain dosage information if a higher concentration of nitroglycerin or a longer duration of infusion is desired. Aseptically transfer the required volume from the ampoules to 250 ml of either 5% Dextrose Injection, USP or 0.9% Sodium Chloride Injection, USP.
If the concentration is adjusted, it is imperative to flush or replace the Nitrostat IV infusion set before a new concentration is utilized. The dead space of the set is approximately 15 ml and, depending on the flow rate, it could take from 9 minutes to 3 hours for the new concentration to reach the patient if the set were not flushed or replaced.

RATE OF ADMINISTRATION
(microdrops per minute or milliliters per hour)

Desired Dose (mcg/min)	20 ml in 250 ml = 60 mcg/ml (approx) Microdrops Per Minute	ml/hour
5	5	5
10	10	10
15	15	15
20	20	20
30	30	30
40	40	40
50	50	50
60	60	60
80	80	80
100	100	100

Desired Dose (mcg/min)	30 ml in 250 ml = 85 mcg/ml (approx)	
	Microdrops Per Minute	ml/hour
5	3	3.529
10	7	7.058
15	10	10.588
20	14	14.117
30	21	21.176
40	28	28.235
50	35	35.294
60	42	42.352
80	56	56.47
100	70	70.588

Dosage: *IMPORTANT NOTICE:* Dosage is affected by the type of container used as well as the type of infusion set used (See Warnings). Although the usual starting adult dose range reported in clinical studies was 25 mcg/min or more, those studies used *PVC TUBING. The use of nonabsorbing tubing will result in the need to use reduced doses.*

The recommended dosage when using the nonabsorbing Nitrostat IV Intravenous Infusion Set should initially be 5 mcg/min delivered through an infusion pump capable of exact and constant delivery of the drug. Subsequent titration must be adjusted to the clinical situation, with dose increments becoming more cautious as partial response is seen. Initial titration should be 5 mcg/min increments, with increases every 3 to 5 minutes until some response is noted. If no response is seen at 20 mcg/min, increments of 10 and later 20 mcg/min can be used. Once a partial blood pressure response is observed, the dose increase should be reduced and the interval between increments should be lengthened.

Patients with normal or low left ventricular filling pressure or pulmonary capillary wedge pressure (eg, angina patients without other complications) may be hypersensitive to the effects of nitroglycerin and may respond fully to doses as small as 5 mcg/min. These patients require especially careful titration and monitoring.

There is no fixed optimum dose of nitroglycerin. Due to variations in the responsiveness of individual patients to the drug, each patient must be titrated to the desired level of hemodynamic function. Therefore, continuous monitoring of physiologic parameters (blood pressure and heart rate in all patients, other measurements such as pulmonary capillary wedge pressure, as appropriate) MUST BE PERFORMED to achieve the correct dose. Adequate systemic blood pressure and coronary perfusion pressure must be maintained.

Directions For Preparing Nitrostat IV Infusion Set:

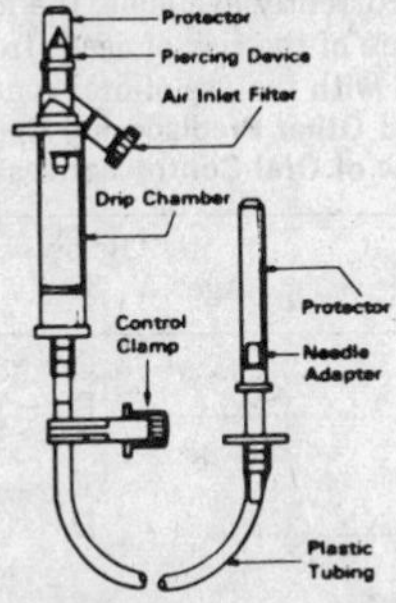

Caution—The fluid path and areas under the protectors of the intravenous infusion set are sterile. Do not use if damaged or if end protectors are not in place.

1. Position control clamp 6 to 8 inches from the needle adapter end of set, then close clamp. (To close clamp, rotate screw stem clockwise.)
2. With IV solution bottle in the upright position,
   a) remove plastic protector from the piercing device,
   b) THRUST the piercing device STRAIGHT DOWN through the CENTER of the target area in the rubber stopper (push straight down, do not twist).
   c) squeeze drip chamber and hold.
3. Invert the bottle and suspend from suitable stand.
4. Release pressure from drip chamber.
5. Remove needle adapter protector by pulling straight off (do not twist off).

If required, place needle on needle adapter. Hold this end of the tubing above the level of the nitroglycerin solution in the bottle. Loosen the control clamp and allow the solution to run into and to fill the tubing and needle. Displace the air in the entire injection set by raising or lowering the intravenous needle end of tubing until all the air bubbles are expelled.

(NOTE: Drip chamber should not be completely filled.)

6. Attach the infusion set to a suitable mechanical infusion control device.
7. Tighten control clamp and proceed with venipuncture or connect to needle.
8. Adjust infusion control device for precise measurement of flow rate.

HOW SUPPLIED

N 0071-4572-35 Nitrostat IV Infusion Kit containing one 10-ml ampoule of Nitrostat IV, 8 mg (0.8 mg/ml) and one disposable intravenous infusion set.

N 0071-4572-10 Carton of 10 × 10-ml ampoules of Nitrostat IV.

Store at controlled room temperature 15°–30° C (59°–86° F).

4572G022

Shown in Product Identification Section, page 421

NORLESTRIN® 21 1/50 ℞

[nōr″lĕs′trĭn]

(Each tablet contains 1 mg norethindrone acetate and 50 mcg ethinyl estradiol.)

NORLESTRIN® 21 2.5/50 ℞

(Each tablet contains 2.5 mg norethindrone acetate and 50 mcg ethinyl estradiol.)

NORLESTRIN® Fe 1/50 ℞

(Each yellow tablet contains 1 mg norethindrone acetate and 50 mcg ethinyl estradiol. Each brown tablet contains 75 mg ferrous fumarate, USP.)

NORLESTRIN® Fe 2.5/50 ℞

(Each pink tablet contains 2.5 mg norethindrone acetate and 50 mcg ethinyl estradiol. Each brown tablet contains 75 mg ferrous fumarate, USP.)

NORLESTRIN® 28 1/50 ℞

(Each yellow tablet contains 1 mg norethindrone acetate and 50 mcg ethinyl estradiol. Each white tablet is inert.)

Each yellow tablet contains: norethindrone acetate (17 alpha-ethinyl-19-nortestosterone acetate), 1 mg; ethinyl estradiol (17 alpha-ethinyl-1,3,5(10)-estratriene-3, 17 beta-diol), 50 mcg.

Each pink tablet contains: norethindrone acetate (17 alpha-ethinyl-19-nortestosterone acetate). 2.5 mg; ethinyl estradiol (17 alpha-ethinyl-1,3,5(10)-estratriene-3, 17 beta-diol), 50 mcg.

Each brown tablet contains 75 mg ferrous fumarate, USP.

Each white tablet is inert.

DESCRIPTION

Norlestrin is a progestogen-estrogen combination.

Norlestrin **Fe** 1/50 and 2.5/50 provides a continuous dosage regimen consisting of 21 oral contraceptive tablets and seven ferrous fumarate tablets. The ferrous fumarate tablets are present to facilitate ease of drug administration via a 28-day regimen and are not intended to serve any therapeutic purpose.

Norlestrin **28** 1/50 provides a continuous dosage regimen consisting of 21 oral contraceptive tablets and 7 inert tablets.

CLINICAL PHARMACOLOGY

Combination oral contraceptives act primarily through the mechanism of gonadotropin suppression due to the estrogenic and progestational activity of the ingredients. Although the primary mechanism of action is inhibition of ovulation, alterations in the genital tract, including changes in the cervical mucus (which increase the difficulty of sperm penetration) and the endometrium (which reduce the likelihood of implantation) may also contribute to contraceptive effectiveness.

INDICATIONS AND USAGE

Norlestrin is indicated for the prevention of pregnancy in women who elect to use oral contraceptives as a method of contraception.

Oral contraceptives are highly effective. The pregnancy rate in women using conventional combination oral contraceptives (containing 35 mcg or more of ethinyl estradiol or 50 mcg or more of mestranol) is generally reported as less than one pregnancy per 100 woman-years of use. Slightly higher rates (somewhat more than 1 pregnancy per 100 woman-years of use) are reported for some combination products containing 35 mcg or less of ethinyl estradiol, and rates on the order of 3 pregnancies per 100 woman-years are reported for the progestogen-only oral contraceptives.

These rates are derived from separate studies conducted by different investigators in several population groups and cannot be compared precisely. Furthermore, pregnancy rates tend to be lower as clinical studies are continued, possibly due to selective retention in the longer studies of those patients who accept the treatment regimen and do not discontinue as a result of adverse reactions, pregnancy, or other reasons.

In clinical trials with Norlestrin 1/50, 1,156 patients completed 25,983 cycles and a total of one pregnancy was reported. This represents a pregnancy rate of 0.05 per 100 woman-years.

In clinical trials with Norlestrin 2.5/50, 3,829 patients completed 96,388 cycles and a total of 18 pregnancies were reported. This represents a pregnancy rate of 0.22 per 100 woman-years based upon data that include the cases where patients failed to comply with the dosage regimen. The pregnancy rate in patients who adhered to the dosage regimen was 0.02 per 100 woman-years (two pregnancies in these trials).

Table 1 gives ranges of pregnancy rates reported in the literature[1] for other means of contraception. The efficacy of these means of contraception (except the IUD) depends upon the degree of adherence to the method.

Table 1 Pregnancies per 100 Woman-Years

IUD, less than 1–6; Diaphragm with spermicidal products (creams or jellies), 2–20; Condom, 3–36; Aerosol foams, 2–29; Jellies and creams, 4–36; Periodic abstinence (rhythm) all types, less than 1–47; *1. Calendar method, 14–47; 2. Temperature method, 1–20; 3. Temperature method—intercourse only in post-ovulatory phase, less than 1–7; 4. Mucus method, 1–25;* No contraception, 60–80.

Dose-Related Risk of Thromboembolism from Oral Contraceptives

Two studies have shown a positive association between the dose of estrogens in oral contraceptives and the risk of thromboembolism.[2,3] For this reason, it is prudent and in keeping with good principles of therapeutics to minimize exposure to estrogen. The oral contraceptive product prescribed for any given patient should be that product which contains the least amount of estrogen that is compatible with an acceptable pregnancy rate and patient acceptance. It is recommended that new acceptors of oral contraceptives be started on preparations containing 0.05 mg or less of estrogen.

CONTRAINDICATIONS

Oral contraceptives should not be used in women with any of the following conditions.

1. Thrombophlebitis or thromboembolic disorders
2. A past history of deep vein thrombophlebitis or thromboembolic disorders
3. Cerebral vascular or coronary artery disease
4. Known or suspected carcinoma of the breast
5. Known or suspected estrogen-dependent neoplasia
6. Undiagnosed abnormal genital bleeding
7. Known or suspected pregnancy (see Warning No. 5)
8. Benign or malignant liver tumor which developed during the use of oral contraceptives or other estrogen-containing products.

WARNINGS

Cigarette smoking increases the risk of serious cardiovascular side effects from oral contraceptive use. This risk increases with age and with heavy smoking (15 or more cigarettes per day) and is quite marked in women over 35 years of age. Women who use oral contraceptives should be strongly advised not to smoke.

The use of oral contraceptives is associated with increased risk of several serious conditions including thromboembolism, stroke, myocardial infarction, hepatic adenoma, gallbladder disease, and hypertension. Practitioners prescribing oral contraceptives should be familiar with the following information relating to these risks.

1. *Thromboembolic Disorders and Other Vascular Problems.* An increased risk of thromboembolic and thrombotic disease associated with the use of oral contraceptives is well established. Three principal studies in Great Britain[4–6] and three in the United States[7–10] have demonstrated an increased risk of fatal and nonfatal venous thromboembolism and stroke, both hemorrhagic and thrombotic. These studies estimate that users of oral contraceptives are 4 to 11 times more likely than nonusers to develop these diseases without evident cause (Table 2).

Cerebrovascular Disorders

In a collaborative American study[9,10] of cerebrovascular disorders in women with and without predisposing causes, it was estimated that the risk of hemorrhagic stroke was 2.0 times greater in users than nonusers and the risk of thrombotic stroke was 4 to 9.5 times greater in users than in nonusers (Table 2).

Table 2

Summary of relative risk of thromboembolic disorders and other vascular problems in oral contraceptive users compared to nonusers

	Relative risk, times greater
Idiopathic thromboembolic disease	4–11
Postsurgery thromboembolic complications	4–6
Thrombotic stroke	4–9.5
Hemorrhagic stroke	2
Myocardial infarction	2–12

Continued on next page

This product information was prepared in August, 1986. On these and other Parke-Davis Products, information may be obtained by addressing PARKE-DAVIS, Division of Warner-Lambert Company, Morris Plains, New Jersey 07950.

Parke-Davis—Cont.

Myocardial Infarction

An increased risk of myocardial infarction associated with the use of oral contraceptives has been reported[11-13] confirming a previously suspected association. These studies, conducted in the United Kingdom, found, as expected, that the greater the number of underlying risk factors for coronary artery disease (cigarette smoking, hypertension, hypercholesterolemia, obesity, diabetes, history of preeclamptic toxemia) the higher the risk of developing myocardial infarction, regardless of whether the patient was an oral contraceptive user or not. Oral contraceptives, however, were found to be a clear additional risk factor.

In terms of relative risk, it has been estimated[52] that oral contraceptive users who do not smoke (smoking is considered a major predisposing condition to myocardial infarction) are about twice as likely to have a fatal myocardial infarction as nonusers who do not smoke. Oral contraceptive users who are also smokers have about a 5-fold increased risk of fatal infarction compared to users who do not smoke, but about a 10- to 12-fold increased risk compared to nonusers who do not smoke. Furthermore, the amount of smoking is also an important factor. In determining the importance of these relative risks, however, the baseline rates for various age groups, as shown in Table 3, must be given serious consideration. The importance of other predisposing conditions mentioned above in determining relative and absolute risks has not yet been quantified; it is quite likely that the same synergistic action exists, but perhaps to a lesser extent.

[See table below].

Table 3

Estimated annual mortality rate per 100,000 women from myocardial infarction by use of oral contraceptives, smoking habits, and age (in years)

Risk of Dose

Persistence of Risk

In confirmation of earlier reports,[53,54] two studies have suggested that an increased risk may persist for as long as 6 years after discontinuation of oral contraceptive use for cerebrovascular disease[55] and 9 years for myocardial infarction[56]. In addition, a prospective study suggested the persistence of risk for subarachnoid hemorrhage.[57]

In an analysis of data derived from several national adverse reaction reporting systems,[2] British investigators concluded that the risk of thromboembolism, including coronary thrombosis, is directly related to the dose of estrogen used in oral contraceptives. Preparations containing 100 mcg or more of estrogen were associated with a higher risk of thromboembolism than those containing 50 to 80 mcg of estrogen. Their analysis did suggest, however, that the quantity of estrogen may not be the sole factor involved. This finding has been confirmed in the United States. Careful epidemiological studies to determine the degree of thromboembolic risk associated with progestogen-only oral contraceptives have not been performed. Cases of thromboembolic disease have been reported in women using these products, and they should not be presumed to be free of excess risk.

Estimate of Excess Mortality from Circulatory Diseases

A large prospective study [53] carried out in the U.K. estimated the mortality rate per 100,000 women per year from diseases of the circulatory system for users and nonusers of oral contraceptives according to age, smoking habits, and duration of use. The overall excess death rate annually from circulatory diseases for oral contraceptive users was estimated to be 20 per 100,000 (ages 15 to 34—5/100,000; ages 35 to 44—33/100,000; ages 45 to 49—140/100,000), the risk being concentrated in older women, in those with a long duration of use, and in cigarette smokers. It was not possible, however, to examine the interrelationships of age, smoking, and duration of use, nor to compare the effects of continuous versus intermittent use. Although the study showed a 10-fold increase in death due to circulatory diseases in users for 5 or more years, all of these deaths occurred in women 35 or older. Until larger numbers of women under 35 with continuous use for 5 or more years are available, it is not possible to assess the magnitude of the relative risk for this younger age group.

Figure 1. Estimated annual number of deaths associated with control of fertility and no control per 100,000 nonsterile women, by regimen of control and age of woman.

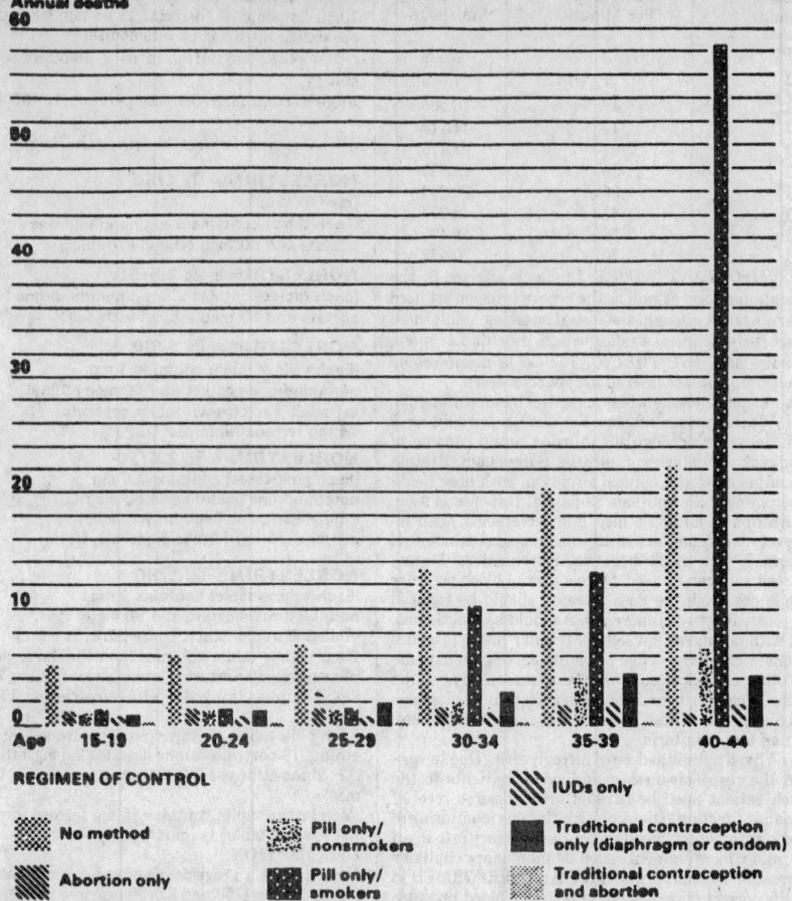

The available data from a variety of sources have been analyzed[14] to estimate the risk of death associated with various methods of contraception. The estimates of risk of death for each method include the combined risk of the contraceptive method (eg, thromboembolic and thrombotic disease in the case of oral contraceptives) plus the risk attributable to pregnancy or abortion in the event of method failure. This latter risk varies with the effectiveness of the contraceptive method. The findings of this analysis are shown in Figure 1 which follows.[14] The study concluded that the mortality associated with all methods of birth control is low and below that associated with childbirth, with the exception of oral contraceptives in women over 40 who smoke. (The rates given for pill only/smokers for each age group are for smokers as a class. For "heavy" smokers [more than 15 cigarettes a day] the rates given would be about double, for "light" smokers [less than 15 cigarettes a day] about 50 percent.) The lowest mortality is associated with the condom or diaphragm backed up by early abortion.

[See Figure 1 above].

The risk of thromboembolic and thrombotic disease associated with oral contraceptives increases with age after approximately age 30 and, for myocardial infarction, is further increased by hypertension, hypercholesterolemia, obesity, diabetes, or history of preeclamptic toxemia and especially by cigarette smoking.

Based on the data currently available, the following chart gives a gross estimate of the risk of death from circulatory disorders associated with the use of oral contraceptives.

Smoking Habits and Other Predisposing Conditions—Risk Associated with Use of Oral Contraceptives

Age:	Below 30	30–39	40+
Heavy smokers	C	B	A
Light smokers	D	C	B
Nonsmokers (no predisposing conditions)	D	C,D	C
Nonsmokers (other predisposing conditions)	C	C,B	B,A

A—Use associated with very high risk
B—Use associated with high risk
C—Use associated with moderate risk
D—Use associated with low risk

The physician and the patient should be alert to the earliest manifestations of thromboembolic and thrombotic disorders (eg, thrombophlebitis, pulmonary embolism, cerebrovascular insufficiency, coronary occlusion, retinal thrombosis, and mesenteric thrombosis). Should any of these occur or be suspected, the drug should be discontinued immediately.

A four- to six-fold increased risk of postsurgery thromboembolic complications has been reported in oral contraceptive users.[15,16] If feasible, oral contraceptives should be discontinued at least 4 weeks before surgery of a type associated with an increased risk of thromboembolism or prolonged immobilization.

2. *Ocular Lesions.* There have been reports of neuro-ocular lesions, such as optic neuritis or retinal thrombosis, associated with the use of oral contraceptives. Discontinue oral contraceptive medication if there is unexplained, sudden or gradual, partial or complete loss of vision; onset of proptosis or diplopia; papilledema; or retinal vascular lesions and institute appropriate diagnostic and therapeutic measures.

3. *Carcinoma.* Long-term continuous administration of either natural or synthetic estrogen in certain animal species increases the frequency of carcinoma of the breast, cer-

Norlestrin

	Myocardial infarction			
	Women aged 30–39		Women aged 40–44	
Smoking habits	Users	Nonusers	Users	Nonusers
All smokers	10.2	2.6	62.0	15.9
Heavy*	13.0	5.1	78.7	31.3
Light	4.7	0.9	28.6	5.7
Nonsmokers	1.8	1.2	10.7	7.4
Smokers and nonsmokers	5.4	1.9	32.8	11.7

*Heavy smoker: 15 or more cigarettes per day. From Jain, A.K., Studies in Family Planning 8:50, 1977.

vix, vagina, and liver. Certain synthetic progestogens, none currently contained in oral contraceptives, have been noted to increase the incidence of mammary nodules, benign and malignant, in dogs.

In humans, three case control studies have reported an increased risk of endometrial carcinoma associated with the prolonged use of exogenous estrogen in post-menopausal women.[17–19] One publication[20] reported on the first 21 cases submitted by physicians to a registry of cases of adenocarcinoma of the endometrium in women under 40 on oral contraceptives. Of the cases found in women without predisposing risk factors for adenocarcinoma of the endometrium (eg, irregular bleeding at the time oral contraceptives were first given, polycystic ovaries), nearly all occurred in women who had used a sequential oral contraceptive. These products are no longer marketed. No evidence has been reported suggesting an increased risk of endometrial cancer in users of conventional-combination or progestogen-only oral contraceptives.

Several studies[8,21–24] have found no increase in breast cancer in women taking oral contraceptives or estrogens. One study,[25] however, while also noting no overall increased risk of breast cancer in women treated with oral contraceptives, found an excess risk in the subgroups of oral contraceptive users with documented benign breast disease. A reduced occurrence of benign breast tumors in users of oral contraceptives has been well-documented.[8,21,25–27]

In summary, there is at present no confirmed evidence from human studies of an increased risk of cancer associated with oral contraceptives. Close clinical surveillance of all women taking oral contraceptives is, nevertheless, essential. In all cases of undiagnosed persistent or recurrent abnormal vaginal bleeding, appropriate diagnostic measures should be taken to rule out malignancy. Women with a strong family history of breast cancer or who have breast nodules, fibrocystic disease, or abnormal mammograms, should be monitored with particular care if they elect to use oral contraceptives instead of other methods of contraception.

4. *Hepatic Tumors.* Benign hepatic adenomas have been found to be associated with the use of oral contraceptives.[28–30,46] One study[46] showed that oral contraceptive formulations with high hormonal potency were associated with a higher risk than lower potency formulations. Although benign, hepatic adenomas may rupture and may cause death through intra-abdominal hemorrhage. This has been reported in short-term as well as long-term users of oral contraceptives. Two studies relate risk with duration of use of the contraceptive, the risk being much greater after 4 or more years of oral contraceptive use.[30,46] While hepatic adenoma is a rare lesion, it should be considered in women presenting abdominal pain and tenderness, abdominal mass or shock.

A few cases of hepatocellular carcinoma have been reported in women taking oral contraceptives. The relationship of these drugs to this type of malignancy is not known at this time.

5. *Use in or Immediately Preceding Pregnancy, Birth Defects in Offspring, and Malignancy in Female Offspring.* The use of female sex hormones— both estrogenic and progestational agents—during early pregnancy may seriously damage the offspring. It has been shown that females exposed *in utero* to diethylstilbestrol, a nonsteroidal estrogen, have an increased risk of developing in later life a form of vaginal or cervical cancer that is ordinarily extremely rare.[31,32] This risk has been estimated to be of the order of 1 in 1,000 exposures or less.[33,47] Although there is no evidence at the present time that oral contraceptives further enhance the risk of developing this type of malignancy, such patients should be monitored with particular care if they elect to use oral contraceptives instead of other methods of contraception. Furthermore, a high percentage of such exposed women (from 30% to 90%) have been found to have epithelial changes of the vagina and cervix.[34–38] Although these changes are histologically benign, it is not known whether this condition is a precursor of vaginal malignancy. Male children so exposed may develop abnormalities of the urogenital tract.[48–50] Although similar data are not available with the use of other estrogens, it cannot be presumed that they would not induce similar changes.

An increased risk of congenital anomalies, including heart defects and limb defects, has been reported with the use of sex hormones, including oral contraceptives, in pregnancy.[39–42,51] One case control study[42] has estimated a 4.7-fold increase in risk of limb-reduction defects in infants exposed *in utero* to sex hormones (oral contraceptives, hormonal withdrawal tests for pregnancy or attempted treatment for threatened abortion). Some of these exposures were very short and involved only a few days of treatment. The data suggest that the risk of limb-reduction defects in exposed fetuses is somewhat less than 1 in 1,000 live births.

In the past, female sex hormones have been used during pregnancy in an attempt to treat threatened or habitual abortion. There is considerable evidence that estrogens are ineffective for these indications, and there is no evidence from well-controlled studies that progestogens are effective for these uses.

There is some evidence that triploidy and possibly other types of polyploidy are increased among abortuses from women who become pregnant soon after ceasing oral contraceptives.[43] Embryos with these anomalies are virtually always aborted spontaneously. Whether there is an overall increase in spontaneous abortion of pregnancies conceived soon after stopping oral contraceptives is unknown.

It is recommended that for any patient who has missed two consecutive periods, pregnancy should be ruled out before continuing the contraceptive regimen. If the patient has not adhered to the prescribed schedule, the possibility of pregnancy should be considered at the time of the first missed period, and further use of oral contraceptives should be withheld until pregnancy has been ruled out. If pregnancy is confirmed, the patient should be apprised of the potential risks to the fetus and the advisability of continuation of the pregnancy should be discussed in the light of these risks.

It is also recommended that women who discontinue oral contraceptives with the intent of becoming pregnant use an alternate form of contraception for a period of time before attempting to conceive. Many clinicians recommend 3 months although no precise information is available on which to base this recommendation.

The administration of progestogen-only or progestogen-estrogen combinations to induce withdrawal bleeding should not be used as a test of pregnancy.

6. *Gallbladder Disease.* Studies[8,23,26] report an increased risk of surgically confirmed gallbladder disease in users of oral contraceptives and estrogens. In one study, an increased risk appeared after 2 years of use and doubled after 4 or 5 years of use. In one of the other studies, an increased risk was apparent between 6 and 12 months of use.

7. *Carbohydrate and Lipid Metabolic Effects.* A decrease in glucose tolerance has been observed in a significant percentage of patients on oral contraceptives. For this reason, prediabetic and diabetic patients should be carefully observed while receiving oral contraceptives.

An increase in triglycerides and total phospholipids has been observed in patients receiving oral contraceptives.[44] The clinical significance of this finding remains to be defined.

8. *Elevated Blood Pressure.* An increase in blood pressure has been reported in patients receiving oral contraceptives.[26] In some women, hypertension may occur within a few months of beginning oral contraceptive use. In the first year of use, the prevalence of women with hypertension is low in users and may be no higher than that of a comparable group of nonusers. The prevalence in users increases, however, with longer exposure, and in the fifth year of use is two and a half to three times the reported prevalence in the first year. Age is also strongly correlated with the development of hypertension in oral contraceptive users. Women who previously have had hypertension during pregnancy may be more likely to develop elevation of blood pressure when given oral contraceptives. Hypertension that develops as a result of taking oral contraceptives usually returns to normal after discontinuing the drug.

9. *Headache.* The onset or exacerbation of migraine or development of headache of a new pattern which is recurrent, persistent, or severe, requires discontinuation of oral contraceptives and evaluation of the cause.

10. *Bleeding Irregularities.* Breakthrough bleeding, spotting and amenorrhea are frequent reasons for patients discontinuing oral contraceptives. In breakthrough bleeding, as in all cases of irregular bleeding from the vagina, nonfunctional causes should be borne in mind. In undiagnosed persistent or recurrent abnormal bleeding from the vagina, adequate diagnostic measures are indicated to rule out pregnancy or malignancy. If pathology has been excluded, time or a change to another formulation may solve the problem. Changing to an oral contraceptive with a higher estrogen content, while potentially useful in minimizing menstrual irregularity, should be done only if necessary since this may increase the risk of thromboembolic disease.

Women with a past history of oligomenorrhea or secondary amenorrhea or young women without regular cycles may have a tendency to remain anovulatory or to become amenorrheic after discontinuation of oral contraceptives. Women with these preexisting problems should be advised of this possibility and encouraged to use other contraceptive methods. Post-use anovulation, possibly prolonged, may also occur in women without previous irregularities.

11. *Ectopic Pregnancy.* Ectopic as well as intrauterine pregnancy may occur in contraceptive failures. However, in progestogen-only oral contraceptive failures, the ratio of ectopic to intrauterine pregnancies is higher than in women who are not receiving oral contraceptives, since the drugs are more effective in preventing intrauterine than ectopic pregnancies.

12. *Breast-Feeding.* Oral contraceptives given in the postpartum period may interfere with lactation. There may be a decrease in the quantity and quality of the breast milk. Furthermore, a small fraction of the hormonal agents in oral contraceptives has been identified in the milk of mothers receiving these drugs.[45] The effects, if any, on the breast-fed child have not been determined. If feasible, the use of oral contraceptives should be deferred until the infant has been weaned.

PRECAUTIONS

General

1. A complete medical and family history should be taken prior to the initiation of oral contraceptives. The pretreatment and periodic physical examinations should include special reference to blood pressure, breasts, abdomen and pelvic organs, including Papanicolaou smear and relevant laboratory tests. As a general rule, oral contraceptives should not be prescribed for longer than 1 year without another physical examination being performed.
2. Under the influence of estrogen-progestogen preparations preexisting uterine leiomyomata may increase in size.
3. Patients with a history of psychic depression should be carefully observed and the drug discontinued if depression recurs to a serious degree. Patients becoming significantly depressed while taking oral contraceptives should stop the medication and use an alternate method of contraception in an attempt to determine whether the symptom is drug related.
4. Oral contraceptives may cause some degree of fluid retention. They should be prescribed with caution, and only with careful monitoring, in patients with conditions which might be aggravated by fluid retention, such as convulsive disorders, migraine syndrome, asthma, or cardiac or renal insufficiency.
5. Patients with a past history of jaundice during pregnancy have an increased risk of recurrence of jaundice while receiving oral contraceptive therapy. If jaundice develops in any patient receiving such drugs, the medication should be discontinued.
6. Steroid hormones may be poorly metabolized in patients with impaired liver function and should be administered with caution in such patients.
7. Oral contraceptive users may have disturbances in normal tryptophan metabolism which may result in a relative pyridoxine deficiency. The clinical significance of this is yet to be determined.
8. Serum folate levels may be depressed by oral contraceptive therapy. Since the pregnant woman is predisposed to the development of folate deficiency and the incidence of folate deficiency increases with increasing gestation, it is possible that if a woman becomes pregnant shortly after stopping oral contraceptives, she may have a greater chance of developing folate deficiency and complications attributed to this deficiency.
9. The pathologist should be advised of oral contraceptive therapy when relevant specimens are submitted.
10. Certain endocrine and liver function tests and blood components may be affected by estrogen-containing oral contraceptives:

a. Increased sulfobromophthalein retention
b. Increased prothrombin and factors VII, VIII, IX, and X; decreased antithrombin 3; increased norepinephrine-induced platelet aggregability
c. Increased thyroid binding globulin (TBG) leading to increased circulating total thyroid hormone, as measured by protein-bound iodine (PBI), T4 by column, or T4 by radioimmunoassay. Free T3 resin uptake is decreased, reflecting the elevated TBG, free T4 concentration is unaltered
d. Decreased pregnanediol excretion
e. Reduced response to metyrapone test

Information For The Patient: See Patient Labeling printed following the reference section.

DRUG INTERACTIONS

Reduced efficacy and increased incidence of breakthrough bleeding have been associated with concomitant use of rifampin. A similar association has been suggested with barbiturates, phenylbutazone, phenytoin sodium, tetracycline, and ampicillin.

Carcinogenesis: See Warnings section for information on the carcinogenic potential of oral contraceptives.

Pregnancy: Pregnancy category X. See Contraindications and Warnings.

Nursing Mothers: See Warnings.

ADVERSE REACTIONS

An increased risk of the following serious adverse reactions has been associated with the use of oral contraceptives (see Warnings):

Thrombophlebitis
Pulmonary embolism
Coronary thrombosis
Cerebral thrombosis
Cerebral hemorrhage

Continued on next page

This product information was prepared in August, 1986. On these and other Parke-Davis Products, information may be obtained by addressing PARKE-DAVIS, Division of Warner-Lambert Company, Morris Plains, New Jersey 07950.

Parke-Davis—Cont.

Hypertension
Gallbladder disease
Benign hepatomas
Congenital anomalies

There is evidence of an association between the following conditions and the use of oral contraceptives, although additional confirmatory studies are needed:

Mesenteric thrombosis
Neuro-ocular lesions, eg, retinal thrombosis and optic neuritis

The following adverse reactions have been reported in patients receiving oral contraceptives and are believed to be drug related:

Nausea and/or vomiting, usually the most common adverse reactions, occur in approximately 10 percent or less of patients during the first cycle. Other reactions, as a general rule, are seen much less frequently or only occasionally.

Gastrointestinal symptoms (such as abdominal cramps and bloating)
Breakthrough bleeding
Spotting
Change in menstrual flow
Dysmenorrhea
Amenorrhea during and after treatment
Temporary infertility after discontinuance of treatment
Edema
Chloasma or melasma which may persist
Breast changes: tenderness, enlargement and secretion
Change in weight (increase or decrease)
Change in cervical erosion and cervical secretion
Possible diminution in lactation when given immediately postpartum
Cholestatic jaundice
Migraine
Increase in size of uterine leiomyomata
Rash (allergic)
Mental depression
Reduced tolerance to carbohydrates
Vaginal candidiasis
Change in corneal curvature (steepening)
Intolerance to contact lenses

The following adverse reactions have been reported in users of oral contraceptives, and the association has been neither confirmed nor refuted:

Premenstrual-like syndrome
Cataracts
Changes in libido
Chorea
Changes in appetite
Cystitis-like syndrome
Headache
Nervousness
Dizziness
Hirsutism
Loss of scalp hair
Erythema multiforme
Erythema nodosum
Hemorrhagic eruption
Vaginitis
Porphyria

ACUTE OVERDOSE

Serious ill effects have not been reported following acute ingestion of large doses of oral contraceptives by young children. Overdosage may cause nausea, and withdrawal bleeding may occur in females.

Dosage and Administration For 21-Day Dosage Regimen: To achieve maximum contraceptive effectiveness, Norlestrin must be taken exactly as directed and at intervals not exceeding 24 hours. Norlestrin **21** provides the patient with a convenient tablet schedule of "3 weeks on—1 week off."

The first day of menstrual flow is considered Day 1. Initially, the patient begins taking tablets on Day 5 and takes one tablet daily for 21 days. She then takes no tablets for seven days. After the seven days during which no tablets are taken, the patient begins a new course of one tablet daily for 21 days. Each course of tablets will begin on the same day of the week as the first course. Likewise, the interval of no tablets will always start on the same day of the week.

Tablets should be taken regularly with a meal or at bedtime. It should be stressed that efficacy of medication depends on strict adherence to the dosage schedule.

Special Notes on Administration

Menstruation usually begins two or three days, but may begin as late as the fourth or fifth day, after discontinuing medication.

If spotting occurs while on the usual regimen of one tablet daily, the patient should continue medication without interruption.

If a patient forgets to take one or more tablets, the following is suggested: If one tablet is missed, take it as soon as remembered, or take two tablets the next day. If two consecutive tablets are missed, take two tablets daily for the next two days, then resume the regular schedule. If three consecutive tablets are missed, begin a new compact of tablets, starting seven days after the last tablet was taken.

The possibility of ovulation occurring increases with each successive day that scheduled tablets are missed. When three consecutive tablets are missed the patient should use an alternate means of contraception, other than oral tablets, until the start of the next menstrual period.

While there is little likelihood of ovulation occurring if only one tablet is missed, the possibility of spotting or bleeding is increased. This is particularly likely to occur if two or more consecutive tablets are missed.

In the rare case of bleeding which resembles menstruation, the patient should be advised to discontinue medication and then begin taking tablets from a new compact on the fifth day (Day 5). Persistent bleeding which is not controlled by this method indicates the need for re-examination of the patient at which time nonfunctional causes should be borne in mind.

Dosage and Administration For 28-Day Dosage Regimen: To achieve maximum contraceptive effectiveness, Norlestrin must be taken exactly as directed and at intervals not exceeding 24 hours.

Norlestrin **Fe** and **28** provides a continuous administration regimen consisting of 21 *light-colored* tablets of Norlestrin and 7 brown tablets of ferrous fumarate or 7 white inert tablets. There is no need for the patient to count days between cycles because there are no "off-tablet days."

The dosage schedule is one *light-colored* tablet daily for 21 days, starting initially on Day 5 of the menstrual cycle, followed without interruption by one brown or white tablet daily for 7 days. The first day of menstrual flow is considered Day 1. Upon completion of this first course of tablets, a second course of tablets is started without interruption. All subsequent courses also are taken without interruption.

Tablets should be taken regularly with a meal or at bedtime. It should be stressed that efficacy of medication depends on strict adherence to the dosage schedule.

Special Notes on Administration

Menstruation usually begins two or three days, but may begin as late as the fourth or fifth day, after the brown or white tablets have been started. In any event, the next course of tablets should be started without interruption. There should never be a day when the patient is not taking a tablet.

If spotting occurs while the patient is taking *light-colored* tablets, continue medication without interruption.

If a patient forgets to take one or more *light-colored* tablets, the following is suggested: If one *light-colored* tablet is missed, take it as soon as remembered, or take two *light-colored* tablets the next day. If two consecutive *light-colored* tablets are missed, take two *light-colored* tablets daily for the next two days, then resume the regular schedule. If three consecutive *light-colored* tablets are missed, begin a new compact of tablets, starting seven days after the last *light-colored* tablet was taken.

The possibility of ovulation occurring increases with each successive day that scheduled *light-colored* tablets are missed. When three consecutive *light-colored* tablets are missed, the patient should use an alternate means of contraception, other than oral tablets, until the start of the next menstrual period.

While there is little likelihood of ovulation occurring if only one *light-colored* tablet is missed, the possibility of spotting or bleeding is increased. This is particularly likely to occur if two or more consecutive *light-colored* tablets are missed.

If one or more brown or white tablets are missed, the *light-colored* tablets should be started no later than the eighth day after the last *light-colored* tablet was taken. The possibility of conception occurring is not increased if brown or white tablets are missed.

In the rare case of bleeding which resembles menstruation, the patient should be advised to discontinue medication and then begin taking tablets from a new compact on the fifth day (Day 5). Persistent bleeding which is not controlled by this method indicates the need for re-examination of the patient, at which time nonfunctional causes should be borne in mind.

Use of oral contraceptives in the event of a missed menstrual period:

1. If the patient has not adhered to the prescribed dosage regimen, the possibility of pregnancy should be considered after the first missed period and oral contraceptives should be withheld until pregnancy has been ruled out.
2. If the patient has adhered to the prescribed regimen and misses two consecutive periods, pregnancy should be ruled out before continuing the contraceptive regimen.

After several months on treatment, bleeding may be reduced to a point of virtual absence. This reduced flow may occur as a result of medication, in which event it is not indicative of pregnancy.

HOW SUPPLIED

Norlestrin **21** 1/50 is available in compacts each containing 21 tablets. Each tablet contains 1 mg of norethindrone acetate and 50 mcg of ethinyl estradiol. Available in packages of five compacts and packages of five refills.

Norlestrin **21** 2.5/50 is available in compacts each containing 21 tablets. Each tablet contains 2.5 mg of norethindrone acetate and 50 mcg of ethinyl estradiol. Available in packages of five compacts and packages of five refills.

Norlestrin **Fe** 1/50 is available in compacts each containing 21 yellow tablets and 7 brown tablets. Each yellow tablet contains 1 mg of norethindrone acetate and 50 mcg of ethinyl estradiol. Each brown tablet contains 75 mg ferrous fumarate, USP. Available in packages of five compacts and packages of five refills.

Norlestrin **Fe** 2.5/50 is available in compacts each containing 21 pink tablets and 7 brown tablets. Each pink tablet contains 2.5 mg of norethindrone acetate and 50 mcg of ethinyl estradiol. Each brown tablet contains 75 mg ferrous fumarate, USP. Available in packages of five compacts and packages of five refills.

Norlestrin **28** 1/50 is available in compacts each containing 21 yellow tablets and 7 white inert tablets. Each yellow tablet contains 1 mg of norethindrone acetate and 50 mcg of ethinyl estradiol. Available in packages of five compacts and packages of five refills.

References:

1. "*Population Reports,*" Series H, Number 2, May 1974; Series 1, Number 1, June 1974; Series B, Number 2, January 1975; Series H, Number 3, 1975; Series H, Number 4, January 1976 (published by the Population Information Program, The George Washington University Medical Center, 2001 S. St. NW., Washington, D.C.)
2. Inman, W. H. W., M. P. Vessey, B. Westerholm, and A. Engelund. "Thromboembolic disease and the steroidal content of oral contraceptives. A report to the Committee on Safety of Drugs," *Brit Med J* 2:203–209, 1970.
3. Stolley, P.D., J. A. Tonascia, M. S. Tockman, P. E. Sartwell, A. H. Rutledge, and M. P. Jacobs, "Thrombosis with low-estrogen oral contraceptives," *Am J Epidemiol* 102: 197–208, 1975.
4. Royal College of General Practitioners, "Oral contraception and thromboembolic disease," *J Coll Gen Pract* 13:267–279, 1967.
5. Inman, W. H. W. and M. P. Vessey, "Investigation of deaths from pulmonary, coronary and cerebral thrombosis and embolism in women of childbearing age," *Brit Med. J* 2-193–199, 1968.
6. Vessey, M. P. and R. Doll, "Investigation of relation between use of oral contraceptives and thromboembolic disease. A further report," *Brit Med J* 2:651–657, 1969.
7. Sartwell, P. E., A. T. Masi, F. G. Arthes, G. R. Greene, and H. E. Smith, "Thromboembolism and oral contraceptives an epidemiological case control study," *Am J Epidemiol* 90:365–380, 1969.
8. Boston Collaborative Drug Surveillance Program. "Oral contraceptives and venous thromboembolic disease, surgically confirmed gallbladder disease and breast tumors," *Lancet* 1:1399–1404, 1973.
9. Collaborative Group for the Study of Stroke in Young Women, "Oral contraception and increased risk of cerebral ischemia or thrombosis," *N Engl J Med* 288:871–878, 1973.
10. Collaborative Group for the Study of Stroke in Young Women, "Oral contraceptives and stroke in young women: associated risk factors," *JAMA* 231:718–722, 1975.
11. Mann, J. I., and W. H. W. Inman, "Oral contraceptives and death from myocardial infarction," *Brit Med J* 2:245–248, 1975.
12. Mann, J. I., W. H. W. Inman, and M. Thorogood, "Oral contraceptive use in older women and fatal myocardial infarction," *Brit Med J* 2:445–447, 1976.
13. Mann, J. I., M. P. Vessey, M. Thorogood and R. Doll, "Myocardial infarction in young women with special reference to oral contraceptive practice," *Brit Med J* 2:241–245, 1975.
14. Tietze, C., "New Estimates of Mortality Associated with Fertility Control," *Family Planning Perspectives,* 9:74–76, 1977.
15. Vessey, M. P., R. Doll, A. S. Fairbairn, and G. Glober, "Post-operative thromboembolism and the use of oral contraceptives," *Brit Med J* 3:123–126, 1970.
16. Greene, G. R., P. E. Sartwell, "Oral contraceptive use in patients with thromboembolism following surgery, trauma or infection," *Am J Pub Health* 62:680–685, 1972.
17. Smith, D. C., R. Prentice, D. J. Thompson and W. L. Herrmann, "Association of exogenous estrogen and endometrial carcinoma," *N Engl J Med* 293:1164–1167, 1975.
18. Ziel, H. K., and W. D. Finkle, "Increased risk of endometrial carcinoma among users of conjugated estrogens," *N Engl J Med* 293: 1167–1170, 1975.
19. Mack, T. N., M. C. Pike, B. E. Henderson, R. I. Pfeffer, V. R. Gerkins, M. Arthur and S. E. Brown, "Estrogens and endometrial cancer in a retirement community," *N Engl J Med* 294: 1262–1267, 1976.
20. Silverberg, S. G., and E. L. Makowski, "Endometrial carcinoma in young women taking oral contraceptive agents," *Obstet Gynecol* 46:503–506, 1975.
21. Vessey, M. P., R. Doll, and P. M. Sutton, "Oral contraceptives and breast neoplasia: a retrospective study," *Brit Med J* 3:719–724, 1972.

22. Vessey, M. P., R. Doll, and K. Jones, "Oral contraceptives and breast cancer. Progress report of an epidemiological study," *Lancet* 1:941–943, 1975.
23. Boston Collaborative Drug Surveillance Program, "Surgically confirmed gallbladder disease, venous thromboembolism and breast tumors in relation to postmenopausal estrogen therapy," *N Engl J Med* 290:14–19, 1974.
24. Arthes, F. G., P. E. Sartwell, and E. F. Lewison, "The pill, estrogens, and the breast, Epidemiologic aspects," *Cancer* 28:1391–1394, 1971.
25. Fasal, E., and R. S. Paffenbarger, "Oral contraceptives as related to cancer and benign lesions of the breast." *J Natl Cancer Inst* 55:767–773, 1975.
26. Royal College of General Practitioners, "Oral Contraceptives and Health," London, Pitman, 1974.
27. Ory, H., P. Cole, B. MacMahon, and R. Hoover, "Oral contraceptives and reduced risk of benign breast diseases," *N Engl J Med* 294:419–422, 1976.
28. Baum, J., F. Holtz, J. J. Bookstein, and E. W. Klein, "Possible association between benign hepatomas and oral contraceptives," *Lancet* 2:926–928, 1973.
29. Mays, E. T., W. M. Christopherson, M. M. Mahr, and H. C. Williams, "Hepatic changes in young women ingesting contraceptive steroids. Hepatic hemorrhage and primary hepatic tumors," *JAMA* 235:730–732, 1976.
30. Edmondson, H. A., B. Henderson, and B. Benton, "Liver-cell adenomas associated with use of oral contraceptives," *N Engl J Med* 294:470–472, 1976.
31. Herbst, A. L., H. Ulfelder, and D. C. Poskanzer, "Adenocarcinoma of the vagina," *N Engl J Med* 284:878–881, 1971.
32. Greenwald, P., J. J. Barlow, P. C. Nasca and W. Burnett, "Vaginal cancer after maternal treatment with synthetic estrogens," *N Engl J Med* 285: 390–392, 1971.
33. Lanier, A. P., K. L. Noller, D. G. Decker, L. Elveback, and L. T. Kurland, "Cancer and stilbestrol. A follow-up of 1719 persons exposed to estrogens in utero and born 1943–1959," *Mayo Clin Pro* 48:793–799, 1973.
34. Herbst, A. L., R. J. Kurman, and R. E. Scully, "Vaginal and cervical abnormalities after exposure to stilbestrol in utero," *Obstet Gynecol* 40:287–298, 1972.
35. Herbst, A. L., S. J. Robboy, G. J. Macdonald, and R. E. Scully, "The effects of local progesterone on stilbestrol-associated vaginal adenosis," *Am J. Obstet Gynecol* 118:607–615, 1974.
36. Herbst, A. L., D. C. Poskanzer, S. J. Robboy, L. Friedlander, and R. E. Scully, "Prenatal exposure to stilbestrol: a prospective comparison of exposed female offspring with unexposed controls," *N Engl J Med* 292:334–339, 1975.
37. Stafl, A., R. F. Mattingly, D. V. Foley, W. Fetherston, "Clinical diagnosis of vaginal adenosis," *Obstet Gynecol* 43:118–128, 1974.
38. Sherman, A. I., M. Goldrath, A. Berlin, V. Vakhariya, F. Banooni, W. Michaels, P. Goodman, and S. Brown, "Cervical-vaginal adenosis after in utero exposure to synthetic estrogens," *Obstet Gynecol* 44:531–545, 1974.
39. Gal, I., B. Kirman, and J. Stern, "Hormone pregnancy tests and congenital malformation," *Nature* 216:83, 1967.
40. Levy, E. P., A. Cohen, and F. C. Fraser, "Hormone treatment during pregnancy and congenital heart defects," *Lancet* 1:611, 1973.
41. Nora, J. J., and A. H. Nora, "Birth defects and oral contraceptives," *Lancet* 1:941–942, 1973.
42. Janerich, D. T., J. M. Piper, and D. M. Glebatis, "Oral contraceptives and congenital limb-reduction defects," *N Engl J Med* 291:697–700, 1974.
43. Carr, D. H., "Chromosome studies in selected spontaneous abortions: I. Conception after oral contraceptives," *Canad Med Assoc J* 103:343–348, 1970.
44. Wynn, V., J. W. H. Doar, and G. L. Mills, "Some effects of oral contraceptives on serum-lipid and lipoprotein levels," *Lancet* 2:720–723, 1966.
45. Laumas, K. R., P. K. Malkani, S. Bhatnagar, and V. Laumas, "Radioactivity in the breast milk of lactating women after oral administration of 3 H-norethynodrel," *Amer J Obstet Gynecol* 98:411–413, 1967.
46. Center for Disease Control, "Increased Risk of Hepatocellular Adenoma in Women with Long-term use of Oral Contraceptives," *Morbidity and Mortality Weekly Report* 26:293–294, 1977.
47. Herbst, A. L., P. Cole, T. Colton, S. J. Robboy, R. E. Scully, "Age-incidence and Risk of Diethylstilbestrol-related Clear Cell Adenocarcinoma of the Vagina and Cervix," *Am J. Obstet Gynecol* 128:43–50, 1977.
48. Bibbo, M., M. Al-Naqeeb, I. Baccarini, W. Gill, M. Newton, K. M. Sleeper, M. Sonek, G. L. Wied, "Follow-Up Study of Male and Female Offspring of DES-treated Mothers. A Preliminary Report," *Jour of Repro Med* 15:29–32, 1975.
49. Gill, W. B., G. F. B. Schumacher, M. Bibbo, "Structural and Functional Abnormalities in the Sex Organs of Male Offspring of Mothers Treated with Diethylstilbestrol (DES)," *Jour of Repro Med* 16:147–153, 1976.
50. Henderson, B. E., B. Benton, M. Cosgrove, J. Baptista, J. Aldrich, D. Townsend, W. Hart, T. Mack, "Urogenital Tract Abnormalities in Sons of Women Treated with Diethylstilbestrol," *Pediatrics* 58:505–507, 1976.
51. Heinonen, O. P., D. Slone, R. R. Nonson, E. B. Hook, S. Shapiro, "Cardiovascular Birth Defects and Antenatal Exposure to Female Sex Hormones," *N Engl J Med* 296:67–70, 1977.
52. Jain, A. K., "Mortality Risk Associated with the Use of Oral Contraceptives," *Studies in Family Planning* 8:50–54, 1977.
53. Beral, V., "Mortality Among Oral Contraceptive Users," *Lancet* 2:727–731, 1977.
54. Layde, P.M., et al.: *Lancet 1:541–546, 1981.*
55. Royal College of General Practitioners *J Coll Gen Pract* 33:75, 19.
56. Slone, D., et al.: *NEJM* 305:4, 1981.
57. Petitti, D.B., et al.: *Lancet* 2:234, 1978.

The patient labeling for oral contraceptive drug products is set forth below:

Brief Summary Patient Package Insert

> Cigarette smoking increases the risk of serious adverse effects on the heart and blood vessels from oral contraceptive use. This risk increases with age and with heavy smoking (15 or more cigarettes per day) and is quite marked in women over 35 years of age. Women who use oral contraceptives should not smoke.

Oral contraceptives taken as directed are about 99% effective in preventing pregnancy. (The mini-pill, however is somewhat less effective.) Forgetting to take your pills increases the chance of pregnancy. Various drugs, such as antibiotics, may also decrease the effectiveness of oral contraceptives.

Women who have or have had clotting disorders, cancer of the breast or sex organs, unexplained vaginal bleeding, a stroke, heart attack, angina pectoris, or who suspect they may be pregnant should not use oral contraceptives.

Most side effects of the pill are not serious. The most common side effects are nausea, vomiting, bleeding between menstrual periods, weight gain, and breast tenderness. However, proper use of oral contraceptives requires that they be taken under your doctor's continuous supervision, because they can be associated with serious side effects which may be fatal. Fortunately, these occur very infrequently.

The serious side effects are:

1. Blood clots in the legs, lungs, brain, heart or other organs and hemorrhage into the brain due to bursting of a blood vessel. Certain of these effects may occur after pill use has been stopped
2. Liver tumors, which may rupture and cause severe bleeding
3. Birth defects if the pill is taken while you are pregnant
4. High blood pressure
5. Gallbladder disease

The symptoms associated with these serious side effects are discussed in the detailed leaflet given you with your supply of pills. Notify your doctor if you notice any unusual physical disturbance while taking the pill.

The estrogen in oral contraceptives has been found to cause breast cancer and other cancers in certain animals. These findings suggest that oral contraceptives may also cause cancer in humans. However, studies to date in women taking currently marketed oral contraceptives have not confirmed that oral contraceptives cause cancer in humans.

The detailed leaflet describes more completely the benefits and risks of oral contraceptives. It also provides information on other forms of contraception. Read it carefully. If you have any questions, consult your doctor.

Caution: Oral contraceptives are of no value in the prevention or treatment of venereal disease.

Detailed Patient Labeling

What You Should Know About Oral Contraceptives

Oral contraceptives ("the pill") are the most effective way (except for sterilization) to prevent pregnancy . They are also convenient and, for most women, free of serious or unpleasant side effects. Oral contraceptives must always be taken under the continuous supervision of a physician.

It is important that any woman who considers using an oral contraceptive understand the risks involved. Although the oral contraceptives have important advantages over other methods of contraception, they have certain risks that no other method has, and some of these risks may continue after you have stopped using the pill. Only you can decide whether the advantages are worth these risks. This leaflet will tell you about the most important risks. It will explain how you can help your doctor prescribe the pill as safely as possible by telling him about yourself and being alert for the earliest signs of trouble. And it will tell you how to use the pill properly, so that it will be as effective as possible. There is more detailed information available in the leaflet prepared for doctors. Your pharmacist can show you a copy; you may need your doctor's help in understanding parts of it.

Who Should Not Use Oral Contraceptives

A. If you have any of the following conditions you should not use the pill:

1. Clots in the legs or lungs
2. Angina pectoris
3. Known or suspected cancer of the breast or sex organs
4. Unusual vaginal bleeding that has not yet been diagnosed
5. Known or suspected pregnancy

B. If you have had any of the following conditions you should not use the pill:

1. Heart attack or stroke
2. Clots in the legs or lungs

> C. Cigarette smoking increases the risk of serious adverse effects on the heart and blood vessels from oral contraceptive use. This risk increases with age and with heavy smoking (15 or more cigarettes per day) and is quite marked in women over 35 years of age. Women who use oral contraceptives should not smoke.

D. If you have scanty or irregular periods or are a young woman without a regular cycle, you should use another method of contraception because, if you use the pill, you may have difficulty becoming pregnant or may fail to have menstrual periods after discontinuing the pill.

Deciding To Use Oral Contraceptives

If you do not have any of the conditions listed above and are thinking about using oral contraceptives, to help you decide, you need information about the advantages and risks of oral contraceptives and of other contraceptive methods as well. This leaflet describes the advantages and risks of oral contraceptives. Except for sterilization, the IUD and abortion, which have their own exclusive risks, the only risks of other methods of contraception are those due to pregnancy should the method fail. Your doctor can answer questions you may have with respect to other methods of contraception. He can also answer any questions you may have after reading this leaflet on oral contraceptives.

1. What Oral Contraceptives Are and How They Work.-

Oral contraceptives are of two types. The most common, often simply called "the pill," is a combination of an estrogen and a progestogen, the two kinds of female hormones. The amount of estrogen and progestogen can vary, but the amount of estrogen is most important because both the effectiveness and some of the dangers of oral contraceptives are related to the amount of estrogen. This kind of oral contraceptive works principally by preventing release of an egg from the ovary. When the amount of estrogen is 50 micrograms or more, and the pill is taken as directed, oral contraceptives are more than 99% effective (ie, there would be less than one pregnancy if 100 women used the pill for 1 year). Pills that contain 20 to 35 micrograms of estrogen vary slightly in effectiveness, ranging from 98% to more than 99% effective. Norlestrin was shown in clinical trials to be more than 99% effective.

The second type of oral contraceptive, often called the "mini-pill," contains only a progestogen. It works in part by preventing release of an egg from the ovary but also by keeping sperm from reaching the egg and by making the uterus (womb) less receptive to any fertilized egg that reaches it. The mini-pill is less effective than the combination oral contraceptive, about 97% effective.

In addition, the progestogen-only pill has a tendency to cause irregular bleeding which may be quite inconvenient, or cessation of bleeding entirely. The progestogen-only pill is used despite its lower effectiveness in the hope that it will prove not to have some of the serious side effects of the estrogen-containing pill (which follows) but it is not yet certain that the mini-pill does in fact have fewer serious side effects. The discussion which follows, while based mainly on information about the combination pills, should be considered to apply, as well, to the mini-pill.

2. Other Nonsurgical Ways to Prevent Pregnancy. As this leaflet will explain, oral contraceptives have several serious risks. Other methods of contraception have lesser risks or none at all. They are also less effective than oral contraceptives but, used properly, may be effective enough for many women. The following gives reported pregnancy rates (the number of women out of 100 who would become pregnant in 1 year) for these methods:

Pregnancies Per 100 Women Per Year

Intrauterine device (IUD), less than 1-6; Diaphragm with spermicidal products (creams or jellies), 2-20; Condom (rubber), 3-36; Aerosol foams, 2-29; Jellies and creams, 4-36; Periodic abstinence (rhythm) all types, less than 1-47; 1. *Calendar method, 14-47; 2. Temperature method, 1-20; 3. Temperature method—intercourse only in post-ovulatory phase, less than 1-7; 4. Mucus method, 1-25;* No contraception, 60-80.

Continued on next page

This product information was prepared in August, 1986. On these and other Parke-Davis Products, information may be obtained by addressing PARKE-DAVIS, Division of Warner-Lambert Company, Morris Plains, New Jersey 07950.

Parke-Davis—Cont.

The figures (except for the IUD) vary widely because people differ in how well they use each method. Very faithful users of the various methods obtain very good results except for users of the calendar method of periodic abstinence (rhythm). Except for the IUD, effective use of these methods requires somewhat more effort than simply taking a single pill every morning, but it is an effort that many couples undertake successfully. Your doctor can tell you a great deal more about these methods of contraception.

3. The Dangers of Oral Contraceptives.

a. *Circulatory disorders (abnormal blood clotting and stroke due to hemorrhage).* Blood clots (in various blood vessels of the body) are the most common of the serious side effects of oral contraceptives. A clot can result in a stroke (if the clot is in the brain), a heart attack (if the clot is in a blood vessel of the heart), or a pulmonary embolus (a clot which forms in the legs or pelvis, then breaks off and travels to the lungs). Any of these can be fatal. Clots also occur rarely in the blood vessels of the eye, resulting in blindness or impairment of vision in that eye. There is evidence that the risk of clotting increases with higher estrogen doses. It is, therefore, important to keep the dose of estrogen as low as possible, so long as the oral contraceptive used has an acceptable pregnancy rate and doesn't cause unacceptable changes in the menstrual pattern. Furthermore, cigarette smoking by oral contraceptive users increases the risk of serious adverse effects on the heart and blood vessels. This risk increases with age and with heavy smoking (15 or more cigarettes per day) and begins to become quite marked in women over 35 years of age. For this reason, women who use oral contraceptives should not smoke.

The risk of abnormal clotting increases with age in both users and nonusers of oral contraceptives, but the increased risk from the contraceptives appears to be present at all ages. For oral contraceptive users in general, it has been estimated that in women between the ages of 15 and 34 the risk of death due to a circulatory disorder is about 1 in 12,000 per year, whereas for nonusers the rate is about 1 in 50,000 per year. In the age group 35 to 44, the risk is estimated to be about 1 in 2,500 per year for oral contraceptive users and about 1 in 10,000 per year for nonusers.

Even without the pill the risk of having a heart attack increases with age and is also increased by such heart attack risk factors as high blood pressure, high cholesterol, obesity, diabetes, and cigarette smoking. Without any risk factors present, the use of oral contraceptives alone may double the risk of heart attack. However, the combination of cigarette smoking, especially heavy smoking, and oral contraceptive use greatly increases the risk of heart attack. Oral contraceptive users who smoke are about 5 times more likely to have a heart attack than users who do not smoke and about 10 times more likely to have a heart attack than nonusers who do not smoke. It has been estimated that users between the ages of 30 and 39 who smoke have about a 1 in 10,000 chance each year of having a fatal heart attack compared to about a 1 in 50,000 chance in users who do not smoke, and about a 1 in 100,000 chance in nonusers who do not smoke. In the age group 40 to 44, the risk is about 1 in 1,700 per year for users who smoke compared to about 1 in 10,000 for users who do not smoke and to about 1 in 14,000 per year for nonusers who do not smoke. Heavy smoking (about 15 cigarettes or more a day) further increases the risk. If you do not smoke and have none of the other heart attack risk factors described above, you will have a smaller risk than listed. If you have several heart attack risk factors, the risk may be considerably greater than listed.

In addition to blood-clotting disorders, it has been estimated that women taking oral contraceptives are twice as likely as nonusers to have a stroke due to rupture of a blood vessel in the brain.

b. *Formation of tumors.* Studies have found that when certain animals are given the female sex hormone estrogen, which is an ingredient of oral contraceptives, continuously for long periods, cancers may develop in the breast, cervix, vagina, and liver.

These findings suggest that oral contraceptives may cause cancer in humans. However, studies to date in women taking currently marketed oral contraceptives have not confirmed that oral contraceptives cause cancer in humans. Several studies have found no increase in breast cancer in users, although one study suggested oral contraceptives might cause an increase in breast cancer in women who already have benign breast disease (eg, cysts).

Women with a strong family history of breast cancer or who have breast nodules, fibrocystic disease, or abnormal mammograms or who were exposed to DES (diethylstilbestrol), an estrogen, during their mother's pregnancy must be followed very closely by their doctors if they choose to use oral contraceptives instead of another method of contraception. Many studies have shown that women taking oral contraceptives have less risk of getting benign breast disease than those who have not used oral contraceptives. Recently, strong evidence has emerged that estrogens (one component of oral contraceptives), when given for periods of more than one year to women after the menopause, increase the risk of cancer of the uterus (womb). There is also some evidence that a kind of oral contraceptive which is no longer marketed, the sequential oral contraceptive, may increase the risk of cancer of the uterus. There remains no evidence, however, that the oral contraceptives now available increase the risk of this cancer.

Oral contraceptives do cause, although rarely, a benign (nonmalignant) tumor of the liver. These tumors do not spread, but they may rupture and cause internal bleeding, which may be fatal. A few cases of cancer of the liver have been reported in women using oral contraceptives, but it is not yet known whether the drug caused them.

c. *Dangers to a developing child if oral contraceptives are used in or immediately preceding pregnancy.* Oral contraceptives should not be taken by pregnant women because they may damage the developing child. An increased risk of birth defects, including heart defects and limb defects, has been associated with the use of sex hormones, including oral contraceptives, in pregnancy. In addition, the developing female child whose mother has received DES (diethylstilbestrol), an estrogen, during pregnancy has a risk of getting cancer of the vagina or cervix in her teens or young adulthood. This risk is estimated to be about 1 in 1,000 exposures or less. Abnormalities of the urinary and sex organs have been reported in male offspring so exposed. It is possible that other estrogens, such as the estrogens in oral contraceptives, could have the same effect in the child if the mother takes them during pregnancy.

If you stop taking oral contraceptives to become pregnant, your doctor may recommend that you use another method of contraception for a short while. The reason for this is that there is evidence from studies in women who have had "miscarriages" soon after stopping the pill, that the lost fetuses are more likely to be abnormal. Whether there is an overall increase in "miscarriage" in women who become pregnant soon after stopping the pill, as compared with women who do not use the pill, is not known, but it is possible that there may be. If, however, you do become pregnant soon after stopping oral contraceptives, and do not have a miscarriage, there is no evidence that the baby has an increased risk of being abnormal.

d. *Gallbladder disease.* Women who use oral contraceptives have a greater risk than nonusers of having gallbladder disease requiring surgery. The increased risk may first appear within 1 year of use and may double after 4 or 5 years of use.

e. *Other side effects of oral contraceptives.* Some women using oral contraceptives experience unpleasant side effects that are not dangerous and are not likely to damage their health. Some of these may be temporary. Your breasts may feel tender, nausea and vomiting may occur, you may gain or lose weight, and your ankles may swell. A spotty darkening of the skin, particularly of the face, is possible and may persist. You may notice unexpected vaginal bleeding or changes in your menstrual period. Irregular bleeding is frequently seen when using the mini-pill or combination oral contraceptives containing less than 50 micrograms of estrogen.

More serious side effects include worsening of migraine, asthma, epilepsy, and kidney or heart disease because of a tendency for water to be retained in the body when oral contraceptives are used. Other side effects are growth of preexisting fibroid tumors of the uterus, mental depression, and liver problems with jaundice (yellowing of the skin). Your doctor may find that levels of sugar and fatty substances in your blood are elevated; the long-term effects of these changes are not known. Some women develop high blood pressure while taking oral contraceptives, which ordinarily returns to the original levels when the oral contraceptive is stopped.

Other reactions, although not proved to be caused by oral contraceptives, are occasionally reported. These include more frequent urination and some discomfort when urinating, nervousness, dizziness, some loss of scalp hair, an increase in body hair, an increase or decrease in sex drive, appetite changes, cataracts, and a need for a change in contact lens prescription or inability to use contact lenses.

After you stop using oral contraceptives there may be a delay before you are able to become pregnant or before you resume having menstrual periods. This is especially true of women who had irregular menstrual cycles prior to the use of oral contraceptives. As discussed previously, your doctor may recommend that you wait a short while after stopping the pill before you try to become pregnant. During this time, use another form of contraception. You should consult your physician before resuming use of oral contraceptives after childbirth, especially if you plan to nurse your baby. Drugs in oral contraceptives are known to appear in the milk, and the long-range effect on infants is not known at this time. Furthermore, oral contraceptives may cause a decrease in your milk supply as well as in the quality of the milk.

4. Comparison of the Risks of Oral Contraceptives and Other Contraceptive Methods. The many studies on the risks and effectiveness of oral contraceptives and other methods of contraception have been analyzed to estimate the risk of death associated with various methods of contraception. This risk has two parts: (a) the risk of the method itself (eg, the risk that oral contraceptives will cause death due to abnormal clotting); and (b) the risk of death due to pregnancy or abortion in the event the method fails. The results of this analysis are shown in the following bar graph. The height of the bars is the number of deaths per 100,000 women each year. There are six sets of bars, each set referring to a specific age group of women. Within each set of bars, there is a single bar for each of the different contraceptive methods. For oral contraceptives, there are two bars—one for smokers and the other for nonsmokers. The analysis is based on present knowledge and new information could, of course, alter it. The analysis shows that the risk of death from all methods of birth control is low and below that associated with childbirth, except for oral contraceptives in women over 40 who smoke. It shows that the lowest risk of death is associated with the condom or diaphragm (traditional contraception) backed up by early abortion in case of failure of the condom or diaphragm to prevent pregnancy. Also, at any age the risk of death (due to unexpected pregnancy) from the use of traditional contraception, even without a backup of abortion, is generally the same as or less than that from use of oral contraceptives.

[See Figure 1 on next page].

How to Use Oral Contraceptives As Safely and Effectively As Possible, Once You Have Decided to Use Them

1. What to Tell your Doctor.

You can make use of the pill as safely as possible, by telling your doctor if you have any of the following:

a. Conditions that mean you should not use oral contraceptives:

Clots in the legs or lungs
Clots in the legs or lungs in the past
A stroke, heart attack, or angina pectoris
Known or suspected cancer of the breast or sex organs
Unusual vaginal bleeding that has not yet been diagnosed
Known or suspected pregnancy

b. Conditions that your doctor will want to watch closely or which might cause him to suggest another method of contraception:

A family history of breast cancer
Breast nodules, fibrocystic disease of the breast, or an abnormal mammogram
Diabetes
High blood pressure
High cholesterol
Cigarette smoking
Migraine headaches
Heart or kidney disease
Epilepsy
Mental depression
Fibroid tumors of the uterus
Gallbladder disease

c. Once you are using oral contraceptives, you should be alert for signs of a serious adverse effect and call your doctor if they occur:

Sharp pain in the chest, coughing blood, or sudden shortness of breath (indicating possible clots in the lungs)
Pain in the calf (possible clot in the leg)
Crushing chest pain or heaviness (indicating possible heart attack)
Sudden severe headache or vomiting, dizziness or fainting, disturbance of vision or speech, or weakness or numbness in an arm or leg (indicating a possible stroke)
Sudden partial or complete loss of vision (indicating a possible clot in the eye)
Breast lumps (you should ask your doctor to show you how to examine your own breasts)
Severe pain in the abdomen (indicating a possible ruptured tumor of the liver)
Severe depression
Yellowing of the skin (jaundice)

2. How to Take the Pill So That It Is Most Effective.

Reduced effectiveness and an increased incidence of breakthrough bleeding have been associated with the use of oral contraceptives with antibiotics such as rifampin, ampicillin, and tetracycline or with certain other drugs, such as barbiturates, phenylbutazone or phenytoin sodium. You should use an additional means of contraception during any cycle in which any of these drugs are taken.

Directions For 21-Day Dosage Regimen

a. The first day of your period is Day 1. On the fifth day (Day 5), start taking a tablet daily, beginning with the tablet in the upper left corner of the Petipac. In the space provided, write the day you start. To remove a tablet, press down on it with your thumb or finger. The tablet will drop through a hole in the bottom of the Petipac. Do not press on the tablet with your thumbnail or fingernail, or any other sharp object.

If your period begins on:	Start taking tablets on:
Sunday	Thursday
Monday	Friday
Tuesday	Saturday
Wednesday	Sunday
Thursday	Monday
Friday	Tuesday
Saturday	Wednesday

b. Continue to take one tablet daily until all the tablets have been taken.
c. After you have taken all 21 tablets, stop and don't take any tablets for the next seven days. You should have a menstrual period one to three days after you stop taking tablets; sometimes, it may take a day or so longer.
d. After seven days, during which you take no tablets, put a new refill in your Petipac and begin a new course of tablets, taking one tablet daily for 21 days. You will always start each new course of 21 tablets on the same day of the week. Likewise, the interval of no tablets will always start on the same day of the week.
e. If spotting should occur at an unexpected time, continue to take your tablets as directed. Spotting is usually temporary and without significance. However, if bleeding should occur at an unexpected time, consult your physician. Call your physician regarding any problem or change in your general health that may concern you.
f. If you forget to take a tablet, take it as soon as you remember, even if it is the next day. Then take the next scheduled tablet at the usual time. If you miss two consecutive tablets, take two tablets daily for the next two days. Then resume the regular schedule. While there is little likelihood of pregnancy occurring if you miss only one or two tablets, the possibility of pregnancy increases with each successive day that tablets are missed. If you miss three consecutive tablets, discard any tablets remaining and begin a new course of tablets, starting seven days after the last tablet was taken, even if you are still menstruating. You should use an alternate means of contraception, other than oral tablets, until the start of your next menstrual period.

Directions For 28-Day Dosage Regimen

a. The first day of your period is Day 1. On the fifth day (Day 5), start taking one *light-colored* tablet daily, beginning with the tablet in the upper left corner of the Petipac. In the space provided, write the day you start. Take all the tablets in the top row first, followed by the second row, and so on. To remove a tablet, press down on it with your thumb or finger. The tablet will drop through a hole in the bottom of the Petipac. Do not press on the tablet with your thumbnail or fingernail, or any other sharp object.

If your period begins on:	Start taking tablets on:
Sunday	Thursday
Monday	Friday
Tuesday	Saturday
Wednesday	Sunday
Thursday	Monday
Friday	Tuesday
Saturday	Wednesday

b. On the day after taking the last *light-colored* tablet, begin taking one *brown* or *white* tablet daily until all the tablets have been taken.
c. When the last tablet has been taken, put a new refill in your Petipac and, without interruption, begin a new course of tablets by taking the *light-colored* tablets first, followed by the *brown* or *white* tablets. There should never be a day when you are not taking a tablet.
d. Continue taking *light-colored* tablets without interruption whether or not your period has occurred or is still in progress. Your period will usually occur during the time you are taking *brown* or *white* tablets.
e. If spotting should occur at an unexpected time, continue to take your tablets as directed. Spotting is usually temporary and without significance. However, if bleeding should occur at an unexpected time, consult your physician. Call your physician regarding any problem or change in your general health that may concern you.
f. If you forget to take a *light-colored* tablet, take it as soon as you remember, even if it is the next day. Then take the next scheduled *light-colored* tablet at the usual time. If you miss two consecutive *light-colored* tablets, take two *light-colored* tablets daily for the next two days. Then resume the regular schedule. While there is little likelihood of pregnancy occurring if you miss only one or two *light-colored* tablets, the possibility of pregnancy increases with each successive day that scheduled *light-colored* tablets are missed. If you miss three consecutive *light-colored* tablets, discard any tablets remaining and begin a new course of tablets, starting seven days after the last *light-colored* tablet was taken, even if you are still menstruating. You should use an alternate means of contraception, other than oral tablets, until the start of your next menstrual period.
g. If you miss one or more *brown* or *white* tablets discard the remainder and begin a new course of tablets no later than the eighth day after you took the last *light-colored* tablet. Under no circumstances should you substitute a *brown* or *white* tablet for a *light-colored* one, or take any *brown* or *white* tablets before you have taken all the *light-colored* tablets, unless your physician advises you to do so.

Missed Menstrual Period For Both Dosage Regimens: At times there may be no menstrual period after a cycle of pills. Therefore, if you miss one menstrual period but have taken the pills *exactly as your were supposed to,* continue as usual into the next cycle. If you have not taken the pills correctly and miss a menstrual period, *you may be pregnant* and should stop taking oral contraceptives until your doctor determines whether or not you are pregnant. Until you can get to your doctor, use another form of contraception. If two consecutive menstrual periods are missed, you should stop taking pills until it is determined whether you are pregnant. If you do become pregnant while using oral contraceptives, you should discuss the risks to the developing child with your doctor.

Periodic Examination

Your doctor will take a complete medical and family history before prescribing oral contraceptives. At that time and about once a year thereafter, he will generally examine your blood pressure, breasts, abdomen, and pelvic organs (including a Papanicolaou smear, ie, test for cancer).

Figure 1. Estimated annual number of deaths associated with control of fertility and no control per 100,000 nonsterile women, by regimen of control and age of woman.

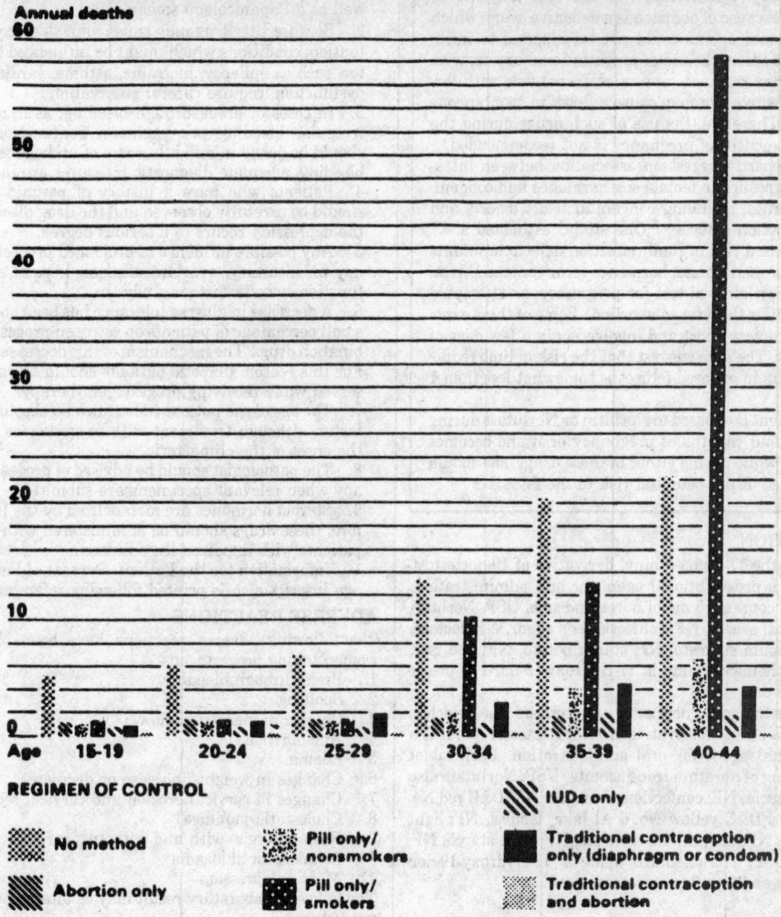

SUMMARY

Oral contraceptives are the most effective method, except sterilization, for preventing pregnancy. Other methods, when used conscientiously, are also very effective and have fewer risks. Although the serious risks of oral contraceptives are uncommon, some of the risks may persist after you stop using the pill. On the other hand, the "pill" is a very convenient method of preventing pregnancy.

If you have certain conditions or have had these conditions in the past, you should not use oral contraceptives because the risk is too great. These conditions are listed in this leaflet. If you do not have these conditions, and decide to use the "pill," please read this leaflet carefully so that you can use the "pill" most safely and effectively.

Based on his or her assessment of your medical needs, your doctor has prescribed this drug for you. Do not give this drug to anyone else.

0907G131

Shown in Product Identification Section, page 421

NORLUTIN® ℞
[*nōr"lū'tĭn*]
(norethindrone tablets, USP)*
NORLUTATE® ℞
[*nōr"lū'tāte*]
(norethindrone acetate tablets, USP)*

*Product of Warner-Lambert Inc

WARNING

THE USE OF PROGESTATIONAL AGENTS DURING THE FIRST FOUR MONTHS OF PREGNANCY IS NOT RECOMMENDED.

Progestational agents have been used beginning with the first trimester of pregnancy in an attempt to prevent habitual abortion or to treat threatened abortion. There is no adequate evidence that such use is effective and there is evidence of potential harm to the fetus when such drugs are given during the first four months

Continued on next page

This product information was prepared in August, 1986. On these and other Parke-Davis Products, information may be obtained by addressing PARKE-DAVIS, Division of Warner-Lambert Company, Morris Plains, New Jersey 07950.

Parke-Davis—Cont.

of pregnancy. Furthermore, in the vast majority of women, the cause of abortion is a defective ovum, which progestational agents could not be expected to influence. In addition, the use of progestational agents, with their uterine-relaxant properties, in patients with fertilized defective ova may cause a delay in spontaneous abortion. Therefore, the use of such drugs during the first four months of pregnancy is not recommended.

Several reports suggest an association between intrauterine exposure to female sex hormones and congenital anomalies, including congenital heart defects and limb reduction defects.[1-5] One study[4] estimated a 4.7 fold increased risk of limb reduction defects in infants exposed *in utero* to sex hormones (oral contraceptives, hormone withdrawal test for pregnancy, or attempted treatment for threatened abortion). Some of these exposures were very short and involved only a few days of treatment. The data suggest that the risk of limb reduction defects in exposed fetuses is somewhat less than 1 in 1,000.

If the patient is exposed to Norlutin or Norlutate during the first four months of pregnancy or if she becomes pregnant while taking either of these drugs, she should be apprised of the potential risk to the fetus.

DESCRIPTION

Norlutin is the 17 alpha-ethinyl derivative of 19-nortestosterone. It is a progestational agent for oral administration. Each tablet contains 5 mg of norethindrone, USP. Norlutin also contains: acacia, NF; confectioner's sugar, NF; lactose, NF; magnesium stearate, NF; starch potato, NF; and talc, USP. The chemical name is 17-Hydroxy-19-nor-17α-pregn-4-en-20-yn-3-one.

Norlutate is the acetic acid ester of norethindrone, which is the 17 alpha-ethinyl derivative of 19-nortestosterone. It is a progestational agent for oral administration. Each tablet contains 5 mg of norethindrone acetate, USP. Norlutate also contains: acacia, NF; confectioner's sugar, NF; D&C red No. 30 Al lake; FD&C yellow No. 6 Al lake; lactose, NF; light mineral oil, NF; magnesium stearate, NF; corn starch, NF; and talc, USP. The chemical name is 17-Hydroxy-19-nor-17α-pregn-4-en-20-yn-3-one acetate.

ACTIONS

Transforms proliferative endometrium into secretory endometrium

Inhibits (at the usual dosage range) the secretion of pituitary gonadotropins, which in turn prevents follicular maturation and ovulation.

May also demonstrate some estrogenic, anabolic, or androgenic activity but should not be relied upon.

INDICATIONS

Norlutin and Norlutate are indicated in amenorrhea; in abnormal uterine bleeding due to hormonal imbalance in the absence of organic pathology, such as submucous fibroids or uterine cancer; and in endometriosis.

CONTRAINDICATIONS

1. Thrombophlebitis, thromboembolic disorders, cerebral apoplexy, or patients with a past history of these conditions
2. Known or suspected carcinoma of the breast
3. Undiagnosed vaginal bleeding
4. Missed abortion
5. As a diagnostic test for pregnancy

WARNINGS

1. Discontinue medication pending examination if there is a sudden partial or complete loss of vision, or if there is sudden onset of proptosis, diplopia, or migraine. If examination reveals papilledema or retinal vascular lesions, medication should be withdrawn.
2. Detectable amounts of progestogens have been identified in the milk of mothers receiving them. The effect of this on the nursing infant has not been determined.
3. Because of the occasional occurrence of thrombophlebitis and pulmonary embolism in patients taking progestogens, the physician should be alert to the earliest manifestations of the disease.
4. Masculinization of the female fetus has occurred when progestogens have been used in pregnant women.
5. Some beagle dogs treated with medroxyprogesterone acetate developed mammary nodules. Although nodules occasionally appeared in control animals, they were intermittent in nature, whereas nodules in treated animals were larger and more numerous, and persisted. There is no general agreement as to whether the nodules are benign or malignant. Their significance with respect to humans has not been established.

PRECAUTIONS

1. The pretreatment physical examination should include special reference to breasts and pelvic organs, as well as a Papanicolaou smear.
2. Because this drug may cause some degree of fluid retention, conditions which might be influenced by this factor, such as epilepsy, migraine, asthma, cardiac or renal dysfunction, require careful observation.
3. In cases of breakthrough bleeding, as in all cases of irregular bleeding per vaginam, nonfunctional causes should be borne in mind. In cases of undiagnosed vaginal bleeding, adequate diagnostic measures are indicated.
4. Patients who have a history of psychic depression should be carefully observed and the drug discontinued if the depression recurs to a serious degree.
5. Any possible influence of prolonged progestogen therapy on pituitary, ovarian, adrenal, hepatic, or uterine functions awaits further study.
6. A decrease in glucose tolerance has been observed in a small percentage of patients on estrogen-progestogen combination drugs. The mechanism of this decrease is obscure. For this reason, diabetic patients should be carefully observed while receiving progestogen therapy.
7. The age of the patient constitutes no absolute limiting factor, although treatment with progestogens may mask the onset of the climacteric.
8. The pathologist should be advised of progestogen therapy when relevant specimens are submitted.
9. Steroid hormones are metabolized by the liver, therefore, these drugs should be administered with caution in patients with impaired liver function.
10. Information for the Patient. See text of Patient Package Insert which is printed following references.

ADVERSE REACTIONS

The following adverse reactions have been observed in women taking progestogens.

1. Breakthrough bleeding
2. Spotting
3. Change in menstrual flow
4. Amenorrhea
5. Edema
6. Changes in weight (increase or decrease)
7. Changes in cervical erosion and cervical secretions
8. Cholestatic jaundice
9. Rash (allergic) with and without pruritus
10. Melasma or chloasma
11. Mental depression

The following laboratory result may be altered by the use of progestogens:

Pregnanediol determination.

In addition, the following laboratory results may be altered by the concomitant use of estrogens with progestogens.

1. Hepatic function
2. Coagulation tests: increase in prothrombin, factors VII, VIII, IX, and X
3. Increase in PBI, BEI, and a decrease in T3 uptake
4. Metyrapone test

A statistically significant association has been demonstrated between use of estrogen-progestogen combination drugs and the following serious adverse reactions: thrombophlebitis; pulmonary embolism, and cerebral thrombosis and embolism. For this reason, patients on progestogen therapy should be carefully observed.

Although available evidence is suggestive of an association, such a relationship has been neither confirmed nor refuted for the following serious adverse reactions:

Neuro-ocular lesions, eg, retinal thrombosis and optic neuritis.

The following adverse reactions have been observed in patients receiving estrogen-progestogen combination drugs.

1. Rise in blood pressure in susceptible individuals
2. Premenstrual-like syndrome
3. Changes in libido
4. Changes in appetite
5. Cystitis-like syndrome
6. Headache
7. Nervousness
8. Dizziness
9. Fatigue
10. Backache
11. Hirsutism
12. Loss of scalp hair
13. Erythema multiforme
14. Erythema nodosum
15. Hemorrhagic eruption
16. Itching

In view of these observations, patients on progestogen therapy should be carefully observed for their occurrence.

DOSAGE AND ADMINISTRATION

Norlutin (norethindrone tablets, USP): *Therapy with Norlutin must be adapted to the specific indications and therapeutic response of the individual patient.*

This dosage schedule assumes the interval between menses to be 28 days.

Amenorrhea, abnormal uterine bleeding due to hormonal imbalance in the absence of organic pathology: 5 to 20 mg Norlutin starting with the fifth day of the menstrual cycle and ending on the 25th day.

Endometriosis: Initial daily dosage of 10 mg Norlutin for two weeks with increments of 5 mg per day of Norlutin every two weeks until 30 mg per day of Norlutin is reached. Therapy may be held at this level for from six to nine months or until annoying breakthrough bleeding demands temporary termination.

Norlutate (norethindrone acetate tablets, USP): *Therapy with Norlutate must be adapted to the specific indications and therapeutic response of the individual patient.*

This dosage schedule assumes the interval between menses to be 28 days.

Amenorrhea, abnormal uterine bleeding due to hormonal imbalance in the absence of organic pathology: 2.5 to 10 mg Norlutate starting with the fifth day of the menstrual cycle and ending on the 25th day.

Endometriosis: Initial daily dosage of 5 mg Norlutate for two weeks, with increments of 2.5 mg per day of Norlutate every two weeks until 15 mg per day of Norlutate is reached. Therapy may be held at this level for from six to nine months or until annoying breakthrough bleeding demands temporary termination.

HOW SUPPLIED

N 0710-0882-19 (Tablet 882)—Norlutin is supplied as 5-mg scored tablets in bottles of 50. **0882G011**

Shown in Product Identification Section, page 421

N 0710-0918-19 (Tablet 918)—Norlutate is supplied as 5-mg scored tablets in bottles of 50.

AHFS 68:32 **0918G032**

Shown in Product Identification Section, page 421

PATIENT LABELING FOR PROGESTOGENS

WARNING FOR WOMEN

There is an increased risk of birth defects in children whose mothers take these drugs during the first four months of pregnancy.

Norlutin and Norlutate are similar to the progesterone hormones naturally produced by the body. Progesterone and progesterone-like drugs are used to treat menstrual disorders, to test if the body is producing certain hormones, and to treat some forms of cancer in women.

These drugs have been used as a test for pregnancy but such use is no longer considered safe because of possible damage to a developing baby. Also, more rapid methods for testing for pregnancy are now available.

These drugs have also been used to prevent miscarriage in the first few months of pregnancy. No adequate evidence is available to show that they are effective for this purpose and there is evidence of an increased risk of birth defects, such as heart or limb defects, if these drugs are taken during the first four months of pregnancy. Furthermore, most cases of early miscarriage are due to causes which could not be helped by these drugs.

The exact risk of taking these drugs early in pregnancy and having a baby with a birth defect is not known. However, one study found that babies born to women who had taken sex hormones (such as progesterone-like drugs) during the first three months of pregnancy were 4 to 5 times more likely to have abnormalities of the arms or legs than if their mothers had not taken such drugs. Some of these women had taken these drugs for only a few days. The chance that an infant whose mother had taken this drug will have this type of defect is about 1 in 1,000.

If you take Norlutin or Norlutate and later find you were pregnant when you took it, be sure to discuss this with your doctor as soon as possible.

OPHTHOCHLOR® ℞

[*ŏph 'thō "chlōr*]

(chloramphenicol ophthalmic solution)

0.5%

WARNING

Bone marrow hypoplasia including aplastic anemia and death has been reported following local application of chloramphenicol. Chloramphenicol should not be used when less potentially dangerous agents would be expected to provide effective treatment.

DESCRIPTION

Ophthochlor (Chloramphenicol Ophthalmic Solution, USP), 0.5%, is a sterile, buffered solution containing 0.5% (5 mg/ml) of chloramphenicol. It contains no preservatives.

The chemical names for chloramphenicol are:

(1) Acetamide,2,2-dichloro-*N*-[2-hydroxy-1- (hydroxymethyl)-2-(4-nitrophenyl) ethyl]-, and

(2) D-*threo*-(–)-2,2-Dichloro-*N*-[β-hydroxy- α-(hydroxymethyl)-*p*-nitrophenethyl] acetamide

CLINICAL PHARMACOLOGY

Chloramphenicol is a broad-spectrum antibiotic originally isolated from *Streptomyces venezuelae.* It is primarily bacteriostatic and acts by inhibition of protein synthesis by interfering with the transfer of activated amino acids from soluble RNA to ribosomes. It has been noted that chloramphenicol is found in measurable amounts in the aqueous humor following local application to the eye. Development of resistance to chloramphenicol can be regarded as minimal for staphylococci and many other species of bacteria.

INDICATIONS AND USAGE

Chloramphenicol should be used only in those serious infections for which less potentially dangerous drugs are ineffective or contraindicated. Bacteriological studies should be performed to determine the causative organisms and their sensitivity to chloramphenicol (See Box Warning).

Ophthochlor (chloramphenicol ophthalmic solution) 0.5% is indicated for the treatment of surface ocular infections involving the conjunctiva and/or cornea caused by chloramphenicol-susceptible organisms.

The particular antiinfective drug in this product is active against the following common bacterial eye pathogens:

Staphylococcus aureus
Streptococci, including *Streptococcus pneumoniae*
Escherichia coli
Haemophilus influenzae
Klebsiella/Enterobacter species
Moraxella lacunata (Morax-Axenfeld bacillus)
Neisseria species

The product does not provide adequate coverage against:

Pseudomonas aeruginosa
Serratia marcescens

CONTRAINDICATIONS

This product is contraindicated in persons sensitive to any of its components.

WARNINGS

SEE BOX WARNING

PRECAUTIONS

The prolonged use of antibiotics may occasionally result in overgrowth of nonsusceptible organisms, including fungi. If new infections appear during medication, the drug should be discontinued and appropriate measures should be taken. In all serious infections the topical use of chloramphenicol should be supplemented by appropriate systemic medication.

ADVERSE REACTIONS

Blood dyscrasias have been reported in association with the use of chloramphenicol (See WARNINGS).

DOSAGE AND ADMINISTRATION

Two drops applied to the affected eye every three hours or more frequently if deemed advisable by the prescribing physician. Administration should be continued day and night for the first 48 hours, after which the interval between applications may be increased. Treatment should be continued for at least 48 hours after the eye appears normal.

HOW SUPPLIED

N 0071-3395-11 15 ml bottle.

Ophthochlor (Chloramphenicol Ophthalmic Solution, USP), 0.5% is supplied in plastic dropper bottles and contains no preservatives. Each ml contains 5 mg chloramphenicol in a boric acid-sodium borate buffer solution. Sodium hydroxide may have been added for adjustment of pH. To protect it from light, the solution should be dispensed in the carton. This product should be stored in a refrigerator until dispensed. Discard solution within 21 days from date dispensed.

AHFS Category 52:04.04 **3395G011**

Shown in Product Identification Section, page 421

OPHTHOCORT® ℞

[*ŏph 'thō "cōrt*]

(Chloramphenicol, Polymyxin B Sulfate, and Hydrocortisone Acetate Ophthalmic Ointment, USP)

WARNING

Bone marrow hypoplasia including aplastic anemia and death has been reported following local application of chloramphenicol. Chloramphenicol should not be used when less potentially dangerous agents would be expected to provide effective treatment.

DESCRIPTION

Ophthocort® (Chloramphenicol, Polymyxin B Sulfate, and Hydrocortisone Acetate Ophthalmic Ointment, USP) is a sterile antibiotic/antiinflammatory ointment for ophthalmic administration. Each gram of Ophthocort contains 10 mg chloramphenicol, 10,000 units polymyxin B (as the sulfate), and 5 mg hydrocortisone acetate in a special base of liquid petrolatum and polyethylene. It contains no preservatives.

CLINICAL PHARMACOLOGY

Corticoids suppress the inflammatory response to a variety of agents and they probably delay or slow healing. Since corticoids may inhibit the body's defense mechanism against infection, a concomitant antimicrobial drug may be used when this inhibition is considered to be clinically significant in a particular case.

The antiinfective components in this combination are included to provide action against specific organisms susceptible to them. Chloramphenicol is considered active against a wide spectrum of gram-negative and gram-positive organisms such as *Escherichia coli, Hemophilus influenzae, Staphylococcus aureus, Streptococcus hemolyticus,* and *Moraxella lacunata* (Morax-Axenfeld bacillus). Development of resistance to chloramphenicol can be regarded as minimal for staphylococci and many other species of bacteria. Chloramphenicol is primarily bacteriostatic and acts by inhibition of protein synthesis by interfering with the transfer of activated amino acids from soluble RNA to ribosomes. It has been noted that chloramphenicol is found in measurable amounts in the aqueous humor following local application to the eye.

Polymyxin B sulfate has a bactericidal action against almost all gram-negative bacilli except the *Proteus* group. All gram-positive bacteria, fungi, and the gram-negative cocci, *Neisseria gonorrhoeae* and *N meningitidis,* are resistant.

When a decision to administer both a corticoid and an antimicrobial is made, the administration of such drugs in combination has the advantage of greater patient compliance and convenience, with the added assurance that the appropriate dosage of both drugs is administered, plus assured compatibility of ingredients when both types of drug are in the same formulation and, particularly, that the correct volume of drug is delivered and retained.

The relative potency of corticosteroids depends on the molecular structure, concentration, and release from the vehicle.

INDICATIONS AND USAGE

Chloramphenicol should be used only in those serious infections for which less potentially dangerous drugs are ineffective or contraindicated. Bacteriological studies should be performed to determine the causative organisms and their sensitivity to chloramphenicol (See Box Warning).

For steroid-responsive inflammatory ocular conditions for which a corticosteroid is indicated and where bacterial infection or a risk of bacterial ocular infection exists.

Ocular steroids are indicated in inflammatory conditions of the palpebral and bulbar conjunctiva, cornea, and anterior segment of the globe where the inherent risk of steroid use in certain infective conjunctivitides is accepted to obtain a diminution in edema and inflammation. They are also indicated in chronic anterior uveitis and corneal injury from chemical radiation, thermal burns, or penetration of foreign bodies.

The use of a combination drug with an antiinfective component is indicated where the risk of infection is high or where there is an expectation that potentially dangerous numbers of bacteria will be present in the eye.

The particular antiinfective drugs in this product are active against the following common bacterial eye pathogens.

Staphylococcus aureus
Streptococci, including *Streptococcus pneumoniae*
Escherichia coli
Hemophilus influenzae
Klebsiella/Enterobacter species
Neisseria species
Moraxella lacunata (Morax-Axenfeld bacillus)
Pseudomonas aeruginosa

The product does not provide adequate coverage against:

Serratia marcescens

CONTRAINDICATIONS

Epithelial herpes simplex keratitis (dendritic keratitis), vaccinia, varicella, and many other viral diseases of the cornea and conjunctiva. Mycobacterial infection of the eye. Fungal diseases of ocular structures. Hypersensitivity to a component of the medication. (Hypersensitivity to the antibiotic component occurs at a higher rate than for other components.)

The use of these combinations is always contraindicated after uncomplicated removal of a corneal foreign body.

WARNINGS

SEE BOX WARNING

Prolonged use of steroids may result in glaucoma, with damage to the optic nerve, defects in visual acuity and fields of vision, and posterior subcapsular cataract formation. Prolonged use may suppress the host response and thus increase the hazard of secondary ocular infections. In those diseases causing thinning of the cornea or sclera, perforations have been known to occur with the use of topical steroids. In acute purulent conditions of the eye, steroids may mask infection or enhance existing infection. If these products are used for 10 days or longer, intraocular pressure should be routinely monitored even though it may be difficult in children and uncooperative patients.

Employment of steroid medication in the treatment of herpes simplex requires great caution.

Ophthalmic ointments may retard corneal wound healing.

PRECAUTIONS

The initial prescription and renewal of the medication order beyond 8 grams should be made by a physician only after examination of the patient with the aid of magnification, such as slit lamp biomicroscopy and, where appropriate, fluorescein staining.

The possibility of persistent fungal infections of the cornea should be considered after prolonged steroid dosing.

The prolonged use of antibiotics may occasionally result in overgrowth of nonsusceptible organisms, including fungi. If new infections appear during medication, the drug should be discontinued and appropriate measures should be taken.

In all serious infections the topical use of chloramphenicol should be supplemented by appropriate systemic medication.

ADVERSE REACTIONS

There have been reports of punctate staining of the cornea following intensive treatment (every one to two hours during the waking day) of corneal ulcers with Ophthocort. In each reported case, the staining has disappeared after discontinuation of the medication.

Blood dyscrasias have been reported in association with the use of chloramphenicol (See WARNINGS).

Adverse reactions have occurred with steroid/antiinfective combination drugs which can be attributed to the steroid component, the antiinfective component, or the combination. Exact incidence figures are not available since no denominator of treated patients is available.

Reactions occurring most often from the presence of the antiinfective ingredient are allergic sensitizations. The reactions due to the steroid component in decreasing order of frequency are: elevation of intraocular pressure (IOP) with possible development of glaucoma, and infrequent optic nerve damage; posterior subcapsular cataract formation; and delayed wound healing.

Secondary Infection: The development of secondary infection has occurred after use of combinations containing steroids and antimicrobials. Fungal infections of the cornea are particularly prone to develop coincidentally with long-term applications of steroid. The possibility of fungal invasion must be considered in any persistent corneal ulceration where steroid treatment has been used.

Secondary bacterial ocular infection following suppression of host responses also occurs.

DOSAGE AND ADMINISTRATION

Application of a small amount of ointment, placed in the lower conjunctival sac, is made to the affected eye every three hours, or more frequently if deemed advisable by the prescribing physician. Administration should be continued day and night for the first 48 hours, after which the interval between applications may be increased. Treatment should be continued for at least 48 hours after the eye appears normal. Not more than 8 grams should be prescribed initially and the prescription should not be refilled without further evaluation as outlined in Precautions above.

HOW SUPPLIED

N 0071-3079-07 Ophthocort (Chloramphenicol, Polymyxin B Sulfate, and Hydrocortisone Acetate Ophthalmic Ointment, USP); Each gram of ointment contains 10 mg chloramphenicol, 10,000 units polymyxin B (as the sulfate), and 5 mg hydrocortisone acetate in a special base of liquid petrolatum and polyethylene. Supplied in 3.5 g tubes.

AHFS Category 52:04.04 **3079G011**

PARSIDOL® ℞

[*păr 'sĭ-dōl "*]

(Ethopropazine Hydrochloride Tablets, USP)

DESCRIPTION

Parsidol, an orally effective antiparkinsonism drug, is a phenothiazine derivative. The chemical name is: 10H-Phenothiazine-10-ethanamine, N,N-diethyl-α-methyl-,monohydrochloride.

Parsidol (ethopropazine hydrochloride) is available as 10 mg and 50 mg tablets for oral administration. Each tablet also contains: gelatin, NF; lactose, NF; magnesium stearate, NF; methylcellulose, USP; and starch, NF.

ACTIONS

Among a wide variety of pharmacologic effects, Parsidol exerts significant anticholinergic (para-sympatholytic) ac-

Continued on next page

This product information was prepared in August, 1986. On these and other Parke-Davis Products, information may be obtained by addressing PARKE-DAVIS, Division of Warner-Lambert Company, Morris Plains, New Jersey 07950.

Parke-Davis—Cont.

tions. Although its specific mode of action in parkinsonism is unknown, it exerts a marked influence upon the neuromuscular symptoms of the disease. Most of the symptoms of parkinsonism—rigidity, spasms, tremors, sialorrhea, oculogyric crises, and festination—will respond to therapy with this drug. Parsidol is one of the drugs effective against tremor; in certain instances, however, rigidity may respond better to treatment than tremor. It is highly effective given alone or in combination with other drugs such as atropine, stramonium, dextroamphetamine, and antihistamines. Combination therapy with appropriate agents increases its efficacy in the control of specific symptoms in extreme cases, e.g., atropine plus Parsidol in refractory oculogyric crises. Unlike other phenothiazine derivatives, Parsidol does not potentiate central nervous system depressants nor does it have an antiemetic action.

INDICATIONS

Parsidol is effective as an adjunct in the therapy of all forms of parkinsonism (postencephalitic, idiopathic, and arteriosclerotic). Although chemically a phenothiazine derivative, Parsidol is distinct from other drugs of its class and is useful in the control of extrapyramidal disorders due to central nervous system drugs such as reserpine and phenothiazines.

CONTRAINDICATIONS

Glaucoma or prostatic hypertrophy. Hypersensitivity.

WARNING

Safety of use during pregnancy and lactation has not been established. This drug should not be used in pregnant patients unless the expected benefits outweigh the potential risk. Patients receiving this drug should be cautioned against hazardous activities requiring complete mental alertness, such as operating machinery or driving a motor vehicle.

PRECAUTIONS

Use with caution in patients for whom anticholinergic action would be undesirable. Because chronic use may predispose elderly persons toward glaucoma, older patients should be checked periodically for glaucoma.

Antiparkinsonism agents, when used to treat extrapyramidal reactions resulting from phenothiazines or reserpine in patients with mental disorders, may exacerbate mental symptoms and precipitate a toxic psychosis.

Permanent extrapyramidal symptoms have been described with prolonged phenothiazine therapy. The possibility that ethopropazine might mask the development of these symptoms has not been investigated.

ADVERSE REACTIONS

The most common side effects reported to occur with Parsidol are drowsiness and cerebral reaction (this latter effect has been described as fogginess, inability to think, lassitude, forgetfulness and confusion). Additional side effects (dryness of mouth, nausea, vomiting, blurring of vision and diplopia, constipation, and urinary retention—signs of the drug's anticholinergic effects) are rarely severe and either disappear as the drug is continued, or diminish when the dose is reduced.

Less commonly observed side effects include epigastric discomfort, muscular cramping, paresthesia, a sensation of heaviness of the limbs, skin rash and, following high dosages, mild, transient hypotension. Although Parsidol is different from other drugs of the phenothiazine class, the following side effects are theoretically possible with its use: EEG slowing, seizures, ECG abnormalities (e.g., tachycardia), rare hematologic reactions (agranulocytosis, pancytopenia, purpura), certain endocrinologic disturbances, jaundice, pigmentation of the cornea, lens, retina, or skin, and visual hallucinations.

DOSAGE

Initial dosage is usually 50 mg once or twice a day, increase gradually if necessary. Patients with mild-to-moderate symptoms are frequently controlled with 100 to 400 mg daily. Severe cases may require further gradual increase to 500 to 600 mg or more daily.

HOW SUPPLIED

Parsidol Tablets are supplied as:
N 0071-0320-24 10 mg (white) bottles of 100
N 0071-0321-24 50 mg (white, scored) bottles of 100

Caution—Federal law prohibits dispensing without prescription.

0320G011

Shown in Product Identification Section, page 421

PENICILLIN V POTASSIUM, USP ℞

[*pĕ″nĭ-cĭ′llĭn v pō″tă′ssĭ-ŭm*]

(Penapar VK®)

[*pĕ′nă-păr″*]

DESCRIPTION

Penicillin V is the phenoxymethyl analog of penicillin G. Penicillin V Potassium Tablets also contain: lactose, NF; magnesium stearate, NF; microcrystalline cellulose, NF; polyethylene glycol, NF; povidone, USP; sodium laurel sulfate, NF.

Penicillin V Potassium for Oral Solution also contains: aspartame, NF; citric acid, USP; FD&C red No. 40; flavors; primary taste modifier; saccharin sodium, USP; silica gel, USP; sodium citrate, USP; sodium propionate, NF; sucrose NF.

ACTION AND PHARMACOLOGY

Penicillin V exerts a bactericidal action against penicillin-sensitive microorganisms during the stage of active multiplication. It acts through the inhibition of biosynthesis of cell wall mucopeptide. It is not active against the penicillinase-producing bacteria, which include many strains of staphylococci. The drug exerts high *in vitro* activity against staphylococci (except penicillinase-producing strains), streptococci (groups A, C, G, H, L, and M), and pneumococci. Other organisms sensitive *in vitro* to penicillin V are *Corynebacterium diphtheriae, Bacillus anthracis,* Clostridia, *Actinomyces bovis, Streptobacillus moniliformis, Listeria monocytogenes,* Leptospira, and *N gonorrhoeae. Treponema pallidum* is extremely sensitive.

Penicillin V has the distinct advantage over penicillin G in resistance to inactivation by gastric acid. It may be given with meals; however, blood levels are slightly higher when the drug is given on an empty stomach. Average blood levels are two to five times higher than the levels following the same dose of oral penicillin G and also show much less individual variation.

Once absorbed, penicillin V is about 80% bound to serum protein. Tissue levels are highest in the kidneys, with lesser amounts in the liver, skin, and intestines. Small amounts are found in all other body tissues and the cerebrospinal fluid. The drug is excreted as rapidly as it is absorbed in individuals with normal kidney function; however, recovery of the drug from the urine indicates that only about 25% of the dose given is absorbed. In neonates, young infants, and individuals with impaired kidney function, excretion is considerably delayed.

INDICATIONS

Penicillin V is indicated in the treatment of mild to moderately severe infections due to penicillin G-sensitive microorganisms that are sensitive to the low serum levels common to this particular dosage form. Therapy should be guided by bacteriologic studies (including sensitivity tests) and by clinical response.

NOTE: Severe pneumonia, empyema, bacteremia, pericarditis, meningitis, and arthritis should not be treated with penicillin V during the acute stage.

Indicated surgical procedures should be performed.

The following infections will usually respond to adequate dosage of penicillin V:

Streptococcal infections (without bacteremia); mild to moderate infections of the upper respiratory tract, scarlet fever, and mild erysipelas

NOTE: Streptococci in groups A, C, G, H, L, and M are very sensitive to penicillin. Other groups, including group D (enterococcus), are resistant.

Pneumococcal infections. Mild to moderately severe infections of the respiratory tract

Staphylococcal infections —penicillin G-sensitive; mild infections of the skin and soft tissues.

NOTE: Reports indicate an increasing number of strains of staphylococci resistant to penicillin G, emphasizing the need for culture and sensitivity studies in treating suspected staphylococcal infections.

Fusospirochetosis (Vincent's gingivitis and pharyngitis); mild to moderately severe infections of the oropharynx usually respond to therapy with oral penicillin.

NOTE: Necessary dental care should be accomplished in infections involving the gum tissue.

Medical conditions in which oral penicillin therapy is indicated as prophylaxis:

For the prevention of recurrence following rheumatic fever and/or chorea: prophylaxis with oral penicillin on a continuing basis has proved effective in preventing recurrence of these conditions.

Although no controlled clinical efficacy studies have been conducted, penicillin V has been suggested by the American Heart Association and the American Dental Association for use as part of a parenteral-oral regimen and as an alternative oral regimen for prophylaxis against bacterial endocarditis in patients with congenital heart disease or rheumatic or other acquired valvular heart disease when they undergo dental procedures and surgical procedures of the respiratory tract.[1] Since it may happen that *alpha* hemolytic streptococci relatively resistant to penicillin may be found when patients are receiving continuous oral penicillin for secondary prevention of rheumatic fever, prophylactic agents other than penicillin may be chosen for these patients and prescribed in addition to their continuous rheumatic fever prophylactic regimen. Oral penicillin should not be used as adjunctive prophylaxis for genitourinary instrumentation or surgery, lower intestinal tract surgery, sigmoidoscopy, and childbirth.

NOTE: When selecting antibiotics for the prevention of bacterial endocarditis, the physician or dentist should read the full joint statement of the American Heart Association and the American Dental Association.[1]

CONTRAINDICATIONS

A previous hypersensitivity reaction to any penicillin is a contraindication.

WARNING

Serious and occasionally fatal hypersensitivity (anaphylactoid) reactions have been reported in patients on penicillin therapy. Although anaphylaxis is more frequent following parenteral therapy, it has occurred in patients on oral penicillins. These reactions are more apt to occur in individuals with a history of sensitivity to multiple allergens.

There have been well-documented reports of individuals with a history of penicillin hypersensitivity reactions who have experienced severe hypersensitivity reactions when treated with a cephalosporin. Before therapy with a penicillin, careful inquiry should be made concerning previous hypersensitivity reactions to penicillins, cephalosporins, and other allergens. If an allergic reaction occurs, the drug should be discontinued and the patient treated with the usual agents, eg, pressor amines, antihistamines, and corticosteroids.

PRECAUTIONS

Penicillin should be used with caution in individuals with histories of significant allergies and/or asthma.

The oral route of administration should not be relied upon in patients with severe illness, or with nausea, vomiting, gastric dilatation, cardiospasm, or intestinal hypermotility.

Occasional patients will not absorb therapeutic amounts of orally administered penicillin.

In streptococcal infections, therapy must be sufficient to eiiminate the organism (ten days minimum); otherwise, the sequelae of streptococcal disease may occur. Cultures should be taken following completion of treatment to determine whether streptococci have been eradicated.

Prolonged use of antibiotics may promote the overgrowth of nonsusceptible organisms, including fungi. Should superinfection occur, appropriate measures should be taken.

Oral solutions contain aspartame.

Phenylketonurics: contains phenylalanine 4.5 mg per 5 mL.

ADVERSE REACTIONS

Although the incidence of reactions to oral penicillins has been reported with much less frequency than following parenteral therapy, it should be remembered that all degrees of hypersensitivity, including fatal anaphylaxis, have been reported with oral penicillin.

The most common reactions to oral penicillin are nausea, vomiting, epigastric distress, diarrhea, and black hairy tongue. The hypersensitivity reactions reported are skin eruptions (maculopapular to exfoliative dermatitis), urticaria and other serum sickness reactions, laryngeal edema, and anaphylaxis. Fever and eosinophilia may frequently be the only reaction observed. Hemolytic anemia, leukopenia, thrombocytopenia, neuropathy, and nephropathy are infrequent reactions and usually associated with high doses of parenteral penicillin.

DOSAGE AND ADMINISTRATION

The dosage of penicillin V should be determined according to the sensitivity of the causative microorganisms and the severity of the infection, and adjusted to the clinical response of the patient.

The usual dosage recommendations for adults and children 12 years and over are as follows.

Streptococcal infections —mild to moderately severe—of the upper respiratory tract and including scarlet fever and erysipelas: 125 to 250 mg (200,000 to 400,000 units) every six to eight hours for ten days

Pneumococcal infections —mild to moderately severe—of the respiratory tract, including otitis media: 250 mg (400,000 units) every six hours until the patient has been afebrile for at least two days

Staphylococcal infections —mild infections of skin and soft tissue (culture and sensitivity tests should be performed): 250 mg (400,000 units) every six to eight hours

Fusospirochetosis (Vincent's infection) of the oropharynx —mild to moderately severe infections: 250 mg (400,000 units) every six to eight hours

For the prevention of recurrence following rheumatic fever and/or chorea: 125 mg (200,000 units) twice daily on a continuing basis.

NOTE: Therapy for children under 12 years of age is calculated on the basis of body weight. For infants and small chil-

dren, the suggested dosage is 15 to 56 mg (25,000 to 90,000 units) per kg per day in three to six divided doses.
For prophylaxis against bacterial endocarditis[1] in patients with congenital heart disease or rheumatic or other acquired valvular heart disease when undergoing dental procedures or surgical procedures of the upper respiratory tract, one of two regimens may be selected:
(1) For the oral regimen, give 2.0 gm of penicillin V (1.0 gm for children under 60 lbs) ½ to 1 hour before the procedure, and then, 500 mg (250 mg for children under 60 lbs) every 6 hours for 8 doses; or
(2) For the combined parenteral-oral regimen give one million units of aqueous crystalline penicillin G (30,000 units/kg in children) intramuscularly mixed with 600,000 units procaine penicillin G (600,000 units for children) ½ to 1 hour before the procedure, and then oral penicillin V, 500 mg for adults or 250 mg for children under 60 lbs, every 6 hours for 8 doses. Doses for children should not exceed recommendations for adults for a single dose or for a 24 hour period.

HOW SUPPLIED

Penicillin V Tablets are supplied as:
N 0071-0648-24 250 mg—Bottle of 100.
N 0071-0648-32 250 mg—Bottle of 1000.
N 0071-0648-40 250 mg—Unit dose Package of 100 (10 strips of 10).
Each tablet contains penicillin V potassium equivalent to 250 mg (400,000 units) penicillin V.
N 0071-0673-24 500 mg—Bottle of 100.
N 0071-0673-30 500 mg—Bottle of 500.
Each tablet contains penicillin V potassium equivalent to 500 mg (800,000 units) penicillin V.
Shown in Product Identification Section, page 421
Penicillin V For Oral Solution is supplied as:
N 0071-2449-17 125 mg/5 ml—100 ml individual bottles and packs of six.
N 0071-2449-20 125 mg/5 ml—200 ml individual bottles and packs of six.
When reconstituted according to directions, each 5 ml contains penicillin V potassium equivalent to 125 mg (200,000 units) penicillin V.
N 0071-2506-17 250 mg/5 ml—100 ml individual bottles and packs of six.
N 0071-2506-20 250 mg/5 ml—200 ml individual bottles and packs of six.
When reconstituted according to directions, each 5 ml contains penicillin V potassium equivalent to 250 mg (400,000 units) penicillin V.

REFERENCE

1. American Heart Association: Prevention of bacterial endocarditis. *Circulation* 56: 139A-143A, 1977.
Manufactured by John D. Copanos Inc., Baltimore, MD 21225 and distributed by Parke-Davis, Warner-Lambert Co, Morris Plains, NJ 07950
AHFS 8:12.16 **7000G105**

PERITRATE® SA ℞

[*pĕ'rĭ-trāte"*]
(pentaerythritol tetranitrate tablets)
Sustained Action*

PERITRATE® ℞

(pentaerythritol tetranitrate tablets, USP)

DESCRIPTION

Each tablet of Peritrate 40 mg contains pentaerythritol tetranitrate 40 mg.
Each tablet of Peritrate 20 mg contains pentaerythritol tetranitrate 20 mg.
Each tablet of Peritrate 10 mg contains pentaerythritol tetranitrate 10 mg.
Pentaerythritol tetranitrate is a nitric acid ester of a tetrahydric alcohol (pentaerythritol).
Peritrate 10 mg and 20 mg contain alginic acid, NF; D&C yellow No. 10; FD&C blue No. 1; gelatin, NF; lactose, NF; methylcellulose, USP; propylparaben, NF; corn starch, NF; stearic acid, NF; and may also contain magnesium stearate, NF. Peritrate 40 mg contains D&C yellow No. 10 Al lake; D&C red No. 30 Al lake; lactose, NF; povidone, USP; silicon dioxide, NF; corn starch, NF; stearic acid, NF; and confectioner's sugar, NF.
Each tablet of Peritrate SA Sustained Action contains: pentaerythritol tetranitrate 80 mg (20 mg in immediate release layer and 60 mg in sustained release base). Pentaerythritol tetranitrate is a nitric acid ester of a tetrahydric alcohol (pentaerythritol).
Peritrate SA 80 mg also contains D&C yellow No. 10; FD&C blue No. 1; lactose, NF; magnesium stearate, NF; silicon dioxide, NF; confectioner's sugar, NF; and other ingredients.

ACTIONS

The exact cause of angina pectoris (that is, the pain associated with coronary artery disease) remains obscure, despite the numerous and often conflicting hypotheses concerning its pathophysiology. Therapy at the present time, therefore, remains essentially empirical. Customarily, clinical improvement has been measured by: reduction in (1) number, intensity and duration of angina pectoris attacks and (2) necessity for glyceryl trinitrate intake for prevention or relief of anginal attacks. Peritrate SA (pentaerythritol tetranitrate) Sustained Action and Peritrate (pentaerythritol tetranitrate) have been reported in clinical usage to reduce in number and severity the incidence of angina pectoris attacks, with concomitant reduction in glyceryl trinitrate intake.
In the evaluation of Peritrate and Peritrate SA in angina pectoris, clinical improvement has been customarily measured subjectively by: reduction in number and severity of attacks and necessity for glyceryl trinitrate intake for prevention or abortion of anginal attacks. Individual patterns of angina pectoris differ widely as does the symptomatic response to antianginal agents such as pentaerythritol tetranitrate. The published literature contains both favorable and unfavorable clinical reports. In conjunction with total management of the patient with angina pectoris, Peritrate and Peritrate SA have been accepted as safe for prolonged administration and widely regarded as useful.

INDICATIONS

Based on a review of this drug by the National Academy of Sciences—National Research Council and/or other information, FDA has classified the indications as follows:
"Possibly" effective: Peritrate is indicated for the relief of angina pectoris (pain associated with coronary artery disease). It is not intended to abort the acute anginal episode but is widely regarded as useful in the prophylactic treatment of angina pectoris.
Final classification of the less-than-effective indications requires further investigation.

CONTRAINDICATIONS

Peritrate SA and Peritrate are contraindicated in patients who have a history of sensitivity to the drug.

WARNINGS

Data supporting the use of Peritrate or Peritrate SA during the early days of the acute phase of myocardial infarction (the period during which clinical and laboratory findings are unstable) are insufficient to establish safety.
This drug can act as a physiological antagonist to norepinephrine, acetylcholine, histamine, and many other agents.

PRECAUTIONS

Should be used with caution in patients who have glaucoma. Tolerance to this drug and cross-tolerance to other nitrites and nitrates may occur.

ADVERSE REACTIONS

Side effects reported to date have been predominantly related to rash (which requires discontinuation of medication) and headache and gastrointestinal distress, which are usually mild and transient with continuation of medication. In some cases severe persistent headaches may occur. In addition, the following adverse reactions to nitrates such as pentaerythritol tetranitrate have been reported in the literature:
(a) Cutaneous vasodilatation with flushing.
(b) Transient episodes of dizziness and weakness, as well as other signs of cerebral ischemia associated with postural hypotension, may occasionally develop.
(c) An occasional individual exhibits marked sensitivity to the hypotensive effects of nitrite and severe responses (nausea, vomiting, weakness, restlessness, pallor, perspiration and collapse) can occur, even with the usual therapeutic doses. Alcohol may enhance this effect.

DOSAGE

Peritrate may be administered in individualized doses up to 160 mg a day. Dosage can be initiated at one 10 mg or 20 mg tablet q.i.d. and titrated upward to 40 mg (two 20 mg tablets or one 40 mg tablet) q.i.d. one-half hour before or one hour after meals and at bedtime. Tablets can be chewed or swallowed whole. Alternatively, Peritrate SA can be administered on a convenient b.i.d. (on an empty stomach) dosage schedule. One tablet immediately on arising and 1 tablet 12 hours later. Tablets should not be chewed.

SUPPLIED

Peritrate SA Sustained Action 80 mg—double layer, biconvex, dark green/light green tablets in bottles of 100 (N 0710-0004-24) and 1000 (N 0710-0004-32).
Shown in Product Identification Section, page 421
Also in unit dose package of 10 × 10 strips (N 0710-0004-40).
Peritrate 40 mg—coral scored tablets in bottles of 100 (N 0710-0008-24).
Shown in Product Identification Section, page 421
Peritrate 20 mg—light green, scored tablets in bottles of 100 (N 0710-0001-24) and 1000 (N 0710-0001-32).
Shown in Product Identification Section, page 421
Also in unit dose package of 10 × 10 strips (N 0710-0001-40).
Peritrate 10 mg—light green, unscored tablets in bottles of 100 (N 0710-0013-24) and 1000 (N 0710-0013-32).
Shown in Product Identification Section, page 421

ANIMAL PHARMACOLOGY

In a series of carefully designed studies in pigs, Peritrate was administered for 48 hours before an artificially induced occlusion of a major coronary artery and for seven days thereafter. The pigs were sacrificed at various intervals for periods up to six weeks. The result showed a significantly larger number of survivors in the drug-treated group. Damage to myocardial tissue in the drug-treated survivors was less extensive than in the untreated group. Studies in dogs subjected to oligemic shock through progressive bleeding have demonstrated that Peritrate is vasoactive at the postarteriolar level, producing increased blood flow and better tissue perfusion. These animal experiments cannot be translated to the drug's actions in humans.
0001G011/0004G011

PITOCIN® ℞

[*pĭ"tō'cĭn*]
(oxytocin injection, USP) synthetic

IMPORTANT NOTICE

Pitocin is not indicated for the elective induction of labor because available data and information are inadequate to define the benefits-to-risks considerations in the use of the drug product. Elective induction of labor is defined as the initiation of labor in an individual with a term pregnancy who is free of medical indications for the initiation of labor.

DESCRIPTION

Pitocin (oxytocin injection, USP) is a sterile, aqueous solution of synthetic oxytocic hormone standardized to contain 10 units/ml and containing 0.5% Chloretone® (chlorobutanol) (chloroform derivative) as a preservative, with the acidity adjusted with acetic acid. The drug is prepared synthetically to avoid possible contamination with vasopressin (ADH) and its antidiuretic and cardiovascular effects. However, the physician should be cognizant of the fact that even highly purified synthetic oxytocin contains inherent pressor-antidiuretic properties which may become manifest following administration of large doses (see Precautions).

ACTION

Uterine motility is controlled by a variety of biochemical and regulatory processes. Oxytocin appears to act primarily on uterine myofibril activity by increasing the permeability of the cell membranes to sodium ions, thus augmenting the number of contracting myofibrils, and thereby enabling the uterus to produce the necessary number of contractions. The effect depends on the uterine threshold of excitability. The sensitivity of the uterus to oxytocin increases gradually during gestation; then increases sharply before parturition.

INDICATIONS

Antepartum: Pitocin is indicated for the initiation or improvement of uterine contractions, where this is desirable and considered suitable, for the following purposes: induction of labor in patients with a medical indication for the initiation of labor, such as mild preeclampsia at or near term, when delivery is in the best interest of mother and fetus or when membranes are prematurely ruptured and delivery is indicated; stimulation or reinforcement of labor, as in selected cases of uterine inertia; as adjunctive therapy in the management of incomplete or inevitable abortion. In the first trimester, curettage is generally considered primary therapy. In second trimester abortion, oxytocin infusion will often be successful in emptying the uterus. Other means of therapy, however, may be required in such cases.
Postpartum: Pitocin is indicated to produce uterine contractions during the third stage of labor and to control postpartum bleeding or hemorrhage.

CONTRAINDICATIONS

Pitocin is contraindicated in any of the following conditions: significant cephalopelvic disproportion; unfavorable fetal positions or presentations which are undeliverable without conversion prior to delivery (as, for example, transverse lies); in obstetrical emergencies where the benefit-to-risk ratio for either the fetus or the mother favors surgical intervention;

Continued on next page

This product information was prepared in August, 1986. On these and other Parke-Davis Products, information may be obtained by addressing PARKE-DAVIS, Division of Warner-Lambert Company, Morris Plains, New Jersey 07950.

Parke-Davis—Cont.

in cases of fetal distress where delivery is not imminent; prolonged use in uterine inertia or severe toxemia; hypertonic uterine patterns; patients with hypersensitivity to the drug; induction or augmentation of labor in those cases where vaginal delivery is contraindicated, such as invasive cervical carcinoma, cord presentation or prolapse, total placentia previa, and vasa previa.

WARNINGS

Pitocin, when given for induction or stimulation of labor, must be administered only by the intravenous route and with adequate medical supervision in a hospital.

PRECAUTIONS

1. All patients receiving intravenous oxytocin must be under continuous observation by trained personnel with a thorough knowledge of the drug and qualified to identify complications. A physician qualified to manage any complications should be immediately available.
2. When properly administered, oxytocin should stimulate uterine contractions comparable to those seen in normal labor. Overstimulation of the uterus by improper administration can be hazardous to both mother and fetus. Even with proper administration and adequate supervision, hypertonic contractions can occur in patients whose uteri are hypersensitive to oxytocin. This fact must be considered by the physician in exercising judgment regarding patient selection.
3. Except in unusual circumstances, oxytocin should not be administered in the following conditions: fetal distress, partial placenta previa, prematurity, borderline cephalopelvic disproportion, and in any conditions where there is a predisposition for uterine rupture, such as previous major surgery on the cervix or uterus including cesarean section, overdistention of the uterus, grand multiparity, or past history of uterine sepsis or of traumatic delivery. Because of the variability of the combinations of factors which may be present in the conditions listed above, the definition of "unusual circumstances" must be left to the judgment of the physician. The decision can only be made by carefully weighing the potential benefits which oxytocin can provide in a given case against rare but definite potential for the drug to produce hypertonicity or tetanic spasm.
4. Maternal deaths due to hypertensive episodes, subarachnoid hemorrhage, rupture of the uterus, and fetal deaths due to various causes have been reported associated with the use of parenteral oxytocic drugs for induction of labor or for augmentation in the first and second stages of labor.
5. Oxytocin has been shown to have an intrinsic antidiuretic effect, acting to increase water reabsorption from the glomerular filtrate. Consideration should, therefore, be given to the possibility of water intoxication, particularly when oxytocin is administered continuously by infusion and the patient is receiving fluids by mouth.
6. When oxytocin is used for induction or reinforcement of already existent labor, patients should be carefully selected. Pelvic adequacy must be considered and maternal and fetal conditions evaluated before use of the drug.

ADVERSE REACTIONS

Fetal bradycardia, anaphylactic reaction, postpartum hemorrhage, cardiac arrhythmia, and pelvic hematoma have been reported.

Excessive dosage or hypersensitivity to the drug may result in uterine hypertonicity, spasm, tetanic contraction, or rupture.

Side effects that may also occur during spontaneous labor, such as nausea, vomiting, and premature ventricular contractions, have been noted occasionally with oxytocin.

A fatality due to afibrinogenemia has been reported, naming oxytocin injection as a possible cause. The possibility of increased blood loss and afibrinogenemia should be kept in mind when administering the drug.

Severe water intoxication with convulsions and coma has occurred, associated with a slow oxytocin infusion over a 24-hour period. Maternal death due to oxytocin-induced water intoxication has been reported.

DOSAGE AND ADMINISTRATION

Dosage of oxytocin is determined by uterine response. The following dosage information is based upon the various regimens and indications in general use.

A. Induction or Stimulation of Labor

Intravenous infusion (drip method) is the only acceptable method of parenteral administration for the induction or stimulation of labor. Accurate control of the rate of infusion flow is essential. An infusion pump or other such device and at least external electronic monitoring are necessary for the safe administration of oxytocin for the induction or stimulation of labor. If uterine contractions become too powerful, the infusion can be abruptly stopped, and oxytocic stimulation of the uterine musculature will soon wane.

1. An intravenous infusion of non-oxytocin containing solution should be started. (Physiologic electrolyte solution should be used.)
2. To prepare the standard solution for infusion, the contents of one 1-ml ampoule is combined aseptically with 1,000 ml of 0.9% aqueous sodium chloride solution or other nonhydrating diluent. The combined solution (1 ml = 10 milliunits) is rotated in the infusion bottle to insure thorough mixing. Add the container with dilute oxytocic solution to the system through use of a constant infusion pump.
3. The initial dose should be 1 to 2 mU/min- ute. At 15 to 30 minute intervals, the dose should be gradually increased in increments of 1 to 2 mU/ minute until the desired contraction pattern has been established, which should be comparable to that seen in normal labor.
4. The fetal heart rate, resting uterine tone, and the frequency, duration, and force of contractions should be monitored.
5. The oxytocin infusion should be discontinued immediately in the event of uterine hyperactivity or fetal distress. Oxygen should be administered to the mother. The mother and the fetus must be evaluated by the responsible physician.

B. Control of Postpartum Uterine Bleeding

1. Intravenous Infusion (Drip Method)

To control postpartum bleeding, 10 to 40 units of oxytocin may be added to 1,000 ml of 5% dextrose injection and run at a rate necessary to control uterine atony.

2. Intramuscular Administration

1 ml (10 units) of oxytocin can be given after delivery of the placenta.

C. Treatment of Incomplete or Inevitable Abortion:

Intravenous infusion with physiologic saline solution, 500 ml, or 5% dextrose in physiologic saline solution to which 10 units of Pitocin have been added should be infused at a rate of 10 to 20 milliunits (20 to 40 drops) per minute.

HOW SUPPLIED

N 0071-4160-02 (Ampoule 163)
Contains 5 units in a 0.5-ml ampoule, packages of ten
N 0071-4160-03 (Ampoule 160)
Contains 10 units in a 1-ml ampoule, packages of ten
N 0071-4160-40 (Steri-Dose® syringe 1489)
Contains 10 units in a 1-ml sterile disposable syringe, packages of ten
N 0071-4160-10 (Steri-Vial® 1541)
Contains 10 units per milliliter in a 10-ml Steri-Vial (multiple dose vial)
AHFS 76:00

4160G061

PITRESSIN® ℞

[pĭ″trĕ′ssĭn]
(vasopressin injection, USP)
synthetic

DESCRIPTION

Pitressin (vasopressin injection) is a sterile, aqueous solution of synthetic vasopressin (8-arginine vasopressin) of the posterior pituitary gland. It is substantially free from the oxytocic principle and is standardized to contain 20 pressor units/ml. The solution contains 0.5% Chloretone® (chlorobutanol) (chloroform derivative) as a preservative. The acidity of the solution is adjusted with acetic acid.

ACTION

The antidiuretic action of vasopressin is ascribed to increasing reabsorption of water by the renal tubules.

Vasopressin can cause contraction of smooth muscle of the gastrointestinal tract and of all parts of the vascular bed, especially the capillaries, small arterioles and venules, with less effect on the smooth musculature of the large veins. The direct effect on the contractile elements is neither antagonized by adrenergic blocking agents nor prevented by vascular denervation.

CONTRAINDICATION

Anaphylaxis or hypersensitivity to the drug or its components.

INDICATIONS

Pitressin is indicated for prevention and treatment of postoperative abdominal distention, in abdominal roentgenography to dispel interfering gas shadows, and in diabetes insipidus.

WARNINGS

This drug should not be used in patients with vascular disease, especially disease of the coronary arteries, except with extreme caution. In such patients, even small doses may precipitate anginal pain, and with larger doses, the possibility of myocardial infarction should be considered.

Vasopressin may produce water intoxication. The early signs of drowsiness, listlessness, and headaches should be recognized to prevent terminal coma and convulsions.

PRECAUTIONS

Vasopressin should be used cautiously in the presence of epilepsy, migraine, asthma, heart failure, or any state in which a rapid addition to extracellular water may produce hazard for an already overburdened system.

Chronic nephritis with nitrogen retention contraindicates the use of vasopressin until reasonable nitrogen blood levels have been attained.

ADVERSE REACTIONS

Local or systemic allergic reactions may occur in hypersensitive individuals. The following side effects have been reported following the administration of vasopressin: tremor, sweating, vertigo, circumoral pallor, "pounding" in head, abdominal cramps, passage of gas, nausea, vomiting, urticaria, bronchial constriction. Anaphylaxis (cardiac arrest and/ or shock) has been observed shortly after injection of vasopressin.

DOSAGE AND ADMINISTRATION

Pitressin may be administered subcutaneously or intramuscularly.

Ten units of Pitressin (0.5 ml) will usually elicit full physiologic response in adult patients; 5 units will be adequate in many cases. Pitressin should be given intramuscularly at three- or four-hour intervals as needed. The dosage should be proportionately reduced for children. (For an additional discussion of dosage, consult the sections below).

When determining the dose of Pitressin for a given case, the following should be kept in mind.

It is particularly desirable to give a dose not much larger than is just sufficient to elicit the desired physiologic response. Excessive doses may cause undesirable side actions—blanching of the skin, abdominal cramps, nausea—which, though not serious, may be alarming to the patient. Spontaneous recovery from such side actions occurs in a few minutes. It has been found that one or two glasses of water given at the time Pitressin is administered reduces such symptoms.

Abdominal Distention: In the average post- operative adult patient, give 5 units (0.25 ml) initially; increase to 10 units (0.5 ml) at subsequent injections if necessary. It is recommended that Pitressin be given intramuscularly and that injections be repeated at three- or four-hour intervals as required. Dosage to be reduced proportionately for children. Pitressin used in this manner will frequently prevent, or relieve, postoperative distention. These recommendations apply also to distention complicating pneumonia or other acute toxemias.

Abdominal Roentgenography: For the average case, two injections of 10 units each (0.5 ml) are suggested. These should be given two hours and one half hour, respectively, before films are exposed. Many roentgenologists advise giving an enema prior to the first dose of Pitressin.

Diabetes Insipidus: Pitressin may be given by injection or administered intranasally on cotton pledgets, by nasal spray, or by dropper. The dose by injection is 5 to 10 units (0.25 to 0.5 ml) repeated two or three times daily as needed. When Pitressin is administered intranasally by spray or on pledgets, the dosage and interval between treatments must be determined for each patient.

HOW SUPPLIED

Pitressin (vasopressin injection, USP) synthetic is supplied in ampoules as follows.
N 0071-4200-02
0.5 ml (10 pressor units). Packages of 10
N 0071-4200-03
1 ml (20 pressor units). Packages of 10

Note: When ordering Pitressin Ampoules, Synthetic, be sure to state whether the 10- or 20-unit is desired.

4200G041

PITRESSIN® TANNATE IN OIL ℞

[pĭ″trĕ′ssĭn tă′nāte]
(vasopressin tannate)
FOR INTRAMUSCULAR USE ONLY

DESCRIPTION

Pitressin Tannate in Oil (Sterile Vasopressin Tannate Suspension) is a water insoluble chemical compound of vasopressin, the pressor fraction of the posterior lobe of the pituitary gland, and tannic acid. It has antidiuretic activity. It is available as a sterile suspension for intramuscular administration. Vasopressin tannate is substantially free from the oxytocic principle and is standardized to contain 5 pressor units per mL in peanut oil.

CLINICAL PHARMACOLOGY

The antidiuretic action of vasopressin tannate is ascribed to increasing reabsorption of water by the renal tubules.

Vasopressin can cause contraction of smooth muscle of the gastrointestinal tract and of all parts of the vascular bed, especially the capillaries, small arterioles, and venules, with less effect on the smooth musculature of the large veins. These effects are ordinarily not seen to a significant degree with recommended antidiuretic doses of vasopressin tannate. The direct effect on the contractile elements is neither antagonized by adrenergic blocking agents nor prevented by vascular denervation.

INDICATIONS

Pitressin Tannate in Oil is indicated for the control or prevention of the symptoms and complications of diabetes insipidus due to a deficiency of endogenous posterior pituitary antidiuretic hormone.

CONTRAINDICATION

Anaphylaxis or hypersensitivity to the drug or its components.

WARNINGS

This preparation should never be administered intravenously. This drug should not be used in patients with vascular disease, especially disease of the coronary arteries, except with extreme caution. In such patients, even small doses may precipitate anginal pain.

Vasopressin may produce water intoxication. The early signs of drowsiness, listlessness, and headaches should be recognized to prevent terminal coma and convulsions.

PRECAUTIONS

Vasopressin should be used cautiously in the presence of epilepsy, migraine, asthma, heart failure, or any state in which a rapid addition to extracellular water may produce hazard for an already overburdened system.

Chronic nephritis with nitrogen retention contraindicates the use of vasopressin until reasonable nitrogen blood levels have been attained.

ADVERSE REACTIONS

Local or systemic allergic reactions may occur in hypersensitive individuals. The following side effects have been reported following the administration of vasopressin: tremor, sweating, vertigo, circumoral pallor, "pounding" in head, abdominal cramps, passage of gas, nausea, vomiting, urticaria, bronchial constriction, anaphylaxis, cardiac arrest.

DOSAGE AND ADMINISTRATION

Intramuscular —0.3 to 1 ml repeated as required. The duration of action varies with the patient and his condition, and may be as prolonged as 48 to 96 hours.

Shake ampoule thoroughly before use to obtain a uniform suspension. Contents of the ampoules may show a cloudiness, or colorless crystals, of solid fats from the peanut oil vehicle. If this occurs, warm the ampoules to dissolve the solid fats. Warming of the ampoules will also facilitate transfer of product from ampoule to syringe.

HOW SUPPLIED

N 0071-4302-03

Pitressin Tannate in Oil (Sterile Vasopressin Tannate Suspension) is supplied in 1 mL ampoules containing 5 pressor units per mL in peanut oil. Packages of 10.

Store at controlled room temperature 15°–30°C (59°–86°F)

AHFS 68:28

4302G041

PONSTEL® ℞

[pŏn ′stĕl″]

(mefenamic acid)

DESCRIPTION

Ponstel (mefenamic acid) is N-(2,3-xylyl)-anthranilic acid. It is an analgesic agent for oral administration. Ponstel is available in capsules containing 250 mg of mefenamic acid. Each capsule also contains lactose, NF. The capsule shell and/or band contains citric acid, USP; D&C yellow No. 10; FD&C blue No. 1; FD&C red No. 3; FD&C yellow No. 6; gelatin, NF; glycerol monooleate; sodium benzoate, NF; titanium dioxide, USP.

It is a white powder with a melting point of 230–231° C, molecular weight 241.28, and water solubility of 0.004% at pH 7.1.

CLINICAL PHARMACOLOGY

Ponstel is a nonsteroidal agent with demonstrated antiinflammatory, analgesic, and antipyretic activity in laboratory animals.[1,2] The mode of action is not known. In animal studies, Ponstel was found to inhibit prostaglandin synthesis and to compete for binding at the prostaglandin receptor site.[3]

Pharmacologic studies show Ponstel did not relieve morphine abstinence signs in abstinent, morphine-habituated monkeys.[1]

Following a single 1-gram oral dose, peak plasma levels of 10 μg/ml occurred in 2 to 4 hours with a half-life of 2 hours. Following multiple doses, plasma levels are proportional to dose with no evidence of drug accumulation. One gram of Ponstel given four times daily produces peak blood levels of 20 μg/ml by the second day of administration.[4]

Following a single dose, sixty-seven percent of the total dose is excreted in the urine as unchanged drug or as one of two metabolites. Twenty to twenty-five percent of the dose is excreted in the feces during the first three days.[4]

In controlled, double-blind, clinical trials, Ponstel was evaluated for the treatment of primary spasmodic dysmenorrhea. The parameters used in determining efficacy included pain assessment by both patient and investigator; the need for concurrent analgesic medication; and evaluation of change in frequency and severity of symptoms characteristic of spasmodic dysmenorrhea. Patients received either Ponstel, 500 mg (2 capsules) as an initial dose and 250 mg every 6 hours, or placebo at onset of bleeding or of pain, whichever began first. After three menstrual cycles, patients were crossed over to the alternate treatment for an additional three cycles. Ponstel was significantly superior to placebo in all parameters, and both treatments (drug and placebo) were equally tolerated.

INDICATIONS AND USAGE

Ponstel is indicated for the relief of moderate pain[5] when therapy will not exceed one week. Ponstel is also indicated for the treatment of primary dysmenorrhea.[5,6]

Studies in children under 14 years of age have been inadequate to evaluate the safety and effectiveness of Ponstel.

CONTRAINDICATIONS

Ponstel should not be used in patients who have previously exhibited hypersensitivity to it.

Because the potential exists for cross-sensitivity to aspirin or other nonsteroidal antiinflammatory drugs, Ponstel should not be given to patients in whom these drugs induce symptoms of bronchospasm, allergic rhinitis, or urticaria.

Ponstel is contraindicated in patients with active ulceration or chronic inflammation of either the upper or lower gastrointestinal tract.

Ponstel should be avoided in patients with preexisting renal disease.

WARNINGS

In patients with a history of ulceration or chronic inflammation of the upper or lower gastrointestinal tract, Ponstel should be given under close supervision and only after consulting the Adverse Reactions Section.

If diarrhea occurs, the dosage should be reduced or temporarily suspended (see Adverse Reactions and Dosage and Administration). Certain patients who develop diarrhea may be unable to tolerate the drug because of recurrence of the symptoms on subsequent exposure.

PRECAUTIONS

If rash occurs, administration of the drug should be stopped.

A false-positive reaction for urinary bile, using the diazo tablet test, may result after mefenamic acid administration. If biliuria is suspected, other diagnostic procedures, such as the Harrison spot test, should be performed.

Renal Effects: As with other nonsteroidal antiinflammatory drugs, long-term administration of mefenamic acid to animals has resulted in renal papillary necrosis and other abnormal renal pathology. In humans, there have been reports of acute interstitial nephritis with hematuria, proteinuria and occasionally nephrotic syndrome.

A second form of renal toxicity has been seen in patients with prerenal conditions leading to a reduction in renal blood flow or blood volume, where the renal prostaglandins have a supportive role in the maintenance of renal perfusion. In these patients administration of an NSAID may cause a dose-dependent reduction in prostaglandin formation and may precipitate overt renal decompensation. Patients at greatest risk of this reaction are those with impaired renal function, heart failure, liver dysfunction, those taking diuretics, and the elderly Discontinuation of NSAID therapy is typically followed by recovery to the pretreatment state.

Since Ponstel is eliminated primarily by the kidneys, the drug should not be administered to patients with significantly impaired renal functions.

As with other nonsteroidal antiinflammatory drugs, borderline elevations of one or more liver tests may occur in some patients. These abnormalities may progress, may remain essentially unchanged, or may be transient with continued therapy. The SGPT (ALT) test is probably the most sensitive indicator of liver dysfunction. Meaningful (3 times the upper limit of normal) elevations of SGPT or SGOT (AST) occurred in controlled clinical trials in less than 1% of patients. A patient with symptoms and/or signs suggesting liver dysfunction, or in whom an abnormal liver test has occurred, should be evaluated for evidence of the development of more severe hepatic reaction while on therapy with Ponstel. Severe hepatic reactions, including jaundice and cases of fatal hepatitis, have been reported with other nonsteroidal antiinflammatory drugs. Although such reactions are rare, if abnormal liver tests persist or worsen, if clinical signs and symptoms consistent with liver disease develop, or if systemic manifestations occur (eg eosinophilia, rash, etc), Ponstel should be discontinued.

Information for Patients: Patients should be advised that if rash, diarrhea or other digestive problems arise, they should stop the drug and consult their physician.

Patients in whom aspirin or other nonsteroidal antiinflammatory drugs induce symptoms of bronchospasm, allergic rhinitis, or urticaria should be made aware that the potential exists for cross-sensitivity to Ponstel.

The long-term effects, if any, of intermittent Ponstel therapy for dysmenorrhea are not known. Women on such therapy should consult their physician if they should decide to become pregnant.

Drug Interactions: Ponstel may prolong prothrombin time.[5] Therefore, when the drug is administered to patients receiving oral anticoagulant drugs, frequent monitoring of prothrombin time is necessary.

Use in Pregnancy: Pregnancy Category C. Reproduction studies have been performed in rats, rabbits and dogs. Rats given up to 10 times the human dose showed decreased fertility, delay in parturition, and a decreased rate of survival to weaning. Rabbits at 2.5 times the human dose showed an increase in the number of resorptions. There were no fetal anomalies observed in these studies nor in dogs at up to 10 times the human dose.[5]

There are no adequate and well-controlled studies in pregnant women. Because animal reproduction studies are not always predictive of human response, this drug should be used only if clearly needed.

The use of Ponstel in late pregnancy is not recommended because of the effects on the fetal cardiovascular system of drugs of this class.

Nursing Mothers: Trace amounts of Ponstel may be present in breast milk and transmitted to the nursing infant[7]; thus Ponstel should not be taken by the nursing mother because of the effects on the infant cardiovascular system of drugs of this class.

Use in Children: Safety and effectiveness in children below the age of 14 have not been established.

ADVERSE REACTIONS

Gastrointestinal: The most frequently reported adverse reactions associated with the use of Ponstel involve the gastrointestinal tract. In controlled studies for up to eight months, the following disturbances were reported in decreasing order of frequency: diarrhea (approximately 5% of patients), nausea with or without vomiting, other gastrointestinal symptoms, and abdominal pain.

In certain patients, the diarrhea was of sufficient severity to require discontinuation of medication. The occurrence of the diarrhea is usually dose related, generally subsides on reduction of dosage, and rapidly disappears on termination of therapy.

Other gastrointestinal reactions less frequently reported were anorexia, pyrosis, flatulence, and constipation.

Gastrointestinal ulceration with and without hemorrhage has been reported.

Hematopoietic: Cases of autoimmune hemolytic anemia have been associated with the continuous administration of Ponstel for 12 months or longer. In such cases the Coombs test results are positive with evidence of both accelerated RBC production and RBC destruction. The process is reversible upon termination of Ponstel administration.

Decreases in hematocrit have been noted in 2–5% of patients and primarily in those who have received prolonged therapy. Leukopenia, eosinophilia, thrombocytopenic purpura, agranulocytosis, pancytopenia, and bone marrow hypoplasia have also been reported on occasion.

Nervous System: Drowsiness, dizziness, nervousness, headache, blurred vision, and insomnia have occurred.

Integumentary: Urticaria, rash, and facial edema have been reported.

Renal: As with other nonsteroidal antiinflammatory agents, renal failure, including papillary necrosis, has been reported. In elderly patients renal failure has occurred after taking Ponstel for 2–6 weeks. The renal damage may not be completely reversible. Hematuria and dysuria have also been reported with Ponstel.

Other: Eye irritation, ear pain, perspiration, mild hepatic toxicity, and increased need for insulin in a diabetic have been reported. There have been rare reports of palpitation, dyspnea, and reversible loss of color vision.

OVERDOSAGE

Although doses up to 6000 mg/day have been given, no specific information is available on the management of acute massive overdosage.

Should accidental overdosage occur, the stomach should be emptied by inducing emesis or by careful gastric lavage followed by the administration of activated charcoal.[8] Laboratory studies indicate that Ponstel should be adsorbed from the gastrointestinal tract by activated charcoal.[4] Vital functions should be monitored and supported. Because mefenamic acid and its metabolities are firmly bound to plasma proteins, hemodialysis and peritoneal dialysis may be of little value.[4]

Continued on next page

This product information was prepared in August, 1986. On these and other Parke-Davis Products, information may be obtained by addressing PARKE-DAVIS, Division of Warner-Lambert Company, Morris Plains, New Jersey 07950.

Parke-Davis—Cont.

DOSAGE AND ADMINISTRATION

Administration is by the oral route, preferably with food.
The recommended regimen in acute pain for adults and children over 14 years of age is 500 mg as an initial dose followed by 250 mg every six hours as needed, usually not to exceed one week.[5]
For the treatment of primary dysmenorrhea, the recommended dosage is 500 mg as an initial dose followed by 250 mg every 6 hours, starting with the onset of bleeding and associated symptoms. Clinical studies indicate that effective treatment can be initiated with the start of menses and should not be necessary for more than 2 to 3 days.[6]

HOW SUPPLIED

N 0710-0540-24 (P-D 540) Ponstel (mefenamic acid) is available as 250 mg capsules in bottles of 100.

Shown in Product Identification Section, page 421

References:

1. Winder CV, et al: Antiinflammatory, antipyretic and antinociceptive properties of N-(2,3-xylyl) anthranilic acid (mefenamic acid). *J Pharmacol Exp Ther* 138: 405–413, 1962.
2. Wax J, et al: Comparative activities, tolerances and safety of nonsteroidal antiinflammatory agents in rats. *J Pharmacol Exp Ther* 192: 172–178, 1975.
3. Ferreira SH, Vane JR: Aspirin and prostaglandins, in *The Prostaglandins,* Ramwell PW Ed, Plenum Press, NY, vol. 2, 1974, pp 1–47.
4. Glazko AJ: Experimental observations of flufenamic, mefenamic, and meclofenamic acids. Part III. Metabolic disposition, in *Fenamates in Medicine.* A Symposium, London 1966; *Annals of Physical Medicine,* supplement, pp 23–36, 1967.
5. Data on file, Medical Affairs Dept, Parke-Davis.
6. Budoff PW: Use of mefenamic acid in the treatment of primary dysmenorrhea. *JAMA* 241: 2713–2716, 1979.
7. Buchanan RA, et al: The breast milk excretion of mefenamic acid. *Curr Ther Res* 10:592, 1968.
8. Corby DG, Decker WJ: Management of acute poisoning with activated charcoal. *Pediatrics* 54:324, 1974.

Direct Medical Inquiries to: Parke-Davis
Div of Warner-Lambert Inc, 201 Tabor Road
Morris Plains, NJ 07950
Att: Medical Affairs Department

0540G015

Caution—Federal law prohibits dispensing without prescription.

PROCAN® SR ℞

[*prō 'căn"*]
(procainamide hydrochloride tablets)
SUSTAINED RELEASE

> The prolonged administration of procainamide often leads to the development of a positive antinuclear antibody (ANA) test with or without symptoms of lupus erythematosus-like syndrome. If a positive ANA titer develops, the benefit/risk ratio related to continued procainamide therapy should be assessed. This may necessitate consideration of alternative antiarrhythmic therapy.

DESCRIPTION

Each tablet of Procan SR contains procainamide hydrochloride in a tablet matrix specially designed for the prolonged release of the drug in the gastrointestinal tract. Following release of the drug, the expended wax tablet matrix, which is not absorbed, may be detected in the stool.
Procainamide hydrochloride is the amide analogue of procaine hydrochloride. The chemical name is 4-amino-N-[2-(diethylamino)ethyl]benzamide monohydrochloride.
Procan SR is available for oral administration as green, film-coated tablets containing 250 mg procainamide hydrochloride; as yellow, scored, film-coated tablets containing 500 mg procainamide hydrochloride; as orange, scored, film-coated tablets containing 750 mg procainamide hydrochloride; and as red, scored, film-coated tablets containing 1000 mg procainamide hydrochloride.
All strengths of Procan SR contain candelilla wax FCC, colloidal silicon dioxide NF, magnesium stearate NF, titanium dioxide, vanillin NF, and other ingredients. The individual strengths contain additional ingredients as follows.
250 mg: D&C yellow No. 10 Al lake; FD&C blue No. 1 Al lake; FD&C yellow No 6 Al lake; lactose, NF; may also contain methylparaben, NF, and propylparaben, NF, or simethicone emulsion and polysorbate 80.
500 mg: D&C yellow No. 10 Al lake; FD&C blue No. 2 Al lake; FD&C yellow No. 6 Al lake; sucrose NF; may also contain methylparaben, NF; and propylparaben, NF; or simethicone emulsion and polysorbate 80.
750 mg: FD&C yellow No. 6 Al lake; may also contain propylene glycol, USP or simethicone emulsion and polysorbate 80.
1000 mg: FD&C red No. 3 Al lake; FD&C yellow No. 6 Al lake; propylene glycol, USP.

CLINICAL PHARMACOLOGY

Procainamide is a Group 1 antiarrhythmic drug. It suppresses myocardial automaticity, and by increasing the threshold potential for electrical stimulation, it decreases myocardial excitability both in diastole and in the relative refractory period. Conduction velocity is decreased in the atria, ventricles, and His-Purkinje system. Procainamide diminishes membrane responsiveness and thus increases the refractory period in relation to the action's potential duration. The refractory period of the atrium is considerably more prolonged than that of the ventricle.
With therapeutic plasma levels of the drug, contractility of the heart is usually not affected nor is cardiac output decreased unless myocardial damage exists. Procainamide may reduce peripheral resistance and blood pressure as a result of peripheral vasodilation. In the absence of any arrhythmia, the heart rate may occasionally be accelerated by conventional doses, suggesting that procainamide possesses anticholinergic properties.
Procainamide plasma levels of about 4 to 8 mcg/mL are effective in suppressing ventricular arrhythmias in most patients without serious adverse effects. Toxicity begins to appear above 8 mcg/mL, and remains quite low up to 12 mcg/mL, but becomes progressively more frequent with higher concentrations.
After oral administration, procainamide is almost completely absorbed. It is rapidly distributed in the cerebrospinal fluid, liver, kidneys, spleen, lungs, muscles, brain, and heart. About 14% to 23% is bound to plasma proteins. From 7% to 34% is acetylated, presumably in the liver, to form N-acetylprocainamide (NAPA), an active metabolite that can accumulate. Plasma levels of NAPA may represent more than 50% of the total drug in the plasma. The rate of acetylation is genetically determined and varies among individuals, but remains constant for each person. Procainamide and NAPA are excreted in the urine by active tubular secretion and glomerular filtration. The total amount of unchanged procainamide excreted in the urine varies from 40% to 70% of a dose due to differences in acetylator phenotype and in renal excretion. The rate of renal excretion of procainamide and NAPA is not affected by changes in urine pH nor by acetylator phenotype.
Cardiac failure has a marked effect on the absorption, distribution, and clearance of procainamide, and may necessitate modified dosage for oral maintenance. Absorption may be slow and incomplete in patients with acute myocardial infarction. The apparent volume of distribution in patients with cardiac failure is considerably decreased from the approximate 2 L/kg for normal individuals. In patients with congestive heart failure, low cardiac output states, and/or renal insufficiency, clearance of procainamide and NAPA is decreased and plasma concentrations are markedly higher due to the impaired renal function. Procainamide and NAPA can be removed from the circulation by hemodialysis but not by peritoneal dialysis.
The sustained-release characteristic of Procan SR tablets has been demonstrated in studies in human subjects. A multiple-dose study has shown equivalent steady-state plasma levels of Procan SR tablets given every six hours when compared with an equal total daily dose of Pronestyl® (procainamide hydrochloride capsules, E.R. Squibb and Sons) given every three hours.

INDICATIONS AND USAGE

Oral procainamide is indicated in the treatment of premature ventricular contractions, ventricular tachycardia, atrial fibrillation, and paroxysmal atrial tachycardia.

CONTRAINDICATIONS

Hypersensitivity to procainamide is an absolute contraindication. In this connection, cross-sensitivity to procaine and related drugs must be borne in mind.
Procainamide should not be administered to patients with complete atrioventricular heart block. It is also contraindicated in cases of second degree and third degree A-V nodal block unless an electrical pacemaker is operative.
It has been suggested that procainamide be contraindicated in patients with myasthenia gravis.

WARNINGS

Granulocytopenia may follow the use of procainamide, and deaths from sepsis have occurred. Leukocyte changes are most likely to occur during the first three months of therapy. During this time routine blood counts should be done at least every two weeks and thereafter at longer intervals throughout maintenance procainamide therapy. Complaints of malaise and aches (a flu-type syndrome) are often reported in association with the granulocyte depression.
Patients should be instructed to report such symptoms promptly, as well as any soreness of mouth, throat or gums, unexplained fever, or symptoms of an upper respiratory tract infection. If these should occur and a complete blood count indicates a granulocyte depression, procainamide therapy should be discontinued immediately and appropriate treatment instituted. Recovery of leukocyte count usually occurs within a few weeks.
The incidence of granulocytopenia appears to be higher with procainamide sustained-release tablets than with standard tablets.

PRECAUTIONS

General—During administration of the drug, evidence of untoward myocardial responses should be carefully watched for in all patients. In the presence of an abnormal myocardium, procainamide may at times produce untoward responses. In atrial fibrillation or flutter, the ventricular rate may increase suddenly as the atrial rate is slowed. Adequate digitalization reduces, but does not abolish, this danger. If myocardial damage exists, ventricular tachysystole is particularly hazardous. Correction of atrial fibrillation, with resultant forceful contractions of the atrium, may cause a dislodgement of mural thrombi and produce an embolic episode. However, it has been suggested that in a patient who is already discharging emboli, procainamide is more likely to stop than to aggravate the process.
Attempts to adjust the heart rate in a patient who has developed ventricular tachycardia during an occlusive coronary episode should be carried out with extreme caution. Caution is also required in marked disturbances of atrioventricular conduction such as A-V block, bundle branch block, or severe digitalis intoxication, where the use of procainamide may result in additional depression of conduction and ventricular asystole or fibrillation.
Because patients with severe organic heart disease and ventricular tachycardia may also have complete heart block, which is difficult to diagnose under these circumstances, this complication should always be kept in mind when treating ventricular arrhythmias with procainamide. If the ventricular rate is significantly slowed by procainamide without attainment of regular atrioventricular conduction, the drug should be stopped and the patient reevaluated since asystole may result under these circumstances.
In patients receiving normal dosage, but who have both liver and kidney disease, symptoms of overdosage (principally, ventricular tachycardia and severe hypotension) may occur due to drug accumulation.
Serious hypotension can result from peripheral vasodilation and from decreases in cardiac output. At high plasma levels, procainamide may produce sinus tachycardia due to reflex sympathetic response to its hypotensive effect. Large doses may increase cardiac automaticity and can induce complete atrioventricular block, cardiac standstill, or ventricular extrasystoles that may proceed to ventricular fibrillation. These effects on the myocardium are reflected in the electrocardiogram: a widening of the QRS complex occurs most consistently; less regularly, the P-R and Q-T intervals are prolonged; and the QRS and T waves show some decrease in voltage.
Antinuclear antibodies (ANA) are often found in patients receiving long-term procainamide therapy. The induction of ANA appears to be independent of dosage. Patients with procainamide-induced increases in ANA titers may develop a syndrome resembling systemic lupus erythematosus (SLE). The mechanism of this syndrome is uncertain. Polyarthralgia, arthritic symptoms, and pleuritic pain are common symptoms; to a lesser extent fever, myalgia, skin lesions, pleural effusion, pericarditis, headache, fatigue, weakness, nausea and abdominal pain may occur. Rare cases of thrombocytopenia, Coombs positive hemolytic anemia, increased SGOT, SGPT, and serum amylase have been reported which may be related to this SLE-like syndrome.
It is recommended that tests for systemic lupus erythematosus be carried out at regular intervals in patients receiving maintenance procainamide therapy. The drug should be discontinued if there is a rising ANA titer or clinical symptoms of SLE appear. The SLE-like syndrome may be reversible upon discontinuation of the drug. If discontinuation does not cause remission of the symptoms, corticosteroid therapy may be effective. If the SLE-like syndrome develops in a patient with recurrent life-threatening arrhythmias not controllable by other antiarrhythmic agents, corticosteroid suppressive therapy may be used concomitantly with procainamide.
Information for Patient—Practitioners should give the following information and instructions to patients receiving Procan SR.

1. Do not crush or chew these tablets. Swallow them whole.
2. Take this medicine exactly as directed by your doctor. Do not miss any doses and do not take more medicine than ordered. Do not stop taking this medicine without first checking with your doctor.
3. If you miss a dose and remember within one hour or so, take it as soon as possible. Then go back to your regular dosing schedule. Do not take double doses. If you have any questions about this, check with your doctor.
4. Report to your doctor any flu-type symptoms, such as malaise and aches, as well as any soreness of the mouth,

throat or gums, unexplained fever, skin rash, unusual bleeding or bruising, symptoms that resemble arthritis, or symptoms of an upper respiratory tract infection.
5. Do not be concerned if you occasionally notice in your stool something that looks like a tablet. In Procan SR tablets, the drug is 'held' in a wax core that has been specially designed to slowly release the drug for your body to absorb. When this process is completed the empty, nonabsorbable wax core, which looks nearly unchanged, is eliminated from your body.
6. Keep container tightly closed and store in a cool, dry place.

Laboratory Tests—Patients receiving procainamide for extended periods of time, or in whom symptoms suggestive of a lupus-like reaction appear, should have antinuclear antibody titers measured at regular intervals.

Routine blood counts are advisable during maintenance procainamide therapy. See WARNINGS for additional information.

Plasma concentrations of procainamide and NAPA should be monitored in patients with renal disease, hepatic disease, cardiac failure, or low cardiac output states.

Drug Interactions

1. **Antiarrhythmics:** Concurrent use with procainamide may result in additive cardiac effects and/or additive toxic effects.
2. **Anticholinergics:** Procainamide enhances the anticholinergic effects. Extreme caution must be exercised with such a combination.
3. **Anticholinesterases:** Procainamide antagonizes the effect of anticholinesterases in myasthenia gravis, and paralysis returns.
4. **Antihypertensives:** Procainamide may potentiate the hypotensive effects of thiazide diuretics and other antihypertensive agents. Adjustment of dosage may be required.
5. **Cimetidine:** It has been reported that the histamine H_2-antagonist cimetidine reduces renal clearance of procainamide and NAPA, resulting in higher plasma concentrations for longer durations. Caution should be exercised when administering these drugs concurrently, especially in the elderly who have a reduced ability to clear all three. Dosage modification may be required.
6. **Neuromuscular Blocking Agents:** Procainamide potentiates the effects of skeletal muscle relaxants such as succinylcholine. It also may enhance or prolong the neuromuscular blocking activity of bacitracin, colistimethate, dihydrostreptomycin, gentamicin, gramicidin, kanamycin, neomycin, polymyxin B, streptomycin, and viomycin, producing respiratory depression.

Pregnancy—Pregnancy Category C. Animal reproduction studies have not been conducted with procainamide. It is also not known whether procainamide can cause fetal harm when administered to a pregnant woman or can affect reproduction capacity. Procainamide should be given to a pregnant woman only if clearly needed.

Nursing Mothers—It is not known whether this drug is excreted in human milk. Because many drugs are excreted in human milk, caution should be exercised when procainamide is administered to a nursing woman.

ADVERSE REACTIONS

Most frequent, especially with large oral doses:

1. Anorexia
2. Nausea
3. Vomiting
4. Diarrhea
5. Urticaria
6. Pruritus

Less frequent:

1. Reactions in patients on long-term procainamide therapy
   a. Antinuclear antibodies (ANA)
   b. Syndrome resembling systemic lupus erythematosus (SLE) (See PRECAUTIONS)
2. Hypersensitivity reactions
   a. Angioneurotic edema
   b. Maculopapular rash
   c. Fever
   d. Eosinophilia
   e. Hypergammaglobulinemia

Infrequent:

1. Granulocytopenia, sometimes resulting in death (See WARNINGS)
2. Convulsions
3. Psychosis with hallucinations
4. Confusion
5. Mental depression
6. Giddiness
7. Lightheadedness
8. Weakness
9. Bitter taste

Rare:

1. Hypotension
2. A case was reported with fever and chills plus nausea, vomiting, abdominal pain, acute hepatomegaly, and a rise in serum glutamic oxaloacetic transaminase following a single dose of the drug.

OVERDOSAGE

Signs and symptoms: Severe hypotension, ventricular fibrillation, widening of QRS complex, junctional tachycardia, intraventricular conduction delay, oliguria, lethargy, confusion, nausea, and vomiting.

Treatment: If ingestion is recent, emesis, activated charcoal, or gastric lavage may reduce absorption. Dopamine, phenylephrine, or levarterenol may be helpful in reversing severe hypotensive responses.

Management of overdosage includes symptomatic treatment with ECG and blood pressure monitoring. Procainamide toxicity can usually be treated, if necessary, by administering vasopressors after adequate fluid volume replacement. Intravenous infusion of $\frac{1}{6}$ molar sodium lactate injection reportedly reduces the cardiotoxic effects of procainamide.

If procainamide toxicity causes severe hypotension and renal insufficiency, urinary elimination of procainamide and NAPA is decreased, and hemodialysis may be required. Hemodialysis significantly reduces the serum half-life of procainamide, and effectively removes procainamide and NAPA. Peritoneal dialysis is not effective.

It has been reported that one patient who ingested approximately 7 grams of procainamide hydrochloride recovered after treatment consisting of IV levarterenol, IV furosemide, attempted volume expansion with albumin, and hemodialysis. Also reported is the case of an elderly patient who recovered after ingestion of approximately 19 grams of procainamide hydrochloride The patient was treated with IV isoproterenol and IV epinephrine. The latter report suggested that insertion of a ventriular pacing electrode is a reasonable precautionary measure in case high grade A-V block develops.

DOSAGE AND ADMINISTRATION

Procan SR tablets are a sustained-release product form. The duration of action of procainamide hydrochloride supplied in this sustained-release product form allows dosing at intervals of every six hours instead of the more frequent every-three-hour dosing intervals required for standard preparations of oral procainamide hydrochloride. The convenient six-hour dosing schedule may encourage patient compliance. For control of arrhythmias requiring immediate suppression, procainamide hydrochloride injection or other antiarrhythmic therapy is recommended. Following interruption of the arrhythmia, Procan SR may be used for maintenance therapy.

Plasma level determinations are strongly recommended when patients are changed from a standard dosage form to the SR preparation.

Patients should be advised not to break, crush or chew the tablet, as this would interfere with designed dissolution characteristics.

The dosage for each patient must be determined on an individual basis. Therefore, it is recommended that the patient be treated with standard procainamide hydrochloride until the total daily dosage required by that individual is determined.

Once the patient is titrated to the clinically effective dosage with the standard procainamide hydrochloride preparation, maintenance may be continued with Procan SR. The maintenance dosage of Procan SR is equal to the total daily dosage determined for the standard preparation, divided into 4 equal doses and administered at six-hour intervals.

If procainamide therapy is continued for appreciable periods, electrocardiograms should be made occasionally to determine the need for the drug.

Atrial Fibrillation and Paroxysmal Atrial Tachycardia

Suggested Titration Dosage: Initial dose of 1.25 g of standard oral procainamide HCl preparation, followed in one hour by 0.75 g if there have been no electrocardiographic changes, and then given at a dose of 0.5 to 1.0 g every two hours until arrhythmia is interrupted or the limit of tolerance is reached.

Suggested Maintenance Dosage of Procan SR: 50 mg/kg of body weight daily, given in divided doses at six-hour intervals starting 2 to 3 hours after the last dose of standard oral procainamide. Although the dosage for each patient must be determined on an individual basis, the table presented below may be used as a guide for providing the total daily dosage using Procan SR.

Ventricular Tachycardia and Premature Ventricular Contractions

Suggested Titration Dosage: Initial dose of 1 g of standard oral procainamide HCl preparation, followed by total daily dose of 50 mg/kg of body weight, given in divided doses at three-hour intervals, to be increased until arrhythmia is interrupted or the limit of tolerance is reached.

Suggested Maintenance Dosage of Procan SR: 50 mg/kg of body weight daily, given in divided doses at six-hour intervals starting 2 to 3 hours after the last dose of standard oral procainamide. Although the dosage for each patient must be determined on an individual basis, the table presented below may be used as a guide for providing the total daily dosage using Procan SR.

Patient's Weight	Approximate Total Daily Dosage	Dosage with Procan SR
Less than 121 lb (<55 kg)	2000 mg	One 500-mg tablet q6h
121 to 200 lb (55 to 91 kg)	3000 mg	One 750-mg tablet q6h
More than 200 lb (>91 kg)	4000 mg	One 1000-mg tablet q6h

HOW SUPPLIED

Procan SR 250 mg (elliptical, green, film-coated, coded PD 202) is a sustained-release tablet that contains 250 mg of procainamide hydrochloride. It is supplied-as follows:
N 0071-0202-24 Bottles of 100
N 0071-0202-30 Bottles of 500
N 0071-0202-40 Unit-dose packages of 100 (10 strips of 10 tablets each)

Procan SR 500 mg (elliptical, yellow, scored, film-coated coded PD 204) is a sustained-release tablet that contains 500 mg of procainamide hydrochloride. It is supplied as follows:
N 0071-0204-24 Bottles of 100
N 0071-0204-30 Bottles of 500
N 0071-0204-40 Unit-dose packages of 100 (10 strips of 10 tablets each)

Procan SR 750 mg (elliptical, orange, scored, film-coated, coded PD 205) is a sustained-release tablet that contains 750 mg of procainamide hydrochloride. It is supplied as follows:
N 0071-0205-24 Bottles of 100
N 0071-0205-30 Bottles of 500
N 0071-0205-40 Unit-dose packages of 100 (10 strips of 10 tablets each)

Procan SR 1000 mg (oblong, red, scored, film-coated, coded PD 207) is a sustained-release tablet that contains 1000 mg of procainamide hydrochloride. It is supplied as follows:
N 0071-0207-24 Bottles of 100
N 0071-0207-40 Unit-dose packages of 100 (10 strips of 10 tablets each)

Storage Conditions

Protect from moisture.
Store bottles below 30°C (86°F).
Store unit-dose packages at controlled room temperature, 15°–30°C (59°–86°F).

Caution:—Federal law prohibits dispensing without prescription.

0207G072

Shown in Product Identification Section, page 421

PROLOID® ℞

[prō'loid]
(Thyroglobulin Tablets, USP)

DESCRIPTION

Proloid is obtained from a purified extract of hog thyroid. It contains the known calorigenically active components, levothyroxine (T_4) and liothyronine (T_3).

Chromatographic analysis to standardize the levothyroxine and liothyronine content of Proloid is routinely employed. See instructions for use.

Proloid is stable when stored at room temperature.

ACTIONS

The actions of the thyroid hormone(s) involve the maturation and proper function of such organ systems as the endocrine, nervous, skeletal, reproductive, and gastrointestinal. The calorigenic and other actions of thyroid hormone(s) are instrumental in maintaining the normal functional capacity of tissues in organ systems throughout the body.

INDICATIONS

Proloid is thyroid replacement therapy for conditions of inadequate endogenous thyroid production, e.g., cretinism and myxedema. Replacement therapy will be effective only in manifestations of hypothyroidism.

In simple (nontoxic) goiter, Proloid may be tried therapeutically, in nonemergency situations, in an attempt to reduce the size of such goiters.

CONTRAINDICATION

Thyroid preparations are contraindicated in the presence of uncorrected adrenal insufficiency.

Continued on next page

This product information was prepared in August, 1986. On these and other Parke-Davis Products, information may be obtained by addressing PARKE-DAVIS, Division of Warner-Lambert Company, Morris Plains, New Jersey 07950.

Parke-Davis—Cont.

WARNINGS

> Drugs with thyroid hormone activity, alone or together with other therapeutic agents, have been used for the treatment of obesity. In euthyroid patients, doses within the range of daily hormonal requirements are ineffective for weight reduction. Larger doses may produce serious or even life-threatening manifestations of toxicity, particularly when given in association with sympathomimetic amines such as those used for their anorectic effects.

Thyroglobulin should not be used in the presence of cardiovascular disease unless thyroid-replacement therapy is clearly indicated. If the latter exists, low doses should be instituted beginning at 0.5 to 1.0 grain (approximately 32 to 65 mg) and increased by the same amount in increments at two-week intervals. This demands careful clinical judgment. Morphologic hypogonadism and nephroses should be ruled out before the drug is administered. If hypopituitarism is present, the adrenal deficiency must be corrected prior to starting the drug.
Myxedematous patients are very sensitive to thyroid and dosage should be started at a very low level and increased gradually.

PRECAUTION
As with all thyroid preparations this drug will alter results of thyroid function tests.

ADVERSE REACTIONS
Overdosage or too rapid increase in dosage may result in signs and symptoms of hyperthyroidism, such as menstrual irregularities, nervousness, cardiac arrhythmias, and angina pectoris.

DOSAGE AND ADMINISTRATION
Optimal dosage of Proloid is usually determined by the patient's clinical response. Confirmatory tests include BMR $T_3{}^{131}I$ resin sponge uptake, $T_3{}^{131}I$ red cell uptake, Thyro Binding Index (TBI), and Achilles Tendon Reflex Test. Clinical experience has shown that a normal PBI (3.5–8 mcg/100 ml) will be obtained in patients made clinically euthyroid when the content of T_4 and T_3 is adequate. Dosage should be started in small amounts and increased gradually with increments at intervals of one to two weeks. Usual maintenance dose is 0.5 to 3.0 grains (approximately 32 to 200 mg) daily.

Instructions for Use
The following conversion table lists the approximate equivalents of other thyroid preparations to Proloid when changing medication from desiccated thyroid. T_4 (levothyroxine sodium), T_3 (liothyronine sodium), or T_4/T_3 (liotrix).
[See table below].

OVERDOSAGE
Symptoms: Headache, instability, nervousness, sweating, tachycardia, with unusual bowel motility. Angina pectoris or congestive heart failure may be induced or aggravated. Shock may develop. Massive overdosage may result in symptoms resembling thyroid storm. Chronic excessive dosage will produce the signs and symptoms of hyperthyroidism. (Treatment: In shock, supportive measures should be utilized. Treatment of unrecognized adrenal insufficiency should be considered.)

HOW SUPPLIED
Proloid tablets are supplied:

N 0710-0251-24	½ grain (32 mg)	Bottles of 100
N 0710-0251-32	½ grain (32 mg)	Bottles of 1000
N 0710-0252-24	1 grain (65 mg) Scored	Bottles of 100
N 0710-0252-32	1 grain (65 mg) Scored	Bottles of 1000
N 0710-0253-24	1½ grain (100 mg)	Bottles of 100
N 0710-0253-32	1½ grain (100 mg)	Bottles of 1000
N 0710-0257-24	2 grain (130 mg) Scored	Bottles of 100
N 0710-0254-24	3 grain (200 mg)	Bottles of 100
N 0710-0254-32	3 grain (200 mg)	Bottles of 1000

Tablets are gray and uncoated
Store at controlled room temperature 15°–30°C (59°–86°F).
0250G011
Shown in Product Identification Section, page 421

PYRIDIUM® ℞
[py″rĭ′dĭ-ŭm]
(Phenazopyridine Hydrochloride Tablets, USP)

DESCRIPTION
Pyridium (phenazopyridine hydrochloride) is chemically designated 2,6-Pyridinediamine, 3-(phenylazo), monohydrochloride. It is a urinary tract analgesic agent for oral administration. Pyridium tablets contain 100 mg or 200 mg phenazopyridine hydrochloride. Also contains acacia, NF; calcium carbonate; carnauba wax, NF; corn starch, NF; D and C red No. 7; FD and C blue No. 2; FD and C yellow No. 6; gelatin, NF; kaolin, USP; lactose, NF; methylcellulose, USP; sodium starch glycolate, NF; stearic acid, NF; sucrose, NF; talc, USP; titanium dioxide, USP; tragacanth, NF; white wax. NF.

CLINICAL PHARMACOLOGY
Pyridium is excreted in the urine where it exerts a topical analgesic effect on the mucosa of the urinary tract. This action helps to relieve pain, burning, urgency and frequency. The precise mechanism of action is not known.
The pharmacokinetic properties of Pyridium have not been determined. Phenazopyridine is rapidly excreted by the kidneys, with as much as 65% of an oral dose being excreted unchanged in the urine.

INDICATIONS AND USAGE
Pyridium is indicated for the symptomatic relief of pain, burning, urgency, frequency, and other discomforts arising from irritation of the lower urinary tract mucosa caused by infection, trauma, surgery, endoscopic procedures, or the passage of sounds or catheters. The use of Pyridium for relief of symptoms should not delay definitive diagnosis and treatment of causative conditions. Because it provides only symptomatic relief, prompt appropriate treatment of the cause of pain must be instituted and Pyridium should be discontinued when symptoms are controlled.
The analgesic action may reduce or eliminate the need for systemic analgesics or narcotics. It is, however, compatible with antibacterial therapy and can help to relieve pain and discomfort during the interval before antibacterial therapy controls the infection. Treatment of a urinary tract infection with Pyridium should not exceed 2 days because there is a lack of evidence that the combined administration of Pyridium and an antibacterial provides greater benefit than administration of the antibacterial alone after 2 days. (See Dosage and Administration Section.)

CONTRAINDICATIONS
Pyridium should not be used in patients who have previously exhibited hypersensitivity to it. The use of Pyridium is contraindicated in patients with renal insufficiency.

PRECAUTIONS
General: A yellowish tinge of the skin or sclera may indicate accumulation due to impaired renal excretion and the need to discontinue therapy.
The decline in renal function associated with advanced age should be kept in mind.
Information for Patients: Pyridium produces an orange to red color in the urine and may stain fabric.
Laboratory Test Interactions: Due to its properties as an azo dye, Pyridium may interfere with urinalysis based on spectrometry or color reactions.
Carcinogenesis, Mutagenesis, Impairment of Fertility: Long-term administration of phenazopyridine hydrochloride has induced neoplasia in rats (large intestine) and mice (liver). Although no association between phenazopyridine hydrochloride and human neoplasia has been reported, adequate epidemiological studies along these lines have not been conducted.
Pregnancy Category B: Reproduction studies have been performed in rats at doses up to 50 mg/kg/day and have revealed no evidence of impaired fertility or harm to the fetus due to Pyridium. There are, however, no adequate and well controlled studies in pregnant women. Because animal reproduction studies are not always predictive of human response, this drug should be used during pregnancy only if clearly needed.
Nursing Mothers: No information is available on the appearance of Pyridium or its metabolites in human milk.

ADVERSE REACTIONS
Headache, rash and occasional gastrointestinal disturbance. Methemoglobinemia, hemolytic anemia, renal and hepatic toxicity have been described, usually at overdose levels (see Overdosage section). Staining of contact lenses has been reported.

OVERDOSAGE
Exceeding the recommended dose in patients with good renal function or administering the usual dose to patients with impaired renal function (common in elderly patients), may lead to increased serum levels and toxic reactions. Methemoglobinemia generally follows a massive, acute overdose. Methylene blue, 1 to 2 mg/kg body weight intravenously, or ascorbic acid 100 to 200 mg given orally should cause prompt reduction of the methemoglobinemia and disappearance of the cyanosis which is an aid in diagnosis. Oxidative Heinz body hemolytic anemia may also occur, and "bite cells" (degmacytes) may be present in a chronic overdosage situation. Red blood cell G-6-PD deficiency may predispose to hemolysis. Renal and hepatic impairment and occasional failure, usually due to hypersensitivity, may also occur.

DOSAGE AND ADMINISTRATION
100 mg tablets: Adult dosage is two tablets 3 times a day after meals. 200 mg tablets: Adult dosage is one tablet 3 times a day after meals.
When used concomitantly with an antibacterial agent for the treatment of a urinary tract infection, the administration of Pyridium should not exceed 2 days.

HOW SUPPLIED
N 0710-0180-24 100 mg tablets
Bottles of 100
N 0710-0180-32 100 mg tablets
Bottles of 1000
N 0710-0180-40 100 mg tablets Unit dose packages of 100 (10 strips of 10)
Tablets are dark maroon and coated.
N 0710-0181-24 200 mg tablets
Bottles of 100
N 0710-0181-32 200 mg tablets
Bottles of 1000
N 0710-0181-40 200 mg tablets Unit dose packages of 100 (10 strips of 10)
Tablets are dark maroon and coated.
Store at controlled room temperature 15° to 30° C (59° to 86° F).
Direct Medical Inquiries to Parke-Davis, Div Warner-Lambert Company, 201 Tabor Road, Morris Plains, NJ 07950, Attn: Medical Affairs Department
AHFS Category 84:08 **0180G012**
Shown in Product Identification Section, page 421

PYRIDIUM® PLUS Tablets ℞
[py″rĭ′dĭ-ŭm]

DESCRIPTION
Each Pyridium Plus tablet contains:
150 mg phenazopyridine hydrochloride (Pyridium®)
0.3 mg hyoscyamine hydrobromide
15 mg butabarbital
Also contains acacia, NF; calcium carbonate; carnauba wax, NF; corn starch, NF; D and C red No. 7; FD and C blue No. 2; FD and C yellow No. 6; gelatin, NF; guar gum, NF; kaolin, USP; lactose NF; magnesium stearate, NF; methylcellulose, USP; stearic acid, NF; sucrose, NF; talc, USP; titanium dioxide, USP; tragacanth, NF; white wax, NF.

CLINICAL PHARMACOLOGY
Pyridium Plus relieves lower urinary symptoms of pain, frequency, urgency, burning and dysuria arising from inflammation of the urothelium, the mucosal lining of the lower urinary tract.
Lower urinary tract pain can cause reflex spasm of the detrusor. Pain and spasm are often aggravated by apprehension to promote a pain-spasm-apprehension cycle. Each of the three pharmacologic components of Pyridium Plus acts against a phase of this cycle.
Phenazopyridine hydrochloride (Pyridium), excreted in the urine, is a topical analgesic to relieve pain and discomfort. Hyoscyamine hydrobromide, a parasympatholytic, acts to relieve detrusor muscle spasm. Butabarbital, a short-to-intermediate-acting sedative, helps to allay associated anxiety and apprehension.

INDICATIONS AND USAGE
Pyridium Plus is indicated for the symptomatic relief of pain, burning, frequency, urgency, and dysuria, particularly

Conversion Table

Dose of Proloid (thyroglobulin) grain	mg	Dose of Desiccated Thyroid grain	Dose of T_4 (levothyroxine) sodium) mg	Dose of T_3 (liothyronine sodium) mcg	Dose of liotrix (T_4/T_3)
1	(65)	1	0.1	25	#1(60 mcg/15 mcg)
2	(130)	2	0.2	50	#2(120 mcg/30 mcg)
3	(200)	3	0.3	75	#3(180 mcg/45 mcg)
4	(260)	4	0.4	100	
5	(325)	5	0.5	125	

In changing from Thyroid USP to Proloid, substitute the equivalent dose of Proloid. Each patient may still require fine adjustment of dosage because the equivalents are only estimates.

when accompanied by detrusor muscle spasm and apprehension.
These symptoms may arise from infection, trauma, surgery, endoscopic procedures, or passage of sounds or catheters.
Therapy with Pyridium Plus does not interfere with antibacterial therapy and can help to relieve symptoms of pain and discomfort before definitive treatment is effective. The use of Pyridium Plus for symptomatic relief should not delay definitive diagnosis and treatment. Treatment of a urinary tract infection with Pyridium Plus should not exceed 2 days because there is a lack of evidence that the combined administration of phenazopyridine hydrochloride and an antibacterial provides greater benefit than administration of the antibacterial alone after 2 days. (See Dosage and Administration Section.)
In the absence of infection, Pyridium Plus may be the only medication required.

CONTRAINDICATIONS

Pyridium Plus should not be used in patients who have previously exhibited hypersensitivity to any component. The use of Pyridium Plus is contraindicated in patients with renal or hepatic insufficiency, glaucoma, bladder neck obstruction, porphyria.

WARNING

BUTABARBITAL MAY BE HABIT-FORMING. Drowsiness or dizziness may occur. Patients should be instructed to use caution in driving or operating machinery.

PRECAUTIONS

General: A yellowish tinge of the skin or sclera may indicate accumulation due to impaired renal excretion of phenazopyridine (Pyridium) and the need to discontinue therapy.
The decline in renal function asssociated with advanced age should be kept in mind.
Information for Patients: Phenazopyridine hydrochloride produces an orange to red color in the urine and may stain fabric. Butabarbital may cause drowsiness or dizziness, patients should be instructed to use caution in driving or operating machinery.
Laboratory Test Interactions: Due to its properties as an azo dye, phenazopyridine hydrochloride may interfere with urinalysis based on spectrometry or color reactions.
Carcinogenesis, Mutagenesis, Impairment of Fertility: Pyridium Plus has not undergone adequate studies relating to carcinogenesis, mutagenesis, or impairment of fertility; however, the component phenazopyridine hydrochloride has induced neoplasia in rats (large intestine) and mice (liver). Although no association between phenazopyridine hydrochloride and human neoplasia has been reported, adequate epidemiological studies along these lines have not been conducted.
Pregnancy Category C: Animal reproduction studies have not been conducted with Pyridium Plus. It is also not known whether Pyridium Plus can cause fetal harm when administered to a pregnant woman or can affect reproduction capacity. Pyridium Plus should be given to a pregnant woman only if clearly needed.
Nursing Mothers: No information is available on the appearance of the components of Pyridium Plus in human milk.

ADVERSE REACTIONS

Methemoglobinemia, hemolytic anemia, and renal and hepatic toxicity have been described for phenazopyridine, usually at overdosage levels (see Overdosage Section). Staining of contact lenses has been reported.
Hyoscyamine hydrobromide is an atropinic drug that may produce adverse effects characteristic of this class of drugs. Dry mouth, drowsiness, or dizziness is noted in more than one third of patients (and may occur in half of the patients of older age groups). Other atropine-like effects, such as blurred vision, may occur. There may be occasional gastrointestinal disturbances.
Butabarbital is a short- to intermediate-acting barbiturate which has the potential for adverse reactions attributable to barbiturates.

OVERDOSAGE

Pyridium Plus is a combination of three active drugs, and overdosage can be expected to show the effects related to each ingredient. Management includes the usual measures to empty the stomach by emesis or lavage, administration of a charcoal slurry, and supportive measures as needed.
Toxicity and management suggestions relating to the individual ingredients are as follows:
Phenazopyridine Hydrochloride (Pyridium): Exceeding the recommended dose in patients with good renal function or administering the usual dose to patients with impaired renal function (common in elderly patients), may lead to increased serum levels and toxic reactions. Methemoglobinemia generally follows a massive, acute overdose. Methylene blue, 1 to 2 mg/kg body weight intravenously or ascorbic acid 100 to 200 mg given orally should cause prompt reduction of the methemoglobinemia and disappearance of cyanosis which is an aid in diagnosis. Oxidative Heinz body hemolytic anemia may also occur, and "bite cells" (degmacytes) may be present in a chronic overdosage situation. Red blood cell G-6-PD deficiency may predispose to hemolysis. Renal and hepatic impairment and occasional failure, usually due to hypersensitivity, may also occur.
Hyoscyamine Hydrobromide: Overdosage of hyoscyamine, a form of atropine, will cause dilated pupils, blurred vision, rapid pulse, increased intraocular tension, hot, dry, red skin, dry mouth, disorientation, delirium, fever, convulsions, and coma. As an antidote, physostigmine salicylate may be given IV slowly. Dilute 1 mg in 5 ml of saline and use 1 ml of this dilution in children. Repeat every five minutes as needed up to a total of 2 mg in children, or 6 mg in adults every 30 minutes.
Butabarbital: This drug may produce sedation and respiratory depression progressing to coma, depending on the amount ingested. General and supportive measures should be instituted.

DOSAGE AND ADMINISTRATION

Adult Dosage: One tablet four times a day (after meals and at bedtime).
When used concomitantly with an antibacterial agent for the treatment of a urinary tract infection, the administration of Pyridium Plus should not exceed 2 days.

HOW SUPPLIED

N 0710-0182-24 Bottles of 100. Tablets are dark maroon and square.
Store at controlled room temperature 15° to 30°C (59° to 86°F).
Direct Medical Inquiries to: Parke-Davis, Div Warner-Lambert Inc, c/o Warner-Lambert Company, 201 Tabor Road, Morris Plains, NJ 07950. Attn: Medical Affairs Department
AHFS Category 8:12.24 **0182G063**
Shown in Product Identification Section, page 421

SINUBID® ℞

[*sīn ′ū-bĭd ″*]

DESCRIPTION

Each Sinubid tablet contains:
600 mg acetaminophen
100 mg phenylpropanolamine hydrochloride
66 mg phenyltoloxamine citrate
Also contains calcium sulfate, NF; carnauba wax; confectioners sugar, NF; D and C red No. 30 lake; ethylcellulose, NF, 45 cps; FD and C blue No. 2 lake; FD and C yellow No. 6 lake; hydrogenated vegetable oil; hydroxypropyl methylcellulose, USP, 2910; lactose, USP; locust bean gum; magnesium stearate NF; stearic acid, NF; syloid 244 silica gel; talc, USP; titanium dioxide, USP.

CLINICAL PHARMACOLOGY

Sinubid is designed to provide symptomatic relief of coryza and nasal congestion when given twice a day (every 12 hours). Sinubid can provide symptomatic relief of headache, fever, and other symptoms associated with mucosal congestion (nasopharyngeal), general malaise, and irritability associated with the common cold, allergic and vasomotor disorders, sinusitis, and rhinitis.
Sinubid contains an analgesic-antipyretic (acetaminophen) to relieve the pain of sinus headache and nasal congestion. This analgesic-antipyretic is rapidly absorbed and as effective as aspirin in raising the pain threshold, but has the advantage of causing little or no gastric irritation. Sinubid, because it contains no salicylates, can be used by patients who are allergic to aspirin.
Decongestion of the nasopharyngeal mucosa is provided by phenylpropanolamine hydrochloride, a sympathomimetic amine which provides symptomatic relief. Because its vasoconstrictor activity is similar to that of ephedrine, but less likely to cause CNS stimulation, Sinubid may eliminate the need for topical decongestants.
Phenyltoloxamine citrate is a mild antihistamine which may provide symptomatic relief of seasonal and perennial allergic rhinitis, vasomotor rhinitis, nasal and sinus symptoms of sinusitis, and adjunctive therapy for bacterial sinusitis in uncomplicated upper respiratory infections.

INDICATIONS AND USAGE

Sinubid is indicated for the rapid, prolonged, symptomatic relief of nasal congestion in sinus or other frontal headache; allergic and vasomotor manifestations of upper respiratory disorders such as sinusitis, allergic rhinitis, vasomotor rhinitis, coryza; facial pain and "pressure" of acute and chronic sinusitis; and for the relief of accompanying fever. Sinubid is indicated only for intermittent treatment of the above noted acute symptoms.

CONTRAINDICATIONS

This compound should not be used in patients whose oversensitivity to small doses of sympathomimetic amines produces sleeplessness, dizziness, lightheadedness, weakness, tremulousness, or cardiac arrhythmias. The drug is contraindicated in any patient hypersensitive to any of the ingredients of the formulation.

WARNINGS

Instruct patients not to drive or operate machinery if drowsiness occurs. Individuals should not ingest alcoholic beverages, monoamine oxidase inhibitors, or barbiturates while taking this medication.

PRECAUTIONS

General: Individuals with high blood pressure, heart disease, diabetes mellitus, chronic renal disease, or thyroid disease should use only as directed by a physician.
Drug Interactions: See Warnings
Pregnancy: Pregnancy Category C. Animal reproduction studies have not been conducted with Sinubid. It is also not known whether Sinubid can cause fetal harm when administered to a pregnant woman or can affect reproduction capacity. Sinubid should be given to a pregnant woman only if clearly needed.
Nursing mothers: This drug should not be used in nursing mothers.

ADVERSE REACTIONS

The following adverse reactions have been reported for each of the individual or combinations of ingredients: Acetaminophen—urticaria, epigastric distress, dizziness, and palpitation. Phenylpropanolamine HCl—anxiety, restlessness, tension, insomnia, tremor, weakness, headache, vertigo, sweating, arrhythmia, nausea, and vomiting. Phenyltoloxamine Citrate—urticaria, drowsiness, disturbed coordination, inability to concentrate, dizziness, insomnia, tremors, nervousness, palpitation, convulsions, muscular weakness, gastric distress, diarrhea, intestinal cramps, blurred vision, hypotension, urinary retention, dryness of mouth, throat and nose.

DOSAGE AND ADMINISTRATION

Adults: One tablet twice daily (every 12 hours).
Children (6-12 years of age): One-half tablet twice daily (every 12 hours).
Tablets should not be chewed.

HOW SUPPLIED

Sinubid (P-D 177) is an ellipsoid, bi-layered (light pink/pink), scored tablet, supplied in bottles of 100 (N 0071-0177-24).
Store between 15°-30°C (59°-86°F).
0177G021
Shown in Product Identification Section, page 421

SPIRONOLACTONE ℞

[*spĭ-rō ″nō-lăc ′tōne*]
Tablets, USP

> **Warning**
> Spironolactone has been shown to be a tumorigen in chronic toxicity studies in rats. This drug should be used only in those conditions described under INDICATIONS. Unnecessary use of this drug should be avoided.

DESCRIPTION

Spironolactone is a potassium-sparing, diuretic-antihypertensive agent, available in 25 mg strength tablets for oral administration. Tablets also contain calcium stearate, NF; calcium sulfate, NF; microcrystalline cellulose, NF; peppermint oil, NF (or peppermint oil redistilled); polysorbate 80, NF; povidone, USP; pregelatinized starch, NF.
Spironolactone is a synthetic steroidal aldosterone antagonist, occurring as a light cream-colored to light tan, crystalline powder which is practically insoluble in water and soluble in alcohol. Its chemical name is 17-hydroxy-7α-mercapto-3-oxo-17α-pregn-4-ene-21-carboxylic acid γ-lactone acetate; its empirical formula is $C_{24}H_{32}O_4S$.

CLINICAL PHARMACOLOGY

Spironolactone specifically inhibits the physiologic effects of the adrenocortical hormone aldosterone through competitive binding of receptors at the aldosterone-dependent sodium potassium exchange site in the distal convoluted renal tubule, thereby producing increased excretion of sodium, chloride, and water while potassium is retained.
Spironolactone is rapidly and extensively metabolized, primarily to the pharmacologically active derivative canrenone. Peak plasma levels of canrenone occur two to four hours after administration of a single oral dose of spironolactone. After multiple doses, the half-life of canrenone is between 13 and 24 hours. Both spironolactone and canrenone are more than 90% bound to plasma proteins. Spironolac-

Continued on next page

This product information was prepared in August, 1986. On these and other Parke-Davis Products, information may be obtained by addressing PARKE-DAVIS, Division of Warner-Lambert Company, Morris Plains, New Jersey 07950.

Parke-Davis—Cont.

tone metabolites are excreted primarily in urine, but also in bile. After withdrawal of spironolactone, diuresis persists for two to three days.

Spironolactone has diuretic activity only in the presence of aldosterone, with the most pronounced effect in patients with aldosteronism. Through its action in antagonizing the effect of aldosterone, it inhibits the exchange of sodium for potassium in the distal renal tubule and helps to prevent potassium loss.

Spironolactone is also effective in significantly lowering the systolic and diastolic blood pressure in many patients with essential hypertension, even when aldosterone secretion is within normal limits.

INDICATIONS AND USAGE

Spironolactone is indicated in the management of:

1. **Primary hyperaldosteronism** for:
   a. Establishing the diagnosis of primary hyperaldosteronism by therapeutic trial.
   b. Short-term preoperative treatment for patients with primary hyperaldosteronism.
   c. Long-term maintenance therapy for patients with discrete aldosterone-producing adrenal adenomas who are judged to be poor operative risks, or who decline surgery.
   d. Long-term maintenance therapy for patients with bilateral micro- or macro-nodular adrenal hyperplasia (idiopathic hyperaldosteronism).
2. **Edematous conditions** for patients with:
   a. **Congestive heart failure:** For the management of edema and sodium retention when the patient is only partially responsive to, or is intolerant of, other therapeutic measures. Spironolactone is also indicated for patients with congestive heart failure taking digitalis, when other therapies are considered inappropriate.
   b. **Cirrhosis of the liver accompanied by edema and/or ascites:** Aldosterone levels may be exceptionally high in this condition. Spironolactone is indicated for maintenance therapy together with bed rest and restriction of fluid and sodium.
   c. **The nephrotic syndrome:** For nephrotic patients when treatment of the underlying disease, restriction of fluid and sodium intake, and the use of other diuretics do not provide an adequate response.
3. **Essential hypertension:** Usually in combination with other drugs, spironolactone is indicated for patients who cannot be treated adequately with other agents or for whom other agents are considered inappropriate.
4. **Hypokalemia:** For the treatment of patients with hypokalemia when other measures are considered inappropriate or inadequate. Spironolactone is also indicated for the prophylaxis of hypokalemia in patients taking digitalis when other measures are considered inadequate or inappropriate.

Usage in Pregnancy: The routine use of diuretics in an otherwise healthy woman is inappropriate and exposes mother and fetus to unnecessary hazard. Diuretics do not prevent development of toxemia of pregnancy, and there is no satisfactory evidence that they are useful in the treatment of developed toxemia.

Edema during pregnancy may arise from pathological causes or from the physiological and mechanical consequences of pregnancy. Spironolactone is indicated in pregnancy when edema is due to pathological causes just as it is in the absence of pregnancy (however, see PRECAUTIONS below). Dependent edema in pregnancy, resulting from restriction of venous return by the expanded uterus, is properly treated through elevation of the lower extremities and use of support hose; use of diuretics to lower intravascular volume in this case is unsupported and unnecessary. There is hypervolemia during normal pregnancy which is harmful to neither the fetus nor the mother (in the absence of cardiovascular disease), but which is associated with edema, including generalized edema, in the majority of pregnant women. If this edema produces discomfort, increased recumbency will often provide relief. In rare instances, this edema may cause extreme discomfort that is not relieved by rest. In these cases, a short course of diuretics may provide relief and may be appropriate.

CONTRAINDICATIONS

Anuria, acute renal insufficiency, significant impairment of renal function, hyperkalemia.

WARNINGS

Excessive potassium intake may cause hyperkalemia in patients receiving spironolactone (see PRECAUTIONS). Potassium supplementation, either in the form of medication or as a diet rich in potassium, should not ordinarily be given in association with spironolactone.

Spironolactone should not be administered concurrently with other potassium-sparing diuretics.

Spironolactone has been shown to be a tumorigen in chronic toxicity studies performed in rats, with its proliferative effects being manifested on endocrine organs and the liver.

PRECAUTIONS

General: Periodic determinations of serum electrolytes should be performed at appropriate intervals for the purpose of detecting possible fluid and electrolyte imbalance. Serum and urine electrolyte determinations are particularly important when a patient is vomiting excessively or receiving parenteral fluids.

Hyperkalemia may occur in patients with impaired renal function or excessive potassium intake and can cause cardiac irregularities that may be fatal. Consequently, no potassium supplement should ordinarily be given with spironolactone. Hyperkalemia can be treated promptly by the rapid intravenous administration of glucose (20% to 50%) and regular insulin, using 0.25 to 0.5 units of insulin per gram of glucose. This is a temporary measure to be repeated as required. Spironolactone should be discontinued and potassium intake (including dietary potassium) restricted.

Reversible hyperchloremic metabolic acidosis, usually in association with hyperkalemia,, has been reported to occur in some patients with decompensated hepatic cirrhosis, even in the presence of normal renal function.

Spironolactone may cause a transient elevation of BUN. This appears to represent a concentration phenomenon rather than renal toxicity since the BUN returns to normal after the drug is discontinued. Progressive elevation of BUN is suggestive of the presence of preexisting renal impairment. Spironolactone may cause mild acidosis.

Hyponatremia, manifested by dryness of the mouth, thirst, lethargy and drowsiness and confirmed by a low serum level, may be induced or aggravated, especially when spironolactone is administered in combination with other diuretics.

Gynecomastia may develop in association with the use of spironolactone, and physicians should be alert to its possible onset. The development of gynecomastia appears to be related to both dosage levels and duration of therapy and is normally reversible when spironolactone therapy is discontinued. In rare instances some breast enlargement may persist.

DRUG INTERACTIONS

Excessive potassium intake or concurrent administration of other potassium-sparing diuretics may cause hyperkalemia in patients receiving spironolactone.

Spironolactone reduces vascular responsiveness to norepinephrine. Therefore, caution should be used in the management of patients subjected to regional or general anesthesia while they are being treated with spironolactone.

When used in combination with other diuretics or antihypertensive agents, spironolactone potentiates their effects. Therefore, the dosage of such drugs, particularly the ganglionic blocking agents, should be reduced by at least fifty percent when spironolactone is added to the regimen.

Usage in Pregnancy: Spironolactone or its metabolites may cross the placental barrier. Therefore, the use of this drug in pregnant women requires that the anticipated benefit be weighed against possible hazards to the fetus. These hazards include fetal or neonatal jaundice, thrombocytopenia, and other possible adverse reactions that have been reported in the adult. Also see INDICATIONS AND USAGE above.

Nursing Mothers: Canrenone, a metabolite of spironolactone, appears in breast milk. If use of spironolactone is deemed essential, an alternative method of infant feeding should be instituted.

ADVERSE REACTIONS

Adverse reactions are usually reversible upon discontinuation of spironolactone.

A. **Gastrointestinal System**
   1. cramping
   2. diarrhea

B. **Central Nervous System**
   1. drowsiness
   2. lethargy
   3. headache
   4. mental confusion
   5. ataxia

C. **Endocrine System**
   1. gynecomastia
   2. inability to achieve or maintain erection
   3. irregular menses or amenorrhea
   4. postmenopausal bleeding
   5. hirsutism
   6. deepening of the voice
   7. hypochloremic acidosis in cirrhosis

D. **Other**
   1. maculopapular or erythematous cutaneous eruptions
   2. urticaria
   3. drug fever
   4. carcinoma of the breast has been reported in patients taking spironolactone, but a cause-and-effect relationship has not been established.

DOSAGE AND ADMINISTRATION

Spironolactone is administered orally. Therapy should be individualized according to the patient's requirements and response. The response of the patient depends on factors such as the nature and degree of the disease, state of hydration, cardiac output, physical activity, diet, and concurrent administration of other drugs.

Primary hyperaldosteronism. Spironolactone may be employed as an initial diagnostic measure to provide presumptive evidence of primary hyperaldosteronism while patients are on normal diets.

Long test: Administer a daily dosage of 400 mg for three to four weeks. Correction of hypokalemia and hypertension provides presumptive evidence for the diagnosis of primary hyperaldosteronism.

Short test: Administer a daily dosage of 400 mg for four days. If serum potassium increases during spironolactone administration but drops when spironolactone is discontinued, a presumptive diagnosis of primary hyperaldosteronism should be considered.

After establishing the diagnosis of hyperaldosteronism by more definitive testing procedures, administer spironolactone in doses of 100 to 400 mg daily in preparation for surgery. For patients who are considered unsuitable for surgery, spironolactone may be employed for long-term maintenance therapy at the lowest effective dosage determined for the individual patient.

Edema in adults (congestive heart failure, hepatic cirrhosis or nephrotic syndrome). An initial daily dosage of 100 mg spironolactone administered in either single or divided doses is recommended, but may range from one to eight tablets (25 to 200 mg) daily. When given as the sole agent for diuresis, spironolactone should be continued for at least five days at the initial dosage level, after which it may be adjusted to the optimal therapeutic or maintenance level administered in either single or divided daily doses. If after five days an adequate diuretic response to spironolactone has not occurred, a second diuretic that acts more proximally in the renal tubule may be added to the regimen. Because of the additive effect of spironolactone when administered concurrently with such diuretics, an enhanced diuresis usually begins on the first day of combined treatment; combined therapy is indicated when more rapid diuresis is desired. The dosage of spironolactone should remain unchanged when other diuretic therapy is added.

Edema in children: The initial daily dosage should provide approximately 1.5 mg of spironolactone per pound of body weight (3.3 mg/kg) administered in either single or divided doses. For small children, spironolactone tablets may be pulverized and administered as a suspension in Cherry Syrup, NF. When refrigerated, such a suspension is stable for one month.

Essential hypertension: For adults, an initial daily dosage of 50 to 100 mg of spironolactone administered in either single or divided doses is recommended. Spironolactone may also be given with diuretics that act more proximally in the renal tubule or with other antihypertensive agents. Treatment with spironolactone should be continued for at least two weeks, since the maximum response may not occur before this time. Subsequently, dosage should be adjusted according to the response of the patient.

Hypokalemia: Spironolactone in a dosage ranging from 25 to 100 mg daily is useful in treating a diuretic-induced hypokalemia, when oral potassium supplements or other potassium-sparing regimens are considered inappropriate.

HOW SUPPLIED

Spironolactone Tablets, USP, 25 mg (round, white, scored tablets coded P-D 713) are supplied as follows:

N 0071-0713-24 Bottles of 100
N 0071-0713-32 Bottles of 1000
N 0071-0713-40 Unit-dose packages of 100 individually sealed tablets

Store at room temperature below 30°C (86°F).
Protect from moisture and light.
Caution—Federal law prohibits dispensing without prescription.

0713G011

SPIRONOLACTONE WITH HYDROCHLOROTHIAZIDE ℞

[*spī-rō"nō-lăc'tōne with hy"drō-chlō"rō-thī'ă-zīde*]
Tablets

WARNING

Spironolactone has been shown to be a tumorigen in chronic toxicity studies in rats (see WARNINGS). Spironolactone with Hydrochlorothiazide Tablets should be used only in those conditions described under INDICATIONS. Unnecessary use of this drug should be avoided.

Fixed-dose combination drugs are not indicated for initial therapy of edema or hypertension. Edema or hypertension requires therapy titrated to the individual patient. If the fixed combination represents the dosage so determined, its use may be more convenient in patient management. The treatment of hypertension and edema is not static, but must be reevaluated as conditions in each patient warrant.

DESCRIPTION

Spironolactone with Hydrochlorothiazide is a combination of two diuretic agents with different but complementary mechanisms and sites of action, thereby providing additive diuretic and antihypertensive effects. In addition, spironolactone helps to decrease the potassium excretion characteristically induced by hydrochlorothiazide.
Spironolactone with Hydrochlorothiazide is available as tablets for oral administration, with each tablet containing:
Spironolactone ....25 mg
Hydrochlorothiazide ....25 mg
Also contains calcium stearate, NF; calcium sulfate, NF; microcrystalline cellulose, NF; peppermint oil, NF (or peppermint oil redistilled); polysorbate 80, NF; povidone, USP; pregelatinized starch, NF.
Spironolactone is a synthetic steroid aldosterone antagonist, occurring as a light cream-colored to light tan, crystalline powder that is practically insoluble in water and soluble in alcohol. Its chemical name is 17-hydroxy-7α-mercapto-3-oxo-17α-pregn-4-ene-21-carboxylic acid γ-lactone acetate; its empirical formula is $C_{24}H_{32}O_4S$.
Hydrochlorothiazide is a member of the benzothiadiazine (thiazide) family of drugs, closely related to chlorothiazide. It occurs as a white, or practically white, crystalline compound that is slightly soluble in water and soluble in alcohol. Its chemical name is 6-chloro-3,4-dihydro-2*H*-1,2,4-benzothiadiazine-7-sulfonamide 1,1-dioxide; its empirical formula is $C_7H_8ClN_3O_4S_2$.

CLINICAL PHARMACOLOGY

Spironolactone inhibits the physiologic effects of the adrenocortical hormone aldosterone through competitive binding of receptors at the aldosterone-dependent sodium-potassium exchange site in the distal convoluted renal tubule, thereby producing increased excretion of sodium, chloride, and water while potassium is retained. Spironolactone has diurectic activity only in the presence of aldosterone, with the most pronounced effect in patients with aldosteronism.
Spironolactone is rapidly and extensively metabolized, primarily to the pharmacologically active derivative canrenone. Peak plasma levels of canrenone occur two to four hours after administration of a single oral dose of spironolactone. After multiple doses, the half-life of canrenone is between 13 and 24 hours. Both spironolactone and canrenone are more than 90% bound to plasma proteins. Spironolactone metabolites are excreted primarily in urine, but also in bile. After withdrawal of spironolactone, diuresis persists for two to three days.
The diuretic and saluretic effects of hydrochlorothiazide result from a drug-induced inhibition of the renal tubular reabsorption of electrolytes. The excretion is enhanced to a variable degree.
Hydrochlorothiazide is readily absorbed from the gastrointestinal tract. There is significant natriuresis and diuresis within two hours after administration of a single oral dose. These effects reach a peak in about six hours and persist for about twelve hours. Hydrochlorothiazide is excreted unchanged by the kidneys, and excretion is essentially complete within 24 hours.
Spironolactone with Hydrochlorothiazide is effective in significantly lowering the systolic and diastolic blood pressure in many patients with essential hypertension, even when aldosterone secretion is within normal limits.
Both spironolactone and hydrochlorothiazide reduce exchangeable sodium, plasma volume, body weight, and blood pressure. The diuretic and antihypertensive effects of the individual components are potentiated when spironolactone and hydrochlorothiazide are given concurrently.

INDICATIONS AND USAGE

Spironolactone has been shown to be a tumorigen in chronic toxicity studies in rats. Spironolactone with Hydrochlorothiazide Tablets should be used only in those conditions described below. Unnecessary use of this drug should be avoided.

Edematous conditions associated with:

Congestive heart failure: Management of edema and sodium retention when the patient is only partially responsive to or is intolerant of other therapeutic measures. Treatment of diuretic-induced hypokalemia in patients with congestive heart failure when other measures are considered inappropriate. For patients with congestive heart failure who are taking digitalis, when other therapies are considered inadequate or inappropriate.

Cirrhosis of the liver accompanied by edema and /or ascites: Maintenance therapy together with bed rest and restriction of fluid and sodium. Aldosterone levels may be exceptionally high in this condition.

The nephrotic syndrome: For nephrotic patients when treatment of the underlying disease, restriction of fluid and sodium intake, and the use of other diuretics do not provide an adequate response.

Essential hypertension

For patients with essential hypertension in whom other measures are considered inadequate or inappropriate.
For hypertensive patients for the treatment of a diuretic-induced hypokalemia when other measures are considered inappropriate.

Usage in Pregnancy: The routine use of diuretics in an otherwise healthy pregnant woman is inappropriate and exposes mother and fetus to unnecessary hazard. Diuretics do not prevent development of toxemia of pregnancy, and there is no satisfactory evidence that they are useful in the treatment of developed toxemia.
Edema during pregnancy may arise from pathological causes or from physiological and mechanical consequences of pregnancy. This drug is indicated in pregnancy when edema is due to pathological causes, just as it is in the absence of pregnancy (however, see PRECAUTIONS below). Dependent edema in pregnancy, resulting from restriction of venous return by the expanded uterus, is properly treated through elevation of the lower extremities and use of support hose; use of diuretics to lower intravascular volume in this case is illogical and unnecessary. There is hypervolemia during normal pregnancy which is harmful to neither the fetus nor the mother (in the absence of cardiovascular disease), but which is associated with edema, including generalized edema, in the majority of pregnant women. If this edema produces discomfort, increased recumbency will often provide relief. In rare instances, this edema may cause extreme discomfort that is not relieved by rest. In these cases, a short course of diuretics may provide relief and may be appropriate.

CONTRAINDICATIONS

Anuria, acute renal insufficiency, significant impairment of renal function, hyperkalemia, allergy to thiazide diuretics or to other sulfonamide-derived drugs. This drug may also be contraindicated in acute or severe hepatic failure.

WARNINGS

Excessive potassium intake may cause hyperkalemia in patients receiving Spironolactone with Hydrochlorothiazide Tablets (see PRECAUTIONS). Potassium supplementation, either in the form of medication or as a diet rich in potassium, should not ordinarily be given in association with this drug. Spironolactone with Hydrochlorothiazide should not be administered concurrently with other potassium-sparing diuretics.
The possibility of exacerbation or activation of systemic lupus erythematosus has been reported with sulfonamide derivatives, including thiazides.
Spironolactone has been shown to be a tumorigen in chronic toxicity studies performed in rats, with its proliferative effects manifested on endocrine organs and the liver.

PRECAUTIONS

General: Periodic determinations of serum electrolytes should be performed at appropriate intervals for the purpose of detecting possible fluid and electrolyte imbalance. Patients receiving Spironolactone with Hydrochlorothiazide Tablets should be observed for clinical signs of fluid or electrolyte imbalance, namely hyponatremia, hypochloremic alkalosis, hypokalemia and hyperkalemia. Serum and urine electrolyte determinations are particularly important when a patient is vomiting excessively or receiving parenteral fluids. Warning signs of fluid and electrolyte imbalance include dryness of mouth, thirst, weakness, lethargy, drowsiness, restlessness, muscle pains or cramps, muscular fatigue, hypotension, oliguria, tachycardia, and gastrointestinal disturbances such as nausea and vomiting.
Hyperkalemia may occur in patients with impaired renal function or excessive potassium intake and can cause cardiac irregularities that may be fatal. Consequently, no potassium supplement should ordinarily be given with this drug. Hyperkalemia can be treated promptly by the rapid intravenous administration of glucose (20% to 50%) and regular insulin, using 0.25 to 0.5 units of insulin per gram of glucose. This is a temporary measure to be repeated as required. Spironolactone with Hydrochlorothiazide should be discontinued and potassium intake (including dietary potassium) restricted.
Reversible hyperchloremic metabolic acidosis, usually in association with hyperkalemia, has been reported to occur in some patients with decompensated hepatic cirrhosis, even in the presence of normal renal function.
Spironolactone with Hydrochlorothiazide may cause a transient elevation of BUN. This appears to represent a concentration phenomenon rather than renal toxicity since the BUN returns to normal after the drug is discontinued. Progressive elevation of BUN is suggestive of the presence of preexisting renal impairment.
Dilutional hyponatremia, manifested by dryness of the mouth, thirst, lethargy and drowsiness and confirmed by a low serum sodium level, may be induced, especially when Spironolactone with Hydrochlorothiazide is administered in combination with other diuretics. A true low-salt syndrome may rarely develop with Spironolactone with Hydrochlorothiazide therapy and may be manifested by increasing mental confusion similar to that observed with hepatic coma. This syndrome is differentiated from dilutional hyponatremia in that it does not occur with obvious fluid retention. Its treatment requires that diuretic therapy be discontinued and sodium administered.
Gynecomastia may develop in association with the use of spironolactone, and physicians should be alert to its possible onset. The development of gynecomastia appears to be related to both dosage level and duration of therapy and is normally reversible when Spironolactone with Hydrochlorothiazide is discontinued. In rare instances some breast enlargement may persist.
Thiazides have been shown to alter the metabolism of uric acid and carbohydrates, with possible development of hyperuricemia, gout, and decreased glucose tolerance. Thiazides may temporarily exaggerate abnormalities of glucose metabolism in diabetic patients or cause latent diabetes mellitus to become manifest.
The antihypertensive effects of hydrochlorothiazide may be enhanced in patients who have undergone sympathectomy.
Pathologic changes in the parathyroid gland with hypercalcemia and hypophosphatemia have been observed in patients on prolonged thiazide therapy. Thiazides may decrease serum PBI levels without evidence of thyroid disturbance.

DRUG INTERACTIONS

Excessive potassium intake or concurrent administration of other potassium-sparing diuretics may cause hyperkalemia in patients receiving Spironolactone with Hydrochlorothiazide Tablets.
Hypokalemia may develop as a result of brisk diuresis, particularly when loop diuretics, glucocorticoids, or ACTH are given concomitantly with Spironolactone with Hydrochlorothiazide. Hypokalemia may exaggerate the effects of digitalis therapy. Potassium depletion may induce signs of digitalis intoxication at previously tolerated levels.
Both spironolactone and hydrochlorothiazide reduce vascular responsiveness to norepinephrine. Therefore, caution should be used in the management of patients subjected to regional or general anesthesia while they are being treated with Spironolactone with Hydrochlorothiazide.
Thiazides may increase the responsiveness to tubocurarine.

Usage in Pregnancy: Spironolactone or its metabolites may, and hydrochlorothiazide does, cross the placental barrier. Therefore, the use of this combination drug in pregnant women requires that the anticipated benefit be weighed against possible hazards to the fetus. These hazards include fetal or neonatal jaundice, thrombocytopenia and other possible adverse reactions that have been reported in the adult. Also see INDICATIONS AND USAGE above.

Nursing Mothers: Canrenone, a metabolite of spironolactone, and hydrochlorothiazide appear in breast milk. If use of Spironolactone with Hydrochlorothiazide is deemed essential, an alternative method of infant feeding should be instituted.

ADVERSE REACTIONS

Adverse reactions are usually reversible upon discontinuation of Spironolactone with Hydrochlorothiazide.
The following adverse reactions have been reported in association with the use of spironolactone:

A. Gastrointestinal System
1. cramping
2. diarrhea

B. Central Nervous System
1. drowsiness
2. lethargy
3. headache
4. mental confusion
5. ataxia

C. Endocrine System
1. gynecomastia
2. inability to achieve or maintain erection
3. irregular menses or amenorrhea
4. postmenopausal bleeding
5. hirsutism
6. deepening of the voice
7. hypochloremic acidosis in cirrhosis

D. Other
1. maculopapular or erythematous cutaneous eruptions
2. urticaria
3. drug fever
4. Carcinoma of the breast has been reported in patients taking spironolactone, but a cause-and-effect relationship has not been established.

Continued on next page

This product information was prepared in August, 1986. On these and other Parke-Davis Products, information may be obtained by addressing PARKE-DAVIS, Division of Warner-Lambert Company, Morris Plains, New Jersey 07950.

Parke-Davis—Cont.

The following adverse reactions have been reported in association with the use of hydrochlorothiazide:

A. Gastrointestinal System
1. anorexia
2. gastric irritation
3. nausea
4. vomiting
5. cramping
6. diarrhea
7. constipation
8. jaundice (intrahepatic cholestatic jaundice)
9. pancreatitis

B. Central Nervous System
1. dizziness
2. vertigo
3. paresthesias
4. headache
5 xanthopsia

C. Hematologic
1. leukopenia
2. agranulocytosis
3. thrombocytopenia
4. aplastic anemia

D. Dermatologic-Hypersensitivity
1. purpura
2. photosensitivity
3. rash
4. urticaria
5. necrotizing angiitis (vasculitis, cutaneous vasculitis)

E. Cardiovascular
Orthostatic hypotension may occur and may be aggravated by alcohol, barbiturates, or narcotics.

F. Other
1. hyperglycemia
2. glycosuria
3. hyperuricemia
4. muscle spasm
5. weakness
6. restlessness
7. hypercalcemia
8. severe fluid and electrolyte derangements (rare)

DOSAGE AND ADMINISTRATION

Spironolactone with Hydrochlorothiazide is administered orally. Therapy should be individualized according to the patient's requirements and response. The response of the patient depends on factors such as the nature and degree of the disease, state of hydration, cardiac output, physical activity, diet, and concurrent administration of other drugs. Optimal dosage should be established by individual titration of the components (see Box Warning).

Edema in adults (congestive heart failure, hepatic cirrhosis or nephrotic syndrome). The usual maintenance dose is four tablets daily, administered in either single or divided doses, but it may range from one to eight tablets daily, depending on the response to the initial titration. In some instances it may be desirable to administer, in addition to Spironolactone with Hydrochlorothiazide Tablets, separate tablets of either spironolactone or hydrochlorothiazide in order to provide optimal individual therapy.

The onset of diuresis occurs promptly and, due to prolonged effect of the spironolactone component, persists for two to three days after discontinuance of the drug.

Edema in children. The usual daily maintenance dose should be that which provides 0.75 to 1.5 mg of spironolactone per pound of body weight (1.65 to 3.3 mg/kg), administered in either single or divided doses.

Essential hypertension. Although the dosage will vary depending on the results of titration of the individual ingredients, many patients will be found to have an optimal response to the amount of hydrochlorothiazide and spironolactone contained in two to four tablets of Spironolactone with Hydrochlorothiazide Tablets per day, administered in single or divided doses.

Concurrent potassium supplementation is not recommended when this drug is used in the long-term management of hypertension or in the treatment of most edematous conditions, since the spironolactone content is usually sufficient to minimize loss induced by the hydrochlorothiazide component.

HOW SUPPLIED

Spironolactone with Hydrochlorothiazide Tablets (round, white, scored tablets coded P-D 712) are supplied as follows::
N 0071-0712-24 Bottles of 100
N 0071-0712-32 Bottles of 1000
N 0071-0712-40 Unit-dose packages of 100 individually sealed tablets

Store at room temperature below 30°C (86°F).
Protect from moisture and light.
Caution—Federal law prohibits dispensing without prescription.

0712G011

SURITAL® ㉃ ℞

[*sŭ'rĭ-tăl"*]
(thiamylal sodium for injection, USP)

DESCRIPTION

Surital (thiamylal sodium for injection, USP) is sodium-5-allyl-5-(1-methylbutyl)-2-thiobarbiturate.

ACTIONS

Thiamylal sodium is a rapid, ultra-short-acting barbiturate, intravenous, anesthetic agent.

INDICATIONS

Surital is indicated for induction of anesthesia, for supplementing other anesthetic agents, as intravenous anesthesia for short surgical procedures with minimal painful stimuli, or as an agent for inducing a hypnotic state.

CONTRAINDICATIONS

Thiamylal sodium is contraindicated when general anesthesia is contraindicated, in patients with latent or manifest porphyria, or in patients with a known hypersensitivity to barbiturates.

WARNINGS

RESUSCITATIVE EQUIPMENT AND DRUGS SHOULD BE IMMEDIATELY AVAILABLE. This drug should be administered by persons qualified in the use of intravenous anesthetics.

Repeated and continuous infusion may cause cumulative effects resulting in prolonged somnolence, and respiratory and circulatory depression.

Usage in pregnancy: Safe use of thiamylal sodium has not been established with respect to adverse effects upon fetal development. Therefore, thiamylal sodium should not be used in women of childbearing potential, and particularly during early pregnancy, unless, in the judgment of the physician, the expected benefits outweigh the potential hazards.

PRECAUTIONS

Respiratory depression, apnea, or hypotension may occur due to variations in tolerance from individual to individual or to physical status of patient. Caution should be exercised in debilitated patients, or those with impaired function of respiratory, circulatory, renal, hepatic, and endocrine systems.

Thiamylal sodium should be used with extreme caution in patients in status asthmaticus.

Extravascular injection may cause pain, swelling, ulceration, and necrosis. Intra-arterial injection is dangerous and may produce gangrene of an extremity.

ADVERSE REACTIONS

The following adverse reactions have been reported: circulatory depression, thrombophlebitis, pain at injection site, and respiratory depression, including apnea, laryngospasm, bronchospasm, salivation, hiccups, emergence delirium, headache, injury to nerves adjacent to injection site, skin rashes, urticaria, nausea, and emesis.

DOSAGE AND ADMINISTRATION

The dosage is individualized according to the patient's response.

A 2.5% solution is recommended for induction of anesthesia as well as for maintenance by intermittent intravenous injection. A dilute solution (0.3%) may be used by continuous drip for maintenance. The rate of injection during induction should be approximately 1 ml of 2.5% solution every five seconds; an initial injection of 3 to 6 ml of 2.5% solution is generally sufficient to produce short periods of surgical anesthesia.

Sterile Water for Injection is the preferred solvent for preparing Surital (thiamylal sodium for injection, USP) solutions. Initially, Surital solutions are clear, but they may become cloudy on aging. Thiamylal sodium cannot be reconstituted with Ringer's Solution or solutions containing bacteriostatic or buffer agents, because they may tend to cause precipitation. In preparing dilute solutions for continuous drip maintenance, either 5% dextrose or isotonic sodium chloride should be used instead of sterile water for injection to avoid extreme hypotonicity. Dextrose solutions are occasionally sufficiently acid, however, to cause precipitation. Injection of air into the solution should be avoided because this may hasten the development of cloudiness.

Solutions of atropine sulfate, *d*-tubocurarine, or succinylcholine may be given concurrently with Surital, but they should not be mixed prior to administration.

Thiamylal sodium solutions should be prepared under aseptic conditions. Solutions cannot be heated for sterilization. The solutions should be stored in a refrigerator and used within six days. If kept at room temperature, the solution should be used within 24 hours. Only clear solutions should be used; discard if cloudiness or precipitate form. Refrigeration of the reconstituted Surital contributes to the maintenance of a clear solution.

[See table below].

PREPARING *SURITAL* SOLUTIONS

Surital (g)	Amount of solvent required (in ml) for percentage solutions shown								
	0.2%	0.3%	0.4%	2%	2.5%	3%	4%	5%	10%
1	500	333	250	50	40	33.3	25	20	10
5	2,500	1,670	1,250	250	200	167	125	100	50
10	5,000	3,333	2,500	500	400	333	250	200	100

HOW SUPPLIED

Surital is supplied as follows.
N 0071-4064-03 (35-64-25)
1 g, in packages of 25 (Steri-Vial® 64)
N 0071-4122-08 (35-122-10)
5 g, in packages of 10 (Steri-Vial 122)
N 0071-4123-10 (35-123-10)
10 g, in packages of 10 (Steri-Vial 123)
AHFS 28:24 **4064G020**

TABRON® FILMSEAL® ℞

[*tăb'rŏn"*]

Each tablet represents:

Ferrous fumarate (represents 100 mg of elemental iron)	304.2 mg
Vitamin C (ascorbic acid)	500 mg
Vitamin B_1 (thiamine mononitrate)	6 mg
Vitamin B_2 (riboflavin)	6 mg
Vitamin B_6 (pyridoxine hydrochloride)	5 mg
Vitamin B_{12} (cyanocobalamin), crystalline	25 mcg
Folic acid	1 mg
Nicotinamide (niacinamide)	30 mg
Calcium pantothenate	10 mg
Vitamin E (*dl*-alpha tocopheryl acetate)	(30 mg) 30 IU
Docusate sodium	50 mg

Caution—Folic acid in doses above 0.1 mg daily may obscure pernicious anemia in that hematologic remission can occur while neurological manifestations remain progressive.

INDICATIONS

Tabron is a hematinic for the treatment of iron-deficiency anemia and folate deficiency.

DOSAGE

Usual adult dose: One tablet per day.

HOW SUPPLIED

N 0071-0638—Bottles of 100 and unit-dose packages of 100 (ten 10s). Parcode® No. 638

Shown in Product Identification Section, page 421

TEDRAL® ℞

[*tĕd'ral*]
TEDRAL® SUSPENSION
TEDRAL ELIXIR

DESCRIPTION

Tedral Suspension: Each 5 mL teaspoonful of suspension contains 65 mg theophylline (59.1 mg anhydrous), 12 mg ephedrine hydrochloride, and 4 mg phenobarbital. (**Warning**—May be habit forming.) Also contains: benzoic acid, USP; D&C Yellow No. 10; FD&C Yellow No. 6; flavors; saccharin sodium, NF; sugar, invert; tragacanth, USP; water, potable.

Tebral Elixir: Each 5 mL teaspoonful contains 32.5 mg theophylline (29.5 mg anhydrous), 6 mg ephedrine hydrochloride, and 2 mg phenobarbital. (**Warning**—May be habit forming.) The alcohol content is 15%. Also contains: D&C Green No. 5 and Red No. 33; FD&C Red No. 40; flavors; propylene glycol, USP; saccharin sodium, NF; sorbitol solution, USP; water, purified, USP.

ACTIONS

Tedral combines theophylline and ephedrine—widely accepted oral bronchodilators, with differing modes of action—with the sedative phenobarbital.

From experimental evidence,[1] it appears that a combination of a sympathomimetic and methylxanthine is more effective than either drug alone in inhibiting the release of bronchoconstricting mediators (histamine and slow-reacting substance of anaphylaxis) produced by antigen-antibody (IgE) interaction on sensitive cells. The β-adrenergic stimulation

by the sympathomimetics produces cyclic 3'5'-adenosine monophosphate (cAMP), and the degradation of cAMP by the specific enzyme, phosphodiesterase, is inhibited by methylxanthines. Thus, at present, the principal action of the Tedral formulations in the relief or prevention of bronchoconstriction appears to be involved with the cAMP system.
Phenobarbital is incorporated to counteract possible stimulation by ephedrine and to provide a mild, long-acting sedative for the apprehensive asthmatic patient.
Tedral Suspension and Tedral Elixir are convenient formulations for children and other persons who may have difficulty in swallowing tablets.

INDICATIONS
Tedral Suspension and Tedral Elixir are indicated for the symptomatic relief of bronchial asthma, asthmatic bronchitis, and other bronchospastic disorders. They may also be used prophylactically to abort or minimize asthmatic attacks and are of value in managing occasional, seasonal or perennial asthma.
Tedral Suspension and Tedral Elixir are convenient for persons who may have difficulty in swallowing tablets.
These Tedral formulations are adjuncts in the total management of the asthmatic patient. Acute or severe asthmatic attacks may necessitate supplemental therapy with others drugs by inhalation or other parenteral routes.

CONTRAINDICATIONS
Sensitivity to any of the ingredients; porphyria.

WARNINGS
Drowsiness may occur. Phenobarbital may be habit-forming.

PRECAUTIONS
Use with caution in the presence of cardiovascular disease, severe hypertension, hyperthyroidism, prostatic hypertrophy, or glaucoma.

ADVERSE REACTIONS
Mild epigastric distress, palpitation, tremulousness, insomnia, difficulty of micturition, and CNS stimulation have been reported.

DOSAGE AND ADMINISTRATION
Tedral Suspension
Adults—two to four teaspoonfuls every 4 hours.
Children—one teaspoonful per 60 lb body weight, every 4–6 hours. Should be given to children under 2 years of age only with extreme caution.
SHAKE BOTTLE WELL.
Tedral Elixir
Children—one teaspoonful per 30 lb body weight, every 4–6 hours. Should be given to children under 2 years of age only with extreme caution.
Adults—one to two tablespoonfuls every four hours.

HOW SUPPLIED
Tedral Suspension is supplied as a yellow, licorice-flavored suspension in bottles of 8 fl oz (237 ml) (N 0071-2237-20) and in bottles of 16 fl oz (474 ml) (N 0071-2237-23).
Tedral Elixir is supplied as a dark red, cherry-flavored elixir in bottles of 16 fl oz (474 ml) (N 0071-2242-23).
Store between 15°–30°C (59°–86°F).

Reference: 1. Koopman WJ, Orange RP, Austen KF: *J. Immunol* 105:1096, November 1970.

0230G013

Shown in Product Identification Section, page 421

TEDRAL®SA ℞
[tĕd'ral]

DESCRIPTION
Tedral SA: Each tablet contains 180 mg anhydrous theophylline (90 mg in the immediate release layer and 90 mg in the sustained release layer); 48 mg ephedrine hydrochloride (16 mg in the immediate release layer and 32 mg in the sustained release layer); 25 mg phenobarbital in the immediate release layer.
Also contains: D&C red No. 30 and yellow No. 10 Lake; lactose, NF; magnesium stearate, NF; starch; sucrose and other ingredients.

ACTIONS
Tedral SA combines theophylline and ephedrine—widely accepted oral bronchodilators with differing modes of action. From experimental evidence,[1] it appears that a combination of a sympathomimetic and methylxanthine is more effective than either drug alone in inhibiting the release of bronchoconstricting mediators (histamine and slow-reacting substance of anaphylaxis) produced by antigen-antibody (IgE) interaction on sensitive cells. Th β-adrenergic stimulation by the sympathomimetics produces cyclic 3'5'-adenosine monophosphate (cAMP), and the degradation of cAMP by the specific enzyme, phosphodiesterase, is inhibited by methylxanthines. Thus, at present, the principal action of Tedral SA in the relief or prevention of bronchoconstriction appears to be involved with the cAMP system.
Phenobarbital is incorporated into Tedral SA to counteract possible stimulation by ephedrine and to provide a mild, long-acting sedative for the apprehensive asthmatic patient.
Tedral SA provides sustained as well as immediate bronchodilatation for the asthmatic patient, with the convenience of bid dosage.

INDICATIONS
Tedral SA is indicated for the symptomatic relief of bronchial asthma, asthmatic bronchitis, and other bronchospastic disorders. It may also be used prophylactically to abort or minimize asthmatic attacks and is of value in managing occasional, seasonal, or perennial asthma.
Tedral SA (Sustained Action) offers the convenience of bid dosage.
This Tedral formulation is an adjunct in the total management of the asthmatic patient. Acute or severe asthmatic attacks may necessitate supplemental therapy with other drugs by inhalation or other parenteral routes.

CONTRAINDICATIONS
Sensitivity to any of the ingredients; porphyria.

WARNINGS
Drowsiness may occur. Phenobarbital may be habit forming.

PRECAUTIONS
Use with caution in the presence of cardiovascular disease, severe hypertension, hyperthyroidism, prostatic hypertrophy, or glaucoma.

ADVERSE REACTIONS
Mild epigastric distress, palpitation, tremulousness, insomnia, difficulty of micturition, and CNS stimulation have been reported.

DOSAGE AND ADMINISTRATION
Adults—one tablet on arising and one tablet 12 hours later. Tablets should not be chewed.
Children—not established for children under 12.

HOW SUPPLIED
Tedral SA is supplied as double-layered, uncoated, coral/mottled white tablets in bottles of 100 (N 0710-0231-24) and 1000 (N 0710-0231-32).
Store between 15°–30°C (59°–86°F).
Reference: 1. Koopman WJ, Orange RP, Austen KF. *J Immunol* 105:1096, November 1970.
Shown in Product Identification Section, page 421

0231G112

TETRACYCLINE HCl CAPSULES, USP ℞
[tĕ"tră-cy'clīne]
Cyclopar®/Cyclopar® 500

DESCRIPTION
Tetracycline hydrochloride capsules, USP contain the broad-spectrum antibiotic, tetracycline hydrochloride. Also contain lactose, NF; magnesium stearate, NF. The capsule shell and/or band of the 250 mg capsule contains FD and C blue No. 1; FD and C red No. 3; FD and C red No. 40; gelatin, NF; silicon dioxide; sodium lauryl sulfate, NF; titanium dioxide, USP. The capsule shell and/or band of the 500 mg capsule contains FD and C red No. 3; FD and C red No. 40; FD and C yellow No. 6; gelatin, NF; silicon dioxide; sodium lauryl sulfate, NF; titanium dioxide, USP. Tetracycline hydrochloride is a yellow, odorless crystalline powder with the chemical formula $C_{22}H_{24}N_2O_8HCl$.

ACTIONS
The tetracyclines are primarily bacteriostatic and are thought to exert their antimicrobial effect by the inhibition of protein synthesis. Tetracyclines are active against a wide range of gram-negative and gram-positive organisms.
The drugs in the tetracycline class have closely similar antimicrobial spectra, and cross-resistance among them is common. Microorganisms may be considered susceptible if the MIC (minimum inhibitory concentration) is not more than 4.0 mcg/ml, and intermediate if the MIC is 4.0 to 12.5 mcg/ml.
Susceptibility plate testing: A tetracycline disc may be used to determine microbial susceptibility to drugs in the tetracycline class. If the Kirby-Bauer method of disc susceptibility testing is used, a 30-mcg tetracycline disc should give a zone of at least 19 mm when tested against a tetracycline-susceptible bacterial strain.
Tetracyclines are readily absorbed and are bound to plasma proteins in varying degrees. They are concentrated by the liver in the bile and excreted in the urine and feces at high concentrations and in a biologically active form.

INDICATIONS
Tetracycline is indicated in infections caused by the following microorganisms.
Rickettsiae (Rocky Mountain spotted fever, typhus fever and the typhus group, Q fever, rickettsialpox, and tick fevers)
Mycoplasma pneumoniae (PPLO, Eaton agent)
Agents of psittacosis and ornithosis
Agents of lymphogranuloma venereum and granuloma inguinale
The spirochetal agent of relapsing fever *(Borrelia recurrentis)*
The following gram-negative microorganisms:
Haemophilus ducreyi (chancroid)
Pasteurella pestis and *Pasteurella tularensis*
Bartonella bacilliformis
Bacteroides species
Vibrio comma and *Vibrio fetus*
Brucella species (in conjunction with streptomycin)
Because many strains of the following groups of microorganisms have been shown to be resistant to tetracyclines, culture and susceptibility testing is recommended.
Tetracycline is indicated for treatment of infections caused by the following gram-negative microorganisms when bacteriologic testing indicates appropriate susceptibility to the drug.
Escherichia coli
Enterobacter aerogenes (formerly *Aerobacter aerogenes)*
Shigella species
Mima species and *Herellea* species
Haemophilus influenzae (respiratory infections)
Klebsiella species (respiratory and urinary infections)
Tetracycline is indicated for treatment of infections caused by the following gram-positive microorganisms when bacteriologic testing indicates appropriate susceptibility to the drug.
Streptococcus species:
Up to 44 percent of strains of *Streptococcus pyogenes* and 74 percent of *Streptococcus faecalis* have been found to be resistant to tetracycline drugs. Therefore, tetracyclines should not be used for streptococcal disease unless the organism has been demonstrated to be sensitive.
For upper respiratory infections due to group A beta-hemolytic streptococci, penicillin is the usual drug of choice, including prophylaxis of rheumatic fever.
Diplococcus pneumoniae
Staphylococcus aureus
Skin and soft-tissue infections. Tetracyclines are not the drugs of choice in the treatment of any type of staphylococcal infection.
When penicillin is contraindicated, tetracyclines are alternative drugs in the treatment of infections due to:
Neisseria gonorrhoeae,
Treponema pallidum and *Treponema pertenue* (syphilis and yaws),
Listeria monocytogenes,
Clostridium species,
Bacillus anthracis,
Fusobacterium fusiforme (Vincent's infection),
Actinomyces species.
Tetracycline hydrochloride is indicated for the treatment of uncomplicated urethral, endocervical or rectal infections in adults caused by *Chlamydia trachomatis.*[1]
In acute intestinal amebiasis, the tetracyclines may be a useful adjunct to amebicides.
In severe acne, the tetracyclines may be useful adjunctive therapy.
Tetracyclines are indicated in the treatment of trachoma, although the infectious agent is not always eliminated, as judged by immunofluorescence.
Inclusion conjunctivitis may be treated with oral tetracyclines or with a combination of oral and topical agents.

CONTRAINDICATION
This drug is contraindicated in persons who have shown hypersensitivity to any of the tetracyclines.

WARNINGS
THE USE OF DRUGS OF THE TETRACYCLINE CLASS DURING TOOTH DEVELOPMENT (LAST HALF OF PREGNANCY, INFANCY, AND CHILDHOOD TO THE AGE OF 8 YEARS) MAY CAUSE PERMANENT DISCOLORATION OF THE TEETH (YELLOW-GRAY-BROWN). This adverse reaction is more common during long-term use of the drugs but has been observed following repeated short-term courses. Enamel hypoplasia has also been reported. TETRACYCLINE DRUGS, THEREFORE, SHOULD NOT BE USED IN THIS AGE GROUP UNLESS OTHER DRUGS ARE NOT LIKELY TO BE EFFECTIVE OR ARE CONTRAINDICATED.
If renal impairment exists, even usual oral or parenteral doses may lead to excessive systemic accumulation of the drug and possible liver toxicity. Under such conditions,

Continued on next page

This product information was prepared in August, 1986. On these and other Parke-Davis Products, information may be obtained by addressing PARKE-DAVIS, Division of Warner-Lambert Company, Morris Plains, New Jersey 07950.

Parke-Davis—Cont.

lower than usual total doses are indicated and, if therapy is prolonged, serum level determinations of the drug may be advisable.

Photosensitivity manifested by an exaggerated sunburn reaction has been observed in some individuals taking tetracyclines. Patients apt to be exposed to direct sunlight or ultraviolet light should be advised that this reaction can occur with tetracycline drugs, and treatment should be discontinued at the first evidence of skin erythema.

The antianabolic action of the tetracyclines may cause an increase in BUN. While this is not a problem in those with normal renal function, in patients with significantly impaired function, higher serum levels of tetracycline may lead to azotemia, hyperphosphatemia, and acidosis.

Usage in pregnancy. (See above Warnings about use during tooth development).

Results of animal studies indicate that tetracyclines cross the placenta, are found in fetal tissues, and can have toxic effects on the developing fetus (often related to retardation of skeletal development.) Evidence of embryotoxicity has also been noted in animals treated early in pregnancy.

Usage in newborns, infants, and children. (See above Warnings about use during tooth development.)

All tetracyclines form a stable calcium complex in any bone-forming tissue. A decrease in the fibula growth rate has been observed in prematures given oral tetracycline in doses of 25 mg/kg every 6 hours. This reaction was shown to be reversible when the drug was discontinued.

Tetracyclines are present in the milk of lactating women who are taking a drug in this class.

PRECAUTIONS

As with other antibiotic preparations, use of this drug may result in overgrowth of nonsusceptible organisms, including fungi. If superinfection occurs, the antibiotic should be discontinued and appropriate therapy instituted.

In venereal diseases when coexistent syphilis is suspected, darkfield examination should be done before treatment is started and the blood serology repeated monthly for at least four months.

Because tetracyclines have been shown to depress plasma prothrombin activity, patients who are on anticoagulant therapy may require downward adjustment of their anticoagulant dosage.

In long-term therapy, periodic laboratory evaluation of organ systems, including hematopoietic, renal, and hepatic studies, should be performed.

All infections due to Group A beta-hemolytic streptococci should be treated for at least 10 days.

Since bacteriostatic drugs may interfere with the bactericidal action of penicillin, it is advisable to avoid giving tetracycline in conjunction with penicillin.

ADVERSE REACTIONS

Gastrointestinal: anorexia, nausea, vomiting, diarrhea, glossitis, dysphagia, enterocolitis, and inflammatory lesions (with monilial overgrowth) in the anogenital region. These reactions have been caused by both the oral and parenteral administration of tetracyclines.

Skin: maculopapular and erythematous rashes. Exfoliative dermatitis has been reported but is uncommon. Photosensitivity is discussed above. (See Warnings.)

Renal toxicity: rise in BUN has been reported and is apparently dose-related. (See Warnings.)

Hypersensitivity reactions: urticaria, angioneurotic edema, anaphylaxis, anaphylactoid purpura, pericarditis, and exacerbation of systemic lupus erythematosus

Bulging fontanels have been reported in young infants following full therapeutic dosage. This sign disappeared rapidly when the drug was discontinued.

Blood: hemolytic anemia, thrombocytopenia, neutropenia, and eosinophilia have been reported.

When given over prolonged periods, tetracyclines have been reported to produce brown-black microscopic discoloration of thyroid glands. No abnormalities of thyroid function studies are known to occur.

DOSAGE AND ADMINISTRATION

Therapy should be continued for at least 24 to 48 hours after symptoms and fever have subsided.

Concomitant therapy: Antacids containing aluminum, calcium, or magnesium impair absorption and should not be given to patients taking oral tetracycline.

Food and some dairy products also interfere with absorption. Oral forms of tetracycline should be given 1 hour before or 2 hours after meals. Pediatric oral dosage forms should not be given with milk formulas and should be given at least 1 hour prior to feeding.

In patients with renal impairment (See Warnings.): Total dosage should be decreased by reduction of recommended individual doses and/or by extending time intervals between doses.

In the treatment of streptococcal infections, a therapeutic dose of tetracycline should be administered for at least 10 days.

Adults: Usual daily dosage, 1 to 2 grams divided in two or four equal doses, depending on the severity of the infection.

For children above eight years of age: Usual daily dosage, 10 to 20 mg (25 to 50 mg/kg) per pound of body weight divided in four equal doses.

For treatment of brucellosis, 500 mg tetracycline four times daily for three weeks should be accompanied by streptomycin, 1 gram, intramuscularly twice daily the first week and once daily the second week.

For treatment of syphilis, a total of 30 to 40 grams in equally divided doses over a period of 10 to 15 days should be given. Close follow-up, including laboratory tests, is recommended.

For the treatment of acute gonococcal urethritis, a single, initial dose of 1.5 grams followed by 0.5 grams every 4 to 6 hours for 4 to 6 days should be given. Female patients may require more prolonged therapy.

Uncomplicated urethral, endocervical, or rectal infection in adults caused by *Chlamydia trachomatis;* 500 mg, by mouth, 4 times a day for at least 7 days.[1]

HOW SUPPLIED

Tetracycline hydrochloride capsules, USP (Cyclopar)
N 0071-0407-24 250 mg Bottles of 100.
N 0071-0407-32 250 mg Bottles of 1000.
Each capsule contains 250 mg tetracycline hydrochloride.
Tetracycline hydrochloride capsules, USP (Cyclopar 500)
N 0071-0697-24 500 mg Bottles of 100.
Each capsule contains 500 mg tetracycline hydrochloride.

Reference: 1. CDC Sexually Transmitted Diseases Treatment Guidelines 1982.

AHFS 8:12.24 **0407G102**

Shown in Product Identification Section, page 421

THROMBOSTAT® ℞
(Thrombin, USP) Bovine Origin

Thrombostat must not be injected! Apply on the surface of bleeding tissue as a solution or powder.

DESCRIPTION

Thrombostat (Thrombin, USP) is a protein substance produced through a conversion reaction in which prothrombin of bovine origin is activated by tissue thromboplastin in the presence of calcium chloride. It is supplied as a sterile powder that has been freeze-dried in the final container. Also contained in this preparation are calcium chloride, sodium chloride, and aminoacetic acid (glycine) as follows: calcium chloride—3 mg per 1000 unit vial, 5 mg per 5000 unit vial, 10 mg per 10,000 unit vial, and 21 mg per 20,000 unit vial; sodium chloride—4 mg per 1000 unit vial, 8 mg per 5000 unit vial, 15 mg per 10,000 unit vial, and 30 mg per 20,000 unit vial; aminoacetic acid—22 mg per 1000 unit vial, 39 mg per 5000 unit vial, 78 mg per 10,000 unit vial, and 156 mg per 20,000 unit vial. Glycine is included to make the dried product friable and more readily soluble.

A 5 mL, 10 mL, or 20 mL vial of Isotonic Saline is enclosed to be used as a diluent with the 5 mL, 5000 unit; 10 mL, 10,000 unit; or 20 mL, 20,000 unit vial, respectively, of Thrombostat. Isotonic Saline is a sterile, isotonic solution of sodium chloride in Water For Injection, USP. It contains Phemerol® (benzethonium chloride) 0.02 mg per mL as a preservative. (See Dosage and Administration for additional information on diluents which may be used.)

This product is prepared under rigid assay control. A unit is defined as the amount required to clot 1 mL of standardized fibrinogen solution in 15 seconds.

Approximately 2 units are required to clot 1 mL of oxalated human plasma in the same period of time.

CLINICAL PHARMACOLOGY

Thrombostat requires no intermediate physiological agent for its action. It clots the fibrinogen of the blood directly. Failure to clot blood occurs in the rare case where the primary clotting defect is the absence of fibrinogen itself. The speed with which thrombin clots blood is dependent upon its concentration. For example, the contents of a 5000 unit vial of Thrombostat dissolved in 5 mL of saline diluent is capable of clotting an equal volume of blood in less than a second, or 1000 mL in less than a minute.

INDICATIONS AND USAGE

Thrombostat (Thrombin, USP) is indicated as an aid in hemostasis wherever oozing blood from capillaries and small venules is accessible.

In various types of surgery solutions of Thrombostat may be used in conjunction with Absorbable Gelatin Sponge, USP for hemostasis.

CONTRAINDICATIONS

Thrombostat is contraindicated in persons known to be sensitive to any of its components and /or to material of bovine origin.

WARNING

Because of its action in the clotting mechanism, Thrombostat must not be injected or otherwise allowed to enter large blood vessels. Extensive intravascular clotting and even death may result. Thrombostat is an antigenic substance and has caused sensitivity and allergic reactions when injected into animals.

PRECAUTIONS

General: Consult the absorbable gelatin sponge product labeling for complete information for use prior to utilizing the thrombin-saturated sponge procedure.

Pregnancy—

Teratogenic effects: Pregnancy Category C. Animal reproduction studies have not been conducted with Thrombin, Topical (Bovine). It is also not known whether Thrombin, Topical (Bovine) can cause fetal harm when administered to a pregnant woman or can affect reproduction capacity. Thrombin, Topical (Bovine) should be given to a pregnant woman only if clearly indicated.

Pediatric Use: Safety and effectiveness in children have not been established.

ADVERSE REACTIONS

An allergic type reaction following the use of Thrombostat for treatment of epistaxis has been reported. Febrile reactions have also been observed following the use of Thrombostat in certain surgical procedures but no cause-effect relationship has been established.

DOSAGE AND ADMINISTRATION

General: Solutions of Thrombostat may be prepared in sterile distilled water or isotonic saline. The intended use determines the strength of the solution to prepare. For general use in plastic surgery, dental extractions, skin grafting, neurosurgery, etc, solutions containing approximately 100 units per mL are frequently used. For this, 10 mL of diluent added to the 1000 unit package is suitable. Where bleeding is profuse, as from cut surfaces of liver and spleen, concentrations as high as 1000 to 2000 units per mL may be required. For this the 5000 unit vial dissolved in 5 mL or 2.5 mL, respectively, of the diluent supplied in the package is convenient. Intermediate strengths to suit the needs of the case may be prepared by selecting the proper strength package and dissolving the contents in an appropriate volume of diluent. In many situations, it may be advantageous to use Thrombostat in dry form on oozing surfaces.

Caution:

Solutions should be used immediately upon reconstitution. If necessary, refrigerate the solution and use within 3 hours of reconstitution.

The following techniques are suggested for the topical application of Thrombostat.

1. The recipient surface should be sponged (not wiped) free of blood before Thrombostat is applied.
2. A spray may be used or the surface may be flooded using a sterile syringe and small gauge needle. The most effective hemostasis results when the Thrombostat mixes freely with the blood as soon as it reaches the surface.
3. In instances where Thrombostat in dry form is needed, the vial is opened by removing the metal ring by flipping up the plastic cap and tearing counterclockwise. The rubber-diaphragm cap may be easily removed and the dried Thrombostat is then broken up into a powder by means of a sterile glass rod or other suitable sterile instrument.
4. Sponging of treated surfaces should be avoided in order that the clot remain securely in place.

Thrombostat may be used in conjunction with Absorbable Gelatin Sponge, USP as follows:

1. Prepare Thrombostat solution of the desired strength.
2. Immerse sponge strips of the desired size in the Thrombostat solution. Knead the sponge strips vigorously with moistened gloved fingers to remove trapped air, thereby facilitating saturation of the sponge.
3. Apply saturated sponge to bleeding area. Hold in place for 10 to 15 seconds with a pledget of cotton or a small gauze sponge.

Thrombostat Kit: Thrombostat Kit contains one sterile 20,000 unit vial of Thrombostat, one sterile vial of Isotonic Saline Diluent, and one sterile pump sprayer cap. The Kit may be used as follows:

1. Remove the Tyvek blister lid by pulling up at the indicated corner. The sterile inner tray can be lifted out or introduced into the operating field.
2. The cover to the sterile inner tray is removed by pulling up on the finger tab, exposing the sterile contents.
3. Thrombostat solution of the desired strength is prepared and the pump sprayer cap inserted and seated on the Thrombostat solution vial. Note: Several strokes of the pump sprayer will be required before the Thrombostat solution is expelled.
4. Alternatively, when Thrombostat in dry form is needed, the vial is opened as described above and the dried Thrombostat broken up into a powder by means of a sterile glass rod or other suitable sterile instrument.

HOW SUPPLIED

Thrombostat is supplied as:

N 0071-4173-35—Package contains one 5000 unit vial of Thrombostat and one 5 mL vial of Isotonic Saline Diluent with Phemerol, 0.02 mg per mL, as a preservative.

N 0071-4176-35—Package contains one 10,000 unit vial of Thrombostat and one 10 mL vial of Isotonic Saline Diluent with Phemerol, 0.02 mg per mL, as a preservative.

N 0071-4177-01—Package contains one 1000 unit vial of Thrombostat.

N 0071-4180-35—Package contains one 20,000 unit vial of Thrombostat and one 20 mL vial of Isotonic Saline Diluent with Phemerol, 0.02 mg per mL, as a preservative.

N 0071-4180-36—Kit contains one sterile 20,000 unit vial of Thrombostat, one 20 mL vial of Isotonic Saline Diluent with Phemerol, 0.02 mg per mL, as a preservative, and one sterile pump sprayer cap in a sterile tray with a Tyvek lid.

STORAGE

This product should be stored at 2° to 8°C (36° to 46°F).

Caution—Federal law prohibits dispensing without prescription.

Tyvek is a registered trademark of E. I. du Pont de Nemours & Co.

4173G016

UTICORT® ℞

[*ū'tĭ-cōrt"*]

(betamethasone benzoate)

Cream, 0.025%

Gel, 0.025%

Lotion, 0.025%

Ointment, 0.025%

For external use only

Caution: Federal law prohibits dispensing without prescription.

DESCRIPTION

Uticort Gel/Cream/Ointment/ Lotion contain the active fluorinated corticosteroid compound betamethasone benzoate, the 17-benzoate ester of betamethasone, having the chemical formula of 9-fluoro-11β, 17, 21-trihydroxy-16β-methylpregna-1, 4-diene-3, 20-dione 17-benzoate.

Each gram of 0.025% Gel contains 0.25 mg of betamethasone benzoate in a specially formulated gel base consisting of 13.8% (w/w) alcohol, carboxyvinyl polymer, propylene glycol, disodium edetate, diisopropanolamine and purified water. The gel is self-liquefying, clear, greaseless and nonstaining. The active ingredient is completely solubilized and remains in the clear film without crystallization after evaporation of volatile substances.

Each gram of 0.025% Cream contains 0.25 mg of betamethasone benzoate in a water-washable emollient cream base consisting of cetyl alcohol, glyceryl stearate, light mineral oil, propylene glycol, disodium monooleamidosulfosuccinate, citric acid and purified water.

Each gram of 0.025% Ointment contains 0.25 mg of betamethasone benzoate in an emollient ointment base of light mineral oil, glyceryl stearate, food starch-modified and polyethylene.

In this formulation the active ingredient is micronized to provide uniform distribution and optimal activity.

Each gram of 0.025% Lotion contains 0.25 mg of betamethasone benzoate in a water miscible, oil- and fat-free vehicle consisting of cetyl alcohol, stearyl alcohol, propylene glycol, sodium lauryl sulfate, purified water, and propyl-, butyl-, and methylparabens as preservatives.

CLINICAL PHARMACOLOGY

Topical corticosteroids share antiinflammatory, antipruritic and vasoconstrictive actions.

The mechanism of antiinflammatory activity of the topical corticosteroids is unclear. Various laboratory methods, including vasoconstrictor assays, are used to compare and predict potencies and/or clinical efficacies of the topical corticosteroids. There is some evidence to suggest that a recognizable correlation exists between vasoconstrictor potency and therapeutic efficacy in man.

Pharmacokinetics

The extent of percutaneous absorption of topical corticosteroids is determined by many factors including the vehicle, the integrity of the epidermal barrier, and the use of occlusive dressings.

Topical corticosteroids can be absorbed from normal intact skin. Inflammation and/or other disease processes in the skin increase percutaneous absorption.

Occlusive dressings substantially increase the percutaneous absorption of topical corticosteroids. Thus, occlusive dressings may be a valuable therapeutic adjunct for treatment of resistant dermatoses (See *DOSAGE AND ADMINISTRATION.*)

Once absorbed through the skin, topical corticosteroids are handled through pharmacokinetic pathways similar to systemically administered corticosteroids. Corticosteroids are bound to plasma proteins in varying degrees. Corticosteroids are metabolized primarily in the liver and are then excreted by the kidneys. Some of the topical corticosteroids and their metabolites are also excreted into the bile.

INDICATIONS AND USAGE

Topical corticosteroids are indicated for the relief of the inflammatory and pruritic manifestations of corticosteroid-responsive dermatoses.

CONTRAINDICATIONS

Topical corticosteroids are contraindicated in those patients with a history of hypersensitivity to any of the components of the preparation.

PRECAUTIONS

General

Systemic absorption of topical corticosteroids has produced reversible hypothalamic-pituitary-adrenal (HPA) axis suppression, manifestations of Cushing's syndrome, hyperglycemia and glucosuria in some patients.

Conditions which augment systemic absorption include the application of the more potent steroids, use over large surface areas, prolonged use, and the addition of occlusive dressings.

Therefore, patients receiving a large dose of a potent topical steroid applied to a large surface area or under an occlusive dressing should be evaluated periodically for evidence of HPA axis suppression by using the urinary free cortisol and ACTH stimulation tests. If HPA axis suppression is noted, an attempt should be made to withdraw the drug, to reduce the frequency of application, or to substitute a less potent steroid.

Recovery of HPA axis function is generally prompt and complete upon discontinuation of the drug. Infrequently, signs and symptoms of steroid withdrawal may occur, requiring supplemental systemic corticosteroids.

Children may absorb proportionally larger amounts of topical corticosteroids and thus be more susceptible to systemic toxicity (See *PRECAUTIONS—Pediatric Use*).

If irritation develops, topical corticosteroids should be discontinued and appropriate therapy instituted.

In the presence of dermatological infections, the use of an appropriate antifungal or antibacterial agent should be instituted. If a favorable response does not occur promptly, the corticosteroid should be discontinued until the infection has been adequately controlled.

Information for the Patient

Patients using topical corticosteroids should receive the following information and instructions:

1. This medication is to be used as directed by the physician. It is for external use only. Avoid contact with the eyes.
2. Patients should be advised not to use this medication for any disorder other than for which it was prescribed.
3. The treated skin area should not be bandaged or otherwise covered or wrapped as to be occlusive unless directed by the physician.
4. Patients should report any signs of local adverse reactions especially under occlusive dressing.
5. Parents of pediatric patients should be advised not to use tight-fitting diapers or plastic pants on a child being treated in the diaper area, as these garments may constitute occlusive dressings.

Laboratory Tests

The following tests may be helpful in evaluating the HPA axis suppression:

Urinary free cortisol test

ACTH stimulation test

Carcinogenesis, Mutagenesis, and Impairment of Fertility

Long-term animal studies have not been performed to evaluate the carcinogenic potential or the effect on fertility of topical corticosteroids.

Studies to determine mutagenicity with prednisolone and hydrocortisone have revealed negative results.

Pregnancy Category C

Corticosteroids are generally teratogenic in laboratory animals when administered systemically at relatively low dosage levels. The more potent corticosteroids have been shown to be teratogenic after dermal application in laboratory animals. There are no adequate and well-controlled studies in pregnant women on teratogenic effects from topically applied corticosteroids. Therefore, topical corticosteroids should be used during pregnancy only if the potential benefit justifies the potential risk to the fetus. Drugs of this class should not be used extensively on pregnant patients, in large amounts, or for prolonged periods of time.

Nursing Mothers

It is not known whether topical administration of corticosteroids could result in sufficient systemic absorption to produce detectable quantities in breast milk. Systemically administered corticosteroids are secreted into breast milk in quantities *not* likely to have a deleterious effect on the infant. Nevertheless, caution should be exercised when topical corticosteroids are administered to a nursing woman.

Pediatric Use

Pediatric patients may demonstrate greater susceptibility to topical corticosteroid-induced HPA axis suppression and Cushing's syndrome than mature patients because of a larger skin surface area to body weight ratio.

Hypothalamic-pituitary-adrenal (HPA) axis suppression, Cushing's syndrome, and intracranial hypertension have been reported in children receiving topical corticosteroids. Manifestations of adrenal suppression in children include linear growth retardation, delayed weight gain, low plasma cortisol levels, and absence of response to ACTH stimulation. Manifestations of intracranial hypertension include bulging fontanelles, headaches, and bilateral papilledema.

Administration of topical corticosteroids to children should be limited to the least amount compatible with an effective therapeutic regimen. Chronic corticosteroid therapy may interfere with the growth and development of children.

Uticort (Betamethasone Benzoate) Gel/Cream/Ointment/ Lotion are not for ophthalmic use.

ADVERSE REACTIONS

The following local adverse reactions are reported infrequently with topical corticosteroids, but may occur more frequently with the use of occlusive dressings. These reactions are listed in an approximate decreasing order of occurrence.

Burning
Itching
Irritation
Dryness
Folliculitis
Hypertrichosis
Acneiform eruptions
Hypopigmentation
Perioral dermatitis
Allergic contact dermatitis
Maceration of the skin
Secondary infection
Skin atrophy
Striae
Miliaria

OVERDOSAGE

Topically applied corticosteroids can be absorbed in sufficient amounts to produce systemic effects (See *PRECAUTIONS*).

DOSAGE AND ADMINISTRATION

Topical corticosteroids are generally applied to the affected area as a thin film from two to four times daily depending on the severity of the condition.

Occlusive dressings may be used for the management of psoriasis or recalcitrant conditions.

If an infection develops, the use of occlusive dressings should be discontinued and appropriate antimicrobial therapy instituted.

HOW SUPPLIED

Uticort Gel 0.025% is supplied as:

N 0071-3025-11—15 gram tube

N 0071-3025-15—60 gram tube

Each gram of Uticort Gel contains 0.25 mg of betamethasone benzoate

Uticort Cream 0.025% is supplied as:

N 0071-3027-11—15 gram tube

N 0071-3027-15—60 gram tube

Each gram of Uticort Cream contains 0.25 mg of betamethasone benzoate

Uticort Ointment 0.025% is supplied as:

N 0071-3026-11—15 gram tube

N 0071-3026-15—60 gram tube

Each gram of Uticort Ointment contains 0.25 mg of betamethasone benzoate

Uticort Lotion 0.025% is supplied as:

N 0071-3029-11—15 ml plastic bottle

N 0071-3029-15—60 ml plastic bottle

US Patent Nos. 3,529,060 and 3,749,773

Store between 59°-86° F.

3026G010

Shown in Product Identification Section, page 421

VIRA-A® ℞

[*vī"rā ā'*]

(vidarabine concentrate for infusion, USP)

DESCRIPTION

Vira-A is the trade name for vidarabine (also known as adenine arabinoside and Ara-A), an antiviral drug. Vira-A is a purine nucleoside obtained from fermentation cultures of *Streptomyces antibioticus.* Each milliliter of sterile suspen-

Continued on next page

This product information was prepared in August, 1986. On these and other Parke-Davis Products, information may be obtained by addressing PARKE-DAVIS, Division of Warner-Lambert Company, Morris Plains, New Jersey 07950.

Parke-Davis—Cont.

sion contains 200 milligrams of vidarabine monohydrate equivalent to 187.4 milligrams of vidarabine. Each milliliter contains 0.1 milligrams Phemerol® (benzethonium chloride) as a preservative; sodium phosphate, USP, 1.8 milligrams, and sodium biphosphate, USP, 4.8 milligrams, as buffering agents. Hydrochloric acid may have been added to adjust pH. Vira-A is a white, crystalline solid with this empirical formula: $C_{10}H_{13}N_5O_4.H_20$. The molecular weight is 285.2; the solubility is 0.45 mg/ml at 25 C; and the melting point ranges from 260 to 270 C. The chemical name is 9-β-D-arabinofuranosyladenine monohydrate.

CLINICAL PHARMACOLOGY

Following intravenous administration, Vira-A is rapidly deaminated into arabinosylhypoxanthine (Ara-Hx), the principal metabolite, which is promptly distributed into the tissues. Peak Ara-Hx and Ara-A plasma levels ranging from 3 to 6 μg/ml and 0.2 to 0.4 μg/ml, respectively, are attained after slow intravenous infusion of Vira-A doses of 10 mg/kg of body weight. These levels reflect the rate of infusion and show no accumulation across time. The mean half-life of Ara-Hx is 3.3 hours. Ara-Hx penetrates into the cerebrospinal fluid (CSF) to give a CSF/plasma ratio of approximately 1:3.

Excretion of Vira-A is principally via the kidneys. Urinary excretion is constant over 24 hours. Forty-one to 53% of the daily dose is recovered in the urine as Ara-Hx with 1 to 3% appearing as the parent compound. There is no evidence of fecal excretion of drug or metabolites. In patients with impaired renal function Ara-Hx may accumulate in the plasma and reach levels several-fold higher than those described above.

Vira-A possesses *in vitro* and *in vivo* antiviral activity against Herpes simplex virus types 1 and 2, and *in vitro* activity against varicella-zoster virus.

The antiviral mechanism of action has not yet been established. The drug is converted into nucleotides which appear to be involved with the inhibition of viral replication. In KB cells infected with Herpes simplex virus type 1, Vira-A inhibits viral DNA synthesis. Vira-A is rapidly deaminated to Ara-Hx, the principal metabolite, in cell cultures, laboratory animals, and humans.

Ara-Hx also possesses *in vitro* antiviral activity but this activity is significantly less than the activity of Vira-A.

INDICATIONS AND USAGE

Herpes Simplex Virus Encephalitis—Vira-A is indicated in the treatment of Herpes simplex virus encephalitis. Controlled studies indicated that Vira-A therapy will reduce the mortality caused by Herpes simplex virus encephalitis from 70 to 28% 30 days following onset. In a larger uncontrolled study of 75 patients with biopsy-proven herpes simplex encephalitis, the mortality 6 months from onset was 39%, similar to 44% in the initial controlled study at 6 months.

Morbidity from both studies one year after onset was: normal 53%, moderately debilitated 29%, and severely damaged 18%. Vira-A does not appear to alter morbidity and resulting serious neurological sequelae in the comatose patient. Therefore early diagnosis and treatment are essential.

Herpes simplex virus encephalitis should be suspected in patients with a history of an acute febrile encephalopathy associated with disordered mentation, altered level of consciousness and focal cerebral signs.

Studies which may support the suspected diagnosis include examination of cerebrospinal fluid and localization of an intra-cerebral lesion by brain scan, electroencephalography or computerized axial tomography (CAT).

Brain biopsy is required in order to confirm the etiological diagnosis by means of viral isolation in cell cultures.

Detection of Herpes simplex virus in the biopsied brain tissue can also be reliably done by specific fluorescent antibody techniques. Detection of Herpes virus-like particles by electron microscopy or detection of intranuclear inclusions by histopathologic techniques only provides a presumptive diagnosis.

Herpes zoster—Vira-A is indicated in the treatment of herpes zoster (shingles) due to reactivated varicella-zoster virus infections in immunosuppressed patients. Placebo-controlled studies have shown that Vira-A significantly reduced the severity of acute pain, new vesicle formation, time to pustulation and scabbing, cutaneous dissemination inside and outside the primary dermatome(s), and the overall frequency of visceral complications (uveitis or keratitis, hepatitis, encephalitis and peripheral neuropathy). To be effective, Vira-A therapy should be initiated as early as possible, within 72 hours after the appearance of vesicular lesions.

Herpes zoster is recognized by the formation of clear skin vesicles progressing to pustules and scabs along a sensory nerve distribution. The appearance of vesicles may be preceded by fever, local pain and erythema. Varicella-zoster virus can be isolated from vesicular lesions or detected by fluorescent antibody techniques.

CONTRAINDICATIONS

Vira-A is contraindicated in patients who develop hypersensitivity reactions to it.

WARNINGS

Vira-A should not be administered by the intramuscular or subcutaneous route because of its low solubility and poor absorption.

There are no reports available to indicate that Vira-A for infusion is effective in the management of encephalitis due to varicella-zoster or vaccinia viruses. Vira-A is not effective against infections caused by adenovirus or RNA viruses. It is also not effective against bacterial or fungal infections. There are no data to support efficacy of Vira-A against cytomegalovirus, vaccinia virus, or smallpox virus.

PRECAUTIONS

General—Treatment should be discontinued in the patient with a brain biopsy negative for Herpes simplex virus in cell culture.

Special care should be exercised when administering Vira-A to patients susceptible to fluid overloading or cerebral edema. Examples are patients with CNS infections and impaired renal function.

Patients with impaired renal function, such as post-operative renal transplant recipients, may have a slower rate of renal excretion of Ara-Hx. Therefore, the dose of Vira-A may need to be adjusted according to the severity of impairment. These patients should be carefully monitored.

Patients with impaired liver function should also be observed for possible adverse effects.

Although clear evidence of adverse experience in humans from simultaneous Vira-A and allopurinol administration has not been reported, laboratory studies indicate that allopurinol may interfere with Vira-A metabolism. Therefore, caution is recommended when administering Vira-A to patients receiving allopurinol.

Laboratory Tests—Appropriate hematologic tests are recommended during Vira-A administration since hemoglobin, hematocrit, white blood cells, and platelets may be depressed during therapy.

Some degree of immunocompetence must be present in order for Vira-A to achieve clinical response.

Carcinogenesis—Chronic parenteral (IM) studies of vidarabine have been conducted in mice and rats.

In the mouse study, there was a statistically significant increase in liver tumor incidence among the vidarabine-treated females. In the same study, some vidarabine-treated male mice developed kidney neoplasia. No renal tumors were found in the vehicle-treated control mice or the vidarabine-treated female mice.

In the rat study, intestinal, testicular, and thyroid neoplasia occurred with greater frequency among the vidarabine-treated animals than in the vehicle-treated controls. The increases in thyroid adenoma incidence in the high-dose (50 mg/kg) males and the low-dose (30 mg/kg) females were statistically significant.

Hepatic megalocytosis, associated with vidarabine treatment, has been found in short- and long-term rodent (rat and mouse) studies. It is not clear whether or not this represents a preneoplastic change.

In the Balb/3T3 *in vitro* neoplastic transformation assay, used to provide preliminary assessment of potential oncogenicity, vidarabine induced a significant and dose-related increase in transformed foci over the concentration range of 0.5–3.0 μg/ml.

Mutagenesis—Results of *in vitro* experiments indicate that vidarabine can be incorporated into mammalian DNA and can induce mutation in mammalian cells (mouse L5178Y cell line). Thus far, *in vivo* studies have not been as conclusive, but there is some evidence (dominant lethal assay in mice) that vidarabine may be capable of producing mutagenic effects in male germ cells.

It has also been reported that vidarabine causes chromosome breaks and gaps when added to human leukocytes *in vitro*. While the significance of these effects in terms of mutagenicity is not fully understood, there is a well-known correlation between the ability of various agents to produce such effects and their ability to produce heritable genetic damage.

Pregnancy Category C—Vira-A given parenterally is teratogenic in rats and rabbits. Doses of 5 mg/kg or higher given intramuscularly to pregnant rabbits during organogenesis induced fetal abnormalities. Doses of 3 mg/kg or less did not induce teratogenic changes in pregnant rabbits. Vira-A doses ranging from 30 to 250 mg/kg were given intramuscularly to pregnant rats during organogenesis; signs of maternal toxicity were induced at doses of 100 mg/kg or higher and frank fetal anomalies were found at doses of 150 to 250 mg/kg.

A safe dose for the human embryo or fetus has not been established.

There are no adequate and well controlled studies in pregnant women. Vira-A should be used during pregnancy only if the potential benefit justifies the potential risk to the fetus.

Nursing Mothers—It is not known whether Vira-A is excreted in human milk. Because many drugs are excreted in human milk and because of the potential tumorigenicity shown for Vira-A in animal studies, a decision should be made whether to discontinue nursing or to discontinue the drug, taking into account the importance of the drug to the mother.

ADVERSE REACTIONS

The principal adverse reactions involve the gastrointestinal tract and are anorexia, nausea, vomiting, and diarrhea. These reactions are mild to moderate, and seldom require termination of Vira-A therapy.

CNS disturbances have been reported at therapeutic doses. These are tremor, dizziness, hallucinations, confusion, psychosis, ataxia, headache and encephalopathy.

Hematologic clinical laboratory changes noted in controlled and uncontrolled studies were a decrease in hemoglobin or hematocrit, white blood cell count, and platelet count. SGOT elevations were also observed. Other changes occasionally observed were decreases in reticulocyte count and elevated total bilirubin.

Other symptoms which have been reported are weight loss, malaise, pruritus, rash, hematemesis, and pain at the injection site.

OVERDOSAGE

Acute massive overdose of the intravenous form has been reported without any serious evidence of adverse effect. Because of the low solubility of Vira-A, acute water overloading would pose a greater threat to the patient than Vira-A. Doses of Vira-A over 20 mg/kg/day can produce bone marrow depression with concomitant thrombocytopenia and leukopenia. If a massive overdose of the intravenous form occurs, hematologic, liver, and renal functions should be carefully monitored.

DOSAGE AND ADMINISTRATION

CAUTION— THE CONTENTS OF THE VIAL MUST BE DILUTED IN AN APPROPRIATE INTRAVENOUS SOLUTION PRIOR TO ADMINISTRATION. RAPID OR BOLUS INJECTION MUST BE AVOIDED.

Dosage— **Herpes simplex virus encephalitis**—15 mg/kg/day for 10 days.
Herpes zoster—10 mg/kg/day for 5 days.

Method of Preparation—Each 5-ml vial contains 1 gram of Vira-A (200 mg per ml of suspension). The solubility of Vira-A in intravenous infusion fluids is limited. Each one mg of Vira-A requires 2.22 ml of intravenous infusion fluid for complete solubilization. Therefore, each one liter of intravenous infusion fluid will solubilize a maximum of 450 mg of Vira-A.

Any appropriate intravenous solution is suitable for use as a diluent *EXCEPT* biologic or colloidal fluids (e.g., blood products, protein solutions, etc.).

Shake the Vira-A vial well to obtain a homogeneous suspension before measuring and transferring.

Prepare the Vira-A solution for intravenous administration by aseptically transferring the proper dose of Vira-A into an appropriate intravenous infusion fluid. The intravenous infusion fluid used to prepare the Vira-A solution should be prewarmed to 35° to 40°C (95° to 100°F) to facilitate solution of the drug following its transference. Depending on the dose to be given, more than one liter of intravenous infusion fluid may be required. Thoroughly agitate the prepared admixture until *completely* clear. Complete solubilization of the drug, as indicated by a completely clear solution, is ascertained by careful visual inspection. Final filtration with an in-line membrane filter (0.45 μ pore size or smaller) is necessary.

Dilution should be made just prior to administration and used at least within 48 hours. Subsequent agitation, shaking, or inversion of the bottle is unnecessary once the drug is completely in solution. DO NOT REFRIGERATE THE DILUTION.

Administration—Using aseptic technique, slowly infuse the total daily dose by intravenous infusion (prepared as discussed above) at a constant rate over a 12- to 24-hour period.

HOW SUPPLIED

N 0071-4150-08 (Steri-Vial® 4150) Vira-A (Vidarabine Concentrate for Infusion, USP), a sterile suspension containing 200 mg/ml, is supplied in 5 ml Steri-Vials; packages of 10.

ANIMAL PHARMACOLOGY AND TOXICITY

Acute Toxicity: The intraperitoneal LD_{50} for Vira-A ranged from 3,890 to 4,500 mg/kg in mice, and from 2,239 to 2,512 mg/kg in rats, suggesting a low order of toxicity to a single parenteral dose. Hepatic megalocytosis was observed in rats after single, intraperitoneal injections at doses near and exceeding the LD_{50} value. The hepatic megalocytosis appeared to regress completely over several months. Acute intravenous LD_{50} values could not be obtained because of the limited solubility of Vira-A.

Subacute Toxicity: Rats, dogs, and monkeys have been given daily intramuscular injections of Vira-A as a 20% suspension for 28 days. These animal species showed dose related decreases in hemoglobin, hematocrit, and lymphocytes. Bone marrow depression was also observed in monkeys. Except for localized, injection-site injury and weight gain inhibition or loss, rats tolerated daily doses up to 150 mg/kg, and dogs tolerated daily doses up to 50 mg/kg. Megalocytosis was not seen in the rats dosed by the intramuscular route for 28 days. Rhesus monkeys were particularly sensitive to Vira-A. Daily intramuscular doses of 15 mg/kg were tolerable, but doses of 25 mg/kg or higher induced progressively severe clinical signs of CNS toxicity. Three monkeys given slow intravenous infusions of Vira-A in solution at a dose of 15 mg/kg daily for 28 days had no significant adverse reactions.

4150G021

VIRA-A® ℞

[*vī″rā ā′*]

(vidarabine ophthalmic ointment, USP), 3%

DESCRIPTION

VIRA-A is the trade name for vidarabine (also known as adenine arabinoside and Ara-A), an antiviral drug for the topical treatment of epithelial keratitis caused by Herpes simplex virus. The chemical name is 9-β-D-arabinofuranosyladenine. Each gram of the ophthalmic ointment contains 30 mg of vidarabine monohydrate equivalent to 28.11 mg of vidarabine in a sterile, inert, petrolatum base.

CLINICAL PHARMACOLOGY

Vira-A is a purine nucleoside obtained from fermentation cultures of *Streptomyces antibioticus*. Vira-A possesses *in vitro* and *in vivo* antiviral activity against Herpes simplex types 1 and 2, Varicella-Zoster, and Vaccinia viruses. Except for Rhabdovirus and Oncornavirus, Vira-A does not display *in vitro* antiviral activity against other RNA or DNA viruses, including Adenovirus.

The antiviral mechanism of action has not been established. Vira-A appears to interfere with the early steps of viral DNA synthesis. Vira-A is rapidly deaminated to arabinosyl-hypoxanthine (Ara-Hx), the principal metabolite. Ara-Hx also possesses *in vitro* antiviral activity but this activity is less than that of Vira-A. Because of the low solubility of Vira-A, trace amounts of both Vira-A and Ara-Hx can be detected in the aqueous humor only if there is an epithelial defect in the cornea. If the cornea is normal, only trace amounts of Ara-Hx can be recovered from the aqueous humor.

Systemic absorption of Vira-A should not be expected to occur following ocular administration and swallowing lacrimal secretions. In laboratory animals, Vira-A is rapidly deaminated in the gastrointestinal tract to Ara-Hx.

In contrast to topical idoxuridine, Vira-A demonstrated less cellular toxicity in the regenerating corneal epithelium in the rabbit.

INDICATIONS AND USAGE

Vira-A Ophthalmic Ointment, 3%, is indicated for the treatment of acute keratoconjunctivitis and recurrent epithelial keratitis due to Herpes simplex virus types 1 and 2. It is also effective in superficial keratitis caused by Herpes simplex virus which has not responded to topical idoxuridine or when toxic or hypersensitivity reactions to idoxuridine have occurred. The effectiveness of Vira-A Ophthalmic Ointment, 3%, against stromal keratitis and uveitis due to Herpes simplex virus has not been established.

The clinical diagnosis of keratitis caused by Herpes simplex virus is usually established by the presence of typical dendritic or geographic lesions on slit-lamp examination.

In controlled and uncontrolled clinical trials, an average of seven and nine days of continuous Vira-A Ophthalmic Ointment, 3%, therapy was required to achieve corneal re-epithelialization. In the controlled trials, 70 of 81 subjects (86%) re-epithelialized at the end of three weeks of therapy. In the uncontrolled trials, 101 of 142 subjects (71%) re-epithelialized at the end of three weeks. Seventy-five percent of the subjects in these uncontrolled trials had either not healed previously or had developed hypersensitivity to topical idoxuridine therapy.

The following topical antibiotics: gentamicin, erythromycin, and chloramphenicol; or topical steroids: prednisolone or dexamethasone, have been administered concurrently with Vira-A Ophthalmic Ointment, 3%, without an increase in adverse reactions.

CONTRAINDICATION

Vira-A Ophthalmic Ointment, 3%, is contraindicated in patients who develop hypersensitivity reactions to it.

WARNINGS

Normally, corticosteroids alone are contraindicated in Herpes simplex virus infections of the eye. If Vira-A Ophthalmic Ointment, 3%, is administered concurrently with topical corticosteroid therapy, corticosteroid-induced ocular side effects must be considered. These include corticosteroid-induced glaucoma or cataract formation and progression of a bacterial or viral infection.

Vira-A is not effective against RNA virus or adenoviral ocular infections. It is also not effective against bacterial, fungal, or chlamydial infections of the cornea or nonviral trophic ulcers.

Although viral resistance to VIRA-A has not been observed, this possibility may exist.

PRECAUTIONS

General—The diagnosis of keratoconjunctivitis due to Herpes simplex virus should be established clinically prior to prescribing VIRA-A Ophthalmic Ointment, 3%.

Patients should be forewarned that VIRA-A Ophthalmic Ointment, 3%, like any ophthalmic ointment, may produce a temporary visual haze.

Carcinogenesis—Chronic parenteral (IM) studies of vidarabine have been conducted in mice and rats.

In the mouse study, there was a statistically significant increase in liver tumor incidence among the vidarabine-treated females. In the same study some vidarabine-treated male mice developed kidney neoplasia. No renal tumors were found in the vehicle-treated control mice or the vidarabine-treated female mice.

In the rat study, intestinal, testicular, and thyroid neoplasia occurred with greater frequency among the vidarabine-treated animals than in the vehicle-treated controls. The increases in thyroid adenoma incidence in the high dose (50 mg/kg) males and the low dose (30 mg/kg) females were statistically significant.

Hepatic megalocytosis, associated with vidarabine treatment, has been found in short- and long-term rodent (rat and mouse) studies. It is not clear whether or not this represents a preneoplastic change.

The recommended frequency and duration of administration should not be exceeded (See Dosage and Administration).

Mutagenesis—Results of *in vitro* experiments indicate that vidarabine can be incorporated into mammalian DNA and can induce mutation in mammalian cells (mouse L5178Y cell line). Thus far, *in vivo* studies have not been as conclusive, but there is some evidence (dominant lethal assay in mice) that vidarabine may be capable of producing mutagenic effects in male germ cells.

It has also been reported that vidarabine causes chromosome breaks and gaps when added to human leukocytes *in vitro*. While the significance of these effects in terms of mutagenicity is not fully understood, there is a well-known correlation between the ability of various agents to produce such effects and their ability to produce heritable genetic damage.

Pregnancy Category C—VIRA-A parenterally is teratogenic in rats and rabbits. Ten percent VIRA-A ointment applied to 10% of the body surface during organogenesis induced fetal abnormalities in rabbits. When 10% VIRA-A ointment was applied to 2% to 3% of the body surface of rabbits, no fetal abnormalities were found. This dose greatly exceeds the total recommended ophthalmic dose in humans. The possibility of embryonic or fetal damage in pregnant women receiving VIRA-A Ophthalmic Ointment, 3%, is remote. The topical ophthalmic dose is small, and the drug relatively insoluble. Its ocular penetration is very low. However, a safe dose for a human embryo or fetus has not been established. There are no adequate and well controlled studies in pregnant women. VIRA-A should be used during pregnancy only if the potential benefit justifies the potential risk to the fetus.

Nursing Mothers—It is not known whether VIRA-A is secreted in human milk. Because many drugs are excreted in human milk and because of the potential for tumorigenicity shown for VIRA-A in animal studies, a decision should be made whether to discontinue nursing or to discontinue the drug, taking into account the importance of the drug to the mother. However, breast milk excretion is unlikely because VIRA-A is rapidly deaminated in the gastrointestinal tract.

ADVERSE REACTIONS

Lacrimation, foreign body sensation, conjunctival injection, burning, irritation, superficial punctate keratitis, pain, photophobia, punctal occlusion, and sensitivity have been reported with VIRA-A Ophthalmic Ointment, 3%. The following have also been reported but appear disease-related: uveitis, stromal edema, secondary glaucoma, trophic defects, corneal vascularization, and hyphema.

OVERDOSAGE

Acute massive overdosage by oral ingestion of the ophthalmic ointment has not occurred. However, the rapid deamination to arabinosylhypoxanthine should preclude any difficulty. The oral LD_{50} for vidarabine is greater than 5020 mg/kg in mice and rats. No untoward effects should result from ingestion of the entire contents of a tube.

Overdosage by ocular instillation is unlikely because any excess should be quickly expelled from the conjunctival sac. Too frequent administration should be avoided.

DOSAGE AND ADMINISTRATION

Administer approximately one half inch of VIRA-A Ophthalmic Ointment, 3%, into the lower conjunctival sac five times daily at three-hour intervals.

If there are no signs of improvement after 7 days, or complete re-epithelialization has not occurred by 21 days, other forms of therapy should be considered. Some severe cases may require longer treatment.

After re-epithelialization has occurred, treatment for an additional seven days at a reduced dosage (such as twice daily) is recommended in order to prevent recurrence.

HOW SUPPLIED

N 0071-3677-07 (Stock 18-1677-139)

VIRA-A Ophthalmic Ointment, 3%, is supplied sterile in ophthalmic ointment tubes of 3.5 g. The base is a 60:40 mixture of solid and liquid petrolatum.

3677G020

Shown in Product Identification Section, page 421

ZARONTIN® ℞

[*ză″rŏn′tĭn*]

(ethosuximide, USP)

Capsules

DESCRIPTION

Zarontin (ethosuximide) is an anticonvulsant succinimide, chemically designated as alpha-ethyl-alpha-methyl-succinimide.

Each Zarontin capsule contains 250 mg ethosuximide, USP. Also contains: polyethylene glycol 400, NF. The capsule contains D&C yellow No. 10; FD&C red No. 3; gelatin, NF; glycerin, USP; and sorbitol.

ACTION

Ethosuximide suppresses the paroxysmal three-cycle-per-second spike and wave activity associated with lapses of consciousness which is common in absence (petit mal) seizures. The frequency of epileptiform attacks is reduced, apparently by depression of the motor cortex and elevation of the threshold of the central nervous system to convulsive stimuli.

INDICATION

Zarontin is indicated for the control of absence (petit mal) epilepsy.

CONTRAINDICATION

Ethosuximide should not be used in patients with a history of hypersensitivity to succinimides.

WARNINGS

Blood dyscrasias, including some with fatal outcome, have been reported to be associated with the use of ethosuximide; therefore, periodic blood counts should be performed.

Ethosuximide is capable of producing morphological and functional changes in the animal liver. In humans, abnormal liver and renal function studies have been reported.

Ethosuximide should be administered with extreme caution to patients with known liver or renal diseases. Periodic urinalysis and liver function studies are advised for all patients receiving the drug.

Cases of systemic lupus erythematosus have been reported with the use of ethosuximide. The physician should be alert to this possibility.

Usage in Pregnancy: The effects of Zarontin in human pregnancy and nursing infants are unknown.

Recent reports suggest an association between the use of anticonvulsant drugs by women with epilepsy and an elevated incidence of birth defects in children born to these women. Data are more extensive with respect to phenytoin and phenobarbital, but these are also the most commonly prescribed anticonvulsants. Less systematic or anecdotal reports suggest a possible similar association with the use of all known anticonvulsant drugs.

The reports suggesting an elevated incidence of birth defects in children of drug-treated epileptic women cannot be regarded as adequate to prove a definite cause-and-effect relationship. There are intrinsic methodologic problems in obtaining adequate data on drug teratogenicity in humans. The possibility also exists that other factors, eg, genetic factors or the epileptic condition itself, may be more important than drug therapy in leading to birth defects. The great majority of mothers on anticonvulsant medication deliver normal infants. It is important to note that anticonvulsant drugs should not be discontinued in patients in whom the drug is administered to prevent major seizures because of the strong possibility of precipitating status epilepticus with attendant hypoxia and threat to life. In individual cases where the severity and frequency of the seizure disorder are such that the removal of medication does not pose a serious threat to the patient, discontinuation of the drug may be considered prior to and during pregnancy, although it cannot be said with any confidence that even minor seizures do not pose some hazard to the developing embryo or fetus.

Continued on next page

This product information was prepared in August, 1986. On these and other Parke-Davis Products, information may be obtained by addressing PARKE-DAVIS, Division of Warner-Lambert Company, Morris Plains, New Jersey 07950.

Parke-Davis—Cont.

The prescribing physician will wish to weigh these considerations in treating or counseling epileptic women of childbearing potential.

Hazardous Activities: Ethosuximide may impair the mental and/or physical abilities required for the performance of potentially hazardous tasks, such as driving a motor vehicle or other such activity requiring alertness; therefore, the patient should be cautioned accordingly.

PRECAUTIONS

Ethosuximide, when used alone in mixed types of epilepsy, may increase the frequency of grand mal seizures in some patients.

As with other anticonvulsants, it is important to proceed slowly when increasing or decreasing dosage, as well as when adding or eliminating other medication. Abrupt withdrawal of anticonvulsant medication may precipitate absence (petit mal) status.

ADVERSE REACTIONS

Gastrointestinal System: Gastrointestinal symptoms occur frequently and include anorexia, vague gastric upset, nausea and vomiting, cramps, epigastric and abdominal pain, weight loss, and diarrhea.

Hemopoietic System: Hemopoietic complications associated with the administration of ethosuximide have included leukopenia, agranulocytosis, pancytopenia, aplastic anemia, and eosinophilia.

Nervous System: Neurologic and sensory reactions reported during therapy with ethosuximide have included drowsiness, headache, dizziness, euphoria, hiccups, irritability, hyperactivity, lethargy, fatigue, and ataxia. Psychiatric or psychological aberrations associated with ethosuximide administration have included disturbances of sleep, night terrors, inability to concentrate, and aggressiveness. These effects may be noted particularly in patients who have previously exhibited psychological abnormalities. There have been rare reports of paranoid psychosis, increased libido, and increased state of depression with overt suicidal intentions.

Integumentary System: Dermatologic manifestations which have occurred with the administration of ethosuximide have included urticaria, Stevens-Johnson syndrome, systemic lupus erythematosus, and pruritic erythematous rashes.

Miscellaneous: Other reactions reported have included myopia, vaginal bleeding, swelling of the tongue, gum hypertrophy, and hirsutism.

DOSAGE AND ADMINISTRATION

Zarontin Capsules (ethosuximide capsules, USP): Zarontin is administered by the oral route. The initial dose for patients 3 to 6 years of age is one capsule (250 mg) per day; for patients 6 years of age and older, 2 capsules (500 mg) per day. The dose thereafter must be individualized according to the patient's response. Dosage should be increased by small increments. One useful method is to increase the daily dose by 250 mg every four to seven days until control is achieved with minimal side effects. Dosages exceeding 1.5 g daily, in divided doses, should be administered only under the strictest supervision of the physician. The *optimal* dose for most children is 20 mg/kg/day. This dose has given average plasma levels within the accepted therapeutic range of 40 to 100 mcg/ml. Subsequent dose schedules can be based on effectiveness and plasma level determinations.

Zarontin may be administered in combination with other anticonvulsants when other forms of epilepsy coexist with absence (petit mal). The *optimal* dosage for most children is 20 mg/kg/day.

HOWSUPPLIED

N 0071-0237-24 Bottle of 100. Each capsule contains 250 mg ethosuximide.

0237G022

Shown in Product Identification Section, page 422

ZARONTIN® ℞

[*ză″rŏn′tĭn*]

(ethosuximide)

Syrup

DESCRIPTION

Zarontin (ethosuximide) is an anticonvulsant succinimide, chemically designated as alpha-ethyl-alpha-methyl-succinimide.

Each teaspoonful (5 ml), for oral administration, contains 250 mg ethosuximide, USP. Also contains citric acid; anhydrous, USP; FD&C red No. 40; FD&C yellow No. 6; flavor; glycerin, USP; purified water, USP; saccharin sodium, USP; sodium benzoate, NF; sodium citrate, USP; sucrose, NF.

CLINICAL PHARMACOLOGY

Ethosuximide suppresses the paroxysmal three cycle per second spike and wave activity associated with lapses of consciousness which is common in absence (petit mal) seizures. The frequency of epileptiform attacks is reduced, apparently by depression of the motor cortex and elevation of the threshold of the central nervous system to convulsive stimuli.

INDICATION AND USAGE

Zarontin is indicated for the control of absence (petit mal) epilepsy.

CONTRAINDICATION

Ethosuximide should not be used in patients with a history of hypersensitivity to succinimides.

WARNINGS

Blood dyscrasias, including some with fatal outcome, have been reported to be associated with the use of ethosuximide; therefore, periodic blood counts should be performed. Ethosuximide is capable of producing morphological and functional changes in the animal liver. In humans, abnormal liver and renal function studies have been reported.

Ethosuximide should be administered with extreme caution to patients with known liver or renal disease. Periodic urinalysis and liver function studies are advised for all patients receiving the drug.

Cases of systemic lupus erythematosus have been reported with the use of ethosuximide. The physician should be alert to this possibility.

Hazardous Activities: Ethosuximide may impair the mental and/or physical abilities required for the performance of potentially hazardous tasks, such as driving a motor vehicle or other such activity requiring alertness; therefore, the patient should be cautioned accordingly.

Usage in Pregnancy: The effects of Zarontin in human pregnancy and nursing infants are unknown.

Recent reports suggest an association between the use of anticonvulsant drugs by women with epilepsy and an elevated incidence of birth defects in children born to these women. Data are more extensive with respect to phenytoin and phenobarbital, but these are also the most commonly prescribed anticonvulsants; less systematic or anecdotal reports suggest a possible similar association with the use of all known anticonvulsant drugs.

The reports suggesting an elevated incidence of birth defects in children of drug-treated epileptic women cannot be regarded as adequate to prove a definite cause and effect relationship. There are intrinsic methodologic problems in obtaining adequate data on drug teratogenicity in humans; the possibility also exists that other factors, eg. genetic factors or the epileptic condition itself, may be more important than drug therapy in leading to birth defects. The great majority of mothers on anticonvulsant medication deliver normal infants. It is important to note that anticonvulsant drugs should not be discontinued in patients in whom the drug is administered to prevent major seizures because of the strong possibility of precipitating status epilepticus with attendant hypoxia and threat to life. In individual cases where the severity and frequency of the seizure disorder are such that the removal of medication does not pose a serious threat to the patient, discontinuation of the drug may be considered prior to and during pregnancy, although it cannot be said with any confidence that even minor seizures do not pose some hazard to the developing embryo or fetus.

The prescribing physician will wish to weigh these considerations in treating or counseling epileptic women of childbearing potential.

PRECAUTIONS

General: Ethosuximide, when used alone in mixed types of epilepsy, may increase the frequency of grand mal seizures in some patients.

As with other anticonvulsants, it is important to proceed slowly when increasing or decreasing dosage, as well as when adding or eliminating other medication. Abrupt withdrawal of anticonvulsant medication may precipitate absence (petit mal) status.

Information for Patient: Ethosuximide may impair the mental and/or physical abilities required for the performance of potentially hazardous tasks such as driving a motor vehicle or other such activity requiring alertness; therefore, the patient should be cautioned accordingly.

Pregnancy: See WARNINGS

ADVERSE REACTIONS

Gastrointestinal System: Gastrointestinal symptoms occur frequently and include anorexia, vague gastric upset, nausea and vomiting, cramps, epigastric and abdominal pain, weight loss, and diarrhea.

Hemopoietic System: Hemopoietic complications associated with the administration of ethosuximide have included leukopenia, agranulocytosis, pancytopenia, aplastic anemia, and eosinophilia.

Nervous System: Neurologic and sensory reactions reported during therapy with ethosuximide have included drowsiness, headache, dizziness, euphoria, hiccups, irritability, hyperactivity, lethargy, fatigue, and ataxia.

Psychiatric or psychological aberrations associated with ethosuximide administration have included disturbances of sleep, night terrors, inability to concentrate, and aggressiveness. These effects may be noted particularly in patients who have previously exhibited psychological abnormalities. There have been rare reports of paranoid psychosis, increased libido, and increased state of depression with overt suicidal intentions.

Integumentary System: Dermatologic manifestations which have occurred with the administration of ethosuximide have included urticaria, Stevens-Johnson syndrome, systemic lupus erythematosus, and pruritic erythematous rashes.

Miscellaneous: Other reactions reported have included myopia, vaginal bleeding, swelling of the tongue, gum hypertrophy, and hirsutism.

DOSAGE AND ADMINISTRATION

Zarontin is administered by the oral route. The *initial* dose for patients 3 to 6 years of age is one teaspoonful (250 mg) per day; for patients 6 years of age and older, 2 teaspoonfuls (500 mg) per day. The dose thereafter must be individualized according to the patient's response. Dosage should be increased by small increments. One useful method is to increase the daily dose by 250 mg every four to seven days until control is achieved with minimal side effects. Dosages exceeding 1.5 g daily, in divided doses, should be administered only under the strictest supervision of the physician. The *optimal* dose for most children is 20 mg/kg/day. This dose has given average plasma levels within the accepted therapeutic range of 40 to 100 mcg/ml. Subsequent dose schedules can be based on effectiveness and plasma level determinations.

Zarontin may be administered in combination with other anticonvulsants when other forms of epilepsy coexist with absence (petit mal). The optimal dose for most children is 20 mg/kg/day.

HOW SUPPLIED

Zarontin is supplied as:

N0071-2418-23–1 pint bottles. Each 5 ml of syrup contains 250 mg ethosuximide in a raspberry flavored base. Store below 30°C (86°F). Protect from freezing and light.

Zarontin is also supplied in the following form:

N0071-0237-24–Bottle of 100. Each capsule contains 250 mg ethosuximide. Store below 30°C (86°F).

2418G022

Pedinol Pharmacal Inc.

30 BANFI PLAZA NORTH
FARMINGDALE, N.Y. 11735

BREEZEE MIST FOOT POWDER OTC

COMPOSITION

Aluminum Chlorhydrate, Menthol, Undecylenic Acid, contains no Fluorocarbons.

INDICATIONS

Topical treatment for hyperhidrosis, bromidrosis and tinea pedis (athlete's foot).

HOW SUPPLIED

4 oz. aerosol can.

CASTELLANI PAINT ℞

COMPOSITION

Basic Fuchsin, Phenol, Resorcinol, Acetone, Alcohol. Colorless—without Basic Fuchsin.

INDICATIONS

Topical antifungal agent for macerations and ulcerations.

CAUTION

Federal law prohibits dispensing without prescription.

PRECAUTIONS

If irritation or sensitivity develops, discontinue treatment and consult podiatrist or physician.

ADMINISTRATION

Apply to affected areas once or twice a day.

HOW SUPPLIED

1 oz. and 1 pt. plastic bottle.

FUNGOID CREME and SOLUTION ℞

COMPOSITION

Cetyl Pyridinium Chloride, Triacetin, Chloroxylenol, Vanishing Creme Base and Oil Base Solution.

INDICATIONS

Topical treatment for fungus, yeast and bacterial infections of the skin.

CAUTION
Federal law prohibits dispensing without prescription.

PRECAUTIONS
If irritation or sensitivity develops, discontinue treatment and consult podiatrist or physician.

ADMINISTRATION
Apply to affected areas three times a day.

HOW SUPPLIED
1 oz. plastic tube; 15cc plastic bottle with controlled dropper.

FUNGOID TINCTURE ℞

COMPOSITION
Cetyl Pyridinium Chloride, Triacetin, Chloroxylenol.

INDICATIONS
Topical treatment for fungus infections of the nails, tinea unguium (onychomycosis).

CAUTION
Federal law prohibits dispensing without prescription.

PRECAUTIONS
If irritation or sensitivity develops, discontinue treatment and consult podiatrist or physician.

ADMINISTRATION
Apply to affected nails twice a day.

HOW SUPPLIED
1 oz. bottle with brush applicator, 1 pt. bottle.

G-MYTICIN CREME and OINTMENT 0.1% (gentamicin sulfate 0.1%) ℞

COMPOSITION
Creme and ointment—each gram contains gentamicin sulfate equivalent to 1 mg. of gentamicin base.

INDICATIONS
Topical wide-spectrum antibiotic provides highly effective treatment in primary and secondary bacterial infections of the skin. *NOTE:* G-myticin Creme/Ointment is not effective against viruses or fungal skin infections.

ADVERSE REACTIONS
In patients with dermatoses treated with G-myticin erythema and pruritis that did not usually require discontinuance of treatment has been reported in a small percentage of cases.

CONTRAINDICATIONS
G-myticin creme/ointment, is contraindicated in those patients with a history of hypersensitivity to any of the components of this preparation.

CAUTION
Federal law prohibits dispensing without prescription.

PRECAUTIONS
The overgrowth of nonsusceptible organisms, including fungi, occasionally occurs with the use of topical antibiotics. If this occurs, or if irritation, sensitization, or superinfection develops, treatment with G-myticin should be discontinued and consult podiatrist or physician.

ADMINISTRATION
Apply 3 to 4 times daily.

HOW SUPPLIED
G-myticin Creme/Ointment—15 grm tubes.

HYDRISALIC GEL ℞

COMPOSITION
Salicyclic Acid 6%, Isopropanol, Propylene Glycol, Hydroxypropyl Cellulose.

INDICATIONS
Topical treatment for hyperkeratotic skin.

CAUTION
Federal law prohibits dispensing without prescription.

PRECAUTIONS
Use should be limited in children under 12 years of age. If irritation or sensitivity develops, discontinue treatment and consult podiatrist or physician.

ADMINISTRATION
Apply to affected area in the evening. Wash hands thoroughly following application. The medication is washed off the following morning.

HOW SUPPLIED
1 oz. plastic tubes.

HYDRISINOL CREME AND LOTION OTC

COMPOSITION
Sulfonated Hydrogenated Castor Oil, N.F. IX, Hydrogenated Vegetable Oil.

INDICATIONS
Topical emollient to soften dry, cracked, calloused skin.

ADMINISTRATION
Apply as needed.

HOW SUPPLIED
4 oz. and 1 lb. jars;
8 oz. plastic bottle.

LAZER CREME OTC

COMPOSITION
Vitamin E, 3,500 u/oz., Vitamin A, 100,000 u/oz.

INDICATIONS
To enhance post surgical regeneration of skin, revitalize lasered tissue, healing aid for post surgical lesions, keratosis and dryness of the skin.

CAUTION
FOR EXTERNAL USE ONLY. Keep out of reach of children. Keep in cool place.

ADMINISTRATION
Apply topically to affected area as often as needed or as directed by your podiatrist or physician.

HOW SUPPLIED
Available in 2 oz. plastic jar.

LAZERFORMALYDE SOLUTION ℞

COMPOSITION
Formaldehyde 10%, Polysorbate 20, Mint Fragrance, Hydroxyethyl Cellulose, Water.

INDICATIONS
Drying Agent for pre and post surgical removal of warts or for non-surgical laser treatment of warts. Anti-perspirant for treatment of hyperhidrosis and bromidosis of the feet.

CONTRAINDICATIONS
Do not use in patients known to be sensitive to any ingredients in LazerFormalyde Solution.

PRECAUTION
Check skin for sensitivity to Formaldehyde prior to application since it may be irritating and sensitizing to the skin of some patients.
If redness or irritation persists, consult your podiatrist or physician.

CAUTION
FEDERAL LAW PROHIBITS DISPENSING WITHOUT PRESCRIPTION. Keep out of reach of children. For external use only. Avoid contact with eyes or mucous membranes.

ADMINISTRATION
Apply with roll-on applicator once a day to affected areas or as directed by your podiatrist or physician.

HOW SUPPLIED
Available in 3 oz. plastic bottle with roll-on applicator.

LAZERSPORIN-C SOLUTION ℞

COMPOSITION
Neomycin Sulfate equivalent to 3.5 mg., Polymyxin B Sulfate 10,000 U, Hydrocortisone 1%.

INDICATIONS
For post surgical, post non-surgical laser and non-surgical treatment of superficial bacterial infections of the skin, nails and warts susceptible to the action of the antibiotics.

CONTRAINDICATIONS
Do not use in patients known to be sensitive to any ingredients in LazerSporin-C Solution.

WARNINGS
As with other antibiotic preparations, prolonged treatment may result in overgrowth of nonsusceptible organisms and fungi. If the infection is not improved after one week, cultures and susceptibility test should be repeated to verify the identity of the organism and to determine whether therapy should be changed.

PRECAUTION
If redness, irritation or pain and swelling persist, discontinue use and consult your podiatrist or physician.

CAUTION
FEDERAL LAW PROHIBITS DISPENSING WITHOUT A PRESCRIPTION. Keep out of reach of children. For external use only.

ADMINISTRATION
Apply to affected area 3 or 4 times a day or as directed by your podiatrist or physician.

HOW SUPPLIED
10cc bottle with sterile dropper.

OSTI-DERM LOTION OTC

COMPOSITION
Liquified Phenol, Glycerin, Zinc Oxide, Magnesium Carbonate, Aluminum Acetate Solution (Burow's Solution), Camphor Water, in a Hydrated Aluminum Silicate Gel.

INDICATIONS
Topical treatment for bromidrosis, hyperhidrosis, decubitus ulcers, blisters, itching, poison ivy and dermatitis.

PRECAUTIONS
Check skin sensitivity to phenol. If irritation or sensitivity develops, discontinue treatment and consult podiatrist or physician.

ADMINISTRATION
Apply 2–3 times a day.

HOW SUPPLIED
45cc plastic tube.

PEDI-BATH SALTS OTC

COMPOSITION
Colloidal Sulphur, Sodium, Magnesium Sulphate, Potassium Iodide, Sodium Chloride, Sodium Bicarb., Pine Needle Oil, Balsam Peru.

INDICATIONS
Topical foot bath; soak for tired aching feet.

DOSAGE AND ADMINISTRATION
Two capsful in a foot bath.

HOW SUPPLIED
6 oz. plastic bottle.

PEDI-BORO SOAK PAKS OTC

COMPOSITION
Aluminum Sulfate, Calcium Acetate, Coloring Agent.

ACTIONS
A soothing astringent wet dressing of a modified Burow's Solution, buffered.

DOSAGE AND ADMINISTRATION
Dissolve 1 or 2 paks in a pint of water. Prepare fresh daily.

HOW SUPPLIED
Box of 12 and Box of 100.

PEDI-CORT V CREME ℞

COMPOSITION
Hydrocortisone 1%, Iodochlorhydroxyquin 3%.

INDICATIONS
Topical anti-inflammatory antifungal, antibacterial, antipruritic creme for the skin.

CONTRAINDICATIONS
Hypersensitivity to any of the ingredients. Not for use in the presence of tuberculosis, vaccinia, varicella or other viral skin conditions.

CAUTION
Federal law prohibits dispensing without prescription.

PRECAUTIONS
Observe all precautions for using a steroid preparation. If irritation or sensitivity develops, discontinue treatment and consult podiatrist or physician.

ADMINISTRATION
Apply 1–3 times a day.

HOW SUPPLIED
20 gm. tubes.

Continued on next page

Pedinol—Cont.

PEDI-DRI FOOT POWDER ℞

COMPOSITION
Aluminum Chlorhydroxide, Menthol, Zinc Undecylenate, Formaldehyde.

INDICATIONS
Topical treatment for hyperhidrosis, bromidrosis and tinea pedis (athlete's foot).

CAUTION
Federal law prohibits dispensing without prescription.

PRECAUTIONS
External use only. Check for skin sensitivity to formaldehyde. If irritation or sensitivity develops, discontinue treatment and consult podiatrist or physician.

ADMINISTRATION
Apply twice a day.

HOW SUPPLIED
2 oz. plastic bottle.

PEDI-PRO FOOT POWDER OTC

COMPOSITION
Aluminum Chlorhydroxide, Chloroxylenol, Zinc Undecylenate, Menthol, Micro-Kaolin, Starch.

INDICATIONS
Athlete's Foot: Aids in temporary relief of burning, itching and cracking skin in athlete's foot.

CAUTION
External use only. Do not use near eyes or mucous membranes. Keep out of reach of children. Persons with impaired circulation, including diabetes, should consult a podiatrist before using medication. If symptoms persist consult your podiatrist or physician.

CONTRAINDICATIONS
Do not use in patients known to be sensitive to any ingredients in Pedi-Pro Foot Powder.

ADMINISTRATION
Apply twice a day.

HOW SUPPLIED
2 oz. plastic bottle.

PEDI-VIT A CREME OTC

COMPOSITION
Vitamin A, 100,000 u/oz.

INDICATIONS
Topical treatment for irritated, dry, sensitive skin.

ADMINISTRATION
Apply daily as needed.

HOW SUPPLIED
2 oz. jar and 1 lb. jar.

SALACTIC FILM ℞

COMPOSITION
Salicyclic Acid 16.7% U.S.P., Lactic Acid 16.7% U.S.P., Flexible Collodion U.S.P., Coloring Agent.

INDICATIONS
Topical treatment as a keratolytic agent for removal of verrucae.

CONTRAINDICATIONS
Diabetics or patients with impaired blood circulation. Do not use on moles, birthmarks or warts with hair growing from them.

CAUTION
Federal law prohibits dispensing without prescription.

PRECAUTIONS
Highly flammable. Keep bottle tightly capped when not in use. If irritation or sensitivity develops, discontinue treatment and consult podiatrist or physician.

ADMINISTRATION
Apply once daily as directed.

HOW SUPPLIED
½ oz. bottle with brush applicator.

UREACIN-10 LOTION OTC
UREACIN-20 CREME OTC
UREACIN-40 CREME ℞

COMPOSITION
Urea 10%, Urea 20% and 40%, Vegetable Oil Base.

INDICATIONS
Ureacin-10 Lotion, Ureacin-20 Creme is a topical treatment for rough, dry, cracked, calloused skin. Ureacin-40 Creme is indicated for the treatment of nail destruction and dissolution.

CAUTION
For Ureacin-40 Creme—Federal law prohibits dispensing without prescription.

PRECAUTIONS
If irritation or sensitivity develops, discontinue treatment and consult podiatrist or physician.

ADMINISTRATION
Rub in gently two or three times a day to affected area. Ureacin-40 Creme to be applied to diseased nail surface by podiatrist or physician only.

HOW SUPPLIED
8 oz. plastic bottle, 2½ oz. plastic jar, 1 oz. plastic jar.

For further product information please contact Pedinol Pharmacal Inc.

Pennwalt Corp.
Prescription Division
ROCHESTER, NY 14623

ADAPIN® ℞
[*ad'uh-pin"*]
(doxepin HCl)

DESCRIPTION
Adapin (doxepin HCl) is an isomeric mixture of 1-Propanamine,3-dibenz[b,e] oxepin-11 (6H) ylidene -N, N-dimethyl-,hydrochloride.
Other Ingredients in Adapin: Dye, D&C Yellow No. 10; Dye, FD&C Blue No. 1; Dye, FD&C Yellow No. 6; Gelatin; Magnesium Stearate; Sodium Lauryl Sulfate; Starch; Titanium Dioxide.

ACTIONS
Adapin has a variety of pharmacological actions with its predominant action on the central nervous system. While its mechanism of action is not known, studies have demonstrated that it is neither a monoamine oxidase inhibitor nor a primary stimulant of the central nervous system.

INDICATIONS
In controlled clinical evaluations, Adapin has shown marked antianxiety and significant antidepressant effects. Adapin has been found to be well tolerated even in elderly patients. Adapin is indicated for the treatment of patients with:
1. Psychoneurotic anxiety and/or depressive reactions.
2. Mixed symptoms of anxiety and depression.
3. Anxiety and/or depression associated with alcoholism.
4. Anxiety associated with organic disease.
5. Psychotic depressive disorders including involutional depression and manic-depressive reactions.

Target symptoms of psychoneurosis that respond particularly well to Adapin include: anxiety, tension, depression, somatic symptoms and concerns, insomnia, guilt, lack of energy, fear, apprehension and worry.
Because Adapin provides antidepressant as well as antianxiety effects, it is of particular value in patients in whom anxiety masks depression. Patients who have not responded to other antianxiety or antidepressant drugs may benefit from Adapin.

CONTRAINDICATIONS
Because Adapin has an anticholinergic effect, it is contraindicated in patients with glaucoma or a tendency toward urinary retention.
Use of Adapin is contraindicated in patients who have been found hypersensitive to it.

WARNINGS
Usage in Pregnancy: Adapin has not been evaluated in pregnant patients. Therefore, it should not be used during pregnancy unless, in the judgment of the physician, it is essential to the welfare of the patient.
In animal reproduction studies of Adapin, gross and microscopic examination of the offspring gave no evidence of drug-related teratogenic effect. Following doses of up to 25 mg./kg./day for 8 to 9 months, no changes were observed in the number of live births, litter size, or lactation. A decreased rate of conception was observed when male rats were given 25 mg./kg./day for prolonged periods —an effect which has occurred with other psychotropic drugs and has been attributed to drug effect on the central and/or autonomic nervous systems.
Usage in Children: The use of Adapin in children under 12 years of age is not recommended, because safe conditions for its use have not been established.
MAO Inhibitors: Serious side effects and even death have been reported following the concomitant use of certain drugs with MAO inhibitors. Therefore, MAO inhibitors should be discontinued at least two weeks prior to the cautious initiation of therapy with Adapin (doxepin HCl). The exact length of time may vary and is dependent upon the particular MAO inhibitor being used, the length of time it has been administered, and the dosage involved.
Alcohol: In patients who may use alcohol excessively, it should be borne in mind that the potentiation may increase the danger inherent in any suicide attempt or overdosage.

PRECAUTIONS
Drowsiness may occur with Adapin (doxepin HCl); therefore, patients should be warned of its possible occurrence and cautioned against driving a motor vehicle or operating hazardous machinery while taking the drug.
Patients should also be cautioned that the effects of alcoholic beverages may be increased.
Since suicide is an inherent risk in depressed patients and remains a risk through the initial phases of improvement, depressed patients should be closely supervised.
Although Adapin has shown effective tranquilizing activity, the possibility of activating or unmasking latent psychotic symptoms should be kept in mind.
Compounds structurally related to Adapin can block the effects of guanethidine and similarly acting compounds. However, at the usual clinical dosages, 75 mg. to 150 mg. per day, Adapin has been given concomitantly with guanethidine without blocking its antihypertensive effect. But at dosages of 300 mg. per day or higher, Adapin has exerted a significant blocking effect.
When administering cimetidine concurrently with tricyclic antidepressants, close supervision and careful adjustment of dosages are required because of the possibility of producing significant increases or decreases in the plasma concentrations of the tricyclic antidepressant.
Adapin, like other structurally related psychotropic drugs, potentiates norepinephrine response in animals. But this effect has not been observed with Adapin in humans, which is in accord with the low incidence of tachycardia reported clinically.

ADVERSE REACTIONS
Anticholinergic Effects: Dry mouth, blurred vision and constipation have been reported. These are usually mild, and often subside as therapy is continued or dosage reduced.
Central Nervous System Effects: Drowsiness has been observed. It usually occurs early in the course of therapy and tends to subside as therapy continues.
Cardiovascular Effects: Tachycardia and hypotension have been reported infrequently.
Other infrequently reported adverse effects with tricyclic antidepressants include extrapyramidal symptoms, syndrome of inappropriate ADH (antidiuretic hormone) secretion, gastrointestinal reactions, secretory effects such as increased sweating, weakness, dizziness, fatigue, weight gain, edema, paresthesias, flushing, chills, tinnitus, photophobia, decreased libido, rash, and pruritus.
Withdrawal Symptoms: Abrupt cessation of treatment after prolonged administration may produce nausea, headache and malaise. These are not indicative of addiction.

DOSAGE AND ADMINISTRATION
In most patients with mild to moderate anxiety and/or depression: A starting dose of 25 mg. t.i.d. is recommended. Decrease or increase the dosage at appropriate intervals according to individual response. Usual optimum dosage is 75 mg. to 150 mg. per day. As an alternate regimen the total daily dosage, up to 150 mg., may be given at bedtime without loss of effectiveness.
In some patients with mild symptomatology or emotional symptoms accompanying organic disease, dosage as low as 25 mg. to 50 mg. per day has provided effective control.
In more severe anxiety and/or depression: 50 mg. t.i.d. may be required to start—if necessary, gradually increase to 300 mg. per day. Additional effectiveness is rarely obtained by exceeding 300 mg. per day.
Although optimal antidepressant response may not be evident for two to three weeks, antianxiety activity is rapidly apparent.

OVERDOSAGE
Symptoms—An increase of any of the reported adverse reactions, primarily excessive sedation and anticholinergic effects such as blurred vision and dry mouth. Other effects may be: pronounced tachycardia, hypotension and extrapyramidal symptoms. Treatment—Essentially symptomatic; supportive therapy in the case of hypotension and excessive sedation.

HOW SUPPLIED

Each capsule contains doxepin, as the hydrochloride, 10 mg. (NDC 0018-0356), 25 mg. (NDC 0018-0357), 50 mg. (NDC 0018-0358), 75 mg. (NDC 0018-0361) and 100 mg (NDC 0018-0359). Capsules in bottles of 100, and 1000; 25 mg and 50 mg capsules also in bottles of 5000.

Rev 6/85

Shown in Product Identification Section, page 422

HYLOREL® Tablets ℞

[hi'lō-rel"]
(guanadrel sulfate)
10 and 25 mg

DESCRIPTION

HYLOREL Tablets for oral administration contain guanadrel sulfate, an antihypertensive agent belonging to the class of adrenergic neuron blocking drugs. The tablets are available in two strengths: 10 mg and 25 mg. Guanadrel sulfate is (1,4-Dioxaspiro[4.5]dec-2-ylmethyl) guanidine sulfate with a molecular weight of 524.63. It is a white to off-white crystalline powder, which melts with decomposition at about 235°C. It is soluble in water to the extent of 76 mg/ml. HYLOREL Tablets are available in two strengths: 10 mg. and 25 mg. Inactive ingredients: microcrystalline cellulose, corn starch, lactose, magnesium stearate, colloidal silicon dioxide, and talc. The 10 mg tablet also contains FD&C Yellow No 6.

CLINICAL PHARMACOLOGY

Guanadrel sulfate is an orally effective antihypertensive agent that lowers both systolic and diastolic arterial blood pressures. Guanadrel sulfate inhibits sympathetic vasoconstriction by inhibiting norepinephrine release from neuronal storage sites in response to stimulation of the nerve and also causes depletion of norepinephrine from the nerve ending. This results in relaxation of vascular smooth muscle which decreases total peripheral resistance, and decreases venous return, both of which reduce the ability to maintain blood pressure in the upright position. The result is a hypotensive effect that is greater in the standing than in the supine position by about 10 mmHg systolic and 3.5 mmHg diastolic, on the average. Heart rate is also decreased usually by about 5 beats/minute. Fluid retention occurs during treatment with guanadrel, particularly when it is not accompanied by a diuretic. The drug does not inhibit parasympathetic nerve function nor does it enter the central nervous system.

Guanadrel sulfate is rapidly absorbed after oral administration. Plasma concentrations generally peak 1½ to 2 hours after ingestion. The half life is about 10 hours, but individual variability is great. Approximately 85% of the drug is eliminated in the urine. Urinary excretion is approximately 85% complete within 24 hours after administration; about 40% of a dose is excreted as unchanged drug. There is no information available regarding pharmacokinetics in patients with impaired renal function.

Guanadrel sulfate begins to decrease blood pressure within 2 hours and produces maximal decreases in 4 to 6 hours. No significant change in cardiac output accompanies the blood pressure decline in normal individuals.

Because drugs of the adrenergic neuron blocking class are transported into the neuron by the "norepinephrine pump," drugs that compete for the pump may block their effects. Tricyclic antidepressants have been shown to block the norepinephrine-depleting effect of guanadrel sulfate in rats and monkeys, and the blood pressure lowering effect of guanadrel sulfate in monkeys. Similar effects have been seen with guanethidine and inhibition of the antihypertensive effects of guanadrel sulfate by tricyclic antidepressants in humans should be presumed.

Therefore caution is recommended if guanadrel sulfate and a tricyclic antidepressant are used concomitantly. Should patients be on both a tricyclic antidepressant and guanadrel sulfate, caution is advised upon discontinuation of the tricyclic antidepressant, especially if discontinued abruptly, as an enhanced effect of guanadrel sulfate may occur. Chlorpromazine seems to have a similar effect on guanethidine and may affect guanadrel as well. Indirectly acting adrenergic amines are transported into the neuron by the "norepinephrine pump" and may interfere with uptake or may displace blocking agents. Ephedrine rapidly reverses the effects of guanadrel but other agents have not been studied.

Agents of the guanethidine class cause increased sensitivity to circulating norepinephrine, probably by preventing uptake of norepinephrine by adrenergic neurons, the usual mechanism for terminating norepinephrine effects. Agents of this class are thus dangerous in the presence of excess norepinephrine, eg, in the presence of a pheochromocytoma.

In controlled clinical studies comparing guanadrel to guanethidine and methyldopa, involving about 2000 patients exposed to guanadrel, patients with supine blood pressures averaging 160-170/105-110 mmHg had decreases in blood pressure of 20-25/15-20 mmHg in the standing position. The decreases in supine blood pressure were less than the decreases in standing blood pressure by 6-10/2-7 mmHg in different studies. Guanethidine and guanadrel were very similar in effectiveness while methyldopa had a larger effect on supine systolic pressure. Side effects of guanadrel and guanethidine were generally similar in type (see **Adverse Reactions**) while methyldopa had more central nervous system effects (depression, drowsiness) but fewer orthostatic effects and less diarrhea.

Drug No. patients treated Event	Guanadrel 1544 %	Methyldopa 743 %	Guanethidine 330 %
Cardiovascular-Respiratory			
Chest Pain	27.9	37.4	27.3
Coughing	26.9	36.2	21.5
Palpitations	29.5	35.0	24.5
Shortness of breath at rest	18.3	22.3	17.0
Shortness of breath on exertion	45.9	53.2	48.8
Central Nervous System-Special Senses			
Confusion	14.8	22.6	10.9
Depression	1.9	3.9	1.8
Drowsiness	44.6	64.1	28.5
Headache	58.1	69.0	49.7
Paresthesias	25.1	35.1	16.4
Psychological problems	3.8	4.8	3.9
Sleep disorders	2.1	2.3	2.7
Visual disturbances	29.2	35.3	26.1
Gastrointestinal			
Abdominal distress or pain	1.7	1.9	1.5
Anorexia	18.7	23.0	17.6
Constipation	21.0	29.1	20.3
Dry mouth, dry throat	1.7	4.0	0.6
Gas pain	32.0	39.7	29.4
Glossitis	8.4	10.8	4.8
Indigestion	23.7	30.8	18.5
Nausea and/or vomiting	3.9	4.8	3.6
Genitourinary			
Hematuria	2.3	4.2	2.1
Nocturia	48.4	52.4	41.5
Peripheral edema	28.6	37.4	22.7
Urination urgency or frequency	33.6	39.8	27.6
Miscellaneous			
Excessive weight gain	44.3	53.7	42.4
Excessive weight loss	42.2	51.1	41.5
Fatigue	63.6	76.2	57.0
Musculoskeletal			
Aching limbs	42.9	51.7	33.9
Backache or neckache	1.5	1.1	1.8
Joint pain or inflammation	1.7	2.0	2.4
Leg cramps during the day	21.1	26.0	20.0
Leg cramps during the night	25.6	32.6	21.2

INDICATIONS AND USAGE

HYLOREL Tablets are indicated for the treatment of hypertension in patients not responding adequately to a thiazide type diuretic. HYLOREL is Step-2 therapy and should be added to a diuretic regimen for optimum blood pressure control.

CONTRAINDICATIONS

HYLOREL Tablets are contraindicated in known or suspected pheochromocytoma.

HYLOREL should not be used concurrently with, or within one week of, monoamine oxidase inhibitors.

HYLOREL should not be used in patients hypersensitive to the drug.

HYLOREL should not be used in patients with frank congestive heart failure.

WARNINGS

a. Orthostatic Hypotension: Orthostatic hypotension and its consequences (dizziness and weakness) are frequent in people treated with HYLOREL Tablets. Rarely, fainting upon standing or exercise is seen. Careful instructions to the patient can minimize these symptoms, as can recognition by the physician that the supine blood pressure does not constitute an adequate assessment of the effects of this drug. Patients with known regional vascular disease (cerebral, coronary) are at particular risk from marked orthostatic hypotension and HYLOREL should be avoided in them unless drugs with lesser degrees of orthostatic hypotension are ineffective or unacceptable. In such patients hypotensive episodes should be avoided, even if this requires accepting a poorer degree of blood pressure control.

Instructions to patients: Patients should be advised about the risk of orthostatic hypotension and told to sit or lie down immediately at the onset of dizziness or weakness so that they can prevent loss of consciousness. They should be told that postural hypotension is worst in the morning and upon arising and may be exaggerated by alcohol, fever, hot weather, prolonged standing, or exercise.

Surgery: To reduce the possibility of vascular collapse during anesthesia, guanadrel should be discontinued 48-72 hours before elective surgery. If emergency surgery is required, the anesthesiologist should be made aware that the patient has been taking HYLOREL and that preanesthetic and anesthetic agents should be administered cautiously in reduced dosage. If vasopressors are needed they must be used cautiously, as guanadrel can enhance the pressor response to such agents and increase their arrhythmogenicity.

b. Drug Interactions: As discussed above (**Clinical Pharmacology**), tricyclic antidepressants and indirect-acting sympathomimetics such as ephedrine or phenylpropanolamine, and possibly phenothiazines, can reverse the effects of neuronal blocking agents. IN VIEW OF THE PRESENCE OF SYMPATHOMIMETIC AMINES IN MANY NON-PRESCRIPTION DRUGS FOR THE TREATMENT OF COLDS, ALLERGY, OR ASTHMA, PATIENTS GIVEN GUANADREL SHOULD BE SPECIFICALLY WARNED NOT TO USE SUCH PREPARATIONS WITHOUT THEIR PHYSICIAN'S ADVICE.

Guanadrel enhances the activity of direct-acting sympathomimetics, like norepinephrine, by blocking neuronal uptake. Drugs that affect the adrenergic response by the same or other mechanisms would be expected to potentiate the effects of guandrel, causing excessive postural hypotension and bradycardia. These include alpha- or beta-adrenergic blocking agents and reserpine. There is no clinical experience with the combination of HYLOREL with alpha-adrenergic blocking agents or reserpine.

When HYLOREL was added to the treatment regimen in hypertensive patients inadequately controlled with a diuretic and propranolol, no significant adverse effects, including bradycardia, were reported in the 26 patients treated concomitantly with the three drugs.

The use of HYLOREL with vasodilators has not been adequately studied and is not generally recommended because concomitant use may increase the potential for symptomatic orthostatic hypotension.

c. Asthmatic patients: Special care is needed in patients with bronchial asthma, as their condition may be aggravated by catecholamine depletion and sympathomimetic amines may interfere with the hypotensive effect of guanadrel.

PRECAUTIONS

General: Salt and water retention may occur with the use of HYLOREL Tablets. In clinical studies major problems did not arise because of concomitant diuretic use. Patients with heart failure have not been studied on HYLOREL, but guanadrel could interfere with the adrenergic mechanisms that maintain compensation.

In patients with a history of peptic ulcer, which could be aggravated by a relative increase in parasympathetic tone, HYLOREL should be used cautiously.

HYLOREL has not been studied in patients with renal failure.

Continued on next page

Pennwalt—Cont.

Information for patients: See **Warnings** section.
Drug interactions: See **Warnings** section.
Carcinogenesis, mutagenesis, impairment of fertility: No evidence of carcinogenic potential appeared in a 2-year mouse study of guanadrel sulfate. In a 22-month rat study, endometrial fibromatous polyps were observed at a dosage of 100 mg/kg per day. The polyps are common, spontaneous lesions of aged rats, and their relationship to drug therapy is unknown. Salmonella testing (Ames test) showed no evidence of mutagenic activity.
Pregnancy Category B: Teratogenic effects: Reproduction studies have been performed in rats and rabbits at doses up to 12 times the maximum recommended human dose and have revealed no evidence of impaired fertility or harm to the fetus due to guanadrel sulfate. There are, however, no adequate and well-controlled studies in pregnant women. Because animal reproduction studies are not always predictive, HYLOREL should be used in pregnant women only when the potential benefit outweighs the potential risk to mother and infant.
Nursing mothers: Whether guanadrel sulfate is excreted in human milk is not known, but because many drugs are excreted in human milk and because of the potential for serious adverse reactions in nursing infants from guanadrel, a decision should be made whether to discontinue nursing or discontinue the drug, taking into account the importance of the drug to the mother.
Pediatric Use: Safety and effectiveness in children have not been established.

ADVERSE REACTIONS

The adverse reaction data for guanadrel are derived principally from comparative long-term (6 months to 3 years) studies with methyldopa and guanethidine in which side effects were assessed through use of periodic questionnaires, a method that tends to give high adverse reaction rates. In the tables that follow, some of the adverse effects reported may not be drug-related, but in the absence of a placebo-treated group, these cannot be readily distinguished. Comparative results with two well-known drugs, methyldopa and guanethidine, should aid in interpretation of these adverse reaction rates.
The following table displays the frequency of side effects which are believed to be related to sympathetic blocking agents: orthostatic faintness, increased bowel movements and ejaculation disturbances for peripherally acting drugs such as guanadrel and drowsiness for centrally acting drugs such as methyldopa. The frequencies observed were generally higher during the first 8 weeks of therapy. Week 0 frequencies, which were recorded just prior to administration of the antihypertensive drugs while the patients were receiving diuretics, serve as a reference point. Frequency while on therapy is shown for the first 8 weeks and for weeks 9 to 52.
[See table below].
The following paragraph shows the incidence of reactions often associated with adrenergic neuron blockers as the percent of patients who reported the event at least once over the treatment periods of 6 months to 3 years. For such long-term studies these incidence rates of side effects, which are found often in untreated patients, tend to be high and accumulate with time. The incidence rates for two well-known comparison drugs, methyldopa and guanethidine, should aid in interpreting the high rates. It can be seen that the serious consequences of the orthostatic effect of guanadrel, such as syncope, were very uncommon.
1544 guanadrel, 743 methyldopa and 330 guanethidine patients were evaluated in comparison studies. The observed incidence rates of major drug related side effects for guanadrel, methyldopa and guanethidine, respectively, are as follows: orthostatic faintness: 49%, 41% 48%; other faintness: 47%, 46% 45%; increased bowel movements: 31%, 28%, 36%; ejaculation disturbances: 18%, 21%, 22%; impotence: 5.1% 12.2%, 7.2%; syncope: 0.4%, 0.3%, 2%; urine retention: 0.2%, 0%, 0%.
Apart from these adverse effects, many others were reported. Relationship to therapy is less clear, although some (such as peripheral edema with all three drugs, depression with methyldopa) are in part drug related. All adverse effects reported in at least 1% of guanadrel patients are listed in the following table:
[See table on preceding page]

OVERDOSAGE

Overdosage usually produces marked dizziness and blurred vision related to postural hypotension and may progress to syncope on standing. The patient should lie down until these symptoms subside.
If excessive hypotension occurs and persists despite conservative treatment, intensive therapy may be needed to support vital functions. A vasoconstrictor such as phenylephrine will ameliorate the effect of HYLOREL Tablets (guanadrel sulfate), but great care must be used because patients may be hypersensitive to such agents.

DOSAGE AND ADMINISTRATION

As with other sympathetic suppressant drugs, the dose response to HYLOREL Tablets varies widely and must be adjusted for each patient until the therapeutic goal is achieved. With long-term therapy, some tolerance may occur and the dosage may have to be increased.
Because HYLOREL has a substantial orthostatic effect, monitoring both supine and standing pressures is essential, especially while dosage is being adjusted.
HYLOREL should be administered in divided doses. The usual starting dosage for treating hypertension is 10 mg per day, which can be given as 5 mg b.i.d. by breaking the 10 mg tablet. Because the half-life is approximately ten hours, the dosages should be adjusted weekly or monthly until blood pressure is controlled. Most patients will require daily dosage in the range of 20 to 75 mg usually in twice daily doses. For larger doses 3 or 4 times daily dosing may be needed.

HOW SUPPLIED

HYLOREL Tablets are available as follows:
10 mg. scored elliptical tablets (light orange)
Bottles of 100—NDC 0018-0787-71
25 mg. scored elliptical tablets (white)
Bottles of 100—NDC 0018-0788-71
Store at controlled room temperature 15°–30°C (59°–86°F)
Caution: Federal law prohibits dispensing without a prescription.
Rev 8/85 US Patent No. 3,547,951
Mkt by
PENNWALT CORP.
PRESCRIPTION DIVISION
Rochester, NY 14623
Shown in Product Identification Section, page 422

IONAMIN® Ⓒ

[i″on ′uh-min]
(phentermine resin)

DESCRIPTION

Ionamin '15' and Ionamin '30' contain 15 mg. and 30 mg. respectively of phentermine as the cationic exchange resin complex. Phentermine is α, α-dimethyl phenethylamine (phenyl-tertiary-butylamine).
Other Ingredients in Ionamin: Dibasic Calcium Phosphate; Dye, FD&C Yellow No. 6; Dye, D&C Yellow No. 10; Gelatin; Iron Oxides (15 mg capsules only); Lactose; Magnesium Stearate; Titanium Dioxide.

ACTIONS

Ionamin is a sympathomimetic amine with pharmacologic activity similar to the prototype drug of this class used in obesity, amphetamine (d- and *dl*-amphetamine). Actions include central nervous system stimulation and elevation of blood pressure. Tachyphylaxis and tolerance have been demonstrated with all drugs of this class in which these phenomena have been looked for.
Drugs of this class used in obesity are commonly known as "anorectics" or "anorexigenics." It has not been established, however, that the action of such drugs in treating obesity is primarily one of appetite suppression. Other central nervous system actions, or metabolic effects may be involved.
Adult obese subjects instructed in dietary management and treated with "anorectic" drugs, lose more weight on the average than those treated with placebo and diet, as determined in relatively short-term clinical trials.
The magnitude of increased weight loss of drug-treated patients over placebo-treated patients is only a fraction of a pound a week. The rate of weight loss is greatest in the first weeks of therapy for both drug and placebo subjects and tends to decrease in succeeding weeks. The possible origins of the increased weight loss due to the various drug effects are not established. The amount of weight loss associated with the use of an "anorectic" drug varies from trial to trial, and the increased weight loss appears to be related in part to variables other than the drugs prescribed, such as the physician-investigator, the population treated, and the diet prescribed. Studies do not permit conclusions as to the relative importance of the drug and non-drug factors on weight loss.
The natural history of obesity is measured in years, whereas the studies cited are restricted to a few weeks or months duration; thus, the total impact of drug-induced weight loss over that of diet alone must be considered clinically limited.
The bioavailability of Ionamin has been studied in humans in which blood levels of phentermine were measured by a gas-chromatography method. Blood levels obtained with the 15 mg. and 30 mg. resin complex formulations indicated slower absorption with a reduced but prolonged peak concentration and without a significant difference in prolongation of blood levels when compared with the same doses of phentermine hydrochloride. The clinical significance of these differences is not known. In clinical trials establishing the efficacy of Ionamin, a single daily dose produced an effect comparable to that produced by other regimens of "anorectic" drug therapy.

INDICATION

Ionamin is indicated in the management of exogenous obesity as a short-term (a few weeks) adjunct in a regimen of weight reduction based on caloric restriction. The limited usefulness of agents of this class (see ACTIONS) should be measured against possible risk factors inherent in their use such as those described below.

CONTRAINDICATIONS

Advanced arterlosclerosis, symptomatic cardiovascular disease, moderate to severe hypertension, hyperthyroidism,

FREQUENCY OF SIDE EFFECTS
Percent of Clinic Visits in Which Side Effect was Reported

	Guanadrel			Methyldopa			Guanethidine		
	Pre-Drug			Pre-Drug			Pre-Drug		
Week	0	1-8	9-52	0	1-8	9-52	0	1-8	9-52
Number of clinic visits analyzed	470	3003	4260	266	1610	2216	215	1421	2009
Side Effect									
Morning orthostatic faintness	6.6	9.4	6.8	6.8	8.1	7.4	4.6	10.7	7.9
Orthostatic faintness during the day	7.5	10.8	8.5	7.5	8.0	7.8	5.6	8.9	6.3
Other faintness	7.8	4.8	4.5	6.2	3.7	3.8	5.9	2.7	2.0
Increased bowel movements	4.9	7.9	6.1	4.9	5.9	3.8	3.7	7.9	9.4
Drowsiness	15.3	14.4	8.7	13.2	21.2	18.6	10.2	10.3	6.4
Fatigue	25.7	26.6	23.7	32.9	22.6	27.6	21.4	20.5	17.5
Ejaculation disturbance	7.0	17.5	12.0	10.3	13.4	11.5	6.9	16.6	18.2

The frequency of side effects over time may be reduced by the discontinuation of drugs in patients who experience intolerable side effects. Reasons for discontinuation of therapy with guanadrel are shown in the following table.

PERCENT OF PATIENTS WHO DISCONTINUED

	Guanadrel	Methyldopa	Guanethidine
Orthostatic faintness	0.6	0.7	6.0
Syncope	0.4	0.3	2.0
Other faintness	1.2	0.0	0.0
Increased bowel movements	0.8	0.7	1.4
Drowsiness	0.0	1.9*	0.0
Fatigue	0.2	2.6*	0.0
Ejaculation disturbances	0.4	0.0	0.0

*Significantly greater than HYLOREL, $p < 0.003$

known hypersensitivity, or idiosyncrasy to the sympathomimetic amines, glaucoma.
Agitated states.
Patients with a history of drug abuse.
During or within 14 days following the administration of monoamine oxidase inhibitors (hypertensive crises may result).

WARNINGS

If tolerance to the "anorectic" effect develops, the recommended dose should not be exceeded in an attempt to increase the effect: rather, the drug should be discontinued.
Ionamin may impair the ability of the patient to engage in potentially hazardous activities such as operating machinery or driving a motor vehicle; the patient should therefore be cautioned accordingly.
When using CNS active agents, consideration must always be given to the possibility of adverse interactions with alcohol.
Drug Dependence: Ionamin is related chemically and pharmacologically to amphetamine (d- and *dl*- amphetamine) and other stimulant drugs that have been extensively abused. The possibility of abuse of Ionamin should be kept in mind when evaluating the desirability of including a drug as part of a weight reduction program. Abuse of amphetamine (d- and *dl*- amphetamine) and related drugs may be associated with intense psychological dependence and severe social dysfunction. There are reports of patients who have increased the dosage of some of these drugs to many times that recommended. Abrupt cessation following prolonged high dosage administration results in extreme fatigue and mental depression; changes are also noted on the sleep EEG. Manifestations of chronic intoxication with anorectic drugs include severe dermatoses, marked insomnia, irritability, hyperactivity, and personality changes. The most severe manifestation of chronic intoxications is psychosis, often clinically indistinguishable from schizophrenia.
Usage in Pregnancy: Safe use in pregnancy has not been established. Use of Ionamin by women who are or may become pregnant requires that the potential benefit be weighed against the possible hazard to mother and infant.
Usage in Children: Ionamin is not recommended for use in children under 12 years of age.

PRECAUTIONS

Caution is to be exercised in prescribing Ionamin for patients with even mild hypertension. Insulin requirements in diabetes mellitus may be altered in association with the use of Ionamin and the concomitant dietary regimen.
Ionamin may decrease the hypotensive effect of adrenergic neuron blocking drugs.
The least amount feasible should be prescribed or dispensed at one time in order to minimize the possibility of overdosage.

ADVERSE REACTIONS

Cardiovascular: Palpitation, tachycardia, elevation of blood pressure.
Central Nervous System: Overstimulation, restlessness, dizziness, insomnia, euphoria, dysphoria, tremor, headache; rarely psychotic episodes at recommended doses with some drugs in this class.
Gastrointestinal: Dryness of the mouth, unpleasant taste, diarrhea, constipation, other gastrointestinal disturbances.
Allergic: Urticaria.
Endocrine: Impotence, changes in libido.

DOSAGE AND ADMINISTRATION

One capsule daily, before breakfast or 10–14 hours before retiring. For individuals exhibiting greater drug responsiveness, Ionamin '15' will usually suffice. Ionamin '30' is recommended for less responsive patients. Ionamin is not recommended for use in children under 12 years of age.

OVERDOSAGE

Manifestations of acute overdosage may include restlessness, tremor, hyperreflexia, rapid respiration, confusion, assaultiveness, hallucinations, panic states.
Fatigue and depression usually follow the central stimulation.
Cardiovascular effects include arrhythmias, hypertension, or hypotension and circulatory collapse. Gastrointestinal symptoms include nausea, vomiting, diarrhea, and abdominal cramps. Overdosage of pharmacologically similar compounds has resulted in fatal poisoning, usually terminating in convulsions and coma.
Management of acute Ionamin intoxication is largely symptomatic and includes lavage and sedation with a barbiturate. Experience with hemodialysis or peritoneal dialysis is inadequate to permit recommendation in this regard. Intravenous phentolamine (Regitine) has been suggested on pharmacologic grounds for possible acute, severe hypertension, if this complicates overdosage.

HOW SUPPLIED

Two strengths: Ionamin (phentermine resin) 15 mg. (NDC 0018-0903) yellow and gray capsules; Ionamin (phentermine resin) 30 mg. (NDC 0018-0904) yellow capsules. Available on prescription only. Stock bottles of 100 and 400.

Rev 3/85

Shown in Product Identification Section, page 422

PENNTUSS® Ⓒ
(controlled release codeine polistirex with chlorpheniramine polistirex)
[*pĕn 'tuhs*]

DESCRIPTION

Provides 12-hour relief of cough. Each teaspoonful (5 ml.) contains codeine polistirex (warning: may be habit forming) equivalent to 10 mg. of codeine base, plus chlorpheniramine polistirex equivalent to 4 mg. of chlorpheniramine maleate.

INDICATIONS

Temporarily controls cough due to minor throat and bronchial irritation as may occur with the common cold or inhaled irritants. Temporarily alleviates runny nose and relieves sneezing, itching of the nose or throat, and itchy, watery eyes due to hay fever or other upper respiratory allergies (allergic rhinitis). Temporarily relieves runny nose and reduces sneezing associated with the common cold.

WARNINGS

Prescribe with caution to children who have a chronic pulmonary disease, shortness of breath, or who are taking other drugs. Use with caution in patients with persistent or chronic cough such as occurs with smoking, asthma, or emphysema, or if cough is accompanied by excessive phlegm (mucus). Caution is also advised when prescribing this drug to patients with asthma, glaucoma, emphysema, chronic pulmonary disease, shortness of breath, difficulty in breathing, or difficulty in urination due to enlargement of the prostate gland. May cause excitability especially in children. May cause or aggravate constipation. May cause marked drowsiness; alcohol may increase the drowsiness effect. Patients should be advised to avoid alcoholic beverages and to use caution when driving a motor vehicle or operating machinery while taking this product.

DIRECTIONS

SHAKE VIGOROUSLY BEFORE USING. Adults and children 12 years of age and over: 2 to 3 teaspoonsful every 12 hours; not to exceed 6 teaspoonsful in 24 hours, or as directed by a physician. Children 6 to under 12: 1 teaspoonful every 12 hours; not to exceed 2 teaspoonsful in 24 hours, or as directed by a physician. Children under 6: Use only under the advice and supervision of a physician.

HOW SUPPLIED

Pint bottles (NDC# 0018-0818-67)

Antitussive
TUSSIONEX® Ⓒ III
[*tus 'e-uh-nex*]
(Resin Complexes of Hydrocodone and Phenyltoloxamine)

TUSSIONEX® Capsules, Suspension and Tablets

COMPOSITION

Each capsule, teaspoonful (5 ml.) or tablet contains 5 mg. hydrocodone (*Warning:* may be habit-forming), and 10 mg. phenyltoloxamine as cationic resin complexes.
Other Ingredients (Capsules and Tablets): Colloidal Silicon Dioxide, Dibasic Calcium Phosphate, Lactose, Magnesium Stearate, Starch, Sucrose. (Capsules only); Dye, FD&C Blue No. 1 or Green No. 3, Dye, FD&C Yellow No. 6, Dye, D&C Yellow No. 10; Gelatin, Titanium Dioxide.
Other Ingredients (Suspension): Alcohol 0.59%; Dye, FD&C Yellow No. 6; Dye, D&C Yellow No. 10; Glycerin, Methylparaben, Natural Gums; Propylparaben; Propylene Glycol; Sorbitol Solution; Tragacanth; Water.

EFFECTS

An effective antitussive which acts for approximately 12 hours.

DOSAGE

Adults: 1 teaspoonful (5 ml.), capsule or tablet every 8-12 hours. May be adjusted to individual requirements. *Children:* Under 1 year: $\frac{1}{4}$ teaspoonful every 12 hours. From 1-5 years: $\frac{1}{2}$ teaspoonful every 12 hours. Over 5 years: 1 teaspoonful every 12 hours.

SIDE EFFECTS

Negligible, but when encountered may include mild constipation, nausea, facial pruritus, drowsiness, which disappear with adjustment of dose or discontinuance of treatment.

PRECAUTION

In young children the respiratory center is especially susceptible to the depressant action of narcotic cough suppressants. Benefit to risk ratio should be carefully considered especially in children with respiratory embarrassment. Estimation of dosage relative to the age and weight of the child is of great importance.

OVERDOSAGE

Immediately evacuate the stomach. Respiratory depression, if any, can be counteracted by respiratory stimulants. Convulsions, sometimes seen in children, can be controlled by intravenous administration of short-acting barbiturates. Hypothermia can be controlled by the usual supportive methods.

HOW SUPPLIED

Tussionex Suspension, neutral in taste, golden color; 16 oz. and 900 ml. bottles. Tussionex Tablets, light brown, scored; bottles of 100. Tussionex Capsules, green and white; bottles of 50. A prescription for 2 oz. of the Suspension, or 12 Capsules or Tablets, constitutes a 6 day supply in the average case.

Rev 5/85

Diuretic, Antihypertensive
ZAROXOLYN® ℞
[*zar "ox 'uh-lin*]
(Metolazone)

Each ZAROXOLYN Tablet contains $2\frac{1}{2}$, 5, or 10 mg of metolazone.

DESCRIPTION

ZAROXOLYN (metolazone) has the molecular formula $C_{16}H_{16}ClN_3O_3S$ and a molecular weight of 365.84 and its chemical name is 7-chloro-1,2,3,4-tetrahydro-2-methyl-4-oxo-3-o- tolyl-6-quinazolinesulfonamide. Metolazone is only sparingly soluble in water, but more soluble in plasma, blood, alkali, and organic solvents. ZAROXOLYN Tablets also contain magnesium stearate, microcrystalline cellulose and dye: $2\frac{1}{2}$ mg—D&C Red No. 33; 5 mg—FD&C Blue No. 2; 10 mg—D&C Yellow No. 10 and FD&C Yellow No. 6.

ACTIONS

ZAROXOLYN (metolazone) is a diuretic/saluretic/antihypertensive drug. The action of ZAROXOLYN results in an interference with the renal tubular mechanism of electrolyte reabsorption. The mechanism of this action is unknown. ZAROXOLYN acts primarily to inhibit sodium reabsorption at the cortical diluting site and in the proximal convoluted tubule. Sodium and chloride ions are excreted in approximately equivalent amounts. The increased delivery of sodium to the distal-tubular exchange site may result in increased potassium excretion.
DRUG INTERACTION STUDIES: In animals pretreated with ZAROXOLYN, the drug did not alter the characteristic effect of heparin on clotting time nor protamine antagonism; dicumarol on prothrombin time nor Vitamin K antagonism; the response of guanethidine, reserpine and hydralazine to cardiovascular parameters nor the pressor response of the subsequent dose of norepinephrine.
ZAROXOLYN and furosemide, administered concurrently have produced marked diuresis in some patients where edema or ascites was refractory to treatment with maximum recommended doses of these or other diuretics administered alone. The mechanism of this interaction is not known.
In clinical usage, ZAROXOLYN does not inhibit carbonic anhydrase. Its proximal action has been evidenced in humans by increased excretion of phosphate and magnesium ions, by markedly increased fractional excretion of sodium in patients with severely compromised glomerular filtration, and in animals by the results of micropuncture studies. Decrease in calcium ion excretion has not been noted.
At maximum therapeutic dosage ZAROXOLYN is approximately equal to thiazide diuretics in its diuretic potency. However, ZAROXOLYN may produce diuresis in patients with glomerular filtration rates below 20 ml/min.
When ZAROXOLYN is given, diuresis and saluresis usually begin within one hour and persist for 12 to 24 hours depending on dosage. Maximum effect occurs about two hours after administration. At the higher recommended dosages, effect may be prolonged beyond 24 hours. *A single daily dose is recommended.* For most patients the duration of effect can be varied by adjusting the daily dose.
The prolonged duration of action of ZAROXOLYN is attributed to protein-binding and enterohepatic recycling. A small amount of ZAROXOLYN is metabolized and the fraction so changed is nontoxic. The primary route of excretion is renal.
The mechanism whereby diuretics function in the control of hypertension is unknown; both renal and extra-renal actions may be involved. An antihypertensive effect may be seen as early as three to four days after ZAROXOLYN has been started. Administration for three to four weeks, however, is usually required for optimum antihypertensive effect.

INDICATIONS

ZAROXOLYN (metolazone) is indicated in the management of hypertension either as the sole therapeutic agent or to

Continued on next page

Pennwalt—Cont.

enhance the effectiveness of other antihypertensive drugs in the more severe forms of hypertension.
ZAROXOLYN (metolazone) is indicated for the treatment of salt and water retention including
—edema accompanying congestive heart failure
—edema accompanying renal diseases, including the nephrotic syndrome, and states of diminished renal function

Usage in Pregnancy
The routine use of diuretics in an otherwise healthy woman is inappropriate and exposes mother and fetus to unnecessary hazard. Diuretics do not prevent development of toxemia of pregnancy, and there is no satisfactory evidence that they are useful in the treatment of developed toxemia.
Edema during pregnancy may arise from pathological causes or from the physiologic and mechanical consequences of pregnancy. ZAROXOLYN is indicated in pregnancy when edema is due to pathologic causes, just as it is in the absence of pregnancy (however, see Warnings, below). Dependent edema in pregnancy, resulting from restriction of venous return by the expanded uterus, is properly treated through elevation of the lower extremities and use of support hose; use of diuretics to lower intravascular volume in this case is illogical and unnecessary. There is hypervolemia during normal pregnancy which is harmful to neither the fetus nor the mother (in the absence of cardiovascular disease), but which is associated with edema, including generalized edema, in the majority of pregnant women. If this edema produces discomfort, increased recumbency will often provide relief. In rare instances, this edema may cause extreme discomfort which is not relieved by rest. In these cases, a short course of diuretics may provide relief and may be appropriate.

CONTRAINDICATIONS
Anuria.
Hepatic coma or pre-coma; known allergy or hypersensitivity to ZAROXOLYN (metolazone).

WARNINGS
Rarely, the rapid onset of severe hyponatremia and/or hypokalemia has been reported following initial doses of thiazide or non-thiazide diuretics. When symptoms consistent with severe electrolyte imbalance appear rapidly, drug should be discontinued and supportive means should be initiated immediately. Appropriateness of diuretic therapy should be carefully re-evaluated.
While not reported to date, cross-allergy theoretically may occur when ZAROXOLYN (metolazone) is given to patients known to be allergic to sulfonamide-derived drugs, thiazides, or quinethazone.
Hypokalemia may occur, with consequent weakness, cramps, and cardiac dysrhythmias. Hypokalemia is a particular hazard in digitalized patients; dangerous or fatal arrhythmias may be precipitated.
Azotemia and hyperuricemia may be noted or precipitated during the administration of ZAROXOLYN. (Infrequently, gouty attacks have been reported in persons with history of gout.)
If azotemia and oliguria worsen during treatment of patients with severe renal disease, ZAROXOLYN should be discontinued.
Until additional data have been obtained, ZAROXOLYN is not recommended for patients in the pediatric age group.
Unusually large or prolonged effects on volume and electrolytes may result when ZAROXOLYN and furosemide are administered concurrently. It is recommended that concurrent administration of these diuretics for treatment of resistant edema be started under hospital conditions in order to provide for adequate monitoring.
When ZAROXOLYN is used with other antihypertensive drugs, particular care must be taken, especially during initial therapy. Dosage of other antihypertensive agents, especially the ganglionic blockers, should be reduced.
ZAROXOLYN may be given with a potassium-sparing diuretic when indicated. In this circumstance, diuresis may be potentiated and dosages should be reduced. Potassium retention and hyperkalemia may result; the serum potassium should be determined frequently. Potassium supplementation is contraindicated when a potassium-sparing diuretic is given.

Usage in Pregnancy
ZAROXOLYN crosses the placental barrier and appears in cord blood. The use of ZAROXOLYN in pregnant women requires that the anticipated benefit be weighed against possible hazards to the fetus. These hazards include fetal or neonatal jaundice, thrombocytopenia, and possibly other adverse reactions which have occurred in the adult.

Nursing Mothers
ZAROXOLYN appears in breast milk. If use of the drug is deemed essential, the patient should stop nursing.

PRECAUTIONS
Periodic determination of serum electrolytes to detect possible electrolyte imbalance should be performed at appropriate intervals. Blood urea nitrogen, uric acid, and glucose levels should be assessed at intervals during diuretic therapy.
All patients receiving ZAROXOLYN (metolazone) therapy should be observed for clinical signs of fluid and/or electrolyte imbalance; namely, hyponatremia, hypochloremic alkalosis, and hypokalemia. Serum and urine electrolyte determinations are particularly important when the patient is vomiting excessively or receiving parenteral fluids. Medication such as digitalis may also influence serum electrolytes. Warning signs, irrespective of cause, are: dryness of mouth, thirst, weakness, lethargy, drowsiness, restlessness, muscle pains or cramps, muscular fatigue, hypotension, oliguria, tachycardia, and gastrointestinal disturbances such as nausea and vomiting.
The serum potassium should be determined at regular intervals, and potassium supplementation instituted whenever indicated. Hypokalemia will be more common in association with intensive or prolonged diuretic therapy, with concomitant steroid or ACTH therapy, and with inadequate electrolyte intake.
While not reported to date for ZAROXOLYN, related diuretics have increased responsiveness to tubocurarine and decreased arterial responsiveness to norepinephrine. Accordingly, it may be advisable to discontinue ZAROXOLYN three days before elective surgery.
Caution should be observed when administering ZAROXOLYN to hyperuricemic or gouty patients. ZAROXOLYN exerts minimal effects on glucose metabolism; insulin requirements may be affected in diabetics, and hyperglycemia and glycosuria may occur in patients with latent diabetes.
Chloride deficit and hypochloremic alkalosis may occur. In patients with severe edema accompanying cardiac failure or renal disease, a low-salt syndrome may be produced; hot weather and a low-salt diet will contribute.
Caution should be observed when administering ZAROXOLYN to patients with severely impaired renal function. As most of the drug is excreted by the renal route, cumulative effects may be seen in this circumstance.
Orthostatic hypotension may occur, this may be potentiated by alcohol, barbiturates, narcotics, or concurrent therapy with other antihypertensive drugs.
While not reported for ZAROXOLYN, use of other diuretics has been associated on rare occasions with pathological changes in the parathyroid glands and with hypercalcemia. This possibility should be kept in mind with clinical use of ZAROXOLYN.

ADVERSE REACTIONS
Adverse reactions encountered during therapy with potent medications should be considered in two groups: those that represent extensions of the expected pharmacologic actions of the drug, and those which are pharmacologically unexpected, idiosyncratic, specially toxic, due to allergy or hypersensitivity, or due to unexplained causes.
For ZAROXOLYN (metolazone), adverse reactions constituting extensions of the expected pharmacologic actions of this potent diuretic/saluretic/antihypertensive drug may include:
Gastrointestinal reactions: constipation.
Central nervous system reactions: syncope, dizziness, drowsiness.
Cardiovascular reactions: orthostatic hypotension, excessive volume depletion, hemoconcentration, venous thrombosis.
Other reactions: dryness of the mouth, symptomatic and asymptomatic hypokalemia, hyponatremia, hypochloremia; hypochloremic alkalosis, hypophosphatemia, hyperuricemia, hyperglycemia, glycosuria, increase in BUN or creatinine, fatigue, muscle cramps or spasm, weakness, restlessness sometimes resulting in insomnia.
In the second classification, adverse reactions to ZAROXOLYN may include:
Gastrointestinal reactions: nausea, vomiting, anorexia, diarrhea, abdominal bloating, epigastric distress, intrahepatic cholestatic jaundice, hepatitis.
Central nervous system reactions: vertigo, headache, paresthesias.
Hematologic reactions: leukopenia, aplastic anemia.
Dermatologic-hypersensitivity reactions: urticaria and other skin rashes, purpura, necrotizing angiitis (cutaneous vasculitis).
Cardiovascular reactions: palpitation, chest pain.
Other reactions: chills, acute gouty attacks, transient blurred vision.
Adverse reactions which have occurred with other diuretics, but which have not been reported to date for ZAROXOLYN (metolazone), include:
pancreatitis, xanthopsia, agranulocytosis, thrombocytopenia, and photosensitivity. These reactions should be considered as possible occurrences with clinical usage of ZAROXOLYN.
Whenever adverse reactions are moderate or severe, ZAROXOLYN dosage should be reduced or therapy withdrawn.

DOSAGE AND ADMINISTRATION
Therapy should be individualized according to patient response. Programs of therapy with ZAROXOLYN (metolazone) should be titrated to gain a maximal initial therapeutic response, and to determine the minimal dose possible to maintain that therapeutic response.
ZAROXOLYN is a potent drug with a prolonged, 12-to-24-hour duration of action. When an initially-desired therapeutic effect has been obtained, it is ordinarily advisable to reduce the dosage of ZAROXOLYN to a lower maintenance level. The time interval required for the initial higher-dosage regimen may vary from days in edematous states to three or four weeks in the treatment of elevated blood pressure.
The daily dosage depends on the severity of each patient's condition, his sodium intake, and his responsiveness. Therefore, dosage adjustment is usually necessary during the course of therapy. A decision to reduce the daily dosage of ZAROXOLYN from a higher induction level to a lower maintenance level should be based on the results of thorough clinical and laboratory evaluations. If antihypertensive drugs or diuretics are given concurrently with ZAROXOLYN, careful dosage adjustment may be necessary.

Usual single daily dosage schedules
Suitable initial dosages will usually fall in the ranges given:
Mild to moderate essential hypertension: ZAROXOLYN 2½–5 mg. once daily
Edema of cardiac failure: ZAROXOLYN 5–10 mg. once daily
Edema of renal disease: ZAROXOLYN 5–20 mg. once daily
For patients with congestive cardiac failure who tend to experience paroxysmal nocturnal dyspnea, it is usually advisable to employ a dosage near the upper end of the range, to ensure prolongation of diuresis and saluresis for a full 24-hour period.

HOW SUPPLIED
ZAROXOLYN (metolazone) is provided as: pink 2½ mg tablets, blue 5 mg tablets, and yellow 10 mg tablets; in package sizes of 100, 500, 1000 and unit-dose strip packages of 100 (10 × 10's).

Rev 5/85

Shown in Product Identification Section, page 422

Persōn & Covey, Inc.
616 ALLEN AVENUE
GLENDALE, CA 91201

DHS™ Conditioning Rinse

(See 1987 PDR For Nonprescription Drugs)

DHS™ Shampoo
Dermatological Hair and Scalp Shampoo

(See 1987 PDR For Nonprescription Drugs)

DHS™ Tar Shampoo and DHS™ Tar Gel Shampoo (Scented)
Dermatological Hair and Scalp Shampoo

(See 1987 PDR For Nonprescription Drugs)

DHS™ Zinc Dandruff Shampoo
2% Zinc Pyrithione

(See 1987 PDR For Nonprescription Drugs)

DML™ Moisturizing Lotion

(See 1987 PDR For Nonprescription Drugs)

DRYSOL™ ℞

A Solution of:
Aluminum Chloride (Hexahydrate) 20% w/v in Anhydrous Ethyl Alcohol (S.D. Alcohol 40) 93% v/v.

INDICATION
An aid in the management of hyperhidrosis.

DIRECTIONS
Apply Drysol™ to the affected area once a day, **only at bedtime.** To help prevent irritation, the area should be completely dry prior to application. Do not apply Drysol to broken, irritated or recently shaved skin.

FOR MAXIMUM EFFECT
Your doctor may instruct you to cover the treated area with saran wrap held in place by a snug fitting "T" or body shirt, mitten or sock. (Never hold saran in place with tape.) Wash

the treated area the following morning. Excessive sweating may be stopped after two or more treatments. Thereafter, apply Drysol™ once or twice weekly or as needed.

NOTICE

Drysol™ may produce a burning or prickling sensation. Keep cap tightly closed when not in use to prevent evaporation.

WARNING

For external use only. Keep out of the reach of children. Avoid contact with the eyes. If irritation or sensitization occurs, discontinue use or consult with a physician. Drysol™ may be harmful to certain fabrics. Keep away from open flame.

HOW SUPPLIED

37.5 cc polyethylene bottle (NDC 0096-0707-37) and 35 cc bottle with Dab-O-Matic applicator head (NDC 0096-0707-35).

SOLBAR® PF 15 Cream (Paba Free)
SPF 15

(See 1987 PDR For Nonprescription Drugs)

SOLBAR® PF Liquid (Paba Free)
SPF 15

(See 1987 PDR For Nonprescription Drugs)

SOLBAR® PLUS 15 Cream
Sun Protectant Cream
SPF 15

(See 1987 PDR For Nonprescription Drugs)

XERAC®
(alcohol gel)

(See 1987 PDR For Nonprescription Drugs)

XERAC AC™ ℞
Aluminum Chloride Hexahydrate in Anhydrous Ethanol

DESCRIPTION

A solution of Aluminum Chloride (Hexahydrate) 6.25% (w/v) in Anhydrous Ethyl Alcohol (S.D. Alcohol 40) 96% (v/v).

INDICATION

For topical application as an antiperspirant (anhidrotic).

DIRECTIONS

Apply Xerac AC™ to the axillae at bedtime or as directed by physician. To help prevent irritation, the area should be completely dry prior to application. Do not apply Xerac AC to broken or irritated skin. Keep container tightly closed.

ADVERSE REACTIONS

Transient stinging or itching may occur. It is not evidence of contact sensitivity and may be prevented or reduced by applying Xerac AC™ only to skin which is completely dry or by removing the solution with soap and water.

WARNING

For External Use Only. Some users of this product will experience skin irritation. If this occurs, discontinue use. Avoid contact with the eyes. This product may be harmful to certain fabrics. Keep the container tightly closed when not in use to prevent evaporation. Keep this and all medication out of the reach of children. Do not use near open flame.

HOW SUPPLIED

In bottles with Dab-O-Matic applicator head. 35 cc (NDC 0096-0709) and 60 cc (NDC 0096-0709).

XERAC BP5™
XERAC BP10™
(benzoyl peroxide water gel)

(See 1987 PDR For Nonprescription Drugs)

Pfipharmecs Division

PFIZER INC.
235 EAST 42ND STREET
NEW YORK,NY 10017

All Pfipharmecs Division products have been reassigned to other Pfizer divisions as follows:

PFIZER LABORATORIES DIVISION

Antiminth® (pyrantel pamoate) Oral Suspension
Cortil® (hydrocortisone) Topical Ointment 1%
Renese® (polythiazide) Tablets
Renese®-R (polythiazide and reserpine) Tablets
Sustaire® (theophylline [anhydrous]) Tablets
Terramycin® (oxytetracycline HCl) Capsules
Vansil™ (oxamniquine) Capsules

ROERIG DIVISION

Geopen® (carbenicillin disodium) IM/IV
Permapen® Isoject® (pencillin G benzathine in Aqueous Suspension)
Pfizerpen®-AS (penicillin G procaine) IM
Pfizerpen® (penicillin G potassium) for injection
Streptomycin Sulfate
Terra-Cortril® Ophthalmic Suspension
Terramycin® (oxytetracycline) IM Solution
Terramycin® (oxytetracycline HCl with polymyxin B sulfate) Ophthalmic Ointment
Vibramycin® Hyclate (doxycycline hyclate for injection) IV
Vistaril® (hydroxyzine HCl) IM Solution

LEEMING/PACQUIN DIVISION

Bonine® (meclizine HCl) Chewable Tablets
Coryban®-D Capsules
Coryban®-D Cough Syrup
Li-Ban® Spray
Rid®
Terramycin® (oxytetracycline HCl topical ointment with polymyxin B sulfate)
Wart-Off™

Pfizer Laboratories Division

PFIZER INC.
235 EAST 42ND STREET
NEW YORK, NY 10017

Full prescribing information for all Pfizer Laboratories products is available from your Pfizer Laboratories representative.

Product Identification Codes

To provide quick and positive identification of Pfizer Laboratories Division products, we have imprinted the product identification number of the National Drug Code on all tablets and capsules.

In order that you may quickly identify a product by its code number, we have compiled below a numerical list of code numbers with their corresponding product names. We are also listing the code numbers by alphabetical order of products.

NUMERICAL PRODUCT INDEX

Product Identification Code	Product
073	Terramycin® (Oxytetracycline HCl) Capsules 250 mg.
084	Terramycin® (Oxytetracycline) Film Coated Tablets 250 mg.
094	Vibramycin® Hyclate (Doxycycline Hyclate) Capsules 50 mg.
095	Vibramycin® Hyclate (Doxycycline Hyclate) Capsules 100 mg.
099	Vibra-Tabs® (Doxycycline Hyclate) Film Coated Tablets 100 mg.
220	Sustaire Sustained-Release Tablets 100 mg.
221	Sustaire Sustained-Release Tablets 300 mg.
260	Procardia® (Nifedipine) Capsules 10 mg.
261	Procardia® (Nifedipine) Capsules 20 mg.
322	Feldene® (Piroxicam) Capsules 10 mg.
323	Feldene® (Piroxicam) Capsules 20 mg.
375	Renese® (Polythiazide) Tablets 1 mg.
376	Renese® (Polythiazide) Tablets 2 mg.
377	Renese® (Polythiazide) Tablets 4 mg.
393	Diabinese® (Chlorpropamide) Tablets 100 mg.
394	Diabinese® (Chlorpropamide) Tablets 250 mg.
430	Minizide® 1 Capsules (1 mg. Prazosin HCl and 0.5 mg. Polythiazide)
431	Minipress® (Prazosin HCl) Capsules 1 mg.
432	Minizide® 2 Capsules (2 mg. Prazosin HCl and 0.5 mg. Polythiazide)
436	Minizide® 5 Capsules (5 mg. Prazosin HCl and 0.5 mg. Polythiazide)
437	Minipress® (Prazosin HCl) Capsules 2 mg.
438	Minipress® (Prazosin HCl) Capsules 5 mg.
441	Moderil® (Rescinnamine) Tablets 0.25 mg.
442	Moderil® (Rescinnamine) Tablets 0.5 mg.
446	Renese®-R (Polythiazide 2.0 mg. and Reserpine 0.25 mg.) Tablets
541	Vistaril® (Hydroxyzine Pamoate) Capsules 25 mg.
542	Vistaril® (Hydroxyzine Pamoate) Capsules 50 mg.
543	Vistaril® (Hydroxyzine Pamoate) Capsules 100 mg.
641	Vansil™ (Oxamniquine) Capsules 250 mg.

ALPHABETICAL PRODUCT INDEX

Product	Product Identification Code
Diabinese® (Chlorpropamide) Tablets 100 mg.	393
Diabinese® (Chlorpropamide) Tablets 250 mg.	394
Feldene® (Piroxicam) Capsules 10 mg.	322
Feldene® (Piroxicam) Capsules 20 mg.	323
Minipress® (Prazosin HCl) Capsules 1 mg.	431
Minipress® (Prazosin HCl) Capsules 2 mg.	437
Minipress® (Prazosin HCl) Capsules 5 mg.	438
Minizide® 1 Capsules (1 mg. Prazosin HCl and 0.5 mg. Polythiazide)	430
Minizide® 2 Capsules (2 mg. Prazosin HCl and 0.5 mg. Polythiazide)	432
Minizide® 5 Capsules (5 mg. Prazosin HCl and 0.5 mg. Polythiazide)	436
Moderil® (Rescinnamine) Tablets 0.25 mg.	441
Moderil® (Rescinnamine) Tablets 0.5 mg.	442
Procardia® (Nifedipine) Capsules 10 mg.	260
Procardia® (Nifedipine) Capsules 20 mg.	261
Renese® (Polythiazide) Tablets 1 mg.	375
Renese® (Polythiazide) Tablets 2 mg.	376
Renese® (Polythiazide) Tablets 4 mg.	377
Renese®-R (Polythiazide 2.0 mg. and Reserpine 0.25 mg.) Tablets	446
Sustaire Sustained-Release Tablets 100 mg.	220
Sustaire Sustained-Release Tablets 300 mg.	221
Terramycin® (Oxytetracycline HCl) Capsules 250 mg.	073

Continued on next page

Pfizer—Cont.

Terramycin® (Oxytetracycline) Film Coated Tablets 250 mg. 084
Vansil™ (Oxamniquine) Capsules 250 mg. 641
Vibramycin® Hyclate (Doxycycline Hyclate) Capsules 50 mg. 094
Vibramycin® Hyclate (Doxycycline Hyclate) Capsules 100 mg. 095
Vibra-Tabs® (Doxycycline Hyclate) Film Coated Tablets 100 mg. 099
Vistaril® (Hydroxyzine Pamoate) Capsules 25 mg. 541
Vistaril® (Hydroxyzine Pamoate) Capsules 50 mg. 542
Vistaril® (Hydroxyzine Pamoate) Capsules 100 mg. 543

ANTIMINTH® ℞
[*ăn 'tē-minth*]
(pyrantel pamoate)
ORAL SUSPENSION

DESCRIPTION

Pyrantel pamoate is a crystalline, water insoluble salt with the chemical name, (E)-1,4,5,6-tetrahydro-1-methyl-2-[2-(2-thienyl) vinyl] pyrimidine pamoate (1:1).
Antiminth (pyrantel pamoate) Oral Suspension contains the equivalent of 50 mg pyrantel base per ml.

ACTIONS

Antiminth has demonstrated anthelmintic activity against *Enterobius vermicularis* (pinworm) and *Ascaris Lumbricoides* (common roundworm). The anthelmintic action is probably due to the neuromuscular blocking property of the drug.
Antiminth is partially absorbed after an oral dose. Plasma levels of unchanged drug are low. Peak levels (0.05–0.13 μg./ml.) are reached in 1–3 hours. Quantities greater than 50% of administered drug are excreted in feces as the unchanged form, whereas only 7% or less of the dose is found in urine as the unchanged form of the drug and its metabolites.

INDICATIONS

For the treatment of ascariasis (common roundworm infection) and enterobiasis (pinworm infection).

WARNINGS

Usage in Pregnancy
Reproduction studies have been performed in animals and there was no evidence of propensity for harm to the fetus. The relevance to the human is not known.
There is no experience in pregnant women who have received this drug.
This drug has not been extensively studied in children under two years; therefore, in the treatment of children under the age of two years, the relative benefit/risk should be considered.

PRECAUTIONS

Minor transient elevations of SGOT have occurred in a small percentage of patients. Therefore, this drug should be used with caution in patients with pre-existing liver dysfunction.

ADVERSE REACTIONS

The most frequently encountered adverse reactions are related to the gastrointestinal system.
Gastrointestinal and hepatic reactions: anorexia, nausea, vomiting, gastralgia, abdominal cramps, diarrhea and tenesmus, transient elevation of SGOT.
CNS reactions: headache, dizziness, drowsiness, and insomnia.
Skin reactions: rashes.

DOSAGE AND ADMINISTRATION

Children and Adults
Antiminth Oral Suspension (50 mg of pyrantel base/ml) should be administered in a single dose of 11 mg of pyrantel base per kg of body weight (or 5 mg/lb); maximum total dose 1 gram. This corresponds to a simplified dosage regimen of 1 ml of Antiminth per 10 lb of body weight. (One teaspoonful = 5 ml)
Antiminth (pyrantel pamoate) Oral Suspension may be administered without regard to ingestion of food or time of day, and purging is not necessary prior to, during, or after therapy. It may be taken with milk or fruit juices.

HOW SUPPLIED

Antiminth Oral Suspension is available as a pleasant tasting caramel-flavored suspension which contains the equivalent of 50 mg NDC 0995-6400-23 pyrantel base per ml, supplied in 60 ml bottles.
Literature available: Yes
65-1876-00-7 Revised March 1982
Shown in Product Identification Section, page 422

CORTRIL® ℞
[*kor 'trĭl*]
(hydrocortisone)
TOPICAL OINTMENT
1.0%
Not For Ophthalmic Use

DESCRIPTION

Cortril Topical Ointment contains 1.0% (10 mg/g) hydrocortisone in a washable base. Chemically hydrocortisone is Pregn-4-ene-3,20-dione, 11,17,21-trihydrox-, (11β)-. The empirical formula is $C_{21}H_{30}O_5$ and the molecular weight is 362.47.
The base of the ointment contains sodium lauryl sulfate, propylene glycol, stearyl alcohol, cetyl alcohol, cholesterol, white petrolatum, mineral oil, and water. Methylparaben and propylparaben are added as preservatives.

CLINICAL PHARMACOLOGY

Topical corticosteroids share anti-inflammatory, antipruritic and vasoconstrictive actions.
The mechanism of anti-inflammatory activity of the topical corticosteroids is unclear. Various laboratory methods, including vasoconstrictor assays, are used to compare and predict potencies and/or clinical efficacies of the topical corticosteroids. There is some evidence to suggest that a recognizable correlation exists between vasoconstrictor potency and therapeutic efficacy in man.
Pharmacokinetics
The extent of percutaneous absorption of topical corticosteroids is determined by many factors including the vehicle, the integrity of the epidermal barrier, and the use of occlusive dressings.
Topical corticosteroids can be absorbed from normal intact skin. Inflammation and/or other disease processes in the skin increase percutaneous absorption. Occlusive dressings substantially increase the percutaneous absorption of topical corticosteroids. Thus, occlusive dressings may be a valuable therapeutic adjunct for treatment of resistant dermatoses. (See *DOSAGE AND ADMINISTRATION.*)
Once absorbed through the skin, topical corticosteroids are handled through pharmacokinetic pathways similar to systemically administered corticosteroids. Corticosteroids are bound to plasma proteins in varying degrees. Corticosteroids are metabolized primarily in the liver and are then excreted by the kidneys. Some of the topical corticosteroids and their metabolites are also excreted into the bile.

INDICATIONS AND USAGE

Topical corticosteroids are indicated for the relief of the inflammatory and pruritic manifestations of corticosteroid-responsive dermatoses.

CONTRAINDICATIONS

Topical corticosteroids are contraindicated in those patients with a history of hypersensitivity to any of the components of the preparation.

PRECAUTIONS

General
Systemic absorption of topical corticosteroids has produced reversible hypothalamic-pituitary-adrenal (HPA) axis suppression, manifestations of Cushing's syndrome, hyperglycemia, and glucosuria in some patients.
Conditions which augment systemic absorption include the application of the more potent steroids, use over large surface areas, prolonged use, and the addition of occlusive dressings.
Therefore, patients receiving a large dose of a potent topical steroid applied to a large surface area or under an occlusive dressing should be evaluated periodically for evidence of HPA axis suppression by using the urinary free cortisol and ACTH stimulation tests. If HPA axis suppression is noted, an attempt should be made to withdraw the drug, to reduce the frequency of application, or to substitute a less potent steroid.
Recovery of HPA axis function is generally prompt and complete upon discontinuation of the drug. Infrequently, signs and symptoms of steroid withdrawal may occur, requiring supplemental systemic corticosteroids.
Children may absorb proportionally larger amounts of topical corticosteroids and thus be more susceptible to systemic toxicity. (See *PRECAUTIONS—Pediatric Use.)*
If irritation develops, topical corticosteroids should be discontinued and appropriate therapy instituted.
In the presence of dermatological infections, the use of an appropriate antifungal or antibacterial agent should be instituted. If a favorable response does not occur promptly, the corticosteroid should be discontinued until the infection has been adequately controlled.
Information for the Patient
Patients using topical corticosteroids should receive the following information and instructions:

1. This medication is to be used as directed by the physician. It is for external use only. Avoid contact with the eyes.
2. Patients should be advised not to use this medication for any disorder other than that for which it was prescribed.
3. The treated skin area should not be bandaged or otherwise covered or wrapped as to be occlusive unless directed by the physician.
4. Patients should report any signs of local adverse reactions especially under occlusive dressings.
5. Parents of pediatric patients should be advised not to use tight-fitting diapers or plastic pants on a child being treated in the diaper area, as these garments may constitute occlusive dressings.

Laboratory Tests
The following tests may be helpful in evaluating the HPA axis suppression:
Urinary free cortisol test
ACTH stimulation test
Carcinogenesis, Mutagenesis, and Impairment of Fertility
Long term animal studies have not been performed to evaluate the carcinogenic potential or the effect on fertility of topical corticosteroids.
Studies to determine mutagenicity with prednisolone and hydrocortisone have revealed negative results.
Pregnancy Category C
Corticosteroids are generally teratogenic in laboratory animals when administered systemically at relatively low dosage levels. The more potent corticosteroids have been shown to be teratogenic after dermal application in laboratory animals. There are no adequate and well controlled studies in pregnant women on teratogenic effects from topically applied corticosteroids. Therefore, topical corticosteroids should be used during pregnancy only if the potential benefit justifies the potential risk to the fetus. Drugs of this class should not be used extensively on pregnant patients, in large amounts, or for prolonged periods of time.
Nursing Mothers
It is not known whether topical administration of corticosteroids could result in sufficient systemic absorption to produce detectable quantities in breast milk. Systemically administered corticosteroids are secreted into breast milk in quantities *not* likely to have a deleterious effect on the infant. Nevertheless, caution should be exercised when topical corticosteroids are administered to a nursing woman.
Pediatric Use
Pediatric patients may demonstrate greater susceptibility to topical corticosteroid-induced HPA axis suppression and Cushing's syndrome than mature patients because of a larger skin surface area to body weight ratio.
Hypothalamic-pituitary-adrenal (HPA) axis suppression. Cushing's syndrome, and intracranial hypertension have been reported in children receiving topical corticosteroids.
Manifestations of adrenal suppression in children include linear growth retardation, delayed weight gain, low plasma cortisol levels, and absence of response to ACTH stimulation.
Manifestations of intracranial hypertension include bulging fontanelles, headaches, and bilateral papilledema.
Administration of topical corticosteroids to children should be limited to the least amount compatible with an effective therapeutic regimen. Chronic corticosteroid therapy may interfere with the growth and development of children.

ADVERSE REACTIONS

The following local adverse reactions are reported infrequently with topical corticosteroids, but may occur more frequently with the use of occlusive dressings. These reactions are listed in an approximate decreasing order of occurrence:

Burning	Perioral dermatitis
Itching	Allergic contact dermatitis
Irritation	Maceration of the skin
Dryness	Secondary infection
Folliculitis	Skin atrophy
Hypertrichosis	Striae
Acneiform eruptions	Miliaria
Hypopigmentation	

OVERDOSAGE

Topically applied corticosteroids can be absorbed in sufficient amounts to produce systemic effects. (See *PRECAUTIONS.*)

DOSAGE AND ADMINISTRATION

Topical corticosteroids are generally applied to the affected area as a thin film from three to four times daily depending on the severity of the condition.
Occlusive dressings may be used for the management of psoriasis or recalcitrant conditions.
If an infection develops, the use of occlusive dressings should be discontinued and appropriate antimicrobial therapy instituted.

HOW SUPPLIED

Cortril (hydrocortisone) Topical Ointment 1.0%; ½ oz (14.2g) tube containing 10 mg/g of hydrocortisone (NDC 0995-3260-13).
Literature Available: No
23-2434-00-4 Revised Oct. 1982

DIABINESE® ℞
[dī-ab 'in-ees]
(chlorpropamide)
Tablets, USP
For Oral Use

DESCRIPTION

DIABINESE (chlorpropamide), is an oral blood-glucose-lowering drug of the sulfonylurea class. Chlorpropamide is 1-[(p-Chlorophenyl) sulfonyl]-3-propylurea, $C_{10}H_{13}ClN_2O_3S$.

Chlorpropamide is a white crystalline powder, that has a slight odor. It is practically insoluble in water at pH 7.3 (solubility at pH 6 is 2.2 mg/ml). It is soluble in alcohol and moderately soluble in chloroform. The molecular weight of chlorpropamide is 276.74. DIABINESE is available as 100 mg and 250 mg tablets.

CLINICAL PHARMACOLOGY

DIABINESE appears to lower the blood glucose acutely by stimulating the release of insulin from the pancreas, an effect dependent upon functioning beta cells in the pancreatic islets. The mechanism by which DIABINESE lowers blood glucose during long-term administration has not been clearly established. Extra-pancreatic effects may play a part in the mechanism of action of oral sulfonylurea hypoglycemic drugs. While chlorpropamide is a sulfonamide derivative, it is devoid of antibacterial activity.

DIABINESE may also prove effective in controlling certain patients who have experienced primary or secondary failure to other sulfonylurea agents.

A method developed which permits easy measurement of the drug in blood is available on request.

Chlorpropamide does not interfere with the usual tests to detect albumin in the urine.

DIABINESE is absorbed rapidly from the gastrointestinal tract. Within one hour after a single oral dose, it is readily detectable in the blood, and the level reaches a maximum within two to four hours. It undergoes metabolism in humans and it is excreted in the urine as unchanged drug and as hydroxylated or hydrolyzed metabolites. The biological half-life of chlorpropamide averages about 36 hours. Within 96 hours, 80–90% of a single oral dose is excreted in the urine. However, long-term administration of therapeutic doses does not result in undue accumulation in the blood, since absorption and excretion rates become stabilized in about 5 to 7 days after the initiation of therapy.

DIABINESE exerts a hypoglycemic effect in normal humans within one hour, becoming maximal at 3 to 6 hours and persisting for at least 24 hours. The potency of chlorpropamide is approximately six times that of tolbutamide. Some experimental results suggest that its increased duration of action may be the result of slower excretion and absence of significant deactivation.

INDICATIONS AND USAGE

DIABINESE is indicated as an adjunct to diet to lower the blood glucose in patients with non-insulin-dependent diabetes mellitus (type II) whose hyperglycemia cannot be controlled by diet alone.

In initiating treatment for non-insulin-dependent diabetes, diet should be emphasized as the primary form of treatment. Caloric restriction and weight loss are essential in the obese diabetic patient. Proper dietary management alone may be effective in controlling the blood glucose and symptoms of hyperglycemia. The importance of regular physical activity should also be stressed, and cardiovascular risk factors should be identified and corrective measures taken where possible.

If this treatment program fails to reduce symptoms and/or blood glucose, the use of an oral sulfonylurea or insulin should be considered. Use of DIABINESE must be viewed by both the physician and patient as a treatment in addition to diet, and not as a substitute for diet or as a convenient mechanism for avoiding dietary restraint. Furthermore, loss of blood glucose control on diet alone may be transient, thus requiring only short-term administration of DIABINESE.

During maintenance programs, DIABINESE should be discontinued if satisfactory lowering of blood glucose is no longer achieved. Judgments should be based on regular clinical and laboratory evaluations.

In considering the use of DIABINESE in asymptomatic patients, it should be recognized that controlling the blood glucose in non-insulin-dependent diabetes, has not been definitely established to be effective in preventing the long-term cardiovascular or neural complications of diabetes.

CONTRAINDICATIONS

DIABINESE is contraindicated in patients with:

1. Known hypersensitivity to the drug.
2. Diabetic ketoacidosis, with or without coma. This condition should be treated with insulin.

WARNINGS

SPECIAL WARNING ON INCREASED RISK OF CARDIOVASCULAR MORTALITY

The administration of oral hypoglycemic drugs has been reported to be associated with increased cardiovascular mortality as compared to treatment with diet alone or diet plus insulin. This warning is based on the study conducted by the University Group Diabetes Program (UGDP), a long-term prospective clinical trial designed to evaluate the effectiveness of glucose-lowering drugs in preventing or delaying vascular complications in patients with non-insulin-dependent diabetes. The study involved 823 patients who were randomly assigned to one of four treatment groups (*Diabetes,* 19 (supp. 2): 747–830, 1970).

UGDP reported that patients treated for 5 to 8 years with diet plus a fixed dose of tolbutamide (1.5 grams per day) had a rate of cardiovascular mortality approximately 2½ times that of patients treated with diet alone. A significant increase in total mortality was not observed, but the use of tolbutamide was discontinued based on the increase in cardiovascular mortality, thus limiting the opportunity for the study to show an increase in over-all mortality. Despite controversy regarding the interpretation of these results, the findings of the UGDP study provide an adequate basis for this warning. The patient should be informed of the potential risks and advantages of DIABINESE and of alternative modes of therapy.

Although only one drug in the sulfonylurea class (tolbutamide) was included in this study, it is prudent from a safety standpoint to consider that this warning may also apply to other oral hypoglycemic drugs in this class, in view of their close similarities in mode of action and chemical structure.

PRECAUTIONS

General

Hypoglycemia: All sulfonylurea drugs are capable of producing severe hypoglycemia. Proper patient selection, dosage, and instructions are important to avoid hypoglycemic episodes. Renal or hepatic insufficiency may cause elevated blood levels of DIABINESE and the latter may also diminish gluconeogenic capacity, both of which increase the risk of serious hypoglycemic reactions. Elderly, debilitated or malnourished patients, and those with adrenal or pituitary insufficiency are particularly susceptible to the hypoglycemic action of glucose-lowering drugs. Hypoglycemia may be difficult to recognize in the elderly, and in people who are taking beta-adrenergic blocking drugs. Hypoglycemia is more likely to occur when caloric intake is deficient, after severe or prolonged exercise, when alcohol is ingested, or when more than one glucose-lowering drug is used.

Because of the long half-life of chlorpropamide, patients who become hypoglycemic during therapy require careful supervision of the dose and frequent feedings for at least 3 to 5 days. Hospitalization and intravenous glucose may be necessary.

Loss of control of blood glucose: When a patient stabilized on any diabetic regimen is exposed to stress such as fever, trauma, infection, or surgery, a loss of control may occur. At such times, it may be necessary to discontinue DIABINESE and administer insulin.

The effectiveness of any oral hypoglycemic drug, including DIABINESE, in lowering blood glucose to a desired level decreases in many patients over a period of time, which may be due to progression of the severity of the diabetes or to diminished responsiveness to the drug. This phenomenon is known as secondary failure, to distinguish it from primary failure in which the drug is ineffective in an individual patient when first given.

INFORMATION FOR PATIENTS

Patients should be informed of the potential risks and advantages of DIABINESE and of alternative modes of therapy. They should also be informed about the importance of adherence to dietary instructions, of a regular exercise program, and of regular testing of urine and/or blood glucose.

The risks of hypoglycemia, its symptoms and treatment, and conditions that predispose to its development should be explained to patients and responsible family members. Primary and secondary failure should also be explained.

Patients should be instructed to contact their physician promptly if they experience symptoms of hypoglycemia or other adverse reactions.

LABORATORY TESTS

Blood and urine glucose should be monitored periodically. Measurement of glycosylated hemoglobin may be useful.

DRUG INTERACTIONS

The hypoglycemic action of sulfonylurea may be potentiated by certain drugs including nonsteroidal anti-inflammatory agents and other drugs that are highly protein bound, salicylates, sulfonamides, chloramphenicol, probenecid, coumarins, monoamine oxidase inhibitors, and beta-adrenergic blocking agents. When such drugs are administered to a patient receiving DIABINESE, the patient should be observed closely for hypoglycemia. When such drugs are withdrawn from a patient receiving DIABINESE, the patient should be observed closely for loss of control.

Certain drugs tend to produce hyperglycemia and may lead to loss of control. These drugs include the thiazides and other diuretics, corticosteroids, phenothiazines, thyroid products, estrogens, oral contraceptives, phenytoin, nicotinic acid, sympathomimetics, calcium channel blocking drugs, and isoniazid. When such drugs are administered to a patient receiving DIABINESE, the patient should be closely observed for loss of control. When such drugs are withdrawn from a patient receiving DIABINESE, the patient should be observed closely for hypoglycemia.

Since animal studies suggest that the action of barbiturates may be prolonged by therapy with chlorpropamide, barbiturates should be employed with caution. In some patients, a disulfiram-like reaction may be produced by the ingestion of alcohol.

Carcinogenesis, Mutagenesis, Impairment of Fertility: Chronic toxicity studies have been carried out in dogs and rats. Dogs treated for 6, 13, or 20 months with doses of DIABINESE greater than 20 times the human dose, have not shown any gross histological or pathological abnormalities. After treatment with 100 mg/kg of DIABINESE for 20 months, a dog showed no histopathological liver changes.

Rats treated with continuous DIABINESE therapy for 6 to 12 months showed varying degrees of suppression of spermatogenesis at higher dosage levels (up to 125 mg/kg). The extent of suppression seemed to follow that of growth retardation associated with chronic administration of high-dose DIABINESE in rats.

Pregnancy

Teratogenic Effects:

Pregnancy Category C. Animal reproductive studies have not been conducted with DIABINESE. It is also not known whether DIABINESE can cause fetal harm when administered to a pregnant woman or can affect reproduction capacity. DIABINESE should be given to a pregnant woman only if clearly needed.

Because recent information suggests that abnormal blood glucose levels during pregnancy are associated with a higher incidence of congenital abnormalities, many experts recommend that insulin be used during pregnancy to maintain blood glucose levels as close to normal as possible.

Nonteratogenic Effects:

Prolonged severe hypoglycemia (4 to 10 days) has been reported in neonates born to mothers who were receiving a sulfonylurea drug at the time of delivery. This has been reported more frequently with the use of agents with prolonged half-lives. If DIABINESE is used during pregnancy, it should be discontinued at least one month before the expected delivery date.

Nursing Mothers: An analysis of a composite of two samples of human breast milk, each taken five hours after ingestion of 500 mg of chlorpropamide by a patient, revealed a concentration of 5 mcg/ml. For reference, the normal peak blood level of chlorpropamide after a single 250 mg dose is 30 mcg/ml. Therefore, it is not recommended that a woman breast feed while taking this medication.

Use in Children: Safety and effectiveness in children have not been established.

ADVERSE REACTIONS

Hypoglycemia: See PRECAUTIONS and OVERDOSAGE sections.

Gastrointestinal Reactions: Cholestatic jaundice may occur rarely; DIABINESE should be discontinued if this occurs. Gastrointestinal disturbances are the most common reactions; nausea has been reported in less than 5% of patients, and diarrhea, vomiting, anorexia, and hunger in less than 2%. Other gastrointestinal disturbances have occurred in less than 1% of patients including proctocolitis. They tend to be dose related and may disappear when dosage is reduced.

Dermatologic Reactions: Pruritus has been reported in less than 3% of patients. Other allergic skin reactions, e.g., urticaria and maculopapular eruptions, have been reported in approximately 1% or less of patients. These may be transient and may disappear despite continued use of DIABINESE; if skin reactions persist the drug should be discontinued.

Porphyria cutanea tarda and photosensitivity reactions have been reported with sulfonylureas.

Skin eruptions rarely progressing to erythema multiforme and exfoliative dermatitis have also been reported.

Hematologic Reactions: Leukopenia, agranulocytosis, thrombocytopenia, hemolytic anemia, aplastic anemia, pancytopenia, and eosinophilia have been reported with sulfonylureas.

Metabolic Reactions: Hepatic porphyria and disulfiram-like reactions have been reported with DIABINESE. See DRUG INTERACTIONS section.

Endocrine Reactions: On rare occasions, chlorpropamide has caused a reaction identical to the syndrome of inappropriate antidiuretic hormone (ADH) secretion. The features of this syndrome result from excessive water retention and include hyponatremia, low serum osmolality, and high urine osmolality.

OVERDOSAGE

Overdose of sulfonylureas including DIABINESE can produce hypoglycemia. Mild hypoglycemic symptoms without loss of consciousness or neurologic findings should be treated

Continued on next page

Pfizer—Cont.

aggressively with oral glucose and adjustments in drug dosage and/or meal patterns. Close monitoring should continue until the physician is assured that the patient is out of danger. Severe hypoglycemic reactions with coma, seizure, or other neurological impairment occur infrequently, but constitute medical emergencies requiring immediate hospitalization. If hypoglycemic coma is diagnosed or suspected, the patient should be given a rapid intravenous injection of concentrated (50%) glucose solution. This should be followed by a continuous infusion of a more dilute (10%) glucose solution at a rate that will maintain the blood glucose at a level above 100 mg/dL. Patients should be closely monitored for a minimum of 24 to 48 hours since hypoglycemia may recur after apparent clinical recovery.

DOSAGE AND ADMINISTRATION

There is no fixed dosage regimen for the management of diabetes mellitus with DIABINESE or any other hypoglycemic agent. In addition to the usual monitoring of urinary glucose, the patient's blood glucose must also be monitored periodically to determine the minimum effective dose for the patient; to detect primary failure, i.e., inadequate lowering of blood glucose at the maximum recommended dose of medication; and to detect secondary failure, i.e., loss of an adequate blood glucose lowering response after an initial period of effectiveness. Glycosylated hemoglobin levels may also be of value in monitoring the patient's response to therapy.

Short-term administration of DIABINESE may be sufficient during periods of transient loss of control in patients usually controlled well on diet.

The total daily dosage is generally taken at a single time each morning with breakfast. Occasionally cases of gastrointestinal intolerance may be relieved by dividing the daily dosage. A LOADING OR PRIMING DOSE IS NOT NECESSARY AND SHOULD NOT BE USED.

Initial Therapy: 1. The mild to moderately severe, middle-aged, stable, non-insulin-dependent diabetic patient should be started on 250 mg daily. In elderly patients, debilitated or malnourished patients, and patients with impaired renal or hepatic function, the initial and maintenance dosing should be conservative to avoid hypoglycemic reactions (see PRECAUTIONS section). Older patients should be started on smaller amounts of DIABINESE, in the range of 100 to 125 mg daily.

2. No transition period is necessary when transferring patients from other oral hypoglycemic agents to DIABINESE. The other agent may be discontinued abruptly and chlorpropamide started at once. In prescribing chlorpropamide, due consideration must be given to its greater potency.

Many mild to moderately severe, middle-aged, stable non-insulin-dependent diabetic patients receiving insulin can be placed directly on the oral drug and their insulin abruptly discontinued. For patients requiring more than 40 units of insulin daily, therapy with DIABINESE may be initiated with a 50 per cent reduction in insulin for the first few days, with subsequent further reductions dependent upon the response.

During the initial period of therapy with chlorpropamide, hypoglycemic reactions may occasionally occur, particularly during the transition from insulin to the oral drug. Hypoglycemia within 24 hours after withdrawal of the intermediate or long-acting types of insulin will usually prove to be the result of insulin carry-over and not primarily due to the effect of chlorpropamide.

During the insulin withdrawal period, the patient should test his urine for sugar and ketone bodies at least three times daily and report the results frequently to his physician. If they are abnormal, the physician should be notified immediately. In some cases, it may be advisable to consider hospitalization during the transition period.

Five to seven days after the inital therapy, the blood level of chlorpropamide reaches a plateau. Dosage may subsequently be adjusted upward or downward by increments of not more than 50 to 125 mg at intervals of three to five days to obtain optimal control. More frequent adjustments are usually undesirable.

Maintenance Therapy: Most moderately severe, middle-aged, stable non-insulin-dependent diabetic patients are controlled by approximately 250 mg daily. Many investigators have found that some milder diabetics do well on daily doses of 100 mg or less. Many of the more severe diabetics may require 500 mg daily for adequate control. PATIENTS WHO DO NOT RESPOND COMPLETELY TO 500 MG DAILY WILL USUALLY NOT RESPOND TO HIGHER DOSES. MAINTENANCE DOSES ABOVE 750 mg DAILY SHOULD BE AVOIDED.

HOW SUPPLIED

[See table below].

Strength	Tablet Description	Tablet Code	NDC	Package Size
DIABINESE (chlorpropamide) 100 mg	Blue, D-shaped, scored	393	0663-3930-66 0663-3930-73 0663-3930-41	100's 500's 100 (10 × 10) unit dose
DIABINESE (chlorpropamide) 250 mg	Blue, D-shaped, scored	394	0663-3940-66 0663-3940-71 0663-3940-82 0663-3940-41	100's 250's 1000's 100 (10 × 10) unit dose
DIABINESE (chlorpropamide) 250 mg	Blue, D-shaped, scored	394	0663-3940-30	30's D-Pak

RECOMMENDED STORAGE

Store below 86°F (30°C).

CAUTION

Federal law prohibits dispensing without prescription.

Revised Jan. 1985
(70-2141-37-7)

Literature Available: Yes.

Shown in Product Identification Section, page 422

FELDENE® ℞

[fĕl 'deen]
(piroxicam)
CAPSULES
For Oral Use

DESCRIPTION

FELDENE (piroxicam) is 4-Hydroxy-2-methyl-*N*-2-pyridinyl-2*H*-1,2- benzothiazine-3-carboxamide 1,1-dioxide, an oxicam. Members of the oxicam family are not carboxylic acids, but they are acidic by virtue of the enolic 4-hydroxy substituent. FELDENE occurs as a white crystalline solid, sparingly soluble in water, dilute acid and most organic solvents. It is slightly soluble in alcohols and in aqueous alkaline solution. It exhibits a weakly acidic 4-hydroxy proton (pKa 5.1) and a weakly basic pyridyl nitrogen (pKa 1.8).

CLINICAL PHARMACOLOGY

FELDENE has shown anti- inflammatory, analgesic and antipyretic properties in animals. Edema, erythema, tissue proliferation, fever, and pain can all be inhibited in laboratory animals by the administration of FELDENE. It is effective regardless of the etiology of the inflammation. The mode of action of FELDENE is not fully established at this time. However, a common mechanism for the above effects may exist in the ability of FELDENE to inhibit the biosynthesis of prostaglandins, known mediators of inflammation.

It is established that FELDENE does not act by stimulating the pituitary-adrenal axis.

FELDENE is well absorbed following oral administration. Drug plasma concentrations are proportional for 10 and 20 mg doses, generally peak within three to five hours after medication, and subsequently decline with a mean half-life of 50 hours (range of 30 to 86 hours, although values outside of this range have been encountered).

This prolonged half-life results in the maintenance of relatively stable plasma concentrations throughout the day on once daily doses and to significant drug accumulation upon multiple dosing. A single 20 mg dose generally produces peak piroxicam plasma levels of 1.5 to 2 mcg/ml, while maximum drug plasma concentrations, after repeated daily ingestion of 20 mg FELDENE, usually stabilize at 3–8 mcg/ml. Most patients approximate steady state plasma levels within 7 to 12 days. Higher levels, which approximate steady state at two to three weeks, have been observed in patients in whom longer plasma half-lives of piroxicam occurred.

FELDENE and its biotransformation products are excreted in urine and feces, with about twice as much appearing in the urine as the feces. Metabolism occurs by hydroxylation at the 5 position of the pyridyl side chain and conjugation of this product; by cyclodehydration; and by a sequence of reactions involving hydrolysis of the amide linkage, decarboxylation, ring contraction, and N-demethylation. Less than 5% of the daily dose is excreted unchanged.

Concurrent administration of aspirin (3900 mg/day) and FELDENE (20 mg/day), resulted in a reduction of plasma levels of piroxicam to about 80% of their normal values. The use of FELDENE in conjunction with aspirin is not recommended because data are inadequate to demonstrate that the combination produces greater improvement than that achieved with aspirin alone and the potential for adverse reactions is increased. Concomitant administration of antacids had no effect on FELDENE plasma levels. The effects of impaired renal function or hepatic disease on plasma levels have not been established.

FELDENE, like salicylates and other nonsteroidal anti-inflammatory agents, is associated with symptoms of gastrointestinal tract irritation (see ADVERSE REACTIONS). However, in a study utilizing ^{51}Cr-tagged red blood cells, 20 mg of FELDENE administered as a single dose for four days did not result in a significant increase in fecal blood loss and did not detectably affect the gastric mucosa. In the same study a total daily dose of 3900 mg of aspirin, i.e., 972 mg q.i.d., caused a significant increase in fecal blood loss and mucosal lesions as demonstrated by gastroscopy.

In controlled clinical trials, the effectiveness of FELDENE (piroxicam) has been established for both acute exacerbations and long-term management of rheumatoid arthritis and osteoarthritis.

The therapeutic effects of FELDENE are evident early in the treatment of both diseases with a progressive increase in response over several (8–12) weeks. Efficacy is seen in terms of pain relief and, when present, subsidence of inflammation. Doses of 20 mg/day FELDENE display a therapeutic effect comparable to therapeutic doses of aspirin, with a lower incidence of minor gastrointestinal effects and tinnitus.

FELDENE has been administered concomitantly with fixed doses of gold and corticosteroids. The existence of a "steroid-sparing" effect has not been adequately studied to date.

INDICATIONS AND USAGE

FELDENE is indicated for acute or long-term use in the relief of signs and symptoms of the following:

1. osteoarthritis
2. rheumatoid arthritis

Dosage recommendations for use in children have not been established.

CONTRAINDICATIONS

FELDENE should not be used in patients who have previously exhibited hypersensitivity to it, or in individuals with the syndrome comprised of bronchospasm, nasal polyps, and angioedema precipitated by aspirin or other nonsteroidal anti-inflammatory drugs.

WARNINGS

Peptic ulceration, perforation, and G.I. bleeding—sometimes severe, and, in some instances fatal—have been reported with patients receiving FELDENE. If FELDENE must be given to patients with a history of upper gastrointestinal tract disease, the patient should be under close supervision (see ADVERSE REACTIONS). In controlled clinical trials, incidence of peptic ulceration with the maximum recommended FELDENE capsule dose of 20 mg per day was 0.8%. The use of doses higher than the recommended dose is associated with an increase in the incidence of gastrointestinal irritation and ulcers.

PRECAUTIONS

Renal Effects: As with other nonsteroidal anti-inflammatory drugs, long-term administration of piroxicam to animals has resulted in renal papillary necrosis and other abnormal renal pathology. In humans, there have been reports of acute interstitial nephritis with hematuria, proteinuria, and occasionally, nephrotic syndrome.

A second form of renal toxicity has been seen in patients with prerenal conditions leading to a reduction in renal blood flow or blood volume, where the renal prostaglandins have a supportive role in the maintenance of renal perfusion. In these patients administration of an NSAID may cause a dose-dependent reduction in prostaglandin formation and may precipitate overt renal decompensation. Patients at greatest risk of this reaction are those with impaired renal function, heart failure, liver dysfunction, those taking diuretics, and the elderly. Discontinuation of NSAID therapy is typically followed by recovery to the pretreatment state.

Because of extensive renal excretion of piroxicam and its biotransformation products (less than 5% of the daily dose excreted unchanged, see Clinical Pharmacology), lower doses of piroxicam should be anticipated in patients with impaired renal function and they should be carefully monitored.

Although other nonsteroidal anti-inflammatory drugs do not have the same direct effects on platelets that aspirin does, all drugs inhibiting prostaglandin biosynthesis do interfere with platelet function to some degree; therefore, patients who may be adversely affected by such an action should be carefully observed when FELDENE is administered.

Because of reports of adverse eye findings with nonsteroidal anti-inflammatory agents, it is recommended that patients who develop visual complaints during treatment with FELDENE have ophthalmic evaluation.

As with other nonsteroidal anti-inflammatory drugs, borderline elevations of one or more liver tests may occur in up to 15% of patients. These abnormalities may progress, may remain essentially unchanged, or may be transient with continued therapy. The SGPT (ALT) test is probably the most sensitive indicator of liver dysfunction. Meaningful (3 times the upper limit of normal) elevations of SGPT or SGOT (AST) occurred in controlled clinical trials in less than 1% of patients. A patient with symptoms and/or signs suggesting liver dysfunction, or in whom an abnormal liver test has occurred, should be evaluated for evidence of the development of more severe hepatic reaction while on therapy with FELDENE. Severe hepatic reactions, including jaundice and cases of fatal hepatitis, have been reported with FELDENE. Although such reactions are rare, if abnormal liver tests persist or worsen, if clinical signs and symptoms consistent with liver disease develop, or if systemic manifestations occur (e.g. eosinophilia, rash, etc.), FELDENE should be discontinued. (See also ADVERSE REACTIONS.)

Although at the recommended dose of 20 mg/day of FELDENE increased fecal blood loss due to gastrointestinal irritation did not occur (see CLINICAL PHARMACOLOGY), in about 4% of the patients treated with FELDENE alone or concomitantly with aspirin, reductions in hemoglobin and hematocrit values were observed. Therefore, these values should be determined if signs or symptoms of anemia occur.

Peripheral edema has been observed in approximately 2% of the patients treated with FELDENE. Therefore, as with other nonsteroidal anti-inflammatory drugs, FELDENE should be used with caution in patients with heart failure, hypertension or other conditions predisposing to fluid retention, since its usage may be associated with a worsening of these conditions.

A combination of dermatological and/or allergic signs and symptoms suggestive of serum sickness have occasionally occurred in conjunction with the use of FELDENE. These include arthralgias, pruritus, fever, fatigue, and rash including vesiculo bullous reactions and exfoliative dermatitis.

DRUG INTERACTIONS

FELDENE is highly protein bound, and, therefore, might be expected to displace other protein-bound drugs. Although this has not occurred in *in vitro* studies with coumarin-type anticoagulants, interactions with coumarin-type anticoagulants have been reported with FELDENE since marketing, therefore, physicians should closely monitor patients for a change in dosage requirements when administering FELDENE to patients on coumarin-type anticoagulants and other highly protein-bound drugs.

Plasma levels of piroxicam are depressed to approximately 80% of their normal values when FELDENE is administered in conjunction with aspirin (3900 mg/day), but concomitant administration of antacids has no effect on piroxicam plasma levels (see CLINICAL PHARMACOLOGY).

Nonsteroidal anti-inflammatory agents, including FELDENE, have been reported to increase steady state plasma lithium levels. It is recommended that plasma lithium levels be monitored when initiating, adjusting and discontinuing FELDENE (piroxicam).

Carcinogenesis, Chronic Animal Toxicity and Impairment of Fertility

Subacute and chronic toxicity studies have been carried out in rats, mice, dogs, and monkeys.

The pathology most often seen was that characteristically associated with the animal toxicology of anti-inflammatory agents; renal papillary necrosis (see PRECAUTIONS) and gastrointestinal lesions.

In classical studies in laboratory animals piroxicam did not show any teratogenic potential.

Reproductive studies revealed no impairment of fertility in animals.

Pregnancy and Nursing Mothers

Like other drugs which inhibit the synthesis and release of prostaglandins, piroxicam increased the incidence of dystocia and delayed parturition in pregnant animals when piroxicam administration was continued late into pregnancy. Gastrointestinal tract toxicity was increased in pregnant females in the last trimester of pregnancy compared to non-pregnant females or females in earlier trimesters of pregnancy.

FELDENE is not recommended for use in nursing mothers or in pregnant women because of the animal findings and since safety for such use has not been established in humans.

Use in Children

Dosage recommendations and indications for use in children have not been established.

ADVERSE REACTIONS

The incidence of adverse reactions to piroxicam is based on clinical trials involving approximately 2300 patients, about 400 of whom were treated for more than one year and 170 for more than two years. About 30% of all patients receiving daily doses of 20 mg of FELDENE experienced side effects. Gastrointestinal symptoms were the most prominent side effects—occurring in approximately 20% of the patients, which in most instances did not interfere with the course of therapy. Of the patients experiencing gastrointestinal side effects, approximately 5% discontinued therapy with an overall incidence of peptic ulceration of about 1%.

Other than the gastrointestinal symptoms, edema, dizziness, headache, changes in hematological parameters, and rash have been reported in a small percentage of patients. Routine ophthalmoscopy and slit-lamp examinations have revealed no evidence of ocular changes in 205 patients followed from 3 to 24 months while on therapy.

Incidence Greater than 1% The following adverse reactions occurred more frequently than 1 in 100.

Gastrointestinal: stomatitis, anorexia, epigastric distress*, nausea*, constipation, abdominal discomfort, flatulence, diarrhea, abdominal pain, indigestion

Hematological: decreases in hemoglobin* and hematocrit* (see PRECAUTIONS), anemia, leucopenia, eosinophilia

Dermatologic: pruritus, rash

Central Nervous System: dizziness, somnolence, vertigo

Urogenital: BUN and creatinine elevations (see PRECAUTIONS)

Body as a Whole: headache, malaise

Special Senses: tinnitus

Cardiovascular/Respiratory: edema (see PRECAUTIONS)

*Reactions occurring in 3% to 9% of patients treated with FELDENE. Reactions occurring in 1–3% of patients are unmarked.

Incidence Less Than 1% (Causal Relationship Probable) The following adverse reactions occurred less frequently than 1 in 100. The probability exists that there is a causal relationship between FELDENE and these reactions.

Gastrointestinal: liver function abnormalities, jaundice, hepatitis (see PRECAUTIONS), vomiting, hematemesis, melena, gastrointestinal bleeding, perforation and ulceration (see WARNINGS), dry mouth

Hematological: thrombocytopenia, petechial rash, ecchymosis, bone marrow depression including aplastic anemia, epistaxis

Dermatologic: sweating, erythema, bruising, desquamation, exfoliative dermatitis, erythema multiforme, toxic epidermal necrolysis, Stevens-Johnson syndrome, vesiculo bullous reaction, photoallergic skin reactions

Central Nervous System: depression, insomnia, nervousness

Urogenital: hematuria, proteinuria, interstitial nephritis, renal failure, hyperkalemia, glomerulitis, papillary necrosis, nephrotic syndrome (see PRECAUTIONS)

Body as a Whole: pain (colic), fever, flu-like syndrome (see PRECAUTIONS)

Special Senses: swollen eyes, blurred vision, eye irritations

Cardiovascular/Respiratory: hypertension, worsening of congestive heart failure (see PRECAUTIONS), exacerbation of angina

Metabolic: hypoglycemia, hyperglycemia, weight increase, weight decrease

Hypersensitivity: anaphylaxis, bronchospasm, urticaria/angioedema, vasculitis, "serum sickness" (see PRECAUTIONS)

Incidence Less Than 1% (Causal Relationship Unknown) Other adverse reactions were reported with a frequency of less than 1 in 100, but a causal relationship between FELDENE and the reaction could not be determined.

Gastrointestinal: pancreatitis

Dermatologic: onycholysis, loss of hair

Central Nervous System: akathisia, hallucinations, mood alterations, dream abnormalities, mental confusion, paresthesias

Urogenital System: dysuria

Body as a Whole: weakness

Cardiovascular/Respiratory: palpitations, dyspnea

Hypersensitivity: positive ANA

OVERDOSAGE

In the event treatment for overdosage is required the long plasma half-life (see CLINICAL PHARMACOLOGY) of piroxicam should be considered. The absence of experience with acute overdosage precludes characterization of sequelae and recommendation of specific antidotal efficacy at this time. It is reasonable to assume, however, that the standard measures of gastric evacuation and general supportive therapy would apply. In addition to supportive measures, the use of activated charcoal may effectively reduce the absorption and reabsorption of piroxicam. Experiments in dogs have demonstrated that the use of multiple-dose treatments with activated charcoal could reduce the half-life of piroxicam elimination from 27 hours (without charcoal) to 11 hours and reduce the systemic bioavailability of piroxicam by as much as 37% when activated charcoal is given as late as 6 hours after administration of piroxicam.

ADMINISTRATION AND DOSAGE

Rheumatoid Arthritis, Osteoarthritis

It is recommended that FELDENE therapy be initiated and maintained at a single daily dose of 20 mg. If desired the daily dose may be divided. Because of the long half-life of FELDENE, steady-state blood levels are not reached for 7–12 days. Therefore although the therapeutic effects of FELDENE are evident early in treatment, there is a progressive increase in response over several weeks and the effect of therapy should not be assessed for two weeks.

Dosage recommendations and indications for use in children have not been established.

HOW SUPPLIED

FELDENE Capsules for oral administration

Bottles of 100: 10 mg (NDC 0069-3220-66) maroon and blue #322
20 mg (NDC 0069-3230-66) maroon #323

Bottles of 500: 20 mg (NDC 0069-3230-73) maroon #323

Unit dose packages of 100: 20 mg (NDC 0069-3230-41) maroon #323 Revised July 1985

 65-4100-37-8

LITERATURE AVAILABLE

Yes.

Shown in Product Identification Section, page 422

MINIPRESS® CAPSULES ℞

[*min'ē-prēs*]
(prazosin hydrochloride)
For Oral Use

DESCRIPTION

MINIPRESS (prazosin hydrochloride), a quinazoline derivative, is the first of a new chemical class of antihypertensives. It is the hydrochloride salt of 1-(4-amino-6,7-dimethoxy-2-quinazolinyl)-4-(2-furoyl) piperazine.

It is a white, crystalline substance, slightly soluble in water and isotonic saline, and has a molecular weight of 419.87. Each 1 mg capsule of MINIPRESS for oral use contains drug equivalent to 1 mg free base.

CLINICAL PHARMACOLOGY

The exact mechanism of the hypotensive action of prazosin is unknown. Prazosin causes a decrease in total peripheral resistance and was originally thought to have a direct relaxant action on vascular smooth muscle. Recent animal studies, however, have suggested that the vasodilator effect of prazosin is also related to blockade of postsynaptic *alpha*-adrenoceptors. The results of dog forelimb experiments demonstrate that the peripheral vasodilator effect of prazosin is confined mainly to the level of the resistance vessels (arterioles). Unlike conventional *alpha*-blockers, the antihypertensive action of prazosin is usually not accompanied by a reflex tachycardia. Tolerance has not been observed to develop in long term therapy.

Hemodynamic studies have been carried out in man following acute single dose administration and during the course of long term maintenance therapy. The results confirm that the therapeutic effect is a fall in blood pressure unaccompanied by a clinically significant change in cardiac output, heart rate, renal blood flow and glomerular filtration rate. There is no measurable negative chronotropic effect.

In clinical studies to date, MINIPRESS (prazosin hydrochloride) has not increased plasma renin activity.

In man, blood pressure is lowered in both the supine and standing positions. This effect is most pronounced on the diastolic blood pressure.

Following oral administration, human plasma concentrations reach a peak at about three hours with a plasma half-life of two to three hours. The drug is highly bound to plasma protein. Bioavailability studies have demonstrated that the total absorption relative to the drug in a 20% alcoholic solution is 90%, resulting in peak levels approximately 65% of that of the drug in solution. Animal studies indicate that MINIPRESS (prazosin hydrochloride) is extensively metabolized, primarily by demethylation and conjugation, and excreted mainly via bile and feces. Less extensive human studies suggest similar metabolism and excretion in man.

In clinical studies in which lipid profiles were followed, there were generally no adverse changes noted between pre- and post-treatment lipid levels.

INDICATIONS AND USAGE

MINIPRESS (prazosin hydrochloride) is indicated in the treatment of hypertension. As an antihypertensive drug, it is mild to moderate in activity. It can be used as the initial agent or it may be employed in a general treatment program in conjunction with a diuretic and/or other antihypertensive drugs as needed for proper patient response.

Continued on next page

Pfizer—Cont.

CONTRAINDICATIONS

None known.

WARNINGS

MINIPRESS (prazosin hydrochloride) may cause syncope with sudden loss of consciousness. In most cases this is believed to be due to an excessive postural hypotensive effect, although occasionally the syncopal episode has been preceded by a bout of severe tachycardia with heart rates of 120–160 beats per minute. Syncopal episodes have usually occurred within 30 to 90 minutes of the initial dose of the drug; occasionally they have been reported in association with rapid dosage increases or the introduction of another antihypertensive drug into the regimen of a patient taking high doses of MINIPRESS (prazosin hydrochloride). The incidence of syncopal episodes is approximately 1% in patients given an initial dose of 2 mg or greater. Clinical trials conducted during the investigational phase of this drug suggest that syncopal episodes can be minimized by limiting the initial dose of the drug to 1 mg, by subsequently increasing the dosage slowly, and by introducing any additional antihypertensive drugs into the patient's regimen with caution (see DOSAGE AND ADMINISTRATION). Hypotension may develop in patients given MINIPRESS who are also receiving a beta-blocker such as propranolol.

If syncope occurs, the patient should be placed in the recumbent position and treated supportively as necessary. This adverse effect is self-limiting and in most cases does not recur after the initial period of therapy or during subsequent dose titration.

Patients should always be started on the 1 mg capsules of MINIPRESS (prazosin hydrochloride). The 2 and 5 mg capsules are not indicated for initial therapy.

More common than loss of consciousness are the symptoms often associated with lowering of the blood pressure, namely, dizziness and lightheadedness. The patient should be cautioned about these possible adverse effects and advised what measures to take should they develop. The patient should also be cautioned to avoid situations where injury could result should syncope occur during the initiation of MINIPRESS (prazosin hydrochloride) therapy.

PRECAUTIONS

Information for Patients: Dizziness or drowsiness may occur after the first dose of this medicine. Avoid driving or performing hazardous tasks for the first 24 hours after taking this medicine or when the dose is increased. Dizziness, lightheadedness or fainting may occur, especially when rising from a lying or sitting position. Getting up slowly may help lessen the problem. These effects may also occur if you drink alcohol, stand for long periods of time, exercise, or if the weather is hot. While taking MINIPRESS, be careful in the amount of alcohol you drink. Also, use extra care during exercise or hot weather, or if standing for long periods. Check with your physician if you have any questions.

Drug Interactions

MINIPRESS (prazosin hydrochloride) has been administered without any adverse drug interaction in limited clinical experience to date with the following: (1) cardiac glycosides—digitalis and digoxin; (2) hypoglycemics—insulin, chlorpropamide, phenformin, tolazamide, and tolbutamide; (3) tranquilizers and sedatives—chlordiazepoxide, diazepam, and phenobarbital; (4) antigout—allopurinol, colchicine, and probenecid; (5) antiarrhythmics—procainamide, propranolol (see WARNINGS however), and quinidine; and (6) analgesics, antipyretics and antiinflammatories—propoxyphene, aspirin, indomethacin and phenylbutazone.

Addition of a diuretic or other antihypertensive agent to MINIPRESS has been shown to cause an additive hypotensive effect. This effect can be minimized by reducing the MINIPRESS dose to 1 to 2 mg three times a day, by introducing additional anti-hypertensive drugs cautiously and then by retitrating MINIPRESS based on clinical response.

Drug/Laboratory Test Interactions

In a study on five patients given from 12 to 24 mg of prazosin per day for 10 to 14 days, there was an average increase of 42% in the urinary metabolite of norepinephrine and an average increase in urinary VMA of 17%. Therefore, false positive results may occur in screening tests for pheochromocytoma in patients who are being treated with prazosin. If an elevated VMA is found, prazosin should be discontinued and the patient retested after a month.

Laboratory Tests

In clinical studies in which lipid profiles were followed, there were generally no adverse changes noted between pre- and post-treatment lipids levels.

Carcinogenesis, Mutagenesis, Impairment of Fertility: No carcinogenic potential was demonstrated in an 18 month study in rats with MINIPRESS at dose levels more than 225 times the usual maximum recommended human dose of 20 mg per day. MINIPRESS was not mutagenic in *in vivo* genetic toxicology studies. In a fertility and general reproductive performance study in rats, both males and females, treated with 75 mg/kg (225 times the usual maximum recommended human dose), demonstrated decreased fertility while those treated with 25 mg/kg (75 times the usual maximum recommended human dose) did not.

In chronic studies (one year or more) of MINIPRESS in rats and dogs, testicular changes consisting of atrophy and necrosis occurred at 25 mg/kg/day (75 times the usual recommended human dose). No testicular changes were seen in rats or dogs at 10 mg/kg/day (30 times the usual maximum recommended human dose). In view of the testicular changes observed in animals, 105 patients on long term MINIPRESS therapy were monitored for 17-ketosteroid excretion and no changes indicating a drug effect were observed. In addition, 27 males on MINIPRESS for up to 51 months did not have changes in sperm morphology suggestive of drug effect.

Usage in Pregnancy: Pregnancy Category C. MINIPRESS has been shown to be associated with decreased litter size at birth, 1, 4, and 21 days of age in rats when given doses more than 225 times the usual maximum recommended human dose. No evidence of drug-related external, visceral, or skeletal fetal abnormalities were observed. No drug-related external, visceral, or skeletal abnormalities were observed in fetuses of pregnant rabbits and pregnant monkeys at doses more than 225 times and 12 times the usual maximum recommended human dose respectively.

The use of prazosin and a beta-blocker for the control of severe hypertension in 44 pregnant women revealed no drug-related fetal abnormalities or adverse effects. Therapy with prazosin was continued for as long as 14 weeks.[1]

Prazosin has also been used alone or in combination with other hypotensive agents in severe hypertension of pregnancy by other investigators. No fetal or neonatal abnormalities have been reported with the use of prazosin.[2]

There are no adequate and well controlled studies which establish the safety of MINIPRESS (prazosin HCl) in pregnant women. MINIPRESS should be used during pregnancy only if the potential benefit justifies the potential risk to the mother and fetus.

Nursing Mothers: MINIPRESS has been shown to be excreted in small amounts in human milk. Caution should be exercised when MINIPRESS is administered to a nursing woman.

Usage in Children: Safety and effectiveness in children have not been established.

ADVERSE REACTIONS

Clinical trials were conducted on more than 900 patients. During these trials and subsequent marketing experience, the most frequent reactions associated with MINIPRESS therapy are: dizziness 10.3%, headache 7.8%, drowsiness 7.6%, lack of energy 6.9%, weakness 6.5%, palpitations 5.3%, and nausea 4.9%. In most instances side effects have disappeared with continued therapy or have been tolerated with no decrease in dose of drug.

Less frequent adverse reactions which are reported to occur in 1–4% of patients are:

Gastrointestinal: vomiting, diarrhea, constipation.
Cardiovascular: edema, orthostatic hypotension, dyspnea, syncope.
Central Nervous System: vertigo, depression, nervousness.
Dermatologic: rash.
Genitourinary: urinary frequency.
EENT: blurred vision, reddened sclera, epistaxis, dry mouth, nasal congestion.

In addition, fewer than 1% of patients have reported the following (in some instances, exact causal relationships have not been established):

Gastrointestinal: abdominal discomfort and/or pain, liver function abnormalities, pancreatitis.
Cardiovascular: tachycardia.
Central Nervous System: paresthesia, hallucinations.
Dermatologic: pruritus, alopecia, lichen planus.
Genitourinary: incontinence, impotence, priapism.
EENT: tinnitus.
Other: diaphoresis, fever, positive ANA titer, arthralgia.

Single reports of pigmentary mottling and serous retinopathy, and a few reports of cataract development or disappearance have been reported. In these instances, the exact causal relationship has not been established because the baseline observations were frequently inadequate.

In more specific slit-lamp and funduscopic studies, which included adequate baseline examinations, no drug-related abnormal ophthalmological findings have been reported.

OVERDOSAGE

Accidental ingestion of at least 50 mg of MINIPRESS (prazosin hydrochloride) in a two year old child resulted in profound drowsiness and depressed reflexes. No decrease in blood pressure was noted. Recovery was uneventful.

Should overdosage lead to hypotension, support of the cardiovascular system is of first importance. Restoration of blood pressure and normalization of heart rate may be accomplished by keeping the patient in a supine position. If this measure is inadequate, shock should first be treated with volume expanders. If necessary, vasopressors should then be used. Renal function should be monitored and supported as needed. Laboratory data indicate MINIPRESS is not dialysable because it is protein bound.

DOSAGE AND ADMINISTRATION

The dose of MINIPRESS should be adjusted according to the patient's individual blood pressure response. The following is a guide to its administration:

Initial Dose

1 mg two or three times a day. (See Warnings)

Maintenance Dose

Dosage may be slowly increased to a total daily dose of 20 mg given in divided doses. The therapeutic dosages most commonly employed have ranged from 6 mg to 15 mg daily given in divided doses. Doses higher than 20 mg usually do not increase efficacy, however a few patients may benefit from further increases up to a daily dose of 40 mg given in divided doses. After initial titration some patients can be maintained adequately on a twice daily dosage regimen.

Use With Other Drugs

When adding a diuretic or other antihypertensive agent, the dose of MINIPRESS should be reduced to 1 mg or 2 mg three times a day and retitration then carried out.

HOW SUPPLIED

[See table below].

Strength	Capsule Color	Capsule Coder	NDC	Package Size
MINIPRESS 1 mg	White	431	0663-4310-71 0663-4310-82 0663-4310-41	250's 1000's 100 (10×10) Unit Dose
MINIPRESS 2 mg	Pink and White	437	0663-4370-71 0663-4370-82 0663-4370-41	250's 1000's 100 (10×10) Unit Dose
MINIPRESS 5 mg	Blue and White	438	0663-4380-71 0663-4380-73 0663-4380-41	250's 500's 100 (10×10) Unit Dose

REFERENCES

1. Lubbe, WF, and Hodge, JV: *New Zealand Med J* **94** (691) 169–172, 1981.
2. Davey, DA, and Dommisse, J: *S.A. Med J*, Oct 4, 1980 (551–556).

Revised April 1986
60-2318-37-9

Literature Available—Yes.

Shown in Product Identification Section, page 422

MINIZIDE® CAPSULES ℞

[*mĭn 'ē-zīd*]
(prazosin hydrochloride and polythiazide)
FOR ORAL ADMINISTRATION

This fixed combination drug is not indicated for initial therapy of hypertension. Hypertension requires therapy titrated to the individual patient. If the fixed combination represents the dose so determined, its use may be more convenient in patient management. The treatment of hypertension is not static, but must be re-evaluated as conditions in each patient warrant.

DESCRIPTION

MINIZIDE is a combination of MINIPRESS® (prazosin hydrochloride) plus RENESE® (polythiazide).

MINIPRESS (prazosin hydrochloride), a quinazoline derivative, is the first of a new chemical class of antihypertensives.

It is the hydrochloride salt of 1-(4-amino-6,7-dimethoxy-2-quinazolinyl)-4- (2-furoyl) piperazine.
It is a white, crystalline substance, slightly soluble in water and isotonic saline, and has a molecular weight of 419.87.
Each 1 mg capsule of MINIPRESS (prazosin hydrochloride) contains drug equivalent to 1 mg free base.
RENESE (polythiazide) is an orally effective, nonmercurial diuretic, saluretic, and antihypertensive agent.
It is designated chemically as 2*H*-1,2,4-Benzothiadiazine-7-sulfonamide, 6-chloro-3, 4-dihydro-2-methyl-3-[[(2,2,2-trifluoroethyl)thio]methyl]-,1,1- dioxide.
It is a white, crystalline substance insoluble in water, but readily soluble in alkaline solution.

CLINICAL PHARMACOLOGY

MINIZIDE (prazosin hydrochloride/polythiazide)
Minizide produces a more pronounced antihypertensive response than occurs after either prazosin hydrochloride or polythiazide alone in equivalent doses.
MINIPRESS (prazosin hydrochloride)
The exact mechanism of the hypotensive action of prazosin is unknown. Prazosin causes a decrease in total peripheral resistance and was originally thought to have a direct relaxant action on vascular smooth muscle. Recent animal studies, however, have suggested that the vasodilator effect of prazosin is also related to blockade of postsynaptic *alpha*-adrenoceptors. The results of dog forelimb experiments demonstrate that the peripheral vasodilator effect of prazosin is confined mainly to the level of the resistance vessels (arterioles). Unlike conventional *alpha*-blockers, the antihypertensive action of prazosin is usually not accompanied by a reflex tachycardia. Tolerance has not been observed to develop in long term therapy.
Hemodynamic studies have been carried out in man following acute single dose administration and during the course of long term maintenance therapy. The results confirm that the therapeutic effect is a fall in blood pressure unaccompanied by a clinically significant change in cardiac output, heart rate, renal blood flow, and glomerular filtration rate. There is no measurable negative chronotropic effect.
In clinical studies to date, MINIPRESS has not increased plasma renin activity.
In man, blood pressure is lowered in both the supine and standing positions. This effect is most pronounced on the diastolic blood pressure.
Following oral administration, human plasma concentrations reach a peak at about three hours with a plasma half-life of two to three hours. The drug is highly bound to plasma protein. Bioavailability studies have demonstrated that the total absorption relative to the drug in a 20% alcoholic solution is 90%, resulting in peak levels approximately 65% of that of the drug in solution. Animal studies indicate that MINIPRESS is extensively metabolized, primarily by demethylation and conjugation, and excreted mainly via bile and feces. Less extensive human studies suggest similar metabolism and excretion in man.
MINIPRESS has been administered without any adverse drug interaction in limited clinical experience to date with the following: (1) cardiac glycosides—digitalis and digoxin; (2) hypoglycemics—insulin, chlorpropamide, phenformin, tolazamide, and tolbutamide; (3) tranquilizers and sedatives—chlordiazepoxide, diazepam, and phenobarbital; (4) antigout—allopurinol, colchicine, and probenecid; (5) antiarrhythmics—procainamide, propranolol (see WARNINGS however), and quinidine; and (6) analgesics, antipyretics and anti-inflammatories—propoxyphene, aspirin, indomethacin, and phenylbutazone.
RENESE (polythiazide)
RENESE is a member of the benzothiadiazine (thiazide) family of diuretic/antihypertensive agents. Its mechanism of action results in an interference with the renal tubular mechanism of electrolyte reabsorption. At maximal therapeutic dosage all thiazides are approximately equal in their diuretic potency. The mechanism whereby thiazides function in the control of hypertension is unknown. Renese is well absorbed, giving peak human plasma concentrations about 5 hours after oral administration. Drug is removed slowly thereafter with a plasma elimination half-life of approximately 27 hours. One fifth of the drug is recovered unchanged in human urine; the remainder is cleared via feces and as metabolites. Animal studies indicate metabolism occurs by rupture of the thiadiazine ring and loss of the side chain.

INDICATIONS AND USAGE

MINIZIDE is indicated in the treatment of hypertension. (See box warning.)

CONTRAINDICATIONS

RENESE (polythiazide) is contraindicated in patients with anuria, and in patients known to be sensitive to thiazides or to other sulfonamide derivatives.

MINIZIDE CAPSULES
prazosin HCl/polythiazide

STRENGTH	COMPONENTS	COLOR	CAPSULE CODE	PKG. SIZE
MINIZIDE 1	1 mg prazosin + 0.5 mg polythiazide	Blue-Green	430	100's
MINIZIDE 2	2 mg prazosin + 0.5 mg polythiazide	Blue-Green/Pink	432	100's
MINIZIDE 5	5 mg prazosin + 0.5 mg polythiazide	Blue-Green/Blue	436	100's

WARNINGS

MINIPRESS (prazosin hydrochloride)
MINIPRESS may cause syncope with sudden loss of consciousness. In most cases this is believed to be due to an excessive postural hypotensive effect, although occasionally the syncopal episode has been preceded by a bout of severe tachycardia with heart rates of 120–160 beats per minute. Syncopal episodes have usually occurred within 30 to 90 minutes of the initial dose of the drug; occasionally they have been reported in association with rapid dosage increases or the introduction of another antihypertensive drug into the regimen of a patient taking high doses of MINIPRESS. The incidence of syncopal episodes is approximately 1% in patients given an initial dose of 2 mg or greater. Clinical trials conducted during the investigational phase of this drug suggest that syncopal episodes can be minimized by limiting the initial dose of the drug to 1 mg, by subsequently increasing the dosage slowly, and by introducing any additional antihypertensive drugs into the patient's regimen with caution (see DOSAGE AND ADMINISTRATION). Hypotension may develop in patients given MINIPRESS who are also receiving a beta-blocker such as propranolol.
If syncope occurs, the patient should be placed in the recumbent position and treated supportively as necessary. This adverse effect is self-limiting and in most cases does not recur after the initial period of therapy or during subsequent dose titration.
Patients should always be started on the 1 mg capsules of MINIPRESS (prazosin hydrochloride). The 2 and 5 mg capsules are not indicated for initial therapy.
More common than loss of consciousness are the symptoms often associated with lowering of the blood pressure, namely, dizziness and lightheadedness. The patient should be cautioned about these possible adverse effects and advised what measures to take should they develop. The patient should also be cautioned to avoid situations where injury could result should syncope occur during the initiation of MINIPRESS therapy.
RENESE (polythiazide)
RENESE should be used with caution in severe renal disease. In patients with renal disease, thiazides may precipitate azotemia. Cumulative effects of the drug may develop in patients with impaired renal function.
Thiazides should be used with caution in patients with impaired hepatic function or progressive liver disease, since minor alterations of fluid and electrolyte balance may precipitate hepatic coma.
Sensitivity reactions may occur in patients with a history of allergy or bronchial asthma.
The possibility of exacerbation or activation of systemic lupus erythematosus has been reported.
Thiazides may be additive or potentiative of the action of other antihypertensive drugs.
Potentiation occurs with ganglionic or peripheral adrenergic blocking drugs.
Periodic determinations of serum electrolytes to detect possible electrolyte imbalance should be performed at appropriate intervals.
All patients receiving thiazide therapy should be observed for clinical signs of fluid or electrolyte imbalance, namely, hyponatremia, hypochloremic alkalosis, and hypokalemia. Serum and urine electrolyte determinations are particularly important when the patient is vomiting excessively or receiving parenteral fluids. Medications such as digitalis may also influence serum electrolytes. Warning signs, irrespective of cause, are: dryness of mouth, thirst, weakness, lethargy, drowsiness, restlessness, muscle pains or cramps, muscular fatigue, hypotension, oliguria, tachycardia, and gastrointestinal disturbances such as nausea and vomiting.
Hypokalemia may develop with thiazides as with any potent diuretic, especially with brisk diuresis, when severe cirrhosis is present, or during concomitant use of corticosteroids or ACTH.
Interference with adequate oral electrolyte intake will also contribute to hypokalemia. Digitalis therapy may exaggerate the metabolic effects of hypokalemia, especially with reference to myocardial activity.
Any chloride deficit is generally mild and usually does not require specific treatment except under extraordinary circumstances (as in hepatic or renal disease). Dilutional hyponatremia may occur in edematous patients in hot weather; appropriate therapy is water restriction rather than administration of salt, except in rare instances when the hyponatremia is life-threatening. In actual salt depletion, appropriate replacement is the therapy of choice.
Hyperuricemia may occur or frank gout may be precipitated in certain patients receiving thiazide therapy.
Insulin requirements in diabetic patients may be either increased, decreased, or unchanged. Latent diabetes mellitus may become manifest during thiazide administration.
Thiazide drugs may increase responsiveness to tubocurarine.
The antihypertensive effects of the drug may be enhanced in the post-sympathectomy patient.
Thiazides may decrease arterial responsiveness to norepinephrine. This diminution is not sufficient to preclude effectiveness of the pressor agent for therapeutic use.
If progressive renal impairment becomes evident, as indicated by a rising nonprotein nitrogen or blood urea nitrogen, a careful reappraisal of therapy is necessary with consideration given to withholding or discontinuing diuretic therapy.
Thiazides may decrease serum protein-bound iodine levels without signs of thyroid disturbance.

PRECAUTIONS

Drug/Laboratory Test Interactions: In a study on five patients given from 12 to 24 mg of prazosin per day for 10 to 14 days, there was an average increase of 42% in the urinary metabolite of norepinephrine and an average increase in urinary VMA of 17%. Therefore, false positive results may occur in screening tests for pheochromocytoma in patients who are being treated with prazosin. If an elevated VMA is found, prazosin should be discontinued and the patient retested after a month.
Carcinogenesis, Mutagenesis, Impairment of Fertility: No carcinogenic or mutagenic studies have been conducted with MINIZIDE. However, no carcinogenic potential was demonstrated in 18 month studies in rats with either MINIPRESS or RENESE at dose levels more than 100 times the usual maximum human doses. MINIPRESS was not mutagenic in *in vivo* genetic toxicology studies.
MINIZIDE produced no impairment of fertility in male or female rats at 50 and 25 mg/kg/day of MINIPRESS and RENESE respectively. In chronic studies (one year or more) of MINIPRESS in rats and dogs, testicular changes consisting of atrophy and necrosis occurred at 25 mg/kg/day (60 times the usual maximum recommended human dose). No testicular changes were seen in rats or dogs at 10 mg/kg/day (24 times the usual maximum recommended human dose). In view of the testicular changes observed in animals, 105 patients on long term MINIPRESS therapy were monitored for 17-ketosteroid excretion and no changes indicating a drug effect were observed. In addition, 27 males on MINIPRESS alone for up to 51 months did not have changes in sperm morphology suggestive of drug effect.
Use in Pregnancy: Pregnancy Category C. MINIZIDE was not teratogenic in either rats or rabbits when administered in oral doses more than 100 times the usual maximum human dose. Studies in rats indicated that the combination of RENESE (40 times the usual maximum recommended human dose) and MINIPRESS (8 times the usual maximum recommended human dose) caused a greater number of stillbirths, a more prolonged gestation, and a decreased survival of pups to weaning than that caused by MINIPRESS alone. There are no adequate and well controlled studies in pregnant women. Therefore, MINIZIDE should be used in pregnancy only if the potential benefit justifies the potential risk to the fetus.
Nursing Mothers: It is not known whether MINIPRESS or RENESE are excreted in human milk. Thiazides appear in breast milk. Thus, if use of the drug is deemed essential the patient should stop nursing.
Pediatric Use: Safety and effectiveness in children has not been established.

ADVERSE REACTIONS

MINIPRESS (prazosin hydrochloride)
The most common reactions associated with MINIPRESS therapy are: dizziness 10.3%, headache 7.8%, drowsiness 7.6%, lack of energy 6.9%, weakness 6.5%, palpitations 5.3%, and nausea 4.9%. In most instances side effects have

Continued on next page

Pfizer—Cont.

disappeared with continued therapy or have been tolerated with no decrease in dose of drug.
The following reactions have been associated with MINIPRESS, some of them rarely. (In some instances exact causal relationships have not been established.)
Gastrointestinal: vomiting, diarrhea, constipation, abdominal discomfort and/or pain, liver function abnormalities, pancreatitis.
Cardiovascular: edema, dyspnea, syncope, tachycardia.
Central Nervous System: nervousness, vertigo, depression, paresthesia, hallucinations.
Dermatologic: rash, pruritus, alopecia, lichen planus.
Genitourinary: urinary frequency, incontinence, impotence, priapism.
EENT: blurred vision, reddened sclera, epistaxis, tinnitus, dry mouth, nasal congestion.
Other: diaphoresis, fever.
Single reports of pigmentary mottling and serous retinopathy, and a few reports of cataract development or disappearance have been reported. In these instances, the exact causal relationship has not been established because the baseline observations were frequently inadequate.
In more specific slit-lamp and funduscopic studies, which included adequate baseline examinations, no drug-related abnormal ophthalmological findings have been reported.
RENESE (polythiazide)
Gastrointestinal: anorexia, gastric irritation, nausea, vomiting, cramping, diarrhea, constipation, jaundice (intrahepatic cholestatic jaundice), pancreatitis.
Central Nervous System: dizziness, vertigo, paresthesia, headache, xanthopsia.
Hematologic: leukopenia, agranulocytosis, thrombocytopenia, aplastic anemia.
Dermatologic: purpura, photosensitivity, rash, urticaria, necrotizing angiitis, (vasculitis) (cutaneous vasculitis).
Cardiovascular: Orthostatic hypotension may occur and be aggravated by alcohol, barbiturates, or narcotics.
Other: hyperglycemia, glycosuria, hyperuricemia, muscle spasm, weakness, restlessness.

OVERDOSAGE

MINIPRESS (prazosin hydrochloride)
Accidental ingestion of at least 50 mg of MINIPRESS in a two year old child resulted in profound drowsiness and depressed reflexes. No decrease in blood pressure was noted. Recovery was uneventful.
Should overdosage lead to hypotension, support of the cardiovascular system is of first importance. Restoration of blood pressure and normalization of heart rate may be accomplished by keeping the patient in the supine position. If this measure is inadequate, shock should first be treated with volume expanders. If necessary, vasopressors should then be used. Renal function should be monitored and supported as needed. Laboratory data indicate that MINIPRESS is not dialysable because it is protein bound.
RENESE (polythiazide)
Should overdosage with RENESE occur, electrolyte balance and adequate hydration should be maintained. Gastric lavage is recommended, followed by supportive treatment. Where necessary, this may include intravenous dextrose and saline with potassium and other electrolyte therapy, administered with caution as indicated by laboratory testing at appropriate intervals.

DOSAGE AND ADMINISTRATION

MINIZIDE (prazosin hydrochloride/polythiazide)
Dosage: as determined by individual titration of MINIPRESS (prazosin hydrochloride) and RENESE (polythiazide). (See box warning.)
Usual MINIZIDE dosage is one capsule two or three times daily, the strength depending upon individual requirement following titration.
The following is a general guide to the administration of the individual components of MINIZIDE:
MINIPRESS (prazosin hydrochloride)
Initial Dose: 1 mg two or three times a day. (See Warnings.)
Maintenance Dose: Dosage may be slowly increased to a total daily dose of 20 mg given in divided doses. The therapeutic dosages most commonly employed have ranged from 6 mg to 15 mg daily given in divided doses. Doses higher than 20 mg usually do not increase efficacy, however a few patients may benefit from further increases up to a daily dose of 40 mg given in divided doses. After initial titration some patients can be maintained adequately on a twice daily dosage regimen.
Use With Other Drugs: When adding a diuretic or other antihypertensive agent, the dose of MINIPRESS should be reduced to 1 mg or 2 mg three times a day and retitration then carried out.
RENESE (polythiazide)
The usual dose of Renese for antihypertensive therapy is 2 to 4 mg daily.

HOW SUPPLIED

[See table on preceding page]

Revised Oct. 1984
69-2463-37-3

LITERATURE AVAILABLE

Yes.
Shown in Product Identification Section, page 422

MODERIL® ℞

[*mō'dĕr-ĭl*]
(rescinnamine)
TABLETS

DESCRIPTION

Rescinnamine is a pure crystalline alkaloid that has been identified chemically as the 3,4,5-trimethoxycinnamic acid ester of methyl reserpate. Pure rescinnamine occurs as white, needle-shaped crystals that are readily absorbed when ingested.
Moderil is available as oval, scored salmon tablets providing 0.5 mg. of crystalline rescinnamine or as oval, scored yellow tablets providing 0.25 mg. of crystalline rescinnamine.

ACTIONS

Rescinnamine probably produces its antihypertensive effects through depletion of tissue stores of catecholamines (epinephrine and norepinephrine) from peripheral sites. By contrast, its sedative and tranquilizing properties are thought to be related to depletion of 5-hydroxytryptamine from the brain.
Rescinnamine is characterized by slow onset of action and sustained effect. Both its cardiovascular and central nervous system effects may persist following withdrawal of the drug.

INDICATIONS

Indicated in the treatment of mild essential hypertension.

CONTRAINDICATIONS

Do not use in patients with known hypersensitivity, mental depression—especially with suicidal tendencies—active peptic ulcer, and ulcerative colitis. It is also contraindicated in patients receiving electroconvulsive therapy.

WARNINGS

Extreme caution should be exercised in treating patients with a history of mental depression. Discontinue the drug at the first sign of despondency, early morning insomnia, loss of appetite, impotence, or self-depreciation. Drug-induced depression may persist for several months after drug withdrawal and may be severe enough to result in suicide.
Usage in pregnancy: The safety of rescinnamine for use during pregnancy or lactation has not been established. Therefore, the drug should be used in pregnant patients or in women of child-bearing potential only when, in the judgment of the physician, its use is deemed essential to the welfare of the patient. Increased respiratory secretions, nasal congestion, cyanosis, and anorexia may occur in infants born to rescinnamine-treated mothers, since this preparation is known to cross the placental barrier, appearing in cord blood and breast milk.

PRECAUTIONS

Because Rauwolfia preparations increase gastrointestinal motility and secretion, this drug should be used cautiously in patients with a history of peptic ulcer, ulcerative colitis, or gallstones where biliary colic may be precipitated.
Caution should be exercised when treating hypertensive patients with renal insufficiency since they adjust poorly to lowered blood pressure levels.
Use rescinnamine cautiously with digitalis and quinidine since cardiac arrhythmias have occurred with Rauwolfia preparations.
Preoperative withdrawal of rescinnamine does not assure that circulatory instability will not occur. It is important that the anesthesiologist be aware of the patient's drug intake and consider this in the over-all management, since hypotension has occurred in patients receiving Rauwolfia preparations. Anticholinergic and/or adrenergic drugs (metaraminol, norepinephrine) have been employed to treat adverse vagocirculatory effects.

ADVERSE REACTIONS

Rauwolfia preparations have caused gastrointestinal reactions including hypersecretion, nausea and vomiting, anorexia, and diarrhea; cardiovascular reactions including angina-like symptoms, arrhythmias, particularly when used concurrently with digitalis or quinidine, and bradycardia; and central nervous system reactions including drowsiness, depression, nervousness, paradoxical anxiety, nightmares, rare parkinsonian syndrome, C.N.S. sensitization manifested by dull sensorium, deafness, glaucoma, uveitis, and optic atrophy. Nasal congestion is a frequent complaint; and pruritus, rash, dryness of mouth, dizziness, headache, dyspnea, purpura, impotence or decreased libido, dysuria, muscular aches, conjunctival injection, and weight gain have been reported. Extrapyramidal tract symptoms have also occurred. These reactions are usually reversible and disappear when the drug is discontinued.
Water retention with edema in patients with hypertensive vascular disease may occur rarely, but the condition generally clears with cessation of therapy, or with the administration of a diuretic agent.

DOSAGE AND ADMINISTRATION

For adults the average initial dose is 0.5 mg. orally, twice daily. Increase dosage gradually, if necessary. Maintenance doses may vary from 0.25 mg. to 0.5 mg. daily. Higher doses should be used cautiously because serious mental depression and other side effects may be increased considerably.
Concomitant use of rescinnamine and ganglionic blocking agents, guanethidine, veratrum, hydralazine, methyldopa, chlorthalidone, or thiazides necessitates careful titration of dosage with each agent.

SUPPLY

0.25 mg. tablets, oval, scored, yellow (imprinted with code number 441): bottles of 100.
0.5 mg. tablets, oval, scored, salmon (imprinted with code number 442): bottles of 100.

Revised August 1972
60-0695-00-7
Shown in Product Identification Section, page 422

PROCARDIA® ℞

[*pro-car'dē-ă*]
(nifedipine)
CAPSULES
For Oral Use

DESCRIPTION

PROCARDIA (nifedipine) is an antianginal drug belonging to a new class of pharmacological agents, the calcium channel blockers. Nifedipine is 3,5-pyridinedicarboxylic acid, 1,4-dihydro-2,6-dimethyl-4-(2-nitrophenyl)-, dimethyl ester, $C_{17}H_{18}N_2O_6$.
Nifedipine is a yellow crystalline substance, practically insoluble in water but soluble in ethanol. It has a molecular weight of 346.3. PROCARDIA CAPSULES are formulated as soft gelatin capsules for oral administration each containing 10 mg or 20 mg nifedipine.

CLINICAL PHARMACOLOGY

PROCARDIA is a calcium ion influx inhibitor (slow channel blocker or calcium ion antagonist) and inhibits the transmembrane influx of calcium ions into cardiac muscle and smooth muscle. The contractile processes of cardiac muscle and vascular smooth muscle are dependent upon the movement of extracellular calcium ions into these cells through specific ion channels. PROCARDIA selectively inhibits calcium ion influx across the cell membrane of cardiac muscle and vascular smooth muscle without changing serum calcium concentrations.
Mechanism of Action
The precise means by which this inhibition relieves angina has not been fully determined, but includes at least the following two mechanisms:
1) Relaxation and prevention of coronary artery spasm
PROCARDIA dilates the main coronary arteries and coronary arterioles, both in normal and ischemic regions, and is a potent inhibitor of coronary artery spasm, whether spontaneous or ergonovine-induced. This property increases myocardial oxygen delivery in patients with coronary artery spasm, and is responsible for the effectiveness of PROCARDIA in vasospastic (Prinzmetal's or variant) angina. Whether this effect plays any role in classical angina is not clear, but studies of exercise tolerance have not shown an increase in the maximum exercise rate-pressure product, a widely accepted measure of oxygen utilization. This suggests that, in general, relief of spasm or dilation of coronary arteries is not an important factor in classical angina.
2) Reduction of oxygen utilization
PROCARDIA regularly reduces arterial pressure at rest and at a given level of exercise by dilating peripheral arterioles and reducing the total peripheral resistance (afterload) against which the heart works. This unloading of the heart reduces myocardial energy consumption and oxygen requirements and probably accounts for the effectiveness of PROCARDIA in chronic stable angina.
Pharmacokinetics and Metabolism
PROCARDIA is rapidly and fully absorbed after oral administration. The drug is detectable in serum 10 minutes after oral administration, and peak blood levels occur in approximately 30 minutes. Bioavailability is proportional to dose from 10 to 30 mg; half-life does not change significantly with dose. There is little difference in relative bioavailability when PROCARDIA capsules are given orally and either swallowed whole; bitten and swallowed; or, bitten and held sublingually. However, biting through the capsule prior to swallowing does result in slightly earlier plasma concentrations (27 ng/ml 10 minutes after 10 mg) than if capsules are swallowed intact. It is highly bound by serum proteins. PROCARDIA is extensively converted to inactive metabo-

lites and approximately 80 percent of PROCARDIA and metabolites are eliminated via the kidneys. The half-life of nifedipine in plasma is approximately two hours. There is no information on the effects of renal or hepatic impairment on excretion or metabolism of PROCARDIA.

Hemodynamics

Like other slow channel blockers, PROCARDIA exerts a negative inotropic effect on isolated myocardial tissue. This is rarely, if ever, seen in intact animals or man, probably because of reflex responses to its vasodilating effects. In man, PROCARDIA causes decreased peripheral vascular resistance and a fall in systolic and diastolic pressure, usually modest (5–10mm Hg systolic), but sometimes larger. There is usually a small increase in heart rate, a reflex response to vasodilation. Measurements of cardiac function in patients with normal ventricular function have generally found a small increase in cardiac index without major effects on ejection fraction, left ventricular end diastolic pressure (LVEDP) or volume (LVEDV). In patients with impaired ventricular function, most acute studies have shown some increase in ejection fraction and reduction in left ventricular filling pressure.

Electrophysiologic Effects

Although like other members of its class, PROCARDIA decreases sinoatrial node function and atrioventricular conduction in isolated myocardial preparations, such effects have not been seen in studies in intact animals or in man. In formal electrophysiologic studies, predominantly in patients with normal conduction systems, PROCARDIA has had no tendency to prolong atrioventricular conduction, prolong sinus node recovery time, or slow sinus rate.

INDICATIONS AND USAGE

I. Vasospastic Angina

PROCARDIA (nifedipine) is indicated for the management of vasospastic angina confirmed by any of the following criteria: 1) classical pattern of angina at rest accompanied by ST segment elevation, 2) angina or coronary artery spasm provoked by ergonovine, or 3) angiographically demonstrated coronary artery spasm. In those patients who have had angiography, the presence of significant fixed obstructive disease is not incompatible with the diagnosis of vasospastic angina, provided that the above criteria are satisfied. PROCARDIA may also be used where the clinical presentation suggests a possible vasospastic component but where vasospasm has not been confirmed, e.g., where pain has a variable threshold on exertion or in unstable angina where electrocardiographic findings are compatible with intermittent vasospasm, or when angina is refractory to nitrates and/or adequate doses of beta blockers.

II. Chronic Stable Angina (Classical Effort-Associated Angina)

PROCARDIA is indicated for the management of chronic stable angina (effort-associated angina) without evidence of vasospasm in patients who remain symptomatic despite adequate doses of beta blockers and/or organic nitrates or who cannot tolerate those agents.

In chronic stable angina (effort-associated angina) PROCARDIA has been effective in controlled trials of up to eight weeks duration in reducing angina frequency and increasing exercise tolerance, but confirmation of sustained effectiveness and evaluation of long term safety in these patients are incomplete.

Controlled studies in small numbers of patients suggest concomitant use of PROCARDIA and beta blocking agents may be beneficial in patients with chronic stable angina, but available information is not sufficient to predict with confidence the effects of concurrent treatment, especially in patients with compromised left ventricular function or cardiac conduction abnormalities. When introducing such concomitant therapy, care must be taken to monitor blood pressure closely since severe hypotension can occur from the combined effects of the drugs. (See WARNINGS.)

CONTRAINDICATIONS

Known hypersensitivity reaction to PROCARDIA.

WARNINGS

Excessive Hypotension

Although in most patients, the hypotensive effect of PROCARDIA is modest and well tolerated, occasional patients have had excessive and poorly tolerated hypotension. These responses have usually occurred during initial titration or at the time of subsequent upward dosage adjustment, and may be more likely in patients on concomitant beta blockers.

Severe hypotension and/or increased fluid volume requirements have been reported in patients receiving PROCARDIA together with a beta blocking agent who underwent coronary artery bypass surgery using high dose fentanyl anesthesia. The interaction with high dose fentanyl appears to be due to the combination of PROCARDIA and a beta blocker, but the possibility that it may occur with PROCARDIA alone, with low doses of fentanyl, in other surgical procedures, or with other narcotic analgesics cannot be ruled out. In PROCARDIA treated patients where surgery using high dose fentanyl anesthesia is contemplated, the physician should be aware of these potential problems and, if the patient's condition permits, sufficient time (at least 36 hours) should be allowed for PROCARDIA to be washed out of the body prior to surgery.

Increased Angina and/or Myocardial Infarction

Rarely, patients, particularly those who have severe obstructive coronary artery disease, have developed well documented increased frequency, duration and/or severity of angina or acute myocardial infarction on starting PROCARDIA or at the time of dosage increase. The mechanism of this effect is not established.

Beta Blocker Withdrawal

Patients recently withdrawn from beta blockers may develop a withdrawal syndrome with increased angina, probably related to increased sensitivity to catecholamines. Initiation of PROCARDIA treatment will not prevent this occurrence and might be expected to exacerbate it by provoking reflex catecholamine release. There have been occasional reports of increased angina in a setting of beta blocker withdrawal and PROCARDIA initiation. It is important to taper beta blockers if possible, rather than stopping them abruptly before beginning PROCARDIA.

Congestive Heart Failure

Rarely, patients, usually receiving a beta blocker, have developed heart failure after beginning PROCARDIA. Patients with tight aortic stenosis may be at greater risk for such an event, as the unloading effect of PROCARDIA would be expected to be of less benefit to these patients, owing to their fixed impedance to flow across the aortic valve.

PRECAUTIONS

General: Hypotension: Because PROCARDIA decreases peripheral vascular resistance, careful monitoring of blood pressure during the initial administration and titration of PROCARDIA is suggested. Close observation is especially recommended for patients already taking medications that are known to lower blood pressure. (See WARNINGS.)

Peripheral edema: Mild to moderate peripheral edema, typically associated with arterial vasodilation and not due to left ventricular dysfunction, occurs in about one in ten patients treated with PROCARDIA. This edema occurs primarily in the lower extremities and usually responds to diuretic therapy. With patients whose angina is complicated by congestive heart failure, care should be taken to differentiate this peripheral edema from the effects of increasing left ventricular dysfunction.

Laboratory tests: Rare, usually transient, but occasionally significant elevations of enzymes such as alkaline phosphatase, CPK, LDH, SGOT and SGPT have been noted. The relationship to PROCARDIA therapy is uncertain in most cases, but probable in some. These laboratory abnormalities have rarely been associated with clinical symptoms, however, cholestasis with or without jaundice has been reported. Rare instances of allergic hepatitis have been reported.

PROCARDIA, like other calcium channel blockers, decreases platelet aggregation *in vitro*. Limited clinical studies have demonstrated a moderate but statistically significant decrease in platelet aggregation and increase in bleeding time in some PROCARDIA patients. This is thought to be a function of inhibition of calcium transport across the platelet membrane. No clinical significance for these findings has been demonstrated.

Positive direct Coombs test with/without hemolytic anemia has been reported.

Although PROCARDIA has been used safely in patients with renal dysfunction and has been reported to exert a beneficial effect in certain cases, rare, reversible elevations in BUN and serum creatinine have been reported in patients with pre-existing chronic renal insufficiency. The relationship to PROCARDIA therapy is uncertain in most cases but probable in some.

Drug interactions: Beta-adrenergic blocking agents: (See INDICATIONS and WARNINGS.) Experience in over 1400 patients in a non-comparative clinical trial has shown that concomitant administration of PROCARDIA and beta-blocking agents is usually well tolerated, but there have been occasional literature reports suggesting that the combination may increase the likelihood of congestive heart failure, severe hypotension or exacerbation of angina.

Long acting nitrates: PROCARDIA may be safely co-administered with nitrates, but there have been no controlled studies to evaluate the antianginal effectiveness of this combination.

Digitalis: Administration of PROCARDIA with digoxin increased digoxin levels in nine of twelve normal volunteers. The average increase was 45%. Another investigator found no increase in digoxin levels in thirteen patients with coronary artery disease. In an uncontrolled study of over two hundred patients with congestive heart failure during which digoxin blood levels were not measured, digitalis toxicity was not observed. Since there have been isolated reports of patients with elevated digoxin levels, it is recommended that digoxin levels be monitored when initiating, adjusting, and discontinuing PROCARDIA to avoid possible over- or under-digitalization.

Coumarin anticoagulants: There have been rare reports of increased prothrombin time in patients taking coumarin anticoagulants to whom PROCARDIA was administered. However, the relationship to PROCARDIA therapy is uncertain.

Cimetidine: A study in six healthy volunteers has shown a significant increase in peak nifedipine plasma levels (80%) and area-under-the-curve (74%) after a one week course of cimetidine at 1000 mg per day and nifedipine at 40 mg per day. Ranitidine produced smaller, non-significant increases. The effect may be mediated by the known inhibition of cimetidine on hepatic cytochrome P-450, the enzyme system probably responsible for the first-pass metabolism of nifedipine. If nifedipine therapy is initiated in a patient currently receiving cimetidine, cautious titration is advised.

Carcinogenesis, mutagenesis, impairment of fertility: Nifedipine was administered orally to rats for two years and was not shown to be carcinogenic. When given to rats prior to mating, nifedipine caused reduced fertility at a dose approximately 30 times the maximum recommended human dose. *In vivo* mutagenicity studies were negative.

Pregnancy: Pregnancy category C. Nifedipine has been shown to be teratogenic in rats when given in doses 30 times the maximum recommended human dose. Nifedipine was embryotoxic (increased fetal resorptions, decreased fetal weight, increased stunted forms, increased fetal deaths, decreased neonatal survival) in rats, mice and rabbits at doses of from 3 to 10 times the maximum recommended human dose. In pregnant monkeys, doses ⅔ and twice the maximum recommended human dose resulted in small placentas and underdeveloped chorionic villi. In rats, doses three times maximum human dose and higher caused prolongation of pregnancy. There are no adequate and well controlled studies in pregnant women. PROCARDIA should be used during pregnancy only if the potential benefit justifies the potential risk to the fetus.

ADVERSE REACTIONS

In multiple-dose U.S. and foreign controlled studies in which adverse reactions were reported spontaneously, adverse effects were frequent but generally not serious and rarely required discontinuation of therapy or dosage adjustment. Most were expected consequences of the vasodilator effects of PROCARDIA.

Adverse Effect	PROCARDIA (%) (N = 226)	Placebo (%) (N = 235)
Dizziness, lightheadedness, giddiness	27	15
Flushing, heat sensation	25	8
Headache	23	20
Weakness	12	10
Nausea, heartburn	11	8
Muscle cramps, tremor	8	3
Peripheral edema	7	1
Nervousness, mood changes	7	4
Palpitation	7	5
Dyspnea, cough, wheezing	6	3
Nasal congestion, sore throat	6	8

There is also a large uncontrolled experience in over 2100 patients in the United States. Most of the patients had vasospastic or resistant angina pectoris, and about half had concomitant treatment with beta-adrenergic blocking agents. The most common adverse events were:

Incidence Approximately 10% *Cardiovascular:* peripheral edema

Central Nervous System: dizziness or lightheadedness

Gastrointestinal: nausea

Systemic: headache and flushing, weakness

Incidence Approximately 5% *Cardiovascular:* transient hypotension

Incidence 2% or Less *Cardiovascular:* palpitation

Respiratory: nasal and chest congestion, shortness of breath

Gastrointestinal: diarrhea, constipation, cramps, flatulence

Musculoskeletal: inflammation, joint stiffness, muscle cramps

Central Nervous System: shakiness, nervousness, jitteriness, sleep disturbances, blurred vision, difficulties in balance

Other: dermatitis, pruritus, urticaria, fever, sweating, chills, sexual difficulties.

Incidence Approximately 0.5% *Cardiovascular:* syncope. Syncopal episodes did not recur with reduction in the dose of PROCARDIA or concomitant antianginal medication.

Incidence Less Than 0.5% *Hematologic:* thrombocytopenia, anemia, leukopenia, purpura

Gastrointestinal: allergic hepatitis

Oral: gingival hyperplasia

CNS: depression, paranoid syndrome

Special Senses: transient blindness at the peak of plasma level

Other: erythromelalgia, arthritis with ANA (+)

Continued on next page

Pfizer—Cont.

Several of these side effects appear to be dose related. Peripheral edema occurred in about one in 25 patients at doses less than 60 mg per day and in about one patient in eight at 120 mg per day or more. Transient hypotension, generally of mild to moderate severity and seldom requiring discontinuation of therapy, occurred in one of 50 patients at less than 60 mg per day and in one of 20 patients at 120 mg per day or more. Very rarely, introduction of PROCARDIA therapy was associated with an increase in anginal pain, possibly due to associated hypotension.

In addition, more serious adverse events were observed, not readily distinguishable from the natural history of the disease in these patients. It remains possible, however, that some or many of these events were drug related. Myocardial infarction occurred in about 4% of patients and congestive heart failure or pulmonary edema in about 2%. Ventricular arrhythmias or conduction disturbances each occurred in fewer than 0.5% of patients.

In a subgroup of over 1000 patients receiving PROCARDIA with concomitant beta blocker therapy, the pattern and incidence of adverse experiences was not different from that of the entire group of PROCARDIA treated patients. (See PRECAUTIONS.)

In a subgroup of approximately 250 patients with a diagnosis of congestive heart failure as well as angina, dizziness or lightheadedness, peripheral edema, headache or flushing each occurred in one in eight patients. Hypotension occurred in about one in 20 patients. Syncope occurred in approximately one patient in 250. Myocardial infarction or symptoms of congestive heart failure each occurred in about one patient in 15. Atrial or ventricular dysrhythmias each occurred in about one patient in 150.

OVERDOSAGE

Although there is no well documented experience with PROCARDIA overdosage, available data suggest that gross overdosage could result in excessive peripheral vasodilation with subsequent marked and probably prolonged systemic hypotension. Clinically significant hypotension due to PROCARDIA overdosage calls for active cardiovascular support including monitoring of cardiac and respiratory function, elevation of extremities, and attention to circulating fluid volume and urine output. A vasoconstrictor (such as norepinephrine) may be helpful in restoring vascular tone and blood pressure, provided that there is no contraindication to its use. Clearance of PROCARDIA would be expected to be prolonged in patients with impaired liver function. Since PROCARDIA is highly protein-bound, dialysis is not likely to be of benefit.

DOSAGE AND ADMINISTRATION

The dosage of PROCARDIA needed to suppress angina and that can be tolerated by the patient must be established by titration. Excessive doses can result in hypotension.

Therapy should be initiated with the 10 mg capsule. The starting dose is one 10 mg capsule, swallowed whole, 3 times/day. The usual effective dose range is 10–20 mg three times daily. Some patients, especially those with evidence of coronary artery spasm, respond only to higher doses, more frequent administration, or both. In such patients, doses of 20–30 mg three or four times daily may be effective. Doses above 120 mg daily are rarely necessary. More than 180 mg per day is not recommended.

In most cases, PROCARDIA titration should proceed over a 7–14 day period so that the physician can assess the response to each dose level and monitor the blood pressure before proceeding to higher doses.

If symptoms so warrant, titration may proceed more rapidly provided that the patient is assessed frequently. Based on the patient's physical activity level, attack frequency, and sublingual nitroglycerin consumption, the dose of PROCARDIA may be increased from 10 mg t.i.d to 20 mg t.i.d and then to 30 mg t.i.d over a three-day period.

In hospitalized patients under close observation, the dose may be increased in 10 mg increments over four to six-hour periods as required to control pain and arrhythmias due to ischemia. A single dose should rarely exceed 30 mg.

No "rebound effect" has been observed upon discontinuation of PROCARDIA. However, if discontinuation of PROCARDIA is necessary, sound clinical practice suggests that the dosage should be decreased gradually with close physician supervision.

Co-Administration with Other Antianginal Drugs

Sublingual nitroglycerin may be taken as required for the control of acute manifestations of angina, particularly during PROCARDIA titration. See **Precautions, Drug Interactions**, for information on co-administration of PROCARDIA with beta blockers or long acting nitrates.

HOW SUPPLIED

PROCARDIA soft gelatin capsules are supplied in:

Bottles of 100: 10 mg (NDC 0069-2600-66) orange #260;
20 mg (NDC 0069-2610-66) orange and light brown #261

Bottles of 300: 10 mg (NDC 0069-2600-72) orange #260;
20 mg (NDC 0069-2610-72) orange and light brown #261

Unit dose packages of 100: 10 mg (NDC 0069-2600-41) orange #260;
20 mg (NDC 0069-2610-41) orange and light brown #261

The capsules should be protected from light and moisture and stored at controlled room temperature 59° to 77°F (15° to 25°C) in the manufacturer's original container.

 Revised June 1986
65-4027-00-8

LITERATURE AVAILABLE

Yes

Shown in Product Identification Section, page 422

RENESE® ℞

[rĕ-nēsʹ]
(polythiazide)
TABLETS
For Oral Administration

DESCRIPTION

Renese is designated generically as polythiazide, and chemically as 2*H*-1,2,4-Benzothiadiazine-7-sulfonamide, 6-chloro-3,4-dihydro-2-methyl-3[[(2, 2, 2-trifluoroethyl)thio]methyl]-, 1, 1-dioxide. It is a white crystalline substance, insoluble in water but readily soluble in alkaline solution.

ACTION

The mechanism of action results in an interference with the renal tubular mechanism of electrolyte reabsorption. At maximal therapeutic dosage all thiazides are approximately equal in their diuretic potency. The mechanism whereby thiazides function in the control of hypertension is unknown.

INDICATIONS

Renese is indicated as adjunctive therapy in edema associated with congestive heart failure, hepatic cirrhosis, and corticosteroid and estrogen therapy.

Renese has also been found useful in edema due to various forms of renal dysfunction as: Nephrotic syndrome; Acute glomerulonephritis; and Chronic renal failure.

Renese is indicated in the management of hypertension either as the sole therapeutic agent or to enhance the effectiveness of other antihypertensive drugs in the more severe forms of hypertension.

Usage in Pregnancy: The routine use of diuretics in an otherwise healthy woman is inappropriate and exposes mother and fetus to unnecessary hazard. Diuretics do not prevent development of toxemia of pregnancy, and there is no satisfactory evidence that they are useful in the treatment of developed toxemia.

Edema during pregnancy may arise from pathological causes or from the physiologic and mechanical consequences of pregnancy. Thiazides are indicated in pregnancy when edema is due to pathologic causes, just as they are in the absence of pregnancy (however, see Warnings, below). Dependent edema in pregnancy, resulting from restriction of venous return by the expanded uterus, is properly treated through elevation of the lower extremities and use of support hose; use of diuretics to lower intravascular volume in this case is illogical and unnecessary. There is hypervolemia during normal pregnancy which is harmful to neither the fetus nor the mother (in the absence of cardiovascular disease), but which is associated with edema, including generalized edema, in the majority of pregnant women. If this edema produces discomfort, increased recumbency will often provide relief. In rare instances, this edema may cause extreme discomfort which is not relieved by rest. In these cases, a short course of diuretics may provide relief and may be appropriate.

CONTRAINDICATIONS

Anuria. Hypersensitivity to this or other sulfonamide derived drugs.

WARNINGS

Thiazides should be used with caution in severe renal disease. In patients with renal disease, thiazides may precipitate azotemia. Cumulative effects of the drug may develop in patients with impaired renal function.

Thiazides should be used with caution in patients with impaired hepatic function or progressive liver disease, since minor alterations of fluid and electrolyte balance may precipitate hepatic coma.

Thiazides may add to or potentiate the action of other antihypertensive drugs. Potentiation occurs with ganglionic or peripheral adrenergic blocking drugs.

Sensitivity reactions may occur in patients with a history of allergy or bronchial asthma.

The possibility of exacerbation or activation of systemic lupus erythematosus has been reported.

Usage in pregnancy. Thiazides cross the placental barrier and appear in cord blood. The use of thiazides in pregnant women requires that the anticipated benefit be weighed against possible hazards to the fetus. These hazards include fetal or neonatal jaundice, thrombocytopenia, and possibly other adverse reactions which have occurred in the adult.

Nursing Mothers. Thiazides appear in breast milk. If use of the drug is deemed essential, the patient should stop nursing.

PRECAUTIONS

Periodic determination of serum electrolytes to detect possible electrolyte imbalance should be performed at appropriate intervals.

All patients receiving thiazide therapy should be observed for clinical signs of fluid or electrolyte imbalance; namely, hyponatremia, hypochloremic alkalosis, and hypokalemia. Serum and urine electrolyte determinations are particularly important when the patient is vomiting excessively or receiving parenteral fluids. Medication such as digitalis may also influence serum electrolytes. Warning signs, irrespective of cause, are: dryness of mouth, thirst, weakness, lethargy, drowsiness, restlessness, muscle pains or cramps, muscular fatigue, hypotension, oliguria, tachycardia, and gastrointestinal disturbances such as nausea and vomiting.

Hypokalemia may develop with thiazides as with any other potent diuretic, especially with brisk diuresis, when severe cirrhosis is present, or during concomitant use of corticosteroids or ACTH.

Interference with adequate oral electrolyte intake will also contribute to hypokalemia. Digitalis therapy may exaggerate metabolic effects of hypokalemia especially with reference to myocardial activity.

Any chloride deficit is generally mild and usually does not require specific treatment except under extraordinary circumstances (as in liver disease or renal disease). Dilutional hyponatremia may occur in edematous patients in hot weather; appropriate therapy is water restriction, rather than administration of salt except in rare instances when the hyponatremia is life threatening. In actual salt depletion, appropriate replacement is the therapy of choice.

Hyperuricemia may occur or frank gout may be precipitated in certain patients receiving thiazide therapy.

Insulin requirements in diabetic patients may be increased, decreased, or unchanged. Latent diabetes mellitus may become manifest during thiazide administration.

Thiazide drugs may increase the responsiveness to tubocurarine.

The antihypertensive effects of the drug may be enhanced in the postsympathectomy patient.

Thiazides may decrease arterial responsiveness to norepinephrine. This diminution is not sufficient to preclude effectiveness of the pressor agent for therapeutic use.

If progressive renal impairment becomes evident, as indicated by a rising nonprotein nitrogen or blood urea nitrogen, a careful reappraisal of therapy is necessary with consideration given to withholding or discontinuing diuretic therapy.

Thiazides may decrease serum PBI levels without signs of thyroid disturbance.

ADVERSE REACTIONS

A. GASTROINTESTINAL SYSTEM REACTIONS

1. anorexia
2. gastric irritation
3. nausea
4. vomiting
5. cramping
6. diarrhea
7. constipation
8. jaundice (intrahepatic cholestatic jaundice)
9. pancreatitis

B. CENTRAL NERVOUS SYSTEM REACTIONS

1. dizziness
2. vertigo
3. paresthesias
4. headache
5. xanthopsia

C. HEMATOLOGIC REACTIONS

1. leukopenia
2. agranulocytosis
3. thrombocytopenia
4. aplastic anemia

D. DERMATOLOGIC–HYPERSENSITIVITY REACTIONS

1. purpura
2. photosensitivity
3. rash
4. urticaria
5. necrotizing angiitis (vasculitis) (cutaneous vasculitis)

E. CARDIOVASCULAR REACTION

Orthostatic hypotension may occur and may be aggravated by alcohol, barbiturates or narcotics.

F. OTHER

1. hyperglycemia
2. glycosuria
3. hyperuricemia
4. muscle spasm
5. weakness
6. restlessness

Whenever adverse reactions are moderate or severe, thiazide dosage should be reduced or therapy withdrawn.

DOSAGE AND ADMINISTRATION

Therapy should be individualized according to patient response. This therapy should be titrated to gain maximal therapeutic response as well as the minimal dose possible to maintain that therapeutic response. The usual dosage of Renese tablets for diuretic therapy is 1 to 4 mg daily, and for antihypertensive therapy is 2 to 4 mg daily.

HOW SUPPLIED
RENESE (polythiazide) Tablets are available as:
1 mg white, scored tablets (imprinted with code number 375) in bottles of 100 and 1000.
2 mg yellow, scored tablets (imprinted with code number 376) in bottles of 100 and 1000.
4 mg white, scored tablets (imprinted with code number 377) in bottles of 100 and 1000.

Revised Oct. 1982
(69-1116-00-3)

LITERATURE AVAILABLE
Yes.

Shown in Product Identification Section, page 422

RENESE®-R ℞
[*rĕ-nēs'*]
(polythiazide and reserpine)

> **Warning**
> This fixed combination drug is not indicated for initial therapy of hypertension. Hypertension requires therapy titrated to the individual patient. If the fixed combination represents the dosage so determined, its use may be more convenient in patient management. The treatment of hypertension is not static, but must be reevaluated as conditions in each patient warrant.

RENESE-R tablets combine polythiazide and reserpine, two antihypertensive agents with complementary properties. Each blue, scored tablet of RENESE-R provides:
Renese (polythiazide) .... 2.0 mg
Reserpine .... 0.25 mg

ACTIONS
RENESE (polythiazide) is a member of the benzothiadiazine (thiazide) family of diuretic/ antihypertensive agents. RENESE (polythiazide) alone has demonstrated clinical effectiveness in lowering elevated blood pressure in patients without visible edema as well as in edematous hypertensive patients. This antihypertensive action probably comes about through depletion of sodium and fluid accumulation in the blood vessel wall.
RENESE (polythiazide) is 2*H*-1,2,4-Benzothiadiazine-7-sulfonamide, 6-chloro-3,4-dihydro-2- methyl-3-[[(2,2,2-trifluoroethyl)thio]methyl]-, 1, 1- dioxide.
Reserpine, an alkaloid of Rauwolfia serpentina has several complementary actions of benefit to the hypertensive patient, including a calming effect and a slowing of the pulse rate. Its ultimate effect in lowering blood pressure is thought to be due to vasodilatation unaccompanied by reduction in cardiac performance, probably as a result of depletion of norepinephrine from tissue receptor sites.
Since polythiazide reduces or eliminates the sodium and fluid retention frequently associated with hypertension, it enhances the efficacy of reserpine in lowering elevated blood pressure. RENESE-R often has been found to be more effective than equivalent doses of either agent alone. Both the cardiovascular and central nervous system effects may persist following withdrawal of the drug.

INDICATIONS
Hypertension (see box warning).

CONTRAINDICATIONS
A. Related to polythiazide:
1. Advanced renal or hepatic failure.
2. Hypersensitivity to this or other sulfonamide derivatives.
B. Related to reserpine:
1. Demonstrated hypersensitivity.
2. Mental depression.
3. Demonstrated peptic ulcer or ulcerative colitis.

WARNINGS
Serum electrolyte determinations are especially indicated for patients with severe derangement of metabolic processes, e.g., surgery, vomiting, or parenteral fluid therapy. Electrolyte imbalance may be caused by certain diseases such as cirrhosis, or it may result from drug therapy, such as therapy with corticosteroids. Patients with cirrhosis who are continually receiving RENESE-R should be observed carefully for the development of hepatic precoma or coma. Indications of impending hepatic failure are tremor, confusion, drowsiness, and hepatic fetor.
Thiazides may precipitate kidney failure and uremia in patients with pre-existing renal pathology and impaired renal function.
Available information tends to implicate all oral dosage forms of potassium salts ingested in solid form with or without thiazides in the etiology of nonspecific, small bowel lesions consisting of ulceration with or without stenosis, causing obstruction, hemorrhage and perforation, and frequently requiring surgery. Deaths due to these complications have been reported. All oral dosage forms of potassium salts ingested in solid form should be used only when adequate dietary supplementation is not practical and should be discontinued immediately if abdominal pain, distention, nausea, vomiting or gastrointestinal bleeding occur.
RENESE-R does not itself contain enteric-coated potassium.
Electroshock therapy should not be given within one week of cessation of reserpine.
Usage in Pregnancy and the Childbearing Age.
Since thiazides appear in breast milk, the usage of polythiazide is contraindicated in nursing mothers. Thiazides cross the placental barrier and appear in cord blood. The safety of reserpine for use during pregnancy or lactation has not been established. When polythiazide and reserpine are used in women of childbearing age, the potential benefits of this drug combination should be weighed against the possible hazards to the fetus. The hazards include fetal or neonatal jaundice, thrombocytopenia, and possibly other adverse reactions which have occurred in the adult.

PRECAUTIONS
Since all diuretic agents may reduce serum levels of sodium, chloride, and potassium, especially with brisk diuresis or when used concurrently with steroids, patients should be observed regularly for early signs of fluid or electrolyte imbalance and serum electrolyte studies should be performed periodically. Warning signs of possible electrolyte imbalance irrespective of cause include fatigue, muscle cramps, gastrointestinal disturbances, lethargy, oliguria, and tachycardia. In extreme cases, hypotension, shock, and coma may develop. Frequently, serum electrolyte levels do not correlate with signs or symptoms of electrolyte imbalance. Unduly restricted salt intake as well as concurrent administration of digitalis may exaggerate metabolic effects of hypokalemia. A favorable ratio of potassium to sodium excretion lessens the possibility of hypokalemia. However, should this occur or be suspected, foods with a high potassium content (bananas, apricots, citrus fruits, prune juice, etc.) should be given. When necessary, oral potassium supplements may be administered. If other antihypertensive agents are used concurrently, lower than usual doses of RENESE-R and of the other agents should be considered.
Like other thiazide diuretics, polythiazide may cause a rise in serum uric acid levels with or without overt symptoms of gout. Thiazides are known to disturb glucose tolerance in some individuals, even when there is no history of glucose intolerance or diabetes in the individual or his family. Likewise, thiazides may decrease PBI levels without signs of thyroid disturbances.
Thiazide drugs may augment the paralyzing actions of tubocurarine, and may decrease the arterial responsiveness to norepinephrine. Extra precautions may be necessary in patients who may require these drugs or their derivatives, as in surgery. The antihypertensive effects of the drug may be enhanced in the postsympathectomy patient.
Reserpine: Since reserpine may increase gastric acid secretion, it should be used cautiously in patients with a history of peptic ulcer or ulcerative colitis. Extreme caution is needed in patients with a history of mental depression, and reserpine should be discontinued at the first sign of depressive symptoms. Parkinsonism and confusion have been encountered, particularly in psychiatric patients, and constitute an indication for withdrawal of the drug. Caution should be exercised when treating patients with impairment of renal function, as lowered blood pressure may result in further decompensation and embarrassment of function. Reserpine should be used cautiously with digitalis or quinidine as the concurrent use may enhance the appearance of arrhythmias. Discontinue the drug one to two weeks prior to elective surgery since an unexpected degree of hypotension and bradycardia have been reported in patients receiving anesthetic agents concurrently with reserpine, probably due to a reduced responsiveness to norepinephrine. For emergency surgical procedures vagal blocking agents may be given parenterally to prevent or reverse hypotension and/or bradycardia. Reserpine may cause increased appetite and weight gain in some patients.
Animal tumorigenicity: Rodent studies have shown that reserpine is an animal tumorigen, causing an increased incidence of mammary fibroadenomas in female mice, malignant tumors of the seminal vesicles in male mice, and malignant adrenal medullary tumors in male rats. These findings arose in 2 year studies in which the drug was administered in the feed at concentrations of 5 and 10 ppm—about 100 to 300 times the usual human dose. The breast neoplasms are thought to be related to reserpine's prolactin-elevating effect. Several other prolactin-elevating drugs have also been associated with an increased incidence of mammary neoplasia in rodents.
The extent to which these findings indicate a risk to humans is uncertain. Tissue culture experiments show that about one-third of human breast tumors are prolactin-dependent *in vitro*, a factor of considerable importance if the use of the drug is contemplated in a patient with previously detected breast cancer. The possibility of an increased risk of breast cancer in reserpine users has been studied extensively; however, no firm conclusion has emerged. Although a few epidemiologic studies have suggested a slightly increased risk (less than twofold in all studies except one) in women who have used reserpine, other studies of generally similar design have not confirmed this. Epidemiologic studies conducted using other drugs (neuroleptic agents) that, like reserpine, increase prolactin levels and therefore would be considered rodent mammary carcinogens, have not shown an association between chronic administration of the drug and human mammary tumorigenesis. While long-term clinical observation has not suggested such an association, the available evidence is considered too limited to be conclusive at this time. An association of reserpine intake with pheochromocytoma or tumors of the seminal vesicles has not been explored.

ADVERSE REACTIONS
Polythiazide: Side effects such as nausea, vertigo, weakness, paresthesias, and fatigue occur but seldom require cessation of therapy. Most of these can be overcome by reducing the dose or taking measures to improve electrolyte imbalance. Maculopapular skin rash has been reported, as has reversible cholestatic jaundice. Leukopenia (neutropenia) and purpura, with or without thrombocytopenia, have been reported rarely, and agranulocytosis and aplastic anemia have been reported with the older thiazides but not as yet with the newer compounds such as polythiazide. Pancreatitis, photosensitivity reactions, gastrointestinal disturbances, headache, xanthopsia, necrotizing angiitis, orthostatic hypotension, and dizziness have all been reported following the use of the benzothiadiazine class of diuretics.
Reserpine: Gastrointestinal reactions include hypersecretion, nausea and vomiting, anorexia, and diarrhea. Cardiovascular reactions reported include angina-like symptoms, arrhythmias— particularly when used concurrently with digitalis or quinidine—flushing of the skin, and bradycardia. Central nervous system reactions range from drowsiness, depression, nervousness, paradoxical anxiety, nightmares, and a rare Parkinsonian syndrome to C.N.S. sensitization manifested by deafness, glaucoma, uveitis, and optic atrophy. Nasal congestion is a frequent complaint, and pruritus, rash, dryness of mouth, dizziness, headache, purpura, impotence or decreased libido, and miosis have been reported with use of this drug. These reactions are usually reversible and disappear when the drug is discontinued.

DOSAGE
As determined by individual titration (see box warning).
Initial dosages of the combination should conform to those dosages of the individual components established during titration.
Maintenance dosages range from ½ tablet to 2 tablets daily. Dosage of other antihypertensive agents, particularly ganglionic blockers, that are used concomitantly should be reduced.

SUPPLY
RENESE-R tablets (2 mg polythiazide-0.25 mg reserpine) are available as blue, scored tablets (imprinted with code number 446) in bottles of 100 and 1,000.

Revised April 1983
(69-1200-00-9)

Literature Available: Yes.
Shown in Product Identification Section, page 422

SUSTAIRE® ℞
[*sus'tār*]
theophylline (anhydrous)
SUSTAINED RELEASE TABLETS

DESCRIPTION
SUSTAIRE Sustained Release Tablets contain anhydrous theophylline, with no color additives. SUSTAIRE is available in two strengths: 100 mg and 300 mg: each tablet is scored for flexibility of dose. Theophylline, a xanthine compound, is a white, odorless crystalline powder, having a bitter taste.

ACTIONS
The pharmacologic actions of theophylline are as a bronchodilator, pulmonary vasodilator, and smooth muscle relaxant since the drug directly relaxes the smooth muscle of the bronchial airways and pulmonary blood vessels. Theophylline also possesses other actions typical of the xanthine derivatives: coronary vasodilator, diuretic, cardiac stimulant, and skeletal muscle stimulant. The actions of theophylline may be mediated through inhibition of phosphodiesterase and a resultant increase in intracellular cyclic AMP which could mediate smooth muscle relaxation.
No development of tolerance appears to occur with chronic use of theophylline. The half-life is shortened with cigarette smoking and prolonged in alcoholism, reduced hepatic or renal function, congestive heart failure, and in patients receiving certain antibiotics (see DRUG INTERACTIONS). High fever for prolonged periods may decrease theophylline elimination. Children over six months of age have rapid

Continued on next page

Pfizer—Cont.

clearances with average half-lives of approximately 3–5 hours. Newborn infants have extremely slow clearances and half-lives exceeding 24 hours. Older adults with chronic obstructive pulmonary disease, any patients with cor pulmonale or other causes of heart failure, and patients with liver pathology may have much lower clearances with half-lives that exceed 24 hours. The half-life in non-smokers averages 7–9 hours.

In single dose studies, SUSTAIRE, administered at 8 mg/kg body weight, produced mean peak theophylline blood levels of 7.5 ± 1.9 mcg/ml at 9.2 ± 1.9 hours following administration. In the multiple dose, steady-state, 3 and 5 day studies, SUSTAIRE achieved remarkably constant intra-subject theophylline levels with an average peak-trough difference of only 4 mcg/ml. This is indicative of smooth and stable maintenance therapeutic theophylline levels throughout a q12h dosing interval.

INDICATIONS

Symptomatic relief and/or prevention of asthma and reversible bronchospasm associated with chronic bronchitis and emphysema.

CONTRAINDICATIONS

SUSTAIRE is contraindicated in individuals who have shown hypersensitivity to any of its components or xanthine derivatives.

WARNINGS

Excessive theophylline doses may be associated with toxicity; serum theophylline levels should be monitored to assure maximum benefit with minimum risk. Incidence of toxicity increases at serum levels greater than 20 mcg/ml. High blood levels of theophylline resulting from conventional doses are correlated with clinical manifestations of toxicity in patients with lowered body plasma clearances, patients with liver dysfunction or chronic obstructive lung disease, and patients who are older than 55 years of age—particularly males. There are often no early signs of less serious theophylline toxicity such as nausea and restlessness, which may be the first signs of toxicity. Many patients who have higher theophylline serum levels exhibit a tachycardia. Theophylline products may worsen preexisting arrhythmias.

USAGE IN PREGNANCY

Safe use in pregnancy has not been established relative to possible adverse effects on fetal development, but neither have adverse effects on fetal development been established. This is, unfortunately, true for most anti-asthmatic medications. Therefore, use of theophylline in pregnant women should be balanced against the risk of uncontrolled asthma.

PRECAUTIONS

SUSTAIRE TABLETS SHOULD NOT BE CHEWED OR CRUSHED.

Theophylline should not be administered concurrently with other xanthine medications. It should be used with caution in patients with severe cardiac disease, severe hypoxemia, hypertension, hyperthyroidism, acute myocardial injury, cor pulmonale, congestive heart failure, liver disease, in the elderly (particularly males), and in neonates. Great caution should be used in giving theophylline to patients in congestive heart failure since these patients show markedly prolonged theophylline blood level curves. Use theophylline cautiously in patients with history of peptic ulcer. Theophylline may occasionally act as a local irritant to the G.I. tract although gastrointestinal symptoms are more commonly central and associated with high serum concentrations above 20 mcg/ml.

ADVERSE REACTIONS

The most consistent adverse reactions are usually due to overdose and are:

Gastrointestinal: nausea, vomiting, epigastric pain, hematemesis, diarrhea.

Central Nervous System: headaches, irritability, restlessness, insomnia, reflex hyperexcitability, muscle twitching, clonic and tonic generalized convulsions.

Cardiovascular: palpitation, tachycardia, extrasystoles, flushing, hypotension, circulatory failure, life threatening ventricular arrhythmias.

Respiratory: tachypnea

Renal: albuminuria, increased excretion of renal tubular cells and red blood cells; potentiation of diuresis.

Others: hyperglycemia and inappropriate ADH syndrome.

DRUG INTERACTIONS

Drug-Drug:

Drug	Effect
Theophylline with Furosemide	Increased diuresis
Theophylline with Hexamethonium	Decreased chronotropic effect
Theophylline with Reserpine	Tachycardia
Theophylline with Cyclamycin, TAO® (troleandomycin), Erythromycin or Lincomycin	Increased theophylline blood levels

Drug-Food: SUSTAIRE has not been adequately studied to determine whether its bioavailability is altered when it is given with food.

Available data suggest that drug administration at the time of food ingestion may influence the absorption characteristics of some or all theophylline controlled-release products resulting in serum values different from those found after administration in the fasting state.

A drug-food effect, if any, would likely have its greatest clinical significance when high theophylline serum levels are being maintained and/or when large single doses (greater than 13 mg/kg or 900 mg) of a controlled-release theophylline product are given. The influence of the type and amount of food on performance of controlled-release theophylline products is under study at this time.

OVERDOSAGE

Management

A. If potential oral overdose is established and seizure has not occurred:
   1) Induce vomiting.
   2) Administer a cathartic. (This is particularly important if sustained release preparations have been taken.)
   3) Administer activated charcoal.

B. Patient is having a seizure:
   1) Establish an airway.
   2) Administer O_2.
   3) Treat the seizure with intravenous diazepam: 0.1 to 0.3 mg/kg up to 10 mg.
   4) Monitor vital signs. Maintain blood pressure and provide adequate hydration.

C. Post Seizure Coma:
   1) Maintain airway and oxygenation.
   2) If a result of oral medication, follow above recommendations to prevent absorption of drug; but intubation and lavage will have to be performed instead of inducing emesis, and the cathartic and charcoal will need to be introduced via a large bore gastric lavage tube.
   3) Continue to provide full supportive care and adequate hydration while waiting for drug to be metabolized. In general, the drug is metabolized sufficiently rapidly so as to not warrant consideration of dialysis.

DOSAGE AND ADMINISTRATION

Therapeutic serum levels associated with optimal likelihood for benefit and minimal risk of toxicity are considered to be between 10 and 20 mcg/ml. There is a great variation from patient to patient in dosage needed in order to achieve a therapeutic blood level due to variable rates of elimination. Because of this wide variation from patient to patient, and the relatively narrow therapeutic range, dosage must be individualized.

THE AVERAGE INITIAL CHILDREN'S (UNDER 9 YEARS OF AGE) DOSE IS ONE SUSTAIRE 100 mg TABLET q12h.

THE AVERAGE INITIAL CHILDREN'S (AGES 9–12) DOSE IS ONE HALF (150 mg) OF A SUSTAIRE 300 mg TABLET q12h.

THE AVERAGE INITIAL ADOLESCENT (AGES 12–16) DOSE IS TWO SUSTAIRE 100 mg TABLETS q12h.

THE AVERAGE INITIAL ADULT DOSE IS ONE SUSTAIRE 300 mg TABLET q12h.

If the desired response is not achieved with the above AVERAGE INITIAL DOSAGE recommendations and there are no adverse reactions, the dose may be safely increased by 2–3 mg/kg body weight per day at 3 day intervals until the following MAXIMUM DOSE WITHOUT MEASUREMENT OF SERUM CONCENTRATION or a maximum of 900 mg in any 24 hour period, whichever is less, is attained:

SUSTAIRE has not been adequately studied for its bioavailability when administered with food. (See PRECAUTIONS, Drug-Food Interactions.)

MAXIMUM DOSE WITHOUT MEASUREMENT OF SERUM CONCENTRATION

	mg per kg body weight*	dose per interval
Children (under 9)	24 mg per day	12 mg q12h**
Children (9–12)	20 mg per day	10 mg q12h
Adolescents (12–16)	18 mg per day	9 mg q12h
Adults	13 mg per day	6.5 mg q12h

*Use ideal body weight for obese patients.

**Some children under 9 may require 8 mg q8h.

If doses higher than those contained in the above MAXIMUM DOSE WITHOUT MEASUREMENT OF SERUM CONCENTRATION are necessary, it is recommended that serum theophylline levels be monitored. Check serum theophylline levels between 3 and 8 hours after a dose. It is important that the patient will have missed *no* doses during the previous 72 hours and that dosing intervals will have been reasonably typical with *no* added doses during that period of time. DOSAGE ADJUSTMENT BASED ON SERUM THEOPHYLLINE MEASUREMENTS WHEN THESE INSTRUCTIONS HAVE NOT BEEN FOLLOWED, MAY RESULT IN RECOMMENDATIONS THAT PRESENT RISK OF TOXICITY TO THE PATIENT.

HOW SUPPLIED

SUSTAIRE 100 mg and 300 mg Sustained Release Tablets are available in bottles of 100.

STORAGE CONDITIONS: Keep tightly closed. Store at controlled room temperature 15–30°C (59–86°F).

69-3091-00-5

Shown in Product Identification Section, page 422

TERRAMYCIN® ℞

[*tĕra-my'sĭn*]

Capsules
(oxytetracycline HCl)
Film-coated Tablets
(oxytetracycline)

DESCRIPTION

Oxytetracycline is a product of the metabolism of *Streptomyces rimosus* and is one of the family of tetracycline antibiotics.

Oxytetracycline diffuses readily through the placenta into the fetal circulation, into the pleural fluid and, under some circumstances, into the cerebrospinal fluid. It appears to be concentrated in the hepatic system and excreted in the bile, so that it appears in the feces, as well as in the urine, in a biologically active form.

ACTIONS

Oxytetracycline is primarily bacteriostatic and is thought to exert its antimicrobial effect by the inhibition of protein synthesis. Oxytetracycline is active against a wide range of gram-negative and gram-positive organisms. The drugs in the tetracycline class have closely similar antimicrobial spectra, and cross-resistance among them is common. Microorganisms may be considered susceptible if the M.I.C. (minimum inhibitory concentration) is not more than 4.0 mcg/ml and intermediate if the M.I.C. is 4.0 to 12.5 mcg/ml.

Susceptibility plate testing: A tetracycline disc may be used to determine microbial susceptiblity to drugs in the tetracycline class. If the Kirby-Bauer method of disc susceptibility testing is used, a 30 mcg tetracycline disc should give a zone of at least 19 mm when tested against a tetracycline-susceptible bacterial strain.

Tetracyclines are readily absorbed and are bound to plasma proteins in varying degree. They are concentrated by the liver in the bile and excreted in the urine and feces at high concentrations and in a biologically active form.

INDICATIONS

Oxytetracycline is indicated in infections caused by the following microorganisms:

Rickettsiae (Rocky Mountain spotted fever, typhus fever and the typhus group, Q fever, rickettsialpox and tick fevers),

Mycoplasma pneumoniae (PPLO, Eaton Agent), Agents of psittacosis and ornithosis,

Agents of lymphogranuloma venereum and granuloma inguinale,

The spirochetal agent of relapsing fever *(Borrelia recurrentis).*

The following gram-negative microorganisms:

Haemophilus ducreyi (chancroid),

Pasteurella pestis and *Pasteurella tularensis,*

Bartonella bacilliformis,

Bacteroides species,

Vibrio comma and *Vibrio fetus,*

Brucella species (in conjunction with streptomycin).

Because many strains of the following groups of microorganisms have been shown to be resistant to tetracyclines, culture and susceptibility testing are recommended.

Oxytetracycline is indicated for treatment of infections caused by the following gram- negative microorganisms, when bacteriologic testing indicates appropriate susceptibility to the drug:

Escherichia coli,

Enterobacter aerogenes (formerly *Aerobacter aerogenes*),

Shigella species,

Mima species and *Herellea* species,

Haemophilus influenzae (respiratory infections),

Klebsiella species (respiratory and urinary infections).

Oxytetracycline is indicated for treatment of infections caused by the following gram-positive microorganisms when bacteriologic testing indicates appropriate susceptibility to the drug:

Streptococcus species:

Up to 44 percent of strains of *Streptococcus pyogenes* and 74 percent of *Streptococcus faecalis* have been found to be resistant to tetracycline drugs. Therefore, tetracyclines should not be used for streptococcal disease unless the organism has been demonstrated to be sensitive.

For upper respiratory infections due to Group A beta-hemolytic streptococci, penicillin is the usual drug of choice, including prophylaxis of rheumatic fever.

Diplococcus pneumoniae,
Staphylococcus aureus, skin and soft tissue infections. Oxytetracycline is not the drug of choice in the treatment of any type of staphylococcal infections.
When penicillin is contraindicated, tetracyclines are alternative drugs in the treatment of infections due to:
Neisseria gonorrhoeae
In acute intestinal amebiasis, the tetracyclines may be a useful adjunct to amebicides.
In severe acne, the tetracyclines may be useful adjunctive therapy. (This indication is for the oral use only, not for I.M. or I.V.)
Tetracyclines are indicated in the treatment of trachoma, although the infectious agent is not always eliminated, as judged by immunofluorescence.
Inclusion conjunctivitis may be treated with oral tetracyclines or with a combination of oral and topical agents.

CONTRAINDICATIONS
This drug is contraindicated in persons who have shown hypersensitivity to any of the tetracyclines.

WARNINGS
THE USE OF DRUGS OF THE TETRACYCLINE CLASS DURING TOOTH DEVELOPMENT (LAST HALF OF PREGNANCY, INFANCY, AND CHILDHOOD TO THE AGE OF 8 YEARS) MAY CAUSE PERMANENT DISCOLORATION OF THE TEETH (YELLOW-GRAY-BROWN). This adverse reaction is more common during long term use of the drugs but has been observed following repeated short term courses. Enamel hypoplasia has also been reported. *TETRACYCLINE DRUGS, THEREFORE, SHOULD NOT BE USED IN THIS AGE GROUP UNLESS OTHER DRUGS ARE NOT LIKELY TO BE EFFECTIVE OR ARE CONTRAINDICATED.*
When the need for intensive treatment outweighs its potential dangers (mostly during pregnancy or in individuals with known or suspected renal or liver impairment), it is advisable to perform renal and liver function tests before and during therapy. Also, tetracycline serum concentrations should be followed. If renal impairment exists, even usual oral or parenteral doses may lead to excessive systemic accumulation of the drug and possible liver toxicity. Under such conditions, lower than usual total doses are indicated, and if therapy is prolonged, serum level determinations of the drug may be advisable. This hazard is of particular importance in the parenteral administration of tetracyclines to pregnant or postpartum patients with pyelonephritis.
When used under these circumstances, the blood level should not exceed 15 mcg/ml and liver function tests should be made at frequent intervals. Other potentially hepatotoxic drugs should not be prescribed concomitantly.
Photosensitivity manifested by an exaggerated sunburn reaction has been observed in some individuals taking tetracyclines. Patients apt to be exposed to direct sunlight or ultraviolet light should be advised that this reaction can occur with tetracycline drugs, and treatment should be discontinued at the first evidence of skin erythema.
The antianabolic action of the tetracyclines may cause an increase in BUN. While this is not a problem in those with normal renal function, in patients with significantly impaired function, higher serum levels of tetracycline may lead to azotemia, hyperphosphatemia, and acidosis.
Usage in pregnancy. (See above "Warnings" about use during tooth development.)
Results of animal studies indicate that tetracyclines cross the placenta, are found in fetal tissues and can have toxic effects on the developing fetus (often related to retardation of skeletal development). Evidence of embryotoxicity has also been noted in animals treated early in pregnancy.
Usage in newborns, infants, and children. (See above "Warnings" about use during tooth development.)
All tetracyclines form a stable calcium complex in any bone forming tissue. A decrease in the fibula growth rate has been observed in prematures given oral tetracycline in doses of 25 mg/kg every 6 hours. This reaction was shown to be reversible when the drug was discontinued.
Tetracyclines are present in the milk of lactating women who are taking a drug in this class.

PRECAUTIONS
As with other antibiotic preparations, use of this drug may result in overgrowth of nonsusceptible organisms, including fungi. If superinfection occurs, the antibiotic should be discontinued and appropriate therapy instituted.
In venereal diseases when coexistent syphilis is suspected, a dark field examination should be done before treatment is started and the blood serology repeated monthly for at least 4 months.
Because tetracyclines have been shown to depress plasma prothrombin activity, patients who are on anticoagulant therapy may require downward adjustment of their anticoagulant dosage.
In long term therapy, periodic laboratory evaluation of organ systems, including hematopoietic, renal and hepatic studies should be performed.
All infections due to Group A beta-hemolytic streptococci should be treated for at least 10 days.
Since bacteriostatic drugs may interfere with the bactericidal action of penicillin, it is advisable to avoid giving tetracycline in conjunction with penicillin.

ADVERSE REACTIONS
Gastrointestinal: anorexia, nausea, vomiting, diarrhea, glossitis, dysphagia, enterocolitis, and inflammatory lesions (with monilial overgrowth) in the anogenital region. These reactions have been caused by both the oral and parenteral administration of tetracyclines. Rare instances of esophagitis and esophageal ulcerations have been reported in patients receiving capsule and tablet forms of drugs in the tetracycline class. Most of these patients took medications immediately before going to bed. (See Dosage and Administration.)
Skin: maculopapular and erythematous rashes. Exfoliative dermatitis has been reported but is uncommon. Photosensitivity is discussed above. (See "Warnings.")
Renal toxicity: Rise in BUN has been reported and is apparently dose related. (See "Warnings.")
Hypersensitivity reactions: Urticaria, angioneurotic edema, anaphylaxis, anaphylactoid purpura, pericarditis and exacerbation of systemic lupus erythematosus.
Bulging fontanels in infants and benign intracranial hypertension in adults have been reported in individuals receiving full therapeutic dosages. These conditions disappeared rapidly when the drug was discontinued.
Blood: Hemolytic anemia, thrombocytopenia, neutropenia and eosinophilia have been reported.
When given over prolonged periods, tetracyclines have been reported to produce brown-black microscopic discoloration of thyroid glands. No abnormalities of thyroid function studies are known to occur.

DOSAGE AND ADMINISTRATION
Oral: Capsules:
Adults: Usual daily dose, 1–2 g divided in four equal doses, depending on the severity of the infection.
Film-coated Tablets only:
Adults: A dosage schedule providing 2 tablets initially, then 1 tablet every six hours, is the usual average dose. In severe infections a larger dose (2 to 4 grams daily) may be indicated.
The total daily dose should be administered in four equal portions given at six hour intervals.
All Oral Forms:
For children above eight years of age: Usual daily dose, 10–20 mg per pound (25–50 mg/kg) of body weight divided in four equal doses.
Therapy should be continued for at least 24–48 hours after symptoms and fever have subsided. For treatment of brucellosis, 500 mg oxytetracycline four times daily for 3 weeks should be accompanied by streptomycin, 1 gram intramuscularly twice daily the first week, and once daily the second week.
For treatment of uncomplicated gonorrhea, when penicillin is contraindicated, tetracycline may be used for the treatment of both males and females in the following divided dosage schedule: 1.5 grams initially followed by 0.5 gram q.i.d. for a total of 9.0 grams.
For treatment of syphilis, a total of 30–40 grams in equally divided doses over a period of 10–15 days should be given. Close follow-up, including laboratory tests, is recommended.
Administration of adequate amounts of fluid along with capsule and tablet forms of drugs in the tetracycline class is recommended to wash down the drugs and reduce the risk of esophageal irritation and ulceration. (See Adverse Reactions.)
Concomitant therapy: Antacids containing aluminum, calcium, or magnesium impair absorption and should not be given to patients taking oral tetracyclines.
Food and some dairy products also interfere with absorption. Oral forms of tetracyclines should be given 1 hour before or 2 hours after meals. Pediatric oral dosage forms should not be given with milk formulas and should be given at least 1 hour prior to feeding.
In patients with renal impairment: (See "Warnings.") Total dosage should be decreased by reduction of recommended individual doses and/or by extending time intervals between doses.
In the treatment of streptococcal infections, a therapeutic dose of oxytetracycline should be administered for at least 10 days.

HOW SUPPLIED
Oral: Terramycin (oxytetracycline HCl) Capsules are available as opaque, yellow, hard gelatin capsules which contain oxytetracycline HCl equivalent to 250 mg of oxytetracycline, and glucosamine hydrochloride (imprinted with code number 073): bottles of 16, 100, and 500 and unit dose pack of 100 (10 × 10's).
Capsule Shown in Product Identification Section, page 422
Revised Sept. 1981
(Capsule) 60-0755-00-6
(Tablets: Discontinued)

LITERATURE AVAILABLE
Yes

VANSIL™ ℞
[*van'sĭl*]
(Brand of Oxamniquine)
(Capsules of 250 mg)

DESCRIPTION
VANSIL (brand of oxamniquine) is a tetrahydroquinoline derivative for the oral treatment of *Schistosoma mansoni* infections. It is 1, 2, 3, 4,-tetrahydro-2-[[(1- methylethyl) amino]methyl]-7-nitro-6-quinolinemethanol.
Oxamniquine is a yellow-orange crystalline solid which is sparingly soluble in water, but soluble in methanol, acetone, and chloroform.
VANSIL (oxamniquine) capsules contain 250 mg of oxamniquine.

CLINICAL PHARMACOLOGY
Oxamniquine is well absorbed when administered orally. Human plasma concentrations reach a peak at 1 to 1.5 hours after oral administration of therapeutic doses, with a plasma half-life of 1 to 2.5 hours. It is extensively metabolized to inactive acidic metabolites which are largely excreted in the urine.
Male schistosomes are more susceptible than females, but after treatment with oxamniquine the residual female schistosomes cease to lay eggs thus losing the parasitological aspect of their pathological significance. Animal studies with immature *S. mansoni* infections have demonstrated oxamniquine to be highly active in the immediate post-infection phase. Oxamniquine significantly reduces the egg load of *S. mansoni.*

INDICATIONS
Oxamniquine is indicated for all stages of *S. mansoni* infection, including the acute phase and the chronic phase with hepatosplenic involvement.

CONTRAINDICATIONS
At present, there are no known contraindications to the administration of oxamniquine.

WARNINGS
In rare instances epileptiform convulsions have been observed within the first few hours after ingestion of oxamniquine. When a convulsion occurred, it was mostly in a patient with a previous history of a convulsive condition. Oxamniquine should be used with care in such individuals and they should remain under medical supervision with facilities available to treat a convulsion should it occur.

PRECAUTIONS
Pregnancy Cateogry C: Oxamniquine has been shown to have an embryocidal effect in rabbits and mice when given in doses 10 times the human dose.
There are no adequate and well controlled studies in pregnant women. Oxamniquine should be used during pregnancy only if the potential benefit justifies the potential risk to the fetus.
Nursing Mothers: It is not known whether this drug is excreted in human milk.
Because many drugs are excreted in human milk, caution should be exercised when oxamniquine is administered to a nursing mother.

ADVERSE EFFECTS
Oxamniquine is generally well tolerated and toleration is improved if the doses are given after food. Transitory dizziness/drowsiness occurred in approximately one-third of the patients assessed. Other effects observed to a lesser degree are headache, nausea, vomiting, abdominal pain and anorexia. Urticaria has also been reported. In rare instances epileptiform convulsions have been observed (see WARNINGS).
Minor and transient abnormalities in laboratory data have been observed after treatment with oxamniquine which were not considered to be drug-related and were of no clinical significance. They included rare instances of mild to moderate liver enzyme elevations but there was no evidence of hepatotoxicity even in patients with severe hepatosplenic involvement. There was evidence, however, of liver abnormalities in animals with the female rat being uniquely sensitive to relatively low doses.

DOSAGE AND ADMINISTRATION
Adults
The recommended dosage is 12 to 15 mg per kilogram of body weight given as a single oral dose in patients with Western

Continued on next page

Pfizer—Cont.

Hemisphere strains of *S. mansoni*. The recommended capsule dosage according to body weight is as follows:

Body Weight (kg)	No. of Capsules (250 mg)
30– 40	2
41– 60	3
61– 80	4
81–100	5

Children

The recommended dosage for children under 30 kg in weight is 20 mg/kg of body weight given in two divided doses of 10 mg/kg in one day with an interval of 2 to 8 hours between doses. Toleration is improved if the doses are given after food.

HOW SUPPLIED

VANSIL (brand of oxamniquine) is supplied as #1 capsules of 250 mg in dark green opaque (cap) and rich yellow opaque (body), in bottles of 24 each.

68-4058-00-0 Issued June 1980

Literature Available: Yes

Shown in Product Identification Section, page 422

VIBRAMYCIN® Hyclate ℞

[*vī″bra-mī″sĭn*]

(doxycycline hyclate)

CAPSULES

VIBRA-TABS®

[*vī″bra-tabs′*]

(doxycycline hyclate)

FILM COATED TABLETS

VIBRAMYCIN® Calcium

(doxycycline calcium oral suspension)

SYRUP

VIBRAMYCIN® Monohydrate

(doxycycline monohydrate)

FOR ORAL SUSPENSION

DESCRIPTION

Vibramycin is a broad-spectrum antibiotic synthetically derived from oxytetracycline, and is available as Vibramycin Monohydrate (doxycycline monohydrate), Vibramycin Hyclate and Vibra-Tabs (doxycycline hydrochloride hemiethanolate hemihydrate), and Vibramycin Calcium (doxycycline calcium). The chemical designation of this light-yellow crystalline powder is alpha-6-deoxy-5-oxytetracycline. Doxycycline has a high degree of lipoid solubility and a low affinity for calcium binding. It is highly stable in normal human serum. Doxycycline will not degrade into an epianhydro form.

ACTIONS

Doxycycline is primarily bacteriostatic and is thought to exert its antimicrobial effect by the inhibition of protein synthesis. Doxycycline is active against a wide range of gram-positive and gram-negative organisms.

The drugs in the tetracycline class have closely similar antimicrobial spectra, and cross resistance among them is common. Microorganisms may be considered susceptible if the M.I.C. (minimum inhibitory concentration) is less than 4.0 mcg/ml and intermediate if the M.I.C. is 4.0 to 12.5 mcg/ml.

Susceptibility plate testing: If the Kirby-Bauer method of disc susceptibility testing is used, a 30 mcg doxycycline disc should give a zone of at least 16 mm when tested against a doxycycline-susceptible bacterial strain. A tetracycline disc may be used to determine microbial susceptibility. If the Kirby-Bauer method of disc susceptibility testing is used, a 30 mcg tetracycline disc should give a zone of at least 19 mm when tested against a tetracycline-susceptible bacterial strain.

Tetracyclines are readily absorbed and are bound to plasma proteins in varying degree. They are concentrated by the liver in the bile, and excreted in the urine and feces at high concentrations and in a biologically active form. Doxycycline is virtually completely absorbed after oral administration.

Following a 200 mg dose, normal adult volunteers averaged peak serum levels of 2.6 mcg/ml of doxycycline at 2 hours decreasing to 1.45 mcg/ml at 24 hours. Excretion of doxycycline by the kidney is about 40%/72 hours in individuals with normal function (creatinine clearance about 75 ml/min.). This percentage excretion may fall as low as 1–5%/72 hours in individuals with severe renal insufficiency (creatinine clearance below 10 ml/min.). Studies have shown no significant difference in serum half-life of doxycycline (range 18–22 hours) in individuals with normal and severely impaired renal function.

Hemodialysis does not alter serum half-life.

INDICATIONS

Doxycycline is indicated in infections caused by the following microorganisms:

Rickettsiae: Rocky Mountain spotted fever, typhus fever and the typhus group, Q. fever, rickettsialpox, and tick fevers.

Mycoplasma pneumoniae (PPLO, Eaton agent),

Agents of psittacosis and ornithosis,

Agents of lymphogranuloma venereum and granuloma inguinale,

The spirochetal agent of relapsing fever (*Borrelia recurrentis*).

The following gram-negative microorganisms:

Haemophilus ducreyi (chancroid),

Pasteurella pestis, and *Pasteurella tularensis*,

Bartonella bacilliformis,

Bacteroides species,

Vibrio comma and *Vibrio fetus*,

Brucella species (in conjunction with streptomycin).

Because many strains of the following groups of microorganisms have been shown to be resistant to tetracyclines, culture and susceptibility testing are recommended.

Doxycycline is indicated for treatment of infections caused by the following gram-negative microorganisms, when bacteriologic testing indicates appropriate susceptibility to the drug:

Escherichia coli,

Enterobacter aerogenes (formerly *Aerobacter aerogenes*),

Shigella species,

Mima species and *Herellea* species,

Haemophilus influenzae (respiratory infections),

Klebsiella species (respiratory and urinary infections).

Doxycycline is indicated for treatment of infections caused by the following gram-positive microorganisms when bacteriologic testing indicates appropriate susceptibility to the drug:

Streptococcus species:

Up to 44 percent of strains of *Streptococcus pyogenes* and 74 percent of *Streptococcus faecalis* have been found to be resistant to tetracycline drugs. Therefore, tetracyclines should not be used for streptococcal disease unless the organism has been demonstrated to be sensitive.

For upper respiratory infections due to group A beta-hemolytic streptococci, penicillin is the usual drug of choice, including prophylaxis of rheumatic fever.

Diplococcus pneumoniae,

Staphylococcus aureus, respiratory, skin and soft-tissue infections. Tetracyclines are not the drug of choice in the treatment of any type of staphylococcal infection.

When penicillin is contraindicated, doxycycline is an alternative drug in the treatment of infections due to:

Treponema pallidum and *Treponema pertenue* (syphilis and yaws),

Listeria monocytogenes,

Clostridium species,

Bacillus anthracis,

Fusobacterium fusiforme (Vincent's infection),

Actinomyces species.

In acute intestinal amebiasis doxycycline may be a useful adjunct to amebicides.

In severe acne doxycycline may be useful adjunctive therapy.

Doxycycline is indicated in the treatment of trachoma, although the infectious agent is not always eliminated, as judged by immunofluorescence.

Inclusion conjunctivitis may be treated with oral doxycycline alone, or with a combination of topical agents.

Doxycycline is indicated for the treatment of uncomplicated urethral, endocervical, or rectal infections in adults caused by *Chlamydia trachomatis*.[1]

Doxycycline is indicated for the treatment of nongonococcal urethritis caused by *Chlamydia trachomatis* and *Ureaplasma urealyticum* and for the treatment of acute epididymo-orchitis caused by *Chlamydia trachomatis*.[1]

Doxycycline is indicated for the treatment of uncomplicated gonococcal infections in adults (except for anorectal infections in men) and acute epididymo-orchitis caused by *N. gonorrhoeae*.[1]

CONTRAINDICATIONS

This drug is contraindicated in persons who have shown hypersensitivity to any of the tetracyclines.

WARNINGS

THE USE OF DRUGS OF THE TETRACYCLINE CLASS DURING TOOTH DEVELOPMENT (LAST HALF OF PREGNANCY, INFANCY AND CHILDHOOD TO THE AGE OF 8 YEARS) MAY CAUSE PERMANENT DISCOLORATION OF THE TEETH (YELLOW-GRAY-BROWN). This adverse reaction is more common during long term use of the drugs but has been observed following repeated short term courses. Enamel hypoplasia has also been reported. *TETRACYCLINE DRUGS, THEREFORE, SHOULD NOT BE USED IN THIS AGE GROUP UNLESS OTHER DRUGS ARE NOT LIKELY TO BE EFFECTIVE OR ARE CONTRAINDICATED.*

Photosensitivity manifested by an exaggerated sunburn reaction has been observed in some individuals taking tetracyclines. Patients apt to be exposed to direct sunlight or ultraviolet light should be advised that this reaction can occur with tetracycline drugs, and treatment should be discontinued at the first evidence of skin erythema.

The antianabolic action of the tetracyclines may cause an increase in BUN. Studies to date indicate that this does not occur with the use of doxycycline in patients with impaired renal function.

USAGE IN PREGNANCY

(See above "Warnings" about use during tooth development.)

Results of animal studies indicate that tetracyclines cross the placenta, are found in fetal tissues, and can have toxic effects on the developing fetus (often related to retardation of skeletal development). Evidence of embryotoxicity has also been noted in animals treated early in pregnancy.

USAGE IN NEWBORNS, INFANTS, AND CHILDREN:

(See above "Warnings" about use during tooth development.)

As with other tetracyclines, doxycycline forms a stable calcium complex in any bone-forming tissue. A decrease in the fibula growth rate has been observed in prematures given oral tetracycline in doses of 25 mg/kg every six hours. This reaction was shown to be reversible when the drug was discontinued.

Tetracyclines are present in the milk of lactating women who are taking a drug in this class.

PRECAUTIONS

As with other antibiotic preparations, use of this drug may result in overgrowth of nonsusceptible organisms, including fungi. If superinfection occurs, the antibiotic should be discontinued and appropriate therapy should be instituted.

In venereal disease when coexistent syphilis is suspected, a dark field examination should be done before treatment is started and the blood serology repeated monthly for at least four months.

Because the tetracyclines have been shown to depress plasma prothrombin activity, patients who are on anticoagulant therapy may require downward adjustment of their anticoagulant dosage.

In long term therapy, periodic laboratory evaluation of organ systems, including hematopoietic, renal, and hepatic studies should be performed.

All infections due to group A beta-hemolytic streptococci should be treated for at least 10 days.

Since bacteriostatic drugs may interfere with the bactericidal action of penicillin, it is advisable to avoid giving tetracycline in conjunction with penicillin.

ADVERSE REACTIONS

Due to oral doxycycline's virtually complete absorption, side effects of the lower bowel, particularly diarrhea, have been infrequent. The following adverse reactions have been observed in patients receiving tetracyclines:

Gastrointestinal: anorexia, nausea, vomiting, diarrhea, glossitis, dysphagia, enterocolitis, and inflammatory lesions (with monilial overgrowth) in the anogenital region. These reactions have been caused by both the oral and parenteral administration of tetracyclines. Rare instances of esophagitis and esophageal ulcerations have been reported in patients receiving capsule and tablet forms of drugs in the tetracycline class. Most of these patients took medications immediately before going to bed. (See Dosage and Administration.)

Skin: maculopapular and erythematous rashes. Exfoliative dermatitis has been reported but is uncommon. Photosensitivity is discussed above (see "Warnings").

Renal toxicity: Rise in BUN has been reported and is apparently dose related. (See "Warnings.")

Hypersensitivity reactions: urticaria, angioneurotic edema, anaphylaxis, anaphylactoid purpura, pericarditis, and exacerbation of systemic lupus erythematosus.

Bulging fontanels in infants and benign intracranial hypertension in adults have been reported in individuals receiving full therapeutic dosages. These conditions disappeared rapidly when the drug was discontinued.

Blood: Hemolytic anemia, thrombocytopenia, neutropenia, and eosinophilia have been reported with tetracyclines.

When given over prolonged periods, tetracyclines have been reported to produce brown-black microscopic discoloration of thyroid glands. No abnormalities of thyroid function studies are known to occur.

DOSAGE AND ADMINISTRATION

THE USUAL DOSAGE AND FREQUENCY OF ADMINISTRATION OF DOXYCYCLINE DIFFERS FROM THAT OF THE OTHER TETRACYCLINES. EXCEEDING THE RECOMMENDED DOSAGE MAY RESULT IN AN INCREASED INCIDENCE OF SIDE EFFECTS.

Adults: The usual dose of oral doxycycline is 200 mg on the first day of treatment (administered 100 mg every 12 hours) followed by a maintenance dose of 100 mg/day. The maintenance dose may be administered as a single dose or as 50 mg every 12 hours. In the management of more severe infections (particularly chronic infections of the urinary tract), 100 mg every 12 hours is recommended.

For children above eight years of age: The recommended dosage schedule for children weighing 100 pounds or less is 2 mg/lb. of body weight divided into two doses on the first day of treatment, followed by 1 mg/lb. of body weight given as a single daily dose or divided into two doses, on subsequent

days. For more severe infections up to 2 mg/lb. of body weight may be used. For children over 100 lbs. the usual adult dose should be used.
Uncomplicated gonococcal infections in adults (except anorectal infections in men): 100 mg, by mouth, twice a day for 7 days.[1]
As an alternate single visit dose, administer 300 mg stat followed in one hour by a second 300 mg dose. The dose may be administered with food, including milk or carbonated beverage, as required.
Acute epididymo-orchitis caused by *N. gonorrhoeae:* 100 mg, by mouth, twice a day for at least 10 days.[1]
Primary and secondary syphilis: 300 mg a day in divided doses for at least 10 days.
The therapeutic antibacterial serum activity will usually persist for 24 hours following recommended dosage.
When used in streptococcal infections, therapy should be continued for 10 days.
Administration of adequate amounts of fluid along with capsule and tablet forms of drugs in the tetracycline class is recommended to wash down the drugs and reduce the risk of esophageal irritation and ulceration. (See Adverse Reactions.)
If gastric irritation occurs, it is recommended that doxycycline be given with food or milk. The absorption of doxycycline is not markedly influenced by simultaneous ingestion of food or milk.
Uncomplicated urethral, endocervical, or rectal infection in adults caused by *Chlamydia trachomatis:* 100 mg, by mouth, twice a day for at least 7 days.[1]
Nongonococcal urethritis caused by *C. trachomatis* and *U. urealyticum:* 100 mg, by mouth, twice a day for at least 7 days.[1]
Acute epididymo-orchitis caused by *C. trachomatis:* 100 mg, by mouth, twice a day for at least 10 days.[1]
Concomitant therapy: Antacids containing aluminum, calcium, or magnesium impair absorption and should not be given to patients taking oral doxycycline.
Studies to date have indicated that administration of doxycycline at the usual recommended doses does not lead to excessive accumulation of the antibiotic in patients with renal impairment.

HOW SUPPLIED

Vibramycin Hyclate (doxycycline hyclate) is available in capsules containing doxycycline hyclate equivalent to:
50 mg doxycycline (imprinted with code number 094)
bottles of 50
unit-dose pack of 100 (10 x 10's)
X-pack of 50 (5 x 10's)
100 mg doxycycline (imprinted with code number 095)
bottles of 50 and 500
unit-dose pack of 100 (10 x 10's)
V-pack of 25 (5 x 5's)
Nine-Paks (10 x 9's)
Vibra-Tabs (doxycycline hyclate) is available in film coated tablets (imprinted with code number 099) containing doxycycline hyclate equivalent to:
100 mg of doxycycline
bottles of 50 and 500
unit-dose pack of 100 (10 x 10's)
Vibramycin Calcium Syrup (doxycycline calcium oral suspension) is available as a raspberry-apple flavored oral suspension. Each teaspoonful (5 ml) contains doxycycline calcium equivalent to 50 mg of doxycycline: bottles of 1 oz. (30 ml) and 1 Pint (473 ml).
Vibramycin Monohydrate (doxycycline monohydrate) for Oral Suspension is available as a pleasant tasting, raspberry flavored, dry powder for oral suspension. When reconstituted, each teaspoonful (5 ml) contains doxycycline monohydrate equivalent to 25 mg of doxycycline: 2 oz. (60 ml) bottles.
Reference:

1. CDC Sexually Transmitted Diseases Treatment Guidelines 1982.

Revised October 1983
69-1680-00-7

LITERATURE AVAILABLE

Yes.

Shown in Product Identification Section, page 422

VISTARIL® ℞

[*vĭs 'tăr-ĭl*]
(hydroxyzine pamoate)
Capsules and Oral Suspension

DESCRIPTION

Hydroxyzine pamoate is designated chemically as 1-(p-chlorobenzhydryl) 4-[2-(2-hydroxyethoxy) ethyl] diethylenediamine salt of 1,1'- methylene bis (2 hydroxy-3-naphthalene carboxylic acid).

CLINICAL PHARMACOLOGY

Vistaril (hydroxyzine pamoate) is unrelated chemically to the phenothiazines, reserpine, meprobamate, or the benzodiazepines.
Vistaril is not a cortical depressant, but its action may be due to a suppression of activity in certain key regions of the subcortical area of the central nervous system. Primary skeletal muscle relaxation has been demonstrated experimentally. Bronchodilator activity, and antihistaminic and analgesic effects have been demonstrated experimentally and confirmed clinically. An antiemetic effect, both by the apomorphine test and the veriloid test, has been demonstrated. Pharmacological and clinical studies indicate that hydroxyzine in therapeutic dosage does not increase gastric secretion or acidity and in most cases has mild antisecretory activity. Hydroxyzine is rapidly absorbed from the gastrointestinal tract and Vistaril's clinical effects are usually noted within 15 to 30 minutes after oral administration.

INDICATIONS

For symptomatic relief of anxiety and tension associated with psychoneurosis and as an adjunct in organic disease states in which anxiety is manifested.
Useful in the management of pruritus due to allergic conditions such as chronic urticaria and atopic and contact dermatoses, and in histamine-mediated pruritus.
As a sedative when used as premedication and following general anesthesia, **Hydroxyzine may potentiate meperidine (Demerol®) and barbiturates,** so their use in pre-anesthetic adjunctive therapy should be modified on an individual basis. Atropine and other belladonna alkaloids are not affected by the drug. Hydroxyzine is not known to interfere with the action of digitalis in any way and it may be used concurrently with this agent.
The effectiveness of hydroxyzine as an antianxiety agent for long term use, that is more than 4 months, has not been assessed by systematic clinical studies. The physician should reassess periodically the usefulness of the drug for the individual patient.

CONTRAINDICATIONS

Hydroxyzine, when administered to the pregnant mouse, rat, and rabbit, induced fetal abnormalities in the rat and mouse at doses substantially above the human therapeutic range. Clinical data in human beings are inadequate to establish safety in early pregnancy. Until such data are available, hydroxyzine is contraindicated in early pregnancy.
Hydroxyzine pamoate is contraindicated for patients who have shown a previous hypersensitivity to it.

WARNINGS

Nursing Mothers: It is not known whether this drug is excreted in human milk. Since many drugs are so excreted, hydroxyzine should not be given to nursing mothers.

PRECAUTIONS

THE POTENTIATING ACTION OF HYDROXYZINE MUST BE CONSIDERED WHEN THE DRUG IS USED IN CONJUNCTION WITH CENTRAL NERVOUS SYSTEM DEPRESSANTS SUCH AS NARCOTICS, NON-NARCOTIC ANALGESICS AND BARBITURATES. Therefore, when central nervous system depressants are administered concomitantly with hydroxyzine their dosage should be reduced. Since drowsiness may occur with use of the drug, patients should be warned of this possibility and cautioned against driving a car or operating dangerous machinery while taking Vistaril (hydroxyzine pamoate). Patients should be advised against the simultaneous use of other CNS depressant drugs, and cautioned that the effect of alcohol may be increased.

ADVERSE REACTIONS

Side effects reported with the administration of Vistaril are usually mild and transitory in nature.
Anticholinergic: Dry mouth.
Central Nervous System: Drowsiness is usually transitory and may disappear in a few days of continued therapy or upon reduction of the dose. Involuntary motor activity including rare instances of tremor and convulsions has been reported, usually with doses considerably higher than those recommended. Clinically significant respiratory depression has not been reported at recommended doses.

OVERDOSAGE

The most common manifestation of overdosage of Vistaril is hypersedation. As in the management of overdosage with any drug, it should be borne in mind that multiple agents may have been taken.
If vomiting has not occurred spontaneously, it should be induced. Immediate gastric lavage is also recommended. General supportive care, including frequent monitoring of the vital signs and close observation of the patient, is indicated. Hypotension, though unlikely, may be controlled with intravenous fluids and Levophed® (levarterenol) or Aramine® (metaraminol). Do not use epinephrine as Vistaril counteracts its pressor action. Caffeine and Sodium Benzoate Injection, U.S.P., may be used to counteract central nervous system depressant effects.
There is no specific antidote. It is doubtful that hemodialysis would be of any value in the treatment of overdosage with hydroxyzine. However, if other agents such as barbiturates have been ingested concomitantly, hemodialysis may be indicated. There is no practical method to quantitate hydroxyzine in body fluids or tissue after its ingestion or administration.

DOSAGE

For symptomatic relief of anxiety and tension associated with psychoneurosis and as an adjunct in organic disease states in which anxiety is manifested: in adults, 50–100 mg q.i.d.; children under 6 years, 50 mg daily in divided doses and over 6 years, 50–100 mg daily in divided doses.
For use in the management of pruritus due to allergic conditions such as chronic urticaria and atopic and contact dermatoses, and in histamine-mediated pruritus: in adults, 25 mg t.i.d. or q.i.d.; children under 6 years, 50 mg daily in divided doses and over 6 years, 50–100 mg daily in divided doses.
As a sedative when used as a premedication and following general anesthesia: 50–100 mg in adults, and 0.6 mg/kg in children.
When treatment is initiated by the intramuscular route of administration, subsequent doses may be administered orally.
As with all medications, the dosage should be adjusted according to the patient's response to therapy.

SUPPLY

Vistaril Capsules (hydroxyzine pamoate equivalent to hydroxyzine hydrochloride)

25 mg:	100's and 500's, and unit dose (10 × 10's) —two-tone green capsules (imprinted with code number 541).
50 mg:	100's and 500's, and unit dose (10 × 10's) —green and white capsules (imprinted with code number 542).
100 mg:	100's and 500's, and unit dose (10 × 10's) —green and gray capsules (imprinted with code number 543).

Vistaril Oral Suspension (hydroxyzine pamoate equivalent to 25 mg hydroxyzine hydrochloride per teaspoonful-5 ml): 1 pint bottles and 4 ounce (120 ml) bottles in packages of 4.

BIBLIOGRAPHY

Available on request.

Revised April 1979
(60-0846-00-9)

Shown in Product Identification Section, page 422

EDUCATIONAL MATERIAL

Booklets—free
The *Learning to Live With. . . .* series of patient information booklets on the symptoms of specific diseases, preventive measures, techniques for changing lifestyle habits, adherence to diet and drug regimens. This ongoing series includes booklets on angina, osteoarthritis, hypertension and diabetes.
Address requests to:
Communications Program Coordination
Pfizer Pharmaceuticals
235 East 42nd Street
New York, N.Y. 10017

Vibramycin:
Booklet:
MMWR Supplement: 1985 STD Treatment Guidelines, Centers for Disease Control, United States Department of Health and Human Services, Vol. 34, No. 4S, October 18, 1985.
A comprehensive overview of the major sexually transmitted diseases (STD) is presented in this reprint of the *1985 STD Treatment Guidelines.* The booklet presents a description of major STD pathologies, such as AIDS, *Chlamydia trachomatis* infection and PID, and their approved CDC treatments. This booklet is available free to physicians, pharmacists, and allied health practitioners.
Address requests to:
Pfizer Laboratories Medical Department
Professional Services
235 East 42nd Street
New York, N.Y. 10017

Products are cross-indexed by generic and chemical names in the **YELLOW SECTION**

Pharmacia Laboratories,
Pharmacia Inc.
800 CENTENNIAL AVENUE
PISCATAWAY, NJ 08854

AZULFIDINE® (sulfasalazine, USP) ℞
[*ă-zul'fi-dēn"*]
Tablets
AZULFIDINE® (sulfasalazine, USP) ℞
EN-tabs®
AZULFIDINE® (sulfasalazine, USP) ℞
Oral Suspension

DESCRIPTION

Azulfidine® (Sulfasalazine USP) Tablets, 500 mg for Oral Administration
Azulfidine (Sulfasalazine USP) EN-tabs®, 500 mg for Oral Administration
Azulfidine EN-tabs are film coated with cellulose acetate phthalate to prevent disintegration of the tablet in the stomach and thus reduce possible irritation of the gastric mucosa.
Azulfidine® (Sulfasalazine USP) Oral Suspension, 250 mg/5ml for Oral Administration
Therapeutic classification: Anti-inflammatory agent.
Chemical designation: 5-([p-(2-Pyridylsulfamoyl) phenyl] azo) salicylic acid.
Chemical structure:

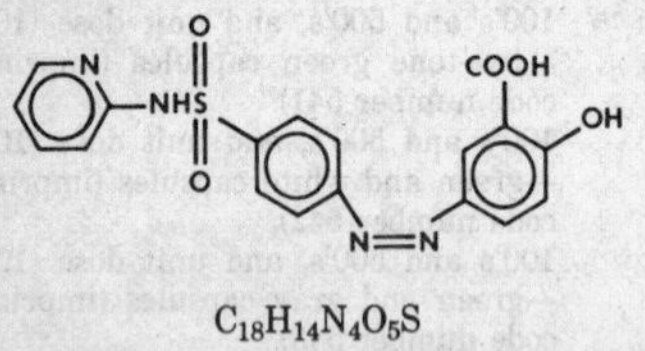

$C_{18}H_{14}N_4O_5S$

CLINICAL PHARMACOLOGY

After oral administration, AZULFIDINE is partially absorbed and extensively metabolized as described below.
About one-third of a given dose of sulfasalazine (SS) is absorbed from the small intestine. The remaining two-thirds pass to the colon where the compound is split (presumably by intestinal bacteria) into its components, 5-aminosalicylic acid (5-ASA) and sulfapyridine (SP). Most of the SP thus liberated is absorbed whereas only about one-third of the 5-ASA is absorbed, the remainder being excreted in the feces. The distribution metabolism and excretion of SS and its two components are as follows:

AZULFIDINE Tablets:

Sulfasalazine (SS): Detectable serum concentrations of SS have been found in healthy subjects within 90 minutes after the ingestion of a single 2 g dose of AZULFIDINE Tablets. Maximum concentrations of SS occur between 1.5 and 6 hours, with the mean peak concentration (14 mcg/ml) occurring at 3 hours. Small amounts of SS are excreted unchanged in the urine.
Sulfapyridine (SP): Following absorption and distribution, SP is acetylated and hydroxylated in the liver, and then conjugated with glucuronic acid. After ingestion of a single 2 g dose of AZULFIDINE Tablets by healthy subjects, SP and its various metabolites appear in the serum within 3 to 6 hours. Maximum concentrations of total SP occur between 6 and 24 hours, with the mean peak concentration (21 mcg/ml) occurring at 12 hours. The total recovery of SS and its SP metabolites from the urine of healthy subjects 3 days after the administration of a single 2 g dose of AZULFIDINE Tablets averaged 91%.
5-Aminosalicylic Acid (5-ASA): The serum concentration of 5-ASA in patients with ulcerative colitis was found to range from 0 to 4 mcg/ml, and to exist mainly in the form of free 5-ASA. The urinary recovery of this compound was mostly in the acetylated form.

AZULFIDINE EN-tabs

Sulfasalazine (SS): Detectable serum concentrations of SS have been found in healthy subjects within 90 minutes after the ingestion of a single 2 g dose of AZULFIDINE EN-tabs. Maximum concentrations of SS occur between 3 and 12 hours, with the mean peak concentration (6 mcg/ml) occurring at 6 hours. Small amounts of SS are excreted unchanged in the urine.
Sulfapyridine (SP): Following absorption and distribution, SP is acetylated and hydroxylated in the liver, and then conjugated with glucuronic acid. After ingestion of a single 2 g dose of AZULFIDINE EN-tabs by healthy subjects, peak concentrations of SP and its various metabolites appear in the serum between 12 and 24 hours, with the peak concentration (13 mcg/ml) occurring at 12 and lasting until 24 hours. The total recovery of SS and its SP metabolites from the urine of healthy subjects 3 days after the administration of a single 2 g dose of AZULFIDINE EN-tabs averaged 81%.
5-Aminosalicylic Acid (5-ASA): The serum concentration of 5-ASA in patients with ulcerative colitis was found to range from 0 to 4 mcg/ml, and to exist mainly in the form of free 5-ASA. The urinary recovery of this compound was mostly in the acetylated form.

AZULFIDINE Oral Suspension

Sulfasalazine (SS): Detectable serum concentrations of SS have been found in healthy subjects within 90 minutes after the injection of a single 2 g dose of AZULFIDINE Oral Suspension. Maximum concentrations of SS occur between 1.5 and 6 hours, with the mean peak concentration (20 mcg/ml) occurring at 3 hours. Small amounts of SS are excreted unchanged in the urine.
Sulfapyridine (SP): Following absorption and distribution, SP is acetylated and hydroxylated in the liver, and then conjugated with glucuronic acid. After ingestion of a single 2 g dose of AZULFIDINE Oral Suspension by healthy subjects, SP and its various metabolites appear in the serum within 3 to 6 hours. Maximum concentrations of total SP occur between 9 and 24 hours with the mean peak concentration (19 mcg/ml) occurring at 12 hours. The total recovery of SS and its SP metabolites from the urine of healthy subjects 3 days after the administration of a single 2 g dose of AZULFIDINE Oral Suspension averaged 75%.
5-Aminosalicylic Acid (5-ASA): The serum concentrations of 5-ASA in patients with ulcerative colitis was found to range from 0 to 4 mcg/ml, and to exist mainly in the form of free 5-ASA. The urinary recovery of this compound was mostly in the acetylated form.
Mean serum concentrations of total SP, i.e. SP and its metabolites, tend to be significantly greater in patients with a slow acetylator phenotype than in those with a fast acetylator phenotype. Total serum sulfapyridine concentrations greater than 50 mcg/ml appear to be associated with an increased incidence of adverse reactions.
The mode of action of AZULFIDINE is still under investigation. It may be related to the immunosuppressant properties that have been observed in animal and **in vitro** models, to its affinity for connective tissue, and/or to the relatively high concentration it reaches in serous fluids, the liver and intestinal walls, as demonstrated in autoradiographic studies in animals. AZULFIDINE has also been described as a highly efficient vehicle for carrying its principal metabolites, SP and 5-ASA, to the colon, where a local action for both of them has been postulated. Recent clinical studies utilizing rectal administration of SS, SP, and 5-ASA have indicated that the major therapeutic action may reside in the 5-ASA moiety.

INDICATIONS AND USAGE

AZULFIDINE is indicated:
a. in the treatment of mild to moderate ulcerative colitis, and as adjunctive therapy in severe ulcerative colitis.
b. for the prolongation of the remission period between acute attacks of ulcerative colitis.
AZULFIDINE EN-tabs are particularly indicated in patients who cannot take the regular AZULFIDINE tablet because of gastrointestinal intolerance, and in whom there is evidence that this intolerance is not primarily due to high blood levels of sulfapyridine and its metabolites, e.g. patients experiencing nausea, vomiting, etc., when taking the first few doses of the drug or patients in whom a reduction in dosage does not alleviate the gastrointestinal side effects.

CONTRAINDICATIONS

Hypersensitivity to sulfasalazine, its metabolites, sulfonamides or salicylates. In infants under 2 years of age. Intestinal and urinary obstruction. Patients with porphyria should not receive sulfonamides as these drugs have been reported to precipitate an acute attack.

WARNINGS

Only after critical appraisal should AZULFIDINE be used in patients with hepatic or renal damage or blood dyscrasias. Deaths associated with the administration of AZULFIDINE have been reported from hypersensitivity reactions, agranulocytosis, aplastic anemia, other blood dyscrasias, renal and liver damage, irreversible neuromuscular and CNS changes, and fibrosing alveolitis. The presence of clinical signs such as sore throat, fever, pallor, purpura, or jaundice may be indications of serious blood disorders. Complete blood counts as well as urinalysis with careful microscopic examination should be done frequently in patients receiving AZULFIDINE. Oligospermia and infertility have been observed in men treated with AZULFIDINE. Withdrawal of the drug appears to reverse these effects.

PRECAUTIONS

General: AZULFIDINE should be given with caution to patients with severe allergy or bronchial asthma. Adequate fluid intake must be maintained in order to prevent crystalluria and stone formation. Patients with glucose-6-phosphate dehydrogenase deficiency should be observed closely for signs of hemolytic anemia. This reaction is frequently dose related. If toxic or hypersensitivity reactions occur, the drug should be discontinued immediately.
Isolated instances have been reported when AZULFIDINE EN-tabs have passed undisintegrated. This may be due to a lack of intestinal esterases in these patients. If this is observed, the administration of AZULFIDINE EN-tabs should be discontinued immediately.
Information for Patients: Patients should be informed of the possibility of adverse reactions and of the need for careful medical supervision. They should also be made aware that ulcerative colitis rarely remits completely, and that the risk of relapse can be substantially reduced by continued administration of AZULFIDINE (at a maintenance dosage). Diabetic patients should be advised that AZULFIDINE Oral Suspension contains sucrose.
Patients should be instructed to take AZULFIDINE in evenly divided doses preferably after meals. Additionally, patients should be advised that AZULFIDINE may produce an orange-yellow discoloration of the urine or skin.
Laboratory Tests: The progress of the disease during treatment can be evaluated by clinical criteria, including the presence of fever, weight changes, degree and frequency of diarrhea and bleeding as well as by sigmoidoscopy and the evaluation of biopsy samples. The determination of serum sulfapyridine levels may be useful since concentrations greater than 50 mcg/ml appear to be associated with an increased incidence of adverse reactions. Complete blood counts, as well as a urinalysis with careful microscopic examination should be done frequently in patients receiving AZULFIDINE.
Drug Interactions: Reduced absorption of folic acid and digoxin have been reported when administered concomitantly with AZULFIDINE.
Drug/Laboratory Test Interactions: The presence of AZULFIDINE or its metabolites in body fluids has not been reported to interfere with laboratory test procedures.
Carcinogenesis, Mutagenesis, Impairment of Fertility: There have been no long-term studies of the carcinogenic or mutagenic potential of AZULFIDINE. Impairment of male fertility was observed in reproductive studies performed in rats and rabbits at doses up to six times the human dose. Oligospermia and infertility have been described in men treated with AZULFIDINE. Withdrawal of the drug appears to reverse these effects (see "**WARNINGS**").
Pregnancy:
Teratogenic Effects:
Pregnancy Category B: Reproduction studies have been performed in rats and rabbits at doses up to 6 times the human dose and have revealed no evidence of impaired female fertility or harm to the fetus due to AZULFIDINE.
There are, however, no adequate and well-controlled studies in pregnant women. Because animal reproduction studies are not always predictive of human response, this drug should be used during pregnancy only if clearly needed. A national survey evaluated the outcome of pregnancies associated with inflammatory bowel disease (IBD). In a group of 186 women treated with AZULFIDINE alone or AZULFIDINE and concomitant steroid therapy, the incidence of fetal morbidity and mortality was comparable to that for 245 untreated IBD pregnancies as well as with population data from the National Center for Health Statistics[1]. Another study of 1,445 pregnancies associated with exposure to sulfonamides in which AZULFIDINE was included indicated that this group of drugs appeared to be devoid of any association with fetal malformation[2]. A review of the medical literature covering 1,155 pregnancies which occurred in women having ulcerative colitis suggested that the outcome was similar to what was expected in the general population[3].
No clinical studies have been performed which indicate the effect of AZULFIDINE on the later growth development and functional maturation of children whose mothers received the drug during pregnancy.
Nonteratogenic Effects: AZULFIDINE and sulfapyridine pass the placental barrier. Although sulfapyridine has been shown to have a poor bilirubin displacing capacity, the potential for kernicterus in newborns should be kept in mind.
Nursing Mothers: Caution should be exercised when AZULFIDINE is administered to a nursing woman. Sulfonamides are excreted in the milk. In the newborn, they compete with bilirubin for binding sites on the plasma proteins and may thus cause kernicterus. Insignificant amounts of uncleaved sulfasalazine have been found in milk, whereas the sulfapyridine levels in milk are about 30–60 per cent of those in the serum. Sulfapyridine has been shown to have a poor bilirubin displacing capacity.
Pediatric Use: Safety and effectiveness in children below the age of two years have not been established.

ADVERSE REACTIONS

The most common adverse reactions associated with AZULFIDINE are anorexia, headache, nausea, vomiting, gastric distress and apparently reversible oligospermia. These occur in about one-third of the patients. Less frequent adverse reactions are skin rash, pruritus, urticaria, fever, Heinz body anemia, hemolytic anemia and cyanosis which may occur at a frequency of one in every thirty patients or less. Experience suggests that with a daily dosage of 4 g or more, or total serum sulfapyridine levels above 50 mcg/ml, the incidence of adverse reactions tends to increase.
Although the listing which follows includes a few adverse reactions which have not been reported with this specific drug, the pharmacological similarities among the sulfona-

mides require that each of these reactions be considered when AZULFIDINE is administered.
Other adverse reactions which occur rarely, in approximately 1 in 1000 patients or less are:
Blood dyscrasias: aplastic anemia, agranulocytosis, leukopenia, megaloblastic (macrocytic) anemia, purpura, thrombocytopenia, hypoprothrombinemia and methemoglobinemia.
Hypersensitivity reactions: erythema multiforme (Stevens Johnson syndrome), exfoliative dermatitis, epidermal necrolysis (Lyell's syndrome) with corneal damage, anaphylaxis, serum sickness syndrome, transient pulmonary changes with eosinophilia and decreased pulmonary function, allergic myocarditis, polyarteritis nodosa, L.E. syndrome, hepatitis with immune complexes, parapsoriasis varioliformis acuta (Mucha Haberman syndrome), photosensitization, arthralgia, periorbital edema, conjuctival and scleral injection and alopecia.
Gastrointestinal reactions: hepatitis, pancreatitis, bloody diarrhea, impaired folic acid absorption, impaired digoxin absorption, stomatitis, diarrhea and abdominal pains.
CNS reactions: transverse myelitis, convulsions, transient lesions of the posterior spinal column, peripheral neuropathy, mental depression, vertigo, hearing loss, insomnia, ataxia, hallucinations, tinnitus and drowsiness.
Renal reactions: toxic nephrosis with oliguria and anuria, nephrotic syndrome, hematuria, crystalluria and proteinuria.
Other reactions: urine discoloration and skin discoloration.
The sulfonamides bear certain chemical similarities to some goitrogens, diuretics, (acetazolamide and the thiazides), and oral hypoglycemic agents. Goiter production, diuresis, and hypoglycemia have occurred rarely in patients receiving sulfonamides. Cross-sensitivity may exist with these agents. Rats appear to be especially susceptible to the goitrogenic effects of sulfonamides and long-term administration has produced thyroid malignancies in this species.

DRUG ABUSE AND DEPENDENCE

None reported.
Overdosage: There is evidence that the incidence and severity of toxicity are directly related to the total serum sulfapyridine concentration. Symptoms of overdosage may include nausea, vomiting, gastric distress and abdominal pains. In more advanced cases, CNS symptoms such as drowsiness, convulsions, etc. may be observed. Serum sulfapyridine concentrations may be used to monitor the progress of recovery from overdosage.
Experience suggests that with a daily dosage of 4 g or more or total serum sulfapyridine levels above 50 mcg/ml the incidence of adverse reactions tends to increase. There are no documented reports of deaths due to ingestion of large single doses of AZULFIDINE.
It has not been possible to determine the oral LD_{50} in laboratory animals such as mice, since the highest daily oral dose which can be given (12 g/Kg) is not lethal. Doses of AZULFIDINE of 16 g per day have been given to patients without mortality.
Instructions for overdosage: Gastric lavage or emesis plus catharsis as indicated. Alkalinize urine. If kidney function is normal, force fluids. If anuria is present, restrict fluids and salt, and treat appropriately. Catheterization of the ureters may be indicated for complete renal blockage by crystals. The low molecular weight of AZULFIDINE and its metabolites may facilitate their removal by dialysis. For agranulocytosis, discontinue the drug immediately, hospitalize the patient and institute appropriate therapy.
For hypersensitivity reactions, discontinue treatment immediately. Such reactions may be controlled with antihistamines and, if necessary, systemic corticosteroids.
When in the physician's opinion, reinstitution of AZULFIDINE is warranted, regimens modeled upon desensitization procedures may be attempted approximately two weeks after AZULFIDINE has been discontinued and symptoms have disappeared (see "**Dosage and Administration**").

DOSAGE AND ADMINISTRATION

Dosage should be adjusted to each individual's response and tolerance. The drug should be given in evenly divided doses over each 24-hour period; intervals between nighttime doses should not exceed 8 hours, with administration after meals recommended when feasible. Experience suggests that with daily dosages of 4 g or more, the incidence of adverse reactions tends to increase; hence, patients receiving these dosages should be instructed about and carefully observed for the appearance of adverse effects.
Various desensitization-like regimens have been reported to be effective in 34 of 53 patients[4], 7 of 8 patients[5] and 19 of 20 patients[6]. Upon reinstituting AZULFIDINE, such regimens comprise a total daily dose of 50 to 250 mg which, every 4 to 7 days thereafter, is doubled until the desired therapeutic level is achieved. Administration of small desensitization doses of AZULFIDINE are achieved most easily through the use of AZULFIDINE Oral Suspension (250 mg/5 ml). If the symptoms of sensitivity recur, AZULFIDINE should be discontinued. Desensitization should not be attempted in patients who have a history of agranulocytosis or who have experienced an anaphylactoid reaction while on a previous course of AZULFIDINE therapy.

USUAL DOSAGE

AZULFIDINE Tablets and AZULFIDINE EN-tabs
Initial therapy: ADULTS: 3-4 g daily in evenly divided doses. In some cases it is advisable to initiate therapy with a small dosage, e.g. 1-2 g daily, to lessen adverse gastrointestinal effects. If daily doses exceeding 4 g are required to achieve desired effects, the increased risk of toxicity should be kept in mind. CHILDREN TWO YEARS OF AGE AND OLDER: 40-60 mg per Kg body weight in each 24-hour period, divided into 3-6 doses.
Maintenance therapy: ADULTS: 2 g daily. CHILDREN TWO YEARS OF AGE AND OLDER: 30 mg per Kg body weight in each 24-hour period, divided into 4 doses.
AZULFIDINE Oral Suspension
[Each 5 ml (one teaspoonful) contains 250 mg of sulfasalazine.]
Initial Therapy:
Adults: 3-4 g daily in evenly divided doses. In some cases it is advisable to initiate therapy with a smaller dosage, e.g. 1-2 g daily, to lessen adverse gastrointestinal effects. If daily doses up to 4 g are required to achieve desired effects, the increased risk of toxicity should be kept in mind.
Children two years of age and older: 40-60 mg per Kg body weight in each 24-hour period, divided into 3-6 doses.
Maintenance Therapy:
Adults: 2 g daily.
Children two years of age and older: 30 mg per kg body weight in each 24-hour period, divided into 4 doses.
Response to therapy and adjustment of dosage should be determined by periodic examination. It is often necessary to continue medication, even when clinical symptoms, including diarrhea, have been controlled. When endoscopic examination confirms satisfactory improvement, dosage is reduced to a maintenance level. If symptoms of gastric intolerance (anorexia, nausea, vomiting, etc.) occur after the first few doses of AZULFIDINE, they are probably due to mucosal irritation and may be alleviated by distributing the total daily dose more evenly over the day or by giving enteric-coated EN-tabs. If diarrhea recurs, dosage should be increased to previous effective levels. If such symptoms occur after the first few days of treatment with AZULFIDINE, they are probably due to increased serum levels of total sulfapyridine, and may be alleviated by halving the dose and subsequently increasing it gradually over several days. If symptoms continue, the drug should be stopped for 5–7 days, then reinstituted at a lower daily dose.

HOW SUPPLIED

AZULFIDINE Tablets are round, gold-colored, scored tablets, monogrammed "101" in the following package sizes:
AZULFIDINE Tablets 500 mg 100's — NDC No. 0016-0101-01
AZULFIDINE Tablets 500 mg 500's — NDC No. 0016-0101-05
AZULFIDINE Unit Dose Tablets
500 mg 100's — NDC No. 0016-0101-11
AZULFIDINE Unit Dose Tablets
500 mg 10 × 100's— NDC No. 0016-0101-10
AZULFIDINE EN-tabs are eliptical, gold colored, film enteric coated tablets, monogrammed "102" in the following package sizes.
AZULFIDINE EN-tabs 500 mg 100's — NDC No. 0016-0102-01
AZULFIDINE EN-tabs 500 mg 500's — NDC No. 0016-0102-05
Storage: Room temperature (15–30°C/59–86°F).
AZULFIDINE Oral Suspension is an orange-yellow, flavored suspension in the following package size.
AZULFIDINE Oral Suspension 250 mg/5 ml — 1 Pint (473 ml) — NDC No. 0016-0103-06
Storage: Room temperature (15–30°C/59–86°F)
Avoid Freezing.
Shake Well Before Use

References:

1. Mogadam M, et al: Pregnancy in inflammatory bowel disease: Effect of sulfasalazine and corticosteroids on fetal outcome *Gastroenterol* 80:72–76, 1981.
2. Kaufman D W (ed): *Birth Defects and Drugs in Pregnancy.* Littleton, MA, Publishing Sciences Group, Inc. 1977, pp 296–313.
3. Jarnerot G: Fertility, sterility and pregnancy in chronic inflammatory bowel disease. *Scand J Gastroenterol* 17:1–4, 1982.
4. Korelitz BI, et al: *Gastroenterol* 82:1104, 1982.
5. Holdsworth C G: *Brit Med J* 282:110, 1981.
6. Taffet S L, Das K M: *Amer J Med* 73:520–524, 1982.

CAUTION

Federal law prohibits dispensing without prescription.
Pharmacia Laboratories,
Pharmacia Inc.
800 Centennial Avenue
Piscataway, New Jersey 08854

Shown in Product Identification Section, page 422

HYSKON® Hysteroscopy Fluid ℞

[his'kon]
32% (W/V) dextran-70 in dextrose

DESCRIPTION

HYSKON Hysteroscopy Fluid is a clear, viscid, sterile, nonpyrogenic solution of dextran-70 (32% W/V) in dextrose (10% W/V). Dextran-70 is that fraction of dextran, a branched polysaccharide composed of glucose units, having a weight average molecular weight of 70,000. The fluid is electrolyte-free and non-conductive. At room temperature HYSKON Hysteroscopy Fluid has a viscosity of 220 cS.
HYSKON has a tendency to crystalize when subjected to temperature variations or when stored for long periods. If flakes of dextran are present, heat at 100°–110° C until complete dissolution is achieved.

INDICATIONS

HYSKON Hysteroscopy Fluid is indicated for use with the hysteroscope as an aid in distending the uterine cavity and in irrigating and visualizing its surfaces.

CONTRAINDICATIONS

HYSKON Hysteroscopy Fluid should not be instilled in patients known to be hypersensitive to dextran. All other contraindications are those related to the hysteroscopic procedure itself, such as pregnancy, endometrial carcinoma, etc.

WARNINGS

It is possible that during hysteroscopy dextran may leak into the peritoneal cavity, the precise amount depending on the volume of HYSKON® used and the infusion pressure. Slow absorption from the peritoneal cavity (peak blood levels are reached in 3–4 days) (1) may result in systemic effects varying from simple plasma volume expansion or a transient prolongation of the bleeding time, to severe, fatal anaphylactic reactions. It is also reported that dextran may enter the pleural cavity through a pathway that has yet to be defined (2). When HYSKON® is employed during diagnostic hysteroscopy adverse effects are rare. In hysteroscopic surgery greater volumes of HYSKON® are infused over a longer period of time and the exposed blood vessels of the freshly traumatized endometrium allow the dextran direct access to the systemic circulation.
There is, therefore, the potential for these patients to rapidly develop adverse systemic effects, in particular pulmonary edema (3). Patients are considered at increased risk of developing pulmonary edema if:

1. They undergo a surgical procedure lasting more than 45 minutes when HYSKON® is being used to distend the uterus.
2. Greater than 500 ml of HYSKON® are infused.
3. Large areas of endometrium are traumatized during surgery.

ADVERSE REACTIONS

The following adverse reactions, although rare, have been reported for HYSKON®: fatal anaphylactic reaction, generalized itching, macular rash, urticaria, nasal congestion, flushing, hypotension, dyspnea, tightness of chest, cyanosis, wheezing, coughing, peripheral edema, pulmonary edema, pleural effusion, ascites, nausea, vomiting, fever, joint pains, oliguria, convulsions and increased clotting time.

DOSAGE AND ADMINISTRATION

The amount of HYSKON Hysteroscopy Fluid required depends on a number of factors, including the type and length of the procedure and whether manipulation or surgery is performed. Usually, the amount of HYSKON instilled into the uterus will be between 50 ml and 100 ml.
HYSKON should be introduced into the uterine cavity through the cannula of a hysteroscope under low pressure (approximately 100 mm Hg) until the uterus is sufficiently distended to permit adequate visualization. During the hysteroscopic examination, HYSKON should be infused at a rate that keeps the cavity suitably distended. To avoid injection of the fluid into the tissues of the uterus and parametria and to prevent unnecessary amounts of the fluid leaking into the peritoneal cavity and backwards along the side of the hysteroscope, infusion pressures should not exceed 150 mm Hg.

HOW SUPPLIED

HYSKON Hysteroscopy Fluid (32% W/V dextran-70 in 10% W/V dextrose) is available as a sterile, nonpyrogenic solution in 100 ml bottles packed 12 to a carton.
(NDC No. 0016-0231-61.)

Continued on next page

Pharmacia—Cont.

and 250 ml bottles packed 6 to a carton
(NDC No. 0016-0231-62)

Store at 20–25°C (68–77°F). Protect from cold.

CAUTION

Federal law restricts this device to sale by or on the order of a physician.
Revised August 1985

MACRODEX® ℞
[mak 'ro-dex]
(Plasma Volume Expander)

6% Dextran 70 in 5% Dextrose Injection. 500 ml.
6% Dextran 70 in 0.9% Sodium Chloride Injection. 500 ml.

RHEOMACRODEX® ℞
[re "o-mak 'ro-dex]
(low molecular weight dextran)

10% Dextran 40 in 5% Dextrose Injection. 500 ml.
10% Dextran 40 in 0.9% Sodium Chloride Injection. 500 ml.

Pharmacraft Division

PENNWALT CORPORATION
755 JEFFERSON ROAD
ROCHESTER, NY 14623

ALLEREST®
[al 'e-rest]
Tablets, Childrens Chewable Tablets, Headache Strength Tablets, Sinus Pain Formula Tablets, Eye Drops, 12 Hour Capsules and 12 Hour Nasal Spray

(See PDR For Nonprescription Drugs)

CaldeCORT®
[kal 'de-cort]
Hydrocortisone Multi-Purpose Anti-Itch Cream and Spray

(See PDR For Nonprescription Drugs)

CaldeCORT Light™
[kal 'de-cort līt]
Hydrocortisone in a Light Moisturizing Creme with Aloe

(See PDR For Nonprescription Drugs)

CALDESENE®
[kal 'de-sēn]
Medicated Baby Powder and Ointment

(See PDR For Nonprescription Drugs)

CRUEX®
[kru 'ex]
Antifungal Powder, Spray Powder and Cream

(See PDR For Nonprescription Drugs)

DESENEX®
[dess 'i-nex]
Antifungal Powder, Spray Powder, Cream, Ointment, Liquid and Penetrating Foam

(See PDR For Nonprescription Drugs)

SINAREST®
[sīn 'a-rest]
Tablets, Extra Strength Tablets and 12 Hour Nasal Spray

(See PDR For Nonprescription Drugs)

Products are
listed alphabetically
in the
PINK SECTION.

Pharmaderm

a division of Altana Inc.
60 BAYLIS ROAD
MELVILLE, NY 11747

BETAMETHASONE VALERATE ℞
[ba "tah-meth 'ah-sōn vah-ler 'āt]
Cream, USP 0.1%
Ointment, USP 0.1%
Lotion, 0.1%
for dermatologic use only—not for ophthalmic use

DESCRIPTION

Betamethasone Valerate Cream, Ointment, and Lotion contain Betamethasone Valerate U.S.P. (Pregna-1, 4-diene-3, 20-dione, 9-fluoro-11, 21-dihydroxy-16-methyl-17-[(1-oxopentyl) oxy]-,(11β, 16β)-); it has an empirical formula of $C_{27}H_{37}FO_6$ and a molecular weight of 476.58 (CAS Registry Number 2152-44-5).

betamethasone valerate cream

Each gram of the 0.1% cream contains 1.2 mg Betamethasone Valerate (equivalent to 1.0 mg Betamethasone) in a soft, white, hydrophilic cream of Water, Mineral Oil, White Petrolatum, Polyethylene Glycol 1000 Monocetyl Ether, Cetostearyl Alcohol, Monobasic Sodium Phosphate and Phosphoric Acid or Sodium Hydroxide; Chlorocresol is present as a preservative. Betamethasone Valerate Cream contains no parabens.

betamethasone valerate ointment

Each gram of the 0.1% ointment contains 1.2 mg Betamethasone Valerate (equivalent to 1.0 mg Betamethasone) in an ointment base of White Petrolatum and Mineral Oil. Betamethasone Valerate Ointment contains no parabens.

betamethasone valerate lotion

Each gram of the 0.1% lotion contains 1.2 mg Betamethasone Valerate (equivalent to 1.0 mg Betamethasone) in a vehicle of Isopropyl Alcohol and Water slightly thickened with Carbomer 934P. Phosphoric Acid or Sodium Hydroxide are used to adjust the pH.

CLINICAL PHARMACOLOGY

Topical corticosteroids share anti-inflammatory, anti-pruritic and vasoconstrictive actions. The mechanism of anti-inflammatory activity of the topical corticosteroids is unclear. Various laboratory methods, including vasoconstrictor assays, are used to compare and predict potencies and/or clinical efficacies of the topical corticosteroids. There is some evidence to suggest that a recognizable correlation exists between vasoconstrictor potency and therapeutic efficacy in man.

Pharmacokinetics: The extent of percutaneous absorption of topical corticosteroids is determined by many factors including the vehicle, the integrity of the epidermal barrier and the use of occlusive dressings. Topical corticosteroids can be absorbed from normal intact skin. Inflammation and/or other disease processes in the skin increase percutaneous absorption. Occlusive dressings substantially increase the percutaneous absorption of topical corticosteroids. Thus, occlusive dressings may be a valuable therapeutic adjunct for treatment of resistant dermatoses (See DOSAGE AND ADMINISTRATION). Once absorbed through the skin, topical corticosteroids are handled through pharmacokinetic pathways similar to systemically administered corticosteroids. Corticosteroids are bound to plasma proteins in varying degrees. Corticosteroids are metabolized primarily in the liver and are then excreted by the kidneys. Some of the topical corticosteroids and their metabolites are also excreted into the bile.

INDICATIONS AND USAGE

Topical corticosteroids are indicated for the relief of the inflammatory and pruritic manifestations of corticosteroid-responsive dermatoses.

CONTRAINDICATIONS

Topical corticosteroids are contraindicated in those patients with a history of hypersensitivity to any of the components of the preparation.

PRECAUTIONS

General: Systemic absorption of topical corticosteroids has produced reversible hypothalamic-pituitary-adrenal (HPA) axis suppression, manifestations of Cushing's syndrome, hyperglycemia, and glucosuria in some patients. Conditions which augment systemic absorption include the application of the more potent steroids, use over large surface areas, prolonged use, and the addition of occlusive dressings. Therefore, patients receiving a large dose of a potent topical steroid applied to a large surface area or under an occlusive dressing should be evaluated periodically for evidence of HPA axis suppression by using the urinary free cortisol and ACTH stimulation tests. If HPA axis suppression is noted, an attempt should be made to withdraw the drug, to reduce the frequency of application, or to substitute a less potent steroid. Recovery of HPA axis function is generally prompt and complete upon discontinuation of the drug. Infrequently, signs and symptoms of steroid withdrawal may occur, requiring supplemental systemic corticosteroids. Children may absorb proportionally larger amounts of topical corticosteroids and thus be more susceptible to systemic toxicity (See PRECAUTIONS-Pediatric use). If irritation develops, topical corticosteroids should be discontinued and appropriate therapy instituted. In the presence of dermatological infections, the use of an appropriate antifungal or antibacterial agent should be instituted. If a favorable response does not occur promptly, the corticosteroid should be discontinued until the infection has been adequately controlled.

Information for the Patient: Patients using topical corticosteroids should receive the following information and instructions:

1. This medication is to be used as directed by the physician. It is for external use only. Avoid contact with the eyes.
2. Patients should be advised not to use this medication for any disorder other than for which it was prescribed.
3. The treated skin area should not be bandaged or otherwise covered or wrapped as to be occlusive unless directed by the physician.
4. Patients should report any signs of local adverse reactions especially under occlusive dressing.
5. Parents of pediatric patients should be advised not to use tight fitting diapers or plastic pants on a child being treated in the diaper area, as these garments may constitute occlusive dressings.

Laboratory Tests: The following tests may be helpful in evaluating the HPA axis suppression: Urinary free cortisol test; ACTH stimulation test.

Carcinogenesis, Mutagenesis, and Impairment of Fertility: Long-term animal studies have not been performed to evaluate the carcinogenic potential or the effect on fertility of topical corticosteroids. Studies to determine mutagenicity with prednisolone and hydrocortisone have revealed negative results.

Pregnancy Category C: Corticosteroids are generally teratogenic in laboratory animals when administered systemically at relatively low dosage levels. The more potent corticosteroids have been shown to be teratogenic after dermal application in laboratory animals. There are no adequate and well-controlled studies in pregnant women on teratogenic effects from topically applied corticosteroids. Therefore, topical corticosteroids should be used during pregnancy only if the potential benefit justifies the potential risk to the fetus. Drugs of this class should not be used extensively on pregnant patients, in large amounts or for prolonged periods of time.

Nursing Mothers: It is not known whether topical administration of corticosteroids could result in sufficient systemic absorption to produce detectable quantities in breast milk. Systemically administered corticosteroids are secreted into breast milk in quantities not likely to have a deleterious effect on the infant. Nevertheless, caution should be exercised when topical corticosteroids are administered to a nursing woman.

Pediatric Use: *Pediatric patients may demonstrate greater susceptibility to topical corticosteroid-induced HPA axis suppression and Cushing's syndrome than mature patients because of larger skin surface area to body weight ratio.* Hypothalamic-pituitary-adrenal (HPA) axis suppression, Cushing's syndrome, and intracranial hypertension have been reported in children receiving topical corticosteroids. Manifestations of adrenal suppression in children include linear growth retardation, delayed weight gain, low plasma cortisol levels, and absence of response to ACTH stimulation. Manifestations of intracranial hypertension include bulging fontanelles, headaches, and bilateral papilledema. Administration of topical corticosteroids to children should be limited to the least amount compatible with an effective therapeutic regimen. Chronic corticosteroid therapy may interfere with the growth and development of children.

ADVERSE REACTIONS

The following local adverse reactions are reported infrequently with topical corticosteroids, but may occur more frequently with the use of occlusive dressings. These reactions are listed in an approximate decreasing order of occurrence. burning, itching, irritation, dryness, folliculitis, hypertrichosis, acneiform eruptions, hypopigmentation, perioral dermatitis, allergic contact dermatitis, maceration of the skin, secondary infection, skin atrophy, striae and miliaria.

OVERDOSAGE

Topically applied corticosteroids can be absorbed in sufficient amounts to produce systemic effects. (See PRECAUTIONS).

DOSAGE AND ADMINISTRATION

Topical corticosteroid ointments and creams are generally applied to the affected area as a thin film two or three times daily depending on the severity of the condition. Lotion: Apply a few drops of Betamethasone Valerate Lotion to the affected area two or three times daily depending on the severity of the condition and massage lightly until it disappears. Occlusive dressings may be used for the management of psoriasis or recalcitrant conditions. If an infection develops, the use of occlusive dressings should be discontinued and appropriate antimicrobial therapy instituted.

HOW SUPPLIED

Betamethasone Valerate Cream U.S.P., 0.1% in 15 gram tubes, NDC 0462-0040-15 and 45 gram tubes, NDC 0462-0040-46.
Betamethasone Valerate Ointment U.S.P., 0.1% in 15 gram tubes, NDC 0462-0033-15 and 45 gram tubes, NDC 0462-0033-46.
Betamethasone Valerate Lotion U.S.P., 0.1% in 60 ml bottles, NDC 0462-0041-60. Shake well before using. Store at controlled room temperature 15°-30°C (59°-86°F).

CAUTION

Federal law prohibits dispensing without prescription.

Other ℞ items available from Pharmaderm are:

BETAMETHASONE DIPROPIONATE CREAM USP		
NDC 0462-0055-15	0.05%	15 gm tube
NDC 0462-0055-46		45 gm tube
BETAMETHASONE DIPROPIONATE OINTMENT USP		
NDC 0462-0056-15	0.05%	15 gm tube
NDC 0462-0056-46		45 gm tube
BETAMETHASONE DIPROPIONATE LOTION USP		
NDC 0462-0057-60	0.05%	60 ml bottle
FLUOCINOLONE ACETONIDE CREAM USP		
NDC 0462-0058-15	0.01%	15 gm tube
NDC 0462-0058-60		60 gm tube
NDC 0462-0060-15	0.025%	15 gm tube
NDC 0462-0060-60		60 gm tube
FLUOCINOLONE ACETONIDE OINTMENT USP		
NDC 0462-0064-15	0.025%	15 gm tube
NDC 0462-0064-60		60 gm tube
FLUOCINOLONE ACETONIDE TOPICAL SOLUTION USP		
NDC 0462-0059-60	0.01%	60 ml bottle
GENTAMICIN SULFATE CREAM USP		
NDC 0462-0071-15	0.1%	15 gm tube
GENTAMICIN SULFATE OINTMENT USP		
NDC 0462-0078-15	0.1%	15 gm tube
HYDROCORTISONE CREAM USP		
NDC 0462-0015-29	1%	20 gm tube
NDC 0462-0015-31		1 oz. tube
NDC 0462-0015-04		4 oz. tube
NDC 0462-0015-16		1 lb. jar
HYDROCORTISONE CREAM USP		
NDC 0462-0080-31	2.5%	30 gm tube
HYDROCORTISONE OINTMENT USP		
NDC 0462-0020-31	1%	1 oz. tube
NDC 0462-0020-16		1 lb. jar
NYSTATIN CREAM 100,000 U/g USP		
NDC 0462-0054-15		15 gm tube
NDC 0462-0054-30		30 gm tube
NYSTATIN OINTMENT 100,000 U/g USP		
NDC 0462-0007-15		15 gm tube
NYSTATIN ORAL SUSPENSION 100,000 U/ml USP		
NDC 0462-0037-60		60 ml bottle
NYSTATIN-TRIAMCINOLONE ACETONIDE CREAM		
NDC 0462-0081-15		15 gm tube
NDC 0462-0081-30		30 gm tube
NDC 0462-0081-60		60 gm tube
NYSTATIN-TRIAMCINOLONE ACETONIDE OINTMENT		
NDC 0462-0089-15		15 gm tube
NDC 0462-0089-30		30 gm tube
NDC 0462-0089-60		60 gm tube
NYSTATIN VAGINAL TABLETS USP		
NDC 0462-0031-15		15 tablets
NDC 0462-0031-30		30 tablets
TRIAMCINOLONE ACETONIDE CREAM USP		
NDC 0462-0003-15	0.025%	15 gm tube
NDC 0462-0003-80		80 gm tube
NDC 0462-0003-16		1 lb. jar
NDC 0462-0004-15	0.1%	15 gm tube
NDC 0462-0004-80		80 gm tube
NDC 0462-0004-16		1 lb. jar
NDC 0462-0002-15	0.5%	15 gm tube
TRIAMCINOLONE ACETONIDE OINTMENT USP		
NDC 0462-0005-15	0.025%	15 gm tube
NDC 0462-0005-80		80 gm tube
NDC 0462-0006-15	0.1%	15 gm tube
NDC 0462-0006-80		80 gm tube
TRIPLE SULFA VAGINAL CREAM (With applicator)		
NDC 0462-0018-33		2.75 oz. tube

SEE PDR FOR OPHTHALMOLOGY FOR A COMPLETE LIST OF OUR OPHTHALMIC PRODUCTS.

Pharmafair, Inc.

110 KENNEDY DRIVE
HAUPPAUGE, NY 11788

NDC 24208 INJECTABLES (prefilled syringe)

-503-50 **GENTAFAIR 60 mg** ℞
(Gentamicin Sulfate, USP)
1.5 ml

-503-52 **GENTAFAIR 80 mg.** ℞
(Gentamicin Sulfate, USP)
2 ml

INJECTABLES (vials)

-523-48 **PROCAINAMIDE HCl PRONESTYL** ℞
500 mg/ml
(Procainamide Hydrochloride)
2 ml

-518-49 **PROCAINAMIDE HCl PRONESTYL** ℞
100 mg/ml
(Procainamide Hydrochloride)
10 ml

TOPICALS

-430-53 **BENZOYL PEROXIDE GEL 5%** OTC
1.5 oz. plastic tube

-435-53 **BENZOYL PEROXIDE GEL 10%** OTC
1.5 oz. plastic tube

-515-04 **CORTIFAIR** ℞
(Hydrocortisone Cream 1% USP)
1 ounce tube

-551-67 **ERYTHROMYCIN 2% TOPICAL SOLUTION** ℞
60 ml bottles

-470-89 **GENTAFAIR CREAM** ℞
(Gentamicin Sulfate Cream USP 0.1%)
15 gram tube

-475-89 **GENTAFAIR OINTMENT** ℞
(Gentamicin Sulfate Ointment USP 0.1%)
15 gram tube

-985-62 **TOLNAFTATE 1% CREAM** OTC
½ oz. tube

-506-62 **TOLNAFTATE 1% SOLUTION** OTC
10 ml bottles

-530- **TOPISPORIN** OTC
(Neomycin and Polymyxin B Sulfates and Bacitracin Zinc Ointment)
-02 ½ ounce tube
-04 1 ounce

OTICS

-561-64 **AURAFAIR OTIC SOLUTION** ℞
(Antipyrine and Benzocaine)
15 ml

-615-77 **BOROFAIR OTIC** ℞
(Acetic Acid 2% in a modified Burow's Solution Sterile)
2 fluid oz.

-531-73 **EAR DROPS** OTC
(Carbamide Peroxide 6.5%)
15 ml

-630-04 **OCTICAIR OTIC SOLUTION** ℞
(Neomycin Sulfate and Polymyxin B Sulfate and Hydrocortisone Otic Solution-Sterile)
10 ml

-635-62 **OCTICAIR OTIC SUSPENSION** ℞
(Neomycin Sulfate and Polymyxin B Sulfate and Hydrocortisone Otic Suspension-Sterile)
10 ml

ORAL PREPARATIONS

-960- **NYSTATIN ORAL SUSPENSION, USP** ℞
100,000 units per ml
-67 60 ml (with calibrated dropper)
-60 5 ml (single use)

-965- **ERYTHROMYCIN ETHYLSUCCINATE ORAL SUSPENSION** ℞
200 mg/5 ml
-64 473 ml (pint)
-39 100 ml bottles

-970- **ERYTHROMYCIN ETHYLSUCCINATE ORAL SUSPENSION** ℞
400 mg/5 ml
-64 473 ml (pint)
-39 100 ml bottles

IRRIGATING SOLUTIONS

-605- **BALANCED SALT SOLUTION** ℞
-64 15 ml plastic bottle
-66 30 ml plastic bottle
-46 300 ml glass bottle
-99 500 ml glass bottle

Please see **PDR FOR OPHTHALMOLOGY** for a complete list of our ophthalmic products

Philips Roxane Laboratories

(See ROXANE LABORATORIES)

Poythress Laboratories, Inc.

16 N. 22nd ST.
POST OFFICE BOX 26946
RICHMOND, VA 23261

ANTROCOL® ℞

[an-trō ′cal]
TABLETS, CAPSULES AND ELIXIR

COMPOSITION

Each tablet or capsule contains atropine sulfate, 0.195 mg.; phenobarbital, 16 mg. (Warning: may be habit-forming). Each lcc of elixir contains atropine sulfate 0.039 mg.; phenobarbital 3 mg., (Warning: May be habit-forming) and 20% alcohol (V/V). Citrus flavored-artificially colored.

HOW SUPPLIED

Yellow uncoated tablets embossed with I.D. #9540, green #4 capsules branded WMP and green liquid.
Bottles of 100 tablets ....NDC 0095-0040-01
Bottles of 500 tablets ....NDC 0095-0040-05
Bottles of 100 capsules ....NDC 0095-0041-01
Bottles of 1 fl. oz (30cc) Elixir ....NDC 0095-0042-01
Containing individually wrapped droppers
Calibrated from 0.5 to lcc for Pediatric use.
Bottles of 16 fl. oz. (475cc)
Elixir ....NDC 0095-0042-16

BENSULFOID® LOTION OTC

[ben ′sul-foid]

COMPOSITION

A greaseless, cosmetic lotion containing Bensulfoid, 6% (33% colloidal sulfur) Zinc Oxide, 6%; thymol, 0.5% as active ingredients. Also contains alcohol (V/V) 12%; methyl salicylate, 5%; perfume; cosmetic colors; preservatives, 0.1%.

HOW SUPPLIED

2 oz. bottles .... **NDC** 0095-0130-02

LODRANE™ ℞

[lo ′drāne]
(theophylline anhydrous)
SUSTAINED RELEASE CAPSULES

COMPOSITION

Lodrane 130 and Lodrane 260:
Each capsule contains 130 mg. or 260 mg. of theophylline anhydrous in a sustained release bead formulation.

HOW SUPPLIED

130 mg. green and white capsules
Bottles of 100 ....NDC 0095-0060-01
260 mg. red and white capsules
Bottles of 100 ....NDC 0095-0065-01
Mfg. for Poythress Laboratories, Inc.

Continued on next page

Poythress—Cont.

LODRANE CR® ℞
[*lo 'drane*]
(theophylline anhydrous)
CONTINUOUS RELEASE TABLETS

COMPOSITION
Lodrane CR 100, 200, 300
Each tablet contains 100, 200 or 300mg. of theophylline anhydrous in a continuous release tablet form.

HOW SUPPLIED
100 mg. white round tablet
bottles of 100 0095-0070-01
200 mg. white oval tablet
bottles of 100 0095-0071-01
300 mg. white capsule shaped tablet
bottles of 100 0095-0072-01
Mfg. for Poythress Laboratories, Inc.

MUDRANE® TABLETS ℞
[*mu 'drāne*]

COMPOSITION
Each tablet contains potassium iodide, 195 mg.; aminophylline (anhydrous), 130 mg. (equivalent to 111 mg. anhydrous theophylline); phenobarbital, 8 mg. (Warning: may be habit-forming); ephedrine HCl, 16 mg.

HOW SUPPLIED
Yellow scored tablet with I.D. #9550.
Bottles of 100 .... NDC 0095-0050-01
Bottles of 1000 .... NDC 0095-0050-10

MUDRANE®-2 TABLETS ℞
[*mu 'drāne*]

COMPOSITION
Each tablet contains potassium iodide, 195 mg.; aminophylline (anhydrous) 130 mg. (Equivalent to 111 mg. Anhydrous theophylline)

HOW SUPPLIED
White scored tablets with I. D. #9532.
Bottles of 100 .... NDC 0095-0032-01

MUDRANE® GG TABLETS ℞
[*mu 'drāne*]

COMPOSITIONS
Each tablet contains aminophylline (anhydrous), 130 mg. (Equivalent to 111 mg. Anhydrous theophylline); ephedrine HCl, 16mg.; phenobarbital, 8 mg. (Warning: may be habit-forming); Guaifenesin, 100 mg.

HOW SUPPLIED
Yellow, mottled, GG embossed tablets with I. D. #9551.
Bottles of 100 .... NDC 0095-0051-01
Bottles of 1000 .... NDC 0095-0051-10

MUDRANE® GG-2 TABLETS ℞
[*mu 'drāne*]

COMPOSITION
Each tablet contains aminophylline (anhydrous), 130 mg. (Eqivalent to 111 mg. Anhydrous theophylline); Guaifenesin, 100 mg.

HOW SUPPLIED
Green, mottled, GG embossed tablets with I. D. #9533.
Bottles of 100 .... NDC 0095-0033-01

MUDRANE® GG ELIXIR ℞
[*mu 'drāne*]

COMPOSITION
Each 5 ml teaspoonful contains theophylline, 20 mg.; ephedrine HCl, 4 mg.; phenobarbital 2.5 mg. (Warning: may be habit-forming); Guaifenesin, 26 mg. The theophylline in the Elixir is in solution. (The theophylline in the tablet is supplied by aminophylline for prompt solubility from the rapid-disintegrating, uncoated tablet) Preserved with 0.1% paraben. Contains 20% alcohol.

HOW SUPPLIED
As a red liquid.
Bottles of 16 fl. ozs. (475 cc) .... NDC 0095-0053-16
Bottles of 64 fl. ozs. (1900 cc) .... NDC 0095-0053-64

PANALGESIC® OTC
[*pan 'al-gesic*]
Liniment and Cream

COMPOSITION
(Liniment) Methyl Salicylate, 55%; Camphor 3.1%; Menthol, 1.25%; mineral oil & color, 18.6%; alcohol, 22% by weight, (Cream) methyl salicylate, 35%; menthol, 4%.

HOW SUPPLIED
Green, non-staining, greaseless liniment.
4 fl. oz. bottles .... NDC 0095-0120-04
16 fl. oz. bottles .... NDC 0095-0120-16
64 fl. oz. bottles .... NDC 0095-0120-14
White, non-staining, greaseless cream
4 oz. jars .... NDC 0095-0021-04
(cream mfg. for Poythress)

SOLFOTON® Ⓒ
[*sulfa-tōne*]
TABLETS AND CAPSULES

COMPOSITION
Each tablet or capsule contains phenobarbital, 16 mg. (Warning: may be habit-forming).

HOW SUPPLIED
Uncoated P embossed tablets with I.D. #9523. Brown and yellow #4 capsules branded WmP and I.D. #9525.
Bottles of 100 Tablets .... NDC 0095-0023-01
Bottles of 500 Tablets .... NDC 0095-0023-05
Bottles of 100 Capsules .... NDC 0095-0025-01
Bottles of 500 Capsules .... NDC 0095-0025-05

URO-PHOSPHATE TABLETS ℞
[*urō 'fos-fāt*]
(Methenamine, Sodium biphosphate)

DESCRIPTION
Uro-Phosphate, a urinary antibacterial agent, is a combination of Methenamine (urinary antiseptic) 300 mg. and sodium biphosphate (urinary acidifier) (sodium phosphate, monobasic) 500 mg.

HOW SUPPLIED
White film coated tablets with I.D. #9531 debossed on one side.
Bottles of 100 .... NDC 0095-0031-01
Bottles of 1000 .... NDC 0095-0031-10
Protect from heat, store at room temperature 60°– 75°F.
Manufactured for Poythress Laboratories Inc., Richmond, Virginia 23261

Princeton Pharmaceutical Products

(A Squibb Company)
P. O. BOX 4000
PRINCETON, NJ 08543-4000

UNILOG®
(Tablet and Capsule Identification Code)
NUMERICAL INDEX

Unilog Number — **Product**

207 Corgard (Nadolol Tablets) 40 mg
208 Corgard (Nadolol Tablets) 120 mg
241 Corgard (Nadolol Tablets) 80 mg
246 Corgard (Nadolol Tablets) 160 mg
283 Corzide (Nadolol-Bendroflumethiazide Tablets) 40 mg-5 mg
284 Corzide (Nadolol-Bendroflumethiazide Tablets) 80 mg-5 mg
431 Pronestyl Tablets
(Procainamide Hydrochloride Tablets) 250 mg
434 Pronestyl Tablets
(Procainamide Hydrochloride Tablets) 375 mg
438 Pronestyl Tablets
(Procainamide Hydrochloride Tablets) 500 mg
539 Rautrax N
(Powdered Rauwolfia Serpentina 50 mg and Bendroflumethiazide 4 mg with Potassium Choride 400 mg)
602 Naturetin c̄K
(Bendroflumethiazide 2.5 mg with Potassium Chloride 500 mg)
605 Naturetin-2.5
(Bendroflumethiazide Tablets USP) 2.5 mg
606 Naturetin-5
(Bendroflumethiazide Tablets USP) 5 mg
608 Naturetin c̄K
(Bendroflumethiazide 5 mg with Potassium Chloride 500 mg)
618 Naturetin-10
(Bendroflumethiazide Tablets USP) 10 mg
685 Rautrax
(Powdered Rauwolfia Serpentina 50 mg and Flumethiazide 400 mg with Potassium Chloride 400 mg)
713 Raudixin
(Rauwolfia Serpentina Tablets USP) 50 mg
756 Pronestyl Capsules
(Procainamide Hydrochloride Capsules USP) 375 mg
757 Pronestyl Capsules
(Procainamide Hydrochloride Capsules USP) 500 mg
758 Pronestyl Capsules
(Procainamide Hydrochloride Capsules USP) 250 mg
769 Rauzide Tablets
(50 mg powdered Rauwolfia serpentina with 4 mg bendroflumethiazide)
775 Pronestyl-SR Tablets
(Procainamide Hydrochloride Tablets) 500 mg
776 Raudixin
(Rauwolfia Serpentina Tablets USP) 100 mg
863 Prolixin Tablets
(Fluphenazine Hydrochloride Tablets USP) 1 mg
864 Prolixin Tablets
(Fluphenazine Hydrochloride Tablets USP) 2.5 mg
877 Prolixin Tablets
(Fluphenazine Hydrochloride Tablets USP) 5 mg
956 Prolixin Tablets
(Fluphenazine Hydrochloride Tablets USP) 10 mg

CORGARD® ℞
[*kor 'gard*]
(Nadolol Tablets)

DESCRIPTION
CORGARD (nadolol) is a synthetic nonselective beta-adrenergic receptor blocking agent designated chemically as 1-(*tert* -butylamino) -3- [(5,6,8-tetrahydro-*cis* -6,7-dihydroxy-1-naphthyl)oxy]-2-propanol.
Nadolol is a white crystalline powder. It is freely soluble in ethanol, soluble in hydrochloride acid, slightly soluble in water and in chloroform, and very slightly soluble in sodium hydroxide.
CORGARD (nadolol) is available for oral administration as 40 mg, 80 mg, 120 mg, and 160 mg tablets. Inactive ingredients: cellulose, colorant (FD&C Blue No. 2), corn starch, magnesium stearate, providone (except 40 mg), and other ingredients.

CLINICAL PHARMACOLOGY
CORGARD (nadolol) is a nonselective beta-adrenergic receptor blocking agent. Clinical pharmacology studies have demonstrated beta-blocking activity by showing (1) reduction in heart rate and cardiac output at rest and on exercise, (2) reduction of systolic and diastolic blood pressure at rest and on exercise, (3) inhibition of isoproterenol-induced tachycardia, and (4) reduction of reflex orthostatic tachycardia.
CORGARD (nadolol) specifically competes with beta-adrenergic receptor agonists for available beta receptor sites; it inhibits both the $beta_1$ receptors located chiefly in cardiac muscle and the $beta_2$ receptors located chiefly in the bronchial and vascular musculature, inhibiting the chronotropic, inotropic, and vasodilator responses to beta-adrenergic stimulation proportionately. CORGARD (nadolol) has no intrinsic sympathomimetic activity and, unlike some other beta-adrenergic blocking agents, nadolol has little direct myocardial depressant activity and does not have an anesthetic-like membrane-stabilizing action. Animal and human studies show that CORGARD (nadolol) slows the sinus rate and depresses AV conduction. In dogs, only minimal amounts of nadolol were detected in the brain relative to amounts in blood and other organs and tissues. CORGARD has low lipophilicity as determined by octanol/water partition coefficient, a characteristic of certain beta-blocking agents that has been correlated with the limited extent to which these agents cross the blood-brain barrier, their low concentration in the brain, and low incidence of CNS-related side effects.
In controlled clinical studies, CORGARD (nadolol) at doses of 40 to 320 mg/day has been shown to decrease both standing and supine blood pressure, the effect persisting for approximately 24 hours after dosing.
The mechanism of the antihypertensive effects of beta-adrenergic receptor blocking agents has not been established; however, factors that may be involved include (1) competitive antagonism of catecholamines at peripheral (non-CNS) adrenergic neuron sites (especially cardiac) leading to decreased cardiac output, (2) a central effect leading to reduced tonic-sympathetic nerve outflow to the periphery, and (3)

suppression of renin secretion by blockade of the beta-adrenergic receptors responsible for renin release from the kidneys.

While cardiac output and arterial pressure are reduced by nadolol therapy, renal hemodynamics are stable, with preservation of renal blood flow and glomerular filtration rate.

By blocking catecholamine-induced increases in heart rate, velocity and extent of myocardial contraction, and blood pressure, CORGARD (nadolol) generally reduces the oxygen requirements of the heart at any given level of effort, making it useful for many patients in the long-term management of angina pectoris. On the other hand, nadolol can increase oxygen requirements by increasing left ventricular fiber length and end diastolic pressure, particularly in patients with heart failure.

Although beta-adrenergic receptor blockade is useful in treatment of angina and hypertension, there are also situations in which sympathetic stimulation is vital. For example, in patients with severely damaged hearts, adequate ventricular function may depend on sympathetic drive. Beta-adrenergic blockade may worsen AV block by preventing the necessary facilitating effects of sympathetic activity on conduction. $Beta_2$-adrenergic blockade results in passive bronchial constriction by interfering with endogenous adrenergic bronchodilator activity in patients subject to bronchospasm and may also interfere with exogenous bronchodilators in such patients.

Absorption of nadolol after oral dosing is variable, averaging about 30 percent. Peak serum concentrations of nadolol usually occur in three to four hours after oral administration and the presence of food in the gastrointestinal tract does not affect the rate or extent of nadolol absorption. Approximately 30 percent of the nadolol present in serum is reversibly bound to plasma protein.

Unlike many other beta-adrenergic blocking agents, nadolol is not metabolized and is excreted unchanged, principally by the kidneys.

The half-life of therapeutic doses of nadolol is about 20 to 24 hours, permitting once-daily dosage. Because nadolol is excreted predominantly in the urine, its half-life increases in renal failure (see PRECAUTIONS and DOSAGE AND ADMINISTRATION). Steady-state serum concentrations of nadolol are attained in six to nine days with once-daily dosage in persons with normal renal function. Because of variable absorption and different individual responsiveness, the proper dosage must be determined by titration.

Exacerbation of angina and, in some cases, myocardial infarction and ventricular dysrhythmias have been reported after abrupt discontinuation of therapy with beta-adrenergic blocking agents in patients with coronary artery disease. Abrupt withdrawal of these agents in patients without coronary artery disease has resulted in transient symptoms, including tremulousness, sweating, palpitation, headache, and malaise. Several mechanisms have been proposed to explain these phenomena, among them increased sensitivity to catecholamines because of increased numbers of beta receptors.

INDICATIONS AND USAGE

Angina Pectoris—CORGARD (nadolol) is indicated for the long-term management of patients with angina pectoris.

Hypertension—CORGARD (nadolol) is indicated in the management of hypertension; it may be used alone or in combination with other antihypertensive agents, especially thiazide-type diuretics.

CONTRAINDICATIONS

Nadolol is contraindicated in bronchial asthma, sinus bradycardia and greater than first degree conduction block, cardiogenic shock, and overt cardiac failure (see WARNINGS).

WARNINGS

Cardiac Failure—Sympathetic stimulation may be a vital component supporting circulatory function in patients with congestive heart failure, and its inhibition by beta-blockade may precipitate more severe failure. Although beta-blockers should be avoided in overt congestive heart failure, if necessary, they can be used with caution in patients with a history of failure who are well-compensated, usually with digitalis and diuretics. Beta-adrenergic blocking agents do not abolish the inotropic action of digitalis on heart muscle.

IN PATIENTS WITHOUT A HISTORY OF HEART FAILURE, continued use of beta-blockers can, in some cases, lead to cardiac failure. Therefore, at the first sign or symptom of heart failure, the patient should be digitalized and/or treated with diuretics, and the response observed closely, or nadolol should be discontinued (gradually, if possible).

Exacerbation of Ischemic Heart Disease Following Abrupt Withdrawal—Hypersensitivity to catecholamines has been observed in patients withdrawn from beta-blocker therapy; exacerbation of angina and, in some cases, myocardial infarction have occurred after *abrupt* discontinuation of such therapy. When discontinuing chronically administered nadolol, particularly in patients with ischemic heart disease, the dosage should be gradually reduced over a period of one to two weeks and the patient should be carefully monitored. If angina markedly worsens or acute coronary insufficiency develops, nadolol administration should be reinstituted promptly, at least temporarily, and other measures appropriate for the management of unstable angina should be taken. Patients should be warned against interruption or discontinuation of therapy without the physician's advice. Because coronary artery disease is common and may be unrecognized, it may be prudent not to discontinue nadolol therapy abruptly even in patients treated only for hypertension.

Nonallergic Bronchospasm (e.g., chronic bronchitis, emphysema)—PATIENTS WITH BRONCHOSPASTIC DISEASES SHOULD IN GENERAL NOT RECEIVE BETA-BLOCKERS. Nadolol should be administered with caution since it may block bronchodilation produced by endogenous or exogenous catecholamine stimulation of $beta_2$ receptors.

Major Surgery—Because beta-blockade impairs the ability of the heart to respond to reflex stimuli and may increase the risks of general anesthesia and surgical procedures, resulting in protracted hypotension or low cardiac output, it has generally been suggested that such therapy should be withdrawn several days prior to surgery. Recognition of the increased sensitivity to catecholamines of patients recently withdrawn from beta-blocker therapy, however, has made this recommendation controversial. If possible, beta-blockers should be withdrawn well before surgery takes place. In the event of emergency surgery, the anesthesiologist should be informed that the patient is on beta-blocker therapy. The effects of nadolol can be reversed by administration of beta-receptor agonists such as isoproterenol, dopamine, dobutamine, or levarterenol. Difficulty in restarting and maintaining the heart beat has also been reported with beta-adrenergic receptor blocking agents.

Diabetes and Hypoglycemia—Beta-adrenergic blockade may prevent the appearance of premonitory signs and symptoms (e.g., tachycardia and blood pressure changes) of acute hypoglycemia. This is especially important with labile diabetics. Beta-blockade also reduces the release of insulin in response to hyperglycemia; therefore, it may be necessary to adjust the dose of antidiabetic drugs.

Thyrotoxicosis—Beta-adrenergic blockade may mask certain clinical signs (e.g., tachycardia) of hyperthyroidism. Patients suspected of developing thyrotoxicosis should be managed carefully to avoid abrupt withdrawal of beta-adrenergic blockade which might precipitate a thyroid storm.

PRECAUTIONS

Impaired Hepatic or Renal Function—Nadolol should be used with caution in patients with impaired hepatic or renal function (see DOSAGE AND ADMINISTRATION).

Information for Patients—Patients, especially those with evidence of coronary artery insufficiency, should be warned against interruption or discontinuation of nadolol therapy without the physician's advice. Although cardiac failure rarely occurs in properly selected patients, patients being treated with beta-adrenergic blocking agents should be advised to consult the physician at the first sign or symptom of impending failure.

Drug Interactions — When administered concurrently, the following drugs may interact with beta-adrenergic receptor blocking agents:

Anesthetics, general—exaggeration of the hypotension induced by general anesthetics (see WARNINGS, Major Surgery).

Antidiabetic drugs (oral agents and insulin)—hypoglycemia or hyperglycemia; adjust dosage of antidiabetic drug accordingly (see WARNINGS, Diabetes and Hypoglycemia).

Catecholamine-depleting drugs (e.g., reserpine)—additive effect; monitor closely for evidence of hypotension and/or excessive bradycardia (e.g., vertigo, syncope, postural hypotension).

Carcinogenesis, Mutagenesis, Impairment of Fertility—In chronic oral toxicologic studies (one to two years) in mice, rats, and dogs, nadolol did not produce any significant toxic effects. In two-year oral carcinogenic studies in rats and mice, nadolol did not produce any neoplastic, preneoplastic, or nonneoplastic pathologic lesions. In fertility and general reproductive performance studies in rats, nadolol caused no adverse effects.

Pregnancy Category C—In animal reproduction studies with nadolol, evidence of embryo- and fetotoxicity was found in rabbits, but not in rats or hamsters, at doses 5 to 10 times greater (on a mg/kg basis) than the maximum indicated human dose. No teratogenic potential was observed in any of these species.

There are no adequate and well-controlled studies in pregnant women. Nadolol should be used during pregnancy only if the potential benefit justifies the potential risk to the fetus. Neonates whose mothers are receiving nadolol at parturition have exhibited bradycardia, hypoglycemia, and associated symptoms.

Nursing Mothers—Nadolol is excreted in human milk. Because of the potential for adverse effects in nursing infants, a decision should be made whether to discontinue nursing or to discontinue therapy taking into account the importance of CORGARD to the mother.

Pediatric Use—Safety and effectiveness in children have not been established.

ADVERSE REACTIONS

Most adverse effects have been mild and transient and have rarely required withdrawal of therapy.

Cardiovascular—Bradycardia with heart rates of less than 60 beats per minute occurs commonly, and heart rates below 40 beats per minute and/or symptomatic bradycardia were seen in about 2 of 100 patients. Symptoms of peripheral vascular insufficiency, usually of the Raynaud type, have occurred in approximately 2 of 100 patients. Cardiac failure, hypotension, and rhythm/conduction disturbances have each occurred in about 1 of 100 patients. Single instances of first degree and third degree heart block have been reported; intensification of AV block is a known effect of beta-blockers (see also CONTRAINDICATIONS, WARNINGS, and PRECAUTIONS).

Central Nervous System—Dizziness or fatigue has been reported in approximately 2 of 100 patients; paresthesias, sedation, and change in behavior have each been reported in approximately 6 of 1000 patients.

Respiratory—Bronchospasm has been reported in approximately 1 of 1000 patients (see CONTRAINDICATIONS and WARNINGS).

Gastrointestinal—Nausea, diarrhea, abdominal discomfort, constipation, vomiting, indigestion, anorexia, bloating, and flatulence have been reported in 1 to 5 of 1000 patients.

Miscellaneous—Each of the following has been reported in 1 to 5 of 1000 patients: rash; pruritus; headache; dry mouth, eyes, or skin; impotence or decreased libido; facial swelling; weight gain; slurred speech; cough; nasal stuffiness; sweating; tinnitus; blurred vision. Reversible alopecia has been reported infrequently.

The following adverse reactions have been reported in patients taking nadolol and/or other beta-adrenergic blocking agents, but no causal relationship to nadolol has been established.

Central Nervous System—Reversible mental depression progressing to catatonia; visual disturbances; hallucinations; an acute reversible syndrome characterized by disorientation for time and place, short-term memory loss, emotional lability with slightly clouded sensorium, and decreased performance on neuropsychometrics.

Gastrointestinal—Mesenteric arterial thrombosis; ischemic colitis; elevated liver enzymes.

Hematologic—Agranulocytosis; thrombocytopenic or nonthrombocytopenic purpura.

Allergic—Fever combined with aching and sore throat; laryngospasm; respiratory distress.

Miscellaneous—Pemphigoid rash; hypertensive reaction in patients with pheochromocytoma; sleep disturbances; Peyronie's disease.

The oculomucocutaneous syndrome associated with the beta-blocker practolol has not been reported with nadolol.

OVERDOSAGE

Nadolol can be removed from the general circulation by hemodialysis.

In addition to gastric lavage, the following measures should be employed, as appropriate. In determining the duration of corrective therapy, note must be taken of the long duration of the effect of nadolol.

Excessive Bradycardia—Administer atropine (0.25 to 1.0 mg). If there is no response to vagal blockade, administer isoproterenol cautiously.

Cardiac Failure—Administer a digitalis glycoside and diuretic. It has been reported that glucagon may also be useful in this situation.

Hypotension—Administer vasopressors, e.g., epinephrine or levarterenol. (There is evidence that epinephrine may be the drug of choice.)

Bronchospasm—Administer a $beta_2$-stimulating agent and/or a theophylline derivative.

DOSAGE AND ADMINISTRATION

DOSAGE MUST BE INDIVIDUALIZED. CORGARD (NADOLOL) MAY BE ADMINISTERED WITHOUT REGARD TO MEALS.

Angina Pectoris—The usual initial dose is 40 mg CORGARD (nadolol) once daily. Dosage should be gradually increased in 40 to 80 mg increments at 3- to 7-day intervals until optimum clinical response is obtained or there is pronounced slowing of the heart rate. The usual maintenance dose range is 40 or 80 mg administered once daily. Doses up to 160 or 240 mg administered once daily may be needed.

The usefulness and safety in angina pectoris of dosage exceeding 240 mg per day have not been established. If treatment is to be discontinued, reduce the dosage gradually over a period of one to two weeks (see WARNINGS).

Hypertension—The usual initial dose is 40 mg CORGARD (nadolol) once daily, whether it is used alone or in addition to diuretic therapy. Dosage may be gradually increased in 40 to

Continued on next page

Princeton—Cont.

80 mg increments until optimum blood pressure reduction is achieved. The usual maintenance dose is 40 or 80 mg administered once daily. Doses up to 240 or 320 mg administered once daily may be needed.

Dosage Adjustment in Renal Failure—Absorbed nadolol is excreted principally by the kidneys and, although nonrenal elimination does occur, dosage adjustments are necessary in patients with renal impairment. The following dose intervals are recommended:

Creatinine Clearance (mL/min/1.73m^2)	Dosage Interval (hours)
>50	24
31–50	24–36
10–30	24–48
<10	40–60

HOW SUPPLIED

CORGARD Tablets (Nadolol Tablets) are supplied as scored tablets containing 40, 80, 120, or 160 mg nadolol per tablet in bottles of 100 and in Unimatic® unit-dose packs of 100 tablets. The 40 mg, 80 mg and 120 mg tablets are also available in bottles of 1000. [Military Depot Item: 40 mg, 100's, NSN 6505-01-113-8345; 40 mg, 1000's, NSN 6505-01-114-9384; 80 mg 100's, NSN 6505-01-114-3090; 80 mg, 1000's, NSN 6505-01-110-1994; 120 mg, 1000's, NSN 6505-01-110-1995.]

Storage: Store at room temperature; avoid excessive heat. Protect from light. Keep bottle tightly closed. Dispense in tight, light-resistant containers.

(J3-527E)

Shown in Product Identification Section, page 422

CORZIDE® 40/5 ℞
CORZIDE® 80/5

[kor'zīd]

Nadolol and Bendroflumethiazide Tablets

DESCRIPTION

CORZIDE (Nadolol and Bendroflumethiazide Tablets) for oral administration combines two antihypertensive agents: CORGARD® (nadolol), a nonselective beta-adrenergic blocking agent, and NATURETIN® (bendroflumethiazide), a thiazide diuretic-antihypertensive. Formulations: 40 mg and 80 mg nadolol per tablet combined with 5 mg bendroflumethiazide. Inactive ingredients: cellulose, colorant (FD&C Blue No. 2), lactose, magnesium stearate, povidone, sodium starch glycolate, and starch.

Nadolol—Nadolol is a white crystalline powder. It is freely soluble in ethanol, soluble in hydrochloric acid, slightly soluble in water and in chloroform, and very slightly soluble in sodium hydroxide.

Nadolol is designated chemically as 1-(*tert*-butylamino) -3-[5,6,7,8,-tetrahydro-*cis* -6,7,-dihydroxy-1-naphthyl)oxy]-2-propanol.

Bendroflumethiazide—Bendroflumethiazide is a white crystalline powder. It is soluble in alcohol and in sodium hydroxide, and insoluble in hydrochloric acid, water, and chloroform.

Bendroflumethiazide is designated chemically as 3-benzyl-3,4,-dihydro-6-(trifluoromethyl)-2*H*-1,2,4- benzothiadiazine-7-sulfonamide 1,1-dioxide.

CLINICAL PHARMACOLOGY

Nadolol—Nadolol is a nonselective beta-adrenergic receptor blocking agent. Clinical pharmacology studies have demonstrated beta-blocking activity by showing (1) reduction in heart rate and cardiac output at rest and on exercise, (2) reduction of systolic and diastolic blood pressure at rest and on exercise, (3) inhibition of isoproterenol-induced tachycardia, and (4) reduction of reflex orthostatic tachycardia.

Nadolol specifically competes with beta-adrenergic receptor agonists for available beta receptor sites; it inhibits both the beta$_1$ receptors located chiefly in cardiac muscle and the beta$_2$ receptors located chiefly in the bronchial and vascular musculature, inhibiting the chronotropic, inotropic, and vasodilator responses to beta-adrenergic stimulation proportionately. Nadolol has no intrinsic sympathomimetic activity and, unlike some other beta-adrenergic blocking agents, nadolol has little direct myocardial depressant activity and does not have an anesthetic-like membrane-stabilizing action. Animal and human studies show that nadolol slows the sinus rate and depresses AV conduction. In dogs, only minimal amounts of nadolol were detected in the brain relative to amounts in blood and other organs and tissues. Nadolol has low lipophilicity as determined by octanol/water partition coefficient, a characteristic of certain beta-blocking agents that has been correlated with the limited extent to which these agents cross the blood-brain barrier, their low concentration in the brain, and low incidence of CNS-related side effects.

In controlled clinical studies, nadolol at doses of 40 to 320 mg/day has been shown to decrease both standing and supine blood pressure, the effect persisting for approximately 24 hours after dosing.

The mechanism of the antihypertensive effects of beta-adrenergic receptor blocking agents has not been established; however, factors that may be involved include (1) competitive antagonism of catecholamines at peripheral (non-CNS) adrenergic neuron sites (especially cardiac) leading to decreased cardiac output, (2) a central effect leading to reduced tonic-sympathetic nerve outflow to the periphery, and (3) suppression of renin secretion by blockade of the beta-adrenergic receptors responsible for renin release from the kidneys.

While cardiac output and arterial pressure are reduced by nadolol therapy, renal hemodynamics are stable, with preservation of renal blood flow and glomerular filtration rate.

By blocking catecholamine-induced increases in heart rate, velocity and extent of myocardial contraction, and blood pressure, nadolol generally reduces the oxygen requirements of the heart at any given level of effort, making it useful for many patients in the long-term management of angina pectoris. On the other hand, nadolol can increase oxygen requirements by increasing left ventricular fiber length and end diastolic pressure, particularly in patients with heart failure.

Although beta-adrenergic receptor blockade is useful in treatment of angina and hypertension, there are also situations in which sympathetic stimulation is vital. For example, in patients with severely damaged hearts, adequate ventricular function may depend on sympathetic drive. Beta-adrenergic blockade may worsen AV block by preventing the necessary facilitating effects of sympathetic activity on conduction. Beta$_2$-adrenergic blockade results in passive bronchial constriction by interfering with endogenous adrenergic bronchodilator activity in patients subject to bronchospasm and may also interfere with exogenous bronchodilators in such patients.

Absorption of nadolol after oral dosing is variable, averaging about 30 percent. Peak serum concentrations of nadolol usually occur in three to four hours after oral administration and the presence of food in the gastrointestinal tract does not affect the rate or extent of nadolol absorption. Approximately 30 percent of the nadolol present in serum is reversibly bound to plasma protein.

Unlike may other beta-adrenergic blocking agents, nadolol is not metabolized by the liver and is excreted unchanged, principally by the kidneys.

The half-life of therapeutic doses of nadolol is about 20 to 24 hours, permitting once-daily dosage. Because nadolol is excreted predominantly in the urine, its half-life increases in renal failure (see PRECAUTIONS, *General,* and DOSAGE AND ADMINISTRATION). Steady state serum concentrations of nadolol are attained in six to nine days with once-daily dosage in persons with normal renal function. Because of variable absorption and different individual responsiveness, the proper dosage must be determined by titration.

Exacerbation of angina and, in some cases, myocardial infarction and ventricular dysrhythmias have been reported after abrupt discontinuation of therapy with beta-adrenergic blocking agents in patients with coronary artery disease. Abrupt withdrawal of these agents in patients without coronary artery disease has resulted in transient symptoms, including tremulousness, sweating, palpitation, headache, and malaise. Several mechamisms have been proposed to explain these phenomena, among them increased sensitivity to catecholamines because of increased numbers of beta receptors.

Bendroflumethiazide—The mechanism of action of bendroflumethiazide results in an interference with the renal tubular mechanism of electrolyte reabsorption. At maximal therapeutic dosage all thiazides are approximately equal in their diuretic potency. The mechamism whereby thiazides function in the control of hypertension is unknown.

INDICATIONS

CORZIDE (Nadolol and Bendroflumethiazide Tablets) is indicated in the management of hypertension.

This fixed combination drug is not indicated for initial therapy of hypertension. If the fixed combination represents the dose titrated to the individual patient's needs, it may be more convenient than the separate components.

CONTRAINDICATIONS

Nadolol—Nadolol is contraindicated in bronchial asthma, sinus bradycardia and greater than first degree conduction block, cardiogenic shock, and overt cardiac failure (see WARNINGS).

Bendroflumethiazide—Bendroflumethiazide is contraindicated in anuria. It is also contraindicated in patients who have previously demonstrated hypersensitivity to bendroflumethiazide or other sulfonamide-derived drugs.

WARNINGS

Nadolol—Cardiac Failure—Sympathetic stimulation may be a vital component supporting circulatory function in patients with congestive heart failure, and its inhibition by beta-blockade may precipitate more severe failure. Although beta-blockers should be avoided in overt congestive heart failure, if necessary, they can be used with caution in patients with a history of failure who are well compensated, usually with digitalis and diuretics. Beta-adrenergic blocking agents do not abolish the inotropic action of digitalis on heart muscle.

IN PATIENTS WITHOUT A HISTORY OF HEART FAILURE, continued use of beta-blockers can, in some cases, lead to cardiac failure. Therefore, at the first sign or symptom of heart failure, the patient should be digitalized and/or treated with diuretics, and the response observed closely, or nadolol should be discontinued (gradually, if possible).

> **Exacerbation of Ischemic Heart Disease Following Abrupt Withdrawal**—Hypersensitivity to catecholamines has been observed in patients withdrawn from beta-blocker therapy; exacerbation of angina and, in some cases, myocardial infarction have occurred after *abrupt* discontinuation of such therapy. When discontinuing chronically administered nadolol, particularly in patients with ischemic heart disease, the dosage should be gradually reduced over a period of one to two weeks and the patient should be carefully monitored. If angina markedly worsens or acute coronary insufficiency develops, nadolol administration should be reinstituted promptly, at least temporarily, and other measures appropriate for the management of unstable angina should be taken. Patients should be warned against interruption or discontinuation of therapy without the physician's advice. Because coronary artery disease is common and may be unrecognized, it may be prudent not to discontinue nadolol therapy abruptly even in patients treated only for hypertension.

Nonallergic Bronchospasm (e.g., chronic bronchitis, emphysema)—PATIENTS WITH BRONCHOSPASTIC DISEASES SHOULD IN GENERAL NOT RECEIVE BETA-BLOCKERS. Nadolol should be administered with caution since it may block bronchodilation produced by endogenous or exogenous catecholamine stimulation of beta$_2$ receptors.

Major Surgery—Because beta blockade impairs the ability of the heart to respond to reflex stimuli and may increase the risks of general anesthesia and surgical procedures, resulting in protracted hypotension or low cardiac output, it has generally been suggested that such therapy should be withdrawn several days prior to surgery. Recognition of the increased sensitivity to catecholamines of patients recently withdrawn from beta-blocker therapy, however, has made this recommendation controversial. If possible, beta-blockers should be withdrawn well before surgery takes place. In the event of emergency surgery, the anesthesiologist should be informed that the patient is on beta-blocker therapy. The effects of nadolol can be reversed by administration of beta-receptor agonists such as isoproterenol, dopamine, dobutamine, or levarterenol. Difficulty in restarting and maintaining the heart beat has also been reported with beta-adrenergic receptor blocking agents.

Diabetes and Hypoglycemia—Beta-adrenergic blockade may prevent the appearance of premonitory signs and syptoms (e.g., tachycardia and blood pressure changes) of acute hypoglycemia. This is especially important with labile diabetics. Beta-blockade also reduces the release of insulin in response to hyperglycemia; therefore, it may be necessary to adjust the dose of antidiabetic drugs.

Thyrotoxicosis—Beta-adrenergic blockage may mask certain clinical signs (e.g., tachycardia) of hyperthyroidism. Patients suspected of developing thyrotoxicosis should be managed carefully to avoid abrupt withdrawal of beta-adrenergic blockade which might precipitate a thyroid storm.

Bendroflumethiazide—Thiazides should be used with caution in severe renal disease. In patients with renal disease, thiazides may precipitate azotemia. Cumulative effects of the drug may develop in patients with impaired renal function.

Thiazides should be used with caution in patients with impaired hepatic function or progressive liver disease, since minor alterations of fluid and electrolyte balance may precipitate hepatic coma.

Sensitivity reactions may occur in patients with a history of allergy or bronchial asthma.

The possibility of exacerbation or activation of systemic lupus erythematosus has been reported.

PRECAUTIONS

General—Nadolol—Nadolol should be used with caution in patients with impaired renal function (see DOSAGE AND ADMINISTRATION).

Bendroflumethiazide—All patients receiving thiazide therapy should be observed for clinical signs or fluid or electrolyte imbalance, namely, hyponatremia, hypochloremic alkalosis, and hypokalemia. Serum and urine electrolyte determinations are particularly important when the patient is vomiting excessively or receiving parenteral fluids. Medication such as digitalis may also influence serum electrolytes. Warning signs, irrespective of cause, are: dryness of the mouth, thirst, weakness, lethargy, drowsiness, restlessess, muscle pains or cramps, muscular fatigue, hypotension, oliguria, tachycardia, and gastrointestinal disturbances, such as nausea and vomiting.

Hypokalemia may develop with thiazides as with any other potent diuretic, especially with brisk diuresis, when severe cirrhosis is present.

Interference with adequate oral electrolyte intake will also contribute to hypokalemia. Hypokalemia can sensitize or exaggerate the response of the heart to the toxic effects of digitalis (e.g., increased ventricular irritability). Hypokalemia may be avoided or treated by use of potassium supplements such as foods with a high potassium content.

Any chloride deficit is generally mild and usually does not require specific treatment except under extraordinary circumstances (as in liver disease or renal disease). Dilutional hyponatremia may occur in edematous patients in hot weather; appropriate therapy is water restriction, rather than administration of salt except in rare instances when the hyponatremia is life threatening. In actual salt depletion, appropriate replacement is the therapy of choice.

Hyperuricemia may occur or frank gout may be precipitated in certain patients receiving thiazide therapy.

Latent diabetes mellitus may become manifest during thiazide administration.

The antihypertensive effects of the drug may be enhanced in the post-sympathectomy patient.

If progressive renal impairment becomes evident, as indicated by rising nonprotein nitrogen or blood urea nitrogen, a careful reappraisal of therapy is necessary with consideration given to withholding or discontinuing diuretic therapy.

Thiazides may decrease serum PBI levels without signs of thyroid disturbances.

Calcium excretion is decreased by thiazides. Pathologic changes in the parathyroid gland with hypercalcemia and hypophosphatemia have been observed in a few patients on prolonged thiazide therapy. The common complications of hyperparathyroidism have not been seen.

Information for Patients—Patients, especially those with evidence of coronary artery insufficiency, should be warned against interruption or discontinuation of therapy without the physician's advice. Although cardiac failure rarely occurs in properly selected patients, patients being treated with beta-adrenergic blocking agents should be advised to consult the physician at the first sign or symptom of impending failure.

The patient should also be advised of a proper course in the event of an inadvertently missed dose.

Laboratory Tests—Serum and urine electrolyte levels should be regularly monitored (see WARNINGS, *Bendroflumethiazide,* also PRECAUTIONS, *General, Bendroflumethiazide*).

Drug Interactions—Nadolol—When administered concurrently the following drugs may interact with beta-adrenergic receptor blocking agents:

Anesthetics, general—exaggeration of the hypotension induced by general anesthetics (see WARNINGS, *Nadolol, Major Surgery*).

Antidiabetic drugs (oral agents and insulin)— hypoglycemia or hyperglycemia; adjust dosage of antidiabetic drug accordingly (see WARNINGS, *Nadolol, Diabetes and Hypoglycemia*).

Catecholamine-depleting drugs (e.g., reserpine) —additive effect; monitor closely for evidence of hypotension and/or excessive bradycardia (e.g., vertigo, syncope, postural hypotension).

Bendroflumethiazide—When administered concurrently the following drugs may interact with thiazide diuretics:

Alcohol, barbiturates, or narcotics—potentiation of orthostatic hypotension may occur.

Antidiabetic drugs (oral agents and insulin)— hyperglycemia induced by thiazide may require dosage adjustment of antidiabetic drug.

Other antihypertensive drugs—additive effect or potentiation of other antihypertensive drugs.

Corticosteroids, ACTH—intensified electrolyte depletion, particularly hypokalemia.

Ganglionic or peripheral adrenergic blocking drugs—potentiated effect of ganglionic or peripheral adrenergic blocking drugs.

Preanesthetic and anesthetic agents—effects of preanesthetic and anesthetic agents may be potentiated; adjust dosage of these agents accordingly.

Pressor amines (e.g., norepinephrine)—possible decreased response to pressor amines but not sufficient to preclude their use.

Skeletal muscle relaxants, nondepolarizing (e.g., tubocurarine)—possible increased responsiveness to the muscle relaxant.

Drug/Laboratory Test Interactions—Thiazides should be discontinued before carrying out tests for parathyroid function (see PRECAUTIONS, *General, Bendroflumethiazide*).

Carcinogenesis, Mutagenesis, Impairment of Fertility—

Nadolol—In chronic oral toxicologic studies (one to two years) in mice, rats, and dogs, nadolol did not produce any significant toxic effects. In two-year oral carcinogenicity studies in rats and mice, nadolol did not produce any neoplastic, preneoplastic, or nonneoplastic pathologic lesions. In fertility and general reproductive performance studies in rats, nadolol caused no adverse effect.

Bendroflumethiazide—Long-term studies in animals have not been performed to evaluate carcinogenic potential, mutagenesis, or whether this drug affects fertility in males or females.

Pregnancy—Teratogenic Effects—Nadolol—Category C. In animal reproduction studies with nadolol, evidence of embryo- and fetotoxicity was found in rabbits, but not in rats or hamsters, at doses 5 to 10 times greater (on a mg/kg basis) than the maximum indicated human dose. No teratogenic potential was observed in any of these species.

There are no adequate and well-controlled studies in pregnant women. Nadolol should be used during pregnancy only if the potential benefit justifies the potential risk to the fetus. Neonates whose mothers are receiving nadolol at parturition have exhibited bradycardia, hypoglycemia, and associated symptoms.

Bendroflumethiazide—Category C. Animal reproduction studies have not been conducted with bendroflumethiazide. It is also not known whether this drug can cause fetal harm when administered to a pregnant woman or can affect reproduction capacity. Bendroflumethiazide should be given to a pregnant woman only if clearly needed.

Pregnancy—Nonteratogenic Effects—Thiazides cross the placental barrier and appear in cord blood. The use of thiazides in pregnant women requires that the anticipated benefit be weighed against possible hazards to the fetus. These hazards include fetal or neonatal jaundice, thrombocytopenia, and possibly other adverse reactions which have occurred in the adult.

Nursing Mothers—Both nadolol and bendroflumethiazide are excreted in human milk. Because of the potential for serious adverse reactions in nursing infants from both drugs, a decision should be made whether to discontinue nursing or to discontinue therapy taking into account the importance of CORZIDE (Nadolol and Bendroflumethiazide Tablets) to the mother.

Pediatric Use—Safety and effectiveness in children have not been established.

ADVERSE REACTIONS

Nadolol—Most adverse effects have been mild and transient and have rarely required withdrawal of therapy.

Cardiovascular—Bradycardia with heart rates of less than 60 beats per minute occurs commonly, and heart rates below 40 beats per minute and/or symptomatic bradycardia were seen in about 2 of 100 patients. Symptoms of peripheral vascular insufficiency, usually of the Raynaud type, have occurred in approximately 2 of 100 patients. Cardiac failure, hypotension, and rhythm/conduction disturbances have each occurred in about 1 of 100 patients. Single instances of first degree and third degree heart block have been reported; intensification of AV block is a known effect of beta-blockers (see also CONTRAINDICATIONS, WARNINGS, and PRECAUTIONS).

Central Nervous System—Dizziness or fatigue has been reported in approximately 2 of 100 patients; paresthesias, sedation, and change in behavior have each been reported in approximately 6 of 1000 patients.

Respiratory—Bronchospasm has been reported in approximately 1 of 1000 patients (see CONTRAINDICATIONS and WARNINGS).

Gastrointestinal—Nausea, diarrhea, abdominal discomfort, constipation, vomiting, indigestion, anorexia, bloating, and flatulence have been reported in 1 to 5 of 1000 patients.

Miscellaneous—Each of the following has been reported in 1 to 5 of 1000 patients: rash; pruritus; headache; dry mouth, eyes, or skin; impotence or decreased libido; facial swelling; weight gain; slurred speech; cough; nasal stuffiness; sweating; tinnitus; blurred vision. Reversible alopecia has been reported infrequently.

The following adverse reactions have been reported in patients taking nadolol and/or other beta-adrenergic blocking agents, but no causal relationship to nadolol has been established.

Central Nervous System—Reversible mental depression progressing to catatonia; visual disturbances; hallucinations; an acute reversible syndrome characterized by disorientation for time and place, short-term memory loss, emotional liability with slightly clouded sensorium, and decreased performance on neuropsychometrics.

Gastrointestinal—Mesenteric arterial thrombosis; ischemic colitis; elevated liver enzymes.

Hematologic—Agranulocytosis; thrombocytopenic or nonthrombocytopenic purpura.

Allergic—Fever combined with aching and sore throat; laryngospasm; respiratory distress.

Miscellaneous—Pemphigoid rash; hypertensive reaction in patients with pheochromocytoma; sleep disturbances; Peyronie's disease.

The oculomucocutaneous syndrome associated with the beta-blocker practolol has not been reported with nadolol.

Bendroflumethiazide — Gastrointestinal System —anorexia, gastric irritation, nausea, vomiting, cramping, diarrhea, constipation, jaundice (intrahepatic cholestatic jaundice), and pancreatitis.

Central Nervous System—dizziness, vertigo, paresthesia, headache, and xanthopsia.

Hematologic—leukopenia, agranulocytosis, thrombocytopenia, and aplastic anemia.

Dermatologic-Hypersensitivity — purpura, photosensitivity, rash, urticaria, and necrotizing angiitis (vasculitis, cutaneous vasculitis).

Cardiovascular—Orthostatic hypotension may occur.

Other—hyperglycemia, glycosuria, occasional metabolic acidosis in diabetic patients, hyperuricemia, allergic glomerulonephritis, muscle spasm, weakness, and restlessness.

Whenever adverse reactions are moderate or severe, thiazide dosage should be reduced or therapy withdrawn.

OVERDOSAGE

In the event of overdosage, nadolol may cause excessive bradycardia, cardiac failure, hypotension, or bronchospasm.

In addition to the expected diuresis, overdosage of thiazides may produce varying degrees of lethargy which may progress to coma within a few hours, with minimal depression of respiration and cardiovascular function and without evidence of serum electrolyte changes or dehydration. The mechanism of thiazide-induced CNS depression is unknown. Gastrointestinal irritation and hypermotility may occur. Transitory increase in BUN has been reported, and serum electrolyte changes may occur, especially in patients with impaired renal function.

Treatment—Nadolol can be removed from the general circulation by hemodialysis. In determining the duration of corrective therapy, note must be taken of the long duration of the effect of nadolol. In addition to gastric lavage, the following measures should be employed, as appropriate.

Excessive Bradycardia—Administer atropine (0.25 to 1.0 mg). If there is no response to vagal blockade, administer isoproterenol cautiously.

Cardiac Failure—Administer a digitalis glycoside and diuretic. It has been reported that glucagon may also be useful in this situation.

Hypotension—Administer vasopressors, e.g., epinephrine or levarterenol. (There is evidence that epinephrine may be the drug of choice.)

Bronchospasm—Administer a beta$_2$-stimulating agent and/ or a theophylline derivative.

Stupor or Coma—Supportive therapy as warranted.

Gastrointestinal Effects—Symptomatic treatment as needed.

BUN and/or Serum Electrolyte Abnormalities —Institute supportive measures as required to maintain hydration, electrolyte balance, respiration, and cardiovascular and renal function.

DOSAGE AND ADMINISTRATION

DOSAGE MUST BE INDIVIDUALIZED (SEE INDICATIONS). CORZIDE (Nadolol and Bendroflumethiazide Tablets) MAY BE ADMINISTERED WITHOUT REGARD TO MEALS.

Bendroflumethiazide is usually given at a dose of 5 mg daily. The usual initial dose of nadolol is 40 mg once daily whether used alone or in combination with a diuretic. Bendroflumethiazide in CORZIDE is 30 percent more bioavailable than that of 5 mg Naturetin (Bendroflumethiazide) tablets. Conversion from 5 mg Naturetin to CORZIDE represents a 30 percent increase in dose of bendroflumethiazide.

The initial dose of CORZIDE (Nadolol and Bendroflumethiazide Tablets) may therefore be the 40 mg/5 mg tablet once daily. When the antihypertensive response is not satisfactory, the dose may be increased by administering the 80 mg/5 mg tablet once daily.

When necessary, another antihypertensive agent may be added gradually beginning with 50 percent of the usual recommended starting dose to avoid an excessive fall in blood pressure.

Dosage Adjustment In Renal Failure—Absorbed nadolol is excreted principally by the kidneys and, although nonrenal elimination does occur, dosage adjustments are necessary in patients with renal impairment. The following dose intervals are recommended:

Creatinine Clearance (ml/min/1.73m^2)	Dosage Interval (hours)
>50	24
31-50	24-36
10-30	24-48
<10	40-60

HOW SUPPLIED

CORZIDE (Nadolol and Bendroflumethiazide Tablets) is available as tablets containing 40 mg nadolol combined with 5 mg bendroflumethiazide and 80 mg nadolol combined with 5 mg bendroflumethiazide in bottles of 100. The round, biconvex tablets are white to bluish white with dark blue specks. Each tablet has a full bisect bar. Tablet identification numbers: 40 mg/5 mg combination, 283; 80 mg/5 mg combination, 284.

Continued on next page

Princeton—Cont.

Storage: Keep bottle tightly closed. Store at room temperature; avoid excessive heat.
(J3-548D)
Shown in Product Identification Section, page 422

HALOG® ℞

[*hā'log*]
(Halcinonide)
CREAM/OINTMENT/SOLUTION/EMOLLIENT BASE

DESCRIPTION

The topical corticosteroids constitute a class of primarily synthetic steroids used as anti-inflammatory and antipruritic agents. The steroids in this class include halcinonide. Halcinonide is designated chemically as 21-Chloro-9-fluoro-11β, 16α, 17-trihydroxypregn-4-ene-3,20-dione cyclic 16,17-acetal with acetone.
Each gram of 0.025% Halog Cream (Halcinonide Cream USP) contains 0.25 mg halcinonide in a specially formulated cream base consisting of glyceryl monostearate NF XII, cetyl alcohol, cetyl esters wax, polysorbate 60, propylene glycol, dimethicone 350, and purified water. Each gram of 0.1% Halog Cream (Halcinonide Cream USP) contains 1 mg halcinonide in a specially formulated cream base consisting of glyceryl monostearate NF XII, cetyl alcohol, isopropyl palmitate, dimethicone 350, polysorbate 60, titanium dioxide, propylene glycol, and purified water.
Each gram of 0.1% Halog Ointment (Halcinonide Ointment) contains 1 mg halcinonide in Plastibase® (Plasticized Hydrocarbon Gel), a polyethylene and mineral oil gel base with polyethylene glycol 400, polyethylene glycol 6000 distearate, polyethylene glycol 300, polyethylene glycol 1450, and butylated hydroxytoluene as an antioxidant.
Each mL of 0.1% Halog Solution (Halcinonide Topical Solution USP) contains 1 mg halcinonide with edetate disodium, polyethylene glycol 300, purified water, and butylated hydroxytoluene as a preservative.
Each gram of 0.1% Halog-E® Cream (Halcinonide Cream USP) contains 1 mg halcinonide in a hydrophilic vanishing cream base consisting of propylene glycol, dimethicone 350, castor oil, ceteary1 alcohol (and) ceteareth-20, propylene glycol stearate, white petrolatum, and purified water. This formulation is water-washable, greaseless, and nonstaining, with moisturizing and emollient properties.

CLINICAL PHARMACOLOGY

Topical corticosteroids share anti-inflammatory, antipruritic and vasoconstrictive actions.
The mechanism of anti-inflammatory activity of the topical corticosteroids is unclear. Various laboratory methods, including vasoconstrictor assays, are used to compare and predict potencies and/or clinical efficacies of the topical corticosteroids. There is some evidence to suggest that a recognizable correlation exists between vasoconstrictor potency and therapeutic efficacy in man.

PHARMACOKINETICS

The extent of percutaneous absorption of topical corticosteroids is determined by many factors including the vehicle, the integrity of the epidermal barrier, and the use of occlusive dressings.
Topical corticosteroids can be absorbed from normal intact skin. Inflammation and/or other disease processes in the skin increase percutaneous absorption. Occlusive dressings substantially increase the percutaneous absorption of topical corticosteroids. Thus, occlusive dressings may be a valuable therapeutic adjunct for treatment of resistant dermatoses (see DOSAGE AND ADMINISTRATION).
Once absorbed through the skin, topical corticosteroids are handled through pharmacokinetic pathways similar to systemically administered corticosteroids. Corticosteroids are bound to plasma proteins in varying degrees. Corticosteroids are metabolized primarily in the liver and are then excreted by the kidneys. Some of the topical corticosteroids and their metabolites are also excreted into the bile.

INDICATIONS AND USAGE

Halog (Halcinonide) preparations are indicated for the relief of the inflammatory and pruritic manifestations of corticosteroid-responsive dermatoses.

CONTRAINDICATIONS

Topical corticosteroids are contraindicated in those patients with a history of hypersensitivity to any of the components of the preparations.

PRECAUTIONS

General: Systemic absorption of topical corticosteroids has produced reversible hypothalamic-pituitary-adrenal (HPA) axis suppression, manifestations of Cushing's syndrome, hyperglycemia, and glucosuria in some patients.
Conditions which augment systemic absorption include the application of the more potent steroids, use over large surface areas, prolonged use, and the addition of occlusive dressings.
Therefore, patients receiving a large dose of any potent topical steroid applied to a large surface area or under an occlusive dressing should be evaluated periodically for evidence of HPA axis suppression by using the urinary free cortisol and ACTH stimulation tests, and for impairment of thermal homeostasis. If HPA axis suppression or elevation of the body temperature occurs, an attempt should be made to withdraw the drug, to reduce the frequency of application, substitute a less potent steroid, or use a sequential approach when utilizing the occlusive technique.
Recovery of HPA axis function and thermal homeostasis are generally prompt and complete upon discontinuation of the drug. Infrequently, signs and symptoms of steroid withdrawal may occur, requiring supplemental systemic corticosteroids. Occasionally, a patient may develop a sensitivity reaction to a particular occlusive dressing material or adhesive and a substitute material may be necessary.
Children may absorb proportionally larger amounts of topical corticosteroids and thus be more susceptible to systemic toxicity (see PRECAUTIONS, Pediatric Use).
If irritation develops, topical corticosteroids should be discontinued and appropriate therapy instituted.
In the presence of dermatological infections, the use of an appropriate antifungal or antibacterial agent should be instituted. If a favorable response does not occur promptly, the corticosteroid should be discontinued until the infection has been adequately controlled.
These preparations are not for ophthalmic use.

Information for the Patient

Patients using topical corticosteroids should receive the following information and instructions:

1. This medication is to be used as directed by the physician. It is for external use only. Avoid contact with the eyes.
2. Patients should be advised not to use this medication for any disorder other than for which it was prescribed.
3. The treated skin area should not be bandaged or otherwise covered or wrapped as to be occlusive unless directed by the physician.
4. Patients should report any signs of local adverse reactions especially under occlusive dressing.
5. Parents of pediatric patients should be advised not to use tight-fitting diapers or plastic pants on a child being treated in the diaper area, as these garments may constitute occlusive dressings.

Laboratory Tests

A urinary free cortisol test and ACTH stimulation test may be helpful in evaluating HPA axis suppression.

Carcinogenesis, Mutagenesis, and Impairment of Fertility

Long-term animal studies have not been performed to evaluate the carcinogenic potential or the effect on fertility of topical corticosteroids. Studies to determine mutagenicity with prednisolone and hydrocortisone showed negative results.

Pregnancy: Teratogenic Effects

Category C. Corticosteroids are generally teratogenic in laboratory animals when administered systemically at relatively low dosage levels. The more potent corticosteroids have been shown to be teratogenic after dermal application in laboratory animals. There are no adequate and well-controlled studies in pregnant women on teratogenic effects from topically applied corticosteroids. Therefore, topical corticosteroids should be used during pregnancy only if the potential benefit justifies the potential risk to the fetus. Drugs of this class should not be used extensively on pregnant patients, in large amounts, or for prolonged periods of time.

Nursing Mothers

It is not known whether topical administration of corticosteroids could result in sufficient systemic absorption to produce detectable quantities in breast milk. Systemically administered corticosteroids are secreted into breast milk in quantities **not** likely to have a deleterious effect on the infant. Nevertheless, caution should be exercised when topical corticosteroids are administered to a nursing woman.

Pediatric Use

Pediatric patients may demonstrate greater susceptibility to topical corticosteroid-induced HPA axis suppression and Cushing's syndrome than mature patients because of a larger skin surface area to body weight ratio.
HPA axis suppression, Cushing's syndrome, and intracranial hypertension have been reported in children receiving topical corticosteroids. Manifestations of adrenal suppression in children include linear growth retardation, delayed weight gain, low plasma cortisol levels, and absence of response to ACTH stimulation. Manifestations of intracranial hypertension include bulging fontanelles, headaches, and bilateral papilledema.
Administration of topical corticosteroids to children should be limited to the least amount compatible with an effective therapeutic regimen. Chronic corticosteroid therapy may interfere with the growth and development of children.

ADVERSE REACTIONS

The following local adverse reactions are reported infrequently with topical corticosteroids, but may occur more frequently with the use of occlusive dressings (reactions are listed in an approximate decreasing order of occurrence): burning, itching, irritation, dryness, folliculitis, hypertrichosis, acneiform eruptions, hypopigmentation, perioral dermatitis, allergic contact dermatitis, maceration of the skin, secondary infection, skin atrophy, striae, and miliaria.

OVERDOSAGE

Topically applied corticosteroids can be absorbed in sufficient amounts to produce systemic effects (see PRECAUTIONS, General).

DOSAGE AND ADMINISTRATION

Halog Cream (Halcinonide Cream USP): Apply the 0.025% or the 0.1% Halog Cream (Halcinonide Cream USP) to the affected area two to three times daily. Rub in gently.
Halog Ointment (Halcinonide Ointment 0.1%): Apply a thin film to the affected area two to three times daily.
Halog Solution (Halcinonide Topical Solution 0.1%): Apply to the affected area two to three times daily.
Halog Cream (Halcinonide Cream USP) 0.1%: Apply to the affected area one to three times daily. Rub in gently.

Occlusive Dressing Technique

Occlusive dressings may be used for the management of psoriasis or other recalcitrant conditions.
Halog Cream (Halcinonide Cream USP) 0.025% and 0.1% and Halog-E Cream (Halcinonide Cream USP) 0.1%: Gently rub a small amount of the cream into the lesion until it disappears. Reapply the preparation leaving a thin coating on the lesion, cover with a pliable nonporous film, and seal the edges. If needed, additional moisture may be provided by covering the lesion with a dampened clean cotton cloth before the nonporous film is applied or by briefly wetting the affected area with water immediately prior to applying the medication. The frequency of changing dressings is best determined on an individual basis. It may be convenient to apply the cream under an occlusive dressing in the evening and to remove the dressing in the morning (i.e., 12-hour occlusion). When utilizing the 12-hour occlusion regimen, additional cream should be applied, without occlusion, during the day. Reapplication is essential at each dressing change. If an infection develops, the use of occlusive dressings should be discontinued and appropriate antimicrobial therapy instituted.
Halog Ointment (Halcinonide Ointment 0.1%): Apply a thin film of the ointment to the lesion, cover with a pliable nonporous film, and seal the edges. If needed, additional moisture may be provided by covering the lesion with a dampened clean cotton cloth before the nonporous film is applied or by briefly wetting the affected area with water immediately prior to applying the medication. The frequency of changing dressings is best determined on an individual basis. It may be convenient to apply the ointment under an occlusive dressing in the evening and to remove the dressing in the morning (i.e., 12-hour occlusion). When utilizing the 12-hour occlusion regimen, additional ointment should be applied, without occlusion, during the day. Reapplication is essential at each dressing change. If an infection develops, the use of occlusive dressings should be discontinued and appropriate antimicrobial therapy instituted.
Halog Solution (Halcinonide Topical Solution 0.1%): Apply the solution to the lesion, cover with a pliable nonporous film, and seal the edges. If needed, additional moisture may be provided by covering the lesion with a dampened clean cotton cloth before the nonporous film is applied or by briefly wetting the affected area with water immediately prior to applying the medication. The frequency of changing dressings is best determined on an individual basis. It may be convenient to apply the solution under an occlusive dressing in the evening and to remove the dressing in the morning (i.e., 12-hour occlusion). When utilizing the 12-hour occlusion regimen, additional solution should be applied, without occlusion, during the day. Reapplication is essential at each dressing change. If an infection develops, the use of occlusive dressings should be discontinued and appropriate antimicrobial therapy instituted.

HOW SUPPLIED

0.025% Cream Tubes of 15 g and 60 g; jars of 240 g (8 oz).
0.1% Cream Tubes of 15 g, 30 g, and 60 g; jars of 240 g (8 oz).
0.1% Ointment Tubes of 15 g, 30 g, and 60 g; jars of 240 g (8 oz). 0.1% Solution—Plastic squeeze bottles of 20 mL and 60 mL.
0.1% Cream (emollient base): Tubes of 15 g, 30 g, and 60 g
Storage: Store the 0.025% and 0.1% Creams at room temperature; avoid excessive heat (104°F). Store the 0.1% Ointment at room temperature; avoid excessive heat (104°F). Store the Solution at room temperature; avoid freezing and temperatures above 104°F. Store the 0.1% Cream (emollient base) at room temperature; avoid freezing and refrigeration.
(J3-552B/553C/554B/643A)

NATURETIN®-2.5 ℞
NATURETIN®-5 ℞
NATURETIN®-10 ℞
[*na"chūr-ē'tin*]
(Bendroflumethiazide Tablets USP)

DESCRIPTION

Naturetin is a benzothiadiazine derivative containing a benzyl and a trifluoromethyl group. It is a potent oral diuretic and antihypertensive agent available as compressed tablets providing 2.5, 5, or 10 mg bendroflumethiazide.
Inactive ingredients: cellulose, colorants [D&C Yellow No. 10; FD&C Blue No. 1 for 2.5 mg and 5 mg only, and Yellow No. 6 for 10 mg only], lactose, magnesium stearate, sodium starch glycolate, and starch.

CLINICAL PHARMACOLOGY

Thiazides affect the renal tubular mechanism of electrolyte reabsorption. At maximal therapeutic dosage all thiazides are approximately equal in their diuretic potency.
Thiazides increase excretion of sodium and chloride in approximately equivalent amounts. Natriuresis causes a secondary loss of potassium and bicarbonate.
The mechanism of the antihypertensive effect of thiazides is unknown. Thiazides do not affect normal blood pressure.
Onset of action of thiazides occurs in two hours and the peak effect at about four hours. Duration of action persists for approximately six to 12 hours. Thiazides are eliminated rapidly by the kidney.

INDICATIONS AND USAGE

Naturetin is indicated as adjunctive therapy in edema associated with congestive heart failure, hepatic cirrhosis, and corticosteroid and estrogen therapy.
Naturetin has also been found useful in edema due to various forms of renal dysfunction such as: nephrotic syndrome, acute glomerulonephritis, and chronic renal failure.
Naturetin (Bendroflumethiazide Tablets USP) tablets are indicated in the management of hypertension either as the sole therapeutic agent or to enhance the effectiveness of other antihypertensive drugs in the more severe forms of hypertension.
Usage in Pregnancy—The routine use of diuretics in an otherwise healthy woman is inappropriate and exposes mother and fetus to unnecessary hazard. Diuretics do not prevent development of toxemia of pregnancy, and there is no satisfactory evidence that they are useful in the treatment of developed toxemia.
Edema during pregnancy may arise from pathological causes or from the physiologic and mechanical consequences of pregnancy. Thiazides are indicated in pregnancy when edema is due to pathologic causes, just as they are in the absence of pregnancy (however, see WARNINGS below). Dependent edema in pregnancy, resulting from restriction of venous return by the expanded uterus, is properly treated through elevation of the lower extremities and use of support hose; use of diuretics to lower intravascular volume in this case is illogical and unnecessary. There is hypervolemia during normal pregnancy which is harmful to neither the fetus nor the mother (in the absence of cardiovascular disease), but which is associated with edema, including generalized edema, in the majority of pregnant women. If this edema produces discomfort, increased recumbency will often provide relief. In rare instances, this edema may cause extreme discomfort which is not relieved by rest. In these cases, a short course of diuretics may provide relief and may be appropriate.

CONTRAINDICATIONS

Bendroflumethiazide is contraindicated in anuria.
It is also contraindicated in patients who have previously demonstrated hypersensitivity to it or other sulfonamide-derived drugs.

WARNINGS

Thiazides should be used with caution in severe renal disease. In patients with renal disease, thiazides may precipitate azotemia. Cumulative effects of the drug may develop in patients with impaired renal function.
Thiazides should be used with caution in patients with impaired hepatic function or progressive liver disease, since minor alterations of fluid and electrolyte balance may precipitate hepatic coma.
Thiazides may be additive or may potentiate the action of other antihypertensive drugs. Potentiation occurs with ganglionic or peripheral adrenergic blocking drugs.
Sensitivity reactions may occur in patients with a history of allergy or bronchial asthma.
The possibility of exacerbation or activation of systemic lupus erythematosus has been reported.
Lithium generally should not be given with diuretics; diuretic agents reduce the renal clearance of lithium and add a high risk of lithium toxicity. Refer to the package insert for lithium preparations before use of such concomitant therapy.
Usage in Pregnancy—Thiazides cross the placental barrier and appear in cord blood. The use of thiazides in pregnant women requires that the anticipated benefit be weighed against possible hazards to the fetus. These hazards include fetal or neonatal jaundice, thrombocytopenia, and possibly other adverse reactions which have occurred in the adult.
Nursing Mothers—Thiazides appear in breast milk. If use of the drug is deemed essential, the patient should stop nursing.

PRECAUTIONS

Periodic determination of serum electrolytes to detect possible electrolyte imbalance should be performed at appropriate intervals.
All patients receiving thiazide therapy should be observed for clinical signs of fluid or electrolyte imbalance; namely, hyponatremia, hypochloremic alkalosis, and hypokalemia. Serum and urine electrolyte determinations are particularly important when the patient is vomiting excessively or receiving parenteral fluids. Warning signs or symptoms of fluid and electrolyte imbalance include: dryness of the mouth, thirst, weakness, lethargy, drowsiness, restlessness, muscle pains or cramps, muscular fatigue, hypotension, oliguria, tachycardia, and gastrointestinal disturbances such as nausea and vomiting.
Hypokalemia may develop, especially with brisk diuresis, when severe cirrhosis is present, or during concomitant use of corticosteroids, ACTH, or after prolonged thiazide therapy.
Interference with adequate oral electrolyte intake will also contribute to hypokalemia.
Hypokalemia can sensitize or exaggerate the response of the heart to the toxic effects of digitalis (e.g., increased ventricular irritability). Concurrent administration of a potassium-sparing diuretic or potassium supplements may be indicated in these patients.
Any chloride deficit is generally mild and usually does not require specific treatment except under extraordinary circumstances (as in liver disease or renal disease). Dilutional hyponatremia may occur in edematous patients in hot weather; appropriate therapy is water restriction, rather than administration of salt, except in rare instances when the hyponatremia is life threatening. In actual salt depletion, appropriate replacement is the therapy of choice.
Hyperuricemia may occur or frank gout may be precipitated in certain patients receiving thiazide therapy.
Insulin requirements in diabetic patients may be increased, decreased, or unchanged. Latent diabetes mellitus may become manifest during thiazide administration.
Thiazide drugs may increase the responsiveness to tubocurarine.
The antihypertensive effects of the drug may be enhanced in the postsympathectomy patient.
Thiazides may decrease arterial responsiveness to norepinephrine. This diminution is not sufficient to preclude effectiveness of the pressor agent for therapeutic use. If emergency surgery is indicated, preanesthetic and anesthetic agents should be administered in reduced dosage.
If progressive renal impairment becomes evident, as indicated by a rising nonprotein nitrogen or blood urea nitrogen, a careful reappraisal of therapy is necessary with consideration given to withholding or discontinuing diuretic therapy.
Thiazides may decrease serum PBI levels without signs of thyroid disturbance.
Calcium excretion is decreased by thiazides. Pathological changes in the parathyroid gland with hypercalcemia and hypophosphatemia have been observed in a few patients on prolonged thiazide therapy. The common complications of hyperparathyroidism such as renal lithiasis, bone resorption, and peptic ulceration have not been seen. Thiazides should be discontinued before carrying out tests for parathyroid function.

ADVERSE REACTIONS

1. *Gastrointestinal system*—anorexia; gastric irritation; nausea; vomiting; cramping; diarrhea; constipation; jaundice (intrahepatic cholestatic jaundice); pancreatitis; sialadenitis.
2. *Central nervous system*—dizziness; vertigo; paresthesia; headache; xanthopsia.
3. *Hematologic-leukopenia;* agranulocytosis; aplastic anemia; hemolytic anemia.
4. *Cardiovascular*—orthostatic hypotension (may be aggravated by alcohol, barbiturates, or narcotics)
5. *Hypersensitivity*—purpura; photosensitivity; rash; urticaria; necrotizing angiitis (vasculitis, cutaneous vasculitis); fever; respiratory distress including pneumonitis; anaphylactic reactions.
6. *Other*—hyperglycemia; glycosuria; hyperuricemia; muscle spasm; weakness; restlessness; transient blurred vision.

Whenever adverse reactions are moderate or severe, thiazide dosage should be reduced or therapy withdrawn.

DOSAGE AND ADMINISTRATION

Therapy should be individualized according to patient response and titrated to obtain maximal therapeutic response as well as the lowest dose possible to maintain that therapeutic response and minimize side effects.
Diuretic: The usual dose is 5 mg once daily, preferably given in the morning. To initiate therapy, doses up to 20 mg may be given once daily or divided into two doses. A single daily dose of 2.5 to 5 mg should suffice for maintenance.
Alternatively, intermittent therapy may be advantageous in many patients. By administering the preparation every other day or on a three to five day per week schedule, electrolyte imbalance is less likely to occur; however, the possibility still exists.
In general, the lowest dosage that achieves the therapeutic response should be employed.
Antihypertensive: The suggested initial dosage is 5 to 20 mg daily. Maintenance dosage may range from 2.5 to 15 mg per day depending on the individual response of the patient. When the diuretic is used with other antihypertensive agents, lower maintenance doses for each drug are usually sufficient.

HOW SUPPLIED

2.5 mg in bottles of 100; 5 mg (scored) in bottles of 100 and 1000; 10 mg (scored) in bottles of 100.
Storage: Store at room temperature; avoid excessive heat. Dispense in tight containers.
(J3-419H)

Shown in Product Identification Section, page 422

PROLIXIN® INJECTION ℞
Fluphenazine Hydrochloride Injection USP
PROLIXIN® TABLETS ℞
Fluphenazine Hydrochloride Tablets USP
PROLIXIN® ELIXIR ℞
Fluphenazine Hydrochloride Elixir USP
PROLIXIN® ORAL CONCENTRATE ℞
Fluphenazine Hydrochloride Oral Solution*

DESCRIPTION

Prolixin is a trifluoromethyl phenothiazine derivative.
Prolixin Injection (Fluphenazine Hydrochloride Injection USP) is available in multiple-dose vials providing 2.5 mg fluphenazine hydrochloride per mL **FOR INTRAMUSCULAR USE ONLY.** The preparation also includes sodium chloride for isotonicity, sodium hydroxide or hydrochloric acid to adjust the pH to 4.8 to 5.2, and 0.1% methylparaben and 0.01% propylparaben as preservatives. At the time of manufacture, the air in the vials is replaced by nitrogen.
Prolixin Tablets (Fluphenazine Hydrochloride Tablets USP) are available for oral administration as tablets providing 1, 2.5, 5, and 10 mg fluphenazine hydrochloride. Inactive ingredients: acacia, calcium carbonate, carnauba wax for 1 and 2.5 mg only, castor oil, colorants [FD&C Blue No. 1 for 5 mg only, Blue No. 2 for 2.5 mg only, Red No. 3 for 1 and 10 mg only, and Yellow No. 5 (tartrazine) for 2.5, 5, and 10 mg only], corn starch, ethylcellulose, gelatin, lactose, magnesium carbonate, magnesium sterate, shellac, sodium benzoate for 1, 2.5, and 5 mg only, sucrose, talc, titanium dioxide, and white wax for 1 and 2.5 mg only.
Prolixin Elixir (Fluphenazine Hydrochloride Elixir USP) is available as an elixir for oral administration which provides 0.5 mg fluphenazine hydrochloride per mL (2.5 mg per 5 mL teaspoonful). Inactive ingredients: alcohol [14% (v/v)], colorant (FD&C Yellow No. 6), flavors, glycerin, polysorbate 40, purified water, sodium benzoate, and sucrose.
Prolixin Oral Concentrate (Fluphenazine Hydrochloride Oral Solution*) contains 5 mg fluphenzine hydrochloride per mL. Inactive ingredients: *alcohol 14% (exceeds the USP monograph 1.2% limit); glycerin; purified water; sodium benzoate.

CLINICAL PHARMACOLOGY

Prolixin (Fluphenazine) has activity at all levels of the central nervous system as well as on multiple organ systems. The mechanism whereby its therapeutic action is exerted is unknown.
Fluphenazine differs from other phenothiazine derivatives in several respects: it is more potent on a milligram basis, it has less potentiating effect on central nervous system depressants and anesthetics than do some of the phenothiazines and appears to be less sedating, and it is less likely than some of the older phenothiazines to produce hypotension (nevertheless, appropriate cautions should be observed—see sections on PRECAUTIONS and ADVERSE REACTIONS).

INDICATIONS AND USAGE

Prolixin (Fluphenazine Hydrochloride) Injection, Tablets, and Elixir are indicated in the management of manifestations of psychotic disorders.
Fluphenazine has not been shown effective in the management of behavorial complications in patients with mental retardation.

CONTRAINDICATIONS

Phenothiazines are contraindicated in patients with suspected or established subcortical brain damage, in patients receiving large doses of hypnotics, and in comatose or severely depressed states. The presence of blood dyscrasia or

Continued on next page

Princeton—Cont.

liver damage precludes the use of fluphenazine. Prolixin (fluphenazine hydrochloride) is contraindicated in patients who have shown hypersensitivity to fluphenazine; cross-sensitivity to phenothiazine derivatives may occur.

WARNINGS

Tardive Dyskinesia: Tardive dyskinesia, a syndrome consisting of potentially irreversible, involuntary, dyskinetic movements may develop in patients treated with neuroleptic (antipsychotic) drugs. Although the prevalence of the syndrome appears to be highest among the elderly, especially elderly women, it is impossible to rely upon prevalence estimates to predict, at the inception of neuroleptic treatment, which patients are likely to develop the syndrome. Whether neuroleptic drug products differ in their potential to cause tardive dyskinesia is unknown.

Both the risk of developing the syndrome and the likelihood that it will become irreversible are believed to increase as the duration of treatment and the total cumulative dose of neuroleptic drugs administered to the patient increase. However, the syndrome can develop, although much less commonly, after relatively brief treatment periods at low doses.

There is no known treatment for established cases of tardive dyskinesia, although the syndrome may remit, partially or completely, if neuroleptic treatment is withdrawn. Neuroleptic treatment, itself, however, may suppress (or partially suppress) the signs and symptoms of the syndrome and thereby may possibly mask the underlying disease process. The effect that symptomatic suppression has upon the long-term course of the syndrome is unknown.

Given these considerations, neuroleptics should be prescribed in a manner that is most likely to minimize the occurrence of tardive dyskinesia. Chronic neuroleptic treatment should generally be reserved for patients who suffer from a chronic illness that, 1) is known to respond to neuroleptic drugs, and, 2) for whom alternative, equally effective, but potentially less harmful treatments are *not* available or appropriate. In patients who do require chronic treatment, the smallest dose and the shortest duration of treatment producing a satisfactory clinical response should be sought. The need for continued treatment should be reassessed periodically.

If signs and symptoms of tardive dyskinesia appear in a patient on neuroleptics, drug discontinuation should be considered. However, some patients may require treatment despite the presence of the syndrome.

(For further information about the description of tardive dyskinesia and its clinical detection, please refer to the sections on PRECAUTIONS, Information for Patients and ADVERSE REACTIONS, Tardive Dyskinesia.)

The use of this drug may impair the mental and physical abilities required for driving a car or operating heavy machinery.

Potentiation of the effects of alcohol may occur with the use of this drug.

Since there is no adequate experience in children who have received this drug, safety and efficacy in children have not been established.

Physicians should be alert to the possibility that severe adverse reactions may occur which require immediate medical attention.

Usage in Pregnancy: The safety for the use of this drug during pregnancy has not been established; therefore, the possible hazards should be weighed against the potential benefits when administering these drugs to pregnant patients.

PRECAUTIONS

General—Because of the possibility of cross-sensitivity, fluphenazine should be used cautiously in patients who have developed cholestatic jaundice, dermatoses or other allergic reactions to phenothiazine derivatives.

Prolixin Tablets (Fluphenazine Hydrochloride Tablets USP) 2.5, 5, and 10 mg contain FD&C Yellow No. 5 (tartrazine) which may cause allergic-type reactions (including bronchial asthma) in certain susceptible individuals. Although the overall incidence of FD&C Yellow No. 5 (tartrazine) sensitivity in the general population is low, it is frequently seen in patients who also have aspirin hypersensitivity.

Psychotic patients on large doses of a phenothiazine drug who are undergoing surgery should be watched carefully for possible hypotensive phenomena. Moreover, it should be remembered that reduced amounts of anesthetics or central nervous system depressants may be necessary.

The effects of atropine may be potentiated in some patients receiving fluphenazine because of added anticholinergic effects.

Fluphenazine should be used cautiously in patients exposed to extreme heat or phosphorus insecticides; in patients with a history of convulsive disorders, since grand mal convulsions have been known to occur; and in patients with special medical disorders, such as mitral insufficiency or other cardiovascular diseases and pheochromocytoma.

The possibility of liver damage, pigmentary retinopathy, lenticular and corneal deposits, and development of irreversible dyskinesia should be remembered when patients are on prolonged therapy.

Neuroleptic drugs elevate prolactin levels; the elevation persists during chronic administration. Tissue culture experiments indicate that approximately one-third of human breast cancers are prolactin dependent *in vitro*, a factor of potential importance if the prescription of these drugs is contemplated in a patient with a previously detected breast cancer. Although disturbances such as galactorrhea, amenorrhea, gynecomastia, and impotence have been reported, the clinical significance of elevated serum prolactin levels is unknown for most patients. An increase in mammary neoplasms has been found in rodents after chronic administration of neuroleptic drugs. Neither clinical studies nor epidemiologic studies conducted to date, however, have shown an association between chronic administration of these drugs and mammary tumorigenesis; the available evidence is considered too limited to be conclusive at this time.

Facilities should be available for periodic checking of hepatic function, renal function and the blood picture. Renal function of patients on long-term therapy should be monitored; if BUN (blood urea nitrogen) becomes abnormal, treatment should be discontinued.

As with any phenothiazine, the physician should be alert to the possible development of "silent pneumonias" in patients under treatment with fluphenazine.

Outside state hospitals or other psychiatric institutions, fluphenazine decanoate should be administered under the direction of a physician experienced in the clinical use of psychotropic drugs, particularly phenothiazine derivatives.

Information for Patients

Given the likelihood that some patients exposed chronically to neuroleptics will develop tardive dyskinesia, it is advised that all patients in whom chronic use is contemplated be given, if possible, full information about this risk. The decision to inform patients and/or their guardians must obviously take into account the clinical circumstances and the competency of the patient to understand the information provided.

Abrupt Withdrawal: In general, phenothiazines do not produce psychic dependence; however, gastritis, nausea and vomiting, dizziness, and tremulousness have been reported following abrupt cessation of high dose therapy. Reports suggest that these symptoms can be reduced if concomitant antiparkinsonian agents are continued for several weeks after the phenothiazine is withdrawn.

ADVERSE REACTIONS

Central Nervous System: The side effects most frequently reported with phenothiazine compounds are extrapyramidal symptoms including pseudoparkinsonism, dystonia, dyskinesia, akathisia, oculogyric crises, opisthotonos, and hyperreflexia. With any given phenothiazine derivative, the incidence and severity of such reactions depend more on individual patient sensitivity than on other factors, but dosage level and patient age are also determinants.

Extrapyramidal reactions may be alarming, and the patient should be forewarned and reassured. These reactions can usually be controlled by administration of antiparkinsonian drugs such as Benztropine Mesylate or intravenous Caffeine and Sodium Benzoate Injection, and by subsequent reduction in dosage.

Tardive Dyskinesia: See WARNINGS. The syndrome is characterized by involuntary choreoathetoid movements which variously involve the tongue, face, mouth, lips, or jaw (e.g., protrusion of the tongue, puffing of cheeks, puckering of the mouth, chewing movements), trunk and extremities. The severity of the syndrome and the degree of impairment produced vary widely.

The syndrome may become clinically recognizable either during treatment, upon dosage reduction, or upon withdrawal of treatment. Early detection of tardive dyskinesia is important. To increase the likelihood of detecting the syndrome at the earliest possible time, the dosage of neuroleptic drug should be reduced periodically (if clinically possible) and the patient observed for signs of the disorder. This maneuver is critical, since neuroleptic drugs may mask the signs of the syndrome.

Other CNS Effects: Rare occurrences of neuroleptic malignant syndrome (NMS) have been reported in patients on neuroleptic therapy. The syndrome is characterized by hyperthermia, muscular rigidity, autonomic instability (labile blood pressure, tachycardia, diaphoresis), akinesia, and altered consciousness, sometimes progressing to stupor or coma. Leukocytosis, elevated CPK, liver function abnormalities, and acute renal failure may also occur. Neuroleptic therapy should be discontinued immediately and vigorous symptomatic treatment implemented since the syndrome is potentially fatal.

Drowsiness or lethargy, if they occur, may necessitate a reduction in dosage; the induction of a catatonic-like state has been known to occur with dosages of fluphenazine far in excess of the recommended amounts. As with other phenothiazine compounds, reactivation or aggravation of psychotic processes may be encountered.

Phenothiazine derivatives have been known to cause, in some patients, restlessness, excitement, or bizarre dreams.

Autonomic Nervous System: Hypertension and fluctuations in blood pressure have been reported with fluphenazine.

Hypotension has rarely presented a problem with fluphenazine. However, patients with pheochromocytoma, cerebral vascular or renal insufficiency, or a severe cardiac reserve deficiency such as mitral insufficiency appear to be particularly prone to hypotensive reactions with phenothiazine compounds, and should therefore be observed closely when the drug is administered. If severe hypotension should occur, supportive measures including the use of intravenous vasopressor drugs should be instituted immediately. Levarterenol Bitartrate Injection is the most suitable drug for this purpose; *epinephrine should not be used* since phenothiazine derivatives have been found to reverse its action, resulting in a further lowering of blood pressure.

Autonomic reactions including nausea and loss of appetite, salivation, polyuria, perspiration, dry mouth, headache, and constipation may occur. Autonomic effects can usually be controlled by reducing or temporarily discontinuing dosage.

In some patients, phenothiazine derivatives have caused blurred vision, glaucoma, bladder paralysis, fecal impaction, paralytic ileus, tachycardia, or nasal congestion.

Metabolic and Endocrine: Weight change, peripheral edema, abnormal lactation, gynecomastia, menstrual irregularities, false results on pregnancy tests, impotency in men and increased libido in women have all been known to occur in some patients on phenothiazine therapy.

Allergic Reactions: Skin disorders such as itching, erythema, urticaria, seborrhea, photosensitivity, eczema and even exfoliative dermatitis have been reported with phenothiazine derivatives. The possibility of anaphylactoid reactions occurring in some patients should be borne in mind.

Hematologic: Routine blood counts are advisable during therapy since blood dyscrasias including leukopenia, agranulocytosis, thrombocytopenic or nonthrombocytopenic purpura, eosinophilia, and pancytopenia have been observed with phenothiazine derivatives. Furthermore, if any soreness of the mouth, gums, or throat, or any symptoms of upper respiratory infection occur and confirmatory leukocyte count indicates cellular depression, therapy should be discontinued and other appropriate measures instituted immediately.

Hepatic: Liver damage as manifested by cholestatic jaundice may be encountered, particularly during the first months of therapy; treatment should be discontinued if this occurs. An increase in cephalin flocculation, sometimes accompanied by alterations in other liver function tests, has been reported in patients receiving fluphenazine hydrochloride and the enanthate ester of fluphenazine (a compound closely related to fluphenazine decanoate) who have had no clinical evidence of liver damage.

Others: Sudden, unexpected and unexplained deaths have been reported in hospitalized psychotic patients receiving phenothiazines. Previous brain damage or seizures may be predisposing factors; high doses should be avoided in known seizure patients. Several patients have shown sudden flare-ups of psychotic behavior patterns shortly before death. Autopsy findings have usually revealed acute fulminating pneumonia or pneumonitis, aspiration of gastric contents, or intramyocardial lesions.

Although this is not a general feature of fluphenazine, potentiation of central nervous system depressants (opiates, analgesics, antihistamines, barbiturates, alcohol) may occur.

The following adverse reactions have also occurred with phenothiazine derivatives: systemic lupus erythematosus-like syndrome, hypotension severe enough to cause fatal cardiac arrest, altered electrocardiographic and electroencephalographic tracings, altered cerebrospinal fluid proteins, cerebral edema, asthma, laryngeal edema and angioneurotic edema; with long-term use—skin pigmentation, and lenticular and corneal opacities.

DOSAGE AND ADMINISTRATION

Parenteral drug products should be inspected visually for particulate matter and discoloration prior to administration, whenever solution and container permit.

Prolixin Injection (Fluphenazine Hydrochloride Injection USP)

Prolixin Injection (Fluphenazine Hydrochloride Injection USP) is useful when psychotic patients are unable or unwilling to take oral therapy.

The average well-tolerated starting dose for adult psychotic patients is 1.25 mg (0.5 mL) intramuscularly. Depending on the severity and duration of symptoms, initial total daily parenteral dosage may range from 2.5 to 10.0 mg and should be divided and given at six- to eight-hour intervals.

The smallest amount that will produce the desired results must be carefully determined for each individual, since optimal dosage levels of this potent drug vary from patient to patient. In general, the parenteral dose for fluphenazine has been found to be approximately ⅓ to ½ the oral dose. Treatment may be instituted with a *low initial dosage*, which

may be increased, if necessary, until the desired clinical effects are achieved. Dosages exceeding 10.0 mg intramuscularly daily should be used with caution.
When symptoms are controlled, oral maintenance therapy can generally be instituted, often with single daily doses. Continued treatment, by the oral route if possible, is needed to achieve maximum therapeutic benefits; further adjustments in dosage may be necessary during the course of therapy to meet the patient's requirements.

Prolixin (Fluphenazine Hydrochloride) Tablets, Elixir and Oral Concentrate

Depending on severity and duration of symptoms, total daily oral dosage for *adult* psychotic patients may range initially from 2.5 to 10.0 mg and should be divided and given at six- to eight-hour intervals.
The smallest amount that will produce the desired results must be carefully determined for each individual since optimal dosage levels of this potent drug vary from patient to patient. In general, the oral dose has been found to be approximately two to three times the parenteral dose of fluphenazine. Treatment is best instituted with a *low initial dosage,* which may be increased, if necessary, until the desired clinical effects are achieved. Therapeutic effect is often achieved with doses under 20 mg daily. Patients remaining severely disturbed or inadequately controlled may require upward titration of dosage. Daily doses up to 40 mg may be necessary; controlled clinical studies have not been performed to demonstrate safety of prolonged administration of such doses.
When symptoms are controlled, dosage can generally be reduced gradually to daily maintenance doses of 1.0 or 5.0 mg, often given as a single daily dose. Continued treatment is needed to achieve maximum therapeutic benefits; further adjustments in dosage may be necessary during the course of therapy to meet the patient's requirements.
For *geriatric* patients, the suggested starting dose is 1.0 to 2.5 mg orally daily, adjusted according to the response of the patient.
When the Oral Concentrate dosage form is to be used, the desired dose (measured by calibrated device only) should be added to at least 60 mL (2 fl oz) of a suitable diluent *just prior to administration* to insure palatability and stability. Suggested diluents include tomato or fruit juice, milk, and uncaffeinated soft drinks. The Oral Concentrate should not be mixed with beverages containing caffeine (coffee, cola), tannics (tea), or pectinates (apple juice) because of potential incompatibility.
For psychotic patients who have been stabilized on a fixed daily dosage of orally administered Prolixin (fluphenazine hydrochloride) dosage forms, conversion to the long-acting injectable Prolixin Decanoate (Fluphenazine Decanoate Injection) may be indicated.

HOW SUPPLIED

Prolixin Injection (Fluphenazine Hydrochloride Injection USP) is available as a sterile, aqueous solution providing 2.5 mg fluphenazine hydrochloride per mL in multiple-dose vials of 10 mL.
Prolixin Tablets (Fluphenazine Hydrochloride Tablets USP) are available for oral administration as sugar-coated tablets providing 1, 2.5, 5, and 10 mg fluphenazine hydrochloride.
Prolixin Elixir (Fluphenazine Hydrochloride Elixir USP) is available as an elixir for oral administration which provides 0.5 mg fluphenazine hydrochloride per mL (2.5 mg per 5 mL teaspoonful).
Prolixin Oral Concentrate (Fluphenazine Hydrochloride Oral Solution) provides 5 mg fluphenazine hydrochloride per mL.
*TABLETS—available in bottles of 50 and 500, and in Unimatic® cartons of 100. ELIXIR—available in dropper-assembly bottles of 60 mL calibrated at 0.5 mL (0.25 mg), 1 mL (0.5 mg), 1.5 mL (0.75 mg), and 2 mL (1 mg); and in bottles of 473 mL (1 pint). ORAL CONCENTRATE—available in bottles of 120 mL with 1 mL safety-cap droppers calibrated at 0.1 mL and in 0.2 mL increments.
Storage: Prolixin Injection (Fluphenazine Hydrochloride Injection USP) should be protected from exposure to light. Parenteral solutions may vary in color from essentially colorless to light amber. If a solution has become any darker than light amber or is discolored in any other way, it should not be used. Store at room temperature; avoid freezing.
Store the tablets, elixir and oral concentrate at room temperature; protect from light; keep tightly closed. Tablets: avoid excessive heat. Elixir and Oral Concentrate: avoid freezing.
(J4-010A/011D/050B)

**Shown in Product Identification Section, page 422*

PROLIXIN DECANOATE® ℞

[pro″lik′sin dek″ah-nō′āt]
(Fluphenazine Decanoate Injection)

DESCRIPTION

Prolixin Decanoate is the decanoate ester of a trifluoromethyl phenothiazine derivative. It is a highly potent behavior modifier with a markedly extended duration of effect. Prolixin Decanoate is available for intramuscular or subcutaneous administration, providing 25 mg fluphenazine decanoate per mL in a sesame oil vehicle with 1.2% (w/v) benzyl alcohol as a preservative. At the time of manufacture, the air in the vials is replaced by nitrogen.

CLINICAL PHARMACOLOGY

The basic effects of fluphenazine decanoate appear to be no different from those of fluphenazine hydrochloride, with the exception of duration of action. The esterification of fluphenazine markedly prolongs the drug's duration of effect without unduly attenuating its beneficial action.
Prolixin Decanoate has activity at all levels of the central nervous system as well as on multiple organ systems. The mechanism whereby its therapeutic action is exerted is unknown.
Fluphenazine differs from other phenothiazine derivatives in several respects: it is more potent on a milligram basis, it has less potentiating effect on central nervous system depressants and anesthetics than do some of the phenothiazines and appears to be less sedating, and it is less likely than some of the older phenothiazines to produce hypotension (nevertheless, appropriate cautions should be observed—see sections on PRECAUTIONS and ADVERSE REACTIONS).

INDICATIONS AND USAGE

Prolixin Decanoate is a long-acting parenteral antipsychotic drug intended for use in the management of patients requiring prolonged parenteral neuroleptic therapy (e.g., chronic schizophrenics).
Fluphenazine decanoate has not been shown effective in the management of behavioral complications in patients with mental retardation.

CONTRAINDICATIONS

Phenothiazines are contraindicated in patients with suspected or established subcortical brain damage.
Phenothiazine compounds should not be used in patients receiving large doses of hypnotics.
Prolixin Decanoate is contraindicated in comatose or severely depressed states.
The presence of blood dyscrasia or liver damage precludes the use of fluphenazine decanoate.
Fluphenazine decanoate is not intended for use in children under 12 years of age.
Prolixin Decanoate (Fluphenazine Decanoate Injection) is contraindicated in patients who have shown hypersensitivity to fluphenazine; cross-sensitivity to phenothiazine derivatives may occur.

Warnings—Tardive Dyskinesia

Tardive dyskinesia, a syndrome consisting of potentially irreversible, involuntary, dyskinetic movements may develop in patients treated with neuroleptic (antipsychotic) drugs. Although the prevalence of the syndrome appears to be highest among the elderly, especially elderly women, it is impossible to rely upon prevalence estimates to predict, at the inception of neuroleptic treatment, which patients are likely to develop the syndrome. Whether neuroleptic drug products differ in their potential to cause tardive dyskinesia is unknown.
Both the risk of developing the syndrome and the likelihood that it will become irreversible are believed to increase as the duration of treatment and the total cumulative dose of neuroleptic drugs administered to the patient increase. However, the syndrome can develop, although much less commonly, after relatively brief treatment periods at low doses.
There is no known treatment for established cases of tardive dyskinesia, although the syndrome may remit, partially or completely, if neuroleptic treatment is withdrawn. Neuroleptic treatment, itself, however, may suppress (or partially suppress) the signs and symptoms of the syndrome and thereby may possibly mask the underlying disease process. The effect that symptomatic suppression has upon the long-term course of the syndrome is unknown.
Given these considerations, neuroleptics should be prescribed in a manner that is most likely to minimize the occurrence of tardive dyskinesia. Chronic neuroleptic treatment should generally be reserved for patients who suffer from a chronic illness that, 1) is known to respond to neuroleptic drugs, and, 2) for whom alternative, equally effective, but potentially less harmful treatments are *not* available or appropriate. In patients who do require chronic treatment, the smallest dose and the shortest duration of treatment producing a satisfactory clinical response should be sought. The need for continued treatment should be reassessed periodically.
If signs and symptoms of tardive dyskinesia appear in a patient on neuroleptics, drug discontinuation should be considered. However, some patients may require treatment despite the presence of the syndrome.
(For further information about the description of tardive dyskinesia and its clinical detection, please refer to the sections on PRECAUTIONS, Information for Patients and ADVERSE REACTIONS, Tardive Dyskinesia.) The use of this drug may impair the mental and physical abilities required for driving a car or operating heavy machinery.
Physicians should be alert to the possibility that severe adverse reactions may occur which require immediate medical attention.
Potentiation of the effects of alcohol may occur with the use of this drug.
Since there is no adequate experience in children who have received this drug, safety and efficacy in children have not been established.
Usage in Pregnancy—The safety for the use of this drug during pregnancy has not been established; therefore, the possible hazards should be weighed against the potential benefits when administering this drug to pregnant patients.

PRECAUTIONS

General—Because of the possibility of cross-sensitivity, fluphenazine decanoate should be used cautiously in patients who have developed cholestatic jaundice, dermatoses, or other allergic reactions to phenothiazine derivatives.
Psychotic patients on large doses of a phenothiazine drug who are undergoing surgery should be watched carefully for possible hypotensive phenomena. Moreover, it should be remembered that reduced amounts of anesthetics or central nervous system depressants may be necessary.
The effects of atropine may be potentiated in some patients receiving fluphenazine because of added anticholinergic effects.
Fluphenazine decanoate should be used cautiously in patients exposed to extreme heat or phosphorus insecticides.
The preparation should be used with caution in patients with a history of convulsive disorders since grand mal convulsions have been known to occur.
Use with caution in patients with special medical disorders such as mitral insufficiency or other cardiovascular diseases and pheochromocytoma.
The possibility of liver damage, pigmentary retinopathy, lenticular and corneal deposits, and development of irreversible dyskinesia should be remembered when patients are on prolonged therapy.
Outside state hospitals or other psychiatric institutions, fluphenazine decanoate should be administered under the direction of a physician experienced in the clinical use of psychotropic drugs, particularly phenothiazine derivatives. Furthermore, facilities should be available for periodic checking of hepatic function, renal function, and the blood picture. Renal function of patients on long-term therapy should be monitored; if BUN (blood urea nitrogen) becomes abnormal, treatment should be discontinued.
As with any phenothiazine, the physician should be alert to the possible development of "silent pneumonias" in patients under treatment with fluphenazine decanoate.
Neuroleptic drugs elevate prolactin levels; the elevation persists during chronic administration. Tissue culture experiments indicate that approximately one-third of human breast cancers are prolactin dependent *in vitro*, a factor of potential importance if the prescription of these drugs is contemplated in a patient with a previously detected breast cancer. Although disturbances such as galactorrhea, amenorrhea, gynecomastia, and impotence have been reported, the clinical significance of elevated serum prolactin levels is unknown for most patients. An increase in mammary neoplasms has been found in rodents after chronic administration of neuroleptic drugs. Neither clinical studies nor epidemiologic studies conducted to date, however, have shown an association between chronic administration of these drugs and mammary tumorigenesis; the available evidence is considered too limited to be conclusive at this time.

Information for Patients

Given the likelihood that a substantial proportion of patients exposed chronically to neuroleptics will develop tardive dyskinesia, it is advised that all patients in whom chronic use is contemplated be given, if possible, full information about this risk. The decision to inform patients and/or their guardians must obviously take into account the clinical circumstances and the competency of the patient to understand the information provided.

ADVERSE REACTIONS

Central Nervous System — The side effects most frequently reported with phenothiazine compounds are extrapyramidal symptoms including pseudoparkinsonism, dystonia, dyskinesia, akathisia, oculogyric crises, opisthotonos, and hyperreflexia. Muscle rigidity sometimes accompanied by hyperthermia has been reported following use of fluphenazine decanoate. Most often these extrapyramidal symptoms are reversible; however, they may be persistent (see below). The frequency of such reactions is related in part to chemical structure: one can expect a higher incidence with fluphenazine decanoate than with less potent piperazine derivatives or with straight-chain phenothiazines such as chlorpromazine. With any given phenothiazine derivative, the incidence and severity of such reactions depend more on individual patient sensitivity than on other factors, but dosage level and patient age are also determinants.

Continued on next page

Princeton—Cont.

Extrapyramidal reactions may be alarming, and the patient should be forewarned and reassured. These reactions can usually be controlled by administration of antiparkinsonian drugs, such as Benztropine Mesylate or intravenous Caffeine and Sodium Benzoate Injection, and by subsequent reduction in dosage.

Tardive Dyskinesia: See WARNINGS. The syndrome is characterized by involuntary choreoathetoid movements which variously involve the tongue, face, mouth, lips, or jaw (e.g., protrusion of the tongue, puffing of cheeks, puckering of the mouth, chewing movements), trunk and extremities. The severity of the syndrome and the degree of impairment produced vary widely.

The syndrome may become clinically recognizable either during treatment, upon dosage reduction, or upon withdrawal of treatment. Early detection of tardive dyskinesia is important. To increase the likelihood of detecting the syndrome at the earliest possible time, the dosage of neuroleptic drug should be reduced periodically (if clinically possible) and the patient observed for signs of the disorder. This maneuver is critical, since neuroleptic drugs may mask the signs of the syndrome.

Other CNS Effects: Rare occurrences of neuroleptic malignant syndrome (NMS) have been reported in patients on neuroleptic therapy. The syndrome is characterized by hyperthermia, muscular rigidity, autonomic instability (labile blood pressure, tachycardia, diaphoresis), akinesia, and altered consciousness, sometimes progressing to stupor or coma. Leukocytosis, elevated CPK, liver function abnormalities, and acute renal failure may also occur. Neuroleptic therapy should be discontinued immediately and vigorous symptomatic treatment implemented since the syndrome is potentially fatal.

Drowsiness or lethargy, if they occur, may necessitate a reduction in dosage; the induction of a catatonic-like state has been known to occur with dosages of fluphenazine far in excess of the recommended amounts. As with other phenothiazine compounds, reactivation or aggravation of psychotic processes may be encountered.

Phenothiazine derivatives have been known to cause, in some patients, restlessness, excitement, or bizarre dreams.

Autonomic Nervous System—Hypertension and fluctuations in blood pressure have been reported with fluphenazine.

Hypotension has rarely presented a problem with fluphenazine. However, patients with pheochromocytoma, cerebral vascular or renal insufficiency, or a severe cardiac reserve deficiency such as mitral insufficiency appear to be particularly prone to hypotensive reactions with phenothiazine compounds, and should therefore be observed closely when the drug is administered. If severe hypotension should occur, supportive measures including the use of intravenous vasopressor drugs should be instituted immediately. Levarterenol Bitartrate Injection is the most suitable drug for this purpose; *epinephrine should not be used* since phenothiazine derivatives have been found to reverse its action, resulting in a further lowering of blood pressure.

Autonomic reactions including nausea and loss of appetite, salivation, polyuria, perspiration, dry mouth, headache, and constipation may occur. Autonomic effects can usually be controlled by reducing or temporarily discontinuing dosage.

In some patients, phenothiazine derivatives have caused blurred vision, glaucoma, bladder paralysis, fecal impaction, paralytic ileus, tachycardia, or nasal congestion.

Metabolic and Endocrine—Weight change, peripheral edema, abnormal lactation, gynecomastia, menstrual irregularities, false results on pregnancy tests, impotency in men and increased libido in women have all been known to occur in some patients on phenothiazine therapy.

Allergic Reactions—Skin disorders such as itching, erythema, urticaria, seborrhea, photosensitivity, eczema and even exfoliative dermatitis have been reported with phenothiazine derivatives. The possibility of anaphylactoid reactions occurring in some patients should be borne in mind.

Hematologic—Routine blood counts are advisable during therapy since blood dyscrasias including leukopenia, agranulocytosis, thrombocytopenic or nonthrombocytopenic purpura, eosinophilia, and pancytopenia have been observed with phenothiazine derivatives. Furthermore, if any soreness of the mouth, gums, or throat, or any symptoms of upper respiratory infection occur and confirmatory leukocyte count indicates cellular depression, therapy should be discontinued and other appropriate measures instituted immediately.

Hepatic—Liver damage as manifested by cholestatic jaundice may be encountered, particularly during the first months of therapy; treatment should be discontinued if this occurs. An increase in cephalin flocculation, sometimes accompanied by alterations in other liver function tests, has been reported in patients receiving the enanthate ester of fluphenazine (a closely related compound) who have had no clinical evidence of liver damage.

Others—Sudden, unexpected and unexplained deaths have been reported in hospitalized psychotic patients receiving phenothiazines. Previous brain damage or seizures may be predisposing factors; high doses should be avoided in known seizure patients. Several patients have shown sudden flare-ups of psychotic behavior patterns shortly before death. Autopsy findings have usually revealed acute fulminating pneumonia or pneumonitis, aspiration of gastric contents, or intramyocardial lesions.

Although this is not a general feature of fluphenazine, potentiation of central nervous system depressants (opiates, analgesics, antihistamines, barbiturates, alcohol) may occur.

The following adverse reactions have also occurred with phenothiazine derivatives: systemic lupus erythematosus-like syndrome, hypotension severe enough to cause fatal cardiac arrest, altered electrocardiographic and electroencephalographic tracings, altered cerebrospinal fluid proteins, cerebral edema, asthma, laryngeal edema, and angioneurotic edema; with long-term use—skin pigmentation and lenticular and corneal opacities.

Injections of fluphenazine decanoate are extremely well tolerated, local tissue reactions occurring only rarely.

DOSAGE AND ADMINISTRATION

Parenteral drug products should be inspected visually for particulate matter and discoloration prior to administration, whenever solution and container permit.

Prolixin Decanoate (Fluphenazine Decanoate Injection) may be given intramuscularly or subcutaneously. A dry syringe and needle of at least 21 gauge should be used. Use of a wet needle or syringe may cause the solution to become cloudy.

To begin therapy with Prolixin Decanoate the following regimens are suggested:

For *most patients,* a dose of 12.5 to 25 mg (0.5 to 1 mL) may be given to initiate therapy. The onset of action generally appears between 24 and 72 hours after injection and the effects of the drug on psychotic symptoms becomes significant within 48 to 96 hours. Subsequent injections and the dosage interval are determined in accordance with the patient's response. When administered as maintenance therapy, a single injection may be effective in controlling schizophrenic symptoms up to four weeks or longer. The response to a single dose has been found to last as long as six weeks in a few patients on maintenance therapy.

It may be advisable that patients who have no history of taking phenothiazines should be treated initially with a shorter-acting form of fluphenazine (see HOW SUPPLIED section for the availability of the shorter-acting fluphenazine hydrochloride dosage forms) before administering the decanoate to determine the patient's response to fluphenazine and to establish appropriate dosage. For psychotic patients who have been stabilized on a fixed daily dosage of Prolixin® Tablets (Fluphenazine Hydrochloride Tablets USP), Elixir (Fluphenazine Hydrochloride Elixir USP), or Oral Concentrate (Fluphenazine Hydrochloride Oral Solution), conversion of therapy from these short-acting oral forms to the long-acting injectable Prolixin Decanoate may be indicated.

Appropriate dosage of Prolixin Decanoate should be individualized for each patient and responses carefully monitored. No precise formula can be given to convert to use of Prolixin Decanoate; however, a controlled multicentered study*, in patients receiving oral doses from 5 to 60 mg fluphenazine hydrochloride daily, showed that 20 mg fluphenazine hydrochloride daily was equivalent to 25 mg (1 mL) Prolixin Decanoate every three weeks. This represents an approximate conversion ratio of 0.5 mL (12.5 mg) of decanoate every three weeks for every 10 mg of fluphenazine hydrochloride daily.

Once conversion to Prolixin Decanoate is made, careful clinical monitoring of the patient and appropriate dosage adjustment should be made at the time of each injection.

Severely agitated patients may be treated with a rapid-acting phenothiazine compound such as Prolixin Injection (Fluphenazine Hydrochloride Injection USP—see package insert accompanying that product for complete information). When acute symptoms have subsided, 25 mg (1 mL) of Prolixin Decanoate may be administered; subsequent dosage is adjusted as necessary.

"Poor risk" patients (those with known hypersensitivity to phenothiazines or with disorders that predispose to undue reactions): Therapy may be initiated cautiously with oral or parenteral fluphenazine hydrochloride (see package inserts accompanying these products for complete information). When the pharmacologic effects and an appropriate dosage are apparent, an equivalent dose of Prolixin Decanoate may be administered. Subsequent dosage adjustments are made in accordance with the response of the patient.

The optimal amount of the drug and the frequency of administration must be determined for each patient, since dosage requirements have been found to vary with clinical circumstances as well as with individual response to the drug.

Dosage should not exceed 100 mg. If doses greater than 50 mg are deemed necessary, the next dose and succeeding doses should be increased cautiously in increments of 12.5 mg.

HOW SUPPLIED

Prolixin Decanoate (Fluphenazine Decanoate Injection) is available in 1 mL Unimatic® single dose preassembled syringes, and 5 mL vials, providing 25 mg fluphenazine decanoate per mL [5 mL vial—Military Depot Item, NSN 6505-01-147-2083, V.A. Depot Item, NSN 6505-00-264-7759A.] Prolixin (fluphenazine) is also available for oral administration as Prolixin Tablets (Fluphenazine Hydrochloride Tablets USP) providing 1, 2.5, 5, and 10 mg fluphenazine hydrochloride per tablet, Prolixin Elixir (Fluphenazine Hydrochloride Elixir USP) providing 0.5 mg fluphenazine hydrochloride per mL (2.5 mg per 5 mL teaspoonful), and Prolixin Oral Concentrate (Fluphenazine Hydrochloride Oral Solution) providing 5 mg fluphenazine hydrochloride per mL.

Storage: Store at room temperature; avoid freezing and excessive heat. Protect from light.

---

*The Initiation of Long-Term Pharmacotherapy in Schizophrenia: Dosage and Side Effect Comparisons Between Oral and Depot Fluphenazine; N.R. Schooler; Pharmakopsych. 9:159-169, 1976.

(J4-014A)

PRONESTYL® INJECTION ℞

Procainamide Hydrochloride Injection USP

PRONESTYL® TABLETS ℞

Procainamide Hydrochloride Tablets

PRONESTYL® CAPSULES ℞

Procainamide Hydrochloride Capsules USP

> The prolonged administration of procainamide often leads to the development of a positive anti-nuclear antibody (ANA) test, with or without symptoms of lupus erythematosus-like syndrome. If a positive ANA titer develops, the benefits versus risks of continued procainamide therapy should be assessed. This may necessitate consideration of alternative antiarrythmic therapy.

DESCRIPTION

Pronestyl (procainamide hydrochloride), a Group 1A cardiac antiarrhythmic drug, is p-amino-N-[2-(diethylamino)ethyl]-benzamide monohydrochloride, molecular weight 271.79.

It differs from procaine which is the p-aminobenzoyl *ester* of 2-(diethylamino)-ethanol. Procainamide as the free base has a pK_a of 9.23; the monohydrochloride is very soluable in water.

Pronestyl Injection is a sterile, aqueous solution for intramuscular or intravenous use providing 100 mg or 500 mg procainamide hydrochloride per mL. The 100 mg/mL potency contains 9 mg/mL of benzyl alcohol and not more than 0.9 mg/mL sodium bisulfite as preservatives; the 500 mg/mL potency contains 1 mg/mL methylparaben and not more than 2 mg sodium bisulfite as preservatives. In both formulations, the pH has been adjusted to 5.0 ± 1.0 with hydrochloric acid and/or sodium hydroxide. At the time of manufacture, the air in the containers is replaced by nitrogen.

Pronestyl is supplied for oral administration as capsules and tablets in potencies of 250, 375, and 500 mg. Inactive ingredients: Tablets—calcium silicate, cellulose, colorants [FD&C Yellow No. 5 (tartrazine) and Yellow No. 6], flavor, povidone, starch, stearic acid, and other ingredients. Capsules—colorants (D&C Yellow No. 10, except 375 mg; FD&C Yellow No. 6), gelatin, lactose (except 500 mg), magnesium stearate, talc, and titanium dioxide.

CLINICAL PHARMACOLOGY

Procainamide (PA) increases the effective refractory period of the atria, and to a lesser extent the bundle of His-Purkinje system and ventricles of the heart. It reduces impulse conduction velocity in the atria, His-Purkinje fibers, and ventricular muscle, but has variable effects on the atrioventricular (A-V) node, a direct slowing action and a weaker vagolytic effect which may speed A-V conduction slightly. Myocardial excitability is reduced in the atria, Purkinje fibers, papillary muscles, and ventricles by an increase in the threshold for excitation, combined with inhibition of ectopic pacemaker activity by retardation of the slow phase of diastolic depolarization, thus decreasing automaticity especially in ectopic sites. Contractility of the undamaged heart is usually not affected by therapeutic concentrations, although slight reduction of cardiac output may occur, and may be significant in the presence of myocardial damage. Therapeutic levels of PA may exert vagolytic effects and produce slight acceleration of heart rate, while high or toxic concentrations may prolong A-V conduction time or induce A-V block, or even cause abnormal automaticity and spontaneous firing, by unknown mechanisms.

The electrocardiogram may reflect these effects by showing slight sinus tachycardia (due to anticholinergic action) and widened QRS complexes and, less regularly, prolonged Q-T and P-R intervals (due to longer systole and slower conduction), as well as some decreases in QRS and T wave amplitude. These direct effects of PA on electrical activity, conduction, responsiveness, excitability and automaticity are characteristic of Group 1A antiarrhythmic agent, the prototype for which is quinidine; PA effects are very similar. However, PA has weaker vagal blocking action than does quinidine, does not induce alpha-adrenergic blockade, and is less depressing to cardiac contractility.

Following intramuscular injection, Pronestyl Injection (Procainamide Hydrochloride Injection USP) is rapidly absorbed into the bloodstream, and plasma levels peak in 15 to 60 minutes, considerably faster than orally administered forms. Intravenous administration of Pronestyl can produce therapeutic procainamide levels within minutes after infusion is started. About 15 to 20 percent of PA is reversibly bound to plasma proteins, and considerable amounts are more slowly and reversibly bound to tissues of the heart, liver, lung, and kidney. The apparent volume of distribution eventually reaches about 2 liters per kilogram body weight with a half-time of approximately five minutes. While PA has been shown in the dog to cross the blood-brain barrier, it did not concentrate in the brain at levels higher than in plasma. It is not known if PA crosses the placenta. Plasma esterases are far less active in hydrolysis of PA than of procaine. The half-time for elimination is three to four hours in patients with normal renal function, but reduced creatinine clearance and advancing age each prolong the renal PA elimination half-time.

Ingested PA is resistant to digestive hydrolysis, and the drug is well absorbed from the entire small intestinal surface, but individual patients vary in their completeness of absorption of PA. Following oral administration of Pronestyl, plasma PA levels reach about 50 percent of peak in 30 minutes, 90 percent at an hour, and peak at about 90 to 120 minutes.

A significant fraction of the circulating PA may be metabolized in hepatocytes to N-acetylprocainamide (NAPA), ranging from 16 to 21 percent of an administered dose in "slow acetylators" to 24 to 33 percent in "fast-acetylators". Since NAPA also has significant antiarrhythmic activity and somewhat slower renal clearance than PA, both hepatic acetylation rate capability and renal function, as well as age, have significant effects on the effective biological half-time of therapeutic action of adminstered PA and the NAPA derivative. Trace amounts may be excreted in the urine as free and conjugated p-aminobenzoic acid, 30 to 60 percent as unchanged PA, and 6 to 52 percent as the NAPA derivative. Both PA and NAPA are eliminated by active tubular secretion as well as by glomerular filtration. Action of PA on the central nervous system is not prominent, but high plasma concentrations may cause tremors. While therapeutic plasma levels for PA have been reported to be 3 to 10 μg/mL, certain patients such as those with sustained ventricular tachycardia may need higher levels for adequate control. This may justify the increased risk of toxicity (see OVERDOSAGE). Where programmed ventricular stimulation has been used to evaluate efficacy of PA in preventing recurrent ventricular tachyarrhythmias, higher plasma levels (mean, 13.6 μg/mL) of PA were found necessary for adequate control.

INDICATIONS AND USAGE

Pronestyl (procainamide hydrochloride) is indicated in the treatment of ventricular premature contractions, and in preventing recurrence of ventricular tachycardia after conversion to sinus rhythm by intravenous drugs or by electrical cardioversion or by other antiarrhythmic therapy; also in preventing recurrence of paroxysmal supraventricular tachycardia, atrial fibrillation or flutter following conversion to sinus rhythm by initial vagotonic maneuvers, digitalis preparations, other pharmaceutical antiarrhythmic agents, or electrical cardioversion. The injection formulation is particularly appropriate in patients who cannot swallow, absorb, or otherwise tolerate oral administration of PA.

CONTRAINDICATIONS

Complete heart block: Procainamide should not be administered to patients with complete heart block because of its effects in suppressing nodal or ventricular pacemakers and the hazard of asystole. It may be difficult to recognize complete heart block in patients with ventricular tachycardia, but if significant slowing of ventricular rate occurs during PA treatment without eivdence of A-V conduction appearing, PA should be stopped. In cases of second degree A-V block or various types of hemiblock, PA should be avoided or discontinued because of the possibility of increased severity of block, unless the ventricular rate is controlled by an electrical pacemaker.

Torsades de Pointes: In the unusual ventricular arrhythmia called "les torsades de pointes" (twistings of the points), characterized by alternation of one or more ventricular premature beats in the directions of the QRS complexes on ECG in persons with prolonged Q-T and often enhanced U waves, Group 1A antiarrhythmic drugs are contraindicated. Administration of PA in such cases may aggravate this special type of ventricular extrasystole or tachycardia instead of suppressing it.

Idiosyncratic hypersensitivity: In patients sensitive to procaine or other ester-type local anesthetics, cross sensitivity to PA is unlikely; however, it should be borne in mind, and PA should not be used if it produces acute allergic dermatitis, asthma, or anaphylactic symptoms.

Lupus Erythematosus: An established diagnosis of systemic lupus erythematosus is a contraindication to PA therapy, since aggravation of symptoms is highly likely.

WARNINGS

Digitalis intoxication—Caution should be exercised in the use of procainamide in arrhythmias associated with digitalis intoxication. Procainamide can suppress digitalis-induced arrhythmias; however, if there is concomitant marked disturbance of atrioventricular conduction, additional depression of conduction and ventricular asystole or fibrillation may result. Therefore, use of procainamide should be considered only if discontinuation of digitalis, and therapy with potassium, lidocaine, or phenytoin are ineffective.

First degree heart block—Caution should be exercised also if the patient exhibits or develops first degree heart block while taking PA, and dosage reduction is advised in such cases. If the block persists despite dosage reduction, continuation of PA administration must be evaluated on the basis of current benefit versus risk of increased heart block.

Predigitalization for atrial flutter or fibrillation—Patients with atrial flutter or fibrillation should be cardioverted or digitalized prior to PA administration to avoid enhancement of A-V conduction which may result in ventricular rate acceleration beyond tolerable limits. Adequate digitalization reduces but does not eliminate the possibility of sudden increase in ventricular rate as the atrial rate is slowed by PA in these arrhythmias.

Congestive heart failure—For patients in congestive heart failure, and those with acute ischemic heart disease or cardiomyopathy, caution should be used in PA therapy, since even slight depression of myocardial contractility may further reduce cardiac output of the damaged heart.

Concurrent other antiarrhythmic agents—Concurrent use of PA with other Group 1A antiarrhythmic agents such as quinidine or disopyramide may produce enhanced prolongation of conduction or depression of contractility and hypotension, especially in patients with cardiac decompensation. Such use should be reserved for patients with serious arrhythmias unresponsive to a single drug and employed only if close observation is possible.

Renal insufficiency—Renal insufficiency may lead to accumulation of high plasma levels from conventional oral doses of PA, with effects similar to those of overdosage (see OVERDOSAGE), unless dosage is adjusted for the individual patient.

Myasthenia gravis—Patients with myasthenia gravis may show worsening of symptoms from PA due to its procaine-like effect on diminishing acetylcholine release at skeletal muscle motor nerve endings, so that PA administration may be hazardous without optimal adjustment of anticholinesterase medications and other precautions.

PRECAUTIONS

Procainamide Hydrochloride Injection USP—Blood-pressure and ECG monitoring: Blood pressure should be monitored with the patient supine during parenteral, especially intravenous, administration of PA (see DOSAGE AND AMINISTRATION). There is a possibility that relatively high although transient plasma levels of PA may be attained and cause hypotension before the PA can be distributed from the plasma volume to its full apparent volume of distribution which is approximately 50 times greater. Therefore, caution should be exercised to avoid overly rapid administration of PA. If the blood pressure falls 15 mm Hg or more, PA administration should be temporarily discontinued. Electrocardiographic (ECG) monitoring is advisable as well, both for observation of the progress and response of the arrhythmia under treatment, and for early detection of any tendency to excessive widening of the QRS complex, prolongation of the P-R interval, or any signs of heart block (see OVERDOSAGE). Parenteral therapy with PA should be limited to use in hospitals in which monitoring and intensive supportive care are available, or to emergency situations in which equivalent observation and treatment can be provided.

General—Immediately after initiation of PA therapy, patients should be closely observed for possible hypersensitivity reactions, especially if procaine or local anesthetic sensitivity is suspected, and for muscular weakness if myasthenia gravis is a possibility. In conversion of atrial fibrillation to normal sinus rhythm by any means, dislodgement of mural thrombi may lead to embolization, which should be kept in mind. In conversion of atrial fibrillation to normal sinus rhythm by any means, dislodgement of mural thrombi may lead to emoblization, which should be kept in mind.

After a day or so, steady state plasma PA levels are produced following regular oral administration of a given dose of Pronestyl (Procainamide Hydrochloride Tablets; Procainamide Hydrochloride Capsules) at set intervals, with peak plasma concentrations at about 90 to 120 minutes after each dose. After achieving and maintaining therapeutic plasma concentrations and satisfactory electrocardiographic and clinical responses, continued frequent periodic monitoring of vital signs and electrocardiograms is advised. If evidence of QRS widening of more than 25 percent or marked prolongation of the Q-T interval occurs, concern for overdosage is appropriate, and reduction in dosage, or interruption of the PA infusion, is advisable if a 50 percent increase occurs. Elevated serum creatinine or urea nitrogen, reduced creatinine clearance, or history of renal insufficiency, as well as use in older patients (over age 50), provide grounds to anticipate that less than the usual dosage and longer time intervals between doses may suffice, since the urinary elimination of PA and NAPA may be reduced, leading to gradual accumulation beyond normally-predicted amounts. If facilities are available for measurement of plasma PA and NAPA, or acetylation capability, individual dose adjustment for optimal therapeutic levels may be easier, but close observation of clinical effectiveness is the most important criterion.

In the longer term, periodic complete blood counts are useful to detect possible idiosyncratic hematologic effects of PA on neutrophil, platelet or red cell homeostasis; agranulocytosis has been reported to occur occasionally in patients on long-term PA therapy. A rising titer of serum ANA may precede clinical symptoms of the lupoid syndrome (see BOX WARNING and ADVERSE REACTIONS). If the lupus erythematosus-like syndrome develops in a patient with recurrent life-threatening arrhythmias not controlled by other agents, corticosteroid suppressive therapy may be used concomitantly with PA. Since the PA-induced lupoid syndrome rarely includes the dangerous pathologic renal changes, PA therapy may not necessarily have to be stopped unless the symptoms of serositis and the possibility of further lupoid effects are of greater risk than the benefit of PA in controlling arrhythmias. Patients with rapid acetylation capability are less likely to develop the lupoid syndrome after prolonged PA therapy.

Pronestyl Tablets (Procainamide Hydrochloride Tablets) contain FD&C Yellow No. 5 (tartrazine) which may cause allergic-type reactions (including bronchial asthma) in certain susceptible individuals. Although the overall incidence of FD&C Yellow No. 5 (tartrazine) sensitivity in the general population is low, it is frequently seen in patients who also have aspirin hypersensitivity.

Information for Patients—The patient should be encouraged to disclose any past history of drug sensitivity, especially to procaine or other local anesthetic agents, or aspirin, and to report any history of kidney disease, congestive heart failure, myasthenia gravis, liver disease, or lupus erythematosus.

The physician is advised to explain to the patient that close cooperation in adhering to the prescribed oral maintainance dosage schedule is of great importance in controlling the cardiac arrhythmia safely. The patient should understand clearly that more medication is not necessarily better and may be dangerous, that skipping doses or increasing intervals between doses to suit personal convenience may lead to loss of control of the heart problem, and that "making up" missed doses by doubling up later may be hazardous.

The patient should be counseled to report promptly any symptoms of arthralgia, myalgia, fever, chills, skin rash, easy bruising, sore throat or sore mouth, infections, dark urine or icterus, wheezing, muscular weakness, chest or abdominal pain, palpitations, nausea, vomiting, anorexia, diarrhea, hallucinations, dizziness, or depression.

Laboratory Tests—Laboratory tests such as complete blood count (CBC), electrocardiogram, and serum creatinine or urea nitrogen may be indicated, depending on the clinical situation, and baseline and periodic rechecking of the CBC and ANA may be helpful in early detection of untoward reactions, especially with long-term PA treatment.

Drug Interactions—If other antiarrhythmic drugs are being used, additive effects on the heart may occur with PA administration, and dosage reduction may be necessary (see WARNINGS). Anticholinergic drugs administered concurrently with PA may produce additive antivagal effects on A-V nodal conduction, although this is not as well documented for PA as for quinidine. Patients taking PA who require neuromuscular blocking agents such as succinylcholine may require less than usual doses of the latter, due to PA effects on reducing acetylcholine release.

Drug/Laboratory Test Interactions—Suprapharmacologic concentrations of lidocaine and meprobamate may inhibit fluorescence of PA and NAPA, and propranolol shows a native fluorescence close to the PA/NAPA peak wavelengths, so that tests which depend on fluorescence measurement may be affected.

Carcinogenesis, Mutagenesis, Impairment of Fertility—Long term studies in animals have not been performed.

Teratogenic Effects: Pregnancy Category C—Animal reproduction studies have not been conducted with PA. It also is not known whether PA can cause fetal harm when administered to a pregnant woman or can affect reproduction capacity. PA should be given to a pregnant woman only if clearly needed.

Continued on next page

Princeton—Cont.

Nursing Mothers—Both PA and NAPA are excreted in human milk, and absorbed by the nursing infant. Because of the potential for serious adverse reactions in nursing infants, a decision to discontinue nursing or the drug should be made, taking into account the importance of the drug to the mother.

Pediatric Use—Safety and effectiveness in children have not been established.

ADVERSE REACTIONS

Cardiovascular system: Hypotension and serious disturbances of cardiorhythm such as ventricular asystole or fibrillation are more common with intravenous administration of PA than with intramuscular administration. Because PA is a peripheral vasodilator in concentrations higher than the usual therapeutic range, transient high plasma levels which may occur especially during intravenous administration may produce temporary but at times severe lowering of blood pressure (see OVERDOSAGE, WARNINGS, and PRECAUTIONS). Hypotension following oral PA administration is rare. Second degree heart block has been reported in 2 of almost 500 patients taking PA orally.

Multisystem effects: A lupus erythematosus-like syndrome of arthralgia, pleural or abdominal pain, and sometimes arthritis, pleural effusion, pericarditis, fever, chills, myalgia, and possibly related hematologic or skin lesions (see below) is fairly common after prolonged PA administration, perhaps more often in patients who are slow acetylators (see BOX WARNING and PRECAUTIONS). While some series have reported less than 1 in 500, others have reported the syndrome in up to 30 percent of patients on long term oral PA therapy. If discontinuation of PA does not reverse the lupoid symptoms, corticosteroid treatment may be effective.

Hematologic system: Neutropenia, thrombocytopenia, or hemolytic anemia may rarely be encountered. Agranulocytosis has occurred after repeated use of PA, and deaths have been reported.

Skin: Angioneurotic edema, urticaria, pruritus, flushing, and maculopapular rash have also occurred occasionally.

Gastrointestinal system: Anorexia, nausea, vomiting, abdominal pain, bitter taste, or diarrhea may occur in 3 to 4 percent of patients taking oral procainamide. Hepatomegaly with increased serum aminotransferase activity have been reported after a single oral dose.

Nervous system: Dizziness or giddiness, weakness, mental depression, and psychosis with hallucinations have been reported occasionally.

OVERDOSAGE

Progressive widening of the QRS complex, prolonged Q-T and P-R intervals, lowering of the R and T waves, as well as increasing A-V block, may be seen with doses which are excessive for a given patient. Increased ventricular extrasystoles, or even ventricular tachycardia or fibrillation may occur. After intravenous administration but seldom after oral therapy, transient high plasma levels of PA may induce hypotension, affecting systolic more than diastolic pressures, especially in hypertensive patients. Such high levels may also produce central nervous depression, tremor, and even respiratory depression.

Plasma levels above 10 μg /mL are increasingly associated with toxic findings, which are seen occasionally in the 10 to 12 μg/mL range, more often in the 12 to 15 μg/mL range, and commonly in patients with plasma levels greater than 15 μg/mL. A single oral dose of 2 g may produce overdosage symptoms, while 3 g may be dangerous, especially if the patient is a slow acetylator, has decreased renal function, or underlying organic heart disease.

Treatment of overdosage or toxic manifestations includes general supportive measures, close observation, monitoring of vital signs and possibly intravenous pressor agents and mechanical cardiorespiratory support. If available, PA and NAPA plasma levels may be helpful in assessing the potential degree of toxicity and response to therapy. Both PA and NAPA are removed from the circulation by hemodialysis but not peritoneal dialysis. No specific antidote for PA is known.

DOSAGE AND ADMINISTRATION

Pronestyl Injection (Procainamide Hydrochloride Injection) is useful for arrhythmias which require immediate suppression and for maintenance of arrhythmia control. Intravenous therapy allows most rapid control of serious arrhythmias, including those following myocardial infarction; it should be carried out in circumstances where close observation and monitoring of the patient are possible, such as in hospital or emergency facilities. Intramuscular administration is less apt to produce temporary high plasma levels but therapeutic plasma levels are not obtained as rapidly as with intravenous administration. Oral procainamide dosage forms are preferable for less urgent arrhythmias as well as for long-term maintenance after initial parenteral PA therapy.

Intramuscular administration may be used as an alternative to the oral route for patients with less threatening arrhythmias but who are nauseated or vomiting, who are ordered to receive nothing by mouth preoperatively, or who may have malabsorptive problems. An initial daily dose of 50 mg per kg body weight may be estimated. This amount should be divided into fractional doses of one eighth to one quarter to be injected intramuscularly every three to six hours until oral therapy is possible. If more than three injections are given, the physician may wish to assess patient factors such as age and renal function (see below), clinical response and, if available, blood levels of PA and NAPA in adjusting further doses for that individual. For treatment of arrhythmias associated with anesthesia or surgical operation, the suggested dose is 100 to 500 mg by intramuscular injection.

Intravenous administration of Pronestyl Injection should be done cautiously to avoid a possible hypotensive response (see PRECAUTIONS and OVERDOSAGE). Initial arrhythmia control, under ECG monitoring, may usually be accomplished safely within a half-hour by either of the two methods which follows:

a) Direct injection into a vein or into tubing of an established infusion line should be done slowly at a rate not to exceed 50 mg per minute. It is advisable to dilute either the 100 mg/mL or the 500 mg/mL concentrations of Pronestyl Injection prior to intravenous injection to facilitate control of dosage rate. Doses of 100 mg may be administered every 5 minutes at this rate until the arrhythmia is suppressed or until 500 mg has been administered, after which it is advisable to wait 10 minutes or longer to allow for more distribution into tissues before resuming.

b) Alternatively, a loading infusion containing 20 mg of Pronestyl per mL (1 g diluted to 50 mL with 5% Dextrose Injection USP) may be administered at a constant rate of 1 mL per minute for 25 to 30 minutes to deliver 500 to 600 mg of PA. Some effects may be seen after infustion of the first 100 or 200 mg; it is unusual to require more than 600 mg to achieve satisfactory antiarrhythmic effects.

The maximum advisable dosage to be given either by repeated bolus injections or such loading infusion is 1 g.

To maintain therapeutic levels, a more dilute intravenous infusion at a concentration of 2 mg/mL is convenient (1 g Pronestyl in 500 mL of 5% Dextrose Injection USP), and may be administered at 1 to 3 mL/minute. If daily total fluid intake must be limited, a 4 mg/mL concentration (1 g of Pronestyl Injection [Procainamide Hydrochloride Injection] in 250 mL of 5% Dextrose Injection USP) administered at 0.5 to 1.5 mL/minute will deliver an equivalent 2 to 6 mg per minute. The amount needed in a given patient to maintain the therapeutic level should be assessed principally from the clinical response, and will depend upon the patient's weight and age, renal elimination, hepatic acetylation rate, and cardiac status, but should be adjusted for each patient based upon close observation. A maintenance infusion rate of 50 μg/min/kg body weight to a person with a normal renal PA elimination half-time of three hours may be expected to produce a plasma level of approximately 6.5 μg/mL.

[See table below].

Since the principal route for elimination of PA and NAPA is renal excretion, reduced excretion will prolong the half-life of elimination and lower the dose rate needed to maintain therapeutic levels. Advancing age reduces the renal excretion of PA and NAPA independently of reductions in creatinine clearance; compared to normal young adults, there is approximately 25 percent reduction at age 50 and 50 percent at age 75.

Intravenous therapy should be terminated if persistent conduction disturbances or hypotension develop. As soon as the patient's basic cardiac rhythm appears to be stabilized, oral antiarrhythmic maintenance therapy is preferable, if indicated and possible. A period of about three to four hours (one half-time for renal elimination, ordinarily) should elapse after the last intraveneous dose before administering the first dose of Pronestyl Tablets or Capsules.

Parenteral drug products should be examined visually for particulate matter and discoloration (see HOW SUPPLIED) prior to administration.

Oral Pronestyl (Procainamide Hydrochloride Tablets; Procainamide Hydrochloride Capsules) therapy is preferred for treatment of arrhythmias which do not require immediate suppression, and for prevention of recurrence of serious arrhythmias after initial control by cardioversion, by intravenous Pronestyl Injection (Procainamide Hydrochloride Injection USP) or by other antiarrhythmic therapy.

Ideally, the oral dose and interval of administration should be adjusted for the individual patient, based on clinical assessment of the degree of underlying myocardial disease, the patient's age, and renal function.

As a general guide, for younger patients with normal renal function, an initial total daily oral dose of up to 50 mg/kg of body weight of Pronestyl Capsules or Tablets may be used, given in divided doses, every three hours, to maintain therapeutic blood levels. For older patients, especially those over 50 years of age, or for patients with renal, hepatic, or cardiac insufficiency, lesser amounts or longer intervals may produce adequate blood levels. The initial total daily dose should be divided for administration at three, four, or six hour intervals as estimated for the patient's needs; then, the dose and interval should be adjusted for the individual.

to provide up to 50 mg per kg of body weight per day:*

Patients weighing:

088–110	(40–50 kg)	250 mg q3 hrs to 500 mg q6 hrs
132–154	(60–70 kg)	375 mg q3 hrs to 750 mg q6 hrs
176–198	(80–90 kg)	500 mg q3 hrs to 1 g q6 hrs
> 220 lb	(> 100 kg)	625 mg q3 hrs to 1.25 g q6 hrs

*Initial dosage schedule guide only, to be adjusted for each patient individually, based on age, cardiorenal function, blood level (if available), and clinical response.

DILUTIONS AND RATES FOR INTRVENOUS INFUSIONS*
PRONESTYL INJECTION (PROCAINAMIDE HYDROCHLORIDE INJECTION)

	Final Concentration	Infusion Volume†	Pronestyl To Be Added	Infusion Rate
Initial Loading Infusion	20 mg/mL	50 mL	1000 mg	1 mL/min (for up to 25–30 min*)
Maintenance infusion	2 mg/mL	500 mL	1000 mg	1 to 3 mL/min
	or			
	4 mg/mL	250 mL	1000 mg	0.5 to 1.5 mL/min

The maintenance infusion rates are calculated to deliver 2 to 6 mg per minute, depending on body weight, renal elimination rate, and steady-state plasma level needed to maintain control of the arrhythmia*. The 4 mg/mL maintenance concentration may be preferred if total infused volume must be limited.

† All infusions should be made up to final volume with 5% Dextrose Injection USP.)
* Please see text under DOSAGE AND ADMINISTRATION for further details. The flow rate of any intravenous procainamide infusion must be monitored closely to avoid transiently high plasma levels and possible hypotension (see PRECAUTIONS).

HOW SUPPLIED

Pronestyl Injection (Procainamide Hydrochloride Injection USP) is available as a sterile, aqueous solution in either 10 mL vials containing 100 mg procainamide hydrochloride per mL or 2 mL vials containing 500 mg procainamide hydrochloride per mL. The solutions, which are clear and colorless initially, may develop a slight yellow color in time. This does not indicate a change which should preclude its use, but a solution any darker than light amber or otherwise discolored should not be used.

*Pronestyl Tablets (Procainamide Hydrochloride Tablets) are available as FILMLOK® tablets: **250 mg** in bottles of 100 and 1000, **375 mg** in bottles of 100, and **500 mg** in bottles of 100. (**FILMLOK** is a Squibb trademark for veneer-coated tablets.) Tablet color and identification numbers: 250 mg yellow, **431**; 375 mg orange, **434**; 500 mg red, **438**.

*Pronestyl Capsules (Procainamide Hydrochloride Capsules USP) are available as two-piece gelatin capsules: **250 mg** in bottles of 100 and 1000, **375 mg** in bottles of 100, and **500 mg** in bottles of 100 and 1000. Unimatic® unit-dose packs containing 100 capsules are also available for each potency. Capsule color and identification numbers: 250 mg yellow, **758**; 375 mg white and orange, **756**; 500 mg yellow and orange, **757**.

Storage: Store Pronestyl Injection between 50° and 80°F (10° and 27°C). Store Pronestyl Tablets and Capsules at room temperature; avoid excessive heat; protect from moisture.
(J3-301E/J4-020A)

Shown in Product Identification Section, page 422

PRONESTYL-SR® TABLETS ℞

[pro″nest′tl es-ahr]
(Procainamide Hydrochloride Tablets)

> The prolonged administration of procainamide often leads to the development of a positive antinuclear antibody (ANA) test with or without symptoms of lupus erythematosus-like syndrome. If a positive ANA titer develops, the benefit/risk ratio related to continued procainamide therapy should be assessed. This may necessitate consideration of alternative antiarrhythmic therapy.

DESCRIPTION

Procainamide hydrochloride is the amide analogue of procaine hydrochloride. Chemically, procainamide hydrochloride is p-Amino-N-[2-(diethylamino)ethyl] benzamide monohydrochloride.
Pronestyl-SR Tablets (Procainamide Hydrochloride Tablets), containing 500 mg procainamide hydrochloride, are for oral administration. The tablet matrix is specially designed for the prolonged release of the drug in the gastrointestinal tract.

CLINICAL PHARMACOLOGY

Procainamide depresses the excitability of cardiac muscle to electrical stimulation and slows conduction in the atrium, the bundle of His, and the ventricle. The refractory period of the atrium is considerably more prolonged than that of the ventricle. Contractility of the heart is usually not affected, nor is cardiac output decreased to any extent unless myocardial damage exists. In the absence of any arrhythmia, the heart rate may occasionally be accelerated by conventional doses, suggesting that the drug possesses anticholinergic properties. Larger doses can induce atrioventricular block and ventricular extrasystoles which may proceed to ventricular fibrillation. These effects on the myocardium are reflected in the electrocardiogram; a widening of the QRS complex occurs most consistently; less regularly, the P-R and Q-T intervals are prolonged, and the QRS and T waves show some decrease in voltage.
Following oral administration q6h, the tablets achieve a mean steady state of procainamide (as well as procainamide plus N-acetylprocainamide) serum concentrations approximately equivalent to those from a comparable dose of Pronestyl® Capsules (Procainamide Hydrochloride Capsules USP) q3h. Pronestyl-SR Tablets (Procainamide Hydrochloride Tablets) have a half-life which is significantly longer than that of the capsules.
The specially-formulated tablet coating and core of Pronestyl-SR (Procainamide Hydrochloride Tablets) was designed to provide the biopharmaceutic characteristics of a sustained and relatively constant rate of release and absorption throughout the entire small intestine.
Therapeutic plasma levels have been reported to be 3 to 10 mcg/mL, with those for the majority of patients in the range of 4 to 8 mcg/mL.
Procainamide is less readily hydrolyzed than procaine, and plasma levels decline slowly—about 10 to 20 percent per hour for standard dosage forms of procainamide. The drug is excreted primarily in the urine, with an average of about 60 percent being excreted unchanged; about 10 percent is excreted as free and conjugated p-aminobenzoic acid. The fate of the remainder is unknown.

INDICATIONS AND USAGE

Pronestyl-SR (Procainamide Hydrochloride Tablets) are indicated in the treatment of premature ventricular contractions and ventricular tachycardia, atrial fibrillation, and paroxysmal atrial tachycardia.

CONTRAINDICATIONS

It has been suggested that procainamide be contraindicated in patients with myasthenia gravis. Hypersensitivity to the drug is an absolute contraindication; in this connection, cross sensitivity to procaine and related drugs must be borne in mind. Procainamide should not be administered to patients with complete atrioventricular heart block. Procainamide is also contraindicated in cases of second degree and third degree A-V block unless an electrical pacemaker is operative.

PRECAUTIONS

During administration of the drug, evidence of untoward myocardial responses should be carefully watched for in all patients. In the presence of an abnormal myocardium, procainamide may at times produce untoward responses. In atrial fibrillation or flutter, the ventricular rate may increase suddenly as the atrial rate is slowed. Adequate digitalization reduces, but does not abolish this danger. If myocardial damage exists, ventricular tachysystole is particularly hazardous. Correction of atrial fibrillation, with resultant forceful contractions of the atrium, may cause a dislodgment of mural thrombi and produce an embolic episode. However, it has been suggested that in a patient who is already discharging emboli, procainamide is more likely to stop than to aggravate the process.
Attempts to adjust the heart rate in a patient who has developed ventricular tachycardia during an occlusive coronary episode should be carried out with extreme caution. Caution is also required in marked disturbances of atrioventricular conduction such as second degree and third degree A-V block, bundle branch block, or severe digitalis intoxication, where the use of procainamide may result in additional depression of conduction and ventricular asystole or fibrillation.
Since patients with severe heart disease and ventricular tachycardia may also have complete heart block which is difficult to diagnose under these circumstances, this complication should always be kept in mind when treating ventricular arrhythmias with procainamide. If the ventricular rate is significantly slowed by procainamide without attainment of regular atrioventricular conduction, the drug should be stopped and the patient reevaluated as asystole may result under these circumstances.
In patients receiving normal dosage, but who have both liver and kidney disease, symptoms of overdosage (principally ventricular tachycardia and severe hypotension) may occur due to drug accumulation.
Instances of a syndrome resembling lupus erythematosus have been reported in connection with oral maintenance procainamide therapy. The mechanism of this syndrome is uncertain. Polyarthralgia, arthritis, and pleuritic pain are common symptoms; to a lesser extent fever, myalgia, skin lesions, pleural effusion and pericarditis may occur. Rare cases of thrombocytopenia or Coombs positive hemolytic anemia have been reported which may be related to this syndrome. Patients receiving procainamide for extended periods of time or in whom symptoms suggestive of lupus-like reaction appear should have anti-nuclear antibody titers measured at regular intervals. If there is a rising titer (anti-nuclear antibody) or clinical symptoms of LE appear, the drug should be discontinued. The LE syndrome may be reversible upon discontinuance of the drug. If discontinuation of the drug does not cause remission of the symptoms, steroid therapy may be effective. If the syndrome develops in a patient with recurrent life-threatening arrhythmias not controllable by other antiarrhythmic agents, steroid suppressive therapy may be used concomitantly with procainamide.

ADVERSE REACTIONS

Hypotension following oral administration is rare. Serious disturbances of cardiac rhythm such as ventricular asystole or fibrillation are more common with intravenous administration.
Large oral doses of procainamide may sometimes produce anorexia, nausea, urticaria, and/or pruritus.
A syndrome resembling lupus erythematosus has been reported in patients on oral maintenance therapy (see PRECAUTIONS). Reactions consisting of fever and chills have also been reported, including a case with fever and chills plus nausea, vomiting, abdominal pain, acute hepatomegaly, and a rise in serum glutamic oxaloacetic transaminase following single doses of the drug. Bitter taste, diarrhea, weakness, mental depression, giddiness, and psychosis with hallucinations have been reported. The possibility of such untoward effects should be borne in mind.
Hypersensitivity reactions such as angioneurotic edema and maculopapular rash have also occurred.
Agranulocytosis has occasionally followed the repeated use of the drug, and deaths have occurred. Therefore, routine blood counts are advisable during maintenance procainamide therapy. The patients should be instructed to report any soreness of the mouth, throat, or gums, unexplained fever or any symptoms of upper respiratory tract infection. If any of these should occur, and leukocyte counts indicate cellular depression, procainamide therapy should be discontinued and appropriate treatment should be instituted immediately.

DOSAGE AND ADMINISTRATION

Initial Therapy:
Pronestyl-SR Tablets (Procainamide Hydrochloride Tablets) are a sustained-release dosage form not intended for initial therapy. For initial therapy by oral administration, conventional oral formulations of Pronestyl (procainamide hydrochloride) are recommended (see HOW SUPPLIED).
The duration of action of procainamide hydrochloride supplied in this sustained release dosage form allows dosing at intervals of every six hours, a schedule which may encourage patient compliance.
For control of arrhythmias requiring immediate suppression, Pronestyl Injection (Procainamide Hydrochloride Injection USP)—see HOW SUPPLIED) or other antiarrhythmic therapy is recommended; following interruption of the arrhythmia, or when the limit of tolerance is reached, Pronestyl-SR is indicated for maintenance.
Maintenance Therapy:
Dosage:
Ventricular Tachycardia and Premature Ventricular Contractions—The suggested maintenance dosage of Pronestyl-SR (Procainamide Hydrochloride Tablets) is 50 mg/kg of body weight daily given in divided doses at six hour intervals.
To provide approximately 50 mg per kg per day: Give patients weighing less than 120 lbs (less than 55 kg) 500 mg q6h; give patients between 120 and 200 lbs (55 to 91 kg) 500 mg or 1 g q6h; and give patients over 200 lbs (more than 91 kg) 1 g q6h. This dosage schedule is for use as a guide for treating the average patient; however, each patient must be considered on an individual basis.
Atrial Fibrillation and Paroxysmal Atrial Tachycardia—The suggested maintenance dosage for Pronestyl-SR is 1 g every six hours.
Administration:
Patients should be advised not to break or chew the tablet, as this would interfere with designed dissolution characteristics. The tablet matrix may be seen in the stool since it does not disintegrate following release of procainamide.

HOW SUPPLIED

Pronestyl-SR Tablets (Procainamide Hydrochloride Tablets) are available as FILMLOK® tablets containing 500 mg procainamide hydrochloride; these tablets are unscored, biconvex, greenish-yellow elongated ovals and are available in bottles of 100 and Unimatic® cartons of 100. (FILMLOK is a Squibb trademark for veneer-coated tablets.)
Also Available: For initial therapy, available oral dosage forms include Pronestyl Capsules (Procainamide Hydrochloride Capsules USP) and conventionally-formulated capsule-shaped FILMLOK Pronestyl Tablets (Procainamide Hydrochloride Tablets); tablets and capsules are available in potencies of 250 mg, 375 mg, and 500 mg procainamide hydrochloride. Consult the common package insert provided with these formulations for complete information.
Pronestyl is also available for parenteral use as Pronestyl Injection (Procainamide Hydrochloride Injection USP) as sterile aqueous solutions in 10 mL vials providing 100 mg procainamide hydrochloride per mL or 2 mL vials providing 500 mg procainamide hydrochloride per mL. Consult the package insert provided with this product for complete information.
Storage: Store Pronestyl-SR Tablets (Procainamide Hydrochloride Tablets) at room temperature; avoid excessive heat.
(J3-498A)

Shown in Product Identification Section, page 422

RAUDIXIN® ℞

[raw″dik′sin]
(Rauwolfia Serpentina Tablets USP)
Whole Root—Biologically Standardized

DESCRIPTION

Raudixin (Rauwolfia Serpentina Tablets USP) contains powdered rauwolfia serpentina USP, an antihypertensive agent for oral administration, prepared from the powdered whole root of *Rauwolfia serpentina* Benth.
Each tablet contains 50 mg or 100 mg powdered rauwolfia serpentina composed of not less than 0.15 percent and not more than 0.2 percent of reserpine-rescinnamine group alkaloids, calculated as reserpine. Inactive ingredients: acacia, calcium carbonate, carnauba wax, castor oil, color additives [FD&C Red No. 3, FD&C Yellow No. 5 (tartrazine), FD&C Yellow No. 6], corn starch, ethylcellulose, flavor, gelatin, lactose, magnesium carbonate, mineral oil, shellac, stearic acid, sucrose, talc, titanium dioxide, and white wax.
Reserpine is a white to slightly yellow, crystalline powder, insoluble in water, very slightly soluble in ether and alcohol, slightly soluble in benzene, and freely soluble in acetic acid and chloroform. It is designated chemically as methyl 18β-hydroxy-11,17α-dimethoxy-3β, 20α-yohimban-16β-carboxylate 3,4,5-trimethoxybenzoate (ester).

CLINICAL PHARMACOLOGY

The rauwolfia alkaloids probably exert their antihypertensive effects through depletion of tissue stores of catecholamines (epinephrine and norepinephrine) from peripheral sites. By contrast, their sedative and tranquilizing properties are thought to be related to depletion of catecholamines and serotonin (5-hydroxytryptamine) from the brain.
Following absorption from the gastrointestinal tract, rauwolfia alkaloids concentrate in tissues with high lipid content. The drug crosses the blood-brain barrier and the placenta.
The rauwolfia alkaloids are characterized by slow onset of action and sustained effect. Both its cardiovascular and central nervous system effects may persist following withdrawal of the drug. The rauwolfia alkaloids are metabolized in the liver to inactive compounds that are excreted primarily in the urine. Unchanged alkaloids are excreted primarily in the feces.

INDICATIONS AND USAGE

Raudixin (Rauwolfia Serpentina Tablets) is indicated in the treatment of mild essential hypertension. It is also useful as

Continued on next page

Princeton—Cont.

adjunctive therapy with other antihypertensive agents in the more severe forms of hypertension.

Raudixin is also indicated for the relief of symptoms in agitated psychotic states (e.g., schizophrenia), primarily in those individuals unable to tolerate phenothiazine derivatives or those who also require antihypertensive medication.

CONTRAINDICATIONS

The preparation is contraindicated in patients who have previously demonstrated hypersensitivity to rauwolfia. It is also contraindicated in patients with mental depression (especially with suicidal tendencies), active peptic ulcer, ulcerative colitis, and in patients receiving electroconvulsive therapy.

WARNINGS

Extreme caution should be exercised in treating patients with a history of mental depression. Discontinue the drug at the first sign of despondency, early morning insomnia, loss of appetite, impotence, or self-deprecation. Drug-induced depression may persist for several months after drug withdrawal and may be severe enough to result in suicide.

Sensitivity reactions may occur in patients with or without a history of allergy or bronchial asthma.

The use of this drug may impair the mental and physical abilities required for the performance of tasks requiring alertness, such as driving or operating heavy machinery.

PRECAUTIONS

General—Because rauwolfia preparations increase gastrointestinal motility and secretion, this drug should be used cautiously in patients with a history of peptic ulcer, ulcerative colitis, or gallstones where biliary colic may be precipitated. Patients on high dosage should be observed carefully at regular intervals to detect possible reactivation of peptic ulcer.

Chronic administration of rauwolfia alkaloids may increase serum prolactin levels and decrease urinary catecholamine and vanilmandelic acid (VMA) excretion. Therefore, any diagnostic tests performed for these determinations should be interpreted with caution.

Caution should be exercised when treating hypertensive patients with renal insufficiency since they adjust poorly to lowered blood pressure levels.

Preoperative withdrawal of rauwolfia serpentina does not insure that circulatory instability will not occur. It is important that the anesthesiologist be aware of the patient's drug intake and consider this in the overall management since hypotension has occurred in patients receiving rauwolfia preparations. Anticholinergic and/or adrenergic drugs (metaraminol, norepinephrine) have been employed to treat adverse vagocirculatory effects.

This product contains FD&C Yellow No. 5 (tartrazine) which may cause allergic-type reactions (including bronchial asthma) in certain susceptible individuals. Although the overall incidence of FD&C Yellow No. 5 (tartrazine) sensitivity in the general population is low, it is frequently seen in patients who also have aspirin hypersensitivity.

Animal tumorigenicity: rodent studies have shown that reserpine is an animal tumorigen, causing an increased incidence of mammary fibroadenomas in female mice, malignant tumors of the seminal vesicles in male mice, and malignant adrenal medullary tumors in male rats. These findings arose in two year studies in which the drug was administered in the feed at concentrations of 5 and 10 ppm—about 100 to 300 times the usual human dose. The breast neoplasms are thought to be related to reserpine's prolactin-elevating effect. Several other prolactin-elevating drugs have also been associated with an increased incidence of mammary neoplasia in rodents.

The extent to which these findings indicate a risk to humans is uncertain. Tissue culture experiments show that about one-third of human breast tumors are prolactin-dependent *in vitro*, a factor of considerable importance if the use of the drug is contemplated in a patient with previously detected breast cancer. The possibility of an increased risk of breast cancer in reserpine users has been studied extensively; however, no firm conclusion has emerged. Although a few epidemiologic studies have suggested a slightly increased risk (less than twofold in all studies except one) in women who have used reserpine, other studies of generally similar design have not confirmed this. Epidemiologic studies conducted using other drugs (neuroleptic agents) that, like reserpine, increase prolactin levels and therefore would be considered rodent mammary carcinogens, have not shown an association between chronic administration of the drug and human mammary tumorigenesis. While long-term clinical observation has not suggested such an association, the available evidence is considered too limited to be conclusive at this time. An association of reserpine intake with pheochromocytoma or tumors of the seminal vesicles has not been explored.

Information for the Patient—Patients should be advised to report any symptoms of potential adverse effects. Patients should be warned against taking this medication for any disorder other than for which it was prescribed, or discontinuing medication unless instructed by the physician. Caution patients that the drug may impair mental and/or physical abilities required for performance of hazardous tasks, such as operating machinery or driving a motor vehicle.

Drug Interactions—When administered concurrently, the following drugs may interact with rauwolfia alkaloids:

Alcohol/CNS Depressants—may increase the CNS depressant effects of these drugs or the rauwolfia alkaloids.

Other Antihypertensives/Diuretics—antihypertensive effects may be potentiated.

Digitalis Glycosides/Quinidine—may result in cardiac arrhythmias.

Levodopa—effects of levodopa may be inhibited.

Methotrimeprazine—may result in increased orthostatic hypotension.

Monamine Oxidase (MAO) Inhibitors—may result in excessive excitation, hypertension, and sympathetic response.

Sympathomimetics (Direct-acting)—rauwolfia alkaloids may prolong their effects; (Indirect-acting)—rauwolfia alkaloids may inhibit their action.

Tricyclic Antidepressants—the antidepressant effects of these drugs and the antihypertensive effects of rauwolfia alkaloids may be decreased.

Drug/Laboratory Test Interactions—Since rauwolfia alkaloids slightly decrease absorbance readings obtained on urinary steroid colorimetric determinations (e.g., modified Glenn-Nelson technique or Holtorff Koch modification of Zimmerman reaction), false low results may be reported.

Carcinogenesis, Mutagenesis, Impairment of Fertility—Animal carcinogenicity studies using reserpine at dosages of 25 to 50 times and 50 to 100 times the average human dose were conducted with rats and mice, respectively. Carcinogenic effects associated with the administration of reserpine were increased incidence of adrenal medullary pheochromocytomas in male rats, undifferentiated carcinomas of the seminal vesicles in male mice, and mammary cancer in female mice; carcinogenic effects were not seen in female rats.

Bacteriological studies to determine mutagenicity using reserpine showed negative results.

Long-term animal studies have not been performed with rauwolfia alkaloids to determine any impairment of fertility in males or females.

Pregnancy: Teratogenic Effects—Category C. Animal reproduction studies have not been conducted with rauwolfia alkaloids. There are no adequte and well-controlled studies in pregnant women. Since rauwolfia alkaloids cross the placental barrier and appear in cord blood, drugs of this class should be used during pregnancy only if the potential benefit justifies the potential risk to the fetus.

Pregnancy: Nonteratogenic Effects—Increased respiratory secretions, nasal congestion, cyanosis and hypothermia, and anorexia are potential hazards in neonates of rauwolfia alkaloid-treated mothers.

Nursing Mothers—Rauwolfia alkaloids are excreted in human milk. Because of the potential for serious adverse reactions in nursing infants from rauwolfia alkaloids, a decision should be made whether to continue nursing or to discontinue therapy taking into account the importance of the drug to the mother.

Pediatric Use—Safety and effectiveness in children have not been established.

ADVERSE REACTIONS

The following adverse reactions (categorized by organ system in decreasing order of severity) have been observed, but there are insufficient data to support an estimate of their frequency. The reactions are usually reversible and disappear when the drug is discontinued.

Cardiovascular: Bradycardia; arrhythmias, particularly when used concurrently with digitalis or quinidine (see PRECAUTIONS, Drug Interactions); angina-like symptoms. Water retention with edema in patients with hypertensive vascular disease may occur rarely, but the condition generally clears with cessation of therapy, or the administration of a diuretic agent.

Central Nervous System: CNS sensitization manifested by optic atrophy, glaucoma, uveitis, deafness, and dull sensorium; extrapyramidal tract symptoms, rare Parkinsonian disease; depression; paradoxical anxiety; nightmares; nervousness; headache; dizziness; drowsiness.

Gastrointestinal: Gastrointestinal bleeding; hypersecretion and increased intestinal motility; diarrhea; vomiting; nausea; anorexia; dryness of mouth.

Respiratory: Dyspnea; epistaxis; nasal congestion.

Hypersensitivity: Purpura; pruritus; rash.

Other: Conjunctival injection; dysuria; muscular aches; weight gain; breast engorgement; pseudolactation; impotence or decreased libido; gynecomastia.

OVERDOSAGE

Signs and symptoms of overdosage include CNS depression ranging from drowsiness to coma, flushing of the skin, bradycardia, hypotension, conjunctival congestion, and pupillary constriction. Hypothermia, central respiratory depression, mental depression, diarrhea, vomiting, ptosis, miosis, and extrapyramidal signs such as stiffness, leg pain, and tremors may also occur.

Treatment is symptomatic. Provided the patient is not comatose or convulsing, evacuation of stomach contents by emesis or gastric lavage is recommended; precautions should be taken to preclude aspiration of contents by the patient, and to protect the airway. An activated charcoal slurry or saline cathartic may then be administered. Bradycardia and parasympathetic effects may be relieved with appropriate anticholinergic medication. Hypotension and coma usually respond to conservative supportive therapy. In cases of severe hypotension, treatment with a vasopressor having direct action upon vascular smooth muscle or a direct-acting sympathomimetic (see PRECAUTIONS, Drug Interactions), is recommended. Rapid infusion of IV solutions intended to raise arterial blood pressure should be avoided, since cardiac status in rauwolfia poisoning is uncertain. Because the effects of rauwolfia alkaloids are long acting, patients should be carefully observed for at least 72 hours.

DOSAGE AND ADMINISTRATION

For adults, the average oral dose is 200 to 400 mg daily, given in divided doses in the morning and evening. Higher doses should be used cautiously because serious mental depression and other side effects may be considerably increased. (Orally, 200 to 300 mg of powdered whole root is equivalent to 0.5 mg of reserpine.) Maintenance doses may vary from 50 to 300 mg per day given as a single dose or as two divided doses.

Concomitant use of rauwolfia serpentina and ganglionic blocking agents, guanethidine, veratrum, hydralazine, methyldopa, chlorthalidone, or thiazides necessitates careful titration of dosage with each agent in order to obtain maximal therapeutic response as well as the lowest dose necessary to maintain that therapeutic response and minimize side effects.

Elderly and severely debilitated patients may require dosage lower than the usual adult dosage.

HOW SUPPLIED

Raudixin (Rauwolfia Serpentina Tablets USP)

50 mg/tablet: bottles of 100 and 1000.

100 mg/tablet: bottles of 100.

Each round, biconvex, red tablet is imprinted with the following identification numbers: 50 mg, **713**; 100 mg, **776**.

Storage: Keep and dispense in tighly closed, light-resistant containers. Store at room temperature; avoid excessive heat.

(J4-017)

Shown in Product Identification Section, page 422

RAUZIDE® ℞

Powdered Rauwolfia Serpentina with Bendroflumethiazide Tablets

WARNING

This fixed combination drug is not indicated for initial therapy of hypertension. Hypertension requires therapy titrated to the individual patient. If the fixed combination represents the dosage so determined, its use may be more convenient in patient management. The treatment of hypertension is not static, but must be reevaluated as conditions in each patient warrant.

DESCRIPTION

Rauzide (Powdered Rauwolfia Serpentina with Bendroflumethiazide Tablets) is an antihypertensive agent for oral administration.

Each tablet contains 50 mg powdered rauwolfia serpentina composed of not less than 0.15 percent and not more than 0.2 percent of reserpine-rescinnamine group alkaloids calculated as reserpine, combined with 4 mg bendroflumethiazide. Inactive ingredients: acacia, calcium carbonate, castor oil, cellulose, color additives [FD&C Blue No. 1, FD&C Yellow No. 5 (tartrazine)], corn starch, ethylcellulose, gelatine, lactose, magnesium carbonate, shellac, stearic acid, sucrose, talc, and titanium dioxide.

Reserpine is a white to slightly yellow crystalline powder, insoluble in water, very slightly soluble in ether and alcohol, slightly soluble in benzene, and freely soluble in acetic acid and chloroform. It is designated chemically as methyl 18β-hydroxy-11, 17α-dimethoxy-3β, 20α-yohimban-16β-carboxylate 3,4,5-trimethoxybenzoate (ester). Bendroflumethiazide is a white to cream crystalline powder, practically insoluble in water, and freely soluble in acetone and alcohol. It is designated chemically as 3-benzyl-3,4-dihydro-6-(trifluoromethyl)-2H-1,2,4-benzothiadazine-7-sulfonamide 1,1-dioxide.

CLINICAL PHARMACOLOGY

Either of the components of Rauzide (Powdered Rauwolfia Serpentine with Bendroflumethiazide Tablets), when administered alone, may produce a reduction of blood pressure in hypertension. When the two agents are administered simultaneously, the action of the one appears to supplement that of the other so that a hypotensive effect may be produced which is greater than that produced by either agent alone. Thus, hypertension which does not adequately respond to either drug alone may frequently respond to the combination of both drugs.

Rauwolfia Serpentina—Rauwolfia serpentina probably exerts its antihypertensive effects through depletion of tissue stores of catecholamines (epinephrine and norepinephrine) from peripheral sites. By contrast, its sedative and tranquilizing properties are thought to be related to depletion of catecholamines and serotonin (5-hydroxytryptamine) from the brain.

Following absorption from the gastrointestinal tract, rauwolfia alkaloids concentrate in tissues with high lipid content. The drug crosses the blood-brain barrier and the placenta.

The rauwolfia alkaloids are characterized by slow onset of action and sustained effect. Cardiovascular and central nervous system effects may persist following discontinuation of therapy. The rauwolfia alkaloids are metabolized in the liver to inactive compounds that are excreted primarily in the urine. Unchanged alkaloids are excreted primarily in the feces.

Bendroflumethiazide—Bendroflumethiazide interferes with the renal tubular mechanism of electrolyte reabsorption. At maximal therapeutic dosage all thiazides are approximately equal in their diuretic potency. Thiazides produce less alteration in the extracellular fluid composition than other diuretic agents. The mechanism whereby thiazides function in the control of hypertension has not been completely elucidated.

Thiazides increase the excretion of sodium and chloride in approximately equivalent amounts. Natriuresis may be accompanied by some loss of potassium, bicarbonate, and other electrolytes. The thiazides are absorbed from the gastrointestinal tract in varying degrees and exhibit a high degree of binding to plasma proteins. They are distributed in the extracellular space and cross the placenta. It has been reported that the diuretic effect of bendroflumethiazide is apparent within one to two hours, the peak effect occurs within 6 to 12 hours, and its diuretic activity persists for approximately 18 to 24 hours. Thiazides are excreted principally by tubular secretion, primarily in unchanged form.

INDICATIONS AND USAGE

Rauzide (Powdered Rauwolfia Serpentina with Bendroflumethiazide Tablets) is indicated for hypertension (see boxed WARNING).

Usage in Pregnancy. The routine use of diuretics in an otherwise healthy woman is inappropriate and exposes mother and fetus to unnecessary hazard. Diuretics do not prevent development of toxemia of pregnancy, and there is no satisfactory evidence that they are useful in the treatment of developed toxemia.

Edema during pregnancy may arise from pathological causes or from the physiologic and mechanical consequences of pregnancy. Thiazides are indicated in pregnancy when edema is due to pathologic causes, just as they are in the absence of pregnancy (however, see PRECAUTIONS below). Dependent edema in pregnancy, resulting from restriction of venous return by the expanded uterus, is properly treated through elevation of the lower extremities and use of support hose; use of diuretics to lower intravascular volume in this case is illogical and unnecessary. There is hypervolemia during normal pregnancy which is harmful to neither the fetus nor the mother (in the absence of cardiovascular disease), but which is associated with edema, including generalized edema, in the majority of pregnant women. If this edema produces discomfort, increased recumbency will often provide relief. In rare instances, this edema may cause extreme discomfort which is not relieved by rest. In these cases, a short course of diuretics may provide relief and may be appropriate.

CONTRAINDICATIONS

Rauwolfia Serpentina—Rauwolfia serpentina is contraindicated in patients who have previously demonstrated hypersensitivity to this agent, those with mental depression (especially with suicidal tendencies), active peptic ulcer, ulcerative colitis, and in patients receiving electroconvulsive therapy.

Bendroflumethiazide—Bendroflumethiazide is contraindicated in anuria and in patients who have previously demonstrated hypersensitivity to thiazides or other sulfonamide-derived drugs.

WARNINGS

Sensitivity reactions may occur in patients with or without a history of allergy or bronchial asthma.

Lithium generally should not be given with diuretics; diuretic agents reduce the renal clearance of lithium and add a high risk of lithium toxicity. Refer to the package insert for lithium preparations before use of such concomitant therapy.

Rauwolfia Serpentina—Extreme caution should be exercised in treating patients with a history of mental depression. Discontinue the drug at the first sign of despondency, early morning insomnia, loss of appetite, impotence, or self-depreciation. Drug-induced depression may persist for several months after drug withdrawal and may be severe enough to result in suicide.

Rauwolfia serpentina may impair the mental and physical abilities required for the performance of tasks requiring alertness, such as driving or operating heavy machinery.

Bendroflumethiazide—In patients with renal disease, thiazides may precipitate azotemia. Cumulative effects of the drug may develop in patients with impaired renal function. Thiazides should be used with caution in patients with impaired hepatic function or progressive liver disease, since minor alterations of fluid and electrolyte balance may precipitate hepatic coma.

The possibility of exacerbation or activation of systemic lupus erythematosus has been reported.

PRECAUTIONS

General—This product contains FD&C Yellow No. 5 (tartrazine) which may cause allergic-type reactions (including bronchial asthma) in certain susceptible individuals. Although the overall incidence of FD&C Yellow No. 5 (tartrazine) sensitivity in the general population is low, it is frequently seen in patients who also have aspirin hypersensitivity.

Rauwolfia Serpentina—Because rauwolfia preparations increase gastrointestinal motility and secretion, this drug should be used cautiously in patients with a history of peptic ulcer, ulcerative colitis, or gallstones where biliary colic may be precipitated. Patients on high dosage should be observed carefully at regular intervals to detect possible reactivation of peptic ulcer.

Chronic administration of rauwolfia alkaloids may increase serum prolactin levels and decrease urinary catecholamine and vanilmandelic acid (VMA) excretion. Therefore, any diagnostic tests performed for these determinations should be interpreted with caution.

Caution should be exercised when treating hypertensive patients with renal insufficiency since they adjust poorly to lowered blood pressure levels.

Preoperative withdrawal of rauwolfia serpentina does not insure that circulatory instability will not occur. It is important that the anesthesiologist be aware of the patient's drug intake and consider this in the overall management since hypotension has occurred in patients receiving rauwolfia preparations. Anticholinergic and/or adrenergic drugs (metaraminol, norepinephrine) have been employed to treat adverse vagocirculatory effects.

Animal tumorigenicity: Rodent studies have shown that reserpine is an animal tumorigen, causing an increased incidence of mammary fibroadenomas in female mice, malignant tumors of the seminal vesicles in male mice, and malignant adrenal medullary tumors in male rats. These findings arose in two year studies in which the drug was administered in the feed at concentrations of 5 and 10 ppm—about 100 to 300 times the usual human dose. The breast neoplasms are thought to be related to reserpine's prolactin-elevating effect. Several other prolactin-elevating drugs have also been associated with an increased incidence of mammary neoplasia in rodents.

The extent to which these findings indicate a risk to humans is uncertain. Tissue culture experiments show that about one-third of human breast tumors are prolactin-dependent *in vitro*, a factor of considerable importance if the use of the drug is contemplated in a patient with previously detected breast cancer. The possibility of an increased risk of breast cancer in reserpine users has been studied extensively; however, no firm conclusion has emerged. Although a few epidemiologic studies have suggested a slightly increased risk (less than twofold in all studies except one) in women who have used reserpine, other studies of generally similar design have not confirmed this. Epidemiologic studies conducted using other drugs (neuroleptic agents) that, like reserpine, increase prolactin levels and therefore would be considered rodent mammary cancinogens, have not shown an association between chronic administration of the drug and human mammary tumorigenesis. While long-term clinical observation has not suggested such an association, the available evidence is considered too limited to be conclusive at this time. An association of reserpine intake with pheochromocytoma or tumors of the seminal vesicles has not been explored.

Bendroflumethiazide—All patients receiving thiazide therapy should be observed for clinical signs of fluid or electolyte imbalance; namely, hyponatremia, hypochloremic alkalosis, and hypokalemia. Serum and urine electrolyte determinations are particularly important when the patient is vomiting excessively or receiving parenteral fluids. Warning signs or symptoms of fluid and electrolyte imbalance include: dryness of the mouth, thirst, weakness, lethargy, drowsiness, restlessness, muscle pains or cramps, muscular fatigue, hypotension, oliguria, tachycardia, and gastrointestinal disturbances such as nausea and vomiting.

Hypokalemia may develop with thiazides as with any other potent diuretic, especially with brisk diuresis, when severe cirrhosis is present, or during concomitant use of corticosteroids, ACTH, digitalis, or after prolonged thiazide therapy. Interference with adequate oral electrolyte intake will also contribute to hypokalemia. Hypokalemia can sensitize or exaggerate the response of the heart to the toxic effects of digitalis (e.g., increased ventricular irritability). Concurrent administration of a potassium-sparing diuretic or potassium supplements may be indicated in these patients.

Any chloride deficit is generally mild and usually does not require specific treatment except under extraordinary circumstances (as in liver disease or renal disease). Dilutional hyponatremia may occur in edematous patients in hot weather; appropriate therapy is water restriction, rather than administration of salt except in rare instances when the hyponatremia is life threatening. In actual salt depletion appropriate replacement is the therapy of choice.

Calcium excretion is decreased by thiazides. Pathological changes in the parathyroid gland with hypophosphatemia have been observed in a few patients on prolonged thiazide therapy. The common complications of hyperparathyroidism such as renal lithiasis, bone resorption, and peptic ulceration have not been seen. Thiazides should be discontinued before carrying out tests for parathyroid function.

Hyperuricemia may occur or frank gout may be precipitated in certain patients receiving thiazide therapy.

Latent diabetes mellitus may become manifest during thiazide administration.

The antihypertensive effects of the drug may be enhanced in the postsympathectomy patient.

If progressive renal impairment becomes evident, as indicated by a rising nonprotein nitrogen or blood urea nitrogen, a careful reappraisal of therapy is necessary with consideration given to withholding or discontinuing diuretic therapy.

Information for the Patient—Patients should be advised to report any symptoms of potential adverse effects.

Patients should be warned against taking this medication for any disorder other than for which it was prescribed, or discontinuing medication unless instructed by the physician.

Caution patients that the drug may impair mental and/or physical abilities required for performance of hazardous tasks, such as operating machinery or driving a motor vehicle.

Laboratory Tests—Serum and urine electrolyte levels should be regularly monitored (see WARNINGS, Bendroflumethiazide, also PRECAUTIONS, General, Bendroflumethiazide).

Drug Interactions: Rauwolfia Serpentina—When administered concurrently, the following drugs may interact with rauwolfia alkaloids:

Alcohol/CNS Depressants—may increase the CNS depressant effects of these drugs or the rauwolfia alkaloids.

Other Antihypertensives/Diuretics—antihypertensive effects may be potentiated.

Digitalis Glycosides/Quinidine—may result in cardiac arrhythmias.

Levodopa—effects of levodopa may be inhibited.

Methotrimeprazine—may result in increased orthostatic hypotension.

Monamine Oxidase (MAO) Inhibitors—may result in excessive excitation, hypertension, and sympathetic response.

Sympathomimetics (Direct-acting)—rauwolfia alkaloids may prolong their effects; (Indirect-acting)—rauwolfia alkaloids may inhibit their action.

Tricyclic Antidepressants—the antidepressant effects of these drugs and the antihypertensive effects of rauwolfia alkaloids may be decreased.

Bendroflumethiazide—When administered concurrently, the following drugs may interact with thiazide diuretics:

Alcohol, Barbiturates, or Narcotics—aggravation of orthostatic hypotension may occur.

Amphotericin B, Corticosteroids, or Corticotropin (ACTH)—may intensify electrolyte imbalance, particularly hypokalemia.

Anticoagulants (oral)—dosage adjustments of anticoagulant medication may be necessary since bendroflumethiazide may decrease their effects.

Antigout medications—dosage adjustments of antigout medication may be necessary since bendroflumethiazide may raise the level of blood uric acid.

Other Antihypertensive medications (e.g., ganglionic or peripheral adrenergic blocking agents)—dosage adjustments may be necessary since bendroflumethiazide may potentiate their effects.

Antidiabetic drugs (oral agents and insulin)—dosage adjustments of antidiabetic agents may be necessary due to the possible hyperglycemic effect of bendroflumethiazide.

Calcium—increased serum calcium levels due to decreased excretion.

Cardiac Glycosides—increased possibility of digitalis toxicity associated with hypokalemia.

Cholestyramine Resin and Colestipol HCL—may delay or decrease absorption of bendroflumethiazide. Sulfonamide

Continued on next page

Princeton—Cont.

diuretics should be taken at least one hour before or four to six hours after these medications.
Diazoxide —possible hyperglycemic, hyperuricemic, and antihypertensive effects.
Lithium —possible lithium toxicity due to reduced renal clearance (see WARNINGS, Bendroflumethiazide).
MAO Inhibitors —dosage adjustments of MAO Inhibitors and/or thiazides may be necessary since hypotensive effects are increased.
Nondepolarizing muscle relaxants, Preanesthetics and Anesthetics used in surgery (e.g., tubocurarine chloride and gallamine triethiodide)—increased responsiveness to muscle relaxants; *Pressor amines* (e.g., norepinephrine)—decreased arterial responsiveness to pressor amines, but not sufficient to preclude effectiveness of the pressor agent for therapeutic use.
Use caution in patients taking any of these medications who undergo surgery. Administer preanesthetic and anesthetic agents in reduced dosage, and if possible, discontinue bendroflumethiazide one week prior to surgery.
Methenamine —possible decreased effectiveness of methenamine due to possible increased alkalinization of the urine from thiazide therapy.
Probenecid or Sulfinpyrazone —increased dosage of these agents may be necessary since bendroflumethiazide may exhibit increased hyperuricemic effects.
Drug/Laboratory Test Interactions: Rauwolfia Serpentina —Since rauwolfia alkaloids slightly decrease absorbance readings obtained on urinary steroid colorimetric determinations (e.g., modified Glenn-Nelson technique or Holtorff Koch modification of Zimmerman reaction), false low results may be obtained.
Bendroflumethiazide —Thiazides may produce false-negative results with the phentolamine and tyramine tests, and may interfere with the phenosulfonphthalein (PSP) test due to decreased excretion of PSP.
Thiazides may decrease serum PBI levels without signs of thyroid disturbance.
Carcinogenesis, Mutagenesis, Impairment of Fertility: Rauwolfia Serpentina —Animal carcinogenicity studies using reserpine at dosages of 25 to 50 times and 50 to 100 times the average human dose were conducted with rats and mice, respectively. Carcinogenic effects associated with the administration of reserpine were increased incidence of adrenal medullary pheochromocytomas in male rats, undifferentiated carcinomas of the seminal vesicles in male mice, and mammary cancer in female mice; carcinogenic effects were not seen in female rats.
Bacteriological studies to determine mutagenicity using reserpine showed negative results.
Long-term studies in animals have not been performed to evaluate mutagenicity, or possible impairment of fertility in males or females.
Bendroflumethiazide —Long-term studies in animals have not been performed to evaluate carcinogenic or mutagenic potential, or possible impairment of fertility in males or females.
Pregnancy: Teratogenic Effects. —Catecory C. Animal reproduction studies have not been conducted with rauwolfia alkaloids or bendroflumethiazide. There are no adequate and well-controlled studies in pregnant women. Since rauwolfia alkaloids and thiazides cross the placental barrier and appear in cord blood, drugs in these classes should be used during pregnancy only if the potential benefit justifies the potential risk to the fetus.
Pregnancy: Nonteratogenic Effects—Rauwolfia Serpentina —Increased respiratory secretions, nasal congestion, cyanosis and hypothermia, and anorexia are potential hazards in neonates of rauwolfia alkaloid-treated mothers.
Bendroflumethiazide —Fetal or neonatal jaundice, thrombocytopenia, and possibly other adverse reactions which have occurred in the adult are potential hazards in fetuses and neonates of thiazide-treated mothers.
Nursing Mothers —Both rauwolfia serpentina and bendroflumethiazide are excreted in human milk. Because of the potential for serious adverse reactions in nursing infants from both drugs, a decision should be made whether to continue nursing or to discontinue therapy taking into account the importance of this preparation to the mother.
Pediatric Use —Safety and effectiveness in children have not been established.

ADVERSE REACTIONS

The following adverse reactions (categorized by organ system in decreasing order of severity) have been observed with bendroflumethiazide and rauwolfia serpentina; there is, however, insufficient data to support an estimate of their frequency.
Rauwolfia Serpentina—*Cardiovascular:* Bradycardia; arrhythmias, particularly when used concurrently with digitalis or quinidine (see PRECAUTIONS, Drug Interactions); angina-like symptoms.
Central Nervous System: CNS sensitization manifested by optic atrophy, glaucoma, uveitis, deafness, and dull sensorium; extrapyramidal tract symptoms; rare parkinsonian disease; depression, paradoxical anxiety; nightmares, nervousness; drowsiness.
Gastrointestinal: Gastrointestinal bleeding; hypersecretion and increased intestinal motility; dryness of mouth.
Respiratory: Dyspnea; epistaxis; nasal congestion.
Other: Conjunctival injection; dysuria; muscular aches; weight gain; breast engorgement; pseudolactation; impotence or decreased libido; gynecomastia.
These reactions are usually reversible and disappear when the drug is discontinued.
Bendroflumethiazide—*Central Nervous System:* Vertigo; paresthesias; xanthopsia; lightheadedness.
Hematologic: Leukopenia (agranulocytopenia); agranulocytosis; thrombocytopenia; aplastic anemia; hemolytic anemia.
Cardiovascular: Orthostatic hypotension (may be aggravated by alcohol, barbiturates, or narcotics—see PRECAUTIONS, Drug Interactions, Bendroflumethiazide).
Gastrointestinal: Gastric irritation; abdominal cramps or bloating; constipation; pancreatitis; sialadenitis.
Hepatic: Jaundice (intrahepatic cholestatic jaundice).
Renal: Allergic glomerulonephritis.
Hypersensitivity: Ecchymosis; skin photosensitivity; exfoliative dermatitis; urticaria; necrotizing angiitis (vasculitis, cutaneous vasculitis); fever; respiratory distress including pneumonitis; anaphylactic reactions.
Other: Hyperglycemia; glycosuria; occasional metabolic acidosis in diabetic patients; hyperuricemia; muscle spasm or cramps; weakness; restlessness; transient blurred vision.
Whenever adverse reactions are moderate or severe, thiazide dosage should be reduced or therapy withdrawn.
Common to Bendroflumethiazide and Rauwolfia Serpentina—*Gastrointestinal:* Anorexia; nausea; vomiting; diarrhea.
Central Nervous System: Headache; dizziness.
Hypersensitivity: Purpura; pruritus; rash.

OVERDOSAGE

Rauwolfia Serpentina —In the event of overdosage, rauwolfia serpentina may cause CNS depression ranging from drowsiness to coma, flushing of the skin, bradycardia, hypotension, conjunctival congestion, and pupillary constriction. Hypothermia, central respiratory depression, mental depression, diarrhea, vomiting, ptosis, miosis, and extrapyramidal signs such as stiffness, leg pain, and tremors may also occur.
Treatment is symptomatic. Provided the patient is not comatose or convulsing, evacuation of stomach contents by emesis or gastric lavage is recommended; precautions should be taken to preclude aspiration of contents by the patient, and to protect the airway. An activated charcoal slurry may then be administered. Bradycardia and parasympathetic effects may be relieved with appropriate anticholinergic medication. Hypotension and coma usually respond to conservative supportive therapy. In cases of severe hypotension, treatment with a vasopressor having direct action upon vascular smooth muscle or a direct-acting sympathomimetic (see PRECAUTIONS, Drug Interactions) is recommended. Rapid infusion of IV solutions intended to raise arterial blood pressure should be avoided, since cardiac status in rauwolfia poisoning is uncertain. Because the effects of rauwolfia alkaloids are long acting, patients should be carefully observed for at least 72 hours.
Bendroflumethiazide —In addition to the expected diuresis, overdosage of thiazides may produce varying degrees of lethargy which may progress to coma within a few hours, with minimal depression of respiration and cardiovascular function and without evidence of serum electrolyte changes or dehydration. The mechanism of thiazide-induced CNS depression is unknown. Gastrointestinal irritation and hypermotility may occur. Transitory increase in BUN has been reported, and serum electrolyte changes may occur, especially in patients with impaired renal function.
In addition to gastric lavage and supportive therapy for stupor or coma, symptomatic treatment of gastrointestinal effects may be needed. Cathartics should be avoided since they tend to enhance the loss of fluid and electrolytes. Measures as required to maintain hydration, electrolyte balance, respiration, and cardiovascular and renal function should be instituted.

DOSAGE AND ADMINISTRATION

As determined by individual titration (see boxed WARNING). Usual dosage may range from one to four tablets daily.

HOW SUPPLIED

Rauzide (Powdered Rauwolfia Serpentina with Bendroflumethiazide Tablets)
Tablets providing 50 mg powdered rauwolfia serpentina with 4 mg bendroflumethiazide are available in bottles of 100 and 1000.
Each dark green, discoid-shaped tablet is imprinted with identification number **769.**
Storage: Keep and dispense in tightly closed containers. Store at room temperature; avoid excessive heat.
(J4-022A)

Shown in Product Identification Section, page 422

Procter & Gamble
P. O. BOX 171
CINCINNATI, OH 45201

HEAD & SHOULDERS®
Antidandruff Shampoo

Head & Shoulders Shampoo offers effective dandruff control and beautiful hair in a formula that is pleasant to use. Independently conducted clinical testing (double-blind and dermatologist-graded) has proved that Head & Shoulders reduces dandruff flaking. Head & Shoulders is also gentle enough to use every day for clean, manageable hair.

ACTIVE INGREDIENT

1.0% pyrithione zinc suspended in an anionic detergent system. Cosmetic ingredients are also included.

INDICATIONS

For effective control of dandruff and seborrheic dermatitis of the scalp.

ACTIONS

Pyrithione zinc is substantive to the scalp and remains after rinsing. Its mechanism of action has not been fully established, but it is believed to control the microorganisms associated with dandruff flaking and itching.

PRECAUTIONS

Not to be taken internally. Keep out of children's reach. Avoid getting shampoo in eyes— if this happens, rinse eyes with water.

DOSAGE AND ADMINISTRATION

For best results in controlling dandruff, Head & Shoulders should be used regularly. It is gentle enough to use for every shampoo. In treating seborrheic dermatitis, a minimum of four shampooings are needed to achieve full effectiveness.

COMPOSITION

Lotion—Normal to Oily Formula: Pyrithione Zinc in a shampoo base of water, Ammonium Laureth Sulfate, Ammonium Lauryl Sulfate, Cocamide MEA, Glycol Distearate, Ammoniumxylenesulfonate, Fragrance, Citric Acid, Methylchloroisothiazolinone, Methylisothiazolinone, and FD&C Blue No. 1. Lotion—Normal to Dry Formula: Pyrithione Zinc in a shampoo base of water, Ammonium Laureth Sulfate, Ammonium Lauryl Sulfate, Cocamide MEA, Glycol Distearate, Ammoniumxylenesulfonate, Propylene Glycol, Fragrance, Citric Acid, Methylchloroisothiazolinone, Methylisothiazolinone, and FD&C Blue No. 1. Cream—Normal to Oily Formula: Pyrithione zinc in a shampoo base of water, sodium cocoglyceryl ether sulfonate, sodium chloride, sodium lauroyl sarcosinate, cocamide DEA, cocoyl sarcosine, fragrance, and FD&C Blue No. 1. Cream—Normal to Dry Formula: Pyrithione zinc in a shampoo base of water, sodium cocoglyceryl ether sulfonate, sodium chloride, sodium lauroyl sarcosinate, cocamide DEA, propylene glycol, cocoyl sarcosine, fragrance, and FD&C Blue No. 1.

HOW SUPPLIED

Lotion avalable in 4.0, 7.0, 11.0, and 15.0 fl. oz. unbreakable plastic bottles. Concentrate cream available in 5.5 oz. tube. Both lotion and concentrate are available in formulas for "Normal to Oily" and "Normal to Dry" hair.

Shown in Product Identification Section, page 422

Regular Flavor
METAMUCIL® Powder
[met"uh-mū'sil]
(psyllium hydrophilic mucilloid)

DESCRIPTION

Regular Flavor Metamucil is a bulk laxative containing refined hydrophilic mucilloid, a highly efficient dietary fiber derived from the husk of the psyllium seed *(Plantago ovata).* Each dose contains approximately 3.4 g of psyllium hydrophilic mucilloid. Inactive ingredients include dextrose (a carbohydrate). Each dose contains about 1 mg of sodium, 31 mg of potassium, and 14 calories. Carbohydrate content is approximately 3.5 g.

ACTIONS

Metamucil provides a bland, nonirritating bulk and promotes normal elimination. It is uniform, instantly miscible, palatable, and nonirritative in the gastrointestinal tract.

INDICATIONS

Metamucil is indicated in the management of chronic constipation, in irritable bowel syndrome, as adjunctive therapy in the constipation of duodenal ulcer and diverticular disease, in the bowel management of patients with hemorrhoids, and for constipation during pregnancy, convalescence, and senility.

CONTRAINDICATIONS
Intestinal obstruction, fecal impaction.

PRECAUTION
May cause allergic reaction in people sensitive to inhaled or ingested psyllium powder.

DOSAGE AND ADMINISTRATION
The usual adult dosage is one rounded teaspoonful (7 g) stirred into a standard 8-oz glass of cool water or other suitable liquid and taken orally one to three times a day, depending on the need and response. It may require continuing use for 2 or 3 days to provide optimal benefit. An additional glass of liquid after each dose is helpful.

HOW SUPPLIED
Powder, containers of 7 oz, 14 oz, and 21 oz (OTC); also available in cartons of 100 single-dose (7g) packets.

IS THIS PRODUCT OTC
Yes. See also PDR for Nonprescription Drugs.

Sugar Free Regular Flavor METAMUCIL® Powder
[met "uh-mū 'sil]
(psyllium hydrophilic mucilloid)

DESCRIPTION
Sugar Free Regular Flavor Metamucil is a bulk laxative containing refined hydrophilic mucilloid, a highly efficient dietary fiber derived from the husk of the psyllium seed (*Plantago ovata*), which has been sweetened with NutraSweet®* brand sweetener (aspartame). It contains no chemical stimulants or sugar. Each dose contains approximately 3.4 g of psyllium hydrophilic mucilloid. Inactive ingredients include aspartame and maltodextrin. Each dose contains about 1 calorie, 1 mg of sodium, 31 mg of potassium and 5 mg of phenylalanine. Carbohydrate content is 0.3 grams.

ACTIONS
Metamucil provides a bland, nonirritating bulk and promotes normal elimination. It is uniform, instantly miscible, palatable, and nonirritative in the gastrointestinal tract.

INDICATIONS
Metamucil is indicated in the management of chronic constipation, in irritable bowel syndrome, as adjunctive therapy in the constipation of duodenal ulcer and diverticular disease, in the bowel management of patients with hemorrhoids, and for constipation during pregnancy, convalescence, and senility.

CONTRAINDICATIONS
Intestinal obstruction, fecal impaction.

WARNING
Phenylketonurics should be aware that Sugar Free Metamucil contains phenylalanine.

PRECAUTION
May cause allergic reaction in people sensitive to inhaled or ingested psyllium powder.

DOSAGE AND ADMINISTRATION
The usual adult dosage is one rounded teaspoonful (3.7 g) stirred into a standard 8-oz glass of cool water or other suitable liquid and taken orally one to three times a day, depending on the need and response. It may require continuing use for 2 or 3 days to provide optimal benefit. An additional glass of liquid after each dose is helpful.

HOW SUPPLIED
Powder, containers of 3.7 oz, 7.4 oz, and 11.1 oz (OTC); also available in cartons of 100 single-dose (3.7 g) packets.

IS THIS PRODUCT OTC
Yes. See also PDR for Nonprescription Drugs.

*NutraSweet is a registered trademark of G.D. Searle & Co.

Orange Flavor METAMUCIL® Powder
[met "uh-mū 'sil]
(psyllium hydrophilic mucilloid)

DESCRIPTION
Orange Flavor Metamucil is a bulk laxative containing refined hydrophilic mucilloid, a highly efficient dietary fiber derived from the husk of the psyllium seed *(Plantago ovata)*. Each dose contains approximately 3.4 g of psyllium hydrophilic mucilloid. Inactive ingredients include citric acid, FD&C Yellow No. 6, flavoring, and sucrose (a carbohydrate). Each dose contains about 1 mg of sodium, 31 mg of potassium, and 30 calories. Carbohydrate content is approximately 7.1 g.

ACTIONS
Metamucil provides a bland, nonirritating bulk and promotes normal elimination. It is uniform, instantly miscible, palatable, and nonirritative in the gastrointestinal tract.

INDICATIONS
Metamucil is indicated in the management of chronic constipation, in irritable bowel syndrome, as adjunctive therapy in the constipation of duodenal ulcer and diverticular disease, in the bowel management of patients with hemorrhoids, and for constipation during pregnancy, convalescence, and senility.

CONTRAINDICATIONS
Intestinal obstruction, fecal impaction.

PRECAUTION
May cause allergic reaction in people sensitive to inhaled or ingested psyllium powder.

DOSAGE AND ADMINISTRATION
The usual adult dose is one rounded tablespoonful (11 g) stirred into a standard 8-oz glass of cool water and taken orally one to three times a day, depending on the need and response. It may require continuing use for 2 or 3 days to provide optimal benefit. An additional glass of liquid after each dose is helpful.

HOW SUPPLIED
Powder, containers of 7 oz, 14 oz, and 21 oz.

IS THIS PRODUCT OTC
Yes. See also PDR for Nonprescription Drugs.

Sugar Free Orange Flavor METAMUCIL® Powder
[met "uh-mū 'sil]
(psyllium hydrophilic mucilloid)

DESCRIPTION
Sugar Free Orange Flavor Metamucil is a bulk laxative containing refined hydrophilic mucilloid, a highly efficient dietary fiber derived from the husk of the psyllium seed (*Plantago ovata*), which has been sweetened with NutraSweet®* brand sweetener (aspartame). It contains no chemical stimulants or sugar. Each dose contains approximately 3.4 g of psyllium hydrophilic mucilloid. Inactive ingredients include aspartame, citric acid, FD&C Yellow No. 6, flavoring, and maltodextrin. Each dose contains about 2 calories, 1 mg of sodium, 31 mg of potassium, and 23 mg of phenylalanine. Carbohydrate content is approximately 0.6 grams.

ACTIONS
Metamucil provides a bland, nonirritating bulk and promotes normal elimination. It is uniform, instantly miscible, palatable, and nonirritative in the gastrointestinal tract.

INDICATIONS
Metamucil is indicated in the management of chronic constipation, in irritable bowel syndrome, as adjunctive therapy in the constipation of duodenal ulcer and diverticular disease, in the bowel management of patients with hemorrhoids, and for constipation during pregnancy, convalescence, and senility.

CONTRAINDICATIONS
Intestinal obstruction, fecal impaction.

WARNING
Phenylketonurics should be aware that Sugar Free Metamucil contains phenylalanine.

PRECAUTIONS
May cause allergic reaction in people sensitive to inhaled or ingested psyllium powder.

DOSAGE AND ADMINISTRATION
The usual adult dosage is one rounded teaspoonful (4.3 g) stirred into a standard 8-oz glass of cool water or other suitable liquid and taken orally one to three times a day, depending on the need and response. It may require continuing use for 2 or 3 days to provide optimal benefit. An additional glass of liquid after each dose is helpful.

HOW SUPPLIED
Powder, containers of 3.7 oz, 7.4 oz, and 11.1 oz (OTC).

IS THIS PRODUCT OTC
Yes. See also PDR for Nonprescription Drugs.

* NutraSweet is a registered trademark of G. D. Searle & Co.

Strawberry Flavor METAMUCIL® Powder
[met "uh-mū 'sil]
(psyllium hydrophilic mucilloid)

DESCRIPTION
Strawberry Flavor Metamucil is a bulk laxative containing refined hydrophilic mucilloid, a highly efficient dietary fiber derived from the husk of the psyllium seed *(Plantago ovata)*. Each dose contains approximately 3.4 g of psyllium hydrophilic mucilloid. Inactive ingredients include citric acid, FD&C Red No. 40, flavoring, and sucrose (a carbohydrate). Each dose contains about 1 mg of sodium, 31 mg of potassium, and 30 calories. Carbohydrate content is approximately 7.1 g.

ACTIONS
Metamucil provides a bland, nonirritating bulk and promotes normal elimination. It is uniform, instantly miscible, palatable, and nonirritative in the gastrointestinal tract.

INDICATIONS
Metamucil is indicated in the management of chronic constipation, in irritable bowel syndrome, as adjunctive therapy in the constipation of duodenal ulcer and diverticular disease, in the bowel management of patients with hemorrhoids, and for constipation during pregnancy, convalescence, and senility.

CONTRAINDICATIONS
Intestinal obstruction, fecal impaction.

PRECAUTION
May cause allergic reaction in people sensitive to inhaled or ingested psyllium powder.

DOSAGE AND ADMINISTRATION
The usual adult dose is one rounded tablespoonful (11 g) stirred into a standard 8-oz glass of cool water and taken orally one to three times a day, depending on the need and response. It may require continuing use for 2 or 3 days to provide optimal benefit. An additional glass of liquid after each dose is helpful.

HOW SUPPLIED
Powder, containers of 7 oz, 14 oz, and 21 oz.

IS THIS PRODUCT OTC
Yes. See also PDR for Nonprescription Drugs.

Sugar Free Lemon-Lime Flavor INSTANT MIX METAMUCIL®
[met "uh-mū 'sil]
(psyllium hydrophilic mucilloid)

DESCRIPTION
Sugar Free Lemon-Lime Flavor Instant Mix Metamucil is a bulk laxative containing refined hydrophilic mucilloid, a highly efficient dietary fiber derived from the husk of the psyllium seed *(Plantago ovata)*, which has been sweetened with NutraSweet®* brand sweetener (aspartame). It contains no chemical stimulants or sugar. Each dose contains approximately 3.4 g of psyllium hydrophilic mucilloid. Inactive ingredients include aspartame, calcium carbonate, citric acid, flavoring, potassium bicarbonate, silicon dioxide, and sodium bicarbonate. Each packet provides less than 1 calorie, 285 mg of potassium, 2 mg of sodium, and 25 mg phenylalanine.

ACTIONS
Instant Mix Metamucil provides a bland, nonirritating bulk and promotes normal elimination. It is effervescent and requires no stirring, and it is uniform, instantly miscible, palatable, and nonirritative in the gastrointestinal tract.

INDICATIONS
Instant Mix Metamucil is indicated in the management of chronic constipation, in irritable bowel syndrome, as adjunctive therapy in the constipation of duodenal ulcer and diverticular disease, in the bowel management of patients with hemorrhoids, and for constipation during pregnancy, convalescence, and senility.

CONTRAINDICATIONS
Intestinal obstruction, fecal impaction.

WARNING
Phenylketonurics should be aware that Sugar Free Instant Mix Metamucil contains phenylalanine.

PRECAUTION
May cause allergic reaction in people sensitive to inhaled or ingested psyllium powder.

DOSAGE AND ADMINISTRATION
The usual adult dosage is the contents of one packet (5.4 g) taken one to three times daily as follows: (1) Entire contents of a packet are poured into a standard 8-oz water glass. (2) The glass is slowly filled with cool water. (3) Entire contents are to be drunk immediately. (An additional glass of liquid after each dose is helpful.)

HOW SUPPLIED
Cartons of 16 and 30 single-dose (5.4 g) packets (OTC); also available in cartons of 100 single-dose (5.4 g) packets.

Continued on next page

Procter & Gamble—Cont.

IS THIS PRODUCT OTC

Yes. See also PDR for Nonprescription Drugs.

* NutraSweet is a registered trademark of G.D. Searle & Co.

Sugar Free Orange Flavor INSTANT MIX METAMUCIL®

[met"uh-mū'sil]

(psyllium hydrophilic mucilloid)

DESCRIPTION

Sugar Free Orange Flavor Instant Mix Metamucil is a bulk laxative containing refined hydrophilic mucilloid, a highly efficient dietary fiber derived from the husk of the psyllium seed (*Plantago ovata*), which has been sweetened with NutraSweet®* brand sweetener (aspartame). It contains no chemical stimulants or sugar. Each dose contains approximately 3.4 g of psyllium hydrophilic mucilloid. Inactive ingredients include aspartame, citric acid, FD&C Yellow No. 6, flavoring, potassium bicarbonate, silicon dioxide, and sodium bicarbonate. Each packet provides less than 1 calorie, 305 mg of potassium, 2 mg of sodium, and 25 mg phenylalanine.

ACTIONS

Instant Mix Metamucil provides a bland, nonirritating bulk and promotes normal elimination. It is effervescent and requires no stirring, and it is uniform, instantly miscible, palatable, and nonirritative in the gastrointestinal tract.

INDICATIONS

Instant Mix Metamucil is indicated in the management of chronic constipation, in irritable bowel syndrome, as adjunctive therapy in the constipation of duodenal ulcer and diverticular disease, in the bowel management of patients with hemorrhoids, and for constipation during pregnancy, convalescence, and senility.

CONTRAINDICATIONS

Intestinal obstruction, fecal impaction.

WARNING

Phenylketonurics should be aware that Sugar Free Instant Mix Metamucil contains phenylalanine.

PRECAUTION

May cause allergic reaction in people sensitive to inhaled or ingested psyllium powder.

DOSAGE AND ADMINISTRATION

The usual adult dosage is the contents of one packet (5.2 g) taken one to three times daily as follows: (1) Entire contents of a packet are poured into a standard 8-oz water glass. (2) The glass is slowly filled with cool water. (3) Entire contents are to be drunk immediately. (An additional glass of liquid after each dose is helpful.)

HOW SUPPLIED

Cartons of 16 and of 30 single-dose (5.2 g) packets.

IS THIS PRODUCT OTC

Yes. See also PDR for Nonprescription Drugs.

* NutraSweet is a registered trademark of G.D. Searle & Co.

PEPTO-BISMOL® LIQUID AND TABLETS

For diarrhea, heartburn, indigestion, upset stomach and nausea.

DESCRIPTION

Each Pepto-Bismol Tablet contains 262 mg bismuth subsalicylate and each tablespoonful (15 ml) of Pepto-Bismol Liquid contains 262 mg bismuth subsalicylate. Each tablet contains 100 mg salicylate and each tablespoonful of liquid contains 130 mg salicylate. Contains no sugar. Tablets are sodium-free (less than 2 mg/tablet) and Liquid is low in sodium (5 mg/tablespoonful). Inactive ingredients include (Tablets): calcium carbonate, FD&C Red. No. 3, aluminum lake, flavor, magnesium stearate, mannitol, povidone, saccharin sodium and talc; (Liquid): FD&C Red No. 40, FD&C Red No 3, flavor, magnesium aluminum silicate, methylcellulose, saccharin sodium, salicylic acid, sodium salicylate and water.

INDICATIONS

Pepto-Bismol controls diarrhea within 24 hours, relieving associated abdominal cramps; soothes heartburn and indigestion without constipating; and relieves nausea and upset stomach.

CAUTION

This product contains salicylates. If taken with aspirin and ringing of the ears occurs, discontinue use. This product does not contain aspirin, but should not be administered to those patients who have a known allergy to aspirin or salicylates. Caution is advised in the administration to patients taking medication for anticoagulation, diabetes and gout.

WARNING

Consult a physician before giving this medication to children, including teenagers, during or after recovery from chicken pox or flu. As with any drug, if you are pregnant or nursing a baby, seek the advice of a health professional before taking this product. KEEP THIS AND ALL MEDICATIONS OUT OF THE REACH OF CHILDREN.

Note: This medication may cause a harmless darkening of the tongue and/or stool. Stool darkening should not be confused with melena.

DOSAGE AND ADMINISTRATION

Tablets:

Adults—Two tablets

Children (according to age)—

9–12 yrs.	1 tablet
6–9 yrs.	$\frac{2}{3}$ tablet
3–6 yrs.	$\frac{1}{3}$ tablet

Chew or dissolve in mouth. Repeat every $\frac{1}{2}$ to 1 hour as needed, to a maximum of 8 doses.

Liquid: Shake well before using.

Adults—2 tablespoonsful

Children (according to age)—

9–12 yrs.	1 tablespoonful
6–9 yrs.	2 teaspoonsful
3–6 yrs.	1 teaspoonful

Repeat dosage every $\frac{1}{2}$ to 1 hour, if needed, to a maximum of 8 doses in a 24-hour period.

For children under 3 years, dose according to weight.

28+ lbs.	1 teaspoonful
14–18 lbs.	$\frac{1}{2}$ teaspoonful

Repeat every 4 hours, if needed, to a maximum of 6 doses in a 24-hour period.

HOW SUPPLIED

Pepto-Bismol Liquid is available in:

NDC 37000-032-01	4 fl. oz. bottle
NDC 37000-032-02	8 fl. oz. bottle
NDC 37000-032-03	12 fl. oz. bottle
NDC 37000-032-04	16 fl. oz. bottle

Pepto-Bismol Tablets are pink triangular chewable tablets imprinted with "Pepto-Bismol" on one side and "NE" on the other. Tablets are available in:

NDC 37000-034-03	box of 24
NDC 37000-033-04	box of 42

PERIDEX® ℞

[per-i-dex]

(chlorhexidine gluconate)

Oral Rinse

PRODUCT OVERVIEW

KEY FACTS

Peridex is an oral rinse containing 0.12% chlorhexidine gluconate. Peridex has been shown to achieve significant reductions in gingival inflammation and associated bleeding. Approximately 30% of the active ingredient, is retained in the oral cavity following a single rinsing. This retained active is slowly released into the oral fluids.

MAJOR USES

Peridex has proved to be clinically effective for use between dental visits as part of a professional program for the treatment of gingivitis as characterized by redness, swelling of the gingivae and gingival bleeding. Therapy should be initiated directly following an oral prophylaxis. Patients using Peridex should be reevaluated and given a thorough prophylaxis at intervals no longer than six months. Recommended use is a 30-second rinse of $\frac{1}{2}$ fluid ounce (marked in cap) twice daily.

SAFETY INFORMATION

The most common side effects associated with chlorhexidine oral rinses are (1) an increase in staining of teeth and other oral sufaces, (2) an increase in supragingival calculus formation, and (3) an alteration in taste perception. No serious systemic adverse reactions associated with use of Peridex were observed in clinical testing.

PRESCRIBING INFORMATION

PERIDEX® ℞

(chlorhexidine gluconate)

Oral Rinse

DESCRIPTION

Peridex is an oral rinse containing 0.12% chlorhexidine gluconate (1, 1′-hexamethylene bis [5-(p-chlorophenyl) biguanide] di-D-gluconate) in a base containing water, 11.6% alcohol, glycerin, PEG-40 sorbitan diisostearate, flavor, sodium saccharin, and FD&C Blue No. 1. Peridex is a near-neutral solution (pH range 5–7). Chlorhexidine gluconate is a salt of chlorhexidine and gluconic acid. Its chemical structure is: [See Chemical Formula at top of next column].

CLINICAL PHARMACOLOGY

Peridex provides microbicidal activity during oral rinsing. The clinical significance of Peridex's antimicrobial activities is not clear. Microbiological sampling of plaque has shown a general reduction of counts of certain assayed bacteria, both aerobic and anaerobic, ranging from 54–97% through six months' use.

Use of Peridex in a six-month clinical study did not result in any significant changes in bacterial resistance, overgrowth of potentially opportunistic organisms or other adverse changes in the oral microbial ecosystem. Three months after Peridex use was discontinued, the number of bacteria in plaque had returned to baseline levels and resistance, of plaque bacteria to chlorhexidine gluconate was equal to that at baseline.

PHARMACOKINETICS

Pharmacokinetic studies with Peridex indicate approximately 30% of the active ingredient, chlorhexidine gluconate, is retained in the oral cavity following rinsing. This retained drug is slowly released into the oral fluids.

Studies conducted on human subjects and animals demonstrate chlorhexidine gluconate is poorly absorbed from the gastrointestinal tract. The mean plasma level of chlorhexidine gluconate reached a peak of 0.206 ug/g in humans 30 minutes after they ingested a 300-mg dose of the drug. Detectable levels of chlorhexidine gluconate were not present in the plasma of these subjects 12 hours after the compound was administered. Excretion of chlorhexidine gluconate occurred primarily through the feces (~90%). Less than 1% of the chlorhexidine gluconate ingested by these subjects was excreted in the urine.

INDICATION

Peridex is indicated for use between dental visits as part of a professional program for the treatment of gingivitis as characterized by redness and swelling of the gingivae, including gingival bleeding upon probing. Peridex has not been tested among patients with acute necrotizing ulcerative gingivitis (ANUG). For patients having coexisting gingivitis and periodontitis, see PRECAUTIONS.

CONTRAINDICATIONS

Peridex should not be used by persons who are known to be hypersensitive to chlorhexidine gluconate.

WARNINGS

The effect of Peridex on periodontitis has not been determined. An increase in supragingival calculus was noted in clinical testing in Peridex users compared with control users. It is not known if Peridex use results in an increase in subgingival calculus. Calculus deposits should be removed by a dental prophylaxis at intervals no greater than six months. Rare hypersensitivity and generalized allergic reactions have also been reported. Peridex should not be used by persons who have a sensitivity to it or its components.

PRECAUTIONS

GENERAL:

1. For patients having coexisting gingivitis and periodontitis, the presence or absence of gingival inflammation following treatment with Peridex should not be used as a major indicator of underlying periodontitis.
2. Peridex can cause staining of oral surfaces, such as tooth surfaces, restorations, and the dorsum of the tongue. Not all patients will experience a visually significant increase in toothstaining. In clinical testing, 56% of Peridex users exhibited a measurable increase in facial anterior stain, compared to 35% of control users after six months; 15% of Peridex users developed what was judged to be heavy stain, compared to 1% of control users after six months. Stain will be more pronounced in patients who have heavier accumulations of unremoved plaque.

   Stain resulting from use of Peridex does not adversely affect health of the gingivae or other oral tissues. Stain can be removed from most tooth surfaces by conventional professional prophylactic techniques. Additional time may be required to complete the prophylaxis.

   Discretion should be used when prescribing to patients with anterior facial restorations with rough surfaces or margins. If natural stain cannot be removed from these surfaces by a dental prophylaxis, patients should be excluded from Peridex treatment if permanent discoloration is unacceptable. Stain in these areas may be difficult to remove by dental prophylaxis and on rare occasions may necessitate replacement of these restorations.
3. Some patients may experience an alteration in taste perception while undergoing treatment with Peridex. Most patients accommodate to this effect with continued use of Peridex. No instances of permanent taste alteration due to Peridex have been reported.

USAGE IN PREGNANCY: Pregnancy Category B. Reproduction and fertility studies with chlorhexidine gluconate have been conducted. No evidence of impaired fertility was observed in rats at doses up to 100 mg/kg/day, and no evidence of harm to the fetus was observed in rats and rabbits at doses up to 300 mg/kg/day and 40 mg/kg/day, respectively. These doses are approximately 100, 300, and 40 times that which would result from a person's ingesting 30 ml (2 capfuls) of Peridex per day. Since controlled studies in pregnant women have not been conducted, the benefits of the drug in pregnant women should be weighed against possible risk to the fetus.

NURSING MOTHERS: It is not known whether this drug is excreted in human milk. Because many drugs are excreted in human milk, caution should be exercised when Peridex is administered to a nursing woman.

In parturition and lactation studies with rats, no evidence of impaired parturition or of toxic effects to suckling pups was observed when chlorhexidine gluconate was administered to dams at doses that were over 100 times greater than that which would result from a person's ingesting 30 ml (2 capfuls) of Peridex per day.

PEDIATRIC USE: Clinical effectiveness and safety of Peridex have not been established in children under the age of 18.

CARCINOGENESIS, MUTAGENESIS: In two mammalian *in vivo* mutagenic studies with chlorhexidine gluconate, mutagenesis was not observed. The highest dose of chlorhexidine gluconate used in a mouse dominant lethal assay was 1000 mg/kg/day and in a hamster cytogenetics test was 250 mg/kg/day, i.e. > 3200 times the amount that would be ingested from the recommended daily dose of Peridex. In a drinking water study in rats, carcinogenesis was not observed. The highest dose of chlorhexidine gluconate used in this study, 38 mg/kg/day, is at least 500 times the amount that would be ingested from the recommended daily dose of Peridex.

ADVERSE REACTIONS

The most common side effects associated with chlorhexidine gluconate oral rinses are (1) an increase in staining of teeth and other oral surfaces, (2) an increase in calculus formation, and (3) an alteration in taste perception; see WARNINGS and PRECAUTIONS. No serious systemic adverse reactions associated with use of Peridex were observed in clinical testing.

Minor irritation and superficial desquamation of the oral mucosa have been noted in patients using Peridex, particularly among children.

Although there have been no reports of parotitis (inflammation or swelling of salivary glands) among Peridex users in controlled clinical studies, transient parotitis has been reported in research studies with chlorhexidine-containing mouthrinses.

OVERDOSAGE

Ingestion of 1 or 2 ounces of Peridex by a small child (~10 kg body weight) might result in gastric distress, including nausea, or signs of alcohol intoxication. Medical attention should be sought if more than 4 ounces of Peridex is ingested by a small child or if signs of alcohol intoxication develop.

DOSAGE AND ADMINISTRATION

Peridex therapy should be initiated directly following a dental prophylaxis. Patients using Peridex should be reevaluated and given a thorough prophylaxis at intervals no longer than six months.

Recommended use is twice daily oral rinsing for 30 seconds, morning and evening after toothbrushing. Usual dosage is ½ fl. oz. (marked in cap) of undiluted Peridex. Peridex is not intended for ingestion and should be expectorated after rinsing.

HOW SUPPLIED

Peridex is supplied as a blue liquid in 1-pint amber plastic bottles with child-resistant dispensing closures. Store above freezing (32°F).

NDC 37000-007- 01

The Purdue Frederick Company

100 CONNECTICUT AVENUE
NORWALK, CT 06856

BETADINE® Microbicides
[*bā 'tăh-dīn"*]

BETADINE Microbicides (povidone-iodine) are available in 22 dosage forms—more than any other antiseptic agent. Formulated for topical, vaginal, and perineal application, these preparations of BETADINE Microbicides are designed especially to meet the varied needs of physicians, nurses and patients.

Of all antiseptic preparations, only povidone-iodine, as in BETADINE Microbicides, is capable of killing the classes of pathogens encountered in nosocomial infections: gram-positive bacteria and gram-negative bacteria (including antibiotic-resistant strains and mycobacteria), fungi/yeasts, viruses, and protozoa. It is the only microbicide with this broad spectrum of activity.

Other advantages: Most bacteria are killed in 15 to 30 seconds. Resistance has not been reported. Not inactivated by blood, pus, mucous secretions, soap and hard water. When used as a surgical scrub, the effect lasts 6 to 8 hours. Vitually nonirritating; washes easily off skin and natural fabrics. BETADINE® Solution and BETADINE® Aerosol Spray are film-forming and may be applied with or without bandages. BETADINE® Ointment and BETADINE® Hēlafoam Solution may be bandaged or covered with gauze.

Note: BETADINE Microbicides should not be heated prior to application. Patients with iodine sensitivity should not use BETADINE preparations.

BETADINE® Microbicides are available for hospital use and home healthcare.

BETADINE® Aerosol Spray
BETADINE® Antiseptic Gauze Pad
BETADINE® Antiseptic Gel
BETADINE® Antiseptic Lubricating Gel
BETADINE® Medicated Douche
BETADINE® Disposable Medicated Douche
BETADINE® Medicated Douche Kit
BETADINE® Hēlafoam Solution
BETADINE® Mouthwash/Gargle
BETADINE® Ointment
BETADINE® Perineal Wash Concentrate Kit
BETADINE® Shampoo
BETADINE® Skin Cleanser
BETADINE® Skin Cleanser Foam
BETADINE® Solution
BETADINE® Solution Swab Aid®
BETADINE® Solution Swabsticks
BETADINE® Surgical Scrub
BETADINE® Surgi-Prep Sponge-Brush
BETADINE® Vaginal Suppositories
BETADINE® Viscous Formula Antiseptic Gauze Pad
BETADINE® Whirlpool Concentrate

BETADINE® Antiseptic Gel
[*bā 'tăh-dīn"*]
(povidone-iodine, 10%)

ACTION AND USES

Applied at bedtime, BETADINE Antiseptic Gel works through the night to provide prompt, soothing, symptomatic relief of minor vaginal irritation, itching and soreness associated with vaginitis due to Candida albicans, Trichomonas vaginalis, and Gardnerella vaginalis. Its active ingredient — the broad-spectrum microbicide povidone-iodine — significantly and rapidly reduces the aerobic and anaerobic count, offering comfort on contact from annoying vaginal symptoms and odor. May also be used for preoperative degerming.

ADVANTAGES

Its gel formulation offers the advantage of prolonged contact with irritated vaginal tissue to help provide long-lasting relief. BETADINE Antiseptic Gel is gentle and virtually nonirritating to delicate vaginal tissue. It is nongreasy and nonsticky.

DIRECTIONS FOR USE

Insert one applicatorful of BETADINE Antiseptic Gel. Leave medication in the vagina overnight. A sanitary napkin should be worn overnight. When external irritation is present, BETADINE Antiseptic Gel may be applied manually to the affected area. Treatment should be continued for seven days. Women with iodine sensitivity should not use this product. BETADINE Antiseptic Gel should not be used during pregnancy except with physician's approval.

HOW SUPPLIED

18 g tubes and 3 oz. tubes, each packaged with a convenient, easy-to-use vaginal applicator.

BETADINE® MEDICATED DOUCHE
[*bā 'tăh-dīn"*]
(povidone-iodine)

A pleasantly scented solution, BETADINE Medicated Douche is clinically effective in the treatment of vaginitis. Also indicated for the prompt symptomatic relief of minor vaginal irritation, itching, and soreness associated with vaginitis due to Candida albicans, Trichomonas vaginalis, and Gardnerella vaginalis. May be used as a cleansing douche.

ADVANTAGES

Low surface tension, with uniform wetting action to assist penetration into vaginal crypts and crevices. Active in the presence of blood, pus, or vaginal secretions. Virtually nonirritating to vaginal mucosa. Will not stain skin or natural fabrics.

DIRECTIONS FOR USE

Suggested Regimen For Therapeutic Use: In the office, swab the cervix and vulvovaginal area with BETADINE Solution. Prescribe BETADINE Medicated Douche: Two tablespoonfuls or two ½ fl. oz. packettes to a quart of lukewarm water once daily, through the entire menstrual cycle. If further therapy is warranted, douching should be continued through the next cycle. The patient may be instructed to return for an office visit following two weeks of therapy.

As a Routine Cleansing Douche: One (1) tablespoonful to a quart of lukewarm water once or twice per week.

As a douche for prompt symptomatic relief of minor vaginal irritation and itching: One (1) tablespoonful to a quart of lukewarm water once daily for five days. Treatment should continue for the full five days, even if symptoms are relieved earlier.

Women with iodine sensitivity should not use this product. BETADINE Medicated Douche preparations should not be used during pregnancy except with physician's approval.

HOW SUPPLIED

1 oz., 4 oz. and 8 oz. plastic bottles. Disposable ½ oz. (1 tablespoonful) packettes.

ALSO AVAILABLE

BETADINE Medicated Douche Kit (2 oz. and 8 oz.) and Disposable BETADINE Medicated Douche (single- and twin-pack).

BETADINE® OINTMENT
[*bā 'tăh-dīn"*]
(povidone-iodine)

ACTION

BETADINE Ointment, in a water-soluble base, is a topical agent active against organisms commonly encountered in skin and wound infections.

INDICATIONS

Therapeutically, BETADINE Ointment may be used as an adjunct to systemic therapy where indicated; for primary or secondary topical infections caused by iodine-susceptible organisms such as, infected surgical incisions, infected decubitus or stasis ulcers, pyodermas, secondarily infected dermatoses, and infected traumatic lesions.

Prophylactically: BETADINE Ointment may be used to prevent microbial contamination in burns, incisions and other topical lesions; for degerming skin in hyperalimentation, catheter care, the umbilical area or circumcision. The use of BETADINE Ointment for abrasions, minor cuts, and wounds, may prevent the development of infections and permit wound healing.

ADMINISTRATION

Apply directly to affected area as needed. May be bandaged.

SUPPLIED

1/32 oz. and ⅛ oz. packettes; 1 oz. tubes; 16 oz. (1 lb.) and 5 lbs.

BETADINE® SKIN CLEANSER
[*bā 'tăh-dīn"*]
(povidone-iodine)

BETADINE Skin Cleanser is a sudsing, antiseptic liquid cleanser which forms a rich, golden lather.

INDICATIONS

BETADINE Skin Cleanser aids in degerming the skin of patients with common pathogens, including *Staphylococcus aureus.* To help prevent the recurrence of acute inflammatory skin infections caused by iodine-susceptible pyogenic bacteria. In pyodermas, as a topical adjunct to systemic antimicrobial therapy. To help prevent spread of infection in acne pimples. Also kills three organisms often associated with acne vulgaris: *Staph. epidermidis, Corynebacterium acnes* and Pityrosporon.

Continued on next page

Purdue Frederick—Cont.

DIRECTIONS FOR USE
Wet the skin and apply a sufficient amount of Skin Cleanser to work up a rich golden lather. Allow lather to remain about 3 minutes. Then rinse. Repeat 2-3 times a day or as needed.

CAUTION
In rare instances of local sensitivity, discontinue use by the individual.

HOW SUPPLIED
1 fl. oz. and 4 fl. oz. plastic bottles.

NOTE
Blue stains on starched linen will wash off with soap and water.

BETADINE® SOLUTION
[*bā 'tăh-dīn "*]
(povidone-iodine)
Topical Antiseptic Microbicide

ACTION AND USES
For preoperative prepping of operative site, including the vagina, and as a general topical microbicide for: disinfection of wounds; emergency treatment of lacerations and abrasions; second– and third–degree burns; as a prophylactic anti-infective agent in hospital and office procedures, including postoperative application to incisions to help prevent infection; oral moniliasis (thrush); bacterial and mycotic skin infections; decubitus and stasis ulcers; preoperatively, in the mouth and throat, as a swab.

ADMINISTRATION
Apply full strength as often as needed as a paint, spray, or wet soak. May be bandaged. Caution: In preoperative prepping, avoid "pooling" beneath the patient. Prolonged exposure to unabsorbed, wet solution may cause irritation.

HOW SUPPLIED
½ oz., 4 oz., 8 oz., 16 oz. (1 pt.), 32 oz. (1 qt.) and 1 gal. plastic bottles and 1 oz. packettes.

ALSO AVAILABLE
BETADINE® Solution Swab Aid® Pads for degerming small areas of skin or mucous membranes prior to injections, aspirations, catheterization and surgery; boxes of 100 packettes. Also: disposable BETADINE® Solution Swabsticks, in packettes of 1's and 3's.

BETADINE® SURGICAL SCRUB
[*bā 'tăh-dīn "*]
(povidone-iodine)
Topical Antiseptic Germicide

ACTION AND USES
An antiseptic, germicidal, sudsing skin cleanser for pre- and postoperative scrubbing or washing by hospital operating room personnel; for preoperative use on patients; and general use as an antiseptic germicide in physician's office. Forms rich, golden lather.

CAUTION
In rare instance of local irritation or sensitivity, discontinue use by individual.

DIRECTIONS FOR USE
A. **For Preoperative Washing by Operating Personnel**

1. Wet hands and forearms with water. Pour about 5 cc. (1 teaspoonful) of BETADINE Surgical Scrub on the palm of the hand and spread over both hands and forearms. Without adding more water, rub the Scrub thoroughly over all areas for about five minutes. Use a brush if desired. Clean thoroughly under fingernails. Add a little water and develop copious suds. Rinse thoroughly under running water.
2. Complete the wash by scrubbing with another 5 cc. of BETADINE Surgical Scrub in the same way.

B. **For Preoperative Use on Patients**

After the skin area is shaved, wet it with water. Apply BETADINE Surgical Scrub (1 cc. is sufficient to cover an area of 20-30 square inches), develop lather and scrub thoroughly for about five minutes. Rinse off by aid of sterile gauze saturated with water. The area may then be painted with BETADINE Solution or sprayed with BETADINE Aerosol Spray and allowed to dry.

C. **For use in the Physician's Office**

Use for washing whenever a germicidal detergent is required. For maximum degerming of the hands proceed as under (A). To prepare the patient's skin proceed as under (B). Note: Blue stains on starched linen will wash off with soap and water.

SUPPLIED
16 oz. (1 pint) plastic bottle with and without pump, 32 oz. (1 quart) and 1 gal. plastic bottles, and ½ oz. packettes.

BETADINE® Vaginal Suppositories
[*bā 'tăh-dīn "*]
(povidone-iodine, 10%)

ACTION AND USES
Applied at bedtime, BETADINE Vaginal Suppositories work through the night to provide prompt symptomatic relief of minor vaginal irritation, itching and soreness associated with vaginitis due to Candida albicans, Trichomonas vaginalis, and Gardnerella vaginalis. Its active ingredient—the broad-spectrum microbicide povidone-iodine—significantly and rapidly reduces the aerobic and anaerobic count, offering soothing, night-long relief from annoying vaginal symptoms and odor.

ADVANTAGES
Each measured-dose BETADINE Vaginal Suppository is easily and quickly inserted to provide prolonged contact with irritated vaginal tissue to help provide long-lasting relief. BETADINE Vaginal Suppositories are gentle and virtually nonirritating to delicate vaginal tissue. Nonstaining to skin and natural fabrics, color can be washed off with soap and water.

DIRECTIONS FOR USE
Unwrap a suppository and gently insert its smaller end into the applicator. Insert the applicator into the vagina and release the suppository. Leave medication in the vagina overnight. A sanitary napkin should be worn overnight. Treatment should be continued for seven days. Women with iodine sensitivity should not use this product. BETADINE Vaginal Suppositories should not be used during pregnancy except with physician's approval.

HOW SUPPLIED
7 Suppositories packaged with a convenient, easy-to-use applicator and patient instruction booklet.

CARDIOQUIN® TABLETS ℞
[*car 'dē "ō-quin*]
(quinidine polygalacturonate)
275 mg
In the treatment of cardiac arrhythmias

DESCRIPTION
Each scored CARDIOQUIN Tablet contains 275 mg quinidine polygalacturonate equivalent in quinidine content to 3 grains (200 mg) of quinidine sulfate.

ACTIONS
The quinidine component slows conduction time, prolongs the refractory period, and depresses the excitability of heart muscle. Polygalaturonate slows ionization of the drug and protects the gastrointestinal tract by its demulcent effect.[1–3]

INDICATIONS
CARDIOQUIN Tablets are indicated as maintenance therapy after spontaneous and electrical conversion of atrial tachycardia, flutter or fibrillation and in the treatment of:

- Premature atrial and ventricular contractions.
- Paroxysmal atrial tachycardia.
- Paroxysmal A-V junctional rhythm.
- Atrial flutter.
- Paroxysmal atrial fibrillation.
- Established atrial fibrillation when therapy is appropriate.
- Paroxysmal ventricular tachycardia when not associated with complete heartblock.

CONTRAINDICATIONS
1. History of hypersensitivity to quinidine manifested by thrombocytopenia, skin eruptions, febrile reactions, etc.
2. Complete A-V block.
3. Complete bundle branch block or other severe intraventricular conduction defects exhibiting marked QRS widening or bizarre complexes.
4. Myasthenia gravis.
5. Arrhythmias associated with digitalis toxicity.

WARNINGS
1. In the treatment of atrial fibrillation with rapid ventricular response, ventricular rate should be controlled with digitalis glycosides *prior* to administration of quinidine.
2. In the treatment of atrial flutter with quinidine, reversion to sinus rhythm may be preceded by progessive reduction in the degree of A-V block to a 1:1 ratio resulting in an extremely high ventricular rate. This potential hazard may be reduced by digitalization prior to administration of quinidine.

Recent reports have described increased, potentially toxic, digoxin plasma levels when quinidine is administered concurrently. When concurrent use is necessary, digoxin dosage should be reduced and plasma concentration should be monitored and patients observed closely for digitalis intoxication.

3. Quinidine cardiotoxicity may be manifested by increased P-R and Q-T intervals, 50% widening of QRS, and/or ventricular ectopic beats or tachycardia. Appearance of these toxic signs during quinidine administration mandates immediate discontinuation of the drug, and/or close clinical and electrocardiographic monitoring. Note: Quinidine effect is enhanced by potassium and reduced in the presence of hypokalemia.
4. Quinidine syncope may occur as a complication of long-term therapy. It is manifested by sudden loss of consciousness and by ventricular arrhythmias with bizarre QRS complexes. This syndrome does not appear to be related to dose or plasma levels but occurs more often with prolonged Q-T intervals.
5. Because quinidine antagonizes the effect of vagal excitation upon the atrium and the A-V node, the administration of parasympathomimetic drugs (choline esters) or the use of any other procedure to enhance vagal activity may fail to termirnate paroxysmal supraventricular tachycardia in patients receiving quinidine.
6. Quinidine should be used with extreme caution in:
   - **a)** The presence of incomplete A-V block, since a complete block and asystole may result.
   - **b)** Quinidine may cause unpredictable abnormalities of rhythm in digitalized hearts. Therefore, it should be used with caution in the presence of digitals intoxication (see 2 above).
   - **c)** Partial bundle branch block.
   - **d)** Severe congestive heart failure and hypotensive states due to the depressant effects of quinidine on myocardial contractility and arterial pressure.
   - **e)** Poor renal function, especially renal tubular acidosis, because of the potential accumulation of quinidine in plasma leading to toxic concentrations.

PRECAUTIONS
1. **Test Dose**—A preliminary test dose of a single tablet of quinidine *sulfate* should be administered prior to the initiation of treatment with CARDIOQUIN Tablets to determine whether the patient has an idiosyncrasy to the quinidine molecule.
2. **Hypersensitivity**—During the first weeks of therapy, hypersensitivity to quinidine, although rare, should be considered (e.g., angioedema, purpura, acute asthmatic episode, vascular collapse).
3. **Long-Term Therapy**—Periodic blood counts and liver and kidney function tests should be performed during long-term therapy, and the drug should be discontinued if blood dyscrasias or signs of hepatic or renal disorders occur.
4. **Large Doses**—ECG monitoring and determination of plasma quinidine levels are recommended when doses greater than 2.5 g/day are administered.
5. **Usage in Pregnancy**—The use of quinidine in pregnancy should be reserved only for those cases where the benefits outweigh the possible hazards to the patient and fetus.
6. **Nursing Mothers**—The drug should be used with extreme caution in nursing mothers because the drug is excreted in breast milk.
7. **General**—In patients exhibiting asthma, muscle weakness and infection with fever *prior* to quindine administration, hypersensitivity reactions to the drug may be masked.

DRUG INTERACTIONS
1. Caution should be used when quinidine and its analogs are administered concurrently with coumarin anticoagulants. This combination may reduce prothrombin levels and cause bleeding.
2. Quinidine, a weak base, may have its half-life prolonged in patients who are concurrently taking drugs that can alkalize the urine, such as thiazide diuretics, sodium bicarbonate, and carbonic anhydrase inhibitors. Quinidine and drugs which alkalize the urine should be used together cautiously.
3. Quinidine exhibits a distinct anticholinergic activity in the myocardial tissues. An additive vagolytic effect may be seen when quinidine and drugs having anticholinergic blocking activity are used together. Drugs having cholinergic activity may be antagonized by quinidine.
4. Quinidine and other antiarrhythmic agents may produce additive cardiac depressant effects when administered together.
5. Quinidine interaction with cardiac glycosides (digoxin). See **Warnings**.
6. Antacids may delay absorption of quindine but appear unlikely to cause incomplete absorption.
7. Phenobarbital and phenytoin may reduce plasma half-life of quinidine by 50%.
8. Quindine may potentiate the neuromuscular blocking effect in ventilatory depression of patients receiving decamethonium, tubocurare or succinylcholine.

ADVERSE REACTIONS

Symptoms of cinchonism (ringing in the ears, headache, disturbed vision) may appear in sensitive patients after a single dose of the drug.

Gastrointestinal: The most common side effects encountered with quinidine are referable to this system. Diarrhea frequently occurs, but it rarely necessitates withdrawal of the drug. Nausea, vomiting and abdominal pain also occur. Some of these effects may be minimized by administering the drug with meals.

Cardiovascular: Widening of QRS complex, cardiac asystole, ventricular ectopic beats, idioventricular rhythms including ventricular tachycardia and fibrillation; paradoxical tachycardia, arterial embolism, and hypotension.

Hematologic: Acute hemolytic anemia, hypoprothrombinemia, thrombocytopenic purpura, agranulocytosis.

CNS: Headache, fever, vertigo, apprehension, excitement, confusion, delirium, and syncope, disturbed hearing (tinnitus, decreased auditory acuity), disturbed vision (mydriasis, blurred vision, disturbed color perception, photophobia, diplopia, night blindness, scotomata), optic neuritis.

Dermatologic: Cutaneous flushing with intense pruritus.

Hypersensitivity Reactions: Angioedema, acute asthmatic episode, vascular collapse, respiratory arrest, hepatic dysfunction.

DOSAGE AND ADMINISTRATION

Each CARDIOQUIN Tablet contains 275 mg quinidine polygalacturonate, equivalent to a 3-grain tablet of quinidine sulfate. Dosage must be adjusted to individual patient's needs, both for conversion and maintenance. An initial dose of 1 to 3 tablets may be used to terminate arrhythmia, and may be repeated in 3–4 hours. If normal sinus rhythm is not restored after 3 or 4 equal doses, the dose may be increased by ½ to 1 tablet (137.5 to 275 mg) and administered three to four times before any further dosage increase. For maintenance, one tablet may be used two or three times a day; generally, one tablet morning and night will be adequate.

Overdosage: Cardiotoxic effects of quinidine may be reversed in part by molar sodium lactate; the hypotension may be reversed by vasoconstrictors and by catecholamines (since vasodilation is partly due to alpha-adrenergic blockage)

SUPPLIED

Uncoated, scored tablets in bottles of 100.

REFERENCES

1. Schwartz, G.: *Angiology* 10:115 (Apr.) 1959.
2. Tricot, R., Nogrette, P.: *Presse med.* 68:1085 (June 4) 1960.
3. Shaftel, N., Halpern, A.: *Am. J. Med. Sci.* 236:184 (Aug.) 1958.

Shown in Product Identification Section, page 423

CERUMENEX® DROPS ℞

[*sĕ-rū ′mĕn-ĕx* ″]
(triethanolamine polypeptide oleate-condensate)

Cerumenolytic agent for effective and easy removal of earwax

COMPOSITION

CERUMENEX Drops contain (10%) Triethanolamine polypeptide oleate-condensate in propylene glycol with chlorbutanol (0.5%), for effective, convenient cerumenolytic action and easy removal of earwax.

Among its properties are:

1. Aqueous-miscible solution—low surface tension and optimal viscosity.
2. Slightly acid pH range to approximate surface of normal ear canal.
3. Hygroscopic — helps absorb aqueous transudates.
4. Antiseptic protection against contamination.

ADVANTAGES

- Usually effective with a single 15-30 minute treatment.
- Excellent results reported in over 90% of about 2,700 adult and pediatric patients.
- Helps avoid painful instrumentation.
- Simple and easy to administer.

ACTION

CERUMENEX Drops are specifically designed as a cerumenolytic agent, to emulsify and disperse excess or impacted earwax for easier removal without painful instrumentation. They are usually effective with a single 15-30 minute treatment, and are simple and easy to administer.

INDICATIONS

Removal of impacted cerumen—including prior to ear examination, prior to otologic therapy, and prior to audiometry.

CONTRAINDICATIONS

- A history of a previous untoward reaction to CERUMENEX Drops.
- A positive patch test (see "Precautions").
- Knowledge or suspicion of a perforated eardrum or otitis media may be considered as a relative contraindication.

PRECAUTIONS

It is recommended that the following precautions be observed in prescribing and administration of this agent:

1. Extreme caution is indicated in patients with demonstrable dermatologic idiosyncrasies or with history of allergic reactions in general.
2. In case of doubt, a patch test should be performed by placing a drop of CERUMENEX Drops on the flexor surface of the arm or forearm and covering it with a small Band-Aid® strip. The results are read and interpreted after 24 hours. Positive reaction indicates the probability of an allergic reaction following instillation in the ear.
3. Exposure of the ear canal to the CERUMENEX Drops should be limited to 15-30 minutes.
4. Patients must be instructed not to exceed the time of exposure, nor to use the medication more frequently than directed by the physician.
5. When administering CERUMENEX Drops, care must be taken to avoid undue exposure of the periaural skin during the instillation and the flushing out of the medication. If the medication comes in contact with the skin, the area should be washed with soap and water. Use of proper technique (see Dosage and Administration) will help avoid such undue exposure.
6. Although introduction of CERUMENEX Drops (triethanolamine polypeptide oleate-condensate) into the middle ear of animals with surgically perforated drums or into patients with ruptured drums has been accomplished without untoward reactions, the use of this medication should be avoided in the presence of underlying disease in the middle ear (otitis media, perforated drum) and it should be used only with caution in certain types of external otitis.
7. Patients should be advised to discontinue the use of the medication in case of a possible reaction and to consult their physician promptly.

ADVERSE REACTIONS

Clinical Reactions of Possible Allergic Origin

Localized dermatitis reactions were reported in about 1% of 2,700 patients treated, ranging from a very mild erythema and pruritus of the external canal to a severe eczematoid reaction involving the external ear and periauricular tissue, generally with duration of 2-10 days. In all cases, complete and uneventful resolution occurred without residual sequelae, sometimes without supplemental therapy. Such therapy may consist of only symptomatic relief in mild cases and may include anti-inflammatory agents when indicated. Thus, while reactions of a possible allergic origin may occur, their incidence is minimal and usually not disproportionate to other commonly used dermatologic agents.

DOSAGE AND ADMINISTRATION

1. Fill ear canal with CERUMENEX Drops with the patient's head tilted at a 45° angle.
2. Insert cotton plug and allow to remain 15-30 minutes.
3. Then gently flush ear with lukewarm water, using soft rubber syringe (avoid excessive pressure). Avoid undue exposure of large skin areas to the drug. If a second application is necessary in unusually hard impactions, the procedure may be repeated.

HOW SUPPLIED

6 ml and 12 ml bottles with cellophane-wrapped, blunt-end dropper.

FIBERMED®

[*fī ′bĕr-mĕd* ″]
High-Fiber Supplements
Fruit Flavor/Original Flavor
Also Fruit Flavor Snacks

DESCRIPTION

FIBERMED High-Fiber Supplements provide a measured quantity of natural dietary fiber in a palatable, ready-to-eat form. FIBERMED Supplements are standardized to provide concentrated dietary fiber in precise amounts—10 grams in two delicious biscuits. Original-Flavor FIBERMED contain natural dietary fiber from corn, wheat and oats. Fruit-Flavor FIBERMED contain natural dietary fiber from six sources: corn, oats, wheat, soy, apple and currants.

Lack of fiber in the diet is a recognized cause of constipation, irritable bowel syndrome, diverticulosis and hemorrhoids. Two FIBERMED High-Fiber Biscuits a day help provide the supplementary bulk that patients may need in their diet to avoid constipation.

FIBERMED also helps curb appetite and may help in weight control programs. Fiber produces feelings of satiety and fullness, and can reduce one's desire for food.

FIBERMED Supplements are superior to other fiber sources because of their uniform high-fiber content, convenience and good taste, qualities which encourage good compliance.

Ready-to-eat FIBERMED Supplements can be eaten any time, any place. Unlike most high-fiber foods or powdered bulks, FIBERMED requires no preparation and no mixing. They can be eaten with milk, coffee, tea, juice, soup or fruit; or dunked in a beverage.

INGREDIENTS

FIBERMED Supplements Original Flavor contain: Corn Bran, Brown Sugar, Wheat Flour, Corn Starch, Wheat Bran, Oat Flakes, Corn Germ Meal, Vegetable Shortening (Partially Hydrogenated Soybean Oil), Sodium Bicarbonate, Natural Vanilla Flavor, Ammonium Bicarbonate, Baking Acid, Salt, Cinnamon and Citric Acid.

FIBERMED Supplements Fruit Flavor contain: Corn Bran, Brown Sugar, Whole Rolled Oats, Soy Flour, Vegetable Shortening (Partially Hydrogenated Soybean Oil), Currants, Wheat Bran, Dried Apple, Ammonium Bicarbonate, Citric Acid, Wheat Flour, Salt, Vanilla, Baking Acid, Cinnamon.

USAGE

FIBERMED Supplements are indicated for those conditions, including constipation, in which it is desirable to regulate gastrointestinal transit time, increase stool weight and make elimination easier. Because of their taste and convenience, FIBERMED Supplements are the product of choice to significantly increase intake of dietary fiber in uniform amounts. Two FIBERMED Supplements a day provide a high level of dietary fiber—10 grams—more dietary fiber than a serving of high-fiber cereal.

DIRECTIONS

Two FIBERMED Biscuits per day provide the extra fiber required by most people. As with any healthful diet, adequate fluid intake is important.

SUPPLIED

FIBERMED Supplements Fruit Flavor, and Original Flavor Biscuits are each supplied in boxes of 14. For most individuals, 14 is a week's supply.

ALSO AVAILABLE

Fruit Flavor FIBERMED® High-Fiber SNACKS. Thirteen bite-size FIBERMED SNACKS provide 5 grams of concentrated natural dietary fiber. Supplied in 8.5 oz. boxes and 1.3 oz. Packs.

MS CONTIN® Ⓒ

[*em es* ″*kŏn* ′*tĕn*]
(morphine sulfate pentahydrate)
30 mg
Controlled-Release Tablets
WARNING: May be habit forming.

DESCRIPTION

Each MS CONTIN Tablet contains 30 mg morphine sulfate in a controlled-release formulation. Chemically, morphine sulfate is 7,8-didehydro-4,5,α-epoxy-17-methyl-morphinan-3,6α-diol sulfate (2:1) (salt) pentahydrate and has the following structural formula:

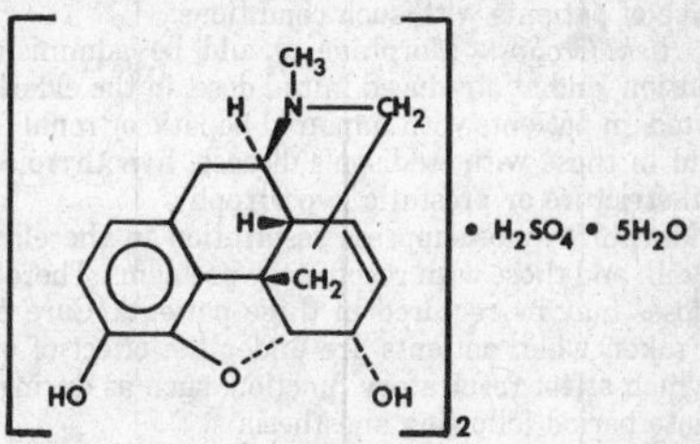

CLINICAL PHARMACOLOGY

Morphine exerts its major effects on the central nervous system and the bowel. Like other opium derivatives, it acts as an agonist, interacting with stereospecific and saturable binding sites or receptors in various tissues, including the brain. Morphine acts directly on the CNS to produce analgesia, drowsiness, mental clouding, and altered mood. Cough suppression is mediated through direct effect on the medullary center. Respiratory depression results from reduced responsiveness of the respiratory center to carbon dioxide. Emesis is a consequence of direct stimulation of the chemoreceptor trigger zone. Biliary tract pressure may result from morphine induced spasm of the Sphincter of Oddi. Constipation is secondary to the narcotic action on bowel wall nerve plexuses.

INDICATIONS AND USAGE

MS Contin is indicated for the prolonged relief of severe pain.

Continued on next page

Purdue Frederick—Cont.

CONTRAINDICATIONS

Contraindications include hypersensitivity to morphine; respiratory depression or insufficiency; bronchial asthma (attack); severe CNS depression; cardiac failure secondary to chronic pulmonary disease; cardiac arrhythmias; increased cerebrospinal or intracranial pressure; head injuries; brain tumor; acute alcoholism; delirium tremens; convulsive disorders and suspected surgical abdomen. Morphine is also contraindicated after biliary tract surgery, following surgical anastomosis, and concomitantly with MAO inhibitors (or within 14 days of such treatment).

As with all oral morphine preparations MS Contin Tablets should be used with caution peri-operatively in abdominal surgery. Should paralytic ileus occur during or after administration of MS Contin Tablets, their use should be immediately discontinued. As with all morphine preparations, patients who are scheduled for cordotomy or other pain-relieving surgical procedures, should not receive MS Contin Tablets within 24 hours prior to surgery.

WARNINGS

Morphine may cause tolerance as well as psychological and physicial dependence. Withdrawal symptoms can occur upon abrupt discontinuation, or on administration of a narcotic antagonist.

Interaction with Other CNS Depressants

Morphine should be used with caution, in reduced dosage, during concurrent administration of other narcotic analgesics, general anesthetics, phenothiazines or other tranquilizers, sedative-hypnotics, tricyclic antidepressants, and other CNS depressants (including alcohol). If not, respiratory depression, hypotension, and profound sedation or coma may result.

PRECAUTIONS

General

Head Trauma and Increased Intracranial Pressure: The respiratory depressant effects of morphine, and the drug's capacity to elevate cerebrospinal fluid pressure, may be greatly exaggerated in the presence of increased intracranial pressure. In addition, narcotics can produce side effects that may obscure the clinical course in case of head injury. In such patients, morphine must be used with caution and only if it is judged essential.

Asthma and Other Respiratory Disorders: Morphine must be used with caution during acute asthmatic attacks, in patients with chronic obstructive lung disease, or cor pulmonale, and in patients with substantially decreased respiratory reserve, preexisting respiratory depression, hypoxia, or hypercapnia. Even commonly prescribed therapeutic doses of narcotics may reduce respiratory drive while simultaneously raising airway resistance to the point of apnea.

Hypotensive Effect: Morphine administration may result in severe hypotension in patients whose ability to maintain adequate blood pressure is already compromised by diminished blood volume or concurrent administration of such drugs as phenothiazines or certain anesthetics.

Acute Abdominal Conditions: The administration of morphine or other narcotics may obscure the diagnosis or clinical course of patients with such conditions.

Special Risk Groups: Morphine should be administered with caution, and at a reduced initial dose, in the elderly or debilitated, in patients with impaired hepatic or renal function, and in those with Addison's disease, hypothyroidism, urethral stricture or prostatic hypertrophy.

Note: Morphine may suppress respiration in the elderly, the very ill, and those with respiratory problems. Therefore, lower doses may be required in these patients. Care must also be taken when patients are under the effect of other drugs which affect respiratory function, such as during the immediate period following anesthesia.

Information for Patients

Ambulatory Patients: Morphine may impair the abilities, mental and/or physical, needed for certain potentially hazardous activities, such as driving a car or operating machinery. The patient should be cautioned accordingly.

Like other narcotics, morphine may cause orthostatic hypotension in ambulatory patients.

Patients should also be cautioned about the combined effects of other CNS depressants with morphine, including those of alcohol and antihistamines.

Drug Interactions

Generally, effects of morphine may be antagonized by acidifying agents and potentiated by alkalizing agents. The analgesic effect of morphine is potentiated by chlorpromazine and methocarbamol. CNS depressants, such as other narcotics, anesthetics, sedatives, hypnotic agents, barbiturates, phenothiazines, chloral hydrate, and glutethimide may enhance the depressant effects of morphine. Monoamine oxidase inhibitors (including procarbazine hydrochloride), furazolidone, antihistamines, "beta blockers" such as propranolol, and alcohol may also enhance the depressant effects of morphine.

Morphine may increase the anticoagulant activity of coumarin and other anticoagulant drugs.

Carcinogenicity/Mutagenicity

No long-term studies of the carcinogenic/mutagenic potential of morphine is available.

Pregnancy Category C: Reproduction studies in animals have not been carried out with morphine. It is also not known whether morphine can cause fetal harm when administered to a pregnant woman or can affect the reproduction capacity. Morphine should be given to a pregnant woman only if clearly needed.

Labor and Delivery

Morphine readily crosses the placental barrier and its administration during labor may lead to respiratory depression in the newborn.

Use by Nursing Mothers

Morphine has been detected in human milk. Caution should therefore be exercised when this drug is administered to a nursing mother.

Pediatric Usage

The safety and effectiveness of morphine in children has not been established.

ADVERSE REACTIONS

THE MAJOR HAZARDS ASSOCIATED WITH MORPHINE, AS WITH OTHER NARCOTIC ANALGESICS, ARE RESPIRATORY DEPRESSION, AND TO A LESSER DEGREE, CIRCULATORY DEPRESSION. RESPIRATORY ARREST, SHOCK, AND CARDIAC ARREST HAVE OCCURRED FOLLOWING ORAL OR PARENTERAL USE OF MORPHINE.

Lightheadedness, sedation, dizziness, nausea, vomiting and excessive sweating are among the most frequently observed adverse reactions. These effects seem to be more prominent in ambulatory patients and in those not experiencing intense pain. In such cases, lower doses are advisable. Some adverse reactions may be alleviated in ambulatory patients if they lie down.

Other adverse reactions observed include the following:

CNS: Weakness, headache, insomnia, disorientation, visual disturbances, agitation, euphoria and dysphoria.

Cardiovascular: Palpitations, bradycardia, faintness/syncope and facial flushing.

Gastrointestinal: Constipation, anorexia, dry mouth and spasm of the biliary tract.

Genitourinary: Urinary retention or hesitancy, antidiurectic effect, reduced libido and/or reduced sexual potency.

Allergic: Pruritus, skin rashes including urticaria, hemorrhagic urticaria (rarely), and edema.

Treatment of the Most Frequent Adverse Effects

Constipation: Ample fluid intake should be encouraged. Concomitant administration of a stool-softener combined with a peristaltic stimulant (e.g., standardized senna concentrate with docusate sodium) can be effective prophylaxis against morphine-induced constipation. If elimination does not occur for two days, an enema should be considered to prevent fecal impaction.

If diarrhea occurs, seepage around an impaction should be evaluated as a possible cause before antidiarrheal measures are used.

Nausea and Vomiting: Phenothiazines or antihistaminic agents can be effective treatments for nausea of medullary or vestibular origin, respectively. However, concomitant therapy with these drugs may potentiate the side effects of morphine.

Sedation: Once pain control is achieved, undesirable drowsiness can be minimized by adjustment of dosage to a level that just maintains a pain-free state or a tolerable level of pain.

DRUG ABUSE AND DEPENDENCE

The narcotic morphine sulfate is a Schedule II controlled substance under the Federal Controlled Substance Act. As with other narcotics, its administration may result in development of physical and psychological dependence by some patients. Such patients may increase dosage without consulting a physician and subsequently may develop a physical dependence on the drug. In cases of this type, abrupt discontinuance may precipitate typical withdrawal symptoms, including convulsions. The drug should therefore be withdrawn gradually from those known to be taking excessive dosages over a prolonged period.

In treating the terminally ill, the benefits of morphine administration may outweigh the risk of drug dependence. The chance of such dependence is substantially reduced under a scheduled narcotic administration program as compared to PRN dosage.

OVERDOSAGE

Signs and Symptoms: Serious morphine overdosage is characterized by respiratory depression (reduced respiratory rate and/or tidal volume; Cheyne-Stokes respiration; cyanosis), extreme somnolence progressing to stupor or coma, flaccidity of skeletal muscle, cold or clammy skin, and sometimes hypotension and bradycardia. Severe overdosage may result in apnea, circulatory collapse, cardia arrest and death.

Treatment: Primary attention should be given to the reestablishment of adequate respiratory exchange through the provision of a patent airway and controlled or assisted ventilation. The narcotic antagonist naloxone hydrochloride is a specific antidote against respiratory depression due to overdosage or as a result of unusual sensitivity to narcotics, including morphine. An appropriate dose of naloxone hydrochloride should therefore be administered, preferably by the intravenous route; the usual initial i.v. adult dose is 0.4 mg. Concomitant efforts at respiratory resuscitation should be carried out. Since the duration of action of morphine may exceed that of the antagonist, the patient should be under continued surveillance and doses of the antagonist should be repeated as needed to maintain adequate respiration.

Do not administer an antagonist in the absence of clinically significant respiratory or cardiovascular depression.

Oxygen, intravenous fluids, vasopressor substances, and other supportive measures should be used as indicated.

Evacuation of gastric contents may be useful in removing unabsorbed drug.

DOSAGE AND ADMINISTRATION

Usual Adult Oral Dose: One 30 mg MS CONTIN (morphine sulfate pentahydrate) Tablet every 12 hours, or as directed by physician. Patients established on an immediate-release oral morphine product may be transferred to MS CONTIN Tablets on a mg- for-mg basis, using the same total daily dose (24 hour) divided for q 12 h administration. If converting a patient from another narcotic to morphine sulfate on the basis of standard equivalence tables, a 1 to 3 ratio of parenteral to oral morphine equivalence is suggested.

MS CONTIN Tablets are to be taken whole, and are not to be broken, chewed or crushed.

Dosage of morphine is a patient-dependent variable, which must be individualized according to the patient's metabolism and response to morphine. Clinical studies* confirm that the majority of patients are adequately maintained with MS CONTIN Tablets administered q 12 h. Other patients will require dosing q 8 h. Due to the long-acting characteristics of MS CONTIN Tablets, dosage is not recommended more frequently than q 8 h.

Each patient should be maintained at the lowest dosage level that will produce acceptable analgesia. As the patient's well-being improves after successful relief of severe pain, periodic reduction of dosage and/or extension of dosing interval should be attempted to minimize exposure to morphine.

CAUTION

DEA Order Form Required.

Federal law prohibits dispensing without prescription.

HOW SUPPLIED

NDC 0034-0515-50: MS CONTIN (morphine sulfate pentahydrate) Tablets, 30 mg are supplied in opaque plastic bottles, containing 50 tablets.

NDC 0034-0515-10: MS CONTIN (morphine sulfate pentahydrate) Tablets, 30 mg are supplied in opaque plastic bottles, containing 100 tablets.

NDC 0034-0515-45: MS CONTIN (morphine sulfate pentahydrate) Tablets, 30 mg are supplied in opaque plastic bottles, containing 250 tablets.

NDC 0034-0515-25: MS CONTIN (morphine sulfate pentahydrate) Tablets, 30 mg are supplied in unit-dose packaging with 25 individually-numbered tablets per card (numbered in descending order for easier counting) and shrink-wrapped in inner packs of 100 tablets (4 cards of 25 tablets per card). One shipper contains 300 tablets (3 inner packs of 100 tablets each). Each individual tablet-unit is labeled "MS CONTIN CII, 30 mg."

Each round, lavender-colored tablet bears the symbol PF on one side and M30 on the other side. Store tablets at controlled room temperature 15 to 30°C (59–86°F).

** Data available on request.*

1-2-86

Shown in Product Identification Section, page 423

MSIR® Oral Solution Ⓒ
[em 'es ĭ"ahr]
(morphine sulfate)
(WARNING: May be habit forming)

MSIR® Oral Solution Concentrate Ⓒ
(morphine sulfate)
(WARNING: May be habit forming)

MSIR® Immediate Release Oral Tablets Ⓒ
(morphine sulfate)
(WARNING: May be habit forming)

DESCRIPTION

Chemically, morphine sulfate is 7,8 didehydro-4,5 α-epoxy-17 methyl-morphinian-3,6 α-diol sulfate (2:1) (salt) pentahydrate and has the following structural formula:

[See Chemical Formula at top of next column].

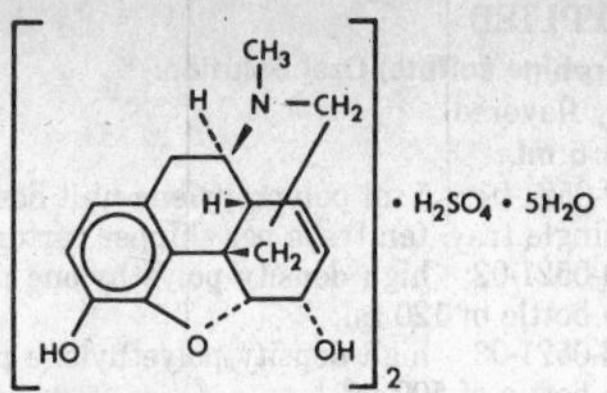

Each 5 ml of MSIR Oral Solution contains:
Morphine Sulfate .... 10 or 20 mg
(WARNING: May be habit forming)
Each 1 ml of MSIR Oral Solution Concentrate contains:
Morphine Sulfate .... 20 mg
(WARNING: May be habit forming)
Each MSIR Tablet for oral administration contains:
Morphine Sulfate .... 15 or 30 mg
(WARNING: May be habit forming)

CLINICAL PHARMACOLOGY

METABOLISM AND PHARMACOKINETICS

MSIR Solutions and Tablets containing morphine sulfate are for oral administration and are conventional immediate release products. Only about 40% of the administered dose reaches the central compartment because of pre-systemic elimination (i.e., metabolism in the gut wall and liver).
Once absorbed, morphine is distributed in skeletal muscle, kidneys, liver, intestinal tract, lungs, spleen and brain. Morphine also crosses the placental membranes and has been found in breast milk.
Although a small fraction (less than 5%) of morphine is demethylated, for all practical purposes, virtually all morphine is converted to glucuronide metabolites; among these, morphine-3-glucuronide is present in the highest plasma concentration following oral administration.
The glucuronide system has a very high capacity and is not easily saturated even in disease. Therefore, the rate of delivery of morphine to the gut and liver does not influence the total and/or the relative quantities of the various metabolites formed.
The following pharmacokinetic parameters show considerable inter-subject variation but are representative of average values reported in the literature. The volume of distribution (Vd) for morphine is 4 liters per kilogram, and the terminal elimination half-life is approximately 2 to 4 hours. Fifty percent of the morphine that will reach the central compartment intact, reaches it within 30 minutes following the administration of conventional oral morphine products.
Variation in the physical/mechanical properties of a formulation of an oral morphine drug product can affect both its absolute bioavailability and its absorption rate constant (k_a). The basic pharmacokinetic parameters (e.g., volume of distribution [Vd], elimination rate constant [k_e], clearance [Cl]) are fundamental properties of morphine in the organism.
While there is no predictable relationship between morphine blood levels and analgesic response, effective analgesia probably will not occur below some minimum blood level in a given patient. The minimum effective blood level for analgesia will vary among patients, especially among patients who have or have not been previously treated with potent mu (μ)agonist opioids. Similarly, there is no predictable relationship between blood morphine concentration and untoward clinical responses; but higher concentrations are more likely to be toxic.
The elimination of morphine occurs primarily as renal excretion of 3-morphine glucuronide. A small amount of the glucuronide conjugate is excreted in the bile, and there is some minor enterohepatic recycling.
The elimination half-life of morphine is reported to vary between 2 and 4 hours. Thus, steady state is probably achieved on most regimens within a day. Because morphine is primarily metabolized to inactive metabolites, the effects of renal disease on morphine's elimination are not likely to be pronounced. However, as with any drug, caution should be taken to guard against unanticipated accumulation if renal and/or hepatic function is seriously impaired.
Individual differences in the metabolism of morphine suggest that MSIR Oral Solutions and Tablets be dosed conservatively according to the dosing initiation and titration recommendations in the Dosage and Administration section.

PHARMACODYNAMICS

The effects described below are common to all morphine-containing products.

Central Nervous System

The principal actions of therapeutic value of morphine are analgesia and sedation.
The precise mechanism of analgesic action is unknown. However, specific CNS opiate receptors and endogenous compounds with morphine-like activity have been identified throughout the brain and spinal cord and are likely to play a role in the expression of analgesic effects.
Morphine produces respiratory depression by direct action on brain stem respiratory centers. The mechanism of respiratory depression involves a reduction in the responsiveness of the brain stem respiratory centers to increases in carbon dioxide tension, and to electrical stimulation.
Morphine depresses the cough reflex by direct effect on the cough center in the medulla. Antitussive effects may occur with doses lower than those usually required for analgesia.
Morphine causes miosis, even in total darkness. Pinpoint pupils are a sign of narcotic overdose but are not pathognomonic (e.g., pontine lesions hemorrhagic or ischemic origins may produce similar findings). Marked mydriasis rather than miosis may be seen with worsening hypoxia.

Gastrointestinal Tract and Other Smooth Muscle

Gastric, biliary and pancreatic secretions are decreased by morphine. Morphine causes a reduction in motility associated with an increase in tone in the antrum of the stomach and duodenum. Digestion of food in the small intestine is delayed and propulsive contractions are decreased. In addition propulsive peristaltic waves in the colon are decreased, while tone is increased to the point of spasm. The end result is constipation. Morphine can cause a marked increase in biliary tract pressure as a result of spasm of the sphincter of Oddi.

Cardiovascular System

Morphine produces peripheral vasodilation which may result in orthostatic hypotension. Release of histamine can occur and may contribute to narcotic-induced hypotension. Manifestations of histamine release and/or peripheral vasodilation may include pruritus, flushing, red eyes and sweating.

INDICATIONS AND USAGE

MSIR Oral Solutions and Tablets are indicated for the relief of moderate to severe pain.

CONTRAINDICATIONS

MSIR Oral Solutions and Tablets are contraindicated in patients with known hypersensitivity to the drug, in patients with respiratory depression in the absence of resuscitative equipment, and in patients with acute or severe bronchial asthma.

WARNINGS: (see also: CLINICAL PHARMACOLOGY)

Impaired Respiration

Respiratory depression is the chief hazard of all morphine preparations although mitigated in the presence of pain. Respiratory depression occurs most frequently in elderly and debilitated patients, and those suffering from conditions accompanied by hypoxia or hypercapnia when even moderate therapeutic doses may dangerously decrease pulmonary ventilation.
Morphine should be used with extreme caution in patients with chronic obstructive pulmonary disease or cor pulmonale, and in patients having a substantially decreased respiratory reserve, hypoxia, hypercapnia, or preexisting respiratory depression. In such patients, even usual therapeutic doses of morphine may decrease respiratory drive while simultaneously increasing airway resistance to the point of apnea.

Head Injury and Increased Intracranial Pressure

The respiratory depressant effects of morphine with carbon dioxide retention and secondary elevation of cerebrospinal fluid pressure may be markedly exaggerated in the presence of head injury, other intracranial lesions, or preexisting increase in intracranial pressure. Morphine produces effects which may obscure neurologic signs of further increase in pressure in patients with head injuries.

Hypotensive Effects

MSIR Oral Solutions and Tablets, like all opioid analgesics, may cause severe hypotension in an individual whose ability to maintain his blood pressure has already been compromised by a depleted blood volume, or a concurrent administration of drugs such as phenothiazines, or general anesthetics. (see also: PRECAUTIONS: Drug Interactions.) MSIR Oral Solutions and Tablets may produce orthostatic hypotension in ambulatory patients.
MSIR Oral Solutions and Tablets, like all opioid analgesics, should be administered with caution to patients in circulatory shock, since vasodilation produced by the drug may further reduce cardiac output and blood pressure.

Interactions with Other CNS Depressants

MSIR Oral Solutions and Tablets, like all opioid analgesics, should be used with great caution and in reduced dosage in patients who are concurrently receiving other central nervous system depressants including sedatives or hypnotics, general anesthetics, phenothiazines, other tranquilizers and alcohol, because respiratory depression, hypotension and profound sedation or coma may result.

Interactions with Mixed Agonist/Antagonist Opioid Analgesics

From a theoretical perspective, agonist/antagonist analgesics (i.e., pentazocine, nalbuphine, butorphanol and buprenorphine) should NOT be administered to a patient who has received or is receiving a course of therapy with a pure agonist opioid analgesic. In these patients, mixed agonist-antagonist analgesics may reduce the analgesic effect or may precipitate withdrawal symptoms.

Drug Dependence

Morphine can produce drug dependence and has a potential for being abused. Tolerance and psychological and physical dependence may develop upon repeated administration. Physical dependence, however, is not of paramount importance in the management of any patient in severe pain. Abrupt cessation or a sudden reduction in dose after prolonged use may result in withdrawal symptoms. After prolonged exposure to opioid analgesics, if withdrawal is necessary, it must be undertaken gradually. (See DRUG ABUSE AND DEPENDENCE.)
Infants born to mothers physically dependent on opioid analgesics may also be physically dependent and exhibit respiratory depression and withdrawal symptoms. (See **DRUG ABUSE AND DEPENDENCE.**)
The development of psychological dependence is relatively rare when morphine is used under medically supervised conditions.

PRECAUTIONS; (See also: CLINICAL PHARMACOLOGY)

General

MSIR Oral Solutions and Tablets are intended for use in patients who require a potent opioid analgesic for relief of moderate to severe pain.
Selection of patients for treatment with MSIR Oral Solutions and Tablets should be governed by the same principles that apply to the use of morphine and other potent opioid analgesics which take in account: the elderly or debilitated and those with the following—severe impairment of hepatic, pulmonary or renal function; myxedema or hypothyroidism; adrenocortical insufficiency (e.g., Addison's Disease); CNS depression or coma; toxic psychoses; prostatic hypertrophy or urethral stricture; acute alcoholism; delirium tremens; or kyphoscoliosis.
The administration of morphine, like all opioid analgesics, may obscure the diagnosis or clinical course in patients with acute abdominal conditions.
Morphine may aggravate preexisting convulsions in patients with convulsive disorders.
Morphine should be used with caution in patients about to undergo surgery of the biliary tract, since it may cause spasm of the sphincter of Oddi. Similarly, morphine should be used with caution in patients with acute pancreatitis secondary to biliary tract disease.

Information for Patients

If clinically advisable, patients receiving MSIR Oral Solutions and Tablets should be given the following instructions by the physician.

1. Morphine may produce physical dependence and may be associated with the development of psychological dependence. For this reason, the dose of the drug should not be adjusted without consulting a physician.
2. Morphine may impair mental and/or physical ability required for the performance of potentially hazardous tasks (e.g., driving, operating machinery).
3. Morphine should not be taken with alcohol or other CNS depressants (sleep aids, tranquilizers) because additive effects including CNS depression may occur. A physician should be consulted if other prescription medications are currently being used or are prescribed for future use.
4. For women of childbearing potential who become or are planning to become pregnant, a physician should be consulted regarding analgesics and other drug use.

Drug Interactions (See also **WARNINGS**)

The concomitant use of other central nervous system depressant including sedatives or hypnotics, general anesthetics, phenothiazines, tranquilizers and alcohol may produce additive depressant effects. Respiratory depression, hypotension and profound sedation or coma may occur. When such combined therapy is contemplated, the dose of one or both agents should be reduced. Opioid analgesics, including MSIR Oral Solutions and Tablets, may enhance the neuromuscular blocking action of skeletal muscle relaxants and produce an increased degree of respiratory depression.

Carcinogenicity/Mutagenicity/Impairment of Fertility

Studies of morphine sulfate in animals to evaluate the drug's carcinogenic and mutagenic potential or the effect on fertility have not been conducted.

Pregnancy

Teratogenic effects—CATEGORY C: There are no well-controlled studies in women, but marketing experience does not include any evidence of adverse effects on the fetus following routine (short-term) clinical use of morphine sulfate products. Although there is no clearly defined risk, such experience cannot exclude the possibility of infrequent or subtle damage to the human fetus. MSIR Oral Solutions and Tablets should be used in pregnant women only when clearly needed. (See also: **PRECAUTIONS: Labor and Delivery,** and **DRUG ABUSE AND DEPENDENCE.**)
Nonteratogenic effects: Infants born from mothers who have been taking morphine chronically may exhibit withdrawal symptoms.

Continued on next page

Purdue Frederick—Cont.

Labor and Delivery

MSIR Oral Solutions and Tablets are not recommended for use in women during and immediately prior to labor. Occasionally, opioid analgesics may prolong labor through actions which temporarily reduce the strength, duration and frequency of uterine contractions. However, this effect is not consistent and may be offset by an increased rate of cervical dilatation which tends to shorten labor.

Neonates whose mothers receive opioid analgesics during labor should be observed closely for signs of respiratory depression. A specific narcotic antagonist, naloxone, should be available for reversal of narcotic-induced respiratory depression in the neonate.

Nursing Mothers

Low levels of morphine sulfate have been detected in human milk. Withdrawal symptoms can occur in breast-feeding infants when maternal administration of morphine sulfate is stopped. Nursing should not be undertaken while a patient is receiving MSIR Oral Solutions and Tablets since morphine may be excreted in the milk.

ADVERSE REACTIONS

The adverse reactions caused by morphine are essentially the same as those observed with other opioid analgesics. They include the following major hazards: respiratory depression, apnea, and to a lesser degree, circulatory depression; respiratory arrest, shock, and cardiac arrest.

Most Frequently Observed

Constipation, lightheadedness, dizziness, sedation, nausea, vomiting, and sweating.

Some of these effects seem to be more prominent in ambulatory patients and in those not experiencing severe pain. Some adverse reactions in ambulatory patients may be alleviated if the patient lies down.

Less Frequently Observed Reactions

Central Nervous System	Weakness, headache, agitation, tremor, uncoordinated muscle movements, seizure, alterations of mood (dysphoria, euphoria, nervousness, apprehension, depression, floating feelings), dreams, muscle rigidity, transient hallucinations and disorientation, visual disturbances, insomnia and increased intracranial pressure.
Gastrointestinal	Dry mouth, biliary tract spasm, anorexia, diarrhea, cramps and taste alterations.
Cardiovascular	Flushing of the face, chills, tachycardia, bradycardia, palpitation, faintness, syncope, hypotension and hypertension.
Genitourinary	Urinary retention or hesitance, reduced libido, and/or impotence.
Dermatologic	Pruritus, urticaria, other skin rashes, and edema.
Other	Antidiuretic effect, paresthesia, muscle tremor, blurred vision, nystagmus, diplopia, miosis and laryngospasm.

DRUG ABUSE AND DEPENDENCE

Opioid analgesics may cause physical dependence and be associated with the development of psychological dependence. (See WARNINGS.) Physical dependence results in withdrawal symptoms in patients who abruptly discontinue the drug or may be precipitated through the administration of drugs with narcotic antagonist activity, e.g., naloxone or mixed agonist/antagonist analgesics (pentazocine, etc.; see also OVERDOSAGE.). Physical dependence usually does not occur to a clinically significant degree until after several weeks of continued narcotic usage. Tolerance, in which increasingly large doses are required in order to produce the same degree of analgesia, is initially manifested by a shortened duration of analgesic effect, and, subsequently, by decreases in the intensity of analgesia. In chronic-pain patients and in narcotic-tolerant cancer patients, the administration of MSIR Oral Solutions and Tablets should be guided by the degree of tolerance manifested. Physical dependence, per se, is not a concern when one is dealing with the cancer patient with moderate to severe pain. The primary objective in this situation is to relieve the patient's pain.

If MSIR Oral Solutions and Tablets are abruptly discontinued, a moderate to severe abstinence syndrome may occur. The opioid agonist abstinence syndrome is characterized by some or all of the following: restlessness, lacrimation, rhinorrhea, yawning, perspiration, cutis anserina, restless sleep known as the "yen"and mydriasis during the first 24 hours. These symptoms often increase in severity and over the next 72 hours may be accompanied by increasing irritability, anxiety, weakness, twitching and spasms of muscles; kicking movements; severe backache, abdominal and leg pains; abdominal and muscle cramps; hot and cold flashes; insomnia; nausea, anorexia, vomiting, intestinal spasm, diarrhea; coryza and repetitive sneezing; and increase in body temperature, blood pressure, respiratory rate and heart rate. Because of excessive loss of fluids through sweating, vomiting and diarrhea, there is usually marked weight loss, dehydration, ketosis, and disturbances in acid-base balance. Cardiovascular collapse can occur. Without treatment, most observable symptoms disappear in 5–14 days; however, there appears to be a phase of secondary or chronic abstinence which may last for 2–6 months, characterized by insomnia, irritability, and muscular aches.

If treatment of physical dependence on MSIR Oral Solutions and Tablets is necessary, the patient may be detoxified by gradual reduction of the dosage. If abstinence symptoms become severe, the patient may be given methadone. Temporary administration of tranquilizers and sedatives may aid in reducing patient anxiety and narcotic craving. Gastrointestinal disturbances or dehydration should be treated accordingly.

OVERDOSAGE

Acute overdosage with morphine is manifested by respiratory depression, somnolence progressing to stupor or coma, skeletal muscle flaccidity, cold and clammy skin, constricted pupils, and, sometimes, bradycardia and hypotension.

In the treatment of overdosage, primary attention should be given to the re-establishment of a patent airway and institution of assisted or controlled ventilation. The pure opioid antagonist, naloxone, is a specific antidote against respiratory depression which results from opioid overdose. Naloxone (usually 0.4 to 2.0 mg) should be administered intravenously; however, because its duration of action is relatively short, the patient must be carefully monitored until spontaneous respiration is reliably reestablished. If the response to naloxone is suboptimal or not sustained, additional naloxone may be re-administered, as needed, or given by continuous infusion to maintain alertness and respiratory function; however, there is no information available about the cumulative dose of naloxone that may be safely administered.

Naloxone should not be administered in the absence of clinically significant respiratory or circulatory depression secondary to morphine overdose. Naloxone should be administered cautiously to persons who are known or suspected to be physically dependent on morphine. In such cases, an abrupt or complete reversal of narcotic effects may precipitate an acute abstinence syndrome.

Note: In an individual physically dependent on opioids, administration of the usual dose of the antagonist will precipitate an acute withdrawal syndrome. The severity of the withdrawal syndrome produced will depend on the degree of physical dependence and the dose of the antagonist administered. Use of a narcotic antagonist in such a person should be avoided. If necessary to treat serious respiratory depression in the physically dependent patient, the antagonist should be administered with extreme care and by titration with smaller than usual doses of the antagonist.

Supportive measures (including oxygen, vasopressors) should be employed in the management of circulatory shock and pulmonary edema accompanying overdose as indicated. Cardiac arrest or arrhythmias may require cardiac massage or defibrillation.

CAUTION

DEA Order Form Required.

Federal law prohibits dispensing without prescription.

DOSAGE AND ADMINISTRATION: (See also: CLINICAL PHARMACOLOGY, WARNINGS AND PRECAUTIONS sections)

Dosage of morphine is a patient-dependent variable, which must be individualized according to patient metabolism, age and disease state and also response to morphine. Each patient should be maintained at the lowest dosage level that will produce acceptable analgesia. As the patient's well-being improves after successful relief of moderate to severe pain, periodic reduction of dosage and/or extension of dosing interval should be attempted to minimize exposure to morphine.

Usual Adult Oral Dose: 5 to 30 mg every four (4) hours or as directed by physician administered either as MSIR Oral Solutions or MSIR Oral Tablets. For control of pain in terminal illness, it is recommended that the appropriate dose of MSIR Oral Solutions or MSIR Oral Tablets be given on a regularly scheduled basis every four hours at the minimum dose to achieve acceptable analgesia. If converting a patient from another narcotic to morphine sulfate on the basis of standard equivalence tables, a 1 to 3 ratio of parenteral to oral morphine equivalence is suggested. This ratio is conservative and may underestimate the amount of morphine required. If this is the case, the dose of MSIR Oral Solutions or MSIR Oral Tablets should be gradually increased to achieve acceptable analgesia and tolerable side effects.

HOW SUPPLIED

MSIR (morphine sulfate) Oral Solution:
(pleasantly flavored)

10 mg per 5 ml.

NDC 0034-0521-01: 5 ml polypropylene unit dose cups, 10 cups per single tray, ten trays per shipper carton.
NDC 0034-0521-02: high density polyethylene plastic metered dose bottle of 120 ml.
NDC 0034-0521-03: high density polyethylene plastic metered dose bottle of 500 ml.

20 mg per 5 ml.

NDC 0034-0522-01: 5 ml polypropylene unit dose cups, 10 cups per single tray, ten trays per shipper carton.
NDC 0034-0522-02: high density polyethylene plastic metered dose bottle of 120 ml.
NDC 0034-0522-03: high density polyethylene plastic metered dose bottle of 500 ml.

MSIR (morphine sulfate) Oral Solution Concentrate:
(unflavored)

20 mg per 1 ml.

NDC 0034-0523-01: high density polyethylene plastic, child resistant closure bottle with child resistant dropper in 30 ml size.
NDC 0034-0523-02: high density polyethylene plastic, child resistant closure bottle with child resistant dropper in 120 ml size.
Discard opened bottle of Oral Solution after 90 days.
Protect from light.

MSIR (morphine sulfate) Immediate Release Oral Tablets:
15 mg round, white scored tablets

NDC 0034-0518-15: opaque plastic bottle, containing 50 tablets. Each tablet bears the symbol PF on the scored side and MI 15 on the other side.

30 mg capsule-shaped, white scored tablets

NDC 0034-0519-30: opaque plastic bottle containing 50 tablets. Each tablet bears the symbol PF on the scored side and MI 30 on the other side.

Store Oral Solutions and Tablets at controlled room temperature 15°to 30°C (59°–86°F).

Shown in Product Identification Section, page 423

SENOKOT® TABLETS/GRANULES

[*sĕn'ō-kŏt*]

(standardized senna concentrate)

ACTION AND USES

Indicated for relief of functional constipation (chronic or occasional). SENOKOT Tablets/Granules contain a natural vegetable derivative, purified and standardized for uniform action. The current theory of the mechanism of action is that glycosides are transported to the colon, where they are changed to aglycones that stimulate Auerbach's plexus to induce peristalsis. This virtually colon-specific action is gentle, effective and predictable, usually inducing comfortable evacuation of well-formed stool within 8-10 hours. Found effective even in many previously intractable cases of functional constipation, SENOKOT preparations may aid in rehabilitation of the constipated patient by facilitating regular elimination. At proper dosage levels, SENOKOT preparations are virtually free of adverse reactions (such as loose stools or abdominal discomfort) and enjoy high patient acceptance. Numerous and extensive clinical studies show their high degree of effectiveness in varieties of functional constipation: chronic, geriatric, antepartum and postpartum, drug-induced, pediatric, as well as in functional constipation concurrent with heart disease or anorectal surgery.

CONTRAINDICATIONS

Acute surgical abdomen.

ADMINISTRATION AND DOSAGE

Preferably at bedtime. GRANULES (deliciously cocoa-flavored): Adults: 1 level tsp. (maximum—2 level tsp. b.i.d.). For older, debilitated, and OB/GYN patients, the physician may consider prescribing ½ the initial adult dose. Children above 60 lb.: ½ level tsp. (maximum—1 level tsp. b.i.d.). TABLETS: Adults: 2 tablets (maximum—4 tablets b.i.d.). For older, debilitated, and OB/GYN patients, the physician may consider prescribing ½ the initial dose. Children above 60 lb.: 1 tablet (maximum—2 tablets b.i.d.). To meet individual requirements, if comfortable bowel movement is not achieved by the second day, decrease or increase daily by ½ level tsp. or 1 tablet (up to maximum) until optimal dose for evacuation is established.

HOW SUPPLIED

Granules: 2, 6, and 12 oz. plastic canisters. Tablets: Box of 20, bottles of 50, 100 and 1000. Unit Strip Packs in boxes of 100 tablets; each tablet individually sealed in see-through pockets.

ALSO AVAILABLE

SENOKOT Syrup (standardized extract of senna fruit) in bottles of 2 and 8 fl. oz.

ADMINISTRATION AND DOSAGE

Preferable at bedtime. Adults: 2 to 3 tsp. (maximum—3 tsp. b.i.d.). For older, debilitated, and OB/GYN patients, the physician may consider prescribing ½ the initial adult dose. Children 5–15 years: 1 to 2 tsp. (maximum—2 tsp. b.i.d.). 1–5 years: ½ to 1 tsp. (maximum—1 tsp. b.i.d.). 1 month to 1 year: ¼ to ½ tsp. (maximum—½ tsp. bi.d.).

SENOKOT-S® Tablets

[sĕn'ō-kŏt-ĕs"]

(standardized senna concentrate and docusate sodium)

Natural Laxative/Stool Softener Combination

ACTION AND USES

SENOKOT-S Tablets are designed to relieve both aspects of functional constipation—bowel inertia and hard, dry stools. They provide a natural neuroperistaltic stimulant combined with a classic stool softener: standardized senna concentrate gently stimulates Auerbach's plexus in the colonic wall, while docusate sodium softens the stool for smoother and easier evacuation. This coordinated dual action of the two ingredients results in colon-specific, predictable laxative effect, usually in 8–10 hours. Administering the tablets at bedtime allows the patient an uninterrupted night's sleep, with a comfortable evacuation in the morning. Flexibility of dosage permits fine adjustment to individual requirements. At proper dosage levels, SENOKOT-S Tablets are virtually free from side effects. SENOKOT-S Tablets are highly suitable for relief of postsurgical and postpartum constipation, and effectively counteract drug-induced constipation. They facilitate regular elimination in impaction-prone and elderly patients, and are indicated in the presence of cardiovascular disease where straining must be avoided, as well as in the presence of hemorrhoids and anorectal disease.

CONTRAINDICATIONS

Acute surgical abdomen.

ADMINISTRATION AND DOSAGE

(Preferably at bedtime). Recommended Initial Dosage: ADULTS—2 tablets (maximum dosage—4 tablets b.i.d.); CHILDREN (above 60 lbs.)—1 tablet (maximum dosage—2 tablets b.i.d.). For older or debilitated patients, the physician may consider prescribing half the initial adult dose. To meet individual requirements, if comfortable bowel movement is not achieved by the second day, dosage may be decreased or increased by 1 tablet, up to maximum, until the most effective dose is established.

SUPPLIED

Bottles of 30, 60 and 1000 Tablets.

TRILISATE® TABLETS/LIQUID ℞

[trī'ĭ-sāt"]

(choline magnesium trisalicylate)

500 mg, 750 mg or 1000 mg salicylate content

DESCRIPTION

TRILISATE Tablets/Liquid are nonsteroidal, anti-inflammatory preparations combining choline salicylate and magnesium salicylate in mixtures which are freely soluble in water.

TRILISATE Tablets are available in scored, pale pink 500 mg tablets; in scored, white, film-coated 750 mg tablets, and in scored, red film-coated 1000 mg tablets. Trilisate Liquid is a cherry cordial-flavored liquid providing 500 mg salicylate content per teaspoonful (5 ml) for oral administration.

Each 500 mg tablet contains 293 mg of choline salicylate combined with 362 mg of magnesium salicylate to provide 500 mg salicylate content. Each 750 mg tablet contains 440 mg of choline salicylate combined with 544 mg of magnesium salicylate to provide 750 mg salicylate content. Each 1000 mg tablet contains 587 mg of choline salicylate combined with 725 mg of magnesium salicylate to provide 1000 mg salicylate content. TRILISATE Liquid contains 293 mg of choline salicylate combined with 362 mg of magnesium salicylate to provide 500 mg salicylate per teaspoonful (5 ml) in a clear amber, cherry cordial-flavored vehicle.

CLINICAL PHARMACOLOGY

TRILISATE Tablets/Liquid contain salicylate with anti-inflammatory, analgesia and antipyretic action. On ingestion of TRILISATE Tablets/Liquid, the salicylate moiety is absorbed rapidly and reaches peak blood levels within an average of one to two hours after single doses of the tablets or liquid. The primary route of excretion is renal: the excretion products are chiefly the glycine and glucuronide conjugates. TRILISATE preparations differ from other non-steroidal anti-arthritic agents and from aspirin in having a more selective action on the prostaglandin pathway.

The bioequivalence of TRILISATE Liquid and Tablets 500 mg/750 mg/1000 mg has been established. With the tablets, a steady-state condition is usually reached after 4 to 5 doses, and the half-life of elimination, on repeated administration of the tablets, is 9 to 17 hours. This permits a maintenance dosage schedule of once or twice daily. Unlike aspirin and certain other non-steroidal anti-inflammatory agents, such as arylpropionic acid derivatives and arylacetic acid derivatives, choline magnesium trisalicylate, at therapeutic dosage levels, does not affect platelet aggregation, as shown in invitro and in-vivo studies.

INDICATIONS AND USAGE

Osteoarthritis, Rheumatoid Arthritis and Acute Painful Shoulder: Salicylates are considered the base therapy of choice in the arthritides; and TRILISATE preparations are indicated for the relief of the signs and symptoms of rheumatoid arthritis, osteoarthritis and other arthritides. TRILISATE Tablets or Liquid are indicated in the long-term management of these diseases and especially in the acute flare of rheumatoid arthritis. TRILISATE Tablets or Liquid are also indicated for the treatment of acute painful shoulder.

TRILISATE preparations are effective and generally well tolerated, and are logical choices whenever salicylate treatment is indicated. They are particularly suitable when a once-a-day or b.i.d. dosage regimen is important to patient compliance; when gastrointestinal intolerance to aspirin is encountered; when gastrointestinal microbleeding or hematolgic effects of aspirin are considered a patient hazard; and when interference (or the risk of interference) with normal platelet function by aspirin or by propionic acid derivatives is considered to be clinically undesirable. Use of TRILISATE Liquid is appropriate when a liquid dosage form is preferred, as in the elderly patient.

The efficacy of TRILISATE preparations has not been studied in those patients who are designated by the American Rheumatism Association as belonging in Functional Class IV (incapacitated, largely or wholly bedridden or confined to a wheelchair, with little or no self-care). Analgesic and Antipyretic Action: TRILISATE Tablets/Liquid are also indicated for the relief of mild to moderate pain and for antipyresis. *In children*, TRILISATE preparations are indicated for conditions requiring anti-inflammatory, analgesic or antipyretic action—such as juvenile rheumatoid arthritis and other appropriate conditions. Used concomitantly with antibiotics, TRILISATE preparations are useful for analgesia and antipyresis in many bacterial or viral infections.

CONTRAINDICATIONS

Patients who are hypersensitive to non-acetylated salicylates should not take TRILISATE Tablets or Liquid.

WARNING

Reye's Syndrome is a rare but serious disease which may develop in children and teenagers who have chicken pox, influenza, or flu symptoms. While the cause of Reye's Syndrome is unknown, some studies suggest a possible association between the development of Reye's Syndrome and the use of medicines containing acetylated salicylates or aspirin. TRILISATE Tablets and Liquid are a combination of choline and magnesium salicylate which are nonacetylated salicylates, and there have been no reported cases associating TRILISATE with Reye's Syndrome. Nevertheless, physicians should exercise caution in the use of any salicylate-containing product and make a risk benefit assessment before prescribing this product for use in children and teenagers with chicken pox, influenza or flu symptoms.

PRECAUTIONS

Like other salicylates, TRILISATE preparations should be used with caution in patients with chronic renal insufficiency or with active erosive gastritis or peptic ulcer.

Reports indicate that when acetylated salicylates are given with steroids, the butazones, or alcohol, the risk of gastrointestinal ulceration is increased. Caution should be exercised in patients requiring coumarin or indandione anticoagulants, or heparin.

While salicylates are not known to be associated with teratogenic potential in man, the usual care should be exercised in the administration of any drug during pregnancy. Because of the possible inhibition of prostaglandin with high doses of salicylates, the use of TRILISATE (choline magnesium trisalicylate) preparations immediately prior to the onset of labor is not recommended.

ADVERSE REACTIONS

Choline magnesium trisalicylate is generally well-tolerated at recommended dosage ranges, and has been shown to be particularly well-tolerated by the gastrointestinal system. Salicylism and/or salicylate intoxication may occur with large doses or with extended therapy.

Tinnitus may be regarded as a therapeutic guide. Should it develop, reduction of dosage is recommended.

DOSAGE

ADULTS: In rheumatoid arthritis, osteoarthritis, the more severe arthritides, and acute painful shoulder, the recommended daily dosage is 3000 mg given once a day (h.s.) or 1500 mg b.i.d. Dosage should be adjusted in accordance with the patient's response.

For mild to moderate pain or for antipyresis, the usual dosage is 2000 mg to 3000 mg daily in divided doses (b.i.d.). Based on patient response or salicylate blood levels, dosage may be adjusted to achieve optimum therapeutic effect. Salicylate blood levels should be in the range of 15 to 30 mg/100 ml for anti-inflammatory effect and 5 to 15 mg/100 ml for analgesia and antipyresis.

Each 500 mg tablet or teaspoonful is equivalent in salicylate content to 10 gr of aspirin; each 750 mg tablet, to 15 gr of aspirin; and each 1000 mg tablet, to 20 gr of aspirin.

If the physician prefers, the recommended daily dosage may be administered on a t.i.d. schedule.

As with other therapeutic agents, individual dosage adjustment is advisable, and a number of patients may require higher or lower dosages than those recommended. Certain patients require 2 to 3 weeks of therapy for optimal effect.

CHILDREN: *Usual total daily dose for children* for anti-inflammatory, analgesic and antipyretic action:

TRILISATE 500 mg Tablets/Liquid and TRILISATE 750 mg and 1000 mg Tablets, 50 mg/kg/day.

Weight (kg)	Total daily dose
12–13	500 mg
14–17	750 mg
18–22	1000 mg
23–27	1250 mg
28–32	1500 mg
33–37	1750 mg

Total daily doses should be administered in divided doses (b.i.d.). Doses of TRILISATE preparations are calculated as the total daily dose of 50 mg/kg/day for children of 37 kg body weight or less and 2250 mg/day for heavier children. TRILISATE Liquid is available for greater convenience in treating younger patients. TRILISATE Liquid may be mixed with fruit juices just before drinking.

CAUTION

Federal law prohibits dispensing without a prescription.

HOW SUPPLIED

NDC 0034-0500-80: TRILISATE 500 mg Tablets (pale pink, scored) supplied in bottles of 100 tablets.

NDC 0034-0500-10: TRILISATE 500 mg Tablets (pale pink, scored) supplied in Unit Dose packaging with 10 tablets per card. Ten cards are packed in each carton; 10 cartons are packed in each shipper.

NDC 0034-0505-80: TRILISATE 750 mg Tablets (scored, white, film-coated) in bottles of 100 tablets.

NDC 0034-0505-10: TRILISATE 750 mg Tablets (scored, white film-coated) supplied in Unit Dose packaging with 10 tablets per card. Ten cards are packed in each carton; 10 cartons are packed in each shipper.

NDC 0034-0510-60: TRILISATE 1000 mg Tablets (scored, red, film-coated) in bottles of 60 tablets.

NDC 0034-0520-80: TRILISATE Liquid in bottles of 8 fl. oz. (237 ml).

Store at controlled room temperature 59° to 86°F (15° to 30°C).

Copyright 1982, 1986. The Purdue Frederick Company

U.S. Patent Numbers 3759980 and 4067974

Shown in Product Identification Section, page 423

UNIPHYL® Tablets ℞

[ū'nĭ-fĭl]

(theophylline, anhydrous)

200 mg

UNICONTIN®

Controlled-Release System

DESCRIPTION

UNIPHYL Tablets contain 200 mg anhydrous theophylline in a controlled-release system. The tablets are scored to facilitate dosage adjustment.

Theophylline anhydrous, a xanthine bronchodilator, is a white, odorless, crystalline powder having a bitter taste. Theophylline has a molecular weight of 180.18, represented by $C_7H_8N_4O_2$ and depicted as:

[chemical structure of theophylline: O, CH_3, N, H, N, O, N, N, CH_3]

CLINICAL PHARMACOLOGY

Theophylline directly relaxes the smooth muscle of the bronchial airways and pulmonary blood vessels. The drug also produces other actions typical of the xanthine derivatives: coronary vasodilation, cardiac stimulation, diuresis, cerebral stimulation, and skeletal muscle stimulation. These

Continued on next page

Purdue Frederick—Cont.

actions may be mediated through inhibition of phosphodiesterase with a resultant increase in intracellular cyclic AMP. *In vitro,* theophylline has been shown to act synergistically with beta agonists that increase intracellular cyclic AMP through the stimulation of adenyl cyclase; but synergism has not been demonstrated in patient studies. More data are needed to determine if theophylline and beta agonists have a clinically important additive effect *in vivo.*

Pharmacokinetics: A single dose randomized crossover bioavailability study in healthy male volunteers compared 200 mg UNIPHYL Tablets with an approved controlled-release BID theophylline product. UNIPHYL 200 mg Tablets were found to be interchangeable on a mg basis according to average AUC (area under curve), C-max (maximum theophylline concentration), T-max (time to maximum concentration), T-max (time to maximum concentration), absorption rate and apparent elimination half-life.

In a multiple dose, steady-state study with UNIPHYL Tablets, a single 400 mg dose produced a peak average serum level of 10.0 mcg/ml within 4 hours. The average trough level was 7.8 mcg/ml during steady-state indicating little fluctuation between C-max and C-min.

Newborns and neonates have extremenly slow clearance rates compared to older infants (over 6 months) and children, and may also have a theophylline half-life of over 24 hours.

The half-life of theophylline in smokers averages 4 to 5 hours contrasted with 7 to 11 hours in non-smokers. Following the cessation of smoking, the effects on theophylline pharmacokinetics may persist for 3 months to 2 years.

Theophylline Elimination Characteristics

	Theophylline Clearance Rates (mean ± S.D.)	Half-Life Average (mean ± S.D.)
Children (over 6 months of age)	1.45 ± 0.58 ml/kg/min	3.7 ± 1.1 hr
Adult non-smokers with uncomplicated asthma	0.65 ± 0.19 ml/kg/min	8.7 ± 2.2 hr

INDICATIONS

UNIPHYL Tablets are indicated for relief and/or prevention of symptoms of asthma and reversible bronchospasm associated with chronic bronchitis and emphysema.

CONTRAINDICATIONS

This product is contraindicated in individuals who have shown hypersensitivity to theophylline.

WARNINGS

Status asthmaticus should be considered a medical emergency and is defined as that degree of bronchospasm which is not rapidly reponsive to usual doses of conventional bronchodilators. Optimal therapy for such patients frequently requires both *additional medication,* parenterally administered, and *close monitoring,* preferably in an intensive care setting.

Excessive theophylline doses may be associated with toxicity. Determination of serum theophylline levels is recommended to assure maximum therapeutic benefit without excessive risk. The incidence of toxicity increases at serum levels greater than 20 mcg/ml.

Optimum therapeutic response occurs in most patients when the serum theophylline concentration is 10 to 20 mcg/ml. In other patients satisfactory results (as determined by both relief of symptoms and improvement in pulmonary function) may be obtained at lower levels. In still others, adequate response may require higher levels. The physician should adjust the desired serum concentration range to the patients' requirements, keeping in mind that *an increased probability of toxicity exists* when levels exceed 20 mcg/ml. Therefore, in order to assure maximum benefit without excessive risk, measurement of serum levels is highly recommended.

Reduced theophylline clearance may result in increased serum levels and potential toxicity in the following patient groups: (1) those with impaired renal or liver function, (2) those over 55 years of age, particularly males and those with chronic lung disease, (3) those with cardiac failure, (4) those receiving macrolide antibiotics or cimetidine and (5) neonates. Decreased theophylline clearance may occur during active influenza infection or following immunization for influenza.

Less serious signs of theophylline toxicity, i.e. nausea and restlessness, may appear. Serious side effects such as ventricular arrhythmias, convulsions or even death may appear as the first sign of toxicity without any previous warning. *Serious toxicity is not reliably preceded by less severe side effects.*

Patients who require theophylline may exhibit tachycardia due to their underlying disease. The possible relationship of elevated serum theophylline concentration to tachycardia may not be recognized.

Theophylline products may cause arrhythmia and/or worsen pre-existing arrhythmia. Any significant change in rate and/ or rhythm warrants monitoring and further investigation.

PRECAUTIONS

General: Use with caution in patients with severe cardiac disease, severe hypoxemia, hypertension, hyperthyroidism, acute myocardial injury, cor pulmonale, liver disease, in the elderly (especially males) and in neonates. Particular caution should be used in giving theophylline to patients with congestive heart failure. Frequently, such patients have markedly prolonged theophylline serum levels with theophylline persisting in serum for long periods following discontinuation of the drug.

Caution should be exercised in patients concurrently receiving other xanthine medications.

Some patients who are rapid metabolizers of theophylline, such as the young, smokers and some nonsmoking adults, may not be suitable candidates for once daily dosing. Dividing the total daily dose into two doses may be indicated for these patients, who may exhibit symptoms of bronchospasm repeatedly, especially near the end of a 24-hour dosing interval. Also, such individuals may have wider peak-to-trough differences than desired.

Theophylline half-life is shorter in smokers than in nonsmokers. Therefore, smokers may require larger or more frequent doses.

Use theophylline cautiously in patients with history of peptic ulcer. Theophylline may occasionally act as a local irritant to the G.I. tract although gastrointestinal symptoms are more commonly centrally mediated and associated with serum drug concentrations over 20 mcg/ml.

Information for Patients: The physician should reinforce the importance of taking only the prescribed dose and observing the time interval between doses. All patients should be asked to report side effects which occur at any time, or recurrence of symptoms, especially toward the end of a dosing interval. UNIPHYL Tablets are not to be chewed or crushed.

Drug Interactions: Toxic synergism with ephedrine has been documented and may occur with other sympathomimetic bronchodilators. Concomitant administration of theophylline with cimetidine, troleandomycin or erythromycin may lead to higher serum theophylline levels. Theophylline may increase the excretion of lithium carbonate and antagonize the effects of propranolol.

Drug-Laboratory Test Interactions: When plasma levels of theophylline are measured by spectrophotometric methods, coffee, tea, cola beverages, chocolate and acetaminophen contribute to falsely high values.

Carcinogenesis, Mutagenesis, and Impairment of Fertility: Long-term animal studies have not been performed to evaluate the carcinogenic potential, mutagenic potential or the effect on fertility of xanthine compounds.

Pregnancy: Category C—Animal reproduction studies have not been conducted with theophylline. It is not known whether theophylline can cause fetal harm when administered to a pregnant woman or can effect reproduction capacity. Xanthines should be given to a pregnant woman only if clearly needed.

Nursing Mothers: It has been reported that theophylline distributed readily into breast milk and may cause adverse effects in the infant. Caution must be used when prescribing xanthines to a mother who is nursing, taking into account the risk-benefit of this therapy.

Pediatric Use: Safety and effectiveness in children under six (6) years of age have not been established with 200 mg UNIPHYL Tablets.

ADVERSE REACTIONS

The most consistent adverse reactions are usually due to overdose and are:

1. *Gastrointestinal:* nausea, vomiting, epigastric pain, hematemesis, diarrhea.
2. *Central Nervous System:* headaches, irritability, restlessness, insomnia, reflex hyperexcitability, muscle twitching, clonic and tonic generalized convulsions.
3. *Cardiovascular:* palpitation, tachycardia, extrasystole, flushing, hypotension, circulatory failure, ventricular arrhythmia.
4. *Respiratory:* tachypnea.
5. *Renal:* albuminuria, microhematuria, potentiation of diuresis.
6. *Others:* hyperglycemia; inappropriate ADH syndrome; rash.

OVERDOSAGE

Management: If potential oral overdose is established and seizure has not occurred:

A. Induce vomiting.

B. Administer a cathartic. This is particularly important with sustained-release drugs.

C. Administer activated charcoal.

If patient is having a seizure:

A. Establish an airway.

B. Administer oxygen.

C. Treat the seizure with intravenous diazepam, 0.1 to 0.3 mg/kg up to 10 mg.

D. Monitor vital signs, maintain blood pressure and provide adequate hydration.

Post Seizure Coma:

A. Maintain airway and oxygenation.

B. If a result of oral medication, follow above recommendations to prevent absorption of the drug, but intubation and lavage will have to be performed instead of inducing emesis, and the cathartic and charcoal will need to be introduced via a large bore gastric lavage tube.

C. Continue to provide full supportive care and adequate hydration while waiting for drug to be metabolized. In general, the drug is metabolized sufficiently rapidly so as not to warrant consideration of dialysis. However, if serum levels exceed 50 mcg/ml, charcoal hemoperfusion may be indicated.

DOSAGE AND ADMINISTRATION

In chronic therapy, theophylline, as found in UNIPHYL Tablets, is a treatment of first choice for the management of chronic asthma and other reversible obstructive pulmonary diseases to prevent and/or relieve symptoms and maintain patent airways.

Monitoring of clinical response and determining serum theophylline concentration is appropriate to guide dosing and minimize risk of toxicity due to overdosing. A serum level of 20 mcg/ml is an important safety reference point to reduce the possibility of toxicity.

There is considerable variation from patient to patient in the dosage required to achieve and maintain therapeutic and safe levels, primarily due to variable rates of elimination and the degree of bronchospasm present. Therefore, it is essential that dosage be individualized to the patient's clinical response and that serum levels be monitored before and after transfer to any sustained-release product.

UNIPHYL, like other controlled-release theophylline products, is intended for patients with relatively continuous or recurring symptoms who have a need to maintain therapeutic serum levels of theophylline. It is not intended for patients experiencing an acute episode of bronchospasm (associated with asthma, chronic bronchitis, or emphysema). Such patients require rapid relief of symptoms and should be treated with an immediate release or intravenous theophylline preparation (or other bronchodilators) and not with controlled-release products.

Effective use of theophylline (i.e., the concentration of drug in the serum associated with optimal benefit and minimal risk of toxicity) is considered to occur when the theophylline concentration is maintained from 10 to 20 mcg/ml. The early studies from which these levels were derived were carried out in patients immediately after or shortly after recovery from acute exacerbations of their disease (some hospitalized with status asthmaticus).

Although the 20 mcg/ml level remains appropriate as a critical value (above which toxicity is more likely to occur) for safety purposes, additional data are now available which indicate that the serum theophylline concentrations required to produce maximum physiologic benefit may, in fact, fluctuate with the degree of bronchospasm present and are variable. Therefore, the physician should individualize the range appropriate to the patient's requirements, based on both symptomatic response and improvement in pulmonary function. It should be stressed that serum theophylline concentrations maintained at the upper level of the 10 to 20 mcg/ml range may be associated with potential toxicity when factors known to reduce theophylline clearance become operative. (See *Precautions,* including *Drug Interactions.)*

Dosage guidelines are approximations only and the wide range of theophylline clearance between individuals (particularly those with concomitant disease) makes indiscriminate usage hazardous. Each patient should be titrated to establish the appropriate dosage, and serum theophylline levels used for any dosage adjustment after transfer to UNIPHYL Tablets. As a practical consideration, it is not always possible to obtain serum level determinations. Under such conditions, restriction of the daily dose of UNIPHYL Tablets (in otherwise healthy adults) to approximately 13 mg/kg/day (or up to 900 mg) will result in relatively few patients exceeding serum levels of 20 mcg/ml and the associated risk of toxicity.

DOSAGE GUIDELINES

When appropriate, dosage should be calculated on the basis of lean body weight where mg/kg doses are to be prescribed, since theophylline does not distribute into fatty tissue.

I. *INITIATION OF THERAPY WITH UNIPHYL TABLETS*

a. *Stabilized Patients*

Individuals who are taking an immediate-release or controlled-release theohylline product may be transferred to twice-daily administration of 200 mg

UNIPHYL Tablets on a mg-for-mg basis. For example, a patient stabilized on 400 mg twice daily (800 mg total daily dose) should be given two 200 mg UNIPHYL Tablets q. 12 h.

It must be recognized that the peak and trough serum theophylline levels produced by the twice-daily dosing may vary from those produced by the previous product and/or regimen.

b. *Initiation of Theophylline Dosing*

Patients not currently receiving theophylline may be initiated on UNIPHYL 200 mg Tablets as follows: THE AVERAGE INITIAL CHILDREN'S (15 TO 25 KG) DOSE IS ONE-HALF (100 MG) OF A UNIPHYL 200 MG TABLE q. 12 h.

THE AVERAGE INITIAL ADULT AND CHILDREN'S (OVER 25 KG) DOSE IS ONE UNIPHYL 200 MG TABLET q. 12 h.

If the desired response is not achieved with the above AVERAGE INITIAL DOSAGE recommendations, the dose may be adjusted as is described below:

II. *TITRATION AND DOSE ADJUSTMENT*

a. *When Serum Levels Are Measured*

After 4 days therapy with UNIPHYL Tablets, steady-state should have been achieved, and peak serum theophylline concentration should be determined from blood samples obtained 8 to 12 hours after the morning dose. Trough concentration should be taken just prior to the administration of the next dose. It is important that the patient not have missed or added any dose during the previous 72 hours, and that the dosing intervals remain relatively constant. DOSAGE ADJUSTMENT BASED ON THE MEASUREMENTS WHEN THESE INSTRUCTIONS HAVE NOT BEEN FOLLOWED MAY RESULT IN TOXICITY.

Peak and trough theophylline serum concentration values allow: 1) maintaining the established dosage schedule if values are within the desired range and the dose is tolerated, 2) increasing the dose, or 3) decreasing the dose.

b. *When Serum Levels Are Not Measured*

In the absence of laboratory facilities for determining serum theophylline concentration levels, clinical judgement should be followed.

- The original total twice-daily dose should continue if it is well-tolerated and the clinical response is satisfactory.
- Minimal improvement with the initial dose usually requires increasing the dose as described below.
- If adverse reactions occur, decrease the dose as stated below.

c. *Increasing the Dose of UNIPHYL Tablets*

If patient response with UNIPHYL Tablets is unsatisfactory and/or the observed serum theophylline concentration range is too low, the dosage may be increased at recommended intervals as follows:

Serum Theophylline (mcg/ml)	*Directions*
7.5 to 10	Increase dose by about 25%* and recheck serum concentrations in 3 days.
5 to 7.5	Increase dose by about 25% to the nearest dose increment and recheck serum theophylline for guidance in further dosage adjustment (another increase will probably be needed, but this provides a safety check).

d. *Decreasing the Dose of UNIPHYL Tablets*

Serum theophylline values above 20 mcg/ml require decreasing the daily dose unless such dose in required to maintain the patient and is well-tolerated. Dosage may be reduced by adjustments as are described below. Peak and trough measurements should be taken 3 days after each decrease in dosage.

Serum Theophylline (mcg/ml)	*Directions*
20 to 25	Decrease dose by about 10%.
25 to 30	Skip next dose and decrease subsequent doses by about 25%.
Over 30	Skip next 2 doses and decrease subsequent doses by 50%.

*Dividing the daily dose into 3 doses administered at 8-hour intervals may be indicated if symptoms occur repeatedly at the end of a dosing interval.

Finer adjustments in dosage may be needed for some patients.

III. *MAINTENANCE THERAPY*

Careful clinical titration is important to assure patient acceptance and safety of the medication. Patients, when stabilized as established by serum theophylline concentration or respiratory function, usually remain controlled without further dosage adjustment. It should be borne in mind, however, that for reasons stated in the Precautions and Warnings sections, dosage adjustments may be necessary. Serum theophylline levels should be measured periodically (at 6- to 12-month intervals) even in clinically controlled patients.

As with all sustained-release theophylline products, UNIPHYL Tablets are for chronic or long-term use only and are not intended for initial treatment in a patient with acute symptoms.

Caution should be exercised for younger childrlen who cannot complain of minor side effects. The elderly as well as patients with congestive heart failure, cor pulmonale, and/or liver disease may have unusually low dosage requirements and thus may experience toxicity even at the dosages recommended above.

It is important that no patient be maintained on any dosage that is not tolerated. In instructing patients to increase dosage according to the schedule above, they should be instructed not to take a subsequent dose if apparent side effects occur and to resume therapy at a lower dose once adverse effects have disappeared.

WARNING: DO NOT MAINTAIN ANY DOSE THAT IS NOT TOLERATED.

CAUTION

Federal law prohibits dispensing without prescription.

HOW SUPPLIED

UNIPHYL (theophylline anhydrous) 200 mg scored Controlled-Release Tablets supplied in white-opaque plastic bottles, containing 100 tablets [NDC 0034-7002-80]. Each round, white tablet bears the symbol PF on one side and is marked U200 on the other side.

U.S. Patent Numbers 3965256 and 4235870

6/14/86 7219 D1494

Shown in Product Identification Section, page 423

UNIPHYL® Tablets ℞

[*ū 'nĭ-fĭl*]

(theophylline, anhydrous)

400 mg

UNICONTIN®

Controlled-Release System

DESCRIPTION

Uniphyl Tablets contain 400 mg anhydrous theophylline in a controlled-release system.

Theophylline anhydrous, a xanthine bronchodilator, is a white, odorless, crystalline powder having a bitter taste. Theophylline has a molecular weight of 180.18, represented by $C_7H_8N_4O_2$ and depicted as:

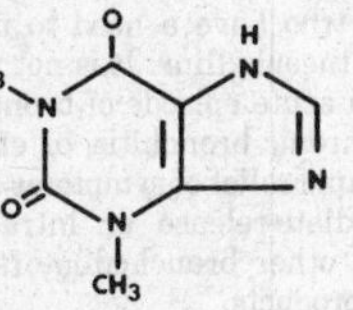

CLINICAL PHARMACOLOGY

Theophylline directly relaxes the smooth muscle of the bronchial airways and pulmonary blood vessels. The drug also produces other actions typical of the xanthine derivatives: coronary vasodilation, cardiac stimulation, diuresis, cerebral stimulation, and skeletal muscle stimulation. These actions may be mediated through inhibition of phosphodiesterase with a resultant increase in intracellular cyclic AMP. *In vitro,* theophylline has been shown to act synergistically with beta agonists that increase intracellular cyclic AMP through the stimulation of adenyl cyclase; but synergism has not been demonstrated in patient studies. More data are needed to determine if theophylline and beta agonists have a clinically important additive effect *in vivo.*

Pharmacokinetics: A single-dose study in 15 normal male volunteers, whose theophylline inherent mean elimination half-life was verified by a liquid theophylline product to be 6.9 ± 2.5 (S.D.) hours were administered two or three 400 mg Uniphyl Tablets. Peak serum theophylline levels occurred at 6.9 ± 5.2 (S.D.) hours, with a normalized (to 800 mg) peak level being 6.2 ± 2.1 (S.D.). The apparent elimination half-life for the 400 mg Uniphyl Tablets was 17.2 ± 5.8 (S.D.) hours.

Steady-state pharmacokinetics were determined in a study of 12 patients with chronic reversible obstructive pulmonary disease. All were dosed with two 400 mg Uniphyl Tablets given once daily in the morning and a widely-used approved controlled- release B.I.D. product administered as two 200 mg tablets given 12 hours apart. The pharmacokinetic parameters obtained for Uniphyl Tablets given at doses of 800 mg once daily in the morning were virtually identical to the corresponding parameters for the reference drug when given as 400 mg B.I.D. In particular, the area-under-curve and highest and lowest mean serum theophylline levels, i.e., the AUC, Cmax and Cmin values, obtained in this study were as follows:

	Uniphyl Tablets 800 mg Q 24 h ± S.D.	Reference Drug 400 mg Q 12 h ± S.D.
AUC (0–24 hours), mcg-hr/ml	288.9 ± 21.5	283.5 ± 38.4
Cmax, mcg/ml	15.7 ± 2.8	15.2 ± 2.1
Cmin, mcg/ml	7.9 ± 1.6	7.8 ± 1.7
Cmax-Cmin diff	7.7 ± 1.5	7.4 ± 1.5

Bioavailability was calculated to be 104 ± 18% (S.D.) for the 24-hour period with Uniphyl Tablets once daily as compared with the reference drug given twice daily, as shown above. The AUC and Cmax are dose-dependent and will increase by upward dosage adjustment with Uniphyl Tablets. Patients who are fast theophylline metabolizers (clearance—greater than 5L/hr) may not be suitable candidates for once-daily dosing. Those patients who are not well-maintained on recommended once-a-day therapy are likely to be better controlled when administered Uniphyl Tablets in divided doses.

The half-life of theophylline is prolonged in patients suffering from chronic alcoholism, impaired hepatic or renal function, congestive heart failure, and in patients receiving macrolide antibiotics and cimetidine. Older adults (over age 55) and patients with chronic obstructive pulmonary disease, with or without cor pulmonale, may also have slower clearance rates of theophylline with half-lives that exceed 24 hours. High fever for prolonged periods may reduce the rate of theophylline elimination.

Newborns and neonates have extremely slow clearance rates compared to older infants (over 6 months) and children, and may also have a theophylline half-life of over 24 hours.

The half-life of theophylline in smokers averages 4 to 5 hours contrasted with 7 to 11 hours in non-smokers. Following the cessation of smoking, the effects on theophylline pharmacokinetics may persist for 3 months to 2 years.

Theophylline Elimination Characteristics

	Theophylline Clearance Rates (mean ± S.D.)	Half-Life Average (mean ± S.D.)
Children (over 6 months of age)	1.45 ± 0.58 ml/kg/min	3.7 ± 1.1 hr
Adult non-smokers with uncomplicated asthma	0.65 ± 0.19 ml/kg/min	8.7 ± 2.2 hr

INDICATIONS

Uniphyl Tablets are indicated for relief and/or prevention of symptoms of asthma and reversible bronchospasm associated with chronic bronchitis and emphysema.

CONTRAINDICATIONS

This product is contraindicated in individuals who have shown hypersensitivity to theophylline.

WARNINGS

Status asthmaticus should be considered a medical emergency and is defined as that degree of bronchospasm which is not rapidly reponsive to usual doses of conventional bronchodilators. Optimal therapy for such patients frequently requires both *additional medication,* parenterally administered, and *close monitoring,* preferably in an intensive-care setting.

Excessive theophylline doses may be associated with toxicity. Determination of serum theophylline levels is recommended to assure maximum therapeutic benefit without excessive risk. The incidence of toxicity increases at serum levels greater than 20 mcg/ml.

Optimum therapeutic response occurs in most patients when the serum theophylline concentration is 10 to 20 mcg/ml. In other patients satisfactory results (as determined by both relief of symptoms and improvement in pulmonary function) may be obtained at lower levels. In still others, adequate response may require higher levels. The physician should adjust the desired serum concentration range to the patients' requirements, keeping in mind that *an increased probability of toxicity exists when levels exceed 20 mcg/ml.* Therefore, in order to assure maximum benefit without excessive risk, measurement of serum levels is highly recommended.

Reduced theophylline clearance may result in increased serum levels and potential toxicity in the following patient groups: (1) those with impaired renal or liver function, (2) those over 55 years of age, particularly males and those with

Continued on next page

Purdue Frederick—Cont.

chronic lung disease, (3) those with cardiac failure, (4) those receiving macrolide antibiotics or cimetidine and (5) neonates. Decreased theophylline clearance may occur during active influenza infection or following immunization for influenza.

Less serious signs of theophylline toxicity, i.e. nausea and restlessness, may appear. Serious side effects such as ventricular arrhythmias, convulsions or even death may appear as the first sign of toxicity without any previous warning. *Serious toxicity is not reliably preceded by less severe side effects.*

Patients who require theophylline may exhibit tachycardia due to their underlying disease. The possible relationship of elevated serum theophylline concentration to tachycardia may not be recognized.

Theophylline products may cause arrhythmia and/or worsen pre-existing arrhythmia. Any significant change in rate and/or rhythm warrants monitoring and further investigation.

PRECAUTIONS

General: Use with caution in patients with severe cardiac disease, severe hypoxemia, hypertension, hyperthyroidism, acute myocardial injury, cor pulmonale, liver disease, in the elderly (especially males) and in neonates. Particular caution should be used in giving theophylline to patients with congestive heart failure. Frequently, such patients have markedly prolonged theophylline serum levels with theophylline persisting in serum for long periods following discontinuation of the drug.

Caution should be exercised in patients concurrently receiving other xanthine medications.

Some patients who are rapid metabolizers of theophylline, such as the young, smokers and some nonsmoking adults, may not be suitable candidates for once daily dosing. Dividing the total daily dose into two doses may be indicated for these patients, who may exhibit symptoms of bronchospasm repeatedly, especially near the end of a 24-hour dosing interval. Also, such individuals may have wider peak-to-trough differences than desired.

Theophylline half-life is shorter in smokers than in nonsmokers. Therefore, smokers may require larger or more frequent doses.

Use theophylline cautiously in patients with history of peptic ulcer. Theophylline may occasionally act as a local irritant to the G.I. tract although gastrointestinal symptoms are more commonly centrally mediated and associated with serum drug concentrations over 20 mcg/ml.

Information for Patients: The physician should reinforce the importance of taking only the prescribed dose and observing the time interval between doses. All patients should be asked to report side effects which occur at any time, or recurrence of symptoms, especially toward the end of a 24-hour dosing interval. Uniphyl Tablets are to be taken whole, and are not to be broken, chewed or crushed.

Drug Interactions: Toxic synergism with ephedrine has been documented and may occur with other sympathomimetic bronchodilators. Concomitant administration of theophylline with cimetidine, troleandomycin or erythromycin may lead to higher serum theophylline levels. Theophylline may increase the excretion of lithium carbonate and antagonize the effects of propranolol.

Drug-Laboratory Test Interactions: When plasma levels of theophylline are measured by spectrophotometric methods, coffee, tea, cola beverages, chocolate and acetaminophen contribute to falsely high values.

Carcinogenesis, Mutagenesis, and Impairment of Fertility: Long-term animal studies have not been performed to evaluate the carcinogenic potential, mutagenic potential or the effect on fertility of xanthine compounds.

Pregnancy: Category C—Animal reproduction studies have not been conducted with theophylline. It is not known whether theophylline can cause fetal harm when administered to a pregnant woman or can effect reproduction capacity. Xanthines should be given to a pregnant woman only if clearly needed.

Nursing Mothers: It has been reported that theophylline distributes readily into breast milk and may cause adverse effects in the infant. Caution must be used when prescribing xanthines to a mother who is nursing, taking into account the risk-benefit of this therapy.

Pediatric Use: Safety and effectiveness in children under 12 years of age have not been established with 400 mg Uniphyl Tablets.

ADVERSE REACTIONS

The most consistent adverse reactions are usually due to overdose and are:

1. *Gastrointestinal:* nausea, vomiting, epigastric pain, hematemesis, diarrhea.
2. *Central Nervous System:* headaches, irritability, restlessness, insomnia, reflex hyperexcitability, muscle twitching, clonic and tonic generalized convulsions.
3. *Cardiovascular:* palpitation, tachycardia, extrasystole, flushing, hypotension, circulatory failure, ventricular arrhythmia.
4. *Respiratory:* tachypnea.
5. *Renal:* albuminuria, microhematuria, potentiation of diuresis.
6. *Others:* hyperglycemia; inappropriate ADH syndrome, rash.

OVERDOSAGE

Management: If potential oral overdose is established and seizure has not occurred:

A. Induce vomiting. **B.** Administer a cathartic. This is particularly important with sustained-release drugs. **C.** Administer activated charcoal.

If patient is having a seizure:

A. Establish an airway. **B.** Administer oxygen. **C.** Treat the seizure with intravenous diazepam, 0.1 to 0.3 mg/kg up to 10 mg. **D.** Monitor vital signs, maintain blood pressure and provide adequate hydration.

Post Seizure Coma:

A. Maintain airway and oxygenation. **B.** If a result of oral medication, follow above recommendations to prevent absorption of the drug, but intubation and lavage will have to be performed instead of inducing emesis, and the cathartic and charcoal will need to be introduced via a large bore gastric lavage tube. **C.** Continue to provide full supportive care and adequate hydration while waiting for drug to be metabolized. In general, the drug is metabolized sufficiently rapidly so as not to warrant consideration of dialysis. However, if serum levels exceed 50 mcg/ml, charcoal hemoperfusion may be indicated.

DOSAGE AND ADMINISTRATION

In chronic therapy, theophylline, as found in Uniphyl Tablets, is a treatment of first choice for the management of chronic asthma and other reversible obstructive pulmonary diseases to prevent and/or relieve symptoms and maintain patent airways.

Monitoring of clinical response and determining serum theophylline concentration is appropriate to guide dosing and minimize risk of toxicity due to overdosing. A serum level of 20 mcg/ml is an important safety reference point to reduce the possibility of toxicity.

There is considerable variation from patient to patient in the dosage required to achieve and maintain therapeutic and safe levels, primarily due to variable rates of elimination and the degree of bronchospasm present. Therefore, it is essential that dosage be individualized to the patient's clinical response and that serum levels be monitored before and after transfer to any sustained-release product.

Uniphyl, like other controlled-release theophylline products, is intended for patients with relatively continuous or recurring symptoms who have a need to maintain therapeutic serum levels of theophylline. It is not intended for patients experiencing an acute episode of bronchospasm (associated with asthma, chronic bronchitis, or emphysema). Such patients require rapid relief of symptoms and should be treated with an immediate-release or intravenous theophylline preparation (or other bronchodilators) and not with controlled-release products.

Until additional data are available to evaluate the rate of absorption and/or clearance rates of theophylline from controlled-release dosage forms administered at night, it is not recommended that Uniphyl Tablets be administered at night when used on a once-daily schedule.

Effective use of theophylline (i.e., the concentration of drug in the serum associated with optimal benefit and minimal risk of toxicity) is considered to occur when the theophylline concentration is maintained from 10 to 20 mcg/ml. The early studies from which these levels were derived were carried out in patients immediately after or shortly after recovery from acute exacerbations of their disease (some hospitalized with status asthmaticus).

Although the 20 mcg/ml level remains appropriate as a critical value (above which toxicity is more likely to occur) for safety purposes, additional data are now available which indicate that the serum theophylline concentrations required to produce maximum physiologic benefit may, in fact, fluctuate with the degree of bronchospasm present and are variable. Therefore, the physician should individualize the range appropriate to the patient's requirements, based on both symptomatic response and improvement in pulmonary function. It should be stressed that serum theophylline concentrations maintained at the upper level of the 10 to 20 mcg/ml range may be associated with potential toxicity when factors known to reduce theophylline clearance become operative. (See *Precautions,* including *Drug Interactions.)*

Uniphyl Tablets taken once daily in the morning at the recommended dosage may provide the required bronchodilation of patients who clear theophylline normally or relatively slowly, e.g., non-smokers. However, certain patients, such as the young, smokers and some non-smoking adults are likely to metabolize theophylline more rapidly and *may require dosing at 12-hour intervals.* Such patients may experience symptoms of bronchospasm toward the end of a once-daily dosing interval and/or require a high daily dose (higher than those recommended in labeling) and are more likely to experience relatively wide peak to trough differences in serum theophylline concentrations.

Dosage guidelines are approximations only and the wide range of theophylline clearance between individuals (particularly those with concomitant disease) makes indiscriminate usage hazardous. Each patient should be titrated to establish the appropriate dosage, and serum theophylline levels used for any dosage adjustment after transfer to Uniphyl Tablets, especially on a once-a-day A.M. schedule. As a practical consideration, it is not always possible to obtain serum level determinations. Under such conditions, restriction of the daily dose of Uniphyl Tablets (in otherwise healthy adults), to approximately 13 mg/kg/day (or up to 900 mg) will result in relatively few patients exceeding serum levels of 20 mcg/ml and the associated risk of toxicity.

DOSAGE GUIDELINES:

Until additional bioavailability data are available, it is recommended that Uniphyl be taken as intact tablets only. When appropriate dosage should be calculated on the basis of lean body weight where mg/kg doses are to be prescribed, since theophylline does not distribute into fatty tissue.

I. *INITIATION OF THERAPY WITH UNIPHYL TABLETS*

a. *Stabilized Patients* (12 years of age or older)

Individuals who are taking an immediate-release or controlled-release theophylline product may be transferred to once-daily administration of 400 mg Uniphyl Tablets on a mg-for-mg basis. For example, a patient stabilized on 400 mg twice daily (800 mg total daily dose) should be given two 400 mg Uniphyl Tablets as a single A.M. daily dose of 800 mg.

It must be recognized that the peak and trough serum theophylline levels produced by the once-daily dosing may vary from those produced by the previous product and/or regimen.

b. *Initiation of Theophylline Dosing*

Adult patients and children 12 years of age and over not currently receiving theophylline may be titrated using an immediate- or sustained-release theophylline product, which can be adjusted in small dosage increments. Patients titrated to a total daily dose approximating 400, 800, or 1200 mg. may be transferred to once-daily dosage with equivalent doses of 400 mg Unihyl Tablets, as is described in (a) above.

II. *TITRATION AND DOSE ADJUSTMENT*

a. *When Serum Levels Are Measured*

After 4 days therapy with Uniphyl Tablets, steady-state should have been achieved, and peak serum theophylline concentration should be determined from blood samples obtained 8 to 12 hours after the morning dose. Trough concentration should be taken just prior to the administration of the next dose. It is important that the patient not have missed or added any dose during the previous 72 hours, and that the dosing intervals remain relatively constant. DOSAGE ADJUSTMENT BASED ON MEASUREMENTS WHEN THESE INSTRUCTIONS HAVE NOT BEEN FOLLOWED MAY RESULT IN TOXICITY.

Peak and trough theophylline serum concentration values allow: 1) maintaining the established dosage schedule if values are within the desired range and the dose is tolerated, 2) increasing the dose, or 3) decreasing the dose.

b. *When Serum Levels Are Not Measured*

In the absence of laboratory facilities for determining serum theophylline concentration levels, clinical judgment should be followed.

- The original total once-daily dose should continue if it is well-tolerated and the clinical response is satisfactory.
- If adverse reactions occur, decrease the dose as stated below.

If a patient is better controlled on another regimen than on a once-daily regimen, the patient should be maintained on the more effective regimen.

c. *Increasing the Dose of Uniphyl Tablets*

If patient response with Uniphyl Tablets is unsatisfactory and/or the observed serum theophylline concentration range is too low, the patient should be transferred to an immediate or controlled release (b.i.d.) theophylline schedule and dosage increased at recommended intervals as follows:

Serum Theophylline (mcg/ml)	*Directions*
7.5 to 10	Increase dose by about 25%* and recheck serum concentrations in 3 days.
5 to 7.5	Increase dose by about 25% to the nearest dose increment and recheck serum theophylline for guidance in further dosage adjustment (another increase will probably be needed, but this provides a safety check).

Patients titrated to a total daily dosage of 800 mg or 1200 mg on a twice-daily schedule, can be transferred to once-daily A.M. dosing, using 400 mg Uniphyl Tablets.

d. *Decreasing the Dose of Uniphyl Tablets*

Serum theophylline values above 20 mcg/ml require decreasing the daily dose unless such dose in required to maintain the patient and is well-tolerated. Dosage may be reduced by transferring the patient to an immediate- or controlled-release (b.i.d.) theophylline product and making adjustments. Peak and trough measurements should be taken 3 days after each decrease in dosage.

Serum Theophylline (mcg/ml)	*Directions*
20 to 25	Decrease dose by about 10%.
25 to 30	Skip next dose and decrease subsequent doses by about 25%.
Over 30	Skip next 2 doses and decrease subsequent doses by 50%.

*Dividing the daily dose into 3 doses administered at 8-hour intervals may be indicated if symptoms occur repeatedly at the end of a dosing interval.

Finer adjustments in dosage may be needed for some patients.

III. *MAINTENANCE THERAPY*

Careful clinical titration is important to assure patient acceptance and safety of the medication. Patients when stabilized, as established by serum theophylline concentration or respiratory function, usually remain controlled without further dosage adjustment. It should be borne in mind, however, that for reasons stated in the Precautions and Warnings sections, dosage adjustments may be necessary. Serum theophylline levels should be measured periodically (at 6- to 12-month intervals) even in clinically controlled patients. As with all sustained-release theophylline products, Uniphyl Tablets are for chronic or long-term use only and are not intended for initial treatment in a patient with acute symptoms.

Caution should be exercised for younger children who cannot complain of minor side effects. The elderly as well as patients with congestive heart failure, cor pulmonale, and/or liver disease may have unusually low dosage requirements and thus may experience toxicity even at the dosages recommended above.

It is important that no patient be maintained on any dosage that is not tolerated. In instructing patients to increase dosage according to the schedule above, they should be instructed not to take a subsequent dose if apparent side effects occur and to resume therapy at a lower dose once adverse effects have disappeared.

WARNING: DO NOT MAINTAIN ANY DOSE THAT IS NOT TOLERATED.

CAUTION

Federal law prohibits dispensing without prescription.

HOW SUPPLIED

Uniphyl (theophylline, anhydrous) 400 mg scored Controlled-Release Tablets supplied in white-opaque plastic bottles, containing 100 tablets [**NDC** 0034-7004-80], or 500 tablets [**NDC** 0034-7004-70] or in unit dose packaging with 10 tablets per card [**NDC** 0034-7004-10]; ten cards are packed in each carton; 10 cartons are packed in each shipper.

Each round, white tablet bears the symbol PF on one side and is marked U400 on the other side.

Store tablets at controlled room temperature 15° to 30° C (59°–86°F).

U.S. Patent Numbers 3965256 and 4235870

6/14/86 G1374

Shown in Product Identification Section, page 423

EDUCATIONAL MATERIAL

Audio Visuals—Booklets—Samples

"Fiber and Your Health" Booklets (Fibermed)

"How You Can Relieve Constipation Naturally" (Senokot-S)

"Coping with Arthritis" patient booklet and exercise chart (Trilisate) plus 750 mg and 1000 mg samples.

Cancer Pain Management Videotape Program (MS Contin)

Pain Assessment Program medical forms and patient booklets (MS Contin)

Cancer Pain Management Slide Program (MS Contin)

"Protect Your Family From Germs" patient aid booklet (English and Spanish). (Betadine)

"Your Betadine Antiseptics Guide to First Aid" patient aid booklet.

Samples of Betadine First Aid and Betadine Feminine Hygiene Products.

RAM Laboratories Corp.

P. O. BOX 559071
MIAMI, FL 33255

ALGISIN Capsules ℞
(chlorzoxazone 250 mg. + acetaminophen 300 mg.)

SUPPLIED

Bottles of 60 capsules.

APETIL Liquid ℞
(Therapeutic Vitamins-Minerals)

SUPPLIED

Bottles 8 ounces.

DIGEPEPSIN ℞
Enteric coated digestant tablets
(pepsin 250 mg. + pancreatin 300 mg. + bile salts 150 mg.)

SUPPLIED

Bottles of 60 tablets.

GEROTON FORTE OTC
Supplement—Stimulant tonic

SUPPLIED

Bottles of 1 pint.

NEUROCHOL Capsules ℞
Dietary Supplement

SUPPLIED

Bottles of 60 capsules.

OTISAN Drops ℞
Otic solution

SUPPLIED

10 ml. plastic dropper.

PASMOL Tablets ℞
(Ethaverine Hydrochloride 100 mg.)

SUPPLIED

Bottles 30 scored tablets.

TUSIBRON OTC
(Guaifenesin 100 mg.)

SUPPLIED

Bottles of 4 ounces.

TUSIBRON-DM OTC
(Guaifenesin w/D-Methorphan Hydrobromide)

SUPPLIED

Bottles of 4 ounces.

ZINCVIT Capsules ℞
Multivitamin and Multimineral Formula
with 1 mg. folic acid and 120 mg. Zinc

SUPPLIED

Bottles 60 capsules.

Important Notice

Before prescribing or administering any product described in PHYSICIANS' DESK REFERENCE always consult the PDR Supplement for possible new or revised information

Reed & Carnrick

1 NEW ENGLAND AVENUE
PISCATAWAY, NJ 08854

COLYTE® ℞
[*kō'līt*]
Colon Electrolyte Lavage Preparation

DESCRIPTION

Colyte® is an orally administered colon electrolyte lavage preparation delivered in the form of separately packaged, water-soluble components for reconstitution. Each Colyte® preparation contains the following, in grams per liter of water on a delivered basis:

Packet A—Polyethylene glycol 3350 ....60 grams
Packet B—Sodium chloride ....1.46 grams
Packet C—Potassium chloride ....0.745 grams
Packet D—Sodium bicarbonate ....1.68 grams
Packet E—Sodium sulfate (anhydrous) ....5.68 grams

It is an isotonic (with respect to colon contents) and isosmotic solution.

CLINICAL PHARMACOLOGY

When administered orally, it cleanses the bowel rapidly by inducing diarrhea. Because the Polyethylene glycol 3350 acts as an osmotic agent, there is virtually no net ion absorption or loss. Water and electrolyte balances do not change significantly when large volumes of Colyte® are ingested.

INDICATIONS AND USAGE

Colyte® is indicated for cleansing the bowel by means of total gut perfusion and whole bowel irrigation in preparation for gastrointestinal examination.

CONTRAINDICATIONS

Colyte® is contraindicated for patients with actual or suspected ileus or gastric outlet obstruction; for patients whose body weight is less than 20 kg; for patients with suspected or actual perforations of the colon and toxic colitis or megacolon.

WARNING

Do not add additional ingredients, flavorings, etc. before administration.

PRECAUTIONS

Pregnancy Category C. Animal reproduction studies have not been conducted with Colyte®, and it is not known whether Colyte® can affect reproductive capacity or harm the fetus when administered to a pregnant patient. Colyte® should be given to a pregnant patient only if clearly needed. If Colyte® is administered to a patient who is in any way prone to aspiration or regurgitation (for example, impaired gag reflex, unconscious), the patient should be observed carefully, particularly in the case of nasogastric intubation.

Safety and effectiveness in children has not been established.

Long term carcinogenic and reproductive studies with animals have not been performed.

ADVERSE REACTIONS

The most frequent adverse reactions to Colyte® are nausea and bloating. Less frequent adverse reactions include vomiting and rectal irritation. These adverse reactions are temporary and generally disappear rapidly.

DOSAGE AND ADMINISTRATION

Preparation of Solution: The preparation is made by dissolving the contents of the five packets, labeled A through E, in a food-grade container, in a sufficient quantity of water to produce the final volume according to package directions. Mix well.

Usual Dosage: Colyte® can be ingested orally or administered via nasogastric intubation. Lavage is complete when fecal discharge is clear. The typical dosage per patient is one gallon (3.785 liters).

Peroral: Drink 200 ml to 300 ml every 10 minutes (7 to 10 ounces).

Recommended ingestion rate ranges from 1.2 liters per hour to 1.8 liters per hour.

Nasogastric intubation: Infuse at a rate of 20 ml per minute to 30 ml per minute.

If possible, patients should fast for three or four hours before ingestion begins. Patients should never be given solid food less than two hours prior to administration. Only clear liquids are permitted during the interval between Colyte® ingestion and examination.

HOW SUPPLIED

Colyte® is supplied in two sizes as five separate packets, each containing one of the five chemicals. The five chemicals are in powdered form for reconstitution to produce a two liter or one gallon (3.785 liters) final solution. The different sizes contain the following:

Continued on next page

Reed & Carnrick—Cont.

1. **Two liter:** (NDC 0021-001-03): polyethylene glycol 3350 120g, sodium chloride 2.92g, potassium chloride 1.49g, sodium bicarbonate 3.36g, sodium sulfate 11.36 g.
2. **One gallon:** (NDC 0021-001-02): polyethylene glycol 3350 227.1g, sodium chloride 5.53g., potassium chloride 2.82g, sodium bicarbonate 6.36g, sodium sulfate 21.5g.

CAUTION

Federal law prohibits dispensing without a prescription. KEEP RECONSTITUTED SOLUTION REFRIGERATED. USE WITHIN 48 HOURS. DISCARD UNUSED PORTION.

Revised June 1986

CORTIFOAM® ℞
(hydrocortisone acetate) 10%

DESCRIPTION

Contains hydrocortisone acetate 10% as the sole active ingredient in 20 g of a foam containing propylene glycol, emulsifying wax, steareth-10, cetyl alcohol, methylparaben and propylparaben, trolamine, water and inert propellants, dichlorodifluoromethane and dichlorotetrafluoroethane.

Each application delivers approximately 900 mg of foam containing 80 mg of hydrocortisone (90 mg of hydrocortisone acetate).

CLINICAL PHARMACOLOGY

CORTIFOAM provides effective topical administration of an anti-inflammatory corticosteroid as adjunctive therapy of ulcerative proctitis.

INDICATIONS

CORTIFOAM is indicated as adjunctive therapy in the topical treatment of ulcerative proctitis of the distal portion of the rectum in patients who cannot retain hydrocortisone or other corticosteroid enemas. Direct observations of methylene blue-containing foam have shown staining about 10 centimeters into the rectum.

CONTRAINDICATIONS

Local contraindications to the use of intrarectal steroids include obstruction, abscess, perforation, peritonitis, fresh intestinal anastomoses, extensive fistulas and sinus tracts. Tuberculosis (active, latent or questionably healed), ocular herpes simplex and acute psychosis are usually considered absolute contraindications to the use of corticosteroids. Relative contraindications include active peptic ulcer, acute glomerulonephritis, myasthenia gravis, osteoporosis, diverticulitis, thrombophlebitis, psychic disturbances, pregnancy, diabetes, hyperthyroidism, acute coronary disease, hypertension, limited cardiac reserve, and local or systemic infections, including fungal or exanthematous diseases. Where these conditions exist, the expected benefits from steroid therapy must be weighed against the risks involved in its use. Pregnancy is a relative contraindication to corticosteroids, particularly during third trimester. If corticosteroids must be administered in pregnancy, watch newborn infant closely for signs of hypoadrenalism, and administer appropriate therapy if needed.

WARNING

Do not insert any part of the aerosol container into the anus. Contents of the container are under pressure, but not flammable. Do not burn or puncture the aerosol container. Store at room temperature but not over 120° F. Because CORTIFOAM is not expelled, systemic hydrocortisone absorption may be greater from CORTIFOAM than from corticosteroid enema formulations. If there is no evidence of clinical or proctologic improvement within two or three weeks after starting CORTIFOAM therapy, or if the patient's condition worsens, discontinue the drug.

PRECAUTIONS

Steroid therapy should be administered with caution in patients with severe ulcerative disease because these patients are predisposed to perforation of the bowel wall. Where surgery is imminent, it is hazardous to wait more than a few days for a satisfactory response to medical treatment. General precautions common to all corticosteroid therapy should be observed during treatment with CORTIFOAM. These include gradual withdrawal of therapy to allow for possible adrenal insufficiency and awareness to possible growth suppression in children. Patients should be kept under close observation, for, as with all drugs, rare individuals may react unfavorably under certain conditions. If severe reactions or idiosyncrasies occur, steroids should be discontinued immediately and appropriate measures instituted. Do not employ in immediate or early postoperative period following ileorectostomy.

ADVERSE REACTIONS

Corticosteroid therapy may produce side effects which include moon face, fluid retention, excessive appetite and weight gain, abnormal fat deposits, mental symptoms, hypertrichosis, acne, ecchymosis, increased sweating, pigmentation, dry scaly skin, thinning scalp hair, thrombophlebitis, decreased resistance to infection, negative nitrogen balance with delayed bone and wound healing, menstrual disorders, neuropathy, peptic ulcer, decreased glucose tolerance, hypopotassemia, adrenal insufficiency, necrotizing angiitis, hypertension, pancreatitis and increased intraocular pressure. In children, suppression of growth may occur. Increased intracranial pressure may occur and possibly account for headache, insomnia and fatigue. Subcapsular cataracts may result from prolonged usage. Long-term use of all corticosteroids results in catabolic effects characterized by negative protein and calcium balance. Osteoporosis, spontaneous fractures and aseptic necrosis of the hip and humerus may occur as part of this catabolic phenomenon. Where hypopotassemia and other symptoms associated with fluid and electrolyte imbalance call for potassium supplementation and salt poor or salt-free diets, these may be instituted and are compatible with diet requirements for ulcerative proctitis.

ADMINISTRATION AND DOSAGE

Usual dose is one applicatorful once or twice daily for two or three weeks, and every second day thereafter, administered rectally. The patient directions packaged with the applicator describe how to use the aerosol container and applicator. Satisfactory response usually occurs within five to seven days marked by a decrease in symptoms. Symptomatic improvement in ulcerative proctitis should not be used as the sole criterion for evaluating efficacy. Sigmoidoscopy is also recommended to judge dosage adjustment, duration of therapy and rate of improvement.

Directions For Use:

1. Shake foam container vigorously for 5–10 seconds. Do not remove cap.
2. Withdraw applicator plunger past the fill line until it stops.
3. Place foam container upright on level surface, insert tip of cap into tip of applicator.
   To fill applicator:
   - Depress cap on foam container-RELEASE.
   - Pause, a few seconds, allowing foam to enter and expand in applicator barrel.
   - Repeat until foam rises to fill applicator to Fill Line.
4. Hold applicator by barrel and gently insert tip into anus. Once in place, push plunger to expel foam, then withdraw applicator.
   Note: Pull applicator apart and wash thoroughly with warm water.

HOW SUPPLIED

CORTIFOAM is supplied in an aerosol container with a special rectal applicator. Each applicator delivers approximately 900 mg of foam containing approximately 80 mg of hydrocortisone as 90 mg of hydrocortisone acetate. When used correctly the aerosol container will deliver a minimum of 14 applications.

LITERATURE AVAILABLE

Patient information available on request.

Shown in Product Identification Section, page 423

DILATRATE®-SR ℞
[dī'lă-trāt]
(Isosorbide Dinitrate)
Sustained Release Capsules
40 mg

DESCRIPTION

Isosorbide dinitrate, an organic nitrate, is a vasodilator with effects on both arteries and veins. Isosorbide dinitrate is available as a 40 mg sustained release capsule. The chemical name for isosorbide dinitrate is 1,4,3,6-dianhydrosorbitol-2, 5-dinitrate and, the compound has the following structural formula:

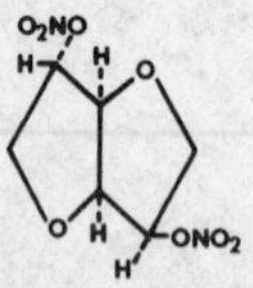

Molecular Weight: 236.14

Isosorbide dinitrate is a white, crystalline, odorless compound which is stable in air and in solution, has a melting point of 70°C and has an optical rotation of +134° (c=1.0, alcohol, 20°C). Isosorbide dinitrate is freely soluble in organic solvents such as acetone, alcohol, and ether, but is only sparingly soluble in water.

CLINICAL PHARMACOLOGY

The principal pharmacological action of isosorbide dinitrate is relaxation of vascular smooth muscle, producing a vasodilatory effect on both peripheral arteries and veins, with predominant effects on the latter. Dilation of the postcapillary vessels, including large veins, promotes peripheral pooling of blood and decreases venous return to the heart, thereby reducing left-ventricular end-diastolic pressure (preload). Arteriolar relaxation reduces systemic vascular resistance and arterial pressure (after-load).

The mechanism by which isosorbide dinitrate relieves angina pectoris is not fully understood. Myocardial oxygen consumption or demand (as measured by the pressure-rate product, tension-time index, and stroke work index) is decreased by both the arterial and venous effects of isosorbide dinitrate and, presumably, a more favorable supply-demand ratio is achieved. While the large epicardial coronary arteries are also dilated by isosorbide dinitrate, the extent to which this contributes to relief of exertional angina is unclear.

Therapeutic doses of isosorbide dinitrate may reduce systolic, diastolic, and mean arterial blood pressures, especially in the upright posture. Effective coronary perfusion is usually maintained. The decrease in systemic blood pressure may result in reflex tachycardia, an effect which results in an unfavorable influence on myocardial oxygen demand. Hemodynamic studies indicate that isosorbide dinitrate may reduce the abnormally elevated left ventricular end-diastolic and pulmonary capillary wedge pressures that occur during an acute episode of angina pectoris.

Isosorbide dinitrate is metabolized by enzymatic denitration to the intermediate products isosorbide-2-mononitrate and isosorbide-5-mononitrate. Both metabolites have biological activity, especially the 5-mononitrate which is also the principal metabolite. The liver is a principal site of metabolism and isosorbide dinitrate is subject to a large first pass effect. The systemic clearance of the drug following intravenous infusion is about 3.4 liters/min. Since the clearance exceeds hepatic blood flow, considerable extra hepatic metabolism must also occur.

The average bioavailability of isosorbide dinitrate is 59 and 22 percent following sublingual and oral administration, respectively. The terminal half-life is about 20 minutes, 60 minutes, and 4 hours following IV, sublingual, and oral administration, respectively. The dependence of half-life on the route of administration is not understood. Over limited ranges of IV dosing, the pharmacokinetics of isosorbide dinitrate appear linear. However, both the 2- and 5-mononitrate metabolites have been shown to decrease the rate of disappearance of the dinitrate from the blood and the half-lives of isosorbide-5-mononitrate and isosorbide-2-mononitrate range from 4.0–5.6 and 1.5–3.1 hours, respectively.

The pharmacokinetics and/or bioavailability of isosorbide dinitrate during multiple dosing have not been well-studied. Because the metabolites influence the clearance of isosorbide dinitrate, prediction of blood levels of parent compound or metabolites from single-dose studies is uncertain.

INDICATIONS AND USAGE

Isosorbide dinitrate is indicated for the treatment and prevention of angina pectoris. Controlled clinical trials have demonstrated that the sublingual, chewable, immediate release, and controlled-release oral dosage forms of isosorbide dinitrate are effective in improving exercise tolerance in patients with angina pectoris. When single sublingual or chewable doses (5mg) of isosorbide dinitrate were administered prophylactically to patients with angina pectoris in various clinical studies, duration of exercise until chest pain or fatigue was significantly improved for at least 45 minutes (and as long as 2 hours in some studies) following dosing. Similar studies after single oral (15 to 120 mg) and oral controlled-released (40 to 80 mg) doses of isosorbide dinitrate have shown significant improvement in exercise tolerance for up to 8 hours following dosing. The exercise electrocardiographic evidence suggests that improved exercise tolerance with isosorbide dinitrate is not at the expense of greater myocardial ischemia. All dosage forms of isosorbide dinitrate may therefore be used prophylactically to decrease frequency and severity of anginal attacks and can be expected to decrease the need for sublingual nitroglycerin.

The sublingual and chewable forms of the drug are indicated for acute prophylaxis of angina pectoris when taken a few minutes before situations likely to provoke anginal attacks. Because of a slower onset of effect, the oral forms of isosorbide dinitrate are not indicated for acute prophylaxis.

In controlled clinical trials chewable and sublingual isosorbide dinitrate were effective in relieving an acute attack of angina pectoris. Relief occurred with a mean time of 2.9 and 3.4 minutes (chewable and sublingual respectively) compared to relief of angina with a mean time of 1.9 minutes following sublingual nitroglycerin. Because of the more rapid relief of chest pain with sublingual nitroglycerin, the use of sublingual or chewable isosorbide dinitrate for aborting an acute anginal attack should be limited to patients intolerant or unresponsive to sublingual nitroglycerin.

CONTRAINDICATIONS

Isosorbide dinitrate is contraindicated in patients who have shown purported hypersensitivity or idiosyncrasy to it or other nitrates or nitrites.

WARNINGS

The benefits of isosorbide dinitrate during the early days of an acute myocardial infarction have not been established. If one elects to use organic nitrates in early infarction hemodynamic monitoring and frequent clinical assessment should be used because of the potential deleterious effects of hypotension.

PRECAUTIONS

General: Severe hypotensive response, particularly with upright posture, may occur with even small doses of isosorbide dinitrate. The drug should therefore be used with caution in subjects who may have blood volume depletion from diuretic therapy or in subjects who have low systolic blood pressure (e.g., below 90 mm Hg). Paradoxical bradycardia and increased angina pectoris may accompany nitrate-induced hypotension.

Nitrate therapy may aggravate the angina caused by hypertrophic cardiomyopathy. Tolerance to this drug and cross-tolerance to other nitrates and nitrites may occur.

Marked symptomatic, orthostatic hypotension has been reported when calcium channel blockers and organic nitrates were used in combination. Dose adjustment of either class of agents may be necessary.

Tolerance to the vascular and antianginal effects of isosorbide dinitrate or nitroglycerin has been demonstrated in clinical trials, experience through occupational exposure, and in isolated tissue experiments in the laboratory. The importance of tolerance to the appropriate use of isosorbide dinitrate in the management of patients with angina pectoris has not been determined. However, one clinical trial using treadmill exercise tolerance (as an endpoint) found an 8 hour duration of action of oral isosorbide dinitrate following the first dose (after a 2 week placebo washout) and only a 2 hour duration of effect of the same dose after 1 week of repetitive dosing a conventional dosing intervals. On the other hand, several trials have been able to differentiate isosorbide dinitrate from placebo after 4 weeks of therapy, and in open trials an effect seems detectable for as long as several months.

Tolerance clearly occurs in industrial workers continuously exposed to nitroglycerin. Moreover, physical dependence also occurs since chest pain, acute myocardial infarction, and even sudden death have occurred during temporary withdrawal of nitroglycerin from the workers. In clinical trials in angina patients, there are reports of anginal attacks being more easily provoked and of rebound in the hemodynamic effects soon after nitrate withdrawal. The relative importance of these observations to the routine, clinical use of isosorbide dinitrate is not known. However, it seems prudent to gradually withdraw patients from isosorbide dinitrate when the therapy is being terminated, rather than stopping the drug abruptly.

Information for Patients: Headache may occur during initial therapy with isosorbide dinitrate. Headache is usually relieved by the use of standard headache remedies, or by lowering the dose, and tends to disappear after the first week or two of use.

Drug Interactions: Alcohol may enhance any marked sensitivity to the hypotensive effect of nitrates. Isosorbide dinitrate acts directly on vascular smooth muscle; therefore, any other agent that depends on vascular smooth muscle as the final common path can be expected to have decreased or increased effect depending on the agent.

Carcinogenesis, Mutagenesis, Impairment of Fertility: No long-term studies in animals have been performed to evaluate the carcinogenic potential of this drug. A modified two-litter reproduction study in rats fed isosorbide dinitrate at 25 or 100 mg/kg/day did not reveal any effects on fertility or gestation or any remarkable growth pathology in any parent or offspring fed isosorbide dinitrate as compared with rats fed a basal controlled diet.

Pregnancy Category C: Isosorbide dinitrate has been shown to cause a dose-related increase in embryotoxicity (increase in mummified pups) in rabbits at oral doses 35 and 150 times the maximum recommended human daily dose. There are no adequate and well-controlled studies in pregnant women. Isosorbide dinitrate should be used during pregnancy only if the potential benefit justifies the potential risk to the fetus.

Nursing Mothers: It is not known whether this drug is excreted in human milk. Because many drugs are excreted in human milk, caution should be exercised when isosorbide dinitrate is administered to a nursing woman.

Pediatric Use: The safety and effectiveness of isosorbide dinitrate in children has not been established.

ADVERSE REACTIONS

Adverse reactions, particularly headache and hypotension, are dose related. In clinical trials at various doses, the following have been observed.

Headache is the most common (reported incidence varies widely, apparently being dose related, with an average occurrence of about 25%) adverse reaction and may be severe and persistent. Cutaneous vasodilation wth flushing may occur. Transient episodes of dizziness and weakness, as well as other signs of cerebral ischemia associated with postural hypotension, may occasionally develop (the incidence of reported symptomatic hypotension ranges from 2% to 36%). An occasional individual will exhibit marked sensitivity to the hypotensive effects of nitrates and severe responses (nausea, vomiting, weakness, restlessness, pallor, perspiration, and collapse) may occur even with the usual therapeutic dose. Drug rash and/or exfoliative dermatitis may occasionally occur. Nausea and vomiting appear to be uncommon.

OVERDOSAGE

Signs and Symptoms: These may include the following: a prompt fall in blood pressure, persistent and throbbing headache, vertigo, palpitation, visual disturbances, flushed and perspiring skin (later becoming cold and cyanotic), nausea and vomiting (possibly with colic and even bloody diarrhea), syncope (especially in the upright position), methemoglobinemia with cyanosis and anoxia, initial hyperpnea, dyspnea and slow breathing, slow pulse (dicrotic and intermittent), heart block, increased intracranial pressure with cerebral symptoms of confusion and moderate fever, paralysis and coma followed by clonic convulsions and possibly death due to circulatory collapse.

It is not known what dose of the drug is associated with symptoms of overdosing or what dose of the drug would be life-threatening. The acute oral LD50 of isosorbide dinitrate in rats was found to be approximately 1100 mg/kg of body weight. These animal experiments indicate that approximately 500 times the usual therapeutic dose would be required to produce such toxic symptoms in humans. It is not known whether the drug is dialyzable.

Treatment of Overdosage: Prompt removal of the ingested material by gastric lavage is reasonable but not documented to be useful. Keep the patient recumbent in a shock position and comfortably warm. Passive movements of the extremities may aid venous return. Administer oxygen and artificial respiration if necessary. If methemoglobinemia is present, administer methylene blue (1% solution), 1 to 2 mg/kg intravenously.

Methemoglobin: Case reports of clinically significant methemoglobinemia are rare at conventional doses of organic nitrates. The formation of methemoglobin is dose related and in the case of genetic abnormalities of hemoglobin that favor methemoglobin formation, even conventional doses of organic nitrate could produce harmful concentrations of methemoglobin.

WARNING

Epinephrine is ineffective in reversing the severe hypotensive events associated with overdose. It and related compounds are contraindicated in this situation.

DOSAGE AND ADMINISTRATION

Because of a slower onset of effect, the oral forms of isosorbide dinitrate are not indicated for acute prophylaxis or for the treament of acute anginal attacks.

Isosorbide dinitrate should be titrated upward until angina is relieved or side effects limit the dose. In ambulatory patients, the magnitude of the incremental dose increase should be guided by measurements of standing blood pressure.

For the treatment of chronic stable angina pectoris, the usual starting dose for controlled-release forms, 40 mg. For maintenance therapy, oral controlled-release doses of 40 to 80 mg given every 8 to 12 hours is generally recommended. The extent to which development of tolerance should modify the dosage program has not been defined. The oral controlled release forms of isosorbide dinitrate should not be chewed.

HOW SUPPLIED

Bottles of 100 (opaque pink and colorless body) capsules.

STORAGE

Store at controlled room temperature 15-30°C (59-86°F) in a dry place.

WARNING

KEEP OUT OF REACH OF CHILDREN.

CAUTION

Federal law prohibits dispensing without prescription.
Manufactured for
Reed & Carnrick
by Vitarine Pharmaceuticals, Inc.
S. Hackensack, NJ 07606

Date of Revision
May 1986

Shown in Product Identification Section, page 423

EPIFOAM® ℞

[*ĕp 'ē-fōm*]
(hydrocortisone acetate 1% and pramoxine hydrochloride 1% topical aerosol)

DESCRIPTION

A topical corticosteroid aerosol foam containing hydrocortisone acetate 1% and pramoxine hydrochloride 1% in a base containing: propylene glycol, cetyl alcohol, glyceryl stearate, PEG-100 stearate, laureth-23, polyoxyl-40 stearate, methylparaben, propylparaben, trolamine or hydrochloric acid to adjust pH, purified water and propellants (inert): butane and propane.

EPIFOAM contains a synthetic steroid used as an anti-inflammatory and anti-pruritic agent, and a local anesthetic.

Molecular weight: Hydrocortisone acetate 404.51. Solubility of hydrocortisone acetate in water: 1 mg/100 ml. Chemical name: Pregn-4-ene, 3,20-dione, 21-(acetyloxy)-11, 17-dihydroxy-, (11B).

$CH_2-O-C(=O)-CH_3$; C=O ; CH_3 ; ...OH ; HO ; CH_3 ; O

Pramoxine Hydrochloride

$CH_3CH_2CH_2CH_2O-C_6H_4-OCH_2CH_2CH_2-N$ (morpholine) OCHL

CLINICAL PHARMACOLOGY

Topical corticosteroids share anti-inflammatory, anti-pruritic and vascoconstrictive actions.

The mechanism of anti-inflammatory activity of the topical corticosteroids is unclear. Various laboratory methods, including vasoconstrictor assays, are used to compare and predict potencies clinical efficacies of the topical corticosteroids. There is some evidence to suggest that a recognizable correlation exists between vasoconstrictor potency and therapeutic efficacy in man.

Pramoxine Hydrochloride: A surface or local anesthetic which is not chemically related to the "caine" types of local anesthetics. Its unique chemical structure is likely to minimize the danger of cross-sensitivity reactions in patients allergic to other local anesthetics.

Pharmacokinetics: The extent of percutaneous absorption of topical corticosteroids is determined by many factors including the vehicle, the integrity of the epidermal barrier, and the use of occlusive dressings.

Topical corticosteroids can be absorbed from normal intact skin. Inflammation and/or other disease processes in the skin increase the percutaneous absorption of topical corticosteroids. Occlusive dressings substantially increase the percutaneous absorption of topical corticosteroids. Thus, occlusive dressings may be a valuable therapeutic adjunct for treatment of resistant dermatoses. (See DOSAGE AND ADMINISTRATION.)

Once absorbed through the skin, topical corticosteroids are handled through pharmacokinetic pathways similar to systemically administered corticosteroids. Corticosteroids are bound to plasma proteins in varying degrees. Corticosteroids are metabolized primarily in the liver and are then excreted by the kidneys. Some of the topical corticosteroids and their metabolites are also excreted in the bile.

INDICATIONS AND USAGE

Topical corticosteroids are indicated for the relief of the inflammatory and pruritic manifestations of corticosteroid-responsive dermatoses.

CONTRAINDICATIONS

Topical corticosteroid products are contraindicated in those patients with a history of hypersensitivity to any of the components of the preparation.

WARNING

Not for prolonged use. If redness, pain, irritation or swelling persists, discontinue use and consult a physician. Contents of the container are under pressure, but not flammable. Do not burn or puncture the aerosol container. Store at temperatures below 120°F. Keep this and all medicines out of the reach of children.

PRECAUTIONS

General: Systemic absorption of topical corticosteroids has produced reversible hypothalamic-pituitary-adrenal (HPA) axis suppression, manifestations of Cushing's syndrome, hyperglycemia and glucosuria in some patients.

Conditions which augment systemic absorption include the application of the more potent steroids, use over large surface areas, prolonged use and the addition of occlusive dressings.

Therefore, patients receiving a large dose of a potent topical steroid applied to a large surface area or under an occlusive dressing should be evaluated periodically for evidence of HPA axis suppression by using the urinary hydrocortisone

Continued on next page

Reed & Carnrick—Cont.

and ACTH stimulation tests. If HPA axis suppression is noted, an attempt should be made to withdraw the drug, to reduce the frequency of application, or to substitute a less potent steroid.
Recovery of HPA axis function is generally prompt and complete upon discontinuation of the drug. Infrequently, signs and symptoms of steroid withdrawal may occur, requiring supplemental systemic corticosteroids.
In children absorption may result in higher blood levels and thus more susceptibility to systemic toxicity. (See PRECAUTIONS—Pediatric Use.)
If irritation develops, topical corticosteroids should be discontinued and appropriate therapy instituted.
In the presence of dermatological infections, the use of an appropriate antifungal or antibacterial agent should be instituted. If a favorable response does not occur promptly, the corticosteroid should be discontinued until the infection has been adequately controlled.
Information for the Patient: Patients using topical corticosteroids should receive the following information and instructions:
1. This medication is to be used as directed by the physician. It is for external use only. Avoid contact with the eyes.
2. Do not use this medication for any disorder other than for which it was prescribed.
3. The treated skin area should not be bandaged or otherwise covered or wrapped as to be occlusive unless directed by physician.
4. Report any signs of local adverse reactions especially under occlusive dressings.
5. Do not use tight fitting diapers or plastic pants on a child being treated in the diaper area, as these garments may constitute occlusive dressings.

Laboratory Tests: The following test may be helpful in evaluating the HPA axis suppression:
Urinary hydrocortisone test
ACTH stimulation test
Carcinogenesis, Mutagenesis, and Impairment of Fertility: Long-term animal studies have not been performed to evaluate the carcinogenic potential or the effect on fertility of topical corticosteroids.
Studies to determine mutagenicity with prednisolone and hydrocortisone have revealed negative results.
Pregnancy Category C: Corticosteroids are generally teratogenic in laboratory animals when administered systemically at relatively low dosage levels. The more potent corticosteroids have been shown to be teratogenic after dermal application in laboratory animals. There are no adequate and well-controlled studies in pregnant women of teratogenic effects from topically applied corticosteroids. Therefore, topical corticosteroids should be used during pregnancy only if the potential benefit justifies the potential risk to the fetus. Drugs of this class should not be used extensively on pregnant patients, in large amounts, or for prolonged periods of time.
Nursing Mothers: It is not known whether topical administration of corticosteroids could result in sufficient systemic absorption to produce detectable quantities in breast milk. Systemically administered corticosteroids are secreted into breast milk in quantities not likely to have a deleterious effect on the infant. Caution should be exercised when any topical corticosteroids are administered to a nursing woman.
Pediatric Use: Pediatric patients may demonstrate greater susceptibility to topical corticosteroid-induced HPA axis suppression and Cushing's syndrome than mature patients because of a larger skin surface area to body weight ratio.
Hypothalamic-pituitary-adrenal (HPA) axis suppression, Cushing's syndrome and intracranial hypertension have been reported in children receiving topical corticosteroids. Manifestations of adrenal suppression in children include linear growth retardation, delayed weight gain, low plasma cortisone levels and absence of response to ACTH stimulation. Manifestations of intracranial hypertension include bulging fontanelles, headaches and bilateral papilladema.
Administration of topical corticosteroids to children should be limited to the least amount compatible with an effective therapeutic regimen. Chronic corticosteroid therapy may interfere with the growth and development of children.

ADVERSE REACTIONS
The following local adverse reactions are reported infrequently with topical corticosteroids, but may occur more frequently with the use of occlusive dressings. These reactions are listed in an approximately decreasing order of occurrence:
Burning
Itching
Irritation
Dryness
Folliculitis
Hypopigmentation
Perioral dermatitis
Allergic contact dermatitis
Maceration of the skin
Secondary infection
Skin atrophy
Striae
Miliaria

OVERDOSAGE
Topically applied corticosteroids can be absorbed in sufficient amounts to produce systemic effects. (See PRECAUTIONS.)

DOSAGE AND ADMINISTRATION
Apply to affected area 3 or 4 times daily.
(NOTE: Refer to the enclosed Directions for Use.):

DIRECTIONS FOR USE
1. Shake foam container vigorously before use.
2. Hold container upright and dispense medication onto a pad by depressing the container cap several times. A small amount of foam is all that is needed on the pad. Apply to affected areas.
Alternatively, the foam may be applied directly to affected areas.
3. The container and cap should be disassembled and rinsed with warm water after use.

NOTE: The aerosol container should never be inserted into the vagina or anus.

HOW SUPPLIED
EPIFOAM (NDC-0021-0740-10) available in 10g pressurized cans.

CAUTION
FEDERAL LAW PROHIBITS DISPENSING WITHOUT PRESCRIPTION.
Reed & Carnrick
1 New England Avenue
Piscataway, NJ 08854
Revised 4/10/84
Shown in Product Identification Section, page 423

KWELL® Cream ℞
[*kwel*]
(lindane) 1%

DESCRIPTION
KWELL Cream (lindane) 1% is an ectoparasiticide and ovicide effective against Sarcoptes scabiei (scabies) and their ova. Inert ingredients: 99% in a pleasantly scented water dispersible cream containing stearic acid, glycerin, lanolin, 2-amino-2-methyl-1-propanol, perfume and purified water. Lindane, which is the highly purified gamma isomer of 1, 2, 3, 4, 5, 6, hexachlorocyclohexane, has the following chemical structure.

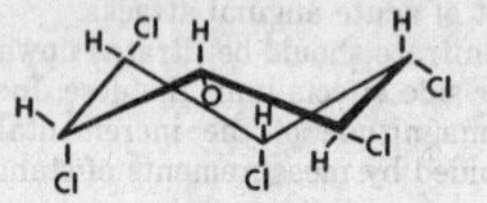

CLINICAL PHARMACOLOGY
KWELL Cream exerts its parasiticidal action by being directly absorbed into the parasites and their ova. Feldmann and Maibach[1] reported approximately 10% absorption of a lindane acetone solution applied to the forearm and left in place to 24 hours. Dale, et al[2] reported a blood level of 290ng/ml associated with convulsions following the accidental ingestion of a lindane containing product. Ginsburg[3] found a mean peak blood level of 28ng/ml 6 hours after total body application of KWELL Lotion to scabietic infants and children. The half-life was determined to be 18 hours.

INDICATIONS AND USAGE
KWELL Cream is indicated for the treatment of patients infested with Sarcoptes scabiei (scabies).

CONTRAINDICATIONS
KWELL Cream is contraindicated for premature neonates because their skin may be more permeable than full term infants and their liver enzymes may not be sufficiently developed. It is also contraindicated for patients with known seizure disorders and for individuals with a known sensitivity to the product or any of its components.

WARNINGS
LINDANE PENETRATES HUMAN SKIN AND HAS THE POTENTIAL FOR CNS TOXICITY (SEE CLINICAL PHARMACOLOGY SECTION). KWELL CREAM SHOULD BE USED ACCORDING TO RECOMMENDED DOSAGE (SEE DIRECTIONS FOR USE) ESPECIALLY ON INFANTS, PREGNANT WOMEN AND NURSING MOTHERS. ANIMAL STUDIES INDICATE THAT POTENTIAL TOXIC EFFECTS OF TOPICALLY APPLIED LINDANE ARE GREATER IN THE YOUNG. Seizures have been reported after excessive use or oral ingestion of lindane. No residual effects of KWELL treatment have been demonstrated, therefore, this product should not be used to ward off a possible infestation. If accidental ingestion occurs prompt gastric lavage is indicated. Because oils may enhance absorption, saline rather than oily cathartics should be used. Central nervous excitation can be controlled by the administration of pentobarbital, phenobarbital or diazepam.

PRECAUTIONS
General
Care should be taken to avoid contact with the eyes. If such contact occurs, eyes should be immediately flushed with water. If irritation or sensitization occurs, the patient should be advised to consult a physician.
Information to Patients
Patients should be instructed on the proper use of the medication. Directions for Use should accompany the prescription.

LABORATORY TESTS
No laboratory tests are needed for the proper use of this medication.

DRUG INTERACTIONS
Oils may enhance absorption, therefore, simultaneous use of creams, ointments or oils should be avoided.

CARCINOGENESIS
Although no studies have been conducted with KWELL Cream, numerous long term feeding studies have been conducted in mice and rats to evaluate the carcinogenic potential of the technical grade of hexachlorocyclohexane (BHC) as well as the alpha, beta, gamma lindane) and delta isomers. Both oral and topical applications have been evaluated. Nagasaki[4], Goto[5] and Hanada[6] found varying amounts of benign and malignant hepatomas associated with BHC and the alpha, delta and epsilon isomers. None reported a carcinogenic potential for lindane. Tumors were found only in the animals which had received the alpha isomer. Weisse and Herbst[7] also evaluated the carcinogenic potential of lindane in mice but could find no evidence of lindane in mice but could find no evidnece of lindane carcinogenicity. The National Cancer Institute[8] also found no evidence of carcinogenicity.
Thorpe and Walker[9] compared beta BHC with lindane, dieldrin, DDT and hexabarbital in mice. Despite the unusually high incidence of tumors in the control group, they concluded that 600 ppm of lindane was associated with a significant increase in the incidence of hepatoma and thus considered it a tumorigen.
Orr[10] and Kashyap, et al[11] evaluated the carcinogenic potential in mice of topically applied BHC. In neither study was there any evidence of a tumorigenic or carcinogenic potential associated with topical application of BHC.
Mutagenicity tests have been used as predictive information about the carcinogenicity of various chemical compounds. Numerous types of mutagenicity tests have been performed with lindane. The results of these tests do not indicate that lindane is mutagenic.

PREGNANCY
Teratogenetic Effects
Pregnancy category B: Reproduction, including multigeneration, studies have been performed in mice, rats, rabbits, pigs, and dogs at doses up to 10 times the human dose and have revealed no evidence of impaired fertility or harm to the fetus due to administered lindane. There are, however, no adequate and well controlled studies in pregnant women. Because animal reproduction studies are not always predictive of human response, the recommended dosage should not be exceeded on pregnant women. They should be treated no more than twice during a pregnancy.

NURSING MOTHERS
Lindane is secreted in human milk in low concentrations. Studies conducted in the United States as well as Europe and South America found levels of lindane in human milk ranging from 0 to 113 ppb, as the result of ingestion of foods which had been treated with lindane. There appeared to be no difference in concentrations between country and urban dwellers. Although the levels of lindane found in blood after topical application with KWELL Cream make it unlikely that amounts of lindane sufficient to cause serious adverse reactions will be excreted in the milk of nursing mothers who have used KWELL Cream, if there is any concern, an alternate method of feeding may be used for 2 days.

PEDIATRIC USE
Refer to the Contraindications and Warning sections.

ADVERSE REACTIONS
Lindane has been reported to cause central nervous stimulation ranging from dizziness to convulsions. Cases of convulsions have been reported in connection with KWELL Cream therapy. However, these incidents were almost always associated with accidental oral ingestion or misuse of the product. Eczematous eruptions due to irritation from this product have also been reported. Incidence of these adverse reactions is relatively infrequent, occurring in less than 1 in 100,000 patients.

DRUG ABUSE AND DEPENDENCE

KWELL Cream is not subject to abuse, nor is there any dependence on the drug.

OVERDOSAGE

Overdosage or oral ingestion of KWELL Cream can cause central nervous system excitation and, if taken in sufficient quantities, convulsions may occur.

If accidental ingestion occurs, prompt gastric lavage should be instituted. However, since oils favor absorption, saline cathartics for intestinal evacuation should be given rather than oil laxatives. If central nervous system manifestations occur they can be antagonized by the administration of pentobarbital, phenobarbital or diazepam.

DOSAGE AND ADMINISTRATION

CAUTION: USE ONLY AS DIRECTED. DO NOT EXCEED RECOMENDED DOSAGE

No residual effects of KWELL treatment have been demonstrated therefore, this product should not be used to ward off a possible infestation.

NOTE: PLEASE READ CAREFULLY.

DIRECTIONS FOR USE

Scabies (sarcoptes scabiei)—The cream should be applied to dry skin in a thin layer and rubbed in thoroughly. If crusted lesions are present, a tepid bath preceding the medication is helpful. If a bath is used, allow the skin to dry before applying the cream. Usually two ounces are sufficient for an adult. A total body application should be made from the neck down including the soles of the feet. Scabies rarely affects the head of children or adults but may occur in infants.

The cream should be left on for 8–12 hours and should then be removed by thorough washing. ONE APPLICATION IS USUALLY CURATIVE.

Sexual contacts should be treated simultaneously.

Avoid unnecessary skin contact. Particularly when applying to more than one patient, those assisting in lindane therapy (especially pregnant and/or nursing women) should wear rubber gloves.

Avoid use on open cuts and extensive excoriations.

Many patients exhibit persistent pruritus after treatment; this is rarely a sign of treatment failure and is not an indication for retreatment unless living mites can be demonstrated.

CAUTION

Federal law prohibits dispensing without prescription.

HOW SUPPLIED

KWELL Cream in tubes of 2 oz (57 g) and jars of 16 oz (454 g).

REFERENCES

1. Feldmann, R.J. and Maibach, H.I., *Toxicol. Applied. Pharmacol.*, 28:126, 1974.
2. Dale, W.E., Curly, A. and Cueto, C. *Life Sci* 5:47, 1966.
3. Ginsburg, C.M., et al., *J. Pediatr.* 91:6, 998–1000, 1977.
4. Nagasaki, T., Tomii, S., Mepa, T., Marugami, M. and Ito, *N. Gann* (Cancer) 63(3):393, 1972.
5. Goto, M. Hattori, M., Miyagawa, T. and Enomoto, M., *Chemosphere* 6:279, 1972.
6. Hanada, M., Yatani, C., Miyaji, T., *Gann* 64:511, 1973.
7. Weisse, I, and Herbst, M., *Toxicol.* 7:233, 1977.
8. Technical Report Series, NCI-CG-TR-14, *HEW PUBLICATIONS*, No. (NIH) 77–814.
9. Thorpe, E., and Walker, A.I.T., *Food Cosmetic Toxicol.* 11:433, 1973.
10. Orr, J.W., *Nature* 162:189, 1948.
11. Kashyap, S.K. et al., *J. Environ, Sci. Health* 14:305–318, 1979.

MANUFACTURED FOR
REED & CARNRICK
Piscataway, NJ 08854
By Reedco Inc., Humacao, PR 00661

Date of Revision
August 1985

KWELL® Lotion ℞
[kwel]
(lindane) 1%

DESCRIPTION

KWELL Lotion (lindane) 1% is an ectoparasiticide and ovicide effective against Sarcoptes scabiei (scabies). In addition to the active ingredient, lindane, it contains glycerol monostearate, cetyl alcohol, stearic acid, trolamine, 2-amino-2-methyl-1 propanol, methyl p-hydroxybenzoate, butyl p-hydroxybenzoate, carrageenan perfume and purified water to form a non-greasy lotion. Lindane, which is the highly purified gamma isomer of 1, 2, 3, 4, 5, 6, hexachlorocyclohexane, has the following chemical structure.

[See Chemical Formula at top of next column].

CLINICAL PHARMACOLOGY

KWELL Lotion exerts its parasiticidal action by being directly absorbed into the parasites and their ova. Feldmann and Maibach[1] reported approximately 10% absorption of a

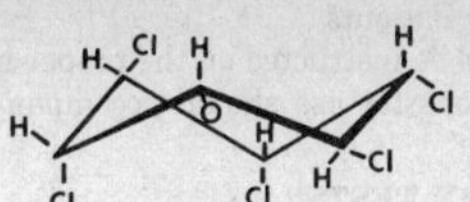

lindane acetone solution applied to the forearm and left in place to 24 hours. Dale, et al[2] reported a blood level of 290ng/ml associated with convulsions following the accidental ingestion of a lindane containing product. Ginsburg[3] found a mean peak blood level of 28ng/ml 6 hours after total body application of KWELL Lotion to scabietic infants and children. The half-life was determined to be 18 hours.

INDICATIONS AND USAGE

KWELL Lotin is indicated for the treatment of patients infested with Sarcoptes scabiei (scabies).

CONTRAINDICATIONS

KWELL Lotion is contraindicated for premature neonates because their skin may be more permeable than full term infants and their liver enzymes may not be sufficiently developed. It is also contraindicated for patients with known seizure disorders and for individuals with a known sensitivity to the product or any of its components.

WARNINGS

LINDANE PENETRATES HUMAN SKIN AND HAS THE POTENTIAL FOR CNS TOXICITY (SEE CLINICAL PHARMACOLOGY SECTION). KWELL CREAM SHOULD BE USED ACCORDING TO RECOMMENDED DOSAGE (SEE DIRECTIONS FOR USE) ESPECIALLY ON INFANTS, PREGNANT WOMEN AND NURSING MOTHERS. ANIMAL STUDIES INDICATE THAT POTENTIAL TOXIC EFFECTS OF TOPICALLY APPLIED LINDANE ARE GREATER IN THE YOUNG. Seizures have been reported after excessive use or oral ingestion of lindane. No residual effects of KWELL treatment have been demonstrated, therefore, this product should not be used to ward off a possible infestation. If accidental ingestion occurs prompt gastric lavage is indicated. Because oils may enhance absorption, saline rather than oily cathartics should be used. Central nervous excitation can be controlled by the administration of pentobarbital, phenobarbital or diazepam.

PRECAUTIONS

General

Care should be taken to avoid contact with the eyes. If such contact occurs, eyes should be immediately flushed with water. If irritation or sensitization occurs, the patient should be advised to consult a physician.

Information to Patients

Patients should be instructed on the proper use of the medication. Directions for Use should accompany the prescription.

LABORATORY TESTS

No laboratory tests are needed for the proper use of this medication.

DRUG INTERACTIONS

Oils may enhance absorption, therefore, simultaneous use of creams, ointments or oils should be avoided.

CARCINOGENESIS

Although no studies have been conducted with KWELL Lotion, numerous long term feeding studies have been conducted in mice and rats to evaluate the carcinogenic potential of the technical grade of hexachlorocyclohexane (BHC) as well as the alpha, beta, gamma lindane) and delta isomers. Both oral and topical applications have been evaluated. Nagasaki[4], Goto[5] and Hanada[6] found varying amounts of benign and malignant hepatomas associated with BHC and the alpha, delta and epsilon isomers. None reported a carcinogenic potential for lindane. Tumors were found only in the animals which had received the alpha isomer. Weisse and Herbst[7] also evaluated the carcinogenic potential of lindane in mice but could find no evidence of lindane in mice but could find no evidnece of lindane carcinogenicity. The National Cancer Institute[8] also found no evidence of carcinogenicity.

Thorpe and Walker[9] compared beta BHC with lindane, dieldrin, DDT and hexabarbital in mice. Despite the unusually high incidence of tumors in the control group, they concluded that 600 ppm of lindane was associated with a significant increase in the incidence of hepatoma and thus considered it a tumorigen.

Orr[10] and Kashyap, et al[11] evaluated the carcinogenic potential in mice of topically applied BHC. In neither study was there any evidence of a tumorigenic or carcinogenic potential associated with topical application of BHC.

Mutagenicity tests have been used as predictive information about the carcinogenicity of various chemical compounds. Numerous types of mutagenicity tests have been performed with lindane. The results of these tests do not indicate that lindane is mutagenic.

PREGNANCY

Teratogenetic Effects

Pregnancy category B: Reproduction, including multigeneration, studies have been performed in mice, rats, rabbits, pigs, and dogs at doses up to 10 times the human dose and have revealed no evidence of impaired fertility or harm to the fetus due to administered lindane. There are, however, no adequate and well controlled studies in pregnant women. Because animal reproduction studies are not always predictive of human response, the recommended dosage should not be exceeded on pregnant women. They should be treated no more than twice during a pregnancy.

NURSING MOTHERS

Lindane is secreted in human milk in low concentrations. Studies conducted in the United States as well as Europe and South America found levels of lindane in human milk ranging from 0 to 113 ppb, as the result of ingestion of foods which had been treated with lindane. There appeared to be no difference in concentrations between country and urban dwellers. Although the levels of lindane found in blood after topical application with KWELL Lotion make it unlikely that amounts of lindane sufficient to cause serious adverse reactions will be excreted in the milk of nursing mothers who have used KWELL Lotion, if there is any concern, an alternate method of feeding may be used for 2 days.

PEDIATRIC USE

Refer to the Contraindications and Warning sections.

ADVERSE REACTIONS

Lindane has been reported to cause central nervous stimulation ranging from dizziness to convulsions. Cases of convulsions have been reported in connection with KWELL Lotion therapy. However, these incidents were almost always associated with accidental oral ingestion or misuse of the product. Ezematous eruptions due to irritation from this product have also been reported. Incidence of these adverse reactions is relatively infrequent, occurring in less than 1 in 100,000 patients.

DRUG ABUSE AND DEPENDENCE

KWELL Lotion is not subject to abuse, nor is there any dependence on the drug.

OVERDOSAGE

Overdosage or oral ingestion of KWELL Lotion can cause central nervous system excitation and, if taken in sufficient quantities, convulsions may occur.

If accidental ingestion occurs, prompt gastric lavage should be instituted. However, since oils favor absorption, saline cathartics for intestinal evacuation should be given rather than oil laxatives. If central nervous system manifestations occur they can be antagonized by the administration of pentobarbital, phenobarbital or diazepam.

DOSAGE AND ADMINISTRATION

CAUTION: USE ONLY AS DIRECTED. DO NOT EXCEED RECOMENDED DOSAGE

No residual effects of KWELL treatment have been demonstrated therefore, this product should not be used to ward off a possible infestation.

NOTE: PLEASE READ CAREFULLY.

DIRECTIONS FOR USE

Scabies (sarcoptes scabiei)—The lotion should be applied to dry skin in a thin layer and rubbed in thoroughly. If crusted lesions are present, a tepid bath preceding the medication is helpful. If a bath is used, allow the skin to dry before applying the lotion. Usually two ounces are sufficient for an adult. A total body application should be made from the neck down including the soles of the feet. Scabies rarely affects the head of children or adults but may occur in infants. The lotion should be left on for 8–12 hours and should then be removed by thorough washing. ONE APPLICATION IS USUALLY CURATIVE.

Sexual contacts should be treated simultaneously.

Avoid unnecessary skin contact. Particularly when applying to more than one patient, those assisting in lindane therapy (especially pregnant and/or nursing women) should wear rubber gloves.

Avoid use on open cuts and extensive excoriations.

Many patients exhibit persistent pruritus after treatment; this is rarely a sign of treatment failure and is not an indication for retreatment unless living mites can be demonstrated.

CAUTION

Federal law prohibits dispensing without prescription.

HOW SUPPLIED

KWELL Lotion in in bottles of 59 ml (2 fl. oz.) and 472 ml (16 fl. oz.) and 3.8 liters (1 gallon).

Continued on next page

Reed & Carnrick—Cont.

REFERENCES
1. Feldmann, R.J. and Maibach, H.I., *Toxicol. Applied. Pharmacol.*, 28:126, 1974.
2. Dale, W.E., Curly, A. and Cueto, C. *Life Sci* 5:47, 1966.
3. Ginsburg, C.M., et al., *J. Pediatr.* 91:6, 998–1000, 1977.
4. Nagasaki, T., Tomii, S., Mepa, T., Marugami, M. and Ito, *N. Gann* (Cancer) 63(3):393, 1972.
5. Goto, M. Hattori, M., Miyagawa, T. and Enomoto, M., *Chemosphere* 6:279, 1972.
6. Hanada, M., Yatani, C., Miyaji, T., *Gann* 64:511, 1973.
7. Weisse, I, and Herbst, M., *Toxicol.* 7:233, 1977.
8. Technical Report Series, NCI-CG-TR-14, *HEW PUBLICATIONS*, No. (NIH) 77–814.
9. Thorpe, E., and Walker, A.I.T., *Food Cosmetic Toxicol.* 11:433, 1973.
10. Orr, J.W., *Nature* 162:189, 1948.
11. Kashyap, S.K. et al., *J. Environ, Sci. Health* 14:305–318, 1979.

MANUFACTURED FOR
REED & CARNRICK
Piscataway, NJ 08854
By Reedco Inc., Humacao, PR 00661

Date of Revision
August 1985

Shown in Product Identification Section, page 423

KWELL® Shampoo ℞
[*kwel*]
(lindane) 1%

DESCRIPTION

KWELL Shampoo (lindane) 1% is an ectoparasiticide and ovicide effective against Pediculosis capitis (head lice), Pediculosis pubis (crab lice) and their ova. In addition to the active ingredient, lindane, it contains Trolamine Lauryl Sulfate, Polysorbate 60, acetone and purified water to form a cosmetically pleasant shampoo. Lindane, which is the highly purified gamma isomer of 1, 2, 3, 4, 5, 6, hexachlorocyclohexane, has the following chemical structure:

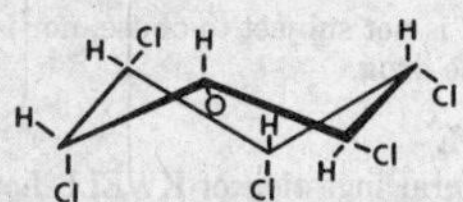

CLINICAL PHARMACOLOGY

KWELL Shampoo exerts its parasiticidal action by being directly absorbed into the parasites and their ova. Dale et al.[1] reported a blood level of 290ng/ml associated with convulsions following the accidental ingestion of a lindane containing product. Analysis of blood taken from subjects before and after the use of KWELL Shampoo showed a mean peak blood level of only 3ng/ml which appeared at six hours and disappeared at eight hours after the shampoo was applied.[2].

INDICATIONS AND USAGE

KWELL Shampoo is indicated for the treatment of patients infested with Pediculus capitis (head lice), Pediculus pubis (crab lice) and their ova.

CONTRAINDICATIONS

KWELL Shampoo is contraindicated for premature neonates because their skin may be more permeable than full term infants and their liver enzymes may not be sufficiently developed. It is also contraindicated for patients with known seizure disorders and for individuals with a known sensitivity to the product or any of its components.

WARNINGS

LINDANE PENETRATES HUMAN SKIN AND HAS THE POTENTIAL FOR CNS TOXICITY (SEE CLINICAL PHARMACOLOGY SECTION). KWELL SHAMPOO SHOULD BE USED ACCORDING TO RECOMMENDED DOSAGE (SEE DIRECTIONS FOR USE) ESPECIALLY ON INFANTS, PREGNANT WOMEN AND NURSING MOTHERS. ANIMAL STUDIES INDICATE THAT POTENTIAL TOXIC EFFECTS OF TOPICALLY APPLIED LINDANE ARE GREATER IN THE YOUNG. Seizures have been reported after excessive use or oral ingestion of lindane. No residual effects of KWELL treatment have been demonstrated, therefore, this product should not be used to ward off a possible infestation.

If accidental ingestion occurs prompt gastric lavage is indicated. Because oils may enhance absorption, saline rather than oily cathartics should be used. Central nervous excitation can be controlled by the administration of pentobarbital, phenobarbital or diazepam.

PRECAUTIONS

General

Care should be taken to avoid contact with the eyes. If such contact occurs, eyes should be immediately flushed with water. If irritation or sensitization occurs, the patient should be advised to consult a physician.

Information to Patients

Patients should be instructed on the proper use of the medication. Directions for use should accompany the prescription.

LABORATORY TESTS

No laboratory tests are needed for the proper use of this medication.

DRUG INTERACTIONS

Oils may enhance absorption, therefore, if an oil-based hair dressing is used, it is recommended that the hair be shampooed, rinsed and dried before application of KWELL Shampoo.

CARCINOGENESIS

Although no studies have been conducted with KWELL Shampoo, numerous long term feeding studies have been conducted in mice and rats to evaluate the carcinogenic potential of the technical grade of hexachlorocyclohexane (BHC) as well as the alpha, beta, gamma (lindane) and delta isomers. Both oral and topical applications have been evaluated. Nagasaki[3], Goto[4] and Hanada[5] found varying amounts of benign and malignant hepatomas associated with BHC and the alpha, delta and epsilon isomers. None reported a carcinogenic potential for lindane. Tumors were found only in the animals which had received the alpha isomer. Weisse and Herbst[6] also evaluated the carcinogenic potential of lindane in mice but could find no evidence of lindane carcinogenicity. The National Cancer Institute[7] had also found no evidence of carcinogenicity.

Thorpe and Walker[8] compared beta BHC with lindane, dieldrin, DDT and hexabarbital in mice. Despite the unusually high incidence of tumors in the control group, they concluded that 600 ppm of lindane was associated with a significant increase in the incidence of hepatoma and thus, considered it a tumorigen.

Orr[9] and Kashyap, et al[10] evaluated the carcinogenic potential in mice of topically applied BHC. In neither study was there any evidence of a tumorigenic or carcinogenic potential associated with topical application of BHC.

Mutagenicity tests have been used as predictive information about the carcinogenicity of various chemical compounds. Numerous types of mutagenicity tests have been performed with lindane. The results of these tests do not indicate that lindane is mutapenic.

PREGNANCY

Teratogenetic Effects

Pregnancy category B: Reproduction, including multigeneration, studies have been performed in mice, rats, rabbits, pigs, and dogs at doses up to 10 times the human dose and have revealed no evidence of impaired fertility or harm to the fetus due to orally administered lindane. There are, however, no adequate and well controlled studies in pregnant women. Because animal reproduction studies are not always predictive of human response, the recommended dosage should not be exceeded on pregnant women. They should be treated no more than twice during a pregnancy.

NURSING MOTHERS

Lindane is secreted in human milk in low concentrations. Studies conducted in the United States as well as Europe and South America found levels of lindane in human milk ranging from 0 to 113 ppb, as the result of ingestion of foods which had been treated with lindane. There appeared to be no difference in concentrations between country and urban dwellers. Although the levels of lindane found in blood after topical application with KWELL Shampoo make it unlikely that amounts of lindane sufficient to cause serious adverse reactions will be excreted in the milk of nursing mothers who have used KWELL Shampoo, if there is any concern, an alternate method of feeding may be used for 2 days.

PEDIATRIC USE

Refer to the Contraindications and Warnings sections.

ADVERSE REACTIONS

Lindane has been reported to cause central nervous stimulation ranging from dizziness to convulsions. Cases of convulsions have been reported in connection with KWELL Shampoo therapy. However, these incidents were almost always associated with accidental oral ingestion or misuse of the product. Eczematous eruptions due to irritation from this product have also been reported. Incidence of these adverse reactions is relatively infrequent, occurring in less than 1 in 100,000 patients.

DRUG ABUSE AND DEPENDENCE

KWELL Shampoo is not subject to abuse nor is there any dependence on the drug.

OVERDOSAGE

Overdosage or oral ingestion of KWELL Shampoo can cause central nervous system excitation and, if taken in sufficient quantities, convulsions may occur.

If accidental ingestion occurs, prompt gastric lavage should be instituted. However, since oils favor absorption, saline cathartics for intestinal evacuation should be given rather than oil laxatives. If central nervous system manifestations occur, they can be antagonized by the administration of pentobarbital, phenobarbital or diazepam.

DOSAGE AND ADMINISTRATION

CAUTION: USE ONLY AS DIRECTED. DO NOT EXCEED RECOMMENDED DOSAGE.

No residual effects of KWELL treatment have been demonstrated, therefore, this product should not be used to ward off a possible infestation.

NOTE: PLEASE READ CAREFULLY

DIRECTIONS FOR USE

Pediculosis capitis (head lice)—1) Apply a sufficient quantity of the shampoo to the dry hair. Approximately 1 oz. (30ml) for short, 1.5 oz. (45 ml) for medium and 2 oz. (60 ml) for long hair. 2) Work thoroughly into the hair and allow to remain in place four minutes. 3) Add small quantities of water until a good lather forms. 4) Rinse thoroughly. Towel briskly. Nits should be removed using a nit comb or tweezers.

Pediculosis pubis (crab lice)—1) Apply a sufficient quantity of the shampoo to the dry hair. 2) Work thoroughly into the hair and allow to remain in place four minutes. 3) Add small quantities of water until a good lather forms. 4) Rinse thoroughly. Towel briskly. Nits should be removed using a nit comb or tweezers.

Retreatment is usually not necessary. Demonstrable living organisms after 7 days indicate that retreatment is necessary.

NOTE

1. If person to be treated uses an oil-based hair dressing, it is recommended that their hair be shampooed and dried before applying KWELL Shampoo.
2. Avoid unnecessary skin contact. Particularly when applying to more than one patient, those assisting in lindane therapy (especially pregnant and/or nursing women) should wear rubber gloves.
3. Avoid use on open cuts and extensive excoriations. Sexual contacts should be treated simultaneously.

CAUTION

Federal law prohibits dispensing without prescription.

HOW SUPPLIED

KWELL Shampoo in bottles of 59 ml (2 fl. oz.) and 472 ml (16 fl. oz.) and 3.8 liters (1 gallon).

REFERENCES
1. Dale, W.E., Curly, A. and Cueto, C. *Life Sci* 5:47, 1966.
2. Data on File at Reed & Carnrick.
3. Nagasaki, T., Tomii, S., Mega, T., Marugami, M. and Ito, N. *Gann* (Cancer) 63(3):373, 1972.
4. Goto, M., Hattori, M., Miyagawa, T. and Enomoto, M., *Chemosphere* 6:279, 1972.
5. Hanada, M., Yatani, C., Miyaji, T., *Gann* 64:511, 1973.
6. Weisse, I. and Herbst, M., *Toxicol.* 7:233, 1977.
7. Technical Report Series, NCI-CG-TR-14, *HEW PUBLICATIONS*, No. (NIH) 77–814.
8. Thorpe, E., and Walker, A.I.T., *Food Cosmetic Toxicol.* 11:433, 1973.
9. Orr, J.W., *Nature* 162:189, 1948.
10. Kashyap, S.K., et al, *J. Environ. Sci. Health* 14:305–318, 1979.

MANUFACTURED FOR
REED & CARNRICK
Piscataway, NJ 08854
By Reedco Inc., Humacao, P.R. 00661

Date of Revision
August 1985

Shown in Product Identification Section, page 423

PHAZYME® OTC
[*fā'zīm*]

DESCRIPTION

A two-phase tablet. Contains specially-activated simethicone, both in the outer layer for release in the stomach and in the inner enteric-coated core for release in the small intestine.

CONTAINS: ACTIVE INGREDIENTS: Specially-activated simethicone, both in the outer layer for release in the stomach and in the inner enteric-coated core for release in the small intestine, a total of 60 mg.

INACTIVE INGREDIENTS: Acacia, Calcium sulfate, Carnauba Wax, Crospovidone, D&C Red No. 7 Lake, FD&C Blue No. 1 Lake, Gelatin, Lactose, Microcrystalline Cellulose, Polyoxyl-40 Stearate, Polyvinyl Acetate Phthalate, Povidone, Pregelatinized Starch, Rice Starch, Sodium Benzoate, Sucrose, Titanium Dioxide.

ACTIONS/CLINICAL PHARMACOLOGY

PHAZYME is the only dual approach to the problem of gastrointestinal gas. Simethicone minimizes gas formation and relieves gas entrapment in both the stomach and lower G.I. tract. This action helps combat pain, due to gastrointestinal gas. Also, for relief of gas distress associated with other functional or organic conditions such as: diverticulitis, spastic colitis, hyperacidity, postcholecystectomy syndrome and chronic cholecystitis.

INDICATIONS AND USAGE

PHAZYME is indicated for the relief of occasional or chronic pain caused by gas entrapped in the stomach or in the lower gastrointestinal tract—resulting from aerophagia, post-operative distention, dyspepsia and food intolerance.

CONTRAINDICATIONS

A known sensitivity to any ingredient.

DOSAGE AND ADMINISTRATION

One or two tablets with each meal and at bedtime, or as directed by a physician.

HOW SUPPLIED

Pink coated two-phase tablet in bottles of 50, 100 and 1,000.

Shown in Product Identification Section, page 423

Revision Date Oct 1985

PHAZYME®–95 Tablets

[fā 'zīm]

DESCRIPTION

CONTAINS: ACTIVE INGREDIENT: Specially-activated simethicone, both in the outer layer for release in the stomach and in the inner enteric-coated core for release in the small intestine, a total of 95 mg.

INACTIVE INGREDIENT: Acacia, Calcium Sulfate, Carnauba Wax, Crospovidone, FD&C Yellow No. 6 Lake, FD&C Red No. 40 Lake, Gelatin, Lactose, Microcrystalline Cellulose, Polyoxyl-40 Stearate, Polyvinyl Acetate Phthalate, Povidone, Pregelatinized Starch, Rice Starch, Sodium Benzoate, Sucrose, Titanium Dioxide.

ACTIONS/CLINICAL PHARMACOLOGY

SEE PHAZYME

INDICATIONS AND USAGE

SEE PHAZYME

DOSAGE AND ADMINISTRATION

One tablet with each meal and at bedtime, or as directed by a physician.

HOW SUPPLIED

Red coated two-phase tablet in 10 pack, bottles of 50, 100 and 500.

Shown in Product Identification Section, page 423

Revision Date Oct 1985

PHAZYME®–125 Capsules

[fā 'zīm]

DESCRIPTION

A red capsule containing the highest dose of simethicone available in a single capsule.

ACTIVE INGREDIENTS: Simethicone.

INACTIVE INGREDIENTS: Soybean oil, gelatin, glycerin, vegetable shortening, polysorbate 80, purified water, hydrogenated soybean oil, yellow wax, lecithin, titanium dioxide, FD&C Red #40, methylparaben, propylparaben.

ACTIONS/CLINICAL PHARMACOLOGY

SEE PHAZYME

INDICATIONS AND USAGE

SEE PHAZYME

DOSAGE AND ADMINISTRATION

One capsule with each meal and at bedtime, or as directed by a physician.

HOW SUPPLIED

Red capsule in bottle of 50.

Shown in Product Identification Section, page 423

Revision Date Oct 1985

PHAZYME®–PB Tablets ℂ ℞

[fā 'zīm]

DESCRIPTION

A yellow coated two-phase tablet. Contains specially activated simethicone both in the outer layer for release in the stomach and in the inner enteric coated core for release in the small intestine, a total of 60 mg. Also in the outer layer for release in the stomach phenobarbital 15 mg (WARNING: MAY BE HABIT FORMING). Inactive ingredients include: lactose, calcium sulfate, sucrose, microcrystalline cellulose, talc, rice starch, acacia, gelatin, D&C Yellow #10 Lake, FD&C Yellow #6 Lake and titanium dioxide, pregelatinized starch, polyvinyl acetate phthalate, povidone, crospovidone, polyoxyl-40 stearate, sodium benzoate, white wax, carnauba wax.

ACTIONS

PHAZYME-PB provides the same advantages of the PHAZYME formula (minimizes gas formation, relieves gas entrapment) and in addition, supplies the calming benefits of phenobarbital to control the emotional component of gastrointestinal gas pain. Also for relief of gas distress associated with other functional or organic conditions such as: diverticulitis, spastic colitis, hyperacidity, post-cholecystectomy syndrome and chronic cholecystitis.

INDICATIONS

PHAZYME-PB is indicated for gas pain associated with anxiety-resulting in aerophagia, post-operative distention, dyspepsia and food intolerance.

CONTRAINDICATIONS

Known sensitivity to barbiturates or any other ingredient.

WARNING

MAY BE HABIT FORMING.

PRECAUTIONS

Excessive use may produce drowsiness.

HOW SUPPLIED

Yellow coated two-phase tablets in bottles of 100.

Shown in Product Identification Section, page 423

PROCTOFOAM®–HC ℞

[prŏc 'tō-fōm]

(hydrocortisone acetate) 1%
(and pramoxine hydrochloride 1%
topical aerosol)

DESCRIPTION

A topical corticosteroid aerosol foam for intrarectal use containing hydrocortisone acetate 1% and pramoxine hydrochloride 1% in a hydrophilic base of: propylene glycol, ethoxylated cetyl and stearyl alcohols, steareth-10, cetyl alcohol, methylparaben, propylparaben, trolamine, purified water and propellants (inert): dichlorodifluoromethane and dichlortetrafluoroethane.

PROTOFOAM®-HC contains a synthetic steroid used as an anti-inflammatory and anti-pruritic agent, and a local anesthetic.

Molecular weight: Hydrocortisone acetate 404.51. Solubility of hydrocortisone acetate in water: 1 mg/100ml.

Chemical name: Pregn-4-ene, 3,20-dione, 21-(acetyloxy)-11, 17-dihydroxy- (11β).

Pramoxine Hydrochloride

$CH_3CH_2CH_2CH_2O$–⬡–$OCH_2CH_2CH_2$–N⬡O·HCl

CLINICAL PHARMACOLOGY

Topical corticosteroids share anti-inflammatory, anti-pruritic and vasoconstrictive actions.

The mechanism of anti-inflammatory activity of the topical corticosteroids is unclear. Various laboratory methods, including vasoconstrictor assays, are used to compare and predict potencies and/or clinical efficacies of the topical corticosteroids. There is some evidence to suggest that a recognizable correlation exists between vasoconstrictor potency and therapeutic efficacy in man.

Pramoxine Hydrochloride: A surface or local anesthetic which is not chemically related to the "caine" types of local anesthetics. Its unique chemical structure is likely to minimize the danger of cross-sensitivity reactions in patients allergic to other local anesthetics.

Pharmacokinetics: The extent of percutaneous absorption of topical corticosteroids is determined by many factors including the vehicle, the integrity of the epidermal barrier, and the use of occlusive dressings.

Topical corticosteroids can be absorbed from normal intact skin. Inflammation and/or other disease processes in the skin increase the percutaneous absorption of topical corticosteroids. Occlusive dressings substantially increase the percutaneous absorption of topical corticosteroids. Thus, occlusive dressings may be a valuable therapeutic adjunct for treatment of resistant dermatoses. (See DOSAGE AND ADMINISTRATION.)

Once absorbed through the skin, topical corticosteroids are handled through pharmacokinetic pathways similar to systemically administered corticosteroids. Corticosteroids are bound to plasma proteins in varying doegrees. Corticosteroids are metabolized primarily in the liver and are then excreted by the kidneys. Some of the topical corticosteroids and their metabolites are also excreted in the bile.

INDICATIONS AND USAGE

Topical corticosteroids are indicated for the relief of the inflammatory and pruritic manifestations of corticosteroid-responsive dermatoses of the anal region.

CONTRAINDICATIONS

Topical corticosteroid products are contraindicated in those patients with a history of hypersensitivity to any of the components of the preparation.

WARNINGS

Do not insert any part of the aerosol container into the anus. Contents of the container are under pressure. Do not burn or puncture the aerosol container. Store at temperatures below 120°F. If there is no evidence of clinical or proctologic improvement within two or three weeks after therapy, or if the patient's condition worsens, discontinue the drug. Keep this and all medicines out of the reach of children.

PRECAUTIONS

General: Systemic absorption of topical corticosteroids has produced reversible hypothalamic-pituitary-adrenal (HPA) axis suppression, manifestations of Cushing's syndrome, hyperglycemia and glucosuria in some patients.

Conditions which augment systemic absorption include the application of the more potent steroids, use over large surface areas, prolonged use and the addition of occlusive dressings.

Therefore, patients receiving a large dose of a potent topical steroid applied to a large surface area or under an occlusive dressing should be evaluated periodically for evidence of HPA axis suppression by using the urinary hydrocortisone and ACTH stimulation tests. If HPA axis suppression is noted, an attempt should be made to withdraw the drug, to reduce the frequency of application, or to substitute a less potent steroid.

Recovery of HPA axis function is generally prompt and complete upon discontinuation of the drug. Infrequently, signs and symptoms of steroid withdrawal may occur, requiring supplemental systemic corticosteroids.

In children absorption may result in higher blood levels and thus more susceptibility to systemic toxicity. (See PRECAUTIONS—Pediatric Use.)

If irritation develops, topical corticosteroids should be discontinued and appropriate therapy instituted.

In the presence of dermatological infections, the use of an appropriate antifungal or antibacterial agent should be instituted. If a favorable response does not occur promptly, the corticosteroid should be discontinued until the infection has been adequately controlled.

Information for the Patient

Patients using topical corticosteroids should receive the following information and instructions.

1. This medication is to be used as directed by the physician. It is for intrarectal or parianual use only. Avoid contact with the eyes.
2. Be advised not to use this medication for any disorder other than for which it has been prescribed.
3. Report any signs of adverse reactions.

Laboratory Tests

The following tests may be helpful in evaluating the HPA axis suppression:

Urinary hydrocortisone test
ACTH stimulation test

Carcinogenesis, Mutagenesis, and Impairment of Fertility

Long-term animal studies have not been performed to evaluate carcinogenic potential or the effect on fertility of topical corticosteroids.

Studies to determine mutagenicity with prednisolone and hydrocortisone have revealed negative results.

Pregnancy Category C

Corticosteroids are generally teratogenic in laboratory animals when administered systemically at relatively low dosage levels. The more potent corticosteroids have been shown to be teratogenic after dermal application in laboratory animals. There are no adequate and well-controlled studies in pregnant women of teratogenic effects from topically applied corticosteroids. Therefore, topical corticosteroids should be used during pregnancy only if the potential benefit justifies the potential risk to the fetus. Drugs of this class should not be used extensively on pregnant patients, in large amounts, or for prolonged periods of time.

Nursing Mothers

It is not known whether topical administration of corticosteroids could result in sufficient systemic absorption to produce detectable quantities in breast milk. Systemically administered corticosteroids are secreted into breast milk in quantities not likely to have a deleterious effect on the infant. Caution should be exercised when any topical corticosteroids are administered to a nursing woman.

Continued on next page

Reed & Carnrick—Cont.

Pediatric Use

Pediatric patients may demonstrate greater susceptibility to topical corticosteroid-induced HPA axis suppression and Cushing's syndrome than mature patients because of a larger skin surface area to body weight ratio.

Hypothalamic-pituitary-adrenal (HPA) axis suppression. Cushing's syndrome and intracranial hypertension have been reported in children receiving topical corticosteroids. Manifestations of adrenal suppression in children include linear growth retardation, delayed weight gain, low plasma cortisone levels and absense of response to ACTH stimulation. Manifestations of intracranial hypertension include bulging fontanelles, headaches and bilateral papilledema. Administration of topical corticosteroids to children should be limited to the least amount compatible with an effective therapeutic regimen. Chronic corticosteroid therapy may interfere with the growth and development of children.

ADVERSE REACTIONS

The following local adverse reactions are reported infrequently with topical corticosteroids, but may occur more frequently with the use of occlusive dressings. These reactions are listed in an approximate decreasing order of occurrence.

Burning	Perioral dermatitis
Itching	Allergic contact dermatitis
Irritation	
Dryness	Maceration of the skin
Folliculitis	Secondary infection
Hypertrichosis	Skin atrophy
Acneiform eruptions	Striae
Hypopigmentation	Miliaria

OVERDOSAGE

Topically applied corticosteroids can be absorbed in sufficient amounts to produce systemic effects. (See PRECAUTIONS.)

DOSAGE AND ADMINISTRATION

(NOTE: SEE INNER PACKAGE FOR FULL DIRECTIONS FOR USE.)

Apply to affected areas 3 or 4 times daily. Use the applicator supplied for rectal application. For perianal use, transfer a small quantity to a tissue and rub in gently.

1. Shake foam container vigorously before use. Hold container upright and insert into opening of the tip of the applicator. Be sure applicator plunger is drawn all the way out. **CONTAINER MUST BE HELD UPRIGHT TO OBTAIN PROPER FLOW OF MEDICATION.**
2. To fill, press down slowly on container cap. Repeat until foam reaches **fill line** in the applicator. CAUTION: The aerosol container should never be inserted directly into the anus.
3. Remove applicator from container. Allow some foam to remain on the applicator tip. Hold applicator by barrel and gently insert tip into the anus. With applicator in place, push plunger in order to expel foam, then withdraw applicator. (Applicator parts should be pulled apart for thorough cleaning with warm water.)

HOW SUPPLIED

PROCTOFOAM®-HC (NDC 0021-0690-10) is supplied in 10 gram aerosol container with a special rectal applicator.

CAUTION

FEDERAL LAW PROHIBITS DISPENSING WITHOUT PRESCRIPTION.

Revised April 1985

Shown in Product Identification Section, page 423

R&C SPRAY® Lice Control Insecticide

DESCRIPTION

Active ingredients: 3-Phenoxy- benzyl d-cis and trans 2,2-dimethyl-3-(2-methylpropenyl)

cyclopropanecarboxylate	0.382%
Other Isomers	0.018%
Petroleum Distillates	4.255%
Inert Ingredients:	95.345%
	100.000%

ACTIONS

R&C SPRAY is specially formulated to kill lice and their nits on inanimate objects.

INDICATIONS

R&C SPRAY is recommended for use only on bedding, mattresses, furniture and other objects infested or possibly infested with lice which cannot be laundered or dry cleaned.

WARNINGS

Contents under pressure. Do not use or store near heat or open flame. Do not puncture or incinerate container. Exposure to temperatures above 130°F may cause bursting.

It is a violation of Federal law to use this product in a manner inconsistent with its labeling.

NOT FOR USE ON HUMANS OR ANIMALS.

CAUTION

Avoid spraying in eyes. Avoid breathing spray mist. Avoid contact with the skin. In case of contact, wash immediately with soap and water. Harmful if swallowed. Vacate room after treatment and ventilate before reoccupying. Avoid contamination of feed and foodstuffs.

Remove pets, birds and cover fish aquariums before spraying.

DIRECTIONS

SHAKE WELL BEFORE AND OCCASIONALLY DURING USE. Spray on an inconspicuous area to test for possible staining or discoloration. Inspect after drying, then proceed to spray entire area to be treated.

Hold container upright with nozzle away from you. Depress valve and spray from a distance of 8 to 10 inches.

Spray each square foot for about three seconds.

For mattresses, furniture, or similar objects (that cannot be laundered or dry cleaned): Spray thoroughly. Do not use article until spray is dry. Repeat treatment as necessary. Do not use in commercial food processing, preparation, storage or serving areas.

STORAGE

Store in a cool area away from heat or open flame.

DISPOSAL

Wrap container and put in trash. Do not incinerate.

HOW SUPPLIED

In 5 oz. and 10 oz. aerosol container.

Reid-Rowell

Corporate Offices and Manufacturing
901 SAWYER ROAD
MARIETTA, GA 30062
Manufacturing
210 MAIN STREET W.
BAUDETTE, MN 56623

BALNEOL®

[*băl 'nē-ŏl*]

Perianal cleansing lotion

(See PDR For Nonprescription Drugs)

CHENIX® ℞

[*kē 'nix*]

Chenodiol Tablets 250 mg

SPECIAL NOTE

Because of the potential hepatotoxicity of chenodiol, poor response rates in some sub-groups of chenodiol-treated patients, and an increased rate of a need for cholecystectomy. In other chenodiol-treated subgroups, chenodiol is not an appropriate treatment for many patients with gallstones. Chenodiol should be reserved for carefully selected patients and treatment must be accompanied by systematic monitoring for liver function alterations. Aspects of patient selection, response rates and risks versus benefits are given in the Insert.

DESCRIPTION

CHENIX® is chenodiol, the nonproprietary name for chenodeoxycholic acid, a naturally occurring human bile acid. It is a bitter-tasting white powder consisting of crystalline and amorphous particles freely soluble in methanol, acetone and acetic acid and practically insoluble in water. Its chemical name is 3α,7α-dihydroxy-5β-cholan-24-oic acid ($C_{24}H_{40}O_4$), it has a molecular weight of 392.58, and its structure is shown below:

COOH
HO OH

Inactive Ingredients: Magnesium stearate, pregelatinized starch, silicon dioxide and sodium starch glycolate. In addition, the tablet film-coating contains carnauba wax, cellulose, cetyl alcohol, dibutyl sebecate, polyethylene glycol and sodium lauryl sulfate.

CLINICAL PHARMACOLOGY

At therapeutic doses, chenodiol suppresses hepatic synthesis of both cholesterol and cholic acid, gradually replacing the latter and its metabolite, deoxycholic acid, in an expanded bile acid pool. These actions contribute to biliary cholesterol desaturation and gradual dissolution of radiolucent cholesterol gallstones in the presence of a gallbladder visualized by oral cholecystography. Chenodiol has no effect on radiopaque (calcified) gallstones or on radiolucent bile pigment stones.

Chenodiol is well absorbed from the small intestine and taken up by the liver, where it is converted to its taurine and glycine conjugates and secreted in bile. Owing to 60% to 80% first-pass hepatic clearance, the body pool of chenodiol resides mainly in the enterohepatic circulation; serum and urinary bile acid levels are not significantly affected during chenodiol therapy.

At steady-state, an amount of chenodiol near the daily dose escapes to the colon and is converted by bacterial action to lithocholic acid. About 80% of the lithocholate is excreted in the feces; the remainder is absorbed and converted in the liver to its poorly absorbed sulfolithocholyl conjugates. During chenodiol therapy there is only a minor increase in biliary lithocholate, while fecal bile acids are increased three- to fourfold.

Chenodiol is unequivocally hepatotoxic in many animal species, including sub-human primates at doses close to the human dose. Although the theoretical cause is the metabolite, lithocholic acid, an established hepatotoxin, and man has an efficient mechanism for sulfating and eliminating this substance, there is some evidence that the demonstrated hepatotoxicity is partly due to chenodiol per se. The hepatotoxicity of lithocholic acid is characterized biochemically and morphologically as cholestatic.

Man has the capacity to form sulfate conjugates of lithocholic acid. Variation in this capacity among individuals has not been well established and a recent published report suggests that patients who develop chenodiol-induced serum aminotransferase elevations are poor sulfators of lithocholic acid (see **WARNINGS** and **ADVERSE REACTIONS**).

General Clinical Results: Both the desaturation of bile and the clinical dissolution of cholesterol gallstones are dose-related. In the National Cooperative Gallstone Study (NCGS) involving 305 patients in each treatment group, placebo and chenodiol dosages of 375 and 750 mg per day were associated with complete stone dissolution in 0.8%, 5.2% and 13.5%, respectively, of enrolled subjects over 24 months of treatment. Uncontrolled clinical trials using higher doses than those used in the NCGS have shown complete dissolution rates of 28 to 38% of enrolled patients receiving body weight doses of from 13 to 16 mg/kg/day for up to 24 months. In a prospective trial using 15 mg/kg/day, 31% enrolled surgical-risk patients treated more than six months (n=86) achieved complete confirmed dissolutions.

Observed stone dissolution rates achieved with chenodiol treatment are higher in subgroups having certain pretreatment characteristics. In the NCGS, patients with small (less than 15 mm in diameter) radiolucent stones, the observed rate of complete dissolution was approximately 20% on 750 mg/day. In the uncontrolled trials using 13 to 16 mg/kg/day doses of chenodiol, the rates of complete dissolution for small radiolucent stones ranged from 42% to 60%. Even higher dissolution rates have been observed in patients with small floatable stones. (See **Floatable versus Nonfloatable Stones,** below.) Some obese patients and occasional normal weight patients fail to achieve bile desaturation even with doses of chenodiol up to 19 mg/kg/day for unknown reasons.

Although dissolution is generally higher with increased dosage of chenodiol, doses that are too low are associated with increased cholecystectomy rates (see **ADVERSE REACTIONS**).

Stones have recurred within five years in about 50% of patients following complete confirmed dissolutions. Although retreatment with chenodiol has proven successful in dissolving some newly formed stones, the indications for and safety of retreatment are not well defined. Serum aminotransferase elevations and diarrhea have been notable in all clinical trials and are dose-related (refer to **ADVERSE REACTIONS** and **WARNINGS** sections for full information).

Floatable versus Nonfloatable Stones: A major finding in clinical trials was a difference between floatable and nonfloatable stones, with respect to both natural history and response to chenodiol. Over the two-year course of the National Cooperative Gallstone Study (NCGS), placebo-treated patients with floatable stones (n=47) had signficantly higher rates of biliary pain and cholecystectomy than patients with nonfloatable stones (n=258) (47% versus 27% and 19% versus 4%, respectively). Chenodiol treatment (750 mg/day) compared to placebo was associated with a significant reduction in both biliary pain and the cholecystectomy rate in the group with floatable stones (27% versus 47% and 1.5% versus 19%, respectively). In an uncontrolled clinical trial using 15 mg/kg/day, 70% of the patients with small (less than 15 mm) floatable stones (n=10) had complete confirmed dissolutions.

In the NCGS in patients with nonfloatable stones, chenodiol produced no reduction in biliary pain and showed a tendency to increase the cholecystectomy rate (8% versus 4%). This finding was more pronounced with doses of chenodiol below 10 mg/kg. The subgroup of patients with nonfloatable stones and a history of biliary pain had the highest rates of cholecystectomy and aminotransferase elevations during chenodiol treatment. Except for the NCGS subgroup with pretreatment biliary pain, dose-related aminotransferase elevations and diarrhea have occurred with equal frequency in patients with floatable or nonfloatable stones. In the uncontrolled clinical trial mentioned above, 27% of the patients with nonfloatable stones (n=59) had complete confirmed dissolutions, including 35% with small (less than 15 mm) (n=40) and only 11% with large, nonfloatable stones (n=19).

Of 916 patients enrolled in NCGS, 17.8% had stones seen in upright films (horizontal X-ray beam) to float in the dye-laden bile during oral cholecystography using iopanoic acid. Other investigators report similar findings. Floatable stones are not detected by ultrasonography in the absence of dye. Chemical analysis has shown floatable stones to be essentially pure cholesterol.

Other Radiographic and Laboratory Features: Radiolucent stones may have rims or centers of opacity representing calcification. Pigment stones and partially calcified radiolucent stones do not respond to chenodiol. Subtle calcification can sometimes be detected in flat film X-rays, if not obvious in the oral cholecystogram. Among nonfloatable stones, cholesterol stones are more apt than pigment stones to be smooth-surfaced, less than 0.6 cm in diameter and to occur in numbers less than 10. As stone size, number and volume increase, the probability of dissolution within 24 months decreases. Hemolytic disorders, chronic alcoholism, biliary cirrhosis and bacterial invasion of the biliary system predispose to pigment gallstone formation. Pigment stones of primary biliary cirrhosis should be suspected in patients with elevated alkaline phosphatase, especially if positive antimitochondrial antibodies are present. The presence of microscopic cholesterol crystals in aspirated gallbladder bile, and demonstration of cholesterol supersaturation by bile lipid analysis, increase the likelihood that the stones are cholesterol stones.

PATIENT SELECTION

Evaluation of Surgical Risk: Surgery offers the advantage of immediate and permanent stone removal, but carries a fairly high risk in some patients. About 5% of cholecystectomized patients have residual symptoms or retained common duct stones. The spectrum of surgical risk varies as a function of age and the presence of disease other than cholelithiasis. Selected tabulation of results from the National Halothane Study (**JAMA, 1966, 197:775–778**) is shown below; the study included 27,600 cholecystectomies.

Mortality per Operation
(Smoothed rates with denominators adjusted to one death)

		Cholecys-tectomy	Cholecystectomy & Common Duct Exploration
Low Risk Patients*			
Women	0–49 yrs	1/1851	1/469
	50–69 yrs	1/357	1/99
Men	0–49 yrs	1/961	1/243
	50–69 yrs	1/185	1/52
High Risk Patients**			
Women	0–49 yrs	1/79	1/21
	50–69 yrs	1/58	1/17
Men	0–49 yrs	1/41	1/11
	50–69 yrs	1/30	1/9

*Includes those with good health or moderate systemic disease, with or without emergency surgery.

**Severe or extreme systemic disease, with or without emergency surgery.

Women in good health, or having only moderate systemic disease, under 49 years of age have the lowest rate (0.054%); men in all categories have a surgical mortality rate twice that of women; common duct exploration quadruples the rates in all categories; the rates rise with each decade of life and increase tenfold or more in all categories with severe or extreme systemic disease.

Relatively young patients requiring treatment might be better treated by surgery than with CHENIX, because treatment with chenodiol, even if successful, is associated with a high rate of recurrence. The long-term consequences of repeated courses of chenodiol in terms of liver toxicity, neoplasia and elevated cholesterol levels are not known.

Watchful waiting has the advantage that no therapy may ever be required. For patients with silent or minimally symptomatic stones, the rate of moderate to severe symptoms or gallstone complications is estimated to be between 2% and 6% per year, leading to a cumulative rate of 7% and 27% in five years. Presumably the rate is higher for patients already having symptoms.

INDICATIONS AND USAGE

CHENIX is indicated for patients with radiolucent stones in well-opacifying gallbladders, in whom elective surgery would be undertaken except for the presence of increased surgical risk due to systemic disease or age. The likelihood of successful disolution is far greater if the stones are floatable or small. For patients with nonfloatable stones, dissolution is less likely and added weight should be given to the risk that more emergent surgery might result from a delay due to unsuccessful treatment. Safety of use beyond 24 months is not established. CHENIX will not dissolve calcified (radiopaque) or radiolucent bile pigment stones.

CONTRAINDICATIONS

Chenodiol is contraindicated in the presence of known hepatocyte dysfunction or bile ductal abnormalities such as intrahepatic cholestasis, primary biliary cirrhosis or sclerosing cholangitis (see **Warnings**); a gallbladder confirmed as nonvisualizing after two consecutive single doses of dye; radiopaque stones; or gallstone complications or compelling reasons for gallbladder surgery including unremitting acute cholecystitis, cholangitis, biliary obstruction, gallstone pancreatitis, or biliary gastrointestinal fistula.

Pregnancy Category X:
Chenodiol may cause fetal harm when administered to a pregnant woman. Serious hepatic, renal and adrenal lesions occurred in fetuses of female Rhesus monkeys given 60 to 90 mg/kg/day (4 to 6 times the maximum recommended human dose, MRHD) from day 21 to day 45 of pregnancy. Hepatic lesions also occurred in neonatal baboons whose mothers had received 18 to 38 mg/kg (1 to 2 times the MRHD), all during pregnancy. Fetal malformations were not observed. Neither fetal liver damage nor fetal abnormalities occurred in reproduction studies in rats and hamsters. No human data are available at this time. Chenodiol is contraindicated in women who are or may become pregnant. If this drug is used during pregnancy, or if the patient becomes pregnant while taking this drug, the patient should be apprised of the potential hazard to the fetus.

WARNINGS

Safe use of chenodiol depends upon selection of patients without preexisting liver disease and upon faithful monitoring of serum aminotransferase levels to detect drug-induced liver toxicity. Aminotransferase elevations over three times the upper limit of normal have required discontinuation of chenodiol in 2% to 3% of patients. Although clinical and biopsy studies have not shown fulminant lesions, the possibility remains that an occasional patient may develop serious hepatic disease.

Three patients with biochemical and histologic pictures of chronic active hepatitis while on chenodiol, 375 mg/day or 750 mg/day, have been reported. The biochemical abnormalities returned spontaneously to normal in two of the patients within 13 to 17 months; and after 17 months' treatment with prednisone in the third. Followup biopsies were not done; and the causal relationship of the drug could not be determined. Another biopsied patient was terminated from therapy because of elevated aminotransferase levels and a liver biopsy was interpreted as showing active drug hepatitis.

One patient with sclerosing cholangitis, biliary cirrhosis and a history of jaundice died during chenodiol treatment for hepatic duct stones. Before treatment, serum aminotransferase and alkaline phosphatase levels were over twice the upper limit of normal; within one month they rose to over 10 times normal. Chenodiol was discontinued at seven weeks when the patient was hospitalized with advanced hepatic failure and E. coli peitonitis; death ensued at the eighth week. A contribution of chenodiol to the fatal outcome could not be ruled out.

Epidemiologic studies suggest that bile acids might contribute to human colon cancer, but direct evidence is lacking. Bile acids, including chenodiol and lithocholic acid, have no carcinogenic potential in animal models, but have been shown to increase the number of tumors when administered with certain known carcinogens. The possibility that chenodiol therapy might contribute to colon cancer in otherwise susceptible individuals cannot be ruled out.

PRECAUTIONS

Information for Patients: Patients should be counseled on the importance of periodic visits for liver function tests and oral cholecystograms (or ultrasonograms) for monitoring stone dissolution; they should be made aware of the symptoms of gallstone complications and be warned to report immediately such symptoms to the physician. Patients should be instructed on ways to facilitate faithful compliance with the dosage regimen throughout the usual long term of therapy, and on temporary dose reduction if episodes of diarrhea occur.

Drug Interactions: Bile acid sequestering agents, such as cholestyramine and colestipol, may interfere with the action of CHENIX by reducing its absorption. Aluminum-based antacids have been shown to absorb bile acids *in vitro* and may be expected to interfere with CHENIX in the same manner as the sequestering agents. Estrogens, oral contraceptives and clofibrate (and perhaps other lipid-lowering drugs) increase biliary cholesterol secretion, and the incidence of cholesterol gallstones hence may counteract the effectiveness of CHENIX.

Carcinogenesis, Mutagenesis, and Impairment of Fertility: A two-year study of chenodiol in rats failed to show a carcinogenic potential at the tested levels of 15 to 60 mg/kg/day (1 to 4 times the maximum recommended human dose, MRHD). It has been reported that chenodiol given in long-term studies at oral doses up to 600 mg/kg/day (40 times the MRHD) to rats and 1000 mg/kg/day (65 times the MRHD) to mice induced benign and malignant liver cell tumors in female rats and cholangiomata in female rats and male mice. Two-year studies of lithocholic acid (a major metabolite of chenodiol) in mice (125 to 250 mg/kg/day) and rats (250 to 500 mg/kg/day) found it not to be carcinogenic. The dietary administration of lithocholic acid to chickens is reported to cause hepatic adenomatous hyperplasia.

Pregnancy Category X: See **CONTRAINDICATIONS.**

Nursing Mothers: It is not known whether chenodiol is excreted in human milk. Because many drugs are excreted in human milk, caution should be exercised when chenodiol is administered to a nursing mother.

Pediatric Use: The safety and effectiveness of chenodiol in children have not been established.

ADVERSE REACTIONS

Hepatobiliary: Dose-related serum aminotransferase (mainly SGPT) elevations, usually not accompanied by rises in alkaline phosphatase or bilirubin, occurred in 30% or more of patients treated with the recommended dose of CHENIX. In most cases, these elevations were minor (1½ to 3 times the upper limit of laboratory normal) and transient, returning to within the normal range within six months despite continued administration of the drug. In 2% to 3% of patients, SGPT levels rose to over three times the upper limit of laboratory normal, recurred on rechallenge with the drug, and required discontinuation of chenodiol treatment. Enzyme levels have returned to normal following withdrawal of chenodiol (see **WARNINGS** section).

Morphologic studies of liver biopsies taken before and after 9 and 24 months' treatment with chenodiol have shown that 63% of the patients prior to chenodiol treatment had evidence of intrahepatic cholestasis. Almost all pretreatment patients had electron microscopic abnormalities. By the ninth month of treatment, reexamination of two-thirds of the patients showed an 89% incidence of the signs of intrahepatic cholestasis. Two of 89 patients at the ninth month had lithocholate-like lesions in the canalicular membrane, although there were no clinical enzyme abnormalities in the face of continued treatment and no change in Type 2 light microscopic parameters.

Increased Cholecystectomy Rates: NCGS patients with a history of biliary pain prior to treatment had higher cholecystectomy rates during the study if assigned to low dosage chenodiol (375 mg/day) than if assigned to either placebo or high dosage chenodiol (750 mg/day). The association with low dosage chenodiol, though not clearly a causal one, suggests that patients unable to take higher doses of chenodiol may be at a greater risk of cholecystectomy.

Gastrointestinal: Dose-related diarrhea has been encountered in 30% to 40% of chenodiol-treated patients and may occur at any time during treatment, but is most commonly encountered when treatment is initiated. Usually, the diarrhea is mild, transient, well-tolerated and does not interfere with therapy. Dose reduction has been required in 10% to 15% of patients, and in a controlled trial about half of these required a permanent reduction in dose. Anti-diarrheal agents have proven useful in some patients. Discontinuation of chenodiol because of failure to control diarrhea is to be expected in approximately 3% of patients treated. Steady epigastric pain with nausea typical of lithiasis (biliary colic) usually is easily distinguishable from the crampy abdominal pain of drug-induced diarrhea.

Other, less frequent, gastrointestinal side effects reported include urgency, cramps, heartburn, constipation, nausea and vomiting, anorexia, epigastric distress, dyspepsia, flatulence and nonspecific abdominal pain.

Serum Lipids: Serum total cholesterol and low-density lipoprotein (LDL) cholesterol may rise 10% or more during administration of chenodiol; no change has been seen in the high-density lipoprotein (HDL) fraction; small decreases in serum triglyceride levels for females have been reported.

Hematologic: Decreases in white cell count, never below 3000, have been noted in a few patients treated with chenodiol; the drug was continued in all patients without incident.

OVERDOSAGE

Accidental or intentional overdoses of chenodiol have not been reported. One patient tolerated 4 gm/day (58 mg/kg/day) for six months without incident.

DOSAGE AND ADMINISTRATION

The recommended dose range for CHENIX is 13 to 16 mg/kg/day in two divided doses, morning and night, starting with 250 mg b.i.d. the first two weeks and increasing by 250 mg/day each week thereafter until the recommended or maximum tolerated dose is reached. If diarrhea occurs during dosage buildup or later in treatment, it usually can be controlled by temporary dosage adjustment until symptoms abate, after which the previous dose usually is tolerated.

Continued on next page

Reid-Rowell—Cont.

Dosage less than 10 mg/kg usually is ineffective and may be associated with increased risk of cholecystectomy, so is not recommended.

Weight/Dosage Guide

Body Weight lb	Body Weight kg	Recommended Tablets /Day	Dose Range mg/kg
100–130	45–58	3	17–13
131–165	59–75	4	17–13
166–200	76–90	5	16–14
201–235	91–107	6	16–14
236–275	108–125	7	16–14

The optimal frequency of monitoring liver function tests is not known. It is suggested that serum aminotransferase levels should be monitored monthly for the first three months and every three months thereafter during CHENIX administration. Under NCGS guidelines, if a minor, usually transient, elevation (1 ½ to 3 times the upper limit of normal) persisted longer than three to six months, chenodiol was discontinued and resumed only after the aminotransferase level returned to normal; however, allowing the elevations to persist over such an interval is not known to be safe. Elevations over three times the upper limit of normal require immediate discontinuation of CHENIX, and usually reoccur on challenge.
Serum cholesterol should be monitored at six-month intervals. It may be advisable to discontinue CHENIX if cholesterol rises above the acceptable age-adjusted limit for a given patient.
Oral cholecystograms or ultrasonograms are recommended at six- to nine-month intervals to monitor response. Complete dissolutions should be confirmed by a repeat test after one to three months'continued CHENIX administration. Most patients who eventually achieve complete dissolution will show partial (or complete) dissolution at the first on-treatment test. If partial dissolution is not seen by nine to 12 months, the likelihood of success of treating longer is greatly reduced; CHENIX should be discontinued if there is no response by 18 months. Safety of use beyond 24 months is not established.
Stone recurrence can be expected within five years in 50% of cases. After confirmed dissolution, treatment generally should be stopped. Serial cholecystograms or ultrasonograms are recommended to monitor for recurrence, keeping in mind that radiolucency and gallbladder function should be established before starting another course of CHENIX. A prophylactic dose is not established; reduced doses cannot be recommended; stones have recurred on 500 mg/day. Low cholesterol or carbohydrate diets, and dietary bran, have been reported to reduce biliary cholesterol; maintenance of reduced weight is recommended to forestall stone recurrence.

CAUTION

Federal law prohibits dispensing without prescription.

HOW SUPPLIED

CHENIX brand chenodiol is available as white, film-coated, 250-mg tablets imprinted "ROWELL 7720" in bottles of 100, NDC 0032-7720.
Shown in Product Identification Section, page 423

COMPAL CAPSULES Ⓒ℞

[*com 'pal*]

DESCRIPTION

Each light aqua and bluish-green capsule contains Dihydrocodeine Bitartrate 16 mg. (Warning: May be habit forming), Acetaminophen 356.4 mg., Caffeine 30 mg.

CLINICAL PHARMACOLOGY

Dihydrocodeine is a semi-synthetic narcotic analgesic related to codeine, with multiple actions qualitatively similar to those of codeine; the most prominent of these involve the central nervous system and organs with smooth muscle components. The principal action of therapeutic value is analgesia.
Compal also contains acetaminophen, a nonopiate, non-salicylate analgesic and antipyretic.

INDICATIONS

For the relief of moderate to moderately severe pain.

CONTRAINDICATIONS

Hypersensitivity to dihydrocodeine, codeine, or acetaminophen.

WARNINGS

Usage in Ambulatory Patients: Dihydrocodeine may impair the mental and/or physical abilities required for the performance of potentially hazardous tasks such as driving a car or operating machinery. The patient using Compal should be cautioned accordingly.
Interactions With Other Central Nervous System Depressants: Patients receiving other narcotic analgesics, general anesthetics, tranquilizers, sedative-hypnotics or other CNS depressants (including alcohol) concomitantly with Compal may exhibit an additive CNS depression. When such combined therapy is contemplated, the dose of one or both agents should be reduced.

PRECAUTIONS

General: Compal should be given with caution to certain patients such as the elderly or debilitated.

DRUG INTERACTIONS

The CNS-depressant effects of dihydrocodeine bitartrate may be additive with that of other CNS depressants. See "Warnings."

USAGE IN PREGNANCY

Reproduction studies have not been performed in animals. There is no adequate information on whether this drug may affect fertility in human males and females or has a teratogenic potential or other adverse effect on the fetus.

USAGE IN CHILDREN

Since there is no experience in children who have received this drug, safety and efficacy in children have not been established.

ADVERSE REACTIONS

The most frequently observed reactions include lightheadedness, dizziness, drowsiness, sedation, nausea, vomiting, constipation, pruritus, and skin reactions.

DRUG ABUSE AND DEPENDENCE

Compal is subject to the provisions of the Controlled Substance Act, and has been placed in Schedule III. Dihydrocodeine can produce drug dependence of the codeine type and therefore has the potential of being abused. Psychic dependence, physical dependence, and tolerance may develop upon repeated administration of dihydrocodeine, and it should be prescribed and administered with the same degree of caution appropriate to the use of other oral narcotic-containing medications.

DOSAGE AND ADMINISTRATION

Dosage should be adjusted according to the severity of the pain and the response of the patient. Compal is given orally. The usual adult dose is two capsules every four (4) hours as needed for pain.

MANAGEMENT OF OVERDOSAGE

Dihydrocodeine:

SIGNS AND SYMPTOMS

Serious overdose with Compal is characterized by respiratory depression (a decrease in respiratory rate and/or tidal volume, Cheyne-Stokes respiration, cyanosis), extreme somnolence progressing to stupor or coma, skeletal muscle flaccidity, cold and clammy skin, and sometimes bradycardia and hypotension. In severe overdosage, apnea, circulatory collapse, cardiac arrest and death may occur.

TREATMENT

Primary attention should be given to the re-establishment of adequate respiratory exchange through provision of a patent airway and the institution of assisted or controlled ventilation. The narcotic antagonist naloxone is a specific antidote against respiratory depression which may result from overdosage or unusual sensitivity to narcotics, including codeine. Therefore, an appropriate dose of naloxone (usual initial adult dose: 0.4 mg.) should be administered, preferably by the intravenous route and simultaneously with efforts at respiratory resuscitation. Since the duration of action of dihydrocodeine may exceed that of the antagonist, the patient should be kept under continued surveillance and repeated doses of the antagonist should be administered as needed to maintain adequate respiration.
An antagonist should not be administered in the absence of clinically significant respiratory or cardiovascular depression.
Oxygen, intravenous fluids, vasopressors and other supportive measures should be employed as indicated.
Gastric emptying may be useful in removing unabsorbed drug.

Acetaminophen:

Signs and Symptoms: Acetaminophen in massive overdosage may cause hepatic toxicity in some patients. In all cases of suspected overdose, immediately call your regional poison center for assistance in diagnosis and for directions in the use of N-acetylcysteine as an antidote. In adults, hepatic toxicity has rarely been reported with acute overdoses of less than 10 grams and fatalities with less than 15 grams. Importantly, young children seem to be more resistant than adults to the hepatotoxic effect of an acetaminophen overdose. Despite this, the measures outlined below should be initiated in any adult or child suspected of having ingested an acetaminophen overdose.
Early symptoms following a potentially hepatotoxic overdose may include: nausea, vomiting, diaphoresis and general malaise. Clincal and laboratory evidence of hepatic toxicity may not be apparent until 48 to 72 hours post-ingestion.

TREATMENT

The stomach should be emptied promptly by lavage or by induction of emesis with syrup of ipecac. Patients' estimates of the quantity of a drug ingested are notoriously unreliable. Therefore, if an acetaminophen overdose is suspected, a serum acetaminophen assay should be obtained as early as possible, but no sooner than four hours following ingestion. Liver function studies should be obtained initially and repeated at 24-hour intervals.
The antidote, N-acetylcysteine, should be administered as early as possible, and within 16 hours of the overdose ingestion for optimal results. Following recovery, there are no residual, structural or functional hepatic abnormalities.

HOW SUPPLIED

Available in light aqua and bluish-green capsules imprinted with REID-PROVIDENT 1290 containing Dihydrocodeine Bitartrate 16 mg. (Warning: May be habit forming). Acetaminophen 356.4 mg., Caffeine 30 mg. Supplied in bottles of 100 capsules (NDC 0063-1290-06).

STORAGE

Store below 25°C (77°F). Dispense in tight, light-resistant containers as defined in the U.S.P. Protect from moisture.
Shown in Product Identification Section, page 423

CORTENEMA® ℞

[*kort "en 'a-ma*]
(Hydrocortisone Retention Enema)
Disposable Unit for Rectal Use Only

Each disposable unit (60 ml.) contains: Hydrocortisone, 100 mg. in an aqueous solution containing carboxypolymethylene, polysorbate 80, and methylparaben, 0.18% as a preservative.

DESCRIPTION

CORTENEMA is a convenient disposable single-dose hydrocortisone enema designed for ease of self-administration. Hydrocortisone is a naturally occurring glucocorticoid (adrenal corticosteroid), which similarly as its acetate and sodium hemisuccinate derivatives, is partially absorbed following rectal administration. Absorption studies in ulcerative colitis patients have shown up to 50% absorption of hydrocortisone administered as CORTENEMA and up to 30% of hydrocortisone acetate administered in an identical vehicle.

ACTIONS

CORTENEMA provides the potent anti-inflammatory effect of hydrocortisone. Because this drug is absorbed from the colon, it acts both topically and systemically. Although rectal hydrocortisone, used as recommended for CORTENEMA, has a low incidence of reported adverse reactions, prolonged use presumably may cause systemic reactions associated with oral dosage forms.

INDICATIONS

CORTENEMA is indicated as adjunctive therapy in the treatment of ulcerative colitis, especially distal forms, including ulcerative proctitis, ulcerative proctosigmoiditis, and left-sided ulcerative colitis. It has proved useful also in some cases involving the transverse and ascending colons.

CONTRAINDICATIONS

Systemic fungal infections; and ileocolostomy during the immediate or early postoperative period.

WARNINGS

In severe ulcerative colitis, it is hazardous to delay needed surgery while awaiting response to medical treatment.
Damage to the rectal wall can result from careless or improper insertion of an enema tip.
In patients on corticosteroid therapy subjected to unusual stress, increased dosage of rapidly acting corticosteroids before, during, and after the stressful situation is indicated.
Corticosteroids may mask some signs of infection, and new infections may appear during their use.
There may be decreased resistance and inability to localize infection when corticosteroids are used.
Prolonged use of corticosteroids may produce posterior subcapsular cataracts, glaucoma with possible damage to the optic nerves, and may enhance the establishment of secondary ocular infections due to fungi or viruses.
Usage in pregnancy: Since adequate human reproduction studies have not been done with corticosteroids, the use of these drugs in pregnancy, nursing mothers or women of childbearing potential requires that the possible benefits of the drug be weighed against the potential hazards to the mother and embryo or fetus. Infants born of mothers who have received substantial doses of corticosteroids during pregnancy, should be carefully observed for signs of hypoadrenalism.
Average and large doses of hydrocortisone or cortisone can cause elevation of blood pressure, salt and water retention, and increased excretion of potassium. These effects are less likely to occur with the synthetic derivatives except when

used in large doses. Dietary salt restriction and potassium supplementation may be necessary. All corticosteroids increase calcium excretion.

While on corticosteroid therapy patients should not be vaccinated against smallpox. Other immunization procedures should not be undertaken in patients who are on corticosteroids, especially on high dose, because of possible hazards of neurological complications and a lack of antibody response. If corticosteroids are indicated in patients with latent tuberculosis or tuberculin reactivity, close observation is necessary as reactivation of the disease may occur. During prolonged corticosteroid therapy, these patients should receive chemoprophylaxis.

PRECAUTIONS

CORTENEMA Hydrocortisone Retention Enema should be used with caution where there is a probability of impending perforation, abscess or other pyogenic infection; fresh intestinal anastomoses; obstruction; or extensive fistulas and sinus tracts. Use with caution in presence of active or latent peptic ulcer; diverticulitis; renal insufficiency; hypertension; osteoporosis; and myasthenia gravis.

Steroid therapy might impair prognosis in surgery by increasing the hazard of infection. If infection is suspected, appropriate antibiotic therapy must be administered, usually in larger than ordinary doses.

Drug-induced secondary adrenocortical insufficiency may occur with prolonged CORTENEMA therapy. This is minimized by gradual reduction of dosage. This type of relative insufficiency may persist for months after discontinuation of therapy; therefore, in any situation of stress occurring during that period, hormone therapy should be reinstituted. Since mineralocorticoid secretion may be impaired, salt and/or a mineralocorticoid should be administered concurrently.

There is an enhanced effect of corticosteroids on patients with hypothyroidism and in those with cirrhosis.

Corticosteroids should be used cautiously in patients with ocular herpes simplex because of possible corneal perforation.

The lowest possible dose of corticosteroid should be used to control the condition under treatment, and when reduction in dosage is possible, the reduction should be gradual.

Psychic derangement may appear when corticosteroids are used, ranging from euphoria, insomnia, mood swings, personality changes, and severe depression, to frank psychotic manifestations. Also, existing emotional instability or psychotic tendencies may be aggravated by corticosteroids. Aspirin should be used cautiously in conjunction with corticosteroids in hypoprothrombinemia.

Growth and development of infants and children on prolonged corticosteroid therapy should be carefully observed.

ADVERSE REACTIONS

Local pain or burning, and rectal bleediing attributed to CORTENEMA have been reported rarely. Apparent exacerbations or sensitivity reactions also occur rarely. The following adverse reactions should be kept in mind whenever corticosteroids are given by rectal administration.

Fluid and Electrolyte Disturbances: Sodium retention; fluid retention; congestive heart failure in susceptible patients; potassium loss; hypokalemic alkalosis; hypertension. Musculoskeletal: Muscle weakness; steroid myopathy; loss of muscle mass; osteoporosis; vertebral compression fractures; aseptic necrosis of femoral and humeral heads; pathologic fracture of long bones. Gastrointestinal: Peptic ulcer with possible perforation and hemorrhage; pancreatitis; abdominal distention; ulcerative esophagitis. Dermatologic: Impaired wound healing, thin fragile skin; petechiae and ecchymoses; facial erythema; increased sweating; may suppress reactions to skin tests. Neurological: Convulsions; increased intracranial pressure with papilledema (pseudo-tumor cerebri) usually after treatment; vertigo; headache. Endocrine: Menstrual irregularities; development of Cushingoid state; suppression of growth in children; secondary adrenocortical and pituitary unresponsiveness, particularly in times of stress, as in trauma, surgery or illness; decreased carbohydrate tolerance; manifestations of latent diabetes mellitus; increased requirements for insulin or oral hypoglycemic agents in diabetics. Ophthalmic: Posterior subcapsular cataracts; increased intraocular pressure; glaucoma; exophthalmos. Metabolic: Negative nitrogen balance due to protein catabolism.

DOSAGE AND ADMINISTRATION

The use of CORTENEMA Hydrocortisone Retention Enema is predicated upon the concomitant use of modern supportive measures such as rational dietary control, sedatives, antidiarrheal agents, antibacterial therapy, blood replacement if necessary, etc.

The usual course of therapy is one CORTENEMA nightly for 21 days, or until the patient comes into remission both clinically and proctologically. Clinical symptoms usually subside promptly within 3 to 5 days. Improvement in the appearance of the mucosa, as seen by sigmoidoscopic examination, may lag somewhat behind clinical improvement. Difficult cases may require as long as 2 or 3 months of CORTENEMA treatment. Where the course of therapy extends beyond 21 days, CORTENEMA should be discontinued gradually by reducing administration to every other night for 2 or 3 weeks.

If clinical or proctologic improvement fail to occur within 2 or 3 weeks after starting CORTENEMA, discontinue its use. Symptomatic improvement, evidenced by decreased diarrhea and bleeding; weight gain; improved appetite; lessened fever; and decrease in leukocytosis, may be misleading and should not be used as the sole criterion in judging efficacy. Sigmoidoscopic examination and X-ray visualization are essential for adequate monitoring of ulcerative colitis. Biopsy is useful for differential diagnosis. Patient instructions for administering CORTENEMA are enclosed in each box of seven units. We recommend that the patient lie on his left side during administraion and for 30 minutes thereafter, so that the fluid will distribute throughout the left colon. Every effort should be made to retain the enema for at least an hour and, preferably, all night. This may be facilitated by prior sedation and/or antidiarrheal medication, especially early in the therapy, when the urge to evacuate is great.

HOW SUPPLIED

CORTENEMA Hydrocortisone 100 mg. Retention Enema is supplied as disposable single-dose bottles with lubricated rectal applicator tips, in boxes of seven × 60 ml. (NDC 0032-1904-82) and boxes of one × 60 ml. (NDC 0032-1904-73).

Shown in Product Identification Section, page 423

CURRETAB® ℞

[kur'e-tab]

Medroxyprogesterone Acetate 10 mg tablets

HOW SUPPLIED

Bottles of 50 (NDC 0063-1007-42).

Shown in Product Identification Section, page 423

ESTRATAB® ℞

[es'trah-tab]

Esterified Estrogens Tablets

0.3 mg., 0.625 mg. 1.25 mg. 2.5 mg.

HOW SUPPLIED

NDC 0063-1014-06 0.3 mg. Bottles of 100
NDC 0063-1022-06 0.625 mg. Bottles of 100
NDC 0063-1022-09 0.625 mg. Bottles of 1000
NDC 0063-1024-06 1.25 mg. Bottles of 100
NDC 0063-1024-09 1.25 mg. Bottles of 1000
NDC 0063-1025-06 2.5 mg. Bottles of 100

Shown in Product Identification Section, page 423

ESTRATEST® ℞

[es'trah-test]

ESTRATEST® H.S. (Half-Strength) ℞

Androgen-Estrogen Therapy

DESCRIPTION

ESTRATEST® Oral Tablets

Each dark green tablet contains:

Esterified Estrogens, U.S.P. .... 1.25 mg
Methyltestosterone, U.S.P. .... 2.5 mg

ESTRATEST® H.S. (Half-Strength) Oral Tablets

Each light green tablet contains:

Esterified Estrogens, U.S.P. .... 0.625 mg
Methyltestosterone, U.S.P. .... 1.25 mg

HOW SUPPLIED

Estratest® NDC 0063-1026-06 bottles of 100
NDC 0063-1026-09 bottles of 1000
Estratest® H.S. NDC 0063-1023-06 bottles of 100

Shown in Product Identification Section, page 423

HISTALET® Syrup ℞
HISTALET® DM Syrup
HISTALET® X Syrup
HISTALET® X Tablets
HISTALET® FORTE Tablets

[hist'ă-let for-tā]

for oral use only

[See table above].

DOSAGE SCHEDULE FOR HISTALET® FAMILY

FORMULA	Per 5 ml: Histalet® Syrup	Histalet® DM Syrup	Histalet® X Syrup	Per tab Histalet® X Tablets
Pseudoephedrine HCl	45 mg	45 mg	45 mg	120 mg
Chlorpheniramine Maleate	3 mg	3 mg		
Dextromethorphan HBr		15 mg		
Guaifenesin			200 mg	400 mg

Histalet® Forte Tablets:

Each tablet contains:

Phenylephrine HCl .... 10 mg.
Phenylpropanolamine HCl .... 50 mg.
Pyrilamine Maleate .... 25 mg.
Chlorpheniramine Maleate .... 4 mg.

DESCRIPTION

Each Histalet Forte tablet contains: Phenylpropanolamine HCl 50 mg, Pyrilamine Maleate 25 mg, Chlorpheniramine Maleate 4 mg and Phenylephrine HCl 10 mg.

CLINICAL PHARMACOLOGY

Phenylpropanolamine Hydrochloride

The drug may directly stimulate adrenergic receptors, but probably indirectly stimulates both alpha (α) and beta (β) adrenergic receptors by releasing norepinephrine from its storage sites. Phenylpropanolamine increases heart rate, force of contraction and cardiac output, and excitability. It acts on alpha receptors in the mucosa of the respiratory tract, producing vasoconstriction which results in shrinkage of swollen mucous membranes, reduction of tissue, hyperemia, edema and nasal congestion, and an increase in nasal airway patency. Phenylpropanolamine causes CNS stimulation and reportedly has an anorexigenic effect.

Phenylephrine Hydrochloride

Phenylephrine acts predominantly by a direct action on alpha (α) adrenergic receptors. In therapeutic doses, the drug has no significant stimulant effect on the beta (β) adrenergic receptors of the heart. Following oral administration, constriction of blood vessels in the nasal mucosa may relieve nasal congestion. In therapeutic doses the drug causes little, if any, central nervous system stimulation.

Chlorpheniramine Maleate

Chlorpheniramine is an antihistamine belonging to the alkylamine class. It possesses anticholinergic and sedative effects. It is considered one of the most effective and least toxic of the histamine antagonists. Chlorpheniramine is an H_1 receptor antagonist. It antagonizes many of the pharmacologic actions of histamine. It prevents released histamine from dilating capillaries and causing edema of the respiratory mucosa. Chlorpheniramine has a duration of action of 4 to 6 hours in clinical studies.

Pyrilamine Maleate

Pyrilamine is an antihistamine belonging to the ethylenediamine class. Pyrilamine is a highly effective H_1 blocker. Pyrilamine is an especially active H_1 blocking drug which possesses local anesthetic activity. Pyrilamine antagonizes most of the smooth muscle stimulating actions of histamine on the H_1 receptors of the gastro-intestinal tract, blood vessels and bronchial muscle. It also antagonizes the actions of histamine that result in increased capillary permeability and the formation of edema. Pyrilamine has a duration of action of 4 to 6 hours in clinical studies.

INDICATIONS AND USAGE

Histalet® Forte is indicated for symptomatic relief in allergic rhinitis, allergic bronchitis, bronchospasm, hay fever, common cold, sinusitis and skin allergies.

CONTRAINDICATIONS

This preparation is contraindicated for individuals sensitive to phenylephrine HCl and antihistamines.

PRECAUTIONS

General Precautions—Administer with caution to patients with hypertension, cardiac or peripheral vascular disease, hyperthyroidism or diabetes. **Information for Patients**—This medication may cause drowsiness. Patients should be advised not to drive a car or operate dangerous machinery while taking this medication.

Usage in Pregnancy: Pregnancy Category C. Animal reproduction studies have not been conducted with Histalet® Forte. It is also not known whether Histalet® Forte can cause fetal harm when administered to a pregnant woman or can affect reproductive capacity. Histalet® Forte should be given to a pregnant woman only if clearly needed.

DESCRIPTION

Each white with greenish dots, scored HISTALET® X Tablet contains: Pseudoephedrine HCl 120 mg, Guaifenesin 400 mg.

Each teaspoonful (5 ml) of HISTALET® X Syrup contains: Pseudoephedrine HCl 45 mg, Guaifenesin 200 mg, Alcohol 15%.

CLINICAL PHARMACOLOGY

Pseudoephedrine, a sympathomimetic amine, acts on alpha-adrenergic receptors in the mucosa of the respiratory tract,

Continued on next page

Reid-Rowell—Cont.

producing vasoconstriction. The medication shrinks swollen nasal mucous membranes, reduces tissue hyperemia, edema, and nasal congestion, and increases nasal airway patency. Also, drainage of sinus secretions is increased and obstructed eustachian ostia may be opened.
Guaifenesin has an expectorant action which increases the output of respiratory tract fluid by reducing adhesiveness and surface tension. The increased flow of less viscid secretions promotes ciliary action, lubricating irritated respiratory tract membranes, and facilitates removal of viscous, inspissated mucus. This changes a dry, unproductive cough to a cough that is more productiive and less frequent.

INDICATIONS

HISTALET® X Tablets and Syrup are indicated for the symptomatic relief of nasal congestion and dry non-productive cough in conditions such as: the common cold, acute bronchitis, allergic asthma, bronchiolitis, croup, emphysema and tracheobronchitis.

CONTRAINDICATIONS

Contraindicated in patients with severe hypertension, severe coronary artery disease and in patients on monoamine oxidase (MAO) inhibitor therapy.
Nursing Mothers: Pseudoephedrine is contraindicated in nursing mothers because of the higher than usual risk for infants from sympathomimetic amines.
Hypersensitivity: This drug is contraindicated in patients with hypersensitivity or idiosyncrasy to its ingredients. Patient idiosyncrasy to adrenergic agents may be manifested by insomnia, dizziness, weakness, tremor or arrhythmias.

WARNINGS

HISTALET® X Tablets and Syrup should be used with considerable caution in patients with increased intraocular pressure (narrow angle glaucoma), symptomatic prostatic hypertrophy, bladder neck obstruction, hypertension, diabetes mellitus, ischemic heart disease, and hyperthyroidism.
Use in Children: As in adults, a sympathomimetic amine can elicit either mild stimulation or mild sedation.
Use in the Elderly (Approximately 60 years or older): The elderly are more likely to exhibit adverse reactions to sympathomimetics. At doses higher than the recommended dose, nervousness, dizziness, or sleeplessness may occur.

PRECAUTIONS

General: DO NOT CRUSH OR CHEW HISTALET® X TABLETS BEFORE INGESTION. As with other sympathomimetic drugs, HISTALET® X Tablets and Syrup should be used with caution in the presence of hypertension, hyperthyroidism, diabetes, heart disease, glaucoma, and prostatic hypertrophy. Tricyclic antidepressants may antagonize the effects of pseudoephedrine.
Drug Interactions: Monoamine oxidase (MAO) inhibitors and beta adrenergic blockers may potentiate the effects of sympathomimetic amines. Sympathomimetic amines may reduce the antihypertensive effects of guanethidine, mecamylamine, methyldopa, reserpine, and veratrum alkaloids.
Drug/Laboratory Test Interactions: Guaifenesin has been shown to produce a color interference with certain clinical laboratory determinations of 5-hydroxyindoleacetic acid (5-HIAA) and vanillylmandelic acid (VMA).
Usage in Pregnancy: Pregnancy Category C. Reproduction studies have not been performed in animals with HISTALET® X Tablets and Syrup. There is no adequate information on whether this drug may affect fertility in males and females or has a teratogenic potential or other adverse effect on the fetus.
Usage in Nursing Mothers: The components of HISTALET® X Tablets and Syrup are excreted in breast milk in small amounts, but the significance of their effect on nursing infants is not known. Because of the potential for serious adverse reactions in nursing infants from maternal ingestion of HISTALET® X Tablets and Syrup, a decision should be made whether to discontinue nursing or to discontinue the drug, taking into account the importance of the drug to the mother.

ADVERSE REACTIONS

Possible adverse reactions include nervousness, insomnia, restlessness, tachycardia, headache, nausea, weakness, dizziness, dry mouth, or urinary retention in patients with prostatic hypertrophy.

DOSAGE AND ADMINISTRATION

Histalet® Syrup, Histalet® DM Syrup and Histalet® X Syrup—ADULTS—2 teaspoonfuls 4 times daily, CHILDREN (6–12)—1 teaspoonful 4 times daily, CHILDREN (2–6)—½ teaspoonful 4 times daily, CHILDREN (under 2)—only as directed by physician.
DO NOT EXCEED 4 DOSES IN 24 HOUR PERIOD
Histalet® X Tablets—ADULTS and Children Over 12—1 tablet every 12 hours, CHILDREN (6–12)—½ tablet every 12 hours. Children (under 6 years)—only as directed by physician. Tablets may be broken in half for ease of administration without affecting release of medication but not crushed or chewed. DO NOT EXCEED RECOMMENDED DOSAGE.
Histalet® Forte Tablets—ADULTS—1 tablet, 2–3 times daily, CHILDREN (6–12)—½ tablet 2–3 times daily. Children (under 6): only as directed by physician.
Do not exceed recommended dosage.

HOW SUPPLIED

Histalet® Syrup NDC 0063-1035-12, pint bottles
Histalet® DM Syrup NDC 0063-1037-12, pint bottles
Histalet® X Syrup NDC 0063-1052-12, pint bottles
Histalet® X Tablets NDC 0063-1050-06, bottles of 100 tablets
Histalet® Forte Tablets NDC 0063-1039-06 bottles of 100 tablets
NDC 0063-1039-07 bottles of 250 tablets. Store at controlled room temperature 15°–30°C (59°–86°F).

Shown in Product Identification Section, page 423

HYDROCIL® INSTANT

[hī'dro-sĭl]

(See PDR For Nonprescription Drugs)

MELFIAT®-105 UNICELLES® Ⓒ℞

[mel'fē-aht 105 ūn'i-sels]
(phendimetrazine tartrate)
105 mg.
Sustained Release Capsules

DESCRIPTION

Chemical name: Phendimetrazine Tartrate (+) 3, 4 Dimethyl-2-phenylmorpholine tartrate. Phendimetrazine Tartrate is a white, odorless powder with a bitter taste. It is soluble in water, methanol and ethanol.

CLINICAL PHARMACOLOGY

Phendimetrazine Tartrate is a sympathomimetic amine with pharmacological activity similar to the prototype drugs of this class used in obesity, the amphetamines. Actions include central nervous system stimulation and elevation of blood pressure. Tachyphylaxis and tolerance have been demonstrated with all drugs of this class in which these phenomena have been looked for.
Drugs of this class used in obesity are commonly known as "anorectics" or "anorexigenics". It has not been established, however, that the action of such drugs in treating obesity is primarily one of appetite suppression. Other central nervous system actions, or metabolic effects, may be involved.
Adult obese subjects instructed in dietary management and treated with anorectic drugs, lose more weight on the average than those treated with placebo and diet, as determined in relatively short-term clinical trials.
The magnitude of increased weight loss of drug-treated patients over placebo-treated patients is only a fraction of a pound a week. The rate of weight loss is greatest in the first weeks of therapy for both drug and placebo subjects and tends to decrease in succeeding weeks. The possible origin of the increased weight loss due to the various drug effects are not established. The amount of weight loss associated with the use of an anorectic drug varies from trial to trial, and the increased weight loss appears to be related in part to variables other than the drug prescribed, such as the physician-investigator, the population treated, and the diet prescribed. Studies do not permit conclusions as to the relative importance of the drug and non-drug factors on weight loss.
The natural history of obesity is measured in years, whereas the studies cited are restricted to a few weeks duration; thus, the total impact of drug-induced weight loss over that of diet alone must be considered clinically limited.

INDICATIONS AND USAGE

MELFIAT®-105 (Phendimetrazine Tartrate) is indicated in the management of exogenous obesity as a short term adjunct (a few weeks) in a regimen of weight reduction based on caloric restriction. The limited usefulness of agents of this class (see CLINICAL PHARMACOLOGY) should be measured against possible risk factors inherent in their use such as those described below.

CONTRAINDICATIONS

Advanced arteriosclerosis, symptomatic cardiovascular disease, moderate to severe hypertension, hyperthyroidism, known hypersensitivity, or idiosyncrasy to the sympathomimetic amines, glaucoma.
Agitated states.
Patients with a history of drug abuse.
Use in patients taking other CNS stimulants including monoamine oxidase inhibitors.

WARNINGS

Tolerance to the anorectic effect usually develops within a few weeks. When this occurs, the recommended dose should not be exceeded in an attempt to increase the effect; rather, the drug should be discontinued.
Use of phendimetrazine within 14 days following the administration of monoamine oxidase inhibitors may result in a hypertensive crisis.
Abrupt cessation of administration following prolonged high dosage, results in extreme fatigue and depression. Because of the effect on the central nervous system, phendimetrazine tartrate may impair the ability of the patient to engage in potentially hazardous activities such as operating machinery or driving a motor vehicle; the patient should be cautioned accordingly.
Usage in Pregnancy: The safety of phendimetrazine tartrate in pregnancy and lactation has not been established. Therefore, Phendimetrazine Tartrate should not be taken by women who are or who may become pregnant, unless, in the opinion of the physician, the potential benefits outweigh the possible hazards.
Usage in Children: Phendimetrazine Tartrate is not recommended for use in children under 12 years of age.

PRECAUTIONS

Caution is to be exercised in prescribing Phendimetrazine Tartrate for patients with even mild hypertension.
Insulin requirements in diabetes mellitus may be altered in association with the use of Phendimetrazine Tartrate and the concomitant dietary regimen. Phendimetrazine Tartrate may decrease the hypotensive effect of guanethidine. The least amount feasible should be prescribed or dispensed at one time in order to minimize the possibility of overdosage.

ADVERSE REACTIONS

Cardiovascular: Palpitation, tachycardia, elevation of blood pressure.
Central Nervous System: Overstimulation, restlessness, dizziness, insomnia, tremor, headache; rarely psychotic episodes at recommended doses, agitation, flushing, sweating, blurring of vision.
Gastrointestinal: Dryness of the mouth, diarrhea, constipation, nausea, stomach pain.
Allergic: Urticaria.
Genitourinary: Changes in libido, urinary frequency, dysuria.

DRUG ABUSE AND DEPENDENCE

Controlled Substance: Phendimetrazine is a Schedule III controlled substance.
Dependence: Phendimetrazine Tartrate is related chemically and pharmacologically to the amphetamines. Amphetamines and related stimulant drugs have been extensively abused, and the possibility of abuse of Phendimetrazine Tartrate should be kept in mind when evaluating the desirability of including a drug as part of a weight reduction program. Abuse of amphetamines and related drugs may be associated with intense psychological dependence and severe social dysfunction. There are reports of patients who have increased the dosage to many times that recommended. Abrupt cessation following prolonged high dosage administration results in extreme fatigue and mental depression; changes are also noted on the sleep EEG. Manifestations of chronic intoxication with anorectic drugs include severe dermatoses, marked insomnia, irritability, hyperactivity, and personality changes. The most severe manifestation of chronic intoxications is psychosis, often clinically indistinguishable from schizophrenia.

OVERDOSAGE

Manifestations of acute overdosage with Phendimetrazine Tartrate include restlessness, tremor, hyperreflexia, rapid respiration, confusion, assaultiveness, hallucinations, panic states.
Fatigue and depression usually follow the central stimulation.
Cardiovascular effects include arrhythmias, hypertension or hypotension and circulatory collapse. Gastrointestinal symptoms include nausea, vomiting, diarrhea, and abdominal cramps. Poisoning may result in convulstions, coma and death. Management of acute Phendimetrazine Tartrate intoxication is largely symptomatic and includes lavage and sedation with a barbiturate. Experience with hemodialysis or peritoneal dialysis is inadequate to permit recommendation in this regard. Acidification of the urine increases Phendimetrazine Tartrate excretion. Intravenous phentolamine (Regitine) has been suggested for possible acute, severe hypertension, if this complicates Phendimetrazine Tartrate overdosage.

DOSAGE AND ADMINISTRATION

Since MELFIAT®-105 (Phendimetrazine Tartrate 105 mg.) is a sustained release dosage form, limit to one sustained release capsule in the morning.
MELFIAT®-105 (Phendimetrazine Tartrate) is not recommended for use in children under 12 years of age.

HOW SUPPLIED

Each orange and clear sustained release capsule contains 105 mg. Phendimetrazine Tartrate in bottles of 100 (NDC 0063-1082-06).

CAUTION

Federal law prohibits dispensing without prescription.

Shown in Product Identification Section, page 423

P-V-TUSSIN® SYRUP ℞

[p-v-tŭs 'in]

P-V-TUSSIN® TABLETS

Antitussive-Antihistamine-Expectorant
Liquid and Tablets

DESCRIPTION

Each teaspoonful (5 ml) of P-V-TUSSIN® Syrup contains: Hydrocodone Bitartrate 2.5 mg (WARNING: May be habit forming), Phenylephrine HCl 5 mg, Pyrilamine Maleate 6 mg, Chlorpheniramine Maleate 2 mg, Phenindamine Tartrate 5 mg, Ammonium Chloride 50 mg; Alcohol 5%
Each Scored P-V-TUSSIN® Tablet contains: Hydrocodone Bitartrate 5 mg (WARNING: May be habit forming), Phenindamine Tartrate 25 mg, Guaifenesin 200 mg.

INDICATIONS AND USAGE

For the symptomatic relief of cough and nasal congestion due to common cold, upper respiratory tract congestion associated with the common cold, influenza, bronchitis and sinusitis.

CONTRAINDICATIONS

P-V-TUSSIN® Syrup and Tablets is contraindicated in patients with a known hypersensitivity to hydrocodone bitartrate, phenylephrine HCl, pyrilamine maleate, chlorpheniramine maleate, phenindamine tartrate, ammonium chloride, or guaifenesin.

WARNING

Hydrocodone should be prescribed and administered with the same degree of caution as all oral medications containing a narcotic analgesic.

PRECAUTIONS

General Precautions—Use with caution in the presence of hypertension, cardiovascular disease, hyperthyroidism, or diabetes.
Information for Patients—Patients should be cautioned against driving a car or engaging in mechanical operations which require alertness, until it is known that they do not respond to the drug by becoming drowsy or dizzy.
Usage in Pregnancy: Pregnancy Category C. Animal reproduction studies have not been conducted with P-V TUSSIN® Syrup or P-V-TUSSIN® Tablets. It is also not known whether P-V TUSSIN® Syrup or P-V TUSSIN® Tablets can cause fetal harm when administered to a pregnant woman or can affect reproductive capacity. P-V TUSSIN® Syrup or P-V TUSSIN® Tablets should be given to a pregnant woman only if clearly needed.
Drug Interactions—Hydrocodone may potentiate the effects of other narcotics, general anesthetics, tranquilizers, sedatives and hypnotics, tricyclic antidepressants, MAO inhibitors, alcohol and other CNS depressants.

ADVERSE REACTIONS

Adverse reactions, when they occur, include sedation, nausea, vomiting and constipation.

DRUG ABUSE AND DEPENDENCE

Controlled Substance—P-V-Tussin® is a schedule III drug.
Dependence—Continued use of hydrocodone may result in true addiction.

DOSAGE AND ADMINISTRATION

P-V-Tussin® Syrup:
Adults, 2 teaspoonfuls every 4 to 6 hours
Children 6 to 12, 1 teaspoonful every 4 to 6 hours
Children 3 to 6, ½ to 1 teaspoonful every 4 to 6 hours.
Children 1 to 3, ½ teaspoonful every 4 to 6 hours.
Dose for children should not be repeated more than 4 times in a 24 hour period.
P-V-Tussin® Tablets:
Adults and children over 12, 1 tablet 4 times daily or as directed by physician. Children 6 to 12, ½ tablet 4 times daily. Should be taken after meals and at bedtime, not less than 4 hours apart. Do not exceed the recommended dosage.

CAUTION

Federal law prohibits dispensing without prescription.

HOW SUPPLIED

P-V-Tussin® Syrup
NDC 0063-1087-12, pint bottles
NDC 0063-1087-13, gallon bottles
P-V-Tussin® Tablets
NDC 0063-1088-06, bottles of 100 tablets
Store at controlled room temperature 15°–30°C (59°–86°F).

Shown in Product Identification Section, page 423

PROCTOCORT™ ℞

[prokt 'o-kort]
(Hydrocortisone Cream USP, 1%)

CAUTION

Federal law prohibits dispensing without prescription.

DESCRIPTION

PROCTOCORT (Hydrocortisone) 1% Cream a topical corticosteroid contains hydrocortisone 1% in a pH-adjusted Cream containing stearyl alcohol, cetyl alcohol, isopropyl palmitate, citric acid anhydrous, polyoxylethylene 40 stearate, dibasic sodium phosphate dried, propylene glycol, water, and benzyl alcohol as a preservative. Hydrocortisone has the chemical name Pregn-4-ene-3,20-dione,11,17,21-trihydroxy-, (11β)-; molecular formula $C_{21}H_{30}O_5$; molecular weight 362.47; Chemical Abstract Service registry number 50-23-7, and has the chemical structure:

CLINICAL PHARMACOLOGY

Topical corticosteroids share anti-inflammatory, antipruritic and vasoconstrictive actions.
The mechanism of anti-inflammatory activity of the topical corticosteroids is unclear. Various laboratory methods, including vasoconstrictor assays, are used to compare and predict potencies and/or clinical efficacies of the topical corticosteroids. There is some evidence to suggest that a recognizable correlation exists between vasoconstrictor potency and therapeutic efficacy in man.
Pharmacokinetics: The extent of percutaneous absorption of topical corticosteroids is determined by many factors including the vehicle, the integrity of the epidermal barrier, and the use of occlusive dressings.
Topical corticosteroids can be absorbed from normal intact skin. Inflammation and/or other disease processes in the skin increase percutaneous absorption. Occlusive dressings substantially increase the percutaneous absorption of topical corticosteroids. Thus, occlusive dressings may be a valuable therapeutic adjunct for treatment of resistant dermatoses (See DOSAGE AND ADMINISTRATION)
Once absorbed through the skin, topical corticosteroids are handled through pharmacokinetic pathways similar to systemically administered corticosteroids. Corticosteroids are bound to plasma proteins in varying degrees. Corticosteroids are metabolized primarily in the liver and are then excreted by the kidneys. Some of the topical corticosteroids and their metabolites are also excreted into the bile.

INDICATION AND USAGE

Topical corticosteroids are indicated for the relief of the inflammatory and pruritic manifestations of corticosteroid-responsive dermatoses.

CONTRAINDICATIONS

Topical corticosteroids are contraindicated in those patients with a history of hypersensitivity to any of the components of the preparation.

PRECAUTIONS

General: Systemic absorption of topical corticosteroids has produced reversible hypothalamic pituitary-adrenal (HPA) axis suppression, manifestations of Cushing's syndrome, hyperglycemia, and glucosuria in some patients.
Conditions which augment systemic absorption include the application of the more potent steroids, use over large surface areas, prolonged use, and the addition of occlusive dressings.
Therefore, patients receiving a large dose of a potent topical steroid applied to a large surface area or under an occlusive dressing should be evaluated periodically for evidence of HPA axis suppression by using the urinary-free cortisol and ACTH stimulation tests. If HPA axis suppression is noted, an attempt should be made to withdraw the drug, to reduce the frequency of application, or to substitute a less potent steroid.
Recovery of HPA axis function is generally prompt and complete upon discontinuation of the drug. Infrequently, signs and symptoms of steroid withdrawal may occur, requiring supplemental systemic corticosteroids.
Children may absorb proportionally larger amounts of topical corticosteroids and thus be more susceptible to systemic toxicity (see PRECAUTIONS—Pediatric Use).
If irritation develops, topical corticosteroids should be discontinued and appropriate therapy instituted. In the presence of dermatological infections, the use of an appropriate antifungal or antibacterial agent should be instituted. If a favorable response does not occur promptly, the corticosteroid should be discontinued until the infection has been adequately controlled.
Information for the Patient: Patients using topical corticosteroids should receive the following information and instructions:

1. This medication is to be used as directed by the physician. It is for external use only. Avoid contact with the eyes.
2. Patients should be advised not to use this medication for any disorder other than for which it was prescribed.
3. The treated skin area should not be bandaged or otherwise covered or wrapped as to be occlusive unless directed by the physician.
4. Patients should report any signs of local adverse reactions especially under occlusive dressing.
5. Parents of pediatric patients should be advised not to use tight-fitting diapers or plastic pants on a child being treated in the diaper area, as these garments may constitute occlusive dressings.

Laboratory Tests: The following tests may be helpful in evaluating the HPA axis suppression:
Urinary-free cortisol test—ACTH stimulation test
Carcinogenesis, Mutagenesis, and Impairment of Fertility: Long-term animal studies have not been performed to evaluate the carcinogenic potential or the effect on fertility of topical corticosteroids. Studies to determine mutagenicity with prednisolone and hydrocortisone have revealed negative results.
Pregnancy Category C: Corticosteroids are generally teratogenic in laboratory animals when administered systemically at relatively low dosage levels. The more potent corticosteroids have been shown to be teratogenic after dermal application in laboratory animals. There are no adequate and well-controlled studies in pregnant women on teratogenic effects from topically applied corticosteroids.
Therefore, topical corticosteroids should be used during pregnancy only if the potential benefit justifies the potential risk to the fetus. Drugs of this class should not be used extensively on pregnant patients, in large amounts, or for prolonged periods of time.
Nursing Mothers: It is not known whether topical administration of corticosteroids could result in sufficient systemic absorption to produce detectable quantities in breast milk. Systemically administered corticosteroids are secreted into breast milk in quantities not likely to have a deleterious effect on the infant. Nevertheless, caution should be exercised when topical corticosteroids are administered to a nursing woman.
Pediatric Use: *Pediatric patients may demonstrate greater susceptibility to topical corticosteroid-induced HPA axis suppression and Cushing's syndrome than mature patients because of a larger skin surface area to body weight ratio.*
Hypothalamic-pituitary-adrenal (HPA) axis suppression, Cushing's syndrome, and intracranial hypertension have been reported in children receiving topical corticosteroids. Manifestations of adrenal suppression in children include linear growth retardation, delayed weight gain, low plasma cortisol levels, and absence of response to ACTH stimulation. Manifestations of intracranial hypertension include bulging fontanelles, headaches, and bilateral papilledema.
Administration of topical corticosteroids to children should be limited to the least amount compatible with an effective therapeutic regimen. Chronic corticosteroid therapy may interfere with the growth and development of children.

ADVERSE REACTIONS

The following local adverse reactions are reported infrequently with topical corticosteroids, but may occur more frequently with the use of occlusive dressings. These reactions are listed in an approximate decreasing order of occurrence:
Burning, Itching, Irritation, Dryness, Folliculitis, Hypertrichosis, Acneiform eruptions, Hypopigmentation, Perioral dermatitis, Allergic contact dermatitis, Maceration of the skin, Secondary infection, Skin atrophy, Striae & Millaria.

OVERDOSAGE

Topically applied corticosteroids can be absorbed in sufficient amounts to produce systemic effects (see PRECAUTIONS).

DOSAGE AND ADMINISTRATION

Topical corticosteroids are generally applied to the affected area as a thin film from three to four times daily depending on the severity of the condition.
Occlusive dressings may be used for the management of psoriasis or recalcitrant conditions. If an infection develops, the use of occlusive dressings should be discontinued and appropriate antimicrobial therapy instituted.

HOW SUPPLIED

PROCTOCORT (Hydrocortisone) 1% Cream is supplied in 30 Gram tubes with tear-off label. A reusable measured dose applicator and 12 finger cots are included with each tube. (NDC 0032-1920-61).
Store at room temperature. Avoid freezing.

Shown in Product Identification Section, page 423

Continued on next page

Reid-Rowell—Cont.

ZENATE® PRENATAL TABLETS ℞
[*zē'nāt*]
Film Coated

CLINICAL ADVANTAGES
Each tablet contains iron that is specifically formulated to minimize gastric irritation.
[See table below].

INDICATIONS AND USES
Vitamin-mineral dietary adjunct in nutritional stress associated with pregnancy and lactation.
Zenate® is a phosphorous free[1] vitamin-mineral dietary supplement, specifically formulated for use during pregnancy and lactation. All ingredients covered by a warning or caution for usage in pregnancy have been formulated so as not to exceed maximum recommended strengths. The formulation includes essential vitamins and minerals, including 300 mg. of elemental calcium, 65 mg. of elemental iron and 20 mg. of elemental zinc. Zenate® also offers 1 mg. of folic acid to aid in the prevention of megaloblastic anemia.

PRECAUTIONS
Folic Acid in doses above 0.1 mg. daily may obscure pernicious anemia in that hematologic remission can occur while neurological manifestations remain progressive. Periodic laboratory studies are considered essential and are recommended. Allergic sensitization has been reported following both oral and parenteral administration of Folic Acid.

DOSAGE AND ADMINISTRATION
As a dietary adjunct in nutritional stress associated with pregnancy and lactation. One tablet daily before the first meal, or as directed by physician.

HOW SUPPLIED
Bottles of 100 baby blue film coated tablets.
NDC 0063-1146-06.

CAUTION
Federal Law Prohibits Dispensing Without Prescription.
Reference: 1. Pitkin, R.M.: Vitamins and Minerals in Pregnancy. *Clinics in Perinatology,* 2:221–232, 1975.
Shown in Product Identification Section, page 423

Research Industries Corporation
Pharmaceutical Division
1847 WEST 2300 SOUTH
SALT LAKE CITY, UTAH 84119

RIMSO®-50 ℞
(brand of dimethyl sulfoxide)

DESCRIPTION
RIMSO®-50, brand of dimethyl sulfoxide ((DMSO)
50% w/w Aqueous Solution for intravesical instillation.
Each ml contains 0.54 gm dimethyl sulfoxide STERILE AND PYROGEN-FREE.
Intravesical instillation for the treatment of interstitial cystitis.
NOT FOR I.M. OR I.V. INJECTION

CAUTION
Federal law prohibits dispensing without a prescription.
The active component of RIMSO®-50 is dimethyl sulfoxide which has the empirical formula C_2H_6OS.
Dimethyl sulfoxide is a clear, colorless and essentially odorless liquid which is miscible with water and most organic solvents. Other physical characteristics include: molecular weight 78.13, melting point 18.4°C, and a specific gravity of 1.1014.

CLINICAL PHARMACOLOGY
Dimethyl sulfoxide is metabolized in man by oxidation to dimethyl sulfone or by reduction to dimethyl sulfide. Dimethyl sulfoxide and dimethyl sulfone are excreted in the urine and feces. Dimethyl sulfide is eliminated through the breath and skin and is responsible for the characteristic odor from patients on dimethyl sulfoxide medication. Dimethyl sulfone can persist in serum for longer than two weeks after a single intravesical instillation. No residual accumulation of dimethyl sulfoxide has occurred in man or lower animals who have received treatment for protracted periods of time. Following topical application, dimethyl sulfoxide is absorbed and generally distributed in the tissues and body fluids.

INDICATIONS AND USAGE
RIMSO®-50 (dimethyl sulfoxide) is indicated for the symptomatic relief of patients with interstitial cystitis. RIMSO®-50 has not been approved as being safe and effective for any other indication. There is no clinical evidence of effectiveness of dimethyl sulfoxide in the treatment of bacterial infections of the urinary tract.

CONTRAINDICATIONS
None known.

WARNINGS
Dimethyl sulfoxide can initiate the liberation of histamine and there has been an occasional hypersensitivity reaction with topical administration of dimethyl sulfoxide. This hypersensitivity has been reported in one patient receiving intravesical RIMSO®-50. The physician should be cognizant of this possibility in prescribing RIMSO®-50. If anaphylactoid symtoms develop, appropriate therapy should be instituted.

PRECAUTIONS
Changes in the refractive index and lens opacities have been seen in monkeys, dogs and rabbits given high doses of dimethyl sulfoxide chronically. Since lens changes were noted in animals, full eye evaluations, including slit lamp examinations are recommended prior to and periodically during treatment.
Approximately every six months patients receiving dimethyl sulfoxide should have a biochemical screening, particularly liver and renal function tests, and complete blood count. Intravesical instillation of RIMSO®-50 may be harmful to patients with urinary tract malignancy because of dimethyl sulfoxide-induced vasodilation.
Some data indicate that dimethyl sulfoxide potentiates other concomitantly administered medications.
Pregnancy Category C. Dimethyl sulfoxide caused teratogenic responses in hamsters, rats and mice when administered intraperitoneally at high doses (2.5–12 gm/kg). Oral or topical doses of dimethyl sulfoxide did not cause problems of reproduction in rats, mice and hamsters. Topical doses (5 gm/kg first two days, then 2.5 gm/kg-last eight days) produced terata in rabbits, but in another study, topical doses of 1.1 gm/kg days 3 through 16 of gestation failed to produce any abnormalities. There are no adequate and well controlled studies in pregnant women. Dimethyl sulfoxide should be used during pregnancy only if the potential benefit justifies the potential risk to the fetus. It is not known whether this drug is excreted in human milk. Because many drugs are excreted in human milk, caution should be exercised when dimethyl sulfoxide is administered to a nursing woman.
Safety and effectiveness in children have not been established.
Information available to be given to the patient is reprinted at the end of this text.

ADVERSE REACTIONS
A garlic-like taste may be noted by the patient within a few minutes after instillation of RIMSO®-50 (dimethyl sulfoxide). This taste may last several hours and because of the presence of metabolites an odor on the breath and skin may remain for 72 hours.
Transient chemical cystitis has been noted following instillation of dimethyl sulfoxide.
The patient may experience moderately severe discomfort on administration. Usually this becomes less prominent with repeated administration.

DRUG ABUSE AND DEPENDENCE
None known.

OVERDOSAGE
The oral LD_{50} of dimethyl sulfoxide in the dog is greater than 10 gm/kg. It is improbable that this dosage level could be obtained with intravesical instillation of RIMSO®-50 in the patient.
In case of accidental oral ingestion, specific measures should be taken to induce emesis. Additional measures which may be considered are gastric lavage, activated charcoal and forced diuresis.

DOSAGE AND ADMINISTRATION
Instillation of 50 ml of RIMSO®-50 (dimethyl sulfoxide) directly into the bladder may be accomplished by catheter or asepto syringe and allowed to remain for 15 minutes. Application of an analgesic lubricant gel such as lidocaine jelly to the urethra is suggested prior to insertion of the catheter to avoid spasm. The medication is expelled by spontaneous voiding. It is recommended that the treatment be repeated every two weeks until maximum symptomatic relief is obtained. Thereafter, time intervals between therapy may be increased appropriately.
Administration of oral analgesic medication or suppositories containing belladonna and opium prior to the instillation of RIMSO®-50 can reduce bladder spasm.
In patients with severe interstitial cystitis with very sensitive bladders, the initial treatment, and possibly the second and third (depending on patient response) should be done under anesthesia. (Saddle block has been suggested).

HOW SUPPLIED
Bottles contain 50 ml of sterile and pyrogen-free RIMSO®-50 (50% w/w dimethyl sulfoxide aqueous solution).
Dimethyl sulfoxide is clear and colorless
Protect from strong light
Store at room temperature (59° to 86°F) (15° to 30°C)
Do not autoclave
NDC #0433-0433-05
For additional information concerning RIMSO®-50, contact the Pharmaceutical Division, Research Industries Corporation. Salt Lake City, Utah
RIMSO®-50 is manufactured by Tera Pharmaceuticals, Inc., Buena Park, California, for the Pharmaceutical Division, Research Industries Corp., Salt Lake City, Utah.

Richardson-Vicks Inc.
Health Care Products Division
TEN WESTPORT ROAD
WILTON, CT 06897

CHILDREN'S CHLORASEPTIC® LOZENGES

ACTIVE INGREDIENTS
Benzocaine 5 mg per lozenge in a grape flavored base.

INACTIVE INGREDIENTS
Color, corn syrup, glycerine, sucrose and water.

INDICATIONS
Children's Chloraseptic Lozenges provide prompt, temporary relief of minor sore throat pain which may accompany conditions such as tonsillitis, pharyngitis and in posttonsillectomy soreness, and discomfort of minor mouth and gum irritations.

DOSAGE AND ADMINISTRATION
Allow one lozenge to dissolve slowly in the mouth. Repeat hourly if needed. Do not take more than 12 lozenges per day.
In addition, consumer labeling carries the following statement:
Warning: Consult physician promptly if sore throat is severe or lasts more than 2 days or is accompanied by high fever, headache, nausea, or vomiting. Do not administer to children under 3 years unless directed by physician or dentist. Discontinue use and consult a physician if irritation persists or increases or a rash appears on the skin.

ZENATE®

Each tablet contains:	ZENATE®	% U.S. RDA Pregnant or Lactating Women
VITAMINS:		
A (as palmitate)	5,000I.U.	62.5
D (as calciferol)	400I.U.	100
E (as dl-alpha tocopheryl acetate)	30I.U.	100
C (ascorbic acid)	80mg.	133
Folic Acid	1mg.	125
Thiamine (as thiamine mononitrate Vitamin B_1)	3mg.	176
Riboflavin (Vitamin B_2)	3mg.	150
Niacin (as niacinamide)	20mg.	100
B_6 (as pyridoxine hydrochloride)	10mg.	400
B_{12} (cyanocobalamin)	12mcg.	150
MINERALS:		
Calcium (from 833mg. calcium carbonate)	300mg.	23
Iodine (from 230mcg. potassium iodide)	175mcg.	117
Iron (from 198mg. ferrous fumarate)	65mg.	361
Magnesium (from 173mg. magnesium oxide)	100mg.	22
Zinc (from 25mg. zinc oxide)	20mg.	133

STORE BELOW 86°F (30°C). PROTECT FROM MOISTURE. KEEP ALL MEDICINES OUT OF REACH OF CHILDREN.

HOW SUPPLIED

Cartons of 18.

CHLORASEPTIC® LIQUID
(oral anesthetic, antiseptic)

ACTIVE INGREDIENTS

Phenol and sodium phenolate (total phenol 1.4%).

INACTIVE INGREDIENTS

Color, flavor, glycerine, saccharin sodium and water.

INDICATIONS

Chloraseptic provides fast, temporary relief of occasional minor sore throat pain and irritations, and discomfort of minor mouth and gum irritations. It is also an effective deodorizing mouthwash for maintaining oral hygiene.

Chloraseptic's anesthetic and antiseptic formula is a valuable adjunct to systemic antibacterial therapy for prompt, temporary relief of minor oral pain and discomfort.

Chloraseptic is indicated for prompt, temporary relief of discomfort due to the following conditions: *Medical:* oropharyngitis and throat infections; acute tonsilitis; and posttonsillectomy soreness; *Dental:* minor irritations or injury of soft tissue of the mouth; minor oral surgery or extractions; irritation caused by dentures or orthodontic appliances; and aphthous ulcers.

ADMINISTRATION AND DOSAGE

Chloraseptic Spray (Pump), Mouthwash and Gargle—*Irritated throat:* Spray 5 times (children 3–12 years of age, 3 times) and swallow. May be used as a gargle. Repeat every 2 hours if necessary. *After oral surgery:* Allow full-strength solution to run over affected areas for 15 seconds without swishing, then expel remainder. Repeat every 2 hours if necessary. *Adjunctive gingival therapy:* Rinse vigorously with full-strength solution for 15 seconds, working between teeth, then expel remainder. Repeat every 2 hours if necessary. *Daily deodorizing mouthwash and gargle:* Dilute with equal parts of water and rinse thoroughly, or spray full strength, then expel remainder.

Chloraseptic Aerosol Spray: *Irritated throat:* Spray throat about 2 seconds (children 3-12 years about 1 second) and swallow. Repeat every 2 hours if necessary. *After oral surgery:* Spray affected area for 1 to 2 seconds, allow solution to remain for 15 seconds without swishing, then expel remainder. Repeat every 2 hours if necessary. *Adjunctive gingival therapy:* Spray affected area for about 2 seconds, swish for 15 seconds working between teeth, then expel remainder. Repeat every 2 hours if necessary. *Daily deodorizing spray:* Spray, rinse thoroughly, and expel remainder.

Consumer labeling contains the following caution statement:

CAUTION

Severe or persistent sore throat or sore throat accompanied by high fever, headache, nausea or vomiting may be serious. Consult your physician. If sore throat persists more than 2 days consult physician. Do not administer to children under 3 years unless directed by physician or dentist.

WARNING

For 1.5 oz. Aerosol Spray—Avoid spraying in eyes. Contents under pressure. Do not puncture or incinerate. (Do not burn or throw in fire, as can will burst). Do not store at temperature above 120°F. (Such high temperatures may cause bursting.) **KEEP ALL MEDICINES OUT OF REACH OF CHILDREN.** To insure product quality, avoid excessive heat (over 104°F or 40°C). See bottom of can for expiration date and control number.

HOW SUPPLIED

Available in Menthol and Cherry flavor in 6 fl. oz bottles with sprayer, 12 fl. oz refill bottles and 1.5 oz nitrogen propelled aerosol sprays.

CHLORASEPTIC® LOZENGES

ACTIVE INGREDIENTS

Phenol and Sodium Phenolate (total phenol 32.5 mg/Lozenge).

INACTIVE INGREDIENTS

Color, corn syrup, flavor, sucrose, water.

INDICATIONS

Chloraseptic Lozenges provide temporary relief of discomfort due to minor sore throat and mouth and gum irritations. They also may be used for topical anesthesia as an adjunct to systemic antibacterial therapy. For prompt temporary relief of pain and discomfort associated with the following conditions: *Medical*—oropharyngitis and throat infections; acute tonsillitis; and posttonsillectomy soreness; *Dental*—minor irritation or injury of soft tissue of the mouth; minor oral surgery; and aphthous ulcers.

ADMINISTRATION AND DOSAGE

Adults and children over 3 years of age: Dissolve 1 lozenge in the mouth every 2 hours. Children under 12 years, do not exceed 8 lozenges per day.

Consumer labeling contains the following caution statement:

WARNING

Consult physician if sore throat is severe or lasts more than 2 days or is accompanied by high fever, headache, nausea or vomiting. Not for children under 3 unless directed by physician or dentist. In case of accidental overdose, seek professional assistance or contact a poison control center immediately.

KEEP ALL MEDICINES OUT OF REACH OF CHILDREN.

Avoid excessive heat (over 104°F or 40°C).

HOW SUPPLIED

Available in menthol or cherry flavor. In packages of 18 and 36.

CREMACOAT™ 1
[*krĕm 'a kōte*]
Throat Coating Cough Medicine

(See PDR For Nonprescription Drugs)

CREMACOAT™ 2
[*krĕm "ă 'kōte*]
Throat Coating Cough Medicine

(See PDR For Nonprescription Drugs)

CREMACOAT™ 3
[*krĕm 'a kōte*]
Throat Coating Cough Medicine

(See PDR For Nonprescription Drugs)

CREMACOAT™ 4
[*krĕm ' a kōte*]
Throat Coating Cough Medicine

(See PDR For Nonprescription Drugs)

DRAMAMINE® Liquid
[*dram 'uh-meen*]
(dimenhydrinate syrup USP)
DRAMAMINE® Tablets

DESCRIPTION

Dimenhydrinate, an antinauseant/antiemetic, is the 8-chlorotheophylline (8-chloro-3,7-dihydro-1,3-dimethyl-1H-purine-2,6-dione) salt of diphenhydramine (2-diphenylmethoxy-N,N-dimethylethanamine). The structural formula of dimenhydrinate is

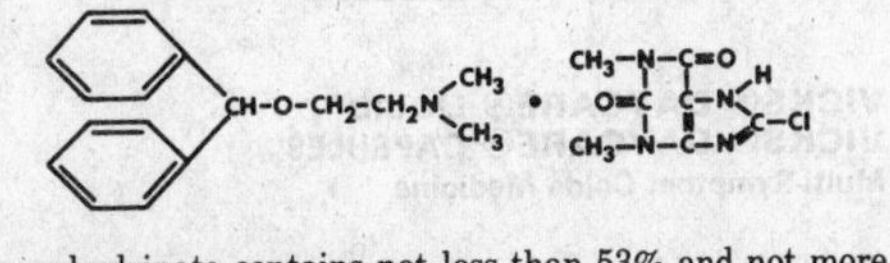

Dimenhydrinate contains not less than 53% and not more than 56% of diphenhydramine, and not less than 44% and not more than 47% of 8-chlorotheophylline, calculated on the dried basis.

CLINICAL PHARMACOLOGY

While the precise mode of action of dimenhydrinate is not known, it has a depressant action on hyperstimulated labyrinthine function.

INDICATIONS AND USAGE

Dramamine is indicated for the prevention and treatment of the nausea, vomiting, or vertigo of motion sickness.

CONTRAINDICATIONS

WARNINGS

Caution should be used when Dramamine is taken in conjunction with certain antibiotics that may cause ototoxicity, since Dramamine is capable of masking ototoxic symptoms and an irreversible state may be reached. As with any drug, pregnant or nursing women should seek the advice of a health professional before using this product.

This drug may impair the mental and/or physical abilities required for the performance of potentially hazardous tasks, such as driving a vehicle or operating machinery. The concomitant use of alcohol or other central nervous system depressants may have an additive effect. Therefore, patients should be warned accordingly.

Dimenhydrinate should be used with caution in patients having conditions which might be aggravated by anticholinergic therapy (ie, prostatic hypertrophy, stenosing peptic ulcer, pyloroduodenal obstruction, bladder neck obstruction, narrow-angle glaucoma, bronchial asthma, or cardiac arrhythmias).

USAGE IN CHILDREN

For infants and children especially, antihistamines in overdosage may cause hallucinations, convulsions, or death.

As in adults, antihistamines may diminish mental alertness in children. In the young child, particularly, they may produce excitation.

PRECAUTIONS

General: Drowsiness may be experienced by some patients, especially with high dosage. This condition frequently is not undesirable in conditions for which the drug is used.

Information for Patients: Because of the potential for drowsiness, patients taking Dramamine should be cautioned against operating automobiles or dangerous machinery. See *Warnings.*

Carcinogenesis, mutagenesis, impairment of fertility: Mutagenicity screening tests performed with dimenhydrinate, diphenhydramine, and 8-chlorotheophylline produced positive results in the bacterial systems and negative results in the mammalian systems. There are no human data that indicate Dramamine is a carcinogen or mutagen or that it impairs fertility.

Pregnancy: Pregnancy Category B. Reproduction studies have been performed in rats at doses up to 20 times the human dose, and in rabbits at doses up to 25 times the human dose (on an mg/kg basis), and have revealed no evidence of impaired fertility or harm to the fetus due to Dramamine. There are no adequate and well-controlled studies in pregnant women. However, clinical studies in pregnant women have not indicated that Dramamine increases the risk of abnormalities when administered in any trimester of pregnancy. It would appear that the possibility of fetal harm is remote when the drug is used during pregnancy. Nevertheless, because the studies in humans cannot rule out the possibility of harm, Dramamine should be used during pregnancy only if clearly needed.

Nursing mothers: Small amounts of dimehydrinate are excreted in breast milk. Because of the potential for adverse reactions in nursing infants from dimenhydrinate, a decision should be made whether to discontinue nursing or to discontinue the drug, taking into account the importance of the drug to the mother.

ADVERSE REACTIONS

The most frequent adverse reaction to Dramamine (dimenhydrinate) is drowsiness. Dizziness may also occur. Symptoms of dry mouth, nose and throat, blurred vision, difficult or painful urination, headache, anorexia, nervousness, restlessness or insomnia (especially in children), skin rash, thickening of bronchial secretions, tachycardia, epigastric distress, lassitude, excitation, and nausea have been reported.

OVERDOSAGE

Drowsiness is the usual clinical side effect. Convulsions, coma, and respiratory depression may occur with massive overdosage. No specific antidote is known. If respiratory depression occurs, mechanically assisted respiration should be initiated and oxygen administered. Convulsions should be treated with appropriate doses of diazepam. Phenobarbital (5 to 6 mg/kg) may be given to control convulsions in children.

The oral LD_{50} in mice and rats is 203 mg/kg and 1320 mg/kg, respectively. The intraperitoneal LD_{50} in mice is 149 mg/kg.

DOSAGE AND ADMINISTRATION

Dramamine Tablets: To prevent motion sickness, the first dose should be taken ½ to 1 hour before starting the activity. Additional medication depends on travel conditions. *Dosage: Adults:* Nausea or vomiting may be expected to be controlled for approximately 4 hours with 50 mg of Dramamine, and prevented by a similar dose every 4 hours. Its administration may be attended by some degree of drowsiness in some patients, and 100 mg every 4 hours may be given in conditions in which drowsiness is not objectionable or is even desirable. The usual adult dosage is 1 to 2 tablets every 4 to 6 hours, not to exceed 8 tablets in 24 hours. *Children 6 to 12 years:* ½ to 1 tablet every 6 to 8 hours, not to exceed 3 tablets in 24 hours. *Children 2 to 6 years:* Up to ½ tablet every 6 to 8 hours, not to exceed 1½ tablets in 24 hours. Children may also be given Dramamine (dimenhydrinate) cherry-flavored liquid in accordance with directions for use. Not for frequent or prolonged use except on advice of a physician. Do not exceed recommended dosage.

Dramamine Liquid: To prevent motion sickness, the first dose should be taken ½ to 1 hour before starting the activity. Additional medication depends on travel conditions. *Dosage: Adults:* 4 to 8 teaspoonfuls (4 ml per teaspoonful) every 4 to 6 hours, not to exceed 32 teaspoonfuls in 24 hours. *Children 6 to 12 years:* 2 to 4 teaspoonfuls (4 ml per teaspoonful) every 6 to 8 hours, not to exceed 12 teaspoonfuls in 24 hours. *Children 2 to 6 years:* 1 to 2 teaspoonfuls every 6 to 8

Continued on next page

Richardson-Vicks—Cont.

hours, not to exceed 6 teaspoonfuls in 24 hours. *Children under 2 years:* Only on advice of a physician.
Not for frequent or prolonged use except on advice of a physician. Do not exceed recommended dosage. Use of a measuring device is recommended for all liquid medication.

HOW SUPPLIED

Dramamine (dimenhydrinate) is supplied in the following dosage forms and package sizes:
For oral use —**tablets**, scored, white, 50 mg, cartons of 12, individual blister-sealed tablets, bottles of 36 and 100 tablets.
liquid, 12.5 mg/ 4 ml, ethyl alcohol 5%, bottles of 3 fl oz.
[Please note: Dramamine Tablets and Liquid are also shown in the PDR For Nonprescription Drugs.]

HEAD & CHEST™
DECONGESTANT/EXPECTORANT COLD MEDICINE

ACTIVE INGREDIENTS

Each tablet and capsule contains:
Phenylpropanolamine HCl .... 25 mg
Guaifenesin .... 200 mg
Inactive ingredients (capsule) include color, silica gel, gelatin, starch, titanium dioxide and zinc stearate; (tablet), maltodextrin, povidone, starch, stearic acid and sucrose.
Each 5 ml (one teaspoonful) liquid contains:
Phenylpropanolamine .... 12.5 mg
Guaifenesin .... 100 mg
Inactive ingredients include alcohol (5%), citric acid, color, flavor, glycerin, saccharin sodium, sodium benzoate, sodium chloride, sorbitol, sucrose and water.

INDICATIONS

HEAD & CHEST is indicated in colds, sinusitis, bronchitis, and other respiratory conditions to reduce nasal congestion and promote drainage of bronchial passageways.

ACTIONS

Phenylpropanolamine HCl is an effective vasoconstrictor that decongests swollen mucous membranes of the respiratory tract. The expectorant guaifenesin enhances the flow of respiratory tract fluid, promotes ciliary action and facilitates removal of viscous, inspissated mucus. As a result, sinus and bronchial drainage is improved, and dry, nonproductive coughs become more productive and less frequent.

WARNINGS

This product should not be taken by persons who are hypersensitive to any of its ingredients or those who have high blood pressure, heart disease, diabetes, thyroid disease or persistent or chronic cough such as occurs with smoking, asthma, or emphysema, or where cough is accompanied by excessive secretions, or by children under 2 years except under the advice and supervision of a physician. If symptoms do not improve within 7 days or are accompanied by fever, rash, or persistent headache, consult a physician before continuing use. Do not exceed recommended dosage because at higher doses nervousness, dizziness or sleeplessness are more likely to occur. Keep all medicines out of reach of children. In case of accidental overdose, seek professional assistance or contact a poison control center immediately. As with any drug, if you are pregnant or nursing a baby, seek the advice of a health professional before using the product.

DRUG INTERACTION PRECAUTION

Do not take this product if you are presently taking a prescription antihypertensive or antidepressant drug containing a monoamine oxidase inhibitor except under the advice and supervision of a physician.

OVERDOSAGE

Treatment of overdosage should be directed toward supporting the patient and reversing the effects of the drug.

DOSAGE

Adults and children over 12 years—2 teaspoonfuls LIQUID or 1 TABLET or 1 CAPSULE
Children 6–12 years—1 teaspoonful LIQUID or ½ tablet
Children 2–6 years—½ teaspoonful LIQUID
Repeat above dosage every 4 hours as needed to maximum of 6 doses in 24 hours.

HOW SUPPLIED

Head & Chest Tablets are white oval-shaped imprinted with the Head & Chest logo on the smooth side and "NE 037" on the scored side. Tablets are available in boxes of 16 and 36
Head & Chest Capsules are blue and white with the Head & Chest logo on one half and "NE 036" on the other half. Capsules are available in boxes of 12 and 24
Head & Chest Liquid is available in 4 fl. oz and 8 fl. oz bottles.

PERCOGESIC®
[pĕr′kō-gē-sĭk]
Analgesic Tablets

ACTIVE INGREDIENTS

Each tablet contains:
Acetaminophen .... 325 mg
Phenyltoloxamine citrate .... 30 mg

INACTIVE INGREDIENTS

Celluose, Color, Flavor, Magnesium Stearate, Povidone, Silica Gel, Starch, Stearic acid, Sucrose.

INDICATIONS

For relief of pain and discomfort due to headache, for temporary relief of pain associated with muscle and joint soreness, neuralgia, sinusitis, minor menstrual cramps, the common cold, toothache, and minor aches and pains of rheumatism and arthritis.

WARNING

If arthritic or rheumatic pain persists for more than 10 days; in the presence of redness or swelling; or in arthritic or rheumatic conditions affecting children under 12 years of age, consult a physician immediately. When used for temporary, symptomatic relief of colds, do not use for more than 3 days, except as directed by a physician. This preparation may cause drowsiness. Do not drive or operate machinery while taking this medication. Do not administer to children under 6 years of age or exceed recommended dosage unless directed by a physician. Keep this and all drugs out of the reach of children. In case of accidental overdosage, seek professional assistance or contact a poison control center immediately. As with any drug, if you are pregnant or nursing a baby, seek the advice of a health professional before using this product. Keep this and all drugs out of reach of children.

DOSAGE AND ADMINISTRATION

ADULTS (12 years and over)—1 or 2 tablets every four hours. Maximum daily dose—8 tablets
CHILDREN (6-12 years)—one-half adult dose. Maximum daily dose—4 tablets
Do not use for more than 10 days unless directed by a physician.
Store at room temperature; avoid excessive heat.

HOW SUPPLIED

Bottles of 24, 50 and 90 tablets.
Shown in Product Identification Section, page 423

VICKS® CHILDRENS COUGH SYRUP
Expectorant, Antitussive Cough Syrup

(See PDR For Nonprescription Drugs)

VICKS® COUGH SILENCERS
Cough Drops

(See PDR For Nonprescription Drugs)

VICKS® DAYCARE® LIQUID
VICKS® DAYCARE® CAPSULES
Multi-Symptom Colds Medicine

(See PDR For Nonprescription Drugs)

VICKS® FORMULA 44® COUGH CONTROL DISCS

(See PDR For Nonprescription Drugs)

VICKS® FORMULA 44® COUGH MIXTURE

(See PDR For Nonprescription Drugs)

VICKS® FORMULA 44D®
DECONGESTANT COUGH MIXTURE

(See PDR For Nonprescription Drugs)

VICKS® FORMULA 44M
Multi-Symptom Cough Mixture

(See PDR For Nonprescription Drugs)

VICKS® INHALER
with decongestant action

(See PDR For Nonprescription Drugs)

VICKS® NYQUIL®
[nī′quĭl]
Nighttime Colds Medicine in oral liquid form.

(See PDR For Nonprescription Drugs)

VICKS® ORACIN COOLING THROAT LOZENGES
[ŏ′ră″sĭn]
VICKS® ORACIN CHERRY FLAVOR COOLING THROAT LOZENGES

(See PDR For Nonprescription Drugs)

VICKS® SINEX™
[sī′nĕx]
Decongestant Nasal Spray

(See PDR For Nonprescription Drugs)

VICKS® SINEX™ LONG-ACTING
[sī′nĕx]
Decongestant Nasal Spray

(See PDR For Nonprescription Drugs)

VICKS® THROAT LOZENGES

(See PDR For Nonprescription Drugs)

VICKS® VAPORUB®
Decongestant Vaporizing Ointment

(See PDR For Nonprescription Drugs)

VICKS® VAPOSTEAM®
[vā′pō″stēm]
Liquid Medication for Hot Steam Vaporizers.

(See PDR For Nonprescription Drugs)

VICKS® VATRONOL®
[vā′trō″nŏl]
Nose Drops

(See PDR For Nonprescription Drugs)

Richardson-Vicks Inc.
Personal Care Products Division
TEN WESTPORT ROAD
WILTON, CT 06897

CLEARASIL® Adult Care™
(Sulfur/Resorcinol)

(See PDR For Nonprescription Drugs)

CLEARASIL® Maximum Strength Medicated Anti-Acne Cream
(10% Benzoyl Peroxide)
Vanishing and Tinted

(See PDR For Nonprescription Drugs)

CLEARASIL® 10% Benzoyl Peroxide
Medicated Anti-Acne Lotion

(See PDR For Nonprescription Drugs)

CLEARASIL® Medicated Astringent
(Salicylic Acid 0.5%)

(See PDR For Nonprescription Drugs)

DENQUEL® Sensitive Teeth Toothpaste
Desensitizing Dentifrice

(See PDR For Nonprescription Drugs)

Products are cross-indexed by generic and chemical names in the **YELLOW SECTION**

Riker Laboratories, Inc.

225-1S-07 3M CENTER
ST. PAUL, MN 55144

[See table right].

ALU-TAB® Tablets
and
ALU-CAP® Capsules

DESCRIPTION
Each green Alu-Tab "swallow" tablet contains dried aluminum hydroxide gel 600 mg. Alu-Tab tablets also contain: acetylated monoglycerides, cellulose, ethylcellulose, hydrogenated vegetable oil, hydroxypropyl cellulose, hydroxypropyl methylcellulose, magnesium stearate, polyethylene glycol, sodium starch glycolate, starch, talc, titanium dioxide, D&C yellow #10, FD&C blue #1, and FD&C yellow #6.
Each red and green Alu-Cap capsule contains dried aluminum hydroxide gel 475 mg. Alu-Cap capsules also contain: cellulose, gelatin, polyethylene glycol, talc, titanium dioxide, FD&C red #40, D&C yellow #10, FD&C blue #1, FD&C green #3, and FD&C yellow #6.

ACTIONS
Antacid actions include neutralization of gastric hyperacidity and mild astringent and absorbent properties. Aluminum hydroxide dried gel increases phosphate excretion in the bowel by the formation of non-absorbable salts.*

INDICATIONS
Treatment in uncomplicated peptic ulcer and gastric hyperacidity.

PRECAUTIONS
Aluminum hydroxide is essentially a nontoxic compound. If constipation occurs, medication should be discontinued and a physician should be consulted. Aluminum hydroxide must be given with care to patients who have recently suffered massive upper gastrointestinal hemorrhage. Do not give this product to any patient presently taking a prescription antibiotic drug containing any form of tetracycline.

DIRECTIONS
Three Alu-Tab "swallow" tablets three times a day or as prescribed by physician. Three Alu-Cap capsules three times a day or as prescribed by physician.

HOW SUPPLIED
Bottles of 250 green film-coated Alu-Tab "swallow" tablets (NDC **0089-0107-25**). Bottles of 100 red and green Alu-Cap capsules (NDC **0089-0106-10**).
*Goodman, L.S., and Gilman, A.: *The Pharmacological Basis of Therapeutics,* 6th ed., Macmillan Publishing Co., Inc. New York, 1980, p. 990.

The following Riker products are available in Military and Veterans Administration depots:

Military Depot Items	**National Stock Number**
Disalcid® Tablets 500's	6505-01-067-2750
Duo-Medihaler® (aerosol) w/adapter 22.5 ml.	6505-00-071-7861
Medihaler-Iso® (aerosol) w/adapter 15 ml.	6505-00-023-6481
Medihaler-Iso® (aerosol) w/adapter 22.5 ml.	6505-00-014-8486
Norflex® Sustained-Release Tablets 100's	6505-00-138-8462
Norgesic® Tablets 500's	6505-00-952-6762
Norgesic® Forte Tablets 500's	6505-01-029-9116
Tepanil® Ten-tab® (controlled-release tablet) 75 mg. 100's	6505-00-082-2684
Urex® Tablets 100's	6505-00-126-3207

Veterans Administration Depot Items	**National Stock Number**
Alu-Cap® Capsules 100's	6505-00-166-7844
Disalcid® Tablets 500's	6505-01-067-2750A
Duo-Medihaler® (aerosol) w/adapter 22.5 ml.	6505-00-071-7861A
Medihaler-Iso® (aerosol) w/adapter 22.5 ml.	6505-00-014-8486A
Norflex® Sustained-Release Tablets 100's	6505-00-138-8462A
Norgesic® Tablets 500's	6505-00-952-6762A
Norgesic® Forte Tablets 500's	6505-01-029-9116A
Theolair™ Tablets 125 mg. 250's	6505-01-075-8307A
Theolair™ Tablets 250 mg. 250's	6505-01-075-8308A
Theolair™-SR Tablets 250 mg. 100's	6505-01-094-1613A
Urex® Tablets 500's	6505-00-443-4501

CALCIUM DISODIUM VERSENATE* ℞
(calcium disodium edetate injection, U.S.P.)
Injection

WARNING
Calcium Disodium Edetate is capable of producing toxic and potentially fatal effects. The dosage schedule should be followed and at no time should the recommended daily dose be exceeded. In lead encephalopathy avoid rapid infusion; intramuscular route is preferred.

DESCRIPTION
Calcium Disodium Versenate Injection (Calcium Disodium Edetate Injection, U.S.P.) is a sterile concentrated solution (20%) containing 200 mg. of calcium disodium edetate per ml. for intravenous infusion or intramuscular injection.

CLINICAL PHARMACOLOGY
The calcium in calcium disodium edetate is readily displaced by heavy metals, such as lead, to form stable complexes. Following parenteral injection, the chelate formed is excreted in the urine, with 50 percent appearing in the first hour after administration.

INDICATIONS AND USAGE
Calcium disodium edetate is indicated for the reduction of blood levels and depot stores of lead in lead poisoning (acute and chronic) and lead encephalopathy.

CONTRAINDICATIONS
Calcium disodium edetate should not be given during periods of anuria.

WARNINGS
See box warning above.
Usage in pregnancy: The safe use of calcium disodium edetate has not been established with respect to possible adverse effects upon fetal development. Therefore, it should not be used in women of child-bearing potential and particularly during early pregnancy unless, in the judgment of the physician, the potential benefits outweigh the possible hazards.

PRECAUTIONS
Severe acute lead poisoning by itself may cause proteinuria and microscopic hematuria. Calcium disodium edetate may produce the same signs of renal damage. Routine urinalysis should be done daily during each course of therapy to determine whether the proteinuria and hematuria is improving or the evidence of renal tubular injury is getting worse. The presence of large renal epithelial cells or increasing numbers of red blood cells in the urinary sediment or greater proteinuria call for immediate stopping of calcium disodium edetate administration. Evidence of renal impairment should be looked for by periodic blood urea nitrogen determinations before and during each course of therapy. The patient should also be monitored for irregularities of cardiac rhythm.

ADVERSE REACTIONS
The principal toxic effect is renal tubular necrosis.

DOSAGE AND ADMINISTRATION
Calcium disodium edetate is equally effective whether administered intravenously, subcutaneously or intramuscularly. Because of convenience in administration and greater safety in treating symptomatic children, many physicians experienced in the treatment of lead poisoning prefer the intramuscular route which is recommended in patients with either overt or incipient lead encephalopathy. Rapid intravenous infusions may be lethal by suddenly increasing intracranial pressure in this group of patients with cerebral edema.
Note: In patients with lead encephalopathy and increased intracranial pressure, excess fluids must be avoided. In such case a 20 percent solution of calcium disodium edetate is mixed with procaine to give a final concentration of 0.5 percent of procaine in the mixture which is administered intramuscularly.
Acutely ill individuals may be dehydrated from vomiting. Since calcium disodium edetate is excreted almost exclusively in the urine, it is very important to establish urine flow by intravenous infusion before the first dose of the chelating agent is given. Once urine flow is established further intravenous fluid is restricted to basal water and electrolyte requirements. Administration of calcium disodium edetate should be stopped whenever there is cessation of urine flow in order to avoid unduly high tissue levels of the drug.
Intravenous Administration: Dilute the 5 ml. (1 gram, 20% solution) from an ampule with 250-500 ml. of Solution Isotonic Sodium Chloride, USP, or sterile 5% dextrose solution in water. In asymptomatic adults, administer this diluted solution over a period of at least one hour. Such doses may be administered twice daily for periods up to 5 days. The therapy should then be interrupted for 2 days and followed by an additional 5 days of treatment, if indicated.
In mildy affected or asymptomatic individuals the dosage of 50 mg./kg. per day should not be exceeded.
In symptomatic adults, fluids should be kept to basal levels and the time of administration increased to two hours. A second daily infusion is to be given six or more hours after the first.
Intramuscular Administration: This is the route of choice for children. The dosage should not exceed 0.5 gram per 30 pounds of body weight twice daily (total, 1.0 gram/30 lbs./day). This is equivalent to 35 mg./kg. twice daily (total, approx. 75 mg./kg./day). In mild cases a dose of 50 mg./kg. per day should not be exceeded. For young children the total daily dose may be given in divided doses every 8 or 12 hours for 3 to 5 days. A second course may be given after a rest period of 4 or more days. Procaine to produce a concentration of 0.5% should be added to minimize pain at injection site. (1 ml. of 1% procaine solution for each ml. of concentrated Calcium Disodium Versenate solution, or crystalline procaine may be used to reduce volume.)
Regardless of method of administration, doses larger than those recommended should not be undertaken.
Lead Encephalopathy: This condition is relatively rare in adults but is quite common in children in whom the mortality rate has been high. Recent reports by Chisolm and by Coffin et al who employed a combination of BAL and calcium disodium edetate, suggest that this may be the preferred treatment, although calcium disodium edetate alone has been used over a longer period of time. Each group administered calcium disodium edetate intramuscularly concurrently with BAL in separate deep I.M. sites. Procaine was added to the 20% solution of calcium disodium edetate to give a procaine concentration of 0.5%. In the studies of Coffin and Chisolm, 125 children with acute lead encephalopathy have been treated with this combined therapy with only one death.

HOW SUPPLIED
Calcium Disodium Versenate Injection, 5 ml. ampules containing 200 mg. of calcium disodium edetate per ml., boxes containing 6 ampules.
(NDC **0089-0510-06**).
*Registered trademark of the Dow Chemical Company

CAUTION
Federal law prohibits dispensing without prescription.

DISALCID® ℞
(salsalate)
Tablets and Capsules

DESCRIPTION
DISALCID (salsalate) is a nonsteroidal anti-inflammatory agent for oral administration. Chemically, salsalate (salicylsalicylic acid or 2-hydroxy-benzoic acid 2-carboxyphenyl ester) is a dimer of salicylic acid.
Each round, aqua, film coated DISALCID tablet contains 500 mg salsalate. Each aqua and white DISALCID capsule contains 500 mg salsalate. Disalcid capsules also contain: colloidal silicon dioxide, gelatin, magnesium stearate, starch, titanium dioxide, FD&C blue #1, and D&C yellow #10. Each capsule-shaped aqua, scored, film coated DISALCID tablet contains 750 mg salsalate. Disalcid tablets also contain: hydroxypropyl methylcellulose, magnesium stearate, microcrystalline cellulose, polyethylene glycol, polysorbate 80, starch, talc, FD&C blue #1, and D&C yellow #10. (See HOW SUPPLIED).

CLINICAL PHARMACOLOGY
DISALCID is insoluble in acid gastric fluids (< 0.1 mg/ml at pH 1.0), but readily soluble in the small intestine where it is partially hydrolyzed to two molecules of salicylic acid. A significant portion of the parent compound is absorbed unchanged and undergoes rapid esterase hydrolysis in the body; its half-life is about one hour. About 13% is excreted through the kidneys as a glucuronide conjugate of the parent compound, the remainder as salicylic acid and its metabolites. Thus, the amount of salicylic acid available from DISALCID is about 15% less than from aspirin, when the two drugs are administered on a salicylic acid molar equivalent basis (3.6 g salsalate/5 g aspirin). Salicylic acid biotransformation is saturated at anti-inflammatory doses of DISAL-

Continued on next page

Riker—Cont.

CID. Such capacity-limited biotransformation results in an increase in the half-life of salicylic acid from 3.5 to 16 or more hours. Thus, dosing with DISALCID twice a day will satisfactorily maintain blood levels within the desired therapeutic range (10 to 30 mg/100 ml) throughout the 12-hour intervals. Therapeutic blood levels continue for up to 16 hours after the last dose. The parent compound does not show capacity-limited biotransformation, nor does it accumulate in the plasma on multiple dosing. Food slows the absorption of all salicylates including DISALCID.

The mode of anti-inflammatory action of DISALCID and other nonsteroidal anti-inflammatory drugs is not fully defined. Although salicylic acid (the primary metabolite of DISALCID) is a weak inhibitor of prostaglandin synthesis **in vitro**, DISALCID appears to selectively inhibit prostaglandin synthesis **in vivo**, providing anti-inflammatory effect equivalent to aspirin, indomethacin, and ibuprofen. Unlike aspirin, DISALCID does not inhibit platelet aggregation.[1]

The usefulness of salicylic acid, the active **in vivo** product of DISALCID, in the treatment of arthritic disorders has been established.[2,3] In contrast to aspirin and the other nonsteroidal anti-inflammatory drugs, DISALCID does not cause gastrointestinal blood loss[4] or peptic disease.[5]

INDICATIONS AND USAGE

DISALCID is indicated for relief of the signs and symptoms of rheumatoid arthritis, osteoarthritis and related rheumatic disorders.

DISALCID can safely be given to aspirin- sensitive patients (and those sensitive to tartrazine, FD&C Yellow No. 5), since it does not induce asthma in such patients.[6]

CONTRAINDICATIONS

DISALCID is contraindicated in patients hypersensitive to salsalate.

WARNINGS

Reye Syndrome may develop in individuals who have chicken pox, influenza, or flu symptoms. Some studies suggest possible association between the development of Reye Syndrome and the use of medicines containing salicylate or aspirin. Disalcid contains a salicylate and therefore is not recommended for use in patients with chicken pox, influenza, or flu symptoms. See PRECAUTIONS.

PRECAUTIONS

General Precautions: Patients on long-term treatment with DISALCID should be warned not to take other salicylates so as to avoid potentially toxic concentrations. Great care should be exercised when DISALCID is prescribed in the presence of chronic renal insufficiency. Protein binding of salicylic acid can be influenced by nutritional status, competitive binding of other drugs, and fluctuations in serum proteins caused by disease (rheumatoid arthritis, etc.).

Laboratory Tests: Plasma salicylic acid concentrations should be periodically monitored during long-term treatment with DISALCID to aid maintenance of therapeutically effective levels: 10 to 30 mg/100 ml. Toxic manifestations are not usually seen until plasma concentrations exceed 30 mg/100 ml (see OVERDOSAGE). Urinary pH should also be regularly monitored: sudden acidification, as from pH 6.5 to 5.5, can double the plasma level, resulting in toxicity.

Drug Interactions: Salicylates antagonize the uricosuric action of drugs used to treat gout. Aspirin and other salicylate drugs will be additive to DISALCID and may increase plasma concentrations of salicylic acid to toxic levels. Drugs and foods that raise urine pH will increase renal clearance and urinary excretion of salicylic acid, thus lowering plasma levels; acidifying drugs or foods will decrease urinary excretion and increase plasma levels. Salicylates may competitively displace anticoagulant drugs from plasma protein binding sites and thereby predispose to systemic bleeding. Salicylates may enhance the hypoglycemic effect of oral antidiabetic drugs of the sulfonylurea class. Salicylate competes with a number of drugs for protein binding sites, notably penicillin, thiopental, thyroxine, triiodothyronine, phenytoin, sulfinpyrazone, naproxen, warfarin, methotrexate, and possibly corticosteroids.

Drug/Laboratory Test Interactions: Salicylate competes with thyroid hormone for binding to plasma proteins, which may be reflected in a depressed plasma T_4 value in some patients; thyroid function and basal metabolism are unaffected.

Carcinogenesis: No long-term animal studies have been performed with DISALCID to evaluate its carcinogenic potential; however, several such studies using aspirin and other salicylates have failed to demonstrate any association of these agents with cancerous cell changes.

Use in Pregnancy: Pregnancy Category C: Salsalate and salicylic acid have been shown to be teratogenic and embryocidal in rats when given in doses 4 to 5 times the usual human dose. These effects were not observed at doses twice as great as the usual human dose. There are no adequate and well-controlled studies in pregnant women. DISALCID should be used during pregnancy only if the potential benefit justifies the potential risk to the fetus.

Labor and Delivery: There exist no adequate and well-controlled studies in pregnant women. Although adverse effects on mother or infant have not been reported with DISALCID use during labor, caution is advised when anti-inflammatory dosage is involved. However, other salicylates have been associated with prolonged gestation and labor, maternal and neonatal bleeding sequelae, potentiation of narcotic and barbiturate effects (respiratory or cardiac arrest in the mother), delivery problems and stillbirth.

Nursing Mothers: It is not known whether salsalate per se is excreted in human milk; salicylic acid, the primary metabolite of DISALCID, has been shown to appear in human milk in concentrations approximating the maternal blood level. Thus the infant of a mother on DISALCID therapy might ingest in mother's milk 30 to 80% as much salicylate per kg body weight as the mother is taking. Accordingly, caution should be exercised when DISALCID is administered to a nursing woman.

Pediatric Use: Safety and effectiveness in children have not been established.

ADVERSE REACTIONS

Auditory system: Tinnitus and temporary hearing loss can occur. Tinnitus probably represents blood salicylic acid levels reaching or exceeding the upper limit of the therapeutic range. It is therefore a helpful guide to dose titration. Temporary hearing loss disappears gradually upon discontinuation of the drug.

Gastrointestinal system: Nausea, dyspepsia and heartburn occur occasionally.

DRUG ABUSE AND DEPENDENCE

Drug abuse and dependence have not been reported with DISALCID.

OVERDOSAGE

No deaths after overdosage have been reported for DISALCID. Death has followed ingestion of 10 to 30 g of other salicylates in adults, but much larger amounts have been ingested without fatal outcome.

The oral LD_{50} for DISALCID in rats is approximately 2000 mg/kg (sixty times the recommended maximum single dose for adults).

Symptoms: The usual symptoms of salicylism —tinnitus, vertigo, headache, confusion, drowsiness, sweating, hyperventilation, vomiting and diarrhea—will occur. More severe intoxication will lead to disruption of electrolyte balance and blood pH, and hyperthermia and dehydration.

Treatment: Further absorption of DISALCID from the G.I. tract should be prevented by emesis (syrup of ipecac) and, if necessary, by gastric lavage.

Fluid and electrolyte imbalance should be corrected by the administration of appropriate I.V. therapy. Adequate renal function should be maintained. Hemodialysis or peritoneal dialysis may be required in extreme cases.

DOSAGE AND ADMINISTRATION

Adults: The usual dosage is 3000 mg daily, given in divided doses as follows: 1) Two doses of two 750 mg tablets; 2) two doses of three 500 mg tablets/ capsules; or 3) three doses of two 500 mg tablets/ capsules. Dosage should be adjusted depending on individual response. Alleviation of symptoms is gradual, and full benefit may not be evident for 3 to 4 days, when plasma salicylate levels have achieved steady state. There is no evidence for development of tissue tolerance (tachyphylaxis), but salicylate therapy may induce increased activity of metabolizing liver enzymes, causing a greater rate of salicyluric acid production and excretion, with a resultant increase in dosage requirement for maintenance of therapeutic serum salicylate levels.

Children: DISALCID has not been evaluated in children. No dosage recommendations can, therefore, be made.

HOW SUPPLIED

750 mg tablets in bottles of 100 (NDC **0089-0151-10**)
750 mg tablets in boxes of 100 in unit-dose blisterstrips (NDC **0089-151-16**)
750 mg tablets in bottles of 500 (NDC **0089-0151-50**)
500 mg tablets in bottles of 100 (NDC **0089-0149-10**)
500 mg tablets in boxes of 100 in unit-dose blisterpacks (NDC **0089-149-16**)
500 mg tablets in bottles of 500 (NDC **0089-0149-50**)
500 mg capsules in bottles of 100 (NDC **0089-0148-10**)

REFERENCES

1. Estes D, Kaplan K: Lack of Platelet Effect With the Aspirin Analog, Salsalate. Arthritis and Rheumatism **23**: 1303, 1980.
2. Dick C, Dick PH, Nuki G, et al: Effect of Anti-inflammatory Drug Therapy on Clearance of ^{133}Xe from Knee Joints of Patients with Rheumatoid Arthritis. British Med. J. 3:278–280, 1969.
3. Dick WC, Grayson MF, Woodburn A, et al: Indices of Inflammatory Activity. Ann. of the Rheum. Dis. **29**:643–648, 1970.
4. Cohen A: Fecal Blood Loss and Plasma Salicylate Study of Salicylsalicylic Acid and Aspirin. J. Clin. Pharmacol. **19**:242–247, 1979.
5. Voltin, RF: Safety of Salsalate in Peptic Disease. Scientific Exhibit, PANLAR, June 6–10, 1982.
6. Simon MR, Salberg DJ, Muller BF, et al: Lack of Adverse Reactions to Salsalate in Asthmatic Subjects. Data on file, Medical Department, Riker Laboratories, Inc.

CAUTION

Federal law prohibits dispensing without prescription.

Shown in Product Identification Section, page 423

DISIPAL® ℞

(orphenadrine hydrochloride)
TABLETS

DESCRIPTION

Each round, green Disipal tablet contains orphenadrine hydrochloride (2-dimethylaminoethyl 2-methylbenzhydryl ether hydrochloride) 50 mg. Disipal tablets also contain: acetylated monoglycerides, colloidal silicon dioxide, ethylcellulose, hydroxypropyl methylcellulose, hydroxypropyl cellulose, lactose, magnesium stearate, microcrystalline cellulose, starch, talc, titanium dioxide, D&C yellow #10, FD&C blue #1, and FD&C yellow #6.

HOW SUPPLIED

Bottles of 100 Tablets (NDC **0089-0161-10**) imprinted "RIKER" on one side and "161" on the other.

DUO-MEDIHALER® ℞

(isoproterenol hydrochloride and phenylephrine bitartrate)

DESCRIPTION

Duo-Medihaler (isoproterenol hydrochloride and phenylephrine bitartrate) is an aerosol device which delivers micronized particles of isoproterenol hydrochloride and phenylephrine bitartrate. Also contains: cetylpyridinium chloride, dichlorodifluoromethane, dichlorotetrafluoroethane, sorbitan trioleate, and trichloromonofluoromethane. This drug-propellant system is contained in a hermetically sealed metal vial. Each valve actuation releases a uniform aerosolized dose of 0.16 mg. isoproterenol hydrochloride (equivalent to 0.137 mg. of isoproterenol base) and 0.24 mg. phenylephrine bitartrate (equivalent to 0.126 mg. of phenylephrine base).

HOW SUPPLIED

Duo-Medihaler with adapter (450 doses, 22.5 ml.) NDC **0089-0732-21.**
Duo-Medihaler refill vial (450 doses, 22.5 ml.) NDC **0089-0732-11.**
Duo-Medihaler with adapter (300 doses, 15 ml.) NDC **0089-0735-21.**
Duo-Medihaler refill (300 doses, 15 ml.) NDC **0089-0735-11.**

MEDIHALER-EPI®

(epinephrine bitartrate)
FOR TEMPORARY RELIEF FROM ACUTE PAROXYSMS OF BRONCHIAL ASTHMA.

FOR ORAL INHALATION THERAPY ONLY

Each inhalation delivers 0.3 mg epinephrine bitartrate equivalent to 0.16 mg of epinephrine base. Also contains: cetylpyridinium chloride, dichlorodifluoromethane, dichlorotetrafluoroethane, sorbitan trioleate, and trichloromonofluoromethane.

HOW SUPPLIED

15 ml. size: Available as a combination package (vial with oral adapter) or as a refill (vial only).

MEDIHALER ERGOTAMINE® ℞

(ergotamine tartrate)

DESCRIPTION

Medihaler Ergotamine (ergotamine tartrate) is an aerosol device which contains a fine particle suspension of 9.0 mg. ergotamine tartrate per ml. in an inert, nontoxic aerosol vehicle. The inert ingredients are dichlorodifluoromethane, dichlorotetrafluoroethane, sorbitan trioleate, and trichloromonofluoromethane. Each depression of the valve delivers a measured dose of 0.36 mg. to the patient.

ACTION

Ergotamine exerts a constrictor action upon the cranial vessels.

INDICATIONS

As therapy to abort vascular headache, e.g., migraine, migraine variants, or so-called "histaminic cephalalgia."

CONTRAINDICATIONS

Ergotamine tartrate should not be used in the presence of coronary artery disease, peripheral vascular disease, hypertension, impaired renal or hepatic function, infectious states or malnutrition.
Ergotamine tartrate is contraindicated in patients with a history of hypersensitivity reactions.
Pregnancy: Ergotamine tartrate is contraindicated in pregnancy.

WARNINGS

Patients who are being treated with Medihaler Ergotamine should be informed adequately of the symptoms of ergotism. Close medical supervision by the physician is recommended so that he may react appropriately should signs of ergotism develop. Six inhalations per day, if continued daily, entail the risk of vasospastic complications. Avoid prolonged administration or in excess of the recommended dosage because of the danger of ergotism and gangrene.
Pediatric Patients: Since there is no experience in children who have received this drug, safety and efficacy in children have not been established.
Nursing Mothers: Whether ergotamine tartrate is excreted in mothers' milk is not known. As a general rule, nursing should not be undertaken while a patient is on a drug (since many drugs are excreted in human milk).

ADVERSE REACTIONS

Ergotamine tartrate may cause nausea and vomiting. Patients with headaches may become nauseated and drug induced distress may be difficult to evaluate.
Ergotamine in large doses raises arterial pressure, produces coronary vasoconstriction and slows the heart both by direct action and its effect on the vagus. Under this condition, ergotamine also has oxytocic and spasmolytic properties. The above conditions are seen as a consequence of overdosage and may be manifested at the dosage recommended for control of headaches.
Vasoconstrictive complications, at times of a serious nature, may occur. These include pulselessness, weakness, muscle pains and paresthesias of the extremities and precordial distress and pain. Although these effects occur most commonly with long term therapy at relatively high doses, they have also been reported with short term or normal doses. Other adverse effects include transient tachycardia or bradycardia, nausea, vomiting, localized edema and itching.

DOSAGE AND ADMINISTRATION

Adults: A single inhalation at the first sign of headache or prodrome. Repeat this procedure in 5 minutes if relief is not obtained. Space any additional inhalations at no less than 5-minute intervals. No more than 6 inhalations should be administered in any 24-hour period, and no more than 15 in a one week period.
Children: A recommended dose for children has not been determined.
Directions For Use: Before each use, remove dust cap and shake Medihaler Ergotamine.

1. Breathe out fully and place mouthpiece well into the mouth, aimed at the back of the throat.
2. As you begin to breathe in deeply, press the vial firmly down into the adapter with the index finger. This releases one dose.
3. Release pressure on vial and remove unit from mouth. Hold the breath as long as possible, then breathe out slowly.

HOW SUPPLIED

Metal vial (2.5 ml.) and adapter. Each depression of the valve delivers 0.36 mg. ergotamine tartrate. (NDC **0089-0762-21**).

CAUTION

Federal law prohibits dispensing without prescription.
Shown in Product Identification Section, page 424

MEDIHALER-ISO® ℞
(isoproterenol sulfate)

DESCRIPTION

Medihaler-Iso (isoproterenol sulfate) is an aerosol device which contains a fine particle suspension of 2.0 mg. per ml. isoproterenol sulfate. Also contains: dichlorodifluoromethane, dichlorotetrafluoroethane, sorbitan trioleate, and trichloromonofluoromethane. Each depression of the valve delivers a measured dose of 0.08 mg. to the patient.

HOW SUPPLIED

Medihaler-Iso (isoproterenol sulfate) with oral adapter (300 doses 15 ml.) NDC **0089-0785-21**.
Medihaler-Iso (isoproterenol sulfate) refill vial only (300 doses 15 ml.) NDC **0089-0785-11**.
Medihaler-Iso (isoproterenol sulfate) with oral adapter (450 doses 22.5 ml.) NDC **0089-0782-21**.
Medihaler-Iso (isoproterenol sulfate) refill vial only (450 doses 22.5 ml.) NDC **0089-0782-11**.

NORFLEX® ℞
(orphenadrine citrate)
Tablets and Injectable

PRODUCT OVERVIEW

KEY FACTS

Norflex sustained-release tablets provide 12 hours relief from the pain of muscle spasm. Also available in injectable form, IV or IM, also given every 12 hours.

MAJOR USES

Norflex is indicated as an adjunct to rest, physical therapy, and other measures for the relief of discomfort associated with painful musculoskeletal disorders.

SAFETY INFORMATION

Contraindicated in patients with glaucoma, pyloric or duodenal obstruction, stenosing peptic ulcers, prostatic hypertrophy or obstruction of the bladder neck, cardiospasm (megaesophagus) and myasthenia gravis. Contraindicated in patients who have a previous sensitivity to the drug.

PRESCRIBING INFORMATION

NORFLEX® ℞
(orphenadrine citrate)
Tablets and Injectable

DESCRIPTION

Orphenadrine citrate is the citrate salt of orphenadrine (2-dimethylaminoethyl 2-methylbenzhydryl ether citrate). It occurs as a white, crystalline powder having a bitter taste. It is practically odorless; sparingly soluble in water, slightly soluble in alcohol.

ACTIONS

The mode of therapeutic action has not been clearly identified, but may be related to its analgesic properties. Orphenadrine citrate also possesses anti-cholinergic actions.

INDICATIONS

Orphenadrine citrate is indicated as an adjunct to rest, physical therapy, and other measures for the relief of discomfort associated with acute painful musculo skeletal conditions. The mode of action of the drug has not been clearly identified, but may be related to its analgesic properties. Orphenadrine citrate does not directly relax tense skeletal muscles in man.

CONTRAINDICATIONS

Contraindicated in patients with glaucoma, pyloric or duodenal obstruction, stenosing peptic ulcers, prostatic hypertrophy or obstruction of the bladder neck, cardio-spasm (megaesophagus) and myasthenia gravis. Contraindicated in patients who have demonstrated a previous hypersensitivity to the drug.

WARNINGS

Some patients may experience transient episodes of lightheadedness, dizziness or syncope. Norflex may impair the ability of the patient to engage in potentially hazardous activities such as operating machinery or driving a motor vehicle; ambulatory patients should therefore be cautioned accordingly.

USAGE IN PREGNANCY

Safe use of orphenadrine has not been established with respect to adverse effects upon fetal development. Therefore, Norflex should be used in women of childbearing potential and particularly during early pregnancy only when in the judgment of the physician the potential benefits outweigh the possible hazards.

USAGE IN CHILDREN

Safety and effectiveness in children have not been established; therefore, this drug is not recommended for use in the pediatric age group.

PRECAUTIONS

Confusion, anxiety and tremors have been reported in few patients receiving propoxyphene and orphenadrine concomitantly. As these symptoms may be simply due to an additive effect, reduction of dosage and/or discontinuation of one or both agents is recommended in such cases.
Orphenadrine citrate should be used with caution in patients with tachycardia, cardiac decompensation, coronary insufficiency, cardiac arrhythmias.
Safety of continuous long-term therapy with orphenadrine has not been established. Therefore, if orphenadrine is prescribed for prolonged use, periodic monitoring of blood, urine and liver function values is recommended.

ADVERSE REACTIONS

Adverse effects of orphenadrine are mainly due to the mild anticholinergic action of orphenadrine, and are usually associated with higher dosage. Dryness of the mouth is usually the first adverse effect to appear. When the daily dose is increased, possible adverse effects include: tachycardia, palpitation, urinary hesitancy or retention, blurred vision, dilatation of pupils, increased ocular tension, weakness, nausea, vomiting, headache, dizziness, constipation, drowsiness, hypersensitivity reactions, pruritus, hallucinations, agitation, tremor, gastric irritation, and rarely urticaria and other dermatoses. Infrequently, an elderly patient may experience some degree of mental confusion. These adverse reactions can usually be eliminated by reduction in dosage. Very rare cases of aplastic anemia associated with the use of orphenadrine tablets have been reported. No causal relationship has been established.
Rare instances of anaphylactic reaction have been reported associated with the intramuscular injection of Norflex injectable.

DOSAGE AND ADMINISTRATION

TABLETS: Adults—Two tablets per day; one in the morning and one in the evening.
INJECTABLE: Adults—One 2 ml. ampul (60 mg.) intravenously or intramuscularly; may be repeated every 12 hours. Relief may be maintained by 1 Norflex tablet twice daily.

HOW SUPPLIED

TABLETS: Bottles of 100 (NDC **0089-0221-10**) and 500 (NDC **0089-0221-50**), each tablet containing 100 mg. of orphenadrine citrate. Norflex tablets also contain: calcium stearate, ethylcellulose, and lactose.
INJECTABLE: Boxes of 6 (NDC **0089-0540-06**) and 50 (NDC **0089-0540-50**) 2 ml. ampuls, each ampul containing 60 mg. of orphenadrine citrate in aqueous solution. Norflex Injectable also contains: water for injection, USP; sodium chloride; sodium bisulfite; and sodium hydroxide.
A.H.F.S. Category 12:08

CAUTION

Federal law prohibits dispensing without prescription.
Shown in Product Identification Section, page 424

NORGESIC® ℞
and
NORGESIC® FORTE ℞

ACTIONS

Orphenadrine citrate is a centrally acting (brain stem) compound which in animals selectively blocks facilitatory functions of the reticular formation. Orphenadrine does not produce myoneural block, nor does it affect crossed extensor reflexes. Orphenadrine prevents nicotine-induced convulsions but not those produced by strychnine.
Chronic administration of Norgesic to dogs and rats has revealed no drug-related toxicity. No blood or urine changes were observed, nor were there any macroscopic or microscopic pathological changes detected. Extensive experience with combinations containing aspirin and caffeine has established them as safe agents. The addition of orphenadrine citrate does not alter the toxicity of aspirin and caffeine.
The mode of therapeutic action of orphenadrine has not been clearly identified, but may be related to its analgesic properties. Orphenadrine citrate also possesses anti-cholinergic actions.

INDICATIONS

1. Symptomatic relief of mild to moderate pain of acute musculo-skeletal disorders.
2. The orphenadrine component is indicated as an adjunct to rest, physical therapy, and other measures for the relief of discomfort associated with acute painful musculo-skeletal conditions.
   The mode of action of orphenadrine has not been clearly identified, but may be related to its analgesic properties. Norgesic and Norgesic Forte do not directly relax tense skeletal muscles in man.

CONTRAINDICATIONS

Because of the mild anticholinergic effect of orphenadrine, Norgesic or Norgesic Forte should not be used in patients with glaucoma, pyloric or duodenal obstruction, achalasia, prostatic hypertrophy or obstructions at the bladder neck. Norgesic or Norgesic Forte is also contraindicated in patients with myasthenia gravis and in patients known to be sensitive to aspirin or caffeine.
The drug is contraindicated in patients who have demonstrated a previous hypersensitivity to the drug.

WARNINGS

Reye Syndrome may develop in individuals who have chicken pox, influenza, or flu symptoms. Some studies suggest possible association between the development of Reye Syndrome and the use of medicines containing salicylate or aspirin. Norgesic and Norgesic Forte contain aspirin and therefore are not recommended for use in patients with chicken pox, influenza, or flu symptoms.
Norgesic Forte may impair the ability of the patient to engage in potentially hazardous activities such as operating machinery or driving a motor vehicle; ambulatory patients should therefore be cautioned accordingly.

Continued on next page

Riker—Cont.

Aspirin should be used with extreme caution in the presence of peptic ulcers and coagulation abnormalities.

USAGE IN PREGNANCY

Since safety of the use of this preparation in pregnancy, during lactation, or in the childbearing age has not been established, use of the drug in such patients requires that the potential benefits of the drug be weighed against its possible hazard to the mother and child.

USAGE IN CHILDREN

The safe and effective use of this drug in children has not been established. Usage of this drug in children under 12 years of age is not recommended.

PRECAUTIONS

Confusion, anxiety and tremors have been reported in few patients receiving propoxyphene and orphenadrine concomitantly. As these symptoms may be simply due to an additive effect, reduction of dosage and/or discontinuation of one or both agents is recommended in such cases.

Safety of continuous long term therapy with Norgesic Forte has not been established; therefore, if Norgesic Forte is prescribed for prolonged use, periodic monitoring of blood, urine and liver function values is recommended.

ADVERSE REACTIONS

Side effects of Norgesic or Norgesic Forte are those seen with aspirin and caffeine or those usually associated with mild anticholinergic agents. These may include tachycardia, palpitation, urinary hesitancy or retention, dry mouth, blurred vision, dilatation of the pupil, increased intraocular tension, weakness, nausea, vomiting, headache, dizziness, constipation, drowsiness, and rarely, urticaria and other dermatoses. Infrequently an elderly patient may experience some degree of confusion. Mild central excitation and occasional hallucinations may be observed. These mild side effects can usually be eliminated by reduction in dosage. One case of aplastic anemia associated with the use of Norgesic has been reported. No causal relationship has been established. Rare G.I. hemorrhage due to aspirin content may be associated with the administration of Norgesic or Norgesic Forte. Some patients may experience transient episodes of light-headedness, dizziness or syncope.

DOSAGE AND ADMINISTRATION

Norgesic: Adults 1 to 2 tablets 3 to 4 times daily.

Norgesic Forte: Adults ½ to 1 tablet 3 to 4 times daily.

HOW SUPPLIED

Norgesic tablets can be identified by their three layers colored light green, white and yellow. Each round tablet contains orphenadrine citrate (2-dimethylaminoethyl 2-methylbenzhydryl ether citrate) 25 mg., aspirin 385 mg., and caffeine 30 mg.

Norgesic Forte tablets are exactly twice the strength of Norgesic. They are identified by their scored capsule shape and by their three layers colored light green, white and yellow. Each capsule shaped tablet contains orphenadrine citrate 50 mg., aspirin 770 mg., and caffeine 60 mg.

Norgesic and Norgesic Forte also contain: lactose, polyethylene glycol, povidone, starch, sucrose, zinc stearate, and D&C yellow #10.

Norgesic: Bottles of 100 (NDC **0089-0231-10**) and 500 tablets (NDC **0089-0231-50**).

Norgesic Forte: Bottles of 100 tablets (NDC **0089-0233-10**) and 500 tablets (NDC **0089-0233-50**).

CAUTION

Federal law prohibits dispensing without prescription.

Shown in Product Identification Section, page 424

RAUWILOID® ℞

(alseroxylon)
tablets

DESCRIPTION

Each tablet contains 2 mg. of the alseroxylon fraction of Rauwolfia serpentina, equivalent to not less than 0.15 mg. and not more than 0.20 mg. reserpine-rescinnamine group alkaloids expressed as reserpine. Rauwiloid tablets also contain: calcium stearate, lactose, starch, sucrose, FD&C yellow #5, FD&C red #3, and FD&C blue #1.

HOW SUPPLIED

Bottle of 100 (NDC **0089-0265-10**) tablets.

TAMBOCOR ℞

[*tăm-ba-kŏr*]
(flecainide acetate)
Tablets

DESCRIPTION

TAMBOCOR® (flecainide acetate) is an antiarrhythmic drug available in tablets of 100 mg for oral administration.

Flecainide acetate is benzamide, N-(2-piperidinylmethyl)-2,5-bis(2,2,2-trifluoroethoxy)-, monoacetate.

Flecainide acetate is a white crystalline substance with a pK_a of 9.3. It has an aqueous solubility of 48.4 mg/ml at 37°C.

TAMBOCOR tablets also contain: hydrogenated vegetable oil, magnesium stearate, microcrystalline cellulose and starch.

CLINICAL PHARMACOLOGY

TAMBOCOR has local anesthetic activity and belongs to the membrane stabilizing (Class I) group of antiarrhythmic agents; it has electrophysiologic effects characteristic of the IC class of antiarrhythmics.

Electrophysiology. In man, TAMBOCOR produces a dose-related decrease in intracardiac conduction in all parts of the heart, with the greatest effect on the His-Purkinje system (H-V conduction). Effects upon atrioventricular (AV) nodal conduction time and intra-atrial conduction times, although present, are less pronounced than those on ventricular conduction velocity. Significant effects on refractory periods were observed only in the ventricle. Sinus node recovery times (corrected) following pacing and spontaneous cycle lengths are somewhat increased. This latter effect may become significant in patients with sinus node dysfunction (see Warnings).

TAMBOCOR causes a dose-related and plasma-level-related decrease in single and multiple PVCs and can suppress recurrence of ventricular tachycardia. In limited studies of patients with a history of ventricular tachycardia, TAMBOCOR has been successful 30–40% of the time in fully suppressing the inducibility of arrhythmias by programmed electrical stimulation. Based on PVC suppression, it appears that plasma levels of 0.2 to 1.0 μg/ml may be needed to obtain the maximal therapeutic effect. It is more difficult to assess the dose needed to suppress serious arrhythmias, but trough plasma levels in patients successfully treated for recurrent ventricular tachycardia were between 0.2 and 1.0 μg/ml. Plasma levels above 0.7–1.0 μg/ml are associated with a higher rate of cardiac adverse experiences such as conduction defects or bradycardia. The relation of plasma levels to proarrhythmic events is not established, but dose reduction in clinical trials of patients with ventricular tachycardia appears to have led to a reduced frequency and severity of such events.

Hemodynamics. TAMBOCOR does not usually alter heart rate, although bradycardia and tachycardia have been reported occasionally.

In animals and isolated myocardium, a negative inotropic effect of flecainide has been demonstrated. Decreases in ejection fraction, consistent with a negative inotropic effect, have been observed after single administration of 200 to 250 mg of the drug in man; both increases and decreases in ejection fraction have been encountered during multidose therapy in patients at usual therapeutic doses (see Warnings).

Metabolism in Humans. Following oral administration, the absorption of TAMBOCOR is nearly complete. Peak plasma levels are attained at about three hours in most individuals (range, 1 to 6 hours). Flecainide does not undergo any consequential presystemic biotransformation (first-pass effect). Food or antacids do not affect absorption.

The apparent plasma half-life averages about 20 hours and is quite variable (range, 12 to 27 hours) after multiple oral doses in patients with premature ventricular contractions (PVCs). With multiple dosing, plasma levels increase because of its long half-life with steady-state levels approached in 3 to 5 days; once at steady-state, no additional (or unexpected accumulation of drug in plasma occurs during chronic therapy. Over the usual therapeutic range, data suggest that plasma levels in an individual are approximately proportional to dose, deviating upwards from linearity only slightly (about 10 to 15% per 100 mg on average).

In healthy subjects, about 30% of a single oral dose (range, 10 to 50%) is excreted in urine as unchanged drug. The two major urinary metabolites are meta-O-dealkylated flecainide (active, but about one fifth as potent) and the meta-O-dealkylated lactam of flecainide (non-active metabolite). These two metabolites (primarily conjugated) account for most of the remaining portion of the dose. Several minor metabolites (3% of the dose or less) are also found in urine; only 5% of an oral dose is excreted in feces. In patients, free (unconjugated) plasma levels of the two major metabolites are very low (less than 0.05 μg/ml).

The elimination of flecainide from the body depends on renal function (i.e. 10 to 50% appears in urine as unchanged drug). With increasing renal impairment, the extent of unchanged drug excretion in urine is reduced and the plasma half-life of flecainide is prolonged. Since flecainide is also extensively metabolized, there is no simple relationship between creatinine clearance and the rate of flecainide elimination from plasma. (See Dosage and Administration.)

In patients with congestive heart failure (NYHA class III), the rate of flecainide elimination from plasma (mean half-life, 19 hours) is moderately slower than for healthy subjects (mean half-life, 14 hours), but similar to the rate for otherwise well patients with PVCs. The extent of unchanged drug excretion in urine is also similar. (See Dosage and Administration.)

The extent of flecainide binding to human plasma proteins is about 40% and is independent of plasma drug level over the range of 0.015 to about 3.4 μg/ml. Thus, clinically significant drug interactions based on protein binding effects would not be expected.

Hemodialysis removes only about 1% of an oral dose as unchanged flecainide.

Small increases in plasma digoxin levels are seen during coadministration of TAMBOCOR with digoxin. Small increases in both flecainide and propranolol plasma levels are seen during coadministration of these two drugs (see Precautions, Drug Interaction).

INDICATIONS AND USAGE

TAMBOCOR is indicated for the treatment of documented life-threatening ventricular arrhythmias, such as sustained ventricular tachycardia.

TAMBOCOR is also indicated for the treatment of patients with symptomatic nonsustained ventricular tachycardia and frequent premature ventricular complexes. Because of the proarrhythmic effects of TAMBOCOR, its use in these less severe arrhythmias should be reserved for patients in whom, in the opinion of the physician, the benefits of treatment outweigh the risks.

For patients with sustained ventricular tachycardia, TAMBOCOR, like other antiarrhythmics, should be initiated in the hospital. Hospitalization may be necessary for certain other patients depending on their cardiac status and underlying cardiac disease (see Dosage and Administration).

The effects of TAMBOCOR in patients with supraventricular arrhythmias and in patients with recent acute myocardial infarction have not been adequately studied.

No antiarrhythmic agent, including TAMBOCOR, has been shown to have a favorable effect on mortality or sudden death.

CONTRAINDICATIONS

TAMBOCOR is contraindicated in patients with preexisting second- or third-degree AV block, or with right bundle branch block when associated with a left hemiblock (bifascicular block), unless a pacemaker is present to sustain the cardiac rhythm should complete heart block occur. TAMBOCOR is also contraindicated in the presence of cardiogenic shock or known hypersensitivity to the drug.

WARNINGS

Proarrhythmic Effects. TAMBOCOR, like other antiarrhythmic agents, can cause new or worsened arrhythmias. Such proarrhythmic effects range from an increase in frequency of PVCs to the development of more severe ventricular tachycardia, e.g., tachycardia that is more sustained or more resistant to conversion to sinus rhythm, with potentially fatal consequences. In studies of TAMBOCOR, three-fourths of proarrhythmic events were new or worsened ventricular tachyarrhythmias, the remainder being increased frequency of PVCs or new supraventricular arrhythmias.

In patients with complex arrhythmias, it is often difficult to distinguish a spontaneous variation in the patient's underlying rhythm disorder from drug-induced worsening, so that the following occurrence rates must be considered approximations. Proarrhythmic effects were reported in 7% of patients treated with TAMBOCOR. Their frequency appears to be related to dose and to the underlying cardiac disease.

Among patients treated for <u>sustained</u> ventricular tachycardia (who frequently also had heart failure, a low ejection fraction, a history of myocardial infarction and/or an episode of cardiac arrest), the incidence of proarrhythmic events was 13% when dosage was initiated at 200 mg/day with slow upward titration, and did not exceed 300 mg/day in most patients. In early studies in patients with <u>sustained</u> ventricular tachycardia utilizing a higher initial dose (400 mg/day) the incidence of proarrhythmic events was 26%; moreover, in about 10% of the patients treated proarrhythmic events resulted in death, despite prompt medical attention. With lower initial doses, the incidence of proarrhythmic events resulting in death decreased to 0.5% of these patients. Accordingly, it is extremely important to follow the recommended dosage schedule (see Dosage and Administration).

Patients with less serious arrhythmias (chronic PVCs and nonsustained ventricular tachycardia) have experienced a lower rate of proarrhythmic events, about 3%, with 0.1% being fatal.

The relatively high frequency of proarrhythmic events in patients with sustained ventricular tachycardia and serious underlying heart disease, and the need for careful titration and monitoring, requires that therapy of patients with sus-

Table 1
Most Common Adverse Effects in Patients Treated With TAMBOCOR in the Multicenter Study

Adverse Effect	Incidence in All 429 Patients at Any Dose	Incidence by Dose During Upward Titration 200 mg/Day (N=426)	300 mg/Day (N=293)	400 mg/Day (N=100)
Dizziness*	18.9%	11.0%	10.6%	13.0%
Visual Disturbance†	15.9%	5.4%	12.3%	18.0%
Dyspnea	10.3%	5.2%	7.5%	4.0%
Headache	9.6%	4.5%	6.1%	9.0%
Nausea	8.9%	4.9%	4.8%	6.0%
Fatigue	7.7%	4.5%	4.4%	3.0%
Palpitation	6.1%	3.5%	2.4%	7.0%
Chest Pain	5.4%	3.1%	3.8%	1.0%
Asthenia	4.9%	2.6%	2.0%	4.0%
Tremor	4.7%	2.4%	3.4%	2.0%
Constipation	4.4%	2.8%	2.1%	1.0%
Edema	3.5%	1.9%	1.4%	2.0%
Abdominal Pain	3.3%	1.9%	2.4%	1.0%

* Dizziness includes reports of dizziness, lightheadedness, faintness, unsteadiness, near syncope, etc.
† Visual disturbance includes reports of blurred vision, difficulty in focusing, spots before eyes, etc.

tained ventricular tachycardia be started in the hospital. Hospitalization should also be considered for other patients with underlying structural heart disease (see Dosage and Administration).

Heart Failure. TAMBOCOR has a negative inotropic effect and may cause or worsen congestive heart failure (CHF), particularly in patients with cardiomyopathy, preexisting severe heart failure (NYHA functional class III or IV) or low ejection fractions (less than 30%). New or worsened CHF which might be attributed to TAMBOCOR therapy occurred in approximately 5% of patients studied in various trials. CHF developed rarely (1%) in patients who had no previous history of CHF. Exacerbation of preexisting CHF occurred more commonly in studies which included patients with class III or IV failure than in studies which excluded such patients. TAMBOCOR should be used cautiously in patients who are known to have a history of congestive heart failure or myocardial dysfunction. The initial dosage in such patients should be no more than 100 mg bid (see Dosage and Administration) and patients should be monitored carefully. Close attention must be given to maintenance of cardiac function, including optimization of digitalis, diuretic, or other therapy. In cases where CHF has developed or worsened during treatment with TAMBOCOR, the time of onset has ranged from a few hours to several months after starting therapy. Some patients who develop evidence of reduced myocardial function while on TAMBOCOR can continue on TAMBOCOR with adjustment of digitalis or diuretics, others may require dosage reduction or discontinuation of TAMBOCOR. When feasible, it is recommended that plasma flecainide levels be monitored. Attempts should be made to keep trough plasma levels below 0.7 to 1.0 μg/ml.

Effects on Cardiac Conduction. TAMBOCOR slows cardiac conduction in most patients to produce dose-related increases in PR, QRS, and QT intervals.

PR interval increases on average about 25% (0.04 seconds) and as much as 118% in some patients. Approximately one-third of patients may develop new first-degree AV heart block (PR interval ≥ 0.20 seconds). The QRS complex increases on average about 25% (0.02 seconds) and as much as 150% in some patients. Many patients develop QRS complexes with a duration of 0.12 seconds or more. In one study, 4% of patients developed new bundle branch block while on TAMBOCOR. The degree of lengthening of PR and QRS intervals does not predict either efficacy or the development of cardiac adverse effects. In clinical trials, it was unusual for PR intervals to increase to 0.30 seconds or more, or for QRS intervals to increase to 0.18 seconds or more. Thus, caution should be used when such intervals occur, and dose reductions may be considered. The QT interval widens about 8%, but most of this widening (about 60% to 90%) is due to widening of the QRS duration. The JT interval (QT minus QRS) only widens about 4% on the average. Significant JT prolongation occurs in less than 2% of patients. There has been one case of Torsade de Pointes-type arrhythmia associated with TAMBOCOR-induced QT prolongation and bradycardia.

Clinically significant conduction changes have been observed at these rates: sinus node dysfunction such as sinus pause, sinus arrest, and symptomatic bradycardia (1.2%), second-degree AV block (0.5%) and third-degree AV block (0.4%). An attempt should be made to manage the patient on the lowest effective dose in an effort to minimize these effects (see Dosage and Administration). If second- or third-degree AV block, or right bundle branch block associated with a left hemiblock occurs, TAMBOCOR therapy should be discontinued unless a temporary or implanted ventricular pacemaker is in place to ensure an adequate ventricular rate.

Sick Sinus Syndrome (Bradycardia-Tachycardia Syndrome). TAMBOCOR should be used only with extreme caution in patients with sick sinus syndrome because it may cause sinus bradycardia, sinus pause, or sinus arrest.

Effects on Pacemaker Thresholds. TAMBOCOR is known to increase endocardial pacing thresholds and may suppress ventricular escape rhythms. These effects are reversible if flecainide is discontinued. It should be used with caution in patients with permanent pacemakers or temporary pacing electrodes and should not be administered to patients with existing poor thresholds or nonprogrammable pacemakers unless suitable pacing rescue is available.

The pacing threshold in patients with pacemakers should be determined prior to instituting therapy with TAMBOCOR, again after one week of administration and at regular intervals thereafter. Generally threshold changes are within the range of multiprogrammable pacemakers and, when these occur, a doubling of either voltage or pulse width is usually sufficient to regain capture.

Electrolyte Disturbances. Hypokalemia or hyperkalemia may alter the effects of Class I antiarrhythmic drugs. Preexisting hypokalemia or hyperkalemia should be corrected before administration of TAMBOCOR.

PRECAUTIONS

Drug Interactions. TAMBOCOR has been administered to patients receiving digitalis preparations or beta-adrenergic blocking agents without adverse effects. During administration of multiple oral doses of TAMBOCOR to healthy subjects stabilized on a maintenance dose of digoxin, a 13% ± 19% increase in plasma digoxin levels occurred at six hours postdose.

In a study involving healthy subjects receiving TAMBOCOR and propranolol concurrently, plasma flecainide levels were increased about 20% and propranolol levels were increased about 30% compared to control values. In this formal interaction study, TAMBOCOR and propranolol were each found to have negative inotropic effects; when the drugs were administered together, the effects were additive. The effects of concomitant administration of TAMBOCOR and propranolol on the PR interval were less than additive. In TAMBOCOR clinical trials, patients who were receiving beta blockers concurrently did not experience an increased incidence of side effects. Nevertheless, the possibility of additive negative inotropic effects of beta blockers and flecainide should be recognized.

Flecainide is not extensively bound to plasma proteins. In vitro studies with several drugs which may be administered concomitantly showed that the extent of flecainide binding to human plasma proteins is either unchanged or only slightly less. Consequently, interactions with other drugs which are highly protein bound (eg, anticoagulants) would not be expected. TAMBOCOR has been used in a large number of patients receiving diuretics without apparent interaction.

There has been little experience with the coadministration of TAMBOCOR and either disopyramide or verapamil. Because both of these drugs have negative inotropic properties and the effects of coadministration with TAMBOCOR are unknown, neither disopyramide nor verapamil should be administered concurrently with TAMBOCOR unless, in the judgement of the physician, the benefits of this combination outweigh the risks. There has been too little experience with the coadministration of TAMBOCOR with nifedipine or diltiazem to recommend concomitant use.

Carcinogenesis, Mutagenesis, Impairment of Fertility. Long-term studies with flecainide in rats and mice at doses up to about eight times the usual human dose of 8 mg/kg/day (assuming patient weight of 50 kg) have not revealed any compound-related carcinogenic effects. Mutagenicity studies (Ames test, mouse lymphoma and in vivo cytogenetics) did not reveal any mutagenic effects. A rat reproduction study at doses up to 50 mg/kg/day (seven times the usual human dose) did not reveal any adverse effect on male or female fertility.

Pregnancy. Pregnancy Category C. Flecainide has been shown to have teratogenic effects (club paws, sternebrae and vertebrae abnormalities, pale hearts with contracted ventricular septum) and an embryotoxic effect (increased resorptions) in one breed of rabbit (New Zealand White) but not in another breed of rabbit (Dutch Belted) when given in doses about four times (but not three times) the usual human dose (assuming a patient weight of 50 kg). No teratogenic effects were observed in rats and mice given doses up to 50 and 80 mg/kg/day, respectively; however, delayed sternebral and vertebral ossification was observed at the high dose in rats. Because there are no adequate and well-controlled studies in pregnant women, TAMBOCOR should be used during pregnancy only if the potential benefit justifies the potential risk to the fetus.

Labor and Delivery. It is not known whether the use of TAMBOCOR during labor or delivery has immediate or delayed adverse effects on the mother or fetus, affects the duration of labor or delivery, or increases the possibility of forceps delivery or other obstetrical intervention.

Nursing Mothers. It is not known whether flecainide is excreted in human milk. Because many drugs are excreted in human milk and because of the drug's potential for serious adverse effects in infants, a decision should be made whether to discontinue nursing or discontinue the drug, taking into account the importance of the drug to the mother.

Pediatric Use. The safety and effectiveness of TAMBOCOR in children less than 18 years of age have not been established.

Use in Patients with Hepatic Impairment. Studies to determine the effect of hepatic impairment upon the elimination of TAMBOCOR have not yet been completed. Because the drug undergoes extensive biotransformation (most likely in the liver), patients with significant hepatic impairment should not receive TAMBOCOR unless the potential benefits clearly outweigh the risks.

ADVERSE EFFECTS

The most serious adverse effects reported for TAMBOCOR, described in detail in Warnings section, were new or exacerbated ventricular arrhythmias which occurred in 7% of patients, and new or worsened congestive heart failure which occurred in approximately 5% of patients. In some patients, TAMBOCOR treatment has been associated with episodes of unresuscitatable ventricular tachycardia or ventricular fibrillation. There have also been instances of second- (0.5%) or third-degree (0.4%) AV block. Patients have developed sinus bradycardia, sinus pause, or sinus arrest, about 1.2% altogether (see Warnings). The frequency of most of these serious adverse events probably increases with higher trough plasma levels, especially when these trough levels exceed 1.0 μg/ml.

There have been rare reports of isolated elevations of serum alkaline phosphatase and isolated elevations of serum transaminase levels. These elevations have been asymptomatic and no cause and effect relationship with TAMBOCOR has been established. In foreign postmarketing surveillance studies, there have been rare reports of hepatic dysfunction, including reports of cholestasis and hepatic failure, and extremely rare report of blood dyscrasias. Although no cause and effect relationship has been established, it is advisable to discontinue TAMBOCOR in patients who develop unexplained jaundice or signs of hepatic dysfunction or blood dyscrasias in order to eliminate TAMBOCOR as the possible causative agent.

Incidence figures for other adverse effects are based on a multicenter efficacy study, utilizing starting doses of 200 mg/day with gradual upward titration to 400 mg/day. Patients were treated for an average of 4.7 months, with some receiving up to 22 months of therapy. In this trial, 5.4% of patients discontinued due to non-cardiac adverse effects. [See table above].

In a trial in ambulatory patients with frequent premature ventricular complexes and nonsustained ventricular tachycardia utilizing a starting dose of 400 mg/day and a maintenance dose of 400–600 mg/day, the incidence of these adverse experiences was similar, except for dizziness (32%) and visual disturbances (28%).

The following additional adverse experiences, possibly related to TAMBOCOR therapy and occurring in 1% to less than 3% of patients, have been reported in acute and chronic studies: Body as a Whole—malaise, fever; Cardiovascular—tachycardia, sinus pause or arrest; Gastrointestinal—vomiting, diarrhea, dyspepsia, anorexia; Skin—rash; Visual—diplopia; Nervous System—hypoesthesia, paresthesia, paresis, ataxia, flushing, increased sweating, vertigo, syncope, somnolence, tinnitus; Psychiatric—anxiety, insomnia, depression.

The following additional adverse experiences, possibly related to TAMBOCOR, have been reported in less than 1% of patients: Body as a While—Swollen lips, tongue and mouth; arthralgia, bronchospasm, myalgia; Cardiovascular—angina pectoris, second-degree and third-degree AV block, bradycardia, hypertension, hypotension; Gastrointestinal—

Continued on next page

Riker—Cont.

flatulence; Urinary System—polyuria, urinary retention; Hematologic—leukopenia, thrombocytopenia; Skin—urticaria, exfoliative dermatitis, pruritis; Visual—eye pain or irritation, photophobia, nystagmus; Nervous System—twitching, weakness, change in taste, dry mouth, convulsions, impotence, speech disorder, stupor; Psychiatric—amnesia, confusion, decreased libido, depersonalization, euphoria, morbid dreams, apathy.

OVERDOSAGE

No specific antidote has been identified for the treatment of TAMBOCOR overdosage. Animal studies suggest that the following events might occur with overdosage: lengthening of the PR interval; increase in the QRS duration, QT interval and amplitude of the T-wave; a reduction in myocardial rate and contractility; conduction disturbances; hypotension; and death from respiratory failure or asystole. Treatment of overdosage should be supportive and may include the following: administration of inotropic agents or cardiac stimulants such as dopamine, dobutamine or isoproterenol; mechanically assisted respiration; circulatory assists such as intra-aortic balloon pumping; and transvenous pacing in the event of conduction block. Because of the long plasma half-life of flecainide (12 to 27 hours in patients receiving usual doses), and the possibility of markedly non-linear elimination kinetics at very high doses, these supportive treatments may need to be continued for extended periods of time. Hemodialysis is not an effective means of removing flecainide from the body.

DOSAGE AND ADMINISTRATION

For patients with sustained ventricular tachycardia, no matter what their cardiac status, TAMBOCOR, like other antiarrhythmics, should be initiated in-hospital with rhythm monitoring. Hospitalization is also recommended for patients with symptomatic congestive heart failure or sinus node dysfunction, even if there is no history of sustained ventricular tachycardia, and would be considered in compensated patients with significant myocardial dysfunction, eg, low ejection fractions (see Warnings).

Flecainide has a long half-life (12 to 27 hours in patients). Steady-state plasma levels, in patients with normal renal and hepatic function, may not be achieved until the patient has received 3 to 5 days of therapy at a given dose. Therefore, **increases in dosage should be made no more frequently than once every four days,** since during the first 2 to 3 days of therapy the optimal effect of a given dose may not be achieved.

For sustained ventricular tachycardia the recommended starting dose is 100 mg every 12 hours. This dose may be increased in increments of 50 mg bid every four days until efficacy is achieved. Most such patients do not require more than 150 mg every 12 hours (300 mg/day), and the maximum dose is 400 mg/day.

For patients with symptomatic nonsustained ventricular tachycardia, couplets, or premature ventricular complexes the recommended starting dose is also 100 mg every 12 hours. This dose may be increased in increments of 50 mg bid every four days until efficacy is achieved. Most of these patients do not require more than 200 mg every 12 hours (400 mg/day). If such a patient is still symptomatic due to the arrhythmia at 400 mg/day, the plasma level is below 0.6 μg/ml, the dosage may be cautiously increased to a maximum of 600 mg/day.

Use of higher initial doses and more rapid dose adjustments have resulted in an increased incidence of proarrhythmic events and congestive heart failure, particularly during the first few days of dosing (see Warnings). Therefore, a loading dose is not recommended.

Intravenous lidocaine has been used occasionally with TAMBOCOR while awaiting the therapeutic effect of TAMBOCOR. No adverse drug interactions were apparent. However, no formal studies have been performed to demonstrate the usefulness of this regimen.

An occasional patient not adequately controlled by (or intolerant to) a dose given at 12-hour intervals may be dosed at eight-hour intervals.

Once adequate control of the arrhythmia has been achieved, it may be possible in some patients to reduce the dose as necessary to minimize side effects or effects on conduction. In such patients, efficacy at the lower dose should be evaluated.

TAMBOCOR should be used cautiously in patients with a history of congestive heart failure or myocardial dysfunction (see Warnings). The initial dose should be no more than 100 mg every 12 hours. If needed to achieve efficacy, the dosage may be increased cautiously in increments of 50 mg bid every four days. The maximum dosage should not exceed 200 mg every 12 hours (400 mg/day) because higher doses are associated with a greater incidence of worsened CHF.

In patients with severe renal impairment (creatinine clearance of 35 ml/min/1.73 square meters or less), the initial dosage should be 100 mg once daily (or 50 mg b.i.d.); when used in such patients, frequent plasma level monitoring is required to guide dosage adjustments (see Plasma Level Monitoring). In patients with less severe renal disease, the initial dosage should be 100 mg every 12 hours; plasma level monitoring may also be useful in these patients during dosage adjustment. In both groups of patients, dosage increases should be made very cautiously when plasma levels have plateaued (after more than four days), observing the patient closely for signs of adverse cardiac effects or other toxicity. It should be borne in mind that in these patients it may take longer than four days before a new steady-state plasma level is reached following a dosage change.

Based on theoretical considerations, rather than experimental data, the following suggestion is made: when transferring patients from another antiarrhythmic drug to TAMBOCOR allow at least two to four plasma half-lives to elapse for the drug being discontinued before starting TAMBOCOR at the usual dosage. In patients where withdrawal of a previous antiarrhythmic agent is likely to produce life-threatening arrhythmias, the physician should consider hospitalizing the patient.

Plasma Level Monitoring: The large majority of patients successfully treated with TAMBOCOR were found to have trough plasma levels between 0.2 and 1.0 μg/ml. The probability of adverse experiences, especially cardiac, may increase with higher trough plasma levels, especially when these exceed 1.0 μg/ml. Periodic monitoring of trough plasma levels may be useful in patient management. Because elimination of flecainide from plasma may be slower in patients with severe chronic renal failure or severe congestive heart failure, plasma level monitoring may be especially helpful in these patients.

HOW SUPPLIED

TAMBOCOR is supplied as white, round, scored tablets containing 100 mg of flecainide acetate and embossed with RIKER on one side and TR 100 on the other side.

TAMBOCOR, 100 mg/tablet, is available in
Bottles of 100—NDC #0089-0307-10.
Unit Dose (blister pack) Box of 100 (strips of 10)—NDC 0089-0307-16

Store at controlled room temperature 15°-30°C (59°-86°F) in a tight, light-resistant container.

Manufactured by: TR-1
Riker Laboratories, Inc./3M
St. Paul, Minnesota 55144-1000

Shown in Product Identification Section, page 424

TEPANIL® Ⓒ℞
(diethylpropion hydrochloride, U.S.P.)
TEPANIL® TEN-TAB® Ⓒ℞
(diethylpropion hydrochloride U.S.P.)
sustained-release tablets

DESCRIPTION

Diethylpropion hydrochloride, a sympathomimetic agent, is 1-phenyl-2-diethylamino-1-propanone hydrochloride. Tepanil tablets also contain: magnesium stearate, mannitol, starch, talc, and tartaric acid.

In Tepanil Ten-Tab tablets, diethylpropion hydrochloride is dispersed in a hydrophilic matrix. On exposure to water the diethylpropion hydrochloride is released at a relatively uniform rate as a result of slow hydration of the matrix. The result is sustained-release of the drug. Tepanil Ten-Tab tablets also contain : carbomer, mannitol, povidone, tartaric acid, and zinc stearate.

HOW SUPPLIED

Tepanil 25 mg.: bottles of 100 (NDC **0089-0351-10**) white tablets, Tepanil Ten-Tab 75 mg.: bottles of 30 (NDC **0089-0353-03**), 100 (NDC **0089-0353-10**), and 250 (NDC **0089-0353-25**) white tablets.

Shown Product Identification Section, page 424

THEOLAIR™ ℞
(theophylline)
TABLETS
THEOLAIR™ ℞
LIQUID
THEOLAIR™-SR ℞
TABLETS

DESCRIPTION

THEOLAIR Tablets contain 125 mg or 250 mg anhydrous theophylline. Theolair tablets also contain: colloidal silicon dioxide, lactose, magnesium stearate, and starch.

THEOLAIR Liquid contains 80 mg theophylline per 15 ml (tablespoonful) in a nonalcoholic solution. Theolair liquid also contains: flavor, methyl & propyl parabens, purified water, sorbitol, and sucrose.

THEOLAIR-SR Tablets contain 200 mg, 250 mg, 300 mg or 500 mg anhydrous theophylline, in a sustained-release formulation. Theolair-SR tablets also contain: cellulose acetate phthalate, lactose, and magnesium stearate.

HOW SUPPLIED

THEOLAIR Tablets:
125 mg tablets—Bottles of 100 (NDC 0089-0342-10) and boxes of 250 unit-dose, aluminum foil, non-child-resistant strips (NDC **0089-0342-26**). Each round, white, scored tablet imprinted with "RIKER" on one side and "342" on the other.
250 mg tablets—Bottles of 100 (NDC **0089-0344-10**) and boxes of 250 unit-dose, aluminum foil, non-child-resistant strips (NDC **0089-0344-26**). Each capsule-shaped, white, scored tablet imprinted with "RIKER" on one side and "THEOLAIR 250" on the other.
STORE AT CONTROLLED ROOM TEMPERATURE 15°-30° C (59°-86° F).

THEOLAIR Liquid:
1 pint bottles (NDC 0089-0960-16)
STORE AT CONTROLLED ROOM TEMPERATURE 15°-30° C (59°-86° F).

THEOLAIR-SR Tablets:
200 mg sustained-release tablets—Bottles of 100 (NDC **0089-0341-10**). Each round white, scored tablet imprinted with "RIKER" on one side and "SR 200" on the other.
250 mg sustained-release tablets—Bottles of 100 (NDC **0089-0345-10**) and bottles of 250 (NDC **0089-0345-25**). Each round, white, scored tablet imprinted with "RIKER" on one side and "SR 250" on the other.
300 mg sustained-release tablets—Bottles of 100 (NDC **0089-0343-10**). Each oval white, scored tablet imprinted with "RIKER" on one side and "SR 300" on the other.
500 mg sustained-release tablets—Bottles of 100 (NDC **0089-0347-10**) and bottles of 250 (NDC **0089-0347-25**). Each capsule-shaped, white, scored tablet imprinted on one side with "RIKER" and "SR 500" on the other.
STORE AT CONTROLLED ROOM TEMPERATURE 15°-30° C (59°-86° F).

Shown in Product Identification Section, page 424

THEOLAIR™-PLUS ℞
TABLETS AND LIQUID

DESCRIPTION

Theolair-Plus contains anhydrous theophylline and guaifenesin and is available in two tablet strengths and as a pleasant tasting liquid.

Theolair-Plus 125—each tablet contains theophylline 125 mg and guaifenesin 100 mg.

Theolair-Plus 250—each tablet contains theophylline 250 mg and guaifenesin 200 mg.

Theolair-Plus tablets also contain: carboxymethylcellulose sodium, magnesium stearate, microcrystalline cellulose, and stearic acid.

Theolair-Plus Liquid—each 15 ml contains theophylline 125 mg and guaifenesin 100 mg. Theolair-Plus liquid also contains: citric acid, menthol, methyl & propyl parabens, peppermint stick, propylene glycol, purified water, sodium citrate, and sucrose.

HOW SUPPLIED

THEOLAIR-PLUS 125 tablets: Bottles of 100 (NDC 0089-0348-10).
THEOLAIR-PLUS 250 tablets: Bottles of 100 (NDC 0089-0349-10).
THEOLAIR-PLUS LIQUID—1 pint (NDC 0089-0962-16).

UREX® ℞
(methenamine hippurate)

DESCRIPTION

Urex (methenamine hippurate) is the hippuric acid salt of methenamine (hexamethylenetetramine). Urex tablets also contain: magnesium stearate, povidone, and saccharin sodium.

HOW SUPPLIED

One gram scored, white tablets, bottles of 100 (NDC **0089-0371-10**) and 500 (NDC **0089-0371-50**).

Shown in Product Identification Section, page 424

EDUCATIONAL MATERIAL

Books, Booklets, Brochures

Exercises for better care of the back, neck, knee and shoulder. Back exercises feature the "Williams Exercises," Free to physicians for distribution to their patients and available through local Riker representatives.

Films, Slides, Videos

Videotapes of current interests are available for viewing and may be obtained through your local Riker representatives.

Samples

Patient starter packets are available by mail and through your local Riker representative.

A. H. Robins Company
PHARMACEUTICAL DIVISION
1407 CUMMINGS DRIVE
RICHMOND, VA 23220

ALLBEE® WITH C CAPSULES
[all-be']

(See PDR For Nonprescription Drugs)

ALLBEE® C-800 TABLETS
ALLBEE® C-800 plus IRON TABLETS
[all-be']

(See PDR For Nonprescription Drugs)

DIMACOL® CAPSULES
DIMACOL® LIQUID
[di'mă-col]

(See PDR For Nonprescription Drugs)

DIMETANE EXTENTABS®
[di'mĕ-tāne eks"tĕn'tabs]
brand of Brompheniramine Maleate, USP
8 mg and 12 mg

(See PDR For Nonprescription Drugs)

DIMETANE®
[di'mĕ-tāne]
brand of Brompheniramine Maleate, USP
Tablets—4 mg
Elixir—2 mg/5 ml
Alcohol, 3%

(See PDR For Nonprescription Drugs)

DIMETANE® DECONGESTANT ELIXIR
[di'mĕ-tāne]
DIMETANE® DECONGESTANT TABLETS

(See PDR For Nonprescription Drugs)

DIMETANE®-DC Ⓒ ℞
COUGH SYRUP
[di'mĕ-tāne]

DESCRIPTION

Dimetane-DC Cough Syrup is a light bluish-pink syrup with a raspberry flavor.

Each 5 mL (1 teaspoonful) contains:
Brompheniramine Maleate, USP .... 2.0 mg
Phenylpropanolamine Hydrochloride, USP .... 12.5 mg
Codeine Phosphate, USP .... 10.0 mg
(Warning: May be habit forming)
Alcohol 0.95 percent
In a palatable aromatic vehicle.

Inactive Ingredients: Citric Acid, FD&C Blue 1, FD&C Red 40, Flavors, Glycerin, Sodium Benzoate, Sorbitol, Water.

Antihistamine/Nasal Decongestant/Antitussive syrup for oral administration.

CLINICAL PHARMACOLOGY

Brompheniramine maleate is a histamine antagonist, specifically an H_1-receptor-blocking agent belonging to the alkylamine class of antihistamines. Antihistamines appear to compete with histamine for receptor sites on effector cells. Brompheniramine also has anticholinergic (drying) and sedative effects. Among the antihistaminic effects, it antagonizes the allergic response (vasodilatation, increased vascular permeability, increased mucus secretion) of nasal tissue. Brompheniramine is well absorbed from the gastrointestinal tract, with peak plasma concentration after a single oral dose of 4 mg reached in 5 hours; urinary excretion is the major route of elimination, mostly as products of biodegradation; the liver is assumed to be the main site of metabolic transformation.

Phenylpropanolamine hydrochloride is a sympathomimetic drug which is readily absorbed from the gastrointestinal tract and produces nasal vasoconstriction (decongestion). Phenylpropanolamine stimulates both α and β-adrenergic receptors, similar to ephedrine. Part of its peripheral action is indirect and is due to the displacement of norepinephrine from storage sites, but it also has direct effect on the adrenergic receptors.

Codeine is an opiate analgesic and antitussive. Codeine calms the cough control center.

INDICATIONS AND USAGE

For relief of coughs and upper respiratory symptoms, including nasal congestion, associated with allergy or the common cold.

CONTRAINDICATIONS

Hypersensitivity to any of the ingredients. Do not use in the newborn, in premature infants, in nursing mothers, in patients with severe hypertension or severe coronary artery disease, or in those receiving monoamine oxidase (MAO) inhibitors.

Antihistamines should not be used to treat lower respiratory tract conditions including asthma.

WARNINGS

Especially in infants and small children, antihistamines in overdosage may cause hallucinations, convulsions, death. Codeine may cause or aggravate constipation.

Antihistamines may diminish mental alertness. In the young child, they may produce excitation.

PRECAUTIONS

General: Because of its antihistamine component, Dimetane-DC Cough Syrup should be used with caution in patients with a history of bronchial asthma, narrow angle glaucoma, gastrointestinal obstruction, or urinary bladder neck obstruction. Because of its sympathomimetic component, Dimetane-DC Cough Syrup should be used with caution in patients with diabetes, hypertension, heart disease, or thyroid disease.

Information for Patients: Patients should be warned about engaging in activities requiring mental alertness, such as driving a car or operating dangerous machinery.

Drug Interactions: Antihistamines have additive effects with alcohol and other CNS depressants (hypnotics, sedatives, tranquilizers, antianxiety agents, etc.). MAO inhibitors prolong and intensify the anticholinergic (drying) effects of antihistamines. MAO inhibitors may enhance the effect of phenylpropanolamine. Sympathomimetics may reduce the effects of antihypertensive drugs.

Carcinogenesis, Mutagenesis: Long-term studies in animals to evaluate carcinogenic and mutagenic potential have not been performed.

Pregnancy Category C: Animal reproduction studies have not been conducted with Dimetane-DC Cough Syrup. It is also not known whether Dimetane-DC Cough Syrup can cause fetal harm when administered to a pregnant woman or can affect reproduction capacity. Dimetane-DC Cough Syrup should be given to a pregnant woman only if clearly needed. Reproduction studies of brompheniramine maleate (one of the components of the Dimetane formulations) in rats and mice at doses up to 16 times the maximum human dose have revealed no evidence of impaired fertility or harm to the fetus.

Nursing Mothers: Because of the higher risk of intolerance of antihistamines in small infants generally, and in newborns and prematures in particular, and the fact that codeine appears in human milk, Dimetane-DC Cough Syrup is contraindicated in nursing mothers.

ADVERSE REACTIONS

The most frequent adverse reactions to Dimetane-DC Cough Syrup are: sedation; dryness of mouth, nose and throat; thickening of bronchial secretions; dizziness. Other adverse reactions may include:

Dermatologic: Urticaria, drug rash, photosensitivity, pruritus.

Cardiovascular System: Hypotension, hypertension, cardiac arrhythmias.

CNS: Disturbed coordination, tremor, irritability, insomnia, visual disturbances, weakness, nervousness, convulsions, headache, euphoria, and dysphoria.

G. U. System: Urinary frequency, difficult urination.

G. I. System: Epigastric discomfort, anorexia, nausea, vomiting, diarrhea, constipation.

Respiratory System: Tightness of chest and wheezing, shortness of breath. At higher doses, codeine has most of the disadvantages of morphine including respiratory depression.

Hematologic System: Hemolytic anemia, thrombocytopenia, agranulocytosis.

DRUG ABUSE AND DEPENDENCE

Codeine can produce drug dependence of the morphine type, and therefore has the potential for being abused. Psychic dependence, physical dependence and tolerance may develop upon repeated administration of this drug, and it should be prescribed and administered with the same degree of caution appropriate to the use of other oral narcotic medications. Dimetane-DC Cough Syrup is subject to the Federal Controlled Substances Act (Schedule V).

OVERDOSAGE

Signs and Symptoms: Serious overdose with codeine is characterized by respiratory depression, extreme somnolence progressing to stupor or coma. In severe overdosage, apnea, circulatory collapse, cardiac arrest and death may occur. The central nervous system effects from overdosage of brompheniramine may vary from depression to stimulation. Anticholinergic effects may also occur. Overdosage of phenylpropanolamine may be associated with tachycardia, hypertension and cardiac arrhythmias.

Toxic Doses: Doses of 800 mg or more of codeine have caused partial loss of consciousness, delirium, restlessness, excitement, tremors, convulsions and collapse; or respiratory paralysis with such sequelae as mydriasis, marked vasodilatation, and finally death. A 2½-year-old child survived a dose of 300–900 mg of brompheniramine; the lethal dose of phenylpropanolamine is in the range of 50 mg/kg.

Treatment: Respiratory depression should be treated promptly. Oxygen, intravenous fluids, vasopressors and other supportive measures should be employed as indicated. If necessary, reestablishment of adequate respiratory exchange through provision of a patent airway and the institution of assisted or controlled ventilation must be provided. The narcotic antagonist, naloxone, is a specific antidote to codeine-induced respiratory depression, and should be administered by the intravenous route if appropriate (see package insert for naloxone). Since the duration of action of codeine may exceed that of the antagonist, the patient should be kept under constant surveillance.

Gastric emptying may be useful in removing unabsorbed drug, either by inducing emesis or lavage; precautions against aspiration must be taken. Stimulants or depressants should be used cautiously and only when specifically indicated. If marked excitement is present, one of the short-acting barbiturates or chloral hydrate may be used.

DOSAGE AND ADMINISTRATION

Adults and children 12 years of age and over: 2 teaspoonfuls every 4 hours. Children 6 to under 12 years: 1 teaspoonful every 4 hours. Children 2 to under 6 years: ½ teaspoonful every 4 hours. Children 6 months to under 2 years: Dosage to be established by physician.

Do not exceed 6 doses during a 24-hour period.

HOW SUPPLIED

Dimetane-DC Cough Syrup is a light bluish-pink syrup containing in each 5 mL (1 teaspoonful): brompheniramine maleate 2 mg, phenylpropanolamine HCl 12.5 mg, and codeine phosphate 10 mg; available in pints (NDC 0031-1833-25) and gallons (NDC 0031-1833-29).

Store at controlled room temperature, between 15°C and 30°C (59°F and 86°F).

Dispense in tight, light-resistant container.

DIMETANE®-DX Cough Syrup ℞
[di'mĕ-tāne]

DESCRIPTION

Dimetane-DX Cough Syrup is a light-red syrup with a butterscotch flavor.

Each 5 mL (1 teaspoonful) contains:
Brompheniramine Maleate, USP .... 2 mg
Pseudoephedrine Hydrochloride, USP .... 30 mg
Dextromethorphan Hydrobromide, USP .... 10 mg
Alcohol 0.95 percent
in a palatable, aromatic vehicle.

Inactive Ingredients: Citric Acid, FD&C Red 40, FD&C Yellow 6, Flavors, Glycerin, Saccharin Sodium, Sodium Benzoate, Sorbitol, Water.

Antihistamine/Nasal Decongestant/Antitussive syrup for oral administration.

CLINICAL PHARMACOLOGY

Brompheniramine maleate is a histamine antagonist, specifically an H_1-receptor-blocking agent belonging to the alkylamine class of antihistamines. Antihistamines appear to compete with histamine for receptor sites on effector cells. Brompheniramine also has anticholinergic (drying) and sedative effects. Among the antihistaminic effects, it antagonizes the allergic response (vasodilatation, increased vascular permeability, increased mucus secretion) of nasal tissue. Brompheniramine is well absorbed from the gastrointestinal tract, with peak plasma concentration after single, oral dose of 4 mg reached in 5 hours; urinary excretion is the major route of elimination, mostly as products of biodegradation; the liver is assumed to be the main site of metabolic transformation.

Pseudoephedrine acts on sympathetic nerve endings and also on smooth muscle, making it useful as a nasal decongestant. The nasal decongestant effect is mediated by the action of pseudoephedrine on α-sympathetic receptors, producing vasoconstriction of the dilated nasal arterioles. Following

Continued on next page

Prescribing information on A. H. Robins products listed here is based on official labeling in effect June 1, 1986, with Indications, Contraindications, Warnings, Precautions, Adverse Reactions, and Dosage stated in full.

Robins—Cont.

oral administration, effects are noted within 30 minutes with peak activity occurring at approximately one hour.
Dextromethorphan acts centrally to elevate the threshold for coughing. It has no analgesic or addictive properties. The onset of antitussive action occurs in 15 to 30 minutes after administration and is of long duration.

INDICATIONS AND USAGE
For relief of coughs and upper respiratory symptoms, including nasal congestion, associated with allergy or the common cold.

CONTRAINDICATIONS
Hypersensitivity to any of the ingredients. Do not use in the newborn, in premature infants, in nursing mothers, in patients with severe hypertension or severe coronary artery disease, or in those receiving monoamine oxidase (MAO) inhibitors.
Antihistamines should not be used to treat lower respiratory tract conditions including asthma.

WARNINGS
Especially in infants and small children, antihistamines in overdosage may cause hallucinations, convulsions, and death.
Antihistamines may diminish mental alertness. In the young child, they may produce excitation.

PRECAUTIONS
General: Because of its antihistamine component, Dimetane-DX Cough Syrup should be used with caution in patients with a history of bronchial asthma, narrow angle glaucoma, gastrointestinal obstruction, or urinary bladder neck obstruction. Because of its sympathomimetic component, Dimetane-DX Cough Syrup should be used with caution in patients with diabetes, hypertension, heart disease, or thyroid disease.
Information for Patients: Patients should be warned about engaging in activities requiring mental alertness, such as driving a car or operating dangerous machinery.
Drug Interactions: Antihistamines have additive effects with alcohol and other CNS depressants (hypnotics, sedatives, tranquilizers, antianxiety agents, etc.) MAO inhibitors prolong and intensify the anticholinergic (drying) effects of antihistamines. MAO inhibitors may enhance the effect of pseudoephedrine. Sympathomimetics may reduce the effects of antihypertensive drugs.
Carcinogenesis, Mutagenesis, Impairment of Fertility
Animal studies of Dimetane-DX Cough Syrup to assess the carcinogenic and mutagenic potential or the effect on fertility have not been performed.
Pregnancy
Teratogenic Effects—Pregnancy Category C
Animal reproduction studies have not been conducted with Dimetane-DX Cough Syrup. It is also not known whether Dimetane-DX Cough Syrup can cause fetal harm when administered to a pregnant woman or can affect reproduction capacity. Dimetane-DX Cough Syrup should be given to a pregnant woman only if clearly needed.
Reproduction studies of brompheniramine maleate (a component of Dimetane-DX Cough Syrup) in rats and mice at doses up to 16 times the maximum human dose have revealed no evidence of impaired fertility or harm to the fetus.
Nursing Mothers: Because of the higher risk of intolerance of antihistamines in small infants generally, and in newborns and prematures in particular. Dimetane-DX Cough Syrup is contraindicated in nursing mothers.

ADVERSE REACTIONS
The most frequent adverse reactions to Dimetane-DX Cough Syrup are: sedation; dryness of mouth, nose and throat; thickening of bronchial secretions; dizziness. Other adverse reactions may include:
Dermatologic: Urticaria, drug rash, photosensitivity, pruritus.
Cardiovascular System: Hypotension, hypertension, cardiac arrhythmias, palpitation.
CNS: Disturbed coordination, tremor, irritability, insomnia, visual disturbances, weakness, nervousness, convulsions, headache, euphoria, and dysphoria.
G. U. System: Urinary frequency difficult urination.
G. I. System: Epigastric discomfort, anorexia, nausea, vomiting, diarrhea, constipation.
Respiratory System: Tightness of chest and wheezing, shortness of breath.
Hematologic System: Hemolytic anemia, thrombocytopenia, agranulocytosis.

OVERDOSAGE
Signs and Symptoms: Central nervous system effects from overdosage of brompheniramine may vary from depression to stimulation, especially in children. Anticholinergic effects may be noted. Toxic doses of pseudoephedrine may result in CNS stimulation, tachycardia, hypertension, and cardiac arrhythmias; signs of CNS depression may occasionally be seen. Dextromethorphan in toxic doses will cause drowsiness, ataxia, nystagmus, opisthotonos, and convulsive seizures.
Toxic Doses: Data suggest that individuals may respond in an unexpected manner to apparently small amounts of a particular drug. A 2½-year-old child survived the ingestion of 21 mg/kg of dextromethorphan exhibiting only ataxia, drowsiness, and fever, but seizures have been reported in 2 children following the ingestion of 13–17 mg/kg. Another 2½-year-old child survived a dose of 300–900 mg of brompheniramine. The toxic dose of pseudoephedrine should be less than that of ephedrine, which is estimated to be 50 mg/kg.
Treatment: Induce emesis if patient is alert and is seen prior to 6 hours following ingestion. Precautions against aspiration must be taken, especially in infants and small children. Gastric lavage may be carried out, although in some instances tracheostomy may be necessary prior to lavage. Naloxone hydrochloride 0.005 mg/kg intravenously may be of value in reversing the CNS depression that may occur from an overdose of dextromethorphan. CNS stimulants may counter CNS depression. Should CNS hyperactivity or convulsive seizures occur, intravenous short-acting barbiturates may be indicated. Hypertensive responses and/or tachycardia should be treated appropriately. Oxygen, intravenous fluids, and other supportive measures should be employed as indicated.

DOSAGE AND ADMINISTRATION
Adults and children 12 years of age and over: 2 teaspoonfuls every 4 hours. Children 6 to under 12 years: 1 teaspoonful every 4 hours. Children 2 to under 6 years: ½ teaspoonful every 4 hours. Children 6 months to under 2 years: Dosage to be established by physician.
Do not exceed 6 doses during a 24-hour period.

HOW SUPPLIED
Dimetane-DX Cough Syrup is a light-red syrup containing in each 5 mL (1 teaspoonful) brompheniramine maleate 2 mg, pseudoephedrine hydrochloride 30 mg and dextromethorphan hydrobromide 10 mg, available in pints (NDC 0031-1836-25).
Store at controlled room temperature, between 15°C and 30°C (59°F and 86°F).
Dispense in tight, light-resistant container.

DIMETAPP® ELIXIR
[di ′mĕ-tap]

(See PDR For Nonprescription Drugs)

DIMETAPP EXTENTABS®
[di ′mĕ-tap eks ″tĕn ′tabs]

(See PDR Nonprescription Drugs)

DONNAGEL®-PG Ⓒ
[don ′nă-gel]

DESCRIPTION
Each fluid ounce (2 tablespoonfuls) contains:
Powdered Opium, USP or equivalent 24.0 mg. (Warning: May be habit forming), Kaolin, USP 6.0 g, Pectin, USP 142.8 mg, Hyoscyamine Sulfate, USP 0.1037 mg, Atropine Sulfate, USP 0.0194 mg, Scopolamine Hydrobromide, USP 0.0065 mg, Sodium Benzoate, NF 60.0 mg (preservative), Alcohol 5.0 per cent.
Inactive Ingredients: Citric Acid, D&C Yellow 10, Flavors, High Fructose Corn Syrup, Sodium Carboxymethylcellulose, Sodium Chloride, Water.
Donnagel-PG combines the effects of kaolin, pectin and the natural belladonna alkaloids with the efficacy of powdered opium (or equivalent). The opium content in one fluid ounce of Donnagel-PG is equivalent to 5 mL of paregoric.

INDICATIONS
Donnagel-PG is indicated for the treatment of diarrhea.

WARNINGS TO PATIENT
Diarrhea may be serious. Do not use for more than two days or in the presence of high fever. Not to be used by persons having glaucoma or excessive pressure within the eye, by elderly persons (where undiagnosed glaucoma or excessive pressure within the eye occurs most frequently), or by children under 6 years of age, unless directed by a physician. Discontinue use if blurring of vision, rapid pulse, or dizziness occurs. Do not exceed recommended dosage. Not for frequent or prolonged use. If dryness of the mouth occurs, decrease dosage. If eye pain occurs, discontinue use and see your physician immediately as this may indicate undiagnosed glaucoma.

RECOMMENDED DOSAGE
Adults and children 12 years of age and over: two tablespoonfuls (one fl. oz.) initially, followed by 1 tablespoonful every 3 hours; Children 6 to under 12 years: two teaspoonfuls initially and 1 or 2 teaspoonfuls every 3 hours thereafter. Do not take more than 4 doses in any 24-hour period.

HOW SUPPLIED
Donnagel-PG (light yellow, banana-flavored suspension) in 6 fl. oz. (NDC 0031-3083-15) and pint (NDC 0031-3083-25).

DONNATAL® TABLETS ℞
DONNATAL® CAPSULES ℞
DONNATAL® ELIXIR ℞
[don ′nă-tal]

PRODUCT OVERVIEW

KEY FACTS
This drug combination provides natural belladonna alkaloids in a specific, fixed ratio combined with phenobarbital to provide peripheral anticholinergic/antispasmodic action and mild sedation.

MAJOR USES
For use as adjunctive therapy in the treatment of irritable bowel syndrome and acute enterocolitis.

SAFETY INFORMATION
The signs and symptoms of overdose are headache, nausea, vomiting, blurred vision, dilated pupils, hot and dry skin, dizziness, dryness of the mouth, difficulty in swallowing, CNS stimulation.

PRESCRIBING INFORMATION

DONNATAL® TABLETS ℞
DONNATAL® CAPSULES ℞
DONNATAL® ELIXIR ℞
[don ′nă-tal]

DESCRIPTION
Each Donnatal tablet, capsule or 5 mL (teaspoonful) of elixir (23% alcohol) contains:

Phenobarbital, USP (¼ gr)	16.2 mg
(Warning: May be habit forming)	
Hyoscyamine Sulfate, USP	0.1037 mg
Atropine Sulfate, USP	0.0194 mg
Scopolamine Hydrobromide, USP	0.0065 mg

Inactive Ingredients:
TABLETS: Dibasic Calcium Phosphate, Magnesium Stearate, Microcrystalline Cellulose, Silicon Dioxide, Sodium Starch Glycolate, Stearic Acid, Sucrose. May contain Corn Starch, Dextrose, or Invert Sugar.
CAPSULES: Corn Starch, Edible Ink, D&C Yellow 10 and FD&C Green 3 or FD&C Blue 1 and FD&C Yellow 6, FD&C Blue 2 Aluminum Lake, Gelatin, Lactose, Sucrose. May contain FD&C Red 40 and Yellow 6 Aluminum Lakes.
ELIXIR: D&C Yellow 10, FD&C Blue 1, FD&C Yellow 6, Flavors, Glucose, Saccharin Sodium, Water.

ACTIONS
This drug combination provides natural belladonna alkaloids in a specific, fixed ratio combined with phenobarbital to provide peripheral anticholinergic/antispasmodic action and mild sedation.

Indications
Based on a review of this drug by the National Academy of Sciences—National Research Council and/or other information, FDA has classified the following indications as "possibly" effective:
For use as adjunctive therapy in the treatment of irritable bowel syndrome (irritable colon, spastic colon, mucous colitis) and acute enterocolitis.
May also be useful as adjunctive therapy in the treatment of duodenal ulcer. IT HAS NOT BEEN SHOWN CONCLUSIVELY WHETHER ANTICHOLINERGIC/ANTISPASMODIC DRUGS AID IN THE HEALING OF A DUODENAL ULCER, DECREASE THE RATE OF RECURRENCES OR PREVENT COMPLICATIONS.

CONTRAINDICATIONS
Glaucoma, obstructive uropathy (for example, bladder neck obstruction due to prostatic hypertrophy); obstructive disease of the gastrointestinal tract (as in achalasia, pyloroduodenal stenosis, etc.); paralytic ileus, intestinal atony of the elderly or debilitated patient; unstable cardiovascular status in acute hemorrhage; severe ulcerative colitis especially if complicated by toxic megacolon; myasthenia gravis; hiatal hernia associated with reflux esophagitis.
Donnatal is contraindicated in patients with known hypersensitivity to any of the ingredients. Phenobarbital is contraindicated in acute intermittent porphyria and in those patients in whom phenobarbital produces restlessness and/or excitement.

WARNINGS

In the presence of a high environmental temperature, heat prostration can occur with belladonna alkaloids (fever and heatstroke due to decreased sweating).

Diarrhea may be an early symptom of incomplete intestinal obstruction, especially in patients with ileostomy or colostomy. In this instance treatment with this drug would be inappropriate and possibly harmful.

Donnatal may produce drowsiness or blurred vision. The patient should be warned, should these occur, not to engage in activities requiring mental alertness, such as operating a motor vehicle or other machinery, and not to perform hazardous work.

Phenobarbital may decrease the effect of anticoagulants, and necessitate larger doses of the anticoagulant for optimal effect. When the phenobarbital is discontinued, the dose of the anticoagulant may have to be decreased.

Phenobarbital may be habit forming and should not be administered to individuals known to be addiction prone or to those with a history of physical and/or psychological dependence upon drugs.

Since barbiturates are metabolized in the liver, they should be used with caution and initial doses should be small in patients with hepatic dysfunction.

PRECAUTIONS

Use with caution in patients with: autonomic neuropathy, hepatic or renal disease, hyperthyroidism, coronary heart disease, congestive heart failure, cardiac arrhythmias, tachycardia, and hypertension.

Belladonna alkaloids may produce a delay in gastric emptying (antral stasis) which would complicate the management of gastric ulcer.

Theoretically, with overdosage, a curare-like action may occur.

Carcinogenesis, mutagenesis. Long-term studies in animals have not been performed to evaluate carcinogenic potential.

Pregnancy Category C. Animal reproduction studies have not been conducted with Donnatal. It is not known whether Donnatal can cause fetal harm when administered to a pregnant woman or can affect reproduction capacity. Donnatal should be given to a pregnant woman only if clearly needed.

Nursing mothers. It is not known whether this drug is excreted in human milk. Because many drugs are excreted in human milk, caution should be exercised when Donnatal is administered to a nursing mother.

ADVERSE REACTIONS

Adverse reactions may include xerostomia; urinary hesitancy and retention; blurred vision; tachycardia; palpitation; mydriasis; cycloplegia; increased ocular tension; loss of taste sense, headache, nervousness; drowsiness; weakness; dizziness; insomnia; nausea; vomiting; impotence; suppression of lactation; constipation; bloated feeling; musculoskeletal pain; severe allergic reaction or drug idiosyncrasies, including anaphylaxis, urticaria and other dermal manifestations; and decreased sweating. Elderly patients may react with symptoms of excitement, agitation, drowsiness, and other untoward manifestations to even small doses of the drug.

Phenobarbital may produce excitement in some patients, rather than a sedative effect. In patients habituated to barbiturates, abrupt withdrawal may produce delirium or convulsions.

DOSAGE AND ADMINISTRATION

The dosage of Donnatal should be adjusted to the needs of the individual patient to assure symptomatic control with a minimum of adverse effects.

Donnatal Tablets or Capsules. Adults: One or two Donnatal tablets or capsules three or four times a day according to condition and severity of symptoms.

Donnatal Elixir. Adults: One or two teaspoonfuls of elixir three or four times a day according to conditions and severity of symptoms.

Children (Elixir)—may be dosed every 4 or 6 hours.:

Body Weight	Starting Dosage q4h	q6h
10 lb (4.5 kg)	0.5 mL	0.75 mL
20 lb (9.1 kg)	1.0 mL	1.5 mL
30 lb (13.6 kg)	1.5 mL	2.0 mL
50 lb (22.7 kg)	½ tsp	¾ tsp
75 lb (34.0 kg)	¾ tsp	1 tsp
100 lb (45.4 kg)	1 tsp	1½ tsp

OVERDOSAGE

The signs and symptoms of overdose are headache, nausea, vomiting, blurred vision, dilated pupils, hot and dry skin, dizziness, dryness of the mouth, difficulty in swallowing, CNS stimulation. Treatment should consist of gastric lavage, emetics, and activated charcoal. If indicated, parenteral cholinergic agents such as physostigmine or bethanechol chloride, should be added.

HOW SUPPLIED

Donnatal Tablets. White, compressed, embossed "R" on one side, scored and engraved 4250 on the reverse side; in bottles of 100 (NDC 0031-4250-63), 1000 (NDC 0031-4250-74) and Dis-Co® Unit Dose Packs of 100 (NDC 0031-4250-64).

Donnatal Capsules. Green and white, monogrammed "AHR" and "4207"; in bottles of 100 (NDC 0031-4207-63) and 1000 (NDC 0031-4207-74).

Donnatal Elixir. Green, citrus flavored, in 4 fl. oz. (NDC 0031-4221-12), pints (NDC 0031-4221-25), gallons (NDC 0031-4221-29) and 5 mL Dis-Co® Unit Dose Packs (4 × 25s) (NDC 0031-4221-13).

Store at controlled room temperature, between 15°C and 30°C (59°F and 86°F).

Dispense in tight, light-resistant container.

Shown in Product Identification Section, page 424

DONNATAL EXTENTABS® ℞

[*don'nă-tal ĕks"tĕn'tabs*]

DESCRIPTION

Each Donnatal Extentabs Tablet contains:

Phenobarbital, USP (¾gr) ....48.6 mg
(Warning: May be habit forming)
Hyoscyamine Sulfate, USP ....0.3111 mg
Atropine Sulfate, USP ....0.0582 mg
Scopolamine Hydrobromide, USP ....0.0195 mg

Each Donnatal Extentabs tablet contains the equivalent of three Donnatal tablets. Extentabs are designed to release the ingredients gradually to provide effects for up to twelve (12) hours.

Inactive Ingredients: Acacia, Acetylated Monoglycerides, Calcium Sulfate, Carnauba Wax, D&C Yellow 10, Edible Ink, FD&C Blue 1, FD&C Blue 2 Aluminum Lake, FD&C Yellow 6, Gelatin, Guar Gum, Magnesium Stearate, Polysorbates, Shellac, Sodium Phosphate, Sucrose, Titanium Dioxide, Wheat Flour, White Wax and other ingredients, one of which is a corn derivative. May include FD&C Red 40 and Yellow 6 Aluminum Lakes.

ACTIONS

This drug combination provides natural belladonna alkaloids in a specific, fixed ratio combined with phenobarbital to provide peripheral anticholinergic/antispasmodic action and mild sedation.

Indications

Based on a review of this drug by the National Academy of Sciences—National Research Council and/or other information, FDA has classified the following indications as "possibly" effective:

For use as adjunctive therapy in the treatment of irritable bowel syndrome (irritable colon, spastic colon, mucous colitis) and acute enterocolitis.

May also be useful as adjunctive therapy in the treatment of duodenal ulcer. IT HAS NOT BEEN SHOWN CONCLUSIVELY WHETHER ANTICHOLINERGIC/ANTISPASMODIC DRUGS AID IN THE HEALING OF A DUODENAL ULCER, DECREASE THE RATE OF RECURRENCES OR PREVENT COMPLICATIONS.

CONTRAINDICATIONS

Glaucoma, obstructive uropathy (for example, bladder neck obstruction due to prostatic hypertrophy); obstructive disease of the gastrointestinal tract (as in achalasia, pyloroduodenal stenosis, etc.); paralytic ileus, intestinal atony of the elderly or debilitated patient; unstable cardiovascular status in acute hemorrhage; severe ulcerative colitis especially if complicated by toxic megacolon; myasthenia gravis, hiatal hernia associated with reflux esophagitis.

Donnatal is contraindicated in patients with known hypersensitivity to any of the ingredients. Phenobarbital is contraindicated in acute intermittent porphyria and in those patients in whom phenobarbital produces restlessness and/or excitement.

WARNINGS

In the presence of a high environmental temperature, heat prostration can occur with belladonna alkaloids (fever and heatstroke due to decreased sweating).

Diarrhea may be an early symptom of incomplete intestinal obstruction, especially in patients with ileostomy or colostomy. In this instance treatment with this drug would be inappropriate and possibly harmful.

Donnatal may produce drowsiness or blurred vision. The patient should be warned, should these occur, not to engage in activities requiring mental alertness, such as operating a motor vehicle or other machinery, and not to perform hazardous work.

Phenobarbital may decrease the effect of anticoagulants and necessitate larger doses of the anticoagulant for optimal effect. When the phenobarbital is discontinued, the dose of the anticoagulant may have to be decreased.

Phenobarbital may be habit forming and should not be administered to individuals known to be addiction prone or to those with a history of physical and/or psychological dependence upon drugs.

Since barbiturates are metabolized in the liver, they should be used with caution and initial doses should be small in patients with hepatic dysfunction.

PRECAUTIONS

Use with caution in patients with: autonomic neuropathy, hepatic or renal disease, hyperthyroidism, coronary heart disease, congestive heart failure, cardiac arrhythmias, tachycardia, and hypertension.

Belladonna alkaloids may produce a delay in gastric emptying (antral stasis) which would complicate the management of gastric ulcer.

Theoretically, with overdosage, a curare-like action may occur.

Carcinogenesis, mutagenesis. Long-term studies in animals have not been performed to evaluate carcinogenic potential.

Pregnancy Category C. Animal reproduction studies have not been conducted with Donnatal. It is not known whether Donnatal can cause fetal harm when administered to a pregnant woman or can affect reproduction capacity. Donnatal should be given to a pregnant woman only if clearly needed.

Nursing mothers. It is not known whether this drug is excreted in human milk. Because many drugs are excreted in human milk, caution should be exercised when Donnatal is administered to a nursing mother.

ADVERSE REACTIONS

Adverse reactions may include xerostomia; urinary hesitancy and retention; blurred vision; tachycardia; palpitation; mydriasis; cycloplegia; increased ocular tension; loss of taste sense; headache; nervousness; drowsiness; weakness; dizziness; insomnia; nausea; vomiting; impotence; suppression of lactation; constipation; bloated feeling; musculoskeletal pain; severe allergic reaction or drug idiosyncrasies, including anaphylaxis, urticaria and other dermal manifestations; and decreased sweating. Elderly patients may react with symptoms of excitement, agitation, drowsiness, and other untoward manifestations to even small doses of the drug.

Phenobarbital may produce excitement in some patients, rather than a sedative effect. In patients habituated to barbiturates, abrupt withdrawal may produce delirium or convulsions.

DOSAGE AND ADMINISTRATION

The dosage of Donnatal Extentabs should be adjusted to the needs of the individual patient to assure symptomatic control with a minimum of adverse reactions. The usual dose is one tablet every twelve (12) hours. If indicated, one tablet every eight (8) hours may be given.

OVERDOSAGE

The signs and symptoms of overdose are headache, nausea, vomiting, blurred vision, dilated pupils; hot and dry skin, dizziness, dryness of the mouth, difficulty in swallowing, CNS stimulation. Treatment should consist of gastric lavage, emetics, and activated charcoal. If indicated, parenteral cholinergic agents such as physostigmine or bethanechol chloride should be added.

HOW SUPPLIED

Pale green, coated tablets, monogrammed AHR and Donnatal Extentab in bottles of 100 (NDC 0031-4235-63) and 500 (NDC 0031-4235-70); and Dis-Co® Unit Dose Packs of 100 (NDC 0031-4235-64).

Store at controlled room temperature, between 15°C and 30°C (59°F and 86°F).

Dispense in well-closed, light-resistant container.

Shown in Product Identification Section, page 424

DONNAZYME® TABLETS ℞

[*don'nă" zīm*]

DESCRIPTION

Donnazyme tablets are available for oral administration. Each tablet contains:

Pancreatin, USP equivalent ....300 mg
Pepsin ....150 mg
Bile Salts ....150 mg
Hyoscyamine Sulfate, USP ....0.0518 mg
Atropine Sulfate, USP ....0.0097 mg
Scopolamine Hydrobromide, USP ....0.0033 mg
Phenobarbital, USP (⅛ gr) ....8.1 mg
(Warning: may be habit forming)

Inactive Ingredients: Acacia, Acetylated Monoglycerides, Calcium Sulfate, Carnauba Wax, Cellulose Acetate Phthalate, Corn Starch, D&C Yellow 10 Aluminum Lake, Diethyl Phthalate, Edible Ink, FD&C Blue 1 Aluminum Lake, FD&C

Continued on next page

Prescribing information on A. H. Robins products listed here is based on official labeling in effect June 1, 1986, with Indications, Contraindications, Warnings, Precautions, Adverse Reactions, and Dosage stated in full.

Robins—Cont.

Yellow 6 Aluminum Lake, Gelatin, Methylparaben, Microcrystalline Cellulose, Polysorbates, Povidone, Propylparaben, Shellac, Sodium Benzoate, Stearic Acid, Sucrose, Tartaric Acid, Titanium Dioxide, Wheat Flour, White Wax. May contain Docusate Sodium.
The combination of anticholinergic/antispasmodic/sedative components with natural digestive enzymes plus bile salts makes it useful for symptomatic relief of functional G.I. disorders.

CLINICAL PHARMACOLOGY

The outer layer of Donnazyme tablets is gastric-soluble and contains the belladonna alkaloids, phenobarbital and pepsin. These ingredients rapidly become available for absorption as the tablet begins disintegrating in the stomach. The pepsin supplements the stomach's digestive secretions by aiding the breakdown of proteins into proteoses and peptones. Spasmolysis and sedation are produced as the belladonna alkaloids and phenobarbital are absorbed.
The core of the tablet contains pancreatin and bile salts. It is designed to disintegrate in the alkaline medium of the duodenum where it releases the active enzyme components of pancreatin (trypsin, amylase and lipase), along with the bile salts. Trypsin breaks down larger protein fractions into peptides; amylase converts starch into maltose; lipase splits fat into fatty acids and glycerin; and bile salts enhance the fat-splitting action of the lipase and aid in the emulsification of fats and the absorption of fatty acids.

INDICATIONS AND USAGE

Donnazyme is indicated for the relief of symptoms associated with "nervous indigestion" and other functional G.I. disorders in the absence of organic pathology. Some of these conditions are chronic pancreatitis, chronic gastritis, post-cholecystectomy syndrome, and chronic biliary disorders. Donnazyme may prove especially useful in patients with decreased digestive enzyme secretory activity, which is frequently suspect in older patients with visceral complaints.

CONTRAINDICATIONS

Glaucoma, obstructive uropathy (for example, bladder neck obstruction due to prostatic hypertrophy); obstructive disease of the gastrointestinal tract (as in achalasia, pyloroduodenal stenosis, etc.); paralytic ileus, intestinal atony of the elderly or debilitated patient, unstable cardiovascular status in acute hemorrhage, severe ulcerative colitis especially if complicated by toxic megacolon; myasthenia gravis; hiatal hernia associated with reflux esophagitis.
Donnazyme is contraindicated in patients with known hypersensitivity to any of the ingredients. Phenobarbital is contraindicated in acute intermittent porphyria and in those patients in whom phenobarbital produces restlessness and /or excitement.

WARNINGS

In the presence of a high environmental temperature, heat prostration can occur with belladonna alkaloids (fever and heatstroke due to decreased sweating).
Diarrhea may be an early symptom of incomplete intestinal obstruction, especially in patients with ileostomy or colostomy. In this instance, treatment with this drug would be inappropriate and possibly harmful.
Donnazyme may produce drowsiness or blurred vision. The patient should be warned, should these occur, not to engage in activities requiring mental alertness, such as operating a motor vehicle or other machinery, and not to perform hazardous work.
Phenobarbital may decrease the effect of anticoagulants and necessitate larger doses of the anticoagulant for optimal effect. When the phenobarbital is discontinued, the dose of the anticoagulant may have to be decreased.
Phenobarbital may be habit forming and should not be administered to individuals known to be addiction prone or to those with a history of physical and/or psychological dependence upon drugs.
Since barbiturates are metabolized in the liver, they should be used with caution and initial small doses in patients with hepatic dysfunction.

PRECAUTIONS

General. Use with caution in patients with autonomic neuropathy, hepatic or renal disease, hyperthyroidism, coronary heart disease, congestive heart failure, cardiac arrhythmias, tachycardia, and hypertension.
Belladonna alkaloids may produce a delay in gastric emptying (antral stasis) which would complicate the management of gastric ulcer.
Theoretically, with overdosage, a curare-like action may occur.
Carcinogenesis, mutagenesis: Long-term studies in animals have not been performed to evaluate carcinogenic potential.
Pregnancy Category C. Animal reproduction studies have not been conducted with Donnazyme. It is not known whether Donnazyme can cause fetal harm when administered to a pregnant woman or can affect reproduction capacity. Donnazyme should be given to a pregnant woman only if clearly needed.
Nursing mothers: It is not known whether this drug is excreted in human milk. Because many drugs are excreted in human milk, caution should be exercised when Donnazyme is administered to a nursing mother.
Pediatric Use: Safety and effectiveness in children have not been established.

ADVERSE REACTIONS

Adverse reactions may include xerostomia; urinary hesitancy and retention; blurred vision; tachycardia; palpitation; mydriasis; cycloplegia; increased ocular tension; loss of taste sense; headache; nervousness; drowsiness; weakness, dizziness, insomnia; nausea; vomiting; impotence; suppression of lactation; constipation; bloated feeling; musculoskeletal pain; severe allergic reaction or drug idiosyncrasies, including "anaphylaxis, urticaria and other dermal manifestations; and decreased sweating." Elderly patients may react with symptoms of excitement, agitation, drowsiness, and other untoward manifestations to even small doses of the drug.
Phenobarbital may produce excitement in some patients, rather than a sedative effect. In patients habituated to barbiturates, abrupt withdrawal may produce delirium or convulsions.

OVERDOSAGE

The signs and symptoms of overdose are headache, nausea, vomiting, blurred vision, dilated pupils, hot and dry skin, dizziness, dryness of the mouth, difficulty in swallowing, CNS stimulation. Treatment should consist of gastric lavage, emetics, and activated charcoal. If indicated, parenteral cholinergic agents, such as physostigmine or bethanechol chloride, should be added.

DOSAGE AND ADMINISTRATION

Adult dosage: Two tablets after each meal.

HOW SUPPLIED

Kelly green tablets in bottles of 100 (NDC 0031-4649-63) and 500 (NDC 0031-4649-70). Store at controlled room temperature, between 15°C and 30°C (59°F and 86°F). Dispense in tight container.

Shown in Product Identification Section, page 424

DOPRAM® INJECTABLE ℞

[do' pram]
brand of Doxapram Hydrochloride Injection, USP

PRODUCT OVERVIEW

KEY FACTS

Dopram Injectable is a clear, colorless, sterile, non-pyrogenic, aqueous solution for intravenous injection. The respiratory stimulant action is manifested by an increase in tidal volume associated with a slight increase in respiratory rate. Due to its benzyl alcohol (preservative) content, Dopram Injectable should not be used in newborns.

MAJOR USES

Post Anesthesia: To stimulate respiration in patients with drug-induced respiratory depression or apnea other than that due to muscle relaxant drugs. To pharmacologically stimulate deep breathing.
Drug-Induced CNS Depression: To stimulate respiration, hasten arousal, and to encourage the return of laryngopharyngeal reflexes.
Chronic Plumonary Disease Associated with Acute Hypercapnia: To aid in the prevention of elevated arterial CO_2 tension during the administration of oxygen; restricted to a short period of time (approximately 2 hours).
Doxapram Hydrochloride is compatible wiith 5% and 10% dextrose in water or normal saline. Admixture of Doxapram with alkaline solutions such as 2.5% thiopental sodium, bicarbonate, or aminophylline will result in precipitation or gas formation.

SAFETY INFORMATION

Dopram Injectable should not be used in patients with convulsive disorders, mechanical disorders of ventilation, head injury, or cardiovascular impairment. Doxapram should not be used in conjunction with mechanical ventilation.

PRESCRIBING INFORMATION

DOPRAM® INJECTABLE ℞

[do'pram]
brand of Doxapram Hydrochloride Injection, USP

DESCRIPTION

Dopram Injectable (Doxapram Hydrochloride Injection, USP) is a clear, colorless, sterile, non-pyrogenic, aqueous solution with pH 3.5—5.0, for intravenous administration.
Each 1 mL contains:

Doxapram Hydrochloride, USP	20 mg.
Benzyl Alcohol, NF (as preservative)	0.9%
Water for Injection, USP	q.s.

Due to its benzyl alcohol content, Dopram Injectable should not be used in newborns.
Dopram Injectable is a respiratory stimulant.
Doxapram hydrochloride is a white to off-white, crystalline powder, sparingly soluble in water, alcohol and chloroform. It has the following chemical name:
1-ethyl-4-[2-(4-morpholinyl)ethyl]-3,3-diphenyl-2-pyrrolidinone monohydrochloride, monohydrate.

CLINICAL PHARMACOLOGY

Doxapram hydrochloride produces respiratory stimulation mediated through the peripheral carotid chemoreceptors. As the dosage level is increased, the central respiratory centers in the medulla are stimulated with progressive stimulation of other parts of the brain and spinal cord.
The onset of respiratory stimulation following the recommended single intravenous injection of doxapram hydrochloride usually occurs in 20–40 seconds with peak effect at 1–2 minutes. The duration of effect may vary from 5–12 minutes. The respiratory stimulant action is manifested by an increase in tidal volume associated with a slight increase in respiratory rate.
A pressor response may result following doxapram administration. Provided there is no impairment of cardiac function, the pressor effect is more marked in hypovolemic than in normovolemic states. The pressor response is due to the improved cardiac output rather than peripheral vasoconstriction. Following doxapram administration an increased release of catecholamines has been noted.
Although opiate induced respiratory depression is antagonized by doxapram, the analgesic effect is not affected.

INDICATIONS

1. ***Post-anesthesia.***
   a. When the possibility of airway obstruction and/or hypoxia have been eliminated, doxapram may be used to stimulate respiration in patients with drug-induced post-anesthesia respiratory depression or apnea other than that due to muscle relaxant drugs.
   b. To pharmacologically stimulate deep breathing in the so-called "stir-up" regimen in the postoperative patient. (Simultaneous administration of oxygen is desirable.)
2. ***Drug-induced central nervous system depression.*** Exercising care to prevent vomiting and aspiration, doxapram may be used to stimulate respiration, hasten arousal, and to encourage the return of laryngopharyngeal reflexes in patients with mild to moderate respiratory and CNS depression due to drug overdosage.
3. ***Chronic pulmonary disease associated with acute hypercapnia.*** Doxaram is indicated as a temporary measure in hospitalized patients with acute respiratory insufficiency superimposed on chronic obstructive pulmonary disease. Its use should be for a short period of time (approximately 2 hours) as an aid in the prevention of elevation of arterial CO_2 tension during the administration of oxygen. It should not be used in conjuction with mechanical ventilation.

CONTRAINDICATIONS

Due to its benzyl alcohol content, Dopram Injectable should not be used in newborns.
Doxapram should not be used in patients with epilepsy or other convulsive disorders.
Doxapram is contraindicated in patients with mechanical disorders of ventilation such as mechanical obstruction, muscle paresis, flail chest, pneumothorax, acute bronchial asthma, pulmonary fibrosis or other conditions resulting in restriction of chest wall, muscles of respiration or alveolar expansion.
Doxapram is contraindicated in patients with evidence of head injury or cerebral vascular accident and in those with significant cardiovascular impairment, severe hypertension, or known hypersensitivity to the drug.

WARNINGS

1. ***Warning in post-anesthetic use.***
   a. Doxapram is neither an antagonist to muscle relaxant drugs nor a specific narcotic antagonist. Adequacy of airway and oxygenation must be assured prior to doxapram administration.
   b. Doxapram should be administered with great care and only under careful supervision to patients with hypermetabolic states such as hyperthyroidism or pheochromocytoma.
   c. Since narcosis may recur after stimulation with doxapram, care should be taken to maintain close observation until the patient has been fully alert for $\frac{1}{2}$ to 1 hour.
2. ***In drug-induced CNS and respiratory depression.*** Doxapram alone may not stimulate adequate spontaneous breathing or provide sufficient arousal in patients who are ***severely*** depressed either due to respiratory failure or to

CNS depressant drugs, but should be used as an adjunct to establish supportive measures and resuscitative techniques.

3. ***In chronic obstructive pulmonary disease.***
   a. Because of the associated increased work of breathing, do not increase the rate of infusion of doxapram in severely ill patients in an attempt to lower pCO_2.
   b. Doxapram should not be used in conjunction with mechanical ventilation.

PRECAUTIONS

1. ***General.***
   a. An adequate airway is essential.
   b. Recommended dosages of doxapram should be employed and maximum total dosages should not be exceeded. In order to avoid side effects, it is advisable to use the minimum effective dosage.
   c. Monitoring of the blood pressure and deep tendon reflexes is recommended to prevent overdosage.
   d. Vascular extravasation or use of a single injection site over an extended period should be avoided since either may lead to thrombophlebitis or local skin irritation.
   e. Rapid infusion may result in hemolysis.
   f. Lowered pCO_2 induced by hyperventilation produces cerebral vasoconstriction and slowing of the cerebral circulation. This should be taken into consideration on an individual basis.
   g. Intravenous short-acting barbiturates, oxygen and resuscitative equipment should be readily available to manage overdosage manifested by excessive central nervous system stimulation. Slow administration of the drug, and careful observation of the patient during administration and for some time subsequently, are advisable. These precautions are to assure that the protective reflexes have been restored and to prevent possible posthyperventilation hypoventilation.
   h. Doxapram should be administered cautiously to patients receiving sympathomimetic or monoamine oxidase inhibiting drugs, since an additive pressor effect may occur.
   i. Blood pressure increases are generally modest but significant increases have been noted in some patients. Because of this doxapram is not recommended for use in severe hypertension (see Contraindications).
   j. If sudden hypotension or dyspnea develops, doxapram should be stopped.
2. ***In postanesthetic use.***
   a. The same consideration to pre-existing disease states should be exercised as in non-anesthetized individuals. See Contraindications and Warnings covering use in hypertension, asthma, disturbances of respiratory mechanics including airway obstruction, CNS disorders including increased cerebrospinal fluid pressure, convulsive disorders, acute agitation, and profound metabolic disorders.
   b. See Drug Interactions.
3. ***In chronic obstructive pulmonary disease.***
   a. Arrhythmias seen in some patients in acute respiratory failure secondary to chronic obstructive pulmonary disease are probably the result of hypoxia. Doxapram should be used with caution in these patients.
   b. Arterial blood gases should be drawn prior to the initiation of doxapram infusion and oxygen administration, then at least every ½ hour. Doxapram administration does not diminish the need for careful monitoring of the patient or the need for supplemental oxygen in patients with acute respiratory failure. Doxapram should be stopped if the arterial blood gases deteriorate, and mechanical ventilation initiated.

Drug Interactions: Administration of doxapram to patients who are receiving sympathomimetic or monoamine oxidase inhibiting drugs may result in an additive pressor effect. (See Precautions).

Table I. Dopram Injectable Dosage for post-anesthetic use—I.V.

I.V. Administration	Recommended dosage mg/kg	mg/lb	Maximum dose per single injection mg/kg	mg/lb	Maximum total dose mg/kg	mg/lb
Single Injection	0.5–1.0	0.25–0.5	1.5	0.70	1.5	0.70
Repeat Injections (5 min. intervals)	0.5–1.0	0.25–0.5	1.5	0.70	2.0	1.0
Infusion	0.5–1.0	0.25–0.5	—	—	4.0	2.0

In patients who have received muscle relaxants, doxapram may temporarily mask the residual effects of muscle relaxant drugs.

In patients who have received anesthetics known to sensitize the myocardium to catecholamines, such as halothane, cyclopropane and enflurane, initiation of doxapram therapy should be delayed for at least 10 minutes following discontinuance of anesthesia, since an increase in epinephrine release has been noted with doxapram.

Carcinogenesis, mutagenesis, impairment of fertility. No carcinoenic or mutagenic studies have been performed using doxapram. Doxapram did not adversely affect the breeding performance of rats.

Pregnancy Category B. Reproduction studies have been performed in rats at doses up to 1.6 times the human dose and have revealed no evidence of impaired fertility or harm to the fetus due to doxapram. There are, however, no adequate and well-controlled studies in pregnant women. Since the animals in the reproduction studies were dosed by the IM and oral routes and animal reproduction studies, in general, are not always predictive of human response, this drug should be used during pregnancy only if clearly needed.

Nursing mothers. It is not known whether this drug is excreted in human milk. Because many drugs are excreted in human milk, caution should be exercised when doxapram hydrochloride is administered to a nursing mother.

Pedatric use. The use of the preservative benzyl alcohol in the newborn has been associated with metabolic, CNS, respiratory, circulatory, and renal dysfunction. Safety and effectiveness in children below the age of 12 years have not been established.

ADVERSE REACTIONS

The following adverse reactions have been reported:

1. ***Central and autonomic nervous systems.***
   Pyrexia, flushing, sweating; pruritus and paresthesia, such as a feeling of warmth, burning, or hot sensation, especially in the area of genitalia and perineum; apprehension, disorientation, pupillary dilatation, headache, dizziness, hyperactivity, involuntary movements, muscle spasticity, increased deep tendon reflexes, clonus, bilateral Babinski, and convulsions.
2. ***Respiratory***
   Dyspnea, cough, tachypnea, laryngospasm, bronchospasm, hiccough, and rebound hypoventilation.
3. ***Cardiovascular.***
   Phlebitis, variations in heart rate, lowered T-waves, arrhythmias, chest pain, tightness in chest. A mild to moderate increase in blood pressure is commonly noted and may be of concern in patients with severe cardiovascular diseases.
4. ***Gastrointestinal.***
   Nausea, vomiting, diarrhea, desire to defecate.
5. ***Genitourinary.***
   Stimulation of urinary bladder with spontaneous voiding; urinary retention.

6. ***Laboratory determinations.***
   A decrease in hemoglobin, hematocrit, or red blood cell count has been observed in postoperative patients. In the presence of pre-existing leukopenia, a further decrease in WBC has been observed following anesthesia and treatment with doxapram hydrochloride. Elevation of BUN and albuminuria have also been observed. As some of the patients cited above had received multiple drugs concomitantly, a cause and effect relationship could not be determined.

OVERDOSAGE

Signs and Symptoms. Symptoms of overdosage are extensions of the pharmacologic effects of the drug. Excessive pressor effect, tachycardia, skeletal muscle hyperactivity, and enhanced deep tendon reflexes may be early signs of overdosage. Therefore, the blood pressure, pulse rate and deep tendon reflexes should be evaluated periodically and the dosage or infusion rate adjusted accordingly.

Convulsive seizures are unlikely at recommended dosages. In unanethetized animals, the convulsant dose is 70 times greater than the respiratory stimulant dose. Intravenous LD_{50} values in the mouse and rat were approximately 75 mg/kg and in the cat and dog were 40–80 mg/kg.

Except for management of chronic obstructive pulmonary disease associated with acute hypercapnia, the maximum recommended dosage is 3 GRAMS/24 HOURS. (See Dosage and Administration.)

Management. There is no specific antidote for doxapram. Management should be symptomatic. Short-acting intravenous barbiturates, oxygen and resuscitative equipment should be used as needed for supportive treatment.

There is no evidence that doxapram is dialyzable; further, the half-life of doxapram makes it unlikely that dialysis would be appropriate in managing overdose with this drug.

DOSAGE AND ADMINISTRATION

1. Doxapram hydrochloride is compatible with 5% and 10% dextrose in water or normal saline. ADMIXTURE OF DOXAPRAM WITH ALKALINE SOLUTIONS SUCH AS 2.5% THIOPENTAL SODIUM, BICARBONATE, OR AMINOPHYLLINE WILL RESULT IN PRECIPITATION OR GAS FORMATION.
2. ***In postanesthetic use.***
   a. By i.v. injection (see Table I. Dosage for postanesthetic use—I.V.) Slow administration of the drug and careful observation of the patient during administration and for some time subsequently are advisable.

[See table above].

   b. By infusion. The solution is prepared by adding 250 mg of doxapram (12.5 mL) to 250 mL of dextrose or saline solution. The infusion is initiated at a rate of approximately 5 mg/minute until a satisfactory respiratory response is observed, and maintained at a rate of 1–3 mg/minute. The rate of infusion should be adjusted to sustain the desired level of respiratory stimulation with a minimum of side effects. The recommended total dosage by infusion is 4 mg/kg (2.0 mg/lb), or approximately 300 mg for the average adult.
3. ***In the management of drug-induced CNS depression.***
   (See Table II. Dosage for drug-induced CNS depression.)

[See table below].

METHOD ONE

Using Single and/or Repeat Single I.V. ***Injections.***

a. Give priming dose of 1.0 mg/lb (2.0 mg/kg) body weight and repeat in 5 minutes.
b. Repeat same dose q1–2h until patient wakens. Watch for relapse into unconsciousness or development of respiratory depression, since Dopram does not affect the metabolism of CNS-depressant drugs.
c. If relapse occurs, resume injections q1–2h until arousal is sustained, or total maximum daily dose (3 grams) is given. Allow patients to sleep until 24 hours have elapsed from

Continued on next page

Prescribing information on A. H. Robins products listed here is based on official labeling in effect June 1, 1986, with Indications, Contraindications, Warnings, Precautions, Adverse Reactions, and Dosage stated in full.

Table II. Dopram Injectable Dosage for drug-induced CNS depression.

Level of Depression	METHOD ONE Priming dose single/repeat i.v. injection mg/kg	mg/lb	METHOD TWO Rate of intermittent i.v. infusion mg/kg/hr	mg/lb/hr
Mild*	1.0	0.5	1.0–2.0	0.5–1.0
Moderate†	2.0	1.0	2.0–3.0	1.0–1.5

*Mild Depression
Class 0: Asleep, but can be aroused and can answer questions.
Class 1: Comatose, will withdraw from painful stimuli, reflexes intact.

†Moderate Depression
Class 2: Comatose, will not withdraw from painful stimuli, reflexes intact.
Class 3: Comatose, reflexes absent, no depression of circulation or respiration.

Robins—Cont.

first injection of Dopram, using assisted or automatic-respiration if necessary.

d. Repeat procedure the following day until patient breathes spontaneously and sustains desired level of consciousness, or until maximum dosage (3 grams) is given.
e. Repetitive doses should be administered only to patients who have shown response to the initial dose.
f. Failure to respond appropriately indicates the need for neurologic evaluation for a possible central nervous system source of sustained coma.

METHOD TWO

By Intermittent I.V. ***Infusion.***

a. Give priming dose as in Method One.
b. If patient wakens, watch for relapse; if no response, continue general supportive treatment for 1–2 hours and repeat Dopram. If some respiratory stimulation occurs, prepare I.V. infusion by adding 250 mg of Dopram (12.5 mL) to 250 mL of saline or dextrose solution. Deliver at rate of 1–3 mg/min (60–180 mL/hr) according to size of patient and depth of coma. Discontinue Dopram if patient begins to waken or at end of 2 hours.
c. Continue supportive treatment for ½ to 2 hours and repeat Step b.
d. Do not exceed 3 grams/day.

4. ***Chronic obstructive pulmonary disease associated with acute hypercapnia.***
   a. One vial of doxapram (400 mg) should be mixed with 180 mL of dextrose or saline solution (concentration of 2.0 mg/mL). The infusion should be started at 1–2 mg/minute (½–1 mL/minute); if indicated, increase to a maximum of 3 mg/minute. Arterial blood gases should be determined prior to the onset of doxapram's administration and at least every half hour during the two hours of infusion to insure against the insidious development of CO_2-RETENTION AND ACIDOSIS. Alteration of oxygen concentration or flow rate may necessitate adjustment in the rate of doxapram infusion.
   b. Predictable blood gas patterns are more readily established with a continuous infusion of doxapram. If the blood gases show evidence of deterioration, the infusion of doxapram should be discontinued.
   c. ADDITIONAL INFUSIONS BEYOND THE SINGLE MAXIMUM TWO HOUR ADMINISTRATION PERIOD ARE NOT RECOMMENDED.

Parenteral drug products should be inspected visually for particulate matter and discoloration prior to administration, whenever solution and container permit.

HOW SUPPLIED

Dopram Injectable (doxapram hydrochloride injection) is available in 20 mL multiple dose vials containing 20 mg of doxapram hydrochloride per mL. with benzyl alcohol 0.9% as the preservative (NDC 0031-4849-83).

Store at Controlled Room Temperature, Between 15°C and 30°C (59°F and 86°F).

Manufactured for Pharmaceutical Division, A. H. Robins Company, Richmond, Virginia 23220 by Elkins-Sinn, Inc., Cherry Hill, New Jersey 08003-4099, a subsidiary of A. H. Robins Co.

Shown in Product Identification Section, page 424

ENTOZYME® TABLETS ℞

[*ĕn 'to-zīm*]

DESCRIPTION

Entozyme tablets are available for oral administration. Each tablet contains:

Pancreatin, USP equivalent ....300 mg
Pepsin ....250 mg
Bile salts ....150 mg

Natural Digestive Enzymes

Inactive Ingredients: Acacia, Acetylated Monoglycerides, Calcium Carbonate, Calcium Sulfate, Carnauba Wax, Cellulose Acetate Phthalate, Corn Starch, Diethyl Phthalate, Edible Ink, FD&C Blue 2 Aluminum Lake, Gelatin, Microcrystalline Cellulose, Polysorbates, Shellac, Stearic Acid, Sucrose, Tartaric Acid, Titanium Dioxide, White Wax. May contain FD&C Red 40 and Yellow 6 Aluminum Lakes.

CONSTRUCTION

Entozyme is a specially constructed tablet. The outer layer dissolves in the stomach and releases pepsin. The "inner tablet" is protected by an enteric coating that disintegrates in the alkaline medium of the small intestine and releases pancreatin and bile salts, thus preserving the digestive potency of the pancreatin as it passes through the stomach.

CLINICAL PHARMACOLOGY

Entozyme should be considered a form of nutritional therapy since it is made up of naturally-occurring digestive enzymes. Entozyme enhances proteolysis by its peptic and tryptic activity, carbohydrate digestion by amylolytic activity, and fat emulsification and transport by lipolytic activity and the action of the bile salts. The components of six Entozyme tablets will digest 60 grams of fat, 48 grams of protein and 48 grams of carbohydrate, amounts of food that yield nearly 1,000 calories (one-third to one-half the daily caloric intake for many patients).

INDICATIONS AND USAGE

Entozyme is indicated for the relief of steatorrhea, pyrosis, flatulence, and belching associated with incomplete digestion of food due to a deficiency of digestive enzymes.

By effectively supplementing the patient's secretion of digestive enzymes, Entozyme promotes more complete digestion of carbohydrates, proteins and fats.

CONTRAINDICATIONS

Biliary tract obstruction or hypersensitivity to any of the ingredients.

WARNINGS

Do not administer to patients who are allergic to pork products.

PRECAUTIONS

Carcinogenesis, mutagenesis. Long-term studies in animals have not been performed to evaluate carcinogenic potential.

Pregnancy Category C. Animal reproduction studies have not been conducted with Entozyme. It is not known whether Entozyme can cause fetal harm when administered to a pregnant woman or can affect reproduction capacity. Entozyme should be given to a pregnant woman only if clearly needed.

Nursing mothers. It is not known whether this drug is excreted in human milk. Because many drugs are excreted in human milk, caution should be exercised when Entozyme is administered to a nursing woman.

Pediatric Use. Safety and effectiveness in children have not been established.

ADVERSE REACTIONS

Skin rash is the most frequently reported adverse reaction to Entozyme, and appears to be associated with hypersensitivity to pork protein in the pancreatin. At high doses, a laxative effect may occur.

OVERDOSAGE

Excessive dosage may produce a laxative effect. Systemic toxicity does not occur.

DOSAGE AND ADMINISTRATION

Two tablets with each meal and 1 or 2 tablets with each snack. The dose may be increased as necessary to achieve adequate digestion. Entozyme tablets should be swallowed whole and not crushed or chewed.

HOW SUPPLIED

White coated tablets, monogrammed "AHR" and 5049 in bottles of 100 (NDC 0031-5049-63) and 500 (NDC 0031-5049-70).

Store at controlled room temperature, between 15°C and 30°C (59°F and 86°F). Dispense in tight container.

Shown in Product Identification Section, page 424

EXNA® TABLETS ℞

[*ĕks'nă*]

brand of Benzthiazide Tablets, USP

DESCRIPTION

Exna (benzthiazide) is a diuretic available in round, yellow, scored tablets engraved AHR and 5449 for oral administration. Each tablet conatins 50 mg benzthiazide.

Inactive Ingredients: Corn Starch, Dibasic Calcium Phosphate, FD&C Yellow 5, Lactose, Magnesium Stearate, Polyethylene Glycol , Sodium Lauryl Sulfate.

Benzthiazide is a white, crystalline powder with a characteristic odor, freely soluble in alkaline solution.

CLINICAL PHARMACOLOGY

Exna is a diuretic and anti-hypertensive. It affects the renal tubular mechanism of electrolyte reabsorption. At maximal therpeutic dosage, all thiazides are approximately equal in their diuretic potency. The mechanism whereby thiazides function in the control of hypertension is unknown. Exna increases excretion of sodium and chloride in approximately equivalent amounts. Natriuresis may be accompanied by some loss of potassium and bicarbonate.

In humans, benzthiazide is excreted in the urine almost entirely unchanged. Following a single oral dose of Exna Tablets or benzthiazide solution, 1% and 4.3% of the respective doses were recovered in the urine in 24 hr. The relative bioavailability of Exna Tablets was determined to be about 25% in reference to benzthiazide solution.

INDICATIONS

Exna (benzthiazide) is indicated as adjunctive therapy in edema associated with congestive heart failure, hepatic cirrhosis and corticosteroid and estrogen therapy.

Exna has also been found useful in edema due to various forms of renal dysfunction as: nephrotic syndrome; acute glomerulonephritis; and chronic renal failure.

Exna is indicated in the management of hypertension either as the sole therapeutic agent or to enhance the effectiveness of other antihypertensive drugs in the more severe forms of hypertension.

Usage in Pregnancy. The routine use of diuretics in an otherwise healthy woman is inappropriate and exposes mother and fetus to unnecessary hazard. Diuretics do not prevent development of toxemia of pregnancy, and there is no satisfactory evidence that they are useful in the treatment of developed toxemia.

Edema during pregnancy may arise from pathological causes or from the physiologic and mechanical consequences of pregnancy. Thiazides are indicated in pregnancy when edema is due to pathologic causes, just as they are in the absence of pregnancy (however, see Warnings). Dependent edema in pregnancy, resulting from restriction of venous return by the expanded uterus, is properly treated through elevation of the lower extremities and use of support hose; use of diuretics to lower intravascular volume in this case is illogical and unnecessary. There is hypervolemia during normal pregnancy which is harmful to neither the fetus nor the mother (in the absence of cardiovascular disease), but which is associated with edema, including generalized edema, in the majority of pregnant women. If this edema produces discomfort, increased recumbency will often provide relief. In rare instances, this edema may cause extreme discomfort which is not relieved by rest. In these cases, a short course of diuretics may provide relief and may be appropriate.

CONTRAINDICATIONS

Anuria. Hypersensitivity to this or other sulfonamide derived drugs.

WARNINGS

Thiazides should be used with caution in severe renal disease. In patients with renal disease, thiazides may precipitate azotemia. Cumulative effects of the drug may develop in patients with impaired renal function.

Thiazides should be used with caution in patients with impaired hepatic function or progressive liver disease, since minor alterations of fluid and electrolyte balance may precipitate hepatic coma.

Sensitivity reactions may occur in patients with a history of allergy or bronchial asthma.

The possibility of exacerbation or activation of systemic lupus erythematosus has been reported.

Latent diabetes mellitus may become manifest during thiazide administration; hyperuricemia or frank gout may also be precipitated in certain patients. The antihypertensive effect of the drug may be enhanced in the postsympathectomy patient.

PRECAUTIONS

General: All patients receiving thiazide therapy should be observed for clinical signs of fluid or electrolyte imbalance; namely, hyponatremis, hypochloremic alkalosis, and hypokelemia.

Dilutional hyponatremia may occur in edematous pateints in hot weather; appropriate therapy is water restriction, rather than administration of salt except in rare instances when hyponatremia is life threatening.

In actual salt depletion, appropriate replacement is the therapy of choice. Any chloride deficit is generally mild and usually does not require specific treatment except under extraordinary circumstances (as in liver disease or renal disease).

Hypokalemia may develop with thiazides as with any other potent diuretic especially with brisk diuresis. Inadequate oral electrolyte intake will also contribute to hypokalemia.

This product contains FD&C Yellow No. 5 (tartazine) which may cause allergic-type reactions (including bronchial asthma) in certain susceptible individuals. Although the over-all incidence of FD&C Yellow No. 5 (tartazine) sensitivity in the general population is low, it is frequently seen in patients who have aspirin hypersensitivity.

Information for patients: Warning signs of electrolyte imbalance are: dryness of mouth, thirst, weakness, lethargy, drowsiness, restlessness, muscle pains or cramps. muscular fatigue, hypotension, oliguria, tachycardia, and gastrointestinal disturbances such as nausea and vomiting.

Laboratory tests: Periodic determination of serum electrolytes to detect possible electrolyte imbalance should be performed at appropriate intervals. When the patient is vomiting excessively or receiving parenteral fluids, serum and urine electrolyte determinations are particularly important. In patients with renal impairment, nonprotein nitrogen or blood urea nitrogen level should be tested periodically; rising values would indicate progressive renal impairment and careful reappraisal of therapy is necessary with consideration given to withholding or discontinuing diuretic therapy.

Drug interaction: Thiazides may add to or potentiate the action of other hypotensive drugs. Potentiation occurs with ganglionic or peripheral adrenegic-blocking drugs.

Thiazides may increase the responsiveness to tubocurarine. Thiazides may decrease arterial responsiveness to norepinephrine. This diminution is not sufficient to preclude effectiveness of the pressor agent for therapeutic use.
Insulin requirement in diabetic patients may be increased, decreased, or unchanged.
Medication such as digitalis may also influence serum electrolytes. Digitalis therapy may exaggerate metabolic effects of hypokalemia especially with reference to myocardial activity.
Drug/Laboratory Test Interactions: Thiazides may decrease serum PBI levels without signs of thyroid disturbance.
Carcinogenesis, mutagenesis, impairment of fertility: No animal carcinogenicity or mutagenesis studies on benzthiazide are known.
Pregnancy-teratogenic effects: Pregnancy Category C. Benzthiazide has an embryocidal effect in rats when given in doses several hundred times the human dose. Exna (benzthiazide) can cause fetal harm when administered to a pregnant woman. Fetal or neonatal jaundice has been reported. Thrombocytopenia and possibly other adverse reactions have occurred in the adult. If this drug is used during pregnancy, or if patient becomes pregnant while taking this drug, the patient should be apprised of the potential hazard to the fetus.
Thiazides cross the placental barrier and appear in cord blood.
Nursing mothers: It is not known whether this drug is excreted in human milk. Because many drugs are excreted in human milk, caution should be exercised when Exna is administered to a nursing mother.
Pediatric use: Safety and effectiveness in children have not been established.

ADVERSE REACTIONS

The following adverse reactions have been observed, but there is not enough systematic collection of data to support an estimate of their frequency.
Gastrointestinal System: jaundice (intrahepatic cholestatic jaundice); pancreatitis; gastric irritation; vomiting; cramping; nausea; anorexia; diarrhea; constipation.
Central Nervous System: dizziness; restlessness; paresthesia; headache; xanthopsia.
Hematologic: aplastic anemia; thrombocytopenia; agranulocytosis; leukopenia.
Dermatologic-Hypersensitivity: necrotizing angiitis (vasculitis) (cutaneous vasculitis); purpura; urticaria; rash; photosensitivity.
Cardiovascular: Orthostatic hypotension may occur and may be aggravated by alcohol, barbiturates or narcotics.
Other: hyperglycemia; glycosuria; hyperuricemia; weakness; muscle spasm.
Whenever adverse reactions are moderate or severe, thiazide dosage should be reduced or therapy withdrawn.

OVERDOSAGE

Symptoms of overdosage include electrolyte imbalance and signs of potassium deficiency such as confusion, dizziness, muscular weakness, and gastrointestinal disturbances. General supportive measures including replacement of fluids and electrolytes may be indicated in treatment of overdosage.

DOSAGE AND ADMINISTRATION

Therapy should be individualized according to patient response. This therapy should be titrated to gain maximal therapeutic response as well as the minimal dose possible to maintain that therapeutic response.

	Diuretic	Antihypertensive
Benzthiazide	50 to 200 mg	50 to 200 mg

Edema: ***Initiation of diuresis:*** 50 to 200 mg daily should be used for several days, or until dry weight is attained. With 100 mg or more daily, it is generally preferable to administer benzthiazide in two doses, following morning and evening meals.
Maintenance of diuresis: 50 to 150 mg daily depending upon the patient's response. To maintain effectiveness, reduction to minimal effective dosage should be gradual.
Hypertension: *Initiation of antihypertensive therapy:* 50 to 100 mg daily is the average dose. It may be given in two doses of 25 mg or 50 mg each after breakfast and after lunch. This dosage may be continued until a therapeutic drop in blood pressure occurs.
Maintenance of antihypertensive therapy: Dosage should be adjusted according to the patient response, either upward to as much as 50 mg q.i.d., or downward to the minimal effective dosage level.

HOW SUPPLIED

Exna (benzthiazide) is supplied in 50 mg yellow, scored monogramed AHR and 5449 tablets, packaged in bottles of 100 (NDC 0031-5449-63).
Store at controlled room temperature, between 15°C and 30°C (59°F and 86°F).
Dispense in tight container.
Shown in Product Identification Section, page 424

MICRO-K EXTENCAPS® ℞
[*mi 'cro "ĕks "tĕn 'tabs*]
MICRO-K 10 EXTENCAPS® ℞
brand of Potassium Chloride

PRODUCT OVERVIEW

KEY FACTS

Each particle of potassium chloride is microencapsulated by a patented process with a polymeric coating which allows for the controlled release of potassium and chloride ions over an eight-to-ten hour period. The dispersibility of the microcapsules and the controlled release of ions are intended to minimize the likelihood of high localized concentration of potassium chloride and resultant mucosal ulceration within the gastrointestinal tract.

MAJOR USES

For therapeutic use in patients with hypokalemia with or without metabolic alkalosis; in digitalis intoxication and in patients with hypokalemic familial periodic paralysis.
For prevention of potassium depletion when the dietary intake of potassium is inadequate.

SAFETY INFORMATION

Potassium supplements are contraindicated in patients with hyperkalemia since a further increase in serum potassium concentration in such patients can produce cardiac arrest. The treatment of potassium depletion, particularly in the presence of cardiac disease, renal disease, or acidosis, requires careful attention to acid-base balance and appropriate monitoring of serum electrolytes, the electrocardiogram and the clinical status of the patient.

PRESCRIBING INFORMATION

MICRO-K EXTENCAPS® ℞
MICRO-K 10 EXTENCAPS® ℞
brand of Potassium Chloride

DESCRIPTION

Micro-K Extencaps are pale orange, hard gelatin capsules, each containing 600 mg of dispersible small crystalline particles of potassium chloride (equivalent to 8 mEq K), monogrammed Micro-K and AHR/5720
Micro-K 10 Extencaps are pale orange and opaque white, hard gelatin capsules, each containing 750 mg of dispersible, small crystalline particles of potassium chloride (equivalent to 10 mEq K) monogrammed Micro-K 10 and AHR/5730.
Each particle of potassium chloride (KCl) is microencapsulated by a patented process with a polymeric coating which allows for the controlled release of potassium and chloride ions over an eight- to ten-hour period. The dispersibility of the microcapsules and the controlled release of ions are intended to minimize the likelihood of high localized concentrations of potassium chloride and resultant mucosal ulceration within the gastrointestinal tract.
The polymeric coating forming the microcapsules functions as a water-permeable membrane. Fluids pass through the membrane and gradually dissolve the potassium chloride within the microcapsules. The resulting potassium chloride solution slowly diffuses outward through the membrane.
Inactive Ingredients: Edible Ink, Ethylcellulose, FD&C Blue 2 Aluminum Lake, FD&C Yellow 6, Gelatin, Magnesium Stearate, Sodium Lauryl Sulfate, Titanium Dioxide. May contain FD&C Red 40 and Yellow 6 Aluminum Lakes.

ACTIONS

Potassium ion is the principal intracellular cation of most body tissues. Potassium ions participate in a number of essential physiological processes, including the maintenance of intracellular tonicity, the transmission of nerve impulses, the contraction of cardiac, skeletal, and smooth muscle and the maintenance of normal renal function.
Potassium depletion may occur whenever the rate of potassium loss through renal excretion and/or loss from the gastrointestinal tract exceeds the rate of potassium intake. Such depletion usually develops slowly as a consequence of prolonged therapy with oral diuretics, primary or secondary hyperaldosteronism, diabetic ketoacidosis, severe diarrhea, or inadequate replacement of potassium in patients on prolonged parenteral nutrition. Potassium depletion due to these causes is usually accompanied by a concomitant deficiency of chloride and is manifested by hypokalemia and metabolic alkalosis. Potassium depletion may produce weakness, fatigue, disturbances of cardiac rhythm (primarily ectopic beats), prominent U-waves in the electrocardiogram, and in advanced cases, flaccid paralysis and/or impaired ability to concentrate urine.
Potassium depletion associated with metabolic alkalosis is managed by correcting the fundamental causes of the deficiency whenever possible and administering supplemental potassium chloride, in the form of high potassium food or potassium chloride solution, capsules or tablets. In rare circumstances (e.g., patients with renal tubular acidosis) potassium depletion may be associated with metabolic acidosis and hyperchloremia. In such patients potassium replacement should be accomplished with potassium salts other than the chloride, such as potassium bicarbonate, potassium citrate, or potassium acetate.

INDICATIONS

BECAUSE OF REPORTS OF INTESTINAL AND GASTRIC ULCERATION AND BLEEDING WITH SLOW-RELEASE POTASSIUM CHLORIDE PREPARATIONS, THESE DRUGS SHOULD BE RESERVED FOR THOSE PATIENTS WHO CANNOT TOLERATE OR REFUSE TO TAKE LIQUID OR EFFERVESCENT POTASSIUM PREPARATIONS OR FOR PATIENTS IN WHOM THERE IS A PROBLEM OF COMPLIANCE WITH THESE PREPARATIONS.

1. For therapeutic use in patients with hypokalemia with or without metabolic alkalosis; in digitalis intoxication and in patients with hypokalemic familial periodic paralysis.
2. For prevention of potassium depletion when the dietary intake of potassium is inadequate in the following conditions: patients receiving digitalis and diuretics for congestive heart failure; hepatic cirrhosis with ascites; states of aldosterone excess with normal renal function; potassium-losing nephropathy, and certain diarrheal states.
3. The use of potassium salts in patients receiving diuretics for uncomplicated essential hypertension is often unnecessary when such patients have a normal dietary pattern. Serum potassium should be checked periodically, however, and, if hypokalemia occurs, dietary supplementation with potassium-containing foods may be adequate to control milder cases. In more severe cases, supplementation with potassium salts may be indicated.

CONTRAINDICATIONS

Potassium supplements are contraindicated in patients with hyperkalemia since a further increase in serum potassium concentration in such patients can produce cardiac arrest. Hyperkalemia may complicate any of the following conditions: chronic renal failure, systemic acidosis such as diabetic acidosis, acute dehydration, extensive tissue breakdown as in severe burns, adrenal insufficiency, or the administration of a potassium-sparing diuretic (e.g., spironolactone, triamterene).
Wax-matrix potassium chloride preparations have produced esophageal ulceration in certain cardiac patients with esophageal compression due to an enlarged left atrium.
All solid dosage forms of potassium supplements are contraindicated in any patient in whom there is cause for arrest or delay in tablet passage through the gastrointestinal tract. In these instances, potassium supplementation should be with a liquid preparation.

WARNINGS

Hyperkalemia. In patients with impaired mechanisms for excreting potassium, the administration of potassium salts can produce hyperkalemia and cardiac arrest. This occurs most commonly in patients given potassium by the intravenous route but may also occur in patients given potassium orally. Potentially fatal hyperkalemia can develop rapidly and be asymptomatic.
The use of potassium salts in patients with chronic renal disease, or any other condition which impairs potassium excretion, requires particularly careful monitoring of the serum potassium concentration and appropriate dosage adjustments.
Interaction with Potassium-Sparing Diuretics. Hypokalemia should not be treated by the concomitant administration of potassium salts and a potassium-sparing diuretic (e.g., spironolactone or triamterene), since the simultaneous administration of these agents can produce severe hyperkalemia.
Gastrointestinal lesions. Potassium chloride tablets have produced stenotic and/or ulcerative lesions of the small bowel and deaths, in addition to upper gastrointestinal bleeding. These lesions are caused by a high localized concentration of potassium ion in the region of a rapidly dissolving tablet which injures the bowel wall and thereby produces obstruction, hemorrhage, or perforation.
Micro-K Extencaps contain microcapsules which disperse upon dissolution of the hard gelatin capsule. The microcapsules are formulated to provide a controlled release of potassium chloride. The dispersibility of the microcapsules and the controlled release of ions from the microcapsules are intended to minimize the possibility of a high local concentration near the gastrointestinal mucosa and the ability of the KCl to cause stenosis or ulceration. Other means of accomplishing this (e.g., incorporation of KCl into a wax matrix) have reduced the frequency of such lesions to less than

Continued on next page

Prescribing information on A. H. Robins products listed here is based on official labeling in effect June 1, 1986, with Indications, Contraindications, Warnings, Precautions, Adverse Reactions, and Dosage stated in full.

Robins—Cont.

one per 100,000 patient years (compared to 40–50 per 100,000 patient years with enteric-coated KCl), but have not eliminated them. The frequency of GI lesions with Micro-K Extencaps is, at present, unknown. Micro-K Extencaps should be discontinued immediately and the possibility of bowel obstruction or perforation considered if severe vomiting, abdominal pain, distention, or gastrointestinal bleeding occurs.
Metabolic Acidosis. Hypokalemia in patients with metabolic *acidosis* should be treated with an alkalinizing potassium salt such as potassium bicarbonate, potassium citrate, or potassium acetate.

PRECAUTIONS

The diagnosis of potassium depletion is ordinarily made by demonstrating hypokalemia in a patient with a clinical history suggesting some cause for potassium depletion. In interpreting the serum potassium level, the physician should bear in mind that acute alkalosis per se can produce hypokalemia in the absence of a deficit in total body potassium, while acute acidosis per se can increase the serum potassium concentration into the normal range even in the presence of a reduced total body potassium. The treatment of potassium depletion, particularly in the presence of cardiac disease, renal disease, or acidosis, requires careful attention to acid-base balance and appropriate monitoring of serum electrolytes, the electrocardiogram, and the clinical status of the patient.

ADVERSE REACTIONS

The most common adverse reactions to oral potassium salts are nausea, vomiting, abdominal discomfort, and diarrhea. These symptoms are due to irritation of the gastrointestinal tract and may be minimized by taking the dose with meals or by reducing the dose.
Intestinal bleeding, ulceration, perforation and obstruction have been reported in patients treated with solid dosage forms of potassium salts and may occur with Micro-K Extencaps (see Contraindications and Warnings).
One of the most severe adverse effects of potassium supplementation is hyperkalemia (see Contraindications, Warnings, and Overdosage).
Skin rash has been reported rarely with potassium preparations.

OVERDOSAGE

The administration of oral potassium salts to persons with normal excretory mechanisms for potassium rarely causes serious hyperkalemia. However, if excretory mechanisms are impaired or if potassium is administered too rapidly intravenously, potentially fatal hyperkalemia can result (see Contraindications and Warnings). It is important to recognize that hyperkalemia is usually asymptomatic and may be manifested only by an increased serum potassium concentration and characteristic electrocardiogram changes (peaking of T-waves, loss of P-wave, depression of S-T segment, and prolongation of the QT interval). Late manifestations include muscle paralysis and cardiovascular collapse from cardiac arrest.
Treatment measures for hyperkalemia include the following: (1) elimination of foods and medications containing potassium and of potassium-sparing diuretics; (2) intravenous administration of 300 to 500 ml/hr of 10% dextrose solution containing 10–20 units of insulin per 1,000 ml; (3) correction of acidosis, if present, with intravenous sodium bicarbonate; (4) use of exchange resins, hemodialysis, or peritoneal dialysis.
In treating hyperkalemia, it should be recalled that in patients who have been stabilized on digitalis, too rapid a lowering of the serum potassium concentration can produce digitalis toxicity.

DOSAGE AND ADMINISTRATION

The usual dietary intake of potassium by the average adult is 40 to 80 mEq per day. Potassium depletion sufficient to cause hypokalemia usually requires the loss of 200 or more mEq of potassium from the total body store.
Dosage must be adjusted to the individual needs of each patient, but typically is around 20 mEq per day for the prevention of hypokalemia and 40 to 100 mEq per day for the treatment of potassium depletion.

	For Prevention	For Treatment
Micro-K Extencaps (8 mEq K)	2 or 3 Extencaps/day (16–24 mEq K)	5 to 12 Extencaps/day (40–96 mEq K)
Micro-K 10 Extencaps (10 mEq K)	2 Extencaps/day (20 mEq K)	4 to 10 Extencaps/day (40–100 mEq K)

If more than 2 Extencaps are prescribed per day, the total daily dosage should be divided into two or more separate doses. Those patients having difficulty swallowing the capsules may be advised to sprinkle the contents onto a spoonful of soft food to facilitate ingestion.

HOW SUPPLIED

Micro-K Extencaps® are pale orange capsules monogrammed Micro-K and AHR/5720, each containing 600 mg microencapsulated potassium chloride (equivalent to 8 mEq K) in bottles of 100 (NDC 0031-5720-63), 500 (NDC 0031-5720-70) and Dis-Co® unit dose packs of 100 (NDC 0031-5720-64).
Micro-K 10 Extencaps® are pale orange and opaque white capsules monogrammed Micro-K 10 and AHR/5730, each containing 750 mg microencapsulated potassium chloride (equivalent to 10 mEq K) in bottles of 100 (NDC 0031-5730-63), 500 (NDC 0031-5730-70) and Dis-Co® unit dose packs of 100 (NDC 0031-5730-64).
Animal Toxicology: The ulcerogenic potential of microencapsulated KCl was studied in anesthetized cats by direct applications on exteriorized gastric mucosa. The microcapsules of KCl were found to be non-ulcerogenic and significantly less irritating than wax-matrix tablets and 20% solution of KCl.
In groups of monkeys (up to 8 monkeys per group) receiving different formulations of potassium chloride at equivalent daily dosage (2400 mg KCl) for four and one-half days, Micro-K Extencaps showed no tendency to cause intestinal ulceration (similar to liquid KCl and a wax-matrix preparation but in contrast to an enteric-coated KCl tablet) and minimal gastric irritation (less than a wax-matrix preparation).

Shown in Product Identification Section, page 424

MITROLAN® TABLETS

[*mī'tro ″lan*]
brand of Calcium Polycarbophil

Each chewable tablet contains:
Calcium Polycarbophil (equivalent to 500 mg Polycarbophil, USP)
Inactive Ingredients: Aminoacetic Acid, Corn Starch, D&C Yellow 10 Aluminum Lake, Flavors, Magnesium Stearate, Mannitol, Povidone, Sucrose.

ACTIONS

Mitrolan (calcium polycarbophil) is a hydrophilic agent. As a bulk laxative, Mitrolan retains free water within the lumen of the intestine, and indirectly opposes dehydrating forces of the bowel, promoting well-formed stools. In diarrhea, when the intestinal mucosa is incapable of absorbing water at normal rates, Mitrolan absorbs free fecal water, forming a gel and producing formed stools. Thus, in both diarrhea and constipation, the drug works by restoring a more normal moisture level and providing bulk in the patient's intestinal tract.

INDICATIONS

For the treatment of constipation or diarrhea, associated with conditions such as irritable bowel syndrome and diverticulosis. Also for the treatment of acute non-specific diarrhea. Restores normal stool consistency by regulating its water and bulk content.

CONTRAINDICATIONS

As with all hydrophilic bulking agents, calcium polycarbophil should not be used in patients with signs of gastrointestinal obstruction.

WARNINGS

As with any drug, if you are pregnant or nursing a baby, seek the advice of a health professional before using this product.

ADVERSE REACTIONS

Abdominal fullness may be noted occasionally. An adjustment of the dosage schedule with smaller doses given more frequently but spaced evenly throughout the day may provide relief of this symptom during continued use of Mitrolan.

DRUG INTERACTION

Antacids containing aluminum, calcium or magnesium impair absorption of tetracycline. Although Mitrolan is not an antacid, it releases free calcium after ingestion and should not be used by any patient who is taking a prescription antibiotic drug containing any form of tetracycline.

Directions of Use:
CHEW TABLETS BEFORE SWALLOWING.
Recommended dosage for OTC use: Adults— Chew and swallow 2 tablets 4 times a day, or as needed. Do not exceed 12 tablets in a 24-hour period. Children (6 to under 12 years)—Chew and swallow 1 tablet 3 times a day, or as needed. Do not exceed 6 tablets in a 24-hour period. Children (3 to under 6 years)—Chew and swallow 1 tablet 2 times a day, or as needed. Do not exceed 3 tablets in a 24-hour period.
For episodes of severe diarrhea, the dose may be repeated every ½ hour, but do not exceed the maximum daily dosage.
Dosage may be adjusted according to individual response.
When using as a laxative, patient should drink a full glass (8 fl. oz.) of water or other liquid with each dose.

Sodium Content: Less than 0.02 mEq (0.46 mg) per tablet.

HOW SUPPLIED

Chewable Tablets—cartons of 36 individually packaged blister units (NDC 0031-1535-57) and bottles of 100 (NDC 0031-1535-63).

Shown in Product Identification Section, page 424

PABALATE® TABLETS

[*păb'ah ″lāt*]

DESCRIPTION

Pabalate® tablets are intended for oral administration.
Each enteric-coated tablet contains:
Sodium Salicylate, USP ....0.3 g
Sodium Aminobenzoate ....0.3 g
Inactive Ingredients: Acacia, Acetylated Monoglycerides, Calcium Carbonate, Calcium Sulfate, Carnauba Wax, Cellulose Acetate Phthalate, D&C Yellow 10, Diethyl Phthalate, Edible Ink, FD&C Blue 2 Aluminum Lake, FD&C Yellow 6, Gelatin, Magnesium Stearate, Polysorbates, Shellac, Stearic Acid, Sucrose, Talc, Titanium Dioxide, Wheat Flour, White Wax. May contain FD&C Red 40 and Yellow 6 Aluminum Lakes.

CLINICAL PHARMACOLOGY

Sodium salicylate is a mild analgesic with antiinflammatory and antipyretic activity. Compared to aspirin, sodium salicylate has substantially less effect on platelet adhesiveness. In large doses, however, it has a hypoprothrombinemic effect. Sodium salicylate in conventional dosage form dissolves in the stomach and is absorbed as un-ionized salicylic acid. However, in Pabalate, the enteric coating delays release of the salicylate until the tablet reaches the alkaline medium of the intestine. After absorption, salicylic acid is extensively bound to plasma protein, and the bound portion is in equilibrium with the free salicylate in the plasma. The action of sodium aminobenzoate in this formulation has not been established.

INDICATIONS

Pabalate tablets are indicated for the temporary relief of mild to moderate pain.

CONTRAINDICATIONS

Hypersensitivity to any of the ingredients. Presence of an active ulcer, hypoprothrombinemia, Vitamin K deficiency, severe hepatic or renal damage, or hemophilia. This product is not recommended for persons on a sodium-restricted diet.

WARNINGS

Children and teenagers should not use this medicine for chicken pox or flu symptoms before a doctor is consulted about Reye syndrome, a rare but serious illness.

PRECAUTIONS

General: Treatment with salicylates may interfere with blood clotting; therefore, salicylate therapy should be stopped at least one week prior to surgery.
Drug Interaction: This product contains sodium aminobenzoate, the aminobenzoic acid portion of which inhibits the bacteriostatic action of sulfonamides when the two are present concurrently.
Carcinogenesis, mutagenesis: Long-term studies in animals have not been performed to evaluate carcinogenic potential.
Pregnancy Category C: Animal reproduction studies have not been conducted with Pabalate.
Safe use of Pabalate has not been established with regard to possible adverse effects upon fetal development. Therefore, Pabalate should not be used in women who are or may become pregnant and particularly during early pregnancy unless in the judgment of the physician the potential benefits outweigh the possible hazards.
Nursing Mothers: Salicylates appear in human milk in moderate amounts. They can produce a bleeding tendency by decreasing the amount of prothrombin in the infant's blood. As a general rule, nursing should not be undertaken while a patient is on this drug.
Pediatric Use: Safety and effectiveness in children below the age of 12 years have not been established.

ADVERSE REACTIONS

The most frequent adverse reactions to products such as Pabalate which contain salicylates are nausea and gastrointestinal upset. Fine rash with or without pruritus and urticaria occurs less frequently. The occasional occurrence of mild salicylism (diarrhea, tinnitus, dizziness) may require an adjustment in dosage.
Overdosage: Mild chronic overdosage, termed salicylism, may cause symptoms such as tinnitus, nausea, headache, hyperventilation, dizziness, drowsiness, mental confusion, dimness of vision, sweating, thirst and occasionally diarrhea. Withdrawal of salicylates and supportive therapy may be sufficient treatment.
A more severe degree of salicylate intoxication may occur with acute massive overdosage or the chronic administration of more moderate overdoses, especially in infants and chil-

dren. CNS effects are more pronounced and may progress to delirium, hallucinations, gereralized convulsions and coma. A variety of cutaneous lesions may be observed.
A most important feature of salicylate intoxication is a disturbance of acid-base balance and plasma electrolytes. Careful monitoring of these laboratory parameters along with plasma glucose concentration is essential. The type and quantity of repair solutions used will depend upon interpretation of the laboratory data. Bicarbonate solution should be administered IV in order to produce alkaline diuresis. Correction of hypoglycemia and ketosis by the administration of glucose is essential.
Since hyperthermia and dehydration are immediate threats to life, external sponging and the administration of adequate quantities of IV fluids are important first steps to correct these conditions and maintain adequate renal function.
If hemorrhagic phenomena (petechiae, thrombocytopenia) occur, whole blood transfusions and vitamin K may be necessary.
The gastrointestinal tract should be emptied either by emesis or purging to remove undissolved tablets in cases of acute ingestion of a large single dose. Since enteric coated tablets do not disintegrate in the stomach, they cannot be removed by lavage.
Rapid and immediate removal of salicylate from the body by alkaline diuresis is essential. In more severe cases, extrarenal measures such as peritoneal dialysis, hemodialysis, hemoperfusion or exchange transfusion may be required.

DOSAGE AND ADMINISTRATION
The average adult dose is two tablets every 4 hours. Due to the enteric coating, tablets should not be taken within one hour of ingesting milk or antacids. For Chicken Pox or Flu, see Warnings.

HOW SUPPLIED
Yellow, enteric-coated tablets, monogrammed AHR and 5816 in bottles of 100 (NDC 0031-5816-63) and 500 (NDC 0031-5816-70).
Store at Controlled Room Temperature, Between 15°C and 30°C (59°F and 86°F).
Shown in Product Identification Section, page 424

PABALATE®-SF TABLETS ℞
[păb'ah"lāt]

DESCRIPTION
Pabalate®-SF tablets are intended for oral administration. Each enteric-coated tablet contains:
Potassium Salicylate .... 0.3 g
Potassium Aminobenzoate .... 0.3 g
Potassium content per tablet:
131.5 mg (3.4 mEq)
Inactive Ingredients: Acacia, Acetylated Monoglycerides, Calcium Carbonate, Calcium Sulfate, Carnauba Wax, Cellulose Acetate Phthalate, Diethyl Phthalate, Docusate Sodium, Edible Ink, FD&C Blue 1 Aluminum Lake, FD&C Blue 2 Aluminum Lake, FD&C Red 3 Aluminum Lake, Gelatin, Magnesium Stearate, Polysorbates, Shellac, Stearic Acid, Sucrose, Talc, Titanium Dioxide, Wheat Flour, White Wax. May contain FD&C Red 40 and Yellow 6 Aluminum Lakes.
Analgesic Drug Product

CLINICAL PHARMACOLOGY
Potassium salicylate is a mild analgesic with antiinflammatory and antipyretic activity. Compared to aspirin, potassium salicylate has substantially less effect on platelet adhesiveness. In large doses, however, it has a hypoprothrombinemic effect. Potassium salicylate in conventional dosage form dissolves in the stomach and is absorbed as un-ionized salicylic acid. However, in Pabalate-SF, the enteric coating delays release of the salicylate until the tablet reaches the alkaline medium of the intestine. After absorption, salicylic acid is extensively bound to plasma protein, and the bound portion is in equilibrium with the free salicylate in the plasma. The action of potassium aminobenzoate in this formulation has not been established.

INDICATIONS
Pabalate-SF tablets are indicated for the temporary relief of mild to moderate pain complicated by conditions in which the restriction of sodium intake may be desirable, such as: congestive heart failure, essential hypertension and glomerulonephritis.

CONTRAINDICATIONS
Hypersensitivity to any of the ingredients. Presence of an active ulcer, hypoprothrombinemia, Vitamin K deficiency, severe hepatic or renal damage, hemophilia, or hyperkalemia. Do not administer to patients who are receiving a potassium-sparing diuretic.

WARNINGS
Salicylates have been reported to be associated with the development of Reye syndrome in children and teenagers with chicken pox, influenza, and influenza-like infections. There have been several reports, published and unpublished, concerning non-specific small bowel lesions consisting of stenosis with or without ulceration, associated with the administration of enteric-coated thiazides with potassium salts. These lesions may occur with enteric-coated potassium tablets alone or when they are used with nonenteric-coated thiazides, or certain other oral diuretics.
These small bowel lesions have caused obstruction, hemorrhage, and perforation. Surgery was frequently required and deaths have occurred.
Based on a large survey of physicians and hospitals, both American and foreign, the incidence of these lesions is low, and a causal relationship in man has not been definitely established.
Available information tends to implicate enteric-coated potassium salts although lesions of this type also occur spontaneously. Therefore, coated potassium-containing formulations should be administered only when indicated, and should be discontinued immediately if abdominal pain, distension, nausea, vomiting, or gastrointestinal bleeding occur.
When prescribing Pabalate-SF for patients who are receiving concurrent potassium supplementation (e.g., to replace potassium excreted during thiazide therapy), it should be kept in mind that each Pabalate-SF tablet contains 131.5 mg (3.4 mEq) of potassium. A decrease in supplemental potassium dosage should be considered in order to avoid hyperkalemia.
The use of potassium salts in patients with chronic renal disease, or any other condition which impairs potassium excretion, requires particularly careful monitoring of the serum potassium concentration and appropriate dosage adjustment.

PRECAUTIONS
General: Treatment with salicylates may interfere with blood clotting; therefore, salicylate therapy should be stopped at least one week prior to surgery.
Drug Interaction: This product contains aminobenzoic acid which inhibits the bacteriostatic action of sulfonamides when the two are administered concurrently.
Carcinogenesis, mutagenesis: Long-term studies in animals have not been performed to evaluate carcinogenic potential.
Pregnancy Category C: Animal reproduction studies have not been conducted with Pabalate-SF.
Safe use of Pabalate-SF has not been established with regard to possible adverse effects upon fetal development. Therefore, Pabalate-SF should not be used in women who are or may become pregnant and particularly during early pregnancy unless in the judgment of the physician the potential benefits outweigh the possible hazards.
Nursing Mothers: Salicylates appear in human milk in moderate amounts. They can produce a bleeding tendency by decreasing the amount of prothrombin in the infant's blood. As a general rule, nursing should not be undertaken while a patient is on this drug.
Pediatric Use: Safety and effectiveness in children below the age of 12 have not been established.

ADVERSE REACTIONS
Hyperkalemia is a potential adverse effect (see Contraindications and Warnings). The most frequent adverse reactions to products such as Pabalate-SF which contain potassium and /or salicylates are nausea and gastrointestinal upset. Fine rash with or without pruritus and urticaria occur less frequently. The occasional occurrence of mild salicylism may require adjustment in dosage.

OVERDOSAGE
Overdose may cause symptoms of hyperkalemia and/or salicylate intoxication. Mild chronic overdosage, termed salicylism, may cause symptoms such as tinnitus, nausea, headache, hyperventilation, dizziness, drowsiness, mental confusion, dimness of vision, sweating, thirst, and occasionally diarrhea. Withdrawal of salicylates and supportive therapy may be sufficient treatment.
A more severe degree of salicylate intoxication may occur with acute massive overdosage or the chronic administration of more moderate overdoses, especially in infants and children. CNS effects are more pronounced and may progress to delirium, hallucinations, generalized convulsions and coma. A variety of cutaneous lesions may be observed.
A most important feature of salicylate intoxication is a disturbance of acid-base balance and plasma electrolytes. Careful monitoring of these laboratory parameters along with plasma glucose concentration is essential. The type and quantity of repair solutions used will depend upon interpretation of the laboratory data. Bicarbonate solution should be administered IV in order to produce alkaline diuresis. Correction of hypoglycemia and ketosis by the administration of glucose is essential.
Since hyperthermia and dehydration are immediate threats to life, external sponging and the administration of adequate quantities of IV fluids are important first steps to correct these conditions and maintain adequate renal function.
If hemorrhagic phenomena (petechiae, thrombocytopenia) occur, whole blood transfusions and vitamin K may be necessary.
The gastrointestinal tract should be emptied either by emesis or purging to remove undissolved tablets in cases of acute ingestion of a large single dose. Since enteric-coated tablets do not disintegrate in the stomach, they cannot be removed by lavage.
Rapid and immediate removal of salicylate from the body by alkaline diuresis is essential. In more severe cases, extrarenal measures such as peritoneal dialysis, hemodialysis, hemoperfusion or exchange transfusion may be required.

DOSAGE AND ADMINISTRATION
The average adult dose is two tablets every 4 hours. Due to the enteric coating, tablets should not be taken within one hour of ingesting milk or antacids. For Chicken Pox or Flu, see Warnings.

HOW SUPPLIED
Persian rose, enteric-coated tablets, monogrammed AHR and 5883 in bottles of 100 (NDC 0031-5883-63) and 500 (NDC 0031-5883-70).
Store at Controlled Room Temperature, Between 15°C and 30°C (59°F and 86°F).
Dispense in well-closed container.
Shown in Product Identification Section, page 424

PHENAPHEN® WITH CODEINE NO. 2 ℞ Ⓒ III
PHENAPHEN® WITH CODEINE NO. 3 ℞ Ⓒ III
PHENAPHEN® WITH CODEINE NO. 4 ℞ Ⓒ III
[fen'ah-fen"]

DESCRIPTION
Each Phenaphen® with Codeine No. 2 capsule contains:
Codeine Phosphate, USP .... 15 mg
(Warning: May be habit forming)
Acetaminophen, USP .... 325 mg
Inactive Ingredients: Corn Starch, D&C Yellow 10, Edible Ink, FD&C Blue 1, FD&C Red 3 or 40, FD&C Yellow 6, Gelatin, Magnesium Stearate, Sodium Starch Glycolate, Stearic Acid.
Each Phenaphen® with Codeine No. 3 capsule contains:
Codeine Phosphate, USP .... 30 mg
(Warning: May be habit forming)
Acetaminophen, USP .... 325 mg
Inactive Ingredients: D&C Yellow 10, Edible Ink, FD&C Blue 1, (FD&C Green 3 *and* Red 40) or Red 3, FD&C Yellow 6, Gelatin, Lactose, Magnesium Stearate, Sodium Starch Glycolate, Stearic Acid.
Each Phenaphen® with Codeine No. 4 capsule contains:
Codeine Phosphate, USP .... 60 mg
(Warning: May be habit forming)
Acetaminophen, USP .... 325 mg
Inactive Ingredients: Corn Starch, D&C Yellow 10, Edible Ink, FD&C Green 3 or Blue 1, FD&C Yellow 6, Gelatin, Lactose, Magnesium Stearate, Sodium Starch Glycolate, Stearic Acid.
Acetaminophen occurs as a white, odorless, crystalline powder possessing a slightly bitter taste. Codeine is an alkaloid, obtained from opium or prepared from morphine by methylation. Codeine phosphate occurs as fine, white, needle-shaped crystals, or white, crystalline powder. It is affected by light.

CLINICAL PHARMACOLOGY
Phenaphen with Codeine combines the analgesic effects of a centrally acting analgesic, codeine, with a peripherally acting analgesic, acetaminophen. Both ingredients are well absorbed orally. The plasma elimination half-life ranges from 1 to 4 hours for acetaminophen, and from 2.5 to 3 hours for codeine.
Codeine retains at least one-half of its analgesic activity when administered orally. A reduced first-pass metabolism of codeine by the liver accounts for the greater oral efficacy of codeine when compared to most other morphine-like narcotics. Following absorption, codeine is metabolized by the liver and metabolic products are excreted in the urine. Approximately 10 percent of the administered codeine is demethylated to morphine, which may account for its analgesic activity.
Acetaminophen is distributed throughout most fluids of the body, and is metabolized primarily in the liver. Little unchanged drug is excreted in the urine, but most metabolic products appear in the urine within 24 hours.

Continued on next page

Prescribing information on A. H. Robins products listed here is based on official labeling in effect June 1, 1986, with Indications, Contraindications, Warnings, Precautions, Adverse Reactions, and Dosage stated in full.

Robins—Cont.

INDICATIONS AND USAGE

Phenaphen with Codeine is indicated for the relief of mild to moderately severe pain.

CONTRAINDICATIONS

Acetaminophen and codeine phosphate should not be administered to patients who have previously exhibited hypersensitivity to codeine or acetaminophen.

PRECAUTIONS

General:

Head injury and increased intracranial pressure. The respiratory depressant effects of narcotics and their capacity to elevate cerebrospinal fluid pressure may be markedly exaggerated in the presence of head injury, other intracranial lesions or a pre-existing increase in intracranial pressure. Furthermore, narcotics produce adverse reactions which may obscure the clinical course of patients with head injuries.

Acute abdominal conditions. The administration of products containing codeine or other narcotics may obscure the diagnosis or clinical course in patients with acute abdominal conditions.

Special risk patients. Acetaminophen with codeine should be given with caution to certain patients such as the elderly or debilitated, and those with severe impairment of hepatic or renal function, hypothyroidism, Addison's disease, and prostatic hypertrophy or urethral stricture.

Information for Patients. Codeine may impair the mental and/or physical abilities required for the performance of potentially hazardous tasks such as driving a car or operating machinery. The patient taking this drug should be cautioned accordingly.

Drug Interactions. Patients receiving other narcotic analgesics, antipsychotics, antianxiety agents, or other CNS depressants (including alcohol) concomitantly with acetaminophen and codeine may exhibit additive CNS depression due to the codeine component. When such therapy is contemplated, the dose of one or both agents should be reduced.

The use of monoamine oxidase inhibitors or tricyclic antidepressants with codeine preparations may increase the effect of either the antidepressant or codeine.

The concurrent use of anticholinergics with codeine may produce paralytic ileus.

Carcinogenesis, Mutagenesis, Impairment of Fertility: No long-term studies in animals have been performed with acetaminophen or codeine to determine carcinogenic potential or effects on fertility.

Acetaminophen and codeine have been found to have no mutagenic potential using the Ames Salmonella-Microsomal Activation test, the Basc test on Drosophila germ cells, and the Micronucleus test on mouse bone marrow.

Teratogenic Effects: Pregnancy Category C. Codeine has been shown to be teratogenic in mice when given in doses 17 times the maximum human daily dose. There are no adequate and well controlled studies in pregnant women. Acetaminophen and codeine phosphate should be used during pregnancy only if the potential benefit justifies the potential risk to the fetus.

Nursing Mothers: It is not known whether the components of this drug are excreted in human milk. Because many drugs are excreted in human milk, caution should be exercised when acetaminophen with codeine is administered to a nursing woman.

ADVERSE REACTIONS

The most frequently observed adverse reactions include lightheadedness, dizziness, sedation; shortness of breath, nausea and vomiting. These effects seem to be more prominent in ambulatory than in nonambulatory patients, and some of these adverse reactions may be alleviated if the patient lies down.

Other adverse reactions include euphoria, dysphoria, constipation and pruritus. At higher doses, codeine has most of the disadvantages of morphine including respiratory depression.

DRUG ABUSE AND DEPENDENCE

Acetaminophen and Codeine Phosphate capsules are a Schedule III controlled substance.

Codeine can produce drug dependence of the morphine type, and therefore has the potential for being abused. Psychic dependence, physical dependence and tolerance may develop upon repeated administration of this drug, and it should be prescribed and administered with the same degree of caution appropriate to the use of other oral narcotic-containing medications.

OVERDOSAGE

Acetaminophen:

Signs and Symptoms: Acetaminophen in massive overdosage may cause hepatic toxicity in some patients. In all cases of suspected overdosage you may wish to call your regional poison center for assistance in diagnosis and for directions in the use of N-acetylcysteine as an antidote.

In adults, hepatic toxicity has rarely been reported with acute overdoses of less than 10 grams and fatalities with less than 15 grams. Importantly, young children seem to be more resistant than adults to the hepatotoxic effect of an acetaminophen overdose. Despite this, the measures outlined below should be initiated in any adult or child suspected of having ingested an acetaminophen overdose.

Early symptoms following a potentially hepatotoxic overdose may include nausea, vomiting, diaphoresis and general malaise. Clinical and laboratory evidence of hepatic toxicity may not be apparent until 48 to 72 hours post-ingestion.

Treatment: The stomach should be emptied promptly by lavage or by induction of emesis with syrup of ipecac. Patient's estimates of the quantity of a drug ingested are notoriously unreliable. Therefore, if an acetaminophen overdose is suspected, a serum acetaminophen assay should be obtained as early as possible, but no sooner than four hours following ingestion. Liver function studies should be obtained initially and repeated at 24-hour intervals.

The antidote, N-acetylcysteine, should be administered as early as possible, and within 16 hours of the overdose ingestion for optimal results, but in any case, within 24 hours. Following recovery, there are no residual, structural or functional hepatic abnormalities.

Codeine:

Signs and Symptoms: Serious overdose with codeine is characterized by respiratory depression (a decrease in respiratory rate and/or tidal volume. Cheyne-Stokes respiration, cyanosis), extreme somnolence progressing to stupor or coma, skeletal muscle flaccidity, cold and clammy skin, and sometimes bradycardia and hypotension. In severe overdosage, apnea, circulatory collapse, cardiac arrest and death may occur.

Treatment: Primary attention should be given to the reestablishment of adequate respiratory exchange through provision of a patent airway and the institution of assisted or controlled ventilation. The narcotic antagonist naloxone is a specific antidote against respiratory depression which may result from overdosage or unusual sensitivity to narcotics, including codeine. Therefore, an appropriate dose of naloxone (see package insert) should be administered, preferably by the intravenous route, and simultaneously with efforts at respiratory resuscitation. Since the duration of action of codeine may exceed that of the antagonist, the patient should be kept under continued surveillance and repeated doses of the antagonist should be administered as needed to maintain adequate respiration.

An antagonist should not be administered in the absence of clinically significant respiratory or cardiovascular depression. Oxygen, intravenous fluids, vasopressors and other supportive measures should be employed as indicated.

Gastric emptying may be useful in removing unabsorbed drug.

DOSAGE AND ADMINISTRATION

Dosage should be adjusted according to severity of pain and response of the patient. The usual dosage is: Adults: Codeine Phosphate 15 mg to 60 mg. Acetaminophen 325 mg to 650 mg. Children: Codeine Phosphate 0.5 mg/kg. Doses may be repeated up to every 4 hours. The usual adult dose for Phenaphen with Codeine No. 2 and Phenaphen with Codeine No. 3 is one or two capsules every 4 hours as required. The usual adult dose for Phenaphen with Codeine No. 4 is one capsule every 4 hours as required.

It should be kept in mind, however, that tolerance to codeine can develop with continued use and that the incidence of untoward effects is dose related.

This product is inappropriate even in high doses for severe or intractable pain. Adult doses of codeine higher than 60 mg fail to give commensurate relief of pain but merely prolong analgesia and are associated with an appreciably increased incidence of undesirable side effects. Equivalently high doses in children would have similar effects.

HOW SUPPLIED

Phenaphen with Codeine No. 2, black and yellow capsules in bottles of 100 (NDC 0031-6242-63) and 500 (NDC 0031-6242-70) and Dis-Co® Unit Dose Packs (4 × 25's) (6242-61).

Phenaphen with Codeine No. 3, black and green capsules in bottles of 100 (NDC 0031-6257-63) and 500 (NDC 0031-6257-70) and Dis-Co® Unit Dose Packs (4 × 25's) (6257-61).

Phenaphen with Codeine No. 4, green and white capsules in bottles of 100 (NDC 0031-6274-63) and 500 (NDC 0031-6274-70) and Dis-Co® Unit Dose Packs (4 × 25's) (6274-61).

Store at controlled room temperature, between 15°C and 30°C (59°F and 86°F).

Dispense capsules in well-closed container.

Also available without codeine as Phenaphen® Capsules containing 325 mg of acetaminophen.

Shown in Product Identification Section, page 424

PHENAPHEN®-650 WITH CODEINE TABLETS ℞ Ⓒ

[fen'ah-fen"]

DESCRIPTION

Each Phenaphen®-650 with Codeine tablet contains:

Codeine Phosphate, USP .... 30 mg

(Warning: May be habit forming)

Acetaminophen, USP .... 650 mg

Inactive Ingredients: Calcium Sulfate, Corn Starch, Microcrystalline Cellulose, Polyethylene Glycol, Povidone, Silicon Dioxide, Sodium Bisulfite, Sodium Starch Glycolate, Stearic Acid.

Acetaminophen occurs as a white, odorless, crystalline powder possessing a slightly bitter taste. Codeine is an alkaloid, obtained from opium or prepared from morphine by methylation. Codeine occurs as colorless or white crystals, effloresces slowly in dry air and is affected by light.

ACTIONS

Acetaminophen is a non-opiate, non-salicylate analgesic and antipyretic. Codeine is an opiate analgesic and antitussive. Codeine retains at least one-half of its analgesic activity when administered orally.

INDICATIONS AND USAGE

Phenaphen-650 with Codeine is indicated for the relief of mild to moderately severe pain.

CONTRAINDICATIONS

Hypersensitivity to acetaminophen or codeine.

WARNINGS

Drug dependence. Codeine can produce drug dependence of the morphine type, and, therefore, has the potential for being abused. Psychic dependence, physical dependence and tolerance may develop upon repeated administration of this drug and it should be prescribed and administered with the same degree of caution appropriate to the use of other oral narcotic medications. This acetaminophen with codeine dosage form is subject to the Federal Controlled Substances Act (Schedule III).

PRECAUTIONS

General:

Head Injury and increased intracranial pressure. The respiratory depressant effects of narcotics and their capacity to elevate cerebrospinal fluid pressure may be markedly exaggerated in the presence of head injury, other intracranial lesions or a pre-existing increase in intracranial pressure. Furthermore, narcotics produce adverse reactions which may obscure the clinical course of patients with head injuries.

Acute abdominal conditions. The administration of products containing codeine or other narcotics may obscure the diagnosis or clinical course in patients with acute abdominal conditions.

Special risk patients. Acetaminophen with codeine should be given with caution to certain patients such as the elderly or debilitated, and those with severe impairment of hepatic or renal function, hypothyroidism, Addison's disease, and prostatic hypertrophy or urethral stricture.

Information for Patients. Codeine may impair the mental and/or physical abilities required for the performance of potentially hazardous tasks such as driving a car or operating machinery. The patient taking this drug should be cautioned accordingly.

Drug Interactions. Patients receiving other narcotic analgesics, antipsychotics, antianxiety agents, or other CNS depressants (including alcohol) concomitantly with acetaminophen and codeine may exhibit additive CNS depression due to the codeine component. When such therapy is contemplated, the dose of one or both agents should be reduced.

The use of monoamine oxidase inhibitors or tricyclic antidepressants with codeine preparations may increase the effect of either the antidepressant or codeine.

The concurrent use of anticholinergics with codeine may produce paralytic ileus.

Usage in Pregnancy. Safe use in pregnancy has not been established relative to possible adverse effects on fetal development. Therefore, acetaminophen and codeine should not be used in pregnant women unless, in the judgment of the physician, the potential benefits outweigh the possible hazards.

Nursing Mothers. It is not known whether the components of this drug are excreted in human milk. Because many drugs are excreted in human milk, caution should be exercised when acetaminophen with codeine is administered to a nursing woman.

ADVERSE REACTIONS

The most frequently observed adverse reactions include lightheadedness, dizziness, sedation; shortness of breath, nausea and vomiting. These effects seem to be more prominent in ambulatory than nonambulatory patients, and some of these adverse reactions may be alleviated if the patient lies down.

Other adverse reactions include euphoria, dysphoria, constipation and pruritus. At higher doses, codeine has most of the disadvantages of morphine including respiratory depression.

OVERDOSAGE

Acetaminophen:

Signs and Symptoms: Acetaminophen in massive overdosage may cause hepatic toxicity in some patients. In all cases of suspected overdose, immediately call your regional poison center or the Rocky Mountain Poison Center's toll-free number (800-525-6115) for assistance in diagnosis and for directions in the use of N-acetylcysteine as an antidote, a use currently restricted to investigational status.

In adults, hepatic toxicity has rarely been reported with acute overdoses of less than 10 grams and fatalities with less than 15 grams. Importantly, young children seem to be more resistant than adults to the hepatotoxic effect of an acetaminophen overdose. Despite this, the measures outlined below should be initiated in any adult or child suspected of having ingested an acetaminophen overdose.

Early symptoms following a potentially hepatotoxic overdose may include: nausea, vomiting, diaphoresis and general malaise. Clinical and laboratory evidence of hepatic toxicity may not be apparent until 48 to 72 hours post-ingestion.

Treatment: The stomach should be emptied promptly by lavage or by induction of emesis with syrup of ipecac. Patient's estimates of the quantity of a drug ingested are notoriously unreliable. Therefore, if an acetaminophen overdose is suspected, a serum acetaminophen assay should be obtained as early as possible, but no sooner than four hours following ingestion. Liver function studies should be obtained initially and repeated at 24-hour intervals.

The antidote, N-acetylcysteine, should be administered as early as possible, and within 16 hours of the overdose ingestion for optimal results. Following recovery, there are no residual, structural or functional hepatic abnormalities.

Codeine:

Signs and Symptoms: Serious overdose with codeine is characterized by respiratory depression (a decrease in respiratory rate and/or tidal volume, Cheyne-Stokes respiration, cyanosis), extreme somnolence progressing to stupor or coma, skeletal muscle flaccidity, cold and clammy skin, and sometimes bradycardia and hypotension. In severe overdosage, apnea, circulatory collapse, cardiac arrest and death may occur.

Treatment: Primary attention should be given to the reestablishment of adequate respiratory exchange through provision of a patent airway and the institution of assisted or controlled ventilation. The narcotic antagonist naloxone is a specific antidote against respiratory depression which may result from overdosage or unusual sensitivity to narcotics, including codeine. Therefore, an appropriate dose of naloxone (see package insert) should be administered, preferably by the intravenous route, and simultaneously with efforts at respiratory resuscitation. Since the duration of action of codeine may exceed that of the antagonist, the patient should be kept under continued surveillance and repeated doses of the antagonist should be administered as needed to maintain adequate respiration.

An antagonist should not be administered in the absence of clinically significant respiratory or cardiovascular depression. Oxygen, intravenous fluids, vasopressors and other supportive measures should be employed as indicated.

Gastric emptying may be useful in removing unabsorbed drug.

DOSAGE AND ADMINISTRATION

Dosage should be adjusted according to severity of pain and response of the patient. However, it should be kept in mind that tolerance to codeine can develop with continued use and that the incidence of untoward effects is dose related. This product is inappropriate even in high doses for severe or intractable pain. Adult doses of codeine higher than 60 mg fail to give commensurate relief of pain but merely prolong analgesia and are associated with an appreciably increased incidence of undesirable side effects. Equivalently high doses in children would have similar effects. The usual adult dose for Phenaphen-650 with Codeine is one tablet every four hours as required.

HOW SUPPLIED

Phenaphen-650 with Codeine is available as a scored, white, capsule-shaped compressed tablet, engraved AHR and 6251 in bottles of 50 (NDC 0031-6251-60) and Dis-Co® Unit Dose Packs (4 × 25's) (6251-61).

Store at controlled room temperature, between 15°C and 30°C (59°F and 86°F).

Dispense tablets in well-closed container.

Shown in Product Identification Section, page 424

PONDIMIN® TABLETS ℞ Ⓒ

[*pŏn 'dĭ-min*]

brand of fenfluramine hydrochloride

Tablets—20 mg

DESCRIPTION

Pondimin (fenfluramine hydrochloride) is an anorectic drug for oral administration. Immediate release tablets containing 20 mg fenfluramine hydrochloride are orange, scored, compressed tablets engraved AHR and 6447.

Inactive Ingredients: Corn Starch, FD&C Yellow 6, Magnesium Stearate, Microcrystalline Cellulose, Silicon Dioxide, Sodium Lauryl Sulfate.

Pondimin is a phenethylamine with the chemical name, N-ethyl-α-methyl-m-(trifluoro- methyl) phenethylamine hydrochloride.

CLINICAL PHARMACOLOGY

Fenfluramine is a sympathomimetic amine, the pharmacologic activity of which differs somewhat from that of the prototype drugs of this class used in obesity, the amphetamines, in appearing to produce more central nervous system depression than stimulation.

The mechanism of action of Pondimin is unclear but may be related to brain levels (or turnover rates) of serotonin or to increased glucose utilization. The antiappetite effects of Pondimin are suppressed by serotonin-blocking drugs and by drugs that lower brain levels of the amine. Furthermore, decreased serotonin levels produced by selective brain lesions suppress the action of Pondimin.

In a study of 20 normal males, fenfluramine increased glucose utilization, resulting in decreased blood glucose levels. Experimental work in animals suggested that increased glucose utilization activated the satiety center and decreased the activity of the feeding center. Perhaps by this mechanism Pondimin inhibits appetite. The relationship between glucose utilization and serotonin has not been clarified.

Fenfluramine is well-absorbed from the gastrointestinal tract, and a maximal anorectic effect is generally seen after 2 to 4 hours. In man, fenfluramine is de-ethylated to norfenfluramine which is subsequently oxidized to m-trifluoromethyl benzoic acid and excreted as the glycine conjugate, m-trifluoromethylhippuric acid. Other compounds found in the urine include unchanged fenfluramine and norfenfluramine.

The rate of excretion of fenfluramine is pH dependent, with much smaller amounts appearing in an alkaline than in an acid urine.

The half-life of fenfluramine is said to be about 20 hours, compared with 5 hours for amphetamines; however, if urinary excretion is rapid and the pH maintained in the acidic range (below pH 5), half-life can be reduced to 11 hours. Fenfluramine and norfenfluramine reach steady state concentrations in plasma within 3 to 4 days following chronic dosage.

The greatest weight loss is seen in those patients who maintain the highest levels of Pondimin. A 2-to-3-kg weight loss over 6 weeks is associated with a plasma level of 0.1 mcg/mL (or 10 mcg/100 mL).

Fenfluramine is widely distributed in almost all body tissues. It is soluble in lipids and crosses the blood-brain barrier. Fenfluramine crosses the placenta readily in monkeys.

INDICATIONS AND USAGE

Pondimin is indicated in the management of exogenous obesity as a short-term (a few weeks) adjunct in a regimen of weight reduction based on caloric restriction.

Drugs of this class used in obesity are commonly known as "anorectics" or "anorexigenics." It has not been established, however, that the action of such drug in treating obesity is primarily one of appetite suppression. Other central nervous system actions or metabolic effects may be involved.

Adult obese subjects instructed in dietary management and treated with "anorectic" drugs, lose more weight on the average than those treated with placebo and diet, as determined in relatively short-term trials.

The average magnitude of increased weight loss of drug-treated patients over placebo-treated is only a fraction of a pound a week. The rate of weight loss is greatest in the first weeks of therapy for both drug and placebo subjects and tends to decrease in succeeding weeks. The possible origins of the increased weight loss due to the various drug effects are not established. The average amount of weight loss associated with the use of an "anorectic" drug varies from trial to trial, and the increased weight loss appears to be related in part to variables other than the drug prescribed such as the physician-investigator, the population treated and the diet prescribed. Studies do not permit conclusions as to the relative importance of the drug and non-drug factors on weight loss.

The natural history of obesity is measured in years, whereas the studies cited are restricted to a few weeks duration; thus, the total impact of drug-induced weight loss over that of diet alone must be considered clinically limited.

CONTRAINDICATIONS

Fenfluramine is contraindicated in patients with glaucoma or with hypersensitivity to fenfluramine or other sympathomimetic amines. Do not administer fenfluramine during or within 14 days following the administration of monoamine oxidase inhibitors, since hypertensive crises may result. Patients with a history of drug abuse should not receive the drug.

Do not administer fenfluramine to patients with alcoholism since psychiatric symptoms (paranoia, depression, psychosis) have been reported in a few such patients who had been administered this drug.

A fatal cardiac arrest has been reported shortly after the induction of anesthesia in a patient who had been taking fenfluramine prior to surgery. Fenfluramine may have a catecholamine-depleting effect when administered for prolonged periods of time; therefore, potent anesthetic agents should be administered with caution to patients taking fenfluramine. If general anesthesia cannot be avoided, full cardiac monitoring and facilities for instant resuscitative measures are a minimum necessity.

WARNINGS

When tolerance to the "anorectic" effect develops, the maximum recommended dose should not be exceeded in an attempt to increase the effect; rather, the drug should be discontinued.

PRECAUTIONS

General. Fenfluramine differs in its pharmacological profile from other "anorectic" drugs with which the prescribing practitioner may be familiar. Correspondingly, there are possible adverse effects not associated with other "anorectics"; such effects include those of diarrhea, sedation, and depression. The possibility of these effects should be weighed against the possible advantage of decreased central nervous system stimulation and/or abuse potential.

Pulmonary hypertension has been reported in two female patients who had been taking fenfluramine (120 mg to 160 mg daily) for over 8 months for weight reduction. All symptoms and evidence of EKG changes associated with pulmonary hypertension disappeared in 3 to 6 weeks after discontinuation of treatment with fenfluramine. In one patient, evidence of pulmonary hypertension recurred after being rechallenged with fenfluramine (80 mg daily for 6 weeks). Patients taking fenfluramine should be advised to report immediately any deterioration in exercise tolerance.

Use only with caution in hypertension, with monitoring of blood pressure, since evidence is insufficient to rule out a possible adverse effect on blood pressure in some hypertensive patients. The drug is not recommended in severely hypertensive patients. The drug is not recommended for patients with symptomatic cardiovascular disease including arrhythmias.

Caution should be exercised in prescribing fenfluramine for patients with a history of mental depression. Further depression of mood may become evident while the patient is on fenfluramine or following withdrawal of fenfluramine. Symptoms of depression occurring immediately following abrupt withdrawal can be readily controlled by reinstituting Pondimin, followed by a gradual tapering off of the daily dose.

Information for Patients. Fenfluramine may impair the ability of the patient to engage in potentially hazardous activities such as operating machinery or driving a motor vehicle (see "Adverse Reactions"); the patient should be cautioned accordingly. Patient should also be advised to avoid alcoholic beverages while taking Pondimin.

Drug Interactions. Fenfluramine may increase slightly the effect of antihypertensive drugs, e.g., guanethidine, methyldopa, reserpine.

Other CNS depressant drugs should be used with caution in patients taking fenfluramine, since the effects may be additive.

Carcinogenesis, Mutagenesis. No carcinogenic studies or mutagenic studies have been undertaken with this drug.

Pregnancy Category C. Pondimin was shown to produce a questionable embryotoxic effect in rats and a reduced conception rate when given in a dose of 20 times the human dose. However, additional reproduction studies in rats, rabbits, mice, and monkeys at doses up to, respectively, 5 times, 20 times, 1 time, and 5 times the human dose yielded negative results.

There are no adequate and well-controlled studies in pregnant women. Pondimin should be used during pregnancy only if the potential benefit justifies the potential risk to the fetus.

Labor and Delivery. The effect of fenfluramine during labor or delivery on the mother and the fetus is unknown. The

Continued on next page

Prescribing information on A. H. Robins products listed here is based on official labeling in effect June 1, 1986, with Indications, Contraindications, Warnings, Precautions, Adverse Reactions, and Dosage stated in full.

Robins—Cont.

effect on later growth, development, and functional maturation of the child is unknown.

Nursing Mothers. It is not known whether this drug is excreted in human milk. Because many drugs are excreted in human milk, caution should be exercised when fenfluramine is administered to a nursing mother.

Pediatric Use. Safety and effectiveness in children below the age of 12 years have not been established.

ADVERSE REACTIONS

The most common adverse reactions of fenfluramine are drowsiness, diarrhea, and dry mouth. Less frequent adverse reactions reported in association with fenfluramine are:

Central nervous system. Dizziness; confusion; incoordination; headache; elevated mood; depression; anxiety, nervousness, or tension; insomnia; weakness or fatigue; increased or decreased libido; agitation, dysarthria.

Gastrointestinal. Constipation; abdominal pain; nausea.

Autonomic. Sweating; chills; blurred vision.

Genitourinary. Dysuria; urinary frequency.

Cardiovascular. Palpitation; hypotension; hypertension; fainting; pulmonary hypertension.

Skin. Rash; urticaria; burning sensation.

Miscellaneous. Eye irritation; myalgia; fever; chest pain; bad taste.

DRUG ABUSE AND DEPENDENCE

Pondimin (fenfluramine hydrochloride) is a controlled substance in Schedule IV. Fenfluramine is related chemically to the amphetamines, although it differs somewhat pharmacologically. The amphetamines and related stimulant drugs have been extensively abused and can produce tolerance and severe psychological dependence, as well as other adverse organic and mental changes. In this regard, there has been a report of abuse of fenfluramine by subjects with a history of abuse of other drugs. Abuse of 80 to 400 milligrams of the drug has been reported to be associated with euphoria, derealization, and perceptual changes. Fenfluramine did not produce signs of dependence in animals and appears to produce sedation more often than CNS stimulation at therapeutic doses. Its abuse potential appears qualitatively different from that of amphetamines. The possibility that fenfluramine may induce dependence should be kept in mind when evaluating the desirability of including the drug in the weight reduction programs of individual patients.

OVERDOSAGE

Signs and Symptoms: Only limited data have been reported concerning clinical effects and management of overdosage of fenfluramine.

Agitation and drowsiness, confusion, flushing, tremor (or shivering), fever, sweating, abdominal pain, hyperventilation, and dilated non-reactive pupils seem frequent in fenfluramine overdosage. Reflexes may be either exaggerated or depressed and some patients may have rotary nystagmus. Tachycardia may be present, but blood pressure may be normal or only slightly elevated. Convulsions, coma, and ventricular extrasystoles, culminating in ventricular fibrillation, and cardiac arrest, may occur at higher dosages.

Human Toxicity. Less than 5 mg/kg are toxic to humans. Five-ten mg/kg may produce coma and convulsions. Reported single overdoses have ranged from 300 to 2000 mg; the lowest reported fatal dose was a few hundred mg in a small child, and the highest reported nonfatal dose was 1800 mg in an adult. Most deaths were apparently due to respiratory failure and cardiac arrest.

Toxic effects will appear within 30 to 60 minutes and may progress rapidly to potentially fatal complications in 90 to 240 minutes. Symptoms may persist for extended periods depending upon the dose ingested.

Management. After overdosage, only a small percentage of the drug is excreted in the urine. Forced acid diuresis has been recommended only in extreme cases in which the patient survives the early hours of intoxication but fails to show decisive improvement from other measures. Hemodialysis and peritoneal dialysis are of theoretical advantage but have not been used clinically.

Reportedly the treatment of fenfluramine intoxication should include:

- ***Gastric lavage*** (but not drug-induced emesis because the patient may become unconscious at a very early stage.)
- In the event that gastric lavage is not feasible due to trismus, consult an anesthesiologist for endotracheal intubation after administration of muscle relaxants; only then gastric evacuation should be tried.
- Administration of activated charcoal after emesis or lavage may reduce absorption of drug.
- ***Monitoring of vital functions.*** If necessary, mechanical respiration, defibrillation, or "cardioversion" should be instituted.
- ***Drug therapy.*** Diazepam or phenobarbital for convulsions or muscular hyperactivity. In the presence of extreme tachycardia; propranolol; in the presence of ventricular extrasystoles; lidocaine; in the presence of hyperpyrexia; chlorpromazine.

Since fenfluramine has been shown to have a slight lowering effect on blood sugar in some patients, the theoretical possibility of hypoglycemia should be borne in mind although this effect has not been reported in cases of clinical overdosage.

DOSAGE AND ADMINISTRATION

The usual dose is one 20 mg tablet three times daily before meals. Depending on the degree of effectiveness and side effects, the dosage may be increased at weekly intervals by one tablet (20 mg) daily until a maximum dosage of two tablets three times daily is attained. Total dosage of fenfluramine should not exceed 120 mg per day.

HOW SUPPLIED

Pondimin is available in 20 mg orange, scored, compressed tablets monogrammed AHR and 6447, in bottles of 100 (NDC 0031-6447-63) and 500 (NDC 0031-6447-70).

Store at controlled room temperature, between 15°C and 30°C (59°F and 86°F).

Dispense in well-closed container.

Shown in Product Identification Section, page 424

QUINIDEX EXTENTABS® ℞

[*kwĭn'ĭ"dĕks ĕks"tĕn'tabs*]

brand of Quinidine Sulfate, USP

PRODUCT OVERVIEW

KEY FACTS

Quinidex Extentabs (300 mg), a long acting form of quinidine sulfate, are constructed to release one-third of their alkaloidal salt, quinidine sulfate (100 mg), on reaching the stomach. The remaining two-thirds (200 mg) is evenly distributed throughout a homogeneous core which slowly dissolves as it moves along the intestinal tract, releasing quinidine sulfate for continuous absorption over an 8–12 hour period.

MAJOR USES

Quinidex Extentabs are indicated in the treatment of atrial and ventricular arrhythmias and may be administered on a BID or TID dosage regimen. G-I symptoms can be minimized by giving the drug with food.

SAFETY INFORMATION

Quinidex Extentabs are contraindicated in pateints with intraventricular conduction defects, A-V block, idiosyncrasy or hypersensitivity.

All precautions applying to regular quinidine therapy apply to Quinidex Extentabs.

PRESCRIBING INFORMATION

QUINIDEX EXTENTABS® ℞

[*kwĭn'ĭ"dĕks ĕks"tĕn'tabs*]

brand of Quinidine Sulfate, USP

300 mg in each Quinidex Extentabs tablet.

DESCRIPTION

Quinidex Extentabs (quinidine sulfate) are constructed to release one-third of their alkaloidal salt, quinidine sulfate (100 mg), on reaching the stomach, to begin absorption in the upper intestinal tract. The remaining two-thirds of the active drug (200 mg) is evenly distributed throughout a homogeneous core which slowly dissolves as it moves along the intestinal tract, releasing the quinidine sulfate for continuous absorption over an 8–12 hour period.

Inactive Ingredients: Acacia, Acetylated Monoglycerides, Calcium Sulfate, Carnauba Wax, Edible Ink, FD&C Blue 2, Gelatin, Guar Gum, Magnesium Oxide, Magnesium Stearate, Polysorbates, Shellac, Sucrose, Titanium Dioxide, White Wax and other ingredients, one of which is a corn derivative. May contain FD&C Red 40 and FD&C Yellow 6.

ACTION

The action of quinidine in preventing aberrant cardiac rhythms of atrial and ventricular origin resides in its ability to (a) depress excitability of cardiac muscle, (b) slow the rate of spontaneous rhythm, (c) decrease vagal tone, and (d) prolong conduction and effective refractory period.

INDICATIONS

Quinidex Extentabs are indicated in the treatment of:

Premature atrial and ventricular contractions.

Paroxysmal atrial tachycardia.

Paroxysmal A-V junctional rhythm.

Atrial flutter.

Paroxysmal atrial fibrillation.

Established atrial fibrillation when therapy is appropriate.

Paroxysmal ventricular tachycardia when not associated with complete heartblock.

Maintenance therapy after electrical conversion of atrial fibrillation and/or flutter.

CONTRAINDICATIONS

Intraventricular conduction defects. A-V block. Idiosyncrasy or hypersensitivity.

Aberrant impulses and abnormal rhythms due to escape mechanisms should not be treated with quinidine.

WARNING

In the treatment of atrial flutter, reversion to sinus rhythm may be preceded by a progressive reduction in the degree of A-V block to a 1:1 ratio and resulting extremely rapid ventricular rate.

PRECAUTIONS

All the precautions applying to regular quinidine therapy apply to this product. Use with care in patients with severe congestive failure, renal insufficiency or with digitalis intoxication.

Patients should be carefully observed for signs of toxicity; e.g., (1) allergy or idiosyncrasy, such as febrile reactions, skin eruptions, and thrombocytopenia (extremely rare); (2) "cinchonism," such as tinnitus, blurred vision, dizziness, lightheadedness, and tremor; (3) G-I symptoms (nausea, vomiting, diarrhea, and colic); (4) cardiotoxic effects such as ventricular extrasystoles occurring at a rate of one or more every 6 normal beats, an increase of the QRS complex of 50% or more, a complete A-V block, or ventricular tachycardia.

NOTE: The development of "cinchonism" is not usually sufficient reason for terminating quinidine therapy. G-I symptoms can also be minimized by giving the drug with food.

ADVERSE REACTIONS

Cases of quinidine-induced hypoprothrombinemic hemorrhage in patients on chronic anticoagulant drug therapy have been reported.

DOSAGE

One or two tablets every 8 to 12 hours.

HOW SUPPLIED

White sugar-coated Extentabs monogrammed Quinidex and AHR in bottles of 100 (NDC 0031-6649-63), 250 (NDC 0031-6649-67), and Dis-Co® unit dose packs of 100 (NDC 0031-6649-64).

Store at controlled room temperature, between 15°C and 30°C (59°F and 86°F).

Dispense tablets in well-closed container.

Shown in Product Identification Section, page 424

REGLAN® ℞

[*rĕg'lan*]

(Metoclopramide Hydrochloride)

Tablets, Syrup and Injectable

PRODUCT OVERVIEW

KEY FACTS

Reglan increases LES pressure and the rate of gastric emptying, providing the pharmacological basis for its use in gastroesophageal reflux and gastric stasis. Its effects on motility in the upper gastrointestinal tract appear to be mediated by sensitizing tissues to acetylcholine and/or antagonizing dopamine. Dopamine antagonism within the chemoreceptor trigger zone may also contribute to the antiemetic activity of Reglan. Reglan is not indicated for long-term use.

MAJOR USES

Reglan tablets are indicated as short-term (4 to 12 weeks) therapy for adults with symptomatic, documented gastroesophageal reflux who fail to respond to conventional therapy. If symptoms are confined to particular situations, such as following the evening meal, use of single doses of Reglan prior to the provocative situation should be considered, rather than continuous therapy. In higher dosages, Reglan Injectable is effective in preventing vomiting associated with emetogenic cancer chemotherapy; especially cisplatin.

SAFETY INFORMATION

The most common side effects are restlessness, drowsiness, fatigue, and lassitude, which occur in approximately 10 percent of pateints receiving the most commonly prescribed dosage of 10 mg qid. Extrapyramidal symptoms may occur in approximately 1 in 500 patients; usually these are manifested as dystonic reactions, but rarely may present as parkinsonism or tardive dyskinesia.

PRESCRIBING INFORMATION

REGLAN® ℞

[*rĕg'lan*]

(Metuclopramide Hydrochloride)

Tablets, Syrup And Injectable

DESCRIPTION

Reglan (metoclopramide hydrochloride) is available in both oral and parenteral forms. Reglan Tablets are pink, scored, capsule-shaped tablets engraved Reglan on one side, and AHR 10 on the opposite side.

Each tablet contains:

Metoclopramide base **10 mg**

(as the monohydrochloride monohydrate)

Inactive Ingredients: FD&C Red 3 Aluminum Lake, FD&C Yellow 6 Aluminum Lake, Magnesium Stearate, Mannitol, Microcrystalline Cellulose, Stearic Acid.

Reglan Syrup is an orange-colored, palatable, aromatic, sugar-free liquid.

Each 5 mL (1 teaspoonful) contains:
Metoclopramide base **5 mg**
(as the monohydrochloride monohydrate)
Inactive Ingredients: Citric Acid, FD&C Yellow 6, Flavors, Glycerin, Methylparaben, Propylparaben, Sorbitol, Water.
Reglan Injectable is a clear, colorless, sterile solution with a pH of 4.5–6.5 for intravenous or intramuscular administration.
2 mL and 10 mL **single dose** vials/ampuls; 30 mL **single dose** vial
Each **1** mL contains:
Metoclopramide base **5 mg**
(as the monohydrochloride monohydrate)
Sodium Chloride, USP 8.5 mg, Water for Injection, USP q.s. pH adjusted, when necessary, with hydrochloric acid and/or sodium hydroxide.

CONTAINS NO PRESERVATIVE.

Metoclopramide hydrochloride is a white crystalline, odorless substance, freely soluble in water. Chemically, it is 4-amino-5-chloro-N-[2-(diethyl-amino)ethyl]-2-methoxy benzamide monohydrochloride monohydrate. Molecular weight: 354.3.

Clinical Pharmacology: Metoclopramide stimulates motility of the upper gastrointestinal tract without stimulating gastric, biliary, or pancreatic secretions. Its mode of action is unclear. It seems to sensitize tissues to the action of acetylcholine. The effect of metoclopramide on motility is not dependent on intact vagal innervation, but it can be abolished by anticholinergic drugs.

Metoclopramide increases the tone and amplitude of gastric (especially antral) contractions, relaxes the pyloric sphincter and the duodenal bulb, and increases peristalsis of the duodenum and jejunum resulting in accelerated gastric emptying and intestinal transit. It increases the resting tone of the lower esophageal sphincter. It has little, if any, effect on the motility of the colon or gallbladder.

In patients with gastroesophageal reflux and low LESP (lower esophageal sphincter pressure), single oral doses of metoclopramide produce dose-related increases in LESP. Effects begin at about 5 mg and increase through 20 mg (the largest dose tested). The increase in LESP from a 5 mg dose lasts about 45 minutes and that of 20 mg lasts between 2 and 3 hours. Increased rate of stomach emptying has been observed with single oral doses of 10 mg.

Like the phenothiazines and related drugs, which are also dopamine antagonists, metoclopramide produces sedation and may produce extrapyramidal reactions, although these are comparatively rare (See Warnings). Metoclopramide inhibits the central and peripheral effects of apomorphine, induces release of prolactin and causes a transient increase in circulating aldosterone levels, which may be associated with transient fluid retention.

The onset of pharmacological action of metoclopramide is 1 to 3 minutes following an intravenous dose, 10 to 15 minutes following intramuscular administration, and 30 to 60 minutes following an oral dose; pharmacological effects persist for 1 to 2 hours.

Pharmacokinetics: Metoclopramide is rapidly and well absorbed. Relative to an intravenous dose of 20 mg, the absolute oral bioavailability of metoclopramide is 80% ± 15.5% as demonstrated in a crossover study of 18 subjects. Peak plasma concentrations occur at about 1–2 hr after a single oral dose. Similar time to peak is observed after individual doses at steady state.

In a single dose study of 12 subjects the area under the drug concentration-time curve increases linearly with doses from 20 to 100 mg. Peak concentrations increase linearly with dose; time to peak concentrations remains the same; whole body clearance is unchanged; and the elimination rate remains the same. The average elimination half-life in individuals with normal renal function is 5–6 hr. Linear kinetic processes adequately describe the absorption and elimination of metoclopramide.

Approximately 85% of the radioactivity of an orally administered dose appears in the urine within 72 hr. Of the 85% eliminated in the urine, about half is present as free or conjugated metoclopramide.

The drug is not extensively bound to plasma proteins (about 30%). The whole body volume of distribution is high (about 3.5 L/kg) which suggests extensive distribution of drug to the tissues.

Renal impairment affects the clearance of metoclopramide. In a study with patients with varying degrees of renal impairment, a reduction in creatinine clearance was correlated with a reduction in plasma clearance, renal clearance, nonrenal clearance, and increase in elimination half-life. The kinetics of metoclopramide in the presence of renal impairment remained linear however. The reduction in clearance as a result of renal impairment suggests that adjustment downward of maintenance dosage should be done to avoid drug cumulation.

INDICATIONS AND USAGE

Symptomatic gastroesophageal reflux: Reglan Tablets are indicated as short-term (4 to 12 weeks) therapy for adults with symptomatic, documented gastroesophageal reflux who fail to respond to conventional therapy.

The principal effect of metoclopramide is on symptoms of postprandial and daytime heartburn with less observed effect on nocturnal symptoms. If symptoms are confined to particular situations, such as following the evening meal, use of metoclopramide as single doses prior to the provocative situation should be considered, rather than using the drug throughout the day. Healing of esophageal ulcers and erosions has been endoscopically demonstrated at the end of a 12-week trial using doses of 15 mg q.i.d. As there is no documented correlation between symptoms and healing of esophageal lesions, patients with documented lesions should be monitored endoscopically.

Diabetic gastroparesis (diabetic gastric stasis). Reglan (metoclopramide hydrochloride) is indicated for the relief of symptoms associated with acute and recurrent diabetic gastric stasis. The usual manifestations of delayed gastric emptying (e.g., nausea, vomiting, heartburn, persistent fullness after meals and anorexia) appear to respond to Reglan within different time intervals. Significant relief of nausea occurs early and continues to improve over a three-week period. Relief of vomiting and anorexia may precede the relief of abdominal fullness by one week or more.

The prevention of nausea and vomiting associated with emetogenic cancer chemotherapy. Reglan Injectable is indicated for the prophylaxis of vomiting associated with emetogenic cancer chemotherapy.

Small bowel intubation. Reglan Injectable may be used to facilitate small bowel intubation in adults and children in whom the tube does not pass the pylorus with conventional maneuvers.

Radiological examination. Reglan Injectable may be used to stimulate gastric emptying and intestinal transit of barium in cases where delayed emptying interferes with radiological examination of the stomach and/or small intestine.

CONTRAINDICATIONS

Metoclopramide should not be used whenever stimulation of gastrointestinal motility might be dangerous, e.g., in the presence of gastrointestinal hemorrhage, mechanical obstruction, or perforation.

Metoclopramide is contraindicated in patients with pheochromocytoma because the drug may cause a hypertensive crisis, probably due to release of catecholamines from the tumor. Such hypertensive crises may be controlled by phentolamine.

Metoclopramide is contraindicated in patients with known sensitivity or intolerance to the drug.

Metoclopramide should not be used in epileptics or patients receiving other drugs which are likely to cause extrapyramidal reactions, since the frequency and severity of seizures or extrapyramidal reactions may be increased.

WARNINGS

Depression bearing a temporal relationship to Reglan adminstration has been reported.

Extrapyramidal symptons, manifested primarily as acute dystonic reactions, occur in approximately 1 in 500 patients treated with the usual adult dosages of 30–40 mg/day of metoclopramide. These usually are seen during the first 24–48 hours of treatment with metoclopramide, occur more frequently in children and young adults, and are even more frequent at the higher doses used in prophylaxis of vomiting due to cancer chemotherapy. These symptoms may include involuntary movements of limbs and facial grimacing, torticollis, oculogyric crisis, rhythmic protrusion of tongue, bulbar type of speech, trismus, or dystonic reactions resembling tetanus. Rarely, dystonic reactions may present as stridor and dyspnea, possibly due to laryngospasm. If these symptoms should occur, inject 50 mg Benadryl® (diphenhydramine hydrochloride) intramuscularly, and they usually will subside. Cogentin® (benztropine mesylate), 1 to 2 mg intramuscularly, may also be used to reverse these reactions.

Parkinsonian-like symptoms have occurred, more commonly within the first 6 months after beginning treatment with metoclopramide, but occasionally after longer periods. These symptoms generally subside within 2–3 months following discontinuance of metoclopramide.

Tardive Dyskinesia: Tardive dyskinesia, a syndrome consisting of potentially irreversible, involuntary, dyskinetic movements may develop in patients treated with metoclopramide. Although the prevalence of the syndrome appears to be highest among the elderly, especially elderly women, it is impossible to predict which pateints are likely to develop the syndrome. Both the risk of developing the syndrome and the likelihood that it will become irreversible are believed to increase with the duration of treatment and the total cumulative dose.

Less commonly, the syndrome can develop after relatively brief treatment periods at low doses; in these cases, symptoms appear more likely to be reversible.

There is no known treatment for established cases of tardive dyskinesia although the syndrome may remit, partially or completely, within several weeks-to-months after metoclopramide is withdrawn. Metoclopramide itself, however, may suppress (or partially suppress) the signs of tardive dyskinesia, thereby making the underlying disease process. The effect of this symptomatic suppression upon the long-term course of the syndrome is unknown. Therefore, the use of metoclopramide for the symptomatic control of tardive dyskenesia is not recommended.

PRECAUTIONS

General. Metoclopramide may impair the mental and/or physical abilities required for the performance of hazardous tasks such as operating machinery or driving a motor vehicle. The ambulatory patient should be cautioned accordingly.

In one study in hypertensive patients, intravenously administered metoclopramide was shown to release catecholamines; hence caution should be exercised when metoclopramide is used in patients with hypertension.

Intravenous injections of undiluted metoclopramide should be made slowly allowing 1- to 2-minutes for 10 mg since a transient but intense feeling of anxiety and restlessness, followed by drowsiness, may occur with rapid administration.

Intravenous administration of Reglan Injectable diluted in a parenteral solution should be made slowly over a period of not less than 15 minutes.

Drug Interactions. The effects of metoclopramide on gastrointestinal motility are antagonized by anti-cholinergic drugs and narcotic analgesics. Additive sedative effects can occur when metoclopramide is given with alcohol, sedatives, hypnotics, narcotics or tranquilizers.

The finding that metoclopramide releases catecholamines in patients with essential hypertension suggests that it should be used cautiously, if at all, in patients receiving monoamine oxidase inhibitors.

Absorption of drugs from the stomach may be diminished (e.g., digoxin) by metoclopramide, whereas absorption of drugs from the small bowel may be accelerated (e.g., acetaminophen, tetracycline, levodopa, ethanol).

Gastroparesis (gastric stasis) may be responsible for poor diabetic control in some patients. Exogenously administered insulin may begin to act before food has left the stomach and lead to hypoglycemia. Because the action of metaclopramide will influence the delivery of food to the intestines and thus the rate of absorption, insulin dosage or timing of dosage may require adjustment.

Carcinogenesis, Mutagenesis, Impairment of Fertility: A 77-week study was conducted in rats in oral doses up to about 40 times the maximum recommended human daily doses. Metoclopramide elevates prolactin levels and the elevation persists during chronic administration. Tissue culture experiments indicate that approximately one-third of human breast cancers are prolactin-dependent *in vitro*, a factor of potential importance if the prescription of metoclopramide is contemplated in a patient with previously detected breast cancer. Although disturbances such as galactorrhea, amenorrhea, gynecomastia, and impotence have been reported wth prolactin-elevating drugs, the clinical significance of elevated serum prolactin levels is unknown for most patients. An increase in mammary neoplasms has been found in rodents after chronic administration of prolactin-stimulating neuroleptic drugs and metoclopramide. Neither clinical studies nor epidemiologic studies conducted to date, however, have shown an association between chronic administration of these drugs and mammary tumorigenesis; the available evidence is too limited to be conclusive at this time. An Ames mutagenicity test performed on metoclopramide was negative.

Pregnancy Category B. Reproduction studies performed in rats, mice, and rabbits by the i.v., i.m., s.c. and oral routes at maximum levels ranging from 12 to 250 times the human dose have demonstrated no impairment of fertility or significant harm to the fetus due to metoclopramide. There are, however, no adequate and well-controlled studies in pregnant women. Because animal reproduction studies are not always predictive of human response, this drug should be used during pregnancy only if clearly needed.

Nursing Mothers. Metoclopramide is excreted in human milk. Caution should be exercised when metoclopramide is administered to a nursing mother.

ADVERSE REACTIONS

In general, the incidence of adverse reactions correlates with the dose and duration of metoclopramide administration. The following reactions have been reported, although in most instances, data do not permit an estimate of frequency.

CNS Effects. Restlessness, drowsiness, fatigue and lassitude occur in approximately 10% of patients receiving the most commonly prescribed dosage of 10 mg q.i.d. (see Precautions). Insomnia, headache, confusion, dizziness or depression (see

Continued on next page

Prescribing information on A. H. Robins products listed here is based on official labeling in effect June 1, 1986, with Indications, Contraindications, Warnings, Precautions, Adverse Reactions, and Dosage stated in full.

Robins—Cont.

Warnings) occur less frequently. In cancer chemotherapy patients being treated with 1–2 mg/kg per dose, incidence of drowsiness is about 70%. There are isolated reports of convulsive seizures without clearcut relationship to metoclopramide. Rarely, hallucinations have been reported.

Extrapyramidal Reactions (EPS). Acute dystonic reactions, the most common type of EPS associated with metoclopramide, occur in approximately 0.2% of patients (1 in 500) treated with 30 to 40 mg of metoclopramide per day. In cancer chemotherapy patients receiving 1–2 mg/kg per dose, the incidence is 2% in patients over the ages of 30–35, and 25% or higher in children and young adults who have not had prophylactic administration of diphenhydramine. Symptoms include involuntary movements of limbs, facial grimacing, torticollis, oculogyric crisis, rhythmic protrusion of tongue, bulbar type of speech, trismus, opisthotonus (tetanus-like reactions) and rarely, stridor and dyspnea possibly due to laryngospasm; ordinarily these symptoms are readily reversed by diphenhydramine (see Warnings).

Parkinsonian-like symptoms may include bradykinesia, tremor, cogwheel rigidity, mask-like facies (see Warnings).

Tardive dyskinesia most frequently is characterized by involuntary movements of the tongue, face, mouth or jaw, and sometimes by involuntary movements of the trunk and/or extremities (see Warnings).

Motor restlessness (akathisia) may consist of feelings of anxiety, agitation, jitteriness, and insomnia, as well as inability to sit still, pacing, foot-tapping. These symptoms may disappear spontaneously or respond to a reduction in dosage.

Endocrine Disturbances. Galactorrhea, amenorrhea, gynecomastia, impotence secondary to hyperprolactinemia (see Precautions). Fluid retention secondary to transient elevation of aldosterone (see Clinical Pharmacology).

Cardiovascular. Hypotension, hypertension and a single instance of supraventricular tachycardia (see Contraindications, Precautions).

Gastrointestinal. Nausea and bowel disturbances, primarily diarrhea.

Renal. Urinary frequency and incontinence.

Hematologic. A few cases of neutropenia, leukopenia, or agranulocytosis, generally without clearcut relationship to metoclopramide.

Allergic Reactions. A few cases of rash, urticaria, or bronchospasm, especially in patients with a history of asthma. Rarely, angioneurotic edema, including glossal or laryngeal edema.

Miscellaneous. Visual disturbances. Porphyria. Rare occurrences of neuroleptic malignant syndrome (NMS) have been reported. This potentially fatal syndrome is comprised of the symptom complex of hyperthermia, altered consciousness, muscular rigidity and autonomic dysfunction.

Transient flushing of the face and upper body, without alterations in vital signs, following high doses intravenously.

OVERDOSAGE

Symptoms of overdosage may include drowsiness, disorientation and extrapyramidal reactions. Anticholinergic or antiparkinson drugs of antihistamines with anticholinergic properties may be helpful in controlling the extrapyramidal reactions. Symptoms are self-limiting and usually disappear within 24 hours.

Hemodialysis removes relatively little metoclopramide, probably because of the small amount of the drug in blood relative to tissues. Similarly, continuous ambulatory peritoneal dialysis does not remove significant amounts of drug. It is unlikely that dosage would need to be adjusted to compensate for losses through dialysis. Dialysis is not likely to be an effective method of drug removal in overdose situations.

Literature reports describe methemoglobinemia in premature and full term neonates who were given metoclopramide intramuscularly, 1–2 mg/kg/day for 3 or more days. Methemoglobinemia has not been reported in similar infants treated with 0.5 mg/kg/day in divided doses. Methemoglobinemia can be reversed by the intravenous administration of methylene blue.

DOSAGE AND ADMINISTRATION

For the relief of symptomatic gastroesophageal reflux: Administer from 10 mg (1 tablet) to 15 mg (1½ tablets) up to q.i.d. 30 minutes before each meal and at bedtime, depending upon symptoms being treated and clinical response (see Clinical Pharmacology and Indications). If symptoms occur only intermittently or at specific times of the day, use of metoclopramide in single doses up to 20 mg prior to the provoking situation may be preferred rather than continuous treatment.

Experience with esophageal erosions and ulcerations is limited, but healing has thus far been documented in one controlled trial using q.i.d. therapy at 15 mg/dose, and this regimen should be used when lesions are present, so long as it is tolerated (see Adverse Reactions). Because of the poor correlation between symptoms and endoscopic appearance of the esophagus, therapy directed at esophageal lesions is best guided by endoscopic evaluation.

Therapy longer than 12 weeks has not been evaluated and cannot be recommended.

For the relief of symptoms associated with diabetic gastroparesis (diabetic gastric stasis): Administer 10 mg of metoclopramide 30 minutes before each meal and at bedtime for two to eight weeks, depending upon response and the likelihood of continued well-being upon drug discontinuation.

The initial route of administration should be determined by the severity of the presenting symptoms. If only the earliest manifestations of diabetic gastric stasis are present, oral administration of Reglan may be initiated. However, if severe symptoms are present, therapy should begin with Reglan Injectable (I.M. or I.V.). Doses of 10 mg may be administered slowly by the intravenous route over a 1-to-2 minute period.

Administration of Reglan Injectable up to 10 days may be required before symptoms subside, at which time oral administration may be instituted. Since diabetic gastric stasis is frequently recurrent, Reglan therapy should be reinstituted at the earliest manifestation.

For the prevention of nausea and vomiting associated with emetogenic cancer chemotherapy: For doses in excess of 10 mg. Reglan Injectable should be diluted in 50 mL of a parenteral solution.

The preferred parenteral solution is Sodium Chloride Injection (normal saline), which when combined with Reglan Injectable, can be stored frozen for up to 4 weeks. Reglan Injectable is degraded when admixed and frozen with Dextrose-5% in Water. Reglan Injectable diluted in Sodium Chloride Injection, Dextrose-5% in Water, Dextrose-5% in 0.45% Sodium Chloride. Ringer's Injection or Lactated Ringer's Injection may be stored up to 48 hours (without freezing) after preparation if protected from light. All dilutions may be stored unprotected from light under normal light conditions up to 24 hours after preparation.

Intravenous infusions should be made slowly over a period of not less than 15 minutes. 30 minutes before beginning cancer chemotherapy and repeated every 2 hours for two doses, then every 3 hours for three doses.

The initial two doses should be 2 mg/kg if highly emetogenic drugs such as cisplatin or dacarbazine are used alone or in combination. For less emetogenic regimes. 1 mg/kg per dose may be adequate.

If extrapyramidal symptoms should occur, inject 50 mg Benadryl® (diphenhydramine hyudrochloride) intramuscularly, and EPS usually will subside.

To facilitate small bowel intubation: If the tube has not passed the pylorus with conventional maneuvers in 10 minutes, a single dose (undiluted) may be administered slowly by the intravenous route over a 1- to 2-minute period.

The recommended single dose is: Adults—10 mg metoclopramide base (2 mL). Children (6-14 years of age)—2.5 to 5 mg metoclopramide base (0.5 to 1 mL); (under 6 years of age)—0.1 mg/kg metoclopramide base.

To aid in radiological examinations: In patients where delayed gastric emptying interferes with radiological examination of the stomach and/or small intestine, a single dose may be administered slowly by the intravenous route over a 1- to 2-minute period.

For dosage, see intubation, above.

Use in Patients with Renal or Hepatic Impairment: Since metoclopramide is excreted principally through the kidneys, in those patients whose creatinine clearance is below 40 mL/min, therapy should be initiated at approximately one-half the recommended dosage. Depending upon clinical efficacy and safety considerations, the dosage may be increased or decreased as appropriate.

See Overdosage section for information regarding dialysis.

Metoclopramide undergoes minimal hepatic metabolism, except for simple conjugation. Its safe use has been described in patients with advanced liver disease whose renal function was normal.

Parenteral drug products should be inspected visually for particulate matter and discoloration prior to administration, whenever solution and container permit.

Parenteral drug products should be inspected visually for particulate matter and discoloration prior to administration, whenever solution and container permit.

Admixture Compatibilities. Reglan (metoclopramide hydrochloride) Injectable is compatible for mixing and injection with the following dosage forms to the extent indicated below:

Physically and Chemically Compatible up to 48 hours. Cimetidine Hydrochloride (SK&F), Mannitol, USP (Abbott), Potassium Acetate, USP (Invenex), Potassium Chloride, USP (ESI), Potassium Phosphate, USP (Invenex).

Physically Compatible up to 48 hours. Ascorbic Acid, USP (Abbott), Benztropine Mesylate, USP (MS&D), Cytarabine, USP (Upjohn), Dexamethasone Sodium Phosphate, USP (ESI, MS&D), Diphenhydramine Hydrochloride, USP (Parke-Davis), Doxorubicin Hydrochloride, USP (Adria), Heparin Sodium, USP (ESI), Hydrocortisone Sodium Phosphate (MS&D), Lidocaine Hydrochloride, USP (ESI), Magnesium Sulfate, USP (ESI), Multi-Vitamin Infusion (must be refrigerated-USV), Vitamin B Complex with Ascorbic Acid (Roche).

Physically Compatible up to 24 hours (Do not use if precipitation occurs). Aminophylline, USP (ESI), Clindamycin Phosphate, USP (Upjohn), Cyclophosphamide, USP (Mead-Johnson), Insulin, USP (Lilly), Methylprednisolone Sodium Succinate, USP (ESI).

Conditionally Compatible (Use Within one hour after mixing or may be infused directly into the same running IV line. Ampicillin Sodium, USP (Bristol), Calcium Gluconate, USP (ESI), Cisplatin (Bristol), Erythromycin Lactobionate, USP (Abbott), Methotrexate Sodium, USP (Lederle), Penicillin G Potassium, USP (Squibb), Tetracycline Hydrochloride, USP (Lederle).

Incompatible (Do Not Mix). Cephalothin Sodium, USP (Lilly), Chloramphenicol Sodium, USP (Parke-Davis), Sodium Bicarbonate, USP (Abbott).

HOW SUPPLIED

Each pink, capsule-shaped, scored Reglan® Tablet contains 10 mg metoclopramide base (as the monohydrochloride monohydrate). Available in bottles of 100 (NDC 0031-6701-63), and 500 tablets (NDC 0031-6701-70) and Dis-Co® Unit Dose Packs of 100 tablets (NDC 0031-6701-64). Dispense tablets in tight container.

Reglan® Syrup, 5 mg metoclopramide base (as the monohydrochloride monohydrate) per 5 mL, available in pints (NDC 0031-6706-25) and 10 mL Dis-Co® Unit Dose Packs (10 × 10s) (NDC 0031-6706-26). Dispense syrup in well-closed container.

Reglan® Injectable, 5 mg metoclopramide base (as the monohydrochloride monohydrate) **per mL;** available in 2 mL single dose vials in cartons of 25 (NDC 0031-6709-72), 10 mL single dose vials in cartons of 25 (NDC 0031-6709-78); 30 mL single dose vials in cartons of 6 (NDC 0031-6709-85) and in cartons of 25 (NDC 0031-6709-24); 2 mL ampuls in cartons of 5 (NDC 0031-6709-90) and 25 (NDC 0031-6709-95); 10 mL ampuls in cartons of 25 (NDC 0031-6709-94).

Store vials/ampuls in carton until used. Do not store open vials/ampuls for later use, **as they contain no preservative. Dilutions may be stored unprotected from light under normal light conditions up to 24 hours after preparation.**

TABLETS, SYRUP AND INJECTABLE SHOULD BE STORED AT CONTROLLED ROOM TEMPERATURE BETWEEN 15°C and 30°C (59°F and 86°F).

Reglan Injectable is manufactured for Pharmaceutical Division, A. H. Robins Company, Richmond, Virginia 23220 by Elkins-Sinn, Inc., Cherry Hill, NJ 08003-4099, a subsidiary of A. H. Robins.

Tablet Shown in Product Identification Section, page 424

ROBAXIN® INJECTABLE ℞

[ro"baks'in]

brand of Methocarbamol Injection, USP

PRODUCT OVERVIEW

KEY FACTS

Robaxin Injectable is a parenteral dosage form containing 100 mg of methocarbamol per mL, for intravenous and intramuscular use.

MAJOR USE

The injectable form of methocarbamol is indicated as an adjunct to rest, physical therapy and other measures for the relief of discomfort associated with acute painful musculoskeletal conditions.

SAFETY INFORMATION

Robaxin Injectable is contraindicated in patients hypersensitive to any of the ingredients. Patients should be cautioned about the combined effects with alcohol and other CNS depressants. Administration to patients with epilepsy is not recommended. The rate of injection should not exceed 3 mL per minute. Vascular extravasation must be avoided.

PRESCRIBING INFORMATION

ROBAXIN® INJECTABLE ℞

[ro"baks'in]

brand of Methocarbamol Injection, USP

DESCRIPTION

Robaxin Injectable is a parenteral dosage form.

Each mL contains:

Methocarbamol, USP **100 mg;** Polyethylene Glycol 300, NF 0.5 mL; Water for Injection, USP q.s. pH adjusted, when necessary, with hydrochloric acid and/or sodium hydroxide. AFTER MIXING WITH I.V. INFUSION FLUIDS, **DO NOT REFRIGERATE.**

ACTIONS

The mechanism of action of methocarbamol in humans has not been established, but may be due to general central nervous system depression. It has no direct action on the contractile mechanism of striated muscle, the motor end plate or the nerve fiber.

INDICATIONS

The injectable form of methocarbamol is indicated as an adjunct to rest, physical therapy, and other measures for the relief of discomfort associated with acute, painful musculoskeletal conditions. The mode of action of this drug has not been clearly identified, but may be related to its sedative properties. Methocarbamol does not directly relax tense skeletal muscles in man.

CONTRAINDICATIONS

Robaxin Injectable should not be administered to patients with known or suspected renal pathology. This caution is necessary because of the presence of polyethylene glycol 300 in the vehicle.

A much larger amount of polyethylene glycol 300 than is present in recommended doses of Robaxin Injectable is known to have increased pre-existing acidosis and urea retention in patients with renal impairment. Although the amount present in this preparation is well within the limits of safety, caution dictates this contraindication.

Robaxin Injectable is contraindicated in patients hypersensitive to any of the ingredients.

WARNINGS

Since methocarbamol may possess a general central nervous system depressant effect, patients receiving Robaxin Injectable (methocarbamol injection) should be cautioned about combined effects with alcohol and other CNS depressants.

Safe use of Robaxin Injectable has not been established with regard to possible adverse effects upon fetal development. Therefore, Robaxin Injectable should not be used in women who are or may become pregnant and particularly during early pregnancy unless in the judgment of the physician the potential benefits outweigh the possible hazards.

PRECAUTIONS

As with other agents administered either intravenously or intramuscularly, careful supervision of dose and rate of injection should be observed. Rate of injection should not exceed 3 mL per minute—i.e., one 10 mL vial in approximately three minutes. Since Robaxin Injectable is hypertonic, vascular extravasation must be avoided. A recumbent position will reduce the likelihood of side reactions.

Blood aspirated into the syringe does not mix with the hypertonic solution. This phenomenon occurs with many other intravenous preparations. The blood may be safely injected with the methocarbamol, or the injection may be stopped when the plunger reaches the blood, whichever the physician prefers.

The total dosage should not exceed 30 mL (three vials) a day for more than three consecutive days except in the treatment of tetanus.

Caution should be observed in using the injectable form in suspected or known epileptic patients.

Safety and effectiveness in children below the age of 12 years have not been established except in tetanus. See special directions for use in tetanus.

It is not known whether this drug is secreted in human milk. As a general rule, nursing should not be undertaken while a patient is on a drug since many drugs are excreted in human milk.

Methocarbamol may cause a color interference in certain screening tests for 5-hydroxyindoleacetic acid (5-HIAA) and vanillylmandelic acid (VMA).

ADVERSE REACTIONS

Dizziness, lightheadedness, drowsiness, vertigo, fainting, syncope, hypotension, gastrointestinal upset, metallic taste, thrombophlebitis, sloughing at the site of injection, pain at the site of injection, anaphylactic reaction, urticaria, pruritus, rash, conjunctivitis with nasal congestion, flushing, nystagmus, diplopia, mild muscular incoordination, bradycardia, blurred vision, headache, fever. In most cases of syncope there was spontaneous recovery. In others, epinephrine, injectable steroids and/or injectable antihistamines were employed to hasten recovery. Certain of these complaints may have been due to any overly rapid rate of intravenous injection.

The onset of convulsive seizures during intravenous administration has been reported, including instances in known epileptics. The psychic trauma of the procedure may have been a contributing factor. Although several observers have reported success in terminating epileptiform seizures with Robaxin Injectable, its administration to patients with epilepsy is not recommended.

DOSAGE AND ADMINISTRATION

For Intravenous and Intramuscular Use Only. Total adult dosage should not exceed 30 mL (3 vials) a day for more than 3 consecutive days except in the treatment of tetanus. A like course may be repeated after a lapse of 48 hours if the condition persists. Dosage and frequency of injection should be based on the severity of the condition being treated and therapeutic response noted.

For the relief of symptoms of moderate degree, 10 mL (one vial) may be adequate. Ordinarily this injection need not be repeated, as the administration of the oral form will usually sustain the relief initiated by the injection. For the severest cases or in postoperative conditions in which oral administration is not feasible, 20 to 30 mL (two to three vials) may be required.

Directions for Intravenous Use. Robaxin Injectable may be administered undiluted directly into the vein at a ***maximum rate of three mL per minute.*** It may also be added to an intravenous drip of Sodium Chloride Injection (Sterile Isotonic Sodium Chloride Solution for Parenteral Use) or five per cent Dextrose Injection (Sterile 5 per cent Dextrose Solution); one vial given as a single dose should not be diluted to more than 250 mL for I. V. infusion. Care should be exercised to avoid vascular extravasation of this hypertonic solution which may result in thrombophlebitis. It is preferable that the patient be in a recumbent position during and for at least 10 to 15 minutes following the injection.

Directions for Intramuscular Use. When the intramuscular route is indicated, not more than five mL (one-half vial) should be injected into each gluteal region. The injections may be repeated at eight hour intervals, if necessary. When satisfactory relief of symptoms is achieved, it can usually be maintained with tablets.

Not Recommended for Subcutaneous Administration.

Special Directions for Use in Tetanus: There is clinical evidence which suggests that methocarbamol may have a beneficial effect in the control of the neuromuscular manifestations of tetanus. It does not, however, replace the usual procedure of debridement, tetanus antitoxin, penicillin, tracheotomy, attention to fluid balance, and supportive care. Robaxin Injectable should be added to the regimen as soon as possible.

For adults: Inject one or two vials directly into the tubing of a previously inserted indwelling needle. An additional 10 mL or 20 mL may be added to the infusion bottle so that a total of up to 30 mL (three vials) is given as the initial dose (note Precautions). This procedure should be repeated every six hours until conditions allow for the insertion of a nasogastric tube. Crushed Robaxin (methocarbamol) tablets suspended in water or saline may then be given through this tube. Total daily oral doses up to 24 grams may be required as judged by patient response.

For children: A minimum initial dose of 15 mg/kg is recommended. This dosage may be repeated every six hours as indicated. The maintenance dosage may be given by injection into the tubing or by I.V. infusion with an appropriate quantity of fluid. See directions for I.V. use.

HOW SUPPLIED

Robaxin Injectable—10 mL single dose vials in packages of 5 (NDC 0031-7409-87) and 25 (NDC 0031-7409-94).

Manufactured for PHARMACEUTICAL DIVISION, A. H. ROBINS CO., Richmond, VA 23220, by ELKINS-SINN, INC. Cherry Hill, NJ 08003-4099 a subsidiary of A. H. Robins.

Shown in Product Identification Section, page 424

ROBAXIN® TABLETS ℞

[*ro"baks'in*]

brand of Methocarbamol Tablets, USP
500 mg per tablet

ROBAXIN®-750 TABLETS ℞

brand of Methocarbamol Tablets, USP
750 mg per tablet

PRODUCT OVERVIEW

KEY FACTS

Robaxin/Robaxin-750 tablets contain 500 mg and 750 mg of methocarbamol, respectively.

MAJOR USE

Robaxin (methocarbamol) is indicated as an adjunct to rest, physical therapy, and other measures for the relief of discomforts associated with acute, painful musculoskeletal conditions.

SAFETY INFORMATION

Robaxin (methocarbamol) is contraindicated in patients hypersensitive to any of the ingredients. Patients should be cautioned about combined effects with alcohol and other CNS depressants

PRESCRIBING INFORMATION

ROBAXIN® TABLETS ℞

[*ro"baks'in*]

brand of Methocarbamol Tablets, USP
500 mg per tablet

ROBAXIN®-750 TABLETS ℞

brand of Methocarbamol Tablets, USP
750 mg per tablet

DESCRIPTION

Inactive Ingredients: ROBAXIN—Corn Starch, FD&C Yellow 6 Aluminum Lake, Hydroxypropyl Cellulose, Hydroxypropyl Methylcellulose, Magnesium Stearate, Polysorbate 20, Povidone, Propylene Glycol, Saccharin Sodium, Sodium Lauryl Sulfate, Sodium Starch Glycolate, Stearic Acid, Titanium Dioxide.

ROBAXIN-750—Corn Starch, D&C Yellow 10 Aluminum Lake, FD&C Yellow 6 Aluminum Lake, Hydroxypropyl Cellulose, Hydroxypropyl Methylcellulose, Magnesium Stearate, Polysorbate 20, Povidone, Propylene Glycol, Saccharin Sodium, Sodium Lauryl Sulfate, Sodium Starch Glycolate, Stearic Acid, Titanium Dioxide.

ACTIONS

The mechanism of action of methocarbamol in humans has not been established, but may be due to general central nervous system depression. It has no direct action on the contractile mechanism of striated muscle, the motor end plate or the nerve fiber.

INDICATIONS

Robaxin (methocarbamol) is indicated as an adjunct to rest, physical therapy, and other measures for the relief of discomforts associated with acute, painful musculoskeletal conditions. The mode of action of this drug has not been clearly identified, but may be related to its sedative properties. Methocarbamol does not directly relax tense skeletal muscles in man.

CONTRAINDICATIONS

Robaxin is contraindicated in patients hypersensitive to any of the ingredients.

WARNINGS

Since methocarbamol may possess a general central nervous system depressant effect, patients receiving Robaxin/Robaxin-750 (methocarbamol tablets) should be cautioned about combined effects with alcohol and other CNS depressants.

Safe use of methocarbamol has not been established with regard to possible adverse effects upon fetal development. Therefore, methocarbamol tablets should not be used in women who are or may become pregnant and particularly during early pregnancy unless in the judgment of the physician the potential benefits outweigh the possible hazards.

PRECAUTIONS

Safety and effectiveness in children below the age of 12 years have not been established.

It is not known whether this drug is secreted in human milk. As a general rule, nursing should not be undertaken while a patient is on a drug since many drugs are excreted in human milk.

Methocarbamol may cause a color interference in certain screening tests for 5-hydroxyindoleacetic acid (5-HIAA) and vanilmandelic acid (VMA).

ADVERSE REACTIONS

Lightheadedness, dizziness, drowsiness, nausea, allergic manifestations such as urticaria, pruritus, rash, conjunctivitis with nasal congestion, blurred vision, headache, fever.

DOSAGE AND ADMINISTRATION

Robaxin (methocarbamol), 500 mg—Adults: initial dosage, 3 tablets q.i.d.; maintenance dosage, 2 tablets q.i.d.

Robaxin-750 (methocarbamol), 750 mg — Adults: initial dosage, 2 tablets q.i.d.; maintenance dosage, 1 tablet q.4h. or 2 tablets t.i.d.

Six grams a day are recommended for the first 48 to 72 hours of treatment. (For severe conditions 8 grams a day may be administered.) Thereafter, the dosage can usually be reduced to approximately 4 grams a day.

HOW SUPPLIED

Robaxin—light orange, round, film-coated tablets monogrammed Robaxin and AHR in bottles of 100 (NDC 0031-7429-63), 500 (NDC 0031-7429-70) and Dis-Co® unit dose packs of 100 (NDC 0031-7429-64).

Robaxin-750—orange, capsule-shaped, film-coated tablets monogrammed Robaxin-750 and AHR in bottles of 100 (NDC 0031-7449-63), 500 (NDC 0031-7449-70) and Dis-Co® unit dose packs of 100 (NDC 0031-7449-64).

Store at Controlled Room Temperature. Between 15°C and 30°C (59°F and 86°F).

Dispense in tight container.

Shown in Product Identification Section, page 424

ROBAXISAL® TABLETS ℞

[*ro"baks'ĭ-sal"*]

PRODUCT OVERVIEW

KEY FACTS

Robaxisal is available as a pink and white laminated tablet containing 400 mg of methocarbamol and 325 mg of aspirin. Robaxisal provides a double approach to the management of discomforts associated with musculoskeletal disorders.

Continued on next page

Prescribing information on A. H. Robins products listed here is based on official labeling in effect June 1, 1986, with Indications, Contraindications, Warnings, Precautions, Adverse Reactions, and Dosage stated in full.

Robins—Cont.

MAJOR USE

Robaxisal is indicated as an adjunct to rest, physical therapy, and other measures for the relief of discomfort associated with acute, painful musculoskeletal conditions.

SAFETY INFORMATION

Robaxisal is contraindicated in patients hypersensitive to aspirin or methocarbamol. Patients should be cautioned about combined effects with alcohol and other CNS depressants.

PRESCRIBING INFORMATION

ROBAXISAL® TABLETS ℞
[*ro"baks'ī-sal"*]

DESCRIPTION

For oral administration, Robaxisal is available as a pink and white laminated tablet containing:

Methocarbamol, USP ....400 mg
Aspirin, USP ....325 mg

Inactive Ingredients: Corn Starch, FD&C Red 3, Magnesium Stearate, Povidone, Sodium Lauryl Sulfate, Sodium Starch Glycolate, Stearic Acid.

ACTIONS

Robaxisal provides a double approach to the management of discomforts associated with musculoskeletal disorders.

Methocarbamol. The mechanism of action of methocarbamol in humans has not been established, but may be due to general central nervous system depression. It has no direct action on the contractile mechanism of striated muscle, the motor end plate or the nerve fiber.

Aspirin. Aspirin is a mild analgesic with anti-inflammatory and antipyretic activity.

INDICATIONS

Robaxisal is indicated as an adjunct to rest, physical therapy, and other measures for the relief of discomfort associated with acute, painful musculoskeletal conditions. The mode of action of methocarbamol has not been clearly identified but may be related to its sedative properties. Methocarbamol does not directly relax tense skeletal muscles in man.

CONTRAINDICATIONS

Hypersensitivity to methocarbamol or aspirin.

WARNINGS

Salicylates have been reported to be associated with the development of Reye syndrome in children and teenagers with chicken pox, influenza, and influenza-like infections. Since methocarbamol may possess a general central nervous system depressant effect, patients receiving Robaxisal should be cautioned about combined effects with alcohol and other CNS depressants.

PRECAUTIONS

Products containing aspirin should be administered with caution to patients with gastritis or peptic ulceration, or those receiving hypoprothrombinemic anticoagulants.

Methocarbamol may cause a color interference in certain screening tests for 5-hydroxyindoleacetic acid (5-HIAA) and vanilmandelic acid (VMA).

Pregnancy. Safe use of Robaxisal has not been established with regard to possible adverse effects upon fetal development. Therefore, Robaxisal should not be used in women who are or may become pregnant and particularly during early pregnancy unless in the judgment of the physician the potential benefits outweigh the possible hazards.

Nursing Mothers. It is not known whether methocarbamol is secreted in human milk; however, aspirin does appear in human milk in moderate amounts. It can produce a bleeding tendency either by interfering with the function of the infant's platelets or by decreasing the amount of prothrombin in the blood. The risk is minimal if the mother takes the aspirin just after nursing and if the infant has an adequate store of vitamin K. As a general rule, nursing should not be undertaken while a patient is on a drug.

Pediatric Use. Safety and effectiveness in children 12 years of age and below have not been established.

Use in Activities Requiring Mental Alertness. Robaxisal may rarely cause drowsiness. Until the patient's response has been determined, he should be cautioned against the operation of motor vehicles or dangerous machinery.

ADVERSE REACTIONS

The most frequent adverse reaction to methocarbamol is dizziness or lightheadedness and nausea. This occurs in about one in 20–25 patients. Less frequent reactions are drowsiness, blurred vision, headache, fever, allergic manifestations such as urticaria, pruritus, and rash.

Adverse reactions that have been associated with the use of aspirin include: nausea and other gastrointestinal discomfort, gastritis, gastric erosion, vomiting, constipation, diarrhea, angio-edema, asthma, rash, pruritus, urticaria.

Gastrointestinal discomfort may be minimized by taking Robaxisal with food.

DOSAGE AND ADMINISTRATION

Adults and children over 12 years of age: Two tablets four times daily. Three tablets four times daily may be used in severe conditions for one to three days in patients who are able to tolerate salicylates. These dosage recommendations provide respectively 3.2 and 4.8 grams of methocarbamol per day. For Chicken Pox or Flu, see Warnings.

OVERDOSAGE

Toxicity due to overdosage of methocarbamol is unlikely; however, acute overdosage of aspirin may cause symptoms of salicylate intoxication.

Treatment of Overdosage. Supportive therapy for 24 hours, as methocarbamol is excreted within that time. If salicylate intoxication occurs, especially in children, the hyperpnea may be controlled with sodium bicarbonate. Judicious use of 5% CO_2 with 95% O_2 may be of benefit. Abnormal electrolyte patterns should be corrected with appropriate fluid therapy.

HOW SUPPLIED

Robaxisal® is supplied as pink and white laminated, compressed tablets monogrammed AHR and Robaxisal in bottles of 100 (NDC 0031-7469-63), 500 (NDC 0031-7469-70) and Dis-Co® Unit Dose Packs of 100 (NDC 0031-7469-64).

Store at controlled room temperature, between 15°C and 30°C (59°F and 86°F).

Dispense in well-closed container.

Shown in Product Identification Section, page 424

ROBINUL® TABLETS ℞
[*ro'bĭ-nul*]

ROBINUL® FORTE TABLETS ℞
brand of Glycopyrrolate Tablets, USP

DESCRIPTION

Robinul and Robinul Forte tablets contain the synthetic anticholinergic, glycopyrrolate. Glycopyrrolate is a quaternary ammonium compound with the following chemical name: 3-[(cyclopentylhydroxyphenylacetyl)oxy]-1,1-dimethylpyrrolidinium bromide.

Robinul tablets are scored, compressed pink tablets engraved AHR and 7824. Each tablet contains:

Glycopyrrolate, USP ....1 mg

Robinul Forte tablets are scored, compressed pink tablets engraved $\frac{AHR}{2}$ on one side and 7840 on the reverse side.

Each tablet contains:

Glycopyrrolate, USP ....2 mg

Inactive Ingredients: Dibasic Calcium Phosphate, FD&C Red 3 Aluminum Lake, Lactose, Magnesium Stearate, Povidone, Sodium Starch Glycolate.

ACTIONS

Glycopyrrolate, like other anticholinergic (antimuscarinic) agents, inhibits the action of acetylcholine on structures innervated by postganglionic cholinergic nerves and on smooth muscles that respond to acetylcholine but lack cholinergic innervation. These peripheral cholinergic receptors are present in the autonomic effector cells of smooth muscle, cardiac muscle, the sino-atrial node, the atrioventricular node, exocrine glands, and, to a limited degree, in the autonomic ganglia. Thus, it diminishes the volume and free acidity of gastric secretions and controls excessive pharyngeal, tracheal, and bronchial secretions.

Glycopyrrolate antagonizes muscarinic symptoms (e.g., bronchorrhea, bronchospasm, bradycardia, and intestinal hypermotility) induced by cholinergic drugs such as the anticholinesterases.

The highly polar quaternary ammonium group of glycopyrrolate limits its passage across lipid membranes, such as the blood-brain barrier, in contrast to atropine sulfate and scopolamine hydrobromide, which are non-polar tertiary amines which penetrate lipid barriers easily.

INDICATIONS

For use as adjunctive therapy in the treatment of peptic ulcer.

CONTRAINDICATIONS

Glaucoma; obstructive uropathy (for example, bladder neck obstruction due to prostatic hypertrophy); obstructive disease of the gastrointestinal tract (as in achalasia, pyloroduodenal stenosis, etc.); paralytic ileus; intestinal atony of the elderly or debilitated patient; unstable cardiovascular status in acute hemorrhage; severe ulcerative colitis; toxic megacolon complicating ulcerative colitis; myasthenia gravis. Robinul (glycopyrrolate) tablets are contraindicated in those patients with a hypersensitivity to glycopyrrolate.

WARNINGS

In the presence of a high environmental temperature, heat prostration (fever and heat stroke due to decreased sweating) can occur with use of Robinul.

Diarrhea may be an early symptom of incomplete intestinal obstruction, especially in patients with ileostomy or colostomy. In this instance treatment with this drug would be inappropriate and possibly harmful.

Robinul (glycopyrrolate) may produce drowsiness or blurred vision. In this event, the patient should be warned not to engage in activities requiring mental alertness such as operating a motor vehicle or other machinery, or performing hazardous work while taking this drug.

Theoretically, with overdosage a curare-like action may occur, i.e., neuromuscular blockade leading to muscular weakness and possible paralysis.

Pregnancy. The safety of this drug during pregnancy has not been established. The use of any drug during pregnancy requires that the potential benefits of the drug be weighed against possible hazards to mother and child. Reproduction studies in rats revealed no teratogenic effects from glycopyrrolate; however, the potent anticholinergic action of this agent resulted in diminished rates of conception and of survival at weaning, in a dose-related manner. Other studies in dogs suggest that this may be due to diminished seminal secretion which is evident at high doses of glycopyrrolate. Information on possible adverse effects in the pregnant female is limited to uncontrolled data derived from marketing experience. Such experience has revealed no reports of teratogenic or other fetus-damaging potential. No controlled studies to establish the safety of the drug in pregnancy have been performed.

Nursing Mothers. It is not known whether this drug is secreted in human milk. As a general rule, nursing should not be undertaken while a patient is on a drug since many drugs are excreted in human milk.

Pediatric Use. Since there is no adequate experience in children who have received this drug, safety and efficacy in children have not been established.

PRECAUTIONS

Use Robinul with caution in the elderly and in all patients with:

- Autonomic neuropathy.
- Hepatic or renal disease.
- Ulcerative colitis—large doses may suppress intestinal motility to the point of producing a paralytic ileus and for this reason may precipitate or aggravate "toxic megacolon," a serious complication of the disease.
- Hyperthyroidism, coronary heart disease, congestive heart failure, cardiac tachyarrhythmias, tachycardia, hypertension and prostatic hypertrophy.
- Hiatal hernia associated with reflux esophagitis, since anticholinergic drugs may aggravate this condition.

ADVERSE REACTIONS

Anticholinergics produce certain effects, most of which are extensions of their fundamental pharmacological actions. Adverse reactions to anticholinergics in general may include xerostomia; decreased sweating; urinary hesitancy and retention; blurred vision; tachycardia, palpitations; dilatation of the pupil; cycloplegia; increased ocular tension; loss of taste; headaches; nervousness; mental confusion; drowsiness; weakness; dizziness; insomnia; nausea; vomiting; constipation; bloated feeling; impotence; suppression of lactation; severe allergic reaction or drug idiosyncrasies including anaphylaxis; urticaria and other dermal manifestations.

Robinul (glycopyrrolate) is chemically a quaternary ammonium compound; hence, its passage across lipid membranes, such as the blood-brain barrier, is limited in contrast to atropine sulfate and scopolamine hydrobromide. For this reason the occurrence of CNS related side effects is lower, in comparison to their incidence following administration of anticholinergics which are chemically tertiary amines that can cross this barrier readily.

OVERDOSAGE

The symptoms of overdosage of glycopyrrolate are peripheral in nature rather than central.

1. To guard against further absorption of the drug—use gastric lavage, cathartics and/or enemas.
2. To combat peripheral anticholinergic effects (residual mydriasis, dry mouth, etc.)—utilize a quaternary ammonium anticholinesterase, such as neostigmine methylsulfate.
3. To combat hypotension—use pressor amines (norepinephrine, metaraminol) i.v.; and supportive care.
4. To combat respiratory depression—administer oxygen; utilize a respiratory stimulant such as Dopram® i.v.; artificial respiration.

DOSAGE AND ADMINISTRATION

The dosage of Robinul or Robinul Forte should be adjusted to the needs of the individual patient to assure symptomatic control with a minimum of adverse reactions. The presently recommended maximum daily dosage of glycopyrrolate is 8 mg.

Robinul (glycopyrrolate, 1 mg) tablets. The recommended initial dosage of Robinul for adults is one tablet three times daily (in the morning, early afternoon, and at bedtime). Some patients may require two tablets at bedtime to assure overnight control of symptoms. For maintenance, a dosage of one tablet twice a day is frequently adequate.

Robinul Forte (glycopyrrolate, 2 mg) tablets. The recommended dosage of Robinul Forte for adults is one tablet two or three times daily at equally spaced intervals.

Robinul tablets are not recommended for use in children under the age of 12 years.

DRUG INTERACTIONS

There are no known drug interactions.

HOW SUPPLIED

Robinul (glycopyrrolate, 1 mg) tablets in bottles of 100 (NDC 0031-7824-63) and 500 (NDC 0031-7824-70).

Robinul Forte (glycopyrrolate, 2 mg) tablets in bottles of 100 (NDC 0031-7840-63).

Shown in Product Identification Section, page 424

ROBINUL® INJECTABLE ℞

[ro 'bĭ-nul]

brand of Glycopyrrolate Injection, USP

PRODUCT OVERVIEW

KEY FACTS

Robinul is a synthetic anticholinergic agent for intramuscular or intravenous administration. The highly polar quaternary ammonium moiety of glycopyrrolate limits its passage across lipid membranes, such as the blood-brain or placental barriers.

MAJOR USES

Robinul Injectable is indicated as a preoperative antimuscarinic to reduce salivary, tracheobronchial and pharyngeal secretions; intraoperatively to counteract drug-induced or vagal traction reflexes with the associated arrhythmias. Postoperatively, Robinul protects against the peripheral muscarinic effects of cholinergic agents given to reverse the neuromuscular blockade due to nondepolarizing muscle relaxants.

SAFETY INFORMATION

Robinul Injectable is contraindicated in patients hypersensitive to glycopyrrolate. It should be used with great caution, if at all, in patients with glaucoma or asthma. Robinul may produce drowsiness or blurred vision.

PRESCRIBING INFORMATION

ROBINUL® INJECTABLE ℞

[ro 'bĭ-nul]

brand of Glycopyrrolate Injection, USP

DESCRIPTION

Robinul (glycopyrrolate) is a synthetic anticholinergic agent. Each 1 mL contains:

Glycopyrrolate, USP .... 0.2 mg
Water for Injection, USP .... q.s.
Benzyl Alcohol, NF (preservative) 0.9%

pH adjusted, when necessary, with hydrochloric acid and/or sodium hydroxide.

For Intramuscular or Intravenous administration.

Unlike atropine, glycopyrrolate is completely ionized at physiological pH values.

Robinul Injectable is a clear, colorless, sterile liquid; pH 2.0–3.0.

CLINICAL PHARMACOLOGY

Glycopyrrolate, like other anticholinergic (antimuscarinic) agents, inhibts the action of acetylcholine on structures innervated by postganglionic cholinergic nerves and on smooth muscles that respond to acetylcholine but lack cholinergic innervation. These peripheral cholinergic receptors are present in the autonomic effector cells of smooth muscle, cardiac muscle, the sinoatrial node, the atrioventricular node, exocrine glands, and, to a limited degree, in the autonomic ganglia. Thus, it diminishes the volume and free acidity of gastric secretions and controls excessive pharyngeal, tracheal, and bronchial secretions.

Glycopyrrolate antagonizes muscarinic symptoms (e.g., bronchorrhea, bronchospasm, bradycardia, and intestinal hypermotility) induced by cholinergic drugs such as the anticholinesterases.

The highly polar quaternary ammonium group of glycopyrrolate limits its passage across lipid membranes, such as the blood-brain barrier, in contrast to atropine sulfate and scopolamine hydrobromide, which are non-polar tertiary amines which penetrate lipid barriers easily.

Peak effects occur approximately 30 to 45 minutes after intramuscular administration. The vagal blocking effects persist for 2 to 3 hours and the antisialagogue effects persist up to 7 hours, periods longer than for atropine. With intravenous injection, the onset of action is generally evident within one minute.

INDICATIONS AND USAGE

In Anesthesia: Robinul (glycopyrrolate) Injectable is indicated for use as a preoperative antimuscarinic to reduce salivary, tracheobronchial, and pharyngeal secretions; to reduce the volume and free acidity of gastric secretions; and, to block cardiac vagal inhibitory reflexes during induction of anesthesia and intubation. When indicated, Robinul Injectable may be used intraoperatively to counteract drug-induced or vagal traction reflexes with the associated arrhythmias. Glycopyrrolate protects against the peripheral muscarinic effects (e.g., bradycardia and excessive secretions) of cholinergic agents such as neostigmine and pyridostigmine given to reverse the neuromuscular blockade due to nondepolarizing muscle relaxants.

In Peptic Ulcer: For use in adults as adjunctive therapy for the treatment of peptic ulcer when rapid anticholinergic effect is desired or when oral medication is not tolerated.

CONTRAINDICATIONS

Known hypersensitivity to glycopyrrolate.

In addition, in the management of ***peptic ulcer*** patients, because of the longer duration of therapy, Robinul Injectable may be contraindicated in patients with concurrent glaucoma; obstructive uropathy (for example, bladder neck obstruction due to prostatic hypertrophy); obstructive disease of the gastrointestinal tract (as in achalasia, pyloroduodenal stenosis, etc.); paralytic ileus, intestinal atony of the elderly or debilitated patient; unstable cardiovascular status in acute hemorrhage; severe ulcerative colitis; toxic megacolon complicating ulcerative colitis; myasthenia gravis.

WARNINGS

This drug should be used with great caution, if at all, in patients with glaucoma or asthma.

In the ambulatory patient. Robinul (glycopyrrolate) may produce drowsiness or blurred vision. The patient should be cautioned regarding activities requiring mental alertness such as operating a motor vehicle or other machinery or performing hazardous work while taking this drug.

In addition, in the presence of a high environmental temperature, heat prostration (fever and heat stroke due to decreased sweating) can occur with use of Robinul (glycopyrrolate).

Diarrhea may be an early symptom of incomplete intestinal obstruction, expecially in patients with ileostomy or colostomy. In this instance treatment with Robinul (glycopyrrolate) would be inappropriate and possibly harmful.

PRECAUTIONS

General.

Investigate any tachycardia before giving glycopyrrolate since an increase in the heart rate may occur.

Use with caution in patients with: coronary artery disease; congestive heart failure; cardiac arrhythmias; hypertension; hyperthyroidism.

In managing ulcer patients, use Robinul with caution in the elderly and in all patients with autonomic neuropathy, hepatic or renal disease, ulcerative colitis or hiatal hernia, since anticholinergic drugs may aggravate these conditions.

With overdosage, a curare-like action may occur.

Drug Interactions. The intravenous administration of any anticholinergic in the presence of cyclopropane anesthesia can result in ventricular arrhythmias; therefore, caution should be observed if Robinul (glycopyrrolate) Injectable is used during cyclopropane anesthesia. If the drug is given in small incremental doses of 0.1 mg or less, the likelihood of producing ventricular arrhythmias is reduced.

Carcinogenesis, mutagenesis, impairment of fertility. Long-term studies in animals have not been performed to evaluate carcinogenic potential. In the teratology studies, diminished rates of conception and of survival at weaning were observed in rats, in a dose-related manner. Studies in dogs suggest that this may be due to diminished seminal secretion which is evident at high doses of glycopyrrolate.

Pregnancy Category B. Reproduction studies have been performed in rats and rabbits up to 1000 times the human dose and have revealed no teratogenic effects from glycopyrrolate. There are, however, no adequate and well-controlled studies in pregnant women. Because animal reproduction studies are not always predictive of human response, this drug should be used during pregnancy only if clearly needed.

Nursing Mothers. It is not known whether this drug is excreted in human milk. Because many drugs are excreted in human milk, caution should be exercised when Robinul is administered to a nursing woman.

Pediatric Use. Safety and effectiveness in children below the age of 12 years have not been established for the management of peptic ulcer.

ADVERSE REACTIONS

Anticholinergics produce certain effects, most of which are extensions of their pharmacologic actions. Adverse reactions to anticholinergics in general may include dry mouth; urinary hesitancy and retention; blurred vision due to mydriasis; increased ocular tension; tachycardia; palpitation; decreased sweating; loss of taste; headache; nervousness; drowsiness; weakness; dizziness; insomnia; nausea; vomiting; impotence; suppression of lactation; constipation; bloated feeling; severe allergic reaction or drug idiosyncrasies incuding anaphylaxis; urticaria and other dermal manifestations; some degree of mental confusion and/or excitement, especially in elderly persons.

Robinul is chemically a quaternary ammonium compound; hence, its passage across lipid membranes, such as the blood-brain barrier is limited in contrast to atropine sulfate and scopolamine hydrobromide. For this reason the occurrence of CNS related side effects is lower, in comparison to their incidence following administration of anticholinergics which are chemically tertiary amines that can cross this barrier readily.

OVERDOSAGE

To combat peripheral anticholinergic effects, a quaternary ammonium anticholinesterase such as neostigmine methylsulfate (which does not cross the blood-brain barrier) may be given intravenously in increments of 0.25 mg in adults. This dosage may be repeated every five to ten minutes until anticholinergic over-activity is reversed or up to a maximum of 2.5 mg. Proportionately smaller doses should be used in children. Indication for repetitive doses of neostigmine should be based on close monitoring of the decrease in heart rate and the return of bowel sounds.

In the unlikely event that CNS symptoms (excitement, restlessness, convulsions, psychotic behavior) occur, physostigmine (which does cross the blood-barrier) should be used. Physostigmine 0.5 to 2 mg should be slowly administered intravenously and repeated as necessary up to a total of 5 mg in adults. Proportionately smaller doses should be used in children.

Fever should be treated symptomatically. In the event of a curare-like effect on respiratory muscles, artificial respiration should be instituted and maintained until effective respiratory action returns.

DOSAGE AND ADMINISTRATION

Robinul (glycopyrrolate) Injectable may be administered intramuscularly, or intravenously, without dilution, in the following indications:

Adults: *Preanesthetic Medication.* The recommended dose of Robinul (glycopyrrolate) Injectable is 0.002 mg (0.01 mL) per pound of body weight by intramuscular injection, given 30 to 60 minutes prior to the anticipated time of induction of anesthesia or at the time the preanesthetic narcotic and/or sedative are administered.

Intraoperative Medication. Robinul (glycopyrrolate) Injectable may be used during surgery to counteract drug induced or vagal traction reflexes with the associated arrhythmias (e.g., bradycardia). It should be administered intravenously as single doses of 0.1 mg (0.5 mL) and repeated, as needed, at intervals of 2–3 minutes. The usual attempts should be made to determine the etiology of the arrhythmia, and the surgical or anesthetic manipulations necessary to correct parasympathetic imbalance should be performed.

Reversal of Neuromuscular Blockade. The recommended dose of Robinul (glycopyrrolate) Injectable is 0.2 mg (1.0 mL) for each 1.0 mg of neostigmine or 5.0 mg of pyridostigmine. In order to minimize the appearance of cardiac side effects, the drugs may be administered simultaneously by intravenous injection and may be mixed in the same syringe.

Children: *Preanesthetic Medication.* The recommended dose of Robinul (glycopyrrolate) Injectable in children to 12 years of age is 0.002 mg (0.01 mL) per pound of body weight intramuscularly, given 30 to 60 minutes prior to the anticipated time of induction of anesthesia or at the time the preanesthetic narcotic and/or sedative are administered.

Children under 2 years of age may require up to 0.004 mg (0.02 mL) per pound of body weight.

Intraoperative Medication. Because of the long duration of action of Robinul (glycopyrrolate) if used as preanesthetic medication, additional Robinul (glycopyrrolate) Injectable for anticholinergic effect intraoperatively is rarely needed; in the event it is required the recommended pediatric dose is 0.002 mg (0.01 mL) per pound of body weight intravenously, not to exceed 0.1 mg (0.5 mL) in a single dose which may be repeated, as needed, at intervals of 2–3 minutes. The usual attempts should be made to determine the etiology of the arrhythmia, and the surgical or anesthetic manipulations necessary to correct parasympathetic imbalance should be performed.

Reversal of Neuromuscular Blockade. The recommended pediatric dose of Robinul (glycopyrrolate) Injectable is 0.2 mg (1.0 mL) for each 1.0 mg of neostigmine or 5.0 mg of pyridostigmine. In order to minimize the appearance of cardiac side effects, the drugs may be administered simultaneously by intravenous injection and may be mixed in the same syringe.

Adults: *Peptic Ulcer.* The usual recommended dose of Robinul Injectable is 0.1 mg (0.5 mL) administered at 4-hour intervals, 3 or 4 times daily intravenously or intramuscularly. Where more profound effect is required, 0.2 mg (1.0 mL) may be given. Some patients may need only a single dose, and frequency of administration should be dictated by patient response up to a maximum of four times daily.

Robinul Injectable is not recommended for peptic ulcers in children under 12 years of age. (See Precautions.)

Continued on next page

Prescribing information on A. H. Robins products listed here is based on official labeling in effect June 1, 1986, with Indications, Contraindications, Warnings, Precautions, Adverse Reactions, and Dosage stated in full.

Robins—Cont.

NOTE: Parenteral drug products should be inspected visually for particulate matter and discoloration prior to administration whenever solution and container permit.

Admixture Compatibilities. Robinul (glycopyrrolate) Injectable is compatible for mixing and injection with the following injectable dosage forms: 5% and 10% glucose in water or saline; atropine sulfate, USP; Antilirium® (physostigmine salicylate); Benadryl® (diphenhydramine HCl); codeine phosphate, USP; Emete-Con® (benzquinamide HCl); hydromorphone HCl, USP; Inapsine® (droperidol); Innovar® (droperidol and fentabyl citrate); Largon® (propiomazine HCl); Levo-Dromoran® (levorphanol tartrate); lidocaine, USP; Mepergan® (meperidine and promethazine HCls); meperidine HCl, USP; Mestinon® /Regonol® (pyridostigmine bromide); morphine sulfate, USP; Nisentil® (alphaprodine HCl); Nubain® (nalbuphine HCl); Numorphan® (oxymorphone HCl); Pantopon® (opium alkaloids HCls); procaine HCl, USP; promethazine HCl, USP; Prostigmin® (neostigmine methylsulfate, USP); scopolamine HBr, USP; Sparine® (promazine HCl); Stadol® (butorphanol tartrate); Sublimaze® (fentanyl citrate); Talwin® (pentazocine lactate); Tigan® (trimethobenzamide HCl); Vesprin® (triflupromazine HCl); and Vistaril® (hydroxyzine HCl).

Robinul Injectable may be administered via the tubing of a running infusion of physiological saline or lactated Ringer's solution.

Since the stability of glycopyrrolate is questionable above a pH of 6.0, do *not* combine Robinul Injectable in the same syringe with Brevital® (methohexital Na); Chloromycetin® (chloramphenicol Na succinate); Dramamine® (dimenhydrinate); Nembutal® (pentobarbital Na); Pentothal® (thiopental Na); Seconal® (secobarbital Na); sodium bicarbonate (Abbott); or Valium® (diazepam). A gas will evolve or a precipitate may form. Mixing with Decadron® (dexamethazone Na phosphate) or a buffered solution of lactated Ringer's solution will result in a pH higher than 6.0. Mixing chlorpromazine HCl, USP, or Compazine® (prochlorperazine) with other agents in a syringe is not recommended by the manufacturer, although the mixture with Robinul Injectable is physically compatible.

HOW SUPPLIED

Robinul (glycopyrrolate) Injectable, 0.2 mg/mL, is available in 1 mL single dose vials packaged in 5's (NDC 0031-7890-87), and 25's (NDC 0031-7890-11), 2 mL single dose vials packaged in 25's (NDC 0031-7890-95), 5 mL multiple dose vials packaged individually (NDC 0031-7890-93) and in 25's (NDC 0031-7890-06), and 20 mL (NDC 0031-7890-83) multiple dose vials.

Store at controlled room temperature, between 15°C and 30°C (59°F and 86°F).

Manufactured for Pharmaceutical Division, A. H. Robins Company, Richmond, Virginia 23220 by Elkins-Sinn, Inc., Cherry Hill, NJ 08003-4099, a subsidiary of A. H. Robins Co.

Shown in Product Identification Section, page 424

ROBITUSSIN®
[*ro"bĭ-tuss'ĭn*]
ROBITUSSIN-CF®
ROBITUSSIN-DM®
ROBITUSSIN-PE®

(See PDR For Nonprescription Drugs)

ROBITUSSIN A-C® Ⓒ
[*ro"bĭ-tuss'ĭn*]

PRODUCT OVERVIEW

KEY FACTS

Guaifenesin enhances the output of lower respiratory tract fluid. Codeine phosphate is favored for its antitussive efficacy in low dosage. As a result, dry, unproductive coughs become more productive and less frequent.

MAJOR USES

Useful in combating coughs associated with the common cold, bronchitis, laryngitis, tracheitis, pharyngitis, pertussis, influenza, and measles.

SAFETY INFORMATION

Use this product with caution in children under two years or in children taking another drug. Prescribe cautiously for patients with persistent or chronic cough.

PRESCRIBING INFORMATION

ROBITUSSIN A-C® Ⓒ
[*ro"bĭ-tuss'ĭn*]

Robitussin and codeine.

Each 5 mL (1 teaspoonful) contains:

Guaifenesin, USP .... 100 mg
Codeine Phosphate, USP .... 10 mg
(Warning: May be habit forming)
Alcohol 3.5 per cent
In a palatable, aromatic syrup

Inactive Ingredients: Caramel, Citric Acid, FD&C Red 40, Flavors, Glycerin, High Fructose Corn Syrup, Saccharin Sodium, Sodium Benzoate, Water.

ACTIONS

Robitussin A-C combines the expectorant, guaifenesin, with the cough suppressant, codeine. Guaifenesin enhances the output of lower respiratory tract fluid (RTF). The enhanced flow of less viscid secretions promotes ciliary action and facilitates the removal of inspissated mucus. As a result, dry, unproductive coughs become more productive and less frequent.

Codeine phosphate is favored for its efficacy in low dosage. Robitussin A-C is especially useful when concurrent expectorant and cough suppressant actions are desired.

INDICATIONS

Robitussin A-C is useful in combating coughs associated with the common cold, bronchitis, laryngitis, tracheitis, pharyngitis, pertussis, influenza, and measles.

CONTRAINDICATIONS

Hypersensitivity to any of the ingredients.

WARNINGS

Use this product with caution in children under 2 years or in children taking another drug. Prescribe cautiously for patients with persistent or chronic cough such as occurs with smoking, asthma, emphysema, or where cough is accompanied by excessive secretions. In patients with chronic pulmonary disease or shortness of breath, this product should be administered with caution. This product may cause or aggravate constipation. As with any drug, if you are pregnant or nursing a baby, seek the advice of a health professional before using this product.

Note: Guaifenesin has been shown to produce a color interference with certain clinical laboratory determinations of 5-hydroxyindoleacetic acid (5-HIAA) and vanillylmandelic acid (VMA).

ADVERSE REACTIONS

Rarely, nausea, gastrointestinal upset, constipation, and drowsiness may occur. No serious side effects from guaifenesin have been reported.

DOSAGE

Adults and children 12 years of age and over: 2 teaspoonfuls every four hours, not to exceed 12 teaspoonfuls in a 24 hour period; children 6 to under 12 years: 1 teaspoonful every four hours, not to exceed 6 teaspoonfuls in a 24 hour period; children 2 to under 6 years: ½ teaspoonful every four hours, not to exceed 3 teaspoonfuls in a 24 hour period; children under 2 years: use as directed by physician.

HOW SUPPLIED

Bottles of 2 ounces (NDC 0031-8674-05), 4 ounces (NDC 0031-8674-12), one pint (NDC 0031-8674-25), and one gallon (NDC 0031-8674-29).

ROBITUSSIN® -DAC Ⓒ
[*ro"bĭ-tuss'ĭn*]

PRODUCT OVERVIEW

KEY FACTS

The expectorant, guaifenesin, relieves irritated membranes in the respiratory passages; the nasal decongestant, pseudoephedrine, reduces the swelling of nasal passages; the antitussive, codeine, calms the cough control center and relieves coughing.

MAJOR USES

For the temporary relief of cough and nasal congestion as may occur with the common cold or with inhaled irritants.

SAFETY INFORMATION

Use this product with caution in children under two years of age or in children taking another drug. Do not exceed recommended dosage since nervousness, dizziness, or sleeplessness may occur. Prescribe cautiously for patients with persistent or chronic cough.

PRESCRIBING INFORMATION

ROBITUSSIN® -DAC Ⓒ
[*ro"bĭ-tuss'ĭn*]

Each 5 mL (1 teaspoonful) contains:

Guaifenesin, USP .... 100 mg
Pseudoephedrine
Hydrochloride, USP .... 30 mg
Codeine Phosphate, USP .... 10 mg
(Warning: May be habit forming)
In a palatable, aromatic syrup
Alcohol 1.4 per cent

Inactive Ingredients: Citric Acid, FD&C Red 40, Flavors, Glucose, Glycerin, High Fructose Corn Syrup, Saccharin Sodium, Sodium Benzoate, Water.

INDICATIONS

For the temporary relief of cough and nasal congestion as may occur with the common cold or with inhaled irritants. Contains the expectorant, guaifenesin, which relieves irritated membranes in the respiratory passageways by preventing dryness through increased mucus flow. The nasal decongestant, pseudoephedrine, reduces the swelling of nasal passages. The antitussive, codeine, calms the cough control center and relieves coughing.

CONTRAINDICATIONS

Hypersensitivity to any of the ingredients, marked hypertension, hyperthyroidism, or in patients who are receiving MAO inhibitors or antihypertensive medication.

WARNINGS

Use this product with caution in children under 2 years or in children taking another drug. Prescribe cautiously for patients with persistent or chronic cough such as comes with smoking, asthma, emphysema, or where cough is accompanied by excessive secretions. Caution should be taken in administering this drug to patients with high blood pressure, heart disease or diabetes. In patients with chronic pulmonary disease or shortness of breath, this product should be administered with caution. As with all products containing sympathomimetic amines, use with caution in patients with prostatic hypertrophy or glaucoma. Do not exceed recommended dosage because at higher doses nervousness, dizziness or sleeplessness may occur. May cause or aggravate constipation. As with any drug, if you are pregnant or nursing a baby, seek the advice of a health professional before using this product.

Note: Guaifenesin has been shown to produce a color interference with certain clinical laboratory determinations of 5-hydroxyindoleacetic acid (5-HIAA) and vanillylmandelic acid (VMA).

ADVERSE REACTIONS

Agitation, dizziness, insomnia, palpitations or nausea may occur. In such instances, reduction in frequency and/or quantity of dose is indicated.

RECOMMENDED DOSAGE

Adults and children 12 years of age and over: 1 or 2 teaspoonfuls every four hours, not to exceed 8 teaspoonfuls in a 24-hour period; children 6 to under 12 years: 1 teaspoonful every four hours, not to exceed 4 teaspoonfuls in a 24-hour period; children 2 to under 6 years: ½ teaspoonful every four hours, not to exceed 2 teaspoonfuls in a 24-hour period; children under 2 years: use as directed by physician.

HOW SUPPLIED

Robitussin-DAC is available in pints (NDC 0031-8680-25).

VIOKASE® ℞
[*vi'o-kās*]
(Pancrelipase, USP)
Tablets
Powder

DESCRIPTION

Viokase (Pancrelipase, USP) is a pancreatic enzyme concentrate of porcine origin containing standardized lipase, protease, and amylase as well as other pancreatic enzymes. Viokase is available in tablet and powder dosage form for oral administration.

The enzyme potencies of the tablets and powder are:

	Each Tablet	Each 0.7g powder (¼ teaspoonful)
Lipase, USP Units	8,000	16,800
Protease, USP Units	30,000	70,000
Amylase, USP Units	30,000	70,000

Inactive Ingredients:
TABLETS—Lactose, Magnesium Stearate, Sodium Chloride, Stearic Acid.
POWDER—Lactose, Sodium Chloride

CLINICAL PHARMACOLOGY

The natural digestive enzymes in Viokase hydrolyze fats into fatty acids and glycerol, split protein into amino acids, and convert carbohydrates to dextrins and short chain sugars. Under conditions of the USP test method (in vitro) Viokase has the following total digestive capacity:

	Each Tablet	Each 0.7g powder
Dietary Fat, grams	28	59
Dietary Protein, grams	30	70
Dietary Starch, grams	30	70

Viokase Tablets are not enteric coated.

The digestive capacity of a pancreatic enzyme concentrate depends on the amount that passes through the stomach unchanged and is available at the site of action in the small intestine.

INDICATIONS

Viokase (Pancrelipase, USP) is indicated as a digestive aid in the treatment of exocrine pancreatic insufficiency as associated with but not limited to cystic fibrosis, chronic pancreatitis, pancreatectomy, or obstruction of the pancreas ducts.

CONTRAINDICATIONS

Do not use in patients hypersensitive to pork protein.

PRECAUTIONS

General: Individuals previously sensitized to trypsin, pancreatin or pancrelipase may have allergic manifestations.

Information for patients: Viokase should not be held in the mouth as the proteolytic action may cause irritation of the mucosa.

Avoid inhalation of the powder when administering Viokase.

Carcinogenesis, Mutagenesis, Impairment of fertility: - Long-term studies in animals have not been performed to evaluate carcinogenic potential.

Pregnancy Category C. Animal reproduction studies have not been conducted with Viokase. It is also not known whether Viokase can cause fetal harm when administered to a pregnant woman or can affect reproduction capacity. Viokase should be given to a pregnant woman only if clearly needed.

Nursing Mothers: It is not known whether this drug is excreted in human milk. Because many drugs are excreted in human milk, caution should be exercised when Viokase is administered to a nursing mother.

ADVERSE REACTIONS

The dust or finely powdered pancreatic enzyme concentrate is irritating to the nasal mucosa and the respiratory tract. It has been documented that inhalation of the airborne powder can precipitate an asthma attack. The literature also contains several references to asthma due to inhalation in patients sensitized to pancreatic enzyme concentrates. Extremely high doses of exogenous pancreatic enzymes have been associated with hyperuricemia and hyperuricosuria. Overdosage of pancreatic enzyme concentrate may cause diarrhea or transient intestinal upset.

OVERDOSAGE

Acute toxicity determinations in animals have not been possible since the maximum dose that could be given orally produced no toxic reaction. In chronic feeding tests. rats developed swollen salivary glands. This is believed due to the proteolytic activity and the mucosal irritation caused by tissue digestion.

No acute toxic reactions have been reported.

DOSAGE AND ADMINISTRATION

Powder: Dosage for patients with cystic fibrosis—¼ teaspoonful (0.7 grams) with meals.

Tablets: Dosage for patients with cystic fibrosis or chronic pancreatitis—1 to 3 tablets with meals or as directed by physician. As a digestive aid in patients with pancreatectomy or obstruction of pancreatic ducts—1 to 2 tablets taken at 2-hour intervals or as directed by physician.

HOW SUPPLIED

Tablets—Tan, round, compressed tablets engraved Viokase/AHR on one side and 9111 on the other side in bottles of 100 (NDC 0031-9111-63) and 500 (NDC 0031-9111-70). *Powder*—Tan powder in bottles of 4 oz. (113.5 grams) (NDC 0031-9115-12) and 8 oz. (227 grams) (NDC 0031-9115-25).

Store in tightly closed container in a dry place at a temperature not exceeding 25°C (77°F).

Dispense tablets and powder in tight container, preferably with a desiccant.

CLINICAL STUDIES

The effectiveness of Viokase as a digestive aid in the treatment of patients with exocrine pancreatic insufficiency has been documented in the literature as follows:

1. Regan, PT, Malagelada J-R, DiMagno EP, Glanzman SL., Go VLW: Comparative effects of antacids, cimetidine and enteric coating on the therapeutic response to oral enzymes in severe pancreatic insufficiency. N. Engl. J. Med. 297:854-8, 1977.

2. Graham DY: Enzyme replacement therapy of exocrine pancreatic insufficiency in man. N. Engl. J. Med. 296:1314-7, 1977.

Shown in Product Identification Section, page 424

Z-BEC®

[zē'bĕk]

(See PDR For Nonprescription Drugs)

Products are cross-indexed by
generic and chemical names in the
YELLOW SECTION

Roche Laboratories

Division of Hoffmann-La Roche Inc.
NUTLEY, NJ 07110

ACCUTANE® ℞

[acc'u-tane]
isotretinoin/Roche
CAPSULES

The following text is complete prescribing information based on official labeling in effect July 1, 1986.

CONTRAINDICATION

Accutane must not be used by females who are pregnant or who intend to become pregnant while undergoing treatment.

Major human fetal abnormalities related to Accutane administration have been reported, including hydrocephalus, microcephalus, abnormalities of the external ear (micropinna, small or absent external auditory canals), microphthalmia and cardiovascular abnormalities.

Women of childbearing potential should not be given Accutane until pregnancy is excluded. It is strongly recommended that a pregnancy test be performed within two weeks prior to Accutane therapy. Accutane therapy should start on the second or third day of the next normal menstrual period. An effective form of contraception should be used for at least one month before and also throughout Accutane therapy. It is recommended that contraception be continued for one month following discontinuation of Accutane therapy.

Females should be fully counseled on the serious risk to the fetus should they become pregnant while undergoing treatment. If pregnancy does occur during treatment, the physician and patient should discuss the desirability of continuing the pregnancy.

DESCRIPTION

Accutane (isotretinoin/Roche), a retinoid which inhibits sebaceous gland function and keratinization, is available in 10-mg, 20-mg and 40-mg soft gelatin capsules for oral administration. Each capsule also contains beeswax, butylated hydroxyanisole, edetate disodium, hydrogenated soybean oil flakes, hydrogenated vegetable oil and soybean oil. Gelatin capsules contain glycerin and parabens (methyl and propyl), with the following dye systems: 10 mg—iron oxide (red) and titanium dioxide; 20 mg—FD&C Red No. 3, FD&C Blue No. 1 and titanium dioxide; 40 mg—FD&C Yellow No. 6, D&C Yellow No. 10 and titanium dioxide.

Chemically, isotretinoin is 13-*cis*-retinoic acid and is related to both retinoic acid and retinol (vitamin A). It is a yellow-orange to orange crystalline powder with a molecular weight of 300.44.

CLINICAL PHARMACOLOGY

The exact mechanism of action of Accutane is unknown.

Cystic Acne: Clinical improvement in cystic acne patients occurs in association with a reduction in sebum secretion. The decrease in sebum secretion is temporary and is related to the dose and duration of treatment with Accutane, and reflects a reduction in sebaceous gland size and an inhibition of sebaceous gland differentiation.[1]

Clinical Pharmacokinetics: The pharmacokinetic profile of isotretinoin is predictable and can be described using linear pharmacokinetic theory.

After oral administration of 80 mg (two 40-mg capsules), peak blood concentrations ranged from 167 to 459 ng/ml (mean 256 ng/ml) and mean time to peak was 3.2 hours in normal volunteers, while in acne patients peak concentrations ranged from 98 to 535 ng/ml (mean 262 ng/ml) with a mean time to peak of 2.9 hours. The drug is 99.9% bound in human plasma almost exclusively to albumin. The terminal elimination half-life of isotretinoin ranged from 10 to 20 hours in volunteers and patients. Following an 80-mg liquid suspension oral dose of ^{14}C-isotretinoin, ^{14}C-activity in blood declined with a half-life of 90 hours. Relatively equal amounts of radioactivity were recovered in the urine and feces with 65% to 83% of the dose recovered.

The major identified metabolite in blood is 4-*oxo*-isotretinoin. Tretinoin and 4-*oxo*-tretinoin were also observed. The terminal elimination of 4-*oxo*-isotretinoin is formation rate limited and therefore the apparent half-life of the 4-*oxo* metabolite is similar to isotretinoin following Accutane administration. After two 40-mg capsules of isotretinoin, maximum concentrations of the metabolite of 87 to 399 ng/ml occurred at 6 to 20 hours. The blood concentration of the major metabolite generally exceeded that of isotretinoin after six hours.

The mean ± SD minimum steady-state blood concentration of isotretinoin was 160 ± 19 ng/ml in ten patients receiving 40-mg *b.i.d.* doses. After single and multiple doses, the mean ratio of areas under the blood concentration:time curves of 4-*oxo*-isotretinoin to isotretinoin was 3 to 3.5.

Tissue Distribution in Animals: Tissue distribution of ^{14}C-isotretinoin in rats after oral dosing revealed high concentrations of radioactivity in many tissues after 15 minutes, with a maximum in one hour, and declining to nondetectable levels by 24 hours in most tissues. After seven days, however, low levels of radioactivity were detected in the liver, ureter, adrenal, ovary and lacrimal gland.

INDICATIONS AND USAGE

Cystic Acne: Accutane is indicated for the treatment of severe recalcitrant cystic acne, and a single course of therapy has been shown to result in complete and prolonged remission of disease in many patients.[1–3] If a second course of therapy is needed, it should not be initiated until at least eight weeks after completion of the first course, since experience has shown that patients may continue to improve while off drug.

Because of significant adverse effects associated with its use, Accutane should be reserved for patients with severe cystic acne who are unresponsive to conventional therapy, including systemic antibiotics.

CONTRAINDICATIONS

Pregnancy: Category X. See boxed Contraindication.

Accutane should not be given to patients who are sensitive to parabens, which are used as preservatives in the gelatin capsule.

WARNINGS

Pseudotumor cerebri: **Accutane use has been associated with a number of cases of pseudotumor cerebri (benign intracranial hypertension). Early signs and symptoms of pseudotumor cerebri include papilledema, headache, nausea and vomiting, and visual disturbances. Patients with these symptoms should be screened for papilledema and, if present, they should be told to discontinue Accutane immediately and be referred to a neurologist for further diagnosis and care.**

Corneal opacities: Corneal opacities have occurred in patients receiving Accutane for acne and more frequently when higher drug dosages were used in patients with disorders of keratinization. All Accutane patients experiencing visual difficulties should discontinue the drug and have an ophthalmological examination. The corneal opacities that have been observed in patients treated with Accutane have either completely resolved or were resolving at follow-up six to seven weeks after discontinuation of the drug. See ADVERSE REACTIONS.

Inflammatory Bowel Disease: Accutane has been temporally associated with inflammatory bowel disease (including regional ileitis) in patients without a prior history of intestinal disorders. Patients experiencing abdominal pain, rectal bleeding or severe diarrhea should discontinue Accutane immediately.

Lipids: Blood lipid determinations should be performed before Accutane is given and then at intervals until the lipid response to Accutane is established, which usually occurs within four weeks. See PRECAUTIONS.

Approximately 25% of patients receiving Accutane experienced an elevation in plasma triglycerides. Approximately 15% developed a decrease in high density lipoproteins and about 7% showed an increase in cholesterol levels. These effects on triglycerides, HDL and cholesterol were reversible upon cessation of Accutane therapy.

Patients with increased tendency to develop hypertriglyceridemia include those with diabetes mellitus, obesity, increased alcohol intake and familial history.

The cardiovascular consequences of hypertriglyceridemia are not well understood, but may increase the patient's risk status. In addition, elevation of serum triglycerides in excess of 800 mg/dl has been associated with acute pancreatitis. Therefore, every attempt should be made to control significant triglyceride elevation.

Some patients have been able to reverse triglyceride elevation by reduction in weight, restriction of dietary fat and alcohol, and reduction in dose while continuing Accutane.[4] An obese male patient with Darier's disease developed elevated triglycerides and subsequent eruptive xanthomas.[5]

Hyperostosis: In clinical trials of disorders of keratinization with a mean dose of 2.24 mg/kg/day, a high prevalence of skeletal hyperostosis was noted. Two children showed x-ray findings suggestive of premature closure of the epiphysis. Additionally, skeletal hyperostosis was noted in six of eight patients in a prospective study of disorders of keratinization.[6] Minimal skeletal hyperostosis has also been observed by x-rays in prospective studies of cystic acne patients treated with a single course of therapy at recommended doses.

Animal Studies: In rats given 32 or 8 mg/kg/day of isotretinoin for 18 months or longer, the incidences of focal cal-

Continued on next page

Roche Labs.—Cont.

cification, fibrosis and inflammation of the myocardium, calcification of coronary, pulmonary and mesenteric arteries and metastatic calcification of the gastric mucosa were greater than in control rats of similar age. Focal endocardial and myocardial calcifications associated with calcification of the coronary arteries were observed in two dogs after approximately six to seven months of treatment with isotretinoin at a dosage of 60 to 120 mg/kg/day.

In dogs given isotretinoin chronically at a dosage of 60 mg/kg/day, corneal ulcers and corneal opacities were encountered at a higher incidence than in control dogs. In general, these ocular changes tended to revert toward normal when treatment with isotretinoin was stopped, but did not completely clear during the observation period.

In rats given isotretinoin at a dosage of 32 mg/kg/day for approximately 15 weeks, long bone fracture has been observed.

PRECAUTIONS

Information for Patients: **Women of childbearing potential should be instructed that they must not be pregnant when Accutane therapy is initiated, and that they should use an effective form of contraception while taking Accutane and for one month after Accutane has been stopped. See boxed Contraindication.**

Because of the relationship of Accutane to vitamin A, patients should be advised against taking vitamin supplements containing vitamin A to avoid additive toxic effects.

Patients should be informed that transient exacerbation of acne has been seen, generally during the initial period of therapy.

Patients should be informed that they may experience decreased tolerance to contact lenses during and after therapy.

Laboratory Tests: The incidence of hypertriglyceridemia is 1 patient in 4 on Accutane therapy. Pretreatment and follow-up blood lipids should be obtained under fasting conditions. After consumption of alcohol at least 36 hours should elapse before these determinations are made. It is recommended that these tests be performed at weekly or biweekly intervals until the lipid response to Accutane is established.

Certain patients receiving Accutane have experienced problems in the control of their blood sugar. Therefore, known or suspected diabetics should have periodic blood sugar determinations performed during Accutane therapy. Some patients undergoing vigorous physical activity while on Accutane therapy have experienced elevated CPK levels; however, the clinical significance is unknown.

Carcinogenesis, Mutagenesis, Impairment of Fertility: In Fischer 344 rats given isotretinoin at dosages of 32 or 8 mg/kg/day for greater than 18 months, there was an increased incidence of pheochromocytoma. The incidence of adrenal medullary hyperplasia was also increased at the higher dosage. The relatively high level of spontaneous pheochromocytomas occurring in the Fischer 344 rat makes it a poor model for study of this tumor, since the increase in adrenal medullary proliferative lesions following chronic treatment with relatively high dosages of isotretinoin may be an accentuation of a genetic predisposition in the Fischer 344 rat, and its relevance to the human population is not clear. In addition, a decreased incidence of liver adenomas, liver angiomas and leukemia was noted at the dose levels of 8 and 32 mg/kg/day.

The Ames test was conducted in two laboratories. The results of the tests in one laboratory were completely negative, while in the second laboratory a weakly positive (less than 1.6 x background) was seen with S. typhimurium TA100. No dose-response effect was seen and all other strains were negative. Additionally, other mutagenicity tests (Chinese hamster cells, mouse micronucleus test and S. cerevisiae) were also negative.

No adverse effects on gonadal function, fertility, conception rate, gestation or parturition were observed at dose levels of 2, 8 or 32 mg/kg/day in male and female rats.

In dogs, testicular atrophy was noted after treatment with isotretinoin for approximately 30 weeks at dosages of 60 or 20 mg/kg/day. In general, there was microscopic evidence for appreciable depression of spermatogenesis but some sperm were observed in all testes examined and in no instance were completely atrophic tubules seen. In studies in 66 human males, 30 of whom were patients with cystic acne, no significant changes were noted in the count or motility of spermatozoa in the ejaculate. Studies further evaluating this in humans are being conducted.

Pregnancy: **Category X. See boxed Contraindication.**

Nursing Mothers: It is not known whether this drug is excreted in human milk. Because of the potential for adverse effects, nursing mothers should not receive Accutane.

ADVERSE REACTIONS

Clinical: Many of the side effects and adverse reactions seen or expected in patients receiving Accutane are similar to those described in patients taking high doses of vitamin A. The percentages of adverse reactions listed below reflect the total experience in Accutane studies, including investigational studies of disorders of keratinization, with the exception of those pertaining to dry skin and mucous membranes. These latter reflect the experience only in patients with cystic acne because reactions relating to dryness are more commonly recognized as adverse reactions in this disease. Included in this category are dry skin, skin fragility, pruritus, epistaxis, dry nose and dry mouth, which may be seen in up to 80% of cystic acne patients.

The most frequent adverse reaction to Accutane is cheilitis, which occurs in over 90% of patients. A less frequent reaction was conjunctivitis (about two patients in five).

Skeletal hyperostosis has been observed on x-rays of patients treated with Accutane. See WARNINGS.

Approximately 16% of patients treated with Accutane developed musculoskeletal symptoms during treatment. In general, these were mild to moderate and have occasionally required discontinuation of drug. Less frequently, transient pain in the chest has also been reported. These symptoms generally cleared rapidly after discontinuation of Accutane, but in rare cases have persisted.

In less than one patient in ten—rash; thinning of hair, which in rare cases has persisted.

In approximately one patient in twenty—peeling of palms and soles, skin infections, nonspecific urogenital findings, nonspecific gastrointestinal symptoms, fatigue, headache and increased susceptibility to sunburn.

Accutane has been associated with a number of cases of pseudotumor cerebri, some of which involved concomitant use of tetracyclines. See WARNINGS.

The following CNS reactions have been reported and may bear no relationship to therapy—seizures, emotional instability, dizziness, nervousness, drowsiness, malaise, weakness, insomnia, lethargy and paresthesias.

Depression has been reported in some patients on Accutane therapy. In some of these patients, this has subsided with discontinuation of therapy and recurred with reinstitution of therapy.

The following reactions have been reported in less than 1% of patients and may bear no relationship to therapy—changes in skin pigment (hypo- and hyperpigmentation), urticaria, bruising, disseminated herpes simplex, edema, hair problems (other than thinning), hirsutism, respiratory infections, weight loss, erythema nodosum, paronychia, nail dystrophy, bleeding and inflammation of the gums, abnormal menses and optic neuritis.

A few isolated reports of Wegener's granulomatosis have been received, but no causal relationship to Accutane therapy has been established.

In Accutane studies to date, of 72 patients who had normal pretreatment ophthalmological examinations, five developed corneal opacities while on Accutane (all five patients had a disorder of keratinization). Corneal opacities have also been reported in cystic acne patients treated with Accutane. See WARNINGS. Dry eyes and decrease in night vision have been reported and in rare instances have persisted. Cataracts and visual disturbances have also been reported.

Accutane has been temporally associated with inflammatory bowel disease. See WARNINGS.

As may be seen with healing cystic acne lesions, an occasional exaggerated healing response, manifested by exuberant granulation tissue with crusting, has also been reported in patients receiving therapy with Accutane.

Laboratory: Accutane therapy induces change in serum lipids in a significant number of treated subjects. Approximately 25% of patients had elevation of plasma triglycerides. Five out of 135 patients treated for cystic acne and 32 out of 298 total subjects treated for all diagnoses showed an elevation of triglycerides above 500 mg percent. About 16% of patients showed a mild to moderate decrease in serum high density lipoprotein (HDL) levels while receiving treatment with Accutane and about 7% of patients experienced minimal elevations of serum cholesterol during treatment. Abnormalities of serum triglycerides, HDL and cholesterol were reversible upon cessation of Accutane therapy.

Approximately 40% of patients receiving Accutane developed elevated sedimentation rates, often from elevated baseline values.

From one in ten to one in five patients showed decreases in red blood cell parameters and white blood cell counts, elevated platelet counts, white cells in the urine, increased alkaline phosphatase, SGOT, SGPT, GGTP or LDH.

Less than one in ten patients showed proteinuria, microscopic or gross hematuria, elevated fasting blood sugar, elevated CPK or hyperuricemia.

Dose Relationship and Duration: Cheilitis and hypertriglyceridemia are usually dose-related.

Most adverse reactions were reversible when therapy was discontinued; however, some have persisted after cessation of therapy. (See WARNINGS and ADVERSE REACTIONS.)

Overdosage: The oral LD_{50} of isotretinoin is greater than 4000 mg/kg in rats and mice and is approximately 1960 mg/kg in rabbits. Overdose has been associated with transient headache, vomiting, facial flushing, cheilosis, abdominal pain, headache, dizziness and ataxia. All symptoms quickly resolved without apparent residual effects.

DOSAGE AND ADMINISTRATION

The recommended dosage range for Accutane is 0.5 to 2 mg/kg given in two divided doses daily for 15 to 20 weeks. In studies comparing 0.1, 0.5, and 1 mg/kg/day,[7] it was found that all doses provided initial clearing of disease but there was a greater need for retreatment with the lower dose(s).

It is recommended that for most patients the initial dose of Accutane be 0.5 to 1 mg/kg/day. Patients whose disease is very severe or is primarily manifest on the body may require up to the maximum recommended dose, 2 mg/kg/day. During treatment, the dose may be adjusted according to response of the disease and/or the appearance of clinical side effects—some of which may be dose-related.

If the total cyst count has been reduced by more than 70 percent prior to completing 15 to 20 weeks of treatment, the drug may be discontinued. After a period of two months or more off therapy, and if warranted by persistent or recurring severe cystic acne, a second course of therapy may be initiated.

ACCUTANE DOSING BY BODY WEIGHT

Body Weight		Total Mg/Day		
kilograms	pounds	0.5 mg/kg	1 mg/kg	2 mg/kg
40	88	20	40	80
50	110	25	50	100
60	132	30	60	120
70	154	35	70	140
80	176	40	80	160
90	198	45	90	180
100	220	50	100	200

HOW SUPPLIED

Soft gelatin capsules, 10 mg (light pink), imprinted ACCUTANE 10 ROCHE; bottles of 100 (NDC-0004-0155-01).

Soft gelatin capsules, 20 mg (maroon), imprinted ACCUTANE 20 ROCHE; bottles of 100 (NDC-0004-0169-01).

Soft gelatin capsules, 40 mg (yellow), imprinted ACCUTANE 40 ROCHE; bottles of 100 (NDC-0004-0156-01).

REFERENCES

1. Peck GL, Olsen TG, Yoder FW, Strauss JS, Downing DT, Pandya M, Butkus D, Arnaud-Battandier J: Prolonged remissions of cystic and conglobate acne with 13-*cis* -retinoic acid. *N Engl J Med 300* :329–333, 1979. 2. Farrell LN, Strauss JS, Stranieri AM: The treatment of severe cystic acne with 13-*cis* -retinoic acid. Evaluation of sebum production and the clinical response in a multiple-dose trial. *J Am Acad Dermatol 3* :602–611, 1980. 3. Jones H, Blanc D, Cunliffe WJ: 13-*cis* -retinoic acid and acne. *Lancet 2* :1048–1049, 1980. 4. Katz RA, Jorgensen H, Nigra TP: Elevation of serum triglyceride levels from oral isotretinoin in disorders of keratinization. *Arch Dermatol 116* :1369–1372, 1980. 5. Dicken CH, Connolly SM: Eruptive xanthomas associated with isotretinoin (13-*cis* -retinoic acid). *Arch Dermatol 116* :951–952, 1980. 6. Ellis CN, Madison KC, Pennes DR, Martel W, Voorhees JJ: Isotretinoin therapy is associated with early skeletal radiographic changes. *J Am Acad Dermatol 10* :1024–1029, 1984. 7. Strauss JS, Rapini RP, Shalita AR, Konecky E, Pochi PE, Comite H, Exner JH: Isotretinoin therapy for acne: Results of a multicenter dose-response study. *J Am Acad Dermatol 10* :490–496, 1984.

Shown in Product Identification Section, page 424

ALURATE® ELIXIR Ⓒⅲ

[al'u-rate]

(aprobarbital/Roche)

The following text is complete prescribing information based on official labeling in effect June 1, 1986.

The following sections contain information specifically applicable to Alurate as well as information pertinent to other barbiturates. The information pertinent to other barbiturates should be considered when administering Alurate.

DESCRIPTION

Alurate (aprobarbital/Roche) is an intermediate-acting barbiturate which is used as a sedative-hypnotic. As with other barbiturates, it acts as a CNS depressant. Alurate is available for oral administration as a red elixir providing 40 mg of aprobarbital per teaspoonful (5 ml) in a vehicle containing 20 percent alcohol, dextrose, saccharin, sorbitol, sucrose, FD&C Yellow No. 6, FD&C Red No. 40, flavors and water. Chemically, aprobarbital is 5-allyl-5-isopropylbarbituric acid. It is a bitter, white crystalline powder with an empirical formula of $C_{10}H_{14}N_2O_3$ and a molecular weight of 210.23.

CLINICAL PHARMACOLOGY

Barbiturates are capable of producing all levels of CNS mood alteration from excitation to mild sedation, hypnosis and deep coma. Overdosage can produce death. In high enough therapeutic doses, barbiturates induce anesthesia.

Barbiturates depress the sensory cortex, decrease motor activity, alter cerebellar function and produce drowsiness, sedation and hypnosis.
Barbiturate-induced sleep differs from physiological sleep. Sleep laboratory studies have demonstrated that barbiturates reduce the amount of time spent in the rapid eye movement (REM) phase of sleep or dreaming stage. Also, Stages III and IV sleep are decreased. Patients may experience markedly increased dreaming, nightmares and/or insomnia if barbiturates are prescribed for a period of time and then abruptly withdrawn. It is recommended that dosage be reduced gradually over a period of 5 or 6 days to lessen REM rebound and disturbed sleep (for example, decrease the dose from 3 to 2 doses a day for 1 week).
In studies, secobarbital sodium and pentobarbital sodium have been found to lose most of their effectiveness for both inducing and maintaining sleep by the end of 2 weeks of continued drug administration, even with the use of multiple doses. Other barbiturates might also be expected to lose their effectiveness for inducing and maintaining sleep after about 2 weeks. Therefore, as sleep medications, the barbiturates are of limited value beyond short-term use.
Barbiturates have little analgesic action at subanesthetic doses. Rather, they may increase the reaction to painful stimuli. All barbiturates exhibit anticonvulsant activity in anesthetic doses; however, only phenobarbital, mephobarbital and metharbital are effective as oral anticonvulsants in subhypnotic doses.
Barbiturates are respiratory depressants; the degree of depression is dose-dependent. With hypnotic doses, respiratory depression produced by barbiturates is similar to that which occurs during physiologic sleep. Hypnotic doses also cause a slight decrease in blood pressure and heart rate.
Studies in laboratory animals have shown that barbiturates cause reduction in the tone and contractility of the uterus, ureters and urinary bladder. However, concentrations of the drugs required to produce this effect in humans are not reached with sedative-hypnotic doses.
Barbiturates do not impair normal hepatic function, but have been shown to induce liver microsomal enzymes, thus altering the metabolism of certain other drugs. (See Precautions — Drug Interactions section.)
Pharmacokinetics: Barbiturates are absorbed in varying degrees following oral administration. The onset of action for oral barbiturate administration varies from 20 to 60 minutes. Duration of action, which is related to the rate at which the barbiturates are redistributed throughout the body, varies among persons and in the same person from time to time. Aprobarbital, which is an intermediate-acting barbiturate, has a duration of action ranging from 6 to 8 hours.
Barbiturates are weak acids that are absorbed and rapidly distributed to all tissues and fluids, with high concentrations in the brain, liver and kidneys. Lipid solubility of the barbiturates is the dominant factor in their distribution throughout the body. Barbiturates are bound to plasma and tissue proteins to a varying degree, with the degree of binding increasing directly as a function of lipid solubility. Aprobarbital is approximately 20 percent plasma protein-bound. The half-life of aprobarbital ranges from 14 to 34 hours with a mean half-life of 24 hours.
Barbiturates are metabolized primarily by the hepatic microsomal enzyme system; the metabolic products are excreted in the urine and, less commonly, in the feces. Approximately 13 to 24 percent of aprobarbital is eliminated unchanged in the urine. The inactive metabolites of the barbiturates are excreted as conjugates of glucuronic acid.

INDICATIONS AND USAGE

Alurate is indicated for sedation and induction of sleep, on a short-term basis, in conditions requiring a sedative-hypnotic.

CONTRAINDICATIONS

Barbiturates are contraindicated in patients with known barbiturate sensitivity. Barbiturates are also contraindicated in patients with a history of manifest or latent porphyria.

WARNINGS

Habit forming: Barbiturates may be habit forming. Tolerance and psychological and physical dependence may occur with continued use. (See Drug Abuse and Dependence section.) Patients who have a psychological dependence on barbiturates may increase the dosage or decrease the dosage interval without consulting a physician and may subsequently develop a physical dependence. To minimize the possibility of overdosage or the development of dependence, the quantity of sedative-hypnotic barbiturates prescribed or dispensed should be limited to the amount required between appointments. Abrupt cessation after prolonged use may result in withdrawal symptoms, including delirium, convulsions and possibly death.
Barbiturates should be withdrawn gradually from any patient known to be taking excessive doses over long periods of time.
Acute or chronic pain: Caution should be exercised when barbiturates are administered to patients with acute or chronic pain, because paradoxical excitement may be induced or important symptoms may be masked.
Use in pregnancy: Barbiturates can cause fetal damage when administered to a pregnant woman. Retrospective case-controlled studies have suggested a connection between maternal consumption of barbiturates and a higher than expected incidence of fetal abnormalities. Following oral administration, barbiturates readily cross the placental barrier and are distributed throughout the placenta and fetal tissues, with highest concentrations found in the liver and brain.
Withdrawal symptoms occur in infants born to mothers who receive barbiturates throughout the last trimester of pregnancy. (See Drug Abuse and Dependence section.) If this drug is used during pregnancy, or if the patient becomes pregnant while taking this drug, the patient should be apprised of the potential hazard to the fetus.
Synergistic effects: The concomitant use of alcohol or other CNS depressants may produce additive CNS-depressant effects.

PRECAUTIONS

General: Barbiturates may be habit forming. Tolerance and psychological and physical dependence may occur with continued use. (See Drug Abuse and Dependence section.) Barbiturates should be administered with caution, if at all, to patients who are mentally depressed, have suicidal tendencies, or a history of drug abuse. Elderly or debilitated patients may react to barbiturates with marked excitement, depression and confusion. In some persons, barbiturates repeatedly produce excitement rather than depression. In patients with hepatic damage, barbiturates should be administered with caution, and initially in reduced doses. Barbiturates should not be administered to patients showing the premonitory signs of hepatic coma.
Information for Patients: The use of barbiturates carries with it an associated risk of psychological and/or physical dependence. The patient should be warned against increasing the dose of the drug without consulting a physician.
Barbiturates may impair mental and/or physical abilities required for the performance of potentially hazardous tasks, such as driving a car or operating machinery.
Alcohol should not be consumed while taking barbiturates. Concurrent use of barbiturates with other CNS depressants (*e.g.,* alcohol, narcotics, tranquilizers, antihistamines) may result in additional CNS depressant effects.
Laboratory Tests: Prolonged therapy with barbiturates should be accompanied by periodic laboratory evaluation of organ systems, including hematopoietic, renal and hepatic systems.
Drug Interactions: Most reports of clinically significant drug interactions occurring with the barbiturates have involved phenobarbital. However, the application of these data to other barbiturates appears valid and warrants serial blood level determinations of the relevant drugs when there are multiple therapies.
1. *Anticoagulants.* Phenobarbital lowers the plasma levels of dicumarol (name previously used: bishydroxycoumarin) and causes a decrease in anticoagulant activity as measured by the prothrombin time. Barbiturates can induce hepatic microsomal enzymes resulting in increased metabolism of and decreased anticoagulant response to oral anticoagulants (*e.g.,* warfarin, acenocoumarol, dicumarol and phenprocoumon). Patients stabilized on anticoagulant therapy may require dosage adjustments if barbiturates are added to or withdrawn from their dosage regimen.
2. *Corticosteroids.* Barbiturates appear to enhance the metabolism of exogenous corticosteroids, probably through the induction of hepatic microsomal enzymes. Patients stabilized on corticosteroid therapy may require dosage adjustments if barbiturates are added to or withdrawn from their dosage regimen.
3. *Griseofulvin.* Phenobarbital appears to interfere with the absorption of orally administered griseofulvin, thus decreasing its blood level. This effect on therapeutic response has not been established; however, it would be preferable to avoid concomitant administration of these drugs.
4. *Doxycycline.* Phenobarbital has been shown to shorten the half-life of doxycycline for as long as two weeks after discontinuance of the barbiturate therapy. This action is probably the result of induction of hepatic microsomal enzymes that metabolize the antibiotic. If phenobarbital and doxycycline are administered concurrently, the clinical response to doxycycline should be monitored closely.
5. *Phenytoin, sodium valproate, valproic acid.* The effect of barbiturates on the metabolism of phenytoin appears to be variable. Some investigators report an accelerating effect, while others report no effect. Because the effect is not predictable, phenytoin and barbiturate blood levels should be monitored more frequently if these drugs are given concurrently. Sodium valproate and valproic acid appear to decrease barbiturate metabolism; therefore, barbiturate blood levels should be monitored and appropriate dosage adjustments made.
6. *Central nervous system depressants.* The concomitant use of other central nervous system depressants, including other sedatives or hypnotics, antihistamines, tranquilizers or alcohol, may produce additive effects.
7. *Monoamine oxidase inhibitors (MAOI).* MAOI prolong the effects of barbiturates, probably because metabolism of the barbiturates is inhibited.
8. *Estradiol, estrone, progesterone and other steroidal hormones.* Pretreatment with or concurrent administration of phenobarbital may decrease the effect of estradiol by increasing its metabolism. There have been reports of patients treated with antiepileptic drugs (*e.g.,* phenobarbital) who became pregnant while taking oral contraceptives. An alternate contraceptive method might be suggested to women taking phenobarbital.
Carcinogenesis: 1. Animal data. Phenobarbital sodium is carcinogenic in mice and rats after lifetime administration. In mice, it produced benign and malignant liver cell tumors. In rats, benign liver cell tumors were observed very late in life.
2. Human data. In a 29-year epidemiological study of 9136 patients who were treated on an anticonvulsant protocol which included phenobarbital sodium, results indicated a higher than normal incidence of hepatic carcinoma. Previously, some of these patients were treated with Thorotrast, a drug which is known to produce hepatic carcinomas. Thus, this study did not provide sufficient evidence that phenobarbital sodium is carcinogenic in humans.
A retrospective study of 84 children with brain tumors matched to 73 normal controls and 78 cancer controls (malignant disease other than brain tumors) suggested an association between exposure to barbiturates prenatally and an increased incidence of brain tumors.
Pregnancy: 1. Teratogenic Effects. Pregnancy Category D. See Warnings section.
2. Nonteratogenic Effects. Reports of infants suffering from long-term barbiturate exposure *in utero* include the acute withdrawal syndrome of seizures and hyperirritability from birth. A delayed onset of the symptoms may be seen for up to 14 days. (See Drug Abuse and Dependence section.)
Labor and Delivery: Hypnotic doses of barbiturates do not appear to significantly impair uterine activity during labor. Full anesthetic doses of barbiturates decrease the force and frequency of uterine contractions. Administration of sedative-hypnotic barbiturates to the mother during labor may result in respiratory depression in the newborn.
Premature infants are particularly susceptible to the depressant effects of barbiturates. If barbiturates are used during labor and delivery, resuscitation equipment should be available.
Data are not currently available to evaluate the effect of these barbiturates when forceps delivery or other intervention is necessary. Also, data are not available to determine the effect of these barbiturates on the later growth, development and functional maturation of the child.
Nursing mothers: Small amounts of barbiturates are excreted in the human milk. Because of the potential for serious adverse reactions in nursing infants from barbiturates, a decision should be made whether to discontinue nursing or to discontinue the drug, taking into account the importance of the drug to the mother.
Pediatric use: Safety and effectiveness in children have not been established.

ADVERSE REACTIONS

The following adverse reactions have been reported following the use of Alurate in an incidence of less than 1 in 100 patients.
Nervous system: Dizziness, nervousness.
Digestive system: Nausea and vomiting.
Other reported reactions: Headache, hypersensitivity reactions (skin rashes) and purpura.
Although the following adverse reactions have not been reported with Alurate, they have been compiled from surveillance of thousands of hospitalized patients receiving barbiturates and should be considered when administering Alurate:
More than 1 in 100 patients. The most common adverse reaction estimated to occur at a rate of 1 to 3 patients per 100 is:
Nervous system: Somnolence.
Less than 1 in 100 patients. Adverse reactions estimated to occur at a rate of less than 1 in 100 patients are listed below, grouped by organ system and by decreasing order of occurrence:
Nervous system: Agitation, confusion, hyperkinesia, ataxia, CNS depression, nightmares, psychiatric disturbances, hallucinations, insomnia, anxiety, thinking abnormality.
Respiratory system: Hypoventilation, apnea.
Cardiovascular system: Bradycardia, hypotension, syncope.
Digestive system: Constipation.
Other reported reactions: Hypersensitivity reactions (angioedema, exfoliative dermatitis), fever, liver damage, megaloblastic anemia following chronic phenobarbital use.

Continued on next page

Roche Labs.—Cont.

DRUG ABUSE AND DEPENDENCE

Alurate is subject to Class III control under the Federal Controlled Substances Act.

Barbiturates may be habit forming. Tolerance, psychological dependence and physical dependence may occur especially following prolonged use of high doses of barbiturates. Daily administration in excess of 400 mg of pentobarbital or secobarbital for approximately 90 days is likely to produce some degree of physical dependence. A dosage of from 600 to 800 mg taken for at least 35 days is sufficient to produce withdrawal seizures. The average daily dose for the barbiturate addict is usually about 1.5 grams. As tolerance to barbiturates develops, the amount needed to maintain the same level of intoxication increases; tolerance to fatal dosage, however, does not increase more than twofold. As this occurs, the margin between an intoxicating dosage and fatal dosage becomes smaller.

Symptoms of acute intoxication with barbiturates include unsteady gait, slurred speech and sustained nystagmus. Mental signs of chronic intoxication include confusion, poor judgment, irritability, insomnia and somatic complaints.

Symptoms of barbiturate dependence are similar to those of chronic alcoholism. If an individual appears to be intoxicated with alcohol to a degree that is radically disproportionate to the amount of alcohol in his or her blood, the use of barbiturates should be suspected. The lethal dose of a barbiturate is far less if alcohol is also ingested.

The symptoms of barbiturate withdrawal can be severe and may cause death. Minor withdrawal symptoms may appear 8 to 12 hours after the last dose of a barbiturate. These symptoms usually appear in the following order: anxiety, muscle twitching, tremor of hands or fingers, progressive weakness, dizziness, distortion in visual perception, nausea, vomiting, insomnia and orthostatic hypotension. Major withdrawal symptoms (convulsions and delirium) may occur within 16 hours and last up to 5 days after abrupt cessation of these drugs. Intensity of withdrawal symptoms gradually declines over a period of approximately 15 days. Individuals susceptible to barbiturate abuse and dependence include alcoholics and opiate abusers, as well as other sedative-hypnotic and amphetamine abusers.

Drug dependence to barbiturates arises from repeated administration of a barbiturate or an agent with barbiturate-like effect on a continuous basis, generally in amounts exceeding therapeutic dosage levels. The characteristics of drug dependence to barbiturates include: (a) a strong desire or need to continue taking the drug; (b) a tendency to increase the dose; (c) a psychic dependence on the effects of the drug related to subjective and individual appreciation of those effects; and (d) a physical dependence on the effects of the drug requiring its presence for maintenance of homeostasis and resulting in a definite, characteristic and self-limited abstinence syndrome when the drug is withdrawn.

Treatment of barbiturate dependence consists of cautious and gradual withdrawal of the drug. Barbiturate-dependent patients can be withdrawn by using a number of different withdrawal regimens. In all cases withdrawal takes an extended period of time. One method involves substituting 30 mg of phenobarbital for each 100 mg of the short-acting barbiturate which the patient has been taking. The total daily amount of phenobarbital is then administered in 4 divided doses, not to exceed 600 mg daily. Should signs of withdrawal occur on the first day of treatment, a loading dose of 200 mg of phenobarbital may be administered IM, and the daily oral dosage increased. After stabilization with phenobarbital is achieved, the total daily dose of phenobarbital is decreased by 30 mg a day as long as withdrawal is proceeding smoothly. An alternative method of treatment is to decrease the daily dosage of the barbiturate which the patient has been taking by 10 percent/day, if tolerated by the patient.

Infants physically dependent on barbiturates may be given phenobarbital 3 to 10 mg/kg/day. After withdrawal symptoms (hyperactivity, disturbed sleep, tremors, hyperreflexia) are relieved, the dosage of phenobarbital should be gradually decreased and completely withdrawn over a 2-week period.

OVERDOSAGE

The toxic dose of barbiturates varies considerably. In general, an oral dose of 1 gram of most barbiturates produces serious poisoning in an adult. Death commonly occurs after ingestion of 2 to 10 grams of barbiturate. Barbiturate intoxication may be confused with alcoholism, bromide intoxication and with various neurological disorders.

Acute overdosage with barbiturates is manifested by CNS and respiratory depression which may progress to Cheyne-Stokes respiration, areflexia, constriction of the pupils to a slight degree (though in severe poisoning they may show paralytic dilation), oliguria, tachycardia, hypotension, lowered body temperature and coma. Typical shock syndrome (apnea, circulatory collapse, respiratory arrest and death) may occur.

In extreme overdose, all electrical activity in the brain may cease, in which case the EEG may be "flat," which does not necessarily indicate clinical death. This effect is fully reversible unless hypoxic damage occurs. Consideration should be given to the possibility of barbiturate intoxication even in situations that appear to involve trauma.

Complications such as pneumonia, pulmonary edema, cardiac arrhythmias, congestive heart failure and renal failure may occur. Uremia may increase CNS sensitivity to barbiturates if renal function is impaired. Differential diagnosis should include hypoglycemia, head trauma, cerebrovascular accidents, convulsive states and diabetic coma. Blood levels from acute overdosage for some barbiturates are listed in the accompanying table.

[See table below].

Treatment of overdosage is mainly supportive and consists of the following:

1. Maintenance of an adequate airway, with assisted respiration and oxygen administration as necessary.
2. Monitoring of vital signs and fluid balance.
3. If the patient is conscious and has not lost the gag reflex, emesis may be induced with ipecac. Care should be taken to prevent pulmonary aspiration of vomitus. After completion of vomiting, 30 grams activated charcoal, in a glass of water, may be administered.
4. If emesis is contraindicated, gastric lavage may be performed with a cuffed endotracheal tube in place with the patient in the face down position. Activated charcoal may be left in the emptied stomach and a saline cathartic administered.
5. Fluid therapy and other standard treatment for shock, if needed.
6. If renal function is normal, forced diuresis may aid in the elimination of the barbiturate. *Alkalinization of the urine increases renal excretion of some barbiturates, especially* phenobarbital, *aprobarbital* and mephobarbital (which is metabolized to phenobarbital).
7. Although not recommended as a routine procedure, hemodialysis may be used in severe barbiturate intoxication or if the patient is anuric or in shock.
8. Patient should be rolled from side to side every 30 minutes.
9. Antibiotics should be given if pneumonia is suspected.
10. Appropriate nursing care to prevent hypostatic pneumonia, decubiti, aspiration and other complications in patients with altered states of consciousness.

Concentration of Barbiturate in the Blood Versus Degree of CNS Depression

Barbiturate	Onset/ duration	Degree of depression in nontolerant persons*				
		1	2	3	4	5
		Barbiturate blood levels in ppm (mcg/ml)				
Pentobarbital	Fast/short	≤2	0.5 to 3	10 to 15	12 to 25	15 to 40
Secobarbital	Fast/short	≤2	0.5 to 5	10 to 15	15 to 25	15 to 40
Amobarbital	Intermediate/ intermediate	≤3	2 to 10	30 to 40	30 to 60	40 to 80
Butabarbital	Intermediate/ intermediate	≤5	3 to 25	40 to 60	50 to 80	60 to 100
Phenobarbital	Slow/long	≤10	5 to 40	50 to 80	70 to 120	100 to 200

*Categories of degree of depression in nontolerant persons:

1. Under the influence and appreciably impaired for purposes of driving a motor vehicle or performing tasks requiring alertness and unimpaired judgment and reaction time.
2. Sedated, therapeutic range, calm, relaxed, and easily aroused.
3. Comatose, difficult to arouse, significant depression of respiration.
4. Compatible with death in aged or ill persons or in presence of obstructed airway, other toxic agents, or exposure to cold.
5. Usual lethal level, the upper end of the range includes those who received some supportive treatment.

DOSAGE AND ADMINISTRATION

Usual Adult Dosage: As a sedative, one 5-ml teaspoonful (40 mg) three times daily; for mild insomnia, one to two 5-ml teaspoonfuls before retiring; for pronounced insomnia, two to four 5-ml teaspoonfuls before retiring.

Special Patient Population: Dosage should be reduced in the elderly or debilitated because these patients may be more sensitive to barbiturates. Dosage should be reduced for patients with impaired renal function or hepatic disease.

HOW SUPPLIED

Elixir (red) providing 40 mg of aprobarbital/Roche per 5 ml in a vehicle containing 20 percent alcohol — bottles of 16 oz (1 pint) (NDC 0004-1000-28).

ANCOBON® ℞

[*an 'co-bon*]

(flucytosine/Roche)

The following text is complete prescribing information based on official labeling in effect June 1, 1986.

> WARNING
>
> Use with extreme caution in patients with impaired renal function. Close monitoring of hematologic, renal and hepatic status of all patients is essential. These instructions should be thoroughly reviewed before administration of Ancobon.

DESCRIPTION

Ancobon is available as capsules containing 250 mg or 500 mg flucytosine. Each capsule also contains corn starch, lactose and talc. Gelatin capsule shells contain parabens (butyl, methyl, propyl) and sodium propionate, with the following dye systems: 250 mg capsules—black iron oxide, FD&C Blue No. 1, FD&C Yellow No. 6, D&C Yellow No. 10 and titanium dioxide; 500 mg capsules—black iron oxide and titanium dioxide.

Flucytosine, an antifungal agent, is a fluorinated pyrimidine chemically related to fluorouracil and floxuridine. Chemically, it is 5-fluorocytosine, a white to off-white crystalline powder, with a molecular weight of 129.1.

ACTIONS

Flucytosine has *in vitro* and *in vivo* activity against Candida and Cryptococcus. The exact mode of action against these fungi is not known. Ancobon is not metabolized significantly when given orally to man.

SUSCEPTIBILITY:

Cryptococcus: Most strains initially isolated from clinical material have shown flucytosine minimal inhibitory concentrations (MIC's) ranging from .46 to 7.8 mcg/ml. Any isolate with an MIC greater than 12.5 mcg/ml is considered resistant. *In vitro* resistance has developed in originally susceptible strains during therapy. It is recommended that clinical cultures for susceptibility testing be taken initially and at weekly intervals during therapy. The initial culture should be reserved as a reference in susceptibility testing of subsequent isolates.

Candida: As high as 40 to 50 percent of the pretreatment clinical isolates of Candida have been reported to be resistant to flucytosine. It is recommended that susceptibility studies be performed as early as possible and be repeated during therapy. An MIC value greater than 100 mcg/ml is considered resistant.

Interference with *in vitro* activity of flucytosine occurs in complex or semisynthetic media. In order to rely upon the recommended *in vitro* interpretations of susceptibility, it is essential that the broth medium and the testing procedure used be that described by Shadomy.[1]

INDICATIONS

Ancobon is indicated only in the treatment of serious infections caused by susceptible strains of Candida and/or Cryptococcus. Candida: septicemia, endocarditis and urinary system infections have been effectively treated with flucytosine. Limited trials in pulmonary infections justify the use of flucytosine. Cryptococcus: meningitis and pulmonary infections have been treated effectively. Studies in septicemias and urinary tract infections are limited, but good responses have been reported.

CONTRAINDICATIONS

Patients with a known hypersensitivity to the drug.

WARNINGS

Ancobon must be given with extreme caution to patients with impaired renal function. Since Ancobon is excreted primarily by the kidneys, renal impairment may lead to accumulation of the drug. Assays for blood levels of Ancobon should be done in order to determine the adequacy of renal excretion in such patients.[1]

Ancobon must be given with extreme caution to patients with bone marrow depression. Patients may be more prone to depression of bone marrow function if they: 1) have a hematologic disease, 2) are being treated with radiation or drugs which depress bone marrow, or 3) have a history of treatment with such drugs or radiation. Frequent monitoring of hepatic function and of the hematopoietic system is indicated during therapy.

Usage in Pregnancy: Safe use of Ancobon in pregnancy has not been established. NOTE: Teratogenic effects have been seen in rats which metabolize flucytosine to fluorouracil. Use of Ancobon in pregnancy, lactation and in women of childbearing age requires that the potential benefits of therapy be weighed against its possible hazards.

PRECAUTIONS

Before therapy with Ancobon is instituted, the hematologic and renal status of the patient should be determined (see WARNINGS), and close monitoring of the patient is essential. Liver enzyme levels (alkaline phosphatase, SGOT, SGPT) should be determined at frequent intervals during therapy, as indicated.

ADVERSE REACTIONS

Nausea, vomiting, diarrhea, rash, anemia, leukopenia, thrombopenia, and elevation of hepatic enzymes, BUN and creatinine have been reported. Less frequently reported were confusion, hallucinations, headache, sedation and vertigo.

DOSAGE AND ADMINISTRATION

The usual dosage is 50 to 150 mg/kg/day at 6-hour intervals. Nausea or vomiting may be reduced or avoided if the capsules are given a few at a time over a 15-minute period. If the BUN or the serum creatinine is elevated, or if there are other signs of renal impairment, the initial dose should be at the lower level (see WARNINGS).

HOW SUPPLIED

Capsules, containing 250 mg flucytosine/Roche, green and gray; containing 500 mg flucytosine/Roche, white and gray; bottles of 100.

REFERENCE

1. Shadomy, S.: *Appl. Microbiol., 17*:871, 1969.

Shown in Product Identification Section, page 424

ARFONAD® ℞

[*ar'fo-nad*]

(trimethaphan camsylate/Roche)

Ampuls

The following text is complete prescribing information based on official labeling in effect June 1, 1986.

DESCRIPTION

A thiophanium derivative, Arfonad is a vasodepressor agent used for inducing controlled hypotension. Chemically, trimethaphan camsylate is (+)-1,3-dibenzyldecahydro-2-oxoimidazo[4,5-c]thieno[1,2-a]-thiolium 2-oxo-10-bornanesulfonate. It has a molecular weight of 596.80.

Arfonad is stable under refrigeration; it should not be frozen, to avoid ampul breakage which may result from ice formation. Each 10-ml ampul contains 500 mg trimethaphan camsylate/Roche compounded with 0.013% sodium acetate and pH adjusted to approximately 5.2 with hydrochloric acid.

ACTIONS

Arfonad is primarily a ganglionic blocking agent. It blocks transmission in autonomic ganglia without producing any preceding or concomitant change in the membrane potentials of the ganglion cells. It does not modify the conduction of impulses in the preganglionic or postganglionic neurones and does not prevent the release of acetylcholine by preganglionic impulses. Arfonad produces ganglionic blockade by occupying receptor sites on the ganglion cells and by stabilizing the postsynaptic membranes against the action of acetylcholine liberated from the presynaptic nerve endings.

In addition to ganglionic blocking, Arfonad may also exert a direct peripheral vasodilator effect. By inducing vasodilation, it causes pooling of blood in the dependent periphery and the splanchnic system. The vasodilation results in a lowering of the blood pressure. Arfonad liberates histamine.

INDICATIONS

Arfonad is indicated for the production of controlled hypotension during surgery; for the short term (acute) control of blood pressure in hypertensive emergencies; in the emergency treatment of pulmonary edema in patients with pulmonary hypertension associated with systemic hypertension.

CONTRAINDICATIONS

Arfonad is contraindicated in those conditions where hypotension may subject the patient to undue risk, e.g., uncorrected anemia, hypovolemia, shock (both incipient and frank), asphyxia, or uncorrected respiratory insufficiency. Inadequate availability of fluids and inability to replace blood for technical reasons may also constitute contraindications.

WARNINGS

Arfonad is a powerful hypotensive drug and should always be diluted before use.

It is recommended that the use of Arfonad to produce hypotension in surgical or medical indications be limited to physicians with proper training in this technique. Adequate facilities, equipment and personnel should be available for vigilant monitoring of the circulation since Arfonad is an extremely potent hypotensive agent. Adequate oxygenation must be assured throughout the treatment period, especially in regard to coronary and cerebral circulation.

Arfonad should be used with extreme caution in patients with arteriosclerosis, cardiac disease, hepatic or renal disease, degenerative disease of the central nervous system, Addison's disease, diabetes and patients who are under treatment with steroids.

USAGE IN PREGNANCY

Induced hypotension may have serious consequences upon the fetus.

PRECAUTIONS

Arfonad should be used with care in patients who have been receiving antihypertensive drugs, since an additive hypotensive effect may occur. It should be used with caution with anesthetic agents, especially spinal anesthetics, which themselves may produce hypotension. Also, use with great caution in the elderly or debilitated, or in children. Because Arfonad liberates histamine, it should be used with caution in allergic individuals. Concomitant therapy with other drugs can modify materially the dose of Arfonad necessary to achieve the desired response.

Diuretic agents may enhance markedly the responses evoked by ganglionic-blocking drugs. NOTE: Pupillary dilation does not necessarily indicate anoxia or the depth of anesthesia, since Arfonad appears to have a specific effect on the pupil.

Some animal studies indicate that aggressive dosage administration may result in respiratory arrest. Rare cases of respiratory arrest in humans have been reported, although a causal relationship has not been established. It is recommended that the patient's respiratory status be monitored closely, particularly if large doses of Arfonad are used.

DOSAGE AND ADMINISTRATION

Arfonad must always be diluted and administered by intravenous infusion. Solutions should be freshly prepared and any unused portions discarded. For this purpose a 0.1 per cent (1 mg/ml) concentration of Arfonad in 5% Dextrose Injection USP should be employed. Use of other diluents is not recommended, since experience with them has not been reported. The infusion fluid used for administration of Arfonad should not be employed as a vehicle for the simultaneous administration of any other drugs. One (1) ampul of Arfonad—10 ml, 50 mg/ml—should be diluted to 500 ml. Since individual response varies, the rate of administration must be adjusted to the requirements of each patient. The patient should be positioned so as to avoid cerebral anoxia and, when used in surgery, adequate anesthesia established. Intravenous drip with Arfonad is started at an average rate of 3 to 4 ml (3 to 4 mg) per minute (see chart below). The rate of administration is then adjusted to maintain the desired level of hypotension. Since there is a marked variation of individual response, **frequent blood pressure determinations are essential to maintain proper control.** Rates from as low as 0.3 ml (0.3 mg) per minute to rates exceeding 6 ml (6 mg) per minute have been found necessary in the experience of clinical investigators of Arfonad.

0.1% (1 mg/ml) CONCENTRATION OF ARFONAD

Delivery System Drops/ml	Drops/Min to Obtain 3–4 ml (3–4 mg) Arfonad
10	30–40
15	45–60
60	180–240

For surgical use, administration of Arfonad should be stopped prior to wound closure in order to permit blood pressure to return to normal. A systolic pressure of 100 mm will usually be attained within 10 minutes after stopping Arfonad.

OVERDOSAGE

Vasopressor agents may be used to correct undesirable low pressures during surgery or to effect a more rapid return to normotensive levels. Phenylephrine HCl or mephentermine sulfate should be tried initially and nonepinephrine should be reserved for refractory cases.

HOW SUPPLIED

Ampuls, 10 ml, boxes of 10.

AZO GANTANOL® ℞

[*a"zo gan'tan-ol*]

The following text is complete prescribing information based on official labeling in effect June 1, 1986.

DESCRIPTION

Azo Gantanol combines the antibacterial effectiveness of sulfamethoxazole (Gantanol®) with the local urinary analgesic activity of phenazopyridine hydrochloride. Each tablet contains 0.5 Gm sulfamethoxazole/Roche and 100 mg phenazopyridine hydrochloride. Each tablet also contains carnauba wax, castor oil, corn starch, docusate sodium, magnesium stearate, polyvinyl acetate, polyvinyl alcohol, pregelatinized starch, shellac and FD&C Red No. 3, and may contain red and brown synthetic iron oxides.

Gantanol (sulfamethoxazole/Roche) is an intermediate-dosage sulfonamide. Sulfamethoxazole is an almost white, odorless, tasteless compound. Chemically, it is N^1-(5-methyl-3-isoxazolyl) sulfanilamide.

Phenazopyridine hydrochloride is a urinary analgesic. Chemically, it is 3-phenylazo-2,6- diaminopyridine hydrochloride.

Sulfonamides exist in the blood as free, conjugated (acetylated and possibly other forms) and protein-bound forms. The "free" form is considered to be the therapeutically active form. It has been shown that approximately 70 per cent of Gantanol is protein bound in the blood;[1] of the unbound portion 80 to 90 per cent is in the nonacetylated form.[2,3] Excretion of sulfonamides is chiefly by the kidneys with glomerular filtration as the primary mechanism.

ACTIONS

The systemic sulfonamides are bacteriostatic agents. The spectrum of activity is similar for all. Sulfonamides competitively inhibit bacterial synthesis of folic acid (pteroylglutamic acid) from para-aminobenzoic acid. Resistant strains are capable of utilizing folic acid precursors or preformed folic acid.

Phenazopyridine hydrochloride has a specific analgesic effect in the urinary tract, promptly relieving pain and burning.

INDICATIONS

For the initial treatment of uncomplicated urinary tract infections caused by susceptible strains of the following microorganisms: *Escherichia coli, Klebsiella* species, *Enterobacter* species, *Proteus mirabilis, Proteus vulgaris* and *Staphylococcus aureus* when relief of symptoms of pain, burning or urgency is needed during the first 2 days of therapy. Treatment with Azo Gantanol should not exceed 2 days. There is a lack of evidence that the combination of sulfamethoxazole and phenazopyridine hydrochloride provides greater benefit than sulfamethoxazole alone after 2 days. Treatment beyond 2 days should only be continued with Gantanol (sulfamethoxazole/ Roche). (See DOSAGE AND ADMINISTRATION section.)

Important note. In vitro sulfonamide sensitivity tests are not always reliable. The test must be carefully coordinated with bacteriologic and clinical response. When the patient is already taking sulfonamides, follow-up cultures should have aminobenzoic acid added to the culture media.

Currently, the increasing frequency of resistant organisms is a limitation of the usefulness of antibacterial agents including the sulfonamides.

Wide variation in blood levels may result with identical doses. Blood levels should be measured in patients receiving sulfonamides for serious infections. Free sulfonamide blood levels of 5 to 15 mg per 100 ml may be considered therapeutically effective for most infections, with blood levels of 12 to 15 mg per 100 ml optimal for serious infections; 20 mg per 100 ml should be the maximum total sulfonamide level, as adverse reactions occur more frequently above this level.

CONTRAINDICATIONS

Children below age 12. Hypersensitivity to sulfonamides. Pregnancy at term and during the nursing period, because sulfonamides pass the placenta and are excreted in the milk and may cause kernicterus.

Because Azo Gantanol contains phenazopyridine hydrochloride it is contraindicated in glomerulonephritis, severe hepatitis, uremia, and pyelonephritis of pregnancy with gastrointestinal disturbances.

WARNINGS

Usage in Pregnancy: The safe use of sulfonamides in pregnancy has not been established. The teratogenicity potential of most sulfonamides has not been thoroughly investigated in either animals or humans. However, a significant increase in the incidence of cleft palate and other bony abnormalities of offspring has been observed when certain sulfonamides of the short, intermediate and long-acting types were given to pregnant rats and mice at high oral doses (7 to 25 times the human therapeutic dose).

Deaths associated with the administration of sulfonamides have been reported from hypersensitivity reactions, hepato-

Continued on next page

Roche Labs.—Cont.

cellular necrosis, agranulocytosis, aplastic anemia and other blood dyscrasias.
The presence of clinical signs such as sore throat, fever, pallor, purpura or jaundice may be early indications of serious blood disorders. Complete blood counts should be done frequently in patients receiving sulfonamides.
The frequency of renal complications is considerably lower in patients receiving the more soluble sulfonamides. Urinalysis with careful microscopic examination should be obtained frequently in patients receiving sulfonamides.

PRECAUTIONS

Sulfonamides should be given with caution to patients with impaired renal or hepatic function and to those with severe allergy or bronchial asthma. In glucose-6-phosphate dehydrogenase-deficient individuals, hemolysis may occur. This reaction is frequently dose-related. Adequate fluid intake must be maintained in order to prevent crystalluria and stone formation.
Carcinogenesis: Azo Gantanol has not undergone adequate trials relating to carcinogenicity; each component, however, has been evaluated separately. Rats appear to be especially susceptible to the goitrogenic effects of sulfonamides, and long-term administration of sulfonamides has resulted in thyroid malignancies in this species. Long-term administration of phenazopyridine hydrochloride has induced neoplasia in rats (large intestine) and mice (liver). Although no association between phenazopyridine hydrochloride and human neoplasia has been reported, adequate epidemiological studies have not been conducted.

ADVERSE REACTIONS

Blood dyscrasias: Agranulocytosis, aplastic anemia, thrombocytopenia, leukopenia, hemolytic anemia, purpura, hypoprothrombinemia and methemoglobinemia.
Allergic reactions: Erythema multiforme (Stevens-Johnson syndrome), generalized skin eruptions, epidermal necrolysis, urticaria, serum sickness, pruritus, exfoliative dermatitis, anaphylactoid reactions, periorbital edema, conjunctival and scleral injection, photosensitization, arthralgia and allergic myocarditis.
Gastrointestinal reactions: Nausea, emesis, abdominal pains, hepatitis, hepatocellular necrosis, diarrhea, anorexia, pancreatitis and stomatitis.
C.N.S. reactions: Headache, peripheral neuritis, mental depression, convulsions, ataxia, hallucinations, tinnitus, vertigo and insomnia.
Miscellaneous reactions: Drug fever, chills, and toxic nephrosis with oliguria and anuria. Polyarteritis nodosa and L.E. phenomenon have occurred.
The sulfonamides bear certain chemical similarities to some goitrogens, diuretics (acetazolamide and the thiazides) and oral hypoglycemic agents. Goiter production, diuresis and hypoglycemia have occurred rarely in patients receiving sulfonamides. Cross-sensitivity may exist with these agents.

DOSAGE AND ADMINISTRATION

Azo Gantanol is intended for the acute, painful phase of urinary tract infections. The usual dosage in adults is 4 tablets initially followed by 2 tablets morning and evening for up to 2 days. Treatment with Azo Gantanol should not exceed 2 days. Treatment beyond 2 days should only be continued with Gantanol (sulfamethoxazole/Roche).
NOTE: Patients should be told that the orange-red dye (phenazopyridine HCl) will color the urine soon after ingestion of the medication.

HOW SUPPLIED

Tablets, red, film-coated, each containing 0.5 Gm sulfamethoxazole/Roche and 100 mg phenazopyridine HCl—bottles of 100 and 500.

REFERENCES

1. Struller, T.: *Antibiot. Chemother., 14:* 179, 1968.
2. Boger, W. P., and Gavin, J. J.: *Antibiotics and Chemother., 10* :572, 1960.
3. Brandman, O., and Engelberg, R.: *Curr. Therap. Res., 2* :364, 1960.

Shown in Product Identification Section, page 424

AZO GANTRISIN® ℞

[a"zo gan 'tris-in]

The following text is complete prescribing information based on official labeling in effect June 1, 1986.

DESCRIPTION

Azo Gantrisin is a combination containing 0.5 Gm of the antibacterial sulfisoxazole/Roche and 50 mg of the urinary analgesic phenazopyridine hydrochloride per tablet for oral administration. Each tablet also contains carnauba wax, castor oil, docusate sodium, hydrogenated cottonseed oil, magnesium stearate, pregelatinized starch, shellac, FD&C Red No. 3 and D&C Red No. 28.
Gantrisin® (sulfisoxazole/Roche), a rapid-acting sulfonamide, is N^1-(3,4-dimethyl-5-isoxazolyl) sulfanilamide. It is a white to slightly yellowish, odorless, slighty bitter, crystalline powder which is soluble in alcohol and very slightly soluble in water. Sulfisoxazole has an empirical formula of $C_{11}H_{13}N_3O_3S$, and a molecular weight of 267.30.
Phenazopyridine hydrochloride, a local urinary analgesic, is 2,6-diamino-3-(phenylazo)-pyridine monohydrochloride. It is a light or dark red to dark violet, odorless, slightly bitter, crystalline powder with an empirical formula of $C_{11}H_{11}N_5 \cdot HCl$, and a molecular weight of 249.70.

CLINICAL PHARMACOLOGY

An oral dose of sulfisoxazole is rapidly and completely absorbed. Sulfonamides are present in the blood as free, conjugated (acetylated and possibly other forms) and protein-bound forms. The amount present as "free" drug is considered to be the therapeutically active form. Approximately 85% of a dose of sulfisoxazole is bound to plasma proteins.
Following a single 2.0-Gm dose of sulfisoxazole, the mean time of peak plasma concentration was 2.5 hours; the mean peak plasma concentration was 169 μg/ml, ranging from 127 to 211 μg/ml. Of the 97% of the original dose excreted in the urine within 0 to 48 hours, 52% was free sulfisoxazole and 45% was the metabolite N^4-acetyl sulfisoxazole. The mean elimination half-life was 5.8 hours, ranging from 4.6 to 7.8 hours.
Sulfonamides are excreted primarily by the kidneys through glomerular filtration. The drug diffuses across the placenta into the fetus and crosses the blood-brain barrier.
Phenazopyridine hydrochloride has a specific local analgesic effect in the urinary tract, promptly relieving pain and burning. No pharmacokinetic data are available on this drug.
Microbiology: The systemic sulfonamides are bacteriostatic agents. The spectrum of activity is similar for all. Sulfonamides competitively inhibit bacterial synthesis of folic acid (pteroylglutamic acid) from *para*-aminobenzoic acid. Resistant strains are capable of utilizing folic acid precursors or preformed folic acid.

INDICATIONS

For the initial treatment of uncomplicated urinary tract infections caused by susceptible strains of the following microorganisms: *Escherichia coli, Klebsiella* species, *Enterobacter* species, *Proteus mirabilis, Proteus vulgaris* and *Staphylococcus aureus* when relief of symptoms of pain, burning or urgency is needed during the first 2 days of therapy. Treatment with Azo Gantrisin should not exceed 2 days. There is a lack of evidence that the combination of sulfisoxazole and phenazopyridine hydrochloride provides greater benefit than sulfisoxazole alone after 2 days. Treatment beyond 2 days should only be continued with Gantrisin (sulfisoxazole/Roche). (See DOSAGE AND ADMINISTRATION section.)
Important Note: In vitro sensitivity tests for sulfonamides are not always reliable, and must be carefully coordinated with bacteriologic and clinical response. When the patient is already taking sulfonamides, follow-up cultures should have aminobenzoic acid added to the culture media.
Currently, the increasing frequency of resistant organisms is a limitation of the usefulness of antibacterial agents, including the sulfonamides.
Wide variation in blood levels may result with identical doses of a sulfonamide. Blood levels should be measured in patients receiving these drugs for serious infections. Free sulfonamide blood levels of 5 to 15 mg/100 ml may be considered therapeutically effective for most infections, with blood levels of 12 to 15 mg/100 ml being optimal for serious infections. The maximum sulfonamide level should be 20 mg/100 ml, since adverse reactions occur more frequently above this concentration.

CONTRAINDICATIONS

Azo Gantrisin is contraindicated in patients with a known sensitivity to either of its components; in children younger than 12 years; and in pregnancy *at term* and during the nursing period, because sulfonamides pass the placenta and are excreted in the milk and may cause kernicterus.
Azo Gantrisin, because it contains phenazopyridine hydrochloride, is also contraindicated in glomerulonephritis, severe hepatitis, uremia, and pyelonephritis of pregnancy with gastrointestinal disturbances.

WARNINGS

Sulfonamides are bacteriostatic and resistance is frequent in organisms responsible for common infections. Sulfa drugs will not eradicate group A streptococci and have not been demonstrated, in these infections, to prevent sequelae such as rheumatic fever and glomerulonephritis.
Deaths associated with the administration of sulfonamides have been reported from hypersensitivity reactions, hepatocellular necrosis, agranulocytosis, aplastic anemia and other blood dyscrasias.
The presence of clinical signs such as sore throat, fever, pallor, purpura or jaundice may be early indications of serious blood disorders. Blood counts and renal function tests are recommended during treatment.

PRECAUTIONS

General: Sulfonamides should be given with caution to patients with impaired renal or hepatic function and to those with severe allergy or bronchial asthma. In glucose-6-phosphate dehydrogenase-deficient individuals, hemolysis may occur; this reaction is frequently dose-related.
The frequency of renal complications is considerably lower in patients receiving the more soluble sulfonamides. Adequate fluid intake must be maintained in order to prevent crystalluria and stone formation.
Information for Patients: Patients should maintain an adequate fluid intake. Patients should also be told that soon after ingestion of this medication, the phenazopyridine HCl component will produce reddish-orange discoloration of the urine.
Laboratory Tests: Urinalysis with careful microscopic examination should be performed at least once a week for patients receiving sulfonamides. Blood counts should be performed regularly in patients receiving sulfonamide therapy for longer than two weeks. Blood levels of a sulfonamide should be measured in patients receiving these drugs for serious infection (see INDICATIONS section).
Drug Interactions: It has been reported that some sulfonamides may displace oral anticoagulants from plasma protein binding sites and thereby increase the anticoagulant effect. Sulfonamides can also displace methotrexate from plasma protein binding sites.
Drug/Laboratory Test Interactions: Both components of Azo Gantrisin have been reported to affect results of liver function tests in isolated cases of hepatitis.
Carcinogenesis, Mutagenesis, Impairment of Fertility:
Carcinogenesis: Azo Gantrisin has not undergone adequate trials relating to carcinogenicity; each component, however, has been evaluated separately. Rats appear to be especially susceptible to the goitrogenic effects of sulfonamides, and long-term administration of sulfonamides has resulted in thyroid malignancies in this species. Long-term administration of phenazopyridine hydrochloride has induced neoplasia in rats (large intestine) and mice (liver). Although no association between phenazopyridine hydrochloride and human neoplasia has been reported, adequate epidemiological studies have not been conducted.
Mutagenesis: There are no studies available that evaluate the mutagenic potential of Azo Gantrisin or either of its components.
Impairment of Fertility: Azo Gantrisin has not undergone adequate trials relating to impairment of fertility; each component, however, has been studied in laboratory animals. In a reproduction study of rats given 800 mg/kg/day sulfisoxazole, no effects were observed regarding mating behavior, conception rate or fertility index (percent pregnant). No effects on fertility were demonstrated in a two-litter reproduction study of rats given 50 mg/kg/day phenazopyridine.
Pregnancy:
Teratogenic Effects: Pregnancy Category C. Each component of Azo Gantrisin has been evaluated in reproduction studies in laboratory animals. At dosages of 800 mg/kg/day, sulfisoxazole was not teratogenic in either rats or rabbits, and had no perinatal or postnatal effects in rats. However, in two other teratogenicity studies, cleft palates developed in both rats and mice after administration of 500 to 1000 mg/kg/day sulfisoxazole (8 to 16 times the therapeutic dose for an individual weighing 143 lbs). In regard to phenazopyridine, no congenital malformations developed in rats given 50 mg/kg/day.
There are no adequate or well-controlled studies of Azo Gantrisin in either laboratory animals or in pregnant women. It is not known whether Azo Gantrisin can cause fetal harm when administered to a pregnant woman or can affect reproduction capacity. Azo Gantrisin should be used during pregnancy only if the potential benefit justifies the potential risk to the fetus.
Nonteratogenic Effects: See **Contraindications** section.
Nursing Mothers: See **Contraindications** section.
Pediatric Use: See **Contraindications** section.

ADVERSE REACTIONS

Included in the listing that follows are adverse reactions that have not been reported with this specific drug; however, the pharmacologic similarities among the sulfonamides require that each of the reactions be considered with Azo Gantrisin administration.
Allergic: Anaphylaxis, generalized allergic reactions, angioneurotic edema, arteritis and vasculitis, myocarditis, serum sickness, conjunctival and scleral injection. In addition, periarteritis nodosa and systemic lupus erythematosus have been reported.
Cardiovascular: Tachycardia, palpitations, syncope and cyanosis.
Dermatologic: Rash, urticaria, pruritus, erythema multiforme, Stevens-Johnson syndrome, toxic epidermal necrolysis, exfoliative dermatitis and photosensitivity.
Endocrine: The sulfonamides bear certain chemical similarities to some goitrogens, diuretics (acetazolamide and the thiazides) and oral hypoglycemic agents. Cross-sensitivity

may exist with these agents. Goiter production, diuresis and hypoglycemia have occurred rarely in patients receiving sulfonamides.
Gastrointestinal: Nausea, emesis, abdominal pain, anorexia, diarrhea, glossitis, stomatitis, flatulence, salivary gland enlargement, G.I. hemorrhage, pseudomembranous enterocolitis, melena and pancreatitis. Hepatic dysfunction, jaundice and hepatocellular necrosis have also been reported following the use of sulfonamides.
Genitourinary: Crystalluria, hematuria, BUN and creatinine elevation, nephritis and toxic nephrosis with oliguria and anuria. Acute renal failure and urinary retention have also been reported.
Hematologic: Leukopenia, agranulocytosis, aplastic anemia, thrombocytopenia, purpura, hemolytic anemia, anemia, eosinophilia, clotting disorders including hypoprothrombinemia and hypofibrinogenemia, sulfhemoglobinemia and methemoglobinemia.
Musculoskeletal: Arthralgia, chest pain and myalgia.
Neurologic: Headache, dizziness, peripheral neuritis, paresthesia, convulsions, tinnitus, vertigo, ataxia and intracranial hypertension.
Psychiatric: Psychosis, hallucinations, disorientation, depression and anxiety.
Miscellaneous: Edema (including periorbital), pyrexia, drowsiness, weakness, fatigue, lassitude, rigors, flushing, hearing loss, insomnia and pneumonitis.

OVERDOSAGE

Signs and symptoms of overdosage with Azo Gantrisin include anorexia, colic, nausea, vomiting, dizziness, drowsiness, and even unconsciousness. Pyrexia, hematuria and crystalluria may be noted. Blood dyscrasias and jaundice are potential late manifestations of overdosage.
General principles of treatment include instituting gastric lavage or emesis; forcing oral fluids; and administering intravenous fluids if urine output is low and renal function is normal. The patient should be monitored with blood counts and appropriate blood chemistries, including electrolytes. If the patient becomes cyanotic, the possibility of methemoglobinemia should be considered and, if present, the condition should be treated appropriately with intravenous 1% methylene blue. If a significant blood dyscrasia or jaundice occurs, specific therapy should be instituted for these complications. The oral LD_{50} of Azo Gantrisin in mice is 4317 mg/kg.

DOSAGE AND ADMINISTRATION

Azo Gantrisin is intended for the acute, painful phase of urinary tract infections. The recommended dosage in adults is 4 to 6 tablets initially, followed by 2 tablets four times daily for up to 2 days. Treatment with Azo Gantrisin should not exceed 2 days. Treatment beyond 2 days should only be continued with Gantrisin (sulfisoxazole/Roche).

HOW SUPPLIED

Each red, film-coated tablet contains 0.5 Gm sulfisoxazole/Roche and 50 mg phenazopyridine HCl. Azo Gantrisin is available in bottles of 100 tablets (NDC-0004-0012-01) and 500 tablets (NDC-0004-0012-14).
Imprint on tablets: AZO GANTRISIN® ROCHE.
Shown in Product Identification Section, page 424

BACTRIM™ I.V. INFUSION ℞

[*bac 'trim*]
(trimethoprim and sulfamethoxazole/Roche)

The following text is complete prescribing information based on official labeling in effect June 1, 1986.

DESCRIPTION

Bactrim (trimethoprim and sulfamethoxazole) I.V. Infusion, a sterile solution for intravenous infusion only, is a synthetic antibacterial combination product. Each 5 ml contains 80 mg trimethoprim (16 mg/ml) and 400 mg sulfamethoxazole (80 mg/ml) compounded with 40% propylene glycol, 10% ethyl alcohol and 0.3% diethanolamine; 1% benzyl alcohol and 0.1% sodium metabisulfite added as preservatives, water for injection, and pH adjusted to approximately 10 with sodium hydroxide.
Trimethoprim is 2,4-diamino-5-(3,4,5-trimethoxybenzyl) pyrimidine. It is a white to light yellow, odorless, bitter compound with a molecular weight of 290.3.
Sulfamethoxazole is N^1-(5-methyl-3-isoxazolyl)sulfanilamide. It is an almost white, odorless, tasteless compound with a molecular weight of 253.28.

CLINICAL PHARMACOLOGY

Following a one-hour intravenous infusion of a single dose of 160 mg trimethoprim and 800 mg sulfamethoxazole to 11 patients whose weight ranged from 105 lbs to 165 lbs (mean, 143 lbs), the peak plasma concentrations of trimethoprim and sulfamethoxazole were 3.4 ± 0.3 μg/ml and 46.3 ± 2.7 μg/ml, respectively. Following repeated intravenous administration of the same dose at eight-hour intervals, the mean plasma concentrations just prior to and immediately after each infusion at steady state were 5.6 ± 0.6 μg/ml and 8.8 ± 0.9 μg/ml for trimethoprim and 70.6 ± 7.3 μg/ml and 105.6 ± 10.9 μg/ml for sulfamethoxazole. The mean plasma half-life was 11.3 ± 0.7 hours for trimethoprim and 12.8 ± 1.8 hours for sulfamethoxazole. All of these 11 patients had normal renal function, and their ages ranged from 17 to 78 years (median, 60 years).[1]
Pharmacokinetic studies in children and adults suggest an age-dependent half-life of trimethoprim, as indicated in the following table.[2]

Age (years)	No. of Patients	Mean TMP Half-life (hours)
<1	2	7.67
1–10	9	5.49
10–20	5	8.19
20–63	6	12.82

Patients with severely impaired renal function exhibit an increase in the half-lives of both components, requiring dosage regimen adjustment (See DOSAGE AND ADMINISTRATION section).
Both trimethoprim and sulfamethoxazole exist in the blood as unbound, protein-bound and metabolized forms; sulfamethazole also exists as the conjugated form. The metabolism of sulfamethoxazole occurs predominately by N_4-acetylation, although the glucuronide conjugate has been identified. The principal metabolites of trimethoprim are the 1- and 3-oxides and the 3'- and 4'-hydroxy derivatives. The free forms of trimethoprim and sulfamethoxazole are considered to be the therapeutically active forms. Approximately 44% of trimethoprim and 70% of sulfamethoxazole are bound to plasma proteins. The presence of 10 mg percent sulfamethoxazole in plasma decreases the protein binding of trimethoprim by an insignificant degree; trimethoprim does not influence the protein binding of sulfamethoxazole.
Excretion of trimethoprim and sulfamethoxazole is primarily by the kidneys through both glomerular filtration and tubular secretion. Urine concentrations of both trimethoprim and sulfamethoxazole are considerably higher than are the concentrations in the blood. The percent of dose excreted in urine over a 12-hour period following the intravenous administration of the first dose of 240 mg of trimethoprim and 1200 mg of sulfamethoxazole on day 1 ranged from 17% to 42.4% as free trimethoprim; 7% to 12.7% as free sulfamethoxazole; and 36.7% to 56% as total (free plus the N_4-acetylated metabolite) sulfamethoxazole. When administered together as Bactrim, neither trimethoprim nor sulfamethoxazole affects the urinary excretion pattern of the other. Both trimethoprim and sulfamethoxazole distribute to sputum and vaginal fluid; trimethoprim also distributes to bronchial secretions, and both pass the placental barrier and are excreted in breast milk.
Microbiology: Sulfamethoxazole inhibits bacterial synthesis of dihydrofolic acid by competing with *para*-aminobenzoic acid (PABA). Trimethoprim blocks the production of tetrahydrofolic acid from dihydrofolic acid by binding to and reversibly inhibiting the required enzyme, dihydrofolate reductase. Thus, Bactrim blocks two consecutive steps in the biosynthesis of nucleic acids and proteins essential to many bacteria.
In vitro studies have shown that bacterial resistance develops more slowly with Bactrim than with either trimethoprim or sulfamethoxazole alone.
In vitro serial dilution tests have shown that the spectrum of antibacterial activity of Bactrim includes common bacterial pathogens with the exception of *Pseudomonas aeruginosa.* The following organisms are usually susceptible: *Escherichia coli, Klebsiella* species, *Enterobacter* species, *Morganella morganii, Proteus mirabilis,* indole-positive *Proteus* species including *Proteus vulgaris, Haemophilus influenzae* (including ampicillin-resistant strains), *Streptococcus pneumoniae, Shigella flexneri* and *Shigella sonnei.* It should be noted, however, that there are little clinical data on the use of Bactrim I.V. Infusion in serious systemic infections due to *Haemophilus influenzae* and *Streptococcus pneumoniae.*
[See table above].

REPRESENTATIVE MINIMUM INHIBITORY CONCENTRATION VALUES FOR BACTRIM-SUSCEPTIBLE ORGANISMS (MIC—μg/ml)

Bacteria	TMP alone	SMX alone	TMP/SMX (1:20) TMP	SMX
Escherichia coli	0.05–1.5	1.0–245	0.05–0.5	0.95–9.5
Proteus species (indole positive)	0.5–5.0	7.35–300	0.05–1.5	0.95–28.5
Morganella morganii	0.5–5.0	7.35–300	0.05–1.5	0.95–28.5
Proteus mirabilis	0.5–1.5	7.35–30	0.05–0.15	0.95–2.85
Klebsiella species	0.15–5.0	2.45–245	0.05–1.5	0.95–28.5
Enterobacter species	0.15–5.0	2.45–245	0.05–1.5	0.95–28.5
Haemophilus influenzae	0.15–1.5	2.85–95	0.015–0.15	0.285–2.85
Streptococcus pneumoniae	0.15–1.5	7.35–24.5	0.05–0.15	0.95–2.85
*Shigella flexneri**	<0.01–0.04	<0.16–>320	<0.002–0.03	0.04–0.625
*Shigella sonnei**	0.02–0.08	0.625–>320	0.004–0.06	0.08–1.25

TMP = trimethoprim SMX = sulfamethoxazole
*Rudoy RC, Nelson JD, Haltalin KC: *Antimicrob Agents Chemother 5*:439–443, May 1974.

The recommended quantitative disc susceptibility method may be used for estimating the susceptibility of bacteria to Bactrim.[3,4] With this procedure, a report from the laboratory of "Susceptible to trimethoprim and sulfamethoxazole" indicates that the infection is likely to respond to therapy with Bactrim. If the infection is confined to the urine, a report of "Intermediate susceptibility to trimethoprim and sulfamethoxazole" also indicates that the infection is likely to respond. A report of "Resistant to trimethoprim and sulfamethoxazole" indicates that the infection is unlikely to respond to therapy with Bactrim.

INDICATIONS AND USAGE

PNEUMOCYSTIS CARINII PNEUMONITIS: Bactrim I.V. Infusion is indicated in the treatment of *Pneumocystis carinii* pneumonitis in children and adults (see PRECAUTIONS section).
SHIGELLOSIS: Bactrim I.V. Infusion is indicated in the treatment of enteritis caused by susceptible strains of *Shigella flexneri* and *Shigella sonnei* in children and adults.
URINARY TRACT INFECTIONS: Bactrim I.V. Infusion is indicated in the treatment of severe or complicated urinary tract infections due to susceptible strains of *Escherichia coli, Klebsiella* species, *Enterobacter* species, *Morganella morganii* and *Proteus* species when oral administration of Bactrim is not feasible and when the organism is not susceptible to single agent antibacterials effective in the urinary tract.
Although appropriate culture and susceptibility studies should be performed, therapy may be started while awaiting the results of these studies.

CONTRAINDICATIONS

Hypersensitivity to trimethoprim or sulfonamides. Patients with documented megaloblastic anemia due to folate deficiency. Pregnancy at term and during the nursing period, because sulfonamides pass the placenta and are excreted in the milk and may cause kernicterus. Infants less than two months of age.

WARNINGS

FATALITIES ASSOCIATED WITH THE ADMINISTRATION OF SULFONAMIDES, ALTHOUGH RARE, HAVE OCCURRED DUE TO SEVERE REACTIONS, INCLUDING STEVENS-JOHNSON SYNDROME, TOXIC EPIDERMAL NECROLYSIS, FULMINANT HEPATIC NECROSIS, AGRANULOCYTOSIS, APLASTIC ANEMIA AND OTHER BLOOD DYCRASIAS.
BACTRIM SHOULD BE DISCONTINUED AT THE FIRST APPEARANCE OF SKIN RASH OR ANY SIGN OF ADVERSE REACTION. Clinical signs, such as rash, sore throat, fever, pallor, purpura or jaundice may be early indications of serious reactions. In rare instances a skin rash may be followed by more severe reactions, such as Stevens-Johnson syndrome, toxic epidermal necrolysis, hepatic necrosis or serious blood disorder. Complete blood counts should be done frequently in patients receiving sulfonamides.
BACTRIM SHOULD NOT BE USED IN THE TREATMENT OF STREPTOCOCCAL PHARYNGITIS. Clinical studies have documented that patients with group A β-hemolytic streptococcal tonsillopharyngitis have a greater incidence of bacteriologic failure when treated with Bactrim than do those patients treated with penicillin, as evidenced by failure to eradicate this organism from the tonsillopharyngeal area.

Continued on next page

Roche Labs.—Cont.

Bactrim I.V. Infusion contains sodium metabisulfite, a sulfite that may cause allergic-type reactions (*e.g.*, hives, itching, wheezing, anaphylaxis) in certain susceptible persons. Although the overall prevalence of sulfite sensitivity in the general population is probably low, it is seen more frequently in asthmatics or in atopic nonasthmatic persons.

PRECAUTIONS

General: Bactrim should be given with caution to patients with impaired renal or hepatic function, to those with possible folate deficiency (*e.g.*, the elderly, chronic alcoholics, patients receiving anticonvulsant therapy, patients with malabsorption syndrome, and patients in malnutrition states) and to those with severe allergies or bronchial asthma. In glucose-6-phosphate dehydrogenase deficient individuals, hemolysis may occur. This reaction is frequently dose-related.

Local irritation and inflammation due to extravascular infiltration of the infusion have been observed with Bactrim I.V. Infusion. If these occur, the infusion should be discontinued and restarted at another site.

Use in the Elderly: There may be an increased risk of severe adverse reactions in elderly patients, particularly when complicating conditions exist, *e.g.*, impaired kidney and/or liver function, or concomitant use of other drugs. Severe skin reactions, generalized bone marrow suppression (see WARNINGS and ADVERSE REACTIONS sections) or a specific decrease in platelets (with or without purpura) are the most frequently reported severe adverse reactions in elderly patients. In those concurrently receiving certain diuretics, primarily thiazides, an increased incidence of thrombocytopenia with purpura has been reported. Appropriate dosage adjustments should be made for patients with impaired kidney function (see DOSAGE AND ADMINISTRATION section).

Use in the Treatment of Pneumocystis Carinii Pneumonitis in Patients with Acquired Immunodeficiency Syndrome (AIDS): Because of their unique immune dysfunction, AIDS patients may not tolerate or respond to Bactrim in the same manner as non-AIDS patients. The incidence of side effects, particularly rash, fever and leukopenia, with Bactrim therapy in AIDS patients who are being treated for *Pneumocystis carinii* pneumonitis has been reported to be greatly increased compared with the incidence normally associated with the use of Bactrim in non-AIDS patients.

Laboratory Tests: Appropriate culture and susceptibility studies should be performed before and throughout treatment. Complete blood counts should be done frequently in patients receiving Bactrim; if a significant reduction in the count of any formed blood element is noted, Bactrim should be discontinued. Urinalyses with careful microscopic examination and renal function tests should be performed during therapy, particularly for those patients with impaired renal function.

Drug Interactions: In elderly patients concurrently receiving certain diuretics, primarily thiazides, an increased incidence of thrombocytopenia with purpura has been reported. It has been reported that Bactrim may prolong the prothrombin time in patients who are receiving the anticoagulant warfarin. This interaction should be kept in mind when Bactrim is given to patients already on anticoagulant therapy, and the coagulation time should be reassessed.

Bactrim may inhibit the hepatic metabolism of phenytoin. Bactrim, given at a common clinical dosage, increased the phenytoin half-life by 39% and decreased the phenytoin metabolic clearance rate by 27%. When administering these drugs concurrently, one should be alert for possible excessive phenytoin effect.

Sulfonamides can also displace methotrexate from plasma protein binding sites, thus increasing free methotrexate concentrations.

Drug/Laboratory Test Interactions: Bactrim, specifically the trimethoprim component, can interfere with a serum methotrexate assay as determined by the competitive binding protein technique (CBPA) when a bacterial dihydrofolate reductase is used as the binding protein. No interference occurs, however, if methotrexate is measured by a radioimmunoassay (RIA).

The presence of trimethoprim and sulfamethoxazole may also interfere with the Jaffé alkaline picrate reaction assay for creatinine, resulting in overestimations of about 10% in the range of normal values.

Carcinogenesis, Mutagenesis, Impairment of Fertility:

Carcinogenesis: Long-term studies in animals to evaluate carcinogenic potential have not been conducted with Bactrim I.V. Infusion.

Mutagenesis: Bacterial mutagenic studies have not been performed with sulfamethoxazole and trimethoprim in combination. Trimethoprim was demonstrated to be nonmutagenic in the Ames assay. No chromosomal damage was observed in human leukocytes cultured *in vitro* with sulfamethoxazole and trimethoprim alone or in combination; the concentrations used exceeded blood levels of these compounds following therapy with Bactrim. Observations of leukocytes obtained from patients treated with Bactrim revealed no chromosomal abnormalities.

Impairment of Fertility: Bactrim I.V. Infusion has not been studied in animals for evidence of impairment of fertility. However, studies in rats at oral dosages as high as 70 mg/kg trimethoprim plus 350 mg/kg sulfamethoxazole daily showed no adverse effects on fertility or general reproductive performance.

Pregnancy: Teratogenic Effects: Pregnancy Category C. In rats, oral doses of 533 mg/kg sulfamethoxazole or 200 mg/kg trimethoprim produced teratological effects manifested mainly as cleft palates.

The highest dose which did not cause cleft palates in rats was 512 mg/kg sulfamethoxazole or 192 mg/kg trimethoprim when administered separately. In two studies in rats, no teratology was observed when 512 mg/kg of sulfamethoxazole was used in combination with 128 mg/kg of trimethoprim. In one study, however, cleft palates were observed in one litter out of nine when 355 mg/kg of sulfamethoxazole was used in combination with 88 mg/kg of trimethoprim.

In some rabbit studies, an overall increase in fetal loss (dead and resorbed and malformed conceptuses) was associated with doses of trimethoprim six times the human therapeutic dose.

While there are no large, well-controlled studies on the use of trimethoprim and sulfamethoxazole in pregnant women, Brumfitt and Pursell,[5] in a retrospective study, reported the outcome of 186 pregnancies during which the mother received either placebo or oral trimethoprim and sulfamethoxazole. The incidence of congenital abnormalities was 4.5% (3 of 66) in those who received placebo and 3.3% (4 of 120) in those receiving trimethoprim and sulfamethoxazole. There were no abnormalities in the 10 children whose mothers received the drug during the first trimester. In a separate survey, Brumfitt and Pursell also found no congenital abnormalities in 35 children whose mothers had received oral trimethoprim and sulfamethoxazole at the time of conception or shortly thereafter.

Because trimethoprim and sulfamethoxazole may interfere with folic acid metabolism, Bactrim I.V. Infusion should be used during pregnancy only if the potential benefit justifies the potential risk to the fetus.

Nonteratogenic Effects: See CONTRAINDICATIONS section.

Nursing Mothers: See CONTRAINDICATIONS section.

Pediatric Use: Bactrim I.V. Infusion is not recommended for infants younger than two months of age (see CONTRAINDICATIONS section).

ADVERSE REACTIONS

The most common adverse effects are gastrointestinal disturbances (nausea, vomiting, anorexia) and allergic skin reactions (such as rash and urticaria). **FATALITIES ASSOCIATED WITH THE ADMINISTRATION OF SULFONAMIDES, ALTHOUGH RARE, HAVE OCCURRED DUE TO SEVERE REACTIONS, INCLUDING STEVENS-JOHNSON SYNDROME, TOXIC EPIDERMAL NECROLYSIS, FULMINANT HEPATIC NECROSIS, AGRANULOCYTOSIS, APLASTIC ANEMIA AND OTHER BLOOD DYSCRASIAS (SEE WARNINGS SECTION).** Local reaction, pain and slight irritation on I.V. administration are infrequent. Thrombophlebitis has rarely been observed.

Hematologic: Agranulocytosis, aplastic anemia, thrombocytopenia, leukopenia, neutropenia, hemolytic anemia, megaloblastic anemia, hypoprothrombinemia, methemoglobinemia, eosinophilia.

Allergic Reactions: Stevens-Johnson syndrome, toxic epidermal necrolysis, anaphylaxis, allergic myocarditis, erythema multiforme, exfoliative dermatitis, angioedema, drug fever, chills, Henoch-Schoenlein purpura, serum sickness-like syndrome, generalized allergic reactions, generalized skin eruptions, conjunctival and scleral injection, photosensitivity, pruritus, urticaria and rash. In addition, periarteritis nodosa and systemic lupus erythematosus have been reported.

Gastrointestinal: Hepatitis (including cholestatic jaundice and hepatic necrosis), elevation of serum transaminase and bilirubin, pseudomembraneous enterocolitis, pancreatitis, stomatitis, glossitis, nausea, emesis, abdominal pain, diarrhea, anorexia.

Genitourinary: Renal failure, interstitial nephritis, BUN and serum creatinine elevation, toxic nephrosis with oliguria and anuria, and crystalluria.

Neurologic: Aseptic meningitis, convulsions, peripheral neuritis, ataxia, vertigo, tinnitus, headache.

Psychiatric: Hallucinations, depression, apathy, nervousness.

Endocrine: The sulfonamides bear certain chemical similarities to some goitrogens, diuretics (acetazolamide and the thiazides) and oral hypoglycemic agents. Cross-sensitivity may exist with these agents. Diuresis and hypoglycemia have occurred rarely in patients receiving sulfonamides.

Musculoskeletal: Arthralgia and myalgia.

Miscellaneous: Weakness, fatigue, insomnia.

OVERDOSAGE

Acute: Since there has been no extensive experience in humans with single doses of Bactrim I.V. Infusion in excess of 25 ml (400 mg trimethoprim and 2000 mg sulfamethoxazole), the maximum tolerated dose in humans is unknown. Signs and symptoms of overdosage reported with sulfonamides include anorexia, colic, nausea, vomiting, dizziness, headache, drowsiness and unconsciousness. Pyrexia, hematuria and crystalluria may be noted. Blood dyscrasias and jaundice are potential late manifestations of overdosage.

Signs of acute overdosage with trimethoprim include nausea, vomiting, dizziness, headache, mental depression, confusion and bone marrow depression.

General principles of treatment include the administration of intraveneous fluids if urine output is low and renal function is normal. Acidification of the urine will increase renal elimination of trimethoprim. The patient should be monitored with blood counts and appropriate blood chemistries, including electrolytes. If a significant blood dyscrasia or jaundice occurs, specific therapy should be instituted for these complications. Peritoneal dialysis is not effective and hemodialysis is only moderately effective in eliminating trimethoprim and sulfamethoxazole.

Chronic: Use of Bactrim I.V. Infusion at high doses and/or for extended periods of time may cause bone marrow depression manifested as thrombocytopenia, leukopenia and/or megaloblastic anemia. If signs of bone marrow depression occur, the patient should be given leucovorin 5 to 15 mg daily until normal hematopoiesis is restored.

Animal Toxicity: The LD_{50} of Bactrim I.V. Infusion in mice is 700 mg/kg or 7.3 ml/kg; in rats and rabbits the LD_{50} is >500 mg/kg or >5.2 ml/kg. The vehicle produced the same LD_{50} in each of these species as the active drug.

The signs and symptoms noted in mice, rats and rabbits with Bactrim I.V. Infusion or its vehicle at the high I.V. doses used in acute toxicity studies included ataxia, decreased motor activity, loss of righting reflex, tremors or convulsions, and/or respiratory depression.

DOSAGE AND ADMINISTRATION

CONTRAINDICATED IN INFANTS LESS THAN TWO MONTHS OF AGE. CAUTION—BACTRIM I.V. INFUSION MUST BE DILUTED IN 5% DEXTROSE IN WATER SOLUTION PRIOR TO ADMINISTRATION. DO NOT MIX BACTRIM I.V. INFUSION WITH OTHER DRUGS OR SOLUTIONS. RAPID INFUSION OR BOLUS INJECTION MUST BE AVOIDED.

Dosage:

Children and Adults:

PNEUMOCYSTIS CARINII PNEUMONITIS: Total daily dose is 15 to 20 mg/kg (based on the trimethoprim component) given in three or four equally divided doses every 6 to 8 hours for up to 14 days. One investigator noted that a total daily dose of 10 to 15 mg/kg was sufficient in ten adult patients with normal renal function.[6]

SEVERE URINARY TRACT INFECTIONS AND SHIGELLOSIS: Total daily dose is 8 to 10 mg/kg (based on the trimethoprim component) given in two to four equally divided doses every 6, 8 or 12 hours for up to 14 days for severe urinary tract infections and five days for shigellosis. The maximum recommended daily dose is 60 ml per day.

For Patients with Impaired Renal Function: When renal function is impaired, a reduced dosage should be employed using the following table:

Creatinine Clearance (ml/min)	Recommended Dosage Regimen
Above 30	Usual standard regimen
15–30	½ the usual regimen
Below 15	Use not recommended

Method of Preparation: Bactrim I.V. Infusion must be diluted. EACH 5 ML SHOULD BE ADDED TO 125 ML OF 5% DEXTROSE IN WATER. After diluting with 5% dextrose in water, the solution should not be refrigerated and should be used within six hours. If a dilution of 5 ml per 100 ml of 5% dextrose in water is desired, it should be used within 4 hours. If upon visual inspection there is cloudiness or evidence of crystallization after mixing, the solution should be discarded and a fresh solution prepared.

Multidose Vials: After initial entry into the vial, the remaining contents must be used within 48 hours.

The following infusion systems have been tested and found satisfactory: unit-dose glass containers; unit-dose polyvinyl chloride and polyolefin containers. No other systems have been tested and therefore no others can be recommended.

Dilution: EACH 5 ML OF BACTRIM I.V. INFUSION SHOULD BE ADDED TO 125 ML OF 5% DEXTROSE IN WATER.

NOTE: *In those instances where fluid restriction is desirable,* each 5 ml may be added to 75 ml of 5% dextrose in water. Under these circumstances the solution should be mixed just prior to use and should be administered within two (2)

REPRESENTATIVE MINIMUM INHIBITORY CONCENTRATION VALUES FOR BACTRIM-SUSCEPTIBLE ORGANISMS (MIC—μg/ml)

Bacteria	TMP alone	SMX alone	TMP/SMX (1:20) TMP	SMX
Escherichia coli	0.05–1.5	1.0–245	0.05–0.5	0.95–9.5
Proteus species (indole positive)	0.5–5.0	7.35–300	0.05–1.5	0.95–28.5
Morganella morganii	0.5–5.0	7.35–300	0.05–1.5	0.95–28.5
Proteus mirabilis	0.5–1.5	7.35–30	0.05–0.15	0.95–2.85
Klebsiella species	0.15–5.0	2.45–245	0.05–1.5	0.95–28.5
Enterobacter species	0.15–5.0	2.45–245	0.05–1.5	0.95–28.5
Haemophilus influenzae	0.15–1.5	2.85–95	0.015–0.15	0.285–2.85
Streptococcus pneumoniae	0.15–1.5	7.35–24.5	0.05–0.15	0.95–2.85
*Shigella flexneri**	<0.01–0.04	<0.16–>320	<0.002–0.03	0.04–0.625
*Shigella sonnei**	0.02–0.08	0.625–>320	0.004–0.06	0.08–1.25

TMP = trimethoprim SMX = sulfamethoxazole

*Rudoy RC, Nelson JD, Haltalin KC: *Antimicrob Agents Chemother 5:* 439–443, May 1974.

hours. If upon visual inspection there is cloudiness or evidence of crystallization after mixing, the solution should be discarded and a fresh solution prepared.

DO NOT MIX BACTRIM I.V. INFUSION—5% DEXTROSE IN WATER WITH DRUGS OR SOLUTIONS IN THE SAME CONTAINER.

Administration: The solution should be given by intravenous infusion over a period of 60 to 90 minutes. Rapid infusion or bolus injection must be avoided. Bactrim I.V. Infusion should not be given intramuscularly.

HOW SUPPLIED

5-ml *ampuls,* containing 80 mg trimethoprim (16 mg/ml) and 400 mg sulfamethoxazole (80 mg/ml) for infusion with 5% dextrose in water. Boxes of 10 (NDC 0004-1943-06).

5-ml *vials,* containing 80 mg trimethoprim (16 mg/ml) and 400 mg sulfamethoxazole (80 mg/ml) for infusion with 5% dextrose in water. Boxes of 10 (NDC 0004-1956-01).

10-ml *vials,* containing 160 mg trimethoprim (16 mg/ml) and 800 mg sulfamethoxazole (80 mg/ml) for infusion with 5% dextrose in water. Boxes of 10 (NDC 0004-1955-01).

30-ml *multidose vials,* each 5 ml containing 80 mg trimethoprim (16 mg/ml) and 400 mg sulfamethoxazole (80 mg/ml) for infusion with 5% dextrose in water. Boxes of 1 (NDC 0004-1958-01).

STORE AT ROOM TEMPERATURE (15°–30°C or 59°–86°F). DO NOT REFRIGERATE.

Bactrim is also available as *DS (double strength) Tablets* (white, notched, capsule shaped), containing 160 mg trimethoprim and 800 mg sulfamethoxazole—bottles of 100 (NDC 0004-0117-01), 250 (NDC 0004-0117-04) and 500 (NDC 0004-0117-14); Tel-E-Dose® packages of 100 (NDC 0004-0117-49); Prescription Paks of 20 (NDC 0004-0117-54). Imprint on tablets: (front) BACTRIM-DS; (back) ROCHE.

Tablets (light green, scored, capsule shaped), containing 80 mg trimethoprim and 400 mg sulfamethoxazole—bottles of 100 (NDC 0004-0050-01) and 500 (NDC 0004-0050-14); Tel-E-Dose® packages of 100 (NDC 0004-0050-49); Prescription Paks of 40 (NDC 0004-0050-34). Imprint on tablets: (front) BACTRIM; (back) ROCHE.

Pediatric Suspension (pink, cherry flavored), containing 40 mg trimethoprim and 200 mg sulfamethoxazole per teaspoonful (5 ml)—bottles of 100 ml (NDC 0004-1033-01) and 16 oz (1 pint) (NDC 0004-1033-28).

Suspension (pink, fruit-licorice flavored), containing 40 mg trimethoprim and 200 mg sulfamethoxazole per teaspoonful (5 ml)—bottles of 16 oz (1 pint) (NDC 0004-1015-28).

REFERENCES

1. Grose WE, Bodey GP, Loo TL: Clinical Pharmacology of Intravenously Administered Trimethoprim-Sulfamethoxazole. *Antimicrob Agents Chemother 15* :447-451, Mar 1979. 2. Siber GR, Gorham C, Durbin W, Lesko L, Levin MJ: Pharmacology of Intravenous Trimethoprim-Sulfamethoxazole in Children and Adults. *Current Chemotherapy and Infectious Diseases,* American Society for Microbiology, Washington, D.C., 1980, Vol. 1, pp. 691-692. 3. Bauer AW, Kirby WMM, Sherris JC, Turck M: Antibiotic Susceptibility Testing by a Standardized Single Disk Method. *Am J Clin Pathol 45* :493-496, Apr 1966. 4. Approved Standard ASM-2 Performance Standards for Antimicrobial Disc Susceptibility Test: National Committee for Clinical Laboratory Standards, 771 East Lancaster Avenue, Villanova, Pennsylvania 19085. 5. Brumfitt W, Pursell R: Trimethoprim/Sulfamethoxazole in the Treatment of Bacteriuria in Women. *J Infect Dis 128* (Suppl): S657-S663, Nov 1973. 6. Winston DJ, Lau WK, Gale RP, Young LS: Trimethoprim-Sulfamethoxazole for the Treatment of *Pneumocystis carinii* pneumonia. *Ann Intern Med 92* :762-769, June 1980.

BACTRIM™ ℞

[bac 'trim]

(trimethoprim and sulfamethoxazole/Roche)
DS (double strength) Tablets
Tablets
Suspension
and
Pediatric Suspension

The following text is complete prescribing information based on official labeling in effect June 1, 1986.

DESCRIPTION

Bactrim (trimethoprim and sulfamethoxazole) is a synthetic antibacterial combination product available in DS (double strength) tablets, tablets, pediatric suspension and suspension for oral administration. Each DS tablet contains 160 mg trimethoprim and 800 mg sulfamethoxazole plus magnesium stearate, pregelatinized starch and sodium starch glycolate. Each tablet contains 80 mg trimethoprim and 400 mg sulfamethoxazole plus magnesium stearate, pregelatinized starch, sodium starch glycolate, FD&C Blue No. 1 lake, FD&C Yellow No. 6 lake and D&C Yellow No. 10 lake. Each teaspoonful (5 ml) of the pediatric suspension or suspension contains 40 mg trimethoprim and 200 mg sulfamethoxazole in a vehicle containing 0.3 percent alcohol, edetate disodium, glycerin, microcrystalline cellulose, parabens (methyl and propyl), polysorbate 80, saccharin sodium, simethicone, sorbitol, sucrose, FD&C Yellow No. 6, FD&C Red No. 40, flavors and water.

Trimethoprim is 2,4-diamino-5-(3,4,5-trimethoxybenzyl) pyrimidine. It is a white to light yellow, odorless, bitter compound with a molecular weight of 290.3.

Sulfamethoxazole is N^1-(5-methyl-3-isoxazolyl) sulfanilamide. It is an almost white, odorless, tasteless compound with a molecular weight of 253.28.

CLINICAL PHARMACOLOGY

Bactrim is rapidly absorbed following oral administration. Both sulfamethoxazole and trimethoprim exist in the blood as unbound, protein-bound and metabolized forms; sulfamethoxazole also exists as the conjugated form. The metabolism of sulfamethoxazole occurs predominately by N_4-acetylation, although the glucuronide conjugate has been identified. The principal metabolites of trimethoprim are the 1- and 3-oxides and the 3'- and 4'-hydroxy derivatives. The free forms of sulfamethoxazole and trimethoprim are considered to be the therapeutically active forms. Approximately 44% of trimethoprim and 70% of sulfamethoxazole are bound to plasma proteins. The presence of 10 mg percent sulfamethoxazole in plasma decreases the protein binding of trimethoprim by an insignificant degree; trimethoprim does not influence the protein binding of sulfamethoxazole.

Peak blood levels for the individual components occur 1 to 4 hours after oral administration. The mean serum half-lives of sulfamethoxazole and trimethoprim are 10 and 8 to 10 hours, respectively. However, patients with severely impaired renal function exhibit an increase in the half-lives of both components, requiring dosage regimen adjustment (see DOSAGE AND ADMINISTRATION section). Detectable amounts of trimethoprim and sulfamethoxazole are present in the blood 24 hours after drug administration. During administration of 160 mg trimethoprim and 800 mg sulfamethoxazole *b.i.d.,* the mean steady-state plasma concentration of trimethoprim was 1.72 μg/ml. The steady-state mean plasma levels of free and total sulfamethoxazole were 57.4 μg/ml and 68.0 μg/ml, respectively. These steady-state levels were achieved after three days of drug administration.[1]

Excretion of sulfamethoxazole and trimethoprim is primarily by the kidneys through both glomerular filtration and tubular secretion. Urine concentrations of both sulfamethoxazole and trimethoprim are considerably higher than are the concentrations in the blood. The average percentage of the dose recovered in urine from 0 to 72 hours after a single oral dose of Bactrim is 84.5% for total sulfonamide and 66.8% for free trimethoprim. Thirty percent of the total sulfonamide is excreted as free sulfamethoxazole, with the remaining as N_4-acetylated metabolite.[2] When administered together as Bactrim, neither sulfamethoxazole nor trimethoprim affects the urinary excretion pattern of the other.

Both trimethoprim and sulfamethoxazole distribute to sputum, vaginal fluid and middle ear fluid; trimethoprim also distributes to bronchial secretion, and both pass the placental barrier and are excreted in breast milk.

Microbiology: Sulfamethoxazole inhibits bacterial synthesis of dihydrofolic acid by competing with *para* -aminobenzoic acid (PABA). Trimethoprim blocks the production of tetrahydrofolic acid from dihydrofolic acid by binding to and reversibly inhibiting the required enzyme, dihydrofolate reductase. Thus, Bactrim blocks two consecutive steps in the biosynthesis of nucleic acids and proteins essential to many bacteria.

In vitro studies have shown that bacterial resistance develops more slowly with Bactrim than with either trimethoprim or sulfamethoxazole alone.

In vitro serial dilution tests have shown that the spectrum of antibacterial activity of Bactrim includes the common urinary tract pathogens with the exception of *Pseudomonas aeruginosa.* The following organisms are usually susceptible: *Escherichia coli, Klebsiella* species, *Enterobacter* species, *Morganella morganii, Proteus mirabilis,* and indole-positive *Proteus* species including *Proteus vulgaris.* The usual spectrum of antimicrobial activity of Bactrim includes the following bacterial pathogens isolated from middle ear exudate and from bronchial secretions: *Haemophilus influenzae,* including ampicillin-resistant strains, and *Streptococcus pneumoniae. Shigella flexneri* and *Shigella sonnei* are usually susceptible.

[See table above].

The recommended quantitative disc susceptibility method may be used for estimating the susceptibility of bacteria to Bactrim.[3,4] With this procedure, a report from the laboratory of "Susceptible to trimethoprim and sulfamethoxazole" indicates that the infection is likely to respond to therapy with Bactrim. If the infection is confined to the urine, a report of "Intermediate susceptibility to trimethoprim and sulfamethoxazole" also indicates that the infection is likely to respond. A report of "Resistant to trimethoprim and sulfamethoxazole" indicates that the infection is unlikely to respond to therapy with Bactrim.

INDICATIONS AND USAGE

Urinary Tract Infections: For the treatment of urinary tract infections due to susceptible strains of the following organisms: *Escherichia coli, Klebsiella* species, *Enterobacter* species, *Morganella morganii, Proteus mirabilis* and *Proteus vulgaris.* It is recommended that initial episodes of uncomplicated urinary tract infections be treated with a single effective antibacterial agent rather than the combination.

Acute Otitis Media: For the treatment of acute otitis media in children due to susceptible strains of *Streptococcus pneumoniae* or *Haemophilus influenzae* when in the judgment of the physician Bactrim offers some advantage over the use of other antimicrobial agents. To date, there are limited data on the safety of repeated use of Bactrim in children under two years of age. Bactrim is not indicated for prophylactic or prolonged administration in otitis media at any age.

Acute Exacerbations of Chronic Bronchitis in Adults: For the treatment of acute exacerbations of chronic bronchitis due to susceptible strains of *Streptococcus pneumoniae* or *Haemophilus influenzae* when in the judgment of the physician Bactrim offers some advantage over the use of a single antimicrobial agent.

Shigellosis: For the treatment of enteritis caused by susceptible strains of *Shigella flexneri* and *Shigella sonnei* when antibacterial therapy is indicated.

***Pneumocystis Carinii* Pneumonitis:** For the treatment of documented *Pneumocystis carinii* pneumonitis (see PRECAUTIONS section).

CONTRAINDICATIONS

Hypersensitivity to trimethoprim or sulfonamides. Patients with documented megaloblastic anemia due to folate deficiency. Pregnancy at term and during the nursing period, because sulfonamides pass the placenta and are excreted in the milk and may cause kernicterus. Infants less than two months of age.

WARNINGS

FATALITIES ASSOCIATED WITH THE ADMINISTRATION OF SULFONAMIDES, ALTHOUGH RARE, HAVE OCCURRED DUE TO SEVERE REACTIONS, INCLUDING STEVENS-JOHNSON SYNDROME, TOXIC EPIDERMAL NECROLYSIS, FULMINANT HEPATIC NECROSIS, AGRANULOCYTOSIS, APLASTIC ANEMIA AND OTHER BLOOD DYSCRASIAS.

BACTRIM SHOULD BE DISCONTINUED AT THE FIRST APPEARANCE OF SKIN RASH OR ANY SIGN OF ADVERSE REACTION. Clinical signs, such as rash, sore throat, fever, pallor, purpura or jaundice may be early indications of serious reactions. In rare instances a skin rash may be followed

Continued on next page

Roche Labs.—Cont.

by more severe reactions, such as Stevens-Johnson syndrome, toxic epidermal necrolysis, hepatic necrosis or serious blood disorder. Complete blood counts should be done frequently in patients receiving sulfonamides.

BACTRIM SHOULD NOT BE USED IN THE TREATMENT OF STREPTOCOCCAL PHARYNGITIS. Clinical studies have documented that patients with group A β-hemolytic streptococcal tonsillopharyngitis have a greater incidence of bacteriologic failure when treated with Bactrim than do those patients treated with penicillin, as evidenced by failure to eradicate this organism from the tonsillopharyngeal area.

PRECAUTIONS

General: Bactrim should be given with caution to patients with impaired renal or hepatic function, to those with possible folate deficiency (*e.g.*, the elderly, chronic alcoholics, patients receiving anticonvulsant therapy, patients with malabsorption syndrome, and patients in malnutrition states) and to those with severe allergies or bronchial asthma. In glucose-6-phosphate dehydrogenase deficient individuals, hemolysis may occur. This reaction is frequently dose-related.

Use in the Elderly: There may be an increased risk of severe adverse reactions in elderly patients, particularly when complicating conditions exist, *e.g.*, impaired kidney and/or liver function, or concomitant use of other drugs. Severe skin reactions, generalized bone marrow suppression (see WARNINGS and ADVERSE REACTIONS sections) or a specific decrease in platelets (with or without purpura) are the most frequently reported severe adverse reactions in elderly patients. In those concurrently receiving certain diuretics, primarily thiazides, an increased incidence of thrombocytopenia with purpura has been reported. Appropriate dosage adjustments should be made for patients with impaired kidney function (see DOSAGE AND ADMINISTRATION section).

Use in the Treatment of Pneumocystis Carinii Pneumonitis in Patients with Acquired Immunodeficiency Syndrome (AIDS): Because of their unique immune dysfunction, AIDS patients may not tolerate or respond to Bactrim in the same manner as non-AIDS patients. The incidence of side effects, particularly rash, fever and leukopenia, with Bactrim therapy in AIDS patients who are being treated for *Pneumocystis carinii* pneumonitis has been reported to be greatly increased compared with the incidence normally associated with the use of Bactrim in non-AIDS patients.

Information for Patients: Patients should be instructed to maintain an adequate fluid intake in order to prevent crystalluria and stone formation.

Laboratory Tests: Complete blood counts should be done frequently in patients receiving Bactrim; if a significant reduction in the count of any formed blood element is noted, Bactrim should be discontinued. Urinalyses with careful microscopic examination and renal function tests should be performed during therapy, particularly for those patients with impaired renal function.

Drug Interactions: In elderly patients concurrently receiving certain diuretics, primarily thiazides, an increased incidence of thrombocytopenia with purpura has been reported. It has been reported that Bactrim may prolong the prothrombin time in patients who are receiving the anticoagulant warfarin. This interaction should be kept in mind when Bactrim is given to patients already on anticoagulant therapy, and the coagulation time should be reassessed.

Bactrim may inhibit the hepatic metabolism of phenytoin. Bactrim, given at a common clinical dosage, increased the phenytoin half-life by 39% and decreased the phenytoin metabolic clearance rate by 27%. When administering these drugs concurrently, one should be alert for possible excessive phenytoin effect.

Sulfonamides can also displace methotrexate from plasma protein binding sites, thus increasing free methotrexate concentrations.

Drug/Laboratory Test Interactions: Bactrim, specifically the trimethoprim component, can interfere with a serum methotrexate assay as determined by the competitive binding protein technique (CBPA) when a bacterial dihydrofolate reductase is used as the binding protein. No interference occurs, however, if methotrexate is measured by a radioimmunoassay (RIA).

The presence of trimethoprim and sulfamethoxazole may also interfere with the Jaffé alkaline picrate reaction assay for creatinine, resulting in overestimations of about 10% in the range of normal values.

Carcinogenesis, Mutagenesis, Impairment of Fertility:

Carcinogenesis: Long-term studies in animals to evaluate carcinogenic potential have not been conducted with Bactrim.

Mutagenesis: Bacterial mutagenic studies have not been performed with sulfamethoxazole and trimethoprim in combination. Trimethoprim was demonstrated to be nonmutagenic in the Ames assay. No chromosomal damage was observed in human leukocytes *in vitro* with sulfamethoxazole and trimethoprim alone or in combination; the concentrations used exceeded blood levels of these compounds following therapy with Bactrim. Observations of leukocytes obtained from patients treated with Bactrim revealed no chromosomal abnormalities.

Impairment of Fertility: No adverse effects on fertility or general reproductive performance were observed in rats given oral dosages as high as 70 mg/kg/day trimethoprim plus 350 mg/kg/day sulfamethoxazole.

Pregnancy: Teratogenic Effects: Pregnancy Category C. In rats, oral doses of 533 mg/kg sulfamethoxazole or 200 mg/kg trimethoprim produced teratologic effects manifested mainly as cleft palates.

The highest dose which did not cause cleft palates in rats was 512 mg/kg sulfamethoxazole or 192 mg/kg trimethoprim when administered separately. In two studies in rats, no teratology was observed when 512 mg/kg of sulfamethoxazole was used in combination with 128 mg/kg of trimethoprim. In one study, however, cleft palates were observed in one litter out of 9 when 355 mg/kg of sulfamethoxazole was used in combination with 88 mg/kg of trimethoprim.

In some rabbit studies, an overall increase in fetal loss (dead and resorbed and malformed conceptuses) was associated with doses of trimethoprim 6 times the human therapeutic dose.

While there are no large, well-controlled studies on the use of trimethoprim and sulfamethoxazole in pregnant women, Brumfitt and Pursell,[5] in a retrospective study, reported the outcome of 186 pregnancies during which the mother received either placebo or trimethoprim and sulfamethoxazole. The incidence of congenital abnormalities was 4.5% (3 of 66) in those who received placebo and 3.3% (4 of 120) in those receiving trimethoprim and sulfamethoxazole. There were no abnormalities in the 10 children whose mothers received the drug during the first trimester. In a separate survey, Brumfitt and Pursell also found no congenital abnormalities in 35 children whose mothers had received oral trimethoprim and sulfamethoxazole at the time of conception or shortly thereafter.

Because trimethoprim and sulfamethoxazole may interfere with folic acid metabolism, Bactrim should be used during pregnancy only if the potential benefit justifies the potential risk to the fetus.

Nonteratogenic Effects: See CONTRAINDICATIONS section.

Nursing Mothers: See CONTRAINDICATIONS section.

Pediatric Use: Bactrim is not recommended for infants younger than two months of age (see INDICATIONS and CONTRAINDICATIONS sections).

ADVERSE REACTIONS

The most common adverse effects are gastrointestinal disturbances (nausea, vomiting, anorexia) and allergic skin reactions (such as rash and urticaria). **FATALITIES ASSOCIATED WITH THE ADMINISTRATION OF SULFONAMIDES, ALTHOUGH RARE, HAVE OCCURRED DUE TO SEVERE REACTIONS, INCLUDING STEVENS-JOHNSON SYNDROME, TOXIC EPIDERMAL NECROLYSIS, FULMINANT HEPATIC NECROSIS, AGRANULOCYTOSIS, APLASTIC ANEMIA AND OTHER BLOOD DYSCRASIAS (SEE WARNINGS SECTION).**

Hematologic: Agranulocytosis, aplastic anemia, thrombocytopenia, leukopenia, neutropenia, hemolytic anemia, megaloblastic anemia, hypoprothrombinemia, methemoglobinemia, eosinophilia.

Allergic Reactions: Stevens-Johnson syndrome, toxic epidermal necrolysis, anaphylaxis, allergic myocarditis, erythema multiforme, exfoliative dermatitis, angioedema, drug fever, chills, Henoch-Schoenlein purpura, serum sickness-like syndrome, generalized allergic reactions, generalized skin eruptions, photosensitivity, conjunctival and scleral injection, pruritus, urticaria and rash. In addition, periarteritis nodosa and systemic lupus erythematosus have been reported.

Gastrointestinal: Hepatitis (including cholestatic jaundice and hepatic necrosis), elevation of serum transaminase and bilirubin, pseudomembranous enterocolitis, pancreatitis, stomatitis, glossitis, nausea, emesis, abdominal pain, diarrhea, anorexia.

Genitourinary: Renal failure, interstitial nephritis, BUN and serum creatinine elevation, toxic nephrosis with oliguria and anuria, and crystalluria.

Neurologic: Aseptic meningitis, convulsions, peripheral neuritis, ataxia, vertigo, tinnitus, headache.

Psychiatric: Hallucinations, depression, apathy, nervousness.

Endocrine: The sulfonamides bear certain chemical similarities to some goitrogens, diuretics (acetazolamide and the thiazides) and oral hypoglycemic agents. Cross-sensitivity may exist with these agents. Diuresis and hypoglycemia have occurred rarely in patients receiving sulfonamides.

Musculoskeletal: Arthralgia and myalgia.

Miscellaneous: Weakness, fatigue, insomnia.

OVERDOSAGE

Acute: The amount of a single dose of Bactrim that is either associated with symptoms of overdosage or is likely to be life-threatening has not been reported. Signs and symptoms of overdosage reported with sulfonamides include anorexia, colic, nausea, vomiting, dizziness, headache, drowsiness and unconsciousness. Pyrexia, hematuria and crystalluria may be noted. Blood dyscrasias and jaundice are potential late manifestations of overdosage.

Signs of acute overdosage with trimethoprim include nausea, vomiting, dizziness, headache, mental depression, confusion and bone marrow depression.

General principals of treatment include the institution of gastric lavage or emesis, forcing oral fluids, and the administration of intravenous fluids if urine output is low and renal function is normal. Acidification of the urine will increase renal elimination of trimethoprim. The patient should be monitored with blood counts and appropriate blood chemistries, including electrolytes. If a significant blood dyscrasia or jaundice occurs, specific therapy should be instituted for these complications. Peritoneal dialysis is not effective and hemodialysis is only moderately effective in eliminating trimethoprim and sulfamethoxazole.

Chronic: Use of Bactrim at high doses and/or for extended periods of time may cause bone marrow depression manifested as thrombocytopenia, leukopenia and/or megaloblastic anemia. If signs of bone marrow depression occur, the patient should be given leucovorin 5 to 15 mg daily until normal hematopoiesis is restored.

DOSAGE AND ADMINISTRATION

Not recommended for use in infants less than two months of age.

URINARY TRACT INFECTIONS AND SHIGELLOSIS IN ADULTS AND CHILDREN, AND ACUTE OTITIS MEDIA IN CHILDREN:

Adults: The usual adult dosage in the treatment of urinary tract infections is one Bactrium DS (double strength) tablet, two Bactrim tablets or four teaspoonfuls (20 ml) of Bactrim Pediatric Suspension or Bactrim Suspension every 12 hours for 10 to 14 days. An identical daily dosage is used for 5 days in the treatment of shigellosis.

Children: The recommended dose for children with urinary tract infections or acute otitis media is 8 mg/kg trimethoprim and 40 mg/kg sulfamethoxazole per 24 hours, given in two divided doses every 12 hours for 10 days. An identical daily dosage is used for 5 days in the treatment of shigellosis. The following table is a guideline for the attainment of this dosage:

Children two months of age or older:

Weight		Dose—every 12 hours	
lb	kg	Teaspoonfuls	Tablets
22	10	1 teasp. (5 ml)	—
44	20	2 teasp. (10 ml)	1 tablet
66	30	3 teasp. (15 ml)	1½ tablets
88	40	4 teasp. (20 ml)	2 tablets or 1 DS tablet

For Patients with Impaired Renal Function: When renal function is impaired, a reduced dosage should be employed using the following table:

Creatinine Clearance (ml/min)	Recommended Dosage Regimen
Above 30	Usual standard regimen
15–30	½ the usual regimen
Below 15	Use not recommended

ACUTE EXACERBATIONS OF CHRONIC BRONCHITIS IN ADULTS:

The usual adult dosage in the treatment of acute exacerbations of chronic bronchitis is one Bactrim DS (double strength) tablet, two Bactrim tablets or four teaspoonfuls (20 ml) of Bactrim Pediatric Suspension or Bactrim Suspension every 12 hours for 14 days.

PNEUMOCYSTIS CARINII PNEUMONITIS:

The recommended dosage for patients with documented *Pneumocystis carinii* pneumonitis is 20 mg/kg trimethoprim and 100 mg/kg sulfamethoxazole per 24 hours given in equally divided doses every 6 hours for 14 days. The following table is a guideline for the attainment of this dosage in children:

Weight		Dose—every six hours	
lb	kg	Teaspoonfuls	Tablets
18	8	1 teasp. (5 ml)	—
35	16	2 teasp. (10 ml)	1 tablet
53	24	3 teasp. (15 ml)	1½ tablets
70	32	4 teasp. (20 ml)	2 tablets or 1 DS tablet

HOW SUPPLIED

DS (double strength) Tablets (white, notched, capsule shaped), containing 160 mg trimethoprim and 800 mg sulfamethoxazole—bottles of 100 (NDC 0004-0117-01), 250 (NDC 0004-0117-04) and 500 (NDC 0004-0117-14); Tel-E-Dose® packages of 100 (NDC 0004-0117-49); Prescription Paks of 20 (NDC 0004-0117-54). Imprint on tablets: (front) BACTRIM-DS; (back) ROCHE.

Tablets (light green, scored, capsule shaped), containing 80 mg trimethoprim and 400 mg sulfamethoxazole—bottles of 100 (NDC 0004-0050-01) and 500 (NDC 0004-0050-14); Tel-E-Dose® packages of 100 (NDC 0004-0050-49); Prescription Paks of 40 (NDC 0004-0050-34). Imprint on tablets: (front) BACTRIM; (back) ROCHE.

Pediatric Suspension (pink, cherry flavored), containing 40 mg trimethoprim and 200 mg sulfamethoxazole per teaspoonful (5 ml)—bottles of 100 ml (NDC 0004-1033-01) and 16 oz (1 pint) (NDC 0004-1033-28).

Suspension (pink, fruit-licorice flavored), containing 40 mg trimethoprim and 200 mg sulfamethoxazole per teaspoonful (5 ml)—bottles of 16 oz (1 pint) (NDC 0004-1015-28).

TABLETS SHOULD BE STORED AT 15°-30°C (59°-86°F) IN A DRY PLACE AND PROTECTED FROM LIGHT.

SUSPENSIONS SHOULD BE STORED AT 15°-30°C (59°-86°F) AND PROTECTED FROM LIGHT.

REFERENCES

1. Kremers P, Duvivier J, Heusghem C: Pharmacokinetic Studies of Co-Trimoxazole in Man after Single and Repeated Doses. *J Clin Pharmacol 14:* 112–117, Feb-Mar 1974. 2. Kaplan SA, *et al:* Pharmacokinetic Profile of Trimethoprim-Sulfamethoxazole in Man. *J Infect Dis 128* (Suppl): S547–S555, Nov 1973. 3. *Federal Register 37:* 20527–20529, 1972. 4. Bauer AW, Kirby WMM, Sherris JC, Turck M: Antibiotic Susceptibility Testing by a Standardized Single Disk Method. *Am J Clin Path 45:* 493–496, Apr 1966. 5. Brumfitt W, Pursell R: Trimethoprim/Sulfamethoxazole in the Treatment of Bacteriuria in Women. *J Infect Dis 128* (Suppl): S657–S663, Nov 1973.

Shown in Product Identification Section, page 424

BEROCCA® ℞

[ber-o'ka]

PARENTERAL NUTRITION

Injectable

Vitamins for Addition to Intravenous Fluids

The following text is complete prescribing information based on official labeling in effect June 1, 1986.

DESCRIPTION

Berocca Parenteral Nutrition is a sterile injectable solution of nine water-soluble and three fat-soluble vitamins for addition to intravenous fluids. Each duplex package contains Solution 1 and Solution 2 in either ampuls or vials. When the contents of both containers are combined, 2 ml of the resulting parenteral multivitamin solution will provide eight B-complex vitamins and vitamins C, A, D and E at levels recommended by the American Medical Association.*

* *Multivitamin Preparations for Parenteral Use: A Statement by the Nutrition Advisory Group.* American Medical Association Department of Foods and Nutrition, 1975. *JPEN 3* :258–269, Jul-Aug 1979.

Each ml of Berocca Parenteral Nutrition Solution 1 provides:

Thiamine hydrochloride (B_1)	3	mg
d-Biotin	60	mcg
Riboflavin (as riboflavin 5'-phosphate sodium) (B_2)	3.6	mg
Niacinamide	40	mg
Pyridoxine hydrochloride (B_6)	4	mg
Dexpanthenol	15	mg
Ascorbic Acid (C)	100	mg

compounded with propylene glycol 40%, gentisic acid ethanolamide 2%, disodium edetate 0.01%, and benzyl alcohol 1% as stabilizers and preservatives; and sodium hydroxide to adjust pH to approximately 5.

Each ml of Berocca Parenteral Nutrition Solution 2 provides:

Vitamin A palmitate	3300 USP units
Vitamin E (*dl*-alpha tocopherol)	10 USP units
Vitamin D_2 (ergocalciferol)	200 USP units
Folic acid	400 mcg
Cyanocobalamin (B_{12})	5 mcg

compounded with polyoxyethylated vegetable oil 10% as solubilizer for vitamins A, D, E; propylene glycol 10%, ethyl alcohol 10%, gentisic acid ethanolamide 2%, sodium citrate 1.7%, benzyl alcohol 1%, and disodium edetate 0.01% as stabilizers and preservatives; and sodium hydroxide and citric acid to adjust pH to approximately 6.5.

CLINICAL PHARMACOLOGY

Vitamins are essential for maintenance of normal metabolic functions including hematopoiesis: The water-soluble vitamins play vital roles in the conversion of carbohydrate, protein and fat into tissue and energy. *Thiamine (B_1)* acts as a coenzyme in carbohydrate metabolism. *Riboflavin (B_2)* functions as a coenzyme in the electron transport system associated with conversion of tissue oxidations into usable energy. *Niacin* serves as a coenzyme in oxidation-reduction reactions in tissue respiration. *Pyridoxine hydrochloride (B_6)* is essential for the metabolism of amino acids. *Pantothenic acid* functions as a coenzyme in various metabolic acetylation reactions and *biotin* in specific carboxylation reactions in lipid metabolism. *Folic acid* and *cyanocobalamin (B_{12})* are metabolically interrelated. They are essential to nucleic acid synthesis and normal maturation of red blood cells. *Ascorbic acid (C)* performs a vital function in the process of cellular respiration, and is involved in both carbohydrate and amino acid metabolism. It is essential for collagen formation and tissue repair.

Vitamin A is necessary for proper functioning of the retina; it appears to be essential to the integrity of epithelial cells. *Vitamin D* is necessary for the absorption of calcium and for the maintenance of bone structure. *Vitamin E* is an antioxidant which preserves essential cellular constituents, including those of the red blood cell. It also serves as protection against lipid peroxidation.

Berocca Parenteral Nutrition provides, in a 2 ml dose, the daily requirements of twelve essential vitamins for nutritional rehabilitation and maintenance of optimal nutritional status in conditions for which parenteral vitamin nutrition is indicated.

INDICATIONS

Berocca Parenteral Nutrition is indicated as daily multivitamin maintenance dosage for adults and children age 11 and above receiving parenteral nutrition. It is also indicated in other situations where administration by the intravenous route is required. Such situations include surgery, excessive burns, fractures and other trauma, severe infectious diseases and comatose states, which may provoke a "stress" situation with profound alterations in the body's metabolic demands and consequent tissue depletion of nutrients.

The physician should not await the development of clinical signs of vitamin deficiency before initiating vitamin therapy. The use of a multivitamin product obviates the need to speculate on the status of individual vitamin nutriture.

Berocca Parenteral Nutrition (administered in intravenous fluids under proper dilution) contributes vitamins, except vitamin K, necessary for maintaining the body's normal resistance and repair processes.

Patients with multiple vitamin deficiencies or with markedly increased requirements may be given multiples of the daily dosage for two or more days as indicated by the clinical status. Berocca Parenteral Nutrition does not contain vitamin K, which may have to be administered separately. Clinical testing indicates that some patients do not maintain adequate levels of certain vitamins when Berocca Parenteral Nutrition in recommended amounts is the sole source of vitamins. No vitamin deficiencies were clinically evident, but blood levels of vitamins A, C, D, E and folic acid declined in a number of subjects who received Berocca Parenteral Nutrition as the only vitamin source for 4 to 6 months. Therefore, in patients for whom total parenteral nutrition will be continued for long periods of time, these vitamins should be monitored. If deficiencies appear to be developing, multiples of the formulation (1.5 to 3 times) may be needed for a period of time. When multiples of the formulation are used for more than a few weeks, vitamins A, D and E should be monitored occasionally to be certain that an excess accumulation of these vitamins is not occurring.

CONTRAINDICATIONS

Berocca Parenteral Nutrition is contraindicated in patients known to be hypersensitive to any of its components and in those with a preexisting hypervitaminosis.

WARNINGS

Allergic reactions, including anaphylaxis, may occur in patients hypersensitive to thiamine or other components of the product; the solubilizer has been associated with anaphylaxis or anaphylactoid reactions.

Patients who have early Leber's disease (hereditary optic nerve atrophy) have been found to suffer severe, acute optic atrophy when treated with vitamin B_{12}. Pyridoxine can decrease the efficacy of levodopa in the treatment of patients with parkinsonism. Folic acid may alter patient response to methotrexate therapy. These facts should be considered before prescribing Berocca Parenteral Nutrition for such patients.

Folic acid in doses above 0.1 mg daily may obscure pernicious anemia. Berocca Parenteral Nutrition is not intended for treatment of pernicious anemia or other megaloblastic anemias where vitamin B_{12} is deficient. Neurologic involvement may develop or progress, despite temporary remission of anemia, in patients with vitamin B_{12} deficiency who receive supplemental folic acid and who are inadequately treated with B_{12}. This product should not be used as primary treatment for specific vitamin deficiencies such as beriberi, pellagra, scurvy, and riboflavin or pyridoxine deficiency.

PRECAUTIONS

Because fat-soluble vitamins can accumulate in the body, toxicity from vitamins A and D is possible, especially if patients are inadvertently administered oral vitamin supplementation in addition to the parenteral regimen.

Berocca Parenteral Nutrition does not contain vitamin K. Supplements of vitamin K may be necessary to meet patients' individual requirements. Patients routinely receiving fat emulsion as part of the total parenteral regimen may have increased requirements for vitamin E.

Most antibiotics, methotrexate and pyrimethamine invalidate diagnostic microbiological blood assays for folic acid and cyanocobalamin.

Safety and effectiveness in children under the age of 11 have not been established.

ADVERSE REACTIONS

Allergic sensitization has been reported following parenteral administration of folic acid and thiamine. Hepatomegaly, leukopenia and projectile vomiting have been reported in the literature as vitamin A toxicity symptoms; elevated serum calcium and multiple areas of tissue calcification have been reported with hypervitaminosis D.

DOSAGE AND ADMINISTRATION

For addition to intravenous fluids. I.V. administration should always be done slowly. Initial administration should only be done when facilities are available to cope with anaphylactic events, if they should occur.

In a recent dog study, histamine-like reactions were induced with infusions given over a two-hour period, at dosages approximately five times the therapeutic human dose.

The recommended daily dose is 2 ml of Berocca Parenteral Nutrition (1 ml of Solution 1 and 1 ml of Solution 2) added to intravenous infusion fluids. **Berocca Parenteral Nutrition should be infused over a period of at least two hours.**

IMPORTANT: DIRECTIONS FOR RECONSTITUTION, ADDITION TO INTRAVENOUS INFUSION SOLUTIONS AND STORAGE:

Ampuls: To prepare solution for single dose administration, mix 1 ml of Berocca Parenteral Nutrition Solution 1 with 1 ml of Berocca Parenteral Nutrition Solution 2. The reconstituted product is ready for addition to intravenous infusion fluids. Or, add the contents of each ampul directly to the intravenous infusion fluid. *Multiple dose vials:* To prepare solution for 10 doses, add 10 ml of Berocca Parenteral Nutrition Solution 2 to 10 ml of Berocca Parenteral Nutrition Solution 1 (20 ml vial, 10 ml fill). To administer single doses, add 2 ml of the reconstituted product to intravenous infusion fluids. Or, add 1 ml of Solution 1 and 1 ml of Solution 2 directly to the intravenous infusion fluid.

BEROCCA PARENTERAL NUTRITION CAN BE USED WITH COMPATIBLE INTRAVENOUS INFUSION SOLUTIONS: 0.9% sterile saline, 5% or 10% sterile glucose or dextrose, lactated Ringer's solution. Two ml of Berocca Parenteral Nutrition (1 ml of Solution 1 and 1 ml of Solution 2) should be added to at least 250 ml of the intravenous infusion solution. Either glass or plastic containers can be used.

Berocca Parenteral Nutrition, like other parenteral vitamins, should not be added to I.V. fluids containing sodium bisulfite as this causes rapid degradation of vitamin B_1 (thiamine). If Berocca Parenteral Nutrition is added to I.V. fluids which do contain the preservative sodium bisulfite, a separate supplemental injection of thiamine should be administered.

Store unreconstituted product in refrigerator (2°- 8°C, 36°-46°F). PROTECT FROM LIGHT. DO NOT STORE AT ROOM TEMPERATURE.

Store reconstituted (mixed) product for no longer than 14 days in refrigerator (2°-8°C, 36°-46°F). PROTECT FROM LIGHT.

Store intravenous fluids with added Berocca Parenteral Nutrition in refrigerator (2°-8°C, 36°-46°F) for no longer than 24 hours. PROTECT FROM LIGHT.

Note: Berocca Parenteral Nutrition contains a soluble form of riboflavin which permits use of a large dose and minimizes pain on injection. This form of riboflavin may result in darkening of the solution and the color change is intensified on prolonged storage. However, the darkening of the solution in no way affects the safety and therapeutic efficacy of the preparation.

Parenteral drug products should be inspected visually for particulate matter prior to administration, whenever solution and container permit.

HOW SUPPLIED

Ampuls: Duplex packages, each containing a 1-ml ampul of Solution 1 and a 1-ml ampul of Solution 2; boxes of 25.

Vials: Duplex packages, each containing a 20-ml vial (10-ml fill) of Solution 1 and a 10-ml vial (10-ml fill) of Solution 2; boxes of 1.

Continued on next page

Roche Labs.—Cont.

BEROCCA® TABLETS ℞

[ber-o'ka]

The following text is complete prescribing information based on official labeling in effect June 1, 1986.
(See accompanying table.)
[See table below].
Each tablet also contains acacia, calcium sulfate, carnauba wax, hydrogenated vegetable oil, magnesium oxide, magnesium stearate, povidone, shellac, sodium benzoate, sugar and talc with the following dyes: FD&C Blue No. 1, FD&C Yellow No. 6, D&C Yellow No. 10 and titanium dioxide.

DESCRIPTION

Berocca is a prescription-only oral multivitamin tablet specially formulated for prophylactic or therapeutic nutritional supplementation in conditions requiring water-soluble vitamins.
Berocca tablets supply *therapeutic* levels of ascorbic acid, vitamins B_1, B_2, B_6, niacin and pantothenic acid and a *supplemental* level of vitamin B_{12}. Berocca tablets also supply a supplemental level of folic acid for pregnant or lactating women and a therapeutic level for adults and children four or more years of age.

CLINICAL PHARMACOLOGY

Vitamins are essential for normal metabolic functions including hematopoiesis. The B-complex vitamins are necessary for the conversion of carbohydrate, protein and fat into tissue and energy.
Ascorbic acid (C) is involved in collagen formation and tissue repair.
The water-soluble vitamins (B-complex and C) are not significantly stored by the body; excess quantities are excreted in the urine. They must be replenished regularly through diet or other means to maintain essential tissue levels. Thus, these vitamins are rapidly depleted in conditions interfering with their intake or absorption.

INDICATIONS AND USAGE

Berocca is indicated for supportive nutritional supplementation in conditions in which water-soluble vitamins are required prophylactically or therapeutically. These include:
Conditions causing depletion, or reduced absorption or bioavailability of water-soluble vitamins—
Gastrointestinal disorders, chronic alcoholism, febrile illnesses, prolonged or wasting diseases, hyperthyroidism or poorly controlled diabetes.
Conditions resulting in increased needs for water-soluble vitamins—
Pregnancy, severe burns, recovery from surgery.

CONTRAINDICATIONS

Berocca is contraindicated in patients known to be hypersensitive to any of its components.

WARNINGS

Berocca is not intended for treatment of pernicious anemia or other megaloblastic anemias where vitamin B_{12} is deficient. Neurologic involvement may develop or progress, despite temporary remission of anemia, in patients with vitamin B_{12} deficiency who receive supplemental folic acid and who are inadequately treated with B_{12}.

PRECAUTIONS

General: Certain conditions listed above may require additional nutritional supplementation. During pregnancy, for instance, supplementation with fat-soluble vitamins and minerals may be required according to the dietary habits of the individual. Berocca is not intended for treatment of severe specific deficiencies.
Information for the Patient: Because toxic reactions have been reported with injudicious use of certain vitamins, urge patients to follow your specific instructions regarding dosage regimen. As with any medication, advise patients to keep Berocca out of reach of children.

Each **Berocca® tablet** contains:	Quantity	U.S. RDA—Adults and children 4 or more years of age	U.S. RDA—Pregnant or lactating women
Vitamin C (ascorbic acid)	500 mg	60 mg	60 mg
Vitamin B_1 (as thiamine mononitrate)	15 mg	1.5 mg	1.7 mg
Vitamin B_2 (riboflavin)	15 mg	1.7 mg	2 mg
Niacin (as niacinamide)	100 mg	20 mg	20 mg
Vitamin B_6 (as pyridoxine HCl)	4 mg	2 mg	2.5 mg
Pantothenic acid (as calcium *d*-pantothenate)	18 mg	10 mg	10 mg
Folic acid	0.5 mg	0.4 mg	0.8 mg
Vitamin B_{12} (cyanocobalamin)	5 mcg	6 mcg	8 mcg

Each **Berocca® Plus** tablet contains:	Quantity	U.S. RDA—Adults and children 4 or more years of age	U.S. RDA—Pregnant or lactating women
Fat-Soluble Vitamins			
Vitamin A (as vitamin A acetate)	5000 IU	5000 IU	8000 IU
Vitamin E (as *dl*-alpha tocopheryl acetate)	30 IU	30 IU	30 IU
Water-Soluble Vitamins			
Vitamin C (ascorbic acid)	500 mg	60 mg	60 mg
Vitamin B_1 (as thiamine mononitrate)	20 mg	1.5 mg	1.7 mg
Vitamin B_2 (riboflavin)	20 mg	1.7 mg	2 mg
Niacin (as niacinamide)	100 mg	20 mg	20 mg
Vitamin B_6 (as pyridoxine HCl)	25 mg	2 mg	2.5 mg
Biotin	0.15 mg	0.30 mg	0.30 mg
Pantothenic acid (as calcium pantothenate)	25 mg	10 mg	10 mg
Folic acid	0.8 mg	0.4 mg	0.8 mg
Vitamin B_{12} (cyanocobalamin)	50 mcg	6 mcg	8 mcg
Minerals			
Iron (as ferrous fumarate)	27 mg	18 mg	18 mg
Chromium (as chromium nitrate)	0.1 mg	0.05–0.2 mg*	
Magnesium (as magnesium oxide)	50 mg	400 mg	450 mg
Manganese (as manganese dioxide)	5 mg	2.5–5 mg*	
Copper (as cupric oxide)	3 mg	2 mg	2 mg
Zinc (as zinc oxide)	22.5 mg	15 mg	15 mg

Each tablet also contains carnauba wax, ethylcellulose, ethyl vanillin, hydroxypropyl methylcellulose, magnesium stearate, povidone, silicon dioxide, stearic acid, triacetin and flavor with the following dyes: yellow iron oxide and titanium dioxide.
*Not established. Estimated by NAS/NRC as safe and adequate daily dietary intake for adults.

Drug and Treatment Interactions: As little as 5 mg pyridoxine daily can decrease the efficacy of levodopa in the treatment of parkinsonism. Therefore, Berocca is not recommended for patients undergoing such therapy.

ADVERSE REACTIONS

Adverse reactions have been reported with specific vitamins, but generally at levels substantially higher than those in Berocca. However, allergic and idiosyncratic reactions are possible at lower levels.

DOSAGE AND ADMINISTRATION

Usual adult dosage: one tablet daily.
Berocca is available on prescription only.

HOW SUPPLIED

Light green, capsule-shaped tablets—bottles of 100 (NDC 0004-0020-01) and 500 (NDC 0004-0020-14).
Imprint on tablets: BEROCCA®
ROCHE
Shown in Product Identification Section, page 424

BEROCCA® PLUS TABLETS ℞

[ber-o'ka]

The following text is complete prescribing information based on official labeling in effect June 1, 1986.
(See accompanying table.)
[See table above].

DESCRIPTION

Berocca Plus is a prescription-only oral multivitamin/mineral tablet specially formulated for prophylactic or therapeutic nutritional supplementation in physiologically stressful conditions.
Berocca Plus supplies: *therapeutic* levels of water-soluble vitamins (ascorbic acid and all B-complex vitamins except biotin); *supplemental* levels of biotin, fat-soluble vitamins (A and E) and minerals (iron, chromium, manganese, copper and zinc); plus magnesium.

CLINICAL PHARMACOLOGY

Vitamins and minerals are essential for normal metabolic functions including hematopoiesis. The B-complex vitamins are necessary for the conversion of carbohydrate, protein and fat into tissue and energy. Ascorbic acid is involved in tissue repair and collagen formation. Vitamin A is necessary for proper functioning of the retina; it appears to be essential to the integrity of epithelial cells. Vitamin E is an antioxidant which preserves essential cellular constituents. Magnesium is a structural component of body tissues; iron, chromium, manganese, copper and zinc serve as catalysts in enzyme systems which perform vital cellular functions.
Water-soluble vitamins (B-complex and C) are not significantly stored by the body and must be replaced continually to maintain essential tissue levels; excess quantities are excreted in urine. These vitamins are rapidly depleted in conditions interfering with their intake or absorption. Berocca Plus supplies therapeutic levels of vitamin C and all B-complex vitamins (except biotin).
Fat-soluble vitamins and several trace minerals, however, can accumulate in the body and do not need replacement as frequently. Therefore, Berocca Plus supplies more conservative levels of vitamins A and E and various essential minerals.
Specifically, Berocca Plus contains an adequate level of vitamin B_6 (25 mg) to normalize the tryptophan metabolism disturbance which has been associated with the use of estrogenic oral contraceptives or other estrogen therapy. It provides zinc (22.5 mg) which facilitates wound healing, the level of folic acid (0.8 mg) recommended during pregnancy, and ascorbic acid (500 mg) which has been demonstrated to improve the absorption of inorganic iron.

INDICATIONS

Berocca Plus is indicated for prophylactic or therapeutic nutritional supplementation in physiologically stressful conditions. These include:
Conditions causing depletion, or reduced absorption or bioavailability of essential vitamins and minerals—
Inadequate intake due to highly restricted or unbalanced diets such as those frequently associated with anorexic conditions and other states of severe malnutrition.
Gastrointestinal disorders, chronic alcoholism, chronic or acute infections (especially those involving febrile illness), prolonged or wasting disease, congestive heart failure, hyperthyroidism, poorly controlled diabetes or other physiologic stress.
Also, patients on estrogenic oral contraceptives or other estrogen therapy, antibacterials which affect intestinal microflora, or other interfering drugs.
Certain conditions resulting from severe B-vitamin or ascorbic acid deficiency—
Cheilosis, gingivitis, stomatitis and certain other classic water-soluble vitamin deficiency syndromes.
Conditions resulting in increased needs for essential vitamins and minerals—
Recovery from surgery or trauma involving severe burns, fractures or other extensive tissue damage.
Also, pregnant women and those with heavy menstrual bleeding.

CONTRAINDICATIONS

Berocca Plus is contraindicated in patients hypersensitive to any of its components.

WARNINGS

Not intended for treatment of pernicious anemia or other megaloblastic anemias where vitamin B_{12} is deficient. Neurologic involvement may develop or progress, despite temporary remission of anemia, in patients with vitamin B_{12} deficiency who receive supplemental folic acid and who are inadequately treated with B_{12}.

PRECAUTIONS

General: Certain conditions listed above may require additional nutritional supplementation. During pregnancy, for instance, supplementation with vitamin D and calcium may be required according to the dietary habits of the individual. Berocca Plus is not intended for treatment of severe specific deficiencies.

Information for the Patient: Because toxic reactions have been reported with injudicious use of certain vitamins and minerals, urge patients to follow your specific instructions regarding dosage regimen. Advise patients to keep Berocca Plus out of reach of children.

Drug and Treatment Interactions: As litte as 5 mg pyridoxine daily can decrease the efficacy of levodopa in the treatment of parkinsonism. Therefore, Berocca Plus is not recommended for patients undergoing such therapy.

ADVERSE REACTIONS

Adverse reactions have been reported with specific vitamins and minerals, but generally at levels substantially higher than those in Berocca Plus. However, allergic and idiosyncratic reactions are possible at lower levels. Iron, even at the usual recommended levels, has been associated with gastrointestinal intolerance in some patients.

DOSAGE AND ADMINISTRATION

Usual adult dosage: one tablet daily. Not recommended for children. *Berocca Plus is available on prescription only.*

HOW SUPPLIED

Golden yellow, capsule-shaped tablets—bottles of 100.
Imprint on tablets: (front) BEROCCA PLUS; (back) ROCHE.

Shown in Product Identification Section, page 424

BUMEX® ℞
[bu 'mex]
(bumetanide/Roche)
TABLETS
INJECTION

The following text is complete prescribing information based on official labeling in effect June 1, 1986.

WARNING

Bumex (bumetanide/Roche) is a potent diuretic which, if given in excessive amounts, can lead to a profound diuresis with water and electrolyte depletion. Therefore, careful medical supervision is required, and dose and dosage schedule have to be adjusted to the individual patient's needs. (See DOSAGE AND ADMINISTRATION.)

DESCRIPTION

Bumex® (bumetanide/Roche) is a loop diuretic, available as scored tablets, 0.5 mg (light green), 1 mg (yellow) and 2 mg (peach) for oral administration; each tablet also contains lactose, magnesium stearate, microcrystalline cellulose, corn starch and talc, with the following dye systems: 0.5 mg—D&C Yellow No. 10 and FD&C Blue No. 1; 1 mg—D&C Yellow No. 10; 2 mg—red iron oxide. Also as 2-ml ampuls, 2-ml vials, 4-ml vials and 10-ml vials (0.25 mg/ml) for intravenous or intramuscular injection as a sterile solution, each 2 ml of which contains 0.5 mg (0.25 mg/ml) bumetanide compounded with 0.85% sodium chloride and 0.4% ammonium acetate as buffers; 0.01% disodium edetate; 1% benzyl alcohol as preservative, and pH adjusted to approximately 7 with sodium hydroxide.

Chemically, bumetanide is 3-(butylamino)-4-phenoxy-5-sulfamoylbenzoic acid. It is a practically white powder having a calculated molecular weight of 364.41.

CLINICAL PHARMACOLOGY

Bumex is a loop diuretic with a rapid onset and short duration of action. Pharmacological and clinical studies have shown that 1 mg Bumex has a diuretic potency equivalent to approximately 40 mg furosemide. The major site of Bumex action is the ascending limb of the loop of Henle.

The mode of action has been determined through various clearance studies in both humans and experimental animals. Bumex inhibits sodium reabsorption in the ascending limb of the loop of Henle, as shown by marked reduction of free-water clearance (C_{H_2O}) during hydration and tubular free-water reabsorption ($T^C_{H_2O}$) during hydropenia. Reabsorption of chloride in the ascending limb is also blocked by Bumex, and Bumex is somewhat more chloruretic than natriuretic.

Potassium excretion is also increased by Bumex, in a dose-related fashion.

Bumex may have an additional action in the proximal tubule. Since phosphate reabsorption takes place largely in the proximal tubule, phosphaturia during Bumex-induced diuresis is indicative of this additional action. This is further supported by the reduction in the renal clearance of Bumex by probenecid, associated with diminution in the natriuretic response. This proximal tubular activity does not seem to be related to an inhibition of carbonic anhydrase. Bumex does not appear to have a noticeable action on the distal tubule.

Bumex decreases uric acid excretion and increases serum uric acid. Following oral administration of Bumex the onset of diuresis occurs in 30 to 60 minutes. Peak activity is reached between 1 and 2 hours. At usual doses (1 to 2 mg) diuresis is largely complete within 4 hours; with higher doses, the diuretic action lasts for 4 to 6 hours. Diuresis starts within minutes following an intravenous injection and reaches maximum levels within 15 to 30 minutes.

Several pharmacokinetic studies have shown that Bumex, administered orally or parenterally, is eliminated rapidly in humans, with a half-life of between 1 and 1½ hours. Plasma protein-binding is in the range of 94% to 96%.

Oral administration of carbon-14 labeled Bumex to human volunteers revealed that 81% of the administered radioactivity was excreted in the urine, 45% of it as unchanged drug. Urinary and biliary metabolites identified in this study were formed by oxidation of the N-butyl side chain. Biliary excretion of Bumex amounted to only 2% of the administered dose.

INDICATIONS AND USAGE

Bumex is indicated for the treatment of edema associated with congestive heart failure, hepatic and renal disease, including the nephrotic syndrome.

Almost equal diuretic response occurs after oral and parenteral administration of Bumex. Therefore, if impaired gastrointestinal absorption is suspected or oral administration is not practical, Bumex should be given by the intramuscular or intravenous route.

Successful treatment with Bumex following instances of allergic reactions to furosemide suggests a lack of cross-sensitivity.

CONTRAINDICATIONS

Bumex is contraindicated in anuria. Although Bumex can be used to induce diuresis in renal insufficiency, any marked increase in blood urea nitrogen or creatinine, or the development of oliguria during therapy of patients with progressive renal disease, is an indication for discontinuation of treatment with Bumex. Bumex is also contraindicated in patients in hepatic coma or in states of severe electrolyte depletion until the condition is improved or corrected. Bumex is contraindicated in patients hypersensitive to this drug.

WARNINGS

1. Volume and electrolyte depletion. The dose of Bumex should be adjusted to the patient's need. Excessive doses or too frequent administration can lead to profound water loss, electrolyte depletion, dehydration, reduction in blood volume and circulatory collapse with the possibility of vascular thrombosis and embolism, particularly in elderly patients.

2. Hypokalemia. Hypokalemia can occur as a consequence of Bumex administration. Prevention of hypokalemia requires particular attention in the following conditions: patients receiving digitalis and diuretics for congestive heart failure, hepatic cirrhosis and ascites, states of aldosterone excess with normal renal function, potassium-losing nephropathy, certain diarrheal states, or other states where hypokalemia is thought to represent particular added risks to the patient, *i.e.*, history of ventricular arrhythmias.

In patients with hepatic cirrhosis and ascites, sudden alterations of electrolyte balance may precipitate hepatic encephalopathy and coma. Treatment in such patients is best initiated in the hospital with small doses and careful monitoring of the patient's clinical status and electrolyte balance. Supplemental potassium and/or spironolactone may prevent hypokalemia and metabolic alkalosis in these patients.

3. Ototoxicity. In cats, dogs and guinea pigs, Bumex has been shown to produce ototoxicity. In these test animals Bumex was 5 to 6 times more potent than furosemide and, since the diuretic potency of Bumex is about 40 to 60 times furosemide, it is anticipated that blood levels necessary to produce ototoxicity will rarely be achieved. The potential exists, however, and must be considered a risk of intravenous therapy, especially at high doses, repeated frequently in the face of renal excretory function impairment. Potentiation of aminoglycoside ototoxicity has not been tested for Bumex. Like other members of this class of diuretics, Bumex probably shares this risk.

4. Allergy to sulfonamides. Patients allergic to sulfonamides may show hypersensitivity to Bumex.

PRECAUTIONS

General: Serum potassium should be measured periodically and potassium supplements or potassium-sparing diuretics added if necessary. Periodic determinations of other electrolytes are advised in patients treated with high doses or for prolonged periods, particularly in those on low salt diets.

Hyperuricemia may occur; it has been asymptomatic in cases reported to date. Reversible elevations of the BUN and creatinine may also occur, especially in association with dehydration and particularly in patients with renal insufficiency. Bumex may increase urinary calcium excretion with resultant hypocalcemia.

Laboratory Tests: Studies in normal subjects receiving Bumex revealed no adverse effects on glucose tolerance, plasma insulin, glucagon and growth hormone levels, but the possibility of an effect on glucose metabolism exists. Periodic determinations of blood sugar should be done, particularly in patients with diabetes or suspected latent diabetes.

Patients under treatment should be observed regularly for possible occurrence of blood dyscrasias, liver damage or idiosyncratic reactions, which have been reported occasionally in foreign marketing experience. The relationship of these occurrences to Bumex use is not certain.

Drug Interactions:

1. Drugs with ototoxic potential (see WARNINGS): Especially in the presence of impaired renal function, the use of parenterally administered Bumex in patients to whom aminoglycoside antibiotics are also being given should be avoided, except in life-threatening conditions.

2. Drugs with nephrotoxic potential: There has been no experience on the concurrent use of Bumex with drugs known to have a nephrotoxic potential. Therefore, the simultaneous administration of these drugs should be avoided.

3. Lithium: Lithium should generally not be given with diuretics (such as Bumex) because they reduce its renal clearance and add a high risk of lithium toxicity.

4. Probenecid: Pretreatment with probenecid reduces both the natriuresis and hyperreninemia produced by Bumex. This antagonistic effect of probenecid on Bumex natriuresis is not due to a direct action on sodium excretion but is probably secondary to its inhibitory effect on renal tubular secretion of bumetanide. Thus, probenecid should not be administered concurrently with Bumex.

5. Indomethacin: Indomethacin blunts the increases in urine volume and sodium excretion seen during Bumex treatment and inhibits the bumetanide-induced increase in plasma renin activity. Concurrent therapy with Bumex is thus not recommended.

6. Antihypertensives: Bumex may potentiate the effect of various antihypertensive drugs, necessitating a reduction in the dosage of these drugs.

7. Digoxin: Interaction studies in humans have shown no effect on digoxin blood levels.

8. Anticoagulants: Interaction studies in humans have shown Bumex to have no effect on warfarin metabolism or on plasma prothrombin activity.

Carcinogenesis, Mutagenesis, Impairment of Fertility: Bumex was devoid of mutagenic activity in various strains of *Salmonella typhimurium* when tested in the presence or absence of an *in vitro* metabolic activation system. An 18-month study showed an increase in mammary adenomas of questionable significance in female rats receiving oral doses of 60 mg/kg/day (2000 times a 2-mg human dose). A repeat study at the same doses failed to duplicate this finding.

Reproduction studies were performed to evaluate general reproductive performance and fertility in rats at oral dose levels of 10, 30, 60 or 100 mg/kg/day. The pregnancy rate was slightly decreased in the treated animals; however, the differences were small and not statistically significant.

Pregnancy: Teratogenic Effects: Pregnancy Category C. Bumex is neither teratogenic nor embryocidal in mice when given in doses up to 3400 times the maximum human therapeutic dose.

Bumex has been shown to be nonteratogenic, but it has a slight embryocidal effect in rats when given in doses of 3400 times the maximum human therapeutic dose and in rabbits at doses of 3.4 times the maximum human therapeutic dose. In one study, moderate growth retardation and increased incidence of delayed ossification of sternebrae were observed in rats at oral doses of 100 mg/kg/day, 3400 times the maximum human therapeutic dose. These effects were associated with maternal weight reductions noted during dosing. No such adverse effects were observed at 30 mg/kg/day (1000 times the maximum human therapeutic dose). No fetotoxicity was observed at 1000 to 2000 times the human therapeutic dose.

In rabbits, a dose-related decrease in litter size and an increase in resorption rate were noted at oral doses of 0.1 and 0.3 mg/kg/day (3.4 and 10 times the maximum human therapeutic dose). A slightly increased incidence of delayed ossification of sternebrae occurred at 0.3 mg/kg/day; however, no such adverse effects were observed at the dose of 0.03 mg/kg/day. The sensitivity of the rabbit to Bumex parallels the marked pharmacologic and toxicologic effects of the drug in this species.

Bumex was not teratogenic in the hamster at an oral dose of 0.5 mg/kg/day (17 times the maximum human therapeutic dose). Bumex was not teratogenic when given intravenously to mice and rats at doses up to 140 times the maximum human therapeutic dose.

There are no adequate and well-controlled studies in pregnant women. A small investigational experience in the United States and marketing experience in other countries to date have not indicated any evidence of adverse effects on the fetus, but these data do not rule out the possibility of harmful effects. Bumex should be given to a pregnant woman only if the potential benefit justifies the potential risk to the fetus.

Continued on next page

Roche Labs.—Cont.

Nursing Mothers: It is not known whether this drug is excreted in human milk. As a general rule, nursing should not be undertaken while the patient is on Bumex since it may be excreted in human milk.
Pediatric Use: Safety and effectiveness in children below the age of 18 have not been established.

ADVERSE REACTIONS

The most frequent clinical adverse reactions considered probably or possibly related to Bumex are muscle cramps (seen in 1.1% of treated patients), dizziness (1.1%), hypotension (0.8%), headache (0.6%), nausea (0.6%), and encephalopathy (in patients with preexisting liver disease) (0.6%). One or more of these adverse reactions have been reported in approximately 4.1% of Bumex-treated patients.
Less frequent clinical adverse reactions to Bumex are impaired hearing (0.5%), pruritus (0.4%), electrocardiogram changes (0.4%), weakness (0.2%), hives (0.2%), abdominal pain (0.2%), arthritic pain (0.2%), musculoskeletal pain (0.2%), rash (0.2%) and vomiting (0.2%). One or more of these adverse reactions have been reported in approximately 2.9% of Bumex-treated patients.
Other clinical adverse reactions, which have each occurred in approximately 0.1% of patients, are vertigo, chest pain, ear discomfort, fatigue, dehydration, sweating, hyperventilation, dry mouth, upset stomach, renal failure, asterixis, itching, nipple tenderness, diarrhea, premature ejaculation and difficulty maintaining an erection.
Laboratory abnormalities reported have included hyperuricemia (in 18.4% of patients tested), hypochloremia (14.9%), hypokalemia (14.7%), azotemia (10.6%), hyponatremia (9.2%), increased serum creatinine (7.4%), hyperglycemia (6.6%), and variations in phosphorus (4.5%), CO_2 content (4.3%), bicarbonate (3.1%) and calcium (2.4%). Although manifestations of the pharmacologic action of Bumex, these conditions may become more pronounced by intensive therapy.
Diuresis induced by Bumex may also rarely be accompanied by changes in LDH (1.0%), total serum bilirubin (0.8%), serum proteins (0.7%), SGOT (0.6%), SGPT (0.5%), alkaline phosphatase (0.4%), cholesterol (0.4%) and creatinine clearance (0.3%). Also reported have been deviations in hemoglobin (0.8%), prothrombin time (0.8%), hematocrit (0.6%), WBC (0.3%), platelet counts (0.2%) and differential counts (0.1%). Increases in urinary glucose (0.7%) and urinary protein (0.3%) have also been seen.

OVERDOSAGE

Overdosage can lead to acute profound water loss, volume and electrolyte depletion, dehydration, reduction of blood volume and circulatory collapse with a possibility of vascular thrombosis and embolism. Electrolyte depletion may be manifested by weakness, dizziness, mental confusion, anorexia, lethargy, vomiting and cramps. Treatment consists of replacement of fluid and electrolyte losses by careful monitoring of the urine and electrolyte output and serum electrolyte levels.

DOSAGE AND ADMINISTRATION

Dosage should be individualized with careful monitoring of patient response.
Oral Administration: The usual total daily dosage of Bumex is 0.5 to 2.0 mg and in most patients is given as a single dose.
If the diuretic response to an initial dose of Bumex is not adequate, in view of its rapid onset and short duration of action, a second or third dose may be given at 4- to 5-hour intervals up to a maximum daily dose of 10 mg. An intermittent dose schedule, whereby Bumex is given on alternate days or for 3 to 4 days with rest periods of 1 to 2 days in between, is recommended as the safest and most effective method for the continued control of edema. In patients with hepatic failure, the dosage should be kept to a minimum, and if necessary, dosage increased very carefully.
Because cross-sensitivity with furosemide has rarely been observed, Bumex can be substituted at approximately a 1:40 ratio of Bumex to furosemide in patients allergic to furosemide.
Parenteral Administration: Bumex may be administered parenterally (IV or IM) to patients in whom gastrointestinal absorption may be impaired or in whom oral administration is not practical.
Parenteral treatment should be terminated and oral treatment instituted as soon as possible.
The usual initial dose is 0.5 to 1.0 mg intravenously or intramuscularly. Intravenous administration should be given over a period of 1 to 2 minutes. If the response to an initial dose is deemed insufficient, a second or third dose may be given at intervals of 2 to 3 hours, but should not exceed a daily dosage of 10 mg.
Miscibility and Parenteral Solutions: The compatibility tests of Bumex injection (0.25 mg/ml, 2-ml ampuls) with 5% dextrose in water, 0.9% sodium chloride, and lactated Ringer's solution in both glass and plasticized PVC (Viaflex) containers have shown no significant absorption effect with either containers, nor a measurable loss of potency due to degradation of the drug. However, solutions should be freshly prepared and used within 24 hours.
Parenteral drug products should be inspected visually for particulate matter and discoloration prior to administration whenever solution and container permit.

HOW SUPPLIED

Tablets: 0.5 mg (light green), bottles of 100 (NDC 0004-0125-01) and 500 (NDC 0004-0125-14); Prescription Paks of 30 (NDC 0004-0125-57); Tel-E-Dose® packages of 100 (NDC 0004-0125-49). 1 mg (yellow), bottles of 100 (NDC 0004-0121-01) and 500 (NDC 0004-0121-14); Prescription Paks of 30 (NDC 0004-0121-57); Tel-E-Dose® packages of 100 (NDC 0004-0121-49). 2 mg (peach), bottles of 100 (NDC 0004-0162-01); Tel-E-Dose® packages of 100 (NDC 0004-0162-07).
Imprint on tablets: 0.5 mg—ROCHE BUMEX 0.5; 1 mg—ROCHE BUMEX 1; 2 mg—ROCHE BUMEX 2.
Ampuls (0.25 mg/ml), 2 ml, boxes of 10 (NDC 0004-1944-06).
Vials (0.25 mg/ml), 2 ml, boxes of 10 (NDC 0004-1968-01); 4 ml, boxes of 10 (NDC 0004-1969-01); 10 ml, boxes of 10 (NDC 0004-1970-01).

Shown in Product Identification Section, page 424

CLONOPIN® Ⓒ ℞
(clonazepam/Roche)

see KLONOPIN™

COACTIN® ℞
[*kō-ak'tin*]
(amdinocillin/Roche)

The following text is complete prescribing information based on official labeling in effect June 1, 1986.

DESCRIPTION

Coactin (amdinocillin) sterile is a semisynthetic penicillin for intramuscular or intravenous administration. Amdinocillin is a 6-β-amidinopenicillanic acid, different from other penicillins which are 6-β-aminopenicillanic acid derivatives. Chemically, amdinocillin is 6-β-[(hexahydro-1H-azepine-1-yl)-methyleneamino]-penicillanic acid, with an empirical formula of $C_{15}H_{23}N_3O_3S$.
Amdinocillin has a molecular weight of 325.43 and is supplied as a white to off-white crystalline powder which is readily soluble in water and methanol. The pKa values are 3.4 and 8.9 corresponding to an isoelectric point of 6.2. The pH of a 10% aqueous solution is 4.0 to 6.2. The reconstituted solutions are clear, almost colorless to yellow.

CLINICAL PHARMACOLOGY

Intravenous Administration: In healthy adult volunteers, mean plasma concentrations of amdinocillin following a 15-minute intravenous infusion of 10 mg/kg are shown below: [See table below].

Amdinocillin Plasma Concentrations (mcg/ml) in Adults
I.V. Infusion

Dose	15 min	30 min	1 hr	2 hr	4 hr
10 mg/kg	61	34	20	7.5	1.4
	(34–80)*	(26–43)	(13–25)	(6–10)	(0.7–1.9)

*Range

Following a 15-minute intravenous infusion of 10 mg/kg every 4 hours for a total of 6 doses in healthy adult volunteers, the mean steady state (after the second dose) maximum plasma concentrations ranged from 47 to 55 mcg/ml and the minimum steady stated plasma concentrations ranged from 1.2 to 2.0 mcg/ml.
Intramuscular Administration: Amdinocillin is rapidly absorbed after intramuscular injection. Mean plasma concentrations following an intramuscular injection of 10 mg/kg in healthy adult volunteers are shown above: [See table above].

Amdinocillin Plasma Concentrations (mcg/ml) in Adults
I.M. Injection

Dose	15 min	30 min	1 hr	2 hr	4 hr
10 mg/kg	18	26	17	11	2
	(7–35)*	(14–44)	(10–29)	(5–22)	(0.8–5)

*Range

General: As with other penicillins, amdinocillin is excreted primarily by glomerular filtration and tubular secretion. In patients with normal renal function, approximately 70% of the administered dose is recovered in the urine within the first 6 hours after dosing. Following an intravenous infusion of 10 mg/kg, average concentrations of active drug in urine usually exceed 1000 mcg/ml within 30 minutes. At 4 to 6 hours after the infusion, average urinary concentrations usually decline to a range of about 97 to 135 mcg/ml. The average plasma elimination half-life of amdinocillin is approximately 51 minutes (range, 39 to 66 minutes) after intravenous administration; and 55 minutes (range, 39 to 64 minutes) after intramuscular administration. The rate of elimination is related to the degree of renal function impairment. In patients with severe renal insufficiency (creatinine clearance less than 10 ml/min), the mean half-life is slightly prolonged (3.3 hours). The drug is partially removed from the serum by hemodialysis and peritoneal dialysis. As with other penicillins, amdinocillin is metabolized only slightly. Following parenteral administration, the drug is present in active form in the serum, urine and bile, as well as in other body fluids and tissues. As with other penicillins, penetration into the cerebrospinal fluid (CSF) is generally poor; however, higher CSF concentrations are obtained in the presence of meningeal inflammation. Protein binding studies indicate that the degree of amdinocillin binding is low (5 to 10%).
Microbiology: Amdinocillin is highly active against gram-negative bacteria. It has low activity against gram-positive bacteria and is not active against *Pseudomonas* species, indole-positive *Proteus* species, anaerobic rods or enterococci.
Amdinocillin is usually active *in vitro* against strains of the following organisms, although clinical efficacy for infections other than those included in the Indications section has not been documented: *Escherichia coli, Klebsiella* species, *Enterobacter* species, *Citrobacter* species, *Shigella* species and *Salmonella* species. Some strains of *Serratia* species are also susceptible.
Amdinocillin is more stable than ampicillin against β-lactamases, including the common plasmid-mediated TEM-1.
Unlike other penicillins that bind to penicillin-binding protein $1B_S$ and 3, amdinocillin binds preferentially to penicillin-binding protein 2, causing the formation of spherical forms of bacteria by preventing cell elongation. This mechanism of action is primarily bacteriostatic; however, the high levels of amdinocillin achieved in the urinary tract provide bactericidal activity. *In vitro* studies have shown that amdinocillin acts synergistically in combination with other β-lactam antibiotics, enhancing their bactericidal activity against strains with diminished susceptibility. Susceptible strains include *E. coli, K. pneumoniae, Klebsiella* species, *Enterobacter* species, *S. marcescens, Serratia* species, *Proteus mirabilis* and *Citrobacter* species, as well as some strains of *Providencia* species, *Morganella morganii* and indole-positive *Proteus* species. To determine the synergistic activity of amdinocillin in combination with another β-lactam antibiotic against a particular microorganism, susceptibility testing should be performed.
Susceptibility Tests: Quantitative methods that require measurement of zone diameters give good estimates of bacterial susceptibility. One such procedure (Bauer AW, Kirby WM, Sherris JC, Turck M: Antibiotic Susceptibility Testing by a Standardized Single Disk Method, *Am J Clin Pathol, 45:* 493–496, 1966; Standardized Disc Susceptibility Test, *Federal Register, 39:* 19182–19184, 1974) has been recommended for use with discs to test suceptibility to antimicrobials.
With this procedure, a report from the laboratory of "Susceptible" indicates that the infecting organism is likely to respond to therapy. A report of "Resistant" indicates that the infecting organism may not respond to therapy and other therapy should be selected.
When the causative organism is tested by the Kirby-Bauer method of disc susceptibility testing, a 10-mcg amdinocillin disc should give a zone of 16 mm or greater to indicate susceptibility. Zone sizes of 15 mm or less indicate resistance.
Standardized procedures require use of control organisms. The 10-mcg amdinocillin disc should give zone diameters between 23 and 29 mm for the reference strain *E. coli* ATCC 25922.
Under certain conditions, it may be desirable to do additional susceptibility testing by broth or agar dilution techniques. An MIC of ≤ 4 mcg/ml can be considered susceptible. *E. coli* ATCC 25922 is the recommended reference strain for controlling amdinocillin dilution tests. Greater than 95% of MIC's for this control organism should fall within the range of 0.125 to 0.5 mcg/ml.
Suggested methods for susceptibility testing of amdinocillin in combination with other β-lactams: The macro-broth disc method is a simple test that can be employed to qualitatively determine the susceptibility of organisms to a combination of amdinocillin and another β-lactam antibiotic. In this test,

an amdinocillin disc (10 mcg) and a standard disc of the other β-lactam antibiotic are added to 2 ml of Mueller-Hinton broth. The tube and a control tube are inoculated with 10 μl of a bacterial suspension prepared as described for the Kirby-Bauer disc test. The tubes are incubated overnight at 37°C. Inhibition of growth is considered to indicate susceptibility. This test is applicable to all organisms tested by the Kirby-Bauer method.
Broth dilution tests can also be carried out to quantitatively determine the susceptibility of organisms to amdinocillin in combination with other β-lactam antibiotics. MIC's are determined by testing the combined agents in ratios based on the mean serum levels achieved after parenteral administration of a standard dose of the individual agents. Organisms are considered susceptible if the MIC of each antibiotic in the combination falls within the range of susceptibility indicated for the individual components.

INDICATIONS AND USAGE

Coactin is indicated for the treatment of *complicated* and *uncomplicated urinary tract infections* caused by susceptible strains of *E. coli, Klebsiella pneumoniae, Klebsiella* species and *Enterobacter* species.
Bacteremia associated with severe urinary tract infection due to *E. coli* has been successfully treated with Coactin.
It has been demonstrated that amdinocillin acts synergistically with other β-lactam antibiotics. Therefore, combination therapy with various other β-lactam antibiotics may be considered in the treatment of more severe urinary tract infections.
Appropriate culture and susceptibility tests should be performed before treatment in order to isolate and identify organisms causing infections and determine their susceptibility to amdinocillin or to its combination with another β-lactam antibiotic. Therapy with Coactin may be initiated before results of these tests are known; once results become available, appropriate therapy should be continued. In certain severe infections when the causative organisms are unknown, Coactin may be administered with another appropriate β-lactam antibiotic as initial therapy. As soon as results of culture and susceptibility tests become available, antimicrobial therapy should be adjusted if indicated. Culture and susceptibility testing, performed periodically during therapy, will provide information on the therapeutic effect of the antimicrobial and will monitor for the possible emergence of bacterial resistance.

CONTRAINDICATIONS

Coactin is contraindicated in patients with a history of hypersensitivity reactions to any of the penicillins.

WARNINGS

Serious and occasionaly fatal hypersensitivity (anaphylactic) reactions have occurred in patients receiving a penicillin. These reactions are more apt to occur in individuals with a history of sensitivity to multiple allergens. There have been reports of individuals with a history of penicillin hypersensitivity reactions experiencing severe hypersensitivity reactions when treated with a cephalosporin. Before therapy with amdinocillin is instituted, careful inquiry should be made to determine whether the patient has had previous hypersensitivity reactions to penicillins, cephalosporins or other drugs. Antibiotics should be used with caution in any patient who has demonstrated some form of allergy, particularly to drugs.
If an allergic reaction occurs during therapy with amdinocillin, the drug should be discontinued. SERIOUS ANAPHYLACTOID REACTIONS REQUIRE EMERGENCY TREATMENT WITH EPINEPHRINE, OXYGEN AND INTRAVENOUS STEROIDS. AIRWAY MANAGEMENT, INCLUDING INTUBATION, SHOULD ALSO BE PROVIDED AS INDICATED.

PRECAUTIONS

General: Although Coactin shares with other penicillins the low potential for toxicity, as with any potent drug, periodic assessment of organ system functions, including renal, hepatic and hematopoietic, is advisable during prolonged therapy.
As with other antibiotics, prolonged use of Coactin may result in overgrowth of nonsusceptible organisms. If this occurs, appropriate measures should be taken.
Drug Interactions: Probenecid interferes with the renal tubular secretion of amdinocillin, thereby increasing serum concentrations and prolonging the serum half-life of the antibiotic.
Carcinogenesis, Mutagenesis, Impairment of Fertility: Considering the maximum duration of treatment and the class of the compound, carcinogenicity or mutagenicity studies with amdinocillin in animals have not been performed. The maximum durations of animal toxicity studies were 3 months parenterally and 6 months orally.
Amdinocillin produced no impairment of fertility in rats at daily doses up to 450 mg/kg, 7.5 times the recommended human dose.
Pregnancy: Pregnancy Category B. Reproduction studies have been performed in rats and mice at doses up to 7.5 times the recommended human dose and have revealed no evidence of harm to the fetus due to Coactin. There are, however, no adequate or well-controlled studies in pregnant women. Because animal reproduction studies are not always predictive of human response, this drug should be used during pregnancy only if clearly needed. Amdinocillin crosses the placenta and is found in low concentrations in cord blood and amniotic fluid.
Nursing Mothers: In limited studies, amdinocillin, following a single dose, has not been detected in the milk of nursing mothers; however, caution should be exercised when Coactin is administered to a nursing woman.
Pediatric Use: Safety and effectiveness in children below the age of 12 have not been established.

ADVERSE REACTIONS

The most frequent adverse reactions to Coactin which occur in about 5% of the patients are:
Hemic and lymphatic systems: Eosinophilia and thrombocytosis.
Hepatic function tests: Elevations of serum aspartate aminotransferase (SGOT) and serum alkaline phosphatase.
Less frequent adverse reactions, which occur in about 1% of the patients, are:
Hypersensitivity: Rash.
Local reactions: Thrombophlebitis.
Gastrointestinal: Diarrhea and nausea.
Central nervous system: Dizziness.
Hemic and lymphatic systems: Anemia, neutropenia and leukopenia.
Other adverse reactions, which occur rarely (in less than 1% of the patients), are itching and/or urticaria, tenderness and/or pain at the injection site, vomiting, drowsiness or lethargy, elevated blood pressure, vaginitis, thrombocytopenia, and elevations of serum alanine aminotransferase (SGPT) or serum bilirubin.

OVERDOSAGE

There has been no experience to date with either deliberate or inadvertent overdoses of amdinocillin. As with other penicillins, Coactin in overdosage has the potential to cause neuromuscular hypersensitivity or convulsive seizures. Hemodialysis, if necessary, will aid in removal of the drug from the blood.

DOSAGE AND ADMINISTRATION

Coactin may be administered intravenously or intramuscularly. For serious infections, the intravenous route of administration is recommended. The recommended adult dosage for serious infections when Coactin is used alone is 60 mg/kg/day, given in divided doses (10 mg/kg every 4 hours). If the drug is to be given in combination with another β-lactam antibiotic, the daily dose of Coactin should be reduced to 40 mg/kg in divided doses (10 mg/kg every 6 hours).
Dosage for any individual patient must take into consideration the severity of infection, the susceptibility of the organisms causing the infection, and the status of the patient's host defense mechanism. The duration of therapy depends on the severity of infection. Generally, Coactin should be continued for at least 2 days after the signs and symptoms of infection have disappeared. The usual duration is 7 to 10 days, but in complicated infections, more prolonged therapy may be required. In patients with moderate to severe renal impairment (creatinine clearance less than 30 ml/min), the dosage should be limited to 10 mg/kg 3 or 4 times daily.
Parenteral drug products should be inspected visually for particulate matter and discoloration prior to administration, whenever solution and container permit. The normal color of Coactin solutions is off-white to yellow.

DIRECTIONS FOR USE

Intravenous Administration: Coactin is administered intravenously by intermittent infusion. Reconstitute powder with Sterile Water for Injection, U.S.P.
Add the required amount of diluent to the drug powder in the vial; shake well and withdraw the entire contents. Further dilute, using aseptic technique, to 50 ml with 5% Dextrose Injection, U.S.P., and infuse the appropriate dose over 15 to 30 minutes. Other appropriate intravenous solutions at concentrations between 5 mg/ml and 100 mg/ml may be used (see Compatibility and Stability section).

Vial Size	Amount of Diluent to be Added	Concentration after Dilution to 50 ml
500 mg	4.8 ml	10 mg/ml
1 gm	9.6 ml	20 mg/ml

The solution of reconstituted drug may be administered by direct infusion or through a Y-type intravenous infusion set which may already be in place. If this method or the "piggyback" method of administration is used, it is advisable to discontinue temporarily the administration of any other solutions during the infusion of Coactin.
When Coactin is given in combination with another antimicrobial, each drug should be given separately (not mixed physically) in accordance with the recommended dosages and routes of administration for each drug.
Intramuscular Administration: For intramuscular administration, use Sterile Water for Injection, U.S.P., or 0.9% Sodium Chloride Injection, U.S.P., for reconstitution.

Vial Size	Amount of Diluent to be Added
500 mg	2.2 ml
1 gm	4.4 ml

Dissolve drug powder in required volume of diluent and shake well. After reconstitution, each milliliter of solution will contain approximately 200 mg of amdinocillin. As with all intramuscular preparations, Coactin should be injected well within the body of a relatively large muscle, such as the upper outer quadrant of the buttocks (*i.e.*, gluteus maximus); aspiration will help avoid unintentional injection into a blood vessel.

COMPATABILITY AND STABILITY

Coactin *intramuscular* solutions (1 gm/4.4 ml) remain stable (loss of potency less than 10%) for 16 hours when stored at room temperature or for 24 hours under refrigerated (5° C) storage condition.
Coactin *intravenous* solutions, at concentrations between 5 mg/ml and 100 mg/ml remain stable (loss of potency less than 10%) for the following time periods:

Diluent	Storage: Room Temperature	Storage: Refrigerated (5°C)
5% Dextrose*	24 hours	3 days
10% Dextrose*	24 hours	3 days
5% Dextrose + 0.45% Sodium Chloride*	24 hours	3 days
5% Dextrose + 0.9% Sodium Chloride†	24 hours	3 days
5% Dextrose in Ringer's†	24 hours	7 days
Lactated Ringer's with 5% Dextrose†	24 hours	7 days
Lactated Ringer's†	24 hours	7 days
Ringer's Injection*	24 hours	3 days
Sodium Lactate*	24 hours	3 days
0.9% Sodium Chloride	24 hours	7 days
0.45% Sodium Chloride†	24 hours	7 days
Sterile Water*	24 hours	3 days
10% Travert*	24 hours	3 days
5% Dextrose + Electrolyte #48	24 hours	3 days
5% Dextrose + Electrolyte #75	24 hours	7 days

* These solutions remain stable for 7 days under refrigerated conditions at 30 mg/ml or lower concentrations.
† These solutions remain stable for 14 days under refrigerated conditions at 30 mg/ml or lower concentrations.
Unused portions of solutions should be discarded after the time periods stated above.
The above stabilities apply to solutions stored in either glass or Viaflex (PVC) containers.

HOW SUPPLIED

Vials containing 500 mg equivalent of amdinocillin as a crystalline powder for reconstitution. Boxes of 10 (NDC 0004-1960-01).
Vials containing 1 gm equivalent of amdinocillin as a crystalline powder for reconstitution. Boxes of 10 (NDC 0004-1961-01).
Coactin vials should be stored at controlled room temperatures (59°F to 86°F).

EFUDEX® ℞
[ef'u-dex]
(fluorouracil/Roche)

The following text is complete prescribing information based on official labeling in effect June 1, 1986.

DESCRIPTION

Efudex solutions and cream are topical preparations containing the fluorinated pyrimidine 5-fluorouracil, an antineoplastic antimetabolite.
Efudex Solution consists of 2% or 5% fluorouracil/Roche on a weight/weight basis, compounded with propylene glycol, tris(hydroxymethyl) aminomethane, hydroxypropyl cellulose, parabens (methyl and propyl) and disodium edetate.
Efudex Cream contains 5% fluorouracil/Roche in a vanishing cream base consisting of white petrolatum, stearyl alcohol, propylene glycol, polysorbate 60 and parabens (methyl and propyl).

ACTIONS

There is evidence that the metabolism of fluorouracil in the anabolic pathway blocks the methylation reaction of deoxyuridylic acid to thymidylic acid. In this fashion fluorouracil interferes with the synthesis of deoxyribonucleic acid (DNA) and to a lesser extent inhibits the formation of ribonucleic acid (RNA). Since DNA and RNA are essential for cell divi-

Continued on next page

Roche Labs.—Cont.

sion and growth, the effect of fluorouracil may be to create a thymine deficiency which provokes unbalanced growth and death of the cell. The effects of DNA and RNA deprivation are most marked on those cells which grow more rapidly and which take up fluorouracil at a more rapid pace. The catabolic metabolism of fluorouracil results in degradative products (e.g., CO_2, urea, α-fluoro-β-alanine) which are inactive. Studies in man with topical application of ^{14}C-labeled Efudex demonstrated insignificant absorption as measured by ^{14}C content of plasma, urine and respiratory CO_2.

INDICATIONS

Efudex is recommended for the topical treatment of multiple actinic or solar keratoses. In the 5% strength it is also useful in the treatment of superficial basal cell carcinomas, when conventional methods are impractical, such as with multiple lesions or difficult treatment sites. The diagnosis should be established prior to treatment, since this new method has not been proven effective in other types of basal cell carcinomas. With isolated, easily accessible lesions, conventional techniques are preferred since success with such lesions is almost 100% with these methods. The success rate with Efudex cream and solution is approximately 93%. This 93% success rate is based on 113 lesions in 54 patients. Twenty-five lesions treated with the solution produced one failure and 88 lesions treated with the cream produced 7 failures.

CONTRAINDICATIONS

Efudex is contraindicated in patients with known hypersensitivity to any of its components.

WARNINGS

If an occlusive dressing is used, there may be an increase in the incidence of inflammatory reactions in the adjacent normal skin. A porous gauze dressing may be applied for cosmetic reasons without increase in reaction.

Prolonged exposure to ultraviolet rays should be avoided while under treatment with Efudex because the intensity of the reaction may be increased.

Usage in Pregnancy: Safety for use in pregnancy has not been established.

PRECAUTIONS

If Efudex is applied with the fingers, the hands should be washed immediately afterward. Efudex should be applied with care near the eyes, nose and mouth. Solar keratoses which do not respond should be biopsied to confirm the diagnosis. Patients should be forewarned that the reaction in the treated areas may be unsightly during therapy, and, in some cases, for several weeks following cessation of therapy.

Follow-up biopsies should be performed as indicated in the management of superficial basal cell carcinoma.

ADVERSE REACTIONS

The most frequently encountered local reactions are pain, pruritus, hyperpigmentation and burning at the site of application. Other local reactions include allergic contact dermatitis, scarring, soreness, tenderness, suppuration, scaling and swelling.

Also reported are alopecia, insomnia, stomatitis, irritability, medicinal taste, photosensitivity, lacrimation, telangiectasia and urticaria, although a causal relationship is remote.

Laboratory abnormalities reported are leukocytosis, thrombocytopenia, toxic granulation and eosinophilia.

DOSAGE AND ADMINISTRATION

When Efudex is applied to a lesion, a response occurs with the following sequence: erythema, usually followed by vesiculation, erosion, ulceration, necrosis and epithelization.

Actinic or solar keratosis: Apply cream or solution twice daily in an amount sufficient to cover the lesions. Medication should be continued until the inflammatory response reaches the erosion, necrosis and ulceration stage, at which time use of the drug should be terminated. The usual duration of therapy is from two to four weeks. Complete healing of the lesions may not be evident for one to two months following cessation of Efudex therapy.

Superficial basal cell carcinomas: **Only the 5% strength is recommended.** Apply cream or solution twice daily in an amount sufficient to cover the lesions. Treatment should be continued for at least three to six weeks. Therapy may be required for as long as 10 to 12 weeks before the lesions are obliterated. As in any neoplastic condition, the patient should be followed for a reasonable period of time to determine if a cure has been obtained.

HOW SUPPLIED

Efudex Solution, 10-ml drop dispensers—containing 2% or 5% fluorouracil/Roche on a weight/weight basis, compounded with propylene glycol, tris(hydroxymethyl)-aminomethane, hydroxypropyl cellulose, parabens (methyl and propyl) and disodium edetate.

Efudex Cream, 25-Gm tubes—containing 5% fluorouracil/Roche in a vanishing cream base consisting of white petrolatum, stearyl alcohol, propylene glycol, polysorbate 60 and parabens (methyl and propyl).

EMCYT® ℞

[em 'sit]

(estramustine phosphate sodium/Roche)
CAPSULES

The following text is complete prescribing information based on official labeling in effect June 1, 1986.

DESCRIPTION

Estramustine phosphate sodium, an antineoplastic agent, is an off-white powder readily soluble in water. Emcyt is available as white opaque capsules, each containing estramustine phosphate sodium equivalent to 140 mg estramustine phosphate, for oral administration. Each capsule also contains magnesium stearate, silicon dioxide, sodium lauryl sulfate and talc. Gelatin capsule shells contain the following dye: titanium dioxide.

Chemically, estramustine phosphate sodium is estra-1, 3, 5(10)-triene -3, 17β- diol-3[bis-(2-chloroethyl)carbamate] 17-(dihydrogen phosphate), disodium salt. It is also referred to as estradiol 3-bis(2-chloroethyl)carbamate 17-(dihydrogen phosphate), disodium salt.

Estramustine phosphate sodium has an empiric formula of $C_{23}H_{30}Cl_2NNa_2O_6P$ and a calculated molecular weight of 582.4.

CLINICAL PHARMACOLOGY

Estramustine phosphate is a molecule combining estradiol and nornitrogen mustard by a carbamate link. The molecule is phosphorylated to make it water soluble.

Estramustine phosphate taken orally is readily dephosphorylated during absorption, and the major metabolites in plasma are estramustine, the estrone analog, estradiol and estrone.

Prolonged treatment with estramustine phosphate produces elevated total plasma concentrations of estradiol that fall within ranges similar to the elevated estradiol levels found in prostatic cancer patients given conventional estradiol therapy. Estrogenic effects, as demonstrated by changes in circulating levels of steroids and pituitary hormones, are similar in patients treated with either estramustine phosphate or conventional estradiol.

The metabolic urinary patterns of the estradiol moiety of estramustine phosphate and estradiol itself are very similar, although the metabolites derived from estramustine phosphate are excreted at a slower rate.

INDICATIONS AND USAGE

Emcyt is indicated in the palliative treatment of patients with metastatic and/or progressive carcinoma of the prostate.

CONTRAINDICATIONS

Emcyt should not be used in patients with any of the following conditions:

1) Known hypersensitivity to either estradiol or to nitrogen mustard.
2) Active thrombophlebitis or thromboembolic disorders, except in those cases where the actual tumor mass is the cause of the thromboembolic phenomenon and the physician feels the benefits of therapy may outweigh the risks.

WARNINGS

It has been shown that there is an increased risk of thrombosis, including nonfatal myocardial infarction, in men receiving estrogens for prostatic cancer. Emcyt should be used with caution in patients with a history of thrombophlebitis, thrombosis or thromboembolic disorders, especially if they were associated with estrogen therapy. Caution should also be used in patients with cerebral vascular or coronary artery disease.

Glucose Tolerance—Because glucose tolerance may be decreased, diabetic patients should be carefully observed while receiving Emcyt.

Elevated Blood Pressure—Because hypertension may occur, blood pressure should be monitored periodically.

PRECAUTIONS

General: Fluid Retention—Exacerbation of preexisting or incipient peripheral edema or congestive heart disease has been seen in some patients receiving Emcyt therapy. Other conditions which might be influenced by fluid retention, such as epilepsy, migraine or renal dysfunction, require careful observation.

Emcyt may be poorly metabolized in patients with impaired liver function and should be administered with caution in such patients.

Because Emcyt may influence the metabolism of calcium and phosphorus, it should be used with caution in patients with metabolic bone diseases that are associated with hypercalcemia or in patients with renal insufficiency.

Information for the Patient: Because of the possibility of mutagenic effects, patients should be advised to use contraceptive measures.

Laboratory Tests: Certain endocrine and liver function tests may be affected by estrogen-containing drugs. Abnormalities of hepatic enzymes and of bilirubin have occurred in patients receiving Emcyt, but have seldom been severe enough to require cessation of therapy. Such tests should be done at appropriate intervals during therapy and repeated after the drug has been withdrawn for two months.

Food/Drug Interaction: Limited data now indicate that milk may impair the absorption of Emcyt. Therefore, consideration should be given to taking Emcyt at least one hour before or two hours after ingestion of milk or milk products.

Carcinogenesis, Mutagenesis, Impairment of Fertility: Long-term continuous administration of estrogens in certain animal species increases the frequency of carcinomas of the breast and liver. Compounds structurally similar to Emcyt are carcinogenic in mice. Carcinogenic studies of Emcyt have not been conducted in man. Although testing by the Ames method failed to demonstrate mutagenicity for estramustine phosphate sodium, it is known that both estradiol and nitrogen mustard are mutagenic. For this reason and because some patients who had been impotent while on estrogen therapy have regained potency while taking Emcyt, the patient should be advised to use contraceptive measures.

ADVERSE REACTIONS

In a randomized, double-blind trial comparing therapy with Emcyt in 93 patients (11.5 to 15.9 mg/kg/day) or diethylstilbestrol (DES) in 93 patients (3.0 mg/day), the following adverse effects were reported:

	EMCYT n=93	DES n=93
CARDIOVASCULAR–RESPIRATORY		
Cardiac Arrest	0	2
Cerebrovascular Accident	2	0
Myocardial Infarction	3	1
Thrombophlebitis	3	7
Pulmonary Emboli	2	5
Congestive Heart Failure	3	2
Edema	19	17
Dyspnea	11	3
Leg Cramps	8	11
Upper Respiratory Discharge	1	1
Hoarseness	1	0
GASTROINTESTINAL		
Nausea	15	8
Diarrhea	12	11
Minor Gastrointestinal Upset	11	6
Anorexia	4	3
Flatulence	2	0
Vomiting	1	1
Gastrointestinal Bleeding	1	0
Burning Throat	1	0
Thirst	1	0
INTEGUMENTARY		
Rash	1	4
Pruritus	2	2
Dry Skin	2	0
Pigment Changes	0	3
Easy Bruising	3	0
Flushing	1	0
Night Sweats	0	1
Fingertip—Peeling Skin	1	0
Thinning Hair	1	1
BREAST CHANGES		
Tenderness	66	64
Enlargement		
Mild	60	54
Moderate	10	16
Marked	0	5
MISCELLANEOUS		
Lethargy Alone	4	3
Depression	0	2
Emotional Lability	2	0
Insomnia	3	0
Headache	1	1
Anxiety	1	0
Chest Pain	1	1
Hot Flashes	0	1
Pain in Eyes	0	1
Tearing of Eyes	1	1
Tinnitus	0	1
LABORATORY ABNORMALITIES		
Hematologic		
Leukopenia	4	2
Thrombopenia	1	2
Hepatic		
Bilirubin Alone	1	5
Bilirubin and LDH	0	1
Bilirubin and SGOT	2	1
Bilirubin, LDH and SGOT	2	0
LDH and/or SGOT	31	28
Miscellaneous		
Hypercalcemia—Transient	0	1

OVERDOSAGE

Although there has been no experience with overdosage to date, it is reasonable to expect that such episodes may produce pronounced manifestations of the known adverse reactions. In the event of overdosage, the gastric contents should be evacuated by gastric lavage and symptomatic therapy should be initiated. Hematologic and hepatic parameters should be monitored for at least six weeks after overdosage of Emcyt.

DOSAGE AND ADMINISTRATION

The recommended daily dose is 14 mg per kg of body weight (*i.e.*, one 140 mg capsule for each 10 kg or 22 lb of body weight), given in 3 or 4 divided doses. Most patients in studies in the United States have been treated at a dosage range of 10 to 16 mg per kg per day.

Patients should be treated for 30 to 90 days before the physician determines the possible benefits of continued therapy. Therapy should be continued as long as the favorable response lasts. Some patients have been maintained on therapy for more than three years at doses ranging from 10 to 16 mg per kg of body weight per day.

HOW SUPPLIED

White opaque capsules, each containing estramustine phosphate sodium equivalent to 140 mg estramustine phosphate—bottles of 100 (NDC 0004-0132-02).

Note: Emcyt should be stored in the refrigerator at 36° to 46°F (2° to 8°C).

Shown in Product Identification Section, page 424

FANSIDAR® ℞

[*fan 'sid-ar*]

(sulfadoxine and pyrimethamine/Roche)

TABLETS

The following text is complete prescribing information based on official labeling in effect June 1, 1986.

WARNING: FATALITIES ASSOCIATED WITH THE ADMINISTRATION OF FANSIDAR HAVE OCCURRED DUE TO SEVERE REACTIONS, INCLUDING STEVENS-JOHNSON SYNDROME AND TOXIC EPIDERMAL NECROLYSIS. FANSIDAR PROPHYLAXIS SHOULD BE DISCONTINUED AT THE FIRST APPEARANCE OF SKIN RASH, IF A SIGNIFICANT REDUCTION IN THE COUNT OF ANY FORMED BLOOD ELEMENTS IS NOTED, OR UPON THE OCCURRENCE OF ACTIVE BACTERIAL OR FUNGAL INFECTIONS.

DESCRIPTION

Fansidar is an antimalarial agent, each tablet containing 500 mg N^1-(5,6-dimethoxy-4-pyrimidinyl) sulfanilamide (sulfadoxine) and 25 mg 2,4-diamino-5-(p-chlorophenyl)-6-ethylpyrimidine (pyrimethamine). Each tablet also contains corn starch, gelatin, lactose, magnesium stearate and talc.

CLINICAL PHARMACOLOGY

Fansidar is an antimalarial agent which acts by reciprocal potentiation of its two components, achieved by a sequential blockade of two enzymes involved in the biosynthesis of folinic acid within the parasites. Fansidar is effective against certain strains of *Plasmodium falciparum* that are resistant to chloroquine.

Both the sulfadoxine and the pyrimethamine of Fansidar are absorbed orally and are excreted mainly by the kidney. Following a single tablet administration, sulfadoxine peak plasma concentrations of 51 to 76 mcg/ml were achieved in 2.5 to 6 hours and the pyrimethamine peak plasma concentrations of 0.13 to 0.4 mcg/ml were achieved in 1.5 to 8 hours. The apparent half-life of elimination of sulfadoxine ranged from 100 to 231 hours with a mean of 169 hours, whereas pyrimethamine half-lives ranged from 54 to 148 hours with a mean of 111 hours. Both drugs appear in breast milk of nursing mothers.

INDICATIONS AND USAGE

Fansidar is indicated for the treatment of *P. falciparum* malaria for those patients in whom chloroquine resistance is suspected. Malaria prophylaxis with Fansidar is indicated for travelers to areas where chloroquine-resistant *P. falciparum* malaria is endemic. However, strains of *P. falciparum* may be encountered which have developed resistance to Fansidar.

CONTRAINDICATIONS

Prophylactic (repeated) use of Fansidar is contraindicated in patients with severe renal insufficiency, marked liver parenchymal damage or blood dyscrasias. Hypersensitivity to pyrimethamine or sulfonamides. Patients with documented megaloblastic anemia due to folate deficiency. Infants less than two months of age. Pregnancy at term and during the nursing period because sulfonamides pass the placenta and are excreted in the milk and may cause kernicterus.

WARNINGS

FATALITIES ASSOCIATED WITH THE ADMINISTRATION OF FANSIDAR HAVE OCCURRED DUE TO SEVERE REACTIONS, INCLUDING STEVENS-JOHNSON SYNDROME AND TOXIC EPIDERMAL NECROLYSIS. FANSIDAR PROPHYLAXIS SHOULD BE DISCONTINUED AT THE FIRST APPEARANCE OF SKIN RASH, IF A SIGNIFICANT REDUCTION IN THE COUNT OF ANY FORMED BLOOD ELEMENTS IS NOTED, OR UPON THE OCCURRENCE OF ACTIVE BACTERIAL OR FUNGAL INFECTIONS.

Fatalities associated with the administration of sulfonamides, although rare, have occurred due to severe reactions, including fulminant hepatic necrosis, agranulocytosis, aplastic anemia and other blood dyscrasias. Fansidar prophylactic regimen has been reported to cause leukopenia during a treatment of two months or longer. This leukopenia is generally mild and reversible.

PRECAUTIONS

1. *General:* Fansidar should be given with caution to patients with impaired renal or hepatic function, to those with possible folate deficiency and to those with severe allergy or bronchial asthma. As with some sulfonamide drugs, in glucose-6-phosphate dehydrogenase-deficient individuals, hemolysis may occur. Urinalysis with microscopic examination and renal function tests should be performed during therapy of those patients who have impaired renal function.

2. *Information for the patient:* Patients should be warned that at the first appearance of a skin rash, they should stop use of Fansidar and seek medical attention immediately. Adequate fluid intake must be maintained in order to prevent crystalluria and stone formation.

Patients should also be warned that the appearance of sore throat, fever, pallor, purpura, jaundice or glossitis may be early indications of serious disorders which require prophylactic treatment to be stopped and medical treatment to be sought.

Females should be cautioned against becoming pregnant and should not breast feed their infants during Fansidar therapy or prophylactic treatment.

Patients should be warned to keep Fansidar out of reach of children.

3. *Laboratory tests:* Periodic blood counts and analysis of urine for crystalluria are desirable during prolonged prophylaxis.

4. *Drug interactions:* There have been reports which may indicate an increase in incidence and severity of adverse reactions when chloroquine is used with Fansidar as compared to the use of Fansidar alone. Fansidar is compatible with quinine and with antibiotics. However, antifolic drugs such as sulfonamides or trimethoprim-sulfamethoxazole combinations should not be used while the patient is receiving Fansidar for antimalarial prophylaxis. Fansidar has not been reported to interfere with antidiabetic agents.

If signs of folic acid deficiency develop, Fansidar should be discontinued. Folinic acid (leucovorin) may be administered in doses of 5 mg to 15 mg intramuscularly daily, for 3 days or longer, for depressed platelet or white blood cell counts in patients with drug-induced folic acid deficiency when recovery is too slow.

5. *Carcinogenesis, mutagenesis, impairment of fertility:* Pyrimethamine was not found carcinogenic in female mice or in male and female rats. The carcinogenic potential of pyrimethamine in male mice could not be assessed from the study because of markedly reduced life-span. Pyrimethamine was found to be mutagenic in laboratory animals and also in human bone marrow following 3 or 4 consecutive daily doses totaling 200 mg to 300 mg. Pyrimethamine was not found mutagenic in the Ames test. Testicular changes have been observed in rats treated with 105 mg/kg/day of Fansidar and with 15 mg/kg/day of pyrimethamine alone. Fertility of male rats and the ability of male or female rats to mate were not adversely affected at dosages of up to 210 mg/kg/day of Fansidar. The pregnancy rate of female rats was not affected following their treatment with 10.5 mg/kg/day, but was significantly reduced at dosages of 31.5 mg/kg/day or higher, a dosage approximately 30 times the weekly human prophylactic dose or higher.

6. *Pregnancy:* Teratogenic effects: Pregnancy Category C. Fansidar has been shown to be teratogenic in rats when given in weekly doses approximately 12 times the weekly human prophylactic dose. Teratology studies with pyrimethamine plus sulfadoxine (1:20) in rats showed the minimum oral teratogenic dose to be approximately 0.9 mg/kg pyrimethamine plus 18 mg/kg sulfadoxine. In rabbits, no teratogenic effects were noted at oral doses as high as 20 mg/kg pyrimethamine plus 400 mg/kg sulfadoxine.

There are no adequate and well-controlled studies in pregnant women. However, due to the teratogenic effect shown in animals and because pyrimethamine plus sulfadoxine may interfere with folic acid metabolism, Fansidar therapy should be used during pregnancy only if the potential benefit justifies the potential risk to the fetus. Women of childbearing potential who are traveling to areas where malaria is endemic should be warned against becoming pregnant.

Nonteratogenic effects: See "CONTRAINDICATIONS" section.

7. *Nursing mothers:* See "CONTRAINDICATIONS" section.

8. *Pediatric use:* Fansidar should not be given to infants less than two months of age because of inadequate development of the glucuronide-forming enzyme system.

ADVERSE REACTIONS

For completeness, all major reactions to sulfonamides and to pyrimethamine are included below, even though they may not have been reported with Fansidar. See "WARNINGS" and "PRECAUTIONS" (Information for the Patient) sections.

Blood dyscrasias: Agranulocytosis, aplastic anemia, megaloblastic anemia, thrombopenia, leukopenia, hemolytic anemia, purpura, hypoprothrombinemia and methemoglobinemia.

Allergic reactions: Erythema multiforme, Stevens-Johnson syndrome, generalized skin eruptions, toxic epidermal necrolysis, urticaria, serum sickness, pruritus, exfoliative dermatitis, anaphylactoid reactions, periorbital edema, conjunctival and scleral injection, photosensitization, arthralgia and allergic myocarditis.

Gastrointestinal reactions: Glossitis, stomatitis, nausea, emesis, abdominal pains, hepatitis, hepatocellular necrosis, diarrhea and pancreatitis.

C.N.S. reactions: Headache, peripheral neuritis, mental depression, convulsions, ataxia, hallucinations, tinnitus, vertigo, insomnia, apathy, fatigue, muscle weakness and nervousness.

Miscellaneous reactions: Drug fever, chills, and toxic nephrosis with oliguria and anuria. Periarteritis nodosa and L. E. phenomenon have occurred.

The sulfonamides bear certain chemical similarities to some goitrogens, diuretics (acetazolamide and the thiazides) and oral hypoglycemic agents. Diuresis and hypoglycemia have occurred rarely in patients receiving sulfonamides. Cross-sensitivity may exist with these agents. Rats appear to be especially susceptible to the goitrogenic effects of sulfonamides, and long-term administration has produced thyroid malignancies in the species.

OVERDOSAGE

Acute intoxication may be manifested by anorexia, vomiting and central nervous system stimulation (including convulsions), followed by megaloblastic anemia, leukopenia, thrombocytopenia, glossitis and crystalluria. In acute intoxication, emesis and gastric lavage followed by purges may be of benefit. The patient should be adequately hydrated to prevent renal damage. The renal and hematopoietic systems should be monitored for at least one month after an overdosage. If the patient is having convulsions, the use of a parenteral barbiturate is indicated. For depressed platelet or white blood cell counts, folinic acid (leucovorin) should be administered in a dosage of 5 mg to 15 mg intramuscularly daily for 3 days or longer.

DOSAGE AND ADMINISTRATION

(See Indications and Usage Section):

(a) *Treatment of acute attack of malaria*

A single dose of the following number of Fansidar Tablets is used in sequence with quinine or alone:

Adults	2 to 3 tablets
9 to 14 years	2 tablets
4 to 8 years	1 tablet
Under 4 years	½ tablet

(b) *Malaria prophylaxis*

The first dose of Fansidar should be taken one or two days before departure to an endemic area; administration should be continued during the stay and for four to six weeks after return.

	Once Weekly	Once Every Two Weeks
Adults	1 tablet	2 tablets
9 to 14 years	¾ tablet	1½ tablets
4 to 8 years	½ tablet	1 tablet
Under 4 years	¼ tablet	½ tablet

HOW SUPPLIED

Scored tablets, containing 500 mg sulfadoxine and 25 mg pyrimethamine—boxes of 25 (NDC-0004-0161-03).

Shown in Product Identification Section, page 424

Continued on next page

Roche Labs.—Cont.

FLUOROURACIL ℞
[flu″ro-u′ra-sil]
INJECTION

The following text is complete prescribing information based on official labeling in effect June 1, 1986.

> WARNING
> It is recommended that FLUOROURACIL be given only by or under the supervision of a qualified physician who is experienced in cancer chemotherapy and who is well versed in the use of potent antimetabolites. Because of the possibility of severe toxic reactions, it is recommended that patients be hospitalized at least during the initial course of therapy.
> These instructions should be thoroughly reviewed before administration of Fluorouracil.

DESCRIPTION
FLUOROURACIL INJECTION/Roche, an antineoplastic antimetabolite, is a sterile nonpyrogenic injectable solution available in 10-ml ampuls for intravenous administration. Each 10-ml ampul contains 500 mg of fluorouracil; pH is adjusted to approximately 9.2 with sodium hydroxide.
Fluorouracil is a fluorinated pyrimidine belonging to the category of antimetabolites. Fluorouracil resembles the natural uracil molecule in structure, except that a hydrogen atom has been replaced by a fluorine atom in the 5 position.

ACTIONS
There is evidence that the metabolism of fluorouracil in the anabolic pathway blocks the methylation reaction of deoxyuridylic acid to thymidylic acid. In this fashion fluorouracil interferes with the synthesis of deoxyribonucleic acid (DNA) and to a lesser extent inhibits the formation of ribonucleic acid (RNA). Since DNA and RNA are essential for cell division and growth, the effect of fluorouracil may be to create a thymine deficiency which provokes unbalanced growth and death of the cell. The effects of DNA and RNA deprivation are most marked on those cells which grow more rapidly and which take up fluorouracil at a more rapid pace. The catabolic metabolism of fluorouracil results in degradative products (e.g., CO_2, urea, α-fluoro-β-alanine) which are inactive.
Following an intravenous injection, no intact drug can be detected in the plasma after three hours. Approximately 15 percent is excreted intact in the urine in six hours, of which over 90 percent is excreted in the first hour. Of the injected intravenous dose 60 to 80 percent is excreted as respiratory CO_2 in 8 to 12 hours.

INDICATIONS
Fluorouracil is effective in the palliative management of carcinoma of the colon, rectum, breast, stomach and pancreas in patients who are considered incurable by surgery or other means.

CONTRAINDICATIONS
Fluorouracil therapy is contraindicated for patients in a poor nutritional state, those with depressed bone marrow function, those with potentially serious infections or those with known hypersensitivity to Fluorouracil.

WARNINGS
THE DAILY DOSE OF FLUOROURACIL IS NOT TO EXCEED 800 MG. IT IS RECOMMENDED THAT PATIENTS BE HOSPITALIZED DURING THEIR FIRST COURSE OF TREATMENT.
Fluorouracil should be used with extreme caution in poor risk patients with a history of high-dose pelvic irradiation, previous use of alkylating agents or who have a widespread involvement of bone marrow by metastatic tumors or impaired hepatic or renal function. The drug is not intended as an adjuvant to surgery. Although severe toxicity is more likely in poor risk patients, fatalities may be encountered occasionally even in patients in relatively good condition.
Usage in Pregnancy: Safe use of Fluorouracil has not been established with respect to adverse effects on fetal development. Therefore, this drug should not be used during pregnancy, particularly in the first trimester, unless in the judgment of the physician the potential benefits to the patient outweigh the hazards.
Because the risk of mutagenesis has not been evaluated, such possible effects on males and females must be considered.
Combination Therapy: Any form of therapy which adds to the stress of the patient, interferes with nutrition or depresses bone marrow function will increase the toxicity of Fluorouracil.

PRECAUTIONS
Fluorouracil is a highly toxic drug with a narrow margin of safety. Therefore, patients should be carefully supervised, since therapeutic response is unlikely to occur without some evidence of toxicity. Patients should be informed of expected toxic effects, particularly oral manifestations. White blood counts with differential are recommended before each dose. Severe hematological toxicity, gastrointestinal hemorrhage and even death may result from the use of Fluorouracil despite meticulous selection of patients and careful adjustment of dosage.
Therapy is to be discontinued promptly whenever one of the following signs of toxicity appears:
Stomatitis or *esophagopharyngitis,* At the first visible sign.
Leukopenia (WBC under 3500), or a *rapidly falling white blood count.*
Vomiting, Intractable.
Diarrhea, Frequent bowel movements or watery stools.
Gastrointestinal ulceration and bleeding.
Thrombocytopenia, Platelets under 100,000.
Hemorrhage from any site.

ADVERSE REACTIONS
Stomatitis and esophagopharyngitis (which may lead to sloughing and ulceration), diarrhea, anorexia, nausea and emesis are commonly seen during therapy. Allergic reactions including anaphylaxis, bronchospasm, urticaria and pruritus have also been reported.
Leukopenia usually follows every course of adequate therapy with Fluorouracil. The lowest white blood cell counts are commonly observed between the 9th and 14th days after the first course of treatment, although uncommonly the maximal depression may be delayed for as long as 20 days. By the 30th day the count has usually returned to the normal range.
Pancytopenia, agranulocytosis, anemia and thrombocytopenia have also been reported.
Alopecia and dermatitis may be seen in a substantial number of cases. Patients should be alerted to the possibility of alopecia as a result of therapy and should be informed that it is a transient effect. The dermatitis most often seen is a pruritic maculopapular rash usually appearing on the extremities and less frequently on the trunk. It is generally reversible and usually responsive to symptomatic treatment. Dry skin and fissuring have also been noted. Photosensitivity, as manifested by erythema or increased pigmentation of the skin, has been observed on occasion. Also noted were photophobia, visual changes, lacrimation, lacimal duct stenosis, epistaxis, euphoria, disorientation, confusion, acute cerebellar syndrome (which may persist following discontinuation of treatment), thrombophlebitis and nail changes, including loss of nails. Myocardial ischemia has also been reported.

DOSAGE AND ADMINISTRATION
General Instructions: Administration of Fluorouracil Injection should be done only intravenously, using care to avoid extravasation. No dilution is required.
All dosages are based on the patient's actual weight. However, the estimated lean body mass (dry weight) is used if the patient is obese or if there has been a spurious weight gain due to edema, ascites or other forms of abnormal fluid retention.
It is recommended that prior to treatment each patient be carefully evaluated in order to estimate as accurately as possible the optimum initial dosage of Fluorouracil.
Dosage: Twelve mg/kg are given intravenously once daily for four successive days. The daily dose should not be more than 800 mg. *If no toxicity is observed,* 6 mg/kg are given on the 6th, 8th, 10th and 12th days unless toxicity occurs. No therapy is given on the 5th, 7th, 9th or 11th days. *Therapy is to be discontinued at the end of the 12th day, even if no toxicity has become apparent.* (See CONTRAINDICATIONS and WARNINGS.)
Poor risk patients or those who are not in an adequate nutritional state (see CONTRAINDICATIONS and WARNINGS) should receive 6 mg/kg/day for three days. *If no toxicity is observed,* 3 mg/kg may be given on the 5th, 7th and 9th days *unless toxicity occurs.* No therapy is given on the 4th, 6th or 8th days. The daily dose should not exceed 400 mg.
A sequence of injections on either schedule constitutes a "course of therapy."
Maintenance Therapy: In instances where toxicity has not been a problem, it is recommended that therapy be continued using either of the following schedules:

1. Repeat dosage of first course every 30 days after the last day of the previous course of treatment.
2. When toxic signs resulting from the initial course of therapy have subsided, administer a maintenance dosage of 10 to 15 mg/kg/week as a single dose. Do not exceed 1 Gm per week.

The amount of the drug to be used should take into account the patient's reaction to the previous course and should be adjusted accordingly. Some patients have received from 9 to 45 courses of treatment during periods which ranged from 12 to 60 months.

HOW SUPPLIED
10-ml ampuls (for intravenous use) containing 500 mg fluorouracil in a colorless to faint yellow aqueous solution, with pH adjusted to approximately 9.2 with sodium hydroxide. Boxes of 10.
Note: Although Fluorouracil solution may discolor slightly during storage, the potency and safety are not adversely affected.
Store at room temperature (59° to 86°F). Protect from light. If a precipitate occurs due to exposure to low temperatures, resolubilize by heating to 140°F with vigorous shaking; allow to cool to body temperature before using.

FUDR ℞
[ef-u-dee-are]
(floxuridine/Roche)

The following text is complete prescribing information based on official labeling in effect June 1, 1986.

FOR INTRA-ARTERIAL INFUSION ONLY

> **WARNING**
> **It is recommended that FUDR be given only by or under the supervision of a qualified physician who is experienced in cancer chemotherapy and intra-arterial drug therapy.**
> **Because of the possibility of severe toxic reactions, all patients should be hospitalized for initiation of treatment.**

DESCRIPTION
Floxuridine is a fluorinated pyrimidine belonging to the category of antimetabolites. It is a white to off-white odorless solid, soluble in alcohol and freely soluble in water. The 2% aqueous solution has a pH of 4.0 to 5.5. Chemically, floxuridine is 2′-deoxy-5-fluorouridine with a molecular weight of 246.19.

ACTIONS
When FUDR is given by intra-arterial injection it is apparently rapidly catabolized to 5-fluorouracil. Thus, rapid injection of FUDR produces the same toxic and antimetabolic effects as does 5-fluorouracil. The primary effect is to interfere with the synthesis of deoxyribonucleic acid (DNA) and to a lesser extent inhibit the formation of ribonucleic acid (RNA). However, when FUDR is given by continuous intra-arterial infusion its direct anabolism to FUDR-monophosphate is enhanced, thus increasing the inhibition of DNA.

INDICATIONS
FUDR is effective in the palliative management of gastrointestinal adenocarcinoma metastatic to the liver, when given by continuous regional intra-arterial infusion in carefully selected patients who are considered incurable by surgery or other means. Patients with known disease extending beyond an area capable of infusion via a single artery should, except in unusual circumstances, be considered for systemic therapy with other chemotherapeutic agents.

CONTRAINDICATIONS
FUDR therapy is contraindicated for patients in a poor nutritional state, those with depressed bone marrow function, or those with potentially serious infections.

WARNINGS
IT IS IMPERATIVE THAT ALL PATIENTS BE HOSPITALIZED FOR INITIATION OF TREATMENT.
FUDR should be used with extreme caution in poor risk patients with impaired hepatic or renal function or a history of high-dose pelvic irradiation or previous use of alkylating agents. The drug is not intended as an adjuvant to surgery.
Usage in Pregnancy: Safe use of FUDR has not been established with respect to adverse effects on fetal development. Therefore, this drug should not be used during pregnancy, particularly in the first trimester, unless in the judgment of the physician the potential benefits to the patient outweigh the hazards.
Because teratogenicity and mutagenicity have been demonstrated in animals, such possible effects on men and women must be considered.
Combination Therapy: Any form of therapy which adds to the stress of the patient, interferes with nutrition, or depresses bone marrow function will increase the toxicity of FUDR.
Therapy is to be discontinued promptly whenever one of the following signs of toxicity appears:
Stomatitis or esophagopharyngitis, At the first visible sign.
Leukopenia (WBC under 3500), or a rapidly falling white blood count.
Vomiting, Intractable.
Diarrhea, Frequent bowel movements or watery stools.
Gastrointestinal ulceration and bleeding.
Thrombocytopenia, Platelets under 100,000.
Hemorrhage from any site.

PRECAUTIONS
FUDR is potentially a highly toxic drug with a narrow margin of safety. Therefore, patients should be carefully supervised since therapeutic response is unlikely to occur without some evidence of toxicity. Patients should be informed of expected toxic effects, particularly oral manifestations. Careful monitoring of the white blood count and platelet

count is recommended. Severe hematological toxicity, gastrointestinal hemorrhage and even death may result from the use of FUDR despite meticulous selection of patients and careful adjustment of dosage. Although severe toxicity is more likely in poor risk patients, fatalities may be encountered occasionally even in patients in relatively good condition.

ADVERSE REACTIONS

The adverse reactions to the arterial infusion of FUDR are generally related to the drug-infused area and can be grouped under the following categories: functional gastrointestinal, mucosal gastrointestinal, hematologic, dermatologic, miscellaneous clinical reactions, laboratory abnormalities and procedural complications of regional arterial infusion.

The more common adverse reactions are nausea, vomiting, diarrhea, enteritis, stomatitis and localized erythema. The more common laboratory abnormalities are anemia, leukopenia, and elevations of alkaline phosphatase, serum transaminase, serum bilirubin and lactic dehydrogenase.

Other adverse reactions are:

Functional gastrointestinal: anorexia, cramps and pain.

Mucosal gastrointestinal: duodenal ulcer, duodenitis, gastritis, gastroenteritis, glossitis and pharyngitis; possible intra- and extrahepatic biliary sclerosis, as well as acalculus cholecystitis.

Dermatological: alopecia, dermatitis, nonspecific skin toxicity and rash.

Other clinical reactions: fever, lethargy, malaise, and weakness.

Laboratory abnormalities: BSP, prothrombin, total proteins, sedimentation rate and thrombopenia.

Procedural complications of regional arterial infusion: arterial aneurysm, arterial ischemia, arterial thrombosis, bleeding at catheter site, catheter blocked, displaced or leaking, embolism, fibromyositis, infection at catheter site, abscesses and thrombophlebitis.

DOSAGE AND ADMINISTRATION

The recommended therapeutic dose schedule of FUDR by continuous arterial infusion is 0.1 to 0.6 mg/kg/day. The higher dose ranges (0.4 to 0.6 mg) are usually employed for hepatic artery infusion because the liver metabolizes the drug, thus reducing the potential for systemic toxicity. Therapy can be given until adverse reactions appear. When these side effects have subsided, therapy may be resumed. The patient should be maintained on therapy as long as response to FUDR continues. The administration of FUDR is best achieved with the use of an appropriate pump to overcome pressure in large arteries and to ensure a uniform rate of infusion.

HOW SUPPLIED

500 mg FUDR (floxuridine/Roche) sterile powder, in a 5-ml vial. This is reconstituted with 5 ml sterile water. Reconstituted vials should be stored under refrigeration (36° to 46°F.) for not more than two weeks.

CLINICAL STUDIES

In 349 evaluable patients treated with continuous arterial infusion of FUDR, 144 obtained significant objective response associated with clinical benefit for at least one month, and an additional 14 patients had objective and subjective benefits for at least one year.

GANTANOL® ℞

[gan'tan-ol]

sulfamethoxazole/Roche

TABLETS • SUSPENSION • DS (double strength) TABLETS

The following text is complete prescribing information based on official labeling in effect July 1, 1986.

DESCRIPTION

Gantanol® (brand of sulfamethoxazole/Roche) is an intermediate-dosage antibacterial sulfonamide available in tablets, DS (double strength) tablets and suspension. Each tablet contains 0.5 Gm sulfamethoxazole plus corn starch, polyvinyl acetate, polyvinyl alcohol, magnesium stearate, FD&C Blue No. 1 Lake, FD&C Yellow No. 6 Lake and D&C Yellow No. 10 Lake. Each DS tablet contains 1 Gm sulfamethoxazole plus magnesium stearate, pregelatinized starch, sodium starch glycolate and FD&C Yellow No. 6 Lake. Each teaspoonful (5 mL) of the suspension contains 0.5 Gm sulfamethoxazole in a vehicle containing carboxyvinyl polymer, citric acid, edetate disodium, methylcellulose, saccharin, saccharin sodium, simethicone, sodium benzoate, sodium citrate, sodium hydroxide, sodium lauryl sulfate, sorbitol, sucrose, FD&C Red. No. 40, flavors and water.

Sulfamethoxazole is N^1-(5-methyl-3-isoxazolyl) sulfanilamide. It is an almost white, odorless, tasteless compound with a molecular weight of 253.28.

CLINICAL PHARMACOLOGY

Sulfamethoxazole is rapidly absorbed following oral administration. It exists in the blood as unbound, protein-bound, metabolized and conjugated forms. The metabolism of sulfamethoxazole occurs predominately by N_4-acetylation, although the glucuronide conjugate has been identified. The free form is considered to be the therapeutically active form. Approximately 70% of sulfamethoxazole is bound to plasma proteins; of the unbound portion, 80% to 90% is in the nonacetylated form.

Following a single 1-Gm oral dose in 12 volunteer male subjects, the mean peak plasma concentration of 38 mcg/mL of intact sulfamethoxazole was achieved by 2 hours. The mean half-life of sulfamethoxazole is approximately 10 hours. However, patients with severely impaired renal function, as shown by a creatinine clearance of less than 30 mL/minute, exhibit an increase of the half-life of sulfamethoxazole, requiring dosage regimen adjustment.

Sulfamethoxazole is excreted primarily by the kidneys chiefly through glomerular filtration but also through tubular secretion. Urine concentrations of sulfamethoxazole are considerably higher than are the concentrations in blood. Eighty percent to 100 percent of the dose is excreted in the urine as total sulfamethoxazole, of which 30% is intact drug with the remaining as the N_4-acetylated metabolite.

Sulfamethoxazole diffuses into cerebrospinal fluid, with peak concentrations occurring at 8 hours and reaching approximately 14% of simultaneous plasma concentrations. The drug has also been shown to distribute to aqueous humor, vaginal fluid and middle ear fluid; it also passes the placental barrier and is excreted in breast milk.

Microbiology: The systemic sulfonamides are bacteriostatic agents and the spectrum of activity is similar for all. Sulfonamides inhibit bacterial synthesis of dihydrofolic acid by competing with *para*-aminobenzoic acid (PABA). Resistant strains are capable of utilizing folic acid precursors or preformed folic acid.

INDICATIONS AND USAGE

Acute, recurrent or chronic urinary tract infections (primarily pyelonephritis, pyelitis and cystitis) due to susceptible organisms (usually *E. coli, Klebsiella-Enterbacter*, staphylococcus, *Proteus mirabilis* and, less frequently, *Proteus vulgaris*) in the absence of obstructive uropathy or foreign bodies.

Meningococcal meningitis prophylaxis when sulfonamide-sensitive group A strains are known to prevail in family groups or larger closed populations. (The prophylactic usefulness of sulfonamides when group B or C infections are prevalent has not been proven and in closed population groups may be harmful.)

Acute otitis media due to *Haemophilus influenzae* when used concomitantly with adequate doses of penicillin.

Trachoma, Inclusion conjunctivitis, Nocardiosis, Chancroid.

Toxoplasmosis as adjunctive therapy with pyrimethamine.

Malaria due to chloroquine-resistant strains of *Plasmodium falciparum*, when used as adjunctive therapy.

Important note: In vitro sulfonamide susceptibility tests are not always reliable. The test must be carefully coordinated with bacteriologic and clinical response. When the patient is already taking sulfonamides, follow-up cultures should have aminobenzoic acid added to the culture media.

Currently, the increasing frequency of resistant organisms is a limitation of the usefulness of antibacterial agents including the sulfonamides, especially in the treatment of chronic and recurrent urinary tract infections.

Wide variation in blood concentrations may result with identical doses. Blood concentrations should be measured in patients receiving sulfonamides for serious infections. Free sulfonamide blood concentrations of 5 to 15 mg/100 mL may be considered therapeutically effective for most infections, with blood concentrations of 12 to 15 mg/100 mL optimal for serious infections; 20 mg/100 mL should be the maximum total sulfonamide concentration, since adverse reactions occur more frequently above this concentration.

CONTRAINDICATIONS

Hypersensitivity to sulfonamides. Infants less than 2 months of age (except in the treatment of congenital toxoplasmosis as adjunctive therapy with pyrimethamine). Pregnancy at term and during the nursing period because sulfonamides pass the placenta and are excreted in the milk and may cause kernicterus.

WARNINGS

The sulfonamides should not be used for the treatment of group A beta-hemolytic streptococcal infections. In an established infection, they will not eradicate the streptococcus, and therefore will not prevent sequelae such as rheumatic fever and glomerulonephritis.

Deaths associated with the administration of sulfonamides have been reported from hypersensitivity reactions, hepatocellular necrosis, agranulocytosis, aplastic anemia and other blood dyscrasias.

The presence of clinical signs such as sore throat, fever, pallor, purpura or jaundice may be early indications of serious blood disorders.

PRECAUTIONS

General: Sulfonamides should be given with caution to patients with impaired renal or hepatic function and to those with severe allergy or bronchial asthma. In glucose-6-phosphate dehydrogenase-deficient individuals, hemolysis may occur. This reaction is frequently dose-related.

Information for patients: Patients should be instructed to maintain an adequate fluid intake in order to prevent crystalluria and stone formation.

Laboratory tests: Complete blood counts should be done frequently in patients receiving sulfonamides. If a significant reduction in the count of any formed blood element is noted, Gantanol should be discontinued. Urinalyses with careful microscopic examination and renal function tests should be performed during therapy, particularly for those patients with impaired renal function.

Drug interactions: In elderly patients concurrently receiving certain diuretics, primarily thiazides, an increased incidence of thrombopenia with purpura has been reported.

It has been reported that sulfamethoxazole may prolong the prothrombin time in patients who are receiving the anticoagulant warfarin. This interaction should be kept in mind when Gantanol is given to patients already on anticoagulant therapy, and the coagulation time should be reassessed.

Sulfamethoxazole may inhibit the hepatic metabolism of phenytoin. At a 1.6 Gm dose, sulfamethoxazole produced a slight but significant increase in the half-life of phenytoin but did not produce a corresponding decrease in the metabolic clearance rate. When administering these drugs concurrently, one should be alert for possible excessive phenytoin effect.

Sulfonamides can also displace methotrexate from plasma protein-binding sites, thus increasing free methotrexate concentrations.

The presence of sulfamethoxazole may interfere with the Jaffé alkaline picrate reaction assay for creatinine, resulting in overestimations of about 10% in the range of normal values.

Carcinogenesis, mutagenesis, impairment of fertility: Carcinogenesis: Sulfamethoxazole has not been adequately tested in animals to permit an evaluation of its carcinogenic potential.

Mutagenesis: Bacterial mutagenic studies have not been performed with sulfamethoxazole. No chromosomal damage was observed in human leukocytes cultured *in vitro* with sulfamethoxazole; the concentrations used exceeded blood levels of sulfamethoxazole following therapy with Gantanol.

Impairment of fertility: No adverse effects on fertility or general reproductive performance were observed in rats given sulfamethoxazole in oral dosages as high as 350 mg/kg/day.

Pregnancy: Teratogenic Effects: Pregnancy Category C. In rats, oral doses of 533 mg/kg of sulfamethoxazole produced teratologic effects manifested mainly as cleft palates. The highest dose which did not cause cleft palates in rats was 512 mg/kg of sulfamethoxazole. In rabbits, 150 to 350 mg/kg/day increased maternal mortality but had no deleterious effects on fetal development.

There are no adequate and well-controlled studies of Gantanol in pregnant women. Gantanol should be used during pregnancy only if the potential benefit justifies the potential risk to the fetus.

Nonteratogenic effects: See CONTRAINDICATIONS section.

Nursing mothers: See CONTRAINDICATIONS section.

Pediatric Use: Gantanol is not recommended in infants under 2 months of age, except in the treatment of congenital toxoplasmosis as adjunctive therapy with pyrimethamine. (See CONTRAINDICATIONS section.) At the present time there are insufficient clinical data on prolonged or recurrent therapy in chronic renal diseases of children under 6 years of age.

ADVERSE REACTIONS

Included in the listing that follows are adverse reactions that have not been reported with this specific drug; however, the pharmacologic similarities among the sulfonamides require that each of the reactions be considered with Gantanol administration.

Hematologic: Agranulocytosis, aplastic anemia, thrombocytopenia, leukopenia, hemolytic anemia, purpura, hypoprothrombinemia, methemoglobinemia, neutropenia, eosinophilia.

Allergic Reactions: Anaphylaxis, allergic myocarditis, serum sickness, conjunctival and scleral injection, generalized allergic reactions. In addition, periarteritis nodosa and systemic lupus erythematosus have been reported.

Dermatologic: Stevens-Johnson syndrome, epidermal necrolysis, erythema multiforme, exfoliative dermatitis, photosensitivity, pruritus, urticaria, rash, generalized skin eruptions.

Gastrointestinal: Hepatitis, hepatocellular necrosis, pseudomembranous enterocolitis, pancreatitis, stomatitis, glossitis, nausea, emesis, abdominal pain, diarrhea, anorexia.

Genitourinary: Creatinine elevation, toxic nephrosis with oliguria and anuria. The frequency of renal complications is considerably lower in patients receiving the more soluble sulfonamides.

Continued on next page

Roche Labs.—Cont.

Neurologic: Convulsions, peripheral neuritis, ataxia, vertigo, tinnitus, headache.
Psychiatric: Hallucinations, depression, apathy.
Endocrine: The sulfonamides bear certain chemical similarities to some goitrogens, diuretics (acetazolamide and the thiazides) and oral hypoglycemic agents. Cross-sensitivity may exist with these agents. Diuresis and hypoglycemia have occurred rarely in patients receiving sulfonamides.
Musculoskeletal: Arthralgia, myalgia.
Miscellaneous: Edema (including periorbital), pyrexia, chills, weakness, fatigue, insomnia.

OVERDOSAGE

Acute: The amount of a single dose of sulfamethoxazole that is either associated with symptoms of overdosage or is likely to be life-threatening has not been reported. Signs and symptoms of overdosage reported with sulfonamides include anorexia, colic, nausea, vomiting, dizziness, headache, drowsiness and unconsciousness. Pyrexia, hematuria and crystalluria may be noted. Blood dyscrasias and jaundice are potential late manifestations of overdosage.
General principles of treatment include the institution of gastric lavage or emesis; forcing oral fluids; and the administration of intravenous fluids if urine output is low and renal function is normal. The patient should be monitored with blood counts and appropriate blood chemistries, including electrolytes. If a significant blood dyscrasia or jaundice occurs, specific therapy should be instituted for these complications. Peritoneal dialysis is not effective and hemodialysis is only moderately effective in eliminating sulfamethoxazole.
Chronic: Use of sulfamethoxazole at high doses and/or for extended periods of time may cause bone marrow depression manifested as thrombocytopenia, leukopenia and/or megaloblastic anemia. If signs of bone marrow depression occur, the patient should be given leucovorin 3 to 6 mg intramuscularly daily for three days, or as required to restore normal hematopoiesis.
Animal Toxicity: The oral LD_{50} of sulfamethoxazole is 2300 mg/kg in mice, 3000 mg/kg in rats and >2000 mg/kg in rabbits.

DOSAGE AND ADMINISTRATION

Systemic sulfonamides are contraindicated in infants under 2 months of age, except in the treatment of congenital toxoplasmosis as adjunctive therapy with pyrimethamine.
The usual dosage schedules are as follows:

Children

Infants (2 Months or Older) and Children	Initial Dose (50–60 mg/kg)	Dose Morning and Evening Daily Thereafter (25–30 mg/kg)
20 lbs	1 tablet or 1 teas. (0.5 Gm)	½ tablet or ½ teasp. (0.25 Gm)
40 lbs	2 tablets or 2 teasp. (1 Gm)	1 tablet or 1 teasp. (0.5 Gm)
60 lbs	3 tablets or 3 teasp. (1.5 Gm)	1½ tablets or 1½ teasp. (0.75 Gm)
80 lbs	2 DS (double strength) tablets or 4 tablets or 4 teasp. (2 Gm)	1 DS (double strength) tablet or 2 tablets or 2 teasp. (1 Gm)

The maximum dose for children should not exceed 75 mg/kg/24 hours.

Adults		
Mild to Moderate Infections	2 DS (double strength) tablets or 4 tablets or 4 teasp. (2 Gm)	1 DS (double strength) tablet or 2 tablets or 2 teasp. (1 Gm)

Note: One teaspoonful equals 5 ml.

Severe Infections: 2 DS (double strength) tablets, or 4 tablets, or 4 teaspoonfuls (2 Gm) initially, followed by 1 DS (double strength) tablet, or 2 tablets, or 2 teaspoonfuls (1 Gm) three times daily thereafter.
Patients with impaired renal function (creatinine clearance below 20 to 30 mL/min) require decreased dosage adjustment.

HOW SUPPLIED

DS (double strength) Tablets (light orange, scored, capsule shaped), containing 1 Gm sulfamethoxazole—bottles of 100 (NDC 0004-0131-01). Imprint on tablets: GANTANOL-DS ROCHE.
Tablets (pale green, scored), containing 0.5 Gm sulfamethoxazole—bottles of 100 (NDC 0004-0010-01) and 500 (NDC 0004-0010-14); Tel-E-Dose® packages of 100 (NDC 0004-0010-49). Imprint on tablets: GANTANOL® ROCHE.
Suspension, 10%, containing 0.5 Gm sulfamethoxazole per teaspoonful (5 mL); cherry-flavored—bottles of 1 pint (473 mL) (NDC 0004-1002-28).

Shown in Product Identification Section, page 425

GANTRISIN® ℞
[gan 'tris-in]
(sulfisoxazole diolamine/Roche)
OPHTHALMIC SOLUTION
OPHTHALMIC OINTMENT

The following text is complete prescribing information based on official labeling in effect June 1, 1986.

DESCRIPTION

GANTRISIN Ophthalmic Ointment and Solution are sulfonamide preparations specifically for topical ophthalmic use. The solution is a sterile, isotonic preparation containing 4% (40 mg/ml) sulfisoxazole/Roche in the form of the diolamine salt and phenylmercuric nitrate 1:100,000 added as a preservative. It has a physiologic pH, and does not cause significant stinging or burning on application. The ointment is a sterile preparation containing 4% sulfisoxazole in the form of the diolamine salt compounded with white petrolatum, mineral oil and phenylmercuric nitrate 1:50,000 added as a preservative. Both dosage forms are stable at room temperature and do not require refrigeration.

ACTIONS

Sulfonamides exert a bacteriostatic effect against a wide range of gram-positive and gram-negative microorganisms by restricting, through competition with para-aminobenzoic acid, the synthesis of folic acid which bacteria require for growth.

INDICATIONS

For the treatment of conjunctivitis, corneal ulcer, and other superficial ocular infections due to susceptible microorganisms, and as an adjunct in systemic sulfonamide therapy of trachoma.

CONTRAINDICATIONS

Hypersensitivity to sulfonamide preparations.

PRECAUTIONS

Gantrisin Ophthalmic Solution and Ointment are incompatible with silver preparations. Ophthalmic ointments may retard corneal healing. Nonsusceptible organisms, including fungi, may proliferate with the use of these preparations. Sulfonamides are inactivated by the para-aminobenzoic acid present in purulent exudates. Should undesirable reactions occur, discontinue administration immediately.

DOSAGE AND ADMINISTRATION

Solution: Instill two to three drops in the eye three or more times daily. Care should be taken not to touch dropper tip to any surface, as contamination of solution may result. Ointment: Instill small amount in the lower conjunctival sac one to three times daily and at bedtime.

HOW SUPPLIED

Solution: ½-oz bottles with dropper. Ointment: ⅛-oz tubes.

GANTRISIN® ℞
[gan 'tris-in]
sulfisoxazole/Roche Tablets
GANTRISIN® ℞
acetyl sulfisoxazole/Roche
Pediatric Suspension and Syrup

The following text is complete prescribing information based on official labeling in effect July 1, 1986.

DESCRIPTION

Gantrisin (brand of sulfisoxazole/Roche) is an antibacterial sulfonamide available in tablets, pediatric suspension and syrup for oral administration. Each tablet contains 0.5 Gm sulfisoxazole with corn starch, gelatin, lactose and magnesium stearate. Each teaspoonful (5 mL) of the pediatric suspension contains the equivalent of approximately 0.5 Gm sulfisoxazole in the form of acetyl sulfisoxazole in a vehicle containing 0.3 percent alcohol, carboxymethylcellulose (sodium), citric acid, methylcellulose, parabens (methyl and propyl), partial invert sugar, sodium citrate, sorbitan monolaurate, sucrose, flavors and water. Each teaspoonful (5 mL) of the syrup contains the equivalent of approximately 0.5 Gm sulfisoxazole in the form of acetyl sulfisoxazole in a vehicle containing 0.9 percent alcohol, benzoic acid, carrageenan, citric acid, cocoa, sodium citrate, sorbitan monolaurate, sucrose, flavors and water.
Sulfisoxazole is N^1-(3,4-dimethyl-5-isoxazoly)sulfanilamide. It is a white to slightly yellowish, odorless, slightly bitter, crystalline powder that is soluble in alcohol and very slightly soluble in water. Sulfisoxazole has a molecular weight of 267.30.
Acetyl sulfisoxazole, the tasteless form of sulfisoxazole, is N^1-acetyl sulfisoxazole and must be distinguished from N^4-acetyl sulfisoxazole, which is a metabolite of sulfisoxazole. Acetyl sulfisoxazole is a white or slightly yellow, crystalline powder that is slightly soluble in alcohol and practically insoluble in water. Acetyl sulfisoxazole has a molecular weight of 309.34.

CLINICAL PHARMACOLOGY

Following oral administration, sulfisoxazole is rapidly and completely absorbed; the small intestine is the major site of absorption, but some of the drug is absorbed from the stomach. Sulfisoxazole exists in the blood as unbound, protein-bound and conjugated forms. Sulfisoxazole is metabolized primarily by acetylation and oxidation in the liver. The free form is considered to be the therapeutically active form. Approximately 85% of sulfisoxazole is bound to plasma proteins, primarily to albumin; of the unbound portion, 65% to 72% is in the nonacetylated form.
Maximum plasma concentrations of intact sulfisoxazole following a single 2-Gm oral dose of sulfisoxazole to healthy adult volunteers ranged from 127 to 211 mcg/mL (mean, 169 mcg/mL) and the time of peak plasma concentration ranged from 1 to 4 hours (mean, 2.5 hours). The half-life of elimination of sulfisoxazole ranged from 4.6 to 7.8 hours after oral administration. The elimination of sulfisoxazole has been shown to be slower in elderly subjects (63 to 75 years) with diminished renal function (creatinine clearance, 37 to 68 mL/min).[1] After multiple dose oral administration of 500 mg Q.I.D. to healthy volunteers, the average steady-state plasma concentrations of intact sulfisoxazole ranged from 49.9 to 88.8 mcg/mL (mean, 63.4 mcg/mL).[2]
N^1-acetyl sulfisoxazole is metabolized to sulfisoxazole by digestive enzymes in the gastrointestinal tract and is absorbed as sulfisoxazole. This enzymatic splitting is presumed to be responsible for slower absorption and lower peak blood concentrations than are attained following administration of an equal oral dose of sulfisoxazole. With continued administration of acetyl sulfisoxazole, blood concentrations approximate those of sulfisoxazole. Following a single 4-Gm dose of acetyl sulfisoxazole to healthy volunteers, maximum plasma concentrations of sulfisoxazole ranged from 122 to 282 mcg/mL (mean, 181 mcg/mL) for the pediatric suspension and from 101 to 202 mcg/mL (mean, 144 mcg/mL) for the syrup, and occurred between 2 and 6 hours postadministration. The half-lives of elimination from plasma ranged from 5.4 to 7.4 and from 5.9 to 8.5 hours, respectively.
Sulfisoxazole and acetylated metabolites are excreted primarily by the kidneys through glomerular filtration. Urine concentrations of sulfisoxazole are considerably higher than are the concentrations in blood. The mean urinary excretion recovery following oral administration of sulfisoxazole is 97% within 48 hours, of which 52% is intact drug, with the remaining as the N^4-acetylated metabolite. Following administration of acetyl sulfisoxazole syrup or suspension, approximately 58% is excreted in the urine as total drug within 72 hours.
Sulfisoxazole is distributed only in extracellular body water. It readily crosses the placental barrier and enters into fetal circulation; it is also secreted in breast milk. It also crosses the blood-brain barrier. In healthy subjects, cerebrospinal fluid concentrations of sulfisoxazole vary; in patients with meningitis, however, concentrations of free drug as high as 94 mcg/mL have been reported.
Microbiology: The systemic sulfonamides are bacteriostatic agents. The spectrum of activity is similar for all. Sulfonamides inhibit bacterial synthesis of dihydrofolic acid by competing with *para*-aminobenzoic acid (PABA). Resistant strains are capable of utilizing folic acid precursors or preformed folic acid.

INDICATIONS AND USAGE

Acute, recurrent or chronic urinary tract infections (primarily pyelonephritis, pyelitis and cystitis) due to susceptible organisms (usually *Escherichia coli, Klebsiella-Enterobacter,* staphylococcus, *Proteus mirabilis* and, less frequently, *Proteus vulgaris*) in the absence of obstructive uropathy or foreign bodies.
Meningococcal meningitis where the organism has been demonstrated to be susceptible. *Haemophilus influenzae* meningitis as adjunctive therapy with parenteral streptomycin.
Meningococcal meningitis prophylaxis when sulfonamide-sensitive group A strains are known to prevail in family groups or larger closed populations. (The prophylactic usefulness of sulfonamides when group B or C infections are prevalent has not been proven and in closed population groups may be harmful.)
Acute otitis media due to *Haemophilus influenzae* when used concomitantly with adequate doses of penicillin or erythromycin (see appropriate labeling for prescribing information).
Trachoma. Inclusion conjunctivitis. Nocardiosis. Chancroid.
Toxoplasmosis as adjunctive therapy with pyrimethamine.
Malaria due to chloroquine-resistant strains of *Plasmodium falciparum,* when used as adjunctive therapy.
Important Note: In vitro sulfonamide susceptibility tests are

not always reliable. The test must be carefully coordinated with bacteriologic and clinical response. When the patient is already taking sulfonamides, follow-up cultures should have aminobenzoic acid added to the culture media.
Currently, the increasing frequency of resistant organisms is a limitation of the usefulness of antibacterial agents including the sulfonamides, especially in the treatment of chronic and recurrent urinary tract infections.
Wide variation in blood concentrations may result with identical doses. Blood concentrations should be measured in patients receiving sulfonamides for serious infections. Free sulfonamide blood concentrations of 5 to 15 mg/100 mL may be considered therapeutically effective for most infections, with blood concentrations of 12 to 15 mg/100 mL optimal for serious infections; 20 mg/100 mL should be the maximum total sulfonamide concentration, since adverse reactions occur more frequently above this concentration.

CONTRAINDICATIONS

Hypersensitivity to sulfonamides. Infants less than 2 months of age (except in the treatment of congenital toxoplasmosis as adjunctive therapy with pyrimethamine). Pregnancy at term and during the nursing period, because sulfonamides pass the placenta and are excreted in the milk and may cause kernicterus.

WARNINGS

The sulfonamides should not be used for the treatment of group A beta-hemolytic streptococcal infections. In an established infection, they will not eradicate the streptococcus, and therefore will not prevent sequelae such as rheumatic fever and glomerulonephritis.
Deaths associated with the administration of sulfonamides have been reported from hypersensitivity reactions, hepatocellular necrosis, agranulocytosis, aplastic anemia and other blood dyscrasias.
The presence of clinical signs such as sore throat, fever, pallor, purpura or jaundice may be early indications of serious blood disorders.

PRECAUTIONS

General: Sulfonamides should be given with caution to patients with impaired renal or hepatic function and to those with severe allergy or bronchial asthma. In glucose-6-phosphate dehydrogenase-deficient individuals, hemolysis may occur. This reaction is frequently dose-related. Patients should be instructed to maintain an adequate fluid intake in order to prevent crystalluria and stone formation.
Laboratory tests: Complete blood counts should be done frequently in patients receiving sulfonamides. If a significant reduction in the count of any formed blood element is noted, Gantrisin should be discontinued. Urinalyses with careful microscopic examination and renal function tests should be performed during therapy, particularly for those patients with impaired renal function.
Drug interactions: It has been reported that sulfisoxazole may prolong the prothrombin time in patients who are receiving the anticoagulant warfarin. This interaction should be kept in mind when Gantrisin is given to patients already on anticoagulant therapy, and the coagulation time should be reassessed.
It has been proposed that sulfisoxazole competes with thiopental for plasma protein binding. In one study involving 48 patients, intravenous sulfisoxazole reduced the amount of thiopental required for anesthesia and shortened the awakening time. It is not known whether chronic oral doses of sulfisoxazole would have a similar effect. Until more is known about this interaction, physicians should be aware that patients receiving sulfisoxazole might require less thiopental for anesthesia.
Sulfonamides can displace methotrexate from plasma protein-binding sites, thus increasing free methotrexate concentrations. Studies in man have shown sulfisoxazole infusions to decrease plasma protein-bound methotrexate by one-fourth.
Sulfisoxazole can also potentiate the blood sugar lowering activity of sulfonylureas.
Carcinogenesis, mutagenesis, impairment of fertility: Carcinogenesis: Sulfisoxazole was not carcinogenic in either sex when administered by gavage for 103 weeks at dosages up to 2000 mg/kg/day to mice or 400 mg/kg/day to rats.
Mutagenesis: Bacterial mutagenic studies have not been performed with sulfisoxazole. However, Gantrisin was not observed to be mutagenic in *E. coli* Sd-4-73 when tested in the absence of a metabolic activating system.
Impairment of fertility: No effects on mating behavior, conception rate or fertility index (percent pregnant) were observed in a reproduction study in rats given 800 mg/kg/day sulfisoxazole.
Pregnancy: Teratogenic effects: Pregnancy Category C. Sulfisoxazole was not teratogenic in either rats or rabbits at dosages of 800 mg/kg/day. However, in another teratogenicity study, cleft palates developed in both rats and mice after administration of 1000 mg/kg/day sulfisoxazole; skeletal defects were also observed in rats. This dose is 9 to 18 times the usual adult dosage for Gantrisin. There are no adequate and well-controlled studies of Gantrisin in pregnant women. Gantrisin should be used during pregnancy only if the potential benefit justifies the potential risk to the fetus.
Nonteratogenic effects: See CONTRAINDICATIONS section.
Nursing mothers: See CONTRAINDICATIONS section.
Pediatric use: Gantrisin is not recommended for use in infants younger than 2 months of age except in the treatment of congenital toxoplasmosis as adjunctive therapy with pyrimethamine. (See CONTRAINDICATIONS section.)

ADVERSE REACTIONS

Included in the listing that follows are adverse reactions that have not been reported with this specific drug; however, the pharmacologic similarities among the sulfonamides require that each of the reactions be considered with the administration of any of the Gantrisin dosage forms.
Hematologic: Agranulocytosis, aplastic anemia, thrombocytopenia, leukopenia, hemolytic anemia, purpura, hypoprothrombinemia, methemoglobinemia, eosinophilia.
Allergic reactions: Anaphylaxis, allergic myocarditis, serum sickness, conjunctival and scleral injection, generalized allergic reactions. In addition, periarteritis nodosa and systemic lupus erythematosus have been reported.
Dermatologic: Stevens-Johnson syndrome, epidermal necrolysis, erythema multiforme, exfoliative dermatitis, photosensitivity, pruritus, urticaria, rash, generalized skin eruptions.
Gastrointestinal: Hepatitis, hepatocellular necrosis, pseudomembranous enterocolitis, pancreatitis, stomatitis, glossitis, nausea, emesis, abdominal pain, diarrhea, anorexia.
Genitourinary: Creatinine elevation, toxic nephrosis with oliguria and anuria. The frequency of renal complications is considerably lower in patients receiving the more soluble sulfonamides.
Neurologic: Convulsions, peripheral neuritis, ataxia, vertigo, tinnitus, headache.
Psychiatric: Hallucinations, depression, apathy.
Endocrine: The sulfonamides bear certain chemical similarities to some goitrogens, diuretics (acetazolamide and the thiazides) and oral hypoglycemic agents. Cross-sensitivity may exist with these agents. Diuresis and hypoglycemia have occurred rarely in patients receiving sulfonamides.
Musculoskeletal: Arthralgia, myalgia.
Miscellaneous: Edema (including periorbital), pyrexia, chills, weakness, fatigue, insomnia.

OVERDOSAGE

The amount of a single dose of sulfisoxazole that is either associated with symptoms of overdosage or is likely to be life-threatening has not been reported. Signs and symptoms of overdosage reported with sulfonamides include anorexia, colic, nausea, vomiting, dizziness, headache, drowsiness and unconsciousness. Pyrexia, hematuria and crystalluria may be noted. Blood dyscrasias and jaundice are potential late manifestations of overdosage.
General principles of treatment include the immediate discontinuation of the drug; institution of gastric lavage or emesis; forcing oral fluids; and the administration of intravenous fluids if urine output is low and renal function is normal. The patient should be monitored with blood counts and appropriate blood chemistries, including electrolytes. If a significant blood dyscrasia or jaundice occurs, specific therapy should be instituted for these complications. Peritoneal dialysis is not effective and hemodialysis is only moderately effective in eliminating sulfonamides.
The acute toxicity of sulfisoxazole in animals is as follows:

Species	$LD_{50}\pm$S.E. (mg/kg)
mouse	5700 ± 235
rats	> 10,000
rabbits	> 2000

DOSAGE AND ADMINISTRATION

Systemic sulfonamides are contraindicated in infants under 2 months of age, except in the treatment of congenital toxoplasmosis as adjunctive therapy with pyrimethamine.
Usual dose for infants over 2 months of age and children: Initial dose: One-half of the 24-hour dose. Maintenance dose: 150 mg/kg/24 hours or 4 Gm/M^2/24 hours—dose to be divided into 4 to 6 doses/24 hours. The maximum dose should not exceed 6 Gm/24 hours.
Usual adult dose: Initial dose: 2 to 4 Gm. Maintenance dose: 4 to 8 Gm/24 hours, divided in 4 to 6 doses/24 hours.

HOW SUPPLIED

Tablets (white, scored), containing 0.5 Gm sulfisoxazole—bottles of 100 (NDC 0004-0009-01), 500 (NDC 0004-0009-14) and 1000 (NDC 0004-0009-13); Tel-E-Dose® packages of 100 (NDC 0004-0009-49); Prescription Paks of 100 (NDC 0004-0009-45). Imprint on tablets: ROCHE GANTRISIN®.
Pediatric Suspension (raspberry flavored), containing acetyl sulfisoxazole equivalent to approximately 0.5 Gm sulfisoxazole per teaspoonful (5 mL)—bottles of 4 oz (NDC 0004-1003-30) and 16 oz (1 pint) (NDC 0004-1003-28).
Syrup (chocolate flavored), containing acetyl sulfisoxazole equivalent to approximately 0.5 Gm sulfisoxazole per teaspoonful (5 mL)—bottles of 16 oz (1 pint) (NDC 0004-1004-28).

REFERENCES

1. Boisvert A, Barbeau G, Belanger PM: Pharmacokinetics of sulfisoxazole in young and elderly subjects. *Gerontology 30:* 125–131, 1984
2. Oie S, Gambertoglio JG, Fleckenstein L: Comparison of the disposition of total and unbound sulfisoxazole after single and multiple dosing. *J Pharmacokinet Biopharm 10:* 157–172, 1982

Shown in Product Identification Section, page 425

KLONOPIN™ ©

[klon 'o-pin]
(clonazepam/Roche)
(formerly known as Clonopin®)

The following text is complete prescribing information based on official labeling in effect June 1, 1986.

DESCRIPTION

Klonopin is available as scored tablets containing 0.5 mg, 1 mg or 2 mg clonazepam/Roche. Each tablet also contains lactose, magnesium stearate, microcrystalline cellulose and corn starch, with the following dye systems: 0.5 mg—FD&C Yellow No. 6; 1 mg—FD&C Blue No. 1 and FD&C Blue No. 2. Chemically, clonazepam is 5-(2-chlorophenyl)-1,3-dihydro-7-nitro-2H-1,4-benzodiazepin-2-one. It is a light yellow crystalline powder. It has a molecular weight of 315.7.

ACTIONS

In laboratory animals, Klonopin exhibits several pharmacologic properties which are characteristic of the benzodiazepine class of drugs. Convulsions produced in rodents by pentylenetetrazol or electrical stimulation are antagonized, as are convulsions produced by photic stimulation in susceptible baboons. A taming effect in aggressive primates, muscle weakness and hypnosis are likewise produced by Klonopin. In humans it is capable of suppressing the spike and wave discharge in absence seizures (petit mal) and decreasing the frequency, amplitude, duration and spread of discharge in minor motor seizures.
Single oral dose administration of Klonopin to humans gave maximum blood levels of drug, in most cases, within one to two hours. The half-life of the parent compound varied from approximately 18 to 50 hours, and the major route of excretion was in the urine. In humans, five metabolites have been identified. In general, the biotransformation of clonazepam followed two pathways: oxidative hydroxylation at the C-3 position and reduction of the 7-nitro function to form 7-amino and/or 7-acetyl-amino derivatives.

INDICATIONS

Klonopin is useful alone or as an adjunct in the treatment of the Lennox-Gastaut syndrome (petit mal variant), akinetic and myoclonic seizures. In patients with absence seizures (petit mal) who have failed to respond to succinimides, Klonopin may be useful.
In some studies, up to 30% of patients have shown a loss of anticonvulsant activity, often within three months of administration. In some cases, dosage adjustment may reestablish efficacy.

CONTRAINDICATIONS

Klonopin should not be used in patients with a history of sensitivity to benzodiazepines, nor in patients with clinical or biochemical evidence of significant liver disease. It may be used in patients with open angle glaucoma who are receiving appropriate therapy, but is contraindicated in acute narrow angle glaucoma.

WARNINGS

Since Klonopin produces CNS depression, patients receiving this drug should be cautioned against engaging in hazardous occupations requiring mental alertness, such as operating machinery or driving a motor vehicle. They should also be warned about the concomitant use of alcohol or other CNS-depressant drugs during Klonopin therapy (see Drug Interactions).
Usage in Pregnancy: The effects of Klonopin in human pregnancy and nursing infants are unknown.
Recent reports suggest an association between the use of anticonvulsant drugs by women with epilepsy and an elevated incidence of birth defects in children born to these women. Data are more extensive with respect to diphenylhydantoin and phenobarbital, but these are also the most commonly prescribed anticonvulsants; less systematic or anecdotal reports suggest a possible similar association with the use of all known anticonvulsant drugs.
The reports suggesting an elevated incidence of birth defects in children of drug-treated epileptic women cannot be re-

Continued on next page

Roche Labs.—Cont.

garded as adequate to prove a definite cause and effect relationship. There are intrinsic methodologic problems in obtaining adequate data on drug teratogenicity in humans; the possibility also exists that other factors, *e.g.,* genetic factors or the epileptic condition itself, may be more important than drug therapy in leading to birth defects. The great majority of mothers on anticonvulsant medication deliver normal infants. It is important to note that anticonvulsant drugs should not be discontinued in patients in whom the drug is administered to prevent seizures because of the strong possibility of precipitating status epilepticus with attendant hypoxia and threat to life. In individual cases where the severity and frequency of the seizure disorder are such that the removal of medication does not pose a serious threat to the patient, discontinuation of the drug may be considered prior to and during pregnancy, although it cannot be said with any confidence that even mild seizures do not pose some hazards to the developing embryo or fetus.
These considerations should be weighed in treating or counseling epileptic women of childbearing potential.
Use of Klonopin in women of childbearing potential should be considered only when the clinical situation warrants the risk. Mothers receiving Klonopin should not breast feed their infants.
In a two-generation reproduction study with Klonopin given orally to rats at 10 or 100 mg/kg/day, there was a decrease in the number of pregnancies and a decrease in the number of offspring surviving until weaning. When Klonopin was administered orally to pregnant rabbits at 0.2, 1.0, 5.0 or 10.0 mg/kg/day, a nondose-related incidence of cleft palates, open eyelids, fused sternebrae and limb defects was observed at the 0.2 and 5.0 mg/kg/day levels. Nearly all of the malformations were seen from one dam in each of the affected dosages.
Usage in Children: Because of the possibility that adverse effects on physical or mental development could become apparent only after many years, a benefit-risk consideration of the long-term use of Klonopin is important in pediatric patients.
Physical and Psychological Dependence: Withdrawal symptoms similar in character to those noted with barbiturates and alcohol have occurred following abrupt discontinuance of benzodiazepine drugs. These symptoms include convulsions, tremor, abdominal and muscle cramps, vomiting and sweating. Addiction-prone individuals, such as drug addicts or alcoholics, should be under careful surveillance when receiving benzodiazepines because of the predisposition of such patients to habituation and dependence.

PRECAUTIONS

When used in patients in whom several different types of seizure disorders coexist, Klonopin may increase the incidence or precipitate the onset of generalized tonic-clonic seizures (grand mal). This may require the addition of appropriate anticonvulsants or an increase in their dosages. The concomitant use of valproic acid and clonazepam may produce absence status.
Periodic blood counts and liver function tests are advisable during long-term therapy with Klonopin.
The abrupt withdrawal of Klonopin, particularly in those patients on long-term, high-dose therapy, may precipitate status epilepticus. Therefore, when discontinuing Klonopin, gradual withdrawal is essential. While Klonopin is being gradually withdrawn, the simultaneous substitution of another anticonvulsant may be indicated. Metabolites of Klonopin are excreted by the kidneys; to avoid their excess accumulation, caution should be exercised in the administration of the drug to patients with impaired renal function.
Klonopin may produce an increase in salivation. This should be considered before giving the drug to patients who have difficulty handling secretions. Because of this and the possibility of respiratory depression, Klonopin should be used with caution in patients with chronic respiratory diseases.

ADVERSE REACTIONS

The most frequently occurring side effects of Klonopin are referable to CNS depression. Experience to date has shown that drowsiness has occurred in approximately 50% of patients and ataxia in approximately 30%. In some cases, these may diminish with time; behavior problems have been noted in approximately 25% of patients. Others, listed by system, are:
Neurologic: Abnormal eye movements, aphonia, choreiform movements, coma, diplopia, dysarthria, dysdiadochokinesis, "glassy-eyed" appearance, headache, hemiparesis, hypotonia, nystagmus, respiratory depression, slurred speech, tremor, vertigo.
Psychiatric: Confusion, depression, forgetfulness, hallucinations, hysteria, increased libido, insomnia, psychosis, suicidal attempt (the behavior effects are more likely to occur in patients with a history of psychiatric disturbances).
Respiratory: Chest congestion, rhinorrhea, shortness of breath, hypersecretion in upper respiratory passages.
Cardiovascular: Palpitations.
Dermatologic: Hair loss, hirsutism, skin rash, ankle and facial edema.
Gastrointestinal: Anorexia, coated tongue, constipation, diarrhea, dry mouth, encopresis, gastritis, hepatomegaly, increased appetite, nausea, sore gums.
Genitourinary: Dysuria, enuresis, nocturia, urinary retention.
Musculoskeletal: Muscle weakness, pains.
Miscellaneous: Dehydration, general deterioration, fever, lymphadenopathy, weight loss or gain.
Hematopoietic: Anemia, leukopenia, thrombocytopenia, eosinophilia.
Hepatic: Transient elevations of serum transaminases and alkaline phosphatase.

DRUG INTERACTIONS

The CNS-depressant action of the benzodiazepine class of drugs may be potentiated by alcohol, narcotics, barbiturates, nonbarbiturate hypnotics, antianxiety agents, the phenothiazines, thioxanthene and butyrophenone classes of antipsychotic agents, monoamine oxidase inhibitors and the tricyclic antidepressants, and by other anticonvulsant drugs.

OVERDOSAGE

Symptoms of Klonopin overdosage, like those produced by other CNS depressants, include somnolence, confusion, coma and diminished reflexes. Treatment includes monitoring of respiration, pulse and blood pressure, general supportive measures and immediate gastric lavage. Intravenous fluids should be administered and an adequate airway maintained. Hypotension may be combated by the use of levarterenol or metaraminol. Methylphenidate or caffeine and sodium benzoate may be given to combat CNS depression. Dialysis is of no known value.

DOSAGE AND ADMINISTRATION

Infants and Children: Klonopin is administered orally. In order to minimize drowsiness, the initial dose for infants and children (up to 10 years of age or 30 kg of body weight) should be between 0.01 and 0.03 mg/kg/day but not to exceed 0.05 mg/kg/day given in two or three divided doses. Dosage should be increased by no more than 0.25 to 0.5 mg every third day until a daily maintenance dose of 0.1 to 0.2 mg/kg of body weight has been reached unless seizures are controlled or side effects preclude further increase. Whenever possible, the daily dose should be divided into three equal doses. If doses are not equally divided, the largest dose should be given before retiring.
Adults: The initial dose for adults should not exceed 1.5 mg/day divided into three doses. Dosage may be increased in increments of 0.5 to 1 mg every three days until seizures are adequately controlled or until side effects preclude any further increase. Maintenance dosage must be individualized for each patient depending upon response. Maximum recommended daily dose is 20 mg.
The use of multiple anticonvulsants may result in an increase of depressant adverse effects. This should be considered before adding Klonopin to an existing anticonvulsant regimen.

HOW SUPPLIED

Scored tablets—0.5 mg, orange; 1 mg, blue; 2 mg, white—Prescription Paks of 100.

Shown in Product Identification Section, page 425

KONAKION®

℞

[ko-nak 'e-on]
(phytonadione/Roche)
INJECTABLE

The following text is complete prescribing information based on official labeling in effect June 1, 1986.

FOR INTRAMUSCULAR USE ONLY

DESCRIPTION

Konakion is an essentially clear, aqueous dispersion of vitamin K_1, available for injection by the intramuscular route only. Slight opalescence may occur in the 10 mg ampuls. However, this does not affect the potency, safety or usefulness of the preparation.
The ingredients are as follows: *0.5-ml ampuls:* Each 0.5 ml contains 1 mg phytonadione (vitamin K_1) compounded with 10 mg polysorbate 80, 0.45% phenol as preservative, 10.4 mg propylene glycol, 0.17 mg sodium acetate and 0.00002 ml glacial acetic acid.
1-ml ampuls: Each ml contains 10 mg phytonadione (vitamin K_1) compounded with 40 mg polysorbate 80, 20.7 mg propylene glycol, 0.8 mg sodium acetate and 0.00006 ml glacial acetic acid.

ACTIONS

Konakion possesses the same type and degree of activity as does naturally occurring vitamin K, which is necessary for the synthesis in the liver of prothrombin (factor II), proconvertin (factor VII), plasma thromboplastin component (factor IX), and Stuart factor (factor X).
The prothrombin test is sensitive to the levels of factors II, VII and X. The mechanism by which vitamin K promotes formation of these clotting factors in the liver is not known.
The action of the aqueous dispersion when administered parenterally is generally detectable within an hour or two, and hemorrhage is usually controlled within 3 to 6 hours. A normal prothrombin level may often be obtained in 12 to 14 hours.
In the prophylaxis and treatment of hemorrhagic disease of the newborn, Konakion has demonstrated a greater margin of safety than that of the water-soluble vitamin K analogs.

INDICATIONS

- anticoagulant-induced prothrombin deficiency;
- prophylaxis and therapy of hemorrhagic disease of the newborn;
- hypoprothrombinemia due to oral antibacterial therapy;
- hypoprothrombinemia secondary to factors limiting absorption or synthesis of vitamin K, *e.g.,* obstructive jaundice, biliary fistula, sprue, ulcerative colitis, celiac disease, intestinal resection, cystic fibrosis of the pancreas and regional enteritis;
- other drug-induced hypoprothrombinemia (such as that due to salicylates) where it is definitely shown that the result is due to interference with vitamin K metabolism.

CONTRAINDICATIONS

Parenteral use in persons who are hypersensitive to the drug.

WARNINGS

Konakion promotes the synthesis of prothrombin by the liver and does not directly counteract the effects of the oral anticoagulants; it takes up to two hours for vitamin K to promote prothrombin synthesis. Fresh plasma or blood transfusions may be required for severe blood loss or lack of response to vitamin K. Phytonadione will not counteract the anticoagulant action of heparin.
When vitamin K_1 is used to correct excessive anticoagulant-induced hypoprothrombinemia, anticoagulant therapy still being indicated, the patient is again faced with the clotting hazards existing prior to starting the anticoagulant therapy. Phytonadione is not a clotting agent, but overzealous therapy with vitamin K may restore conditions which originally permitted thromboembolic phenomena. Dosage, therefore, should be kept as low as possible, and prothrombin time should be checked regularly as clinical conditions indicate.
Repeated large doses of vitamin K are not warranted in liver disease if the response to initial use of the vitamin is unsatisfactory (Koller test). Failure to respond to vitamin K may indicate the presence of a coagulation defect or that the condition being treated is unresponsive to vitamin K.
Effects on reproduction have not been studied in animals. There is no adequate information on whether this drug may affect fertility in human males or females or have a teratogenic potential or other adverse effects on the fetus.

PRECAUTIONS

Store in a dark place and protect from light at all times.
Temporary resistance to prothrombin-depressing anticoagulants may result, especially when larger doses of phytonadione are used. If relatively large doses have been employed, it may be necessary when reinstituting anticoagulant therapy to use somewhat larger doses of the prothrombin-depressing anticoagulant or to use one which acts on a different principle, such as heparin.

ADVERSE REACTIONS

Pain, swelling and tenderness at the injection site have occurred rarely. The possibility of allergic sensitivity, including an anaphylactoid reaction, should be kept in mind.
Although Konakion has a greater margin of safety than the water-soluble vitamin K analogs, hyperbilirubinemia has been reported in the newborn, particularly in prematures when used at 5 to 10 times the recommended dosage. This effect, with its possibility of attendant kernicterus, should be borne in mind if such dosages are deemed necessary.

DOSAGE AND ADMINISTRATION

The human minimum daily requirements for vitamin K have not been established officially. Minimal daily requirements have been estimated at 1 to 5 micrograms per kilogram of body weight for infants and 0.03 micrograms per kilogram for adults. The dietary abundance of vitamin K satisfies the requirements normally except for the neonatal period of 5 to 8 days.

INFANTS

Neonatal hemorrhage due to hypoprothrombinemia:
- *Prophylactic*—1 to 2 mg intramuscularly, immediately after birth.
- *Control*—1 to 2 mg intramuscularly, daily.

ADULTS

Hypoprothrombinemia due to:
- *Anticoagulant therapy* (except of heparin type)—5 to 10 mg I.M. initially; up to 20 mg, if necessary.
- *Antibacterial therapy*—5 to 20 mg I.M.
- *Factors limiting absorption or synthesis*—2 to 20 mg I.M.
- *Other drugs* (*e.g.,* salicylates)—2 to 20 mg I.M.

In older children and adults, injection of Konakion should be in the upper outer quadrant of the buttocks. In infants and young children, the anterolateral aspect of the thighs or the deltoid region is preferred so that danger of sciatic nerve injury is avoided.

STORAGE

Konakion is stable in the air, but is photosensitive, decomposing with loss of potency on exposure to light. Therefore, it should be stored in a dark place and protected from light at all times. Konakion need not be refrigerated. Store at 59° to 86°F.

HOW SUPPLIED

Ampuls, 0.5 ml (boxes of 10). Ampuls, 1 ml (boxes of 10).

LAROBEC® TABLETS ℞

[*lar 'o-bek*]

The following text is complete prescribing information based on official labeling in effect June 1, 1986.

Each Larobec® tablet contains:	Quantity	U.S. RDA—Adults and children 4 or more years of age
Water-Soluble Vitamins		
Vitamin C (ascorbic acid)	500 mg	60 mg
Vitamin B_1 (as thiamine mononitrate)	15 mg	1.5 mg
Vitamin B_2 (riboflavin)	15 mg	1.7 mg
Niacin (as niacinamide)	100 mg	20 mg
Pantothenic acid (as calcium *d*-pantothenate)	18 mg	10 mg
Folic acid	0.5 mg	0.4 mg
Vitamin B_{12} (cyanocobalamin)	5 mcg	6 mcg

Each tablet also contains acacia, calcium sulfate, carnauba wax, hydrogenated vegetable oil, magnesium oxide, magnesium stearate, povidone, shellac, sodium benzoate, sugar and talc with the following dyes: FD&C Yellow No. 6, D&C Yellow No. 10 and titanium dioxide.

DESCRIPTION

Larobec is a prescription-only oral multivitamin tablet specially formulated for patients who require prophylactic or therapeutic nutritional supplementation of water-soluble vitamins and are receiving levodopa therapy for Parkinson's disease and syndrome. Larobec provides *therapeutic* levels of ascorbic acid, vitamins B_1, B_2, niacin, pantothenic acid and folic acid and a *supplemental* level of vitamin B_{12} *without* pyridoxine (vitamin B_6), which has been reported to reduce the clinical benefits of levodopa therapy.

CLINICAL PHARMACOLOGY

Vitamins are essential for maintenance of normal metabolic functions including hematopoiesis. The water-soluble vitamins play vital roles in the conversion of carbohydrate, protein and fat into tissue and energy. *Thiamine (B_1)* acts as a coenzyme in carbohydrate metabolism. *Riboflavin (B_2)* functions as a coenzyme in the electron transport system associated with conversion of tissue oxidations into usable energy. *Niacin* serves as a coenzyme in oxidation-reduction reactions in tissue respiration. *Pantothenic acid* functions as a coenzyme in various metabolic acetylation reactions. *Folic acid* and *cyanocobalamin (B_{12})* are metabolically interrelated. They are essential to nucleic acid synthesis and normal maturation of red blood cells. *Ascorbic acid (C)* performs a vital function in the process of cellular respiration, and is involved in both carbohydrate and amino acid metabolism. It is essential for collagen formation and tissue repair.
The water-soluble vitamins (B-complex and C) are not significantly stored by the body; excess quantities are excreted in the urine. They must be replenished regularly through diet or other means to maintain essential tissue levels. Thus these vitamins are rapidly depleted in conditions interfering with their intake or absorption.

INDICATIONS AND USAGE

Larobec is indicated for supportive nutritional supplementation when a water-soluble vitamin formulation (without pyridoxine) is required prophylactically or therapeutically in patients who are undergoing treatment with levodopa.

CONTRAINDICATIONS

Larobec is contraindicated in patients known to be hypersensitive to any of its components.

WARNINGS

Administration of vitamin B_6 may be required if signs of pyridoxine deficiency develop. Folic acid in doses above 0.1 mg daily may obscure pernicious anemia. Larobec is not intended for treatment of pernicious anemia or other megaloblastic anemias where vitamin B_{12} is deficient. Neurologic involvement may develop or progress, despite temporary remission of anemia, in patients with vitamin B_{12} deficiency who receive supplemental folic acid and who are inadequately treated with B_{12}.

PRECAUTIONS

General: Certain patients may require additional nutritional supplementation with fat-soluble vitamins and minerals according to the dietary habits of the individual. Larobec is not intended for treatment of severe specific vitamin deficiencies.
Information for the Patient: Because toxic reactions have been reported with injudicious use of certain vitamins, urge patients to follow your specific instructions regarding dosage regimen. As with any medication, advise patients to keep Larobec out of reach of children.

ADVERSE REACTIONS

Adverse reactions have been reported with specific vitamins, but generally at levels substantially higher than those in Larobec. However, allergic and idiosyncratic reactions are possible at lower levels.

DOSAGE AND ADMINISTRATION

Usual adult dosage: one tablet daily.
Larobec is available on prescription only.

HOW SUPPLIED

Orange-colored, capsule-shaped tablets—bottles of 100 (NDC 0004-0073-01).
Imprint on tablets: LAROBEC® ROCHE
Shown in Product Identification Section, page 425

LARODOPA® ℞

[*lar "o-do 'pa*]
(levodopa/Roche)

The following text is complete prescribing information based on official labeling in effect June 1, 1986.

In order to reduce the high incidence of adverse reactions, it is necessary to individualize the therapy and to gradually increase the dosage to the desired therapeutic level.

DESCRIPTION

Larodopa is available as tablets and capsules containing 0.1 Gm, 0.25 Gm or 0.5 Gm levodopa. Each tablet also contains corn starch, magnesium stearate, microcrystalline cellulose, povidone, talc and D&C Red No. 7 lake dye. Each capsule also contains corn starch and talc. Gelatin capsule shells have the following dye systems: 100 mg—FD&C Blue No. 1, FD&C Red No. 3, D&C Red No. 33, FD&C Yellow No. 6 and D&C Yellow No. 10; 250 mg—FD&C Blue No. 1, D&C Red No. 33, FD&C Yellow No. 6; 500 mg—D&C Red No. 33, FD&C Yellow No. 6.
Chemically, levodopa is (−)-3-(3,4-dihydroxyphenyl)-*L*-alanine. It is a colorless, crystalline compound, slightly soluble in water and insoluble in alcohol, with a molecular weight of 197.2.

ACTIONS

Evidence indicates that the symptoms of Parkinson's disease are related to depletion of striatal dopamine. Since dopamine apparently does not cross the blood-brain barrier, its administration is ineffective in the treatment of Parkinson's disease. However, levodopa, the levo-rotatory isomer of dihydroxyphenylalanine (dopa) which is the metabolic precursor of dopamine, does cross the blood-brain barrier. Presumably it is converted into dopamine in the basal ganglia. This is generally thought to be the mechanism whereby oral levodopa acts in relieving the symptoms of Parkinson's disease.
The major urinary metabolites of levodopa in man appear to be dopamine and homovanillic acid (HVA). In 24-hour urine samples, HVA accounts for 13 to 42 percent of the ingested dose of levodopa.

INDICATIONS

Larodopa is indicated in the treatment of idiopathic Parkinson's disease (Paralysis Agitans), postencephalitic parkinsonism, symptomatic parkinsonism which may follow injury to the nervous system by carbon monoxide intoxication, and manganese intoxication. It is indicated in those elderly patients believed to develop parkinsonism in association with cerebral arteriosclerosis.

CONTRAINDICATIONS

Monoamine oxidase (MAO) inhibitors and Larodopa should not be given concomitantly and these inhibitors must be discontinued two weeks prior to initiating therapy with Larodopa. Larodopa is contraindicated in patients with known hypersensitivity to the drug and in narrow angle glaucoma.
Because levodopa may activate a malignant melanoma, it should not be used in patients with suspicious, undiagnosed skin lesions or a history of melanoma.

WARNINGS

Larodopa should be administered cautiously to patients with severe cardiovascular or pulmonary disease, bronchial asthma, renal, hepatic or endocrine disease.
Care should be exercised in administering Larodopa to patients with a history of myocardial infarction who have residual atrial, nodal or ventricular arrhythmias. If Larodopa is necessary in this type of patient, it should be used in a facility with a coronary care unit or an intensive care unit.
One must be on the alert for the possibility of upper gastrointestinal hemorrhage in those patients with a past history of active peptic ulcer disease.
All patients should be carefully observed for the development of depression with concomitant suicidal tendencies. Psychotic patients should be treated with caution.
Pyridoxine hydrochloride (vitamin B_6) in oral doses of 10 to 25 mg rapidly reverses the toxic and therapeutic effects of Larodopa. This should be considered before recommending vitamin preparations containing pyridoxine hydrochloride (vitamin B_6).
Usage in Pregnancy: The safety of Larodopa in women who are or who may become pregnant has not been established; hence it should be given only when the potential benefits have been weighed against possible hazards to mother and child. Studies in rodents have shown that levodopa at dosages in excess of 200 mg/kg/day has an adverse effect on fetal and postnatal growth and viability.
Larodopa should not be used in nursing mothers.
Usage in Children: The safety of Larodopa under the age of 12 has not been established.

PRECAUTIONS

Periodic evaluations of hepatic, hematopoietic, cardiovascular and renal function are recommended during extended therapy in all patients.
Patients with chronic wide angle glaucoma may be treated cautiously with Larodopa, provided the intraocular pressure is well controlled and the patient monitored carefully for changes in intraocular pressure during therapy.
Postural hypotensive episodes have been reported as adverse reactions. Therefore, Larodopa should be administered to patients on antihypertensive drug cautiously (for patients receiving pargyline, see note on MAO inhibitors contraindications), and it may be necessary to adjust the dosage of the antihypertensive drugs.

ADVERSE REACTIONS

The most serious adverse reactions associated with the administration of Larodopa having frequent occurrences are: adventitious movements such as choreiform and/or dystonic movements. Other serious adverse reactions with a lower incidence are: cardiac irregularities and/or palpitations, orthostatic hypotensive episodes, bradykinetic episodes (the "on-off" phenomena), mental changes including paranoid ideation and psychotic episodes, depression with or without the development of suicidal tendencies, dementia, and urinary retention.
Rarely, gastrointestinal bleeding, development of duodenal ulcer, hypertension, phlebitis, hemolytic anemia, agranulocytosis, and convulsions have been observed. (The causal relationship between convulsions and Larodopa has not been established.)
Adverse reactions of a less serious nature having a relatively frequent occurrence are the following: anorexia, nausea and vomiting with or without abdominal pain and distress, dry mouth, dysphagia, sialorrhea, ataxia, increased hand tremor, headache, dizziness, numbness, weakness and faintness, bruxism, confusion, insomnia, nightmares, hallucinations and delusions, agitation and anxiety, malaise, fatigue and euphoria. Occurring with a lesser order of frequency are the following: muscle twitching and blepharospasm (which may be taken as an early sign of overdosage; consideration of dosage reduction may be made at this time), trismus, burning sensation of the tongue, bitter taste, diarrhea, constipation, flatulence, flushing, skin rash, increased sweating, bizarre breathing patterns, urinary incontinence, diplopia, blurred vision, dilated pupils, hot flashes, weight gain or loss, dark sweat and/or urine.
Rarely, oculogyric crises, sense of stimulation, hiccups, development of edema, loss of hair, hoarseness, priapism and activation of latent Horner's syndrome have been observed.
Elevations of blood urea nitrogen, SGOT, SGPT, LDH, bilirubin, alkaline phosphatase or protein-bound iodine have been reported; and the significance of this is not known. Occasional reductions in WBC, hemoglobin, and hematocrit have been noted.
Leukopenia has occurred and requires cessation, at least temporarily, of Larodopa administration. The Coombs test has occasionally become positive during extended therapy. Elevations of uric acid have been noted when colorimetric method was used but not when uricase method was used.

Continued on next page

Roche Labs.—Cont.

OVERDOSAGE
For acute overdosage general supportive measures should be employed, along with immediate gastric lavage. Intravenous fluids should be administered judiciously and an adequate airway maintained.
Electrocardiographic monitoring should be instituted and the patient carefully observed for the possible development of arrhythmias; if required, appropriate antiarrhythmic therapy should be given. Consideration should be given to the possibility of multiple drug ingestion by the patient. To date, no experience has been reported with dialysis; hence its value in Larodopa overdosage is not known. Although pyridoxine hydrochloride (vitamin B_6) has been reported to reverse the antiparkinson effects of Larodopa, its usefulness in the management of acute overdosage has not been established.

DOSAGE AND ADMINISTRATION
The optimal daily dose of Larodopa, *i.e.,* the dose producing maximal improvement with tolerated side effects, must be determined and *carefully titrated for each individual patient.* The usual initial dosage is 0.5 to 1 Gm daily, divided in two or more doses with food.
The total daily dosage is then increased gradually in increments not more than 0.75 Gm every three to seven days as tolerated. The usual optimal therapeutic *dosage should not exceed 8 Gm.* The exceptional patient may carefully be given more than 8 Gms as required. In some patients, a significant therapeutic response may not be obtained until six months of treatment.
In the event general anesthesia is required, Larodopa therapy may be continued as long as the patient is able to take fluids and medication by mouth. If therapy is temporarily interrupted, the usual daily dosage may be administered as soon as the patient is able to take oral medication. Whenever therapy has been interrupted for longer periods, dosage should again be adjusted gradually; however, in many cases the patient can be rapidly titrated to his previous therapeutic dosage.

HOW SUPPLIED
Tablets, pink, scored, each containing levodopa/Roche 0.1 Gm, bottles of 100; 0.25 Gm or 0.5 Gm—bottles of 100 and 500.
Capsules, each containing levodopa/Roche 0.1 Gm (pink and scarlet)—bottles of 100; 0.25 Gm (pink and beige) or 0.5 Gm (pink)—bottles of 100 and 500.
Shown in Product Identification Section, page 425

LEVO-DROMORAN® Ⓒ
[lee "vo dro 'mo-ran]
(levorphanol tartrate/Roche)
Ampuls • Vials • Tablets

The following text is complete prescribing information based on official labeling in effect June 1, 1986.

DESCRIPTION
Levo-Dromoran is available as 1-ml ampuls containing 2 mg levorphanol tartrate compounded with 0.2% parabens (methyl and propyl) as preservatives and sodium hydroxide to adjust pH to approximately 4.3; as 10-ml vials containing 2 mg levorphanol tartrate per ml, compounded with 0.45% phenol as preservative and sodium hydroxide to adjust pH to approximately 4.3; and as scored tablets, each containing 2 mg levorphanol tartrate plus lactose, corn starch, stearic acid and talc.
Levo-Dromoran is a highly potent synthetic analgesic with properties and actions similar to those of morphine. It produces a degree of analgesia at least equal to that of morphine and greater than that of meperidine at far smaller doses than either. It is longer acting than either; from 6 to 8 hours of pain relief can be expected with Levo-Dromoran whether given orally or by injection. It is almost as effective orally as it is parenterally. Its safety margin is about equal to that of morphine, but it is less likely to produce nausea, vomiting and constipation.

INDICATIONS
Levo-Dromoran is recommended whenever a narcotic-analgesic is required. It is recommended for the relief of pain whether moderate or severe. For example, it may be used in alleviating pain due to biliary and renal colic, myocardial infarction, and severe trauma; intractable pain due to cancer and other tumors; and for postoperative pain relief. Used preoperatively, it allays apprehension, provides prolonged analgesia, reduces thiopental requirements and shortens recovery-room time. Levo-Dromoran is compatible with a wide range of anesthetic agents. It is a useful supplement to nitrous oxide-oxygen anesthesia. It has been given by slow intravenous injection for special indications.

CONTRAINDICATIONS
As with the use of morphine, Levo-Dromoran is contraindicated in acute alcoholism, bronchial asthma, increased intracranial pressure, respiratory depression and anoxia.

WARNING
May be habit forming. Levo-Dromoran is a narcotic with an addiction liability similar to that of morphine, and for this reason the same precautions should be taken in administering the drug as with morphine. As with all narcotics, Levo-Dromoran should be used in early pregnancy only when expected benefits outweigh risks.

PRECAUTIONS
To counteract narcotic-induced respiratory depression, a narcotic antagonist, such as Narcan (naloxone hydrochloride), is recommended and should be readily available whenever Levo-Dromoran is used by parenteral administration.

ADVERSE REACTIONS
As is true with the use of any narcotic-analgesic, nausea, emesis and dizziness are not uncommon in the ambulatory patient. Respiratory depression, hypotension, urinary retention and various cardiac arrhythmias have been infrequently reported following the use of Levo-Dromoran, primarily in surgical patients. Occasional allergic reactions in the form of skin rash or urticaria have been reported. Pruritus or sweating are rarely observed.

DOSAGE AND ADMINISTRATION
Good medical practice dictates that the dose of any narcotic-analgesic be appropriate to the degree of pain to be relieved. This is especially important during the postoperative period because (a) residual CNS-depressant effects of anesthetic agents may still be present, and (b) later, gradual lessening of pain may not warrant full narcotizing doses. The average adult dose is 2 mg orally or subcutaneously. The dosage may be increased to 3 mg, if necessary.

ANTIDOTE FOR OVERDOSAGE
In the event of overdosage of Levo-Dromoran, an appropriate dose of a narcotic antagonist, such as Narcan (naloxone HCl), should be administered; consult the prescribing information of the specific narcotic antagonist for details about use.

HOW SUPPLIED
Ampuls, 1 ml (boxes of 10). Each ml of solution contains 2 mg levorphanol tartrate/Roche (WARNING: May be habit forming).
Multiple Dose Vials, 10 ml, 2 mg/ml (boxes of 1). Each ml of solution contains 2 mg levorphanol tartrate/Roche (WARNING: May be habit forming).
Oral Tablets, 2 mg, scored (bottles of 100). Each tablet contains 2 mg levorphanol tartrate/Roche (WARNING: May be habit forming).
Narcotic order required.
Shown in Product Identification Section, page 425

MARPLAN® TABLETS ℞
[mar 'plan]
(isocarboxazid/Roche)

The following text is complete prescribing information based on official labeling in effect June 1, 1986.

DESCRIPTION
Marplan (isocarboxazid/Roche), an amine-oxidase inhibitor, is available for oral administration in 10-mg tablets. Each tablet also contains gelatin, lactose, magnesium stearate, corn starch, talc, FD&C Red No. 3 and FD&C Yellow No. 6. Chemically, isocarboxazid is 5-methyl-3-isoxazolecarboxylic acid 2-benzylhydrazide.
Isocarboxazid is a colorless, crystalline substance with very little taste.

ACTIONS
Isocarboxazid, a potent inhibitor of amine-oxidase, exhibits antidepressant activity. *In vivo* and *in vitro* studies demonstrated inhibition of amine-oxidase in the brain, heart and liver.
The oral LD_{50} in mice was 171 mg/kg and in rats, 270 mg/kg. In rats administered 120 mg/kg daily for 6 weeks, isocarboxazid produced a reduction of growth rate and appetite. In chronic tolerance studies of 24 weeks duration, hyperexcitability and depression of growth rate occurred in male rats given oral doses of 5 mg/kg/day and in both sexes of this species given 10 mg/kg/day orally. The relevance of these findings to the clinical use of Marplan is not known. No hematologic changes were observed.
Dogs given 15 mg/kg/day for 2 weeks showed emetic effects and a slight lowering of hemoglobin and hematocrit. No adverse effects were noted, however, at doses of 10 mg/kg/day for 6 weeks. Given as successively increasing daily oral doses to a dog, isocarboxazid was tolerated up to 40 mg/kg.
Monkeys given 20 mg/kg/day orally for 2 weeks tolerated the drug with no apparent adverse effects.
Reproduction studies were carried out in rats given 0.5 and 5 mg/kg/day of isocarboxazid as a dietary mixture for 10 weeks prior to mating and continuing through two mating cycles to the weaning of the second litter. The parent animals remained in good condition throughout the test period. Litters of the treated groups compared favorably with those of the controls. No evidence of teratogenic effects was seen in any of the young.

INDICATIONS: Based on a review of this drug by the National Academy of Sciences—National Research Council and/or other information, FDA has classified the indications as follows:
"Probably" effective for the treatment of depressed patients who are refractory to tricyclic antidepressants or electroconvulsive therapy and depressed patients in whom tricyclic antidepressants are contraindicated.
Final classification of the less-than-effective indications requires further investigation.

Careful selection of candidates for Marplan—with due regard to the symptomatology of the patient and to the properties of the compound—will result in more effective therapy. Complete review of the package insert is advised before initiating treatment.

CONTRAINDICATIONS
Marplan is contraindicated in patients with known hypersensitivity to the drug, severe impairment of liver or renal function, congestive heart failure or pheochromocytoma.
The potentiation of sympathomimetic substances by MAO inhibitors may result in *hypertensive crisis;* therefore, patients taking Marplan should not be given *sympathomimetic drugs* (including amphetamines, methyldopa, levodopa, dopamine, and tryptophan as well as epinephrine and norepinephrine) nor *foods with a high concentration of tryptophan* (broad beans) or *tyramine* (cheese, beers, wines, pickled herring, chicken livers, yeast extract). Excessive amounts of caffeine can also cause hypertensive reactions.
These hypertensive crises can be fatal, due to circulatory collapse or intracranial bleeding. Hypertensive crises are characterized by some or all of the following symptoms: occipital headache which may radiate frontally, neck stiffness or soreness, nausea, vomiting, photophobia, dilated pupils, sweating (sometimes with fever and sometimes with cold, clammy skin) and palpitations. Either tachycardia or bradycardia may be present, and can be associated with constricting chest pain. These crises usually occur within several hours after the ingestion of a contraindicated substance. Marplan should be discontinued immediately upon the occurrence of palpitations or frequent headaches.
Recommended treatment in hypertensive crisis: Marplan should be discontinued and therapy to lower blood pressure should be started immediately. A successful method of treatment is with an alpha-adrenergic blocking agent such as phentolamine, 5 mg, I.V., or pentolinium, 3 mg, subcutaneously. These drugs should be administered slowly to avoid excessive hypotension. Fever should be managed by external cooling.
Marplan should not be administered together with or immediately following other MAO inhibitors or dibenzazepines. Such combinations can produce hypertensive crisis, fever, marked sweating, excitation, delirium, tremor, twitching, convulsions, coma, and circulatory collapse. At least 10 days should elapse between the discontinuation of Marplan and the institution of another antidepressant, or the discontinuation of another MAO inhibitor and the institution of Marplan.
Some other amine-oxidase inhibitors commonly used in this country include: pargyline HCl, phenelzine sulfate and tranylcypromine.
Some antidepressants (dibenzazepine derivatives) commonly used in this country include amitriptyline HCl, desipramine HCl, imipramine HCl, nortriptyline HCl and protriptyline HCl.
Patients taking Marplan should not undergo elective surgery requiring general anesthesia. Should spinal anesthesia be essential, consideration should be given to possible combined hypotensive effects of Marplan and the blocking agent. Also, they should not be given cocaine or local anesthetic solutions containing sympathomimetic vasoconstrictors. Marplan should be discontinued at least 10 days prior to elective surgery.
Marplan should not be used in combination with CNS depressants such as narcotics and ethanol (see PRECAUTIONS for barbiturates). Circulatory collapse and death have been reported from the combination of amine-oxidase inhibitors and a single dose of meperidine. In addition, serious hyperpyrexia can occur following administration of this combination. It is thought that this latter reaction may be mediated by release of 5-hydroxytryptamine, as it does not occur in experimental animals pretreated with inhibitors of 5-HT synthesis.

WARNINGS
Because the most serious reactions to Marplan relate to effects on blood pressure, it is not advisable to use this drug in elderly or debilitated patients or in the presence of hyperten-

sion, cardiovascular or cerebrovascular disease. Patients with severe or frequent headaches should not be considered as candidates for therapy with Marplan because headaches during therapy may be the first symptom of a hypertensive reaction to the drug.

Marplan should be used with caution in combination with antihypertensive drugs including thiazide diuretics since hypotension may result.

In patients who may be suicidal risks, no single form of treatment, such as Marplan, electroshock or other therapy, should be relied on as a sole therapeutic measure. The strictest supervision, and preferably hospitalization, are advised.

Warning to patient: All patients taking Marplan should be warned against self-medication with proprietary cold, hay fever or reducing preparations, since most of these contain sympathomimetic agents. They should be warned against eating the foods previously mentioned that contain high concentrations of tyramine or tryptophan. Beverages containing caffeine should be used in moderation. Patients should be instructed to report promptly the occurrence of headache or other unusual symptoms.

Use in Children: Marplan is not recommended for use in patients under 16 years of age since there are no controlled studies of safety or efficacy in this group.

Use in Pregnancy: Safe use of Marplan during pregnancy or lactation has not yet been established. Before prescribing Marplan in pregnancy, lactation, or in women of childbearing age, the potential benefit of the drug should be weighed against its possible hazard to mother and child. (See ACTIONS.)

PRECAUTIONS

Concomitant use of Marplan and other psychotropic agents is not recommended because of possible potentiating effects and decreased margin of safety. This is especially true in patients who may subject themselves to an overdosage of drugs. If combination therapy is indicated, careful consideration should be given to the pharmacology of all agents to be employed. The effects of Marplan may persist for a substantial period after discontinuation of the drug, and this should be borne in mind when another drug is prescribed following Marplan. To avoid potentiation, the physician wishing to terminate treatment with Marplan and begin therapy with another agent should allow for an interval of 10 days.

Marplan should be used cautiously in hyperactive or agitated patients, as well as schizophrenic patients, because it may cause excessive stimulation. Characteristically, in manic-depressive states there may be a tendency for patients to swing from a depressive to a manic phase. If such a swing should occur during Marplan therapy, brief discontinuation of the drug, followed by resumption of therapy at a reduced dosage, is advised.

Clinical evidence indicates only a low incidence of altered liver function or jaundice in patients treated with Marplan. It is difficult to differentiate most cases of drug-induced hepatocellular jaundice from viral hepatitis since they are histopathologically and biochemically indistinguishable. Moreover, many of the clinical signs and symptoms are identical. While some of the few cases of jaundice reported during Marplan therapy may have been drug-induced, the reaction is rare. Nevertheless, Marplan is an amine-oxidase inhibitor and, as with the use of all these agents, it is advisable to watch for hepatic complications. It is suggested that periodic liver function tests, such as bilirubins, alkaline phosphatase or transaminases, be performed during Marplan therapy; use of the drug should be discontinued at the first sign of hepatic dysfunction or jaundice. In patients with impaired renal function, Marplan should be used cautiously to prevent accumulation.

Marplan appears to have varying effects in epileptic patients; while some have a decrease in frequency of seizures, others have more seizures. Appropriate consideration must be given to the latter possibility if Marplan is prescribed for such patients.

All patients taking Marplan should be watched for symptoms of postural hypotension. If such hypotension occurs, the dose should be reduced or the drug discontinued.

Since the MAO inhibitors, including Marplan, potentiate hexobarbital hypnosis in animals, the dose of barbiturates if given concomitantly should be reduced.

Since the MAO inhibitors inhibit the destruction of serotonin, which is believed to be released from tissue stores by rauwolfia alkaloids, caution should be exercised when these drugs are used together.

There is conflicting evidence as to whether MAO inhibitors affect glucose metabolism or potentiate hypoglycemic agents. This should be considered if Marplan is used in diabetics.

ADVERSE REACTIONS

Marplan is a potent therapeutic agent with a relatively low incidence of adverse reactions. Since Marplan affects many enzyme systems of the body, a variety of side effects may be anticipated. The most frequently noted have been orthostatic hypotension, associated in some patients with falling, disturbances in cardiac rate and rhythm, complaints of dizziness and vertigo, constipation, headache, overactivity, hyperreflexia, tremors and muscle twitching, mania, hypomania, jitteriness, confusion and memory impairment, insomnia, peripheral edema, weakness, fatigue, dryness of the mouth, blurred vision, hyperhidrosis, anorexia and body weight changes, gastrointestinal disturbances, and minor sensitivity reactions such as skin rashes. Isolated cases of akathisia, ataxia, black tongue, coma, dysuria, euphoria, hematologic changes, incontinence, neuritis, photosensitivity, sexual disturbances, spider telangiectases and urinary retention have been reported. These side effects sometimes necessitate discontinuation of therapy. In rare instances, hallucinations have been reported with high dosages, but they have disappeared upon reduction of dosage or discontinuation of therapy. Toxic amblyopia was reported in one psychiatric patient who had received isocarboxazid for about a year; no causal relationship to isocarboxazid was established. Impaired water excretion compatible with the syndrome of inappropriate secretion of antidiuretic hormone (SIADH) has been reported.

DOSAGE AND ADMINISTRATION

As with other potent drugs, for maximum therapeutic effect the dosage of Marplan must be individually adjusted on the basis of careful observation of the patient. The usual starting dose is 30 mg daily, to be given in single or divided doses. Marplan has a cumulative effect; therefore, as soon as clinical improvement is observed, the dosage should be reduced to a maintenance level of 10 to 20 mg daily (or less). Since daily doses larger than 30 mg may cause an increase in the incidence or severity of side effects, it is recommended that this dosage generally not be exceeded. Many patients may show a favorable response to Marplan therapy within a week or less; however, since Marplan acts by directly affecting enzyme metabolism, a beneficial effect may not be seen in some patients for three or four weeks. If no response is obtained by then, continued administration is unlikely to help.

MANAGEMENT OF OVERDOSAGE

The lethal dose of Marplan in man is not known. There has been one report of a fatality in a patient who ingested 400 mg of Marplan together with an unspecified amount of another drug. Major overdosage may be evidenced by symptoms such as tachycardia, hypotension, coma, convulsions, respiratory depression, sluggish reflexes, pyrexia and diaphoresis; these signs may persist for 8 to 14 days. General supportive measures should be employed, along with immediate gastric lavage or emetics. If the latter are given, the danger of aspiration must be borne in mind. An adequate airway should be maintained, with supplemental oxygen if necessary. The mechanism by which amine-oxidase inhibitors produce hypotension is not fully understood, but there is evidence that these agents block the vascular bed response. Thus it is suggested that plasma may be of value in the management of this hypotension. Administration of pressor amines such as Levophed® (levarterenol bitartrate) may be of limited value (note that their effects may be potentiated by Marplan). Continue treatment for several days until homeostasis is restored. Liver function studies are recommended during the 4 to 6 weeks after recovery, as well as at the time of overdosage. As with the management of intentional overdosage with any drug, it should be borne in mind that multiple agents may have been ingested.

HOW SUPPLIED

Tablets, 10 mg isocarboxazid/Roche each, peach-colored, scored—bottles of 100.

Shown in Product Identification Section, page 425

MATULANE® ℞

[mat'u-lane]

procarbazine hydrochloride/Roche

The following text is complete prescribing information based on official labeling in effect July 1, 1986.

WARNING

It is recommended that MATULANE be given only by or under the supervision of a physician experienced in the use of potent antineoplastic drugs. Adequate clinical and laboratory facilities should be available to patients for proper monitoring of treatment.

DESCRIPTION

Matulane (procarbazine hydrochloride/Roche), a hydrazine derivative antineoplastic agent, is available as capsules containing the equivalent of 50 mg procarbazine as the hydrochloride. Each capsule also contains corn starch, mannitol and talc. Gelatin capsule shells contain parabens (methyl and propyl), potassium sorbate, titanium dioxide, FD&C Yellow No. 6 and D&C Yellow No. 10.

Chemically, procarbazine hydrochloride is *N*-isopropyl-*α*-(2-methylhydrazino)-*p*-toluamide monohydrochloride. It is a white to pale yellow crystalline powder which is soluble but unstable in water or aqueous solutions. The molecular weight of procarbazine hydrochloride is 257.76.

CLINICAL PHARMACOLOGY

The precise mode of cytotoxic action of procarbazine has not been clearly defined. There is evidence that the drug may act by inhibition of protein, RNA and DNA synthesis. Studies have suggested that procarbazine may inhibit transmethylation of methyl groups of methionine into t-RNA. The absence of functional t-RNA could cause the cessation of protein synthesis and consequently DNA and RNA synthesis. In addition, procarbazine may directly damage DNA. Hydrogen peroxide, formed during the auto-oxidation of the drug, may attack protein sulfhydryl groups contained in residual protein which is tightly bound to DNA.

Procarbazine is metabolized primarily in the liver and kidneys. The drug appears to be auto-oxidized to the azo derivative with the release of hydrogen peroxide. The azo derivative isomerizes to the hydrazone, and following hydrolysis splits into a benzylaldehyde derivative and methylhydrazine. The methylhydrazine is further degraded to CO_2 and CH_4 and possibly hydrazine, whereas the aldehyde is oxidized to the isopropylamide of terephthalic acid, which is excreted in the urine.

Procarbazine is rapidly and completely absorbed. Following oral administration of 30 mg of ^{14}C-labeled procarbazine, maximum peak plasma radioactive concentrations were reached within 60 minutes.

After intravenous injection, the plasma half-life of procarbazine is approximately 10 minutes. Approximately 70% of the radioactivity is excreted in the urine as *N*-isopropylterephthalamic acid within 24 hours following both oral and intravenous administration of ^{14}C-labeled procarbazine.

Procarbazine crosses the blood-brain barrier and rapidly equilibrates between plasma and cerebrospinal fluid after oral administration.

INDICATIONS AND USAGE

Matulane is indicated for use in combination with other anticancer drugs for the treatment of Stage III and IV Hodgkin's disease. Matulane is used as part of the MOPP (nitrogen mustard, vincristine, procarbazine, prednisone) regimen.

CONTRAINDICATIONS

Matulane is contraindicated in patients with known hypersensitivity to the drug or inadequate marrow reserve as demonstrated by bone marrow aspiration. Due consideration of this possible state should be given to each patient who has leukopenia, thrombocytopenia or anemia.

WARNINGS

To minimize CNS depression and possible potentiation, barbiturates, antihistamines, narcotics, hypotensive agents or phenothiazines should be used with caution. Ethyl alcohol should not be used since there may be an Antabuse (disulfiram)-like reaction. Because Matulane exhibits some monoamine oxidase inhibitory activity, sympathomimetic drugs, tricyclic antidepressant drugs (e.g., amitriptyline HCl, imipramine HCl) and other drugs and foods with known high tyramine content, such as wine, yogurt, ripe cheese and bananas, should be avoided. A further phenomenon of toxicity common to many hydrazine derivatives is hemolysis and the appearance of Heinz-Ehrlich inclusion bodies in erythrocytes.

Pregnancy: Teratogenic effects: Pregnancy Category D. Procarbazine hydrochloride can cause fetal harm when administered to a pregnant woman. While there are no adequate and well-controlled studies with procarbazine hydrochloride in pregnant women, there are case reports of malformations in the offspring of women who were exposed to procarbazine hydrochloride in combination with other antineoplastic agents during pregnancy. Matulane should be used during pregnancy only if the potential benefit justifies the potential risk to the fetus. If this drug is used during pregnancy, or if the patient becomes pregnant while taking this drug, the patient should be apprised of the potential hazard to the fetus. Women of childbearing potential should be advised to avoid becoming pregnant. Procarbazine hydrochloride is teratogenic in the rat when given at doses approximately 4 to 13 times the maximum recommended human therapeutic dose of 6 mg/kg/day.

Nonteratogenic effects: Procarbazine hydrochloride has not been adequately studied in animals for its effect on peri- and postnatal development. However, neurogenic tumors were noted in the offspring of rats given intravenous injections of 125 mg/kg of procarbazine hydrochloride on day 22 of gestation. Compounds which inhibit DNA, RNA and protein synthesis might be expected to have adverse effects on peri- and postnatal development.

Carcinogenesis, mutagenesis and impairment of fertility: Carcinogenesis: The carcinogenicity of procarbazine hydrochloride in mice, rats and monkeys has been reported in a considerable number of studies. Instances of a second nonlymphoid malignancy, including acute myelocytic leukemia, have been reported in patients with Hodgkin's disease

Continued on next page

Roche Labs.—Cont.

treated with procarbazine in combination with other chemotherapy and/or radiation. The International Agency for Research on Cancer (IARC) considers that there is "sufficient evidence" for the human carcinogenicity of procarbazine hydrochloride when it is given in intensive regimens which include other antineoplastic agents but that there is inadequate evidence of carcinogenicity in humans given procarbazine hydrochloride alone.
Mutagenesis: Procarbazine hydrochloride has been shown to be mutagenic in a variety of bacterial and mammalian test systems.
Impairment of fertility: Azoospermia and antifertility effects associated with procarbazine hydrochloride administration in combination with other chemotherapeutic agents for treating Hodgkin's disease have been reported in human clinical studies. Since these patients received multicombinaion therapy, it is difficult to determine to what extent procarbazine hydrochloride alone was involved in the male germ-cell damage. The usual Segment I fertility/reproduction studies in laboratory animals have not been carried out with procarbazine hydrochloride. However, compounds which inhibit DNA, RNA and/or protein synthesis might be expected to have adverse effects on gametogenesis. Unscheduled DNA synthesis in the testis of rabbits and decreased fertility in male mice treated with procarbazine hydrochloride have been reported.

PRECAUTIONS

General: Undue toxicity may occur if Matulane is used in patients with impairment of renal and/or hepatic function. When appropriate, hospitalization for the initial course of treatment should be considered.
If radiation or a chemotherapeutic agent known to have marrow-depressant activity has been used, an interval of one month or longer without such therapy is recommended before starting treatment with Matulane. The length of this interval may also be determined by evidence of bone marrow recovery based on successive bone marrow studies.
Prompt cessation of therapy is recommended if any one of the following occurs:

Central nervous system signs or symptoms such as paresthesias, neuropathies or confusion.
Leukopenia (white blood count under 4000).
Thrombocytopenia (platelets under 100,000).
Hypersensitivity reaction.
Stomatitis—The first small ulceration or persistent spot soreness around the oral cavity is a signal for cessation of therapy.
Diarrhea—Frequent bowel movements or watery stools.
Hemorrhage or bleeding tendencies.

Bone marrow depression often occurs 2 to 8 weeks after the start of treatment. If leukopenia occurs, hospitalization of the patient may be needed for appropriate treatment to prevent systemic infection.
Information for patients: Patients should be warned not to drink alcoholic beverages while on Matulane therapy since there may be an Antabuse (disulfiram)-like reaction. They should also be cautioned to avoid foods with known high tyramine content such as wine, yogurt, ripe cheese and bananas. Over-the-counter drug preparations which contain antihistamines or sympathomimetic drugs should also be avoided. Patients taking Matulane should also be warned against the use of prescription drugs without the knowledge and consent of their physician.
Laboratory tests: Baseline laboratory data should be obtained prior to initiation of therapy. The hematologic status as indicated by hemoglobin, hematocrit, white blood count (WBC), differential, reticulocytes and platelets should be monitored closely—at least every 3 or 4 days.
Hepatic and renal evaluation are indicated prior to beginning therapy. Urinalysis, transaminase, alkaline phosphatase and blood urea nitrogen tests should be repeated at least weekly.
Drug interactions: See WARNINGS section.
No cross-resistance with other chemotherapeutic agents, radiotherapy or steroids has been demonstrated.
Carcinogenesis, mutagenesis and impairment of fertility: See WARNINGS section.
Pregnancy: Pregnancy Category D. See WARNINGS section.
Nursing mothers: It is not known whether Matulane is excreted in human milk. Because of the potential for tumorigenicity shown for procarbazine hydrochloride in animal studies, mothers should not nurse while receiving this drug.

ADVERSE REACTIONS

Leukopenia, anemia and thrombopenia occur frequently. Nausea and vomiting are the most commonly reported side effects.
Other adverse reactions are:
Hematologic: Pancytopenia; eosinophilia; hemolytic anemia; bleeding tendencies such as petechiae, purpura, epistaxis and hemoptysis.
Gastrointestinal: Hepatic dysfunction, jaundice, stomatitis, hematemesis, melena, diarrhea, dysphagia, anorexia, abdominal pain, constipation, dry mouth.
Neurologic: Coma, convulsions, neuropathy, ataxia, paresthesia, nystagmus, diminished reflexes, falling, foot drop, headache, dizziness, unsteadiness.
Cardiovascular: Hypotension, tachycardia, syncope.
Ophthalmic: Retinal hemorrhage, papilledema, photophobia, diplopia, inability to focus.
Respiratory: Pneumonitis, pleural effusion, cough.
Dermatologic: Herpes, dermatitis, pruritus, alopecia, hyperpigmentation, rash, urticaria, flushing.
Allergic: Generalized allergic reactions.
Genitourinary: Hematuria, urinary frequency, nocturia.
Musculoskeletal: Pain, including myalgia and arthralgia; tremors.
Psychiatric: Hallucinations, depressions, apprehension, nervousness, confusion, nightmares.
Endocrine: Gynecomastia in prepubertal and early pubertal boys.
Miscellaneous: Intercurrent infections, hearing loss, pyrexia, diaphoresis, lethargy, weakness, fatigue, edema, chills, insomnia, slurred speech, hoarseness, drowsiness.
Second nonlymphoid malignancies, including acute myelocytic leukemia and malignant myelosclerosis and azoospermia have been reported in patients with Hodgkin's disease treated with procarbazine in combination with other chemotherapy and/or radiation.

OVERDOSAGE

The major manifestations of overdosage with Matulane would be anticipated to be nausea, vomiting, enteritis, diarrhea, hypotension, tremors, convulsions and coma. Treatment should consist of either the administration of an emetic or gastric lavage. General supportive measures such as intravenous fluids are advised. Since the major toxicity of procarbazine hydrochloride is hematologic and hepatic, patients should have frequent complete blood counts and liver function tests throughout their period of recovery and for a minimum of two weeks thereafter. Should abnormalities appear in any of these determinations, appropriate measures for correction and stabilization should be immediately undertaken.
The estimated mean lethal dose of procarbazine hydrochloride in laboratory animals varied from approximately 150 mg/kg in rabbits to 1300 mg/kg in mice.

DOSAGE AND ADMINISTRATION

The following doses are for administration of the drug as a single agent. When used in combination with other anticancer drugs, the Matulane dose should be appropriately reduced, e.g., in the MOPP regimen, the Matulane dose is 100 mg/m^2 daily for 14 days. All dosages are based on the patient's actual weight. However, the estimated lean body mass (dry weight) is used if the patient is obese or if there has been a spurious weight gain due to edema, ascites or other forms of abnormal fluid retention.
Adults —To minimize the nausea and vomiting experienced by a high percentage of patients beginning Matulane therapy, single or divided doses of 2 to 4 mg/kg/day for the first week are recommended. Daily dosage should then be maintained at 4 to 6 mg/kg/day until maximum response is obtained or until the white blood count falls below 4000/cmm or the platelets fall below 100,000/cmm. When maximum response is obtained, the dose may be maintained at 1 to 2 mg/kg/day. Upon evidence of hematologic or other toxicity (see PRECAUTIONS section), the drug should be discontinued until there has been satisfactory recovery. After toxic side effects have subsided, therapy may then be resumed at the discretion of the physician, based on clinical evaluation and appropriate laboratory studies, at a dosage of 1 to 2 mg/kg/day.
Children —Very close clinical monitoring is mandatory. Undue toxicity, evidenced by tremors, coma and convulsions, has occurred in a few cases. Dosage, therefore, should be individualized. The following dosage schedule is provided as a guideline only.
Fifty (50) mg per square meter of body surface per day is recommended for the first week. Dosage should then be maintained at 100 mg per square meter of body surface per day until maximum response is obtained or until leukopenia or thrombocytopenia occurs. When maximum response is attained, the dose may be maintained at 50 mg per square meter of body surface per day. Upon evidence of hematologic or other toxicity (see PRECAUTIONS section), the drug should be discontinued until there has been satisfactory recovery, based on clinical evaluation and appropriate laboratory tests. After toxic side effects have subsided, therapy may then be resumed.

HOW SUPPLIED

Capsules, ivory, containing the equivalent of 50 mg procarbazine as the hydrochloride; bottles of 100 (NDC 0004-0053-01). Imprint on capsules: MATULANE® ROCHE.

Shown in Product Identification Section, page 425

MESTINON® INJECTABLE ℞

[mes'tin-on]
(pyridostigmine bromide/Roche)

The following text is complete prescribing information based on official labeling in effect June 1, 1986.

DESCRIPTION

Mestinon Injectable is an active cholinesterase inhibitor. Chemically, pyridostigmine bromide is 3-hydroxy-1-methylpyridinium bromide dimethylcarbamate.
Each ml contains 5 mg pyridostigmine bromide/ Roche compounded with 0.2% parabens (methyl and propyl) as preservatives, 0.02% sodium citrate and pH adjusted to approximately 5.0 with citric acid and, if necessary, sodium hydroxide.

ACTIONS

Mestinon facilitates the transmission of impulses across the myoneural junction by inhibiting the destruction of acetylcholine by cholinesterase. Pyridostigmine is an analog of neostigmine (Prostigmin®) but differs from it clinically by having fewer side effects. Currently available data indicate that pyridostigmine may have a significantly lower degree and incidence of bradycardia, salivation and gastrointestinal stimulation. Animal studies using the injectable form of pyridostigmine and human studies using the oral preparation have indicated that pyridostigmine has a longer duration of action than does neostigmine measured under similar circumstances.

INDICATIONS

Mestinon Injectable is useful in the treatment of myasthenia gravis and as a reversal agent or antagonist to nondepolarizing muscle relaxants such as curariform drugs and gallamine triethiodide.

CONTRAINDICATIONS

Known hypersensitivity to anticholinesterase agents; intestinal and urinary obstructions of mechanical type.

WARNINGS

Mestinon Injectable should be used with particular caution in patients with bronchial asthma or cardiac dysrhythmias. Transient bradycardia may occur and be relieved by atropine sulfate. Atropine should also be used with caution in patients with cardiac dysrhythmias. When large doses of Mestinon are administered, as during reversal of muscle relaxants, the prior or simultaneous injection of atropine sulfate is advisable. Because of the possibility of hypersensitivity in an occasional patient, atropine and antishock medication should always be readily available.
As is true of all cholinergic drugs, overdosage of Mestinon may result in cholinergic crisis, a state characterized by increasing muscle weakness which, through involvement of the muscles of respiration, may lead to death. Myasthenic crisis due to an increase in the severity of the disease is also accompanied by extreme muscle weakness and thus may be difficult to distinguish from cholinergic crisis on a symptomatic basis. Such differentiation is extremely important, since increases in doses of Mestinon or other drugs in this class in the presence of cholinergic crisis or of a refractory or "insensitive" state could have grave consequences. Osserman and Genkins[1] indicate that the two types of crisis may be differentiated by the use of Tensilon® (edrophonium chloride) as well as by clinical judgment. The treatment of the two conditions obviously differs radically. Whereas the presence of *myasthenic crisis* requires more intensive anticholinesterase therapy, *cholinergic crisis,* according to Osserman and Genkins,[1] calls for the prompt withdrawal of all drugs of this type. The immediate use of atropine in cholinergic crisis is also recommended. A syringe containing 1 mg of atropine sulfate should be immediately available to be given in aliquots intravenously to counteract severe cholinergic reactions.
Atropine may also be used to abolish or obtund gastrointestinal side effects or other muscarinic reactions; but such use, by masking signs of overdosage, can lead to inadvertent induction of cholinergic crisis.
For detailed information on the management of patients with myasthenia gravis, the physician is referred to one of the excellent reviews such as those by Osserman and Genkins,[2] Grob[3] or Schwab.[4,5]
When used as an antagonist to nondepolarizing muscle relaxants, adequate recovery of voluntary respiration and neuromuscular transmission must be obtained prior to discontinuation of respiratory assistance and there should be continuous patient observation. Satisfactory recovery may be defined by a combination of clinical judgment, respiratory measurements and observation of the effects of peripheral nerve stimulation. If there is any doubt concerning the adequacy of recovery from the effects of the nondepolarizing muscle relaxant, artificial ventilation should be continued until all doubt has been removed.
Usage in Pregnancy: The safety of Mestinon during pregnancy or lactation in humans has not been established. Therefore, use of Mestinon in women who may become preg-

nant requires weighing the drug's potential benefits against its possible hazards to mother and child.

ADVERSE REACTIONS

The side effects of Mestinon are most commonly related to overdosage and generally are of two varieties, muscarinic and nicotinic. Among those in the former group are nausea, vomiting, diarrhea, abdominal cramps, increased peristalsis, increased salivation, increased bronchial secretions, miosis and diaphoresis. Nicotinic side effects are comprised chiefly of muscle cramps, fasciculation and weakness. Muscarinic side effects can usually be counteracted by atropine, but for reasons shown in the preceding section the expedient is not without danger. As with any compound containing the bromide radical, a skin rash may be seen in an occasional patient. Such reactions usually subside promptly upon discontinuance of the medication. Thrombophlebitis has been reported subsequent to intravenous administration.

DOSAGE AND ADMINISTRATION

For Myasthenia Gravis—To supplement oral dosage, pre- and postoperatively, during labor and postpartum, during myasthenic crisis, or whenever oral therapy is impractical, approximately 1/30th of the oral dose of Mestinon may be given parenterally, either by intramuscular or *very slow* intravenous injection. *The patient must be closely observed for cholinergic reactions, particularly if the intravenous route is used.*

For details regarding the management of myasthenic patients who are to undergo major surgical procedures, see the article by Foldes.[6]

Neonates of myasthenic mothers may have transient difficulty in swallowing, sucking and breathing. Injectable Mestinon may be indicated—by symptomatology and use of the Tensilon® (edrophonium chloride) test—until Mestinon Syrup can be taken. To date the world literature consists of less than 100 neonate patients.[7] Of these only 5 were treated with injectable pyridostigmine, with the vast majority of the remaining neonates receiving neostigmine. Dosage requirements of Mestinon Injectable are minute, ranging from 0.05 mg to 0.15 mg/kg of body weight given intramuscularly. It is important to differentiate between cholinergic and myasthenic crises in neonates. (See WARNINGS.)

Mestinon given parenterally one hour before completion of second stage labor enables patients to have adequate strength during labor and provides protection to infants in the immediate postnatal state. For further information on the use of Mestinon Injectable in neonates of myasthenic mothers, see the article by Namba.[7]

NOTE: For information on a diagnostic test for myasthenia gravis, and on the evaluation and stabilization of therapy, please see product information on Tensilon® (edrophonium chloride/Roche).

For Reversal of Nondepolarizing Muscle Relaxants: When Mestinon Injectable is given intravenously to reverse the action of muscle relaxant drugs, it is recommended that atropine sulfate (0.6 to 1.2 mg) also be given intravenously immediately prior to the Mestinon. Side effects, notably excessive secretions and bradycardia, are thereby minimized. Usually 10 or 20 mg of Mestinon will be sufficient for antagonism of the effects of the nondepolarizing muscle relaxants. Although full recovery may occur within 15 minutes in most patients, others may require a half hour or more. Satisfactory reversal can be evident by adequate voluntary respiration, respiratory measurements and use of a peripheral nerve stimulator device. It is recommended that the patient be well ventilated and a patent airway maintained until complete recovery of normal respiration is assured. Once satisfactory reversal has been attained, recurarization has not been reported. For additional information on the use of Mestinon for antagonism of nondepolarizing muscle relaxants see the article by Katz[8] and McNall.[9]

Failure of Mestinon Injectable to provide prompt (within 30 minutes) reversal may occur, *e.g.,* in the presence of extreme debilitation, carcinomatosis, or with concomitant use of certain broad spectrum antibiotics or anesthetic agents, notably ether. Under these circumstances ventilation must be supported by artificial means until the patient has resumed control of his respiration.

HOW SUPPLIED

Mestinon is available in 2-ml ampuls (boxes of 10).

REFERENCES

1. K. E. Osserman and G. Genkins, *J.A.M.A. 183:* 97, 1963.
2. K. E. Osserman and G. Genkins, *New York State J. Med., 61:* 2076, 1961.
3. D. Grob, *Arch. Intern. Med., 108:* 615, 1961.
4. R. S. Schwab, *New Eng. J. Med., 268:* 596, 1963.
5. R. S. Schwab, *New Eng. J. Med., 268:* 717, 1963.
6. F. F. Foldes and P. McNall, *Anesthesiology, 23:* 837, 1962.
7. T. Namba *et al., Pediatrics, 45:* 488, 1970.
8. R. L. Katz, *Anesthesiology, 28:* 528, 1967.
9. P. McNall *et al., Anesthesia and Analgesia, 48:* 1026, 1969.

MESTINON® ℞

[mes'tin-on]
(pyridostigmine bromide/Roche)
TABLETS and SYRUP
TIMESPAN® TABLETS

The following text is complete prescribing information based on official labeling in effect June 1, 1986.

DESCRIPTION

Mestinon is an orally active cholinesterase inhibitor. Chemically, pyridostigmine bromide is 3-hydroxy-1-methylpyridinium bromide dimethylcarbamate.

Mestinon is available in the following forms: Syrup containing 60 mg pyridostigmine bromide per teaspoonful in a vehicle containing 5% alcohol, glycerin, lactic acid, sodium benzoate, sorbitol, sucrose, FD&C Red No. 40, FD&C Blue No. 1, flavors and water. *Tablets* containing 60 mg pyridostigmine bromide; each tablet also contains lactose, silicon dioxide and stearic acid. *Timespan Tablets* containing 180 mg pyridostigmine bromide; each tablet also contains carnauba wax, corn-derived proteins, magnesium stearate, silica gel and tribasic calcium phosphate.

ACTIONS

Mestinon inhibits the destruction of acetylcholine by cholinesterase and thereby permits freer transmission of nerve impulses across the neuromuscular junction. Pyridostigmine is an analog of neostigmine (Prostigmin®), but differs from it in certain clinically significant respects; for example, pyridostigmine is characterized by a longer duration of action and fewer gastrointestinal side effects.

INDICATION

Mestinon is useful in the treatment of myasthenia gravis.

CONTRAINDICATIONS

Mestinon is contraindicated in mechanical intestinal or urinary obstruction, and particular caution should be used in its administration to patients with bronchial asthma. Care should be observed in the use of atropine for counteracting side effects, as discussed below.

WARNINGS

Although failure of patients to show clinical improvement may reflect underdosage, it can also be indicative of overdosage. As is true of all cholinergic drugs, overdosage of Mestinon may result in cholinergic crisis, a state characterized by increasing muscle weakness which, through involvement of the muscles of respiration, may lead to death. Myasthenic crisis due to an increase in the severity of the disease is also accompanied by extreme muscle weakness, and thus may be difficult to distinguish from cholinergic crisis on a symptomatic basis. Such differentiation is extremely important, since increases in doses of Mestinon or other drugs of this class in the presence of cholinergic crisis or of a refractory or "insensitive" state could have grave consequences. Osserman and Genkins[1] indicate that the differential diagnosis of the two types of crisis may require the use of Tensilon® (edrophonium chloride/Roche) as well as clinical judgment. The treatment of the two conditions obviously differs radically. Whereas the presence of myasthenic crisis suggests the need for more intensive anticholinesterase therapy, the diagnosis of cholinergic crisis, according to Osserman and Genkins,[1] calls for the prompt *withdrawal* of all drugs of this type. The immediate use of atropine in cholinergic crisis is also recommended.

Atropine may also be used to abolish or obtund gastrointestinal side effects or other muscarinic reactions; but such use, by masking signs of overdosage, can lead to inadvertent induction of cholinergic crisis.

For detailed information on the management of patients with myasthenia gravis, the physician is referred to one of the excellent reviews such as those by Osserman and Genkins,[2] Grob[3] or Schwab.[4,5]

Usage in Pregnancy: The safety of Mestinon during pregnancy or lactation in humans has not been established. Therefore, use of Mestinon in women who may become pregnant requires weighing the drug's potential benefits against its possible hazards to mother and child.

ADVERSE REACTIONS

The side effects of Mestinon are most commonly related to overdosage and generally are of two varieties, muscarinic and nicotinic. Among those in the former group are nausea, vomiting, diarrhea, abdominal cramps, increased peristalsis, increased salivation, increased bronchial secretions, miosis and diaphoresis. Nicotinic side effects are comprised chiefly of muscle cramps, fasciculation and weakness. Muscarinic side effects can usually be counteracted by atropine, but for reasons shown in the preceding section the expedient is not without danger. As with any compound containing the bromide radical, a skin rash may be seen in an occasional patient. Such reactions usually subside promptly upon discontinuance of the medication.

DOSAGE AND ADMINISTRATION

Mestinon is available in three dosage forms:

Syrup—raspberry-flavored, containing 60 mg pyridostigmine bromide per teaspoonful (5 ml). This form permits accurate dosage adjustment for children and "brittle" myasthenic patients who require fractions of 60-mg doses. It is more easily swallowed, especially in the morning, by patients with bulbar involvement.

Conventional tablets—each containing 60 mg pyridostigmine bromide.

Timespan tablets—each containing 180 mg pyridostigmine bromide. This form provides uniformly slow release, hence prolonged duration of drug action; it facilitates control of myasthenic symptoms with fewer individual doses daily. The immediate effect of a 180-mg Timespan tablet is about equal to that of a 60-mg conventional tablet; however, its duration of effectiveness, although varying in individual patients, averages 2½ times that of a 60-mg dose.

Dosage: The size and frequency of the dosage must be adjusted to the needs of the individual patient.

Syrup and conventional tablets—The average dose is ten 60-mg tablets or ten 5-ml teaspoonfuls daily, spaced to provide maximum relief when maximum strength is needed. In severe cases as many as 25 tablets or teaspoonfuls a day may be required, while in mild cases one to six tablets or teaspoonfuls a day may suffice.

Timespan tablets—One to three 180-mg tablets, once or twice daily, will usually be sufficient to control symptoms; however, the needs of certain individuals may vary markedly from this average. The interval between doses should be at least six hours. For optimum control, it may be necessary to use the more rapidly acting regular tablets or syrup in conjunction with Timespan therapy.

Note: For information on a diagnostic test for myasthenia gravis, and for the evaluation and stabilization of therapy, please see product literature on Tensilon® (edrophonium chloride/Roche).

HOW SUPPLIED

Syrup, 60 mg pyridostigmine bromide per teaspoonful (5 ml) and 5% alcohol—bottles of 16 fluid ounces (1 pint).

Tablets, scored, 60 mg pyridostigmine bromide each—bottles of 100 and 500.

Timespan tablets, scored, 180 mg pyridostigmine bromide each—bottles of 100.

Note: Because of the hygroscopic nature of the Timespan tablets, mottling may occur. This does not affect their efficacy.

REFERENCES

1. K. E. Osserman and G. Genkins, *J.A.M.A., 183:* 97, 1963.
2. K. E. Osserman and G. Genkins, *New York State J. Med., 61* :2076, 1961.
3. D. Grob, *Arch. Int. Med., 108* :615, 1961.
4. R. S. Schwab, *New England J. Med., 268* :596, 1963.
5. R. S. Schwab, *New England J. Med., 268* :717, 1963.

Shown in Product Identification Section, page 425

NIPRIDE® ℞

[ny'pryde]
(sodium nitroprusside/Roche)

The following text is complete prescribing information based on official labeling in effect June 1, 1986.

Nipride is to be used only as an infusion with sterile 5% dextrose in water. Not for direct injection.
Nipride should be used only when the necessary facilities and equipment for continuous monitoring of blood pressure are available.
If at infusion rates of up to 10 mcg/kg/minute, an adequate reduction of blood pressure is not obtained within 10 minutes, administration of Nipride should be terminated.
As metabolic acidosis is the earliest and most reliable evidence of cyanide toxicty, blood pH and acid base balance should be determined frequently in all patients and, particularly, if there is increased tolerance to the drug.
The instructions herein should be reviewed thoroughly before administration of Nipride.

DESCRIPTION

Nipride (sodium nitroprusside/Roche), a hypotensive agent, is available as a sterile powder for reconstitution and dilution in sterile 5% dextrose in water to be used only for intravenous infusion. Each 5-ml vial contains the equivalent of 50 mg of sodium nitroprusside dihydrate. Chemically, sodium nitroprusside is disodium pentacyanonitrosylferrate(2-) dihydrate. It is a reddish-brown powder which is soluble in

Continued on next page

Roche Labs.—Cont.

water. In aqueous solution, it is photosensitive and should be protected from light. It has a molecular weight of 297.95.

CLINICAL PHARMACOLOGY

Nipride is a potent immediate-acting, intravenous hypotensive agent. The active component of sodium nitroprusside is the free nitroso (NO) group, not its metabolites. The onset of Nipride's hypotensive activity is observed within 0.5 to 5 minutes of initiation of intravenous infusion. The intensity of the pharmacodynamic response is related to the infusion rate; whereas the duration of action continues only as long as the infusion is maintained. Blood pressure returns to pretreatment levels within one to ten minutes after cessation of the infusion.

It has been demonstrated in animals that sodium nitroprusside acts on the excitation-contraction coupling of vascular smooth muscle by interfering with both influx and the intracellular activation of calcium without affecting cAMP, ATP or the contractile proteins. No relaxation is seen in the smooth muscle of the uterus or duodenum *in situ* in animals.

Nitroprusside is rapidly metabolized to cyanide and thiocyanate through a reaction with hemoglobin, yielding methemoglobin and an unstable intermediate which dissociates, releasing cyanide. The major elimination pathway of cyanide is by conversion in the liver and kidney to thiocyanate which requires the enzyme rhodanase. Other pathways include the formulation of biologically inert cyanmethemoglobin and cyanocobalamin. Cyanocobalamin is formed by the complexing of cyanide with hydroxocobalamin. The rate of conversion from cyanide to thiocyanate is dependent on the availability of sulfur, usually thiosulfate.

Because of its rapid decomposition in the presence of red blood cells, plasma concentrations of nitroprusside cannot be determined. Nitroprusside is not excreted intact. Animal studies indicate that some metabolites are excreted in urine, some are exhaled and others may be present in the feces since the thiocyanate ion can be detected in saliva and gastric juice. Thiocyanate, the major metabolite of sodium nitroprusside, is largely excreted through the kidneys.

The passage of nitroprusside through the blood-brain or placental barriers or excretion in breast milk have not been determined.

Sodium nitroprusside administered by infusion to hypertensive and normotensive patients produced a marked lowering of arterial blood pressure, slight increase in heart rate, a mild decrease in cardiac output and a moderate diminution in calculated total peripheral vascular resistance.

The decrease in calculated total peripheral vascular resistance suggests arteriolar vasodilatation. The decreases in cardiac and stroke index noted may be due to peripheral vascular pooling of blood.

In hypertensive patients, moderate depressor doses induce renal vasodilatation roughly equivalent to the decrease in pressure without an appreciable increase in renal blood flow or a decrease in glomerular filtration.

In normotensive subjects, acute reduction of mean arterial pressure to 60 to 75 mmHg by infusion of sodium nitroprusside caused a significant increase in renin activity of renal venous plasma in correlation with the degree of reduction in pressure. Renal response to reduction in pressure was more striking in renovascular hypertensive patients with significant increase in renin release occurring from the involved kidney at mean arterial pressures ranging from 90 to 137 mmHg. Furthermore, the magnitude of renin release from the involved kidney was significantly greater when compared with that in normotensive subjects, while in the contralateral, uninvolved kidney, no significant release of renin was detected during the reduction of pressure.

INDICATIONS AND USAGE

Nipride is indicated for the immediate reduction of blood pressure of patients in hypertensive crises. Concomitant oral antihypertensive medication should be started while the hypertensive emergency is being brought under control with Nipride. There is no contraindication in using Nipride simultaneously with oral antihypertensive medications.

Nipride is also indicated for producing controlled hypotension during anesthesia in order to reduce bleeding in surgical procedures when the surgeon and anesthesiologist deem it appropriate.

CONTRAINDICATIONS

Nipride should not be used in the treatment of compensatory hypertension, *e.g.,* arteriovenous shunt or coarctation of the aorta.

The use of Nipride to produce controlled hypotension during surgery is contraindicated in patients with known inadequate cerebral circulation. Nipride is not intended for use during emergency surgery in moribund patients (A.S.A. Class 5E).

WARNINGS

> If excessive amounts of Nipride are used and/or sulfur—usually thiosulfate—supplies are depleted, cyanide toxicity can occur. See OVERDOSAGE section.
>
> If sodium nitroprusside infusion is to be extended, particularly if renal impairment is present, close attention should be given to not exceeding the recommended maximum infusion rate of 10 mcg/kg/minute. If in the course of therapy increased tolerance to the drug (as shown by the need for a higher infusion rate) develops, it is essential to monitor blood acid-base balance, as metabolic acidosis is the earliest and most reliable evidence of cyanide toxicity. If signs of metabolic acidosis appear, Nipride should be discontinued and an alternate drug administered.
>
> Plasma thiocyanate concentrations do not reflect cyanide toxicity (see subsequent Warning concerning thiocyanate toxicity).

Some patients may fail to respond to adequate Nipride administration. Since failure to respond to Nipride may represent associated increase in free cyanide, appearance of increased tolerance to the drug constitutes reason for discontinuing Nipride and promptly instituting alternate therapy.

Prolonged use of sodium nitroprusside may result in excessive thiocyanate formation. Thiocyanate accumulation and toxicity can manifest itself as tinnitus, blurred vision, mental confusion, psychotic behavior, convulsions, delirium, lactic acidosis, bone marrow depression, and hypothyroidism. Plasma thiocyanate concentrations should be monitored daily in any patient receiving therapy for longer than 48 hours, especially in patients with renal or hepatic impairment. Plasma thiocyanate levels above 10 mg/100 ml have been considered toxic and levels of 20 mg/100 ml have been judged fatal.

Since cyanide is converted into thiocyanate through the mediation of a hepatic enzyme, rhodanase, Nipride should be used with caution in patients with hepatic insufficiency.

Since thiocyanate inhibits both the uptake and binding of iodine, caution should be exercised in using Nipride in patients with hypothyroidism or severe renal impairment.

Hypertensive patients are more sensitive to the intravenous effect of sodium nitroprusside than are normotensive subjects. Patients who are receiving concomitant antihypertensive medications are more sensitive to the hypotensive effect of sodium nitroprusside and the dosage of Nipride should be adjusted accordingly.

The following warnings apply to the use of Nipride for controlled hypotension during anesthesia:

1. Tolerance to blood loss, anemia and hypovolemia may be diminished. If possible, prexisting anemia and hypovolemia should be corrected prior to employing controlled hypotension.
2. Hypotensive anesthetic techniques may alter pulmonary ventilation perfusion ratio. Patients intolerant of additional dead air space at ordinary oxygen partial pressure may benefit from higher oxygen partial pressure.
3. Extreme caution should be exercised in patients who are especially poor surgical risks (A.S.A. Class 4 and 4E).

Nipride is to be used only as an infusion with sterile 5% dextrose in water. Not for direct injection.

Infusion rates greater than 10 mcg/kg/minute are rarely required. If, at this rate, an adequate reduction in blood pressure is not obtained within 10 minutes, administration of Nipride should be stopped. Tachyphylaxis has been reported during Nipride usage, particularly when used in dosages higher than 10 mcg/kg/minute. Should this occur, immediately discontinue the administration of Nipride.

PRECAUTIONS

General: Adequate facilities, equipment and personnel should be available for frequent and vigilant monitoring of blood pressure, since the hypotensive effect of Nipride occurs rapidly. When the infusion is slowed or stopped, blood pressure usually begins to rise immediately and returns to pretreatment levels within one to ten minutes. It should be used with caution and initially in low doses in elderly patients since they may be more sensitive to the hypotensive effects of the drug. Young, vigorous males may require somewhat larger than ordinary doses of sodium nitroprusside for hypotensive anesthesia; however, the infusion rate of 10 mcg/kg/minute should not be exceeded. Deepening of anesthesia, if indicated, might permit satisfactory conditions to exist within the recommended dosage range.

Because of the rapid onset of action and potency of Nipride, it should preferably be administered with the use of an infusion pump, micro-drip regulator, or any similar device that would allow precise measurement of the flow rate.

Laboratory tests: See WARNINGS section.

Drug interactions: Patients receiving other antihypertensive medications appear to be more sensitive to the effects of sodium nitroprusside and may require lower doses of Nipride.

The hypotensive effect of Nipride is augmented by ganglionic blocking agents, volatile liquid anesthetics (such as halothane and enflurane) and by most other circulatory depressants.

Carcinogenesis, mutagenesis, impairment of fertility: Nipride has not undergone adequate carcinogenicity testing in animals. The mutagenic potential of Nipride has not been assessed. Nipride has not been tested for effects on fertility.

Pregnancy: Teratogenic effects: Pregnancy Category C. There are no adequate or well-controlled studies of Nipride in either laboratory animals or pregnant women. It is not known whether Nipride can cause fetal harm when administered to a pregnant woman or can affect reproductive capacity. Nipride should be given to a pregnant woman only if clearly needed.

Nonteratogenic effects: In three studies in pregnant ewes, nitroprusside was shown to cross the placental barrier. Fetal cyanide levels were shown to be dose-related to maternal levels of nitroprusside. The metabolic transformation of sodium nitroprusside given to pregnant ewes led to fatal levels of cyanide in the fetuses. The infusion of 25 mcg/kg/minute of sodium nitroprusside for one hour in pregnant ewes resulted in the death of all fetuses. Pregnant ewes infused with 1 mcg/kg/minute of sodium nitroprusside for one hour delivered normal lambs.

Nursing mothers: It is not known whether Nipride is excreted in human milk. Because of the potential for serious adverse reactions from Nipride in nursing infants, mothers who require Nipride should not nurse.

ADVERSE REACTIONS

Nausea, retching, diaphoresis, apprehension, headache, restlessness, muscle twitching, retrosternal discomfort, palpitations, dizziness and abdominal pain have been noted when the blood pressure was too rapidly reduced. The symptoms quickly disappeared when the rate of infusion was slowed or the infusion was temporarily discontinued and did not reappear with a continued slower rate of administration.

Other adverse reactions reported are:

Cardiovascular: Bradycardia, electrocardiographic changes, tachycardia.

Dermatologic: Rash.

Hematologic: Methemoglobinemia.

Neurologic: Raised intracranial pressure.

Miscellaneous: Flushing, venous streaking, irritation at the infusion site.

One case of hypothyroidism following prolonged therapy with intravenous sodium nitroprusside has been reported. A patient with severe hypertension with uremia received 3900 mg of sodium nitroprusside intravenously over a period of 21 days. This is one of the longest reported intravenous uses of this agent. There was no tachyphylaxis, but the patient developed evidence of hypothyrodism, together with retention of thiocyanate (9.5 mg/100 ml). With peritoneal dialysis the thiocyanate level diminished and the signs of hypothyroidism subsided.

OVERDOSAGE

The first signs of sodium nitroprusside overdosage are those of profound hypotension. As with instances of depletion of thiosulfate supplies, overdosage may lead to cyanide toxicity. Metabolic acidosis and increasing tolerance to the drug are early indications of overdosage. These may be associated with or followed by dyspnea, headache, vomiting, dizziness, ataxia and loss of consciousness. Sodium nitroprusside should be immediately discontinued. Other signs of cyanide poisoning are coma, imperceptible pulse, absent reflexes, widely dilated pupils, pink color, distant heart sounds and shallow breathing. Oxygen alone will not provide relief. Nitrites should be administered to induce methemoglobin formation. Methemoglobin, in turn, combines with cyanide bound to cytochrome oxidase to liberate cytochrome oxidase and form a nontoxic complex, cyanmethemoglobin. Cyanide then gradually dissociates from the latter and is converted by administration of thiosulfate to sodium thiocyanate in the presence of rhodanase.

Treatment of overdosage: In cases of massive overdosage when signs of cyanide toxicity are present use the following regimen:

1. Discontinue administration of Nipride.
2. Administer amyl nitrite inhalations for 15 to 30 seconds per each minute until a 3% sodium nitrite solution can be prepared for I.V. administration.
3. Inject sodium nitrite 3% solution intravenously at a rate not to exceed 2.5 to 5.0 ml/minute, up to a total dose of 10 to 15 ml. Carefully monitor the blood pressure.
4. Next, inject sodium thiosulfate intravenously, 12.5 gm in 50 ml of 5% dextrose in water, over a ten-minute period.
5. Since signs of overdosage may reappear, the patient must be observed for several hours.
6. If signs of overdosage reappear, repeat sodium nitrite and sodium thiosulfate injections at one-half of the above doses.
7. During the administration of nitrites and later when thiocyanate formation is taking place, blood pressure may drop, but it can be corrected with vasopressor agents.

The acute toxicity of Nipride is as follows:

Species	Route	$LD_{50}\pm$ S.E. (mg/kg)
Mouse	I.V.	8.4 ± 0.3
Rat	I.V.	11.2 ± 1.1
Rabbit	I.V.	2.8 ± 1.1
Dog	I.V.	~5

DOSAGE AND ADMINISTRATION

The contents of a 50-mg Nipride vial should be dissolved in 2 to 3 ml of dextrose in water. No other diluent should be used. Depending on the desired concentration, all of the prepared stock solution should be diluted in 250 to 1000 ml of 5% dextrose in water. Once it is dissolved in solution, Nipride tends to deteriorate in the presence of light. Therefore, the container of the prepared solution should be promptly wrapped with aluminum foil or other opaque material affording protection from light. Both the stock solution and the infusion solution should be freshly prepared and any unused portion discarded. The freshly prepared solution for infusion has a very faint brownish tint. Nipride in aqueous solution yields the nitroprusside ion which reacts with even minute quantities of a wide variety of inorganic and organic substances to form usually highly colored reaction products (blue, green or dark red). If this occurs, the infusion should be replaced. *Once prepared, the solution should not be kept or used for longer than twenty-four hours, while protected from light. The infusion fluid used for the administration of Nipride should not be employed as a vehicle for simultaneous administraion of any other drug.*

In patients who are not receiving antihypertensive drugs, the average dose of Nipride for both adults and children is 3 mcg/kg/minute (range of 0.5 to 10 mcg/kg/minute). Usually, at 3 mcg/kg/minute, blood pressure can be lowered by about 30 to 40 percent below the pretreatment diastolic levels and maintained. In hypertensive patients receiving concomitant antihypertensive medications, smaller doses are required. In order to avoid excessive levels of thiocyanate and lessen the possibility of a precipitous drop in blood pressure, infusion rates greater than 10 mcg/kg/minute should rarely be used. If, at this rate, an adequate reduction of blood pressure is not obtained within 10 minutes, administraion of Nipride should be stopped.

1 Vial (50 mg) Nipride in 1000 ml 5% DW (50 mcg/ml)
1 Vial (50 mg) Nipride in 500 ml 5% DW (100 mcg/ml)
1 Vial (50 mg) Nipride in 250 ml 5% DW (200 mcg/ml)

Dose	mcg/kg/minute
Average	3
Range	0.5 to 10

The intravenous infusion of Nipride should be administered by an infusion pump, micro-drip regulator or any similar device that will allow precise measurement of the flow rate. Care should be taken to avoid extravasation. The rate of administration should be adjusted to maintain the desired antihypertensive or hypotensive effect, as determined by frequent blood pressure determinations. It is recommended that the blood pressure should not be allowed to drop at too rapid a rate and that the systolic pressure should not be allowed to drop below 60 mmHg. In hypertensive emergencies, Nipride infusion may be continued until the patient can safely be treated with oral antihypertensive medications alone.

Parenteral drug products should be inspected visually for particulate matter and discoloration prior to administration, whenever solution and container permit. (See above.)

HOW SUPPLIED

Nipride is supplied in 5-ml amber-colored vials containing the equivalent of 50 mg sodium nitroprusside dihydrate for reconstitution with dextrose in water—boxes of 1 (NDC 0004-1938-08).

NOLUDAR® 300 Ⓒ III

[nol'u-dar]
(methyprylon/Roche)
CAPSULES

NOLUDAR® Ⓒ III

(methyprylon/Roche)
TABLETS

The following text is complete prescribing information based on official labeling in effect June 1, 1986.

DESCRIPTION

Noludar (methyprylon/Roche), a hypnotic, is available for oral use as capsules and tablets. Each capsule contains 300 mg methyprylon plus aluminum hydroxide and calcium carbonate coprecipitate and magnesium stearate; gelatin capsule shells contain methyl and propyl parabens, potassium sorbate, FD&C Blue No. 1 and FD&C Red No. 3. Each tablet contains 50 mg or 200 mg methyprylon with aluminum hydroxide and calcium carbonate coprecipitate, corn starch, magnesium stearate and talc.

Chemically, methyprylon, a piperidine derivative, is 3,3-diethyl-5-methyl-2,4-piperidinedione. Methyprylon is a white crystalline powder, freely soluble in water, with a molecular weight of 183.25.

CLINICAL PHARMACOLOGY

In animal studies, methyprylon has been shown to increase the threshold of the arousal centers in the brainstem. In humans, when taken at bedtime, Noludar usually induces sleep within 45 minutes and provides sleep for 5 to 8 hours.

Methyprylon is rapidly absorbed following oral administration and is approximately 60% bound to plasma proteins. Mean peak plasma concentrations of methyprylon in six subjects following a single 650-mg dose occurred at one to two hours postadministration at concentrations of 5.7 to 10.0 mcg/ml. The concentrations declined to 3.3 to 7.9 mcg/ml at 4 hours. Trace amounts of the dihydro-metabolite were detected in the one- to four-hour plasma specimens. Following administration of 400 mg of Noludar, less than 1% of the dose was recovered as intact drug and approximately 23% as identified metabolites in the 0- to 72-hour urine specimens. Identified metabolites include the dihydro-metabolite, the 6-oxo, the 5-hydroxymethyl and the 5-carboxyl derivatives. Methyprylon is metabolized by two pathways: dehydrogenation with subsequent oxidation to form the alcohol and corresponding acid, and oxidation to form 6-oxymethyprylon.

Therapeutic blood concentrations are approximately 1 mg%. Serum concentrations in excess of 30 mg/l are generally consistent with unconsciousness in the acutely poisoned patient.

INDICATIONS AND USAGE

Noludar is indicated for use as a hypnotic. In the sleep laboratory it has been objectively determined that Noludar is effective for at least 7 consecutive nights of drug administration. Since insomnia is often transient and intermittent, the prolonged use of hypnotics is usually not indicated and should only be undertaken concomitantly with appropriate evaluation of the patient.

CONTRAINDICATIONS

Noludar is contraindicated in patients with known hypersensitivity to the drug.

WARNINGS

Synergistic effects: The concomitant use of alcohol or other CNS depressants may produce additive CNS depressant effects.

PRECAUTIONS

General: Total daily intake should not exceed 400 mg, as greater amounts do not significantly increase hypnotic effects. Caution should be exercised in treating patients with impaired renal or hepatic function. In view of isolated reports associating methyprylon with exacerbation of porphyria, caution should be exercised in prescribing methyprylon to patients suffering from this disease.

Information for patients: Patients receiving Noludar should be cautioned about possible combined effects with alcohol and other CNS depressants. Since Noludar is an effective hypnotic agent, patients should also be cautioned against engaging in hazardous occupations requiring complete mental alertness, such as operating machinery or driving a motor vehicle shortly after ingesting the drug.

Laboratory tests: If Noludar is used repeatedly or over prolonged periods of time, periodic blood counts should be made.

Drug interactions: Noludar stimulates the hepatic microsomal enzyme system. (Also see WARNINGS section.)

Carcinogenesis, mutagenesis, impairment of fertility: Studies sufficient to evaluate the carcinogenic or mutagenic potential of Noludar have not been performed. Noludar had no adverse effects on the reproductive process in rats when administered at dose levels of 5 and 50 mg/kg/day.

Pregnancy: Teratogenic effects: Pregnancy Category B. Reproduction studies have been performed in rats and in rabbits at doses up to approximately 9 times the maximum recommended human dose and have revealed no evidence of teratogenic effects on the fetus due to Noludar. There are, however, no adequate or well-controlled studies in pregnant women. Because animal reproduction studies are not always predictive of human response, this drug should be used in pregnancy only if clearly needed.

Nonteratogenic effects: At a dose of 50 mg/kg/day, Noludar caused an increased incidence of resorptions in the rabbit.

Nursing mothers: It is not known whether this drug is excreted in human milk. Because many drugs are excreted in human milk, caution should be exercised when Noludar is administered to a nursing woman.

Pediatric use: Safety and effectiveness in children below the age of 12 have not been established.

ADVERSE REACTIONS

Neurologic: Convulsions, hallucinations, ataxia, EEG changes, pyrexia, morning drowsiness, headache, dizziness, vertigo.

Psychiatric: Acute brain syndrome and confusion (particularly in elderly patients), paradoxical excitation, anxiety, depression, nightmares, dreaming.

Hematologic: Aplastic anemia, thrombocytopenic purpura, neutropenia.

Cardiovascular: Hypotension, syncope.

Ophthalmic: Diplopia, blurred vision.

Gastrointestinal: Esophagitis, vomiting, nausea, diarrhea, constipation.

Allergic: Generalized allergic reactions.

Dermatologic: Pruritus, rash.

Miscellaneous: Hangover effect.

DRUG ABUSE AND DEPENDENCE

Noludar is subject to Schedule III control under the Federal Controlled Substances Act of 1970. Physical and psychological dependence have been reported in patients receiving Noludar therapy. Withdrawal symptoms, when they occur, tend to resemble those associated with the withdrawal of barbiturates and should be treated in a similar fashion. Caution must be exercised in administering Noludar to individuals known to be addiction-prone or to those whose history suggests that they may increase the dosage on their own initiative. As with all hypnotic agents, good medical practice suggests the desirability of limiting repeated prescriptions without adequate medical supervision.

OVERDOSAGE

Manifestations of Noludar overdosage include somnolence, confusion, coma, shock, constricted pupils, respiratory depression, hypotension, tachycardia, edema and hepatic dysfunction. Blood concentrations of methyprylon associated with serious toxic symptoms in humans have been reported to range from 3 to 6 mg%. Blood concentrations of methyprylon that have been reported to cause death range from 5.3 to 114 mg%. A fatality occurred after ingestion of 6 grams of the drug. Respiration, pulse and blood pressure should be monitored, as in all cases of drug overdosage. General supportive measures should be employed, along with immediate gastric lavage with precautions to prevent pulmonary aspiration. Appropriate intravenous fluids should be administered and an adequate airway maintained. Hypotension may be combated by the use of Levophed® (norepinephrine bitartrate), Aramine (metaraminol bitartrate) or other accepted antihypotensive measures. Several reports clearly indicate that hemodialysis is of value. Therefore, its use should be considered, especially in those cases where supportive measures are failing and adequate urinary output cannot be maintained. There have been occasional reports of excitation and convulsions in patients following methyprylon overdosage, almost invariably during the recovery phase. Should these occur, barbiturates may be used, but only with great caution. As with the management of intentional overdosage of any drug, it should be borne in mind that multiple agents may have been ingested.

The acute toxicity of Noludar is as follows:

Species	Route	$LD_{50}\pm$ S.E. (mg/kg)
Mouse	P.O.	1000 ± 45
Rat	P.O.	400 ± 32
Rabbit	P.O.	340 ± 78

DOSAGE AND ADMINISTRATION

The dosage should be individualized for maximum beneficial effects. The usual adult dosage is one capsule (300 mg) or one or two tablets of 200 mg (200 or 400 mg) before retiring.

Noludar is not recommended for use in children under 12 years of age. In children over 12 years, the effective dosage of Noludar varies greatly and, therefore, should also be individualized. Treatment may be initiated with one 50-mg tablet at bedtime, and increased up to 200 mg, if required.

HOW SUPPLIED

Noludar is available as amethyst and white 300-mg capsules in bottles of 100 (NDC 0004-0019-01) and in bottles of 500 (NDC 0004-0019-14); as 50-mg white, scored tablets in bottles of 100 (NDC 0004-0016-01); and as 200-mg white, scored tablets in bottles of 100 (NDC 0004-0017-01). Imprints on all dosage forms of Noludar are as follows: Noludar 300—NOLUDAR® 300 Roche; Noludar 50-mg tablets—ROCHE 16; Noludar 200-mg tablets—(front) NOLUDAR 200, (back) ROCHE.

Shown in Product Identification Section, page 425

PANTOPON® Ⓒ II

[pan'to-pon]
(hydrochlorides of opium alkaloids/Roche)

The following text is complete prescribing information based on official labeling in effect June 1, 1986.

DESCRIPTION

Pantopon (hydrochlorides of opium alkaloids), a narcotic analgesic, is a sterile injectable preparation for intramuscular and subcutaneous administration. It contains all the al-

Continued on next page

Roche Labs.—Cont.

kaloids of opium in a highly purified form free from inert matter and in approximately the same proportions as they occur in nature.

Hydrochlorides of opium alkaloids is a yellowish-gray powder which is freely soluble in water. The approximate composition of Pantopon is as follows: anhydrous morphine — 50 percent, and bases of secondary opium alkaloids — 29.9 to 34.2 percent. One part of Pantopon is equivalent to five parts of opium, U.S.P.

One ml of Pantopon contains 20 mg hydrochlorides of opium alkaloids compounded with 6% alcohol, 136 mg glycerin, 0.2% parabens (methyl and propyl) as preservatives, and either acetic acid, sodium hydroxide, or both, as necessary to adjust pH to approximately 3.3.

CLINICAL PHARMACOLOGY

The action of Pantopon is essentially that of opium. Pantopon, therefore, exhibits not only the action of morphine but also the actions of codeine, papaverine and other alkaloids present in opium. The other alkaloids in Pantopon enhance the sedative and analgesic effects of morphine and tend to minimize its undesirable side effects. Pharmacokinetic data on Pantopon are not available; however, data are available on morphine, the major component of Pantopon.

Morphine acts as an agonist interacting with stereospecific receptors in the brain and other tissues; the receptor sites are distributed throughout the CNS and are present in highest concentrations in the limbic system, thalamus, striatum, hypothalamus, midbrain and spinal cord. Morphine is well absorbed after subcutaneous and intramuscular administration. When therapeutic concentrations of morphine are present in plasma, approximately one-third of the drug is protein bound. Unbound morphine accumulates in parenchyma tissues (such as lung, liver, kidney and spleen) and skeletal muscle; however, 24 hours following the last dose, concentrations of the drug in these tissues are quite low.

The half-life of morphine in plasma is about 2.5 to 3 hours in young adults; in older patients, the half-life may be more prolonged. The major metabolic pathway for the drug is conjugation with glucuronic acid and the major route of elimination is through glomerular filtration. Ninety percent of the total excretion takes place during the first 24 hours after administration, although traces of the drug are detectable in the urine for well over 48 hours. About 7 to 10% of administered morphine eventually appears in the feces.

INDICATIONS AND USAGE

Pantopon is indicated in conditions in which the analgesic, sedative-hypnotic or narcotic effect of an opiate is needed. It is recommended for the relief of severe pain in place of morphine.

CONTRAINDICATIONS

Pantopon is contraindicated in patients with a known hypersensitivity to this drug or to other opiates.

WARNINGS

Drug Dependence. Pantopon may be habit forming. Pantopon can produce drug dependence of the morphine type and has the potential for being abused. Psychological and physical dependence and tolerance may develop upon repeated administration of Pantopon; it should be prescribed and administered with the same degree of caution appropriate to the use of morphine.

Intravenous Use: Pantopon should not be administered intravenously. Rapid intravenous injection of narcotic analgesics increases the incidence of adverse reactions; severe respiratory depression, apnea, hypotension, peripheral circulatory collapse and cardiac arrest have occurred.

Interaction with Other Central Nervous System Depressants: Pantopon should be used with great caution and in reduced dosage in patients who are concurrently receiving other narcotic analgesics, general anesthetics, tranquilizers (including phenothiazines), sedative-hypnotics (including barbiturates), tricyclic antidepressants, MAO inhibitors and other CNS depressants, including alcohol. Respiratory depression, hypotension and profound sedation or coma may result.

Hypotensive Effects: The administration of Pantopon may result in severe hypotension in the postoperative patient or in any individual whose ability to maintain blood pressure has been compromised by a depleted blood volume or by the administration of drugs, such as phenothiazines or certain anesthetics.

Head Injury: The respiratory depressant effects of Pantopon may be markedly exaggerated in the presence of head injury or other intracranial lesions. Furthermore, narcotics produce adverse reactions which may obscure the clinical course of patients with head injuries. In such patients Pantopon must be used with extreme caution and only if its use is deemed essential.

Asthma and Other Respiratory Conditions: Pantopon should be used with extreme caution in patients with bronchial asthma, chronic obstructive pulmonary disease or *cor pulmonale.* Similarly, it should be used with extreme caution in patients having a decreased respiratory reserve or with preexisting respiratory depression, hypoxia or hypercapnia. In such patients, usual therapeutic doses of narcotics may decrease respiratory drive while simultaneously increasing airway resistance to the point of apnea.

PRECAUTIONS

General: The administration of Pantopon or other narcotics may obscure the diagnosis or clinical course in patients with acute abdominal conditions. Pantopon should be administered with caution and the initial dose should be reduced in patients who are elderly or debilitated and in those patients with severe impairment of hepatic or renal function, hypothyroidism, Addison's disease, toxic psychosis, and prostatic hypertrophy or urethral stricture.

Information for Patients: In the unlikely event that Pantopon would be administered to ambulatory patients, they should be cautioned that Pantopon may impair the mental and/or physical abilities required for the performance of potentially hazardous tasks such as driving a car or operating machinery.

Drug Interactions: See WARNINGS section.

Carcinogenesis, mutagenesis, impairment of fertility: There have been no studies performed with Pantopon to permit an evaluation of its carcinogenic or mutagenic potential. Studies have not been performed to determine the effect of Pantopon on fertility and reproduction.

Pregnancy:

Teratogenic Effects. Pregnancy Category C. Animal studies have demonstrated the teratogenicity of morphine, the major component of Pantopon, in rats, mice and hamsters. There are no adequate or well-controlled studies of Pantopon in either laboratory animals or in pregnant women. It is also not known whether Pantopon can cause fetal harm when administered to a pregnant woman or if it can affect reproductive capacity. Pantopon should be used during pregnancy only if the potential benefit justifies the potential risk to the fetus.

Nursing Mothers: It has been reported that morphine is excreted in human milk in microgram amounts. Because of the potential for serious adverse reactions from Pantopon in nursing infants, a decision should be made whether to discontinue nursing or to discontinue the drug, taking into account the importance of the drug to the mother.

Pediatric Use: Safety and effectiveness in children have not been established.

ADVERSE REACTIONS

Note: Included in this listing are adverse reactions which have not been reported with this specific drug; however, the pharmacologic similarities among the narcotics require that each of the reactions be considered with Pantopon administration.

Neurologic: Respiratory depression and arrest, pinpoint pupils, visual disturbances, coma, sedation, dizziness, headache, tremors, uncoordinated muscle movements. Inadvertent injection in close proximity to a nerve may result in a sensory-motor paralysis which is usually, though not always, transitory.

Psychiatric: Delirium, euphoria, dysphoria, weakness, agitation, hallucinations.

Cardiovascular: Hypotension, collapse, tachycardia, bradycardia, palpitation.

Dermatologic: Rash, urticaria (local and generalized), pruritus.

Gastrointestinal: Nausea, emesis, constipation, dry mouth, biliary tract spasm.

Genitourinary: Urinary retention.

Miscellaneous: Diaphoresis, flushing, pain at the site of injection, anaphylactoid reactions.

DRUG ABUSE AND DEPENDENCE

Pantopon is subject to Schedule II control under the Federal Controlled Substances Act of 1970. This drug can produce drug dependence of the morphine type and, therefore, has the potential for being abused. Psychological and physical dependence and tolerance may develop upon repeated administration of Pantopon, and consequently the same precautions should be taken in administering the drug as with morphine. A narcotic order is required.

OVERDOSAGE

Serious overdosage with Pantopon is characterized by respiratory depression (a decrease in respiratory rate and/or tidal volume, Cheyne-Stokes respiration, cyanosis), extreme somnolence progressing to stupor or coma, skeletal muscle flaccidity, cold and clammy skin, and sometimes bradycardia and hypotension. In severe overdosage, apnea, circulatory collapse, cardiac arrest and death may occur. The triad of coma, pinpoint pupils and depressed respiration strongly suggests opioid poisoning.

Primary attention should be given to the reestablishment of adequate respiratory exchange through provision of a patent airway and through the institution of assisted or controlled ventilation. The narcotic antagonist, naloxone hydrochloride (Narcan), is a specific antidote against respiratory depression resulting from narcotic overdosage or unusual sensitivity to narcotics. An appropriate dose of this antagonist should be administered, preferably by the intravenous route, simultaneously with efforts at respiratory resuscitation.

An antagonist should not be administered in the absence of clinically significant respiratory or cardiovascular depression.

Oxygen, intravenous fluids, vasopressors and other supportive measures should be employed if needed.

NOTE

The administration of the usual dose of a narcotic antagonist will precipitate an acute withdrawal syndrome in patients physically dependent on narcotics. The severity of this syndrome will depend on the degree of physical dependence and the dose of the antagonist administered. The use of narcotic antagonists in such patients should be avoided if possible. If a narcotic antagonist must be used in physically dependent patients to treat serious respiratory depression, the antagonist should be administered with extreme care using only one-fifth to one-tenth the usual initial dose.

The intravenous LD_{50} of Pantopon in mice is 96 to 99 mg/kg.

DOSAGE AND ADMINISTRATION

One-third grain (20 mg) of Pantopon with a morphine content of 1/6 grain (10 mg) is therapeutically equivalent to and is usually administered where 1/4 grain (15 mg) of morphine is indicated.

Usual Adult Dosage:

5 to 20 mg (1/12 to 1/3 grain) approximately every 4 to 5 hours according to the individual needs and severity of pain. Administer only by intramuscular or subcutaneous injection.

Parenteral drug products should be inspected visually for particulate matter and discoloration prior to administration, whenever solution and container permit.

HOW SUPPLIED

Pantopon is supplied in 1-ml ampuls each containing 20 mg (1/3 grain) hydrochlorides of opium alkaloids/Roche — boxes of 10 (NDC 0004-1918-06).

PROSTIGMIN® ℞

[pro-stig'min]

(neostigmine methylsulfate/Roche)

INJECTABLE

The following text is complete prescribing information based on official labeling in effect June 1, 1986.

DESCRIPTION

Prostigmin (neostigmine methylsulfate/Roche) Injectable, an anticholinesterase agent, is a sterile aqueous solution intended for intramuscular, intravenous or subcutaneous administration.

Prostigmin Injectable is available in the following concentrations:

Prostigmin 1:2000 Ampuls — each ml contains 0.5 mg neostigmine methylsulfate compounded with 0.2% parabens (methyl and propyl) as preservatives and sodium hydroxide to adjust pH to approximately 5.9.

Prostigmin 1:4000 Ampuls — each ml contains 0.25 mg neostigmine methylsulfate compounded with 0.2% parabens (methyl and propyl) as preservatives and sodium hydroxide to adjust pH to approximately 5.9.

Prostigmin 1:1000 Multiple Dose Vials — each ml contains 1 mg neostigmine methylsulfate compounded with 0.45% phenol as preservative, 0.2 mg sodium acetate, and acetic acid and sodium hydroxide to adjust pH to approximately 5.9.

Prostigmin 1:2000 Multiple Dose Vials — each ml contains 0.5 mg neostigmine methylsulfate compounded with 0.45% phenol as preservative, 0.2 mg sodium acetate, and acetic acid and sodium hydroxide to adjust pH to approximately 5.9.

Chemically, neostigmine methylsulfate is (*m*-hydroxyphenyl)trimethylammonium methylsulfate dimethylcarbamate. It has a molecular weight of 334.39.

CLINICAL PHARMACOLOGY

Neostigmine inhibits the hydrolysis of acetylcholine by competing with acetylcholine for attachment to acetylcholinesterase at sites of cholinergic transmission. It enhances cholinergic action by facilitating the transmission of impulses across neuromuscular junctions. It also has a direct cholinomimetic effect on skeletal muscle and possibly on autonomic ganglion cells and neurons of the central nervous system.

Neostigmine undergoes hydrolysis by cholinesterase and is also metabolized by microsomal enzymes in the liver. Protein binding to human serum albumin ranges from 15 to 25 percent.

Following intramuscular administration, neostigmine is rapidly absorbed and eliminated. In a study of five patients with myasthenia gravis, peak plasma levels were observed at 30 minutes, and the half-life ranged from 51 to 90 minutes. Approximately 80 percent of the drug was eliminated in urine within 24 hours; approximately 50 percent as the unchanged drug, and 30 percent as metabolites. Following intravenous administration, plasma half-life ranges from 47 to

60 minutes have been reported with a mean half-life of 53 minutes.
The clinical effects of neostigmine usually begin within 20 to 30 minutes after intramuscular injection and last from 2.5 to 4 hours.

INDICATIONS AND USAGE

Prostigmin is indicated for:
— the symptomatic control of myasthenia gravis when oral therapy is impractical.
— the prevention and treatment of postoperative distention and urinary retention after mechanical obstruction has been excluded.
— reversal of effects of nondepolarizing neuromuscular blocking agents (*e.g.,* tubocurarine, metocurine, gallamine, or pancuronium) after surgery.

CONTRAINDICATIONS

Prostigmin is contraindicated in patients with known hypersensitivity to the drug. It is also contraindicated in patients with peritonitis or mechanical obstruction of the intestinal or urinary tract.

WARNINGS

Prostigmin should be used with caution in patients with epilepsy, bronchial asthma, bradycardia, recent coronary occlusion, vagotonia, hyperthyroidism, cardiac arrhythmias or peptic ulcer. When large doses of Prostigmin are administered, the prior or simultaneous injection of atropine sulfate may be advisable. Separate syringes should be used for the Prostigmin and atropine. Because of the possibility of hypersensitivity in an occasional patient, atropine and antishock medication should always be readily available.

PRECAUTIONS

General: It is important to differentiate between myasthenic crisis and cholinergic crisis caused by overdosage of Prostigmin. Both conditions result in extreme muscle weakness but require radically different treatment. (See OVERDOSAGE section.)
Drug Interactions: Prostigmin does not antagonize, and may in fact prolong, the Phase I block of *depolarizing* muscle relaxants such as succinylcholine or decamethonium. Certain antibiotics, especially neomycin, streptomycin and kanamycin, have a mild but definite nondepolarizing blocking action which may accentuate neuromuscular block. These antibiotics should be used in the myasthenic patient only where definitely indicated, and then careful adjustment should be made of the anticholinesterase dosage. Local and some general anesthetics, antiarrhythmic agents and other drugs that interfere with neuromuscular transmission should be used cautiously, if at all, in patients with myasthenia gravis; the dose of Prostigmin may have to be increased accordingly.
Carcinogenesis, Mutagenesis and Impairment of Fertility: There have been no studies with Prostigmin which would permit an evaluation of its carcinogenic or mutagenic potential. Studies on the effect of Prostigmin on fertility and reproduction have not been performed.
Pregnancy:
Teratogenic Effects: Pregnancy Category C. There are no adequate or well-controlled studies of Prostigmin in either laboratory animals or in pregnant women. It is not known whether Prostigmin can cause fetal harm when administered to a pregnant woman or can affect reproductive capacity. Prostigmin should be given to a pregnant woman only if clearly needed.
Nonteratogenic Effects: Anticholinesterase drugs may cause uterine irritability and induce premature labor when given intravenously to pregnant women near term.
Nursing Mothers: It is not known whether Prostigmin is excreted in human milk. Because many drugs are excreted in human milk and because of the potential for serious adverse reactions from Prostigmin in nursing infants, a decision should be made whether to discontinue nursing or to discontinue the drug, taking into account the importance of the drug to the mother.
Pediatric Use: Safety and effectiveness in children have not been established.

ADVERSE REACTIONS

Side effects are generally due to an exaggeration of pharmacological effects of which salivation and fasciculation are the most common. Bowel cramps and diarrhea may also occur. The following additional adverse reactions have been reported following the use of either neostigmine bromide or neostigmine methylsulfate:
Allergic: Allergic reactions and anaphylaxis.
Neurologic: Dizziness, convulsions, loss of consciousness, drowsiness, headache, dysarthria, miosis and visual changes.
Cardiovascular: Cardiac arrhythmias (including bradycardia, tachycardia, A-V block and nodal rhythm) and nonspecific EKG changes have been reported, as well as cardiac arrest, syncope and hypotension. These have been predominantly noted following the use of the injectable form of Prostigmin.
Respiratory: Increased oral, pharyngeal and bronchial secretions, dyspnea, respiratory depression, respiratory arrest and bronchospasm.
Dermatologic: Rash and urticaria.
Gastrointestinal: Nausea, emesis, flatulence and increased peristalsis.
Genitourinary: Urinary frequency.
Musculoskeletal: Muscle cramps and spasms, arthralgia.
Miscellaneous: Diaphoresis, flushing and weakness.

OVERDOSAGE

Overdosage of Prostigmin can cause cholinergic crisis, which is characterized by increasing muscle weakness, and through involvement of the muscles of respiration, may result in death. Myasthenic crisis, due to an increase in the severity of the disease, is also accompanied by extreme muscle weakness and may be difficult to distinguish from cholinergic crisis on a symptomatic basis. However, such differentiation is extremely important because increases in the dose of Prostigmin or other drugs in this class, in the presence of cholinergic crisis or of a refractory or "insensitive" state, could have grave consequences. The two types of crises may be differentiated by the use of Tensilon® (edrophonium chloride/ Roche) as well as by clinical judgment.
Treatment of the two conditions differs radically. Whereas the presence of *myasthenic crisis* requires more intensive anticholinesterase therapy, *cholinergic crisis* calls for the prompt withdrawal of all drugs of this type. The immediate use of atropine in cholinergic crisis is also recommended.
Atropine may also be used to abolish or minimize gastrointestinal side effects or other muscarinic reactions; but such use, by masking signs of overdose, can lead to inadvertent induction of cholinergic crisis.
The LD_{50} of neostigmine methylsulfate in mice is 0.3 ± 0.02 mg/kg intravenously, 0.54 ± 0.03 mg/kg subcutaneously, and 0.395 ± 0.025 mg/kg intramuscularly; in rats the LD_{50} is 0.315 ± 0.019 mg/kg intravenously, 0.445 ± 0.032 mg/kg subcutaneously, and 0.423 ± 0.032 mg/kg intramuscularly.

DOSAGE AND ADMINISTRATION

Symptomatic control of myasthenia gravis: One ml of the 1:2000 solution (0.5 mg) subcutaneously or intramuscularly. Subsequent doses should be based on the individual patient's response. In most patients, however, oral treatment with Prostigmin (neostigmine bromide) tablets, 15 mg each, is adequate for control of symptoms.
Prevention of postoperative distention and urinary retention: One ml of the 1:4000 solution (0.25 mg) subcutaneously or intramuscularly as soon as possible after operation; repeat every 4 to 6 hours for two or three days.
Treatment of postoperative distention: One ml of the 1:2000 solution (0.5 mg) subcutaneously or intramuscularly, as required.
Treatment of urinary retention: One ml of the 1:2000 solution (0.5 mg) subcutaneously or intramuscularly. If urination does not occur within an hour, the patient should be catheterized. After the patient has voided, or the bladder has been emptied, continue the 0.5 mg injections every three hours for at least 5 injections.
Reversal of Effects of Nondepolarizing Neuromuscular Blocking Agents: When Prostigmin is administered intravenously, it is recommended that atropine sulfate (0.6 to 1.2 mg) also be given intravenously using separate syringes. Some authorities have recommended that the atropine be injected several minutes before the Prostigmin rather than concomitantly. The usual dose is 0.5 to 2 mg Prostigmin given by *slow* intravenous injection, repeated as required. Only in exceptional cases should the total dose of Prostigmin exceed 5 mg. It is recommended that the patient be well ventilated and a patent airway maintained until complete recovery of normal respiration is assured. The optimum time for administration of the drug is during hyperventilation when the carbon dioxide level of the blood is low. It should never be administered in the presence of high concentrations of halothane or cyclopropane. In cardiac cases and severely ill patients, it is advisable to titrate the exact dose of Prostigmin required, using a peripheral nerve stimulator device. In the presence of bradycardia, the pulse rate should be increased to about 80/minute with atropine before administering Prostigmin.
Parenteral drug products should be inspected visually for particulate matter and discoloration prior to administration, whenever solution and container permit.

HOW SUPPLIED

Prostigmin 1:2000 (0.5 mg neostigmine methylsulfate/ml), 1-ml ampuls — boxes of 10 (NDC 0004-1919-06).
Prostigmin 1:4000 (0.25 mg neostigmine methylsulfate/ml), 1-ml ampuls — boxes of 10 (NDC 0004-1920-06).
Prostigmin 1:1000 (1 mg neostigmine methylsulfate/ml), 10-ml multiple dose vials — boxes of 10 (NDC 0004-1921-01).
Prostigmin 1:2000 (0.5 mg neostigmine methylsulfate/ml), 10-ml multiple dose vials — boxes of 10 (NDC 0004-1922-01).

PROSTIGMIN® ℞
[*pro-stig'min*]
(neostigmine bromide/Roche)
TABLETS

The following text is complete prescribing information based on official labeling in effect June 1, 1986.

DESCRIPTION

Prostigmin (neostigmine bromide/Roche), an anticholinesterase agent, is available for oral administration in 15-mg tablets. Each tablet also contains gelatin, lactose, corn starch, stearic acid, sugar and talc.
Chemically, neostigmine bromide is (*m*-hydroxyphenyl)-trimethylammonium bromide dimethylcarbamate. It is a white, crystalline, bitter powder, soluble 1:1 in water, with a molecular weight of 303.20.

CLINICAL PHARMACOLOGY

Neostigmine inhibits the hydrolysis of acetylcholine by competing with acetylcholine for attachment to acetylcholinesterase at sites of cholinergic transmission. It enhances cholinergic action by facilitating the transmission of impulses across neuromuscular junctions. It also has a direct cholinomimetic effect on skeletal muscle and possibly on autonomic ganglion cells and neurons of the central nervous system.
Neostigmine undergoes hydrolysis by cholinesterase and is also metabolized by microsomal enzymes in the liver. Protein binding to human serum albumin ranges from 15 to 25 percent.
Neostigmine bromide is poorly absorbed from the gastrointestinal tract following oral administration. As a rule, 15 mg of neostigmine bromide orally is equivalent to 0.5 mg of neostigmine methylsulfate parenterally, due to poor absorption of the tablet from the intestinal tract. In a study in fasting myasthenic patients, the extent of absorption was estimated to be 1 to 2 percent of the ingested 30-mg single oral dose. Peak concentrations in plasma occurred 1 to 2 hours following drug ingestion, with considerable individual variations. The half-life ranged from 42 to 60 minutes with a mean half-life of 52 minutes.

INDICATIONS AND USAGE

Prostigmin is indicated for the symptomatic treatment of myasthenia gravis. Its greatest usefulness is in prolonged therapy where no difficulty in swallowing is present. In acute myasthenic crisis where difficulty in breathing and swallowing is present, the parenteral form (neostigmine methylsulfate) should be used. The patient can be transferred to the oral form as soon as it can be tolerated.

CONTRAINDICATIONS

Prostigmin is contraindicated in patients with known hypersensitivity to the drug. Because of the presence of the bromide ion, it should not be used in patients with a previous history of reaction to bromides. It is contraindicated in patients with peritonitis or mechanical obstruction of the intestinal or urinary tract.

WARNINGS

Prostigmin should be used with caution in patients with epilepsy, bronchial asthma, bradycardia, recent coronary occlusion, vagotonia, hyperthyroidism, cardiac arrhythmias or peptic ulcer. As a rule, 15 mg of neostigmine bromide orally is equivalent to 0.5 mg of neostigmine methylsulfate parenterally, due to poor absorption of the tablet from the intestinal tract. Large doses should be avoided in situations where there might be an increased absorption rate from the intestinal tract. It should be used with caution when co-administered with anticholinergic drugs, in order to avoid reduction of intestinal motility.

PRECAUTIONS

General: It is important to differentiate between myasthenic crisis and cholinergic crisis caused by overdosage of Prostigmin. Both conditions result in extreme muscle weakness but require radically different treatment. (See OVERDOSAGE section.)
Drug Interactions: Certain antibiotics, especially neomycin, streptomycin and kanamycin, have a mild but definite nondepolarizing blocking action which may accentuate neuromuscular block. These antibiotics should be used in the myasthenic patient only where definitely indicated, and then careful adjustment should be made of adjunctive anticholinesterase dosage.
Local and some general anesthetics, antiarrhythmic agents and other drugs that interfere with neuromuscular transmission should be used cautiously, if at all, in patients with myasthenia gravis; the dose of Prostigmin may have to be increased accordingly.
Carcinogenesis, Mutagenesis and Impairment of Fertility: There have been no studies with Prostigmin which would permit an evaluation of its carcinogenic or mutagenic potential. Studies on the effect of Prostigmin on fertility and reproduction have not been performed.

Continued on next page

Roche Labs.—Cont.

Pregnancy:
Teratogenic Effects: Pregnancy Category C. There are no adequate or well-controlled studies of Prostigmin in either laboratory animals or in pregnant women. It is not known whether Prostigmin can cause fetal harm when administered to a pregnant woman or can affect reproductive capacity. Prostigmin should be given to a pregnant woman only if clearly needed.
Nonteratogenic Effects: Anticholinesterase drugs may cause uterine irritability and induce premature labor when given intravenously to pregnant women near term.
Nursing Mothers: It is not known whether Prostigmin is excreted in human milk. Because many drugs are excreted in human milk and because of the potential for serious adverse reactions from Prostigmin in nursing infants, a decision should be made whether to discontinue nursing or to discontinue the drug, taking into account the importance of the drug to the mother.
Pediatric Use: Safety and effectiveness in children have not been established.

ADVERSE REACTIONS

Side effects are generally due to an exaggeration of pharmacological effects of which salivation and fasciculation are the most common. Bowel cramps and diarrhea may also occur.
The following additional adverse reactions have been reported following the use of either neostigmine bromide or neostigmine methylsulfate:
Allergic: Allergic reactions and anaphylaxis.
Neurologic: Dizziness, convulsions, loss of consciousness, drowsiness, headache, dysarthria, miosis and visual changes.
Cardiovascular: Cardiac arrhythmias (including bradycardia, tachycardia, A-V block and nodal rhythm) and nonspecific EKG changes have been reported, as well as cardiac arrest, syncope and hypotension. These have been predominantly noted following the use of the injectable form of Prostigmin.
Respiratory: Increased oral, pharyngeal and bronchial secretions, and dyspnea. Respiratory depression, respiratory arrest and bronchospasm have been reported following the use of the injectable form of Prostigmin.
Dermatologic: Rash and urticaria.
Gastrointestinal: Nausea, emesis, flatulence and increased peristalsis.
Genitourinary: Urinary frequency.
Musculoskeletal: Muscle cramps and spasms, arthralgia.
Miscellaneous: Diaphoresis, flushing and weakness.

OVERDOSAGE

Overdosage of Prostigmin can cause cholinergic crisis, which is characterized by increasing muscle weakness, and through involvement of the muscles of respiration, may result in death. Myasthenic crisis, due to an increase in the severity of the disease, is also accompanied by extreme muscle weakness and may be difficult to distinguish from cholinergic crisis on a symptomatic basis. However, such differentiation is extremely important because increases in the dose of Prostigmin or other drugs in this class, in the presence of cholinergic crisis or of a refractory or "insensitive" state, could have grave consequences. The two types of crises may be differentiated by the use of Tensilon® (edrophonium chloride/ Roche) as well as by clinical judgment.
Treatment of the two conditions differs radically. Whereas the presence of *myasthenic crisis* requires more intensive anticholinesterase therapy, *cholinergic crisis* calls for the prompt withdrawal of all drugs of this type. The immediate use of atropine in cholinergic crisis is also recommended. Atropine may also be used to abolish or minimize gastrointestinal side effects or other muscarinic reactions; but such use, by masking signs of overdosage, can lead to inadvertent induction of cholinergic crisis.
The LD_{50} of neostigmine methylsulfate in mice is 0.3 ± 0.02 mg/kg intravenously, 0.54 ± 0.03 mg/kg subcutaneously, and 0.395 ± 0.025 mg/kg intramuscularly; in rats the LD_{50} is 0.315 ± 0.019 mg/kg intravenously, 0.445 ± 0.032 mg/kg subcutaneously, and 0.423 ± 0.032 mg/kg intramuscularly.

DOSAGE AND ADMINISTRATION

The onset of action of Prostigmin given orally is slower than when given parenterally, but the duration of action is longer and the intensity of action more uniform. Dosage requirements for optimal results vary from 15 mg to 375 mg per day. In some instances it may be necessary to exceed these dosages, but the possibility of cholinergic crisis must be recognized. The average dose is 10 tablets (150 mg) administered over a 24-hour period. The interval between doses is of paramount importance. The dosage schedule should be adjusted for each patient and changed as the need arises. Frequently, therapy is required day and night. Larger portions of the total daily dose may be given at times when the patient is more prone to fatigue (afternoon, mealtimes, etc.). The patient should be encouraged to keep a daily record of his or her condition to assist the physician in determining an optimal therapeutic regimen.

HOW SUPPLIED

Scored, white tablets containing 15 mg neostigmine bromide — bottles of 100 (NDC 0004-0035-01) and 1000 (NDC 0004-0035-13). Imprint on tablets: (front) PROSTIGMIN; (back) ROCHE.

Shown in Product Identification Section, page 425

ROCALTROL® ℞

[ro-cal 'trol]
(calcitriol/Roche)
CAPSULES

The following text is complete prescribing information based on official labeling in effect June 1, 1986.

DESCRIPTION

Rocaltrol (calcitriol/Roche) is a synthetic vitamin D analog which is active in the regulation of the absorption of calcium from the gastrointestinal tract and its utilization in the body. It is available in capsules containing 0.25 mcg or 0.5 mcg calcitriol/Roche. Each capsule also contains butylated hydroxyanisole (BHA), butylated hydroxytoluene (BHT) and fractionated triglyceride of coconut oil. Gelatin capsule shells contain glycerin, parabens (methyl and propyl) and sorbitol, with the following dye systems: 0.25 mcg—FD&C Yellow No. 6 and titanium dioxide; 0.5 mcg—FD&C Red No. 3, FD&C Yellow No. 6 and titanium dioxide.
Calcitriol is a colorless, crystalline compound which occurs naturally in humans. It has a calculated molecular weight of 416.65 and is soluble in organic solvents but relatively insoluble in water. Chemically, calcitriol is 9,10-seco(5Z,7E)-5,7,10(19)-cholestatriene-1α, 3β, 25-triol.
The other names frequently used for calcitriol are 1α,25-dihydroxycholecalciferol, 1,25-dihydroxyvitamin D_3, 1,25-DHCC, 1,25$(OH)_2D_3$ and 1,25-diOHC.

CLINICAL PHARMACOLOGY

Man's natural supply of vitamin D depends mainly on exposure to the ultraviolet rays of the sun for conversion of 7-dehydrocholesterol in the skin to vitamin D_3 (cholecalciferol). Vitamin D_3 must be metabolically activated in the liver and the kidney before it is fully active as a regulator of calcium and phosphorus metabolism at target tissues. The initial transformation of vitamin D_3 is catalyzed by a vitamin D_3-25-hydroxylase enzyme (25-OHase) present in the liver, and the product of this reaction is 25-hydroxyvitamin D_3 [25-$(OH)D_3$]. Hydroxylation of 25-$(OH)D_3$ occurs in the mitochondria of kidney tissue, activated by the renal 25-hydroxyvitamin D_3-1 alpha-hydroxylase (alpha-OHase), to produce 1,25-$(OH)_2D_3$ (calcitriol), the active form of vitamin D_3. Several metabolites of calcitriol have been identified which include:
1α, 25, $(OH)_2$-24-oxo-D_3
1α, 23,25$(OH)_3$-24-oxo-D_3
1α, 24R,25$(OH)_3D_3$
1α, 25R$(OH)_2$-26-23S-lactone D_3
1α, 25S,26$(OH)_3D_3$
1α, 25$(OH)_2$-23-oxo-D_3
1α, 25R,26$(OH)_3$-23-oxo-D_3
1α, (OH)24,25,26,27-tetranor-COOH-D_3
The two known sites of action of calcitriol are intestine and bone. A calcitriol receptor-binding protein appears to exist in the mucosa of human intestine. Additional evidence suggests that calcitriol may also act on the kidney and the parathyroid glands. Calcitriol is the most active known form of vitamin D_3 in stimulating intestinal calcium transport. In acutely uremic rats calcitriol has been shown to stimulate intestinal calcium absorption. The kidneys of uremic patients cannot adequately synthesize calcitriol, the active hormone formed from precursor vitamin D. Resultant hypocalcemia and secondary hyperparathyroidism are a major cause of the metabolic bone disease of renal failure. However, other bone-toxic substances which accumulate in uremia (*e.g.,* aluminum) may also contribute.
The beneficial effect of Rocaltrol in renal osteodystrophy appears to result from correction of hypocalcemia and secondary hyperparathyroidism. It is uncertain whether Rocaltrol produces other independent beneficial effects.
Calcitriol is rapidly absorbed from the intestine. Peak serum concentrations (above basal values) were reached within 3 to 6 hours following oral administration of single doses of 0.25 to 1.0 mcg of Rocaltrol. The half-life of calcitriol elimination from serum was found to range from 3 to 6 hours. Following a single oral dose of 0.5 mcg, mean serum concentrations of calcitriol rose from a baseline value of 40.0 ± 4.4 (S.D.) pg/ml to 60.0 ± 4.4 pg/ml at 2 hours, and declined to 53.0 ± 6.9 at 4 hours, 50 ± 7.0 at 8 hours, 44 ± 4.6 at 12 hours and 41.5 ± 5.1 at 24 hours. The duration of pharmacologic activity of a single dose of calcitriol is about 3 to 5 days.
Calcitriol and other vitamin D metabolites are transported in blood, bound to specific plasma proteins. Enterohepatic recycling and biliary excretion of calcitriol occurs. Following intravenous administration of radiolabeled calcitriol in normal subjects, approximately 27% and 7% of the radioactivity appeared in the feces and urine, respectively, within 24 hours. When a 1-mcg oral dose of radiolabeled calcitriol was administered to normals, approximately 10% of the total radioactivity appeared in urine within 24 hours. Cumulative excretion of radioactivity on the sixth day following intravenous administration of radiolabeled calcitriol averaged 16% in urine and 49% in feces.
There is evidence that maternal calcitriol may enter the fetal circulation. It is not known if calcitriol is excreted in human milk.

INDICATIONS AND USAGE

Rocaltrol is indicated in the management of hypocalcemia and the resultant metabolic bone disease in patients undergoing chronic renal dialysis. In these patients, Rocaltrol administration enhances calcium absorption, reduces serum alkaline phosphatase levels and may reduce elevated parathyroid hormone levels and the histological manifestations of osteitis fibrosa cystica and defective mineralization.
Rocaltrol is also indicated in the management of hypocalcemia and its clinical manifestations in patients with postsurgical hypoparathyroidism, idiopathic hypoparathyroidism, and pseudohypoparathyroidism.

CONTRAINDICATIONS

Rocaltrol should not be given to patients with hypercalcemia or evidence of vitamin D toxicity.

WARNINGS

Since Rocaltrol is the most potent metabolite of vitamin D available, pharmacologic doses of vitamin D and its derivatives should be withheld during Rocaltrol treatment to avoid possible additive effects and hypercalcemia.
Both appropriate oral phosphate-binders and a low phosphate diet should be used to control serum phosphate levels in patients undergoing dialysis.
Magnesium-containing antacids and Rocaltrol should not be used concomitantly in patients on chronic renal dialysis because such use may lead to the development of hypermagnesemia.
Overdosage of any form of vitamin D is dangerous (see also OVERDOSAGE). Progressive hypercalcemia due to overdosage of vitamin D and its metabolites may be so severe as to require emergency attention. Chronic hypercalcemia can lead to generalized vascular calcification, nephrocalcinosis and other soft-tissue calcification. **The serum calcium times phospate (Ca × P) product should not be allowed to exceed 70.** Radiographic evaluation of suspect anatomical regions may be useful in the early detection of this condition.

PRECAUTIONS

General: Excessive dosage of Rocaltrol induces hypercalcemia and in some instances hypercalciuria; therefore, early in treatment during dosage adjustment, serum calcium should be determined twice weekly. In dialysis patients, a fall in serum alkaline phosphatase levels usually antedates the appearance of hypercalcemia and may be an indication of impending hypercalcemia. Should hypercalcemia develop, the drug should be discontinued immediately. Rocaltrol should be given cautiously to patients on digitalis, because hypercalcemia in such patients may precipitate cardiac arrhythmias.
In patients with normal renal function, chronic hypercalcemia may be associated with an increase in serum creatinine. While this is usually reversible, it is important in such patients to pay careful attention to those factors which may lead to hypercalcemia. Rocaltrol therapy should always be started at the lowest possible dose and should not be increased without careful monitoring of the serum calcium. An estimate of daily dietary calcium intake should be made and the intake adjusted when indicated.
Patients with normal renal function taking Rocaltrol should avoid dehydration. Adequate fluid intake should be maintained.
Information for the patient: The patient and his or her parents or spouse should be informed about compliance with dosage instructions, adherence to instructions about diet and calcium supplementation and avoidance of the use of unapproved nonprescription drugs. Patients should also be carefully informed about the symptoms of hypercalcemia (see ADVERSE REACTIONS section).
Laboratory tests: For dialysis patients, serum calcium, phosphorus, magnesium and alkaline phosphatase should be determined periodically. For hypoparathyroid patients, serum calcium, phosphorus and 24-hour urinary calcium should be determined periodically.
Drug interactions: Cholestyramine has been reported to reduce intestinal absorption of fat-soluble vitamins; as such it may impair intestinal absorption of Rocaltrol. (Also see WARNINGS and PRECAUTIONS [General] sections.)
Carcinogenesis, mutagenesis, impairment of fertility: Long-term studies in animals have not been conducted to evaluate the carcinogenic potential of Rocaltrol. There was no evidence of mutagenicity as studied by the Ames method. No significant effects of Rocaltrol on fertility and/or general reproductive performances were reported.
Pregnancy: Teratogenic effects: Pregnancy Category C. Rocaltrol has been found to be teratogenic in rabbits

when given in doses 4 and 15 times the dose recommended for human use. All 15 fetuses in 3 litters at these doses showed external and skeletal abnormalities. However, none of the other 23 litters (156 fetuses) showed significant abnormalities compared with controls. Teratogenicity studies in rats showed no evidence of teratogenic potential. There are no adequate and well-controlled studies in pregnant women. Rocaltrol should be used during pregnancy only if the potential benefit justifies the potential risk to the fetus.
Nonteratogenic effects: In the rabbit, dosages of 0.3 mcg/kg/day administered on days 7 to 18 of gestation resulted in 19% maternal mortality, a decrease in mean fetal body weight and a reduced number of newborn surviving to 24 hours. A study of peri- and postnatal development in rats resulted in hypercalcemia in the offspring of dams given Rocaltrol at doses of 0.08 or 0.3 mcg/kg/day, hypercalcemia and hypophosphatemia in dams at doses of 0.08 or 0.3 mcg/kg/day, and increased serum urea nitrogen in dams given Rocaltrol at a dose of 0.3 mcg/kg/day. In another study in rats, maternal weight gain was slightly reduced at a dose of 0.3 mcg/kg/day administered on days 7 to 15 of gestation. The offspring of a woman administered 17 to 36 mcg/day of Rocaltrol (17 to 144 times the recommended dose) during pregnancy manifested mild hypercalcemia in the first two days of life which returned to normal at day 3.
Nursing mothers: It is not known whether calcitriol is excreted in human milk. Because many drugs are excreted in human milk and because of the potential for serious adverse reactions from Rocaltrol in nursing infants, a mother should not nurse while taking this drug.
Pediatric use: Safety and efficacy of Rocaltrol in children undergoing dialysis have not been established.

ADVERSE REACTIONS

Since Rocaltrol is believed to be the active hormone which exerts vitamin D activity in the body, adverse effects are, in general, similar to those encountered with excessive vitamin D intake. The early and late signs and symptoms of vitamin D intoxication associated with hypercalcemia include:
Early: Weakness, headache, somnolence, nausea, vomiting, dry mouth, constipation, muscle pain, bone pain and metallic taste.
Late: Polyuria, polydipsia, anorexia, weight loss, nocturia, conjunctivitis (calcific), pancreatitis, photophobia, rhinorrhea, pruritus, hyperthermia, decreased libido, elevated BUN, albuminuria, hypercholesterolemia, elevated SGOT and SGPT, ectopic calcification, hypertension, cardiac arrhythmias and, rarely, overt psychosis.
In clinical studies on hypoparathyroidism and pseudohypoparathyroidism, hypercalcemia was noted on at least one occasion in about 1 in 3 patients and hypercalciuria in about 1 in 7. Elevated serum creatinine levels were observed in about 1 in 6 patients (approximately one half of whom had normal levels at baseline).
One case of erythema multiforme was confirmed by rechallenge.

OVERDOSAGE

Administration of Rocaltrol to patients in excess of their daily requirements can cause hypercalcemia, hypercalciuria and hyperphosphatemia. High intake of calcium and phosphate concomitant with Rocaltrol may lead to similar abnormalities. High levels of calcium in the dialysate bath may contribute to the hypercalcemia.
Treatment of Hypercalcemia and Overdosage: General treatment of hypercalcemia (greater than 1 mg/dl above the upper limit of the normal range) consists of immediate discontinuation of Rocaltrol therapy, institution of a low calcium diet and withdrawal of calcium supplements. Serum calcium levels should be determined daily until normocalcemia ensues. Hypercalcemia frequently resolves in two to seven days. When serum calcium levels have returned to within normal limits, Rocaltrol therapy may be reinstituted at a dose of 0.25 mcg/day less than prior therapy. Serum calcium levels should be obtained at least twice weekly after all dosage changes and subsequent dosage titration. In dialysis patients, persistent or markedly elevated serum calcium levels may be corrected by dialysis against a calcium-free dialysate.
Treatment of Accidental Overdosage of Rocaltrol: The treatment of acute accidental overdosage of Rocaltrol should consist of general supportive measures. If drug ingestion is discovered within a relatively short time, induction of emesis or gastric lavage may be of benefit in preventing further absorption. If the drug has passed through the stomach, the administration of mineral oil may promote its fecal elimination. Serial serum electrolyte determinations (especially calcium), rate of urinary calcium excretion and assessment of electrocardiographic abnormalities due to hypercalcemia should be obtained. Such monitoring is critical in patients receiving digitalis. Discontinuation of supplemental calcium and a low calcium diet are also indicated in accidental overdosage. Due to the relatively short duration of the pharmacological action of calcitriol, further measures are probably unnecessary. Should, however, persistent and markedly elevated serum calcium levels occur, there are a variety of therapeutic alternatives which may be considered, depending on the patient's underlying condition. These include the use of drugs such as phosphates and corticosteroids as well as measures to induce an appropriate forced diuresis. The use of peritoneal dialysis against a calcium-free dialysate has also been reported.
The oral toxicity of calcitriol is as follows:

Species	LD_{50} (mg/kg)
mouse	2.0
rat	>5.0

DOSAGE AND ADMINISTRATION

The optimal daily dose of Rocaltrol must be carefully determined for each patient.
The effectiveness of Rocaltrol therapy is predicated on the assumption that each patient is receiving an adequate daily intake of calcium. The U.S. RDA for calcium in adults is 800 to 1200 mg. To ensure that each patient receives an adequate daily intake of calcium, the physician should either prescribe a calcium supplement or instruct the patient in proper dietary measures.
Dialysis patients: The recommended initial dose of Rocaltrol is 0.25 mcg/day. If a satisfactory response in the biochemical parameters and clinical manifestations of the disease state is not observed, dosage may be increased by 0.25 mcg/day at four- to eight-week intervals. During this titration period, serum calcium levels should be obtained at least twice weekly, and if hypercalcemia is noted, the drug should be immediately discontinued until normocalcemia ensues.
Patients with normal or only slightly reduced serum calcium levels may respond to Rocaltrol doses of 0.25 mcg every other day. Most patients undergoing hemodialysis respond to doses between 0.5 and 1 mcg/day.
Oral Rocaltrol may normalize plasma ionized calcium in some uremic patients, yet fail to suppress parathyroid hyperfunction. In these individuals with autonomous parathyroid hyperfunction, oral Rocaltrol may be useful to maintain normocalcemia, but has not been shown to be adequate treatment for hyperparathyroidism.
Hypoparathyroidism: The recommended initial dose of Rocaltrol is 0.25 mcg/day given in the morning. If a satisfactory response in the biochemical parameters and clinical manifestations of the disease is not observed, the dose may be increased at two- to four-week intervals. During the dosage titration period, serum calcium levels should be obtained at least twice weekly and, if hypercalcemia is noted, Rocaltrol should be immediately discontinued until normocalcemia ensues. Careful consideration should also be given to lowering the dietary calcium intake.
Most adult patients and pediatric patients age 6 years and older have responded to dosages in the range of 0.5 to 2 mcg daily. Pediatric patients in the 1–5 year age group with hypoparathyroidism have usually been given 0.25 to 0.75 mcg daily. The number of treated patients with pseudohypoparathyroidism less than 6 years of age is too small to make dosage recommendations.

HOW SUPPLIED

0.25 mcg calcitriol/Roche in soft gelatin, light orange, oval capsules, imprinted ROCALTROL 0.25 ROCHE; bottles of 30, (NDC 0004-0143-23), and bottles of 100, (NDC 0004-0143-01).
0.5 mcg calcitriol/Roche in soft gelatin, dark orange, oblong capsules, imprinted ROCALTROL 0.5 ROCHE; bottles of 100, (NDC 0004-0144-01).
Rocaltrol should be protected from heat and light.
Shown in Product Identification Section, page 425

ROCEPHIN® ℞

[ro-sef'in]
(ceftriaxone sodium/Roche)

The following text is complete prescribing information based on official labeling in effect June 1, 1986.

DESCRIPTION

Rocephin* (ceftriaxone sodium/ Roche) is a sterile, semisynthetic, broad-spectrum cephalosporin antibiotic for intravenous or intramuscular administration. Ceftriaxone sodium is 5-Thia-1-azabicyclo[4.2.0]oct-2-ene-2-carboxylic acid, 7-[[(2-amino-4-thiazolyl)(methoxyimino) acetyl amino]-8-oxo-3-[[(1, 2, 5, 6-tetrahydro-2-methyl-5, 6-dioxo-1, 2, 4-triazin-3-yl)thio]methyl]-, disodium salt, [6R-[6α,7β(Z)]]-.
The chemical formula of ceftriaxone sodium is $C_{18}H_{16}N_8Na_2O_7S_3 3.5\ H_2O$. It has a calculated molecular weight of 661.59.
Rocephin is a white to yellowish-orange crystalline powder which is readily soluble in water, sparingly soluble in methanol and very slightly soluble in ethanol. The pH of a 1% aqueous solution is approximately 6.7. The color of Rocephin solutions ranges from light yellow to amber, depending on the length of storage, concentration and diluent used.
Rocephin contains approximately 83 mg (3.6 mEq) of sodium per gram of ceftriaxone activity.

CLINICAL PHARMACOLOGY

Average plasma concentrations of ceftriaxone following a single 30-minute intravenous (I.V.) infusion of a 0.5, 1 or 2 gm dose and intramuscular (I.M.) administration of a single 0.5 or 1 gm dose in healthy subjects are presented in Table 1.
[See table above].

TABLE 1
Ceftriaxone Plasma Concentrations After Single Dose Administration

Dose/Route	Average Plasma Concentrations (mcg/ml)								
	0.5 hr	1 hr	2 hr	4 hr	6 hr	8 hr	12 hr	16 hr	24 hr
0.5 gm I.V.*	82	59	48	37	29	23	15	10	5
0.5 gm I.M.	30	41	43	39	31	25	16	ND†	ND
1 gm I.V.*	151	111	88	67	53	43	28	18	9
1 gm I.M.	40	68	76	68	56	44	29	ND	ND
2 gm I.V.*	257	192	154	117	89	74	46	31	15

* I.V. doses were infused at a constant rate over 30 minutes.
† ND = Not determined.

Ceftriaxone was completely absorbed following I.M. administration with mean maximum plasma concentrations occurring between two and three hours postdosing. Multiple I.V. or I.M. doses ranging from 0.5 to 2 gm at 12 to 24-hour intervals resulted in 15 to 36% accumulation of ceftriaxone above single dose values.
Ceftriaxone concentrations in urine are high, as shown in Table 2.
[See table left].

TABLE 2
Urinary Concentrations of Ceftriaxone After Single Dose Administration

Dose/Route	Average Urinary Concentrations (mcg/ml)					
	0–2 hr	2–4 hr	4–8 hr	8–12 hr	12–24 hr	24–48 hr
0.5 gm I.V.	526	366	142	87	70	15
0.5 gm I.M.	115	425	308	127	96	28
1 gm I.V.	995	855	293	147	132	32
1 gm I.M.	504	628	418	237	ND*	ND
2 gm I.V.	2692	1976	757	274	198	40

*ND = Not determined.

Thirty-three to 67% of a ceftriaxone dose was excreted in the urine as unchanged drug and the remainder was secreted in the bile and ultimately found in the feces as microbiologically inactive compounds. After a 1 gm I.V. dose, average concentrations of ceftriaxone, determined from one to three hours after dosing, were 581 mcg/ml in the gallbladder bile, 788 mcg/ml in the common duct bile, 898 mcg/ml in the cystic duct bile, 78.2 mcg/gm in the gallbladder wall and 62.1 mcg/ml in the concurrent plasma.
Over a 0.15 to 3 gm dose range in healthy adult subjects, the values of elimination half-life ranged from 5.8 to 8.7 hours; apparent volume of distribution from 5.78 to 13.5 L; plasma clearance from 0.58 to 1.45 L/hour; and renal clearance from 0.32 to 0.73 L/hour. Ceftriaxone is reversibly bound to hu-

Continued on next page

Roche Labs.—Cont.

man plasma proteins, and the binding decreased from a value of 95% bound at plasma concentrations of <25 mcg/ml to a value of 85% bound at 300 mcg/ml.

The average values of maximum plasma concentration, elimination half-life, plasma clearance and volume of distribution after a 50 mg/kg I.V. dose and after a 75 mg/kg I.V. dose in pediatric patients suffering from bacterial meningitis are shown in Table 3. Ceftriaxone penetrated the inflamed meninges of infants and children; CSF concentrations after a 50 mg/kg I.V. dose and after a 75 mg/kg I.V. dose are also shown in Table 3.

TABLE 3
Average Pharmacokinetic Parameters of Ceftriaxone in Pediatric Patients with Meningitis

	50 mg/kg I.V.	75 mg/kg I.V.
Maximum Plasma Concentrations (mcg/ml)	216	275
Elimination Half-life (hr)	4.6	4.3
Plasma Clearance (ml/hr/kg)	49	60
Volume of Distribution (ml/kg)	338	373
CSF Concentration—inflamed meninges (mcg/ml)	5.6	6.4
Range (mcg/ml)	1.3–18.5	1.3–44
Time after dose (hr)	3.7 (± 1.6)	3.3 (± 1.4)

Compared to that in healthy adult subjects, the pharmacokinetics of ceftriaxone were only minimally altered in elderly subjects and in patients with renal impairment or hepatic dysfunction (Table 4); therefore, dosage adjustments are not necessary for these patients with ceftriaxone dosages up to 2 gm per day. Ceftriaxone was not removed to any significant extent from the plasma by hemodialysis. In 6 of 26 dialysis patients, the elimination rate of ceftriaxone was markedly reduced, suggesting that plasma concentrations of ceftriaxone should be monitored in these patients to determine if dosage adjustments are necessary.

[See table below].

MICROBIOLOGY: The bactericidal activity of ceftriaxone results from inhibition of cell wall synthesis. Ceftriaxone has a high degree of stability in the presence of beta-lactamases, both penicillinases and cephalosporinases, of gram-negative and gram-positive bacteria. Ceftriaxone is usually active against the following microorganisms *in vitro* and in clinical infections (see Indications and Usage):

GRAM-NEGATIVE AEROBES: Enterobacter aerogenes, Enterobacter cloacae, Escherichia coli, Haemophilus influenzae (including ampicillin-resistant strains), *H. parainfluenzae, Klebsiella* species (including *K. pneumoniae*), *Neisseria gonorrhoeae* (including penicillinase and nonpenicillinase producing strains), *Neisseria meningitidis, Proteus mirabilis, Proteus vulgaris, Morganella morganii* and *Serratia marcescens.*

Note: Many strains of the above organisms that are multiply resistant to other antibiotics, *e.g.,* penicillins, cephalosporins and aminoglycosides, are susceptible to ceftriaxone sodium.

Ceftriaxone is also active against many strains of *Pseudomonas aeruginosa.*

GRAM-POSITIVE AEROBES: Staphylococcus aureus (including penicillinase-producing strains) and *Staphylococcus epidermidis* (Note: methicillin-resistant staphylococci are resistant to cephalosporins, including ceftriaxone), *Streptococcus pyogenes* (Group A beta-hemolytic streptococci), *Streptococci agalactiae* (Group B streptococci) and *Streptococcus pneumoniae.* (Note: Most strains of enterococci, *Streptococcus faecalis* and Group D streptococci are resistant.)

Ceftriaxone also demonstrates *in vitro* activity against the following microorganisms, although the clinical significance is unknown:

GRAM-NEGATIVE AEROBES: Citrobacter freundii, Citrobacter diversus, Providencia species (including *Providencia rettgeri*), *Salmonella* species (including *S. typhi*), *Shigella* species and *Acinetobacter calcoaceticus.*

ANAEROBES: Bacteroides species, *Clostridium* species (Note: most strains of *C. difficile* are resistant).

SUSCEPTIBILITY TESTING: Standard susceptibility disk method. Quantitative methods that require measurement of zone diameters give the most precise estimate of antibiotic susceptibility. One such procedure (Bauer AW, Kirby WMM, Sherris JC, Turck M: Antibiotic Susceptibility Testing by a Standardized Single Disk Method, *Am J Clin Pathol 45*:493–496, 1966; Standardized Disk Susceptibility Test, *Federal Register 39*: 19182–19184, 1974; National Committee for Clinical Laboratory Standards, Approved Standard: ASM-2, Performance Standards for Antimicrobial Disk Susceptibility Tests, July 1975.) has been recommended for use with disks to test susceptibility to ceftriaxone.

Laboratory results of the standardized single-disk susceptibility test using a 30-mcg ceftriaxone disk should be interpreted according to the following three criteria:

1. Susceptible organisms produce zones of 18 mm or greater, indicating that the tested organism is likely to respond to therapy.
2. Organisms that produce zones of 14 to 17 mm are expected to be susceptible if a high dosage (not to exceed 4 gm per day) is used or if the infection is confined to tissues and fluids (*e.g.,* urine), in which high antibiotic levels are attained.
3. Resistant organisms produce zones of 13 mm or less, indicating that other therapy should be selected.

Organisms should be tested with the ceftriaxone disk, since ceftriaxone has been shown by *in vitro* tests to be active against certain strains found resistant to cephalosporin class disks.

Organisms having zones of less than 18 mm around the cephalothin disk are not necessarily of intermediate susceptibility or resistant to ceftriaxone.

Standardized procedures require use of control organisms. The 30-mcg ceftriaxone disk should give zone diameters between 29 and 35 mm, 22 and 28 mm and 17 and 23 mm for the reference strains *E. coli* ATCC 25922, *S. aureus* ATCC 25923 and *P. aeruginosa* ATCC 27853, respectively.

DILUTION TECHNIQUES: Based on the pharmacokinetic profile of ceftriaxone, a bacterial isolate may be considered susceptible if the MIC value for ceftriaxone is not more than 16 mcg/ml. Organisms are considered resistant to ceftriaxone if the MIC is equal to or greater than 64 mcg/ml. Organisms having an MIC value of less than 64 mcg/ml, but greater than 16 mcg/ml, are expected to be susceptible if a high dosage (not to exceed 4 gm per day) is used or if the infection is confined to tissues and fluids (*e.g.,* urine), in which high antibiotic levels are attained.

E. coli ATCC 25922, *S. aureus* ATCC 25923 and *P. aeruginosa* ATCC 27853 are also the recommended reference strains for controlling ceftriaxone dilution tests. Greater than 95% of MICs for the *E. coli* strain should fall within the range of 0.016 to 0.5 mcg/ml. The range for the *S. aureus* strain should be 1 to 2 mcg/ml, while for the *P. aeruginosa* strain the range should be 8 to 64 mcg/ml.

INDICATIONS AND USAGE

Rocephin is indicated for the treatment of the following infections when caused by susceptible organisms.

LOWER RESPIRATORY TRACT INFECTIONS caused by *Strep. pneumoniae, Streptococcus* species (excluding enterococci), *Staph. aureus, H. influenzae, H. parainfluenzae, Klebsiella* species (including *K. pneumoniae*), *E. coli, E. aerogenes, Proteus mirabilis* and *Serratia marcescens.*

SKIN AND SKIN STRUCTURE INFECTIONS caused by *Staph. aureus, Staph. epidermidis, Streptococcus* species (excluding enterococci), *E. cloacae, Klebsiella* species (including *K. pneumoniae*), *Proteus mirabilis* and *Pseudomonas aeruginosa.*

URINARY TRACT INFECTIONS (complicated and uncomplicated) caused by *E. coli, Proteus mirabilis, Proteus vulgaris, M. morganii* and *Klebsiella* species (including *K. pneumoniae*).

TABLE 4
Average Pharmacokinetic Parameters of Ceftriaxone in Humans

Subject Group	Elimination Half-Life (hr)	Plasma Clearance (L/hr)	Volume of Distribution (L)
Healthy Subjects	5.8–8.7	0.58–1.45	5.8–13.5
Elderly Subjects (mean age, 70.5 yr)	8.9	0.83	10.7
Patients with renal impairment			
Hemodialysis patients (0–5 ml/min)*	14.7	0.65	13.7
Severe (5–15 ml/min)	15.7	0.56	12.5
Moderate (16–30 ml/min)	11.4	0.72	11.8
Mild (31–60 ml/min)	12.4	0.70	13.3
Patients with liver disease	8.8	1.1	13.6

*Creatinine clearance.

UNCOMPLICATED GONORRHEA (cervical/urethral and rectal) caused by *Neisseria gonorrhoeae,* including both penicillinase and nonpenicillinase producing strains.

PELVIC INFLAMMATORY DISEASE caused by *N. gonorrhoeae.*

BACTERIAL SEPTICEMIA caused by *Staph. aureus, Strep. pneumoniae, E. coli, H. influenzae* and *K. pneumoniae.*

BONE AND JOINT INFECTIONS caused by *Staph. aureus, Strep. pneumoniae, Streptococcus* species (excluding enterococci), *E. coli, P. mirabilis, K. pneumoniae* and *Enterobacter* species.

INTRA-ABDOMINAL INFECTIONS caused by *E. coli* and *K. pneumoniae.*

MENINGITIS caused by *H. influenzae, N. meningitidis* and *Strep. pneumoniae.* Ceftriaxone has also been used successfully in a limited number of cases of meningitis and shunt infections caused by *Staph. epidermidis* and *E. coli.*

PROPHYLAXIS: The administration of a single dose of ceftriaxone preoperatively may reduce the incidence of postoperative infections in patients undergoing coronary artery bypass surgery. Although ceftriaxone has been shown to have been as effective as cefazolin in the prevention of infection following coronary artery bypass surgery, no placebo-controlled trials have been conducted to evaluate any cephalosporin antibiotic in the prevention of infection following coronary artery bypass surgery.

SUSCEPTIBILITY TESTING: Before instituting treatment with Rocephin, appropriate specimens should be obtained for isolation of the causative organism and for determination of its susceptibility to the drug. Therapy may be instituted prior to obtaining results of susceptibility testing.

CONTRAINDICATIONS

Rocephin is contraindicated in patients with known allergy to the cephalosporin class of antibiotics.

WARNINGS

BEFORE THERAPY WITH ROCEPHIN IS INSTITUTED, CAREFUL INQUIRY SHOULD BE MADE TO DETERMINE WHETHER THE PATIENT HAS HAD PREVIOUS HYPERSENSITIVITY REACTIONS TO CEPHALOSPORINS, PENICILLINS OR OTHER DRUGS. THIS PRODUCT SHOULD BE GIVEN CAUTIOUSLY TO PENICILLIN-SENSITIVE PATIENTS. ANTIBIOTICS SHOULD BE ADMINISTERED WITH CAUTION TO ANY PATIENT WHO HAS DEMONSTRATED SOME FORM OF ALLERGY, PARTICULARLY TO DRUGS. SERIOUS ACUTE HYPERSENSITIVITY REACTIONS MAY REQUIRE THE USE OF SUBCUTANEOUS EPINEPHRINE AND OTHER EMERGENCY MEASURES.

Pseudomembranous colitis has been reported with the use of cephalosporins (and other broad-spectrum antibiotics); therefore, it is important to consider its diagnosis in patients who develop diarrhea in association with antibiotic use.

Treatment with broad-spectrum antibiotics alters the normal flora of the colon and may permit overgrowth of clostridia. Studies indicate a toxin produced by *Clostridium difficile* is one primary cause of antibiotic-associated colitis. Cholestyramine and colestipol resins have been shown to bind to the toxin *in vitro.*

Mild cases of colitis respond to drug discontinuance alone. Moderate to severe cases should be managed with fluid, electrolyte and protein supplementation as indicated.

When the colitis is not relieved by drug discontinuance or when it is severe, oral vancomycin is the treatment of choice for antibiotic-associated pseudomembranous colitis produced by *C. difficile.* Other causes of colitis should also be considered.

PRECAUTIONS

GENERAL: Although transient elevations of BUN and serum creatinine have been observed, at the recommended dosages, the nephrotoxic potential of Rocephin is similar to that of other cephalosporins.

Ceftriaxone is excreted via both biliary and renal excretion (see Clinical Pharmacology). Therefore, patients with renal failure normally require no adjustment in dosage when usual doses of Rocephin are administered, but concentrations of drug in the serum should be monitored periodically. If evidence of accumulation exists, dosage should be decreased accordingly.

Dosage adjustments should not be necessary in patients with hepatic dysfunction; however, in patients with both hepatic dysfunction and significant renal disease, Rocephin dosage should not exceed 2 gm daily without close monitoring of serum concentrations.

Alterations in prothrombin times have occurred rarely in patients treated with Rocephin. Patients with impaired vitamin K synthesis or low vitamin K stores (*e.g.,* chronic hepatic disease and malnutrition) may require monitoring of prothrombin time during Rocephin treatment. Vitamin K administration (10 mg weekly) may be necessary if the prothrombin time is prolonged before or during therapy.

Prolonged use of Rocephin may result in overgrowth of nonsusceptible organisms. Careful observation of the patient is essential. If superinfection occurs during therapy, appropriate measures should be taken.

Rocephin should be prescribed with caution in individuals with a history of gastrointestinal disease, especially colitis.

CARCINOGENESIS, MUTAGENESIS, IMPAIRMENT OF FERTILITY:

Carcinogenesis: Considering the maximum duration of treatment and the class of the compound, carcinogenicity studies with ceftriaxone in animals have not been performed. The maximum duration of animal toxicity studies was six months.

Mutagenesis: Genetic toxicity tests included the Ames test, a micronucleus test and a test for chromosomal aberrations in human lymphocytes cultured *in vitro* with ceftriaxone. Ceftriaxone showed no potential for mutagenic activity in these studies.

Impairment of Fertility: Ceftriaxone produced no impairment of fertility when given intravenously to rats at daily doses up to 586 mg/kg/day, approximately 20 times the recommended clinical dose of 2 gm/day.

PREGNANCY: Teratogenic Effects: Pregnancy Category B. Reproductive studies have been performed in mice and rats at doses up to 20 times the usual human dose and have no evidence of embryotoxicity, fetotoxicity or teratogenicity. In primates, no embryotoxicity or teratogenicity was demonstrated at a dose approximately three times the human dose. There are, however, no adequate and well-controlled studies in pregnant women. Because animal reproductive studies are not always predictive of human response, this drug should be used during pregnancy only if clearly needed.

Nonteratogenic Effects: In rats, in the Segment I (fertility and general reproduction) and Segment III (perinatal and postnatal) studies with intravenously administered ceftriaxone, no adverse effects were noted on various reproductive parameters during gestation and lactation, including postnatal growth, functional behavior and reproductive ability of the offspring, at doses of 586 mg/kg/day or less.

NURSING MOTHERS: Low concentrations of ceftriaxone are excreted in human milk. Caution should be exercised when Rocephin is administered to a nursing woman.

PEDIATRIC USE: Safety and effectiveness of Rocephin in neonates, infants and children have been established for the dosages described in the Dosage and Administration section.

ADVERSE REACTIONS

Rocephin is generally well tolerated. In clinical trials, the following adverse reactions, which were considered to be related to Rocephin therapy or of uncertain etiology, were observed:

LOCAL REACTIONS—pain, induration or tenderness at the site of injection (1%). Less frequently reported (less than 1%) was phlebitis after I.V. administration.

HYPERSENSITIVITY—rash (1.7%). Less frequently reported (less than 1%) were pruritus, fever or chills.

HEMATOLOGIC—eosinophilia (6%), thrombocytosis (5.1%) and leukopenia (2.1%). Less frequently reported (less than 1%) were anemia, neutropenia, lymphopenia, thrombocytopenia and prolongation of the prothrombin time.

GASTROINTESTINAL—diarrhea (2.7%). Less frequently reported (less than 1%) were nausea or vomiting, and dysgeusia.

HEPATIC—elevations of SGOT (3.1%) or SGPT (3.3%). Less frequently reported (less than 1%) were elevations of alkaline phosphatase and bilirubin.

RENAL—elevations of the BUN (1.2%). Less frequently reported (less than 1%) were elevations of creatinine and the presence of casts in the urine.

CENTRAL NERVOUS SYSTEM—headache or dizziness were reported occasionally (less than 1%).

GENITOURINARY—moniliasis or vaginitis were reported occasionally (less than 1%).

MISCELLANEOUS—diaphoresis and flushing were reported occasionally (less than 1%).

Other rarely observed adverse reactions (less than 0.1%) include leukocytosis, lymphocytosis, monocytosis, basophilia, a decrease in the prothrombin time, jaundice, glycosuria, hematuria, bronchospasm, serum sickness, abdominal pain, colitis, flatulence, dyspepsia, palpitations and epistaxis.

DOSAGE AND ADMINISTRATION

Rocephin may be administered intravenously or intramuscularly. The usual adult daily dose is 1 to 2 gm given once a day (or in equally divided doses twice a day) depending on the type and severity of the infection. The total daily dose should not exceed 4 grams.

For the treatment of serious miscellaneous infections in children, other than meningitis, the recommended total daily dose is 50 to 75 mg/kg (not to exceed 2 grams), given in divided doses every 12 hours.

Generally, Rocephin therapy should be continued for at least two days after the signs and symptoms of infection have disappeared. The usual duration is 4 to 14 days; in complicated infections longer therapy may be required.

In the treatment of meningitis, a daily dose of 100 mg/kg (not to exceed 4 grams), given in divided doses every 12 hours, should be administered with or without a loading dose of 75 mg/kg.

For the treatment of uncomplicated gonococcal infections, a single intramuscular dose of 250 mg is recommended.

For preoperative use (surgical prophylaxis), a single dose of 1 gm administered ½ to 2 hours before surgery is recommended.

When treating infections caused by *Streptococcus pyogenes*, therapy should be continued for at least ten days.

No dosage adjustment is necessary for patients with impairment of renal or hepatic function; however, blood levels should be monitored in patients with severe renal impairment (*e.g.,* dialysis patients) and in patients with both renal and hepatic dysfunctions.

DIRECTIONS FOR USE

INTRAMUSCULAR ADMINISTRATION: Reconstitute Rocephin powder with the appropriate diluent (see Compatibility-Stability section).

Vial Dosage Size	Amount of Diluent to be Added
250 mg	0.9 ml
500 mg	1.8 ml
1 gm	3.6 ml
2 gm	7.2 ml

After reconstitution, each 1 ml of solution contains approximately 250 mg equivalent of ceftriaxone. If required, more dilute solutions could be utilized. As with all intramuscular preparations, Rocephin should be injected well within the body of a relatively large muscle; aspiration helps to avoid unintentional injection into a blood vessel.

INTRAVENOUS ADMINISTRATION: Rocephin should be administered intravenously by intermittent infusion. Concentrations between 10 mg/ml and 40 mg/ml are recommended; however, lower concentrations may be used if desired. Reconstitute vials or "piggyback" bottles with an appropriate I.V. diluent (see Compatibility-Stability section).

Vial Dosage Size	Amount of Diluent to be Added
250 mg	2.4 ml
500 mg	4.8 ml
1 gm	9.6 ml
2 gm	19.2 ml

After reconstitution, each 1 ml of solution contains approximately 100 mg equivalent of ceftriaxone. Withdraw entire contents and dilute to the desired concentration with the appropriate I.V. diluent.

Piggyback Bottle Dosage Size	Amount of Diluent to be Added
1 gm	10 ml
2 gm	20 ml

After reconstitution, further dilute to 50 ml or 100 ml volumes with the appropriate I.V. diluent.

10 gm Bulk Pharmacy Container: This dosage size is *NOT FOR DIRECT ADMINISTRATION.* Reconstitute powder with 95 ml of an appropriate I.V. diluent. Before parenteral administration, withdraw the required amount, then further dilute to the desired concentration.

Diluent	Storage Room Temp. (25°C)	Refrigerated (4°C)
Sterile Water	3 days	10 days
0.9% Sodium Chloride Solution	3 days	10 days
5% Dextrose Solution	3 days	10 days
10% Dextrose Solution	3 days	10 days
5% Dextrose + 0.9% Sodium Chloride Solution*	3 days	Incompatible
5% Dextrose + 0.45% Sodium Chloride Solution	3 days	Incompatible

*Data available for 10–40 mg/ml concentrations in this diluent in PVC containers only.

Diluent	Concentration mg/ml	Storage Room Temp. (25°C)	Refrigerated (4°C)
Sterile Water for Injection	100	3 days	10 days
	250	24 hours	3 days
0.9% Sodium Chloride Solution	100	3 days	10 days
	250	24 hours	3 days
5% Dextrose Solution	100	3 days	10 days
	250	24 hours	3 days
Bacteriostatic Water + 0.9% Benzyl Alcohol	100	24 hours	10 days
	250	24 hours	3 days
1% Lidocaine Solution (without epinephrine)	100	24 hours	10 days
	250	24 hours	3 days

COMPATIBILITY AND STABILITY

Rocephin sterile powder should be stored at room temperature—77°F (25°C)—or below and protected from light. After reconstitution, protection from normal light is not necessary. The color of solutions ranges from light yellow to amber, depending on the length of storage, concentration and diluent used.

Rocephin *intramuscular* solutions remain stable (loss of potency less than 10%) for the following time periods:

[See table above].

Rocephin *intravenous* solutions, at concentrations of 10, 20 and 40 mg/ml, remain stable (loss of potency less than 10%) for the following time periods stored in glass or PVC containers:

[See table below left].

Similarly, Rocephin *intravenous* solutions, at concentrations of 100 mg/ml, remain stable in the I.V. piggyback glass containers for the above specified time periods.

The following *intravenous* Rocephin solutions are stable at room temperature (25°C) for 24 hours, at concentrations between 10 mg/ml and 40 mg/ml: Sodium Lactate (PVC container), 10% Invert Sugar (glass container), 5% Sodium Bicarbonate (glass container), Freamine III (glass container), Normosol-M in 5% Dextrose (glass and PVC containers), Ionosol-B in 5% Dextrose (glass container), 5% Mannitol (glass container), 10% Mannitol (glass container).

After the indicated stability time periods, unused portions of solutions should be discarded.

Rocephin reconstituted with 5% Dextrose or 0.9% Sodium Chloride solution at concentrations between 10 mg/ml and 40 mg/ml, and then stored in frozen state (−20°C) in PVC (Viaflex) or polyolefin containers, remains stable for 26 weeks.

Frozen solutions should be thawed at room temperature before use. After thawing, unused portions should be discarded. Do not refreeze.

Rocephin solutions should *not* be physically mixed with or piggybacked into solutions containing other antimicrobial drugs or into diluent solutions other than those listed above, due to possible incompatibility.

ANIMAL PHARMACOLOGY

Concretions consisting of the precipitated calcium salt of ceftriaxone have been found in the gallbladder bile of dogs and baboons treated with ceftriaxone.

These appeared as a gritty sediment in dogs that received 100 mg/kg/day for four weeks. A similar phenomenon has been observed in baboons but only after a protracted dosing period (6 months) at higher dose levels (335 mg/kg/day or more). The likelihood of this occurrence in humans is considered to be low, since ceftriaxone has a greater plasma half-life in humans, the calcium salt of ceftriaxone is more soluble in human gallbladder bile and the calcium content of human gallbladder bile is relatively low.

HOW SUPPLIED

Rocephin (ceftriaxone sodium/Roche) is supplied as a sterile crystalline powder in glass vials and piggyback bottles. The following packages are available:

Vials containing 250 mg equivalent of ceftriaxone. Boxes of 10 (NDC 0004-1962-01).

Vials containing 500 mg equivalent of ceftriaxone. Boxes of 10 (NDC 0004-1963-01).

Vials containing 1 gm equivalent of ceftriaxone. Boxes of 10 (NDC 0004-1964-01).

Piggyback bottles containing 1 gm equivalent of ceftriaxone. Boxes of 10 (NDC 0004-1964-03).

Vials containing 2 gm equivalent of ceftriaxone. Boxes of 10 (NDC 0004-1965-01).

Piggyback bottles containing 2 gm equivalent of ceftriaxone. Boxes of 10 (NDC 0004-1965-03).

Bulk pharmacy containers, containing 10 gm equivalent of ceftriaxone. Boxes of 1 (NDC 0004-1971-01). NOT FOR DIRECT ADMINISTRATION.

Continued on next page

Roche Labs.—Cont.

ROFERON®-A ℞

[ro-fear'on]

(Interferon alfa-2a, recombinant/Roche)

The following text is complete prescribing information based on official labeling in effect July 1, 1986.

DESCRIPTION

Roferon®-A (Interferon alfa-2a, recombinant/Roche) is a sterile protein product for use by injection. Roferon-A is manufactured by recombinant DNA technology that employs a genetically engineered *E. coli* bacterium containing DNA that codes for the human protein. Interferon alfa-2a, recombinant/Roche is a highly purified protein containing 165 amino acids, and it has an approximate molecular weight of 19,000 daltons. The purification procedure includes affinity chromatography using a murine monoclonal antibody. Roferon-A is supplied as an injectable solution. The solution is colorless and contains Interferon alfa-2a, recombinant/Roche, phenol as a preservative, sodium chloride for isotonicity and human serum albumin as a stabilizer. Fermentation is carried out in a defined nutrient medium containing the antibiotic tetracycline hydrochloride, 5 mg/liter. However, the presence of the antibiotic is not detectable in the final product.

Each vial of Roferon-A contains 3 million or 18 million international units (IU) of Interferon alfa-2a, recombinant/Roche. The specific activity of Interferon alfa-2a, recombinant/Roche is 2×10^8 IU/mg protein. The route of administration is subcutaneous or intramuscular.

CLINICAL PHARMACOLOGY

The mechanism by which Interferon alfa-2a, recombinant/Roche, or any other interferon, exerts antitumor activity is not clearly understood. However, it is believed that direct antiproliferative action against tumor cells and modulation of the host immune response play important roles in the antitumor activity.

The biological activities of Interferon alfa-2a, recombinant/Roche are species-restricted, *i.e.*, they are expressed in a very limited number of species other than humans. As a consequence, preclinical evaluation of Interferon alfa-2a, recombinant/Roche has involved *in vitro* experiments with human cells and some *in vivo* experiments. [1] Using human cells in culture, Interferon alfa-2a, recombinant/Roche has been shown to have antiproliferative and immunomodulatory activities that are very similar to those of the mixture of interferon alfa subtypes produced by human leukocytes. *In vivo*, Interferon alfa-2a, recombinant/Roche has been shown to inhibit the growth of several human tumors growing in immunocompromised (nude) mice. Because of its species-restricted activity, it has not been possible to demonstrate antitumor activity in immunologically intact syngeneic tumor model systems, where effects on the host immune system would be observable. However, such antitumor activity has been repeatedly demonstrated with, for example, mouse interferon-alfa in transplantable mouse tumor systems. The clinical significance of these findings is unknown.

The metabolism of Interferon alfa-2a, recombinant/Roche is consistent with that of alfa interferons in general. Alfa interferons are totally filtered through the glomeruli and undergo rapid proteolytic degradation during tubular reabsorption, rendering a negligible reappearance of intact alfa interferon in the systemic circulation. Small amounts of radiolabeled Interferon alfa-2a, recombinant/Roche appear in the urine of isolated rat kidneys, suggesting near complete reabsorption of Interferon alfa-2a, recombinant/Roche catabolites. Liver metabolism and subsequent biliary excretion are considered minor pathways of elimination for alfa interferons.

The serum concentrations of Interferon alfa-2a, recombinant/Roche reflected a large intersubject variation in both healthy volunteers and patients with disseminated cancer.

In healthy people, Interferon alfa-2a, recombinant/Roche exhibited an elimination half-life of 3.7 to 8.5 hours (mean 5.1 hours), volume of distribution at steady-state of 0.223 to 0.748 L/kg (mean 0.400 L/kg) and a total body clearance of 2.14 to 3.62 mL/min/kg (mean 2.79 mL/min/kg) after a 36 million IU (2.2×10^8 pg) intravenous infusion. After intramuscular and subcutaneous administrations of 36 million IU, peak serum concentrations ranged from 1500 to 2580 pg/mL (mean 2020 pg/mL) at a mean time to peak of 3.8 hours and from 1250 to 2320 pg/mL (mean 1730 pg/mL) at a mean time to peak of 7.3 hours, respectively. The apparent fraction of the dose absorbed after intramuscular injection was greater than 80%.

The pharmacokinetics of Interferon alfa-2a, recombinant/Roche after single intramuscular doses to patients with disseminated cancer were similar to those found in healthy volunteers. Dose proportional increases in serum concentrations were observed after single doses up to 198 million IU. There were no changes in the distribution or elimination of Interferon alfa-2a, recombinant/Roche during twice daily (0.5 to 36 million IU), once daily (1 to 54 million IU), or three times weekly (1 to 136 million IU) dosing regimens up to 28 days of dosing. Multiple intramuscular doses of Interferon alfa-2a, recombinant/Roche resulted in an accumulation of 2 to 4 times the single dose serum concentrations. Pharmacokinetic information in patients with hairy cell leukemia is presently unknown.

The acute parenteral toxicity of Interferon alfa-2a, recombinant/Roche has been studied in mice, rats, rabbits and ferrets at doses up to 30 million IU/kg intravenously, and 500 million IU/kg intramuscularly. No treatment-related mortality was noted in any species given Interferon alfa-2a, recombinant/Roche by any of the routes of administration.

Effects on Hairy Cell Leukemia: During the first one to two months of treatment of patients with hairy cell leukemia, significant depression of hematopoiesis was likely to occur. Subsequently, there was improvement in circulating blood cell counts.

Of the 75 patients who were evaluable for efficacy following at least 16 weeks of therapy, 46 (61%) achieved complete or partial response. Twenty-one patients (28%) had a minor remission, eight (11%) remained stable, and none had worsening of disease. All patients who achieved either a complete or partial response had complete or partial normalization of all peripheral blood elements including hemoglobin level, white blood cell, neutrophil, monocyte and platelet counts with a concomitant decrease in peripheral blood and bone marrow hairy cells. Responding patients also exhibited a marked reduction in red blood cell and platelet transfusion requirements, a decrease in infectious episodes and improvement in performance status. The probability of survival for two years in patients receiving Roferon-A (94%) was statistically increased compared to a historical control group (75%).

INDICATIONS AND USAGE

Roferon-A is indicated for use in the treatment of hairy cell leukemia in people 18 years of age or older. Studies have shown that Roferon-A can produce clinically meaningful regression or stabilization of this disease, both in previously splenectomized and nonsplenectomized patients.[2,3]

Prior to initiation of therapy, tests should be performed to quantitate peripheral blood hemoglobin, platelets, granulocytes and hairy cells and bone marrow hairy cells. These parameters should be monitored periodically (*e.g.*, monthly) during treatment to determine whether response to treatment has occurred. If a patient does not respond within six months, treatment should be discontinued. If a response to treatment does occur, treatment should be continued until no further improvement is observed and these laboratory parameters have been stable for about three months. It is not known whether continued treatment after that time is beneficial. Studies are in progress to evaluate this question.

CONTRAINDICATIONS

Roferon-A is contraindicated in patients with known hypersensitivity to alfa interferon, mouse immunoglobulin or any component of the product.

WARNINGS

Roferon-A should be administered under the guidance of a qualified physician. (See DOSAGE AND ADMINISTRATION.) Appropriate management of the therapy and its complications is possible only when adequate diagnostic and treatment facilities are readily available.

Roferon-A should be used with caution in patients with severe preexisting cardiac disease, severe renal or hepatic disease, seizure disorders and/or compromised central nervous system function.

Because of the possibility of severe or even fatal adverse reactions, patients should be informed not only of the benefits of therapy but also of the risks involved.

Roferon-A should be administered with caution to patients with cardiac disease or with any history of cardiac illness. No direct cardiotoxic effect has been demonstrated, but it is likely that acute, self-limited toxicities (*i.e.*, fever, chills) frequently associated with Roferon-A administration may exacerbate preexisting cardiac conditions. Rarely, myocardial infarction has occurred in patients receiving Roferon-A.

Caution should be exercised when administering Roferon-A to patients with myelosuppression.

Central nervous system adverse reactions have been reported in a number of patients. These reactions included decreased mental status, exaggerated central nervous system function, and dizziness. More severe obtundation and coma have been rarely observed. Most of these abnormalities were mild and reversible within a few days to three weeks upon dose reduction or discontinuation of Roferon-A therapy. Careful periodic neuropsychiatric monitoring of all patients is recommended.

Leukopenia and elevation of hepatic enzymes occurred frequently but were rarely dose-limiting. Thrombocytopenia occurred less frequently. Proteinuria and increased cells in urinary sediment were also seen infrequently. Rarely, significant hepatic, renal and myelosuppressive toxicities were noted.

PRECAUTIONS

General: In all instances where the use of Roferon-A is considered for chemotherapy, the physician must evaluate the need and usefulness of the drug against the risk of adverse reactions. Most adverse reactions are reversible if detected early. If severe reactions occur, the drug should be reduced in dosage or discontinued and appropriate corrective measures should be taken according to the clinical judgment of the physician. Reinstitution of Roferon-A therapy should be carried out with caution and with adequate consideration of the further need for the drug and alertness as to possible recurrence of toxicity.

The minimum effective dose of Roferon-A for treatment of hairy cell leukemia has not been established.

Information for Patient: Patients should be cautioned not to change brands of Interferon without medical consultation, as a change in dosage may result. Patients should be informed regarding the potential benefits and risks attendant to the use of Roferon-A. If home use is determined to be desirable by the physician, instructions on appropriate use should be given, including review of the contents of the enclosed Patient Information Sheet. Patients should be well hydrated, especially during the initial stages of treatment.

Laboratory Tests: Periodic complete blood counts and liver function tests should be performed during the course of Roferon-A treatment. They should be performed prior to therapy and at appropriate periods during therapy. Since responses of hairy cell leukemia are not generally observed for one to three months after initiation of treatment, very careful monitoring for severe depression of blood cell counts is warranted during the initial phase of treatment.

Those patients who have preexisting cardiac abnormalities and/or are in advanced stages of cancer should have electrocardiograms taken prior to and during the course of treatment.

Carcinogenesis, Mutagenesis and Impairment of Fertility:

Carcinogenesis: Roferon-A has not been tested for its carcinogenic potential.

Mutagenesis: A. Internal studies—Ames tests using six different tester strains, with and without metabolic activation, were performed with Roferon-A up to a concentration of 1920 μg/plate. There was no evidence of mutagenicity.

Human lymphocyte cultures were treated *in vitro* with Roferon-A at noncytotoxic concentrations. No increase in the incidence of chromosomal damage was noted.

B. Published studies—There are no published studies on the mutagenic potential of Roferon-A. However, a number of studies on the genotoxicity of human leukocyte interferon have been reported.

A chromosomal defect following the addition of human leukocyte interferon to lymphocyte cultures from a patient suffering from a lymphoproliferative disorder has been reported.

In contrast, other studies have failed to detect chromosomal abnormalities following treatment of lymphocyte cultures from healthy volunteers with human leukocyte interferon.

It has also been shown that human leukocyte interferon protects primary chick embryo fibroblasts from chromosomal aberrations produced by gamma rays.

Impairment of Fertility: Roferon-A has been studied for its effect on fertility in Macaca mulatta (rhesus monkeys). Nonpregnant rhesus females treated with Roferon-A at doses of 5 and 25 million IU/kg/day have shown menstrual cycle irregularities, including prolonged or shortened menstrual periods and erratic bleeding; these cycles were considered to be anovulatory. These monkeys returned to a normal menstrual rhythm following discontinuation of treatment.

Drug Interactions: Interactions between Roferon-A and other drugs have not been fully evaluated.

PREGNANCY

Teratogenic Effects: Pregnancy Category C. Roferon-A has been shown to demonstrate a statistically significant increase in abortifacient activity in rhesus monkeys when given at approximately 20 to 500 times the human dose. A study in pregnant rhesus monkeys treated with 1, 5, or 25 million IU/kg/day of Roferon-A in their early to mid-fetal period (days 22 to 70 of gestation) has failed to demonstrate teratogenic activity for Roferon-A.

There are no adequate and well-controlled studies in pregnant women.

Nonteratogenic Effects: Dose-related abortifacient activity was observed in pregnant rhesus monkeys treated with 1, 5 or 25 million IU/kg/day of Roferon-A in their early to mid-fetal period (days 22 to 70 of gestation). A late-fetal study (days 79 to 100 of gestation) is in progress and as yet there have been no reports of any increased rate of abortion.

Usage in Pregnancy: Safe use in human pregnancy has not been established. Therefore, Roferon-A should be used during pregnancy only if the potential benefit justifies the potential risk to the fetus. Information from primate studies showed dose-related menstrual irregularities and an increased incidence of spontaneous abortions. Therefore, fertile women should not receive Roferon-A unless they are using effective contraception during the therapy period.

Male fertility and teratologic evaluations have yielded no significant adverse effects to date.

Nursing Mothers: It is not known whether this drug is excreted in human milk. Because many drugs are excreted in human milk and because of the potential for serious adverse reactions in nursing infants from Roferon-A, a decision should be made whether to discontinue nursing or to discontinue the drug, taking into account the importance of the drug to the mother.

Pediatric Use: Safety and effectiveness in children under 18 years of age have not been established.

ADVERSE REACTIONS

The following data on adverse reactions are based on the subcutaneous or intramuscular administration of Roferon-A as a single agent for the treatment of 63 patients with hairy cell leukemia during investigational trials in the United States.

Flu-like syndromes consisting of fatigue (89%), fever (98%), chills (64%), myalgias (73%) and headache (71%) occurred in the majority of patients and tended to diminish with continuing therapy. Other side effects such as anorexia (46%), nausea (32%), emesis (10%), diarrhea (29%), dizziness (21%), rash (18%), change in taste (13%), dryness or inflammation of the oropharynx (16%), dry skin or pruritus (13%) and weight loss (14%) were observed with moderate frequency. Less commonly, diaphoresis (8%), paresthesias (6%), numbness (6%), partial alopecia (8%), reactivation of herpes labialis (8%), transient impotence (6%) and arthralgias (5%) were also observed. Rarely (< 3%), central nervous system effects including decreased mental status, depression, visual disturbances, sleep disturbances and nervousness, as well as cardiac adverse events, including hypertension, chest pain, arrhythmias and palpitations, were reported. Adverse experiences which occurred rarely and may have been related to underlying disease, included epistaxis, bleeding gums, ecchymosis and petechiae. Miscellaneous adverse events, such as night sweats, urticaria, conjunctivitis and inflammation at the site of injection, were also rarely observed.

Roferon-A has also been evaluated for the treatment of many other types of cancer under investigational trials in the United States. These studies generally utilized higher doses (12 to 50 million IU/m^2). All of the previously described adverse reactions which occurred in patients with hairy cell leukemia were also observed in patients receiving higher doses. The incidence of most adverse reactions was similar between the two groups, but tended to be more severe in patients who received higher doses of Roferon-A. Some additional adverse effects which occurred in these patients included confusion (10%), hypotension (6%), lethargy (3%) and edema (3%). Adverse experiences occurring in less than 1% of these patients and observed only in patients with malignancies other than hairy cell leukemia are as follows: *Gastrointestinal*—abdominal fullness, hypermotility and hepatitis; *Central Nervous System*—gait disturbance, poor coordination, hallucinations, syncope, seizures, encephalopathy, psychomotor retardation, coma, stroke, transient ischemic attacks, aphasia, aphonia, dysarthria, dysphasia, forgetfulness, amnesia, sedation, apathy, anxiety, emotional lability, irritability, hyperactivity, involuntary movements, claustrophobia and loss of libido; *Peripheral Nervous System*—muscle contractions; *Cardiovascular*—congestive heart failure, pulmonary edema, myocardial infarction, Raynaud's phenomenon and hot flashes; *Pulmonary*—bronchospasm and tachypnea; *Miscellaneous*—excessive salivation and flushing of skin.

Abnormal Laboratory Test Values: The percentage of patients with hairy cell leukemia or with other types of malignancies who experienced a significant abnormal laboratory test value at least once during their treatment is shown in the following table:

ABNORMAL LABORATORY TEST VALUES

	Hairy Cell Leukemia (n=63)	Overall Safety Summary* (n=1019)
Hematologic		
Leukopenia	59%	69%
Neutropenia	39%	58%
Thrombocytopenia	42%	42%
Decreased Hemoglobin	36%	6.3%
Decreased Hematocrit	43%	12.5%
Mean Time to Nadir		
WBC	38 days	22 days
Platelets	19 days	17 days
Hepatic		
SGOT	47%	78%
Alkaline Phosphatase	18%	48%
LDH	12%	47%
Bilirubin	1.6%	31%
Renal/Urinary		
BUN	2%	10%
Serum Creatinine	3%	10%
Uric Acid†	6%	15%
Proteinuria†	10%	25%
Other Chemistry Tests		
Hypocalcemia	10%	51%
Elevated FBS‡	33%	39%
Elevated Serum Phosphorus	2%	17%

* Patients with hairy cell leukemia are included in this overall summary.

† The majority of abnormal uric acid values and proteinuria were of minimal severity. Since these abnormalities are commonly observed in patients with advanced malignancy, it is difficult to ascertain their relationship to Roferon-A treatment.

‡ Random glucose determination.

Neutralizing antibodies to Roferon-A were detected in approximately 27% of all patients (3.4% for patients with hairy cell leukemia). No clinical sequelae of their presence have been documented thus far. Antibodies to human leukocyte interferon may occur spontaneously in certain clinical conditions (cancer, systemic lupus erythematosus, herpes zoster) in patients who have never received exogenous interferon.[4]

DOSAGE AND ADMINISTRATION

Hairy Cell Leukemia—The induction dose of Roferon-A is 3 million IU daily for 16 to 24 weeks, administered as a subcutaneous or intramuscular injection. Subcutaneous administration is particularly advisable for, but not limited to, thrombocytopenic patients (platelet count < 50,000) or for patients at risk for bleeding. The recommended maintenance dose is 3 million IU, three times per week. Dosage reduction by one-half or withholding of individual doses may be needed when severe adverse reactions occur. The use of doses higher than 3 million IU is not recommended.

Patients should be treated for approximately six months before the physician determines whether to continue therapy in patients who respond or discontinue therapy in patients who did not respond. Patients with hairy cell leukemia have been treated for up to 20 consecutive months. The optimal duration of treatment for this disease has not been determined.

If severe reactions occur, dosage should be modified (50% reduction) or therapy should be temporarily discontinued until the adverse reactions abate. The need for dosage reduction should take into account the effects of prior X-ray therapy or chemotherapy that may be have compromised bone marrow reserve. The minimum effective dose of Roferon-A has not been established.

DIRECTIONS FOR USE

The subcutaneous or intramuscular routes of administration should be used. Subcutaneous administration is particularly suggested for, but not limited to, patients who are thrombocytopenic (platelet count < 50,000) or who are at risk for bleeding.

Injectable Solution:

3 million IU Roferon-A per vial—Each 1 mL contains 3 million IU of Interferon alfa-2a, recombinant/Roche, 9 mg sodium chloride for isotonicity, 5 mg human serum albumin as a stabilizer and 3 mg phenol as a preservative.

18 million IU Roferon-A per vial (for multiple-dose use)—Each 1 mL contains 6 million IU of Interferon alfa-2a, recombinant/Roche, 9 mg sodium chloride for isotonicity, 5 mg human serum albumin as a stabilizer and 3 mg phenol as a preservative. Each 0.5 mL contains 3 million IU of Interferon alfa-2a, recombinant/Roche.

The injectable solution should be stored in the refrigerator at 36° to 46°F (2° to 8°C). Do *not* freeze. Do not shake.

Parenteral drug products should be inspected visually for particulate matter and discoloration prior to administration, whenever solution and container permit.

HOW SUPPLIED

Sterile Roferon-A is supplied as single and multiple-dose vials:

Roferon-A Injectable Solution: Vials containing 3 million IU Interferon alfa-2a, recombinant/Roche (3 million IU/mL). Boxes of 10. (NDC 0004-1987-01).

Roferon-A Injectable Solution: Multiple-dose vials containing 18 million IU Interferon alfa-2a, recombinant/Roche (3 million IU/0.5 mL). Boxes of 1. (NDC 0004-1988-09).

REFERENCES

1. Trown PW *et al: Cancer 57* (Suppl.):1648–1656, 1986.
2. Foon KA *et al: Blood 64* (Suppl. 1):164a, 1984.
3. Quesada JR *et al: Cancer 57* (Suppl.):1678–1680, 1986.
4. Jones GJ, Itri LM: *Cancer 57* (Suppl.):1709–1715, 1986.

SOLATENE® ℞

[sol 'a-teen]

(beta-carotene/Roche)

capsules

The following text is complete prescribing information based on official labeling in effect June 1, 1986.

DESCRIPTION

Solatene (beta-carotene) is available in capsules for oral administration. Each capsule is composed of beadlets containing 30 mg beta-carotene, gelatin, sucrose, ascorbyl palmitate, butylated hydroxyanisole, butylated hydroxytoluene, hydrogenated coconut oil, parabens (methyl and propyl), sodium benzoate, sodium carbonate and/or sodium bicarbonate, sorbic acid and starch (modified food grade); nonpareil seeds containing starch and sucrose; and magnesium stearate. Gelatin capsule shells may contain parabens (methyl and propyl), potassium sorbate, FD&C Blue No. 1, FD&C Yellow No. 10, FD&C Red No. 3, FD&C Green No. 3 and titanium dioxide.

Beta-carotene, precursor of vitamin A, is a carotenoid pigment occurring naturally in green and yellow vegetables. Chemically, beta-carotene has the empirical formula $C_{40}H_{56}$ and a calculated molecular weight of 536.85. Trans-beta-carotene is a red, crystalline compound which is insoluble in water.

CLINICAL PHARMACOLOGY

Beta-carotene, a provitamin A, belongs to the class of carotenoid pigments. In terms of its vitamin activity, 6 μg of dietary beta-carotene is considered equivalent to 1 μg of vitamin A (retinol). Bioavailability of beta-carotene depends on the presence of fat in the diet to act as a carrier, and bile in the intestinal tract for its absorption. Beta-carotene is metabolized, primarily in the intestine, to vitamin A at a rate of approximately 50% to 60% of normal dietary intake and falls off rapidly as intake goes up. In humans, an appreciable amount of unchanged beta-carotene is absorbed and stored in various tissues, especially the depot fat. Small amounts may be converted to vitamin A in the liver. The vitamin A derived from beta-carotene follows the same metabolic pathway as that from dietary sources. The major route of elimination is fecal excretion. Excessive ingestion of carotenes is not harmful, but it may cause yellow coloration of the skin, which disappears upon reduction or cessation of intake.

INDICATIONS AND USAGE

Solatene is used to reduce the severity of photosensitivity reactions in patients with erythropoietic protoporphyria (EPP).

CONTRAINDICATIONS

Solatene is contraindicated in patients with known hypersensitivity to the drug.

WARNINGS

Solatene has not been shown to be effective as a sunscreen.

PRECAUTIONS

General: Solatene should be used with caution in patients with impaired renal or hepatic function because safe use in the presence of these conditions has not been established.

Information for Patients: Patients receiving Solatene should be advised against taking supplementary vitamin A since Solatene administration will fulfill normal vitamin A requirements. They should be cautioned to continue sun protection, and forewarned that their skin may appear slightly yellow while receiving Solatene.

Carcinogenesis, Mutagenesis, Impairment of Fertility: Long-term studies in animals to determine carcinogenesis have not been completed. *In vitro* and *in vivo* studies to evaluate mutagenic potential were negative. No effects on fertility in male rats were observed at doses as high as 500 mg/kg/day (100 times the recommended human dose).

Pregnancy: Teratogenic Effects: Pregnancy Category C. Beta-carotene has been shown to be fetotoxic (*i.e.*, cause an increase in resorption rate), but not teratogenic when given to rats at doses 300 to 400 times the maximum recommended human dose. No such fetotoxicity was observed at 75 times the maximum recommended human dose or less. A three-generation reproduction study in rats receiving beta-carotene at a dietary concentration of 0.1% (1000 ppm) has revealed no evidence of impaired fertility or effect on the fetus. There are no adequate and well-controlled studies in pregnant women. Solatene should be used during pregnancy only if the potential benefit justifies the potential risk to the fetus.

Nursing Mothers: It is not known whether this drug is excreted in human milk. Because many drugs are excreted in human milk, caution should be exercised when Solatene is administered to a nursing mother.

ADVERSE REACTIONS

Some patients may have occasional loose stools while taking Solatene. This reaction is sporadic and may not require discontinuance of medication. Other reactions which have been reported rarely are ecchymoses and arthralgia.

OVERDOSAGE

There are no reported cases of overdosage. The oral LD_{50} of beta-carotene (suspended in 5% gum acacia solution) in mice and rats is greater than 20,000 mg/kg. No lethality was observed in mice following administration of 30-mg beadlet capsules (ground and suspended in 5% gum acacia) at a dose of 1200 mg/kg beta-carotene.

DOSAGE AND ADMINISTRATION

Solatene may be administered either as a single daily dose or in divided doses, preferably with meals.

Continued on next page

Roche Labs.—Cont.

Usage in Children: The usual dosage for children under 14 is 30 to 150 mg (1 to 5 capsules) per day. Capsules may be opened and the contents mixed in orange juice or tomato juice to aid administration.
Usage in Adults: The usual adult dosage is 30 to 300 mg (1 to 10 capsules) per day.
Dosage should be adjusted depending on the severity of the symptoms and the response of the patient. Several weeks of therapy are necessary to accumulate enough Solatene in the skin to exert its effect. Patients should be instructed not to increase exposure to sunlight until they appear carotenemic (first seen as yellowness of palms and soles). This usually occurs after two to six weeks of therapy. Exposure to the sun may then be increased gradually. The protective effect is not total and each patient should establish his or her own limits of exposure.

HOW SUPPLIED

Solatene is available in blue and green capsules, each containing 30 mg of beta-carotene—bottles of 100 (NDC 0004-0115-01). Imprint on capsules: SOLATENE ROCHE.

Shown in Product Identification Section, page 425

SYNKAYVITE® ℞

(menadiol sodium diphosphate/Roche)
INJECTABLE

The following text is complete product information based on official labeling in effect June 1, 1986.

DESCRIPTION

Synkayvite (menadiol sodium diphosphate/Roche) Injectable, a synthetic water-soluble derivative of menadione (vitamin K_3), is a sterile aqueous solution intended for intramuscular, intravenous or subcutaneous administration. Synkayvite Injectable is available in the following concentrations:
1-ml Ampuls, 5 mg/ml—each ml contains 5 mg menadiol sodium diphosphate compounded with 2.5 mg sodium metabisulfite, 0.45% phenol as preservative, 0.4% sodium chloride for isotonicity and sodium hydroxide to adjust pH to approximately 8.0.
1-ml Ampuls, 10 mg/ml—each ml contains 10 mg menadiol sodium diphosphate compounded with 2.5 mg sodium metabisulfite, 0.45% phenol as preservative, 0.4% sodium chloride for isotonicity and sodium hydroxide to adjust pH to approximately 8.0.
2-ml Ampuls, 75 mg/2 ml—each 2 ml contains 75 mg menadiol sodium diphosphate compounded with 5 mg sodium metabisulfite, 0.45% phenol as preservative, 0.4% sodium chloride for isotonicity and sodium hydroxide to adjust pH to approximately 8.0.
Chemically, menadiol sodium diphosphate is 2-methyl-1,4-naphthalenediol bis (dihydrogen phosphate) tetrasodium salt, hexahydrate. It is a white to pink hygroscopic powder with a characteristic odor and is very soluble in water and insoluble in alcohol. It has a molecular weight of 530.18.

CLINICAL PHARMACOLOGY

Synkayvite is converted *in vivo* to menadione (vitamin K_3). Its potency is approximately one-half that of menadione. Synkayvite is similar in activity to naturally occurring vitamin K, which is necessary for the synthesis in the liver of blood coagulation factors prothrombin (factor II), proconvertin (factor VII), thromboplastin (factor IX) and Stuart factor (factor X). The prothrombin test is sensitive to the concentrations of factors II, VII and X. The mechanism by which vitamin K_1 promotes formation of these clotting factors is not known, but animal data suggest that it acts as an enzyme or catalyst upon a substrate within the liver or combines with an apoenzyme (AE) to form an active enzyme (AE-K) which then is involved in prothrombin synthesis.
Pharmacokinetic data are unavailable because there is no acceptable assay procedure for the determination of menadiol in biological specimens. The physiochemical properties of menadiol sodium diphosphate indicate a negligible potential for absorption problems. The action of menadiol sodium diphosphate is generally detectable within one to two hours following parenteral administration; the prothrombin time often returns to normal in 8 to 24 hours. Vitamin K appears to pass through the placenta.

INDICATIONS AND USAGE

Synkayvite Injectable is indicated for the treatment of hypoprothrombinemia secondary to factors limiting absorption or synthesis of vitamin K, *e.g.,* obstructive jaundice, biliary fistula, sprue, ulcerative colitis, celiac disease, intestinal resection, cystic fibrosis of the pancreas, regional enteritis and antibacterial therapy.
It is also indicated in hypoprothrombinemia secondary to administration of salicylates.
Synkayvite Injectable may also be used as a liver function test, although newer methods are available.

CONTRAINDICATIONS

Vitamin K, or any of its synthetic analogs, should not be administered to the mother during the *last few weeks of pregnancy* as a prophylactic measure against physiologic hypoprothrombinemia or hemorrhagic disease of the newborn.
Synkayvite is contraindicated in patients with known hypersensitivity to the drug.

WARNINGS

Synkayvite Injectable should not be used in the prophylaxis and treatment of hemorrhagic disease of the newborn, because phytonadione/Roche (Konakion®) is safer than the water-soluble vitamin K analogs.
Synkayvite and other water-soluble vitamin K analogs are ineffective in the treatment of oral anticoagulant-induced hypoprothrombinemia and, therefore, should not be used in its treatment. Synkayvite will not counteract the anticoagulant action of heparin.

PRECAUTIONS

General: Temporary resistance to prothrombin-depressing anticoagulants may result, especially when larger doses of Synkayvite are used. If relatively large doses have been employed, it may be necessary when reinstituting anticoagulant therapy to use somewhat larger doses of prothrombin-depressing anticoagulant or one which has a different mode of action, such as heparin.
Since the liver is the site of metabolic synthesis of prothrombin, hypoprothrombinemia resulting from hepatocellular damage is not corrected by administration of vitamin K. Repeated large doses of vitamin K are not warranted in liver disease if the response to initial use of the vitamin is unsatisfactory (Koller test).
Failure to respond to vitamin K may indicate that a coagulation defect is present or that the condition being treated is unresponsive to vitamin K.
Laboratory Tests: The dose, route and frequency of administration and duration of treatment depend on the severity of the prothrombin deficiency and should be regulated by repeated determinations of prothrombin time.
Drug Interactions: Patients being treated with coumarin and indandione derivative anticoagulants are extremely sensitive to changes in available vitamin K. Therefore, large doses of menadione or menadiol sodium diphosphate may decrease patient sensitivity to oral anticoagulants, although these vitamin K analogs are ineffective in treating anticoagulant overdosage.
Drug/Laboratory Test Interactions: Menadione has been reported to interfere with the modified Reedy, Jenkins, Thorn procedure for determining urinary 17-hydroxycorticosteroids, producing falsely elevated levels.
Carcinogenesis, Mutagenesis and Impairment of Fertility: Synkayvite has not undergone adequate animal testing to evaluate carcinogenic potential. The mutagenicity of Synkayvite has not been evaluated in the Ames test. Synkayvite has not been evaluated for effects on fertility.
Pregnancy: Teratogenic Effects: Pregnancy Category C. Segment II reproduction studies have not been conducted with menadiol. However, menadione (vitamin K_3) was nonteratogenic in rats at doses of 15 and 150 mg/day. The 150 mg/day dose in rats is approximately 872 times the maximum human therapeutic dose of 30 mg daily for the treatment of hypoprothrombinemia and 350 times the human dose of 75 mg for the liver function test. It is not known whether Synkayvite can cause fetal harm when administered to a pregnant woman or can affect reproductive capacity. Synkayvite should be given to a pregnant woman only if clearly needed.
Nonteratogenic effects: Retardation of skeletal ossification and an increase in fetal resorptions have been reported in rats with menadione (vitamin K_3).
Menadione and its derivatives have been implicated in producing hemolytic anemia, hyperbilirubinemia and kernicterus in the newborn, especially in premature infants, when administered to the mother prior to delivery or to the newborn. A marked hyperbilirubinemia has been reported in premature infants of mothers given menadione 2 to 112 hours prior to delivery. Synkayvite given parenterally during labor caused an elevation in prothrombin levels in 16 of 22 infants. (Also see **Contraindications** section.)
Nursing Mothers: A study has shown that vitamin K is excreted in human milk. This should be considered if it is necessary to administer Synkayvite to a nursing mother.
Pediatric Use: See **Warnings** section.

ADVERSE REACTIONS

In adults, bromsulfalein retention and prolongation of prothrombin time have been reported after maximum doses of vitamin K analogs. In infants (particularly premature babies), excessive doses of vitamin K analogs may cause increased bilirubinemia in the first few days of life. This, in turn, may result in kernicterus, which may lead to brain damage or even death. Immaturity is apparently an important factor in the appearance of toxic reactions to vitamin K analogs as full-term and larger premature infants demonstrate greater tolerance than smaller premature infants. (Also see **Warnings** section.)
Menadione can induce erythrocyte hemolysis in persons having a genetic deficiency of glucose-6-phosphate dehydrogenase in their red blood cells.
In patients with severe hepatic disease, large doses of menadione may further depress liver function. Paradoxically, the administration of excessive doses of vitamin K or its analogs in an attempt to correct the hypoprothrombinemia associated with severe hepatitis or cirrhosis may actually result in a further depression of the concentration of prothrombin. (Also see **Precautions,** *General,* section.)
Occasional allergic reactions, such as skin rash and urticaria, have been reported.

OVERDOSAGE

There are no data available on overdosage of Synkayvite in man. The administration of large doses of menadione and its derivatives to animals has resulted in the production of anemia, polycythemia, splenomegaly, renal and hepatic damage and death.
The acute intravenous toxicity of Synkayvite is as follows:

	$LD_{50} \pm$ S.D.
Mouse	500 $\pm$ 55 mg/kg
Rat	400 $\pm$ 65 mg/kg

DOSAGE AND ADMINISTRATION

The U.S. Recommended Daily Allowances for vitamin K in humans have not been established officially. The adequate daily dietary intake of vitamin K for adults has been estimated to be 70 to 140 mcg; for infants 10 to 20 mcg; for children and adolescents 15 to 100 mcg. The dietary abundance of vitamin K normally satisfies the requirements except for the neonatal period of 5 to 8 days.
Synkayvite may be injected subcutaneously, intramuscularly or intravenously. The response after intravenous administration may be more prompt, but more sustained action follows intramuscular or subcutaneous use.
Duration of treatment and frequency of dosage should be governed by blood prothrombin-time determination. In the absence of impaired liver function, a single dose usually corrects hypoprothrombinemia in 8 to 24 hours. Injections should be repeated in 12 hours if tests at this time show no evidence of improvement.
Following are the usual recommended dosages:

	ADULTS	CHILDREN
For treatment of hypoprothrombinemia	5 to 15 mg once or twice daily	5 to 10 mg once or twice daily
For liver function test	75 mg intravenously	

Parenteral drug products should be inspected visually for particulate matter and discoloration prior to administration, whenever solution and container permit. Synkayvite Injectable is incompatible with protein hydrolysate.

HOW SUPPLIED

1-ml Ampuls (5 mg menadiol sodium diphosphate/ml) —boxes of 10 (NDC 0004-1923-06).
1-ml Ampuls (10 mg menadiol sodium diphosphate/ml) —boxes of 10 (NDC 0004-1924-06).
2-ml Ampuls (75 mg menadiol sodium diphosphate/2 ml) —boxes of 10 (NDC 0004-1925-06).
Store at room temperature (15° to 30°C or 59° to 86°F).
Synkayvite need not be refrigerated.

SYNKAYVITE® ℞

(menadiol sodium diphosphate/Roche)
TABLETS

The following text is complete product information based on official labeling in effect June 1, 1986.

DESCRIPTION

Synkayvite (menadiol sodium diphosphate/Roche), a synthetic, water-soluble derivative of menadione (vitamin K_3), is available for oral administration in 5-mg tablets. Each tablet also contains gelatin, lactose, magnesium stearate, corn starch and talc. Chemically, menadiol sodium diphosphate is 2-methyl-1,4-naphthalenediol bis (dihydrogen phosphate) tetrasodium salt, hexahydrate. It is a white to pink hygroscopic powder with a characteristic odor and is very soluble in water and insoluble in alcohol. It has a molecular weight of 530.18.

CLINICAL PHARMACOLOGY

Synkayvite is converted *in vivo* to menadione (vitamin K_3). Its potency is approximately one-half that of menadione. Synkayvite is similar in activity to naturally occurring vitamin K, which is necessary for the synthesis in the liver of blood coagulation factors prothrombin (factor II), proconvertin (factor VII), thromboplastin (factor IX) and Stuart factor (factor X). The prothrombin test is sensitive to the concentrations of factors II, VII and X. The mechanism by which vitamin K_1 promotes formation of these clotting factors is not known, but animal data suggest that it acts as an enzyme or catalyst upon a substrate within the liver or combines with

an apoenzyme (AE) to form an active enzyme (AE-K) which then is involved in prothrombin synthesis.
Pharmacokinetic data are unavailable because there is no acceptable assay procedure for the determination of menadiol in biological specimens. The physiochemical properties of menadiol sodium diphosphate indicate a negligible potential for absorption problems. The onset and duration of action following oral administration are not known. Vitamin K appears to pass through the placenta.

INDICATIONS AND USAGE

Synkayvite Tablets are indicated for:
—vitamin K deficiency secondary to the administration of antibacterial therapy;
—hypoprothrombinemia secondary to obstructive jaundice and biliary fistulas;
—hypoprothrombinemia secondary to administration of salicylates.

CONTRAINDICATIONS

Vitamin K, or any of its synthetic analogs, should not be administered to the mother *during the last few weeks of pregnancy* as a prophylactic measure against physiologic hypoprothrombinemia or hemorrhagic disease of the newborn.
Synkayvite is contraindicated in patients with known hypersensitivity to the drug.

WARNINGS

Synkayvite and other water-soluble vitamin K analogs are ineffective in the treatment of oral anticoagulant-induced hypoprothrombinemia and should, therefore, not be used in its treatment. Synkayvite will not counteract the anticoagulant action of heparin.

PRECAUTIONS

General: Temporary resistance to prothrombin-depressing anticoagulants may result, especially when larger doses of Synkayvite are used. If relatively large doses have been employed, it may be necessary when reinstituting anticoagulant therapy to use somewhat larger doses of the prothrombin-depressing anticoagulant or one which has a different mode of action, such as heparin.
Since the liver is the site of metabolic synthesis of prothrombin, hypoprothrombinemia resulting from hepatocellular damage is not corrected by administration of vitamin K. Repeated large doses of vitamin K are not warranted in liver disease if the response to initial use of the vitamin is unsatisfactory (Koller test).
Failure to respond to vitamin K may indicate that a coagulation defect is present or that the condition being treated is unresponsive to vitamin K.
Information for Patients: To assure safe and effective use of this drug, the following information and instructions should be given to the patient:

1. Take this medication exactly as directed by your doctor. Do not increase or decrease the prescribed dosage, or take it more often, or take it for a longer period of time than instructed.
2. If you miss a dose, take it as soon as possible, and then continue with your normal dosing schedule. Do not take the missed dose if it is almost time for your next dose; continue on your normal schedule and inform your doctor about any doses that you miss. If you have any questions about this, ask your doctor or pharmacist.
3. Inform all doctors and pharmacists that you are taking this medication; other medicines may affect the way this medicine works.
4. Before starting or stopping any other medications, including nonprescription drugs such as aspirin, check with your doctor or pharmacist.
5. A blood test should be performed at regular intervals to determine how this medicine is working. This will help your doctor decide the best dosing schedule for you.
6. Inform your doctor if you are pregnant or become pregnant while using this drug, even though vitamin K has not been shown to cause birth defects or other problems. Also inform your doctor if you are nursing.

Laboratory Tests: The dose, route and frequency of administration and duration of treatment depend on the severity of the prothrombin deficiency and should be regulated by repeated determinations of prothrombin time.
Drug Interactions: Patients being treated with coumarin and indandione derviative anticoagulants are extremely sensitive to changes in available vitamin K. Therefore, large doses of menadione or menadiol sodium diphosphate may decrease patient sensitivity to oral anticoagulants, although these vitamin K analogs are ineffective in treating anticoagulant overdosage.
Drug/Laboratory Test Interactions: Menadione has been reported to interfere with the modified Reddy, Jenkins, Thorn procedure for determining urinary 17-hydroxycorticosteroids, producing falsely elevated levels.
Carcinogenesis, Mutagenesis and Impairment of Fertility: Synkayvite has not undergone adequate animal testing to evaluate carcinogenic potential. The mutagenicity of Synkayvite has not been evaluated in the Ames test. Synkayvite has not been evaluated for effects on fertility.
Pregnancy: Teratogenic Effects: Pregnancy Category C. Segment II reproduction studies have not been conducted with menadiol. However, menadione (vitamin K_3) was nonteratogenic in rats at doses of 15 and 150 mg/day. The 150 mg/day dose in rats is approximately 2640 times the maximum human therapeutic dose of 10 mg daily. It is not known whether Synkayvite can cause fetal harm when administered to a pregnant woman or can affect reproductive capacity. Synkayvite should be given to a pregnant woman only if clearly needed.
Nonteratogenic Effects: Retardation of skeletal ossification and an increase in fetal resorptions have been reported in rats with menadione (vitamin K_3).
Menadione and its derivatives have been implicated in producing hemolytic anemia, hyperbilirubinemia and kernicterus in the newborn, especially in premature infants, when administered to the mother prior to delivery or to the newborn. A marked hyperbilirubinemia has been reported in premature infants of mothers given menadione 2 to 112 hours prior to delivery. Synkayvite given parenterally during labor caused an elevation in prothrombin levels in 16 of 22 infants. (Also see **Contraindications** section.)
Nursing Mothers: A study has shown that vitamin K is excreted in human milk. This should be considered if it is necessary to administer Synkayvite to a nursing mother.

ADVERSE REACTIONS

Bromsulfalein retention and prolongation of prothrombin time have been reported after maximum doses of vitamin K analogs.
Menadione can induce erythrocyte hemolysis in persons having a genetic deficiency of glucose-6-phosphate dehydrogenase in their red blood cells.
In patients with severe hepatic disease, large doses of menadione may further depress liver function. Paradoxically, the administration of excessive doses of vitamin K or its analogs in an attempt to correct the hypoprothrombinemia associated with severe hepatitis or cirrhosis may actually result in a further depression of the concentration of prothrombin. (Also see **Precautions,** *General,* section.)
Occasional allergic reactions, such as skin rash and urticaria, have been reported. There have also been minor instances of gastric disturbance.

OVERDOSAGE

There are no data on overdosage of Synkayvite in man. The administration of large doses of menadione and its derivatives to animals has resulted in the production of anemia, polycythemia, splenomegaly, renal and hepatic damage and death.
The acute oral toxicity of Synkayvite is as follows:

	$LD_{50} \pm$ S.D.
Mouse	6172 $\pm$ 966 mg/kg
Rat	5250 $\pm$ 740 mg/kg

DOSAGE AND ADMINISTRATION

The U.S. Recommended Daily Allowances for vitamin K in humans have not been established officially. The adequate daily dietary intake of vitamin K for adults has been estimated to be 70 to 140 mcg. The dietary abundance of vitamin K normally satisfies these requirements.
Following are the usual recommended dosages:

For hypoprothrombinemia secondary to obstructive jaundice and biliary fistulas	5 mg daily
For hypoprothrombinemia secondary to the administration of antibacterials or salicylates	5 to 10 mg daily

HOW SUPPLIED

White tablets containing 5 mg menadiol sodium diphosphate—bottls of 100 (NDC 0004-0037-01). Imprint on tablets: (front) SYNKAYVITE 5; (back) ROCHE.
Note: Slight pink discoloration of tablets does not affect the safety and efficacy of Synkayvite.
Store at room temperature (15° to 30° C or 59° to 86° F).
Shown in Product Identification Section, page 425

TARACTAN® ℞
[*tar-ac'tan*]
(chlorprothixene/Roche)
TABLETS

TARACTAN® ℞
(chlorprothixene lactate and HCl/Roche)
CONCENTRATE

TARACTAN® ℞
(chlorprothixene HCl/Roche)
AMPULS

The following text is complete prescribing information based on official labeling in effect June 1, 1986.

DESCRIPTION

Tablets—each containing 10 mg, 25 mg, 50 mg or 100 mg chlorprothixene; each tablet also contains acacia, corn starch, dibasic calcium phosphate, gelatin, magnesium stearate, shellac, sugar, talc, hydrogenated vegetable oil, wax (beeswax and carnauba) and other ingredients, with the following dye systems: 10-mg, 25-mg and 50-mg tablets—FD&C Blue No. 2, FD&C Red No. 3, FD&C Yellow No. 5 and FD&C Yellow No. 6; 100-mg tablets—FD&C Blue No. 2, FD&C Red No. 3 and FD&C Yellow No. 5. Concentrate—100 mg/5 ml as the lactate and hydrochloride, fruit flavored; also contains benzoic acid, edetate disodium, glycerin, hydrochloric acid, lactic acid, magnesium aluminum silicate, parabens (methyl and propyl), polyoxyethylene (8) stearate, silicone emulsion, sodium hydroxide, sorbitol, sucrose, FD&C Red No. 40, FD&C Blue No. 1, FD&C Yellow No. 6, flavors and water. Ampuls—25 mg/2 ml as the hydrochloride, with 0.2% parabens (methyl and propyl) added as preservatives and pH adjusted to approximately 3.4 with HCl.
Taractan (chlorprothixene/Roche) is a thioxanthene derivative. Chemically, it is the alpha isomer of 2-chloro-*N, N*-dimethylthioxanthene-Δ^9, γ-propylamine. In chemical structure chlorprothixene resembles the phenothiazines; however, in place of the nitrogen (N) in the phenothiazine ring, chlorprothixene carries a carbon atom with a double bond to a side chain.

ACTIONS

EEG changes following the injection of Taractan into cats suggest that it acts on the brain stem. Effects demonstrated were the synchronization of the EEG tracings during rest, a shortening of cortical activation obtained by stimulation of the reticular formation, and modifications of elicited potentials.

INDICATIONS

Taractan is indicated for the management of manifestations of psychotic disorders. Taractan has not been shown effective in the management of behavioral complications in patients with mental retardation.

CONTRAINDICATIONS

Circulatory collapse, comatose states due to central depressant drugs (alcohol, hypnotics, opiates, etc.) and known sensitivity to the drug are contraindications.

WARNINGS

Tardive Dyskinesia: Tardive dyskinesia, a syndrome consisting of potentially irreversible, involuntary, dyskinetic movements, may develop in patients treated with neuroleptic (antipsychotic) drugs. Although the prevalence of the syndrome appears to be highest among the elderly, especially elderly women, it is impossible to rely upon prevalence estimates to predict, at the inception of neuroleptic treatment, which patients are likely to develop the syndrome. Whether neuroleptic drug products differ in their potential to cause tardive dyskinesia is unknown.
Both the risk of developing the syndrome and the likelihood that it will become irreversible are believed to increase as the duration of treatment and the total cumulative dose of neuroleptic drugs increase. However, the syndrome can develop, although much less commonly, after relatively brief treatment periods at low doses.
There is no known treatment for established cases of tardive dyskinesia, although the syndrome may remit, partially or completely, if neuroleptic treatment is withdrawn. Neuroleptic treatment itself, however, may suppress (or partially suppress) the signs and symptoms of the syndrome and thereby may possibly mask the underlying disease process. The effect that symptomatic suppression has upon the long-term course of the syndrome is unknown.
Given these considerations, neuroleptics should be prescribed in a manner that is most likely to minimize the occurrence of tardive dyskinesia. Chronic neuroleptic treatment should generally be reserved for patients who suffer from a chronic illness that 1) is known to respond to neuroleptic drugs, and 2) for whom alternative, equally effective, but potentially less harmful treatments are not available or appropriate. In patients who do require chronic treatment, the smallest dose and the shortest duration of treatment producing a satisfactory clinical response should be sought. The need for continued treatment should be reassessed periodically.
If signs and symptoms of tardive dyskinesia appear in a patient on neuroleptics, drug discontinuation should be considered. However, some patients may require treatment despite the presence of the syndrome.
(For further information about the description of tardive dyskinesia and its clinical detection, please refer to the sections on Information for Patients and Adverse Reactions.)
Usage in Pregnancy: The safety of Taractan during pregnancy or lactation in humans has not been established. Therefore, use of Taractan in women who may become pregnant requires weighing the drug's potential benefits against its possible hazards to mother and child. For the results of reproductive and teratogenic studies in rats and rabbits see **Animal Pharmacology and Toxicology.**
This drug may impair the mental and/or physical abilities required for the performance of hazardous tasks such as op-

Continued on next page

Roche Labs.—Cont.

erating machinery or driving a motor vehicle; therefore, the patient should be cautioned accordingly.

As in the case of other CNS-acting drugs, patients receiving Taractan should be cautioned about possible combined effects with alcohol.

The safety and efficacy of Taractan have not been established for oral administration in children under age 6 or for parenteral use in those under age 12.

PRECAUTIONS

Because of its structural similarity to the phenothiazines, all of the precautions associated with phenothiazine therapy should be considered when patients receive Taractan. Therefore, Taractan should be used with caution in patients who:

—are receiving barbiturates or narcotics, because of additive effects of central nervous system depressants. The dosage of the narcotic or barbiturate should be reduced when given concomitantly with Taractan.

—are receiving atropine or related drugs, because of additive anticholinergic effects.

—have a history of epilepsy. When necessary, Taractan may be used concomitantly with anticonvulsant drugs. However, use of Taractan may lower the convulsive threshold; therefore, an adequate dosage of the anticonvulsant should be maintained.

—are exposed to extreme heat or phosphorous insecticides.

—have cardiovascular disease.

—have respiratory impairment due to acute pulmonary infections or chronic respiratory disorders such as severe asthma or emphysema.

The concurrent use of Taractan and electroshock treatment should be reserved for those patients for whom it is essential, but the hazards may be increased.

Taractan may augment or interfere with the absorption, metabolism or therapeutic activity of other psychotropic drugs and vice versa.

The appearance of signs of blood dyscrasias requires immediate discontinuance of the drug and the institution of appropriate therapy.

The possibility of liver damage, variations in thyroid function, pigmentary retinopathy, lenticular or corneal deposits and development of irreversible dyskinesias should be kept in mind when patients are on prolonged therapy.

When used in the treatment of agitated states accompanying depression, the usual precautions indicated with such patients are necessary, particularly the recognition that a suicidal tendency may be present and protective measures necessary.

Taractan tablets contain FD&C Yellow No. 5 (tartrazine) which may cause allergic-type reactions (including bronchial asthma) in certain susceptible individuals. Although the overall incidence of FD&C Yellow No. 5 (tartrazine) sensitivity in the general population is low, it is frequently seen in patients who also have aspirin hypersensitivity.

Information for Patients: Given the likelihood that some patients exposed chronically to neuroleptics will develop tardive dyskinesia, it is advised that all patients in whom chronic use is contemplated be given, if possible, full information about this risk. The decision to inform patients and/or their guardians must obviously take into account the clinical circumstances and the competency of the patient to understand the information provided.

Abrupt Withdrawal: Taractan is not known to produce physical dependence. However, gastritis, nausea and vomiting, dizziness and tremulousness have been reported following abrupt cessation of high-dose therapy.

Neuroleptic drugs elevate prolactin levels; the elevation persists during chronic administration. Tissue culture experiments indicate that approximately one-third of human breast cancers are prolactin-dependent *in vitro*, a factor of potential importance if the prescription of these drugs is contemplated in a patient with a previously detected breast cancer. Although disturbances such as galactorrhea, amenorrhea, gynecomastia and impotence have been reported, the clinical significance of elevated serum prolactin levels is unknown for most patients. An increase in mammary neoplasms has been found in rodents after chronic administration of neuroleptic drugs. Neither clinical studies nor epidemiologic studies conducted to date, however, have shown an association between chronic administration of these drugs and mammary tumorigenesis; the available evidence is considered too limited to be conclusive at this time.

ADVERSE REACTIONS

General Introduction: Untoward events reported in association with a drug's use can be classified into three general categories: 1) those which are more or less predictable extensions of the pharmacological activity of the drug; 2) those which are caused by the drug, but in an unpredictable and/or idiosyncratic manner (*e.g.*, jaundice, agranulocytosis, etc.); and 3) those which have occurred in circumstances where evidence of a causal link to the drug's use is inconclusive. The first section describes the neurological events that are commonly seen in association with the use of neuroleptics, regardless of mechanism. The second and third sections present events that have been reported in association with the use of Taractan and of phenothiazine derivatives, respectively.

Common Reactions Linked to the Use of Neuroleptics: Untoward Neurological Events: The following section details events that have been reported to occur in association with the use of neuroleptics or drugs which share the ability to block CNS dopamine receptors.

The common acute neurological untoward effects of neuroleptics consist of dystonia, akathisia and pseudoparkinsonism.

Chronic use of neuroleptics, including Taractan, may be associated with the development of tardive dyskinesia. The salient features of this syndrome are described below and in the WARNINGS section. Additional details about the common acute neurological impairments also follow.

Tardive Dyskinesia: Clinical picture and detection. The syndrome is characterized by involuntary choreoathetoid movements which variously involve the tongue, face, mouth, lips or jaw (*e.g.*, protrusion of the tongue, puffing of the cheeks, puckering of the mouth, chewing movements), trunk and extremities. The severity of the syndrome and the degree of impairment produced vary widely.

The syndrome may become clinically recognizable either during treatment, upon dosage reduction, or upon withdrawal of treatment. Movements may decrease in intensity and may disappear altogether if further treatment with neuroleptics is withheld. It is generally believed that reversibility is more likely after short- rather than long-term neuroleptic exposure. Consequently, early detection of tardive dyskinesia is important. To increase the likelihood of detecting the syndrome at the earliest possible time, the dosage of neuroleptic drug should be reduced periodically (if clinically possible) and the patient observed for signs of the disorder. This maneuver is critical, for neuroleptic drugs may mask the signs of the syndrome.

Acute Neurological Effects:

1. Dystonia. This may present as acute, reversible torticollis, opisthotonos, carpopedal spasm, trismus, dysphagia, respiratory difficulty, oculogyric crisis, and protrusion of the tongue. Treatment consists of the parenteral administration of either an anticholinergic antiparkinsonism agent or diphenhydramine.
2. Akathisia. Akathisia presents as constant motor restlessness. It is often confused with agitation and the differential diagnosis can be difficult. One feature that may permit a distinction is that the patient with akathisia often complains, *when asked*, about his or her inability to stop moving. The importance of the differential diagnosis is that akathisia should *not* be treated with an increased dose of neuroleptic. In the treatment of akathisia, the dose of antipsychotic may be lowered until the motor restlessness has subsided. The efficacy of anticholinergic treatment of this side effect is unestablished.
3. Pseudoparkinsonism. Pseudoparkinsonism refers to a drug-induced state similar to the classic syndrome. Its features include a generalized increase in muscle tone, often accompanied by "cogwheeling," tremor, and other signs and symptoms of the spontaneously occurring syndrome (*i.e.*, bradyphrenia, bradykinesia, masked facies, drooling, difficulty initiating movements, lack of associated movements, micrographia, etc.). Generally, anticholinergic antiparkinsonism agents (*i.e.*, benztropine, biperiden, procyclidine, or trihexyphenidyl) and amantadine are helpful in alleviating symptoms that cannot be managed by neuroleptic dose reduction. The value of prophylactic antiparkinsonism drug therapy has not been established. The need for continued use of antiparkinsonism medication should be reevaluated periodically.

Adverse Reactions Associated with Taractan: See **Warnings** and **Adverse Reactions:** *Common Reactions Linked to the Use of Neuroleptics: Untoward Neurological Events.*

Note: Sudden death has occasionally been reported in patients who have received phenothiazines. In some cases death was apparently due to cardiac arrest; in others the cause appeared to be asphyxia due to failure of the cough reflex. In some patients the cause could not be determined nor could it be established that death was due to the phenothiazine.

Taractan commonly causes sedation and hypotension.

The following adverse reactions have been reported with Taractan:

Central Nervous System: The most frequently occurring effect is initial drowsiness which usually disappears with or without dose adjustments. Hyperactivity or stimulation can occur, sometimes requiring discontinuation of the medication. Convulsions, particularly in patients with a history of EEG abnormalities, have been reported. Ataxia.

Autonomic Nervous System: Dry mouth, nasal stuffiness, visual changes and constipation have been occasionally reported. Headache. Gastric upset.

Cardiovascular System: Postural hypotension, tachycardia (especially with sudden marked increase in dosage) and dizziness have been reported. In the event that a vasoconstrictor is required, Levophed® (levarterenol) or Aramine (metaraminol) are the most suitable. Other pressor agents, including epinephrine, should not be used, as a paradoxical further lowering of the blood pressure may ensue.

EKG changes—particularly nonspecific, usually reversible Q and T wave distortions—have been observed in some patients receiving phenothiazine tranquilizers. Their relationship to myocardial damage has not been confirmed.

Skin: Dermatitis and urticarial type skin reactions have been observed infrequently. Photosensitivity is rare but undue exposure to the sun should be avoided.

Hepatotoxicity: Jaundice has been reported occasionally.

Hematological Disorders: Agranulocytosis, eosinophilia, leukopenia, hemolytic anemia, thrombocytopenic purpura and pancytopenia have been reported very rarely.

Endocrine Disorders: Galactorrhea and increased libido have been reported in isolated cases.

Other: Excessive weight gain and excessive thirst have occasionally been reported. Hyperpyrexia, paradoxical exacerbation of psychotic symptoms and ocular changes may also occur. Insomnia. Weakness.

Adverse Reactions Associated with Phenothiazine Derivatives: See **Warnings** and **Adverse Reactions:** *Common Reactions Linked to the Use of Neuroleptics: Untoward Neurological Events.*

Adverse Reactions Associated with Phenothiazine Derivatives: The following adverse reactions have not been reported specifically for Taractan nor have they been observed with every phenothiazine derivative; however, because of pharmacological similarities of Taractan to the various phenothiazine derivatives, they should be considered when administering drugs of this class.

Central Nervous System: Extrapyramidal symptoms (opisthotonos, oculogyric crisis, hyperreflexia); grand mal convulsions; altered cerebrospinal fluid proteins; cerebral edema; intensification and prolongation of the action of central nervous system depressants (opiates, analgesics, antihistamines, barbiturates, alcohol), atropine, exposure to extreme heat or organophosphorus insecticides.

Autonomic Nervous System: Obstipation; adynamic ileus; inhibition of ejaculation.

Cardiovascular System: Cardiac arrest; bradycardia; faintness.

Hepatotoxicity: Biliary stasis.

Endocrine Disorders: Lactation; gynecomastia; menstrual irregularities; moderate breast engorgement; hyperglycemia, hypoglycemia, glycosuria.

Allergic Reactions: Itching; erythema; eczema up to exfoliative dermatitis; asthma; laryngeal edema; angioneurotic edema; anaphylactoid reactions.

Other: Enlargement of the parotid gland; catatonic-like states; peripheral edema, reversed epinephrine effect; systemic lupus erythematosus-like syndrome; pigmentary retinopathy; with prolonged administration of substantial doses—skin pigmentation, epithelial keratopathy, and lenticular and corneal deposits.

DOSAGE AND ADMINISTRATION

Dosage should be individually adjusted according to diagnosis and severity of the condition. In general, small doses should be used initially, and increased to the optimal effective level as rapidly as possible based on therapeutic response. When higher dosage is required, greater sedation may be encountered; therefore, patients should be closely supervised. Lethargy and drowsiness are readily controlled by dosage reduction. Initially, lower doses (10 to 25 mg three or four times daily) should be used for elderly or debilitated patients.

For convenience in prescribing and dispensing, all recommended dosages are expressed as strengths of the active moiety, chlorprothixene.

Taractan may be administered orally as tablets or concentrate. The concentrate, containing 100 mg of the drug per 5 ml teaspoonful, is pleasantly flavored and may be administered alone or in milk, water, fruit juices, coffee and carbonated beverages.

ORAL	AVERAGE DAILY DOSE
Adults:	Initially, 25 to 50 mg three or four times daily; to be increased as needed. Dosages exceeding 600 mg daily are rarely required.
Children (over 6 years of age):	10 to 25 mg three or four times daily.
PARENTERAL Not to be used in children under the age of 12.	25 to 50 mg I.M. up to three or four times daily.

Pain or induration at the site of injection is minimal. Since postural hypotension may occur in some patients, injection should be given with the patient seated or recumbent. If hypotension does occur, recovery is usually spontaneous; however, the patient should be observed until symptoms of weakness or dizziness pass.

As soon as the acutely agitated patient is brought under control, oral medication should be instituted. The changeover should be made gradually, with oral and parenteral doses being given alternately on the same day, then oral doses only, adjusted to the required maintenance level.

OVERDOSAGE

Taractan can be fatal in overdosage in the range of 2.5 to 4 Gm or above. Manifestations of overdosage or drowsiness, coma, respiratory depression, hypotension (which may appear after a delay of several hours and may persist for two to three days), tachycardia, pyrexia and constricted pupils. Convulsions, hyperactivity and hematuria may be seen in the recovery period.

Treatment is essentially symptomatic. Early gastric lavage is recommended, along with supportive measures such as I.V. fluids and the maintenance of an adequate airway. Severe hypotension usually responds to the use of levarterenol or metaraminol. Should coma be prolonged, caffeine and sodium benzoate, or ethamivan may be used, but the possibility must be borne in mind that these may lead to a convulsive episode. Should convulsions occur, the judicious use of sodium amytal is recommended. **Epinephrine must not be used in these patients.**

HOW SUPPLIED

Tablets — 10 mg chlorprothixene/ Roche—bottles of 100; 25 mg, 50 mg or 100 mg chlorprothixene/Roche—bottles of 100 and 500.

Concentrate—containing, in each teaspoonful, chlorprothixene/Roche 100 mg base (as the lactate and hydrochloride)—bottles of 16 fluid ounces (1 pint).

Ampuls—containing chlorprothixene/Roche 25 mg/2 ml as the hydrochloride—boxes of 10.

Animal Pharmacology and Toxicology: In mice, the oral LD_{50} of the two oral dosage forms of chlorprothixene were 350 ± 27 mg/kg (as the 2 per cent concentrate) and 220 ± 24 mg/kg (as the tablet form ground and suspended in 5 per cent gum acacia). For the injectable form the intramuscular LD_{50} in mice was greater than 125 mg/kg.

Reproduction Studies: Reproductive and teratological studies in rats and rabbits were performed at levels of 12 and 24 mg/kg. In the rats, a decreased conception rate and an increased incidence of stillborns was noted at both levels. An increased number of resorptions was noted only at the high dose level. There was a decrease in the number of implantation sites at both doses. The number of live fetuses per litter and the mean fetal body weights were reduced slightly at 12 mg/kg and more so at 24 mg/kg. No teratological effects were observed. No deleterious effects on reproduction were seen in rabbits nor were any teratological findings noted.

Shown in Product Identification Section, page 425

TEL-E-DOSE®

Tel-E-Dose is a unit package designed by Roche for convenience in dispensing medications in the hospital and nursing home. Each unit, sealed against contamination and moisture, is clearly identified by product name and strength and carries the control number and expiration date.

Currently available in this package form are the following products: Bactrim™ (80 mg trimethoprim and 400 mg sulfamethoxazole) tablets; Bactrim™ DS (160 mg trimethoprim and 800 mg sulfamethoxazole) tablets; Bumex® (bumetanide HCl) tablets, 0.5 mg, 1 mg, 2 mg; Gantanol® (sulfamethoxazole) tablets, 0.5 Gm; Gantrisin® (sulfisoxazole) tablets, 0.5 Gm; Trimpex® (trimethoprim) tablets, 100 mg.

Shown in Product Identification Section, page 425

TENSILON® ℞

[ten'sil-on]

(edrophonium chloride/Roche)

Injectable Solution

ampuls • vials

The following text is complete prescribing information based on official labeling in effect June 1, 1986.

DESCRIPTION

Tensilon is a short and rapid-acting cholinergic drug. Chemically, edrophonium chloride is ethyl (*m*-hydroxyphenyl)-dimethylammonium chloride.

10-ml vials: Each ml contains, in a sterile solution, 10 mg edrophonium chloride/Roche compounded with 0.45% phenol and 0.2% sodium sulfite as preservatives, buffered with sodium citrate and citric acid, and pH adjusted to approximately 5.4.

1-ml ampuls: Each ml contains, in a sterile solution, 10 mg edrophonium chloride/Roche compounded with 0.2% sodium sulfite, buffered with sodium citrate and citric acid, and pH adjusted to approximately 5.4.

ACTIONS

Tensilon is an anticholinesterase drug. Its pharmacological action is due primarily to the inhibition or inactivation of acetylcholinesterase at sites of cholinergic transmission. Its effect is manifest within 30 to 60 seconds after injection and lasts an average of 10 minutes.

INDICATIONS

Tensilon is recommended for the differential diagnosis of myasthenia gravis and as an adjunct in the evaluation of treatment requirements in this disease. It may also be used for evaluating emergency treatment in myasthenic crises. Because of its brief duration of action, it is not recommended for maintenance therapy in myasthenia gravis.

Tensilon is also useful whenever a curare antagonist is needed to reverse the neuromuscular block produced by curare, tubocurarine, gallamine triethiodide or dimethyl-tubocurarine. It is *not* effective against decamethonium bromide and succinylcholine chloride. It may be used adjunctively in the treatment of respiratory depression caused by curare overdosage.

CONTRAINDICATIONS

Known hypersensitivity to anticholinesterase agents; intestinal and urinary obstructions of mechanical type.

WARNINGS

Whenever anticholinesterase drugs are used for testing, a syringe containing 1 mg of atropine sulfate should be immediately available to be given in aliquots intravenously to counteract severe cholinergic reactions which may occur in the hypersensitive individual, whether he is normal or myasthenic. Tensilon should be used with caution in patients with bronchial asthma or cardiac dysrhythmias. The transient bradycardia which sometimes occurs can be relieved by atropine sulfate. Isolated instances of cardiac and respiratory arrest following administration of Tensilon have been reported. It is postulated that these are vagotonic effects.

Usage in Pregnancy: The safety of Tensilon during pregnancy or lactation in humans has not been established. Therefore, use of Tensilon in women who may become pregnant requires weighing the drug's potential benefits against its possible hazards to mother and child.

PRECAUTIONS

Patients may develop "anticholinesterase insensitivity" for brief or prolonged periods. During these periods the patients should be carefully monitored and may need respiratory assistance. Dosages of anticholinesterase drugs should be reduced or withheld until patients again become sensitive to them.

ADVERSE REACTIONS

Careful observation should be made for severe cholinergic reactions in the hyperreactive individual. The myasthenic patient in crisis who is being tested with Tensilon should be observed for bradycardia or cardiac standstill and cholinergic reactions if an overdose is given. The following reactions common to anticholinesterase agents may occur, although not all of these reactions have been reported with the administration of Tensilon, probably because of its short duration of action and limited indications: **Eye:** Increased lacrimation, pupillary constriction, spasm of accommodation, diplopia, conjunctival hyperemia. **CNS:** Convulsions, dysarthria, dysphonia, dysphagia. **Respiratory:** Increased tracheobronchial secretions, laryngospasm, bronchiolar constriction, paralysis of muscles of respiration, central respiratory paralysis. **Cardiac:** Arrhythmias (especially bradycardia), fall in cardiac output leading to hypotension. **G.I.:** Increased salivary, gastric and intestinal secretion, nausea, vomiting, increased peristalsis, diarrhea, abdominal cramps. **Skeletal Muscle:** Weakness, fasciculations. **Miscellaneous:** Increased urinary frequency and incontinence, diaphoresis.

DOSAGE AND ADMINISTRATION

Tensilon Test in the Differential Diagnosis of Myasthenia Gravis:[1-8]

Intravenous Dosage (Adults): A tuberculin syringe containing 1 ml (10 mg) of Tensilon is prepared with an intravenous needle, and 0.2 ml (2 mg) is injected intravenously within 15 to 30 seconds. The needle is left *in situ*. *Only* if no reaction occurs after 45 seconds is the remaining 0.8 ml (8 mg) injected. If a cholinergic reaction (muscarinic side effects, skeletal muscle fasciculations and increased muscle weakness) occurs after injection of 0.2 ml (2 mg), the test is discontinued and atropine sulfate 0.4 mg to 0.5 mg is administered intravenously. After one-half hour the test may be repeated.

Intramuscular Dosage (Adults): In adults with inaccessible veins, dosage for intramuscular injection is 1 ml (10 mg) of Tensilon. Subjects who demonstrate hyperreactivity to this injection (cholinergic reaction), should be retested after one-half hour with 0.2 ml (2 mg) of Tensilon intramuscularly to rule out false-negative reactions.

Dosage (Children): The intravenous testing dose of Tensilon in children weighing up to 75 lbs is 0.1 ml (1 mg); above this weight, the dose is 0.2 ml (2 mg). If there is no response after 45 seconds, it may be titrated up to 0.5 ml (5 mg) in children under 75 lbs, given in increments of 0.1 ml (1 mg) every 30 to 45 seconds and up to 1 ml (10 mg) in heavier children. In infants, the recommended dose is 0.05 ml (0.5 mg). Because of technical difficulty with intravenous injection in children, the intramuscular route may be used. In children weighing up to 75 lbs, 0.2 ml (2 mg) is injected intramuscularly. In children weighing more than 75 lbs, 0.5 ml (5 mg) is injected intramuscularly. All signs which would appear with the intravenous test appear with the intramuscular test except that there is a delay of two to ten minutes before a reaction is noted.

Tensilon Test for Evaluation of Treatment Requirements in Myasthenia Gravis: The recommended dose is 0.1 ml to 0.2 ml (1 mg to 2 mg) of Tensilon, administered intravenously one hour after oral intake of the drug being used in treatment.[1-5] Response will be myasthenic in the undertreated patient, adequate in the controlled patient, and cholinergic in the overtreated patient. Responses to Tensilon in myasthenic and nonmyasthenic individuals are summarized in the accompanying chart.[2]

[See table above].

Responses to Tensilon in Myasthenic and Nonmyasthenic Individuals

	Myasthenic*	Adequate†	Cholinergic‡
Muscle Strength (ptosis, diplopia, dysphonia, dysphagia, dysarthria, respiration, limb strength)	Increased	No change	Decreased
Fasciculations (orbicularis oculi, facial muscles, limb muscles)	Absent	Present or absent	Present or absent
Side reactions (lacrimination, diaphoresis, salivation, abdominal cramps, nausea, vomiting, diarrhea)	Absent	Minimal	Severe

*Myasthenic Response—occurs in untreated myasthenics and may serve to establish diagnosis; in patients under treatment, indicates that therapy is inadequate.

†Adequate Response—observed in treated patients when therapy is stabilized; a typical response in normal individuals. In addition to this response in nonmyasthenics, the phenomenon of forced lid closure is often observed in psychoneurotics.[1]

‡Cholinergic Response—seen in myasthenics who have been overtreated with anticholinesterase drugs.

Tensilon Test in Crisis: The term *crisis* is applied to the myasthenic whenever severe respiratory distress with objective ventilatory inadequacy occurs and the response to medication is not predictable. This state may be secondary to a sudden increase in severity of myasthenia gravis (myasthenic crisis), or to overtreatment with anticholinesterase drugs (cholinergic crisis).

When a patient is apneic, controlled ventilation must be secured immediately in order to avoid cardiac arrest and irreversible central nervous system damage. No attempt is made to test with Tensilon until respiratory exchange is adequate. *Dosage used at this time is most important:* If the patient is cholinergic, Tensilon will cause increased oropharyngeal secretions and further weakness in the muscles of respiration. If the crisis is myasthenic, the test clearly improves respiration and the patient can be treated with longer-acting intravenous anticholinesterase medication. When the test is performed, there should not be more than 0.2 ml (2 mg) Tensilon in the syringe. An intravenous dose of 0.1 ml (1 mg) is given initially. The patient's heart action is carefully observed. If, after an interval of one minute, this dose does not further impair the patient, the remaining 0.1 ml (1 mg) can be injected. If no clear improvement of respiration occurs after 0.2 ml (2 mg) dose, it is usually wisest to discontinue all anticholinesterase drug therapy and secure controlled ventilation by tracheostomy with assisted respiration.[5]

For Use as a Curare Antagonist: Tensilon should be administered by intravenous injection in 1 ml (10 mg) doses given slowly over a period of 30 to 45 seconds so that the onset of cholinergic reaction can be detected. This dosage may be repeated whenever necessary. The maximal dose for any one patient should be 4 ml (40 mg). Because of its brief effect, Tensilon should not be given prior to the administration of curare, tubocurarine, gallamine triethiodide or dimethyl-tubocurarine; it should be used at the time when its effect is needed. When given to counteract curare overdosage, the effect of each dose on the respiration should be carefully ob-

Continued on next page

Roche Labs.—Cont.

served before it is repeated, and assisted ventilation should always be employed.

DRUG INTERACTIONS

Care should be given when administering this drug to patients with symptoms of myasthenic weakness who are also on anticholinesterase drugs. Since symptoms of anticholinesterase overdose (cholinergic crisis) may mimic underdosage (myasthenic weakness), their condition may be worsened by the use of this drug. (See OVERDOSAGE section for treatment.)

OVERDOSAGE

With drugs of this type, muscarine-like symptoms (nausea, vomiting, diarrhea, sweating, increased bronchial and salivary secretions and bradycardia) often appear with overdosage (cholinergic crisis). An important complication that can arise is obstruction of the airway by bronchial secretions. These may be managed with suction (especially if tracheostomy has been performed) and by the use of atropine. Many experts have advocated a wide range of dosages of atropine *(for Tensilon, see atropine dosage below)*, but if there are copious secretions, up to 1.2 mg intravenously may be given initially and repeated every 20 minutes until secretions are controlled. Signs of atropine overdosage such as dry mouth, flush and tachycardia should be avoided as tenacious secretions and bronchial plugs may form. A total dose of atropine of 5 to 10 mg or even more may be required. The following steps should be taken in the management of overdosage of Tensilon:

1. Adequate respiratory exchange should be maintained by assuring an open airway, and the use of assisted respiration augmented by oxygen.
2. Cardiac function should be monitored until complete stabilization has been achieved.
3. Atropine sulfate in doses of 0.4 to 0.5 mg should be administered intravenously. This may be repeated every 3 to 10 minutes. Because of the short duration of action of Tensilon the total dose required will seldom exceed 2 mg.
4. Pralidoxime chloride (a cholinesterase reactivator) may be given intravenously at the rate of 50 to 100 mg per minute; usually the total dose does not exceed 1000 mg. Extreme caution should be exercised in the use of pralidoxime chloride when the cholinergic symptoms are induced by double-bond phosphorous anticholinesterase drugs.[9]
5. If convulsions or shock is present, appropriate measures should be instituted.

HOW SUPPLIED

Multiple Dose Vials, 10 ml, boxes of 10. *Ampuls,* 1 ml, boxes of 10.

REFERENCES

1. Osserman, K.E. and Kaplan, L.I., *J.A.M.A., 150:* 265, 1952.
2. Osserman, K.E., Kaplan, L.I. and Besson, G., *J. Mt. Sinai Hosp., 20:* 165, 1953.
3. Osserman, K.E. and Kaplan, L.I., *Arch. Neurol. & Psychiat., 70:* 385, 1953.
4. Osserman, K.E. and Teng, P., *J.A.M.A., 160:* 153, 1956.
5. Osserman, K.E. and Genkins, G., *Ann. N.Y. Acad. Sci., 135:* 312, 1966.
6. Tether, J.E., Second International Symposium Proceedings, Myasthenia Gravis, 1961, p. 444.
7. Tether, J.E., in H.F. Conn: *Current Therapy 1960,* Philadelphia, W. B. Saunders Company, p. 551.
8. Tether, J.E., in H.F. Conn: *Current Therapy 1965,* Philadelphia, W. B. Saunders Company, p. 556.
9. Grob, D. and Johns, R.J., *J.A.M.A., 166:* 1855, 1958.

TRIMPEX® ℞

[trim 'pex]
(trimethoprim/Roche)
TABLETS

The following text is complete prescribing information based on official labeling in effect June 1, 1986.

DESCRIPTION

Trimpex (trimethoprim/Roche) is a synthetic antibacterial available as 100-mg tablets for oral administration. Each tablet also contains lactose, magnesium stearate, sodium starch glycolate and pregelatinized starch.

Trimethoprim is 2,4-diamino-5-(3,4,5-trimethoxybenzyl)-pyrimidine. It is a white to light yellow, odorless, bitter compound with a molecular weight of 290.3.

CLINICAL PHARMACOLOGY

Trimethoprim is rapidly absorbed following oral administration. It exists in the blood as unbound, protein-bound and metabolized forms. Ten to twenty percent of trimethoprim is metabolized, primarily in the liver; the remainder is excreted unchanged in the urine. The principal metabolites of trimethoprim are the 1- and 3-oxides and the 3'- and 4'-hydroxy derivatives. The free form is considered to be the therapeutically active form. Approximately 44% of trimethoprim is bound to plasma proteins.

Mean peak plasma concentrations of approximately 1.0 mcg/ml occur 1 to 4 hours after oral administration of a single 100-mg dose. A single 200-mg dose will result in plasma concentrations approximately twice as high. The half-life of trimethoprim ranges from 8 to 10 hours. However, patients with severely impaired renal function exhibit an increase in the half-life of trimethoprim, which requires either dosage regimen adjustment or not using the drug in such patients (see DOSAGE AND ADMINISTRATION section). During a 13-week study of trimethoprim administered at a dosage of 50 mg *q.i.d.,* the mean minimum steady-state concentration of the drug was 1.1 mcg/ml. Steady-state concentrations were achieved within 2 to 3 days of chronic administration and were maintained throughout the experimental period.

Excretion of trimethoprim is primarily by the kidneys through glomerular filtration and tubular secretion. Urine concentrations of trimethoprim are considerably higher than are the concentrations in the blood. After a single oral dose of 100 mg, urine concentrations of trimethoprim ranged from 30 to 160 mcg/ml during the 0- to 4-hour period and declined to approximately 18 to 91 mcg/ml during the 8- to 24-hour period. A 200-mg single oral dose will result in trimethoprim urine concentrations approximately twice as high. After oral administration, 50% to 60% of trimethoprim is excreted in urine within 24 hours, approximately 80% of this being unmetabolized trimethoprim.

Since normal vaginal and fecal flora are the source of most pathogens causing urinary tract infections, it is relevant to consider the distribution of trimethoprim into these sites. Concentrations of trimethoprim in vaginal secretions are consistently greater than those found simultaneously in the serum, being typically 1.6 times the concentrations of simultaneously obtained serum samples. Sufficient trimethoprim is excreted in the feces to markedly reduce or eliminate trimethoprim-susceptible organisms from the fecal flora. The dominant non-*Enterobacteriaceae* fecal organisms, *Bacteroides* spp. and *Lactobacillus* spp., are not susceptible to trimethoprim concentrations obtained with the recommended dosage.

Trimethoprim also passes the placental barrier and is excreted in breast milk.

Microbiology: Trimpex blocks the production of tetrahydrofolic acid from dihydrofolic acid by binding to and reversibly inhibiting the required enzyme, dihydrofolate reductase. This binding is very much stronger for the bacterial enzyme than for the corresponding mammalian enzyme. Thus, Trimpex selectively interferes with bacterial biosynthesis of nucleic acids and proteins.

In vitro serial dilution tests have shown that the spectrum of antibacterial activity of Trimpex includes the common urinary tract pathogens with the exception of *Pseudomonas aeruginosa.*

Representative Minimum Inhibitory Concentrations for Trimethoprim-Susceptible Organisms

Bacteria	Trimethoprim MIC—mcg/ml (Range)
Escherichia coli	0.05—1.5
Proteus mirabilis	0.5—1.5
Klebsiella pneumoniae	0.5—5.0
Enterobacter species	0.5—5.0
Staphylococcus species (coagulase-negative)	0.15—5.0

The recommended quantitative disc susceptibility method[1,2] may be used for estimating the susceptibility of bacteria to Trimpex. With this procedure, reports from the laboratory giving results using the 5-mcg trimethoprim disc should be interpreted according to the following criteria: Organisms producing zones of 16 mm or greater are classified as susceptible, whereas those producing zones of 11 to 15 mm are classified as having intermediate susceptibility. A report from the laboratory of "Susceptible to trimethoprim" or "Intermediate susceptibility to trimethoprim" indicates that the infection is likely to respond when, as in uncomplicated urinary tract infections, effective therapy is dependent upon the urine concentration of trimethoprim. Organisms producing zones of 10 mm or less are reported as resistant, indicating that other therapy should be selected.

Dilution methods for determining susceptibility are also used, and results are reported as the minimum drug concentration inhibiting microbial growth (MIC).[3] If the MIC is 8 mcg per ml or less, the microorganism is considered "susceptible." If the MIC is 16 mcg per ml or greater, the microorganism is considered "resistant."

INDICATIONS AND USAGE

For the treatment of initial episodes of uncomplicated urinary tract infections due to susceptible strains of the following organisms: *Escherichia coli, Proteus mirabilis, Klebsiella pneumoniae, Enterobacter* species and coagulase-negative *Staphylococcus* species, including *S. saprophyticus.*

Cultures and susceptibility tests should be performed to determine the susceptibility of the bacteria to trimethoprim. Therapy may be initiated prior to obtaining the results of these tests.

CONTRAINDICATIONS

Trimpex is contraindicated in individuals hypersensitive to trimethoprim and in those with documented megaloblastic anemia due to folate deficiency.

WARNINGS

Experience with trimethoprim alone is limited, but it has been reported rarely to interfere with hematopoiesis, especially when administered in large doses and/or for prolonged periods.

The presence of clinical signs such as sore throat, fever, pallor or purpura may be early indications of serious blood disorders.

PRECAUTIONS

General: Trimethoprim should be given with caution to patients with possible folate deficiency. Folates may be administered concomitantly without interfering with the antibacterial action of trimethoprim. Trimethoprim should also be given with caution to patients with impaired renal or hepatic function. If any clinical signs of a blood disorder are noted in a patient receiving trimethoprim, a complete blood count should be obtained and the drug discontinued if a significant reduction in the count of any formed blood element is found.

Drug interactions: Trimpex may inhibit the hepatic metabolism of phenytoin. Trimethoprim, given at a common clinical dosage, increased the phenytoin half-life by 51% and decreased the phenytoin metabolic clearance rate by 30%. When administering these drugs concurrently, one should be alert for possible excessive phenytoin effect.

Drug/laboratory test interactions: Trimethoprim can interfere with a serum methotrexate assay as determined by the competitive binding protein technique (CBPA) when a bacterial dihydrofolate reductase is used as the binding protein. No interference occurs, however, if methotrexate is measured by a radioimmunoassay (RIA).

The presence of trimethoprim may also interfere with the Jaffé alkaline picrate reaction assay for creatinine resulting in overestimations of about 10% in the range of normal values.

Carcinogenesis, mutagenesis, impairment of fertility:

Carcinogenesis: Long-term studies in animals to evaluate carcinogenic potential have not been conducted with trimethoprim.

Mutagenesis: Trimethoprim was demonstrated to be non-mutagenic in the Ames assay. No chromosomal damage was observed in human leukocytes cultured *in vitro* with trimethoprim; the concentration used exceeded blood levels following therapy with Trimpex.

Impairment of fertility: No adverse effects on fertility or general reproductive performance were observed in rats given trimethoprim in oral dosages as high as 70 mg/kg/day for males and 14 mg/kg/day for females.

Pregnancy: Teratogenic effects: Pregnancy Category C. Trimethoprim has been shown to be teratogenic in the rat when given in doses 40 times the human dose. In some rabbit studies, the overall increase in fetal loss (dead and resorbed and malformed conceptuses) was associated with doses 6 times the human therapeutic dose.

While there are no large well-controlled studies on the use of trimethoprim in pregnant women, Brumfitt and Pursell,[4] in a retrospective study, reported the outcome of 186 pregnancies during which the mother received either placebo or trimethoprim in combination wih sulfamethoxazole. The incidence of congenital abnormalities was 4.5% (3 of 66) in those who received placebo and 3.3% (4 of 120) in those receiving trimethoprim plus sulfamethoxazole. There were no abnormalities in the 10 children whose mothers received the drug during the first trimester. In a separate survey, Brumfitt and Pursell also found no congenital abnormalities in 35 children whose mothers had received trimethoprim plus sulfamethoxazole at the time of conception or shortly thereafter.

Because trimethoprim may interfere with folic acid metabolism, Trimpex should be used during pregnancy only if the potential benefit justifies the potential risk to the fetus.

Nonteratogenic effects: The oral administration of trimethoprim to rats at a dose of 70 mg/kg/day commencing with the last third of gestation and continuing through parturition and lactation caused no deleterious effects on gestation or pup growth and survival.

Nursing mothers: Trimethoprim is excreted in human milk. Because trimethoprim may interfere with folic acid metabolism, caution should be exercised when Trimpex is administered to a nursing woman.

Pediatric use: The safety of trimethoprim in infants under two months of age has not been demonstrated. The effectiveness of trimethoprim has not been established in children under 12 years of age.

ADVERSE REACTIONS

The adverse effects encountered most often with trimethoprim were rash and pruritus. Other adverse effects reported involved the gastrointestinal and hematopoietic systems.
Dermatologic reactions: Rash, pruritus and exfoliative dermatitis. At the recommended dosage regimens of 100 mg *b.i.d.* or 200 mg *q.d.*, each for 10 days, the incidence of rash is 2.9% to 6.7%. In clinical studies which employed high doses of Trimpex, an elevated incidence of rash was noted. These rashes were maculopapular, morbilliform, pruritic and generally mild to moderate, appearing 7 to 14 days after the initiation of therapy.
Gastrointestinal reactions: Epigastric distress, nausea, vomiting and glossitis.
Hematologic reactions: Thrombocytopenia, leukopenia, neutropenia, megaloblastic anemia and methemoglobinemia.
Miscellaneous reactions: Fever, elevation of serum transaminase and bilirubin, and increases in BUN and serum creatinine levels.

OVERDOSAGE

Acute: Signs of acute overdosage with trimethoprim may appear following ingestion of 1 gram or more of the drug and include nausea, vomiting, dizziness, headaches, mental depression, confusion and bone marrow depression (see CHRONIC OVERDOSAGE).
Treatment consists of gastric lavage and general supportive measures. Acidification of the urine will increase renal elimination of trimethoprim. Peritoneal dialysis is not effective and hemodialysis only moderately effective in eliminating the drug.
Chronic: Use of trimethoprim at high doses and/ or for extended periods of time may cause bone marrow depression manifested as thrombocytopenia, leukopenia and/or megaloblastic anemia. If signs of bone marrow depression occur, trimethoprim should be discontinued and the patient should be given leucovorin, 3 to 6 mg intramuscularly daily for three days, or as required to restore normal hematopoiesis.

DOSAGE AND ADMINISTRATION

The usual oral adult dosage is 100 mg (one tablet) every 12 hours or 200 mg (two tablets) every 24 hours, each for 10 days. The use of trimethoprim in patients with a creatinine clearance of less than 15 ml/min is not recommended. For patients with a creatinine clearance of 15 to 30 ml/min, the dose should be 50 mg every 12 hours.
The effectiveness of trimethoprim has not been established in children under 12 years of age.

HOW SUPPLIED

100-mg tablets (white, elliptical, scored)—bottles of 100 (NDC 0004-0127-01); Tel-E-Dose® packages of 100 (NDC 0004-0127-49). Imprint on tablets: TRIMPEX 100 ROCHE.

REFERENCES

1. Bauer AW, Kirby WMM, Sherris JC, Turck M: Antibiotic Susceptibility Testing by Standardized Single Disk Method, *Am J Clin Pathol 45*:493–496, 1966.
2. Approved Standard ASM-2 Performance Standards for Antimicrobial Disc Susceptibility Test; National Committee for Clinical Laboratory Standards, 771 East Lancaster Avenue, Villanova, Pennsylvania 19085.
3. Ericsson HM, Sherris JC: Antibiotic Sensitivity Testing. Report of an International Collaborative Study. *Acta Pathol Microbiol Scand* [B] (Suppl 217): 1–90, 1971.
4. Brumfitt W, Pursell R: Trimethoprim/Sulfamethoxazole in the Treatment of Bacteriuria in Women, *J Infect Dis 128* (Suppl): S657–S663, 1973.

Shown in Product Identification Section, page 425

VALRELEASE® ℞

[*val 're-lease*]
(diazepam/Roche)
CAPSULES
A slow-release dosage form of Valium® (diazepam/Roche)

The following text is complete prescribing information based on official labeling in effect June 1, 1986.

DESCRIPTION

Diazepam is a benzodiazepine derivative developed through original Roche research. Chemically, diazepam is 7-chloro-1,3-dihydro-1-methyl-5-phenyl-2*H*-1, 4-benzodiazepin-2- one. It is a colorless crystalline compound, insoluble in water and has a molecular weight of 284.74.
Valrelease capsules provide the actions of Valium® (diazepam/Roche) in a slow-release dosage form.

PHARMACOLOGY

In animals, diazepam appears to act on parts of the limbic system, the thalamus and hypothalamus, and induces calming effects. Diazepam, unlike chlorpromazine and reserpine, has no demonstrable peripheral autonomic blocking action, nor does it produce extrapyramidal side effects; however, animals treated with diazepam do have a transient ataxia at higher doses. Diazepam was found to have transient cardiovascular depressor effects in dogs. Long-term experiments in rats revealed no disturbances of endocrine function.
Oral LD_{50} of diazepam is 720 mg/kg in mice and 1240 mg/kg in rats. Intraperitoneal administration of 400 mg/kg to a monkey resulted in death on the sixth day.
Reproduction Studies: A series of rat reproduction studies was performed with diazepam in oral doses of 1, 10, 80 and 100 mg/kg. At 100 mg/kg there was a decrease in the number of pregnancies and surviving offspring in these rats. Neonatal survival of rats at doses lower than 100 mg/kg was within normal limits. Several neonates in these rat reproduction studies showed skeletal or other defects. Further studies in rats at doses up to and including 80 mg/kg/day did not reveal teratological effects on the offspring.
In humans, measurable blood levels of diazepam were obtained in maternal and cord blood, indicating placental transfer of the drug.
The administration of one 15-mg Valrelease capsule results in blood levels of diazepam over a 24-hour period which are comparable to those of 5-mg Valium tablets given three times daily.
The mean time to maximum plasma diazepam concentrations after administration of 15-mg Valrelease capsules to eleven fasted subjects was 5.3 hours. The harmonic mean half-life of diazepam was 36 hours. The range of average minimum steady-state plasma diazepam concentrations during once daily administration of 15-mg Valrelease capsules to eleven normal subjects was 196 to 341 ng/ml.

INDICATIONS

Valrelease is indicated for the management of anxiety disorders or for the short-term relief of the symptoms of anxiety. Anxiety or tension associated with the stress of everyday life usually does not require treatment with an anxiolytic.
In acute alcohol withdrawal, Valrelease may be useful in the symptomatic relief of acute agitation, tremor, impending or acute delirium tremens and hallucinosis.
Valrelease is a useful adjunct for the relief of skeletal muscle spasm due to reflex spasm to local pathology (such as inflammation of the muscles or joints, or secondary to trauma); spasticity caused by upper motor neuron disorders (such as cerebral palsy and paraplegia); athetosis; and stiff-man syndrome.
Valrelease may be used adjunctively in convulsive disorders, although it has not proved useful as the sole therapy.
The effectiveness of diazepam in long-term use, that is, more than 4 months, has not been assessed by systematic clinical studies. The physician should periodically reassess the usefulness of the drug for the individual patient.

CONTRAINDICATIONS

Valrelease is contraindicated in patients with a known hypersensitivity to this drug and, because of lack of sufficient clinical experience, in children under 6 months of age. It may be used in patients with open angle glaucoma who are receiving appropriate therapy, but is contraindicated in acute narrow angle glaucoma.

WARNINGS

Valrelease is not of value in the treatment of psychotic patients and should not be employed in lieu of appropriate treatment. As is true of most preparations containing CNS-acting drugs, patients receiving Valrelease should be cautioned against engaging in hazardous occupations requiring complete mental alertness such as operating machinery or driving a motor vehicle.
As with other agents which have anticonvulsant activity, when Valrelease is used as an adjunct in treating convulsive disorders, the possibility of an increase in the frequency and/ or severity of grand mal seizures may require an increase in the dosage of standard anticonvulsant medication. Abrupt withdrawal of Valrelease in such cases may also be associated with a temporary increase in the frequency and/or severity of seizures.
Since Valrelease has a central nervous system depressant effect, patients should be advised against the simultaneous ingestion of alcohol and other CNS-depressant drugs during Valrelease therapy.
Physical and Psychological Dependence: Withdrawal symptoms (similar in character to those noted with barbiturates and alcohol) have occurred following abrupt discontinuance of diazepam (convulsions, tremor, abdominal and muscle cramps, vomiting and sweating). These were usually limited to those patients who had received excessive doses over an extended period of time. Although infrequently seen, milder withdrawal symptoms have also been reported following abrupt discontinuance of benzodiazepines taken continuously, generally at higher therapeutic levels, for at least several months. Consequently, after extended therapy, abrupt discontinuation should be generally avoided and a gradual tapering in dosage followed. Particularly addiction-prone individuals (such as drug addicts or alcoholics) should be under careful surveillance when receiving diazepam or other psychotropic agents because of the predisposition of such patients to habituation and dependence.

Usage in Pregnancy: **An increased risk of congenital malformations associated with the use of minor tranquilizers (diazepam, meprobamate and chlordiazepoxide) during the first trimester of pregnancy has been suggested in several studies. Because use of these drugs is rarely a matter of urgency, their use during this period should almost always be avoided. The possibility that a woman of childbearing potential may be pregnant at the time of institution of therapy should be considered. Patients should be advised that if they become pregnant during therapy or intend to become pregnant they should communicate with their physicians about the desirability of discontinuing the drug.**
Management of Overdosage: Manifestations of diazepam overdosage include somnolence, confusion, coma and diminished reflexes. Respiration, pulse and blood pressure should be monitored, as in all cases of drug overdosage, although, in general, these effects have been minimal following overdosage. General supportive measures should be employed, along with immediate gastric lavage. Intravenous fluids should be administered and an adequate airway maintained. Hypotension may be combated by the use of Levophed® (levarterenol) or Aramine (metaraminol). Dialysis is of limited value. As with the management of intentional overdosage with any drug, it should be borne in mind that multiple agents may have been ingested.

PRECAUTIONS

If Valrelease is to be combined with other psychotropic agents or anticonvulsant drugs, careful consideration should be given to the pharmacology of the agents to be employed—particularly with known compounds which may potentiate the action of diazepam, such as phenothiazines, narcotics, barbiturates, MAO inhibitors and other antidepressants.
The usual precautions are indicated for severely depressed patients or those in whom there is any evidence of latent depression; particularly the recognition that suicidal tendencies may be present and protective measures may be necessary. The usual precautions in treating patients with impaired renal or hepatic function should be observed.
In elderly and debilitated patients, it is recommended that the dosage be limited to the smallest effective amount to preclude the development of ataxia or oversedation (2 mg to 2½ mg once or twice daily, initially, to be increased gradually as needed and tolerated).
The clearance of Valium and certain other benzodiazepines can be delayed in association with Tagamet (cimetidine) administration. The clinical significance of this is unclear.

ADVERSE REACTIONS

Side effects most commonly reported were drowsiness, fatigue and ataxia. Infrequently encountered were confusion, constipation, depression, diplopia, dysarthria, headache, hypotension, incontinence, jaundice, changes in libido, nausea, changes in salivation, skin rash, slurred speech, tremor, urinary retention, vertigo and blurred vision. Paradoxical reactions such as acute hyperexcited states, anxiety, hallucinations, increased muscle spasticity, insomnia, rage, sleep disturbances and stimulation have been reported; should these occur, use of the drug should be discontinued.
Because of isolated reports of neutropenia and jaundice, periodic blood counts and liver function tests are advisable during long-term therapy. Minor changes in EEG patterns, usually low-voltage fast activity, have been observed in patients during and after diazepam therapy and are of no known significance.

DOSAGE AND ADMINISTRATION

Dosage should be individualized for maximum beneficial effect. While the usual daily dosages given below will meet the needs of most patients, there will be some who may require higher doses. In such cases dosage should be increased cautiously to avoid adverse effects.
Whenever oral Valium® (diazepam/Roche), 5 mg t.i.d., would be considered the appropriate dosage, one 15-mg Valrelease capsule daily may be used.
Note: If 1 mg or 2½ mg is the desired dose, scored Valium (diazepam/Roche) tablets should be used.
Valrelease 15-mg capsules are recommended for elderly or debilitated patients and children only when it has been determined that 5 mg oral Valium t.i.d. is the optimal daily dose. Oral Valium is not recommended for children under 6 months of age.

Adults:	USUAL DAILY DOSE
Management of Anxiety Disorders and Relief of Symptoms of Anxiety.	Depending upon severity of symptoms—1 or 2 (15 to 30 mg) capsules once daily
Symptomatic Relief in Acute Alcohol Withdrawal	2 capsules (30 mg) the first 24 hours, followed by 1 capsule (15 mg) daily as needed.

Continued on next page

Roche Labs.—Cont.

Adults:	USUAL DAILY DOSE
Adjunctively for Relief of Skeletal Muscle Spasm.	1 or 2 capsules (15 to 30 mg) once daily
Adjunctively in Convulsive Disorders.	1 or 2 capsules (15 to 30 mg) once daily

HOW SUPPLIED

For oral administration, Valrelease (diazepam/Roche) capsules—15 mg (yellow and blue)—bottles of 100; Prescription Paks of 30.

Shown in Product Identification Section, page 425

VERSED® Ⓒ
[*ver-sed'*]
midazolam HCl/Roche
INJECTION

The following text is complete prescribing information based on official labeling in effect June 1, 1986.

DESCRIPTION

VERSED (brand of midazolam hydrochloride/Roche) is a water-soluble benzodiazepine available as a sterile parenteral dosage form for intravenous or intramuscular injection. Each ml contains midazolam hydrochloride equivalent to 5 mg midzaolam compounded with 0.8% sodium chloride and 0.01% disodium edetate, with 1% benzyl alcohol as preservative; the pH is adjusted to approximately 3 with hydrochloric acid and, if necessary, sodium hydroxide.

Midazolam is a white to light yellow crystalline compound, insoluble in water. The hydrochloride salt of midazolam, which is formed *in situ*, is soluble in aqueous solutions. Chemically, midazolam HCl is 8-chloro-6-(2-fluorophenyl)-1-methyl-4*H*-imidazo[1,5-a][1,4]benzodiazepine hydrochloride. Midazolam hydrochloride has a calculated molecular weight of 362.25.

CLINICAL PHARMACOLOGY

VERSED is a short-acting benzodiazepine central nervous system depressant.

The effects of VERSED on the CNS are dependent on the dose administered, the route of administration, and the presence or absence of other premedications. Onset time of sedative effects after IM administration was 15 minutes, with peak sedation occurring 30 to 60 minutes following injection. In one study, when tested the following day, 73% of the patients who received VERSED intramuscularly had no recall of memory cards shown 30 minutes following drug administration; 40% had no recall of the memory cards shown 60 minutes following drug administration.

Sedation after IV injection was achieved within 3 to 5 minutes; the time of onset is affected by total dose administered and the concurrent administration of narcotic premedication. Seventy-one percent of the patients in the endoscopy studies had no recall of introduction of the endoscope; 82% of the patients had no recall of withdrawal of the endoscope.

When VERSED is given intravenously as an anesthetic induction agent, induction of anesthesia occurs in approximately 1.5 minutes when narcotic premedication has been administered and in 2 to 2.5 minutes without narcotic premedication or with sedative premedication. Some impairment in a test of memory was noted in 90% of the patients studied.

VERSED, used as directed, does not delay awakening from general anesthesia. Gross tests of recovery after awakening (orientation, ability to stand and walk, suitability for discharge from the recovery room, return to baseline Trieger competency) usually indicate recovery within 2 hours but recovery may take up to 6 hours in some cases. When compared with patients who received thiopental, patients who received midazolam generally recovered at a slightly slower rate. Reaction time under stress (operating automobiles or other hazardous machinery) has not been studied. (See **Warnings**.)

The intravenous administration of VERSED decreases the minimum alveolar concentration (MAC) of halothane required for general anesthesia. This decrease correlates with the dose of VERSED administered.

In patients without intracranial lesions, induction with VERSED is associated with a moderate decrease in cerebrospinal fluid pressure (lumbar puncture measurements), similar to that seen following use of thiopental. Preliminary data in intracranial surgical patients with normal intracranial pressure but decreased compliance (subarachnoid screw measurements) show comparable elevations of intracranial pressure with VERSED and with thiopental during intubation.

Measurements of intraocular pressure in patients without eye disease show a moderate lowering following induction with VERSED; patients with glaucoma have not been studied.

Usual intramuscular premedicating doses of VERSED do not depress the ventilatory response to carbon dioxide stimulation to a clinically significant extent. Induction doses of VERSED depress the ventilatory response to carbon dioxide stimulation for 15 minutes or more beyond the duration of ventilatory depression following administration of thiopental. Impairment of ventilatory response to carbon dioxide is more marked in patients with chronic obstructive pulmonary disease (COPD). Sedation with intravenous VERSED does not adversely affect the mechanics of respiration (resistance, static recoil, most lung volume measurements); total lung capacity and peak expiratory flow decrease significantly but static compliance and maximum expiratory flow at 50% of awake total lung capacity (Vmax) increase.

In cardiac hemodynamic studies, induction with VERSED was associated with a slight to moderate decrease in mean arterial pressure, cardiac output, stroke volume and systemic vascular resistance. Slow heart rates (less than 65/minute), particularly in patients taking propranolol for angina, tended to rise slightly; faster heart rates (*e.g.,* 85/minute) tended to slow slightly.

The following preliminary pharmacokinetic data for midazolam have been reported. In normal subjects and healthy patients intravenous midazolam exhibited an elimination half-life of 1.2 to 12.3 hours, a large volume of distribution (0.95 to 6.6 L/kg) and a plasma clearance of 0.15 to 0.77 L/hr/kg.

Following intravenous administration, less than 0.03% of the dose is excreted in the urine as intact midazolam. Midazolam is rapidly metabolized to 1-hydroxymethyl midazolam, which is conjugated, with subsequent excretion in the urine. Approimxately 45% to 57% of the dose is excreted in the urine as the conjugate of 1-hydroxymethyl midazolam, the major metabolite of midazolam. The half-life of elimination of 1-hydroxymethyl midazolam is similar to the parent compound. The concentration of midazolam is 10- to 30-fold greater than that of 1-hydroxymethyl midazolam after single IV administration.

Clinical effects of VERSED do not directly correlate with the blood concentrations of midazolam.

In a small group of patients (n = 11) with congestive heart failure, there appeared to be a 2- to 3-fold increase in the elimination half-life and volume of distribution of midazolam; however, the total body clearance of midazolam appeared to remain unchanged at a single 5-mg intravenous dose. There was no apparent change in the pharmacokinetic profile following the intravenous administration of 5 mg of midazolam to a small group of patients (n = 12) with hepatic dysfunction. There was a 1.5- to 2-fold increase in elimination half-life, total body clearance and volume of distribution in a small group of patients (n = 15) with chronic renal failure.

In a small group (n = 12) of surgical patients, aged 49 to 60 years old, given 0.2 mg/kg midazolam intravenously, there appeared to be a small increase in the volume of distribution and elimination half-life with little change in total body clearance compared to an equal number of younger surgical patients (aged 18 to 30).

The mean absolute bioavailability of midazolam following intramuscular administration is greater than 90%. The mean time of maximum midazolam plasma concentrations following intramuscular dosing occurs within 45 minutes postadministration. Peak concentrations of midazolam as well as 1-hydroxymethyl midazolam after intramuscular administration are about one-half of those achieved after equivalent intravenous doses. The pharmacokinetic profile of elimination after intramuscularly administered midazolam is comparable to that observed following intravenous administration of the drug. Dose-linearity relationships have not been adequately defined.

Midazolam is approximately 97% plasma protein-bound in normal subjects and patients with renal failure. In animals, midazolam has been shown to cross the blood-brain barrier. In animals and in humans, midazolam has been shown to cross the placenta and enter into fetal circulation. It is not known whether midazolam is excreted in human milk.

INDICATIONS

Injectable VERSED is indicated—

- Intramuscularly for preoperative sedation (induction of sleepiness or drowsiness and relief of apprehension) and to impair memory of perioperative events;
- intravenously as an agent for conscious sedation prior to short diagnostic or endoscopic procedures, such as bronchoscopy, gastroscopy, cystoscopy, coronary angiography and cardiac catheterization, either alone or with a narcotic;
- intravenously for induction of general anesthesia, before administration of other anesthetic agents. With the use of narcotic premedication, induction of anesthesia can be attained within a relatively narrow dose range and in a short period of time. Intravenous VERSED can also be used as a component of intravenous supplementation of nitrous oxide and oxygen (balanced anesthesia) *for short surgical procedures;* longer procedures have not been studied.

When used intravenously, VERSED is associated with a high incidence of partial or complete impairment of recall for the next several hours. (See **Clinical Pharmacology**.)

CONTRAINDICATIONS

Injectable VERSED is contraindicated in patients with a known hypersensitivity to the drug. Benzodiazepines are contraindicated in patients with acute narrow angle glaucoma. Benzodiazepines may be used in patients with open angle glaucoma only if they are receiving appropriate therapy. (See **Clinical Pharmacology**.)

WARNINGS

PRIOR TO THE INTRAVENOUS ADMINISTRAITON OF VERSED IN ANY DOSE, THE IMMEDIATE AVAILABILITY OF OXYGEN AND RESUSCITATIVE EQUIPMENT FOR THE MAINTENANCE OF A PATENT AIRWAY AND SUPPORT OF VENTILATION SHOULD BE ENSURED.

Because intravenous VERSED depresses respiration (see **Clinical Pharmacology**) and because opioid agonists and other sedatives can add to this depression, VERSED should be administered as an induction agent only by a person trained in general anesthesia and should be used in conscious sedation only when a person skilled in maintaining a patent airway and supporting ventilation is present.

Injectable VERSED should not be administered to patients in shock or coma, or in acute alcohol intoxication with depression of vital signs.

The hazards of intra-arterial injection of VERSED solutions in humans are unknown; therefore, extreme precautions against unintended intra-arterial injection should be taken. Extravasation should also be avoided.

Higher risk sugical patients or debilitated patients require lower dosages for induction of anesthesia, whether premedicated or not. Patients with chronic obstructive pulmonary disease are unusually sensitive to the respiratory depressant effect of VERSED. Patients with chronic renal failure have a 1.5- to 2-fold increase in elimination half-life, total body clearance and volume of distribution of midazolam. Patients with congestive heart failure have a 2- to 3-fold increase in the elimination half-life and volume of distribution of midazolam. Patients over the age of 55 years require lower dosages for induction of anesthesia, whether premedicated or not. Because elderly patients frequently have inefficient function of one or more organ systems, and because dosage requirements have been shown to decrease with age, reduced initial dosage of VERSED is recommended and the possibility of profound and/or prolonged effect should be considered.

Concomitant use of barbiturates, alcohol or other central nervous system depressants may increase the risk of underventilation or apnea and may contribute to profound and/or prolonged drug effect. Narcotic premedication also depresses the ventilatory response to carbon dioxide stimulation.

Hypotension occurred more frequently in the conscious sedation studies in patients premedicated with a narcotic.

The decision as to when patients who have received injectable VERSED, particularly on an outpatient basis, may again engage in activities requiring complete mental alertness, operate hazardous machinery or drive a motor vehicle must be individualized. Gross tests of recovery from the effects of VERSED (see **Clinical Pharmacology**) cannot be relied upon alone to predict reaction time under stress. This drug is never used alone during anesthesia and the contribution of other perioperative drugs and events can vary. It is recommended that no patient operate hazardous machinery or a motor vehicle until the effects of the drug, such as drowsiness, have subsided or until the day after anesthesia and surgery, whichever is longer.

Usage in Pregnancy: An increased risk of congenital malformations associated with the use of benzodiazepine drugs (diazepam and chlordiazepoxide) has been suggested in several studies. If this drug is used during pregnancy, the patient should be apprised of the potential hazard to the fetus.

PRECAUTIONS

General: Because an increase in cough reflex and laryngospasm may occur with peroral endoscopic procedures, the use of a topical anesthetic agent and the availability of necessary countermeasures are recommended. The use of narcotic premedication is recommended for bronchoscopies.

Intravenous doses of VERSED should be decreased by 25% to 30% for elderly and debilitated patients. (See **Warnings and Dosage and Administration.**) These patients will also probably take longer to recover completely after VERSED administration for the induction of anesthesia.

VERSED does not protect against the increase in intracranial pressure or circulatory effects noted following administration of succinylcholine.

VERSED does not protect against the increase in intracranial pressure or against the heart rate rise and/or blood pressure rise associated with endotracheal intubation under light general anesthesia.

Informtion for patients: To assure safe and effective use of benzodiazepines, the following information and instructions should be communicated to the patient when appropriate:

1. Inform your physician about any alcohol consumption and medicine you are now taking, including drugs you buy without a prescription. Alcohol has an increased effect when consumed with benzodiazepines; therefore, caution

should be exercised regarding simultaneous ingestion of alcohol during benzodiazepine treatment.

2. Inform you physician if you are pregnant or are planning to become pregnant.
3. Inform you physician if you are nursing.

Drug Interactions: The hypnotic effect of intravenous VERSED is accentuated by premedication, particularly narcotics (*e.g.,* morphine, meperidine and fentanyl) and also secobarbital and Innovar (fentanyl and droperidol). Consequently, the dosage of VERSED should be adjusted according to the type and amount of premedication administered. (See **Dosage and Administration**.)

A moderate reduction in induction dosage requirements of theiopental (about 15%) has been noted following use of intramuscular VERSED for premedication.

The use of VERSED as an induction agent may result in a reduction of the inhalation anesthetic requirement during maintenance of anesthesia. (See **Clinical Pharmacology**.)

Although the possibility of minor interactive effects has not been fully studied, VERSED and pancuronium have been used together in patients without noting clinically significant changes in dosage, onset or duration. VERSED does not protect against the characteristic circulatory changes noted after administration of succinylcholine or pancuronium and does not protect against the increased intracranial pressure noted following administration of succinylcholine. VERSED does not cause a clinically significant change in dosage, onset or duration of a single intubating dose of succinylcholine.

No significant adverse interactions with commonly used premedications or drugs used during anesthesia and surgery (including atropine, scopolamine, glycopyrrolate, diazepam, hydroxyzine, d-tubocurarine, succinylcholine and non-depolarizing muscle relaxants) or topical local anesthetics (including lidocaine, dyclonine HCl and Cetacaine) have been observed.

Drug/laboratory test interactions: Midazolam has not been shown to interfere with results obtained in clinical laboratory tests.

Carcinogenesis, mutagenesis, impairment of fertility:

Carcinogenesis: Midazolam maleate was administered with diet in mice and rats for two years at dosages of 1, 9 and 80 mg/kg/day. In female mice in the highest dose group there was a marked increase in the incidence of hepatic tumors. In high dose male rats there was a small but statistically significant increase in benign thyroid follicular cell tumors. Dosages of 9 mg/kg/day of midazolam maleate (25 times a human dose of 0.35 mg/kg) do not increase the incidence of tumors. The pathogenesis of induction of these tumors is not known. These tumors were found after chronic administration, whereas human use will ordinarily be of single or several doses.

Mutagenesis: Midazolam did not have mutagenic activity in *Salmonella typhimurium* (5 bacterial strains), Chinese hamster lung cells (V79), human lymphocytes, or in the micronucleus test in mice.

Impairment of fertility: A reproduction study in male and female rats did not show any impairment of fertility at dosages up to ten times the human IV dose of 0.35 mg/kg.

Pregnancy: Teratogenic effects: pregnancy Category D. See **Warnings** section.

Segment II teratology studies, performed with midazolam maleate injectable in rabbits and rats at 5 and 10 times the human dose of 0.35 mg/kg, did not show evidence of teratogenicity.

Nonteratogenic effects: Studies in rats showed no adverse effects on reproductive parameters during gestation and lactation. Dosages tested were approximately 10 times the human dose of 0.35 mg/kg.

Labor and delivery: In humans, measurable levels of midazolam were found in maternal venous serum, umbilical venous and arterial serum and amniotic fluid, indicating placental transfer of the drug. Following intramuscular administration of 0.05 mg/kg of midazolam, both the venous and the umbilical arterial serum concentrations were lower than maternal concentrations.

The use of injectable VERSED In obstetrics has not been evaluated in clinical studies. Because midazolam is transfered transplacentally and because other benzodiazepines given in the last weeks of pregnancy have resulted in neonatal CNS depression, VERSED is not recommended for obstetrical use.

Nursing mothers: It is not known whether midazolam is excreted in human milk. Because many drugs are excreted in human milk, caution should be exercised when injectable VERSED is administered to a nursing woman.

Pediatric use: Safety and effectiveness of VERSED In children below the age of 18 have not been established.

ADVERSE REACTIONS

Fluctuations in vital signs were the most frequently seen findings following parenteral administration of VERSED and included decreased tidal volume and/or respiratory rate decrease (23.3% of patients following IV and 10.8% of patients following IM administration) and apnea (15.4% of patients following IV administration), as well as variations in blood pressure and pulse rate. These are common occurrences during anesthesia and surgery and are affected by the lightening or deepening of anesthesia, instrumentation, intubation and use of concomitant drugs.

In the conscious sedation studies, hypotension occurred more frequently after IV administration of VERSED in patients concurrently premedicated with meperidine. It should especially be noted that VERSED does not modify the circulatory effects of neuromuscular blocking agents or the tachycardia and blood pressure rises seen during endotracheal intubation under light general anesthesia. During the clinical investigations, three cases (0.2%) of transient fall in blood pressure greater than 50% were reported during the induction phase.

The following adverse reactions were reported after intramuscular administration:

headache (1.3%)	*Local effects at IM Injection site*
	pain (3.7%)
	induration (0.5%)
	redness (0.5%)
	muscle stiffness (0.3%)

The following adverse reactions were reported subsequent to intravenous administration:

hiccoughs (3.9%)	*Local effects at the IV site*
nausea (2.8%)	tenderness (5.6%)
vomiting (2.6%)	pain during injection (5.0%)
coughing (1.3%)	redness (2.6%)
"oversedation" (1.6%)	induration (1.7%)
headache (1.5%)	phlebitis (0.4%)
drowsiness (1.2%)	

Other adverse experiences, observed mainly following IV injection and occurring at an incidence of less than 1.0%, are as follows:

Respiratory: Laryngospasm, bronchospasm, dyspnea, hyperventilation, wheezing, shallow respirations, airway obstruction, tachypnea.

Cardiovascular: Bigeminy, premature ventricular contractions, vasovagal episode, tachycardia, nodal rhythm.

Gastrointestinal: Acid taste, excessive salivation, retching.

CNS/Neuromuscular: Retrograde amnesia, euphoria, confusion, argumentativeness, nervousness, agitation, anxiety, grogginess, restlessness, emergence delirium or agitation, prolonged emergence from anesthesia, dreaming during emergence, sleep disturbance, insomnia, nightmares, tonic/clonic movements, muscle tremor, involuntary movements, athetoid movements, ataxia, dizziness, dysphoria, slurred speech, dysphonia, paresthesia.

Special Sense: Blurred vision, diplopia, nystagmus, pinpoint pupils, cyclic movements of eyelids, visual disturbance, difficulty focusing eyes, ears blocked, loss of balance, lightheadedness.

Integumentary: Hives, hive-like elevation at injection site, swelling or feeling of burning, warmth or coldness at injection site, rash, pruritus.

Miscellaneous: Yawning, lethargy, chills, weakness, toothache, faint feeling, hematoma.

DRUG ABUSE AND DEPENDENCE

Midazolam is subject to Schedule IV control under the controlled Substances Act of 1970.

Midazolam was actively self-administered in primate models used to assess the positive reinforcing effects of psychoactive drugs.

Midazolam produced physical dependence of a mild to moderate intensity in cynomolgus monkeys after 5 to 10 weeks of administraiton. Available data concerning the drug abuse and dependence potential of midazolam suggest that its abuse potential is at least equivalent to that of diazepam.

OVERDOSAGE

There have been no reports of injectable VERSED overdosage. The manifestations of VERSED overdosage are expected to be similar to those observed with other benzodiazepines and include sedation, somnolence, confusion, impaired coordination, diminished reflexes, coma and untoward effects on vital signs. No evidence of specific organ toxicity from VERSED overdosage would be expected.

Treatment of overdosage: Treatment of injectable VERSED overdosage is the same as that followed for overdosage with other benzodiazepines. Respiration, pulse rate and blood pressure should be monitored and general supportive measures should be employed. Attention should be given to the maintenance of a patent airway and support of ventilation. An intravenous infusion should be started. Should hypotension develop, treatment may include intravenous fluid therapy, repositioning, judicious use of vasopressors appropriate to the clinical situation, if indicated, and other appropriate countermeasures. There is no information as to whether peritoneal dialysis, forced diuresis or hemodialysis are of any value in the treatment of midazolam overdosage.

DOSAGE AND ADMINISTRATION

Dosage should be individualized. In general, lower doses are required in elderly or debilitated patients. The dosage of intravenous VERSED administered should be adjusted according to the type and amount of premedication used. When intravenous use is indicated, oxygen, resuscitative equipment and personnel resources for the maintenance of a patent airway should be immediately available. (See **Warnings**).

Injectable VERSED may be mixed in the same syringe with the following frequently used premedications: morphine sulfate, meperidine, atropine sulfate or scopolamine. Injectable VERSED is compatible with 5% dextrose in water, 0.9% sodium chloride, and lactated Ringer's solution.

For *intramuscular* use, VERSED should be injected deep in a large muscle mass. *Intravenous* VERSED for conscious sedation should be administered slowly; rapid injection may cause respiratory depression or apnea requiring assisted or controlled ventilation. For induction of general anesthesia, the initial dose should be administered over 20 to 30 seconds for optimum effect. Extreme care should be taken to avoid intra-arterial injection or extravasation (see **Warnings**).

INTRAMUSCULARLY	USUAL ADULT DOSE
For preoperative sedation (induction of sleepiness or drowsiness and relief of apprehension) and to impair memory of perioperative events.	For premedication the recommended dose of VERSED is 0.07 to 0.08 mg/kg IM (approximately 5 mg IM for an average adult) approximately one hour before surgery. Onset is within 15 minutes, peaking at 30 to 60 minutes. It can be administered concomitantly with atropine sulfate or scopolamine hydrochloride and reduced doses of narcotics.
INTRAVENOUSLY	
Endoscopic or Cardiovascular Procedures For conscious sedation, VERSED can be used either alone or together with a narcotic immediately before the procedure, with supplemental doses of VERSED to maintain the desired level of sedation, throughout the procedure For peroral procedures. the use of an appropriate topical anesthetic is recommended. For bronchoscopic procedures, the use of narcotic premedication is recommended.	VERSED should be administered immediately prior to the procedure in small increments and titrated slowly until the desired sedative effect, *i.e.,* the initiation of slurred speech, is reached. An initial titration with a small dose, such as 2 to 2.5 mg (0.035 mg/kg) (½ ml), is suggested for an average healthy adult. The dosage may then be further titrated to the desired effect; generally a dose of 0.1 to 0.15 mg/kg is adequate as a *total dose* when administered over a 2 to 3 minute period. In rare cases, a total dose of up to 0.2 mg/kg may be necessary, particularly when concomitant narcotics are omitted. Doses in excess of 0.15 mg/kg may result in increased risk of respiratory depression or drowsiness in elderly or debilitated patients. Additional maintenance doses may be given in increments of 25% of the initial dose to maintain the desired level of sedation. Narcotic premedication results in less variability in patient response. Dosage should be lowered by about 25% to 30% if narcotic premedication is used. Patients 60 years or older may require lower doses (by about 30%) than younger patients.
Induction of Anesthesia: For induction of general anesthesia, before administration of other anesthetic agents.	Individual response to the drug is variable, particularly when a narcotic premedication is not used. The dosage should be titrated to the desired effect according to the patient's age and clinical status. *Unpremedicated Patients* In the absence of premedication, an average adult under the age of 55 years will usually require an initial dose of 0.3 to 0.35 mg/kg for induction, administered over 20 to 30 seconds and allowing 2 minutes for effect. If needed to complete induction, increments of approximately 25% of the patient's initial dose may be used; induction may instead be completed with

Continued on next page

Roche Labs.—Cont.

volatile liquid inhalational anesthetics. In resistant cases, up to 0.6 mg/kg total dose may be used for induction, but such larger doses may prolong recovery.

Unpremedicated patients over the age of 55 years usually require less VERSED for induction; an initial dose of 0.3 mg/kg is recommended.

Unpremedicated patients with severe systemic disease or other debilitation usually require less VERSED for induction. An initial dose of 0.2 to 0.25 mg/kg will usually suffice; in some cases, as little as 0.15 mg/kg may suffice.

Premedicated Patients

When the patient has received sedative or narcotic premedication, particularly narcotic premedication, the range of recommended doses is 0.15 to 0.35 mg/kg.

In average adults below the age of 55 years, a dose of 0.25 mg/kg, administered over 20 to 30 seconds and allowing 2 minutes for effect, will usually suffice.

The initial dose of 0.2 mg/kg is recommended for good risk (ASA I & II) surgical patients over the age of 55 years.

In some patients with severe systemic disease or debilitation, as little as 0.15 mg/kg may suffice.

Narcotic premedication frequently used during clinical trials included fentanyl (1.5 to 2 μg/kg IV, administered five minutes before induction), morphine (dosage individualized, up to 0.15 mg/kg IM), meperidine (dosage individualized, up to 1 mg/kg IM) and Innovar (0.02 ml/kg IM). Sedative premedications were hydroxyzine pamoate (100 mg orally) and sodium secobarbital (200 mg orally). Except for intravenous fentanyl, all other premedications should be administered approximately one hour prior to the time anticipated for VERSED induction.

Injectable VERSED can also be used during maintenance of anesthesia, *for short surgical procedures*, as a component of balanced anethesia. Effective narcotic premedication is especially recommended in such cases. Long surgical procedures have not been studied.

Incremental injections of approximately 25% of the induction dose should be given in response to signs of lightening of anesthesia and repeated as necessary.

Note: Parenteral drug products should be inspected visually for particulate matter and discoloration prior to administration, whenever solution and container permit.

HOW SUPPLIED

All package configurations contain midazolam hydrochloride equivalent to 5 mg midazolam/ml.
1 ml vials (5 mg)—boxes of 10 (NDC 0004-1974-01);
2 ml vials (10 mg)—boxes of 10 (NDC 0004-1973-01);
5 ml vials (25 mg)—boxes of 10 (NDC 0004-1975-01);
10 ml vials (50 mg)—boxes of 10 (NDC 0004-1946-01);
2 ml Tel-E-Ject® disposable syringes (10 mg)—boxes of 10 (NDC 0004-1947-01).

VI-PENTA® F CHEWABLES ℞

[*vy-pen 'ta*]

The following text is complete prescribing information based on official labeling in effect June 1, 1986.

DESCRIPTION

Vi-Penta F Chewables is a prescription-only chewable multivitamin tablet containing eleven vitamins and dietary fluoride. Vi-Penta F Chewables is specially formulated to provide daily nutritional support and aid in the prevention of tooth decay in children three years of age and older. Vi-Penta F Chewables is available as green, yellow, pink, purple and orange tablets. Each fruit-flavored tablet contains less than one calorie and will not interfere with the appetite.

Each chewable tablet contains:

Fat-Soluble Vitamins

Vitamin A (as vitamin A acetate) .... 5000 IU
Vitamin D_2 (ergocalciferol) .... 400 IU
Vitamin E (as *dl*-alpha-tocopheryl acetate) .... 2 IU

Water-Soluble Vitamins

Vitamin C (as ascorbic acid and sodium ascorbate) .... 60 mg
Vitamin B_1 (as thiamine mononitrate) .... 1.2 mg
Vitamin B_2 (riboflavin) .... 1.5 mg
Niacin (as niacinamide) .... 10 mg
Vitamin B_6 (as pyridoxine HCl) .... 1 mg
d-biotin .... 40 mcg
Pantothenic acid (as calcium *d*-pantothenate) .... 9 mg
Vitamin B_{12} (cyanocobalamin) .... 3 mcg

Trace Elements

Fluoride (as sodium fluoride) .... 1 mg

Each tablet also contains cottonseed oil, magnesium stearate, mannitol, sodium chloride, sodium saccharin, stearic acid, talc, titanium dioxide and flavors, with the following dye systems: green—FD&C Blue No. 1, D&C Yellow No. 10, FD&C Yellow No. 6; yellow—D&C Yellow No. 10, FD&C Yellow No. 6; pink—FD&C Red No. 3; purple—FD&C Blue No. 1, D&C Yellow No. 10, FD&C Yellow No. 6, FD&C Red No. 3; orange—FD&C Yellow No. 6.

CLINICAL PHARMACOLOGY

Vitamins are necessary for maintenance of normal metabolic functions including hematopoiesis. *Vitamin A* is necessary for proper functioning of the retina; it appears to be essential to the integrity of epithelial cells. *Vitamin D* is necessary for the absorption of calcium and for the proper development and maintenance of bone structure. *Vitamin E* is an antioxidant which preserves essential cellular constituents, including those of the red blood cell. It also serves as protection against lipid peroxidation.

The water-soluble vitamins play vital roles in the conversion of carbohydrate, protein and fat into tissue and energy. *Thiamine (B_1)* acts as a coenzyme in carbohydrate metabolism. *Riboflavin (B_2)* functions as a coenzyme in the electron transport system associated with conversion of tissue oxidations into usable energy. *Niacin* serves as a coenzyme in oxidation-reduction reactions in tissue respiration. *Pyridoxine (B_6)* is essential for the metabolism of amino acids. *Pantothenic acid* functions as a coenzyme in various metabolic acetylation reactions and *biotin* in specific carboxylation reactions in lipid metabolism. *Cyanocobalamin (B_{12})* is essential to nucleic acid synthesis and normal maturation of red blood cells. *Ascorbic acid (C)* performs a vital function in the process of cellular respiration, and is involved in both carbohydrate and amino acid metabolism. It is essential for collagen formation and tissue repair.

Fluorine is an essential trace element that renders the dentine and enamel of teeth more resistant to acid.

There is ample evidence that the fluoridation of drinking water leads to a substantial decrease in the incidence of dental caries in childhood. This effect is greatest when fluoride is ingested during the first 9 to 10 years of life when teeth are developing. However, in areas where drinking water is devoid of natural or artificially controlled fluoride, or where fluoridation is not feasible, a single daily dose of fluoride as a dietary supplement is recommended as an effective substitute.

Recognizing the merits of dietary fluoride supplements, the Council on Dental Therapeutics of the American Dental Association strongly urges: "*Such administration should be consistent and continuous over long periods of time if substantial benefit is to be anticipated.*"

INDICATIONS AND USAGE

Vi-Penta F Chewable Tablets are indicated for supportive nutritional supplementation and as an aid in the prevention of tooth decay in children three years of age and older who reside in areas where the fluoride content of drinking water is known to be less than 0.7 parts per million.

CONTRAINDICATIONS

Vi-Penta F Chewables is contraindicated in patients known to be hypersensitive to any of its components.

WARNINGS

This preparation should not be used in areas where the fluoride content of drinking water is known to be 0.7 parts per million or greater. The recommended dose of Vi-Penta F Chewables should not be exceeded, since dental fluorosis may result from continued ingestion of excessive amounts of fluoride.

PRECAUTIONS

General: Certain patients may require nutritional supplementation with folic acid as well as other nutrients according to the dietary needs of the individual. Vi-Penta F Chewables is not intended for treatment of pernicious anemia or other severe specific vitamin deficiencies.

Information for the Patient: Because dental fluorosis may result from continued ingestion of excessive amounts of fluoride and toxic reactions have been reported with injudicious use of certain vitamins, urge patients to follow your specific instructions regarding dosage regimen. As with any medication, advise patients to keep Vi-Penta F Chewables out of reach of children.

ADVERSE REACTIONS

Adverse reactions have been reported with specific vitamins, but generally at levels substantially higher than those in Vi-Penta F Chewables. However, allergic and idiosyncratic reactions are possible at lower levels.

DOSAGE AND ADMINISTRATION

Usual dosage for children three years of age and over: one tablet daily, chewed or crushed.

Vi-Penta F Chewables is available on prescription only.

HOW SUPPLIED

Green, yellow, pink, purple and orange shield-shaped, biconvex tablets, engraved ROCHE 51—bottles of 100 chewable tablets (NDC 0004-0051-01).

Shown in Product Identification Section, page 425

VI-PENTA® F INFANT DROPS ℞

[*vy-pen 'ta*]

The following text is complete prescribing information based on official labeling in effect June 1, 1986.

DESCRIPTION

Vi-Penta F Infant Drops is a prescription-only liquid multivitamin preparation containing ascorbic acid, dietary fluoride and fat-soluble vitamins A, D and E in a vehicle containing caramel, glycerin, parabens (methyl and propyl), polysorbate 80, sodium hydroxide, flavors and water. It is specially formulated to provide daily nutritional support and aid in the prevention of tooth decay in infants from birth. Vi-Penta F Infant Drops is a fruit-flavored, liquid preparation in an aqueous nonalcoholic vehicle that may be administered by dropping directly on the tongue or mixing with liquids or food.

Each 0.6 ml provides:

Fat-Soluble Vitamins

Vitamin A (as vitamin A palmitate) .... 5000 IU
Vitamin D_2 (ergocalciferol) .... 400 IU
Vitamin E (as *dl*-alpha-tocopheryl acetate) .... 2 IU

Water-Soluble Vitamins

Vitamin C (ascorbic acid) .... 50 mg

Trace Elements

Fluoride (as sodium fluoride) .... 0.5 mg

CLINICAL PHARMACOLOGY

Vitamins are necessary for maintenance of normal metabolic functions including hematopoiesis. *Vitamin A* is necessary for proper functioning of the retina; it appears to be essential to the integrity of epithelial cells. *Vitamin D* is necessary for the absorption of calcium and for the proper development and maintenance of bone structure. *Vitamin E* is an antioxidant which preserves essential cellular constituents, including those of the red blood cell. It also serves as protection against lipid peroxidation. *Vitamin C* performs a vital function in the process of cellular respiration, and is involved in both carbohydrate and amino acid metabolism. It is essential for collagen formation and tissue repair.

Fluorine is an essential trace element that renders the dentine and enamel of teeth more resistant to acid.

There is ample evidence that the fluoridation of drinking water leads to a substantial decrease in the incidence of dental caries in childhood. This effect is greatest when fluoride is ingested during the first 9 to 10 years of life when teeth are developing. However, in areas where drinking water is devoid of natural or artificially controlled fluoride, or where fluoridation is not feasible, a single daily dose of fluoride as a dietary supplement is recommended as an effective substitute.

Recognizing the merits of dietary fluoride supplements, the Council on Dental Therapeutics of the American Dental Association strongly urges: "*Such administration should be consistent and continuous over long periods of time if substantial benefit is to be anticipated.*"

INDICATIONS AND USAGE

Vi-Penta F Infant Drops is indicated for supportive nutritional supplementation and as an aid in the prevention of tooth decay in infants from birth who reside in areas where the fluoride content of drinking water is known to be less than 0.7 parts per million.

CONTRAINDICATIONS

Vi-Penta F Infant Drops is contraindicated in patients known to be hypersensitive to any of its components.

WARNINGS

This preparation should not be used in areas where the fluoride content of drinking water is known to be 0.7 parts per million or greater. The recommended dose of Vi-Penta F Infant Drops should not be exceeded, since dental fluorosis may result from continued ingestion of excessive amounts of fluoride.

PRECAUTIONS

General: Certain patients may require nutritional supplementation with the B-complex vitamins as well as other nutrients according to the dietary needs of the individual. Vi-Penta F Infant Drops is not intended for treatment of severe specific vitamin deficiencies.

Information for the Patient: Because dental fluorosis may result from continued ingestion of excessive amounts of fluoride and toxic reactions have been reported with injudicious use of certain vitamins, urge patients to follow your specific instructions regarding dosage regimen. As with any medication, advise patients to keep Vi-Penta F Infant Drops out of reach of children. Vi-Penta F Infant Drops should be stored under refrigeration.

ADVERSE REACTIONS

Adverse reactions have been reported with specific vitamins, but generally at levels substantially higher than those in Vi-Penta F Infant Drops. However, allergic and idiosyncratic reactions are possible at lower levels.

DOSAGE AND ADMINISTRATION

Usual dosage for infants from birth: 0.6 ml daily, as measured by the dropper. Vi-Penta F Infant Drops may be administered by dropping directly on the tongue or mixing with liquids or food.

Vi-Penta F Infant Drops is available on prescription only.

HOW SUPPLIED

Fruit-flavored liquid in bottle of 30 ml, packaged with a calibrated dropper (NDC 0004-1012-23).

NOTE TO THE PHARMACIST: Vi-Penta F Infant Drops should be dispensed in the original special plastic containers, since contact with glass leads to instability and precipitation. Preparation should be stored under refrigeration.

VI-PENTA® F ℞
[*vy-pen 'ta*]
MULTIVITAMIN DROPS

The following text is complete prescribing information based on official labeling in effect June 1, 1986.

DESCRIPTION

Vi-Penta F Multivitamin Drops is a prescription-only liquid multivitamin preparation containing ten vitamins and dietary fluoride in a vehicle containing glycerin, parabens (methyl and propyl), polysorbate 80, sodium saccharin, flavors and water. It is specially formulated to provide daily nutritional support and aid in the prevention of tooth decay in infants and children. Vi-Penta F Multivitamin Drops is a fruit-flavored, liquid preparation in an aqueous nonalcoholic vehicle that may be administered by dropping directly on the tongue or mixing with liquids or food.

Each 0.6 ml provides:	
Fat-Soluble Vitamins	
Vitamin A (as vitamin A palmitate)	5000 IU
Vitamin D_2 (ergocalciferol)	400 IU
Vitamin E (as *dl*-alpha-tocopheryl acetate)	2 IU
Water-Soluble Vitamins	
Vitamin C (ascorbic acid)	50 mg
Vitamin B_1 (as thiamine HCl)	1 mg
Vitamin B_2 (as riboflavin-5′-phosphate sodium)	1 mg
Niacin (as niacinamide)	10 mg
Vitamin B_6 (as pyridoxine HCl)	0.8 mg
d-Biotin	30 mcg
Pantothenic acid (as dexpanthenol)	10 mg
Trace Elements	
Fluoride (as sodium fluoride)	0.5 mg

CLINICAL PHARMACOLOGY

Vitamins are necessary for maintenance of normal metabolic functions including hematopoiesis. *Vitamin A* is necessary for proper functioning of the retina; it appears to be essential to the integrity of epithelial cells. *Vitamin D* is necessary for the absorption of calcium and for the proper development and maintenance of bone structure. *Vitamin E* is an antioxidant which preserves essential cellular constituents, including those of the red blood cell. It also serves as protection against lipid peroxidation.

The water-soluble vitamins play vital roles in the conversion of carbohydrate, protein and fat into tissue and energy. *Thiamine (B_1)* acts as a coenzyme in carbohydrate metabolism. *Riboflavin (B_2)* functions as a coenzyme in the electron transport system associated with conversion of tissue oxidations into usable energy. *Niacin* serves as a coenzyme in oxidation-reduction reactions in tissue respiration. *Pyridoxine (B_6)* is essential for the metabolism of amino acids. *Pantothenic acid* functions as a coenzyme in various metabolic acetylation reactions and *biotin* in specific carboxylation reactions in lipid metabolism. *Ascorbic acid (C)* performs a vital function in the process of cellular respiration, and is involved in both carbohydrate and amino acid metabolism. It is essential for collagen formation and tissue repair.

Fluorine is an essential trace element that renders the dentine and enamel of teeth more resistant to acid.

There is ample evidence that the fluoridation of drinking water leads to a substantial decrease in the incidence of dental caries in childhood. This effect is greatest when fluoride is ingested during the first 9 to 10 years of life when teeth are developing. However, in areas were drinking water is devoid of natural or artificially controlled fluoride, or where fluoridation is not feasible, a single daily dose of fluoride as a dietary supplement is recommended as an effective substitute. Recognizing the merits of dietary fluoride supplements, the Council on Dental Therapeutics of the American Dental Association strongly urges: "*Such administration should be consistent and continuous over long periods of time if substantial benefit is to be anticipated.*"

INDICATIONS AND USAGE

Vi-Penta F Multivitamin Drops is indicated for supportive nutritional supplementation and as an aid in the prevention of tooth decay in infants and children who reside in areas where the fluoride content of drinking water is known to be less than 0.7 parts per million.

CONTRAINDICATIONS

Vi-Penta F Multivitamin Drops is contraindicated in patients known to be hypersensitive to any of its components.

WARNINGS

This preparation should not be used in areas where the fluoride content of drinking water is known to be 0.7 parts per million or greater. The recommended dose of Vi-Penta F Multivitamin Drops should not be exceeded, since dental fluorosis may result from continued ingestion of excessive amounts of fluoride.

PRECAUTIONS

General: Certain patients may require nutritional supplementation with folic acid and vitamin B_{12} as well as other nutrients according to the dietary needs of the individual. Vi-Penta F Multivitamin Drops is not intended for treatment of severe specific vitamin deficiencies.

Information for the Patient: Because dental fluorosis may result from continued ingestion of excessive amounts of fluoride and toxic reactions have been reported with injudicious use of certain vitamins, urge patients to follow your specific instructions regarding dosage regimen. As with any medication, advise patients to keep Vi-Penta F Multivitamin drops out of reach of children. Vi-Penta F Multivitamin Drops should be stored under refrigeration.

ADVERSE REACTIONS

Adverse reactions have been reported with specific vitamins, but generally at levels substantially higher than those in Vi-Penta F Multivitamin Drops. However, allergic and idiosyncratic reactions are possible at lower levels.

DOSAGE AND ADMINISTRATION

Usual dosage for infants and children: 0.6 ml daily, as measured by the dropper. Vi-Penta F Multivitamin Drops may be administered by dropping directly on the tongue or mixing with liquids or food.

Vi-Penta F Multivitamin Drops is available on prescription only.

HOW SUPPLIED

Fruit-flavored liquid in bottles of 30 ml, packaged with a calibrated dropper (NDC 0004-1014-23).

NOTE TO THE PHARMACIST: Vi-Penta F Multivitamin Drops should be dispensed in the original special plastic containers, since contact with glass leads to instability and precipitation. Preparation should be stored under refrigeration.

Vi-Penta Composition Table

Each 0.6 cc of Vi-Penta Infant Drops Provides:		% minimum daily requirements (MDR) Infants (under 1 year)	Young Children (1–6 years)
Vitamin A (as the palmitate)	5000 U.S.P. Units	333%	166%
Vitamin D_2	400 U.S.P. Units	100%	100%
Vitamin C	50 mg	500%	250%
Vitamin E (as *dl*-α-tocopheryl acetate)	2 Int. Units	*	*

Each 0.6 cc of Vi-Penta Multivitamin Drops provides:		% minimum daily requirements (MDR) Infants (under 1 year)	Children (1–6 years)	(6–12 years)
Vitamin A (as the palmitate)	5000 U.S.P. Units	333%	166%	166%
Vitamin D_2	400 U.S.P. Units	100%	100%	100%
Vitamin C	50 mg	500%	250%	250%
Vitamin B_1 (as hydrochloride)	1 mg	400%	200%	133%
Vitamin B_2 (as riboflavin-5′-phosphate sodium)	1 mg	166%	111%	111%
Vitamin B_6	1 mg	*	*	*
Vitamin E (as *dl*-α-tocopheryl acetate)	2 Int. Units	*	*	*
d-Biotin	30 mcg	†	†	†
Niacinamide	10 mg	*	200%	133%
Dexpanthenol (equiv. to 11.6 mg calcium pantothenate)	10 mg	†	†	†

*MDR for these vitamins has not been determined.

†The need for these vitamins in human nutrition has not been established.

VI-PENTA® INFANT DROPS
VI-PENTA® MULTIVITAMIN DROPS
[*vy-pen 'ta*]

The following text is complete prescribing information based on official labeling in effect June 1, 1986.

COMPOSITION

Vi-Penta Infant Drops and Vi-Penta Multivitamin Drops are designed to fill the vitamin needs of specific age groups. (See Composition Table above.)

ACTION AND USES

Vi-Penta Drops are water miscible and can be mixed with food or infant formula, or placed directly on the tongue.

Vi-Penta Infant Drops—a selective formula for prevention of vitamin deficiencies in infants and young children. *Vi-Penta Multivitamin Drops*—a comprehensive formula for daily nutritional support in adults as well as children of all ages. It is an especially convenient dosage form when a small volume liquid vitamin supplement is desired, such as to supplement the diets of those patients with conditions which permanently or temporarily impair their ability to swallow, chew or consume normal amounts and/or kinds of food.

DOSAGE

The average daily dose is 0.6 cc; therapeutic doses should be given according to the needs of the patient.

HOW SUPPLIED

Vi-Penta Infant Drops and Vi-Penta Multivitamin Drops—fruit flavored, 50-cc bottles packaged with calibrated dropper.

EDUCATIONAL MATERIAL

Please contact your Roche representative concerning availability of educational programs and material.

Products are cross-indexed
by product classifications
in the
BLUE SECTION

Roche Products Inc.
MANATI, PUERTO RICO 00701

DALMANE® C
[dal 'mane]
(flurazepam hydrochloride/Roche)
Capsules

The following text is complete prescribing information based on official labeling in effect June 1, 1986.

DESCRIPTION
Dalmane is available as capsules containing 15 mg or 30 mg fluazepam hydrochloride/Roche. Each 15-mg capsule also contains corn starch, lactose, magnesium stearate and talc; gelatin capsule shells may contain methyl and propyl parabens and potassium sorbate, with the following dye system: FD&C Red No. 3, FD&C Yellow No. 6 and D&C Yellow No. 10. Each 30-mg capsule also contains corn starch, lactose and magnesium stearate; gelatin capsule shells may contain methyl and propyl parabens and potassium sorbate, with the following dye systems: FD&C Blue No. 1, FD&C Yellow No. 6, D&C Yellow No. 10 and either FD&C Red No. 3 or FD&C Red No. 40.
Flurazepam hydrochloride is chemically 7-chloro-1-[2-(diethylamino) ethyl]-5-(o -fluorophenyl) -1, 3-dihydro-2*H* -1, 4-benzodiazepin-2-one dihydrochloride. It is a pale yellow, crystalline compound, freely soluble in U.S.P. alcohol and very soluble in water. It has a molecular weight of 460.826.

CLINICAL PHARMACOLOGY
Flurazepam hydrochloride is rapidly absorbed from the G.I. tract. Flurazepam is rapidly metabolized and is excreted primarily in the urine. Following a single oral dose, peak flurazepam plasma concentrations ranging from 0.5 to 4.0 ng/ml occur at 30 to 60 minutes post-dosing. The harmonic mean apparent half-life of flurazepam is 2.3 hours. The blood level profile of flurazepam and its major metabolites was determined in man following the oral administration of 30 mg daily for 2 weeks. The N_1-hydroxyethyl-flurazepam was measurable only during the early hours after a 30-mg dose and was not detectable after 24 hours. The major metabolite in blood was N_1-desalkyl-flurazepam, which reached steady-state (plateau) levels after 7 to 10 days of dosing, at levels approximately five- to sixfold greater than the 24-hour levels observed on Day 1. The half-life of elimination of N_1-desalkyl-flurazepam ranged from 47 to 100 hours. The major urinary metabolite is conjugated N_1-hydroxyethyl-flurazepam which accounts for 22 to 55 percent of the dose. Less than 1% of the dose is excreted in the urine as N_1-desalkyl-flurazepam.
This pharmacokinetic profile may be responsible for the clinical observation that flurazepam is increasingly effective on the second or third night of consecutive use and that for one or two nights after the drug is discontinued both sleep latency and total wake time may still be decreased.

INDICATIONS
Dalmane is a hypnotic agent useful for the treatment of insomnia characterized by difficulty in falling asleep, frequent nocturnal awakenings, and/or early morning awakening. Dalmane can be used effectively in patients with recurring insomnia or poor sleeping habits, and in acute or chronic medical situations requiring restful sleep. Sleep laboratory studies have objectively determined that Dalmane is effective for at least 28 consecutive nights of drug administration. Since insomnia is often transient and intermittent, short-term use is usually sufficient. Prolonged use of hypnotics is usually not indicated and should only be undertaken concomitantly with appropriate evaluation of the patient.

CONTRAINDICATIONS
Dalmane is contraindicated in patients with known hypersensitivity to the drug.
Usage in Pregnancy: Benzodiazepines may cause fetal damage when administered during pregnancy. An increased risk of congenital malformations associated with the use of diazepam and chlordiazepoxide during the first trimester of pregnancy has been suggested in several studies.
Dalmane is contraindicated in pregnant women. Symptoms of neonatal depression have been reported; a neonate whose mother received 30 mg of Dalmane nightly for insomnia during the 10 days prior to delivery appeared hypotonic and inactive during the first four days of life. Serum levels of N_1-desalkyl-flurazepam in the infant indicated transplacental circulation and implicate this long-acting metabolite in this case. If there is a likelihood of the patient becoming pregnant while receiving flurazepam, she should be warned of the potential risks to the fetus. Patients should be instructed to discontinue the drug prior to becoming pregnant. The possibility that a woman of childbearing potential may be pregnant at the time of institution of therapy should be considered.

WARNINGS
Patients receiving Dalmane should be cautioned about possible combined effects with alcohol and other CNS depressants. Also, caution patients that an additive effect may occur if alcoholic beverages are consumed during the day following the use of Dalmane for nighttime sedation. The potential for this interaction continues for several days following discontinuance of flurazepam, until serum levels of psychoactive metabolites have declined.
Patients should also be cautioned about engaging in hazardous occupations requiring complete mental alertness such as operating machinery or driving a motor vehicle after ingesting the drug, including potential impairment of the performance of such activities which may occur the day following ingestion of Dalmane.
Usage in Children: Clinical investigations of Dalmane have not been carried out in children. Therefore, the drug is not currently recommended for use in persons under 15 years of age.
Physical and Psychological Dependence: Withdrawal symptoms similar in character to those noted with barbiturates and alcohol have been reported following abrupt discontinuance of benzodiazepines taken continuously, generally at higher therapeutic levels, for at least several months. Withdrawal symptoms have rarely been reported with Dalmane. If it is determined that a patient has been taking Dalmane for a prolonged period of time, particularly at excessive doses, abrupt discontinuation should generally be avoided and a gradual tapering of dosage followed. Also, as with any hypnotic, caution must be exercised in administering Dalmane to individuals known to be addiction-prone or those whose history suggests they may increase the dosage on their own initiative.

PRECAUTIONS
Since the risk of the development of oversedation, dizziness, confusion and/or ataxia increases substantially with larger doses in elderly and debilitated patients, it is recommended that in such patients the dosage be limited to 15 mg. If Dalmane is to be combined with other drugs having known hypnotic properties or CNS-depressant effects, due consideration should be given to potential additive effects.
The usual precautions are indicated for severely depressed patients or those in whom there is any evidence of latent depression; particularly the recognition that suicidal tendencies may be present and protective measures may be necessary.
The usual precautions should be observed in patients with impaired renal or hepatic function and chronic pulmonary insufficiency.

ADVERSE REACTIONS
Dizziness, drowsiness, light-headedness, staggering, ataxia and falling have occurred, particularly in elderly or debilitated persons. Severe sedation, lethargy, disorientation and coma, probably indicative of drug intolerance or overdosage, have been reported.
Also reported were headache, heartburn, upset stomach, nausea, vomiting, diarrhea, constipation, gastrointestinal pain, nervousness, talkativeness, apprehension, irritability, weakness, palpitations, chest pains, body and joint pains and genitourinary complaints. There have also been rare occurrences of leukopenia, granulocytopenia, sweating, flushes, difficulty in focusing, blurred vision, burning eyes, faintness, hypotension, shortness of breath, pruritus, skin rash, dry mouth, bitter taste, excessive salivation, anorexia, euphoria, depression, slurred speech, confusion, restlessness, hallucinations, and elevated SGOT, SGPT, total and direct bilirubins, and alkaline phosphatase. Paradoxical reactions, *e.g.,* excitement, stimulation and hyperactivity, have also been reported in rare instances.

DOSAGE AND ADMINISTRATION
Dosage should be individualized for maximal beneficial effects. The usual adult dosage is 30 mg before retiring. In some patients, 15 mg may suffice. In elderly and /or debilitated patients, 15 mg is usually sufficient for a therapeutic response and it is therefore recommended that therapy be initiated with this dosage.

OVERDOSAGE
Manifestations of Dalmane overdosage include somnolence, confusion and coma. Respiration, pulse and blood pressure should be monitored as in all cases of drug overdosage. General supportive measures should be employed, along with immediate gastric lavage. Intravenous fluids should be administered and an adequate airway maintained. Hypotension and CNS depression may be combated by judicious use of appropriate therapeutic agents. The value of dialysis has not been determined. If excitation occurs in patients following Dalmane overdosage, barbiturates should not be used. As with the management of intentional overdosage with any drug, it should be borne in mind that multiple agents may have been ingested.

HOW SUPPLIED
Dalmane (flurazepam hydrochloride/Roche) capsules—15 mg, orange and ivory; 30 mg, red and ivory—bottles of 100 and 500; Tel-E-Dose® packages of 100, available in boxes containing 10 strips of 10, in trays of 4 boxes each containing a reverse-numbered roll of 25 and in boxes of 4 reverse-numbered cards of 25; Prescription Paks of 30, available in trays of 10.
Shown in Product Identification Section, page 424

ENDEP® ℞
[en 'dep]
(amitriptyline HCl/Roche)
TABLETS

The following text is complete prescribing information based on official labeling in effect June 1, 1986.

DESCRIPTION
Endep (amitriptyline HCl/Roche), a tricyclic antidepressant, is available as 10-mg, 25-mg, 50-mg, 75-mg, 100-mg and 150-mg tablets for oral administration. Each tablet also contains corn starch, ethylcellulose, hydroxypropyl methylcellulose, lactose, magnesium stearate, microcrystalline cellulose, povidone, talc and triacetin, with the following dye systems: 10 mg, 25 mg, 50 mg and 75 mg—FD&C Yellow No. 6 and D&C Yellow No. 10; 100 mg and 150 mg—D&C Red No. 30 and FD&C Yellow No. 6.
Amitriptyline HCl, a dibenzocycloheptadiene derivative, is a white crystalline compound that is readily soluble in water. It is designated chemically as 10, 11-dihydro-*N,N* -dimethyl-5*H* -dibenzo[*a,d*]cycloheptene-$\Delta^{5,\gamma}$ -propylamine hydrochloride. The molecular weight is 313.87. The empirical formula is $C_{20}H_{23}N \cdot HCl$.

CLINICAL PHARMACOLOGY
Endep is an antidepressant with sedative effects. Its mechanism of action in man is not known. It is not a monoamine oxidase inhibitor, and it does not act primarily by stimulation of the central nervous system.
Amitriptyline inhibits the membrane pump mechanism responsible for uptake of norepinephrine and serotonin in adrenergic and serotonergic neurons. Pharmacologically this action may potentiate or prolong neuronal activity, since reuptake of these biogenic amines is important physiologically in terminating its transmitting activity. This interference with reuptake of norepinephrine and/or serotonin is believed by some to underlie the antidepressant activity of amitriptyline.
Amitriptyline undergoes extensive metabolism primarily through N-demethylation to nortriptyline, an active metabolite, followed by extensive hydroxylation to their respective 10-hydroxy metabolites which are eliminated as glucuronide conjugates.
Following a single oral dose of 75 mg of amitriptyline HCl, the mean maximum plasma concentrations of 39.4 ng/ml of amitriptyline and 16.1 ng/ml of nortriptyline were reached in approximately 4 and 10 hours, respectively. The average minimum steady-state plasma concentrations in patients receiving 50 mg of amitriptyline HCl, three times a day for an average of 32 days, were 81 ng/ml for amitriptyline, 71 ng/ml for nortriptyline, 12 ng/ml for 10-hydroxyamitriptyline, 91 ng/ml for conjugated 10-hydroxyamitriptyline, 82 ng/ml for 10-hydroxynortriptyline and 176 ng/ml for conjugated 10-hydroxynortriptyline. Steady-state plasma concentrations are usually reached by day 14. The mean apparent half-life of elimination of amitriptyline is 22.4 hours and the apparent half-life of elimination of nortriptyline is 26.0 hours. Amitriptyline is approximately 96% bound to plasma proteins.
Amitriptyline has been shown to cross the blood-brain barrier in cats, mice and rats. It has also been shown to pass the placental barrier and to enter fetal circulation in mice after intramuscular and intravenous administration. Amitriptyline is excreted in human breast milk.

INDICATIONS AND USAGE
Endep is indicated for the relief of symptoms of depression. Endogenous depression is more likely to be alleviated than are other depressive states.

CONTRAINDICATIONS
Endep is contraindicated in patients who have shown prior hypersensitivity to this agent; cross-sensitivity to other tricyclic antidepressants can occur.
Endep is not recommended for use during the acute recovery phase following myocardial infarction.
Endep should not be given concomitantly with a monoamine oxidase inhibitor. Hyperpyretic crises, severe convulsions and deaths have occurred in patients receiving tricyclic antidepressant and monoamine oxidase inhibiting drugs simultaneously. When it is desired to replace a monoamine oxidase inhibitor with Endep, a minimum of 14 days should be allowed to elapse after the former is discontinued. Endep should then be initiated cautiously with gradual increase in dosage until optimum response is achieved.

WARNINGS
Endep should be used with caution in patients with a history of seizures and, because of its atropine-like action, in patients with a history of urinary retention, angle-closure glaucoma or increased intraocular pressure. In patients with

angle-closure glaucoma, even average doses may precipitate an attack.
Patients with cardiovascular disorders should be watched closely. Tricyclic antidepressant drugs, including Endep, particularly when given in high doses, have been reported to produce arrhythmias, sinus tachycardia and prolongation of the conduction time. Myocardial infarction and stroke have been reported with drugs of this class.
Close supervision is required when Endep is given to hyperthyroid patients or those receiving thyroid medication.
Amitriptyline HCl may enhance the response to alcohol and the effects of barbiturates and other CNS depressants. In patients who may use alcohol excessively, it should be borne in mind that the potentiation may increase the danger inherent in any suicide attempt or overdosage.

PRECAUTIONS

General: Schizophrenic patients may develop increased symptoms of psychosis; patients with paranoid symptomatology may have an exaggeration of such symptoms; manic depressive patients may experience a shift to the manic phase. In these circumstances, the dose of Endep may be reduced or a major tranquilizer such as perphenazine may be administered concurrently.
The possibility of suicide in depressed patients remains during treatment and until significant remission occurs. Potentially suicidal patients should not have access to large quantities of this drug. Prescriptions should be written for the smallest amount feasible.
Concurrent administration of Endep and electroshock therapy may increase the hazards associated with such therapy. Such treatment should be limited to patients for whom it is essential.
Amitriptyline HCl should be used with caution in patients with impaired liver function.
Both elevation and lowering of blood sugar levels have been reported.
The drug should be discontinued several days before elective surgery, if possible.
Information for Patients: Patients should be cautioned about engaging in hazardous occupations requiring complete mental alertness such as operating machinery or driving a motor vehicle after ingesting the drug.
Patients receiving amitriptyline HCl should also be cautioned about the possible combined effects with alcohol, barbiturates and other CNS depressants.
Drug Interactions: MAO inhibitors—see CONTRAINDICATIONS section. Thyroid medications; alcohol, barbiturates and other CNS depressants—see WARNINGS section.
Endep may block the antihypertensive action of guanethidine or similarly acting compounds.
When Endep is given with anticholinergic agents or sympathomimetic drugs, including epinephrine combined with local anesthetics, close supervision and careful adjustment of dosages are required.
Paralytic ileus may occur in patients taking tricyclic antidepressants in combination with anticholinergic-type drugs.
Caution is advised if patients receive large doses of ethchlorvynol concurrently. Transient delirium has been reported in patients who were treated with one gram of ethchlorvynol and 75 to 150 mg of amitriptyline HCl.
Carcinogenesis, Mutagenesis, Impairment of Fertility: Carcinogenesis: Amitriptyline HCl has not been adequately studied in animals to permit an evaluation of its carcinogenic potential. However, in a study during which relatively small numbers of rats received amitriptyline HCl as a dietary admixture at dosages up to 100 mg/kg/day for 78 weeks, no increase in the incidence of any tumor was reported.
Mutagenesis: Amitriptyline HCl was tested in a bacterial mutagenesis assay (Ames test) in the presence and absence of activating enzymes. No evidence for mutagenicity was found using *Salmonella* tester strains TA 1535, TA 100, TA 98 and TA 1537 at concentrations up to 5000 mcg/plate.
Impairment of Fertility: Amitriptyline HCl was studied in a Segment I fertility and general reproduction study in rats at dosages up to 20 mg/kg/day. There were no adverse effects on fertility, fetal growth and development, litter size, pup survival or pup growth. Similarly, no adverse effects were reported in a rat litter test in which amitriptyline HCl was administered at dosages up to 20 mg/kg/day.
Pregnancy: Teratogenic Effects: Pregnancy Category C. Animal reproduction studies have been inconclusive, and clinical experience has been limited. Amitriptyline HCl was tested in rats and in rabbits for teratogenic potential at dosages up to 20 mg/kg/day. Although stunting and increased neonatal mortality were observed in rabbits, there was no evidence for teratogenicity in either rats or rabbits. In a brief report, amitriptyline HCl was shown to be teratogenic in the hamster at dosages up to 100 mg/kg administered intraperitoneally on day 8 of gestation. In a more detailed study, amitriptyline HCl was shown to produce malformations in the rabbit at dosages of 15 to 60 mg/kg/day and in the mouse at dosages of 14 to 56 mg/kg/day. In another study, amitriptyline HCl was shown to be teratogenic in JBT/Jd and JBT/Ju strains of mice at dosages of 60 to 65 mg/kg, respectively; these dosages are near the litter LD_{50}. The dosages which were teratogenic in animals ranged from 10.5 to 70 times the maximum recommended adult maintenance dosage of 100 mg/day of Endep and from 3.5 to 23 times the maximum recommended initial dosage for hospitalized patients (300 mg/day).
There are no adequate or well-controlled studies of Endep in pregnant women. Endep should be used during pregnancy only if the potential benefit justifies the potential risk to the fetus.
Nonteratogenic Effects: Amitriptyline HCl was tested in rats in a Segment II study at dosages up to 20 mg/kg/day. No significant adverse effects were observed in the peri- or postnatal development and growth of pups.
Nursing Mothers: Amitriptyline and its metabolite, nortriptyline, are excreted in breast milk. Because of the potential for serious adverse reactions from Endep in nursing infants, a decision should be made whether to discontinue nursing or to discontinue the drug, taking into account the importance of the drug to the mother.
Pediatric Use: Safety and effectiveness in children below the age of 12 have not been established.

ADVERSE REACTIONS

Note: Included in this listing which follows are a few adverse reactions which have not been reported with this specific drug. However, pharmacological similarities among the tricyclic antidepressant drugs require that each of the reactions be considered when Endep is administered.
Cardiovascular: Hypotension, hypertension, tachycardia, palpitation, myocardial infarction, arrhythmias, heart block, stroke.
CNS and Neuromuscular: Confusional states; disturbed concentration; disorientation; delusions; hallucinations; excitement; anxiety; restlessness; insomnia; nightmares; numbness; tingling and paresthesias of the extremities; peripheral neuropathy; incoordination; ataxia; tremors; seizures; alteration in EEG patterns; extrapyramidal symptoms; tinnitus.
Anticholinergic: Dry mouth, blurred vision, disturbance of accommodation, constipation, paralytic ileus, urinary retention, dilatation of urinary tract.
Allergic: Skin rash, urticaria, photosensitization, edema of face and tongue.
Hematologic: Bone marrow depression including agranulocytosis, leukopenia, eosinophilia, purpura, thrombocytopenia.
Gastrointestinal: Nausea, epigastric distress, vomiting, anorexia, stomatitis, peculiar taste, diarrhea, parotid swelling, black tongue. Rarely, hepatitis (including altered liver function and jaundice).
Endocrine: Testicular swelling and gynecomastia in the male, breast enlargement and galactorrhea in the female, increased or decreased libido, elevation and lowering of blood sugar levels, syndrome of inappropriate ADH (antidiuretic hormone) secretion.
Other: Dizziness, weakness, fatigue, headache, weight gain or loss, increased perspiration, urinary frequency, mydriasis, drowsiness, alopecia.
Withdrawal Symptoms: Abrupt cessation of treatment after prolonged administration may produce nausea, headache and malaise. These are not indicative of addiction.

OVERDOSAGE

Manifestations: High doses may cause temporary confusion, disturbed concentration or transient visual hallucinations. Overdosage may cause drowsiness; hypothermia; tachycardia and other arrhythmic abnormalities, such as bundle branch block; ECG evidence of impaired conduction; congestive heart failure; dilated pupils; convulsions; severe hypotension; stupor and coma. Other symptoms may be agitation, hyperactive reflexes, muscle rigidity, vomiting, hyperpyrexia or any of those listed in the ADVERSE REACTIONS section.
Treatment: **All patients suspected of having taken an overdosage should be admitted to a hospital as soon as possible.** Treatment is symptomatic and supportive. Empty the stomach as quickly as possible by emesis followed by gastric lavage upon arrival at the hospital. Following gastric lavage, activated charcoal may be administered. Twenty to 30 Gm of activated charcoal may be given every four to six hours during the first 24 to 48 hours after ingestion. An ECG should be taken and close monitoring of cardiac function instituted if there is any sign of abnormality. Maintain an open airway and adequate fluid intake; regulate body temperature.
The intravenous administration of 1 to 3 mg of physostigmine salicylate has been reported to reverse the symptoms of tricyclic antidepressant poisoning. Because physostigmine is rapidly metabolized, the dosage of physostigmine should be repeated as required, particularly if life-threatening signs such as arrhythmias, convulsions and deep coma recur or persist after the initial dosage of physostigmine. Because physostigmine itself may be toxic, it is not recommended for routine use.
Standard measures should be used to manage circulatory shock and metabolic acidosis. Cardiac arrhythmias may be treated with neostigmine, pyridostigmine or propranolol. Should cardiac failure occur, the use of digitalis should be considered. Close monitoring of cardiac function for not less than five days is advisable. Anticonvulsants may be given to control convulsions. Amitriptyline increases the CNS depressant action but not the anticonvulsant action of barbiturates; therefore, an inhalation anesthetic, diazepam or paraldehyde is recommended for control of convulsions.
Dialysis is of no value because of low plasma concentrations of the drug.
Since overdosage is often deliberate, patients may attempt suicide by other means during the recovery phase.
Deaths by deliberate or accidental overdosage have occurred with this class of drugs.
The acute oral toxicity of amitriptyline HCl is as follows:

Species	$LD_{50} \pm$ S.E. (mg/kg)
Mouse	260 ± 16
Rat	617 ± 50
Rabbit	446 ± 32
Dog	≈ 290

DOSAGE AND ADMINISTRATION

Oral Dosage: Dosage should be initiated at a low level and increased gradually, noting carefully the clinical response and any evidence of intolerance.
Initial Dosage for Adults: Twenty-five mg 3 times a day usually is satisfactory for outpatients. If necessary, this may be increased to a total of 150 mg a day. Increases are made preferably in the late afternoon and/or bedtime doses. A sedative effect may be apparent before the antidepressant effect is noted, but an adequate therapeutic effect may take as long as 30 days to develop.
An alternative method of initiating therapy in outpatients is to begin with 50 to 100 mg amitriptyline HCl at bedtime. This may be increased by 25 to 50 mg as necessary in the bedtime dose to a total of 150 mg per day.
Hospitalized patients may require 100 mg a day initially. This can be increased gradually to 200 mg a day if necessary. A small number of hospitalized patients may need as much as 300 mg a day.
Adolescent and Elderly Patients: In general, lower dosages are recommended for these patients. Ten mg 3 times a day with 20 mg at bedtime may be satisfactory in adolescent and elderly patients who do not tolerate higher dosages.
Maintenance: The usual maintenance dosage of amitriptyline HCl is 50 to 100 mg per day. In some patients 40 mg per day is sufficient. For maintenance therapy the total daily dosage may be given in a single dose preferably at bedtime. When satisfactory improvement has been reached, dosage should be reduced to the lowest amount that will maintain relief of symptoms. It is appropriate to continue maintenance therapy 3 months or longer to lessen the possibility of relapse.
Usage in Children: In view of the lack of experience in children, this drug is not recommended at the present time for patients under 12 years of age.

HOW SUPPLIED

10-mg tablets, orange, round, film-coated, scored—bottles of 100 (NDC 0140-0106-01); Tel-E-Dose® packages of 100 (NDC 0140-0106-49). Imprint on tablets: ENDEP 10 ROCHE.
25-mg tablets, orange, round, film-coated, scored—bottles of 100 (NDC 0140-0107-01) and 500 (NDC 0140-0107-14); Tel-E-Dose® packages of 100 (NDC 0140-0107-49). Imprint on tablets: ENDEP 25 ROCHE.
50-mg tablets, orange, round, film-coated, scored—bottles of 100 (NDC 0140-0109-01) and 500 (NDC 0140-0109-14); Tel-E-Dose® packages of 100 (NDC 0140-0109-49). Imprint on tablets: ENDEP 50 ROCHE.
75-mg tablets, yellow, round, film-coated, scored—bottles of 100 (NDC 0140-0114-01); Tel-E-Dose® packages of 100 (NDC 0140-0114-49). Imprint on tablets: ENDEP 75 ROCHE.
100-mg tablets, peach, round, film-coated, scored—bottles of 100 (NDC 0140-0116-01); Tel-E-Dose® packages of 100 (NDC 0140-0116-49). Imprint on tablets: ENDEP 100 ROCHE.
150-mg tablets, salmon, round, film-coated, scored—bottles of 100 (NDC 0140-0124-01). Imprint on tablets: ENDEP 150 ROCHE.

Shown in Product Identification Section, page 424

LIBRAX® ℞

[lib ′rax]

The following text is complete prescribing information based on official labeling in effect June 1, 1986.

COMPOSITION

Each capsule contains 5 mg chlordiazepoxide hydrochloride (Librium®) and 2.5 mg clidinium bromide (Quarzan®).

DESCRIPTION

Librax combines in a single capsule formulation the antianxiety action of Librium (chlordiazepoxide hydrochloride/Roche) and the anticholinergic/spasmolytic effects of Quar-

Continued on next page

Roche Products—Cont.

zan (clidinium bromide/Roche), both exclusive developments of Roche research.

Each Librax capsule contains 5 mg chlordiazepoxide hydrochloride and 2.5 clidinium bromide. Each capsule also contains corn starch, lactose and talc. Gelatin capsule shells may contain methyl and propyl parabens and potassium sorbate, with the following dye systems: D&C Yellow No. 10 and either FD&C Blue No. 1 or FD&C Green No. 3.

Librium (chlordiazepoxide hydrochloride/Roche) is a versatile therapeutic agent of proven value for the relief of anxiety and tension. It is indicated when anxiety, tension or apprehension are significant components of the clinical profile. It is among the safer of the effective psychopharmacologic compounds.

Chlordiazepoxide hydrochloride is 7-chloro-2-methylamino-5-phenyl-3H-1, 4-benzodiazepine 4-oxide hydrochloride. A colorless, crystalline substance, it is soluble in water. It is unstable in solution and the powder must be protected from light. The molecular weight is 336.22.

Quarzan (clidinium bromide/Roche) is a synthetic anticholinergic agent which has been shown in experimental and clinical studies to have a pronounced antispasmodic and antisecretory effect on the gastrointestinal tract.

ANIMAL PHARMACOLOGY

Chlordiazepoxide hydrochloride has been studied extensively in many species of animals and these studies are suggestive of action on the limbic system of the brain,[1,2,3] which recent evidence indicates is involved in emotional responses.[4,5]

Hostile monkeys were made tame by oral drug doses which did not cause sedation. Chlordiazepoxide hydrochloride revealed a "taming" action with the elimination of fear and aggression.[6] The taming effect of chlordiazepoxide hydrochloride was further demonstrated in rats made vicious by lesions in the septal area of the brain. The drug dosage which effectively blocked the vicious reaction was well below the dose which caused sedation in these animals.[6]

The oral LD_{50} of single doses of chlordiazepoxide hydrochloride, calculated according to the method of Miller and Tainter,[7] is 720 $\pm$ 51 mg/kg as determined in mice observed over a period of five days following dosage.

Clidinium bromide is an effective anticholinergic agent with activity approximating that of atropine sulfate against acetylcholine-induced spasms in isolated intestinal strips. On oral administration in mice it proved an effective antisialagogue in preventing pilocarpine-induced salivation. Spontaneous intestinal motility in both rats and dogs is reduced following oral dosing with 0.1 to 0.25 mg/kg. Potent cholinergic ganglionic blocking effects (vagal) are produced with intravenous usage in anesthetized dogs.

Oral doses of 2.5 mg/kg to dogs produced signs of nasal dryness and slight pupillary dilation. In two other species, monkeys and rabbits, doses of 5 mg/kg, p.o., given three times daily for 5 days did not produce apparent secretory or visual changes.

The oral LD_{50} of single doses of clidinium bromide is 860$\pm$57 mg/kg as determined in mice observed over a period of 5 days following dosage; the calculations were made according to the method of Miller and Tainter.[7]

Effects on Reproduction: Reproduction studies in rats fed chlordiazepoxide hydrochloride, 10, 20 and 80 mg/kg daily, and bred through one or two matings showed no congenital anomalies, nor were there adverse effects on lactation of the dams or growth of the newborn. However, in another study at 100 mg/kg daily there was noted a significant decrease in the fertilization rate and a marked decrease in the viability and body weight of offspring which may be attributable to sedative activity, thus resulting in lack of interest in mating and lessened maternal nursing and care of the young.[8,9] One neonate in each of the first and second matings in the rat reproduction study at the 100 mg/kg dose exhibited major skeletal defects. Further studies are in progress to determine the significance of these findings.

Two series of reproduction experiments with clidinium bromide were carried out in rats, employing dosages of 2.5 and 10 mg/kg daily in each experiment. In the first experiment clidinium bromide was administered for a 9-week interval prior to mating; no untoward effect on fertilization or gestation was noted. The offspring were taken by caesarean section and did not show a significant incidence of congenital anomalies when compared to control animals. In the second experiment adult animals were given clidinium bromide for ten days prior to and through two mating cycles. No significant effects were observed on fertility, gestation, viability of offspring or lactation, as compared to control animals, nor was there a significant incidence of congenital anomalies in the offspring derived from these experiments.

A reproduction study of Librax was carried out in rats through two successive matings. Oral daily doses were administered in two concentrations: 2.5 mg/kg chlordiazepoxide hydrochloride with 1.25 mg/kg clidinium bromide, or 25 mg/kg chlordiazepoxide hydrochloride with 12.5 mg/kg clidinium bromide. In the first mating no significant differences were noted between the control or the treated groups, with the exception of a slight decrease in the number of animals surviving during lactation among those receiving the highest dosage. As with all anticholinergic drugs, an inhibiting effect on lactation may occur. In the second mating similar results were obtained except for a slight decrease in the number of pregnant females and in the percentage of offspring surviving until weaning. No congenital anomalies were observed in both matings in either the control or treated groups. Additional animal reproduction studies are in progress.

INDICATIONS

Based on a review of this drug by the National Academy of Sciences—National Research Council and/or other information, FDA has classified the indications as follows:

"Possibly" effective: as adjunctive therapy in the treatment of peptic ulcer and in the treatment of the irritable bowel syndrome (irritable colon, spastic colon, mucous colitis) and acute enterocolitis.

Final classification of the less-than-effective indications requires further investigation.

CONTRAINDICATIONS

Librax is contraindicated in the presence of glaucoma (since the anticholinergic component may produce some degree of mydriasis) and in patients with prostatic hypertrophy and benign bladder neck obstruction. It is contraindicated in patients with known hypersensitivity to chlordiazepoxide hydrochloride and/or clidinium bromide.

WARNINGS

As in the case of other preparations containing CNS-acting drugs, patients receiving Librax should be cautioned about possible combined effects with alcohol and other CNS depressants. For the same reason, they should be cautioned against hazardous occupations requiring complete mental alertness such as operating machinery or driving a motor vehicle.

Physical and Psychological Dependence: Physical and psychological dependence have rarely been reported in persons taking recommended doses of Librium (chlordiazepoxide hydrochloride/Roche). However, caution must be exercised in administering Librium to individuals known to be addiction-prone or those whose history suggests they may increase the dosage on their own initiative. Withdrawal symptoms following discontinuation of chlordiazepoxide hydrochloride have been reported.[10] These symptoms (including convulsions) are similar to those seen with barbiturates.

***Usage in Pregnancy:* An increased risk of congenital malformations associated with the use of minor tranquilizers (chlordiazepoxide, diazepam and meprobamate) during the first trimester of pregnancy has been suggested in several studies. Because use of these drugs is rarely a matter of urgency, their use during this period should almost always be avoided. The possibility that a woman of childbearing potential may be pregnant at the time of institution of therapy should be considered. Patients should be advised that if they become pregnant during therapy or intend to become pregnant they should communicate with their physicians about the desirability of discontinuing the drug.**

As with all anticholinergic drugs, an inhibiting effect on lactation may occur. (See Animal Pharmacology.)

Management of Overdosage: Manifestations of Librium (chlordiazepoxide hydrochloride/Roche) overdosage include somnolence, confusion, coma and diminished reflexes. Respiration, pulse and blood pressure should be monitored, as in all cases of drug overdosage, although, in general, these effects have been minimal following Librium overdosage.

While the signs and symptoms of Librax overdosage may be produced by either of its components, usually such symptoms will be overshadowed by the anticholinergic actions of Quarzan (clidinium bromide/Roche). The symptoms of overdosage of Quarzan are excessive dryness of mouth, blurring of vision, urinary hesitancy and constipation.

General supportive measures should be employed, along with immediate gastric lavage. Administer physostigmine (Antilirium) 0.5 to 2 mg at a rate of no more than 1 mg per minute. This may be repeated in 1 to 4 mg doses if arrhythmias, convulsions or deep coma recur. Intravenous fluids should be administered and an adequate airway maintained. Hypotension may be combated by the use of Levophed® (levarterenol) or Aramine (metaraminol). Ritalin (methylphenidate) or caffeine and sodium benzoate may be given to combat CNS-depressive effects. Dialysis is of limited value. Should excitation occur, barbiturates should not be used. As with the management of intentional overdosage with any drug, it should be borne in mind that multiple agents may have been ingested.

PRECAUTIONS

In elderly and debilitated patients, it is recommended that the dosage be limited to the smallest effective amount to preclude the development of ataxia, oversedation, or confusion (not more than two Librax capsules per day initially, to be increased gradually as needed and tolerated). In general, the concomitant administration of Librax and other psychotropic agents is not recommended. If such combination therapy seems indicated, careful consideration should be given to the pharmacology of the agents to be employed—particularly when the known potentiating compounds such as the MAO inhibitors and phenothiazines are to be used. The usual precautions in treating patients with impaired renal or hepatic function should be observed.

Paradoxical reactions to chlordiazepoxide hydrochloride, *e.g.,* excitement, stimulation and acute rage, have been reported in psychiatric patients and should be watched for during Librax therapy. The usual precautions are indicated when chlordiazepoxide hydrochloride is used in the treatment of anxiety states where there is any evidence of impending depression; it should be borne in mind that suicidal tendencies may be present and protective measures may be necessary. Although clinical studies have not established a cause and effect relationship, physicians should be aware that variable effects on blood coagulation have been reported very rarely in patients receiving oral anticoagulants and Librium (chlordiazepoxide hydrochloride).

ADVERSE REACTIONS

[11] No side effects or manifestations not seen with either compound alone have been reported with the administration of Librax. However, since Librax contains chlordiazepoxide hydrochloride and clidinium bromide, the possibility of untoward effects which may be seen with either of these two compounds cannot be excluded.

When chlordiazepoxide hydrochloride has been used alone the necessity of discontinuing therapy because of undesirable effects has been rare.[12] Drowsiness,[13] ataxia[14] and confusion[9] have been reported in some patients—particularly the elderly and debilitated.[9] While these effects can be avoided in almost all instances by proper dosage adjustment, they have occasionally been observed at the lower dosage ranges. In a few instances syncope has been reported.[15]

Other adverse reactions reported during therapy with Librium (chlordiazepoxide hydrochloride/Roche) include isolated instances of skin eruptions,[13] edema,[16] minor menstrual irregularities,[13] nausea and constipation,[17] extrapyramidal symptoms,[9] as well as increased and decreased libido. Such side effects have been infrequent and are generally controlled with reduction of dosage. Changes in EEG patterns (low-voltage fast activity) have been observed in patients during and after Librium treatment.[18]

Blood dyscrasias,[11] including agranulocytosis,[19] jaundice and hepatic dysfunction[20] have occasionally been reported during therapy with Librium. When Librium treatment is protracted, periodic blood counts and liver function tests are advisable.

Adverse effects reported with use of *Librax* are those typical of anticholinergic agents, *i.e.,* dryness of the mouth, blurring of vision, urinary hesitancy and constipation. Constipation has occurred most often when Librax therapy has been combined with other spasmolytic agents and/or a low residue diet.

DOSAGE

Because of the varied individual responses to tranquilizers and anticholinergics, the optimum dosage of Librax varies with the diagnosis and response of the individual patient. The dosage, therefore, should be individualized for maximum beneficial effects. The usual maintenance dose is 1 or 2 capsules, 3 or 4 times a day administered before meals and at bedtime.

HOW SUPPLIED

Librax is available in green capsules, each containing 5 mg chlordiazepoxide hydrochloride (Librium®) and 2.5 mg clidinium bromide (Quarzan®)—bottles of 100 (NDC 0140-0007-01) and 500 (NDC 0140-0007-14); Tel-E-Dose® packages of 100 (NDC 0140-0007-49).

REFERENCES

1. Schallek, W., *et al:* Arch. Int. Pharmacodyn. *149*:467-483, 1964.
2. Himwich, H. E., *et al:* J. Neuropsych. *3* (Suppl. 1):S15-S26, August 1962.
3. Morillo, A., *et al:* Psychopharmacologia *3* (No. 5):386-394, 1962.
4. MacLean, P. D.: Psychosomatic Med. *17:* 355-366, September 1955.
5. Morgan, C. T.: Physiological Psychology, 3rd Ed.; New York, McGraw-Hill, 1965.
6. Randall, L. O. *et al:* J. Pharm. Exper. Therap. *129*:163-171, June 1960.
7. Miller, L. C. and Tainter, M. C.: Proc. Soc. Exp. Biol. & Med. 57:261, 1944.
8. Zbinden, G., *et al:* Toxicology and Applied Pharmacology *3*:619-637, November 1961.
9. Data on file, Hoffmann-La Roche Inc., Nutley, New Jersey.

10. Hollister, L. E., *et al:* Psychopharmacologia *2*:63-68, 1961.
11. Bibliography and References available on request from Roche Laboratories.
12. Rickels, K. *et al:* Med. Times *93*:238-245, March 1965.
13. Tobin, J. M. *et al:* J. Amer. Med. Assoc. *174:* 1242-1249, November 1960.
14. Jenner, F. A., *et al:* J. Ment. Sci. *107*:575-582, May 1961.
15. Robinson, R. C. V.: Dis. Nerv. System *21*:43-45, March 1960.
16. Rose, J. T.: Amer. J. Psychiat. *120*:899-900, March 1964.
17. Hines, L. R.: Curr. Therap. Res. *2*:227-236, June 1960.
18. Gibbs, F. A. and Gibbs, E. L.: J. Neuropsych., 3 (Suppl. 1):S73-S78, August 1962.
19. Kaelbling, R., *et al:* J. Amer. Med. Assoc. *174*:1863-1865, December 1960.
20. Cacioppo, J., *et al:* Amer. J. Psychiat. *117*:1040-1041, May 1961.

Shown in Product Identification Section, page 425

LIBRIUM® CAPSULES Ⓒ
[*lib'ree-um*]
(chlordiazepoxide HCl/Roche)
LIBRITABS® Ⓒ
[*lib'rit-abs*]
(chlordiazepoxide/Roche)

The following text is complete prescribing information based on official labeling in effect June 1, 1986.

DESCRIPTION

Librium (the original chlordiazepoxide HCl) and Libritabs (the original chlordiazepoxide), prototypes for the benzodiazepine compounds, were synthesized and developed at Hoffmann-La Roche Inc. They are versatile therapeutic agents of proven value for the relief of anxiety, and are among the safer of the effective psychopharmacologic compounds available, as demonstrated by extensive clinical evidence.

Librium is available as capsules containing 5 mg, 10 mg or 25 mg chlordiazepoxide HCl. Each capsule also contains corn starch, lactose and talc. Gelatin capsule shells may contain methyl and propyl parabens and potassium sorbate, with the following dye systems: 5-mg capsules—FD&C Yellow No. 6 plus D&C Yellow No. 10 and either FD&C Blue No. 1 or FD&C Green No. 3. 10-mg capsules—FD&C Yellow No. 6 plus D&C Yellow No. 10 and either FD&C Blue No. 1 plus FD&C Red No. 3 or FD&C Green No. 3 plus FD&C Red No. 40. 25-mg capsules—D&C Yellow No. 10 and either FD&C Green No. 3 or FD&C Blue No. 1.

Chlordiazepoxide hydrochloride is 7-chloro-2-(methylamino)-5-phenyl-3H-1,4-benzodiazepine 4-oxide hydrochloride. A white to practically white crystalline substance, it is soluble in water. It is unstable in solution and the powder must be protected from light. The molecular weight is 336.22.

Libritabs is available as tablets containing 5 mg, 10 mg or 25 mg chlordiazepoxide. Each tablet also contains corn starch, ethylcellulose, hydroxypropyl methylcellulose, lactose, magnesium stearate, microcrystalline cellulose and triacetin; with FD&C Blue No. 1, D&C Yellow No. 10 and FD&C Yellow No. 6 dyes.

Chlordiazepoxide is 7-chloro-2-(methylamino)-5-phenyl-3H-1,4-benzodiazepine 4-oxide. A yellow crystalline substance, it is insoluble in water. The powder must be protected from light. The molecular weight is 299.76.

ACTIONS

Librium (chlordiazepoxide HCl/Roche) and Libritabs (chlordiazepoxide/Roche) have antianxiety, sedative, appetite-stimulating and weak analgesic actions. The precise mechanism of action is not known. The drugs block EEG arousal from stimulation of the brain stem reticular formation. It takes several hours for peak blood levels to be reached and the half-life of the drugs is between 24 and 48 hours. After Librium or Libritabs is discontinued plasma levels decline slowly over a period of several days. Chlordiazepoxide is excreted in the urine, with 1 to 2% unchanged and 3 to 6% as a conjugate.

INDICATIONS

Librium and Libritabs are indicated for the management of anxiety disorders or for the short-term relief of symptoms of anxiety, withdrawal symptoms of acute alcoholism, and preoperative apprehension and anxiety. Anxiety or tension associated with the stress of everyday life usually does not require treatment with an anxiolytic.

The effectiveness of Librium or Libritabs in long-term use, that is, more than 4 months, has not been assessed by systematic clinical studies. The physician should periodically reassess the usefulness of the drug for the individual patient.

CONTRAINDICATIONS

Librium and Libritabs are contraindicated in patients with known hypersensitivity to the drug.

WARNINGS

Chlordiazepoxide HCl and chlordiazepoxide may impair the mental and/or physical abilities required for the performance of potentially hazardous tasks such as driving a vehicle or operating machinery. Similarly, they may impair mental alertness in children. The concomitant use of alcohol or other central nervous system depressants may have an additive effect. PATIENTS SHOULD BE WARNED ACCORDINGLY.

Physical and Psychological Dependence: Physical and psychological dependence have rarely been reported in persons taking recommended doses of chlordiazepoxide HCl or chlordiazepoxide. However, caution must be exercised in administering chlordiazepoxide HCl or chlordiazepoxide to individuals known to be addiction-prone or those whose histories suggest they may increase the dosage on their own initiative. Withdrawal symptoms following abrupt discontinuation of chlordiazepoxide HCl or chlordiazepoxide have been reported in patients receiving excessive doses over extended periods of time. These symptoms (including convulsions) are similar to those seen with barbiturates. Although infrequently seen, milder withdrawal symptoms have also been reported following abrupt discontinuance of benzodiazepines taken continuously, generally at higher therapeutic levels, for at least several months. Consequently, after extended therapy, abrupt discontinuation should generally be avoided and a gradual tapering in dosage followed.

Usage in Pregnancy: An increased risk of congenital malformations associated with the use of minor tranquilizers (chlordiazepoxide, diazepam and meprobamate) during the first trimester of pregnancy has been suggested in several studies. Because use of these drugs is rarely a matter of urgency, their use during this period should almost always be avoided. The possibility that a woman of childbearing potential may be pregnant at the time of institution of therapy should be considered. Patients should be advised that if they become pregnant during therapy or intend to become pregnant they should communicate with their physicians about the desirability of discontinuing the drug.

PRECAUTIONS

In elderly and debilitated patients, it is recommended that the dosage be limited to the smallest effective amount to preclude the development of ataxia or oversedation (10 mg or less per day initially, to be increased gradually as needed and tolerated). In general, the concomitant administration of Librium or Libritabs and other psychotropic agents is not recommended. If such combination therapy seems indicated, careful consideration should be given to the pharmacology of the agents to be employed — particularly when the known potentiating compounds such as the MAO inhibitors and phenothiazines are to be used. The usual precautions in treating patients with impaired renal or hepatic function should be observed.

Paradoxical reactions, *e.g.,* excitement, stimulation and acute rage, have been reported in psychiatric patients and in hyperactive aggressive children, and should be watched for during Librium or Libritabs therapy. The usual precautions are indicated when Librium or Libritabs is used in the treatment of anxiety states where there is any evidence of impending depression; it should be borne in mind that suicidal tendencies may be present and protective measures may be necessary. Although clinical studies have not established a cause and effect relationship, physicians should be aware that variable effects on blood coagulation have been reported very rarely in patients receiving oral anticoagulants and Librium or Libritabs. In view of isolated reports associating chlordiazepoxide HCl and chlordiazepoxide with exacerbation of porphyria, caution should be exercised in prescribing these agents to patients suffering from this disease.

ADVERSE REACTIONS

The necessity of discontinuing therapy because of undesirable effects has been rare. Drowsiness, ataxia and confusion have been reported in some patients — particularly the elderly and debilitated. While these effects can be avoided in almost all instances by proper dosage adjustment, they have occasionally been observed at the lower dosage ranges. In a few instances syncope has been reported.

Other adverse reactions reported during therapy include isolated instances of skin eruptions, edema, minor menstrual irregularities, nausea and constipation, extrapyramidal symptoms, as well as increased and decreased libido. Such side effects have been infrequent and are generally controlled with reduction of dosage. Changes in EEG patterns (low-voltage fast activity) have been observed in patients during and after Librium or Libritabs treatment.

Blood dyscrasias (including agranulocytosis), jaundice and hepatic dysfunction have occasionally been reported during therapy. When Librium or Libritabs treatment is protracted, periodic blood counts and liver function tests are advisable.

OVERDOSAGE

Manifestations of Librium or Libritabs overdosage include somnolence, confusion, coma and diminished reflexes. Respiration, pulse and blood pressure should be monitored, as in all cases of drug overdosage, although, in general, these effects have been minimal following Librium or Libritabs overdosage. General supportive measures should be employed, along with immediate gastric lavage. Intravenous fluids should be administered and an adequate airway maintained. Hypotension may be combated by the use of Levophed® (norepinephrine) or Aramine (metaraminol). Dialysis is of limited value. There have been occasional reports of excitation in patients following chlordiazepoxide HCl or chlordiazepoxide overdosage; if this occurs barbiturates should not be used. As with the management of intentional overdosage with any drug, it should be borne in mind that multiple agents may have been ingested.

DOSAGE AND ADMINISTRATION

Because of the wide range of clinical indications for Librium and Libritabs, the optimum dosage varies with the diagnosis and response of the individual patient. The dosage, therefore, should be individualized for maximum beneficial effects.

ADULTS	Usual Daily Dose
Relief of mild and moderate anxiety disorders and symptoms of anxiety	5 mg or 10 mg, 3 or 4 times daily
Relief of severe anxiety disorders and symptoms of anxiety	20 mg or 25 mg, 3 or 4 times daily
Geriatric patients, or in the presence of debilitating disease	5 mg, 2 to 4 times daily

Preoperative apprehension and anxiety:
On days preceding surgery, 5 to 10 mg orally, 3 or 4 times daily. If used as preoperative medication, 50 to 100 mg I.M.* one hour prior to surgery.

CHILDREN	Usual Daily Dose
Because of the varied response of children to CNS-acting drugs, therapy should be initiated with the lowest dose and increased as required. Since clinical experience in children under 6 years of age is limited, the use of the drug in this age group is not recommended.	5 mg, 2 to 4 times daily (may be increased in some children to 10 mg, 2 or 3 times daily)

For the relief of withdrawal symptoms of acute alcoholism, the parenteral form* is usually used initially. If the drug is administered orally, the suggested initial dose is 50 to 100 mg, to be followed by repeated doses as needed until agitation is controlled — up to 300 mg per day. Dosage should then be reduced to maintenance levels.

* See package insert for injectable Librium (chlordiazepoxide HCl/Roche).

HOW SUPPLIED

Librium (chlordiazepoxide HCl/Roche) capsules — 5 mg, green and yellow; 10 mg, green and black; 25 mg, green and white — bottles of 100 and 500; Tel-E-Dose® packages of 100, available in trays of 4 reverse-numbered cards of 25, and in boxes containing 10 strips of 10.

Libritabs (chlordiazepoxide/Roche) tablets — 5 mg or 10 mg— bottles of 100 and 500; 25 mg—bottles of 100.

Shown in Product Identification Section, page 425

LIBRIUM® INJECTABLE Ⓒ
[*lib'ree-um*]
(chlordiazepoxide HCl/Roche)

Librium Injectable is manufactured by Hoffmann-La Roche Inc., Nutley, N.J. 07110 and distributed by Roche Products Inc., Manati, P.R. 00701.

The following text is complete prescribing information based on official labeling in effect June 1, 1986.

DESCRIPTION

Librium is a versatile therapeutic agent of proven value for the relief of anxiety and tension.

Librium is the first of a new class, unrelated chemically and pharmacologically to other types of tranquilizers. Librium promptly relieves anxiety and is among the safer of the effective psychopharmacologic compounds available.

Chlordiazepoxide HCl is 7-chloro-2-methylamino-5-phenyl-3H-1,4-benzodiazepine 4-oxide hydrochloride. A colorless, crystalline substance, it is soluble in water. It is unstable in solution and the powder must be protected from light. The molecular weight is 336.22.

Continued on next page

Roche Products—Cont.

ANIMAL PHARMACOLOGY

The drug has been studied extensively in many species of animals and these studies are suggestive of action on the limbic system of the brain, which recent evidence indicates is involved in emotional responses.

Hostile monkeys were made tame by oral drug doses which did not cause sedation. Librium revealed a "taming" action with the elimination of fear and aggression. The taming effect of Librium was further demonstrated in rats made vicious by lesions in the septal area of the brain. The drug dosage which effectively blocked the vicious reaction was well below the dose which caused sedation in these animals.

The LD_{50} of parenterally administered chlordiazepoxide HCl was determined in mice (72 hours) and rats (5 days), and calculated according to the method of Miller and Tainter, with the following results: mice, I.V., 123 ± 12 mg/kg; mice, I.M., 366 ± 7 mg/kg; rats, I.V., 120 ± 7 mg/kg; rats, I.M., > 160 mg/kg.

Effects on Reproduction: Reproduction studies in rats fed 10, 20 and 80 mg/kg daily and bred through one or two matings showed no congenital anomalies, nor were there adverse effects on lactation of the dams or growth of the newborn. However, in another study at 100 mg/kg daily there was noted a significant decrease in the fertilization rate and a marked decrease in the viability and body weight of offspring which may be attributable to sedative activity, thus resulting in lack of interest in mating and lessened maternal nursing and care of the young. One neonate in each of the first and second matings in the rat reproduction study at the 100 mg/kg dose exhibited major skeletal defects. Further studies are in progress to determine the significance of these findings.

INDICATIONS

Injectable Librium is indicated for the management of anxiety disorders or for the short-term relief of symptoms of anxiety, withdrawal symptoms of acute alcoholism, and preoperative apprehension and anxiety. Anxiety or tension associated with the stress of everyday life usually does not require treatment with an anxiolytic.

CONTRAINDICATIONS

Librium is contraindicated in patients with known hypersensitivity to the drug.

WARNINGS

As in the case of other CNS-acting drugs, patients receiving Librium should be cautioned about possible combined effects with alcohol and other CNS depressants.

As is true of all preparations containing CNS-acting drugs, patients receiving Librium should be cautioned against hazardous occupations requiring complete mental alertness such as operating machinery or driving a motor vehicle.

Physical and Psychological Dependence: Physical and psychological dependence have rarely been reported in persons taking recommended doses of Librium. However, caution must be exercised in administering Librium to individuals known to be addiction-prone or those whose history suggests they may increase the dosage on their own initiative. Withdrawal symptoms following abrupt discontinuation of chlordiazepoxide HCl have been reported in patients receiving excessive doses over extended periods of time. These symptoms (including convulsions) are similar to those seen with barbiturates. Although infrequently seen, milder withdrawal symptoms have also been reported following abrupt discontinuance of benzodiazepines taken continuously, generally at higher therapeutic levels, for at least several months. Consequently, after extended therapy, abrupt discontinuation should generally be avoided and a gradual tapering in dosage followed.

***Usage in Pregnancy:* An increased risk of congenital malformations associated with the use of minor tranquilizers (chlordiazepoxide, diazepam and meprobamate) during the first trimester of pregnancy has been suggested in several studies. Because use of these drugs is rarely a matter of urgency, their use during this period should almost always be avoided. The possibility that a woman of childbearing potential may be pregnant at the time of institution of therapy should be considered. Patients should be advised that if they become pregnant during therapy or intend to become pregnant they should communicate with their physicians about the desirability of discontinuing the drug.**

Management of Overdosage: Manifestations of Librium overdosage include somnolence, confusion, coma and diminished reflexes. Respiration, pulse and blood pressure should be monitored, as in all cases of drug overdosage, although, in general, these effects have been minimal following Librium overdosage. General supportive measures should be employed, along with immediate gastric lavage. Intravenous fluids should be administered and an adequate airway maintained. Hypotension may be combated by the use of Levophed® (levarterenol) or Aramine (metaraminol). Dialysis is of limited value. There have been occasional reports of excitation in patients following Librium overdosage; if this occurs barbiturates should not be used. As with the management of intentional overdosage with any drug, it should be borne in mind that multiple agents may have been ingested.

PRECAUTIONS

Injectable Librium (intramuscular or intravenous) is indicated primarily in acute states, and patients receiving this form of therapy should be kept under observation, preferably in bed, for a period of up to three hours. Ambulatory patients should not be permitted to operate a vehicle following an injection. Injectable Librium should not be given to patients in shock or comatose states. Reduced dosage (usually 25 to 50 mg) should be used for elderly or debilitated patients, and for children age twelve or older. In general, the concomitant administration of Librium and other psychotropic agents is not recommended. If such combination therapy seems indicated, careful consideration should be given to the pharmacology of the agents to be employed—particularly when the known potentiating compounds such as the MAO inhibitors and phenothiazines are to be used. The usual precautions in treating patients with impaired renal or hepatic function should be observed.

Paradoxical reactions, *e.g.,* excitement, stimulation and acute rage, have been reported in psychiatric patients and in hyperactive aggressive children, and should be watched for during Librium therapy. The usual precautions are indicated when Librium is used in the treatment of anxiety states where there is any evidence of impending depression; it should be borne in mind that suicidal tendencies may be present and protective measures may be necessary. Although clinical studies have not established a cause and effect relationship, physicians should be aware that variable effects on blood coagulation have been reported very rarely in patients receiving oral anticoagulants and Librium. In view of isolated reports associating chlordiazepoxide with exacerbation of porphyria, caution should be exercised in prescribing chlordiazepoxide to patients suffering from this disease.

ADVERSE REACTIONS

The necessity of discontinuing therapy because of undesirable effects has been rare. Drowsiness, ataxia and confusion are more commonly seen in the elderly and debilitated.

Other adverse reactions reported during therapy include isolated instances of syncope, hypotension, tachycardia, skin eruptions, edema, minor menstrual irregularities, nausea and constipation, extrapyramidal symptoms, blurred vision, as well as increased and decreased libido. Such side effects have been infrequent and are generally controlled with reduction of dosage. Similarly, hypotension associated with spinal anesthesia has occurred. Pain following intramuscular injection has been reported. Changes in EEG patterns (low-voltage fast activity) have been observed in patients during and after Librium treatment.

Blood dyscrasias (including agranulocytosis), jaundice and hepatic dysfunction, have occasionally been reported during therapy. When Librium treatment is protracted, periodic blood counts and liver function tests are advisable.

PREPARATION AND ADMINISTRATION OF SOLUTIONS

Solutions of Librium for intramuscular or intravenous use should be prepared aseptically. Sterilization by heating should not be attempted.

Intramuscular: Add 2 ml of *Special Intramuscular Diluent* to contents of 5-ml dry-filled amber ampul of Librium Sterile Powder (100 mg). Avoid excessive pressure in injecting this special diluent into the ampul containing the powder since bubbles will form on the surface of the solution. Agitate gently until completely dissolved. Solution should be prepared immediately before administration. Any unused solution should be discarded. Deep intramuscular injection should be given *slowly* into the upper outer quadrant of the gluteus muscle.

Caution: Librium solution made with the Special Intramuscular Diluent should not be given intravenously because of the air bubbles which form when the intramuscular diluent is added to the Librium powder. Do not use diluent solution if it is opalescent or hazy.

Intravenous: In most cases, intramuscular injection is the preferred route of administration of Injectable Librium since beneficial effects are usually seen within 15 to 30 minutes. When, in the judgment of the physician, even more rapid action is mandatory, Injectable Librium may be administered intravenously. A suitable solution for intravenous administration may be prepared as follows: Add 5 ml of *sterile physiological saline* or *sterile water for injection* to contents of 5-ml dry-filled amber ampul of Librium Sterile Powder (100 mg). Agitate gently until thoroughly dissolved. Solution should be prepared immediately before administration. Any unused portion should be discarded. *Intravenous injection should be given slowly over a one-minute period.*

Caution: Librium solution made with physiological saline or sterile water for injection should not be given intramuscularly because of pain on injection.

DOSAGE

Dosage should be individualized according to the diagnosis and the response of the patient. While 300 mg may be given during a 6-hour period, this dose should not be exceeded in any 24-hour period.

INDICATION	ADULT DOSAGE*
Withdrawal Symptoms of Acute Alcoholism	50 to 100 mg I.M. or I.V. initially; repeat in 2 to 4 hours, if necessary
Acute or Severe Anxiety Disorders or Symptoms of Anxiety	50 to 100 mg I.M. or I.V. initially; then 25 to 50 mg 3 or 4 times daily, if necessary
Preoperative Apprehension and Anxiety	50 to 100 mg I.M. one hour prior to surgery

* Lower doses (usually 25 to 50 mg) should be used for elderly or debilitated patients, and for older children. Since clinical experience in children under 12 years of age is limited, the use of the drug in this age group is not recommended.

In most cases, acute symptoms may be rapidly controlled by parenteral administration so that subsequent treatment, if necessary, may be given orally. (See package insert for Oral Librium.)

HOW SUPPLIED

For Parenteral Administration: Ampuls—Duplex package consisting of a 5-ml dry-filled ampul containing 100 mg chlordiazepoxide HCl in dry crystalline form, and a 2-ml ampul of Special Intramuscular Diluent (for intramuscular administration) compounded with 1.5% benzyl alcohol, 4% polysorbate 80, 20% propylene glycol, 1.6% maleic acid and sodium hydroxide to adjust pH to approximately 3.0. Boxes of 10.

CAUTION

Before preparing solution for intramuscular or intravenous administration, please read instructions for PREPARATION AND ADMINISTRATION OF SOLUTIONS.

LIMBITROL® ℂ

[lim 'bit-roll]

(chlordiazepoxide and amitriptyline HCl/Roche)
DS (double strength) Tablets
Tablets

The following text is complete prescribing information based on official labeling in effect June 1, 1986.

DESCRIPTION

Limbitrol combines for oral administration, chlordiazepoxide, an agent for the relief of anxiety and tension, and amitriptyline, an antidepressant. It is available in DS (double strength) white, film-coated tablets, each containing 10 mg chlordiazepoxide and 25 mg amitriptyline (as the hydrochloride salt); and in blue, film-coated tablets, each containing 5 mg chlordiazepoxide and 12.5 mg amitriptyline (as the hydrochloride salt). Each tablet also contains corn starch, ethylcellulose, hydroxypropyl methylcellulose, lactose, magnesium stearate, povidone and triacetin; Limbitrol tablets contain the following dye: FD&C Blue No. 1; Limbitrol DS tablets contain no dye.

Chlordiazepoxide is a benzodiazepine with the formula 7-chloro-2-(methylamino)-5-phenyl-3*H*-1,4-benzodiazepine 4-oxide. It is a slightly yellow crystalline material and is insoluble in water. The molecular weight is 299.76.

Amitriptyline is a dibenzocycloheptadiene derivative. The formula is 10,11-dihydro-*N,N*-dimethyl-5H-dibenzo [a, d] cycloheptene-$\Delta^{5,\gamma}$-propylamine hydrochloride. It is a white or practically white crystalline compound that is freely soluble in water. The molecular weight is 313.87.

ACTIONS

Both components of Limbitrol exert their action in the central nervous system. Extensive studies with chlordiazepoxide in many animal species suggest action in the limbic system. Recent evidence indicates that the limbic system is involved in emotional response. Taming action was observed in some species. The mechanism of action of amitriptyline in man is not known, but the drug appears to interfere with the reuptake of norepinephrine into adrenergic nerve endings. This action may prolong the sympathetic activity of biogenic amines.

INDICATIONS

Limbitrol is indicated for the treatment of patients with moderate to severe depression associated with moderate to severe anxiety.

The therapeutic response to Limbitrol occurs earlier and with fewer treatment failures than when either amitriptyline or chlordiazepoxide is used alone.

Symptoms likely to respond in the first week of treatment include: insomnia, feelings of guilt or worthlessness, agitation, psychic and somatic anxiety, suicidal ideation and anorexia.

CONTRAINDICATIONS

Limbitrol is contraindicated in patients with hypersensitivity to either benzodiazepines or tricyclic antidepressants. It should not be given concomitantly with a monoamine oxidase inhibitor. Hyperpyretic crises, severe convulsions and deaths have occurred in patients receiving a tricyclic antidepressant and a monoamine oxidase inhibitor simultaneously. When it is desired to replace a monoamine oxidase inhibitor with Limbitrol, a minimum of 14 days should be allowed to elapse after the former is discontinued. Limbitrol should then be initiated cautiously with gradual increase in dosage until optimum response is achieved.

This drug is contraindicated during the acute recovery phase following myocardial infarction.

WARNINGS

Because of the atropine-like action of the amitriptyline component, great care should be used in treating patients with a history of urinary retention or angle-closure glaucoma. In patients with glaucoma, even average doses may precipitate an attack. Severe constipation may occur in patients taking tricyclic antidepressants in combination with anticholinergic-type drugs.

Patients with cardiovascular disorders should be watched closely. Tricyclic antidepressant drugs, particularly when given in high doses, have been reported to produce arrhythmias, sinus tachycardia and prolongation of conduction time. Myocardial infarction and stroke have been reported in patients receiving drugs of this class.

Because of the sedative effects of Limbitrol, patients should be cautioned about combined effects with alcohol or other CNS depressants. The additive effects may produce a harmful level of sedation and CNS depression.

Patients receiving Limbitrol should be cautioned against engaging in hazardous occupations requiring complete mental alertness, such as operating machinery or driving a motor vehicle.

Usage in Pregnancy: Safe use of Limbitrol during pregnancy and lactation has not been established. Because of the chlordiazepoxide component, please note the following:

> **An increased risk of congenital malformations associated with the use of minor tranquilizers (chlordiazepoxide, diazepam and meprobamate) during the first trimester of pregnancy has been suggested in several studies. Because use of these drugs is rarely a matter of urgency, their use during this period should almost always be avoided. The possibility that a woman of childbearing potential may be pregnant at the time of institution of therapy should be considered. Patients should be advised that if they become pregnant during therapy or intend to become pregnant they should communicate with their physicians about the desirability of discontinuing the drug.**

Physical and Psychological Dependence: Experience with Limbitrol is as yet too limited to reasonably assess the combination's potential for physical and psychological dependence. However, since physical and psychological dependence to chlordiazepoxide have been reported rarely, caution must be exercised in administering Limbitrol to individuals known to be addiction-prone or to those whose history suggests they may increase the dosage on their own initiative. In the so far limited experience with Limbitrol withdrawal symptoms have not been reported. However, withdrawal symptoms following abrupt cessation of prolonged therapy with either component alone have been reported. With amitriptyline, these have been noted to consist of nausea, headache and malaise; for chlordiazepoxide, the symptoms (including convulsions) are similar to those seen with barbiturates.

PRECAUTIONS

General: Use with caution in patients with a history of seizures.

Close supervision is required when Limbitrol is given to hyperthyroid patients or those on thyroid medication.

The usual precautions should be observed when treating patients with impaired renal or hepatic function.

Patients with suicidal ideation should not have easy access to large quantities of the drug. The possibility of suicide in depressed patients remains until significant remission occurs.

Essential Laboratory Tests: Patients on prolonged treatment should have periodic liver function tests and blood counts.

Drug and Treatment Interactions: Because of its amitriptyline component, Limbitrol may block the antihypertensive action of guanethidine or compounds with a similar mechanism of action.

The effects of concomitant administration of Limbitrol and other psychotropic drugs have not been evaluated. Sedative effects may be additive.

Cimetidine is reported to reduce hepatic metabolism of certain tricyclic antidepressants and benzodiazepines, thereby delaying elimination and increasing steady state concentrations of these drugs. Clinically significant effects have been reported with the tricyclic antidepressants when used concomitantly with cimetidine (Tagamet).

The drug should be discontinued several days before elective surgery.

Concurrent administration of ECT and Limbitrol should be limited to those patients for whom it is essential.

Pregnancy: See WARNINGS section.

Nursing Mothers: It is not known whether this drug is excreted in human milk. As a general rule, nursing should not be undertaken while a patient is on a drug, since many drugs are excreted in human milk.

Pediatric Use: Safety and effectiveness in children below the age of 12 years have not been established.

Elderly Patients: In elderly and debilitated patients it is recommended that dosage be limited to the smallest effective amount to preclude the development of ataxia, oversedation, confusion or anticholinergic effects.

ADVERSE REACTIONS

Adverse reactions to Limbitrol are those associated with the use of either component alone. Most frequently reported were drowsiness, dry mouth, constipation, blurred vision, dizziness and bloating. Other side effects occurring less commonly included vivid dreams, impotence, tremor, confusion and nasal congestion. Many symptoms common to the depressive state, such as anorexia, fatigue, weakness, restlessness and lethargy, have been reported as side effects of treatment with both Limbitrol and amitriptyline.

Granulocytopenia, jaundice and hepatic dysfunction of uncertain etiology have also been observed rarely with Limbitrol. When treatment with Limbitrol is prolonged, periodic blood counts and liver function tests are advisable.

Note: Included in the listing which follows are adverse reactions which have not been reported with Limbitrol. However, they are included because they have been reported during therapy with one or both of the components or closely related drugs.

Cardiovascular: Hypotension, hypertension, tachycardia, palpitations, myocardial infarction, arrhythmias, heart block, stroke.

Psychiatric: Euphoria, apprehension, poor concentration, delusions, hallucinations, hypomania and increased or decreased libido.

Neurologic: Incoordination, ataxia, numbness, tingling and paresthesias of the extremities, extrapyramidal symptoms, syncope, changes in EEG patterns.

Anticholinergic: Disturbance of accommodation, paralytic ileus, urinary retention, dilatation of urinary tract.

Allergic: Skin rash, urticaria, photosensitization, edema of face and tongue, pruritus.

Hematologic: Bone marrow depression including agranulocytosis, eosinophilia, purpura, thrombocytopenia.

Gastrointestinal: Nausea, epigastric distress, vomiting, anorexia, stomatitis, peculiar taste, diarrhea, black tongue.

Endocrine: Testicular swelling and gynecomastia in the male, breast enlargement, galactorrhea and minor menstrual irregularities in the female, elevation and lowering of blood sugar levels, and syndrome of inappropriate ADH (antidiuretic hormone) secretion.

Other: Headache, weight gain or loss, increased perspiration, urinary frequency, mydriasis, jaundice, alopecia, parotid swelling.

OVERDOSAGE

There has been limited experience with Limbitrol overdosage *per se;* the manifestations of overdosage and recommendations for treatment are based on clinical experience with its components. Primary concern should be with the dangers associated with amitriptyline overdosage. Deaths by deliberate or accidental overdosage have occurred with this class of drugs.

All patients suspected of having an overdosage of Limbitrol should be admitted to a hospital as soon as possible.

Manifestations: High doses may cause drowsiness, temporary confusion, disturbed concentration or transient visual hallucinations. Overdosage may cause hypothermia, tachycardia and other arrhythmias, ECG evidence of impaired conduction (such as bundle branch block), congestive heart failure, dilated pupils, convulsions, severe hypotension, stupor and coma. Other symptoms may be agitation, hyperactive reflexes, muscle rigidity, vomiting, hyperpyrexia or any of those listed under Adverse Reactions.

Treatment: Empty the stomach as quickly as possible by emesis or lavage. In the comatose patient a cuff endotracheal tube should be placed in position prior to either of these measures. The instillation of activated charcoal into the stomach also should be considered. If the patient is stuporous but responds to stimuli, only close observation and nursing care may be required. It is essential to maintain an adequate airway and fluid intake. Body temperature should be watched closely and appropriate measures taken should deviations occur.

The intramuscular or slow intravenous administration of 1 to 3 mg in adults (or 0.5 mg in children) of physostigmine salicylate (Antilirium)[1–3] has been reported to reverse the manifestations of amitriptyline overdosage. Because of its relatively short half-life, additional doses may be needed at intervals of 30 minutes to 2 hours.

Convulsions may be treated by the use of an inhalation anesthetic rather than the use of barbiturates. Cardiac monitoring is advisable, and the cautious use of digitalis or other antiarrhythmic agents should be considered if serious cardiovascular abnormalities occur. Serum potassium levels should be monitored and kept within normal limits by the use of appropriate I.V. fluids. Standard measures including oxygen, I.V. fluids, plasma expanders and corticosteroids may be used to control circulatory shock.

Dialysis is unlikely to be of value, as it has not proven useful in overdosages of either amitriptyline or chlordiazepoxide. Since many suicidal attempts involve multiple drugs including barbiturates, the possibility of dialysis being beneficial for removal of other drugs should not be overlooked.

Treatment should be continued for at least 48 hours, along with cardiac monitoring in patients who do not respond to therapy promptly. Since relapses are frequent, patients should be hospitalized until their conditions remain stable without physostigmine for at least 24 hours.

Since overdosage is often deliberate, patients may attempt suicide by other means during the recovery phase.

References:

1. Granacher RP, Baldessarini RJ: Physostigmine: Its use in acute anticholinergic syndrome with antidepressant and antiparkinson drugs. *Arch Gen Psychiatry* *32*:375–380, March 1975.

2. Burks JS, Walker JE, Rumack BH, Ott JE: Tricyclic antidepressant poisoning: Reversal of coma, choreoathetosis, and myoclonus by physostigmine. *JAMA 230*:1405–1407, Dec. 9, 1974.

3. Snyder BD, Blonde L, McWhirter WR: Reversal of amitriptyline intoxication by physostigmine. *JAMA 230*:1433–1434, Dec. 9, 1974.

DOSAGE AND ADMINISTRATION

Optimum dosage varies with the severity of the symptoms and the response of the individual patient. When a satisfactory response is obtained, dosage should be reduced to the smallest amount needed to maintain the remission. The larger portion of the total daily dose may be taken at bedtime. In some patients, a single dose at bedtime may be sufficient. In general, lower dosages are recommended for elderly patients.

Limbitrol DS (double strength) Tablets are recommended in an initial dosage of three or four tablets daily in divided doses; this may be increased to six tablets daily as required. Some patients respond to smaller doses and can be maintained on two tablets daily.

Limbitrol Tablets in an initial dosage of three or four tablets daily in divided doses may be satisfactory in patients who do not tolerate higher doses.

HOW SUPPLIED

DS (double strength) Tablets, containing 10 mg chlordiazepoxide and 25 mg amitriptyline (as the hydrochloride salt)—bottles of 100 and 500; Tel-E-Dose® packages of 100; Prescription Paks of 50.

Tablets, containing 5 mg chlordiazepoxide and 12.5 mg amitriptyline (as the hydrochloride salt)—bottles of 100 and 500; Tel-E-Dose® packages of 100; Prescription Paks of 50.

Shown in Product Identification Section, page 425

MENRIUM® 5-2 ℞

[men 'ree-um]

Each tablet contains 5 mg chlordiazepoxide and 0.2 mg water-soluble esterified estrogens.

MENRIUM® 5-4

Each tablet contains 5 mg chlordiazepoxide and 0.4 mg water-soluble esterified estrogens.

MENRIUM® 10-4

Each tablet contains 10 mg chlordiazepoxide and 0.4 mg water-soluble esterified estrogens.

Menrium tablets are manufactured by Hoffmann-La Roche Inc., Nutley, N.J. 07110 and distributed by Roche Products Inc., Manati, P.R. 00701.

The following text is complete prescribing information based on official labeling in effect July 1, 1986.

> Since estrogens are a component of Menrium, please note:
>
> 1. ESTROGENS HAVE BEEN REPORTED TO INCREASE THE RISK OF ENDOMETRIAL CARCINOMA.
>
> Three independent case control studies have shown an increased risk of endometrial cancer in postmenopausal women exposed to exogenous estrogens for prolonged periods.[1–3] This risk was independent of the other known risk factors for endometrial cancer. These studies are further supported by the finding that incidence rates of endometrial cancer have increased sharply since 1969 in eight different areas of the United States with population-based cancer reporting systems, an

Continued on next page

Roche Products—Cont.

increase which may be related to the rapidly expanding use of estrogens during the last decade.[4] The three case control studies reported that the risk of endometrial cancer in estrogen users was about 4.5 to 13.9 times greater than in nonusers. The risk appears to depend on both duration of treatment[1] and on estrogen dose.[3] In view of these findings, when estrogens are used for the treatment of menopausal symptoms, the lowest dose that will control symptoms should be utilized and medication should be discontinued as soon as possible. When prolonged treatment is medically indicated, the patient should be reassessed on at least a semiannual basis to determine the need for continued therapy. Although the evidence must be considered preliminary, one study suggests that cyclic administration of low doses of estrogen may carry less risk than continuous administration;[3] it therefore appears prudent to utilize such a regimen.

Close clinical surveillance of all women taking estrogens is important. In all cases of undiagnosed persistent or recurring abnormal vaginal bleeding, adequate diagnostic measures should be undertaken to rule out malignancy.

There is no evidence at present that "natural" estrogens are more or less hazardous than "synthetic" estrogens at equiestrogenic doses.

2. ESTROGENS SHOULD NOT BE USED DURING PREGNANCY

The use of female sex hormones, both estrogens and progestogens, during early pregnancy may seriously damage the offspring. It has been shown that females exposed in utero to diethylstilbestrol, a nonsteroidal estrogen, have an increased risk of developing, in later life, a form of vaginal or cervical cancer that is ordinarily extremely rare.[5,6] This risk has been estimated as not greater than 4 per 1000 exposures.[7] Furthermore, a high percentage of such exposed women (from 30 to 90 percent) have been found to have vaginal adenosis,[8–12] epithelial changes of the vagina and cervix. Although these changes are histologically benign, it is not known whether they are precursors of malignancy. Although similar data are not available with the use of other estrogens, it cannot be presumed they would not induce similar changes.

Several reports suggest an association between intrauterine exposure to female sex hormones and congenital anomalies, including congenital heart defects and limb reduction defects.[13–16] One case control study[16] estimated a 4.7-fold increased risk of limb reduction defects in infants exposed in utero to sex hormones (oral contraceptives, hormone withdrawal tests for pregnancy, or attempted treatment for threatened abortion). Some of these exposures were very short and involved only a few days of treatment. The data suggest that the risk of limb reduction defects in exposed fetuses is somewhat less than 1 per 1,000. In the past, female sex hormones have been used during pregnancy in an attempt to treat threatened or habitual abortion. There is considerable evidence that estrogens are ineffective for these indications, and there is no evidence from well-controlled studies that progestogens are effective for these uses.

If Menrium is used during pregnancy, or if the patient becomes pregnant while taking this drug, she should be apprised of the potential risks to the fetus, and the advisability of pregnancy continuation.

DESCRIPTION

Menrium tablets are available in three strengths: Menrium 5-2, containing 5 mg chlordiazepoxide and 0.2 mg water-soluble esterified estrogens; Menrium 5-4, containing 5 mg chlordiazepoxide and 0.4 mg water-soluble esterified estrogens; and Menrium 10-4, containing 10 mg chlordiazepoxide and 0.4 mg water-soluble esterified estrogens. Each tablet also contains acacia, calcium stearate, calcium sulfate, carnauba wax, corn starch, lactose, pregelatinized starch, sodium bicarbonate, sucrose and flavor, with the following dye systems: Menrium 5-2 and Menrium 5-4—FD&C Blue 1, FD&C Yellow No. 6 and D&C Yellow No. 10; Menrium 10-4—FD&C Blue No. 1 and FD&C Red No. 3.

Menrium affords in a single formulation the psychotropic action of Librium® (chlordiazepoxide/Roche) and hormonal replacement in the form of water-soluble esterified estrogens (expressed in terms of sodium estrone sulfate) to provide comprehensive management of the menopausal syndrome or the climacteric.

Librium (chlordiazepoxide/Roche) is a versatile therapeutic agent of proven value for the relief of anxiety and tension. It is indicated when anxiety, tension or apprehension are significant components of the clinical profile. It is among the safer of the effective psychopharmacologic compounds.

Chlordiazepoxide is 7-chloro-2-methylamino-5-phenyl-3H-1, 4-benzodiazepine 4-oxide. It is a slightly yellow, crystalline material and is insoluble in water. The molecular weight is 299.75.

Water-soluble esterified estrogens provide hormonal replacement in the menopausal patient, the need for which is widely recognized and accepted. Esterified estrogens is a mixture of the sodium salts of the sulfate esters of the estrogenic substances, principally estrone, that are of the type excreted by pregnant mares. It is a white to buff-colored, amorphous powder, odorless or having a slight, characteristic odor.

CLINICAL PHARMACOLOGY

The estrogenic component of Menrium is water-soluble esterified estrogens—steroidal compounds—which occur naturally. The action of this substance is substantially equal to the action of both conjugated estrogens, also naturally occurring, and synthetic estrogenic substances.

Menopausal changes, such as atrophic changes of the genital tract and breasts due to a slow decline in estrogen secretion, may be reversed by substitution therapy with estrogenic substances.

Estrogens are, in general, completely absorbed following oral administration. Estrogens are detoxified by the liver, and excretion occurs by way of the urine and the feces.

Librium (chlordiazepoxide HCl/Roche) has antianxiety and sedative actions. The drug has been studied extensively in many species of animals and these studies are suggestive of action on the limbic system of the brain, which recent evidence indicates is involved in emotional responses. However, the precise mechanism of action in man is not known. The drug blocks EEG arousal from stimulation of the brain stem reticular formation. The mean $\pm$S.E. plasma peak time is 1.4 ($\pm$0.3) hours, and the half-life ranges between 7.1 and 19.8 hours with a mean $\pm$S.E. half-life of 12.0 ($\pm$0.7) hours. After the drug is discontinued, plasma levels are usually at the lowest quantitatively detectable amounts by 48 to 72 hours. Chlordiazepoxide HCl is excreted in urine with 1% or less unchanged and 12 to 34% recoverable as conjugates.

INDICATIONS

Menrium is indicated in the management of the manifestations generally associated with the menopausal syndrome—anxiety and tension, vasomotor complaints and hormonal deficiency states.

MENRIUM HAS NOT BEEN SHOWN TO BE EFFECTIVE FOR ANY PURPOSE DURING PREGNANCY AND ITS USE MAY CAUSE SEVERE HARM TO THE FETUS (SEE BOXED WARNING).

The lowest effective dose appropriate for the specific indication should be utilized. Studies of the addition of a progestin for seven or more days of a cycle of estrogen administration have reported a lowered incidence of endometrial hyperplasia. Morphological and biochemical studies of endometrium suggest that 10 to 13 days of progestin are needed to provide maximal maturation of the endometrium and to eliminate any hyperplastic changes. Whether this will provide protection from endometrial carcinoma has not been clearly established. There are possible additional risks which may be associated with the inclusion of progestin in estrogen replacement regimens. The potential risks include adverse effects on carbohydrate and lipid metabolism. The choice of progestin and dosage may be important in minimizing these adverse effects.

CONTRAINDICATIONS

Menrium is contraindicated in patients with known hypersensitivity to chlordiazepoxide and/or esterified estrogens.

Estrogens should not be used in women (or men) with any of the following conditions:

1. Known or suspected cancer of the breast except in appropriately selected patients being treated for metastatic disease.
2. Known or suspected estrogen-dependent neoplasia.
3. Known or suspected pregnancy. (See Boxed Warning.)
4. Undiagnosed abnormal genital bleeding.
5. Active thrombophlebitis or thromboembolic disorders.
6. A past history of thrombophlebitis, thrombosis, or thromboembolic disorders associated with previous estrogen use.

WARNINGS

1. *Induction of malignant neoplasms.* Long term continuous administration of natural and synthetic estrogens in certain animal species increases the frequency of carcinomas of the breast, cervix, vagina, and liver. There is now evidence that estrogens increase the risk of carcinoma of the endometrium in humans. (See Boxed Warning.)

At the present time there is no satisfactory evidence that estrogens given to postmenopausal women increase the risk of cancer of the breast,[17] although a recent long-term followup of a single physician's practice has raised this possibility.[18] Because of the animal data, there is a need for caution in prescribing estrogens for women with a strong family history of breast cancer or who have breast nodules, fibrocystic disease, or abnormal mammograms.

2. *Gall bladder disease.* A recent study has reported a 2- to 3-fold increase in the risk of surgically confirmed gall bladder disease in women receiving postmenopausal estrogens,[17] similar to the 2-fold increase previously noted in users of oral contraceptives.[19,24] In the case of oral contraceptives the increased risk appeared after two years of use.[24]

3. *Effects similar to those caused by estrogen-progestogen oral contraceptives.* There are several serious adverse effects of oral contraceptives, most of which have not, up to now, been documented as consequences of postmenopausal estrogen therapy. This may reflect the comparatively low doses of estrogen used in postmenopausal women. It would be expected that the larger doses of estrogen used to treat prostatic or breast cancer or postpartum breast engorgement are more likely to result in these adverse effects, and, in fact, it has been shown that there is an increased risk of thrombosis in men receiving estrogens for prostatic cancer and women for postpartum breast engorgement.[20-23]

a. *Thromboembolic disease.* It is now well established that users of oral contraceptives have an increased risk of various thromboembolic and thrombotic vascular diseases, such as thrombophlebitis, pulmonary embolism, stroke, and myocardial infarction.[24–31] Cases of retinal thrombosis, mesenteric thrombosis, and optic neuritis have been reported in oral contraceptive users. There is evidence that the risk of several of these adverse reactions is related to the dose of the drug.[32,33] An increased risk of postsurgery thromboembolic complications has also been reported in users of oral contraceptives.[34,35] If feasible, estrogen should be discontinued at least 4 weeks before surgery of the type associated with an increased risk of thromboembolism, or during periods of prolonged immobilization.

While an increased rate of thromboembolic and thrombotic disease in postmenopausal users of estrogens has not been found,[17,36] this does not rule out the possibility that such an increase may be present or that subgroups of women who have underlying risk factors or who are receiving relatively large doses of estrogens may have increased risk. Therefore, estrogens should not be used in persons with active thrombophlebitis or thromboembolic disorders, and they should not be used in persons with a history of such disorders in association with estrogen use. They should be used with caution in patients with cerebral vascular or coronary artery disease and only for those in whom estrogens are clearly needed.

Large doses of estrogen (5 mg conjugated estrogens per day), comparable to those used to treat cancer of the prostate and breast, have been shown in a large prospective clinical trial in men[37] to increase the risk of nonfatal myocardial infarction, pulmonary embolism and thrombophlebitis. When estrogen doses of this size are used, any of the thromboembolic and thrombotic adverse effects associated with oral contraceptive use should be considered a clear risk.

b. *Hepatic adenoma.* Benign hepatic adenomas appear to be associated with the use of oral contraceptives.[38–40] Although benign, and rare, these may rupture and may cause death through intra-abdominal hemorrhage. Such lesions have not yet been reported in association with other estrogen or progestogen preparations but should be considered in estrogen users having abdominal pain and tenderness, abdominal mass, or hypovolemic shock. Hepatocellular carcinoma has also been reported in women taking estrogen-containing oral contraceptives.[39] The relationship of this malignancy to these drugs is not known at this time.

c. *Elevated blood pressure.* Increased blood pressure is not uncommon in women using oral contraceptives. There is now a report that this may occur with the use of estrogens in the menopause[41] and blood pressure should be monitored with estrogen use, especially if high doses are used.

d. *Glucose tolerance.* A worsening of glucose tolerance has been observed in a significant percentage of patients on estrogen-containing oral contraceptives. For this reason, diabetic patients should be carefully observed while receiving estrogen.

4. *Hypercalcemia.* Administration of estrogens may lead to severe hypercalcemia in patients with breast cancer and bone metastases. If this occurs, the drug should be stopped and appropriate measures taken to reduce the serum calcium level.

As in the case of other preparations containing CNS-acting drugs, patients receiving Menrium should be cautioned about possible combined effects with alcohol and other CNS depressants. Other causes of manifestations of the menopausal syndrome, such as pregnancy, should be excluded. As is true of all preparations containing CNS-acting drugs, patients receiving Menrium should be cautioned against hazardous occupations requiring complete mental alertness such as operating machinery or driving a motor vehicle.

Physical and Psychological Dependence: Withdrawal symptoms have not been observed in more than 1300 subjects during clinical trials with Menrium. Physical and psychological dependence have rarely been reported in persons taking recommended doses of Librium (chlordiazepoxide/ Roche). However, caution must be exercised in administering Librium to individuals known to be addiction-prone or those whose history suggests they may increase the dosage on their own initiative. Withdrawal symptoms following discontinuation of chlordiazepoxide hydrochloride have been reported. These symptoms (including convulsions) are similar to those seen with barbiturates.

PRECAUTIONS

A. General Precautions.

1. A complete medical and family history should be taken prior to the initiation of any estrogen therapy. The pretreatment and periodic physical examinations should include special reference to blood pressure, breasts, abdomen, and pelvic organs, and should include a Papanicolaou smear. As a general rule, estrogen should not be prescribed for longer than one year without another physical examination being performed.

2. Fluid retention—Because estrogens may cause some degree of fluid retention, conditions which might be influenced by this factor, such as epilepsy, migraine, and cardiac or renal dysfunction, require careful observation.

3. Certain patients may develop undesirable manifestations of excessive estrogenic stimulation, such as abnormal or excessive uterine bleeding, mastodynia, etc.

4. Oral contraceptives appear to be associated with an increased incidence of mental depression.[24] Although it is not clear whether this is due to the estrogenic or progestogenic component of the contraceptive, patients with a history of depression should be carefully observed.

5. Preexisting uterine leiomyomata may increase in size during estrogen use.

6. The pathologist should be advised of estrogen therapy when relevant specimens are submitted.

7. Patients with a past history of jaundice during pregnancy have an increased risk of recurrence of jaundice while receiving estrogen-containing oral contraceptive therapy. If jaundice develops in any patient receiving estrogen, the medication should be discontinued while the cause is investigated.

8. Estrogens may be poorly metabolized in patients with impaired liver function and they should be administered with caution in such patients.

9. Because estrogens influence the metabolism of calcium and phosphorus, they should be used with caution in patients with metabolic bone diseases that are associated with hypercalcemia or in patients with renal insufficiency.

10. Because of the effects of estrogens on epiphyseal closure, they should be used judiciously in young patients in whom bone growth is not complete.

11. Certain endocrine and liver function tests may be affected by estrogen-containing oral contraceptives. The following similar changes may be expected with larger doses of estrogen:

a. Increased sulfobromophthalein retention.

b. Increased prothrombin and factors VII, VIII, IX, and X; decreased antithrombin 3; increased norepinephrine-induced platelet aggregability.

c. Increased thyroid binding globulin (TBG) leading to increased circulating total thyroid hormone, as measured by PBI, T4 by column, or T4 by radioimmunoassay. Free T3 resin uptake is decreased, reflecting the elevated TBG; free T4 concentration is unaltered.

d. Impaired glucose tolerance.

e. Decreased pregnanediol excretion.

f. Reduced response to metyrapone test.

g. Reduced serum folate concentration.

h. Increased serum triglyceride and phospholipid concentration.

B. Information for the Patient.

See Text of Patient Package Insert which follows below.

WHAT YOU SHOULD KNOW ABOUT ESTROGENS

Estrogens are female hormones produced by the ovaries. The ovaries make several different kinds of estrogens. In addition, scientists have been able to make a variety of synthetic estrogens. As far as we know, all these estrogens have similar properties and therefore much the same usefulness, side effects, and risks. This leaflet is intended to help you understand what estrogens are used for, the risks involved in their use, and how to use them as safely as possible.

This leaflet includes the most important information about estrogens, but not all the information. If you want to know more, you can ask your doctor or pharmacist to let you read the package insert prepared for the doctor.

USES OF ESTROGEN

Estrogens are prescribed by doctors for a number of purposes, including:

1. To provide estrogen during a period of adjustment when a woman's ovaries no longer produce it, in order to prevent certain uncomfortable symptoms of estrogen deficiency. (All women normally stop producing estrogens, generally between the ages of 45 and 55; this is called the menopause.)

2. To prevent symptoms of estrogen deficiency when a woman's ovaries have been removed surgically before the natural menopause.

3. To prevent pregnancy. (Estrogens are given along with a progestogen, another female hormone; these combinations are called oral contraceptives or birth control pills. Patient labeling is available to women taking oral contraceptives and they will not be discussed in this leaflet.)

4. To treat certain cancers in women and men.

5. To prevent painful swelling of the breasts after pregnancy in women who choose not to nurse their babies.

THERE IS NO PROPER USE OF ESTROGENS IN A PREGNANT WOMAN.

ESTROGENS IN THE MENOPAUSE

In the natural course of their lives, all women eventually experience a decrease in estrogen production. This usually occurs between ages 45 and 55 but may occur earlier or later. Sometimes the ovaries may need to be removed before natural menopause by an operation, producing a "surgical menopause."

When the amount of estrogen in the blood begins to decrease, many women may develop typical symptoms: Feelings of warmth in the face, neck, and chest or sudden intense episodes of heat and sweating throughout the body (called "hot flashes" or "hot flushes"). These symptoms are sometimes very uncomfortable. A few women eventually develop changes in the vagina (called "atrophic vaginitis") which cause discomfort, especially during and after intercourse.

Estrogens can be prescribed to treat these symptoms of the menopause. It is estimated that considerably more than half of all women undergoing the menopause have only mild symptoms or no symptoms at all and therefore do not need estrogens. Other woman may need estrogens for a few months, while their bodies adjust to lower estrogen levels. Sometimes the need will be for periods longer than six months. In an attempt to avoid overstimulation of the uterus (womb), estrogens are usually given cyclically during each month of use, that is three weeks of pills followed by one week without pills.

Sometimes women experience nervous symptoms or depression during menopause. There is no evidence that estrogens are effective for such symptoms and they should not be used to treat them, although other treatment may be needed.

You may have heard that taking estrogens for long periods (years) after the menopause will keep your skin soft and supple and keep you feeling young. There is no evidence that this is so, however, and such long-term treatment carries important risks.

Estrogens to Prevent Swelling of the Breasts After Pregnancy: If you do not breast feed your baby after delivery, your breasts may fill up with milk and become painful and engorged. This usually begins about 3 to 4 days after delivery and may last for a few days to up to a week or more. Sometimes the discomfort is severe, but usually it is not and can be controlled by pain relieving drugs such as aspirin and by binding the breasts up tightly. Estrogens can be used to try to prevent the breasts from filling up. While this treatment is sometimes successful, in many cases the breasts fill up to some degree in spite of treatment. The dose of estrogens needed to prevent pain and swelling of the breasts is much larger than the dose needed to treat symptoms of the menopause and this may increase your chances of developing blood clots in the legs or lungs (see below). Therefore, it is important that you discuss the benefits and the risks of estrogen use with your doctor if you have decided not to breast feed your baby.

The Dangers of Estrogens:

1. *Cancer of the uterus.* If estrogens are used in the postmenopausal period for more than a year, there is an increased risk of *endometrial cancer* (cancer of the uterus). Women taking estrogens have roughly 5 to 10 times as great a chance of getting this cancer as women who take no estrogens. To put this another way, while a postmenopausal woman not taking estrogens has 1 chance in 1,000 each year of getting cancer of the uterus, a woman taking estrogens has 5 to 10 chances in 1,000 each year. For this reason *it is important to take estrogens only when you really need them.*

The risk of this cancer is greater the longer estrogens are used and also seems to be greater when larger doses are taken. For this reason *it is important to take the lowest dose of estrogen that will control symptoms and to take it only as long as it is needed.* If estrogens are needed for longer periods of time, your doctor will want to reevaluate your need for estrogens at least every six months.

Women using estrogens should report any irregular vaginal bleeding to their doctors; such bleeding may be of no importance, but it can be an early warning of cancer of the uterus. If you have undiagnosed vaginal bleeding, you should not use estrogens until a diagnosis is made and you are certain there is no cancer of the uterus.

If you have had your uterus completely removed (total hysterectomy), there is no danger of developing cancer of the uterus.

2. *Other possible cancers.* Estrogens can cause development of other tumors in animals, such as tumors of the breast, cervix, vagina, or liver, when given for a long time. At present there is no good evidence that women using estrogen in the menopause have an increased risk of such tumors, but there is no way yet to be sure they do not; and one study raises the possibility that use of estrogens in the menopause may increase the risk of breast cancer many years later. This is a further reason to use estrogens only when clearly needed. While you are taking estrogens, it is important that you go to your doctor at least once a year for a physical examination. Also, if members of your family have had breast cancer or if you have breast nodules or abnormal mammograms (breast x-rays), your doctor may wish to carry out more frequent examinations of your breasts.

3. *Gall bladder disease.* Women who use estrogens after menopause are more likely to develop gall bladder disease needing surgery as women who do not use estrogens. Birth control pills have a similar effect.

4. *Abnormal blood clotting.* Oral contraceptives increase the risk of blood clotting in various parts of the body. This can result in a stroke (if the clot is in the brain), a heart attack (clot in a blood vessel of the heart), or a pulmonary embolus (a clot which forms in the legs or pelvis, then breaks off and travels to the lungs). Any of these can be fatal.

At this time use of estrogens in the menopause is not known to cause such blood clotting, but this has not been fully studied and there could still prove to be such a risk. It is recommended that if you have had clotting in the legs or lungs or a heart attack or stroke while you were using estrogens or birth control pills, you should not use estrogens (unless they are being used to treat cancer of the breast or prostate). If you have had a stroke or heart attack or if you have angina pectoris, estrogens should be used with great caution and only if clearly needed (for example, if you have severe symptoms of the menopause).

The larger doses of estrogen used to prevent swelling of the breasts after pregnancy have been reported to cause clotting in the legs and lungs.

Special Warning About Pregnancy: You should not receive estrogen if you are pregnant. If this should occur, there is a greater than usual chance that the developing child will be born with a birth defect, although the possibility remains fairly small. A female child may have an increased risk of developing cancer of the vagina or cervix later in life (in the teens or twenties). Every possible effort should be made to avoid exposure to estrogens during pregnancy. If exposure occurs, see your doctor.

Other Effects of Estrogens: In addition to the serious known risks of estrogens described above, estrogens have the following side effects and potential risks:

1. *Nausea and vomiting.* The most common side effect of estrogen therapy is nausea. Vomiting is less common.

2. *Effects on breasts.* Estrogens may cause breast tenderness or enlargement and may cause the breasts to secrete a liquid. These effects are not dangerous.

3. *Effects on the uterus.* Estrogens may cause benign fibroid tumors of the uterus to get larger.

Some women will have menstrual bleeding when estrogens are stopped. But if the bleeding occurs on days you are still taking estrogens you should report this to your doctor.

4. *Effects on liver.* Women taking oral contraceptives develop on rare occasions a tumor of the liver which can rupture and bleed into the abdomen. So far, these tumors have not been reported in women using estrogens in the menopause, but you should report any swelling or unusual pain or tenderness in the abdomen to your doctor immediately.

Women with a past history of jaundice (yellowing of the skin and white parts of the eyes) may get jaundice again during estrogen use. If this occurs, stop taking estrogens and see your doctor.

5. *Other effects.* Estrogens may cause excess fluid to be retained in the body. This may make some conditions worse, such as epilepsy, migraine, heart disease, or kidney disease.

SUMMARY

Estrogens have important uses, but they have serious risks as well. You must decide, with your doctor, whether the risks are acceptable to you in view of the benefits of treatment. Except where your doctor has prescribed estrogens for use in special cases of cancer of the breast or prostate, you should not use estrogens if you have cancer of the breast or uterus, are pregnant, have undiagnosed abnormal vaginal bleeding, clotting in the legs or lungs, or have had a stroke, heart attack or angina, or clotting in the legs or lungs in the past while you were taking estrogens.

You can use estrogens as safely as possible by understanding that your doctor will require regular physical examinations while you are taking them and will try to discontinue the drug as soon as possible and use the smallest dose possible. Be alert for signs of trouble including:

1. Abnormal bleeding from the vagina.

2. Pains in the calves or chest or sudden shortness of breath, or coughing blood (indicating possible clots in the legs, heart, or lungs).

3. Severe headache, dizziness, faintness, or changes in vision (indicating possible developing clots in the brain or eye).

4. Breast lumps (you should ask your doctor how to examine your own breasts).

Continued on next page

Roche Products—Cont.

5. Jaundice (yellowing of the skin).
6. Mental depression.

Based on his or her assessment of your medical needs, your doctor has prescribed this drug for you. Do not give the drug to anyone else.

C. Pregnancy: See Contraindications and Box Warning.
D. Nursing Mothers: As a general principle, the administration of any drug to nursing mothers should be done only when clearly necessary since many drugs are excreted in human milk.

In elderly and debilitated patients, it is recommended that the dosage be limited to the smallest effective amount to preclude the development of ataxia or oversedation (10 mg chlordiazepoxide or less per day initially, to be increased gradually as needed and tolerated). In general, the concomitant administration of Menrium and other psychotropic agents is not recommended. If such combination therapy seems indicated, careful consideration should be given to the pharmacology of the agents to be employed—particularly when the known potentiating compounds such as the MAO inhibitors and phenothiazines are to be used. The usual precautions in treating patients with impaired renal or hepatic function should be observed.

Paradoxical reactions to chlordiazepoxide, e.g., excitement, stimulation and acute rage, have been reported in psychiatric patients and should be watched for during Menrium therapy. The usual precautions are indicated when chlordiazepoxide is used in the treatment of anxiety states where there is any evidence of impending depression; it should be borne in mind that suicidal tendencies may be present and protective measures may be necessary. Although clinical studies have not established a cause and effect relationship, physicians should be aware that variable effects on blood coagulation have been reported very rarely in patients receiving oral anticoagulants and Librium (chlordiazepoxide/Roche).

ADVERSE REACTIONS

No side effects or manifestations not seen with either compound alone have been reported with the administration of Menrium. However, since Menrium contains chlordiazepoxide and water-soluble esterified estrogens, the possibility of untoward effects which may be seen with either of these two compounds cannot be excluded.

(See Warnings regarding induction of neoplasia, adverse effects on the fetus, increased incidence of gall bladder disease, and adverse effects similar to those of oral contraceptives, including thromboembolism.) The following additional adverse reactions have been reported with estrogenic therapy, including oral contraceptives:

1. *Genitourinary system.*
Breakthrough bleeding, spotting, change in menstrual flow.
Dysmenorrhea.
Premenstrual-like syndrome.
Amenorrhea during and after treatment.
Increase in size of uterine fibromyomata.
Vaginal candidiasis.
Change in cervical eversion and in degree of cervical secretion.
Cystitis-like syndrome.
2. *Breasts.*
Tenderness, enlargement, secretion.
3. *Gastrointestinal.*
Nausea, vomiting.
Abdominal cramps, bloating.
Cholestatic jaundice.
4. *Skin.*
Chloasma or melasma which may persist when drug is discontinued.
Erythema multiforme.
Erythema nodosum.
Hemorrhagic eruption.
Loss of scalp hair.
Hirsutism.
5. *Eyes.*
Steepening of corneal curvature.
Intolerance to contact lenses.
6. *CNS.*
Headache, migraine, dizziness.
Mental depression.
Chorea.
7. *Miscellaneous.*
Increase or decrease in weight.
Reduced carbohydrate tolerance.
Aggravation of porphyria.
Edema.
Changes in libido.

When chlordiazepoxide has been used alone the necessity of discontinuing therapy because of undesirable effects has been rare. Drowsiness, ataxia and confusion have been reported in some patients—particularly the elderly and debilitated. While these effects can be avoided in almost all instances by proper dosage adjustment, they have occasionally been observed at the lower dosage ranges. In a few instances syncope has been reported.

Other adverse reactions reported during therapy include isolated instances of skin eruptions, edema, minor menstrual irregularities, nausea and constipation, extrapyramidal symptoms, as well as increased and decreased libido. Such side effects have been infrequent and are generally controlled with reduction of dosage. Changes in EEG patterns (low-voltage fast activity) have been observed in patients during and after Librium (chlordiazepoxide/Roche) treatment.

Blood dyscrasias, including agranulocytosis, jaundice and hepatic dysfunction have occasionally been reported during therapy. When Librium treatment is protracted, periodic blood counts and liver function tests are advisable.

Management of Overdosage: Numerous reports of ingestion of large doses of estrogen-containing oral contraceptives by young children indicate that serious ill effects do not occur. Overdosage of estrogen may cause nausea, and withdrawal bleeding may occur in females. Manifestations of Librium (chlordiazepoxide/Roche) overdosage include somnolence, confusion, coma and diminished reflexes. Respiration, pulse and blood pressure should be monitored, as in all cases of drug overdosage, although, in general, these effects have been minimal following Librium overdosage. General supportive measures should be employed, along with immediate gastric lavage. Intravenous fluids should be administered and an adequate airway maintained. Hypotension may be combated by the use of Levophed® (levarterenol) or Aramine (metaraminol). Dialysis is of limited value. There have been occasional reports of excitation in patients following chlordiazepoxide overdosage; if this occurs barbiturates should not be used. As with the management of intentional overdosage with any drug, it should be borne in mind that multiple agents may have been ingested.

DOSAGE

The lowest dose that will control symptoms should be chosen and medication should be discontinued as promptly as possible.

MENRIUM 5-2—for the majority of patients with the menopausal syndrome or the climacteric having anxiety and tension and hormonal deficiency states requiring estrogen replacement—One tablet, t.i.d.

MENRIUM 5-4—for patients with the menopausal syndrome or the climacteric with anxiety and tension and more severe vasomotor manifestations —One tablet, t.i.d.

MENRIUM 10-4—for patients with the menopausal syndrome or the climacteric with pronounced anxiety and tension and marked vasomotor complaints—One tablet, t.i.d.

Therapy should be continued for 21-day courses, followed by one-week rest periods. While these dosage schedules will prove generally satisfactory, individual adjustment of dosage is desirable, since some patients may obtain satisfactory relief with as little as one tablet daily of Menrium 5-2.

Treated patients with an intact uterus should be monitored closely for signs of endometrial cancer and appropriate diagnostic measures should be taken to rule out malignancy in the event of persistent or recurring abnormal vaginal bleeding.

HOW SUPPLIED

Menrium 5-2, light green tablets; Menrium 5-4, dark green tablets; and Menrium 10-4, purple tablets—bottles of 100.

PHYSICIAN REFERENCES

1. Ziel HK, Finkel WD: *N Engl J Med 293*:1167–1170, 1975
2. Smith DC, *et al: N Engl J Med 293*:1164–1167, 1975
3. Mack TM, *et al: N Engl J Med 294*:1262–1267, 1976
4. Weiss NS, Szekely DR, Austin DF: *N Engl J Med 294*:1259–1262, 1976
5. Herbst AL, Ulfelder H, Poskanzer DC: *N Engl J Med 284*:878–881, 1971
6. Greenwald P, *et al: N Engl J Med 285*:390–392, 1971
7. Lanier A, *et al: Mayo Clin Proc 48*:793–799, 1973
8. Herbst A, Kurman R, Scully R: *Obstet Gynecol 40*:287–298, 1972
9. Herbst A, *et al: Am J Obstet Gynecol 118*:607–615, 1974
10. Herbst, A, *et al: N Engl J Med 292*:334–339, 1975
11. Stafl A, *et al: Obstet Gynecol 43*:118–128, 1974
12. Sherman AI, *et al: Obstet Gynecol 44*:531–545, 1974
13. Gal I, Kirman B, Stern J: *Nature 216*:83, 1967
14. Levy EP, Cohen A, Fraser FC: *Lancet 1*:611, 1973
15. Nora J, Nora A: *Lancet 1*:941–942, 1973
16. Janerich DT, Piper JM, Glebatis DM: *N Engl J Med 291*:697–700, 1974
17. Boston Collaborative Drug Surveillance Program: *N Engl J Med 290*:15–19, 1974
18. Hoover R, *et al: N Engl J Med 295*:401–405, 1976
19. Boston Collaborative Drug Surveillance Program: *Lancet 1*:1399–1404, 1973
20. Daniel DG, Campbell H, Turnbull AC: *Lancet 2*:287–289, 1967
21. The Veterans Administration Cooperative Urological Research Group: *J Urol 98*:516–522, 1967
22. Bailar JC: *Lancet 2*:560, 1967
23. Blackard C, *et al: Cancer 26*:249–256, 1970
24. Royal College of General Practitioners: *J Coll Gen Pract 13*:267–279, 1967
25. Inman WHW, Vessey MP: *Br Med J 2*:193–199, 1968
26. Vessey MP, Doll R: *Br Med J 2*:651–657, 1969
27. Sartwell PE, *et al: Am J Epidemiol 90*:365–380, 1969
28. Collaborative Group for the Study of Stroke in Young Women: *N Engl J Med 288*:871–878, 1973
29. Collaborative Group for the Study of Stroke in Young Women: *JAMA 231*:718–722, 1975
30. Mann JI, Inman WHW: *Br Med J 2*:245–248, 1975
31. Mann JI, *et al: Br Med J 2*:241–245, 1975
32. Inman WHW, *et al: Br Med J 2*:203–209, 1970
33. Stolley PD, *et al: Am J Epidemiol 102*:197–208, 1975
34. Vessey MP, *et al: Br Med J 3*:123–126, 1970
35. Greene GR, Sartwell PE: *Am J Public Health 62*:680–685, 1972
36. Rosenberg L, Armstrong MB, Jick H: *N Engl J Med 294*:1256–1259, 1976
37. Coronary Drug Project Research Group: *JAMA 214*:1303–1313, 1970
38. Baum J, *et al: Lancet 2*:926–928, 1973
39. Mays ET, *et al: JAMA 235*:730–732, 1976
40. Edmondson HA, Henderson B, Benton B: *N Engl J Med 294*:470–472, 1976
41. Pfeffer RI, Van Den Noort S: *Am J Epidemiol 103*:445–456, 1976

Shown in Product Identification Section, page 425

QUARZAN® ℞

[*kwar'zan*]
(clidinium bromide/Roche)
CAPSULES

The following text is complete prescribing information based on official labeling in effect June 1, 1986.

DESCRIPTION

Clidinium bromide is 3-hydroxy-1-methylquinuclidinium bromide benzilate. A white or nearly white crystalline compound, it is soluble in water and has a calculated molecular weight of 432.36.

Clidinium bromide is a quaternary ammonium compound with anticholinergic and antispasmodic activity. Quarzan is available as green and red opaque capsules each containing 2.5 mg clidinium bromide, and green and grey opaque capsules each containing 5 mg clidinium bromide. Each capsule also contains corn starch, lactose and talc. Gelatin capsule shells contain methyl and propyl parabens and potassium sorbate, with the following dye systems: 2.5-mg capsules—FD&C Blue No. 1, FD&C Green No. 3, FD&C Red No. 3, D&C Red No. 33 and D&C Yellow No. 10. 5-mg capsules—FD&C Green No. 3, D&C Red No. 33, FD&C Yellow No. 6 and D&C Yellow No. 10.

ACTIONS

Quarzan inhibits gastrointestinal motility and diminishes gastric acid secretion. Its anticholinergic activity approximates that of atropine sulfate and propantheline bromide.

INDICATIONS

Quarzan is effective as adjunctive therapy in peptic ulcer disease. **Quarzan has not been shown to be effective in contributing to the healing of peptic ulcer, decreasing the rate of recurrence or preventing complications.**

CONTRAINDICATIONS

Known hypersensitivity to clidinium bromide or to other anticholinergic drugs, glaucoma, obstructive uropathy (for example, bladder neck obstruction due to prostatic hypertrophy), obstructive disease of the gastrointestinal tract (for example, pyloroduodenal stenosis), paralytic ileus, intestinal atony of the elderly or debilitated patient, unstable cardiovascular status in acute hemorrhage, severe ulcerative colitis, toxic megacolon complicating ulcerative colitis, myasthenia gravis.

WARNINGS

Quarzan may produce drowsiness or blurred vision. The patient should be cautioned regarding activities requiring mental alertness such as operating a motor vehicle or other machinery or performing hazardous work while taking this drug. In the presence of high environmental temperature, heat prostration (fever and heat stroke) may occur with the use of anticholinergics due to decreased sweating. Diarrhea may be an early symptom of incomplete intestinal obstruction, especially in patients with ileostomy or colostomy. Use of anticholinergics in patients with suspected intestinal obstruction would be inappropriate and possibly harmful. With overdosage, a curare-like action may occur, *i.e.*, neuromuscular blockade leading to muscular weakness and possible paralysis.

Usage in Pregnancy: No controlled studies in humans have been performed to establish the safety of the drug in pregnancy. Uncontrolled data derived from clinical usage have failed to show abnormalities attributable to its use. Reproduction studies in rats have failed to show any impaired fertility or abnormality in the fetuses that might be associated with the use of Quarzan. Use of any drug in pregnancy or in women of childbearing potential requires that the potential benefit of the drug be weighed against the possible hazards to mother and fetus.

Nursing Mothers: As with all anticholinergic drugs, Quarzan may be secreted in human milk and may inhibit lactation. As a general rule, nursing should not be undertaken while a patient is on Quarzan, or the drug should not be used by nursing mothers.

Pediatric Use: Since there is no adequate experience in children who have received this drug, safety and efficacy in children have not been established.

PRECAUTIONS

Use Quarzan with caution in the elderly and in all patients with autonomic neuropathy, hepatic or renal disease, ulcerative colitis— large doses may suppress intestinal motility to the point of producing a paralytic ileus and for this reason precipitate or aggravate "toxic megacolon," a serious complication of the disease; hyperthyroidism; coronary heart disease; congestive heart failure; cardiac tachy-arrhythmias; tachycardia; hypertension; prostatic hypertrophy; hiatal hernia associated with reflux esophagitis, since anticholinergic drugs may aggravate this condition.

ADVERSE REACTIONS

As with other anticholinergic drugs, the most frequently reported adverse effects are dryness of mouth, blurring of vision, urinary hesitancy and constipation. Other adverse effects reported with the use of anticholinergic drugs include decreased sweating, urinary retention, tachycardia, palpitations, dilatation of the pupils, cycloplegia, increased ocular tension, loss of taste, headaches, nervousness, mental confusion, drowsiness, weakness, dizziness, insomnia, nausea, vomiting, bloated feeling, impotence, suppression of lactation and severe allergic reactions or drug idiosyncrasies including anaphylaxis, urticaria and other dermal manifestations.

OVERDOSAGE

The symptoms of overdosage with Quarzan progress from an intensification of the usual side effects to CNS disturbances (from restlessness and excitement to psychotic behavior), circulatory changes (flushing, tachycardia, fall in blood pressure, circulatory failure), respiratory failure, paralysis and coma.

Treatment should consist of: *General measures* —(1) gastric lavage, (2) maintenance of adequate airway, using artificial respiration if needed, (3) administration of i.v. fluids, and (4) for fever: alcohol sponging or ice packs.

Specific measures—(1) Antidotes: physostigmine (Antilirium) 0.5 to 2 mg, i.v., repeated as needed up to a total of 5 mg; or pilocarpine, 5 mg, s.c. at intervals until mouth is moist; neostigmine may also be useful. (2) Against excitement: sodium pentothal 2% may be given i.v. or chloral hydrate (100 to 200 ml, 2% solution) *rectally.* (3) Against hypotension and circulatory collapse: levarterenol (Levophed®) or metaraminol (Aramine) infusions. (4) Against CNS depression: caffeine and sodium benzoate.

The usefulness of dialysis is not known.

DOSAGE AND ADMINISTRATION

For maximum efficacy, dosage should be individualized according to severity of symptoms and occurrence of side effects. The usual dosage is 2.5 to 5 mg three or four times daily before meals and at bedtime. Dosage in excess of 20 mg daily is usually not required to obtain maximum effectiveness. For the aged or debilitated, one 2.5-mg capsule three times daily before meals is recommended. The desired pharmacological effect of the drug is unlikely to be attained without occasional side effects.

DRUG INTERACTIONS

No specific drug interactions are known.

HOW SUPPLIED

Opaque capsules, 2.5 mg, green and red—bottles of 100 (NDC 0140-0119-01); 5 mg, green and grey—bottles of 100 (NDC 0140-0120-01).

Shown in Product Identification Section, page 425

TEL–E–DOSE®

Tel-E-Dose is a unit package designed by Roche for convenience in dispensing medications in the hospital and nursing home. Each unit, sealed against contamination and moisture, is clearly identified by product name and strength and carries the control number and expiration date.

Currently available in this package form are the following products: Dalmane® (flurazepam HCl) capsules, 15 mg, 30 mg; Endep® (amitriptyline HCl) tablets, 10 mg, 25 mg, 50 mg, 75 mg, 100 mg; Librax® (5 mg chlordiazepoxide HCl and 2.5 mg clidinium Br) capsules; Librium® (chlordiazepoxide HCl) capsules, 5 mg, 10 mg, 25 mg; Limbitrol® (5 mg chlordiaxepoxide and 12.5 mg amitriptyline HCl) tablets; Limbitrol® DS (10 mg chlordiazepoxide and 25 mg amitriptyline HCl) tablets; Valium® (diazepam) tablets, 2 mg, 5 mg, 10 mg.

Shown in Product Identification Section, page 425

VALIUM® Injectable ℭ

[val 'ee-um]
(diazepam/Roche)

Valium Injectable is manufactured by Hoffmann-La Roche Inc., Nutley, N.J. 07110 and distributed by Roche Products Inc., Manati, P.R. 00701.

The following text is complete prescribing information based on official labeling in effect June 1, 1986.

DESCRIPTION

Each ml contains 5 mg diazepam/Roche compounded with 40% propylene glycol, 10% ethyl alcohol, 5% sodium benzoate and benzoic acid as buffers, and 1.5% benzyl alcohol as preservative.

Diazepam is a benzodiazepine derivative developed through original Roche research. Chemically, diazepam is 7-chloro-1, 3-dihydro-1-methyl-5-phenyl-2H-1,4-benzodiazepin-2-one. It is a colorless crystalline compound, insoluble in water and has a molecular weight of 284.74.

ACTIONS

In animals, diazepam appears to act on parts of the limbic system, the thalamus and hypothalamus, and induces calming effects. Diazepam, unlike chlorpromazine and reserpine, has no demonstrable peripheral autonomic blocking action, nor does it produce extrapyramidal side effects; however, animals treated with diazepam do have a transient ataxia at higher doses. Diazepam was found to have transient cardiovascular depressor effects in dogs. Long-term experiments in rats revealed no disturbances of endocrine function. Injections into animals have produced localized irritation of tissue surrounding injection sites and some thickening of veins after intravenous use.

INDICATIONS

Valium is indicated for the management of anxiety disorders or for the short-term relief of the symptoms of anxiety. Anxiety or tension associated with the stress of everyday life usually does not require treatment with an anxiolytic.

In acute alcohol withdrawal, Valium may be useful in the symptomatic relief of acute agitation, tremor, impending or acute delirium tremens and hallucinosis.

As an adjunct prior to endoscopic procedures if apprehension, anxiety or acute stress reactions are present, and to diminish the patient's recall of the procedures. (See WARNINGS.)

Valium is a useful adjunct for the relief of skeletal muscle spasm due to reflex spasm to local pathology (such as inflammation of the muscles or joints, or secondary to trauma); spasticity caused by upper motor neuron disorders (such as cerebral palsy and paraplegia); athetosis; stiff-man syndrome; and tetanus.

Injectable Valium is a useful adjunct in status epilepticus and severe recurrent convulsive seizures.

Valium is a useful premedication (the I.M. route is preferred) for relief of anxiety and tension in patients who are to undergo surgical procedures. Intravenously, prior to cardioversion for the relief of anxiety and tension and to diminish the patient's recall of the procedure.

CONTRAINDICATIONS

Injectable Valium is contraindicated in patients with a known hypersensitivity to this drug; acute narrow angle glaucoma; and open angle glaucoma unless patients are receiving appropriate therapy.

WARNINGS

When used intravenously, the following procedures should be undertaken to reduce the possibility of venous thrombosis, phlebitis, local irritation, swelling, and, rarely, vascular impairment: the solution should be injected slowly, taking at least one minute for each 5 mg (1 ml) given; do not use small veins, such as those on the dorsum of the hand or wrist; extreme care should be taken to avoid intra-arterial administration or extravasation.

Do not mix or dilute Valium with other solutions or drugs in syringe or infusion flask. If it is not feasible to administer Valium directly I.V., it may be injected slowly through the infusion tubing as close as possible to the vein insertion.

Extreme care must be used in administering Injectable Valium, particularly by the I.V. route, to the elderly, to very ill patients and to those with limited pulmonary reserve because of the possibility that apnea and/or cardiac arrest may occur. Concomitant use of barbiturates, alcohol or other central nervous system depressants increases depression with increased risk of apnea. Resuscitative equipment including that necessary to support respiration should be readily available.

When Valium is used with a narcotic analgesic, the dosage of the narcotic should be reduced by at least one-third and administered in small increments. In some cases the use of a narcotic may not be necessary.

Injectable Valium should not be administered to patients in shock, coma, or in acute alcoholic intoxication with depression of vital signs. As is true of most CNS-acting drugs, patients receiving Valium should be cautioned against engaging in hazardous occupations requiring complete mental alertness, such as operating machinery or driving a motor vehicle.

Tonic status epilepticus has been precipitated in patients treated with I.V. Valium for petit mal status or petit mal variant status.

Physical and Psychological Dependence: Withdrawal symptoms (similar in character to those noted with barbiturates and alcohol) have occurred following abrupt discontinuance of diazepam (convulsions, tremor, abdominal and muscle cramps, vomiting and sweating). These were usually limited to those patients who had received excessive doses over an extended period of time. Although infrequently seen, milder withdrawal symptoms have also been reported following abrupt discontinuance of benzodiazepines taken continuously, generally at higher therapeutic levels, for at least several months. Consequently, after extended therapy, abrupt discontinuation should generally be avoided and a gradual tapering in dosage followed. Particularly addiction-prone individuals (such as drug addicts or alcoholics) should be under careful surveillance when receiving diazepam or other psychotropic agents because of the predisposition of such patients to habituation and dependence.

***Usage in Pregnancy:* An increased risk of congenital malformations associated with the use of minor tranquilizers (diazepam, meprobamate and chlordiazepoxide) during the first trimester of pregnancy has been suggested in several studies. Because use of these drugs is rarely a matter of urgency, their use during this period should almost always be avoided. The possibility that a woman of childbearing potential may be pregnant at the time of institution of therapy should be considered. Patients should be advised that if they become pregnant during therapy or intend to become pregnant they should communicate with their physicians about the desirability of discontinuing the drug.**

In humans, measurable amounts of diazepam were found in maternal and cord blood, indicating placental transfer of the drug. Until additional information is available, Valium Injectable is not recommended for obstetrical use.

Use in Children: Efficacy and safety of parenteral Valium has not been established in the neonate (30 days or less of age).

Prolonged central nervous system depression has been observed in neonates, apparently due to inability to biotransform Valium into inactive metabolites.

In pediatric use, in order to obtain maximal clinical effect with the minimum amount of drug and thus to reduce the risk of hazardous side effects, such as apnea or prolonged periods of somnolence, it is recommended that the drug be given slowly over a three-minute period in a dosage not to exceed 0.25 mg/kg. After an interval of 15 to 30 minutes the initial dosage can be safely repeated. If, however, relief of symptoms is not obtained after a third administration, adjunctive therapy appropriate to the condition being treated is recommended.

PRECAUTIONS

Although seizures may be brought under control promptly, a significant proportion of patients experience a return to seizure activity, presumably due to the short-lived effect of Valium after I.V. administration. The physician should be prepared to re-administer the drug. However, Valium is not recommended for maintenance, and once seizures are brought under control, consideration should be given to the administration of agents useful in longer term control of seizures.

If Valium is to be combined with other psychotropic agents or anticonvulsant drugs, careful consideration should be given to the pharmacology of the agents to be employed—particularly with known compounds which may potentiate the action of Valium, such as phenothiazines, narcotics, barbiturates, MAO inhibitors and other antidepressants. In highly anxious patients with evidence of accompanying depression, particularly those who may have suicidal tendencies, protective measures may be necessary. The usual precautions in treating patients with impaired hepatic function should be observed. Metabolites of Valium are excreted by the kidney; to avoid their excess accumulation, caution should be exercised in the administration to patients with compromised kidney function.

Since an increase in cough reflex and laryngospasm may occur with peroral endoscopic procedures, the use of a topical anesthetic agent and the availability of necessary countermeasures are recommended.

Until additional information is available, injectable diazepam is not recommended for obstetrical use.

Injectable Valium has produced hypotension or muscular weakness in some patients particularly when used with narcotics, barbiturates or alcohol.

Continued on next page

Roche Products—Cont.

Lower doses (usually 2 mg to 5 mg) should be used for elderly and debilitated patients.
The clearance of Valium and certain other benzodiazepines can be delayed in association with Tagamet (cimetidine) administration. The clinical significance of this is unclear.

ADVERSE REACTIONS

Side effects most commonly reported were drowsiness, fatigue and ataxia; venous thrombosis and phlebitis at the site of injection. Other adverse reactions less frequently reported include: *CNS:* confusion, depression, dysarthria, headache, hypoactivity, slurred speech, syncope, tremor, vertigo. *G.I.:* constipation, nausea. *G.U.:* incontinence, changes in libido, urinary retention. *Cardiovascular:* bradycardia, cardiovascular collapse, hypotension. *EENT:* blurred vision, diplopia, nystagmus. *Skin:* urticaria, skin rash. *Other:* hiccups, changes in salivation, neutropenia, jaundice. Paradoxical reactions such as acute hyperexcited states, anxiety, hallucinations, increased muscle spasticity, insomnia, rage, sleep disturbances and stimulation have been reported; should these occur, use of the drug should be discontinued. Minor changes in EEG patterns, usually low-voltage fast activity, have been observed in patients during and after Valium therapy and are of no known significance.
In peroral endoscopic procedures, coughing, depressed respiration, dyspnea, hyperventilation, laryngospasm and pain in throat or chest have been reported.
Because of isolated reports of neutropenia and jaundice, periodic blood counts and liver function tests are advisable during long-term therapy.

DOSAGE AND ADMINISTRATION

Dosage should be individualized for maximum beneficial effect. The usual recommended dose in older children and adults ranges from 2 mg to 20 mg I.M. or I.V., depending on the indication and its severity. In some conditions, e.g., tetanus, larger doses may be required. (See dosage for specific indications.) In acute conditions the injection may be repeated within one hour although an interval of 3 to 4 hours is usually satisfactory. Lower doses (usually 2 mg to 5 mg) and slow increase in dosage should be used for elderly or debilitated patients and when other sedative drugs are administered. (See WARNINGS and ADVERSE REACTIONS.)
For dosage in infants above the age of 30 days and children, see the specific indications below. When intravenous use is indicated, facilities for respiratory assistance should be readily available.
Intramuscular: Injectable Valium should be injected deeply into the muscle.
Intravenous use: (See WARNINGS, particularly for use in children.) The solution should be injected slowly, taking at least one minute for each 5 mg (1 ml) given. Do not use small veins, such as those on the dorsum of the hand or wrist. Extreme care should be taken to avoid intra-arterial administration or extravasation. Do not mix or dilute Valium with other solutions or drugs in syringe or infusion flask. If it is not feasible to administer Valium directly I.V., it may be injected slowly through the infusion tubing as close as possible to the vein insertion.
[See table right].
Once the acute symptomatology has been properly controlled with Injectable Valium, the patient may be placed on oral therapy with Valium if further treatment is required.

Management of Overdosage:
Manifestations of Valium overdosage include somnolence, confusion, coma, and diminished reflexes. Respiration, pulse and blood pressure should be monitored, as in all cases of drug overdosage, although, in general, these effects have been minimal. General supportive measures should be employed, along with intravenous fluids, and an adequate airway maintained. Hypotension may be combated by the use of Levophed® (levarterenol) or Aramine (metaraminol). Dialysis is of limited value.

HOW SUPPLIED

Ampuls, 2 ml, boxes of 10; Vials, 10 ml, boxes of 1 and 10; Tel-E-Ject® (disposable syringes), 2 ml, boxes of 10.

ANIMAL PHARMACOLOGY

Oral LD_{50} of diazepam is 720 mg/kg in mice and 1240 mg/kg in rats. Intraperitoneal administration of 400 mg/kg to a monkey resulted in death on the sixth day.

Reproduction Studies: A series of rat reproduction studies was performed with diazepam in oral doses of 1, 10, 80 and 100 mg/kg given for periods ranging from 60–228 days prior to mating. At 100 mg/kg there was a decrease in the number of pregnancies and surviving offspring in these rats. These effects may be attributable to prolonged sedative activity, resulting in lack of interest in mating and lessened maternal nursing and care of the young. Neonatal survival of rats at doses lower than 100 mg/kg was within normal limits. Several neonates, both controls and experimentals, in these rat reproduction studies showed skeletal or other defects. Further studies in rats at doses up to and including 80 mg/kg/day did not reveal significant teratological effects on the offspring. Rabbits were maintained on doses of 1, 2, 5 and 8 mg/kg from day 6 through day 18 of gestation. No adverse effects on reproduction and no teratological changes were noted.

RECOMMENDED DOSAGE FOR *INJECTABLE VALIUM* ® (diazepam/Roche)

	USUAL ADULT DOSAGE	DOSAGE RANGE IN CHILDREN **(I.V. administration should be made slowly)**
Moderate Anxiety Disorders and Symptoms of Anxiety	2 mg to 5 mg, I.M. or I.V. Repeat in 3 to 4 hours, if necessary.	
Severe Anxiety Disorders and Symptoms of Anxiety	5 mg to 10 mg, I.M. or I.V. Repeat in 3 to 4 hours, if necessary.	
Acute Alcohol Withdrawal: As an aid in symptomatic relief of acute agitation, tremor, impending or acute delirium tremens and hallucinosis.	10 mg, I.M. or I.V. initially, then 5 mg to 10 mg in 3 to 4 hours, if necessary.	
Endoscopic Procedures: Adjunctively, if apprehension, anxiety or acute stress reactions are present prior to endoscopic procedures. Dosage of narcotics should be reduced by at least a third and in some cases may be omitted. See *Precautions* for peroral procedures.	Titrate I.V. dosage to desired sedative response, such as slurring of speech, with slow administration immediately prior to the procedure. Generally 10 mg or less is adequate, but up to 20 mg I.V. may be given, particularly when concomitant narcotics are omitted. If I.V. cannot be used, 5 mg to 10 mg I.M. approximately 30 minutes prior to the procedure.	
Muscle Spasm: Associated with local pathology, cerebral palsy, athetosis, stiff-man syndrome or tetanus.	5 mg to 10 mg, I.M. or I.V. initially, then 5 mg to 10 mg in 3 to 4 hours, if necessary. For tetanus, larger doses may be required.	For tetanus in infants over 30 days of age, 1 mg to 2 mg I.M. or I.V., slowly, repeated every 3 to 4 hours as necessary. In children 5 years or older, 5 mg to 10 mg repeated every 3 to 4 hours may be required to control tetanus spasms. Respiratory assistance should be available.
Status Epilepticus and Severe Recurrent Convulsive Seizures: In the convulsing patient, the I.V. route is by far preferred. This injection should be administered slowly. However, if I.V. administration is impossible, the I.M. route may be used.	5 mg to 10 mg initially (I.V. preferred). This injection may be repeated if necessary at 10 to 15 minute intervals up to a maximum dose of 30 mg. If necessary, therapy with Valium (diazepam) may be repeated in 2 to 4 hours; however, residual active metabolites may persist, and readministration should be made with this consideration. Extreme caution must be exercised with individuals with chronic lung disease or unstable cardiovascular status.	Infants over 30 days of age and children under 5 years, 0.2 mg to 0.5 mg slowly every 2 to 5 minutes up to a maximum of 5 mg (I.V. preferred). Children 5 years or older, 1 mg every 2 to 5 minutes up to a maximum of 10 mg (slow I.V. administration preferred). Repeat in 2 to 4 hours if necessary. EEG monitoring of the seizure may be helpful.
Preoperative Medication: To relieve anxiety and tension. (If atropine, scopolamine or other premedications are desired, they must be administered in separate syringes.)	10 mg, I.M. (preferred route), before surgery.	
Cardioversion: To relieve anxiety and tension and to reduce recall of procedure.	5 mg to 15 mg, IV., within 5 to 10 minutes prior to the procedure.	

Shown in Product Identification Section, page 425

VALIUM® TABLETS ℞

[val 'ee-um]
(diazepam/Roche)

The following text is complete prescribing information based on official labeling in effect June 1, 1986.

DESCRIPTION

Valium (brand of diazepam/Roche) is a benzodiazepine derivative developed through original Roche research. Chemically, diazepam is 7- chloro - 1,3 - dihydro - 1 - methyl - 5 - phenyl - 2H-1,4-benzodiazepin-2-one. It is a colorless crystalline compound, insoluble in water and has a molecular weight of 284.74.

PHARMACOLOGY

In animals Valium appears to act on parts of the limbic system, the thalamus and hypothalamus, and induces calming effects. Valium, unlike chlorpromazine and reserpine, has no demonstrable peripheral autonomic blocking action, nor does it produce extrapyramidal side effects; however, animals treated with Valium do have a transient ataxia at higher doses. Valium was found to have transient cardiovascular depressor effects in dogs. Long-term experiments in rats revealed no disturbances of endocrine function.

Oral LD_{50} of diazepam is 720 mg/kg in mice and 1240 mg/kg in rats. Intraperitoneal administration of 400 mg/kg to a monkey resulted in death on the sixth day.

Reproduction Studies: A series of rat reproduction studies was performed with diazepam in oral doses of 1, 10, 80 and 100 mg/kg. At 100 mg/kg there was a decrease in the number of pregnancies and surviving offspring in these rats. Neonatal survival of rats at doses lower than 100 mg/kg was within normal limits. Several neonates in these rat reproduction studies showed skeletal or other defects. Further studies in rats at doses up to and including 80 mg/kg/day did not reveal teratological effects on the offspring.

In humans, measurable blood levels of Valium were obtained in maternal and cord blood, indicating placental transfer of the drug.

INDICATIONS

Valium is indicated for the management of anxiety disorders or for the short-term relief of the symptoms of anxiety. Anxiety or tension associated with the stress of everyday life usually does not require treatment with an anxiolytic.

In acute alcohol withdrawal, Valium may be useful in the symptomatic relief of acute agitation, tremor, impending or acute delirium tremens and hallucinosis.

Valium is a useful adjunct for the relief of skeletal muscle spasm due to reflex spasm to local pathology (such as inflammation of the muscles or joints, or secondary to trauma); spasticity caused by upper motor neuron disorders (such as cerebral palsy and paraplegia); athetosis; and stiff-man syndrome.

Oral Valium may be used adjunctively in convulsive disorders, although it has not proved useful as the sole therapy.

The effectiveness of Valium in long-term use, that is, more than 4 months, has not been assessed by systematic clinical studies. The physician should periodically reassess the usefulness of the drug for the individual patient.

CONTRAINDICATIONS

Valium is contraindicated in patients with a known hypersensitivity to this drug and, because of lack of sufficient clinical experience, in children under 6 months of age. It may be used in patients with open angle glaucoma who are receiving appropriate therapy, but is contraindicated in acute narrow angle glaucoma.

WARNINGS

Valium is not of value in the treatment of psychotic patients and should not be employed in lieu of appropriate treatment.

As is true of most preparations containing CNS-acting drugs, patients receiving Valium should be cautioned against engaging in hazardous occupations requiring complete mental alertness such as operating machinery or driving a motor vehicle.

As with other agents which have anticonvulsant activity, when Valium is used as an adjunct in treating convulsive disorders, the possibility of an increase in the frequency and/or severity of grand mal seizures may require an increase in the dosage of standard anticonvulsant medication. Abrupt withdrawal of Valium in such cases may also be associated with a temporary increase in the frequency and/or severity of seizures.

Since Valium has a central nervous system depressant effect, patients should be advised against the simultaneous ingestion of alcohol and other CNS-depressant drugs during Valium therapy.

Physical and Psychological Dependence: Withdrawal symptoms (similar in character to those noted with barbiturates and alcohol) have occurred following abrupt discontinuance of diazepam (convulsions, tremor, abdominal and muscle cramps, vomiting and sweating). These were usually limited to those patients who had received excessive doses over an extended period of time. Although infrequently seen, milder withdrawal symptoms have also been reported following abrupt discontinuance of benzodiazepines taken continuously, generally at higher therapeutic levels, for at least several months. Consequently, after extended therapy, abrupt discontinuation should generally be avoided and a gradual tapering in dosage followed. Particularly addiction-prone individuals (such as drug addicts or alcoholics) should be under careful surveillance when receiving diazepam or other psychotropic agents because of the predisposition of such patients to habituation and dependence.

Usage in Pregnancy: **An increased risk of congenital malformations associated with the use of minor tranquilizers (diazepam, meprobamate and chlordiazepoxide) during the first trimester of pregnancy has been suggested in several studies. Because use of these drugs is rarely a matter of urgency, their use during this period should almost always be avoided. The possibility that a woman of childbearing potential may be pregnant at the time of institution of therapy should be considered. Patients should be advised that if they become pregnant during therapy or intend to become pregnant they should communicate with their physicians about the desirability of discontinuing the drug.**

Management of Overdosage: Manifestations of Valium overdosage include somnolence, confusion, coma and diminished reflexes. Respiration, pulse and blood pressure should be monitored, as in all cases of drug overdosage, although, in general, these effects have been minimal following overdosage. General supportive measures should be employed, along with immediate gastric lavage. Intravenous fluids should be administered and an adequate airway maintained. Hypotension may be combated by the use of Levophed® (levarterenol) or Aramine (metaraminol). Dialysis is of limited value. As with the management of intentional overdosage with any drug, it should be borne in mind that multiple agents may have been ingested.

PRECAUTIONS

If Valium is to be combined with other psychotropic agents or anticonvulsant drugs, careful consideration should be given to the pharmacology of the agents to be employed—particularly with known compounds which may potentiate the action of Valium, such as phenothiazines, narcotics, barbiturates, MAO inhibitors and other antidepressants. The usual precautions are indicated for severely depressed patients or those in whom there is any evidence of latent depression; particularly the recognition that suicidal tendencies may be present and protective measures may be necessary. The usual precautions in treating patients with impaired renal or hepatic function should be observed.

In elderly and debilitated patients, it is recommended that the dosage be limited to the smallest effective amount to preclude the development of ataxia or oversedation (2 mg to 2½ mg once or twice daily, initially, to be increased gradually as needed and tolerated).

The clearance of Valium and certain other benzodiazepines can be delayed in association with Tagamet (cimetidine) administration. The clinical significance of this is unclear.

ADVERSE REACTIONS

Side effects most commonly reported were drowsiness, fatigue and ataxia. Infrequently encountered were confusion, constipation, depression, diplopia, dysarthria, headache, hypotension, incontinence, jaundice, changes in libido, nausea, changes in salivation, skin rash, slurred speech, tremor, urinary retention, vertigo and blurred vision. Paradoxical reactions such as acute hyperexcited states, anxiety, hallucinations, increased muscle spasticity, insomnia, rage, sleep disturbances and stimulation have been reported; should these occur, use of the drug should be discontinued.

Because of isolated reports of neutropenia and jaundice, periodic blood counts and liver function tests are advisable during long-term therapy. Minor changes in EEG patterns, usually low-voltage fast activity, have been observed in patients during and after Valium therapy and are of no known significance.

DOSAGE AND ADMINISTRATION

Dosage should be individualized for maximum beneficial effect. While the usual daily dosages given below will meet the needs of most patients, there will be some who may require higher doses. In such cases dosage should be increased cautiously to avoid adverse effects.

	USUAL DAILY DOSE
Adults:	
Management of Anxiety Disorders and Relief of Symptoms of Anxiety	Depending upon severity of symptoms—2 mg to 10 mg, 2 to 4 times daily
Symptomatic Relief in Acute Alcohol Withdrawal.	10 mg, 3 or 4 times during the first 24 hours, reducing to 5 mg, 3 or 4 times daily as needed
Adjunctively for Relief of Skeletal Muscle Spasm.	2 mg to 10 mg, 3 or 4 times daily
Adjunctively in Convulsive Disorders.	2 mg to 10 mg, 2 to 4 times daily
Geriatric Patients, or in the presence of debilitating disease.	2 mg to 2½ mg, 1 or 2 times daily initially; increase gradually as needed and tolerated
Children:	
Because of varied responses to CNS-acting drugs, initiate therapy with lowest dose and increase as required. Not for use in children under 6 months.	1 mg to 2½ mg, 3 or 4 times daily initially; increase gradually as needed and tolerated

HOW SUPPLIED

For oral administration, round, scored tablets with a cut out "V" design—2 mg, white; 5 mg, yellow; 10 mg, blue—bottles of 100 and 500; Prescription Paks of 50, available in trays of 10. Tel-E-Dose® packages of 100, available in boxes of 4 reverse-numbered cards of 25, and in boxes containing 10 strips of 10.

Imprint on tablets:

2 mg:
2 VALIUM® (front)
ROCHE (scored side)

5 mg:
5 VALIUM® (front)
ROCHE (scored side)

10 mg:
10 VALIUM® (front)
ROCHE (scored side)

Shown in Product Identification Section, page 425

Roerig

A division of Pfizer Pharmaceuticals
235 EAST 42nd STREET
NEW YORK, NY 10017

Product Identification Codes

To provide quick and positive identification of Roerig Division products, we have imprinted the product identification number of the National Drug Code on most tablets and capsules.

In order that you may quickly identify a product by its code number, we have compiled below a numerical list of code numbers with their corresponding product names. We are also listing the code numbers by alphabetical order of products.

Numerical Listing

Product Ident. Number	Product
035	**Spectrobid® (bacampicillin HCl) Tablets, 400 mg., equivalent to 280 mg. ampicillin**
092	**Urobiotic®-250 (oxytetracycline HCl 250 mg. with sulfamethizole 250 mg. and phenazopyridine 50 mg.) Capsules**
143	**Geocillin® (carbenicillin indanyl sodium) Tablets, equivalent to 382 mg. carbenicillin**
159	**TAO® (troleandomycin) Capsules, 250 mg.**
210	**Antivert® (meclizine HCl) Tablets, 12.5 mg.**
211	**Antivert® /25 (meclizine HCl) Tablets, 25 mg.**
212	**Antivert® /25 (meclizine HCl) Chewable Tablets**
214	**Antivert® /50 (meclizine HCl) Tablets, 50 mg.**
254	**Marax® (ephedrine sulfate, 25 mg; theophylline, 130 mg; and Atarax® [hydroxyzine HCl], 10 mg) Tablets**
411	**Glucotrol® (glipizide) Tablets, 5 mg.**
412	**Glucotrol® (glipizide) Tablets, 10 mg.**
504	**Heptuna® plus (iron plus vitamins and minerals), Capsules.**
534	**Sinequan® (doxepin HCl) Capsules 10 mg.**
535	**Sinequan® (doxepin HCl) Capsules 25 mg.**
536	**Sinequan® (doxepin HCl) Capsules 50 mg.**
537	**Sinequan® (doxepin HCl) Capsules 150 mg.**
538	**Sinequan® (doxepin HCl) Casules 100 mg.**
539	**Sinequan® (doxepin HCl) Capsules 75 mg.**
214	**Antivert® /50 (meclizine HCl) Tablets, 50 mg.**
560	**Atarax® (hydroxyzine HCl) Tablets, 10 mg.**

Continued on next page

Roerig—Cont.

561 Atarax® (hydroxyzine HCl) Tablets, 25 mg.
562 Atarax® (hydroxyzine HCl) Tablets, 50 mg.
563 Atarax® (hydroxyzine HCl) Tablets, 100 mg.
571 Navane® (thiothixene) Capsules, 1 mg.
572 Navane® (thiothixene) Capsules, 2 mg.
573 Navane® (thiothixene) Capsules, 5 mg.
574 Navane® (thiothixene) Capsules, 10 mg.
577 Navane® (thiothixene) Capsules, 20 mg.

Alphabetical Listing

Prod. Ident. Number	Product
210	Antivert® (meclizine HCl) Tablets, 12.5 mg.
211	Antivert® /25 (meclizine HCl) Tablets, 25 mg.
212	Antivert® /25 (meclizine HCl) Chewable Tablets
214	Antivert® /50 (meclizine HCl) Tablets, 50 mg.
560	Atarax® (hydroxyzine HCl) Tablets, 10 mg.
561	Atarax® (hydroxyzine HCl) Tablets, 25 mg.
562	Atarax® (hydroxyzine HCl) Tablets, 50 mg.
563	Atarax® (hydroxyzine HCl) Tablets, 100 mg.
143	Geocillin® (carbenicillin indanyl sodium) Tablets equivalent to 382 mg. carbenicillin
411	Glucotrol® (glipizide) Tablets, 5 mg.
412	Glucotrol® (glipizide) Tablets, 10 mg.
504	Heptuna® plus (iron plus vitamins and minerals), Capsules.
254	Marax® (ephedrine sulfate, 25 mg; theophylline, 130 mg; and Atarax® [hydroxyzine HCl], 10 mg) Tablets
571	Navane® (thiothixene) Capsules, 1 mg.
572	Navane® (thiothixene) Capsules, 2 mg.
573	Navane® (thiothixene) Capsules, 5 mg.
574	Navane® (thiothixene) Capsules, 10 mg.
577	Navane® (thiothixene) Capsules, 20 mg.
534	Sinequan® (doxepin HCl) Capsules 10 mg.
535	Sinequan® (doxepin HCl) Capsules 25 mg.
536	Sinequan® (doxepin HCl) Capsules 50 mg.
539	Sinequan® (doxepin HCl) Capsules 75 mg.
538	Sinequan® (doxepin HCl) Capsules 100 mg.
537	Sinequan® (doxepin HCl) Capsules 150 mg.
035	Spectrobid® (bacampicillin HCl) Tablets, 400 mg., equivalent to 280 mg. ampicillin
159	TAO® (troleandomycin) Capsules, 250 mg.
092	Urobiotic®-250 (oxytetracycline HCl 250 mg. with sulfamethizole 250 mg. and phenazopyridine 50 mg.) Capsules

ANTIVERT® TABLETS ℞
[*ăn 'tĭ-vert "*]
(12.5 mg. meclizine HCl)
ANTIVERT®/25 TABLETS ℞
(25 mg. meclizine HCl)
ANTIVERT®/25 CHEWABLE TABLETS ℞
(25 mg. meclizine HCl)
ANTIVERT®/50 TABLETS ℞
(50 mg. meclizine HCl)

DESCRIPTION
Chemically, Antivert (meclizine HCl) is 1-(*p*-chloro-α-phenylbenzyl)-4-(*m*-methylbenzyl) piperazine dihydrochloride monohydrate.

ACTIONS
Antivert is an antihistamine which shows marked protective activity against nebulized histamine and lethal doses of intravenously injected histamine in guinea pigs. It has a marked effect in blocking the vasodepressor response to histamine, but only a slight blocking action against acetylcholine. Its activity is relatively weak in inhibiting the spasmogenic action of histamine on isolated guinea pig ileum.

INDICATIONS
Based on a review of this drug by the National Academy of Sciences-National Research Council and/or other information, FDA has classified the indications as follows:
Effective: Management of nausea and vomiting, and dizziness associated with motion sickness.
Possibly Effective: Management of vertigo associated with diseases affecting the vestibular system.
Final classification of the less than effective indications requires further investigation.

CONTRAINDICATIONS
Meclizine HCl is contraindicated in individuals who have shown a previous hypersensitivity to it.

WARNINGS
Since drowsiness may, on occasion, occur with use of this drug, patients should be warned of this possibility and cautioned against driving a car or operating dangerous machinery.
Patients should avoid alcoholic beverages while taking the drug. Due to its potential anticholinergic action, this drug should be used with caution in patients with asthma, glaucoma, or enlargement of the prostate gland.
USAGE IN CHILDREN:
Clinical studies establishing safety and effectiveness in children have not been done; therefore, usage is not recommended in children under 12 years of age.
USAGE IN PREGNANCY:
Pregnancy Category B. Reproduction studies in rats have shown cleft palates at 25–50 times the human dose. Epidemiological studies in pregnant women, however, do not indicate that meclizine increases the risk of abnormalities when administered during pregnancy. Despite the animal findings, it would appear that the possibility of fetal harm is remote. Nevertheless, meclizine, or any other medication, should be used during pregnancy only if clearly necessary.

ADVERSE REACTIONS
Drowsiness, dry mouth and, on rare occasions, blurred vision have been reported.

DOSAGE AND ADMINISTRATION
Vertigo:
For the control of vertigo associated with diseases affecting the vestibular system, the recommended dose is 25 to 100 mg. daily, in divided dosage, depending upon clinical response.
Motion Sickness:
The initial dose of 25 to 50 mg. of Antivert should be taken one hour prior to embarkation for protection against motion sickness. Thereafter, the dose may be repeated every 24 hours for the duration of the journey.

HOW SUPPLIED
Antivert—12.5 mg. tablets: Bottles of 100, 1000 and unit dose 100's.
Antivert/25—25 mg. tablets: Bottles of 100, 1000 and unit dose 100's.
Antivert/25 Chewable Tablets—25 mg. pink scored tablets: Bottles of 100 and 500.
Antivert/50—50 mg. tablets: Bottles of 100.

69-2148-37-6

Shown in Product Identification Section, page 425

ATARAX® ℞
[*ăt 'ă-raks "*]
(hydroxyzine hydrochloride)
TABLETS AND SYRUP

DESCRIPTION
Hydroxyzine hydrochloride is designated chemically as 1-(p-chlorobenzhydryl) 4-[2-(2-hydroxyethoxy)-ethyl] piperazine dihydrochloride.

CLINICAL PHARMACOLOGY
Atarax is unrelated chemically to the phenothiazines, reserpine, meprobamate, or the benzodiazepines.
Atarax is not a cortical depressant, but its action may be due to a suppression of activity in certain key regions of the subcortical area of the central nervous system. Primary skeletal muscle relaxation has been demonstrated experimentally. Bronchodilator activity, and antihistaminic and analgesic effects have been demonstrated experimentally and confirmed clinically. An antiemetic effect, both by the apomorphine test and the veriloid test, has been demonstrated. Pharmacological and clinical studies indicate that hydroxyzine in therapeutic dosage does not increase gastric secretion or acidity and in most cases has mild antisecretory activity. Hydroxyzine is rapidly absorbed from the gastrointestinal tract and Atarax's clinical effects are usually noted within 15 to 30 minutes after oral administration.

INDICATIONS
For symptomatic relief of anxiety and tension associated with psychoneurosis and as an adjunct in organic disease states in which anxiety is manifested.
Useful in the management of pruritus due to allergic conditions such as chronic urticaria and atopic and contact dermatoses, and in histamine-mediated pruritus.
As a sedative when used as premedication and following general anesthesia. **Hydroxyzine may potentiate meperidine (Demerol®) and barbiturates,** so their use in pre-anesthetic adjunctive therapy should be modified on an individual basis. Atropine and other belladonna alkaloids are not affected by the drug. Hydroxyzine is not known to interfere with the action of digitalis in any way and it may be used concurrently with this agent.
The effectiveness of hydroxyzine as an antianxiety agent for long term use, that is more than 4 months, has not been assessed by systematic clinical studies. The physician should reassess periodically the usefulness of the drug for the individual patient.

CONTRAINDICATIONS
Hydroxyzine, when administered to the pregnant mouse, rat, and rabbit, induced fetal abnormalities in the rat and mouse at doses substantially above the human therapeutic range. Clinical data in human beings are inadequate to establish safety in early pregnancy. Until such data are available, hydroxyzine is contraindicated in early pregnancy.
Hydroxyzine is contraindicated for patients who have shown a previous hypersensitivity to it.

WARNINGS
Nursing Mothers: It is not known whether this drug is excreted in human milk. Since many drugs are so excreted, hydroxyzine should not be given to nursing mothers.

PRECAUTIONS
THE POTENTIATING ACTION OF HYDROXYZINE MUST BE CONSIDERED WHEN THE DRUG IS USED IN CONJUNCTION WITH CENTRAL NERVOUS SYSTEM DEPRESSANTS SUCH AS NARCOTICS, NON-NARCOTIC ANALGESICS AND BARBITURATES. Therefore when central nervous system depressants are administered concomitantly with hydroxyzine their dosage should be reduced. Since drowsiness may occur with use of this drug, patients should be warned of this possibility and cautioned against driving a car or operating dangerous machinery while taking Atarax. Patients should be advised against the simultaneous use of other CNS depressant drugs, and cautioned that the effect of alcohol may be increased.

ADVERSE REACTIONS
Side effects reported with the administration of Atarax (hydroxyzine hydrochloride) are usually mild and transitory in nature.
Anticholinergic: Dry mouth.
Central Nervous System: Drowsiness is usually transitory and may disappear in a few days of continued therapy or upon reduction of the dose. Involuntary motor activity including rare instances of tremor and convulsions have been reported, usually with doses considerably higher than those recommended. Clinically significant respiratory depression has not been reported at recommended doses.

OVERDOSAGE
The most common manifestation of Atarax overdosage is hypersedation. As in the management of overdosage with any drug, it should be borne in mind that multiple agents may have been taken.

If vomiting has not occurred spontaneously, it should be induced. Immediate gastric lavage is also recommended. General supportive care, including frequent monitoring of the vital signs and close observation of the patient, is indicated. Hypotension, though unlikely, may be controlled with intravenous fluids and Levophed® (levarterenol), or Aramine® (metaraminol). Do not use epinephrine as Atarax counteracts its pressor action.

There is no specific antidote. It is doubtful that hemodialysis would be of any value in the treatment of overdosage with hydroxyzine. However, if other agents such as barbiturates have been ingested concomitantly, hemodialysis may be indicated. There is no practical method to quantitate hydroxyzine in body fluids or tissue after its ingestion or administration.

DOSAGE

For symptomatic relief of anxiety and tension associated with psychoneurosis and as an adjunct in organic disease states in which anxiety is manifested: in adults, 50–100 mg q.i.d.: children under 6 years, 50 mg daily in divided doses and over 6 years, 50–100 mg daily in divided doses.

For use in the management of pruritus due to allergic conditions such as chronic urticaria and atopic and contact dermatoses, and in histamine-mediated pruritus: in adults, 25 mg t.i.d. or q.i.d.; children under 6 years, 50 mg daily in divided doses and over 6 years, 50–100 mg daily in divided doses.

As a sedative when used as a premedication and following general anesthesia: 50–100 mg in adults, and 0.6 mg/kg in children.

When treatment is initiated by the intramuscular route of administration, subsequent doses may be administered orally.

As with all medications, the dosage should be adjusted according to the patient's response to therapy.

SUPPLY

Atarax Tablets

10 mg: 100's (NDC 0049-5600-66), 500's (NDC 0049-5600-73), Unit Dose 10 × 10's (NDC 0049-5600-41), and Unit of Use 40's (NDC 0049-5600-43)—orange tablets

25 mg: 100's (NDC 0049-5610-66), 500's (NDC 0049-5610-73), Unit Dose 10 × 10's (NDC 0049-5610-41), and Unit of Use 40's (NDC 0049-5610-43)—green tablets

50 mg: 100's (NDC 0049-5620-66), 500's (NDC 0049-5620-73), and Unit Dose 10 × 10's (NDC 0049-5620-41)—yellow tablets

Atarax 100 Tablets

100 mg: 100's (NDC 0049-5630-66), and Unit Dose 10 × 10's (NDC 0049-5630-41)—red tablets

Atarax Syrup

10 mg per teaspoon (5 ml): 1 pint bottles (NDC 0049-5590-93)

Alcohol Content—Ethyl Alcohol—0.5% v/v

BIBLIOGRAPHY

Available on request.

60-0618-00-3

Shown in Product Identification Section, page 425

CEFOBID® ℞

[sĕf'ō-bĭd]

(cefoperazone sodium and cefoperazone sodium injection)

For Intravenous or Intramuscular Use

DESCRIPTION

CEFOBID (cefoperazone sodium) is a sterile, semisynthetic, broad-spectrum, parenteral cephalosporin antibiotic for intravenous or intramuscular administration. It is the sodium salt of 7-[D(-)-α-(4-ethyl-2,3-dioxo-1-piperazine-carboxamido)-α-(4-hydroxyphenyl)acetamido]-3-[(1-methyl-1H-tetrazol-5-yl)thiomethyl]-3-cephem-4-carboxylic acid. Its chemical formula is $C_{25}H_{26}N_9NaO_8S_2$ with a molecular weight of 667.65. The structural formula is given below:

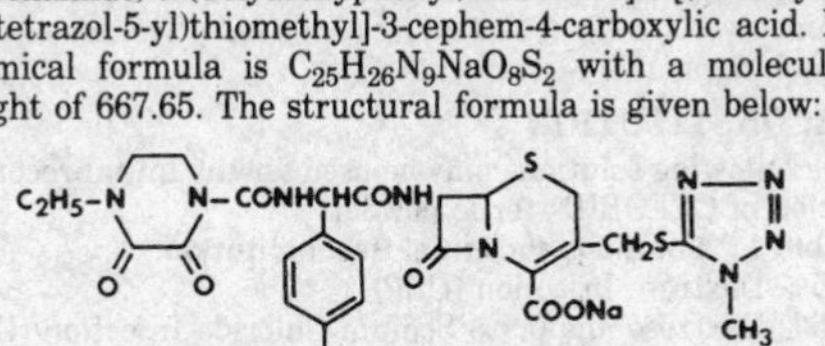

CEFOBID contains 34 mg sodium (1.5 mEq) per gram. CEFOBID is a white powder which is freely soluble in water. The pH of a 25% (w/v) freshly reconstituted solution varies between 4.5–6.5 and the solution ranges from colorless to straw yellow depending on the concentration.

CEFOBID in crystalline form is supplied in vials equivalent to 1 g or 2 g of cefoperazone and in Piggyback Units for intravenous administration equivalent to 1 g or 2 g cefoperazone. CEFOBID is also supplied premixed as a frozen, sterile, nonpyrogenic, iso-osmotic solution equivalent to 2 g cefoperazone in plastic containers. After thawing, the solution is intended for intravenous use.

The plastic container is fabricated from specially formulated polyvinyl chloride. Solutions in contact with the plastic container can leach out certain of its chemical components in very small amounts within the expiration period, e.g., di 2-ethylhexyl phthalate (DEHP), up to 5 parts per million. However, the safety of the plastic has been confirmed in tests in animals according to the USP biological tests for plastic containers, as well as by tissue culture toxicity studies.

TABLE 1. Cefoperazone Serum Concentrations

	Mean Serum Concentrations (mcg/ml)							
Dose/Route	0*	0.5 hr	1 hr	2 hr	4 hr	8 hr	12 hr
1 g IV	153	114	73	38	16	4	0.5
2 g IV	252	153	114	70	32	8	2
3 g IV	340	210	142	89	41	9	2
4 g IV	506	325	251	161	71	19	6
1 g IM	32**	52	65	57	33	7	1
2 g IM	40**	69	93	97	58	14	4

*Hours post-administration, with 0 time being the end of the infusion.
**Values obtained 15 minutes post-injection.

CLINICAL PHARMACOLOGY

High serum and bile levels of CEFOBID are attained after a single dose of the drug. Table 1 demonstrates the serum concentrations of CEFOBID in normal volunteers following either a single 15-minute constant rate intravenous infusion of 1, 2, 3 or 4 grams of the drug, or a single intramuscular injection of 1 or 2 grams of the drug.

[See table above].

The mean serum half-life of CEFOBID is approximately 2.0 hours, independent of the route of administration.

In vitro studies with human serum indicate that the degree of CEFOBID reversible protein binding varies with the serum concentration from 93% at 25 mcg/ml of CEFOBID to 90% at 250 mcg/ml and 82% at 500 mcg/ml.

CEFOBID achieves therapeutic concentrations in the following body tissues and fluids:

Tissue or Fluid	Dose	Concentration
Ascitic Fluid	2 g	64 mcg/ml
Cerebrospinal Fluid (in patients with inflamed meninges)	50 mg/kg	1.8 mcg/ml to 8.0 mcg/ml
Urine	2 g	3,286 mcg/ml
Sputum	3 g	6.0 mcg/ml
Endometrium	2 g	74 mcg/g
Myometrium	2 g	54 mcg/g
Palatine Tonsil	1 g	8 mcg/g
Sinus Mucous Membrane	1 g	8 mcg/g
Umbilical Cord Blood	1 g	25 mcg/ml
Amniotic Fluid	1 g	4.8 mcg/ml
Lung	1 g	28 mcg/g
Bone	2 g	40 mcg/g

CEFOBID is excreted mainly in the bile. Maximum bile concentrations are generally obtained between one and three hours following drug administration and exceed concurrent serum concentrations by up to 100 times. Reported biliary concentrations of CEFOBID range from 66 mcg/ml at 30 minutes to as high as 6000 mcg/ml at 3 hours after an intravenous bolus injection of 2 grams.

Following a single intramuscular or intravenous dose, the urinary recovery of CEFOBID over a 12-hour period averages 20–30%. No significant quantity of metabolites has been found in the urine. Urinary concentrations greater than 2200 mcg/ml have been obtained following a 15-minute infusion of a 2 g dose. After an IM injection of 2 g, peak urine concentrations of almost 1000 mcg/ml have been obtained, and therapeutic levels are maintained for 12 hours.

Repeated administration of CEFOBID at 12-hour intervals does not result in accumulation of the drug in normal subjects. Peak serum concentrations, areas under the curve (AUC's), and serum half-lives in patients with severe renal insufficiency are not significantly different from those in normal volunteers. In patients with hepatic dysfunction, the serum half-life is prolonged and urinary excretion is increased. In patients with combined renal and hepatic insufficiencies, CEFOBID may accumulate in the serum.

CEFOBID has been used in pediatrics, but the safety and effectiveness in children have not been established. The half-life of CEFOBID in serum is 6–10 hours in low birth-weight neonates.

Microbiology

CEFOBID is active *in vitro* against a wide range of aerobic and anaerobic, gram-positive and gram-negative pathogens. The bactericidal action of CEFOBID results from the inhibition of bacterial cell wall synthesis. CEFOBID has a high degree of stability in the presence of beta-lactamases produced by most gram-negative pathogens. CEFOBID is usually active against organisms which are resistant to other beta-lactam antibiotics because of beta-lactamase production. CEFOBID is usually active against the following organisms *in vitro* and in clinical infections:

Gram-Positive Aerobes:

Staphylococcus aureus, penicillinase and non-penicillinase-producing strains
Staphylococcus epidermidis
Streptococcus pneumoniae (formerly *Diplococcus pneumoniae*)
Streptococcus pyogenes (Group A beta-hemolytic streptococci)
Streptococcus agalactiae (Group B beta-hemolytic streptococci)
Enterococcus (*Streptococcus faecalis, S. faecium* and *S. durans*)

Gram-Negative Aerobes:

Escherichia coli
Klebsiella species (including *K. pneumoniae*)
Enterobacter species
Citrobacter species
Haemophilus influenzae
Proteus mirabilis
Proteus vulgaris
Morganella morganii (formerly *Proteus morganii*)
Providencia stuartii
Providencia rettgeri (formerly *Proteus rettgeri*)
Serratia marcescens
Pseudomonas aeruginosa
Pseudomonas species
Some strains of *Acinetobacter calcoaceticus*
Neisseria gonorrhoeae

Anaerobic Organisms:

Gram-positive cocci (including *Peptococcus* and *Peptostreptococcus*)
Clostridium species
Bacteroides fragilis
Other *Bacteroides* species

CEFOBID is also active *in vitro* against a wide variety of other pathogens although the clinical significance is unknown. These organisms include: *Salmonella* and *Shigella* species, *Serratia liquefaciens, N. meningitidis, Bordetella pertussis, Yersinia enterocolitica, Clostridium difficile, Fusobacterium* species, *Eubacterium* species and beta-lactamase producing strains of *H. influenzae* and *N. gonorrhoeae.*

Susceptibility Testing:

Diffusion Technique. For the disk diffusion method of susceptibility testing, a 75 mcg CEFOBID diffusion disk should be used. Organisms should be tested with the CEFOBID 75 mcg disk since CEFOBID has been shown *in vitro* to be active against organisms which are found to be resistant to other beta-lactam antibiotics.

Tests should be interpreted by the following criteria:

Zone Diameter	Interpretation
Greater than or equal to 21 mm	Susceptible
16–20 mm	Moderately Susceptible
Less than or equal to 15 mm	Resistant

Quantitative procedures that require measurement of zone diameters give the most precise estimate of susceptibility. One such method which has been recommended for use with the CEFOBID 75 mcg disk is the NCCLS approved standard. (Performance Standards for Antimicrobic Disc Susceptibility Tests. Second Information Supplement Vol. 2 No. 2 pp. 49–69. Publisher—National Committee for Clinical Laboratory Standards, Villanova, Pennsylvania.)

A report of "susceptible" indicates that the infecting organism is likely to respond to CEFOBID therapy and a report of "resistant" indicates that the infecting organism is not likely to respond to therapy. A "moderately susceptible" report suggests that the infecting organism will be susceptible to CEFOBID if a higher than usual dosage is used or if the infection is confined to tissues and fluids (e.g., urine or bile) in which high antibiotic levels are attained.

Dilution Techniques. Broth or agar dilution methods may be used to determine the minimal inhibitory concentration (MIC) of CEFOBID. Serial twofold dilutions of CEFOBID should be prepared in either broth or agar. Broth should be inoculated to contain 5×10^5 organisms/ml and agar "spotted" with 10^4 organisms.

Continued on next page

Roerig—Cont.

MIC test results should be interpreted in light of serum, tissue, and body fluid concentrations of CEFOBID. Organisms inhibited by CEFOBID at 16 mcg/ml or less are considered susceptible, while organisms with MIC's of 17–63 mcg/ml are moderately susceptible. Organisms inhibited at CEFOBID concentrations of greater than or equal to 64 mcg/ml are considered resistant, although clinical cures have been obtained in some patients infected by such organisms.

INDICATIONS AND USAGE

CEFOBID is indicated for the treatment of the following infections when caused by susceptible organisms:

Respiratory Tract Infections caused by *S. pneumoniae, H. influenzae, S. aureus* (penicillinase and non-penicillinase producing strains), *S. pyogenes* (Group A beta-hemolytic streptococci), *P. aeruginosa, Klebsiella pneumoniae, E. coli, Proteus* species (indole-positive and indole-negative), and *Enterobacter* species.

Peritonitis and Other Intra-abdominal Infections caused by *E. coli, P. aeruginosa*, enterococci, anaerobic gram-positive cocci, and anaerobic gram-positive and gram-negative bacilli (including *Bacteroides fragilis*).

Bacterial Septicemia caused by *S. pneumoniae, S. pyogenes, S. agalactiae, S. aureus*, enterococci, *H. influenzae, Pseudomonas aeruginosa, E. coli, Klebsiella* spp., *Proteus* species (indole-positive and indole-negative), *Clostridium* spp. and anaerobic gram-positive cocci.

Infections of the Skin and Skin Structures caused by *S. aureus* (penicillinase and non-penicillinase producing strains), *S. pyogenes* and *P. aeruginosa.*

Pelvic Inflammatory Disease, Endometritis, and Other Infections of the Female Genital Tract caused by *N. gonorrhoeae, S. aureus* and *S. epidermidis, S. agalactiae, E. coli, Clostridium* spp., *Bacteroides* species (including *Bacteroides fragilis*) and anaerobic gram-positive cocci.

Urinary Tract Infections caused by *Enterococcus, Escherichia coli*, and *Pseudomonas aeruginosa.*

Susceptibility Testing

Before instituting treatment with CEFOBID, appropriate specimens should be obtained for isolation of the causative organism and for determination of its susceptibility to the drug. Treatment may be started before results of susceptibility testing are available.

Combination Therapy

Synergy between CEFOBID and aminoglycosides has been demonstrated with many gram-negative bacilli. However, such enhanced activity of these combinations is not predictable. If such therapy is considered, *in vitro* susceptibility tests should be performed to determine the activity of the drugs in combination, and renal function should be monitored carefully. (See PRECAUTIONS, and DOSAGE AND ADMINISTRATION sections).

CONTRAINDICATIONS

CEFOBID is contraindicated in patients with known allergy to the cephalosporin-class of antibiotics.

WARNINGS

BEFORE THERAPY WITH CEFOBID IS INSTITUTED, CAREFUL INQUIRY SHOULD BE MADE TO DETERMINE WHETHER THE PATIENT HAS HAD PREVIOUS HYPERSENSITIVITY REACTIONS TO CEPHALOSPORINS, PENICILLINS OR OTHER DRUGS. THIS PRODUCT SHOULD BE GIVEN CAUTIOUSLY TO PENICILLIN-SENSITIVE PATIENTS. ANTIBIOTICS SHOULD BE ADMINISTERED WITH CAUTION TO ANY PATIENT WHO HAS DEMONSTRATED SOME FORM OF ALLERGY, PARTICULARLY TO DRUGS. SERIOUS ACUTE HYPERSENSITIVITY REACTIONS MAY REQUIRE THE USE OF SUBCUTANEOUS EPINEPHRINE AND OTHER EMERGENCY MEASURES.

PSEUDOMEMBRANOUS COLITIS HAS BEEN REPORTED WITH THE USE OF CEPHALOSPORINS (AND OTHER BROAD-SPECTRUM ANTIBIOTICS); THEREFORE, IT IS IMPORTANT TO CONSIDER ITS DIAGNOSIS IN PATIENTS WHO DEVELOP DIARRHEA IN ASSOCIATION WITH ANTIBIOTIC USE.

Treatment with broad-spectrum antibiotics alters normal flora of the colon and may permit overgrowth of clostridia. Studies indicate a toxin produced by *Clostridium difficile* is one primary cause of antibiotic-associated colitis. Cholestyramine and colestipol resins have been shown to bind the toxin *in vitro*.

Mild cases of colitis may respond to drug discontinuance alone.

Moderate to severe cases should be managed with fluid, electrolyte, and protein supplementation as indicated.

When the colitis is not relieved by drug discontinuance or when it is severe, oral vancomycin is the treatment of choice for antibiotic-associated pseudomembranous colitis produced by *C. difficile*. Other causes of colitis should also be considered.

PRECAUTIONS

Although transient elevations of the BUN and serum creatinine have been observed, CEFOBID alone does not appear to cause significant nephrotoxicity. However, concomitant administration of aminoglycosides and other cephalosporins has caused nephrotoxicity.

CEFOBID is extensively excreted in bile. The serum half-life of CEFOBID is increased 2–4 fold in patients with hepatic disease and/or biliary obstruction. In general, total daily dosage above 4 g should not be necessary in such patients. If higher dosages are used, serum concentrations should be monitored.

Because renal excretion is not the main route of elimination of CEFOBID (see CLINICAL PHARMACOLOGY), patients with renal failure require no adjustment in dosage when usual doses are administered. When high doses of CEFOBID are used, concentrations of drug in the serum should be monitored periodically. If evidence of accumulation exists, dosage should be decreased accordingly.

The half-life of CEFOBID is reduced slightly during hemodialysis. Thus, dosing should be scheduled to follow a dialysis period. In patients with both hepatic dysfunction and significant renal disease, CEFOBID dosage should not exceed 1–2 g daily without close monitoring of serum concentrations.

As with other antibiotics, vitamin K deficiency has occurred rarely in patients treated with CEFOBID. The mechanism is most probably related to the suppression of gut flora which normally synthesize this vitamin. Those at risk include patients with a poor nutritional status, malabsorption states (e.g., cystic fibrosis), alcoholism, and patients on prolonged hyper-alimentation regimens (administered either intravenously or via a naso-gastric tube). Prothrombin time should be monitored in these patients and exogenous vitamin K administered as indicated.

A disulfram-like reaction characterized by flushing, sweating, headache, and tachycardia has been reported when alcohol (beer, wine) was ingested within 72 hours after CEFOBID administration. Patients should be cautioned about the ingestion of alcoholic beverages following the administration of CEFOBID. A similar reaction has been reported with other cephalosporins.

Prolonged use of CEFOBID may result in the overgrowth of nonsusceptible organisms. Careful observation of the patient is essential. If superinfection occurs during therapy, appropriate measures should be taken.

CEFOBID should be prescribed with caution in individuals with a history of gastrointestinal disease, particularly colitis.

Drug Laboratory Test Interactions

A false-positive reaction for glucose in the urine may occur with Benedict's or Fehling's solution.

Carcinogenesis, Mutagenesis, Impairment of Fertility

Long term studies in animals have not been performed to evaluate carcinogenic potential. The maximum duration of CEFOBID animal toxicity studies is six months. In none of the *in vivo* or *in vitro* genetic toxicology studies did CEFOBID show any mutagenic potential at either the chromosomal or subchromosomal level. CEFOBID produced no impairment of fertility and had no effects on general reproductive performance or fetal development when administered subcutaneously at daily doses up to 500 to 1000 mg/kg prior to and during mating, and to pregnant female rats during gestation. These doses are 10 to 20 times the estimated usual single clinical dose. CEFOBID had adverse effects on the testes of prepubertal rats at all doses tested. Subcutaneous administration of 1000 mg per kg per day (approximately 16 times the average adult human dose) resulted in reduced testicular weight, arrested spermatogenesis, reduced germinal cell population and vacuolation of Sertoli cell cytoplasm. The severity of lesions was dose dependent in the 100 to 1000 mg/kg per day range; the low dose caused a minor decrease in spermatocytes. This effect has not been observed in adult rats. Histologically the lesions were reversible at all but the highest dosage levels. However, these studies did not evaluate subsequent development of reproductive function in the rats. The relationship of these findings to humans is unknown.

Usage in Pregnancy

Pregnancy Category B: Reproduction studies have been performed in mice, rats, and monkeys at doses up to 10 times the human dose and have revealed no evidence of impaired fertility or harm to the fetus due to CEFOBID. There are, however, no adequate and well controlled studies in pregnant women. Because animal reproduction studies are not always predictive of human response, this drug should be used during pregnancy only if clearly needed.

Usage in Nursing Mothers

Only low concentrations of CEFOBID are excreted in human milk. Although CEFOBID passes poorly into breast milk of nursing mothers, caution should be exercised when CEFOBID is administered to a nursing woman.

Pediatric Use

Safety and effectiveness in children have not been established. For information concerning testicular changes in prepubertal rats (see Carcinogenesis, Mutagenesis, Impairment of Fertility).

ADVERSE REACTIONS

In clinical studies the following adverse effects were observed and were considered to be related to CEFOBID therapy or of uncertain etiology:

Hypersensitivity: As with all cephalosporins, hypersensitivity manifested by skin reactions (1 patient in 45), drug fever (1 in 260), or a change in Coombs' test (1 in 60) has been reported. These reactions are more likely to occur in patients with a history of allergies, particularly to penicillin.

Hematology: As with other beta-lactam antibiotics, reversible neutropenia may occur with prolonged administration. Slight decreases in neutrophil count (1 patient in 50) have been reported. Decreased hemoglobins (1 in 20) or hematocrits (1 in 20) have been reported, which is consistent with published literature on other cephalosporins. Transient eosinophilia has occurred in 1 patient in 10.

Hepatic: Of 1285 patients treated with cefoperazone in clinical trials, one patient with a history of liver disease developed significantly elevated liver function enzymes during CEFOBID therapy. Clinical signs and symptoms of nonspecific hepatitis accompanied these increases. After CEFOBID therapy was discontinued, the patient's enzymes returned to pre-treatment levels and the symptomatology resolved. As with other antibiotics that achieve high bile levels, mild transient elevations of liver function enzymes have been observed in 5–10% of the patients receiving CEFOBID therapy. The relevance of these findings, which were not accompanied by overt signs or symptoms of hepatic dysfunction, has not been established.

Gastrointestinal: Diarrhea or loose stools has been reported in 1 in 30 patients. Most of these experiences have been mild or moderate in severity and self-limiting in nature. In all cases, these symptoms responded to symptomatic therapy or ceased when cefoperazone therapy was stopped. Nausea and vomiting have been reported rarely.

Symptoms of pseudomembranous colitis can appear during or for several weeks subsequent to antibiotic therapy (see WARNINGS).

Renal Function Tests: Transient elevations of the BUN (1 in 16) and serum creatinine (1 in 48) have been noted.

Local Reactions: CEFOBID is well tolerated following intramuscular administration. Occasionally, transient pain (1 in 140) may follow administration by this route. When CEFOBID is administered by intravenous infusion some patients may develop phlebitis (1 in 120) at the infusion site.

DOSAGE AND ADMINISTRATION

The usual adult daily dose of CEFOBID is 2 to 4 grams per day administered in divided doses every 12 hours.

In severe infections or infections caused by less sensitive organisms, the total daily dose and/or frequency may be increased. Patients have been successfully treated with a total daily dosage of 6–12 grams divided into 2, 3 or 4 administrations ranging from 1.5 to 4 grams per dose.

In a pharmacokinetic study, a total daily dose of 16 grams was administered to severely immunocompromised patients by constant infusion without complications. Steady state serum concentrations were approximately 150 mcg/ml in these patients.

When treating infections caused by *Streptococcus pyogenes*, therapy should be continued for at least 10 days.

Solutions of CEFOBID and aminoglycoside should not be directly mixed, since there is a physical incompatibility between them. If combination therapy with CEFOBID and an aminoglycoside is contemplated (see INDICATIONS) this can be accomplished by sequential intermittent intravenous infusion provided that separate secondary intravenous tubing is used, and that the primary intravenous tubing is adequately irrigated with an approved diluent between doses. It is also suggested that CEFOBID be administered prior to the aminoglycoside. *In vitro* testing of the effectiveness of drug combination(s) is recommended.

RECONSTITUTION

The following solutions may be used for the initial reconstitution of CEFOBID sterile powder:

Table 1. Solutions for Initial Reconstitution.

5% Dextrose Injection (USP)
5% Dextrose and 0.9% Sodium Chloride Injection (USP)
5% Dextrose and 0.2% Sodium Chloride Injection (USP)
10% Dextrose Injection (USP)
Bacteriostatic Water for Injection [Benzyl Alcohol or Parabens] (USP)*†
0.9% Sodium Chloride Injection (USP)
Normosol® M and Dextrose Injection
Normosol® R
Sterile Water for Injection*

* Not to be used as a vehicle for intravenous infusion
† Preparations containing Benzyl Alcohol should not be used in neonates.

General Reconstitution Procedures

CEFOBID sterile powder for intravenous or intramuscular use may be initially reconstituted with any compatible solution mentioned above in Table 1. Solutions should be allowed to stand after reconstitution to allow any foaming to dissipate to permit visual inspection for complete solubilization.

Vigorous and prolonged agitation may be necessary to solubilize CEFOBID in higher concentrations (above 333 mg cefoperazone/ml). The maximum solubility of CEFOBID sterile powder is approximately 475 mg cefoperazone/ml of compatible diluent.

Preparation For Intravenous Use

General. CEFOBID concentrations between 2 mg/ml and 50 mg/ml are recommended for intravenous administration.

Preparation of Vials. Vials of CEFOBID sterile powder may be initially reconstituted with a minimum of 2.8 ml per gram of cefoperazone of any compatible reconstituting solution appropriate for intravenous administration listed above in Table 1. For ease of reconstitution the use of 5 ml of compatible solution per gram of CEFOBID is recommended. The entire quantity of the resulting solution should then be withdrawn for further dilution and administration using any of the following vehicles for intravenous infusion:

Table 2. Vehicles for Intravenous Infusion.

- 5% Dextrose Injection (USP)
- 5% Dextrose and Lactated Ringer's Injection
- 5% Dextrose and 0.9% Sodium Chloride Injection (USP)
- 5% Dextrose and 0.2% Sodium Chloride Injection (USP)
- 10% Dextrose Injection (USP)
- Lactated Ringer's Injection (USP)
- 0.9% Sodium Chloride Injection (USP)
- Normosol® M and 5% Dextrose Injection
- Normosol® R

Preparation of Piggy Back Units. CEFOBID sterile powder in Piggy Back Units for intravenous use may be prepared by adding between 20 ml and 40 ml of any appropriate diluent listed in Table 2 per gram of cefoperazone. If 5% Dextrose and Lactated Ringer's Injection or Lactated Ringer's Injection (USP) is the chosen vehicle for administration the CEFOBID sterile powder should initially be reconstituted using 2.8–5 ml per gram of any compatible reconstituting solution listed in Table 1 prior to the final dilution.

The resulting intravenous solution should be administered in one of the following manners:

Intermittent Infusion: Solutions of CEFOBID should be administered over a 15–30 minute time period.

Continuous Infusion: CEFOBID can be used for continuous infusion after dilution to a final concentration of between 2 and 25 mg cefoperazone per ml.

Preparation For Intramuscular Injection

Any suitable solution listed above may be used to prepare CEFOBID sterile powder for intramuscular injection. When concentrations of 250 mg/ml or more are to be administered, a lidocaine solution should be used. These solutions should be prepared using a combination of Sterile Water for Injection and 2% Lidocaine Hydrochloride Injection (USP) that approximates a 0.5% Lidocaine Hydrochloride Solution. A two-step dilution process as follows is recommended: First, add the required amount of Sterile Water for Injection and agitate until CEFOBID powder is completely dissolved. Second, add the required amount of 2% lidocaine and mix.

[See table above].

	Final Cefoperazone Concentration	Step 1 Volume of Sterile Water	Step 2 Volume of 2% Lidocaine	Withdrawable Volume*†
1 g vial	333 mg/ml	2.0 ml	0.6 ml	3 ml
	250 mg/ml	2.8 ml	1.0 ml	4 ml
2 g vial	333 mg/ml	3.8 ml	1.2 ml	6 ml
	250 mg/ml	5.4 ml	1.8 ml	8 ml

When a diluent other than Lidocaine HCl Injection (USP) is used reconstitute as follows:

	Cefoperazone Concentration	Volume of Diluent to be Added	Withdrawable Volume*
1 g vial	333 mg/ml	2.6 ml	3 ml
	250 mg/ml	3.8 ml	4 ml
2 g vial	333 mg/ml	5.0 ml	6 ml
	250 mg/ml	7.2 ml	8 ml

* There is sufficient excess present to allow for withdrawal of the stated volume.

† Final lidocaine concentration will approximate that obtained if a 0.5% Lidocaine Hydrochloride Solution is used as diluent.

DIRECTIONS FOR USE OF CEFOBID (cefoperazone sodium) INJECTION IN PLASTIC CONTAINERS

CEFOBID supplied premixed as a frozen, sterile, iso-osmotic solution in plastic containers is to be administered either as continuous or intermittent infusion.

Thaw container at room temperature. After thawing, check for minute leaks by squeezing bag firmly. If leaks are found, discard solution as sterility may be impaired. Additives should not be introduced into this solution. Do not use if the solution is cloudy or precipitated or if the seal is not intact. After thawing, the solution is stable for 10 days if stored under refrigeration (5°C) and for 48 hours at room temperature. DO NOT REFREEZE. Use sterile equipment.

CAUTION: Do not use plastic container in series connections. Such use could result in air embolism due to residual air being drawn from the primary container before administration of the fluid from the secondary container is complete.

Preparation for administration

1. Suspend container from eyelet support.
2. Remove plastic protector from outlet port at bottom of container.
3. Attach administration set. Refer to complete directions accompanying set.

Storage and Stability: CEFOBID sterile powder is to be stored at or below 25°C (77°F) and protected from light prior to reconstitution. After reconstitution, protection from light is not necessary.

The following parenteral diluents and approximate concentrations of CEFOBID provide stable solutions under the following conditions for the indicated time periods. (After the indicated time periods, unused portions of solutions should be discarded.)

[See table below].

Controlled Room Temperature (15°–25°C/59°–77°F) 24 Hours	**Approximate Concentrations**
Bacteriostatic Water for Injection [Benzyl Alcohol or Parabens] (USP)	300 mg/ml
5% Dextrose Injection (USP)	2 mg to 50 mg/ml
5% Dextrose and Lactated Ringer's Injection	2 mg to 50 mg/ml
5% Dextrose and 0.9% Sodium Chloride Injection (USP)	2 mg to 50 mg/ml
5% Dextrose and 0.2% Sodium Chloride Injection (USP)	2 mg to 50 mg/ml
10% Dextrose Injection (USP)	2 mg to 50 mg/ml
Lactated Ringer's Injection (USP)	2 mg/ml
0.5% Lidocaine Hydrochloride Injection (USP)	300 mg/ml
0.9% Sodium Chloride Injection (USP)	2 mg to 300 mg/ml
Normosol® M and 5% Dextrose Injection	2 mg to 50 mg/ml
Normosol® R	2 mg to 50 mg/ml
Sterile Water for Injection	300 mg/ml

Reconstituted CEFOBID solutions may be stored in glass or plastic syringes, or in glass or flexible plastic parenteral solution containers.

Refrigerator Temperature (2°–8°C/36°–46°F) 5 Days	**Approximate Concentrations**
Bacteriostatic Water for Injection [Benzyl Alcohol or Parabens] (USP)	300 mg/ml
5% Dextrose Injection (USP)	2 mg to 50 mg/ml
5% Dextrose and 0.9% Sodium Chloride Injection (USP)	2 mg to 50 mg/ml
5% Dextrose and 0.2% Sodium Chloride Injection (USP)	2 mg to 50 mg/ml
Lactated Ringer's Injection (USP)	2 mg/ml
0.5% Lidocaine Hydrochloride Injection (USP)	300 mg/ml
0.9% Sodium Chloride Injection (USP)	2 mg to 300 mg/ml
Normosol® M and 5% Dextrose Injection	2 mg to 50 mg/ml
Normosol® R	2 mg to 50 mg/ml
Sterile Water for Injection	300 mg/ml

Reconstituted CEFOBID solutions may be stored in glass or plastic syringes, or in glass or flexible plastic parenteral solution containers.

Freezer Temperature (−20° to −10°C/−4° to 14°F)	**Approximate Concentrations**
3 Weeks	
5% Dextrose Injection (USP)	50 mg/ml
5% Dextrose and 0.9% Sodium Chloride Injection (USP)	2 mg/ml
5% Dextrose and 0.2% Sodium Chloride Injection (USP)	2 mg/ml
5 Weeks	
0.9% Sodium Chloride Injection (USP)	300 mg/ml
Sterile Water for Injection	300 mg/ml

Reconstituted CEFOBID solutions may be stored in plastic syringes, or in flexible plastic parenteral solution containers. Frozen samples should be thawed at room temperature before use. After thawing, unused portions should be discarded. Do not refreeze.

HOW SUPPLIED

CEFOBID sterile powder is available in vials containing cefoperazone sodium equivalent to 1 gram cefoperazone × 10 (NDC 0049-1201-83), and 2 gram cefoperazone × 10 (NDC 0049-1202-83) for intramuscular and intravenous administration.

CEFOBID sterile powder is available in Piggyback Units containing cefoperazone sodium equivalent to 1 gram cefoperazone × 10 (NDC 0049-1211-83), and 2 gram cefoperazone × 10 (NDC 0049-1212-83) for intravenous administration.

CEFOBID (cefoperazone sodium) injection is supplied premixed as a frozen, sterile, nonpyrogenic, iso-osmotic solution in plastic containers. Each 50 ml unit contains cefoperazone sodium equivalent to 2 g cefoperazone with approximately 1.8 g dextrose hydrous USP added. The solution is iso-osmotic (approximately 300 mOsmol/L), and solution pH may have been adjusted with sodium hydroxide and/or hydrochloric acid. Do not store above −20°C.

CEFOBID supplied as a frozen, sterile, nonpyrogenic, iso-osmotic solution in 50 ml plastic containers (NDC 0049-1215-18) is manufactured for Roerig Division of Pfizer Pharmaceuticals by Travenol Laboratories, Inc., Deerfield, IL 60015.

70-4169-00-9

EMETE-CON® ℞

[ă-mĕt ′ă-kŏn ″]

(benzquinamide hydrochloride)

For Intramuscular and Intravenous Use

DESCRIPTION

Benzquinamide is a non-amine-depleting benzoquinolizine derivative, chemically unrelated to the phenothiazines and to other antiemetics.

Chemically, Emete-con (benzquinamide hy- drochloride) is N,N-diethyl-1,3,4,6,7,11b-hex- ahydro-2-hydroxy-9, 10-dimethoxy- 2H -benzo-[a]quinolizine-3-carboxamide acetate hydrochloride. The empirical formula is $C_{22}H_{32}N_2O_5$. HCl and the molecular weight is 441.

Emete-con for injection contains benzquinamide hydrochloride equivalent to 50 mg/vial of benzquinamide. When reconstituted with 2.2 ml of proper diluent, each vial yields 2 ml of a solution containing benzquinamide hydrochloride equivalent to 25 mg/ml of benzquinamide. When reconstituted this product maintains its potency for 14 days at room temperature.

ACTIONS

Benzquinamide HCl exhibited antiemetic, antihistaminic, mild anticholinergic and sedative action in animals. Studies conducted in dogs and human volunteers have demonstrated suppression of apomorphine-induced vomiting; however, relevance to clinical efficacy has not been established. The mechanism of action in humans is unknown. The onset of antiemetic activity in humans usually occurs within 15 minutes.

Benzquinamide metabolism has been studied in animals and in man. In both species, 5-10% of an administered dose is excreted unchanged in the urine. The remaining drug undergoes metabolic transformation in the liver by at least three pathways to a spectrum of metabolites which are excreted in the urine and in the bile, from which the more polar metabolites are not reabsorbed but are excreted in the feces. The half-life in plasma of Emete-con is about 40 minutes. More than 95% of an administered dose was excreted within 72 hours in animal studies using C14-labeled benzquinamide. In blood, benzquinamide is about 58% bound to plasma protein.

INDICATIONS

Emete-con is indicated for the prevention and treatment of nausea and vomiting associated with anesthesia and surgery.

Continued on next page

Roerig—Cont.

Since the incidence of postoperative and postanesthetic vomiting has decreased with the adoption of modern techniques and agents, the prophylactic use of Emete-con should be restricted to those patients in whom emesis would endanger the results of surgery or result in harm to the patient.

CONTRAINDICATIONS

Emete-con is contraindicated in individuals who have demonstrated hypersensitivity to the drug.

WARNINGS

Use in Pregnancy

No teratogenic effects of benzquinamide were demonstrated in reproduction studies in chick embryos, mice, rats and rabbits. The relevance of these data to the human is not known. However, safe use of this drug in pregnancy has not been established and its use in pregnancy is not recommended.

Use in Children

As the data available at present are insufficient to establish proper dosage in children, the use of Emete-con in children is not recommended.

Intravenous use

Sudden increase in blood pressure and transient arrhythmias (premature ventricular and auricular contractions) have been reported following intravenous administration of benzquinamide. Until a more predictable pattern of the effect of intravenous benzquinamide has been established, the intramuscular route of administration is considered preferable. The intravenous route of administration should be restricted to patients without cardiovascular disease and receiving no pre-anesthetic and/or concomitant cardiovascular drugs.

If patients receiving pressor agents or epinephrine-like drugs are also given benzquinamide, the latter should be given in fractions of the normal dose. Blood pressure should be monitored. Safeguards against hypertensive reactions are particularly important in hypertensive patients.

PRECAUTIONS

Benzquinamide, like other antiemetics, may mask signs of overdosage of toxic drugs or may obscure diagnosis of such conditions as intestinal obstruction and brain tumor.

ADVERSE REACTIONS

The following adverse reactions have been reported in subjects who have received benzquinamide. However, drowsiness appears to be the most common reaction. One case of pronounced allergic reaction has been encountered, characterized by pyrexia and urticaria.

System Affected

Autonomic Nervous System: Dry mouth, shivering, sweating, hiccoughs, flushing, salivation, blurred vision.

Cardiovascular System: Hypertension, hypotension, dizziness, atrial fibrillation, premature auricular and ventricular contractions.

Hypertensive episodes have occurred after IM and IV administration.

Central Nervous System: Drowsiness, insomnia, restlessness, headache, excitement, nervousness.

Gastrointestinal System: Anorexia, nausea.

Musculoskeletal System: Twitching, shaking/ tremors, weakness.

Skin: Hives/rash.

Other Systems: Fatigue, shaking chills, increased temperature.

DOSAGE AND ADMINISTRATION

Intramuscular: 50 mg (0.5 mg/kg–1.0 mg/kg)

First dose may be repeated in one hour with subsequent doses every 3-4 hours, as necessary. The precautions applicable to all intramuscular injections should be observed. Emete-con should be injected well within the mass of a larger muscle. The deltoid area should be used only if well developed. Injections should not be made into the lower and mid-thirds of the upper arm. Aspiration of the syringe should be carried out to avoid inadvertent intravascular injection. Therapeutic blood levels and demonstrable antiemetic activity appear within fifteen minutes of intramuscular administration. When the objective of therapy is the prevention of nausea and vomiting, intramuscular administration is recommended at least fifteen minutes prior to emergence from anesthesia.

Intravenous: 25 mg (0.2 mg/kg–0.4 mg/kg as a single dose) administered slowly (1 ml per 0.5 to 1 minute). Subsequent doses should be given intramuscularly.

The intravenous route of administration should be restricted to patients without cardiovascular disease (See WARNINGS). If it is necessary to use Emete-con intravenously in elderly or debilitated patients, benzquinamide should be administered cautiously and the lower dose range is recommended.

This preparation must be initially reconstituted with 2.2 ml of Sterile Water for Injection, Bacteriostatic Water for Injection with benzyl alcohol or with methylparaben and propylparaben. This procedure yields 2 ml of a solution equivalent to 25 mg benzquinamide/ml, which maintains its potency for 14 days at room temperature.

OVERDOSAGE

Manifestations: On the basis of acute animal toxicology studies, gross Emete-con overdosage in humans might be expected to manifest itself as a combination of Central Nervous System stimulant and depressant effects. This speculation is derived from experimental studies in which intravenous doses of benzquinamide, at least 150 times the human therapeutic dose, were administered to dogs.

Treatment: There is no specific antidote for Emete-con overdosage. General supportive measures should be instituted, as indicated. Atropine may be helpful. Although there has been no direct experience with dialysis, it is not likely to be of value, since benzquinamide is extensively bound to plasma protein.

HOW SUPPLIED

Emete-con for IM/IV use is available in a vial containing benzquinamide HCl equivalent to 50 mg of benzquinamide in packages of 10 vials.

CAUTION

Federal law prohibits dispensing without prescription.

60-1787-00-4

Geocillin

DRUG	DOSE	Mean Urine Concentration of Carbenicillin mcg/ml Hours After Initial Dose 0–3	3–6	6–24
Geocillin	1 tablet q.6 hr.	1130	352	292
Geocillin	2 tablets q.6 hr.	1428	789	809

Mean serum concentrations of carbenicillin in this study for these dosages are:

DRUG	DOSE	Mean Serum Concentration mcg/ml Hours After Initial Dose ½	1	2	4	6	24	25	26	28
Geocillin	1 tablet q.6 hr.	5.1	6.5	3.2	1.9	0.0	0.4	8.8	5.4	0.4
Geocillin	2 tablets q.6 hr.	6.1	9.6	7.9	2.6	0.4	0.8	13.2	12.8	3.8

GEOCILLIN® ℞

[gē′ō-sil-in]

(carbenicillin indanyl sodium)

TABLETS

For Oral Use

DESCRIPTION

Geocillin (carbenicillin indanyl sodium), a semisynthetic penicillin, is the sodium salt of the indanyl ester of Geopen® (carbenicillin disodium). Geocillin is acid stable and well absorbed following oral administration.

ACTIONS

Microbiology

The antibacterial activity of Geocillin is due to its rapid conversion to carbenicillin by hydrolysis. Though Geocillin provides substantial *in vitro* activity against a variety of both gram-positive and gram-negative microorganisms, the most important aspect of its profile is in its antipseudomonal and antiproteus activity. Because of the high urine levels obtained following administration, Geocillin has demonstrated clinical efficacy in urinary infections due to susceptible strains of:

Escherichia coli
Proteus mirabilis
Proteus morgani
Proteus rettgeri
Proteus vulgaris
Pseudomonas
Enterobacter
Enterococci

In addition, *in vitro* data, not substantiated by clinical studies, indicate the following pathogens to be usually susceptible to Geocillin:

Staphylococcus (non-penicillinase producing)
Streptococcus

Most *Klebsiella* species are often resistant to the action of Geocillin. Some strains of *Pseudomonas* have developed resistance to carbenicillin.

Susceptibility Testing

Geopen (carbenicillin disodium) Susceptibility Powder or 100 mcg. Geopen Susceptibility Discs may be used to determine microbial susceptibility to Geocillin.

Interpretations:

[See table below left].

Geocillin	Susceptible	Intermediate	Resistant
Pseudomonas aeruginosa and Enterococci			
Inhibition Zone	17 mm or greater*	16 mm–14 mm	13 mm or less
MIC	125 mcg/ml or less	greater than 125 mcg/ml less than 250 mcg/ml	250 mcg/ml or greater
Escherichia coli, Proteus species, and Enterobacter.			
Inhibition Zone	23 mm or greater	22 mm–18 mm	17 mm or less
MIC	15 mcg/ml or less	greater than 20 mcg/ml less than 40 mcg/ml	greater than 40 mcg/ml

*Zone diameter interpretations apply only to results obtained by the Bauer, Kirby, Sherris and Turck method of Susceptibility Testing Am. J. Clin. Path. 45:493, 1966.

Interpretations of susceptible, intermediate, and resistant correlate zone size diameters with MIC values. A laboratory report of "susceptible" indicates that the suspected causative microorganism most likely will respond to therapy with carbenicillin. A laboratory report of "resistant" indicates that the infecting microorganism most likely will not respond to therapy. A laboratory report of "intermediate" indicates that the microorganism is most likely susceptible if a high dosage of carbenicillin is used, or if the infection is such that high levels of carbenicillin may be attained as in urine.

Pharmacology

Geocillin is acid stable and well absorbed following oral administration. After absorption, Geocillin is rapidly hydrolyzed to carbenicillin, which is primarily excreted in the urine. In a study utilizing volunteers with normal renal function, the following mean urine levels of carbenicillin were achieved:

[See table above].

INDICATIONS

Geocillin (carbenicillin indanyl sodium) is indicated in the treatment of acute and chronic infections of the upper and lower urinary tract and in asymptomatic bacteriuria due to susceptible strains of the following organisms:

Escherichia coli
Proteus mirabilis
Proteus morgani
Proteus rettgeri
Proteus vulgaris
Pseudomonas
Enterobacter
Enterococci

Geocillin is also indicated in the treatment of prostatitis due to susceptible strains of the following organisms:

Escherichia coli
Enterococcus *(S. faecalis)*
Proteus mirabilis
Enterobacter sp.

WHEN HIGH RAPID BLOOD AND URINE LEVELS OF ANTIBIOTIC ARE INDICATED, THERAPY WITH GEOPEN (CARBENICILLIN DISODIUM) SHOULD BE INITIATED BY PARENTERAL ADMINISTRATION FOLLOWED, AT THE PHYSICIAN'S DISCRETION, BY ORAL THERAPY.

NOTE: Susceptibility testing should be performed prior to and during the course of therapy to detect the possible emergence of resistant organisms which may develop.

CONTRAINDICATIONS

Geocillin is ordinarily contraindicated in patients who have a known penicillin allergy.

WARNINGS

Serious and occasionally fatal hypersensitivity (anaphylactic) reactions have been reported in patients on oral penicillin therapy. These reactions are more apt to occur in individuals with a history of sensitivity to multiple allergens.

There have been reports of individuals with a history of penicillin hypersensitivity who have experienced severe hypersensitivity reactions when treated with a cephalosporin, and vice versa. Therefore, before therapy with a penicillin, careful inquiry should be made concerning previous hypersensitivity reactions to penicillins, cephalosporins, and other allergens.

SERIOUS ANAPHYLACTOID REACTIONS REQUIRE IMMEDIATE EMERGENCY TREATMENT WITH EPINEPHRINE. OXYGEN, INTRAVENOUS STEROIDS AND AIRWAY MANAGEMENT, INCLUDING INTUBATION, SHOULD ALSO BE ADMINISTERED AS INDICATED.

Usage in Children: Since only limited clinical data is available to date in children, the safety of Geocillin administration in this age group has not yet been established.

Usage in Pregnancy: Safety for use in pregnancy has not been established.

PRECAUTIONS

Periodic assessment of organ system function including renal, hepatic and hematopoietic systems is recommended during prolonged therapy.

Long term use of Geocillin may result in the overgrowth of nonsensitive organisms. If superinfection occurs during therapy, appropriate measures should be taken.

Since carbenicillin is excreted by the kidney, patients with severe renal impairment (creatinine clearance of less than 10 ml/min.) will not achieve therapeutic urine levels of carbenicillin.

ADVERSE REACTIONS

The following adverse reactions may occur during therapy with Geocillin:

Gastrointestinal Disturbances: Nausea, vomiting, and diarrhea.

Hypersensitivity Reactions: Skin rashes, urticaria, or pruritus have been reported infrequently.

Blood, Hepatic and Renal Studies: As with other penicillins, anemia, thrombocytopenia, leukopenia, neutropenia, and eosinophilia may occur.

Mild SGOT elevations have been observed following Geocillin administration.

Other reactions that have been reported are flatulence, dry mouth, furry tongue, vaginitis, and abdominal cramps.

DOSAGE AND ADMINISTRATION

Geocillin is available as a coated tablet, to be administered orally.

Usual Adult Dose

URINARY TRACT INFECTIONS	
Escherichia coli, Proteus species, and *Enterobacter*	1-2 tablets 4 times daily
Pseudomonas and Enterococci	2 tablets 4 times daily
PROSTATITIS	
Escherichia coli, Proteus mirabilis, Enterobacter and Enterococcus	2 tablets 4 times daily

CARBENICILLIN BLOOD LEVELS AND URINARY EXCRETION

DOSAGE	ROUTE	SERUM LEVELS mcg/ml ¼ hr.	½ hr.	1 hr.	2 hr.	3 hr.	4 hr.	6 hr.	8 hr.	Urinary excretion of administered dose 0–9 hours
500 mg.	IM	8	10	13	9.8	6.5	3.2	0	—	85%
1000 mg.	IM	—	13	18	15	12	7.5	1.7	0.7	74.6%*
2000 mg.	IM	26	38	47	37	25	15	5.9	1.2	79%
1000 mg.	IV	71	45	31	14	8.2	3	0	—	73%
1000 mg.+	IV									
1 g probenecid	Oral	72	55	40	26	17	12	6.5	2.0	74%

*0–24 hr. collection

HOW SUPPLIED

Geocillin is available as film-coated tablets in bottles of 100's, and unit-dose packages of 100 (10 × 10s). Each tablet contains carbenicillin indanyl sodium equivalent to 382 mg of carbenicillin.

69-1970-00-7

Shown in Product Identification Section, page 425

GEOPEN® ℞

[gē'ō-pen"]

sterile carbenicillin disodium

For Intramuscular and Intravenous Use

DESCRIPTION

Geopen (carbenicillin disodium) is a new semisynthetic injectable penicillin.

Geopen is a benzylpenicillin derivative with substitution by an ionizable functional group in the alpha position.

ACTIONS

Microbiology

Though Geopen has substantial *in vitro* activity against a variety of both gram-positive and gram-negative microorganisms the most important aspect of its profile is in its antipseudomonal and antiproteus effect.

Organisms found to be susceptible to Geopen *in vitro* include the following:

Staphylococcus aureus
(Non-penicillinase producing)
Staphylococcus albus
Streptococcus pneumoniae
Beta-hemolytic Streptococci
Streptococcus faecalis
Hemophilus influenzae
Neisseria species
Enterobacter species
Proteus mirabilis
Proteus morgani
Proteus rettgeri
Proteus vulgaris
Escherichia coli
Salmonella species
Pseudomonas aeruginosa
Anaerobic bacteria, including:
Bacteroides species
Peptostreptococcus species
Peptococcus species
Clostridium species
Fusobacterium species

In vitro synergism between Geopen and gentamicin sulfate in certain strains of *Pseudomonas aeruginosa* has been demonstrated.

Geopen is not stable in the presence of penicillinase.

Most *Klebsiella* species are resistant to the action of Geopen. Some of the newly emerging pathogenic strains of such microorganisms as *Herellea, Mima, Citrobacter* and *Serratia* have shown susceptibility to Geopen.

Some strains of *Pseudomonas* have developed resistance to Geopen fairly rapidly.

Pharmacology

Geopen is not absorbed orally, hence, it must be administered by the intramuscular or intravenous routes.

Following intramuscular injection, peak blood levels are obtained within 1–2 hours. The administration of probenecid results in somewhat higher and more prolonged serum levels as noted in the table above.

The MIC for many strains of *Pseudomonas* and *Bacteroides fragilis* is relatively high; serum levels of 100 mcg/ml or greater are required. However, the low degree of toxicity of carbenicillin permits the use of doses large enough to achieve adequate levels for these strains.

Other susceptible organisms usually require serum levels in the range of 10–25 mcg/ml. Geopen is not highly bound to serum proteins and is excreted unchanged in high concentrations in the urine. After a 0.5 to 2 grams I.M. dose, a urine concentration of 1,000 to 5,000 mcg/ml may be achieved.

INDICATIONS

Geopen is primarily indicated in the treatment of infections due to susceptible *Pseudomonas aeruginosa, Proteus* species (particularly indole positive strains) and certain strains of *Escherichia coli.*

By virtue of the very high urinary levels achieved, Geopen is particularly effective in urinary tract infections due to one or more of the above mentioned organisms.

Clinical studies have demonstrated the effectiveness of Geopen in the following infections when due to these organisms:

1. Severe systemic infections and septicemia including meningitis due to *Hemophilus influenzae* and *Streptococcus pneumoniae.* Although Geopen possesses *in vitro* activity against many ampicillin-resistant *H. influenzae,* clinical data are insufficient to recommend its use for treatment of meningitis due to ampicillin-resistant strains.
2. Genitourinary tract infections including those due to *Neisseria gonorrhoeae, Enterobacter* and *Streptococcus faecalis* (enterococcus).
3. Acute and chronic respiratory infections. Though clinical improvement has been shown, bacteriologic cures cannot be expected in patients with chronic respiratory disease and cystic fibrosis.
4. Soft tissue infections.

Geopen is also indicated in the treatment of the following infections due to susceptible anaerobic bacteria:

1. Septicemia.
2. Lower respiratory tract infections such as empyema, anaerobic pneumonitis and lung abscess.
3. Intra-abdominal infections such as peritonitis and intra-abdominal abscess. (Typically resulting from anaerobic organisms resident in the normal gastrointestinal tract.)
4. Infections of the female pelvis and genital tract such as endometritis, pelvic inflammatory disease, pelvic abscess and salpingitis.
5. Skin and soft tissue infections.

Although Geopen (carbenicillin disodium) is indicated primarily in gram-negative infections, its activity against gram-positive organisms should be kept in mind when both gram-positive and gram-negative organisms are isolated (see Actions).

In the treatment of infections due to certain susceptible strains of *Pseudomonas aeruginosa,* clinical efficacy may be enhanced by the use of combined therapy with Geopen (carbenicillin disodium) and gentamicin sulfate in full therapeutic dosages. For additional prescribing information, see the gentamicin sulfate package insert.

NOTE: During therapy, sensitivity testing should be repeated frequently to detect the possible emergence of resistant organisms which may develop, particularly if a suboptimal dose regimen is used.

CONTRAINDICATIONS

Geopen is ordinarily contraindicated in patients who have a known penicillin allergy.

WARNINGS

Serious and occasional fatal hypersensitivity (anaphylactic) reactions have been reported in patients on penicillin therapy. These reactions are more apt to occur in individuals with a history of sensitivity to multiple allergens.

Patients with renal impairment should be observed for bleeding manifestations. Such patients should be dosed strictly according to recommendations (see Dosage and Administration section). If bleeding manifestations appear, the antibiotic should be discontinued and appropriate therapy be instituted.

There have been reports of individuals with a history of penicillin hypersensitivity reactions who have experienced severe hypersensitivity reactions when treated with a cephalosporin. Before therapy with a penicillin, careful inquiry should be made concerning previous hypersensitivity reactions to penicillins, cephalosporins, and other allergens. If an allergic reaction occurs, appropriate therapy should be instituted and discontinuance of carbenicillin therapy considered, unless, in the opinion of the physician the condition being treated is life threatening and amenable only to carbenicillin therapy. The usual agents (antihistamines, pressor amines and corticosteroids) should be readily available.

SERIOUS ANAPHYLACTOID REACTIONS REQUIRE IMMEDIATE EMERGENCY TREATMENT WITH EPINEPHRINE. OXYGEN AND INTRAVENOUS CORTICOSTEROIDS SHOULD ALSO BE ADMINISTERED AS INDICATED.

Continued on next page

Roerig—Cont.

Usage in Pregnancy
Safety for use in pregnancy has not been established.

PRECAUTIONS

While Geopen (carbenicillin disodium) exhibits the characteristic low toxicity of the penicillin group of antibiotics, as with any other potent agent, it is advisable to check periodically for organ system dysfunction, including renal, hepatic and hematopoietic systems, during prolonged therapy.
Emergence of resistant organisms, such as *Klebsiella* spp., and *Serratia* spp., which may cause superinfection, should be kept in mind.

Geopen is a disodium salt of carboxybenzylpenicillin and hence each gram of Geopen contains 4.7 mEq. of sodium. In patients where sodium restriction is necessary, such as cardiac patients, periodic electrolyte determinations and monitoring of cardiac status should be made.
In a few patients receiving high doses of Geopen, hypokalemia has been reported. Periodic serum potassium determinations should be made and corrective measures should be implemented when necessary.
As with any penicillin preparation, an allergic response, including anaphylaxis, may occur particularly in a hypersensitive individual.
Cases of gonorrhea with a suspected primary lesion of syphilis should have dark field examinations before treatment. In all other cases where concomitant syphilis is suspected, monthly serological tests should be made for a minimum of 4 months.

ADVERSE REACTIONS

The following adverse reactions may occur:
Hypersensitivity reactions: Skin rashes, pruritus, urticaria, drug fever, and anaphylactic reactions.
Gastrointestinal disturbances: Nausea
Hemic and Lymphatic Systems: As with other penicillins, anemia, thrombocytopenia, leukopenia, neutropenia, and eosinophilia may occur.
Blood, Hepatic and Renal Studies: As with other semisynthetic penicillins, SGOT and SGPT elevations have been observed after Geopen administration (particularly in children). In all studies to date, no clinical manifestations of hepatic or renal disorders have been demonstrated.
CNS: As with other penicillins, convulsions or neuromuscular irritability could occur with excessively high serum levels.
Other: Pain at the site of injection after intramuscular and intravenous administration has been reported but is rarely accompanied by induration.
Several uremic patients receiving high doses (24 grams/day) have developed hemorrhagic manifestations associated with abnormalities of coagulation tests such as clotting time and prothrombin time. On withdrawal of the antibiotic, the bleeding ceased. The exact relationship of these findings to carbenicillin therapy is not clear.
Vein Irritation and Phlebitis have been reported occasionally, particularly when undiluted solution was directly injected into the vein.

DOSAGE AND ADMINISTRATION

Indication: Clinical experience indicates that in serious urinary tract and systemic infections intravenous therapy in the higher doses should be used. The recommended maximum dose is 40g per day. Intramuscular injections should not exceed 2g per injection.
[See table left].
Seriously ill patients should receive the higher doses. Geopen has proved to be useful in infections in which protective mechanisms are impaired, such as in acute leukemia and during therapy with immunosuppressive or oncolytic drugs.

Intramuscular Use
As with all intramuscular preparations, Geopen should be injected well within the body of a relatively large muscle.
Adults: The preferred site is the upper outer quadrant of the buttock (i.e., gluteus maximus), or the mid-lateral thigh.
Children: It is recommended that intramuscular injections be given preferably in the midlateral muscles of the thigh. In infants and small children the periphery of the upper outer quadrant of the gluteal region should be used only when necessary, such as in burn patients, in order to minimize the possibility of damage to the sciatic nerve.
The deltoid area should be used only if well developed such as in certain adults and older children, and then only with caution to avoid radial nerve injury. Intramuscular injections should not be made into the lower and mid-third of the upper arm. As with all intramuscular injections, aspiration is necessary to help avoid inadvertent injection into a blood vessel.

Intravenous Use
As with all intravenous administrations, particular attention should be directed to insure that the drug is injected only into a vein (including aspiration and proper anatomical site selection) to avoid either intra-arterial injection or extravasation.

Preparation of Solutions When Using the 1g, 2g, 5g, IM/IV Serum Vials:
For Intramuscular Use—The 1 g vial should be reconstituted with 2.0 ml of Sterile Water for Injection. In order to facilitate reconstitution, up to 3.6 ml of Sterile Water for Injection can be used.

Amount of Diluent to be Added to the 1 g Vial	Volume to be Withdrawn for a 1 g Dose
2.0 ml	2.5 ml
2.5 ml	3.0 ml
3.6 ml	4.0 ml

The 2 g vial should be reconstituted with 4.0 ml of Sterile Water for Injection. In order to facilitate reconstitution, up to 7.2 ml of Sterile Water for Injection can be used.

Amount of Diluent to be Added to the 2 g Vial	Volume to be Withdrawn for a 1 g Dose
4.0 ml	2.5 ml
5.0 ml	3.0 ml
7.2 ml	4.0 ml

The 5 g vial should be reconstituted with 9.5 ml of Sterile Water for Injection. In order to facilitate reconstitution, up to 17 ml of Sterile Water for Injection can be used.

ADULTS:	*Pseudomonas*	*Proteus and E. coli*	*Enterobacter and S. faecalis*	*Anaerobes*	*H. influenzae and S. pneumoniae*
Urinary Tract Infections					
Serious	200 mg/kg/ day by I.V. drip	200 mg/kg/ day by I.V. drip	200 mg/kg/ day by I.V. drip		
Uncomplicated	1–2 g I.M. or I.V. every 6 hours	1–2 g I.M. or I.V. every 6 hours	1–2 g I.M. or I.V. every 6 hours		
Severe Systemic Infections, Septicemia, Respiratory Infections, Soft Tissue Infections	400–500 mg/ kg/day (30–40 grams) I.V. in divided doses or continuously	300–400 mg/ kg/day (20–30 grams) I.V. in divided doses or continuously		400–500 mg/ kg/day (30–40 grams) I.V. in divided doses or continuously	
Infections complicated by renal insufficiency (Creatinine clearance less than 5 ml/min)		2 g I.V.[1] every 8–12 hours			
ADULTS:	*Pseudomonas*	*Proteus and E. coli*	*Enterobacter and S. faecalis*	*Anaerobes*	*H. influenzae and S. pneumoniae*
Meningitis				400–500 mg/kg/day (30–40 grams) I.V. in divided doses or continuously	
During peritoneal dialysis		2 g I.V. every 6 hours			
During hemodialysis		2 g I.V. every 4 hours			

(1) The serum half-life of Geopen in patients with severe renal failure is 12.5 hours. As a consequence 2 grams of Geopen administered intravenously to these patients every 8–12 hours will give Geopen serum levels of approximately 100 mcg/ml, a level notably free of any untoward effects while adequate for treatment of a majority of the infections amenable to Geopen therapy.

Treatment of gonorrhea[2]; acute uncomplicated ano-genital and urethral infections due to ***N. gonorrhoeae.***
SINGLE 4 g I.M. injection, divided between 2 sites.

(2) Probenecid in a dosage of 1 gram may be administered orally about 30 minutes prior to the I.M. treatment of acute gonorrhoeal infections. For complete information and dosage of probenecid, refer to manufacturer's product information.

CHILDREN:	*Pseudomonas*	*Proteus and E. coli*	*Enterobacter and S. faecalis*	*Anaerobes*	*H. influenzae and S. pneumoniae*
Urinary Tract Infections	50–200 mg/ kg/day in divided doses every 4–6 hours I.M. or I.V.	50–100 mg/ kg/day in divided doses every 4–6 hours I.M. or I.V.	50–200 mg/ kg/day in divided doses every 4–6 hours I.M. or I.V.		
Severe Systemic Infections, Septicemia, Respiratory Infections, Soft Tissue Infections	400–500 mg/ kg/day I.V. in divided doses or by continuous drip	300–400 mg/ kg/day I.M. or I.V. in divided doses		400–500 mg/ kg/day I.V. in divided doses or by continuous drip	
Infections complicated by renal insufficiency (Creatinine clearance less than 5 ml/min)		Clinical data is insufficient to recommend an optimum dose			
Meningitis				400–500 mg/kg/day in divided doses or by continuous drip	

NEONATES: In the neonate, for severe systemic infections (sepsis) due to susceptible strains of ***Pseudomonas, Proteus, E. coli, H. influenzae*** and ***S. pneumoniae,*** the following Geopen (carbenicillin disodium) dosages may be given I.M. or by fifteen (15) minute I.V. infusion:
Infants under 2000 g body weight.
Initial dose: 100 mg/kg
Subsequent doses during first week: 75 mg/kg/8 hrs (225 mg/kg/day)
After 7 days of age: 100 mg/kg/6 hrs (400 mg/kg/day)
Infants over 2000 g body weight.
Initial dose: 100 mg/kg
Subsequent doses during first 3 days: 75 mg/kg/6 hrs (300 mg/kg/day)
After 3 days of age: 100 mg/kg/6 hrs (400 mg/kg/day)
NOTE: This dosage schedule should give maximum serum levels of approximately 150–175 mcg/ml and minimum levels of approximately 50–75 mcg/ml of Geopen.
Gentamicin may be used concurrently with carbenicillin for initial therapy until results of culture and susceptibility studies are known.

Amount of Diluent to be Added to the 5 g Vial	Volume to be Withdrawn for a 1 g Dose
9.5 ml	2.5 ml
12.0 ml	3.0 ml
17.0 ml	4.0 ml

After reconstitution, no significant loss of potency occurs for 24 hours at room temperature, and for 72 hours if refrigerated. Discard unused portions held longer than these time periods.

For Direct Intravenous Injection—Following reconstitution, each gram should be further diluted by no less than 5 ml of Sterile Water for Injection. In order to avoid vein irritation, the solution should be administered as slowly as possible.

For Intravenous Infusion—Following reconstitution according to directions, Geopen (carbenicillin disodium) may be added to the desired volume of usual intravenous infusion solutions.

When Using The 5g, 10g Piggyback Units or Bulk Pharmacy Package:

Intravenous Use

As with all intravenous administrations, particular attention should be directed to insure that the drug is injected only into a vein (including aspiration and proper anatomical site selection) to avoid either intra-arterial injection or extravasation.

Direct Intravenous Injection

The 5 gram vial should be reconstituted with a minimum of 50 ml Sterile Water for Injection.

Amount of Diluent	Concentration of Solution
100 ml	1 g/20 ml
50 ml	1 g/10 ml

The 10 gram vial should be reconstituted with a minimum of 95 ml of Sterile Water for Injection.

Amount of Diluent	Concentration of Solution
95 ml	1 g/10 ml

After reconstitution with Sterile Water for Injection, no significant loss of potency occurs for 72 hours at room temperature and for 14 days if refrigerated. Discard unused portions held longer than these time periods.

In order to avoid vein irritation, the solution should be administered as slowly as possible. A dilution of 1 g/20 ml or more will further reduce the incidence of vein irritation.

Bulk Pharmacy Package

The 30 gram vial should be reconstituted by adding 80 ml of water in two separate 40 ml aliquots. Add 40 ml, shake 25 seconds and add the last 40 ml aliquot and shake for final solution. The resulting solution will contain 300 mg/ml of carbenicillin. Transfer recommended dosage to appropriate intravenous infusion solution.

Reconstituted bulk solution should not be used for direct infusion.

After reconstitution of the Bulk Pharmacy Package, no significant loss of potency occurs for 24 hours at room temperature and for 72 hours if refrigerated. Discard unused portions held longer than these time periods.

For Continuous Intravenous Infusion

After reconstitution as directed, Geopen (carbenicillin disodium) may be added to the desired volume of usual intravenous infusion solutions.

Studies of Geopen at concentrations of 10 mg/ml and 100 mg/ml in the following intravenous infusion diluents indicate no significant loss of potency when stored at room temperature and under refrigeration (5°C) for the time periods stated:

[See table above].

It is recommended that Geopen and gentamicin sulfate not be mixed together in the same IV solution due to the gradual inactivation of gentamicin sulfate under these circumstances. The therapeutic effect of the two drugs remains unimpaired when administered separately.

For Intramuscular Use Only

Geopen for intramuscular injection ONLY may be diluted with one of the following:

1. 0.5% Lidocaine Hydrochloride (without epinephrine).
2. Bacteriostatic Water containing 0.9% Benzyl Alcohol.

For reconstitution of Geopen with these diluents for intramuscular use ONLY, follow the directions for the amount of diluent in the **PREPARATION OF SOLUTION, For Intramuscular Use** section.

Geopen may be diluted with these solutions and stored for 24 hours at room temperature or for 72 hours when refrigerated. Discard unused solutions stored longer than these time periods.

For full product information, refer to the package insert for Lidocaine Hydrochloride (without epinephrine).

HOW SUPPLIED

Geopen is available in 1 g (NDC 0995-1410-83), 2 g (NDC 0995-1417-83), and 5 g (NDC 0995-1419-83) vials for intramuscular/intravenous use.

Intravenous Solution	Stability: *Room Temperature*	Stability: *Refrigerated*
Sterile water for injection	72 hours	14 days
Sodium chloride injection, USP	72 hours	14 days
Dextrose injection, USP (5%)	72 hours	14 days
Ringer's injection, USP	72 hours	14 days
Dextrose 5% with 0.255% sodium chloride	24 hours	3 days
Lactated Ringer's injection, USP	24 hours	3 days
5% dextrose with electrolyte #48	24 hours	3 days
5% Levugen (fructose) with electrolyte #75	24 hours	3 days
Invert sugar 10% in water	24 hours	3 days
Dextrose 5% and 0.45% sodium chloride, USP	24 hours	3 days
5% alcohol, 5% dextrose in water	24 hours	3 days
5% alcohol, 5% dextrose in 0.9% sodium chloride	24 hours	3 days
5% dextrose in alcohol	24 hours	3 days
Maintenance electrolyte solution (electrolyte #75)	24 hours	3 days
Pediatric maintenance electrolyte solution (electrolyte #48)	24 hours	3 days

Discard any unused solutions after the time periods outlined above.

Geopen is available in 5 g (NDC 0995-1320-83), 10 g (NDC 0995-1320-07) Piggyback Units, and 30 g (NDC 0995-1322-83) Bulk Pharmacy Package for intravenous use.

70-1856-00-7

GLUCOTROL® ℞

[glu 'kă-trōl]
(glipizide)
TABLETS
For Oral Use

DESCRIPTION

GLUCOTROL (glipizide) is an oral blood-glucose-lowering drug of the sulfonylurea class.

The Chemical Abstracts name of glipizide is 1-cyclohexyl-3-[[p-[2-(5-methylpyrazinecarboxamido)ethyl]phenyl]sulfonyl]urea. The molecular formula is $C_{21}H_{27}N_5O_4S$; the molecular weight is 445.55; the structural formula is shown below:

Glipizide is a whitish, odorless powder with a pKa of 5.9. It is insoluble in water and alcohols, but soluble in 0.1 *N* NaOH; it is freely soluble in dimethylformamide. GLUCOTROL tablets for oral use are available in 5 and 10 mg strengths.

CLINICAL PHARMACOLOGY

Mechanism of Action: The primary mode of action of GLUCOTROL in experimental animals appears to be the stimulation of insulin secretion from the beta cells of pancreatic islet tissue and is thus dependent on functioning beta cells in the pancreatic islets. In humans GLUCOTROL appears to lower the blood glucose acutely by stimulating the release of insulin from the pancreas, an effect dependent upon functioning beta cells in the pancreatic islets. The mechanism by which GLUCOTROL lowers blood glucose during long-term administration has not been clearly established. In man, stimulation of insulin secretion by GLUCOTROL in response to a meal is undoubtedly of major importance. Fasting insulin levels are not elevated even on long-term GLUCOTROL administration, but the postprandial insulin response continues to be enhanced after at least 6 months of treatment. The insulinotropic response to a meal occurs within 30 minutes after an oral dose of GLUCOTROL in diabetic patients, but elevated insulin levels do not persist beyond the time of the meal challenge. Extrapancreatic effects may play a part in the mechanism of action of oral sulfonylurea hypoglycemic drugs.

Blood sugar control persists in some patients for up to 24 hours after a single dose of GLUCOTROL, even though plasma levels have declined to a small fraction of peak levels by that time (see Pharmacokinetics below).

Some patients fail to respond initially, or gradually lose their responsiveness to sulfonylurea drugs, including GLUCOTROL. Alternatively, GLUCOTROL may be effective in some patients who have not responded or have ceased to respond to other sulfonylureas.

Other Effects: It has been shown that GLUCOTROL therapy was effective in controlling blood sugar without deleterious changes in the plasma lipoprotein profiles of patients treated for NIDDM.

In a placebo-controlled, crossover study in normal volunteers, GLUCOTROL had no anti-diuretic activity, and, in fact, led to a slight increase in free water clearance.

Pharmacokinetics: Gastrointestinal absorption of GLUCOTROL in man is uniform, rapid, and essentially complete. Peak plasma concentrations occur 1–3 hours after a single oral dose. The half-life of elimination ranges from 2–4 hours in normal subjects, whether given intravenously or orally. The metabolic and excretory patterns are similar with the two routes of administration, indicating that first-pass metabolism is not significant. GLUCOTROL does not accumulate in plasma on repeated oral administration. Total absorption and disposition of an oral dose was unaffected by food in normal volunteers, but absorption was delayed by about 40 minutes. Thus GLUCOTROL was more effective when administered about 30 minutes before, rather than with, a test meal in diabetic patients. Protein binding was studied in serum from volunteers who received either oral or intravenous GLUCOTROL and found to be 98–99% one hour after either route of administration. The apparent volume of distribution of GLUCOTROL after intravenous administration was 11 liters, indicative of localization within the extracellular fluid compartment. In mice no GLUCOTROL or metabolites were detectable autoradiographically in the brain or spinal cord of males or females, nor in the fetuses of pregnant females. In another study, however, very small amounts of radioactivity were detected in the fetuses of rats given labelled drug.

The metabolism of GLUCOTROL is extensive and occurs mainly in the liver. The primary metabolites are inactive hydroxylation products and polar conjugates and are excreted mainly in the urine. Less than 10% unchanged GLUCOTROL is found in the urine.

INDICATIONS AND USAGE

GLUCOTROL is indicated as an adjunct to diet for the control of hyperglycemia and its associated symptomatology in patients with non-insulin-dependent diabetes mellitus (NIDDM; type II), formerly known as maturity-onset diabetes, after an adequate trial of dietary therapy has proved unsatisfactory.

In initiating treatment for non-insulin-dependent diabetes, diet should be emphasized as the primary form of treatment. Caloric restriction and weight loss are essential in the obese diabetic patient. Proper dietary management alone may be effective in controlling the blood glucose and symptoms of hyperglycemia. The importance of regular physical activity should also be stressed, and cardiovascular risk factors should be identified, and corrective measures taken where possible.

If this treatment program fails to reduce symptoms and/or blood glucose, the use of an oral sulfonylurea or insulin should be considered. Use of GLUCOTROL must be viewed by both the physician and patient as a treatment in addition to diet, and not as a substitute for diet or as a convenient mechanism for avoiding dietary restraint. Furthermore, loss of blood glucose control on diet alone also may be transient, thus requiring only short-term administration of GLUCOTROL.

During maintenance programs, GLUCOTROL should be discontinued if satisfactory lowering of blood glucose is no longer achieved. Judgments should be based on regular clinical and laboratory evaluations.

In considering the use of GLUCOTROL in asymptomatic patients, it should be recognized that controlling blood glucose in non-insulin-dependent diabetes has not been definitely established to be effective in preventing the long-term cardiovascular or neural complications of diabetes.

CONTRAINDICATIONS

GLUCOTROL is contraindicated in patients with:

1. Known hypersensitivity to the drug.
2. Diabetic ketoacidosis, with or without coma. This condition should be treated with insulin.

WARNINGS

SPECIAL WARNING ON INCREASED RISK OF CARDIOVASCULAR MORTALITY: The administration of oral hypoglycemic drugs has been reported to be associated with increased cardiovascular mortality as compared to treatment with diet alone or diet plus insulin. This warning is based on the study conducted by the University Group Diabetes Program (UGDP), a long-term prospective clinical trial

Continued on next page

Roerig—Cont.

designed to evaluate the effectiveness of glucose-lowering drugs in preventing or delaying vascular complications in patients with non-insulin-dependent diabetes. The study involved 823 patients who were randomly assigned to one of four treatment groups (*Diabetes,* 19, supp. 2: 747–830, 1970).

UGDP reported that patients treated for 5 to 8 years with diet plus a fixed dose of tolbutamide (1.5 grams per day) had a rate of cardiovascular mortality approximately 2½ times that of patients treated with diet alone. A significant increase in total mortality was not observed, but the use of tolbutamide was discontinued based on the increase in cardiovascular mortality, thus limiting the opportunity for the study to show an increase in overall mortality. Despite controversy regarding the interpretation of these results, the findings of the UGDP study provide an adequate basis for this warning. The patient should be informed of the potential risks and advantages of GLUCOTROL and of alternative modes of therapy.

Although only one drug in the sulfonylurea class (tolbutamide) was included in this study, it is prudent from a safety standpoint to consider that this warning may also apply to other oral hypoglycemic drugs in this class, in view of their close similarities in mode of action and chemical structure.

PRECAUTIONS

General

Renal and Hepatic Disease: The metabolism and excretion of GLUCOTROL may be slowed in patients with impaired renal and/or hepatic function. If hypoglycemia should occur in such patients, it may be prolonged and appropriate management should be instituted.

Hypoglycemia: All sulfonylurea drugs are capable of producing severe hypoglycemia. Proper patient selection, dosage, and instructions are important to avoid hypoglycemic episodes. Renal or hepatic insufficiency may cause elevated blood levels of GLUCOTROL and the latter may also diminish gluconeogenic capacity, both of which increase the risk of serious hypoglycemic reactions. Elderly, debilitated or malnourished patients, and those with adrenal or pituitary insufficiency are particularly susceptible to the hypoglycemic action of glucose-lowering drugs. Hypoglycemia may be difficult to recognize in the elderly, and in people who are taking beta-adrenergic blocking drugs. Hypoglycemia is more likely to occur when caloric intake is deficient, after severe or prolonged exercise, when alcohol is ingested, or when more than one glucose-lowering drug is used.

Loss of Control of Blood Glucose: When a patient stabilized on any diabetic regimen is exposed to stress such as fever, trauma, infection, or surgery, a loss of control may occur. At such times, it may be necessary to discontinue GLUCOTROL and administer insulin.

The effectiveness of any oral hypoglycemic drug, including GLUCOTROL, in lowering blood glucose to a desired level decreases in many patients over a period of time, which may be due to progression of the severity of the diabetes or to diminished responsiveness to the drug. This phenomenon is known as secondary failure, to distinguish it from primary failure in which the drug is ineffective in an individual patient when first given.

Laboratory Tests: Blood and urine glucose should be monitored periodically. Measurement of glycosylated hemoglobin may be useful.

Information for Patients: Patients should be informed of the potential risks and advantages of GLUCOTROL and of alternative modes of therapy. They should also be informed about the importance of adhering to dietary instructions, of a regular exercise program, and of regular testing of urine and/or blood glucose.

The risks of hypoglycemia, its symptoms and treatment, and conditions that predispose to its development should be explained to patients and responsible family members. Primary and secondary failure should also be explained.

Drug Interactions: The hypoglycemic action of sulfonylureas may be potentiated by certain drugs including nonsteroidal anti-inflammatory agents and other drugs that are highly protein bound, salicylates, sulfonamides, chloramphenicol, probenecid, coumarins, monoamine oxidase inhibitors, and beta-adrenergic blocking agents. When such drugs are administered to a patient receiving GLUCOTROL, the patient should be observed closely for hypoglycemia. When such drugs are withdrawn from a patient receiving GLUCOTROL, the patient should be observed closely for loss of control. *In vitro* binding studies with human serum proteins indicate that GLUCOTROL binds differently than tolbutamide and does not interact with salicylate or dicumarol. However, caution must be exercised in extrapolating these findings to the clinical situation and in the use of GLUCOTROL with these drugs.

Certain drugs tend to produce hyperglycemia and may lead to loss of control. These drugs include the thiazides and other diuretics, corticosteroids, phenothiazines, thyroid products, estrogens, oral contraceptives, phenytoin, nicotinic acid, sympathomimetics, calcium channel blocking drugs, and isoniazid. When such drugs are administered to a patient receiving GLUCOTROL, the patient should be closely observed for loss of control. When such drugs are withdrawn from a patient receiving GLUCOTROL, the patient should be observed closely for hypoglycemia.

A potential interaction between oral miconazole and oral hypoglycemic agents leading to severe hypoglycemia has been reported. Whether this interaction also occurs with the intravenous, topical, or vaginal preparations of miconazole is not known.

Carcinogenesis, Mutagenesis, Impairment of Fertility: A twenty month study in rats and an eighteen month study in mice at doses up to 75 times the maximum human dose revealed no evidence of drug-related carcinogenicity. Bacterial and *in vivo* mutagenicity tests were uniformly negative. Studies in rats of both sexes at doses up to 75 times the human dose showed no effects on fertility.

Pregnancy: Pregnancy Category C: GLUCOTROL (glipizide) was found to be mildly fetotoxic in rat reproductive studies at all dose levels (5–50 mg/kg). This fetotoxicity has been similarly noted with other sulfonylureas, such as tolbutamide and tolazamide. The effect is perinatal and believed to be directly related to the pharmacologic (hypoglycemic) action of GLUCOTROL. In studies in rats and rabbits no teratogenic effects were found. There are no adequate and well controlled studies in pregnant women. GLUCOTROL should be used during pregnancy only if the potential benefit justifies the potential risk to the fetus.

Because recent information suggests that abnormal blood glucose levels during pregnancy are associated with a higher incidence of congenital abnormalities, many experts recommend that insulin be used during pregnancy to maintain blood glucose levels as close to normal as possible.

Nonteratogenic Effects: Prolonged severe hypoglycemia (4 to 10 days) has been reported in neonates born to mothers who were receiving a sulfonylurea drug at the time of delivery. This has been reported more frequently with the use of agents with prolonged half-lives. If GLUCOTROL is used during pregnancy, it should be discontinued at least one month before the expected delivery date.

Nursing Mothers: Although it is not known whether GLUCOTROL is excreted in human milk, some sulfonylurea drugs are known to be excreted in human milk. Because the potential for hypoglycemia in nursing infants may exist, a decision should be made whether to discontinue nursing or to discontinue the drug, taking into account the importance of the drug to the mother. If the drug is discontinued and if diet alone is inadequate for controlling blood glucose, insulin therapy should be considered.

Pediatric Use: Safety and effectiveness in children have not been established.

ADVERSE REACTIONS

In U.S. and foreign controlled studies, the frequency of serious adverse reactions reported was very low. Of 702 patients, 11.8% reported adverse reactions and in only 1.5% was GLUCOTROL discontinued.

Hypoglycemia: See PRECAUTIONS and OVERDOSAGE sections.

Gastrointestinal: Gastrointestinal disturbances are the most common reactions. Gastrointestinal complaints were reported with the following approximate incidence: nausea and diarrhea, one in seventy; constipation and gastralgia, one in one hundred. They appear to be dose-related and may disappear on division or reduction of dosage. Cholestatic jaundice may occur rarely with sulfonylureas: GLUCOTROL should be discontinued if this occurs.

Dermatologic: Allergic skin reactions including erythema, morbilliform or maculopapular eruptions, urticaria, pruritus, and eczema have been reported in about one in seventy patients. These may be transient and may disappear despite continued use of GLUCOTROL; if skin reactions persist, the drug should be discontinued. Porphyria cutanea tarda and photosensitivity reactions have been reported with sulfonylureas.

Hematologic: Leukopenia, agranulocytosis, thrombocytopenia, hemolytic anemia, aplastic anemia, and pancytopenia have been reported with sulfonylureas.

Metabolic: Hepatic porphyria and disulfiram-like reactions have been reported with sulfonylureas. In the mouse, GLUCOTROL pretreatment did not cause an accumulation of acetaldehyde after ethanol administration. Clinical experience to date has shown that GLUCOTROL has an extremely low incidence of disulfiram-like alcohol reactions.

Endocrine Reactions: Cases of hyponatremia and the syndrome of inappropriate antidiuretic hormone (SIADH) secretion have been reported with this and other sulfonylureas.

Miscellaneous: Dizziness, drowsiness, and headache have each been reported in about one in fifty patients treated with GLUCOTROL. They are usually transient and seldom require discontinuance of therapy.

Laboratory Tests: The pattern of laboratory test abnormalities observed with GLUCOTROL was similar to that for other sulfonylureas. Occasional mild to moderate elevations of SGOT, LDH, alkaline phosphatase, BUN and creatinine were noted. One case of jaundice was reported. The relationship of these abnormalities to GLUCOTROL is uncertain, and they have rarely been associated with clinical symptoms.

OVERDOSAGE

There is no well documented experience with GLUCOTROL overdosage. The acute oral toxicity was extremely low in all species tested (LD_{50} greater than 4 g/kg).

Overdosage of sulfonylureas including GLUCOTROL can produce hypoglycemia. Mild hypoglycemic symptoms without loss of consciousness or neurologic findings should be treated aggressively with oral glucose and adjustments in drug dosage and/or meal patterns. Close monitoring should continue until the physician is assured that the patient is out of danger. Severe hypoglycemic reactions with coma, seizure, or other neurological impairment occur infrequently, but constitute medical emergencies requiring immediate hospitalization. If hypoglycemic coma is diagnosed or suspected, the patient should be given a rapid intravenous injection of concentrated (50%) glucose solution. This should be followed by a continuous infusion of a more dilute (10%) glucose solution at a rate that will maintain the blood glucose at a level above 100 mg/dL. Patients should be closely monitored for a minimum of 24 to 48 hours since hypoglycemia may recur after apparent clinical recovery. Clearance of GLUCOTROL from plasma would be prolonged in persons with liver disease. Because of the extensive protein binding of GLUCOTROL, dialysis is unlikely to be of benefit.

DOSAGE AND ADMINISTRATION

There is no fixed dosage regimen for the management of diabetes mellitus with GLUCOTROL or any other hypoglycemic agent. In addition to the usual monitoring of urinary glucose, the patient's blood glucose must also be monitored periodically to determine the minimum effective dose for the patient; to detect primary failure, i.e., inadequate lowering of blood glucose at the maximum recommended dose of medication; and to detect secondary failure, i.e., loss of an adequate blood-glucose-lowering response after an initial period of effectiveness. Glycosylated hemoglobin levels may also be of value in monitoring the patient's response to therapy.

Short-term administration of GLUCOTROL may be sufficient during periods of transient loss of control in patients usually controlled well on diet.

In general, GLUCOTROL should be given approximately 30 minutes before a meal to achieve the greatest reduction in postprandial hyperglycemia.

Initial Dose: The recommended starting dose is 5 mg, given before breakfast. Geriatric patients or those with liver disease may be started on 2.5 mg.

Titration: Dosage adjustments should ordinarily be in increments of 2.5–5 mg, as determined by blood glucose response. At least several days should elapse between titration steps. If response to a single dose is not satisfactory, dividing that dose may prove effective. The maximum recommended once daily dose is 15 mg. Doses above 15 mg should ordinarily be divided and given before meals of adequate caloric content. The maximum recommended total daily dose is 40 mg.

Maintenance: Some patients may be effectively controlled on a once-a-day regimen, while others show better response with divided dosing. Total daily doses above 15 mg should ordinarily be divided. Total daily doses above 30 mg have been safely given on a b.i.d. basis to long-term patients.

In elderly patients, debilitated or malnourished patients, and patients with impaired renal or hepatic function, the initial and maintenance dosing should be conservative to avoid hypoglycemic reactions (see PRECAUTIONS section).

Patients Receiving Insulin: As with other sulfonylurea-class hypoglycemics, many stable non-insulin-dependent diabetic patients receiving insulin may be safely placed on GLUCOTROL. When transferring patients from insulin to GLUCOTROL, the following general guidelines should be considered:

For patients whose daily insulin requirement is 20 units or less, insulin may be discontinued and GLUCOTROL therapy may begin at usual dosages. Several days should elapse between GLUCOTROL titration steps.

For patients whose daily insulin requirement is greater than 20 units, the insulin dose should be reduced by 50% and GLUCOTROL therapy may begin at usual dosages. Subsequent reductions in insulin dosage should depend on individual patient response. Several days should elapse between GLUCOTROL titration steps.

During the insulin withdrawal period, the patient should test urine samples for sugar and ketone bodies at least three times daily. Patients should be instructed to contact the prescriber immediately if these tests are abnormal. In some cases, especially when patient has been receiving greater than 40 units of insulin daily, it may be advisable to consider hospitalization during the transition period.

Patients Receiving Other Oral Hypoglycemic Agents: As with other sulfonylurea-class hypoglycemics, no transition period is necessary when transferring patients to GLUCOTROL. Patients should be observed carefully (1–2 weeks) for hypoglycemia when being transferred from longer half-life sulfonylureas (e.g., chlorpropamide) to GLUCOTROL due to potential overlapping of drug effect.

HOW SUPPLIED

GLUCOTROL tablets are white, dye-free, scored, diamond-shaped, and imprinted as follows:

5 mg—Pfizer 411; 10 mg—Pfizer 412.

5 mg Bottles: 100's (NDC 0049-4110-66); (NDC 0662-4110-66); 500's (NDC 0049-4110-73); (NDC 0662-4110-73); Unit Dose 100's (NDC 0049-4110-41); (NDC 0662-4110-41)

10 mg Bottles: 100's (NDC 0049-4120-66); (NDC 0662-4120-66); Unit Dose 100's (NDC 0049-4120-41); (NDC 0662-4120-41)

Recommended Storage: Store below 86°F (30°C).

Caution: Federal law prohibits dispensing without prescription.

69-4227-00-4

Shown in Product Identification Section, page 426

HEPTUNA® PLUS ℞

[hep-tū'na]

CAPSULES

(Hard Gelatin)

Fortified Oral Hematopoietic Formulation

Each capsule contains:

HEMATOPOIETIC FACTORS

Ferrous Sulfate, dried, U.S.P. (provides 100 mg of elemental iron) ....311 mg
Desiccated Liver (undefatted) ....50 mg
Vitamin B_{12}, cobalamin concentrate NF (as Stablets®) ....5 mcg
With intrinsic factor concentrate (non-inhibitory) ....25 mg

VITAMINS

B_1 (thiamine mononitrate, U.S.P.) ....3.1 mg
B_2 (riboflavin, U.S.P.) ....2 mg
B_6 (pyridoxine hydrochloride, U.S.P.) ....1.6 mg
Vitamin C (from sodium ascorbate) ....150 mg
Niacin (niacinamide, U.S.P.) ....15 mg
Pantothenic Acid (calcium pantothenate, U.S.P.) ....0.9 mg

MINERALS

Copper (from copper sulfate) ....1 mg
Molybdenum (from sodium molybdate) ....0.2 mg
Calcium (from dibasic calcium phosphate) ....37.4 mg
Iodine (from potassium iodide) ....0.05 mg
Manganese (from manganese sulfate) ....0.033 mg
Magnesium (from magnesium sulfate) ....2 mg
Phosphorus (from dibasic calcium phosphate) ....29 mg
Potassium (from potassium sulfate) ....1.7 mg
Stablets® U.S. Pat. No. 2.830.933

INDICATIONS

Heptuna Plus is a multicomponent preparation effective in the treatment of those anemias amenable to oral hematinic therapy. These include pernicious anemia and other megaloblastic anemias, and also iron deficiency anemia. Heptuna Plus also contains balanced amounts of vitamin B complex, vitamin C, and minerals as nutritional supplements.

CLINICAL PHARMACOLOGY

Hematopoietic Factors

Vitamin B_{12}: Exogenous sources of B_{12} are required for normal growth and maintenance of normal erythropoiesis as well as nucleo-protein synthesis, myelin synthesis, and cell reproduction. Vitamin B_{12} is irregularly absorbed from the intact gastrointestinal tract. Free vitamin B_{12} is bound to intrinsic factor which is normally secreted by the gastric mucosal tissue, and acts as a carrier protein for active transport through the gastrointestinal tract. This normal active transport system is usually saturated by 1.5 to 3 mg of vitamin B_{12}. Under conditions of functional or anatomical derangements of the stomach or ileum, where secretion of intrinsic factor is abnormally low, absorption of vitamin B_{12} will proceed poorly, if at all. Megaloblastic anemias may develop after gastrectomy, in Addinsonian permicious anemia, and in fish tapeworm (*Diphyllobothrium latum)* infection; treatment to free the host of competing bacteria and parasites is required. Other causes of B_{12}deficiency are strict vegetarianism, surgical compromise of gastric or ileum activity, gastric atrophy due to multiple sclerosis or iron deficiency or malabsorption syndromes of various etiologies; in this last case parenteral therapy or oral therapy with massive doses of vitamin B_{12} may be necessary for successful treatment. The megaloblastic anemias of malabsorption syndromes may be due to a deficiency of folate—which is not contained in Heptuna Plus, as well as to B_{12} deficiency, and combined therapy may be warranted.

Desiccated Liver: Desiccated Liver is an extract of mammalian livers used in Heptuna Plus as a source of naturally occurring riboflavin, nicotinic acid, and choline as a nutritional supplement. Desiccated liver (undefatted) 50 mg. provides approximately 2.5 mcg riboflavin, 12.5 mcg nicotinic acid, and 0.5 mg choline.

Ferrous Sulfate: As compared to other sources of iron, ferrous sulfate provides the highest amounts of elemental iron for utilization in patients with hypochronic anemias. Iron is a constituent of hemoglobin and its administration usually corrects erythropoietic abnormalities, and may reverse esophageal and gastrointestinal tissue changes associated with iron deficiency.

Approximately 25% of an orally administered dose of ferrous sulfate will be utilizable iron. The primary sites of iron absorption are the duodenum, the jejunum, the stomach, and the proximal portion of the ileum. The ferrous species of iron is the most readily absorbed fraction. While the exact mechanism of absorption is not known, the absorption, metabolism, and excretion of iron appear to be related to body requirements for this mineral. The excretion of iron as ferritin is by way of epithelial cells sloughed from the skin and gastrointestinal tract. There may be trace losses in bile, and cell-free sweat.

Vitamins

Vitamin C: It is known that an acidic environment favors the maintenance of iron in the ferrous state, retards formation of insoluble complexes of iron with food or other substrates, and will thus promote gastric absorption of ferrous iron. The vitamin C content of Heptuna Plus, in addition to contributing to the overall acidic environment of gastric fluids, may also be useful as a supplement to deficiency states. Prolonged and severe vitamin C deficiency is associated with an anemia which is usually hypochronic but occasionally megaloblastic. Vitamin C is also utilized in intracellular reactions such as conversion of folic acid and carbohydrate synthesis.

Vitamin B Complex (B_1, B_2, B_6, Niacin, Pantothenic Acid): These are provided in Heptuna Plus as nutritional supplements. Vitamin B complex is essential for the metabolism of carbohydrates and protein. Administration of these water-soluble vitamins may be useful in deficiency states associated with febrile diseases, severe burns, gastrointestinal disorders interfering with absorption of these vitamins, in prolonged or wasting diseases, or in nutritional deficiency. One capsule of Heptuna Plus provides the following approximate percentage of the U.S. Recommended Adult Daily Allowances (U.S. RDA):

	% U.S. RDA
B_1	221.4
B_2	125
B_6	80
Vitamin C	333.3
Niacin	83.3
Pantothenic Acid	9

Minerals

One capsule of Heptuna Plus provides the following approximate percentages of U.S. Recommended Adult Daily Allowances (U.S. RDA):

	% U.S. RDA
Copper	50
Molybdenum	*
Calcium	4.25
Iodine	38.46
Manganese	*
Magnesium	0.57
Phosphorous	3.63
Potassium	*

*U.S. RDA not yet established.

The precise role of minerals in human nutritional maintenance has yet to be defined. However, several trace elements (including copper, molybdenum, calcium, iodine, manganese) have been identified as being essential for animal life.

Copper: Copper has been identified as a component of several amine oxidases. Copper depletion in experimental animals results in failure to utilize ferritin iron and is accompanied by increases in hepatic iron concentration sometimes with clear evidence of hemosiderosis. Copper-dependent enzyme systems may be intimately involved in tissue iron mobilization.

Molybdenum: Molybdenum has been identified as a component of xanthine oxidase (involved in purine oxidation and possibly in the release of iron from ferritin), aldehydeoxidase, and sulfite oxidase.

Calcium: In addition to this element's well known important roles in maintenance of bone, neurologic, and muscular tissue integrity, calcium may also play a role in maintaining the integrity of cell membrance structures.

Iodine: As the central element of thyroid activity, iodine intake may influence carbohydrate and cholesterol metabolism, functions of the central nervous system, catecholamine secretion, and skeletal growth and maturation. Its exact role in the hematopoietic process, if any, has not been determined.

Manganese: The main manifestations of manganese deficiency in laboratory animals are impaired growth, disturbed or depressed reproductive function, skeletal abnormalities, and nervous disorders. Its exact role in the hematopoietic process, if any, has not been determined.

Magnesium: Magnesium plays a fundamental role in most reactions that include phosphate transfer, and it is believed to be essential for the structural stabilization of nucleic acids. Magnesium depletion has been known to impair homeostasis of potassium and calcium. Deficiency of magnesium almost always occurs as a consequence of some underlying disease, including malabsorption syndromes.

Phosphorus: Hypophosphatemia may cause a marked decrease in erythrocytic concentrations of ATP and of 2,3 diphosphoglycerate. Acute hemolytic-type anemia may develop in severe deficiency states.

Potassium: Potassium is an essential mineral in electrolyte maintenance and in maintaining electrical excitability of cells and acid-base homeostasis. Its exact role in the hematopoietic process, if any, has not been determined.

CONTRAINDICATIONS

Hemachromatosis and hemosiderosis are contraindications to iron therapy. Previous hypersensitivity to any of the components of Heptuna Plus contraindicates its use.

PRECAUTIONS

Anemia is a manifestation of an underlying disease process. While Heptuna Plus provides components useful in the management of certain anemias, appropriate attention should be directed to an etiological diagnosis and treatment of the underlying causes of the anemia.

Resistance to the effects of exogenous intrinsic factor has been reported. Local intestinal antibodies which render exogenous intrinsic factor inactive have been noted to develop in approximately 50% of patients treated within one year of continuous oral therapy. If resistance develops, parenteral therapy or oral therapy with large doses of vitamin B_{12} may be necessary to circumvent normal active transport mechanisms and adequately treat the patient.

Although this product contains vitamin B_{12} (as Stablets®) with intrinsic factor concentrate (non-inhibitory) and desiccated liver, it is not as reliable as parenterally administered cyanocobalamin (vitamin B_{12}) in the management of pernicious anemia. Some patients with pernicious anemia may not respond to orally ingested cobalamin concentrate (vitamin B_{12}). There is no known way to predict which patients will respond or which patients may cease to respond.

Information for Patients: As Heptuna Plus contains substantial amounts of iron, patients should be advised that gastrointestinal reactions such as diarrhea or constipation may occur with usage. Patients should be cautioned against concomitant usage of Heptuna Plus and tetracycline, or its analogs, so as to avoid a chelation interaction which would reduce the amounts of antibiotic and iron or divalent ions available for gastrointestinal absorption.

Laboratory Tests: Periodic clinical and laboratory monitoring are considered essential to proper use of hematopoietics. The following laboratory tests may be useful in evaluating patients' response to therapy: peripheral blood smears, reticulocyte count, serum iron, iron binding capacity, serum B_{12}, serum folic acid, hemoglobin and hematocrit, mean corpuscular volume.

Drug Interactions: The following drug/drug interactions may occur with the use of Heptuna Plus.

Agent	Interaction
Tetracycline and derivatives	Complexation of antibiotic and iron or divalent ions (such as calcium) decrease availability of component for gastric absorption. This may be avoided by administration of Heptuna Plus at least one hour before tetracycline-type agent.
Levodopa	Doses of pyridoxine of approximately 5 mg (three capsules Heptuna Plus provide 4.8 mg B_6) or more per day may reduce the beneficial effects of levodopa in parkinsonian disease. This is thought to be due to increased transamination of levodopa. Patients receiving this combination should be carefully observed for unwanted variations in parkinson control.
Lithium	The presence of iodine in Heptuna Plus may enhance the hypothyroid and goiterogenic potential of these two components. Patients receiving lithium and Heptuna Plus should have baseline and periodic thyroid status checks.

Laboratory Interactions: Heptuna Plus contains iodine 0.05 mg (as potassium iodide) as an active component and the iodinated dye tetraiodofluorescein (FD and C#3) in the capsule shell. These agents may interfere with I^{131} or other diagnostic radioiodine neucleotide testing procedures. Other than changes induced from the therapeutic effects of the

Continued on next page

Roerig—Cont.

components of Heptuna Plus, no other interferences with laboratory testing procedures have been identified.

Carcinogenesis, Mutagenesis, Impairment of Fertility: The potential for Heptuna Plus to impair fertility or act as a carcinogen or a mutagen has not been studied *in vivo* or *in vitro.*

Use in Pregnancy

Category C: Animal reproductive studies have not been conducted with Heptuna Plus. It is also not known whether Heptuna Plus can cause fetal harm when administered to a pregnant woman or can affect reproductive capacity. Heptuna Plus should be given to a pregnant woman only if clearly needed.

Nursing Mothers: It is not known whether this drug is excreted in human milk. Because many drugs are excreted in human milk, caution should be exercised when Heptuna Plus is administered to a nursing woman.

Pediatric Use: Safety and effectiveness in children have not been established.

ADVERSE REACTIONS

Ferrous Sulfate: The most frequent adverse reactions to Heptuna Plus are those associated with oral iron therapy. An incidence of gastrointestinal discomfort in 19.5% to 27% of patients receiving "iron placebo" tablets has been reported. The gastrointestinal complaints usually noted are diarrhea, constipation, nausea, epigastric pain, ructus, vomiting, and black staining of stools. Reduction in dosage or administration with meals may minimize these effects.

In extremely rare instances, skin rash suggesting allergy has been noted following the oral administration of desiccated liver preparations.

Iodine: Allergic reactions, including angioedema, rashes, lymphadenopathy, eosinophilia, arteritis, and febrile reactions have been reported with iodine usage. Also, acne, swelling of salivary glands, iodine coryza, and stomach upsets have been reported. Iodine use may precipitate hypo- or hyperthyroid activity and goiter.

B Complex Vitamins: Adverse reactions to these water-soluble vitamins are rare:

—Thiamine; Hypersensitivity reactions are rare and have been reported mostly with parenteral administration.

—Pyridoxine; Allergic reactions have been reported, but are rare.

—Cyanocobalamine/Cobalamine; Mild forms of polycythemia, and peripheral vascular thrombosis during recovery from pernicious anemia treated with B_{12} have been observed. Use of high dose oral vitamin B_{12} has been associated with the appearance of acne.

Minerals: No adverse reactions other than those specified for iodine have been reported with orally administered minerals as supplied in Heptuna Plus.

OVERDOSAGE

Acute Toxicity: Toxicity may result from overdosage due to ingestion of ferrous sulfate. In young children 300 mg of elemental iron may be fatal. The remainder of the ingredients are essentially nontoxic (water-soluble vitamins) or present in such small amounts as to be nontoxic even with overdosage.

Symptoms: Symptoms may occur 30 to 60 minutes after ingestion. Danger may exist for 24-48 hours. Acute gastroenteritis, vomiting, diarrhea, dehydration, collapse, and coma ending in death may occur. A severe acidosis may also be present. The diarrhea may initially be watery, becoming bloody and then tarry.

Dialyzability: It is known that iron, magnesium, potassium, iodide, and phosphate are dialyzable. Dialysis may not be effective in removing vitamin B_{12} or copper. The effect of dialysis on the other components in Heptuna Plus is not certain.

Management: Management should be directed primarily at the treatment of iron toxicity. Acute toxicity may occur in young children after ingestion of 1 gram of ferrous sulfate (equivalent to 3 capsules of Heptuna Plus). In adults iron toxicity is rare and is most likely to occur only after ingestion of more than 50 grams of ferrous sulfate (equivalent to 150 capsules of Heptuna Plus). Treatment involves gastric lavage and/or use of absorbents. A 1% sodium bicarbonate lavage fluid may be useful to prevent further iron absorption. Lavage must be performed with caution after the first hour of an overdosage because of the potential for gastric necrosis and perforation. Shock and acid-base imbalances should be treated with standard methods. Serum iron levels should be monitored and deferoxamine mesylate therapy initiated if necessary. Other chelating agents should be used only if deferoxamine mesylate is not available or otherwise contraindicated, as it may form toxic complexes with iron.

DOSAGE AND ADMINISTRATION

For many patients one capsule of Heptuna Plus daily will provide sufficient amounts of hematopoietic factors for therapeutic results. If the severity and etiology of the anemia so indicate, 1 capsule three times a day (approximately every six hours) may be prescribed. Therapy with Heptuna Plus may be continued until patient response indicates discontinuation of therapy.

HOW SUPPLIED

Heptuna Plus capsules are available as red and white gelatin capsules, in bottles of 100.

68-0331-00-7

Shown in Product Identification Section, page 426

MARAX® ℞

[*mă'rax*]

(ephedrine sulfate, theophylline, hydroxyzine HCl)

TABLETS AND DF SYRUP

CONTENTS

	Each Tablet Contains:	Each Teaspoon (5 ml.) Syrup Contains:
Ephedrine Sulfate	25 mg.	6.25 mg.
Theophylline	130 mg.	32.50 mg.
Atarax® (hydroxyzine HCl)	10 mg.	2.5 mg.
Alcohol (Ethyl Alcohol)		5% v/v.

ACTIONS

The action of ephedrine as a vasoconstrictor is well known. It is therefore of significant benefit in symptomatic relief of the congestion occurring in bronchial asthma. As a bronchodilator, it has a slower onset but longer duration of action than does epinephrine, which, in contrast to ephedrine, is not effective upon oral administration.

The diverse actions of theophylline—broncho- spasmolytic, cardiovascular, and diuretic—are well established, and make it a particularly useful drug in the treatment of bronchial asthma, both in the acute attack and in the prophylactic therapy of the disease.

Atarax (hydroxyzine HCl) modifies the central stimulatory action of ephedrine preventing excessive excitation in patients on Marax therapy.

In animal studies Atarax (hydroxyzine HCl) has demonstrated antiserotonin activity and antispasmodic potency of a nonspecific nature.

Marax-DF Syrup produces an expectorant action wherein the tenacity of the sputum is decreased and the ease of expectoration is increased.

Indications

Based on a review of this drug by the National Academy of Sciences-National Research Council and/or other information, FDA has classified the indications as follows:

"Possibly" Effective: For controlling bronchospastic disorders.

Final classification of the less than effective indication requires further investigation.

CONTRAINDICATIONS

Because of the ephedrine, Marax is contraindicated in cardiovascular disease, hyperthyroidism, and hypertension. This drug is contraindicated in individuals who have shown hypersensitivity to the drug or its components.

Hydroxyzine, when administered to the pregnant mouse, rat, and rabbit induced fetal abnormalities in the rat at doses substantially above the human therapeutic range. Clinical data in human beings are inadequate to establish safety in early pregnancy. Until such data are available, hydroxyzine is contraindicated in early pregnancy.

PRECAUTIONS

Because of the ephedrine component this drug should be used with caution in elderly males or those with known prostatic hypertrophy.

The potentiating action of hydroxyzine, although mild, must be taken into consideration when the drug is used in conjunction with central nervous system depressants; and when other central nervous system depressants are administered concomitantly with hydroxyzine their dosage should be reduced. Patients should be cautioned that hydroxyzine can increase the effect of alcohol.

Patients should be warned—because of the hydroxyzine component—of the possibility of drowsiness occurring and cautioned against driving a car or operating dangerous machinery while taking this drug.

ADVERSE REACTIONS

With large doses of ephedrine, excitation, tremulousness, insomnia, nervousness, palpitation, tachycardia, precordial pain, cardiac arrhythmias, vertigo, dryness of the nose and throat, headache, sweating, and warmth may occur. Because ephedrine is a sympathomimetic agent some patients may develop vesical sphincter spasm and resultant urinary hesitation, and occasionally acute urinary retention. This should be borne in mind when administering preparations containing ephedrine to elderly males or those with known prostatic hypertrophy. At the recommended dose for Marax, a side effect occasionally reported is palpitation, and this can be controlled with dosage adjustment, additional amounts of concurrently administered Atarax (hydroxyzine HCl), or discontinuation of the medication. When ephedrine is given three or more times daily patients may develop tolerance after several weeks of therapy.

Theophylline when given on an empty stomach frequently causes gastric irritation accompanied by upper abdominal discomfort, nausea, and vomiting. Administration of the medication after meals will serve to minimize this side effect. Theophylline may cause diuresis and cardiac stimulation.

The amount of Atarax (hydroxyzine HCl) present in Marax has not resulted in disturbing side effects. When used alone specifically as a tranquilizer in the normal dosage range (25 to 50 mg. three or four times a day), side effects are infrequent; even at these higher doses, no serious side effects have been reported and confirmed to date. Those which do occasionally occur when Atarax (hydroxyzine HCl) is used alone are drowsiness, xerostomia and, at extremely high doses, involuntary motor activity, unsteadiness of gait, neuromuscular weakness, all of which may be controlled by reduction of the dosage or discontinuation of the medication.

With the relatively low dose of Atarax (hydroxyzine HCl) in Marax, these effects are not likely to occur. In addition, the ataractic action of Atarax (hydroxyzine HCl) may modify the cardiac stimulatory action of ephedrine, and concurrently, increasing the amount of Atarax (hydroxyzine HCl) may control or abolish this undesirable effect of ephedrine.

DOSAGE AND ADMINISTRATION

The dosage of Marax should be adjusted according to the severity of complaints, and the patient's individual toleration.

Tablets: In general, an adult dose of 1 tablet, 2 to 4 times daily, should be sufficient. Some patients are controlled adequately with ½ to 1 tablet at bedtime. The time interval between doses should not be shorter than four hours. The dosage for children over 5 years of age and for adults who are sensitive to ephedrine, is one-half the usual adult dose. Clinical experience to date has been confined to ages above 5 years.

Syrup: The dose for children over 5 years of age is 1 teaspoon (5 ml.), 3 to 4 times daily. Dosage for children 2 to 5 years of age is ½ to 1 teaspoon (2.5-5 ml.), 3 to 4 times daily. Not recommended for children under 2 years of age.

HOW SUPPLIED

Marax Tablets are available as scored, dye free, m-shaped tablets in bottles of 100 and 500.

Marax-DF Syrup is available in pints and gallons as a colorless syrup free of all coal tar dyes, and should be dispensed in tight, light-resistant containers (USP).

67-0928-00-6
65-2265-00-3

Shown in Product Identification Section, page 426

NAVANE® ℞

[*nah'vān*]

(thiothixene) CAPSULES

NAVANE®

(thiothixene hydrochloride) CONCENTRATE

DESCRIPTION

Navane (thiothixene) is a thioxanthene derivative. Specifically, it is the *cis* isomer of N,N-dimethyl-9-[3-(4-methyl-1-piperazinyl)-propylidene] thioxanthene-2-sulfonamide.

The thioxanthenes differ from the phenothiazines by the replacement of nitrogen in the central ring with a carbon-linked side chain fixed in space in a rigid structural configuration. An N,N-dimethyl sulfonamide functional group is bonded to the thioxanthene nucleus.

ACTIONS

Navane is a psychotropic agent of the thioxanthene series. Navane possesses certain chemical and pharmacological similarities to the piperazine phenothiazines and differences from the aliphatic group of phenothiazines.

INDICATIONS

Navane is effective in the management of manifestations of psychotic disorders. Navane has not been evaluated in the management of behavioral complications in patients with mental retardation.

CONTRAINDICATIONS

Navane is contraindicated in patients with circulatory collapse, comatose states, central nervous system depression due to any cause, and blood dyscrasias. Navane is contraindicated in individuals who have shown hypersensitivity to the drug. It is not known whether there is a cross sensitivity between the thioxanthenes and the phenothiazine derivatives, but this possibility should be considered.

WARNINGS

Tardive Dyskinesia—Tardive dyskinesia, a syndrome consisting of potentially irreversible, involuntary, dyskinetic movements may develop in patients treated with neuroleptic (antipsychotic) drugs. Although the prevalence of the syndrome appears to be highest among the elderly, especially elderly women, it is impossible to rely upon prevalence estimates to predict, at the inception of neuroleptic treatment, which patients are likely to develop the syndrome. Whether neuroleptic drug products differ in their potential to cause tardive dyskinesia is unknown.

Both the risk of developing the syndrome and the likelihood that it will become irreversible are believed to increase as the duration of treatment and the total cumulative dose of neuroleptic drugs administered to the patient increase. However, the syndrome can develop, although much less commonly, after relatively brief treatment periods at low doses.

There is no known treatment for established cases of tardive dyskinesia, although the syndrome may remit, partially or completely, if neuroleptic treatment is withdrawn. Neuroleptic treatment, itself, however, may suppress (or partially suppress) the signs and symptoms of the syndrome and thereby may possibly mask the underlying disease process. The effect that symptomatic suppression has upon the long-term course of the syndrome is unknown.

Given these considerations, neuroleptics should be prescribed in a manner that is most likely to minimize the occurrence of tardive dyskinesia. Chronic neuroleptic treatment should generally be reserved for patients who suffer from a chronic illness that, 1) is known to respond to neuroleptic drugs, and 2) for whom alternative, equally effective, but potentially less harmful treatments are *not* available or appropriate. In patients who do require chronic treatment, the smallest dose and the shortest duration of treatment producing a satisfactory clinical response should be sought. The need for continued treatment should be reassessed periodically.

If signs and symptoms of tardive dyskinesia appear in a patient on neuroleptics, drug discontinuation should be considered. However, some patients may require treatment despite the presence of the syndrome.

(For further information about the description of tardive dyskinesia and its clinical detection, please refer to the section on Adverse Reactions.)

Usage in Pregnancy—Safe use of Navane during pregnancy has not been established. Therefore, this drug should be given to pregnant patients only when, in the judgment of the physician, the expected benefits from the treatment exceed the possible risks to mother and fetus. Animal reproduction studies and clinical experience to date have not demonstrated any teratogenic effects.

In the animal reproduction studies with Navane, there was some decrease in conception rate and litter size, and an increase in resorption rate in rats and rabbits. Similar findings have been reported with other psychotropic agents. After repeated oral administration of Navane to rats (5 to 15 mg/kg/day), rabbits (3 to 50 mg/kg/day), and monkeys (1 to 3 mg/kg/day) before and during gestation, no teratogenic effects were seen.

Usage in Children—The use of Navane in children under 12 years of age is not recommended because safe conditions for its use have not been established.

As is true with many CNS drugs, Navane may impair the mental and/or physical abilities required for the performance of potentially hazardous tasks such as driving a car or operating machinery, especially during the first few days of therapy. Therefore, the patient should be cautioned accordingly.

As in the case of other CNS-acting drugs, patients receiving Navane (thiothixene) should be cautioned about the possible additive effects (which may include hypotension) with CNS depressants and with alcohol.

PRECAUTIONS

An antiemetic effect was observed in animal studies with Navane; since this effect may also occur in man, it is possible that Navane may mask signs of overdosage of toxic drugs and may obscure conditions such as intestinal obstruction and brain tumor.

In consideration of the known capability of Navane and certain other psychotropic drugs to precipitate convulsions, extreme caution should be used in patients with a history of convulsive disorders or those in a state of alcohol withdrawal, since it may lower the convulsive threshold. Although Navane potentiates the actions of the barbiturates, the dosage of the anticonvulsant therapy should not be reduced when Navane is administered concurrently.

Though exhibiting rather weak anticholinergic properties, Navane should be used with caution in patients who might be exposed to extreme heat or who are receiving atropine or related drugs.

Use with caution in patients with cardiovascular disease.

Caution as well as careful adjustment of the dosages is indicated when Navane is used in conjunction with other CNS depressants.

Also, careful observation should be made for pigmentary retinopathy, and lenticular pigmentation (fine lenticular pigmentation has been noted in a small number of patients treated with Navane for prolonged periods). Blood dyscrasias (agranulocytosis, pancytopenia, thrombocytopenic purpura), and liver damage (jaundice, biliary stasis), have been reported with related drugs.

Neuroleptic drugs elevate prolactin levels; the elevation persists during chronic administration. Tissue culture experiments indicate that approximately one-third of human breast cancers are prolactin dependent *in vitro*, a factor of potential importance if the prescription of these drugs is contemplated in a patient with a previously detected breast cancer. Although disturbances such as galactorrhea, amenorrhea, gynecomastia, and impotence have been reported, the clinical significance of elevated serum prolactin levels is unknown for most patients. An increase in mammary neoplasms has been found in rodents after chronic administration of neuroleptic drugs. Neither clinical studies nor epidemiologic studies conducted to date, however, have shown an association between chronic administration of these drugs and mammary tumorigenesis; the available evidence is considered too limited to be conclusive at this time.

ADVERSE REACTIONS

NOTE: Not all of the following adverse reactions have been reported with Navane. However, since Navane has certain chemical and pharmacologic similarities to the phenothiazines, all of the known side effects and toxicity associated with phenothiazine therapy should be borne in mind when Navane is used.

Cardiovascular effects: Tachycardia, hypotension, lightheadedness, and syncope. In the event hypotension occurs, epinephrine should not be used as a pressor agent since a paradoxical further lowering of blood pressure may result. Nonspecific EKG changes have been observed in some patients receiving Navane. These changes are usually reversible and frequently disappear on continued Navane therapy. The incidence of these changes is lower than that observed with some phenothiazines. The clinical significance of these changes is not known.

CNS effects: Drowsiness, usually mild, may occur although it usually subsides with continuation of Navane therapy. The incidence of sedation appears similar to that of the piperazine group of phenothiazines but less than that of certain aliphatic phenothiazines. Restlessness, agitation and insomnia have been noted with Navane. Seizures and paradoxical exacerbation of psychotic symptoms have occurred with Navane infrequently.

Hyperreflexia has been reported in infants delivered from mothers having received structurally related drugs.

In addition, phenothiazine derivatives have been associated with cerebral edema and cerebrospinal fluid abnormalities.

Extrapyramidal symptoms, such as pseudo-parkinsonism, akathisia and dystonia have been reported. Management of these extrapyramidal symptoms depends upon the type and severity. Rapid relief of acute symptoms may require the use of an injectable antiparkinson agent. More slowly emerging symptoms may be managed by reducing the dosage of Navane and/or administering an oral antiparkinson agent.

Persistent Tardive Dyskinesia: As with all antipsychotic agents tardive dyskinesia may appear in some patients on long term therapy or may occur after drug therapy has been discontinued. The syndrome is characterized by rhythmical involuntary movements of the tongue, face, mouth or jaw (e.g., protrusion of tongue, puffing of cheeks, puckering of mouth, chewing movements). Sometimes these may be accompanied by involuntary movements of extremities.

Since early detection of tardive dyskinesia is important, patients should be monitored on an ongoing basis. It has been reported that fine vermicular movement of the tongue may be an early sign of the syndrome. If this or any other presentation of the syndrome is observed, the clinician should consider possible discontinuation of neuroleptic medication. (See Warnings section.)

Hepatic effects: Elevations of serum transaminase and alkaline phosphatase, usually transient, have been infrequently observed in some patients. No clinically confirmed cases of jaundice attributable to Navane have been reported.

Hematologic effects: As is true with certain other psychotropic drugs, leukopenia and leucocytosis, which are usually transient, can occur occasionally with Navane. Other antipsychotic drugs have been associated with agranulocytosis, eosinophilia, hemolytic anemia, thrombocytopenia and pancytopenia.

Allergic reactions: Rash, pruritus, urticaria, photosensitivity and rare cases of anaphylaxis have been reported with Navane. Undue exposure to sunlight should be avoided. Although not experienced with Navane, exfoliative dermatitis and contact dermatitis (in nursing personnel), have been reported with certain phenothiazines.

Endocrine disorders: Lactation, moderate breast enlargement and amenorrhea have occurred in a small percentage of females receiving Navane (thiothixene). If persistent, this may necessitate a reduction in dosage or the discontinuation of therapy. Phenothiazines have been associated with false positive pregnancy tests, gynecomastia, hypoglycemia, hyperglycemia and glycosuria.

Autonomic effects: Dry mouth, blurred vision, nasal congestion, constipation, increased sweating, increased salivation and impotence have occurred infrequently with Navane therapy. Phenothiazines have been associated with miosis, mydriasis, and adynamic ileus.

Other adverse reactions: Hyperpyrexia, anorexia, nausea, vomiting, diarrhea, increase in appetite and weight, weakness or fatigue, polydipsia, and peripheral edema.

Although not reported with Navane, evidence indicates there is a relationship between phenothiazine therapy and the occurrence of a systemic lupus erythematosus-like syndrome.

NOTE: Sudden deaths have occasionally been reported in patients who have received certain phenothiazine derivatives. In some cases the cause of death was apparently cardiac arrest or asphyxia due to failure of the cough reflex. In others, the cause could not be determined nor could it be established that death was due to phenothiazine administration.

DOSAGE AND ADMINISTRATION

Dosage of Navane should be individually adjusted depending on the chronicity and severity of the condition. In general, small doses should be used initially and gradually increased to the optimal effective level, based on patient response.

Some patients have been successfully maintained on once-a-day Navane therapy.

The use of Navane in children under 12 years of age is not recommended because safe conditions for its use have not been established.

In milder conditions, an initial dose of 2 mg. three times daily. If indicated, a subsequent increase to 15 mg./day total daily dose is often effective.

In more severe conditions, an initial dose of 5 mg. twice daily. The usual optimal dose is 20 to 30 mg. daily. If indicated, an increase to 60 mg./day total daily dose is often effective. Exceeding a total daily dose of 60 mg. rarely increases the beneficial response.

OVERDOSAGE

Manifestations include muscular twitching, drowsiness and dizziness. Symptoms of gross overdosage may include CNS depression, rigidity, weakness, torticollis, tremor, salivation, dysphagia, hypotension, disturbances of gait, or coma.

Treatment: Essentially symptomatic and supportive. Early gastric lavage is helpful. Keep patient under careful observation and maintain an open airway, since involvement of the extrapyramidal system may produce dysphagia and respiratory difficulty in severe overdosage. If hypotension occurs, the standard measures for managing circulatory shock should be used (I.V. fluids and/or vasoconstrictors).

If a vasoconstrictor is needed, levarterenol and phenylephrine are the most suitable drugs. Other pressor agents, including epinephrine, are not recommended, since phenothiazine derivatives may reverse the usual pressor action of these agents and cause further lowering of blood pressure.

If CNS depression is present, recommended stimulants include amphetamine, dextroamphetamine, or caffeine and sodium benzoate. Stimulants that may cause convulsions (e. g. picrotoxin or pentylenetetrazol) should be avoided. Extrapyramidal symptoms may be treated with antiparkinson drugs.

There are no data on the use of peritoneal or hemodialysis, but they are known to be of little value in phenothiazine intoxication.

HOW SUPPLIED

Navane (thiothixene) Capsules

Bottles of 100's: 1 mg (NDC 0049-5710-66); 2 mg (NDC 0049-5720-66); 5 mg (NDC 0049-5730-66); 10 mg (NDC 0049-5740-66); 20 mg (NDC 0049-5770-66). 1000's: 2 mg (NDC 0049-5720-82); 5 mg (NDC 0049-5730-82); 10 mg (NDC 0049-5740-82). 500's 20 mg (NDC 0049-5770-73).

Unit Doses of: 1 mg (NDC 0049-5710-41); 2 mg (NDC 0049-5720-41); 5 mg (NDC 0049-5730-41); 10 mg (NDC 0049-5740-41); and 20 mg (NDC 0049-5770-41).

Navane (thiothixene hydrochloride) Concentrate is available in 120 ml (4 oz.) bottles (NDC 0049-5750-47) with an accompanying dropper calibrated at 2 mg, 3 mg, 4 mg, 5 mg, 6 mg, 8 mg, and 10 mg and in 30 ml (1 oz.) bottles (NDC 0049-5750-51) with an accompanying dropper calibrated at 2 mg, 3 mg, 4 mg, and 5 mg. Each ml. contains thiothixene hydrochloride equivalent to 5 mg. of thiothixene. Contains alcohol, U.S.P. 7.0% v/v. (small loss unavoidable).

70-1655-00-3

Shown in Product Identification Section, page 426

Continued on next page

Roerig—Cont.

NAVANE® ℞
[*nah 'vān*]
(thiothixene hydrochloride)
Intramuscular
2 mg./ml. 5 mg./ml. †

DESCRIPTION

Navane (thiothixene hydrochloride) is a thioxanthene derivative. Specifically, it is the *cis* isomer of N,N-dimethyl-9-[3-(4-methyl-1- piperazinyl)-propylidene] thioxanthene-2-sulfonamide.

The thioxanthenes differ from the phenothiazines by the replacement of nitrogen in the central ring with a carbon-linked side chain fixed in space in a rigid structural configuration. An N,N-dimethyl sulfonamide functional group is bonded to the thioxanthene nucleus. †Navane Intramuscular contains in each ml. thiothixene HCl equivalent to 2 mg. of thiothixene, dextrose 5% w/v, benzyl alcohol 0.9% w/v, and propyl gallate 0.02% w/v.

Navane (thiothixene hydrochloride) Intramuscular For Injection, when reconstituted with 2.2 ml of Sterile Water for Injection, contains in each ml thiothixene hydrochloride equivalent to 5 mg of thiothixene, and 59.6 mg of mannitol.

ACTIONS

Navane is a psychotropic agent of the thioxanthene series. Navane possesses certain chemical and pharmacological similarities to the piperazine phenothiazines and differences from the aliphatic group of phenothiazines. Navane's mode of action has not been clearly established.

INDICATIONS

Navane is effective in the management of manifestations of psychotic disorders. Navane has not been evaluated in the management of behavioral complications in patients with mental retardation.

CONTRAINDICATIONS

Navane is contraindicated in patients with circulatory collapse, comatose states, central nervous system depression due to any cause, and blood dyscrasias. Navane is contraindicated in individuals who have shown hypersensitivity to the drug. It is not known whether there is a cross sensitivity between the thioxanthenes and the phenothiazine derivatives, but this possibility should be considered.

WARNINGS

Tardive Dyskinesia—Tardive dyskinesia, a syndrome consisting of potentially irreversible, involuntary, dyskinetic movements may develop in patients treated with neuroleptic (antipsychotic) drugs. Although the prevalence of the syndrome appears to be highest among the elderly, especially elderly women, it is impossible to rely upon prevalence estimates to predict, at the inception of neuroleptic treatment, which patients are likely to develop the syndrome. Whether neuroleptic drug products differ in their potential to cause tardive dyskinesia is unknown.

Both the risk of developing the syndrome and the likelihood that it will become irreversible are believed to increase as the duration of treatment and the total cumulative dose of neuroleptic drugs administered to the patient increase. However, the syndrome can develop, although much less commonly, after relatively brief treatment periods at low doses.

There is no known treatment for established cases of tardive dyskinesia, although the syndrome may remit, partially or completely, if neuroleptic treatment is withdrawn. Neuroleptic treatment, itself, however, may suppress (or partially suppress) the signs and symptoms of the syndrome and thereby may possibly mask the underlying disease process. The effect that symptomatic suppression has upon the long-term course of the syndrome is unknown.

Given these considerations, neuroleptics should be prescribed in a manner that is most likely to minimize the occurrence of tardive dyskinesia. Chronic neuroleptic treatment should generally be reserved for patients who suffer from a chronic illness that, 1) is known to respond to neuroleptic drugs, and, 2) for whom alternative, equally effective, but potentially less harmful treatments are *not* available or appropriate. In patients who do require chronic treatment, the smallest dose and the shortest duration of treatment producing a satisfactory clinical response should be sought. The need for continued treatment should be reassessed periodically.

If signs and symptoms of tardive dyskinesia appear in a patient on neuroleptics, drug discontinuation should be considered. However, some patients may require treatment despite the presence of the syndrome.

(For further information about the description of tardive dyskinesia and its clinical detection, please refer to the section on Adverse Reactions.)

Usage in Pregnancy—Safe use of Navane during pregnancy has not been established. Therefore, this drug should be given to pregnant patients only when, in the judgment of the physician, the expected benefits from treatment exceed the possible risks to mother and fetus. Animal reproductive studies and clinical experience to date have not demonstrated any teratogenic effects.

In the animal reproduction studies with Navane, there was some decrease in conception rate and litter size, and an increase in resorption rate in rats and rabbits, changes which have been similarly reported with other psychotropic agents. After repeated oral administration of Navane to rats (5 to 15 mg./kg./day), rabbits (3 to 50 mg./kg./day), and monkeys (1 to 3 mg./kg./day) before and during gestation, no teratogenic effects were seen. (See Precautions).

Usage in Children—The use of Navane in children under 12 years of age is not recommended because safety and efficacy in the pediatric age group have not been established.

As is true with many CNS drugs, Navane may impair the mental and/or physical abilities required for the performance of potentially hazardous tasks such as driving a car or operating machinery, especially during the first few days of therapy. Therefore, the patient should be cautioned accordingly.

As in the case of other CNS-acting drugs, patients receiving Navane should be cautioned about the possible additive effects (which may include hypotension) with CNS depressants and with alcohol.

PRECAUTIONS

An antiemetic effect was observed in animal studies with Navane (thiothixene hydrochloride); since this effect may also occur in man, it is possible that Navane may mask signs of overdosage of toxic drugs and may obscure conditions such as intestinal obstruction and brain tumor.

In consideration of the known capability of Navane and certain other psychotropic drugs to precipitate convulsions, extreme caution should be used in patients with a history of convulsive disorders, or those in a state of alcohol withdrawal since it may lower the convulsive threshold. Although Navane potentiates the actions of the barbiturates, the dosage of the anticonvulsant therapy should not be reduced when Navane is administered concurrently.

Caution as well as careful adjustment of the dosage is indicated when Navane is used in conjunction with other CNS depressants other than anticonvulsant drugs.

Though exhibiting rather weak anticholinergic properties, Navane should be used with caution in patients who are known or suspected to have glaucoma, or who might be exposed to extreme heat, or who are receiving atropine or related drugs.

Use with caution in patients with cardiovascular disease.

Also, careful observation should be made for pigmentary retinopathy, and lenticular pigmentation (fine lenticular pigmentation has been noted in a small number of patients treated with Navane for prolonged periods). Blood dyscrasias (agranulocytosis, pancytopenia, thrombocytopenic purpura), and liver damage (jaundice, biliary stasis), have been reported with related drugs.

Undue exposure to sunlight should be avoided. Photosensitive reactions have been reported in patients on Navane.

As with all intramuscular preparations, Navane Intramuscular should be injected well within the body of a relatively large muscle. The preferred sites are the upper outer quadrant of the buttock (i.e., gluteus maximus) and the mid-lateral thigh.

The deltoid area should be used only if well developed such as in certain adults and older children, and then only with caution to avoid radial nerve injury. Intramuscular injections should not be made into the lower and mid-thirds of the upper arm. As with all intramuscular injections, aspiration is necessary to help avoid inadvertent injection into a blood vessel.

Neuroleptic drugs elevate prolactin levels; the elevation persists during chronic administration. Tissue culture experiments indicate that approximately one-third of human breast cancers are prolactin dependent *in vitro*, a factor of potential importance if the prescription of these drugs is contemplated in a patient with a previously detected breast cancer. Although disturbances such as galactorrhea, amenorrhea, gynecomastia, and impotence have been reported, the clinical significance of elevated serum prolactin levels is unknown for most patients. An increase in mammary neoplasms has been found in rodents after chronic administration of neuroleptic drugs. Neither clinical studies nor epidemiologic studies conducted to date, however, have shown an association between chronic administration of these drugs and mammary tumorigenesis; the available evidence is considered too limited to be conclusive at this time.

ADVERSE REACTIONS

NOTE: Not all of the following adverse reactions have been reported with Navane. However, since Navane has certain chemical and pharmacologic similarities to the phenothiazines, all of the known side effects and toxicity associated with phenothiazine therapy should be borne in mind when Navane is used.

Cardiovascular effects: Tachycardia, hypotension, lightheadedness, and syncope. In the event hypotension occurs, epinephrine should not be used as a pressor agent since a paradoxical further lowering of blood pressure may result. Nonspecific EKG changes have been observed in some patients receiving Navane. These changes are usually reversible and frequently disappear on continued Navane therapy. The clinical significance of these changes is not known.

CNS effects: Drowsiness, usually mild, may occur although it usually subsides with continuation of Navane therapy. The incidence of sedation appears similar to that of the piperazine group of phenothiazines, but less than that of certain aliphatic phenothiazines. Restlessness, agitation and insomnia have been noted with Navane. Seizures and paradoxical exacerbation of psychotic symptoms have occurred with Navane infrequently.

Hyperreflexia has been reported in infants delivered from mothers having received structurally related drugs.

In addition, phenothiazine derivatives have been associated with cerebral edema and cerebrospinal fluid abnormalities.

Extrapyramidal symptoms, such as pseudo-parkinsonism, akathisia, and dystonia have been reported. Management of these extrapyramidal symptoms depends upon the type and severity. Rapid relief of acute symptoms may require the use of an injectable antiparkinson agent. More slowly emerging symptoms may be managed by reducing the dosage of Navane and/or administering an oral antiparkinson agent.

Persistent Tardive Dyskinesia: As with all antipsychotic agents tardive dyskinesia may appear in some patients on long term therapy or may occur after drug therapy has been discontinued. The syndrome is characterized by rhythmical involuntary movements of the tongue, face, mouth or jaw (e.g., protrusion of tongue, puffing of cheeks, puckering of mouth, chewing movements). Sometimes these may be accompanied by involuntary movements of extremities.

Since early detection of tardive dyskinesia is important, patients should be monitored on an ongoing basis. It has been reported that fine vermicular movement of the tongue may be an early sign of the syndrome. If this or any other presentation of the syndrome is observed, the clinician should consider possible discontinuation of neuroleptic medication. (See Warnings section.)

Hepatic effects: Elevations of serum transaminase and alkaline phosphatase, usually transient, have been infrequently observed in some patients. No clinically confirmed cases of jaundice attributable to Navane (thiothixene hydrochloride) have been reported.

Hematologic effects: As is true with certain other psychotropic drugs, leukopenia and leucocytosis, which are usually transient, can occur occasionally with Navane. Other antipsychotic drugs have been associated with agranulocytosis, eosinophilia, hemolytic anemia, thrombocytopenia and pancytopenia.

Allergic reactions: Rash, pruritus, urticaria, and rare cases of anaphylaxis have been reported with Navane. Undue exposure to sunlight should be avoided. Although not experienced with Navane, exfoliative dermatitis, contact dermatitis (in nursing personnel), have been reported with certain phenothiazines.

Endocrine disorders: Lactation, moderate breast enlargement and amenorrhea have occurred in a small percentage of females receiving Navane. If persistent, this may necessitate a reduction in dosage or the discontinuation of therapy. Phenothiazines have been associated with false positive pregnancy tests, gynecomastia, hypoglycemia, hyperglycemia, and glycosuria.

Autonomic effects: Dry mouth, blurred vision, nasal congestion, constipation, increased sweating, increased salivation, and impotence have occurred infrequently with Navane therapy. Phenothiazines have been associated with miosis, mydriasis, and adynamic ileus.

Other adverse reactions: Hyperpyrexia, anorexia, nausea, vomiting, diarrhea, increase in appetite and weight, weakness or fatigue, polydipsia and peripheral edema.

Although not reported with Navane, evidence indicates there is a relationship between phenothiazine therapy and the occurrence of a systemic lupus erythematosus-like syndrome.

NOTE: Sudden deaths have occasionally been reported in patients who have received certain phenothiazine derivatives. In some cases the cause of death was apparently cardiac arrest or asphyxia due to failure of the cough reflex. In others, the cause could not be determined nor could it be established that death was due to phenothiazine administration.

DOSAGE AND ADMINISTRATION

Preparation

Navane (thiothixene hydrochloride) Intramuscular Solution is ready for use as supplied.

Navane (thiothixene hydrochloride) Intramuscular For Injection must be reconstituted with 2.2 ml of Sterile Water for Injection.

For Intramuscular Use Only

Dosage of Navane should be individually adjusted depending on the chronicity and severity of the condition. In general, small doses should be used initially and gradually increased to the optimal effective level, based on patient response.

Usage in children under 12 years of age is not recommended. Where more rapid control and treatment of acute behavior is desirable, the intramuscular form of Navane may be indicated. It is also of benefit where the very nature of the patient's symptomatology, whether acute or chronic, renders oral administration impractical or even impossible.

For treatment of acute symptomatology or in patients unable or unwilling to take oral medication, the usual dose is 4 mg. of Navane Intramuscular administered 2 to 4 times daily. Dosage may be increased or decreased depending on response. Most patients are controlled on a total daily dosage of 16 to 20 mg. The maximum recommended dosage is 30 mg./day. An oral form should supplant the injectable form as soon as possible. It may be necessary to adjust the dosage when changing from the intramuscular to oral dosage forms. Dosage recommendations for Navane Capsules and Concentrate can be found in the Navane oral package insert.

OVERDOSAGE

Manifestations include muscular twitching, drowsiness, and dizziness. Symptoms of gross overdosage may include CNS depression, rigidity, weakness, torticollis, tremor, salivation, dysphagia, hypotension, disturbances of gait, or coma.

Treatment: Essentially symptomatic and supportive. Keep patient under careful observation and maintain an open airway, since involvement of the extrapyramidal system may produce dysphagia and respiratory difficulty in severe overdosage. If hypotension occurs, the standard measures for managing circulatory shock should be used (I.V. fluids and/or vasoconstrictors).

If a vasoconstrictor is needed, levarterenol and phenylephrine are the most suitable drugs. Other pressor agents, including epinephrine, are not recommended, since phenothiazine derivatives may reverse the usual pressor elevating action of these agents and cause further lowering of blood pressure.

If CNS depression is present and specific therapy is indicated, recommended stimulants include amphetamine, dextroamphetamine, or caffeine and sodium benzoate. Picrotoxin or pentylenetetrazol should be avoided. Extrapyramidal symptoms may be treated with antiparkinson drugs.

There are no data on the use of peritoneal or hemodialysis, but they are known to be of little value in phenothiazine intoxication.

HOW SUPPLIED

Navane (thiothixene hydrochloride) Intramuscular Solution is available in a 2 ml. amber glass vial in packages of 10 vials. Each ml. contains thiothixene hydrochloride equivalent to 2 mg. of thiothixene, dextrose 5% w/v, benzyl alcohol 0.9% w/v, and propyl gallate 0.02% w/v.

Navane (thiothixene hydrochloride) Intramuscular For Injection is available in amber glass vials in packages of 10 vials. When reconstituted with 2.2 ml of Sterile Water for Injection, each ml contains thiothixene hydrochloride equivalent to 5 mg of thiothixene, and 59.6 mg of mannitol. The reconstituted solution of Navane Intramuscular For Injection may be stored for 48 hours at room temperature before discarding.

70-1865-00-0
70-4177-00-1

Buffered
PFIZERPEN® ℞
(penicillin G potassium)
for Injection

DESCRIPTION

Buffered Pfizerpen (penicillin G potassium) for Injection is a sterile, pyrogen-free powder which is stable for 36 months when stored at room temperature.

Each million units contains approximately 6.8 milligrams of sodium (0.3 mEq.) and 65.6 milligrams of potassium (1.68 mEq.).

ACTIONS AND PHARMACOLOGY

Penicillin G exerts a bactericidal action against penicillin-sensitive microorganisms during the stage of active multiplication. It acts through the inhibition of biosynthesis of cell wall mucopeptide. It is not active against the penicillinase-producing bacteria, which include many strains of staphylococci. Penicillin G exerts high *in vitro* activity against staphylococci (except penicillinase-producing strains), streptococci (groups A, C, G, H, L, and M) and pneumococci. Other organisms sensitive to penicillin G are *N. gonorrhoeae, Corynebacterium diphtheriae, Bacillus anthracis,* Clostridia, *Actinomyces bovis, Streptobacillus moniliformis, Listeria monocytogenes* and Leptospira. *Treponema pallidum* is extremely sensitive to the bactericidal action of penicillin G. Some species of gram-negative bacilli are sensitive to moderate to high concentrations of the drug obtained with intravenous administration. These include most strains of *Escherichia coli,* all strains of *Proteus mirabilis,* Salmonella and Shigella and some strains of *Aerobacter aerogenes* and *Alcaligenes fecalis.*

Sensitivity Plate Testing: If the Kirby-Bauer method of disc sensitivity is used, a 10 unit penicillin disc should give a zone greater than 28 mm when tested against a penicillin-sensitive bacterial strain.

Aqueous penicillin G is rapidly absorbed following both intramuscular and subcutaneous injection. Approximately 60 percent of the total dose of 300,000 units is excreted in the urine within this 5-hour period. For this reason high and frequent doses are required to maintain the elevated serum levels desirable in treating certain severe infections in individuals with normal kidney function. In neonates and young infants and in individuals with impaired kidney function, excretion is considerably delayed.

INDICATIONS

Aqueous penicillin G (parenteral) is indicated in the therapy of severe infections caused by penicillin G-sensitive microorganisms when rapid and high penicillinemia is required. Therapy should be guided by bacteriological studies (including sensitivity tests) and by clinical response.

The following infections will usually respond to adequate dosage of aqueous penicillin G (parenteral):

Streptococcal infections.

NOTE: Streptococci in groups A, C, H, G, L, and M are very sensitive to penicillin G. Some group D organisms are sensitive to the high serum levels obtained with aqueous penicillin G.

Aqueous penicillin (parenteral) is the penicillin dosage form of choice for bacteremia, empyema, severe pneumonia, pericarditis, endocarditis, meningitis and other severe infections caused by sensitive strains of the gram-positive species listed above.

Pneumococcal infections.
Staphylococcal infections —penicillin G sensitive.
Other infections:
Anthrax.
Actinomycosis.
Clostridial infections (including tetanus).
Diphtheria (to prevent carrier state).
Erysipeloid (*Erysipelothrix insidiosa*) endocarditis.

Fusospirochetal infections—severe infections of the oropharynx (Vincent's), lower respiratory tract and genital area due to *Fusobacterium fusiformisans* spirochetes.

Gram-negative bacillary infections (bateremias)—(*E. coli, A. aero genes, A. faecalis,* Salmonella, Shigella and *P. mirabilis*).

Listeria infections (*Listeria monocytogenes*).
Meningitis and endocarditis.
Pasteurella infections (*Pasteurella multocida*).
Bacteremia and meningitis.
Rat-bite fever (*Spirillum minus* or *Streptobacillus moniliformis*).
Gonorrheal endocarditis and arthritis (*N. gonorrhoeae*).
Syphilis (*T. pallidum*) including congenital syphilis.
Meningococcic meningitis.

Although no controlled clinical efficacy studies have been conducted, aqueous crystalline penicillin G for injection and penicillin G procaine suspension have been suggested by the American Heart Association and the American Dental Association for use as part of a combined parenteral-oral regimen for prophylaxis against bacterial endocarditis in patients with congenital heart disease or rheumatic, or other acquired valvular heart disease when they undergo dental procedures and surgical procedures of the upper respiratory tract.[1] Since it may happen that *alpha* hemolytic streptococci relatively resistant to penicillin may be found when patients are receiving continuous oral penicillin for secondary prevention of rheumatic fever, prophylactic agents other than penicillin may be chosen for these patients and prescribed in addition to their continuous rheumatic fever prophylactic regimen.

NOTE: When selecting antibiotics for the prevention of bacterial endocarditis the physician or dentist should read the full joint statement of the American Heart Association and the American Dental Association.[1]

CONTRAINDICATIONS

A history of a previous hypersensitivity reaction to any of the penicillins is a contraindication.

WARNINGS

Serious and occasionally fatal hypersensitivity (anaphylactoid) reactions have been reported in patients on penicillin therapy. Although anaphylaxis is more frequent following parenteral therapy it has occurred in patients on oral penicillins. These reactions are more apt to occur in individuals with a history of sensitivity to multiple allergens.

There have been well documented reports of individuals with a history of penicillin hypersensitivity reactions who have experienced severe hypersensitivity reactions when treated with a cephalosporin. Before therapy with a penicillin, careful inquiry should be made concerning previous hypersensitivity reactions to penicillins, cephalosporins, and other allergens. If an allergic reaction occurs, the drug should be discontinued and the patient treated with the usual agents, e.g., pressor amines, antihistamines, and corticosteroids.

PRECAUTIONS

Penicillin should be used with caution in individuals with histories of significant allergies and/or asthma.

In streptococcal infections, therapy must be sufficient to eliminate the organism (10 days minimum) otherwise the sequelae of streptococcal disease may occur. Cultures should be taken following the completion of treatment to determine whether streptococci have been eradicated.

Aqueous penicillin G by the intravenous route in high doses (above 10 million units), should be administered slowly because of the adverse effects of electrolyte imbalance from either the potassium or sodium content of the penicillin. The patient's renal, cardiac and vascular status should be evaluated and if impairment of function is suspected or known to exist a reduction in the total dosage should be considered. Frequent evaluation of electrolyte balance, renal and hematopoietic function is recommended during therapy when high doses of intravenous aqueous penicillin G are used.

Prolonged use of antibiotics may promote overgrowth of nonsusceptible organisms, including fungi. Should superinfection occur, appropriate measures should be taken. Indwelling intravenous catheters encourage superinfections and should be avoided whenever possible.

Therapy of susceptible infections should be accompanied by any indicated surgical procedures.

ADVERSE REACTIONS

Penicillin is a substance of low toxicity but does have a significant index of sensitization. The following hypersensitivity reactions have been reported: skin rashes ranging from maculopapular eruptions to exfoliative dermatitis: urticaria and reactions resembling serum sickness, including chills, fever, edema, arthralgia and prostration. Severe and occasionally fatal anaphylaxis has occurred (see "Warnings").

Hemolytic anemia, leucopenia, thrombocytopenia, nephropathy, and neuropathy are rarely observed adverse reactions and are usually associated with high intravenous dosage. Patients given continuous intravenous therapy with penicillin G potassium in high dosage (10 million to 100 million units daily) may suffer severe or even fatal potassium poisoning, particularly if renal insufficiency is present. Hyperreflexia, convulsions and coma may be indicative of this syndrome.

Cardiac arrhythmias and cardiac arrest may also occur. (High dosage of penicillin G sodium may result in congestive heart failure due to high sodium intake.)

The Jarisch-Herxheimer reaction has been reported in patients treated for syphilis.

ADMINISTRATION AND DOSAGE

Severe infections due to Susceptible Strains of Streptococci, Pneumococci and Staphylococci —bacteremia, pneumonia, endocarditis, pericarditis, empyema, meningitis and other severe infections—a minimum of 5 million units daily.

Syphilis —Aqueous penicillin G may be used in the treatment of acquired and congenital syphilis, but because of the necessity of frequent dosage, hospitalization is recommended. Dosage and duration of therapy will be determined by age of patient and stage of the disease.

Gonorrheal endocarditis —a minimum of 5 million units daily.

Meningococcic meningitis —1–2 million units intramuscularly every 2 hours, or continuous I.V. drip of 20–30 million units/day.

Actinomycosis —1–6 million units/day for cervico-facial cases; 10–20 million units/day for thoracic and abdominal disease.

Clostridial infections —20 million units/day; penicillin is adjunctive therapy to antitoxin.

Fusospirochetal infections —severe infections of oropharynx, lower respiratory tract and genital area—5–10 million units/day.

Rat-bite fever (*Spirillum minus* or *Streptobacillus moniliformis*)—12–15 million units/day for 3–4 weeks.

Listeria infections (*Listeria monocytogenes*).
Neonates—500,000 to 1 million units/day.
Adults with meningitis—15–20 million units/ day for 2 weeks.
Adults with endocarditis—15–20 million units/ day for 4 weeks.

Pasteurella infections (*Pasteurella multocida*).
Bacteremia and meningitis—4–6 million units/ day for 2 weeks.

Erysipeloid (*Erysipelothrix insidiosa*).
Endocarditis—2–20 million units/day for 4–6 weeks.

Gram-negative bacillary infections (*E. coli, A. aerogenes, A. faecalis,* Salmonella, Shigella and *Proteus mirabilis*).
Bacteremia—20–80 million units/day.

Diphtheria (carrier state)—300,000–400,000 units of penicillin/day in divided doses for 10–12 days.

Anthrax —a minimum of 5 million units of penicillin/day in divided doses until cure is effected.

For prophylaxis against bacterial endocarditis[1] in patients with congenital heart disease or rheumatic, or other ac-

Continued on next page

Roerig—Cont.

quired valvular heart disease when undergoing dental procedures or surgical procedures of the upper respiratory tract, use a combined parenteral-oral regimen. One million units of aqueous crystalline penicillin G (30,000 units/kg in children) intramuscularly mixed with 600,000 units procaine penicillin G (600,000 units for children) should be given one-half to one hour before the procedure. Oral penicillin V (phenoxymethyl penicillin), 500 mg for adults or 250 mg for children less than 60 lb, should be given every 6 hours for 8 doses. Doses for children should not exceed recommendations for adults for a single dose or for a 24 hour period.
The following table shows the amount of solvent required for solution of various concentrations.
[See table below].
When the required volume of solvent is greater than the capacity of the vial, the penicillin can be dissolved by first injecting only a portion of the solvent into the vial, then withdrawing the resultant solution and combining it with the remainder of the solvent in a larger sterile container.
Buffered Pfizerpen (penicillin G potassium) for Injection is highly water soluble. It may be dissolved in small amounts of Water for Injection, or Sterile Isotonic Sodium Chloride Solution for Parenteral Use. All solutions should be stored in a refrigerator. When refrigerated, penicillin solutions may be stored for seven days without significant loss of potency.
Buffered Pfizerpen (penicillin G potassium) for Injection may be given intramuscularly or by continuous intravenous drip for dosages of 500,000, 1,000,000, or 5,000,000 units. It is also suitable for intrapleural, intraarticular, and other local instillations.
THE 20,000,000 UNIT DOSAGE MAY BE ADMINISTERED BY INTRAVENOUS INFUSION ONLY.
(1) Intramuscular Injection: Keep total volume of injection small. The intramuscular route is the preferred route of administration. Solutions containing up to 100,000 units of penicillin per ml of diluent may be used with a minimum of discomfort. Greater concentration of penicillin G per ml is physically possible and may be employed where therapy demands. When large dosages are required, it may be advisable to administer aqueous solutions of penicillin by means of continuous intravenous drip.
(2) Continuous Intravenous Drip: Determine the volume of fluid and rate of its administration required by the patient in a 24-hour period in the usual manner for fluid therapy, and add the appropriate daily dosage of penicillin to this fluid. For example, if an adult patient requires 2 liters of fluid in 24 hours and a daily dosage of 10 million units of penicillin, add 5 million units to 1 liter and adjust the rate of flow so that the liter will be infused in 12 hours.
(3) Intrapleural or Other Local Infusion: If fluid is aspirated, give infusion in a volume equal to ¼ or ½ the amount of fluid aspirated, otherwise, prepare as for intramuscular injection.
(4) Intrathecal Use: The intrathecal use of penicillin in meningitis must be highly individualized. It should be employed only with full consideration of the possible irritating effects of penicillin when used by this route. The preferred route of therapy in bacterial meningitides is intravenous, supplemental by intramuscular injection.

HOW SUPPLIED

Buffered Pfizerpen (penicillin G potassium) for Injection is available in vials containing respectively 1,000,000 units × 10's (NDC 0995-0510-83), 1,000,000 units × 100's (NDC 0995-0510-95), 5,000,000 units × 10's (NDC 0995-0520-83), 5,000,000 units × 100's (NDC 0995-0520-95), 20,000,000 units × 1's (NDC 0995-0530-28) and a bulk pharmacy package of 20,000,000 units × 10 's (NDC 0995-0530-83) of dry powder for reconstitution; buffered with sodium citrate and citric acid to an optimum pH.
Each million units contains approximately 6.8 milligrams of sodium (0.3 mEq.) and 65.6 milligrams of potassium (1.68 mEq.).

Reference:

1. American Heart Association. 1977. Prevention of bacterial endocarditis. Circulation. **56**:139A- 143A.

Pfizerpen

Desired Concentration (units/ml)	Approx. Volume (ml) 1,000,000 units	Solvent for Vial of 5,000,000 units	Infusion Only 20,000,000 units
50,000	19.6	...	...
100,000	9.6	...	...
250,000	3.6	18.2	74.2
500,000	1.6	8.2	32.4
750,000	...	4.8	...
1,000,000	...	3.2	11.5

PFIZERPEN®–AS ℞
(penicillin G procaine)
in Aqueous Suspension
For Intramuscular Use Only

DESCRIPTION

Pfizerpen-AS (penicillin G procaine) is a highly potent antibacterial agent effective against a wide variety of pathogenic organisms. It is an equimolecular compound of procaine and penicillin G in aqueous suspension for intramuscular administration.

ACTIONS AND PHARMACOLOGY

Penicillin G exerts a bactericidal action against penicillin-sensitive micoorganisms during the stage of active multiplication. It acts through the inhibition of biosynthesis of cell wall mucopeptide. It is not active against the penicillinase-producing bacteria, which include many strains of staphylococci. Penicillin G exerts high in vitro activity against staphylococci (except penicillinase-producing strains), streptococci (groups A.C.G.H.L. and M.) and pneumococci. Other organisms sensitive to penicillin G are *N. gonorrhoeae, Corvnebacterium diphtheriae, Bacillus anthracis,* Clostrida, *Actinomyces bovis, Streptobacillus moniliformis, Listera monocytogenes* and Leptospira. *Treponemia pallidum* is extremely sensitive to the bactericidal action of penicillin G.
Sensitivity plate testing: If the Kirby-Bauer method of disc sensitivity is used, a 10-unit penicillin disc should give a zone greater than 28 mm when tested against a penicillin-sensitive bacterial strain.
Penicillin G procaine is an equimolecular compound of procaine and penicillin G administered intramuscularly as a suspension. It dissolves slowly at the site of injection, giving a plateau type of blood level at about 4 hours which falls slowly over a period of the next 15-20 hours.
Approximately 60% of penicillin G is bound to serum protein. The drug is distributed throughout the body tissues in widely varying amounts. Highest levels are found in the kidneys with lesser amounts in the liver, skin and intestines. Penicillin G penetrates into all other tissues to a lesser degree with a very small level found in the cerebrospinal fluid. With normal kidney function the drug is excreted rapidly by tubular excretion. In neonates and young infants and in individuals with impaired kidney functions, excretion is considerably delayed. Approximately 60-90% of a dose of parenteral penicillin G is excreted in the urine within 24-36 hours.

INDICATIONS

Penicillin G procaine is indicated in the treatment of moderately severe infections due to penicillin G-sensitive microorganisms that are sensitive to the low and persistent serum levels common to this paritcular dosage form. Therapy should be guided by bacteriological studies (including sensitivity tests) and by clinical response.
NOTE: When high sustained serum levels are required, aqueous penicillin G either IM or IV should be used.
The following infections will usually respond to adequate dosages of intramuscular penicillin G procaine.
Streptococcal infections: Group A (without bacteremia). Moderately severe to severe infections of the upper respiratory tract (including middle ear infections—otitis media), skin and soft tissue infections, scarlet fever, and erysipelas.
NOTE: Streptococci in groups A.C.H.G.L. and M are very sensitive to penicillin G. Other groups, including group D (enterococcus) are resistant. Aqueous penicillin is recommended for streptococcal infections with bacteremia.
Pneumococcal infections: Moderately severe infections of the respiratory tract (including middled ear infections—otitis media).
NOTE: Severe pneumonia, empyema, bacteremia, pericarditis, meningitis, peritonitis, and purulent or septic arthritis of pneumococcal etiology are better treated with aqueous penicillin G during the acute stage.
Staphylococcal infections: penicillin G-sensitive. Moderately severe infections of the skin and soft tissues.
NOTE: Reports indicate an increasing number of strains of staphylococci resistant to penicillin G emphasizing the need for culture and sensitivity studies in treating suspected staphylococcal infections.
Indicated surgical procedures should be performed.
Fusospirochetosis (Vincent's gingivitis and pharyngitis). Moderately severe infections of the oropharynx respond to therapy with penicillin G procaine.
NOTE: Necessary dental care should be accomplished in infections involving the gum tissue.
Treponema pallidum (syphilis): all stages.
N. gonorrhoeae; acute and chronic (without bacteremia).
Yaws, Bejel, Pinta.
C. diphtheriae —penicillin G procaine as an adjunct to antitoxin for prevention of the carrier stage.
Anthrax.
Streptobacillus monoliformis and *Spirillum minus* infections (rat bite fever).
Erysipeloid.
Subacute bacterial endocarditis (group A streptococcus) only in extremely sensitive infections.
Prophylaxis Against Bacterial Endocarditis—Although no controlled clinical efficacy studies have been conducted, aqueous crystalline penicillin G for injection and penicillin G procaine suspension have been suggested by the American Heart Association and the American Dental Association for use as part of a combined parenteral-oral regimen for prophylaxis against bacterial endocarditis in patients with congenital heart disease or rheumatic, or other acquired valvular heart disease when they undergo dental procedures and surgical procedures of the upper respiratory tract.[1] Since it may happen that *alpha* hemolytic streptococci relatively resistant to penicillin may be found when patients are receiving continuous oral penicillin for secondary prevention of rheumatic fever, prophylactic agents other than penicillin may be chosen for these patients and prescribed in addition to their continuous rheumatic fever prophylactic regimen.
NOTE: When selecting antibiotics for the prevention of bacterial endocarditis the physician or dentist should read the full joint statement of the American Heart Association and the American Dental Association.[1]

CONTRAINDICATIONS

A previous hypersensitivity reaction to any penicillin or procaine is a contraindication.

WARNINGS

Serious and occasionally fatal hypersensitivity (anaphylactoid) reactions have been reported in patients on penicillin therapy. Although anaphylaxis is more frequent following parenteral therapy it has occurred in patients on oral penicillins. These reactions are more apt to occur in individuals with a history of sensitivity to multiple allergens.
There have been well documented reports of individuals with a history of penicillin hypersensitivity reactions who have experienced severe hypersensitivity reactions when treated with a cephalosporin. Before therapy with a penicillin, careful inquiry should be made concerning previous hypersensitivity reactions to penicillins, cephalosporins, and other allergens. If an allergic reaction occurs, the drug should be discontinued and the patient treated with the usual agents *e.g.,* pressor amines, antihistamines and corticosteroids.
Immediate toxic reactions to procaine may occur in some individuals, particularly when a large single dose is administered in the treatment of gonorrhea (4.8 million units). These reactions may be manifested by mental disturbances including anxiety, confusion, agitation, depression, weakness, seizures, hallucinations, combativeness, and expressed "fear of impending death". The reactions noted in carefully controlled studies occurred in approximately one in 500 patients treated for gonorrhea. Reactions are transient, lasting from 15-30 minutes.

PRECAUTIONS

Penicillin should be used with caution in individuals with histories of significant allergies and/or asthma.
In intramuscular therapy, care should be taken to avoid accidental intravenous administration.
As with all intramuscular preparations, Pfizerpen-AS (penicillin G procaine) should be injected well within the body of a relatively large muscle. ADULTS: The preferred site is the upper outer quadrant of the buttock, (i.e., gluteus maximus), or the mid-lateral thigh. CHILDREN: It is recommended that intramuscular injections be given preferably in the mid-lateral muscles of the thigh. In infants and small children the periphery of the upper outer quadrant of the gluteal region should only be used when necessary, such as in burn patients, in order to minimize the possibility of damage to the sciatic nerve.
The deltoid area should be used only if well developed such as in certain adults and older children, and then only with caution to avoid radial nerve injury. Intramuscular injections should not be made into the lower and mid-third of the upper arm. As with all intramuscualr injections, aspiration is necessary to help avoid inadvertent injection into a blood vessel.
In suspected staphylococcal infections, proper laboratory studies, including sensitivity tests, should be performed.
A small percentage of patients are sensitive to procaine. If there is a history of sensitivity make the usual test: Inject intradermally 0.1 ml of a 1 to 2 percent procaine solution. Development of an erythema, wheal, flare or eruption indicates procaine sensitivity. Sensitivity should be treated by the usual methods, including barbiturates, and penicillin G

procaine preparations should not be used. Antihistamines appear beneficial in treatment of procaine reactions.
The use of antibiotics may result in overgrowth of nonsusceptible organisms. Constant observation of the patient is essential. If new infections due to bacteria or fungi appear during therapy, the drug should be discontinued and appropriate measures taken. Whenever allergic reactions occur, penicillin should be withdrawn unless, in the opinion of the physician, the condition being treated is life threatening and amenable only to penicillin therapy.
In prolonged therapy with penicillin, and particularly with high dosage schedules, periodic evaluation of the renal and hematopoietic systems are recommended.
When treating gonococcal infections in which primary or secondary syphilis may be suspected, proper diagnostic procedures, including dark field examinations should be done. In all cases in which concomitant syphilis is suspected, monthly serological tests should be made for at least four months.

ADVERSE REACTIONS

Penicillin is a substance of low toxicity, but does possess a significant index of sensitization. The following hypersensitivity reactions associated with use of penicillin have been reported: skin rashes, ranging from maculopapular eruptions to exfoliative dermatitis; urticaria; serum sickness-like reactions, including chills, fever, edema, arthralgia and prostration. Severe and often fatal anaphylaxis has been reported (see "Warnings"). As with other treatments for syphilis, the Jarisch-Herxheimer reaction has been reported.
Procaine toxicity manifestations have been reported (see Warnings). Procaine hypersensitivity reactions have not been reported with this drug.

ADMINISTRATION AND DOSAGE

Pediatric Dosage Schedules: In children under 3 months of age, the absorption of aqueous penicillin G produces such high and sustained levels that penicillin G procaine dosage forms offer no advantages and are usually unnecessary.
In children under 12 years of age, dosage should be adjusted in accordance with the age and weight of the child and the severity of the infection.
Under 2 years of age, the dose may be divided between the two buttocks if necessary.
Penicillin G procaine (aqueous) is for intramuscular injection only.
Recommended dosage for penicillin G procaine aqueous:
Pneumonia (pneumococcal), moderately severe (uncomplicated): 600,000-1,000,000 units daily.
Streptococcal infections (group A), moderately severe to severe tonsillitis, erysipelas, scarlet fever, upper respiratory tract, skin and soft tissue: 600,000-1,000,000 units daily for 10 day minimum.
Staphylococcal infections, moderately severe to severe: 600,000-1,000,000 units daily.
Bacterial endocarditis (group A streptococci) only in extremely sensitive infections: 600,000-1,000,000 units daily.
To prevent bacterial endocarditis in patients with rheumatic or congenital heart lesions who are to undergo dental or upper respiratory tract surgery or instrumentation:
600,000 units penicillin G procaine aqueous the day of the procedure.
600,000 units aqueous penicillin G 1-2 hours before surgery.
600,000 units penicillin G procaine aqueous daily for 2 days following surgery.
Syphilis
Primary, secondary and latent with a negative spinal fluid in adults and children over 12 years of age: 600,000 units daily for 8 days—total 4,800,000 units.
Late (tertiary, neurosyphilis and latent syphilis with positive spinal fluid examination or no spinal fluid examination): 600,000 units daily for 10-15 days—total 6-9 million units.
Congenital syphilis (early and late) under 70 lb. body weight 50,000 units/kg/day for 10 days.
Yaws, Bejel, and Pinta—Treatment as syphilis in corresponding stage of disease.
Gonorrheal infections (uncomplicated): Men or women—4.8 million units intramuscularly divided into at least two doses and injected at different sites at one visit, together with 1 gram of oral probenecid, preferably given at least 30 minutes prior to the injection.
NOTE: gonorrheal endocarditis should be treated intensively with aqueous penicillin G.
Diphtheria-adjunctive therapy with antitoxin: 300,000-600,000 units daily.
Diphtheria carrier state—300,000 units daily for 10 days.
Anthrax-cutaneous: 600,000-1,000,000 units/day.
Vincent's infection (fusopirochetosis): 600,000-1,000,000 units/day.
Erysipeloid: 600,000-1,000,000 units/day.
Streptobacillus moniliformis and spirillum minus (rat bite fever). 600,000-1,000,000 units/day.

HOW SUPPLIED

Pfizerpen-AS (penicillin G procaine) in Aqueous Suspension is supplied in 10 ml vials (3,000,000 units)—packages of 5 (NDC 0995-0540-77), packages of 100 (NDC 0995-0540-95).
Each ml contains 300,000 units penicillin G as penicillin G procaine; and as w/v: 0.8% sodium citrate; 0.15% sodium carboxymethylcellulose; 25% of sorbitol solution U.S.P.; 0.06% polyvinylpyrrolidone, and 0.6% lecithin.
Preservatives: 0.103% methylparaben; 0.011% propylparaben.

REFERENCE

1. American Heart Association. 1977. Prevention of bacterial endocarditis. Circulation. **56**:139A-143A.

SINEQUAN® ℞
[sin 'a-kwon]
(doxepin HCl)
Capsules
Oral Concentrate

DESCRIPTION

SINEQUAN (doxepin hydrochloride) is one of a class of psychotherapeutic agents known as dibenzoxepin tricyclic compounds. The molecular formula of the compound is $C_{19}H_{21}NO \cdot HCl$ having a molecular weight of 316. It is a white crystalline solid readily soluble in water, lower alcohols and chloroform.

CHEMISTRY

SINEQUAN (doxepin HCl) is a dibenzoxepin derivative and is the first of a family of tricyclic psychotherapeutic agents. Specifically, it is an isomeric mixture of 1-Propanamine, 3-dibenz[*b,e*]oxepin-11(6*H*)ylidene-*N,N*-dimethyl-, hydrochloride.

ACTIONS

The mechanism of action of SINEQUAN (doxepin HCl) is not definitely known. It is not a central nervous system stimulant nor a monoamine oxidase inhibitor. The current hypothesis is that the clinical effects are due, at least in part, to influences on the adrenergic activity at the synapses so that deactivation of norepinephrine by reuptake into the nerve terminals is prevented. Animal studies suggest that doxepin HCl does not appreciably antagonize the antihypertensive action of guanethidine. In animal studies anticholinergic, antiserotonin and antihistamine effects on smooth muscle have been demonstrated. At higher than usual clinical doses, norepinephrine response was potentiated in animals. This effect was not demonstrated in humans.
At clinical dosages up to 150 mg per day, SINEQUAN can be given to man concomitantly with guanethidine and related compounds without blocking the antihypertensive effect. At dosages above 150 mg per day blocking of the antihypertensive effect of these compounds has been reported.
Sinequan is virtually devoid of euphoria as a side effect. Characteristic of this type of compound, Sinequan has not been demonstrated to produce the physical tolerance or psychological dependence associated with addictive compounds.

INDICATIONS

SINEQUAN is recommended for the treatment of:

1. Psychoneurotic patients with depression and/ or anxiety.
2. Depression and/or anxiety associated with alcoholism (not to be taken concomitantly with alcohol).
3. Depression and/or anxiety associated with organic disease (the possibility of drug interaction should be considered if the patient is receiving other drugs concomitantly).
4. Psychotic depressive disorders with associated anxiety including involutional depression and manic-depressive disorders.

The target symptoms of psychoneurosis that respond particularly well to SINEQUAN include anxiety, tension, depression, somatic symptoms and concerns, sleep disturbances, guilt, lack of energy, fear, apprehension and worry.
Clinical experience has shown that SINEQUAN is safe and well-tolerated even in the elderly patient. Owing to lack of clinical experience in the pediatric population, SINEQUAN is not recommended for use in children under 12 years of age.

CONTRAINDICATIONS

SINEQUAN is contraindicated in individuals who have shown hypersensitivity to the drug. Possibility of cross sensitivity with other dibenzoxepines should be kept in mind.
SINEQUAN is contraindicated in patients with glaucoma or a tendency to urinary retention. These disorders should be ruled out, particularly in older patients.

WARNINGS

The once-a-day dosage regimen of SINEQUAN in patients with intercurrent illness or patients taking other medications should be carefully adjusted. This is especially important in patients receiving other medications with anticholinergic effects.
Usage in Geriatrics
The use of SINEQUAN on a once-a-day dosage regimen in geriatric patients should be adjusted carefully based on the patient's condition.
Usage in Pregnancy
Reproduction studies have been performed in rats, rabbits, monkeys and dogs and there was no evidence of harm to the animal fetus. The relevance to humans is not known. Since there is no experience in pregnant women who have received this drug, safety in pregnancy has not been established. There are no data with respect to the secretion of the drug in human milk and its effect on the nursing infant.
Usage in Children
The use of SINEQUAN in children under 12 years of age is not recommended because safe conditions for its use have not been established.

DRUG INTERACTIONS

MAO Inhibitors
Serious side effects and even death have been reported following the concomitant use of certain drugs with MAO inhibitors. Therefore, MAO inhibitors should be discontinued at least two weeks prior to the cautious initiation of therapy with SINEQUAN. The exact length of time may vary and is dependent upon the particular MAO inhibitor being used, the length of time it has been administered, and the dosage involved.
Cimetidine
Cimetidine has been reported to produce clinically significant fluctuations in steady-state serum concentrations of various tricyclic antidepressants. Serious anticholinergic symptoms (i.e., severe dry mouth, urinary retention and blurred vision) have been associated with elevations in the serum levels of tricyclic antidepressant when cimetidine therapy is initiated. Additionally, higher than expected tricyclic antidepressant levels have been observed when they are begun in patients already taking cimetidine. In patients who have been reported to be well controlled on tricyclic antidepressants receiving concurrent cimetidine therapy, discontinuation of cimetidine has been reported to decrease established steady-state serum tricyclic antidepressant levels and compromise their therapeutic effects.
Alcohol
It should be borne in mind that alcohol ingestion may increase the danger inherent in any intentional or unintentional SINEQUAN overdosage. This is especially important in patients who may use alcohol excessively.

PRECAUTIONS

Since drowsiness may occur with the use of this drug, patients should be warned of the possibility and cautioned against driving a car or operating dangerous machinery while taking the drug. Patients should also be cautioned that their response to alcohol may be potentiated.
Since suicide is an inherent risk in any depressed patient and may remain so until significant improvement has occurred, patients should be closely supervised during the early course of therapy. Prescriptions should be written for the smallest feasible amount.
Should increased symptoms of psychosis or shift to manic symptomatology occur, it may be necessary to reduce dosage or add a major tranquilizer to the dosage regimen.

ADVERSE REACTIONS

NOTE: Some of the adverse reactions noted below have not been specifically reported with SINEQUAN use. However, due to the close pharmacological similarities among the tricyclics, the reactions should be considered when prescribing SINEQUAN (doxepin HCl).
Anticholinergic Effects: Dry mouth, blurred vision, constipation, and urinary retention have been reported. If they do not subside with continued therapy, or become severe, it may be necessary to reduce the dosage.
Central Nervous System Effects: Drowsiness is the most commonly noticed side effect. This tends to disappear as therapy is continued. Other infrequently reported CNS side effects are confusion, disorientation, hallucinations, numbness, paresthesias, ataxia, and extrapyramidal symptoms and seizures.
Cardiovascular: Cardiovascular effects including hypotension and tachycardia have been reported occasionally.
Allergic: Skin rash, edema, photosensitization, and pruritus have occasionally occurred.
Hematologic: Eosinophilia has been reported in a few patients. There have been occasional reports of bone marrow depression manifesting as agranulocytosis, leukopenia, thrombocytopenia, and purpura.
Gastrointestinal: Nausea, vomiting, indigestion, taste disturbances, diarrhea, anorexia, and aphthous stomatitis have been reported. (See anticholinergic effects.)
Endocrine: Raised or lowered libido, testicular swelling, gynecomastia in males, enlargement of breasts and galactorrhea in the female, raising or lowering of blood sugar levels have been reported with tricyclic administration.
Other: Dizziness, tinnitus, weight gain, sweating, chills, fatigue, weakness, flushing, jaundice, alopecia, and headache have been occasionally observed as adverse effects.
Withdrawal Symptoms: The possibility of development of withdrawal symptoms upon abrupt cessation of treatment

Continued on next page

Roerig—Cont.

after prolonged Sinequan administration should be borne in mind. These are not indicative of addiction and gradual withdrawal of medication should not cause these symptoms.

DOSAGE AND ADMINISTRATION

For most patients with illness of mild to moderate severity, a starting daily dose of 75 mg is recommended. Dosage may subsequently be increased or decreased at appropriate intervals and according to individual response. The usual optimum dose range is 75 mg/day to 150 mg/day.

In more severely ill patients higher doses may be required with subsequent gradual increase to 300 mg/day if necessary. Additional therapeutic effect is rarely to be obtained by exceeding a dose of 300 mg/day.

In patients with very mild symptomatology or emotional symptoms accompanying organic disease, lower doses may suffice. Some of these patients have been controlled on doses as low as 25-50 mg/day.

The total daily dosage of SINEQUAN may be given on a divided or once-a-day dosage schedule. If the once-a-day schedule is employed the maximum recommended dose is 150 mg/day. This dose may be given at bedtime. **The 150 mg capsule strength is intended for maintenance therapy only and is not recommended for initiation of treatment.**

Anti-anxiety effect is apparent before the antidepressant effect. Optimal antidepressant effect may not be evident for two to three weeks.

OVERDOSAGE

A. Signs and Symptoms
   1. Mild: Drowsiness, stupor, blurred vision, excessive dryness of mouth.
   2. Severe: Respiratory depression, hypotension, coma, convulsions, cardiac ar- rhythmias and tachycardias.

   Also: urinary retention (bladder atony), decreased gastrointestinal motility (paralytic ileus), hyperthermia (or hypothermia), hypertension, dilated pupils, hyperactive reflexes.

B. Management and Treatment
   1. Mild: Observation and supportive therapy is all that is usually necessary.
   2. Severe: Medical management of severe SINEQUAN overdosage consists of aggressive supportive therapy. If the patient is conscious, gastric lavage, with appropriate precautions to prevent pulmonary aspiration, should be performed even though SINEQUAN is rapidly absorbed. The use of activated charcoal has been recommended, as has been continuous gastric lavage with saline for 24 hours or more. An adequate airway should be established in comatose patients and assisted ventilation used if necessary. EKG monitoring may be required for several days, since relapse after apparent recovery has been reported. Arrhythmias should be treated with the appropriate antiarrhythmic agent. It has been reported that many of the cardiovascular and CNS symptoms of tricyclic antidepressant poisoning in adults may be reversed by the slow intravenous administration of 1 mg to 3 mg of physostigmine salicylate. Because physostigmine is rapidly metabolized, the dosage should be repeated as required. Convulsions may respond to standard anticonvulsant therapy, however, barbiturates may potentiate any respiratory depression. Dialysis and forced diuresis generally are not of value in the management of overdosage due to high tissue and protein binding of SINEQUAN.

SUPPLY

SINEQUAN is available as capsules containing doxepin HCl equivalent to: 10 mg, 75 mg, and 100 mg doxepin; bottles of 100, 1000, and unit-dose packages of 100 (10 × 10's).

25 mg and 50 mg doxepin: bottles of 100, 1000, 5000, and unit-dose packages of 100 (10 × 10's).

150 mg doxepin: bottles of 50, 500, and unit-dose packages of 100 (10 × 10's).

SINEQUAN Oral Concentrate is available in 120 ml bottles with an accompanying dropper calibrated at 5 mg, 10 mg, 15 mg, 20 mg, and 25 mg. Each ml contains doxepin HCl equivalent to 10 mg doxepin. Just prior to administration, SINEQUAN Oral Concentrate should be diluted with approximately 120 ml of water, whole or skimmed milk, or orange, grapefruit, tomato, prune or pineapple juice. SINEQUAN Oral Concentrate is not physically compatible with a number of carbonated beverages. For those patients requiring antidepressant therapy who are on methadone maintenance, SINEQUAN Oral Concentrate and methadone syrup can be mixed together with Gatorade®, lemonade, orange juice, sugar water, Tang®, or water; but not with grape juice. Preparation and storage of bulk dilutions is not recommended.

Literature Available: Yes.

69-2135-37-3

Shown in Product Identification Section, page 426

SPECTROBID®

[spek 'trō-bid]

(bacampicillin HCl)

TABLETS and POWDER for ORAL SUSPENSION

DESCRIPTION

SPECTROBID (bacampicillin HCl) is a member of the ampicillin class of semi-synthetic penicillins derived from the basic penicillin nucleus: 6-aminopenicillanic acid. SPECTROBID, as well as ampicillin and other ampicillin analogues, is acid resistant and suitable for oral administration. SPECTROBID is the hydrochloride salt of 1-ethoxycarbonyloxyethyl ester of ampicillin, available either as tablets or as a microencapsulated oral suspension. During the process of absorption from the gastrointestinal tract, SPECTROBID is hydrolyzed rapidly to ampicillin, a well characterized and effective antibacterial agent. Each 400 mg tablet of SPECTROBID is chemically equivalent to 280 mg of ampicillin, and 125 mg/5 ml of the oral suspension is chemically equivalent to 87.5 mg of ampicillin.

Chemically, SPECTROBID is 1'-ethoxycarbonyloxyethyl-6-(D-α aminophenylacetamide)-penicillinate hydrochloride. It has a molecular weight of 501.96.

ACTIONS

Clinical Pharmacology

SPECTROBID is characterized by its more complete and more rapid absorption from the GI tract than ampicillin. SPECTROBID tablets of 400 mg, 800 mg, and 1600 mg have provided ampicillin peak serum concentrations of 7.9, 12.9, and 20.1 mcg/ml. These peak levels are approximately three times the levels obtained with administration of equivalent amounts of ampicillin. The areas-under-the-serum-concentration curves obtained during the first 6 hours were 24.8 and 12.9 mcg/ml/hr., when bacampicillin HCl 800 mg and ampicillin 500 mg were administered to adults. (See Graph 1.) Graph 2 shows the serum ampicillin curves following a 28 mg/kg dose of bacampicillin HCl and a 25 mg/kg dose of ampicillin in infants and young children. The areas-under-the-serum-concentration-curves were 28.2 and 13.1 respectively.

The absorption of the SPECTROBID oral suspension was shown to be equivalent to that of the 400 mg tablet in fasting adult volunteers. A 400 mg dose of suspension gave a peak serum ampicillin concentration of 7.6 mcg/ml and the tablet gave a peak of 7.2 mcg/ml. In fasting pediatric patients a 12.5 mg/kg dose provided a peak of 8.4 mcg/ml.

After oral administration of SPECTROBID tablet or suspension, ampicillin activity in serum peaks at 0.7–0.9 hours (compared to 1.5–2.0 hours after administration of ampicillin). Serum ampicillin half-life is 1.1 hours after either SPECTROBID or ampicillin administration.

Peak tissue and body fluid ampicillin concentrations also are higher after administration of SPECTROBID. Utilizing a special skin window technique to determine ampicillin levels, therapeutic levels in the interstitial fluid were higher and more prolonged after SPECTROBID than after ampicillin administration. SPECTROBID is stable in the presence of gastric acid. SPECTROBID oral suspension absorption is affected by food. Food does not retard absorption of SPECTROBID tablets which may be given without regard to meals. SPECTROBID has been shown to be rapidly and well absorbed after oral administration, with about 75% of a given dose being recoverable in the urine as active ampicillin within 8 hours of administration. Urinary excretion can be delayed by concurrent administration of probenecid. The active moiety of SPECTROBID (i.e., ampicillin) diffuses readily into most body tissues and fluids. In serum, ampicillin is only 20% protein-bound, compared to 60–90% for other penicillins.

Microbiology

SPECTROBID per se has no *in vitro* antibacterial activity and owes its *in vivo* bactericidal activity to the parent compound, ampicillin. The ampicillin class of penicillins (including SPECTROBID) has a broad spectrum of activity against many gram-negative and gram-positive bacteria. Like other penicillins, the ampicillin class of penicillins inhibits the synthesis of cell wall mucopeptide.

Ampicillin class antibiotics are inactivated by β-lactamases produced by certain strains of *Enterobacter, Citrobacter, Haemophilus influenzae,* and *Escherichia coli,* and by most strains of staphylococci and indole-positive *Proteus* spp. Ampicillin class antibiotics are not active against *Pseudomonas, Klebsiella,* or *Serratia* spp.

Susceptibility Testing:

Elution Technique: For the automated method of susceptibility testing (i.e., Autobac™), gram-negative organisms should be tested with the 4.5 mcg ampicillin elution disk, while gram-positive organisms should be tested with the 0.22 mcg disk.

Diffusion Technique: For the Kirby-Bauer method of susceptibility testing, a 10 mcg ampicillin diffusion disk should be used. With this procedure, a laboratory report of "susceptible" indicates that the infecting organism is likely to respond to SPECTROBID therapy, and a report of "resistant" indicates that the infecting organism is not likely to respond to therapy. An "intermediate susceptibility" report suggests that the infecting organism would be susceptible to SPECTROBID if a high dosage is used or if the infection is confined to tissues and fluids (e.g., urine) in which high antibiotic levels are attained.

Dilution Techniques: Broth or agar dilution methods may be used to determine the minimal inhibitory concentration (MIC) value for susceptibility of bacterial isolates to SPECTROBID. Since SPECTROBID per se has no *in vitro* activity, ampicillin powder should be used in a twofold concentration series of the antibiotic prepared in either broth (in tubes) or agar (in petri plates). Tubes should be inoculated to contain 10^4 to 10^5 organisms/ml or plates "spotted" with 10^3 to 10^4 organisms.

INDICATIONS AND USAGE

SPECTROBID is indicated for the treatment of the following infections when caused by ampicillin-susceptible organisms:

1. Upper and Lower Respiratory Tract Infections (including acute exacerbations of chronic bronchitis) due to streptococci (β-hemolytic streptococci, *Streptococcus pyogenes*), pneumococci (*Streptococcus pneumoniae*), nonpenicillinase-producing staphylococci and *H. influenzae;*
2. Urinary Tract Infections due to *E. coli, Proteus mirabilis,* and *Streptococcus faecalis* (enterococci);
3. Skin and Skin Structure Infections due to streptococci and susceptible staphylococci;
4. Gonorrhea (acute uncomplicated urogenital infections) due to *Neisseria gonorrhoeae.*

Bacteriological studies to determine the causative organisms and their suspectibility to SPECTROBID (i.e., ampicillin) should be performed. Therapy may be instituted prior to obtaining results of susceptibility testing. Indicated surgical procedures should be performed.

CONTRAINDICATIONS

The use of ampicillin class antibiotics is contraindicated in individuals with a history of an allergic reaction to any of the penicillin antibiotics and/or cephalosporins.

WARNINGS

Serious and occasional fatal hypersensitivity (anaphylactic) reactions have been reported in patients on penicillin therapy. Although anaphylaxis is more frequent following parenteral therapy, it has occurred in patients on oral penicillins. These reactions are more apt to occur in individuals with a history of penicillin hypersensitivity and/or hypersensitivity to multiple allergens.

There have been reports of individuals with a history of penicillin hypersensitivity who have experienced severe reactions when treated with cephalosporins. Before therapy with a penicillin, careful inquiry should be made concerning previous hypersensitivity reactions to penicillins, cephalosporins, and other allergens.

IF AN ALLERGIC REACTION OCCURS, THE DRUG SHOULD BE DISCONTINUED AND THE APPROPRIATE THERAPY INSTITUTED. SERIOUS ANAPHYLACTOID REACTIONS REQUIRE IMMEDIATE EMERGENCY TREATMENT WITH EPINEPHRINE. OXYGEN, INTRAVENOUS STEROIDS, AND AIRWAY MANAGEMENT, INCLUDING INTUBATION, SHOULD ALSO BE ADMINISTERED AS INDICATED.

PRECAUTIONS

1. General: The possibility of superinfections with mycotic or bacterial pathogens should be kept in mind during therapy. If superinfections occur (usually involving *Aerobacter, Pseudomonas,* or *Candida*), the drug should be discontinued and appropriate therapy instituted.

As with any potent agent, it is advisable to check periodically for organ system dysfunction during prolonged therapy. This includes renal, hepatic, and hematopoietic systems and is particularly important in prematures, neonates, and patients with liver or renal impairments.

A high percentage of patients with mononucleosis who receive ampicillin develop a skin rash. Thus, ampicillin class antibiotics should not be administered to patients with mononucleosis.

2. Clinically Significant Drug Interactions: The concurrent administration of allopurinol and ampicillin increases substantially the incidence of rashes in patients receiving both drugs as compared to patients receiving ampicillin alone. It is not known whether this potentiation of ampicillin rashes is due to allopurinol or the hyperuricemia present in these patients. There are no data available on the incidence of rash in patients treated concurrently with SPECTROBID (bacampicillin HCl) and allopurinol. SPECTROBID should not be coadministered with Antabuse (disulfiram).

3. Drug and Laboratory Test Interactions: When testing for the presence of glucose in urine using Clinitest™, Benedict's Solution, or Fehling's Solution, high urine concentrations of ampicillin may result in false-positive reactions. Therefore, it is recommended that glucose tests based on enzymatic glucose oxidase reactions (such as Clinistix™ or Testape™) be used.

Following administration of ampicillin to pregnant women a

transient decrease in plasma concentration of total conjugated estriol, estriol-glucuronide, conjugated estrone and estradiol, has been noted.

4. Pregnancy Category B: Reproduction studies have been performed in mice and rats at SPECTROBID doses of up to 750 mg/kg (more than 25 times the human dose) and have revealed no evidence of impaired fertility or harm to the fetus due to SPECTROBID.

There are, however, no adequate and well controlled studies in pregnant women. Because animal reproduction studies are not always predictive of human response, this drug should be used during pregnancy only if clearly needed.

5. Carcinogenesis, Mutagenesis, Impairment of Fertility: No carcinogenicity or mutagenicity studies were conducted. No impairment of fertility and no significant effect on general reproductive performance was observed in rats administered oral doses of up to 750 mg/kg of bacampicillin HCl per day prior to and during mating and gestation. In addition, bacampicillin HCl caused no drug-related effects on the reproductive organs of rats or dogs receiving daily oral doses of up to 800 and 650 mg/kg respectively for 6 months.

6. Labor and Delivery: Oral ampicillin class antibiotics are generally poorly absorbed during labor. Studies in guinea pigs showed that intravenous administration of ampicillin decreased the uterine tone, frequency of contractions, height of contractions, and duration of contractions. However, it is not known whether use of SPECTROBID in humans during labor or delivery has immediate or delayed adverse effects on the fetus, prolongs the duration of labor, or increases the likelihood that forceps delivery or other obstetrical intervention or resuscitation of the newborn will be necessary.

7. Nursing Mothers: Ampicillin class antibiotics are excreted in milk; therefore, caution should be exercised when ampicillin class antibiotics are administered to a nursing woman.

8. Pediatric Use: SPECTROBID tablets are indicated for children weighing 25 kg or more. The SPECTROBID oral suspension is indicated for children and infants weighing less than 25 kg or in those children not able to swallow a tablet.

ADVERSE REACTIONS

As with other penicillins, it may be expected that untoward reactions will be essentially limited to sensitivity phenomena. They are more likely to occur in individuals who have previously demonstrated hypersensitivity to penicillins and in those with a history of allergy, asthma, hay fever, or urticaria.

In well controlled clinical trials conducted in the U.S. the most frequent adverse reactions to SPECTROBID were epigastric upset (2%) and diarrhea (2%). Increased dosage may result in an increased incidence of diarrhea. In the same clinical trials the most frequent adverse effects for amoxicillin were diarrhea (4%) and nausea (2%).

The following adverse reactions have been reported for ampicillin.

Gastrointestinal: diarrhea, gastritis, stomatitis, nausea, vomiting, glossitis, black "hairy" tongue, enterocolitis, and pseudomembranous colitis.

Hypersensitivity Reactions: skin rashes, urticaria, erythema multiforme, and an occasional case of exfoliative dermatitis. These reactions may be controlled with antihistamines and, if necessary, systemic corticosteroids. Whenever such reactions occur, the drug should be discontinued, unless the opinion of the physician dictates otherwise.

Serious and occasional fatal hypersensitivity (anaphylactic) reactions can occur with oral penicillins. (See Warnings).

Liver: A moderate rise in serum glutamic oxaloacetic transaminase (SGOT) has been noted in some ampicillin treated patients, but the significance of this finding is unknown. In well controlled clinical trials no difference was noted between ampicillin and SPECTROBID with regard to the incidence of liver function test abnormalities.

Hemic and Lymphatic Systems: Anemia, thrombocytopenia, thrombocytopenic purpura, eosinophilia, leukopenia, and agranulocytosis have been reported during therapy with penicillins. These reactions are usually reversible on discontinuation of therapy and are believed to be hypersensitivity phenomena.

DOSAGE AND ADMINISTRATION

SPECTROBID tablets may be given without regard to meals. SPECTROBID oral suspension should be administered to fasting patients.

UPPER RESPIRATORY TRACT INFECTIONS (including otitis media) due to streptococci, pneumococci, nonpenicillinase-producing staphylococci and *H. influenzae;*

URINARY TRACT INFECTIONS due to *E. coli, Proteus mirabilis,* and *Streptococcus faecalis;*

SKIN AND SKIN STRUCTURES INFECTIONS due to streptococci and susceptible staphylococci;

Usual Dosage

Adults: 1 × 400 mg tablet every 12 hours (for patients weighing 25 kg or more).

Children: 25 mg/kg per day in 2 equally divided doses at 12 hour intervals.

IN SEVERE INFECTIONS OR THOSE CAUSED BY LESS SUSCEPTIBLE ORGANISMS:

Usual Dosage

Adults: 2 × 400 mg tablets every 12 hours (for patients weighing 25 kg or more).

Children: 50 mg/kg per day in 2 equally divided doses at 12 hour intervals.

LOWER RESPIRATORY TRACT INFECTIONS due to streptococci, pneumococci, nonpenicillinase-producing staphylococci, and *H. influenzae:*

Usual Dosage

Adults: 2 × 400 mg tablets every 12 hours (for patients weighing 25 kg or more).

Children: 50 mg/kg per day in 2 equally divided doses at 12 hour intervals.

GONORRHEA—acute uncomplicated urogenital infections due to *N. gonorrhoeae* (males and females):

1.6 grams (4 × 400 mg tablet plus 1 gram probenecid) as a single oral dose.

No pediatric dosage has been established.

Cases of gonorrhea with a suspected lesion of syphilis should have dark field examination before receiving SPECTROBID and monthly serological tests for a minimum of four months. Larger doses may be required for stubborn or severe infections.

It should be recognized that in the treatment of chronic urinary tract infections, frequent bacteriological and clinical appraisals are necessary. Smaller doses than those recommended above should not be used. In stubborn infections, therapy may be required for several weeks. It may be necessary to continue clinical and/or bacteriological follow-up for several months after cessation of therapy. Except for gonorrhea, treatment should be continued for a minimum of 48 to 72 hours beyond the time that the patient becomes asymptomatic or evidence of bacterial eradication has been obtained.

IT IS RECOMMENDED THAT THERE BE AT LEAST 10 DAYS' TREATMENT FOR ANY INFECTION CAUSED BY HEMOLYTIC STREPTOCOCCI TO PREVENT THE OCCURRENCE OF ACUTE RHEUMATIC FEVER OR GLOMERULONEPHRITIS.

Directions for Mixing Oral Suspension:

Prepare suspension at the time of dispensing as follows: Prior to reconstitution, tap bottle to thoroughly loosen powder. Add the required amount (see table below) of water to the contents of the bottle in approximately two equally divided portions and SHAKE WELL after each addition. Let stand at least 30 minutes and SHAKE WELL just prior to administering each dose. Each level teaspoon (5 ml) will contain 125 mg of bacampicillin HCl.

Final Volume after reconstitution	Amount of Water Required for reconstitution
70 ml	53 ml
100 ml	75 ml

Reconstituted suspension *must be stored under refrigeration and discarded after 10 days.*

GRAPH 1.
Comparison of Bacampicillin HCl 800 mg, Ampicillin 500 mg, and Amoxicillin 500 mg

Serum Antibiotic Concentration (mcg/ml)

Bacampicillin HCl 800 mg* (n = 96)
Amoxicillin 500 mg (n = 20)
Ampicillin 500 mg (n = 47)

Hours Post Dosing

*800 mg Bacampicillin HCl is chemically equivalent to 560 mg of Ampicillin

GRAPH 2.
Crossover Comparison of Bacampicillin HCl Oral Suspension (28 mg/kg)* with Ampicillin Oral Suspension (25 mg/kg) in Fasted Infants and Children (n = 7).

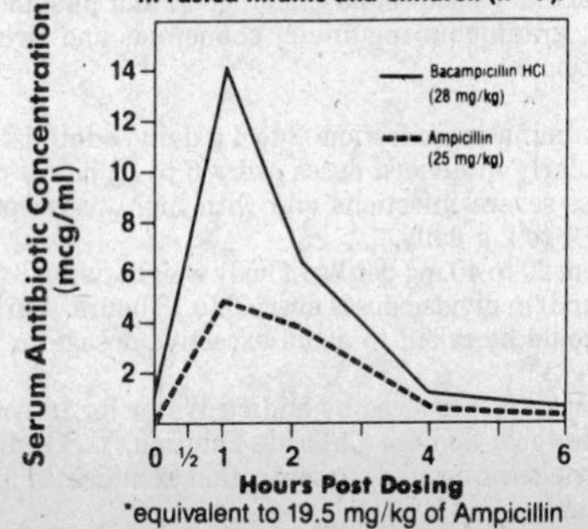

*equivalent to 19.5 mg/kg of Ampicillin

HOW SUPPLIED

SPECTROBID (bacampicillin HCl) Tablets

400 mg (NDC 0049-0350-66): white, film-coated, oblong, unscored are available in bottles of 100.

SPECTROBID (bacampicillin HCl) Powder for Oral Suspension.

Each 5 ml of reconstituted suspension contains 125 mg of bacampicillin HCl.

Bottles containing the following volumes are available: 70 ml (NDC 0049-0357-37), 100 ml (NDC 0049-0357-44).

67-4092-00-3

Shown in Product Identification Section, page 426

STREPTOMYCIN SULFATE ℞

Dry Powder: Vials of 1 g and 5 g

WARNING

THE RISK OF SEVERE NEUROTOXIC REACTIONS IS SHARPLY INCREASED IN PATIENTS WITH IMPAIRED KIDNEY FUNCTION OR PRERENAL AZOTEMIA. THESE INCLUDE DISBURBANCES OF THE AUDITORY NERVE, OPTIC NERVE, PERIPHERAL NEURITIS, ARACHNOIDITIS, AND ENCEPHALOPATHY. RENAL FUNCTION SHOULD BE CAREFULLY DETERMINED AND PATIENTS WITH RENAL DAMAGE AND NITROGEN RETENTION SHOULD HAVE REDUCED DOSAGE. THE PEAK SERUM CONCENTRATION IN INDIVIDUALS WITH KIDNEY DAMAGE SHOULD NOT EXCEED 20 TO 25 MCG PER MILLILITER.

THE CONCURRENT OR SEQUENTIAL USE OF OTHER NEUROTOXIC AND/OR NEPHROTOXIC DRUGS WITH STREPTOMYCIN SULFATE, PARTICULARLY NEOMYCIN, KANAMYCIN, GENTAMICIN, CEPHALORIDINE, PAROMOMYCIN, VIOMYCIN, POLYMYXIN B, COLISTIN, AND TOBRAMYCIN SHOULD BE AVOIDED.

THE NEUROTOXICITY OF STREPTOMYCIN CAN RESULT IN RESPIRATORY PARALYSIS FROM NEUROMUSCULAR BLOCKADE, ESPECIALLY WHEN THE DRUG IS GIVEN SOON AFTER ANESTHESIA AND THE USE OF MUSCLE RELAXANTS.

THE ADMINISTRATION OF STREPTOMYCIN IN PARENTERAL FORM SHOULD BE RESERVED FOR PATIENTS WHERE ADEQUATE LABORATORY FACILITIES ARE AVAILABLE AND CONSTANT SUPERVISION OF THE PATIENT IS POSSIBLE.

DESCRIPTION

Streptomycin is a water-soluble aminoglycoside derived from *Streptomyces griseus.* It is marketed as the sulfate salt of streptomycin.

ACTIONS

Streptomycin sulfate is a bactericidal antibiotic in therapeutic dosage. The mode of action is the interference with normal protein synthesis and production of "faulty proteins." Following intramuscular injection of 1 g of the drug, a peak serum level of 25 to 50 mcg per milliliter is reached within 1 hour, diminishing slowly to about 50 percent after 5 to 6 hours. Appreciable concentrations are found in all organ tissues except the brain. Significant amounts have been found in pleural fluid and tuberculous cavities. Streptomycin passes through the placenta with serum levels in the cord blood similar to maternal levels. Small amounts are excreted in milk, saliva, and sweat.

Streptomycin is excreted rapidly in the urine by glomerular filtration. In patients with normal kidney function, between 29 and 89 percent of a single 0.6 g dose is excreted within 24 hours. Any reduction of glomerular activity results in decreased excretion of the drug and concurrent rise in serum and tissue levels.

Sensitivity plate testing: If the Kirby-Bauermethod of disc sensitivity is used, a 10 mcg streptomycin disc should give a zone of over 15 millimeters when tested against a streptomycin-sensitive bacterial strain.

INDICATIONS

1. Mycobacterium tuberculosis: Streptomycin may be indicated for all forms of this infection when the infecting organisms are susceptible. It should be used only in combination with other antituberculosis drugs. The common combined drug therapy is streptomycin, PAS, and, isoniazid; this com-

Continued on next page

Roerig—Cont.

bination is effective only where the organisms are susceptible to the drugs being used in combination.
2. Nontuberculosis infections: Streptomycin should be used only in those serious nontuberculosis infections caused by organisms shown by *in vitro* sensitivity studies to be susceptible to it and when less potentially hazardous therapeutic agents are ineffective or contraindicated.
a. *Pasteurella pestis* (plague).
b. *Pasteurella tularensis* (tularemia).
c. *Brucella.*
d. *Donovanosis* (granuloma inguinale).
e. *H. ducreyi* (chancroid).
f. *H. influenzae* (in respiratory, endocardial, and meningeal infections—concomitantly with another antibacterial agent).
g. *K. pneumoniae* pneumonia (concomitantly with another antibacterial agent).
h. *E. coli, Proteus, A. aerogenes, K. pneumoniae,* and *Streptococcus faecalis* in urinary tract infections.
i. *Strep. viridans, Strep. faecalis* (in endocardial infections—concomitantly with penicillin).
j. Gram-negative bacillary bacteremia (concomitantly with another antibacterial agent).
Note: The use of streptomycin should be limited to the treatment of infections caused by bacteria which have been shown to be susceptible to the antibacterial effects of streptomycin and which are not amenable to therapy with less potentially toxic agents.

CONTRAINDICATIONS

Streptomycin is contraindicated in those individuals who have shown previous toxic or hypersensitivity reaction to it.

WARNINGS

Ototoxicity: Streptomycin may frequently affect the vestibular branch of the auditory nerve causing severe nausea, vomiting, and vertigo. The incidence is directly proportional to duration and amount of the drug administered. Advanced age and renal impairment predispose to ototoxicity. Symptoms subside and recovery is usually complete following discontinuance of the drug.
Loss of hearing has been reported following long term therapy; however, ototoxic effect on the auditory branch of the eighth nerve is infrequent and usually is preceded by vestibular symptoms. Hearing loss, when extensive, is usually permanent.
USAGE IN PREGNANCY: Since streptomycin readily crosses the placental barrier, caution in use of the drug is important to prevent ototoxicity in the fetus.

PRECAUTIONS

Baseline and periodic caloric stimulation tests and audiometric tests are advisable with extended streptomycin therapy. Tinnitus, roaring noises, or a sense of fullness in the ears indicates need for audiometric examination or termination of streptomycin therapy or both.
Care should be taken by individuals handling or preparing streptomycin for injection to avoid skin sensitivity reactions.
As with all intramuscular preparations, Streptomycin Sulfate Injection should be injected well within the body of a relatively large muscle. ADULTS: The preferred site is the upper outer quadrant of the buttock, (i.e., gluteus maximus), or the mid-lateral thigh. CHILDREN: It is recommended that intramuscular injections be given preferably in the mid-lateral muscles of the thigh. In infants and small children the periphery of the upper outer quadrant of the gluteal region should be used only when necessary, such as in burn patients, in order to minimize the possibility of damage to the sciatic nerve.
The deltoid area should be used only if well developed such as in certain adults and older children, and then only with caution to avoid radial nerve injury. Intramuscular injections should not be made into the lower and mid-third of the upper arm. As with all intramuscular injections, aspiration is necessary to help avoid inadvertent injection into a blood vessel.
Injection sites should be alternated, and solutions of concentration greater than 500 mg/ml are not recommended.
As higher doses or more prolonged therapy with streptomycin may be indicated for more severe or fulminating infections (endocarditis, meningitis, etc.), the physician should always take adequate measures to be immediately aware of any toxic signs or symptoms occurring in the patient as a result of streptomycin therapy.
While disturbances in renal function due to streptomycin have been reported in the past, purification of the drug has minimized this side effect. In the presence of pre-existing renal insufficiency, however, extreme caution must be exercised in the administration of streptomycin. Since in severely uremic patients a single dose may produce reasonably high blood levels for several days, the cumulative effect may produce ototoxic sequelae. When streptomycin must be given for prolonged periods of time, alkalinization of the urine may minimize or prevent renal irritation.
A syndrome of apparent central nervous system depression, characterized by stupor and flaccidity, at times to the extent of coma and deep respiratory depression, has been reported in very young infants in whom streptomycin dosage had materially exceeded the recommended limits. Thus, infants should not receive streptomycin in excess of the recommended dosage.
In the treatment of venereal infections such as granuloma inguinale, and chancroid, if concomitant syphilis is suspected, suitable laboratory procedures such as a dark field examination should be performed before the start of treatment, and monthly serologic tests should be done for at least four months.
As with other antibiotics, use of this drug may result in overgrowth of nonsusceptible organisms, including fungi. If superinfection occurs, appropriate therapy should be instituted.

ADVERSE REACTIONS

The following reactions are common: ototoxicity—nausea, vomiting, and vertigo; paresthesia of face; rash; fever; urticaria; angioneurotic edema; and eosinophilia.
The following reactions are less frequent: deafness, exfoliative dermatitis, anaphylaxis, azotemia, leucopenia, thrombocytopenia, pancytopenia, hemolytic anemia, muscular weakness, and amblyopia.
Vestibular dysfunction resulting from the parenteral administration of streptomycin is cumulatively related to the total daily dose. When 1.8 to 2.0 g/day are given, symptoms are likely to develop in the large percentage of patients—especially in the elderly or patients with impaired renal function—within four weeks. Therefore, it is recommended that caloric and audiometric tests be done prior to, during, and following intensive therapy with streptomycin in order to facilitate detection of any vestibular dysfunction and/or impairment of hearing which may occur.
Vestibular symptoms generally appear early and usually are reversible with early detection and cessation of administration of the drug. After two to three months, gross vesibular symptoms usually disappear, except for the relative inability to walk in total darkness or on very rough terrain.
Clinical judgment as to termination of therapy must be exercised when side effects occur.

DOSAGE AND ADMINISTRATION

Intramuscular Route Only
1. Tuberculosis: All forms when organisms are known or believed to be drug susceptible.
Adult, combined therapy: Streptomycin—1 g daily with PAS 5 g t.i.d. and isoniazid 200 to 300 mg daily. Elderly patients should have a smaller daily dose of streptomycin, based on age, renal function, and eighth nerve function. Ultimately the streptomycin should be discontinued or reduced in dosage to 1 g 2 to 3 times weekly. Therapy with streptomycin may be terminated when toxic symptoms have appeared, when impending toxicity is feared, when organisms become resistant, or when full treatment effect has been obtained.
The total period of drug treatment of tuberculosis is a minimum of 1 year; however, indications for terminating therapy with streptomycin may occur at any time as noted above.
2. Tularemia: One to 2 g daily in divided doses for 7 to 10 days until the patient is afebrile for 5 to 7 days.
3. Plague: Two to 4 g daily in divided doses until the patient is afebrile for at least 3 days.
4a. Bacterial endocarditis: In penicillin-sensitive alpha and nonhemolytic streptococcal endocarditis (penicillin sensitive to 0.1 mcg per milliliter or less), streptomycin may be used for 2-week treatment concomitantly with penicillin. Streptomycin dosage is 1 g b.i.d. for 1 week, and 0.5 g b.i.d. for the 2d week. If the patient is over 60 years of age, the dosage should be 0.5 g b.i.d. for the entire 2-week period.
b. Enterococcal endocarditis: Streptomycin in doses of 1 g b.i.d. for 2 weeks and 0.5 g b.i.d. for 4 weeks is given in combination with penicillin. Ototoxicity may require termination of the streptomycin prior to completion of the 6-week course of treatment.
5. For use concomitantly with other agents to which the infecting organism is also sensitive. Streptomycin in these conditions is considered as a drug of secondary choice: gram-negative bacillary bacteremia, meningitis, and pneumonia; brucellosis; granuloma inguinale; chancroid, and urinary tract infection.
For adults:
a. Severe fulminating infection: 2 to 4 g daily, administered intramuscularly in divided doses every 6 to 12 hours.
b. With less severe infections and with highly susceptible organisms: 1 to 2 g daily.
For children: 20 to 40 mg per kg of body weight daily (8 to 20 mg per pound) in divided doses every 6 to 12 hours. (Particular care should be taken to avoid excessive dosage in children.)
The dry powder is dissolved by adding Water for Injection, U.S.P. or Isotonic Sodium Chloride Solution, U.S.P. in an amount to yield the desired concentration as indicated in the following table:

Approx. Conc. (mg/ml)	Volume (ml) of Solvent 1 g Vial	5 g Vial
200	4.2	—
250	3.2	—
400	1.8	9.0

Sterile reconstituted solutions may be stored at room temperature for four weeks without significant loss of potency.

SUPPLY

Streptomycin Sulfate is supplied as a sterile powder in packages of 100 vials, each vial containing streptomycin sulfate equivalent to 1.0 g and 5.0 g of streptomycin base.

TAO® ℞

[tă'ō]
(troleandomycin)
Capsules and Oral Suspension

DESCRIPTION

TAO (troleandomycin) is a synthetically derived acetylated ester of oleandomycin, an antibiotic elaborated by a species of *Streptomyces antibioticus.* It is a white crystalline compound, insoluble in water, but readily soluble and stable in the presence of gastric juice. The compound has a molecular weight of 814 and corresponds to the empirical formula $C_{41}H_{67}NO_{15}$.

ACTIONS

TAO is an antibiotic shown to be active *in vitro* against the following gram-positive organisms:
Streptococcus pyogenes
Diplococcus pneumoniae
Susceptibility plate testing: If the Kirby-Bauer method of disc sensitivity is used, a 15 mcg. oleandomycin disc should give a zone of over 18 mm. when tested against a troleandomycin sensitive bacterial strain.

INDICATIONS

Diplococcus pneumoniae
Pneumococcal pneumonia due to susceptible strains.
Streptococcus pyogenes
Group A beta-hemolytic streptococcal infections of the upper respiratory tract.
Injectable benzathine penicillin G is considered by the American Heart Association to be the drug of choice in the treatment and prevention of streptococcal pharyngitis and in long term prophylaxis of rheumatic fever.
Troleandomycin is generally effective in the eradication of streptococci from the nasopharynx. However, substantial data establishing the efficacy of TAO in the subsequent prevention of rheumatic fever are not available at present.

CONTRAINDICATIONS

Troleandomycin is contraindicated in patients with known hypersensitivity to this antibiotic.

WARNINGS

Usage in Pregnancy: Safety for use in pregnancy has not been established.
The administration of troleandomycin has been associated with an allergic type of cholestatic hepatitis. Some patients receiving troleandomycin for more than two weeks or in repeated courses have shown jaundice accompanied by right upper quadrant pain, fever, nausea, vomiting, eosinophilia, and leukocytosis. The changes have been reversible on discontinuance of the drug. Liver function tests should be monitored in patients on such dosage, and the drug discontinued if abnormalities develop. Reports in the literature have suggested that the concurrent use of ergotamine-containing drugs and troleandomycin may induce ischemic reactions. Therefore, the concurrent use of ergotamine-containing drugs and troleandomycin should be avoided. Troleandomycin should be administered with caution to patients concurrently receiving estrogen containing oral contraceptives.
Studies in chronic asthmatic patients have suggested that the concurrent use of theophylline and troleandomycin may result in elevated serum concentrations of theophylline. Therefore, it is recommended that patients receiving such concurrent therapy be observed for signs of theophylline toxicity, and that therapy be appropriately modified if such signs develop.

PRECAUTIONS

Troleandomycin is principally excreted by the liver.
Caution should be exercised in administering the antibiotic to patients with impaired hepatic function.

ADVERSE REACTIONS

The most frequent side effects of troleandomycin preparations are gastrointestinal, such as abdominal cramping and discomfort, and are dose related. Nausea, vomiting, and diarrhea occur infrequently with usual oral doses.
During prolonged or repeated therapy, there is a possibility of overgrowth of nonsusceptible bacteria or fungi. If such infections occur, the drug should be discontinued and appropriate therapy instituted.

Mild allergic reactions such as urticaria and other skin rashes have occurred. Serious allergic reactions, including anaphylaxis, have been reported.

DOSAGE AND ADMINISTRATION

Clinical judgment based on the type of infection and its severity should determine dosage within the below listed ranges.
Adults: 250 to 500 mg. 4 times a day
Children: 125 to 250 mg. (3-5 mg./lb. or 6.6 to 11 mg./kg.) every 6 hours
When used in streptococcal infection, therapy should be continued for ten days.

HOW SUPPLIED

TAO is supplied as:
Capsules 250 mg.: Each capsule contains troleandomycin equivalent to 250 mg. of oleandomycin; bottle of 100 capsules.

69-1800-00-6

Shown in Product Identification Section, page 426

TERRA-CORTRIL® ℞

Terramycin ® (oxytetracycline HCl)
—Cortril® (hydrocortisone acetate)
OPHTHALMIC SUSPENSION

DESCRIPTION

Terra-Cortril suspension combines the antibiotic, oxytetracycline HCl ($C_{22}H_{24}N_2O_9 \cdot HCl$) and the adrenocorticoid, hydrocortisone acetate ($C_{23}H_{32}O_6$). **Each ml of Terra-Cortril contains Terramycin (oxytetracycline HCl) equivalent to 5 mg of oxytetracycline, and 15 mg of Cortril (hydrocortisone acetate) incorporated in mineral oil with aluminum tristearate.**

For Ophthalmic Use Only.

CLINICAL PHARMACOLOGY

Corticosteroids suppress the inflammatory response to a variety of agents and they probably delay or slow healing. Since corticoids may inhibit the body's defense mechanism against infection, a concomitant antimicrobial drug may be used when this inhibition is considered to be clinically significant in a particular case.
The anti-infective component in the combination is included to provide action against specific organisms suspectible to it. Terramycin is considered active against the following microorganisms:
Rickettsiae (Rocky Mountain spotted fever, typhus fever and the typhus group, Q fever, rickettsialpox and tick fevers),
Mycoplasma pneumoniae (PPLO, Eaton Agent),
Agents of psittacosis and ornithosis,
Agents of lymphogranuloma venereum and granuloma inguinale,
The spirochetal agent of relapsing fever (*Borrelia recurrentis*).
The following gram-negative microorganisms:
Haemophilus ducreyi (chancroid),
Pasteurella pestis and *Pasteurella tularensis,*
Bartonella bacilliformis,
Bacteroides species,
Vibrio comma and *Vibrio fetus,*
Brucella species (in conjunction with streptomycin).
Because many strains of the following groups of microorganisms have been shown to be resistant to tetracyclines, culture and suspectibility testing are recommended.
Oxytetracycline is indicated for treatment of infections caused by the following gram-negative microorganisms, when bacteriologic testing indicates appropriate susceptibility to the drug:
Escherichia coli,
Enterobacter aerogenes (formerly *Aerobacter aerogenes*),
Shigella species,
Mima species and *Herellea* species,
Haemophilus influenzae (respiratory infections),
Klebsiella species (respiratory and urinary infections).
Oxytetracycline is indicated for treatment of infections caused by the following gram-positive microorganisms when bacteriologic testing indicates appropriate suspectibility to the drug:
Streptococcus species:
Up to 44 percent of strains of *Streptococcus pyogenes* and 74 percent of *Streptococcus faecalis* have been found to be resistant to tetracycline drugs. Therefore, tetracyclines should not be used for streptococcal disease unless the organism has been demonstrated to be sensitive.
For upper respiratory infections due to Group A beta-hemolytic streptococci, pencillin is the usual drug of choice, including prophylaxis of rheumatic fever.
Diplococcus pneumoniae,
Staphylococcus aureus, skin and soft tissue infections. Oxytetracycline is not the drug of choice in the treatment of any type of staphylococcus infections.
When penicillin is contraindicated, tetracyclines are alternative drugs in the treatment of infections due to:

Terramycin Intramuscular
contents per ml (w/v)

Ingredient	2 ml Single Dose Ampules and isoject		10 ml/Vial Multidose
	100 mg/2 ml	250 mg/2 ml	50 mg/ml 10 ml (5 × 2 ml Doses)
oxytetracycline	50 mg	25 mg	50 mg
lidocaine	2.0%	2.0%	2.0%
magnesium chloride hexahydrate	2.5%	6.0%	2.5%
sodium formaldehyde sulfoxylate	0.5%	0.5%	0.3%
α-monothioglycerol	—	—	1.0%
monoethanolamine	approx. 1.7%	approx. 4.2%	approx. 2.6%
citric acid			1.0%
propyl gallate	—	—	0.02%
propylene glycol	75.2%	67.0%	74.1%
water	18.8%	16.8%	18.5%

Neisseria gonorrhoeae,
Treponema pallidum and *Treponema pertenue* (syphilis and yaws),
Listeria monocytogenes,
Clostridium species,
Bacillus anthracis,
Fusobacterium fusiforme (Vincent's infection),
Actinomyces species.
Tetracyclines are indicated in the treatment of trachoma, although the infectious agent is not always eliminated, as judged by immunofluorescence.
Inclusion conjunctivitis may be treated with oral tetracyclines or with a combination of oral and topical agents.
When a decision to administer both a corticoid and an antimicrobial is made, the administration of such drugs in combination has the advantage of greater patient compliance and convenience, with the added assurance that the appropriate dosage of both drugs is administered, plus assured compatibility of ingredients when both types of drug are in the same formulation and, particularly, that the correct volume of drug is delivered and retained.
The relative potency of corticosteroids depends on the molecular structure, concentration, and release from the vehicle.

INDICATIONS AND USAGE

A steroid/anti-infective combination is indicated in ocular inflammation when concurrent use of an antimicrobial is judged necessary.

CONTRAINDICATIONS

Epithelial herpes simplex keratitis (dendritic keratitis), vaccinia, varicella, and many other viral diseases of the cornea and conjunctiva. Mycobacterial infection of the eye. Fungal diseases of ocular structures. Hypersensitivity to a component of the medication. (Hypersensitivity to the antibiotic component occurs at a higher rate than for other components.)
The use of these combinations is always contraindicated after uncomplicated removal of a corneal foreign body.

WARNINGS

Prolonged use may result in glaucoma, with damage to the optic nerve, defects in visual acuity and fields of vision, and posterior subcapsular cataract formation. Prolonged use may suppress the host response and thus increase the hazard of secondary ocular infections. In those diseases causing thinning of the cornea or sclera, perforations have been known to occur with the use of topical steroids. In acute purulent conditions of the eye, steroids may mask infection or enhance existing infection. If these products are used for 10 days or longer, intraocular pressure should be routinely monitored even though it may be difficult in children and uncooperative patients.
Employment of steroid medication in the treatment of herpes simplex requires great caution.

PRECAUTIONS

The initial prescription and renewal of the medication order beyond 20 milliliters should be made by a physician only after examination of the patient with the aid of magnification, such as slit lamp biomicroscopy and, where appropriate, fluorescein staining.
The possibility of persistent fungal infections of the cornea should be considered after prolonged steroid dosing.

ADVERSE REACTIONS

Adverse reactions have occurred with steroid/anti-infective combination drugs which can be attributed to the steroid component, the anti-infective component, or the combination. Exact incidence figures are not available since no denominator of treated patients is available.
Reactions occurring most often from the presence of the anti-infective ingredient are allergic sensitizations. The reactions due to the steroid component in decreasing order of frequency are: elevation of intraocular pressure (IOP) with possible development of glaucoma, and infrequent optic nerve damage; posterior subcapsular cataract formation; and delayed wound healing.

Secondary Infection: The development of secondary infection has occurred after use of combinations containing steroids and antimicrobials. Fungal infections of the cornea are particularly prone to develop coincidentally with long-term applications of steroid. The possibility of fungal invasion must be considered in any persistent corneal ulceration where steroid treatment has been used.
Secondary bacterial ocular infection following suppression of host responses also occurs.

DOSAGE AND ADMINISTRATION

Instill 1 or 2 drops of Terra-Cortril Ophthalmic Suspension into the affected eye three times daily.
Not more than 20 milliliters should be prescribed initially and the prescription should not be refilled without further evaluation as outlined in "Precautions" above.

HOW SUPPLIED

Terra-Cortril Ophthalmic Suspension is supplied in 5 ml vials with separate sterile dropper.

TERRAMYCIN® ℞

(oxytetracycline)
INTRAMUSCULAR SOLUTION*
FOR INTRAMUSCULAR USE ONLY
contains 2% lidocaine

DESCRIPTION

Oxytetracycline is a product of the metabolism of *Streptomyces rimosus* and is one of the family of tetracycline antibiotics.
Oxytetracycline diffuses readily through the placenta into the fetal circulation, into the pleural fluid and, under some circumstances, into the cerebrospinal fluid. It appears to be concentrated in the hepatic system and excreted in the bile, so that it appears in the feces, as well as in the urine, in a biologically active form.

COMPOSITION

[See table above].

ACTIONS

Oxytetracycline is primarily bacteriostatic and is thought to exert its antimicrobial effect by the inhibition of protein synthesis. Oxytetracycline is active against a wide range of gram-negative and gram-positive organisms.
The drugs in the tetracycline class have closely similar antimicrobial spectra, and cross resistance among them is common. Microorganisms may be considered susceptible if the M.I.C. (minimum inhibitory concentration) is not more than 4.0 mcg/ml and intermediate if the M.I.C. is 4.0 to 12.5 mcg/ml.
Susceptibility plate testing: A tetracycline disc may be used to determine microbial susceptibility to drugs in the tetracycline class. If the Kirby-Bauer method of disc susceptibility testing is used, a 30 mcg tetracycline disc should give a zone of at least 19 mm when tested against an oxytetracycline-susceptible bacterial strain.
Tetracyclines are readily absorbed and are bound to plasma proteins in varying degree. They are concentrated by the liver in the bile and excreted in the urine and feces at high concentrations and in a biologically active form.

INDICATIONS

Oxytetracycline is indicated in infections caused by the following microorganisms:
Rickettsiae (Rocky Mountain spotted fever, typhus fever and the typhus group, Q fever, rickettsialpox and tick fevers).
Mycoplasma pneumoniae (PPLO, Eaton agent),
Agents of psittacosis and ornithosis,
Agents of lymphogranuloma venereum and granuloma inguinale,
The spirochetal agent of relapsing fever *(Borrelia recurrentis).*

Continued on next page

Roerig—Cont.

The following gram-negative microorganisms:
Haemophilus ducreyi (chancroid),
Pasteurella pestis and *Pasteurella tularensis*,
Bartonella bacilliformis,
Bacteroides species,
Vibrio comma and *Vibrio fetus*,
Brucella species (in conjunction with streptomycin).

Because many strains of the following groups of microorganisms have been shown to be resistant to tetracyclines, culture and susceptibility testing are recommended.

Oxytetracycline is indicated for treatment of infections caused by the following gram-negative microorganisms, when bacteriologic testing indicates appropriate susceptibility to the drug:
Escherichia coli,
Enterobacter aerogenes (formerly *Aerobacter aerogenes*),
Shigella species,
Mima species and *Herellea* species,
Haemophilus influenzae (respiratory infections),
Klebsiella species (respiratory and urinary infections).

Oxytetracycline is indicated for treatment of infections caused by the following gram-positive microorganisms when bacteriologic testing indicates appropriate susceptibility to the drug: Streptococcus species;

Up to 44 percent of strains of *Streptococcus pyogenes* and 74 percent of *Streptococcus faecalis* have been found to be resistant to tetracycline drugs. Therefore, tetracyclines should not be used for streptococcal disease unless the organism has been demonstrated to be sensitive.

For upper respiratory infections due to Group A beta-hemolytic streptococci, penicillin is the usual drug of choice, including prophylaxis of rheumatic fever.
Diplococcus pneumoniae,
Staphylococcus aureus, skin and soft tissue infections. Oxytetracycline is not the drug of choice in the treatment of any type of staphylococcal infections.

When penicillin is contraindicated, tetracyclines are alternative drugs in the treatment of infections due to:
Neisseria gonorrhoeae,
Treponema pallidum and *Treponema pertenue* (syphilis and yaws),
Listeria monocytogenes,
Clostridium species,
Bacillus anthracis,
Fusobacterium fusiforme (Vincent's infection),
Actinomyces species.

In acute intestinal amebiasis, the tetracyclines may be a useful adjunct to amebicides.

Tetracyclines are indicated in the treatment of trachoma, although the infectious agent is not always eliminated, as judged by immunofluorescence.

Inclusion conjunctivitis may be treated with oral tetracyclines or with a combination of oral and topical agents.

CONTRAINDICATIONS

This drug is contraindicated in persons who have shown hypersensitivity to any of the tetracyclines.

WARNINGS

THE USE OF TETRACYCLINES DURING TOOTH DEVELOPMENT (LAST HALF OF PREGNANCY, INFANCY, AND CHILDHOOD TO THE AGE OF 8 YEARS) MAY CAUSE PERMANENT DISCOLORATION OF THE TEETH (YELLOW-GRAY-BROWN).

This adverse reaction is more common during long term use of the drugs but has been observed following repeated short term courses. Enamel hypoplasia has also been reported. *TETRACYCLINES, THEREFORE, SHOULD NOT BE USED IN THIS AGE GROUP UNLESS OTHER DRUGS ARE NOT LIKELY TO BE EFFECTIVE OR ARE CONTRAINDICATED.*

If renal impairment exists, even usual oral or parenteral doses may lead to excessive systemic accumulation of the drug and possible liver toxicity. Under such conditions, lower than usual total doses are indicated and, if therapy is prolonged, serum level determinations of the drug may be advisable. This hazard is of particular importance in the parenteral administration of tetracyclines to pregnant or postpartum patients with pyelonephritis. When used under these circumstances, the blood level should not exceed 15 mcg/ml and liver function tests should be made at frequent intervals. Other potentially hepatotoxic drugs should not be prescribed concomitantly.

(In the presence of renal dysfunction, particularly in pregnancy, intravenous tetracycline therapy in daily doses exceeding 2 grams has been associated with deaths due to liver failure.)

Photosensitivity manifested by an exaggerated sunburn reaction has been observed in some individuals taking tetracyclnes. Patients apt to be exposed to direct sunlight or ultraviolet light should be advised that this reaction can occur with tetracycline drugs, and treatment should be discontinued at the first evidence of skin erythema.

The antianabolic action of the tetracyclines may cause an increase in BUN. While this is not a problem in those with normal renal function, in patients with significantly impaired function, higher serum levels of this drug may lead to azotemia, hyperphosphatemia, and acidosis.

Usage in pregnancy. (See above "Warnings" about use during tooth development.)

Results of animal studies indicate that tetracyclines cross the placenta, are found in fetal tissues and can have toxic effects on the developing fetus (often related to retardation of skeletal development). Evidence of embryotoxicity has also been noted in animals treated early in pregnancy.

Usage in newborns, infants, and children. (See above "Warnings" about use during tooth deveopment).

All tetracyclines form a stable calcium complex in any bone-forming tissue. A decrease in the fibula growth rate has been observed in prematures given oral tetracyclne in doses of 25 mg/kg every 6 hours. This reaction was shown to be reversible when the drug was discontinued.

Tetracyclines are present in the milk of lactating women who are taking a drug in this class.

PRECAUTIONS

As with all intramuscular preparations, Terramycin (oxytetracycline) Intramuscular Solution should be injected well within the body of a relatively large muscle. ADULTS: The preferred sites are the upper outer quadrant of the buttock, (i.e., gluteus maximus), and the mid-lateral thigh. CHILDREN: It is recommended that intramuscular injections be given preferably in the mid-lateral muscles of the thigh. In infants and small children the periphery of the upper outer quadrant of the gluteal region should be used only when necessary, such as in burn patients, in order to minimize the possibility of damage to the sciatic nerve.

The deltoid area should be used only if well developed such as in certain adults and older children, and then only with caution to avoid radial nerve injury. Intramuscular injections should not be made into the lower and mid-thirds of the upper arm. As with all intramuscular injections, aspiration is necessary to help avoid inadvertent injection into a blood vessel.

As with other antibiotic preparations, use of this drug may result in overgrowth of nonsusceptible organisms, including fungi. If superinfection occurs, the antibiotic should be discontinued and appropriate therapy instituted.

In venereal diseases when coexistent syphilis is suspected, a dark field examination should be done before treatment is started and the blood serology repeated monthly for at least 4 months.

Because tetracyclines have been shown to depress plasma prothrombin activity, patients who are on anticoagulant therapy may require downward adjustment of their anticoagulant dosage.

In long term therapy, periodic laboratory evaluation of organ systems, including hematopoietic, renal and hepatic studies should be performed.

All infections due to Group A beta-hemolytic streptococci should be treated for at least 10 days.

Since bacteriostatic drugs may interfere with the bactericidal action of penicillin, it is advisable to avoid giving tetracycline in conjunction with penicillin.

ADVERSE REACTIONS

Local irritation may be present after intramuscular injection. The injection should be deep, with care taken not to injure the sciatic nerve nor inject intravascularly.

Gastrointestinal: anorexia, nausea, vomiting, diarrhea, glossitis, dyphagia, enterocolitis, and inflammatory lesions (with monilial overgrowth) in the anogenital region. These reactions have been caused by both the oral and parenteral administration of tetracyclines.

Skin: maculopapular and erythematous rashes. Exfoliative dermatitis has been reported but is uncommon. Photosensitivity is discussed above. (See "Warnings").

Renal toxicity: Rise in BUN has been reported and is apparently dose related. (See "Warnings").

Hypersensitivity reactions: Urticaria, angioneurotic edema, anaphylaxis, anaphylactoid purpura, pericarditis, and exacerbation of systemic lupus erythematosus.

Bulging fontanels in infants and benign intracranial hypertension in adults have been reported in individuals receiving full therapeutic dosages. These conditions disappeared rapidly when the drug was discontinued.

Blood: Hemolytic anemia, thrombocytopenia, neutropenia, and eosinophilia have been reported.

When given over prolonged periods, tetracyclines have been reported to produce brown-black microscopic discoloration of thyroid glands. No abnormalities of thyroid function studies are known to occur.

DOSAGE AND ADMINISTRATION

Intramuscular Administration:

Adults: The usual daily dose is 250 mg administered once every 24 hours or 300 mg given in divided doses at 8 to 12 hour intervals.

For children above eight years of age: 15–25 mg/kg body weight up to a maximum of 250 mg per single daily injection. Dosage may be divided and given at 8 to 12 hour intervals.

Intramuscular therapy should be reserved for situations in which oral therapy is not feasible.

The intramuscular administration of oxytetracycline produces lower blood levels than oral administration in the recommended dosages. Patients placed on intramuscular oxytetracycline should be changed to the oral dosage form as soon as possible. If rapid, high blood levels are needed, oxytetracycline should be administered intravenously.

In patients with renal impairment: (See "Warnings") Total dosage should be decreased by reduction of recommended individual doses and/or by extending time intervals between doses.

HOW SUPPLIED

Terramycin (oxytetracycline) Intramuscular Solution is available as follows:

250 mg/2 ml—in 2 ml pre-scored glass ampules, packages of 5 (NDC 0995-0770-09).

100 mg/2 ml—in 2 ml pre-scored glass ampules, packages of 5 (NDC 0995-0760-09).

50 mg/ml—in 10 ml multiple dose vials, packages of 5 (NDC 0995-0750-77).

*U.S. Pat. Nos. 3,017,323 and 3,026,248

TERRAMYCIN® ℞

(oxytetracycline HCl with polymyxin B sulfate)
OPHTHALMIC OINTMENT
STERILE

DESCRIPTION

Each gram of sterile ointment contains oxytetracycline HCl equivalent to 5 mg oxytetracycline, 10,000 units of polymyxin B sulfate, white petrolatum, and liquid petrolatum.

ACTIONS

Terramycin® (oxytetracycline HCl) is a widely used antibiotic with clinically proved activity against gram-positive and gram-negative bacteria, rickettsiae, spirochetes, large viruses, and certain protozoa.

Polymyxin B Sulfate, one of a group of related antibiotics derived from *Bacillus polymyxa*, is rapidly bactericidal. This action is exclusively against gram-negative organisms. It is particularly effective against *Pseudomonas aeruginosa (B. pyocyaneus)* and Koch-Weeks bacillus, frequently found in local infections of the eye.

There is thus made available a particularly effective antimicrobial combination of the broad-spectrum antibiotic Terramycin as well as polymyxin B sulfate against primarily causative or secondarily infecting organisms.

INDICATIONS

The sterile preparation, Terramycin with Polymyxin B Sulfate Ophthalmic Ointment, is indicated for the treatment of superficial ocular infections involving the conjunctiva and/or cornea caused by Terramycin with Polymyxin B Sulfate-susceptible organisms.

It may be administered topically alone, or as an adjunct to systemic therapy.

It is effective in infections caused by susceptible strains of staphylococci, streptococci, pneumococci, *Hemophilus influenzae, Pseudomonas aeruginosa*, Koch-Weeks bacillus, and *Proteus.*

CONTRAINDICATIONS

This drug is contraindicated in individuals who have shown hypersensitivity to any of its components.

PRECAUTIONS

As with all antibiotic preparations, use of this drug may result in overgrowth of nonsusceptible organisms, including fungi. If super-infection occurs, the antibiotic should be discontinued and appropriate specific therapy should be instituted.

ADVERSE REACTIONS

Terramycin with Polymyxin B Sulfate Ophthalmic Ointment is well tolerated by the epithelial membranes and other tissues of the eye. Allergic or inflammatory reactions due to individual hypersensitivity are rare.

DOSAGE AND ADMINISTRATION

Approximately ½ inch of the ointment is squeezed from the tube onto the lower lid of the affected eye two to four times daily.

The patient should be instructed to avoid contamination of the tip of the tube when applying the ointment.

HOW SUPPLIED

Terramycin with Polymyxin B Sulfate Ophthalmic Ointment is supplied in ⅛ oz., (3.5 g) tubes.

UROBIOTIC®-250 ℞
[*u″rō-bī-ot′ik*]

Each capsule contains
Oxytetracycline hydrochloride equivalent to 250 mg. oxytetracycline
Sulfamethizole ....250 mg.
Phenazopyridine hydrochloride ....50 mg.

CAPSULES

ACTIONS
Urobiotic-250 is a product designed for use specifically in urinary tract infections. Terramycin (oxytetracycline HCl) is a widely used antibiotic with clinically proved activity against gram-positive and gram-negative bacteria, rickettsiae, spirochetes, large viruses, and certain protozoa. Terramycin is well tolerated and well absorbed after oral administration. It diffuses readily through the placenta and is present in the fetal circulation. It diffuses into the pleural fluid, and under some circumstances, into the cerebrospinal fluid. Oxytetracycline HCl appears to be concentrated in the hepatic system and is excreted in the bile. It is excreted in the urine and in the feces, in high concentrations, in a biologically active form.
Sulfamethizole is a chemotherapeutic agent active against a number of important gram-positive and gram-negative bacteria. This sulfonamide is well absorbed, has a low degree of acetylation, and is extremely soluble. Because of these features and its rapid renal excretion, sulfamethizole has a low order of toxicity and provides prompt and high concentrations of the active drug in the urinary tract.
Phenazopyridine is an orally absorbed agent which produces prompt and effective local analgesia and relief of urinary symptoms by virtue of its rapid excretion in the urinary tract. These effects are confined to the genitourinary system and are not accompanied by generalized sedation or narcosis.

Indications
Based on a review of this drug by the National Academy of Sciences-National Research Council and/or other information, FDA has classified the indications as follows:
"Lacking substantial evidence of effectiveness as a fixed combination":
Urobiotic-250 is indicated in the therapy of a number of genitourinary infections caused by susceptible organisms. These infections include the following: pyelonephritis, pyelitis, ureteritis, cystitis, prostatitis, and urethritis.
Since both Terramycin and sulfamethizole provide effective levels in blood, tissue, and urine, Urobiotic-250 provides a multiple antimicrobial approach at the site of infection. Both antibacterial components are active against the most common urinary pathogens, including *Escherichia coli, Pseudomonas aeruginosa, Aerobacter aerogenes, Streptococcus faecalis, Streptococcus hemolyticus, and Micrococcus pyogenes.* Urobiotic-250 is particularly useful in the treatment of infections caused by bacteria more sensitive to the combination than to either component alone. The combination is also of value in those cases with mixed infections, and in those instances where the causative organism is unknown pending laboratory isolation.
Final classification of the less than effective indications require further investigation. Clinical studies to substantiate the efficacy of Urobiotic-250 are ongoing. Completion of these ongoing studies will provide data for final classification of these indications.

CONTRAINDICATIONS
This drug is contraindicated in individuals who have shown hypersensitivity to any of its components.
This drug, because of the sulfonamide component, should not be used in patients with a history of sulfonamide sensitivities, and in pregnant females at term.

WARNINGS
If renal impairment exists, even usual oral or parenteral doses may lead to excessive systemic accumulation of the drug and possible liver toxicity. Under such conditions, lower than usual doses are indicated and if therapy is prolonged, tetracycline serum level determinations may be advisable.
Oxytetracycline HCl, which is one of the ingredients of Urobiotic-250, may form a stable calcium complex in any bone-forming tissue with no serious harmful effects reported thus far in humans. However, use of oxytetracycline during tooth development (last trimester of pregnancy, neonatal period and early childhood) may cause discoloration of the teeth (yellow-grey-brownish). This effect occurs mostly during long term use of the drug but it also has been observed in usual short treatment courses.
Because of its sulfonamide content, this drug should be used only after critical appraisal in patients with liver damage, renal damage, urinary obstruction, or blood dyscrasias. Deaths have been reported from hypersensitivity reactions, agranulocytosis, aplastic anemia, and other blood dyscrasias associated with sulfonamide administration. When used intermittently, or for a prolonged period, blood counts and liver and kidney function tests should be performed.
Certain hypersensitive individuals may develop a photodynamic reaction precipitated by exposure to direct sunlight during the use of this drug. This reaction is usually of the photoallergic type which may also be produced by other tetracycline derivatives. Individuals with a history of photosensitivity reactions should be instructed to avoid exposure to direct sunlight while under treatment with this or other tetracycline drugs, and treatment should be discontinued at first evidence of skin discomfort.
NOTE: Reactions of a photoallergic nature are exceedingly rare with Terramycin (oxytetracycline HCl). Phototoxic reactions are not believed to occur with Terramycin.

PRECAUTIONS
As with all antibiotic preparations, use of this drug may result in overgrowth of nonsusceptible organisms, including fungi. If superinfection occurs, the antibiotic should be discontinued and appropriate specific therapy should be instituted. This drug should be used with caution in persons having histories of significant allergies and/or asthma.

ADVERSE REACTIONS
Glossitis, stomatitis, proctitis, nausea, diarrhea, vaginitis, and dermatitis, as well as reactions of an allergic nature, may occur during oxytetracycline HCl therapy, but are rare. If adverse reactions, individual idiosyncrasy, or allergy occur, discontinue medication. Rare instances of esophagitis and esophageal ulcerations have been reported in patients receiving capsule forms of drugs in the tetracycline class. Most of these patients took medications immediately before going to bed. (See Dosage and Administration.)
With oxytetracycline therapy bulging fontanels in infants and benign intracranial hypertension in adults have been reported in individuals receiving full therapeutic dosages. These conditions disappeared rapidly when the drug was discontinued.
As in all sulfonamide therapy, the following reactions may occur: nausea, vomiting, diarrhea, hepatitis, pancreatitis, blood dyscrasias, neuropathy, drug fever, skin rash, infection of the conjunctiva and sclera, petechiae, purpura, hematuria and crystalluria. The dosage should be decreased or the drug withdrawn, depending upon the severity of the reaction.

DOSAGE AND ADMINISTRATION
Urobiotic-250 is recommended in adults only. A dose of 1 capsule four times daily is suggested. In refractory cases 2 capsules four times a day may be used.
Therapy should be continued for a minimum of seven days or until bacteriologic cure in acute urinary tract infections.
Administration of adequate amounts of fluid along with capsule forms of drugs in the tetracycline class is recommended to wash down the drugs and reduce the risk of esophageal irritation and ulceration. (See Adverse Reactions.)
To aid absorption of the drug, it should be given at least one hour before or two hours after eating. Aluminum hydroxide gel given with antibiotics has been shown to decrease their absorption and is contraindicated.

SUPPLY
Urobiotic-250 capsules: bottles of 50, and unit dose packages of 100 (10 x 10's).

LITERATURE AVAILABLE
Yes.

23-1636-00-6

Shown in Product Identification Section, page 426

VIBRAMYCIN® Hyclate ℞
[*vī″bra-mī′sin*]
(doxycycline hyclate for injection)
INTRAVENOUS
For Intravenous Use Only

DESCRIPTION
Vibramycin (doxycycline hyclate for injection) Intravenous is a broad–spectrum antibiotic synthetically derived from oxytetracycline, and is available as Vibramycin Hyclate (doxycycline hydrochloride hemiethanolate hemihydrate). The chemical designation of this light-yellow crystalline powder is alpha-6-deoxy-5-oxytetracycline. Doxycycline has a high degree of lipoid solubility and a low affinity for calcium binding. It is highly stable in normal human serum.

ACTIONS
Doxycycline is primarily bacteriostatic and thought to exert its antimicrobial effect by the inhibition of protein synthesis. Doxycycline is active against a wide range of gram-positive and gram-negative organisms.
The drugs in the tetracycline class have closely similar antimicrobial spectra, and cross resistance among them is common. Microorganisms may be considered susceptible to doxycycline (likely to respond to doxycycline therapy) if the minimum inhibitory concentration (M.I.C.) is not more than 4.0 mcg/ml. Microorganisms may be considered intermediate (harboring partial resistance) if the M.I.C. is 4.0 to 12.5 mcg/ml and resistant (not likely to respond to therapy) if the M.I.C. is greater than 12.5 mcg/ml.
Susceptibility plate testing: If the Kirby-Bauer method of disc susceptibility testing is used, a 30 mcg doxycycline disc should give a zone of at least 16 mm when tested against a doxycycline-susceptible bacterial strain. A tetracycline disc may be used to determine microbial susceptibility. If the Kirby-Bauer method of disc susceptibility testing is used, a 30 mcg tetracycline disc should give a zone of at least 19 mm when tested against a tetracycline-susceptible bacterial strain.
Tetracyclines are readily absorbed and are bound to plasma proteins in varying degree. They are concentrated by the liver in the bile, and excreted in the urine and feces at high concentrations and in a biologically active form.
Following a single 100 mg dose administered in a concentration of 0.4 mg/ml in a one-hour infusion, normal adult volunteers average a peak of 2.5 mcg/ml, while 200 mg of a concentration of 0.4 mg/ml administered over two hours averaged a peak of 3.6 mcg/ml.
Excretion of doxycycline by the kidney is about 40 percent/72 hours in individuals with normal function (creatinine clearance about 75 ml/min.). This percentage excretion may fall as low as 1-5 percent/72 hours in individuals with severe renal insufficiency (creatinine clearance below 10 ml/min.). Studies have shown no significant difference in serum half-life of doxycycline (range 18-22 hours) in individuals with normal and severely impaired renal function.
Hemodialysis does not alter this serum half-life of doxycycline.

INDICATIONS
Doxycycline is indicated in infections caused by the following microorganisms:
Rickettsiae (Rocky Mountain spotted fever, typhus fever, and the typhus group, Q fever, rickettsialpox and tick fevers).
Mycoplasma pneumoniae (PPLO, Eaton Agent).
Agents of psittacosis and ornithosis.
Agents of lymphogranuloma venereum and granuloma inguinale.
The spirochetal agent of relapsing fever *(Borrelia recurrentis).*
The following gram-negative microorganisms:
Haemophilus ducreyi (chancroid),
Pasteurella pestis and *Pasteurella tularensis,*
Bartonella bacilliformis,
Bacteroides species,
Vibrio comma and *Vibrio fetus,*
Brucella species (in conjunction with streptomycin).
Because many strains of the following groups of microorganisms have been shown to be resistant to tetracyclines, culture and susceptibility testing are recommended.
Doxycycline is indicated for treatment of infections caused by the following gram-negative microorganisms when bacteriologic testing indicates appropriate susceptibility to the drug:
Escherichia coli,
Enterobacter aerogenes (formerly *Aerobacter aerogenes),*
Shigella species,
Mima species and *Herellea* species,
Haemophilus influenzae (respiratory infections),
Klebsiella species (respiratory and urinary infections).
Doxycycline is indicated for treatment of infections caused by the following gram-positive microorganisms when bacteriologic testing indicates appropriate susceptibility to the drug:
Streptococcus species:
Up to 44 percent of strains of *Streptococcus pyogenes* and 74 percent of *Streptococcus faecalis* have been found to be resistant to tetracycline drugs. Therefore, tetracyclines should not be used for streptococcal disease unless the organism has been demonstrated to be sensitive.
For upper respiratory infections due to group A beta-hemolytic streptococci, penicillin is the usual drug of choice, including prophylaxis of rheumatic fever.
Diplococcus pneumoniae,
Staphylococcus aureus, respiratory, skin and soft tissue infections. Tetracyclines are not the drugs of choice in the treatment of any type of staphylococcal infections.
When penicillin is contraindicated, doxycycline is an alternative drug in the treatment of infections due to:
Neisseria gonorrhoeae and *N. meningitidis,*
Treponema pallidum and *Treponema per- tenue* (syphilis and yaws),
Listeria monocytogenes,
Clostridium species,
Bacillus anthracis,

Continued on next page

Roerig—Cont.

Fusobacterium fusiforme (Vincent's infection),
Actinomyces species.

In acute intestinal amebiasis, doxycycline may be a useful adjunct to amebicides.

Doxycycline is indicated in the treatment of trachoma, although the infectious agent is not always eliminated, as judged by immunofluorescence.

CONTRAINDICATIONS

This drug is contraindicated in persons who have shown hypersensitivity to any of the tetracyclines.

WARNINGS

THE USE OF DRUGS OF THE TETRACYCLINE CLASS DURING TOOTH DEVELOPMENT (LAST HALF OF PREGNANCY, INFANCY AND CHILDHOOD TO THE AGE OF 8 YEARS) MAY CAUSE PERMANENT DISCOLORATION OF THE TEETH (YELLOW-GRAY-BROWN). This adverse reaction is more common during long-term use of the drugs but has been observed following repeated short-term courses. Enamel hypoplasia has also been reported. *TETRACYCLINE DRUGS, THEREFORE, SHOULD NOT BE USED IN THIS AGE GROUP UNLESS OTHER DRUGS ARE NOT LIKELY TO BE EFFECTIVE OR ARE CONTRAINDICATED.*

Photosensitivity manifested by an exaggerated sunburn reaction has been observed in some individuals taking tetracyclines. Patients apt to be exposed to direct sunlight or ultraviolet light should be advised that this reaction can occur with tetracycline drugs, and treatment should be discontinued at the first evidence of skin erythema.

The antianabolic action of the tetracyclines may cause an increase in BUN. Studies to date indicate that this does not occur with the use of doxycycline in patients with impaired renal function.

Usage in Pregnancy

(See above "Warnings" about use during tooth development.) Vibramycin (doxycycline hyclate for injection) Intravenous has not been studied in pregnant patients. It should not be used in pregnant women unless, in the judgment of the physician, it is essential for the welfare of the patient.

Results of animal studies indicate that tetracyclines cross the placenta, are found in fetal tissues and can have toxic effects on the developing fetus (often related to retardation of skeletal development). Evidence of embryotoxicity has also been noted in animals treated early in pregnancy.

Usage in Children

The use of Vibramycin Intravenous in children under 8 years is not recommended because safe conditions for its use have not been established.

(See above "Warnings" about use during tooth development.) As with other tetracyclines, doxycycline forms a stable calcium complex in any bone-forming tissue. A decrease in the fibula growth rate has been observed in prematures given oral tetracycline in doses of 25 mg/kg every 6 hours. This reaction was shown to be reversible when the drug was discontinued.

Tetracyclines are present in the milk of lactating women who are taking a drug in this class.

PRECAUTIONS

As with other antibiotic preparations, use of this drug may result in overgrowth of nonsusceptible organisms, including fungi. If superinfection occurs, the antibiotic should be discontinued and appropriate therapy instituted.

In venereal diseases when coexistent syphilis is suspected, a dark field examination should be done before treatment is started and the blood serology repeated monthly for at least 4 months.

Because tetracyclines have been shown to depress plasma prothrombin activity, patients who are on anticoagulant therapy may require downward adjustment of their anticoagulant dosage.

In long-term therapy, periodic laboratory evaluation of organ systems, including hematopoietic, renal, and hepatic studies should be performed.

All infections due to group A beta-hemolytic streptococci should be treated for at least 10 days.

Since bacteriostatic drugs may interfere with the bactericidal action of penicillin, it is advisable to avoid giving tetracycline in conjunction with penicillin.

ADVERSE REACTIONS

Gastrointestinal: anorexia, nausea, vomiting, diarrhea, glossitis, dysphagia, enterocolitis, and inflammatory lesions (with monilial overgrowth) in the anogenital region. These reactions have been caused by both the oral and parenteral administration of tetracyclines.

Skin: maculopapular and erythematous rashes. Exfoliative dermatitis has been reported but is uncommon. Photosensitivity is discussed above. (See "Warnings.")

Renal toxicity: Rise in BUN has been reported and is apparently dose related. (See "Warnings.")

Hypersensitivity reactions: urticaria, angioneurotic edema, anaphylaxis, anaphylactoid purpura, pericarditis and exacerbation of systemic lupus erythematosus.

Bulging fontanels in infants and benign intracranial hypertension in adults have been reported in individuals receiving full therapeutic dosages. These conditions disappeared rapidly when the drug was discontinued.

Blood: Hemolytic anemia, thrombocytopenia, neutropenia and eosinophilia have been reported.

When given over prolonged periods, tetracyclines have been reported to produce brown-black microscopic discoloration of thyroid glands. No abnormalities of thyroid function studies are known to occur.

DOSAGE AND ADMINISTRATION

Note: Rapid administration is to be avoided. Parenteral therapy is indicated only when oral therapy is not indicated. Oral therapy should be instituted as soon as possible. If intravenous therapy is given over prolonged periods of time, thrombophlebitis may result.

THE USUAL DOSAGE AND FREQUENCY OF ADMINISTRATION OF VIBRAMYCIN I.V. (100-200 MG/DAY) DIFFERS FROM THAT OF THE OTHER TETRACYCLINES (1-2 G/DAY). EXCEEDING THE RECOMMENDED DOSAGE MAY RESULT IN AN INCREASED INCIDENCE OF SIDE EFFECTS.

Studies to date have indicated that Vibramycin at the usual recommended doses does not lead to excessive accumulation of the antibiotic in patients with renal impairment.

Adults: The usual dosage of Vibramycin (doxycycline hyclate for injection) I.V. is 200 mg on the first day of treatment administered in one or two infusions. Subsequent daily dosage is 100 to 200 mg depending upon the severity of infection, with 200 mg administered in one or two infusions.

In the treatment of primary and secondary syphilis, the recommended dosage is 300 mg daily for at least 10 days.

For children above eight years of age: The recommended dosage schedule for children weighing 100 pounds or less is 2 mg/lb. of body weight on the first day of treatment, administered in one or two infusions. Subsequent daily dosage is 1 to 2 mg/lb. of body weight given as one or two infusions, depending on the severity of the infection. For children over 100 pounds the usual adult dose should be used. (See "Warning" Section for Usage in Children.)

General: The duration of infusion may vary with the dose (100 to 200 mg per day), but is usually one to four hours. A recommended minimum infusion time for 100 mg of a 0.5 mg/ml solution is one hour. Therapy should be continued for at least 24-48 hours after symptoms and fever have subsided. The therapeutic antibacterial serum activity will usually persist for 24 hours following recommended dosage.

Intravenous solutions should not be injected intramuscularly or subcutaneously. Caution should be taken to avoid the inadvertent introduction of the intravenous solution into the adjacent soft tissue.

PREPARATION OF SOLUTION

To prepare a solution containing 10 mg/ml, the contents of the vial should be reconstituted with 10 ml (for the 100 mg/vial container) or 20 ml (for the 200 mg/vial container) of Sterile Water for Injection or any of the ten intravenous infusion solutions listed below. Each 100 mg of Vibramycin (i.e., withdraw entire solution from the 100 mg vial) is further diluted with 100 ml to 1000 ml of the intravenous solutions listed below. Each 200 mg of Vibramycin (i.e., withdraw entire solution from the 200 mg vial) is further diluted with 200 ml to 2000 ml of the following intravenous solutions:

1. Sodium Chloride Injection, USP
2. 5% Dextrose Injection, USP
3. Ringer's Injection, USP
4. Invert Sugar, 10% in Water
5. Lactated Ringer's Injection, USP
6. Dextrose 5% in Lactated Ringer's
7. Normosol-M® in D5-W (Abbott)
8. Normosol-R® in D5-W (Abbott)
9. Plasma-Lyte® 56 in 5% Dextrose (Travenol)
10. Plasma-Lyte® 148 in 5% Dextrose (Travenol)

This will result in desired concentrations of 0.1 to 1.0 mg/ml. Concentrations lower than 0.1 mg/ml or higher than 1.0 mg/ml are not recommended.

Stability:

Vibramycin IV is stable for 48 hours in solution when diluted with Sodium Chloride Injection, USP, or 5% Dextrose Injection, USP, to concentrations between 1.0 mg/ml and 0.1 mg/ml and stored at 25°C. Vibramycin IV in these solutions is stable under fluorescent light for 48 hours, but must be protected from direct sunlight during storage and infusion. Reconstituted solutions (1.0 to 0.1 mg/ml) may be stored up to 72 hours prior to start of infusion if refrigerated and protected from sunlight and artificial light. Infusion must then be completed within 12 hours. Solutions must be used within these time periods or discarded.

Vibramycin IV, when diluted with Ringer's Injection, USP, or Invert Sugar, 10% in Water, or Normosol-M® in D5-W (Abbott), or Normosol-R®in D5-W (Abbott), or Plasma-Lyte® 56 in 5% Dextrose (Travenol), or Plasma-Lyte® 148 in 5% Dextrose (Travenol) to a concentration between 1.0 mg/ml and 0.1 mg/ml, must be completely infused within 12 hours after reconstitution to ensure adequate stability. During infusion, the solution must be protected from direct sunlight. Reconstituted solutions (1.0 to 0.1 mg/ml) may be stored up to 72 hours prior to start of infusion if refrigerated and protected from sunlight and artifical light. Infusion must then be completed within 12 hours. Solutions must be used within these time periods or discarded.

When diluted with Lactated Ringer's Injection, USP, or Dextrose 5% in Lactated Ringer's, infusion of the solution (ca. 1.0 mg/ml) or lower concentrations (not less than 0.1 mg/ml) must be completed within six hours after reconstitution to ensure adequate stability. During infusion, the solution must be protected from direct sunlight. Solutions must be used within this time period or discarded.

Solutions of Vibramycin (doxycycline hyclate for injection) at a concentration of 10 mg/ml in Sterile Water for Injection, when frozen immediately after reconstitution are stable for 8 weeks when stored at −20°C. If the product is warmed, care should be taken to avoid heating it after the thawing is complete. Once thawed the solution should not be refrozen.

HOW SUPPLIED

Vibramycin (doxycycline hyclate for injection) Intravenous is available as a sterile powder in a vial containing doxycycline hyclate equivalent to 100 mg of doxycycline with 480 mg of ascorbic acid, packages of 5; and in individually packaged vials containing doxycycline hyclate equivalent to 200 mg of doxycycline with 960 mg of ascorbic acid.

(23-1940-00-8)

LITERATURE AVAILABLE

Yes.

VISTARIL® ℞

(hydroxyzine hydrochloride)
Intramuscular Solution
For Intramuscular Use Only

CHEMISTRY

Hydroxyzine hydrochloride is designated chemically as 1-(p-chlorobenzhydryl) 4-[2-(2-hydroxyethoxy) ethyl] piperazine dihydrochloride.

ACTIONS

VISTARIL (hydroxyzine hydrochloride) is unrelated chemically to phenothiazine, reserpine, and meprobamate. Hydroxyzine has demonstrated its clinical effectiveness in the chemotherapeutic aspect of the total management of neuroses and emotional disturbances manifested by anxiety, tension, agitation, apprehension or confusion.

Hydroxyzine has been shown clinically to be a rapid-acting true ataraxic with a wide margin of safety. It induces a calming effect in anxious, tense, psychoneurotic adults and also in anxious, hyperkinetic children without impairing mental alertness. It is not a cortical depressant, but its action may be due to a suppression of activity in certain key regions of the subcortical area of the central nervous system.

Primary skeletal muscle relaxation has been demonstrated experimentally.

Hydroxyzine has been shown experimentally to have antispasmodic properties, apparently mediated through interference with the mechanism that reponds to spasmogenic agents such as serotonin, acetylcholine, and histamine.

Antihistaminic effects have been demonstrated experimentally and confirmed clinically.

An antiemetic effect, both by the apomorphine test and the veriloid test, has been demonstrated. Pharmacological and clinical studies indicate that hydroxyzine in therapeutic dosage does not increase gastric secretion or acidity and in most cases provides mild antisecretory benefits.

INDICATIONS

The total management of anxiety, tension, and psychomotor agitation in conditions of emotional stress requires in most instances a combined approach of psychotherapy and chemotherapy. Hydroxyzine has been found to be particularly useful for this latter phrase of therapy in its ability to render the disturbed patient more amenable to psychotherapy in long term treatment of the psychoneurotic and psychotic, although it should not be used as the sole treatment of psychosis or of clearly demonstrated cases of depression.

Hydroxyzine is also useful in alleviating the manifestations of anxiety and tension as in the preparation for dental procedures and in acute emotional problems. It has also been recommended for the management of anxiety associated with organic disturbances and as adjunctive therapy in alcoholism and allergic conditions with strong emotional overlay, such as in asthma, chronic urticaria, and pruritus.

VISTARIL (hydroxyzine hydrochloride) Intramuscular Solution is useful in treating the following types of patients when intramuscular administration is indicated:
1. The acutely disturbed or hysterical patient.
2. The acute or chronic alcoholic with anxiety withdrawal symptoms or delirium tremens.
3. As pre- and postoperative and pre- and postpartum adjunctive medication to permit reduction in narcotic dosage, allay anxiety and control emesis.

VISTARIL (hydroxyzine hydrochloride) has also demonstrated effectiveness in controlling nausea and vomiting, excluding nausea and vomiting of pregnancy. (See Contraindications.)
In prepartum states, the reduction in narcotic requirement effected by hydroxyzine is of particular benefit to both mother and neonate.
Hydroxyzine benefits the cardiac patient by its ability to allay the associated anxiety and apprehension attendant to certain types of heart disease. Hydroxyzine is not known to interfere with the action of digitalis in any way and may be used concurrently with this agent.
The effectiveness of hydroxyzine in long term use, that is, more than 4 months, has not been assessed by systematic clinical studies. The physician should reassess periodically the usefulness of the drug for the individual patient.

CONTRAINDICATIONS
Hydroxyzine hydrochloride intramuscular solution is intended only for intramuscular administration and should not, under any circumstances, be injected subcutaneously, intra-arterially, or intravenously.
This drug is contraindicated for patients who have shown a previous hypersensitivity to it.
Hydroxyzine, when administered to the pregnant mouse, rat, and rabbit, induced fetal abnormalities in the rat at doses substantially above the human therapeutic range. Clinical data in human beings are inadequate to establish safety in early pregnancy. Until such data are available, hydroxyzine is contraindicated in early pregnancy.

PRECAUTIONS
THE POTENTIATING ACTION OF HYDROXYZINE MUST BE CONSIDERED WHEN THE DRUG IS USED IN CONJUNCTION WITH CENTRAL NERVOUS SYSTEM DEPRESSANTS SUCH AS NARCOTICS, BARBITURATES, AND ALCOHOL. Therefore when central nervous system depressants are administered concomitantly with hydroxyzine their dosage should be reduced up to 50 per cent. The efficacy of hydroxyzine as adjunctive pre- and postoperative sedative medication has also been well established, especially as regards its ability to allay anxiety, control emesis, and reduce the amount of narcotic required.
HYDROXYZINE MAY POTENTIATE NARCOTICS AND BARBITURATES, so their use in preanesthetic adjunctive therapy should be modified on an individual basis. Atropine and other belladonna alkaloids are not affected by the drug. When hydroxyzine is used preoperatively or prepartum, narcotic requirements may be reduced as much as 50 per cent. Thus, when 50 mg of VISTARIL (hydroxyzine hydrochloride) Intramuscular Solution is employed, meperidine dosage may be reduced from 100 mg to 50 mg. The administration of meperidine may result in severe hypotension in the postoperative patient or any individual whose ability to maintain blood pressure has been compromised by a depleted blood volume. Meperidine should be used with great caution and in reduced dosage in patients who are receiving other pre- and/or postoperative medications and in whom there is a risk of respiratory depression, hypotension, and profound sedation or coma occurring. Before using any medications concomitant with hydroxyzine, the manufacturer's prescribing information should be read carefully.
Since drowsiness may occur with the use of this drug, patients should be warned of this possibility and cautioned against driving a car or operating dangerous machinery while taking this drug.
As with all intramuscular preparations, VISTARIL Intramuscular Solution should be injected well within the body of a relatively large muscle. Inadvertent subcutaneous injection may result in significant tissue damage.
ADULTS: The preferred site is the upper outer quadrant of the buttock, (i.e., gluteus maximus), or the mid-lateral thigh.
CHILDREN: It is recommended that intramuscular injections be given preferably in the mid-lateral muscles of the thigh. In infants and small children the periphery of the upper outer quadrant of the gluteal region should be used only when necessary, such as in burn patients, in order to minimize the possibility of damage to the sciatic nerve.
The deltoid area should be used only if well developed such as in certain adults and older children, and then only with caution to avoid radial nerve injury. Intramuscular injections should not be made into the lower and mid-third of the upper arm. As with all intramuscular injections, aspiration is necessary to help avoid inadvertent injection into a blood vessel.

ADVERSE REACTIONS
Therapeutic doses of hydroxyzine seldom produce impairment of mental alertness. However, drowsiness may occur; if so, it is usually transitory and may disappear in a few days of continued therapy or upon reduction of the dose. Dryness of the mouth may be encountered at higher doses. Extensive clinical use has substantiated the absence of toxic effects on the liver or bone marrow when administered in the recommended doses for over four years of uninterrupted therapy. The absence of adverse effects has been further demonstrated in experimental studies in which excessively high doses were administered.
Involuntary motor activity, including rare instances of tremor and convulsions, has been reported, usually with doses considerably higher than those recommended. Continuous therapy with over one gram per day has been employed in some patients without these effects having been encountered.

DOSAGE AND ADMINISTRATION
The recommended dosages for VISTARIL (hydroxyzine hydrochloride) Intramuscular Solution are:

For adult psychiatric and emotional emergencies, including acute alcoholism.	I.M.: 50–100 mg stat., and q. 4–6h., p.r.n.
Nausea and vomiting excluding nausea and vomiting of pregnancy.	Adults: 25–100 mg I.M. Children: 0.5 mg/lb. body weight I.M.
Pre- and postoperative adjunctive medication.	Adults: 25–100 mg I.M. Children: 0.5 mg/lb. body weight I.M.
Pre- and postpartum adjunctive therapy.	25–100 mg I.M.

As with all potent medications, the dosage should be adjusted according to the patient's response to therapy.
FOR ADDITIONAL INFORMATION ON THE ADMINISTRATION AND SITE OF SELECTION SEE PRECAUTIONS SECTION. NOTE: VISTARIL (hydroxyzine hydrochloride) Intramuscular Solution may be administered without further dilution.
Patients may be started on intramuscular therapy when indicated. They should be maintained on oral therapy whenever this route is practicable.

SUPPLY
Vistaril IM is an aqueous solution containing either 25 mg or 50 mg hydroxyzine HCl per ml, 0.9% benzyl alcohol and sodium hydroxide to adjust to optimum pH.
Multi-Dose Vials
25 mg per ml, 10 ml vials
50 mg per ml, 10 ml vials
Unit Dose Vials: Packages of 10 vials
50 mg per vial, 1 ml fill
75 mg per vial, 1.5 ml fill
100 mg per vial, 2 ml fill

ROERIG EDUCATIONAL MATERIALS

Printed Material
1. *Comprehensive Product Information* (Glucotrol)—a 50-page Roerig publication describing the chemistry, pharmacokinetics, pharmacology, clinical experience, and other important information about Glucotrol. Free to physicians.
2. *Glipizide: A Worldwide Review*—a 300-page monograph published by Excerpta Medica. Covers Glucotrol's pathology and physiology, clinical pharmacology, and clinical experience. Free to physicians.
3. *The Efficacy and Safety of Cefoperazone—A Two-Year Review*—Proceedings of a symposium reviewing two years of clinical and safety data associated with the use of cefoperazone. Free to physicians.
4. *The Cost of Antibiotic Therapy*—Results of a multicenter trial examining the cost components of antibiotic therapy and the impact different regimens have on length of therapy and length of hospital stay. Free to physicians and pharmacists.
5. *Discussion on Depression: Patient Perspectives*—a 14-page patient information booklet for people suffering from depression. Free to physicians and their patients.

Films
1. "New Perspectives in NIDDM"—30-minute film. Covers NIDDM, effect of sulfonylureas, especially 2nd-generation and glipizide. Narrated by Drs. Lebovitz and Reaven. A 7-minute edited version is also available.
2. "Risk Factors in Non-Insulin-Dependent Diabetes Mellitus"—21-minute color film. Reviews lipid metabolism, the lipid abnormalities found in the Type II diabetic patient, and the associated atherosclerotic complications. Clinical research on lipid metabolism that demonstrates the effect of GLUCOTROL (glipizide) is presented. Narrated by Drs. Castelli, Krall, and Reaven.
3. "Organ Transplantation: A Miracle Kept Waiting"—a 30-minute film describing transplantation of the heart and lung, liver transplantation, and surgical construction of a bladder for a patient faced with a lifetime of incontinence. Narrated by Drs. Cooley, Starzl, and Olsson.
4. "Update: The Management of Surgical Infection in the 1980s."—A discussion of factors contributing to infection following surgery and approaches to its management. Narrated by Harlan Stone, MD. 20 Minutes.

Interactive Videodiscs
1. "Nephrostolithotomy—The Percutaneous Route" Free to physicians.
2. "Urodynamics in Clinical Practice" Free to physicians.

Audiotapes
"Dialogues in Urology." Free to physicians.

Samples
Antivert (meclizine HCl) Tablets—25 mg, 50 mg
Atarax (hydroxyzine HCl) Tablets—10 mg, 25 mg
Atarax Syrup
Geocillin (carbenicillin indanyl sodium) Tablets (equivalent to 382 mg carbenicillin)
Glucotrol (glipizide) Tablets—5 mg
Navane (thiothixene) Capsules—2 mg, 5 mg, 10 mg, 20 mg
Navane Oral Concentrate
Sinequan (doxepin HCl) Capsules—25 mg, 50 mg, 75 mg
Spectrobid (bacampicillin HCl) Tablets—400 mg (equivalent to 280 mg ampicillin)

William H. Rorer, Inc.
500 VIRGINIA DRIVE
FORT WASHINGTON, PA 19034

ALGICON™

(See PDR For Nonprescription Drugs)
Shown in Product Identification Section, page 426

ASCRIPTIN® Tablets

(See PDR For Nonprescription Drugs)
Shown in Product Identification Section, page 426

ASCRIPTIN® A/D Tablets

(See PDR For Nonprescription Drugs)
Shown in Product Identification Section, page 426

ASCRIPTIN® WITH CODEINE Ⓒ℞
[*a-scrip'tin"*]
for the relief of severe pain...
with the protection of Maalox®

DESCRIPTION—Tablets for Oral Use:
Ascriptin® with Codeine No. 2. Each white tablet contains aspirin 325 mg, codeine phosphate 15 mg and Maalox® (magnesium-aluminum hydroxide) 150 mg. Inactive Ingredients: lactose, magnesium stearate, microcrystalline cellulose, starch, talc.
Ascriptin® with Codeine No. 3. Each white tablet contains aspirin 325 mg, codeine phosphate 30 mg and Maalox® (magnesium-aluminum hydroxide) 150 mg. Inactive Ingredients: lactose, magnesium stearate, microcrystalline cellulose, starch, talc.
Ascriptin® with Codeine is an analgesic, antipyretic, and anti-inflammatory designed to give effective relief from severe pain with minimal aspirin-induced gastric distress.
Aspirin, a salicylate, occurs as a white, odorless, crystalline powder which possesses a slightly bitter taste. Aspirin is an analgesic, anti-inflammatory and antipyretic.
Codeine is an alkaloid obtained from opium (or prepared from morphine by methylation) and occurs as colorless or white crystals. Codeine effloresces slowly in dry air and is affected by light. Codeine is an analgesic and an antitussive.
Chemical Names and Structural Formulas

COOH
OCOCH₃

Aspirin
$C_9H_8O_4$ 180.16
Benzoic acid 2-(acetyloxy)-
salicylic acid acetate [*50-78-2*]

Continued on next page

This product information was prepared in August 1986. Information concerning these products may be obtained by addressing William H. Rorer, Inc., 500 Virginia Drive, Fort Washington, PA 19034.

Rorer—Cont.

Codeine Phosphate

$C_{18}H_{21}NO_3 \cdot H_3PO_4 \cdot \frac{1}{2}H_2O$ 406.37

Morphinan-6-ol, 7.8-didehydro-4,5-epoxy-3-methoxy-17-methyl-,-(5α,6α)-,phosphate (1:1) (salt), hemihydrate.

7,8 Didehydro-4,5α-epoxy-3-methoxy-17-methylmorphinan-6α-ol phosphate (1:1) (salt) hemihydrate[*4144-62-6*]

Anhydrous 397.36 [*52-28-8*]

Codeine Phosphate

In addition, Maalox® is added to the formula to help reduce gastric distress caused by aspirin. Studies show that the addition of Maalox® has no effect on the bioavailability of the two active drugs.

CLINICAL PHARMACOLOGY

Aspirin alleviates pain both centrally and peripherally. Orally ingested salicylates are absorbed rapidly, partly from the stomach but mostly from the small intestine. Appreciable concentrations are found in plasma in less than 30 minutes; after a single dose, a peak value is reached in about 2 hours and then gradually declines. Rate of absorption is determined by many factors, particularly the disintegration and dissolution rates if tablets are given, the pH at the mucosal surfaces, and gastric emptying time.

In man, the absorption half-time for unbuffered aspirin is about 30 minutes, for buffered aspirin about 20 minutes, and for an aspirin solution only slightly less. What differences do exist probably have no therapeutic significance, since the rate-limiting factor in the onset of effects is accumulation of these drugs at their sites of action. The presence of food delays absorption of salicylates.

The biotransformation of aspirin takes place mainly in the liver and normally follows first-order kinetics. Salicylates are excreted mainly by the kidney.

Codeine is a narcotic analgesic. Once absorbed, it is metabolized by the liver and excreted chiefly in the urine, largely in inactive forms. A small fraction (approximately 10%) of administered codeine is demethylated to form morphine, and both free and conjugated morphine can be found in the urine after therapeutic doses of codeine. Codeine has an exceptionally low affinity for the opioid receptor, and the analgesic effect of codeine may be due to its conversion to morphine. The half-life of codeine in plasma is 2.5 to 3 hours.

Maalox® provides neutralization of gastric acid, thus increasing the likelihood of G.I. tolerance with the aspirin component.

INDICATIONS

Ascriptin® with Codeine No. 2 and Ascriptin® with Codeine No. 3 are indicated for the relief of pain of all degrees of severity up to that which requires morphine.

CONTRAINDICATIONS

Hypersensitivity or allergy to aspirin or codeine.

WARNINGS

Children and teenagers should not use this medicine for chicken pox or flu symptoms before a doctor is consulted about Reye's Syndrome, a rare but serious illness.

Usage in ambulatory patients. Ascriptin® with Codeine may impair the mental and/or physical abilities required for the performance of potentially hazardous tasks such as driving a car or operating machinery. The patient using this drug should be cautioned accordingly.

Interaction with other central nervous system depressants. Patients receiving other narcotic analgesics, general anesthetics, phenothiazines, tranquilizers, sedative-hynotics or other CNS depressants (including alcohol) concomitantly with **Ascriptin® with Codeine** may exhibit an additive CNS depression. When such combined therapy is contemplated, the dose of one or both agents should be reduced.

Do not use if patient is taking a tetracycline antibiotic.

PRECAUTIONS

Usage in pregnancy. PREGNANCY CATEGORY C—Animal reproduction studies have not been conducted with **Ascriptin® with Codeine.** It is also not known whether **Ascriptin® with Codeine** can cause fetal harm when administered to pregnant women or can affect reproduction capacity. **Ascriptin® with Codeine** should be given to a pregnant woman only if clearly needed.

It is not known whether this drug is excreted in human milk. Because many drugs are excreted in human milk, caution should be exercised when **Ascriptin® with Codeine** is administered to nursing women.

Head injury and increased intracranial pressure: The respiratory depressant effects of narcotics and their capability to elevate cerebrospinal fluid pressure may be markedly exaggerated in the presence of head injury, other intracranial lesions or a pre-existing increase in intracranial pressure. Furthermore, narcotics produce adverse reactions which may obscure the clinical course of patients with head injuries.

Acute abdominal condition: The administration of **Ascriptin® with Codeine** or other narcotics may obscure the diagnosis or clinical course in patients with acute abdominal conditions.

History of allergy: Patients who have a history of allergies may also be hypersensitive or intolerant to aspirin. A history of reaction to other chemicals, asthma or the occurrence of nasal polyps are warning signs. Epinephrine is the drug of choice to treat a reaction should one occur.

Special risk patients: Codeine should be given with caution to certain patients such as the elderly or debilitated and those with severe impairment of hepatic or renal function, hypothyroidism, Addison's disease, and prostatic hypertrophy or urethral stricture. Long-term animal studies to determine carcinogenicity of the ingredients in **Ascriptin® with Codeine** have not been carried out.

Safety and effectiveness in children under 12 years of age have not been established.

ADVERSE REACTIONS

The most frequently observed adverse reactions to codeine include lightheadedness, dizziness, sleepiness, nausea and vomiting. These effects seem to be more prominent in ambulatory than in nonambulatory patients, and some of these adverse reactions may be alleviated if the patient lies down. Less frequent adverse reactions include euphoria, dysphoria, constipation and pruritus.

The most frequently observed reactions to aspirin include headache, vertigo, ringing in the ears, mental confusion, drowsiness, sweating, thirst, nausea, and vomiting. Occasionally, patients experience gastric irritation and bleeding with aspirin. Some patients are unable to take salicylates without developing nausea and vomiting. Hypersensitivity may be manifested by a skin rash or even an anaphylactic reaction. Most of the side effects of aspirin occur only after repeated administration of large doses.

DRUG ABUSE AND DEPENDENCE

Codeine can produce drug dependence of the morphine type, and therefore, has the potential for being abused. Psychic dependence, physical dependence and tolerance may develop upon repeated administration of this drug and it should be prescribed and administered with the same degree of caution appropriate to the use of other oral narcotic-containing medications. Like other narcotic-containing medications, the drug is subject to the Federal Controlled Substances Act.

MANAGEMENT OF OVERDOSAGE

Signs and Symptoms: Serious overdose with **Ascriptin® with Codeine** is characterized by respiratory depression (a decrease in respiratory rate and/or tidal volume, Cheyne-Stokes respiration, cyanosis), extreme somnolence progressing to stupor or coma, skeletal muscle flaccidity, cold and clammy skin, and sometimes bradycardia and hypotension. In severe overdosage, apnea, circulatory collapse, cardiac arrest and death may occur. The ingestion of very large amounts of this drug may, in addition, result in acute hepatic toxicity.

Treatment: Primary attention should be given to the reestablishment of adequate respiratory exchange through provision of a patent airway and the institution of assisted or controlled ventilation. The narcotic antagonist, naloxone, is a specific antidote against respiratory depression which may result from overdosage or unusual sensitivity to narcotics, including codeine. Therefore, an appropriate dose of naloxone (usual initial adult dose: 0.4 mg) should be administered, preferably by the intravenous route, and simultaneously with efforts at respiratory resuscitation. Since the duration of action of codeine may exceed that of the antagonist, the patient should be kept under continued surveillance and repeated doses of the antagonist should be administered as needed to maintain adequate respiration.

An antagonist should not be administered in the absence of clinically significant respiratory or cardiovascular depression.

Oxygen, intravenous fluids, vasopressors and other supportive measures should be employed as indicated.

Gastric emptying may be useful in removing unabsorbed drug.

Salicylate poisoning represents an acute medical emergency. The treatment is largely symptomatic. From 10 to 30 g of aspirin has caused death in adults, but much larger amounts (130 g of aspirin, in one case) have been ingested without fatal outcome.

Initial therapy must be directed to correction of hyperthermia, dehydration and maintenance of adequate renal function. Intravenous fluids should be administered promptly, the type and amount based on interpretation of laboratory data on acid-base balance.

Measures to rid the body rapidly of salicylate should be immediately undertaken. Sodium bicarbonate administration is effective and rapid, if an alkaline urine can be produced. Forced diuresis with alkalinizing solution appears to be better than alkali alone; acetazolamide can be added to this combination if a more rapid effect is necessary and only if systemic acidosis is avoided. Potassium should be administered with the bicarbonate to prevent further depletion of intracellular potassium.

In severe intoxication, extrarenal measures such as exchange transfusion, peritoneal dialysis, hemodialysis, and hemoperfusion are the most effective measures available for the removal of salicylate. Hemodialysis in adults and older children and exchange transfusion or peritoneal dialysis in infants should be considered seriously in all salicylate-intoxicated patients whose clinical condition is deteriorating despite otherwise appropriate therapy and in those who have associated serious disease.

DOSAGE AND ADMINISTRATION

Dosage should be adjusted according to the severity of the pain and the response of the patient. It may occasionally be necessary to exceed the usual dosage recommended below in cases of more severe pain or in those patients who have become tolerant to the analgesic effect of narcotics.

Ascriptin® with Codeine is given orally.

Usual Adult Dose: Ascriptin® with Codeine No. 2—two tablets every 3 to 4 hours when necessary. **Ascriptin® with Codeine No. 3**—one or two tablets every 3 to 4 hours as necessary.

DRUG INTERACTIONS

The CNS depressant effect of **Ascriptin® with Codeine** may be additive with that of other CNS depressants. (See WARNINGS.)

HOW SUPPLIED

Ascriptin® with Codeine No. 2: (Aspirin 325 mg, Maalox® 150 mg, codeine phosphate 15 mg) is available in bottles of 100 tablets. Tablets are marked on one side with the name Rorer and the Identification Number 142; the other side displays the number 2. (NDC 0067-0142-68)

Ascriptin® with Codeine No. 3: (Aspirin 325 mg, Maalox® 150 mg, codeine phosphate 30 mg) in bottles of 100 tablets. Tablets are marked on one side with the name Rorer and the Identification Number 143; the other side displays the number 3. (NDC 0067-0143-68)

DEA number required.

Prescription only.

AZMACORT™ ℞

[*ăz 'ma-kort*]

(triamcinolone acetonide)

inhaler

For Oral Inhalation Only

DESCRIPTION

Azmacort™ (triamcinolone acetonide) is an anti-inflammatory steroid having the chemical name 9α-fluoro-11β, 21-dihydroxy-16α, 17α-isopropylidenedioxy-1, 4-pregnadiene-3, 20-dione ($C_{24}H_{31}FO_6$).

Azmacort™ inhaler is a metered-dose aerosol unit containing a microcrystalline suspension of triamcinolone acetonide in the propellant dichlorodifluoromethane and dehydrated alcohol USP 1% w/w. Each canister contains 60 mg triamcinolone acetonide. Each actuation releases approximately 200 mcg triamcinolone acetonide, of which approximately 100 mcg are delivered from the unit (*in vitro* testing). There are at least 240 oral inhalations in one **Azmacort™** inhaler canister. The device should not be used after 240 inhalations, since the amount delivered thereafter per actuation may be less than consistent.

CLINICAL PHARMACOLOGY

The precise mechanism of the action of the inhaled drug is unknown. However, use of the inhaler makes it possible to provide effective local steroid activity with minimal systemic effect.

Triamcinolone acetonide is a very potent derivative of triamcinolone. Although triamcinolone itself is 1–2 times as potent as prednisone in animal models of inflammation, triamcinolone acetonide is much more potent.

Pharmacokinetic studies with radiolabeled triamcinolone acetonide have been carried out by the oral route and intravenous route in several species. The pharmacokinetic behavior of the triamcinolone acetonide was similar in all species within each route of administration. The major portion of the dose was eliminated in the feces irrespective of route of administration with only one species (rabbit) showing significant urinary excretion of radioactivity.
The results of studies in which triamcinolone acetonide was administered as an aerosol showed rapid disappearance of radioactivity from the lungs comparable to that observed following oral administration with peak blood levels occurring in one to two hours. Virtually no radioactivity was present in the lung and trachea 24 hours after dosing.
Three metabolites of triamcinolone acetonide have been identified. They are: 6β-hydroxy-triamcinolone acetonide, 21-carboxy-triamcinolone acetonide, and 21-carboxy-6β-hydroxytriamcinolone acetonide. There appeared to be some quantitative differences in the metabolites among species. No differences were detected in metabolic pattern related to route of administration.

INDICATIONS

Azmacort™ (triamcinolone acetonide) inhaler is indicated only for patients who require chronic treatment with corticosteroids for the control of the symptoms of bronchial asthma. Such patients would include those already receiving systemic corticosteroids and selected patients who are inadequately controlled on a non-steroid regimen and in whom steroid therapy has been withheld because of concern over potential adverse effects.
Azmacort™ inhaler is *NOT* indicated:

1. For relief of asthma which can be controlled by bronchodilators and other non-steroid medications.
2. In patients who require systemic corticosteroid treatment infrequently.
3. In the treatment of non-asthmatic bronchitis.

CONTRAINDICATIONS

Azmacort™ inhaler is contraindicated in the primary treatment of status asthmaticus or other acute episodes of asthma where intensive measures are required.
Hypersensitivity to any of the ingredients of this preparation contraindicates its use.

WARNINGS

Particular care is needed in patients who are transferred from systemically active corticosteroids to **Azmacort™** inhaler because deaths due to adrenal insufficiency have occurred in asthmatic patients during and after transfer from systemic corticosteroids to aerosolized steroids in recommended doses. After withdrawal from systemic corticosteroids, a number of months is usually required for recovery of hypothalamic-pituitary-adrenal (HPA) function. For some patients who have received large doses of oral steroids for long periods of time before therapy with **Azmacort™** inhaler is initiated, recovery may be delayed for one year or longer. During this period of HPA suppression, patients may exhibit signs and symptoms of adrenal insufficiency when exposed to trauma, surgery or infections, particularly gastroenteritis or other conditions with acute electrolyte loss. Although **Azmacort™** inhaler may provide control of asthmatic symptoms during these episodes; in recommended doses it supplies only normal physiological amounts of corticosteroid systemically and does NOT provide the increased systemic steroid which is necessary for coping with these emergencies.
During periods of stress or a severe asthmatic attack, patients who have been recently withdrawn from systemic corticosteroids should be instructed to resume systemic steroids (in large doses) immediately and to contact their physician for further instruction. These patients should also be instructed to carry a warning card indicating that they may need supplementary systemic steroids during periods of stress or a severe asthma attack.

Localized infections with *Candida albicans* have occurred infrequently in the mouth and pharynx. These areas should be examined by the treating physician at each patient visit. The percentage of positive mouth and throat cultures for *Candida albicans* did not change during a year of continuous therapy. The incidence of clinically apparent infection is low (2.5%). These infections may disappear spontaneously or may require treatment with appropriate antifungal therapy or discontinuance of treatment with **Azmacort™** inhaler.
Azmacort™ inhaler is not to be regarded as a bronchodilator and is not indicated for rapid relief of bronchospasm.
Patients should be instructed to contact their physician immediately when episodes of asthma which are not responsive to bronchodilators occur during the course of treatment with **Azmacort™** inhaler. During such episodes, patients may require therapy with systemic corticosteroids.
There is no evidence that control of asthma can be achieved by the administration of **Azmacort™** inhaler in amounts greater than the recommended doses, which appear to be the therapeutic equivalent of approximately 10 mg/day of oral prednisone.
Theoretically, the use of inhaled corticosteroids with alternate day prednisone oral therapy should be accompanied by more HPA suppression than a therapeutically equivalent regimen of either alone.
Transfer of patients from systemic steroid therapy to **Azmacort™** inhaler may unmask allergic conditions previously suppressed by the systemic steroid therapy, e.g., rhinitis, conjunctivitis, and eczema.

PRECAUTIONS

During withdrawal from oral steroids, some patients may experience symptoms of systemically active steroid withdrawal, e.g., joint and/or muscular pain, lassitude and depression, despite maintenance or even improvement of respiratory function (See DOSAGE AND ADMINISTRATION for details). Although steroid withdrawal effects are usually transient and not severe, severe and even fatal exacerbation of asthma can occur if the previous daily oral corticosteroid requirement had significantly exceeded 10 mg/day of prednisone or equivalent.
In responsive patients, inhaled corticosteroids will often permit control of asthmatic symptoms with less suppression of HPA function than therapeutically equivalent oral doses of prednisone. Since triamcinolone acetonide is absorbed into the circulation and can be systemically active, the beneficial effects of **Azmacort™** inhaler in minimizing or preventing HPA dysfunction may be expected only when recommended dosages are not exceeded.
Suppression of HPA function has been reported in volunteers who received 4000 mcg daily of triamcinolone acetonide. In addition, suppression of HPA function has been reported in some patients who have received recommended doses for as little as 6–12 weeks. Since the response of HPA function to inhaled corticosteroids is highly individualized, the physician should consider this information when treating patients.
Because of the possibility of systemic absorption of inhaled corticosteroids, patients treated with these drugs should be observed carefully for any evidence of systemic corticosteroid effects including suppression of growth in children. Particular care should be taken in observing patients post-operatively or during periods of stress for evidence of a decrease in adrenal function.
The long-term effects of triamcinolone acetonide inhaler in human subjects are not completely known, although patients have received **Azmacort™** inhaler on a continuous basis for periods of two years or longer. While there has been no clinical evidence of adverse experiences, the local effects of the agent on developmental or immunologic processes in the mouth, pharynx, trachea and lung are also unknown.
The potential effects of **Azmacort™** inhaler on acute, recurrent, or chronic pulmonary infections, including active or quiescent tuberculosis, are not known. For this reason, since systemic administration of corticosteroids may mask some signs of fungal, bacterial, or viral infection, the same caution should be observed when treating patients with **Azmacort™** inhaler. The potential effects of long-term administration of **Azmacort™** inhaler on lung or other tissues are unknown. However, pulmonary infiltrates with eosinophilia have occurred in patients receiving other inhaled corticosteroids.
Pregnancy: Pregnancy Category D. **Azmacort™** (triamcinolone acetonide) has been shown to be teratogenic in rats and rabbits when given in doses comparable to the highest dose recommended for human use (approximately 0.032 mg/kg/day). Administration of aerosol inhalation to pregnant rats and rabbits produced embryotoxic and fetotoxic effects which were comparable to those produced by administration by other routes.
Teratogenic effects in both species included a low incidence of cleft palate and/or internal hydrocephaly and axial skeletal defects. These findings represent known effects of glucocorticoids in laboratory animals.
There are no well-controlled studies in pregnant women. Experience with other dosage forms of triamcinolone acetonide does not include any positive evidence of adverse effects on the fetus. However, since such experience cannot exclude possibility of fetal damage, **Azmacort™** inhaler should be used during pregnancy only if the benefit clearly justifies the potential risk to the fetus. Infants born to mothers who have received substantial doses of corticosteroids during pregnancy should be carefully observed for hypoadrenalism.
Nursing mothers: It is not known whether this drug is excreted in human milk. Because of the potential for tumorigenicity shown for triamcinolone acetonide in animal studies, a decision should be made whether to discontinue nursing or to discontinue the drug, taking into account the importance of the drug to the mother.

ADVERSE REACTIONS

A few cases of oral candidiasis have been reported (see WARNINGS). In addition, some patients receiving **Azmacort™** inhaler have experienced hoarseness, dry throat, irritated throat and dry mouth. Increased wheezing and cough have been reported infrequently as has facial edema. These adverse effects have generally been mild and transient.

DOSAGE AND ADMINISTRATION

All patients should be instructed that the **Azmacort™** inhaler must be used on a regular daily basis rather than prn. Reliable dosage delivery cannot be assured after 240 actuations and patients should be cautioned against longer use of individual canisters.
Good oral hygiene including rinsing of the mouth after inhalation is recommended.
Adults: The usual dosage is two inhalations (approximately 200 mcg) given three to four times a day. The maximal daily intake should not exceed 16 inhalations (1600 mcg) in adults. Higher initial doses (12–16 inhalations per day) may be advisable in patients with more severe asthma, the dosage then being adjusted downward according to the response of the patient. In some patients maintenance can be accomplished when the total daily dose is given on a twice a day schedule.
Children 6 to 12 years of age: The usual dosage is one or two inhalations (100 to 200 mcg) given three to four times a day according to the response of the patient. The maximal daily intake should not exceed 12 inhalations (1200 mcg) in children 6 to 12 years of age. Insufficient clinical data exist with respect to the administration of **Azmacort™** inhaler in children below the age of 6. The long-term effects of inhaled steroids on growth are still under evaluation.
Patients receiving bronchodilators by inhalation should be advised to use the bronchodilator before **Azmacort™** inhaler in order to enhance penetration of triamcinolone acetonide into the bronchial tree. After use of an aerosol bronchodilator, several minutes should elapse before use of the **Azmacort™** inhaler to reduce the potential toxicity from the inhaled fluorocarbon propellants in the two aerosols.
Different considerations must be given to the following groups of patients in order to obtain the full therapeutic benefit of **Azmacort™** inhaler:
Patients not receiving systemic steroids: The use of **Azmacort™** inhaler is straightforward in patients who are inadequately controlled with non-steroid medications but in whom systemic steroid therapy has been withheld because of concern over potential adverse reactions. In patients who respond to **Azmacort™**, an improvement in pulmonary functon is usually apparent within one to two weeks after the start of **Azmacort™** inhaler.
Patients receiving systemic steroids: In those patients dependent on systemic steroids, transfer to **Azmacort™** inhaler and subsequent management may be more difficult because recovery from impaired adrenal function is usually slow. Such suppression has been known to last for up to 12 months or longer. Clinical studies, however, have demonstrated that **Azmacort™** inhaler may be effective in the management of these asthmatic patients and may permit replacement or significant reduction in the dosage of systemic corticosteroids.
The patient's asthma should be reasonably stable before treatment with **Azmacort™** inhaler is started. Initially the inhaler should be used concurrently with the patient's usual maintenance dose of systemic steroid. After approximately one week, gradual withdrawal of the systemic steroid is started by reducing the dose. The next reduction is made after an interval of one or two weeks, depending on the response of the patient. Generally, these decrements should not exceed 2.5 mg of prednisone or its equivalent. A slow rate of withdrawal cannot be overemphasized. During withdrawal, some patients may experience symptoms of systemically active steroid withdrawal, e.g., joint and/or muscular pain, lassitude and depression, despite maintenance or even improvement of respiratory function. Such patients should be encouraged to continue with the inhaler but should be watched carefully for objective signs of adrenal insufficiency, such as hypotension and weight loss. If evidence of adrenal insufficiency occurs, the systemic steroid dose should be boosted temporarily and thereafter further withdrawal should continue more slowly. No clinical studies have been conducted evaluating **Azmacort™** with alternate day prednisone regimens. However, based on the results of such a study with another inhaled corticosteroid, inhaled corticosteroids generally are not recommended for chronic use with alternate day prednisone regimens (see WARNINGS).
During periods of stress or a severe asthma attack, transfer patients will require supplementary treatment with systemic steroids. Exacerbations of asthma which occur during the course of treatment with **Azmacort™** inhaler should be

Continued on next page

This product information was prepared in August 1986. Information concerning these products may be obtained by addressing William H. Rorer, Inc., 500 Virginia Drive, Fort Washington, PA 19034.

Rorer—Cont.

treated with a short course of systemic steroid which is gradually tapered as these symptoms subside. There is no evidence that control of asthma can be achieved by administration of **Azmacort™** inhaler in amounts greater than the recommended doses.

Directions for Use: An illustrated leaflet of patient instructions for proper use accompanies each package of **Azmacort™** inhaler.

Contents Under Pressure: Do not puncture. Do not use or store near heat or open flame. Exposure to temperatures above 120°F may cause bursting. Never throw container into fire or incinerator. Keep out of reach of children.

HOW SUPPLIED

Azmacort™ inhaler contains 60 mg triamcinolone acetonide in a 20-gram package which delivers at least 240 oral inhalations. It is supplied with an oral adapter and patient's leaflet of instructions: box of one.
NDC 0067-0060-37

Caution: Federal law prohibits dispensing without prescription.

Shown in Product Identification Section, page 426

CAMALOX® Suspension and Tablets

(See PDR For Nonprescription Drugs)

EMETROL® Solution

(See PDR For Nonprescription Drugs)

FERMALOX® Tablets

(See PDR For Nonprescription Drugs)

MAALOX® Suspension and Tablets

(See PDR For Nonprescription Drugs)
Shown in Product Identification Section, page 426

Double Strength MAALOX® Tablets

(See 1987 PDR For Nonprescription Drugs)
Shown in Product Identification Section, page 426

MAALOX® PLUS Suspension and Tablets

(See PDR For Nonprescription Drugs)
Shown in Product Identification Section, page 426

MAALOX® TC Suspension and Tablets

(See PDR For Nonprescription Drugs)
Shown in Product Identification Section, page 426

NITROL® OINTMENT ℞

[nī'trôl]
2% nitroglycerin ointment

DESCRIPTION

NITROL® Ointment contains 2% nitroglycerin in a special absorptive base formulated to provide a controlled release of active ingredient. Inactive ingredients: Lactose, lanolin, purified water, white petrolatum. Each inch, as squeezed from the tube, contains approximately 15 mg of nitroglycerin.

ACTION

When the ointment is spread on the skin, the active ingredient (nitroglycerin) is continuously absorbed through the skin into the circulation, thus exerting prolonged vasodilator effect. Nitroglycerin ointment is effective in the control of angina pectoris when applied to the trunk or to the proximal parts of extremities.

Nitroglycerin relaxes smooth muscles, principally in the smaller blood vessels and dilates the arterioles and capillaries, especially in the coronary circulation. NITROL Ointment reduces the workload of the heart by virtue of its smooth muscle relaxation. This results predominantly in peripheral venous dilatation which reduces preload, but also to a lesser degree in peripheral arteriolar dilatation which reduces afterload. These hemodynamic effects have been advanced as explanations for the beneficial actions of nitroglycerin ointment in angina pectoris. Nitroglycerin exerts a favorable influence on myocardial oxygen consumption, resulting in increased myocardial efficiency and significant improvement in left ventricular function. Computerized digital plethysmographic studies have shown the duration of action of NITROL Ointment (2 inches applied to the chest) to be eight hours in comparison to placebo; the onset of action occurred within thirty minutes of administration. Controlled clinical studies have demonstrated that nitroglycerin ointment increased measured exercise tolerance in patients with angina pectoris up to three hours after application (the maximal time interval studied).

INDICATIONS

> This drug product has been conditionally approved by the FDA for the prevention and treatment of angina pectoris due to coronary artery disease. The conditional approval reflects a determination that the drug may be marketed pending FDA evaluation of data submitted in support of its effectiveness. A final evaluation of the effectiveness of the product will be announced by the FDA.

CONTRAINDICATIONS

In patients known to be intolerant of the organic nitrate drugs.

WARNINGS

In acute myocardial infarction or congestive heart failure, NITROL Ointment should be used under careful clinical and/or hemodynamic monitoring.

PRECAUTIONS

NITROL Ointment should not be used for treatment of acute anginal attacks. Symptoms of hypotension, particularly when suddenly arising from the recumbent position, are signs of overdosage. When they occur, the dosage should be reduced.

ADVERSE REACTIONS

Transient headaches are the most common side effect, especially at higher dosages. Headaches should be treated with mild analgesics and NITROL Ointment continued. Only with untreatable headaches should the dosage be reduced. Although uncommon, hypotension, an increase in heart rate, faintness, flushing, dizziness, and nausea may occur. These are all attributable to the pharmacologic effects of nitroglycerin on the cardiovascular system, and are symptoms of overdosage. When they occur and persist, the dosage should be reduced. Occasionally, contact dermatitis has been reported with continuous use of topical nitroglycerin. Such incidences may be reduced by changing the site of application.

MANAGEMENT OF OVERDOSAGE

Severe hypotension may result from overdosage of nitroglycerin ointment. Should hypotension develop, quickly remove the ointment. The patient should be placed in a recumbent position with the legs elevated. In case of persistent hypotension, an IV infusion of 5% dextrose should be started.

DOSAGE AND ADMINISTRATION

Using Conventional Appli-Rulers™ When applying the ointment, use the Appli-Ruler™ dose determining applicator supplied with the package and squeeze the necessary amount of ointment from the tube onto the applicator. Then place the applicator with the ointment side down onto the desired area of skin, usually the chest (although other areas can be used). Spread the ointment over at least a $2\frac{1}{4} \times 3\frac{1}{2}$ inch area in a thin uniform layer using the applicator. Cover the area with plastic wrap which can be held in place by adhesive tape. The Appli-Ruler allows the patient to measure the necessary amount of ointment and to spread it without being absorbed through the fingers while applying it to the skin surface.

Using TSAR™ Kit (Tape-Surrounded Appli-Rulers™) Measure the desired dosage of NITROL Ointment onto the Tape-Surrounded Appli-Ruler. Spread the ointment by carefully folding the Tape-Surrounded Appli-Ruler. Be careful not to spread any ointment onto the outer lined border. Bend the Tape-Surrounded Appli-Ruler at the star, peel off and discard the outer lined border. Apply the Tape-Surrounded Appli-Ruler to the desired body area and press the adhesive border firmly to the skin. To assure proper ointment contact, gently press the entire Tape-Surrounded Appli-Ruler.

The usual therapeutic dose is 1 to 2 inches (2.5 to 5.0 cm) applied every eight hours, although some patients may require as much as 4 to 5 inches (10 to 12.5 cm) and/or application every four hours.

Start at ½ inch (1.25 cm) every eight hours and increase the dose by ½ inch (1.25 cm) with each successive application to achieve the desired clinical effects. The optimal dosage should be selected based upon the clinical responses, side effects and the effects of therapy upon blood pressure. The greatest attainable decrease in resting blood pressure which is not associated with clinical symptoms of hypotension especially during orthostasis indicates the optimal dosage. To decrease adverse reactions, the dose and frequency of application should be tailored to the individual patient's needs.

The three gram titratable unit dose is a convenient hospital package. The tube has the same orifice as that of a larger NITROL tube and any prescribed dose up to four inches may be dispensed from the tube using the instructions described above.

Keep tube tightly closed and store at room temperature 59° to 86°F (15° to 30°C).

HOW SUPPLIED

(NDC 0067-5617-31)	30 gram tube
(NDC 0067-5617-02)	60 gram tube
(NDC 0067-5617-61)	30 gram 6 Pack
(NDC 0067-5617-62)	60 gram 6 Pack
(NDC 0067-5617-53)	Titratable Unit Dose— 50 × 3g Tubes

NITROL Ointment TSAR™ Kits (Packages include a supply of Tape-Surrounded Appli-Rulers for convenient application)

(NDC 0067-5617-90)	30 gram tube TSAR Kit
(NDC 0067-5617-91)	60 gram tube TSAR Kit
(NDC 0067-5617-89)	Titratable Unit Dose— 50 × 3g tubes TSAR Kit

Manufactured by
PACO PHARMACEUTICAL SERVICES, INC.
Lakewood, NJ 08701
For
WILLIAM H. RORER, INC.
Fort Washington, PA, U.S.A. 19034
Shown in Product Identification Section, page 426

NITROL® IV Concentrate ℞

[nī'trôl]
(nitroglycerin)

For intravenous use only: Not for direct intravenous injection (must be diluted). Nitrol IV Concentrate must be diluted in dextrose (5%) injection, USP or sodium chloride (0.9%) injection, USP before intravenous administration. The administration set used for infusion may affect the amount of Nitrol IV Concentrate delivered to the patient (see WARNINGS and DOSAGE AND ADMINISTRATION sections).

CAUTION

Several preparations of nitroglycerin for injection are available. They differ in concentration and/or volume per vial. When switching from one product to another, attention must be paid to the dilution and dosage and administration instructions.

DESCRIPTION

Nitrol IV Concentrate (nitroglycerin) is a clear, practically colorless additive solution for intravenous infusion after dilution. Each mL contains 5 mg nitroglycerin in dehydrated alcohol. The solution is sterile, nonpyrogenic and nonexplosive. **Nitrol IV Concentrate**, an organic nitrate, is a vasodilator. The chemical name for nitroglycerin is 1,2,3-propanetriol trinitrate and its chemical structure is:

$$\begin{array}{l} CH_2-ONO_2 \\ | \\ CH-ONO_2 \\ | \\ CH_2-ONO_2 \end{array}$$

$C_3H_5N_3O_9$ Mol. Wt. 227.09

CLINICAL PHARMACOLOGY

Relaxation of vascular smooth muscle is the principal pharmacologic action of **Nitrol IV Concentrate** (nitroglycerin). Although venous effects predominate, nitroglycerin produces, in a dose-related manner, dilation of both arterial and venous beds. Dilation of the postcapillary vessels, including large veins, promotes peripheral pooling of blood and decreases venous return to the heart, reducing left ventricular end-diastolic pressure (preload). Arteriolar relaxation reduces systemic vascular resistance and arterial pressure (afterload). Myocardial oxygen consumption or demand (as measured by the pressure-rate product, tension-time index and stroke-work index) is decreased by both the arterial and venous effects of nitroglycerin and a more favorable supply-demand ratio can be achieved.

Therapeutic doses of intravenous nitroglycerin reduce systolic, diastolic, and mean arterial blood pressure. Effective coronary perfusion pressure is usually maintained, but can be compromised if blood pressure falls excessively or increased heart rate decreases diastolic filling time.

Elevated central venous and pulmonary capillary wedge pressures, pulmonary vascular resistance, and systemic vascular resistance are also reduced by nitroglycerin therapy. Heart rate is usually slightly increased, presumably a reflex response to the fall in blood pressure. Cardiac index may be increased, decreased, or unchanged. Patients with elevated left ventricular filling pressure and systemic vascular resistance values in conjunction with a depressed cardiac index are likely to experience an improvement in cardiac index. On the other hand, when filling pressures and cardiac index are normal, cardiac index may be slightly reduced by intravenous nitroglycerin.

Nitroglycerin is widely distributed in the body with an apparent volume of distribution of approximately 200 liters in adult male subjects, and is rapidly metabolized to dinitrates and mononitrates with a short half-life estimated at 1 to 4 minutes. This results in a low plasma concentration after intravenous infusion. At plasma concentrations of between 50 and 500 ng/mL, the binding of nitroglycerin to plasma proteins is approximately 60% while that of 1,2-dinitroglycerin and 1,3-dinitroglycerin is 60% and 30%, respectively. The activity and half-life of the nitroglycerin metabolites are not well characterized. The mononitrate is not active.

INDICATIONS AND USAGE

Nitrol IV Concentrate is indicated for:

1. Control of blood pressure in perioperative hypertension, i.e. hypertension associated with surgical procedures, especially cardiovascular procedures, such as the hypertension seen during intratracheal intubation, anesthesia, skin incision, sternotomy, cardiac bypass, and in the immediate post-surgical period.
2. Congestive heart failure associated with acute myocardial infarction.
3. Treatment of angina pectoris in patients who have not responded to recommended doses of organic nitrates and/or a beta blocker.
4. Production of controlled hypotension during surgical procedures.

CONTRAINDICATIONS

Nitrol IV Concentrate should not be administered to individuals with:

1. A known hypersensitivity to nitroglycerin or a known idiosyncratic reaction to organic nitrates.
2. Hypotension or uncorrected hypovolemia, as the use of **Nitrol IV Concentrate** is such states could produce severe hypotension or shock.
3. Increased intracranial pressure (e.g., head trauma or cerebral hemorrhage).
4. Inadequate cerebral circulation.
5. Constrictive pericarditis and pericardial tamponade.

WARNINGS

1. Nitroglycerin readily migrates into many plastics. To avoid absorption of nitroglycerin into plastic parenteral solution containers, the dilution and storage of **Nitrol IV Concentrate** for intravenous infusion should be made only in glass parenteral solution bottles.
2. Some filters absorb nitroglycerin; they should be avoided.
3. Forty percent (40%) to eighty percent (80%) of the total amount of nitroglycerin in the final diluted solution for infusion is absorbed by the polyvinyl chloride (PVC) tubing of the intravenous administration sets currently in general use. The higher rates of absorption occur when flow rates are low, nitroglycerin concentrations are high, and tubing is long. Although the rate of loss is highest during the early phase of infusion (when flow rates are lowest), the loss is neither constant nor self-limiting; consequently, no simple calculation or correction can be performed to convert the theoretical infusion rate (based on the concentration of the infusion solution) to the actual delivery rate.
4. Because of the problem of nitroglycerin absorption by polyvinyl chloride (PVC) tubing, **Nitrol IV Concentrate** should be used with the least absorptive infusion tubing (i.e., non-PVC tubing) available.

Dosage instructions must be followed with care. It should be noted that when the appropriate infusion sets are used, the calculated dose will be delivered to the patient because the loss of nitroglycerin due to absorption in standard PVC tubing will be kept to a minimum. Note that the dosages commonly used in published studies utilized general-use PVC infusion sets and recommended doses based on this experience are too high if the low absorbing infusion sets are used.

5. A potential safety problem exists with the combined use of some infusion pumps and some non-PVC infusion sets. Because the special tubing required to prevent the absorption of nitroglycerin tends to be less pliable than the conventional PVC tubing normally used with such infusion pumps, the pumps may fail to occlude the infusion sets completely. The results may be excessive flow at low infusion rate settings, causing alarms, or unregulated gravity flow when the infusion pump is stopped; this could lead to over-infusion of nitroglycerin. All infusion pumps should be tested with the infusion sets to ensure their ability to deliver nitroglycerin accurately at low flow rates, and to occlude the infusion sets properly when the infusion is stopped.

PRECAUTIONS

Nitrol IV Concentrate should be used with caution in patients with severe hepatic or renal disease.

Excessive hypotension, especially for prolonged periods of time, must be avoided because of possible deleterious effects on the brain, heart, liver, and kidney from poor perfusion and the attendant risk of ischemia, thrombosis, and altered function of these organs. Paradoxical bradycardia and increased angina pectoris may accompany nitroglycerin-induced hypotension. Patients with normal or low pulmonary capillary wedge pressure are especially sensitive to the hypotensive effects of nitroglycerin. If pulmonary capillary wedge pressure is being monitored, it will be noted that a fall in wedge pressure precedes the onset of arterial hypotension, and the pulmonary capillary wedge pressure is thus a useful guide to safe titration of the drug.

Carcinogenesis, Mutagenesis, Impairment of Fertility: No long-term studies in animals were performed to evaluate carcinogenic potential of **Nitrol IV Concentrate.**

Pregnancy: Category C. Animal reproduction studies have not been conducted with **Nitrol IV Concentrate.** It is not known whether **Nitrol IV Concentrate** can cause fetal harm when administered to a pregnant woman or can affect reproduction capacity. **Nitrol IV Concentrate** should be given to a pregnant woman only if clearly needed.

Nursing mothers: It is not known whether nitroglycerin is excreted in human milk. Because many drugs are excreted in human milk, caution should be exercised when **Nitrol IV Concentrate** is administered to a nursing woman.

Pediatric use: The safety and effectiveness of **Nitrol IV Concentrate** in children have not been established.

ADVERSE REACTIONS

The most frequent adverse reaction in patients treated with **Nitrol IV Concentrate** is headache which occurs in approximately 2% of patients. Other adverse reactions occurring in less than 1% of patients are the following: tachycardia, nausea, vomiting, apprehension, restlessness, muscle twitching, retrosternal discomfort, palpitations, dizziness, and abdominal pain.

The following additional adverse reactions have been reported with the oral and/or topical use of nitroglycerin: cutaneous flushing, weakness, and occasionally drug rash or exfoliative dermatitis.

OVERDOSAGE

Accidental overdosage of **Nitrol IV Concentrate** may result in severe hypotension and reflex tachycardia which can be treated by elevating the legs and decreasing or temporarily terminating the infusion until the patient's condition stabilizes. Since the duration of the hemodynamic effects following **Nitrol IV Concentrate** administration is quite short, additional corrective measures are usually not required. However, if further therapy is indicated, administration of an intravenous alpha adrenergic agonist (e.g., methoxamine or phenylephrine) should be considered.

DOSAGE AND ADMINISTRATION

Not for direct intravenous injection.

Nitrol IV Concentrate is a concentrated, potent drug which must be diluted in dextrose (5%) injection, USP or sodium chloride (0.9%) injection, USP prior to its infusion. Nitrol IV Concentrate should not be admixed with other drugs.

Dilution:

Nitrol IV Concentrate is supplied in 5 mg/mL solution. A dilution and administration scheme for **Nitrol IV Concentrate** (nitroglycerin) is shown in Table 1 above:

1. Initial Dilution:

Aseptically transfer the contents of one **Nitrol IV Concentrate** ampul (containing 50 mg of nitroglycerin) into a 500 mL glass bottle of either dextrose (5%) injection, USP or sodium chloride (0.9%) injection, USP. This yields a final concentration of 100 μg/mL. Invert the glass parenteral bottle several times following admixture to assure uniform dilution of **Nitrol IV Concentrate.**

2. Maintenance Dilution:

It is important to consider the fluid requirements of the patient as well as the expected duration of infusion in selecting the appropriate dilution of **Nitrol IV Concentrate.**

After the initial dosage titration, the concentration of the admixture may be increased, if necessary, to limit fluids given to the patient. The concentration of the infusion solution should not exceed 400 μg/mL of nitroglycerin.

Table 1: Dilution and Administration Scheme for Nitrol IV Concentrate (nitroglycerin)

Each 10 mL Nitrol IV Concentrate Amp = 50 mg Nitroglycerin

	Dilute		
	1 amp in 500 mL	1 amp in 250 mL or 2 amps in 500 mL	2 amps in 250 mL or 4 amps in 500 mL
Flow Rate micro drops/min* ml/Hr	100 μg/mL	200 μg/mL	400 μg/mL
	Nitrol IV Concentrate Administration Rate μg nitroglycerin/min		
3	5	10	20
6	10	20	40
12	20	40	80
24	40	80	160
48	80	160	320
72	120	240	480
96	160	320	640

*60 microdrops = 1 mL

If the concentration is adjusted, it is imperative to flush or replace the infusion set before a new concentration is utilized. Depending upon the infusion set used and the flow rate, it could take from 1–2 minutes to 10 hours for the new concentration to reach the patient if the set were not flushed or replaced.

DOSAGE

Dosage is affected by the type of infusion set used (see WARNINGS). Although the usual starting adult dose range reported in clinical studies was 25 μg/min or more, these studies used **PVC administration sets. The use of non-absorbing tubing will result in the need to use reduced doses.**

When using a non-absorbing infusion set, initial dosage should be 5 μg/min delivered through an infusion pump capable of exact and constant delivery of the drug. Subsequent titration must be adjusted to the clinical situation, with dose increments becoming more cautious as partial response is seen. Initial titration should be in 5 μg/min increments, with increases every 3–5 minutes until some response is noted. If no response is seen at 20 μg/min, increments of 10 and later 20 μg/min can be used. Once a partial blood pressure response is observed, the dose increase should be reduced and the interval between increments should be lengthened. Patients with normal or low left ventricular filling pressure or pulmonary capillary wedge pressure (e.g., angina patients without other complications), may be hypersensitive to the effects of nitroglycerin and may respond fully to doses as small as 5 μg/min. These patients require especially careful titration and monitoring.

There is no fixed optimum dose of nitroglycerin. Due to variations in the responsiveness of individual patients to the drug, each patient must be titrated to the desired level of hemodynamic function. Therefore, continuous monitoring of physiologic parameters (e.g., blood pressure, heart rate, and pulmonary capillary wedge pressure), **must be performed** to achieve the correct dose. Adequate systemic blood pressure and coronary perfusion pressure must be maintained. Parenteral drug products should be inspected visually for particulate matter and discoloration prior to administration whenever solution and container permit.

HOW SUPPLIED

10-mL (50-mg) ampul—Box of 10—NDC 0067-0802-53

Protect from freezing. Protect from light by retaining product in carton until ready to use.

Manufactured by
Pharma Hameln GmbH
D-3250 Hameln, West Germany
for
G. POHL-BOSKAMP GmbH & Co.
D-2214 Hohenlockstedt
West Germany
Distributed by
WILLIAM H. RORER, INC.
Fort Washington, PA, U.S.A. 19034

Shown in Product Identification Section, page 426

NITROLINGUAL® SPRAY ℞

(nitroglycerin lingual aerosol)

0.4 mg/metered dose

DESCRIPTION

Nitroglycerin, an organic nitrate, is a vasodilator which has effects on both arteries and veins. The chemical name for nitroglycerin is 1,2,3 propanetriol trinitrate ($C_3H_5N_3O_9$).

Continued on next page

This product information was prepared in August 1986. Information concerning these products may be obtained by addressing William H. Rorer, Inc., 500 Virginia Drive, Fort Washington, PA 19034.

Rorer—Cont.

The compound has a molecular weight of 227.09. The chemical structure is:

$$\begin{array}{l} CH_2-ONO_2 \\ | \\ CH\ -ONO_2 \\ | \\ CH_2-ONO_2 \end{array}$$

Nitrolingual Spray (nitroglycerin lingual aerosol 0.4 mg) is a metered dose aerosol containing nitroglycerin in propellants (dichlorodifluoromethane and dichlorotetrafluoroethane). Each metered dose of Nitrolingual Spray delivers 0.4 mg of nitroglycerin per spray emission. This product delivers nitroglycerin in the form of spray droplets onto or under the tongue. Inactive ingredients: caprylic/capric/diglyceryl succinate, ether, flavors.

CLINICAL PHARMACOLOGY

The principal pharmacological action of nitroglycerin is relaxation of vascular smooth muscle, producing a vasodilator effect on both peripheral arteries and veins with more prominent effects on the latter. Dilation of the post-capillary vessels, including large veins, promotes peripheral pooling of blood and decreases venous return to the heart, thereby reducing left ventricular end-diastolic pressure (pre-load). Arteriolar relaxation reduces systemic vascular resistance and arterial pressure (after-load).

The mechanism by which nitroglycerin relieves angina pectoris is not fully understood. Myocardial oxygen consumption or demand (as measured by the pressure-rate product, tension-time index, and stroke-work index) is decreased by both the arterial and venous effects of nitroglycerin and presumably, a more favorable supply-demand ratio is achieved. While the large epicardial coronary arteries are also dilated by nitroglycerin, the extent to which this action contributes to relief of exertional angina is unclear.

Nitroglycerin is rapidly metabolized *in vivo*, with a liver reductase enzyme having primary importance in the formation of glycerol nitrate metabolites and inorganic nitrate. Two active major metabolites, 1, 2- and 1,3-dinitroglycerols, the products of hydrolysis, although less potent as vasodilators, have longer plasma half-lives than the parent compound. The dinitrates are further metabolized to mononitrates (considered biologically inactive with respect to cardiovascular effects) and ultimately glycerol and carbon dioxide.

Therapeutic doses of nitroglycerin may reduce systolic, diastolic, and mean arterial blood pressure. Effective coronary perfusion pressure is usually maintained, but can be compromised if blood pressure falls excessively or increased heart rate decreases diastolic filling time.

Elevated central venous and pulmonary capillary wedge pressures, pulmonary vascular resistance, and systemic vascular resistance are also reduced by nitroglycerin therapy. Heart rate is usually slightly increased, presumably a reflex response to the fall in blood pressure. Cardiac index may be increased, decreased, or unchanged. Patients with elevated left ventricular filling pressure and systemic vascular resistance values in conjunction with a depressed cardiac index are likely to experience an improvement in cardiac index. On the other hand, when filling pressures and cardiac index are normal, cardiac index may be slightly reduced.

A pharmacokinetic study in 13 healthy men showed no statistically significant differences between the mean values for maximum plasma concentration and time to achieve maximum plasma level with equal doses (0.8 mg) of Nitrolingual Spray and sublingual nitroglycerin tablets. Peak plasma concentration after 0.8 mg of Nitrolingual occurred within 4 minutes and the apparent plasma half-life was approximately 5 minutes. In a randomized, double-blind study in patients with exertional angina pectoris dose-related in increases in exercise tolerance were seen following doses of 0.2, 0.4, and 0.8 mg delivered by metered spray.

INDICATIONS AND USAGE

Nitrolingual Spray is indicated for acute relief of an attack or prophylaxis of angina pectoris due to coronary artery disease.

CONTRAINDICATIONS

Nitrolingual Spray is contraindicated in patients who have shown purported hypersensitivity or idiosyncracy to it or other nitrates or nitrites.

WARNINGS

The use of any form of nitroglycerin during the early days of acute myocardial infarction requires particular attention to hemodynamic monitoring and clinical status.

PRECAUTIONS

General—Severe hypotension, particularly with upright posture, may occur even with small doses of nitroglycerin. The drug, therefore, should be used with caution in subjects who may have volume depletion from diuretic therapy or in patients who have low systolic blood pressure (e.g. below 90 mm Hg). Paradoxical bradycardia and increased angina pectoris may accompany nitroglycerin-induced hypotension.

Nitrate therapy may aggravate the angina caused by hypertrophic cardiomyopathy.

Tolerance to this drug and cross-tolerance to other nitrates and nitrites may occur. Tolerance to the vascular and antianginal effects of nitrates has been demonstrated in clinical trials, experience through occupational exposure, and in isolated tissue experiments in the laboratory.

In industrial workers continuously exposed to nitroglycerin, tolerance clearly occurs. Moreover, physical dependence also occurs since chest pain, acute myocardial infarction, and even sudden death have occurred during temporary withdrawal of nitroglycerin from the workers. In various clinical trials in angina patients, there are reports of anginal attacks being more easily provoked and of rebound in the hemodynamic effects soon after nitrate withdrawal. The relative importance of these observations to the routine, clinical use of nitroglycerin is not known.

Drug Interactions: Alcohol may enhance sensitivity to the hypotensive effects of nitrates. Nitroglycerin acts directly on vascular muscle. Therefore, any other agents that depend on vascular smooth muscle as the final common path can be expected to have decreased or increased effect depending upon the agent.

Marked symptomatic orthostatic hypotension has been reported when calcium channel blockers and oral controlled-release nitroglycerin were used in combination. Dose adjustments of either class of agents may be necessary.

Carcinogenesis, Mutagenesis, Impairment of Fertility: No long-term studies in animals have been performed to evaluate carcinogenic potential of Nitrolingual Spray.

Pregnancy: Pregnancy Category C—Animal reproduction studies have not been conducted with Nitrolingual Spray. It is not known whether nitroglycerin can cause fetal harm when administered to a pregnant woman or can affect reproduction capacity. Nitroglycerin should be given to a pregnant woman only if clearly needed.

Nursing Mothers: It is not known whether nitroglycerin is excreted in human milk. Because many drugs are excreted in human milk, caution should be exercised when Nitrolingual Spray is administered to a nursing woman.

Pediatric Use: The safety and effectiveness of nitroglycerin in children have not been established.

ADVERSE REACTIONS

Adverse reaction to Nitrolingual Spray, particularly headache and hypotension, is generally dose-related. In clinical trials at various doses of nitroglycerin, the following adverse effects have been observed:

Headache, which may be severe and persistent, is the most commonly reported side effect of nitroglycerin with an incidence on the order of about 50% in some studies. Cutaneous vasodilation with flushing may occur. Transient episodes of dizziness and weakness, as well as other signs of cerebral ischemia associated with postural hypotension, may occasionally develop. An occasional individual may exhibit marked sensitivity to the hypotensive effects of nitrates and severe responses (nausea, vomiting, weakness, restlessness, pallor, perspiration, and collapse) may occur even with therapeutic doses. Drug rash and/or exfoliative dermatitis have been reported in patients receiving nitrate therapy. Nausea and vomiting appear to be uncommon.

OVERDOSAGE

Signs and Symptoms:

Nitrate overdosage may result in: severe hypotension; persistent throbbing headache; vertigo; palpitation; visual disturbance; flushing and perspiring skin (later becoming cold and cyanotic); nausea and vomiting (possibly with colic and even bloody diarrhea); syncope (especially in the upright posture); methemoglobinemia with cyanosis and anorexia; initial hypernea, dyspnea, and slow breathing; slow pulse (dicrotic and intermittent); heart block; increased intracranial pressure with cerebral symptoms of confusion and moderate fever, paralysis and coma followed by clonic convulsions, and possibly death due to circulatory collapse.

Treatment of Overdosage:

Keep the patient recumbent in a shock position and comfortably warm. Gastric lavage may be of use if the medication has only recently been swallowed. Passive movement of the extremities may aid venous return. Administer oxygen and artificial ventilation, if necessary. If methemoglobinemia is present, administration of methylene blue (1% solution), 1–2 mg per kilogram of body weight intravenously, may be required.

Methemoglobinemia:

Case reports of clinically significant methemoglobinemia are rare at conventional doses of organic nitrates. The formation of methemoglobin is dose-related and in the case of genetic abnormalities of hemoglobin that favor methemoglobin formation, even conventional doses of organic nitrates could produce harmful concentrations of methemoglobin.

WARNING

Epinephrine is ineffective in reversing the severe hypotensive events associated with overdosage. It and related compounds are contraindicated in this situation.

DOSAGE AND ADMINISTRATION

At the onset of an attack, one or two metered doses should be sprayed onto or under the tongue. No more than three metered doses are recommended within a 15-minute period. If the chest pain persists, prompt medical attention is recommended. Nitrolingual Spray may be used prophylactically five to ten minutes prior to engaging in activities which might precipitate an acute attack.

During application the patient should rest, ideally in the sitting position. The canister should be held vertically with the valve head uppermost and the spray orifice as close to the mouth as possible. The dose should preferably be sprayed onto the tongue by pressing the button firmly and the mouth should be closed immediately after each dose. THE SPRAY SHOULD NOT BE INHALED. Patients should be instructed to familiarize themselves with the position of the spray orifice, which can be identified by the finger rest on top of the valve, in order to facilitate orientation for administration at night.

HOW SUPPLIED

Nitrolingual Spray, 13.8g (Net Contents) containing 200 metered doses, box of one. (NDC 0067-0820-80)

Do not expose to heat or store at temperatures above 120°F (49°C).

Shown in Product Identifcation Section, page 426

PAREPECTOLIN® Ⓒ
Antidiarrheal

Contains opium (¼ grain) 15 mg per fluid ounce. *(Warning: may be habit forming.)*

FORMULA

Each fluid ounce contains:

Paregoric (equivalent) ....(1 fl dram) 3.7 mL
Pectin ....(2½ grains) 162 mg
Kaolin ....(85 grains) 5.5 g

INACTIVE INGREDIENTS

Benzoic acid, carboxymethylcellulose sodium, ethyl, ethylparaben, flavors, glycerin, propylparaben, saccharin sodium, purified water, alcohol 0.69%.

INDICATIONS

For symptomatic relief of diarrhea.

ACTIONS

The kaolin adsorbs irritants and forms a protective coating on intestinal mucosa. Pectin acts to consolidate the stool. Paregoric is very useful in diarrhea because it has a soothing action and allays griping pains.

ADVANTAGES

Because Parepectolin contains paregoric (equivalent), it effectively controls both diarrhea and colicky cramps. It is a stable suspension that tastes good.

Usual Adult Dose: One or two tablespoonfuls after each loose bowel movement for no more than four doses in twelve hours.

Usual Children's Dose: One or two teaspoonfuls after each loose bowel movement for no more than four doses in twelve hours.

Usual Pediatric Dose:

Three years	1½ teaspoonfuls
Six years	2 teaspoonfuls

after each loose bowel movement for no more than four doses in twelve hours.

WARNING

Keep this and all drugs out of the reach of children. In case of accidental overdose, seek professional assistance or contact a poison control center immediately.

Supplied: Bottles of 4 (118 mL) (NDC 0067-0660-60) and 8 (237 mL) (NDC 0067-0660-66) fluid ounces.

PERDIEM® Granules

(See PDR For Nonprescription Drugs)
Shown in Product Identification Section, page 426

PERDIEM® PLAIN Granules

(See PDR For Nonprescription Drugs)
Shown in Product Identification Section, page 426

SLO-BID™ ℞

[slō'bid"]

(theophylline, anhydrous)

50 mg, 100 mg, 200 mg, and 300 mg

Gyrocaps®

Timed Release Capsules

DESCRIPTION

Slo-bid™ Gyrocaps® contain 50 mg, 100 mg, 200 mg, or 300 mg theophylline, anhydrous in the form of long-acting beads within a dye-free hard gelatin capsule and are intended for oral administration. Theophylline is a bronchodilator and is a member of the xanthine class of chemical compounds related to both theobromine and caffeine.

Theophylline is *1H*-Purine-2,6-dione,3,7-dihydro-1,3-dimethyl represented by the following structural formula.

Theophylline is a white, odorless, crystalline powder having a bitter taste.

CLINICAL PHARMACOLOGY

Theophylline directly relaxes the smooth muscle of the bronchial airways and pulmonary blood vessels thus acting as a bronchodilator and smooth muscle relaxant. The drug also produces other actions typical of the xanthine derivatives: cardiac stimulation, coronary vasodilatation, stimulation of skeletal muscle, cerebral stimulation, and diuresis. The action of theophylline may be mediated through inhibition of phosphodiesterase and a resultant increase in intracellular cyclic AMP.

In vitro, theophylline has been shown to act synergistically with beta agonists that increase intracellular cyclic AMP through the stimulation of adenyl cyclase but synergism has not been demonstrated in patient studies. More data are needed to determine if the theophylline and beta agonists have a clinically important additive effect *in vivo.* Apparently, no development of tolerance occurs with chronic use of theophylline.

Pharmacokinetics: The half-life of theophylline is influenced by a number of known variables. It is prolonged in patients suffering from chronic alcoholism, impaired hepatic or renal function, congestive heart failure, and in patients receiving macrolide antibiotics and cimetidine. Older adults (over age 55) and patients with chronic obstructive pulmonary disease, with or without cor pulmonale, may also have much slower clearance rates. For such patients, the theophylline half-life may exceed 24 hours.

Newborns and neonates have extremely slow clearance rates compared to older infants (over 6 months) and children, and may also have a theophylline half-life of over 24 hours. High fever for prolonged periods may also reduce the rate of theophylline elimination.

Representative Theophylline Serum Half-Lives	**Half-Life (hours)**
Adults	
non-smokers	7–9
smokers	4–5
congestive heart failure	24
Children (6–16 years)	3–5

The half-life of theophylline in smokers (1 to 2 packs/day) averages 4–5 hours, much shorter than the half-life in non-smokers which averages 7–9 hours. The increase in theophylline clearance caused by smoking is probably the result of induction of drug-metabolizing enzymes that do not readily normalize after cessation of smoking. It appears that between 3 months and 2 years may be necessary for normalization of the effect of smoking on theophylline pharmacokinetics.

In a single-dose bioavailability study in 18 normal subjects, 300 mg sustained-release Slo-bid™ Gyrocaps® produced mean peak serum concentrations of 3.5 ± 0.7 μg/mL at a mean time of 7.8 ± 1.8 hours after dosing. Subjects fasted overnight before dosing and four hours after the dose. At steady state in a multiple dose bioavailability study in 18 normal subjects with q12h dosing (600–1000 mg/day) the mean peak-trough variation was 3.5 ± 0.9 μg/mL. The mean C_{max} and C_{min} were 12.9 ± 3.0 and 9.4 ± 2.5 μg/mL, respectively. The mean percent fluctuation $[(C_{max}-C_{min}/C_{min}) \times 100]$ was $40 \pm 15\%$. Subjects fasted 12 hours before the dose and 4 hours after the dose was administered on the days that the blood samples were drawn. A multiple dose bioequivalence study with 15 asthmatic children, ages 9–16, comparing Slo-bid™ Gyrocaps® administered as intact capsules and as the beaded contents sprinkled on applesauce with b.i.d. dosing (150–600 mg/dose) indicated no significant differences in maximum and minimum theophylline concentrations, time to achieve peak concentration, and peak-trough differences. The bioavailability as measured by comparing area under the curves, (AUC 0–12 hours granules /AUC 0–12 hours capsules) was 0.990 ± 0.214.

INDICATIONS AND USAGE

For relief and/or prevention of symptoms from asthma and reversible bronchospasm associated with chronic bronchitis and emphysema.

CONTRAINDICATIONS

Slo-bid™ is contraindicated in individuals who have shown hypersensitivity to any of the components of this product.

WARNINGS

Status asthmaticus should be considered a medical emergency and is defined as that degree of bronchospasm which is not rapidly responsive to usual doses of conventional bronchodilators. Optimal therapy for such patients frequently requires both *additional medication,* parenterally administered, and *close monitoring,* preferably in an intensive care setting.

Although increasing the dose of theophylline may bring about relief, such treatment may be associated with toxicity. The likelihood of such toxicity developing increases significantly when the serum theophylline concentration exceeds 20 μg/mL. Therefore, determination of serum theophylline levels is recommended to assure maximal benefit without excessive risk.

Serum levels above 20 μg/mL are rarely found after appropriate administration of the recommended doses. However, in individuals in whom theophylline plasma clearance is reduced *for any reason,* even conventional doses may result in increased serum levels and potential toxicity. Reduced theophylline clearance has been documented in the following readily identifiable groups: (1) patients with impaired renal or liver function, (2) patients over 55 years of age, particularly males and those with chronic lung disease, (3) those with cardiac failure from any cause, (4) neonates, and (5) those patients taking certain drugs (macrolide antibiotics and cimetidine). Decreased clearance of theophylline may be associated with either influenza immunization or active infection with influenza.

Reduction of dosage and laboratory monitoring is especially appropriate in the above individuals.

Less serious signs of theophylline toxicity, i.e. nausea and restlessness, may appear in up to 50% of patients.

Unfortunately, however, serious side effects such as ventricular arrhythmias, convulsions, or even death may appear as the first sign of toxicity without any previous warning. Stated differently, *serious toxicity is not reliably preceded by less severe side effects.*

Many patients who require theophylline may exhibit tachycardia due to their underlying disease process so that the cause/effect relationship to elevated serum theophylline concentrations may not be appreciated.

Theophylline products may cause dysrhythmia and/or worsen preexisting arrhythmias and any significant change in rate and/or rhythm warrants monitoring and further investigation.

The occurrence of arrhythmias and sudden death (with histological evidence of necrosis of the myocardium) has been recorded in laboratory animals (minipigs, rodents, and dogs) when theophylline and beta agonists were administered concomitantly, although not when either was administered alone. The significance of these findings when applied to human usage is currently unknown.

PRECAUTIONS

General: Mean half-life in smokers is shorter than non-smokers. Therefore, smokers may require larger or more frequent doses of theophylline. Morphine and curare should be used with caution in patients with airway obstruction as they may suppress respiration and stimulate histamine release. Alternative drugs should be used when possible.

Theophylline should not be administered concurrently with other xanthine preparations. Use with caution in patients with severe cardiac disease, severe hypoxemia, hypertension, hyperthyroidism, acute myocardial injury, cor pulmonale, congestive heart failure, alcoholism, liver disease, and in the elderly, especially males, and neonates. Great caution should be used in giving theophylline to patients with congestive heart failure. Frequently, such patients have shown markedly prolonged theophylline blood levels with theophylline persisting in serum for long periods following discontinuation of the drug. Use theophylline cautiously in patients with a history of peptic ulcer. Theophylline may occasionally act as a local gastrointestinal irritant, although GI symptoms are more commonly centrally mediated and associated with serum drug concentrations over 20 μg/mL.

Information for Patients: The physician should reinforce the importance of taking only the prescribed dose at the prescribed time intervals. The patient should alert the physician if symptoms occur repeatedly, especially near the end of a dosing interval. When prescribing administration by the sprinkle method, details of the proper technique should be explained to the patient.

Drug Interactions: Drug-Drug:

Toxic synergism with ephedrine has been documented and may occur with some other sympathomimetic bronchodilators. In addition, the following drug interactions have been demonstrated:

Drug	**Effect**
Aminophylline with lithium carbonate	Increased excretion of lithium carbonate
Aminophylline with propranolol	Increased theophylline serum concentrations. Antagonism of propranolol effects
Theophylline with troleandomycin or erythromycin	Increased theophylline serum concentrations
Theophylline with cimetidine	Increased theophylline serum concentrations

Drug-Food: Slo-bid™ Gyrocaps® have not been adequately studied to determine whether their bioavailability is altered when they are given with food.

Available data suggest that drug administration at the time of food ingestion may influence the absorption characteristics of some or all theophylline controlled-release products resulting in serum values different from those found after administration in the fasting state.

A drug-food effect, if any, would likely have its greatest clinical significance when high theophylline serum levels are being maintained and/or when large single doses (greater than 13 mg/kg or 900 mg) of a controlled-release theophylline product are given. The influence of the type and amount of food on performance of controlled-release theophylline products is under study at this time.

Drug/Laboratory Test Interactions:

When plasma levels of theophylline are measured by spectrophotometric methods, coffee, tea, cola beverages, chocolate, and acetaminophen contribute falsely high values.

Carcinogenesis, Mutagenesis, Impairment of Fertility: Long-term animal studies have not been performed to evaluate the carcinogenic potential, mutagenic potential, or the effect on fertility by xanthine compounds.

Pregnancy: Pregnancy Category C

Animal reproduction studies have not been conducted with theophylline. It is not known whether theophylline can cause fetal harm when administered to a pregnant woman or can affect reproduction capacity. Theophylline should be given to a pregnant woman only if clearly needed.

Nursing Mothers: It has been reported that theophylline distributes readily into breast milk and may cause adverse effects in the infant. Caution must be used if prescribing xanthines to a mother who is nursing, taking into account the risk-benefit of this therapy.

Pediatric Use: Safety and effectiveness in children under 6 years of age have not been established with this product.

ADVERSE REACTIONS

The most consistent adverse reactions are usually due to overdose and are:

Gastrointestinal: nausea, vomiting, epigastric pain, hematemesis, and diarrhea.

Central Nervous System: headaches, irritability, restlessness, insomnia, reflex hyperexcitability, muscle twitching, and clonic and tonic generalized convulsions.

Cardiovascular: palpitation, tachycardia, extrasystoles, flushing, hypotension, circulatory failure, and ventricular arrhythmias.

Respiratory: tachypnea

Renal: albuminuria, increased excretion of renal tubular cells and red blood cells, potentiation of diuresis.

Other: hyperglycemia, inappropriate ADH syndrome, and rash.

OVERDOSAGE

Management:

A. If potential overdose is established and seizure has not occurred
   1. Induce vomiting
   2. Administer a cathartic (this is particularly important if sustained-release preparations have been taken)
   3. Administer activated charcoal
   4. Monitor vital signs, maintain blood pressure and provide adequate hydration

B. If patient is having a seizure
   1. Establish an airway
   2. Administer oxygen
   3. Treat the seizure with intravenous diazepam 0.1 to 0.3 mg/kg up to a total dose of 10 mg
   4. Monitor vital signs, maintain blood pressure, and provide adequate hydration

Continued on next page

This product information was prepared in August 1986. Information concerning these products may be obtained by addressing William H. Rorer, Inc., 500 Virginia Drive, Fort Washington, PA 19034.

Rorer—Cont.

C. Post-Seizure Coma
1. Maintain airway and oxygenation
2. If a result of oral medication, follow above recommendations to prevent absorption of drug, but intubation and lavage will have to be performed instead of inducing emesis and the cathartic and charcoal will need to be introduced via a large bore gastric lavage tube
3. Continue to provide full supportive care and adequate hydration while waiting for drug to be metabolized. In general, the drug is metabolized sufficiently rapidly so as not to warrant consideration of dialysis; however, if serum levels exceed 50 μg/mL, charcoal hemoperfusion may be indicated.

DOSAGE AND ADMINISTRATION

Slo-Bid™ Gyrocaps® have not been adequately studied for their bioavailability when administered with food (See PRECAUTIONS, Drug-Food Interactions.)

For most patients, *effective use* of theophylline, i.e. associated with optimal likelihood of benefit combined with minimal risk of toxicity, is considered to occur when serum levels are maintained between 10 and 20 μg/mL. Levels above 20 μg/mL may produce toxicity, and in a small number of patients, toxicity may even be seen with serum levels between 15–20 μg/mL, particularly during initiation of therapy.

There is considerable variation from patient to patient in the dosage required to achieve and maintain therapeutic and safe levels, primarily due to variable rates of elimination. Therefore, it is essential that not only must dosage be individualized, but titration and monitoring of serum levels be utilized where available. When serum concentration cannot be obtained, restriction of dosage to the amounts and intervals recommended in the guidelines listed below becomes essential. Dosage should be calculated on the basis of lean (ideal) body weight where mg/kg doses are presented. Theophylline does not distribute into fatty tissue.

Frequency of Dosing: When immediate-release products with rapid absorption (such as tablets or liquid) are used, dosing to maintain serum levels generally requires administration every 6 hours. This is particularly true in children, but dosing intervals up to 8 hours may be satisfactory in adults since they eliminate the drug at a slower rate. Some children, and adults requiring higher than average doses (those having rapid rates of clearance, e.g. half-lives of under 6 hours) may benefit and be more effectively controlled during chronic therapy when given products with sustained-release characteristics since these provide longer dosing intervals and/or less fluctuation in serum concentration between dosing. Those sustained-release products which provide flexibility in dosage through formulations of varying strengths are also helpful in controlling serum levels. Dosage guidelines are approximations only and the wide range of theophylline clearance between individuals (particularly those with concomitant disease) make indiscriminate usage hazardous.

As a practical consideration, it is not always possible to obtain serum level determinations. Under such conditions, restriction of the daily dose (*in otherwise healthy adults*) to not greater than 13 mg/kg/day (or up to 900 mg) of anhydrous theophylline in divided doses will result in relatively few patients exceeding serum levels of 20 μg/mL and the resultant risk of toxicity.

Dosage Guidelines:

I. Acute Symptoms
Slo-bid™ is not intended for patients experiencing an acute episode of bronchospasm (associated with asthma, chronic bronchitis, or emphysema). Such patients require *rapid* relief of symptoms and should be treated with an immediate-release or intravenous theophylline preparation (or other bronchodilators) and not with controlled-release products.

II. Chronic Therapy
A. Initiating Therapy with an Immediate-Release Product
It is recommended that the appropriate dosage be established using an immediate-release preparation. Slow clinical titration is generally preferred to help assure acceptance and safety of the medication, and to allow the patient to develop tolerance to transient caffeine-like side effects. Then, if the total 24-hour dose can be given by use of the available strengths of this product, the patient can usually be switched to Slo-bid™ giving one-third of the daily dose at 8-hour intervals or one-half the daily dose at 12-hour intervals. Patients who metabolize theophylline rapidly, such as the young, smokers, and some non-smoking adults are the most likely candidates for dosing at 8-hour intervals. Such patients can generally be identified as having trough serum concentrations lower than desired or repeatedly exhibiting symptoms near the end of a dosing interval.

B. Initiating Therapy with Slo-bid™ Gyrocaps®
Alternatively, therapy can be initiated with Slo-bid™ Gyrocaps® since they are available in dosage strengths which permit titration and adjustments of dosage (in adults and older children). Children weighing less than 25 kg should have their daily dosage requirements established with Slo-Phyllin® 80 mg Syrup to permit small dosage increments.

Initial Dose: 16 mg/kg/24 hours or 400 mg/24 hours (whichever is less) of anhydrous theophylline in 2- or 3-divided doses at 8- or 12-hour intervals.

Increasing Dose: The above dosage may be increased in approximately 25 percent increments at 3-day intervals so long as the drug is tolerated. Following each adjustment, if the clinical response is satisfactory and serum levels can be measured, then such measurements should be obtained as directed under section IV (below). If serum levels cannot be obtained, then that dosage level should be maintained. Dosage increases may be made in this manner until the maximum dose indicated in section III (below) is reached.

C. Sprinkling Contents on Food
Slo-bid™ Gyrocaps® may be administered by carefully opening the capsule and sprinkling the beaded contents on a spoonful of soft food such as applesauce or pudding; the soft food should be swallowed immediately without chewing and followed with a glass of cool water or juice to ensure complete swallowing of the beads. It is recommended that the food used should not be hot and should be soft enough to be swallowed without chewing. Any bead/food mixture should be used immediately and not stored for future use. SUBDIVIDING THE CONTENTS OF A CAPSULE IS NOT RECOMMENDED.

III. Maximum Dose of Theophylline Where the Serum Concentration is Not Measured:

Warning: DO NOT ATTEMPT TO MAINTAIN ANY DOSE THAT IS NOT TOLERATED.

Not to exceed the following:
[See table below].

IV. Measurement of Serum Theophylline Concentrations During Chronic Therapy:
If the above maximum doses are to be maintained or exceeded, serum theophylline measurement is recommended. The serum sample should be obtained at the time of peak absorption, 1 to 2 hours after administration for immediate-release products and 5 hours after dosing for Slo-bid™ Gyrocaps®. It is important that the patient will have missed *no* doses during the previous 48 hours and that dosing intervals will have been reasonably typical with no added doses during that period of time. DOSAGE ADJUSTMENT BASED ON SERUM THEOPHYLLINE MEASUREMENTS WHEN THESE INSTRUCTIONS HAVE NOT BEEN FOLLOWED MAY RESULT IN RECOMMENDATIONS THAT PRESENT RISK OF TOXICITY TO THE PATIENT.

V. Final adjustment of Dosage: (see Table 1)

Table 1—Dosage adjustment after serum theophylline measurement.

If serum theophylline is:		*Directions:*
Within normal limits	10 to 20 μg/mL	Maintain dosage if tolerated. Recheck serum theophylline concentration at 6- to 12-month intervals.*
Too high	20 to 25 μg/mL	Decrease doses by about 10%. Recheck serum theophylline concentration at 6- to 12-month intervals.*
	25 to 30 μg/mL	Skip next dose and decrease subsequent doses by about 25%.
	Over 30 μg/mL	Skip next 2 doses and decrease subsequent doses by 50%. Recheck serum theophylline.
Too low	7.5 to 10 μg/mL	Increase dose by about 25%.** Recheck serum theophylline concentration at 6- to 12-month intervals.*
	5 to 7.5 μg/mL	Increase dose by about 25% to the nearest dose increment and recheck serum theophylline for guidance in further dosage adjustment (another increase will probably be needed, but this provides a safety check).

*Finer adjustments in dosage may be needed for some patients.

**Dividing the daily dose into 3 doses administered at 8-hour intervals may be indicated if symptoms occur repeatedly at the end of a dosing interval.

From the *Journal of Respiratory Diseases* 2 (7):16, 1981
Caution should be exercised for younger children who cannot complain of minor side effects. Older adults, those with cor pulmonale, congestive heart failure, and/or liver disease may have unusually low dosage requirements and thus may experience toxicity at the maximal dosage recommended above.

It is important that no patient be maintained on any dosage that is not tolerated. In instructing the patients to increase dosage according to the schedule above, they should be instructed not to take a subsequent dose if apparent side effects occur and to resume therapy at a lower dose once adverse effects have disappeared.

HOW SUPPLIED

Slo-bid™ Gyrocaps® 50 mg are available in bottles of 100 (NDC 0067-0057-68), bottles of 1000 (NDC 0067-0057-82) and in unit dose 10×10 (NDC 0067-0057-01), Slo-bid™ Gyrocaps® 100 mg are available in bottles of 100 (NDC 0067-0100-68), bottles of 1000 (NDC 0067-0100-82) and in unit dose 10×10 (NDC 0067-0100-01), Slo-bid™ Gyrocaps® 200 mg are available in bottles of 100 (NDC 0067-0200-68), bottles of 1000 (NDC 0067-0200-82) and in unit dose 10×10 (NDC 0067-0200-01), and Slo-bid™ Gyrocaps® 300 mg are available in bottles of 100 (NDC 0067-0300-68), bottles of 1000 (NDC 0067-0300-82) and in unit dose 10×10 (NDC 0067-0300-01).

Slo-bid™ Gyrocaps® are identified as follows:
50 mg—Clear (cap) and opaque white (body) capsule with WHR 50 mg printed in red on cap and body
100 mg—Clear capsule with WHR 100 printed in red on cap and body
200 mg—Opaque white (cap) and clear (body) capsule with WHR 200 printed in red on cap and body
300 mg—Opaque white capsule with WHR 300 printed in red on cap and body

STORAGE CONDITIONS

Store at room temperature. Protect from excessive heat, light, and moisture.

CAUTION

Federal law prohibits dispensing without prescription. Keep this and all medications out of the reach of children.
Jointly Manufactured by
WILLIAM H. RORER, INC.
AND PACO PHARMACEUTICAL SERVICES, INC.
Lakewood, NJ 08701
for
WILLIAM H. RORER, INC.
Fort Washington, PA, U.S.A. 19034
Printed in U.S.A.

Shown in Product Identification Section, page 426

SLO-PHYLLIN® ℞

(theophylline, anhydrous) SYRUP, TABLETS, (immediate release)
GYROCAPS® (timed release capsules)
[*slō"fil'in*]

DESCRIPTION

Slo-Phyllin® Gyrocaps® contain 60 mg, 125 mg, or 250 mg theophylline, anhydrous, in the form of long acting dye-free beads with a hard gelatin capsule and are intended for oral administration.

Slo-Phyllin® Tablets (theophylline, anhydrous) are scored, dye-free tablets providing 100 mg or 200 mg of theophylline, anhydrous.

Slo-Phyllin® 80 mg Syrup (theophylline, anhydrous) is a nonalcoholic, sugar-free solution containing per 15 mL theophylline, anhydrous, 80 mg with sodium benzoate, NF, 18 mg, and methylparaben, NF, 3 mg added as preservatives.

Theophylline is a bronchodilator and is a member of the xanthine class of chemical compounds related to both theobromine and caffeine.

Theophylline is a white odorless crystalline powder having a bitter taste.

Theophylline is 1-*H*-Purine-2,6-dione,3,7-dihydro-1,3-dimethyl, represented by the following structural formula:
[See Chemical Formula at top of next page].

			Dose per 8 hours	**Dose per 12 hours**
Age	6–9 years	24 mg/kg/day	8.0 mg/kg	12.0 mg/kg
Age	9–12 years	20 mg/kg/day	6.7 mg/kg	10.0 mg/kg
Age	12–16 years	18 mg/kg/day	6.0 mg/kg	9.0 mg/kg
Age	over 16 years	13 mg/kg/day OR 900 mg (*WHICHEVER IS LESS*)	4.3 mg/kg	6.5 mg/kg

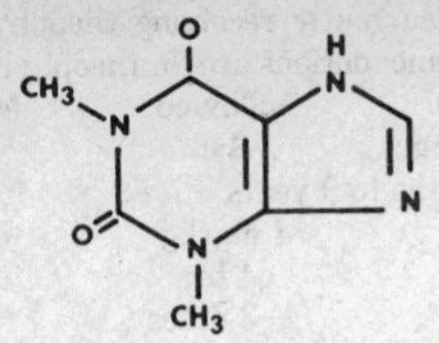

INACTIVE INGREDIENTS

Inactive ingredients in all strengths of Slo-Phyllin Gyrocaps are: FD&C Blue No. 1, gelatin, pharmaceutical glaze, silicon dioxide, sodium bisulfite, sodium lauryl sulfate, starch, sucrose, talc, titanium dioxide. The 60 mg gyrocaps also contain D & C Yellow No. 10, FD&C Red No. 40, FD&C Blue No. 2, iron oxide, propylene glycol. The 125 mg gyrocaps also contain D & C Yellow No. 10, D & C Red No. 28, FD&C Red No. 40, dimethylpolysiloxane, methylparaben, propylparaben, may contain soyalicithin. The 250 mg gyrocaps also contain D & C Red No. 28, dimethylpolysiloxane, may contain soya lecithin.

Syrup inactive ingredients are citric acid, FD&C Red No. 3, FD&C Yellow No. 6, flavors, glycerin, methylparaben, propylene glycol, sodium benzoate, saccharin sodium, sorbitol, purified water.

Tablets: 100 mg inactive ingredients are lactose, magnesium stearate, microcrystalline cellulose, sodium starch glycolate; 200 mg inactive ingredients are magnesium stearate, microcrystalline cellulose, sodium starch glycolate.

CLINICAL PHARMACOLOGY

Theophylline directly relaxes the smooth muscle of the bronchial airways and pulmonary blood vessels, thus acting mainly as a brochodilator and smooth muscle relaxant. The drug also produces other actions typical of the xanthine derivatives: cardiac stimulation, coronary vasodilatation, stimulation of skeletal muscle, cerebral stimulation, and diuresis. The action of theophylline may be mediated through inhibition of phosphodiesterase and a resultant increase in intracellular cyclic AMP.

In vitro, theophylline has been shown to act synergistically with beta agonists that increase intracellular cyclic AMP through the stimulation of adenyl cyclase but synergism has not been demonstrated in patient studies. More data are needed to determine if theophylline and beta agonists have a clinically important additive effect *in vivo.* Apparently, no development of tolerance occurs with chronic use of theophylline.

PHARMACOKINETICS

The half-life of theophylline is influenced by a number of known variables. It is prolonged in patients suffering from chronic alcoholism, impaired hepatic or renal function, congestive heart failure, and in patients receiving macrolide antibiotics and cimetidine. Older adults (over age 55) and patients with chronic obstructive pulmonary disease, with or without cor pulmonale, may also have much slower clearance rates. For such patients, the theophylline half-life may exceed 24 hours.

Newborns and neonates have extremely slow clearance rates compared to older infants (over 6 months) and children, and may also have a theophylline half-life of over 24 hours. High fever for prolonged periods may also reduce the rate of theophylline elimination.

Representative Theophylline Serum Half-Lives	Half-Life (hours)
Adults	
non-smokers	7-9
smokers	4-5
congestive heart failure	24
Children (6 months-16 years)	3-5

The half-life of theophylline in smokers (1 to 2 packs/day) averages 4-5 hours, much shorter than the half-life in non-smokers which averages 7-9 hours. The increase in theophylline clearance caused by smoking is probably the result of induction of drug-metabolizing enzymes that do not readily normalize after cessation of smoking. It appears that between 3 months and 2 years may be necessary for normalization of the effect of smoking on theophylline pharmacokinetics.

In single-dose bioavailability studies in normal volunteers, 300 mg Slo-Phyllin Syrup produced mean peak serum concentrations of 7.90 ± 1.67 μg/mL at a mean time of 1.43 ± 0.87 hours after dosing. At steady state in multiple dose bioavailability studies with four times a day dosing (600-1000 mg/day), the mean peak-trough variation was 4.39 ± 0.77 μg/mL.

In a single-dose three-way cross-over bioavailability study, 400 mg each of the 100 mg Slo-Phyllin tablet, the 200 mg tablet and Slo-Phyllin Syrup were given to 19 volunteers. The respective means ± standard error for the bioequivalence parameters were: peak concentration (C_{max}) 11.18 ± 0.38, 10.91 ± 0.39 and 11.17 ± 0.40 μg/mL; time of peak concentration (T_{max}) 1.67 ± 0.17, 1.84 ± 0.17 and 2.18 ± 0.21 hours; area under the curve, 0 to infinity ($AUC_{0-\infty}$) 120.53 ± 9.80, 121.29 ± 9.61 and 127.37 ± 9.40. There were no statistical differences between the formulations with regards to C_{max}, T_{max} or $AUC_{0-\infty}$. Bioavailability relative to the Syrup was 95% for the 100 mg tablet and 96% for the 200 mg tablet.

In a single-dose bioavailability study in 20 normal subjects, sustained-release Slo-Phyllin Gyrocaps were compared to the immediate-release Slo-Phyllin 80 Syrup. The mean bioavailability of the three strengths of Slo-Phyllin Gyrocaps ranged between 90 and 95%. A dose of 250 mg Slo-Phyllin Gyrocaps produced a mean peak serum concentration of 4.0 ± 0.8 μg/mL at a mean time of 4.8 hours after a single dose. At steady state in a multiple dose bioavailability study, Slo-Phyllin Gyrocaps were compared to Slo-Phyllin 80 Syrup. Doses of 2.6 to 5.6 mg/kg (mean dose of 4.2 mg/kg) of Slo-Phyllin Gyrocaps were administered q8h in 17 normal subjects. The mean peak serum concentration was 17.4 ± 0.9 μg/mL and the mean trough was 10.4 ± 0.7 μg/mL. In both of these studies, subjects fasted overnight before dosing and four hours after the first dose.

A multiple-dose bioequivalence study with 14 asthmatic children, ages 10–12, comparing Slo-Phyllin Gyrocaps administered as intact capsules and as the beaded contents sprinkled on applesauce with q8h dosing (125–250 mg/day) indicated no significant differences in maximum and minimum theophylline concentrations, time to achieve peak concentration, and peak-trough differences. The bioavailability as measured by comparing area under the curves ($AUC_{0-8\ hours}$ granules/$AUC_{0-8\ hours}$ capsules) was 0.999 ± 0.324.

INDICATIONS AND USE

For relief and/or prevention of symptoms of asthma and reversible bronchospasm associated with chronic bronchitis and emphysema.

CONTRAINDICATIONS

Slo-Phyllin Tablets, Syrup, and Gyrocaps are contraindicated in individuals who have shown hypersensitivity to any of their components.

WARNINGS

Status asthmaticus should be considered a medical emergency and is defined as that degree of bronchospasm which is not rapidly responsive to usual doses of conventional bronchodilators. Optimal therapy for such patients frequently requires both *additional medication,* parenterally administered, and *close monitoring,* preferably in an intensive care setting. Although increasing the dose of theophylline may bring about relief, such treatment may be associated with toxicity. The likelihood of such toxicity developing increases significantly when the serum theophylline concentration exceeds 20 μg/mL. Therefore, determination of serum theophylline levels is recommended to assure maximal benefit without excessive risk.

Serum levels above 20 μg/mL are rarely found after appropriate administration of the recommended doses. However, in individuals in whom theophylline plasma clearance is reduced *for any reason,* even conventional doses may result in increased serum levels and potential toxicity. Reduced theophylline clearance has been documented in the following readily identifiable groups: 1) patients with impaired renal or liver function, 2) patients over 55 years of age, particularly males and those with chronic lung disease, 3) those with cardiac failure from any cause, 4) neonates, and 5) those patients taking certain drugs (macrolide antibiotics and cimetidine). Decreased clearance of theophylline may be associated with either influenza immunization or active infection with influenza.

Reduction of dosage and laboratory monitoring is especially appropriate in the above individuals.

Less serious signs of theophylline toxicity, i.e. nausea and restlessness, may appear in up to 50% of patients.

Unfortunately, however, serious side effects such as ventricular arrhythmias, convulsions, or even death may appear as the first sign of toxicity without any previous warning. Stated differently, *serious toxicity is not reliably preceded by less severe side effects.*

Many patients who require theophylline may exhibit tachycardia due to their underlying disease process so that the cause/effect relationship to elevated serum theophylline concentrations may not be appreciated.

Theophylline products may cause dysrhythmia and/or worsen preexisting arrhythmias and any significant change in rate and/or rhythm warrants monitoring and further investigation.

The occurrence of arrhythmias and sudden death (with histological evidence of necrosis of the myocardium) has been recorded in laboratory animals (minipigs, rodents, and dogs) when theophylline and beta agonists were administered concomitantly, although not when either was administered alone. The significance of these findings when applied to human usage is currently unknown.

PRECAUTIONS

General: Mean half-life in smokers is shorter than non-smokers. Therefore, smokers may require larger or more frequent doses of theophylline. Morphine and curare should be used with caution in patients with airway obstruction as they may suppress respiration and stimulate histamine release. Alternative drugs should be used when possible.

Theophylline should not be administered concurrently with other xanthine preparations. Use with caution in patients with severe cardiac disease, severe hypoxemia, hypertension, hyperthyroidism, acute myocardial injury, cor pulmonale, congestive heart failure, alcoholism, liver disease, and in the elderly, especially males, and neonates. Great caution should be used in giving theophylline to patients with congestive heart failure. Frequently such patients have shown markedly prolonged theophylline blood levels with theophylline persisting in serum for long periods following discontinuation of the drug. Use theophylline cautiously in patients with a history of peptic ulcer. Theophylline may occasionally act as a local gastrointestinal irritant, although GI symptoms are more commonly centrally mediated and associated with serum drug concentrations over 20 μg/mL.

INFORMATION FOR PATIENTS

The physician should reinforce the importance of taking only the prescribed dose at the prescribed time intervals. The patient should alert the physician if symptoms occur repeatedly, especially near the end of a dosing interval.

DRUG INTERACTIONS

Drug-Drug: Toxic synergism with ephedrine has been documented and may occur with some other sympathomimetic bronchodilators. In addition, the following drug interactions have been demonstrated:

DRUG	EFFECT
Aminophylline with lithium carbonate	Increased excretion of lithium carbonate
Aminophylline with propranolol	Increased theophylline serum concentrations. Antagonism of propranolol effects
Theophylline with troleandomycin or erythromycin	Increased theophylline serum concentrations
Theophylline with cimetidine	Increased theophylline serum concentrations

Drug-Food: Slo-Phyllin Gyrocaps has not been adequately studied to determine whether its bioavailability is altered when it is given with food.

Available data suggest that drug administration at the time of food ingestion may influence the absorption characteristics of some or all theophylline controlled-release products resulting in serum values different from those found after administration in the fasting state.

A drug-food effect, if any, would likely have its greatest clinical significance when high theophylline serum levels are being maintained and/or when large single doses (greater than 13 mg/kg or 900 mg) of a controlled-release product are given. The influence of the type and amount of food on performance of controlled-release theophylline products is under study at this time.

Drug/Laboratory Test Interactions: When plasma levels of theophylline are measured by spectrophotometric methods, coffee, tea, cola beverages, chocolate, and acetaminophen contribute falsely high values.

Carcinogenesis, Mutagenesis, Impairment of Fertility: Long-term animal studies have not been performed to evaluate the carcinogenic potential, mutagenic potential, or the effect on fertility of xanthine compounds.

Pregnancy: Pregnancy Category C—Animal reproduction studies have not been conducted with theophylline. It is not known whether theophylline can cause fetal harm when administered to a pregnant woman or can affect reproduction capacity. Theophylline should be given to a pregnant woman only if clearly needed.

Nursing Mothers: It has been reported that theophylline distributes readily into breast milk and may cause adverse effects in the infant. Caution must be used if prescribing xanthines to a mother who is nursing, taking into account the risk-benefit of this therapy.

Pediatric Use: Due to the marked variation in theophylline metabolism in infants under 6 months of age, theophylline is not recommended for this age group.

Safety and effectiveness in children under 6 years of age have not been established with controlled-release theophylline products.

Continued on next page

This product information was prepared in August 1986. Information concerning these products may be obtained by addressing William H. Rorer, Inc., 500 Virginia Drive, Fort Washington, PA 19034.

Rorer—Cont.

ADVERSE REACTIONS

The most consistent adverse reactions are usually due to overdose and are:

Gastrointestinal: nausea, vomiting, epigastric pain, hematemesis, and diarrhea.

Central nervous system: headaches, irritability, restlessness, insomnia, reflex hyperexcitability, muscle twitching, and clonic and tonic generalized convulsions.

Cardiovascular: palpitation, tachycardia, extrasystoles, flushing, hypotension, circulatory failure, and ventricular arrhythmias.

Respiratory: tachypnea.

Renal: albuminuria, increased excretion of renal tubular cells and red blood cells, potentiation of diuresis.

Other: hyperglycemia, inappropriate ADH syndrome and rash.

OVERDOSAGE

Management: A. If potential oral overdose is established and seizure has not occurred

1. Induce vomiting
2. Administer a cathartic (this is particularly important if sustained-release preparations have been taken)
3. Administer activated charcoal
4. Monitor vital signs, maintain blood pressure, and provide adequate hydration

B. If patient is having a seizure:

1. Establish an airway
2. Administer oxygen
3. Treat the seizure with intravenous diazepam 0.1 to 0.3 mg/kg up to a total dose of 10 mg
4. Monitor vital signs, maintain blood pressure and provide adequate hydration

C. Post-seizure Coma:

1. Maintain airway and oxygenation
2. If a result of oral medication, follow above recommendations to prevent absorption of drug, but intubation and lavage will have to be performed instead of inducing emesis and the cathartic and charcoal will need to be introduced via a large bore gastric lavage tube.
3. Continue to provide full supportive care and adequate hydration while waiting for drug to be metabolized. In general, the drug is metabolized sufficiently rapidly so as to not warrant consideration of dialysis. However, if serum levels exceed 50 μg/mL, charcoal hemoperfusion may be indicated.

DOSAGE AND ADMINISTRATION

Studies to determine the bioavailability of Slo-Phyllin Gyrocaps when administered with food are being initiated. (See PRECAUTIONS, Drug-Food Interactions.)

For most patients, *effective use* of theophylline, i.e. associated with optimal likelihood of benefit combined with minimal risk of toxicity, is considered to occur when serum levels are maintained between 10 and 20 μg/mL. Levels above 20 μg/ml may produce toxicity, and in a small number of patients, toxicity may even be seen with serum levels between 15–20 μg/mL, particularly during initiation of therapy.

There is considerable variation from patient to patient in the dosage required to achieve and maintain therapeutic and safe levels, primarily due to variable rates of elimination. Therefore, it is essential that not only must dosage be individualized, but titration and monitoring of serum levels be utilized where available. When serum concentration cannot be obtained, restriction of dosage to the amounts and intervals recommended in the guidelines listed below becomes essential. Dosage should be calculated on the basis of lean (ideal) body weight where mg/kg doses are presented. Theophylline does not distribute into fatty tissue. Giving immediate-release theophylline with food may prevent some local gastric irritation and though absorption is slower, it is still complete.

Frequency of Dosing: When immediate-release products with rapid absorption (such as tablets or liquid) are used, dosing to maintain serum levels generally requires administration every 6 hours. This is particularly true in children, but dosing intervals up to 8 hours may be satisfactory in adults since they eliminate the drug at a slower rate. Some children, and adults requiring higher than average doses (those having rapid rates of clearance, e.g. half-lives of under 6 hours) may benefit and be more effectively controlled during chronic therapy when given products with sustained-release characteristics since these provide longer dosing intervals and/or less fluctuation in serum concentration between dosing. Those sustained-release products which provide flexibility in dosage through formulations of varying strengths are also helpful in controlling serum levels. Dosage guidelines are approximations only and the wide range of theophylline clearance between individuals (particularly those with concomitant disease) make indiscriminate usage hazardous.

As a practical consideration, it is not always possible to obtain serum level determinations. Under such conditions, restriction of the daily dose (*in otherwise healthy adults*) to not greater than 13 mg/kg/day (or up to 900 mg) of anhydrous theophylline in divided doses will result in relatively few patients exceeding serum levels of 20 μg/mL and the resultant risk of toxicity.

Dosage Guidelines:

Slo-Phyllin® Gyrocaps®

I. Acute Symptoms

Slo-Phyllin Gyrocaps are not intended for patients experiencing an acute episode of bronchospasm (associated with asthma, chronic bronchitis, or emphysema). Such patients require *rapid* relief of symptoms and should be treated with an immediate-release or intravenous theophylline preparation (or other bronchodilators) and not with controlled-release products.

II. Chronic Therapy

A. Initiating Therapy with an Immediate-Release Product

It is recommended that the appropriate dosage be established using an immediate-release preparation. Children weighing less than 25 kg should have their daily dosage requirements established with Slo-Phyllin 80 mg Syrup to permit small dosage increments. Slow clinical titration is generally preferred to help assure acceptance and safety of the medication. Then, if the total 24-hour dose can be given by use of the sustained-release product, the patient can usually be switched to Slo-Phyllin Gyrocaps, giving one-third of the daily dose at 8-hour intervals or one-half the daily dose at 12-hour intervals. Patients who metabolize theophylline rapidly, such as the young, smokers, and some non-smoking adults are the most likely candidates for dosing at 8-hour intervals. Such patients can generally be identified as having trough serum concentrations lower than desired, or repeatedly exhibiting symptoms near the end of a dosing interval.

B. Initiating Therapy with Slo-Phyllin Gyrocaps

Alternatively, therapy can be initiated with Slo-Phyllin Gyrocaps since they are available in dosage strengths which permit titration and adjustments of dosage (in adults and older children).

Initial Dose:

16 mg/kg/24 hours of 400 mg/24 hours (whichever is less) of anhydrous theophylline in 2- or 3-divided doses at 8- or 12-hour intervals.

Increasing Dose:

The above dosage may be increased in approximately 25 percent increments at 3-day intervals so long as the drug is tolerated, until the maximum dose indicated in section III (below) is reached.

C. Sprinkling Contents on Food

Slo-Phyllin Gyrocaps may be administered by carefully opening the capsule and sprinkling the beaded contents on a spoonful of soft food such as applesauce or pudding; the soft food should be swallowed immediately without chewing and followed with a glass of cool water or juice to ensure complete swallowing of the beads. It is recommended that the food used should not be hot and should be soft enough to be swallowed without chewing. Any bead/food mixture should be used immediately and not stored for future use. Until additional bioavailability data are available, it is recommended that dosing using the sprinkling technique be at intervals up to 8 hours. It is recommended that dosing not take place at mealtime until a study is completed to show the effect of taking Slo-Phyllin Gyrocaps with food as compared to the fasting state.

III. Maximum Dose of Theophylline Where the Serum Concentration is Not Measured:

[See table below].

Slo-Phyllin® Tablets and Syrup

1. Acute Symptoms of Asthma Requiring Rapid Theophyllinization.

WARNING do not attempt to maintain any dose that is not tolerated. Not to exceed the following:

				Dose per 8 hours	*Dose per 12 hours*
Age	6–9	years	24 mg/kg /day	8.0 mg/kg	12.0 mg/kg
Age	9–12	years	20 mg/kg/day	6.7 mg/kg	10.0 mg/kg
Age	12–16	years	18 mg/kg/day	6.0 mg/kg	9.0 mg/kg
Age	over 16	years	13 mg/kg/day OR 900 mg (WHICHEVER IS LESS)	4.3 mg/kg	6.5 mg/kg

A. Patients not currently receiving theophylline products. Dosage recommendations are for theophylline anhydrous.

	Oral Loading:	Followed By:	Maintenance:
Children 6 months to 9 years	6 mg/kg	4 mg/kg q4 hrs × 3 doses	4 mg/kg q6 hrs
Children age 9–16 years and young adult smokers	6 mg/kg	3 mg/kg q4 hrs × 3 doses	3 mg/kg q6 hrs
Otherwise healthy non-smoking adults	6 mg/kg	3 mg/kg q6 hrs × 2 doses	3 mg/kg q8 hrs
Older patients and patients with cor pulmonale	6 mg/kg	2 mg/kg q6 hrs × 2 doses	2 mg/kg q8 hrs
Patients with congestive heart failure	6 mg/kg	2 mg/kg q8 hrs × 2 doses	1–2 mg/kg q12 hrs

B. Patients currently receiving theophylline products: Determine, where possible, the time, amount, dosage form, and route of administration of the patient's last dose.

The loading dose for theophylline is based on the principle that each 0.5 mg/kg of theophylline administered as a loading dose will result in a 1.0 μg/mL increase in serum theophylline concentration. Ideally, the loading dose should be deferred if a serum theophylline concentration can be obtained rapidly.

If this is not possible, the clinician must exercise his judgment in selecting a dose based on the potential for benefit and risk. Where there is sufficient respiratory distress to warrant a small risk, then 2.5 mg/kg of theophylline administered in rapidly absorbed form is likely to increase serum concentration by approximately 5 μg/mL. If the patient is not experiencing theophylline toxicity, this is likely to result in dangerous adverse affects.

Subsequent to the decision regarding modification of the loading dose for this group of patients, the maintenance dosage recommendations are the same as those described above.

II. Chronic Therapy

Theophylline administration is a treatment of first choice for the management of chronic asthma (to prevent symptoms and maintain patent airways). Slow clinical titration is generally preferred to assure acceptance and safety of the medications.

INITIAL DOSE

16 mg/kg/24 hours or 400 mg/24 hours (whichever is less) of anhydrous theophylline in 3- to 4-divided doses at 6- or 8-hour intervals.

INCREASING DOSE

The above dosage may be increased in approximately 25-percent increments at 2- to 3-day intervals so long as the drug is tolerated, until the maximum dose indicated in section III (below) is reached.

III. Maximum Dose of Theophylline Where the Serum Concentration is Not Measured:

WARNING DO NOT ATTEMPT TO MAINTAIN ANY DOSE THAT IS NOT TOLERATED.

Not to exceed the following:

	Dose per 6 hours	Dose per 8 hours
Age <9 years 24 mg/kg/day	6.0 mg/kg	8.0 mg/kg
Age 9–12 years 20 mg/kg/day	5.0 mg/kg	6.7 mg/kg
Age 12–16 years 18 mg/kg/day	4.5 mg/kg	6.0 mg/kg
Age >16 years 13 mg/kg/day OR 900 mg (WHICHEVER IS LESS)	3.5 mg/kg	4.3 mg/kg

IV. Measurement of Serum Theophylline Concentrations During Chronic Therapy:

If the above maximum doses are to be maintained or exceeded, serum theophylline measurement is recommended. The serum sample should be obtained at the time of peak absorption, 1 to 2 hours after administration for immediate-release products and 4 hours after dosing for Slo-Phyllin® Gyrocaps®. It is important that the patient will have missed *no* doses during the previous 48 hours and that dosing intervals will have been reasonably typical with no added doses during that period of time. DOSAGE ADJUSTMENT BASED ON SERUM THEOPHYLLINE MEASUREMENTS WHEN THESE INSTRUCTIONS HAVE NOT BEEN FOL-

LOWED MAY RESULT IN RECOMMENDATIONS THAT PRESENT RISK OF TOXICITY TO THE PATIENT.

V. Final Adjustment of Dosage: (see Table 1)

Table 1—Dosage adjustment after serum theophylline measurement

If serum theophylline is:		*Directions:*
Within normal limits	10 to 20 μg/mL	Maintain dosage if tolerated. Recheck serum theophylline concentration at 6- to 12-month intervals.*
Too high	20 to 25 μg/mL	Decrease doses by about 10%. Recheck serum theophylline concentration at 6- to 12-month intervals.*
	25 to 30 μg/mL	Skip next dose and decrease subsequent doses by about 25%.
	Over 30 μg/mL	Skip next 2 doses and decrease subsequent doses by 50%. Recheck serum theophylline concentration.
Too low	7.5 to 10 μg/mL	Increase dose by about 25%.** Recheck serum theophylline concentration at 6- to 12-month intervals.*
	5 to 7.5 μg/mL	Increase dose by about 25% to the nearest dose increment and recheck serum theophylline for guidance in further dosage adjustment (another increase will probably be needed, but this provides a safety check).

*Finer adjustments in dosage may be needed for some patients

**The total daily dose may need to be administered at more frequent intervals if symptoms occur repeatedly at the end of dosing interval.

From the *Journal of Respiratory Diseases* 2 (7):16, 1981

Caution should be exercised for younger children who cannot complain of minor side effects. Older adults, those with cor pulmonale, congestive heart failure, and/or liver disease may have unusually low dosage requirements and thus may experience toxicity at the maximal dosage recommended above. It is important that no patient be maintained on any dosage that is not tolerated. In instructing the patients to increase dosage according to the schelule above, they should be instructed not to take a subsequent dose if apparent side effects occur and to resume therapy at a lower dose once adverse effects have disappeared.

HOW SUPPLIED

Slo-Phyllin 100 mg Tablets (theophylline, anhydrous) scored, dye-free, white, round, convex tablet, imprinted "WHR 351" in bottles of 100 (NDC-0067-0351-68) and 1000 (NDC-0067-0351-82), and in unit dose packages of 100 tablets (NDC-0067-0351-01).

Slo-Phyllin 200 mg Tablets (theophylline, anhydrous), scored, dye-free, white, flat faced tablet, imprinted "WHR 352" in bottles of 100 (NDC-0067-0352-68) and 1000 (NDC-0067-0352-82), and in unit dose packages of 100 tablets (NDC 0067-0352-01).

Slo-Phyllin® 80 mg Syrup theophylline, anhydrous 80 mg per 15 mL nonalcoholic, orange color in 4 fl oz (NDC-0067-0354-60), pint (NDC-0067-0354-16) and gallon (NDC-0067-0354-28) bottles, and 15 mL unit dose cups (NDC-0067-0354-15).

Slo-Phyllin® Gyrocaps® 60 mg are available in bottles of 100 (NDC-0067-1354-68) and 1000 (NDC-0067-1354-82). Slo-Phyllin® Gyrocaps® 125 mg are available in bottles of 100 (NDC-0067-1355-68), 1000 (NDC-0067-1355-82) and unit dose strip packages (NDC-0067-1355-01). Slo-Phyllin® Gyrocaps® 250 mg are available in bottles of 100 (NDC-0067-1356-68), 1000 (NDC-0067-1356-82) and unit dose strip packages (NDC-0067-1356-01).

Slo-Phyllin® Gyrocaps® are identified as follows:

60 mg—white capsule with WHR 1354 printed in black on body and cap, containing dye-free beads

125 mg—brown capsule with WHR 1355 printed in white on body and cap, containing dye-free beads.

250 mg—purple capsule with WHR 1356 printed in white on body and cap, containing dye-free beads.

Theophylline Elimination Characteristics

	Theophylline Clearance Rates (mean±S.D.)	Half-life Average (mean±S.D.)
Children (over 6 months of age):	1.45±.58 mL/kg/min	3.7±1.1 hours
Adult non-smokers with uncomplicated asthma:	.65±.19 mL/kg/min	8.7±2.2 hours

STORAGE CONDITIONS

Store at room temperature. Protect from excessive heat, light, and moisture.

CAUTION

Federal law prohibits dispensing without prescription. Keep this and all medications out of the reach of children.

Slo-Phyllin® Gyrocaps® are manufactured by
CORD LABORATORIES, INC.
Broomfield, CO 80020
For
WILLIAM H. RORER, INC.
Fort Washington, PA, USA 19034
Slo-Phyllin® Tablets and Syrup are manufactured by
WILLIAM H. RORER, INC.
Fort Washington, PA, USA 19034

Shown in Product Identification Section, page 426

SLO-PHYLLIN® GG CAPSULES, SYRUP

℞

[*slō"fĭl'in*]
(theophylline—Guaifenesin)

DESCRIPTION

Each **Slo-Phyllin® GG** soft gelatin capsule or tablespoonful (15 mL) of liquid contains 150 mg of theophylline (anhydrous) and 90 mg of guaifenesin, as an oral bronchodilator-expectorant. Theophylline (1-*H*-Purine-2,6-dione,3,7-dihydro-1, 3-dimethyl-), a xanthine compound, is a white, odorless crystalline powder, with a bitter, aromatic taste. Guaifenesin (3-[2-methoxyphenoxy] 1,2-Propanediol), a guaiacol compound, is a white to slightly yellow crystalline powder with a bitter, aromatic taste.

Inactive Ingredients: Slo-Phyllin® GG Capsules: black iron oxide, dimethylpolysiloxane, FD&C Blue No. 1, gelatin, glycerin, lecithin, methylparaben, pharmaceutical glaze, polyethylene glycol, propylparaben, sorbitol, titanium dioxide. Slo-Phyllin® GG Syrup: citric acid, flavors, glycerin, methylparaben, propylene glycol, saccharin sodium, sodium benzoate, sorbitol solution, sucrose, purified water.

CLINICAL PHARMACOLOGY

Theophylline: Theophylline directly relaxes the smooth muscle of the bronchial airways and pulmonary blood vessels, thus acting mainly as a bronchodilator, pulmonary vasodilator and smooth muscle relaxant. The drug also possesses other actions typical of the xanthine derivatives: coronary vasodilator, diuretic, cardiac stimulant, cerebral stimulant, and skeletal muscle stimulant. The actions of theophylline may be mediated through inhibition of phosphodiesterase and a resultant increase in intracellular cyclic AMP, which could mediate smooth muscle relaxation. At concentrations higher than attained *in vivo*, theophylline also inhibits the release of histamine by mast cells.

In vitro, theophylline has been shown to react synergistically with beta agonists that increase intracellular cyclic AMP through the stimulation of adenyl cyclase (isoproterenol), but synergism has not been demonstrated in patient studies and more data are needed to determine if theophylline and beta agonists have clinically important additive effects *in vivo*. Apparently, no development of tolerance occurs with chronic use of theophylline.

The half-life is shortened with cigarette smoking. The half-life is prolonged in alcoholism, reduced hepatic or renal function, congestive heart failure, and in patients receiving antibiotics such as TAO (troleandomycin), erthromycin and clindamycin. High fever for prolonged periods may decrease theophylline elimination.

[See table above].

Newborn infants have extremely slow clearances and half-lives exceeding 24 hours which approach those seen for older children after about 3-6 months.

Older adults with chronic obstructive pulmonary disease, any patients with cor pulmonale or other causes of heart failure, and patients with liver pathology may have much lower clearances with half-lives that may exceed 24 hours.

The half-life of theophylline in smokers (1 to 2 packs/day) averaged 4 to 5 hours among various studies, much shorter than the half-life in non-smokers who averaged about 7 to 9 hours. The increase in theophylline clearance caused by smoking is probably the result of induction of drug-metabolizing enzymes that do not readily normalize after cessation of smoking. It appears that between 3 months and 2 years may be necessary for normalization of the effect of smoking on theophylline pharmacokinetics.

Guaifenesin: Guaifenesin increases respiratory tract secretions, possibly by stimulating the Goblet cells. Guaifenesin appears to be well absorbed, but its pharmacokinetics have not been thoroughly studied.

INDICATIONS AND USAGE

For relief and/or prevention of symptoms of asthma and reversible bronchospasm associated with chronic bronchitis and emphysema.

CONTRAINDICATIONS

In individuals who have shown hypersensitivity to any of the components.

WARNINGS

Status asthmaticus is a medical emergency. Optimal therapy frequently requires additional medication including corticosteroids when the patient is not rapidly responsive to bronchodilators.

Excessive theophylline doses may be associated with toxicity. Therefore, monitoring of serum theophylline levels is recommended to assure maximal benefit without excessive risk. Incidence of toxicity increases at levels greater than 20 μg/mL. Morphine, curare, and stilbamidine should be used with caution in patients with airflow obstruction since they stimulate histamine release and can induce asthmatic attacks. They may also suppress respiration leading to respiratory failure. Alternative drugs should be chosen whenever possible.

There is an excellent correlation between high blood levels of theophylline resulting from conventional doses and associated clinical manifestations of toxicity in (1) patients with lowered body plasma clearances (due to transient cardiac decompensation), (2) patients with liver dysfunction or chronic obstructive lung disease, (3) patients who are older than 55 years of age, particularly males. There are often no early signs of less serious theophylline toxicity such as nausea and restlessness, which may appear in up to 50 percent of patients prior to onset of convulsions. Ventricular arrhythmias or seizures may be the first signs of toxicity.

Many patients who have higher theophylline serum levels exhibit tachycardia.

Theophylline products may worsen pre-existing arrhythmias.

PRECAUTIONS

General: Theophylline.

Mean half-life in smokers is shorter than non-smokers, therefore, smokers may require larger doses of theophylline. Theophylline should not be administered concurrently with other xanthine medications. Use with caution in patients with severe cardiac disease, severe hypoxemia, hypertension, hyperthyroidism, acute myocardial injury, cor pulmonale, congestive heart failure, liver disease, and in the elderly (especially males) and in neonates. Great caution should especially be used in giving theophylline to patients in congestive heart failure. Such patients have shown markedly prolonged theophylline blood level curves with theophylline persisting in serum for long periods following discontinuation of the drug.

Use theophylline cautiously in patients with history of peptic ulcer. Theophylline may occasionally act as a local irritant to the G.I. tract although gastrointestinal symptoms are more commonly central and associated with serum concentrations over 20 μg/mL.

DRUG INTERACTIONS

Toxic synergism with ephedrine has been documented and may occur with some other sympathomimetic bronchodilators.

DRUG	EFFECT
Aminophylline with Lithium Carbonate	Increased excretion of Lithium Carbonate
Aminophylline with Propranolol	Antagonism of Propranolol effect

Continued on next page

This product information was prepared in August 1986. Information concerning these products may be obtained by addressing William H. Rorer, Inc., 500 Virginia Drive, Fort Washington, PA 19034.

Rorer—Cont.

Theophylline with Furosemide	Increased diuresis of Furosemide
Theophylline with Hexamethonium	Decreased Hexamethonium-induced chronotropic effect
Theophylline with Reserpine	Reserpine-induced Tachycardia
Theophylline with Chlordiazepoxide	Chlordiazepoxide-induced fatty acid mobilization
Theophylline with Cyclamycin (TAO= troleandomycin): erythromycin, clindamycin, lincomycin	Increased Theophylline plasma levels

Drug/Laboratory Test Interactions: Theophylline may increase uric acid levels and urinary catecholamines. Metabolites of guaifenesin may contribute to increased urinary 5-hydroxy-indoleacetic acid readings, when determined with nitrosonaphthol reagent.

Carcinogenicity, Mutagenesis, Impairment of Fertility: Long-term animal studies have not been performed to evaluate the carcinogenic potential, mutagenic potential, or the effect on fertility by xanthine compounds.

USAGE IN PREGNANCY

Teratogenic effects:

Pregnancy Category C—Animal reproduction studies have not been conducted with **Slo-Phyllin® GG.** It is also not known whether **Slo-Phyllin® GG** can cause fetal harm when administered to a pregnant woman or can affect reproduction capacity. Therefore, it should be given to a pregnant woman only if clearly needed.

Nonteratogenic effects:

Theophylline may be excreted in the milk and cause irritability in the nursing infant. Therefore, caution should be exercised when **Slo-Phyllin® GG** is administered to a nursing mother.

ADVERSE REACTIONS

The frequency of adverse reactions is related to serum theophylline levels and is usually not a problem at levels below 20 μg/mL. The most consistent adverse reactions are usually due to overdosage and, while all have not been reported with **Slo-Phyllin® GG,** the following reactions may be considered when theophylline is administered. Central nervous system: clonic and tonic generalized convulsions, muscle twitching, reflex hyperexcitability, headaches, insomnia, restlessness, and irritability. Cardiovascular: circulatory failure, life threatening ventricular ar- rhythmias, hypotension, extrasystoles, tachycardia, palpitation, and flushing. Gastrointestinal: hematemesis, vomiting, diarrhea, epigastric pain, and nausea. Renal: increased excretion of renal tubular cells and red blood cells, albuminuria, and potentiation of diuresis. Respiratory: tachypnea. Other: hyperglycemia and inappropriate ADH syndrome.

OVERDOSAGE

Symptoms

Nervousness, agitation, headache, insomnia, vomiting, tachycardia, extrasystoles, hyperreflexia, fasciculations and clonic and tonic convulsions. Children may be particularly prone to restlessness and hyperactivity that can proceed to convulsions.

Management

A. If potential oral overdose is established and seizure has not occurred.
   1. Induce vomiting.
   2. Administer a cathartic (this is particularly important if sustained-release preparations have been taken).
   3. Administer activated charcoal.
   4. Monitor vital signs, maintain blood pressure and provide adequate hydration.

B. If patient is having a seizure.
   1. Establish an airway.
   2. Administer oxygen.
   3. Treat the seizure with intravenous diazepam 0.1 to 0.3 mg/kg up to 10 mg.
   4. Monitor vital signs, maintain blood pressure and provide adequate hydration.

C. Post-seizure coma.
   1. Maintain airway and oxygenation.
   2. If a result of oral medication, follow above recommendations to prevent absorption of drug, but intubation and lavage will have to be performed instead of inducing emesis and the cathartic and charcoal will need to be introduced via a large bore gastric lavage tube.
   3. Continue to provide full supportive care and adequate hydration while waiting for drug to be metabolized. In general, the drug is metabolized sufficiently rapidly enough so as to not warrant consideration of dialysis.

D. Animal studies suggest that phenobarbital may decrease theophylline toxicity. There are as yet, however, insufficient data to recommend pretreatment of an overdosage with phenobarbital.

General

The oral LD_{50} of the theophylline in mice is 350 mg/kg. The oral LD_{50} of guaifenesin in mice is 1725 mg/kg. In humans, adverse reactions often occur when serum theophylline levels exceed 20 μg/mL. Information of physiological variables which influence excretion of theophylline can be found under the heading "Clinical Pharmacology."

DOSAGE AND ADMINISTRATION

General

Therapeutic serum levels associated with optimal likelihood for benefit and minimal risk of toxicity are considered to be between 10 μg/mL and 20 μg/mL. Levels above 20 μg/mL may produce toxic effects. There is great variation from patient to patient in dosage needed in order to achieve a therapeutic blood level because of variable rates of elimination. Because of this wide variation from patient to patient and the relatively narrow therapeutic blood level range, dosage must be individualized and monitoring of serum theophylline levels is highly recommended.

Dosage should be calculated on the basis of lean (ideal) body weight where mg/kg doses are stated. Theophylline does not distribute into fatty tissue.

Giving theophylline with food may prevent the rare case of stomach irritation and, although absorption may be slower, it is still complete.

When rapidly absorbed products such as solutions and soft gelatin capsules with rapid dissolution are used, dosing to maintain "around the clock" blood levels generally requires administration every 6 hours to obtain the greatest efficacy for clinical use in children; dosing intervals up to 8 hours may be satisfactory for adults because of their slower elimination. Children and adults requiring higher than average doses may benefit from products with slower absorption which may allow longer dosing intervals and/or less fluctuation in serum concentration over a dosing interval during chronic therapy.

Acute symptoms of asthma requiring rapid theophyllinization

Note: Due to their slower rate of absorption, sustained release theophylline products are not designed for use in conditions requiring rapid theophyllinization.

I. Not currently receiving theophylline products. [See table below].

II. Those currently receiving theophylline products: Determine, where possible, the time, amount, route of administration and form of the patient's last dose.

The loading dose for theophylline will be based on the principle that each .5 mg/kg of theophylline administered as a loading dose will result in a 1 μg/mL increase in serum theophylline concentration. Ideally, then, the loading dose should be deferred if a serum theophylline concentration can be rapidly obtained. If this is not possible, the clinician must exercise for judgment and select a dose based on the potential for benefit and risk. When there is sufficient respiratory distress to warrant a small risk, 2.5 mg/kg of theophylline is likely to increase the serum concentration when administered as a loading dose in rapidly absorbed form by only about 5 μg/mL. If the patient is not already experiencing theophylline toxicity, this is unlikely to result in dangerous adverse effects.

Subsequent to the modified decision regarding the loading dose in this group of patients, subsequent maintenance dosage recommendations are the same as those described above.

Comments: To achieve optimal therapeutic theophylline dosage, it is recommended to monitor serum theophylline concentrations. However, it is not always possible or practical to obtain a serum theophylline level.

Patients should be closely monitored for signs of toxicity. The present data suggest that the above dosage recommendations will achieve therapeutic serum concentrations with minimal risk of toxicity for most patients. However, some risk of toxic serum concentration is still present. Adverse reactions to theophylline often occur when serum theophylline levels exceed 20 μg/mL.

Chronic Asthma: Theophyllinization is a treatment of first choice for the management of chronic asthma (to prevent symptoms and maintain patent airways). Slow clinical titration is generally preferred to assure acceptance and safety of the medication.

Initial dose: 16 mg/kg/day or 400 mg/day (whichever is lower) in 3 to 4 divided doses at 6-to 8-hour intervals for the Syrup and Capsules.

Increased dose: The above dosage may be increased in approximately 25 percent increments at 2-to 3-day intervals so long as no intolerance is observed, until the maximum indicated below is reached.

Maximum dose without measurement of serum concentration:

Not to exceed the following: **(WARNING: DO NOT ATTEMPT TO MAINTAIN ANY DOSE THAT IS NOT TOLERATED.)**

Age 6 months to 9 years .... 24 mg/kg/day
Age 9 to 12 years .... 20 mg/kg/day
Age 12 to 16 years .... 18 mg/kg/day
Age > 16 years .... 13 mg/kg/day or 900 mg/day (WHICHEVER IS LESS)

Note: Use ideal body weight for obese patients.

Measurement of serum theophylline concentration during chronic therapy:

If the above maximum doses are to be maintained or exceeded, serum theophylline measurement is recommended. This should be obtained at the approximate time of peak absorption during chronic therapy for the product used (1 to 2 hours for liquids, soft gelatin capsules, and plain uncoated tablets that undergo rapid dissolution, 3 to 5 hours for sustained-release preparations). It is important that the patient will have missed *no* doses during the previous 48 hours and that dosing intervals will have been reasonably typical with no added doses during that period of time. **DOSAGE ADJUSTMENT BASED ON SERUM THEOPHYLLINE MEASUREMENTS WHEN THESE INSTRUCTIONS HAVE NOT BEEN FOLLOWED MAY RESULT IN RECOMMENDATIONS THAT PRESENT RISK OF TOXICITY TO THE PATIENT.**

Final Dosage Adjustment: Caution should be exercised for younger children who cannot complain of minor side effects. Older adults, those with cor pulmonale, congestive heart failure, and/or liver disease may have unusually low dosage requirements and thus may experience toxicity at the maximal dosage recommended above.

It is important that no patient be maintained on any dosage that he is not tolerating. In instructing patients to increase dosage according to the schedule above, they should be instructed not to take a subsequent dose if apparent side effects occur and to resume therapy at a lower dose once adverse effects have disappeared.

[See table on top next page].

KEEP THIS AND ALL MEDICATION OUT OF THE REACH OF CHILDREN.

HOW SUPPLIED

Slo-Phyllin® GG Syrup is lemon-vanilla flavored, nonalcoholic, dye-free, and each 15 mL tablespoonful contains theophylline, anhydrous, 150 mg and guaifenesin 90 mg. Available in 16 oz. bottles (NDC 0067-0357-16).

Slo-Phyllin® GG Capsules are white, liquid filled, and each soft gelatin capsule contains theophylline, anhydrous, 150 mg and guaifenesin 90 mg. Available in bottles of 100 capsules (NDC 0067-2358-68).

Slo-Phyllin® GG Capsules
Manufactured by
R. P. Scherer Corporation
Troy, MI 48084
For
WILLIAM H. RORER, INC.
Fort Washington, PA, USA 19034
Slo-Phyllin® GG Syrup
Manufactured by
WILLIAM H. RORER, INC.
Fort Washington, PA, USA 19034

Slo-Phyllin® GG Capsules Shown in Product Identification Section, page 426

Slo-Phyllin GG Group	Oral Loading Dose (Theophylline)	Maintenance Dose for Next 12 hours (Theophylline)	Maintenance Dose Beyond 12 hours (Theophylline)
1. Children 6 months to 9 years	6 mg/kg	4 mg/kg q4hrs.	4 mg/kg q6hrs
2. Children age 9–16 and young adult smokers	6 mg/kg	3 mg/kg q4hrs.	3 mg/kg q6hrs
3. Otherwise healthy non-smoking adults	6 mg/kg	3 mg/kg q6hrs	3 mg/kg q8hrs
4. Older patients and patients with cor pulmonale	6 mg/kg	2 mg/kg q6hrs	2 mg/kg q8hrs
5. Patients with congestive heart failure, liver failure	6 mg/kg	2 mg/kg q8hrs	1–2 mg/kg q12hrs

Body Weight		Dosage of *Slo-Phyllin®* GG Syrup Calculated at Approximately:		
Kilos	Expressed in Lbs	3mg Per Kilo	4mg Per Kilo	5mg Per Kilo
9	20	½ tsp	¾ tsp	1 tsp
18	40	1 tsp	1½ tsp	2 tsp
27	60	1½ tsp	2 tsp	2¾ tsp
36	79	2 tsp	3 tsp	3½ tsp
45	99	2¾ tsp	3½ tsp	4½ tsp
54	118	3¼ tsp	4½ tsp	5½ tsp

Administered every six (6) hours.

Ross Laboratories
COLUMBUS, OH 43216

ADVANCE®
[ad-vans']
Nutritional Beverage With Iron

USAGE
As a fortified milk/soy-based feeding more appropriate than 2% lowfat milk for older babies and toddlers.

Features:
- A more appropriate distribution of calories from protein, fat, and carbohydrate than 2% lowfat milk.
- Recommended levels of vitamins and minerals to complement the solid food diet of older infants.
- 1.8 mg of iron (as ferrous sulfate) per 100 Calories to help avoid iron deficiency.
- A combination of heat-treated soy and cow's milk proteins to help reduce the risk of cow's-milk-induced enteric blood loss.
- 16 Calories per fluid ounce.

AVAILABILITY
Concentrated Liquid: 13-fl-oz cans; 12 per case; No. 3313.
Ready To Feed: (Prediluted, 16 Cal/fl oz) 32-fl-oz cans; 6 per case; No. 3301.

PREPARATION
Concentrated Liquid: Standard dilution (16 Cal/fl oz) is one part Concentrated Liquid to one part water. **Ready To Feed:** Do not dilute.
For hospital use, Ready To Feed Advance in disposable nursing bottles is available in the Ross Hospital Formula System.

COMPOSITION
Concentrated Liquid

INGREDIENTS
Ⓤ-D Water, corn syrup, nonfat milk, soy oil, soy protein isolate, corn oil, mono- and diglycerides, soy lecithin, minerals (calcium phosphate tribasic, potassium citrate, magnesium chloride, ferrous sulfate, zinc sulfate, cupric sulfate, manganese sulfate), vitamins (ascorbic acid, alpha-tocopheryl acetate, niacinamide, calcium pantothenate, vitamin A palmitate, thiamine chloride hydrochloride, pyridoxine hydrochloride, riboflavin, folic acid, phylloquinone, vitamin D_3, cyanocobalamin), carrageenan and taurine.
6.3 fl oz provide 100 Cal when prepared as directed. 1 liter of prepared formula provides 540 Cal.

Nutrients:	**Per 100 Cal**	
Protein	3.7	g
Fat	5.0	g
Carbohydrate	10.2	g
Water	170	g
Linoleic Acid	2300	mg
Vitamins:		
Vitamin A	400	IU
Vitamin D	75	IU
Vitamin E	3.7	IU
Vitamin K	10	mcg
Thiamine (Vit. B_1)	140	mcg
Riboflavin (Vit. B_2)	170	mcg
Vitamin B_6	110	mcg
Vitamin B_{12}	0.5	mcg
Niacin	1850	mcg
Folic Acid (Folacin)	19	mcg
Pantothenic Acid	740	mcg
Vitamin C (Ascorbic Acid)	9	mg
Minerals:	**Per 100 Cal**	
Calcium	94	mg
Phosphorus	72	mg
Magnesium	12	mg
Iron	1.8	mg*
Zinc	0.9	mg
Manganese	6	mcg
Copper	110	mcg
Iodine	11	mcg
Sodium	37	mg
Potassium	170	mg
Chloride	95	mg

(FAN 414-02)

COMPOSITION
Ready To Feed

INGREDIENTS
Ⓤ-D Water, corn syrup, nonfat milk, soy oil, soy protein isolate, corn oil, mono- and diglycerides, soy lecithin, minerals (calcium phosphate tribasic, potassium citrate, magnesium chloride, ferrous sulfate, zinc sulfate, cupric sulfate, manganese sulfate), vitamins (ascorbic acid, alpha-tocopheryl acetate, niacinamide, calcium pantothenate, vitamin A palmitate, thiamine chloride hydrochloride, pyridoxine hydrochloride, riboflavin, folic acid, phylloquinone, vitamin D_3, cyanocobalamin), carrageenan and taurine.
6.3 fl oz provide 100 Cal; 1 liter provides 540 Cal.

Nutrients:	**Per 100 Cal**	
Protein	3.7	g
Fat	5.0	g
Carbohydrate	10.2	g
Water	170	g
Linoleic Acid	2300	mg
Vitamins:		
Vitamin A	400	IU
Vitamin D	75	IU
Vitamin E	3.7	IU
Vitamin K	10	mcg
Thiamine (Vit. B_1)	140	mcg
Riboflavin (Vit. B_2)	170	mcg
Vitamin B_6	110	mcg
Vitamin B_{12}	0.5	mcg
Niacin	1850	mcg
Folic Acid (Folacin)	19	mcg
Pantothenic Acid	740	mcg
Vitamin C (Ascorbic Acid)	9	mg
Minerals:		
Calcium	94	mg
Phosphorus	72	mg
Magnesium	12	mg
Iron	1.8	mg*
Zinc	0.9	mg
Manganese	6	mcg
Copper	110	mcg
Iodine	11	mcg
Sodium	37	mg
Potassium	170	mg
Chloride	95	mg

*The addition of iron to this beverage conforms to the recommendation of the Committee on Nutrition of the American Academy of Pediatrics.
(FAN 414-02)

CLEAR EYES® OTC
[klēr īz]
Naphazoline HCl Eye Redness Reliever

PRODUCT OVERVIEW

KEY FACTS
Clear Eyes is a sterile, buffered, isotonic ophthalmic vasoconstrictor solution containing the eye redness reliever naphazoline hydrochloride (0.012%). Clear Eyes soothes, refreshes, and moisturizes while removing redness due to minor eye irritations. Clear Eyes can be used up to 4 times daily.

MAJOR USES
Clear Eyes removes redness due to minor eye irritation.

SAFETY INFORMATION
Clear Eyes should only be used to relieve redness due to minor eye irritation. If eye pain, changes in vision, continued redness, or irritation of the eye occurs, or if the eye condition worsens or persists for more than 72 hours, discontinue use and consult a physician. Not for use by glaucoma patients unless under physician advice and supervision. Overuse of this product may produce increased redness of the eye. Do not use while contact lenses are being worn.

PRESCRIBING INFORMATION

CLEAR EYES® OTC
[klēr īz]
Naphazoline HCl Eye Redness Reliever

DESCRIPTION
Clear Eyes is a sterile isotonic buffered solution containing the active ingredient naphazoline hydrochloride 0.012%, as well as boric acid, sodium borate, and water. Edetate disodium 0.1% and benzalkonium chloride 0.01% are added as preservatives. (Contains vasoconstrictor.)

INDICATIONS
Clear Eyes is a decongestant ophthalmic solution specially designed to soothe, refresh, moisturize and remove redness due to minor eye irritation caused by dust, smoke, smog, sun glare, wearing contact lenses, colds, allergies, swimming, reading, driving, TV or close work. Clear Eyes contains laboratory tested, and scientifically blended ingredients including an effective vasoconstrictor which narrows swollen blood vessels and rapidly whitens reddened eyes in a formulation which produces a refreshing, soothing effect. Clear Eyes is a sterile, isotonic solution compatible with the natural fluids of the eye.

WARNING
To avoid contamination of this product, do not touch tip of container to any surface. Replace cap after using. If you experience eye pain, changes in vision, continued redness or irritation of the eye, or if the condition worsens or persists for more than 72 hours, discontinue use and consult a physician. If you have glaucoma, do not use this product except under the advice and supervision of a physician. Overuse of this product may produce increased redness of the eye. If solution changes color or becomes cloudy, do not use. Remove contact lenses before using. Keep this and all medicines out of the reach of children.

DOSAGE AND ADMINISTRATION
One or two drops in eye(s) up to 4 times daily or as directed by physician.

HOW SUPPLIED
In 0.5-fl-oz and 1.0-fl-oz plastic dropper bottle.
(FAN 2070-02)

EAR DROPS BY MURINE OTC
See Murine Ear Wax Removal System/Murine Ear Drops

ENRICH®
[en-rich']
Liquid Nutrition with Fiber

USAGE
As a high-fiber liquid food providing complete, balanced nutrition. Enrich is for patients who can benefit from increased bulk provided by a high-fiber formula. The dietary fiber level in Enrich (3.4 g per 8 oz can) helps patients maintain normal bowel function, and may be useful for patients with intolerance to low-residue feedings (ie, diarrhea or constipation). Enrich can be used as a full liquid diet, liquid supplement or tube feeding.

Features:
- Complete, balanced nutrition—Enrich can be used as a sole source of nutrition. Caloric distribution: 14.5% protein, 30.5% fat, 55.0% carbohydrate (includes soy polysaccharide, a source of dietary fiber). 1530 Calories meets or surpasses 100% of the U.S. RDA for vitamins and minerals.
- Calorie/nitrogen ratio of 173:1—Assures that protein will be spared for tissue restoration and growth.
- Contains dietary fiber—One serving provides 3.4 g dietary fiber (5 g soy polysaccharide). Six servings provide 20 g of dietary fiber, a level comparable to a typical self-selected diet.
- High-quality protein—Amino acid profile meets the standard of high-quality proteins set by the National Academy of Sciences.
- Good nutrient absorption—Nitrogen balance, fat absorption and mineral balance (in the normally functioning gut) are not compromised by fiber.
- Lactose free—Enrich will not contribute to lactose-associated diarrhea.
- Low osmolality (480 mosm/kg water)—Will not contribute to osmotically induced diarrhea.
- Good taste—Pleasant flavor is readily accepted by most patients. Ready To Use Enrich is available in Vanilla and

Continued on next page

Ross—Cont.

Chocolate flavors. In addition, Vari-Flavors® Flavor Pacs (Pecan, Cherry, Strawberry, Lemon, Orange) mix easily with vanilla to offer patients a greater variety of flavors.

DOSAGE AND ADMINISTRATION

Ready To Use: Shake well. Enrich is ready to use and does not require dilution with water. Enrich may be stored (unopened) and fed at room temperature. Once opened, any unused Enrich should be covered and refrigerated; discard if not used within 48 hours.

Oral Feeding: Enrich may be used for total nutrition, or with and between meals for added nutritional support. Enrich may be fed at room temperature or chilled.

Tube Feeding: Follow physician's instructions. Adjust flow rate, volume and dilution according to patient's condition and tolerance. Avoid contamination during preparation and use. Lower temperatures increase the viscosity of Enrich. Therefore, the product should be at room temperature for tube feeding.

Additional fluid requirements should be met by giving water with or after feedings.

Enrich is not recommended for situations requiring a low-residue feeding.

Not for parenteral use.

[See table below].

AVAILABILITY

Ready To Use:

8-fl-oz cans; 4 six-packs per case; Vanilla, No. 759; Chocolate, No. 756. 32-fl-oz cans; 6 per case; Vanilla, No. 706.

COMPOSITION

Ready To Use Vanilla (Chocolate flavor has similar composition. For specific information, see product label.)

INGREDIENTS

Ⓤ-D Water, hydrolyzed corn starch, sucrose, sodium and calcium caseinates, corn oil, soy polysaccharide (a source of dietary fiber), minerals (potassium citrate, magnesium chloride, calcium phosphate tribasic, sodium citrate, potassium chloride, zinc sulfate, ferrous sulfate, manganese sulfate, cupric sulfate), soy protein isolate, natural and artificial flavor, soy lecithin and vitamins (choline chloride, ascorbic acid, alpha-tocopheryl acetate, niacinamide, calcium pantothenate, thiamine chloride hydrochloride, pyridoxine hydrochloride, riboflavin, vitamin A palmitate, folic acid, biotin, phylloquinone, cyanocobalamin, vitamin D_3).

Nutrients (Grams/8 fl oz): Protein, 9.4; Fat, 8.8; Carbohydrate, 38.3†; Minerals (Ash), 1.9; Water, 196. Calories per fl oz, 32.5; Calories per mL, 1.1.

† Contains 5 g soy polysaccharide/8 fl oz (a source of dietary fiber that contributes 10 Calories/8 fl oz).

Vitamin/Mineral Content of Enrich (Ready To Use)

Vitamins/Minerals	Per 8 Fl Oz		Percent U.S. RDA* (Per 8 Fl Oz)
Vitamin A	850	I.U.	17
Vitamin D	68	I.U.	17
Vitamin E	7.7	I.U.	25.6
Vitamin K_1	12	mcg	**
Vitamin C	51	mg	85
Folic Acid	102	mcg	25.5
Thiamine (Vit. B_1)	0.39	mg	26
Riboflavin (Vit. B_2)	0.44	mg	25.8
Vitamin B_6	0.51	mg	25.5
Vitamin B_{12}	1.6	mcg	26.6
Niacin	5.1	mg	25.5
Choline	102	mg	**
Biotin	77	mcg	25.6
Pantothenic Acid	2.55	mg	25.5
Sodium	200	mg	**
Potassium	370	mg	**
Chloride	340	mg	**
Calcium	170	mg	17
Phosphorus	170	mg	17
Magnesium	68	mg	17
Iodine	25.5	mcg	17
Manganese	0.85	mg	**
Copper	0.34	mg	17
Zinc	3.83	mg	25.5
Iron	3.06	mg	17

*For adults and children 4 or more years of age.
**U.S. RDA not established.
(FAN 366-02)

Sample Administration Schedule for ENRICH

Continuous Drip Schedule

Day	Time	Strength	Rate (mL/h)	Volume (mL)	Calories
1	1st 8 hours	Full	50	400	440
	2nd 8 hours	Full	75	600	660
	3rd 8 hours	Full	100	800	880
					1980 *Total Calories*
2	24 hours	Full	100–125	2400–3000	2640–3300 *Total Calories*

Intermittent Drip Schedule

Day	Time	Strength	Rate (5–10 mL/min)	Volume (mL)	Calories
1	7am–11pm	Full	100 mL q 2 h (7am, 9am)	200	220
			150 mL q 2 h (11am, 1pm, 3pm)	450	495
			200 mL q 2 h (5pm, 7pm, 9pm, 11pm)	800	880
					1595 *Total Calories*
2	7am–11pm	Full	250 mL q 2 h (8 feedings) up to	2000	2200 *Total Calories*
			400 mL q 3 h (5 feedings)	2000	2200 *Total Calories*

- Always tube-feed the product at room temperature.
- When gavage feeding, use a size 10 French or larger tube. Smaller tubes can be used for pump delivery.
- Check gastric residuals before every intermittent feeding or every 2–4 hours during continuous feeding.
- If intolerance develops (such as nausea, abdominal cramps, severe distention or diarrhea), return to previously tolerated rate.
- Rinsing the tube with water (eg, 25–100 mL) after each intermittent feeding or every 3 to 6 hours during continuous feeding will help avoid clogging and provide additional water.

ENSURE®

[en-shur']
Liquid Nutrition

USAGE

For complete, balanced nutrition. Ensure can be used as a full liquid diet, liquid supplement or tube feeding (nasogastric, nasoduodenal, jejunal). Ensure is useful whenever the patient's medical, surgical or psychological state precludes normal food intake and/or leads to inadequate nutrition. Two quarts (2000 Calories) of Ensure meets or surpasses 100% of the U.S. RDA for vitamins and minerals for adults and children 4 or more years of age.

Features:

- Complete, balanced nutrition—1.06 Calories per mL. 250 Calories per 8-fl-oz feeding. 1000 Calories per quart from a balanced distribution of protein, fat, and carbohydrate (caloric distribution: protein, 14.0%; fat, 31.5%; carbohydrate, 54.5%).
- High biologic value protein—Ensure provides high-quality protein (sodium and calcium caseinates and soy protein isolate) at a level appropriate for most hospitalized patients. Ensure provides 14% of the total calories as protein.
- Lactose free—Ensure will not contribute to lactose-associated diarrhea. Corn syrup and sucrose are carbohydrate sources.
- Fat source—A good source of essential fatty acids. Cholesterol is low (<20 mg/L). The fat source is polyunsaturated corn oil.
- Low-residue liquid feeding—The amount of fecal residue produced by Ensure is comparable to that produced by a chemically defined, elemental diet. Therefore, Ensure is appropriate for use in situations where low residue is the primary consideration.
- Low osmolality (470 mosm/kg water)—The osmolality of Ensure is low and will not contribute to osmotically induced diarrhea when proper feeding techniques are used.
- Good taste—Pleasant flavors are readily accepted by most patients. Ready To Use Ensure is available in a variety of flavors (Vanilla, Chocolate, Black Walnut, Coffee, Strawberry and Eggnog). In addition, Vari-Flavors® Flavor Pacs (Pecan, Cherry, Strawberry, Lemon, Orange) mix easily with Ensure Vanilla to offer patients a greater variety of flavors.
- Convenient—Available as a Ready To Use Liquid and Easy To Mix Powder. Ensure Powder mixes readily with water.

[See table on top next page].

DOSAGE AND ADMINISTRATION

Ready To Use: Shake well. May be stored unopened at room temperature. Once opened, Ensure should be covered and refrigerated; discard if not used within 48 hours. Ensure may be fed at room temperature or chilled.

Powder: To prepare an 8-fl-oz glassful; put ¾ cup of cold water in a glass. Gradually stir in ½ cup Ensure Powder and mix until dissolved. Reconstituted Ensure should be used promptly or covered, refrigerated and used within 24 hours. Opened can should be covered with overcap and stored in a cool, dry place, but not refrigerated. Once opened, use contents within 3 weeks.

Oral Feeding: May be used for total nutrition, or with and between meals.

Tube Feeding: Follow physician's instructions. Adjust flow rate, volume and dilution according to patient's condition and tolerance. Additional fluid requirements should be met by giving water with or after feedings. Avoid contamination during preparation and use.

Not for parenteral use.

AVAILABILITY

Ready To Use:

8-fl-oz bottles; 24 per case; Vanilla, No. 708.
8-fl-oz cans; 4 six-packs per case; Chocolate, No. 701; Black Walnut, No. 703; Coffee, No. 704; Strawberry, No. 705; Eggnog, No. 710; Vanilla, No. 711.
32-fl-oz cans; 6 per case; Vanilla, No. 733; Chocolate, No. 799.

Powder:

14-oz (400 g) cans; 6 per case; Vanilla, No. 750.

COMPOSITION

Ready To Use Vanilla (Other Ready To Use flavors and Vanilla Powder at standard dilution have similar composition and nutrient values. For specific information, see product labels.)

INGREDIENTS

Ⓤ-D Water, corn syrup, sucrose, sodium and calcium caseinates, corn oil, minerals (potassium citrate, magnesium chloride, calcium phosphate tribasic, sodium citrate, potassium chloride, zinc sulfate, ferrous sulfate, manganese sulfate, cupric sulfate, potassium iodide), soy protein isolate, soy lecithin, natural and artificial flavor, vitamins (choline chloride, ascorbic acid, alpha-tocopheryl acetate, niacinamide, calcium pantothenate, thiamine chloride hydrochloride, pyridoxine hydrochloride, riboflavin, vitamin A palmitate, folic acid, biotin, phylloquinone, cyanocobalamin, vitamin D_3) and carrageenan.

Nutrients (Grams/8 fl oz): Protein, 8.8; Fat, 8.8; Carbohydrate, 34.3; Water, 200. Calories per mL, 1.06; Calories per fl oz, 31.3.

Vitamin/Mineral Content of Ensure (Ready To Use)

Vitamins/Minerals	Per 8 Fl Oz		Percent U.S. RDA* (Per 8 Fl Oz)
Vitamin A	625	I.U.	12.5
Vitamin D	50	I.U.	12.5
Vitamin E	5.63	I.U.	18.7
Vitamin K_1	9	mcg	**
Vitamin C	37.5	mg	62.5
Folic Acid	100	mcg	25
Thiamine (Vit. B_1)	0.38	mg	25.3
Riboflavin (Vit. B_2)	0.43	mg	25.3
Vitamin B_6	0.50	mg	25
Vitamin B_{12}	1.5	mcg	25
Niacin	5.0	mg	25

Choline	75	mg	**
Biotin	75	mcg	25
Pantothenic Acid	2.5	mg	25
Sodium	200	mg	**
Potassium	370	mg	**
Chloride	340	mg	**
Calcium	125	mg	12.5
Phosphorus	125	mg	12.5
Magnesium	50	mg	12.5
Iodine	18.8	mcg	12.5
Manganese	0.62	mg	**
Copper	0.25	mg	12.5
Zinc	2.82	mg	18.8
Iron	2.25	mg	12.5

*For adults and children 4 or more years of age.
**U.S. RDA not established.
(FAN 432-03)

Sample Administration Schedule For ENSURE

Continuous Drip Schedule

Day	Time	Strength	Rate (mL/hr)	Volume (mL)	Calories
1	1st 8 hours	Full	50	400	400
	2nd 8 hours	Full	75	600	600
	3rd 8 hours	Full	100	800	800
					1800 *Total Calories*
2	24 hours	Full	100–125	2400–3000	2400–3000 *Total Calories*

Intermittent Drip Schedule

Day	Time	Strength	Rate (5–10 mL/min)	Volume (mL)	Calories
1	7am–11pm	Full	100 mL q 2 hr (7am, 9am)	200	200
			150 mL q 2 hr (11am, 1pm, 3pm)	450	450
			200 mL q 2 hr (5pm, 7pm, 9pm, 11pm)	800	800
					1450 *Total Calories*
2	7am–11pm	Full	250 mL q 2 hr (8 feedings) up to	2000	2000 *Total Calories*
			400 mL q 3 hr (5 feedings)	2000	2000 *Total Calories*

- Check gastric residuals before every intermittent feeding or every 2–4 hours during continuous feeding.
- If intolerance develops (such as nausea, abdominal cramps, distention or diarrhea), switch to full strength OSMOLITE or ENRICH or feed ENSURE at half strength. After tolerance to half strength ENSURE is established, continue feeding schedule using half strength ENSURE until desired rate is achieved. Then switch to full strength. Do not alter rate and strength at the same time.
- Rinsing the tube with water (eg, 25–100 mL) after each intermittent feeding or every 3 to 6 hours during continuous feeding will help avoid clogging and provide additional water.

ENSURE® HN

[en-shur′]

High Nitrogen Liquid Nutrition

USAGE

As an all-purpose, high-nitrogen, low-residue liquid food, Ensure HN provides complete, balanced nutritional support for patients with a decreased caloric intake or for those with increased protein needs. Ensure HN can be used as a full liquid diet, liquid supplement or tube feeding (nasogastric, nasoduodenal, jejunal).

Features:

- Complete, balanced nutrition—1.06 Calories per mL, 250 Calories per 8 fl oz, 1000 Calories per quart from a balanced distribution of protein, fat and carbohydrate (caloric distribution: protein, 16.7%; fat, 30.1%; carbohydrate, 53.2%). 1400 Calories of Ensure HN provide at least 100% of the U.S. RDA for vitamins and minerals for adults and children 4 or more years of age.
- High levels of nitrogen—Ensure HN has a total calorie/nitrogen ratio of 150:1, indicated for the stressed patient with increased nitrogen losses.
- High biologic value protein—Ensure HN provides high quality protein at a level appropriate for the stressed patient—10.5 g/8 fl oz (1.68 g nitrogen/8 fl oz). 16.7% of the total calories of Ensure HN are protein.
- Lactose free—Ensure HN will not contribute to lactose-associated diarrhea. Corn syrup and sucrose are the carbohydrate sources.
- Low-residue feeding—Ensure HN is appropriate in situations in which low residue is a consideration.
- Low osmolality (470 mosm/kg water)—Ensure HN will decrease the risk of osmotically induced diarrhea when proper feeding techniques are used.

DOSAGE AND ADMINISTRATION

Ready To Use: Shake well. May be stored unopened at room temperature. Once opened, Ensure HN should be covered and refrigerated; discard if not used within 48 hours. Ensure HN may be fed at room temperature or chilled.

Oral Feeding: May be used for total nutrition, or with and between meals.

Tube Feeding: Follow physician's instructions. Adjust flow rate, volume and dilution according to patient's condition and tolerance. Additional fluid requirements should be met by giving water with or after feedings. Avoid contamination during preparation and use.

Not for parenteral use.

[See table below].

AVAILABILITY

Ready To Use:

8-fl-oz cans; 4 six-packs per case; Chocolate, No. 712; Vanilla, No. 719.

32-fl-oz cans; 6 per case; Vanilla, No. 732.

COMPOSITION

Ready To Use Vanilla (Other flavors have similar composition. For specific information, see product labels.)

Ingredients: Ⓤ-D Water, corn syrup, sodium and calcium caseinates, sucrose, corn oil, minerals (magnesium chloride, potassium citrate, calcium phosphate tribasic, sodium citrate, potassium phosphate dibasic, potassium chloride, zinc sulfate, ferrous sulfate, manganese sulfate, cupric sulfate), soy protein isolate, soy lecithin, natural and artificial flavor, vitamins (choline chloride, ascorbic acid, alpha-tocopheryl acetate, niacinamide, calcium pantothenate, thiamine chloride hydrochloride, pyridoxine hydrochloride, riboflavin, vitamin A palmitate, folic acid, biotin, phylloquinone, cyanocobalamin, vitamin D_3) and carrageenan.

Nutrients (Grams/8 fl oz): Protein, 10.5; Fat, 8.4; Carbohydrate, 33.4; Minerals (Ash), 1.9; Water, 199. Calories per mL, 1.06; Calories per fl oz, 31.3.

Vitamin/Mineral Content of Ensure HN (Ready To Use)

Vitamins/Minerals	Per 8 Fl Oz		Percent U.S. RDA* (Per 8 Fl Oz)
Vitamin A	893	I.U.	17.8
Vitamin D	72	I.U.	18
Vitamin E	8.1	I.U.	27
Vitamin K_1	13	mcg	**
Vitamin C	53.6	mg	89.3
Folic Acid	108	mcg	27
Thiamine (Vit. B_1)	0.41	mg	27.3
Riboflavin (Vit. B_2)	0.46	mg	27
Vitamin B_6	0.54	mg	27
Vitamin B_{12}	1.7	mcg	28.3
Niacin	5.36	mg	26.8
Choline	107	mg	**
Biotin	81	mcg	27
Pantothenic Acid	2.68	mg	26.8
Sodium	220	mg	**
Potassium	370	mg	**
Chloride	340	mg	**
Calcium	179	mg	17.9
Phosphorus	179	mg	17.9
Magnesium	71.5	mg	17.8
Iodine	26.8	mcg	17.8
Manganese	0.89	mg	**
Copper	0.36	mg	18
Zinc	4.02	mg	26.8
Iron	3.22	mg	17.8

*For adults and children 4 or more years of age.
**U.S. RDA not established.
(FAN 366-02)

Sample Administration Schedule For ENSURE HN

Continuous Drip Schedule

Day	Time	Strength	Rate (mL/h)	Volume (mL)	Calories
1	1st 8 hours	Full	50	400	400
	2nd 8 hours	Full	75	600	600
	3rd 8 hours	Full	100	800	800
					1800 *Total Calories*
2	24 hours	Full	100-125	2400-3000	2400-3000 *Total Calories*

Intermittent Drip Schedule

Day	Time	Strength	Rate (5-10 mL/min)	Volume (mL)	Calories
1	7am-11pm	Full	100 mL q 2 h (7am, 9am)	200	200
			150 mL q 2 h (11am, 1pm, 3pm)	450	450
			200 mL q 2 h (5pm, 7pm, 9pm, 11pm)	800	800
					1450 *Total Calories*
2	7am-11pm	Full	250 mL q 2 h (8 feedings) up to	2000	2000 *Total Calories*
			400 mL q 3 h (5 feedings)	2000	2000 *Total Calories*

- Check gastric residuals before every intermittent feeding or every 2–4 hours during continuous feeding.
- If intolerance develops, switch to full strength OSMOLITE® HN or feed ENSURE® HN at half strength. After tolerance to half strength ENSURE® HN is established, continue feeding schedule using half strength ENSURE® HN until desired rate is achieved. Then switch to full strength. Do not alter rate and strength at the same time.
- Rinsing the tube with water (eg, 25–100 mL) after each intermittent feeding or every 3 to 6 hours during continuous feeding will help avoid clogging and provide additional water.

Continued on next page

Ross—Cont.

ENSURE PLUS®

[en-shur']

High Calorie Liquid Nutrition

USAGE

As a high-calorie liquid food providing complete, balanced nutrition. Caloric density is 1500 Calories per liter, 50% greater than most other liquid feedings. Ensure Plus is intended for use when extra calories and correspondingly higher concentrations of protein and most other nutrients are needed to achieve a required calorie intake in a limited volume. When used to provide total nutrition, Ensure Plus can deliver the high-calorie intakes required by patients who are nutritionally depleted, and who may not be able to tolerate large-volume intakes. As a dietary supplement, Ensure Plus can supply extra calories and protein for those patients unable or unwilling to consume adequate nutrition.

Features:

- Complete nutrition—1.5 Cal per mL, 355 Cal per 8 fl oz, from a balanced distribution of protein, fat and carbohydrate (caloric distribution: protein, 14.7%; fat, 32.0%; carbohydrate, 53.3%). 2130 Cal (six 8-oz servings) of Ensure Plus meets or surpasses 100% of the U.S. RDA for vitamins and minerals for adults and children 4 or more years of age.
- 1500 Calories per liter—The use of Ensure Plus will reduce the volume necessary to meet the caloric needs of debilitated patients.
- 55 grams of protein per liter—Ensure Plus provides sufficient protein to meet demands of the nutritionally compromised patient. Appropriate levels of carbohydrate and fat are provided to spare protein for anabolic purposes, tissue synthesis and repair.
- Lactose free—Ensure Plus will not contribute to lactose-associated diarrhea. Corn syrup and sucrose are carbohydrate sources.
- Osmolality (690 mosm/kg water)—Ensure Plus will not contribute to osmotic diarrhea when proper feeding techniques are used.
- Good taste—Pleasant flavor is readily accepted by most patients. Ready To Use Ensure Plus is available in a variety of flavors (Vanilla, Chocolate, Coffee, Strawberry and Eggnog). In addition, Vari-Flavors® Flavor Pacs (Pecan, Cherry, Strawberry, Lemon, Orange) mix easily with Ensure Plus Vanilla to offer patients a greater variety of flavors.
- Convenient—Ensure Plus is ready to use. Potential for contamination during preparation is reduced. Unopened, Ensure Plus can be stored at room temperature.

DOSAGE AND ADMINISTRATION

Ready To Use: Shake well. May be stored unopened at room temperature. Once opened, Ensure Plus should be covered and refrigerated; discard if not used within 48 hours. Ensure Plus may be fed at room temperature or chilled.

Oral Feeding: May be used for total nutrition, or with and between meals.

Tube Feeding: Follow physician's instructions. Adjust flow rate, volume and dilution according to patient's condition and tolerance. Additional fluid requirements should be met by giving water with or after feedings. Avoid contamination during preparation and use.

Not for parenteral use.

[See table below].

AVAILABILITY

8-fl-oz bottles; 24 per case; Vanilla, No. 741.

8-fl-oz cans; 4 six-packs per case; Chocolate, No. 702; Vanilla, No. 707; Eggnog, No. 716; Coffee, No. 717; Strawberry, No. 718.

32-fl-oz cans; 6 per case; Vanilla, No.688; Chocolate, No 698.

COMPOSITION

Ready To Use Vanilla (Other flavors have similar composition. For specific information, see product labels.)

Sample Administration Schedule For ENSURE PLUS

Continuous Drip Schedule

Day	Time	Strength	Rate (mL/hr)	Volume (mL)	Calories
1	1st 8 hours	½	50	400	300
	2nd 8 hours	½	75	600	450
	3rd 8 hours	½	100	800	600
					1350 *Total Calories*
2	1st 8 hours	½	125	1000	750
	2nd 8 hours	Full	100–125	800–1000	1200–1500
	3rd 8 hours	Full	100–125	800–1000	1200–1500
					3150–3750 *Total Calories*
3	24 hours	Full	100–125	2400–3000	3600–4500 *Total Calories*

Intermittent Drip Schedule

Day	Time	Strength	Rate (5–10 mL/min)	Volume (mL)	Calories
1	7am–11pm	½	100 mL q 2 hr (7am, 9am)	200	150
		½	150 mL q 2 hr (11am, 1pm, 3pm)	450	338
		½	200 mL q 2 hr (5pm, 7pm, 9pm, 11pm)	800	600
					1088 *Total Calories*
2	7am–11pm	½	250 mL q 2 hr (7am, 9am, 11am)	750	563
		Full	250 mL q 2 hr (1pm, 3pm, 5pm, 7pm, 9pm, 11pm)	1500	2250
					2813 *Total Calories*
3	7am–11pm	Full	250 mL q 2 hr (8 feedings) up to	2000	3000 *Total Calories*
			400 mL q 3 hr (5 feedings)	2000	3000 *Total Calories*

- Check gastric residuals before every intermittent feeding or every 2–4 hours during continuous feeding.
- If intolerance develops (such as nausea, abdominal cramps, distention, or diarrhea), return to previously tolerated strength and rate. When tolerance is again established, proceed with feeding schedule as indicated. Do not alter rate and strength at the same time.
- Rinsing the tube with water (eg, 25–100 mL) after each intermittent feeding or every 3 to 6 hours during continuous feeding will help avoid clogging and provide additional water.

INGREDIENTS

Ⓤ-D Water, corn syrup, sodium and calcium caseinates, corn oil, sucrose, minerals (magnesium chloride, potassium citrate, calcium phosphate tribasic, sodium citrate, potassium chloride, zinc sulfate, ferrous sulfate, manganese sulfate, cupric sulfate), soy protein isolate, soy lecithin, vitamins (choline chloride, ascorbic acid, alpha-tocopheryl acetate, niacinamide, calcium pantothenate, thiamine chloride hydrochloride, pyridoxine hydrochloride, riboflavin, vitamin A palmitate, folic acid, biotin, phylloquinone, cyanocobalamin, vitamin D_3), natural and artificial flavor and carrageenan.

Nutrients (Grams/8 fl oz): Protein, 13.0; Fat, 12.6; Carbohydrate, 47.3; Ash, 2.2; Water, 182. Calories per mL, 1.5; Calories per fl oz, 44.4.

Vitamin/Mineral Content of Ensure Plus (Ready To Use)

Vitamins/Minerals	Per 8 Fl Oz		Percent U.S. RDA* (Per 8 Fl Oz)
Vitamin A	834	I.U.	16.6
Vitamin D	67	I.U.	16.7
Vitamin E	7.5	I.U.	25
Vitamin K_1	12	mcg	**
Vitamin C	50	mg	83.3
Folic Acid	134	mcg	33.5
Thiamine (Vit. B_1)	0.50	mg	33.3
Riboflavin (Vit. B_2)	0.57	mg	33.5
Vitamin B_6	0.67	mg	33.5
Vitamin B_{12}	2.0	mcg	33.3
Niacin	6.67	mg	33.3
Biotin	100	mcg	33.3
Choline	100	mg	**
Pantothenic Acid	3.34	mg	33.4
Sodium	270	mg	**
Potassium	500	mg	**
Chloride	470	mg	**
Calcium	167	mg	16.7
Phosphorus	167	mg	16.7
Magnesium	67	mg	16.7
Manganese	0.83	mg	**
Iodine	25	mcg	16.6
Copper	0.34	mg	17
Iron	3.0	mg	16.6
Zinc	3.75	mg	25

*For adults and children 4 or more years of age.

**U.S. RDA not established.

(FAN 366-02)

ENSURE PLUS® HN

[en-shur']

High Calorie, High Nitrogen Liquid Nutrition

USAGE

As a high-calorie, high-nitrogen liquid food, Ensure Plus HN provides complete, balanced nutrition. It is most appropriate for patients with increased calorie and protein needs, or for those patients whose volume intake is limited. Ensure Plus HN can be used as a full liquid diet, liquid supplement or tube feeding (nasogastric or nasoduodenal).

Features:

- Complete, balanced nutrition—1.5 Calories per mL, 355 Calories per 8 fl oz, 1500 Calories per liter from a balanced distribution of protein, fat and carbohydrate (caloric distribution: protein, 16.7%; fat, 30.0%; and carbohydrate, 53.3%). 1420 Calories of Ensure Plus HN meets or surpasses 100% of the U.S. RDA for vitamins and minerals for adults and children 4 or more years of age.
- High levels of nitrogen—Ensure Plus HN has a total calorie/nitrogen ratio of 150:1, indicated for the stressed patient because of increased nitrogen losses.
- Concentrated nutrition—Ensure Plus HN will reduce the volume necessary to meet the protein and caloric needs of the debilitated patient (62.6 g of protein per liter, 1500 Calories per liter).
- Lactose free—Ensure Plus HN will not contribute to lactose-associated diarrhea. Hydrolyzed corn starch and sucrose are the carbohydrate sources.
- Moderate osmolality (650 mosm/kg water)—Ensure Plus HN will decrease the potential for osmotically induced diarrhea.

DOSAGE AND ADMINISTRATION

Ready To Use: Shake well. May be stored unopened at room temperature. Once opened, Ensure Plus HN should be covered and refrigerated; discard if not used within 48 hours. Ensure Plus HN may be fed at room temperature or chilled.

Oral Feeding: May be used for total nutrition, or with and between meals.

Tube Feeding: Follow physician's instructions. Adjust flow rate, volume and dilution according to patient's condition and tolerance. Additional fluid requirements should be met by giving water with or after feedings. Avoid contamination during preparation and use.

Not for parenteral use.
[See table right].

AVAILABILITY

Ready To Use:
8-fl-oz cans; 4 six-packs per case; Vanilla, No. 721.

COMPOSITION

Ready To Use Vanilla

INGREDIENTS

Ⓤ-D Water, corn syrup, sodium and calcium caseinates, corn oil, sucrose, minerals (magnesium chloride, potassium citrate, calcium phosphate tribasic, sodium citrate, zinc sulfate, ferrous sulfate, manganese sulfate, cupric sulfate), soy protein isolate, soy lecithin, vitamins (choline chloride, ascorbic acid, alpha-tocopheryl acetate, niacinamide, calcium pantothenate, thiamine chloride hydrochloride, pyridoxine hydrochloride, riboflavin, vitamin A palmitate, folic acid, biotin, phylloquinone, cyanocobalamin, vitamin D_3), natural and artificial flavor, and carrageenan.

Nutrients (Grams/8 fl oz): Protein, 14.8; Fat, 11.8; Carbohydrate, 47.3; Minerals (Ash), 2.3; Water, 182. Calories per mL, 1.5; Calories per fl oz, 44.4.

Vitamin/Mineral Content of Ensure Plus HN (Ready To Use)

Vitamins/Minerals	Per 8 Fl Oz		Percent U.S. RDA* (Per 8 Fl Oz)
Vitamin A	1,250	I.U.	25
Vitamin D	100	I.U.	25
Vitamin E	11.3	I.U.	37.6
Vitamin K_1	18	mcg	**
Vitamin C	75	mg	125
Folic Acid	200	mcg	50
Thiamine (Vit. B_1)	0.75	mg	50
Riboflavin (Vit. B_2)	0.85	mg	50
Vitamin B_6	1.0	mg	50
Vitamin B_{12}	3.0	mcg	50
Niacin	10	mg	50
Choline	150	mg	**
Biotin	150	mcg	50
Pantothenic Acid	5.0	mg	50
Sodium	280	mg	**
Potassium	430	mg	**
Chloride	380	mg	**
Calcium	250	mg	25
Phosphorus	250	mg	25
Magnesium	100	mg	25
Iodine	37.5	mcg	25
Manganese	1.25	mg	**
Copper	0.50	mg	25
Zinc	5.63	mg	37.5
Iron	4.5	mg	25

* For adults and children 4 or more years of age.
** U.S. RDA not established.
(FAN 366-02)

Sample Administration Schedule For ENSURE PLUS HN

Continuous Drip Schedule

Day	Time	Strength	Rate (mL/h)	Volume (mL)	Calories
1	1st 8 hours	½	50	400	300
	2nd 8 hours	½	75	600	450
	3rd 8 hours	½	100	800	600
					1350 *Total Calories*
2	1st 8 hours	½	125	1000	750
	2nd 8 hours	Full	100-125	800-1000	1200-1500
	3rd 8 hours	Full	100-125	800-1000	1200-1500
					3150-3750 *Total Calories*
3	24 hours	Full	100-125	2400-3000	3600-4500 *Total Calories*

Intermittent Drip Schedule

Day	Time	Strength	Rate (5-10 mL/min)	Volume (mL)	Calories
1	7am-11pm	½	100 mL q 2 h (7am, 9am)	200	150
		½	150 mL q 2 h (11am, 1pm, 3pm)	450	338
		½	200 mL q 2 h (5pm, 7pm, 9pm, 11pm)	800	600
					1088 *Total Calories*
2	7am-11pm	½	250 mL q 2 h (7am, 9am, 11am)	750	563
		Full	250 mL q 2 h (1pm, 3pm, 5pm, 7pm, 9pm, 11pm)	1500	2250
					2813 *Total Calories*
3	7am-11pm	Full	250 mL q 2 h (8 feedings)	2000	3000 *Total Calories*
			up to 400 mL q 3 h (5 feedings)	2000	3000 *Total Calories*

- Check gastric residuals before every intermittent feeding or every 2–4 hours during continuous feeding.
- If intolerance develops, return to previously tolerated strength and rate. When tolerance is again established, proceed with feeding schedule as indicated. Do not alter rate and strength at the same time.
- Rinsing the tube with water (eg, 25–100 mL) after each intermittent feeding or every 3 to 6 hours during continuous feeding will help avoid clogging and provide additional water.

ENSURE™ PUDDING

[en-shur']

USAGE

To provide balanced nutrition in a delicious, easy-to-eat form. Ensure Pudding is appropriate for any patient who is able to eat semisolid or solid food. It may be particularly useful for patients with impaired swallowing. Each 5-oz serving provides at least 17% of the U.S. RDA for vitamins and minerals for adults and children 4 or more years of age.

Features:

- High caloric density—50 Cal/oz (250 Calories per 5-oz serving).
- Balanced caloric distribution—for patients who can benefit from increased nutrient intake, not just more calories.
- Moderate sodium content—240 mg per serving of Vanilla Ensure Pudding*—appropriate for diets requiring mild to moderate sodium restriction.
- Easy-open 5-oz cans are ready to serve—at room temperature or chilled.
- Four delicious flavors (Vanilla, Chocolate, Butterscotch, Tapioca) satisfy each patient's preference—and provide taste and texture variety.
- Colorful label design brightens the meal tray and enhances compliance.

*(For sodium levels of other flavors, see product packaging).

AVAILABILITY

Ready To Eat: 5-oz cans; 12 four-packs per case; Chocolate, No. 790; Vanilla, No. 792; Tapioca, No. 794; Butterscotch, No. 798.

COMPOSITION

Vanilla (Other flavors have similar composition. For specific information, see product packaging.)

INGREDIENTS

K DAIRY Nonfat milk, water, sucrose, partially hydrogenated soybean oil, modified food starch, minerals (magnesium sulfate, sodium phosphate dibasic, zinc sulfate, ferrous sulfate, manganese sulfate, cupric sulfate), sodium stearoyl lactylate, artificial flavor, vitamins (ascorbic acid, choline chloride, alpha-tocopheryl acetate, niacinamide, calcium pantothenate, vitamin A palmitate, thiamine chloride hydrochloride, pyridoxine hydrochloride, riboflavin, folic acid, biotin, phylloquinone, vitamin D_3, cyanocobalamin) and artificial color (including FD&C yellow #5).

Nutrients Per 5-oz Serving: Protein, 6.8 g; Fat, 9.7 g; Carbohydrate, 34.0 g; Minerals (Ash), 0.6 g; Water, 91 g. Calories per serving, 250.

Vitamin/Mineral Content of Ensure Pudding

Vitamins/Minerals	Per Can (5 Oz)		Percent U.S. RDA* 250 Calories
Vitamin A	850	I.U.	17
Vitamin D	68	I.U.	17
Vitamin E	7.7	I.U.	25.6
Vitamin K_1	12	mcg	**
Vitamin C	15.4	mg	25.6
Folic Acid	68	mcg	17
Thiamine (Vit. B_1)	0.26	mg	17.3
Riboflavin (Vit. B_2)	0.29	mg	17
Vitamin B_6	0.34	mg	17
Vitamin B_{12}	1.1	mcg	18.3
Niacin	3.4	mg	17
Choline	25	mg	**
Biotin	51	mcg	17
Pantothenic Acid	1.7	mg	17
Sodium	240	mg	**
Potassium	330	mg	**
Chloride	220	mg	**
Calcium	200	mg	20
Phosphorus	200	mg	20
Magnesium	68	mg	17
Iodine	60	mcg	40
Manganese	0.85	mg	**
Copper	0.34	mg	17
Zinc	3.83	mg	25.5
Iron	3.06	mg	17

*For adults and children 4 or more years of age.
**U.S. RDA not established.
(FAN 422-02)

FLEXIFLO® ENTERAL DELIVERY SYSTEM

[fleks'ă-flō"]

A complete delivery system specially designed for enteral feeding.

FLEXIFLO® Enteral Feeding Tube

8 French (45" length)
Tungsten/C-FLEX® weighted bolus

USAGE

For administration of enteral feedings via the nasogastric or nasoenteric route.

AVAILABILITY

Enteral feeding tube; 12 individually packed tubes per case; No. 53.

FLEXIFLO® Enteral Feeding Tube

8 French w/Stylet (45" length)
Tungsten/C-FLEX® weighted bolus

USAGE

For administration of enteral feedings via the nasogastric or nasoenteric route.

AVAILABILITY

Enteral feeding tube; 12 individually packed tubes per case; No. 54.

FLEXIFLO® Enteral Feeding Tube

12 French (36" length)

USAGE

For administration of enteral feedings via the nasogastric route.

AVAILABILITY

Enteral feeding tube; 12 individually packed tubes per case; No. 55.

FLEXIFLO® Enteral Nutrition Pump

Peristaltic pump with constant-speed motor allows accurate flow control from 50 to 200 mL/hr (25-mL increments). The Flexiflo Pump, designed for enteral feeding, is simple to operate, reliable, and cost effective.

AVAILABILITY

Pump; 1 pump per case; retail unit, No. 64; lease unit, No. 72.

FLEXIFLO® Enteral Pump Set

USAGE

For use with the Flexiflo Enteral Nutrition Pump, Nos. 64 and 72. The set has a 40mm screw cap, a specially formulated insert, sight chamber, color coded flow regulation tabs and a tip adapter compatible with most indwelling feeding tubes.

AVAILABILITY

Pump set; 24 individually packed sets per case; No. 65.

Continued on next page

Ross—Cont.

FLEXIFLO® Pump Set with Piercing Pin
USAGE
For use with the Flexiflo Enteral Nutrition Pump, Nos. 64 and 72. The set has a piercing pin which allows hookup to a variety of enteral nutrition containers with spike ports.
AVAILABILITY
Pump set; 24 individually packed sets per case; No. 60.

FLEXIFLO®-II Portable Enteral Nutrition Pump
USAGE
Provides maximum versatility for the delivery of enteral feedings. Suitable for the ambulatory patient.
Features:
- Flow rates of 20, 30, 40, 50, 60, 75, 100, 125, 150, 175, 200, 250 mL/hr.
- Portable with a battery life of at least 8 hours. Alarm override system prevents disturbing alarms when patient is ambulating.
- Ideal for the ambulatory patient, especially when used with shoulder strap. Lightweight. Expensive IV stand not necessary, but can be used if desired.
- Safety—Visual and audible alarm system signals tube occlusion, empty container and low battery.

AVAILABILITY
Pump; 1 pump per case; retail unit, No. 51; lease unit, No. 58.

FLEXIFLO®-II Enteral Pump Set
USAGE
For use with the Flexiflo-II Portable Enteral Nutrition Pump, Nos. 51 and 58. The set has a 40mm screw cap, a specially formulated insert, sight chamber, and a tip adapter compatible with most indwelling feeding tubes.
AVAILABILITY
Pump set; 24 individually packed sets per case; No. 66.

FLEXIFLO®-II Pump Set with Piercing Pin
USAGE
For use with the Flexiflo-II Portable Enteral Nutrition Pump, Nos. 51 and 58. The set has a piercing pin which allows hookup to a variety of enteral nutrition containers with spike ports.
AVAILABILITY
Pump set; 24 individually packed sets per case; No. 57.

FLEXIFLO®-III Enteral Nutrition Pump
USAGE
For controlled, accurate delivery of enteral feedings. Microprocessor controlled rotary peristaltic pump. Flow rates of 1–300 mL/hr in 1 mL increments. Battery life of at least 8 hours. Visual and audible alarms that warn of tube occlusion or empty container, low battery, and completed dose.
AVAILABILITY
Pump; 1 pump per case; retail unit, No. 76; lease unit, No. 82.

FLEXIFLO®-III Enteral Pump Set
USAGE
For use with the Flexiflo-III Enteral Nutrition Pump, Nos. 76 and 82. The set has a 40mm screw cap, a specially formulated insert, sight chamber, and a tip adapter compatible with most indwelling feeding tubes.
AVAILABILITY
Pump set; 24 individually packed sets per case; No. 77.

FLEXIFLO®-III Pump Set with Piercing Pin
USAGE
For use with the Flexiflo-III Enteral Nutrition Pump, Nos. 76 and 82. The set has a piercing pin which allows hookup to a variety of enteral nutrition containers with spike ports.
AVAILABILITY
Pump set; 24 individually packed sets per case; No. 78.

FLEXIFLO® Gravity Gavage Set
USAGE
For use with the Flexitainer Enteral Nutrition Container, Flexitainer 500 Enteral Nutrition Container, or with 8-fl-oz bottles for controlled enteral feeding. Set is composed of a 40mm screw cap, clear plastic sight chamber, air vent protected by bacteria-retentive filter, CAIR® clamp flow regulator (roller clamp), and tip adapter compatible with most indwelling feeding tubes.
AVAILABILITY
Gavage set; 24 individually packed sets per case; No. 61.

FLEXIFLO® Gravity Feeding Set with Piercing Pin
USAGE
For use with Ross Top-Fill Bag #90 and a variety of enteral nutrition containers with spike ports.
AVAILABILITY
Gavage set; 24 individually packed sets per case; No. 59.

FLEXITAINER® Enteral Nutrition Container
Ready-to-use, large-volume, one-liter container combining the best features of a bottle and a bag... collapsible with a rigid neck and a large opening for easy filling, and graduated measurements for both filling and delivery.
AVAILABILITY
Container; 24 per case; No. 69.

FLEXITAINER® 500 Enteral Nutrition Container
USAGE
For convenient administration of small-volume enteral feedings.
AVAILABILITY
Container; 24 per case; No. 68.

FLEXIFLO® Top-Fill Enteral Nutrition System
USAGE
For convenient top-fill administration of large-volume enteral feedings. One-liter bag with rigid neck for easy handling and filling, wide filling port with twist-on cap to prevent leakage, and rigid hanging ring for use with an IV pole. (Use with any Flexiflo Enteral Pump Set or Gravity Set with Piercing Pin.)
AVAILABILITY
Individual bag; 24 per case; No. 90.

FLEXIFLO® Top-Fill Enteral Nutrition System with Preattached Flexiflo Pump Set
USAGE
For convenient top-fill administration of large-volume enteral feedings. Features one-liter bag with rigid neck for easy handling and filling, wide filling port with twist-on cap to prevent leakage, and rigid hanging ring for use with an IV pole. (No assembly needed. Use with Flexiflo Enteral Nutrition Pump, Nos. 64 and 72.)
AVAILABILITY
Individual bag with Preattached Flexiflo Pump Set; 24 per case; No. 91.

FLEXIFLO® Top-Fill Enteral Nutrition System with Preattached Flexiflo-II Pump Set
USAGE
For convenient top-fill administration of large-volume enteral feedings. Features one-liter bag with rigid neck for easy handling and filling, wide filling port with twist-on cap to prevent leakage, and rigid hanging ring for use with an IV pole. (No assembly needed. Use with Flexiflo-II Portable Enteral Nutrition Pump, Nos. 51 and 58.)
AVAILABILITY
Individual bag with Preattached Flexiflo-II Pump Set; 24 per case; No. 92.

FLEXIFLO® Top-Fill Enteral Nutrition System with Preattached Flexiflo-III Pump Set
USAGE
For convenient top-fill administration of large-volume enteral feedings. Features one-liter bag with rigid neck for easy handling and filling, wide filling port with twist-on cap to prevent leakage, and rigid hanging ring for use with an IV pole. (No assembly needed. Use with Flexiflo-III Enteral Nutrition Pump, Nos. 76 and 82.)
AVAILABILITY
Individual bag with Preattached Flexiflo-III Pump Set; 24 per case; No. 93.

FLEXIFLO® Top-Fill Enteral Nutrition System with Preattached Gravity Gavage Set
USAGE
For convenient top-fill administration of large-volume, gravity-fed enteral feedings. (No assembly needed).
AVAILABILITY
Individual bag with Preattached Gravity Gavage Set; 24 per case; No. 89.

ISOMIL®
[*ī'sō-mil*]
Soy Protein Formula With Iron

USAGE
As a beverage for infants, children and adults with an allergy or sensitivity to cow's milk protein. A feeding for patients with disorders where lactose should be avoided: lactase deficiency, lactose intolerance and galactosemia. A feeding following diarrhea.

AVAILABILITY
Powder: 14-oz cans; measuring scoop enclosed; 6 per case; No. 00107.
Concentrated Liquid: 13-fl-oz cans; 24 per case; No. 02110.
Ready To Feed: (Prediluted, 20 Cal/fl oz)
32-fl-oz cans; 6 per case; No. 00230.
8-fl-oz cans; 4 six-packs per case; No. 00173.
For hospital use, Ready To Feed Isomil in disposable nursing bottles is available in the Ross Hospital Formula System.

PREPARATION
Powder: Standard dilution (20 Cal/fl oz) is one level, unpacked scoop of Powder (8.7 g) for each 2 fl oz of warm water.
Concentrated Liquid: Standard dilution (20 Cal/fl oz) is one part Concentrated Liquid to one part water.
Ready To Feed: Do not dilute.
Note: All forms of Isomil should be shaken well before feeding.

COMPOSITION
Powder

INGREDIENTS
(Pareve, Ⓤ) 30.7% corn syrup solids, 20.5% sucrose, 16.1% soy protein isolate, 14.0% corn oil, 14.0% coconut oil, minerals (1.6% calcium phosphate tribasic, 0.9% potassium citrate, 0.3% potassium chloride, 0.3% magnesium chloride, 0.2% sodium chloride, calcium carbonate, ferrous sulfate, zinc sulfate, cupric sulfate, manganese sulfate, potassium iodide), vitamins (ascorbic acid, choline chloride, alpha-tocopheryl acetate, niacinamide, calcium pantothenate, vitamin A palmitate, thiamine chloride hydrochloride, riboflavin, pyridoxine hydrochloride, phylloquinone, folic acid, biotin, vitamin D_3, cyanocobalamin), L-methionine, taurine and L-carnitine.
5 fl oz provide 100 Cal when prepared as directed. 1 liter of prepared formula provides 676 Cal.

Nutrients:	Per 100 Cal	
Protein	2.66	g
Fat	5.46	g
Carbohydrate	10.1	g
Water	133	g
Linoleic Acid	1300	mg
Vitamins:		
Vitamin A	300	IU
Vitamin D	60	IU
Vitamin E	2.5	IU
Vitamin K	15	mcg
Thiamine (Vit. B_1)	60	mcg
Riboflavin (Vit. B_2)	90	mcg
Vitamin B_6	60	mcg
Vitamin B_{12}	0.45	mcg
Niacin	1350	mcg
Folic Acid (Folacin)	15	mcg
Pantothenic Acid	750	mcg
Biotin	4.5	mcg
Vitamin C (Ascorbic Acid)	9	mg
Choline	8	mg
Inositol	5	mg
Minerals:	**Per 100 Cal**	
Calcium	105	mg
Phosphorus	75	mg
Magnesium	7.5	mg
Iron	1.8	mg*
Zinc	0.75	mg
Manganese	30	mcg
Copper	75	mcg
Iodine	15	mcg
Sodium	47	mg
Potassium	115	mg
Chloride	88	mg

Standard dilution is one level scoop of Isomil Powder for each 2 fl oz of warm water, or 131.5 g of Powder diluted to 1 liter. (FAN 382-04)

COMPOSITION
Concentrated Liquid

INGREDIENTS
(Pareve, Ⓤ) 74% water, 7.2% corn syrup, 5.8% sucrose, 4.1% soy oil, 3.8% soy protein isolate, 2.7% coconut oil, 1.0% modified corn starch, minerals (calcium phosphate tribasic, potassium citrate, potassium chloride, magnesium chloride, sodium chloride, ferrous sulfate, zinc sulfate, cupric sulfate, manganese sulfate, potassium iodide), mono- and diglycerides, soy lecithin, vitamins (ascorbic acid, choline chloride, alpha-tocopheryl acetate, niacinamide, calcium pantothenate, vitamin A palmitate, thiamine chloride hydrochloride, riboflavin, pyridoxine hydrochloride, phylloquinone, folic acid, biotin, vitamin D_3, cyanocobalamin), L-methionine, carrageenan, taurine and L-carnitine.
5 fl oz provide 100 Cal when prepared as directed. 1 liter of prepared formula provides 676 Cal.

Nutrients:	Per 100 Cal	
Protein	2.66	g
Fat	5.46	g
Carbohydrate	10.1	g
Water	133	g
Linoleic Acid	1300	mg
Vitamins:		
Vitamin A	300	IU
Vitamin D	60	IU
Vitamin E	3.0	IU
Vitamin K	15	mcg
Thiamine (Vit. B_1)	60	mcg
Riboflavin (Vit. B_2)	90	mcg
Vitamin B_6	60	mcg
Vitamin B_{12}	0.45	mcg
Niacin	1350	mcg

Folic Acid (Folacin)	15	mcg
Pantothenic Acid	750	mcg
Biotin	4.5	mcg
Vitamin C (Ascorbic Acid)	9	mg
Choline	8	mg
Inositol	5	mg

Minerals:	**Per 100 Cal**	
Calcium	105	mg
Phosphorus	75	mg
Magnesium	7.5	mg
Iron	1.8	mg*
Zinc	0.75	mg
Manganese	30	mcg
Copper	75	mcg
Iodine	15	mcg
Sodium	47	mg
Potassium	115	mg
Chloride	88	mg

Standard dilution is equal amounts Isomil Concentrated Liquid and water. (FAN 382-03)

COMPOSITION

Ready To Feed

INGREDIENTS

(Pareve, ⓤ) 86.4% water, 4.1% corn syrup, 3.2% sucrose, 2.1% soy oil, 2.0% soy protein isolate, 1.4% coconut oil, minerals (calcium citrate, calcium phosphate tribasic, potassium phosphate monobasic, potassium chloride, potassium citrate, magnesium chloride, potassium phosphate dibasic, sodium chloride, ferrous sulfate, zinc sulfate, cupric sulfate, manganese sulfate, potassium iodide), mono- and diglycerides, soy lecithin, vitamins (ascorbic acid, choline chloride, alpha-tocopheryl acetate, niacinamide, calcium pantothenate, vitamin A palmitate, thiamine chloride hydrochloride, riboflavin, pyridoxine hydrochloride, phylloquinone, folic acid, biotin, vitamin D_3, cyanocobalamin), carrageenan, L-methionine, taurine and L-carnitine.
5 fl oz provide 100 Cal; 1 liter provides 676 Cal.

Nutrients:	**Per 100 Cal**	
Protein	2.66	g
Fat	5.46	g
Carbohydrate	10.1	g
Water	133	g
Linoleic Acid	1300	mg

Vitamins:		
Vitamin A	300	IU
Vitamin D	60	IU
Vitamin E	3.0	IU
Vitamin K	15	mcg
Thiamine (Vit. B_1)	60	mcg
Riboflavin (Vit. B_2)	90	mcg
Vitamin B_6	60	mcg
Vitamin B_{12}	0.45	mcg
Niacin	1350	mcg
Folic Acid (Folacin)	15	mcg
Pantothenic Acid	750	mcg
Biotin	4.5	mcg
Vitamin C (Ascorbic Acid)	9	mg
Choline	8	mg
Inositol	5	mg

Minerals:	**Per 100 Cal**	
Calcium	105	mg
Phosphorus	75	mg
Magnesium	7.5	mg
Iron	1.8	mg*
Zinc	0.75	mg
Manganese	30	mcg
Copper	75	mcg
Iodine	15	mcg
Sodium	47	mg
Potassium	140	mg
Chloride	65	mg

*The addition of iron to this formula conforms to the recommendation of the Committee on Nutrition of the American Academy of Pediatrics.
(FAN 382-03)

ISOMIL® SF

[ī'sō-mil]

Sucrose-Free Soy Protein Formula With Iron

USAGE

As a beverage for infants, children and adults with an allergy or sensitivity to cow's milk protein or an intolerance to sucrose. A feeding for patients with disorders where lactose and sucrose should be avoided. A feeding following acute diarrhea.

AVAILABILITY

Concentrated Liquid: 13-fl-oz cans; 12 per case; No. 00119.
Ready To Feed: (Prediluted, 20 Cal/fl oz)
32-fl-oz cans; 6 per case; No. 00128.
For hospital use, Ready To Feed Isomil SF in disposable nursing bottles is available in the Ross Hospital Formula System.

PREPARATION

Concentrated Liquid: Standard dilution (20 Cal/fl oz) is one part Concentrated Liquid to one part water.
Ready To Feed: Do not dilute.
Note: All forms of Isomil SF should be shaken well before feeding.

COMPOSITION

Concentrated Liquid

INGREDIENTS

(Pareve, ⓤ) 75.7% water, 13.2% corn syrup solids, 4.2% soy protein isolate, 4.0% soy oil, 2.6% coconut oil, minerals (calcium phosphate tribasic, potassium citrate, potassium chloride, magnesium chloride, calcium carbonate, sodium chloride, ferrous sulfate, zinc sulfate, cupric sulfate, manganese sulfate, potassium iodide), mono- and diglycerides, soy lecithin, vitamins (ascorbic acid, choline chloride, alpha-tocopheryl acetate, niacinamide, calcium pantothenate, vitamin A palmitate, thiamine chloride hydrochloride, riboflavin, pyridoxine hydrochloride, phylloquinone, folic acid, biotin, vitamin D_3, cyanocobalamin), L-methionine, taurine and L-carnitine.
5 fl oz provide 100 Cal when prepared as directed. 1 liter of prepared formula provides 676 Cal.

Nutrients:	**Per 100 Cal**	
Protein	2.96	g
Fat	5.33	g
Carbohydrate	10.1	g
Water	133	g
Linoleic Acid	1300	mg

Vitamins:		
Vitamin A	300	IU
Vitamin D	60	IU
Vitamin E	3.0	IU
Vitamin K	15	mcg
Thiamine (Vit. B_1)	60	mcg
Riboflavin (Vit. B_2)	90	mcg
Vitamin B_6	60	mcg
Vitamin B_{12}	0.45	mcg
Niacin	1350	mcg
Folic Acid (Folacin)	15	mcg
Pantothenic Acid	750	mcg
Biotin	4.5	mcg
Vitamin C (Ascorbic Acid)	9	mg
Choline	8	mg
Inositol	5	mg

Minerals:	**Per 100 Cal**	
Calcium	105	mg
Phosphorus	75	mg
Magnesium	7.5	mg
Iron	1.8	mg*
Zinc	0.75	mg
Manganese	30	mcg
Copper	75	mcg
Iodine	15	mcg
Sodium	47	mg
Potassium	115	mg
Chloride	88	mg

Standard dilution is equal amounts Isomil SF Concentrated Liquid and water. (FAN 382-02)

COMPOSITION

Ready To Feed

INGREDIENTS

(Pareve, ⓤ) 87.3% water, 6.7% corn syrup solids, 2.3% soy protein isolate, 2.0% soy oil, 1.4% coconut oil, minerals (calcium phosphate dibasic, potassium citrate, calcium carbonate, potassium chloride, calcium phosphate monobasic, magnesium chloride, ferrous sulfate, sodium chloride, zinc sulfate, cupric sulfate, manganese sulfate, potassium iodide), mono- and diglycerides, soy lecithin, vitamins (ascorbic acid, choline chloride, alpha-tocopheryl acetate, niacinamide, calcium pantothenate, vitamin A palmitate, thiamine chloride hydrochloride, riboflavin, pyridoxine hydrochloride, phylloquinone, folic acid, biotin, vitamin D_3, cyanocobalamin), carrageenan, L-methionine, taurine and L-carnitine.
5 fl oz provide 100 Cal; 1 liter provides 676 Cal.

Nutrients:	**Per 100 Cal**	
Protein	2.96	g
Fat	5.33	g
Carbohydrate	10.1	g
Water	133	g
Linoleic Acid	1300	mg

Vitamins:		
Vitamin A	300	IU
Vitamin D	60	IU
Vitamin E	3.0	IU
Vitamin K	15	mcg
Thiamine (Vit. B_1)	60	mcg
Riboflavin (Vit. B_2)	90	mcg
Vitamin B_6	60	mcg
Vitamin B_{12}	0.45	mcg
Niacin	1350	mcg
Folic Acid (Folacin)	15	mcg
Pantothenic Acid	750	mcg
Biotin	4.5	mcg
Vitamin C (Ascorbic Acid)	9	mg
Choline	8	mg
Inositol	5	mg

Minerals:	**Per 100 Cal**	
Calcium	105	mg
Phosphorus	75	mg
Magnesium	7.5	mg
Iron	1.8	mg*
Zinc	0.75	mg
Manganese	30	mcg
Copper	75	mcg
Iodine	15	mcg
Sodium	47	mg
Potassium	115	mg
Chloride	88	mg

*The addition of iron to this formula conforms to the recommendation of the Committee on Nutrition of the American Academy of Pediatrics.
(FAN 382-02)

MURINE® REGULAR FORMULA — OTC

[mur'ēn]

Eye Lubricant

PRODUCT OVERVIEW

KEY FACTS

Murine Eye Lubricant is a sterile, buffered, isotonic moisturizing solution formulated to match the natural fluid of the eye. It contains glycerin to moisturize and prevent dryness of the eye. Does not contain vasoconstrictors and can be used as needed.

MAJOR USES

Provides relief from minor eye irritation while moisturizing and preventing dryness.

SAFETY INFORMATION

Should only be used to relieve minor eye irritation, burning, and dryness. If eye pain, changes in vision, continued redness, or irritation of the eye occurs, or if any eye condition worsens or persists for more than 72 hours, discontinue use. Not for use while contact lenses are being worn.

PRESCRIBING INFORMATION

MURINE® REGULAR FORMULA — OTC

[mur'ēn]

Eye Lubricant

DESCRIPTION

Murine eye lubricant is a sterile isotonic buffered solution containing the active ingredient glycerin as well as potassium chloride, sodium chloride, sodium phosphate (monobasic and dibasic), and water. Edetate disodium 0.05% and benzalkonium chloride 0.01% are added as preservatives. (No vasoconstrictor.)

INDICATIONS

Murine is a non-staining, clear solution formulated to closely match the natural fluid of the eye for gentle, soothing relief from minor eye irritation while moisturizing and preventing dryness. Use as desired to temporarily relieve minor eye irritation, dryness and burning due to dust, smoke, smog, sun glare, wearing contact lenses, colds, allergies, swimming, reading, driving, TV or close work.

WARNING

To avoid contamination of this product, do not touch tip of container to any other surface. Replace cap after using. If you experience eye pain, changes in vision, continued redness or irritation of the eye, or if the condition worsens or persists for more than 72 hours, discontinue use and consult a physician. If solution changes color or becomes cloudy, do not use. Remove contact lenses before using. Keep this and all medicines out of the reach of children.

Continued on next page

Ross—Cont.

DOSAGE AND ADMINISTRATION

Tilt head back and squeeze 2 or 3 drops into each eye as needed.

HOW SUPPLIED

In 0.5-fl-oz and 1.0-fl-oz plastic dropper bottle.
(FAN 2070-02)

MURINE® PLUS OTC

[mur'ēn]
Tetrahydrozoline HCl Eye Redness Reliever

PRODUCT OVERVIEW

KEY FACTS

Murine Plus is a sterile buffered isotonic ophthalmic vasoconstrictor solution containing the eye redness reliever tetrahydrozoline HCl (.05%). It soothes, cools, and comforts while removing redness due to minor eye irritation. Can be used up to 4 times daily to remove redness.

MAJOR USE

Removes redness due to minor eye irritation.

SAFETY INFORMATION

Should only be used to relieve redness due to minor eye irritation. If eye pain, changes in vision, continued redness, or irritation of the eye occurs, or if the eye condition worsens or persists for more than 72 hours, discontinue use and consult a physician. Not for use by glaucoma patients unless under physician advice or supervision. Overuse of this product may produce increased redness of the eye. Not for use while contact lenses are being worn.

PRESCRIBING INFORMATION

MURINE® PLUS OTC

[mur'ēn]
Tetrahydrozoline HCl Eye Redness Reliever

DESCRIPTION

Murine Plus is a sterile isotonic buffered solution containing the active ingredient tetrahydrozoline hydrochloride 0.05%, as well as boric acid, sodium borate, and water. Edetate disodium 0.1% and benzalkonium chloride 0.01% are added as preservatives. (Contains vasoconstrictor.)

INDICATIONS

Murine Plus is a sterile, isotonic decongestant ophthalmic solution, compatible with the natural fluids of the eye. Its active ingredient is a sympathomimetic agent, tetrahydrozoline hydrochloride, which produces local vasoconstriction in the eye. Thus, the drug effectively narrows swollen blood vessels locally and provides symptomatic relief of edema and hyperemia of conjunctival tissues due to eye allergies, minor local irritations and conjunctivitis. Use up to 4 times daily, to remove redness due to minor eye irritation caused by dust, smoke, smog, sun glare, wearing contact lenses, colds, allergies, swimming, reading, driving, TV or close work. The effect of Murine Plus is prompt (apparent within minutes) and sustained.

WARNING

To avoid contamination of this product, do not touch tip of container to any surface. Replace cap after using. If you experience eye pain, changes in vision, continued redness or irritation of the eye, or if the condition worsens or persists for more than 72 hours, discontinue use and consult a physician. If you have glaucoma, do not use this product except under the advice and supervision of a physician. Overuse of this product may produce increased redness of the eye. If solution changes color or becomes cloudy, do not use. Remove contact lenses before using. Keep this and all medicines out of the reach of children.

DOSAGE AND ADMINISTRATION

Tilt head back and squeeze 1 or 2 drops into each eye, up to 4 times daily, or as directed by physician.

HOW SUPPLIED

In 0.5-fl-oz and 1.0-fl-oz plastic dropper bottles.
(FAN 2070-03)

MURINE® EAR WAX REMOVAL SYSTEM/MURINE® EAR DROPS OTC

[mur'ēn]

PRODUCT OVERVIEW

KEY FACTS

Murine Ear Drops contain carbamide peroxide 6.5% and alcohol 6.3% in anhydrous glycerin. The Murine Ear Wax Removal System also contains a soft bulb ear syringe. Application of the ear drops followed by warm water irrigation with the ear syringe is an effective, medically recommended method to help loosen and remove hardened ear wax.

MAJOR USES

Murine Ear Wax System/Murine Ear Drops is indicated for adults and children over 12 years of age as an aid in the removal of hardened or tightly packed ear wax from the ear canal.

SAFETY INFORMATION

For use in ears only. Do not use in eyes. If accidental eye contact occurs, wash eyes with water. If redness, tenderness, pain, dizziness, or ear drainage are present or develop, the medication should not be used. This medication should not be used if eardrum is known to be perforated.

PRESCRIBING INFORMATION

MURINE® EAR WAX REMOVAL SYSTEM/MURINE® EAR DROPS OTC

[mur'ēn]

DESCRIPTION

Active Ingredient: Carbamide Peroxide 6.5%. Also Contains: Alcohol (6.3%), Glycerin, Polysorbate 20 and other ingredients. A 1.0 fl oz soft bulb ear washer is also included. The Murine Ear Wax Removal System is the only self-treatment method on the market for ear wax removal. Application of carbamide peroxide drops followed by warm water irrigation is an effective, medically recommended way to help loosen hardened ear wax.

COMPOSITION

Contains the active ingredient carbamide peroxide, 6.5%. Also contains alcohol (6.3%), glycerin, polysorbate 20 and other ingredients.

ACTIONS

The carbamide peroxide formula in Murine Ear Drops is an aid in the removal of hardened cerumen from the ear canal. Anhydrous glycerin penetrates and softens wax while the release of oxygen from carbamide peroxide provides a mechanical action resulting in the loosening of the softened wax accumulation. It is usually necessary to remove the loosened wax by gently flushing the ear with warm water using the soft bulb ear washer provided.

INDICATIONS

The Murine Ear Wax Removal System is indicated as an aid in the removal of hardened or tightly packed cerumen from the ear canal.

CAUTION

If irritation, rash, dizziness, ear pain or drainage is present or develops, discontinue use and consult a doctor. Do not use if eardrum is known to be perforated.

DOSAGE AND ADMINISTRATION

For wax removal —Adults and children over 12 years: Tilt head sideways and place 5 to 10 drops into ear. Tip of bottle should not enter ear canal. Keep drops in ear for several minutes by keeping head tilted or placing cotton in ear. Wax remaining after treatment may be removed by gently flushing ear with warm water, using soft bulb ear washer placed on edge of ear canal. Use twice daily, up to 4 days if needed, or as directed by a doctor. Children under 12 years: Consult a doctor.

Used regularly, the Murine Ear Wax Removal System helps keep the ear canal free from blockage due to accumulated ear wax.

HOW SUPPLIED

The Murine Ear Wax Removal System contains 0.5-fl-oz drops and a 1.0-fl-oz soft bulb ear washer.

Also available in 0.5-fl-oz drops only, Murine Ear Drops.
(FAN 2014-02)

OSMOLITE®

[oz'mō-līt]
Isotonic Liquid Nutrition

USAGE

As an isotonic liquid food providing complete, balanced nutrition. Osmolite has been designed for patients particularly sensitive to hyperosmotic feedings. Osmolite may be used as a tube feeding (nasogastric, nasoduodenal or jejunal) or as an oral feeding. Two quarts (2000 Calories) of Osmolite meets or surpasses 100% of the U.S. RDA for vitamins and minerals for adults and children 4 or more years of age.

Features:

- Complete, balanced nutrition—1.06 Calories per mL, 250 Calories per 8-fl-oz feeding, 1000 Calories per quart from a balanced distribution of protein, fat and carbohydrate (caloric distribution: protein, 14.0%; fat, 31.4%; carbohydrate, 54.6%).
- Isotonic formulation—The osmolality is 300 mosm/kg water, equaling the osmotic pressure of plasma.
- Carbohydrate source—Osmolite is lactose-free and will not contribute to lactose-associated diarrhea. Glucose Polymers are the carbohydrate source, a readily available and easily digested source of calories.
- High biologic value protein—Osmolite provides a full complement of amino acids to meet the National Research Council's profile for high-quality proteins and has a calorie/nitrogen ratio of 178:1.
- Fat source—Osmolite contains a high level of essential fatty acids from corn and soy oils, as well as medium-chain triglycerides as 15% of total calories (50% of fat calories) to facilitate rapid, effective absorption of fat calories.
- Low-residue feeding—The amount of fecal residue produced by Osmolite is comparable to that produced by a chemically defined, elemental diet. Therefore, Osmolite is appropriate for use in situations where low residue is a primary consideration.
- Low electrolyte levels—Osmolite is appropriate for use with moderate electrolyte-restricted diets, yet provides electrolyte levels adequate for most hospitalized patients.
- Unflavored—The mild, acceptable taste makes Osmolite particularly appropriate for use with patients experiencing altered or heightened taste perceptions (eg, individuals undergoing radiation or chemotherapy treatment).
- Convenient—Osmolite is ready to use. No mixing is required. Potential for contamination during preparation is reduced.

DOSAGE AND ADMINISTRATION

Ready To Use: Shake well. May be stored unopened at room temperature. Once opened, Osmolite should be covered and refrigerated; discard if not used within 48 hours. Osmolite may be fed at room temperature or chilled.

Oral Feeding: May be used for total nutrition, or with and between meals.

Tube Feeding: Follow physician's instructions. Adjust flow rate, volume and dilution according to patient's condition and tolerance. Additional fluid requirements should be met by giving water with or after feedings. Avoid contamination during preparation and use.

Not for parenteral use.

[See table on top next page].

AVAILABILITY

Ready To Use:
8-fl-oz bottles; 24 per case; No. 715.
8-fl-oz cans; 4 six-packs per case; No. 709.
32-fl-oz cans; 6 per case; No. 738.

COMPOSITION

Ingredients: ⓤ-D Water, hydrolyzed corn starch, sodium and calcium caseinates, medium-chain triglycerides (fractionated coconut oil), corn oil, soy protein isolate, minerals (potassium citrate, calcium phosphate tribasic, magnesium sulfate, magnesium chloride, zinc sulfate, ferrous sulfate, manganese sulfate, cupric sulfate), soy oil, soy lecithin, vitamins (choline chloride, ascorbic acid, alpha-tocopheryl acetate, niacinamide, calcium pantothenate, thiamine chloride hydrochloride, pyridoxine hydrochloride, riboflavin, vitamin A palmitate, folic acid, biotin, phylloquinone, cyanocobalamin, vitamin D_3) and carrageenan.

Nutrients (Grams/8 fl oz): Protein, 8.8; Fat, 9.1; Carbohydrate, 34.3; Ash, 1.3; Water, 199. Calories per mL, 1.06; Calories per fl oz, 31.3.

Vitamin/Mineral Content of Osmolite (Ready To Use)

Vitamins/Minerals	Per 8 Fl Oz		Percent U.S. RDA* (Per 8 Fl Oz)
Vitamin A	625	I.U.	12.5
Vitamin D	50	I.U.	12.5
Vitamin E	5.63	I.U.	18.7
Vitamin K_1	9	mcg	**
Vitamin C	37.5	mg	62.5
Folic Acid	100	mcg	25
Thiamine (Vit. B_1)	0.38	mg	25.3
Riboflavin (Vit. B_2)	0.43	mg	25.3
Vitamin B_6	0.50	mg	25
Vitamin B_{12}	1.5	mcg	25
Niacin	5.0	mg	25
Choline	75	mg	**
Biotin	75	mcg	25
Pantothenic Acid	2.5	mg	25
Sodium	150	mg	**
Potassium	240	mg	**
Chloride	200	mg	**
Calcium	125	mg	12.5
Phosphorus	125	mg	12.5
Magnesium	50	mg	12.5
Iodine	18.8	mcg	12.5
Manganese	0.62	mg	**
Copper	0.25	mg	12.5
Zinc	2.82	mg	18.8
Iron	2.25	mg	12.5

*For adults and children 4 or more years of age.
**U.S. RDA not established.
(FAN 366-02)

Sample Administration Schedule for OSMOLITE

Continuous Drip Schedule

Day	Time	Strength	Rate (mL/hr)	Volume (mL)	Calories
1	1st 8 hours	Full	50	400	400
	2nd 8 hours	Full	75	600	600
	3rd 8 hours	Full	100	800	800
					1800 *Total Calories*
2	24 hours	Full	100–125	2400–3000	2400–3000 *Total Calories*

Intermittent Drip Schedule

Day	Time	Strength	Rate (5–10 mL/min)	Volume (mL)	Calories
1	7am–11pm	Full	100 mL q 2 hr (7am, 9am)	200	200
		Full	150 mL q 2 hr (11am, 1pm, 3pm)	450	450
		Full	200 mL q 2 hr (5pm, 7pm, 9pm, 11pm)	800	800
					1450 *Total Calories*
2	7am–11pm	Full	250 mL q 2 hr (8 feedings) up to	2000	2000 *Total Calories*
			400 mL q 3 hr (5 feedings)	2000	2000 *Total Calories*

- Check gastric residuals before every intermittent feeding or every 2–4 hours during continuous feeding.
- If intolerance develops (such as nausea, abdominal cramps, distention, or diarrhea) return to previously tolerated rate, or dilute formula to half strength. After tolerance to half strength OSMOLITE is established, continue feeding schedule using half strength OSMOLITE until desired rate is achieved. Then switch to full strength. Do not alter strength and volume at the same time.
- Rinsing the tube with water (eg, 25–100 mL) after each intermittent feeding or every 3 to 6 hours during continuous feeding will help avoid clogging and provide additional water.

OSMOLITE® HN

[oz 'mō-līt]

High Nitrogen Isotonic Liquid Nutrition

USAGE

As a high-nitrogen, isotonic liquid food providing complete, balanced nutrition. Osmolite HN is most appropriate for use in patients with decreased caloric intakes or increased protein needs, with intolerance to hyperosmolar feedings or with fat maldigestion/malabsorption. Osmolite HN may be used as a tube feeding (nasogastric, nasoduodenal, or jejunal) or as an oral feeding.

Features:

- Complete, balanced nutrition—1.06 Calories per mL, 250 Calories per 8 fl oz, 1000 Calories per quart from a balanced distribution of protein, fat and carbohydrate (caloric distribution: protein, 16.7%; fat, 30.0%; carbohydrate, 53.3%). 1400 Calories of Osmolite HN meets or surpasses 100% of the U.S. RDA for vitamins and minerals for adults and children 4 or more years of age.
- High protein level—10.5 g high-quality protein per 8-fl-oz serving (1.68 g nitrogen/8 fl oz).
- Total calorie/nitrogen ratio of 150:1—Appropriate for the stressed patient.
- Lactose-free—Osmolite HN will not contribute to lactose-associated diarrhea. Glucose Polymers is the carbohydrate source.
- Isotonic formulation—The osmolality is 300 mosm/kg water.
- Fat source—Osmolite HN contains a high level of essential fatty acids from corn and soy oils, as well as medium-chain triglycerides as 15% of total calories (50% of fat calories) to facilitate rapid, effective absorption of fat calories.
- Low-residue feeding—Osmolite HN is appropriate for use in situations where low residue is a consideration.
- Unflavored—The mild, acceptable taste makes Osmolite HN particularly appropriate for use with patients experiencing altered or heightened taste perceptions (eg, individuals undergoing radiation or chemotherapy treatment).
- Convenient—Osmolite HN is ready to use. No mixing is required. Potential for contamination during preparation is reduced.

DOSAGE AND ADMINISTRATION

Ready To Use: Shake well. May be stored unopened at room temperature. Once opened, Osmolite HN should be covered and refrigerated; discard if not used within 48 hours. Osmolite HN may be fed at room temperature or chilled.

Oral Feeding: May be used for total nutrition, or with and between meals.

Tube Feeding: Follow physician's instructions. Adjust flow rate, volume and dilution according to patient's condition and tolerance. Additional fluid requirements should be met by giving water with or after feedings. Avoid contamination during preparation and use.

Not for parenteral use.
[See table below].

AVAILABILITY

Ready To Use:
8-fl-oz bottles; 24 per case; No. 736.
8-fl-oz cans; 4 six-packs per case; No. 735.
32-fl-oz cans; 6 per case; No. 739.

COMPOSITION

Ingredients: Ⓤ-D Water, hydrolyzed corn starch, sodium and calcium caseinates, medium-chain triglycerides (fractionated coconut oil), corn oil, minerals (magnesium chloride, potassium citrate, calcium phosphate tribasic, sodium citrate, potassium phosphate dibasic, potassium chloride, zinc sulfate, ferrous sulfate, manganese sulfate, cupric sulfate), soy protein isolate, soy oil, soy lecithin, vitamins (choline chloride, ascorbic acid, alpha-tocopheryl acetate, niacinamide, calcium pantothenate, thiamine chloride hydrochloride, pyridoxine hydrochloride, riboflavin, vitamin A palmitate, folic acid, biotin, phylloquinone, cyanocobalamin, vitamin D_3) and carrageenan.

Nutrients (Grams/8 fl oz): Protein, 10.5; Fat, 8.7; Carbohydrate, 33.4; Minerals (Ash), 1.9; Water, 199. Calories per mL, 1.06; Calories per fl oz, 31.3.

Vitamin/Mineral Content of Osmolite HN (Ready To Use)

Vitamins/Minerals	Per 8 Fl Oz		Percent U.S. RDA* (Per 8 Fl Oz)
Vitamin A	893	I.U.	17.8
Vitamin D	72	I.U.	18
Vitamin E	8.1	I.U.	27
Vitamin K_1	13	mcg	**
Vitamin C	53.6	mg	89.3
Folic Acid	108	mcg	27
Thiamine (Vit. B_1)	0.41	mg	27.3
Riboflavin (Vit. B_2)	0.46	mg	27
Vitamin B_6	0.54	mg	27
Vitamin B_{12}	1.7	mcg	28.3
Niacin	5.36	mg	26.8
Choline	107	mg	**
Biotin	81	mcg	27
Pantothenic Acid	2.68	mg	26.8
Sodium	220	mg	**
Potassium	370	mg	**
Chloride	340	mg	**
Calcium	179	mg	17.9
Phosphorus	179	mg	17.9
Magnesium	71.5	mg	17.8
Iodine	26.8	mcg	17.8
Manganese	0.89	mg	**
Copper	0.36	mg	18
Zinc	4.02	mg	26.8
Iron	3.22	mg	17.8

*For adults and children 4 or more years of age.
**U.S. RDA not established.
(FAN 378-02)

Sample Administration Schedule For OSMOLITE HN

Continuous Drip Schedule

Day	Time	Strength	Rate (mL/h)	Volume (mL)	Calories
1	1st 8 hours	Full	50	400	400
	2nd 8 hours	Full	75	600	600
	3rd 8 hours	Full	100	800	800
					1800 *Total Calories*
2	24 hours	Full	100-125	2400-3000	2400-3000 *Total Calories*

Intermittent Drip Schedule

Day	Time	Strength	Rate (5-10 mL/min)	Volume (mL)	Calories
1	7am-11pm	Full	100 mL q 2 h (7am, 9am)	200	200
		Full	150 mL q 2 h (11am, 1pm, 3pm)	450	450
		Full	200 mL q 2 h (5pm, 7pm, 9pm, 11pm)	800	800
					1450 *Total Calories*
2	7am-11pm	Full	250 mL q 2 h (8 feedings) up to	2000	2000 *Total Calories*
			400 mL q 3 h (5 feedings)	2000	2000 *Total Calories*

- Check gastric residuals before every intermittent feeding or every 2–4 hours during continuous feeding.
- If intolerance develops, return to previously tolerated rate, or dilute formula to half strength. After tolerance to half strength OSMOLITE HN is established, continue feeding schedule using half strength OSMOLITE HN until desired rate is achieved. Then switch to full strength. Do not alter strength and volume at the same time.
- Rinsing the tube with water (eg, 25–100 mL) after each intermittent feeding or every 3 to 6 hours during continuous feeding will help avoid clogging and provide additional water.

Continued on next page

Ross—Cont.

PEDIAFLOR® Drops ℞

[*pē'dē-a-flor"*]

Sodium Fluoride Oral Solution, USP

DESCRIPTION

One dropperful (1.0 mL) provides:

Fluoride ....0.5 mg

(as sodium fluoride ....1.1mg)

Inactive Ingredients: Alcohol less than 0.5%, citric acid, methylparaben, propylparaben, sorbitol, water, artificial flavoring and other ingredients.

INDICATIONS AND USAGE

As an aid in the prevention of dental caries in infants and children.

CONTRAINDICATIONS

Should be used only where the fluoride content of the drinking water supply is known to be 0.7 parts per million or less.

PRECAUTIONS

The recommended dosage should not be exceeded since chronic overdosage of fluoride may result in mottling of tooth enamel and osseous changes.

OVERDOSAGE

In children, acute ingestion of 10 to 20 mg of sodium fluoride may cause excessive salivation and gastrointestinal disturbances; 500 mg may be fatal. Oral and/or intravenous fluids containing calcium may be indicated.

DOSAGE AND ADMINISTRATION

Daily dosage —under 2 years of age, one-half dropperful or less daily; 2 years of age, one dropperful daily; 3 years of age or older, two dropperfuls or less daily; or as directed by physician or dentist.

AVAILABILITY

50-mL bottles, calibrated dropper enclosed; Rx; **NDC** 0074-0101-50.

PEDIALYTE®

[*pē'dē-ah-līt"*]

Oral Electrolyte Maintenance Solution

USAGE

For maintenance of water and electrolytes during mild or moderate diarrhea in infants and children; for maintenance of water and electrolytes following corrective parenteral therapy for severe diarrhea.

Features:

- Ready to use—no mixing or dilution necessary.
- Balanced electrolytes to replace usual stool losses and provide maintenance requirements.
- Provides glucose to promote sodium and water absorption.
- Fruit-flavored form available to enhance compliance in older infants and children.
- Plastic quart bottles are resealable and easy to pour.
- Fluid volume markings on bottles in fl oz and mL for easy measurement.
- No coloring added.
- Widely available in grocery, drug and convenience stores.

AVAILABILITY

32-fl-oz plastic bottles; 8 per case; Unflavored, No. 336—NDC 0074-6470-32; Fruit-flavored, No. 365—NDC 0074-6471-32. 8-fl-oz bottles; 4 six-packs per case; Unflavored, No. 160—NDC 0074-6470-08. For hospital use, Pedialyte is available in the Ross Hospital Formula System.

DOSAGE

See Administration Guide for maintenance of body water and electrolytes in mild or moderate diarrhea (Pedialyte Unflavored or Fruit-Flavored) and management of mild to moderate dehydration secondary to moderate to severe diarrhea (Pedialyte® RS).

Pedialyte, Unflavored or Fruit-Flavored, or Pedialyte RS should be offered frequently in amounts tolerated. Total daily intake should be adjusted to meet individual needs, based on thirst and response to therapy. The suggested intakes for maintenance found in Administration Guide are based on water requirements for ordinary energy expenditure.[1] The suggested intakes for replacement are based on fluid losses of 5% or 10% of body weight, including maintenance requirement.

[See table below].

COMPOSITION

Unflavored Pedialyte (Flavored Pedialyte has similar composition and nutrient value. For specific information, see product label.)

INGREDIENTS

(Pareve, Ⓤ) Water, dextrose, potassium citrate, sodium chloride and sodium citrate.

Provides:	Per 8 Fl Oz	Per Liter	Per 32 Fl Oz
Sodium (mEq)	10.6	45	42.4
Potassium (mEq)	4.7	20	18.8
Chloride (mEq)	8.3	35	33.2
Citrate (mEq)	7.1	30	28.4
Dextrose (g)	5.9	25	23.6
Calories	24	100	96

(FAN 384-01)

Pedialyte, Pedialyte RS Administration Guide

For Infants and Young Children

Age	2 Weeks	3	6 Months	9	1	1½	2	2½ Years	3	3½	4
Approximate Weight[2] (lb)	7	13	17	20	23	25	28	30	32	35	38
(kg)	3.2	6.0	7.8	9.2	10.2	11.4	12.6	13.6	14.6	16.0	17.0
PEDIALYTE UNFLAVORED or FRUIT-FLAVORED fl oz/day for maintenance*	13 to 16	28 to 32	34 to 40	38 to 44	41 to 46	45 to 50	48 to 53	51 to 56	54 to 58	56 to 60	57 to 62
PEDIALYTE RS fl oz/day for Replacement for 5% Dehydration (including maintenance)*	18 to 21	38 to 42	47 to 53	53 to 59	58 to 63	64 to 69	69 to 74	74 to 79	78 to 82	83 to 87	85 to 90
PEDIALYTE RS fl oz/day for Replacement for 10% Dehydration (including maintenance)*	23 to 26	48 to 52	60 to 66	68 to 74	75 to 80	83 to 88	90 to 95	97 to 102	102 to 106	110 to 114	113 to 118

Administration Guide does not apply to infants less than 1 week of age. For children over 4 years, maintenance intakes may exceed 2 qt daily.

1. Extrapolated from Barness L: Nutrition and nutritional disorders, in Behrman RE, Vaughan VC III; *Nelson Textbook of Pediatrics*, ed 12. Philadelphia: WB Saunders Co, 1983, pp 136-138.
2. Weight based on the 50th percentile of weight for age of the National Center for Health Statistics (NCHS) reference data: Hamill PVV, Drizd TA, Johnson CL, et al: Physical growth: National Center for Health Statistics percentiles. *Am J Clin Nutr* 32:607-629, 1979.

* Fluid intakes do not take into account ongoing stool losses. Fluid loss in the stool should be replaced by consumption of an extra amount of Pedialyte or Pedialyte RS equal to stool losses in addition to the amounts given in this Administration Guide.

PEDIALYTE® RS

[*pē'dē-ah-līt"*]

Oral Electrolyte Rehydration Solution

USAGE

For replacement of water and electrolytes during moderate to severe diarrhea.

Features:

- Ready to use—no mixing or dilution necessary.
- Safe, economical alternative to IV therapy.
- 75 mEq of sodium per liter for effective replacement of deficits.
- 2½% glucose solution to promote sodium and water absorption and provide energy.
- Widely available in pharmacies.

AVAILABILITY

8-fl-oz bottles; 4 six-packs per case; No. 162; NDC 0074-6472-08.

DOSAGE

(See Administration Guide under Pedialyte)

INGREDIENTS

(Pareve, Ⓤ) Water, dextrose, sodium chloride, potassium citrate and sodium citrate.

Provides:	Per 8 Fl Oz	Per Liter
Sodium (mEq)	17.7	75
Potassium (mEq)	4.7	20
Chloride (mEq)	15.4	65
Citrate (mEq)	7.1	30
Dextrose (g)	5.9	25
Calories	24	100

(FAN 384-01)

PEDIAMYCIN® ℞

[*pē"dē-e-mī'san*]

erythromycin ethylsuccinate

DESCRIPTION

Erythromycin is produced by a strain of *Streptomyces erythraeus* and belongs to the macrolide group of antibiotics. It is basic and readily forms salts with acids. The base, the stearate salt and the esters are poorly soluble in water. Erythromycin ethylsuccinate is an ester of erythromycin suitable for oral administration. The premixed suspension, granules and drops for oral administration are intended primarily for pediatric use but can also be used in adults.

Pediamycin 400 (erythromycin ethylsuccinate oral suspension), 400 mg erythromycin activity per teaspoonful (5 ml), is a premixed suspension with an appealing cherry flavor, supplied in pint (16 fl oz) bottles. Its form and flavor make it especially suitable for older children unwilling or unable to swallow capsules or tablets.

Inactive Ingredients: Alcohol less than 0.1%, citric acid, DC Red No. 33, FDC Red No. 40, methylparaben, polysorbate 60, propylparaben, sodium chloride, sodium citrate, sucrose, water, xanthan gum, natural & artificial flavoring and other ingredients.

Pediamycin Liquid (erythromycin ethylsuccinate oral suspension), 200 mg erythromycin activity per teaspoonful (5 ml), is a premixed suspension with an appealing cherry flavor, supplied in pint (16 fl oz) bottles. Its form and flavor make it especially suitable for infants and children, and for older children unwilling or unable to swallow capsules or tablets.

Inactive Ingredients: Alcohol less than 0.1%, citric acid, DC Red No. 33, FDC Red No. 3, methylparaben, polysorbate 60, propylparaben, sodium chloride, sodium citrate, sucrose, water, xanthan gum, natural & artificial flavoring and other ingredients.

Pediamycin Suspension and *Pediamycin Drops* (erythromycin ethylsuccinate for oral suspension), 200 mg erythromycin activity per teaspoonful (5 ml), 100 mg erythromycin activity per dropperful (2.5 ml), are pleasant-tasting cherry-flavored oral suspensions, dispensed as granules of erythromycin ethylsuccinate reconstituted with water. Pediamycin granules are packaged in 100-ml and 150-ml (Suspension), and 50-ml (Drops) bottles. A calibrated dropper is supplied with the 50-ml bottles.

Inactive Ingredients: Citric acid, FDC Red No. 3, magnesium aluminum silicate, sodium carboxymethylcellulose, sodium citrate, sucrose, artificial flavoring and other ingredients.

ACTIONS

Microbiology

Biochemical tests demonstrate that erythromycin inhibits protein synthesis of the pathogen without directly affecting nucleic acid synthesis. Antagonism has been demonstrated between clindamycin and erythromycin.

NOTE: Many strains of *Hemophilus influenzae* are resistant to erythromycin alone but are susceptible to erythromycin and sulfonamides together. Staphylococci resistant to erythromycin may emerge during a course of erythromycin therapy. Culture and susceptibility testing should be performed.

Disc Susceptibility Tests

Quantitative methods that require measurement of zone diameters give the most precise estimates of antibiotic susceptibility. One recommended procedure (21 CFR section 460.1) uses erythromycin class discs for testing susceptibility; interpretations correlate zone diameters of this disc test with MIC values for erythromycin. With this procedure, a report from the laboratory of "susceptible" indicates that the infective organism is likely to respond to therapy. A report of "resistant" indicates that the infective organism is not likely to respond to therapy. A report of "intermediate susceptibility" suggests that the organism would be susceptible if higher doses were used.

CLINICAL PHARMACOLOGY

Erythromycin binds to the 50 S ribosomal subunits of susceptible bacteria and suppresses protein synthesis.

Orally administered erythromycin ethylsuccinate suspensions are readily and reliably absorbed. Comparable serum levels of erythromycin are achieved in the fasting and the nonfasting states.

Erythromycin diffuses readily into most body fluids. Only low concentrations are normally achieved in the spinal fluid, but passage of the drug across the blood-brain barrier increases in meningitis. In the presence of normal hepatic function, erythromycin is concentrated in the liver and excreted in the bile; the effect of hepatic dysfunction on excretion of erythromycin by the liver into the bile is not known. Less than 5 percent of the orally administered dose of erythromycin is excreted in active form in the urine.

Erythromycin crosses the placental barrier and is excreted in breast milk.

INDICATIONS

Streptococcus pyogenes (Group A beta-hemolytic streptococcus): Upper and lower respiratory tract, skin, and soft tissue infections of mild to moderate severity.

Injectable benzathine penicillin G is considered by the American Heart Association to be the drug of choice in the treatment and prevention of streptococcal pharyngitis and in long-term prophylaxis of rheumatic fever.

When oral medication is preferred for treatment of the above conditions, penicillin G or V, or erythromycin is the alternate drug of choice.

When oral medication is given, the importance of strict adherence by the patient to the prescribed dosage regimen must be stressed. A therapeutic dose should be administered for at least 10 days.

Alpha-hemolytic streptococci (viridans group): Although no controlled clinical efficacy trials have been conducted, oral erythromycin has been suggested by the American Heart Association and American Dental Association for use in a regimen for prophylaxis against bacterial endocarditis in patients hypersensitive to penicillin who have congenital heart disease, or rheumatic or other acquired valvular heart disease when they undergo dental procedures and surgical procedures of the upper respiratory tract.[1] Erythromycin is not suitable prior to genitourinary or gastrointestinal tract surgery. NOTE: When selecting antibiotics for the prevention of bacterial endocarditis the physician or dentist should read the full joint statement of the American Heart Association and the American Dental Association.[1]

Staphylococcus aureus: Acute infections of skin and soft tissue of mild to moderate severity. Resistant organisms may emerge during treatment.

Streptococcus (Diplococcus) pneumoniae: Upper respiratory tract infections (e.g., otitis media, pharyngitis) and lower respiratory tract infections (e.g., pneumonia) of mild to moderate degree.

Mycoplasma pneumoniae (Eaton agent, PPLO): For respiratory infections due to this organism.

Hemophilus influenzae: For upper respiratory tract infections of mild to moderate severity when used concomitantly with adequate doses of sulfonamides. (See sulfonamide labeling for appropriate prescribing information.) The concomitant use of the sulfonamides is necessary since not all strains of *Hemophilus influenzae* are susceptible to erythromycin at the concentrations of the antibiotic achieved with usual therapeutic doses.

Chlamydia trachomatis: For the treatment of urethritis in adult males due to *Chlamydia trachomatis.*

Ureaplasma urealyticum: For the treatment of urethritis in adult males due to *Ureaplasma urealyticum.*

Treponema pallidum: Erythromycin is an alternate choice of treatment for primary syphilis in patients allergic to the penicillins. In treatment of primary syphilis, spinal fluid examinations should be done before treatment and as part of follow-up after therapy.

Corynebacterium diphtheriae: As an adjunct to antitoxin, to prevent establishment of carriers, and to eradicate the organism in carriers.

Corynebacterium minutissimum: For the treatment of erythrasma.

Entamoeba histolytica: In the treatment of intestinal amebiasis only. Extra-enteric amebiasis requires treatment with other agents.

Listeria monocytogenes: Infections due to this organism.

Bordetella pertussis: Erythromycin is effective in eliminating the organism from the nasopharynx of infected individuals, rendering them non-infectious. Some clinical studies suggest that erythromycin may be helpful in the prophylaxis of pertussis in exposed susceptible individuals.

Legionnaire's disease: Although no controlled clinical efficacy studies have been conducted, *in vitro* and limited preliminary clinical data suggest that erythromycin may be effective in treating Legionnaire's disease.

CONTRAINDICATIONS

Erythromycin is contraindicated in patients with known hypersensitivity to this antibiotic.

PRECAUTIONS

Erythromycin is principally excreted by the liver. Caution should be exercised in administering the antibiotic to patients with impaired hepatic function. There have been reports of hepatic dysfunction, with or without jaundice occurring in patients receiving oral erythromycin products.

Areas of localized infection may require surgical drainage in addition to antibiotic therapy.

Recent data from studies of erythromycin reveal that its use in patients who are receiving high doses of theophylline may be associated with an increase of serum theophylline levels and potential theophylline toxicity. In case of theophylline toxicity and/or elevated serum theophylline levels, the dose of theophylline should be reduced while the patient is receiving concomitant erythromycin therapy.

Usage during pregnancy and lactation: The safety of erythromycin for use during pregnancy has not been established. Erythromycin crosses the placental barrier. Erythromycin also appears in breast milk.

ADVERSE REACTIONS

The most frequent side effects of oral erythromycin preparations are gastrointestinal, such as abdominal cramping and discomfort, and are dose related. Nausea, vomiting and diarrhea occur infrequently with usual oral doses.

During prolonged or repeated therapy, there is a possibility of overgrowth of nonsusceptible bacteria or fungi. If such infections occur, the drug should be discontinued and appropriate therapy instituted.

Allergic reactions ranging from urticaria and mild skin eruptions to anaphylaxis have occurred.

There have been isolated reports of reversible hearing loss occurring chiefly in patients with renal insufficiency and in patients receiving high doses of erythromycin.

DOSAGE AND ADMINISTRATION

Erythromycin ethylsuccinate suspensions may be administered without regard to meals.

Children: Age, weight and severity of the infection are important factors in determining the proper dosage. In mild to moderate infections the usual dosage of erythromycin ethylsuccinate for children is 30 to 50 mg/kg/day in equally divided doses. For more severe infections this dosage may be doubled.

Adults: 400 mg erythromycin ethylsuccinate every 6 hours is the usual dose. Dosage may be increased up to 4 g per day according to the severity of the infections.

If twice-a-day dosage is desired in either adults or children, one-half of the total daily dose may be given every 12 hours. Doses may also be given three times daily if desired by administering one-third of the total daily dose every 8 hours.

The following approximate dosage schedule is suggested for using *Pediamycin Liquid* (erythromycin ethylsuccinate oral suspension), *Pediamycin Suspension* and *Pediamycin Drops* (erythromycin ethylsuccinate for oral suspension) in the treatment of mild to moderate infections by susceptible organisms.

Body Weight	Dose	Frequency	Approximate Daily Dosage
Under 10 lbs (4.5 kg)	40 mg/kg/day (20 mg/lb/day) in divided doses		
10–15 lbs (4.5 to 6.8 kg)	½ dropperful (50 mg)	4 times/day	200 mg
	or 1 dropperful (100 mg)	2 times/day	
15–25 lbs (6.8 to 11.3 kg)	1 dropperful (100 mg) ½ teaspoonful (100 mg)	4 times/day	400 mg
	or 2 dropperfuls (200 mg) 1 teaspoonful (200 mg)	2 times/day	
25–50 lbs (11.3 to 22.7 kg)	1 teaspoonful (200 mg)	4 times/day	800 mg
	or 2 teaspoonfuls (400 mg)	2 times/day	
50–100 lbs (22.7 to 45.4 kg)	1½ teaspoonfuls (300 mg)	4 times/day	1200 mg
	or 3 teaspoonfuls (600 mg)	2 times/day	
over 100 lbs (45.4 kg)	2 teaspoonfuls (400 mg)	4 times/day	1600 mg
	or 4 teaspoonfuls (800 mg)	2 times/day	

The following approximate dosage schedule is suggested for using *Pediamycin 400* (erythromycin ethylsuccinate oral suspension) in the treatment of mild to moderate infections by susceptible organisms.

Body Weight	Dose	Frequency	Approximate Daily Dosage
25–50 lbs (11.3 to 22.7 kg)	1 teaspoonful (400 mg)	2 times/day	800 mg
50–100 lbs (22.7 to 45.4 kg)	1½ teaspoonfuls (600 mg)	2 times/day	1200 mg
over 100 lbs (45.4 kg)	2 teaspoonfuls (800 mg)	2 times/day	1600 mg

The total daily dosage must be administered in equally divided doses.

In the treatment of streptococcal infections, a therapeutic dosage of erythromycin ethylsuccinate should be administered for at least 10 days. In continuous prophylaxis against recurrences of streptococcal infections in persons with a history of rheumatic heart disease, the usual dosage is 400 mg twice a day.

For prophylaxis against bacterial endocarditis[1] in patients with congenital heart disease, or rheumatic or other acquired valvular heart disease when undergoing dental procedures or surgical procedures of the upper respiratory tract, give 1.6 g (20 mg/kg for children) orally 1½ to 2 hours before the procedure, and then, 800 mg (10 mg/kg for children) orally every 6 hours for 8 doses.

For treatment of urethritis due to *C. trachomatis* or *U. urealyticum:* 800 mg three times a day for 7 days.

For treatment of primary syphilis: Adults: 48 to 64 g given in divided doses over a period of 10 to 15 days.

For intestinal amebiasis: Adults: 400 mg four times daily for 10 to 14 days. Children: 30 to 50 mg/kg/day in divided doses for 10 to 14 days.

For use in pertussis: Although optimal dosage and duration have not been established, doses of erythromycin utilized in reported clinical studies were 40 to 50 mg/kg/day, given in divided doses for 5 to 14 days.

For treatment of Legionnaire's disease: Although optimal doses have not been established, doses utilized in reported clinical data were 1.6 to 4 g daily in divided doses.

HOW SUPPLIED

Pediamycin 400 (erythromycin ethylsuccinate oral suspension, USP) is supplied in 1 pint bottles (**NDC** 0074-0211-16). It provides erythromycin ethylsuccinate equivalent to 400 mg erythromycin per teaspoonful (5 ml).

Pediamycin Liquid (erythromycin ethylsuccinate oral suspension, USP) is supplied in 1 pint bottles (**NDC** 0074-0202-16). It provides erythromycin ethylsuccinate equivalent to 200 mg erythromycin per teaspoonful (5 ml).

Pediamycin Suspension (erythromycin ethylsuccinate for oral suspension, USP) is available for teaspoon dosage in 100-ml (**NDC** 0074-0206-13) and 150-ml (**NDC** 0074-0206-09) bot-

Continued on next page

Ross—Cont.

tles, in the form of granules to be reconstituted with 77 ml and 115 ml of water, respectively. It provides erythromycin ethylsuccinate equivalent to 200 mg erythromycin per teaspoonful (5 ml).

Pediamycin Drops (erythromycin ethylsuccinate for oral suspension, USP) is available for dropper dosage in 50-ml bottles (**NDC** 0074-0207-50), in the form of granules to be reconstituted with 38 ml of water, providing 100 mg of erythromycin activity per dropperful (2.5 ml). Dropper marked for 100 mg (dropperful), 75 mg and 50 mg (half dropperful) doses is enclosed in the carton.

Pediamycin Liquid and *Pediamycin 400* require refrigeration to preserve taste. Refrigeration by patient is not required if used within 14 days.

REFERENCE

1. American Heart Association, 1977. Prevention of bacterial endocarditis. Circulation 56:139A-143A.

(.5880)

PEDIAZOLE® ℞

[*pē 'dē-e-zōl ″*]

erythromycin ethylsuccinate and sulfisoxazole acetyl for oral suspension

PRODUCT OVERVIEW

KEY FACTS

Pediazole Suspension provides a combination of erythromycin ethylsuccinate and sulfisoxazole acetyl in a convenient single prescription. This strawberry-banana flavored suspension provides 200 mg erythromycin activity and the equivalent of 600 mg of sulfisoxazole per teaspoonful (5 ml). Pediazole is available in 100 ml, 150 ml and 200 ml bottles.

MAJOR USES

Pediazole is indicated for the treatment of acute otitis media in children that is caused by susceptible strains of Hemophilus influenzae (including ampicillin-resistant strains).

SAFETY INFORMATION

Pediazole Suspension is contraindicated for patients with known hypersensitivity to erythromycin or sulfonamides. It is also contraindicated for use in infants less than 2 months of age and for women who are pregnant or nursing. Fatalities associated with the administration of sulfonamides have occurred due to severe reactions. Pediazole should be discontinued at the first appearance of skin rash or any sign of adverse reaction. Complete blood counts should be done frequently in patients receiving sulfonamide therapy.

Erythromycin therapy in patients receiving high doses of theophylline may be associated with an increase of serum theophylline levels and potential theophylline toxicity. Caution should be exercised in use of sulfonamide therapy in those patients with impaired renal or hepatic function, history of severe allergy or bronchial asthma, or a deficiency in the glucose 6 phosphate dehydrogenase. Adequate fluid intake must be maintained during Pediazole therapy.

PRESCRIBING INFORMATION

PEDIAZOLE® ℞

[*pē 'dē-e-zōl ″*]

erythromycin ethylsuccinate and sulfisoxazole acetyl for oral suspension

DESCRIPTION

Pediazole is a combination of erythromycin ethylsuccinate, USP and sulfisoxazole acetyl, USP. When reconstituted with water as directed on the label, the granules form a white, strawberry-banana flavor suspension which provides 200 mg erythromycin activity and the equivalent of 600 mg of sulfisoxazole per teaspoonful (5 ml).

Erythromycin is produced by a strain of *Streptomyces erythraeus* and belongs to the macrolide group of antibiotics. It is basic and readily forms salts and esters. Erythromycin ethylsuccinate is an ester of erythromycin.

Sulfisoxazole acetyl or N^1-acetyl sulfisoxazole is an ester of sulfisoxazole. Chemically, sulfisoxazole is N^1-(3,4-dimethyl-5-isoxazolyl) sulfanilamide.

Inactive Ingredients: Citric acid, magnesium aluminum silicate, poloxamer, sodium carboxymethylcellulose, sodium citrate, sucrose, artificial flavoring and other ingredients.

ACTIONS

Clinical Pharmacology: Orally administered erythromycin ethylsuccinate suspension is reliably and readily absorbed and serum levels are comparable when administered to patients in either the fasting or non-fasting state. After absorption, erythromycin diffuses readily into most body fluids. In the presence of normal hepatic function, erythromycin is concentrated in the liver and excreted in the bile; the effect of hepatic dysfunction on excretion of erythromycin by the liver into the bile is not known. After oral administration, less than 5 percent of the activity of the administered dose can be recovered in the urine.

Erythromycin crosses the placental barrier but fetal plasma levels are generally low.

Sulfisoxazole acetyl is deacetylated by enzymatic hydrolysis in the gastrointestinal tract from which it is readily absorbed as sulfisoxazole. Sulfisoxazole exists in the blood primarily bound to serum proteins as well as conjugated and in the active or free form. Metabolic pathways include N^4-acetylation and oxidation with approximately 80 percent of an administered dose being excreted by the kidney within 24 hours.

Serum half-life for total erythromycin and free sulfisoxazole is about 1.5 and 6 hours, respectively.

Microbiology: Pediazole has been formulated to contain sulfisoxazole for concomitant use with erythromycin. The mode of action of erythromycin is by inhibition of protein synthesis without affecting nucleic acid synthesis. Sulfonamides, including sulfisoxazole, possess bacteriostatic activity. This bacteriostatic agent acts by means of competitively inhibiting bacterial synthesis of folic acid (pteroylglutamic acid) from para-aminobenzoic acid. Resistance to erythromycin blood levels ordinarily achieved has been demonstrated by some strains of *Hemophilus influenzae.* Pediazole is usually active against *Hemophilus influenzae in vitro,* including ampicillin-resistant strains.

Quantitative methods that require measurements of zone diameters give the most precise estimates of antibiotic susceptibility. One such standardized procedure, the ASM-2 method published by the National Committee for Clinical Laboratory Standards (NCCLS), has been recommended for use with discs to test susceptibility to erythromycin and sulfisoxazole. Interpretation involves correlation of the diameters obtained in the disc test with Minimal Inhibitory Concentrations (MIC) values for erythromycin and sulfisoxazole. If the standardized ASM-2 procedure of disc susceptibility is used, a 15 mcg erythromycin disc should give a zone diameter of at least 18 mm when tested against an erythromycin-susceptible bacterial strain and a 250-300 mcg sulfisoxazole disc should give a zone diameter of at least 17 mm when tested against a sulfisoxazole-susceptible bacterial strain.

In vitro sulfonamide sensitivity tests are not always reliable because media containing excessive amounts of thymidine are capable of reversing the inhibitory effect of sulfonamides which may result in false resistant reports. The tests must be carefully coordinated with bacteriological and clinical responses. When the patient is already taking sulfonamides follow-up cultures should have aminobenzoic acid added to the isolation media but not to subsequent susceptibility test media.

INDICATION

For treatment of ACUTE OTITIS MEDIA in children that is caused by susceptible strains of *Hemophilus influenzae.*

CONTRAINDICATIONS

Known hypersensitivity to either erythromycin or sulfonamides.

Infants less than 2 months of age.

Pregnancy at term and during the nursing period, because sulfonamides pass into the placental circulation and are excreted in human breast milk and may cause kernicterus in the infant.

WARNINGS

FATALITIES ASSOCIATED WITH THE ADMINISTRATION OF SULFONAMIDES, ALTHOUGH RARE, HAVE OCCURRED DUE TO SEVERE REACTIONS INCLUDING STEVENS-JOHNSON SYNDROME, TOXIC EPIDERMAL NECROLYSIS, FULMINANT HEPATIC NECROSIS, AGRANULOCYTOSIS, APLASTIC ANEMIA, AND OTHER BLOOD DYSCRASIAS.

Clinical signs such as sore throat, fever, pallor, rash, purpura, or jaundice may be early indications of serious reactions.

PEDIAZOLE SHOULD BE DISCONTINUED AT THE FIRST APPEARANCE OF SKIN RASH OR ANY SIGN OF ADVERSE REACTION. In some instances a skin rash may be followed by a more severe reaction, such as Stevens-Johnson syndrome, toxic epidermal necrolysis, hepatic necrosis and serious blood disorders.

COMPLETE BLOOD COUNT SHOULD BE DONE FREQUENTLY IN PATIENTS RECEIVING SULFONAMIDES.

Usage in Pregnancy (SEE ALSO: CONTRAINDICATIONS): The safe use of erythromycin or sulfonamides in pregnancy has not been established. The teratogenic potential of most sulfonamides has not been thoroughly investigated in either animals or humans. However, a significant increase in the incidence of cleft palate and other bony abnormalities of offspring has been observed when certain sulfonamides of the short, intermediate and long-acting types were given to pregnant rats and mice at high oral doses (7 to 25 times the human therapeutic dose).

The frequency of renal complications is considerably lower in patients receiving the most soluble sulfonamides such as sulfisoxazole. Urinalysis with careful microscopic examination should be obtained frequently in patients receiving sulfonamides.

PRECAUTIONS

Erythromycin is principally excreted by the liver. Caution should be exercised in administering the antibiotic to patients with impaired hepatic function. There have been reports of hepatic dysfunction, with or without jaundice occurring in patients receiving oral erythromycin products.

Recent data from studies of erythromycin reveal that its use in patients who are receiving high doses of theophylline may be associated with an increase of serum theophylline levels and potential theophylline toxicity. In case of theophylline toxicity and/or elevated serum theophylline levels, the dose of theophylline should be reduced while the patient is receiving concomitant erythromycin therapy.

Surgical procedures should be performed when indicated.

Sulfonamide therapy should be given with caution to patients with impaired renal or hepatic function and in those patients with a history of severe allergy or bronchial asthma. In the presence of a deficiency in the enzyme glucose-6-phosphate dehydrogenase, hemolysis may occur. This reaction is frequently dose-related. Adequate fluid intake must be maintained in order to prevent crystalluria and renal stone formation.

ADVERSE REACTIONS

The most frequent side effects of oral erythromycin preparations are gastrointestinal, such as abdominal cramping and discomfort, and are dose-related. Nausea, vomiting and diarrhea occur infrequently with usual oral doses. During prolonged or repeated therapy, there is a possibility of overgrowth of nonsusceptible bacteria or fungi. If such infections occur, the drug should be discontinued and appropriate therapy instituted. The overall incidence of these latter side effects reported for the combined administration of erythromycin and a sulfonamide is comparable to those observed in patients given erythromycin alone. Mild allergic reactions such as urticaria and other skin rashes have occurred. Serious allergic reactions, including anaphylaxis, have been reported with erythromycin.

There have been isolated reports of reversible hearing loss occurring chiefly in patients with renal insufficiency and in patients receiving high doses of erythromycin.

The following untoward effects have been associated with the use of sulfonamides:

Blood Dyscrasias: Agranulocytosis, aplastic anemia, thrombocytopenia, leukopenia, hemolytic anemia, purpura, hypoprothrombinemia and methemoglobinemia.

Allergic Reactions: Erythema multiforme (Stevens-Johnson syndrome), generalized skin eruptions, epidermal necrolysis, urticaria, serum sickness, pruritus, exfoliative dermatitis, anaphylactoid reactions, periorbital edema, conjunctival and scleral injection, photosensitization, arthralgia and allergic myocarditis.

Gastrointestinal Reactions: Nausea, emesis, abdominal pains, hepatitis, diarrhea, anorexia, pancreatitis and stomatitis.

CNS Reactions: Headache, peripheral neuritis, mental depression, convulsions, ataxia, hallucinations, tinnitus, vertigo and insomnia.

Miscellaneous Reactions: Drug fever, chills and toxic nephrosis with oliguria or anuria. Periarteritis nodosa and LE phenomenon have occurred.

The sulfonamides bear certain chemical similarities to some goitrogens, diuretics (acetazolamide and the thiazides) and oral hypoglycemic agents. Goiter production, diuresis and hypoglycemia have occurred rarely in patients receiving sulfonamides. Cross-sensitivity may exist with these agents. Rats appear to be especially susceptible to the goitrogenic effects of sulfonamides, and long-term administration has produced thyroid malignancies in the species.

DOSAGE AND ADMINISTRATION

PEDIAZOLE SHOULD NOT BE ADMINISTERED TO INFANTS UNDER 2 MONTHS OF AGE BECAUSE OF CONTRAINDICATIONS OF SYSTEMIC SULFONAMIDES IN THIS AGE GROUP.

For Acute Otitis Media in Children: The dose of Pediazole can be calculated based on the erythromycin component (50 mg/kg/day) or the sulfisoxazole component (150 mg/kg/day to a maximum of 6 g/day). Pediazole should be administered in equally divided doses four times a day for 10 days. It may be administered without regard to meals.

The following approximate dosage schedule is recommended for using Pediazole:

Children: Two months of age or older

Weight	Dose—every 6 hours
Less than 8 kg (18 lb)	Adjust dosage by body weight
8 kg (18 lb)	½ teaspoonful (2.5 ml)
16 kg (35 lb)	1 teaspoonful (5 ml)
24 kg (53 lb)	1½ teaspoonfuls (7.5 ml)
Over 45 kg (over 100 lb)	2 teaspoonfuls (10 ml)

HOW SUPPLIED

Pediazole Suspension is available for teaspoon dosage in 100-ml (**NDC** 0074-8030-13), 150-ml (**NDC** 0074-8030-43) and 200-ml (**NDC** 0074-8030-53) bottles, in the form of granules to be reconstituted with water. The suspension provides erythromycin ethylsuccinate equivalent to 200 mg erythromycin activity and sulfisoxazole acetyl equivalent to 600 mg sulfisoxazole per teaspoonful (5 ml).
(.5870)

POLYCOSE®

[pol 'ē-kōs]
Glucose Polymers

USAGE

As a source of calories (derived solely from carbohydrate) for persons with increased caloric needs or those unable to meet their caloric needs with their normal diet. Polycose is particularly useful in supplying carbohydrate calories for protein-, electrolyte- and fat-restricted diets.

Features:

- Mixes readily with most foods and beverages.
- Minimal sweetness increases patient acceptance.
- Absorbed as rapidly as equal concentrations of glucose.
- Low electrolyte levels.
- Low osmolality (900 mosm/kg water),—compared to other carbohydrate sources of similar concentration, Polycose helps reduce potential for osmotic diarrhea.

DOSAGE AND ADMINISTRATION

Polycose may be added to tube feeding formulas and most foods and beverages, or mixed in water, in amounts determined by taste, caloric requirement and tolerance. Small, frequent feedings are more desirable than large amounts given infrequently. Polycose may be used for extended periods with diets containing all other essential nutrients, or as an oral adjunct to intravenous administration of nutrients. Polycose is nutritionally incomplete and should not be used as the sole source of nutrition. Undiluted Polycose should not be fed without physician supervision.

Refrigerate dissolved Polycose Powder and opened Polycose Liquid and discard unused portion after 24 hours. Concentrated solutions become more viscous when cold; thus serving Polycose at room temperature is advised.

NOT FOR PARENTERAL USE.

Precaution (For Infant Use): Not to be fed undiluted. Use only as specifically directed by a physician.

AVAILABILITY

Powder: 12.3 oz (350g) cans; 6 per case; No. 746.
Liquid: (43% solution): 4-fl-oz bottles; 48 per case; No. 749.

COMPOSITION

Powder: (Pareve, Ⓤ) Glucose polymers derived from controlled hydrolysis of corn starch.

Nutrients (per 100 grams):

Carbohydrate		94	g
Water		6	g
Calcium	Does not exceed	30	mg (1.5 mEq)
Sodium	Does not exceed	110	mg (4.8 mEq)
Potassium	Does not exceed	10	mg (0.3 mEq)
Chloride	Does not exceed	223	mg (6.3 mEq)
Phosphorus	Does not exceed	5	mg

Approximate Caloric Equivalents:

1 level teaspoonful (2 g) = 8 Calories; 1 level tablespoonful (6 g) = 23 Calories; 1/4 cup (25 g) = 95 Calories; 1/3 cup (33 g) = 125 Calories; 1/2 cup (50 g) = 190 Calories; 1 cup (100 g) = 380 Calories.
(FAN 366-01)

COMPOSITION

Liquid: (Pareve, Ⓤ) Water and glucose polymers derived from controlled hydrolysis of corn starch.

Nutrients (per 100 mL):

Carbohydrate		50	g
Water		70	g
Calcium	Does not exceed	20	mg (1.0 mEq)
Sodium	Does not exceed	70	mg (3.0 mEq)
Potassium	Does not exceed	6	mg (0.15 mEq)
Chloride	Does not exceed	140	mg (3.9 mEq)
Phosphorus	Does not exceed	3	mg

Approximate Caloric Equivalents:

1 mL = 2 Calories; 1 fl oz = 60 Calories; 100 mL = 200 Calories.
(FAN 366-01)

PRAMET® FA ℞

[pram 'et]
Vitamin/Mineral Prescription
For Expectant and
New Mothers

PRODUCT OVERVIEW

KEY FACTS

Pramet FA is a vitamin/mineral preparation containing 1 mg folic acid for use during pregnancy and lactation. The Gradumet® dosage form provides controlled-release of iron from the inert wax/polymer matrix to minimize gastrointestinal irritation.

MAJOR USES

Pramet FA is effective in helping to prevent vitamin and mineral deficiencies during pregnancy and for treatment of megaloblastic anemias.

SAFETY INFORMATION

Allergic sensitization has been reported following oral administration of folic acid. Folic acid alone is improper therapy for treatment of pernicious anemia and other megaloblastic anemias where vitamin B_{12} is deficient.

PRESCRIBING INFORMATION

PRAMET® FA ℞

[pram 'et]
Vitamin/Mineral Prescription
For Expectant and
New Mothers

DESCRIPTION

Each Pramet FA Filmtab® Film-Sealed oral tablet provides:

Vitamins		
Vitamin A (as acetate and palmitate) 1.2 mg	4000	I.U.
Vitamin D (cholecalciferol, 10 mcg)	400	I.U.
Vitamin C (ascorbic acid)	100	mg
Folic Acid	1	mg
Vitamin B_1 (thiamine mononitrate)	3	mg
Vitamin B_2 (riboflavin)	2	mg
Niacinamide	10	mg
Vitamin B_6 (pyridoxine hydrochloride)	5	mg
Vitamin B_{12} (cyanocobalamin)	3	mcg
Pantothenic Acid (as calcium pantothenate)	0.92	mg
Minerals		
Calcium (as calcium carbonate)	250	mg
Iodine (as calcium iodate)	100	mcg
Elemental Iron* (300 mg ferrous sulfate USP)	60	mg
Copper (as cupric chloride)	0.15	mg

* In controlled-release form—Gradumet®

Inactive Ingredients: Cellulosic polymers, corn starch, DC Yellow No. 10, FDC Blue No. 1, magnesium stearate, methyl acrylate-methyl methacrylate copolymer, microcrystalline cellulose, polyethylene glycols, povidone, talc, titanium dioxide and other ingredients.

INDICATIONS AND USAGE

To help prevent vitamin and mineral deficiencies during and after pregnancy and for treatment of megaloblastic anemias. One mg of folic acid has been found to be effective therapy for megaloblastic anemias of pregnancy and lactation.

WARNING

Folic acid alone is improper therapy in the treatment of pernicious anemia and other megaloblastic anemias where vitamin B_{12} is deficient.

PRECAUTION

Folic acid may mask the presence of pernicious anemia in that hematologic remission may occur while neurologic manifestations remain progressive.

ADVERSE REACTION

Allergic sensitization has been reported following both oral and parenteral administration of folic acid.

OVERDOSAGE

Acute overdosage of iron may cause nausea and vomiting and, in severe cases, cardiovascular collapse and death. The estimated lethal dose of orally ingested elemental iron is 300 mg per kg body weight. Serum iron and total iron-binding capacity may be used as guides for use of chelating agents such as deferoxamine.

DOSAGE AND ADMINISTRATION

One tablet daily, or as directed by physician.

HOW SUPPLIED

100-tablet bottles; ℞; **NDC** 0074-0147-01.
Shown in Product Identification Section, page 426
(.5850)

PRAMILET® FA ℞

[pram 'e-let "]
Prenatal
Vitamin/Mineral Preparation

DESCRIPTION

Each Pramilet FA Filmtab® Film-Sealed oral tablet provides:

Vitamins		
Vitamin A (as acetate and palmitate) 1.2 mg	4000	I.U.
Vitamin D (cholecalciferol, 10 mcg)	400	I.U.
Vitamin C (as sodium ascorbate)	60	mg
Folic Acid	1	mg
Vitamin B_1 (thiamine mononitrate)	3	mg
Vitamin B_2 (riboflavin)	2	mg
Niacinamide	10	mg
Vitamin B_6 (pyridoxine hydrochloride)	3	mg
Vitamin B_{12} (cyanocobalamin)	3	mcg
Calcium Pantothenate	1	mg
Minerals		
Calcium (as calcium carbonate)	250	mg
Iodine (as calcium iodate)	100	mcg
Elemental Iron (as ferrous fumarate)	40	mg
Magnesium (as magnesium oxide)	10	mg
Copper (as cupric chloride)	0.15	mg
Zinc (as zinc oxide)	0.085	mg

Inactive Ingredients: Carmine No. 40, cellulosic polymers, corn starch, crospovidone, FDC Blue No. 1, propylene glycol, magnesium stearate, povidone, sorbic acid, sorbitan monooleate, titanium dioxide, vanillin and other ingredients.

INDICATIONS AND USAGE

To help prevent vitamin and mineral deficiencies during and after pregnancy and for treatment of megaloblastic anemias. One mg of folic acid has been found to be effective therapy for megaloblastic anemias of pregnancy and lactation.

WARNING

Folic acid alone is improper therapy in the treatment of pernicious anemia and other megaloblastic anemias where vitamin B_{12} is deficient.

PRECAUTION

Folic acid may mask the presence of pernicious anemia in that hematologic remission may occur while neurologic manifestations remain progressive.

ADVERSE REACTION

Allergic sensitization has been reported following both oral and parenteral administration of folic acid.

OVERDOSAGE

Acute overdosage of iron may cause nausea and vomiting and, in severe cases, cardiovascular collapse and death. The estimated lethal dose of orally ingested elemental iron is 300 mg per kg body weight. Serum iron and total iron-binding capacity may be used as guides for use of chelating agents such as deferoxamine.

DOSAGE AND ADMINISTRATION

One tablet daily, or as directed by physician.

HOW SUPPLIED

100-tablet bottles; ℞; **NDC** 0074-0121-01.
Shown in Product Identification Section, page 426
(.5860)

PROMOD™

[prō 'mod]
Protein Supplement

USAGE

For providing extra protein to individuals who have increased protein needs and those who are unable to meet their protein needs with a normal diet. ProMod may be added to an oral supplement, an enteral tube feeding or prepared foods. It may also be useful in controlling protein intake in protein-restricted diets when the protein level of regular food or enteral products is inappropriate.

Features:

- Concentrated—High-quality whey protein. 45 g of protein—100% of U.S. RDA in 9 scoops.
- Increase protein intake—May be added to an oral supplement, enteral tube feeding or solid foods to increase protein intake.
- Mixes readily—Formulated to mix easily with both foods and beverages.
- Unflavored—Designed with a bland taste, will not dramatically alter the flavor of foods.

Continued on next page

Ross—Cont.

- Very low lactose—About 0.4 g/scoop.
- Scoop included—For measuring convenience.

DOSAGE AND ADMINISTRATION

Instructions for Use: Designed to be added to an enteral formula, food or beverage. Use the enclosed scoop or standard household measures to add the recommended amount of protein (see table). Opened can should be covered with overcap and stored in a cool, dry place but not refrigerated. Once opened, use contents within 1 month. After mixing, enteral nutritional products should be used promptly, or covered, refrigerated and used within 24 hours. When mixed with prepared foods, use promptly or store appropriately.

Mixing with Liquids: For best results, mix ProMod with a small amount of the liquid or water to make a smooth paste, then gradually add the remaining liquid to the mixture while stirring. For blender mixing, combine ProMod with the desired amount of liquid and briefly blend at the lowest speed to minimize foaming.

Mixing with Foods: ProMod may be mixed directly into prepared foods such as mashed potatoes, oatmeal, gravy or soup.
ProMod is not a balanced diet and should not be used as a sole source of nutrition. ProMod is for enteral use only and should be used as directed by a physician or other health care professional.
Not for parenteral use.

PRECAUTION (For Infant Use)

Use only as directed by a physician.
Availability:
Powder: 9.7 oz (275 g) cans; 6 per case; No. 775.
Composition:
Ingredients: Ⓤ-D Whey protein concentrate and soy lecithin.

Nutrients:		**Per 5 g Protein (one scoop)**
Protein		5.0 g
Fat	Does not exceed	0.60 g
Carbohydrate	Does not exceed	0.67 g
Water	Does not exceed	0.60 g
Calcium	Does not exceed	23 mg (1.15 mEq)
Sodium	Does not exceed	13 mg (0.57 mEq)
Potassium	Does not exceed	65 mg (1.66 mEq)
Phosphorus	Does not exceed	22 mg
Calories		28

Approximate Protein Equivalents:

Amount of ProMod Protein Supplement	Amount of Protein
1 scoop (6.6 g)	5 g
1 level teaspoonful (1.3 g)	1 g
1 level tablespoonful (4.0 g)	3 g
1/4 cup (16 g)	12 g
1/3 cup (22 g)	16 g
1/2 cup (32 g)	24 g
1 cup (64 g)	48 g

Typical Amino Acid Composition Per 100 g Protein*—
Essential Amino Acids: Histidine, 1.9 g; Isoleucine, 6.2 g; Leucine, 10.8 g; Lysine, 9.3 g; Methionine, 2.2 g; Phenylalanine, 3.6 g; Threonine, 7.3 g; Tryptophan, 1.9 g; Valine, 6.0 g.
Non-Essential Amino Acids:
Alanine, 5.3 g; Arginine, 2.6 g; Aspartic Acid, 11.2 g; Cystine, 2.6 g; Glutamic Acid, 18.2 g; Glycine, 2.1 g; Proline, 6.5 g; Serine, 5.6 g; Tyrosine, 3.4 g.
*100 grams of ProMod protein yields approximately 105 grams of individual amino acids.
(FAN 395-01)

PULMOCARE®

[pul 'mō-kăr]
Specialized Nutrition for Pulmonary Patients

USAGE

For the dietary management of respiratory insufficiency, the high-fat and low-carbohydrate content of Pulmocare is designed to reduce carbon dioxide production. Pulmocare can be used for enteral tube-feeding or for oral supplementation and is appropriate for ambulatory or ventilator-dependent patients.
Features:

- The high-fat, low-carbohydrate content is designed to reduce carbon dioxide (CO_2) production. Caloric distribution: 16.7% protein, 55.2% fat, 28.1% carbohydrate.
- 1420 Calories (947 mL) of Pulmocare provide at least 100% of the U.S. RDA for vitamins and minerals.
- Concentrated nutrition (1500 Calories per liter)—Beneficial for patients requiring fluid restriction.
- High levels of nitrogen—Total calorie/nitrogen ratio of 150:1, meets the needs of the stressed patient.
- High-quality protein—The amino acid profile meets the standard for high-quality protein set by the National Academy of Sciences.
- Lactose-free—Pulmocare will not contribute to lactose-associated diarrhea. Hydrolyzed corn starch and sucrose are the carbohydrate sources.
- Moderate osmolality (490 mosm/kg water)—Pulmocare will decrease the potential for osmotically induced diarrhea.

Sample Administration Schedule For PULMOCARE

Continuous Drip Schedule

Day	Time	Strength	Rate (mL/hr)	Volume (mL)	Calories
1	1st 8 hours	1/2	50	400	300
	2nd 8 hours	1/2	75	600	450
	3rd 8 hours	1/2	100	800	600
					1350 *Total Calories*
2	1st 8 hours	1/2	100	800	600
	2nd 8 hours	Full	100	800	1200
	3rd 8 hours	Full	100	800	1200
					3000 *Total Calories*
3	24 hours	Full	100	2400	3600 *Total Calories*

Intermittent Drip Schedule

Day	Time	Strength	Rate (5–10 mL/min)	Volume (mL)	Calories
1	7am–11pm	1/2	100 mL q 2 hr (7am, 9am)	200	150
		1/2	150 mL q 2 hr (11am, 1pm, 3pm)	450	338
		1/2	200 mL q 2 hr (5pm, 7pm, 9pm, 11pm)	800	600
					1088 *Total Calories*
2	7am–11pm	1/2	250 mL q 2 hr (7am, 9am, 11am)	750	563
		Full	250 mL q 2 hr (1pm, 3pm, 5pm, 7pm, 9pm, 11pm)	1500	2250
					2813 *Total Calories*
3	7am–11pm	Full	250 mL q 2 hr (8 feedings)	2000	3000 *Total Calories*
			up to 400 mL q 3 hr (5 feedings)	2000	3000 *Total Calories*

- Check gastric residuals before every intermittent feeding or every 2–4 hours during continuous feeding.
- If signs of intolerance develop, return to previously tolerated strength and rate. When tolerance is again established, proceed with feeding schedule as indicated. Do not alter rate and strength at the same time.
- Rinse the tube with water (eg, 25–100 mL) after each intermittent feeding or every 3 to 6 hours during continuous feeding. This will help avoid clogging and provide additional water.
- Pulmocare should be administered at room temperature, since low temperatures increase the viscosity of the product.

DOSAGE AND ADMINISTRATION

Ready To Use: Shake well. May be stored unopened at room temperature. Once opened, Pulmocare should be covered and refrigerated; discard if not used within 48 hours. Pulmocare may be fed at room temperature or chilled.
Oral Feeding: May be used as total or supplemental nutrition for patients on a low-carbohydrate diet.
Tube Feeding: Follow physician's instructions. Adjust flow rate, volume and dilution according to patient's condition and tolerance. Additional fluid requirements should be met by giving water with or after feedings. Avoid contamination during preparation and use.
Not for parenteral use.
[See table below left].

AVAILABILITY

8-fl-oz cans; 4 six-packs per case; Vanilla, No. 699.

COMPOSITION

Ready To Use Vanilla.

INGREDIENTS

Ⓤ-D Water, corn oil, sodium and calcium caseinates, sucrose, hydrolyzed corn starch, minerals (magnesium chloride, potassium citrate, calcium phosphate tribasic, sodium citrate, potassium phosphate dibasic, sodium chloride, zinc sulfate, ferrous sulfate, manganese sulfate, cupric sulfate), soy lecithin, vitamins (choline chloride, ascorbic acid, alpha-tocopheryl acetate, niacinamide, calcium pantothenate, thiamine chloride hydrochloride, pyridoxine hydrochloride, riboflavin, vitamin A palmitate, folic acid, biotin, phylloquinone, cyanocobalamin, vitamin D_3), artificial flavor and carrageenan.
Nutrients (Grams/8 fl oz): Protein, 14.8; Fat, 21.8; Carbohydrate, 25.0; Minerals (Ash), 2.3; Water, 186. Calories per mL, 1.5; Calories per fl oz, 44.4.

Vitamin/Mineral Content of Pulmocare (Ready To Use)

Vitamins/Minerals	Per 8 Fl Oz		Percent U.S. RDA* (Per 8 Fl Oz)
Vitamin A	1250	I.U.	25
Vitamin D	100	I.U.	25
Vitamin E	11.3	I.U.	37.6
Vitamin K_1	18	mcg	**
Vitamin C	75	mg	125
Folic Acid	200	mcg	50
Thiamine (Vit. B_1)	0.75	mg	50
Riboflavin (Vit. B_2)	0.85	mg	50
Vitamin B_6	1.0	mg	50
Vitamin B_{12}	3.0	mcg	50
Niacin	10	mg	50
Choline	150	mg	**
Biotin	150	mcg	50
Pantothenic Acid	5.0	mg	50
Sodium	310	mg	**
Potassium	450	mg	**
Chloride	400	mg	**
Calcium	250	mg	25
Phosphorus	250	mg	25
Magnesium	100	mg	25
Iodine	37.5	mcg	25
Manganese	1.25	mg	**
Copper	0.50	mg	25
Zinc	5.63	mg	37.5
Iron	4.5	mg	25

*For adults and children 4 or more years of age.
**U.S. RDA not established.
(FAN 386-02)

RCF®

Ross Carbohydrate Free
Low-Iron Soy Protein Formula Base

USAGE

For use in the dietary management of persons unable to tolerate the type or amount of carbohydrate in milk or conventional infant formulas: many of these patients have intractable diarrhea and are not able to tolerate other formulas. This product has been formulated to contain no carbohydrate, which must be added before feeding.

AVAILABILITY

Concentrated Liquid only: 13-fl-oz cans; 12 per case; No. 108.

PREPARATION

RCF is for use only under the supervision of a physician. Physician's instructions must include the type and amount of carbohydrate and the amount of water to be added to RCF. Standard dilution is one part Formula Base to one part prescribed carbohydrate and water solution. If a physician specifies other types or amounts of carbohydrate or other amounts of water to be added to RCF, those instructions should be followed completely.

A full-strength formula, 20 Calories per fluid ounce, may be prepared with one of the following typical carbohydrates: [See table right].

COMPOSITION
Concentrated Liquid

INGREDIENTS
(Pareve, ⓤ) 87% water, 4.4% soy protein isolate, 4.2% soy oil, 2.8% coconut oil, minerals (calcium phosphates [mono- and tribasic], potassium citrate, potassium chloride, magnesium chloride, calcium carbonate, sodium chloride, zinc sulfate, cupric sulfate, potassium iodide), carrageenan, mono- and diglycerides, soy lecithin, vitamins (ascorbic acid, choline chloride, alpha-tocopheryl acetate, niacinamide, calcium pantothenate, vitamin A palmitate, riboflavin, thiamine chloride hydrochloride, pyridoxine hydrochloride, phylloquinone, biotin, folic acid, vitamin D_3, cyanocobalamin), L-methionine, taurine and L-carnitine.
4.2 fl oz of RCF, without added carbohydrate or water, provide 100 Cal (81 Cal/100 mL). 5 fl oz of 20 Cal/fl oz formula provide 100 Cal; see directions.

Nutrients:	Without Carbohydrate Per 100 Cal		With Carbohydrate* Per 100 Cal	
Protein	4.95	g	2.96	g
Fat	8.91	g	5.33	g
Carbohydrate	0.01	g	10.1	g
Water	110	g	133	g
Linoleic Acid	2170	mg	1300	mg
Vitamins:				
Vitamin A	500	IU	300	IU
Vitamin D	100	IU	60	IU
Vitamin E	5	IU	3.0	IU
Vitamin K	25	mcg	15	mcg
Thiamine (Vit. B_1)	100	mcg	60	mcg
Riboflavin (Vit. B_2)	150	mcg	90	mcg
Vitamin B_6	100	mcg	60	mcg
Vitamin B_{12}	0.75	mcg	0.45	mcg
Niacin	2230	mcg	1350	mcg
Folic Acid (Folacin)	25	mcg	15	mcg
Pantothenic Acid	1240	mcg	750	mcg
Biotin	7.5	mcg	4.5	mcg
Vitamin C (Ascorbic Acid)	13.6	mg	9	mg
Choline	13	mg	8	mg
Inositol	8	mg	5	mg
Minerals:				
Calcium	173	mg	105	mg
Phosphorus	124	mg	75	mg
Magnesium	12.4	mg	7.5	mg
Iron	0.37	mg†	0.22	mg†
Zinc	1.24	mg	0.75	mg
Manganese	50	mcg	30	mcg
Copper	124	mcg	75	mcg
Iodine	25	mcg	15	mcg
Sodium	80	mg	47	mg
Potassium	190	mg	115	mg
Chloride	145	mg	88	mg

* When 52 g of carbohydrate are mixed with 13 fl oz of RCF. Varies depending on quantity of carbohydrate and water used. If carbohydrate is not added to this product, a 1:1 dilution with water provides approximately 12 Cal/fl oz (40.5 Cal/100 mL).
† This product is deficient in iron; additional iron should be supplied from other sources.
(FAN 407-03)

RONDEC® Oral Drops ℞
[ron 'dek]
RONDEC® Syrup ℞
RONDEC® Tablet ℞
RONDEC–TR® Tablet ℞

PRODUCT OVERVIEW

KEY FACTS
Rondec products contain the antihistamine carbinoxamine maleate and the decongestant pseudoephedrine hydrochloride. Rondec Oral Drops, Rondec Syrup, and Rondec Tablets are immediate release dosage forms. Rondec-TR Tablet uses a gradual release mechanism allowing twice daily dosing.

MAJOR USES
Rondec products provide symptomatic relief of seasonal and perennial allergic rhinitis and vasomotor rhinitis.

SAFETY INFORMATION
Use with caution in patients with hypertension or ischemic heart disease, persons over age 60, and nursing mothers. Safety for use in pregnancy has not been established.

PRESCRIBING INFORMATION

RONDEC® Oral Drops ℞
[ron 'dek]
RONDEC® Syrup ℞
RONDEC® Tablet ℞
RONDEC-TR® Tablet ℞

DESCRIPTION
Antihistamine/Decongestant for oral use.

RCF

Type of Carbohydrate	Amount of Carbohydrate*	Water	RCF Formula Base
Table Sugar (sucrose)	4 level tablespoonfuls	12 fl oz	one 13-fl-oz can
Dextrose Powder (hydrous)	6 level tablespoonfuls	12 fl oz	one 13-fl-oz can
Polycose® Glucose Polymers Powder	9 level tablespoonfuls	12 fl oz	one 13-fl-oz can

* Approximately the 52 grams needed for 20 Cal/fl oz formula.

For infants
RONDEC® Oral Drops
Each dropperful (1 ml) contains carbinoxamine maleate, 2 mg, pseudoephedrine hydrochloride, 25 mg.
Inactive Ingredients: DC Red No. 33, FDC Yellow No. 6, glycerin, liquid glucose, methylparaben, propylparaben, sodium benzoate, sucrose, water, artificial flavoring and other ingredients.

For young children
RONDEC® Syrup
Each teaspoonful (5 ml) contains carbinoxamine maleate, 4 mg, pseudoephedrine hydrochloride, 60 mg.
Inactive Ingredients: DC Red No. 33, FDC Yellow No. 6, glycerin, liquid glucose, methylparaben, propylparaben, sodium benzoate, sucrose, water, artificial flavoring and other ingredients.

For adults and children 6 years and over
RONDEC® Tablet
Each Filmtab® tablet contains carbinoxamine maleate, 4 mg; pseudoephedrine hydrochloride, 60 mg.
Inactive Ingredients: Castor oil, cellulosic polymers, FDC Yellow No. 6, lactose, polacrilin potassium, povidone, stearic acid, titanium dioxide, vanillin and other ingredients.

For adults and children 12 years and over
RONDEC-TR® Tablet
Each timed-release Filmtab tablet contains carbinoxamine maleate, 8 mg; pseudoephedrine hydrochloride, 120 mg.
Inactive Ingredients: Castor oil, cellulosic polymers, confectioner's sugar, corn starch, FDC Blue No. 1, lactose, magnesium stearate, methyl acrylate-methyl methacrylate copolymer, microcrystalline cellulose, povidone, sorbitan monooleate, titanium dioxide and other ingredients.
Carbinoxamine maleate (2-[p-Chloro-α-[2-(dimethylamino) ethoxy] benzyl] pyridine maleate) is one of the ethanolamine class of H_1 antihistamines.
Pseudoephedrine hydrochloride (Benzenemethanol, α-[1-(methylamino)ethyl]-, [S-(R*, R*)]-, hydrochloride) is the hydrochloride of pseudoephedrine, a naturally occurring dextrorotatory stereoisomer of ephedrine.

CLINICAL PHARMACOLOGY
Antihistaminic and decongestant actions.
Carbinoxamine maleate possesses H_1 antihistaminic activity and mild anticholinergic and sedative effects. Serum half-life for carbinoxamine is estimated to be 10 to 20 hours. Virtually no intact drug is excreted in the urine.
Pseudoephedrine hydrochloride is an oral sympathomimetic amine which acts as a decongestant to respiratory tract mucous membranes. While its vasoconstrictor action is similar to that of ephedrine, pseudoephedrine has less pressor effect in normotensive adults. Serum half-life for pseudoephedrine is 6 to 8 hours. Acidic urine is associated with faster elimination of the drug. About one half of the administered dose is excreted in the urine.

INDICATIONS AND USAGE
For symptomatic relief of seasonal and perennial allergic rhinitis and vasomotor rhinitis.
Rondec Oral Drops, Rondec Syrup and Rondec Tablet are immediate-release dosage forms allowing titration of dose up to four times a day.
Rondec-TR Tablet utilizes a gradual-release mechanism providing approximately a 12-hour therapeutic effect, thus allowing twice-daily dosage.

CONTRAINDICATIONS
Patients with hypersensitivity or idiosyncrasy to any ingredients, patients taking monoamine oxidase (MAO) inhibitors, patients with narrow-angle glaucoma, urinary retention, peptic ulcer, severe hypertension or coronary artery disease, or patients undergoing an asthmatic attack.

WARNINGS
Use in Pregnancy: Safety for use during pregnancy has not been established.
Nursing Mothers: Use with caution in nursing mothers.
Special Risk Patients: Use with caution in patients with hypertension or ischemic heart disease, and persons over 60 years.

PRECAUTIONS
Use with caution in patients with hypertension, heart disease, asthma, hyperthyroidism, increased intraocular pressure, diabetes mellitus and prostatic hypertrophy.
Information for Patients: Avoid alcohol and other CNS depressants while taking these products. Patients sensitive to antihistamines may experience moderate to severe drowsiness. Patients sensitive to sympathomimetic amines may note mild CNS stimulation. While taking these products, exercise care in driving or operating appliances, machinery, etc.
Drug Interactions: Antihistamines may enhance the effects of tricyclic antidepressants, barbiturates, alcohol, and other CNS depressants. MAO inhibitors prolong and intensify the anticholinergic effects of antihistamines. Sympathomimetic amines may reduce the antihypertensive effects of reserpine, veratrum alkaloids, methyldopa and mecamylamine. Effects of sympathomimetics are increased with MAO inhibitors and beta-adrenergic blockers.
Pregnancy Category C.: Animal reproduction studies have not been conducted with these products. It is also not known whether these products can cause fetal harm when administered to a pregnant woman or affect reproduction capacity. Give to pregnant women only if clearly needed.

ADVERSE REACTIONS
Antihistamines: Sedation, dizziness, diplopia, vomiting, diarrhea, dry mouth, headache, nervousness, nausea, anorexia, heartburn, weakness, polyuria and dysuria and, rarely, excitability in children.
Sympathomimetic Amines: Convulsions, CNS stimulation, cardiac arrhythmias, respiratory difficulty, increased heart rate or blood pressure, hallucinations, tremors, nervousness, insomnia, weakness, pallor and dysuria.

OVERDOSAGE
No information is available as to specific results of an overdose of these products. The signs, symptoms and treatment described below are those of H_1 antihistamine and ephedrine overdose.
Symptoms: Should antihistamine effects predominate, central action constitutes the greatest danger. In the small child, symptoms include excitation, hallucination, ataxia, incoordination, tremors, flushed face and fever. Convulsions, fixed and dilated pupils, coma and death may occur in severe cases. In the adult, fever and flushing are uncommon, excitement leading to convulsions and postictal depression is often preceded by drowsiness and coma. Respiration is usually not seriously depressed; blood pressure is usually stable.
Should sympathomimetic symptoms predominate, central effects include restlessness, dizziness, tremor, hyperactive reflexes, talkativeness, irritability and insomnia. Cardiovascular and renal effects include difficulty in micturition, headache, flushing, palpitation, cardiac arrhythmias, hypertension with subsequent hypotension and circulatory collapse. Gastrointestinal effects include dry mouth, metallic taste, anorexia, nausea, vomiting, diarrhea and abdominal cramps.
Treatment: *a*) Evacuate stomach as condition warrants. Activated charcoal may be useful. *b*) Maintain a nonstimulating environment. *c*) Monitor cardiovascular status. *d*) Do not give stimulants. *e*) Reduce fever with cool sponging. *f*) Support respiration. *g*) Use sedatives or anticonvulsants to control CNS excitation and convulsions. *h*) Physostigmine may reverse anticholinergic symptoms. *i*) Ammonium chloride may acidify the urine to increase excretion of pseudoephedrine. *j*) Further care is symptomatic and supportive.

DOSAGE AND ADMINISTRATION
Dosage:
Rondec Oral Drops
for oral use only

Age	Dose*	Frequency*
1–3 months	¼ dropperful (¼ ml)	q.i.d.
3–6 months	½ dropperful (½ ml)	q.i.d.
6–9 months	¾ dropperful (¾ ml)	q.i.d.
9–18 months	1 dropperful (1 ml)	q.i.d.

Continued on next page

Ross—Cont.

Rondec Syrup and Rondec Tablet		
18 months–6 years	½ teaspoonful (2.5 ml)	q.i.d.
adults and children 6 years and over	1 teaspoonful (5 ml) or 1 tablet	q.i.d.
Rondec-TR Tablet adults and children		
12 years and over	1 tablet	b.i.d.

*In mild cases or in particularly sensitive patients, less frequent or reduced doses may be adequate.

HOW SUPPLIED

Rondec Oral Drops, berry-flavored, in 30-ml bottles for dropper dosage, **NDC** 0074-5783-30. Calibrated shatterproof dropper enclosed in each carton. Container meets safety closure requirements. Avoid exposure to excessive heat.

Rondec Syrup, berry-flavored, in 16-fl-oz (1-pint) bottles, **NDC** 0074-5782-16; and 4-fl-oz bottles, **NDC** 0074-5782-04. Dispense in USP tight glass container. Avoid exposure to excessive heat.

Rondec Tablet, Filmtab tablets, in bottles of 100, **NDC** 0074-5726-13; and bottles of 500, **NDC** 0074-5726-53. Each orange-colored tablet marked with Ross "R" and the number 5726 for professional identification. Dispense in USP tight container.

Rondec-TR Tablet, Filmtab tablets, in bottles of 100, **NDC** 0074-6240-13. Each blue-colored tablet marked with Ross "R" and the number 6240 for professional identification. Dispense in USP tight container.

Shown in Product Identification Section, page 426

(.5850)

RONDEC®-DM Syrup ℞
[ron'dek]
RONDEC®-DM Oral Drops ℞

PRODUCT OVERVIEW

KEY FACTS

Rondec-DM products contain the antihistamine carbinoxamine maleate, the decongestant pseudoephedrine hydrochloride, and the nonnarcotic antitussive dextromethorphan hydrobromide.

MAJOR USES

Rondec-DM products are indicated for relief of cough and upper respiratory symptoms, including nasal congestion, associated with allergy or the common cold.

SAFETY INFORMATION

Use with caution in patients with hypertension or ischemic heart disease, persons over 60, and nursing mothers. Safety for use during pregnancy has not been established.

PRESCRIBING INFORMATION

RONDEC®-DM Syrup ℞
[ron'dek]
RONDEC®-DM Oral Drops ℞

DESCRIPTION

Antihistamine/Decongestant/Antitussive for oral use.

Rondec®-DM Syrup

Each teaspoonful (5 ml) contains carbinoxamine maleate, 4 mg; pseudoephedrine hydrochloride, 60 mg; dextromethorphan hydrobromide, 15 mg; less than 0.6% alcohol.

Inactive Ingredients: Alcohol less than 0.6%, DC Red No. 33, FDC Blue No. 1, glycerin, liquid glucose, menthol, sodium benzoate, sucrose, water, natural & artificial flavoring and other ingredients.

Rondec®-DM Oral Drops

Each dropperful (1 ml) contains carbinoxamine maleate, 2 mg; pseudoephedrine hydrochloride, 25 mg; dextromethorphan hydrobromide, 4 mg; less than 0.6% alcohol.

Inactive Ingredients: Alcohol less than 0.6%, DC Red No. 33, FDC Blue No. 1, glycerin, liquid glucose, menthol, sodium benzoate, sucrose, water, natural & artificial flavoring and other ingredients.

Carbinoxamine maleate (2-[p-Chloro-α-[2-(dimethylamino) ethoxy]benzyl]pyridine maleate) is one of the ethanolamine class of H_1 antihistamines.

Pseudoephedrine hydrochloride (Benzenemethanol,α-[1-(methylamino) ethyl]-, [S-(R*, R*)]-, hydrochloride) is the hydrochloride of pseudoephedrine, a naturally occurring dextrorotatory stereoisomer of ephedrine.

Dextromethorphan hydrobromide (Morphinan, 3-methoxy-17-methyl-, (9α, 13α, 14α)-, hydrobromide, monohydrate) is the hydrobromide of d-form racemethorphan.

CLINICAL PHARMACOLOGY

Antihistaminic, decongestant and antitussive actions.

Carbinoxamine maleate possesses H_1 antihistaminic activity and mild anticholinergic and sedative effects. Serum half-life for carbinoxamine is estimated to be 10 to 20 hours. Virtually no intact drug is excreted in the urine.

Pseudoephedrine hydrochloride is an oral sympathomimetic amine which acts as a decongestant to respiratory tract mucous membranes. While its vasoconstrictor action is similar to that of ephedrine, pseudoephedrine has less pressor effect in normotensive adults. Serum half-life for pseudoephedrine is 6 to 8 hours. Acidic urine is associated with faster elimination of the drug. About one half of the administered dose is excreted in the urine.

Dextromethorphan hydrobromide is a nonnarcotic antitussive with effectiveness equal to codeine. It acts in the medulla oblongata to elevate the cough threshold. Dextromethorphan does not produce analgesia or induce tolerance, and has no potential for addiction. At usual doses, it will not depress respiration or inhibit ciliary activity. Dextromethorphan is rapidly metabolized, with trace amounts of the parent compound in blood and urine. About one half of the administered dose is excreted in the urine as conjugated metabolites.

INDICATIONS AND USAGE

For relief of coughs and upper respiratory symptoms, including nasal congestion, associated with allergy or the common cold.

CONTRAINDICATIONS

Patients with hypersensitivity or idiosyncrasy to any ingredients, patients taking monoamine oxidase (MAO) inhibitors, patients with narrow-angle glaucoma, urinary retention, peptic ulcer, severe hypertension or coronary artery disease, or patients undergoing an asthmatic attack.

WARNINGS

Use in Pregnancy: Safety for use during pregnancy has not been established.

Nursing Mothers: Use with caution in nursing mothers.

Special Risk Patients: Use with caution in patients with hypertension or ischemic heart disease, and persons over 60 years.

PRECAUTIONS

Before prescribing medication to suppress or modify cough, identify and provide therapy for the underlying cause of cough.

Use with caution in patients with hypertension, heart disease, asthma, hyperthyroidism, increased intraocular pressure, diabetes mellitus and prostatic hypertrophy.

Information for Patients: Avoid alcohol and other CNS depressants while taking these products. Patients sensitive to antihistamines may experience moderate to severe drowsiness. Patients sensitive to sympathomimetic amines may note mild CNS stimulation. While taking these products, exercise care in driving or operating appliances, machinery, etc.

Drug Interactions: Antihistamines may enhance the effects of tricyclic antidepressants, barbiturates, alcohol, and other CNS depressants. MAO inhibitors prolong and intensify the anticholinergic effects of antihistamines. Sympathomimetic amines may reduce the antihypertensive effects of reserpine, veratrum alkaloids, methyldopa and mecamylamine. Effects of sympathomimetics are increased with MAO inhibitors and beta-adrenergic blockers. The cough suppressant action of dextromethorphan and narcotic antitussives are additive.

Pregnancy Category C.: Animal reproduction studies have not been conducted with Rondec-DM. It is also not known whether these products can cause fetal harm when administered to a pregnant woman or affect reproduction capacity. Give to pregnant women only if clearly needed.

ADVERSE REACTIONS

Antihistamines: Sedation, dizziness, diplopia, vomiting, diarrhea, dry mouth, headache, nervousness, nausea, anorexia, heartburn, weakness, polyuria and dysuria and, rarely, excitability in children.

Sympathomimetic Amines: Convulsions, CNS stimulation, cardiac arrhythmias, respiratory difficulty, increased heart rate or blood pressure, hallucinations, tremors, nervousness, insomnia, weakness, pallor and dysuria.

Dextromethorphan: Drowsiness and GI disturbance.

OVERDOSAGE

No information is available as to specific results of an overdose of these products. The signs, symptoms and treatment described below are those of H_1 antihistamine, ephedrine and dextromethorphan overdose.

Symptoms: Should antihistamine effects predominate, central action constitutes the greatest danger. In the small child, predominant symptoms are excitation, hallucination, ataxia, incoordination, tremors, flushed face and fever. Convulsions, fixed and dilated pupils, coma, and death may occur in severe cases. In the adult, fever and flushing are uncommon; excitement leading to convulsions and postictal depression is often preceded by drowsiness and coma. Respiration is usually not seriously depressed; blood pressure is usually stable.

Should sympathomimetic symptoms predominate, central effects include restlessness, dizziness, tremor, hyperactive reflexes, talkativeness, irritability and insomnia. Cardiovascular and renal effects include difficulty in micturition, headache, flushing, palpitation, cardiac arrhythmias, hypertension with subsequent hypotension and circulatory collapse. Gastrointestinal effects include dry mouth, metallic taste, anorexia, nausea, vomiting, diarrhea and abdominal cramps.

Dextromethorphan may cause respiratory depression with a large overdose.

Treatment: *a*) Evacuate stomach as condition warrants. Activated charcoal may be useful. *b*) Maintain a nonstimulating environment. *c*) Monitor cardiovascular status. *d*) Do not give stimulants. *e*) Reduce fever with cool sponging. *f*) Treat respiratory depression with naloxone if dextromethorphan toxicity is suspected. *g*) Use sedatives or anticonvulsants to control CNS excitation and convulsions. *h*) Physostigmine may reverse anticholinergic symptoms. *i*) Ammonium chloride may acidify the urine to increase urinary excretion of pseudoephedrine. *j*) Further care is symptomatic and supportive.

DOSAGE AND ADMINISTRATION

Dosage:

Age	Dose*	Frequency*
Rondec-DM Syrup		
18 months–6 years	½ teaspoonful (2.5 ml)	q.i.d.
adults and children 6 years and over	1 teaspoonful (5 ml)	q.i.d.
Rondec-DM Oral Drops for oral use only		
1–3 months	¼ dropperful (¼ ml)	q.i.d.
3–6 months	½ dropperful (½ ml)	q.i.d.
6–9 months	¾ dropperful (¾ ml)	q.i.d.
9–18 months	1 dropperful (1 ml)	q.i.d.

*In mild cases or in particularly sensitive patients, less frequent or reduced doses may be adequate.

HOW SUPPLIED

Rondec-DM Syrup, grape-flavored, in 16-fl-oz (1-pint) bottles, **NDC** 0074-5640-16; and 4-fl-oz bottles, **NDC** 0074-5640-04. Dispense in USP tight, light-resistant, glass container. Avoid exposure to excessive heat.

Rondec-DM Oral Drops, grape-flavored, in 30-ml bottles for dropper dosage. Calibrated, shatterproof dropper enclosed in each carton. Container meets safety closure requirements. **NDC** 0074-5639-30. Avoid exposure to excessive heat.

(.5860)

ROSS HOSPITAL FORMULA SYSTEM
Products for hospital nursery use

SIMILAC® 13, Ready To Feed, 13 Cal/fl oz
Availability:
4-fl-oz nursing bottles; 48 per case; No. 408.

SIMILAC® 20, Ready To Feed, 20 Cal/fl oz
Availability:
4-fl-oz nursing bottles; 48 per case; No. 415.
8-fl-oz nursing bottles; 24 per case; No. 841.

SIMILAC® 24, Ready To Feed, 24 Cal/fl oz
Availability:
4-fl-oz nursing bottles; 48 per case; No. 404.

SIMILAC® 24 LBW, Ready To Feed, 24 Cal/fl oz
Availability:
4-fl-oz nursing bottles; 48 per case; No. 422.

SIMILAC® 27, Ready To Feed, 27 Cal/fl oz
Availability:
4-fl-oz nursing bottles; 48 per case; No. 427.

SIMILAC® WITH IRON 13, Ready To Feed, 13 Cal/fl oz
Availability:
4-fl-oz nursing bottles; 48 per case; No. 413.

SIMILAC® WITH IRON 20, Ready To Feed, 20 Cal/fl oz
Availability:
4-fl-oz nursing bottles; 48 per case; No. 426.
8-fl-oz nursing bottles; 24 per case; No. 858.

SIMILAC® WITH IRON 24, Ready To Feed, 24 Cal/fl oz
Availability:
4-fl-oz nursing bottles; 48 per case; No. 403.

SIMILAC® WITH WHEY + IRON 20, Ready To Feed, 20 Cal/fl oz
Availability:
4-fl-oz nursing bottles; 48 per case; No. 442.

SIMILAC® PM 60/40, Ready To Feed, 20 Cal/fl oz
Availability:
4-fl-oz nursing bottles; 48 per case; No. 424.

SIMILAC® SPECIAL CARE™ 20, Ready To Feed, 20 Cal/fl oz
Availability:
4-fl-oz nursing bottles; 48 per case; No. 439.

SIMILAC® SPECIAL CARE™ 24, Ready To Feed, 24 Cal/fl oz
Availability:
4-fl-oz nursing bottles; 48 per case; No. 433.

SIMILAC NATURAL CARE®, Human Milk Fortifier, Ready To Use, 24 Cal/fl oz
Availability:
4-fl-oz nursing bottles; 48 per case; No. 443.
ISOMIL® 20, Ready To Feed, 20 Cal/fl oz
Availability:
4-fl-oz nursing bottles; 48 per case; No. 406.
8-fl-oz nursing bottles; 24 per case; No. 871.
ISOMIL® SF 20, Ready To Feed, 20 Cal/fl oz
Availability:
8-fl-oz nursing bottles; 24 per case; No. 801.
PEDIALYTE®, Ready To Use; unflavored;
NDC 0074-6470-08
Availability:
8-fl-oz nursing bottles; 24 per case; No. 806.
ADVANCE®, Ready To Feed, 16 Cal/fl oz
Availability:
8-fl-oz nursing bottles; 24 per case; No. 804.
5% GLUCOSE WATER, Ready To Feed
Availability:
4-fl-oz nursing bottles; 48 per case; No. 405.
10% GLUCOSE WATER, Ready To Feed
Availability:
4-fl-oz nursing bottles; 48 per case; No. 410.
STERILIZED WATER, Ready To Feed
Availability:
4-fl-oz nursing bottles; 48 per case; No. 432.
8-fl-oz nursing bottles; 24 per case; No. 879.
VOLU-FEED®, Ross Volumetric Feeding System
Availability:
Volu-Feed Nursers; 100 per case; No. 180.
Volu-Feed Dispensing Caps; 250 per case; No. 081.
Component Nipple System
Availability:
Regular Nipple; 250 per case; No. 079.
Premature Nipple; 250 per case; No. 094.
Special Care Nipple; 250 per case; No. 095.
NUK® Nipple; 350 per case; No. 098.
Ross Cleft Palate Assembly
Availability:
Cleft Palate Nipple; supplied in packets of 3 nipple assemblies; No. 70.

ROSS SLD®
Surgical Liquid Diet

USAGE
A low-residue formula for patients requiring a clear liquid diet (ie, pre- and post-surgery, prior to diagnostic testing), and as a low-fat diet. Provides calories, high-quality protein, vitamins and minerals in a delicious-tasting fruit-punch flavor. Ross SLD may also be useful as a high-protein, vitamin and mineral supplement for patients receiving enteral nutritional support.

FEATURES
- Provides 100% of the U.S. RDA for protein, vitamins and minerals in 840 Calories—A concentrated source of nutrients to better meet the needs of patients restricted to clear liquid diets.
- Low residue—Ross SLD is appropriate for use in situations where low-residue is the primary consideration.
- Total calorie/nitrogen ratio of 117:1—A protein-sparing caloric distribution.
- High-quality protein from egg white solids—45 g (6 servings) meets 100% of the U.S. RDA.
- Small, frequent servings enhance patient compliance—Each 6½-fl-oz serving of Ross SLD helps improve nutrient intake yet avoids unnecessary waste.
- Low fat—Provides a concentrated source of nutrients for patients with maldigestion/malabsorption of fat.
- Lactose free/Gluten free—Appropriate for use in a variety of patient populations without the risk of intolerance commonly associated with lactose or gluten.
- Good taste—Delicious fruit-punch flavor enhances patient acceptance.

DOSAGE AND ADMINISTRATION
Instructions for Use: For one serving: pour 6 fl oz (¾ cup) water into a container. Add ⅓ level measuring cup or one packet of SLD and stir until powder dissolves. (If using a blender, low speed is recommended to reduce foaming.) The contents of one can will make approximately 10 servings. To prepare, mix entire contents of can with 7½ cups water. Use within 6 hours or store covered in refrigerator and use within 48 hours. Stir before use. STORAGE: Opened can should be covered with overcap and stored in a cool, dry place but not refrigerated. Once the can is opened, use contents within 1 month. Store unopened powder in a cool, dry place.
CAUTION: Ross SLD is a low-fat product that should be used only under medical supervision. This product and other clear liquid diets should not be used as the sole source of nutrition for extended periods of time. Not intended for infants.
NOT FOR PARENTERAL USE.
Availability: 13.5 oz (383 g) cans; 6 per case; Fruit-punch flavor, No. 674.
1.3 oz (37.8 g) packets; 6 packets per carton; 4 cartons per case; Fruit-punch flavor, No. 673.

COMPOSITION
Powder

INGREDIENTS
Ⓤ Sugar (sucrose), egg white solids, hydrolyzed corn starch, minerals (calcium glycerophosphate, magnesium carbonate, ammonium phosphate dibasic, potassium citrate, sodium citrate, potassium chloride, ferrous sulfate, zinc sulfate, manganese glycerophosphate, copper gluconate, potassium iodide), citric acid, vitamins (choline bitartrate, ascorbic acid, alpha-tocopheryl acetate, niacinamide, calcium pantothenate, pyridoxine hydrochloride, vitamin A palmitate, thiamine mononitrate, riboflavin, folic acid, biotin, phylloquinone, vitamin D_3, cyanocobalamin), natural and artificial flavor, and artificial color.

Nutrients:	Per 140 Calories (1 Serving)	Per 840 Calories (6 Servings)
Protein, g	7.5	45
Fat, g	0.1	0.6
Carbohydrate, g	27.3	163.8
Moisture, g	1.5	9.0

Vitamins/Minerals	Per 140 Calories (1 Serving)	Per 840 Calories (6 Servings)	Percent U.S. RDA* (840 Calories)
Vitamin A, IU	834	5000	100
Vitamin D, IU	67	400	100
Vitamin E, IU	7.5	45	150
Vitamin K_1, mcg	6	36	**
Vitamin C, mg	15	90	150
Folic Acid, mcg	100	600	150
Thiamine (Vit. B_1), mg	0.39	2.3	150
Riboflavin (Vit. B_2), mg	0.43	2.6	150
Vitamin B_6, mg	0.50	3.0	150
Vitamin B_{12}, mcg	1.5	9.0	150
Niacin, mg	5	30	150
Biotin, mcg	75	450	150
Pantothenic Acid, mg	2.5	15	150
Choline, mg	75	450	**
Calcium, mg	167	1000	100
Phosphorus, mg	167	1000	100
Sodium, mg	167	1000	**
Potassium, mg	167	1000	**
Chloride, mg	200	1200	**
Magnesium, mg	67	400	100
Iodine, mcg	25	150	100
Manganese, mg	0.84	5	**
Copper, mg	0.33	2	100
Zinc, mg	3.8	23	150
Iron, mg	3.0	18	100

*For adults and children 4 or more years of age.
**U.S. RDA not established.
(FAN 412-01)

SELSUN BLUE® OTC
[*sel 'sen blü*]
Dandruff Shampoo
(selenium sulfide lotion, 1%)

Selsun Blue is a non-prescription anti-dandruff shampoo containing the active ingredient selenium sulfide, 1%, in a freshly scented, pH balanced formula to leave hair clean and manageable. Available in Dry, Oily, Normal, Extra Conditioning and Extra Medicated formulas (contains 0.5% menthol).

INACTIVE INGREDIENTS
Normal formula: Ammonium laureth sulfate, ammonium lauryl sulfate, bentonite, citric acid, cocamide DEA, cocamidopropyl betaine, DMDM hydantoin, FD&C blue No. 1, fragrance, magnesium aluminum silicate, titanium dioxide, TEA-lauryl sulfate, water and other ingredients.
Dry formula: Acetylated lanolin alcohol, ammonium laureth sulfate, ammonium lauryl sulfate, cetyl acetate, citric acid, cocamide DEA, cocamidopropyl betaine, DMDM hydantoin, FD&C blue No. 1, fragrance, hydroxypropyl methylcellulose, magnesium aluminum silicate, polysorbate 80, titanium dioxide, TEA-lauryl sulfate, water and other ingredients.
Oily formula: Ammonium laureth sulfate, ammonium lauryl sulfate, bentonite, citric acid, cocamide DEA, cocamidopropyl betaine, DMDM hydantoin, FD&C blue No. 1, fragrance, magnesium aluminum silicate, sodium lauryl sulfate, titanium dioxide, TEA-lauryl sulfate, water and other ingredients.
Extra Conditioning formula: Acetylated Lanolin Alcohol, Aloe, Ammonium Laureth Sulfate, Ammonium Lauryl Sulfate, Cetyl Acetate, Citric Acid, Cocamide DEA, Cocamidopropyl Betaine, DMDM Hydantoin, FD&C Blue No. 1, Fragrance, Glycol Distearate, Hydroxypropyl Methylcellulose, Magnesium Aluminum Silicate, Polysorbate 80, Propylene Glycol, Sodium Chloride, TEA-Lauryl Sulfate, Titanium Dioxide, Water and other ingredients.
Extra Medicated formula: Ammonium Laureth Sulfate, Ammonium Lauryl Sulfate, Citric Acid, Cocamide DEA, Cocamidopropyl Betaine, DMDM Hydantoin, D&C Red No. 33, FD&C Blue No. 1, Fragrance, Hydroxypropyl Methylcellulose, Magnesium Aluminum Silicate, Sodium Chloride, TEA-Lauryl Sulfate, Water and other ingredients.

Clinical testing has shown Selsun Blue to be as safe and effective as other leading shampoos in helping control dandruff symptoms with regular use.

DIRECTIONS
Shake well before using. Lather, rinse thoroughly and repeat. Use regularly, once or twice weekly, for effective dandruff control.

CAUTION
For external use only. Keep out of eyes—if this happens, rinse thoroughly with water. If used just before or after bleaching, tinting or permanent waving, rinse hair for at least five minutes in cool running water. If irritation occurs, discontinue use.

WARNING
Keep out of the reach of children.

HOW SUPPLIED
4-, 7- and 11-fl-oz plastic bottles.
(FAN 2064)

SIMILAC®
[*sim 'e-lak*]
Low-Iron Infant Formula

USAGE
When an infant formula is needed: if the decision is made to discontinue breastfeeding before age 1 year, if a supplement to breastfeeding is needed, or as a routine feeding if breastfeeding is not adopted.

AVAILABILITY
Powder: 1-lb cans, measuring scoop enclosed; 6 per case; No. 03139.
Concentrated Liquid: 13-fl-oz cans; 24 per case; No. 00264.
Ready To Feed: (Prediluted, 20 Cal/fl oz)
32-fl-oz cans; 6 per case; No. 00232.
8-fl-oz cans; 4 six-packs per case; No. 00177.
4-fl-oz nursing bottles; 6 per carry-home carton, 8 cartons per case; No. 00480.
8-fl-oz nursing bottles; 6 per carry-home carton, 4 cartons per case; No. 00880.
For hospital use, Ready To Feed Similac in disposable nursing bottles is available in the Ross Hospital Formula System.

PREPARATION
Powder: Standard dilution (20 Cal/fl oz) is one level, unpacked scoop Powder (8.7 g) for each 2 fl oz water.
Concentrated Liquid: Standard dilution (20 Cal/fl oz) is one part Concentrated Liquid to one part water.
Ready To Feed: Do not dilute.

COMPOSITION
Powder
Ingredients: Ⓤ-D Nonfat milk, lactose, corn oil, coconut oil, vitamins (ascorbic acid, alpha-tocopheryl acetate, niacinamide, calcium pantothenate, vitamin A palmitate, thiamine chloride hydrochloride, pyridoxine hydrochloride, riboflavin, folic acid, phylloquinone, vitamin D_3, cyanocobalamin), minerals (zinc sulfate, ferrous sulfate, cupric sulfate, manganese sulfate) and taurine.
5 fl oz provide 100 Cal when prepared as directed. 1 liter of prepared formula provides 676 Cal.

Nutrients:	Per 100 Cal	
Protein	2.22	g
Fat	5.37	g
Carbohydrate	10.7	g
Water	133	g
Linoleic Acid	1300	mg
Vitamins:		
Vitamin A	300	IU
Vitamin D	60	IU
Vitamin E	2.5	IU
Vitamin K	8	mcg
Thiamine (Vit. B_1)	100	mcg
Riboflavin (Vit. B_2)	150	mcg

Continued on next page

Ross—Cont.

Vitamin B_6	60	mcg
Vitamin B_{12}	0.25	mcg
Niacin	1050	mcg
Folic Acid (Folacin)	15	mcg
Pantothenic Acid	450	mcg
Vitamin C (Ascorbic Acid)	9	mg
Minerals:		
Calcium	75	mg
Phosphorus	58	mg
Magnesium	6	mg
Iron	0.22	mg*
Zinc	0.75	mg
Manganese	5	mcg
Copper	90	mcg
Iodine	15	mcg
Sodium	32	mg
Potassium	120	mg
Chloride	75	mg

*Standard dilution is one level scoop of Similac Powder for each 2 fluid ounces of warm water, or 131.7 g of Powder diluted to 1 liter.
(FAN 382-02)

COMPOSITION

Concentrated Liquid

Ingredients: Ⓤ-D Water, nonfat milk, lactose, soy oil, coconut oil, mono- and diglycerides, soy lecithin, vitamins (ascorbic acid, alpha-tocopheryl acetate, niacinamide, calcium pantothenate, vitamin A palmitate, thiamine chloride hydrochloride, pyridoxine hydrochloride, riboflavin, folic acid, phylloquinone, vitamin D_3, cyanocobalamin), carrageenan, minerals (zinc sulfate, ferrous sulfate, cupric sulfate, manganese sulfate) and taurine.

5 fl oz provide 100 Cal when prepared as directed. 1 liter of prepared formula provides 676 Cal.

Nutrients:	**Per 100 Cal**	
Protein	2.22	g
Fat	5.37	g
Carbohydrate	10.7	g
Water	133	g
Linoleic Acid	1300	mg
Vitamins:		
Vitamin A	300	IU
Vitamin D	60	IU
Vitamin E	3.0	IU
Vitamin K	8	mcg
Thiamine (Vit. B_1)	100	mcg
Riboflavin (Vit. B_2)	150	mcg
Vitamin B_6	60	mcg
Vitamin B_{12}	0.25	mcg
Niacin	1050	mcg
Folic Acid (Folacin)	15	mcg
Pantothenic Acid	450	mcg
Vitamin C (Ascorbic Acid)	9	mg
Minerals:		
Calcium	75	mg
Phosphorus	58	mg
Magnesium	6	mg
Iron	0.22	mg*
Zinc	0.75	mg
Manganese	5	mcg
Copper	90	mcg
Iodine	15	mcg
Sodium	32	mg
Potassium	120	mg
Chloride	75	mg

Standard dilution is equal parts Similac Concentrated Liquid and water.
(FAN 382-02)

COMPOSITION

Ready To Feed

Ingredients: Ⓤ-D Water, nonfat milk, lactose, soy oil, coconut oil, mono- and diglycerides, soy lecithin, vitamins (ascorbic acid, alpha-tocopheryl acetate, niacinamide, calcium pantothenate, vitamin A palmitate, thiamine chloride hydrochloride, pyridoxine hydrochloride, riboflavin, folic acid, phylloquinone, vitamin D_3, cyanocobalamin), carrageenan, minerals (zinc sulfate, ferrous sulfate, cupric sulfate, manganese sulfate) and taurine.

5 fl oz provide 100 Cal; 1 liter provides 676 Cal.

Nutrients:	**Per 100 Cal**	
Protein	2.22	g
Fat	5.37	g
Carbohydrate	10.7	g
Water	133	g
Linoleic Acid	1300	mg
Vitamins:		
Vitamin A	300	IU
Vitamin D	60	IU
Vitamin E	3.0	IU
Vitamin K	8	mcg
Thiamine (Vit. B_1)	100	mcg
Riboflavin (Vit. B_2)	150	mcg
Vitamin B_6	60	mcg
Vitamin B_{12}	0.25	mcg
Niacin	1050	mcg
Folic Acid (Folacin)	15	mcg
Pantothenic Acid	450	mcg
Vitamin C (Ascorbic Acid)	9	mg
Minerals:		
Calcium	75	mg
Phosphorus	58	mg
Magnesium	6	mg
Iron	0.22	mg*
Zinc	0.75	mg
Manganese	5	mcg
Copper	90	mcg
Iodine	15	mcg
Sodium	32	mg
Potassium	120	mg
Chloride	75	mg

*This product, like milk, is deficient in iron; additional iron should be supplied from other sources.

(FAN 382-01)

SIMILAC® PM 60/40

[sim 'e-lak]

Low-Iron Infant Formula

USAGE

For infants in the lower range of homeostatic capacity; those who are predisposed to hypocalcemia; and those whose renal, digestive or cardiovascular functions would benefit from lowered mineral levels.

AVAILABILITY

Powder only: 1-lb cans, measuring scoop enclosed; 6 per case; No. 00850.

For hospital use, Ready To Feed Similac PM 60/40 in disposable nursing bottles is available in the Ross Hospital Formula System. (Ready To Feed has similar composition and nutrient values as Powder. For specific information see bottle tray.)

PREPARATION

Standard dilution (20 Cal/fl oz) is one level, unpacked scoop (8.6 g) Powder for each 2 fl oz of warm water.

Higher caloric feedings are prepared by adding 8.56g (one level, unpacked scoopful) of Similac PM 60/40 to the following amounts of water:

For:	Water:	Yields:
24 Cal/oz	48 mL	55 mL (1.8 fl oz)
27 Cal/oz	42 mL	49 mL (1.6 fl oz)
30 Cal/oz	37 mL	44 mL (1.5 fl oz)

INGREDIENTS

Ⓤ-D Lactose, corn oil, coconut oil, whey protein concentrate, sodium caseinate, minerals (calcium phosphate tribasic, potassium citrate, potassium chloride, magnesium chloride, sodium chloride, calcium carbonate, zinc sulfate, ferrous sulfate, cupric sulfate, manganese sulfate, potassium iodide), vitamins (m-inositol, ascorbic acid, choline chloride, alpha-tocopheryl acetate, niacinamide, calcium pantothenate, vitamin A palmitate, thiamine chloride hydrochloride, riboflavin, pyridoxine hydrochloride, folic acid, phylloquinone, vitamin D_3, biotin, cyanocobalamin), taurine and L-carnitine.

5 fl oz provide 100 Cal when prepared as directed. 1 liter of prepared formula provides 676 Cal.

Nutrients:	**Per 100 Cal**	
Protein	2.22	g
Fat	5.59	g
Carbohydrate	10.2	g
Water	134	g
Linoleic Acid	1300	mg
Vitamins:		
Vitamin A	300	IU
Vitamin D	60	IU
Vitamin E	2.5	IU
Vitamin K	8	mcg
Thiamine (Vit. B_1)	100	mcg
Riboflavin (Vit. B_2)	150	mcg
Vitamin B_6	60	mcg
Vitamin B_{12}	0.25	mcg
Niacin	1050	mcg
Folic Acid (Folacin)	15	mcg
Pantothenic Acid	450	mcg
Biotin	4.5	mcg
Vitamin C (Ascorbic Acid)	9	mg
Choline	12	mg
Inositol	24	mg
Minerals:		
Calcium	56	mg
Phosphorus	28	mg
Magnesium	6	mg
Iron	0.22	mg*
Zinc	0.75	mg
Manganese	5	mcg
Copper	90	mcg
Iodine	6	mcg
Sodium	24	mg
Potassium	86	mg
Chloride	59	mg

*This product, like milk, is deficient in iron; additional iron should be supplied from other sources.

Standard dilution is one level scoop of Similac PM 60/40 Powder for each 2 fl oz of water, or 131.7 g of Powder diluted to 1 liter.

PRECAUTIONS

In conditions where the infant is losing abnormal quantities of one or more electrolytes, it may be necessary to supply electrolytes from sources other than the formula. It may be necessary to supply infants weighing less than 1500 g at birth additional calcium, phosphorus and sodium during periods of rapid growth.
(FAN 415-03)

SIMILAC® WITH IRON

[sim 'e-lak]

Infant Formula

USAGE

When an iron-fortified infant formula is needed: if the decision is made to discontinue breastfeeding before age 1 year, if a supplement to breastfeeding is needed, or as a routine feeding if breastfeeding is not adopted.

AVAILABILITY

Powder: 1-lb cans, measuring scoop enclosed; 6 per case; No. 03360.

Concentrated Liquid: 13-fl-oz cans; 24 cans per case; No. 00414.

Ready To Feed: (Prediluted, 20 Cal/fl oz)
32-fl-oz cans; 6 per case; No. 00241.
8-fl-oz cans; 4 six-packs per case; No. 00179.
4-fl-oz nursing bottles; 6 per carry-home carton, 8 cartons per case; No. 06201.
8-fl-oz nursing bottles; 6 per carry-home carton, 4 cartons per case; No. 06202.

For hospital use, Ready To Feed Similac With Iron in disposable nursing bottles is available in the Ross Hospital Formula System.

PREPARATION

Powder: Standard dilution (20 Cal/fl oz) is one level, unpacked scoop Powder (8.7 g) for each 2 fl oz of warm water.

Concentrated Liquid: Standard dilution (20 Cal/fl oz) is one part Concentrated Liquid to one part water.

Ready To Feed: Do not dilute.

COMPOSITION

Powder

INGREDIENTS

Ⓤ-D Nonfat milk, lactose, corn oil, coconut oil, vitamins (ascorbic acid, alpha-tocopheryl acetate, niacinamide, calcium pantothenate, vitamin A palmitate, thiamine chloride hydrochloride, pyridoxine hydrochloride, riboflavin, folic acid, phylloquinone, vitamin D_3, cyanocobalamin), minerals (ferrous sulfate, zinc sulfate, cupric sulfate, manganese sulfate) and taurine.

5 fl oz provide 100 Cal when prepared as directed. 1 liter of prepared formula provides 676 Cal.

Nutrients:	**Per 100 Cal**	
Protein	2.22	g
Fat	5.37	g
Carbohydrate	10.7	g
Water	133	g
Linoleic Acid	1300	mg
Vitamins:		
Vitamin A	300	IU
Vitamin D	60	IU
Vitamin E	2.5	IU
Vitamin K	8	mcg
Thiamine (Vit. B_1)	100	mcg
Riboflavin (Vit. B_2)	150	mcg
Vitamin B_6	60	mcg
Vitamin B_{12}	0.25	mcg
Niacin	1050	mcg
Folic Acid (Folacin)	15	mcg
Pantothenic Acid	450	mcg
Vitamin C (Ascorbic Acid)	9	mg

Minerals:		
Calcium	75	mg
Phosphorus	58	mg
Magnesium	6	mg
Iron	1.8	mg*
Zinc	0.75	mg
Manganese	5	mcg
Copper	90	mcg
Iodine	15	mcg
Sodium	32	mg
Potassium	120	mg
Chloride	75	mg

*Standard dilution is one level scoop of Similac With Iron Powder for each 2 fl oz of warm water, or 131.7 g of Powder diluted to 1 liter.
(FAN 382-02)

COMPOSITION

Concentrated Liquid

Ingredients: ⓤ-D Water, nonfat milk, lactose, soy oil, coconut oil, mono- and diglycerides, soy lecithin, vitamins (ascorbic acid, alpha-tocopheryl acetate, niacinamide, calcium pantothenate, vitamin A palmitate, thiamine chloride hydrochloride, pyridoxine hydrochloride, riboflavin, folic acid, phylloquinone, vitamin D_3, cyanocobalamin), carrageenan, minerals (ferrous sulfate, zinc sulfate, cupric sulfate, manganese sulfate) and taurine.

5 fl oz provide 100 Cal when prepared as directed. 1 liter of prepared formula provides 676 Cal.

Nutrients:	Per 100 Cal	
Protein	2.22	g
Fat	5.37	g
Carbohydrate	10.7	g
Water	133	g
Linoleic Acid	1300	mg
Vitamins:		
Vitamin A	300	IU
Vitamin D	60	IU
Vitamin E	3.0	IU
Vitamin K	8	mcg
Thiamine (Vit. B_1)	100	mcg
Riboflavin (Vit. B_2)	150	mcg
Vitamin B_6	60	mcg
Vitamin B_{12}	0.25	mcg
Niacin	1050	mcg
Folic Acid (Folacin)	15	mcg
Pantothenic Acid	450	mcg
Vitamin C (Ascorbic Acid)	9	mg
Minerals:		
Calcium	75	mg
Phosphorus	58	mg
Magnesium	6	mg
Iron	1.8	mg*
Zinc	0.75	mg
Manganese	5	mcg
Copper	90	mcg
Iodine	15	mcg
Sodium	32	mg
Potassium	120	mg
Chloride	75	mg

Standard dilution is equal amounts Similac With Iron Concentrated Liquid and water.
(FAN 382-02)

COMPOSITION

Ready To Feed

Ingredients: ⓤ-D Water, nonfat milk, lactose, soy oil, coconut oil, mono- and diglycerides, soy lecithin, vitamins (ascorbic acid, alpha-tocopheryl acetate, niacinamide, calcium pantothenate, vitamin A palmitate, thiamine chloride hydrochloride, pyridoxine hydrochloride, riboflavin, folic acid, phylloquinone, vitamin D_3, cyanocobalamin), carrageenan, minerals (ferrous sulfate, zinc sulfate, cupric sulfate, manganese sulfate) and taurine.
5 fl oz provide 100 Cal; 1 liter provides 676 Cal.

Nutrients:	Per 100 Cal	
Protein	2.22	g
Fat	5.37	g
Carbohydrate	10.7	g
Water	133	g
Linoleic Acid	1300	mg
Vitamins:		
Vitamin A	300	IU
Vitamin D	60	IU
Vitamin E	3.0	IU
Vitamin K	8	mcg
Thiamine (Vit. B_1)	100	mcg
Riboflavin (Vit. B_2)	150	mcg
Vitamin B_6	60	mcg
Vitamin B_{12}	0.25	mcg
Niacin	1050	mcg
Folic Acid (Folacin)	15	mcg
Pantothenic Acid	450	mcg
Vitamin C (Ascorbic Acid)	9	mg

Minerals:		
Calcium	75	mg
Phosphorus	58	mg
Magnesium	6	mg
Iron	1.8	mg*
Zinc	0.75	mg
Manganese	5	mcg
Copper	90	mcg
Iodine	15	mcg
Sodium	32	mg
Potassium	120	mg
Chloride	75	mg

*The addition of iron to this formula conforms to the recommendation of the Committee on Nutrition of the American Academy of Pediatrics.
(FAN 382-01)

TRONOLANE® OTC

[tron 'e-lān]
Cream:
(pramoxine hydrochloride 1%)
Suppositories:
(pramoxine 1% as pramoxine and pramoxine HCl)

PRODUCT OVERVIEW

KEY FACTS

Tronolane Cream and Suppositories are indicated for temporary relief of hemorrhoidal symptoms. Tronolane products contain the topical anesthetic pramoxine hydrochloride 1%.

MAJOR USES

Tronolane Cream and Suppositories are indicated for temporary relief of pain, burning, itching and discomfort associated with hemorrhoids.

SAFETY INFORMATION

If bleeding is present, consult physician. Certain persons can develop allergic reactions to ingredients in this product. During treatment, if condition worsens or persists 7 days, consult physician. For children under 12, use only as directed by a physician. As with any drug, if you are pregnant or nursing a baby seek the advice of a health professional before using this product.

PRESCRIBING INFORMATION

TRONOLANE® OTC

[tron 'e-lān]
Cream:
(pramoxine hydrochloride 1%)
Suppositories:
(pramoxine 1% as pramoxine and pramoxine HCl)

DESCRIPTION

The active ingredient in Tronolane is a topical anesthetic agent (pramoxine HCl), chemically unrelated to the benzoate esters of the "caine" type, which is chemically designated as a 4-n-butoxyphenyl gammamorpholinopropyl- ether hydrochloride. The cream contains the following inactive ingredients: Beeswax, cetyl alcohol, cetyl esters wax, glycerin, methylparaben, propylparaben, sodium lauryl sulfate, water and zinc oxide. The suppository contains the following inactive ingredients: Hydrogenated cocoa glycerides and zinc oxide.

INDICATIONS

Tronolane is a topical anesthetic indicated for the temporary relief of the pain, burning, itching and discomfort that accompany hemorrhoids. It has a soothing, lubricant action on mucous membranes.

Tronolane contains a rapidly acting topical anesthetic producing analgesia that lasts up to 5 hours. Because the drug is chemically unrelated to other anesthetics, cross-sensitization is unlikely. Patients who are already sensitized to the "caine" anesthetics can generally use Tronolane.

The emollient/emulsion base of Tronolane cream provides soothing lubrication making bowel movements more comfortable. Tronolane cream is in a nondrying base that is nongreasy and nonstaining to undergarments.

WARNINGS

If bleeding is present, consult physician. Certain persons can develop allergic reactions to ingredients in this product. During treatment, if condition worsens or persists 7 days, consult physician. For children under 12 years, use only as directed by physician. Keep out of the reach of children. As with any drug, if you are pregnant or nursing a baby, we recommend that you seek the advice of a health professional before using this product.

DOSAGE AND ADMINISTRATION

CREAM: Apply up to five times daily, especially morning, night, and after bowel movements, or as directed by physician.

External—Apply liberally to affected area. *Intrarectal*—Remove cap from tube and attach clean applicator. Remove protective cover from clean applicator. Squeeze tube to fill applicator and lubricate tip with cream. Gently insert applicator into rectum and squeeze tube again. Thoroughly cleanse applicator after use.

DOSAGE AND ADMINISTRATION

SUPPOSITORIES: Use up to five times daily, especially morning, night, and after bowel movements, or as directed by physician. Detach one suppository from pack. Tear notch at pointed end and remove wrapper before insertion. Insert suppository into the rectum, pointed end first.

HOW SUPPLIED

Tronolane is available in 1-oz and 2-oz cream tubes and 10 and 20 count suppository boxes.
(FAN 2061-02)

TWOCAL® HN

[tü 'kal]
High Nitrogen Liquid Nutrition

USAGE

As a high-calorie, high-nitrogen liquid food, TwoCal HN delivers 100% of the U.S. RDA for vitamins and minerals in only 950 mL (1 quart). TwoCal HN is most appropriate for use in severely hypermetabolic and fluid-restricted patients. As a concentrated source of nutrition, TwoCal HN is an excellent dietary supplement when voluntary food intake is inadequate to meet nutrient needs.

Features:

- Complete, balanced nutrition—2.0 Calories per mL, 475 Calories per 8 fl oz, 2000 Calories per liter from a balanced distribution of protein, fat and carbohydrate (caloric distribution: protein, 16.7%; fat, 40.1%; and carbohydrate, 43.2%). 1900 Calories of TwoCal HN provide at least 100% of the U.S. RDA for vitamins and minerals for adults and children 4 or more years of age.
- High nitrogen—TwoCal HN has a total calorie/nitrogen ratio of 150:1, indicated for the stressed patient to meet increased nitrogen needs.
- Concentrated nutrition—TwoCal HN will reduce the volume necessary to meet the protein and calorie needs of the hypermetabolic or fluid-restricted patient (83.7g of protein per liter, 2000 Calories per liter).
- Lactose free—TwoCal HN will not contribute to lactose-associated diarrhea. Hydrolyzed corn starch and sucrose are the carbohydrate sources.

DOSAGE AND ADMINISTRATION

Ready To Use: Shake well. May be stored unopened at room temperature. Once opened, TwoCal HN should be covered and refrigerated; discard if not used within 48 hours. TwoCal HN may be fed at room temperature or chilled.

Oral Feeding: May be used for total nutrition, or with and between meals.

Tube Feeding: Follow physician's instructions. Adjust flow rate, volume and dilution according to patient's condition and tolerance. When used as the sole source of nutrition, products containing 2 Cal/mL may provide inadequate water for many patients.

Monitor hydration status; additional fluid requirements should be met by giving water with or after feedings or by parenteral routes. Avoid contamination during preparation and use.

NOT FOR PARENTERAL USE.

[See table on bottom next page].

AVAILABILITY

Ready To Use: 8-fl-oz cans; 4 six-packs per case; Vanilla, No. 729.

COMPOSITION

Ready To Use Vanilla

INGREDIENTS

ⓤ-D Water, hydrolyzed corn starch, corn oil, sodium caseinate, sucrose, sodium calcium caseinate, medium-chain triglycerides (fractionated coconut oil), minerals (potassium citrate, magnesium chloride, calcium phosphate tribasic, sodium citrate, zinc sulfate, ferrous sulfate, manganese sulfate, cupric sulfate), natural and artificial flavors, soy lecithin and vitamins (choline chloride, ascorbic acid, alpha-tocopheryl acetate, niacinamide, calcium pantothenate, pyridoxine hydrochloride, vitamin A palmitate, thiamine chloride hydrochloride, riboflavin, folic acid, biotin, phylloquinone, vitamin D_3, cyanocobalamin).

Nutrients (grams/8 fl oz): Protein, 19.8; Fat, 21.5; Carbohydrate, 51.4; Minerals (Ash), 2.4; Moisture, 169. Calories per mL, 2.0; Calories per fl oz, 59.4.

Vitamin/Mineral Content of TwoCal HN (Ready To Use)

Vitamins/Minerals	Per 8 Fl Oz		Percent U.S. RDA* (Per 8 Fl Oz)
Vitamin A	1250	I.U.	25
Vitamin D	100	I.U.	25
Vitamin E	11.25	I.U.	37.5

Continued on next page

Ross—Cont.

Vitamin K_1	18	mcg	**
Vitamin C	75	mg	125
Folic Acid	160	mcg	40
Thiamine (Vit. B_1)	0.60	mg	40
Riboflavin (Vit. B_2)	0.68	mg	40
Vitamin B_6	0.80	mg	40
Vitamin B_{12}	2.4	mcg	40
Niacin	8.0	mg	40
Choline	150	mg	**
Biotin	120	mcg	40
Pantothenic Acid	4.0	mg	40
Sodium	250	mg	**
Potassium	550	mg	**
Chloride	370	mg	**
Calcium	250	mg	25
Phosphorus	250	mg	25
Magnesium	100	mg	25
Iodine	37.5	mcg	25
Manganese	1.25	mg	**
Copper	0.50	mg	25
Zinc	5.63	mg	37.5
Iron	4.5	mg	25

*For adults and children 4 or more years of age.
**U.S. RDA not established.
(FAN 366-04)

VARI-FLAVORS® Flavor Pacs
[var 'ē-flā "verz]

USAGE
To provide flavor variety for patients receiving full liquid diets and liquid supplements.

Features:
- Five flavors (Pecan, Cherry, Lemon, Orange, Strawberry) offer patients variety and encourage acceptance of liquid diets and liquid supplements.
- Vari-Flavors Flavor Pacs mix readily with Ross Medical Nutritional products to suit individual flavor preferences.
- Flavor Pacs may be stored for use in the dietary department, at nursing stations or by patient's bedside.

AVAILABILITY
One-gram packets; 24 per dispenser carton; Pecan, No. 720; Cherry, No. 722; Lemon, No. 724; Orange, No. 726; Strawberry, No. 728; Assorted flavors, No. 730.

INSTRUCTIONS FOR USE
Tap Pac lightly to shake contents to bottom. Tear off corner of packet. Pour contents into suitable dry serving container. Add 8 ounces of one of the Ross Medical Nutritional products. Allow flavor to dissolve for a few seconds. Stir until flavor is mixed and serve.

COMPOSITION
Dextrose, artificial flavor and color (Strawberry, Cherry, Orange). Dextrose and artificial flavor (Pecan). Dextrose, artificial flavor and FD & C Yellow #5 (Lemon).
When used as directed, Vari-Flavors contribute trace amounts of minerals and less than 1 gram of dextrose. The addition of a single Vari-Flavors Pac (1 gram) to one of the Ross Medical Nutritional products increases total calories per 8-oz serving by approximately 4 Calories.
(FAN 242)

VI-DAYLIN® ADC VITAMINS Drops
[vī "dā 'lin]
Dietary Supplement of Vitamins A, D and C

DESCRIPTION
One dropperful (1.0 mL) provides:

Vitamins		% U.S. RDA*	% U.S. RDA**
Vitamin A	1500 I.U.	100	60
Vitamin D	400 I.U.	100	100
Vitamin C	35 mg	100	87

INGREDIENTS
Propylene glycol, polysorbate 80, ascorbic acid, methylparaben (preservative), vitamin A palmitate, propylparaben (preservative), and ergocalciferol in corn oil, in a glycerin-water vehicle with added artificial pineapple-fruit flavoring and caramel coloring. Contains only a trace (less than ½%) of alcohol.
Contains no sugar.
*% U.S. Recommended Daily Allowance for infants.
**% U.S. Recommended Daily Allowance for children under 4 years of age.

INDICATIONS AND USAGE
Dietary supplement of vitamins A, D and C for infants and children under 4 years of age.

DOSAGE AND ADMINISTRATION
One dropperful daily, or as directed by physician.

HOW SUPPLIED
50-mL Spil-gard® bottles, calibrated dropper enclosed; OTC; **NDC** 0074-0105-04.

VI-DAYLIN® MULTIVITAMIN Drops
[vī "dā 'lin]
Multivitamin Supplement

DESCRIPTION
One dropperful (1.0 mL) provides:

Vitamins			% U.S. RDA*	% U.S. RDA**
Vitamin A	1500	I.U.	100	60
Vitamin D	400	I.U.	100	100
Vitamin E	5	I.U.	100	50
Vitamin C	35	mg	100	87
Thiamine (Vitamin B_1)	0.5	mg	100	71
Riboflavin (Vitamin B_2)	0.6	mg	100	75
Niacin	8	mg	100	88
Vitamin B_6	0.4	mg	100	57
Vitamin B_{12}	1.5	mcg	75	50

INGREDIENTS
Ascorbic acid, d-alpha tocopheryl acid succinate, niacinamide, benzoic acid (preservative), ferric ammonium citrate (stabilizer), vitamin A palmitate, riboflavin-5'-phosphate sodium, methylparaben (preservative), thiamine hydrochloride, pyridoxine hydrochloride, ergocalciferol in corn oil, disodium edetate (stabilizer) and cyanocobalamin in a glycerin-water vehicle with added artificial flavoring. Contains only a trace (less than ½%) of alcohol.
Contains no sugar.
*% U.S. Recommended Daily Allowance for infants.
**% U.S. Recommended Daily Allowance for children under 4 years of age.

INDICATIONS AND USAGE
Multivitamin supplement for infants and children under 4 years of age.

DOSAGE AND ADMINISTRATION
One dropperful daily, or as directed by physician.

HOW SUPPLIED
50-mL Spil-gard® bottles, calibrated dropper enclosed; OTC; **NDC** 0074-0103-04.

VI-DAYLIN®/F ADC VITAMINS Drops With Fluoride ℞
[vī "dā 'lin]
ADC Vitamins/Fluoride

DESCRIPTION
One dropperful (1.0 mL) provides:
Fluoride 0.25 mg

Vitamins			% U.S. RDA*	% U.S. RDA**
Vitamin A	1500	I.U.	100	60
Vitamin D	400	I.U.	100	100
Vitamin C	35	mg	100	87

Active Ingredients: Ascorbid acid, vitamin A palmitate, sodium fluoride and ergocalciferol.
Inactive Ingredients: Alcohol approximately 0.3%, caramel coloring, corn oil, glycerin, methylparaben, polysorbate 80, propylene glycol, propylparaben, water, artificial and natural flavoring, and other ingredients.
Contains no sugar.
*% U.S. Recommended Daily Allowance for infants.
**% U.S. Recommended Daily Allowance for children under 4 years of age.

INDICATIONS AND USAGE
As an aid in the prevention of dental caries in infants and children, and in the prophylaxis of vitamin A, D and C deficiencies.

CONTRAINDICATIONS
Should be used only where the fluoride content of the drinking water supply is known to be 0.7 parts per million or less.

PRECAUTIONS
The recommended dosage should not be exceeded since chronic overdosage of fluoride may result in mottling of tooth enamel and osseous changes.

OVERDOSAGE
In children, acute ingestion of 10 to 20 mg of sodium fluoride may cause excessive salivation and gastrointestinal disturbances; 500 mg may be fatal. Oral and/or intravenous fluids containing calcium may be indicated.

Sample Administration Schedule for TwoCal HN

Continuous Drip Schedule

Day	Time	Strength	Rate (mL/hr)	Volume (mL)	Calories
1	1st 8 hours	½	50	400	400
	2nd 8 hours	½	50	400	400
	3rd 8 hours	½	75	600	600
					1400 *Total Calories*
2	1st 8 hours	½	75–100	600–800	600–800
	2nd 8 hours	½	75–100	600–800	600–800
	3rd 8 hours	½	75–100	600–800	600–800
					1800–2400 *Total Calories*
3	24 hours	Full	75–100	1800–2400	3600–4800 *Total Calories*

Intermittent Drip Schedule

Day	Time	Strength	Rate (5–10 mL/min)	Volume (mL)	Calories
1	7am–11pm	½	100 mL q 2 hr (7am, 9am)	200	200
		½	150 mL q 2 hr (11am, 1pm, 3pm)	450	450
		½	200 mL q 2 hr (5pm, 7pm, 9pm, 11pm)	800	800
					1450 *Total Calories*
2	7am–10pm	½	250 mL q 2 hr (7am, 9am, 11am)	750	750
		Full	250 mL q 3 hr (1pm, 4pm, 7pm, 10pm)	1000	2000
					2750 *Total Calories*
3	7am–10pm	Full	250 mL q 3 hr* in 5–8 feedings/day	1250–2000	2500–4000 *Total Calories*

*Preferable to q 2 hr
- Check gastric residuals before every intermittent feeding or every 2 –4 hours during continuous feeding.
- If intolerance develops, return to previously tolerated strength and rate. When tolerance is again established, proceed with feeding schedule as indicated. Do not alter rate and strength at the same time.
- Rinsing the tube with water (eg, 25–100 mL) after each intermittent feeding or every 3 to 6 hours during continuous feeding will help avoid clogging and provide additional water.

DOSAGE AND ADMINISTRATION
One dropperful daily, or as directed by physician or dentist.

HOW SUPPLIED
50-mL Spil-gard® bottles, calibrated dropper enclosed; Rx; **NDC** 0074-1106-50.

VI-DAYLIN®/F ADC VITAMINS + IRON ℞
Drops With Fluoride
[vī"dā'lin]
ADC Vitamins/Fluoride/Iron Supplement

DESCRIPTION
One dropperful (1.0 mL) provides:
Fluoride 0.25 mg

		% U.S. RDA*	% U.S. RDA**
Vitamins			
Vitamin A	1500 I.U.	100	60
Vitamin D	400 I.U.	100	100
Vitamin C	35 mg	100	87
Minerals			
Iron	10 mg	66	100

Active Ingredients: Ascorbic acid, ferrous sulfate, vitamin A palmitate, sodium fluoride and ergocalciferol.
Inactive Ingredients: Benzoic acid, caramel coloring, glycerin, methylparaben, polysorbate 80, water, artificial flavoring and other ingredients.
Contains no sugar.
*% U.S. Recommended Daily Allowance for infants.
**% U.S. Recommended Daily Allowance for children under 4 years of age.

INDICATIONS AND USAGE
As an aid in the prevention of dental caries in infants and children, and in the prophylaxis of iron and vitamin A, D and C deficiencies.

CONTRAINDICATIONS
Should be used only where the fluoride content of the drinking water supply is known to be 0.7 parts per million or less.

PRECAUTIONS
The recommended dosage should not be exceeded since chronic overdosage of fluoride may result in mottling of tooth enamel and osseous changes. In infants, oral iron-containing preparations may cause temporary darkening of the membrane covering the teeth.

OVERDOSAGE
In children, acute ingestion of 10 to 20 mg of sodium fluoride may cause excessive salivation and gastrointestinal disturbances; 500 mg may be fatal. Oral and/or intravenous fluids containing calcium may be indicated.
Acute overdosage of iron may cause nausea and vomiting and, in severe cases, cardiovascular collapse and death. The estimated lethal dose of orally ingested elemental iron is 300 mg per kg body weight. Serum iron and total iron-binding capacity may be used as guides for use of chelating agents such as deferoxamine.

DOSAGE AND ADMINISTRATION
One dropperful daily, or as directed by physician or dentist.

HOW SUPPLIED
50-mL Spil-gard® bottles, calibrated dropper enclosed; ℞; **NDC** 0074-8929-50.

VI-DAYLIN®/F MULTIVITAMIN Drops With Fluoride ℞
[vī"dā'lin]
Multivitamins/Fluoride

DESCRIPTION
One dropperful (1.0 mL) provides:
Fluoride 0.25 mg

			% U.S. RDA*	% U.S. RDA**
Vitamins				
Vitamin A	1500	I.U.	100	60
Vitamin D	400	I.U.	100	100
Vitamin E	5	I.U.	100	50
Vitamin C	35	mg	100	87
Thiamine (Vitamin B_1)	0.5	mg	100	71
Riboflavin (Vitamin B_2)	0.6	mg	100	75
Niacin	8	mg	100	88
Vitamin B_6	0.4	mg	100	57

Active Ingredients: Ascorbic acid, niacinamide, d-alpha tocopheryl acid succinate, riboflavin-5'-phosphate sodium, sodium fluoride, vitamin A palmitate, thiamine hydrochloride, pyridoxine hydrochloride and ergocalciferol.
Inactive Ingredients: Alcohol less than 0.1%, benzoic acid, caramel coloring, corn oil, glycerin, methylparaben, water, natural flavoring and other ingredients. No artificial sweeteners.
Contains no sugar.
*% U.S. Recommended Daily Allowance for infants.
**% U.S. Recommended Daily Allowance for children under 4 years of age.

INDICATIONS AND USAGE
As an aid in the prevention of dental caries in infants and children, and in the prophylaxis of certain vitamin deficiencies.

CONTRAINDICATIONS
Should be used only where the fluoride content of the drinking water supply is known to be 0.7 parts per million or less.

PRECAUTIONS
The recommended dosage should not be exceeded since chronic overdosage of fluoride may result in mottling of tooth enamel and osseous changes.

OVERDOSAGE
In children, acute ingestion of 10 to 20 mg of sodium fluoride may cause excessive salivation and gastrointestinal disturbances; 500 mg may be fatal. Oral and/or intravenous fluids containing calcium may be indicated.

DOSAGE AND ADMINISTRATION
One dropperful daily, or as directed by physician or dentist.

HOW SUPPLIED
50-mL Spil-gard® bottles, calibrated dropper enclosed; Rx; **NDC** 0074-1104-50.

VI-DAYLIN®/F MULTIVITAMIN + IRON Drops With Fluoride ℞
[vī"dā'lin]
Multivitamins/Fluoride/Iron Supplement

DESCRIPTION
One dropperful (1.0 mL) provides:
Fluoride 0.25 mg

			% U.S. RDA*	% U.S. RDA**
Vitamins				
Vitamin A	1500	I.U.	100	60
Vitamin D	400	I.U.	100	100
Vitamin E	5	I.U.	100	50
Vitamin C	35	mg	100	87
Thiamine (Vitamin B_1)	0.5	mg	100	71
Riboflavin (Vitamin B_2)	0.6	mg	100	75
Niacin	8	mg	100	88
Vitamin B_6	0.4	mg	100	57
Minerals				
Iron	10	mg	66	100

Active Ingredients: Ascorbic acid, ferrous sulfate, niacinamide, d-alpha tocopheryl acid succinate, vitamin A palmitate, riboflavin-5'-phosphate sodium, thiamine hydrochloride, sodium fluoride, pyridoxine hydrochloride and ergocalciferol.
Inactive Ingredients: Alcohol less than 0.1%, benzoic acid, caramel coloring, corn oil, glycerin, methylparaben, water, natural flavoring and other ingredients.
Contains no sugar.
*% U.S. Recommended Daily Allowance for infants.
**% U.S. Recommended Daily Allowance for children under 4 years of age.

INDICATIONS AND USAGE
As an aid in the prevention of dental caries in infants and children and in the prophylaxis of iron and certain vitamin deficiencies.

CONTRAINDICATIONS
Should be used only where the fluoride content of the drinking water supply is known to be 0.7 parts per million or less.

PRECAUTIONS
The recommended dosage should not be exceeded since chronic overdosage of fluoride may result in mottling of tooth enamel and osseous changes. In infants, oral iron-containing preparations may cause temporary darkening of the membrane covering the teeth.

OVERDOSAGE
In children, acute ingestion of 10 to 20 mg of sodium fluoride may cause excessive salivation and gastrointestinal disturbances; 500 mg may be fatal. Oral and/or intravenous fluids containing calcium may be indicated.
Acute overdosage of iron may cause nausea and vomiting and, in severe cases, cardiovascular collapse and death. The estimated lethal dose of orally ingested elemental iron is 300 mg per kg body weight. Serum iron and total iron-binding capacity may be used as guides for use of chelating agents such as deferoxamine.

DOSAGE AND ADMINISTRATION
One dropperful daily, or as directed by physician or dentist.

HOW SUPPLIED
50-mL Spil-gard® bottles, calibrated dropper enclosed; ℞; **NDC** 0074-8928-50.

VI-DAYLIN® MULTIVITAMIN + IRON Drops
[vī"dā'lin]
Multivitamin/Iron Supplement

DESCRIPTION
One dropperful (1 mL) provides:

			% U.S. RDA*	% U.S. RDA**
Vitamins				
Vitamin A	1500	I.U.	100	60
Vitamin D	400	I.U.	100	100
Vitamin E	5	I.U.	100	50
Vitamin C	35	mg	100	87
Thiamine (Vitamin B_1)	0.5	mg	100	71
Riboflavin (Vitamin B_2)	0.6	mg	100	75
Niacin	8	mg	100	88
Vitamin B_6	0.4	mg	100	57
Minerals				
Iron	10	mg	66	100

INGREDIENTS
Ferrous sulfate, ascorbic acid, d-alpha-tocopheryl acid succinate, niacinamide, vitamin A palmitate, benzoic acid (preservative), riboflavin-5'-phosphate sodium, thiamine hydrochloride, methylparaben (preservative), pyridoxine hydrochloride, and ergocalciferol in corn oil, in a glycerin-water vehicle with added artificial coloring and flavoring. Contains only a trace (less than ½%) of alcohol.
Contains no sugar.
*% U.S. Recommended Daily Allowance for infants.
**% U.S. Recommended Daily Allowance for children under 4 years of age.

INDICATIONS AND USAGE
Multivitamin supplement with iron for infants and children under 4 years of age.

ADMINISTRATION AND DOSAGE
One dropperful daily, or as directed by physician.

HOW SUPPLIED
50-mL Spil-gard® bottles, calibrated dropper enclosed; OTC; **NDC** 0074-0116-01.

VI-DAYLIN® ADC VITAMINS + IRON Drops
[vī"dā'lin]
Dietary Supplement of Vitamins A, D and C with Iron

DESCRIPTION
One dropperful (1.0 mL) provides:

		% U.S. RDA*	% U.S. RDA**
Vitamins			
Vitamin A	1500 I.U.	100	60
Vitamin D	400 I.U.	100	100
Vitamin C	35 mg	100	87
Minerals			
Iron	10 mg	66	100

INGREDIENTS
Polysorbate 80, ferrous sulfate, ascorbic acid, vitamin A palmitate, benzoic acid (preservative), methylparaben (preservative), and ergocalciferol in a glycerin-water vehicle with added artificial flavoring and coloring.
Contains no sugar.
*% U.S. Recommended Daily Allowance for infants.
** % U.S. Recommended Daily Allowance for children under 4 years of age.

INDICATIONS AND USAGE
Dietary supplement of vitamins A, D and C with iron for infants and children under 4 years of age.

DOSAGE AND ADMINISTRATION
One dropperful daily, or as directed by physician.

HOW SUPPLIED
50-mL Spil-gard® bottles; calibrated dropper enclosed; OTC; **NDC** 0074-0117-01.

Continued on next page

Ross—Cont.

VI-DAYLIN® MULTIVITAMIN Chewable Tablets

[*vī″dā′lin*]

Multivitamin Supplement

DESCRIPTION

Each chewable tablet provides:

Vitamins			%U.S. RDA*	%U.S. RDA**
Vitamin A	2500	I.U.	100	50
Vitamin D	400	I.U.	100	100
Vitamin E	15	I.U.	150	50
Vitamin C	60	mg	150	100
Folic Acid	0.3	mg	150	75
Thiamine (Vitamin B_1)	1.05	mg	150	70
Riboflavin (Vitamin B_2)	1.2	mg	150	70
Niacin	13.5	mg	150	67
Vitamin B_6	1.05	mg	150	52
Vitamin B_{12}	4.5	mcg	150	75

INGREDIENTS

Sucrose and dextrins, sodium ascorbate, niacinamide, dl-alpha tocopheryl acetate, ascorbic acid, vitamin A palmitate, riboflavin, pyridoxine hydrochloride, thiamine mononitrate, cholecalciferol, folic acid and cyanocobalamin. Made with natural sweeteners, artificial flavoring and artificially colored with natural ingredients.

*% U.S. Recommended Daily Allowance for children under 4 years of age.

**% U.S. Recommended Daily Allowance for adults and children 4 or more years of age.

INDICATIONS AND USAGE

Multivitamin supplement for children and adults.

DOSAGE AND ADMINISTRATION

One chewable tablet daily, or as directed by physician.

HOW SUPPLIED

100-tablet bottles; OTC; **NDC** 0074-4519-13.

Shown in Product Identification Section, page 426

VI-DAYLIN®/F MULTIVITAMIN Chewable Tablets With Fluoride ℞

[*vī″dā′lin*]

Multivitamins/Fluoride

DESCRIPTION

Each chewable tablet provides:

Fluoride (as sodium fluoride) 1 mg

Vitamins			%U.S. RDA*	%U.S. RDA**
Vitamin A (as palmitate, 0.75 mg)	2500	I.U.	100	50
Vitamin D (cholecalciferol, 10 mcg)	400	I.U.	100	100
Vitamin E (dl-alpha tocopheryl acetate)	15	I.U.	150	50
Vitamin C (as sodium ascorbate, 40 mg; ascorbic acid, 20 mg)	60	mg	150	100
Folic Acid	0.3	mg	150	75
Vitamin B_1(as thiamine mononitrate)	1.05	mg	150	70
Vitamin B_2 (as riboflavin)	1.2	mg	150	70
Niacin (as niacinamide)	13.5	mg	150	67
Vitamin B_6 (as pyridoxine hydrochloride)	1.05	mg	150	52
Vitamin B_{12} (as cyano-cobalamin)	4.5	mcg	150	75

*% U.S. Recommended Daily Allowance for children under 4 years of age.

**% U.S. Recommended Daily Allowance for adults and children 4 or more years of age.

INACTIVE INGREDIENTS

Cellulosic polymers, citric acid, corn starch, DC Yellow No. 10, dextrin, FDC Yellow No. 6, magnesium stearate, sucrose, artificial flavoring and other ingredients.

INDICATIONS AND USAGE

As an aid in the prevention of dental caries in children, and in the prophylaxis of certain vitamin deficiencies.

CONTRAINDICATIONS

Should not be used where the fluoride content of the drinking water supply is known to be greater than 0.7 parts per million.

PRECAUTIONS

The recommended use and dosage of Vi-Daylin/F Chewable should not be exceeded, since chronic overdosage of fluoride may result in mottling of tooth enamel and osseous changes.

OVERDOSAGE

In children, acute ingestion of 10 to 20 mg of sodium fluoride may cause excessive salivation and gastrointestinal disturbances; 500 mg may be fatal. Oral and/or intravenous fluids containing calcium may be indicated.

DOSAGE AND ADMINISTRATION

Children 3 years of age or older, 1 chewable tablet daily; age 2 to 3 years, ½ chewable tablet daily; or as directed by physician or dentist.

HOW SUPPLIED

100-tablet bottles; Rx; **NDC** 0074-7626-13.

Shown in Product Identification Section, page 426

(.5860)

VI-DAYLIN®/F MULTIVITAMIN + IRON ℞

Chewable Tablets With Fluoride

[*vī″dā′lin*]

Multivitamins/Fluoride/Iron

DESCRIPTION

Each chewable tablet provides:

Fluoride (as sodium fluoride) 1 mg

Vi-Daylin/F Multivitamin + Iron Chewable Tablets With Fluoride

Vitamins			% U.S. RDA*	% U.S. RDA**
Vitamin A (as palmitate, 0.75 mg)	2500	I.U.	100	50
Vitamin D (as cholecalciferol, 10 mcg)	400	I.U.	100	100
Vitamin E (as dl-alpha tocopheryl acetate)	15	I.U.	150	50
Vitamin C (as sodium ascorbate, 40 mg; ascorbic acid, 20 mg)	60	mg	150	100
Folic Acid	0.3	mg	150	75
Vitamin B_1(as thiamine mononitrate)	1.05	mg	150	70
Vitamin B_2 (as riboflavin)	1.2	mg	150	70
Niacin (as niacinamide)	13.5	mg	150	67
Vitamin B_6 (as pyridoxine hydrochloride)	1.05	mg	150	52
Vitamin B_{12} (as (cyanocobalamin)	4.5	mcg	150	75
Minerals				
Iron (as ferrous fumarate)	12	mg	120	66

*% U.S. Recommended Daily Allowance for children under 4 years of age.

**% U.S. Recommended Daily Allowance for adults and children 4 or more years of age.

INACTIVE INGREDIENTS

Carmine No. 40, cellulosic polymers, citric acid, corn starch, dextrin, FDC Yellow No. 6, magnesium stearate, mannitol, sodium chloride, sucrose, tricalcium phosphate, artificial flavoring and other ingredients.

INDICATIONS AND USAGE

As an aid in the prevention of dental caries in children, and in the prophylaxis of iron and certain vitamin deficiencies.

CONTRAINDICATIONS

Should be used only where the fluoride content of the drinking water supply is known to be 0.7 parts per million or less.

PRECAUTIONS

The recommended dosage should not be exceeded since chronic overdosage of fluoride may result in mottling of tooth enamel and osseous changes.

DOSAGE AND ADMINISTRATION

Children 3 years of age or older, one chewable tablet daily; age 2-3 years, ½ chewable tablet daily; or as directed by physician or dentist.

OVERDOSAGE

In children, acute ingestion of 10 to 20 mg of sodium fluoride may cause excessive salivation and gastrointestinal disturbances; 500 mg may be fatal. Oral and/or intravenous fluids containing calcium may be indicated.

Acute overdosage of iron may cause nausea and vomiting and, in severe cases, cardiovascular collapse and death. The estimated lethal dose of orally ingested elemental iron is 300 mg per kg body weight. Serum iron and total iron-binding capacity may be used as guides for use of chelating agents such as deferoxamine.

HOW SUPPLIED

100-tablet bottles; ℞; **NDC** 0074-7621-13.

Shown in Product Identification Section, page 426

(.5860)

VI-DAYLIN® MULTIVITAMIN + IRON

Chewable Tablets

[*vī″dā′lin*]

Multivitamin/Iron Supplement

DESCRIPTION

Each chewable tablet provides:

Vitamins			% U.S. RDA*	% U.S. RDA**
Vitamin A	2500	I.U.	100	50
Vitamin D	400	I.U.	100	100
Vitamin E	15	I.U.	150	50
Vitamin C	60	mg	150	100
Folic Acid	0.3	mg	150	75
Thiamine (Vitamin B_1)	1.05	mg	150	70
Riboflavin (Vitamin B_2)	1.2	mg	150	70
Niacin	13.5	mg	150	67
Vitamin B_6	1.05	mg	150	52
Vitamin B_{12}	4.5	mcg	150	75
Minerals				
Iron	12	mg	120	66

INGREDIENTS

Sucrose and dextrins, mannitol, sodium ascorbate, niacinamide, ferrous fumarate, dl-alpha tocopheryl acetate, ascorbic acid, vitamin A palmitate, riboflavin, pyridoxine hydrochloride, thiamine mononitrate, cholecalciferol, folic acid and cyanocobalamin. Made with natural sweeteners, artificial flavoring and coloring.

*% U.S. Recommended Daily Allowance for children under 4 years of age.

**% U.S. Recommended Daily Allowance for adults and children 4 or more years of age.

INDICATIONS AND USAGE

Multivitamin supplement with iron for children and adults.

DOSAGE AND ADMINISTRATION

One tablet daily, or as directed by physician.

HOW SUPPLIED

100-tablet bottles; OTC; **NDC** 0074-4520-13.

Shown in Product Identification Section, page 426

VI-DAYLIN® MULTIVITAMIN Liquid

[*vī″dā′lin*]

Multivitamin Supplement

DESCRIPTION

One teaspoonful (5.0 mL) provides:

Vitamins			% U.S. RDA*	% U.S. RDA**
Vitamin A	2500	I.U.	100	50
Vitamin D	400	I.U.	100	100
Vitamin E	15	I.U.	150	50
Vitamin C	60	mg	150	100
Thiamine (Vitamin B_1)	1.05	mg	150	70
Riboflavin (Vitamin B_2)	1.2	mg	150	70
Niacin	13.5	mg	150	67
Vitamin B_6	1.05	mg	150	52
Vitamin B_{12}	4.5	mcg	150	75

*% U.S. Recommended Daily Allowance for children under 4 years of age.

**% U.S. Recommended Daily Allowance for adults and children 4 or more years of age.

INGREDIENTS

Glucose, sucrose, ascorbic acid, polysorbate 80, d-alpha tocopheryl acetate, niacinamide, acacia, cysteine hydrochloride (stabilizer), benzoic acid (preservative), vitamin A palmitate, methylparaben (preservative), pyridoxine hydrochloride, riboflavin, thiamine hydrochloride, ergocalciferol in corn oil, and cyanocobalamin in an aqueous vehicle with added natural citrus flavor and artificial color. Contains only a trace of alcohol (not more than ½%).

INDICATIONS AND USAGE

Multivitamin supplement for children and adults.

DOSAGE AND ADMINISTRATION

One teaspoonful daily, or as directed by physician.

HOW SUPPLIED

16-fl-oz (pint) bottles; OTC; **NDC** 0074-3606-03.

8-fl-oz bottles; OTC; **NDC** 0074-3606-02.

VI-DAYLIN® MULTIVITAMIN + IRON Liquid

[*vī″dā′lin*]
Multivitamin/Iron Supplement

DESCRIPTION

One teaspoonful (5.0 mL) provides:

Vitamins			**% U.S. RDA***	**% U.S. RDA****
Vitamin A	2500	I.U.	100	50
Vitamin D	400	I.U.	100	100
Vitamin E	15	I.U.	150	50
Vitamin C	60	mg	150	100
Thiamine (Vitamin B_1)	1.05	mg	150	70
Riboflavin (Vitamin B_2)	1.2	mg	150	70
Niacin	13.5	mg	150	67
Vitamin B_6	1.05	mg	150	52
Vitamin B_{12}	4.5	mcg	150	75
Minerals				
Iron	10	mg	100	55

*% U.S. Recommended Daily Allowance for children under 4 years of age.
**% U.S. Recommended Daily Allowance for adults and children 4 or more years of age.

INGREDIENTS

Glucose, sucrose, ascorbic acid, ferrous gluconate, polysorbate 80, d-alpha tocopheryl acetate, citric acid, niacinamide, acacia, cysteine hydrochloride (stabilizer), benzoic acid (preservative), methylparaben (preservative), vitamin A palmitate, riboflavin-5′-phosphate sodium, pyridoxine hydrochloride, thiamine hydrochloride, propylparaben (preservative), ergocalciferol in corn oil, and cyanocobalamin in an aqueous vehicle with added natural citrus flavor and artificial color. Contains only a trace of alcohol (not more than ½%).

INDICATIONS AND USAGE

Multivitamin supplement with iron for children and adults.

DOSAGE AND ADMINISTRATION

One teaspoonful daily, or as directed by physician.

HOW SUPPLIED

16-fl-oz (pint) bottles; OTC; **NDC** 0074-6992-03.
8-fl-oz bottles; OTC; **NDC** 0074-6992-02.

VITAL® HIGH NITROGEN

[*vī′tel*]
Nutritionally Complete
Partially Hydrolyzed Diet

USAGE

As a source of total or supplemental nutrition for patients with impaired gastrointestinal function (limited digestion and/or absorption). VITAL HIGH NITROGEN may be used as a tube feeding (nasogastric, nasoduodenal or jejunal) or as an oral feeding. Five servings (1500 Calories) meets or surpasses 100% of the daily U.S. RDA for vitamins and minerals for adults and children 4 or more years of age.

Features:

- Complete nutrition—In standard dilution, Vital High Nitrogen provides 1 Calorie per mL and 300 Calories per serving (1 packet). Caloric distribution: protein, 16.7%; fat, 9.4%; carbohydrate, 73.9%.
- High levels of nitrogen—Vital High Nitrogen provides 62.5 g of protein (10 g nitrogen) in 1500 Calories, with a total Calorie-to-nitrogen ratio of 150:1. Vital High Nitrogen provides partially hydrolyzed whey and meat, and soy fortified with essential amino acids, designed to maximize nitrogen absorption.
- Good taste—Vital High Nitrogen is significantly more palatable and acceptable than diets composed solely of crystalline amino acids. The mild, appealing vanilla flavor assures better patient acceptance of an elemental feeding with no disturbing aftertaste.
- High fat absorption—45% of fat from medium-chain triglycerides.
- Low osmolality—The osmolality of Vital High Nitrogen (500 mosm/kg water) may help to avoid the gastrointestinal distress and dumping syndrome commonly associated with elemental feedings.
- Low fecal residue—The fecal residue produced by Vital High Nitrogen is comparable to that produced by traditional elemental diets.
- Low electrolyte levels—The electrolyte levels are appropriate for diets moderately restricted in electrolytes, yet adequate for most hospitalized patients.

Sample Administration Schedule VITAL HIGH NITROGEN

Continuous Drip Schedule (See dilution rates below)

Day	Time	Strength	Rate (mL/hr)	Volume (mL)	Calories
1	1st 8 hours	½	50	400	200
	2nd 8 hours	½	75	600	300
	3rd 8 hours	½	100	800	400
					900 *Total Calories*
2	1st 8 hours	¾	100	800	600
	2nd 8 hours	¾	100	800	600
	3rd 8 hours	¾	100	800	600
					1800 *Total Calories*
3	1st 8 hours	Full	100	800	800
	2nd 8 hours	Full	100–125	800–1000	800–1000
	3rd 8 hours	Full	100–125	800–1000	800–1000
					2400–2800 *Total Calories*

Intermittent Drip Schedule (See dilution rates below)

Day	Time	Strength	Rate (5–10 mL/min)	Volume (mL)	Calories
1	7am–11pm	½	100 mL q 2 hr (7am, 9am, 11am)	300	150
		½	200 mL q 2 hr (1pm, 3pm, 5pm)	600	300
		½	300 mL q 2 hr (7pm, 9pm, 11pm)	900	450
					900 *Total Calories*
2	7am–11pm	¾	300 mL q 2 hr (7am, 9am, 11am, 1pm, 3pm, 5pm, 7pm, 9pm, 11pm)	2700	2025 *Total Calories*
3	7am–11pm	Full	300 mL q 3 hr (5 feedings) up to 300 mL q 2 hr (8 feedings)	1500–2400	1500–2400 *Total Calories*

- Check gastric residuals before every intermittent feeding or every 2–4 hours during continuous feeding.
- If intolerance develops, return to previously tolerated rate and strength. When tolerance is again established, proceed with feeding schedule as indicated. Do not alter rate and strength at the same time.
- Rinsing the tube with water (eg, 25–100 mL) periodically or after intermittent feedings will help avoid clogging and provide additional water.

Dilution Schedule*

Dilution Cal/mL	Vital Pouch (79 g)	Water mL	Total Volume mL
.50	1	555	600
.75	1	355	400
1.00	1	255	300
1.50	1	155	200
2.00	1	105	150

*Controlling the flow rate of viscous dilutions is facilitated by an enteral feeding pump.

DOSAGE AND ADMINISTRATION

Instructions for Use: [Standard Dilution—One packet of powder (79 g) mixed in 255 mL (8.5 fl oz) of water yields approximately 300 mL.] Pour 255 mL (8.5 fl oz) of cold water into a container. Empty contents of one packet into container and mix until powder dissolves. Prepare only the amount intended for a single day's feeding. Refrigerate after preparation. Store unopened powder in a cool, dry place.

Oral Feeding: Serving Vital High Nitrogen chilled enhances its flavor and increases palatability. May be used for total nutrition, or with and between meals.

Tube Feeding: Follow physician's instructions. Adjust flow rate, volume and dilution according to patient's condition and tolerance. Additional fluid requirements should be met by giving water orally with or after feedings. Avoid contamination during preparation and use.

Not for parenteral use.

AVAILABILITY

Powder: 2.79 oz (79 g) packets; 24 packets per case; Vanilla, No. 766.

COMPOSITION

Ingredients: Hydrolyzed corn starch, protein components (partially hydrolyzed whey and meat, and soy), sucrose, minerals (potassium phosphate dibasic, calcium phosphate tribasic, magnesium sulfate, magnesium chloride, sodium chloride, zinc sulfate, ferrous sulfate, manganese sulfate, cupric sulfate), safflower oil, amino acids (L-tyrosine, L-leucine, L-valine, L-isoleucine, L-phenylalanine, L-histidine, L-methionine, L-threonine, L-tryptophan), medium-chain triglycerides (fractionated coconut oil), artificial and natural flavor, vitamins (choline chloride, ascorbic acid, alpha-tocopheryl acetate, niacinamide, calcium pantothenate, vitamin A palmitate, riboflavin, pyridoxine hydrochloride, thiamine chloride hydrochloride, folic acid, biotin, phylloquinone, vitamin D_3, cyanocobalamin), mono- and diglycerides, and soy lecithin.

Nutrients: (grams)	**Per 300 Calories*** (1 packet)	**Per 1500 Calories*** (5 packets)
Protein	12.5	62.5
Fat	3.25	16.25
Carbohydrate	55.4	277
Minerals (Ash)	1.6	8.0
Water (Max)	5.2	26.0

Vitamins/Minerals	**Per 300 Calories*** (1 Packet)		**Per 1500 Calories*** (5 Packets)		**% U.S. RDA**** (1500 Calories)
Vitamin A	1000	I.U.	5000	I.U.	100
Vitamin D	80	I.U.	400	I.U.	100
Vitamin E	9	I.U.	45	I.U.	150
Vitamin K_1	14	mcg	70	mcg	***
Vitamin C	60	mg	300	mg	500
Folic Acid	160	mcg	800	mcg	200
Thiamine (Vit. B_1)	0.60	mg	3.0	mg	200
Riboflavin (Vit. B_2)	0.68	mg	3.4	mg	200
Vitamin B_6	0.80	mg	4.0	mg	200
Vitamin B_{12}	2.4	mcg	12	mcg	200
Niacin	8	mg	40	mg	200
Choline	120	mg	600	mg	***
Biotin	120	mcg	600	mcg	200
Pantothenic Acid	4.0	mg	20	mg	200
Sodium	140	mg	700	mg	***

Continued on next page

Ross—Cont.

Potassium	400	mg	2000	mg	***
Chloride	270	mg	1350	mg	***
Calcium	200	mg	1000	mg	100
Phosphorus	200	mg	1000	mg	100
Magnesium	80	mg	400	mg	100
Iodine	30	mcg	150	mcg	100
Manganese	1.0	mg	5.0	mg	***
Copper	0.4	mg	2.0	mg	100
Zinc	4.5	mg	22.5	mg	150
Iron	3.6	mg	18	mg	100

*In standard dilution (79 g of Vital High Nitrogen Powder mixed in 255 mL of water).
**For adults and children 4 or more years of age.
***U.S. RDA not established.
(FAN 366-02)

EDUCATIONAL MATERIAL

A complete program of educational services for health professionals and patients is available.
Contact your local Ross representative.

Roxane Laboratories, Inc.
P.O. 16532
COLUMBUS, OH 43216

HOSPITAL UNIT DOSE

Hospital Unit Dose—Roxane, was developed to aid in improved drug distribution and administration. With Hospital Unit Dose, each single unit of medication moves from our quality controlled production lines to the patient's bedside in tamper resistant containers, labeled for positive identification, thus protecting dosage integrity to the point of administration.

The following products are currently available in Hospital Unit Dose:

Acetaminophen Elixir USP (lime) 160mg/5ml, 325mg/10.15ml, 650mg/20.3ml
Acetaminophen Elixir USP (cherry) 160mg/5ml, 325mg/10.15ml, 650mg/20.3ml
Acetaminophen Suppositories 120mg, 650mg
Acetaminophen Tablets USP 325mg, 500mg, 650mg
Acetaminophen 120mg and Codeine Phosphate 12mg Elixir
Acetaminophen 300mg and Codeine Phosphate 30mg Tablets
Acetaminophen 300mg and Codeine Phosphate 60mg Tablets
Aluminum Hydroxide Gel USP (Flavored) 2400mg/30ml
Aluminum Hydroxide, Concentrate, 2400mg/20ml, 3600mg/30ml
Aluminum Hydroxide Tablets 500mg
Aluminum and Magnesium Hydroxides with Simethicone I 15ml, 30ml
Aluminum and Magnesium Hydroxides with Simethicone II 15ml, 30ml
Aminophylline Tablets USP 100mg, 200mg
Aminophylline Oral Solution 210mg/10ml, 315mg/15ml
Amitriptyline Hydrochloride Tablets USP 10mg, 25mg, 50mg, 75mg, 100mg, 150mg
Aromatic Cascara Fluidextract USP 5ml
Aromatic Castor Oil USP 30ml, 60ml
Ascorbic Acid Tablets USP 250mg, 500mg
Aspirin Suppositories USP 300mg, 600mg
Bisacodyl Suppositories USP 10mg
Bisacodyl Tablets USP 5mg
Bisacodyl Patient Pack
Calcium Carbonate Tablets USP 1250mg
Calcium Carbonate Tablets USP, Chewable 420mg, 750mg, 1250mg
Calcium Carbonate Oral Suspension 1250mg/5ml
Calcium Gluconate Tablets USP 500mg
Castor Oil USP 30ml, 60ml
Chloral Hydrate Syrup USP 500mg/10ml, 1g/10ml
Chloral Hydrate Capsules USP 500mg
Chlorpheniramine Maleate Tablets USP 4mg
Cocaine Hydrochloride Topical Solution 4%/4ml, 10%/4ml
Codeine Sulfate Tablets USP 15mg, 30mg, 60mg
Dexamethasone Oral Solution 0.5mg/5ml, 2mg/20ml
Dexamethasone Tablets USP 0.5mg, 0.75mg, 1mg, 1.5mg, 2mg, 4mg, 6mg
Diazepam Tablets USP 2mg, 5mg, 10mg
Dihydrotachysterol Tablets USP 0.125mg, 0.2mg
Diluent (Flavored) for Oral Use 15ml
Diphenhydramine Hydrochloride Elixir USP 25mg/10ml
Diphenhydramine Hydrochloride Capsules USP 50mg
Diphenoxylate Hydrochloride 2.5mg and Atropine Sulfate 0.025mg Tablets USP
Diphenoxylate Hydrochloride and Atropine Sulfate Oral Solution USP 4ml, 10ml
Docusate Sodium Capsules USP 50mg, 100mg, 250mg
Docusate Sodium Syrup USP 50mg/15ml, 100mg/30ml
Docusate Sodium 100mg with Casanthranol 30mg Capsules
Ferrous Sulfate Oral Solution 300mg/5ml
Ferrous Sulfate Tablets USP 300mg
Furosemide Oral Solution 10mg/ml, 40mg/5ml
Furosemide Tablets USP 20mg, 40mg, 80mg
Guaifenesin Syrup USP 100mg/5ml, 200mg/10ml, 300mg/15ml
Hydrochlorothiazide Tablets USP 25mg, 50mg
Hydrochlorothiazide Oral Solution 50mg/5ml
Hydromorphone Hydrochloride Tablets USP 2mg, 4mg
Imipramine Hydrochloride Tablets USP 10mg, 25mg, 50mg
Indomethacin Capsules USP 25mg, 50mg
Ipecac Syrup USP 15ml, 30ml
Isoetharine Hydrochloride 0.1%, 2.5ml
Isoetharine Hydrochloride 0.125%, 4ml
Isoetharine Hydrochloride 0.167%, 3ml
Isoetharine Hydrochloride 0.2%, 2.5ml
Isoetharine Hydrochloride 0.25%, 2ml
Isoxsuprine Hydrochloride Tablets USP 10mg, 20mg
Kaolin-Pectin Suspension 30ml
Lidocaine Viscous 2% 20ml
Lithium Carbonate Capsules USP 150mg, 300mg, 600mg
Lithium Carbonate Tablets USP 300mg
Lithium Citrate Syrup 8 mEq per 5ml, 16 mEq per 10ml
Magaldrate Oral Suspension USP 30ml
Magnesia and Alumina Oral Suspension USP 30ml
Methadone Hydrochloride Tablets USP 5mg, 10mg
Methyldopa Tablets USP 125mg, 250mg, 500mg
Milk of Magnesia USP 15ml, 30ml
Milk of Magnesia Concentrated Flavored 10ml, 15ml, 20ml
Milk of Magnesia—Cascara Suspension Concentrated 15ml
Milk of Magnesia—Mineral Oil Emulsion 30ml
Milk of Magnesia—Mineral Oil Emulsion (Flavored) 30ml
Mineral Oil-Light Sterile 10ml, 30ml
Mineral Oil USP 30ml
Morphine Sulfate Tablets 15mg, 30mg
Morphine Sulfate Oral Solution 10mg/5ml, 20mg/10ml
Neomycin Sulfate Tablets USP 500mg
Paregoric USP 5ml
Phenobarbital Elixir USP 20mg/5ml, 30mg/7.5ml
Phenobarbital Tablets USP 15mg, 30mg, 60mg, 100mg
Potassium Chloride Oral Solution USP 10% (15mEq/11.25ml)
Potassium Chloride Oral Solution USP 10% (20mEq/15ml)
Potassium Chloride Oral Solution USP 10% (30mEq/22.5ml)
Potassium Chloride Oral Solution USP 10% (40mEq/30ml)
Potassium Chloride USP Powder Unflavored 20mEq/1.5g
Potassium Gluconate Elixir USP 20mEq/15ml
Potassium Phosphates Oral Solution, 30ml
Prednisolone Tablets USP 5mg
Prednisone Oral Solution 5mg/5ml, 10mg/10ml, 20mg/20ml
Prednisone Tablets USP 1mg, 2.5mg, 5mg, 10mg, 20mg, 25mg, 50mg
Propantheline Bromide Tablets USP 15mg
Propoxyphene Hydrochloride Capsules USP 65mg
Propranolol Hydrochloride Tablets USP 10mg, 20mg, 40mg, 60mg, 80mg, 90mg
Pseudoephedrine Hydrochloride Tablets USP 30mg, 60mg
Pseudoephedrine Hydrochloride Syrup USP 60mg/10ml
Quinidine Gluconate Sustained Release Tablets 324mg
Quinidine Sulfate Tablets USP 200mg, 300mg
Roxanol SR Tablets (morphine sulfate sustained release tablets) 30mg
Roxicet Oral Solution (oxycodone hydrochloride 5mg and acetaminophen 325mg/5ml)
Roxicet Tablets (oxycodone hydrochloride 5mg and acetaminophen 325mg)
Roxicodone Oral Solution (oxycodone hydrochloride 5mg/5ml)
Roxicodone Tablets (oxycodone hydrochloride 5mg)
Roxiprin Tablets (oxycodone hydrochloride 4.5mg, oxycodone terephalate 0.38mg, and aspirin 325mg)
Sodium Chloride Inhalation USP (Normal Saline) Sterile 0.9% 3ml, 5ml
Sodium Phosphates Oral Solution USP 30ml
Sodium Polystyrene Sulfonate Suspension 60ml, and 120ml Enema Package
Terpin Hydrate and Codeine Elixir USP 5ml
Theophylline Oral Solution 80mg/15ml, 100mg/18.75ml, 160mg/30ml
Thioridazine Hydrochloride Tablets USP 10mg, 25mg, 50mg, 100mg
Triprolidine 2.5mg and Pseudoephedrine Hydrochlorides 60mg Tablets USP
Triprolidine 2.5mg and Pseudoephedrine Hydrochlorides 60mg/10ml Syrup

As research continues, new Roxane Laboratories' products will be available in Hospital Unit Dose packages.

DHT™ ℞
Dihydrotachysterol Tablets USP

DESCRIPTION

Each tablet contains:
Dihydrotachysterol .... 0.125 mg, 0.2 mg; or 0.4 mg

Dihydrotachysterol is a synthetic reduction product of tachysterol, a close isomer of vitamin D. Chemically Dihydrotachysterol is *9, 10- Secoergosta-5,7,22-tri-en-3β- ol.* Dihydrotachysterol acts as a blood calcium regulator.

CLINICAL PHARMACOLOGY

Dyhydrotachysterol is hydroxylated in the liver to 25-hydroxydihydrotachysterol, which is the major circulating active form of the drug. It does not undergo further hydroxylation by the kidney and therefore is the analogue of 1,25-dihydroxyvitamin D. Dihydrotachysterol is effective in the elevation of serum calcium by stimulating intestinal calcium absorption and mobilizing bone calcium in the absence of parathyroid hormone and of functioning renal tissue. Dihydrotachysterol also increases renal phosphate excretion. In contrast to parathyroid extract, Dihydrotachysterol is active when taken orally, exerts a slow but persistent effect, and may be used for long periods without increasing the dosage or causing tolerance. Dihydrotachysterol is faster-acting than pharmacologic doses of vitamin D and is less persistent after cessation of treatment, thus decreasing the risk of accumulation and of hypercalcemia.

INDICATIONS AND USAGE

Dihydrotachysterol is indicated for the treatment of acute, chronic, and latent forms of postoperative tetany, idiopathic tetany, and hypoparathyroidism.

CONTRAINDICATIONS

Contraindicated in patients with hypercalcemia, abnormal sensitivity to the effects of vitamin D, and hypervitaminosis D.

PRECAUTIONS

General: The difference between therapeutic dose and intoxicating dose may be small in any patient and therefore dosage must be individualized and periodically reevaluated.
In patients with renal osteodystrophy accompanied by hyperphosphatemia, maintenance of a normal serum phosphorus level by dietary phosphate restriction and/or administration of aluminum gels as intestinal phosphate binders is essential to prevent metastatic calcification.
Because of its effect on serum calcium, Dihydrotachysterol should be administered to pregnant patients or to patients with renal stones only when, in the judgment of the physician, the potential benefits outweigh the possible hazards.
Laboratory tests: **To prevent hypercalcemia, treatment should always be controlled by regular determinations of blood calcium level, which should be maintained within the normal range.**
Drug interactions: Administration of thiazide diuretics to hypoparathyroid patients who are concurrently being treated with Dihydrotachysterol may cause hypercalcemia.
Pregnancy: Teratogenic effects —Pregnancy Category C: Animal reproduction studies have shown fetal abnormalities in several species associated with hypervitaminosis D. These are similar to the supravalvular aortic stenosis syndrome described in infants by Black in England (1963). This syndrome was characterized by supravalvular aortic stenosis, elfin facies, and mental retardation.
There are no adequate and well-controlled studies in pregnant women. Dihydrotachysterol should be used during pregnancy only if the potential benefit justifies the potential risk to the fetus.
Nursing mothers: It is not known whether this drug is excreted in human milk. Because many drugs are excreted in human milk, caution should be exercised when Dihydrotachysterol is administered to a nursing woman.

OVERDOSAGE

The effects of Dihydrotachysterol can persist for up to one month after cessation of treatment.
Manifestations: Toxicity associated with Dihydrotachysterol is similar to that seen with large doses of vitamin D. Overdosage is manifested by symptoms of hypercalcemia, i.e., weakness, headache, anorexia, nausea, vomiting, abdominal cramps, diarrhea, constipation, vertigo, tinnitus, ataxia, hypotonia, lethargy, depression, amnesia, disorientation, hallucinations, syncope, and coma. Impairment of renal function may result in polyuria, polydipsia, and albuminuria. Widespread calcification of soft tissues, including heart, blood vessels, kidneys, and lungs, can occur. Death can result from cardiovascular or renal failure.
Treatment: Treatment of overdosage consists of withdrawal of Dihydrotachysterol, bed rest, liberal intake of fluids, a low-calcium diet, and administration of a laxative. Hypercalcemic crisis with dehydration, stupor, coma, and azotemia requires more vigorous treatment. The first step should be hydration of the patient. Intravenous saline may quickly and significantly increast urinary calcium excretion. A loop di-

uretic (furosemide or ethacrynic acid) may be given with the saline infusion to further increase renal calcium excretion. Other reported therapeutic measures include dialysis or the administration of citrates, sulfates, phosphates, corticosteroids, EDTA (ethylenediaminetetraacetic acids), and mithramycin via appropriate regimens.

DOSAGE AND ADMINISTRATION

The dosage depends on the nature and seriousness of the disorder and should be adapted to each individual patient. Serum calcium levels should be maintained between 9 to 10 mg per 100 ml.

The following dosage schedule will serve as a guide:

Initial dose: 0.8 mg to 2.4 mg daily for several days.

Maintenance dose: 0.2 mg to 1.0 mg daily as required for normal serum calcium levels. The average maintenance dose is 0.6 mg daily. This dose may be supplemented with 10 to 15 grams of calcium lactate or gluconate by mouth daily.

HOW SUPPLIED

0.125 mg white tablets.

NDC 0054-8172-25: Unit dose, 10 tablets per strip, 10 strips per shelf pack, 10 shelf packs per shipper.

NDC 0054-4190-19: Bottles of 50 tablets.

0.2 mg pink tablets.

NDC 0054-8182-25: Unit dose, 10 tablets per strip, 10 strips per shelf pack, 10 shelf packs per shipper.

NDC 0054-4189-25: Bottles of 100 tablets.

0.4 mg white tablets.

NDC 0054-4191-19: Bottles of 50 tablets.

Oral Solution 0.2 mg/5 ml

NDC 0054-3171-63: 500 ml

Intensol 0.2 mg/ml

NDC 0054-3170-44: Bottles of 30 ml with calibrated dropper (graduated 0.25 ml to 1.0 ml)

LITHIUM CARBONATE ℞

CAPSULES 150 mg, 300 mg, and 600 mg
TABLETS 300 mg

WARNING

Lithium toxicity is closely related to serum lithium levels, and can occur at doses close to therapeutic levels. Facilities for prompt and accurate serum lithium determinations should be available before initiating therapy.

DESCRIPTION

Each tablet for oral administration contains:

Lithium Carbonate .... 300 mg

Each capsule for oral administration contains:

Lithium Carbonate .... 150 mg, 300 mg, or 600 mg

Lithium Carbonate is a white, light alkaline powder with molecular formula Li_2CO_3 and molecular weight 73.89. Lithium is an element of the alkali-metal group with atomic number 3, atomic weight 6.94 and an emission line at 671 nm on the flame photometer. Lithium acts as an antimanic.

CLINICAL PHARMACOLOGY

Preclinical studies have shown that lithium alters sodium transport in nerve and muscle cells and effects a shift toward intraneuronal metabolism of catecholamines, but the specific biochemical mechanism of lithium action in mania is unknown.

INDICATIONS AND USAGE

Lithium carbonate is indicated in the treatment of manic episodes of Bipolar Disorder. Bipolar Disorder, Manic (DSM-III) is equivalent to Manic Depressive illness, Manic, in the older DSM-II terminology.

Lithium is also indicated as a maintenance treatment for individuals with a diagnosis of Bipolar Disorder. Maintenance therapy reduces the frequency of manic episodes and diminishes the intensity of those episodes which may occur.

Typical symptoms of mania include pressure of speech, motor hyperactivity, reduced need for sleep, flight of ideas, grandiosity, or poor judgment, aggressiveness, and possibly hostility. When given to a patient experiencing a manic episode, lithium may produce a normalization of symptomatology within 1 to 3 weeks.

CONTRAINDICATIONS

Lithium should generally not be given to patients with significant renal or cardiovascular disease, severe debilitation or dehydration, or sodium depletion, and to patients receiving diuretics, since the risk of lithium toxicity is very high in such patients. If the psychiatric indication is life-threatening, and if such a patient fails to respond to other measures, lithium treatment may be undertaken with extreme caution, including daily serum lithium determinations and adjustment to the usualy low doses ordinarily tolerated by these individuals. In such instances, hospitlization is a necessity.

WARNINGS

Lithium may cause fetal harm when administered to a pregnant woman. There have been reports of lithium having adverse effects on nidation in rats, embryo viability in mice, and metabolism in-vitro of rat testis and human spermatozoa have been attributed to lithium, as have teratogenicity in submammalian species and cleft palates in mice. Studies in rats, rabbits and monkeys have shown no evidence of lithium-induced teratology. Data from lithium birth registries suggest an increase in cardiac and other anomalies, especially Ebstein's anomaly. If the patient becomes pregnant while taking lithium, she should be apprised of the potential risk to the fetus. If possible, lithium should be withdrawn for at least the first trimester unless it is determined that this would seriously endanger the mother.

Chronic lithium therapy may be associated with diminution of renal concentrating ability, occasionally presenting as nephrogenic diabetes insipidus, with polyuria and polydipsia. Such patients should be carefully managed to avoid dehydration with resulting lithium retention and toxicity. This condition is usually reversible when lithium is discontinued.

Morphologic changes with glomerular and interstitial fibrosis and nephron-atrophy have been reported in patients on chronic lithium therapy. Morphologic changes have been seen in bipolar patients never exposed to lithium. The relationship between renal functional and morphologic changes and their association with lithium therapy has not been established. To date, lithium in therapeutic doses has not been reported to cause end-stage renal disease.

When kidney function is assessed, for baseline data prior to starting lithium therapy or thereafter, routine urinalysis and other tests may be used to evaluate tubular function (e.g., urine specific gravity or osmolality following a period of water deprivation, or 24-hour urine volume) and glomerular function (e.g., serum creatinine or creatinine clearance). During lithium therapy, progressive or sudden changes in renal function, even within the normal range, indicate the need for reevaluation of treatment.

Lithium toxicity is closely related to serum lithium levels, and can occur at doses close to therapeutic levels (see DOSAGE AND ADMINISTRATION).

PRECAUTIONS

General: The ability to tolerate lithium is greater during the acute manic phase and decreases when manic symptoms subside (See DOSAGE AND ADMINISTRATION).

The distribution space of lithium approximates that of total body water. Lithium is primarily excreted in urine with insignificant excretion in feces. Renal excretion of lithium is proportional to its plasma concentration. The half-life of elimination of lithium is approximately 24 hours. Lithium decreases sodium reabsorption by the renal tubules which could lead to sodium depletion. Therefore, it is essential for the patient to maintain a normal diet, including salt, and an adequate fluid intake (2500-3000 ml) at least during the initial stabilization period. Decreased tolerance to lithium has been reported to ensue from protracted sweating or diarrhea and, if such occur, supplemental fluid and salt should be administered.

In addition to sweating and diarrhea, concomitant infection with elevated temperatures may also necessitate a temporary reduction or cessation of medication.

Previously existing underlying thyroid disorders do not necessarily constitute a contraindication to lithium treatment; where hypothyroidism exists, careful monitoring of thyroid function during lithium stabilization and maintenance allows for correction of changing thyroid parameters, if any. Where hypothyroidism occurs during lithium stabilization and maintenance, supplemental thyroid treatment may be used.

Information for the patients: Outpatients and their families should be warned that the patient must discontinue lithium therapy and contact his physician if such clinical signs of lithium toxicity as diarrhea, vomiting, tremor, mild ataxia, drowsiness, or muscular weakness occur.

Lithium may impair mental and/or physical abilities. Caution patients about activities requiring alertness (e.g., operating vehicles or machinery).

Drug interactions: Combined use of haloperidol and lithium: An encephalopathic syndrome (characterized by weakness, lethargy, fever, tremulousness and confusion, extrapyramidal symptoms, leucocytosis, elevated serum enzymes, BUN and FBS) followed by irreversible brain damage has occurred in a few patients treated with lithium plus haloperidol. A causal relationship between these events and the concomitant administration of lithium and haloperidol has not been established; however, patients receiving such combined therapy should be monitored closely for early evidence of neurological toxicity and treatment discontinued promptly if such signs appear.

The possibility of similar adverse interactions with other antipsychotic medication exists.

Lithium may prolong the effects of neuromuscular blocking agents. Therefore, neuromuscular blocking agents should be given with caution to patients receiving lithium.

Indomethacin and piroxicam have been reported to increase significantly steady state plasma lithium levels. In some cases lithium toxicity has resulted from such interactions. There is also evidence that other non-steroidal, anti-inflammatory agents may have a similar effect. When such combinations are used, increased plasma lithium level monitoring is recommended.

Pregnancy: Teratogenic effects—Pregnancy Category D, See "Warnings" section.

Nursing mothers: Lithium is excreted in human milk. Nursing should not be undertaken during lithium therapy except in rare and unusual circumstances where, in the view of the physician, the potential benefits to the mother outweigh possible hazards to the child.

Usage in Children: Since information regarding the safety and effectiveness of lithium in children under 12 years of age is not available, its use in such patients is not recommended at this time. There has been a report of a transient syndrome of acute dystonia and hyperreflexia occurring in a 15 kg child who ingested 300 mg lithium carbonate.

ADVERSE REACTIONS

Lithium toxicity: The likelihood of toxicity increases with increasing serum lithium levels. Serum lithium levels greater than 1.5 mEq/l carry a greater risk than lower levels. However, patients sensitive to lithium may exhibit toxic signs at serum levels below 1.5 mEq/l.

Diarrhea, vomiting, drowsiness, muscular weakness and lack of coordination may be early signs of lithium toxicity, and can occur at lithium levels below 2.0 mEq/l. At higher levels, giddiness, ataxia, blurred vision, tinnitus and a large output of dilute urine may be seen. Serum lithium levels above 3.0 mEq/l may produce a complex clinical picture involving multiple organs and organ systems. Serum lithium levels should not be permitted to exceed 2.0 mEq/l during the acute treatment phase.

Fine hand tremor, polyuria and mild thirst may occur during initial therapy for the acute manic phase, and may persist throughout treatment. Transient and mild nausea and general discomfort may also appear during the first few days of lithium administration.

These side effects are an inconvenience rather than a disabling condition, and usually subside with continued treatment or a temporary reduction or cessation of dosage. If persistent, a cessation of dosage is indicated.

The following adverse reactions have been reported and do not appear to be directly related to serum lithium levels.

Neuromuscular: tremor, muscle hyperirritability (fasciculations, twitching, clonic movements of whole limbs), ataxia, choreo-athetotic movements, hyperactive deep tendon reflexes.

Central Nervous System: Blackout spells, epileptiform seizures, slurred speech, dizziness, vertigo, incontinence of urine or feces, somnolence, psychomotor retardation, restlessness, confusion, stupor, coma, acute dystonia, downbeat nystagmus.

Cardiovascular: cardiac arrhythmia, hypotension, peripheral circulatory collapse.

Gastrointestinal: anorexia, nausea, vomiting, diarrhea.

Genitourinary: albuminuria, oliguria, polyuria, glycosuria.

Dermatologic: drying and thinning of hair, anesthesia of skin, chronic folliculitis, xerosis cutis, alopecia and exacerbation of psoriasis.

Autonomic Nervous System: blurred vision, dry mouth.

Miscellaneous: fatigue, lethargy, tendency to sleep, dehydration, weight loss, transient scotomata.

Thyroid Abnormalities: euthyroid goiter and/ or hypothyroidism (including myxedema) accompanied by lower T_3 and T_4. Iodine 131 uptake may be elevated. (See PRECAUTIONS). Paradoxically, rare cases of hyperthyroidism have been reported.

EEG Changes: diffuse slowing, widening of frequency spectrum, potentiation and disorganization of background rhythm.

EKG Changes: reversible flattening, isoelectricity or inversion of T-waves.

Miscellaneous: fatigue, lethargy, transient scotomata, dehydration, weight loss, tendency to sleep.

Miscellaneous reactions unrelated to dosage are: transient electroencephalographic and electrocardiographic changes, leucocytosis, headache, diffuse nontoxic goiter with or without hypothyroidism, transient hyperglycemia, generalized pruritis with or without rash, cutaneous ulcers, albuminuria, worsening of organic brain syndromes, excessive weight gain, edematous swelling of ankles or wrists, and thirst or polyuria, sometimes resembling diabetes insipidus, and metallic taste.

A single report has been received of the development of painful discoloration of fingers and toes and coldness of the extremities within one day of the starting of treatment of lithium. The mechanism through which these symptoms (resembling Raynaud's Syndrome) developed is not known. Recovery followed discontinuance.

OVERDOSAGE

The toxic levels for lithium are close to the therapeutic levels. It is therefore important that patients and their families be cautioned to watch for early symptoms and to discontinue

Continued on next page

Roxane—Cont.

the drug and inform the physician should they occur. Toxic symptoms are listed in detail under ADVERSE REACTIONS.

Treatment: No specific antidote for lithium poisoning is known. Early symptoms of lithium toxicity can usually be treated by reduction or cessation of dosage of the drug and resumption of the treatment at a lower dose after 24 to 48 hours. In severe cases of lithium poisoning, the first and foremost goal of treatment consists of elimination of this ion from the patient.

Treatment is essentially the same as that used in barbiturate poisoning: 1) gastric lavage, 2) correction of fluid and electrolyte imbalance and 3) regulation of kidney functioning. Urea, mannitol, and aminophylline all produce significant increases in lithium excretion. Hemodialysis is an effective and rapid means of removing the ion from the severely toxic patient. Infection prophylaxis, regular chest X-rays, and preservation of adequate respiration are essential.

DOSAGE AND ADMINISTRATION

Acute Mania: Optimal patient response to Lithium Carbonate usually can be established and maintained with 600 mg t.i.d. Such doses will normally produce an effective serum lithium level ranging between 1.0 and 1.5 mEq/l. Dosage must be individualized according to serum levels and clinical response. Regular monitoring of the patient's clinical state and of serum lithium levels is necessary. Serum levels should be determined twice per week during the acute phase, and until the serum level and clinical condition of the patient have been stabilized.

Long-term Control: The desirable serum lithium levels are 0.6 to 1.2 mEq/l. Dosage will vary from one individual to another, but usually 300 mg t.i.d. or q.i.d. will maintain this level. Serum lithium levels in uncomplicated cases receiving maintenance therapy during remission should be monitored at least every two months.

Patients abnormally sensitive to lithium may exhibit toxic signs at serum levels of 1.0 to 1.5 mEq/l. Elderly patients often respond to reduced dosage, and may exhibit signs of toxicity at serum levels ordinarily tolerated by other patients.

N.B.: Blood samples for serum lithium determination should be drawn immediately prior to the next dose when lithium concentrations are relatively stable (i.e., 8–12 hours after the previous dose.) Total reliance must not be placed on serum levels alone. Accurate patient evaluation requires both clinical and laboratory analysis.

HOW SUPPLIED

Lithium Carbonate Tablets USP

300 mg white, scored tablets (Identified 54 452)

NDC 0054-8528-25: Unit dose, 10 tablets per strip, 10 strips per shelf pack, 10 shelf packs per shipper.
(For Institutional Use Only).
NDC 0054-4527-25: Bottles of 100 tablets.
NDC 0054-4527-31: Bottles of 1000 tablets.

Lithium Carbonate Capsules USP

150 mg white opaque colored capsules (size 4) (Identified 54 213).

NDC 0054-8526-25: Unit dose, 10 capsules per strip, 10 strips per shelf pack, 10 shelf packs per shipper.
(For Institutional Use Only).
NDC 0054-2526-25: Bottles of 100 capsules.
NDC 0054-2526-31: Bottles of 1000 capsules.

300 mg flesh-colored capsules (size 2) (Identified 54 463).

NDC 0054-8527-25: Unit dose, 10 capsules per strip, 10 strips per shelf pack, 10 shelf packs per shipper.
(For Institutional Use Only).
NDC 0054-2527-25: Bottles of 100 capsules.
NDC 0054-2527-31: Bottles of 1000 capsules.

600 mg white opaque/flesh colored capsules (size 0) (Identified 54 702).

NDC 0054-8531-25: Unit dose, 10 capsules per strip, 10 strips per shelf pack, 10 shelf packs per shipper.
(For Institutional Use Only.)
NDC 0054-2531-25: Bottles of 100 capsules.
NDC 0054-2531-31: Bottles of 1000 capsules.

LITHIUM CITRATE SYRUP USP ℞

8 mEq of Lithium per 5 ml, 16mEq of Lithium per 10 ml
SUGAR FREE
FOR ORAL ADMINISTRATION ONLY

DESCRIPTION

Lithium Citrate Syrup is a palatable oral dosage form of lithium ion. Lithium citrate is prepared in solution from lithium hydroxide and citric acid in a ratio approximating di-lithium citrate:

Each 5 ml of Lithium Citrate Syrup contains 8 mEq of lithium ion (Li+), equivalent to the amount of lithium in 300 mg of lithium carbonate and alcohol 0.3% v/v. Lithium is an element of the alkali-metal group with atomic number 3, atomic weight 6.94, and an emission line at 671nm on the flame photometer.

HOW SUPPLIED

Lithium Citrate Syrup, 8 mEq per 5 ml

NDC 0054-8529-04: Unit dose Patient Cup™ filled to deliver 5 ml, ten 5 ml Patient Cups™ per shelf pack, ten shelf packs per shipper. (For Institutional Use Only).
NDC 0054-3527-63: Bottles of 500 ml.

Lithium Citrate Syrup, 10 mEq per 10 ml

NDC 0054-8530-04: Unit dose Patient Cup™ filled to deliver 10 ml, ten 10 ml Patient Cups™ per shelf pack, ten shelf packs per shipper. (For Institutional Use Only).

Refer to Lithium Carbonate Capsules and Tablets heading for complete text.

MARINOL® Ⓒ ℞
(Dronabinol)

(WARNING: May be habit forming)

DESCRIPTION

Each capsule for oral administration contains:
Dronabinol .... 2.5 mg, 5 mg, or 10 mg
(**Warning:** May be habit forming)

MARINOL brand of dronabinol (delta-9-tetrahydrocannabinol, THC), [(6a*R-trans*)-6a,7,8,10a-tetrahydro-6,6,9-trimethyl-3-pentyl-6*H*-dibenzo[*b,d*]pyran-1-ol] is the principal psychoactive substance present in *Cannabis sativa L.* (marijuana). It has the empirical formula $C_{21}H_{30}O_2$ with the molecular weight of 314.45. It has the following structural formula:

MARINOL is chemically synthesized and formulated in sesame oil and encapsulated in round soft gelatin capsules for oral administration.

CLINICAL PHARMACOLOGY

Non-therapeutic Effects

Dronabinol, commonly known as delta-9-THC, is one of the major active substances in marijuana. For practical purposes, the non-therapeutic effects of dronabinol may be considered essentially identical to those of marijuana and other centrally active cannabinoids. MARINOL is highly abusable and can produce both physical and psychological dependence.

Dronabinol has complex effects upon the central nervous system. Subjects using cannabis may experience changes in mood (euphoria, detachment, depression, anxiety, panic, paranoia, etc.), decrements in cognitive performance and memory, a decreased ability to control drives and impulses, and alterations in the experience of reality (e.g., distortions in the perception of objects and the sense of time, hallucinations, etc.). These latter phenomena appear to be more common when larger doses of dronabinol are administered; however, a full blown picture of psychosis (psychotic organic brain syndrome) may occur in patients receiving doses within the lower portion of the therapeutic range.

Reliable information on the behavioral effects of chronic dronabinol use is not available; however, it has been reported that chronic use of cannabis may be associated with decrements in motivation, cognition, judgment, etc. (Whether these impairments reflect the underlying character of individuals chronically abusing cannabis or are a result of the use of cannabis is not known.)

Dronabinol, used within or slightly above the recommended dose range, has several systemic effects of interest. It characteristically causes an increase in heart rate and conjunctival injection. Its effects on blood pressure are inconsistent, but occasional subjects have experienced orthostatic hypotension and/or fainting upon standing. In one study, a slight, but consistent, decrease in oral temperature was recorded.

The potential of dronabinol to cause tolerance and physical dependence was examined in a 30 day rising dose tolerance study. Following thirty days of use, tolerance developed to the cardiovascular and subjective effects of dronabinol administered at doses up to 210 mg/day. An initial tachycardia induced by dronabinol was replaced successively by normal sinus rhythm and then bradycardia. A fall in supine blood pressure, made worse by standing, was also observed initially. Within days, however, these effects disappeared, indicating the development of tolerance.

A withdrawal syndrome, consisting of irritability, insomnia, and restlessness, was observed in some subjects within 12 hours following abrupt withdrawal of dronabinol. The syndrome reached its peak intensity at 24 hours when subjects exhibited "hot flashes", sweating, rhinorrhea, loose stools, hiccoughs and anorexia. The syndrome was essentially complete within 96 hours.

Electroencephalographic changes recorded following dronabinol discontinuation were consistent with a withdrawal syndrome. While on drug, dronabinol produced a decrease in REM sleep. Following discontinuation, a marked rebound of REM sleep occurred. Several subjects reported impressions of disturbed sleep for several weeks after discontinuing high dose dronabinol. Dronabinol is not an opioid, and does not cause opioid-like effects upon respiration or pupil size.

Metabolism and Pharmacokinetics

Reliable information on the pharmacokinetics of MARINOL is not yet available. The following summary highlights important aspects of the literature concerning the absorption, distribution, metabolism and elimination of dronabinol; however, differences in the preparation, formulation and method of administration make it difficult to extrapolate this information directly to the drug product, MARINOL.

Following oral administration, dronabinol has a systemic availability of 10 to 20% relative to an I.V. dose, indicating that the drug undergoes extensive first pass metabolism. Numerous metabolites have been identified, including 11-hydroxy-tetrahydrocannabinol, which is psychoactive. Dronabinol has a volume of distribution about 100 times as large as the plasma volume.

The maximum plasma concentrations of dronabinol, the 11-hydroxy metabolite, and several other metabolites occur approximately 2 to 3 hours after oral dosing. Biliary excretion is the major route of elimination. Within 72 hours following oral administration, approximately 50% of the dose is recovered in feces; another ten to fifteen percent appears in the urine either unchanged or as a metabolite. Renal clearance in normals is approximately one-tenth of the glomerular filtration rate.

The elimination phase of dronabinol exhibits biphasic kinetics with an alpha half-life of about 4 hours and a terminal half-life of 25 to 36 hours. The principal active metabolite, 11-OH-delta-9-THC, appears in the plasma in roughly the same mg quantities as its parent. The terminal plasma half-life for the 11-OH-delta-9-THC is approximately 15–18 hours. Thus, extended use of MARINOL at the doses recommended in this labeling may cause the accumulation of toxic amounts of dronabinol and its metabolites.

INDICATIONS AND USAGE

MARINOL is indicated for the treatment of the nausea and vomiting associated with cancer chemotherapy in patients who have failed to respond adequately to conventional antiemetic treatments. This restriction is required because a substantial proportion of patients treated with MARINOL can be expected to experience disturbing psychotomimetic reactions not observed with other antiemetic agents.

Because of its potential to alter the mental state, MARINOL is intended for use under circumstances that permit close supervision of the patient by a responsible individual.

MARINOL is highly abusable and controlled under Schedule II of the Controlled Substances Act. Prescriptions of MARINOL should be limited to the amount necessary for a single cycle of chemotherapy (i.e., a few days).

Evidence supporting the efficacy of MARINOL in the treatment of nausea and vomiting induced by cancer chemotherapy was obtained from a variety of sources. The most persuasive evidence was obtained in subjects being treated with MOPP for Hodgkin's and non-Hodgkin's lymphomas. Other evidence supports the conclusion that MARINOL is effective against nausea and vomiting induced by other cancer chemotherapy regimens employed in the treatment of a wide variety of tumor types.

CONTRAINDICATIONS

MARINOL is contraindicated in patients whose nausea and vomiting arises from any cause other than cancer chemotherapy.

MARINOL is contraindicated in any patient known to be hypersensitive to either dronabinol or sesame oil.

WARNINGS

Because of its profound effects on the mental status, patients should be warned not to drive, operate complex machinery, or engage in any activity requiring sound judgment and unimpaired coordination while receiving treatment with MARINOL. The effects of MARINOL may persist for a variable and unpredictable period of time following its oral administration. Dronabinol is highly lipid soluble and its metabolites may persist in tissues, including plasma, for days.

Because of individual variation in response and tolerance to the effects of MARINOL, the physician should determine on clinical grounds the period of patient supervision required. Patients receiving MARINOL should be closely observed, if possible within an inpatient setting. This is especially important during the treatment of naive patients. However, even patients experienced with MARINOL (or cannabis) may have serious untoward responses not predicted by prior uneventful exposures. Because a psychotic patient is a potential danger to him/herself and/or others, any patient who has a psychotic experience with MARINOL should be closely

observed in an appropriate setting until his/her mental state returns to normal. The patient should not be given additional doses of MARINOL until he/she has been examined, and the circumstances evaluated, by a physician. If the clinical situation warrants it, a lower dose of MARINOL may be administered under very close supervision. The patient should be counseled about the experience and should share in the decision about further use of MARINOL.
MARINOL should not be taken with alcohol, sedatives, hypnotics, or other psychotomimetic substances.

PRECAUTIONS

General: Because it may cause a general increase in central sympathomimetic activity, MARINOL should be used with caution in persons with hypertension or heart disease. MARINOL should be used cautiously in manic, depressive, or schizophrenic patients as the symptoms of these disease states may be unmasked by the use of cannabinoids.
MARINOL should be used with caution in individuals receiving other psychoactive drugs.
Information for Patients: Persons taking MARINOL should be alerted to the additive central nervous system depression resulting from simultaneous use of MARINOL and alcohol or barbiturates. This combination should be avoided. Operation of machinery or a motor vehicle should be avoided during MARINOL therapy. Patients using MARINOL should be made aware of possible changes in mood and other adverse behavioral effects of the drug so as to avoid panic in the event of such manifestations. Patients should remain under supervision of a responsible adult while using MARINOL.
Drug Interactions: The effects of MARINOL on blood ethanol levels are complex. During sub-chronic MARINOL administration (60 mg/day) for ten days, absorption of ethanol was delayed, resulting in lower and delayed peak blood alcohol levels. Metabolism of ethanol was increased in some subjects and decreased in others. The overall rate of ethanol disappearance was decreased by about ten percent.
Carcinogenesis, Mutagenesis, and Impairment of Fertility: Carcinogenicity studies have not been performed with MARINOL. Reproductive studies in mice (approximately 32–400 times the human dose) and rats (approximately 8–32 times the human dose) demonstrate that MARINOL causes a decrease in pregnancy rate. In a long-term rat study (77 days), oral administration of MARINOL at doses 3–17 times the human dose reduced ventral prostate, seminal vesicle and epididymal weights and caused a decrease in seminal fluid volume. Decreases in spermatogenesis, number of developing germ cells, and number of Leydig cells in the testis were also observed. However, sperm count, mating success and testosterone levels were not affected. The significance of these animal findings in humans is not known.
Pregnancy: Pregnancy Category B. Reproduction studies have been performed in mice, rats and rabbits at doses up to 400 times, 32 times, and 10 times the human dose, respectively, and have revealed no evidence of teratogenicity due to MARINOL. At these dose levels in mice and rats, which produced substantial reductions in maternal weight gain, MARINOL caused a decrease in the number of viable pups, an increase in fetal mortality and an increase in early resorptions. Such effects were dose dependent and less apparent at lower doses which produced less maternal toxicity. There are, however, no adequate and well-controlled studies in pregnant women. Because animal reproduction studies are not always predictive of human response, this drug should be used during pregnancy only if clearly needed.
Nursing Mothers: MARINOL is concentrated and secreted in human milk and is absorbed by the nursing baby. Because the effects on the infant of chronic exposure to MARINOL and its metabolites are unknown, nursing mothers should not use MARINOL.

ADVERSE REACTIONS

In controlled clinical trials, the most frequently reported adverse reactions involved the central nervous system. In decreasing order of frequency these events were drowsiness, dizziness, muddled thinking and brief impairment of coordination, sensory and perceptual functions. Easy laughing, elation and heightened awareness, often termed a "high", was observed in 24% of MARINOL patients.
The incidences listed in the following table are derived from comparative double-blind, crossover or parallel design trials in which patients received MARINOL, an active control drug (usually prochlorperazine) or placebo.
The figures cited cannot be used to predict precisely the incidence of untoward events in the course of usual medical practice where patient characteristics and other factors often differ from those obtained in the clinical trials. Furthermore, these figures should not be compared with those obtained in other clinical studies involving related drug products and placebo, as each group of drug trials are conducted under a different set of conditions.

FREQUENCY OF ADVERSE EFFECTS FROM CONTROLLED STUDIES

Body System/ Adverse Reaction	MARINOL (n=317) %	Control (n=263) %	Placebo (n=68) %
CENTRAL NERVOUS SYSTEM:			
Drowsiness	48	33	49
Dizziness	21	5	1
Anxiety	16	3	24
Muddled Thinking	12	1	1
Perceptual Difficulties	11	1	0
Coordination Impairment	9	2	10
Irritability/Weird Feeling	7	3	0
Depression	7	3	15
Weak, Sluggish	6	3	1
Headache	6	4	4
Hallucinations	5	0	0
Memory Lapse	5	1	0
Unsteadiness, Ataxia	4	1	0
Paranoia	2	0	0
Depersonalization	2	0	0
Disorientation, Confusion	1	0	2
AUTONOMIC NERVOUS SYSTEM:			
Dry Mouth	3	1	1
Paresthesia	3	0	1
Visual Distortions	3	0	0
CARDIOVASCULAR:			
Tachycardia	1	1	0
Postural Hypotension	1	0	0

In addition to the events enumerated above, the following have been reported at a frequency below one percent: CENTRAL NERVOUS SYSTEM: tinnitus, nightmares; AUTONOMIC NERVOUS SYSTEM: speech difficulty, facial flushing, perspiring; CARDIOVASCULAR: syncope; GASTROINTESTINAL: diarrhea, fecal incontinence; MUSCULOSKELETAL: muscular pains.

DRUG ABUSE AND DEPENDENCE

MARINOL is highly abusable and controlled as delta-9-tetrahydrocannabinol under Schedule II of the Controlled Substances Act. Prescriptions of MARINOL should be limited to the amount necessary for a single cycle of chemotherapy (i.e., a few days).
It is not known what proportion of individuals exposed chronically to MARINOL or other cannabinoids will develop either psychological or physical dependence. Long-term use of these compounds has been associated with disorders of motivation, judgment, and cognition. It is not clear, though, if this is a manifestation of the underlying personalities of chronic users of this class of drugs, or if cannabinoids are directly responsible for these effects. An abstinence syndrome has been reported following discontinuation of high doses of delta-9-THC (210 mg per day). The acute phase was characterized by psychic distress, insomnia, and signs of autonomic hyperactivity (sweating, rhinorrhea, loose stools, hiccoughs). A protracted abstinence phase may have occurred as subjects reported sleep disturbances for several weeks after delta-9-THC discontinuation.

OVERDOSAGE

Signs and symptoms of overdosage are an extension of the psychotomimetic and physiologic effects of MARINOL, and, therefore, the clinical picture of overdosage may vary widely from patient to patient. Overdosages may be considered to be of two types: those at therapeutic doses, and those at higher, non-therapeutic doses.

Overdosage at Prescribed Dosages

Overdosage may be considered to have occurred even at prescribed dosages if disturbing psychiatric symptoms have occurred. In these cases, the patient should be observed in a quiet environment and supportive measures, including reassurance, should be used. Subsequent doses should be held until the patient has returned to baseline; routine dosing may then be resumed if clinically indicated, though this should be at a lower dosage. In controlled clinical trials, all such disturbing reactions spontaneously disappeared within 24 hours without specific medical therapy.
Particular attention should be paid to the vital signs in these patients, as tachycardia and both hyper- and hypotension are common adverse reactions. These signs should be monitored and treated, if necessary, in the usual manner according to the judgment of the physician.

Overdosage at Multiples of Prescribed Dosages

No cases of overdosage in multiples of prescribed dosages were reported in the controlled clinical studies. Few deaths have been reported from the use of dronabinol in any of its many forms (e.g., hashish, marijuana, etc.). Two incidents of death following the ingestion of large overdoses of Indian Hemp have been reported, while one death resulting from smoking cannabis herb and/or resin has appeared. No estimate of actual dosages was provided in either case. However, from a case of severe coma due to cannabis in a young French soldier, who recovered with conventional supportive therapy (intubation, I.V. fluids), it has been estimated that the acute lethal intravenous dose of dronabinol would be on the order of 1000–2000 mg total dose. Although this is a crude extrapolation at best, it represents a five to ten-fold multiple of the maximum oral dose recommended for MARINOL in a twenty-four hour period.

DOSAGE AND ADMINISTRATION

MARINOL is best administered at an initial dose of 5 mg/M^2, given 1–3 hours prior to the administration of chemotherapy, then every 2–4 hours after chemotherapy is given, for a total of 4–6 doses/day. Should the 5 mg/M^2 dose prove to be ineffective, and in the absence of significant side effects, the dose may be escalated by 2.5 mg/M^2 increments to a maximum of 15 mg/M^2 per dose. Caution should be exercised, however, as the incidence of disturbing psychiatric symptoms increases significantly at this maximum dose.

HOW SUPPLIED

MARINOL CAPSULES (Dronabinol solution in soft gelatin capsules).
2.5 mg white capsules (Identified UM).
NDC 0054-2601-11: Bottles of 25 capsules.
5 mg dark brown capsules (Identifed UM)
NDC 0054-2602-11: Bottles of 25 capsules.
10 mg orange capsules (Identifed UM)
NDC 0054-2603-11: Bottles of 25 capsules.
MARINOL capsules should be preserved in a well sealed container, and stored in a cool place
MARINOL® is a registered trademark of Unimed, Inc.
DEA ORDER FORM REQUIRED.
Shown in Product Identification Section, page 426

METHADONE HYDROCHLORIDE ORAL SOLUTION USP

Ⓒ II ℞

(WARNING: May be habit forming)

CONDITIONS FOR DISTRIBUTION AND USE OF METHADONE PRODUCTS:
Code of Federal Regulations,
Title 21, Sec. 291.505

METHADONE PRODUCTS, WHEN USED FOR TREATMENT OF NARCOTIC ADDITION IN DETOXIFICATION OR MAINTENANCE PROGRAMS, SHALL BE DISPENSED ONLY BY APPROVED HOSPITAL PHARMACIES, APPROVED COMMUNITY PHARMACIES, AND MAINTENANCE PROGRAMS APPROVED BY THE FOOD AND DRUG ADMINISTRATION AND THE DESIGNATED STATE AUTHORITY.
APPROVED MAINTENANCE PROGRAMS SHALL DISPENSE AND USE METHADONE IN ORAL FORM ONLY AND ACCORDING TO THE TREATMENT REQUIREMENTS STIPULATED IN THE FEDERAL METHADONE REGULATIONS (21 CFR 291.505).
FAILURE TO ABIDE BY THE REQUIREMENTS IN THESE REGULATIONS MAY RESULT IN CRIMINAL PROSECUTION, SEIZURE OF THE DRUG SUPPLY, REVOCATION OF THE PROGRAM APPROVAL, AND INJUNCTION PRECLUDING OPERATION OF THE PROGRAM.
A METHADONE PRODUCT, WHEN USED AS AN ANALGESIC, MAY BE DISPENSED IN ANY LICENSED PHARMACY.

DESCRIPTION

Each 5 ml of Methadone Hydrochloride Oral Solution contains:
Methadone Hydrochloride .... 5 mg or 10 mg
(Warning: May be habit forming)
Alcohol 8%
Chemically, Methadone Hydrochloride is 3-Heptanone, 6-(dimethylamino)-4,4-diphenyl-, hydrochloride, which can be represented by the following structural formula:

CH_2CH_3
CO CH_3
C—$CH_2CHN(CH_3)_2 \cdot HCl$

Methadone Hydrochloride acts as a narcotic analgesic.

CLINICAL PHARMACOLOGY

Methadone Hydrochloride is a synthetic narcotic analgesic with multiple actions quantitatively similar to those of morphine, the most prominent of which involve the central nervous system and organs composed of smooth muscle. The principal actions of therapeutic value are analgesia and sedation and detoxification or temporary maintenance in narcotic addiction. The methadone abstinence syndrome, although qualitatively similar to that of morphine, differs in

Continued on next page

Roxane—Cont.

that the onset is slower, the course is more prolonged, and the symptoms are less severe.
When administered orally, methadone is approximately one-half as potent as when given parenterally. Oral administration results in a delay of the onset, a lowering of the peak, and an increase in the duration of analgesic effect.

INDICATIONS AND USAGE

Methadone Hydrochloride is indicated for relief of severe pain, for detoxification treatment of narcotic addiction, and for temporary maintenance treatment of narcotic addiction.

Note

If methadone is administered for treatment of heroin dependence for more than three weeks, the procedure passes from treatment of the acute withdrawal syndrome (detoxification) to maintenance therapy. Maintenance treatment is permitted to be undertaken only by approved methadone programs. This does not preclude the maintenance treatment of an addict who is hospitalized for medical conditions other than addiction and who requires temporary maintenance during the critical period of his stay or whose enrollment has been verified in a program which has approval for maintenance treatment with methadone.

CONTRAINDICATIONS

Hypersensitivity to methadone.

WARNINGS

Methadone Hydrochloride, a narcotic, is a Schedule II controlled substance under the Federal Controlled Substances Act.
DRUG DEPENDENCE — METHADONE CAN PRODUCE DRUG DEPENDENCE OF THE MORPHINE TYPE AND, THEREFORE, HAS THE POTENTIAL FOR BEING ABUSED. PSYCHIC DEPENDENCE, PHYSICAL DEPENDENCE, AND TOLERANCE MAY DEVELOP UPON REPEATED ADMINISTRATION OF METHADONE, AND IT SHOULD BE PRESCRIBED AND ADMINISTERED WITH THE SAME DEGREE OF CAUTION APPROPRIATE TO THE USE OF MORPHINE.
Interaction with Other Central-Nervous-System Depressants —Methadone should be used with caution and in reduced dosage in patients who are concurrently receiving other narcotic analgesics, general anesthetics, phenothiazines, other tranquilizers, sedative-hypnotics, tricyclic antidepressants, and other C.N.S. depressants (including alcohol). Respiratory depression, hypotension, and profound sedation or coma may result.
Anxiety —Since methadone, as used by tolerant subjects at a constant maintenance dosage, is not a tranquilizer, patients who are maintained on this drug will react to life problems and stresses with the same symptoms of anxiety as do other individuals. The physician should not confuse such symptoms with those of narcotic abstinence and should not attempt to treat anxiety by increasing the dosage of methadone. The action of methadone in maintenance treatment is limited to the control of narcotic symptoms and is ineffective for relief of general anxiety.
Head Injury and Increased Intracranial Pressure —The respiratory depressant effects of methadone and its capacity to elevate cerebrospinal-fluid pressure may be markedly exaggerated in the presence of increased intracranial pressure. Furthermore, narcotics produce side effects that may obscure the clinical course of patients with head injuries. In such patients, methadone must be used with caution and only if it is deemed essential.
Asthma and Other Respiratory Conditions — Methadone should be used with caution in patients having an acute asthmatic attack, in those with chronic obstructive pulmonary disease or cor pulmonale, and in individuals with a substantially decreased respiratory reserve, preexisting respiratory depression, hypoxia, or hypercapnia. In such patients, even usual therapeutic doses of narcotics may decrease respiratory drive while simultaneously increasing airway resistance to the point of apnea.
Hypotensive Effect —The administration of methadone may result in severe hypotension in an individual whose ability to maintain his blood pressure has already been compromised by a depleted blood volume or concurrent administration of such drugs as the phenothiazines or certain anesthetics.
Use in Ambulatory Patients —Methadone may impair the mental and/or physical abilities required for the performance of potentially hazardous tasks, such as driving a car or operating machinery. The patient should be cautioned accordingly.
Methadone, like other narcotics, may produce orthostatic hypotension in ambulatory patients.
Use in Pregnancy —Safe use in pregnancy has not been established in relation to possible adverse effects on fetal development. Therefore, methadone should not be used in pregnant women unless, in the judgment of the physician, the potential benefits outweigh the possible hazards.
Methadone is not recommended for obstetric analgesia because its long duration of action increases the probability of respiratory depression in the newborn.
Use in Children —Methadone is not recommended for use as an analgesic in children, since documented clinical experience has been insufficient to establish a suitable dosage regimen for the pediatric age group.

PRECAUTIONS

***Interaction with Pentazocine* —Patients who are addicted to heroin or who are on the methadone maintenance program may experience withdrawal symptoms when given pentazocine.**
Interaction with Rifampin —The concurrent administration of rifampin may possibly reduce the blood concentration of methadone. The mechanism by which rifampin may decrease blood concentrations of methadone is not fully understood, although enhanced microsomal drug-metabolized enzymes may influence drug disposition.
Acute Abdominal Conditions —The administration of methadone or other narcotics may obscure the diagnosis or clinical course in patients with acute abdominal conditions.
Interaction with Monoamine Oxidase (MAO) Inhibitors — Therapeutic doses of meperidine have precipitated severe reactions in patients concurrently receiving monoamine oxidase inhibitors or those who have received such agents within 14 days. Similar reactions thus far have not been reported with methadone; but if the use of methadone is necessary in such patients, a sensitivity test should be performed in which repeated small incremental doses are administered over the course of several hours while the patient's condition and vital signs are under careful observation.
Special-Risk Patients —Methadone should be given with caution and the initial dose should be reduced in certain patients, such as the elderly or debilitated and those with severe impairment of hepatic or renal function, hypothyroidism, Addison's disease, prostatic hypertrophy, or urethral stricture.

ADVERSE REACTIONS

THE MAJOR HAZARDS OF METHADONE, AS OF OTHER NARCOTIC ANALGESICS, ARE RESPIRATORY DEPRESSION AND, TO A LESSER DEGREE, CIRCULATORY DEPRESSION. RESPIRATORY ARREST, SHOCK, AND CARDIAC ARREST HAVE OCCURRED.
The most frequently observed adverse reactions include lightheadedness, dizziness, sedation, nausea, vomiting, and sweating. These effects seem to be more prominent in ambulatory patients and in those who are not suffering severe chronic pain. In such individuals, lower doses are advisable. Some adverse reactions may be alleviated in the ambulatory patient if he lies down.
Other adverse reactions include the following:
Central Nervous System —Euphoria, dysphoria, weakness, headache, insomnia, agitation, disorientation, and visual disturbances.
Gastrointestinal —Dry mouth, anorexia, constipation, and biliary tract spasm.
Cardiovascular —Flushing of the face, bradycardia, palpitation, faintness, and syncope.
Genitourinary —Urinary retention or hesitancy, antidiuretic effect, and reduced libido and/or potency.
Allergic —Pruritus, urticaria, other skin rashes, edema, and, rarely, hemorrhagic urticaria.

ADMINISTRATION AND DOSAGE

For relief of Severe Pain —Dosage should be adjusted according to the severity of the pain and the response of the patient. Occasionally it may be necessary to exceed the usual dosage recommended in cases of exceptionally severe chronic pain or in those patients who have become tolerant to the analgesic effect of narcotics.
For severe acute pain, the usual adult dose is 2.5 mg to 10 mg every three to four hours as necessary.
For severe chronic pain, the usual adult dose is 5 mg to 20 mg every six to eight hours.
For Detoxification Treatment —THE DRUG SHALL BE ADMINISTERED DAILY UNDER CLOSE SUPERVISION AS FOLLOWS:
A detoxification treatment course shall not exceed 21 days and may not be repeated earlier than four weeks after completion of the preceding course.
The oral form of administration is preferred. However, if the patient is unable to ingest oral medication, he may be started on the parenteral form initially.
In detoxification, the patient may receive methadone when there are significant symptoms of withdrawal. The dosage schedules indicated below are recommended but could be varied in accordance with clinical judgment. Initially, a single dose of 15 to 20 mg of methadone will often be sufficient to suppress withdrawal symptoms. Additional methadone may be provided if withdrawal symptoms are not suppressed or if symptoms reappear. When patients are physically dependent on high doses, it may be necessary to exceed these levels. Forty mg per day in single or divided doses will usually constitute an adequate stabilizing dosage level. Stabilization can be continued for two to three days, and then the amount of methadone normally will be gradually decreased. The rate at which methadone is decreased will be determined separately for each patient. The dose of methadone can be decreased on a daily basis or at two-day intervals, but the amount of intake shall always be sufficient to keep withdrawal symptoms at a tolerable level. In hospitalized patients, a daily reduction of 20 percent of the total dose may be tolerated and may cause little discomfort. In ambulatory patients, a somewhat slower schedule may be needed. If methadone is administered for more than three weeks, the procedure is considered to have progressed from detoxification or treatment of the acute withdrawal syndrome to maintenance treatment, even though the goal and intent may be eventual total withdrawal.

OVERDOSAGE

Symptoms —Serious overdosage of methadone is characterized by respiratory depression (a decrease in respiratory rate and/or tidal volume, Cheyne-Stokes respiration, cyanosis), extreme somnolence progressing to stupor or coma, maximally constricted pupils, skeletal-muscle flaccidity, cold and clammy skin, and sometimes, bradycardia and hypotension. In severe overdosage, particularly by the intravenous route, apnea, circulatory collapse, cardiac arrest, and death may occur.
Treatment —Primary attention should be given to the reestablishment of adequate respiratory exchange through provision of a patent airway and institution of assisted or controlled ventilation. If a nontolerant person, especially a child, takes a large dose of methadone, effective narcotic antagonists are available to counteract the potentially lethal respiratory depression. **The physician must remember, however, that methadone is a long-acting depressant (36 to 48 hours), whereas the antagonists act for much shorter periods (one to three hours).** The patient must, therefore, be monitored continuously for recurrence of respiratory depression and treated repeatedly with the narcotic antagonist as needed. If the diagnosis is correct and respiratory depression is due only to overdosage of methadone, the use of other respiratory stimulants is not indicated.
An antagonist should not be administered in the absence of clinically significant respiratory or cardiovascular depression. Intravenously administered narcotic antagonists (naloxone, nalorphine, and levallorphan) are the drugs of choice to reverse signs of intoxication. These agents should be given repeatedly until the patient's status remains satisfactory. The hazard that the narcotic agent will further depress respiration is less likely with the use of naloxone.
Oxygen, intravenous fluids, vasopressors, and other supportive measures should be employed as indicated.

Note

IN AN INDIVIDUAL PHYSICALLY DEPENDENT ON NARCOTICS, THE ADMINISTRATION OF THE USUAL DOSE OF A NARCOTIC ANTAGONIST WILL PRECIPITATE AN ACUTE WITHDRAWAL SYNDROME. THE SEVERITY OF THIS SYNDROME WILL DEPEND ON THE DEGREE OF PHYSICAL DEPENDENCE AND THE DOSE OF THE ANTAGONIST ADMINISTERED. THE USE OF A NARCOTIC ANTAGONIST IN SUCH A PERSON SHOULD BE AVOIDED IF POSSIBLE. IF IT MUST BE USED TO TREAT SERIOUS RESPIRATORY DEPRESSION IN THE PHYSICALLY DEPENDENT PATIENT, THE ANTAGONIST SHOULD BE ADMINISTERED WITH EXTREME CARE AND BY TITRATION WITH SMALLER THAN USUAL DOSES OF THE ANTAGONIST.

HOW SUPPLIED

Methadone Hydrochloride Oral Solution USP
5 mg per 5 ml
NDC 0054-3555-63: Bottles of 500 ml.
10 mg per 5 ml
NDC 0054-3556-63: Bottles of 500 ml.
Methadone Hydrochloride Tablets USP
5 mg white, scored identified (54/210) tablets.
NDC 0054-4570-25: Bottle of 100 tablets.
NDC 0054-8553-24: Unit dose, 25 tablets per card (reverse numbered), 4 cards per shipper.
10 mg white, scored identified (54/142) tablets.
NDC 0054-4571-25: Bottle of 100 tablets.
NDC 0054-8554-24: Unit dose, 25 tablets per card (reverse numbered), 4 cards per shipper.
Control Pack, Unit Dose

MORPHINE SULFATE ORAL SOLUTION Ⓒ℞
(WARNING: May be habit forming.)
MORPHINE SULFATE TABLETS Ⓒ℞
(WARNING: May be habit forming.)

DESCRIPTION
Each 5 ml of Morphine Sulfate Oral Solution contains:
Morphine Sulfate .... 10 or 20 mg
(WARNING: May be habit forming.)
Alcohol 10%
Each tablet for oral administration contains:
Morphine Sulfate .... 15 or 30 mg
(WARNING: May be habit forming.)

HOW SUPPLIED
Morphine Sulfate Oral Solution
(Unflavored).
10 mg per 5 ml.
NDC 0054-8585-04: Unit dose Patient Cup™ filled to deliver 5 ml (10 mg Morphine Sulfate), ten 5 ml Patient Cups™ per shelf pack, ten shelf packs per shipper.
NDC 0054-8586-04: Unit dose Patient Cup™ filled to deliver 10 ml (20 mg Morphine Sulfate), ten 10 ml Patient Cups™ per shelf pack, ten shelf packs per shipper.
NDC 0054-3785-49: 100 ml "Unit of use" calibrated bottle.
NDC 0054-3785-63: Bottles of 500 ml.
20 mg per 5 ml.
NDC 0054-3786-49: 100 ml "Unit of Use" calibrated bottle.
NDC 0054-3786-63: Bottles of 500 ml.
Tablets
15 mg white scored, identified (54/733) tablets.
NDC 0054-8582-24: Unit dose, 25 tablets per card (reverse numbered), 4 cards per shipper.
NDC 0054-4582-25: Bottles of 100 tablets.
30 mg white scored, identified (54/262) tablets.
NDC 0054-8583-24: Unit dose, 25 tablets per card (reverse numbered), 4 cards per shipper.
NDC 0054-4583-25: Bottles of 100 Tablets.
DEA Order Form Required

POTASSIUM CHLORIDE ORAL SOLUTION USP, and POTASSIUM CHLORIDE POWDER USP ℞

DESCRIPTION
Potassium Chloride Oral Solution: 10 or 20%:
Each 30 ml 10% solution contains potassium 40 mEq and chloride 40 mEq
Each 30 ml 20% solution contains potassium 80 mEq and chloride 80 mEq
The 10% solution is cocoanut flavored, and the 20% solution is grapefruit flavored. Alcohol 5%.
Potassium Chloride Powder, 1.5 g packet (for oral solution). Potassium Chloride is chemically KCl. Potassium Chloride is an electrolyte replenisher.

HOW SUPPLIED
POTASSIUM CHLORIDE ORAL SOLUTIION USP, 10%
15 mEq of potassium per 11.25 ml
NDC 0054-8711-04: Unit dose Patient Cups™ filled to deliver 11.25 ml, ten 11.25 ml Patient Cups™ per shelf pack, ten shelf packs per shipper.
20 mEq of potassium per 15 ml
NDC 0054-8714-04: Unit dose Patient Cups™ filled to deliver 15ml, ten 15ml patient Cups™ per shelf pack, ten shelf packs per shipper.
30 mEq of potassium per 22.5 ml
NDC 0054-8712-04: Unit dose Patient Cups™ filled to deliver 22.5 ml, ten 22.5 ml Patient Cups™ per shelf pack, ten shelf packs per shipper.
40 mEq potassium pr 30 ml
NDC 0054-8713-04: Unit dose Patient Cups™ filled to deliver 30ml, ten 30ml Patient Cups™ per shelf pack, ten shelf packs per shipper.
NDC 0054-3716-54: Bottles of 180 ml.
NDC 0054-3716-63: Bottles of 500 ml.
NDC 0054-3716-68: Bottles of 1 liter.
NDC 0054-3716-75: Bottles of 5 liter.
POTASSIUM CHLORIDE ORAL SOLUTION USP, 20%
80 mEq of potassium per 30 ml
NDC 0054-3714-54: Bottles of 180 ml.
NDC 0054-3714-63: Bottles of 500 ml.
NDC 0054-3714-68: Bottles of 1 liter.
NDC 0054-3714-75: Bottles of 5 liter.
POTASSIUM CHLORIDE POWDER USP
20 mEq of potassium per 1.5 g (unflavored)
NDC 0054-8490-13: Unit dose, 1.5 g packets, 30 packets per carton.
NDC 0054-8490-25: Unit dose, 1.5 g packets, 100 packets per carton.

PREDNISONE TABLETS USP ℞
1 mg, 2.5 mg, 5 mg, 10 mg, 20 mg, 25 mg, or 50 mg

HOW SUPPLIED
1 mg white, scored tablets.
NDC 0054-8739-25: Unit dose, 10 tablets per strip, 10 strips per shelf pack, ten shelf packs per shipper.
NDC 0054-4741-25: Bottles of 100 tablets.
NDC 0054-4741-31: Bottles of 1000 tablets.
2.5 mg white, scored tablets.
NDC 0054-8740-25: Unit dose, 10 tablets per strip, 10 strips per shelf pack, 10 shelf packs per shipper.
NDC 0054-4742-25: Bottles of 100 tablets.
NDC 0054-4742-31: Bottles of 1000 tablets.
5 mg white, scored tablets.
NDC 0054-8724-25: Unit dose, 10 tablets per strip, 10 strips per shelf pack, ten shelf packs per shipper.
NDC 0054-4728-25: Bottles of 100 tablets.
NDC 0054-4728-31: Bottles of 1000 tablets.
10 mg white, scored tablets.
NDC 0054-8725-25: Unit dose, 10 tablets per strip, 10 strips per shelf pack, 10 shelf packs per shipper.
NDC 0054-4730-25: Bottles of 100 tablets.
NDC 0054-4730-29: Bottles of 500 tablets.
20 mg white, scored tablets.
NDC 0054-8726-25: Unit dose, 10 tablets per strip, 10 strips per shelf pack, 10 shelf packs per shipper.
NDC 0054-4729-25: Bottles of 100 tablets.
NDC 0054-4729-29: Bottles of 500 tablets.
25 mg white, scored tablets.
NDC 0054-8747-25: Unit dose, 10 tablets per strip, 10 strips per shelf pack, 10 shelf packs per shipper.
NDC 0054-4747-25: Bottles of 100 tablets.
50 mg white, scored tablets.
NDC 0054-8729-25: Unit dose, 10 tablets per strip, 10 strips per shelf pack, 10 shelf packs per shipper.
NDC 0054-4733-25: Bottles of 100 tablets.

ROXANOL™ Ⓒ℞
[rok 'sĕ-nŭl]
Morphine Sulfate Immediate Release, Concentrated Oral Solution
20 mg per ml

(WARNING: May be habit forming.)
ROXANOL 100™
Morphine Sulfate Immediate Release, Concentrated Oral Solution
100 mg per 5 ml
(WARNING: May be be habit forming.)

DESCRIPTION
Each ml of Roxanol™ contains:
Morphine Sulfate .... 20 mg
(Warning: May be habit forming.)
Each 5 ml of Roxanol 100™ contains:
Morphine Sulfate .... 100 mg
(Warning: May be habit forming.)
Chemically, Morphine Sulfate is, Morphinan3,6-diol, 7,8-didehydro-4,5-epoxy-17-methyl-, (5α,6α)-, sulfate (2:1) (salt), pentahydrate, which can be represented by the following structural formula:

$[\ldots]_2 \cdot H_2SO_4 \cdot 5H_2O$

Morphine Sulfate acts as a narcotic analgesic.

CLINICAL PHARMACOLOGY
The major effects of morphine are on the central nervous system and the bowel. Opioids act as agonists, interacting with stereospecific and saturable binding sites or receptors in the brain and other tissues.
Morphine is about two-thirds absorbed from the gastrointestinal tract with the maximum analgesic effect occurring 60 minutes post administration.

INDICATIONS AND USAGE
Morphine is indicated for the relief of severe acute and severe chronic pain.

CONTRAINDICATIONS
Hypersensitivity to morphine; respiratory insufficiency or depression; severe CNS depression; attack of bronchial asthma; heart failure secondary to chronic lung disease; cardiac arrhythmias; increased intracranial or cerebrospinal pressure; head injuries; brain tumor; acute alcoholism; delirium tremens; convulsive disorders; after biliary tract surgery; suspected surgical abdomen; surgical anastomosis; concomitantly with MAO inhibitors or within 14 days of such treatment.

WARNINGS
Morphine can cause tolerance, psychological and physical dependence. Withdrawal will occur on abrupt discontinuation or administration of a narcotic antagonist.
Interaction with Other Central-Nervous-System Depressants—Morphine should be used with caution and in reduced dosage in patients who are concurrently receiving other narcotic analgesics, general anesthetics, phenothiazines, other tranquilizers, sedative-hypnotics, tricyclic antidepressants, and other CNS depressants (including alcohol). Respiratory depression, hypotension, and profound sedation or coma may result.

PRECAUTIONS
General:
Head Injury and Increased Intracranial Pressure—The respiratory depressant effects of morphine and its capacity to elevate cerebrospinal-fluid pressure may be markedly exaggerated in the presence of increased intracranial pressure. Furthermore, narcotics produce side effects that may obscure the clinical course of patients with head injuries. In such patients, morphine must be used with caution and only if it is deemed essential.
Asthma and Other Respiratory Conditions—Morphine should be used with caution in patients having an acute asthmatic attack, in those with chronic obstructive pulmonary disease or cor pulmonale, and in individuals with a substantially decreased respiratory reserve, preexisting respiratory depression, hypoxia, or hypercapnia. In such patients, even usual therapeutic doses of narcotics may decrease respiratory drive while simultaneously increasing airway resistance to the point of apnea.
Hypotensive Effect—The administration of morphine may result in severe hypotension in an individual whose ability to maintain his blood pressure has already been compromised by a depleted blood volume or concurrent administration of such drugs as the phenothiazines or certain anesthetics.
Special-Risk Patients—Morphine should be given with caution and the initial dose should be reduced in certain patients, such as the elderly or debilitated and those with severe impairment of hepatic or renal function, hypothyroidism, Addison's disease, prostatic hypertrophy, or urethral stricture.
Acute Abdominal Conditions—The administration of morphine or other narcotics may obscure the diagnosis or clinical course in patients with acute abdominal conditions.
Information for patients:
Use in Ambulatory Patients—Morphine may impair the mental and/or physical abilities required for the performance of potentially hazardous tasks, such as driving a car or operating machinery. The patient should be cautioned accordingly.
Morphine, like other narcotics, may produce orthostatic hypotension in ambulatory patients.
Patients should be cautioned about the combined effects of alcohol or other central nervous system depressants with morphine.
Drug interactions:
Generally, effects of morphine may be potentiated by alkalizing agents and antagonized by acidifying agents. Analgesic effect of morphine is potentiated by chlorpromazine and methocarbamol. CNS depressants such as anaesthetics, hypnotics, barbiturates, phenothiazines, chloral hydrate, glutethimide, sedatives, MAO inhibitors (including procarbazine hydrochloride), antihistamines, β-blockers (propranolol), alcohol, furazolidone and other narcotics may enhance the depressant effects of morphine.
Morphine may increase anticoagulant activity of coumarin and other anticoagulants.
Carcinogenicity/Mutagenicity:
Long-term studies to determine the carcinogenic and mutagenic potential of morphine are not available.
Pregnancy:
Teratogenic Effects—Pregnancy Category C: Animal production studies have not been conducted with morphine. It is also not known whether morphine can cause fetal harm when administered to a pregnant woman or can affect reproduction capacity. Morphine should be given to a pregnant woman only if clearly needed.
Labor and Delivery:
Morphine readily crosses the placental barrier and, if administered during labor, may lead to respiratory depression in the neonate.
Nursing Mothers:
Morphine has been detected in human milk. For this reason, caution should be exercised when morphine is administered to a nursing woman.

Continued on next page

Roxane—Cont.

Pediatric Usage:
Safety and effectiveness in children have not been established.

ADVERSE REACTIONS
THE MAJOR HAZARDS OF MORPHINE AS OF OTHER NARCOTIC ANALGESICS, ARE RESPIRATORY DEPRESSION AND, TO A LESSER DEGREE, CIRCULATORY DEPRESSION, RESPIRATORY ARREST, SHOCK, AND CARDIAC ARREST HAVE OCCURRED.
The most frequently observed adverse reactions include lightheadedness, dizziness, sedation, nausea, vomiting, and sweating. These effects seem to be more prominent in ambulatory patients and in those who are not suffering severe pain. In such individuals, lower doses are advisable. Some adverse reactions may be alleviated in the ambulatory patient if he lies down.
Other adverse reactions include the following:
Central Nervous System—Euphoria, dysphoria, weakness, headache, insomnia, agitation, disorientation, and visual disturbances.
Gastrointestinal—Dry mouth, anorexia, constipation, and biliary tract spasm.
Cardiovascular—Flushing of the face, bradycardia, palpitation, faintness, and syncope.
Genitourinary—Urinary retention or hesitancy, anti-diuretic effect, and reduced libido and/or potency.
Allergic—Pruritus, urticaria, other skin rashes, edema, and, rarely hemorrhagic urticaria.
Treatment of the most frequent adverse reactions:
Constipation—Ample intake of water or other liquids should be encouraged. Concommitant administration of a stool softener and a peristaltic stimulant with the narcotic analgesic can be an effective preventive measure for those patients in need of therapeutics. If elimination does not occur for two days, an enema should be administered to prevent impaction.
In the event diarrhea occurs, seepage around a fecal impaction is a possible cause to consider before antidiarrheal measures are employed.
Nausea and Vomiting—Phenothiazines and antihistamines can be effective treatments for nausea of the medullary and vestibular sources respectively. However, these drugs may potentiate the side effects of the narcotics or the antinauseant.
Drowsiness (sedation)—Once pain control is achieved, undesirable sedation can be minimized by titrating the dosage to a level that just maintains a tolerable pain or pain free state.

DRUG ABUSE AND DEPENDENCE
Morphine Sulfate, narcotic, is a Schedule II controlled substance under the Federal Controlled Substance Act. As with other narcotics, some patients may develop a physical and psychological dependence on morphine. They may increase dosage without consulting a physician and subsequently may develop a physical dependence on the drug. In such cases, abrupt discontinuance may precipitate typical withdrawal symptoms, including convulsions. Therefore the drug should be withdrawn gradually from any patient known to be taking excessive dosages over a long period of time.
In treating the terminally ill patient the benefit of pain relief may outweigh the possibility of drug dependence. ***The chance of drug dependence is substantially reduced when the patient is placed on scheduled narcotic programs instead of a "pain to relief-of-pain" cycle typical of a PRN regimen.***

OVERDOSAGE
Signs and Symptoms: Serious overdose with morphine is characterized by respiratory depression (a decrease in respiratory rate and/or tidal volume, Cheyne-Stokes respiration, cyanosis), extreme somnolence progressing to stupor or coma, skeletal muscle flaccidity, cold or clammy skin, and sometimes bradycardia and hypotension. In severe overdosage, apnea, circulatory collapse, cardiac arrest and death may occur.
Treatment: Primary attention should be given to the reestablishment of adequate respiratory exchange through provision of a patent airway and the institution of assisted or controlled ventilation. The narcotic antagonist naloxone is a specific antidote against respiratory depression which may result from overdosage or unusual sensitivity to narcotics, including morphine. Therefore, an appropriate dose of naloxone (usual initial adult dose: 0.4 mg) should be administered, preferably by the intravenous route and simultaneously with efforts at respiratory resuscitation. Since the duration of action of morphine may exceed that of the antagonist, the patient should be kept under continued surveillance and repeated doses of the antagonist should be administered as needed to maintain adequate respiration.
An antagonist should not be administered in the absence of clinically significant respiratory or cardiovascular depression.
Oxygen, intravenous fluids, vasopressors and other supportive measures should be employed as indicated.
Gastric emptying may be useful in removing unabsorbed drug.

DOSAGE AND ADMINISTRATION
ROXANOL™ and ROXANOL 100™—Usual Adult Oral Dose: 10 to 30 mg every 4 hours or as directed by physician. Dosage is a patient dependent variable, therefore increased dosage may be required to achieve adequate analgesia.
For control of chronic, agonizing pain in patients with certain terminal disease, this drug should be administered on a regularly scheduled basis, every 4 hours, at the lowest dosage level that will achieve adequate analgesia.
Note: Medication may suppress respiration in the elderly, the very ill, and those patients with respiratory problems, therefore lower doses may be required.
Morphine Dosage Reduction: During the first two to three days of effective pain relief, the patient may sleep for many hours. This can be misinterpreted as the effect of excessive analgesic dosing rather than the first sign of relief in a pain exhausted patient. The dose, therefore, should be maintained for at least three days before reduction, if respiratory activity and other vital signs are adequate.
Following successful relief of severe pain, periodic attempts to reduce the narcotic dose should be made. Smaller doses or complete discontinuation of the narcotic analgesic may become feasible due to a physiologic change or the improved mental state of the patient.

HOW SUPPLIED
Roxanol™
(Morphine Sulfate Immediate Release, Concentrated Oral Solution)
20 mg per ml
NDC 0054-3751-44: Bottle of 30 ml with calibrated dropper.
NDC 0054-3751-50: Bottle of 120 ml with calibrated dropper.
Roxanol 100™
(Morphine Sulfate Immediate Release, Concentrated Oral Solution)
100 mg per 5 ml
NDC 0054-3751-58: Bottle of 240 ml with calibrated patient spoon.
DEA Order Form Required

ROXANOL SR™ Ⓒ℞
[rok'sĕ-nŭl]
(MORPHINE SULFATE)

Sustained Release Tablets
(WARNING: May be habit forming.)

NOTE
THIS IS A SUSTAINED RELEASE DOSAGE FORM. TABLET MUST BE SWALLOWED WHOLE. DO NOT BREAK THE TABLET IN HALF. DO NOT CRUSH OR CHEW.
THE SUSTAINED RELEASE OF DRUG FROM THE DOSAGE FORM SHOULD BE TAKEN INTO CONSIDERATION IN EVENT OF ADVERSE REACTIONS OR OVERDOSAGE.

DESCRIPTION
Each tablet for oral administration contains:
Morphine Sulfate .... 30 mg
(WARNING: May be habit forming.)
In a tablet that provides for sustained release of the medication.

INDICATIONS AND USAGE
Morphine is indicated for the relief of severe chronic pain.

ADVERSE REACTIONS
NOTE: THE SUSTAINED RELEASE OF THE DRUG FROM THE DOSAGE FORM SHOULD BE TAKEN INTO CONSIDERATION IN THE EVENT OF OCCURRING ADVERSE REACTIONS.

DOSAGE AND ADMINISTRATION
ROXANOL SR™ Tablets—The usual starting dose for patients with severe chronic pain is 30 mg every 8 hours. Patients with terminal cancer may require higher doses for adequate relief. The dose and/or dosage interval should be adjusted according to the severity of pain, as well as the patient's underlying disease, age, and size.
Note: Medication may suppress respiration in the elderly, the very ill, and those patients with respiratory problems, therefore lower doses or longer dosing intervals may be required.
NOTE: TABLET MUST BE SWALLOWED WHOLE. DO NOT BREAK THE TABLET IN HALF. DO NOT CRUSH OR CHEW.

HOW SUPPLIED
ROXANOL SR™ (Morphine Sulfate)
Sustained Release Tablets
30 mg white tablets (Identified 54 090).
NDC 0054-8780-24: Unit dose, 25 tablets per card (reverse numbered), 4 cards per shipper.
NDC 0054-4780-19: Bottles of 50 tablets.
NDC 0054-4780-27: Bottles of 250 tablets.
Refer to Roxanol™ (morphine sulfate concentrated oral solution) 20 mg/ml for the complete text.
Shown in Product Identification Section, page 426

ROXICODONE Ⓒ℞
(oxycodone hydrochloride)
Tablets and Oral Solution

DESCRIPTION
Each tablet contains:
Oxycodone Hydrochloride .... 5 mg
(WARNING: May be habit forming)
Each 5 ml Oral Solution contains:
Oxycodone Hydrochloride .... 5 mg
(WARNING: May be habit forming)
Oxycodone is 14-hydroxydihydrocodeinone, a white odorless crystalline powder which is derived from the opium alkaloid, thebaine.

ACTIONS
The analgesic ingredient, oxycodone, is a semisynthetic narcotic with multiple actions qualitatively similar to those of morphine; the most prominent of these involve the central nervous system and organs composed of smooth muscle. The principal actions of therapeutic value of oxycodone are analgesia and sedation.
Oxycodone is similar to codeine and methadone in that it retains at least one half of its analgesic activity when administered orally.

INDICATIONS
For the relief of moderate to moderately severe pain.

CONTRAINDICATIONS
Hypersensitivity to oxycodone.

WARNINGS
Drug Dependence: Oxycodone can produce drug dependence of the morphine type, and therefore, has the potential for being abused. Psychic dependence, physical dependence and tolerance may develop upon repeated administration of this drug, and it should be prescribed and administered with the same degree of caution appropriate to the use of other oral narcotic-containing medications. Like other narcotic-containing medications, this drug is subject to the Federal Controlled Substances Act.
Usage in ambulatory patients: Oxycodone may impair the mental and/or physical abilities required for the performance of potentially hazardous tasks such as driving a car or operating machinery. The patient using this drug should be cautioned accordingly.
Interaction with other central nervous system depressants: Patients receiving other narcotic analgesics, general anesthetics, phenothiazines, other tranquilizers, sedative-hypnotics or other CNS depressants (including alcohol) concomitantly with oxycodone hydrochloride may exhibit an additive CNS depression. When such combined therapy is contemplated, the dose of one or both agents should be reduced.
Usage in pregnancy: Safe use in pregnancy has not been established relative to possible adverse effects on fetal development. Therefore, this drug should not be used in pregnant women unless, in the judgment of the physician, the potential benefits outweigh the possible hazards.
Usage in children: This drug should not be administered to children.

PRECAUTIONS
Head injury and increased intracranial Pressure: The respiratory depressant effects of narcotics and their capacity to elevate cerebrospinal fluid pressure may be markedly exaggerated in the presence of head injury, other intracranial lesions or a pre-existing increase in intracranial pressure. Furthermore, narcotics produce adverse reactions which may obscure the clinical course of patients with head injuries.
Acute abdominal conditions: The administration of this drug or other narcotics may obscure the diagnosis or clinical course in patients with acute abdominal conditions.
Special risk patients: This drug should be given with caution to certain patients such as the elderly, or debilitated, and those with severe impairment of hepatic or renal function, hypothyroidism, Addison's disease and prostatic hypertrophy or urethral stricture.

ADVERSE REACTIONS
The most frequently observed adverse reactions include light headedness, dizziness, sedation, nausea and vomiting. These effects seem to be more prominent in ambulatory than in

nonambulatory patients, and some of these adverse reactions may be alleviated if the patient lies down.
Other adverse reactions include euphoria, dysphoria, constipation, skin rash and pruritus.

DOSAGE AND ADMINISTRATION

Dosage should be adjusted to the severity of the pain and the response of the patient. It may occasionally be necessary to exceed the usual dosage recommended below in cases of more severe pain or in those patients who have become tolerant to the analgesic effects of narcotics. This drug is given orally. The usual adult dose is one 5 mg tablet or 5 ml every 6 hours as needed for pain.

DRUG INTERACTIONS

The CNS depressant effects of oxycodone hydrochloride may be additive with that of other CNS depressants. See WARNINGS.

MANAGEMENT OF OVERDOSAGE

Signs and Symptoms: Serious overdose of oxycodone hydrochloride is characterized by respiratory depression (a decrease in respiratory rate and/or tidal volume, Cheyne-Stokes respiration, cyanosis), extreme somnolence progessing to stupor or coma, skeletal muscle flaccidity, cold and clammy skin, and sometimes bradycardia and hypotension. In severe overdosage, apnea, circulatory collapse, cardiac arrest and death may occur.

Treatment: Primary attention should be given to the reestablishment of adequate respiratory exchange through provision of a patent airway and the institution of assisted or controlled ventilation. The narcotic antagonist naloxone is a specific antidote against respiratory depression which may result from overdosage or unusual sensitivity to narcotics, including oxycodone. Therefore, an appropriate dose of naloxone (usual initial adult dose: 0.4 mg) should be administered, preferably by the intravenous route, simultaneously with efforts at respiratory resuscitation. Since the duration of action of oxycodone may exceed that of the antagonist, the patient should be kept under continued surveillance and repeated doses of the antagonist should be administered as needed to maintain adequate respiration.
An antagonist should not be administered in the absence of clinically significant respiratory or cardiovascular depression.
Oxygen, intravenous fluids, vasopressors and other supportive measures should be employed as indicated.
Gastric emptying may be useful in removing unabsorbed drug.

HOW SUPPLIED

5 mg white scored tablets. (Identified 54/582).
NDC 0054-8657-24: Unit dose, 25 tablets per card (reverse numbered), 4 cards per shipper.
NDC 0054-4657-25: Bottles of 100 tablets.
5 mg per 5 ml oral solution.
NDC 0054-3682-63: Bottles of 500 ml.
DEA Order Form Required

SODIUM POLYSTYRENE SULFONATE SUSPENSION ℞

DESCRIPTION

Each 60 ml contains:
Sodium Polystyrene Sulfonate USP .... 15 g
Sorbitol Solution USP .... 21.5 ml
Alcohol 0.3%
The suspension is cherry-flavored and also contains propylene glycol USP, Veegum®, sodium saccharin USP, methylparaben NF, propylparaben NF, flavors, and purified water USP.
This concentration of resin gives a sodium content of 1.5 g (65 mEq) per 60 ml. It is a brown, slightly viscous suspension which has an exchange capacity of approximately 3 mEq of potassium per 4 ml (per gram of resin) of suspension in vitro. This product may be administered either orally or rectally.

ACTION

The action of this product is to partially release sodium ions from the resin, and replace them by potassium ions as the resin passes along the intestine or is retained in the colon after administration by enema. For the most part, this action occurs in the large intestine, which excretes potassium ions to a greater degree than does the small intestine. The efficiency of this process is limited and unpredictably variable. It commonly approximates the order of 33%, but the range is so large that definitive indices of electrolyte balance must be clearly monitored. Frequent serum potassium determinations, at least once every 24 hours, should be done in order to adjust the individual dosage. The action of this product can be accomplished by either oral administration or by retention enema.

INDICATION

Sodium Polystyrene Sulfonate suspension is indicated for treatment of hyperkalemia.

WARNINGS

Since the effective lowering of serum potassium with this product may take hours to days, treatment with this drug alone may be insufficient to rapidly correct severe hyperkalemia associated with states of rapid tissue breakdown (e.g., burns and renal failure) or hyperkalemia so marked as to constitute a medical emergency. Therefore, other definitive measures, including dialysis, should always be considered and may be imperative. Serious potassium deficiency can occur from Sodium Polystyrene Sulfonate therapy. The effect must be carefully controlled by frequent serum potassium determinations within each 24 hour period. Since intracellular potassium deficiency is not always reflected by serum potassium levels, the level at which treatment with this product should be discontinued must be determined individually for each patient. Important aids in making this determination are the patient's clinical condition and electrocardiogram. Early clinical signs of severe hypokalemia include a pattern of irritable confusion and delayed thought processes. Electrocardiographically, severe hypokalemia is often associated with a lengthened Q-T interval, widening, flattening, or inversion of the T wave, and prominant U waves. Also, cardiac arrhythmias may occur, such as premature atrial, nodal, and ventricular contractions, and supraventricular and ventricular tachycardias. The toxic effects of digitalis are likely to be exaggerated. Marked hypokalemia can also be manifested by severe muscle weakness, at times extending into frank paralysis.
Like all cation-exchange resins, Sodium Polystyrene Sulfonate is not totally selective (for potassium) in its actions, and small amounts of other cations such as magnesium and calcium can also be lost during treatment. Accordingly, patients receiving the product should be monitored for all applicable electrolyte disturbances. Systemic alkalosis has been reported after cation-exchange resins were administered orally in combination with nonabsorbable cation-donating antacids and laxatives such as magnesium hydroxide and aluminum carbonate. Magnesium hydroxide should not be administered with the product. One case of grand mal seizure has been reported in a patient with chronic hypocalemia of renal failure who was given Sodium Polystyrene Sulfonate with magnesium hydroxide as a laxative. Also, the simultaneous oral administration of the product with nonabsorbable cation-donating antacids and laxatives may reduce the resin's potassium exchange capacity.

PRECAUTIONS

Caution is advised when the product is administered to patients who cannot tolerate even a small increase in sodium loads (i.e., severe congestive heart failure, severe hypertension, or marked edema). In such instances compensatory restriction of sodium intake from other sources may be indicated.
If constipation occurs, patients should be treated with sorbital (from 10 to 20 ml of 70% syrup every 2 hours or as needed to produce 1 or 2 watery stools daily), a measure which also reduces any tendency to fecal impaction.

ADVERSE REACTIONS

The product may cause some degree of gastric irritation. Anorexia, nausea, vomiting, and constipation may occur especially if high doses are given. Also, hypokalemia, hypocalcemia, and significant sodium retention may occur. Occasionally diarrhea develops. Large doses in elderly individuals may cause fecal impaction (see Precautions). This effect may be obviated through usage of the resin in enemas as described under Dosage and Administration. Intestinal obstruction due to concretions of aluminum hydroxide, when used in combination with the product, has been reported.

DOSAGE AND ADMINISTRATION

Oral Administration
The recommended oral adult dose is 60 ml (4 tablespoonfuls) of suspension (15 g of resin) given one to four times a day. This should be accompanied by frequent serum potassium determinations.
A lower dose of the resin is recommended for children.
Rectal Administration
The suspension may be given as a retention enema, but due to less effective potassium exchange, it is recommended that 120 to 180 ml of suspension be used (30 to 45 g of resin). The suspension should be administered following a cleansing enema. The suspension is administered at body temperature.
120 ml enema bottle (retention enema)
Directions—the following steps should be performed for the proper rectal use of enema bottle.

1. Insert a proper tipped rubber tube catheter) into the rectum for a distance of about 20 cm, so that the catheter tip is well into the sigmoid colon.
2. Shake bottle well.
3. Remove safety shield from enema tip.
4. **Insert tip into outer opening of the catheter.**
5. Squeeze bottle to expel drug suepension.
6. Remove tip from bottle.

Proceed, as directed below, with cleansing enemas, insertion of proper rubber tubing, and retention of drug suspension.
The suspension should be administered following a cleansing enema. The suspension is administered at body temperature, into the sigmoid colon by the use of a tipped rubber tube and left in the colon for several hours, if possible. The hip may be elevated on pillows to prevent back leakage if necessary. The colon is then irrigated with a nonsodium containing solution at body temperature to remove the resin. The returns are drained through a Y-tube connection with as much as two quarts of flushing solution possibly needed.
The duration of treatment will depend on the determined serum potassium levels in the individual patient.
The product should not be heated, for to do so may alter the exchange properties of the resin.

HOW SUPPLIED

NDC 0054-8814-11: Unit dose bottle filled to deliver 60 ml, 10 bottles per shipper.
NDC 0054-8813-01: Unit dose enema bottle filled to contain 120 ml (for use in delivering the suspension rectally through appropriate tubing).
NDC 0054-3804-63: Bottle of 500 ml.

EDUCATIONAL MATERIAL

Booklets
"Cancer Pain Management—A Dialogue," Selections from Opioid Analgesics in the Management of Clinical Pain, free to Physicians and Pharmacists
"Oral Morphine in Advanced Cancer," Robert G. Twycross and Sylvia A. Lack, Practical guidelines on the considerations which must be taken into account when initiating oral morphine therapy, free to Physicians and Pharmacists

Russ Pharmaceuticals, Inc.
P.O. BOX 20507
BIRMINGHAM, AL 35216

LORTAB® LIQUID Ⓒ ℞
[lŏr'tab]

DESCRIPTION

Palatable tropical punch flavored, colored green. Each 15 ml contains:
Hydrocodone Bitartrate* .... 5 mg
*WARNING: May be habit forming
Acetaminophen .... 500 mg

HOW SUPPLIED

Bottles of one pint (NDC 50474-906-16).

LORTAB® 5 Tablets Ⓒ ℞
[lŏr'tab]

DESCRIPTION

Each scored white with blue specks tablet contains:
Hydrocodone Bitartrate* .... 5 mg
*WARNING: May be habit forming
Acetaminophen .... 500 mg

HOW SUPPLIED

Bottles of 100 tablets (NDC 50474-902-01), bottles of 500 tablets (NDC 50474-902-50) and in hospital unit dose package of 100 tablets (NDC 50474-902-60).
Shown in Product Identification Section, page 427

LORTAB® ASA Tablets Ⓒ ℞
[lŏr'tab ăsā]

DESCRIPTION

Each tablet contains:
Hydrocodone Bitartrate* .... 5 mg
*WARNING: May be habit forming
Aspirin .... 500 mg

HOW SUPPLIED

Bottles of 100 tablets (NDC 50474-500-01) and in hospital unit dose package of 100 tablets (NDC 50474-500-60).
Shown in Product Identification Section, page 427

Continued on next page

Russ—Cont.

PRECARE® FA Tablets ℞
[*prē-care*]

DESCRIPTION
Each tablet contains:

		% of U.S. RDA*
Vitamin A Acetate	8,000 I.U.	(100%)
Vitamin D	400 I.U.	(100%)
Vitamin C (Ascorbic Acid)	90 mg	(150%)
Folic Acid	1 mg	(125%)
Thiamine (as Thiamine Mononitrate—Vitamin B_1)	3 mg	(224%)
Riboflavin (Vitamin B_2)	3 mg	(150%)
Niacin (as Niacinamide)	20 mg	(100%)
Vitamin B_6 (as Pyridoxine Hydrochloride)	4 mg	(160%)
Vitamin B_{12} (Cyanocobalamin)	12 mcg	(150%)
Calcium (as Calcium Sulfate)	200 mg	(15%)
Iodine (as Potassium Iodide)	150 mcg	(100%)
Iron (as Ferrous Fumarate)	66 mg	(367%)
Magnesium (as Magnesium Oxide)	100 mg	(22%)
Copper (as Cupric Oxide)	2 mg	(100%)
Zinc (as Zinc Sulfate)	15 mg	(100%)

*For pregnant or lactating women.

HOW SUPPLIED
In bottles of 100 tablets (NDC 50474-071-01).

PROMIST® HD Liquid Ⓒ℞
[*prō-mist*]

DESCRIPTION
Each 5cc (one teaspoonful) contains:

Hydrocodone Bitartrate*	2.5 mg
*WARNING: May be habit forming	
Pseudoephedrine Hydrochloride	30 mg
Chlorpheniramine Maleate	2 mg
Alcohol	5%

HOW SUPPLIED
In bottles of one pint (50474-921-16).

PROMIST® LA Tablets ℞
[*prō-mist*]

DESCRIPTION
Each long acting tablet contains:

Pseudoephedrine HCl	120 mg
Guaifenesin	500 mg

HOW SUPPLIED
In bottles of 100 tablets (NDC 50474 -918-01).

Rydelle Laboratories, Inc.
Subsidiary of S. C. Johnson & Son, Inc.
1525 HOWE STREET
RACINE, WI 53403

FIBERALL™ Natural Flavor
[*fī'ber-al*]

DESCRIPTION
Fiberall is a bulk forming non-irritant laxative which contains no sugar. The active ingredient is refined hydrophilic mucilloid, a recognized dietary fiber, extracted from the seed husk of blond psyllium seed (Plantago ovata). The smooth gelatinous bulk formed by Fiberall encourages peristaltic activity and a more normal elimination of the bowel contents.
The recommended dose of one slightly rounded teaspoonful (5g) contains 3.4g of psyllium hydrophilic mucilloid, wheat bran, less than 10mg of sodium, less than 60mg of potassium, and provides less than 6 calories.

INDICATIONS
Fiberall is indicated for the management of chronic constipation, temporary constipation caused by illness or pregnancy, in irritable bowel syndrome, and for constipation related to duodenal ulcer or diverticulosis. Fiberall is also indicated for stool softening in patients with hemorrhoids after anorectal surgery.

ACTIONS
The homogenous, high fiber formula of Fiberall is readily dispersed in liquids and acts without irritants or stimulants in the gastrointestinal tract.

DOSAGE AND ADMINISTRATION
The recommended daily dosage for adults is one slightly rounded teaspoonful (5g) stirred into an 8 oz. glass of cool water or other liquid and taken orally one to three times daily according to the individual response. An additional glass of liquid is recommended and generally provides optimal response. Maximum benefits are usually obtained after two or three days of regular use of Fiberall.

CONTRAINDICATIONS
Fecal impaction or intestinal obstruction.

HOW SUPPLIED
Powder, in 5, 10, and 15 oz. containers.

FIBERALL™ Fiber Wafers OTC
[*fī'ber-al*]
Oatmeal Raisin and Fruit & Nut flavors

DESCRIPTION
Fiberall Fiber Wafers are a bulk forming non-irritant laxative. The active ingredient is refined hydrophilic mucilloid, a recognized dietary fiber extracted from the seed husk of blond psyllium seed (Plantago ovata). The smooth gelatinous bulk formed by Fiberall Fiber Wafers encourages peristaltic activity and a more normal elimination of the bowel contents.
The recommended dose of (1) Fiberall Fiber Wafer contains 3.4g of psyllium hydrophilic mucilloid in a good tasting wafer form which includes wheat bran, oats, sucrose and other ingredients. Oatmeal Raisin Fiberall Fiber Wafers contain approximately 117 calories and 42mg of sodium per serving. Fruit & Nut flavor Fiberall Fiber Wafers contain approximately 79 calories and 54mg of sodium per serving.

INDICATIONS
Fiberall Fiber Wafers are indicated for the management of chronic constipation, temporary constipation caused by illness or pregnancy, irritable bowel syndrome, and for constipation related to duodenal ulcer or diverticulosis. Fiberall Wafers are also indicated for stool softening in patients with hemorrhoids after anorectal surgery.

ACTIONS
The homogenous high fiber formula of Fiberall Fiber Wafers is readily eaten with 8 oz. of an additional beverage of the patient's choice. Fiberall Wafers act without irritants or stimulants in the gastrointestinal tract.

DOSAGE AND ADMINISTRATION
The recommended daily dosage for adults is one Fiberall Fiber Wafer with a full 8 oz. glass of water or other liquid taken one to three times daily according to the individual response. An additional glass of liquid is recommended and generally provides optimal response. Maximum benefits are usually obtained after two or three days of regular use of Fiberall Fiber Wafers.

CONTRAINDICATIONS
Fecal impaction or intestinal obstruction.

HOW SUPPLIED
Boxes containing 14 wafers.
3/4/85

FIBERALL™ Orange Flavor
[*fī'ber-al*]

DESCRIPTION
Fiberall is a bulk forming non-irritant laxative which contains no sugar. The active ingredient is refined hydrophilic mucilloid, a recognized dietary fiber, extracted from the seed husk of blond psyllium seed (Plantago ovata). The smooth gelatinous bulk formed by Fiberall encourages peristaltic activity and a more normal elimination of the lower bowel contents.
The recommended dose of one slightly rounded teaspoonful (5.9g) contains 3.4g of psyllium hydrophilic mucilloid, wheat bran, natural and artificial flavor, less than 40mg of saccharin, citric acid, yellow #6 Lake and beta-carotene (coloring agents) less than 10mg of sodium, less than 60mg of potassium, and provides less than 10 calories.

INDICATIONS
Fiberall is indicated for the management of chronic constipation, temporary constipation caused by illness or pregnancy, in irritable bowel syndrome, and for constipation related to duodenal ulcer or diverticulosis. Fiberall is also indicated for stool softening in patients with hemorrhoids after anorectal surgery.

ACTIONS
The homogenous, high fiber formula of Fiberall is readily dispersed in liquids and acts without irritants or stimulants in the gastrointestinal tract.

DOSAGE AND ADMINISTRATION
The recommended daily dosage for adults is one slightly rounded teaspoonful (5.9g) stirred into an 8 oz. glass of cool water or other liquid and taken orally one to three times daily according to the individual response. An additional glass of liquid is recommended and generally provides optimal response. Maximum benefits are usually obtained after two or three days of regular use of Fiberall.

CONTRAINDICATIONS
Fecal impaction or intestinal obstruction.

HOW SUPPLIED
Powder, in 5, 10, and 15 oz. containers.

EDUCATIONAL MATERIAL

Books-Booklets-Brochures
"The Importance of Fiber" pamphlet provides a brief explanation of fiber for patients. Available free to physicians and pharmacists.
Recipe Book
Fiberall's recipe book in full color provides 44 different recipes that can be used with Fiberall natural and orange powder to improve patient compliance. Available free to physicians and pharmacists.
Samples
Fiberall Powder single dose samples are available to physicians.
Fiberall Fiber Wafer samples are available in three dose sample packages.

Rystan Company, Inc.
47 CENTER STREET
P.O. BOX 214
LITTLE FALLS, NJ 07424-0214

CHLORESIUM®
[*klor-eez'ium*]
Ointment and Solution
Healing and Deodorizing Agent

COMPOSITION
Ointment: 0.5% water-soluble chlorophyll derivatives (Chlorophyllin Copper Complex (Rystan brand, 100% concentration) in a hydrophilic base. Solution: 0.2% chlorophyll derivatives (Chlorophyllin Copper Complex) in isotonic saline solution.

ACTIONS AND USES
To promote normal healing, relieve pain and inflammation and reduce malodors in wounds, burns, surface ulcers, cuts, abrasions and skin irritations.

ADMINISTRATION AND DOSAGE
Ointment: Apply generously and cover with gauze, linen or other appropriate dressing. Dressings preferably changed no more often than every 48 to 72 hours. Solution: Apply full strength as continuous wet dressing, or instill directly into sinus tracts, fistulae, deep ulcers or cavities. As a mouthwash, use half strength.

SIDE EFFECTS
CHLORESIUM Ointment and Solution are soothing and nontoxic. Sensitivity reactions are extremely rare, and only a few instances of slight itching or irritation have been reported.

HOW SUPPLIED
Ointment: 1 oz. (NDC 0263-5158-08 and -32) and 4 oz. tubes, 1 lb. jars (NDC 0263-5155-01 and -04, -16). Solution: 8 oz. and 32 oz. bottles.

DERIFIL® Tablets
[*der'ah-fil*]
Internal Deodorant

COMPOSITION
100 mg water-soluble chlorophyll derivatives (chlorophyllin copper complex, 100% by NNR Assay) per tablet.

ACTIONS AND USES

Oral tablet for the control of fecal and urinary odor associated with incontinence and ostomy conditions, body odors, and odor of surface lesions.

ADMINISTRATION AND DOSAGE

Adults and children 12 years of age and over: Oral dosage is one to two tablets daily. Children under 12 years of age: Consult a doctor. In ostomies, tablets may be either taken by mouth or placed in the appliance.

SIDE EFFECTS

No toxic effects have been reported from use of DERIFIL Tablets at the recommended dosage over long periods. A temporary mild laxative effect may be noted, and the fecal discharge is commonly stained dark green.

HOW SUPPLIED

Bottles of 30 (NDC 0263-5001-03), 100 (NDC 0263-5001-10), and 1000 tablets (NDC 0263-5001-11).

PANAFIL® Ointment ℞
[pan 'ah-fil]
PANAFIL®—WHITE Ointment ℞

DESCRIPTION

PANAFIL® Ointment is an enzymatic debriding-healing ointment which contains standardized papain 10%, urea U.S.P. 10% and water-soluble chlorophyll derivatives (chlorophyllin copper complex) 0.5% in a hydrophilic base. Inactive ingredients are: White Petrolatum, U.S.P.; Propylene Glycol, U.S.P.; Stearyl Alcohol, N.F.; Sorbitan Monostearate, N.F.; Polyoxyl 40 Stearate, N.F.; Boric Acid, N.F.; Sodium Borate, N.F.; Chlorobutanol (Anhydrous), N.F. as a preservative. PANAFIL-WHITE is identical except that the chlorophyll derivatives (Chlorophyllin Copper Complex) are omitted.

CLINICAL PHARMACOLOGY

Papain, the proteolytic enzyme derived from the fruit of carica papaya, is a potent digestant of nonviable protein matter, but is harmless to viable tissue. It has the unique advantage of being active over a wide pH range, 3 to 12. Despite its recognized value as a digestive agent, papain is relatively ineffective when used alone as a debriding agent, primarily because it requires the presence of activators or exert its digestive function.

Urea is combined with papain to provide two supplementary chemical actions: 1) to expose by solvent action the activators of papain (sulfhydryl groups) which are always present, but not necessarily accessible, in the nonviable tissue or debris of lesions, and 2) to denature the nonviable protein matter in lesions and thereby render it more susceptible to enzymatic digestion. In pharmacologic studies involving digestion of beef powder, Miller[1] showed that the combination of papain and urea produced twice as much digestion as papin alone.

Water-soluble chlorophyll derivatives (chlorophyllin copper complex) add healing action to the cleansing action of the proteolytic papain-urea combination. The basic wound-healing properties of chlorophyll derivatives (chlorophyllin copper complex) are promotion of healthy granulations, control of local inflammation and reduction of wound odors.[2] Specifically, chlorophyll derivatives (chlorophyllin copper complex) inhibit the hemagglutinating and inflammatory properties of protein degradation products in the wound, including the products of enzymatic digestion, thus providing an additional protective factor.[1,3] The incorporation of chlorophyll derivatives (chlorophyllin copper complex) in PANAFIL® Ointment permits its continuous use for as long as desired to help produce and then maintain a clean wound base and to promote healing.

INDICATIONS AND USES

Ointment is suggested for treatment of acute and chronic lesions such as varicose, diabetic and decubitus ulcers, burns, postoperative wounds, pilonidal cyst wounds, carbuncles and miscellaneous traumatic or infected wounds.

Ointment is applied continuously throughout treatment of these conditions (1) for enzymatic debridement of necrotic tissue and liquefaction of fibrinous, purulent debris, (2) to **keep** the wound clean, and simultaneously (3) to promote normal healing.

CONTRAINDICATIONS

None known.

PRECAUTIONS

See Dosage and Administration.
Not to be used in eyes.

ADVERSE REACTIONS

Ointment is generally well tolerated and nonirritating. A small percentage of patients may experience a transient "burning" sensation on application of the ointment. Occasionally, the profuse exudate resulting from enzymatic digestion may cause irritation. In such cases, more frequent changes of dressings until exudate diminishes will alleviate discomfort.

DOSAGE AND ADMINISTRATION

Apply Ointment directly to lesion and cover with gauze or linen dressing. When practicable, daily or twice daily changes of dressings are preferred. Longer intervals between redressings (two or three days) have proved satisfactory, and Ointment may be applied under pressure dressings. At each redressing, the lesion should be irrigated with isotonic saline solution or other mild cleansing solution (except hydrogen peroxide solution, which may inactivate the papain) to remove any accumulation of liquefied necrotic material.

NOTE

Papain may also be inactivated by the salts of heavy metals (lead, silver, mercury, etc.) Contact with medications containing these metals should be avoided.

HOW SUPPLIED

PANAFIL—1 oz. tubes, (NDC 0263-5145-01).
1 lb. jars, (NDC 0263-5145-16).
PANAFIL-WHITE—1 oz. tubes, (NDC-0263-5145-01)

REFERENCES

1. Miller, J.M.: The Interaction of Papain, Urea and Water-Soluble Chlorophyll in a Proteolytic Ointment for Infected Wounds, Surgery 43:939, 1958.
2. Smith, L.W.: The Present Status of Topical Chlorophyll Therapy, New York J. Med. 55:2041, 1955.
3. Barnard, R.D.: Elucidation of Chemically Defined Haptenes For Competitive Inhibition of Aggression Activity, Immunol 8:78, 1954.

PROPHYLLIN®
[pro-fil 'in]
Wet Dressing Powder and Ointment

COMPOSITION

Each 2.3 gm. powder packet (or teaspoonful of bulk powder) in 8 ounces of water makes a solution containing 1% sodium propionate and 0.0025% water-soluble chlorophyll derivatives (Chlorophyllin Copper Complex) (Rystan brand, 100% concentration). Ointment: 5% sodium propionate and 0.0125% chlorophyll derivatives (Chlorophyllin Copper Complex) in an emollient base.

ACTION AND USES

Antifungal, antibacterial, antipruritic, antiinflammatory. Solution is nonastringent, nonirritating (even around eyes). Useful in dermatophytosis, contact dermatoses, eczemas, vulvovaginitis, minor burns.

ADMINISTRATION AND DOSAGE

Use solution as wet dressing, soak, mouthwash or douche. Half-strength solution (one packet in 16 oz. water) may be preferred for footbath or in severe inflammation. Ointment: Apply liberally several times daily and on retiring.

HOW SUPPLIED

Powder: Cartons of 12 packets and in 4 oz. jars (NDC 0263-5182-12 and 04). Ointment: 1 oz. tubes (NDC 0263-5185-01).

Sandoz Pharmaceuticals Corp.
ROUTE 10
EAST HANOVER, NJ 07936

ASBRON G® ELIXIR and ℞
[az 'bron]
ASBRON G® INLAY-TABS®

The following prescribing information is based on official labeling in effect on June 1, 1986.

DESCRIPTION

Each ASBRON G INLAY-TAB and tablespoonful (15 ml) of ASBRON G Elixir contains: theophylline sodium glycinate 300 mg (equivalent to 150 mg theophylline), guaifenesin 100 mg. The elixir supplies the active ingredients in a solution containing 15% alcohol. ASBRON G contains a bronchodilator and an expectorant.

Theophylline sodium glycinate, a methylxanthine, is a white crystalline powder that is freely soluble in water, has a slight ammoniacal odor and a bitter taste. It is an equimolar mixture of theophylline sodium and glycine buffered by an additional mole of the essential amino acid, glycine.

The expectorant component is guaifenesin (formerly called glyceryl guaiacolate) which helps loosen and thus clear the bronchial passageways of bothersome, thickened mucus. Guaifenesin, 3-(o-methoxyphenoxy)-1,2-propanediol, occurs as a fine, white powder having a bitter, aromatic taste and a slight odor of guaiacol. The powder tends to become lumpy on storage. It is freely soluble in alcohol and soluble in water.

Asbron-G Elixir
Active Ingredients: Guaifenesin USP and Theophylline Sodium Glycinate USP
Inactive Ingredients: Alcohol, Benzoic Acid, Citric Acid, Yellow 10, Blue 1, Natural and Artificial Flavorings, Purified Water, Saccharin, Saccharin Sodium, Sodium Chloride, Sorbitol, Sucrose, Yellow 10

Asbron-G Inlay Tabs
Active Ingredients: Guaifenesin USP and Theophylline Sodium Glycinate USP
Inactive Ingredients: Blue 1, Calcium Stearate, Calcium Sulfate, Colloidal Silicon Dioxide, Starch, Stearic Acid, Sodium Starch Glycolate, Sucrose and Yellow 10

CLINICAL PHARMACOLOGY

Theophylline sodium glycinate is more stable in the presence of hydrochloric acid due to the buffering action of glycine with subsequent reduction of the chance of theophylline precipitation in the stomach. This and the high solubility of the product are suggested as the reasons why this product has better gastric tolerance than aminophylline.

Theophylline, the active ingredient of theophylline sodium glycinate, accounts for 50% of the weight of this compound.

Theophylline sodium glycinate is highly effective in relaxing the smooth muscle of the bronchioles and the pulmonary blood vessels, thus acting primarily as a bronchodilator, pulmonary vasodilator and smooth muscle relaxant. Like other xanthines, theophylline sodium glycinate is a coronary vasodilator, a diuretic, a cerebral, cardiac and skeletal muscle stimulant.

Theophylline acts by inhibiting phosphodiesterase which causes an increase in intracellular cyclic AMP. This action produces smooth muscle relaxation and inhibits the release of histamine and other bronchoconstricting mediators from mast cells.

In vitro, using human white blood cells, theophylline has been shown to react synergistically with beta agonists to increase intracellular cyclic AMP. More data is required to clearly establish if theophylline and the beta agonists are synergistic or additive in vivo.

Even after prolonged therapy, it has not been possible to demonstrate the development of tolerance to theophylline sodium glycinate.

The half-life of theophylline varies from individual to individual. Since effective bronchodilatation depends upon maintaining serum theophylline levels between 10-20 mg/dl (10-20 mcg/ml), the determination of serum theophylline can be of value.

The half-life of theophylline is prolonged in alcoholism, in patients with reduced hepatic or renal function, congestive heart failure and in patients receiving antibiotics such as triacetyloleandomycin, erythromycin, clindamycin and lincomycin. Fever can also prolong theophylline half-life.

Cigarette smoking (1-2 packs per day) enhances theophylline elimination. The half-life of theophylline is shortened with cigarette smoking. This effect is probably related to the induction of enzymes and requires between three months and two years to normalize after stopping tobacco usage.

By increasing respiratory tract fluid, guaifenesin reduces the viscosity of tenacious secretions and acts as an expectorant. The drug is effective in productive as well as nonproductive cough, but is of particular value in dry, nonproductive cough which tends to injure the mucous membranes of the air passages.

[See table below].

THEOPHYLLINE ELIMINATION CHARACTERISTICS

	Group	Theophylline Renal Clearance Rates	Half-Life Average
1.	Children	1.4 ml/kg/min	3.5 hours
2.	Adults with uncomplicated asthma	1.2 ml/kg/min	7 hours
3.	Older adults with chronic obstructive pulmonary disease	0.6 ml/kg/min	up to 24 hours
4.	Adults with chronic obstructive pulmonary disease and cor pulmonale or other causes of heart failure and liver pathology	0.6 ml/kg/min and less	may exceed 24 hours
5.	Young smokers	Not available	4.3 hours

Continued on next page

Sandoz—Cont.

INDICATIONS AND USAGE

For relief of acute bronchial asthma and for reversible bronchospasm associated with chronic bronchitis and emphysema.

CONTRAINDICATIONS

ASBRON G® INLAY-TABS® and ASBRON G® Elixir are contraindicated in individuals who have shown hypersensitivity to any of the components.

WARNINGS

There is an excellent correlation between high theophylline blood levels and the clinical manifestations of toxicity in (1) patients with lowered body plasma clearances (due to transient cardiac decomposition), (2) chronic obstructive lung disease or patients with liver dysfunction, (3) patients who are older than 55 years of age, particularly males.

There are often no early signs of theophylline toxicity such as nausea and restlessness which may appear in up to 50% of patients. Convulsions or ventricular arrhythmias may be the first signs of toxicity.

Excessive doses of theophylline sodium glycinate may be expected to be toxic and serum theophylline levels are recommended to monitor therapy. The incidence of toxicity increases significantly at levels greater than 20 mcg/ml. Many patients who have higher theophylline serum levels exhibit tachycardia. Theophylline products often worsen preexisting arrhythmias.

ASBRON G® INLAY-TABS®, ASBRON G® Elixir and other oral theophylline compounds should never be used to treat status asthma.

PRECAUTIONS

General: Theophylline should be used with caution in patients with severe cardiovascular disease, severe hypoxemia, hypertension, hyperthyroidism, acute myocardial injury, obstructive lung disease, liver disease, in the elderly and in neonates.

Great caution should be used in giving theophylline to patients in congestive heart failure. Such patients have markedly prolonged theophylline blood levels which have persisted for long periods after discontinuation of the drug.

Smokers have a shorter mean half-life of theophylline than nonsmokers and may require larger doses of theophylline.

Theophylline sodium glycinate should not be administered concurrently with other theophylline containing products.

Theophylline should be given with caution to patients with a history of peptic ulcer. Theophylline may act as a local irritant in the gastrointestinal tract.

Information for Patients: The importance of adherence to the prescribed dosage regimen should be stressed. Patients should be informed of symptoms associated with theophylline toxicity such as nausea and restlessness.

Laboratory Tests: There is great patient-to-patient variation in the serum half-life of theophylline. Therefore, when possible, serum theophylline levels should be measured to assist in titration of dosage.

Drug Interactions: The use of theophylline sodium glycinate with ephedrine and other sympathomimetic bronchodilators may result in a significant increase in side effects. [See table above right].

Drug	Effect
Aminophylline with Lithium Carbonate	Increased excretion of Lithium Carbonate
Aminophylline with Propranolol	Antagonism of Propranolol effect
Theophylline with Furosemide	Increased Diuresis
Theophylline with Hexamethonium	Decreased Hexamethonium-induced chronotropic effect
Theophylline with Reserpine	Reserpine-induced Tachycardia
Theophylline with Cimetidine	Increased theophylline blood levels
Theophylline with clindamycin, troleandomycin, erythromycin, lincomycin	Increased theophylline blood levels

Drug/Laboratory Test Interactions

Theophylline has been shown to increase the urinary excretion of catecholamines. The VMA test for catechols may be falsely elevated by guaifenesin. Theophylline may increase the apparent serum uric acid in certain manual or automated chemical procedures by being treated as if it were uric acid. Guaifenesin may increase renal clearance for urate and thereby lower the serum uric acid. It may also falsely elevate the level of urinary 5HIAA in certain serotonin metabolite chemical tests.

Carcinogenesis, Mutagenesis, Impairment of Fertility: No data are available on the long-term potential for carcinogenicity, mutagenicity or impairment of fertility in animals or humans.

Pregnancy: *Pregnancy Category C*—Animal reproduction studies have not been conducted with ASBRON-G. Safe use in pregnancy has not been established relative to possible adverse effects on fetal development. Therefore, theophylline should not be used in pregnant patients unless, in the judgment of the physician, the potential benefits outweigh possible hazards.

Nursing Mothers: It is not known whether this drug is excreted in human milk. Because many drugs are excreted in human milk, caution should be observed when ASBRON G® INLAY-TABS® or ASBRON-G® Elixir is administered to a nursing mother.

Pediatric Use: See Dosage and Administration Section for mg/kg dosage in pediatric patients.

ADVERSE REACTIONS

Included in this listing which follows are adverse reactions, some of which may have been reported with theophylline sodium glycinate. However, pharmacological similarities among the xanthine drugs require that each of the reactions be considered when theophylline is administered. The most consistent adverse reactions are usually due to overdosage of theophylline sodium glycinate and are:

1. Gastrointestinal: nausea, vomiting, epigastric pain, hematemesis, diarrhea.
2. Central Nervous System: headaches, irritability, restlessness, insomnia, reflex hyperexcitability, muscle twitching, clonic and tonic generalized convulsions.
3. Cardiovascular: palpitation, tachycardia, extrasystoles, flushing hypotension, circulatory failure, life-threatening ventricular arrhythmias.
4. Respiratory: tachypnea.
5. Renal: albuminuria, increased excretion of renal tubular cells and red blood cells; potentiation of diuresis.
6. Others: hyperglycemia and inappropriate ADH syndrome.

Overdosage (Management):

A. If potential oral overdose is established and seizure has not occurred: (1) induce vomiting and resort to gastric lavage if the patient fails to vomit within 20-30 minutes; (2) administer a cathartic (this is particularly important if sustained-release preparations have been taken) and activated charcoal after successful vomiting has been induced or adequate gastric lavage performed.

B. If patient is having a seizure: (1) establish an airway; (2) administer O_2; (3) treat the seizure with intravenous diazepam 0.1 to 0.3 mg/kg up to 10 mg; (4) monitor vital signs, maintain blood pressure and provide adequate hydration.

C. Postseizure Coma: (1) maintain airway and oxygenation; (2) if a result of oral medication, follow above recommendations to prevent absorption of drug, but tracheal intubation and lavage will have to be performed instead of inducing emesis, and the cathartic and charcoal will need to be introduced via a large bore gastric lavage tube; (3) continue to provide full supportive care and adequate hydration while waiting for drug to be metabolized. In general, the drug is metabolized sufficiently rapidly so as to not warrant consideration of dialysis.

DOSAGE AND ADMINISTRATION

Therapeutic serum levels associated with optimal likelihood for benefit and minimal risk of toxicity are between 10-20 mcg/ml. There is great variation from patient to patient in the dosage of theophylline needed to achieve a therapeutic blood level because of variable rates of elimination. Because of this and because of the relatively narrow therapeutic blood level range associated with optimal results, the monitoring of serum theophylline levels is highly recommended. (See Laboratory Tests)

Usual Dosage: Adults—1 or 2 tablets or tablespoonfuls (15-30 ml), 3 or 4 times daily. Children 6 to 12—2 or 3 teaspoonfuls (10-15 ml), 3 or 4 times daily. Children 3 to 6—1 to 1½ teaspoonfuls (5-7.5 ml), 3 or 4 times daily. Children 1 to 3—½ to 1 teaspoonful (2.5-5 ml), 3 or 4 times daily.

Dosage Titration:

A. FOR PATIENTS NOT CURRENTLY RECEIVING THEOPHYLLINE PRODUCTS:

[See table below left].

	Oral Loading Dose (Theophylline Sodium Glycinate)	Maintenance Dose For Next 12 Hours (Theophylline Sodium Glycinate)	Maintenance Dose Beyond 12 Hours (Theophylline Sodium Glycinate)
1. Infants	8 mg/kg *(4 mg/kg)	3-8 mg/kg q6h *(1.5-4.0 mg/kg q6h)	4-6 mg/kg q6h *(2-3 mg/kg q6h)**
2. Children 6 months to 9 years	12 mg/kg *(6 mg/kg)	8 mg/kg q4h *(4 mg/kg q4h)	8 mg/kg q6h *(4 mg/kg q6h)
3. Children age 9-16 and young adult Smokers	12 mg/kg *(6 mg/kg)	6 mg/kg q4h *(3 mg/kg q4h)	6 mg/kg q6h *(3 mg/kg q6h)
4. Otherwise healthy nonsmoking adults	12 mg/kg *(6 mg/kg)	6 mg/kg q6h *(3 mg/kg q6h)	6 mg/kg q8h *(3 mg/kg q8h)
5. Older patients and patients with cor pulmonale	12 mg/kg *(6 mg/kg)	4 mg/kg q6h *(2 mg/kg q6h)	4 mg/kg q8h *(2 mg/kg q8h)
6. Patients with congestive heart failure, liver failure	12 mg/kg *(6 mg/kg)	4 mg/kg q8h *(2 mg/kg q8h)	2-4 mg/kg q12h *(1-2 mg/kg q12h)

Equivalent theophylline dosage indicated in parenthesis and marked with an asterisk (*).

** PEDIATRICS, Vol. 55, No. 5, May 1975.

B. FOR PATIENTS CURRENTLY RECEIVING THEOPHYLLINE PRODUCTS: Determine, where possible, the time, amount, route of administration and form of the patient's last dose of theophylline.

The loading dose of theophylline will be based on the principle that each 0.5 mg/kg of theophylline administered as a loading dose will result in a 1 mcg/ml increase in serum theophylline concentration. Ideally, then, the loading dose should be deferred if a serum theophylline concentration can be rapidly obtained. If this is not possible, the clinician must exercise his judgment in selecting a dose based on the potential for benefit and risk. When there is sufficient respiratory distress to warrant a small risk, 2.5 mg/kg of theophylline is likely to increase the serum concentration when administered as a loading dose in rapidly absorbed form by only about 5 mcg/ml. If the patient is not already experiencing theophylline toxicity, this is unlikely to result in dangerous adverse effects.

Measurement of serum theophylline concentration during chronic therapy:

Blood for peak theophylline determinations should be obtained 1-2 hours after a dose of theophylline sodium glycinate. When determining theophylline serum concentrations in patients who have received chronic therapy, it is essential to establish that no doses were omitted in the 48 hours prior to the determination. Missed doses could result in recommendations of future doses that would cause serious toxicity due to overdosage.

DOSAGE ADJUSTMENT BASED ON SERUM THEOPHYLLINE MEASUREMENTS WHEN THESE INSTRUCTIONS HAVE NOT BEEN FOLLOWED MAY RESULT IN RECOMMENDATIONS THAT PRESENT RISK OF TOXICITY TO THE PATIENT.

PATIENTS SHOULD NEVER BE MAINTAINED ON A DOSAGE OF THEOPHYLLINE THAT IS NOT WELL TOLERATED. Patients experiencing toxic side effects should be instructed to skip the next regular dose and to resume theophylline therapy at a lower dosage when all side effects have disappeared.

Maximum Dose Without Measurement of Serum Concentration: Not to exceed the following: (WARNING: DO NOT ATTEMPT TO MAINTAIN ANY DOSAGE THAT IS NOT WELL TOLERATED.)

[See table on top next page].

Use ideal (lean) body weight for obese patients in computing dosage.

Dosage should always be calculated on the basis of ideal (lean) body weight when mg/kg doses are stated. Theophylline does not distribute into fatty tissues. NEVER ATTEMPT TO MAINTAIN A DOSAGE THAT IS NOT WELL TOLERATED BY THE PATIENT.

HOW SUPPLIED

ASBRON G® INLAY-TABS® (green, round, with white inlay) in bottles of 100. ASBRON G® Elixir (green) in pint bottles.

Company's Product Identification Mark(s): Tablets imprinted "Asbron G" on one side, "78-202" on the other.

[ASB-Z2 Issued October 1, 1985]

Shown in Product Identification Section, page 427

Age	Theophylline Sodium Glycinate	Equivalent Theophylline
Under 9 years	48 mg/kg/day	24 mg/kg/day
9-12 years	40 mg/kg/day	20 mg/kg/day
12-16 years	36 mg/kg/day	18/mg/kg/day
Over 16 years	26 mg/kg/day or 1800 mg/day (WHICHEVER IS LESS)	13 mg/kg/day or 900 mg/day (WHICHEVER IS LESS)

BELLADENAL® Tablets ℞
[bel-ad 'in-ol]
BELLADENAL-S® Tablets

The following prescribing information is based on official labeling in effect on July 15, 1986.

COMPOSITION

Each Belladenal® Tablet and Belladenal-S® Tablet contains 0.25 mg Bellafoline® (levorotatory alkaloids of belladonna, as malates), and 50 mg phenobarbital, USP. (Warning: May be habit forming.)

Belladenal Tablets
Active Ingredients: levorotatory alkaloids of belladonna and phenobarbital, USP
Inactive Ingredients: gelatin, lactose, malic acid, starch, stearic acid, and sucrose

Belladenal-S Tablets
Active Ingredients: levorotatory alkaloids of belladonna and phenobarbital, USP
Inactive Ingredients: colloidal silicon dioxide, FD&C Red #40, FD&C Yellow #1, FD&C Yellow #5, FD&C Yellow #6, gelatin, malic acid, polyvinyl acetate resins, lactose, stearic acid, and sucrose

PROPERTIES AND THERAPEUTICS

Superior antispasmodic/ anticholinergic. The natural levorotatory alkaloids of belladonna (Bellafoline) in Belladenal give the antispasmodic-anticholinergic action of belladonna with only minimal central side effects. One Belladenal Tablet or Belladenal-S Tablet has the antispasmodic-anticholinergic action of 27 minims of tincture belladonna. Both Belladenal Tablets and Belladenal-S Tablets are scored to permit dosage adjustments necessary for optimal control of symptoms.

Indications

Based on a review of this drug by the National Academy of Sciences—National Research Council and/or other information, FDA has classified the indications as follows:
"Possibly" effective: As adjunctive therapy in the treatment of peptic ulcer and in the treatment of the irritable bowel syndrome (irritable colon, spastic colon, mucous colitis) and acute enterocolitis.
Final classification of the less-than-effective indications requires further investigation.

CONTRAINDICATIONS

Glaucoma, elevated intraocular pressure, advanced hepatic or renal disease. Hypersensitivity to any of the components.

PRECAUTIONS

Due to presence of barbiturate, may be habit forming. Caution is advised in the elderly.
Belladenal-S® Tablets contain FD&C Yellow No. 5 (tartrazine) which may cause allergic-type reactions (including bronchial asthma) in certain susceptible individuals. Although the overall incidence of FD&C Yellow No. 5 (tartrazine) sensitivity in the general population is low, it is frequently seen in patients who also have aspirin hypersensitivity.

SIDE EFFECTS

Urinary retention, blurred vision, dry mouth, flushing or drowsiness may occur.

USUAL DOSAGE

Belladenal® Tablets— Adults: 2 to 4 tablets per day, in divided dose of ¼ to ½ tablet.* Children: ¼ to ½ tablet* one to four times daily, according to age.* Tablets are scored so that they can be divided easily.
Belladenal-S Tablets—Adults: One tablet in the morning and one at night.

HOW SUPPLIED

Belladenal Tablets (compressed, white, scored) in bottles of 100. Belladenal-S Tablets (compressed, scored tablets of tricolored pattern: salmon pink, emerald green and white) in bottles of 100.
Company's Product Identification Mark(s): Belladenal Tablets embossed 78-28 on one side and scored on reverse side. Belladenal-S Tablets embossed 78-27 on one side and scored on reverse side.

[BED-Z15 Issued July 15, 1986]
Shown in Product Identification Section, page 427

BELLERGAL-S® Tablets ℞
[bel 'er-gal]

The following prescribing information is based on official labeling in effect on October 15, 1986.

DESCRIPTION

Bellergal S-Tablets
Each BELLERGAL-S Tablet contains: phenobarbital, USP, (Warning: may be habit forming), 40 mg; ergotamine tartrate, USP, 0.6 mg; Bellafoline® (levorotatory alkaloids of belladonna) 0.2 mg.
Inactive Ingredients: Colloidal silicon dioxide, FD&C Blue #1, FD&C Red #40, FD&C Yellow #5, FD&C Yellow #6, gelatin, lactose, magnesium stearate, malic acid, polyvinyl acetate resins, stearic acid, sucrose and tartaric acid.

CLINICAL PHARMACOLOGY

Based on the concept that functional disorders frequently involve hyperactivity of both the sympathetic and parasympathetic nervous systems, the ingredients in BELLERGAL-S are combined to provide a balanced preparation designed to correct imbalance of the autonomic nervous system. The integrated action of BELLERGAL-S is effected through the combined administration of ergotamine and the levorotatory alkaloids of belladonna, specific inhibitors of the sympathetic and parasympathetic respectively, reinforced by the synergistic action of phenobarbital in dampening the cortical centers. It should be noted that on a weight basis the levorotatory alkaloids of belladonna have approximately twice the pharmacological effect as do the usual racemic mixtures.

INDICATIONS AND USAGE

BELLERGAL-S is employed in the management of disorders characterized by nervous tension and exaggerated autonomic response: *Menopausal disorders* with hot flushes, sweats, restlessness and insomnia. *Cardiovascular disorders* with palpitation, tachycardia, chest oppression and vasomotor disturbances. *Gastrointestinal disorders* with hypermotility, hypersecretion, "nervous stomach," and alternately diarrhea and constipation.
Interval treatment of *recurrent, throbbing headache.*

CONTRAINDICATIONS

Peripheral vascular disease, coronary heart disease, hypertension, impaired hepatic or renal function, sepsis, pregnancy, nursing mothers and glaucoma. The concomitant administration of ergotamine and dopamine should be avoided, due to the increased potential for ischemic vasoconstriction. Phenobarbital is contraindicated in patients with a history of manifest or latent porphyria. Phenobarbital is contraindicated in those patients in whom the drug produces restlessness and/or excitement. BELLERGAL-S is contraindicated in patients with a demonstrated hypersensitivity to any of the components.

WARNINGS

Total weekly dosage of ergotamine tartrate should not exceed 10 mg. (This dosage corresponds to 16 BELLERGAL-S Tablets). Due to presence of a barbituate, may be habit forming.

PRECAUTIONS

Even though the ergotamine tartrate content of this product is low and untoward effects have been rare and of minor significance, caution should be exercised if large or prolonged dosage is contemplated, and physicians should be alert to possible peripheral vascular complications in patients sensitive to ergot. Due to the presence of the anticholinergic agent, special caution should be excersised in the use of this drug in patients with bronchial asthma or obstructive uropathy.
BELLERGAL-S contains FD&C Yellow No. 5 (tartrazine) which may cause allergic-type reactions (including bronchial asthma) in certain susceptible individuals. Although the overall incidence of FD&C Yellow No. 5 (tartrazine) sensitivity in the general population is low, it is frequently seen in patients who also have aspirin hypersensitivity.
Information for patients: Patients on large or prolonged dosage should be asked to report numbness or tingling of extremities, claudication or other symptoms of peripheral vasoconstriction.
Drug Interactions:

1. *Oral Anticoagulants:* Phenobarbital may lower the plasma levels of dicumarol (name previously used: bishydroxycoumarin) and may cause a decrease in anticoagulant activity as measured by the prothrombin time. More frequent monitoring of prothrombin time responses is indicated whenever phenobarbital is initiated or discontinued, and the dosage of anticoagulants should be adjusted accordingly.
2. *CNS depressants:* Combined administration of phenobarbital and CNS depressants such as alcohol, tricyclic antidepressants, phenothiazines and narcotic analgesics may result in a potentiation of the depressant action.
3. *Beta adrenergic blocking agents:* Although proof is lacking, several reports in the literature suggest a possible interaction between ergot alkaloids and beta adrenergic blocking agents. This interaction may result in excessive vasoconstriction. Although many patients can apparently take propranolol and ergot alkaloids without ill effects, there is enough evidence of an interaction to dictate closer surveillance of patients so treated.
4. *Hepatic metabolism:* Through the mechanism of enzyme induction caused by phenobarbital, a number of substances have been shown to be metabolized at an increased rate. In these cases, clinical responses should be closely monitored and appropriate dosage adjustments made. Included are such substances as griseofulvin, quinidine, doxycycline and estrogen. Although the meaning of published reports regarding the effects of phenobarbital on estrogen metabolism are unclear at this time, if avoidance of pregnancy is critical, consideration should be given to alternative methods of contraception.
5. *Phenytoin, sodium valproate, valproic acid:* The effect of barbiturates on the metabolism of phenytoin appears to be variable. Some investigators report an accelerating effect, while others report no effect. Because the effect of barbiturates on the metabolism of phenytoin is not predictable, phenytoin and barbiturate blood levels should be monitored more frequently if these drugs are given concurrently. Sodium valproate and valproic acid appear to decrease barbiturate metabolism; therefore, barbiturate blood levels should be monitored and appropriate dosage adjustments made as indicated.
6. *Tricyclic antidepressants:* Due to the presence of levorotatory alkaloids of belladonna, concomitant administration of tricyclic antidepressants may result in additive anticholinergic effects.

Carcinogenesis: No data are available on the long-term potential for carcinogenicity in animals or humans.

Pregnancy: *Pregnancy Category X*—due to the potential uterotonic effects of the ergot alkaloids, the use of BELLERGAL-S® during pregnancy is contraindicated. See "Contraindications" section.

Nursing Mothers: A number of ergot alkaloids inhibit the secretion of prolactin. Therefore, BELLERGAL-S is contraindicated in nursing mothers. See "Contraindications" section.

Pediatric Use: Safety and effectiveness in children have not been established.

ADVERSE REACTIONS

Tingling and other paresthesias of the extremities, blurred vision, palpitations, dry mouth, decreased sweating, decreased gastrointestinal motility, urinary retention, tachycardia, flushing, drowsiness occur rarely.

DRUG ABUSE AND DEPENDENCE

Barbiturates may be habit-forming. Tolerance, psychological dependence, and physical dependence may occur especially following prolonged use of high doses. Daily administration in excess of 400 mg of pentobarbital or secobarbital for approximately 90 days is likely to produce some degree of physical dependence. By way of comparison, the phenobarbital component of BELLERGAL-S at the highest recommended daily dosage amounts to 80 mg.

OVERDOSAGE

Management of Overdosage: While severe symptoms of overdosage with BELLERGAL-S have not been reported, theoretically they could occur. It is imperative to note that overdosage symptoms with BELLERGAL-S may be attributable to any one or more of the three active ingredients. Which toxic manifestation might predominate in any individual case would be impossible to predict but one should be alert to the various possibilities. When anticholinergic/antispasmodic drugs are taken in sufficient overdose to produce such severe symptoms, prompt treatment should be instituted. Gastric lavage and other measures to limit intestinal absorption should be initiated without delay.
Cholinesterase inhibitors administered parenterally may be necessary for treatment of the serious manifestation of anticholinergic overdosage. Additionally, symptomatic therapy,

Continued on next page

Sandoz—Cont.

including oxygen, sedatives and control of hyperthermia may be necessary.
Acute barbiturate overdosage symptoms with BELLERGAL-S, while possible, have not been reported. While the usual procedures for handling barbiturate poisoning should be employed, keep in mind the possibility of anticholinergic overdosing effects.
Acute ergot overdosage symptoms with BELLERGAL-S, while possible, have not been reported. The usual procedures for handling ergot overdosage include the administration of a peripheral vasodilator to counteract the vasospasm.

DOSAGE AND ADMINISTRATION

One in the morning and one in the evening.

HOW SUPPLIED

Compressed tablets of tri-colored pattern: dark green, orange and light lemon yellow, in bottles of 100.
Company's Product Identification Mark(s):
BELLERGAL-S Tablets scored on one side, embossed "78-31" other side.

[BEG-Z13 Issued October 15, 1986]
Shown in Product Identification Section, page 427

CAFERGOT® ℞

[kaf'er-got]
(ergotamine tartrate and caffeine) tablets, USP
(ergotamine tartrate and caffeine) suppositories, USP
CAFERGOT® P-B
Tablets and Suppositories
FOR NON-NARCOTIC RELIEF OF ENTIRE MIGRAINE SYNDROME AND OTHER VASCULAR HEADACHES

The following prescribing information is based on official labeling in effect on June 1, 1986.

DESCRIPTION

CAFERGOT®—
Tablet:
ergotamine tartrate, USP .... 1 mg
caffeine, USP .... 100 mg
Inactive Ingredients: acacia, carnauba wax, lactose, methyl paraben, povidone, propyl paraben, sodium benzoate, sorbitol, starch, stearic acid, sucrose, synthetic black ferric oxide, synthetic red ferric oxide, synthetic yellow ferric oxide, talc, tartaric acid and titanium dioxide.
Suppository:
ergotamine tartrate, USP .... 2 mg
caffeine, USP .... 100 mg
Inactive Ingredients: tartaric acid, NF, and cocoa butter, NF
CAFERGOT® P-B—
Tablet:
ergotamine tartrate, USP .... 1 mg
caffeine, USP .... 100 mg
Bellafoline® (levorotatory alkaloids
of belladonna) .... 0.125 mg
pentobarbital sodium, USP .... 30 mg
Warning: May be habit forming.
Inactive Ingredients: acacia, carnauba wax, D&C Yellow #10, FD&C Blue #1, FD&C Yellow #6, lactose, malic acid, mixed parabens, povidone, sodium benzoate, starch, stearic acid, sucrose, talc, tartaric acid and titanium dioxide
Suppository:
ergotamine tartrate, USP .... 2 mg
caffeine, USP .... 100 mg
Bellafoline® (levorotatory alkaloids
of belladonna) .... 0.25 mg
pentobarbital, USP .... 60 mg
Warning: May be habit forming.
Inactive Ingredients: tartaric acid, NF, malic acid, NF, and cocoa butter, NF
Cafergot Suppositories and Cafergot P-B Suppositories are *sealed* in foil to afford protection from cocoa butter leakage. If an unavoidable period of exposure to heat softens the suppository, it should be chilled in ice-cold water to solidify it before removing the foil.

ACTIONS

Ergotamine is an alpha adrenergic blocking agent with a direct stimulating effect on the smooth muscle of peripheral and cranial blood vessels and produces depression of central vasomotor centers. The compound also has the properties of serotonin antagonism. In comparison to hydrogenated ergotamine, the adrenergic blocking actions are less pronounced and vasoconstrictive actions are greater.
Caffeine, also a cranial vasoconstrictor, is added to further enhance the vasoconstrictive effect without the necessity of increasing ergotamine dosage.
For individuals experiencing excessive nausea and vomiting during migraine attacks the further addition of the anticholinergic and antiemetic alkaloids of belladonna and pentobarbital for reduction of nervous tension has been provided.
Many migraine patients experience excessive nausea and vomiting during attacks, making it impossible for them to retain any oral medication. In such cases, therefore, the only practical means of medication is through the rectal route where medication may reach the cranial vessels directly, evading the splanchnic vasculature and the liver.

INDICATIONS

Cafergot
Indicated as therapy to abort or prevent vascular headache, e.g., migraine, migraine variants, or so-called "histaminic cephalalgia".
Cafergot P-B
Indicated as therapy to abort or prevent vascular headache complicated by tension and gastrointestinal disturbances.

CONTRAINDICATIONS

Peripheral vascular disease, coronary heart disease, hypertension, impaired hepatic or renal function, sepsis and pregnancy. Hypersensitivity to any of the components.

PRECAUTIONS

Although signs and symptoms of ergotism rarely develop even after long term intermittent use of the orally or rectally administered drugs, care should be exercised to remain within the limits of recommended dosage.

ADVERSE REACTIONS

Vasoconstrictive complications, at times of a serious nature, may occur. These include pulselessness, weakness, muscle pains and paresthesias of the extremities and precordial distress and pain. Although these effects occur most commonly with long-term therapy at relatively high doses, they have also been reported with short-term or normal doses. Other adverse effects include transient tachycardia or bradycardia, nausea, vomiting, localized edema and itching. Drowsiness may occur with Cafergot P-B.

DOSAGE AND ADMINISTRATION

Procedure: For the best results, dosage should start at the first sign of an attack. Adults: *Orally*—2 tablets at start of attack; 1 additional tablet every ½ hour, if needed for full relief (maximum 6 tablets per attack, 10 per week). *Rectally*—1 suppository at start of attack; second suppository after 1 hour, if needed for full relief (maximum 2 suppositories per attack, 5 per week).

MAXIMUM ADULT DOSAGE

Orally: Total dose for any one attack should not exceed 6 tablets.
Rectally: Two suppositories is the maximum dose for an individual attack.
Total weekly dosage should not exceed 10 tablets or 5 suppositories.
In carefully selected patients, with due consideration of maximum dosage recommendations, administration of the drug at bedtime may be an appropriate short-term preventive measure.

OVERDOSAGE

The toxic effects of an acute overdosage of Cafergot® (ergotamine tartrate and caffeine) are due primarily to the ergotamine component. The amount of caffeine is such that its toxic effects will be overshadowed by those of ergotamine. Symptoms include vomiting; numbness, tingling, pain and cyanosis of the extremities associated with diminished or absent peripheral pulses; hypertension or hypotension; drowsiness, stupor, coma, convulsions and shock. A case has been reported of reversible bilateral papillitis with ring scotomata in a patient who received five times the recommended daily adult dose over a period of 14 days.
Treatment consists of removal of the offending drug by induction of emesis, gastric lavage, and catharsis. Maintenance of adequate pulmonary ventilation, correction of hypotension, and control of convulsions are important considerations. Treatment of peripheral vasospasm should consist of warmth, but not heat, and protection of the ischemic limbs. Vasodilators may be used with benefit but caution must be exercised to avoid aggravating an already existent hypotension.

HOW SUPPLIED

Cafergot Tablets shell pink colored, sugar coated. Bottles of 250 and cartons of three SigPak® (dispensing unit) packages, each containing 30 tablets in individual blisters. Cafergot Suppositories (sealed in fuchsia-colored aluminum foil) in boxes of 12. Cafergot P-B Tablets bright green, sugar coated. Bottles of 250 and cartons of three SigPak® (dispensing unit) packages, each containing 30 tablets in individual blisters. Cafergot P-B Suppositories (sealed in blue aluminum foil) in boxes of 12.

Company's Product Identification Mark(s): Cafergot Tablets imprinted "CAFERGOT" on one side, triangle (S) other side.
Cafergot P-B Tablets imprinted "78-36" on one side, triangle (S) other side.
Cafergot Suppositories imprinted "triangle (S) CAFERGOT SUPPOSITORY 78-33 SANDOZ".
Cafergot P-B Suppositories imprinted "triangle (S) CAFERGOT P-B SUPPOSITORY 78-35 SANDOZ".

[CAF-Z22 Issued January 15, 1986]
Shown in Product Identification Section, page 427

CEDILANID® -D ℞

[sē-de-lan 'id]
(deslanoside) injection, USP

The following prescribing information is based on official labeling in effect on July 15, 1986.

DESCRIPTION

The cardiac (or digitalis) glycosides are a closely related group of drugs having in common specific and powerful effects on the myocardium. These drugs are found in a number of plants. The term "digitalis" is used to designate the whole group. Typically, the glycosides are composed of three portions, a steroid nucleus, a lactone ring, and a sugar (hence "glycosides").
Cedilanid-D (deslanoside) is provided as ampul solution containing the cardioactive glycoside, desacetyl lanatoside C. This agent is prepared by controlled alkaline hydrolysis of lanatoside C, a glycoside obtained from digitalis lanata.
Supplied in ampuls of 2 ml. Each 2 ml contains:
deslanoside, USP .... 0.4 mg
citric acid, USP, q.s. to .... pH 6.2±0.3
sodium phosphate, USP .... 10.6 mg
alcohol, USP .... 9.8% by vol.
glycerin, USP .... 15% by wt.
water for injection, USP, q.s. to 2 ml

ACTION

The digitalis glycosides have qualitatively the same therapeutic effect on the heart. They (1) increase the force of myocardial contraction, (2) increase the refractory period of the atrioventricular (A-V) node, and (3) to a lesser degree, affect the sinoatrial (S-A) node and conduction system via the parasympathetic and sympathetic nervous systems.
Cedilanid-D (deslanoside) has its onset of action in about 5 minutes after intravenous administration and reaches peak effect in 2-4 hours. Therapeutic action persists for 2 to 5 days.

INDICATIONS

1. "Congestive heart failure," all degrees, is the primary indication. The increased cardiac output results in diuresis and general amelioration of the disturbances characteristic of right (venous congestion, edema) and left (dyspnea, orthopnea, cardiac asthma) heart failure.
   Digitalis, generally, is most effective in "low output" failure and less effective in "high output" (bronchopulmonary insufficiency, infection, hyperthyroidism) heart failure.
   Digitalis should be continued after failure is abolished unless some known precipitating factor is corrected.
2. "Atrial fibrillation"—especially when the ventricular rate is elevated. Digitalis rapidly reduces ventricular rates and eliminates the pulse deficit. Palpitation, precordial distress or weakness are relieved and any concomitant congestive failure ameliorated.
   Digitalis is continued in doses necessary to maintain the desired ventricular rate and other clinical effects.
3. "Atrial flutter" digitalis slows the heart and regular sinus rhythm may appear. Frequently the flutter is converted to atrial fibrillation with a slow ventricular rate. Stopping digitalis at this point may be followed by restoration of sinus rhythm, especially if the flutter was of the paroxysmal type. It is preferable, however, to continue digitalis if failure ensues or if atrial flutter is a frequent occurrence.
4. "Paroxysmal atrial tachycardia" digitalis may be used, especially if it is resistant to lesser measures. Depending on the urgency, a more rapid acting parenteral preparation may be preferable to initiate digitalization, although if failure has ensued or paroxysms recur frequently, digitalis is maintained by oral administration.
   Digitalis is not indicated in sinus tachycardia or premature systoles in the absence of heart failure.

"Cardiogenic shock"—the value of digitalis is not established, but the drug is often employed, especially when the condition is accompanied by pulmonary edema. Digitalis seems to adversely affect shock due to infections.

CONTRAINDICATIONS

The presence of toxic effects (See "Overdosage") induced by any digitalis preparation is an absolute contraindication to all of the glycosides.
"Allergy," though rare, does occur. It may not extend to all preparations and another may be tried.
"Ventricular Fibrillation"
"Ventricular tachycardia," unless congestive failure supervenes after a protracted episode not itself due to digitalis.

WARNINGS

Many of the arrhythmias for which digitalis is advised are identical with those reflecting digitalis intoxication. If the possibility of digitalis intoxication cannot be excluded, car-

diac glycosides should be temporarily withheld if permitted by the clinical situation.
The patient with congestive heart failure may complain of nausea and vomiting. These symptoms may also be indications of digitalis intoxication. A clinical determination of the cause of these symptoms must be attempted before further drug administration.

PRECAUTIONS

"Potassium depletion" sensitizes the myocardium to digitalis and toxicity is apt to develop even with usual dosage. Hypokalemia also tends to reduce the positive inotropic effect of digitalis.
Potassium wastage may result from diuretic, corticosteroid, hemodialysis and other therapy. It is apt to accompany malnutrition, old age and long - standing congestive heart failure.
"Acute myocardial infarction," severe pulmonary disease, or far advanced heart failure are apt to be more sensitive to digitalis and more prone to disturbances of rhythm.
"Calcium" affects contractility and excitability of the heart in a manner similar to that of digitalis. Calcium may produce serious arrhythmias in digitalized patients.
"Myxedema"—Digitalis requirements are less because excretion rate is decreased and blood levels are significantly higher.
"Incomplete AV block," especially patients subject to Stokes Adams attacks, may develop advanced or complete heart block. Heart failure in these patients can usually be controlled by other measures and by increasing the heart rate.
"Chronic constrictive pericarditis," is apt to respond unfavorably.
"Idiopathic hypertrophic subaortic stenosis" must be managed extremely carefully. Unless cardiac failure is severe it is doubtful whether digitalis should be employed.
"Renal insufficiency" delays the excretion of digitalis and dosage must be adjusted accordingly in patients with renal disease.
NOTE: This applies also to potassium administration should it become necessary.
Electrical conversion of arrhythmias may require adjustment of digitalis dosage.

ADVERSE REACTIONS

Gynecomastia, uncommon.
Overdosage, Toxic Effects: "Gastrointestinal" anorexia, nausea, vomiting, diarrhea—are the most common early symptoms of overdosages in the adult.
Uncontrolled heart failure may also produce such symptoms.
"Central Nervous System"—headache, weakness, apathy, visual disturbances.
"Cardiac Disturbances"——
Arrhythmias —"ventricular premature beats" is the most common.
Paroxysmal and nonparoxysmal nodal rhythms, atrioventricular (inference) dissociation and paroxysmal atrial tachycardia (PAT) with block are also common arrhythmias due to digitalis overdosage.
Conduction Disturbances—excessive slowing of the pulse is a clinical sign of digitalis overdosage. Atrioventricular block of increasing degree, may proceed to complete heart block.
NOTE: The electrocardiogram is fundamental in determining the presence and nature of these toxic disturbances. Digitalis may also induce other changes (as of the ST segment), but these provide no measure of the degree of digitalization.
TREATMENT OF TOXIC ARRHYTHMIAS: Digitalis is discontinued until after all signs of toxicity are abolished. This may be all that is necessary if toxic manifestations are not severe and appear after the time for peak effect of the drug.
Potassium salts are commonly used. Potassium chloride in divided doses totaling 4 to 6 gm. for adults provided renal function is adequate.
When correction of the arrhythmia is urgent, potassium is administered intravenously in a solution of 5 percent dextrose in water, a total of 40-100 mEq. (40 mEq. per 500 ml.) at the rate of 40 mEq. per hour unless limited by pain due to local irritation.
Additional amounts may be given if the arrhythmia is uncontrolled and the potassium well tolerated.
Electrocardiographic monitoring is indicated to avoid potassium toxicity, e.g. peaking of T waves.
CAUTION: Potassium should not be used and may be dangerous for severe or complete heart block due to digitalis and not related to any tachycardia.
Chelating agents to bind calcium may also be used to counteract the arrhythmia effect of digitalis toxicity, hypokalemia and of elevated serum calcium which may also precipitate digitalis toxicity.
Four grams (0.8 percent solution) of the disodium salt of EDTA is dissolved in 500 ml of 5 percent dextrose in water (50 mg per ml) and administered over a period of 2 hours unless the arrhythmia is controlled before the infusion is completed.
A continuous electrocardiogram should be observed so that the infusion may be promptly stopped when the desired effect is achieved.
Other counteracting agents are: Quinidine, procainamide, and beta adrenergic blocking agents.

DOSAGE AND ADMINISTRATION

"Parenteral" administration should be used only when the drug cannot be taken orally, or rapid digitalization is very urgent.
Parenteral digitalization can be obtained within 12 hours by giving 8 ml (1.6 mg) *either intramuscularly* or *intravenously.* By the I.V. route the dose may be given as one injection or in portions of 4 ml each. By I.M. route, 4 ml portions are injected at each of 2 sites.
After parenteral digitalization with Cedilanid-D (deslanoside) maintenance therapy may be accomplished by starting administration of an oral preparation, within 12 hours.

HOW SUPPLIED

Ampuls, 2 ml size (2 ml contains 0.4 mg deslanoside, USP) Boxes of 20 ampuls.
Being chemically pure and of constant potency, deslanoside, USP is standardized by weight; the ampul solution of Cedilanid-D (deslanoside) contains in each 2 ml:

deslanoside, USP .... 0.4 mg
citric acid, USP q.s. to .... pH 6.2±0.3
sodium phosphate, USP .... 10.6 mg
alcohol, USP .... 9.8% by vol.
glycerin, USP .... 15% by wt.
water for injection, USP, q.s. to 2 ml

[CED-Z18 Issued July 15, 1986]

D.H.E. 45® Injection ℞
(dihydroergotamine mesylate) injection, USP

The following prescribing information is based on official labeling in effect on July 15, 1986.

DESCRIPTION

DHE-45® is hydrogenated ergotamine as the mesylate. It is a clear, colorless, stable ampul solution containing per ml:

dihydroergotamine
mesylate, USP .... 1 mg
methanesulfonic acid/sodium
hydroxide .... q.s. to pH 3.75±0.5
alcohol, USP .... 6.1% by vol.
glycerin, USP .... 15% by wt.
water for injection, USP, q.s. to .... 1 ml

ACTIONS

Dihydroergotamine is an alpha adrenergic blocking agent with a direct stimulating effect on the smooth muscle of peripheral and cranial blood vessels, and produces depression of central vasomotor centers. The compound also has the properties of serotonin antagonism. In comparison to ergotamine, the adrenergic blocking actions are more pronounced, the vasoconstrictive actions somewhat less pronounced, and there is reduced incidence and degree of nausea and vomiting.
Onset of action occurs in 15 to 30 minutes following intramuscular administration and persists for 3-4 hours.
Repeated dosage at 1 hour intervals up to 3 hours may be required to obtain maximal effect.

INDICATIONS

As therapy to abort or prevent vascular headache, e.g., migraine, migraine variants, or so-called "histaminic cephalalgia" when rapid control is desired or when other routes of administration are not feasible.

CONTRAINDICATIONS

Peripheral vascular disease, coronary heart disease, hypertension, impaired hepatic or renal function, sepsis and pregnancy. Hypersensitivity.

ADVERSE REACTIONS

Numbness and tingling of fingers and toes, muscle pains in the extremities, weakness in the legs, precordial distress and pain, transient tachycardia or bradycardia, nausea, vomiting, localized edema and itching.

DOSAGE AND ADMINISTRATION

For vascular headache, 1 ml intramuscularly at first warning sign of headache, repeated at 1 hour intervals to a total of 3 ml. Optimal results are obtained by titrating the dose for several headaches to find the minimal effective dose for each patient and this dose should then be employed at onset of subsequent attacks. Where more rapid effect is desired, the intravenous route may be employed to a maximum of 2 ml. Total weekly dosage should not exceed 6 ml.

OVERDOSAGE

Failure to observe the upper limits of repeated parenteral dosage may result in eventual onset of the peripheral toxic signs and symptoms of ergotism. Treatment includes discontinuance of the drug, warmth, vasodilators, and good nursing care to prevent tissue damage.

HOW SUPPLIED

As a clear, colorless and stable solution in ampuls containing:

dihydroergotamine
mesylate, USP .... 1 mg
methanesulfonic acid/sodium
hydroxide .... q.s. to pH 3.75±0.5
alcohol, USP .... 6.1% by vol.
glycerin, USP .... 15% by wt.
water for injection, USP, q.s. to .... 1 ml

Ampuls, 1 ml size—boxes of 20.
To assure constant potency, protect the ampuls from light and heat. In the event the ampul solution becomes discolored, it should not be used.

[D.H.E.-Z17 Issued July 15, 1986]

DIAPID® Nasal Spray ℞
[dī'a-pid"]
(lypressin)
nasal solution, USP

The following prescribing information is based on official labeling in effect on July 15, 1986.

DESCRIPTION

Diapid® (lypressin) Nasal Spray contains synthetic lysine-8-vasopressin with an activity of 50 USP Posterior Pituitary (Pressor) Units per ml (0.185 mg/ml). Lysine-8-vasopressin is a polypeptide and is one of the two known naturally occurring molecular forms of mammalian posterior pituitary antidiuretic hormone. This synthetic polypeptide is present as a protein-free substance in Diapid Nasal Spray. Unlike preparations of posterior pituitary antidiuretic hormone of animal origin, Diapid Nasal Spray is completely free of oxytocin and foreign proteins. The molecular formula of lysine-8-vasopressin is $C_{46}H_{65}N_{13}O_{12}S_2$.

ACTION

The principal pharmacologic action of lysine-8-vasopressin, the active ingredient of Diapid (lypressin) Nasal Spray, is similar to that of arginine-8-vasopressin, the posterior pituitary antidiuretic hormone occurring in man. Diapid Nasal Spray increases the rate of reabsorption of solute free water from the distal renal tubules, without significantly modifying the rate of glomerular filtration, producing a fall in free water clearance and an increase in urinary osmolality. The rates of solute and creatinine excretion noted with therapeutic doses of Diapid Nasal Spray suggest that sodium clearance and glomerular filtration rates are essentially unaltered by this hormone. Diapid Nasal Spray is relatively free of oxytocic activity when used within the recommended therapeutic dose levels.
It possesses little pressor activity, the ratio of pressor to antidiuretic activity being in the range of 1:1000.
The antidiuretic effect produced by Diapid Nasal Spray begins rapidly and usually reaches a peak within 30 to 120 minutes. Its usual duration of action is 3 to 8 hours.

INDICATIONS

Diapid Nasal Spray is indicated for the control or prevention of the symptoms and complications of diabetes insipidus due to deficiency of endogenous posterior pituitary antidiuretic hormone. These symptoms and complications include polydipsia, polyuria, and dehydration. It is particularly useful in patients with diabetes insipidus who have become unresponsive to other forms of therapy or who experience various types of local and/or systemic reactions, allergic reactions, or other undesirable effects (e.g., excessive fluid retention) from preparations of posterior pituitary antidiuretic hormone of animal origin.

CONTRAINDICATIONS

There are no known contraindications to the use of Diapid (lypressin) Nasal Spray.

WARNINGS

The safety of this drug in pregnancy has not been established. The possibility of risk to the mother and unborn child should be weighed against potential benefits before the drug is administered to women of child-bearing age.

PRECAUTIONS

Cardiovascular pressor effects with Diapid Nasal Spray are minimal or absent when it is administered as a nasal spray in therapeutic doses. Nevertheless, it should be used with caution in patients for whom such effects would not be desirable because mild blood pressure elevation has been noted in unanesthetized subjects who received lypressin intravenously. Large doses intranasally may cause coronary artery constriction and caution should be observed in treating patients with coronary artery disease.
The effectiveness of Diapid (lypressin) Nasal Spray may be lessened in patients with nasal congestion, allergic rhinitis, and upper respiratory infections because these conditions may interfere with absorption of the drug by the nasal mu-

Continued on next page

Sandoz—Cont.

cosa. In this event, larger doses of Diapid Nasal Spray, or adjunctive therapy, may be needed.
Patients with a known sensitivity to anti-diuretic hormone should be tested for sensitivity to Diapid Nasal Spray.

ADVERSE REACTIONS

With clinical use of Diapid (lypressin) Nasal Spray, adverse reactions have been infrequent and mild. To date, such reactions have included rhinorrhea, nasal congestion, irritation and pruritus of the nasal passages, nasal ulceration, headache, conjunctivitis, heartburn secondary to excessive nasal administration with drippage into the pharynx, and abdominal cramps and increased bowel movements. Periorbital edema with itching has been reported. Inadvertent inhalation of Diapid Nasal Spray has resulted in substernal tightness, coughing, and transient dyspnea. In one patient, an overdose of Diapid Nasal Spray caused marked, but transient, fluid retention. Tolerance or tachyphylaxis to Diapid Nasal Spray has not been reported to date.
Hypersensitivity manifested by a positive skin test.

DOSAGE AND ADMINISTRATION

Patients should be instructed to administer 1 or 2 sprays of Diapid® (lypressin) Nasal Spray to one or both nostrils whenever frequency of urination becomes increased or significant thirst develops. (One spray provides approximately 2 USP Posterior Pituitary [Pressor] Units.) The usual dosage for adults and children is 1 or 2 sprays in each nostril 4 times daily. An additional dose at bedtime is often helpful to eliminate nocturia, if it is not controlled with the regular daily dosage. For patients requiring more than 2 sprays per nostril every 4 to 6 hours, it is recommended that the time interval between doses be reduced rather than increasing the number of sprays at each dose. (More than 2 or 3 sprays in each nostril usually results in wastage because the unabsorbed excess will drain posteriorly, by way of the nasopharynx, into the digestive tract where it will be inactivated.)
Diapid Nasal Spray permits individualization of dosage necessary to control the symptoms of diabetes insipidus. Patients quickly learn to regulate their dosage in accordance with their degree of polyuria and thirst, and once determined, daily requirements remain fairly stable for months or years. Although most patients require 1 or 2 sprays of Diapid (lypressin) Nasal Spray in each nostril 4 times daily, dosage has ranged from 1 spray per day at bedtime to 10 sprays in each nostril every 3-4 hours. Requirements of the larger doses may represent greater severity of disease or other phenomena, such as poor nasal absorption. A seeming requirement for large doses of lypressin may be due to the presence of mixed hypothalamic-hypophyseal and nephrogenic diabetes insipidus, the latter condition being unresponsive to administration of antidiuretic hormone.
Diapid (lypressin) Nasal Spray is conveniently administered, from a compact and portable, plastic squeeze bottle, by inserting the nozzle of the bottle into the nostril and squeezing once firmly to deliver each short spray.
NOTE: To assure that a uniform, well-diffused spray is delivered, the bottle of Diapid Nasal Spray should be held upright and the patient should be in a vertical position with head upright.

SUPPLIED

Diapid Nasal Spray is supplied in a plastic bottle that contains 8 ml of solution. Each ml of solution contains lypressin (0.185 mg) equivalent to 50 USP Posterior Pituitary (Pressor) Units and the following: propylparaben, NF, methylparaben, NF, sodium phosphate, USP, citric acid, USP, sodium chloride, USP, sorbitol solution, USP, glycerin, USP, sodium acetate, USP, acetic acid, NF, chlorobutanol, NF, (0.1%-0.002%), purified water, USP.
This product has an expiration date of 36 months.
[DIA-Z13 Issued July 15, 1986]

EMBOLEX® ℞

[*em-bō 'lex*]
(dihydroergotamine mesylate and heparin sodium; with lidocaine HCl)
INJECTION

The following prescribing information is based on official labeling in effect on August 28, 1986.

DESCRIPTION

Embolex® (dihydroergotamine mesylate and heparin sodium; with lidocaine HCl) Injection is a sterile solution of DHE (dihydroergotamine mesylate) and heparin sodium, for administration by deep subcutaneous (intrafat) injection. DHE, known chemically as Ergotaman-3′,6′,18-trione, 9, 10-dihydro-12′-hydroxy-2′-methyl-5′-(phenylmethyl) -, (5′α)-,monomethanesulfonate, is an α-adrenergic blocking agent also possessing venoconstrictor properties.
The heparin sodium in Embolex (dihydroergotamine mesylate and heparin sodium; with lidocaine HCl) Injection is derived from porcine intestinal mucosa and is standardized for anticoagulant activity. Its potency is determined by a biological assay using a USP reference standard based on units of heparin activity per milligram.
Heparin is a heterogeneous group of straight-chain anionic mucopolysaccharides, called glycosaminoglycans, having anticoagulant properties. Although others may be present, the main sugars occurring in heparin are: (1) α-L-iduronic acid 2-sulfate, (2) 2-deoxy-2-sulfamino-α-D-glucose 6-sulfate, (3) β-D-glucuronic acid, (4) 2-acetamido-2-deoxy-α-D-glucose, and (5) α-L-iduronic acid. These sugars are present in decreasing amounts, usually in the order (2) > (1) > (4) > (3) > (5), and are joined by glycosidic linkages, forming polymers of varying sizes. Heparin is strongly acidic because of its content of covalently linked sulfate and carboxylic acid groups. In heparin sodium, the acidic protons of the sulfate units are partially replaced by sodium ions.
Embolex (dihydroergotamine mesylate and heparin sodium; with lidocaine HCl) Injection is available in ampuls for deep subcutaneous (intrafat) injection.
Each ampul contains 0.7 ml sterile solution consisting of:

dihydroergotamine mesylate, USP	0.5 mg
heparin sodium, USP	5000 USP units
lidocaine hydrochloride, USP	7.46 mg
edetate calcium disodium, USP	1.55 mg
glycerin, USP	32.2 mg
propylene glycol, USP	322 mg
water for injection, USP, qs ad	749.2 mg
methanesulfonic acid 10%, qs to	pH 5.75 ± .75

Lidocaine hydrochloride, USP (1.0% w/v) is added to each ampul to act as a local anaesthetic at the injection site against pain, burning, itching, or other local irritation (see ADVERSE REACTIONS).

CLINICAL PHARMACOLOGY

Pharmacodynamics: DHE is an α-adrenergic blocking agent with a direct stimulating effect on the smooth muscle of peripheral blood vessels. It also produces depression of central vasomotor centers and exhibits properties of serotonin antagonism. The primary pharmacological effect on the venous side of the circulation is a dose-dependent constriction of the capacitance vessels with little effect on precapillary sphincter tone and only a small and variable effect on arterial resistance. Its thromboprophylactic effect is based upon the principle of accelerated venous return and thus inhibition of, or reduction in, venostasis.
Heparin inhibits reactions that lead to the clotting of blood and the formation of fibrin clots both *in vitro* and *in vivo* by acting at multiple sites in the normal coagulation system. Small amounts of heparin in combination with antithrombin III (heparin cofactor) can inhibit thrombosis by inactivating activated Factor X and inhibiting the conversion of prothrombin to thrombin. Once active thrombosis has developed, larger amounts of heparin can inhibit further coagulation by inactivating thrombin and preventing the conversion of fibrinogen to fibrin. Heparin also prevents the formation of a stable fibrin clot by inhibiting the activation of the fibrin stabilizing factor.
Bleeding time is usually unaffected by heparin. Clotting time, while prolonged by full therapeutic doses of heparin, is not measurably affected by low doses of heparin in most cases.
Heparin does not have fibrinolytic activity; therefore, it will not lyse existing clots.
Following subcutaneous injection of Embolex® (dihydroergotamine mesylate and heparin sodium; with lidocaine HCl) solution (1.5 mg DHE and 15,000 IU heparin), a peak plasma level of 0.3 IU heparin occurred in about 4 hours and a peak plasma level of 2.1 ng/ml dihydroergotamine occurred in about 0.9 hours. The terminal half lives, at these doses, were estimated at between 3 to 5 hours and 1 to 2 hours for DHE and heparin respectively.
Co-administration of DHE and heparin, compared to administration of each separately, decreases the peak plasma level and increases the time-to-peak for DHE without changing the area under the curve. The heparin plasma profile is not affected.
Clinical Trials: When compared to either DHE or heparin alone in controlled clinical investigations, Embolex (dihydroergotamine mesylate and heparin sodium; with lidocaine HCl) Injection, given just prior to and after surgery, significantly reduced the incidence of postoperative DVT, identified by radioactive fibrinogen uptake tests. In a multicenter study of 744 patients conducted in the United States, this reduction in incidence of DVT amounted to 44.0% for the combination of DHE with 5,000 units of heparin (DVT incidence = 9.4%) when compared to 5,000 units of heparin alone (DVT incidence = 16.8%) and 61.5% when this same combination was compared to placebo treated patients (DVT incidents = 24.4%). A reduction in incidence of DVT amounting to 51.5% was observed when the combination of DHE with 5000 units of heparin was compared to the DHE treatment group (DVT incidence = 19.4%). The combination of DHE with 2,500 units of heparin (DVT incidence = 16.8%), equal in effectiveness with 5,000 units of heparin given alone, showed a reduction in incidence of DVT amounting to 31.1% when compared to placebo treated patients.
In comparable European studies, the mean reductions in incidence of DVT for the combination of DHE with 5,000 units of heparin, when compared to 5,000 units of heparin alone or untreated controls, were 60.3% and 85.7% respectively.
These results are shown in the following figures:

DATA FROM U.S. STUDY
(Total N = 744)

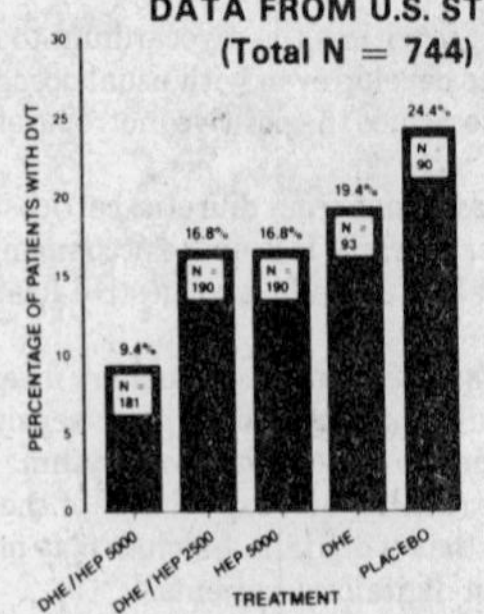

COMBINED DATA, NINE EUROPEAN STUDIES
(Total N = 3073)

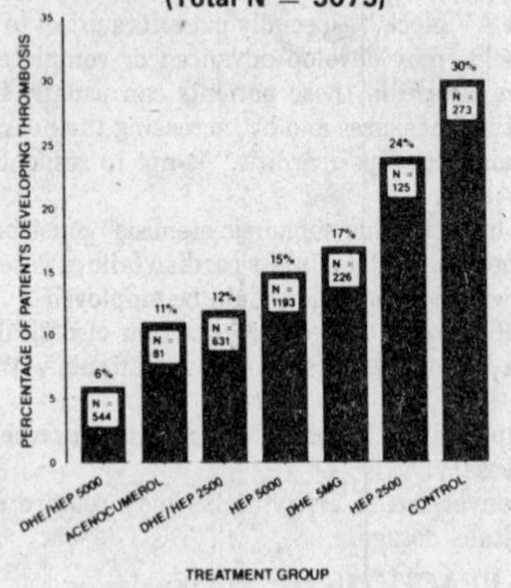

INDICATIONS AND USAGE

Embolex® (dihydroergotamine mesylate and heparin sodium; with lidocaine HCl) Injection (a low-dose regimen) is indicated for the prevention of postoperative deep venous thrombosis and pulmonary embolism in patients undergoing major abdominal, thoracic, or pelvic surgery (see DOSAGE AND ADMINISTRATION).
Such prophylaxis should generally be reserved for patients over the age of 40 who are undergoing major surgery.

CONTRAINDICATIONS

Embolex (dihydroergotamine mesylate and heparin sodium; with lidocaine HCl) treatment is contraindicated in patients who have previously shown hypersensitivity to heparin, ergot alkaloids, or lidocaine.
This combination is also contraindicated in patients with known peripheral arterial disease, coronary artery disease (in particular, unstable or vasospastic angina), uncontrolled hypertension, impaired hepatic or renal function, sepsis, severe thrombocytopenia, or in patients receiving oral anticoagulant therapy.
Embolex (dihydroergotamine mesylate and heparin sodium; with lidocaine HCl) Injection should not be administered to patients with uncontrolled active bleeding or to patients having abnormal coagulation parameters.
DHE possesses oxytocic properties. Therefore, Embolex® (dihydroergotamine mesylate and heparin sodium; with lidocaine HCl) Injection should not be administered during pregnancy.

WARNINGS

Need to Rule Out Bleeding Disorders: All patients should be screened prior to administration of Embolex (dihydroergotamine mesylate and heparin sodium; with lidocaine HCl) prophylaxis to rule out bleeding disorders; appropriate coagulation tests should be repeated just prior to surgery. Test values should be normal or only slightly elevated at these times.
Caution in Disease States in Which There is an Increased Danger of Hemorrhage: Embolex (dihydroergotamine mesylate and heparin sodium; with lidocaine HCl) Injection should be used with extreme caution in disease states in which there is increased danger of hemorrhage. The potential for increased bleeding both during and after surgery should be considered. Some of the conditions in which increased danger of hemorrhage exists are:
Cardiovascular: Subacute bacterial endocarditis; uncontrolled hypertension.
Surgical: During and immediately following (a) spinal tap or spinal anesthesia or (b) major surgery, especially involving the brain, spinal cord, or eye.

Hematologic: Conditions associated with increased bleeding tendencies, such as hemophilia, thrombocytopenia, and some vascular purpuras.
Gastrointestinal: Ulcerative lesions and continuous tube drainage of the stomach or small intestine; liver disease with impaired hemostasis.
Thrombocytopenia: Thrombocytopenia has been reported to occur in patients receiving heparin with a reported incidence of 0 to 30%. Mild thrombocytopenia (count greater than 100,000/mm^3) may remain stable or reverse even if heparin is continued. However, thrombocytopenia of any degree should be monitored closely. If the count falls below 100,000/mm^3 or if recurrent thrombosis develops (see White Clot Syndrome, PRECAUTIONS), Embolex (dihydroergotamine mesylate and heparin sodium; with lidocaine HCl) administration should be discontinued.
Embolex (dihydroergotamine mesylate and heparin sodium; with lidocaine HCl) Injection does not have fibrinolytic activity; therefore it will not lyse pre-existing or established deep-vein-thrombi. If clinical evidence of thromboembolism develops despite Embolex (dihydroergotamine mesylate and heparin sodium; with lidocaine HCl) prophylaxis, this should be discontinued and full therapeutic doses of anticoagulants administered unless contraindicated.
Arterial Spasm: DHE, like other ergot alkaloids, can cause vasospastic reactions, including angina, although it seems to do so less commonly than other ergots. This action appears to be dose-related; however, some patients may demonstrate individual sensitivity to the agent.
Vasospastic reactions are manifested by intense arterial vasoconstriction, producing signs and symptoms of peripheral vascular ischemia (e.g., muscle pains, numbness, coldness and pallor of the digits), angina or unusual syndromes such as mesenteric ischemia. Because persistent vasospasm can result in serious morbidity (gangrene) or death, Embolex®(dihydroergotamine mesylate and heparin sodium; with lidocaine HCl) should be discontinued immediately if signs or symptoms of vasoconstriction develop.
In worldwide experience with Embolex (dihydroergotamine mesylate and heparin sodium; with lidocaine HCl), representing about 3.74 million exposures, there have been 107 reports of vasospasm, most in severely traumatized patients or patients with a severe debilitating condition such as sepsis. In most cases, cessation of Embolex (dihydroergotamine mesylate and heparin sodium; with lidocaine HCl) and institution of vasodilator therapy reversed the vasospasm.
In clinical trials of Embolex (dihydroergotamine mesylate and heparin sodium; with lidocaine HCl) there were two instances of mesenteric ischemia, one of which progressed to bowel necrosis, that may have been related to DHE.

PRECAUTIONS

This combination should be used with caution in patients with uncontrolled hypertension.
"White Clot Syndrome": Rare patients on heparin may develop new thrombus formation in association with thrombocytopenia resulting from irreversible aggregation of platelets induced by heparin, the so-called "white clot syndrome." The process may lead to severe thromboembolic complications like skin necrosis, gangrene of the extremities, myocardial infarction, pulmonary embolism and stroke. Embolex (dihydroergotamine mesylate and heparin sodium; with lidocaine HCl) administration should be promptly discontinued if a patient develops new thrombosis in association with thrombocytopenia.
Heparin Resistance: Increased resistance to heparin has been frequently encountered in fever, thrombosis, thrombophlebitis, infections with thrombosing tendencies, myocardial infarction, cancer and in postsurgical patients.
Increased Risk in Older Women: With full dose heparin, a higher incidence of bleeding has been reported in women over 60 years of age.
Laboratory Tests: Periodic platelet counts, hematocrits, and tests for occult blood in stool are recommended during the entire course of heparin therapy, regardless of the route of administration.
Drug Interactions: Agents of the ergot alkaloid class, of which DHE is a member, have been shown to interact with antibiotics of the macrolide class, resulting in increased plasma levels of the unchanged alkaloid.
Platelet aggregation is the main hemostatic defense of heparinized patients. Drugs which interfere with platelet aggregation reactions (such as acetylsalicylic acid, dextran, phenylbutazone, ibuprofen, indomethacin, dipyridamdole, hydroxychloroquine and others) may induce bleeding and should be used with extreme caution in patients receiving Embolex (dihydroergotamine mesylate and heparin sodium; with lidocaine HCl) Injection prophylaxis.
Digitalis, tetracyclines, nicotine, or antihistamines may partially counteract the anticoagulant action of heparin sodium.
Drug/Laboratory Test Interactions: Hyperaminotransferasemia: Significant elevations of aminotransferase (SGOT S-AST and SGPT S-ALT) levels have been reported in a high percentage of patients (and healthy subjects) who have received heparin. Since aminotransferase determinations are important in the differential diagnosis of myocardial infarction, liver disease, and pulmonary emboli, elevations that may be caused by drugs [like Embolex® (dihydroergotamine mesylate and heparin sodium; with lidocaine HCl) Injection] should be interpreted with caution.
Carcinogenesis, Mutagenesis, Impairment of Fertility: Studies have not been conducted to evaluate the carcinogenic or mutagenic potential of either DHE or heparin, or the potential of these compounds to affect fertility adversely.
Pregnancy: Pregnancy Category X, See CONTRAINDICATIONS.
Nursing Mothers: Heparin is not excreted in human milk. It is not known whether DHE is excreted in human milk. Because many drugs are excreted in human milk, caution should be exercised when Embolex (dihydroergotamine mesylate and heparin sodium; with lidocaine HCl) Injection is administered to a nursing woman.
Pediatric Use: Safety and effectiveness of DHE in children has not been established.

ADVERSE REACTIONS

Hemorrhage: Hematoma at the injection site is the chief complication that may result from Embolex (dihydroergotamine mesylate and heparin sodium; with lidocaine HCl) administration. While hemorrhage is the chief complication that may result from administration of full therapeutic doses of heparin, it should be noted that Embolex (dihydroergotamine mesylate and heparin sodium; with lidocaine HCl) utilizes only low-dose heparin as one of its components, and that excessive postoperative hemorrhage has not been observed in patients given Embolex (dihydroergotamine mesylate and heparin sodium; with lidocaine HCl) Injection.
Deep subcutaneous administration of Embolex (dihydroergotamine mesylate and heparin sodium; with lidocaine HCl) Injection may produce local irritation, mild pain, ecchymosis, or hematoma at the injection site. These complications are much more common after intramuscular use, and such use is not recommended.
[See table above].

HEMORRHAGIC COMPLICATIONS—U.S. STUDY
Number and Percentage of Patients

Complication	TREATMENT GROUP EMBOLEX®	DHE/HEP 2500	HEP 5000	Placebo
Excessive Postoperative Bleeding	N = 212 4 (2%)	N = 227 8 (4%)	N = 220 7 (3%)	N = 106 2 (2%)
Mean Change in Hemoglobin Levels in Gm/100 ml Pretreatment vs. Day 5 Postop	N = 165 −1.3	N = 169 −1.4	N = 173 −1.2	N = 81 −1.5
Wound Hematomas	N = 208 6 (3%)	N = 219 4 (2%)	N = 216 7 (3%)	N = 109 2 (2%)
Hematoma at Injection Site	N = 209 24 (11%)	N = 225 27 (12%)	N = 221 26 (12%)	N = 109 7 (6%)
Microscopic Hematuria-Day 5-All Patients-Catheterized & Uncatheterized	N = 156 38 (24%)	N = 157 43 (27%)	N = 159 41 (26%)	N = 77 28 (36%)

Other Adverse Effects: DHE is known to produce a number of reactions on occasion, including: numbness and tingling of fingers and toes, muscle pain in the extremities, weakness in the legs, precordial distress and pain, transient tachycardia and bradycardia, nausea, vomiting, and localized itching and edema.
Generalized hypersensitivity reactions have been reported in patients receiving heparin therapy. The most common symptoms associated with such reactions are: chills, fever, and urticaria. Asthma, rhinitis, lacrimation, headache, nausea and vomiting, and anaphylactoid reactions, including shock, have also been reported more rarely. Itching and burning, especially on the plantar side of the feet, may occur. Thrombocytopenia has been reported to occur in patients receiving heparin with a reported incidence of 0–30%. While often mild and of no obvious clinical significance, such thrombocytopenia can be accompanied by severe thromboembolic complications such as skin necrosis, gangrene of the extremities, myocardial infarction, pulmonary embolism, and stroke. (See WARNINGS, PRECAUTIONS).
In preliminary studies with normal volunteers, doses of DHE of 2–3 mg resulted in an increased frequency of headache, leg cramps and soreness, nausea and vomiting; these were relatively uncommon in domestic and foreign controlled trials in surgical patients, where DHE was used at the recommended dose of 0.5 mg. The following table shows the frequency of adverse reactions reported in controlled trials for all treatment groups pooled:
[See table on next page].

OVERDOSAGE

Excessive doses of Embolex® (dihydroergotamine mesylate and heparin sodium; with lidocaine HCl) Injection may lead to symptoms associated with overdosage of the components. Excessive doses of DHE may result in peripheral signs and symptoms of **ergotism.** Treatment includes discontinuance of the drug, local application of warmth to the affected area, vasodilators, and nursing care to prevent tissue damage.
Bleeding is the chief sign of heparin overdosage. Nosebleeds, blood in urine or tarry stools may be noted as the first sign of bleeding. Easy bruising or petechial formations may precede frank bleeding.
Treatment: Neutralization of heparin effect. When clinical circumstances (bleeding) require reversal of heparinization, protamine sulfate (1% solution) by slow infusion will neutralize heparin sodium. **No more than 50 mg** should be administered, **very slowly,** in any 10 minute period. Each mg of protamine sulfate neutralizes approximately 100 USP heparin units. The amount of protamine required decreases over time as heparin is metabolized. Although the metabolism of heparin is complex, it may, for the purpose of choosing a protamine dose, be assumed to have half-life of about ½ hour after intravenous injection.
Administration of protamine sulfate can cause severe hypotensive and anaphylactoid reactions. Because fatal reactions often resembling anaphylaxis have been reported, the drug should be given only when resuscitation techniques and treatment of anaphylactoid shock are readily available.
For additional information the labeling of Protamine Sulfate Injection, USP products should be consulted.
The value of dialysis in Embolex® (dihydroergotamine mesylate and heparin sodium; with lidocaine HCl) overdosage has not been determined.
The oral LD_{50} for DHE is > 2000 mg/kg in mice and rats, and > 1000 mg/kg in rabbits. The subcutaneous LD_{50} for DHE is > 625 mg/kg in mice, > 500 mg/kg in rats, and 95 mg/kg in rabbits.

DOSAGE AND ADMINISTRATION

Embolex (dihydroergotamine mesylate and heparin sodium; with lidocaine HCl) Injection should be administered two hours preoperatively and subsequent injections given every twelve hours thereafter for a period of five to seven days.
Parenteral drug products should be inspected visually for particulate matter and discoloration prior to administration. If particulate matter and/or discoloration is observed, the product should be discarded.
Using standard aseptic techniques and a fine (25 or 26 gauge) needle in order to minimize tissue trauma, Embolex® (dihydroergotamine mesylate and heparin sodium; with lidocaine HCl) Injection should be administered by deep subcutaneous (intrafat) injection into a fold in the anterior abdominal wall above the iliac crest. (In the case of abdominal surgery, an alternative injection site may be used.)
Well-controlled clinical investigations have shown that Embolex (dihydroergotamine mesylate and heparin sodium; with lidocaine HCl) Injection is effective in reducing the incidence of postoperative deep vein thrombosis in the legs, as measured by the I-125 fibrinogen technique.

Continued on next page

Sandoz—Cont.

INSTANCES OF ADVERSE EFFECTS*
U.S. EMBOLEX® (dihydroergotamine mesylate and heparin sodium; with lidocaine HCl) CLINICAL TRIALS

Complication by Body System	EMBOLEX® N = 478	DHE/HEP 2500 N = 236	HEP 5000 N = 232	Placebo N = 197
GASTROINTESTINAL				
Nausea	11 (2.3%)		1 (0.4%)	2 (1.0%)
Vomiting	11 (2.3%)			2 (1.0%)
Abdominal Discomfort	3 (0.6%)			
GI Bleeding		3 (1.3%)		
Miscellaneous	4 (0.8%)			
CARDIOVASCULAR				
Chest Pain	7 (1.5%)			2 (1.0%)
Hypertension	2 (0.4%)	2 (0.8%)		
Myocardial Infarction	2 (0.4%)	1 (0.4%)	1 (0.4%)	
Shortness of Breath	2 (0.4%)			
Tachycardia	2 (0.4%)	1 (0.4%)		
Miscellaneous	6 (1.3%)	2 (0.8%)	2 (0.9%)	
CNS				
Pyrexia	3 (0.6%)			
Miscellaneous	5 (1.0%)		1 (0.4%)	2 (1.0%)
SKIN				
Rash	8 (1.7%)	1 (0.4%)	1 (0.4%)	2 (1.0%)
Miscellaneous	9 (1.9%)	1 (0.4%)		2 (1.0%)

*Not all of the adverse reactions can be attributed to Embolex (dihydroergotamine mesylate and heparin sodium; with lidocaine HCl) as these post-surgical patients received other drugs.

Patients with bleeding disorders and those having brain or spinal cord surgery, spinal anesthesia, eye surgery, or potentially sanguineous operations should be excluded, as should patients receiving oral anticoagulants or platelet-active drugs.
Efficacy in hip surgery has not been established.
The intramuscular route of administration should be avoided because of the frequent occurrence of hematoma at the injection site.
Parenteral drug products should be inspected visually for particulate matter and discoloration prior to administration. If particulate matter and/or discoloration is observed, the product should be discarded.
Embolex® (dihydroergotamine mesylate and heparin sodium; with lidocaine HCl) Injection is not effective by oral administration.

HOW SUPPLIED

Embolex (dihydroergotamine mesylate and heparin sodium; with lidocaine HCl) Injection is available as a single ampul in packages of 20 and 100 as follows:
Package of 20 ampuls (NDC 0078-0119-03).
Package of 100 ampuls (NDC 0078-0119-05).
Store and dispense: Store below 77°F (25°C), dispense in light-resistant containers.

Manufactured By Sandoz, Ltd.,
Basle, Switzerland For
SANDOZ PHARMACEUTICALS CORPORATION
East Hanover, N.J. 07936
[EMB-Z4 Issued August 28, 1986]

FIOGESIC® Tablets

[fē-ō-je′zik]

The following prescribing information is based on official labeling in effect on June 1, 1986.

COMPOSITION

Each Tablet contains Calurin® (calcium carbaspirin) 382 mg, equivalent to 300 mg aspirin; phenylpropanolamine hydrochloride, USP 25 mg; pheniramine maleate 12.5 mg; pyrilamine maleate, USP 12.5 mg.

INDICATIONS

For prompt, temporary relief of headache, sinus and nasal congestion, pain and fever due to sinusitis, common cold, or influenza. FIOGESIC® promotes sinus and nasal decongestion and drainage with phenylpropanolamine, an orally used alpha adrenergic sympathomimetic approximately equal in potency to ephedrine but with less CNS stimulation, plus two antihistamines, pheniramine maleate and pyrilamine maleate. Calurin®, a freely soluble aspirin complex, alleviates pain and fever.

CONTRAINDICATIONS

Sensitivity to any of the ingredients.

CAUTION

Not for children under 6. Individuals with high blood pressure, heart disease, diabetes, or thyroid disease should use only as directed by a physician. This preparation may cause drowsiness. Do not drive or operate machinery while taking this medication.

SIDE EFFECTS

Drowsiness, blurred vision, cardiac palpitations, flushing, dizziness, nervousness, or gastrointestinal upsets may occur occasionally.

DOSAGE

Adults—Two tablets followed by one or two tablets every four hours, up to six per day. Children (6 to 12 years)—one-half to one tablet every four hours up to four tablets per day.

SUPPLIED

Fiogesic Oblong Inlay-Tablets (white with yellow inlay) in bottles of 100.
Company's Product Identification Mark(s): Tablets embossed FIOGESIC on one side, SANDOZ other side.
Shown in Product Identification Section, page 427

FIORICET® ℞

[fē″or′i-set]
TABLETS

The following prescribing information is based on offical labeling in effect on July 1, 1986.

DESCRIPTION

Each Fioricet® tablet for oral administration contains: butalbital, USP 50 mg (Warning: May be habit forming); acetaminophen, USP, 325 mg; caffeine, USP, 40 mg.
Butalbital, 5-allyl-5-isobutyl-barbituric acid, a white odorless crystalline powder; is a short- to intermediate-acting barbiturate. Its molecular weight is 224.26 and its empirical formula is $C_{11}H_{16}N_2O_3$.
Active Ingredients: acetaminophen, USP, butalbital, USP, and caffeine, USP
Inactive Ingredients: crospovidone, FD&C Blue #1, magnesium stearate, microcrystalline cellulose, povidone, pregelatinized starch, and stearic acid

ACTIONS

Pharmacologically, Fioricet combines the analgesic properties of acetaminophen-caffeine with the anxiolytic and muscle relaxant properties of butalbital.

INDICATIONS

Fioricet is indicated for the relief of the symptom complex of tension (or muscle contraction) headache.

CONTRAINDICATIONS

Hypersensitivity to acetaminophen, caffeine or barbiturates. Patients with porphyria.

PRECAUTIONS

General: Barbiturates should be administered with caution, if at all, to patients who are mentally depressed, have suicidal tendencies, or a history of drug abuse.
Elderly or debilitated patients may react to barbiturates with marked excitement, depression, and confusion. In some persons, barbiturates repeatedly produce excitement rather than depression.
Information for the Patient: Practitioners should give the following information and instructions to patients receiving barbiturates.

1. The use of barbiturates carries with it an associated risk of psychological and/or physical dependence. The patient should be warned against increasing the dose of the drug without consulting a physician.
2. Barbiturates may impair mental and/or physical abilities required for the performance of potentially hazardous tasks (e.g., driving, operating machinery, etc.).
3. Alcohol should not be consumed while taking barbiturates. Concurrent use of the barbiturates with other CNS depressants (e.g., alcohol, narcotics, tranquilizers, and antihistamines) may result in additional CNS depressant effects.

Drug Interactions: Patients receiving narcotic analgesics, antipsychotics, antianxiety agents, or other CNS depressants (including alcohol) concomitantly with Fioricet may exhibit additive CNS depressant effects.

DRUGS	EFFECT
Butalbital w/coumarin anticoagulants	Decreased effect of anticoagulant because of increased metabolism resulting from enzyme induction.
Butalbital w/tricycle antidepressants	Decreased blood levels of the depressant.

Usage in Pregnancy: Adequate studies have not been performed in animals to determine whether this drug affects fertility in males or females, has teratogenic potential or has other adverse effects on the fetus. There are no well-controlled studies in pregnant women. Although there is no clearly defined risk, one cannot exclude the possibility of infrequent or subtle damage to the human fetus. Fioricet should be used in pregnant women only when clearly needed.
Nursing Mothers: The effects of Fioricet on infants of nursing mothers are not known. Barbiturates are excreted in the breast milk of nursing mothers. The serum levels in infants are believed to be insignificant with therapeutic doses administered to the mother.
Pediatric Use: Safety and effectiveness in children below the age of 12 have not been established.

ADVERSE REACTIONS

The most frequent adverse reactions are drowsiness and dizziness. Less frequent adverse reactions are light-headedness and gastrointestinal disturbances including nausea, vomiting, and flatulence. Mental confusion or depression can occur due to intolerance or overdosage of butalbital.

DRUG ABUSE AND DEPENDENCE

Prolonged use of barbiturate can produce drug dependence, characterized by psychic dependence and tolerance. The abuse liability of Fiorcet is similar to that of other barbiturate-containing drug combinations. Caution should be exercised when prescribing medication for patients with a known propensity for taking excessive quantities of drugs, which is not uncommon in patients with chronic tension headache.

OVERDOSAGE

The toxic effects of acute overdosage of Fioricet are attributable mainly to its barbiturate component, and, to a lesser extent, acetaminophen. Because toxic effects of caffeine occur in very high dosages only, the possibility of significant caffeine toxicity from Fioricet overdosage is unlikely.
Barbiturate Poisoning
Symptoms: Drowsiness, confusion, coma; respiratory depression; hypotension; shock.
Treatment:

1. Maintenance of an adequate airway, with assisted respiration and oxygen administration as necessary.
2. Monitoring of vital signs and fluid balance.
3. If the patient is conscious and has not lost the gag reflex, emesis may be induced with ipecac. Care should be taken to prevent pulmonary aspiration of vomitus. After completion of vomiting, 30 grams activated charcoal in a glass of water may be administered.
4. If emesis is contraindicated, gastric lavage may be performed with a cuffed endotracheal tube in place with the patient in the face-down position. Activated charcoal may be left in the emptied stomach and a saline cathartic administered.
5. Fluid therapy and other standard treatment for shock, if needed.
6. If renal function is normal, forced diuresis may aid in the elimination of the barbiturate. Alkalinization of the urine increases renal excretion of some barbiturates, especially phenobarbital.

7. Although not recommended as a routine procedure, hemodialysis may be used in severe barbiturate intoxications or if the patient is anuric or in shock.

Acetaminophen Poisoning

Symptoms: Acetaminophen in massive overdosage may cause hepatic toxicity in some patients. In cases of suspected overdose, you may wish to call your regional poison center for assistance in diagnosis and for directions in the use of N-acetylcysteine as an antidote.

In adults, hepatic toxicity has rarely been reported with acute overdoses of less than 10 grams and fatalities with less than 15 grams. Importantly, young children seem to be more resistant than adults to the hepatotoxic effect of an acetaminophen overdose.

Early symptoms following a potentially hepatotoxic overdose may include: nausea, vomiting, diaphoresis and general malaise. Clinical and laboratory evidence of hepatic toxicity may not be apparent until 48 to 72 hours post-ingestion.

Treatment: The stomach should be emptied promptly by lavage or by induction of emesis with syrup of ipecac. Patients' estimates of the quantity of a drug ingested are notoriously unreliable. Therefore, if an acetaminophen overdose is suspected, a serum acetaminophen assay should be obtained as early as possible, but no sooner than four hours following ingestion. Liver function studies should be obtained initially and repeated at 24-hour intervals.

The antidote, N-acetylcysteine, should be administered as early as possible, preferably within 16 hours of the overdose ingestion for optimal results, but in any case, within 24 hours. Following recovery, there are no residual, structural or functional hepatic abnormalities.

DOSAGE AND ADMINISTRATION

Oral: One or two tablets every four hours as needed. Do not exceed 6 tablets per day.

HOW SUPPLIED

Light-blue, round compressed tablet, embossed "FIORICET" and triangle "S" on one side, three-head profile on other side. Bottles of 100 (NDC 0078-0084-05) and 500 (NDC 0078-0084-08).

SandoPak® (unit-dose) packages of 100, 10 blisters strips of 10 tablets (NDC 0078-0084-06).

Store and dispense: Below 86°F; tight container.

[FCT-Z6 Issued July 1, 1986]

Shown in Product Identification Section, page 427

FIORINAL® Ⓒ

[fē-ŏr 'ĭ-nol]

Tablets and Capsules

The following prescribing information is based on official labeling in effect on July 15, 1986.

DESCRIPTION

Each Fiorinal® tablet or capsule for oral administration contains: butalbital, USP, 50 mg (Warning: May be habit forming); aspirin, USP, 325 mg; caffeine, USP, 40 mg.

Butalbital, 5-allyl-5-isobutyl-barbituric acid, a white odorless crystalline powder; is a short- to intermediate-acting barbiturate.

Tablets

Active Ingredients: aspirin, USP, butalbital, USP, and caffeine, USP

Inactive Ingredients: lactose, microcrystalline cellulose, povidone, and stearic acid

Capsules

Active Ingredients: aspirin, USP, butalbital, USP, and caffeine, USP

Inactive Ingredients: D&C Yellow #10, gelatin, microcrystalline cellulose, starch, sodium lauryl sulfate, and talc.

May Also Include: benzyl alcohol, butyl paraben, edetate calcium disodium, FD&C Blue #1, FD&C Yellow #6, FD&C Green #3, methyl paraben, propyl paraben, sodium bisulfite, silicon dioxide, and sodium propionate

ACTIONS

Pharmacologically, Fiorinal combines the analgesic properties of aspirin with the anxiolytic and muscle relaxant properties of butalbital.

The clinical effectiveness of Fiorinal in tension headache has been established in double-blind, placebo-controlled, multiclinic trials. A factorial design study compared Fiorinal with each of its major components. This study demonstrated that each component contributes to the efficacy of Fiorinal in the treatment of the target symptoms of tension headache (headache pain, psychic tension, and muscle contraction in the head, neck and shoulder region). For each symptom and the symptom complex as a whole, Fiorinal was shown to have significantly superior clinical effects to either component alone.

INDICATIONS

Fiorinal is indicated for the relief of the symptom complex of tension (or muscle contraction) headache.

CONTRAINDICATIONS

Hypersensitivity to aspirin, caffeine, or barbiturates. Patients with porphyria.

WARNINGS

Drug Dependency: Prolonged use of barbiturates can produce drug dependence, characterized by psychic dependence, and less frequently, physical dependence and tolerance. The abuse liability of Fiorinal is similar to that of other barbiturate-containing drug combinations. Caution should be exercised when prescribing medication for patients with a known propensity for taking excessive quantities of drugs, which is not uncommon in patients with chronic tension headache.

Use in Ambulatory Patients: Fiorinal may impair the mental and/or physical abilities required for the performance of potentially hazardous tasks, such as driving a car or operating machinery. The patient should be cautioned accordingly. Central Nervous System depressant effects of butalbital may be additive with those of other CNS depressants. Concurrent use with other sedative-hypnotics or alcohol should be avoided. When such combined therapy is necessary, the dose of one or more agents may need to be reduced.

Use in Pregnancy: Adequate studies have not been performed in animals to determine whether this drug affects fertility in males or females, has teratogenic potential, or has other adverse effects on the fetus. While there are no well-controlled studies in pregnant women, over twenty years of marketing and clinical experience does not include any positive evidence of adverse effects on the fetus. Although there is no clearly defined risk, such experience cannot exclude the possibility of infrequent or subtle damage to the human fetus. Fiorinal should be used in pregnant women only when clearly needed.

Nursing Mothers: The effects of Fiorinal on infants of nursing mothers are not known. Salicylates and barbiturates are excreted in the breast milk of nursing mothers. The serum levels in infants are believed to be insignificant with therapeutic doses.

PRECAUTIONS

Salicylates should be used with extreme caution in the presence of peptic ulcer or coagulation abnormalities.

Pediatric Use: Safety and effectiveness in children below the age of 12 have not been established.

ADVERSE REACTIONS

The most frequent adverse reactions are drowsiness and dizziness. Less frequent adverse reactions are lightheadedness and gastrointestinal disturbances including nausea, vomiting, and flatulence.

OVERDOSAGE

The toxic effects of acute overdosage of Fiorinal are attributable mainly to its barbiturate component, and, to a lesser extent, aspirin. Because toxic effects of caffeine occur in very high dosages only, the possibility of significant caffeine toxicity from Fiorinal overdosage is unlikely. Symptoms attributable to *acute barbiturate poisoning* include drowsiness, confusion, and coma; respiratory depression; hypotension; shock. Symptoms attributable to *acute aspirin poisoning* include hyperpnea; acid-base disturbances with development of metabolic acidosis; vomiting and abdominal pain; tinnitus; hyperthermia; hypoprothrombinemia; restlessness; delirium; convulsions. *Acute caffeine poisoning* may cause insomnia, restlessness, tremor, and delirium; tachycardia and extrasystoles. *Treatment* consists primarily of management of barbiturate intoxication and the correction of the acid-base imbalance due to salicylism. Vomiting should be induced mechanically or with emetics in the conscious patient. Gastric lavage may be used if the pharyngeal and laryngeal reflexes are present and if less than four hours have elapsed since ingestion. A cuffed endotracheal tube should be inserted before gastric lavage of the unconscious patient and when necessary to provide assisted respiration. Diuresis, alkalinization of the urine, and correction of electrolyte disturbances should be accomplished through administration of intravenous fluids such as 1% sodium bicarbonate in 5% dextrose in water. Meticulous attention should be given to maintaining adequate pulmonary ventilation. Correction of hypotension may require the administration of levarterenol bitartrate or phenylephrine hydrochloride by intravenous infusion. In severe cases of intoxication, peritoneal dialysis, hemodialysis, or exchange transfusion may be lifesaving. Hypoprothrombinemia should be treated with Vitamin K, intravenously.

DOSAGE AND ADMINISTRATION

One or two tablets or capsules every four hours. Total daily dose should not exceed six tablets or capsules.

HOW SUPPLIED

Fiorinal Capsules: Color is bright Kelly green and lime green, in packages of 100 and 500. Also available in ControlPak® package, 25 capsules (continuous reverse numbered roll of sealed blisters). Fiorinal Tablets: White, compressed tablet 11 mm diameter, 5.5 mm thickness, in packages of 100 and 1000.

Company's Product Identification Mark(s): Tablets imprinted "FIORINAL" on one side, "SANDOZ" on other side, and Capsules imprinted "FIORINAL 78–103" on each half of capsule.

[FIO-ZZ23 Issued July 15, 1986]

Shown in Product Identification Section, page 427

FIORINAL® with CODEINE Ⓒ

[fē-or 'ĭ-nol]

Capsules

No. 1, 2 and 3

The following prescribing information is based on official labeling in effect on June 1, 1986.

DESCRIPTION

Contents per capsule in three dosage strengths: codeine phosphate, USP

Warning: May be habit forming.

No. 1	No. 2	No. 3
7.5 mg	15 mg	30 mg
(1/8 gr)	(1/4 gr)	(1/2 gr)

butalbital, USP .... 50 mg

Warning: May be habit forming.

caffeine, USP .... 40 mg

aspirin, USP .... 325 mg

Butalbital, 5-allyl-5-isobutyl-barbituric acid, a white odorless crystalline powder, is a short- to intermediate-acting barbiturate. Its molecular weight is 224.26 and its empirical formula is $C_{11}H_{16}N_2O_3$.

No. 1 Capsules

Inactive Ingredients: D&C Yellow #10, FD&C Blue #1, FD&C Yellow #6, FD&C Red #3, gelatin, microcrystalline cellulose, sodium lauryl sulfate, starch, talc, titanium dioxide.

May Also include: benzyl alcohol, butyl paraben, edetate calcium disodium, FD&C Red #40, glycerin, methyl paraben, propyl paraben, silicon dioxide, sodium propionate.

No. 2 Capsules

Inactive Ingredients: D&C Yellow #10, FD&C Yellow #6, gelatin, microcrystalline cellulose, sodium lauryl sulfate, starch, synthetic black ferric oxide, synthetic red ferric oxide, talc, titanium dioxide.

May Also Include: benzyl alcohol, butyl paraben, carboxymethylcellulose sodium, edetate calcium disodium, glycerin, methyl paraben, propyl paraben, silicon dioxide, sodium propionate.

No. 3 Capsules

Inactive Ingredients: D&C Yellow #10, FD&C Blue #1, FD&C Red #3, FD&C Yellow #6, gelatin, microcrystalline cellulose, sodium lauryl sulfate, starch, talc, titanium dioxide.

May Also Include: benzyl alcohol, butyl paraben, edetate calcium disodium, glycerin, methyl paraben, propyl paraben, silicon dioxide, sodium propionate.

CLINICAL PHARMACOLOGY

Fiorinal® with Codeine combines the analgesic properties of aspirin and codeine with the anxiolytic and muscle relaxant properties of butalbital.

Pharmacokinetics

Aspirin

The systemic availability of aspirin after an oral dose is highly dependent on the dosage form, the presence of food, the gastric emptying time, gastric pH, antacids, buffering agents and particle size. These factors affect not necessarily the extent of absorption of total salicylates but more the stability of aspirin prior to absorption.

During the absorption process and after absorption, aspirin is mainly hydrolyzed to salicylic acid and distributed to all body tissues and fluids, including fetal tissues, breast milk and the central nervous system (CNS). Highest concentrations are found in plasma, liver, renal cortex, heart and lung. In plasma, about 50 to 80 percent of the salicylic acid and its metabolites are loosely bound to plasma proteins.

The clearance of total salicylates is subject to saturable kinetics; however, first-order elimination kinetics are still a good approximation for doses up to 650 mg. The plasma half-life for aspirin is about 12 minutes and for salicylic acid and/or total salicylates is about 3.0 hours.

The elimination of therapeutic doses is through the kidneys either as salicylic acid or other biotransformation products. The renal clearance is greatly augmented by an alkaline urine as is produced by concurrent administration of sodium bicarbonate or potassium citrate.

The biotransformation of aspirin occurs primarily in the hepatocytes. The major metabolites are salicyluric acid (75%), the phenolic and acyl glucuronides of salicylate (15%), and gentisic and gentisuric acid (<1%).

The bioavailability of the aspirin component for Fiorinal with Codeine capsules is equivalent to that of a solution showing only a slightly slower rate of absorption. Peak concentrations are achieved about 30 minutes after a dose.

Continued on next page

Sandoz—Cont.

See *Overdosage Section* for toxic information.

Codeine

Codeine is readily absorbed from the gastrointestinal tract, and is rapidly distributed from blood to body tissues. During distribution it is taken up preferentially by parenchymatous organs such as liver, spleen and kidney. It passes the blood-brain barrier and is found in fetal tissue and breast milk. The drug is not bound to plasma proteins nor does it accumulate in body tissues.

The elimination of codeine is primarily through the kidney. The plasma half-life is about 2.9 hours. The urinary excretion products represent about 90% of the dose within 24 hours and consist of free and glucuronide-conjugated codeine (about 70%), free and conjugated norcodeine (about 10%), free and conjugated morphine (about 10%), normorphine (under 4%) and hydrocodone (< 1%). The remainder of the dose appears in the feces.

At therapeutic doses, the analgesic effect reaches peak within 2 hours and persists for 4–6 hours. Blood concentrations causing CNS depression begin at 50–190 ng/mL.

The bioavailability of the codeine component for Fiorinal with Codeine capsules is equivalent to that of a solution. Peak concentrations of 198 ng/mL were obtained at 1 hour after a 60 mg dose.

See *Overdosage Section* for toxic information.

Butalbital

Butalbital is well absorbed from the gastrointestinal tract and is expected to distribute to most of the tissues in the body. Barbiturates in general may appear in milk and readily cross the placental barrier. They are bound to plasma and tissue proteins to a varying degree and binding increases directly as a function of lipid solubility.

Elimination of butalbital is primarily via the kidney (59–88% of the dose) as unchanged drug or metabolites. The plasma half-life is about 35 hours. Urinary excretion products included parent drug (about 3.6% of the dose), 5-isobutyl-5-(2,3-dihydroxypropyl)barbituric acid (about 24% of the dose), 5-allyl-5(3-hydroxy-2-methyl-1-propyl)barbituric acid (about 4.8% of dose), products with the barbituric acid ring hydrolyzed with excretion of urea (about 14% of the dose) as well as unidentified materials. Of the material excreted in the urine, 32% was conjugated.

The bioavailability of the butalbital component for Fiorinal with Codeine capsules is equivalent to that of a solution except for a decrease in the rate of absorption. A peak concentration of 2020 ng/mL is obtained at about 1.5 hours after a 100 mg dose.

See *Overdosage Section* for toxic information.

Caffeine

Like most xanthines, caffeine is rapidly absorbed and distributed in all body tissues and fluids, including the CNS, fetal tissues and breast milk.

Caffeine is cleared rapidly through metabolism and excretion in the urine. The plasma half-life is about 3 hours. Hepatic biotransformation prior to excretion results in about equal amounts of 1-methyl-xanthine and 1-methyluric acid. Of the 70% of the dose that has been recovered in the urine, only 3% was unchanged drug.

The bioavailability of the caffeine component for Fiorinal with Codeine capsules is equivalent to that of a solution except for a slightly longer time to peak. A peak concentration of 1660 ng/mL was obtained in less than an hour for an 80 mg dose.

See *Overdosage Section* for toxic information.

INDICATIONS

Fiorinal with Codeine raises the threshold of pain and discomfort and can be used in a great variety of painful conditions short of those which require morphine.

Fiorinal with Codeine is indicated for all types of pain associated with medical and surgical aftercare, postpartum pain, dysmenorrhea, neuritis, pleurisy, sciatica, neuralgia, sinusitis, pharyngitis, tonsillitis, otitis, febrile diseases, dental pain following extractions, headache, bursitis, arthritis, rheumatism, low back pain, dislocations, strains, sprains, fractures, etc.

CONTRAINDICATIONS

Fiorinal with Codeine is contraindicated under the following conditions:

1) hypersensitivity or intolerance to aspirin, caffeine, butalbital or codeine
2) peptic ulcer or other serious gastrointestinal lesions, and
3) patients with porphyria.

WARNINGS

Care should be taken when administering salicylates to persons with known allergies. Hypersensitivity to aspirin is particularly likely in patients with nasal polyps, and relatively common in those with asthma.

PRECAUTIONS

Information for Patients

Take medication with food or full glass of water or milk to minimize gastrointestinal irritation.

Fiorinal® with Codeine may impair the mental and/or physical abilities required for performance of potentially dangerous tasks such as driving a car or operating machinery. The patient should be cautioned accordingly.

Central Nervous System depressant effects of butalbital and codeine may be additive with those of other CNS depressants. Concurrent use with sedative-hypnotics or alcohol should be avoided. When such combined therapy is necessary, the dose of one or more agents may need to be reduced.

Codeine and butalbital may be habit-forming when used over long periods or in high doses. Patients should take Fiorinal with Codeine only for as long as prescribed, in the amounts prescribed, and no more frequently than prescribed.

Keep medication out of reach of children; overdose is especially dangerous in young children.

Usage in Pregnancy

Category C. Adequate studies have not been performed in animals to determine whether this drug affects fertility in males or females, has teratogenic potential, or has other adverse effects on the fetus. While there are no well-controlled studies in pregnant women, over twenty years of marketing and clinical experience does not include any positive evidence of adverse effects on the fetus. Although there is no clearly defined risk, such experience cannot exclude the possibility of infrequent or subtle damage to the human fetus. Fiorinal with Codeine capsules should be used in pregnant women only when clearly needed.

Nursing Mothers

The effects of Fiorinal with Codeine capsules on infants or nursing mothers are not known. Salicylates, codeine, caffeine, and barbiturates are excreted in the breast milk of nursing mothers. Caution should be exercised when Fiorinal with Codeine is administered to a nursing woman.

Pediatric Use

Safety and effectiveness in children below the age of 12 have not been established.

ADVERSE REACTIONS

Nausea, vomiting, constipation, dizziness, weakness, drowsiness, and lethargy are the most common side effects. Overdosage is primarily manifested by drowsiness.

DRUG ABUSE AND DEPENDENCE

Fiorinal with Codeine is controlled by the Drug Enforcement Administration and is classified under Schedule III.

Codeine

Codeine can produce drug dependence of the morphine type, and therefore has the potential for being abused. Psychic dependence, physical dependence and tolerance may develop upon repeated administration and it should be prescribed and administered with the same degree of caution appropriate to the use of other oral narcotic medications.

Butalbital

Barbiturates may be habit forming: Tolerance, psychological dependence, and physical dependence may occur especially following prolonged use of high doses of barbiturates. The average daily dose for the barbiturate addict is usually about 1,500 mg. As tolerance to barbiturates develops, the amount needed to maintain the same level of intoxication increases; tolerance to a fatal dosage, however, does not increase more than two-fold. As this occurs, the margin between an intoxication dosage and fatal dosage becomes smaller. The lethal dose of a barbiturate is far less if alcohol is also ingested. Major withdrawal symptoms (convulsions and delirium) may occur within 16 hours and last up to 5 days after abrupt cessation of these drugs. Intensity of withdrawal symptoms gradually declines over a period of approximately 15 days.

Treatment of barbiturate dependence consists of cautious and gradual withdrawal of the drug. Barbiturate-dependent patients can be withdrawn by using a number of different withdrawal regimens. One method involves initiating treatment at the patient's regular dosage level and gradually decreasing the daily dosage as tolerated by the patient.

OVERDOSAGE

The toxic effects of acute overdosage of Fiorinal with Codeine capsules are attributable mainly to its barbiturate component, and, to a lesser extent, codeine and aspirin. Because toxic effects of caffeine occur in very high dosages only, the possibility of significant caffeine toxicity from Fiorinal with Codeine overdosage is unlikely.

Signs and Symptoms

Symptoms attributable to *acute barbiturate poisoning* include drowsiness, confusion, and coma; respiratory depression; hypotension; shock. Symptoms attributable to *acute aspirin poisoning* include hyperpnea; acid-base disturbances with development of metabolic acidosis; vomiting and abdominal pain; tinnitus, hyperthermia; hypoprothrombinemia; restlessness; delirium; convulsions. Symptoms of *acute codeine poisoning* include the triad of: pinpoint pupils, marked depression of respiration, and loss of consciousness. Convulsions may occur.

Treatment

Treatment consists primarily of management of barbiturate intoxication, reversal of the effects of codeine, and the correction of the acid-base imbalance due to salicylism. Vomiting should be induced mechanically or with emetics in the conscious patient. Gastric lavage may be used if the pharyngeal and laryngeal reflexes are present and if less than four hours have elapsed since ingestion. A cuffed endotracheal tube should be inserted before gastric lavage of the unconscious patient and when necessary to provide assisted respiration. Diuresis, alkalinization of the urine, and correction of electrolyte disturbances should be accomplished through administration of intravenous fluids such as 1% sodium bicarbonate in 5% dextrose in water.

Meticulous attention should be given to maintaining adequate pulmonary ventilation. The narcotic antagonist naloxone is a specific antidote for respiratory depression which may result from overdosage or unusual sensitivity to narcotics. A narcotic antagonist should not be administered in the absence of clinically significant respiratory or cardiovascular depression. NOTE: Respiratory depression caused by barbiturates will *not* respond to narcotic antagonists. Unwitting overdosage with narcotic antagonists may occur in an attempt to reverse respiratory depression caused by mixed barbiturate-codeine intoxication.

Correction of hypotension may require the administration of levarterenol bitartrate or phenylephrine hydrochloride by intravenous infusion. In severe cases of intoxication, peritoneal dialysis, hemodialysis, or exchange transfusion may be lifesaving. Hypoprothrombinemia should be treated with vitamin K, intravenously. Methemoglobinemia over 30% should be treated with methylene blue administered slowly intravenously.

Toxic and Lethal Doses

Butalbital: toxic dose 1.0 g (adult); lethal dose 2.0–5.0 g
Aspirin: toxic blood level > 30 mg/100 ml; lethal dose 10–30g (adult)
Caffeine: toxic dose > 1.0 g; lethal dose unknown
Codeine: lethal dose 0.5–1.0 g (adult)

DOSAGE AND ADMINISTRATION

One or two capsules, repeated if necessary up to six capsules per day, or as directed by physician.

HOW SUPPLIED

Fiorinal with Codeine Capsules

7.5 mg (1/8 gr) imprinted "F-C#1" on one half, "SANDOZ 78-105" other half, color is red and yellow; 15 mg (1/4 gr) imprinted "F-C#2" on one half, "SANDOZ 78-106" other half, color is gray and yellow; 30 mg (1/2 gr) imprinted "F-C#3" on one half, "SANDOZ 78-107" other half, color is blue and yellow.

Packaging

Fiorinal with Codeine No. 1 (1/8 gr), No. 2 (1/4 gr) and No. 3 (1/2 gr) in bottles of 100 capsules.

Fiorinal with Codeine No. 3 (1/2 gr) also in ControlPak® package, 25 capsules (continuous reverse-numbered roll of sealed blisters).

[FWC-Z19 Issued March 17, 1986]

Shown in Product Identification Section, page 427

HYDERGINE® ℞

[*hī'der-jēn*]

(ergoloid mesylates) tablets, USP (ORAL)
(ergoloid mesylates) tablets, USP (SUBLINGUAL)
(ergoloid mesylates) liquid

HYDERGINE® LC

(ergoloid mesylates) liquid capsules

The following prescribing information is based on official labeling in effect on June 1, 1986.

DESCRIPTION AND TYPE

Hydergine tablet 1 mg, Hydergine sublingual tablet 1 mg and Hydergine LC (liquid capsule) 1 mg, each contains ergoloid mesylates USP as follows: dihydroergocomine mesylate 0.333 mg, dihydroergocristine mesylate 0.333 mg, and dihydroergocryptine (dihydro-alpha-ergocryptine and dihydro-beta-ergocryptine in the proportion of 2:1) mesylate 0.333 mg, representing a total of 1 mg.

Inactive Ingredients:

1 mg, Oral Tablets: lactose, povidone, starch, stearic acid, and talc

1 mg, Sublingual Tablets: gelatin, mannitol, starch, stearic acid, and sucrose

Liquid Capsules: ascorbic acid, gelatin, glycerin, methyl paraben, polyethylene glycol, propyl paraben, propylene glycol, sorbitol, and titanium dioxide

Hydergine sublingual tablet 0.5 mg, each contains ergoloid mesylates USP as follows: dihydroergocomine mesylate 0.167 mg, dihydroergocristine mesylate 0.167 mg, and dihydroergocryptine (dihydro-alpha-ergocryptine and dihydro-

beta-ergocryptine in the proportion of 2:1) mesylate 0.167 mg, representing a total of 0.5 mg.
Inactive Ingredients: gelatin, mannitol, starch, stearic acid, and sucrose.
Hydergine liquid 1 mg/ml, each ml contains ergoloid mesylates USP as follows: dihydroergocornine mesylate 0.333 mg, dihydroergocristine mesylate 0.333 mg, and dihydroergocryptine (dihydro-alpha-ergocryptine and dihydro-beta-ergocryptine in the proportion of 2:1) mesylate 0.333 mg, representing a total of 1 mg; alcohol, USP, 30% by volume.
Inactive Ingredients: alcohol, glycerin, propylene glycol, and purified water

Pharmacokinetic Properties

Pharmacokinetic studies have been performed in normal volunteers with the help of radiolabelled drug as well as employing a specific radioimmunoassay technique. From the urinary excretion quotient of orally and intravenously administered tritium-labelled Hydergine (ergoloid mesylates) the absorption of ergoloid was calculated to be 25%. Following oral administration, peak levels of 0.5 ng Eq/ml/mg were achieved within 1.5-3 hr. Bioavailability studies with the specific radioimmunoassay confirm that ergoloid is rapidly absorbed from the gastrointestinal tract, with mean peak levels of 0.05-0.13 ng/ml/mg (with extremes of 0.03 and 0.18 ng/ml/mg) achieved within 0.6-1.3 hr. (with extremes of 0.4 and 2.8 hrs.). The finding of lower peak levels of ergoloid compared to the total drug-metabolite composite is consistent with a considerable first pass liver metabolism, with less than 50% of the therapeutic moiety reaching the systemic circulation. The elimination of radioactivity, representing ergoloid plus metabolites bearing the radiolabel, was biphasic with half-lives of 4 and 13 hr. The mean half-life of unchanged ergoloid in plasma is about 2.6-5.1 hr; after 3 half-lives ergoloid plasma levels are less than 10% of radioactivity levels, and by 24 hr no ergoloid is detectable.
Bioequivalence studies were performed comparing Hydergine oral tablets (administered orally) with Hydergine sublingual tablets (administered sublingually), Hydergine oral tablets with Hydergine liquid and Hydergine oral tablets with Hydergine LC (liquid capsules). The oral tablet, sublingual tablet and liquid capsule oral forms were shown to be bioequivalent. Within the bioequivalence limits, the liquid capsule showed a statistically significant (12%) greater bioavailability than the oral tablet. In the study comparing the oral tablet and liquid forms, both forms tested showed an equivalent rate of absorption and an equivalent peak plasma concentration (C_{max}).

ACTIONS

There is no specific evidence which clearly establishes the mechanism by which Hydergine® (ergoloid mesylates) preparations produce mental effects, nor is there conclusive evidence that the drug particularly affects cerebral arteriosclerosis or cerebrovascular insufficiency.

INDICATIONS

A proportion of individuals over sixty who manifest signs and symptoms of an idiopathic decline in mental capacity (i.e., cognitive and interpersonal skills, mood, self-care, apparent motivation) can experience some symptomatic relief upon treatment with Hydergine (ergoloid mesylates) preparations. The identity of the specific trait(s) or condition(s), if any, which would usefully predict a response to Hydergine (ergoloid mesylates) therapy is not known. It appears, however, that those individuals who do respond come from groups of patients who would be considered clinically to suffer from some ill-defined process related to aging or to have some underlying dementing condition (i.e., primary progressive dementia, Alzheimer's dementia, senile onset, multi-infarct dementia).
Before prescribing Hydergine (ergoloid mesylates), the physician should exclude the possibility that the patient's signs and symptoms arise from a potentially reversible and treatable condition. Particular care should be taken to exclude delirium and dementiform illness secondary to systemic disease, primary neurological disease, or primary disturbance of mood. Hydergine (ergoloid mesylates) preparations are not indicated in the treatment of acute or chronic psychosis, regardless of etiology (see CONTRAINDICATIONS section).
The decision to use Hydergine (ergoloid mesylates) in the treatment of an individual with a symptomatic decline in mental capacity of unknown etiology should be continually reviewed since the presenting clinical picture may subsequently evolve sufficiently to allow a specific diagnosis and a specific alternative treatment. In addition, continued clinical evaluation is required to determine whether any initial benefit conferred by Hydergine (ergoloid mesylates) therapy persist with time.
The efficacy of Hydergine (ergoloid mesylates) was evaluated using a special rating scale known as the SCAG (Sandoz Clinical Assessment-Geriatric). The specific items on this scale on which modest but statistically significant changes were observed at the end of twelve weeks include: mental alertness, confusion, recent memory, orientation, emotional lability, self-care, depression, anxiety/fears, cooperation, sociability, appetite, dizziness, fatigue, bothersome(ness), and an overall impression of clinical status.

CONTRAINDICATIONS

Hydergine (ergoloid mesylates) preparations are contraindicated in individuals who have previously shown hypersensitivity to the drug. Hydergine (ergoloid mesylates) preparations are also contraindicated in patients who have psychosis, acute or chronic, regardless of etiology.

PRECAUTIONS

Practitioners are advised that because the target symptoms are of unknown etiology, careful diagnosis should be attempted before prescribing Hydergine (ergoloid mesylates) preparations.

ADVERSE REACTIONS

Hydergine (ergoloid mesylates) preparations have not been found to produce serious side effects. Some sublingual irritation with the sublingual tablets, transient nausea, and gastric disturbances have been reported. Hydergine (ergoloid mesylates) preparations do not possess the vasoconstrictor properties of the natural ergot alkaloids.

DOSAGE AND ADMINISTRATION

1 mg three times daily.
Alleviation of symptoms is usually gradual and results may not be observed for 3-4 weeks.

HOW SUPPLIED

Hydergine tablets (for oral use):
1 mg, round, white, embossed "HYDERGINE 1" on one side, triangle (S) other side. Packages of 100 and 500.
Hydergine sublingual tablets:
1 mg, oval, white, packages of 100 and 1000.
0.5 mg, round, white, packages of 100 and 1000.
Hydergine liquid:
1 mg/ml. Bottles of 100 ml with an accompanying dropper graduated to deliver 1 mg.
Hydergine LC (liquid capsule):
1 mg, oblong, off-white, packages of 100 and 500. (Encapsulated by R. P. Scherer, N.A., Clearwater, Florida 33518)
Company's Product Identification Mark(s): Hydergine Tablets (for oral use): embossed "HYDERGINE" on one side, triangle (S) other side.
Hydergine Sublingual Tablets: 1 mg, embossed "HYDERGINE" on one side, "78-77" other side. 0.5 mg., embossed "HYDERGINE 0.5" on one side, triangle (S) other side.
Hydergine LC (liquid capsules): branded "HYDERGINE LC 1 mg" on one side, triangle (S) other side.

[HYD-ZZ25 Issued October 1, 1985

Shown in Product Identification Section, page 427

KLORVESS® EFFERVESCENT GRANULES, and ℞
[*klor 'ves "*]
KLORVESS® (potassium chloride) 10% LIQUID

The following prescribing information is based on official labeling in effect on June 1, 1986.

DESCRIPTION

KLORVESS® EFFERVESCENT GRANULES: Each packet (2.8 g) contains 20 mEq each of potassium and chloride supplied by potassium chloride 1.125 g, potassium bicarbonate 0.5 g, lysine hydrochloride 0.913 g in a sodium-, sugar- and carbohydrate-free effervescent formulation. Dissolution of the packet contents in water provides the potassium and chloride available for oral ingestion as potassium chloride, potassium bicarbonate, potassium citrate and lysine hydrochloride.
Active Ingredients: lysine hydrochloride, potassium bicarbonate USP and potassium chloride USP
Inactive Ingredients: citric acid, flavorings, polyethylene glycol and saccharin
KLORVESS (potassium chloride) 10% LIQUID: Each tablespoonful (15 ml) contains 20 mEq of potassium chloride (provided by potassium chloride 1.5 g), in a palatable, cherry and pit flavored vehicle, alcohol 0.75%.
Active Ingredient: potassium chloroide USP
Inactive Ingredients: alcohol, malic acid, natural flavor, purified water, saccharin sodium, sodium benzoate and sucrose

INDICATIONS

For the prevention and treatment of potassium depletion and hypokalemic-hypochloremic alkalosis. Deficits of body potassium and chloride can occur as a consequence of therapy with potent diuretic agents and adrenal corticosteroids.

CONTRAINDICATIONS

Severe renal impairment characterized by azotemia or oliguria, untreated Addison's disease, Familial Periodic Paralysis, acute dehydration, heat cramps, patients receiving aldosterone-inhibiting or potassium-sparing diuretic agents, or hyperkalemia from any cause.

PRECAUTIONS

In response to a rise in the concentration of body potassium, renal excretion of the ion is increased. In the presence of normal renal function and hydration, it is difficult to produce potassium intoxication by oral potassium salt supplements.
Since the extent of potassium deficiency cannot be accurately determined, it is prudent to proceed cautiously in undertaking potassium replacement. Periodic evaluations of the patient's clinical status, serum electrolytes and the EKG should be carried out when replacement therapy is undertaken. This is particularly important in patients with cardiac disease and those patients receiving digitalis.
High serum concentrations of potassium may cause death through cardiac depression, arrhythmia or cardiac arrest.
To minimize gastrointestinal irritation associated with potassium chloride preparations, patients should dissolve the packet contents of KLORVESS EFFERVESCENT GRANULES in 3 to 4 ounces of cold water, fruit juice, or other liquid, or dilute each tablespoonful of KLORVESS (potassium chloride) 10% LIQUID in 3 to 4 ounces of cold water. Both of these solutions should be ingested slowly with or immediately after meals.

ADVERSE REACTIONS

Abdominal discomfort, diarrhea, nausea and vomiting may occur with the use of potassium salts.
The symptoms and signs of potassium intoxication include paresthesias, heaviness, muscle weakness and flaccid paralysis of the extremities. Potassium intoxication can produce listlessness, mental confusion, a fall in blood pressure, shock, cardiac arrhythmias, heart block and cardiac arrest.
The EKG picture of hyperkalemia is characterized by the early appearance of tall, peaked T waves. The R wave is decreased in amplitude and the S wave deepens; the QRS complex widens progressively. The P wave widens and decreases in amplitude until it disappears. Occasionally, an apparent elevation of the RS-T junction and a cove plane RS-T segment and T wave will be noted in AVL.

DOSAGE AND ADMINISTRATION

KLORVESS EFFERVESCENT GRANULES: Adults—One packet (20 mEq each of potassium and chloride) completely dissolved in 3 to 4 ounces of cold water, fruit juice or other liquid 2 to 4 times daily depending upon the requirements of the patient.
KLORVESS (potassium chloride) 10% LIQUID: Adults —One tablespoonful (15 ml) of KLORVESS LIQUID (20 mEq of potassium chloride) completely diluted in 3 to 4 ounces of cold water 2 to 4 times daily depending upon the requirements of the patient.
Both of these solutions should be ingested slowly with meals or immediately after eating. Deviations from these recommended dosages may be indicated in certain cases of hypokalemia based upon the patient's status. The average total daily dosage must be governed by the patient's response as determined by frequent evaluation of serum electrolytes, EKG and clinical status.

OVERDOSAGE

Potassium intoxication may result from overdosage of potassium or from therapeutic dosage in conditions stated under "Contraindications." Hyperkalemia, when detected, must be treated immediately because lethal levels can be reached in a few hours.

Treatment of Hyperkalemia:

1. Dextrose solution, 10 or 25% containing 10 units of crystalline insulin per 20 g dextrose, given IV in a dose of 300 to 500 ml in an hour.
2. Absorption and exchange of potassium using sodium or ammonium cycle cation exchange resins, orally and as retention enema. (Caution: Ammonium compounds should not be used in patients with hepatic cirrhosis.)
3. Hemodialysis and peritoneal dialysis.
4. The use of potassium-containing foods or medicaments must be eliminated.

In digitalized patients too rapid a lowering of plasma potassium concentration can cause digitalis toxicity.

HOW SUPPLIED

KLORVESS® EFFERVESCENT GRANULES—packages of 30 packets (2.8 g each). KLORVESS (potassium chloride) 10% LIQUID (dark red) – as a cherry and pit flavored liquid in pint bottles.

[KLO-Z4 Issued February 20, 1986]

KLORVESS® ℞
[*klor 'ves "*]
EFFERVESCENT TABLETS

The following prescribing information is based on official labeling in effect on June 1, 1986.

Continued on next page

Sandoz—Cont.

DESCRIPTION
Each dry, sodium- and sugar-free effervescent tablet contains 20 mEq each of potassium and chloride supplied by potassium chloride 1.125 g, potassium bicarbonate 0.5 g, lysine hydrochloride 0.913 g. Dissolution of the tablet in water provides the potassium and chloride available for oral ingestion as potassium chloride, potassium bicarbonate, potassium citrate and lysine hydrochloride
Active Ingredients: lysine hydrochloride, potassium bicarbonate USP and potassium chloride USP
Inactive Ingredients: citric acid, flavorings, polyethylene glycol and saccharin

INDICATIONS
For the prevention and treatment of potassium depletion and hypokalemic-hypochloremic alkalosis. Deficits of body potassium and chloride can occur as a consequence of therapy with potent diuretic agents and adrenal corticosteroids.

CONTRAINDICATIONS
Severe renal impairment characterized by azotemia or oliguria, untreated Addison's disease, Familial Periodic Paralysis, acute dehydration, heat cramps, patients receiving aldosterone-inhibiting or potassium-sparing diuretic agents, or hyperkalemia from any cause.

PRECAUTIONS
In response to a rise in the concentration of body potassium, renal excretion of the ion is increased. In the presence of normal renal function and hydration, it is difficult to produce potassium intoxication by oral potassium salt supplements.
Since the extent of potassium deficiency cannot be accurately determined, it is prudent to proceed cautiously in undertaking potassium replacement. Periodic evaluations of the patient's clinical status, serum electrolytes and the EKG should be carried out when replacement therapy is undertaken. This is particularly important in patients with cardiac disease and those patients receiving digitalis.
High serum concentrations of potassium may cause death through cardiac depression, arrhythmia or cardiac arrest.
To minimize gastrointestinal irritation associated with potassium chloride preparations, patients should dissolve each Klorvess® Effervescent Tablet in 3 or 4 ounces of water or fruit juice. This solution should be ingested slowly with or immediately after meals.

ADVERSE REACTIONS
Abdominal discomfort, diarrhea, nausea and vomiting may occur with the use of potassium salts.
The symptoms and signs of potassium intoxication include paresthesias, heaviness, muscle weakness and flaccid paralysis of the extremities. Potassium intoxication can produce listlessness, mental confusion, a fall in blood pressure, shock, cardiac arrhythmias, heart block and cardiac arrest.
The EKG picture of hyperkalemia is characterized by the early appearance of tall, peaked T waves. The R wave is decreased in amplitude and the S wave deepens; the QRS complex widens progressively. The P wave widens and decreases in amplitude until it disappears. Occasionally, an apparent elevation of the RS-T junction and a cove-plane RS-T segment and T wave will be noted in AVL.

DOSAGE AND ADMINISTRATION
Adults—One Klorvess Effervescent Tablet (20 mEq each of potassium and chloride) completely dissolved in 3 to 4 ounces of cold water or fruit juice 2 to 4 times daily depending upon the requirements of the patient.
The solution should be ingested slowly with meals or immediately after eating. Deviations from these recommended dosages may be indicated in certain cases of hypokalemia based upon the patient's status. The average total daily dosage must be governed by the patient's response as determined by frequent evaluation of serum electrolytes, EKG and clinical status.

OVERDOSAGE
Potassium intoxication may result from overdosage of potassium or from therapeutic dosage in conditions stated under "Contraindications." Hyperkalemia, when detected, must be treated immediately because lethal levels can be reached in a few hours.

Treatment of Hyperkalemia:
1. Dextrose solution, 10 or 25% containing 10 units of crystalline insulin per 20 g dextrose, given I.V. in a dose of 300 to 500 ml in an hour.
2. Adsorption and exchange of potassium using sodium or ammonium cycle cation exchange resins, orally and as retention enema. (Caution: Ammonium compounds should not be used in patients with hepatic cirrhosis.)
3. Hemodialysis and peritoneal dialysis.
4. The use of potassium-containing foods or medicaments must be eliminated.

In digitalized patients too rapid a lowering of plasma potassium concentration can cause digitalis toxicity.

HOW SUPPLIED
Klorvess Effervescent Tablets (white)—60 tablets. Each tablet is individually foil wrapped. Klorvess® Tablets are also available in institutional packages of 30 and 1000 tablets.
[KLO-ZZ3 Issued February 20, 1986
Shown in Product Identification Section, page 427

MELLARIL® ℞
[mel'ah-ril"]
(thioridazine) HCl tablets, USP
(thioridazine) HCl oral solution, USP
MELLARIL-S®
(thioridazine) oral suspension, USP

The following prescribing information is based on official labeling in effect on June 16, 1986.

DESCRIPTION
Mellaril® (thioridazine) is 2- methylmercapto -10- [2 - (N-methyl -2- piperidyl) ethyl] phenothiazine.
The presence of a thiomethyl radical ($S\text{-}CH_3$) in position 2, conventionally occupied by a halogen, is unique and could account for the greater toleration obtained with recommended doses of thioridazine as well as a greater specificity of psychotherapeutic action.
10 mg, 15 mg, 25 mg, 50 mg, 100 mg, 150 mg, 200 mg Tablets
Active Ingredient: thioridazine HCl, USP
10 mg, Tablets
Inactive Ingredients: acacia, calcium sulfate dihydrate, carnauba wax, D&C Yellow #10, FD&C Blue #1, FD&C Yellow #6, gelatin, lactose, mixed parabens, povidone, sodium benzoate, starch, stearic acid, sucrose, talc, titanium dioxide, and another ingredient
15 mg Tablets
Inactive Ingredients: acacia, calcium sulfate dihydrate, carnauba wax, D&C Red #7, gelatin, lactose, mixed parabens, povidone, starch, stearic acid, sucrose, talc, titanium dioxide, and another ingredient
25 mg, Tablets
Inactive Ingredients: acacia, calcium sulfate dihydrate, carnauba wax, gelatin, lactose, methylparaben, povidone, propylparaben, sodium benzoate, starch, stearic acid, sucrose, synthetic iron oxide, talc, titanium dioxide, and another ingredient
50 mg Tablets
Inactive Ingredients: acacia, calcium sulfate dihydrate, carnauba wax, gelatin, lactose, sodium benzoate, starch, stearic acid, sucrose, talc, titanium dioxide, and other ingredients
100 mg, Tablets
Inactive Ingredients: acacia, calcium sulfate dihydrate, carnauba wax, D&C Yellow #10, FD&C Blue #1, FD&C Blue #2, FD&C Yellow #6 lactose, povidone, sodium benzoate, sorbitol, starch, stearic acid, sucrose, talc, titanium dioxide, and other ingredients
150 mg, Tablets
Inactive Ingredients: acacia, calcium sulfate dihydrate, carnauba wax, D&C Yellow #10, FD&C Green #3, FD&C Yellow #6, lactose, methylparaben, povidone, propylparaben, sodium benzoate, starch, steric acid, sucrose, talc, titanium dioxide, and other ingredients
200 mg, Tablets
Inactive Ingredients: acacia, calcium sulfate dihydrate, carnauba wax, D&C Red #7, gelatin, lactose, magnesium stearate, mixed parabens, povidone, starch, stearic acid, sucrose, talc, titanium dioxide, and other ingredients
30 mg, and 100 mg, Concentrate
Active Ingredient: thioridazine HCl, USP
30 mg, Concentrate
Inactive Ingredients: alcohol, 3.0%, flavor, mixed parabens, purified water, and sorbitol solution
100 mg, Concentrate
Inactive Ingredients: alcohol 4.2%, flavor, glycerin, mixed parabens, purified water, sorbitol solution, and sucrose. May contain sodium hydroxide or hydrochloric acid to adjust pH.
25 mg, and 100 mg, Suspension
Active Ingredient: thioridazine base
25 mg, Suspension
Inactive Ingredients: carbopol, flavor, polysorbate, purified water, sodium hydroxide, and sucrose
100 mg, Suspension
Inactive Ingredients: carbopol, D&C Yellow #10, FD&C Yellow #6, flavor, polysorbate, purified water, sodium hydroxide, and sucrose

CLINICAL PHARMACOLOGY
Mellaril (thioridazine) is effective in reducing excitement, hypermotility, abnormal initiative, affective tension and agitation through its inhibitory effect on psychomotor functions. Successful modification of such symptoms is the prerequisite for, and often the beginning of, the process of recovery in patients exhibiting mental and emotional disturbances.
Thioridazine's basic pharmacological activity is similar to that of other phenothiazines, but certain specific qualities have come to light which support the observation that the clinical spectrum of this drug shows significant differences from those of the other agents of this class. Minimal antiemetic activity and minimal extrapyramidal stimulation, notably pseudoparkinsonism, are distinctive features of this drug.

INDICATIONS
For the management of manifestations of psychotic disorders.
For the short-term treatment of moderate to marked depression with variable degrees of anxiety in adult patients and for the treatment of multiple symptoms such as agitation, anxiety, depressed mood, tension, sleep disturbances, and fears in geriatric patients.
For the treatment of severe behavioral problems in children marked by combativeness and/or explosive hyperexcitable behavior (out of proportion to immediate provocations), and in the short-term treatment of hyperactive children who show excessive motor activity with accompanying conduct disorders consisting of some or all of the following symptoms: impulsivity, difficulty sustaining attention, aggressivity, mood lability, and poor frustration tolerance.

CONTRAINDICATIONS
In common with other phenothiazines, Mellaril (thioridazine) is contraindicated in severe central nervous system depression or comatose states from any cause. It should also be noted that hypertensive or hypotensive heart disease of extreme degree is a contraindication of phenothiazine administration.

WARNINGS
Tardive Dyskinesia: Tardive dyskinesia, a syndrome consisting of potentially irreversible, involuntary, dyskinetic movements may develop in patients treated with neuroleptic (antipsychotic) drugs. Although the prevalence of the syndrome appears to be highest among the elderly, especially elderly women, it is impossible to rely upon prevalence estimates to predict, at the inception of neuroleptic treatment, which patients are likely to develop the syndrome. Whether neuroleptic drug products differ in their potential to cause tardive dyskinesia is unknown.
Both the risk of developing the syndrome and the likelihood that it will become irreversible are believed to increase as the duration of treatment and the total cumulative dose of neuroleptic drugs administered to the patient increase. However, the syndrome can develop, although much less commonly, after relatively brief treatment periods at low doses.
There is no known treatment for established cases of tardive dyskinesia, although the syndrome may remit, partially or completely, if neuroleptic treatment is withdrawn. Neuroleptic treatment, itself, however, may suppress (or partially suppress) the signs and symptoms of the syndrome and thereby may possibly mask the underlying disease process. The effect that symptomatic suppression has upon the long-term course of the syndrome is unknown.
Given these considerations, neuroleptics should be prescribed in a manner that is most likely to minimize the occurrence of tardive dyskinesia. Chronic neuroleptic treatment should generally be reserved for patients who suffer from a chronic illness that, 1) is known to respond to neuroleptic drugs, and, 2) for whom alternative, equally effective, but potentially less harmful treatments are *not* available or appropriate. In patients who do require chronic treatment, the smallest dose and the shortest duration of treatment producing a satisfactory clinical response should be sought. The need for continued treatment should be reassessed periodically.
If signs and symptoms of tardive dyskinesia appear in a patient on neuroleptics, drug discontinuation should be considered. However, some patients may require treatment despite the presence of the syndrome.
(For further information about the description of tardive dyskinesia and its clinical detection, please refer to the sections on Information for Patients and Adverse Reactions.)
It has been suggested in regard to phenothiazines in general, that people who have demonstrated a hypersensitivity reaction (e.g. blood dyscrasias, jaundice) to one may be more prone to demonstrate a reaction to others. Attention should be paid to the fact that phenothiazines are capable of potentiating central nervous system depressants (e.g. anesthetics, opiates, alcohol, etc.) as well as atropine and phosphorus insecticides. Physicians should carefully consider benefit versus risk when treating less severe disorders.
Reproductive studies in animals and clinical experience to date have failed to show a teratogenic effect with Mellaril (thioridazine). However, in view of the desirability of keeping the administration of all drugs to a minimum during pregnancy. Mellaril (thioridazine) should be given only when the benefits derived from treatment exceed the possible risks to mother and fetus.

PRECAUTIONS
Leukopenia and/or agranulocytosis and convulsive seizures have been reported but are infrequent. Mellaril (thioridazine) has been shown to be helpful in the treatment of behav-

ioral disorders in epileptic patients, but anticonvulsant medication should also be maintained. Pigmentary retinopathy, which has been observed primarily in patients taking larger than recommended doses, is characterized by diminution of visual acuity, brownish coloring of vision, and impairment of night vision; examination of the fundus discloses deposits of pigment. The possibility of this complication may be reduced by remaining within the recommended limits of dosage.

Where patients are participating in activities requiring complete mental alertness (e.g., driving) it is advisable to administer the phenothiazines cautiously and to increase the dosage gradually. Female patients appear to have a greater tendency to orthostatic hypotension than male patients. The administration of epinephrine should be avoided in the treatment of drug-induced hypotension in view of the fact that phenothiazines may induce a reversed epinephrine effect on occasion. Should a vasoconstrictor be required, the most suitable are levarterenol and phenylephrine.

Neuroleptic drugs elevate prolactin levels; the elevation persists during chronic administration. Tissue culture experiments indicate that approximately one-third of human breast cancers are prolactin dependent in vitro, a factor of potential importance if the prescription of these drugs is contemplated in a patient with a previously detected breast cancer. Although disturbances such as galactorrhea, amenorrhea, gynecomastia, and impotence have been reported, the clinical significance of elevated serum prolactin levels is unknown for most patients. An increase in mammary neoplasms has been found in rodents after chronic administration of neuroleptic drugs. Neither clinical studies nor epidemiologic studies conducted to date, however, have shown an association between chronic administration of these drugs and mammary tumorigenesis; the available evidence is considered too limited to be conclusive at this time.

It is recommended that a daily dose in excess of 300 mg. be reserved for use only in severe neuropsychiatric conditions.

Information for Patients: Given the likelihood that some patients exposed chronically to neuroleptics will develop tardive dyskinesia, it is advised that all patients in whom chronic use is contemplated be given, if possible, full information about this risk. The decision to inform patients and/or their guardians must obviously take into account the clinical circumstances and the competency of the patient to understand the information provided.

ADVERSE REACTIONS

In the recommended dosage ranges with Mellaril (thioridazine), most side effects are mild and transient.

Central Nervous System: Drowsiness may be encountered on occasion, especially where large doses are given early in treatment. Generally, this effect tends to subside with continued therapy or a reduction in dosage. Pseudoparkinsonism and other extrapyramidal symptoms may occur but are infrequent. Nocturnal confusion, hyperactivity, lethargy, psychotic reactions, restlessness and headache have been reported but are extremely rare.

Autonomic Nervous System: Dryness of mouth, blurred vision, constipation, nausea, vomiting, diarrhea, nasal stuffiness, and pallor have been seen.

Endocrine System: Galactorrhea, breast engorgement, amenorrhea, inhibition of ejaculation and peripheral edema have been described.

Skin: Dermatitis and skin eruptions of the urticarial type have been observed infrequently. Photosensitivity is extremely rare.

Cardiovascular System: ECG changes have been reported (see Phenothiazine Derivatives: Cardiovascular Effects).

Other: Rare cases described as parotid swelling have been reported following administration of Mellaril (thioridazine).

Phenothiazine Derivatives: It should be noted that efficacy, indications and untoward effects have varied with the different phenothiazines. It has been reported that old age lowers the tolerance for phenothiazines. The most common neurological side effects in these patients are parkinsonism and akathisia. There appears to be an increased risk of agranulocytosis and leukopenia in the geriatric population. The physician should be aware that the following have occurred with one or more phenothiazines and should be considered whenever one of these drugs is used:

Autonomic Reactions: Miosis, obstipation, anorexia, paralytic ileus.

Cutaneous Reactions: Erythema, exfoliative dermatitis, contact dermatitis.

Blood Dyscrasias: Agranulocytosis, leukopenia, eosinophilia, thrombocytopenia, anemia, aplastic anemia, pancytopenia.

Allergic Reactions: Fever, laryngeal edema, angioneurotic edema, asthma.

Hepatotoxicity: Jaundice, biliary stasis.

Cardiovascular Effects: Changes in the terminal portion of the electrocardiogram, including prolongation of the Q-T interval, lowering and inversion of the T-wave and appearance of a wave tentatively identified as a bifid T or a U wave have been observed in some patients receiving the phenothiazine tranquilizers, including Mellaril (thioridazine). To date, these appear to be due to altered repolarization and not related to myocardial damage. They appear to be reversible. While there is no evidence at present that these changes are in any way precursors of any significant disturbance of cardiac rhythm, it should be noted that several sudden and unexpected deaths apparently due to cardiac arrest have occurred in patients previously showing characteristic electrocardiographic changes while taking the drug. The use of periodic electrocardiograms has been proposed but would appear to be of questionable value as a predictive device. Hypotension, rarely resulting in cardiac arrest.

Extrapyramidal Symptoms: Akathisia, agitation, motor restlessness, dystonic reactions, trismus, torticollis, opisthotonus, oculogyric crises, tremor, muscular rigidity, akinesia.

Tardive Dyskinesia: Chronic use of neuroleptics may be associated with the development of tardive dyskinesia. The salient features of this syndrome are described in the WARNINGS section and below.

The syndrome is characterized by involuntary choreoathetoid movements which variously involve the tongue, face, mouth, lips, or jaw (e.g. protrusion of the tongue, puffing of cheeks, puckering of the mouth, chewing movements), trunk and extremities. The severity of the syndrome and the degree of impairment produced vary widely.

The syndrome may become clinically recognizable either during treatment, upon dosage reduction, or upon withdrawal of treatment. Movements may decrease in intensity and may disappear altogether if further treatment with neuroleptics is withheld. It is generally believed that reversibility is more likely after short rather than long-term neuroleptic exposure. Consequently, early detection of tardive dyskinesia is important. To increase the likelihood of detecting the syndrome at the earliest possible time, the dosage of neuroleptic drug should be reduced periodically (if clinically possible) and the patient observed for signs of the disorder. This maneuver is critical, for neuroleptic drugs may mask the signs of the syndrome.

Endocrine Disturbances: Menstrual irregularities, altered libido, gynecomastia, lactation, weight gain, edema. False positive pregnancy tests have been reported.

Urinary Disturbances: Retention, incontinence.

Others: Hyperpyrexia. Behavioral effects suggestive of a paradoxical reaction have been reported. These include excitement, bizarre dreams, aggravation of psychoses, and toxic confusional states. More recently, a peculiar skin-eye syndrome has been recognized as a side effect following long-term treatment with phenothiazines. This reaction is marked by progressive pigmentation of areas of the skin or conjunctiva and/or accompanied by discoloration of the exposed sclera and cornea. Opacities of the anterior lens and cornea described as irregular or stellate in shape have also been reported. Systemic lupus erythematosus-like syndrome.

DOSAGE

Dosage must be individualized according to the degree of mental and emotional disburbance. In all cases, the smallest effective dosage should be determined for each patient.

Adults: *Psychotic manifestations:* The usual starting dose is 50 to 100 mg. three times a day, with a gradual increment to a maximum of 800 mg. daily if necessary. Once effective control of symptoms has been achieved, the dosage may be reduced gradually to determine the minimum maintenance dose. The total daily dosage ranges from 200 to 800 mg, divided into two to four doses.

For the short-term treatment of moderate to marked depression with variable degrees of anxiety in adult patients and for the treatment of multiple symptoms such as agitation, anxiety, depressed mood, tension, sleep disturbances, and fears in geriatric patients: The usual starting dose is 25 mg three times a day. Dosage ranges from 10 mg two to four times a day in milder cases to 50 mg three or four times a day for more severely disturbed patients. The total daily dosage range is from 20 mg to a maximum of 200 mg.

Children: Mellaril (thioridazine) is not intended for children under 2 years of age. For children aged 2 to 12 the dosage of thioridazine hydrochloride ranges from 0.5 mg to a maximum of 3.0 mg/Kg per day. For children with moderate disorders 10 mg two or three times a day is the usual starting dose. For hospitalized, severely disturbed, or psychotic children, 25 mg two or three times daily is the usual starting dose. Dosage may be increased gradually until optimum therapeutic effect is obtained or the maximum has been reached.

HOW SUPPLIED

MELLARIL (thioridazine) HCl

Tablets: 10 mg, 15 mg, 25 mg, 50 mg, 100 mg, 150 mg and 200 mg thioridazine hydrochloride, USP. Packages of 100 and 1000 tablets. Also, for wholly tax-supported institutions only, packages of 4800 (48 × 100) and 5000 tablets.

Concentrate—30 mg/ml: Each ml contains 30 mg thioridazine hydrochloride, USP, alcohol, USP, 3.0% by volume. Immediate containers: Amber glass bottles of 4 fl. oz (118 ml) as follows:

4 fl. oz bottles, in cartons of 12 bottles, with an accompanying dropper graduated to deliver 10 mg, 25 mg and 50 mg of thioridazine hydrochloride, USP. Also, for wholly tax-supported institutions only, gallon cartons of 32 x 4 oz. bottles, each with the same dropper.

Concentrate—100 mg/ml: Each ml contains 100 mg thioridazine hydrochloride, USP, alcohol, 4.2% by volume, *4 fl. oz bottles,* in cartons of 12 bottles, with an accompanying dropper graduated to deliver 100 mg, 150 mg and 200 mg of thioridazine hydrochloride.

REMARKS

Store and dispense: Below 86°F; tight, amber glass bottle. The Concentrate may be diluted with distilled water, acidified tap water, or suitable juices. Each dose should be so diluted just prior to administration—preparation and storage of bulk dilutions is not recommended.

MELLARIL-S (thioridazine)

Suspension—25 mg/5 ml: Each 5 ml contains thioridazine, USP, equivalent to 25 mg thioridazine hydrochloride, USP. Buttermint-flavored in pint bottles.

Suspension—100 mg/5 ml: Each 5 ml contains thioridazine, USP, equivalent to 100 mg thioridazine hydrochloride, USP. Buttermint-flavored in pint bottles.

Store and dispense: Below 77°F; tight, amber glass bottle. Additional information available to physicians.

Company's Product Identification Mark(s): 10 mg and 15 mg tablets branded with NDC number on one side, triangle (S) other side. All other tablet strengths branded MELLARIL on one side, triangle (S) other side.

[MEL-Z39 Issued June 16, 1986]

Shown in Product Identification Section, page 427

MESANTOIN® Tablets ℞

[meh-san 'toyn]

(mephenytoin) tablets, USP

The following prescribing information is based on official labeling in effect on October 15, 1986.

DESCRIPTION

Mesantoin® (mephenytoin) is 3- methyl 5,5-phenyl-ethyl-hydantoin. It may be considered to be the hydantoin homolog of the barbiturate mephobarbital.

Active Ingredient: mephenytoin, USP

Inactive Ingredients: D&C Red #7, gelatin, lactose, starch, stearic acid and sucrose

ACTIONS

Mephenytoin exhibits pharmacologic effects similar to both diphenylhydantoin and the barbiturates in antagonizing experimental seizures in laboratory animals. Mephenytoin produces behavioral and electroencephalographic effects in man which are similar to those produced by barbiturates.

INDICATIONS

For the control of grand mal, focal, Jacksonian, and psychomotor seizures in those patients who have been refractory to less toxic anticonvulsants.

CONTRAINDICATIONS

Hypersensitivity to hydantoin products.

WARNINGS

Mephenytoin should be used only after safer anticonvulsants have been given an adequate trial and have failed.

As with all anticonvulsants, dose reduction must be gradual so as to minimize the risk of precipitating seizures.

Patients should be cautioned about possible additive effects of alcohol and other CNS depressants. Acute alcohol intoxication may increase the anticonvulsant effect due to decreased metabolic breakdown. Chronic alcohol abuse may result in decreased anticonvulsant effect due to enzyme induction.

USAGE IN PREGNANCY

The effects of mephenytoin in human pregnancy and nursing infants are unknown.

Recent reports suggest an association between the use of anticonvulsant drugs by women with epilepsy and an elevated incidence of birth defects in children born to these women. Data are more extensive with respect to diphenylhydantoin and phenobarbital, but these are also the most commonly prescribed anticonvulsants; less systematic or anecdotal reports suggest a possible similar association with the use of all known anticonvulsant drugs.

The reports suggesting an elevated incidence of birth defects in children of drug-treated epileptic women cannot be regarded as adequate to prove a definite cause and effect relationship. There are intrinsic methodologic problems in obtaining adequate data on drug teratogenicity in humans; the possibility also exists that other factors, e.g., genetic factors or the epileptic condition itself, may be more important than drug therapy in leading to birth defects. The great majority of mothers on anticonvulsant medication deliver normal infants. It is important to note that anticonvulsant drugs should not be discontinued in patients in whom the drug is administered to prevent major seizures because of the strong

Continued on next page

Sandoz—Cont.

possibility of precipitating status epilepticus with attendant hypoxia and threat to life. In individual cases where the severity and frequency of the seizure disorder are such that the removal of medication does not pose a serious threat to the patient, discontinuation of the drug may be considered prior to and during pregnancy, although it cannot be said with any confidence that even minor seizures do not pose some hazards to the developing embryo or fetus.
The prescribing physician will wish to weigh these considerations in treating or counseling epileptic women of childbearing potential.

PRECAUTIONS

The patient taking Mesantoin® (mephenytoin) must be kept under close medical supervision at all times since serious adverse reactions may emerge.
Because the primary site of degradation is the liver, it is recommended that screening tests of liver function precede introduction of the drug.
Some patients may show side reactions as the result of individual sensitivity. These reactions can be broken down into three types respectively according to severity: 1) blood dyscrasias; 2) skin and mucous membrane manifestations; and 3) central effects. The blood, skin and mucous membrane manifestations are the more important since they can be more serious in nature. Since mephenytoin has been reported to produce blood dyscrasia in certain instances, the patient must be instructed that in the event any unusual symptoms develop (e.g. sore throat, fever, mucous membrane bleeding, glandular swelling, cutaneous reaction), he must discontinue the drug and report for examination immediately. It is recommended that blood examinations be made (total white cell count and differential count) during the initial phase of administration. Such tests are best made: a) before starting medication; b) after 2 weeks on a low dosage; c) again after 2 weeks when full dosage is reached; d) thereafter, monthly for a year; e) from then on, every 3 months. If the neutrophils drop to between 2500 and 1600/cu.mm., counts are made every 2 weeks. Stop medication if the count drops to 1600.

ADVERSE REACTIONS

A number of side effects and toxic reactions have been reported with Mesantoin (mephenytoin) as well as with other hydantoin compounds. Many of these appear to be dose related while others seem to be a manifestation of a hypersensitivity reaction to these drugs.

Blood Dyscrasias
Leukopenia, neutropenia, agranulocytosis, thrombocytopenia and pancytopenia have occurred. Eosinophilia, monocytosis, and leukocytosis have been described. Simple anemia, hemolytic anemia, megaloblastic anemia and aplastic anemia have occurred but are uncommon.

Skin and Mucous Membrane Manifestations
Maculopapular, morbilliform, scarlatiniform, urticarial, purpuric (associated with thrombocytopenia) and non-specific skin rashes have been reported. Exfoliative dermatitis, erythema multiforme (Stevens-Johnson Syndrome), toxic epidermal necrolysis and fatal dermatitides have been described on rare occasions. Skin pigmentation and rashes associated with a lupus erythematosus syndrome have also been reported.

Central Effects
Drowsiness is dose-related and may be reduced by a reduction in dose. Ataxia, diplopia, nystagmus, dysarthria, fatigue, irritability, choreiform movements, depression and tremor have been encountered.
Nervousness, nausea, vomiting, sleeplessness and dizziness may occur during the initial stages of therapy. Generally, these symptoms are transient, often disappearing with continued treatment.
Mental confusion and psychotic disturbances and increased seizures have been reported, but a definite causal relationship with the drug is uncertain.

Miscellaneous
Hepatitis, jaundice and nephrosis have been reported but a definite cause and effect relationship between the drug and these effects has not been established.
Alopecia, weight gain, edema, photophobia, conjunctivitis and gum hyperplasia have been encountered.
Polyarthropathy, pulmonary fibrosis, lupus erythematosus syndrome, and lymphadenopathy which simulates Hodgkin's Disease have also been observed.

DOSAGE AND ADMINISTRATION

Dosage of antiepileptic therapy should be adjusted to the needs of the individual patient. Maintenance dosage is that smallest amount of antiepileptic necessary to suppress seizures completely or reduce their frequency. Optimum dosage is attained by starting with ½ or 1 tablet of Mesantoin (mephenytoin) per day during the first week and thereafter increasing the daily dose by ½ or 1 tablet at weekly intervals. No dose should be increased until it has been taken for at least one week.
The average dose of Mesantoin for adults ranges from 2 to 6 tablets (0.2 to 0.6 Gm.) daily. In some instances it may be necessary to administer as much as 8 tablets or more daily in order to obtain full seizure control. Children usually require from 1 to 4 tablets (0.1 Gm. to 0.4 Gm.) according to nature of seizures and age.
When the physician wishes to replace the anticonvulsant now being employed with Mesantoin (mephenytoin), he should give ½ or 1 tablet of Mesantoin daily during the first week and gradually increase the daily dose at weekly intervals while gradually reducing that of the drug being discontinued. The transition can be made smoothly over a period of three to six weeks. If seizures are not completely controlled with the dose so attained, the daily dose should then be increased by a one-tablet increment at weekly intervals to the point of maximum effect. If the patient had also been receiving phenobarbital, it is well to continue it until the transition is completed, at which time gradual withdrawal of the phenobarbital may be tried.

HOW SUPPLIED

Each tablet contains 100 mg mephenytoin and is scored to permit half-tablet dosage. Packages of 100 tablets. (Pale pink, compressed, scored).
Company's Product Identification Mark(s): Tablets embossed 78-52 and scored on one side, triangle S SANDOZ other side.

[MES—Z16 Issued October 15, 1986]
Shown in Product Identification Section, page 427

METAPREL® ℞

(metaproterenol sulfate USP)
Syrup—10 mg/5 ml
Tablets 10 mg; 20 mg
Oral Bronchodilator

The following prescribing information is based on official labeling in effect on August 1, 1986.

DESCRIPTION

Syrup: Each 5 ml of Metaprel (metaproterenol sulfate) syrup contains metaproterenol sulfate USP 10 mg. Inactive Ingredients: edetate disodium, flavor, hydroxyethyl cellulose, methylparaben, propylparaben, purified water, Red 40, saccharin, sorbitol.
Tablets: Each Metaprel (metaproterenol sulfate) tablet, 10 mg and 20 mg, contains metaproterenol sulfate USP 10 mg and 20 mg respectively.
Other Ingredients: colloidal silicon dioxide, dibasic calcium phosphate, lactose, magnesium stearate, starch.
Chemically, Metaprel (metaproterenol sulfate) is 1-(3, 5-dihydroxyphenyl)-2-isopropyl-aminoethanol sulfate, a white, crystalline, racemic mixture of two optically active isomers. It differs from isoproterenol hydrochloride by having two hydroxyl groups attached at the meta positions on the benzene ring rather than one at the meta and one at the para position.

ACTIONS

Metaprel (metaproterenol sulfate) is a potent beta-adrenergic stimulator. It is postulated that beta-adrenergic stimulants produce many of their pharmacological effects by activation of adenyl cyclase, the enzyme which catalyzes the conversion of adenosine triphosphate to cyclic adenosine monophosphate.
Absorption, biotransformation and excretion studies in humans following oral administration, have indicated that an average of 40 percent of the drug is absorbed; it is not metabolized by catechol-O-methyltransferase or sulfatase enzymes in the gut but is excreted primarily as glucuronic acid conjugates.
Syrup: When administered orally, Metaprel (metaproterenol sulfate) decreases reversible bronchospasm. Pulmonary function tests performed after the administration of Metaprel (metaproterenol sulfate) usually show improvement, e.g., an increase in the one-second forced expiratory volume (FEV_1), an increase in maximum expiratory flow rate, an increase in peak expiratory flow rate, an increase in forced vital capacity, and/or a decrease in airway resistance. The decrease in airway obstruction may relieve the dyspnea associated with bronchospasm. Pulmonary function has been monitored in controlled single-and multiple-dose studies. The duration of effect of a single dose of Metaprel (metaproterenol sulfate) Syrup (that is, the period of time during which there is a 15 percent or greater increase in mean FEV_1) was up to four hours.
Tablets: When administered orally, Metaprel (metaproterenol sulfate) decreases reversible bronchospasm. Pulmonary function tests performed concomitantly usually show improvement following Metaprel (metaproterenol sulfate) administration, e.g., an increase in the one-second forced expiratory volume (FEV_1), an increase in maximum expiratory flow rate, an increase in forced vital capacity, and/or a decrease in airway resistance. The resultant decrease in airway obstruction may relieve the dyspnea associated with bronchospasm.
Controlled single- and multiple-dose studies have been performed with pulmonary function monitoring. The mean duration of effect of a single dose of 20 mg of Metaprel (metaproterenol sulfate) (that is, the period of time during which there is a 15 percent or greater increase in FEV_1) was up to four hours. Four controlled multiple-dose 60-day studies, comparing the effectiveness of metaproterenol sulfate tablets with ephedrine tablets, have been performed. Because of difficulties in study design, only one study was available which could be analyzed in depth. This study showed a loss of efficacy with time for both metaproterenol sulfate and ephedrine. Therefore, the physician should take this phenomenon into account in evaluating the individual patient's overall management. Further studies are in progress to adequately explain these results.
Recent studies in laboratory animals (minipigs, rodents and dogs), recorded the occurrence of cardiac arrhythmias and sudden death (with histologic evidence of myocardial necrosis) when beta agonists and methylxanthines were administered concurrently. The significance of these findings when applied to humans is currently unknown.

INDICATIONS

Metaprel (metaproterenol sulfate) is indicated as a bronchodilator for bronchial asthma, and for reversible bronchospasm which may occur in association with bronchitis and emphysema.

CONTRAINDICATIONS

Use in patients with cardiac arrhythmias associated with tachycardia is contraindicated.
Although rare, immediate hypersensitivity reactions can occur. Therefore, Metaprel (metaproterenol sulfate) is contraindicated in patients with a history of hypersensitivity to any of its components.

PRECAUTIONS

Extreme care must be exercised with respect to the administration of additional sympathomimetic agents. A sufficient interval of time should elapse prior to administration of another sympathomimetic agent.
Because metaproterenol sulfate is a sympathomimetic drug, it should be used with great caution in patients with hypertension, coronary artery disease, congestive heart failure, hyperthyroidism and diabetes, or when there is sensitivity to sympathomimetic amines.
Usage in Pregnancy: Safety in pregnancy has not been established. Metaproterenol should not be used except with caution during pregnancy, weighing the drug's benefit to the patient against potential risk to the fetus. Studies of metaproterenol in mice, rats and rabbits have revealed no significant teratogenic effects at oral doses up to 50 mg/kg (31 times the recommended daily human oral dose). In rabbits, fetal loss and teratogenic effects have been observed at and above oral doses of 50 and 100 mg/kg, respectively.

ADVERSE REACTIONS

Adverse reactions such as tachycardia, hypertension, palpitations, nervousness, tremor, nausea and vomiting have been reported. These reactions are similar to those noted with other sympathomimetic agents.

DOSAGE AND ADMINISTRATION

Syrup: Children aged 6–9 years or weight under 60 lbs—one teaspoonful three or four times a day. Children over 9 years or weight over 60 lbs—two teaspoonfuls three or four times a day. Experience in children under the age of six is limited to seventy-eight children. Of this number, forty were treated with metaproterenol sulfate for at least one month. In this group, daily doses of approximately 1.3 to 2.6 mg/kg were well tolerated. Adults—two teaspoonfuls three or four times a day.
Tablets: The usual adult dose is 20 mg three or four times a day. Children aged 6–9 years or weight under 60 lbs—10 mg three or four times a day. Over 9 years or weight over 60 lbs—20 mg three or four times a day. Metaprel tablets are not recommended for use in children under 6 years at this time. (Please refer to the Actions section for further information on clinical experience with this product.)
If Metaprel (metaproterenol sulfate) is administered before or after other sympathomimetic bronchodilators, caution should be exercised with respect to possible protentiation of adrenergic effects.

SYMPTOMS OF OVERDOSAGE

The symptoms of overdosage are those of excessive beta-adrenergic stimulation listed under Adverse Reactions.

HOW SUPPLIED

Syrup: Metaprel (metaproterenol sulfate) is available as a cherry-flavored syrup, 10 mg per teaspoonful (5 ml), in pint bottles.
Tablets: Metaprel (metaproterenol sulfate) Tablets, 10 mg, white, scored, round, imprinted "78-212" on one side, "10" on the other. Metaprel (metaproterenol sulfate) Tablets, 20 mg, white, scored, round, imprinted "78-213" on one side, "20" on the other. Both strengths are available in bottles of 100.
Metaprel is also available as a micronized powder in 15 cc metered dose inhalers and as a 5% inhalant solution in bot-

tles of 10 ml. For details on Metaprel (metaproterenol sulfate) Metered Dose Inhalers and Metaprel (metaproterenol sulfate) Inhalant Solution 5% please refer to separate Product Information.

CAUTION

Federal law prohibits dispensing without prescription.
Under license from
Boehringer Ingelheim Pharmaceuticals, Inc.
[MTP-Z2 Issued August 1, 1986]
Shown in Product Identification Section, page 427

METHERGINE® ℞

[meth 'er-gin]
(methylergonovine maleate) injection, USP
(methylergonovine maleate) tablets, USP

The following prescribing information is based on official labeling in effect on June 1, 1986.

DESCRIPTION

Each Methergine® (methylergovine maleate) *Tablet* contains 0.2 mg (1/320 gr.) methylergonovine maleate, USP Methergine *Injection* contains per ml: 0.2 mg (1/320 gr.) methylergonovine maleate, USP; 0.25 mg tartaric acid, NF; 3 mg sodium chloride, USP; and water for injection, USP, q.s. to 1 ml.
Methergine (methylergonovine maleate) is the first semisynthetic ergot alkaloid available for therapeutic application—the prevention and control of postpartum hemmorhage.
Active Ingredient: methylergonovine maleate, USP
Inactive Ingredients: D&C Red #7, FD&C Blue #1, lactose, mixed parabens, providone, sodium benzoate, starch, stearic acid, sucrose, talc, and titanium dioxide

ACTION

Methergine (methylergovine maleate) induces a rapid and sustained tetanic uterotonic effect which shortens the third stage of labor and reduces blood loss. The onset of action after i.v. administration is immediate; after i.m. administration, 2 to 5 minutes, and after oral administration, 5 to 10 minutes.

INDICATIONS

For routine management after delivery of the placenta; postpartum atony and hemorrhage; subinvolution. Under full obstetric supervision, it may be given in the second stage of labor following delivery of the anterior shoulder.

CONTRAINDICATIONS

Hypertension; toxemia; pregnancy; and hypersensitivity.

WARNING

This drug should not be administered i.v. routinely because of the possibility of inducing sudden hypertensive and cerebrovascular accidents. If i.v. administration is considered essential as a lifesaving measure, Methergine (methylergovine maleate) should be given slowly over a period of no less than 60 seconds with careful monitoring of blood pressure.

PRECAUTIONS

Caution should be exercised in the presence of sepsis, obliterative vascular disease, hepatic or renal involvement.

ADVERSE REACTIONS

Nausea; vomiting; transient hypertension; dizziness; headache; tinnitus; diaphoresis and palpitation; temporary chest pain; and dyspnea.

DOSAGE AND ADMINISTRATION

Intramuscularly: One ml, 0.2 mg (1/320 grain) after delivery of the anterior shoulder, after delivery of the placenta, or during the puerperium. May be repeated as required, at intervals of 2-4 hours. **Intravenously:** *SEE WARNING SECTION.* Dosage same as intramuscular. **Orally:** One tablet, 0.2 mg (1/320 grain) 3 or 4 times daily in the puerperium for a maximum of 1 week.

SUPPLIED

Tablets in packages of 100 and 1000; Injection in 1 ml ampuls, boxes of 20 and 100.

REMARKS

Methergine injection is a clear and colorless solution. In the event the ampul solution becomes discolored, it should not be used.
Company's Product Identification Mark(s): Tablets imprinted 78-54 on one side, SANDOZ other side.
[Met-Z17 Issued October 1, 1984]
Shown in Product Identification Section, page 427

NEO-CALGLUCON® SYRUP

[nē'ō cal"glū'kon]
(glubionate calcium)
Palatable and Readily Absorbable Calcium Supplement.

The following prescribing information is based on official labeling in effect on June 1, 1986.

DESCRIPTION

Each teaspoonful (5 ml) of NEO-CALGLUCON® (glubionate calcium) Syrup contains: glubionate calcium 1.8 g (calcium content 115 mg—providing the same amount as 1.2 g calcium gluconate), benzoic acid, USP (as preservative) 5 mg.
Adequate calcium intake is particularly important during periods of bone growth in childhood and adolescence, during pregnancy and lactation. An adequate supply of calcium is considered necessary in adults, especially those over 40, to prevent a negative calcium balance which may contribute to the development of osteoporosis. The following are the US Government Recommended Daily Allowances (US RDA) of calcium.

Age Period	Calcium Requirements
Infants	0.6 g
Children under 4 years	0.8 g
Adults and children over 4	1.0 g
Pregnant and lactating women	1.3 g

Eight ounces of whole milk provide approximately 267 mg of calcium. One tablespoonful (15 ml) of NEO-CALGLUCON Syrup contains 345 mg of calcium.

INDICATIONS

1. As a *dietary supplement* where calcium intake may be inadequate:
   a. childhood and adolescence
   b. pregnancy
   c. lactation
   d. postmenopausal females and in the aged
2. In the *treatment* of calcium deficiency states which may occur in diseases such as:
   a. tetany of the newborn*
   b. hypoparathyroidism, acute* and chronic
   c. pseudohypoparathyroidism
   d. postmenopausal and senile osteoporosis
   e. rickets and osteomalacia

*As a supplement to parenterally administered calcium.

CONTRAINDICATIONS

Patients with renal calculi.

WARNINGS

Certain dietary substances interfere with the absorption of calcium. These include oxalic acid (found in large quantities in rhubarb and spinach), phytic acid (bran and whole cereals) and phosphorus (milk and other dairy products).
Administration of corticosteroids may interfere with calcium absorption.

PRECAUTIONS

When calcium is administered in therapeutic amounts for prolonged periods, hypercalcemia and hypercalciuria may result. This is most likely to occur in patients with hypoparathyroidism who are receiving high doses of Vitamin D. It can be avoided by frequent checks of plasma and urine calcium levels. Urine calcium levels may rise before plasma calcium levels. The former may be checked by determining 24-hour calcium excretion or by the Sulkowitch test.

ADVERSE REACTIONS

NEO-CALGLUCON (glubionate calcium) Syrup is exceptionally well tolerated. Gastrointestinal disturbances are exceedingly rare. A fatal case of hypercalcemia associated with an overdose of NEO-CALGLUCON Syrup has been reported in a two pound neonate. Symptoms of hypercalcemia include anorexia, nausea, vomiting, constipation, abdominal pain, dryness of the mouth, thirst and polyuria.

DOSAGE AND ADMINISTRATION

NEO-CALGLUCON (glubionate calcium) Syrup should be administered before meals to enhance absorption.
[See table on next page].

HOW SUPPLIED

NEO-CALGLUCON Syrup (straw yellow) in pint bottles.

PAMELOR® ℞

[pam 'ah-lar"]
(nortriptyline HCl), capsules, USP
(nortriptyline HCl) oral solution, USP

The following prescribing information is based on official labeling in effect on July 15, 1986.

DESCRIPTION

Pamelor® (nortriptyline HCl) is 5-(3-methylaminopropylidene)-10, 11-dihydro-5H-dibenzo [a,d] cycloheptene hydrochloride. Its molecular weight is 299.8, and its empirical formula is $C_{19}H_{21}N \cdot HCl$.
10 mg, 25 mg, 50 mg and 75 mg, Capsules
Active Ingredient: nortriptyline HCl, USP
Inactive Ingredients: D&C Yellow #10, FD&C Yellow #6, gelatin, silicon fluid, sodium lauryl sulfate, starch, and titanium dioxide
10 mg, 25 mg, and 75 mg, Capsules
May Also Include: benzyl alcohol, butyl paraben, D&C Yellow #10, edetate calcium disodium, FD&C Yellow #6, methyl paraben, propyl paraben, silicon dioxide, sodium lauryl sulfate, sodium propionate, and titanium dioxide
50 mg, Capsules
Inactive Ingredients: gelatin, silicon fluid, sodium lauryl sulfate, starch, and titanium dioxide
May Also Include: benzyl alcohol, butyl paraben, edetate calcium disodium, methyl paraben, propyl paraben, silicon dioxide, sodium bisulfite, sodium lauryl sulfate, sodium propionate, and titanium dioxide
Solution
Active Ingredient: nortriptyline HCl, USP
Inactive Ingredients: alcohol, benzoic acid, flavoring, purified water, and sorbitol

ACTIONS

The mechanism of mood elevation by tricyclic antidepressants is at present unknown. Pamelor (nortriptyline HCl) is not a monoamine oxidase inhibitor. It inhibits the activity of such diverse agents as histamine, 5-hydroxytryptamine, and acetylcholine. It increases the pressor effect of norepinephrine but blocks the pressor response of phenethylamine. Studies suggest that Pamelor (nortriptyline HCl) interferes with the transport, release, and storage of catecholamines. Operant conditioning techniques in rats and pigeons suggest that Pamelor (nortriptyline HCl) has a combination of stimulant and depressant properties.

INDICATIONS

Pamelor (nortriptyline HCl) is indicated for the relief of symptoms of depression. Endogenous depressions are more likely to be alleviated than are other depressive states.

CONTRAINDICATIONS

The use of Pamelor (nortriptyline HCl) or other tricyclic antidepressants concurrently with a monoamine oxidase (MAO) inhibitor is contraindicated. Hyperpyretic crises, severe convulsions, and fatalities have occurred when similar tricyclic antidepressants were used in such combinations. It is advisable to have discontinued the MAO inhibitor for at least two weeks before treatment with Pamelor (nortriptyline HCl) is started. Patients hypersensitive to Pamelor (nortriptyline HCl) should not be given the drug.
Cross-sensitivity between Pamelor® (nortriptyline HCl) and other dibenzazepines is a possibility.
Pamelor (nortriptyline HCl) is contraindicated during the acute recovery period after myocardial infarction.

WARNINGS

Patients with cardiovascular disease should be given Pamelor (nortriptyline HCl) only under close supervision because of the tendency of the drug to produce sinus tachycardia and to prolong the conduction time. Myocardial infarction, arrhythmia, and strokes have occurred. The antihypertensive action of guanethidine and similar agents may be blocked. Because of its anticholinergic activity, Pamelor (nortriptyline HCl) should be used with great caution in patients who have glaucoma or a history of urinary retention. Patients with a history of seizures should be followed closely when Pamelor (nortriptyline HCl) is administered, inasmuch as this drug is known to lower the convulsive threshold. Great care is required if Pamelor (nortriptyline HCl) is given to hyperthyroid patients or to those receiving thyroid medication, since cardiac arrhythmias may develop.
Pamelor (nortriptyline HCl) may impair the mental and/or physical abilities required for the performance of hazardous tasks, such as operating machinery or driving a car; therefore, the patient should be warned accordingly.
Excessive consumption of alcohol in combination with nortriptyline therapy may have a potentiating effect, which may lead to the danger of increased suicidal attempts or overdosage, especially in patients with histories of emotional disturbances or suicidal ideation.
Use in Pregnancy—Safe use of Pamelor (nortriptyline HCl) during pregnancy and lactation has not been established; therefore, when the drug is administered to pregnant patients, nursing mothers, or women of childbearing potential, the potential benefits must be weighed against the possible hazards. Animal reproduction studies have yielded inconclusive results.
Use in Children—This drug is not recommended for use in children, since safety and effectiveness in the pediatric age group have not been established.

PRECAUTIONS

The use of Pamelor (nortriptyline HCl) in schizophrenic patients may result in an exacerbation of the psychosis or may activate latent schizophrenic symptoms. If the drug is given to overactive or agitated patients, increased anxiety and agitation may occur. In manic-depressive patients, Pamelor (nortriptyline HCl) may cause symptoms of the manic phase to emerge.

Continued on next page

Sandoz—Cont.

Administration of reserpine during therapy with a tricyclic antidepressant has been shown to produce a "stimulating" effect in some depressed patients.
Troublesome patient hostility may be aroused by the use of Pamelor (nortriptyline HCl). Epileptiform seizures may accompany its administration, as is true of other drugs of its class.
Close supervision and careful adjustment of the dosage are required when Pamelor (nortriptyline HCl) is used with other anticholinergic drugs and sympathomimetic drugs.
Concurrent administration of cimetidine and tricyclic antidepressants can produce clinically significant increases in the plasma concentrations of the tricyclic antidepressant.
The patient should be informed that the response to alcohol may be exaggerated.
When it is essential, the drug may be administered with electroconvulsive therapy, although the hazards may be increased. Discontinue the drug for several days, if possible, prior to elective surgery.
The possibility of a suicidal attempt by a depressed patient remains after the initiation of treatment; in this regard, it is important that the least possible quantity of drug be dispensed at any given time.
Both elevation and lowering of blood sugar levels have been reported.

ADVERSE REACTIONS

Note: Included in the following list are a few adverse reactions that have not been reported with this specific drug. However, the pharmacologic similarities among the tricyclic antidepressant drugs require that each of the reactions be considered when nortriptyline is administered.
Cardiovascular — Hypotension, hypertension, tachycardia, palpitation, myocardial infarction, arrhythmias, heart block, stroke.
Psychiatric —Confusional states (especially in the elderly) with hallucinations, disorientation, delusions; anxiety, restlessness, agitation; insomnia, panic, nightmares; hypomania; exacerbation of psychosis.
Neurologic —Numbness, tingling, paresthesias of extremities; incoordination, ataxia, tremors; peripheral neuropathy; extrapyramidal symptoms; seizures, alteration in EEG patterns; tinnitus.
Anticholinergic —Dry mouth and, rarely, associated sublingual adenitis; blurred vision, disturbance of accommodation, mydriasis; constipation, paralytic ileus; urinary retention, delayed micturition, dilation of the urinary tract.
Allergic —Skin rash, petechiae, urticaria, itching, photosensitization (avoid excessive exposure to sunlight); edema (general or of face and tongue), drug fever, cross-sensitivity with other tricyclic drugs.
Hematologic —Bone-marrow depression, including agranulocytosis; eosinophilia; purpura; thrombocytopenia.
Gastrointestinal —Nausea and vomiting, anorexia, epigastric distress, diarrhea, peculiar taste, stomatitis, abdominal cramps, black-tongue.
Endocrine —Gynecomastia in the male, breast enlargement and galactorrhea in the female; increased or decreased libido, impotence; testicular swelling; elevation or depression of blood sugar levels; syndrome of inappropriate ADH (antidiuretic hormone) secretion.
Other —Jaundice (simulating obstructive); altered liver function; weight gain or loss; perspiration; flushing; urinary frequency, nocturia; drowsiness, dizziness, weakness, fatigue; headache; parotid swelling; alopecia.
Withdrawal Symptoms —Though these are not indicative of addiction, abrupt cessation of treatment after prolonged therapy may produce nausea, headache, and malaise.

DOSAGE AND ADMINISTRATION

Pamelor (nortriptyline HCl) is not recommended for children.
Pamelor (nortriptyline HCl) is administered orally in the form of capsules or liquid. Lower than usual dosages are recommended for elderly patients and adolescents. Lower dosages are also recommended for outpatients than for hospitalized patients who will be under close supervision. The physician should initiate dosage at a low level and increase it gradually, noting carefully the clinical response and any evidence of intolerance. Following remission, maintenance medication may be required for a longer period of time at the lowest dose that will maintain remission.
If a patient develops minor side effects, the dosage should be reduced. The drug should be discontinued promptly if adverse effects of a serious nature or allergic manifestations occur.
Usual Adult Dose —25 mg three or four times daily; dosage should begin at a low level and be increased as required. As an alternate regimen, the total daily dosage may be given once-a-day. When doses above 100 mg daily are administered, plasma levels of nortriptyline should be monitored and maintained in the optimum range of 50-150 ng/ml. Doses above 150 mg per day are not recommended.
Elderly and Adolescent Patients —30 to 50 mg per day, in divided doses, or the total daily dosage may be given once-a-day.

OVERDOSAGE

Toxic overdosage may result in confusion, restlessness, agitation, vomiting, hyperpyrexia, muscle rigidity, hyperactive reflexes, tachycardia, ECG evidence of impaired conduction, shock, congestive heart failure, stupor, coma, and C.N.S. stimulation with convulsions followed by respiratory depression. Deaths have occurred following overdosage with drugs of this class.
No specific antidote is known. General supportive measures are indicated, with gastric lavage. Respiratory assistance is apparently the most effective measure when indicated. The use of C.N.S. depressants may worsen the prognosis.
The administration of barbiturates for control of convulsions alleviates an increase in the cardiac work load but should be undertaken with caution to avoid potentiation of respiratory depression.
Intramuscular paraldehyde or diazepam provides anticonvulsant activity with less respiratory depression than do the barbiturates; diazepam seems to be preferred.
The use of digitalis and/or physostigmine may be considered in case of serious cardiovascular abnormalities or cardiac failure.
The value of dialysis has not been established.

HOW SUPPLIED

Solution: Pamelor® (nortriptyline HCl) USP, equivalent to 10 mg base per 5 ml is supplied in 16-fluid-ounce bottles. Alcohol content 4%.
Capsules: Pamelor (nortriptyline HCl) USP, equivalent to 10 mg, 25 mg, 50 mg and 75 mg base, are supplied in bottles of 100 and 500 and in boxes of 100 individually labeled blisters, each containing one capsule.
10 mg capsules branded "SANDOZ 78–86" on one half, "PAMELOR 10 mg" other half; 25 mg capsules branded "SANDOZ 78–87" on one half, "PAMELOR 25 mg" other half; 50 mg capsules branded "SANDOZ 78–78" on one half, "PAMELOR 50 mg" other half; and 75 mg capsules branded "SANDOZ 78–79" on one half, "PAMELOR 78 mg" other half.

[PAM-Z13 Issued July 15, 1986]
Shown in Product Identification Section, page 427

NEO-CALGLUCON	Grams of Supplemental Calcium Provided Daily	Percentage of US Recommended Daily Allowance (US RDA)
I. As a Dietary Supplement: Adults and children 4 or more years of age—1 tablespoonful 3 times daily.	1.0 g	104
Pregnant or lactating women—1 tablespoonful 4 times daily.	1.4 g	106
Children under 4 years of age—2 teaspoonfuls 3 times daily.	0.7 g	86
Infants—1 teaspoonful 5 times daily (may be taken undiluted, mixed with infant's formula or fruit juice). (Part of need is supplied by diet)	0.6 g	96

NEO-CALGLUCON	Grams of Supplemental Ca Provided Daily
II. In the treatment of Calcium Deficiency States: *Tetany of the Newborn* (Tetany of the newborn appears to be a transient physiologic hypoparathyroidism related to the maturation of the parathyroid glands. Adequate parathyroid gland function usually occurs within one week after birth.) Serum calcium should be determined before therapy is instituted. Hypocalcemia is defined as a serum calcium below 8 mg/100 ml or 4 mEq/liter. It is advisable to lower the solute and phosphorus loads in the feeding as well as to provide extra calcium. Intravenous administration of calcium solutions may be necessary for prompt relief of symptoms. Dose: Infants with confirmed hypocalcemia may be benefited by the oral administration of calcium salts so as to provide ELEMENTAL CALCIUM in a dosage of 50 to 150 mg/kg/day divided into three or more doses. (NEO-CALGLUCON contains 115 mg ELEMENTAL CALCIUM per 5 ml teaspoon.) The lower dosage range should be employed if calcium is also being provided by the parenteral route. Whole milk formulas which are high in phosphorus should be eliminated in order to increase the calcium/phosphorus ratio. Supplemental oral calcium should be gradually reduced over a period of two or three weeks after the condition has completely stabilized.	See left-hand column
Hypoparathyroidism	
Acute: Intravenous administration of calcium solutions may be necessary for prompt correction of hypocalcemia. Supplementary calcium should be given orally as soon as possible. Dose: 1–3 tablespoonfuls 3 times daily	1.0–3.1
Chronic: Dose: 1–3 tablespoonfuls daily	0.3–1.0
Pseudohypoparathyroidism: Dose: 1–3 tablespoonfuls daily	0.3–1.0
Osteoporosis, postmenopausal and senile: Dose: 1–2 tablespoonfuls 3 times daily	1.0–2.1

Rickets and Osteomalacia
Treatment of these disorders consists of the administration of Vitamin D orally. The addition of calcium to the therapeutic regimen may be desirable to provide calcium needed for remineralization and to avoid hypocalcemia which occurs not infrequently in the early days of treatment. Dosages should be those recommended above under Dietary Supplement.

PARLODEL® ℞
[*par 'lō-del "*]
(bromocriptine mesylate) tablets, USP
(bromocriptine mesylate) capsules

The following prescribing information is based on official labeling in effect June 10, 1986.

DESCRIPTION

Parlodel® (bromocriptine mesylate) is an ergot derivative with potent dopamine receptor agonist activity. This activity represents new therapeutic uses for specific peptide ergot alkaloid derivatives. Each Parlodel (bromocriptine mesylate) tablet for oral administration contains 2½ mg and each capsule contains 5 mg bromocriptine (as the mesylate). Parlodel (bromocriptine mesylate) is chemically designated as (1) Ergotaman-3′,6′,18-trione,2-bromo-12′-hydroxy-2′- (1-methylethyl) -5′- (2-methylpropyl)-,(5′α) monomethanesulfonate (salt); (2) 2-bromoergocryptine monomethanesulfonate (salt).*

2.5 mg, Tablets
Active Ingredient: bromocriptine mesylate, USP
Inactive Ingredients: colloidal silicon dioxide, lactose, magnesium stearate, povidone, starch and another ingredient

5 mg, Capsules
Active Ingredient: bromocriptine mesylate, USP
Inactive Ingredients: colloidal silicon dioxide, gelatin, lactose, magnesium stearate, red iron oxide, silicon dioxide, sodium bisulfite, sodium lauryl sulfate, starch, titanium dioxide, yellow iron oxide, and another ingredient

CLINICAL PHARMACOLOGY

Parlodel (bromocriptine mesylate) is a dopamine receptor agonist, which activates post-synaptic dopamine receptors. The dopaminergic neurons in the tuberoinfundibular process modulate the secretion of prolactin from the anterior pituitary by secreting a prolactin inhibitory factor (thought to be dopamine); in the corpus striatum the dopaminergic neurons are involved in the control of motor function. Clinically, Parlodel (bromocriptine mesylate) significantly reduces plasma levels of prolactin in patients with physiologically elevated prolactin as well as in patients with hyperprolactinemia. The inhibition of physiological lactation as well as galactorrhea in pathological hyperprolactinemic states is obtained at dose levels that do not affect secretion of other tropic hormones from the anterior pituitary. Experiments have demonstrated that bromocriptine induces long lasting stereotyped behavior in rodents and turning behavior in rats having unilateral lesions in the substantia nigra. These actions, characteristic of those produced by dopamine, are inhibited by dopamine antagonists and suggest a direct action of bromocriptine on striatal dopamine receptors.

Parlodel (bromocriptine mesylate) is a nonhormonal, nonestrogenic agent that inhibits the secretion of prolactin in humans, with little or no effect on other pituitary hormones, except in patients with acromegaly, where it lowers elevated blood levels of growth hormone in the majority of patients.

In about 75% of cases of amenorrhea and galactorrhea, Parlodel (bromocriptine mesylate) therapy suppresses the galactorrhea completely, or almost completely, and reinitiates normal ovulatory menstrual cycles.

Menses are usually reinitiated prior to complete suppression of galactorrhea; the time for this on average is 6–8 weeks. However, some patients respond within a few days, and others may take up to 8 months.

Galactorrhea may take longer to control depending on the degree of stimulation of the mammary tissue prior to therapy. At least a 75% reduction in secretion is usually observed after 8–12 weeks. Some patients may fail to respond even after 12 months of therapy.

Parlodel (bromocriptine mesylate), by virtue of its ability to inhibit prolactin secretion, acts to prevent physiological lactation in women when therapy is started after delivery and continued for two to three weeks. There is no evidence that Parlodel (bromocriptine mesylate) acts on the mammary tissues to prevent lactation, as is the case with estrogen-containing preparations.

In many acromegalic patients, Parlodel (bromocriptine mesylate) produces a prompt and sustained reduction in circulating levels of serum growth hormone.

Parlodel (bromocriptine mesylate) produces its therapeutic effect in the treatment of Parkinson's disease, a clinical condition characterized by a progressive deficiency in dopamine synthesis in the substantia nigra, by directly stimulating the dopamine receptors in the corpus striatum. In contrast, levodopa exerts its therapeutic effect only after conversion to dopamine by the neurons of the substantia nigra, which are known to be numerically diminished in this patient population.

PHARMACOKINETICS

The pharmacokinetics and metabolism of bromocriptine in human subjects were studied with the help of radioactively labeled drug. 28% of an oral dose was absorbed from the gastrointestinal tract. The blood levels following a 2½ mg dose were in the range of 2–3 ng equivalents/ml. Plasma levels were in the range of 4–6 ng equivalents/ml indicating that the red blood cells did not contain appreciable amounts of drug and/or metabolites. *In vitro* experiments showed that the drug was 90–96% bound to serum albumin.

Bromocriptine was completely metabolized prior to excretion. The major route of excretion of absorbed drug was via the bile. Only 2.5–5.5% of the dose was excreted in the urine. Almost all (84.6%) of the administered dose was excreted in the feces in 120 hours.

INDICATIONS AND USAGE

Hyperprolactinemia-associated Dysfunctions

Parlodel (bromocriptine mesylate) is indicated for the treatment of dysfunctions associated with **hyperprolactinemia** including **amenorrhea** with or without **galactorrhea, infertility or hypogonadism.** Parlodel (bromocriptine mesylate) treatment is indicated in patients with **prolactin-secreting adenomas,** which may be the basic underlying endocrinopathy contributing to the above clinical presentations. **Reduction in tumor size** has been demonstrated in both male and female patients with macroadenomas. In cases where adenectomy is elected, a course of Parlodel (bromocriptine mesylate) therapy may be used to reduce the tumor mass prior to surgery.

Prevention of Physiological Lactation

Parlodel (bromocriptine mesylate) tablets are indicated for the prevention of physiological lactation, (secretion, congestion, and engorgement) occurring:

1. After parturition when the mother elects not to breast feed the infant, or when breast feeding is contraindicated.
2. After stillbirth or abortion.

The physician should keep in mind that the incidence of significant painful engorgement is low and usually responsive to appropriate supportive therapy. In contrast with supportive therapy, Parlodel (bromocriptine mesylate) prevents the secretion of prolactin, thus inhibiting lactogenesis and the subsequent development of secretion, congestion and engorgement.

Once Parlodel (bromocriptine mesylate) therapy is stopped, 18% to 40% of patients experience rebound of breast secretion, congestion or engorgement, which is usually mild to moderate in severity.

Acromegaly

Parlodel (bromocriptine mesylate) therapy is indicated in the treatment of acromegaly. Parlodel (bromocriptine mesylate) therapy, alone or as adjunctive therapy with pituitary irradiation or surgery, reduces serum growth hormone by 50% or more in approximately one-half of patients treated, although not usually to normal levels.

Since the effects of external pituitary radiation may not become maximal for several years, adjunctive therapy with Parlodel (bromocriptine mesylate) offers potential benefit before the effects of irradiation are manifested.

Parkinson's Disease

Parlodel (bromocriptine mesylate) tablets or capsules are indicated in the treatment of the signs and symptoms of idiopathic or postencephalitic Parkinson's disease. As adjunctive treatment to levodopa (alone or with a peripheral decarboxylase inhibitor), Parlodel (bromocriptine mesylate) therapy may provide additional therapeutic benefits in those patients who are currently maintained on optimal dosages of levodopa, those who are beginning to deteriorate (develop tolerance) to levodopa therapy, and those who are experiencing "end of dose failure" on levodopa therapy. Parlodel (bromocriptine mesylate) therapy may permit a reduction of the maintenance dose of levodopa and, thus may ameliorate the occurence and/or severity of adverse reactions associated with long-term levodopa therapy such as abnormal involuntary movements (e.g. dyskinesias) and the marked swings in motor function ("on-off" phenomenon). Continued efficacy of Parlodel (bromocriptine mesylate) therapy during treatment of more than two years has not been established.

Data are insufficient to evaluate potential benefit from treating newly diagnosed Parkinson's disease with Parlodel (bromocriptine mesylate). Studies have shown, however, significantly more adverse reactions (notably nausea, hallucinations, confusion and hypotension) in Parlodel (bromocriptine mesylate) treated patients than in levodopa/carbidopa treated patients. Patients unresponsive to levodopa are poor candidates for Parlodel (bromocriptine mesylate) therapy.

CONTRAINDICATIONS

Sensitivity to any ergot alkaloids.

WARNINGS

Since hyperprolactinemia with amenorrhea/galactorrhea and infertility has been found in patients with pituitary tumors a complete evaluation of the pituitary is indicated before treatment with Parlodel (bromocriptine mesylate).

If pregnancy occurs during Parlodel (bromocriptine mesylate) administration, careful observation of these patients throughout pregnancy is mandatory. Prolactin-secreting adenomas may expand and compression of the optic or other cranial nerves may occur, emergency pituitary surgery becoming necessary. In most cases, the compression resolves following delivery. Reinitiation of Parlodel (bromocriptine mesylate) treatment has been reported to produce improvement in the visual fields of patients in whom nerve compression has occurred during pregnancy. The safety of Parlodel (bromocriptine mesylate) treatment during pregnancy to the mother and fetus has not been established.

Symptomatic hypotension can occur in patients treated with Parlodel (bromocriptine mesylate) for any indication.

In postpartum studies with Parlodel (bromocriptine mesylate), decreases in supine systolic and diastolic pressures of greater than 20 mm and 10 mm Hg, respectively, have been observed in almost 30% of patients receiving Parlodel (bromocriptine mesylate). On occasion, the drop in supine systolic pressure was as much as 50–59 mm of Hg. Since decreases in blood pressure are frequently noted during the puerperium independent of drug therapy, it is likely that many of these decreases in blood pressure observed with Parlodel (bromocriptine mesylate) therapy were not drug induced. **However, Parlodel (bromocriptine mesylate) is known to cause hypotension in some patients, and rarely may cause hypertension in selected patients; therefore, Parlodel (bromocriptine mesylate) therapy for prevention of postpartum lactation should not be initiated until the vital signs have been stabilized and no sooner than four hours after delivery. Particular attention should be paid to patients with toxemia, and to those who have received within the preceding 24 hours other ergot alkaloids or other drugs which can alter the blood pressure.** Periodic monitoring of the blood pressure, particularly during the first few days of therapy, is advisable. Furthermore, care should be exercised when Parlodel (bromocriptine mesylate) is administered concomitantly with other medications known to lower blood pressure.

Long-term treatment (6–36 months) with Parlodel (bromocriptine mesylate) in doses ranging from 20–100 mg/day has been associated with pulmonary infiltrates, pleural effusion and thickening of the pleura in a few patients. In those instances in which Parlodel (bromocriptine mesylate) treatment was terminated, the changes slowly reverted towards normal.

PRECAUTIONS

General

Safety and efficacy of Parlodel (bromocriptine mesylate) have not been established in patients with renal or hepatic disease. Care should be exercised when administering Parlodel (bromocriptine mesylate) therapy concomitantly with other medications known to lower blood pressure.

Hyperprolactinemic States

The relative efficacy of Parlodel (bromocriptine mesylate) versus surgery in preserving visual fields is not known. Patients with rapidly progressive visual field loss should be evaluated by a neurosurgeon to help decide on the most appropriate therapy. Since pregnancy is often the therapeutic objective in many hyperprolactinemic patients presenting with amenorrhea/galactorrhea and hypogonadism (infertility) a careful assessment of the pituitary is essential to detect the presence of a prolactin secreting adenoma. Patients not seeking pregnancy, or those harboring large adenomas, should be advised to use contraceptive measures, other than the oral contraceptives, during treatment with Parlodel® (bromocriptine mesylate). Since pregnancy may occur prior to reinitiation of menses, a pregnancy test is recommended at least every four weeks during the amenorrheic period, and, once menses are reinitiated, every time a patient misses a menstrual period. Treatment with Parlodel (bromocriptine mesylate) tablets or capsules should be discontinued as soon as pregnancy has been established. Patients must be monitored closely throughout pregnancy for signs and symptoms that may signal the enlargement of a previously undetected or existing prolactin-secreting tumor. Discontinuation of Parlodel (bromocriptine mesylate) treatment in patients with known macroadenomas has been associated with rapid regrowth of tumor and increase in serum prolactin in most cases.

Use in Pregnancy

In human studies with Parlodel (bromocriptine mesylate) there have been 1276 reported pregnancies, which have yielded 1109 live and 4 stillborn infants from women who took Parlodel (bromocriptine mesylate) during pregnancy. The majority of these patients received Parlodel (bromocriptine mesylate) therapy during the first two to three weeks of pregnancy and several received the drug for up to three months and 5 were treated for the entire period of gestation. Several studies in the literature reported on the use of Parlodel (bromocriptine mesylate) during the final week of pregnancy to reduce plasma levels of prolactin in cases where possible pituitary tumor expansion occurred. Among the 1113 infants, 37 cases of congenital anomalies have been reported. There were 9 major malformations which included 3 limb reduction defects and 28 minor malformations which include 8 hip dislocations. The total incidence of malformatins (3.3%) and the incidence of spontaneous abortions (11%) in this group of pregnancies does not exceed that generally

Continued on next page

Sandoz—Cont.

reported for the population at large. There were three hydatidiform moles, two of which occurred in the same patient.

Physiological Lactation

Decreases in blood pressure are common during the puerperium and, since Parlodel (bromocriptine mesylate) therapy is known to produce hypotension in some patients, the drug should not be administered until the vital signs have been stabilized.

Acromegaly

Cold sensitive digital vasospasm has been observed in some acromegalic patients treated with Parlodel (bromocriptine mesylate). The response, should it occur, can be reversed by reducing the dosage of Parlodel (bromocriptine mesylate) and may be prevented by keeping the fingers warm. Cases of severe gastrointestinal bleeding from peptic ulcers have been reported, some fatal. Although there is no evidence that Parlodel (bromocriptine mesylate) increases the incidence of peptic ulcers in acromegalic patients, symptoms suggestive of peptic ulcer should be investigated thoroughly and treated appropriately.

Possible tumor expansion while receiving Parlodel (bromocriptine mesylate) therapy has been reported in a few patients. Since the natural history of growth hormone secreting tumors is unknown, all patients should be carefully monitored and, if evidence of tumor expansion develops, discontinuation of treatment and alternative procedures considered.

Parkinson's Disease

Safety during long-term use for more than two years at the doses required for parkinsonism has not been established.

As with any chronic therapy, periodic evaluation of hepatic, hematopoietic, cardiovascular, and renal function is recommended. Symptomatic hypotension can occur and, therefore, caution should be exercised when treating patients receiving antihypertensive drugs.

High doses of Parlodel (bromocriptine mesylate) may be associated with confusion and mental disturbances. Since parkinsonian patients may manifest mild degrees of dementia, caution should be used when treating such patients.

Parlodel (bromocriptine mesylate) administered alone or concomitantly with levodopa may cause hallucinations (visual or auditory). Hallucinations usually resolve with dosage reduction; occasionally, discontinuation of Parlodel (bromocriptine mesylate) is required. Rarely, after high doses, hallucinations have persisted for several weeks following discontinuation of Parlodel (bromocriptine mesylate).

As with levodopa, caution should be exercised when administering Parlodel (bromocriptine mesylate) to patients with a history of myocardial infarction who have a residual atrial, nodal, or ventricular arrhythmia.

Nursing Mothers

Since it prevents lactation, Parlodel (bromocriptine mesylate) should not be administered to mothers who elect to breast feed their infants.

Pediatric Use

Safety and efficacy of Parlodel (bromocriptine mesylate) have not been established in children under the age of 15.

INFORMATION FOR PATIENTS

When initiating therapy, all patients receiving Parlodel (bromocriptine mesylate) should be cautioned with regard to engaging in activities requiring rapid and precise responses, such as driving an automobile or operating machinery since dizziness (8–16%), drowsiness (8%), faintness, fainting (8%), and syncope (less than 1%) have been reported early in the course of therapy. Patients receiving Parlodel (bromocriptine mesylate) for hyperprolactinemic states associated with macroadenoma or those who have had previous transsphenoidal surgery, should be told to report any persistent watery nasal discharge to their physician. Patients receiving Parlodel (bromocriptine mesylate) for treatment of a macroadenoma should be told that discontinuation of drug may be associated with rapid regrowth of the tumor and recurrence of their original symptoms.

DRUG INTERACTIONS

Lack or decrease in efficacy may occur in patients receiving Parlodel (bromocriptine mesylate) when they are treated concurrently with drugs which have dopamine antagonist activity e.g. phenothiazines, butyrophenones. This may be a problem particularly for patients treated with Parlodel (bromocriptine mesylate) for macroadenomas.

ADVERSE REACTIONS

Hyperprolactinemic Indications

The incidence of adverse effects is quite high (69%) but these are generally mild to moderate in degree. Therapy was discontinued in approximately 5% of patients because of adverse effects. These in decreasing order of frequency are: nausea 49%, headache 19%, dizziness 17%, fatigue 7%, lightheadedness 5%, vomiting 5%, abdominal cramps 4%, nasal congestion 3%, constipation 3%, diarrhea 3% and drowsiness 3%.

A slight hypotensive effect may accompany Parlodel (bromocriptine mesylate) treatment. The occurence of adverse reactions may be lessened by temporarily reducing dosage to one-half tablet two or three times daily. A few cases of cerebrospinal fluid rhinorrhea have been reported in patients receiving Parlodel (bromocriptine mesylate) for treatment of large prolactinomas. This has occurred rarely, usually only in patients who have received previous transsphenoidal surgery, pituitary radiation, or both, and who were receiving Parlodel (bromocriptine mesylate) for tumor recurrence. It may also occur in previously untreated patients whose tumor extends into the sphenoid sinus.

Physiological Lactation

23% of patients treated within the recommended dosage range for the prevention of physiological lactation had at least one side effect, but they were generally mild to moderate in degree. Therapy was discontinued in approximately 3% of patients. The most frequently occurring adverse reactions were: headache 10%, dizziness 8%, nausea 7%, vomiting 3%, fatigue 1.0%, syncope 0.7%, diarrhea 0.4% and cramps 0.4%. Decreases in blood pressure (≥ 20 mmHg systolic and ≥ 10 mmHg diastolic) occurred in 28% of patients at least once during the first three postpartum days; these were usually of a transient nature. Two reports of fainting in the puerperium may possibly be related to this effect. However, 6 cases of isolated hypertension, 3 cases of hypertension and stroke (including 1 fatal cerebral hemorrhage), 3 cases of hypertension and seizures, and 3 cases of isolated seizures have been reported. Some of these patients had toxemia (including postpartum eclampsia), and some received concomitantly other ergot alkaloids or other drugs which can raise the blood pressure, so that the relationship between these adverse reactions and Parlodel (bromocriptine mesylate) is not certain.

Acromegaly

The most frequent adverse reactions encountered in acromegalic patients treated with Parlodel (bromocriptine mesylate) were: nausea (18%), constipation (14%), postural/orthostatic hypotension (6%), anorexia (4%), dry mouth/nasal stuffiness (4%), indigestion/dyspepsia (4%), digital vasospasm (3%), drowsiness/tiredness (3%) and vomiting (2%).

Less frequent adverse reactions (less than 2%) were: gastrointestinal bleeding, dizziness, exacerbation of Raynaud's Syndrome, headache and syncope. Rarely (less than 1%) hair loss, alcohol potentiation, faintness, lightheadedness, arrhythmia, ventricular tachycardia, decreased sleep requirement, visual hallucinations, lassitude, shortness of breath, bradycardia, vertigo, paresthesia, sluggishness, vasovagal attack, delusional psychosis, paranoia, insomnia, heavy headedness, reduced tolerance to cold, tingling of ears, facial pallor and muscle cramps have been reported.

Parkinson's Disease

In clinical trials in which bromocriptine was administered with concomitant reduction in the dose of levodopa/carbidopa, the most common newly appearing adverse reactions were: nausea, abnormal involvuntary movements, hallucinations, confusion, "on-off" phenomenon, dizziness, drowsiness, faintness/fainting, vomiting, asthenia, abdominal discomfort, visual disturbance, ataxia, insomnia, depression, hypotension, shortness of breath, constipation, and vertigo.

Less common adverse reactions which may be encountered include: anorexia, anxiety, blepharospasm, dry mouth, dysphagia, edema of the feet and ankles, erythromelalgia, epileptiform seizure, fatigue, headache, lethargy, mottling of skin, nasal stuffiness, nervousness, nightmares, paresthesia, skin rash, urinary frequency, urinary incontinence, urinary retention, and rarely, signs and symptoms of ergotism such as tingling of fingers, cold feet, numbness, muscle cramps of feet and legs or exacerbation of Raynaud's syndrome.

Abnormalities in laboratory tests may include elevations in blood urea nitrogen, SGOT, SGPT, GGPT, CPK, alkaline phosphatase and uric acid, which are usually transient and not of clinical significance.

DOSAGE AND ADMINISTRATION

General

It is recommended that Parlodel (bromocriptine mesylate) be taken with food. Patients should be evaluated frequently during dose escalation to determine the lowest dosage that produces a therapeutic response.

Hyperprolactinemic Indications

The initial dosage of Parlodel (bromocriptine mesylate) is one-half to one $2\frac{1}{2}$ mg tablet daily. An additional $2\frac{1}{2}$ mg tablet may be added to the treatment regimen as tolerated every 3–7 days until an optimal therapeutic response is achieved. The therapeutic dosage usually is 5–7.5 mg and ranges from 2.5–15 mg/day.

In order to reduce the likelihood of prolonged exposure to Parlodel (bromocriptine mesylate) should an unsuspected pregnancy occur, a mechanical contraceptive should be used in conjunction with Parlodel (bromocriptine mesylate) therapy until normal ovulatory menstrual cycles have been restored. Contraception may then be discontinued in patients desiring pregnancy.

Thereafter, if menstruation does not occur within 3 days of the expected date, Parlodel (bromocriptine mesylate) therapy should be discontinued and a pregnancy test performed.

Prevention of Physiological Lactation

Therapy should be started only after the patient's vital signs have been stabilized and no sooner than four hours after delivery. The recommended therapeutic dosage is one $2\frac{1}{2}$ mg tablet of Parlodel (bromocriptine mesylate) twice daily. The usual dosage range is 2.5–7.5 mg daily. Parlodel (bromocriptine mesylate) therapy should be continued for 14 days; however, therapy may be given for up to 21 days if necessary.

Acromegaly

Virtually all acromegalic patients receiving therapeutic benefit from Parlodel (bromocriptine mesylate) also have reductions in circulating levels of growth hormone. Therefore periodic assessment of circulating levels of growth hormone will, in most cases, serve as a guide in determining the therapeutic potential of Parlodel (bromocriptine mesylate). If, after a brief trial with Parlodel (bromocriptine mesylate) therapy, no significant reduction in growth hormone levels has taken place, careful assessment of the clinical features of the disease should be made, and if no change has occurred, dosage adjustment or discontinuation of therapy should be considered.

The initial recommended dosage is $\frac{1}{2}$ to one $2\frac{1}{2}$ mg Parlodel (bromocriptine mesylate) tablet on retiring (with food) for 3 days. An additional $\frac{1}{2}$ to 1 tablet should be added to the treatment regimen as tolerated every 3–7 days until the patient obtains optimal therapeutic benefit. Patients should be reevaluated monthly and the dosage adjusted based on reductions of growth hormone or clinical response. The usual optimal therapeutic dosage range of Parlodel (bromocriptine mesylate) varies from 20 to 30 mg per day in most patients. The maximal dosage should not exceed 100 mg per day.

Patients treated with pituitary irradiation should be withdrawn from Parlodel (bromocriptine mesylate) therapy on a yearly basis to assess both the clinical effects of radiation on the disease process as well as the effects of Parlodel (bromocriptine mesylate) therapy. Usually a four to eight week withdrawal period is adequate for this purpose. Recurrence of the signs/symptoms or increases in growth hormone indicate the disease process is still active and further courses of Parlodel (bromocriptine mesylate) should be considered.

Parkinson's Disease

The basic principle of Parlodel (bromocriptine mesylate) therapy is to initiate treatment at a low dosage and, on an individual basis, increase the daily dosage slowly until a maximum therapeutic response is achieved. The dosage of levodopa during this introductory period should be maintained, if possible. The initial dose of Parlodel (bromocriptine mesylate) is one-half of a $2\frac{1}{2}$ mg tablet twice daily with meals. Assessments are advised at two week intervals during dosage titration to ensure that the lowest dosage producing an optimal therapeutic response is not exceeded. If necessary, the dosage may be increased every 14 to 28 days by $2\frac{1}{2}$ mg per day with meals. Should it be advisable to reduce the dosage of levodopa because of adverse reactions, the daily dosage of Parlodel (bromocriptine mesylate), if increased, should be accomplished gradually in small ($2\frac{1}{2}$ mg) increments.

The safety of Parlodel (bromocriptine mesylate) has not been demonstrated in dosages exceeding 100 mg per day.

HOW SUPPLIED

Tablets, $2\frac{1}{2}$ mg

Round, white, scored tablets, each containing $2\frac{1}{2}$ mg bromocriptine (as the mesylate) in packages of 30 (NDC 0078-0017-15).

Capsules, 5 mg

Caramel and white capsules, each containing 5 mg bromocriptine (as the mesylate) in packages of 30 (NDC 0078-0102-15) and 100 (NDC 0078-0102-05).

Company's Product Identification Mark(s): Tablets embossed "PARLODEL $2\frac{1}{2}$" on one side and scored on reverse side.

Capsules imprinted "PARLODEL 5 mg" on one half and triangle (S) on other half.

Store and dispense: Below 77°F; tight, light-resistant container.

[PAR-Z15 Issues June 10, 1986]

Shown in Product Identification Section, page 427

RESTORIL® Ⓒ

[*res 'tah-ril"*]

(temazepam) capsules

The following prescribing information is based on official labeling in effect on July 15, 1986.

DESCRIPTION

Restoril® (temazepam) is a benzodiazepine hypnotic agent. The chemical name is 7-chloro-1,3-dihydro-3-hydroxy-1-methyl-5-phenyl-2H-1,4-benzodiazepin-2-one.

Temazepam is a white, crystalline substance, very slightly soluble in water and sparingly soluble in alcohol USP. It has a molecular weight of 300.7.

Restoril (temazepam) capsules, 15 mg and 30 mg, are for oral administration.

15 mg, and 30 mg Capsules

Active Ingredient: temazepam

15 mg. Capsules

Inactive Ingredients: FD&C Blue #1, FD&C Red #3, gelatin, lactose, magnesium stearate, sodium lauryl sulfate, synthetic red ferric oxide, and titanium dioxide

May Also Include: benzyl alcohol, butyl paraben, edetate calcium disodium, methyl paraben, propyl paraben, silicon dioxide, sodium bisulfite, sodium propionate, and another ingredient

30 mg, Capsules

Inactive Ingredients: gelatin, FD&C Blue #1, FD&C Red #3, lactose, magnesium stearate, sodium lauryl sulfate, titanium dioxide, and another ingredient

May Also Include: benzyl alcohol, butyl paraben, edetate, calcium disodium, methyl paraben, propyl paraben, silicon dioxide, sodium bisulfite, sodium propionate, and another ingredient

CLINICAL PHARMACOLOGY

Restoril (temazepam) improved sleep parameters in clinical studies. Residual medication effects ("hangover") were essentially absent. Early morning awakening, a particular problem in the geriatric patient, was significantly reduced.

In sleep laboratory studies, Restoril (temazepam) significantly improved sleep maintenance parameters [e.g., wake time after sleep onset, total sleep time and the number of nocturnal awakenings]. There was no significant reduction in sleep latency. REM sleep was essentially unchanged, slow wave sleep was decreased and no rebound effects occurred in these sleep stages. Transient sleep disturbance, mainly during the first night, occurred after withdrawal of the drug. In these studies, there was no evidence of tolerance when patients were given Restoril (temazepam) nightly for approximately one month.

A single and a multiple dose absorption, distribution, metabolism and excretion (ADME) study using ^{3}H-labeled drug, as well as a bioavailability study, were carried out in normal volunteers. Absorption was complete and detectable blood levels were achieved at 20-40 minutes; peak concentration was reached at 2-3 hours. There was minimal (approximately 8%) first pass metabolism.

The only significant metabolite present in blood was the O-conjugate. The unchanged drug was 96% bound to plasma proteins. The blood level decline of the parent drug was biphasic with the short half-life ranging from 0.4-0.6 hours and the terminal half-life from 9.5-12.4 hours (mean: 10 hours), depending on the study population and method of determination. Metabolites were formed with a half-life of 10 hours and excreted with a half-life of approximately 2 hours. Thus, formation of the major metabolite is the rate limiting step in the biodisposition of temazepam. There is no accumulation of metabolites. The area under the blood concentration/time curve was directly proportional to the dose in the 0-45 mg range.

Temazepam was completely metabolized prior to excretion; 80-90% of the dose appeared in the urine. The major metabolite was the O-conjugate of temazepam (90%); the O-conjugate of N-demethyl temazepam was a minor metabolite (7%). There were no active metabolites.

At a dose of 30 mg once-a-day for 8 weeks, no evidence of enzyme induction was found in man.

The steady state plasma concentration measured under therapeutic sleep laboratory conditions was 382 ± 192 ng/ml, 2.5 hours after a 30 mg dose, and 26 ng/ml at 24 hours. On a once-a-day regimen, steady state was attained on the third day.

INDICATIONS AND USAGE

Restoril (temazepam) is indicated for the relief of insomnia associated with the complaints of difficulty in falling asleep, frequent nocturnal awakenings, and/or early morning awakenings. In clinical trials there is a perception by patients that Restoril (temazepam) decreases sleep latency, but sleep laboratory studies have not confirmed such an effect when the drug was administered within 30 minutes of retiring.

Since insomnia is often transient and intermittent, the prolonged administration of Restoril (temazepam) is generally not necessary or recommended. Restoril (temazepam) has been employed for sleep maintenance for up to 35 consecutive nights of drug administration in sleep laboratory studies.

Since insomnia may be a symptom of several other disorders, the possibility that the complaint may be related to a condition for which there is more specific treatment should be considered.

CONTRAINDICATIONS

Benzodiazepines may cause fetal damage when administered during pregnancy. An increased risk of congenital malformations associated with the use of diazepam and chlordiazepoxide during the first trimester of pregnancy has been suggested in several studies. Transplacental distribution has resulted in neonatal CNS depression following the ingestion of therapeutic doses of a benzodiazepine hypnotic during the last weeks of pregnancy.

Reproduction studies in animals with temazepam were performed in rats and rabbits. In a perinatal-postnatal study in rats, oral doses of 60 mg/kg/day resulted in increasing nursling mortality. Teratology studies in rats demonstrated increased fetal resorptions at doses of 30 and 120 mg/kg in one study and increased occurrence of rudimentary ribs, which are considered skeletal variants, in a second study at doses of 240 mg/kg or higher. In rabbits, occasional abnormalities such as exencephaly and fusion or asymmetry of ribs were reported without dose relationship. Although these abnormalities were not found in the concurrent control group, they have been reported to occur randomly in historical controls. At doses of 40 mg/kg or higher, there was an increased incidence of the 13th rib variant when compared to the incidence in concurrent and historical controls.

Restoril® (temazepam) is contraindicated in pregnant women. If there is a likelihood of the patient becoming pregnant while receiving temazepam, she should be warned of the potential risk to the fetus. Patients should be instructed to discontinue the drug prior to becoming pregnant. The possibility that a woman of childbearing potential may be pregnant at the time of institution of therapy should be considered.

WARNINGS

Patients receiving Restoril (temazepam) should be cautioned about possible combined effects with alcohol and other CNS depressants.

PRECAUTIONS

General

Since the risk of the development of oversedation, dizziness, confusion and/or ataxia increases, substantially with larger doses of benzodiazepines in elderly and debilitated patients, 15 mg of Restoril (temazepam) is recommended as the initial dosage for such patients.

Restoril (temazepam) should be administered with caution in severely depressed patients or those in whom there is any evidence of latent depression; it should be recognized that suicidal tendencies may be present and protective measures may be necessary.

If Restoril (temazepam) is to be combined with other drugs having known hypnotic properties or CNS-depressant effects, consideration should be given to potential additive effects.

Information for Patients

Patients receiving Restoril (temazepam) should be cautioned about possible combined effects with alcohol and other CNS depressants. Patients should be cautioned not to operate machinery or drive a motor vehicle after ingesting the drug. Patients should also be advised that they may experience disturbed nocturnal sleep for the first or second night after discontinuing the drug.

Laboratory Tests

The usual precautions should be observed in patients with impaired renal or hepatic function. Abnormal liver function tests as well as blood dyscrasias have been reported with benzodiazepines.

Carcinogenesis, Impairment of Fertility

No carcinogenic potential was demonstrated in long-term studies in mice and rats. Fertility in male and female rats was not adversely affected by Restoril (temazepam).

Pregnancy

Pregnancy Category X. See Contraindications.

Nursing Mothers

It is not known whether this drug is excreted in human milk. Because many drugs are excreted in human milk, caution should be exercised when Restoril (temazepam) is administered to a nursing woman.

Pediatric Use

Safety and effectiveness in children below the age of 18 years have not been established.

ADVERSE REACTIONS

During clinical studies in which 795 patients received Restoril (temazepam), the drug was well tolerated. Side effects were usually mild and transient. These 795 patients included 175 subjects who received Restoril (temazepam) during daytime waking hours, sometimes in excess of recommended therapeutic dosage, in studies to evaluate dosage levels for safety and pharmacokinetic profiles.

The most common adverse reactions were drowsiness (17%), dizziness (7%), and lethargy (5%).

Other side effects include confusion, euphoria and relaxed feeling (2-3%). Less commonly reported were weakness, anorexia and diarrhea (1-2%). Rarely reported were tremor, ataxia, lack of concentration, loss of equilibrium, falling and palpitations (less than 1%).

Hallucinations, horizontal nystagmus and paradoxical reactions, including excitement, stimulation and hyperactivity were rare (less than 0.5%).

DRUG ABUSE AND DEPENDENCE

Controlled Substance

Restoril (temazepam) is a controlled substance in Schedule IV.

Abuse and Dependence

Withdrawal symptoms following abrupt discontinuation of benzodiazepines have been reported in patients receiving excessive doses over extended periods of time. These symptoms (including convulsions) are similar to those seen after barbiturate withdrawal. Although infrequently seen, milder withdrawal symptoms have also been reported following abrupt discontinuance of benzodiazepines taken continuously, generally at higher therapeutic levels, for at least several months. As with any hypnotic, caution must be exercised in administering Restoril® (temazepam) to individuals known to be addiction-prone or those whose history suggests they may increase the dosage on their own initiative. It is desirable to limit repeated prescriptions without adequate medical supervision.

OVERDOSAGE

Manifestations of acute overdosage of Restoril (temazepam) can be expected to reflect the CNS effects of the drug and include somnolence, confusion and coma, with reduced or absent reflexes, respiratory depression and hypotension. If the patient is conscious, vomiting should be induced mechanically or with emetics. Gastric lavage should be employed utilizing concurrently a cuffed endotracheal tube if the patient is unconscious to prevent aspiration and pulmonary complications. Maintenance of adequate pulmonary ventilation is essential. The use of pressor agents intravenously may be necessary to combat hypotension. Fluids should be administered intravenously to encourage diuresis. The value of dialysis has not been determined. If excitation occurs, barbiturates should not be used. It should be borne in mind that multiple agents may have been ingested.

The oral LD_{50} was 1963 mg/kg in mice, 1833 mg/kg in rats and >2400 mg/kg in rabbits.

DOSAGE AND ADMINISTRATION

The recommended usual adult dose is 30 mg before retiring. In some patients, 15 mg may be sufficient. As with all medications, dosage should be individualized for maximal beneficial effects. In elderly and/or debilitated patients it is recommended that therapy be initiated with 15 mg until individual responses are determined.

HOW SUPPLIED

Restoril (temazepam) capsules-15 mg, maroon and pink, 30 mg, maroon and blue. Packages of 30, 100, 500 and Control-Pak® packages of 25 capsules (continuous reverse-numbered roll of sealed blisters).

Company's Product Information Mark(s): Restoril Capsules, 15 mg, imprinted "RESTORIL 15 mg" on each half. Restoril Capsules, 30 mg, imprinted "RESTORIL 30 mg" on each half.

[RES-Z6 Issued July 15, 1986]

Shown in Product Identification Section, page 427

SANDIMMUNE® Oral Solution ℞

[san 'di-mewn]

(cyclosporine)

SANDIMMUNE® I.V. ℞

(cyclosporine)

The following prescribing information is based on official labeling in effect on June 2, 1986.

WARNING

Only physicians experienced in immunosuppressive therapy and management of organ transplant patients should prescribe Sandimmune® (cyclosporine) Oral Solution and I.V. Patients receiving the drug should be managed in facilities equipped and staffed with adequate laboratory and supportive medical resources. The physician responsible for maintenance therapy should have complete information requisite for the follow-up of the patient.

Sandimmune (cyclosporine) Oral Solution and I.V. should be administered with adrenal corticosteroids but not with other immunosuppressive agents. Increased susceptibility to infection and the possible development of lymphoma may result from immunosuppression.

The absorption of cyclosporine during chronic administration of Sandimmune Oral Solution was found to be erratic. It is recommended that patients taking the oral solution over a period of time be monitored at repeated intervals for cyclosporine blood levels and subsequent dose adjustments be made in order to avoid toxicity due to high levels and possible organ rejection due to low

Continued on next page

Sandoz—Cont.

absorption of cyclosporine. This is of special importance in liver transplants. See Dosage and Administration section.

DESCRIPTION

Cyclosporine, the active principle in Sandimmune is a cyclic polypeptide immunosuppressant agent consisting of 11 amino acids. It is produced as a metabolite by the fungus species Tolypocladium inflatum Gams.

Chemically, cyclosporine is designated as [R-[R*,R*-(E)]]-cyclic-(L-alanyl-D-alanyl-N-methyl-L-leucyl-N-methyl- L-leucyl-N-methyl-L-valyl-3-hydroxy-N,4-dimethyl-L-2-amino-6-octenoyl-L-α-amino-butyryl-N-methylglycyl-N-methyl-L-leucyl-L-valyl-N-methyl-L-leucyl).

Sandimmune (cyclosporine) Oral Solution is available in 50 ml bottles.

Each ml contains:

cyclosporine ..... 100 mg
alcohol, Ph. Helv. ..... 12.5% by volume

dissolved in an olive oil, Ph. Helv./Labrafil® M 1944CS (polyoxyethylated oleic glycerides) vehicle which must be further diluted with milk, chocolate milk or orange juice before oral administration.

Sandimmune (cyclosporine) I.V. is available in a 5 ml sterile ampul for I.V. administration.

Each ml contains:

cyclosporine ..... 50 mg
*Cremophor® EL ..... 650 mg
(polyoxyethylated castor oil)
alcohol, Ph. Helv. ..... 32.9% by volume
nitrogen ..... qs

which must be diluted further with 0.9% Sodium Chloride Injection or 5% Dextrose Injection before use.

* Cremophor is the registered trademark of BASF Aktiengesellschaft.

CLINICAL PHARMACOLOGY

Sandimmune (cyclosporine) is a potent immunosuppressive agent which in animals prolongs survival of allogeneic transplants involving skin, heart, kidney, pancreas, bone marrow, small intestine and lung. Sandimmune (cyclosporine) has been demonstrated to suppress some humoral immunity and to a greater extent, cell-mediated reactions such as allograft rejection, delayed hypersensitivity, experimental allergic encephalomyelitis, Freund's adjuvant arthritis and graft vs. host disease in many animal species for a variety of organs.

Successful kidney, liver and heart allogeneic transplants have been performed in man using Sandimmune (cyclosporine).

The exact mechanism of action of Sandimmune (cyclosporine) is not known. Experimental evidence suggests that the effectiveness of cyclosporine is due to specific and reversible inhibition of immunocompetent lymphocytes in the G_0 or G_1-phase of the cell cycle. T-lymphocytes are preferentially inhibited. The T-helper cell is the main target, although the T-suppressor cell may also be suppressed. Sandimmune (cyclosporine) also inhibits lymphokine production and release including interleukin-2 or T-cell growth factor (TCGF).

No functional effects on phagocytic (changes in enzyme secretions not altered, chemotactic migration of granulocytes, macrophage migration, carbon clearance *in vivo*) or tumor cells (growth rate, metastasis) can be detected in animals. Sandimmune (cyclosporine) does not cause bone marrow suppression in animal models or man.

The absorption of cyclosporine from the gastrointestinal tract is incomplete and variable. Peak concentrations (C_{max}) in blood and plasma are achieved at about 3.5 hours. C_{max} and area under the plasma or blood concentration/time curve (AUC) increase with the administered dose; for blood the relationship is curvilinear (parabolic) between 0 and 1400 mg. As determined by a specific assay, C_{max} is approximately 1.0 ng/mL/mg of dose for plasma and 2.7 to 1.4 ng/mL/mg of dose for blood (for low to high doses). Compared to an intravenous infusion, the absolute bioavailability of the oral solution is approximately 30% based upon the results in two patients.

Cyclosporine is distributed largely outside the blood volume. In blood the distribution is concentration dependent. Approximately 33–47% is in plasma, 4–9% in lymphocytes, 5–12% in granulocytes and 41–58% in erythrocytes. At high concentrations, the uptake by leukocytes and erythrocytes becomes saturated. In plasma, approximately 90% is bound to proteins, primarily lipoproteins.

The disposition of cyclosporine from blood is biphasic with a terminal half-life of approximately 19 hours (range: 10–27 hours). Elimination is primarily biliary with only 6% of the dose excreted in the urine.

Cyclosporine is extensively metabolized but there is no major metabolic pathway. Only 0.1% of the dose is excreted in the urine as unchanged drug. Of 15 metabolites characterized in human urine, 7 have been assigned structures. The major pathways consist of hydroxylation of the Cγ-carbon of two of the leucine residues, Cη-carbon hydroxylation and cyclic ether formation (with oxidation of the double bond) in the side chain of the amino acid 3-hydroxyl-N,4-dimethyl-L-2-amino-6-octenoic acid and N-demethylation of N-methyl leucine residues. Hydrolysis of the cyclic peptide chain or conjugation of the above metabolites do not appear to be important biotransformation pathways.

INDICATIONS AND USAGE

Sandimmune® (cyclosporine) Oral Solution and I.V. are indicated for the prophylaxis of organ rejection in kidney, liver and heart allogeneic transplants. They are always to be used with adrenal corticosteroids. The drug may also be used in the treatment of chronic rejection in patients previously treated with other immunosuppressive agents.

Because of the risk of anaphylaxis, Sandimmune I.V. should be reserved for patients who are unable to take the oral solution.

CONTRAINDICATIONS

Sandimmune (cyclosporine) I.V. is contraindicated in patients with a hypersensitivity to cyclosporine and/or Cremophor® EL (polyoxyethylated castor oil).

WARNINGS

SEE BOXED WARNINGS ABOVE

Sandimmune (cyclosporine), when used in high doses, can cause hepatotoxicity and nephrotoxicity.

It is not unusual for serum creatinine and BUN levels to be elevated during Sandimmune (cyclosporine) therapy. These elevations in renal transplant patients do not necessarily indicate rejection, and each patient must be fully evaluated before dosage adjustment is initiated.

Nephrotoxicity has been noted in 25% of cases of renal transplantation, 38% of cases of cardiac transplantation and 37% of cases of liver transplantation. Mild nephrotoxicity was generally noted two to three months after transplant and consisted of an arrest in the fall of the pre-operative elevations of BUN and creatinine at a range of 35–45 mg/dl and 2.0–2.5 mg/dl respectively. These elevations were often responsive to dosage reduction.

More overt nephrotoxicity was seen early after transplantation and was characterized by a rapidly rising BUN and creatinine. Since these events are similar to rejection episodes care must be taken to differentiate between them. This form of nephrotoxicity is usually responsive to Sandimmune (cyclosporine) dosage reduction.

Impaired renal function at any time requires close monitoring, and frequent dosage adjustment may be indicated. In patients with persistent high elevations of BUN and creatinine who are unresponsive to dosage adjustments, consideration should be given to switching to other immunosuppressive therapy. In the event of severe and unremitting rejection, it is preferable to allow the kidney transplant to be rejected and removed rather than increase the Sandimmune (cyclosporine) dosage to a very high level in an attempt to reverse the rejection. Occasionally patients have developed a syndrome of thrombocytopenia and microangiopathic hemolytic anemia which may result in graft failure. Neither the pathogenesis nor the management of this syndrome is clear.

Significant hyperkalemia and hyperuricemia have been seen occasionally in individual patients.

Hepatotoxicity has been noted in 4% of cases of renal transplantation, 7% of cases of cardiac transplantation and 4% of cases of liver transplantation. This was usually noted during the first month of therapy when high doses of Sandimmune (cyclosporine) were used and consisted of elevations of hepatic enzymes and bilirubin. The chemistry elevations usually decreased with a reduction in dosage.

Lymphomas have developed in patients receiving Sandimmune (cyclosporine) and other forms of immunosuppressive therapy after transplantation though no causal relationship has been established. With Sandimmune (cyclosporine), some patients have developed a lymphoproliferative disorder which regresses when the drug is discontinued.

There have been reports of convulsions in adult and pediatric patients receiving cyclosporine, particularly in combination with high dose methylprednisolone.

Rarely (approximately 1 in 1000), patients receiving Sandimmune (cyclosporine) I.V. have experienced anaphylactic reactions. Although the exact cause of these reactions is unknown, it is believed to be due to the Cremophor® EL (polyoxyethylated castor oil) used as the vehicle for the I.V. formulation. These reactions have consisted of flushing of the face and upper thorax, acute respiratory distress with dyspnea and wheezing, blood pressure changes and tachycardia. One patient died after respiratory arrest and aspiration pneumonia. In some cases, the reaction subsided after the infusion was stopped.

Patients receiving Sandimmune I.V. should be under continuous observation for at least the first 30 minutes following start of the infusion and at frequent intervals thereafter. If anaphylaxis occurs, the infusion should be stopped. An aqueous solution of epinephrine 1:1000 should be available at the bedside as well as a source of oxygen.

Anaphylactic reactions have not been reported with the Oral Solution which lacks Cremophor® EL. In fact, patients experiencing anaphylactic reactions have been treated subsequently with the Oral Solution without incident.

Sandimmune (cyclosporine) Oral Solution and I.V. should not be used concomitantly with other immunosuppressive agents except adrenal corticosteroids. Immunosuppression can lead to increased susceptibility to infection and the possible development of lymphoma. [See Boxed Warning.]

Care should be taken in using Sandimmune (cyclosporine) with nephrotoxic drugs. [See Precautions.]

PRECAUTIONS

General: Patients with malabsorption may have difficulty in achieving therapeutic levels with Sandimmune (cyclosporine) Oral Solution. Given its hyperkalemic effect, cyclosporine should not be used concomitantly with potassium-sparing diuretics.

Hypertension is a fairly common side effect of Sandimmune therapy (see Adverse Reactions). In some patients with cardiac transplants antihypertensive therapy was required.

Information for Patients: Patients should be informed of the necessity of repeated laboratory tests while they are receiving the drug. They should be given careful dosage instructions, advised of the potential risks during pregnancy and informed of the increased risk of neoplasia.

Laboratory Tests: Renal and liver functions should be assessed repeatedly by measurement of BUN, serum creatinine, serum bilirubin and liver enzymes.

Drug Interactions: Care should be taken using Sandimmune (cyclosporine) with nephrotoxic drugs since potential synergies of nephrotoxicity may occur. Drugs which have been reported to increase the hepatic metabolism of cyclosporine and *decrease* its plasma levels include rifampin, phenytoin, phenobarbital and I.V. sulfatrimethoprim; drugs which have been reported to *increase* the plasma concentration of cyclosporine by decreasing its metabolism include high dose methylprednisolone, erythromycin and the antifungal agents, ketoconazole and amphotericin B. Monitoring of plasma or blood levels of cyclosporine and appropriate dosage adjustment are essential when these drugs are used concomitantly.

Carcinogenesis, Mutagenesis and Impairment of Fertility: Cyclosporine gave no evidence of mutagenic or teratogenic effects in appropriate test systems. Only at dose levels toxic to dams, were adverse effects seen in reproduction studies in rats. [See Pregnancy.]

Carcinogenicity studies were carried out in male and female rats and mice. In the 78 week mouse study, at doses of 1, 4 and 16 mg/kg/day, evidence of a statistically significant trend was found for lymphocytic lymphomas in females, and the incidence of hepatocellular carcinomas in mid-dose males significantly exceeded the control value. In the 24 month rat study, conducted at 0.5, 2 and 8 mg/kg/day, pancreatic islet cell adenomas significantly exceeded the control rate in the low dose level. The hepatocellular carcinomas and pancreatic islet cell adenomas were not dose related.

No impairment in fertility was demonstrated in studies in male and female rats.

Pregnancy: Pregnancy Category C. Sandimmune® (cyclosporine) Oral Solution has been shown to be embryo- and fetotoxic in rats and rabbits when given in doses 2–5 times the human dose. At toxic doses (rats at 30 mg/kg/day and rabbits at 100 mg/kg/day), Sandimmune (cyclosporine) Oral Solution was embryo- and fetotoxic as indicated by increased pre- and postnatal mortality and reduced fetal weight together with related skeletal retardations. In the well-tolerated dose range (rats at up to 17 mg/kg/day and rabbits at up to 30 mg/kg/day), Sandimmune (cyclosporine) Oral Solution proved to be without any embryolethal or teratogenic effects.

There are no adequate and well-controlled studies in pregnant women. Sandimmune (cyclosporine) should be used during pregnancy only if the potential benefit justifies the potential risk to the fetus.

Nursing Mothers: Since Sandimmune (cyclosporine) is excreted in human milk, nursing should be avoided.

Pediatric Use: Although no adequate and well-controlled studies have been conducted in children, patients as young as 6 months of age have received the drug with no unusual adverse effects.

ADVERSE REACTIONS

The principal adverse reactions of Sandimmune (cyclosporine) therapy are renal dysfunction, tremor, hirsutism, hypertension and gum hyperplasia.

The following reactions occurred in 3% or greater of 892 patients involved in clinical trials of kidney, heart and liver transplants:

[See table on top next page].

The following reactions occurred in 2% or less of patients: allergic reactions, anemia, anorexia, confusion, conjunctivitis, edema, fever, brittle fingernails, gastritis, hearing loss, hiccups, hyperglycemia, muscle pain, peptic ulcer, thrombocytopenia, tinnitus.

The following reactions occurred rarely: anxiety, chest pain, constipation, depression, hair breaking, hematuria, joint pain, lethargy, mouth sores, myocardial infarction, night sweats, pancreatitis, pruritus, swallowing difficulty, tingling, upper GI bleeding, visual disturbance, weakness, weight loss.

[See table below].

Body System/ Adverse Reaction	Randomized Kidney Patients		All Sandimmune Patients		
	Sandimmune (N=227) %	Azathioprine (N=228) %	Kidney (N=705) %	Heart (N=112) %	Liver (N=75) %
Genitourinary					
Renal Dysfunction	32	6	25	38	37
Cardiovascular					
Hypertension	26	18	13	53	27
Cramps	4	<1	2	<1	0
Skin					
Hirsutism	21	<1	21	28	45
Acne	6	8	2	2	1
Central Nervous System					
Tremor	12	0	21	31	55
Convulsions	3	1	1	4	5
Headache	2	<1	2	15	4
Gastrointestinal					
Gum Hyperplasia	4	0	9	5	16
Diarrhea	3	<1	3	4	8
Nausea/Vomiting	2	<1	4	10	4
Hepatotoxicity	<1	<1	4	7	4
Abdominal Discomfort	<1	0	<1	7	0
Autonomic Nervous System					
Paresthesia	3	0	1	2	1
Flushing	<1	0	4	0	4
Hematopoietic					
Leukopenia	2	19	<1	6	0
Lymphoma	<1	0	1	6	1
Respiratory					
Sinusitis	<1	0	4	3	7
Miscellaneous					
Gynecomastia	<1	0	<1	4	3

Cremophor® EL is known to cause hyperlipemia and electrophoretic abnormalities of lipoproteins. These effects are reversible upon discontinuation of treatment but are usually not a reason to stop treatment.

OVERDOSAGE

There is a minimal experience with overdosage. Because of the slow absorption of Sandimmune (cyclosporine) Oral Solution, forced emesis would be of value up to 2 hours after administration. Transient hepatotoxicity and nephrotoxicity may occur which should resolve following drug withdrawal. General supportive measures and symptomatic treatment should be followed in all cases of overdosage. Sandimmune (cyclosporine) is not dialyzable to any great extent, nor is it cleared well by charcoal hemoperfusion. The oral LD_{50} is 2329 mg/kg in mice, 1480 mg/kg in rats, and > 1000 mg/kg in rabbits. The I.V. LD_{50} is 148 mg/kg in mice, 104 mg/kg in rats, and 46 mg/kg in rabbits.

DOSAGE AND ADMINISTRATION

Sandimmune Oral Solution

The initial dose of Sandimmune (cyclosporine) Oral Solution should be given 4–12 hours prior to transplantation as a single dose of 15 mg/kg per day (14–18 mg/kg per day were used in most clinical trials). This daily single dose is continued postoperatively for one to two weeks and then tapered by 5% per week to a maintenance level of 5–10 mg/kg per day. In several studies pediatric patients tolerated and required higher doses of cyclosporine. Some centers have successfully tapered the cyclosporine dose to as low as 3 mg/kg in selected renal transplant patients without an apparent rise in rejection rate.

In one large controlled study in renal transplantation, a lower initial dose of 10 mg/kg/day was used after a preoperative oral dose of 20 mg/kg. In this study, however, dosage was adjusted to achieve specific *plasma* levels as determined by radioimmunoassay (RIA). During the first few weeks after transplant, trough *plasma* levels of 150–250 ng/ml were sought. By three months post-transplant, trough *plasma* levels of 50–150 ng/ml were sought. These values correspond to trough *whole blood* levels of 450–750 ng/ml and 150–450 ng/ml. Overt nephrotoxicity was uncommon in that trial (although BUN and creatinine were somewhat increased on the average), perhaps because of the lower dose. Such a dose should not be considered, however, unless cyclosporine level monitoring can be obtained.

Adjunct steroid therapy is to be used. Study centers used prednisone in different tapering schedules with seemingly similar results. One center started with 2.0 mg/kg/day for days 0–4, tapered to 1.0 mg/kg/day by 1 week, 0.6 mg/kg/day by 2 weeks, 0.3 mg/kg/day by 1 month and reached a maintenance dose of 0.15 mg/kg/day by 2 months. Another center started with a 200 mg dose initially, tapered by 40 mg/day until reaching 20 mg/day and continued at this level for 60 days. A further reduction to 10 mg/day was made during the following months. In all centers adjustments in dosage were made according to the clinical situation.

To make Sandimmune® (cyclosporine) Oral Solution more palatable, the oral solution may be diluted with milk, chocolate milk, or orange juice preferably at room temperature. Take the prescribed amount of Sandimmune (cyclosporine) from the container using the pipette supplied, after removal from the protective cover, and transfer the solution to a glass of milk, chocolate milk, or orange juice. Stir well and drink at once. Do not allow to stand before drinking. It is best to use a glass container and rinse it with more diluent to ensure that the total dose is taken. After use, dry the outside of the pipette with a clean towel and replace it in the protective cover. To avoid turbidity, do not rinse the pipette with water or other cleaning agents.

Sandimmune I.V. Note: Anaphylactic reactions have occurred with Sandimmune (cyclosporine) I.V. See WARNINGS above.

Patients unable to take Sandimmune (cyclosporine) Oral Solution pre- or postoperatively may be treated with the I.V. concentrate. **Sandimmune I.V. concentrate is administered at one third the oral dose.** The initial dose of Sandimmune (cyclosporine) I.V. should be given 4–12 hours prior to transplantation as a single I.V. dose of 5–6 mg/kg per day. This daily single dose is continued postoperatively until the patient can tolerate the oral solution. Patients should be switched to Sandimmune (cyclosporine) Oral Solution as soon as possible after surgery. In pediatric usage, the same dose and dosing regimen may be used.

Adjunct steroid therapy is to be used. (See above.)

Immediately before use, the I.V. concentrate should be diluted 1 ml Sandimmune (cyclosporine) I.V. in 20 ml to 100 ml 0.9% Sodium Chloride Injection or 5% Dextrose Injection and given in a slow intravenous infusion over approximately 2 to 6 hours.

The Cremophor® EL contained in the concentrate for intravenous infusion can cause phthalate stripping from PVC.

Parenteral drug products should be inspected visually for particulate matter and discoloration prior to administration, whenever solution and container permit.

Blood Level Monitoring: Several study centers have found blood level monitoring of cyclosporine useful in patient management. While no fixed relationships have yet been established, 24 hour trough values of 250–800 ng/ml (whole blood, RIA) or 50–300 ng/ml (plasma, RIA) appear to minimize side effects and rejection events. Blood level monitoring is not a replacement for renal function monitoring with serum creatinines, creatinine clearance or tissue biopsies.

HOW SUPPLIED

Sandimmune (cyclosporine) Oral Solution is supplied in 50 ml bottles containing 100 mg of cyclosporine per ml (NDC 0078-0110-22). A graduated pipette for dispensing is provided. Sandimmune (cyclosporine) Oral Solution should be stored and dispensed in the original container at temperatures below 86°F (30°C). Do not store in the refrigerator. Once opened, the contents must be used within 2 months.

Sandimmune (cyclosporine) I.V. for intravenous infusion is supplied as a 5 ml sterile ampul containing 50 mg of cyclosporine per ml, in boxes of 10 ampuls (NDC 0078-0109-01). Sandimmune I.V. should be stored at temperatures below 86°F (30°C) and protected from light.

Protect from freezing.

Manufactured by SANDOZ Ltd.
Basle, Switzerland for
SANDOZ, Pharmaceuticals Corporation
East Hanover, N.J. 07936

[SDI-Z6(B) Issued June 2, 1986]

RENAL TRANSPLANT PATIENTS IN WHOM THERAPY WAS DISCONTINUED

Reason for Discontinuation	Randomized Patients		All Sandimmune Patients
	Sandimmune (N=227) %	Azathioprine (N=228) %	(N=705) %
Renal Toxicity	5.7	0	5.4
Infection	0	0.4	0.9
Lack of Efficacy	2.6	0.9	1.4
Acute Tubular Necrosis	2.6	0	1.0
Lymphoma/ Lymphoproliferative Disease	0.4	0	0.3
Hypertension	0	0	0.3
Hematological Abnormalities	0	0.4	0
Other	0	0	0.7

Sandimmune® (cyclosporine) was discontinued on a temporary basis and then restarted in 18 additional patients.

INFECTIOUS COMPLICATIONS IN THE RANDOMIZED RENAL TRANSPLANT PATIENTS

Complication	Cyclosporine Treatment N=227 % of Complications	Standard Treatment* N=228 % of Complications
Septicemia	5.3	4.8
Abcesses	4.4	5.3
Systemic Fungal Infection	2.2	3.9
Local Fungal Infection	7.5	9.6
Cytomegalovirus	4.8	12.3
Other Viral Infections	15.9	18.4
Urinary Tract Infections	21.1	20.2
Wound and Skin Infections	7.0	10.1
Pneumonia	6.2	9.2

* Some patients also received ALG.

IMMUNE GLOBULIN INTRAVENOUS (HUMAN) SANDOGLOBULIN® ℞

[san 'dō-glob "ū-lin]

Lyophilized Preparation

The following prescribing information is based on official labeling in effect on June 1, 1986.

DESCRIPTION

Immune Globulin Intravenous* (Human) (Sandoglobulin®) is a polyvalent antibody product containing in concentrated

Continued on next page

Sandoz—Cont.

form all the IgG antibodies which regularly occur in the donor population. This immunoglobulin preparation is produced by cold alcohol precipitation from large pools of human venous plasma. Before pooling, the single donor units of plasma have been found non-reactive for hepatitis B surface antigen (HBsAg) using test procedures of third-generation sensitivity. Sandoglobulin (IGIV) is made suitable for intravenous use by treatment at acid pH in the presence of trace amounts of pepsin (1, 2). The preparation contains at least 96% of IgG and upon reconstitution has a pH of 6.6 ± 0.2. Most of the immunoglobulins are monomeric (7 S) IgG; the remainder consists of dimeric IgG and a small amount of polymeric IgG, traces of IgA and IgM and immunoglobulin fragments (3). The distribution of the IgG subclasses corresponds to that of normal serum (4, 5, 6). Final container lyophilized units are prepared so as to contain 1, 3 or 6 g protein and 1.67, 5 or 10 g sucrose, respectively, as well as small quantities of NaCl. The lyophilized powder reconstitutes with 0.9% saline to a sterile 3% or 6% protein solution containing 5% or 10% sucrose, devoid of any preservatives.
*Hereinafter referred to as IGIV.

CLINICAL PHARMACOLOGY

This product contains a broad spectrum of antibody specificities against bacterial and viral antigens, that are capable of both opsonization and neutralization of microbes and toxins. The 3 week half-life of Immune Globulin Intravenous, (Human) (Sandoglobulin) corresponds to that of Immune Globulin (Human) for intramuscular use, although individual variations in half-time have been observed (7, 8). Appropriate doses of Sandoglobulin (IGIV) restore abnormally low immunoglobulin G levels to the normal range. 100% of the infused dose is available in the recipient's circulation immediately after infusion. After approximately 6 days an equilibrium is reached between the intra- and extravascular compartments. This is distributed approximately 50% intravascular and 50% extravascular. In comparison, after the intramuscular injection of an intramuscular immune globulin, the IgG requires 2–5 days to reach its maximum concentration in the intravascular compartment. This concentration corresponds to about 40% of the injected dose (8).
While Sandoglobulin (IGIV) has been shown to be effective in some cases of idiopathic thrombocytopenic purpura (ITP) (see INDICATIONS AND USAGE), the mechanism of action in ITP has not been fully elucidated.
Toxicity from overdose has not been observed on regimens of 0.4 g per kg body weight each day for 5 days (9, 10, 11). Sucrose is added to Sandoglobulin (IGIV) for reasons of stability, solubility and safety.
The intravenous administration of the sucrose used for stabilizing Immune Globulin Intravenous (Sandoglobulin) is considered to be innocuous (12). Because sucrose is excreted unchanged in the urine when given intravenously, Sandoglobulin (IGIV) may be given to diabetics, without compensatory changes in insulin dosage regimen.

INDICATIONS AND USAGE

Immunodeficiency:
Sandoglobulin (IGIV) is indicated for the substitution treatment of patients who are unable to produce sufficient amounts of IgG antibodies, e.g. in common variable immunodeficiency (10, 13, 14, 15). Sandoglobulin (IGIV) is preferable to intramuscular Immune Globulin (Human) preparations in treating patients who require an immediate and high increase in the intravascular immunoglobulin level (8), in patients with limited muscle mass, and in patients with bleeding tendencies for whom intramuscular injections are contraindicated. The infusions must be repeated at regular intervals. Sandoglobulin (IGIV) may also be used in severe combined immunodeficiency and in primary immunoglobulin deficiency syndromes such as X-linked agammaglobulinemia.

Idiopathic Thrombocytopenic Purpura
A controlled study was performed in which Sandoglobulin (IGIV) was compared with steroids for the treatment of acute (defined as less than 6 months duration) ITP in patients aged 13 years and younger. In this study, Sandoglobulin (IGIV) was as effective as steroids in increasing the platelet count (9, 17). However, it should be noted that many cases of acute ITP in childhood resolve spontaneously. The use of Immune Globulin (Intravenous (Human) in the treatment of acute ITP in patients 14 years of age or older has not been subjected to prospectively controlled clinical trials (19, 21, 22).
Some children and adults with chronic (defined as greater than 6 months duration) ITP have also shown an increase (albeit temporary) in platelet counts upon administration of Immune Globulin Intravenous (Sandoglobulin®) (18, 20, 23). Therefore, in situations that require a rapid, temporary rise in platelet count, for example prior to surgery or in control of excessive bleeding, use of Sandoglobulin (IGIV) should be considered. However, it should be noted that not all patients will respond. Even in those patients who do respond, this treatment should not be considered to be curative.

CONTRAINDICATIONS

As with all blood products containing IgA, Sandoglobulin (IGIV) is contraindicated in patients with selective IgA deficiency, who possess antibody to IgA. It may also be contraindicated in patients who have had severe systemic reactions to the intravenous or intramuscular administration of human immune globulin.

WARNINGS

Patients with agamma- or extreme hypogammaglobulinemia who have never before received immunoglobulin substitution treatment or whose time from last treatment is greater than 8 weeks, may be at risk of developing inflammatory reactions on rapid infusion of Sandoglobulin (IGIV) (over 20 drops [1 ml] per minute). These reactions are manifested by a rise in temperature, chills, nausea and vomiting. The patient's vital signs should be monitored continuously and he should be carefully observed throughout the infusion, since these reactions on rare occasions may lead to shock. Epinephrine should be available for treatment of an acute anaphylactic reaction. Particular care should be exercised when Immune Globulin Intravenous (Sandoglobulin) is administered to patients with paraproteins (15).

PRECAUTIONS

It is generally advisable not to dilute plasma derivatives with other infusable drugs. Sandoglobulin (IGIV) should be given by a separate infusion line. No other medications or fluids should be mixed with the Sandoglobulin (IGIV) preparation.
Pregnancy: Pregnancy Category C. Animal reproduction studies have not been conducted with Sandoglobulin (IGIV). It is also not known whether Sandoglobulin (IGIV) can cause fetal harm when administered to a pregnant woman or can affect reproduction capacity. Sandoglobulin (IGIV) should be given to a pregnant woman only if clearly needed (22).
Pediatric use: High dose administration of Sandoglobulin (IGIV) in children with acute or chronic idiopathic thrombocytopenic purpura or in preterm neonates did not reveal any pediatric-specific hazard (9, 16).

ADVERSE REACTIONS

Adverse reactions to Sandoglobulin (IGIV) are rare and occur in less than 1% of patients who are not immunodeficient. Agammaglobulinemic and hypogammaglobulinemic patients who have never received immunoglobulin substitution therapy before or whose time from last treatment is greater than 8 weeks may show adverse reactions if the initial infusion flow rate exceeds 20 drops (1 ml) per minute. This occurs in approximately 10% of the cases.
These reactions, which generally become apparent only 30 minutes to one hour after the beginning of the infusion, are as follows: flushing of the face, feelings of tightness in the chest, chills, fever, dizziness, nausea, diaphoresis and hypotension. In such cases the infusion should be temporarily stopped until the symptoms have subsided. Immediate anaphylactoid and hypersensitivity reactions due to previous sensitization of the recipient to certain antigens, most commonly IgA, may be observed in exceptional cases, described under CONTRAINDICATIONS (10, 11, 24).

DOSAGE AND ADMINISTRATION

Adult and child substitution therapy: The usual dose of Immune Globulin Intravenous (Sandoglobulin) in immunodeficiency syndromes is 0.2 g per kg of body weight administered once a month by intravenous infusion. If the clinical response is inadequate or the level of serum IgG achieved is insufficient (minimum serum level of 300 mg per dl), the dose may be increased to 0.3 g per kg of body weight or the infusion may be repeated more frequently than once a month (10, 13, 14, 15).
The first infusion of Sandoglobulin (IGIV) in previously untreated agammaglobulinemic or hypogammaglobulinemic patients must be given as a 3% immunoglobulin solution (use the total volume of fluid provided to reconstitute the lyophilized product). Start with a flow rate of 10 to 20 drops (0.5 to 1.0 ml) per minute. After 15–30 minutes the rate of infusion may be further increased to 30 to 50 drops (1.5 to 2.5 ml) per minute. Subsequent infusions may be administered at a rate of 40 to 50 drops (2.0 to 2.5 ml) per minute.
If high doses have to be administered repeatedly after the first dose, a 6% solution may be used (use half the volume of fluid provided to reconstitute the lyophilized product). In this case the initial rate of infusion should be 20 to 30 drops (1.0 to 1.5 ml) per minute, increased after 15–30 minutes to a maximum of 50 drops (2.5 ml) per minute.
Recent investigations confirm that Immune Globulin Intravenous (Sandoglobulin®) is well tolerated and not likely to produce side effects when infused at these rates (11). However, the first infusion of Sandoglobulin (IGIV) in previously untreated agammaglobulinemic and hypogammaglobulinemic patients may lead to systemic side effects. Some of the effects may occur as a result of the reaction between the antibodies administered and free antigens in the blood and tissues of the immunodeficient recipient (11, 24). When free antigen is no longer present, further administration of Sandoglobulin (IGIV) to immunodeficient patients as well as to normal individuals usually does not cause further untoward side effects.
Therapy of idiopathic thrombocytopenic purpura (ITP): 0.4 g per kg of body weight on 5 consecutive days.
Reconstitution: Preparation of a 3% or 6% solution
For a 3% solution:

1. Tear off the protective caps from the bottles containing the solvent and the Sandoglobulin (IGIV). Disinfect both rubber stoppers with alcohol.
2. Remove the protective cover from one end of the transfer set and insert the needle through the rubber stopper into the bottle containing the solvent.
3. Remove the cover from the other needle and plunge the inverted Sandoglobulin (IGIV) bottle onto it, as shown in 3.
4. Invert the two bottles, so that the solvent flows into the Sandoglobulin (IGIV) bottle.
5. Discard the empty solvent bottle and the transfer set.

For a 6% solution*:

1. Follow steps 1–3 above.
2. Invert the two bottles, so that the solvent flows into the Immune Globulin Intravenous (Sandoglobulin) bottle. Use half the solvent by removing the solvent bottle with transfer needle as soon as the fluid reaches the 6% mark printed on the Sandoglobulin (IGIV) label.
Note: The 6% mark is printed on the label only to provide general guidance in preparing a solution containing approximately 6 g protein per 100 ml. If an exact dosage of a 6% solution is required, reconstitute with diluent by using a hypodermic needle and syringe; e.g.,
for 1 g vial use 16.5 ml diluent,
for 3 g vial use 50 ml diluent,
for 6 g vial use 100 ml diluent.
3. Discard any unused solvent and the transfer set.
Sandoglobulin (IGIV) normally dissolves within a few minutes, though in exceptional cases it may take up to 20 minutes.

DO NOT SHAKE!
Any undissolved particles should respond to careful rotation of the bottle. Avoid frothing.
PROCEED WITH INFUSION ONLY IF SOLUTION IS CLEAR AND AT APPROXIMATELY BODY TEMPERATURE!
Parenteral drug products should be inspected visually for particulate matter and discoloration prior to administration, whenever solution and container permit.

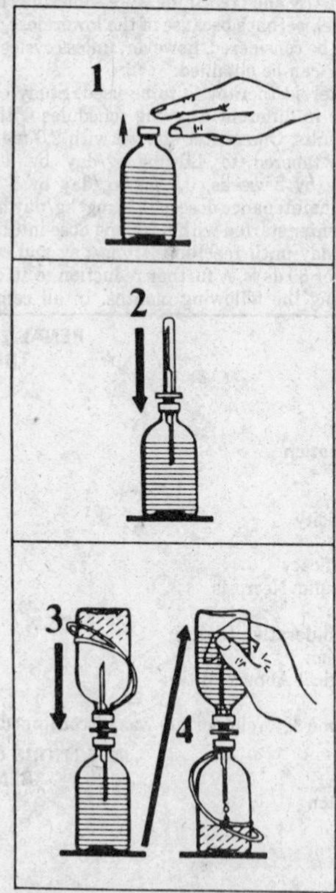

HOW SUPPLIED

Immune Globulin Intravenous (Sandoglobulin) is supplied as a kit containing the lyophilized preparation, sterile Sodium Chloride Injection USP, one double-ended spike for reconstitution and complete directions for use.
Sandoglobulin (IGIV) is available in three package sizes:

- 1 g Sandoglobulin (IGIV) and 33 ml reconstitution fluid
- 3 g Sandoglobulin (IGIV) and 100 ml reconstitution fluid
- 6 g Sandoglobulin (IGIV) and 200 ml reconstitution fluid

STORAGE—Sandoglobulin (IGIV) should be stored at a temperature not exceeding 25°C (77°F).

The preparation should not be used after the expiration date printed on the label.
—Begin administration promptly after reconstitution.
—Partially used vials should be discarded.

CAUTION

U.S. Federal law prohibits dispensing without prescription.

REFERENCES

1. Römer, J., Morgenthaler, J.J., Scherz, R., and F. Skvaril: Characterization of various Immunoglobulin-Preparations for intravenous Application. I. Protein composition and antibody content. Vox. Sang. 42:62–73 (1982).
2. Römer, J., Späth, P.J., Skvaril, F., and U.E. Nydegger: Characterization of various Immunoglobulin Preparations for intravenous Application. II. Complement Activation and Binding to Staphylococcus Protein A. Vox. Sang. 42:74–80 (1982).
3. Römer, J. and P.J. Späth: Molecular Composition of Immunoglobulin Preparations and its Relation to Complement Activation. In Nydegger, U.E. (Editor): Immunohemotherapy: A Guide to Immunoglobulin Prophylaxis and Therapy. Academic Press, London, p. 123 (1981).
4. Skvaril, F., Roth-Wicky, B., and S. Barandun: IgG Subclasses in Human-γ-Globulin Preparations for Intravenous Use and their Reactivity with Staphylococcus Protein A. Vox. Sang. 38:147 (1980).
5. Skvaril, F.: Qualitative and Quantitative Aspects of IgG Subclasses in i.v. Immunoglobulin Preparations. In Nydegger, U.E. (Editor): Immunohemotherapy: A Guide to Immunoglobulin Prophylaxis and Therapy. Academic Press, London p. 113 (1981).
6. Skvaril, F., and S. Barandun: In vitro Characterization of Immunoglobulins for Intravenous Use. In: Immunoglobulins: Characteristics and Uses of Intravenous Preparations. Alving, B.M. and J.S. Finlayson (Eds.). DHHS Publication No. (FDA)-80-9005, Washington: U.S. Government Printing Office, 1980, pp. 201–206.
7. Morell, A., and F. Skvaril: Struktur und biologische Eigenschaften von Immunoglobulinen und γ-Globulin-Präparaten. II. Eigenschaften von γ-Globulin-Präparaten. Schweiz. Med. Wschr. 110:80 (1980).
8. Morell, A., Schürch, B., Ryser, D., Hofer, F., Skvaril, F., and S. Barandun: In vivo Behaviour of Gamma Globulin Preparations. Vox. Sang. 38:272 (1980).
9. Imbach, P., Barandun, S., d'Apuzzo, V., Baumgartner, C., Hirt, A., Morell, A., Rossi, E., Schöni, M., Vest, M., and H.P. Wagner: High-dose Intravenous Gammaglobulin for Idiopathic Thrombocytopenic Purpura in Childhood. The Lancet, June 6: 1228 (1981).
10. Barandun, S., Morell, A., and F. Skvaril: Clinical Experiences with Immunoglobulin for Intravenous Use. In: Immunoglobulins: Characteristics and Uses of Intravenous Preparations. Alving, B.M., and J.S. Finlayson (Eds.). DHHS Publication No. (FDA)-80-9005, Washington: U.S. Government Printing Office, 1980, pp. 31–35.
11. Barandun, S., and A. Morell: Adverse Reactions to Immunoglobulin Preparations. In Nydegger, U.E. (Editor): Immunohemotherapy: A Guide to Immunoglobulin Prophylaxis and Therapy. Academic Press, London, p. 223 (1981).
12. Martindale: The Extra Pharmacopoeia, 27th Edition, ed. by Wade, A., p. 65 (1979). The Pharmaceutical Press, London.
13. Joller, P.W., Barandun, S., and W.H. Hitzig: Neue Möglichkeiten der Immunoglobulin-Ersatztherapie bei Antikörpermangel. Syndrom. Schweiz. Med. Wschr. 110:1451 (1980).
14. Barandun, S., Imbach, P., Morell, A., and H.P. Wagner: Clinical Indications for Immunoglobulin Infusion. In Nydegger, U.E. (Editor): Immunohemotherapy: A Guide to Immunoglobulin Prophylaxis and Therapy. Academic Press, London, p. 275 (1981).
15. Cunningham-Rundles, C., Smithwick, E.M., Siegal, F.P., Day, N.K. et al.: Treatment of Primary Humoral Immunodeficiency Disease with Intravenous (pH 4.0 Treated) Gammaglobulin. In: Nydegger, U.E. (Editor): Immunohemotherapy: A Guide to Immunoglobulin Prophylaxis and Therapy. Academic Press, London, p. 283 (1981).
16. Von Muralt, G., and D. Sidiropoulos: Intravenous IgG Substitution Therapy in the Treatment of Septicemia in Preterm Neonates. In: Nydegger, U.E. (Editor): Immunohemotherapy: A Guide to Immunoglobulin Prophylaxis and Therapy. Academic Press, London, p. 313 (1981).
17. Imbach, P.: A Comparison of Intravenous Immunoglobulin and Oral Corticosteroids in the Treatment of Acute Idiopathic Thrombocytopenia (ITP): A Cooperative, Randomized Study at Swiss and German Paediatric Hospitals/Hospital Departments. Data on File, Sandoz, Inc., East Hanover, N.J.
18. Bussel, J.B., Kimberly, R. P., Inman, R. D., Schulman, I., Cunningham-Rundles, C., Smithwick, E.M., O'Malley, J., Barandun, S., Polk, J.R., Cheung, N., and M.W. Hilgartner: Intravenous Gammaglobulin for Chronic Idiopathic Thrombocytopenic Purpura. Blood 62(2):480–486(Aug) 1983.
19. Fehr, J., Hofmann, V., and U. Kappeler: Transient Reversal of Thrombocytopenia in Idiopathic Thrombocytopenic Purpura by High-Dose Intravenous Gamma Globulin. N. Engl. J. Med. 306:1254 (1982).
20. Abe, T., Matsuda, J., Kawasugi, K., Joshimuro, Y., Kinoshita, T., and M. Kazama: Clinical Effect of Intravenous Immunoglobulin in Chronic Idiopathic Thrombocytopenic Purpura. Blut 47 (2):69–75 (Aug) 1983.
21. Mueller-Eckhardt, C., Küenzler, E., Thilo-Körner, D., and H. Pralle: High-Dose Intravenous Immunoglobulin for Posttransfusion Purpura. N. Engl. J. Med. 308 (5):287 (Feb. 3) 1983.
22. Wenske, G., Gaedicke, G., Küenzler, E. Heyes, H., Mueller-Eckhardt, C., Kleihauer, E., and G. Lauritzen: Treatment of Idiopathic Thrombocytopenic Purpura in Pregnancy by High-Dose Intravenous Immunoglobulin. Blut 46:347–353 (1983).
23. Newland, A.C., Treleaven, J.G., Minchinton, B., and A.H. Waters: High-Dose Intravenous IgG in Adults with Autoimmune Thrombocytopenia. Lancet I :84–87 (Jan. 15) 1983.
24. Cunningham-Rundles, C., Day, N.K., Wahn, V., Smithwick, E.M., Siegal, F.P., Gupta, S., and R.A. Good: Reactions To Intravenous Gammaglobulin Infusions And Immune Complex Formation. In Nydegger, U.E. (Editor): Immunohemotherapy: A Guide to Immunoglobulin Prophylaxis and Therapy. Academic Press, London, p. 447 (1981).

Manufactured by:
CENTRAL LABORATORY
BLOOD TRANSFUSION SERVICE
SWISS RED CROSS
Wankdorfstrasse 10
3000 Berne 22
Switzerland
U.S. License No. 647
Distributed by:
SANDOZ, Pharmaceuticals Corporation
East Hanover, N.J. 07936
[SGL-Z4 Issued: January 21, 1986]

SANOREX® Ⓒ

[san'ō-rex"]
(mazindol) tablets, USP

The following prescribing information is based on official labeling in effect on July 15, 1986.

DESCRIPTION

Sanorex® (mazindol) is an imidazoiso-indole anorectic agent. It is chemically designated as 5-p-chloro-phenyl-5-hydroxy-2, 3- dihydro-5H-imidazo (2,1-a) isoindole, a tautomeric form of 2-[2'-(p-chlorobenzoyl) phenyl]-2-imidazoline.
1 mg. and 2 mg, Tablets
Active Ingredient: mazindol, USP
Inactive Ingredients: calcium sulfate dihydrate, lactose, magnesium stearate, povidone, starch and talc

ACTIONS

Sanorex, (mazindol), although an isoindole, has pharmacologic activity similar in many ways to the prototype drugs used in obesity, the amphetamines. Actions include central nervous system stimulation in humans and animals, as well as such amphetamine-like effects in animals as the production of stereotyped behavior. Animal experiments also suggest certain differences from phenethylamine anorectic drugs, e.g., amphetamine, with respect to site and mechanism of action; for example, mazindol appears to exert its primary effects on the limbic system. The significance of these differences for humans is uncertain. It does not cause brain norepinephrine depletion in animals; on the other hand, it does appear to inhibit storage site uptake of norepinephrine as is suggested by its marked potentiation of the effect of exogenous norepinephrine on blood pressure in dogs (see WARNINGS) and on smooth muscle contraction *in vitro.*
Tolerance has been demonstrated with all drugs of this class in which this phenomenon has been studied.
Drugs used in obesity are commonly known as "anorectics" or "anorexigenics." It has not been established, however, that the action of such drugs in treating obesity is exclusively one of appetite suppression. Other central nervous system actions, or metabolic effects may be involved as well.
Adult obese subjects instructed in dietary management and treated with anorectic drugs, lose more weight on the average than those treated with placebo and diet, as determined in relatively short-term clinical trials.
The average magnitude of increased weight loss of drug-treated patients over placebo-treated patients in studies of anorectics in general is ordinarily only a fraction of a pound a week. The rate of weight loss is greatest in the first weeks of therapy for both drug and placebo subjects and tends to decrease in succeeding weeks.
The amount of weight loss associated with the use of Sanorex (mazindol), as with other anorectic drugs, varies from trial to trial, and the increased weight loss appears to be related in part to variables other than the drugs prescribed, such as the interaction between physician-investigator and the patient, the population treated, and the diet prescribed. The importance of non-drug factors in such weight loss has not been elucidated.
The natural history of obesity is measured in years, whereas, most studies cited are restricted to a few weeks' duration; thus, the total impact of drug-induced weight loss over that of diet alone must be considered clinically limited.

INDICATION

Sanorex® (mazindol) is indicated in the management of exogenous obesity as a short-term (a few weeks) adjunct in a regimen of weight reduction based on caloric restriction. The limited usefulness of agents of this class (see ACTIONS) should be measured against possible risk factors inherent in their use, such as those described below.

CONTRAINDICATIONS

Glaucoma; hypersensitivity or idiosyncrasy to Sanorex (mazindol).
Agitated states.
Patients with a history of drug abuse.
During or within 14 days following the administration of monoamine oxidase inhibitors, (hypertensive crises may result).

WARNINGS

Tolerance to the effect of many anorectic drugs may develop within a few weeks; if this occurs, the recommended dose should not be exceeded in an attempt to increase the effect; rather, the drug should be discontinued.
Sanorex (mazindol) may impair the ability of the patient to engage in potentially hazardous activities such as operating machinery or driving a motor vehicle; the patient should therefore be cautioned accordingly.
Drug Interactions: Sanorex (mazindol) may decrease the hypotensive effect of guanethidine; patients should be monitored accordingly.
Sanorex (mazindol) may markedly potentiate the pressor effect of exogenous catecholamines. If it should be necessary to give a pressor amine agent (e.g., levarterenol or isoproterenol) to a patient in shock (e.g., from a myocardial infarction) who has recently been taking Sanorex (mazindol) extreme care should be taken in monitoring blood pressure at frequent intervals and initiating pressor therapy with a low initial dose and careful titration.
Drug Dependence: Sanorex (mazindol) shares important pharmacologic properties with amphetamines. Amphetamines and related stimulant drugs have been extensively abused and can produce tolerance and severe psychologic dependence. In this regard, the manifestations of chronic overdosage or withdrawal of Sanorex (mazindol) have not been determined in humans. Abstinence effects have been observed in dogs after abrupt cessation for prolonged periods. There was some self-administration of the drug in monkeys. EEG studies and "liking" scores in human subjects yielded equivocal results. While the abuse potential of Sanorex (mazindol) has not been further defined, the possibility of dependence should be kept in mind when evaluating the desirability of including Sanorex (mazindol) as part of a weight reduction program.
Usage in Pregnancy: Sanorex (mazindol) was studied in reproduction experiments in rats and rabbits and an increase in neonatal mortality and a possible increased incidence of rib anomalies in rats were observed at relatively high doses. Although these studies have not indicated important adverse effects, use of mazindol by women who are or may become pregnant requires that the potential benefit be weighed against the possible hazard to mother and infant.
Usage in Children: Sanorex (mazindol) is not recommended for use in children under 12 years of age.

PRECAUTIONS

Insulin requirements in diabetes mellitus may be altered in association with the use of mazindol and the concomitant dietary regimen.
The least amount feasible should be prescribed or dispensed at one time in order to minimize the possibility of overdosage.
Use only with caution in hypertension with monitoring of blood pressure, since evidence is insufficient to rule out a possible adverse effect on blood pressure in some hypertensive patients. The drug is not recommended in severely hypertensive patients. The drug is not recommended for patients with symptomatic cardiovascular disease including arrhythmias.

ADVERSE REACTIONS

The most common adverse effects of Sanorex (mazindol) are dry mouth, tachycardia, constipation, nervousness and insomnia.
Cardiovascular: Palpitation, tachycardia.
Central Nervous System: Overstimulation, restlessness, dizziness, insomnia, dysphoria, tremor, headache, depression, drowsiness, weakness.
Gastrointestinal: Dryness of the mouth, unpleasant taste, diarrhea, constipation, nausea, other gastrointestinal disturbances.

Continued on next page

Sandoz—Cont.

Skin: Rash, excessive sweating, clamminess.
Endocrine: Impotence, changes in libido have rarely been observed with Sanorex (mazindol).
Eye: Treatment of dogs with high doses of Sanorex (mazindol) for long periods resulted in some corneal opacities, reversible on cessation of medication. No such effect has been observed in humans.

DOSAGE AND ADMINISTRATION

Usual dosage is 1 mg three times daily, one hour before meals, or 2 mg once daily, one hour before lunch. The lowest effective dose should be used. To determine the lowest effective dose, therapy with Sanorex (mazindol) may be initiated at 1 mg once a day, and adjusted to the need and response of the patient. Should G.I. discomfort occur, Sanorex (mazindol) may be taken with meals.

OVERDOSAGE

There are no data as yet on acute overdosage with Sanorex (mazindol) in humans.
Manifestations of acute overdosage with amphetamines and related substances include restlessness, tremor, rapid respiration, dizziness. Fatigue and depression may follow the stimulatory phase of overdosage. Cardiovascular effects include tachycardia, hypertension and circulatory collapse. Gastrointestinal symptoms include nausea, vomiting and abdominal cramps. While similar manifestations of overdosage may be seen with Sanorex (mazindol), their exact nature has yet to be determined. The management of acute intoxication is largely symptomatic. Data are not available on the treatment of acute intoxication with Sanorex (mazindol) by hemodialysis or peritoneal dialysis, but the substance is poorly soluble except at very acid pH.

HOW SUPPLIED

Sanorex (mazindol) is available in 1 mg elliptical, white tablets and in 2 mg round, white scored tablets, in packages of 100.
Company's Product Indentification Mark(s): 1 mg tablets embossed SANOREX on one side, 78-71 other side. 2 mg tablets scored 78-66 on one side, SANDOZ other side.
[SNX-Z13 Issued July 15, 1986]
Shown in Product Identification Section, page 427

SANSERT® ℞

[san'surt]
(methysergide maleate) tablets, USP

The following prescribing information is based on official labeling in effect on July 15, 1986.

> **WARNING**
> Retroperitoneal Fibrosis, Pleuropulmonary Fibrosis and Fibrotic Thickening of Cardiac Valves May Occur in Patients Receiving Long-term Methysergide Maleate Therapy. Therefore, This Preparation Must be Reserved for Prophylaxis in Patients Whose Vascular Headaches Are Frequent and/or Severe and Uncontrollable and Who Are Under Close Medical Supervision.
> *(See Also "Warnings" Section.)*

DESCRIPTION

Sansert® (methysergide maleate) is a partially synthetic compound structurally related to lysergic acid butanolamide, well-known as methylergonovine in obstetrical practice as an oxytocic agent.
Methylation in the number 1 position of the ring structure enormously enhances the antagonism to serotonin which is present to a much lesser degree in the partially methylated compound (methylergonovine maleate) as well as profoundly altering other pharmacologic properties.
Active Ingredient: methysergide maleate, USP
Inactive Ingredients: acacia, carnauba wax, colloidal silicon dioxide, FD&C Blue #1, FD&C Yellow #5, gelatin, lactose, malic acid, povidone, sodium benzoate, starch, stearic acid, sucrose, talc, and titanium dioxide

ACTIONS

Sansert (methysergide maleate) has been shown, *in vitro* and *in vivo*, to inhibit or block the effects of serotonin, a substance which may be involved in the mechanism of vascular headaches. Serotonin has been variously described as a central neurohumoral agent or chemical mediator, as a "headache substance" acting directly or indirectly to lower pain threshold (others in this category include tyramine; polypeptides, such as bradykinin; histamine; and acetylcholine), as an intrinsic "motor hormone" of the gastrointestinal tract, and as a "hormone" involved in connective tissue reparative processes. Suggestions have been made by investigators as to the mechanism whereby methysergide produces its clinical effects, but this has not been finally established.

INDICATIONS

For the prevention or reduction of intensity and frequency of vascular headaches in the following kinds of patients:

1. Patients suffering from one or more severe vascular headaches per week.
2. Patients suffering from vascular headaches that are uncontrollable or so severe that preventive therapy is indicated regardless of the frequency of the attack.

CONTRAINDICATIONS

Pregnancy, peripheral vascular disease, severe arteriosclerosis, severe hypertension, coronary artery disease, phlebitis or cellulitis of the lower limbs, pulmonary disease, collagen diseases or fibrotic processes, impaired liver or renal function, valvular heart disease, debilitated states and serious infections.

WARNINGS

With long-term, uninterrupted administration, retroperitoneal fibrosis or related conditions—pleuropulmonary fibrosis and cardiovascular disorders with murmurs or vascular bruits have been reported. Patients must be warned to report immediately the following symptoms: cold, numb, and painful hands and feet; leg cramps on walking; any type of girdle, flank, or chest pain, or any associated symptomatology. Should any of these symptoms develop, methysergide should be discontinued. Continuous administration should not exceed 6 months. There must be a drug-free interval of 3-4 weeks after each 6-month course of treatment. The dosage should be reduced gradually during the last 2-3 weeks of each treatment course to avoid "headache rebound."
The drug is not recommended for use in children.

PRECAUTIONS

All patients receiving Sansert (methysergide maleate) should remain under constant supervision of the physician and be examined regularly for the development of fibrotic or vascular complications. (See Adverse Reactions).
The manifestations of retroperitoneal fibrosis, pleuropulmonary fibrosis, and vascular shutdown have shown a high incidence of regression once Sansert (methysergide maleate) is withdrawn. These facts should be borne in mind to avoid unnecessary surgical intervention. Cardiac murmurs, which may indicate endocardial fibrosis, have shown varying degrees of regression, with complete disappearance in some and persistence in others.
Sansert (methysergide maleate) has been specifically designed for the prophylaxis of vascular headache and has no place in the management of the acute attack.
Sansert tablets contain FD&C Yellow No. 5 (tartrazine) which may cause allergic-type reactions (including bronchial asthma) in certain susceptible individuals. Although the overall incidence of FD&C Yellow No. 5 (tartrazine) sensitivity in the general population is low, it is frequently seen in patients who also have aspirin hypersensitivity.

ADVERSE REACTIONS

Within the recommended dose levels, the following side effects have been reported:

1) Fibrotic Complications
Fibrotic changes have been observed in the retroperitoneal, pleuropulmonary, cardiac, and other tissues, either singly or, very rarely, in combination.
Retroperitoneal Fibrosis: This non-specific fibrotic process is usually confined to the retroperitoneal connective tissue above the pelvic brim and may present clinically with one or more symptoms such as general malaise, fatigue, weight loss, backache, low grade fever (elevated sedimentation rate), urinary obstruction (girdle or flank pain, dysuria, polyuria, oliguria, elevated BUN), vascular insufficiency of the lower limbs (leg pain, Leriche syndrome, edema of legs, thrombophlebitis). The single most useful diagnostic procedure in suspected cases of retroperitoneal fibrosis is intravenous pyelography. Typical deviation and obstruction of one or both ureters may be observed.
Pleuropulmonary Complications: A similar nonspecific fibrotic process, limited to the pleural and immediately subjacent pulmonary tissues, usually presents clinically with dyspnea, tightness and pain in the chest, pleural friction rubs, and pleural effusion. These findings may be confirmed by chest X-ray.
Cardiac Complications: Nonrheumatic fibrotic thickenings of the aortic root and of the aortic and mitral valves usually present clinically with cardiac murmurs and dyspnea.
Other Fibrotic Complications: Several cases of fibrotic plaques, simulating Peyronie's disease have been described.

2) Cardiovascular Complications
Encroachment of retroperitoneal fibrosis on the aorta, inferior vena cava and their common iliac branches may result in vascular insufficiency of the lower limbs, the presenting features of which are mentioned under retroperitoneal fibrosis.
Intrinsic vasoconstriction of large and small arteries, involving one or more vessels or merely a segment of a vessel, may occur at any stage of therapy. Depending on the vessel involved, this complication may present with chest pain, abdominal pain, or cold, numb, painful extremities with or without paresthesias and diminished or absent pulses. Progression to ischemic tissue damage has rarely been reported. Prompt withdrawal of the drug at the first signs of impaired circulation is recommended (See Warnings) to obviate such effects.
Postural hypotension and tachycardia have also been observed.

3) Gastrointestinal Symptoms
Nausea, vomiting, diarrhea, heartburn, abdominal pain. These effects tend to appear early and can frequently be obviated by gradual introduction of the medication and by administration of the drug with meals.
Constipation and elevation of gastric HCl have also been reported.

4) CNS Symptoms
Insomnia, drowsiness, mild euphoria, dizziness, ataxia, lightheadedness, hyperesthesia, unworldly feelings (described variously as "dissociation," "hallucinatory experiences," etc.). Some of these symptoms may be associated with vascular headaches, per se, and may, therefore, be unrelated to the drug.

5) Dermatological Manifestations
Facial flush, telangiectasia, and nonspecific rashes have rarely been reported. Increased hair loss may occur, but in many instances the tendency has abated despite continued therapy.

6) Edema
Peripheral edema, and more rarely, localized brawny edema may occur.
Dependent edema has responded to lowered doses, salt restriction, or diuretics.

7) Weight Gain
Weight gain may be a reason to caution patients regarding their caloric intake.

8) Hematological Manifestations
Neutropenia, eosinophilia.

9) Miscellaneous
Weakness, arthralgia, myalgia.

DOSAGE AND ADMINISTRATION

Usual adult dose 4 to 8 mg daily. Tablets to be given with meals.
Note: There must be a medication-free interval of 3-4 weeks after every 6-month course of treatment (see WARNINGS).
No pediatric dosage has been established.
If, after a 3-week trial period, efficacy has not been demonstrated, longer administration of Sansert (methysergide maleate) is unlikely to be of benefit.

HOW SUPPLIED

Bottles of 100 tablets, each tablet containing 2 mg of methysergide maleate, USP.
Company's Product Identification Mark(s): Imprinted 78-58 on one side, SANDOZ other side.
[SAN-Z21 Issued July 15, 1986]
Shown in Product Identification Section, page 427

SYNTOCINON® INJECTION ℞

[sin"tō'si-non]
(oxytocin injection, USP)

The following prescribing information is based on official labeling in effect on July 15, 1986.

DESCRIPTION

Syntocinon® (oxytocin) injection is a synthetic nonapeptide. For intravenous or intramuscular administration.
Each 1 ml of Syntocinon solution contains 10 USP or International Units of oxytocin and the following inactive ingredients:

sodium acetate, USP	1 mg
sodium chloride, USP	0.017 mg
chlorobutanol, NF	0.5%
alcohol, USP	0.61% by vol.
acetic acid, NF, qs to	pH 4 ± .3
water for injection, USP, qs to	1 ml

The Syntocinon solution in each ampul is sterile.
Syntocinon (oxytocin) is a cyclic (1–6) nonapeptide with the following chemical name.
Glycinamide, L-cysteinyl-L-tyrosyl-L-isoleucyl-L-glutaminyl-L-asparaginyl-L-cysteinyl-L-prolyl-L-leucyl-, cyclic (1–6)-disulfide
Its Chemical Abstract Registry number is: 50-56-6.

CLINICAL PHARMACOLOGY

The pharmacologic and clinical properties of Syntocinon (oxytocin) are identical with the naturally occurring oxytocic principle of the posterior lobe of the pituitary. Syntocinon (oxytocin) injection does not contain the amino acids characteristic of vasopressin, and therefore has fewer and less severe cardiovascular effects. Syntocinon (oxytocin) exerts a selective action on the smooth musculature of the uterus, particularly toward the end of pregnancy, during labor and immediately following delivery. Oxytocin stimulates rhythmic contractions of the uterus, increases the frequency of existing contractions, and raises the tone of the uterine musculature.

Syntocinon (oxytocin), when given in appropriate doses during pregnancy, is capable of eliciting graded increases in uterine motility from a moderate increase in the rate and force of spontaneous motor activity to sustained tetanic contraction.
Syntocinon (oxytocin) is promptly effective after parenteral administration. Following intramuscular injection, the myotonic effect on the uterus appears in 3–7 minutes, and persists for 30–60 minutes. With intravenous injection, the uterine effect appears within one minute and is of more brief duration.

INDICATIONS AND USAGE

IMPORTANT NOTICE
Syntocinon (oxytocin) injection is indicated for the medical rather than the elective induction of labor. Available data and information are inadequate to define the benefits to risks considerations in the use of the drug product for elective induction. Elective induction of labor is defined as the initiation of labor for convenience in an individual with a term pregnancy who is free of medical indications.

Antepartum: Syntocinon® (oxytocin) is indicated for the initiation or improvement of uterine contractions, where this is desirable and considered suitable, in order to achieve early vaginal delivery for fetal or maternal reasons. It is indicated for (1) induction of labor in patients with a medical indication for the initiation of labor, such as Rh problems, maternal diabetes, pre-eclampsia at or near term, when delivery is in the best interest of mother and fetus or when membranes are prematurely ruptured and delivery is indicated; (2) stimulation or reinforcement of labor, as in selected cases of uterine inertia; (3) as adjunctive therapy in the management of incomplete or inevitable abortion. In the first trimester currettage is generally considered primary therapy. In the second trimester abortion, oxytocin infusion will often be successful in emptying the uterus. Other means of therapy, however, may be required in such cases.
Postpartum: Syntocinon (oxytocin) injection is indicated to produce uterine contractions during the third stage of labor and to control postpartum bleeding or hemorrhage.

CONTRAINDICATIONS

Syntocinon (oxytocin) injection is contraindicated in any of the following conditions: Significant cephalopelvic disproportion; unfavorable fetal positions or presentations which are undeliverable without conversion prior to delivery, (transverse lies); i.e., in obstetrical emergencies where the benefit-to-risk ratio for either the fetus or the mother favors surgical intervention; in cases of fetal distress where delivery is not imminent; prolonged use in uterine inertia or severe toxemia; hypertonic uterine patterns; patients with hypersensitivity to the drug; induction or augmentation of labor in those cases where vaginal delivery is contraindicated, such as cord presentation or prolapse, total placenta previa, and vasa previa.

WARNINGS

Syntocinon (oxytocin) when given for induction or stimulation of labor, must be administered only by the intravenous route and with adequate medical supervision in a hospital.

PRECAUTIONS

General: **All patients receiving intravenous oxytocin must be under continuous observation by trained personnel with a thorough knowledge of the drug and qualified to identify complications. A physician qualified to manage any complications should be immediately available.**
When properly administered, oxytocin should stimulate uterine contractions similar to those seen in normal labor. Overstimulation of the uterus by improper administration can be hazardous to both mother and fetus. Even with proper administration and adequate supervision, hypertonic contractions can occur in patients whose uteri are hypersensitive to oxytocin.
Except in unusual circumstances, oxytocin should not be administered in the following conditions: prematurity, borderline cephalopelvic disproportion, previous major surgery on the cervix or uterus including cesarean section, over-distention of the uterus, grand multiparity, or invasive cervical carcinoma. Because of the variability of the combinations of factors which may be present in the conditions listed above, the definition of "unusual circumstances" must be left to the judgment of the physician. The decision can only be made by carefully weighing the potential benefits which oxytocin can provide in a given case against rare but definite potential for the drug to produce hypertonicity or tetanic spasm.
Maternal deaths due to hypertensive episodes, subarchnoid hemorrhage, rupture of the uterus, and fetal deaths due to various causes have been reported associated with the use of parental oxytocic drugs for induction of labor or for augmentation in the first and second stages of labor.
Oxytocin has been shown to have an intrinsic antidiuretic effect, acting to increase water reabsorption from the glomerular filtrate. Consideration should, therefore, be given to the possibility of water intoxication, particularly when oxytocin is administered continuously by infusion and the patient is receiving fluids by mouth.
Drug Interactions: Severe hypertension has been reported when oxytocin was given three to four hours following prophylactic administration of a vasoconstrictor in conjunction with caudal block anesthesia. Cyclopropane anesthesia may modify oxytocin's cardiovascular effects, so as to produce unexpected results such as hypotension. Maternal sinus bradycardia with abnormal atrioventricular rhythms has also been noted when oxytocin was used concomitantly with cyclopropane anesthesia.
Carcinogenesis, Mutagenesis, Impairment of Fertility: - There are no animal or human studies on the carcinogenicity and mutagenicity of this drug, nor is there any information on its effect on fertility.
Pregnancy: Teratogenic Effects. Animal reproduction studies have not been conducted with oxytocin. There are no known indications for use in the first trimester of pregnancy other than in relation to spontaneous or induced abortion. Based on the wide experience with this drug and its chemical structure and pharmacological properties, it would not be expected to present a risk of fetal abnormalities when used as indicated.
Nonteratogenic Effects. See **ADVERSE REACTIONS** in the fetus or infant.
Labor and Delivery: see **INDICATIONS AND USAGE.**
Nursing Mothers: Syntocinon® (oyxtocin) may be found in small quantities in mother's milk. If a patient requires the drug postpartum to control severe bleeding, she should not commence nursing until the day after Syntocinon has been discontinued.
Pediatric Use: Syntocinon (oxytocin) is not intended for use in children.

ADVERSE REACTIONS

The following adverse reactions have been reported in the mother.

- Anaphylactic reaction
- Postpartum hemorrhage
- Cardiac arrhythmia
- Fatal afibrinogenemia
- Nausea
- Vomiting
- Premature ventricular contractions
- Pelvic hematoma
- Excessive dosage or hypersensitivity to the drug may result in uterine hypertonicity, spasm, tetanic contraction, or rupture of the uterus.

The possibility of increased blood loss and afibrinogenemia should be kept in mind when administering the drug.
Severe water intoxication with convulsions and coma has occurred, associated with a slow oxytocin infusion over a 24-hour period. Maternal death due to oxytocin-induced water intoxication has been reported.
The following adverse reactions have been reported in the fetus or infant:
Due to induced uterine motility:

- Bradycardia
- Premature ventricular contractions and other arrhythmias
- Permanent CNS or brain damage
- Fetal death

Due to use of oxytocin in the mother:

- Low Apgar scores at 5 minutes
- Neonatal jaundice
- Neonatal retinal hemorrhage

DRUG ABUSE AND DEPENDENCE

There is no evidence that Syntocinon (oxytocin) has been abused or has provoked drug dependence.

OVERDOSAGE

Overdosage with oxytocin depends essentially on uterine hyperactivity, whether or not due to hypersensitivity to this agent. Hyperstimulation with strong (hypertonic) or prolonged (tetanic) contractions, or a resting tone of 15 to 20 mm H_2O or more between contractions can lead to tumultuous labor, uterine rupture, cervical and vaginal lacerations, postpartum hemorrhage, uteroplacental hypoperfusion, and variable deceleration of fetal heart, fetal hypoxia, hypercapnia or death. Water intoxication with convulsions, which is caused by the inherent antidiuretic effect of oxytocin, is a serious complication that may occur if large doses (40 to 50 ml/minute) are infused for long periods. Treatment of water intoxication consists of discontinuation of oxytocin, restriction of fluid intake, diuresis, IV hypertonic saline solution, correction of electrolyte imbalance, control of convulsions with judicious use of a barbiturate, and special nursing care for the comatose patient.

DOSAGE AND ADMINISTRATION

Dosage of oxytocin is determined by uterine response. The following dosage information is based upon the various regimens and indications in general use. Parenteral drug products should be inspected visually for particulate matter and discoloration prior to administration, wherever solution and container permit.

A. Induction or Stimulation of Labor
Intravenous infusion (drip method) is the only acceptable method of administration for the induction or stimulation of labor.
Accurate control of the rate of infusion flow is essential. An infusion pump or other such device and frequent monitoring of strength of contractions and fetal heart rate are necessary for the safe administration of oxytocin for the induction or stimulation of labor. If uterine contractions become too powerful, the infusion can be abruptly stopped, and oxytocic stimulation of the uterine musculature will soon wane.
1. An intravenous infusion of non-oxytocin containing solution should be started. Physiologic electrolyte solution should be used except under unusual circumstances.
2. To prepare the usual solution for infusion, the contents of one 1-ml ampul are combined aseptically with 1,000 ml of nonhydrating diluent. The combined solution, rotated in the infusion bottle to insure thorough mixing contains 10 mU/ml. Add the container with dilute oxytocic solution to the system through use of a constant infusion pump or other such device, to control accurately the rate of infusion.
3. The initial dose should be no more than 1–2 mU/minute. The dose may be gradually increased in increments of no more than 1 to 2 mU/minute until a contraction pattern has been established, which is similar to normal labor.
4. The fetal heart rate, resting uterine tone, and the frequency, duration, and force of contractions should be monitored.
5. The oxytocin infusion should be discontinued immediately in the event of uterine hyperactivity or fetal distress. Oxygen should be administered to the mother. The mother and the fetus must be evaluated by the responsible physician.

B. Control of Postpartum Uterine Bleeding
1. *Intravenous Infusion (Drip Method):* To control postpartum bleeding, 10–40 units of oxytocin may be added to 1,000 ml of a nonhydrating diluent and run at a rate necessary to control uterine atony.
2. *Intramuscular Administration:* 1 ml (10 units) of oxytocin can be given after delivery of the placenta.

C. Treatment of Incomplete or Inevitable Abortion
Intravenous infusion with physiologic saline solution, 500 ml, or 5% dextrose in physiologic saline solution to which 10 units of Syntocinon® (oxytocin) have been added should be infused at a rate of 20–40 drops/per minute.

HOW SUPPLIED

Ampuls: 1 ml (10 USP units) size, boxes of 20 (NDC 0078-0060-03), 50 (NDC 0078-0060-04) and 100 (NDC 0078-0060-05).
Store and dispense: Below 77°F; DO NOT FREEZE
[SYT-Z20 Issued July 15, 1986]

SYNTOCINON® NASAL SPRAY ℞

[sin"tō'si-non]
(oxytocin nasal solution, USP)

The following prescribing information is based on official labeling in effect on July 15, 1986.

DESCRIPTION

Each ml. contains 40 USP Units (International Units) Syntocinon® (oxytocin) and the following: dried sodium phosphate, USP, citric acid, USP, sodium chloride, USP, glycerin, USP, sorbitol solution, USP, methylparaben, NF, propylparaben, NF, chlorobutanol, NF max. 0.05%, purified water, USP.
Oxytocin is one of the polypeptide hormones of the posterior lobe of the pituitary gland. The pharmacologic and clinical properties of Syntocinon (oxytocin) are identical with *the oxytocic and the galactokinetic* principle of the natural hormone. Syntocinon was synthesized on a commercial scale by Sandoz, and was introduced for clinical use in 1957.
Since oxytocin, a polypeptide, is subject to inactivation by the proteolytic enzymes of the alimentary tract, it is *not absorbed from the gastrointestinal tract.* Intranasal application of the spray preparation, however, is a practical and effective method of administration.

ACTION

Syntocinon Nasal Spray acts specifically on the myoepithelial elements surrounding the alveoli of the breast, causing them to contract and thus force milk into the larger ducts where it is more readily available to the baby.

INDICATION

Initial milk let-down.

CONTRAINDICATIONS

Pregnancy; hypersensitivity.

DOSAGE AND ADMINISTRATION

One spray into one or both nostrils 2 to 3 minutes before nursing or pumping of breasts.

Continued on next page

Sandoz—Cont.

Note: The squeeze bottle should be held in upright position when administering drug to the nose and patient should be in a sitting position rather than lying down. If preferred, the solution can be instilled in drop form by inverting the squeeze bottle and exerting very gentle pressure on its walls.

SUPPLIED

Syntocinon (oxytocin) Nasal Spray in squeeze bottles containing 2 ml oxytocin solution or 5 ml oxytocin solution.

[SYT-ZZ12 Issued July 15, 1986]

TAVIST® ℞
(clemastine fumarate)
Syrup

The following prescribing information is based on official labeling in effect on June 1, 1986.

DESCRIPTION

Each teaspoonful (5 ml) of Tavist® (clemastine fumarate) Syrup for oral administration contains clemastine 0.5 mg (present as clemastine fumarate 0.67 mg). Other ingredients: alcohol 5.5%, flavors, methylparaben, propylene glycol, propylparaben, purified water, saccharin sodium, sorbitol in a buffered solution. Tavist (clemastine fumarate) belongs to the benzhydryl ether group of antihistaminic compounds. The chemical name is (+)-(2R)-2-[2-[[(R)-p-Chloro-α-methyl-α-phenylbenzyl]-oxy] ethyl]-1-methylpyrrolidine fumarate.
Clemastine fumarate occurs as a colorless to faintly yellow, practically odorless, crystalline powder. Tavist (clemastine fumarate) Syrup has an approximate pH of 6.2.

CLINICAL PHARMACOLOGY

Tavist (clemastine fumarate) is an antihistamine with anticholinergic (drying) and sedative side effects. Antihistamines competitively antagonize various physiological effects of histamine including increased capillary permeability and dilatation, the formation of edema, the "flare" and "itch" response, and gastrointestinal and respiratory smooth muscle constriction. Within the vascular tree, H_1-receptor antagonists inhibit both the vasoconstrictor and vasodilator effects of histamine. Depending on the dose, H_1- receptor antagonists can produce CNS stimulation or depression. Most antihistamines exhibit central and /or peripheral anticholinergic activity. Antihistamines act by competitively blocking H_1-receptor sites. Antihistamines do not pharmacologically antagonize or chemically inactivate histamine, nor do they prevent the release of histamine.

PHARMACOKINETICS

Antihistamines are well-absorbed following oral administration. Chlorpheniramine maleate, clemastine fumarate, and diphenhydramine hydrochloride achieve peak blood levels within 2–5 hours following oral administration. The absorption of antihistamines is often partially delayed by the use of controlled release dosage forms. In these instances, plasma concentrations from identical doses of the immediate and controlled release dosage forms will not be similar.
Tissue distribution of the antihistamines in humans has not been established.
Antihistamines appear to be metabolized in the liver chiefly via mono- and didemethylation and glucuronide conjugation. Antihistamine metabolites and small amounts of unchanged drug are excreted in the urine. Small amounts of the drugs may also be excreted in breast milk.
In normal human subjects who received histamine injections over a 24-hour period, the antihistaminic activity of Tavist (clemastine fumarate) reached a peak at 5–7 hours, persisted for 10–12 hours and, in some cases, for as long as 24 hours. Pharmacokinetic studies in man utilizing ^3H and ^{14}C labeled compound demonstrates that: Tavist (clemastine fumarate) is rapidly absorbed from the gastrointestinal tract, peak plasma concentrations are attained in 2–4 hours, and urinary excretion is the major mode of elimination.

INDICATIONS AND USAGE

Tavist (clemastine fumarate) Syrup is indicated for the relief of symptoms associated with allergic rhinitis such as sneezing, rhinorrhea, pruritus and lacrimation. Tavist (clemastine fumarate) Syrup is indicated for use in pediatric populations (age 6 years through 12) and adults (see *DOSAGE AND ADMINISTRATION*).
It should be noted that Tavist® (clemastine fumarate) is indicated for the relief of mild uncomplicated allergic skin manifestations of urticaria and angioedema at the 2 mg dosage level only.

CONTRAINDICATIONS

Antihistamines are contraindicated in patients hypersensitive to the drug or to other antihistamines of similar chemical structure (see *PRECAUTIONS— Drug Interactions*).
Antihistamines *should not* be used *in newborn or premature infants.* Because of the higher risk of antihistamines for infants generally and for newborns and prematures in particular, antihistamine therapy is contraindicated in *nursing mothers* (See *PRECAUTIONS—Nursing Mothers*).

WARNINGS

Antihistamines should be used with considerable caution in patients with: narrow angle glaucoma, stenosing peptic ulcer, pyloroduodenal obstruction, symptomatic prostatic hypertrophy, and bladder neck obstruction.
Use with CNS Depressants: Tavist (clemastine fumarate) has additive effects with alcohol and other CNS depressants (hypnotics, sedatives, tranquilizers, etc.)
Use in Activities Requiring Mental Alertness: Patients should be warned about engaging in activities requiring mental alertness such as driving a car or operating appliances, machinery, etc.
Use in the Elderly (approximately 60 years or older): Antihistamines are more likely to cause dizziness, sedation, and hypotension in elderly patients.

PRECAUTIONS

General: Tavist (clemastine fumarate) should be used with caution in patients with: history of bronchial asthma, increased intraocular pressure, hyperthyroidism, cardiovascular disease, and hypertension.
Information for Patients:
Patients taking antihistamines should receive the following information and instructions:

1. Antihistamines are prescribed to reduce allergic symptoms.
2. Patients should be questioned regarding a history of glaucoma, peptic ulcer, urinary retention, or pregnancy before starting antihistamine therapy.
3. Patients should be told not to take alcohol, sleeping pills, sedatives, or tranquilizers while taking antihistamines.
4. Antihistamines may cause drowsiness, dizziness, dry mouth, blurred vision, weakness, nausea, headache, or nervousness in some patients.
5. Patients should avoid driving a car or working with hazardous machinery until they assess the effects of this medicine.
6. Patients should be told to store this medicine in a tightly closed container in a dry, cool place away from heat or direct sunlight and out of the reach of children.

Drug Interactions:
Additive CNS depression may occur when antihistamines are administered concomitantly with other CNS depressants including barbiturates, tranquilizers, and alcohol. Patients receiving antihistamines should be advised against the concurrent use of other CNS depressant drugs.
Monoamine oxidase (MAO) inhibitors prolong and intensify the anticholinergic effects of antihistamines.
Carcinogenesis, Mutagenesis, Impairment of Fertility:
Carcinogenesis and Mutagenesis: In a 2-year oral study in the rat at a dose of 84 mg/kg (about 500 times the adult human dose) and an 85-week oral study in the mouse at 206 mg/kg (about 1300 times the adult human dose), clemastine fumarate showed no evidence of carcinogenesis. No mutagenic studies have been conducted with clemastine fumarate.
Impairment of Fertility: Oral doses of clemastine fumarate in the rat produced a decrease in mating ability of the male at 312 times the adult human dose. This effect was not found at 156 times the adult human dose.
Pregnancy—*Pregnancy Category B:* Oral reproduction studies performed with clemastine fumarate in rats and rabbits at doses up to 312 and 188 times the adult human doses respectively, have revealed no evidence of teratogenic effects.
There are no adequate and well-controlled studies of Tavist (clemastine fumarate) Syrup in pregnant women. Because animal reproduction studies are not always predictive of human response, this drug should be used in pregnancy only if clearly needed.
Nursing Mothers:
Although quantitative determinations of antihistaminic drugs in breast milk have not been reported, qualitative tests have documented the excretion of diphenhydramine, pyrilamine, and tripelennamine in human milk.
Because of the potential for adverse reactions in nursing infants from antihistamines, a decision should be made whether to discontinue nursing or to discontinue the drug.
Pediatric Use: The safety and efficacy of Tavist (clemastine fumarate) Syrup has been confirmed in the pediatric population (age 6 years through 12). Safety and dose tolerance studies have confirmed children 6 through 11 years tolerated dosage ranges of 0.75 to 2.25 mg clemastine. In infants and children particularly, antihistamines in overdosage may produce hallucinations, convulsions, and death. Symptoms of antihistamine toxicity in children may include fixed dilated pupils, flushed face, dry mouth, fever, excitation, hallucinations, ataxia, incoordination, athetosis, tonicclonic convulsions, and postictal depression (see *OVERDOSAGE*).

ADVERSE REACTIONS

The most frequent adverse reactions are underlined:
Nervous System: <u>Sedation, sleepiness, dizziness, disturbed coordination,</u> fatigue, confusion, restlessness, excitation, nervousness, tremor, irritability, insomnia, euphoria, paresthesia, blurred vision, diplopia, vertigo, tinnitus, acute labyrinthitis, hysteria, neuritis, convulsions.
Gastrointestinal System: <u>Epigastric distress,</u> anorexia, nausea, vomiting, diarrhea, constipation.
Respiratory System: <u>Thickening of bronchial secretions,</u> tightness of chest and wheezing, nasal stuffiness.
Cardiovascular System: Hypotension, headache, palpitations, tachycardia, extrasystoles.
Hematologic System: Hemolytic anemia, thrombocytopenia, agranulocytosis.
Genitourinary System: Urinary frequency, difficult urination, urinary retention, early menses.
General: Urticaria, drug rash, anaphylactic shock, photosensitivity, excessive perspiration, chills, dryness of mouth, nose, and throat.

OVERDOSAGE

Antihistamine overdosage reactions may vary from central nervous system depression to stimulation. In children, stimulation predominates initially in a syndrome which may include excitement, hallucinations, ataxia, incoordination, muscle twitching, athetosis, hyperthermia, cyanosis convulsions, tremors, and hyperreflexia followed by postictal depression and cardio-respiratory arrest. Convulsions in children may be preceded by mild depression. Dry mouth, fixed, dilated pupils, flushing of the face, and fever are common. In adults, CNS depression, ranging from drowsiness to coma, is more common. The convulsant dose of antihistamines lies near the lethal dose. Convulsions indicate a poor prognosis.
In both children and adults, coma and cardiovascular collapse may occur. Deaths are reported especially in infants and children.
There is no specific therapy for acute overdosage with antihistamines. The latent period from ingestion to appearance of toxic effects is characteristically short (½–2 hours). General symptomatic and supportive measures should be instituted promptly and maintained for as long as necessary.
Since overdoses of other classes of drugs (i.e., tricyclic antidepressants) may also present anticholinergic symptomatology, appropriate toxicological analysis should be performed as soon as possible to identify the causative agent.
In the conscious patient, vomiting should be induced even though it may have occured spontaneously. If vomiting cannot be induced, gastric lavage is indicated. Adequate precautions must be taken to protect against aspiration, especially in infants and children. Charcoal slurry or other suitable agents should be instilled into the stomach after vomiting or lavage. Saline cathartics or milk of magnesia may be of additional benefit.
In the unconscious patient, the airway should be secured with a cuffed endotracheal tube before attempting to evacuate the gastric contents. Intensive supportive and nursing care is indicated, as for any comatose patient.
If breathing is significantly impaired, maintenance of an adequate airway and mechanical support of respiration is the most effective means of providing adequate oxygenation.
Hypotension is an early sign of impending cardiovascular collapse and should be treated vigorously. Although general supportive measures are important, specific treatment with intravenous infusion of a vasopressor titrated to maintain adequate blood pressure may be necessary.
Do not use with CNS stimulants.
Convulsions should be controlled by careful administration of diazepam or a short-acting barbiturate, repeated as necessary. Physostigmine may also be considered for use in controlling centrally mediated convulsions.
Ice packs and cooling sponge baths, not alcohol, can aid in reducing the fever commonly seen in children.
A more detailed review of antihistamine toxicology and overdose management is available in Gosselin, R.E., et al., "Clinical Toxicology of Commercial Products."

DOSAGE AND ADMINISTRATION

DOSAGE SHOULD BE INDIVIDUALIZED ACCORDING TO THE NEEDS AND RESPONSE OF THE PATIENT.
Pediatric: Children aged 6 to 12 years:
For Symptoms of Allergic Rhinitis—The starting dose is 1 teaspoonful (0.5 mg clemastine) twice daily. Since since doses of up to 2.25 mg clemastine were well tolerated by this age group, dosage may be increased as required, but not to exceed 6 teaspoonsful daily (3 mg clemastine).
For Urticaria and Angioedema—The starting dose is 2 teaspoonsful (1 mg clemastine) twice daily, not to exceed 6 teaspoonsful daily (3 mg clemastine).
Adults and Children 12 Years and Over:
For Symptoms of Allergic Rhinitis—The starting dose is 2 teaspoonsful (1.0 mg clemastine) twice daily. Dosage may be increased as required, but not to exceed 12 teaspoonsful daily (6 mg clemastine).
For Urticaria and Angioedema—The starting dose is 4 teaspoonsful (2 mg clemastine) twice daily, not to exceed 12 teaspoonsful daily (6 mg clemastine).

HOW SUPPLIED

Tavist (clemastine fumarate) Syrup: clemastine 0.5 mg/5 ml (present as clemastine fumarate 0.67 mg/5 ml). A clear, colorless liquid with a citrus flavor, in 4 fl. oz. bottle (NDC 0078-0222-31).

STORE AND DISPENSE

Below 77°F (25°C) tight, amber glass bottle. Store in an upright position.

[TAS-Z3 Issued April 1, 1986]

TAVIST-1® (clemastine fumarate) ℞
[*tav 'ist*]
Tablets, USP 1.34 mg
TAVIST® (clemastine fumarate)
Tablets, USP 2.68 mg

The following prescribing information is based on official labeling in effect on July 15, 1986.

DESCRIPTION

TAVIST® (clemastine fumarate) belongs to the benzhydryl ether group of antihistaminic compounds. The chemical name is (+)-2- [2- [(p- chloro-α-methyl-α-phenylbenzyl) oxy] ethyl]-1-methylpyrrolidine hydrogen fumarate.
1.34 mg and 2.68 mg, Tablets
Active Ingredient: clemastine fumarate, USP
Inactive Ingredients: lactose, povidone, starch, stearic acid, and talc

ACTIONS

TAVIST is an antihistamine with anticholinergic (drying) and sedative side effects. Antihistamines appear to compete with histamine for cell receptor sites on effector cells. The inherently long duration of antihistaminic effects of TAVIST has been demonstrated in wheal and flare studies. In normal human subjects who received histamine injections over a 24-hour period, the antihistaminic activity of TAVIST reached a peak at 5–7 hours, persisted for 10–12 hours and, in some cases, for as long as 24 hours. Pharmacokinetic studies in man utilizing ^3H and ^{14}C labeled compound demonstrates that: TAVIST (clemastine fumarate) is rapidly and nearly completely absorbed from the gastrointestinal tract, peak plasma concentrations are attained in 2–4 hours, and urinary excretion is the major mode of elimination.

INDICATIONS

TAVIST-1 Tablets 1.34 mg are indicated for the relief of symptoms associated with allergic rhinitis such as sneezing, rhinorrhea, pruritus and lacrimation.
TAVIST Tablets 2.68 mg are indicated for the relief of symptoms associated with allergic rhinitis such as sneezing, rhinorrhea, pruritus, and lacrimation. TAVIST Tablets 2.68 mg are also indicated for the relief of mild, uncomplicated allergic skin manifestations of urticaria and angioedema.
It should be noted that TAVIST (clemastine fumarate) is indicated for the dermatologic indications at the 2.68 mg dosage level only.

CONTRAINDICATIONS

Use in Nursing Mothers: Because of the higher risk of antihistamines for infants generally and for newborns and prematures in particular, antihistamine therapy is contraindicated in nursing mothers.
Use in Lower Respiratory Disease: Antihistamines *should not* be used to treat lower respiratory tract symptoms including asthma.
Antihistamines are also contraindicated in the following conditions:
Hypersensitivity to TAVIST (clemastine fumarate) or other antihistamines of similar chemical structure.
Monamine oxidase inhibitor therapy (see Drug Interaction Section).

WARNINGS

Antihistamines should be used with considerable caution in patients with: narrow angle glaucoma, stenosing peptic ulcer, pyloroduodenal obstruction, symptomatic prostatic hypertrophy, and bladder neck obstruction.
Use in Children: Safety and efficacy of TAVIST have not been established in children under the age of 12.
Use in Pregnancy: Experience with this drug in pregnant women is inadequate to determine whether there exists a potential for harm to the developing fetus.
Use with CNS Depressants: TAVIST has additive effects with alcohol and other CNS depressants (hypnotics, sedatives, tranquilizers, etc.)
Use in Activities Requiring Mental Alertness: Patients should be warned about engaging in activities requiring mental alertness such as driving a car or operating appliances, machinery, etc.
Use in the Elderly (approximately 60 years or older): Antihistamines are more likely to cause dizziness, sedation, and hypotension in elderly patients.

PRECAUTIONS

TAVIST (clemastine fumarate) should be used with caution in patients with: history of bronchial asthma, increased intraocular pressure, hyperthyroidism, cardiovascular disease, and hypertension.

Drug Interactions: MAO inhibitors prolong and intensify the anticholinergic (drying) effects of antihistamines.

ADVERSE REACTIONS

Transient drowsiness, the most common adverse reaction associated with TAVIST (clemastine fumarate), occurs relatively frequently and may require discontinuation of therapy in some instances.
Antihistaminic Compounds: It should been noted that the following reactions have occurred with one or more antihistamines and, therefore, should be kept in mind when prescribing drugs belonging to this class, including TAVIST. The most frequent adverse reactions are underlined.

1. *General:* Urticaria, drug rash, anaphylactic shock, photosensitivity, excessive perspiration, chills, dryness of mouth, nose, and throat.
2. *Cardiovascular System:* Hypotension, headache, palpitations, tachycardia, extrasystoles.
3. *Hematologic System:* Hemolytic anemia, thrombocytopenia, agranulocytosis.
4. *Nervous System:* Sedation, sleepiness, dizziness, disturbed coordination, fatigue, confusion, restlessness, excitation, nervousness, tremor, irritability, insomnia, euphoria, paresthesias, blurred vision, diplopia, vertigo, tinnitus, acute labyrinthitis, hysteria, neuritis, convulsions.
5. *GI System:* Epigastric distress, anorexia, nausea, vomiting, diarrhea, constipation.
6. *GU System:* Urinary frequency, difficult urination, urinary retention, early menses.
7. *Respiratory System:* Thickening of bronchial secretions, tightness of chest and wheezing, nasal stuffiness.

OVERDOSAGE

Antihistamine overdosage reactions may vary from central nervous system depression to stimulation. Stimulation is particularly likely in children. Atropine-like signs and symptoms: dry mouth; fixed, dilated pupils; flushing; and gastrointestinal symptoms may also occur.
If vomiting has not occurred spontaneously the conscious patient should be induced to vomit. This is best done by having him drink a glass of water or milk after which he should be made to gag. Precautions against aspiration must be taken, especially in infants and children.
If vomiting is unsuccessful gastric lavage is indicated within 3 hours after ingestion and even later if large amounts of milk or cream were given beforehand. Isotonic and ½ isotonic saline is the lavage solution of choice.
Saline cathartics, such as milk of magnesia, by osmosis draw water into the bowel and therefore, are valuable for their action in rapid dilution of bowel content.
Stimulants should *not* be used.
Vasopressors may be used to treat hypotension.

DOSAGE AND ADMINISTRATION

DOSAGE SHOULD BE INDIVIDUALIZED ACCORDING TO THE NEEDS AND RESPONSE OF THE PATIENT.
TAVIST-1 Tablets 1.34 mg: The recommended starting dose is one tablet twice daily. Dosage may be increased as required, but not to exceed six tablets daily.
TAVIST Tablets 2.68 mg: The maximum recommended dosage is one tablet three times daily. Many patients respond favorably to a single dose which may be repeated as required, but not to exceed three tablets daily.

HOW SUPPLIED

TAVIST-1 Tablets: 1.34 mg clemastine fumarate. White, oval compressed, scored tablet, packages of 100.
TAVIST Tablets: 2.68 mg clemastine fumarate. White, round compressed tablet, packages of 100.
Company's Product Identification Mark(s): Tavist-1 Tablets: 1.34 mg, embossed "78-75" on one side, "TAVIST 1" on the other.
Tavist Tablets: 2.68 mg, embossed "78/72" and scored on one side, "TAVIST" on the other.

[TAV-Z3 Issued July 15, 1986]

Shown in Product Identification Section, page 427

TAVIST-D® ℞
[*tav 'ist*]
(clemastine fumarate USP
phenylpropanolamine HCl USP)
Tablets

The following prescribing information is based on official labeling in effect on June 1, 1986.

DESCRIPTION

Each TAVIST-D (clemastine fumarate/phenylpropanolamine HCl) Tablet contains 1.34 mg clemastine fumarate (equivalent to 1 mg of the free base) and 75 mg phenylpropanolamine hydrochloride. The clemastine fumarate is in the outer shell of the tablet and is immediately released upon dissolution. The tablet's core is a sustained-release matrix which releases the phenylpropanolamine hydrochloride over a 12-hour period at a rate that produces blood levels bioequivalent to those obtained by the administration of 25 mg standard release tablets of phenylpropanolamine hydrochloride every four hours for three doses. Clemastine fumarate belongs to the benzhydryl ether group of antihistaminic compounds. The chemical name is (+)-2-[2-[(p-chloro-α-methyl-α-phenyl benzyl) oxy] ethyl]-1-methylpyrrolidine hydrogen fumarate.
Phenylpropanolamine hydrochloride is a sympathomimetic, orally effective nasal decongestant. Sympathomimetic compounds, whether catecholamines or noncatecholamines, can be regarded as compounds produced by substitution on the phenylethylamine nucleus common to all these sympathomimetic products, whether their action is on the Alpha receptors of the sympathetic nervous system or on Beta-1 or Beta-2 receptors. The chemical name for phenylpropanolamine hydrochloride is α-(1-Aminoethyl)benzenemethanol hydrochloride.
Active Ingredient: clemastine fumarate, USP phenylpropanolamine HCl, USP
Inactive Ingredients: colloidal silicon dioxide, D&C Yellow #10, dibasic calcium phosphate dihydrate, lactose, magnesium stearate, methylcellulose, polyethylene glycol, povidone, starch, synthetic polymers, and titanium dioxide

CLINICAL PHARMACOLOGY

Clemastine fumarate is an antihistamine with anticholinergic (drying) and sedative side effects. Antihistamines appear to compete with histamine for cell receptor sites on effector cells. The inherently long duration of antihistaminic effects of clemastine fumarate has been demonstrated in wheal and flare studies. In normal human subjects who received intradermal histamine injections over a 24-hour period, the antihistaminic activity of clemastine fumarate, as demonstrated by inhibition of the wheal and flare reaction, reached a peak at 5–7 hours, persisted for 10–12 hours and, in some cases, for as long as 24 hours. Pharmacokinetic studies in man utilizing ^3H and ^{14}C labeled compound demonstrate that clemastine fumarate is rapidly and nearly completely absorbed from the gastrointestinal tract, peak plasma concentrations are attained in 2–4 hours, and urinary excretion is the major mode of elimination.
Phenylpropanolamine hydrochloride is an Alpha adrenergic stimulator producing nasal decongestion by constriction of arterioles and precapillary arterioles in the nasal mucosa. Phenylpropanolamine hydrochloride is one of the most widely used oral nasal decongestants; it is similar in action to ephedrine, but produces less central nervous system stimulation.
In adult subjects who were given one TAVIST-D® (clemastine fumarate/phenylpropanolamine HCl) Tablet, the average peak plasma concentration of phenylpropanolamine was 85.4 ng/ml $\pm$ 13.1 (S.D.) which occurred at about 4.3 hours. In this crossover study these same subjects were given a 25 mg phenylpropanolamine hydrochloride tablet every 4 hours for 3 consecutive doses plus a single dose of a TAVIST-1 Tablet (clemastine fumarate 1.34 mg). The average peak concentration of phenylpropanolamine was found to be 67.6 ng/ml $\pm$ 11.6 (S.D.) which occurred at about 8.2 hours.
In another study, adult subjects received TAVIST-D Tablets every 12 hours for 4 consecutive days. The average peak concentration of phenylpropanolamine was found to be 117.29 ng/ml $\pm$ 14.52 (S.D.) which occurred at about 6.2 hours after the morning dose. In this crossover study these same subjects received a 25 mg phenylpropanolamine hydrochloride tablet every 4 hours for 4 consecutive days. In addition they received a TAVIST-1 Tablet (clemastine fumarate 1.34 mg) every 12 hours for 4 consecutive days. The average peak concentration of phenylpropanolamine was found to be 107.92 ng/ml $\pm$ 15.97 (S.D.) which occurred at about 4.8 hours after the first dose in the morning.

INDICATIONS AND USAGE

TAVIST-D (clemastine fumarate/phenylpropanolamine HCl) Tablets are indicated for the relief of symptoms associated with allergic rhinitis such as sneezing, rhinorrhea, pruritus of the eyes, nose or throat, lacrimation and nasal congestion.

CONTRAINDICATION

Tavist-D Tablets are contraindicated in patients hypersensitive to any of the components. Antihistamines should not be used in newborn or premature infants or in nursing mothers. Antihistamines should not be used to treat lower respiratory tract symptoms including asthma. Tavist-D Tablets are contraindicated in patients receiving monoamine oxidase inhibitors (see PRECAUTIONS—Drug Interactions) and in patients with severe hypertension or severe coronary artery disease.

WARNINGS

Antihistamines such as clemastine fumarate should be used with considerable caution in patients with narrow angle glaucoma, stenosing peptic ulcer, pyloroduodenal obstruction, symptomatic prostatic hypertrophy, and bladder neck obstruction. Sympathomimetic drugs such as phenylpropanolamine hydrochloride should be used with caution in hy-

Continued on next page

Sandoz—Cont.

pertension, cardiovascular disease, diabetes mellitus, and uncontrolled hyperthyroidism.

Use with CNS Depressants: Antihistamines have additive effects with alcohol and other CNS depressants (hypnotics, sedatives, tranquilizers, etc.).

Use in Activities Requiring Mental Alertness: Patients should be warned about engaging in activities requiring mental alertness such as driving a car or operating appliances, machinery, etc.

Use in the Elderly (approximately 60 years or older): Antihistamines are more likely to cause dizziness, sedation and hypotension in elderly patients. Overdosages of sympathomimetics in this age group may cause hallucinations, convulsions, CNS depression and death in elderly patients.

Use in Children: Safety and effectiveness of TAVIST-D® (clemastine fumarate/phenylpropanolamine HCl) have not been established in children under the age of 12. In infants and children, especially, antihistamines in *overdosage* may cause hallucinations, convulsions or death. As in adults antihistamines may diminish mental alertness, but they may also produce excitation, particularly in young children.

PRECAUTIONS

General: TAVIST-D (clemastine fumarate/ phenylpropanolamine HCl) Tablets should be used with caution in patients with: History of bronchial asthma, increased intraocular pressure, hyperthyroidism, cardiovascular disease, hypertension, diabetes mellitus, and prostate disease. (See WARNINGS.)

Information for Patients: Patients should be informed of the potential for sedation or drowsiness and warned about driving or operating machinery. The concomitant consumption of alcoholic beverages or other sedative drugs should be avoided.

Due to the inherently long-acting nature of clemastine fumarate and due to the sustained-release of phenylpropanolamine hydrochloride from the tablet's core, TAVIST-D Tablets provide prolonged symptomatic relief (10–14 hours).

Drug Interactions:

(1) Monoamine oxidase inhibitors; MAO inhibitors prolong and intensify the anticholinergic effects of antihistamines and potentiate the pressor effects of sympathomimetics.

(2) Alcohol and CNS depressants: These agents potentiate the sedative effects of antihistamines.

(3) Certain antihypertensives: Sympathomimetics may reduce the antihypertensive effects of methyldopa, mecamylamine, reserpine and veratrum alkaloids.

Carcinogenesis and Mutagenesis: Carcinogenic studies have not been conducted on the drug combination of clemastine fumarate/phenylpropanolamine hydrochloride. In a two-year oral study in the rat at a dose of 84 mg/Kg (about 1500 times the human dose) and an 85-week oral study in the mouse at 206 mg/Kg (about 3800 times the human dose), clemastine fumarate showed no evidence of carcinogenesis. No mutagenic studies have been conducted with clemastine fumarate, phenylpropanolamine hydrochloride or the drug combination.

Impairment of Fertility: Oral doses of clemastine fumarate alone in the rat produced a decrease in mating ability of the male at 933 times the human dose. This effect was not found at 466 times the human dose.

Pregnancy—*Pregnancy Category B:* Oral reproduction studies performed with clemastine fumarate alone in rats and rabbits at doses up to 933 and 560 times the human dose, respectively, have revealed no evidence of teratogenic effects. Reproduction studies have not been conducted with phenylpropanolamine hydrochloride alone.

Oral reproduction studies on the drug combination in a ratio of 1 part of clemastine fumarate to 49 parts of phenylpropanolamine hydrochloride in rats and rabbits at doses up to 100 and 67 times the human dose, respectively, have revealed no evidence of teratogenic effects. Adverse reactions attributed to the pharmacological effects of phenylpropanolamine were as follows: Rats—Impaired weight gain and deaths in dams at 33 times the human dose and a slight increase in pre-implantation loss and prenatal deaths, and reduced fetal weights at 100 times the human dose. Rabbits—Increased maternal deaths at 20 times the human dose, and increased maternal deaths and weight loss plus a slight increase in prenatal deaths (within normal limits) at 67 times the human dose.

There are no adequate and well controlled studies of TAVIST-D® (clemastine fumarate/phenylpropanolamine HCl) Tablets in pregnant women. Because animal reproductive studies are not always predictive of human response, this drug should be used in pregnancy only if clearly needed.

Nursing Mothers: See CONTRAINDICATIONS:

ADVERSE REACTIONS

Antihistaminic Compounds: It should be noted that the following reactions have occurred with one or more antihistamines and, therefore, should be kept in mind when prescribing drugs belonging to this class, including clemastine fumarate. The most frequent adverse reactions reported with clemastine fumarate are underlined.

1. *General:* Urticaria, drug rash, anaphylactic shock, photosensitivity, excessive perspiration, chills, dryness of mouth, nose and throat.
2. *Cardiovascular System:* Hypotension, headache, palpitations, tachycardia, extrasystoles.
3. *Hematologic System:* Hemolytic anemia, thrombocytopenia, agranulocytosis.
4. *Nervous System:* Sedation, sleepiness, dizziness, disturbed coordination, fatigue, confusion, restlessness, excitation, nervousness, tremor, irritability, insomnia, euphoria, paresthesias, blurred vision, diplopia, vertigo, tinnitus, acute labyrinthitis, hysteria, neuritis, convulsions.
5. *GI System:* Epigastric distress, anorexia, nausea, vomiting, diarrhea, constipation.
6. *GU System:* Urinary frequency, difficult urination, urinary retention, early menses.
7. *Respiratory System:* Thickening of bronchial secretions, tightness of chest and wheezing, nasal stuffiness.

Sympathomimetic Compounds:

Nervous System: At higher doses may cause drowsiness, dizziness, nervousness, or sleeplessness, and especially in children may cause excitability. Phenylpropanolamine hydrochloride may cause elevated blood pressure and tachyarrhythmias, especially in hyperthyroid patients.

OVERDOSAGE

Antihistamine overdosage reactions may vary from central nervous system depression to stimulation. Stimulation is particularly likely in children. Atropine-like signs and symptoms: dry mouth; fixed, dilated pupils; flushing; and gastrointestinal symptoms may also occur.

Overdosage of the phenylpropanolamine hydrochloride may produce tachycardia, pupillary dilatation, excitation and arrhythmias.

If vomiting has not occurred spontaneously the conscious patient should be induced to vomit. This is best done by having the patient drink a glass of water or milk along with an appropriate amount of Syrup of Ipecac. Precautions against aspiration must be taken, especially in infants and children.

If vomiting is unsuccessful in 20 minutes, gastric lavage is indicated within 3 hours after ingestion and even later if large amounts of milk or cream were given beforehand. Isotonic and ½ isotonic saline is the lavage solution of choice.

Saline cathartics, such as milk of magnesia, by osmosis draw water into the bowel and therefore are valuable for their action in rapid dilution of bowel content.

Stimulants should *not* be used.

Activated charcoal has been demonstrated to interfere with phenylpropanolamine absorption.

The value of dialysis has not been established.

The concentration of phenylpropanolamine hydrochloride or clemastine fumarate in biological fluids associated with toxicity is not known.

The amount of TAVIST-D® in single doses associated with significant signs of overdose or death is not known.

The oral LD_{50} for a mixture containing 50 mg phenylpropanolamine hydrochloride and 1.34 mg clemastine fumarate is 1277 mg/Kg in mice, 602 mg/Kg in rats and 634 mg/Kg in rabbits.

DOSAGE AND ADMINISTRATION

Adults and children twelve years and over: One tablet swallowed whole every twelve hours.

HOW SUPPLIED

TAVIST-D (clemastine fumarate/phenylpropanolamine HCl) Tablets: containing 1.34 mg clemastine fumarate (equivalent to 1 mg of the free base) and 75 mg phenylpropanolamine hydrochloride. White, round, film-coated multiple compressed tablet, packages of 100 (NDC 0078-0221-05). TAVIST-D Tablets should be stored and dispensed below 86°F in a tight, light-resistant container.

Company's Product Identification Mark(s): Tavist-D Tablets embossed "TAVIST-D" on one side and "78-221" on the other.

[TAD-Z4 Issued April 15, 1986]

Shown in Product Identification Section, page 427

VISKEN® ℞

[vis'kin]

(pindolol) tablets

The following prescribing information is based on official labeling in effect on July 15, 1986.

DESCRIPTION

Visken® (pindolol), a synthetic beta-adrenergic receptor blocking agent with intrinsic sympathomimetic activity is 4-(2-hydroxy-3-isopropylaminopropoxy)-indole.

5 mg. and 10 mg. Tablets

Active Ingredients: pindolol

Inactive Ingredients: colloidal silicon dioxide, magnesium stearate, microcrystalline cellulose, and pregelatinized starch

CLINICAL PHARMACOLOGY

Visken (pindolol) is a non-selective beta-adrenergic antagonist (beta-blocker) which possesses intrinsic sympathomimetic activity (ISA) in therapeutic dosage ranges but does not possess quinidine-like membrane stabilizing activity.

PHARMACODYNAMICS

In standard pharmacologic tests in man and animals, Visken (pindolol) attenuates increases in heart rate, systolic blood pressure, and cardiac output resulting from exercise and isoproterenol administration, thus confirming its beta-blocking properties. The ISA or partial agonist activity of Visken (pindolol) is mediated directly at the adrenergic receptor sites and may be blocked by other beta-blockers. In catecholamine depleted animal experiments, ISA is manifested as an increase in the inotropic and chronotropic activity of the myocardium. In man, ISA is manifested by a smaller reduction in the resting heart rate (4–8 beats/min) than is seen with drugs lacking ISA. There is also a smaller reduction in resting cardiac output. The clinical significance of this observation has not been evaluated and there is no evidence, or reason to believe, that exercise cardiac output is less affected by Visken (pindolol).

Visken (pindolol) has been shown in controlled, double-blind clinical studies to be an effective antihypertensive agent when used as monotherapy, or when added to therapy with thiazide-type diuretics. Divided dosages in the range of 10 mg—60 mg daily have been shown to be effective. As monotherapy, Visken (pindolol) is as effective as propranolol, α-methyldopa, hydrochlorothiazide and chlorthalidone in reducing systolic and diastolic blood pressure. The effect on blood pressure is not orthostatic, i.e. Visken (pindolol) was equally effective in reducing the supine and standing blood pressure.

In open, long term studies up to four (4) years, no evidence of diminution of the blood pressure lowering response was observed.

An average 3 pound increase in body weight has been noted in patients treated with Visken (pindolol) alone, a larger increase than was observed with propranolol or placebo. The weight gain appeared unrelated to blood pressure response and was not associated with an increased risk of heart failure, although edema was more common than in control patients. Visken (pindolol) does not have a consistent effect on plasma renin activity.

The mechanism of the antihypertensive effects of beta-blocking agents has not been established, but several mechanisms have been postulated: 1) an effect on the central nervous system resulting in a reduced sympathetic outflow to the periphery, 2) competitive antagonism of catecholamines at peripheral (especially cardiac) adrenergic receptor sites, leading to decreased cardiac output, 3) an inhibition of renin release. These mechanisms appear less likely for pindolol than other beta-blockers in view of the modest effect on resting cardiac output and renin.

Beta-blockade therapy is useful when it is necessary to suppress the effects of beta-adrenergic agonists in order to achieve therapeutic goals. However, in certain clinical situations, (e.g., cardiac failure, heart block, bronchospasm) the preservation of an adequate sympathetic tone may be necessary to maintain vital functions. Although a beta-antagonist with ISA such as Visken® (pindolol) does not eliminate sympathetic tone entirely, there is no controlled evidence that it is safer than other beta-blockers in such conditions as heart failure, heart block, or bronchospasm or is less likely to cause those conditions. In single dose studies of the effects of beta-blockers on FEV_1, Visken (pindolol) was indistinguishable from other non-cardioselective agents in its reduction of FEV_1, and its reduction in the effectiveness of an exogenous beta agonist.

Exacerbation of angina and, in some cases, myocardial infarction and ventricular dysrhythmias have been reported after abrupt discontinuation of therapy with beta-adrenergic blocking agents in patients with coronary artery disease. Abrupt withdrawal of these agents in patients without coronary artery disease has resulted in transient symptoms, including tremulousness, sweating, palpitation, headache, and malaise. Several mechanisms have been proposed to explain these phenomena, among them increased sensitivity to catecholamines because of increased numbers of beta receptors.

Pharmacokinetics and Metabolism: Visken (pindolol) is rapidly and reproducibly absorbed (greater than 95%), achieving peak plasma concentrations within one hour of drug administration. Visken (pindolol) has no significant first-pass effect. The blood concentrations are proportional in a linear manner to the administered dose in the range of 5–20 mg. Upon repeated administration to the same subject, variation is minimal. After a single dose, intersubject variation for peak plasma concentrations was about 4 fold (e.g. 45–167 ng/ml for a 20 mg dose). Upon multiple dosing, intersubject variation decreased to 2–2.5 fold. Visken (pindolol) is only 40% bound to plasma proteins and is evenly distributed between plasma and red cells. The volume of distribution in healthy subjects is about 2 L/kg.

Visken (pindolol) undergoes extensive metabolism in animals and man. In man, 35–40% is excreted unchanged in the urine and 60–65% is metabolized primarily to hydroxy-metabolites which are excreted as glucuronides and ethereal sulfates. The polar metabolites are excreted with a half-life of approximately 8 hours and thus multiple dosing therapy (q.8H) results in a less than 50% accumulation in plasma. About 6–9% of an administered intravenous dose is excreted by the bile into the feces.

The disposition of Visken (pindolol) after oral administration is monophasic with a half-life in healthy subjects or hypertensive patients with normal renal function of approximately 3–4 hours. Following t.i.d. administration (q.8H), no significant accumulation of Visken (pindolol) is observed.

In elderly hypertensive patients with normal renal function the half-life of Visken (pindolol) is more variable, averaging about 7 hours, but with values as high as 15 hours.

In hypertensive patients with renal diseases, the half-life is within the range expected for healthy subjects. However, a significant decrease (50%) in volume of distribution (V_D) is observed in uremic patients and V_D appears to be directly correlated to creatinine clearance. Therefore, renal drug clearance is significantly reduced in uremic patients, resulting in a significant decrease in urinary excretion of unchanged drug. Uremic patients with a creatinine clearance of less than 20 ml/min generally excreted less than 15% of the administered dose unchanged in the urine.

In patients with histologically diagnosed cirrhosis of the liver, the elimination of Visken (pindolol) was more variable in rate and generally significantly slower than in healthy subjects. The total body clearance of Visken (pindolol) in cirrhotic patients ranged from about 50 ml/min to 300 ml/min and was directly correlated to antipyrine clearance. The half-life ranged from 2.5 hours to greater than 30 hours. These findings strongly suggest that caution should be exercised in dosage adjustments of Visken (pindolol) in such patients.

The bioavailability of Visken (pindolol) is not significantly affected by co-administration of food, hydralazine, hydrochlorothiazide or aspirin. Visken (pindolol) has no effect on warfarin activity or the clinical effectiveness of digoxin, although small transient decreases in plasma digoxin concentrations were noted.

INDICATIONS AND USAGE

Visken (pindolol) is indicated in the management of hypertension. It may be used alone or concomitantly with other antihypertensive agents, particularly with a thiazide type diuretic.

CONTRAINDICATIONS

Visken (pindolol) is contraindicated in: 1) bronchial asthma; 2) overt cardiac failure; 3) cardiogenic shock; 4) second and third degree heart block; 5) severe bradycardia; (see Warnings).

WARNINGS

Cardiac Failure: Sympathetic stimulation may be a vital component supporting circulatory function in patients with congestive heart failure, and its inhibition by beta-blockade may precipitate more severe failure. Although beta-blockers should be avoided in overt congestive heart failure, if necessary, Visken (pindolol) can be used with caution in patients with a history of failure who are well-compensated, usually with digitalis and diuretics. Beta-adrenergic blocking agents do not abolish the inotropic action of digitalis on heart muscle.

In Patients Without A History of Cardiac Failure: In patients with latent cardiac insufficiency, continued depression of the myocardium with beta-blocking agents over a period of time can in some cases lead to cardiac failure. At the first sign or symptom of impending cardiac failure, patients should be fully digitalized and/or be given a diuretic, and the response observed closely. If cardiac failure continues, despite adequate digitalization and diuretic, Visken (pindolol) therapy should be withdrawn (gradually if possible).

Exacerbation of Ischemic Heart Disease Following Abrupt Withdrawal: Hypersensitivity to catecholamines has been observed in patients withdrawn from beta-blocker therapy; exacerbation of angina and, in some cases, myocardial infarction have occurred after *abrupt* discontinuation of such therapy. When discontinuing chronically administered Visken® (pindolol), particularly in patients with ischemic heart disease, the dosage should be gradually reduced over a period of one to two weeks and the patient should be carefully monitored. If angina markedly worsens or acute coronary insufficiency develops, Visken (pindolol) administration should be reinstituted promptly, at least temporarily, and other measures appropriate for the management of unstable angina should be taken. Patients should be warned against interruption or discontinuation of therapy without the physician's advice. Because coronary artery disease is common and may be unrecognized, it may be prudent not to discontinue Visken (pindolol) therapy abruptly even in patients treated only for hypertension.

Nonallergic Bronchospasm (e.g., chronic bronchitis, emphysema)—Patients with Bronchospastic Diseases Should in General Not Receive Beta-Blockers: Visken (pindolol) should be administered with caution since it may block bronchodilation produced by endogenous or exogenous catecholamine stimulation of $beta_2$ receptors.

Major Surgery: Because beta blockade impairs the ability of the heart to respond to reflex stimuli and may increase the risks of general anesthesia and surgical procedures, resulting in protracted hypotension or low cardiac output, it has generally been suggested that such therapy should be withdrawn several days prior to surgery. Recognition of the increased sensitivity to catecholamines of patients recently withdrawn from beta-blocker therapy, however, has made this recommendation controversial. If possible, beta-blockers should be withdrawn well before surgery takes place. In the event of emergency surgery, the anesthesiologist should be informed that the patient is on beta-blocker therapy. The effects of Visken (pindolol) can be reversed by administration of beta-receptor agonists such as isoproterenol, dopamine, dobutamine, or levarterenol. Difficulty in restarting and maintaining the heart beat has also been reported with beta-adrenergic receptor blocking agents.

Diabetes and Hypoglycemia: Beta-adrenergic blockade may prevent the appearance of premonitory signs and symptoms (e.g., tachycardia and blood pressure changes) of acute hypoglycemia. This is especially important with labile diabetics. Beta-blockade also reduces the release of insulin in response to hyperglycemia; therefore, it may be necessary to adjust the dose of antidiabetic drugs.

Thyrotoxicosis: Beta-adrenergic blockade may mask certain clinical signs (e.g., tachycardia) of hyperthyroidism. Patients suspected of developing thyrotoxicosis should be managed carefully to avoid abrupt withdrawal of beta-blockade which might precipitate a thyroid crisis.

PRECAUTIONS

Impaired Renal or Hepatic Function: Beta-blocking agents should be used with caution in patients with impaired hepatic or renal function. Poor renal function has only minor effects on Visken (pindolol) clearance, but poor hepatic function may cause blood levels of Visken (pindolol) to increase substantially.

Information for Patients: Patients, especially those with evidence of coronary artery insufficiency, should be warned against interruption or discontinuation of Visken® (pindolol) therapy without the physician's advice. Although cardiac failure rarely occurs in properly selected patients, patients being treated with beta-adrenergic blocking agents should be advised to consult the physician at the first sign or symptom of impending failure.

Drug Interactions: Catecholamine-depleting drugs (e.g., reserpine) may have an additive effect when given with beta-blocking agents. Patients receiving Visken (pindolol) plus a catecholamine depleting agent should, therefore, be closely observed for evidence of hypotension and/or marked bradycardia which may produce vertigo, syncope, or postural hypotension.

Visken (pindolol) has been used with a variety of antihypertensive agents, including hydrochlorothiazide, hydralazine, and guanethidine without unexpected adverse interactions.

Carcinogenesis, Mutagenesis, Impairment of Fertility: In chronic oral toxicologic studies (one to two years) in mice, rats, and dogs, Visken (pindolol) did not produce any significant toxic effects. In two-year oral carcinogenicity studies in rats and mice in doses as high as 59 mg/kg/day and 124 mg/kg/day (50 and 100 times the maximum recommended human dose), respectively, Visken (pindolol) did not produce any neoplastic, preneoplastic, or nonneoplastic pathologic lesions. In fertility and general reproductive performance studies in rats, Visken (pindolol) caused no adverse effects at a dose of 10 mg/kg.

In the male fertility and general reproductive performance test in rats, definite toxicity characterized by mortality and decreased weight gain was observed in the group given 100 mg/kg/day. At 30 mg/kg/day, decreased mating was associated with testicular atrophy and /or decreased spermatogenesis. This response is not clearly drug related, however, as there was no dose response relationship within this experiment and no similar effect on testes of rats administered Visken (pindolol) as a dietary admixture for 104 weeks. There appeared to be an increase in prenatal mortality in males given 100 mg/kg but development of offspring was not impaired.

In females administered Visken (pindolol) prior to mating through day 21 of lactation, mating behavior was decreased at 100 mg/kg and 30 mg/kg. At these dosages there also was increased mortality of offspring. Prenatal mortality was increased at 10 mg/kg but there was not a clear dose response relationship in this experiment. There was an increased resorption rate at 100 mg/kg observed in females necropsied on the 15th day of gestation.

Pregnancy—Category B: Studies in rats and rabbits exceeding 100 times the maximum recommended human doses, revealed no embryotoxicity or teratogenicity. Since there are no adequate and well-controlled studies in pregnant women, and since animal reproduction studies are not always predictive of human response, Visken (pindolol), as with any drug, should be employed during pregnancy only if the potential benefit justifies the potential risk to the fetus.

Nursing Mothers: Since Visken (pindolol) is secreted in human milk, nursing should not be undertaken by mothers receiving the drug.

Pediatric Use: Safety and effectiveness in children have not been established.

CLINICAL LABORATORY

Minor persistent elevations in serum transaminases (SGOT, SGPT) have been noted in 7% of patients during Visken (pindolol) administration, but progressive elevations were not observed and liver injury has not been reported in the medical literature over a ten (10) year period of marketing. Alkaline phosphatase, lactic acid dehydrogenase (LDH) and uric acid are also elevated on rare occasions. The significance of these findings is unknown.

ADVERSE REACTIONS

Most adverse reactions have been mild. The incidences listed in the following table are derived from 12 week comparative double-blind, parallel design trials in hypertensive patients given Visken (pindolol) as monotherapy, given various active control drugs as monotherapy, or given placebo. Data for Visken (pindolol) and the positive controls were pooled from several trials because no striking differences were seen in the individual studies, with one exception. The frequency of edema was noticeably higher in positive control trials (16% Visken (pindolol) vs 9% positive control) than in placebo controlled trials (6% Visken (pindolol) vs 3% placebo). The table includes adverse reactions reported in greater than 2% of Visken (pindolol) patients and other selected important reactions.

[See table on next page].

The following selected (potentially important) adverse reactions were seen in 2% or fewer patients and their relationship to Visken® (pindolol) is uncertain. AUTONOMIC NERVOUS SYSTEM: hyperhidrosis; CARDIOVASCULAR: bradycardia, claudication, cold extremities, heart block, hypotension, syncope, tachycardia; GASTROINTESTINAL: diarrhea, vomiting; RESPIRATORY: wheezing; UROGENITAL: impotence, pollakiuria; MISCELLANEOUS: eye discomfort or burning eyes.

POTENTIAL ADVERSE EFFECTS

In addition, other adverse effects not listed above have been reported with other beta-adrenergic blocking agents and should be considered potential adverse effects of Visken (pindolol).

Central Nervous System: Reversible mental depression progressing to catatonia; an acute reversible syndrome characterized by disorientation for time and place, short-term memory loss, emotional lability, slightly clouded sensorium, and decreased performance on neuropsychometrics.

Cardiovascular: Intensification of AV block. See CONTRAINDICATIONS.

Allergic: Erythematous rash; fever combined with aching and sore throat; laryngospasm; respiratory distress.

Hematologic: Agranulocytosis; thrombocytopenic and nonthrombocytopenic purpura.

Gastrointestinal: Mesenteric arterial thrombosis; ischemic colitis.

Miscellaneous: Reversible alopecia; Peyronie's disease.

The oculomucocutaneous syndrome associated with the beta-blocker practolol has not been reported with Visken (pindolol) during investigational use and extensive foreign experience amounting to over 4 million patient-years.

OVERDOSAGE

No specific information on emergency treatment of overdosage is available. Therefore, on the basis of the pharmacologic actions of Visken (pindolol), the following general measures should be employed as appropriate in addition to gastric lavage:

Excessive Bradycardia: administer atropine; if there is no response to vagal blockade, administer isoproterenol cautiously.

Cardiac Failure: digitalize the patient and/or administer diuretic. It has been reported that glucagon may be useful in this situation.

Hypotension: administer vasopressors, e.g., epinephrine or levarterenol, with serial monitoring of blood pressure. (There is evidence that epinephrine may be the drug of choice.)

Bronchospasm: administer a $beta_2$ stimulating agent such as isoproterenol and/or a theophylline derivative.

A case of an acute overdosage has been reported with an intake of 500 mg of Visken® (pindolol) by a hypertensive patient. Blood pressure increased and heart rate was ≥ 80 beat/ min. Recovery was uneventful. In another case 250 mg of Visken (pindolol) was taken with 150 mg diazepam and 50

Continued on next page

Sandoz—Cont.

Body System/Adverse Reaction	Visken (pindolol) (N = 322) %	Total (Volunteered and Elicited) Active Controls* (N = 188) %	Placebo (N = 78) %
Central Nervous System			
Anxiety	4	<1	1
Bizarre or Many Dreams	8	3	8
Dizziness	17	23	8
Fatigue	15	19	12
Hallucinations	1	0	0
Insomnia	19	8	12
Lethargy	3	6	4
Nervousness	11	5	9
Weakness	7	5	4
Autonomic Nervous System			
Paresthesia	5	2	8
Visual Disturbances	4	3	4
Cardiovascular			
Dyspnea	9	8	9
Edema	11	9	3
Heart Failure	2	<1	0
Palpitations	2	2	0
Weight Gain	3	5	0
Musculo-Skeletal			
Chest Pain	5	3	5
Joint Pain	11	6	8
Muscle Cramps	8	2	0
Muscle Pain	12	12	9
Gastrointestinal			
Abdominal Discomfort	7	7	5
Nausea	7	4	1
Skin			
Pruritus	2	<1	0
Rash	2	3	3

*Active Controls: Patients received either propranolol, α-methyldopa or a diuretic (hydrochlorothiazide or chlorthalidone).

mg nitrazepam, producing coma and hypotension. The patient recovered in 24 hours.

DOSAGE AND ADMINISTRATION

The dosage of Visken (pindolol) should be individualized. The recommended initial dose of Visken (pindolol) is 5 mg b.i.d. alone or in combination with other antihypertensive agents. An antihypertensive response usually occurs within the first week of treatment. Maximal response, however, may take as long as or occasionally longer than two weeks. If a satisfactory reduction in blood pressure does not occur within 3–4 weeks, the dose may be adjusted in increments of 10 mg per day at these intervals up to a maximum of 60 mg per day.

HOW SUPPLIED

White, round, scored tablets: 5 mg (NDC 0078-0111-05) and 10 mg (NDC 0078-0073-05), packages of 100.

Company's Product Identification Mark(s): 5 mg tablets embossed "VISKEN 5" on one side, and "78-111" and scored on other side.

10 mg tablets embossed "VISKEN 10" on one side, and "78-73" and scored on other side.

[VIS-Z5 Issued July 15, 1986]

Shown in Product Identification Section, page 427

Savage Laboratories

a division of Altana Inc.
60 BAYLIS ROAD
POST OFFICE BOX 2006
MELVILLE, NY 11747

ALPHATREX® ℞

[al"fah-trex']
(betamethasone dipropionate)
Cream, U.S.P. 0.05%
Ointment, U.S.P. 0.05%
Lotion, U.S.P. 0.05%
For Dermatologic Use Only–Not for Ophthalmic Use

DESCRIPTION

Alphatrex Cream, Ointment and Lotion contain Betamethasone Dipropionate U.S.P. (Pregna-1, 4-diene-3, 20-dione, 9-fluoro-11-hydroxy-16-methyl-17, 21-bis (1-oxopropoxy)-(11β, 16β)-); it has a molecular formula of $C_{28}H_{37}FO_7$, and a molecular weight of 504.59 (CAS Registry Number 5593-20-4).

Each gram of the 0.05% Cream contains 0.64 mg betamethasone dipropionate (equivalent to 0.5 mg betamethasone) in a soft, white, hydrophilic cream of purified water, mineral oil, white petrolatum, polyethylene glycol 1000 monocetyl ether, cetostearyl alcohol, monobasic sodium phosphate and phosphoric acid or sodium hydroxide; chlorocresol is present as a preservative. Betamethasone Dipropionate Cream contains no parabens.

Each gram of the 0.05% Ointment contains 0.64 mg betamethasone dipropionate (equivalent to 0.5 mg betamethasone) in an ointment base of mineral oil and white petrolatum. Betamethasone Dipropionate Ointment contains no parabens.

Each gram of the 0.05% Lotion contains 0.64 mg of betamethasone dipropionate (equivalent to 0.5 mg betamethasone) in a vehicle of isopropyl alcohol and purified water slightly thickened with carbomer 934P. Phosphoric acid or sodium hydroxide is used to adjust pH.

CLINICAL PHARMACOLOGY

Topical corticosteroids share anti-inflammatory, anti-pruritic and vasoconstrictive actions. The mechanism of anti-inflammatory activity of the topical corticosteroids is unclear. Various laboratory methods, including vasoconstrictor assays, are used to compare and predict potencies and/or clinical efficacies of the topical corticosteroids. There is some evidence to suggest that a recognizable correlation exists between vasoconstrictor potency and therapeutic efficacy in man.

Pharmacokinetics: The extent of percutaneous absorption of topical corticosteroids is determined by many factors including the vehicle, the integrity of the epidermal barrier, and the use of occlusive dressings. Topical corticosteroids can be absorbed from normal intact skin. Inflammation and/or other disease processes in the skin increase percutaneous absorption. Occlusive dressings substantially increase the percutaneous absorption of topical corticosteroids. (See DOSAGE AND ADMINISTRATION) Once absorbed through the skin, topical corticosteroids are handled through pharmacokinetic pathways similar to systemically administered corticosteroids. Corticosteroids are bound to plasma proteins in varying degrees. Corticosteroids are metabolized primarily in the liver and are then excreted by the kidneys. Some of the topical corticosteroids and their metabolites are also excreted into the bile.

INDICATIONS AND USAGE

Topical corticosteroids are indicated for the relief of the inflammatory and pruritic manifestations of corticosteroid-responsive dermatoses.

CONTRAINDICATIONS

Topical corticosteroids are contraindicated in those patients with a history of hypersensitivity to any of the components of the preparation.

PRECAUTIONS

General: Systemic absorption of topical corticosteroids has produced reversible hypothalamic-pituitary-adrenal (HPA) axis suppression, manifestations of Cushing's syndrome, hyperglycemia, and glucosuria in some patients. Conditions which augment systemic absorption include the application of the more potent steroids, use over large surface areas, prolonged use, and the addition of occlusive dressings. (See DOSAGE AND ADMINISTRATION) Therefore, patients receiving a large dose of a potent topical steroid applied to a large surface area should be evaluated periodically for evidence of HPA axis suppression by using the urinary free cortisol and ACTH stimulation tests. If HPA axis suppression is noted, an attempt should be made to withdraw the drug, to reduce the frequency of application, or to substitute a less potent steroid. Recovery of HPA axis function is generally prompt and complete upon discontinuation of the drug. Infrequently, signs and symptoms of steroid withdrawal may occur, requiring supplemental systemic corticosteroids. Children may absorb proportionally larger amounts of topical corticosteroids and thus be more susceptible to systemic toxicity (See PRECAUTIONS-Pediatric Use). If irritation develops topical corticosteroids should be discontinued and appropriate therapy instituted. In the presence of dermatological infections, the use of an appropriate antifungal or antibacterial agent should be instituted. If a favorable response does not occur promptly, the corticosteroid should be discontinued until the infection has been adequately controlled.

Information for the Patient: Patients using topical corticosteroids should receive the following information and instructions:

1. This medication is to be used as directed by the physician. It is for external use only. Avoid contact with the eyes.
2. Patients should be advised not to use this medication for any disorder other than for which it was prescribed.
3. The treated skin area should not be bandaged or otherwise covered or wrapped as to be occlusive. (See DOSAGE AND ADMINISTRATION)
4. Patients should report any signs of local adverse reactions.
5. Parents of pediatric patients should be advised not to use tight fitting diapers or plastic pants on a child being treated in the diaper area, as these garments may constitute occlusive dressings. (See DOSAGE AND ADMINISTRATION)

Laboratory Tests: The following tests may be helpful in evaluating the HPA axis suppression: Urinary free cortisol test; ACTH stimulation test.

Carcinogenesis, Mutagenesis, and Impairment of Fertility: Long-term animal studies have not been performed to evaluate the carcinogenic potential or the effect on fertility of topical corticosteroids. Studies to determine mutagenicity with prednisolone and hydrocortisone have revealed negative results.

Pregnancy Category C: Corticosteroids are generally teratogenic in laboratory animals when administered systemically at relatively low dosage levels. The more potent corticosteroids have been shown to be teratogenic after dermal application in laboratory animals. There are no adequate and well-controlled studies in pregnant women on teratogenic effects from topically applied corticosteroids. Therefore, topical corticosteroids should be used during pregnancy only if the potential benefit justifies the potential risk to the fetus. Drugs of this class should not be used extensively on pregnant patients, in large amounts, or for prolonged periods of time.

Nursing Mothers: It is not known whether topical administration of corticosteroids could result in sufficient systemic absorption to produce detectable quantities in breast milk. Systemically administered corticosteroids are secreted into breast milk in quantities *not* likely to have a deleterious effect on the infant. Nevertheless, caution should be exercised when topical corticosteroids are administered to a nursing woman.

Pediatric Use: *Pediatric patients may demonstrate greater susceptibility to topical corticosteroid-induced HPA axis suppression and Cushing's syndrome than mature patients because of a larger skin surface area to body weight ratio.* Hypothalamic-pituitary-adrenal (HPA) axis suppression, Cushing's syndrome, and intracranial hypertension have been reported in children receiving topical corticosteroids. Manifestations of adrenal suppression in children include linear growth retardation, delayed weight gain, low plasma cortisol levels, and absence of response to ACTH stimulation. Manifestations of intracranial hypertension include bulging fontanelles, headaches, and bilateral papilledema. Administration of topical corticosteroids to children should be limited to the least amount compatible with an effective therapeutic regimen. Chronic corticosteroid therapy may interfere with the growth and development of children.

ADVERSE REACTIONS

The following local adverse reactions are reported infrequently when Alphatrex products are used as recommended in the DOSAGE AND ADMINISTRATION section. These reactions are listed in an approximate decreasing order of occurrence: burning, itching, irritation, dryness, folliculitis, hypertrichosis, acneiform eruptions, hypopigmentation, perioral dermatitis, allergic contact dermatitis, maceration of the skin, secondary infection, skin atrophy, striae and miliaria.

Systemic absorption of topical corticosteroids has produced reversible hypothalamic-pituitary-adrenal (HPA) axis suppression, manifestations of Cushing's syndrome, hyperglycemia and glucosuria in some patients.

OVERDOSAGE

Topically applied corticosteroids can be absorbed in sufficient amounts to produce systemic effects (See PRECAUTIONS).

DOSAGE AND ADMINISTRATION

Alphatrex Cream and Ointment are applied to the affected skin areas as a thin film once daily. In some cases, twice daily dosage may be necessary.

Apply a few drops of Alphatrex Lotion to the affected skin areas and massage lightly until it disappears. Apply twice daily, in the morning and night. If an infection develops, appropriate antimicrobial therapy should be instituted.

Alphatrex products should not be used with occlusive dressings.

HOW SUPPLIED

Alphatrex Cream, U.S.P. 0.05%
NDC 0281-0055-15, 15 gram tube
NDC 0281-0055-46, 45 gram tube
Alphatrex Ointment, U.S.P. 0.05%
NDC 0281-0056-15, 15 gram tube
NDC 0281-0056-46, 45 gram tube
Alphatrex Lotion, U.S.P. 0.05%
NDC 0281-0057-60, 60 ml bottle
Shake well before using.

Caution: Federal law prohibits dispensing without prescription.

BETATREX™ ℞

[ba "tah-trex']
(betamethasone valerate)
Cream, U.S.P. 0.1%
Ointment, U.S.P. 0.1%
Lotion, U.S.P. 0.1%
For Dermatologic Use Only—Not for Ophthalmic Use

DESCRIPTION

Betatrex Cream, Ointment and Lotion contain Betamethasone Valerate USP (Pregna-1, 4-diene-3, 20-dione, 9-fluoro-11, 21-dihydroxy-16-methyl-17-[(1-oxopentyl)oxy]-, (11β, 16β)-); it has an empirical formula of $C_{27}H_{37}FO_6$ and a molecular weight of 476.58 (CAS Registry Number 2152-44-5).

Each gram of the 0.1% cream contains 1.2 mg Betamethasone Valerate (equivalent to 1.0 mg Betamethasone) in a soft, white hydrophilic cream of Water, Mineral Oil, White Petrolatum, Polyethylene Glycol 1000 Monocetyl Ether, Cetostearyl Alcohol, Monobasic Sodium Phosphate and Phosphoric Acid or Sodium Hydroxide; Chlorocresol is present as a preservative. Betamethasone Valerate Cream contains no parabens.

Each gram of the 0.1% ointment contains 1.2 mg Betamethasone Valerate (equivalent to 1.0 mg Betamethasone) in an ointment base of White Petrolatum and Mineral Oil. Betamethasone Valerate Ointment contains no parabens.

Each gram of the 0.1% lotion contains 1.2 mg Betamethasone Valerate (equivalent to 1.0 mg Betamethasone) in a vehicle of Isopropyl Alcohol and Water slightly thickened with Carbomer 934P. Phosphoric Acid or Sodium Hydroxide are used to adjust the pH.

CLINICAL PHARMACOLOGY

Topical corticosteroids share anti-inflammatory, anti-pruritic and vasoconstrictive actions. The mechanism of anti-inflammatory activity of the topical corticosteroids is unclear. Various laboratory methods, including vasoconstrictor assays, are used to compare and predict potencies and/or clinical efficacies of the topical corticosteroids. There is some evidence to suggest that a recognizable correlation exists between vasoconstrictor potency and therapeutic efficacy in man.

Pharmacokinetics: The extent of percutaneous absorption of topical corticosteroids is determined by many factors including the vehicle, the integrity of the epidermal barrier, and the use of occlusive dressings. Topical corticosteroids can be absorbed from normal intact skin. Inflammation and/or other disease processes in the skin increase percutaneous absorption. Occlusive dressings substantially increase the percutaneous absorption of topical corticosteroids. Thus occlusive dressings may be a valuable therapeutic adjunct for treatment of resistant dermatoses (See DOSAGE AND ADMINISTRATION). Once absorbed through the skin, topical corticosteroids are handled through pharmacokinetic pathways similar to systemically administered corticosteroids. Corticosteroids are bound to plasma proteins in varying degrees. Corticosteroids are metabolized primarily in the liver and are then excreted by the kidneys. Some of the topical corticosteroids and their metabolites are also excreted into the bile.

INDICATIONS AND USAGE

Topical corticosteroids are indicated for the relief of the inflammatory and pruritic manifestations of corticosteroid-responsive dermatoses.

CONTRAINDICATIONS

Topical corticosteroids are contraindicated in those patients with a history of hypersensitivity to any of the components of the preparation.

PRECAUTIONS

General: Systemic absorption of topical corticosteroids has produced reversible hypothalamic-pituitary-adrenal (HPA) axis suppression, manifestations of Cushing's syndrome, hyperglycemia, and glucosuria in some patients. Conditions which augment systemic absorption include the application of the more potent steroids, use over large surface areas, prolonged use, and the addition of occlusive dressings. Therefore, patients receiving a large dose of a potent topical steroid applied to a large surface area or under an occlusive dressing should be evaluated periodically for evidence of HPA axis suppression by using the urinary free cortisol and ACTH stimulation tests. If HPA axis suppression is noted, an attempt should be made to withdraw the drug, to reduce the frequency of application, or to substitute a less potent steroid. Recovery of HPA axis function is generally prompt and complete upon discontinuation of the drug. Infrequently, signs and symptoms of steroid withdrawal may occur, requiring supplemental systemic corticosteroids. Children may absorb proportionally larger amounts of topical corticosteroids and thus be more susceptible to systemic toxicity (See PRECAUTIONS-Pediatric Use). If irritation develops, topical corticosteroids should be discontinued and appropriate therapy instituted. In the presence of dermatological infections, the use of an appropriate antifungal or antibacterial agent should be instituted. If a favorable response does not occur promptly, the corticosteroid should be discontinued until the infection has been adequately controlled.

Information for the Patient: Patients using topical corticosteroids should receive the following information and instructions:

1. This medication is to be used as directed by the physician. It is for external use only. Avoid contact with the eyes.
2. Patients should be advised not to use this medication for any disorder other than for which it was prescribed.
3. The treated skin area should not be bandaged or otherwise covered or wrapped as to be occlusive unless directed by the physician.
4. Patients should report any signs of local adverse reactions especially under occlusive dressing.
5. Parents of pediatric patients should be advised not to use tight fitting diapers or plastic pants on a child being treated in the diaper area, as these garments may constitute occlusive dressings.

Laboratory Tests: The following tests may be helpful in evaluating the HPA axis suppression: Urinary free cortisol test. ACTH stimulation test.

Carcinogenesis, Mutagenesis, and Impairment of Fertility: Long-term animal studies have not been performed to evaluate the carcinogenic potential or the effect on fertility of topical corticosteroids. Studies to determine mutagenicity with prednisolone and hydrocortisone have revealed negative results.

Pregnancy Category C: Corticosteroids are generally teratogenic in laboratory animals when administered systemically at relatively low dosage levels. The more potent corticosteroids have been shown to be teratogenic after dermal application in laboratory animals. There are no adequate and well-controlled studies in pregnant women on teratogenic effects from topically applied corticosteroids. Therefore, topical corticosteroids should be used during pregnancy only if the potential benefit justifies the potential risk to the fetus. Drugs of this class should not be used extensively on pregnant patients, in large amounts, or for prolonged periods of time.

Nursing Mothers: It is not known whether topical administration of corticosteroids could result in sufficient systemic absorption to produce detectable quantities in breast milk. Systemically administered corticosteroids are secreted into breast milk in quantities not likely to have a deleterious effect on the infant. Nevertheless, caution should be exercised when topical corticosteroids are administered to a nursing woman.

Pediatric Use: *Pediatric patients may demonstrate greater susceptibility to topical corticosteroid-induced HPA axis suppression and Cushing's syndrome than mature patients because of a larger skin surface area to body weight ratio.* Hypothalamic-pituitary-adrenal (HPA) axis suppression. Cushing's syndrome, and intracranial hypertension have been reported in children receiving topical corticosteroids. Manifestations of adrenal suppression in children include linear growth retardation, delayed weight gain, low plasma cortisol levels, and absence of response to ACTH stimulation. Manifestations of intracranial hypertension include bulging fontanelles, headaches, and bilateral papilledema. Administration of topical corticosteroids to children should be limited to the least amount compatible with an effective therapeutic regimen. Chronic corticosteroid therapy may interfere with the growth and development of children.

ADVERSE REACTIONS

The following local adverse reactions are reported infrequently with topical corticosteroids, but may occur more frequently with the use of occlusive dressings. These reactions are listed in an approximate decreasing order of occurrence: burning, itching, irritation, dryness, folliculitis, hypertrichosis, acneiform eruptions, hypopigmentation, perioral dermatitis, allergic contact dermatitis, maceration of the skin, secondary infection, skin atrophy, striae and miliaria.

OVERDOSAGE

Topically applied corticosteroids can be absorbed in sufficient amounts to produce systemic effects (See PRECAUTIONS)

DOSAGE AND ADMINISTRATION

Betatrex Cream: Apply a thin film of Betatrex Cream 0.1% to the affected area two or three times daily depending on the severity of the condition.

Betatrex Ointment: Apply a thin film of Betatrex Ointment 0.1% to the affected area two or three times daily depending on the severity of the condition.

Betatrex Lotion: Apply a few drops of Betatrex Lotion 0.1% to the affected area two or three times daily depending on the severity of the condition and massage lightly until it disappears. Shake well before using. Store at controlled room temperature 15–30°C (59°–86°F).

Occlusive dressings may be used for the management of psoriasis or recalcitrant conditions. If an infection develops, the use of occlusive dressings should be discontinued and appropriate antimicrobial therapy instituted.

HOW SUPPLIED

Betatrex Cream U.S.P., 0.1%
NDC 0281-3510-44, 15 gram tube
NDC 0281-3510-50, 45 gram tube
Betatrex Ointment U.S.P., 0.1%
NDC 0281-3516-44, 15 gram tube
NDC 0281-3516-50, 45 gram tube
Betatrex Lotion U.S.P., 0.1%
NDC 0281-3519-46, 60 ml bottle

CAUTION

Federal law prohibits dispensing without prescription.

BREXIN® E.X. OTC

[brex 'in]
Tablets and Liquid

DESCRIPTION

Tablets: Pseudoephedrine hydrochloride 60 mg and guaifenesin 400 mg.

Liquid: Pseudoephedrine hydrochloride 30 mg and guaifenesin 200 mg.

BREXIN® L.A. Capsules ℞

[brex 'in]
(chlorpheniramine maleate, pseudoephedrine hydrochloride)

DESCRIPTION

Each red and clear colored capsule contains chlorpheniramine maleate USP 8 mg. and pseudoephedrine hydrochloride USP 120 mg. in a specially prepared base containing benzyl alcohol, butyl paraben, carboxymethylcellulose sodium, edetate calcium disodium, FD&C blue #1, FD&C red #3, FD&C red #40, gelatin, methylparaben, pharmaceutical glaze, propylparaben, sodium lauryl sulfate, sodium propionate, starch, sucrose and other ingredients.

HOW SUPPLIED

NDC 0281-1934-53, bottle of 100 capsules.
Distributed by Savage Laboratories

Shown in Product Identification Section, page 427

CHROMAGEN® CAPSULES ℞

[kro "mah-jen]

COMPOSITION

Each maroon soft gelatin capsule contains ferrous fumarate USP 200 mg, ascorbic acid USP 250 mg, cyanocobalamin USP 10 mcg, desiccated stomach substance 100 mg.

INDICATIONS

For the treatment of all anemias responsive to oral iron therapy, such as hypochromic anemia associated with pregnancy, chronic or acute blood loss, dietary restriction, metabolic disease and post-surgical convalescence.

Continued on next page

Savage—Cont.

ADMINISTRATION AND DOSAGE
Usual adult dose is 1 soft gelatin capsule daily.

CONTRAINDICATIONS
Hemochromatosis and hemosiderosis are contraindications to iron therapy.

SIDE EFFECTS
Average capsule doses in sensitive individuals or excessive dosage may cause nausea, skin rash, vomiting, diarrhea, precordial pain, or flushing of the face and extremities.

SUPPLY
NDC 0281-4285-53, bottle of 100.
NDC 0281-4285-56, bottle of 500.
Distributed by Savage Laboratories
Shown in Product Identification Section, page 427

CHROMAGEN® OB — OTC
[*kro"mah-jen*]

DESCRIPTION
A phosphorus-free pre-natal vitamin and mineral supplement for use during pregnancy and lactation.
Each 2 capsules contain:

			% U.S. R.D.A.*
Vitamin A (Palmitate)	8,000	IU	100%
Vitamin D (Ergocalciferol)	400	IU	100%
Vitamin E (*dl*-Alpha Tocopheryl Acetate)	30	IU	100%
Vitamin C (Ascorbic Acid and partially supplied by Sodium Ascorbate)	150	mg	250%
Folic Acid	800	mcg	100%
Thiamine (from Thiamine Mononitrate)	3	mg	176%
Riboflavin	3.4	mg	170%
Niacin (Niacinamide)	20	mg	100%
Vitamin B_6 (from Pyridoxine Hydrochloride)	10	mg	400%
Vitamin B_{12} (from Cyanocobalamin)	12	mcg	150%
Calcium (from Calcium Carbonate)	250	mg	19%
Iodine (from Potassium Iodide)	300	mcg	200%
Iron (from Ferrous Fumarate)	66	mg	366%
Magnesium (from Magnesium Oxide)	25	mg	6%
Copper (from Copper Oxide)	2	mg	100%
Zinc (from Zinc Sulfate)	25	mg	166%
Docusate Sodium†	50	mg	—

* Percentage of U.S. Recommended Daily Allowance for Pregnant or lactating women.
† Added to counteract the constipating effect of iron.
Recommended daily dosage: 2 capsules or as prescribed by a physician.
Store at controlled room temperature 15° to 30° C (59°–86° F).

HOW SUPPLIED
NDC 0281-0763-53, 100 Capsules.
Distributed by Savage Laboratories
Shown in Product Identification Section, page 427

DILOR® Tablets ℞
[*dī'lor*]
(dyphylline)

COMPOSITION
Each blue, scored tablet contains dyphylline (dihydroxypropyl theophylline) 200 mg. and the following inactive ingredients: colloidal silicon dioxide, corn starch, food starch, povidone, sodium lauryl sulfate, stearic acid and artificial coloring.
Each white scored tablet contains dyphylline (dihydroxypropyl theophylline) 400 mg and the following inactive ingredients: colloidal silicon dioxide, corn starch, food starch, povidone, sodium lauryl sulfate and stearic acid.

DESCRIPTION
Dyphylline [7-(2,3-Dihydroxypropyl) theophylline] [$C_{10}H_{14}N_4O_4$] is a white, extremely bitter, amorphous solid, freely soluble in water and soluble to the extent of 2 gm in 100 ml alcohol.

ACTIONS
As a xanthine derivative, dyphylline possesses the peripheral vasodilator and bronchodilator actions characteristic of theophylline. It has diuretic and myocardial stimulant effects, and is effective orally. Dyphylline may show fewer side effects than aminophylline, but its blood levels and possibly its activity are also lower.

INDICATIONS
For relief of acute bronchial asthma and for reversible bronchospasm associated with chronic bronchitis and emphysema.

CONTRAINDICATIONS
In individuals who have shown hypersensitivity to any of its components. Dyphylline should not be administered concurrently with other xanthine preparations.

WARNINGS
Status asthmaticus is a medical emergency. Excessive doses may be expected to be toxic. In children treated with dyphylline elixir, the alcoholic vehicle of the drug product poses a truly significant factor of drug dependence including all three components of tolerance, physical dependence and compulsive abuse.
Usage in Pregnancy: Safe use in pregnancy has not been established relative to possible adverse effects on fetal development. Therefore, dyphylline should not be used in pregnant women unless, in the judgment of the physician, the potential benefits outweigh the possible hazards.

PRECAUTIONS
Use with caution in patients with severe cardiac disease, hypertension, hyperthyroidism, or acute myocardial injury. Particular caution in dose administration must be exercised in patients with peptic ulcers, since the condition may be exacerbated. Chronic oral administration in high doses (500 to 1,000 mg.) is usually associated with gastrointestinal irritation. Great caution should be used in giving dyphylline to patients in congestive heart failure. Such patients have shown markedly prolonged blood level curves which have persisted for long periods following discontinuation of the drug.

ADVERSE REACTIONS
Note: Included in this listing which follows are a few adverse reactions which may not have been reported with this specific drug. However, pharmacological similarities among the xanthine drugs require that each of the reactions be considered when dyphylline is administered. The most consistent adverse reactions are: 1. Gastrointestinal irritation: nausea, vomiting, and epigastric pain, generally preceded by headache, hematemesis, diarrhea. 2. Central nervous system stimulation: irritability, restlessness, insomnia, reflex hyperexcitability, muscle twitching, clonic and tonic generalized convulsions, agitation. 3. Cardiovascular: palpitation, tachycardia, extra systoles, flushing, marked hypotension, and circulatory failure. 4. Respiratory: tachypnea, respiratory arrest. 5. Renal: albuminuria, increased excretion of renal tubule and red blood cells. 6. Others: fever, dehydration.

OVERDOSAGE
Symptoms:
In infants and small children: agitation, headache, hyperreflexia, fasciculations, and clonic and tonic convulsions.
In adults: nervousness, insomnia, nausea, vomiting, tachycardia and extra systoles.
Therapy:
Discontinue drug immediately.
No specific treatment.
Ipecac syrup for oral ingestion.
Avoid sympathomimetics.
Supportive treatment for hypotension, seizure, arrhythmias and dehydration.
Sedatives such as short acting barbiturates will help control central nervous system stimulation.
Restore the acid-base balance with lactate or bicarbonate.
Oxygen and antibiotics provide supportive treatment as indicated.

DRUG INTERACTIONS
Toxic synergism with ephedrine and other sympathomimetic bronchodilator drugs may occur.
Recent controlled studies suggest that the addition of ephedrine to adequate dosage regimens of dyphylline produces no increase in effectiveness over that of dyphylline alone, but does produce an increase in toxic effects.

DOSAGE AND ADMINISTRATION
When administered orally it produces less nausea than aminophylline and other alkaline theophylline compounds. Absorption orally appears to be faster on an empty stomach; preferably the drug is to be given at six hour intervals.
Adults: Usual Adult Dose: 15 mg/kg every 6 hours up to 4 times a day. The dosage should be individualized by titration to the condition and response of the patient.
Pulmonary functional measurements before and after a period of treatment allow an objective assessment of whether or not therapy should be continued in patients with chronic bronchitis and emphysema.

HOW SUPPLIED
Tablets
200 mg– NDC 0281-1115-53, Bottle of 100.
NDC 0281-1115-57, Bottle of 1000.
NDC 0281-1115-63, Unit dose, Box of 100
400 mg– NDC 0281-1116-53, Bottle of 100.
NDC 0281-1116-57, Bottle of 1000.
NDC 0281-1116-63, Unit dose, Box of 100

ALSO AVAILABLE
Dilor Elixir, dyphylline 160 mg/15 ml; and Dilor Injectable, dyphylline 250 mg/ml.
Shown in Product Identification Section, page 427

DILOR-G® ℞
[*dī'lor*]
(dyphylline, guaifenesin USP)

COMPOSITION
Each pink, scored tablet contains dyphylline 200 mg, guaifenesin USP 200 mg and the following inactive ingredients: colloidal silicon dioxide, corn starch, food starch, povidone, stearic acid and artificial coloring.
Each teaspoonful (5 ml) of the liquid contains dyphylline 100 mg, guaifenesin USP 100 mg, in a mint flavored base of citric acid, glycerin, saccharin sodium, sorbitol, sucrose, artificial coloring and flavoring, purified water, veltol and sodium hydroxide to adjust pH. Methylparaben and propylparaben are added as preservatives. Contains no alcohol.

HOW SUPPLIED
Tablets
NDC 0281-1124-53, bottle of 100.
NDC 0281-1124-57, bottle of 1000.
NDC 0281-1124-63, unit dose, box of 100.
Liquid
NDC 0281-1127-74, pint.
NDC 0281-1127-76, gallon.
Shown in Product Identification Section, page 427

DITATE®-DS ℞
[*dī'tāt*]
(testosterone enanthate USP and estradiol valerate USP injection)

Each ml contains: testosterone enanthate USP 180 mg, estradiol valerate USP 8 mg, benzyl alcohol NF 2% in sesame oil NF.

HOW SUPPLIED
NDC 0281-5807-32, box of ten 2 ml single-dose vials.
NDC 0281-5807-43, box of ten 2 ml single-dose syringes.

ETHIODOL® ℞
[*ĕ-thī'ō'dŏl*]
(brand of ethiodized oil injection)

DESCRIPTION
Ethiodol, brand of ethiodized oil, is a sterile injectable radio-opaque diagnostic agent for use in hysterosalpingography and lymphography. It contains 37% iodine (475 mg/ml) organically combined with ethyl esters of fatty acids (primarily as ethyl monoidostearate and ethyl diiodostearate) of poppyseed oil. Stabilized with poppyseed oil, 1%. The precise structure of Ethiodol is unknown at this time. Ethiodol is a straw to amber colored, oil fluid, which because of simplified molecular structure, possesses a greatly reduced viscosity (1.280 specific gravity at 15°C yields viscosity of 0.5 to 1.0 poise). This high fluidity provides a new flexibility for radiographic exploration.

HOW SUPPLIED
Ethiodol (brand of ethiodized oil for injection) is supplied in a box of two 10 ml ampules, NDC 0281-7062-37.

MYTREX® F ℞
[*my"trex'*]
(nystatin-triamcinolone acetonide)
Cream Ointment

For Dermatologic Use Only
Not for Ophthalmic Use

DESCRIPTION
MYTREX® F (nystatin-triamcinolone acetonide) Cream and Ointment contain the antifungal agent Nystatin and the synthetic corticosteroid Triamcinolone Acetonide.
Nystatin is a polyene antimycotic obtained from *Streptomyces noursei.* It is a yellow to light tan powder with a cereal-like odor, very slightly soluble in water, and slightly to sparingly soluble in alcohol. It has an empirical formula of $C_{47}H_{75}NO_{17}$ and a molecular weight of 926.13 (CAS Registry Number 1400-61-9).
Triamcinolone Acetonide is designated chemically as Pregna-1, 4-diene-3, 20-dione, 9-fluoro-11, 21-dihydroxy-16,17-[(1-methylethylidene)bis(oxy)]-, (11β, 16α)-; The white to cream crystalline powder has a slight odor, is practically insoluble in water, and very soluble in alcohol. It has an empirical formula of $C_{24}H_{31}FO_6$ and a molecular weight of 434.50 (CAS Registry Number 76-25-5).

Each gram of MYTREX F (nystatin-triamcinolone acetonide) Cream contains 100,000 units of nystatin and 1.0 mg of triamcinolone acetonide in a cream base containing polyoxyethylene fatty alcohol ether, white petrolatum, glyceryl monostearate, polyethylene glycol 400 monostearate, sorbitol solution, fragrance, simethicone emulsion, ethylenediamine, hydrochloric acid, propylene glycol, sorbic acid, aluminum hydroxide gel, polysorbate 60, titanium dioxide, and purified water with methylparaben and propylparaben as preservatives.

Each gram of MYTREX F (nystatin-triamcinolone acetonide) Ointment contains 100,000 units of nystatin and 1.0 mg of triamcinolone acetonide in a base of polyethylene and mineral oil.

CLINICAL PHARMACOLOGY

NYSTATIN

Nystatin exerts its antifungal activity against a variety of pathogenic and nonpathogenic yeasts and fungi by binding to sterols in the cell membrane. The binding process renders the cell membrane incapable of functioning as a selective barrier. Nystatin provides specific anticandidal activity to *Candida* (Monilia) *albicans* and other *Candida* species, but it is not active against bacteria, protozoa, trichomonads, or viruses. Nystatin is not absorbed from intact skin or mucous membranes.

TRIAMCINOLONE ACETONIDE

Triamcinolone Acetonide is primarily effective because of its anti-inflammatory, anti-pruritic and vasoconstrictive actions, characteristic of the topical corticosteroid class of drugs. The pharmacological effects of the topical corticosteroids are well known; however, mechanism of their dermatologic actions are unclear. Various laboratory methods, including vasoconstrictor assays, are used to compare and predict potencies and/or clinical efficacies of the topical corticosteroids. There is some evidence to suggest that a recognizable correlation exists between vasoconstrictor potency and therapeutic efficacy in man.

Pharmacokinetics: The extent of percutaneous absorption of topical corticosteroids is determined by many factors including the vehicle, the integrity of the epidermal barrier and the use of occlusive dressings (see DOSAGE AND ADMINISTRATION). Topical corticosteroids can be absorbed from normal intact skin. Inflammation and/or other disease processes in the skin increase percutaneous absorption. Occlusive dressings substantially increase the percutaneous absorption of topical corticosteroids (see DOSAGE AND ADMINISTRATION). Once absorbed through the skin, topical corticosteroids are handled through pharmacokinetic pathways similar to systemically administered corticosteroids. Corticosteroids are bound to plasma proteins in varying degrees. Corticosteroids are metabolized primarily in the liver and then excreted by the kidneys. Some of the topical corticosteroids and their metabolites are also excreted into the bile.

NYSTATIN and TRIAMCINOLONE ACETONIDE

Patients having mild to severe manifestations of cutaneous candidiasis, treated with combined nystatin and triamcinolone acetonide show a faster and more pronounced clearing of erythema and pruritis than patients treated with nystatin or triamcinolone acetonide alone.

INDICATIONS AND USAGE

MYTREX F (nystatin-triamcinolone acetonide) Cream and Ointment is indicated for the treatment of cutaneous candidiasis; it has been demonstrated that the nystatin-steroid combination provides greater benefit than the nystatin component alone during the first few days of treatment.

CONTRAINDICATIONS

This preparation is contraindicated in those patients with a history of hypersensitivity to any of its components.

PRECAUTIONS

General: Systemic absorption of topical corticosteroids has produced reversible hypothalamic-pituitary-adrenal (HPA) axis suppression, manifestations of Cushing's syndrome, hyperglycemia, and glucosuria in some patients. Conditions which augment systemic absorption include the application of the more potent steroids, use over large surface areas, prolonged use, and the addition of occlusive dressings (see DOSAGE AND ADMINISTRATION). Therefore, patients receiving a large dose of any potent topical steroid applied to a large surface area should be evaluated periodically for evidence of HPA axis suppression by using the urinary free cortisol and ACTH stimulation tests, and for impairment of thermal homeostasis. If HPA axis suppression or elevation of the body temperature occurs, an attempt should be made to withdraw the drug, to reduce the frequency of application, or to substitute a less potent steroid. Recovery of HPA axis function and thermal homeostasis are generally prompt and complete upon discontinuation of the drug. Infrequently, signs and symptoms of steroid withdrawal may occur, requiring supplemental systemic corticosteroids. Children may absorb proportionally larger amounts of topical corticosteroids and thus be more susceptible to systemic toxicity (See PRECAUTIONS, Pediatric Use). If irritation or hypersensitivity develops with the combination nystatin and triamcinolone acetonide, treatment should be discontinued and appropriate therapy instituted.

Information for the Patient: Patients using this medication should receive the following information and instructions:

1. This medication is to be used as directed by the physician. It is for external use only. Avoid contact with the eyes.
2. Patients should be advised not to use this medication for any disorder other than for which it was prescribed.
3. The treated skin area should not be bandaged or otherwise covered or wrapped as to be occluded (see DOSAGE AND ADMINISTRATION).
4. Patients should report any signs of local adverse reactions.
5. When using this medication in the inguinal area, patients should be advised to apply cream or ointment sparingly and to wear loose fitting clothing.
6. Parents of pediatric patients should be advised not to use tight-fitting diapers or plastic pants on a child being treated in the diaper area, as these garments may constitute occlusive dressings.
7. Patients should be advised on preventive measures to avoid reinfection.

Laboratory Tests: If there is a lack of therapeutic response, appropriate microbiological studies (e.g., KOH smears and/or cultures) should be repeated to confirm the diagnosis and rule out other pathogens, before instituting another course of therapy. The following tests may be helpful in evaluating hypothalamic-pituitary-adrenal (HPA) axis suppression due to the corticosteroid: Urinary free cortisol test; ACTH stimulation test.

Carcinogenesis, Mutagenesis, and Impairment of Fertility: Long-term animal studies have not been performed to evaluate the carcinogenic or mutagenic potential or possible impairment of fertility in males or females.

Pregnancy Category C: There are no teratogenic studies with combined nystatin and triamcinolone acetonide. Corticosteroids are generally teratogenic in laboratory animals when administered systemically at relatively low dosage levels. The more potent corticosteroids have been shown to be teratogenic after dermal application in laboratory animals. Therefore, any topical corticosteroid preparation should be used during pregnancy only if the potential benefit justifies the potential risk to the fetus. Topical preparations containing corticosteroids should not be used extensively on pregnant patients, in large amounts, or for prolonged periods of time.

Nursing Mothers: It is not known whether any component of this preparation is excreted in human milk. Because many drugs are excreted in human milk, caution should be exercised during use of this preparation by a nursing woman.

Pediatric Use: In clinical studies of a limited number of pediatric patients ranging in age from 2 months through twelve years, Nystatin-Triamcinolone Acetonide Cream cleared or significantly ameliorated the disease state in most patients. *Pediatric patients may demonstrate greater susceptibility to topical corticosteroid-induced hypothalamic-pituitary-adrenal (HPA) axis suppression and Cushing's syndrome than mature patients because of a larger skin surface area to body weight ratio.* HPA axis suppression, Cushing's syndrome, and intracranial hypertension have been reported in children receiving topical corticosteroids. Manifestations of adrenal suppression in children include linear growth retardation, delayed weight gain, low plasma cortisol levels, and absence of response to ACTH stimulation. Manifestations of intracranial hypertension include bulging fontanelles, headaches and bilateral papilledema. Administration of topical corticosteroids to children should be limited to the least amount compatible with an effective therapeutic regimen. Chronic corticosteroid therapy may interfere with the growth and development of children.

ADVERSE REACTIONS

A single case (approximately one percent of patients studied) of acneiform eruption occurred with the use of combined nystatin and triamcinolone acetonide in clinical studies.

Nystatin is virtually nontoxic and nonsensitizing and is well tolerated by all age groups, even during prolonged use. Rarely, irritation may occur.

The following local adverse reactions are reported infrequently with topical corticosteroids. These reactions are listed in an approximate decreasing order of occurrence: burning, itching, irritation, dryness, folliculitis, hypertrichosis, acneiform eruptions, hypopigmentation, perioral dermatitis, allergic contact dermatitis, maceration of the skin, secondary infection, skin atrophy, striae and miliaria.

OVERDOSAGE

Topically applied corticosteroids can be absorbed in sufficient amounts to produce systemic effects (see PRECAUTIONS, General). However, acute overdosage and serious adverse effects with dermatologic use are unlikely.

DOSAGE AND ADMINISTRATION

Apply MYTREX F (nystatin-triamcinolone acetonide) Cream to the affected area twice daily in the morning and the evening by gently and thoroughly massaging the preparation into the skin. A thin film of MYTREX F Ointment is usually applied to the affected areas twice daily in the morning and evening. The cream or ointment should be discontinued if symptoms persist after 25 days of therapy. (See PRECAUTIONS, Laboratory Tests). MYTREX F (nystatin-triamcinolone acetonide) Cream and Ointment should not be used with occlusive dressings.

HOW SUPPLIED

MYTREX F Cream
15 Gram Tube—NDC 0281-0081-15
30 Gram Tube—NDC 0281-0081-30
60 Gram Tube—NDC 0281-0081-60

Shown in Product Identification Section, page 427

MYTREX F Ointment
15 gram tube—NDC 0281-0089-15
30 gram tube—NDC 0281-0089-30
60 gram tube—NDC 0281-0089-60

Store at room temperature. Avoid freezing.

CAUTION

Federal law prohibits dispensing without prescription.

NYSTEX™ ℞

[*nī'stex*]
(nystatin cream USP and ointment USP)

DESCRIPTION

NYSTEX (nystatin USP) Cream contains the antifungal antibiotic nystatin at a concentration of 100,000 units per gram in an aqueous, perfumed vanishing cream base containing polysorbate 60, aluminum hydroxide compressed gel, titanium dioxide, glyceryl monostearate, polyethylene glycol monostearate 400, simethicone, sorbic acid, propylene glycol, ethylenediamine, polyoxyethylene fatty alcohol ether, sorbitol solution, methyl paraben, propyl paraben, hydrochloric acid, white petrolatum, and purified water.

NYSTEX (nystatin USP) Nystatin Ointment contains 100,000 units nystatin per gram in a polyethylene and mineral oil base.

HOW SUPPLIED

NYSTEX Cream
NDC 0281-3208-44, 15 gram tube
NDC 0281-3208-45, 30 gram tube
NYSTEX Ointment
NDC 0281-3212-44, 15 gram tube

NYSTEX™ ℞

[*nī'stex*]
(nystatin oral suspension U.S.P.)

DESCRIPTION

Nystatin is an antifungal antibiotic that is both fungistatic and fungicidal in vitro against a wide variety of yeasts and yeastlike fungi. It is a polyene antibiotic of undetermined structural formula that is obtained from *Streptomyces noursei.* Nystex Oral Suspension contains 100,000 units nystatin per ml in a vehicle containing alcohol USP (not more than 1% by volume), cherry flavoring, dibasic sodium phosphate USP, glycerin USP, peppermint oil, purified water USP, silicon dioxide, sucrose NF (50%) and methylparaben NF (0.12%) and propylparaben NF (0.03%) as preservatives.

HOW SUPPLIED

Nystex Oral Suspension (NDC 0281-0037-60) is available as a pleasant-tasting, ready-to-use suspension containing 100,000 units nystatin per ml in 60 ml bottles (each supplied with a calibrated dropper).

STORAGE

Store at room temperaure; avoid freezing.

SĀTRIC™ Tablets ℞

[*sā'trik*]
(metronidazole USP)
[*me-troe-ni'da-zole*]

WARNING

Sātric has been shown to be carcinogenic in mice and rats. (*See Warnings*). Unnecessary use of this drug should be avoided. Its use should be reserved for the conditions described in the *Indications And Usage* section below.

DESCRIPTION

Sātric is a 1-(β-hydroxyethyl)-2-methyl-5-nitroimidazole. Sātric is classified therapeutically as an antiprotozoal (Trichomonas), and antibacterial (antianaerobic) agent. It occurs as pale yellow crystals that are slightly soluble in water and alcohol. Metronidazole has the following structural formula: [See Chemical Formula at top of next page].

Continued on next page

Savage—Cont.

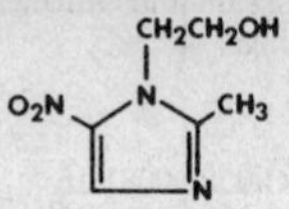

CLINICAL PHARMACOLOGY

Metronidazole is usually well absorbed after oral administration, with peak plasma concentrations occurring between one and two hours. An average elimination half-life is 8 hours in healthy humans. Plasma concentrations of metronidazole are proportional to the administered dose. Oral administration of 250 mg., 500 mg., or 2,000 mg. produced peak plasma concentration of 6 mcg/ml, 12 mcg/ml, and 40 mcg/ml, respectively. Studies reveal no significant bioavailability differences between males and females, however, because of weight differences, the resulting plasma levels in males are generally lower.

Metronidazole is a major component appearing in the plasma, with lesser quantities of the 2-hydroxymethyl metabolite also being present. Less than 20% of the circulating metronidazole is bound to plasma proteins. Both the parent compound and the metabolite possess *in vitro* trichomonacidal activity and *in vitro* bactericidal activity against most strains of anaerobic bacteria.

The major route of elimination of metronidazole and its metabolites is via the urine (60–80% of the dose), with fecal excretion accounting for 6–15% of the dose. The metabolites that appear in the urine result primarily from side-chain oxidation [1-(β-hydroxyethyl)-2-hydroxymethyl-5-nitroimidazole and 2-methyl-5-nitroimidazole-1-yl-acetic acid] and glucuronide conjugation, with unchanged metronidazole accounting for approximately 20% of the total. Renal clearance of metronidazole is approximately 10 ml/min/1.73 m^2.

Decreased renal function does not alter the single-dose pharmacokinetics of metronidazole. However, plasma clearance of metronidazole is decreased in patients with decreased liver function.

Metronidazole appears in cerebrospinal fluid, saliva, and breast milk in concentrations similar to those found in plasma. Bactericidal concentrations of metronidazole have also been detected in pus from hepatic abscesses.

Microbiology: Metronidazole possesses direct trichomonacidal and amebacidal activity against *Trichomonas vaginalis* and *Entamoeba histolytica*. The *in vitro* minimal inhibitory concentration (MIC) for most strains of these organisms is 1 mcg/ml or less. Metronidazole's mechanism of antiprotozoal action is unknown.

Anaerobic Bacteria: Metronidazole is active *in vitro* against obligate anaerobes, but does not appear to possess any clinically relevant activity against facultative anaerobes or obligate aerobes. Against susceptible organisms, Metronidazole is generally bactericidal at concentrations equal to or slightly higher than the minimal inhibitory concentrations (MIC). Metronidazole has been shown to have *in vitro* and clinical activity against the following organisms:

Anaerobic gram-negative bacilli, including:
Bacteroides species, including the *Bacteroides fragilis* group (*B. fragilis, B. distasonis, B. ovatus, B. thetaiotaomicron, B. vulgatus*)
Fusobacterium species
Anaerobic gram-positive bacilli, including:
Clostridium species and susceptible strains of *Eubacterium*
Anaerobic gram-positive cocci, including:
Peptococcus species
Peptostreptococcus species

Susceptibility tests: Bacteriologic studies should be performed to determine the causative organisms and their susceptibility to metronidazole; however, the rapid, routine susceptibility testing of individual isolates of anaerobic bacteria is not always practical, and therapy may be started while awaiting these results.

Quantitative methods give the most precise estimates of susceptibility to antibacterial drugs. A standardized agar dilution method and a broth microdilution method are recommended.[1]

Control strains are recommended for standardized susceptibility testing. Each time the test is performed, one or more of the following strains should be included: *Clostridium perfringens* ATCC 13124, *Bacteroides fragilis* ATCC 25285, and *Bacteroides thetaiotaomicron* ATCC 29741. The mode metronidazole MIC's for those three strains are reported to be 0.25, 0.25, and 0.5 mcg/ml, respectively.

A clinical laboratory is considered under acceptable control if the results of the control strains are within one doubling dilution of the mode MIC's reported for metronidazole.

A bacterial isolate may be considered susceptible if the MIC value for Metronidazole is not more than 16 mcg/ml. An organism is considered resistant if the MIC is greater than 16 mcg/ml. A report of "resistant" from the laboratory indicates that the infecting organism is not likely to respond to therapy.

INDICATIONS AND USAGE

Symptomatic Trichomoniasis: Sātric is indicated for the treatment of symptomatic trichomoniasis in females and males when the presence of trichomonad has been confirmed by appropriate laboratory procedures (wet smears and/or cultures).

Asymptomatic Trichomoniasis: Sātric is indicated in the treatment of asymptomatic females when the organism is associated with endocervicitis, cervicitis, or cervical erosion. Since there is evidence that presence of the trichomonad can interfere with accurate assessment of abnormal cytological smears, additional smears should be performed after eradication of the parasite.

Treatment of Asymptomatic Consorts: *T. vaginalis* infection is a venereal disease. Therefore, asymptomatic sexual partners of treated patients should be treated simultaneously if the organism has been found to be present in order to prevent reinfection of the partner. The decision as to whether to treat an asymptomatic male partner with a negative culture or one in whom no culture has been attempted is an individual one. In making this decision, it should be noted that there is evidence that women may become reinfected if the consort is not treated. Also, since there can be considerable difficulty in isolating the organism from the asymptomatic male carrier, negative smears and cultures cannot be relied upon in this regard. In any event, the consort should be treated with Sātric in cases of reinfection.

Amebiasis: Sātric is indicated in the treatment of acute intestinal amebiasis (amebic dysentery) and amebic liver abscess.

In amebic liver abscess, Sātric therapy does not obviate the need for aspiration or drainage of pus.

Anaerobic Bacterial Infections: Sātric is indicated in the treatment of serious infections caused by susceptible anaerobic bacteria. Indicated surgical procedures should be performed in conjunction with metronidazole therapy. In a mixed aerobic and anaerobic infection, antibiotics appropriate for the treatment of aerobic infection should be used in addition to metronidazole. In the treatment of most serious anaerobic infections the intravenous form of metronidazole is usually administered initially. This may be followed by oral therapy with metronidazole at the discretion of the physician.

INTRA-ABDOMINAL INFECTION, including peritonitis, intra-abdominal abscess, and liver abscess, caused by *Bacteroides* species including the *B. fragilis* group (*B. fragilis, B. distasonis, B. ovatus, B. thetaoitaomicron, B. vulgatus*), *Clostridium* species, *Eubacterium* species, *Peptococcus* species, and *Peptostreptococcus* species.

SKIN AND SKIN STRUCTURE INFECTIONS caused by *Bacteroides* species including the *B. fragilis* group, *Clostridium* species, *Peptococcus* species, *Peptostreptococcus* species, and *Fusobacterium* species.

GYNECOLOGIC INFECTIONS, including endometritis, endomyometritis, tubo-ovarian abscess, and post-surgical vaginal cuff infection, caused by *Bacteroides* species including the *B. fragilis* group, *Clostridium* species, *Peptococcus* species, and *Peptostreptococcus* species.

BACTERIAL SEPTICEMIA caused by *Bacteroides* species including the *B. fragilis* group, and *Clostridium* species.

BONE AND JOINT INFECTIONS, as adjunctive therapy, caused by *Bacteroides* species including the *B. fragilis* group.

CENTRAL NERVOUS SYSTEM (CNS) INFECTIONS, including meningitis and brain abscess, caused by *Bacteroides* species including the *B. fragilis* group.

LOWER RESPIRATORY TRACT INFECTIONS, including pneumonia, empyema, and lung abscess, caused by *Bacteroides* species including the *B. fragilis* group.

ENDOCARDITIS caused by *Bacteroides* species including the *B. fragilis* group.

CONTRAINDICATIONS

Sātric is contraindicated in patients with a prior history of hypersensitivity to metronidazole, or other nitroimidazole derivatives. In patients with trichomoniasis, Sātric is contraindicated during the first trimester of pregnancy. *(See Warnings).*

WARNINGS

Convulsive Seizures and Peripheral Neuropathy: Convulsive seizures and peripheral neuropathy, the latter characterized mainly by numbness or paresthesia of an extremity, have been reported in patients treated with metronidazole. The appearance of abnormal neurologic signs demands the prompt discontinuation of Sātric therapy. Sātric should be administered with caution to patients with central nervous system diseases.

Tumorigenicity Studies in Rodents: Metronidazole has shown evidence of carcinogenic activity in a number of studies involving chronic, oral administration in mice and rats. Prominent among the effects in the mouse was the promotion of pulmonary tumorigenesis. This has been observed in all six reported studies in that species, including one study in which the animals were dosed on an intermittent schedule (administration during every fourth week only). At very high dose levels (approx. 500 mg/kg/day) there was a statistically significant increase in the incidence of malignant liver tumors in males. Also, the published results of one of the mouse studies indicated an increase in the incidence of malignant lymphomas as well as pulmonary neoplasms associated with lifetime feeding of the drug. All these effects are statistically significant.

Several long-term oral dosing studies in the rats have been completed. There was a statistically significant increase in the incidence of various neoplasms, particularly in mammary and hepatic tumors, among female rats administered metronidazole over those noted in the concurrent female control groups.

Two lifetime tumorigenicity studies in hamsters have been performed and reported to be negative.

Mutagenicity Studies: Although metronidazole has shown mutagenic activity in a number of *in vitro* assay systems, studies in mammals (*in vivo*) have failed to demonstrate a potential for genetic damage.

PRECAUTIONS

General: Patients with severe hepatic disease metabolize metronidazole slowly, with resultant accumulation of metronidazole and its metabolites in the plasma. Accordingly, for such patients, doses below those usually recommended should be administered cautiously.

Known or previously unrecognized candidiasis may present more prominent symptoms during therapy with Sātric and requires treatment with a candicidal agent.

Laboratory Tests: Sātric (metronidazole) is a nitroimidazole and should be used with care in patients with evidence of, or history of blood dyscrasia. A mild leukopenia has been observed during its administration; however, no persistent hematologic abnormalities attributable to metronidazole have been observed in clinical studies. Total and differential leukocyte counts are recommended before and after therapy for trichomoniasis and amebiasis, especially if a second course of therapy is necessary, and before and after therapy for anaerobic infection.

Drug Interactions: Metronidazole has been reported to potentiate the anticoagulant effect of coumarin and warfarin resulting in a prolongation of prothrombin time. This possible drug interaction should be considered when Sātric is prescribed for patients on this type of anti-coagulant therapy.

Alcoholic beverages should not be consumed during Sātric therapy because abdominal cramps, nausea, vomiting, headache, and flushing may occur.

Drug/Laboratory Test Interactions: Metronidazole may interfere with certain chemical analyses for serum glutamic oxalacetic transaminase, resulting in decreased values. Values of zero may be observed.

Carcinogenesis: *(See Warnings.)*

Pregnancy: *Teratogenic Effects—Pregnancy Category B:* Metronidazole crosses the placental barrier and enters the fetal circulation rapidly. Reproduction studies have been performed in rabbits and rats at doses up to five times the human dose and have revealed no evidence of impaired fertility or harm to the fetus due to Metronidazole. There are, however, no adequate and well-controlled studies in pregnant women. Because animal reproduction studies are not always predictive of human response, and because metronidazole is a carcinogen in rodents, this drug should be used during pregnancy only if clearly needed. *(See Contraindications).*

Use of Sātric for trichomoniasis in the second and third trimesters should be restricted to those in whom local palliative treatment has been inadequate to control symptoms.

Nursing Mothers: Because of the potential for tumorigenicity shown for metronidazole in mouse and rat studies, a decision should be made whether to discontinue nursing or to discontinue the drug, taking into account the importance of the drug to the mother. Metronidazole is secreted in breast milk in concentrations similar to those found in plasma.

Pediatric Use: Safety and effectiveness in children have not been established, except for the treatment of amebiasis.

ADVERSE REACTIONS

The two most serious adverse reactions reported in patients treated with metronidazole have been convulsive seizures and peripheral neuropathy, the latter characterized mainly by numbness or paresthesia of an extremity. Since persistent peripheral neuropathy has been reported in some patients receiving prolonged administration of metronidazole, patients should be specifically warned about these reactions and should be told to stop the drug and report immediately to their physicians if any neurologic symptoms occur.

The most common adverse reactions reported have been referable to the gastrointestinal tract, particularly nausea, sometimes accompanied by headache, anorexia, and occasionally vomiting; diarrhea; epigastric distress; and abdominal cramping. Constipation has also been reported.

The following reactions have also been reported during the treatment with metronidazole.

Mouth: A sharp, unpleasant metallic taste is not unusual. Furry tongue, glossitis, and stomatitis have oc-

curred; these may be associated with a sudden overgrowth of *Candida* which may occur during effective therapy.
Hematopoietic: Reversible neutropenia (leukopenia). Cardiovascular: Flattening of the T-wave may be seen in electrocardiographic tracings.
Central Nervous System: Convulsive seizures, peripheral neuropathy, dizziness, vertigo, incoordination, ataxia, confusion, irritability, depression, weakness, and insomnia.
Hypersensitivity: Urticaria, erythematous rash, flushing, nasal congestion, dryness of the mouth (or vagina or vulva) and fever.
Renal: Dysuria, cystitis, polyuria, incontinence, and a sense of pelvic pressure. Instances of darkened urine have been reported, and this manifestation has been the subject of a special investigation. Although the pigment which is probably responsible for this phenomenon has not been positively identified, it is almost certainly a metabolite of metronidazole and seems to have no clinical significance.
Other: Proliferation of *Candida* in the vagina, dyspareunia, decrease of libido, proctitis, and fleeting joint pains sometimes resembling "serum sickness." If patients receiving Sātric drink alcoholic beverages, they may experience abdominal distress, nausea, vomiting, flushing, or headache. A modification of the taste of alcoholic beverages has also been reported.

OVERDOSAGE

Single oral doses of metronidazole, up to 15 g. have been reported in suicide attempts and accidental overdoses. Symptoms reported include nausea, vomiting, and ataxia. Oral metronidazole has been studied as a radiation sensitizer in the treating of malignant tumors. Neurotoxic effects, including seizures and peripheral neuropathy, have been reported after 5 to 7 days of doses of 6 to 10.4 g every other day.
Treatment: There is no specific antidote for Sātric overdose; therefore, management of the patient should consist of symptomatic and supportive therapy.

DOSAGE AND ADMINISTRATION

Trichomoniasis: In the Female: One-day treatment—two grams of Sātric given either as a single dose or in two divided doses of one gram each given in the same day.
Seven-day course of treatment—250 mg three times daily for seven consecutive days. There is some indication from controlled comparative studies that cure rates as determined by vaginal smears, signs and symptoms, may be higher after a seven-day course of treatment than after a one-day treatment regimen.
The dosage regimen should be individualized. Single-dose treatment can assure compliance, especially if administered under supervision, in those patients who cannot be relied on to continue the seven-day regimen.
A seven-day course of treatment may minimize reinfection of the female long enough to treat sexual contacts. Further, some patients may tolerate one course of therapy better than the other. Pregnant patients should not be treated during the first trimester with either regimen. If treated during the second or third trimester, the one-day course of therapy should not be used, as it results in higher serum levels which reach the fetal circulation. *(See Contraindications and Precautions).*
When repeated courses of the drug are required, it is recommended that an interval of four to six weeks elapse between courses and that the presence of the trichomonad be reconfirmed by appropriate laboratory measures. Total and differential leukocyte counts should be made before and after treatment.
In the Male: Treatment should be individualized as for the female.
Amebiasis: Adults: For Acute Intestinal Amebiasis (Acute Amebic Dysentery): 750 mg orally 3 times daily for 5 to 10 days.
For Amebic Liver Abscess: 500 mg or 750 mg orally 3 times daily for 5 to 10 days.
Children: 35 to 50 mg/kg of body weight/24 hours divided into 3 doses, orally for 10 days.
Anaerobic Bacterial Infections:
In the treatment of most serious anaerobic infections the intravenous form of metronidazole is usually administered initially.
Following intravenous therapy, oral metronidazole may be used when conditions warrant based upon the severity of the disease and the response of the patient to intravenous treatment.
The usual adult *oral* dosage is 7.5 mg/kg every six hours (approximately 500 mg for a 70 kg adult). A maximum of 4.0 g should not be exceeded during a 24 hour period.
The usual duration of therapy is 7 to 10 days; however, infections of the bone and joint, lower respiratory tract, and endocardium may require longer treatment.
Patients with severe hepatic disease metabolize metronidazole slowly, with resultant accumulation of metronidazole and its metabolites in the plasma. Accordingly, for such patients, doses below those usually recommended should be administered cautiously. Close monitoring of plasma metronidazole levels[2] and toxicity is recommended.
The dose of metronidazole should not be specifically reduced in anuric patients since accumulated metabolites may be rapidly removed by dialysis.

HOW SUPPLIED

Available in tablets containing 250 mg and 500 mg of metronidazole USP. Each tablet of 250 mg is imprinted 3681. It is a white, to off-white round, convex tablet, packaged in bottles of 100 and 250 tablets. Each tablet of 500 mg is imprinted 3688. It is a white to off-white oblong, convex tablet, packaged in bottles of 60.
NDC **0281-3681-53**, bottle of 100
NDC **0281-3681-55**, bottle of 250
NDC **0281-3688-52**, bottle of 60
Dispense in well closed, light resistant containers as defined in the USP.
Store below 86°F (30°C).

CAUTION

Federal law prohibits dispensing without prescription.

1. Proposed standard: PSM-11—Proposed Reference Dilution Procedure for Antimicrobic Susceptibility Testing of Anaerobic Bacteria, National Committee for Clinical Laboratory Standards, and Sutter, et al: Collaborative Evaluation of a Proposed Reference Dilution Method of Susceptibility Testing of Anaerobic Bacteria, Antimicrob. Agents Chemother. *16*:495–502 (Oct.) 1979; and Talley, et al: *In Vitro* Activity of Thienamycin, Antimicrob. Agents Chemother. *14*:436–438 (Sept.) 1978.
2. Ralph, E.D. and Kirby, W.M.M.: Bioassay of Metronidazole With Either Anaerobic or Aerobic Incubation, J. Infect. Dis. *132*:587–591 (Nov.) 175; or Gulaid, et al: Determination of Metronidazole and Its Major Metabolities in Biological Fluids by High Pressure Liquid Chromatography, Br. J. Clin. Pharmacol. *6*:430–432, 1978.

9/84

Distributed by
SAVAGE LABORATORIES
a division of Altana Inc.
Melville, NY 11747
Shown in Product Identification Section, page 427

TRYMEX ℞

[trī′mex]
(triamcinolone acetonide)
Cream U.S.P. and Ointment U.S.P.

DESCRIPTION

Trymex contains Triamcinolone Acetonide [Pregna-1, 4-diene-3, 20-dione, 9-fluoro-11, 21-dihydroxy-16, 17-[(1-methylethylidene) bis (oxy)]-, (11B, 16A)-], with the empirical formula $C_{24}H_{31}FO_6$ and molecular weight 434.50. CAS 76-25-5.

HOW SUPPLIED

Trymex Cream U.S.P., 0.025%
NDC 0281-3622-44, 15 gram tube
NDC 0281-3622-48, 80 gram tube
Trymex Cream U.S.P., 0.1%
NDC 0281-3625-44, 15 gram tube
NDC 0281-3625-48, 80 gram tube
NDC 0281-3625-87, 1 pound jar
Trymex Ointment U.S.P., 0.025%
NDC 0281-3633-44, 15 gram tube
Trymex Ointment U.S.P., 0.1%
NDC 0281-3636-44, 15 gram tube
For External Use Only.
Caution: Federal law prohibits dispensing without prescription.

TRYSUL® ℞

[trī′sul]
(triple sulfa vaginal cream)

DESCRIPTION

Active Ingredients: sulfathiazole 3.42%, sulfacetamide 2.86%, sulfabenzamide 3.70% and urea 0.64%
In a Base Containing: Glyceryl monostearate, cetyl alcohol, stearic acid, lecithin, peanut oil, diethylaminoethyl steramide, phosphoric acid, propylene glycol, ethoxylated cholesterol, methyl paraben 0.15% and propyl paraben 0.05% as preservatives, and purified water.

HOW SUPPLIED

NDC 0281-3790-47, 78 g tube with measured dose applicator.

Products are cross-indexed by
generic and chemical names in the
YELLOW SECTION

Schering Corporation

GALLOPING HILL ROAD
KENILWORTH, NJ 07033

Product Identification Codes

To provide quick and positive identification of Schering Products, we have imprinted the product identification number of the National Drug Code on most tablets and capsules. In some cases, identification letters also appear.
Additionally, the following telephone numbers are provided for inquires:

Professional Services Department
9:00 AM to 5:00 PM EST
1-800-526-4099

After regular hours and on weekends: (201) 558-4000
For convenience, a complete list of all Schering products and their identification codes, where appropriate, follow:

Product Listing

Product	Code
A&D™ Hand Cream•	OTC
A&D™ Ointment•	OTC
AFRIN®•	OTC
oxymetazoline HCl	
Nasal Spray 0.05%	
Menthol Nasal Spray 0.05%	
Nose Drops 0.05%	
Pediatric Nose Drops 0.025%	
AFRINOL®•	OTC
pseudoephedrine sulfate	
Repetabs Tablets Long-Acting Nasal Decongestant	258
CELESTONE®	℞
betamethasone, USP	
Phosphate Injection	
Soluspan® Suspension	
Syrup	
Tablets 0.6 mg	011/BDA
CHLOR-TRIMETON®•	OTC
chlorpheniramine maleate	
Allergy Syrup	
Allergy Tablets 4 mg	080/TW
Long-Acting Allergy Repetabs® Tablets 8 mg	374
Maximum Strength Allergy Repetabs® Tablets 12 mg	009/AAE
CHLOR-TRIMETON®•	OTC
chlorpheniramine maleate/ pseudoephedrine sulfate	
Decongestant Tablets	901
Long-Acting Decongestant Repetabs® Tablets	
CHLOR-TRIMETON® †	℞
chlorpheniramine maleate, USP	
Injection 10 mg/ml	
COD LIVER OIL CONCENTRATE•	OTC
Capsules	
Tablets	
Tablets with Vitamin C	
CORICIDIN®•	OTC
Cough Syrup	
D® Decongestant Tablets	307
DEMILETS® Tablets	
Nasal Mist	
Sinus Headache Tablets (Extra Strength)	
Tablets	522
DEMAZIN®•	OTC
Timed-Release Tablets	751
Syrup	
DERMOLATE®	OTC
hydrocortisone 0.5%	
Anti-Itch Cream	
Anal-Itch Ointment	
Anti-Itch Spray	
Scalp-Itch Lotion	
DIPROLENE®	℞
betamethasone dipropionate, USP	
Cream 0.05%	
Ointment 0.05%	
DIPROSONE®	℞
betamethasone dipropionate, USP	
Aerosol 0.1%	
Cream 0.05%	
Lotion 0.05%	
Ointment 0.05%	
DISOPHROL®•	OTC
CHRONOTAB® Tablets	85-WMH/ 231

Continued on next page

Information on Schering products appearing on these pages is effective as of September 30, 1986.

Schering—Cont.

DISOPHROL® † WBS/866 OTC
Tablets
DRIXORAL®* Sustained-Action Tablets OTC
DRIXORAL Syrup OTC
EMKO®* OTC
BECAUSE® Contraceptor®*
PRE-FIL® Vaginal Contraceptive Foam
Vaginal Contraceptive Foam
ESTINYL® Tablets ℞
estinyl estradiol, USP
0.02 mg 298/ER
0.05 mg 070/EM
0.5 mg 150/EP
ETRAFON® Tablets ℞
perphenazine, USP-amitriptyline hydrochloride, USP
Tablets (2-10) ANA/287
Tablets (2-25) ANC/598
A Tablets (4-10) ANB/119
Forte Tablets (4-25) ANE/720
FIBRE TRIM® Tablets OTC
FULVICIN® P/G Tablets ℞
ultramicrosize griseofulvin, USP
125 mg 228
165 mg 654
250 mg 507
330 mg 352
FULVICIN U/F® Tablets ℞
griseofulvin, (microsize), USP
250 mg AUF/948
500 mg AUG/496
GARAMYCIN® Injectables ℞
gentamicin sulfate, USP
Disposable Syringes 1.5 ml (60 mg)
Disposable Syringes 2.0 ml (80 mg)
Injectable 2 ml vial (80 mg)
Injectable 20 ml vial (800 mg)
Intrathecal 2 ml (4 mg) ampul
Pediatric Injectable 2 ml vial (20 mg)
I.V. Piggyback Injection–60 ml (60 mg), 80 ml (80 mg)
GARAMYCIN® Topicals ℞
gentamicin sulfate, USP
Cream
Ointment
Ophthalmic Ointment
Ophthalmic Solution
GYNE-LOTRIMIN® ℞
clotrimazole, USP
Vaginal Cream 1%
Vaginal Tablets 100 mg 734
Vaginal Tablets 500 mg 396
HYPERSTAT® I.V. Injection ℞
diazoxide, USP
INTRON® A ℞
Interferon alfa-2b, recombinant Injection
LOTRIMIN® ℞
clotrimazole, USP
Cream 1%
Lotion 1%
Solution 1%
LOTRISONE® Cream ℞
clotrimazole, USP, betamethasone dipropionate, USP
METICORTEN® Tablets† ℞
prednisone, USP
1 mg KEM/843
METIMYD® ℞
prednisolone acetate, USP/sulfacetamide sodium, USP
Ophthalmic Ointment
Ophthalmic Solution
MIRADON® Tablets ℞
anisindione, USP
MOL-IRON®* OTC
Tablets
Tablets with Vitamin C
NAQUA® Tablets ℞
trichlormethiazide, USP
2 mg AHG/822
4 mg AHH/547
NAQUIVAL® Tablets ℞
trichlormethiazide, USP/reserpine, USP AHT/394
NETROMYCIN® ℞
netilmicin sulfate
Injection 100 mg/ml
Pediatric Injection 25 mg/ml
NORMODYNE® ℞
labetalol HCl
Tablets 100 mg 244
200 mg 752
300 mg 438
Injection 5 mg/ml
OPTIMINE® Tablets ℞
azatadine maleate, USP 282
OPTIMYD® Ophthalmic Solution† ℞
prednisolone sodium phosphate, USP/sulfacetamide sodium, USP
ORETON® ℞
methyltestosterone, USP
Methyl Tablets 10 mg JD/311
25 mg JE/499
Methyl Buccal Tablets BE/970
OTOBIOTIC® Otic Solution ℞
polymyxin B sulfate, USP and hydrocortisone, USP
PAXIPAM® Tablets Ⓒ ℞
halazepam
20 mg 251
40 mg 538
PERMITIL® ℞
fluphenazine hydrochloride, USP
Oral Concentrate
2.5 mg WDR/442
5 mg WFF/550
10 mg WFG/316
POLARAMINE® ℞
dexchlorpheniramine maleate, USP
Expectorant†
Repetabs® Tablets 4 mg AGA/095
6 mg AGB/148
Syrup
Tablets 2 mg AGT/820
PROVENTIL® ℞
albuterol
Inhaler
PROVENTIL® ℞
albuterol sulfate
Syrup
Tablets 2 mg 252
4 mg 573
RELA® Tablets† ℞
carisoprodol AHR/160
SEBIZON® Lotion† ℞
sulfacetamide sodium, USP 10%
SODIUM SULAMYD® ℞
sulfacetamide sodium, USP
Ophthalmic Ointment 10%
Ophthalmic Solution 10%
Ophthalmic Solution 30% w/v
SOLGANAL® Suspension ℞
aurothioglucose, USP
THEOVENT® Long-Acting Capsules ℞
theophylline anhydrous, USP
125 mg 402
250 mg 753
TINACTIN®* OTC
tolnaftate, USP
Cream 1%
Jock Itch Cream
Jock Itch Spray Powder
Liquid 1% Aerosol
Powder 1%
Powder 1% Aerosol
Solution 1%
TINDAL® Tablets† BBA/968 ℞
acetophenazine maleate, USP
TRILAFON® ℞
perphenazine, USP
Concentrate
Injection
Repetabs® Tablets ADX/141
Tablets 2 mg ADH/705
4 mg ADK/940
8 mg ADJ/313
16 mg ADM/077
TRINALIN® Long-Acting Antihistamine/Decongestant ℞
Repetabs® Tablets 703
VALISONE® ℞
betamethasone valerate, USP
Cream 0.1%
Lotion 0.1%
Ointment 0.1%
Reduced Strength Cream 0.01%
VANCENASE® Nasal Inhaler ℞
beclomethasone dipropionate, USP
VANCERIL® Oral Inhaler ℞
beclomethasone dipropionate, USP

* For complete prescribing information see PDR for Nonprescription Drugs.
† For complete prescribing information contact the Schering Professional Services Department.

CELESTONE® ℞
[se-les'tōn]
brand of betamethasone
Tablets, USP
Syrup, USP

DESCRIPTION

Glucocorticoids are adrenocortical steroids, both naturally occurring and synthetic, that are readily absorbed from the gastrointestinal tract. A derivative of prednisolone, CELESTONE has a 16β-methyl group that enhances the anti-inflammatory action of the molecule and reduces the sodium- and water-retaining properties of the fluorine atom bound at carbon 9.
The formula for betamethasone is $C_{22}H_{29}FO_5$ and has a molecular weight of 392.47. Chemically, it is 9-fluoro-11β, 17,21-trihydroxy-16β-methylpregna-1,4-diene-3,20-dione.
Betamethasone is a white to practically white, odorless, crystalline powder. It melts at about 240°C with some decomposition. Betamethasone is sparingly soluble in acetone, alcohol, dioxane, and methanol; very slightly soluble in chloroform and ether; and is insoluble in water.
Each CELESTONE **Tablet** contains 0.6 mg betamethasone, USP. The inactive ingredients for Celestone Tablets include: corn starch, FD&C Red No. 40, lactose and magnesium stearate.
CELESTONE **Syrup** contains 0.6 mg betamethasone, USP in each 5 ml. The inactive ingredients for Celestone Syrup include: alcohol (less than 1%), citric acid, FD&C Red No. 40, FD&C Yellow No. 6, flavors, propylene glycol, sodium benzoate, sodium chloride, sorbitol, sugar and water.

ACTIONS

Naturally occurring glucocorticoids (hydrocortisone and cortisone), which also have salt-retaining properties, are used as replacement therapy in adrenocortical deficiency states. Their synthetic analogs, such as betamethasone, are primarily used for their potent anti-inflammatory effects in disorders of many organ systems.
Glucocorticoids, such as betamethasone, cause profound and varied metabolic effects. In addition, they modify the body's immune response to diverse stimuli.

INDICATIONS

Endocrine disorders: primary or secondary adrenocortical insufficiency (hydrocortisone or cortisone is the first choice; synthetic analogs may be used in conjunction with mineralocorticoids where applicable; in infancy mineralocorticoid supplementation is of particular importance).
congenital adrenal hyperplasia
nonsuppurative thyroiditis
hypercalcemia associated with cancer
Rheumatic disorders: as adjunctive therapy for short-term administration (to tide the patient over an acute episode or exacerbation) in:
psoriatic arthritis
rheumatoid arthritis, including juvenile rheumatoid arthritis (selected cases may require low-dose maintenance therapy)
ankylosing spondylitis
acute and subacute bursitis
acute nonspecific tenosynovitis
acute gouty arthritis
post-traumatic osteoarthritis
synovitis of osteoarthritis
epicondylitis
Collagen diseases: during an exacerbation or as maintenance therapy in selected cases of:
systemic lupus erythematosus
acute rheumatic carditis
Dermatologic diseases:
pemphigus
bullous dermatitis herpetiformis
severe erythema multiforme (Stevens-Johnson syndrome)
exfoliative dermatitis
mycosis fungoides
severe psoriasis
severe seborrheic dermatitis
Allergic states: control of severe or incapacitating allergic conditions intractable to adequate trials of conventional treatment:
seasonal or perennial allergic rhinitis
serum sickness
bronchial asthma
contact dermatitis
atopic dermatitis
drug hypersensitivity reactions
Ophthalmic diseases: severe acute and chronic allergic and inflammatory processes involving the eye and its adnexa, such as:
allergic conjunctivitis
keratitis
allergic corneal marginal ulcers
herpes zoster ophthalmicus
iritis and iridocyclitis
chorioretinitis

anterior segment inflammation
diffuse posterior uveitis and choroiditis
optic neuritis
sympathetic ophthalmia
Respiratory diseases:
symptomatic sarcoidosis
Löffler's syndrome not manageable by other means
berylliosis
fulminating or disseminated pulmonary tuberculosis when used concurrently with appropriate antituberculous chemotherapy
aspiration pneumonitis
Hematologic disorders:
idiopathic thrombocytopenic purpura in adults
secondary thrombocytopenia in adults
acquired (autoimmune) hemolytic anemia
erythroblastopenia (RBC anemia)
congenital (erythroid) hypoplastic anemia
Neoplastic diseases: for palliative management of:
leukemias and lymphomas in adults
acute leukemia of childhood
Edematous states: to induce a diuresis or remission of proteinuria in the nephrotic syndrome, without uremia, of the idiopathic type or that due to lupus erythematosus.
Gastrointestinal diseases: to tide the patient over a critical period of the disease in:
ulcerative colitis
regional enteritis
Miscellaneous: tuberculous meningitis with subarachnoid block or impending block when used concurrently with appropriate antituberculous chemotherapy; trichinosis with neurologic or myocardial involvement.

CONTRAINDICATIONS

CELESTONE **Tablets** and **Syrup** are contraindicated in systemic fungal infections.

WARNINGS

In patients on corticosteroid therapy subjected to unusual stress, increased dosage of rapidly acting corticosteroids before, during, and after the stressful situation is indicated.
Corticosteroids may mask some signs of infection, and new infections may appear during their use. There may be decreased resistance and inability to localize infection when corticosteroids are used.
Prolonged use of corticosteroids may produce posterior subcapsular cataracts, glaucoma with possible damage to the optic nerves, and may enhance the establishment of secondary ocular infections due to fungi or viruses.
Average and large doses of hydrocortisone or cortisone can cause elevation of blood pressure, salt and water retention, and increased excretion of potassium. These effects are less likely to occur with the synthetic derivatives except when used in large doses. Dietary salt restrictions and potassium supplementation may be necessary. All corticosteroids increase calcium excretion.
While on corticosteroid therapy, patients should not be vaccinated against smallpox. Other immunization procedures should not be undertaken in patients who are on corticosteroids, especially on high doses, because of possible hazards of neurological complications and a lack of antibody response.
The use of CELESTONE **Syrup** and **Tablets** in active tuberculosis should be restricted to those cases of fulminating or disseminated tuberculosis in which the corticosteroid is used for the management of the disease in conjunction with an appropriate antituberculous regimen.
If corticosteroids are indicated in patients with latent tuberculosis or tuberculin reactivity, close observation is necessary as reactivation of the disease may occur. During prolonged corticosteroid therapy, these patients should receive chemoprophylaxis.
Usage in pregnancy: Since adequate human reproduction studies have not been done with corticosteroids, the use of these drugs in pregnancy, nursing mothers or women of childbearing potential requires that the possible benefits of the drug be weighed against the potential hazards to the mother and embryo or fetus. Infants born of mothers who have received substantial doses of corticosteroids during pregnancy should be carefully observed for signs of hypoadrenalism.

PRECAUTIONS

Drug-induced secondary adrenocortical insufficiency may be minimized by gradual reduction of dosage. This type of relative insufficiency may persist for months after discontinuation of therapy; therefore, in any situation of stress occurring during that period, hormone therapy should be reinstituted. Since mineralocorticoid secretion may be impaired, salt and /or a mineralocorticoid should be administered concurrently.
There is an enhanced effect of corticosteroids on patients with hypothyroidism and in those with cirrhosis.
Corticosteroids should be used cautiously in patients with ocular herpes simplex because of possible corneal perforation.
The lowest possible dose of corticosteroid should be used to control the condition under treatment, and when reduction in dosage is possible, the reduction should be gradual.
Psychic derangements may appear when corticosteroids are used, ranging from euphoria, insomnia, mood swings, personality changes, and severe depression to frank psychotic manifestations. Also, existing emotional instability or psychotic tendencies may be aggravated by corticosteroids.
Aspirin should be used cautiously in conjunction with corticosteroids in hypoprothrombinemia.
Steroids should be used with caution in nonspecific ulcerative colitis, if there is a probability of impending perforation, abscess or other pyogenic infection; diverticulitis; fresh intestinal anastomoses; active or latent peptic ulcer; renal insufficiency; hypertension; osteoporosis; and myasthenia gravis.
Growth and development of infants and children on prolonged corticosteroid therapy should be carefully observed.

ADVERSE REACTIONS

Fluid and electrolyte disturbances: sodium retention, fluid retention, congestive heart failure in susceptible patients, potassium loss, hypokalemic alkalosis, hypertension.
Musculoskeletal: muscle weakness, steroid myopathy, loss of muscle mass, osteoporosis, vertebral compression fractures, aseptic necrosis of femoral and humeral heads, pathologic fracture of long bones; tendon rupture.
Gastrointestinal: peptic ulcer with possible perforation and hemorrhage, pancreatitis, abdominal distention, ulcerative esophagitis.
Dermatologic: impaired wound healing, thin fragile skin, petechiae and ecchymoses, facial erythema, increased sweating, may suppress reactions to skin tests.
Neurological: convulsions, increased intracranial pressure with papilledema (pseudotumor cerebri) usually after treatment, vertigo, headache.
Endocrine: menstrual irregularities; development of Cushingoid state; suppression of growth in children; secondary adrenocortical and pituitary unresponsiveness, particularly in times of stress, as in trauma, surgery or illness; decreased carbohydrate tolerance; manifestations of latent diabetes mellitus; increased requirements of insulin or oral hypoglycemic agents in diabetics.
Ophthalmic: posterior subcapsular cataracts, increased intraocular pressure, glaucoma, exophthalmos.
Metabolic: negative nitrogen balance due to protein catabolism.

DOSAGE AND ADMINISTRATION

The initial dosage of CELESTONE may vary from 0.6 mg to 7.2 mg per day depending on the specific disease entity being treated. In situations of less severity lower doses will generally suffice, while in selected patients higher initial doses may be required. The initial dosage should be maintained or adjusted until a satisfactory response is noted. If after a reasonable period of time there is a lack of satisfactory clinical response, betamethasone should be discontinued and the patient transferred to other appropriate therapy. IT SHOULD BE EMPHASIZED THAT DOSAGE REQUIREMENTS ARE VARIABLE AND MUST BE INDIVIDUALIZED ON THE BASIS OF THE DISEASE UNDER TREATMENT AND THE RESPONSE OF THE PATIENT. After a favorable response is noted, the proper maintenance dosage should be determined by decreasing the initial drug dosage in small decrements at appropriate time intervals until the lowest dosage which will maintain an adequate clinical response is reached. It should be kept in mind that constant monitoring is needed in regard to drug dosage. Included in the situations which may make dosage adjustments necessary are changes in clinical status secondary to remissions or exacerbations in the disease process, the patient's individual drug responsiveness, and the effect of patient exposure to stressful situations not directly related to the disease entity under treatment; in this latter situation it may be necessary to increase the dosage of betamethasone for a period of time consistent with the patient's condition. If after long-term therapy the drug is to be stopped, it is recommended that it be withdrawn gradually rather than abruptly.

HOW SUPPLIED

CELESTONE **Tablets,** 0.6 mg pink, compressed, scored tablets impressed with the Schering trademark and product identification letters, BDA, or numbers, 011; bottles of 100 (NDC 0085-0011-05) and 500 (NDC 0085-0011-07). Also available, CELESTONE Tablet Pack (For Six Day Therapy), 0.6 mg, 21 tablets (NDC 0085-0011-01) and CELESTONE **Syrup,** 0.6 mg per 5 ml, orange-red colored liquid; 4 oz. bottle (118 ml) (NDC 0085-0942-05).
Store **Tablets** between 2° and 30°C (36° and 86°F). Additionally, protect the **21 Tablet Pack** from excessive moisture. Protect **Syrup** from light.
Store **Syrup** between 2° and 30° C (36° and 86° F).

Revised 3/86
Shown in Product Identification Section, page 427

CELESTONE® Phosphate ℞

[*se-les'tōn*]
brand of betamethasone sodium phosphate, USP
Injection

DESCRIPTION

CELESTONE Phosphate Injection is a sterile, aqueous solution containing in each ml: 4.0 mg betamethasone sodium phosphate, USP equivalent to 3.0 mg betamethasone alcohol; 10 mg dibasic sodium phosphate; 0.1 mg edetate disodium; 3.2 mg sodium bisulfite; and 5.0 mg phenol as preservative. The pH is adjusted to approximately 8.5 with sodium hydroxide.
The formula for betamethasone sodium phosphate is $C_{22}H_{28}FNa_2O_8P$ and has a molecular weight of 516.41. Chemically, it is 9-fluoro-11β,17,21- trihydroxy -16β-methylpregna-1,4- diene-3,20-dione 21-(disodium phosphate).
Betamethasone sodium phosphate is a white to practically white, odorless powder, and is hygroscopic. Betamethasone sodium phosphate is freely soluble in water and methanol and is practically insoluble in acetone and chloroform.

ACTIONS

Naturally occurring glucocorticoids (hydrocortisone), which also have salt-retaining properties, are used as replacement therapy in adrenocortical deficiency states. Their synthetic analogs are primarily used for their potent anti-inflammatory effects in disorders of many organ systems.
Glucocorticoids cause profound and varied metabolic effects. In addition, they modify the body's immune responses to diverse stimuli.

INDICATIONS

When oral therapy is not feasible and the strength, dosage form, and route of administration of the drug reasonably lend the preparation to the treatment of the condition, the **intravenous or intramuscular use** of CELESTONE Phosphate Injection is indicated as follows:
Endocrine disorders:
Primary or secondary adrenocortical insufficiency (hydrocortisone or cortisone is the drug of choice; synthetic analogs may be used in conjunction with mineralocorticoids where applicable; in infancy, mineralocorticoid supplementation is of particular importance).
Acute adrenocortical insufficiency (hydrocortisone or cortisone is the drug of choice; mineralocorticoid supplementation may be necessary, particularly when synthetic analogs are used).
Preoperatively and in the event of serious trauma or illness, in patients with known adrenal insufficiency or when adrenocortical reserve is doubtful.
Shock unresponsive to conventional therapy if adrenocortical insufficiency exists or is suspected.
Congenital adrenal hyperplasia.
Nonsuppurative thyroiditis.
Hypercalcemia associated with cancer.
Rheumatic disorders: As adjunctive therapy for short-term administration (to tide the patient over an acute episode or exacerbation) in:
Post-traumatic osteoarthritis.
Synovitis of osteoarthritis.
Rheumatoid arthritis, including juvenile rheumatoid arthritis (selected cases may require low-dose maintenance therapy).
Acute and subacute bursitis.
Epicondylitis.
Acute nonspecific tenosynovitis.
Acute gouty arthritis.
Psoriatic arthritis.
Ankylosing spondylitis.
Collagen diseases: During an exacerbation or as maintenance therapy in selected cases of:
Systemic lupus erythematosus.
Acute rheumatic carditis.
Dermatologic diseases:
Pemphigus.
Severe erythema multiforme (Stevens-Johnson syndrome).
Exfoliative dermatitis.
Bullous dermatitis herpetiformis.
Severe seborrheic dermatitis.
Severe psoriasis.
Mycosis fungoides.
Allergic states. Control of severe or incapacitating allergic conditions intractable to adequate trials of conventional treatment in:
Bronchial asthma.
Contact dermatitis.
Atopic dermatitis.
Serum sickness.

Continued on next page

Information on Schering products appearing on these pages is effective as of September 30, 1986.

Schering—Cont.

Seasonal or perennial allergic rhinitis.
Drug hypersensitivity reactions.
Urticarial transfusion reactions.
Acute noninfectious laryngeal edema (epinephrine is the drug of first choice).
Ophthalmic diseases: Severe, acute and chronic allergic and inflammatory processes involving the eye, such as:
Herpes zoster ophthalmicus.
Iritis, iridocyclitis.
Chorioretinitis.
Diffuse posterior uveitis and choroiditis.
Optic neuritis.
Sympathetic ophthalmia.
Anterior segment inflammation.
Allergic conjunctivitis.
Allergic corneal marginal ulcers.
Keratitis.
Gastrointestinal diseases: To tide the patient over a critical period of disease in:
Ulcerative colitis—(systemic therapy).
Regional enteritis—(systemic therapy).
Respiratory diseases:
Symptomatic sarcoidosis.
Berylliosis.
Fulminating or disseminated pulmonary tuberculosis when used concurrently with appropriate antituberculous chemotherapy.
Loffler's syndrome not manageable by other means.
Aspiration pneumonitis.
Hematologic disorders:
Acquired (autoimmune) hemolytic anemia.
Idiopathic thrombocytopenic purpura in adults (I.V. only; I.M. administration is contraindicated).
Secondary thrombocytopenia in adults.
Erythroblastopenia (RBC anemia).
Congenital (erythroid) hypoplastic anemia.
Neoplastic diseases: For palliative management of:
Leukemias and lymphomas in adults.
Acute leukemia of childhood.
Edematous states. To induce diuresis or remission of proteinuria in the nephrotic syndrome, without uremia, of the idiopathic type or that due to lupus erythematosus.
Miscellaneous:
Tuberculous meningitis with subarachnoid block or impending block when used concurrently with appropriate antituberculous chemotherapy.
Trichinosis with neurologic or myocardial involvement.
When the strength and dosage form of the drug lend the preparation to the treatment of the condition, the **intra-articular or soft tissue administration** of CELESTONE Phosphate Injection is indicated as adjunctive therapy for short-term administration (to tide the patient over an acute episode or exacerbation) in:
Synovitis of osteoarthritis.
Rheumatoid arthritis.
Acute and subacute bursitis.
Acute gouty arthritis.
Epicondylitis.
Acute nonspecific tenosynovitis.
Post-traumatic osteoarthritis.
When the strength and dosage form of the drug lend the preparation to the treatment of the condition, the **intralesional administration** of CELESTONE Phosphate Injection is indicated for:
Keloids.
Localized hypertrophic, infiltrated, inflammatory lesions of: lichen planus, psoriatic plaques, granuloma annulare, and lichen simplex chronicus (neurodermatitis).
Discoid lupus erythematosus.
Necrobiosis lipoidica diabeticorum.
Alopecia areata.
CELESTONE Phosphate injection may also be useful in cystic tumors of an aponeurosis or tendon (ganglia).

CONTRAINDICATIONS

CELESTONE Phosphate Injection is contraindicated in systemic fungal infections.

WARNINGS

In patients on corticosteroid therapy subjected to any unusual stress, increased dosage of rapidly acting corticosteroids before, during, and after the stressful situation is indicated.
Corticosteroids may mask some signs of infection, and new infections may appear during their use. There may be decreased resistance and inability to localize infection when corticosteroids are used.
Prolonged use of corticosteroids may produce posterior subcapsular cataracts, glaucoma with possible damage to the optic nerves, and may enhance the establishment of secondary ocular infections due to fungi or viruses.
Average and large doses of cortisone or hydrocortisone can cause elevation of blood pressure, salt and water retention, and increased excretion of potassium. These effects are less likely to occur with the synthetic derivatives except when used in large doses. Dietary salt restriction and potassium supplementation may be necessary. All corticosteroids increase calcium excretion.
While on Corticosteroid Therapy Patients Should Not Be Vaccinated Against Smallpox. Other Immunization Procedures Should Not Be Undertaken in Patients Who are on Corticosteroids, Especially in High Doses, Because of Possible Hazards of Neurological Complications and Lack of Antibody Response.
The use of CELESTONE Phosphate Injection in active tuberculosis should be restricted to those cases of fulminating or disseminated tuberculosis in which the corticosteroid is used for the management of the disease in conjunction with appropriate antituberculous regimen.
If corticosteroids are indicated in patients with latent tuberculosis or tuberculin reactivity, close observation is necessary as reactivation of the disease may occur. During prolonged corticosteroid therapy, these patients should receive chemoprophylaxis.
Because rare instances of anaphylactoid reactions have occurred in patients receiving parenteral corticosteroid therapy, appropriate precautionary measures should be taken prior to administration, especially when the patient has a history of allergy to any drug.
Usage in pregnancy: Since adequate human reproduction studies have not been done with corticosteroids, the use of these drugs in pregnancy, nursing mothers, or women of childbearing potential requires that the possible benefits of the drug be weighed against the potential hazards to the mother and embryo or fetus. Infants born to mothers who have received substantial doses of corticosteroids during pregnancy should be carefully observed for signs of hypoadrenalism.

PRECAUTIONS

Drug-induced secondary adrenocortical insufficiency may be minimized by gradual reduction of dosage. This type of relative insufficiency may persist for months after discontinuation of therapy; therefore, in any situation of stress occurring during that period, hormone therapy should be reinstituted. Since mineralocorticoid secretion may be impaired, salt and /or a mineralocorticoid should be administered concurrently.
There is an enhanced effect of corticosteroids in patients with hypothyroidism and in those with cirrhosis.
Corticosteroids should be used cautiously in patients with ocular herpes simplex for fear of corneal perforation.
The lowest possible dose of corticosteroid should be used to control the condition under treatment, and when reduction in dosage is possible, the reduction must be gradual.
Psychic derangements may appear when corticosteroids are used, ranging from euphoria, insomnia, mood swings, personality changes, and severe depression to frank psychotic manifestations. Also, existing emotional instability or psychotic tendencies may be aggravated by corticosteroids.
Aspirin should be used cautiously in conjunction with corticosteroids in hypoprothrombinemia.
Steroids should be used with caution in nonspecific ulcerative colitis, if there is a probability of impending perforation, abscess or other pyogenic infection, also in diverticulitis, fresh intestinal anastomoses, active or latent peptic ulcer, renal insufficiency, hypertension, osteoporosis, and myasthenia gravis. Growth and development of infants and children on prolonged corticosteroid therapy should be carefully followed.
The following additional precautions also apply for parenteral corticosteroids. Intra-articular injection of a corticosteroid may produce systemic as well as local effects.
Appropriate examination of any joint fluid present is necessary to exclude a septic process.
A marked increase in pain accompanied by local swelling, further restriction of joint motion, fever, and malaise are suggestive of septic arthritis. If this complication occurs and the diagnosis of sepsis is confirmed, appropriate antimicrobial therapy should be instituted.
Local injection of a steroid into a previously infected joint is to be avoided.
Corticosteroids should not be injected into unstable joints.
The slower rate of absorption by intramuscular administration should be recognized.

ADVERSE REACTIONS

Fluid and electrolyte disturbances: sodium retention; fluid retention; congestive heart failure in susceptible patients; potassium loss; hypokalemic alkalosis; hypertension.
Musculoskeletal: muscle weakness; steroid myopathy; loss of muscle mass; osteoporosis; vertebral compression fractures; aseptic necrosis of femoral and humeral heads; pathologic fracture of long bones.
Gastrointestinal: peptic ulcer with possible subsequent perforation and hemorrhage; pancreatitis; abdominal distention; ulcerative esophagitis.
Dermatologic: impaired wound healing; thin fragile skin; petechiae and ecchymoses; facial erythema; increased sweating; may suppress reactions to skin tests.
Neurological: convulsions; increased intracranial pressure with papilledema (pseudotumor cerebri) usually after treatment; vertigo; headache.
Endocrine: menstrual irregularities; development of Cushingoid state; suppression of growth in children; secondary adrenocortical and pituitary unresponsiveness, particularly in times of stress, as in trauma, surgery or illness; decreased carbohydrate tolerance; manifestations of latent diabetes mellitus; increased requirements for insulin or oral hypoglycemic agents in diabetics.
Ophthalmic: posterior subcapsular cataracts; increased intraocular pressure; glaucoma; exophthalmos.
Metabolic: negative nitrogen balance due to protein catabolism.
The following *additional* adverse reactions are also related to parenteral corticosteroid therapy: rare instances of blindness associated with intralesional therapy around the face and head; hyperpigmentation or hypopigmentation; subcutaneous and cutaneous atrophy; sterile abscess; post-injection flare (following intra-articular use); charcot-like arthropathy.

DOSAGE AND ADMINISTRATION

The initial dosage of parenterally administered betamethasone may vary up to 9.0 mg per day depending on the specific disease entity being treated. In situations of less severity, lower doses will generally suffice while in selected patients higher initial doses may be required. Usually the parenteral dosage ranges are one-third to one-half the 12-hourly oral dose. However, in certain overwhelming, acute, life-threatening situations, administration in dosages exceeding the usual dosages may be justified and may be in multiples of the oral dosages.
The initial dosage should be maintained or adjusted until a satisfactory response is noted. If after a reasonable period of time there is a lack of satisfactory clinical response, CELESTONE Phosphate Injection should be discontinued and the patient transferred to other appropriate therapy. *It Should Be Emphasized that Dosage Requirements are Variable and Must Be Individualized on the Basis of the Disease Under Treatment and the Response of the Patient.* After a favorable response is noted, the proper maintenance dosage should be determined by decreasing the initial drug dosage in small decrements at appropriate time intervals until the lowest dosage which will maintain an adequate clinical response is reached. It should be kept in mind that constant monitoring is needed in regard to drug dosage. Included in the situations which may make dosage adjustments necessary are changes in clinical status secondary to remissions or exacerbations in the disease process, the patient's individual drug responsiveness, and the effect of patient exposure to stressful situations not directly related to the disease entity under treatment; in this latter situation it may be necessary to increase dosage of CELESTONE Phosphate Injection for a period of time consistent with the patient's condition. If after long-term therapy the drug is to be stopped, it is recommended that it be withdrawn gradually rather than abruptly.

HOW SUPPLIED

CELESTONE Phosphate Injection, 4.0 mg per ml (equivalent to 3.0 mg per ml betamethasone alcohol), 5 ml multiple-dose vials, box of one (NDC 0085-0879-05).
Protect from freezing.
Protect from light.

Revised 7/83

CELESTONE® SOLUSPAN® • ℞

[*se-les'tōn*]
Suspension
brand of sterile betamethasone sodium phosphate
and betamethasone acetate suspension, USP
6 mg per ml

DESCRIPTION

Each ml of CELESTONE SOLUSPAN• Suspension contains: 3.0 mg betamethasone as betamethasone sodium phosphate; 3.0 mg betamethasone acetate; 7.1 mg dibasic sodium phosphate; 3.4 mg monobasic sodium phosphate; 0.1 mg edetate disodium; and 0.2 mg benzalkonium chloride. It is a sterile, aqueous suspension with a pH between 6.8 and 7.2.
The formula for betamethasone sodium phosphate is $C_{22}H_{28}FNa_2O_8P$ with a molecular weight of 516.41. Chemically it is 9-Fluoro-11β, 17,21-trihydroxy-16β-methylpregna-1,4-diene-3,20-dione 21-(disodium phosphate).
The formula for betamethasone acetate is $C_{24}H_{31}FO_6$ with a molecular weight of 434.50. Chemically it is 9-Fluoro-

11β,17,21-trihydroxy-16β-methylpregna-1, 4-diene-3, 20-dione 21-acetate.

Betamethasone sodium phosphate is a white to practically white, odorless powder, and is hygroscopic. It is freely soluble in water and in methanol, but is practically insoluble in acetone and in chloroform.

Betamethasone acetate is a white to creamy white, odorless powder that sinters and resolidifies at about 165°C, and remelts at about 200°C–220°C with decomposition. It is practically insoluble in water, but freely soluble in acetone, and is soluble in alcohol and in chloroform.

*brand of rapid and repository injectable.

ACTIONS

Naturally occurring glucocorticoids (hydrocortisone), which also have salt-retaining properties, are used as replacement therapy in adrenocortical deficiency states. Their synthetic analogs are primarily used for their potent anti-inflammatory effects in disorders of many organ systems.

Betamethasone sodium phosphate, a soluble ester, provides prompt activity, while betamethasone acetate is only slightly soluble and affords sustained activity.

Glucocorticoids cause profound and varied metabolic effects. In addition, they modify the body's immune responses to diverse stimuli.

INDICATIONS

When oral therapy is not feasible and the strength, dosage form, and route of administration of the drug reasonably lend the preparation to the treatment of the condition, CELESTONE SOLUSPAN Suspension for **intramuscular use** is indicated as follows:

Endocrine disorders: Primary or secondary adrenocortical insufficiency (hydrocortisone or cortisone is the drug of choice; synthetic analogs may be used in conjunction with mineralocorticoids where applicable; in infancy, mineralocorticoid supplementation is of particular importance).

Acute adrenocortical insufficiency (hydrocortisone or cortisone is the drug of choice; mineralocorticoid supplementation may be necessary, particularly when synthetic analogs are used). Preoperatively and in the event of serious trauma or illness, in patients with known adrenal insufficiency or when adrenocortical reserve is doubtful. Shock unresponsive to conventional therapy if adrenocortical insufficiency exists or is suspected. Congenital adrenal hyperplasia. Nonsuppurative thyroiditis. Hypercalcemia associated with cancer.

Rheumatic disorders: As adjunctive therapy for short-term administration (to tide the patient over an acute episode or exacerbation) in: post-traumatic osteoarthritis; synovitis of osteoarthritis; rheumatoid arthritis; acute and subacute bursitis; epicondylitis; acute nonspecific tenosynovitis; acute gouty arthritis; psoriatic arthritis; ankylosing spondylitis; juvenile rheumatoid arthritis (selected cases may require low-dose maintenance therapy).

Collagen disease: During an exacerbation or as maintenance therapy in selected cases of: systemic lupus erythematosus; acute rheumatic carditis.

Dermatologic diseases: Pemphigus: severe erythema multiforme (Stevens-Johnson syndrome); exfoliative dermatitis; bullous dermatitis herpetiformis; severe seborrheic dermatitis; severe psoriasis; mycosis fungoides.

Allergic states: Control of severe or incapacitating allergic conditions intractable to adequate trials of conventional treatment in: bronchial asthma; contact dermatitis; atopic dermatitis; serum sickness; seasonal or perennial allergic rhinitis; drug hypersensitivity reactions; urticarial transfusion reactions; acute noninfectious laryngeal edema (epinephrine is the drug of first choice).

Ophthalmic diseases: Severe, acute and chronic allergic and inflammatory processes involving the eye, such as: herpes zoster ophthalmicus; iritis, iridocyclitis; chorioretinitis; diffuse posterior uveitis and choroiditis; optic neuritis; sympathetic ophthalmia; anterior segment inflammation; allergic conjunctivitis; allergic corneal marginal ulcer; keratitis.

Gastrointestinal diseases: To tide the patient over a critical period of disease in: ulcerative colitis—(systemic therapy); regional enteritis—(systemic therapy).

Respiratory diseases: Symptomatic sarcoidosis; berylliosis; fulminating or disseminated pulmonary tuberculosis, when concurrently with appropriate antituberculous chemotherapy; aspiration pneumonitis; Loffler's syndrome not manageable by other means.

Hematologic disorders: Acquired (autoimmune) hemolytic anemia. Secondary thrombocytopenia in adults. Erythroblastopenia (RBC anemia). Congenital (erythroid) hypoplastic anemia.

Neoplastic diseases: For palliative management of:- leukemias and lymphomas in adults; acute leukemia of childhood.

Edematous state: To induce diuresis or remission of proteinuria in the nephrotic syndrome, without uremia, of the idiopathic type or that due to lupus erythematosus.

Miscellaneous: Tuberculous meningitis with subarachnoid block or impending block when used concurrently with appropriate antituberculous chemotherapy. Trichinosis with neurologic or myocardial involvement.

When the strength and dosage form of the drug lend the preparation to the treatment of the condition, the **intra-articular or soft tissue administration** of CELESTONE SOLUSPAN Suspension is indicated as adjunctive therapy for short-term administration (to tide the patient over an acute episode or exacerbation) in: synovitis of osteoarthritis; rheumatoid arthritis; acute and subacute bursitis; acute gouty arthritis; epicondylitis; acute nonspecific tenosynovitis; post-traumatic osteoarthritis.

When the strength and dosage form of the drug lend the preparation to the treatment of the condition, the **intralesional administration** of CELESTONE SOLUSPAN Suspension is indicated for: keloids; localized hypertrophic, infiltrated, inflammatory lesions of lichen planus, psoriatic plaques, granuloma annulare, and lichen simplex chronicus (neurodermatitis); discoid lupus erythematosus; necrobiosis lipoidica diabeticorum; alopecia areata.

CELESTONE SOLUSPAN Suspension may also be useful in cystic tumors of an aponeurosis or tendon (ganglia).

CONTRAINDICATIONS

CELESTONE SOLUSPAN Suspension is contraindicated in systemic fungal infections.

WARNINGS

CELESTONE SOLUSPAN should not be administered intravenously.

In patients on corticosteroid therapy subjected to any unusual stress, increased dosage of rapidly acting corticosteroids before, during, and after the stressful situation is indicated.

Corticosteroids may mask some signs of infection, and new infections may appear during their use. There may be decreased resistance and inability to localize infection when corticosteroids are used.

Prolonged use of corticosteroids may produce posterior subcapsular cataracts, glaucoma with possible damage to the optic nerves, and may enhance the establishment of secondary ocular infections due to fungi or viruses.

CELESTONE SOLUSPAN contains two betamethasone esters one of which, betamethasone sodium phosphate, disappears rapidly from the injection site. The potential for systemic effect produced by the soluble portion of CELESTONE SOLUSPAN should therefore be taken into account by the physician when using the drug.

Average and large doses of cortisone or hydrocortisone can cause elevation of blood pressure, salt and water retention, and increased excretion of potassium. These effects are less likely to occur with the synthetic derivatives except when used in large doses. Dietary salt restriction and potassium supplementation may be necessary. All corticosteroids increase calcium excretion.

While on Corticosteroid Therapy Patients Should Not Be Vaccinated Against Smallpox. Other Immunization Procedures Should Not Be Undertaken in Patients Who Are on Corticosteroids, Especially in High Doses, Because of Possible Hazards of Neurological Complications and Lack of Antibody Response.

The use of CELESTONE SOLUSPAN Suspension in active tuberculosis should be restricted to those cases of fulminating or disseminated tuberculosis in which the corticosteroid is used for the management of the disease in conjunction with appropriate antituberculous regimen.

If corticosteroids are indicated in patients with latent tuberculosis or tuberculin reactivity, close observation is necessary as reactivation of the disease may occur. During prolonged corticosteroid therapy, these patients should receive chemoprophylaxis.

Because rare instances of anaphylactoid reactions have occurred in patients receiving parenteral corticosteroid therapy, appropriate precautionary measures should be taken prior to administration, especially when the patient has a history of allergy to any drug.

Usage in pregnancy: Since adequate human reproduction studies have not been done with corticosteroids, the use of these drugs in pregnancy, nursing mothers, or women of childbearing potential requires that the possible benefits of the drug be weighed against the potential hazards to the mother and embryo or fetus. Infants born of mothers who have received substantial doses of corticosteroids during pregnancy should be carefully observed for signs of hypoadrenalism.

PRECAUTIONS

Drug-induced secondary adrenocortical insufficiency may be minimized by gradual reduction of dosage. This type of relative insufficiency may persist for months after discontinuation of therapy; therefore, in any situation of stress occurring during that period, hormone therapy should be reinstituted. Since mineralocorticoid secretion may be impaired, salt and /or a mineralocorticoid should be administered concurrently.

There is an enhanced effect of corticosteroids in patients with hypothyroidism and in those with cirrhosis.

Corticosteroids should be used cautiously in patients with ocular herpes simplex for fear of corneal perforation.

The lowest possible dose of corticosteroid should be used to control the condition under treatment, and when reduction in dosage is possible, the reduction must be gradual.

Psychic derangements may appear when corticosteroids are used, ranging from euphoria, insomnia, mood swings, personality changes, and severe depression to frank psychotic manifestations. Also, existing emotional instability or psychotic tendencies may be aggravated by corticosteroids.

Aspirin should be used cautiously in conjunction with corticosteroids in hypoprothrombinemia.

Steroids should be used with caution in nonspecific ulcerative colitis, if there is a probability of impending perforation, abscess or other pyogenic infection, also in diverticulitis, fresh intestinal anastomoses, active or latent peptic ulcer, renal insufficiency, hypertension, osteoporosis, and myasthenia gravis.

Growth and development of infants and children on prolonged corticosteroid therapy should be carefully followed.

The following additional precautions also apply for parenteral corticosteroids. **Intra-articular injection of a corticosteroid may produce systemic as well as local effects.**

Appropriate examination of any joint fluid present is necessary to exclude a septic process.

A marked increase in pain accompanied by local swelling, further restriction of joint motion, fever, and malaise are suggestive of septic arthritis. If this complication occurs and the diagnosis of sepsis is confirmed, appropriate antimicrobial therapy should be instituted.

Local injection of a steroid into a previously infected joint is to be avoided.

Corticosteroids should not be injected into unstable joints.

The slower rate of absorption by intramuscular administration should be recognized.

ADVERSE REACTIONS

Fluid and electrolyte disturbances: sodium retention; fluid retention; congestive heart failure in susceptible patients; potassium loss; hypokalemic alkalosis; hypertension.

Musculoskeletal: muscle weakness; steroid myopathy; loss of muscle mass; osteoporosis; vertebral compression fractures; aseptic necrosis of femoral and humeral heads; pathologic fracture of long bones.

Gastrointestinal: peptic ulcer with possible subsequent perforation and hemorrhage; pancreatitis; abdominal distention; ulcerative esophagitis.

Dermatologic: impaired wound healing; thin fragile skin; petechiae and ecchymoses; facial erythema; increased sweating; may suppress reactions to skin tests.

Neurological: convulsions; increased intracranial pressure with papilledema (pseudotumor cerebri) usually after treatment; vertigo; headache.

Endocrine: menstrual irregularities; development of Cushingoid state; suppression of growth in children; secondary adrenocortical and pituitary unresponsiveness, particularly in times of stress, as in trauma, surgery, or illness; decreased carbohydrate tolerance; manifestations of latent diabetes mellitus; increased requirements for insulin or oral hypoglycemic agents in diabetics.

Ophthalmic: posterior subcapsular cataracts; increased intraocular pressure; glaucoma; exophthalmos.

Metabolic: negative nitrogen balance due to protein catabolism.

The following *additional* adverse reactions are related to parenteral corticosteroid therapy: rare instances of blindness associated with intralesional therapy around the face and head; hyperpigmentation or hypopigmentation; subcutaneous and cutaneous atrophy; sterile abscess; post-injection flare (following intra-articular use); charcot-like arthropathy.

DOSAGE AND ADMINISTRATION

The initial dosage of CELESTONE SOLUSPAN Suspension may vary from 0.5 to 9.0 mg per day depending on the specific disease entity being treated. In situations of less severity, lower doses will generally suffice while in selected patients higher initial doses may be required. Usually the parenteral dosage ranges are one-third to one-half the oral dose given every 12 hours. However, in certain overwhelming, acute, life-threatening situations, administration in dosages exceeding the usual dosages may be justified and may be in multiples of the oral dosages.

The initial dosage should be maintained or adjusted until a satisfactory response is noted. If after a reasonable period of time there is a lack of satisfactory clinical response, CELESTONE SOLUSPAN Suspension should be discontinued and the patient transferred to other appropriate therapy. *It Should Be Emphasized That Dosage Requirements Are Variable and Must Be Individualized on the Basis of the Disease Under Treatment and the Response of the Patient.* After a favorable response is noted, the proper maintenance dosage

Continued on next page

Information on Schering products appearing on these pages is effective as of September 30, 1986.

Schering—Cont.

should be determined by decreasing the initial drug dosage in small decrements at appropriate time intervals until the lowest dosage which will maintain an adequate clinical response is reached. It should be kept in mind that constant monitoring is needed in regard to drug dosage. Included in the situations which may make dosage adjustments necessary are changes in clinical status secondary to remissions or exacerbations in the disease process, the patient's individual drug responsiveness, and the effect of patient exposure to stressful situations not directly related to the disease entity under treatment; in this latter situation it may be necessary to increase the dosage of CELESTONE SOLUSPAN Suspension for a period of time consistent with the patient's condition. If after long-term therapy the drug is to be stopped, it is recommended that it be withdrawn gradually rather than abruptly.

If coadministration of a local anesthetic is desired, CELESTONE SOLUSPAN Suspension may be mixed with 1% or 2% lidocaine hydrochloride, using the formulations which do not contain parabens. Similar local anesthetics may also be used. Diluents containing methylparaben, propylparaben, phenol, etc., should be avoided since these compounds may cause flocculation of the steroid. The required dose of CELESTONE SOLUSPAN Suspension is first withdrawn from the vial into the syringe. The local anesthetic is then drawn in, and the syringe shaken briefly. **Do not inject local anesthetics into the vial of CELESTONE SOLUSPAN Suspension.**

Bursitis, tenosynovitis, peritendinitis. In acute subdeltoid, subacromial, olecranon, and prepatellar bursitis, one intrabursal injection of 1.0 ml CELESTONE SOLUSPAN Suspension can relieve pain and restore full range of movement. Several intrabursal injections of corticosteroids are usually required in recurrent acute bursitis and in acute exacerbations of chronic bursitis. Partial relief of pain and some increase in mobility can be expected in both conditions after one or two injections. Chronic bursitis may be treated with reduced dosage once the acute condition is controlled. In tenosynovitis and tendinitis, three or four local injections at intervals of one to two weeks between injections are given in most cases. Injections should be made into the affected tendon sheaths rather than into the tendons themselves. In ganglions of joint capsules and tendon sheaths, injection of 0.5 ml directly into the ganglion cysts has produced marked reduction in the size of the lesions. *Rheumatoid arthritis and osteoarthritis.* Following intra-articular administration of 0.5 to 2.0 ml of CELESTONE SOLUSPAN Suspension, relief of pain, soreness, and stiffness may be experienced. Duration of relief varies widely in both diseases. Intra-articular Injection—CELESTONE SOLUSPAN Suspension is well tolerated in joints and periarticular tissues. There is virtually no pain on injection, and the "secondary flare" that sometimes occurs a few hours after intra-articular injection of corticosteroids has not been reported with CELESTONE SOLUSPAN Suspension. Using sterile technique, a 20- to 24-gauge needle on an empty syringe is inserted into the synovial cavity, and a few drops of synovial fluid are withdrawn to confirm that the needle is in the joint. The aspirating syringe is replaced by a syringe containing CELESTONE SOLUSPAN Suspension and injection is then made into the joint.

Recommended Doses for Intra-articular Injection

Size of joint	Location	Dose (ml)
Very Large	Hip	1.0-2.0
Large	Knee, Ankle, Shoulder	1.0
Medium	Elbow, Wrist	0.5-1.0
Small (Metacarpophalangeal, interphalangeal) (Sternoclavicular)	Hand Chest	0.25-0.5

A portion of the administered dose of CELESTONE SOLUSPAN Suspension is absorbed systemically following intra-articular injection. In patients being treated concomitantly with oral or parenteral corticosteroids, especially those receiving large doses, the systemic absorption of the drug should be considered in determining intra-articular dosage. *Dermatologic conditions.* In intralesional treatment, 0.2 ml/sq. cm. of CELESTONE SOLUSPAN Suspension is injected intradermally (not subcutaneously) using a tuberculin syringe with a 25-gauge, ½-inch needle. Care should be taken to deposit a uniform depot of medication intradermally. A total of no more than 1.0 ml. at weekly intervals is recommended. *Disorders of the foot.* A tuberculin syringe with a 25-gauge, ¾-inch needle is suitable for most injections into the foot. The following doses are recommended at intervals of three days to a week.

Diagnosis	CELESTONE SOLUSPAN Suspension Dose (ml)
Bursitis	
under heloma durum or heloma molle	0.25-0.5
under calcaneal spur	0.5
over hallux rigidus or digiti quinti varus	0.5
Tenosynovitis, periostitis of cuboid	0.5
Acute gouty arthritis	0.5-1.0

HOW SUPPLIED

CELESTONE SOLUSPAN Suspension, 5 ml multiple-dose vial, box of one (NDC-0085-0566-05). **Shake well before using. Store between 2° and 25°C (36° and 77°F). Protect from light.**

Revised 7/83

DIPROLENE® ℞

[*dī'pro-lēn*]

brand of betamethasone dipropionate

Cream, USP 0.05%

(potency expressed as betamethasone)

For Dermatologic Use Only—

Not For Ophthalmic Use

DESCRIPTION

DIPROLENE® Cream contains betamethasone dipropionate, USP, a synthetic adrenocorticosteroid, for dermatologic use. Betamethasone, an analog of prednisolone, has a high degree of corticosteroid activity and a slight degree of mineralocorticoid activity. Betamethasone dipropionate is the 17, 21-dipropionate ester of betamethasone.

Chemically, betamethasone dipropionate is 9-fluoro-11β, 17, 21-trihydroxy-16β-methylpregna-1,4-diene-3, 20-dione 17,21-dipropionate, with the empirical formula $C_{28}H_{37}FO_7$, and a molecular weight of 504.6.

Betamethasone dipropionate is a white to creamy white, odorless crystalline powder, insoluble in water.

Each gram of DIPROLENE Cream 0.05% contains: 0.64 mg betamethasone dipropionate, USP (equivalent to 0.5 mg betamethasone), in an improved cream base of purified water, propylene glycol, carbomer 940, sodium hydroxide and titanium dioxide.

CLINICAL PHARMACOLOGY

The corticosteroids are a class of compounds comprising steroid hormones secreted by the adrenal cortex and their synthetic analogs. In pharmacologic doses, corticosteroids are used primarily for their anti-inflammatory and/or immunosuppressive effects.

Topical corticosteroids, such as betamethasone dipropionate, are effective in the treatment of corticosteroid-responsive dermatoses primarily because of their anti-inflammatory, anti-pruritic, and vasoconstrictive actions. However, while the physiologic, pharmacologic, and clinical effects of the corticosteroids are well-known, the exact mechanisms of their actions in each disease are uncertain. Betamethasone dipropionate, a corticosteroid, has been shown to have topical (dermatologic) and systemic pharmacologic and metabolic effects characteristics of this class of drugs.

Pharmacokinetics: The extent of percutaneous absorption of topical corticosteroids is determined by many factors including the vehicle, the integrity of the epidermal barrier, and the use of occlusive dressings. (See **Dosage and Administration** section.) Topical corticosteroids can be absorbed from normal intact skin. Inflammation and or other disease processes in the skin may increase percutaneous absorption. Occlusive dressings substantially increase the percutaneous absorption of topical corticosteroids. (See **Dosage and Administration** section.)

Once absorbed through the skin, topical corticosteroids enter pharmacokinetic pathways similar to systemically administered corticosteroids. Corticosteroids are bound to plasma proteins in varying degrees. Corticosteroids are metabolized primarily in the liver and are then excreted by the kidneys. Some of the topical corticosteroids and their metabolites are also excreted into the bile.

At 14 g per day (applied as 7 g twice daily), DIPROLENE Cream depressed the plasma levels of adrenal cortical hormones following application for 8 days to diseased skin in patients with psoriasis. Adrenal output in these patients returned to normal shortly after treatment cessation. At 7 g per day (applied once daily or as 3.5 g twice daily), DIPROLENE Cream was shown to cause inhibition of the hypothalamic-pituitary-adrenal (HPA) axis following application for one, two, or three weeks to diseased skin, in patients with psoriasis or atopic dermatitis. HPA axis inhibition in these patients was transient, and returned to normal during treatment, or shortly after treatment cessation.

INDICATIONS AND USAGE

DIPROLENE Cream is intended for short-term treatment of the inflammatory and pruritic manifestations of moderate to severe corticosteroid-responsive dermatoses.

Treatment beyond two weeks is not recommended, and the total dosage should not exceed 45 g per week because of the potential for the drug to suppress the hypothalamic-pituitary-adrenal (HPA) axis.

This product is not recommended for use in children under 12 years of age.

CONTRAINDICATIONS

DIPROLENE Cream is contraindicated in patients who are hypersensitive to betamethasone dipropionate, to other corticosteroids, or to any ingredient in this preparation.

PRECAUTIONS

General: DIPROLENE Cream is a highly potent topical corticosteroid that has been shown to suppress the HPA axis at doses as low as 7 g per day. Systemic absorption of topical corticosteroids has produced reversible HPA axis suppression, manifestations of Cushing's syndrome, hyperglycemia, and glucosuria in some patients.

Conditions which augment systemic absorption include the application of the more potent corticosteroids, use over large surface areas, prolonged use, and the addition of occlusive dressings. (See **Dosage and Administration** section.)

Therefore, patients receiving a large dose of a potent topical steroid applied to a large surface area should be evaluated periodically for evidence of HPA axis suppression by using the urinary free cortisol and ACTH stimulation tests. If HPA axis suppression is noted, an attempt should be made to withdraw the drug, to reduce the frequency of application, or to substitute a less potent steroid.

Recovery of HPA axis function is generally prompt and complete upon discontinuation of the drug. Infrequently, signs and symptoms of steroid withdrawal may occur, requiring supplemental systemic corticosteroids.

Children may absorb proportionally larger amounts of topical corticosteroids and thus be more susceptible to systemic toxicity. (See **Precautions—Pediatric use.**)

If irritation develops, topical corticosteroids should be discontinued and appropriate therapy instituted.

In the presence of dermatological infections, the use of an appropriate antifungal or antibacterial agent should be instituted. If a favorable response does not occur promptly, the corticosteroid should be discontinued until the infection has been adequately controlled.

Information for Patients: Patients using topical corticosteroids should receive the following information and instructions. This information is intended to aid in the safe and effective use of this medication. It is not a disclosure of all possible adverse or intended effects.

1. This medication is to be used as directed by the physician and should not be used longer than the prescribed time period. It is for external use only. Avoid contact with the eyes.
2. Patients should be advised not to use this medication for any disorder or apply it to any skin areas other than that for which it was prescribed.
3. The treated skin area should not be bandaged or otherwise covered or wrapped as to be occlusive. (See **Dosage and Administration** section.)
4. Patients should report any sign of local adverse reactions.

Laboratory Tests: The following tests may be helpful in evaluating HPA axis suppression.

Urinary free cortisol test
ACTH stimulation test

Carcinogenesis, Mutagenesis, and Impairment of Fertility: Long-term animal studies have not been performed to evaluate the carcinogenic potential or the effect on fertility of topically applied corticosteroids.

Studies to determine mutagenicity with prednisolone and hydrocortisone have revealed negative results.

Pregnancy Category C: Corticosteroids are generally teratogenic in laboratory animals when administered systemically at relatively low dosage levels. The more potent corticosteroids have been shown to be teratogenic after dermal application in laboratory animals. There are no adequate and well-controlled studies of the teratogenic effects of topically applied corticosteroids in pregnant women. Therefore, topical corticosteroids should be used during pregnancy only if the potential benefit justifies the potential risk to the fetus. Drugs of this class should not be used extensively on pregnant patients, in large amounts, or for prolonged periods of time.

Nursing Mothers: It is not known whether topical administration of corticosteroids can result in sufficient systemic absorption to produce detectable quantities in breast milk. Systemically administered corticosteroids are secreted into breast milk in quantities not likely to have a deleterious effect on the infant. Nevertheless, caution should be exercised when topical corticosteroids are prescribed for a nursing woman.

Pediatric Use: Use of DIPROLENE Cream in children under 12 years is not recommended.

Pediatric patients may demonstrate greater susceptibility to topical corticosteroid-induced HPA axis supression and Cushing's syndrome than mature patients because of a larger skin surface area to body weight ratio.

Hypothalamic-pituitary-adrenal (HPA) axis suppression, Cushing's syndrome, and intracranial hypertension have been reported in children receiving topical corticosteroids. Manifestations of adrenal suppression in children include linear growth retardation, delayed weight gain, low plasma cortisol levels, and absence of response to ACTH stimulation. Manifestations of intracranial hypertension include bulging fontanelles, headaches, and bilateral papilledema. Chronic corticosteroid therapy may interfere with the growth and development of children.

ADVERSE REACTIONS

The overall incidence of drug-related adverse reactions in the DIPROLENE Cream clinical studies was 10%. The local adverse reactions that were reported to be possibly or probably related to treatment with DIPROLENE Cream during controlled clinical studies involving 815 patients were as follows: burning/stinging 6%, dry skin 4%, pruritus 2%, irritation 1%, telangiectasia, erythema, cracking/tightening of the skin, follicular rash, and skin atrophy each occurred in less than 1% of patients.

The following local adverse reactions are reported infrequently when topical corticosteroids are used as recommended. These reactions are listed in approximate decreasing order of occurrence: burning, itching, irritation, dryness, folliculitis, hypertrichosis, acneiform eruptions, hypopigmentation, perioral dermatitis, allergic contact dermatitis, maceration of the skin, secondary infection, skin atrophy, striae, miliaria.

Systemic absorption of topical corticosteroids has produced reversible HPA axis suppression, manifestations of Cushing's syndrome, hyperglycemia, and glucosuria in some patients.

OVERDOSAGE

Topically applied corticosteroids can be absorbed in sufficient amounts to produce systemic effects. (See **Precautions.**)

DOSAGE AND ADMINISTRATION

Apply a thin film of DIPROLENE Cream to the affected skin areas once or twice daily. DIPROLENE Cream is potent; therefore, treatment must be limited to 14 days, and amounts greater than 45 g per week should not be used.

DIPROLENE Cream is not to be used with occlusive dressings.

HOW SUPPLIED

DIPROLENE Cream 0.05% is supplied in 15- (NDC 0085-0728-01), and 45-gram (NDC 0085-0728-02) tubes, boxes of one.

Store between 2° and 30°C (36° and 86°F).

1/86

DIPROLENE® ℞

[*dī 'pro-lēn*]

brand of betamethasone dipropionate Ointment, USP 0.05% (potency expressed as betamethasone)

For Dermatologic Use Only–Not for Ophthalmic Use

DESCRIPTION

DIPROLENE Ointment contains betamethasone dipropionate, USP, a synthetic adrenocorticosteroid, for dermatologic use. Betamethasone, an analog of prednisolone, has a high degree of corticosteroid activity and a slight degree of mineralocorticoid activity. Betamethasone dipropionate is the 17,21-dipropionate ester of betamethasone.

Chemically, betamethasone dipropionate is 9- fluoro-11β, 17, 21-trihydroxy-16β-methylpregna-1,4- diene -3,20- dione 17, 21- dipropionate, with the empirical formula $C_{28}H_{37}FO_7$, and a molecular weight of 504.6.

Betamethasone dipropionate is a white to creamy white, odorless crystalline powder, insoluble in water.

Each gram of DIPROLENE Ointment 0.05% contains: 0.64 mg betamethasone dipropionate, USP (equivalent to 0.5 mg betamethasone), in ACTIBASE™, an optimized vehicle of propylene glycol, propylene glycol stearate, white wax and white petrolatum.

CLINICAL PHARMACOLOGY

The corticosteroids are a class of compounds comprising steroid hormones secreted by the adrenal cortex and their synthetic analogs. In pharmacologic doses, corticosteroids are used primarily for their anti-inflammatory and/or immunosuppressive effects.

Topical corticosteroids, such as betamethasone dipropionate, are effective in the treatment of corticosteroid-responsive dermatoses primarily because of their anti-inflammatory, anti-pruritic, and vasoconstrictive actions. However, while the physiologic, pharmacologic, and clinical effects of the corticosteroids are well-known, the exact mechanisms of their actions in each disease are uncertain. Betamethasone dipropionate, a corticosteroid, has been shown to have topical (dermatologic) and systemic pharmacologic and metabolic effects characteristic of this class of drugs.

Pharmacokinetics: The extent of percutaneous absorption of topical corticosteroids is determined by many factors including the vehicle, the integrity of the epidermal barrier, and the use of occlusive dressings. (See **DOSAGE AND ADMINISTRATION** section.)

Topical corticosteroids can be absorbed from normal intact skin. Inflammation and/or other disease processes in the skin may increase percutaneous absorption. Occlusive dressings substantially increase the percutaneous absorption of topical corticosteroids. (See **DOSAGE AND ADMINISTRATION** section.)

Once absorbed through the skin, topical corticosteroids enter pharmacokinetic pathways similar to systemically administered corticosteroids. Corticosteroids are bound to plasma proteins in varying degrees. Corticosteroids are metabolized primarily in the liver and are then excreted by the kidneys. Some of the topical corticosteroids and their metabolites are also excreted into the bile.

At 14 g per day, DIPROLENE Ointment was shown to depress the plasma levels of adrenal cortical hormones following repeated application to diseased skin in patients with psoriasis. Adrenal depression in these patients was transient, and rapidly returned to normal upon cessation of treatment. At 7 g per day (3.5 g bid), DIPROLENE Ointment was shown to cause minimal inhibition of the hypothalamic-pituitary-adrenal (HPA) axis when applied two times daily for two to three weeks, in normal patients and in patients with psoriasis and eczematous disorders.

INDICATIONS AND USAGE

DIPROLENE Ointment is indicated for relief of the inflammatory and pruritic manifestations of corticosteroid-responsive dermatoses.

CONTRAINDICATIONS

DIPROLENE Ointment is contraindicated in patients who are hypersensitive to betamethasone dipropionate, to other corticosteroids, or to any ingredient in this preparation.

PRECAUTIONS

General: Systemic absorption of topical corticosteroids has produced reversible HPA axis suppression, manifestations of Cushing's syndrome, hyperglycemia, and glucosuria in some patients.

Conditions which augment systemic absorption include the application of the more potent corticosteroids, use over large surface areas, prolonged use, and the addition of occlusive dressings. (See **DOSAGE AND ADMINISTRATION** section.)

Therefore, patients receiving a large dose of a potent topical steroid applied to a large surface area should be evaluated periodically for evidence of HPA axis suppression by using the urinary free cortisol and ACTH stimulation tests. If HPA axis suppression is noted, an attempt should be made to withdraw the drug, to reduce the frequency of application, or to substitute a less potent steroid.

Recovery of HPA axis function is generally prompt and complete upon discontinuation of the drug. Infrequently, signs and symptoms of steroid withdrawal may occur, requiring supplemental systemic corticosteroids.

Children may absorb proportionally larger amounts of topical corticosteroids and thus be more susceptible to systemic toxicity. (See **PRECAUTIONS–Pediatric Use.**)

If irritation develops, topical corticosteroids should be discontinued and appropriate therapy instituted.

In the presence of dermatological infections, the use of an appropriate antifungal or antibacterial agent should be instituted. If a favorable response does not occur promptly, the corticosteroid should be discontinued until the infection has been adequately controlled.

Information for Patients: Patients using topical corticosteroids should receive the following information and instructions:

1. This medication is to be used as directed by the physician and should not be used longer than the prescribed time period. It is for external use only. Avoid contact with the eyes.
2. Patients should be advised not to use this medication for any disorder other than that for which it was prescribed.
3. The treated skin area should not be bandaged or otherwise covered or wrapped as to be occlusive. (See **DOSAGE AND ADMINISTRATION** section.)
4. Patients should report any signs of local adverse reactions.

Laboratory Tests: The following tests may be helpful in evaluating HPA axis suppression:

Urinary free cortisol test
ACTH stimulation test

Carcinogenesis, Mutagenesis, and Impairment of Fertility: Long-term animal studies have not been performed to evaluate the carcinogenic potential or the effect on fertility of topically applied corticosteroids.

Studies to determine mutagenicity with prednisolone have revealed negative results.

Pregnancy Category C: Coticosteroids are generally teratogenic in laboratory animals when administered systemically at relatively low dosage levels. The more potent corticosteroids have been shown to be teratogenic after dermal application in laboratory animals. There are no adequate and well-controlled studies of the teratogenic effects of topically applied corticosteroids in pregnant women. Therefore, topical corticosteroids should be used during pregnancy only if the potential benefit justifies the potential risk to the fetus. Drugs of this class should not be used extensively on pregnant patients, in large amounts, or for prolonged periods of time.

Nursing Mothers: It is not known whether topical administration of corticosteroids could result in sufficient systemic absorption to produce detectable quantities in breast milk. Systemically administered corticosteroids are secreted into breast milk in quantities not likely to have a deleterious effect on the infant. Nevertheless, caution should be exercised when topical corticosteroids are prescribed for a nursing woman.

Pediatric Use: Use of DIPROLENE Ointment in children under 12 years is not recommended.

Pediatric patients may demonstrate greater susceptibility to topical corticosteroid-induced HPA axis suppression and Cushing's syndrome than mature patients because of a larger skin surface area to body weight ratio.

Hypothalamic-pituitary-adrenal (HPA) axis supression, Cushing's syndrome, and intracranial hypertension have been reported in children receiving topical corticosteroids. Manifestations of adrenal suppression in children include linear growth retardation, delayed weight gain, low plasma cortisol levels, and absence of response to ACTH stimulation. Manifestations of intracranial hypertension include bulging fontanelles, headaches, and bilateral papilledema.

Administration of topical corticosteroids to children should be limited to the least amount compatible with an effective therapeutic regimen. Chronic corticosteroid therapy may interfere with the growth and development of children.

ADVERSE REACTIONS

The local adverse reactions that were reported with DIPROLENE Ointment during clinical studies are as follows: folliculitis, 2 per 500 patients; erythema, 2 per 500 patients; pruritus, 1 per 500 patients; vesiculation, 1 per 500 patients.

The following local adverse reactions are reported infrequently when topical corticosteroids are used as recommended. These reactions are listed in an approximate decreasing order of occurrence: burning, itching, irritation, dryness, folliculitis, hypertrichosis, acneiform eruptions, hypopigmentation, perioral dermatitis, allergic contact dermatitis, maceration of the skin, secondary infection, skin atrophy, striae, miliaria.

Systemic absorption of topical corticosteroids has produced reversible HPA axis suppression, manifestations of Cushing's syndrome, hyperglycemia, and glucosuria in some patients.

OVERDOSAGE

Topically applied corticosteroids can be absorbed in sufficient amounts to produce systemic effects. (See **PRECAUTIONS.**)

DOSAGE AND ADMINISTRATION

Apply a thin film of DIPROLENE Ointment to the affected skin areas twice daily once in the morning and once at night. Treatment with DIPROLENE Ointment should be limited to 45 g per week.

DIPROLENE Ointment is not to be used with occlusive dressings.

HOW SUPPLIED

DIPROLENE Ointment 0.05% is supplied in 15-(NDC 0085-0575-02), and 45-gram (NDC 0085-0575-03) tubes; boxes of one.

Store between 2° and 30°C (36° and 86°F).

Revised 8/84

Continued on next page

Information on Schering products appearing on these pages is effective as of September 30, 1986.

Schering—Cont.

DIPROSONE® ℞
[dī-pro 'sōn]
brand of betamethasone dipropionate
Cream, USP 0.05%
Ointment, USP 0.05%
Lotion, USP 0.05% w/w
Topical Aerosol, USP 0.1% w/w
(potency expressed as betamethasone)
For Dermatologic Use Only—
Not for Ophthalmic Use

DESCRIPTION

DIPROSONE **Cream, Ointment, Lotion,** and **Topical Aerosol** contain betamethasone dipropionate, USP, a synthetic adrenocorticosteroid, for dermatologic use. Betamethasone, an analog of prednisolone, has high corticosteroid activity and slight mineralocorticoid activity. Betamethasone dipropionate is the 17,21-dipropionate ester of betamethasone.

Chemically, betamethasone dipropionate is 9-Fluoro-11β, 17, 21-trihydroxy-16β -methylpregna-1, 4-diene-3, 20-dione 17, 21-dipropionate, with the empirical formula $C_{28}H_{37}FO_7$, a molecular weight of 504.6.

Betamethasone dipropionate is a white to creamy white, odorless crystalline powder, insoluble in water.

Each gram of DIPROSONE **Cream** 0.05% contains: 0.64 mg betamethasone dipropionate, USP (equivalent to 0.5 mg betamethasone), in a hydrophilic emollient cream consisting of purified water, mineral oil, white petrolatum, ceteareth-30, cetearyl alcohol, monobasic sodium phosphate, and phosphoric acid; chlorocresol and propylene glycol as preservatives.

Each gram of DIPROSONE **Ointment** 0.05% contains: 0.64 mg betamethasone dipropionate, USP (equivalent to 0.5 mg betamethasone), in an ointment base of mineral oil and white petrolatum.

Each gram of DIPROSONE **Lotion** 0.05% w/w contains: 0.64 mg betamethasone dipropionate, USP (equivalent to 0.5 mg betamethasone), in a lotion base of isopropyl alcohol (46.8%) and purified water slightly thickened with carbomer 934P; the pH is adjusted to approximately 4.7 with sodium hydroxide.

DIPROSONE **Topical Aerosol** 0.1% w/w contains: 6.4 mg betamethasone dipropionate, USP (equivalent to 5.0 mg betamethasone), in a vehicle of mineral oil and caprylic/capric triglyceride; also containing 10% isopropyl alcohol and sufficient inert hydrocarbon (propane and isobutane) propellant to make 85 grams. The aerosol spray deposits betamethasone dipropionate equivalent to approximately 0.1% betamethasone in a non-volatile, almost invisible film. A three-second spray delivers betamethasone dipropionate equivalent to approximately 0.06 mg betamethasone.

CLINICAL PHARMACOLOGY

The corticosteroids are a class of compounds comprising steroid hormones secreted by the adrenal cortex and their synthetic analogs. In pharmacologic doses corticosteroids are used primarily for their anti-inflammatory and/or immunosuppressive effects.

Topical corticosteroids, such as betamethasone dipropionate, are effective in the treatment of corticosteroid-responsive dermatoses primarily because of their anti-inflammatory, anti-pruritic, and vasoconstrictive actions. However, while the physiologic, pharmacologic, and clinical effects of the corticosteroids are well-known, the exact mechanisms of their actions in each disease are uncertain. Betamethasone dipropionate, a corticosteroid, has been shown to have topical (dermatologic) and systemic pharmacologic and metabolic effects characteristic of this class of drugs.

Pharmacokinetics: The extent of percutaneous absorption of topical corticosteroids is determined by many factors including the vehicle, the integrity of the epidermal barrier, and the use of occlusive dressings. (See **DOSAGE AND ADMINISTRATION** section.)

Topical corticosteroids can be absorbed from normal intact skin. Inflammation and/or other disease processes in the skin increase percutaneous absorption. Occlusive dressings substantially increase the percutaneous absorption of topical corticosteroids. (See **DOSAGE AND ADMINISTRATION** section.)

Once absorbed through the skin, topical corticosteroids are handled through pharmacokinetic pathways similar to systemically administered corticosteroids. Corticosteroids are bound to plasma proteins in varying degrees. Corticosteroids are metabolized primarily in the liver and are then excreted by the kidneys. Some of the topical corticosteroids and their metabolites are also excreted into the bile.

INDICATIONS AND USAGE

DIPROSONE **Cream, Ointment, Lotion,** and **Topical Aerosol** are indicated for relief of the inflammatory and pruritic manifestations of corticosteroid-responsive dermatoses.

CONTRAINDICATIONS

DIPROSONE **Cream, Ointment, Lotion,** and **Topical Aerosol** are contraindicated in patients who are hypersensitive to betamethasone dipropionate, to other corticosteroids, or to any ingredient in these preparations.

PRECAUTIONS

General: Systemic absorption of topical corticosteroids has produced reversible hypothalamic-pituitary-adrenal (HPA) axis suppression, manifestations of Cushing's syndrome, hyperglycemia, and glucosuria in some patients.

Conditions which augment systemic absorption include the application of the more potent steroids, use over large surface areas, prolonged use, and the addition of occlusive dressings. (See **DOSAGE AND ADMINISTRATION** section.)

Therefore, patients receiving a large dose of a potent topical steroid applied to a large surface area should be evaluated periodically for evidence of HPA axis suppression by using the urinary free cortisol and ACTH stimulation tests. If HPA axis suppression is noted, an attempt should be made to withdraw the drug, to reduce the frequency of application, or to substitute a less potent steroid.

Recovery of HPA axis function is generally prompt and complete upon discontinuation of the drug. Infrequently, signs and symptoms of steroid withdrawal may occur, requiring supplemental systemic corticosteroids.

Children may absorb proportionally larger amounts of topical corticosteroids and thus be more susceptible to systemic toxicity. (See **PRECAUTIONS-Pediatric Use.**)

If irritation develops, topical corticosteroids should be discontinued and appropriate therapy instituted.

In the presence of dermatological infections, the use of an appropriate antifungal or antibacterial agent should be instituted. If a favorable response does not occur promptly, the corticosteroid should be discontinued until the infection has been adequately controlled.

Information for Patients: Patients using topical corticosteroids should receive the following information and instructions:

1. This medication is to be used as directed by the physician. It is for external use only. Avoid contact with the eyes.
2. Patients should be advised not to use this medication for any disorder other than for which it was prescribed.
3. The treated skin area should not be bandaged or otherwise covered or wrapped as to be occlusive. (See **DOSAGE AND ADMINISTRATION** section.)
4. Patients should report any signs of local adverse reactions.
5. Parents of pediatric patients should be advised not to use tight-fitting diapers or plastic pants on a child being treated in the diaper area, as these garments may constitute occlusive dressing. (See **DOSAGE AND ADMINISTRATION** section.)
6. When using DIPROSONE **Topical Aerosol,** the patient should be advised of the following:
   - the spray should be kept away from the eyes or other mucous membranes
   - avoid freezing tissues by not spraying for more than three seconds, at a distance of not less than six inches between the nozzle and the skin
   - use only as directed; intentional misuse by deliberately concentrating and inhaling the container contents can be harmful or fatal
   - the container contents are under pressure; do not puncture the container
   - the container mixture is flammable; do not use or store the container near heat or an open flame; exposure to temperatures above 120° Fahrenheit may cause bursting; never throw container into a fire or incinerator
   - keep out of the reach of children

Laboratory Tests: The following tests may be helpful in evaluating HPA axis suppression:

Urinary free cortisol test
ACTH stimulation test

Carcinogenesis, Mutagenesis, and Impairment of Fertility: Long-term animal studies have not been performed to evaluate the carcinogenic potential or the effect on fertility of topical corticosteroids.

Studies to determine mutagenicity with prednisolone have revealed negative results.

Pregnancy Category C: Corticosteroids are generally teratogenic in laboratory animals when administered systemically at relatively low dosage levels. The more potent corticosteroids have been shown to be teratogenic after dermal application in laboratory animals. There are no adequate and well-controlled studies in pregnant women on teratogenic effects from topically applied corticosteroids. Therefore, topical corticosteroids should be used during pregnancy only if the potential benefit justifies the potential risk to the fetus. Drugs of this class should not be used extensively on pregnant patients, in large amounts, or for prolonged periods of time.

Nursing Mothers: It is not known whether topical administration of corticosteroids could result in sufficient systemic absorption to produce detectable quantities in breast milk. Systemically administered corticosteroids are secreted into breast milk in quantities not likely to have a deleterious effect on the infant. Nevertheless, caution should be exercised when topical corticosteroids are prescribed for a nursing woman.

Pediatric Use: Pediatric patients may demonstrate greater susceptibility to topical corticosteroid-induced HPA axis suppression and Cushing's syndrome than mature patients because of a larger skin surface area to body weight ratio.

Hypothalamic-pituitary-adrenal (HPA) axis suppression, Cushing's syndrome, and intracranial hypertension have been reported in children receiving topical corticosteroids. Manifestations of adrenal suppression in children include linear growth retardation, delayed weight gain, low plasma cortisol levels, and absence of response to ACTH stimulation. Manifestations of intracranial hypertension include bulging fontanelles, headaches, and bilateral papilledema.

Administration of topical corticosteroids to children should be limited to the least amount compatible with an effective therapeutic regimen. Chronic corticosteroid therapy may interfere with the growth and development of children.

ADVERSE REACTIONS

The following local adverse reactions are reported infrequently when DIPROSONE Products are used as recommended in the **DOSAGE AND ADMINISTRATION** section. These reactions are listed in an approximate decreasing order of occurrence: burning; itching; irritation; dryness; folliculitis; hypertrichosis; acneiform eruptions; hypopigmentation; perioral dermatitis; allergic contact dermatitis; maceration of the skin; secondary infection; skin atrophy; striae; miliaria.

Systemic absorption of topical corticosteroids has produced reversible hypothalamic-pituitary-adrenal (HPA) axis suppression, manifestations of Cushing's syndrome, hyperglycemia, and glucosuria in some patients.

OVERDOSAGE

Topically applied corticosteroids can be absorbed in sufficient amounts to produce systemic effects. (See **PRECAUTIONS.**)

DOSAGE AND ADMINISTRATION

DIPROSONE **Cream:** Apply a thin film of DIPROSONE **Cream** 0.05% to the affected skin areas once daily. In some cases, a twice daily dosage may be necessary.

DIPROSONE **Ointment:** Apply a thin film of DIPROSONE **Ointment** to the affected skin areas once daily. In some cases, a twice daily dosage may be necessary.

DIPROSONE **Lotion:** Apply a few drops of DIPROSONE **Lotion** to the affected area and massage lightly until it disappears. Apply twice daily, in the morning and at night. For the most effective and economical use, apply nozzle very close to affected area and gently squeeze bottle.

DIPROSONE **Topical Aerosol:** Apply sparingly to the affected skin area three times a day. The container may be held upright or inverted during use. The spray should be directed onto the affected area from a distance of not less than six inches and applied for only three seconds. For the most effective and economical use, a three-second spray is sufficient to cover an area about the size of the hand.

DIPROSONE Products are not to be used with occlusive dressings.

HOW SUPPLIED

DIPROSONE **Cream** 0.05% is supplied in 15-gram (NDC-0085-0853-02), 45-gram (NDC-0085-0853-03) tubes; boxes of one.

DIPROSONE **Lotion** 0.05% w/w is available in 20 ml (18.7 g) (NDC-0085-0028-04); and 60 ml (56.2 g) (NDC-0085-0028-06) plastic squeeze bottles; boxes of one. **Protect from light. Store in carton until contents are used.**

DIPROSONE **Ointment** 0.05% is supplied in 15-gram (NDC 0085-0510-04) and 45- gram (NDC-0085-0510-06) tubes; boxes of one.

DIPROSONE **Topical Aerosol** 0.1% w/w is supplied as an 85-gram spray can. (NDC-0085-0475-06)

Store all DIPROSONE preparations between 2° and 30°C (36° and 86°F).

Revised 12/85

ESTINYL® ℞
[es 'tĭ-nil]
brand of ethinyl estradiol,
Tablets, USP

WARNINGS

1. ESTROGENS HAVE BEEN REPORTED TO INCREASE THE RISK RATIO OF ENDOMETRIAL CARCINOMA.

Three independent case control studies have reported an increased risk ratio of endometrial cancer in postmenopausal women exposed to exogenous estrogens for

prolonged periods.[1-3] This risk ratio was independent of the other risk factors for endometrial cancer. These studies are further supported by the report that incidence rates of endometrial cancer have increased sharply since 1969 in eight different areas of the United States with population-based cancer reporting systems, an increase which may be related to the rapidly expanding use of estrogens during the last decade.[4]
The three case control studies reported that the risk ratio of endometrial cancer in estrogen users was about 4.5 to 13.9 times greater than in nonusers. The risk ratio appears to depend on both duration of treatment[1] and on estrogen dose.[3] In view of these reports, when estrogens are used for the treatment of menopausal symptoms, the lowest dose that will control symptoms should be utilized and medication should be discontinued as soon as possible. When prolonged treatment is medically indicated, the patient should be reassessed on at least a semiannual basis to determine the need for continued therapy. Although the evidence must be considered preliminary, one study suggests that cyclic administration of low doses of estrogen may carry less risk than continuous administration[3]; it therefore appears prudent to utilize such a regimen.
Close clinical surveillance of all women taking estrogens is important. In all cases of undiagnosed persistent or recurring abnormal vaginal bleeding, adequate diagnostic measures should be undertaken to rule out malignancy.
There is no evidence at present that "natural" estrogens are more or less hazardous than "synthetic" estrogens at equiestrogenic doses.
2. ESTROGENS SHOULD NOT BE USED DURING PREGNANCY.
The use of estrogens during early pregnancy may seriously damage the offspring. It has been reported that females exposed in utero to diethylstilbestrol, a nonsteroidal estrogen, may have an increased risk of developing in later life a form of vaginal or cervical cancer that is ordinarily extremely rare.[5,6] This risk has been estimated statistically as not greater than 4 per 1000 exposures.[7] In certain studies, a high percentage of such exposed women (from 30 to 90 percent) have been found to have vaginal adenosis,[8-11] epithelial changes of the vagina and cervix. Although these changes are histologically benign, it is not known whether they are precursors of malignancy. Although similar data are not available with the use of other estrogens, it cannot be presumed they would not induce similar changes. Exposure to diethylstilbestrol has also been associated with adverse effects on reproductive performance, including increased rates of spontaneous abortion, ectopic pregnancy, premature deliveries, and perinatal deaths.
Several reports suggest an association between intrauterine fetal exposure to female sex hormones and congenital anomalies, including congenital heart defects and limb reduction defects.[12-15] One case control study[15] estimated a 4.7 fold increased risk of limb reduction defects in infants exposed in utero to sex hormones (oral contraceptives, hormone withdrawal tests for pregnancy, or attempted treatment for threatened abortion). Some of these exposures were very short and involved only a few days of treatment. The data suggest that the risk of limb reduction defects in exposed fetuses is somewhat less than 1 per 1000.
In the past, estrogens have been used during pregnancy in an attempt to treat threatened or habitual abortion. There is considerable evidence that estrogens are ineffective for these indications.
If ESTINYL Tablets are used during pregnancy, or if the patient becomes pregnant while taking this drug, she should be apprised of the potential risks to the fetus, and the advisability of pregnancy continuation.

DESCRIPTION

ESTINYL Tablets contain ethinyl estradiol, USP, a potent synthetic estrogen having the chemical name, 19-Nor-17α-pregna-1,3,5(10)-trien-20-yne-3,17-diol; the chemical formula $C_{20}H_{24}O_2$; and a molecular weight of 296.41.
Ethinyl estradiol is a white to creamy white, odorless, crystalline powder. It is insoluble in water, soluble in alcohol, chloroform, ether and vegetable oils.
Biologically, estrogens may be defined as compounds capable of stimulating female secondary sex characteristics. Chemically, there are different groups of estrogens, depending on whether they are natural or synthetic, steroidal or nonsteroidal. Natural human estrogens are ultimately formed from either androstenedione or testosterone as immediate precursors. Ethinyl estradiol is a synthetic, steroidal estrogen.
ESTINYL, for oral administration, is available in tablets containing 0.02, 0.05, or 0.5 mg ethinyl estradiol, USP.
The inactive ingredients for ESTINYL Tablets 0.02 mg include: acacia, butylparaben, calcium phosphate, calcium sulfate, carnauba wax, corn starch, gelatin, FD&C Blue No. 2 Al Lake, FD&C Yellow No. 5, FD&C Yellow No. 5 Al Lake, FD&C Yellow No. 6 Al Lake, lactose, magnesium stearate, potato starch, sodium phosphate, sugar, and white wax. May also contain talc.
The inactive ingredients for ESTINYL Tablets 0.05 mg include: acacia, butylparaben, calcium phosphate, calcium sulfate, carnauba wax, corn starch, FD&C Blue No. 1, FD&C Red No. 3, gelatin, lactose, magnesium stearate, potato starch, sodium phosphate, and white wax. May also contain talc.
The inactive ingredients for ESTINYL Tablets 0.5 mg include: corn starch, FD&C Yellow No. 6, lactose, magnesium stearate, and sodium phosphate.

CLINICAL PHARMACOLOGY

Ethinyl estradiol is a synthetic derivative of the natural estrogen, estradiol.
Ethinyl estradiol, like estradiol, promotes growth of the endometrium and thickening, stratification and cornification of the vagina. It causes growth of the ducts of the mammary glands, but inhibits lactation. It also inhibits the anterior pituitary and causes capillary dilatation, fluid retention and protein anabolism.
Estradiol is the major estrogen in premenopausal women, with up to 100 to 600 mcg being secreted daily by the ovary. Natural estrogens are poorly effective when given by mouth. Apparently this is due to rapid clearance of the endogenous hormone from blood, along with a "first-pass-effect" after oral administration. The addition of a 17-alpha-ethinyl group to estradiol increases potency and enhances oral activity by impeding hepatic degradation. The oral efficacy of ethinyl estradiol is related to slower elimination than estradiol from the circulation. A part of ingested ethinyl estradiol is excreted in glucuronide form via urine in animals and in man, but also extensive metabolism of the steroid nucleus occurs. The major metabolism takes place mainly in the liver. Large amounts of ethinyl estradiol metabolites are excreted via human bile, much similar to what has been reported for estradiol. However, unlike estradiol, ethinyl estradiol metabolites do not exclusively leave via urine. Urinary recovery is much less than that of estradiol and substantial amounts of ethinyl estradiol metabolites appear in human feces. Quantitatively, the major metabolic pathway for ethinyl estradiol, both in rats and in humans, is aromatic hydroxylation, as it is for the natural estrogens.
Rapid and complete absorption follows oral intake of ethinyl estradiol. Elimination of ethinyl estradiol from plasma proceeds slower than that of estradiol. After oral administration, an initial peak occurs in plasma at 2 to 3 hours, with a secondary peak at about 12 hours after dosing; the second peak is interpreted as evidence for extensive enterohepatic circulation of ethinyl estradiol.

INDICATIONS AND USAGE

ESTINYL Tablets are indicated in the treatment of: 1) Moderate to severe *vasomotor* symptoms associated with the menopause. (There is no evidence that estrogens are effective for nervous symptoms or depression which might occur during menopause, and they should not be used to treat these conditions.) 2) Female hypogonadism. 3) Prostatic carcinoma—palliative therapy of advanced disease. 4) Breast cancer (for palliation only) in appropriately selected women, such as those who are more than 5 years postmenopausal with progressing inoperable or radiation-resistant disease.
ETHINYL ESTRADIOL HAS NOT BEEN SHOWN TO BE EFFECTIVE FOR ANY PURPOSE DURING PREGNANCY AND ITS USE MAY CAUSE SEVERE HARM TO THE FETUS (SEE BOXED **WARNINGS**).
The lowest effective dose appropriate for the specific indication should be utilized. Studies of the addition of a progestin for seven or more days of a cycle of estrogen administration have reported a lowered incidence of endometrial hyperplasia. Morphological and biochemical studies of endometrium suggest that 10 to 13 days of progestin are needed to provide maximal maturation of the endometrium and to eliminate any hyperplastic changes. Whether this will provide protection from endometrial carcinoma has not been clearly established. There are possible additional risks which may be associated with the inclusion of progestin in estrogen replacement regimens. The potential risks include adverse effects on carbohydrate and lipid metabolism. The choice of progestin and dosage may be important to minimizing these adverse effects.

CONTRAINDICATIONS

Estrogens should not be used in women (or men) with any of the following conditions:
1. Known or suspected cancer of the breast except in appropriately selected patients being treated for metastatic disease.
2. Known or suspected estrogen-dependent neoplasia.
3. Known or suspected pregnancy (see boxed **WARNINGS**).
4. Undiagnosed abnormal genital bleeding.
5. Active thrombophlebitis or thromboembolic disorders.
6. A past history of thrombophlebitis, thrombosis or thromboembolic disorders associated with previous estrogen use (except when used in treatment of breast or prostatic malignancy).

WARNINGS

1. *Induction of malignant neoplasms.* Long-term continuous administration of natural and synthetic estrogens in certain animal species increases the frequency of carcinomas of the breast, cervix, vagina, and liver. There is now evidence that estrogens increase the risk of carcinoma of the endometrium in humans. (See boxed **WARNINGS**.)
At the present time there is no satisfactory evidence that estrogens given to postmenopausal women increase the risk of cancer of the breast,[16] although a recent long-term followup of a single physician's practice has raised this possibility.[17] Because of the animal data, there is a need for caution in prescribing estrogens for women with a strong family history of breast cancer or who have breast nodules, fibrocystic disease, or abnormal mammograms.
Estrogens have been reported to be associated with carcinoma of the male breast and suspicious lesions in males receiving estrogen therapy should be investigated accordingly.
2. *Gallbladder disease.* A recent study has reported a 2- to 3-fold increase in the risk of surgically confirmed gallbladder disease in women receiving postmenopausal estrogens,[16] similar to the 2-fold increase previously noted in users of oral contraceptives.[18,22] In the case of oral contraceptives, the increased risk appeared after two years of use.[22]
3. *Effects similar to those caused by estrogen-progestagen oral contraceptives.* There are several serious adverse effects of oral contraceptives, most of which have not, up to now, been documented as consequences of postmenopausal estrogen therapy. This may reflect the comparatively low doses of estrogen used in postmenopausal women. It would be expected that the larger doses of estrogen used to treat prostatic or breast cancer are more likely to result in these adverse effects, and, in fact, it has been shown that there is an increased risk of thrombosis in men receiving estrogens for prostatic cancer.[19-22]
a. *Thromboembolic disease* It is now well established that users of oral contraceptives have an increased risk of various thromboembolic and thrombotic vascular diseases, such as thrombophlebitis, pulmonary embolism, stroke and myocardial infarction.[22-29] Cases of retinal thrombosis, mesenteric thrombosis, and optic neuritis have been reported in oral contraceptive users. There is evidence that the risk of several of these adverse reactions is related to the dose of the drug.[30,31] An increased risk of postsurgery thromboembolic complications has also been reported in users of oral contraceptives.[32,33] If feasible, estrogen should be discontinued at least 4 weeks before surgery of the type associated with an increased risk of thromboembolism, or during periods of immobilization.
While an increased rate of thromboembolic and thrombotic disease in postmenopausal users of estrogen has not been found,[16,34] this does not rule out the possibility that such an increase may be present or that subgroups of women who have underlying risk factors or who are receiving relatively large doses of estrogens may have increased risk. Therefore, estrogens should not be used in persons with active thrombophlebitis or thromboembolic disorders, and they should not be used (except in treatment of malignancy) in persons with a history of such disorders in association with estrogen use. They should be used with caution in patients with cerebral vascular or coronary artery disease and only for those in whom estrogens are clearly needed.
Large doses of estrogen (5 mg conjugated estrogens per day), comparable to those used to treat cancer of the prostate and breast, have been shown in a large prospective clinical trial in men[35] to increase the risk of nonfatal myocardial infarction, pulmonary embolism and thrombophlebitis. When estrogen doses of this size are used, any of the thromboembolic and thrombotic adverse effects associated with oral contraceptive use should be considered a clear risk.
b. *Hepatic adenoma* Benign hepatic adenomas appear to be associated with the use of oral contraceptives.[36-38] Although benign, and rare, these may rupture and may cause death through intra-abdominal hemorrhage. Such lesions have not yet been reported in association with other estrogen or progestagen preparations but should be considered in estrogen users having abdominal pain and tenderness, abdominal mass, or hypovolemic shock. Hepatocellular carcinoma has also been reported in women taking estrogen-containing oral contraceptives.[37] The relationship of this malignancy to these drugs is not known at this time.
c. *Elevated blood pressure* Increased blood pressure is not uncommon in women using oral contraceptives. There is now a report that this may occur with use of estrogens in the menopause[39] and blood pressure should be monitored with estrogen use, especially if high doses are used.

Continued on next page

Information on Schering products appearing on these pages is effective as of September 30, 1986.

Schering—Cont.

d. *Glucose tolerance* A worsening of glucose tolerance has been observed in a significant percentage of patients on estrogen-containing oral contraceptives. For this reason, diabetic patients should be carefully observed while receiving estrogen.

4. *Hypercalcemia.* Administration of estrogens may lead to severe hypercalcemia in patients with breast cancer and bone metastases. If this occurs, the drug should be stopped and appropriate measures taken to reduce the serum calcium level.

PRECAUTIONS

General Precautions:

1. A complete medical and family history should be taken prior to the initiation of any estrogen therapy. The pretreatment and periodic physical examinations should include special reference to blood pressure, breasts, abdomen, and pelvic organs, and should include a Papanicolaou smear. As a general rule, estrogen should not be prescribed for longer than one year without another physical examination being performed.
2. Fluid retention—Because estrogens may cause some degree of fluid retention, conditions which might be influenced by this factor, such as epilepsy, migraine, and cardiac or renal dysfunction, require careful observation.
3. Certain patients may develop undesirable manifestations of excessive estrogenic stimulation, such as abnormal or excessive uterine bleeding, mastodynia, etc.
4. Oral contraceptives appear to be associated with an increased incidence of mental depression.[22] Although it is not clear whether this is due to the estrogenic or progestagenic component of the contraceptive, patients with a history of depression should be carefully observed.
5. Preexisting uterine leiomyomata may increase in size during estrogen use.
6. The pathologist should be advised of estrogen therapy when relevant specimens are submitted.
7. Patients with a past history of jaundice during pregnancy have an increased risk of recurrence of jaundice while receiving estrogen-containing oral contraceptive therapy. If jaundice develops in any patient receiving estrogen, the medication should be discontinued while the cause is investigated.
8. Estrogens may be poorly metabolized in patients with impaired liver function and they should be administered with caution in such patients.
9. Because estrogens influence the metabolism of calcium and phosphorus, they should be used with caution in patients with metabolic bone diseases that are associated with hypercalcemia or in patients with renal insufficiency.
10. Because of the effects of estrogens on epiphyseal closure, they should be used judiciously in young patients in whom bone growth is not complete.
11. ESTINYL Tablets, .02 mg contain FD&C Yellow No. 5 (tartrazine) which may cause allergic-type reactions (including bronchial asthma) in certain susceptible individuals. Although the overall incidence of FD&C Yellow No. 5 (tartrazine) sensitivity in the general population is low, it is frequently seen in patients who also have aspirin hypersensitivity.

Information for the Patient: See text of Patient Package Insert.

Drug/Laboratory Test Interactions: Certain endocrine and liver function tests may be affected by estrogen-containing oral contraceptives. The following similar changes may be expected with larger doses of estrogen:
Increased sulfobromophthalein retention; increased prothrombin and factors VII, VIII, IX, and X; decreased antithrombin 3; increased norepinephrine-induced platelet aggregation; increased thyroid binding globulin (TBG) leading to increased circulating total thyroid hormone, as measured by PBI, T4 by column, or T4 by radioimmunoassay. Free T3 resin uptake is decreased, reflecting the elevated TBG; free T4 concentration is unaltered; impaired glucose tolerance; decreased pregnanediol excretion; reduced response to metyrapone test; reduced serum folate concentration; increased serum triglyceride and phospholipid concentration.

Carcinogenesis, Mutagenesis, Impairment of Fertility: See boxed **WARNINGS.**

Pregnancy Category X. See **CONTRAINDICATIONS** and boxed **WARNINGS.**

Nursing Mothers: Because of the potential for tumorigenicity shown for ethinyl estradiol in animal and human studies, a decision should be made whether to discontinue nursing or to discontinue the drug, taking into account the importance of the drug to the mother.

Pediatric Use: Safety and effectiveness in children have not been established.

ADVERSE REACTIONS

(See **WARNINGS** regarding induction of neoplasia, adverse effects on the fetus, increased incidence of gallbladder disease, and adverse effects similar to those of oral contraceptives, including thromboembolism.) The following additional adverse reactions have been reported with estrogenic therapy, including oral contraceptives:

Genitourinary system: Breakthrough bleeding, spotting, change in menstrual flow; dysmenorrhea; premenstrual-like syndrome; amenorrhea during and after treatment; increase in size of uterine fibromyomata; vaginal candidiasis; change in cervical eversion and in degree of cervical secretion; cystitis-like syndrome.

Breasts: Tenderness, enlargement, secretion.

Gastrointestinal: Nausea, vomiting; abdominal cramps, bloating; cholestatic jaundice.

Skin: Chloasma or melasma which may persist when drug is discontinued; erythema multiforme; erythema nodosum; hemorrhagic eruption; loss of scalp hair; hirsutism.

Eyes: Steepening of corneal curvature; intolerance to contact lenses.

CNS: Headache, migraine, dizziness; mental depression; chorea.

Miscellaneous: Increase or decrease in weight; reduced carbohydrate tolerance; aggravation of porphyria; edema; changes in libido.

ACUTE OVERDOSAGE

Numerous reports of ingestion of large doses of estrogen-containing oral contraceptives by young children indicate that serious ill effects do not occur. Overdosage of estrogen may cause nausea, and withdrawal bleeding may occur in females.

DOSAGE AND ADMINISTRATION

1. *Given cyclically for short-term use only.*

For treatment of moderate to severe *vasomotor* symptoms associated with the menopause: The lowest dose that will control symptoms should be chosen and medication should be discontinued as promptly as possible. Administration should be cyclic (e.g., 3 weeks on and 1 week off). Attempts to discontinue or taper medication should be made at 3- to 6-month intervals. The usual dosage range is one 0.02 mg or 0.05 mg tablet daily. In some instances, the effective dose may be as low as one 0.02 mg tablet every other day. A useful dosage schedule for early menopause, while spontaneous menstruation continues, is 0.05 mg once a day for twenty-one days and then a rest period for seven days. For the initial treatment of the late menopause, the same regimen is indicated with the 0.02 mg ESTINYL Tablet for the first few cycles, after which the 0.05 mg dosage may be substituted. In more severe cases, such as those due to surgical and roentgenologic castration, one 0.05 mg tablet may be administered three times daily at the start of treatment. With adequate clinical improvement, usually obtainable in a few weeks, the dosage may be reduced to one 0.05 mg tablet daily and the patient continued thereafter on a maintenance dosage as in the average case.

2. *Given cyclically.*

Female hypogonadism: One 0.05 mg tablet is given one to three times daily during the first two weeks of a theoretical menstrual cycle. This is followed by progesterone during the last half of the arbitrary cycle. This regimen is continued for three to six months. The patient is then allowed to go untreated for two months to determine whether or not she can maintain the cycle without hormonal therapy. If not, additional courses of therapy may be prescribed.

3. *Given chronically.*

Inoperable progressing prostatic cancer: From three 0.05 mg to four 0.5 mg tablets may be administered daily for palliation.

Inoperable progressing breast cancer in appropriately selected postmenopausal women (See **INDICATIONS AND USAGE**): Two 0.5 mg tablets three times daily for palliation. Treated patients with an intact uterus should be monitored closely for signs of endometrial cancer and appropriate diagnostic measures should be taken to rule out malignancy in the event of persistent or recurring abnormal vaginal bleeding.

HOW SUPPLIED

ESTINYL Tablets 0.02 mg, beige, sugar-coated tablets branded in black with the Schering trademark and either product identification number, 298, or letters, ER; bottles of 100 (NDC 0085-0298-03) and 250 (NDC 0085-0298-06).

ESTINYL Tablets 0.05 mg, pink, sugar-coated tablets branded in black with the Schering trademark and either product identification number, 070, or letters, EM; bottles of 100 (NDC 0085-0070-03) and 250 (NDC 0085-0070-06).

ESTINYL Tablets 0.5 mg, peach-colored, compressed, scored tablets impressed with the Schering trademark and either product identification number, 150, or letters, EP; bottle of 100 (NDC 0085-0150-03).

Store between 2° and 30° C (36° and 86° F).

Patient package inserts are being dispensed with this product. They are available to physicians upon request. Physician references available on request.

Rev. 1/86

Shown in Product Identification Section, page 428

ETRAFON® ℞

[ĕ'trah-fon]

brand of perphenazine, USP—amitriptyline hydrochloride, USP

ETRAFON 2-10 TABLETS (2-10)
ETRAFON TABLETS (2-25)
ETRAFON-A TABLETS (4-10)
ETRAFON-FORTE TABLETS (4-25)

DESCRIPTION

ETRAFON Tablets contain perphenazine, USP and amitriptyline hydrochloride, USP. Perphenazine is a piperazinyl phenothiazine having the chemical formula, $C_{21}H_{26}ClN_3OS$. Amitriptyline hydrochloride is a dibenzocycloheptadiene derivative having the chemical formula, $C_{20}H_{23}N.HCl$.

ETRAFON Tablets are available in multiple strengths to afford dosage flexibility for optimum management. They are available as ETRAFON 2-10 Tablets, 2 mg perphenazine and 10 mg amitriptyline hydrochloride; ETRAFON Tablets, 2 mg perphenazine and 25 mg amitriptyline hydrochloride. ETRAFON-A Tablets, 4 mg perphenazine and 10 mg amitriptyline hydrochloride; and ETRAFON-FORTE Tablets, 4 mg perphenazine and 25 mg amitriptyline hydrochloride.

The inactive ingredients for ETRAFON 2-10 Tablets (2-10) include: acacia, butylparaben, calcium phosphate, calcium sulfate, carnauba wax, corn starch, D&C Yellow No. 10 Al Lake, FD&C Yellow No. 6 Al Lake, gelatin, lactose, magnesium stearate, potato starch, sugar, and white wax. May also contain talc.

The inactive ingredients for ETRAFON Tablets (2-25) include: acacia, butylparaben, calcium phosphate, calcium sulfate, carnauba wax, corn starch, D&C Red No. 30 Al Lake, FD&C Yellow No. 6 Al Lake, gelatin, lactose, magnesium stearate, potato starch, sugar, and white wax. May also contain talc.

The inactive ingredients for ETRAFON-A Tablets (4-10) include: acacia, butylparaben, calcium phosphate, calcium sulfate, carnauba wax, corn starch, FD&C Yellow No. 6, gelatin, lactose, magnesium stearate, potato starch, sugar, and white wax. May also contain talc.

The inactive ingredients for ETRAFON-FORTE Tablets (4-25) include: acacia, butylparaben, calcium phosphate, calcium sulfate, carnauba wax, corn starch, FD&C Red No. 40 Al Lake, FD&C Yellow No. 6 Al Lake, gelatin, lactose, magnesium stearate, potato starch, sugar, and white wax. May also contain talc.

ACTIONS

ETRAFON combines the tranquilizing action of perphenazine with the antidepressant properties of amitriptyline hydrochloride. Perphenazine acts on the central nervous system and has a greater behavioral potency than other phenothiazine derivatives whose side chains do not contain a piperazine moiety. Amitriptyline hydrochloride is a tricyclic antidepressant. It is not a monoamine oxidase inhibitor, but its mechanism of action in man is not known, it does not act primarily by stimulation of the central nervous system.

INDICATIONS

ETRAFON Tablets are indicated for the treatment of patients with moderate to severe anxiety and/or agitation and depressed mood; patients with depression in whom anxiety and/or agitation are moderate or severe; patients with anxiety and depression associated with chronic physical disease; patients in whom depression and anxiety cannot be clearly differentiated.

Schizophrenic patients who have associated symptoms of depression should be considered for therapy with ETRAFON.

CONTRAINDICATIONS

ETRAFON Tablets are contraindicated in comatose or greatly obtunded patients and in patients receiving large doses of central nervous system depressants (barbiturates, alcohol, narcotics, analgesics, or antihistamines); in the presence of existing blood dyscrasias, bone marrow depression, or liver damage; and in patients who have shown hypersensitivity to ETRAFON Tablets, its components, or related compounds.

ETRAFON Tablets are also contraindicated in patients with suspected or established subcortical brain damage, with or without hypothalamic damage, since a hyperthermic reaction with temperatures in excess of 104°F may occur in such patients, sometimes not until 14 to 16 hours after drug administration. Total body ice-packing is recommended for such a reaction; antipyretics may also be useful.

ETRAFON should not be given concomitantly with a monoamine oxidase inhibiting compound. Hyperpyretic crises, severe convulsions and deaths have occurred in patients receiving tricyclic antidepressant and monoamine oxidase inhibiting drugs simultaneously. In patients who have been receiving a monoamine oxidase inhibitor, it is recommended that two weeks or longer elapse before the start of treatment with ETRAFON Tablets to permit recovery from the effects of the MAO inhibitor and to avoid possible potentiation. Treatment with ETRAFON Tablets should be initiated cau-

tiously in such patients, with gradual increase in dosage until a satisfactory response is obtained.
Amitriptyline hydrochloride is not recommended for use during the acute recovery phase following myocardial infarction.

WARNINGS

Tardive dyskinesia, a syndrome consisting of potentially irreversible, involuntary, dyskinetic movements, may develop in patients treated with neuroleptic (antipsychotic) drugs. Although the prevalence of the syndrome appears to be highest among the elderly, especially elderly women, it is impossible to rely upon prevalence estimates to predict, at the inception of neuroleptic treatment, which patients are likely to develop the syndrome. Whether neuroleptic drug products differ in their potential to cause tardive dyskinesia is unknown.
Both the risk of developing the syndrome and the likelihood that it will become irreversible are believed to increase as the duration of treatment and the total cumulative dose of neuroleptic drugs administered to the patient increase. However, the syndrome can develop, although much less commonly, after relatively brief treatment periods at low doses.
There is no known treatment for established cases of tardive dyskinesia, although the syndrome may remit, partially or completely, if neuroleptic treatment is withdrawn. Neuroleptic treatment itself, however, may suppress (or partially suppress) the signs and symptoms of the syndrome, and thereby may possibly mask the underlying disease process. The effect that symptomatic suppression has upon the long-term course of the syndrome is unknown.
Given these considerations, neuroleptics should be prescribed in a manner that is most likely to minimize the occurrence of tardive dyskinesia. Chronic neuroleptic treatment should generally be reserved for patients who suffer from a chronic illness that, 1) is known to respond to neuroleptic drugs, and, 2) for whom alternative, equally effective, but potentially less harmful treatments are not available or appropriate. In patients who do require chronic treatment, the smallest dose and the shortest duration of treatment producing a satisfactory clinical response should be sought. The need for continued treatment should be reassessed periodically.
If signs and symptoms of tardive dyskinesia appear in a patient on neuroleptics, drug discontinuation should be considered. However, some patients may require treatment despite the presence of the syndrome.
(For further information about the description of tardive dyskinesia and its clinical detection, please refer to **Information for Patients** and **Adverse Reactions.**)
Patients with cardiovascular disorders should be watched closely. Tricyclic antidepressant drugs, including amitriptyline hydrochloride, particularly when given in high doses, have been reported to produce arrhythmias, sinus tachycardia, and prolongation of the conduction time. Myocardial infarction and stroke have been reported with drugs of this class.
ETRAFON should not be given concomitantly with guanethidine or similarly acting compounds, since amitriptyline, like other tricyclic antidepressants, may block the antihypertensive effect of these compounds.
If hypotension develops, epinephrine should not be administered, since its action is blocked and partially reversed by perphenazine. If a vasopressor is needed, norepinephrine may be used. Severe, acute hypotension has occurred with the use of phenothiazines and is particularly likely to occur in patients with mitral insufficiency or pheochromocytoma. Rebound hypertension may occur in pheochromocytoma patients.
Perphenazine can lower the convulsive threshold in susceptible individuals; it should be used with caution in alcohol withdrawal and in patients with convulsive disorders. If the patient is being treated with an anticonvulsant agent, increased dosage of that agent may be required when ETRAFON Tablets are used concomitantly.
Because of the anticholinergic activity of amitriptyline hydrochloride, ETRAFON should be used with caution in patients with glaucoma, increased intraocular pressure, and those in whom urinary retention is present or anticipated. In patients with angle-closure glaucoma, even average doses may precipitate an attack.
Close supervision is required when amitriptyline hydrochloride is given to hyperthyroid patients or those receiving thyroid medication.
ETRAFON Tablets may impair the mental and/or physical abilities required for the performance of potentially hazardous tasks, such as driving a car or operating machinery, the patient should be warned accordingly.
Usage in Children: Since a dosage for children has not been established, ETRAFON is not recommended for use in children.
Usage in Pregnancy: Safe use of ETRAFON Tablets during pregnancy and lactation has not been established; therefore, in administering the drug to pregnant patients, nursing mothers, or women who may become pregnant, the possible benefits must be weighed against the possible hazards to mother and child.

PRECAUTIONS

The possibility of suicide in depressed patients remains during treatment and until significant remission occurs. This type of patient should not have access to large quantities of this drug.

Perphenazine

As with all phenothiazine compounds, perphenazine should not be used indiscriminately. Caution should be observed in giving it to patients who have previously exhibited severe adverse reactions to other phenothiazines. Some of the untoward actions of perphenazine tend to appear more frequently when high doses are used. However, as with other phenothiazine compounds, patients receiving perphenazine in any dosage should be kept under close supervision.
Neuroleptic drugs elevate prolactin levels; the elevation persists during chronic administration. Tissue culture experiments indicate that approximately one-third of human breast cancers are prolactin dependent *in vitro*, a factor of potential importance if the prescription of these drugs is contemplated in a patient with a previously detected breast cancer. Although disturbances such as galactorrhea, amenorrhea, gynecomastia, and impotence have been reported, the clinical significance of elevated serum prolactin levels is unknown for most patients. An increase in mammary neoplasms has been found in rodents after chronic administration of neuroleptic drugs. Neither clinical studies nor epidemiologic studies conducted to date, however, have shown an association between chronic administration of these drugs and mammary tumorigenesis; the available evidence is considered too limited to be conclusive at this time.
The antiemetic effect of perphenazine may obscure signs of toxicity due to overdosage of other drugs, or render more difficult the diagnosis of disorders such as brain tumors or intestinal obstruction.
A significant, not otherwise explained, rise in body temperature may suggest individual intolerance to perphenazine, in which case ETRAFON should be discontinued.
Patients on large doses of a phenothiazine drug who are undergoing surgery should be watched carefully for possible hypotensive phenomena. Moreover, reduced amounts of anesthetics or central nervous system depressants may be necessary.
Since phenothiazines and central nervous system depressants (opiates, analgesics, antihistamines, barbiturates) can potentiate each other, less than the usual dosage of the added drug is recommended, and caution is advised, when they are administered concomitantly.
Use with caution in patients who are receiving atropine or related drugs because of additive anticholinergic effects and also in patients who will be exposed to extreme heat or organic phosphate insecticides.
The use of alcohol should be avoided, since additive effects and hypotension may occur. Patients should be cautioned that their response to alcohol may be increased while they are being treated with ETRAFON Tablets. The risk of suicide and the danger of overdose may be increased in patients who use alcohol excessively due to its potentiation of the drug's effect.
Blood counts and hepatic and renal functions should be checked periodically. The appearance of signs of blood dyscrasias requires the discontinuance of the drug and institution of appropriate therapy. If abnormalities in hepatic tests occur, phenothiazine treatment should be discontinued. Renal function in patients on long-term therapy should be monitored; if blood urea nitrogen (BUN) becomes abnormal, treatment with the drug should be discontinued.
The use of phenothiazine derivatives in patients with diminished renal function should be undertaken with caution.
Use with caution in patients suffering from respiratory impairment due to acute pulmonary infections, or in chronic respiratory disorders such as severe asthma or emphysema.
In general, phenothiazines do not produce psychic dependence. Gastritis, nausea and vomiting, dizziness, and tremulousness have been reported following abrupt cessation of high-dose therapy. Reports suggest that these symptoms can be reduced by continuing concomitant antiparkinson agents for several weeks after the phenothiazine is withdrawn.
The possibility of liver damage, corneal and lenticular deposits, and irreversible dyskinesias should be kept in mind when patients are on long-term therapy.
Because photosensitivity has been reported, undue exposure to the sun should be avoided during phenothiazine treatment.
Information for Patients: This information is intended to aid in the safe and effective use of this medication. It is not a disclosure of all possible adverse or intended effects.
Given the likelihood that a substantial proportion of patients exposed chronically to neuroleptics will develop tardive dyskinesia, it is advised that all patients in whom chronic use is contemplated be given, if possible, full information about this risk. The decision to inform patients and/or their guardians must obviously take into account the clinical circumstances and the competency of the patients to understand the information provided.

Amitriptyline Hydrochloride

In manic-depressive psychosis, depressed patients may experience a shift toward the manic phase if they are treated with an antidepressant drug. Patients with paranoid symptomatology may have an exaggeration of such symptoms. The tranquilizing effect of ETRAFON has seemed to reduce the likelihood of this effect.
When amitriptyline hydrochloride is given with anticholinergic agents or sympathomimetic drugs, including epinephrine combined with local anesthetics, close supervision and careful adjustment of dosages are required.
Paralytic ileus may occur in patients taking tricyclic antidepressants in combination with anticholinergic-type drugs.
Concurrent use of large doses of ethchlorvynol should be used with caution, since transient delirium has been reported in patients receiving this drug in combination with amitriptyline hydrochloride.
This drug may enhance the response to alcohol and the effects of barbiturates and other CNS depressants.
Concurrent administration of amitriptyline hydrochloride and electroshock therapy may increase the hazards of therapy. Such treatment should be limited to patients for whom it is essential.
Discontinue the drug several days before elective surgery, if possible.
Both elevation and lowering of blood sugar levels have been reported.
The usefulness of amitriptyline in the treatment of depression has been amply demonstrated; however, it should be realized that abuse of amitriptyline among a narcotic-dependent population is not uncommon.
Concurrent administration of cimetidine and tricyclic antidepressants can produce clinically significant increases in the plasma concentrations of the tricyclic antidepressant. Serious anticholinergic symptoms (severe dry mouth, urinary retention, blurred vision) have been associated with elevations in the serum levels of the tricyclic antidepressant when cimetidine is added to the drug regimen. Additionally, higher than expected steady-state serum concentrations of the tricyclic antidepressant have been observed when therapy is initiated in patients taking cimetidine.
Alternatively, decreases in the steady-state serum concentration of the tricyclic antidepressant have been reported in well-controlled patients on concurrent therapy upon discontinuance of cimetidine. The therapeutic efficacy of the tricyclic antidepressant may be compromised in these patients as the cimetidine is discontinued.

ADVERSE REACTIONS

Adverse reactions to ETRAFON Tablets are the same as those to its components, perphenazine and amitriptyline hydrochloride. There have been no reports of effects peculiar to the combination of these components in ETRAFON Tablets.

Perphenazine

Not all of the following adverse reactions have been reported with perphenazine; however, pharmacological similarities among various phenothiazine derivatives require that each be considered. With the piperazine group (of which perphenazine is an example), the extrapyramidal symptoms are more common, and others (e.g., sedative effects, jaundice, and blood dyscrasias) are less frequently seen.
CNS Effects: *Extrapyramidal reactions:* opisthotonus, trismus, torticollis, retrocollis, aching and numbness of the limbs, motor restlessness, oculogyric crisis, hyperreflexia, dystonia, including protrusion, discoloration, aching and rounding of the tongue, tonic spasm of the masticatory muscles, tight feeling in the throat, slurred speech, dysphagia, akathisia, dyskinesia, parkinsonism, and ataxia. Their incidence and severity usually increase with an increase in dosage, but there is considerable individual variation in the tendency to develop such symptoms. Extrapyramidal symptoms can usually be controlled by the concomitant use of effective antiparkinsonian drugs, such as benztropine mesylate, and/or by reduction in dosage.
In some instances, however, these extrapyramidal reactions may persist after discontinuation of treatment with perphenazine.
Persistent tardive dyskinesia: As with all antipsychotic agents, tardive dyskinesia may appear in some patients on long-term therapy or may appear after drug therapy has been discontinued. Although the risk appears to be greater in elderly patients on high-dose therapy, especially females it may occur in either sex and in children. The symptoms are persistent and in some patients appear to be irreversible. The syndrome is characterized by rhythmical, involuntary movements of the tongue, face, mouth or jaw (eg, protrusion of tongue, puffing of cheeks, puckering of mouth, chewing

Continued on next page

Information on Schering products appearing on these pages is effective as of September 30, 1986.

Schering—Cont.

movements). Sometimes these may be accompanied by involuntary movements of the extremities. There is no known effective treatment for tardive dyskinesia; antiparkinsonism agents usually do not alleviate the symptoms of this syndrome. It is suggested that all antipsychotic agents be discontinued if these symptoms appear. Should it be necessary to reinstitute treatment, or increase the dosage of the agent, or switch to a different antipsychotic agent, the syndrome may be masked. It has been reported that fine, vermicular movements of the tongue may be an early sign of the syndrome, and if the medication is stopped at that time the syndrome may not develop.

Other CNS effects include cerebral edema; abnormality of cerebrospinal fluid proteins; convulsive seizures, particularly in patients with EEG abnormalities or a history of such disorders; and headaches.

Neuroleptic malignant syndrome has been reported in patients treated with neuroleptic drugs. It is a relatively uncommon, potentially lethal syndrome, characterized by severe extrapyramidal dysfunction, with rigidity and eventual stupor or coma; hyperthermia; and autonomic disturbances, including cardiovascular effects. There is no specific treatment; the neuroleptic drug should be stopped immediately.

Drowsiness may occur, particularly during the first or second week, after which it generally disappears. If troublesome, lower the dosage. Hypnotic effects appear to be minimal, especially in patients who are permitted to remain active.

Adverse behavioral effects include paradoxical exacerbation of psychotic symptoms, catatonic-like states, paranoid reactions, lethargy, paradoxical excitement, restlessness, hyperactivity, nocturnal confusion, bizarre dreams, and insomnia. Hyperreflexia has been reported in the newborn when a phenothiazine was used during pregnancy.

Autonomic Effects: dry mouth or salivation, nausea, vomiting, diarrhea, anorexia, constipation, obstipation, fecal impaction, urinary retention, frequency or incontinence, polyuria, bladder paralysis, nasal congestion, pallor, myosis, mydriasis, blurred vision, glaucoma, perspiration, hypertension, hypotension, and a change in pulse rate occasionally may occur. Significant autonomic effects have been infrequent in patients receiving less than 24 mg perphenazine daily.

Adynamic ileus occasionally occurs with phenothiazine therapy and if severe can result in complications and death. It is of particular concern in psychiatric patients, who may fail to seek treatment of the condition.

Allergic Effects: urticaria, erythema, eczema, exfoliative dermatitis, pruritus, photosensitivity, asthma, fever, anaphylactoid reactions, laryngeal edema, and angioneurotic edema; contact dermatitis in nursing personnel administering the drug; and in extremely rare instances, individual idiosyncrasy or hypersensitivity to phenothiazines has resulted in cerebral edema, circulatory collapse, and death.

Endocrine Effects: lactation, galactorrhea, moderate breast enlargement in females and gynecomastia in males on large doses, disturbances in the menstrual cycle, amenorrhea, changes in libido, inhibition of ejaculation, false positive pregnancy tests, hyperglycemia, hypoglycemia, glycosuria, syndrome of inappropriate ADH (antidiuretic hormone) secretion.

Cardiovascular Effects: Postural hypotension, tachycardia (especially with sudden marked increase in dosage), bradycardia, cardiac arrest, faintness, and dizziness. Occasionally the hypotensive effect may produce a shock-like condition. ECG changes, nonspecific, (quinidine-like effect) usually reversible, have been observed in some patients receiving phenothiazine tranquilizers.

Sudden death has occasionally been reported in patients who have received phenothiazines. In some cases the death was apparently due to cardiac arrest; in others the cause appeared to be asphyxia due to failure of the cough reflex. In some patients, the cause could not be determined nor could it be established that the death was due to the phenothiazine.

Hematological Effects: agranulocytosis, eosinophilia, leukopenia, hemolytic anemia, thrombocytopenic purpura, and pancytopenia. Most cases of agranulocytosis have occurred between the fourth and tenth weeks of therapy. Patients should be watched closely especially during that period for the sudden appearance of sore throat or signs of infection. If white blood cell and differential cell counts show significant cellular depression, discontinue the drug and start appropriate therapy. However, a slightly lowered white count is not in itself an indication to discontinue the drug.

Other Effects: Special considerations in long-term therapy include pigmentation of the skin, occurring chiefly in the exposed areas; ocular changes consisting of deposition of fine particulate matter in the cornea and lens, progressing in more severe cases to star-shaped lenticular opacities; epithelial keratopathies; and pigmentary retinopathy. Also noted: peripheral edema, reversed epinephrine effect, increase in PBI not attributable to an increase in thyroxine, parotid swelling (rare), hyperpyrexia, systemic lupus erythematosus-like syndrome, increases in appetite and weight, polyphagia, photophobia, and muscle weakness.

Liver damage (biliary stasis) may occur. Jaundice may occur, usually between the second and fourth weeks of treatment, and is regarded as a hypersensitivity reaction. Incidence is low. The clinical picture resembles infectious hepatitis but with laboratory features of obstructive jaundice. It is usually reversible; however, chronic jaundice has been reported.

Amitriptyline Hydrochloride

Although activation of latent schizophrenia has been reported with antidepressant drugs, including amitriptyline hydrochloride, it may be prevented with ETRAFON Tablets in some cases because of the antipsychotic effect of perphenazine. A few instances of epileptiform seizures have been reported in chronic schizophrenic patients during treatment with amitriptyline hydrochloride.

Note: Included in the listing which follows are a few adverse reactions which have not been reported with this specific drug. However, pharmacological similarities among the tricyclic antidepressant drugs require that each of the reactions be considered when amitriptyline hydrochloride is administered.

Allergic: Rash, pruritus, urticaria, photosensitization, edema of face and tongue.

Anticholinergic: Dry mouth, blurred vision, disturbance of accommodation, constipation, paralytic ileus, urinary retention, dilatation of urinary tract.

Cardiovascular: Hypotension, hypertension, tachycardia, palpitations, myocardial infarction, arrhythmias, heart block, stroke.

CNS and Neuromuscular: Confusional states, disturbed concentration, disorientation, delusions, hallucinations, excitement, jitteriness, anxiety, restlessness, insomnia, nightmares, numbness, tingling, and paresthesias of the extremities, peripheral neuropathy, incoordination, ataxia, tremors, seizures, alteration in EEG patterns, extrapyramidal symptoms, tinnitus.

Endocrine: Testicular swelling and gynecomastia in the male, breast enlargement and galactorrhea in the female, increased or decreased libido, elevation and lowering of blood sugar levels, syndrome of inappropriate ADH (antidiuretic hormone secretion).

Gastrointestinal: Nausea, epigastric distress, heartburn, vomiting, anorexia, stomatitis, peculiar taste, diarrhea, jaundice, parotid swelling, black tongue. Rarely hepatitis has occurred (including altered liver function and jaundice).

Hematologic: Bone marrow depression including agranulocytosis, leukopenia, eosinophilia, purpura, thrombocytopenia.

Other: Dizziness, weakness, fatigue, headache, weight gain or loss, increased perspiration, urinary frequency, mydriasis, drowsiness, alopecia.

Withdrawal Symptoms: Abrupt cessation of treatment after prolonged administration may produce nausea, headache, and malaise. These are not indicative of addiction.

DOSAGE AND ADMINISTRATION

Initial Dosage

In psychoneurotic patients whose anxiety and depression warrant combined therapy, one ETRAFON Tablet (2–25) or one ETRAFON-FORTE Tablet (4–25) three or four times a day is recommended.

In elderly patients, adolescents and other patients as indicated, one ETRAFON-A Tablet (4–10) may be administered three or four times a day as initial dosage. This dosage may be adjusted as required to produce an adequate response.

In more severely ill patients with schizophrenia, two ETRAFON-FORTE Tablets (4–25) three times a day are recommended as the initial dosage. If necessary, a fourth dose may be given at bedtime. The total daily dosage should not exceed eight tablets of any strength.

Maintenance Dosage

Depending on the condition being treated, the onset of therapeutic response may vary from a few days to a few weeks or even longer. After a satisfactory response is noted, dosage should be reduced to the smallest dose which is effective for relief of the symptoms for which ETRAFON Tablets are being administered. A useful maintenance dosage is one ETRAFON Tablet (2–25) or one ETRAFON-FORTE Tablet (4–25) two to four times a day. In some patients, maintenance dosage is required for many months.

ETRAFON 2–10 Tablets (2–10) and ETRAFON-A Tablets (4–10) can be used to increase flexibility in adjusting maintenance dosage to the lowest amount consistent with relief of symptoms.

OVERDOSAGE

In the event of overdosage, emergency treatment should be started immediately. All patients suspected of having taken an overdose should be hospitalized as soon as possible.

Manifestations: Overdosage of perphenazine primarily involves the extrapyramidal mechanism and produces the same side effects described under ADVERSE REACTIONS, but to a more marked degree. It is usually evidenced by stupor or coma; children may have convulsive seizures.

High doses of ETRAFON Tablets may cause temporary confusion, disturbed concentration, or transient visual hallucinations. Overdosage may cause drowsiness; hypothermia; tachycardia and other arrhythmic abnormalities—for example, bundle branch block; ECG evidence of impaired conduction; congestive heart failure; dilated pupils; convulsions; severe hypotension; stupor; and coma. Other symptoms may be agitation, hyperactive reflexes, muscle rigidity, vomiting, hyperpyrexia, or any of the adverse reactions listed for perphenazine or amitriptyline hydrochloride.

Overdosage with tricyclic antidepressants (TCAs), such as imipramine, doxepin, or amitriptyline may result in plasma TCA levels of 1,000 ng/ml or higher. Such levels more accurately define patients who are at risk for major medical complications of overdosage than does the amount of drug ingested based on patient history. In one study, all patients with TCA levels of this magnitude had a QRS duration of 100 msec or more on a routine ECG within the first 24 hours following overdose.

In the absence of TCA blood level determinations, a QRS of 100 msec or more suggests a greater likelihood of serious complications.

Oculomotor paresis (loss of conjugate movement in the so-called doll's eyes maneuver) as a manifestation of amitriptyline overdosage has been reported as being significant in the differential diagnosis of a patient in light coma.

Treatment: Treatment is symptomatic and supportive. There is no specific antidote. The patient should be induced to vomit even if emesis has occurred spontaneously. Pharmacologic vomiting by the administration of ipecac syrup is a preferred method. It should be noted that ipecac has a central mode of action in addition to its local gastric irritant properties, and the central mode of action may be blocked by the antiemetic effect of ETRAFON Tablets. Vomiting should not be induced in patients with impaired consciousness. The action of ipecac is facilitated by physical activity and by the administration of 8 to 12 fluid ounces of water. If emesis does not occur within 15 minutes, the dose of ipecac should be repeated. Precautions against aspiration must be taken, especially in infants and children. Following emesis, any drug remaining in the stomach may be adsorbed by activated charcoal administered as a slurry with water. If vomiting is unsuccessful or contraindicated, gastric lavage should be performed. Isotonic and one-half isotonic saline are the lavage solutions of choice. Saline cathartics, such as milk of magnesia, draw water into the bowel by osmosis and therefore may be valuable for their action in rapid dilution of bowel content.

Standard measures (oxygen, intravenous fluids, corticosteroids) should be used to manage circulatory shock or metabolic acidosis. An open airway and adequate fluid intake should be maintained. Body temperature should be regulated. Hypothermia is expected, but severe hyperthermia may occur and must be treated vigorously. (See CONTRAINDICATIONS.)

An electrocardiogram should be taken and close monitoring of cardiac function instituted if there is any sign of abnormality. Cardiac arrhythmias may be treated with neostigmine, pyridostigmine, or propranolol. Digitalis should be considered for cardiac failure. Close monitoring of cardiac function is advisable for not less than five days.

Vasopressors such as norepinephrine may be used to treat hypotension, but epinephrine should NOT be used.

The intravenous administration of 1 to 3 mg physostigmine salicylate has been reported to reverse the symptoms of tricyclic antidepressant poisoning and therefore, should be considered in the symptomatic treatment of the central anticholinergic effects due to overdosage with ETRAFON Tablets. Because physostigmine is rapidly metabolized, it should be re-administered as required, especially if life-threatening signs, such as arrhythmias, convulsions, or deep coma recur or persist.

Anticonvulsants (an inhalation anesthetic, diazepam, or paraldehyde) are recommended for control of convulsions, since perphenazine increases the central nervous system depressant action, but not the anticonvulsant action of barbiturates.

If acute parkinson-like symptoms result from perphenazine intoxication, benztropine mesylate or diphenhydramine may be administered.

Central nervous system depression may be treated with nonconvulsant doses of CNS stimulants. Avoid stimulants that may cause convulsions (e.g., picrotoxin and pentylenetetrazol).

Signs of arousal may not occur for 48 hours.

Dialysis is of no value because of low plasma concentrations of the drug.

Since overdosage is often deliberate, patients may attempt suicide by other means during the recovery phase. Deaths by deliberate or accidental overdosage have occurred with this class of drugs.

HOW SUPPLIED

ETRAFON 2–10 Tablets (perphenazine 2 mg and amitriptyline hydrochloride 10 mg): deep yellow, sugar-coated tablets branded in blue-black with the Schering trademark and ei-

ther product identification letters, ANA, or number, 287; bottles of 100 (NDC 0085-0287-04) and 500 (NDC 0085-0287-07) and box of 100 for unit-dose dispensing (10 strips of 10 tablets each) (NDC 0085-0287-08).
ETRAFON Tablets (perphenazine 2 mg and amitriptyline hydrochloride 25 mg): pink, sugar-coated tablets branded in red with the Schering trademark and either product identification letters, ANC or number, 598; bottles of 100 (NDC 0085-0598-04) and 500 (NDC 0085-0598-07) and box of 100 for unit-dose dispensing (10 strips of 10 tablets each) (NDC 0085-0598-08).
ETRAFON-A Tablets (perphenazine 4 mg and amitriptyline hydrochloride 10 mg): orange, sugar-coated tablets branded in blue-black with the Schering trademark and either product identification letters, ANB, or number, 119; bottles of 100 (NDC 0085-0119-04) and 500 (NDC 0085-0119-07) and box of 100 for unit-dose dispensing (10 strips of 10 tablets each) (NDC 0085-0119-08).
ETRAFON-FORTE Tablets (perphenazine 4 mg and amitriptyline hydrochloride 25 mg): red, sugar-coated tablets branded in blue with the Schering trademark and either product identification letters, ANE, or number, 720; bottles of 100 (NDC 0085-0720-04) and 500 (NDC 0085-0720-07) and box of 100 for unit-dose dispensing (10 strips of 10 tablets each) (NDC 0085-0720-08).
Store ETRAFON 2-10, 4-10, 2-25 and 4-25 Tablets between 2° and 30°C (36° and 86°F). In addition, protect unit-dose packages from excessive moisture.
Revised 9/86

Shown in Product Identification Section, page 428

FULVICIN® P/G ℞

[ful 'vĭ-sin]
brand of ultramicrosize griseofulvin, USP
Tablets

DESCRIPTION

FULVICIN P/G Tablets contain ultramicrosize crystals of griseofulvin, an antibiotic derived from a species of *Penicillium.* Griseofulvin crystals are partly dissolved in polyethylene glycol 6000 and partly dispersed throughout the tablet matrix.
Each FULVICIN P/G Tablet contains 125 mg or 250 mg griseofulvin ultramicrosize.

ACTIONS

Microbiology Griseofulvin is fungistatic with *in vitro* activity against various species of *Microsporum, Epidermophyton,* and *Trichophyton.* It has no effect on bacteria or on other genera of fungi.
Human Pharmacology: Following oral administration, griseofulvin is deposited in the keratin precursor cells and has a greater affinity for diseased tissue. The drug is tightly bound to the new keratin which becomes highly resistant to fungal invasions.
The efficiency of gastrointestinal absorption of ultramicrocrystalline griseofulvin is approximately one and one-half times that of the conventional microsized griseofulvin. This factor permits the oral intake of two-thirds as much ultramicrocrystalline griseofulvin as the microsize form. However, there is currently no evidence that this lower dose confers any significant clinical differences with regard to safety and/or efficacy.

INDICATIONS

FULVICIN P/G Tablets are indicated for the treatment of ringworm infections of the skin, hair, and nails, namely: tinea corporis, tinea pedis, tinea cruris, tinea barbae, tinea capitis, tinea unguium (onychomycosis) when caused by one or more of the following genera of fungi: *Trichophyton rubrum, Trichophyton tonsurans, Trichophyton mentagrophytes, Trichophyton interdigitale, Trichophyton verrucosum, Trichophyton megninii, Trichophyton gallinae, Trichophyton crateriforme, Trichophyton sulphureum, Trichophyton schoenleinii, Microsporum audouinii, Microsporum canis, Microsporum gypseum,* and *Epidermophyton floccosum.*
Note: Prior to therapy, the type of fungi responsible for the infection should be identified.
The use of this drug is not justified in minor or trivial infections which will respond to topical agents alone.
Griseofulvin is not effective in the following: bacterial infections, candidiasis (moniliasis), histoplasmosis, actinomycosis, sporotrichosis, chromoblastomycosis, coccidioidomycosis, North American blastomycosis, cryptococcosis (torulosis), tinea versicolor, and nocardiosis.

CONTRAINDICATIONS

This drug is contraindicated in patients with porphyria, hepatocellular failure, and in individuals with a history of hypersensitivity to griseofulvin.

WARNINGS

Prophylactic Usage: Safety and efficacy of griseofulvin for prophylaxis of fungal infections have not been established.
Animal Toxicology: Chronic feeding of griseofulvin, at levels ranging from 0.5–2.5% of the diet, resulted in the development of liver tumors in several strains of mice, particularly in males. Smaller particle sizes result in an enhanced effect. Lower oral dosage levels have not been tested. Subcutaneous administration of relatively small doses of griseofulvin once a week during the first three weeks of life has also been reported to induce hepatomata in mice. Thyroid tumors, mostly adenomas but some carcinomas, have been reported in male rats receiving griseofulvin at levels of 2.0%, 1.0%, and 0.2% of the diet, and in female rats receiving the two higher dose levels. Although studies in other animal species have not yielded evidence of tumorigenicity, these studies were not of adequate design to form a basis for conclusions in this regard.
In subacute toxicity studies, orally administered griseofulvin produced hepatocellular necrosis in mice, but this has not been seen in other species. Disturbances in porphyrin metabolism have been reported in griseofulvin-treated laboratory animals. Griseofulvin has been reported to have a colchicine-like effect on mitosis and cocarcinogenicity with methylcholanthrene in cutaneous tumor induction in laboratory animals.
Usage in Pregnancy: The safety of this drug during pregnancy has not been established.
Animal Reproduction Studies: It has been reported in the literature that griseofulvin was found to be embryotoxic and teratogenic on oral administration to pregnant rats. Pups with abnormalities have been reported in the litters of a few bitches treated with griseofulvin.
Suppression of spermatogenesis has been reported to occur in rats, but investigation in man failed to confirm this.

PRECAUTIONS

Patients on prolonged therapy with any potent medication should be under close observation. Periodic monitoring of organ system function, including renal, hepatic, and hematopoietic, should be done.
Since griseofulvin is derived from species of *Penicillium,* the possibility of cross-sensitivity with penicillin exists; however, known penicillin-sensitive patients have been treated without difficulty.
Since a photosensitivity reaction is occasionally associated with griseofulvin therapy, patients should be warned to avoid exposure to intense natural or artificial sunlight.
Lupus erythematosus or lupus-like syndromes have been reported in patients receiving griseofulvin.
Griseofulvin decreases the activity of warfarin-type anticoagulants so that patients receiving these drugs concomitantly may require dosage adjustment of the anticoagulant during and after griseofulvin therapy.
Barbiturates usually depress griseofulvin activity, and concomitant administration may require a dosage adjustment of the antifungal agent.
The effects of alcohol may be potentiated by griseofulvin, producing such effects as tachycardia and flush.

ADVERSE REACTIONS

When adverse reactions occur, they are most commonly of the hypersensitivity type, such as skin rashes, urticaria, and rarely, angioneurotic edema, and may necessitate withdrawal of therapy and appropriate countermeasures. Paresthesias of the hands and feet have been reported rarely after extended therapy. Other side effects reported occasionally are oral thrush, nausea, vomiting, epigastric distress, diarrhea, headache, fatigue, dizziness, insomnia, mental confusion, and impairment of performance of routine activities.
Proteinuria and leukopenia have been reported rarely. Administration of the drug should be discontinued if granulocytopenia occurs.
When rare, serious reactions occur with griseofulvin, they are usually associated with high dosages, long periods of therapy, or both.

DOSAGE AND ADMINISTRATION

Accurate diagnosis of the infecting organism is essential. Identification should be made either by direct microscopic examination of a mounting of infected tissue in a solution of potassium hydroxide or by culture on an appropriate medium.
Medication must be continued until the infecting organism is completely eradicated as indicated by appropriate clinical or laboratory examination. Representative treatment periods are tinea capitis, 4 to 6 weeks; tinea corporis, 2 to 4 weeks; tinea pedis, 4 to 8 weeks; tinea unguium—depending on rate of growth—fingernails, at least 4 months; toenails, at least 6 months.
General measures in regard to hygiene should be observed to control sources of infection or reinfection. Concomitant use of appropriate topical agents is usually required particularly in treatment of tinea pedis. In some forms of athlete's foot, yeasts and bacteria may be involved as well as fungi. Griseofulvin will not eradicate the bacterial or monilial infection.
Adults: Daily administration of 375 mg (as a single dose or in divided amounts) will give a satisfactory response in most patients with tinea corporis, tinea cruris, and tinea capitis. For those fungus infections more difficult to eradicate, such as tinea pedis and tinea unguium, a divided daily dose of 750 mg is recommended.
Children: Approximately 3.3 mg per pound of body weight per day of ultramicrosize griseofulvin is an effective dose for most children. On this basis, the following dosage schedule is suggested: Children weighing 35 to 60 pounds—125 mg to 187.5 mg daily. Children weighing over 60 pounds—187.5 mg to 375 mg daily.
Children 2 years of age and younger—dosage has not been established.
Clinical experience with griseofulvin in children with tinea capitis indicates that a single daily dose is effective. Clinical relapse will occur if the medication is not continued until the infecting organism is eradicated.

HOW SUPPLIED

FULVICIN P/G Tablets, 125 mg, white, compressed, scored tablets impressed with the Schering trademark and product identification numbers, 228; bottle of 100.
FULVICIN P/G Tablets, 250 mg, white, compressed, scored tablets impressed with the Schering trademark and product identification numbers, 507; bottle of 100.
Store at controlled room temperature 59°F to 86°F (15°C to 30°C).
Revised 2/82

Shown in Product Identification Section, page 428

FULVICIN® P/G 165 and 330 ℞

[ful 'vĭ-sin]
brand of ultramicrosize griseofulvin
Tablets, USP

DESCRIPTION

FULVICIN P/G Tablets contain ultramicrosize crystals of griseofulvin, an antibiotic derived from a species of *Penicillium.* Griseofulvin crystals are partly dissolved in polyethylene glycol 8000 and partly dispersed throughout the tablet matrix.
Each FULVICIN P/G Tablet contains 165 mg or 330 mg ultramicrosize griscofulvin, USP.

ACTIONS

Microbiology: Griseofulvin is fungistatic with *in vitro* activity against various species of *Microsporum, Epidermophyton,* and *Trichophyton.* It has no effect on bacteria or on other genera of fungi.
Human Pharmacology: Following oral administration, griseofulvin is deposited in the keratin precursor cells and has a greater affinity for diseased tissue. The drug is tightly bound to the new keratin which becomes highly resistant to fungal invasions.
The efficiency of gastrointestinal absorption of ultramicrocrystalline griseofulvin is approximately one and one-half times that of the conventional microsize griseofulvin. This factor permits the oral intake of two-thirds as much ultramicrocrystalline griseofulvin as the microsize form. However, there is currently no evidence that this lower dose confers any significant clinical differences with regard to safety and/or efficacy.

INDICATIONS

FULVICIN P/G Tablets are indicated for the treatment of ringworm infections of the skin, hair, and nails, namely: tinea corporis, tinea pedis, tinea cruris, tinea barbae, tinea capitis, tinea unguium (onychomycosis) when caused by one or more of the following genera of fungi: *Trichophyton rubrum, Trichophyton tonsurans, Trichophyton mentagrophytes, Trichophyton interdigitale, Trichophyton verrucosum, Trichophyton megninii, Trichophyton gallinae, Trichophyton crateriforme, Trichophyton sulphureum, Trichophyton schoenleinii, Microsporum audouinii, Microsporum canis, Microsporum gypseum,* and *Epidermophyton floccosum.*
Note: Prior to therapy, the type of fungi responsible for the infection should be identified.
The use of this drug is not justified in minor or trivial infections which will respond to topical agents alone.
Griseofulvin is not effective in the following: bacterial infections, candidiasis (moniliasis), histoplasmosis, actinomycosis, sporotrichosis, chromoblastomycosis, coccidioidomycosis, North American blastomycosis, cryptococcosis (torulosis), tinea versicolor, and nocardiosis.

CONTRAINDICATIONS

This drug is contraindicated in patients with porphyria, hepatocellular failure, and in individuals with a history of hypersensitivity to griseofulvin.

Continued on next page

Information on Schering products appearing on these pages is effective as of September 30, 1986.

Schering—Cont.

WARNINGS

Prophylactic Usage: Safety and efficacy of griseofulvin for prophylaxis of fungal infections have not been established.
Animal Toxicology: Chronic feeding of griseofulvin, at levels ranging from 0.5–2.5% of the diet, resulted in the development of liver tumors in several strains of mice, particularly in males. Smaller particle sizes result in an enhanced effect. Lower oral dosage levels have not been tested. Subcutaneous administration of relatively small doses of griseofulvin once a week during the first three weeks of life has also been reported to induce hepatomata in mice. Thyroid tumors, mostly adenomas but some carcinomas, have been reported in male rats receiving griseofulvin at levels of 2.0%, 1.0%, and 0.2% of the diet, and in female rats receiving the two higher dose levels. Although studies in other animal species have not yielded evidence of tumorigenicity, these studies were not of adequate design to form a basis for conclusions in this regard.
In subacute toxicity studies, orally administered griseofulvin produced hepatocellular necrosis in mice, but this has not been seen in other species. Disturbances in porphyrin metabolism have been reported in griseofulvin-treated laboratory animals. Griseofulvin has been reported to have a colchicine-like effect on mitosis and cocarcinogenicity with methylcholanthrene in cutaneous tumor induction in laboratory animals.
Usage in Pregnancy: The safety of this drug during pregnancy has not been established.
Animal Reproduction Studies: It has been reported in the literature that griseofulvin was found to be embryotoxic and teratogenic on oral administration to pregnant rats. Pups with abnormalities have been reported in the litters of a few bitches treated with griseofulvin.
Suppression of spermatogenesis has been reported to occur in rats, but investigation in man failed to confirm this.

PRECAUTIONS

Patients on prolonged therapy with any potent medication should be under close observation. Periodic monitoring of organ system function, including renal, hepatic, and hematopoietic, should be done.
Since griseofulvin is derived from species of *Penicillium*, the possibility of cross-sensitivity with penicillin exists; however, known penicillin-sensitive patients have been treated without difficulty.
Since a photosensitivity reaction is occasionally associated with griseofulvin therapy, patients should be warned to avoid exposure to intense natural or artificial sunlight.
Lupus erythematosus or lupus-like syndromes have been reported in patients receiving griseofulvin.
Griseofulvin decreases the activity of warfarin-type anticoagulants so that patients receiving these drugs concomitantly may require dosage adjustment of the anticoagulant during and after griseofulvin therapy.
Barbiturates usually depress griseofulvin activity, and concomitant administration may require a dosage adjustment of the antifungal agent.
The effects of alcohol may be potentiated by griseofulvin, producing such effects as tachycardia and flush.

ADVERSE REACTIONS

When adverse reactions occur, they are most commonly of the hypersensitivity type, such as skin rashes, urticaria, and rarely, angioneurotic edema, and may necessitate withdrawal of therapy and appropriate countermeasures. Paresthesias of the hands and feet have been reported rarely after extended therapy. Other side effects reported occasionally are oral thrush, nausea, vomiting, epigastric distress, diarrhea, headache, fatigue, dizziness, insomnia, mental confusion, and impairment of performance of routine activities.
Proteinuria and leukopenia have been reported rarely. Administration of the drug should be discontinued if granulocytopenia occurs.
When rare, serious reactions occur with griseofulvin, they are usually associated with high dosages, long periods of therapy, or both.

DOSAGE AND ADMINISTRATION

Accurate diagnosis of the infecting organism is essential. Identification should be made either by direct microscopic examination of a mounting of infected tissue in a solution of potassium hydroxide or by culture on an appropriate medium.
Medication must be continued until the infecting organism is completely eradicated as indicated by appropriate clinical or laboratory examination. Representative treatment periods are tinea capitis, 4 to 6 weeks, tinea corporis, 2 to 4 weeks, tinea pedis, 4 to 8 weeks, tinea unguium—depending on rate of growth—fingernails, at least 4 months; toenails, at least 6 months.
General measures in regard to hygiene should be observed to control sources of infection or reinfection. Concomitant use of appropriate topical agents is usually required particularly in treatment of tinea pedis. In some forms of athlete's foot, yeasts and bacteria may be involved as well as fungi. Griseofulvin will not eradicate the bacterial or monilial infection.
Adults: Daily administration of 330 mg (as a single dose or in divided amounts) will give a satisfactory response in most patients with tinea corporis, tinea cruris, and tinea capitis. For those fungus infections more difficult to eradicate, such as tinea pedis and tinea unguium, a divided daily dosage of 660 mg is recommended.
Children: Approximately 3.3 mg per pound of body weight per day is an effective dose for most children. On this basis, the following dosage schedule is suggested: Children weighing 30 to 50 pounds—82.5 mg to 165 mg daily. Children weighing over 50 pounds—165 mg to 330 mg daily.
Children 2 years of age and younger—dosage has not been established.
Clinical experience with griseofulvin in children with tinea capitis indicates that a single daily dose is effective. Clinical relapse will occur if the medication is not continued until the infecting organism is eradicated.

HOW SUPPLIED

FULVICIN P/G 165 Tablets, 165 mg, off-white, oval, compressed, scored tablets impressed with the product name (FULVICIN P/G) and product identification numbers, 654; bottle of 100.
FULVICIN P/G 330 Tablets, 330 mg, off-white, oval, compressed, scored tablets impressed with the product name (FULVICIN P/G) and product identification numbers, 352; bottle of 100.
Store between 2° and 30°C (36° and 86°F).
Revised 9/83

Shown in Product Identification Section, page 428

FULVICIN-U/F® ℞

[ful'vĭ-sin]
brand of griseofulvin, USP
Tablets

DESCRIPTION

FULVICIN-U/F Tablets contain microsize crystals of griseofulvin, an antibiotic derived from a species of *Penicillium.*

ACTIONS

Microbiology: Griseofulvin is fungistatic with *in vitro* activity against various species of *Microsporum, Epidermophyton,* and *Trichophyton.* It has no effect on bacteria or on other genera of fungi.
Human Pharmacology: Griseofulvin absorption from the gastrointestinal tract varies considerably among individuals mainly because of insolubility of the drug in aqueous media of the upper G.I. tract. The peak serum level found in fasting adults given 0.5 g occurs at about four hours and ranges between 0.5 to 1.5 mcg/ml. The serum level may be increased by giving the drug with a meal with a high fat content.
Griseofulvin is deposited in the keratin precursor cells and has a greater affinity for diseased tissue. The drug is tightly bound to the new keratin which becomes highly resistant to fungal invasions.

INDICATIONS

FULVICIN-U/F Tablets are indicated for the treatment of ringworm infections of the skin, hair, and nails, namely: tinea corporis, tinea pedis, tinea cruris, tinea barbae, tinea capitis, tinea unguium (onychomycosis) when caused by one or more of the following genera of fungi: *Trichophyton rubrum, Trichophyton tonsurans, Trichophyton mentagrophytes, Trichophyton interdigitale, Trichophyton verrucosum, Trichophyton megninii, Trichophyton gallinae, Trichophyton crateriforme, Trichophyton sulphureum, Trichophyton schoenleinii, Microsporum audouinii, Microsporum canis, Microsporum gypseum,* and *Epidermophyton floccosum.*
Note: Prior to therapy, the type of fungi responsible for the infection should be identified.
The use of this drug is not justified in minor or trivial infections which will respond to topical agents alone.
Griseofulvin is not effective in the following: bacterial infections, candidiasis (moniliasis), histoplasmosis, actinomycosis, sporotrichosis, chromoblastomycosis, coccidioidomycosis, North American blastomycosis, cryptococcosis (torulosis), tinea versicolor, and nocardiosis.

CONTRAINDICATIONS

This drug is contraindicated in patients with porphyria, hepatocellular failure, and in individuals with a history of hypersensitivity to griseofulvin.

WARNINGS

Prophylactic usage: Safety and efficacy of griseofulvin for prophylaxis of fungal infections have not been established.
Animal toxicology: Chronic feeding of griseofulvin, at levels ranging from 0.5-2.5% of the diet, resulted in the development of liver tumors in several strains of mice, particularly in males. Smaller particle sizes result in an enhanced effect. Lower oral dosage levels have not been tested. Subcutaneous administration of relatively small doses of griseofulvin, once a week, during the first three weeks of life has also been reported to induce hepatomata in mice. Thyroid tumors, mostly adenomas but some carcinomas, have been reported in male rats receiving griseofulvin at levels of 2.0%, 1.0%, and 0.2% of the diet, and in female rats receiving the two higher dose levels. Although studies in other animal species have not yielded evidence of tumorigenicity, these studies were not of adequate design to form a basis for conclusions in this regard.
In subacute toxicity studies, orally administered griseofulvin produced hepatocellular necrosis in mice, but this has not been seen in other species. Disturbances in porphyrin metabolism have been reported in griseofulvin-treated laboratory animals. Griseofulvin has been reported to have a colchicine-like effect on mitosis and cocarcinogenicity with methylcholanthrene in cutaneous tumor induction in laboratory animals.
Usage in pregnancy: The safety of this drug during pregnancy has not been established.
Animal reproduction studies: It has been reported in the literature that griseofulvin was found to be embryotoxic and teratogenic on oral administration to pregnant rats. Pups with abnormalities have been reported in the litters of a few bitches treated with griseofulvin.
Suppression of spermatogenesis has been reported to occur in rats, but investigation in man failed to confirm this.

PRECAUTIONS

Patients on prolonged therapy with any potent medication should be under close observation. Periodic monitoring of organ system functions, including renal, hepatic, and hematopoietic, should be done.
Since griseofulvin is derived from species of *Penicillium,* the possibility of cross sensitivity with penicillin exists; however, known penicillin-sensitive patients have been treated without difficulty.
Since a photosensitivity reaction is occasionally associated with griseofulvin therapy, patients should be warned to avoid exposure to intense natural or artificial sunlight.
Lupus erythematosus or lupus-like syndromes have been reported in patients receiving griseofulvin.
Griseofulvin decreases the activity of warfarin-type anticoagulants so that patients receiving these drugs concomitantly may require dosage adjustment of the anticoagulant during and after griseofulvin therapy.
Barbiturates usually depress griseofulvin activity and concomitant administration may require a dosage adjustment of the antifungal agent.
The effects of alcohol may be potentiated by griseofulvin, producing such effects as tachycardia and flush.

ADVERSE REACTIONS

When adverse reactions occur, they are most commonly of the hypersensitivity type, such as skin rashes, urticaria, and rarely, angioneurotic edema, and may necessitate withdrawal of therapy and appropriate countermeasures. Paresthesias of the hands and feet have been reported rarely after extended therapy. Other side effects reported occasionally are oral thrush, nausea, vomiting, epigastric distress, diarrhea, headache, fatigue, dizziness, insomnia, mental confusion, and impairment of performance of routine activities.
Proteinuria and leukopenia have been reported rarely. Administration of the drug should be discontinued if granulocytopenia occurs.
When rare, serious reactions occur with griseofulvin, they are usually associated with high dosages, long periods of therapy, or both.

DOSAGE AND ADMINISTRATION

Accurate diagnosis of the infecting organism is essential. Identification should be made either by direct microscopic examination of a mounting of infected tissue in a solution of potassium hydroxide or by culture on an appropriate medium.
Medication must be continued until the infecting organism is completely eradicated as indicated by appropriate clinical or laboratory examination. Representative treatment periods are for tinea capitis, four to six weeks; tinea corporis, two to four weeks; tinea pedis, four to eight weeks; tinea unguium, depending on the rate of growth, fingernails, at least four months; toenails, at least six months.
General measures in regard to hygiene should be observed to control sources of infection or reinfection. Concomitant use of appropriate topical agents is usually required, particularly in treatment of tinea pedis. In some forms of athlete's foot, yeasts and bacteria may be involved as well as fungi. Griseofulvin will not eradicate the bacterial or monilial infection.
Adults: Daily administration of 500 mg (as a single dose or in divided amounts), will give a satisfactory response in most patients with tinea corporis, tinea cruris, and tinea capitis. For those fungus infections more difficult to eradicate, such as tinea pedis and tinea unguium, daily dosage of 1.0 g is recommended.

Children: Approximately 5 mg per pound of body weight per day is an effective dose for most children. On this basis the following dosage schedule for children is suggested:
Children weighing 30 to 50 pounds—125 mg to 250 mg daily.
Children weighing over 50 pounds—250 mg to 500 mg daily.
Clinical experience with griseofulvin in children with tinea capitis indicates that a single daily dose is effective. Clinical relapse will occur if the medication is not continued until the infecting organism is eradicated.

HOW SUPPLIED

FULVICIN-U/F Tablets, 250 mg: white, compressed, scored tablets impressed with the Schering trademark and product identification letters, AUF, or numbers, 948; bottles of 60 and 250.
FULVICIN-U/F Tablets, 500 mg: white, compressed, scored tablets impressed with the Schering trademark and product identification letters, AUG, or numbers, 496; bottles of 60 and 250.
Store between 2° and 30° C (36° and 86° F).
Revised 8/80

Shown in Product Identification Section, page 428

GARAMYCIN® ℞
[gar-ah-mī'sin]
brand of gentamicin sulfate
Cream, USP 0.1%
Ointment, USP 0.1%
For Dermatologic Use only
Not For Ophthalmic Use

DESCRIPTION

Each gram of GARAMYCIN **Cream** 0.1% contains 1.7 mg gentamicin sulfate, USP equivalent to 1.0 mg gentamicin base, with 1.0 mg methylparaben and 4.0 mg butylparaben as preservatives, in a bland emulsion-type vehicle composed of stearic acid, propylene glycol stearate, isopropyl myristate, propylene glycol, polysorbate 40, sorbitol solution and purified water.
Each gram of GARAMYCIN **Ointment** 0.1% contains 1.7 mg gentamicin sulfate, USP equivalent to 1.0 mg gentamicin base, with 0.5 mg methylparaben and 0.1 mg propylparaben as preservatives in a bland, unctuous petrolatum base.

ACTIONS

GARAMYCIN, a wide-spectrum antibiotic, provides highly effective topical treatment in primary and secondary bacterial infections of the skin. GARAMYCIN may clear infections that have not responded to other topical antibiotic agents. In impetigo contagiosa and other primary skin infections, treatment three or four times daily with GARAMYCIN usually clears the lesions promptly. In secondary skin infections, GARAMYCIN facilitates the treatment of the underlying dermatosis by controlling the infection. Bacteria susceptible to the action of GARAMYCIN include sensitive strains of streptococci (group A beta-hemolytic, alpha-hemolytic), *Staphylococcus aureus* (coagulase-positive, coagulase-negative, and some penicillinase-producing strains), and the gram-negative bacteria, *Pseudomonas aeruginosa, Aerobacter aerogenes, Escherichia coli, Proteus vulgaris,* and *Klebsiella pneumoniae.*

INDICATIONS

Primary skin infections: Impetigo contagiosa, superficial folliculitis, ecthyma, furunculosis, sycosis barbae, and pyoderma gangrenosum. *Secondary skin infections:* Infectious eczematoid dermatitis, pustular acne, pustular psoriasis, infected seborrheic dermatitis, infected contact dermatitis (including poison ivy), infected excoriations, and bacterial superinfections of fungal or viral infections. Note: GARAMYCIN is a bactericidal agent that is not effective against viruses or fungi in skin infections. GARAMYCIN is useful in the treatment of infected skin cysts and certain other skin abscesses when preceded by incision and drainage to permit adequate contact between the antibiotic and the infecting bacteria. Good results have been obtained in the treatment of infected stasis and other skin ulcers, infected superficial burns, paronychia, infected insect bites and stings, infected lacerations and abrasions, and wounds from minor surgery. Patients sensitive to neomycin can be treated with gentamicin, although regular observation of patients sensitive to topical antibiotics is advisable when such patients are treated with any topical antibiotic. GARAMYCIN **Ointment** helps retain moisture and has been useful in infection on dry eczematous or psoriatic skin. GARAMYCIN **Cream** is recommended for wet, oozing primary infections, and greasy, secondary infections, such as pustular acne or infected seborrheic dermatitis. If a water-washable preparation is desired, GARAMYCIN **Cream** is preferable. GARAMYCIN **Ointment** and **Cream** have been used successfully in infants over one year of age as well as in adults and children.

CONTRAINDICATIONS

This drug is contraindicated in individuals with a history of sensitivity reactions to any of its components.

PRECAUTIONS

Use of topical antibiotics occasionally allows overgrowth of nonsusceptible organisms, including fungi. If this occurs, or if irritation, sensitization, or superinfection develops, treatment with gentamicin should be discontinued and appropriate therapy instituted.

ADVERSE REACTIONS

In patients with dermatoses treated with gentamicin, irritation (erythema and pruritus) that did not usually require discontinuance of treatment has been reported in a small percentage of cases. There was no evidence of irritation or sensitization, however, in any of these patients patch-tested subsequently with gentamicin on normal skin. Possible photosensitization has been reported in several patients but could not be elicited in these patients by reapplication of gentamicin followed by exposure to ultraviolet radiation.

DOSAGE AND ADMINISTRATION

A small amount of GARAMYCIN **Cream** or **Ointment** should be applied gently to the lesions three or four times daily. The area treated may be covered with a gauze dressing if desired. In impetigo contagiosa, the crusts should be removed before application of GARAMYCIN to permit maximum contact between the antibiotic and the infection. Care should be exercised to avoid further contamination of the infected skin. Infected stasis ulcers have responded well to GARAMYCIN under gelatin packing.

HOW SUPPLIED

GARAMYCIN **Cream** 0.1% (NDC-0085-0008-05) and GARAMYCIN **Ointment** 0.1% (NDC-0085-0343-05), 15 g tubes.
Store between 2° and 30° C (36° and 86° F).
Rev. 8/85

GARAMYCIN® ℞
[gar-ah-mī'sin]
brand of gentamicin sulfate
Ophthalmic Solution, USP—Sterile
Ophthalmic Ointment, USP—Sterile
Each ml or gram contains gentamicin sulfate, USP equivalent to 3.0 mg gentamicin

DESCRIPTION

Gentamicin sulfate is a water-soluble antibiotic of the aminoglycoside group active against a wide variety of pathogenic gram-negative and gram-positive bacteria.
GARAMYCIN **Ophthalmic Solution** is a sterile, aqueous solution buffered to approximately pH 7 for use in the eye. Each ml. contains gentamicin sulfate, USP (equivalent to 3.0 mg gentamicin), disodium phosphate, monosodium phosphate, sodium chloride, and benzalkonium chloride as a preservative.
GARAMYCIN **Ophthalmic Ointment** is a sterile ointment, each gram containing gentamicin sulfate, USP (equivalent to 3.0 mg gentamicin) in a bland base of white petrolatum, with methylparaben and propylparaben as preservatives.

ACTIONS

The gram-positive bacteria against which gentamicin sulfate is active include coagulase-positive and coagulase-negative staphylococci, including certain strains that are resistant to penicillin; Group A beta-hemolytic and nonhemolytic streptococci; and *Diplococcus pneumoniae.* The gram-negative bacteria against which gentamicin sulfate is active include certain strains of *Pseudomonas aeruginosa,* indole-positive and indole-negative *Proteus* species, *Escherichia coli, Klebsiella pneumoniae* (Friedlander's bacillus), *Haemophilus influenza* and *Haemophilus aegyptius* (Koch-Weeks bacillus), *Aerobacter aerogenes, Moraxella lacunata* (diplobacillus of Morax-Axenfeld), and *Neisseria* species, including *Neisseria gonorrhoeae.* Although significant resistant organisms have not been isolated from patients treated with gentamicin at the present time, this may occur in the future as resistance has been produced with difficulty *in vitro* by repeated exposures.

INDICATIONS

GARAMYCIN **Ophthalmic Solution** and **Ointment** are indicated in the topical treatment of infections of the external eye and its adnexa caused by susceptible bacteria. Such infections embrace conjunctivitis, keratitis and keratoconjunctivitis, corneal ulcers, blepharitis and blepharoconjunctivitis, acute meibomianitis, and dacryocystitis.

CONTRAINDICATIONS

GARAMYCIN **Ophthalmic Solution** and **Ointment** are contraindicated in patients with known hypersensitivity to any of the components.

WARNINGS

GARAMYCIN **Ophthalmic Solution** is not for injection. It should never be injected subconjunctivally, nor should it be directly introduced into the anterior chamber of the eye.

PRECAUTIONS

Prolonged use of topical antibiotics may give rise to overgrowth of nonsusceptible organisms, such as fungi. Should this occur, or if irritation or hypersensitivity to any component of the drug develops, discontinue use of the preparation and institute appropriate therapy.
Ophthalmic ointments may retard corneal healing.

ADVERSE REACTIONS

Transient irritation has been reported with the use of GARAMYCIN **Ophthalmic Solution.**
Occasional burning or stinging may occur with the use of GARAMYCIN **Ophthalmic Ointment.**

DOSAGE AND ADMINISTRATION

GARAMYCIN **Ophthalmic Solution:** instill one or two drops into the affected eye every four hours. In severe infections, dosage may be increased to as much as two drops once every hour.
GARAMYCIN **Ophthalmic Ointment:** apply a small amount to the affected eye two to three times a day.

HOW SUPPLIED

GARAMYCIN **Ophthalmic Solution—Sterile,** 5 ml. plastic dropper bottle, box of one (NDC 0085-0899-05).
GARAMYCIN **Ophthalmic Ointment—Sterile,** 3.5 g, box of one (NDC 0085-0151-05).
Store GARAMYCIN Ophthalmic Ointment and Solution between 2° and 30°C (36° and 86°F).
Revised 8/85

GARAMYCIN® Injectable ℞
[gar-ah-mī'sin]
brand of gentamicin sulfate injection, USP
40 mg per ml
Each ml contains gentamicin sulfate, USP equivalent to 40 mg gentamicin.
For Parenteral Administration

WARNINGS

Patients treated with aminoglycosides should be under close clinical observation because of the potential toxicity associated with their use.
As with other aminoglycosides, GARAMYCIN Injectable is potentially nephrotoxic. The risk of nephrotoxicity is greater in patients with impaired renal function and in those who receive high dosage or prolonged therapy.
Neurotoxicity manifested by ototoxicity, both vestibular and auditory, can occur in patients treated with GARAMYCIN Injectable primarily in those with preexisting renal damage and in patients with normal renal function treated with higher doses and/or for longer periods than recommended. Aminoglycoside-induced ototoxicity is usually irreversible. Other manifestations of neurotoxicity may include numbness, skin tingling, muscle twitching and convulsions.
Renal and eighth cranial nerve function should be closely monitored, especially in patients with known or suspected reduced renal function at onset of therapy, and also in those whose renal function is initially normal but who develop signs of renal dysfunction during therapy. Urine should be examined for decreased specific gravity, increased excretion of protein, and the presence of cells or casts. Blood urea nitrogen, serum creatinine, or creatinine clearance should be determined periodically. When feasible, it is recommended that serial audiograms be obtained in patients old enough to be tested, particularly high-risk patients. Evidence of ototoxicity (dizziness, vertigo, tinnitus, roaring in the ears or hearing loss) or nephrotoxicity requires dosage adjustment or discontinuance of the drug. As with the other aminoglycosides, on rare occasions changes in renal and eighth cranial nerve function may not become manifest until soon after completion of therapy.
Serum concentrations of aminoglycosides should be monitored when feasible to assure adequate levels and to avoid potentially toxic levels. When monitoring gentamicin peak concentrations, dosage should be adjusted so that prolonged levels above 12 mcg/ml are avoided. When monitoring gentamicin trough concentrations,

Continued on next page

Schering—Cont.

dosage should be adjusted so that levels above 2 mcg/ml are avoided. Excessive peak and/ or trough serum concentrations of aminoglycosides may increase the risk of renal and eighth cranial nerve toxicity. In the event of overdose or toxic reactions, hemodialysis may aid in the removal of gentamicin from the blood, especially if renal function is, or becomes, compromised. The rate of removal of gentamicin is considerably less by peritoneal dialysis than by hemodialysis.
Concurrent and/or sequential systemic or topical use of other potentially neurotoxic and/or nephrotoxic drugs, such as cisplatin, cephaloridine, kanamycin, amikacin, neomycin, polymyxin B, colistin, paromomycin, streptomycin, tobramycin, vancomycin, and viomycin, should be avoided. Other factors which may increase patient risk of toxicity are advanced age and dehydration.
The concurrent use of gentamicin with potent diuretics, such as ethacrynic acid or furosemide, should be avoided, since certain diuretics by themselves may cause ototoxicity. In addition, when administered intravenously, diuretics may enhance aminoglycoside toxicity by altering the antibiotic concentration in serum and tissue.

DESCRIPTION

Gentamicin sulfate, USP, a water-soluble antibiotic of the aminoglycoside group, is derived from *Micromonospora purpurea*, an actinomycete. GARAMYCIN Injectable is a sterile, aqueous solution for parenteral administration. Each ml contains gentamicin sulfate, USP equivalent to 40 mg gentamicin base, 1.8 mg methylparaben and 0.2 mg propylparaben as preservatives, 3.2 mg sodium bisulfite, and 0.1 mg edetate disodium.

CLINICAL PHARMACOLOGY

After intramuscular administration of GARAMYCIN Injectable, peak serum concentrations usually occur between 30 and 60 minutes and serum levels are measurable for six to eight hours. When gentamicin is administered by intravenous infusion over a two-hour period, the serum concentrations are similar to those obtained by intramuscular administration.
In patients with normal renal function, peak serum concentrations of gentamicin (mcg/ml) are usually up to four times the single intramuscular dose (mg/kg); for example, a 1.0 mg/kg injection in adults may be expected to result in a peak serum concentration up to 4 mcg/ml; a 1.5 mg/kg dose may produce levels up to 6 mcg/ml. While some variation is to be expected due to a number of variables such as age, body temperature surface area and physiologic differences, the individual patient given the same dose tends to have similar levels in repeated determinations. Gentamicin administered at 1.0 mg/kg every eight hours for the usual 7- to 10-day treatment period to patients with normal renal function does not accumulate in serum.
Gentamicin, like all aminoglycosides, may accumulate in the serum and tissues of patients treated with higher doses and/ or for prolonged periods, particularly in the presence of impaired renal function. In adult patients, treatment with gentamicin dosages of 4 mg/kg/day or higher for seven to ten days may result in a slight, progressive rise in both peak and trough concentrations. In patients with impaired renal function, gentamicin is cleared from the body more slowly than in patients with normal renal function. The more severe the impairment, the slower the clearance. (Dosage must be adjusted.)
Since gentamicin is distributed in extracellular fluid, peak serum concentrations may be lower than usual in adult patients who have a large volume of this fluid. Serum concentrations of gentamicin in febrile patients may be lower than those in afebrile patients given the same dose. When body temperature returns to normal, serum concentrations of the drug may rise. Febrile and anemic states may be associated with a shorter than usual serum half-life. (Dosage adjustment is usually not necessary.) In severely burned patients, the half-life may be significantly decreased and resulting serum concentrations may be lower than anticipated from the mg/kg dose.
Protein-binding studies have indicated that the degree of gentamicin binding is low; depending upon the methods used for testing, this may be between 0 and 30%.
After initial administration to patients with normal renal function, generally 70% or more of the gentamicin dose is recoverable in the urine in 24 hours; concentrations in urine above 100 mcg/ml may be achieved. Little, if any, metabolic transformation occurs; the drug is excreted principally by glomerular filtration. After several days of treatment, the amount of gentamicin excreted in the urine approaches the daily dose administered. As with other aminoglycosides, a small amount of the gentamicin dose may be retained in the tissues, especially in the kidneys. Minute quantities of aminoglycosides have been detected in the urine weeks after drug administration was discontinued. Renal clearance of gentamicin is similar to that of endogenous creatinine.
In patients with marked impairment of renal function, there is a decrease in the concentration of aminoglycosides in urine and in their penetration into defective renal parenchyma. This decreased drug excretion, together with the potential nephrotoxicity of aminoglycosides, should be considered when treating such patients who have urinary tract infections.
Probenecid does not affect renal tubular transport of gentamicin.
The endogenous creatinine clearance rate and the serum creatinine level have a high correlation with the half-life of gentamicin in serum. Results of these tests may serve as guides for adjusting dosage in patients with renal impairment (see DOSAGE AND ADMINISTRATION).
Following parenteral administration, gentamicin can be detected in serum, lymph, tissues, sputum, and in pleural, synovial, and peritoneal fluids. Concentrations in renal cortex sometimes may be eight times higher than the usual serum levels. Concentrations in bile, in general, have been low and have suggested minimal biliary excretion. Gentamicin crosses the peritoneal as well as the placental membranes. Since aminoglycosides diffuse poorly into the subarachnoid space after parenteral administration, concentrations of gentamicin in cerebrospinal fluid are often low and dependent upon dose, rate of penetration, and degree of meningeal inflammation. There is minimal penetration of gentamicin into ocular tissues following intramuscular or intravenous administration.

Microbiology: *In vitro* tests have demonstrated that gentamicin is a bactericidal antibiotic which acts by inhibiting normal protein synthesis in susceptible microorganisms. It is active against a wide variety of pathogenic bacteria including *Escherichia coli*, *Proteus* species, (indole-positive and indole-negative), *Pseudomonas aeruginosa*, species of the *Klebsiella-Enterobacter-Serratia* group. *Citrobacter* species and *Staphylococcus* species (including penicillin- and methicillin-resistant strains). Gentamicin is also active *in vitro* against species of *Salmonella* and *Shigella*. The following bacteria are usually resistant to aminoglycoside: *Streptococcus pneumoniae*, most species of streptococci, particularly group D and anaerobic organisms, such as *Bacteroides* species or *Clostridium* species.
In vitro studies have shown that an aminoglycoside combined with an antibiotic that interferes with cell wall synthesis may act synergistically against some group D streptococcal strains. The combination of gentamicin and penicillin G has a synergistic bactericidal effect against virtually all strains of *Streptococcus faecalis* and its varieties (*S. faecalis* var. *liquifaciens*, *S. faecalis* var. *zymogenes*), *S. faecium* and *S. durans*. An enhanced killing effect against many of these strains has also been shown *in vitro* with combinations of gentamicin and ampicillin, carbenicillin, nafcillin, or oxacillin.
The combined effect of gentamicin and carbenicillin is synergistic for many strains of *Pseudomonas aeruginosa*. *In vitro* synergism against other gram-negative organisms has been shown with combinations of gentamicin and cephalosporins.
Gentamicin may be active against clinical isolates of bacteria resistant to other aminoglycosides. Bacteria resistant to one aminoglycoside may be resistant to one or more other aminoglycosides. Bacterial resistance to gentamicin is generally developed slowly.

Susceptibility Testing: If the disc method of susceptibility testing used is that described by Bauer *et al.* (*Am J Clin Path* 45:493, 1966; *Federal Register* 37:20525-20529, 1972), a disc containing 10 mcg of gentamicin should give a zone of inhibition of 15mm or more to indicate susceptibility of the infecting organism. A zone of 12mm or less indicates that the infecting organism is likely to be resistant. Zones greater than 12mm and less than 15mm indicate intermediate susceptibility. In certain conditions it may be desirable to do additional susceptibility testing by the tube or agar dilution method; gentamicin substance is available for this purpose.

INDICATIONS AND USAGE

GARAMYCIN Injectable is indicated in the treatment of serious infections caused by susceptible strains of the following microorganisms: *Pseudomonas aeruginosa*, *Proteus* species (indole-positive and indole-negative), *Escherichia coli*, *Klebsiella-Enterobacter-Serratia* species, *Citrobacter* species and *Staphylococcus* species (coagulase-positive and coagulase-negative).
Clinical studies have shown GARAMYCIN Injectable to be effective in bacterial neonatal sepsis; bacterial septicemia; and serious bacterial infections of the central nervous system (meningitis), urinary tract, respiratory tract, gastrointestinal tract (including peritonitis), skin, bone and soft tissue (including burns). Aminoglycosides, including gentamicin, are not indicated in uncomplicated initial episodes of urinary tract infections unless the causative organisms are susceptible to these antibiotics and are not susceptible to antibiotics having less potential for toxicity.
Specimens for bacterial culture should be obtained to isolate and identify causative organisms and to determine their susceptibility to gentamicin.
GARAMYCIN may be considered as initial therapy in suspected or confirmed gram-negative infections, and therapy may be instituted before obtaining results of susceptibility testing. The decision to continue therapy with this drug should be based on the results of susceptibility tests, the severity of the infection, and the important additional concepts contained in the "WARNINGS Box" above. If the causative organisms are resistant to gentamicin, other appropriate therapy should be instituted.
In serious infections when the causative organisms are unknown, GARAMYCIN may be administered as initial therapy in conjunction with a penicillin-type or cephalosporin-type drug before obtaining results of susceptibility testing. If anaerobic organisms are suspected as etiologic agents, consideration should be given to using other suitable antimicrobial therapy in conjunction with gentamicin. Following identification of the organism and its susceptibility, appropriate antibiotic therapy should then be continued.
GARAMYCIN has been used effectively in combination with carbenicillin for the treatment of life-threatening infections caused by *Pseudomonas aeruginosa*. It has also been found effective when used in conjunction with a penicillin-type drug for the treatment of endocarditis caused by group D streptococci.
GARAMYCIN Injectable has also been shown to be effective in the treatment of serious staphylococcal infections. While not the antibiotic of first choice, GARAMYCIN Injectable may be considered when penicillins or other less potentially toxic drugs are contraindicated and bacterial susceptibility tests and clinical judgment indicate its use. It may also be considered in mixed infections caused by susceptible strains of staphylococci and gram-negative organisms.
In the neonate with suspected bacterial sepsis or staphylococcal pneumonia, a penicillin-type drug is also usually indicated as concomitant therapy with gentamicin.

CONTRAINDICATIONS

Hypersensitivity to gentamicin is a contraindication to its use. A history of hypersensitivity or serious toxic reactions to other aminoglycosides may contraindicate use of gentamicin because of the known cross-sensitivity of patients to drugs in this class.

WARNINGS

(See boxed **WARNINGS.**) Aminoglycosides can cause fetal harm when administered to a pregnant woman. Aminoglycoside antibiotics cross the placenta, and there have been several reports of total irreversible bilateral congenital deafness in children whose mothers received streptomycin during pregnancy. Serious side effects to mother, fetus, or newborn have not been reported in the treatment of pregnant women with other aminoglycosides. Animal reproduction studies conducted on rats and rabbits did not reveal evidence of impaired fertility or harm to the fetus due to gentamicin sulfate.
It is not known whether gentamicin sulfate can cause fetal harm when administered to a pregnant woman or can affect reproduction capacity. If gentamicin is used during pregnancy or if the patient becomes pregnant while taking gentamicin, she should be apprised of the potential hazard to the fetus.

PRECAUTIONS

Neurotoxic and nephrotoxic antibiotics may be absorbed in significant quantities from body surfaces after local irrigation or application. The potential toxic effect of antibiotics administered in this fashion should be considered.
Increased nephrotoxicity has been reported following concomitant administration of aminoglycoside antibiotics and cephalosporins.
Neuromuscular blockade and respiratory paralysis have been reported in the cat receiving high doses (40 mg/kg) of gentamicin. The possibility of these phenomena occurring in man should be considered if aminoglycosides are administered by any route to patients receiving anesthetics, or to patients receiving neuromuscular blocking agents, such as succinylcholine, tubocurarine, or decamethonium, or in patients receiving massive transfusions of citrate-anticoagulated blood. If neuromuscular blockade occurs, calcium salts may reverse it.
Aminoglycosides should be used with caution in patients with neuromuscular disorders, such as myasthenia gravis, since these drugs may aggravate muscle weakness because of their potential curare-like effects on the neuromuscular junction. During or following gentamicin therapy, paresthesias, tetany, positive Chvostek and Trousseau signs, and mental confusion have been described in patients with hypomagnesemia, hypocalcemia, and hypokalemia. When this has occurred in infants, tetany and muscle weakness have been described. Both adults and infants required appropriate corrective electrolyte therapy.
Elderly patients may have reduced renal function which may not be evident in the results of routine screening tests, such as BUN or serum creatinine. A creatinine clearance

determination may be more useful. Monitoring of renal function during treatment with gentamicin, as with other aminoglycosides, is particularly important in such patients. A Fanconi-like syndrome, with aminoaciduria and metabolic acidosis, has been reported in some adults and infants being given gentamicin injections.

Cross-allergenicity among aminoglycosides has been demonstrated.

Patients should be well hydrated during treatment.

Although the *in vitro* mixing of gentamicin and carbenicillin results in a rapid and significant inactivation of gentamicin, this interaction has not been demonstrated in patients with normal renal function who received both drugs by different routes of administration. A reduction in gentamicin serum half-life has been reported in patients with severe renal impairment receiving carbenicillin concomitantly with gentamicin.

Treatment with gentamicin may result in overgrowth of nonsusceptible organisms. If this occurs, appropriate therapy is indicated.

See "WARNINGS Box" regarding concurrent use of potent diuretics and regarding concurrent and /or sequential use of other neurotoxic and/or nephrotoxic antibiotics and for other essential information.

Usage in Pregnancy—Safety for use in pregnancy has not been established.

ADVERSE REACTIONS

Nephrotoxicity Adverse renal effects, as demonstrated by the presence of casts, cells, or protein in the urine or by rising BUN, NPN, serum creatinine or oliguria, have been reported. They occur more frequently in patients with a history of renal impairment and in patients treated for longer periods or with larger dosage than recommended.

Neurotoxicity Serious adverse effects on both vestibular and auditory branches of the eighth cranial nerves have been reported, primarily in patients with renal impairment (especially if dialysis is required), and in patients on high doses and/or prolonged therapy. Symptoms include dizziness, vertigo, tinnitus, roaring in the ears and hearing loss, which, as with the other aminoglycosides, may be irreversible. Hearing loss is usually manifested initially by diminution of high-tone acuity. Other factors which may increase the risk of toxicity include excessive dosage, dehydration and previous exposure to other ototoxic drugs.

Peripheral neuropathy or encephalopathy, including numbness, skin tingling, muscle twitching, convulsions, and a myasthenia gravis-like syndrome, have been reported.

Note: The risk of toxic reactions is low in patients with normal renal function who do not receive GARAMYCIN Injectable at higher doses or for longer periods of time than recommended.

Other reported adverse reactions possibly related to gentamicin include: respiratory depression, lethargy, confusion, depression, visual disturbances, decreased appetite, weight loss, and hypotension and hypertension; rash, itching, urticaria, generalized burning, laryngeal edema, anaphylactoid reactions, fever, and headache, nausea, vomiting, increased salivation, and stomatitis; purpura, pseudotumor cerebri, acute organic brain syndrome, pulmonary fibrosis, alopecia, joint pain, transient hepatomegaly, and splenomegaly.

Laboratory abnormalities possibly related to gentamicin include: increased levels of serum transaminase (SGOT, SGPT), serum LDH and bilirubin; decreased serum calcium, magnesium, sodium and potassium; anemia, leukopenia, granulocytopenia, transient agranulocytosis, eosinophilia, increased and decreased reticulocyte counts, and thrombocytopenia. While clinical laboratory test abnormalities may be isolated findings, they may also be associated with clinically related signs and symptoms. For example, tetany and muscle weakness may be associated with hypomagnesemia, hypocalcemia, and hypokalemia.

While local tolerance of GARAMYCIN Injectable is generally excellent, there has been an occasional report of pain at the injection site. Subcutaneous atrophy or fat necrosis suggesting local irritation has been reported rarely.

OVERDOSAGE

In the event of overdose or toxic reactions, hemodialysis may aid in the removal of gentamicin from the blood, and is especially important if renal function is, or becomes, compromised. The rate of removal of gentamicin is considerably less by peritoneal dialysis than it is by hemodialysis.

DOSAGE AND ADMINISTRATION

GARAMYCIN Injectable may be given intramuscularly or intravenously. The patient's pretreatment body weight should be obtained for calculation of correct dosage. The dosage of aminoglycosides in obese patients should be based on an estimate of the lean body mass. It is desirable to limit the duration of treatment with aminoglycosides to short term.

DOSAGE FOR PATIENTS WITH NORMAL RENAL FUNCTION

Adults: The recommended dosage of GARAMYCIN Injectable for patients with serious infections and normal renal function is 3 mg/kg/day, administered in three equal doses every eight hours (Table I).

For patients with life-threatening infections, dosages up to 5 mg/kg/day may be administered in three or four equal doses. This dosage should be reduced to 3 mg/kg/day as soon as clinically indicated (Table I).

It is desirable to measure periodically both peak and trough serum concentrations of gentamicin when feasible during therapy to assure adequate but not excessive drug levels. For example, the peak concentration (at 30 to 60 minutes after intramuscular injection) is expected to be in the range of 4 to 6 mcg/ml. When monitoring peak concentrations after intramuscular or intravenous administration, dosage should be adjusted so that prolonged levels above 12 mcg/ml are avoided. When monitoring trough concentrations (just prior to the next dose), dosage should be adjusted so that levels above 2 mcg/ml are avoided. Determination of the adequacy of a serum level for a particular patient must take into consideration the susceptibility of the causative organism, the severity of the infection, and the status of the patient's host-defense mechanisms.

In patients with extensive burns, altered pharmacokinetics may result in reduced serum concentrations of aminoglycosides. In such patients treated with gentamicin, measurement of serum concentrations is recommended as a basis for dosage adjustment.

TABLE I
DOSAGE SCHEDULE GUIDE FOR ADULTS WITH NORMAL RENAL FUNCTION
(Dosage at Eight-Hour Intervals)
40 mg per ml

Patient's Weight* kg	(lb)	Usual Dose For Serious Infections 1 mg/kg q8h (3 mg/kg/day) mg/dose q8h	ml/dose	Dose for Life-Threatening Infections (Reduce as Soon as Clinically Indicated) 1.7 mg/kg q8h** (5 mg/kg/day) mg/dose q8h	ml/dose
40	(88)	40	1.0	66	1.6
45	(99)	45	1.1	75	1.9
50	(110)	50	1.25	83	2.1
55	(121)	55	1.4	91	2.25
60	(132)	60	1.5	100	2.5
65	(143)	65	1.6	108	2.7
70	(154)	70	1.75	116	2.9
75	(165)	75	1.9	125	3.1
80	(176)	80	2.0	133	3.3
85	(187)	85	2.1	141	3.5
90	(198)	90	2.25	150	3.75
95	(209)	95	2.4	158	4.0
100	(220)	100	2.5	166	4.2

* The dosage of aminoglycosides in obese patients should be based on an estimate of the lean body mass.

** For q6h schedules, dosage should be recalculated.

Children: 6 to 7.5 mg/kg/day. (2.0 to 2.5 mg/kg administered every 8 hours.)

Infants and Neonates: 7.5 mg/kg/day. (2.5 mg/kg administered every 8 hours.)

Premature or Full-Term Neonates One Week of Age or Less: 5 mg/kg/day. (2.5 mg/kg administered every 12 hours).

For further information concerning the use of gentamicin in infants and children, see GARAMYCIN Pediatric Injectable Product Information.

The usual duration of treatment for all patients is seven to ten days. In difficult and complicated infections, a longer course of therapy may be necessary. In such cases, monitoring of renal, auditory, and vestibular functions is recommended, since toxicity is more apt to occur with treatment extended for more than ten days. Dosage should be reduced if clinically indicated.

For Intravenous Administration

The intravenous administration of gentamicin may be particularly useful for treating patients with bacterial septicemia or those in shock. It may also be the preferred route of administration for some patients with congestive heart failure, hematologic disorders, severe burns, or those with reduced muscle mass. For intermittent intravenous administration in adults, a single dose of GARAMYCIN Injectable may be diluted in 50 to 200 ml of sterile isotonic saline solution or in a sterile solution of dextrose 5% in water; in infants and children, the volume of diluent should be less. The solution may be infused over a period of one-half to two hours.

The recommended dosage for intravenous and intramuscular administration is identical.

GARAMYCIN Injectable should not be physically premixed with other drugs, but should be administered separately in accordance with the recommended route of administration and dosage schedule.

DOSAGE FOR PATIENTS WITH IMPAIRED RENAL FUNCTION

Dosage must be adjusted in patients with impaired renal function to assure therapeutically adequate, but not excessive, blood levels. Whenever possible, serum concentrations of gentamicin should be monitored. One method of dosage adjustment is to increase the interval between administration of the usual doses. Since the serum creatinine concentration has a high correlation with the serum half-life of gentamicin, this laboratory test may provide guidance for adjustment of the interval between doses. The interval between doses (in hours) may be approximated by multiplying the serum creatinine level (mg/100 ml) by 8. For example, a patient weighing 60 kg with a serum creatinine level of 2.0 mg/100 ml could be given 60 mg (1 mg/kg) every 16 hours (2 × 8).

In patients with serious systemic infections and renal impairment, it may be desirable to administer the antibiotic more frequently but in reduced dosage. In such patients, serum concentrations of gentamicin should be measured so that adequate but not excessive levels result. A peak and trough concentration measured intermittently during therapy will provide optimal guidance for adjusting dosage. After the usual initial dose, a rough guide for determining reduced dosage at eight-hour intervals is to divide the normally recommended dose by the serum creatinine level (Table II). For example, after an initial dose of 60 mg (1 mg/kg), a patient weighing 60 kg with a serum creatinine level of 2.0 mg/100 ml could be given 30 mg every eight hours (60 ÷ 2). It should be noted that the status of renal function may be changing over the course of the infectious process. It is important to recognize that deteriorating renal function may require a greater reduction in dosage than that specified in the above guidelines for patients with stable renal impairment.

TABLE II
DOSAGE ADJUSTMENT GUIDE FOR PATIENTS WITH RENAL IMPAIRMENT
(Dosage at Eight-Hour Intervals After the Usual Initial Dose)

Serum Creatinine (mg %)	Approximate Creatinine Clearance Rate ($ml/min/1.73M^2$)	Percent of Usual Doses Shown in Table I
≤ 1.0	> 100	100
1.1–1.3	70–100	80
1.4–1.6	55–70	65
1.7–1.9	45–55	55
2.0–2.2	40–45	50
2.3–2.5	35–40	40
2.6–3.0	30–35	35
3.1–3.5	25–30	30
3.6–4.0	20–25	25
4.1–5.1	15–20	20
5.2–6.6	10–15	15
6.7–8.0	< 10	10

In adults with renal failure undergoing hemodialysis, the amount of gentamicin removed from the blood may vary depending upon several factors including the dialysis method used. An eight-hour hemodialysis may reduce serum concentrations of gentamicin by approximately 50%. The recommended dosage at the end of each dialysis period is 1 to 1.7 mg/kg depending upon the severity of infection. In children, a dose of 2 mg/kg may be administered.

The above dosage schedules are not intended as rigid recommendations but are provided as guides to dosage when the measurement of gentamicin serum levels is not feasible.

A variety of methods are available to measure gentamicin concentrations in body fluids; these include microbiologic, enzymatic and radioimmunoassay techniques.

HOW SUPPLIED

GARAMYCIN Injectable, 40 mg per ml, for parenteral administration, is supplied in 2 ml (80 mg) vials, boxes of 25 (NDC 0085-0069-04); 20 ml vials, box of 5 (NDC 0085-0069-08); and in 1.5 ml (60 mg) (NDC 0085-0069-05) and 2 ml (80 mg) (NDC 0085-0069-06) disposable syringes, each in boxes of 1 and 10.

Also available, GARAMYCIN Pediatric Injectable, 10 mg per ml, for parenteral administration, supplied in 2 ml (20 mg) vials, box of one (NDC 0085-0013-05).

GARAMYCIN Injectable is a clear, stable solution that requires no refrigeration.

Continued on next page

Information on Schering products appearing on these pages is effective as of September 30, 1986.

Schering—Cont.

Store between 2° and 30°C (36° and 86°F).
Schering Pharmaceutical Corporation (PR)
Manati, Puerto Rico 00701
An Affiliate of Schering Corporation
Kenilworth, NJ 07033

Revised 2/86

GARAMYCIN® PEDIATRIC ℞
[gar-ah-mī'sin]
Injectable
brand of gentamicin sulfate injection, USP
10 mg per ml
Each ml contains gentamicin sulfate, USP equivalent to 10 mg gentamicin.
For Parenteral Administration

WARNINGS

Patients treated with aminoglycosides should be under close clinical observation because of the potential toxicity associated with their use.
As with other aminoglycosides, GARAMYCIN Pediatric Injectable is potentially nephrotoxic. The risk of nephrotoxicity is greater in patients with impaired renal function and in those who receive high dosage or prolonged therapy.
Neurotoxicity manifested by ototoxicity, both vestibular and auditory, can occur in patients treated with GARAMYCIN Pediatric Injectable, primarily in those with pre-existing renal damage and in patients with normal renal function treated with higher doses and/or for longer periods than recommended. Aminoglycoside-induced ototoxicity is usually irreversible. Other manifestations of neurotoxicity may include numbness, skin tingling, muscle twitching, and convulsions.
Renal and eighth cranial nerve function should be closely monitored, especially in patients with known or suspected reduced renal function at onset of therapy, and also in those whose renal function is initially normal but who develop signs of renal dysfunction during therapy. Urine should be examined for decreased specific gravity, increased excretion of protein, and the presence of cells or casts. Blood urea nitrogen, serum creatinine, or creatinine clearance should be determined periodically. When feasible, it is recommended that serial audiograms be obtained in patients old enough to be tested, particularly high-risk patients. Evidence of ototoxicity (dizziness, vertigo, tinnitus, roaring in the ears or hearing loss) or nephrotoxicity requires dosage adjustment or discontinuance of the drug.
As with the other aminoglycosides, on rare occasions changes in renal and eighth cranial nerve function may not become manifest until soon after completion of therapy.
Serum concentrations of aminoglycosides should be monitored when feasible to assure adequate levels and to avoid potentially toxic levels. When monitoring gentamicin peak concentrations, dosage should be adjusted so that prolonged levels above 12 mcg/ml are avoided. When monitoring gentamicin trough concentrations, dosage should be adjusted so that levels above 2 mcg/ml are avoided. Excessive peak and/or trough serum concentrations of aminoglycosides may increase the risk of renal and eighth cranial nerve toxicity. In the event of overdose or toxic reactions, hemodialysis may aid in the removal of gentamicin from the blood, especially if renal function is, or becomes, compromised. The rate of removal of gentamicin is considerably less by peritoneal dialysis than by hemodialysis.
In the newborn infant, exchange transfusions may also be considered.
Concurrent and/or sequential systemic or topical use of other potentially neurotoxic and/or nephrotoxic drugs, such as cisplatin, cephaloridine, kanamycin, amikacin, neomycin, polymyxin B, colistin, paromomycin, streptomycin, tobramycin, vancomycin, and viomycin, should be avoided. Another factor which may increase patient risk of toxicity is dehydration.
The concurrent use of gentamicin with potent diuretics, such as ethacrynic acid or furosemide, should be avoided, since certain diuretics by themselves may cause ototoxicity. In addition, when administered intravenously, diuretics may enhance aminoglycoside toxicity by altering the antibiotic concentration in serum and tissue.

DESCRIPTION

Gentamicin sulfate, USP, a water-soluble antibiotic of the aminoglycoside group, is derived from *Micromonospora purpurea*, an actinomycete. GARAMYCIN Pediatric Injectable is a sterile, aqueous solution for parenteral administration. Each ml contains gentamicin sulfate, USP equivalent to 10 mg gentamicin base, 1.3 mg methylparaben and 0.2 mg propylparaben as preservatives, 3.2 mg sodium bisulfite and 0.1 mg edetate disodium.

CLINICAL PHARMACOLOGY

After intramuscular administration of GARAMYCIN Pediatric Injectable, peak serum concentrations usually occur between 30 and 60 minutes and serum levels are measurable for 6 to 12 hours. In infants, a single dose of 2.5 mg/kg usually provides a peak serum level in the range of 3 to 5 mcg/ml. When gentamicin is administered by intravenous infusion over a two-hour period, the serum concentrations are similar to those obtained by intramuscular administration. Age markedly affects the peak concentrations: in one report, a 1 mg/kg dose produced mean peak concentrations of 1.58, 2.03, and 2.81 mcg/ml in patients 6 months to 5 years old, 5 to 10 years old, and over 10 years old, respectively.
In infants one week to six months of age, the half-life is 3 to 3½ hours. In full-term and large premature infants less than one week old, the approximate serum half-life of gentamicin is 5½ hours. In small premature infants, the half-life is inversely related to birth weight. In premature infants weighing less than 1500 grams, the half-life is 11½ hours; in those weighing 1500 to 2000 grams, the half-life is 8 hours; in those weighing over 2000 grams, the half-life is approximately 5 hours. While some variation is to be expected due to a number of variables such as age, body temperature, surface area and physiologic differences, the individual patient given the same dose tends to have similar levels in repeated determinations.
Gentamicin, like all aminoglycosides, may accumulate in the serum and tissues of patients treated with higher doses and/or for prolonged periods, particularly in the presence of impaired or immature renal function. In patients with immature or impaired renal function, gentamicin is cleared from the body more slowly than in patients with normal renal function. The more severe the impairment, the slower the clearance. (Dosage must be adjusted.)
Since gentamicin is distributed in extracellular fluid, peak serum concentrations may be lower than usual in patients who have a large volume of this fluid. Serum concentrations of gentamicin in febrile patients may be lower than those in afebrile patients given the same dose. When body temperature returns to normal, serum concentrations of the drug may rise. Febrile and anemic states may be associated with a shorter than usual serum half-life. (Dosage adjustment is usually not necessary.) In severely burned patients, the half-life may be significantly decreased and resulting serum concentrations may be lower than anticipated from the mg/kg/dose.
Protein-binding studies have indicated that the degree of gentamicin binding is low, depending upon the methods used for testing, this may be between 0 and 30%.
In neonates less than 3 days old, approximately 10% of the administered dose is excreted in 12 hours; in infants 5 to 40 days old, approximately 40% is excreted over the same period. Excretion of gentamicin correlates with postnatal age and creatinine clearance. Thus, with increasing postnatal age and concomitant increase in renal maturity, gentamicin is excreted more rapidly. Little, if any metabolic transformation occurs; the drug is excreted principally by glomerular filtration. After several days of treatment, the amount of gentamicin excreted in the urine approaches, but does not equal, the daily dose administered. As with other aminoglycosides, a small amount of the gentamicin dose may be retained in the tissues, especially in the kidneys. Minute quantities of aminoglycosides have been detected in the urine of some patients weeks after drug administration was discontinued. Renal clearance of gentamicin is similar to that of endogenous creatinine.
In patients with marked impairment of renal function, there is a decrease in the concentration of aminoglycosides in urine and in their penetration into defective renal parenchyma. This decreased drug excretion, together with the potential nephrotoxicity of aminoglycosides, should be considered when treating such patients who have urinary tract infections.
Probenecid does not affect renal tubular transport of gentamicin.
The endogenous creatinine clearance rate and the serum creatinine level have a high correlation with the half-life of gentamicin in serum. Results of these tests may serve as guides for adjusting dosage in patients with renal impairment (see DOSAGE AND ADMINISTRATION).
Following parenteral administration, gentamicin can be detected in serum, lymph, tissues, sputum and in pleural, synovial, peritoneal fluids. Concentrations in renal cortex sometimes may be eight times higher than the usual serum levels. Concentrations in bile, in general, have been low and have suggested minimal biliary excretion. Gentamicin crosses the peritoneal as well as the placental membranes. Since aminoglycosides diffuse poorly into the subarachnoid space after parenteral administration, concentrations of gentamicin in cerebrospinal fluid are often low and dependent upon dose, rate of penetration, and degree of meningeal inflammation. There is minimal penetration of gentamicin into ocular tissues following intramuscular or intravenous administration.
Microbiology: *In vitro* tests have demonstrated that gentamicin is a bactericidal antibiotic which acts by inhibiting normal protein synthesis in susceptible microorganisms. It is active against a wide variety of pathogenic bacteria including *Escherichia coli*, *Proteus* species (indole-positive and indole-negative), *Pseudomonas aeruginosa*, species of *Klebsiella-Enterobacter-Serratia* group, *Citrobacter* species, and *Staphylococcus* species (including penicillin- and methicillin-resistant strains). Gentamicin is also active *in vitro* against species of *Salmonella* and *Shigella*. The following bacteria are usually resistant to aminoglycosides: *Streptococcus pneumoniae*, most species of streptococci, particularly group D and anaerobic organisms, such as *Bacteroides* species or *Clostridium* species.
In vitro studies have shown that an aminoglycoside combined with an antibiotic that interferes with cell wall synthesis may act synergistically against some group D streptococcal strains. The combination of gentamicin and penicillin G has a synergistic bactericidal effect against virtually all strains of *Streptococcus faecalis* and its varieties *(S. faecalis* var. *liquifaciens, S. faecalis* var. *zymogenes), S. faecium* and *S. durans*. An enhanced killing effect against many of these strains has also been shown *in vitro* with combinations of gentamicin and ampicillin, carbenicillin, nafcillin, or oxacillin.
The combined effect of gentamicin and carbenicillin is synergistic for many strains of *Pseudomonas aeruginosa*. *In vitro* synergism against other gram-negative organisms has been shown with combinations of gentamicin and cephalosporins.
Gentamicin may be active against clinical isolates of bacteria resistant to other aminoglycosides. Bacteria resistant to one aminoglycoside may be resistant to one or more other aminoglycosides. Bacterial resistance to gentamicin is generally developed slowly.
Susceptibility Testing: If the disc method of susceptibility testing used is that described by Bauer *et al* (*Am J Clin Path* 45:493, 1966; *Federal Register* 37:20525–20529, 1972), a disc containing 10 mcg of gentamicin should give a zone of inhibition of 15 mm or more to indicate susceptibility of the infecting organism. A zone of 12 mm or less indicates that the infecting organism is likely to be resistant. Zones greater than 12mm and less than 15mm indicate intermediate susceptibility. In certain conditions it may be desirable to do additional susceptibility testing by the tube or agar dilution method; gentamicin substance is available for this purpose.

INDICATIONS AND USAGE

GARAMYCIN Pediatric Injectable is indicated in the treatment of serious infections caused by susceptible strains of the following microorganisms: *Pseudomonas aeruginosa*, *Proteus* species (indole-positive and indole-negative), *Escherichia coli*, *Klebsiella-Enterobacter-Serratia* species, *Citrobacter* species, and *Staphyloccous* species (coagulase-positive and coagulase-negative).
Clinical studies have shown GARAMYCIN Pediatric Injectable to be effective in bacterial neonatal sepsis; bacterial septicemia; and serious bacterial infections of the central nervous system (meningitis), urinary tract, respiratory tract, gastrointestinal tract (including peritonitis), skin, bone and soft tissue (including burns).
Aminoglycosides, including gentamicin, are not indicated in uncomplicated initial episodes of urinary tract infections unless the causative organisms are susceptible to these antibiotics and are not susceptible to antibiotics having less potential for toxicity.
Specimens for bacterial culture should be obtained to isolate and identify causative organisms and to determine their susceptibility to gentamicin.
GARAMYCIN may be considered as initial therapy in suspected or confirmed gram-negative infections, and therapy may be instituted before obtaining results of susceptibility testing. The decision to continue therapy with this drug should be based on the results of susceptibility tests, the severity of the infection, and the important additional concepts contained in the "WARNINGS Box" above. If the causative organisms are resistant to gentamicin, other appropriate therapy should be instituted.
In serious infections when the causative organisms are unknown, GARAMYCIN may be administered as initial therapy in conjunction with a penicillin-type or cephalosporin-type drug before obtaining results of susceptibility testing. If anaerobic organisms are suspected as etiologic agents, consideration should be given to using other suitable antimicrobial therapy in conjunction with gentamicin. Following identification of the organism and its susceptibility, appropriate antibiotic therapy should then be continued.
GARAMYCIN has been used effectively in combination with carbenicillin for the treatment of life-threatening infections caused by *Pseudomonas aeruginosa*. It has also been found effective when used in conjunction with a penicillin-type

drug for the treatment of endocarditis caused by group D streptococci.
GARAMYCIN Pediatric Injectable has also been shown to be effective in the treatment of serious staphylococcal infections. While not the antibiotic of first choice, GARAMYCIN Pediatric Injectable may be considered when penicillins or other less potentially toxic drugs are contraindicated and bacterial susceptibility tests and clinical judgment indicate its use. It may also be considered in mixed infections caused by susceptible strains of staphylococci and gram-negative organisms.
In the neonate with suspected bacterial sepsis or staphylococcal pneumonia, a penicillin-type drug is also usually indicated as concomitant therapy with gentamicin.

CONTRAINDICATIONS

Hypersensitivity to gentamicin is a contraindication to its use. A history of hypersensitivity or serious toxic reactions to other aminoglycosides may contraindicate use of gentamicin because of the known cross-sensitivity of patients to drugs in this class.

WARNINGS

(See boxed **WARNINGS.**) Aminoglycosides can cause fetal harm when administered to a pregnant woman. Aminoglycoside antibiotics cross the placenta, and there have been several reports of total irreversible bilateral congenital deafness in children whose mothers received streptomycin during pregnancy. Serious side effects to mother, fetus, or newborn have not been reported in the treatment of pregnant women with other aminoglycosides. Animal reproduction studies conducted on rats and rabbits did not reveal evidence of impaired fertility or harm to the fetus due to gentamicin sulfate.
It is not known whether gentamicin sulfate can cause fetal harm when administered to a pregnant woman or can affect reproduction capacity. If gentamicin is used during pregnancy or if the patient becomes pregnant while taking gentamicin, she should be apprised of the potential hazard to the fetus.

PRECAUTIONS

Neurotoxic and nephrotoxic antibiotics may be absorbed in significant quantities from body surfaces after local irrigation or application. The potential toxic effect of antibiotics administered in this fashion should be considered.
Increased nephrotoxicity has been reported following concomitant administration of aminoglycoside antibiotics and cephalosporins.
Neuromuscular blockade and respiratory paralysis have been reported in the cat receiving high doses (40 mg/kg) of gentamicin. The possibility of these phenomena occurring in man should be considered if aminoglycosides are administered by any route to patients receiving anesthetics, or to patients receiving neuromuscular blocking agents, such as succinylcholine, tubocurarine, or decamethonium, or in patients receiving massive transfusions of citrate-anticoagulated blood. If neuromuscular blockade occurs, calcium salts may reverse it.
Aminoglycosides should be used with caution in patients with neuromuscular disorders, such as myasthenia gravis, since these drugs may aggravate muscle weakness because of their potential curare-like effects on the neuromuscular junction. During or following gentamicin therapy, paresthesias, tetany, positive Chvostek and Trousseau signs, and mental confusion have been described in patients with hypomagnesemia, hypocalcemia, and hypokalemia. When this has occurred in infants, tetany and muscle weakness have been described. Both adults and infants required appropriate corrective electrolyte therapy.
A Fanconi-like syndrome, with aminoaciduria and metabolic acidosis, has been reported in some adults and infants being given gentamicin injections.
Cross-allergenicity among aminoglycosides has been demonstrated.
Patients should be well hydrated during treatment.
Although the *in vitro* mixing of gentamicin and carbenicillin results in a rapid and significant inactivation of gentamicin, this interaction has not been demonstrated in patients with normal renal function who received both drugs by different routes of administration. A reduction in gentamicin serum half-life has been reported in patients with severe renal impairment receiving carbenicillin concomitantly with gentamicin.
Treatment with gentamicin may result in overgrowth of nonsusceptible organisms. If this occurs, appropriate therapy is indicated.
See "WARNINGS Box" regarding concurrent use of potent diuretics and regarding concurrent and/or sequential use of other neurotoxic and/or nephrotoxic antibiotics and for other essential information.
Usage in Pregnancy—Safety for use in pregnancy has not been established.

ADVERSE REACTIONS

Nephrotoxicity Adverse renal effects, as demonstrated by the presence of casts, cells or protein in the urine or by rising BUN, NPN, serum creatinine or oliguria, have been reported. They occur more frequently in patients treated for longer periods or with larger dosages than recommended.
Neurotoxicity Serious adverse effects on both vestibular and auditory branches of the eighth cranial nerves have been reported, primarily in patients with renal impairment (especially if dialysis is required), and in patients on high doses and/or prolonged therapy. Symptoms include dizziness, vertigo, tinnitus, roaring in the ears and hearing loss, which, as with the other aminoglycosides, may be irreversible. Hearing loss is usually manifested initially by diminution of high-tone acuity. Other factors which may increase the risk of toxicity include excessive dosage, dehydration and previous exposure to other ototoxic drugs.
Peripheral neuropathy or encephalopathy, including numbness, skin tingling, muscle twitching, convulsions, and a myasthenia gravis-like syndrome, have been reported.
Note: The risk of toxic reactions is low in neonates, infants and children with normal renal function who do not receive GARAMYCIN Pediatric Injectable at higher doses or for longer periods of time than recommended.
Other reported adverse reactions possibly related to gentamicin include: respiratory depression, lethargy, confusion, depression, visual disturbances, decreased appetite, weight loss and hypotension and hypertension; rash, itching, urticaria, generalized burning, laryngeal edema, anaphylactoid reactions, fever, and headache; nausea, vomiting, increased salivation, and stomatitis; purpura, pseudotumor cerebri, acute organic brain syndrome, pulmonary fibrosis, alopecia, joint pain, transient hepatomegaly, and splenomegaly.
Laboratory abnormalities possibly related to gentamicin include: increased levels of serum transaminase (SGOT, SGPT), serum LDH and bilirubin; decreased serum calcium, magnesium, sodium, and potassium; anemia, leukopenia, granulocytopenia, transient agranulocytosis, eosinophilia, increased and decreased reticulocyte counts, and thrombocytopenia.
While clinical laboratory test abnormalities may be isolated findings, they may also be associated with clinically related signs and symptoms. For example, tetany and muscle weakness may be associated with hypomagnesemia, hypocalcemia, and hypokalemia.
While local tolerance of GARAMYCIN Pediatric Injectable is generally excellent, there has been an occasional report of pain at the injection site. Subcutaneous atrophy or fat necrosis suggesting local irritation has been reported rarely.

OVERDOSAGE

In the event of overdose or toxic reactions, hemodialysis may aid in the removal of gentamicin from the blood, and is especially important if renal function is, or becomes, compromised. The rate of removal of gentamicin is considerably less by peritoneal dialysis than it is by hemodialysis. In the newborn infant, exchange transfusions may also be considered.

DOSAGE AND ADMINISTRATION

GARAMYCIN Pediatric Injectable may be given intramuscularly or intravenously. The patient's pretreatment body weight should be obtained for calculation of correct dosage. The dosage of aminoglycosides in obese patients should be based on an estimate of the lean body mass. It is desirable to limit the duration of treatment with aminoglycosides to short term.

DOSAGE FOR PATIENTS WITH NORMAL RENAL FUNCTION

Children: 6 to 7.5 mg/kg/day. (2.0 to 2.5 mg/kg administered every 8 hours.)
Infants and Neonates: 7.5 mg/kg/day. (2.5 mg/kg administered every 8 hours.)
Premature or Full-Term Neonates One Week of Age or Less: 5 mg/kg/day. (2.5 mg/kg administered every 12 hours.)
It is desirable to measure periodically both peak and trough serum concentrations of gentamicin when feasible during therapy to assure adequate but not excessive drug levels. For example, the peak concentration (at 30 to 60 minutes after intramuscular injection) is expected to be in the range of 3 to 5 mcg/ml. When monitoring peak concentrations after intramuscular or intravenous administration, dosage should be adjusted so that prolonged levels above 12 mcg/ml are avoided. When monitoring trough concentrations (just prior to the next dose), dosage should be adjusted so that levels above 2 mcg/ml are avoided. Determination of the adequacy of a serum level for a particular patient must take into consideration the susceptibility of the causative organism, the severity of the infection, and the status of the patient's host-defense mechanisms.
In patients with extensive burns, altered pharmacokinetics may result in reduced serum concentrations of aminoglycosides. In such patients treated with gentamicin, measurement of serum concentrations is recommended as a basis for dosage adjustment.
The usual duration of treatment is seven to ten days. In difficult and complicated infections, a longer course of therapy may be necessary. In such cases monitoring of renal, auditory, and vestibular functions is recommended, since toxicity is more apt to occur with treatment extended for more than ten days. Dosage should be reduced if clinically indicated.

For Intravenous Administration

The intravenous administration of gentamicin may be particularly useful for treating patients with bacterial septicemia or those in shock. It may also be the preferred route of administration for some patients with congestive heart failure, hematologic disorders, severe burns, or those with reduced muscle mass.
For intermittent intravenous administration, a single dose of GARAMYCIN Pediatric Injectable may be diluted in sterile isotonic saline solution or in a sterile solution of dextrose 5% in water. The solution may be infused over a period of one-half to two hours.
The recommended dosage of intravenous and intramuscular administration is identical.
GARAMYCIN Pediatric Injectable should not be physically premixed with other drugs, but should be administered separately in accordance with the recommended route of administration and dosage schedule.

DOSAGE FOR PATIENTS WITH IMPAIRED RENAL FUNCTION

Dosage must be adjusted in patients with impaired renal function to assure therapeutically adequate, but not excessive, blood levels. Whenever possible, serum concentrations of gentamicin should be monitored. One method of dosage adjustment is to increase the interval between administration of the usual doses. Since the serum creatinine concentration has a high correlation with the serum half-life of gentamicin, this laboratory test may provide guidance for adjustment of the interval between doses. In adults, the interval between doses (in hours) may be approximated by multiplying the serum creatinine level (mg/100 ml) by 8. For example, a patient weighing 60 kg with a serum creatinine level of 2.0 mg/100 ml could be given 60 mg (1 mg/kg) every 16 hours (2×8). These guidelines may be considered when treating infants and children with serious renal impairment.
In patients with serious systemic infections and renal impairment, it may be desirable to administer the antibiotic more frequently but in reduced dosage. In such patients, serum concentrations of gentamicin should be measured so that adequate but not excessive levels result.
A peak and trough concentration measured intermittently during therapy will provide optimal guidance for adjusting dosage. After the usual initial dose, a rough guide for determining reduced dosage at eight-hour intervals is to divide the normally recommended dose by the serum creatinine level (Table 1). For example, after an initial dose of 20 mg (2.0 mg/kg), a child weighing 10 kg with a serum creatinine level of 2.0 mg/100 ml could be given 10 mg every eight hours ($20 \div 2$). It should be noted that the status of renal function may be changing over the course of the infectious process. It is important to recognize that deteriorating renal function may require a greater reduction in dosage than that specified in the above guidelines for patients with stable renal impairment.

TABLE 1
DOSAGE ADJUSTMENT GUIDE FOR PATIENTS WITH RENAL IMPAIRMENT
(Dosage at Eight-Hour Intervals After the Usual Initial Dose)

Serum Creatinine (mg %)	Approximate Creatinine Clearance Rate (ml/min/1.73M^2)	Percent of Usual Doses Shown Above
≤ 1.0	> 100	100
1.1–1.3	70–100	80
1.4–1.6	55–70	65
1.7–1.9	45–55	55
2.0–2.2	40–45	50
2.3–2.5	35–40	40
2.6–3.0	30–35	35
3.1–3.5	25–30	30
3.6–4.0	20–25	25
4.1–5.1	15–20	20
5.2–6.6	10–15	15
6.7–8.0	< 10	10

In patients with renal failure undergoing hemodialysis, the amount of gentamicin removed from the blood may vary depending upon several factors including the dialysis method used. An eight-hour hemodialysis may reduce serum concentrations of gentamicin by approximately 50%. In children, the recommended dose at the end of each dialysis period is 2.0 to 2.5 mg/kg depending upon the severity of infection.

Continued on next page

Schering—Cont.

The above dosage schedules are not intended as rigid recommendations but are provided as guides to dosage when the measurement of gentamicin serum levels is not feasible.
A variety of methods are available to measure gentamicin concentrations in body fluids; these include microbiologic, enzymatic and radioimmunoassay techniques.

HOW SUPPLIED

GARAMYCIN Pediatric Injectable, 10 mg per ml, for parenteral administration, supplied in 2 ml (20 mg) vials; box of one (NDC 0085-0013-05).
Also available, GARAMYCIN Injectable, 40 mg per ml, for parenteral administration, supplied in 2 ml (80 mg) vials, boxes of 25 (NDC 0085-0069-04); 20 ml vials, box of 5 (NDC 0085-0069-08); and in 1.5 ml (60 mg) (NDC 0085-0069-05) and 2 ml (80 mg) (NDC 0085-0069-06) disposable syringes, boxes of 1.
GARAMYCIN Pediatric Injectable is a clear, stable solution that requires no refrigeration.
Store between 2° and 30°C (36° and 86°F).

Schering Pharmaceutical Corporation (PR)
Manati, Puerto Rico 00701
An Affiliate of Schering Corporation
Kenilworth, NJ 07033

Revised 12/85

GARAMYCIN® I.V. ℞

[gar-ah-mī'sin]
Piggyback Injection **Sterile**
brand of gentamicin sulfate, USP
1 mg per ml
Each ml contains gentamicin sulfate, USP equivalent to 1 mg gentamicin.
For Intermittent Intravenous Infusion

WARNINGS

Patients treated with aminoglycosides should be under close clinical observation because of the potential toxicity associated with their use.
As with other aminoglycosides, gentamicin sulfate is potentially nephrotoxic. The risk of nephrotoxicity is greater in patients with impaired renal function and in those who receive high dosage or prolonged therapy.
Neurotoxicity manifested by ototoxicity, both vestibular and auditory, can occur in patients treated with gentamicin sulfate, primarily in those with preexisting renal damage and in patients with normal renal function treated with higher doses and/or for longer periods than recommended. Aminoglycoside-induced ototoxicity is usually irreversible. Other manifestations of neurotoxicity may include numbness, skin tingling, muscle twitching and convulsions.
Renal and eighth cranial nerve function should be closely monitored, especially in patients with known or suspected reduced renal function at onset of therapy, and also in those whose renal function is initially normal but who develop signs of renal dysfunction during therapy. Urine should be examined for decreased specific gravity, increased excretion of protein, and the presence of cells or casts. Blood urea nitrogen, serum creatinine, or creatinine clearance should be determined periodically. When feasible, it is recommended that serial audiograms be obtained in patients old enough to be tested, particularly high-risk patients. Evidence of ototoxicity (dizziness, vertigo, tinnitus, roaring in the ears or hearing loss) or nephrotoxicity requires dosage adjustment or discontinuance of the drug. As with the other aminoglycosides, on rare occasions changes in renal and eighth cranial nerve function may not become manifest until soon after completion of therapy.
Serum concentrations of aminoglycosides should be monitored when feasible to assure adequate levels and to avoid potentially toxic levels. When monitoring gentamicin peak concentrations, dosage should be adjusted so that prolonged levels above 12 mcg/ml are avoided. When monitoring gentamicin trough concentrations, dosage should be adjusted so that levels above 2 mcg/ml are avoided. Excessive peak and/or trough serum concentrations of aminoglycosides may increase the risk of renal and eighth cranial nerve toxicity. In the event of overdose or toxic reactions, hemodialysis may aid in the removal of gentamicin from the blood, especially if renal function is, or becomes, compromised. The rate of removal of gentamicin is considerably less by peritoneal dialysis than by hemodialysis.
Concurrent and/or sequential systemic or topical use of other potentially neurotoxic and/or nephrotoxic drugs, such as cisplatin, cephaloridine, kanamycin, amikacin, neomycin, polymyxin B, colistin, paromomycin, tobramycin, vancomycin, and viomycin, should be avoided. Other factors which may increase patient risk of toxicity are advanced age and dehydration.
The concurrent use of gentamicin with potent diuretics, such as ethacrynic acid or furosemide, should be avoided, since certain diuretics by themselves may cause ototoxicity. In addition, when administered intravenously, diuretics may enhance aminoglycoside toxicity by altering the antibiotic concentration in serum and tissue.

DESCRIPTION

Gentamicin sulfate, USP, a water-soluble antibiotic of the aminoglycoside group, is derived from *Micromonospora purpurea,* an actinomycete. GARAMYCIN I.V. Piggyback Injection is a sterile, aqueous solution for intravenous infusion. Each ml contains gentamicin sulfate, USP, equivalent to 1 mg gentamicin base; and 8.9 mg sodium chloride. It does not contain preservatives.

CLINICAL PHARMACOLOGY

When gentamicin sulfate is administered by intravenous infusion over a two-hour period, the serum concentrations are similar to those obtained by intramuscular administration. Peak serum concentrations following intravenous administration occur 30 to 60 minutes following cessation of infusion. Serum levels are measurable for 6 to 8 hours.
In patients with normal renal function, peak serum concentrations of gentamicin (mcg/ml) are usually up to four times the single intramuscular dose (mg/kg); for example, a 1.0 mg/kg injection in adults may be expected to result in a peak serum concentration up to 4 mcg/ml; a 1.5 mg/kg dose may produce levels up to 6 mcg/ml. While some variation is to be expected due to a number of variables such as age, body temperature, surface area, and physiologic differences, the individual patient given the same dose tends to have similar levels in repeated determinations. Gentamicin administered at 1.0 mg/kg every eight hours for the usual 7- to 10-day treatment period to patients with normal renal function does not accumulate in the serum.
Gentamicin, like all aminoglycosides, may accumulate in the serum and tissues of patients treated with higher doses and/or for prolonged periods, particularly in the presence of impaired renal function. In adult patients, treatment with gentamicin dosages of 4 mg/kg/day or higher for seven to ten days may result in a slight, progressive rise in both peak and trough concentrations. In patients with impaired renal function, gentamicin is cleared from the body more slowly than in patients with normal renal function. The more severe the impairment, the slower the clearance. (Dosage must be adjusted.)
Since gentamicin is distributed in extracellular fluid, peak serum concentrations may be lower than usual in adult patients who have a large volume of this fluid. Serum concentrations of gentamicin in febrile patients may be lower than those in afebrile patients given the same dose. When body temperature returns to normal, serum concentrations of the drug may rise. Febrile and anemic states may be associated with a shorter than usual serum half-life. (Dosage adjustment is usually not necessary.) In severely burned patients, the half-life may be significantly decreased and resulting serum concentrations may be lower than anticipated from the mg/kg dose.
Protein-binding studies have indicated that the degree of gentamicin binding is low; depending upon the methods used for testing, this may be between 0 and 30%.
After initial administration to patients with normal renal function, generally 70% or more of the gentamicin dose is recoverable in the urine in 24 hours; concentrations in urine above 100 mcg/ml may be achieved. Little, if any, metabolic transformation occurs; the drug is excreted principally by glomerular filtration. After several days of treatment, the amount of gentamicin excreted in the urine approaches the daily dose administered. As with other aminoglycosides, a small amount of the gentamicin dose may be retained in the tissues, especially in the kidneys. Minute quantities of aminoglycosides have been detected in the urine weeks after drug administration was discontinued. Renal clearance of gentamicin is similar to that of endogenous creatinine.
In patients with marked impairment of renal function, there is a decrease in the concentration of aminoglycosides in urine and in their penetration into defective renal parenchyma. This decreased drug excretion, together with the potential nephrotoxicity of aminoglycosides, should be considered when treating such patients who have urinary tract infections.
Probenecid does not affect renal tubular transport of gentamicin.
The endogenous creatinine clearance rate and the serum creatinine level have a high correlation with the half-life of gentamicin in serum. Results of these tests may serve as guides for adjusting dosage in patients with renal impairment (see DOSAGE AND ADMINISTRATION).
Following parenteral administration, gentamicin can be detected in serum, lymph, tissues, sputum, and in pleural, synovial, and peritoneal fluids. Concentrations in renal cortex sometimes may be eight times higher than the usual serum levels. Concentrations in bile, in general, have been low and have suggested minimal biliary excretion. Gentamicin crosses the peritoneal as well as the placental membranes. Since aminoglycosides diffuse poorly into the subarachnoid space after parenteral administration, concentrations of gentamicin in cerebrospinal fluid are often low and dependent upon dose, rate of penetration, and degree of meningeal inflammation. There is minimal penetration of gentamicin into ocular tissues following intramuscular or intravenous administration.
Microbiology: *In vitro* tests have demonstrated that gentamicin is a bactericidal antibiotic which acts by inhibiting normal protein synthesis in susceptible microorganisms. It is active against a wide variety of pathogenic bacteria including *Escherichia coli, Proteus* species (indole-positive and indole-negative), *Pseudomonas aeruginosa,* species of the *Klebsiella-Enterobacter-Serratia* group, *Citrobacter* species and *Staphylococcus* species (including penicillin- and methicillin-resistant strains). Gentamicin is also active *in vitro* against species of *Salmonella* and *Shigella.* The following bacteria are usually resistant to aminoglycosides: *Streptococcus pneumoniae,* most species of streptococci, particularly group D and anaerobic organisms, such as *Bacteroides* species or *Clostridium* species.
In vitro studies have shown that an aminoglycoside combined with an antibiotic that interferes with cell wall synthesis may act synergistically against some group D streptococcal strains. The combination of gentamicin and penicillin G has a synergistic bactericidal effect against virtually all strains of *Streptococcus faecalis* and its varieties *(S. faecalis* var. *liquifaciens, S. faecalis* var. *zymogenes), S. faecium* and *S. durans.* An enhanced killing effect against many of these strains has also been shown *in vitro* with combinations of gentamicin and ampicillin, carbenicillin, nafcillin, or oxacillin.
The combined effect of gentamicin and carbenicillin is synergistic for many strains of *Pseudomonas aeruginosa. In vitro* synergism against other gram-negative organisms has been shown with combinations of gentamicin and cephalosporins.
Gentamicin may be active against clinical isolates of bacteria resistant to other aminoglycosides.
Bacteria resistant to one aminoglycoside may be resistant to one or more other aminoglycosides. Bacterial resistance to gentamicin is generally developed slowly.
Susceptibility Testing: If the disc method of susceptibility testing used is that described by Bauer *et al* (*Am J Clin Path* 45:493, 1966; *Federal Register* 37:20525-20529, 1972), a disc containing 10 mcg of gentamicin should give a zone of inhibition of 15mm or more to indicate susceptibility of the infecting organism. A zone of 12mm or less indicates that the infecting organism is likely to be resistant. Zones greater than 12mm and less than 15mm indicate intermediate susceptibility. In certain conditions it may be desirable to do additional susceptibility testing by the tube or agar dilution method; gentamicin substance is available for this purpose.

INDICATIONS AND USAGE

GARAMYCIN I.V. Piggyback Injection is indicated in the treatment of serious infections caused by susceptible strains of the following microorganisms: *Pseudomonas aeruginosa, Proteus* species (indole-positive and indole-negative), *Escherichia coli, Klebsiella-Enterobacter-Serratia* species, *Citrobacter* species and *Staphylococcus* species (coagulase-postive and coagulase-negative).
Clinical studies have shown GARAMYCIN to be effective in bacterial neonatal sepsis; bacterial septicemia; and serious bacterial infections of the central nervous system (meningitis), urinary tract, respiratory tract, gastrointestinal tract (including peritonitis), skin, bone and soft tissue (including burns). Aminoglycosides, including gentamicin, are not indicated in uncomplicated initial episodes of urinary tract infections unless the causative organisms are susceptible to these antibiotics and are not susceptible to antibiotics having less potential for toxicity.
Specimens for bacterial culture should be obtained to isolate and identify causative organisms and to determine their susceptibility to gentamicin.
GARAMYCIN may be considered as initial therapy in suspected or confirmed gram-negative infections, and therapy may be instituted before obtaining results of susceptibility testing. The decision to continue therapy with this drug should be based on the results of susceptibility tests, the severity of the infection, and the important additional concepts contained in the "WARNINGS Box" above. If the causative organisms are resistant to gentamicin, other appropriate therapy should be instituted.
In serious infections when the causative organisms are unknown, GARAMYCIN may be administered as initial therapy in conjunction with a penicillin-type or cephalosporin-type drug before obtaining results of susceptibility testing. If anaerobic organisms are suspected as etiologic agents, consideration should be given to using other suitable antimicro-

bial therapy in conjunction with gentamicin. Following identification of the organism and its susceptibility, appropriate antibiotic therapy should then be continued. GARAMYCIN has been used effectively in combination with carbenicillin for the treatment of life-threatening infections caused by *Pseudomonas aeruginosa*. It has also been found effective when used in conjunction with a penicillin-type drug for the treatment of endocarditis caused by group D streptococci.
GARAMYCIN has also been shown to be effective in the treatment of serious staphylococcal infections. While not the antibiotic of first choice, GARAMYCIN may be considered when penicillins or other less potentially toxic drugs are contraindicated and bacterial susceptibility tests and clinical judgment indicate its use. It may also be considered in mixed infections caused by susceptible strains of staphylococci and gram-negative organisms.
In the neonate with suspected bacterial sepsis or staphylococcal pneumonia, a penicillin-type drug is also usually indicated as concomitant therapy with gentamicin.

CONTRAINDICATIONS

Hypersensitivity to gentamicin is a contraindication to its use. A history of hypersensitivity or serious toxic reactions to other aminoglycosides may contraindicate use of gentamicin because of the known cross-sensitivity of patients to drugs in this class.

WARNINGS

(See boxed **WARNINGS.**) Aminoglycosides can cause fetal harm when administered to a pregnant woman. Aminoglycoside antibiotics cross the placenta, and there have been several reports of total irreversible bilateral congenital deafness in children whose mother received streptomycin during pregnancy. Serious side effects to mother, fetus, or newborn have not been reported in the treatment of pregnant women with other aminoglycosides. Animal reproduction studies conducted on rats and rabbits did not reveal evidence of impaired fertility or harm to the fetus due to gentamicin sulfate.
It is not known whether gentamicin sulfate can cause fetal harm when administered to a pregnant woman or can affect reproduction capacity. If gentamicin is used during pregnancy or if the patient becomes pregnant while taking gentamicin, she should be apprised of the potential hazard to the fetus.

PRECAUTIONS

Neurotoxic and nephrotoxic antibiotics may be absorbed in significant quantities from body surfaces after local irrigation or application. The potential toxic effect of antibiotics administered in this fashion should be considered.
Increased nephrotoxicity has been reported following concomitant administration of aminoglycoside antibiotics and cephalosporins. Neuromuscular blockade and respiratory paralysis have been reported in the cat receiving high doses (40 mg/kg) of gentamicin. The possibility of these phenomena occurring in man should be considered if aminoglycosides are administered by any route to patients receiving anesthetics, or to patients receiving neuromuscular blocking agents, such as succinylcholine, tubocurarine, or decamethonium, or in patients receiving massive transfusions of citrate-anticoagulated blood. If neuromuscular blockade occurs, calcium salts may reverse it. Aminoglycosides should be used with caution in patients with neuromuscular disorders, such as myasthenia gravis, since these drugs may aggravate muscle weakness because of their potential curare-like effects on the neuromuscular junction. During or following gentamicin therapy, paresthesias, tetany, positive Chvostek and Trousseau signs, and mental confusion have been described in patients with hypomagnesemia, hypocalcemia, and hypokalemia. When this has occurred in infants, tetany and muscle weakness have been described. Both adults and infants required appropriate corrective electrolyte therapy.
Elderly patients may have reduced renal function which may not be evident in the results of routine screening tests, such as BUN or serum creatinine. A creatinine clearance determination may be more useful. Monitoring of renal function during treatment with gentamicin, as with other aminoglycosides, is particularly important in such patients. A Fanconi-like syndrome, with aminoaciduria and metabolic acidosis, has been reported in some adults and infants being given gentamicin injections.
Cross-allergenicity among aminoglycosides has been demonstrated.
Patients should be well hydrated during treatment.
Although the *in vitro* mixing of gentamicin and carbenicillin results in a rapid and significant inactivation of gentamicin, this interaction has not been demonstrated in patients with normal renal function who received both drugs by different routes of administration. A reduction in gentamicin serum half-life has been reported in patients with severe renal impairment receiving carbenicillin concomitantly with gentamicin.
Treatment with gentamicin may result in overgrowth of nonsusceptible organisms. If this occurs, appropriate therapy is indicated. See "WARNINGS Box" regarding concurrent use of potent diuretics and regarding concurrent and/or sequential use of other neurotoxic and/or nephrotoxic antibiotics and for other essential information.
Usage in Pregnancy—Safety for use in pregnancy has not been established.

ADVERSE REACTIONS

Nephrotoxicity Adverse renal effects, as demonstrated by the presence of casts, cells, or protein in the urine or by rising BUN, NPN, serum creatinine or oliguria, have been reported. They occur more frequently in patients with a history of renal impairment and in patients treated for longer periods or with larger dosage than recommended.
Neurotoxicity Serious adverse effects on both vestibular and auditory branches of the eighth nerve have been reported, primarily in patients with renal impairment (especially if dialysis is required), and in patients on high doses and/or prolonged therapy. Symptoms include dizziness, vertigo, tinnitus, roaring in the ears and hearing loss, which, as with the other aminoglycosides, may be irreversible. Hearing loss is usually manifested initially by diminution of high-tone acuity. Other factors which may increase the risk of toxicity include excessive dosage, dehydration and previous exposure to other ototoxic drugs.
Peripheral neuropathy or encephalopathy, including numbness, skin tingling, muscle twitching, convulsions, and a myasthenia gravis-like syndrome, have been reported.
Note: The risk of toxic reactions is low in patients with normal renal function who do not receive GARAMYCIN at higher doses or for longer periods of time than recommended. Other reported adverse reactions possibly related to gentamicin include: respiratory depression, lethargy, confusion, depression, visual disturbances, decreased appetite, weight loss, and hypotension and hypertension; rash, itching, urticaria, generalized burning, laryngeal edema, anaphylactoid reactions, fever, and headache; nausea, vomiting, increased salivation, and stomatitis; purpura, pseudotumor cerebri, acute organic brain syndrome, pulmonary fibrosis, alopecia, joint pain, transient hepatomegaly, and splenomegaly.
Laboratory abnormalities possibly related to gentamicin include: increased levels of serum transaminase (SGOT, SGPT), serum LDH and bilirubin; decreased serum calcium, magnesium, sodium and potassium; anemia, leukopenia, granulocytopenia, transient agranulocytosis, eosinophilia, increased and decreased reticulocyte counts, and thrombocytopenia. While clinical laboratory test abnormalities may be isolated findings, they may also be associated with clinically related signs and symptoms. For example, tetany and muscle weakness may be associated with hypomagnesemia, hypocalcemia, and hypokalemia.
While local tolerance of GARAMYCIN is generally excellent, there has been an occasional report of pain at the injection site. Subcutaneous atrophy or fat necrosis suggesting local irritation has been reported rarely.

OVERDOSAGE

In the event of overdose or toxic reactions, hemodialysis may aid in the removal of gentamicin from the blood, and is especially important if renal function is, or becomes, compromised. The rate of removal of gentamicin is considerably less by peritoneal dialysis than it is by hemodialysis.

DOSAGE AND ADMINISTRATION

GARAMYCIN I.V. Piggyback Injection should only be administered intravenously. This product does not contain a preservative system; the contents must be used promptly after the seal is broken. Any unused portion must be discarded. DO NOT RETAIN FOR LATER USE.
It is desirable to limit the duration of treatment with aminoglycosides to short-term.
The usual duration of treatment for all patients is seven to ten days. In difficult and complicated infections, a longer course of therapy may be necessary. In such cases monitoring of renal, auditory, and vestibular functions is recommended, since toxicity is more apt to occur with treatment extended for more than ten days. Dosage should be reduced if clinically indicated.
The patient's pretreatment body weight should be obtained for calculation of correct dosage. The dosage of aminoglycosides in obese patients should be based on an estimate of the lean body mass.
In patients with extensive burns, altered pharmacokinetics may result in reduced serum concentrations of aminoglycosides. In such patients treated with gentamicin, measurement of serum concentrations is recommended as a basis for dosage adjustment.
It is desirable to measure periodically both peak and trough serum concentrations of gentamicin when feasible during therapy to assure adequate but not excessive drug levels. For example, the peak concentrations (at 30 to 60 minutes following cessation of infusion) is expected to be in the range of 4 to 6 mcg/ml. When monitoring peak concentrations, dosage should be adjusted so that prolonged levels above 12 mcg/ml are avoided. When monitoring trough concentrations (just prior to the next dose), dosage should be adjusted so that levels above 2 mcg/ml are avoided. Determination of the adequacy of a serum level for a particular patient must take into consideration the susceptibility of the causative organism, the severity of the infection, and the status of the patient's host-defense mechanisms.
The intravenous administration of gentamicin may be particularly useful for treating patients with bacterial septicemia or those in shock. It may also be the preferred route of administration for some patients with congestive heart failure, hematologic disorders, severe burns, or those with reduced muscle mass. The solution may be infused over a period of one-half to two hours.
GARAMYCIN I.V. Piggyback Injection should not be physically premixed with other drugs but should be administered separately in accordance with the recommended route of administration and dosage schedule.
The dosage recommendations which follow are not intended as rigid schedules, but are provided as guides for initial therapy or when the measurement of gentamicin serum levels during therapy is not feasible.

DOSAGE FOR PATIENTS WITH NORMAL RENAL FUNCTION

Adults: The recommended dosage of GARAMYCIN I.V. Piggyback Injection for patients with serious infections and normal renal function is 3 mg/kg/day, administered in three equal doses every eight hours (Table I).
For patients with life-threatening infections, dosages up to 5 mg/kg/day may be administered in three or four equal doses. This dosage should be reduced to 3 mg/kg/day as soon as clinically indicated (Table I).
[See table on bottom next page].
Children: 6 to 7.5 mg/kg/day (2.0 to 2.5 mg/kg administered every 8 hours.)
Infants and Neonates: 7.5 mg/kg/day (2.5 mg/kg administered every 8 hours).
Premature or Full-Term Neonates one week of age or less: 5 mg/kg/day (2.5 mg/kg administered every 12 hours).
Note: For further information concerning the use of gentamicin in infants and children, see GARAMYCIN Pediatric Injectable Product Information.

DOSAGE FOR PATIENTS WITH IMPAIRED RENAL FUNCTION

Dosage must be adjusted in patients with impaired renal function to assure therapeutically adequate, but not excessive, blood levels. Whenever possible, serum concentrations of gentamicin should be monitored. One method of dosage adjustment is to increase the interval between administration of the usual doses. Since the serum creatinine concentration has a high correlation with the serum half-life of gentamicin, this laboratory test may provide guidance for adjustment of the interval between doses. The interval between doses (in hours) may be approximated by multiplying the serum creatinine level (mg/100 ml) by 8. For example, a patient weighing 60 kg with a serum creatinine level of 2.0 mg/100 ml could be given 60 mg (1 mg/kg every 16 hours (2×8).
In patients with serious systemic infections and renal impairment, it may be desirable to administer the antibiotic more frequently but in reduced dosage. In such patients, serum concentrations of gentamicin should be measured so that adequate but not excessive levels result. A peak and trough concentration measured intermittently during therapy will provide optimal guidance for adjusting dosage. After the usual initial dose, a rough guide for determining reduced dosage at eight-hour intervals is to divide the normally recommended dose by the serum creatinine level (Table II). For example, after an initial dose of 60 mg (1 mg/kg), a patient weighing 60 kg with a serum creatinine level of 2.0 mg/100 ml could be given 30 mg every eight hours ($60 \div 2$).
It should be noted that the status of renal function may be changing over the course of the infectious process.
It is important to recognize that deteriorating renal function may require a greater reduction in dosage than that specified in the above guidelines for patients with stable renal impairment.
[See table on top next page].
In adults with renal failure undergoing hemodialysis, the amount of gentamicin removed from the blood may vary depending upon several factors including the dialysis method used. An eight-hour hemodialysis may reduce serum concentrations of gentamicin by approximately 50%. The recommended dosage at the end of each dialysis period is 1 to 1.7 mg/kg depending upon the severity of infection. In children, a dose of 2 mg/kg may be administered.
A variety of methods are available to measure gentamicin concentrations in body fluids; these include microbiologic, enzymatic and radio-immunoassay techniques.
INSTRUCTIONS FOR THE ADMINISTRATION OF GARAMYCIN I.V. PIGGYBACK INJECTION (For proper apparatus setup see Instruction Sheet).

Continued on next page

Schering—Cont.

THIS PRODUCT IS IN A READY-TO-USE FORM AND IS INTENDED FOR USE ONLY AS AN I.V. PIGGYBACK.

If the prescribed dose is exactly 60 or 80 mg, use the appropriate unit; if the prescribed dose is higher or lower than that of the supplied unit, adjustments can be made in either piggyback unit. If the dose is higher that the contents of the 80 mg unit, the additional amount should be removed from a vial of GARAMYCIN Injectable (40 mg/ml) and added to the 80 mg piggyback unit. If the prescribed dose is less, decrements can be made by removing and discarding the appropriate amount from either unit. **It should be kept in mind that each ml of the piggyback unit contains 1 mg of gentamicin.**

The following are specific examples of dosage adjustment:

- to prepare a 90 mg dose, remove ¼ ml from a vial of GARAMYCIN Injectable (40 mg/ml) and add to the 80 mg piggyback unit.
- to prepare a 70 mg dose, either remove and discard 10 ml from the 80 mg piggyback unit or add the 10 ml from the 80 mg piggyback unit to the 60 mg piggyback unit.
- to prepare a 40 mg dose, remove and discard 20 ml from the 60 mg piggyback unit.

Observe all precautions for sterile technique when adding or removing contents of these units.

HOW SUPPLIED

GARAMYCIN I.V. Piggyback Injection, 1 mg per ml, for intravenous infusion, is supplied in 60 ml (60 mg) (NDC 0085-0527-03) and 80 ml (80 mg) (NDC 0085-0527-04) units; boxes of one.

Store between 2° and 30°C (36° and 86°F).

Also available, GARAMYCIN Injectable, 40 mg per ml, for parenteral administration, is supplied in 2 ml (80 mg) vials, boxes of 25 (NDC 0085-0069-04); and 20 ml vials, box of 5 (NDC 0085-0069-08); and in 1.5 ml (60 mg) NDC 0085-0069-05) and 2 ml (80 mg) (NDC 0085-0069-06) disposable syringes, each in boxes of 1 and 10.

GARAMYCIN Pediatric Injectable, 10 mg per ml, for parenteral administration, supplied in 2 ml (20 mg) vials; box of one (NDC 0085-0013-05).

GARAMYCIN Products are clear, stable solutions that require no refrigeration.

Schering Pharmaceutical
Corporation (P.R.),
Manati, Puerto Rico 00701
An Affiliate of Schering
Corporation, Kenilworth,
N.J. 07033 USA

Revised 2/86

Garamycin I.V.

TABLE II
DOSAGE ADJUSTMENT GUIDE FOR PATIENTS WITH RENAL IMPAIRMENT
(Dosage at Eight-Hour Intervals After the Usual Initial Dose)

Serum Creatinine (mg %)	Approximate Creatinine Clearance Rate (ml/min/1.73M²)	Percent of Usual Doses Shown in Table I
≤1.0	>100	100
1.1-1.3	70-100	80
1.4-1.6	55-70	65
1.7-1.9	45-55	55
2.0-2.2	40-45	50
2.3-2.5	35-40	40
2.6-3.0	30-35	35
3.1-3.5	25-30	30
3.6-4.0	20-25	25
4.1-5.1	15-20	20
5.2-6.6	10-15	15
6.7-8.0	<10	10

GARAMYCIN® Intrathecal ℞

[*gar-ah-mī'sin*]
brand of gentamicin sulfate, USP
Injection 2.0 mg/ml
FOR DIRECT ADMINISTRATION INTO THE CEREBROSPINAL FLUID SPACES OF THE CENTRAL NERVOUS SYSTEM

WARNINGS

GARAMYCIN Intrathecal Injection is intended as adjunctive therapy in patients with central nervous system infections.

Since patients considered for treatment with GARAMYCIN Intrathecal Injection will usually be receiving concomitant treatment with intramuscular or intravenous gentamicin sulfate, all warnings and precautions for this or other concomitantly administered agents must be observed. Moreover, when the drug is administered by more than one route, additive effects must be considered. (See GARAMYCIN Injectable or GARAMYCIN Pediatric Injectable Product Information.) Laboratory studies in animals have shown that gentamicin sulfate, when administered directly into the central nervous system, has caused neurologic disturbances, including adverse effects on the eighth cranial nerve. The risk of direct administration of a potentially neurotoxic drug into the cerebrospinal fluid spaces of the central nervous system must be weighed against the potential benefit to be derived from this route of administration.

DESCRIPTION

Gentamicin sulfate, USP, a water-soluble antibiotic of the aminoglycoside group, is derived from *Micromonospora purpurea*, an actinomycete. GARAMYCIN Intrathecal Injection is a sterile, aqueous solution for direct administration into the cerebrospinal fluid spaces of the central nervous system. Each ml contains: gentamicin sulfate, USP equivalent to 2.0 mg gentamicin base; and 8.5 mg sodium chloride.

CLINICAL PHARMACOLOGY

Since gentamicin sulfate and other aminoglycosides diffuse poorly into the subarachnoid space after systemic administration, concentrations of these antibiotics in the lumbar or ventricular cerebrospinal fluid (CSF) are often low. Following intramuscular or intravenous administration of the usual doses, gentamicin concentrations in CSF in the absence of infection are usually less than 1 mcg/ml. In acute meningitis, slightly higher concentrations are obtained but these vary and are usually well below the peak serum concentration. CSF concentrations which are attained following intravenous or intramuscular administration of gentamicin sulfate tend to become lower as meningeal inflammation subsides. GARAMYCIN Intrathecal Injections are intended to increase the concentration of gentamicin in the CSF when used as part of the management of patients with central nervous system infections.

When GARAMYCIN Intrathecal Injection is given concomitantly with systemically administered gentamicin sulfate, the CSF levels are substantially increased depending upon the location of the injection. Peak CSF concentrations which follow intralumbar administration generally occur at 1 to 6 hours after injection.

Factors which affect the concentration of gentamicin in the CSF following injection into cerebrospinal fluid spaces are the dose administered, the site of the injection (intralumbar, intraventricular), the volume in which the dose is diluted, and the presence or absence of obstruction to the CSF flow. There appears to be considerable inter-patient variation.

The half-life of gentamicin in the CSF of adults who received intralumbar injections is approximately 5.5 hours; this is somewhat longer than that in serum.

In one pharmacokinetic study in adults, a 3 to 4 mg intralumbar injection resulted in a mean CSF concentration of 6.2 mcg/ml 24 hours after injection. The mean CSF concentration was noted to decrease with time; during days 1 through 6 of treatment with GARAMYCIN Intrathecal Injection by the intralumbar route, the mean 24-hour concentration was 9.9 mcg/ml, while during days 7 through 13, the mean concentration was 3.7 mcg/ml.

In another study in adults, CSF levels were measured at varying intervals after intralumbar administration of gentamicin sulfate. During days 1 through 6 of treatment, a 4 mg dose produced a mean CSF level of 2.4 mcg/ml 24 hours after injection, while during days 7 through 13, the same dose produced a mean 24-hour level of 0.5 mcg/ml.

Following intralumbar administration there may be limited upward diffusion of the drug, presumably because of the direction of the CSF flow. Intraventricular administration produces high concentrations in the ventricles and throughout the central nervous system. Adequate levels will usually result from dosing every 24 hours, but it is desirable to manage each patient's infection with serial monitoring of gentamicin serum and CSF concentrations.

Microbiology: *In vitro* tests have demonstrated that gentamicin is a bactericidal antibiotic which acts by inhibiting normal protein synthesis in susceptible microorganisms. It is active against a wide variety of pathogenic bacteria including *Escherichia coli, Proteus* species (indole-positive and indole-negative), *Pseudomonas aeruginosa*, species of the *Klebsiella-Enterobacter-Serratia* group, *Citrobacter* species, and *Staphylococcus* species (including penicillin- and methicillin-resistant strains). Gentamicin is also active *in vitro* against species of *Salmonella* and *Shigella.* The following bacteria are usually resistant to aminoglycosides: *Streptococcus pneumoniae*, most species of streptococci, particularly group D and anaerobic organisms, such as *Bacteroides* species or *Clostridium* species.

Garamycin I.V.

TABLE I
DOSAGE SCHEDULE GUIDE FOR ADULTS WITH NORMAL RENAL FUNCTION
(Dosage at Eight-Hour Intervals)
1 mg/ml

Patient's Weight* kg	(lb)	Usual Dose for Serious Infections 1 mg/kg q8h (3 mg/kg/day) mg/dose	Dose for Life-Threatening Infections (Reduce As Soon As Clinically Indicated) 1.7 mg/kg q8h** (5 mg/kg/day) mg/dose
40	(88)	40	66
45	(99)	45	75
50	(110)	50	83
55	(121)	55	91
60	(132)	60	100
65	(143)	65	108
70	(154)	70	116
75	(165)	75	125
80	(176)	80	133
85	(187)	85	141
90	(198)	90	150
95	(209)	95	158
100	(220)	100	166

* The dosage of aminoglycosides in obese patients should be based on an estimate of the lean body mass.
** For q6h schedules, dosage should be recalculated.

In vitro studies have shown that an aminoglycoside combined with an antibiotic that interferes with cell wall synthesis may act synergistically against some group D streptococcal strains. The combination of gentamicin sulfate and penicillin G has a synergistic bactericidal effect against virtually all strains of *Streptococcus faecalis* and its varieties (*S. faecalis* var. *liquifaciens, S. faecalis* var. *zymogenes), S. faecium* and *S. durans*. An enhanced killing effect against many of these strains has also been shown *in vitro* with combinations of gentamicin and ampicillin, carbenicillin, nafcillin, or oxacillin.
The combined effect of gentamicin and carbenicillin is synergistic for many strains of *Pseudomonas aeruginosa*.
Gentamicin may be active against clinical isolates of bacteria resistant to other aminoglycosides. However, bacteria resistant to one aminoglycoside may be resistant to one or more other aminoglycosides.
Susceptibility Testing: If the disc method of susceptibility testing used is that described by Bauer *et al* (*Am J Clin Path* **45**:493, 1966; *Federal Register* **37**:20525–20529, 1972), a disc containing 10 mcg of gentamicin, when tested against a bacterial strain susceptible to gentamicin, should give a zone of inhibition of $\geq$ 15mm. A zone of $\leq$ 12 mm indicates that the infecting organism is likely to be resistant. Zones greater than 12mm and less than 15mm indicate intermediate susceptibility. In certain conditions it may be desirable to do additional susceptibility testing by the broth or agar dilution method; gentamicin substance is available for this purpose.

INDICATIONS AND USAGE
GARAMYCIN Intrathecal Injection is indicated as adjunctive therapy to systemically administered gentamicin sulfate in the treatment of serious central nervous system infections (meningitis, ventriculitis) caused by susceptible *Pseudomonas* species.
Bacteriologic tests should be performed to determine that the causative organisms are *Pseudomonas* species susceptible to gentamicin.

CONTRAINDICATIONS
Hypersensitivity to gentamicin sulfate is a contraindication to its use. A history of hypersensitivity or serious toxic reactions to aminoglycosides may also contraindicate use of gentamicin sulfate because of the known cross-sensitivity of patients to drugs in this class.

WARNINGS
(See "WARNINGS Box" above and the WARNINGS listed in the Product Information for GARAMYCIN Injectable and GARAMYCIN Pediatric Injectable.)

PRECAUTIONS
(See PRECAUTIONS listed in the Product Information for GARAMYCIN Injectable and GARAMYCIN Pediatric Injectable.)
In a patient with a seven-year history of multiple sclerosis who was treated with gentamicin sulfate by intralumbar injection, disseminated microscopic lesions of the brain stem were reported at autopsy. Lesions observed were: tissue rarefaction with loss and marked swelling of axis cylinders with occasional calcification, loss of oligodendroglia and astroglia, and a poor inflammatory response.
Safety and efficacy in children below the age of three months have not been established.

ADVERSE REACTIONS
Local tolerance to GARAMYCIN Intrathecal Injection has been good. Local reactions of arachnoiditis or burning at the injection site have been reported rarely.
Because the recommended dosage of GARAMYCIN Intrathecal Injection is low, the potential for systemic adverse effects is minimal. However, GARAMYCIN Intrathecal Injection is recommended as adjunctive therapy with other antibiotics, such as parenteral gentamicin sulfate, which should be administered in full therapeutic dosages. Evidence of eighth nerve dysfunction, changes in renal function, leg cramps, rash, fever, convulsions, and an increase in cerebrospinal fluid protein have been reported in patients who were treated concomitantly with GARAMYCIN Intrathecal Injection and the parenteral preparation of gentamicin.
Administration of excessive (40 to 160 mg) doses of the parenteral formulation of gentamicin sulfate (which contains a preservative system) by the various intrathecal routes has been reported to produce neuromuscular disturbances, e.g., ataxia, paresis, and incontinence.

DOSAGE AND ADMINISTRATION
GARAMYCIN Intrathecal Injection is intended for administration directly into the cerebrospinal fluid spaces of the central nervous system.
The dosage will vary depending upon factors, such as age and weight of the patient, site of injection, degree of obstruction to cerebrospinal fluid flow and the amount of cerebrospinal fluid estimated to be present. In general, the recommended dose for infants 3 months of age and older (see PRECAUTIONS) and children is 1 to 2 mg once a day. For adults, 4 to 8 mg may be administered once a day.
Administration of GARAMYCIN Intrathecal Injection should be continued as long as sensitive organisms are demonstrated in the cerebrospinal fluid. Since the intralumbar or intraventricular dose is administered immediately after specimens are taken for laboratory study, treatment should usually be continued for at least one day after negative results have been obtained from CSF cultures and/or stained smears.
The suggested method for administering GARAMYCIN Intrathecal Injection into the lumbar area is as follows: the desired quantity of GARAMYCIN Intrathecal Injection is drawn up carefully from the ampule into a 5- or 10-ml sterile syringe. After the lumbar puncture is performed and a specimen of the spinal fluid is removed for laboratory tests, the syringe containing GARAMYCIN Intrathecal Injection is inserted into the hub of the spinal needle. A quantity of cerebrospinal fluid (approximately 10% of the estimated total CSF volume) is allowed to flow into the syringe and mix with the GARAMYCIN Intrathecal Injection. The resultant solution is then injected over a period of 3 to 5 minutes with the bevel of the needle directed upward.
If the cerebrospinal fluid is grossly purulent, or if it is unobtainable, GARAMYCIN Intrathecal Injection may be diluted with sterile normal saline before injection.
GARAMYCIN Intrathecal Injection may also be administered directly into the subdural space or directly into the ventricles, including administration by use of an implanted reservoir.

HOW SUPPLIED
GARAMYCIN Intrathecal Injection, 2.0 mg per ml, is supplied in 2 ml ampules; box of 25.
Store below 30°C (86°F).
NOTE: This preparation does not contain any preservative. Once opened, contents should be used immediately and unused portions should be discarded.

ANIMAL PHARMACOLOGY AND TOXICOLOGY
In dogs, an 8-hour perfusion of the ventriculosubarachnoid system with a solution containing 40 mcg/ml (~5 mg or ~0.3 mg/kg) gentamicin produced no seizure activity or change in vital signs during administration. No morphological changes were observed when the dogs were sacrificed at 10 and 90 days following infusion.
The effects of repeated intrathecal injections of gentamicin at 0.1 and 0.3 mg/kg were evaluated in tranquilized beagle puppies. Transient flaccid paralysis was observed on the first day when the drug was administered rapidly (i.e., in less than 5 seconds), but no adverse effects were observed thereafter when the drug was administered less rapidly (i.e., over a period of approximately 30 seconds). No drug-related changes were found on histological examination of the cerebellum, brain stem or cephalic cord. In cats, gentamicin administered intracisternally at one-hour intervals in doses of up to 50 mg/kg did not produce any abnormalities in the electroencephalogram. In another study in cats, gentamicin sulfate given daily by the intracisternal route for up to 7 days caused neurologic disturbances, including adverse effects on the eighth cranial nerve.
In rabbits intracisternal injection of gentamicin at doses 50 and 100 times the therapeutic dose produced peak CSF concentrations of 160 and 180 mcg/ml, respectively. These doses were associated with changes in the myelin sheath predominantly of the lateral columns of the upper cervical cord, and some changes in glial cells and lesions in the medulla oblongata. In addition to a high incidence of mortality, the animals demonstrated weakness, ataxia and paralysis. At doses of one and ten times the therapeutic dose (providing peak levels of 16.5 and 40 mcg/ml CSF), no morphologic changes occurred and there were no drug-related symptoms identified.

Schering Pharmaceutical Corporation (PR)
Manati, Puerto Rico 00701
An Affiliate of Schering Corporation
Kenilworth, New Jersey 07033

Revised 7/83

GYNE–LOTRIMIN® ℞
[*gī″ne-lo′trim-in*]
brand of clotrimazole
Vaginal Tablets, USP
Vaginal Cream, USP 1%

DESCRIPTION
GYNE-LOTRIMIN is clotrimazole [1-(*o*-Chloro-α, α-diphenylbenzyl) imidazole], a synthetic antifungal agent having the chemical formula $C_{22}H_{17}ClN_2$.
Each GYNE-LOTRIMIN **Vaginal Tablet** contains 100 mg clotrimazole, USP dispersed in lactose, povidone, corn starch, and magnesium stearate.
Each applicatorful of GYNE-LOTRIMIN **Vaginal Cream** contains approximately 50 mg clotrimazole, USP dispersed in sorbitan monostearate, polysorbate 60, cetyl esters wax, cetearyl alcohol, 2-octyldodecanol, purified water, and as preservative, benzyl alcohol (1%).

ACTIONS
Clotrimazole is a broad-spectrum antifungal agent that inhibits the growth of pathogenic yeasts. Clotrimazole exhibits fungicidal activity *in vitro* against *Candida albicans* and other species of the genus *Candida*.
No single-step or multiple-step resistance to clotrimazole has developed during successive passages of *Candida albicans*.

INDICATIONS
GYNE-LOTRIMIN **Vaginal Cream** and **Tablets** are indicated for the local treatment of patients with vulvovaginal candidiasis (moniliasis). The diagnosis should be confirmed by KOH smears and/or cultures. Other pathogens commonly associated with vulvovaginitis (*Trichomonas* and *Hemophilus vaginalis*) should be ruled out by appropriate laboratory methods.
The 3-day regimen of GYNE-LOTRIMIN **Vaginal Tablets** did not prove to be effective in pregnant patients.
Studies with clotrimazole cream have shown that women taking oral contraceptives had a cure rate similar to those not taking oral contraceptives.

CONTRAINDICATIONS
GYNE-LOTRIMIN **Vaginal Tablets** and **Vaginal Cream** are contraindicated in women who have shown hypersensitivity to any of the components of the preparation.

PRECAUTIONS
Laboratory Tests: If there is a lack of response to GYNE-LOTRIMIN, appropriate microbiological studies should be repeated to confirm the diagnosis and rule out other pathogens before instituting another course of antimycotic therapy.
Application of ^{14}C-labeled clotrimazole has shown negligible absorption (peak of 0.03 mcg/ml of serum 24 hours after insertion of a 100 mg tablet; peak serum level of 0.01 mcg/ml 24 hours after insertion of vaginal cream containing 50 mg of active drug) from both normal and inflamed human vaginal mucosa.
Usage in Pregnancy: While GYNE-LOTRIMIN **Vaginal Tablets** and **Vaginal Cream** have not been studied in the first trimester of pregnancy, use in the second and third trimesters has not been associated with ill effects. Follow-up reports now available on 71 neonates of 177 pregnant patients treated with GYNE-LOTRIMIN **Vaginal Tablets** reveal no adverse effects or complications attributable to GYNE-LOTRIMIN therapy.

ADVERSE REACTIONS
Eighteen (1.6%) of the 1116 patients treated with GYNE-LOTRIMIN **Vaginal Tablets** in double-blind studies reported complaints during therapy that were possibly drug-related. Mild burning occurred in six patients while other complaints, such as skin rash, itching, vulval irritation, lower abdominal cramps and bloating, slight cramping, slight urinary frequency, and burning or irritation in the sexual partner, occurred rarely.
Three (0.5%) of the 653 patients treated with GYNE-LOTRIMIN **Vaginal Cream** reported complaints during therapy that were possibly drug-related. Vaginal burning occurred in one patient; erythema, irritation and burning in another; intercurrent cystitis was reported in the third.

DOSAGE AND ADMINISTRATION
GYNE-LOTRIMIN **Vaginal Cream** has been found to be effective when used from seven to fourteen days; studies have shown that patients treated for fourteen days had a significantly higher cure rate. The recommended dose is one applicatorful of cream (approximately 5 grams) inserted intravaginally for seven to fourteen consecutive days, preferably at bedtime.
GYNE-LOTRIMIN **Vaginal Tablets**: Two tablets inserted intravaginally at bedtime for three nights or one tablet inserted intravaginally at bedtime for seven nights.
In the event of treatment failure, other pathogens commonly responsible for vaginitis should be ruled out before instituting another course of antimycotic therapy.

HOW SUPPLIED
GYNE-LOTRIMIN **Vaginal Tablets,** 100 mg, white, uncoated tablets impressed with the trademark GYNE-LOTRIMIN and/or the Schering trademark and product identification number, 734; carton of six tablets for three-day treatment regimen and carton of seven tablets for seven-day treatment regimen; with plastic applicator and patient instructions.
Store between 2° and 30°C (36° and 86°F).
GYNE-LOTRIMIN **Vaginal Cream 1%** is supplied in 45-gram tubes with a measured-dose applicator; box of one for seven-day treatment; box of two for fourteen-day treatment.

Continued on next page

Information on Schering products appearing on these pages is effective as of September 30, 1986.

Schering—Cont.

Store between 2° and 30°C (36° and 86°F).

Rev. 8/82
Shown in Product Identification Section, page 428

GYNE-LOTRIMIN® 500 mg ℞
[*gī″ne-lo′trim-in*]
brand of clotrimazole
Vaginal Tablets

DESCRIPTION
Each GYNE-LOTRIMIN 500 mg Vaginal Tablet contains 500 mg clotrimazole (the active ingredient) dispersed in lactose, microcrystalline cellulose, lactic acid, corn starch, crospovidone, calcium lactate, magnesium stearate, silicon dioxide and hydroxypropyl methylcellulose. Chemically, clotrimazole is [1-(o-Chloro-α, α-diphenylbenzyl) imidazole], a synthetic antifungal agent having the chemical formula $C_{22}H_{17}ClN_2$, and a molecular weight of 344.84.
Clotrimazole is an odorless, white crystalline substance, practically insoluble in water, sparingly soluble in ether, soluble in carbon tetrachloride, and very soluble in ethanol and chloroform.

CLINICAL PHARMACOLOGY
Serum levels and levels in vaginal secretions of clotrimazole were measured in six healthy volunteers who had one 500 mg vaginal tablet inserted. Although serum levels of clotrimazole were higher than those in other volunteers given 100 mg and 200 mg vaginal tablets, these levels did not exceed 10 nanograms/ml. It has been estimated that three to ten percent of a vaginal dose of clotrimazole may be absorbed, but the drug rapidly and efficiently degrades to microbiologically inactive metabolites. The clotrimazole concentrations remaining in vaginal secretions were still in the mg/ml range for 48 hours and in two of the six subjects at 72 hours.
The findings of high clotrimazole concentrations in vaginal secretions for up to 72 hours and low concentrations in the serum suggest that nearly all the clotrimazole given in the 500 mg vaginal tablet remains in the vagina for 48 hours, and in some cases 72 hours, in fungicidal concentrations.
Clotrimazole is a broad-spectrum antifungal agent. It has been postulated that the compound affects the permeability characteristics of the membrane allowing the leakage of essential intracellular components with a consequent inhibition of the synthesis of such macromolecules as protein, lipid, DNA, and polysaccharides.
At concentrations as low as 2–5 μg/ml, clotrimazole exhibits fungicidal activity *in vitro* against *Candida albicans* and other species of the genus Candida.
No single-step or multiple-step resistance to clotrimazole has developed during successive passages of *Candida albicans.*

INDICATIONS
GYNE-LOTRIMIN 500 mg Vaginal Tablets are indicated for the local treatment of vulvovaginal candidiasis when one day therapy is felt warranted in the case of severe vulvovaginitis due to candidiasis, longer antimycotic therapy is recommended. The diagnosis should be confirmed by KOH smears and/or cultures. Other pathogens commonly associated with vulvovaginitis, *Trichomonas* and *Gardnerella (Haemophilus) vaginalis,* should be ruled out by appropriate laboratory methods.

CONTRAINDICATIONS
GYNE-LOTRIMIN 500 mg Vaginal Tablets are contraindicated in women who have shown hypersensitivity to any components of the preparation.

WARNINGS
None

PRECAUTIONS
If there is a lack of response to GYNE-LOTRIMIN 500 mg Vaginal Tablets, appropriate microbiological studies should be repeated to confirm the diagnosis and rule out other pathogens before instituting another course of antimycotic therapy.
Carcinogenesis: No long term studies in animals have been performed to evaluate the carcinogenic potential of GYNE-LOTRIMIN 500 mg Vaginal Tablets intravaginally. A long term study in rats (Wistar strains) where clotrimazole was administered orally provided no indication of carcinogenicity.
Usage in Pregnancy: Pregnancy Category B: The disposition of ^{14}C-clotrimazole has been studied in humans and animals. Clotrimazole is poorly absorbed following intravaginal administration to humans whereas it is rather well absorbed after oral administration.
In clinical trials, use of vaginally applied clotrimazole in pregnant women in their second and third trimesters has not been associated with ill effects. There are, however, no adequate and well-controlled studies in pregnant women during the first trimester of pregnancy.
Studies in pregnant rats given repeated intravaginal doses up to 100 mg/kg/day have revealed no evidence of harm to the fetus due to clotrimazole.
Repeated high oral doses of clotrimazole in rats and mice ranging from 50 to 120 mg/kg resulted in embryotoxicity (possibly secondary to maternal toxicity), impairment of mating, decreased litter size and number of viable young and decreased pup survival to weaning. However, clotrimazole was not teratogenic in mice, rabbits and rats at oral doses up to 200, 180 and 100 mg/kg, respectively. Oral absorption in the rat amounts to approximately 90% of the administered dose.
Because animal reproduction studies are not always predictive of human response, this drug should be used only if clearly indicated during the first trimester of pregnancy.

ADVERSE REACTIONS
Of 297 patients in double-blind studies with the 500 mg vaginal tablet, 3 of 149 patients treated with active drug and 3 of 148 patients treated with placebo reported complaints during therapy that were possibly drug related. In the active drug group, vomiting occurred in one patient, vaginal soreness with coitus in another, and complaints of vaginal irritation, itching, burning and dyspareunia in the third patient. In the placebo group, clitoral irritation occurred in one patient and dysuria, described as remotely related to drug, in the other. A third patient in the placebo group developed bacterial vaginitis which the investigator classed as possibly related to drug.
Eighteen (1.6%) of the 1116 patients treated with GYNE-LOTRIMIN in other formulations in double-blind studies reported complaints during therapy that were possibly drug-related. Mild burning occurred in six patients while other complaints such as skin rash, itching, vulval irritation, lower abdominal cramps and bloating, slight cramping, slight urinary frequency, and burning or irritation in the sexual partner, occurred rarely.

OVERDOSAGE
No data available.

DRUG ABUSE AND DEPENDENCE
Drug abuse and dependence with GYNE-LOTRIMIN 500 mg Vaginal Tablets has not been reported.

DOSAGE AND ADMINISTRATION
The recommended dose is one tablet inserted intravaginally one time only, preferably at bedtime. In the event of treatment failure, that is, persistence of signs and symptoms of vaginitis after five days, other pathogens commonly responsible for vaginitis should be ruled out before instituting another course of antimycotic therapy.

HOW SUPPLIED
GYNE-LOTRIMIN 500 mg Vaginal Tablets are white, bullet shaped, uncoated tablets, coded with Schering on one side and 396 on the other, supplied as a single 500 mg tablet with plastic applicator and patient instructions (NDC 0085-0396-01).
Store below 30°C (86°F).
March 1986

Shown in Product Identification Section, page 428

HYPERSTAT® I.V. ℞
[*hi′per-stat*]
brand of diazoxide, USP
Injection
For Intravenous Use In
Hospitalized Patients Only

DESCRIPTION
HYPERSTAT I.V. Injection is a nondiuretic benzothiadiazine antihypertensive agent. Each ampule (20 ml) contains 300 mg diazoxide, USP, in a clear, sterile, colorless aqueous solution; the pH is adjusted to approximately 11.6 with sodium hydroxide.
Diazoxide is 7-chloro-3-methyl-2*H*-1,2,4-benzothiadiazine 1,1-dioxide, with the empirical formula $C_8H_7ClN_2O_2S$, and the molecular weight 230.7. It is a white crystalline powder practically insoluble to sparingly soluble in water.

CLINICAL PHARMACOLOGY
HYPERSTAT I.V. Injection produces a prompt reduction of blood pressure in man by relaxing smooth muscle in the peripheral arterioles. Cardiac output is increased as blood pressure is reduced. Studies in animals demonstrate that coronary blood flow is maintained, while renal blood flow is increased after an initial decrease.
Transient hyperglycemia occurs in the majority of patients treated with HYPERSTAT, but usually requires treatment only in patients with diabetes mellitus. It will respond to the usual management measures, including insulin.
Blood glucose levels should be monitored especially in patients with diabetes and in those requiring multiple injections of diazoxide. Cataracts have been observed in a few animals receiving repeated daily doses of intravenous diazoxide.
Since diazoxide causes sodium retention, repeated injections may precipitate edema and congestive heart failure. Increased volume of extracellular fluid may be a cause of treatment failure in nonresponsive patients. The increase in fluid volume characteristically responds to diuretic agents if adequate renal function exists. Concurrently administered thiazide diuretics may be expected to potentiate the antihypertensive and hyperuricemic actions of diazoxide. (See **Drug Interactions.**)
Diazoxide is extensively bound to serum protein (>90%). The plasma half-life is 28 ± 8.3 hours; however, the duration of its antihypertensive effect is variable, generally lasting less than 12 hours.

INDICATIONS AND USAGE
HYPERSTAT I.V. Injection is indicated for short-term use in the emergency reduction of blood pressure in severe, nonmalignant and malignant hypertension in hospitalized adults; and in acute severe hypertension in hospitalized children, when prompt and urgent decrease of diastolic pressure is required. Treatment with orally effective antihypertensive agents should not be instituted until blood pressure has stabilized. The use of HYPERSTAT I.V. Injection for longer than 10 days is not recommended.
HYPERSTAT I.V. Injection is ineffective against hypertension due to pheochromocytoma.

CONTRAINDICATIONS
HYPERSTAT I.V. Injection should not be used in the treatment of compensatory hypertension, such as that associated with aortic coarctation or arteriovenous shunt, and should not be used in patients hypersensitive to diazoxide, other thiazides, or other sulfonamide-derived drugs.

WARNINGS
Rapid decrease of blood pressure Caution must be observed when reducing severely elevated blood pressure. Diazoxide should only be administered utilizing the new 150 mg minibolus dosage. The use of a 300 mg intravenous dose of diazoxide has been associated with angina and with myocardial and cerebral infarction. One instance of optic nerve infarction was reported when a 100 mmHg reduction in diastolic pressure occurred over ten minutes following a single 300 mg bolus. In one prospective trial conducted in patients with severe hypertension and coexistent coronary artery disease, a 50% incidence of ischemic changes in the electrocardiogram was observed following single 300 mg bolus injections of diazoxide. The desired blood pressure lowering should therefore be achieved over as long a period of time as is compatible with the patient's status. At least several hours and preferably one or two days is tentatively recommended. Improved safety with equal efficacy can be achieved by administering HYPERSTAT I.V. Injection as a mini-bolus dose (1 to 3 mg/kg every 5 to 15 minutes up to a maximum of 150 mg in a single injection) until a diastolic blood pressure below 100 mmHg is achieved. HYPERSTAT I.V. Injection should not be administered in a bolus dose of 300 mg since this mode of administration is less predictable and less controllable than the minibolus dosage. If hypotension severe enough to require therapy results from the reduction in blood pressure, it will usually respond to the Trendelenberg maneuver. If necessary, sympathomimetic agents such as dopamine or norepinephrine may be administered.
Special attention is required for patients with diabetes mellitus and those in whom retention of salt and water may present serious problems.
Myocardial Lesions in Animals Intravenous administration of diazoxide in dogs has induced subendocardial necrosis and necrosis of papillary muscles. These lesions, which are also produced by other vasodilator drugs (i.e., hydralazine, minoxidil) and by catecholamines, are presumed to be related to anoxia resulting from a combination of reflex tachycardia and decreased perfusion.

PRECAUTIONS
General: HYPERSTAT (diazoxide) I.V. Injection is an effective antihypertensive agent requiring close monitoring of the patient's blood pressure at frequent intervals. Its administration may occasionally cause hypotension requiring treatment with sympathomimetic drugs. Therefore, HYPERSTAT, I.V. Injection should be used primarily in the hospital or where adequate facilities exist to treat such untoward responses.
HYPERSTAT I.V. Injection should be administered only into a peripheral vein. Because the alkalinity of the solution is irritating to tissue, avoid extravascular injection or leakage. Subcutaneous administration has produced inflammation and pain without subsequent necrosis. If leakage into subcutaneous tissue occurs, the area should be treated with warm compresses and rest.
HYPERSTAT I.V. Injection should be used with care in patients who have impaired cerebral or cardiac circulation,

that is, patients in whom abrupt reduction in blood pressure might be detrimental or those in whom mild tachycardia or decreased blood perfusion may be deleterious (see **Warnings**). Prolonged hypotension should be avoided so as not to aggravate preexisting renal failure.

Information for Patients: During and immediately following intravenous, injection of HYPERSTAT I.V. Injection, the patient should remain supine.

Laboratory Tests: Diagnostic laboratory tests necessary to establish the patient's condition and status should be carried out prior to treatment with HYPERSTAT I.V. Injection. During and following treatment with HYPERSTAT I.V. Injection, laboratory tests to monitor the effects of treatment with this drug and the patient's condition should be done. Among the tests (not necessarily inclusive) are: hematologic (hematocrit, hemoglobin, white blood cell and platelet counts); metabolic (glucose, uric acid, total protein, albumin); electrolyte (sodium, potassium) and osmolality; renal function (creatinine, urine-protein); electrocardiogram.

Drug Interactions: Diazoxide is highly bound to serum protein. It can be expected to displace other substances which are also bound to protein, such as bilirubin or coumarin and its derivatives, resulting in higher blood levels of these substances.

An undesirable hypotension may result when diazoxide is administered to patients who have received other antihypertensive medication within six hours.

One patient in a clinical study exhibited excessive hypotension after concomitant administration of HYPERSTAT with hydralazine and methyldopa. An episode of maternal hypotension and fetal bradycardia occurred in a patient in labor who received both reserpine and hydralazine prior to administration of diazoxide. Neonatal hyperglycemia following intrapartum administration of HYPERSTAT I.V. Injection has also been reported.

HYPERSTAT I.V. Injection should not be administered within six hours of the administration of: hydralazine, reserpine, alphaprodine, methyldopa, beta-blockers, prazosin, minoxidil, the nitrites and other papaverine-like compounds. Concomitant administration with thiazides or other commonly used diuretics may be expected to potentiate the hyperuricemic and antihypertensive effects of diazoxide.

Drug/Laboratory Test Interactions: The hyperglycemic and hyperuricemic effects of diazoxide preclude proper assessment of these metabolic states. Increased renin secretion, IgG concentrations and decreased cortisol secretion have also been noted. Diazoxide inhibits glucagon-stimulated insulin release and will cause a false-negative insulin response to glucagon. In the rat, dog and monkey, diazoxide increased serum free fatty acids and decreased plasma insulin levels.

Carcinogenesis, Mutagenesis, Impairment of Fertility: No long-term animal dosing study has been done to evaluate the carcinogenic potential of diazoxide. No laboratory studies of mutagenic potential or animal studies of effects on fertility have been done.

Pregnancy Category C: Diazoxide has been shown to reduce fetal and/or pup survival; and to reduce fetal growth in rats, rabbits, and dogs at daily doses of 30, 21, or 10 mg/kg, respectively. In rats treated at term, diazoxide, at doses of 10 mg/kg and above, prolonged parturition.

The safety of HYPERSTAT I.V. Injection in pregnancy has not been established.

Non-teratogenic Effects: Diazoxide crosses the placental barrier and appears in cord blood. When given to the mother prior to delivery the drug may produce fetal or neonatal hyperbilirubinemia, thrombocytopenia, altered carbohydrate metabolism, and possibly other side effects that have occurred in adults.

Labor and Delivery: HYPERSTAT I.V. Injection is not indicated for use in pregnancy. Intravenous administration of the drug during labor may cause cessation of uterine contractions, requiring administration of an oxytocic agent.

Nursing Mothers: Information is not available concerning the passage of HYPERSTAT in breast milk. Because many drugs are excreted in human milk and because of the potential for adverse reactions in nursing infants from diazoxide, a decision should be made whether to discontinue nursing or to discontinue the drug, taking into account the importance of the drug to the mother.

Pediatric Use: See **Indications and Usage.**

ADVERSE REACTIONS

It is reasonable to speculate that the currently recommended mini-bolus dosing regimen, which has replaced the 300 mg bolus dose in clinical practice, will result in adverse effects which are of similar character but of lesser frequency and severity.

In clinical experience with the rapid bolus administration of 300 mg, the most common adverse reactions reported were: hypotension (7%); nausea and vomiting (4%); dizziness and weakness (2%). Additional adverse reactions reported with bolus administration of 300 mg were as follows:

Cardiovascular: sodium and water retention after repeated injections, especially important in patients with impaired cardiac reserve; hypotension to shock levels; myocardial ischemia, usually transient and manifested by angina, atrial and ventricular arrhythmias, and marked electrocardiographic changes, but occasionally leading to myocardial infarction; optic nerve infarction following too rapid decrease in severely elevated blood pressure; supraventricular tachycardia and palpitation; bradycardia; chest discomfort or nonanginal "tightness in the chest."

Central Nervous System: cerebral ischemia, usually transient but occasionally leading to infarction and manifested by unconsciousness, convulsions, paralysis, confusion, or focal neurological deficit such as numbness of the hands; vasodilative phenomena, such as orthostatic hypotension, sweating, flushing, and generalized or localized sensations of warmth; various transient neurological findings secondary to alteration in regional blood flow to brain, such as headache (sometimes throbbing), dizziness, lightheadedness, sleepiness (also reported as lethargy, somnolence or drowsiness), euphoria or "funny feeling," ringing in the ears and momentary hearing loss, and weakness of short duration; apprehension or anxiety.

Gastrointestinal: rarely, acute pancreatitis; nausea, vomiting and/or abdominal discomfort, anorexia; alteration in taste, parotid swelling; salivation; dry mouth; lacrimation; ileus; constipation and diarrhea.

Other: hyperglycemia in diabetic patients, especially after repeated injections; hyperosmolar coma in an infant; transient hyperglycemia in nondiabetic patients; transient retention of nitrogenous wastes; various respiratory findings secondary to the relaxation of smooth muscle, such as dyspnea, cough and choking sensation; warmth or pain along the injected vein; cellulitis without sloughing and/or phlebitis at the injection site of extravasation; back pain and increased nocturia; hypersensitivity reactions, such as rash, leukopenia and fever; papilledema induced by plasma volume expansion secondary to the administration of diazoxide reported in a patient who had received eleven injections (300 mg/dose) over a 22-day period; malaise and blurred vision; transient cataract in an infant; hirsutism , and decreased libido.

OVERDOSAGE

Overdosage of HYPERSTAT I.V. Injection may cause an undesirable hypotension. Usually, this can be controlled with the Trendelenberg maneuver. If necessary, sympathomimetic agents, such as dopamine or norepinephrine, may be administered. Failure of blood pressure to rise in response to such agents suggests that the hypotension may have been caused by something other than diazoxide. Excessive hyperglycemia resulting from overdosage will respond to conventional therapy of hyperglycemia.

DOSAGE AND ADMINISTRATION

HYPERSTAT I.V. Injection was originally recommended for use by bolus administration of 300 mg. Recent studies have shown that minibolus administration of HYPERSTAT I.V. Injection i.e., doses of 1 to 3 mg/kg repeated at intervals of 5 to 15 minutes is as effective in reducing blood pressure. Minibolus administration usually provides a more gradual reduction in blood pressure and thus may be expected to reduce the circulatory and neurological risks associated with acute hypotension.

HYPERSTAT I.V. Injection is administered undiluted and rapidly by intravenous injections of 1 to 3 mg/kg up to a maximum of 150 mg in a single injection. This dose may be repeated at intervals of 5 to 15 minutes until a satisfactory reduction in blood pressure (diastolic pressure below 100 mmHg) has been achieved.

With the patient recumbent, the calculated dose of HYPERSTAT I.V. Injection is administered intravenously in 30 seconds or less.

HYPERSTAT I.V. Injection should only be given into a peripheral vein. Do no administer it intramuscularly, subcutaneously, or into body cavities. Avoid extravasation of the drug into subcutaneous tissues.

Following the use of HYPERSTAT I.V. Injection, the blood pressure should be monitored closely until it has stabilized. Thereafter, measurements taken hourly during the balance of the effect should indicate any unusual response. A further decrease in blood pressure 30 minutes or more after injection should be investigated for causes other than the action of HYPERSTAT I.V. Injection. It is preferable that the patient remain supine for at least one hour after injection. In ambulatory patients, the blood pressure should also be measured with the patient standing before surveillance is ended.

Repeated administration of HYPERSTAT I.V. Injection at intervals of 4 to 24 hours usually will maintain the blood pressure below pretreatment levels until a regimen of oral antihypertensive medication can be instituted. The interval between injections may be adjusted by the duration of the response to each injection. It is usually unnecessary to continue treatment with HYPERSTAT I.V. Injection for more than four to five days.

Since repeated administration of HYPERSTAT I.V. Injection can lead to sodium and water retention, administration of a diuretic may be necessary both for maximal blood pressure reduction and to avoid congestive heart failure. (See **Clinical Pharmacology.**)

Parenteral drug products should be inspected visually for particulate matter and discoloration prior to administration whenever solution & container permit.

HOW SUPPLIED

HYPERSTAT I.V. Injection is supplied in a 20 ml. ampule, containing 300 mg diazoxide, in a clear, sterile, colorless aqueous solution; box of one ampule. (NDC 0085-0201-05).

Protect from light and freezing. Store between 36° and 86°F (2° and 30°C).

Revised 2/85

INTRON® A ℞

Interferon alfa-2b recombinant
For Injection

DESCRIPTION

INTRON A Interferon alfa-2b, recombinant for Injection is a purified sterile, lyophilized recombinant interferon formulated for use by intramuscular or subcutaneous injection (see **PRECAUTIONS**).

INTRON A is a water soluble protein with a molecular weight of 19,271 daltons produced by recombinant DNA techniques. Interferon alfa-2b is obtained from the bacterial fermentation of a strain of *Escherichia coli* bearing a genetically engineered plasmid containing an interferon alfa-2b gene from human leukocytes. The fermentation is carried out in a defined nutrient medium containing the antibiotic tetracycline hydrochloride at a concentration of 5 to 10 mg/L; the presence of this antibiotic is not detectable in the final product. The specific activity of INTRON A is approximately 2×10^8 IU/mg protein.

The content of INTRON A is expressed in terms of International Units (IU). International Units are determined by comparison of the antiviral activity of the interferon alfa-2b, recombinant with the activity of the international reference preparation of human leukocyte interferon established by the World Health Organization (WHO).

Each vial of INTRON A contains either 3 million, 5 million, 10 million, or 25 million IU of interferon alfa-2b, recombinant; glycine, sodium phosphate dibasic, sodium phosphate monobasic, and human albumin are also present. Based on the specific activity of INTRON A as approximately 2×10^8 IU/mg protein, the corresponding mg quantities of interferon alfa-2b, recombinant in the vials described above are approximately 0.015 mg, 0.025 mg, 0.05 mg and 0.125 mg protein, respectively. Prior to administration, the lyophilized powder is to be reconstituted with Diluent for INTRON A Interferon alfa-2b, recombinant (bacteriostatic water for injection) provided (see diluent label for preservative). (See **DOSAGE AND ADMINISTRATION.**)

Lyophilized INTRON A is a white to cream colored powder.

CLINICAL PHARMACOLOGY

General: The interferons are a family of naturally occurring, small protein molecules with molecular weights of approximately 15,000 to 21,000 daltons. They are produced and secreted by cells in response to viral infections or to various synthetic and biological inducers. Three major classes of interferons have been identified: alpha, beta, and gamma. These three classes are not homogeneous, and each may contain several different molecular species of interferon. As an example, at least 14 genetically distinct human alpha interferons have been identified thus far. INTRON A has been classified as an alfa interferon.

Interferons exert their cellular activities by binding to specific membrane receptors on the cell surface. Preliminary studies to characterize these membrane receptors and to determine the subsequent fate of the human interferon-receptor complex have been carried out using ^{125}I-labeled interferon alfa-2b, recombinant. Human interferon receptors, as isolated from human lymphoblastoid (Daudi) cells, appear to be highly asymmetric membrane proteins. They exhibit selectivity for human but not murine interferons, suggesting species-specificity. Studies with other interferons have demonstrated varying degrees of species-specificity.

The results of several studies suggest that once bound to the cell membrane, interferon initiates a complex sequence of intracellular events that include the induction of certain enzymes. It is thought that this process, at least in part, is responsible for the various cellular responses to interferon, including inhibition of virus replication in virus-infected cells, suppression of cell proliferation, and such immunomodulating activities as enhancement of the phago-

Continued on next page

Information on Schering products appearing on these pages is effective as of September 30, 1986.

Schering—Cont.

cytic activity of macrophages and augmentation of the specific cytotoxicity of lymphocytes for target cells. Any of these activities might contribute to interferon's therapeutic effects.

Preclinical Pharmacology: INTRON A has exhibited antiproliferative effects in preclinical studies employing both cell culture systems and human tumor xenografts in animals, and has demonstrated significant immunomodulatory activity *in vitro*. The clinical significance of these findings is unknown.

The antiproliferative activity of INTRON A Interferon alfa-2b, recombinant for Injection was evaluated *in vitro* using mouse and human leukemia cell lines, and human osteosarcoma, melanoma, and normal amnion cells. No activity was seen in mouse leukemia cells, which again suggests species-specificity.

The immunomodulating activity of INTRON A was demonstrated *in vitro* by its augmentation of the spontaneous "natural killer" activity of human lymphocytes and its enhancement of the tumoricidal activity of human monocytes against human tumor cells. These effects appear to be dose-dependent.

In vivo studies of INTRON A showed inhibition of tumor growth. INTRON A injected *intralesionally* (0.2 million or 0.8 million IU once daily for 7 days) delayed the development and reduced the volume of human osteosarcoma implants in athymic mice. The effect was dose-related. Additionally, *subcutaneous* administration of INTRON A at a dose of 0.2 million IU/day inhibited the growth of implanted human breast tumor xenografts in athymic mice by about 50% after 23 days. INTRON A has not been shown to be effective in the treatment of osteosarcoma or carcinoma of the breast in humans.

Pharmacokinetics: The pharmacokinetics of INTRON A were studied in healthy male volunteers following single 10 million IU doses administered intramuscularly, subcutaneously, and as a 30 minute intravenous infusion. The mean serum level concentrations of interferon following intramuscular and subcutaneous injections were comparable. The maximum serum levels obtained via the intramuscular and subcutaneous routes were approximately 150 to 180 IU/ml, 6 to 8 hours after administration. The elimination half-lives of interferon following both intramuscular and subcutaneous injections were approximately 6 to 7 hours. Serum levels were below the detection limit of 25 IU/ml 24 hours after the injections. After intravenous administration, serum levels of interferon peaked (546 IU/ml) by the end of the infusion, then declined rapidly with time, becoming undetectable 4 hours after the infusion.

Following a single dose of 10 million IU of INTRON A, by any of the three routes of administration, interferon could not be detected in urine. Preliminary studies with isolated and perfused rabbit kidneys have shown that the kidney may be the main site of interferon catabolism; in addition, the kidney is important in catabolizing proteins with molecular weights below 50,000 daltons.

Hairy Cell Leukemia: In clinical trials in patients with hairy cell leukemia, there was depression of circulating red blood cells, white blood cells and platelets during the first one to two months of treatment with INTRON A. Subsequently, both splenectomized and non-splenectomized patients with hairy cell leukemia, treated with INTRON A achieved substantial and sustained improvements in granulocytes, platelets, and hemoglobin levels in 75% of treated patients and at least some improvement (minor responses) occurred in 90%. For the entire study group median platelet counts were within the normal range after 2 months, median hemoglobin levels were in the normal range after 4 months and median granulocyte counts were in the normal range after 5 months of treatment. Responses of blood cell elements were similar in splenectomized and non-splenectomized patients except that median platelet counts after maximum response was to a level of 100,000/mm^3 in the latter group.

Treatment with INTRON A resulted in a decrease in bone marrow hypercellularity and hairy cell infiltrates. The hairy cell index (HCl), which represents the percent of bone marrow cellularity times the percent of hairy cell infiltrate, was greater than or equal to 50% at the beginning of the study in 87% of patients. The percentage of patients with such an HCl decreased to 25% after six months and to 14% after one year. These results indicate that even though hematologic improvement had occurred earlier, prolonged treatment with INTRON A may be required to obtain maximal reduction in tumor cell infiltrates in the bone marrow.

The percentage of patients with hairy cell leukemia who required red blood cell or platelet transfusions decreased significantly during treatment with INTRON A. Additionally, the percentage of patients with confirmed and serious infections declined during treatment with INTRON A as granulocyte counts improved.

The responses observed in non-splenectomized patients included reversal of splenomegaly and of abnormalities in blood cell counts attributable to hypersplenism. In some cases there was reversal of clinically significant hypersplenism that may have resulted in need for splenectomy.

Reduced risk of major complications of hairy cell leukemia (serious infections, bleeding diatheses, transfusion requirements) were apparent within 3 months of initiation of treatment in comparisons of INTRON A Interferon alfa-2b, recombinant for Injection treated patients to a control group. No deaths occurred in patients treated with INTRON A during the subsequent 9 months of treatment and follow up, while the mortality rate in the control group was 20% in the same time interval based on probability of survival analysis. During the initial 3 months of treatment, there may be interferon-mediated suppression of hematopoiesis.

In a multicenter controlled clinical trial involving 145 hairy cell leukemia patients, no serum neutralizing activity was detected in the 87 patients evaluated. Serum neutralizing activity was detected in some patients treated with higher doses of INTRON A in malignancies other than hairy cell leukemia. The clinical significance of these findings is unknown.

INDICATIONS AND USAGE

INTRON A for Injection is indicated for the treatment of patients 18 years of age or older with hairy cell leukemia. Studies have shown that INTRON A can produce clinically meaningful regression or stabilization of this disease, both in previously splenectomized and non-splenectomized patients.

Prior to initiation of therapy, tests should be performed to quantitate peripheral blood hemoglobin, platelets, granulocytes and hairy cells and bone marrow hairy cells. These parameters should be monitored periodically during treatment to determine whether response to treatment has occurred. If a patient does not respond within 6 months, treatment should be discontinued. If a response to treatment does occur, treatment usually should be continued until no further improvement is observed and these laboratory parameters have been stable for about 3 months (see **DOSAGE AND ADMINISTRATION**). It is not known whether continued treatment after that time point is beneficial. Studies are in progress to evaluate this question.

CONTRAINDICATIONS

INTRON A is contraindicated in patients with a history of hypersensitivity to interferon alfa or any component of the injection.

WARNINGS

Moderate to severe adverse experiences may require modification of the patient's dosage regimen, or in some cases, termination of therapy with INTRON A.

Because of the fever and other "flu-like" symptoms associated with INTRON A administration, it should be used cautiously in patients with debilitating medical conditions, such as those with a history of cardiovascular disease (e.g., unstable angina, uncontrolled congestive heart failure), pulmonary disease (e.g., chronic obstructive pulmonary disease), or diabetes mellitus prone to ketoacidosis. Caution should also be observed in patients with coagulation disorders (e.g., thrombophlebitis, pulmonary embolism) or severe myelosuppression.

Patients with platelet counts of less than 50,000/mm^3 should not be administered INTRON A intramuscularly, but instead by subcutaneous administration.

Cardiovascular adverse experiences which include significant hypotension, arrhythmia, or tachycardia of 150 beats per minute or greater, were observed in approximately 3% of the patients studied who had various malignancies and were treated at doses higher than those for hairy cell leukemia. The incidence of these complications in patients with preexisting heart disease is unknown. Hypotension may occur during administration, or up to two days post therapy, and may require supportive therapy including fluid replacement to maintain intravascular volume. Supraventricular arrhythmias occurred rarely and appeared to be correlated with preexisting conditions, and prior therapy with cardiotoxic agents. These adverse experiences were controlled by modifying the dose or discontinuing treatment, but may require specific additional therapy.

Those patients with a recent history of myocardial infarction and/or previous or current arrhythmic disorder, who require INTRON A therapy, should be closely monitored (see **Laboratory Tests**).

Central nervous system effects manifested by depression, confusion and other alterations of mental status were observed in about 2% of hairy cell leukemia patients treated with INTRON A. The overall incidence in a larger patient population with other malignancies treated with higher doses of INTRON A was 10%. More significant obtundation and coma have been observed in some patients, usually elderly, treated at higher doses for other malignant diseases. These effects are usually rapidly reversible. In a few severe episodes, full resolution of symptoms has taken up to three weeks. Patients should be closely monitored until resolution of these effects. Discontinuation of INTRON A Interferon alfa-2b, recombinant for Injection therapy may be required. Narcotics, hypnotics, or sedatives may be used concurrently with caution.

Acute serious hypersensitivity reactions (e.g., urticaria, angioedema, bronchoconstriction, anaphylaxis, etc.) have not been observed in patients receiving INTRON A; however, if such an acute reaction develops, the drug should be discontinued immediately and appropriate medical therapy instituted. Transient cutaneous rashes have occurred in some patients following injection, but have not necessitated treatment interruption.

Laboratory abnormalities which occurred in hairy cell leukemia patients included elevated SGOT and SGPT, which occurred in 4% and 13% of patients, respectively. The overall incidences of laboratory abnormalities in a larger patient population with other malignancies, and treated at higher doses were somewhat higher. These included elevated liver function tests (SGOT, SGPT in 10% of patients) and reductions in granulocyte (20% of patients) and platelet counts (18% of patients) (see **Laboratory Tests**). These abnormalities are usually mild to moderate and transient. Severe abnormalities of these laboratory parameters are usually rapidly reversible upon cessation or reduction of INTRON A therapy.

PRECAUTIONS

Information for Patients: Patients being treated with INTRON A should be directed in its appropriate use, informed of benefits and risks associated with treatment and referred to the Patient Information Sheet. This information is intended to aid in the safe and effective use of this medication. It is not a disclosure of all possible adverse or intended effects.

Patients should be cautioned not to change brands of Interferon without medical consultation as a change in dosage may result.

The most common adverse experiences occurring with INTRON A therapy are "flu-like" symptoms, such as fever, headache, fatigue, anorexia, nausea, or vomiting (see **ADVERSE REACTIONS** section) and appear to decrease in severity as treatment continues. Some of these "flu-like" symptoms may be minimized by bedtime adminstration. Acetaminophen may be used to prevent or partially alleviate the fever and headache.

It is advised that patients be well hydrated especially during the initial stages of treatment.

Laboratory Tests: In addition to those tests normally required for monitoring patients with hairy cell leukemia, the following laboratory tests are recommended for all patients on INTRON A therapy, prior to beginning treatment and then periodically thereafter:

- Standard hematologic tests—including complete blood counts and differential as well as platelet counts.
- Blood chemistries—electrolytes and liver function tests.

Those patients who have preexisting cardiac abnormalities and/or are in advanced stages of cancer, should have electrocardiograms taken prior to and during the course of treatment.

Carcinogenesis, Mutagenesis, Impairment of Fertility: Studies with INTRON A have not been performed to determine carcinogenicity, or the effect on fertility. Inteferon may impair fertility. Mutagenicity studies with INTRON A revealed no adverse effects.

Studies in mice, rats, and monkeys injected with INTRON A for up to one month have revealed no evidence of toxicity. However, due to the known species-specificity of interferon, the effects in animals are unlikely to be predictive of those in man.

Pregnancy Category C: Animal reproduction studies have not been conducted with INTRON A. It is also not known whether INTRON A can cause fetal harm when administered to a pregnant woman or can affect reproduction capacity. INTRON A should be given to a pregnant woman only if clearly needed. Another interferon alfa preparation has been shown to have abortifacient effects in *Macaca mulatta* (rhesus monkeys) when given at 20 to 500 times the human dose. Therefore, INTRON A should be used during pregnancy only if the potential benefit justifies the potential risk to the fetus. In studies of interferon use in non-human primates, abnormalities of the menstrual cycle have been observed.

INTRON A Interferon alfa-2b, recombinant for Injection should be used with caution in fertile men and women.

Nursing Mothers: It is not known whether this drug is excreted in human milk. However, studies in mice have shown that mouse interferons are excreted into the milk. Because of the potential for serious adverse reactions from INTRON A in nursing infants, a decision should be made whether to discontinue nursing or to discontinue the drug, taking into account the importance of the drug to the mother.

Pediatric Use: Safety and effectiveness have not been established in patients below the age of 18 years.

ADVERSE REACTIONS

Adverse reactions to INTRON A are dose-related. In studies of patients with malignancies other than hairy cell leukemia, hematologic and hepatic toxicities were more common in patients receiving individual injections greater than 10 million IU, than in patients receiving less than this amount. Hematologic, hepatic, cardiovascular and neurologic toxicities were more common in patients receiving more than 30 million IU per injection than in patients receiving less than that amount.

The following adverse reactions were reported to be possibly or probably related to INTRON A therapy during clinical trials. The most frequently reported adverse reactions were flu-like symptoms, primarily fever, fatigue, and chills which occurred in almost all patients treated. Other organ systems in which reactions occurred in more than 5% of the patients are:

General—Taste alteration, anorexia and weight decrease occurred uncommonly.

Cardiovascular—Mild hypotension was frequently recorded although it was rarely symptomatic. Hypertension also occurred less commonly. Tachycardias occurred uncommonly usually in association with high fevers.

Gastrointestinal System—Nausea was common, although vomiting occurred rarely. Mild diarrhea was reported less commonly.

Hematologic—Mild thrombocytopenia and transient granulocytopenia occurred commonly.

Musculo-Skeletal System—Myalgia and arthralgia occurred commonly, usually in association with other flu-like symptoms.

Nervous System—Headache, somnolence, confusion, and dizziness occurred uncommonly. Ataxia and paresthesia were rare.

Psychiatric—Anxiety, depression and nervousness occurred uncommonly.

Skin and Appendages—Mild pruritus occurred uncommonly. Mild alopecia was uncommon. Various transient, mild skin rashes were seen frequently in patients with hairy cell leukemia.

Other Adverse Reactions—The following adverse reactions were reported with an incidence of 5% or less: leg cramps, constipation, insomnia, herpetic eruptions, non-herpetic cold sores, urticaria, hot flashes, supraventricular arrhythmias, epistaxis, stomatitis, paralytic ileus, dehydration, coagulation disorder (elevated PT and PTT), abnormal vision, tremor, emotional lability, chest pain, pharyngitis and syncope.

Adverse reactions reported rarely (less than 1%) were dyspepsia, purpura, dyspnea, sneezing, oculomotor paralysis, nasal congestion, flatulence, increased saliva, hyperglycemia, and ulcerative stomatitis.

Laboratory Value Changes—Those patient laboratory values which were normal to moderately abnormal (WHO grades 0–2) at baseline that worsened to either severe or life-threatening abnormalities (WHO grades 3 or 4) during some phase of treatment included: WBC, platelets, granulocytes, SGOT, creatinine, SGPT, LDH, and alkaline phosphatase.

DOSAGE AND ADMINISTRATION

The recommended dosage of INTRON A for Injection for the treatment of hairy cell leukemia is 2 million IU/m^2 administered intramuscularly (see **WARNINGS**) or subcutaneously 3 times a week. Higher doses are not recommended. The normalization of one or more hematologic variables usually begins within 2 months of initiation of therapy. Improvement in all three hematologic variables may require 6 months or more of therapy.

This dosage regimen should be maintained unless the disease progresses rapidly, or severe intolerance is manifested. If severe adverse reactions develop, the dosage should be modified (50% reduction) or therapy should be temporarily discontinued until the adverse reactions abate. If persistent or recurrent intolerance develops following adequate dosage adjustment, or disease progresses, treatment with INTRON A Interferon alfa-2b, recombinant for Injection should be discontinued. The minimum effective dose of INTRON-A has not been established.

At the discretion of the physician, the patient may self-administer the dose. The medication may be administered at bedtime.

Preparation and Administration of INTRON A

Reconstitution of lyophilized INTRON A for Injection Using a sterile syringe and needle, inject the amount of Diluent for INTRON A Interferon alfa-2b, recombinant (bacteriostatic water for injection) stated in the chart below, into the vial of INTRON A. Agitate gently to hasten complete dissolution of the powder. The appropriate dose of INTRON A should then be withdrawn with a sterile syringe and injected intramuscularly or subcutaneously.

Vial Strength	*ml Diluent*	*Final Concentration*
3 million IU	1	3 million IU/ml
5 million IU	1	5 million IU/ml
10 million IU	2	5 million IU/ml
25 million IU	5	5 million IU/ml

Stability: After reconstitution with Diluent for INTRON A Interferon alfa-2b, recombinant (bacteriostatic water for injection) the solution is stable for one month at 2° to 8°C (36° to 46°F). The reconstituted solution is clear and colorless to light yellow.

Parenteral drug products should be inspected visually for particulate matter and discoloration prior to adminstration, whenever solution and container permit.

INTRON A may be administered using either sterilized glass or plastic disposable syringes.

HOW SUPPLIED

INTRON A Interferon alfa-2b, recombinant for Injection, 3 million IU per vial and Diluent for INTRON A Interferon alfa-2b, recombinant (bacteriostatic water for injection) 1 ml per vial; boxes containing 1 vial of INTRON A for Injection and 1 vial of Diluent for INTRON A Interferon alfa-2b, recombinant (bacteriostatic water for injection) (NDC 0085-0647-03).

INTRON A Interferon alfa-2b, recombinant for Injection, 5 million IU per vial and Diluent for INTRON A Interferon alfa-2b, recombinant (bacteriostatic water for injection) 1 ml per vial; boxes containing 1 vial of INTRON A for Injection and 1 vial of Diluent for INTRON A Interferon alfa-2b, recombinant (bacteriostatic water for injection) (NDC 0085-0120-02).

INTRON A Interferon alfa-2b, recombinant for Injection, 10 million IU per vial and Diluent for INTRON A Interferon alfa-2b, recombinant (bacteriostatic water for injection) 2 ml per vial; boxes containing 1 vial of INTRON A for Injection and 1 vial of Diluent for INTRON A Interferon alfa-2b, recombinant (bacteriostatic water for injection) (NDC 0085-0571-02).

INTRON A Interferon alfa-2b, recombinant for Injection, 25 million IU per vial and Diluent for INTRON A Interferon alfa-2b, recombinant (bacteriostatic water for injection) 5 ml per vial; boxes containing 1 vial of INTRON A for Injection and 1 vial of Diluent for INTRON A Inteferon alfa-2b, recombinant (bacteriostatic water for injection) (NDC 0085-0285-02).

Store INTRON A for Injection, both before and after reconstitution, between 2° and 8°C (36° and 46°F).

5/86 B-13762805

U.S. Pat. 4,530,901

LOTRIMIN® ℞

[lo'trim-in]

brand of clotrimazole

Cream, USP 1%
Lotion 1%
Solution, USP 1%

For Dermatologic Use Only—
Not For Ophthalmic Use

DESCRIPTION

LOTRIMIN products contain clotrimazole, USP, a synthetic antifungal agent having the chemical name [1-(o-Chloro-α,α-diphenylbenzyl)imidazole]; the empirical formula, $C_{22}H_{17}ClN_2$; and a molecular weight of 344.84.

Clotrimazole is an odorless, white crystalline substance. It is practically insoluble in water, sparingly soluble in ether and very soluble in polyethylene glycol 400, ethanol and chloroform.

Each gram of LOTRIMIN **Cream** contains 10 mg clotrimazole, USP in a vanishing cream base of sorbitan monostearate, polysorbate 60, cetyl esters wax, cetearyl alcohol, 2-octyldodecanol, purified water and, as preservative, benzyl alcohol (1%).

Each gram of LOTRIMIN **Lotion** contains 10 mg clotrimazole, USP dispersed in an emulsion vehicle composed of sorbitan monostearate, polysorbate 60, cetyl esters wax, cetearyl alcohol, 2-octyldodecanol, purified water; benzyl alcohol (1%) as preservative; sodium phosphate dibasic and sodium biphosphate to adjust pH.

Each ml of LOTRIMIN **Solution** contains 10 mg clotrimazole, USP in a nonaqueous vehicle of polyethylene glycol 400.

CLINICAL PHARMACOLOGY

Clotrimazole is a broad-spectrum antifungal agent that is used for the treatment of dermal infections caused by various species of pathogenic dermatophytes, yeasts, and *Malassezia furfur.* The primary action of clotrimazole is against dividing and growing organisms.

In vitro, clotrimazole exhibits fungistatic and fungicidal activity against isolates of *Trichophyton rubrum, Trichophyton mentagrophytes, Epidermophyton floccosum, Microsporum canis,* and *Candida* species, including *Candida albicans.* In general, the *in vitro* activity of clotrimazole corresponds to that of tolnaftate and griseofulvin against the mycelia of dermatophytes (*Trichophyton, Microsporum,* and *Epidermophyton*), and to that of the polyenes (amphotericin B and nystatin) against budding fungi (*Candida*). Using an *in vivo* (mouse) and an *in vitro* (mouse kidney homogenate) testing system, clotrimazole and miconazole were equally effective in preventing the growth of the pseudomycelia and mycelia of *Candida albicans.*

Strains of fungi having a natural resistance to clotrimazole are rare. Only a single isolate of *Candida guilliermondi* has been reported to have primary resistance to clotrimazole.

No single-step or multiple-step resistance to clotrimazole has developed during successive passages of *Candida albicans* and *Trichophyton mentagrophytes.* No appreciable change in sensitivity was detected after successive passages of isolates of *C. albicans, C. krusei,* or *C. pseudotropicalis* in liquid or solid media containing clotrimazole. Also, resistance could not be developed in chemically induced mutant strains of polyene-resistant isolates of *C. albicans.* Slight, reversible resistance was noted in three isolates of *C. albicans* tested by one investigator. There is a single report that records the clinical emergence of a *C. albicans* strain with considerable resistance to flucytosine and miconazole, and with cross-resistance to clotrimazole; the strain remained sensitive to nystatin and amphotericin B.

In studies of the mechanism of action, the minimum fungicidal concentration of clotrimazole caused leakage of intracellular phosphorus compounds into the ambient medium with concomitant breakdown of cellular nucleic acids and accelerated potassium efflux. Both these events began rapidly and extensively after addition of the drug.

Clotrimazole appears to be well absorbed in humans following oral administration and is eliminated mainly as inactive metabolites. Following topical and vaginal administration, however, clotrimazole appears to be minimally absorbed.

Six hours after the application of radioactive clotrimazole 1% cream and 1% solution onto intact and acutely inflamed skin, the concentration of clotrimazole varied from 100 mcg/cm^3 in the stratum corneum to 0.5 to 1 mcg/cm^3 in the stratum reticulare, and 0.1 mcg/cm^3 in the subcutis. No measurable amount of radioactivity ($\leq$0.001 mcg/ml) was found in the serum within 48 hours after application under occlusive dressing of 0.5 ml of the solution or 0.8 g of the cream. Only 0.5% or less of the applied radioactivity was excreted in the urine.

Following intravaginal administration of 100 mg ^{14}C-clotrimazole vaginal tablets to nine adult females, an average peak serum level, corresponding to only 0.03 μg equivalents/ml of clotrimazole, was reached one to two days after application. After intravaginal administration of 5 g of 1% ^{14}C-clotrimazole vaginal cream, containing 50 mg active drug, to five subjects (one with candidal colpitis), serum levels corresponding to approximately 0.01 μg equivalents/ml were reached between 8 and 24 hours after application.

INDICATIONS AND USAGE

LOTRIMIN products are indicated for the topical treatment of the following dermal infections: tinea pedis, tinea cruris, and tinea corporis due to *Trichophyton rubrum, trichophyton mentagrophytes, Epidermophyton floccosum,* and *Microsporum canis;* candidiasis due to *Candida albicans;* and tinea versicolor due to *Malassezia furfur.*

CONTRAINDICATIONS

LOTRIMIN products are contraindicated in individuals who have shown hypersensitivity to any of their components.

WARNINGS

LOTRIMIN products are not for ophthalmic use.

PRECAUTIONS

General: If irritation or sensitivity develops with the use of clotrimazole, treatment should be discontinued and appropriate therapy instituted.

Information For Patients:

This information is intended to aid in the safe and effective use of this medication. It is not a disclosure of all possible adverse or intended effects.

The patient should be advised to:

1. Use the medication for the full treatment time even though the symptoms may have improved. Notify the physician if there is no improvement after four weeks of treatment.
2. Inform the physician if the area of application shows signs of increased irritation (redness, itching, burning, blistering, swelling, oozing) indicative of possible sensitization.
3. Avoid sources of infection or reinfection.

Laboratory Tests: If there is lack of response to clotrimazole, appropriate microbiological studies should be repeated to confirm the diagnosis and rule out other pathogens before instituting another course of antimycotic therapy.

Drug Interactions: Synergism or antagonism between clotrimazole and nystatin, or amphotericin B, or flucytosine against strains of *C. albicans* has not been reported.

Carcinogenesis, Mutagenesis, Impairment of Fertility: An 18-month oral dosing study with clotrimazole in rats has not revealed any carcinogenic effect.

Continued on next page

Information on Schering products appearing on these pages is effective as of September 30, 1986.

Schering—Cont.

In tests for mutagenesis, chromosomes of the spermatophores of Chinese hamsters which had been exposed to clotrimazole were examined for structural changes during the metaphase. Prior to testing, the hamsters had received five oral clotrimazole doses of 100 mg/kg body weight. The results of this study showed that clotrimazole had no mutagenic effect.

Usage in Pregnancy: Pregnancy Category B: The disposition of ^{14}C-clotrimazole has been studied in humans and animals. Clotrimazole is very poorly absorbed following dermal application or intravaginal administration to humans. (See **Clinical Pharmacology.**)

In clinical trials, use of vaginally applied clotrimazole in pregnant women in their second and third trimesters has not been associated with ill effects. There are, however, no adequate and well-controlled studies in pregnant women during the first trimester of pregnancy.

Studies in pregnant rats with intravaginal doses up to 100 mg/kg have revealed no evidence of harm to the fetus due to clotrimazole.

High oral doses of clotrimazole in rats and mice ranging from 50 to 120 mg/kg resulted in embryotoxicity (possibly secondary to maternal toxicity), impairment of mating, decreased litter size and number of viable young and decreased pup survival to weaning. However, clotrimazole was not teratogenic in mice, rabbits and rats at oral doses up to 200, 180 and 100 mg/kg, respectively. Oral absorption in the rat amounts to approximately 90% of the administered dose.

Because animal reproduction studies are not always predictive of human response, this drug should be used only if clearly indicated during the first trimester of pregnancy.

Nursing Mothers: It is not known whether this drug is excreted in human milk. Because many drugs are excreted in human milk, caution should be exercised when clotrimazole is used by a nursing woman.

Pediatric Use: Safety and effectiveness in children have been established for clotrimazole when used as indicated and in the recommended dosage.

ADVERSE REACTIONS

The following adverse reactions have been reported in connection with the use of clotrimazole: erythema, stinging, blistering, peeling, edema, pruritus, urticaria, burning, and general irritation of the skin.

OVERDOSAGE

Acute overdosage with topical application of clotrimazole is unlikely and would not be expected to lead to a life-threatening situation.

DOSAGE AND ADMINISTRATION

Gently massage sufficient LOTRIMIN into the affected and surrounding skin areas twice a day, in the morning and evening.

Clinical improvement, with relief of pruritus, usually occurs within the first week of treatment with LOTRIMIN. If the patient shows no clinical improvement after four weeks of treatment with LOTRIMIN, the diagnosis should be reviewed.

HOW SUPPLIED

LOTRIMIN Cream 1% is supplied in 15, 30, 45 and 90-g tubes (NDC 0085-0613-02, 05, 04, 03, respectively); boxes of one.

LOTRIMIN Lotion 1% is supplied in 30 ml bottles (NDC 0085-0707-02); boxes of one.

Shake well before using.

LOTRIMIN Solution 1% is supplied in 10 ml and 30 ml plastic bottles (NDC 0085-0182-02, 04, respectively); boxes of one.

Store LOTRIMIN products between 2° and 30°C (36° and 86°F).

Rev. 2/85

LOTRISONE® ℞

[lō 'trĭ-sōn]

brand of clotrimazole, USP and betamethasone dipropionate, USP Cream

For Dermatologic Use Only— Not for Ophthalmic Use

DESCRIPTION

LOTRISONE Cream contains a combination of clotrimazole, USP, a synthetic antifungal agent, and betamethasone dipropionate, USP, a synthetic corticosteroid, for dermatologic use.

Chemically, clotrimazole is 1-(*o* -Chloro-α,α-diphenyl benzyl) imidazole, with the empirical formula $C_{22}H_{17}ClN_2$ and a molecular weight of 344.8.

Clotrimazole is an odorless, white crystalline powder, insoluble in water and soluble in ethanol.

Betamethasone dipropionate has the chemical name 9-Fluoro-11β, 17,21-trihydroxy-16β-methylpregna-1,4-diene-3,20-dione 17,21-dipropionate, with the empirical formula $C_{28}H_{37}FO_7$ and a molecular weight of 504.6.

Betamethasone dipropionate is a white to creamy white, odorless crystalline powder, insoluble in water.

Each gram of LOTRISONE Cream contains 10.0 mg clotrimazole, USP, and 0.64 mg betamethasone dipropionate, USP (equivalent to 0.5 mg betamethasone), in a hydrophilic emollient cream consisting of purified water, mineral oil, white petrolatum, cetearyl alcohol, ceteareth-30, propylene glycol, sodium phosphate monobasic, and phosphoric acid; benzyl alcohol as preservative.

LOTRISONE is a smooth, uniform, white to off-white cream.

CLINICAL PHARMACOLOGY

Clotrimazole

Clotrimazole is a broad-spectrum, antifungal agent that is used for the treatment of dermal infections caused by various species of pathogenic dermatophytes, yeasts, and *Malassezia furfur.* The primary action of clotrimazole is against dividing and growing organisms.

In vitro, clotrimazole exhibits fungistatic and fungicidal activity against isolates of *Trichophyton rubrum, Trichophyton mentagrophytes, Epidermophyton floccosum* and *Microsporum canis.* In general, the *in vitro* activity of clotrimazole corresponds to that of tolnaftate and griseofulvin against the mycelia of dermatophytes (*Trichophyton, Microsporum,* and *Epidermophyton*).

In vivo studies in guinea pigs infected with *Trichophyton mentagrophytes* have shown no measurable loss of clotrimazole activity due to combination with betamethasone dipropionate.

Strains of fungi having a natural resistance to clotrimazole have not been reported.

No single-step or multiple-step resistance to clotrimazole has developed during successive passages of *Trichophyton mentagrophytes.*

In studies of the mechanism of action in fungal cultures, the minimum fungicidal concentration of clotrimazole caused leakage of intracellular phosphorous compounds into the ambient medium with concomitant breakdown of cellular nucleic acids, and accelerated potassium efflux. Both of these events began rapidly and extensively after addition of the drug to the cultures.

Clotrimazole appears to be minimally absorbed following topical application to the skin. Six hours after the application of radioactive clotrimazole 1% cream and 1% solution onto intact and acutely inflamed skin, the concentration of clotrimazole varied from 100 mcg/cm^3 in the stratum corneum, to 0.5 to 1 mcg/cm^3 in the stratum reticulare, and 0.1 mcg/cm^3 in the subcutis. No measureable amount of radioactivity (<0.001 mcg/ml) was found in the serum within 48 hours after application under occlusive dressing of 0.5 ml of the solution or 0.8 g of the cream.

Betamethasone dipropionate

Betamethasone dipropionate, a corticosteroid, is effective in the treatment of corticosteroid-responsive dermatoses primarily because of its anti-inflammatory, antipruritic, and vasoconstrictive actions. However, while the physiologic, pharmacologic, and clinical effects of corticosteroids are well-known, the exact mechanisms of their actions in each disease are uncertain. Betamethasone dipropionate, a corticosteroid, has been shown to have topical (dermatologic) and systemic pharmacologic and metabolic effects characteristic of this class of drugs.

Pharmacokinetics: The extent of percutaneous absorption of topical corticosteroids is determined by many factors including the vehicle, the integrity of the epidermal barrier, and the use of occlusive dressings. (See **Dosage and Administration** section.)

Topical corticosteroids can be absorbed from normal intact skin. Inflammation and/or other disease processes in the skin increase percutaneous absorption. Occlusive dressings substantially increase the percutaneous absorption of topical corticosteroids. (See **Dosage and Administration** section.)

Once absorbed through the skin, topical corticosteroids are handled through pharmacokinetic pathways similar to systemically administered corticosteroids. Corticosteroids are bound to plasma proteins in varying degrees. Corticosteroids are metabolized primarily in the liver and are then excreted by the kidneys. Some of the topical corticosteroids and their metabolities are also excreted into the bile.

Clotrimazole and betamethasone dipropionate

In clinical studies of tinea corporis, tinea cruris and tinea pedis, patients treated with LOTRISONE Cream showed a better clinical response at the first return visit, than patients treated with clotrimazole cream. In tinea corporis and tinea cruris, the patient returned three days after starting treatment, and in tinea pedis, after one week. Mycological cure rates observed in patients treated with LOTRISONE Cream were as good as or better than in those patients treated with clotrimazole cream.

In these same clinical studies, patients treated with LOTRISONE Cream showed statistically significantly better clinical responses and mycological cure rates when compared with patients treated with betamethasone dipropionate cream.

INDICATIONS AND USAGE

LOTRISONE Cream is indicated for the topical treatment of the following dermal infections: tinea pedis, tinea cruris, and tinea corporis due to *Trichophyton rubrum, Trichophyton mentagrophytes, Epidermophyton floccosum,* and *Microsporum canis.*

CONTRAINDICATIONS

LOTRISONE Cream is contraindicated in patients who are sensitive to clotrimazole, betamethasone dipropionate, other corticosteroids or imidazoles, or to any ingredient in this preparation.

PRECAUTIONS

General: Systemic absorption of topical corticosteroids has produced reversible hypothalamic-pituitary-adrenal (HPA) axis suppression, manifestations of Cushing's syndrome, hyperglycemia, and glucosuria in some patients.

Conditions which augment systemic absorption include the application of the more potent steroids, use over large surface areas, prolonged use, and the addition of occlusive dressings. (See **Dosage and Administration** section.)

Therefore, patients receiving a large dose of a potent topical steroid applied to a large surface area should be evaluated periodically for evidence of HPA axis suppression by using the urinary free cortisol and ACTH stimulation tests. If HPA axis suppression is noted, an attempt should be made to withdraw the drug, to reduce the frequency of application, or to substitute a less potent steroid.

Recovery of HPA axis function is generally prompt and complete upon discontinuation of the drug. Infrequently, signs and symptoms of steroid withdrawal may occur, requiring supplemental systemic corticosteroids.

Children may absorb proportionally larger amounts of topical corticosteroids and thus be more susceptible to systemic toxicity. (See **Precautions-Pediatric Use.**)

If irritation or hypersensitivity develops with the use of LOTRISONE Cream, treatment should be discontinued and appropriate therapy instituted.

Information for Patients Patients using LOTRISONE Cream should receive the following information and instructions:

1. This medication is to be used as directed by the physician. It is for external use only. Avoid contact with the eyes.
2. The medication is to be used for the full prescribed treatment time, even though the symptoms may have improved. Notify the physician if there is no improvement after one week of treatment for tinea cruris or tinea corporis, or after two weeks for tinea pedis.
3. Patients should be advised not to use this medication for any disorder other than for which it was prescribed.
4. The treated skin areas should not be bandaged or otherwise covered or wrapped as to be occluded. (See **Dosage and Administration** section.)
5. When using this medication in the groin area, patients should be advised to use the medication for two weeks only, and to apply the cream sparingly. The physician should be notified if the condition persists after two weeks. Patients should also be advised to wear loose fitting clothing. (See **Dosage and Administration** section.)
6. Patients should report any signs of local adverse reactions.
7. Parents of pediatric patients should be advised not to use tight-fitting diapers or plastic pants on a child being treated in the diaper area, as these garments may constitute occlusive dressing. (See **Dosage and Administration** section.)
8. Patients should avoid sources of infection or reinfection.

Laboratory Tests: If there is a lack of response to LOTRISONE Cream, appropriate microbiological studies should be repeated to confirm the diagnosis and rule out other pathogens before instituting another course of antimycotic therapy.

The following tests may be helpful in evaluating HPA axis suppression due to the corticosteroid component:

Urinary free cortisol test
ACTH stimulation test

Carcinogenesis, Mutagenesis, Impairment of Fertility: There are no animal or laboratory studies with the combination clotrimazole and betamethasone dipropionate to evaluate carcinogenesis, mutagenesis or impairment of fertility.

An 18-month oral dosing study with clotrimazole in rats has not revealed any carcinogenic effect.

In tests for mutagenesis, chromosomes of the spermatophores of Chinese hamsters which have been exposed to clotrimazole were examined for structural changes during the metaphase. Prior to testing, the hamsters had received five oral clotrimazole doses of 100 mg/kg body weight. The results of this study showed that clotrimazole had no mutagenic effect.

Pregnancy Category C: There have been no teratogenic studies performed with the combination clotrimazole and betamethasone dipropionate.

Studies in pregnant rats with intravaginal doses up to 100 mg/kg have revealed no evidence of harm to the fetus due to clotrimazole.
High oral doses of clotrimazole in rats and mice ranging from 50 to 120 mg/kg resulted in embryotoxicity (possibly secondary to maternal toxicity), impairment of mating, decreased litter size and number of viable young and decreased pup survival to weaning. However, clotrimazole was not teratogenic in mice, rabbits and rats at oral doses up to 200, 180 and 100 mg/kg, respectively. Oral absorption in the rat amounts to approximately 90% of the administered dose.
Corticosteroids are generally teratogenic in laboratory animals when administered systemically at relatively low dosage levels. The more potent corticosteroids have been shown to be teratogenic after dermal application in laboratory animals.
There are no adequate and well-controlled studies in pregnant women on teratogenic effects from a topically applied combination of clotrimazole and betamethasone dipropionate. Therefore, LOTRISONE Cream should be used during pregnancy only if the potential benefit justifies the potential risk to the fetus.
Drugs containing corticosteroids should not be used extensively on pregnant patients, in large amounts, or for prolonged periods of time.
Nursing Mothers: It is not known whether this drug is excreted in human milk. Because many drugs are excreted in human milk, caution should be exercised when LOTRISONE Cream is used by a nursing woman.
Pediatric Use: Safety and effectiveness in children below the age of 12 have not been established with LOTRISONE Cream. However, dosage forms containing concentrations of clotrimazole and of betamethasone dipropionate found in LOTRISONE Cream have been demonstrated to be safe and effective when used as indicated and in the recommended dosages.
Pediatric patients may demonstrate greater susceptibility to topical corticosteroid-induced HPA axis suppression and Cushing's syndrome than mature patients because of a larger skin surface area to body weight ratio.
Hypothalamic-pituitary-adrenal (HPA) axis suppression, Cushing's syndrome, and intracranial hypertension have been reported in children receiving topical corticosteroids. Manifestations of adrenal suppression in children include linear growth retardation, delayed weight gain, low plasma cortisol levels, and absence of response to ACTH stimulation. Manifestations of intracranial hypertension include bulging fontanelles, headaches, and bilateral papilledema.
Administration of topical dermatologics containing a corticosteroid to children should be limited to the least amount compatible with an effective therapeutic regimen. Chronic corticosteroid therapy may interfere with the growth and development of children.

ADVERSE REACTIONS

The following adverse reactions have been reported in connection with the use of LOTRISONE Cream: paresthesia in 5 of 270 patients, maculopapular rash, edema, and secondary infection, each in 1 of 270 patients.
Adverse reactions reported with the use of clotrimazole are as follows: erythema, stinging, blistering, peeling, edema, pruritus, urticaria, and general irritation of the skin.
The following local adverse reactions are reported infrequently when topical corticosteroids are used as recommended. These reactions are listed in an approximate decreasing order of occurrence: burning, itching, irritation, dryness, folliculitis, hypertrichosis, acneiform eruptions, hypopigmentation, perioral dermatitis, allergic contact dermatitis, maceration of the skin, secondary infection, skin atrophy, striae, and miliaria.

OVERDOSAGE

Acute overdosage with topical application of LOTRISONE Cream is unlikely and would not be expected to lead to a life-threatening situation.
Topically applied corticosteroids can be absorbed in sufficient amounts to produce systemic effects. (See **Precautions.**)

DOSAGE AND ADMINISTRATION

Gently massage sufficient LOTRISONE Cream into the affected and surrounding skin areas twice a day, in the morning and evening for two weeks in tinea cruris and tinea corporis, and for four weeks in tinea pedis. The use of LOTRISONE Cream for longer than four weeks is not recommended.
Clinical improvement, with relief of erythema and pruritus, usually occurs within three to five days of treatment. If a patient with tinea cruris and tinea corporis shows no clinical improvement after one week of treatment with LOTRISONE Cream, the diagnosis should be reviewed. In tinea pedis, the treatment should be applied for two weeks prior to making that decision.
Treatment with LOTRISONE Cream should be discontinued if the condition persists after two weeks in tinea cruris and tinea corporis, and after four weeks in tinea pedis. Alternate therapy may then be instituted with LOTRIMIN Cream, a product containing an antifungal only.
LOTRISONE Cream should not be used with occlusive dressings.

HOW SUPPLIED

LOTRISONE Cream is supplied in 15-gram (NDC 0085-0924-01), and 45-gram tubes (NDC 0085-0924-02); boxes of one.
Store between 2° and 30°C (36° and 86°F).
Revised 12/85

METIMYD® ℞

[met 'ĭ-mid]
brand of prednisolone acetate, USP and sulfacetamide sodium, USP
Ophthalmic Suspension–Sterile
Ophthalmic Ointment–Sterile

DESCRIPTION

METIMYD Ophthalmic **Suspension** is a steroid/anti-infective sterile preparation having a pH range of 7.0 to 7.4. Each ml contains: 5 mg prednisolone acetate, USP; 100 mg sulfacetamide sodium, USP; sodium phosphate dibasic, sodium phosphate monobasic, tyloxapol, sodium thiosulfate, edetate disodium, and purified water; 5 mg phenylethyl alcohol and 0.25 mg benzalkonium chloride as preservatives.
METIMYD Ophthalmic **Ointment** is a steroid/ anti-infective sterile preparation containing in each gram: 5 mg prednisolone acetate, USP and 100 mg sulfacetamide sodium, USP; 0.5 mg methylparaben and 0.1 mg propylparaben as preservatives, in a bland, unctuous base of mineral oil and white petrolatum.
The empirical formula for prednisolone acetate, a 1-unsaturated analog of hydrocortisone acetate, is $C_{23}H_{30}O_6$. The molecular weight is 402.49. Chemically it is 11β,17,21-trihydroxypregna-1,4-diene-3,20-dione 21-acetate.
Prednisolone acetate is a nearly odorless, white to practically white, crystalline powder. It is slightly soluble in acetone, alcohol, and chloroform, and practically insoluble in water.
Sulfacetamide sodium, $C_8H_9N_2NaO_3S \cdot H_2O$, is a sulfonamide antibacterial agent with a molecular weight of 254.24. Chemically it is *N*-[(4-aminophenyl)sulfonyl]-, acetamide, monosodium salt, monohydrate.
Sulfacetamide sodium is an odorless, white, crystalline powder. It is freely soluble in water, sparingly soluble in alcohol and practically insoluble in benzene, chloroform, and ether.

CLINICAL PHARMACOLOGY

Corticosteroids suppress the inflammatory response to a variety of agents and they probably delay or slow healing. Since corticosteroids may inhibit the body's defense mechanism against infection, a concomitant antimicrobial drug may be used when this inhibition is considered to be clinically significant in a particular case.
The anti-infective component in the combination is included to provide action against specific organisms susceptible to it. When a decision is made to administer both a corticoid and an antimicrobial, the administration of such drugs in combination has the advantages of greater patient compliance and convenience and added assurance that the appropriate dosage of both drugs is administered. There is also assured compatibility of ingredients when both types of drug are in the same formulation and, particularly, that the correct volume of drug is delivered and retained.
The relative potency of corticosteroids depends on the molecular structure, concentration, and release from the vehicle.

INDICATIONS AND USAGE

METIMYD Ophthalmic Suspension or **Ointment** is indicated for steroid-responsive inflammatory ocular conditions for which a corticosteroid is indicated and where bacterial infection or a risk of bacterial ocular infection exists.
Ocular steroids are indicated in inflammatory conditions of the palpebral and bulbar conjunctivae, cornea, and anterior segment of the globe where the inherent risk of steroid use in certain infective conjunctivitides is accepted to obtain a diminution in edema and inflammation. They are also indicated in chronic anterior uveitis and corneal injury from chemical, radiation, or thermal burns, or penetration of foreign bodies.
The use of a combination drug with an anti-infective component is indicated where the risk of infection is high or where there is an expectation that potentially dangerous numbers of bacteria will be present in the eye.
The particular anti-infective drug in this product is active against the following common bacterial eye pathogens: *Pseudomonas* species. *Hemophilus influenzae, Klebsiella* species, *Staphylococcus aureus, Streptococcus pneumoniae, Streptococcus* (Viridans group), *Escherichia coli,* and *Enterobacter* species.
This product does not provide adequate coverage against: *Neisseria* species and *Serratia marcescens.*

CONTRAINDICATIONS

METIMYD is contraindicated in: epithelial herpes simplex keratitis (dendritic keratitis), vaccinia, varicella, and many other viral diseases of the cornea or conjunctiva; mycobacterial infection of the eye; and fungal diseases of ocular structures. METIMYD is contraindicated in individuals with known or suspected hypersensitivity to any of the ingredients of the preparation, or to other sulfonamides, or other corticosteroids. (Hypersensitivity to the antibacterial component occurs at a higher rate than for other components.) The use of these combinations is always contraindicated after uncomplicated removal of a corneal foreign body.

WARNINGS

Prolonged use may result in glaucoma, with damage to the optic nerve, defects in visual acuity and fields of vision, and in posterior subcapsular cataract formation. Prolonged use may suppress the host response and thus increase the hazard of secondary ocular infections. In those diseases causing thinning of the cornea or sclera, perforations have been known to occur with the use of topical steroids. In acute purulent conditions of the eye, steroids may mask infection or enhance existing infection. If these products are used for 10 days or longer, intraocular pressure should be routinely monitored even though this may be difficult in children and uncooperative patients.
Employment of steroid medication in the treatment of herpes simplex requires great caution.
A significant percentage of staphylococcal isolates are completely resistant to sulfonamides.

PRECAUTIONS

The initial prescription and renewal of the medication order beyond 20 ml of METIMYD Ophthalmic **Suspension** or beyond 8 g of the **Ointment** should be made by a physician only after examination of the patient with the aid of magnification, such as slitlamp biomicroscopy and where appropriate, fluorescein staining.
The possibility of fungal infections of the cornea should be considered after prolonged steroid dosing.
Sensitization may recur when a sulfonamide is readministered irrespective of the route of administration and cross-sensitivity among different sulfonamides may occur. (See ADVERSE REACTIONS.) Cross-allergenicity among corticosteroids has been demonstrated. If signs of hypersensitivity or other untoward reactions occur, discontinue use of the preparation.

ADVERSE REACTIONS

Adverse reactions have occurred which can be attributed to the steroid component, the anti-infective component, or the combination. Exact incidence figures are not available since no denominator of treated patients is available.
Reactions occurring most often from the presence of the anti-infective ingredient are allergic sensitizations. Instances of Stevens-Johnson syndrome and systemic lupus erythematosus (in one case producing a fatal outcome) have been reported following the use of ophthalmic sulfonamide containing preparations.
The reactions due to the steroid component in decreasing order of frequency are: elevation of intraocular pressure (IOP) with possible development of glaucoma, and infrequent optic nerve damage; posterior subcapsular cataract formation; and delayed wound healing.
Corticosteroid-containing preparations can also cause acute anterior uveitis or perforation of the globe. Mydriasis, loss of accommodation, and ptosis have occasionally been reported following local use of corticosteroids.
Secondary Infection: The development of secondary infection has occurred after use of combinations containing steroids and antimicrobials. Fungal infections of the cornea are particularly prone to develop coincidentally with long-term applications of the steroid. The possibility of fungal invasion must be considered in any persistent corneal ulceration where steroid treatment has been used.
Secondary bacterial ocular infection following suppression of host responses also occurs.

DOSAGE AND ADMINISTRATION

METIMYD Ophthalmic Suspension: Two or three drops should be instilled into the conjunctival sac every one to two hours during the day and at bedtime until a favorable response is obtained.
METIMYD Ophthalmic Ointment: A thin film should be applied three or four times daily and once at bedtime until a favorable response is obtained.
The initial prescription of METIMYD Ophthalmic should *not* be more than 20 ml of the **Suspension** or 8 g of the **Ointment** and the prescription should not be refilled without further evaluation as outlined in PRECAUTIONS.

Continued on next page

Information on Schering products appearing on these pages is effective as of September 30, 1986.

Schering—Cont.

Dosage should be adjusted according to the specific needs of the patient. METIMYD Ophthalmic **Suspension** or **Ointment** dosage may be reduced, but care should be taken not to discontinue therapy prematurely. In chronic conditions, withdrawal of treatment should be carried out by gradually decreasing the frequency of application.

HOW SUPPLIED

METIMYD Ophthalmic Suspension, 5 ml dropper bottle; box of one; NDC 0085-0074-05. **Store between 2° and 30°C (36° and 86°F). Clumping may occur on long standing at high temperatures. Shake well before using. Protect from light.**
METIMYD Ophthalmic Ointment, 3.5 g applicator tube; box of one; NDC 0085-0695-05. **Store between 2° and 30°C (36° and 86°F).**
Revised 1/83

NAQUA® ℞
[*nak'wah*]
brand of trichlormethiazide, USP
Tablets

DESCRIPTION

NAQUA Tablets contain trichlormethiazide, USP for use as an antihypertensive and diuretic drug. They are to be taken orally.
Trichlormethiazide is a member of a class of antihypertensive and diuretic drugs known as benzothiadiazines. The empirical formula is $C_8H_8Cl_3N_3O_4S_2$, with a molecular weight of 380.65; the chemical name is 6-Chloro-3-(dichloromethyl)-3,4-dihydro-2*H*-1,2,4-benzothiadiazine-7-sulfonamide 1,1-dioxide.
Trichlormethiazide is a white or practically white crystalline powder. It is very slightly soluble in water and sparingly soluble in alcohol.
Each NAQUA Tablet contains 2 mg or 4 mg trichlormethiazide, USP.
The inactive ingredients for NAQUA Tablets 2 mg include corn starch, FD&C Red No. 40, lactose, and magnesium stearate.
The inactive ingredients for NAQUA Tablets 4 mg include corn starch, D&C Yellow No. 10 Al Lake, FD&C Blue No. 1 Al Lake, lactose, and magnesium stearate.

CLINICAL PHARMACOLOGY

The thiazide (benzothiadiazine) diuretics are a class of drug products that have close structural similarity and many similar pharmacological, physiochemical, and pharmocokinetic properties. The thiazide diuretics, including trichlormethiazide, are used generally as adjunctive medication to control the edema associated with various diseases and in the management of hypertension. (See **INDICATIONS AND USAGE.**)
Thiazide diuretics enhance the renal excretion of sodium chloride and water by interfering with the transport of sodium ions across the renal tubular epithelium, primarily in the cortical diluting segment of the nephron. The thiazides also evoke a significant augmentation of potassium excretion, possibly due to the increased amount of sodium reaching the distal tubular site of sodium-potassium exchange. Long-term thiazide therapy can cause mild metabolic alkalosis associated with hypokalemia and hypochloremia.
The glomerular filtration rate is decreased by thiazides. This is of little significance in affecting primary drug action, but may be of clinical importance in patients with diminished renal reserve, contributing to decreased diuretic efficacy. When the glomerular filtration rate falls below 20 ml per minute, the thiazides may not be effective.
Thiazides may decrease uric acid excretion in man, thus increasing the plasma uric acid concentration.
Thiazides may induce hyperglycemia, aggravate existing diabetes mellitus, or precipitate diabetes in prediabetic patients. The exact mechanism of action causing these effects is not certain.
The excretion of certain other ions is affected by the thiazide diuretics: magnesium excretion is enhanced, leading to hypomagnesemia; calcium excretion is decreased relative to that of sodium; iodide and bromide excretion occurs by renal mechanisms similar to those for chloride, possibly leading to slight iodide depletion and allowing chloruretic agents to be useful in the management of bromide intoxication.
Thiazide diuretics have antihypertensive activity per se in hypertensive patients and also may augment the actions of other antihypertensive drugs. The full mechanism of antihypertensive action is not known. Therapy for hypertension is often initiated with a thiazide diuretic which induces diuresis, natriuresis, depletion of extracellular fluid, and reduction of cardiac output. Direct arteriolar dilatation may play a role.
Plasma renin activity is elevated during thiazide therapy. The aldosterone secretion rate is increased slightly but significantly; this contributes to the hypokalemia caused by thiazides.
Paradoxically, thiazides decrease urine volume in patients with diabetes insipidus, and thirst and water consumption decrease.
At maximal therapeutic dosages, all thiazides are approximately equal in their diuretic and antihypertensive activities. The comparative effective daily dose range for chlorothiazide is 250 to 2000 mg; for hydrochlorothiazide 20 to 150 mg; and for trichlormethiazide 2 to 8 mg.
Thiazides are absorbed rapidly from the gastrointestinal tract. Most show demonstrable diuresis within an hour, and peak effects occur 3 to 6 hours after oral administration. Distribution is essentially limited to the extracellular fluid space, with little, if any, accumulation in tissues other than the kidneys. The duration of diuretic action of thiazides is determined by the rate of excretion. Chlorothiazide and hydrochlorothiazide act for six to 12 hours; trichlormethiazide for 24 hours. In general, thiazides with relatively long durations of action show proportionately high degrees of plasma protein-binding. Most thiazides are excreted primarily as unchanged drug in the urine.
Thiazides pass readily through the placenta to the fetus, and also appear in the milk of nursing mothers.

INDICATIONS AND USAGE

NAQUA Tablets are indicated as adjunctive therapy in edema associated with congestive heart failure, hepatic cirrhosis, and corticosteroid and estrogen therapy.
NAQUA Tablets are indicated for the treatment of edema due to various forms of renal dysfunction, such as nephrotic syndrome, acute glomerulonephritis, and chronic renal failure.
NAQUA Tablets are indicated in the management of hypertension either as the sole therapeutic agent or as adjunctive therapy to enhance the effectiveness of other antihypertensive drugs in the management of the more severe forms of hypertension.
NAQUA Tablets are indicated in pregnancy only when the edema is due to pathologic causes. (See **PRECAUTIONS, Pregnancy Category B** and **PRECAUTIONS, Nonteratogenic Effects.**) The routine use of diuretics in an otherwise healthy woman is inappropriate and exposes the mother and fetus to unnecessary hazard. Diuretics do not prevent development of toxemia of pregnancy, and there is no satisfactory evidence that they are useful in the treatment of toxemia.
Edema during pregnancy may arise from pathologic causes or from the physiologic and mechanical consequences of pregnancy. Dependent edema in pregnancy, resulting from restriction of venous return by the expanded uterus, is properly treated through elevation of the lower extremities and use of support hose; use of diuretics to lower intravascular volume in this case is illogical and unnecessary. During normal pregnancy there is hypervolemia which is harmful to neither the fetus nor the mother (in the absence of cardiovascular disease), but which is associated with edema, including generalized edema, in the majority of pregnant women. If this edema produces discomfort, increased recumbency will often provide relief. In rare instances, this edema may cause extreme discomfort which is not relieved by rest. In these cases a short course of diuretics may be appropriate and may provide relief.

CONTRAINDICATIONS

NAQUA Tablets are contraindicated in patients with anuria and in those who are allergic to this drug, to other thiazides or to other sulfonamide-derived drugs. The routine use of thiazides is contraindicated in otherwise healthy pregnant women with mild edema. (See **INDICATIONS AND USAGE** and **PRECAUTIONS, Pregnancy Category B.**)

WARNINGS

Thiazides should be used with caution in severe renal disease. In patients with renal disease thiazides may precipitate azotemia. Cumulative effects of the drug may develop in patients with impaired renal function.
Thiazides should be used with caution in patients with impaired hepatic function or progressive liver disease because minor alterations of fluid and electrolyte balance may precipitate hepatic coma.
Thiazides may add to or potentiate the action of other antihypertensive drugs. Potentiation occurs with ganglionic or peripheral adrenergic blocking drugs.
Hypersensitivity reactions may occur in patients with a history of allergy, including aspirin sensitivity or bronchial asthma.
The exacerbation and activation of systemic lupus erythematosus have been reported.
Lithium generally should not be given with diuretics because the latter reduce its renal clearance and increase the risk of lithium toxicity.

PRECAUTIONS

General: Periodic determinations of serum electrolytes should be done at appropriate intervals. Serum and urine electrolyte determinations are particularly important when the patient is vomiting excessively, having diarrhea, or receiving parenteral fluids. Thiazides may cause hyponatremia, hypochloremic alkalosis, hypokalemia, hypomagnesemia, and changes in serum and urine calcium. All patients receiving thiazide therapy should be observed for the clinical warning signs of fluid or electrolyte imbalance, irrespective of cause, including dryness of mouth, thirst, weakness, lethargy, drowsiness, restlessness, muscular pains, fatigue, or cramps, hypotension, tachycardia, oliguria, and gastrointestinal disturbances such as nausea and vomiting.
Hypokalemia may develop with trichlormethiazide as with other potent diuretics, including other thiazides, especially when the diuresis is brisk, when severe cirrhosis is present, or during concomitant use of corticosteroids or ACTH. Hypokalemia poses an increased risk in digitalized patients and patients with cirrhosis, since decreases in the serum potassium concentration can precipitate serious arrhythmias during digitalis therapy, and in cirrhotic patients low potassium levels may precipitate hepatic coma. Thiazides should be discontinued immediately if signs of impending hepatic coma appear.
Chloride deficits are usually mild and usually do not require treatment except under extraordinary circumstances, as in liver or renal disease. Hypochloremic alkalosis may occur with hypokalemia, especially if patients are losing additional potassium and chloride from vomiting, diarrhea, gastrointestinal disease, or potassium-losing renal diseases.
Dilutional hyponatremia may occur or be aggravated during thiazide therapy in edematous patients especially in hot weather. Appropriate therapy is water restriction; salt should not be administered unless the hyponatremia is life threatening. In actual body salt depletion, appropriate replacement is the therapy of choice, however.
Serum and urine electrolyte determinations are particularly important to diagnose and treat electrolyte disturbances.
Hyperuricemia may occur in patients receiving thiazides or related diuretics. While usually asymptomatic, frank gout may occur in patients with a history of gout, a familial predisposition to gout, or chronic renal failure.
Insulin or oral hypoglycemic drug requirements may be altered in patients with diabetes mellitus because thiazides and related diuretics can produce hyperglycemia and glycosuria. Latent diabetes mellitus may become manifest during thiazide administration. Reversible oculomotor paresis has occurred as a manifestation of thiazide-induced glucose intolerance.
The antihypertensive effects of thiazides may be enhanced in post-sympathectomy patients.
If progressive renal impairment becomes evident during thiazide therapy, careful reappraisal of therapy is necessary with consideration given to withholding or discontinuing diuretic dosing. Nonprotein nitrogen, blood urea nitrogen, or serum creatinine levels should be determined since these will be increased in renal impairment.
Information for Patients: Physicians should give the following information and instructions to patients receiving thiazide diuretics. This information is intended to aid in the safe and effective use of this medication. It is not a disclosure of all possible adverse or intended effects.

1. This drug must be taken on a regular schedule to be effective. Take as prescribed. Do not skip doses; if a dose is missed, do not double the dose. Do not take extra doses.
2. Use of this drug with other medications should be done only with a physician's advice. If other drugs are required for control of edema or hypertension, the patient should understand the need for compliance with the total therapeutic program.
3. This drug should be used only by the patient for whom it is prescribed. Do not allow anyone else to take this medication.
4. Pregnancy or plans for pregnancy should be discussed with the physician.
5. Since thiazides appear in breast milk, it is recommended that the baby not be breast fed.
6. The patient should be alerted to the possibilities of various side effects which might occur during thiazide therapy, including particularly, changes in the control or severity of concurrent illnesses, such as liver or kidney disease, diabetes mellitus, systemic lupus erythematosus, and gout.
7. The patient should be alerted to the effects of diuresis, including excessive losses of sodium, chloride and especially potassium, and how to provide for replacement.
8. Dietary instructions should be provided.
9. As required, return for laboratory tests.

Laboratory Tests: Since thiazides affect many organ functions, the safe and effective use of these drugs may require pretreatment and periodic laboratory tests. They may be helpful: in following the patient's initial response or status after prolonged therapy; in avoiding or identifying possible adverse reactions, as in patients who are vomiting or who have serious diseases such as severe hepatic disease, renal disease, diabetes mellitus, or gout; in patients who are receiving concomitant medications, such as digitalis glycosides or corticosteroids. The following procedures (not necessarily inclusive) should be considered in patient monitoring:

- serum electrolyte determinations, especially sodium, potassium, chloride, and bicarbonate
- serum uric acid and blood glucose
- serum creatinine or blood urea nitrogen
- liver function tests, including serum transaminases, alkaline phosphatase, and bilirubin levels
- electrocardiograms, especially in patients on digitalis glycosides.

Drug Interactions: The following are generally recognized potential thiazide drug interactions (not necessarily inclusive):

Digitalis glycosides: Thiazides may produce hypokalemia, hypomagnesemia, and hypercalcemia which may predispose the patient to digitalis toxicity. Periodic serum electrolyte determinations may be required, and correction of electrolyte abnormalities, particularly hypokalemia, should be undertaken, either prophylactically or therapeutically. Electrocardiographic monitoring of the patient may be required to evaluate the patient's cardiac status initially and to control treatment.

Corticosteroids (and ACTH): Concomitant use with thiazides may enhance potassium loss. Periodic serum electrolyte determinations may be required, and correction of electrolyte abnormalities, particularly hypokalemia, should be undertaken.

Insulin preparations and oral sulfonylureas: Thiazides may antagonize the hypoglycemic effects of these agents. Dosage adjustment may be necessary.

Diazoxide: Concomitant use of thiazides and diazoxide may potentiate the hyperglycemic, hyperuricemic, and antihypertensive effects of both drugs.

Methyldopa, reserpine, guanethidine sulfate, prazosin hydrochloride, and beta-adrenergic receptor blockers: Concomitant use of a thiazide with most other antihypertensive drugs produces a more pronounced antihypertensive response than when either drug is used as the sole therapeutic agent. Severe postural hypotension may result if a thiazide is added to the regimen of a patient stabilized on certain hypotensive agents, such as methyldopa, guanethidine sulfate, or prazosin.

Cholestyramine: Cholestyramine may bind thiazides in the gut. Thiazides should be taken at least one hour before cholestyramine.

Lithium carbonate: Lithium toxicity has been reported in patients receiving thiazides. Renal clearance of lithium is decreased in patients on long-term thiazide treatment, and lithium therapy has been reported in some cases to be associated with morphological changes in the kidneys. Serum lithium concentrations should be measured frequently in such patients also on thiazides.

Tubocurarine and gallamine: Thiazides may cause prolonged neuromuscular blockade in patients receiving nondepolarizing neuromuscular blocking agents, such as turbocurarine chloride or gallamine.

Probenecid: Thiazide-induced uric acid retention is blocked by probenecid.

Fenfluramine: Fenfluramine has been reported to enhance the blood pressure lowering effect and plasma norepinephrine levels resulting from use with hydrochlorothiazide in obese patients.

Indomethacin: The concomitant administration of indomethacin to hypertensive patients being treated with thiazide diuretics has resulted in partial loss of control of the lowered blood pressure. A possible explanation is inhibition of prostacyclin biosynthesis by indomethacin.

Anticholinergics: Drugs with significant anticholinergic effects on the gastrointestinal tract may delay gastric emptying and enhance the absorption of thiazides.

Sympathomimetic agents: A decrease in arterial responsiveness to vasopressors (norepinephrine, phenylephrine), of uncertain clinical significance, has been reported during thiazide therapy.

Drug/Laboratory Test Interactions: Thiazides can affect the laboratory test values for electrolytes, such as sodium potassium, chloride, calcium, magnesium, and iodide, and for glucose, uric acid, blood urea nitrogen, and serum creatinine. Thiazides also may interfere with diagnostic testing as follows:

(a) due to pharmacologic or metabolic effects

- thiazides may cause false-negative results with the phentolamine and the tyramine tests for pheochromocytoma by attenuating the hypertensive response to tyramine.
- thiazides may compete with phenolsulfonphthalein (PSP) for renal tubular secretion, resulting in decreased urinary excretion of PSP.
- thiazides may cause sulfobromophthalein (BSP) retention, probably due to a reduction in plasma volume and a resultant decrease in hepatic blood flow.
- thiazides may decrease urinary cortisol excretion, possibly due to changes in cortisol secretion, renal handling or metabolism.
- thiazides may decrease serum protein-bound iodine, although usually not to subnormal levels, without signs of thyroid disturbance.
- thiazides may cause increases in serum amylase levels, some reported increases being up to two times pretreatment levels. However, the fact that acute pancreatitis has occurred in patients on thiazides should also be kept in mind.

(b) due to interference with laboratory analysis procedures

- thiazides, except for chlorothiazide, may interefere with assays of total urinary estrogens and of estriol.
- thiazides may interfere with urinary 17-hydroxycorticosteroids measurements.

Carcinogenesis, Mutagenesis, Impairment of Fertility: Long-term dosing studies have not been done with trichlormethiazide to determine whether this drug has carcinogenic potential. No study has been done to determine whether trichlormethiazide is mutagenic.

Pregnancy Category B: Reproduction studies have been performed with trichlormethiazide in rats at doses 250 to 1250 times the recommended human daily dose and have revealed no evidence of impaired fertility or harm to the fetus. There are, however, no adequate and well-controlled studies in pregnant women. Since thiazides cross the placental barrier, their use may expose the fetus to other possible hazards, such as fetal or neonatal jaundice or thrombocytopenia. NAQUA Tablets should be used during pregnancy only if clearly needed and when the potential benefits to the mother justify the potential risks to the infant.

Nonteratogenic Effects: Thiazides cross the placenta and appear in cord blood. Infants born to mothers treated with diuretics have shown changes in body water and electrolytes, although not of apparent clinical significance. Fetal or neonatal jaundice and thrombocytopenia have been reported in newborn infants of women receiving thiazides. There is an unconfirmed report of neonatal hemolysis in two infants attributed to maternal thiazide therapy.

Nursing Mothers: Thiazides can decrease milk production. Additionally, thiazides appear in breast milk. Thrombocytopenia can occur in the nursing infant when the mother is taking a thiazide diuretic. Because of the potential for unwanted adverse effects in nursing infants from NAQUA Tablets, a decision should be made whether to discontinue nursing or to discontinue the drug, taking into account the importance of the drug to the mother.

Pediatric Use: Thiazide diuretics have been shown to be effective and safe in children when used as recommended. (See **INDICATIONS AND USAGE** and **DOSAGE AND ADMINISTRATION.)**

ADVERSE REACTIONS

The following adverse reactions have been observed, but there is not enough systematic data collection to support an estimate of their frequency.

Gastrointestinal System: pancreatitis; jaundice (intrahepatic cholestatic jaundice); acute cholecystitis; vomiting; diarrhea; nausea; gastric irritation; anorexia; cramping; constipation.

Central Nervous System: vertigo; headache; xanthopsia; dizziness; paresthesias.

Hematologic: aplastic anemia; thrombocytopenia; agranulocytosis; leukopenia.

Dermatologic-Hypersensitivity: anaphylactoid reactions; necrotizing angiitis (vasculitis, cutaneous vasculitis); purpura; photosensitivity; urticaria; rash.

Cardiovascular: orthostatic hypotension may occur and may be aggravated by alcohol, barbiturates, or narcotics.

Other: hyperuricemia; hyperglycemia; glycosuria; muscle spasm; weakness; restlessness.

Whenever adverse reactions are moderate or severe, the dosage should be reduced or therapy withdrawn.

OVERDOSAGE

Accidental or suicidal poisoning with thiazide diuretics has been reported infrequently.

Manifestations: Diuresis is to be expected; lethargy of varying degree may appear and may progress to coma within a few hours, with minimal depression of respiration and cardiovascular function and without significant serum electrolyte changes or dehydration. The mechanism of CNS depression with thiazide overdosage is unknown. GI irritation and hypermotility may occur; temporary elevation of BUN has been reported and serum electrolyte changes can occur, especially in patients with impaired renal function.

Treatment: Evacuate gastric contents, taking care to prevent aspiration, especially in the stuporous or comatose patient. GI effects are usually of short duration but may require symptomatic treatment.

Monitor serum electrolyte and renal function; institute supportive measures as required individually to maintain hydration, electrolyte balance, respiration, and cardiovascular-renal functions.

DOSAGE AND ADMINISTRATION

Therapy should be individualized according to patient response. Dosage should be titrated to seek maximal therapeutic response and to establish the minimal dose necessary to maintain that response.

Adults: *Edematous Conditions:* The usual oral dosage of NAQUA Tablets for diuretic effect is 1 to 4 mg daily.

Hypertension The usual oral dosage of NAQUA Tablets for antihypertensive effect is 2 to 4 mg daily.

Children: *Edematous Conditions or Hypertension* The usual oral dosage of NAQUA Tablets for children over 6 months of age is determined as follows: 0.07 mg/kg/24 hr or 2 mg/sqM/24 hr orally as a single dose or divided into two doses.

HOW SUPPLIED

NAQUA Tablets, 2 mg, pink, clover-shaped, compressed tablets impressed with the letter S and either product identification letter, AHG, or numbers, 822; bottles of 100 (NDC 0085-0822-03).

NAQUA Tablets, 4 mg, aqua, clover-shaped, compressed tablets impressed with the letter S and either product identification letters, AHH, or numbers, 547; bottles of 100 (NDC 0085-0547-03) and 1000 (NDC 0085-0547-06).

Dispense in tight containers.

Revised 7/85

Shown in Product Identification Section, page 428

NAQUIVAL® ℞

[nak'kwiv-al]

brand of trichlormethiazide, USP—reserpine, USP

Tablets

> **Warning**
>
> This fixed combination drug is not indicated for initial therapy of hypertension. Hypertension requires therapy titrated to the individual patient. If the fixed combination represents the dosage so determined, its use may be more convenient in patient management. The treatment of hypertension is not static, but must be re-evaluated as conditions in each patient warrant.

DESCRIPTION

Each NAQUIVAL Tablet contains 4 mg NAQUA® (brand of trichlormethiazide, USP) and 0.1 mg reserpine, USP. Trichlormethiazide is an antihypertensive agent and diuretic of the benzothiadiazine series having the chemical formula, $C_8H_8Cl_3N_3O_4S_2$. The antihypertensive agent, reserpine, is a rauwolfia alkaloid having the chemical formula, $C_{33}H_{40}N_2O_9$.

ACTIONS

NAQUIVAL Tablets combine the antihypertensive and diuretic properties of trichlormethiazide with the antihypertensive actions of reserpine; maximum antihypertensive effects are achieved with minimal doses of each ingredient.

INDICATIONS

NAQUIVAL Tablets are indicated for the treatment of hypertension (see box warning).

CONTRAINDICATIONS

NAQUIVAL Tablets are contraindicated in patients with anuria.

Hypersensitivity to this or other sulfonamide-derived drugs is a contraindication to the use of this product.

The routine use of diuretics in an otherwise healthy pregnant woman with or without mild edema is contraindicated and possibly hazardous.

The presence of an active peptic ulcer, ulcerative colitis, or severe depression contraindicates the use of reserpine.

WARNINGS

NAQUIVAL Tablets should be withdrawn at least three weeks prior to elective surgery or electroconvulsive therapy because of the reserpine activity.

If parenteral antihypertensive therapy is indicated for a patient receiving NAQUIVAL Tablets, the physician should be alert to the possible synergism of reserpine and trichlormethiazide with such drugs, especially those administered by rapid infusion, e.g., diazoxide.

Sympathomimetics should be used with caution in patients who are receiving reserpine, since its antihypertensive effects may be reduced.

NAQUIVAL Tablets should be used with caution in severe renal disease. In patients with renal disease, thiazides may precipitate azotemia. Cumulative effects of the drug may develop in patients with impaired renal function.

Continued on next page

Schering—Cont.

Thiazides should be used with caution in patients with impaired hepatic function or progressive liver disease, since minor alterations of fluid and electrolyte balance may precipitate hepatic coma.
Thiazides may be additive or potentiative of the action of other antihypertensive drugs. Potentiation occurs with ganglionic or peripheral adrenergic blocking drugs or vasodilators.
Hypersensitivity reactions may occur in patients with a history of allergy or bronchial asthma.
The possibility of exacerbation or activation of systemic lupus erythematosus has been reported.
Usage in Pregnancy Usage of thiazides in women of childbearing age requires that the potential benefits of the drug be weighed against its possible hazards to the fetus. These hazards include fetal or neonatal jaundice, thrombocytopenia, and possibly other adverse reactions which have occurred in the adult.
The safety of reserpine for use during pregnancy or lactation has not been established; therefore, it should be used in pregnant patients or in women of childbearing age only when, in the judgment of the physician, its use is deemed essential to the welfare of the patient.
Nursing Mothers Thiazides cross the placental barrier and appear in cord blood and breast milk.

PRECAUTIONS

Periodic determination of serum electrolytes to detect possible electrolyte imbalance should be performed at appropriate intervals.
All patients receiving thiazide therapy should be observed for clinical signs of fluid or electrolyte imbalance, namely, hyponatremia, hypochloremic alkalosis, hypokalemia, hypomagnesemia, and changes in serum and urinary calcium. Serum and urine electrolyte determinations are particularly important when the patient is vomiting excessively or receiving parenteral fluids. Medications such as digitalis derivatives are sensitive to changes in serum electrolytes. Warning signs, irrespective of cause, are: dryness of mouth, thirst, weakness, lethargy, drowsiness, restlessness, muscle pains or cramps, muscular fatigue, hypotension, oliguria, tachycardia, and gastrointestinal disturbances such as nausea and vomiting.
Hypokalemia may develop with thiazides as with any other potent diuretic, especially with brisk diuresis, when severe cirrhosis is present, or during concomitant use of corticosteroids or ACTH.
Interference with adequate oral electrolyte intake will also contribute to hypokalemia. Digitalis therapy may exaggerate metabolic effects of hypokalemia especially with reference to myocardial activity.
Any chloride deficit is generally mild and usually does not require specific treatment except under extraordinary circumstances (as in liver disease or renal disease). Dilutional hyponatremia may occur in edematous patients in hot weather; appropriate therapy is water restriction, rather than administration of salt, except in rare instances when the hyponatremia is life-threatening. In actual salt depletion, appropriate replacement is the therapy of choice.
Hyperuricemia may occur or frank gout may be precipitated in certain patients receiving thiazide therapy.
Insulin requirements in diabetic patients may be increased, decreased, or unchanged. Latent diabetes mellitus may become manifest during thiazide administration; diabetic complications such as reversible oculomotor paresis may occur.
Thiazide drugs may increase the responsiveness to tubocurarine.
The antihypertensive effects of the drug may be enhanced in the post-sympathectomy patient.
Thiazides may decrease arterial responsiveness to norepinephrine. This diminution is not sufficient to preclude effectiveness of the pressor agent for therapeutic use.
If progressive renal impairment becomes evident, as indicated by a rising nonprotein nitrogen or blood urea nitrogen, a careful reappraisal of therapy is necessary with consideration given to withholding or discontinuing diuretic therapy.
Thiazides may decrease serum PBI levels without signs of thyroid disturbance.
Reserpine may augment secretory and motor activity of the gastrointestinal tract, and gastric hyperacidity, peptic ulceration, and mucous colitis may develop. Patients undergoing emergency surgery should be watched for precipitous falls in blood pressure; vasopressor agents such as levarterenol should be available.
Reserpine may precipitate biliary colic in patients with gallstones.
Because of the decreased sympathetic tone caused by reserpine catecholamine depletion, special care should be exercised in treating patients with a history of bronchial asthma.
NAQUIVAL Tablets contain FD&C Yellow No. 5 (tartrazine) which may cause allergic-type reactions (including bronchial asthma) in certain susceptible individuals. Although the overall incidence of FD&C Yellow No. 5 (tartrazine) sensitivity in the general population is low, it is frequently seen in patients who also have aspirin hypersensitivity.
Animal Tumorigenicity Rodent studies have shown that reserpine is an animal tumorigen, causing an increased incidence of mammary fibroadenomas in female mice, malignant tumors of the seminal vesicles in male mice, and malignant adrenal medullary tumors in male rats. These findings arose in 2 year studies in which the drug was administered in the feed at concentrations of 5 and 10 ppm-about 100 to 300 times the usual human dose. The breast neoplasms are thought to be related to reserpine's prolactin-elevating effect. Several other prolactin-elevating drugs have also been associated with an increased incidence of mammary neoplasia in rodents.
The extent to which these findings indicate a risk to humans is uncertain. Tissue culture experiments show that about one-third of human breast tumors are prolactin-dependent *in vitro*, a factor of considerable importance if the use of the drug is contemplated in a patient with previously detected breast cancer. The possibility of an increased risk of breast cancer in reserpine users has been studied extensively; however, no firm conclusion has emerged. Although a few epidemiologic studies have suggested a slightly increased risk (less than twofold in all studies except one) in women who have used reserpine, other studies of generally similar design have not confirmed this. Epidemiologic studies conducted using other drugs (neuroleptic agents) that, like reserpine, increase prolactin levels and therefore would be considered rodent mammary carcinogens, have not shown an association between chronic administration of the drug and human mammary tumorigenesis. While long-term clinical observation has not suggested such an association, the available evidence is considered too limited to be conclusive at this time. An association of reserpine intake with pheochromocytoma or tumors of the seminal vesicles has not been explored.

ADVERSE REACTIONS

Autonomic Reactions: nasal stuffiness; dryness of the mouth; blurred vision; flushing of the face.
Gastrointestinal System Reactions: anorexia; gastric irritation; nausea; vomiting; cramping; diarrhea; constipation; jaundice (intrahepatic cholestatic jaundice); pancreatitis.
Central Nervous System Reactions: dizziness; vertigo; paresthesias; headache; xanthopsia; depression; central nervous system sensitization manifested as dull sensorium, deafness, glaucoma, uveitis, and optic atrophy.
Hematologic Reactions: leukopenia; agranulocytosis; thrombocytopenia; aplastic anemia.
Dermatologic—Hypersensitivity Reactions: purpura; photosensitivity; rash; urticaria; necrotizing angiitis (vasculitis, cutaneous vasculitis).
Cardiovascular Reactions: Ectopic cardiac rhythms, particularly when used concurrently with digitalis; orthostatic hypotension may occur and may be aggravated by alcohol, barbiturates or narcotics.
Other: hyperglycemia; glycosuria; hyperuricemia; muscle spasm; weakness; restlessness; drowsiness; weight gain; dyspnea; dyskinesia; impotence and decreased libido; conjunctival injection.
Whenever adverse reactions are moderate or severe, NAQUIVAL dosage should be reduced or therapy withdrawn.

DOSAGE AND ADMINISTRATION

The dosage of NAQUIVAL should be determined by individual titration (see box warning).
Initial dosage with NAQUIVAL is frequently one tablet twice a day, with reduction to maintenance levels as therapeutic benefits become manifest. When NAQUIVAL is used with ganglionic blocking agents, careful downward adjustment of these drugs should be made to avoid precipitous blood pressure falls.

HOW SUPPLIED

NAQUIVAL Tablets: peach-colored, scored, compressed tablets impressed with the Schering Trademark and product identification letters, AHT or numbers, 394; bottles of 100 (NDC 0085-0394-03) and 500 (NDC 0085-0394-06).
Store between 2° and 30°C (36° and 86°F).
Revised 6/83

Shown in Product Identification Section, page 428

NETROMYCIN® ℞

[*nĕ"trō-mī'sin*]
brand of netilmicin sulfate
Injection, USP 100 mg/ml
Pediatric Injection, USP 25 mg/ml
Neonatal Injection, USP 10 mg/ml

WARNINGS

Patients treated with aminoglycosides should be under close clinical observation because of the potential toxicity associated with the use of these drugs.
Netilmicin has potent neuromuscular blocking potential. Neuromuscular blockade and respiratory paralysis have been reported in animals receiving netilmicin. The possibility of these phenomena occurring in man should be considered if aminoglycosides are administered by any route to patients receiving neuromuscular blocking agents, such as succinylcholine, tubocurarine, or decamethonium, or to patients receiving massive transfusions of citrate-anticoagulated blood. If neuromuscular blockade occurs, calcium salts may lessen it, but mechanical respiratory assistance may also be necessary.
As with other aminoglycosides, netilmicin sulfate injection is potentially nephrotoxic. The risk is greater in patients with impaired renal function, in those who receive high dosage or prolonged therapy, and in the elderly.
Neurotoxicity manifested by ototoxicity, both vestibular and auditory, can occur in patients treated with netilmicin, primarily in those with preexisting renal damage and in patients, treated with higher doses and/or for longer periods than recommended. Aminoglycoside-induced ototoxicity is usually irreversible. Other manifestations of aminoglycoside-induced neurotoxicity include numbness, skin tingling, muscle twitching, and convulsions.
Renal and eighth cranial nerve function should be closely monitored, especially in patients with known or suspected impairment of renal function either at onset of therapy or during therapy. Urine should be examined for increased excretion of protein, the presence of cells or casts, and decreased specific gravity. Serum creatinine concentration or blood urea nitrogen should be determined periodically. A more precise measure of glomerular filtration rate is a carefully conducted determination of creatinine clearance rate or, often more practically, an estimate of creatinine clearance based on published nomograms or equations. (See DOSAGE AND ADMINISTRATION.) When feasible it is recommended that serial audiograms be obtained in patients old enough to be tested, particularly in high-risk patients.
The dosage of netilmicin should be reduced or administration discontinued if evidence of drug-induced auditory or vestibular toxicity (vertigo, tinnitus, nystagmus, or hearing loss) develops during therapy. If evidence of nephrotoxicity occurs, dosage should be adjusted. (See DOSAGE AND ADMINISTRATION, Dosage for Impaired Renal Function.) As with the other aminoglycosides, on rare occasions changes in renal and eighth cranial nerve functions may not become manifest until soon after completion of therapy.
Serum concentrations of aminoglycosides should be monitored when feasible to assure adequate levels and to avoid potentially toxic levels. After administration of an appropriate dose of netilmicin, peak serum concentrations occur approximately 30 to 60 minutes after an intramuscular injection or at the end of a one hour intravenous infusion. Dosage should be adjusted so that prolonged peak serum concentrations above 16 mcg/ml are avoided.
When monitoring trough concentrations, dosage should be adjusted so that levels above 4 mcg/ml are avoided.
Excessive peak and/or trough serum concentrations of aminoglycosides may increase the risk of renal and eighth cranial nerve toxicity. In the event of overdose or toxic reactions, hemodialysis may aid in removal of netilmicin from the blood, especially if renal function is, or becomes, compromised. Removal of netilmicin by peritoneal dialysis is at a rate considerably less than by hemodialysis.
Concurrent and/or sequential systemic or topical use of other potentially neurotoxic and/or nephrotoxic drugs, such as: cephaloridine, amphotericin B, streptomycin, kanamycin, gentamicin, tobramycin, amikacin, neomycin, vancomycin, bacitracin, polymyxin B, colistin, paromomycin, viomycin, or cisplatin should be avoided. The concurrent use of aminoglycosides with potent diuretics, such as ethacrynic acid or furosemide, should be avoided since certain diuretics by themselves may cause ototoxicity. In addition, when administered intravenously, diuretics may enhance aminoglycoside toxicity by altering the antibiotic concentration in the serum and tissues. Other factors which may increase patient risk of toxicity are advanced age and dehydration.

DESCRIPTION

NETROMYCIN Injection, NETROMYCIN Pediatric Injection, and NETROMYCIN Neonatal Injection contain netilmicin sulfate in clear, sterile, aqueous solution with a pH range of 3.5 to 6.0 for intramuscular or intravenous administration. Netilmicin is a semisynthetic, water-soluble antibiotic of the aminoglycoside group, derived from sisomicin. Its chemical name is: *O*-3-Deoxy-4-*C*-methyl-3-(methylamino)-β-L-arabinopyranosyl(1→4)-*O*-[2,6-diamino-2,3,4,6-tetradeoxy-α-D-*glycero*-hex-4-enopyranosyl-(1→6)]-2-deoxy-N^3-ethyl-L-streptamine sulfate (2:5) (salt).

Each ml of NETROMYCIN Injection contains netilmicin sulfate equivalent to 100 mg netilmicin; 10 mg benzyl alcohol as a preservative; 0.1 mg edetate disodium; 2.4 mg sodium metabisulfite; 0.8 mg sodium sulfite; and water for injection, q.s. Each ml of NETROMYCIN Pediatric Injection contains netilmicin sulfate equivalent to 25 mg netilmicin; 0.2 mg propylparaben and 1.3 mg methylparaben as preservatives; 0.1 mg edetate disodium; 2.6 mg sodium sulfate; 2.1 mg sodium metabisulfite; 1.2 mg of sodium sulfite; and water for injection, q.s. NETROMYCIN Neonatal Injection contains in each ml netilmicin sulfate equivalent to 10 mg netilmicin; 2.4 mg sodium metabisulfite; 0.8 mg sodium sulfite; 6.5 mg sodium chloride; and water for injection, q.s.

CLINICAL PHARMACOLOGY

Netilmicin is rapidly and completely absorbed after intramuscular injection. Peak serum levels, after intramuscular injection, usually occur within 30 to 60 minutes and levels are measurable for 12 hours. In adult volunteers with normal renal function, peak serum concentrations of netilmicin in mcg/ml are usually about 3 to 3.5 times the single intramuscular dose in mg/kg. For example, a dose of 2.0 mg/kg may be expected to result in a peak serum concentration of approximately 7 mcg/ml. At eight or more hours after administration of a dose in the recommended range, serum levels are usually less than 3 mcg/ml. When a single dose of netilmicin is administered by 60-minute intravenous infusion, the peak serum concentrations are similar to those obtained by intramuscular administration. Following a rapid intravenous injection of netilmicin, levels in serum may be transiently 2 to 3 times higher than those of the 60-minute infusion. Netilmicin rapidly distributes to tissues.

The half-life of netilmicin after single doses is usually 2 to 2.5 hours, a half-life which is very similar to that of gentamicin, and is independent of the route of administration. The half-life increases as the dose increases (e.g., 2.2 hours after a 1 mg/kg dose to 3 hours after a 3 mg/kg dose). Approximately 80% of the administered dose is excreted in the urine within 24 hours; the urine netilmicin concentration after a dose often exceeds 100 mcg/ml. There is no evidence of metabolic transformation of netilmicin. The drug is excreted principally by glomerular filtration. Probenecid does not affect tubular transport of aminoglycosides. The volume of distribution of netilmicin is approximately 20% of body weight; total body clearance is about 80 ml/min and renal clearance is about 60 ml/min. In multiple-dose studies in volunteers when the drug was administered every 12 hours at doses ranging from 1.0 to 4.0 mg/kg, steady-state levels were obtained by the second day.

The serum levels at steady-state were less than 20% higher than those of the first dose. As with other aminoglycosides, the half-life of netilmicin increases, and its renal clearance decreases with decreasing renal function.

The endogenous creatinine clearance rate and the serum creatinine level have a high correlation with the half-life of netilmicin. Results of these tests can serve as a guide for adjusting dosage in patients with renal impairment.

In patients with marked impairment of renal function, there is a decrease in the concentration of aminoglycosides in urine and in their penetration into defective renal parenchyma. This should be considered when treating patients with urinary tract infections. In one study of adults with renal failure undergoing hemodialysis, netilmicin serum levels were reduced by approximately 63% over an 8-hour dialysis session. Shorter dialysis sessions will remove less drug. No hemodialysis information is available for children. Aminoglycosides are also removed by peritoneal dialysis but at a rate considerably less than by hemodialysis.

Since netilmicin is distributed in extracellular fluid, peak serum concentrations may be lower than usual in patients whose extracellular fluid volume is expanded (e.g., patients with edema or ascites). Serum concentrations of aminoglycosides in febrile patients may be lower than those in afebrile patients given the same dose. When body temperature returns to normal, serum concentrations of the drug may rise. Both febrile and anemic states may be associated with a shorter than usual half-life. (Dosage adjustment is usually not necessary.)

In severely burned patients, the half-life of aminoglycosides may be significantly decreased, and serum concentrations resulting from a particular dose may be lower than anticipated.

The elimination half-life of netilmicin in neonates during the first week of life is inversely correlated with body weight, ranging from approximately 8 hours for neonates weighing 1.5 to 2.0 kg to approximately 4.5 hours for 3.0 to 4.0 kg neonates. The elimination half-life of infants and children 6 weeks of age and older is 1.5 to 2.0 hours.

Following parenteral administration, aminoglycosides can be detected in serum, tissues, and sputum and in pericardial, pleural, synovial, and peritoneal fluids. A variety of methods are available to measure netilmicin concentrations in body fluids; these include microbiologic, enzymatic, and radioimmunoassay techniques. Concentrations in renal cortex may be markedly higher than the usual serum levels.

Minute quantities of aminoglycosides have been detected in the urine for up to 30 days after discontinuing administration. Hepatic secretion is minimal. As with all aminoglycosides, netilmicin diffuses poorly into the subarachnoid space after parenteral administration. Concentrations of netilmicin in cerebrospinal fluid are often low and dependent upon dose and the degree of meningeal inflammation. Netilmicin crosses the placenta and has been detected in cord blood and in the fetus. Studies in nursing mothers indicate that small amounts of the drug are excreted in breast milk. Netilmicin is poorly absorbed from the intact gastrointestinal tract after oral administration. As with other aminoglycosides, the binding of netilmicin to serum proteins is low (0–30%).

Microbiology: Netilmicin is a rapidly acting, broad-spectrum bactericidal antibiotic which appears to act by inhibiting normal protein synthesis in susceptible microorganisms. Netilmicin is active *in vitro* against a wide variety of pathogenic bacteria, primarily gram-negative bacilli and also a few gram-positive organisms, including *Citrobacter, Enterobacter, Escherichia coli, Klebsiella* species, *Proteus mirabilis, Pseudomonas aeruginosa, Salmonella* species, *Shigella species,* and *Staphylococcus* species (penicillin- and methicillin-resistant strains).

Netilmicin is also active *in vitro* against some isolates of *Acinetobacter* and *Neisseria* species, indole-positive *Proteus* species, *Pseudomonas* and *Serratia* species. In addition, netilmicin is active *in vitro* against many strains which have acquired resistance to other aminoglycosides. Such resistance is usually caused by aminoglycoside modifying (inactivating) enzymes. In general, netilmicin is active against organisms which inactivate aminoglycosides by either phosphorylation or adenylation; it has variable activity against acetylating strains, depending on the specific type. For example, the susceptibility of *Serratia* species producing a combination of adenylating and acetylating enzymes varies according to the level of acetylating enzyme present. Netilmicin is active *in vitro* against certain strains of gram-negative bacteria resistant to gentamicin and tobramycin: *Citrobacter, Enterobacter* species, *Escherichia coli, Klebsiella, Proteus* (indole-positive), *Pseudomonas, Salmonella,* and *Shigella* species. Netilmicin is active *in vitro* against certain staphylococci resistant to amikacin and tobramycin. Like other aminoglycosides, netilmicin is not active against bacteria with reduced permeability to this class of antibiotics.

Most species of streptococci and anaerobic organisms, such as *Bacteroides* and *Clostridium* species, are resistant to aminoglycosides.

The effects of media pH, protein content, divalent cation concentration, and of inoculum size on the *in vitro* activity of netilmicin are similar to those of other aminoglycosides.

Netilmicin acts synergistically *in vitro* with members of the penicillin class of antibiotics against *Streptococcus faecalis.* It also acts synergistically with those pencillins which are active alone against many strains of *Pseudomonas.* In addition, many, but not all isolates of *Serratia* which are resistant to multiple antibiotics, are inhibited by synergistic combinations of netilmicin with carbenicillin, azlocillin, mezlocillin, cefamandole, cefotaxime, or moxalactam. Tests for antibiotic synergy are necessary.

Susceptibility Testing: Quantitative methods that require measurements of zone diameters give the most precise estimates of antibiotic susceptibility. One such procedure has been recommended for use with discs to test susceptibility to netilmicin. Interpretation involves correlation of the diameters obtained in the disc test with minimal inhibitory concentration (MIC) values for netilmicin.

Reports from the laboratory giving results of the standardized single disc susceptibility test (Bauer, et al. Am J Clin Path 1966; 45:493 and Federal Register 37:20525-20529, 1972), using a 30 mcg netilmicin disc should be interpreted according to the following criteria:

Organisms producing zones of 15 mm or greater, or MIC's of 8.0 mcg or less are considered susceptible, indicating that the tested organism is likely to respond to therapy.

Resistant organisms produce zones of 12 mm or less or MIC's of 16 mcg or greater. A report of "resistant" from the laboratory indicates that the infecting organism is not likely to respond to therapy.

Zones greater than 12 mm and less than 15 mm, or MIC's of greater than 8.0 mcg and less than 16 mcg, indicate intermediate susceptibility. A report of "intermediate" susceptibility suggests that the organism would be susceptible if the infection is confined to tissues and fluids (e.g., urine), in which high antibiotic levels are attained.

Control organisms are recommended for susceptibility testing. Each time the test is performed one or more of the following organisms should be included: *Escherichia coli* ATCC 25922, *Staphylococcus aureus* ATCC 25923, and *Pseudomonas aeruginosa* ATCC 27853. The control organisms should produce zones of inhibition within the following ranges:

Escherichia coli (ATCC 25922) 22–30 mm
Staphylococcus aureus (ATCC 25923)
22–31 mm
Pseudomonas aeruginosa (ATCC 27853) 17–23 mm

In certain circumstances, particularly with strains of *Pseudomonas aeruginosa,* it may be desirable to do additional susceptibility testing by the tube or agar dilution method. Netilmicin sulfate powder, a diagnostic reagent, is available for this purpose.

The MIC values of netilmicin for the control strains are the following:

Escherichia coli (ATCC 25922)
0.25–0.5 mcg/ml
Staphylococcus aureus (ATCC 25923) 0.125–0.25 mcg/ml
Pseudomonas aeruginosa (ATCC 27853)
4–8 mcg/ml in media supplemented with calcium and magnesium.

INDICATIONS AND USAGE

Netilmicin sulfate injection is indicated for the short-term treatment of patients of all ages, including neonates, infants, and children with serious or life-threatening bacterial infections caused by susceptible strains of the designated microorganisms in the diseases listed below:

COMPLICATED URINARY TRACT infections caused by *Escherichia coli, Klebsiella pneumoniae, Pseudomonas aeruginosa, Enterobacter species, Proteus mirabilis, Proteus* species (indole-positive), *Serratia** and *Citrobacter* species, and *Staphylococcus aureus***.

SEPTICEMIA caused by *Escherichia coli, Klebsiella pneumoniae, Pseudomonas aeruginosa, Enterobacter* and *Serratia** species, and *Proteus mirabilis.*

SKIN AND SKIN STRUCTURE infections caused by *Escherichia coli, Klebsiella pneumoniae, Pseudomonas aeruginosa, Enterobacter* and *Serratia** species, *Proteus mirabilis, Proteus* species (indole-positive), and *Staphylococcus aureus*** (penicillinase- and non-penicillinase-producing strains).

INTRA-ABDOMINAL infections including peritonitis and intra-abdominal abscess caused by *Escherichia coli, Klebsiella pneumoniae, Psuedomonas aeruginosa, Enterobacter* species, *Proteus mirabilis, Proteus* species (indole-positive), and *Staphylococcus aureus*** (penicillinase- and non-penicillinase-producing strains).

LOWER RESPIRATORY TRACT infections caused by *Escherichia coli, Klebsiella pneumoniae, Pseudomonas aeruginosa, Enterobacter* and *Serratia** species, *Proteus mirabilis, Proteus* species (indole-positive), and *Staphylococcus aureus*** (penicillinase- and non-penicillinase-producing strains).

*(See **Microbiology** Section.)

**While not the antibiotic class of first choice, aminoglycosides, including netilmicin, may be considered for the treatment of serious staphylococcal infections when penicillins or other less potentially toxic drugs are contraindicated and bacterial susceptibility tests and clinical judgment indicate their use. They may also be considered in mixed infections caused by susceptible strains of staphylococci and gram-negative organisms.

Aminoglycosides are indicated for those infections for which less potentially toxic antimicrobial agents are ineffective or contraindicated. They are not indicated in the treatment of uncomplicated initial episodes of urinary tract infection unless the causative organisms are resistant to antimicrobial agents having less potential toxicity.

Netilmicin sulfate injection may be considered as initial therapy in suspected or confirmed gram-negative infections, and therapy may be instituted before obtaining results of susceptibility testing. The decision to continue therapy with netilmicin should be based on the results of susceptibility tests, the severity of the infection, and the important additional concepts contained in the "WARNINGS Box" above. If the causative organisms are resistant to netilmicin, other appropriate therapy should be instituted.

In serious infections when the causative organisms are unknown, netilmicin may be administered as initial therapy in conjunction, with a penicillin-type or cephalosporin-type drug before obtaining results of susceptibility testing. In neonates with suspected sepsis, a penicillin-type drug is also usually indicated as concomitant therapy with netilmicin. If anaerobic organisms are suspected as etiologic agents, other suitable antimicrobial therapy should also be given. Following identification of the organism and its susceptibility, appropriate antibiotic therapy should then be continued.

Netilmicin sulfate injection has been used effectively in combination with carbenicillin or ticarcillin for the treatment of life-threatening infections caused by *Pseudomonas aeruginosa.*

Clinical studies have shown that netilmicin has been effective in the treatment of serious infections caused by some organisms resistant to other aminoglycosides, *i.e.,* gentamicin, tobramycin, and/or amikacin.

Specimens for bacterial culture should be obtained to isolate and identify causative organisms and to determine their susceptibility to netilmicin.

Continued on next page

Information on Schering products appearing on these pages is effective as of September 30, 1986.

Schering—Cont.

CONTRAINDICATION

Hypersensitivity to netilmicin or to any of the ingredients of the preparation is a contraindication to its use. See WARNINGS if patient is hypersensitive to another aminoglycoside.

WARNINGS

(See "WARNINGS Box" above.)

If the patient has a history of hypersensitivity or serious toxic reaction to another aminoglycoside, netilmicin should be used very cautiously, if at all, because cross-sensitivity to drugs in this class has been reported.

Aminoglycosides can cause fetal harm when administered to a pregnant woman. Aminoglycoside antibiotics cross the placenta and there have been several reports of total irreversible bilateral congenital deafness in children whose mothers received streptomycin during pregnancy. Although serious side effects to fetus or newborn have not been reported in the treatment of pregnant women with other aminoglycosides, the potential for harm exists. Reproduction studies of netilmicin have been performed in rats and rabbits using intramuscular and subcutaneous doses approximately 13–15 times the highest adult human dose and have revealed no evidence of impairment of fertility or harm to the fetus. Moreover, there was no evidence of ototoxicity in the offspring of rats treated subcutaneously with netilmicin throughout pregnancy and during the subsequent lactation period. However, if this drug is used during pregnancy, or if the patient becomes pregnant while taking this drug, the patient should be apprised of the potential hazard to the fetus.

PRECAUTIONS

General: Neurotoxic and nephrotoxic antibiotics may be almost completely absorbed from body surfaces (except the urinary bladder) after local irrigation and after topical application during surgical procedures. The potential toxic effects of antibiotics administered in this fashion (neuromuscular blockade, respiratory paralysis, oto- and nephrotoxicity) should be considered. (See "WARNINGS Box".)

Increased nephrotoxicity has been reported following concomitant administration of aminoglycoside antibiotics with some cephalosporins.

Aminoglycosides should be used with caution in patients with neuromuscular disorders, such as myasthenia gravis, parkinsonism, or infant botulism, since these drugs may aggravate muscle weakness because of their potential curare-like effect on the neuromuscular junction.

Elderly patients may have reduced renal function which may not be evident in the results of routine screening tests, such as BUN or serum creatinine levels. Determination of creatinine clearance or an estimate based on published nomograms or equations may be more useful. Monitoring of renal function during treatment with netilmicin, as with other aminoglycosides, is particularly important in such patients.

Patients should be well hydrated during treatment.

Treatment with netilmicin may result in overgrowth of nonsusceptible organisms. If this occurs, appropriate therapy is indicated.

Laboratory Tests: *Test of renal function:* Urine should be examined periodically for increased excretion of protein and the presence of cells and casts, keeping in mind the effects of the primary illness on these tests. One or more of the following laboratory measurements should be obtained at the onset of therapy, periodically during therapy, and at, or shortly after, the end of therapy;

- creatinine clearance rate (either carefully measured or estimated from published nomograms or equations based on the patient's age, sex, body weight, and serum creatinine concentration) (preferred over BUN);
- serum creatinine concentration (preferred over BUN);
- blood urea nitrogen (BUN).

More frequent testing is desirable if renal functon is changing.

See also "PRECAUTIONS, **General**" above regarding elderly patients.

Test of eighth cranial nerve function: Serial audiometric tests are suggested, particularly when renal function is impaired and/or prolonged aminoglycoside therapy is required; such tests should also be repeated periodically after treatment if there is evidence of a hearing deficit or vestibular abnormality before or during therapy, or when consecutive or concomitant use of other potentially ototoxic drugs is unavoidable.

Drug Interactions: *In vitro* mixing of an aminoglycoside with beta-lactam-type antibiotics (penicillins or cephalosporins) may result in a significant mutual inactivation. Even when an aminoglycoside and a penicillin-type drug are administered separately by different routes, a reduction in aminoglycoside serum half-life or serum levels has been reported in patients with impaired renal function and in some patients with normal renal function. Usually, such inactivation of the aminoglycoside is clinically significant only in patients with severely impaired renal function. (See also "**Drug/Laboratory test interactions.**") See "WARNINGS Box" regarding concurrent use of potent diuretics, concurrent and/or sequential use of other neurotoxic and/or nephrotoxic antibiotics, and for other essential information.

See also "PRECAUTIONS, **General.**"

Drug/Laboratory test interactions: Concomitant cephalosporin therapy may spuriously elevate creatinine determinations.

The inactivation between aminoglycosides and beta-lactam antibiotics described in "Drug Interactions" may continue in specimens of body fluids collected for assay, resulting in inaccurate, false low aminoglycoside readings. Such specimens should be properly handled, *i.e.*, assayed promptly, frozen, or treated with beta-lactamase.

Carcinogenesis, mutagenesis, impairment of fertility: Lifetime carcinogenicity tests have been undertaken in the mouse and rat and no drug-related tumors were observed. Similarly, mutagenesis tests with netilmicin have proven negative, and no impairment in fertility has been observed in the rat.

Pregnancy Category D: (See WARNINGS Section.)

Nursing mothers: Clinical studies in nursing mothers indicate that small amounts of netilmicin are excreted in breast milk. Because of the potential for serious adverse reactions from aminoglycosides in nursing infants, a decision should be made whether to discontinue nursing or to discontinue the drug, taking into account the importance of the drug to the mother.

Pediatric Use: Aminoglycosides should be used with caution in prematures and neonates because of the renal immaturity of these patients and the resulting prolongation of serum half-life of these drugs.

ADVERSE REACTIONS

Nephrotoxicity—Adverse renal effects due to netilmicin were reported in 7 per 100 patients.

They were demonstrated by a rise in serum creatinine and may have been accompanied by oliguria; the presence of casts, cells or protein in the urine; by rising levels of BUN; or by decreasing creatinine clearance rates. These effects occurred more frequently in the elderly, in patients with a history of renal impairment, and in patients treated for longer periods or with larger doses than recommended. While permanent impairment of renal function may occur following aminoglycoside therapy, observed renal impairment associated with netilmicin was usually mild and reversible after treatment ended while the drug was being excreted.

Neurotoxicity—Adverse effects on both the auditory and vestibular branches of the eighth cranial nerve have been reported.

Audiometric changes associated with netilmicin occurred in approximately 4 per 100 patients. Subjective netilmicin-related hearing loss occurred in about 1 per 250 patients. Vestibular abnormalities related to netilmicin were seen in 1 per 150 patients. Factors which may increase the risk of aminoglycoside-induced ototoxicity include renal impairment (especially if hemodialysis is required), excessive dosage, dehydration, concomitant administration of ethacrynic acid or furosemide, or previous exposure to other ototoxic drugs. Symptoms include vertigo, tinnitus, nystagmus, and hearing loss. Aminoglycoside-induced ototoxicity is usually irreversible. Cochlear damage is usually manifested initially by small changes in audiometric test results at the higher frequencies and may not be associated with subjective hearing loss. Vestibular dysfunction is usually manifested by nystagmus, vertigo, nausea, vomiting, or acute Meniere's syndrome.

The risk of toxic reactions is low in patients with normal renal function who do not receive netilmicin injection at higher doses or for longer periods of time than recommended. Some patients who have had previous neurotoxic reactions to other aminoglycosides have been treated with netilmicin without further neurotoxicity.

Neuromuscular blockade manifested as acute muscular paralysis and apnea can occur following treatment with aminoglycosides. (See "WARNINGS Box".)

The approximate incidence of other reported adverse reactions to netilmicin injection follows: increased levels of serum transaminase (SGOT or SGPT), alkaline phosphatase, or bilirubin in 15 patients per 1000; rash or itching in 4 or 5 patients per 1000; eosinophilia in 4 patients per 1000; thrombocytosis in 2 patients per 1000; prolonged prothrombin time in 1 patient per 1000; fever in 1 patient per 1000.

Fewer than one patient per 1000 was reported to have netilmicin-related anemia, leukopenia, thrombocytopenia, leukemoid reaction, immature circulating white blood cells, hyperkalemia, vomiting, diarrhea, palpitations, hypotension, headache, disorientation, blurred vision, or paresthesias.

Local tolerance to intramuscular injection and intravenous infusion of netilmicin is generally excellent, but approximately four patients per 1000 have had severe pain, and similar numbers had induration or hematomas.

OVERDOSAGE

In the event of overdosage or toxic reaction, netilmicin can be removed from the blood by hemodialysis, especially if renal function is, or becomes compromised. Although there is no specific information concerning removal of netilmicin by peritoneal dialysis, other aminoglycosides are known to be removed by this method but at a rate considerably less than by hemodialysis.

DOSAGE AND ADMINISTRATION

Netilmicin injection may be given intramuscularly or intravenously. (See CLINICAL PHARMACOLOGY.) The recommended dosage for both methods of administration is identical.

The patient's pretreatment body weight should be obtained for calculation of correct dosage. The dosage of aminoglycosides in obese patients should be based on an estimate of the lean body mass.

The status of renal function should be estimated by measurement of the serum creatinine concentration or calculation of the endogenous creatinine clearance rate. The blood urea nitrogen (BUN) level is much less reliable for this purpose. Reassessment of renal function should be made periodically during therapy.

In patients with extensive body surface burns, altered pharmacokinetics may result in reduced serum concentrations of aminoglycosides. Measurement of netilmicin serum concentrations is particularly important as a basis for dosage adjustment in such patients.

Duration of Treatment: It is desirable to limit the duration of treatment with aminoglycosides to short-term whenever feasible. The usual duration of treatment for all patients is seven to fourteen days. In complicated infections, a longer course of therapy may be necessary. Although prolonged courses of netilmicin injection have been well tolerated, it is particularly important that patients treated for longer than the usual period be carefully monitored for changes in renal, auditory, and vestibular functions. Dosage should be adjusted if clinically indicated.

Measurement of serum concentrations: It is desirable to measure both peak and trough serum concentrations of netilmicin to determine the adequacy and safety of the administered dosage.

When such measurements are feasible, they should be carried out periodically during therapy. Peak serum concentrations are expected to range from 4 to 12 mcg/ml. Dosage should be adjusted to attain the desired peak and trough concentrations and to avoid prolonged peak serum concentrations above 16 mcg/ml. When monitoring trough concentrations (just prior to the next dose), dosage should be adjusted so that levels above 4 mcg/ml are avoided. Inter-patient variation of aminoglycoside serum concentrations occurs in patients with normal or abnormal renal function. Generally, desirable peak and trough concentrations will be in the range of 6–10 and 0.5–2 mcg/ml, respectively.

Determination of the adequacy of a serum level for a particular patient must take into consideration the susceptibility of the causative organism, the severity of the infection, and the status of the patient's host-defense mechanisms.

The dosage recommendations which follow are not intended as rigid schedules, but are provided as guides for initial therapy, or for when the measurement of netilmicin serum levels during therapy is not feasible.

DOSAGE FOR PATIENTS WITH NORMAL RENAL FUNCTION

Table I shows the recommended dosage of netilmicin injection for patients of various ages with normal renal function. [See table on top next page].

DOSAGE FOR PATIENTS WITH IMPAIRED RENAL FUNCTION

Dosage must be individualized in patients with impaired renal function to ensure therapeutic levels are attained. There are several methods of doing this; however, dosage adjustment based upon the measurement of serum drug concentrations during treatment is the most accurate.

If netilmicin serum concentrations are not available and renal function is stable, serum creatinine and creatinine clearance values are the most reliable, readily available indicators of the degree of renal impairment for use as a guide for dosage adjustment.

It is also important to recognize that deteriorating renal function may require a greater reduction in dosage than that specified in the guidelines given below for patients with stable renal impairment.

The initial or loading dose is the same as that for a patient with normal renal function. A number of methods are available to adjust the total daily dosage for the degree of renal impairment. Three suggested methods are:

1) Divide the suggested dosage value for patients with normal renal function from Table I above by the serum creatinine level to obtain the adjusted size of each dose.
2) If the creatinine clearance rate is known or can be estimated from the serum creatinine levels using the formula given below; the adjusted daily dose of netilmicin

may be determined by multiplying the dose given in Table I by:

$$\frac{\text{Patient's Creatinine Clearance Rate}}{\text{Normal Creatinine Clearance Rate}}$$

3) Alternatively, the following graph may be used to obtain the percentage of the dose selected from Table I, which should be administered at 8-hour intervals:

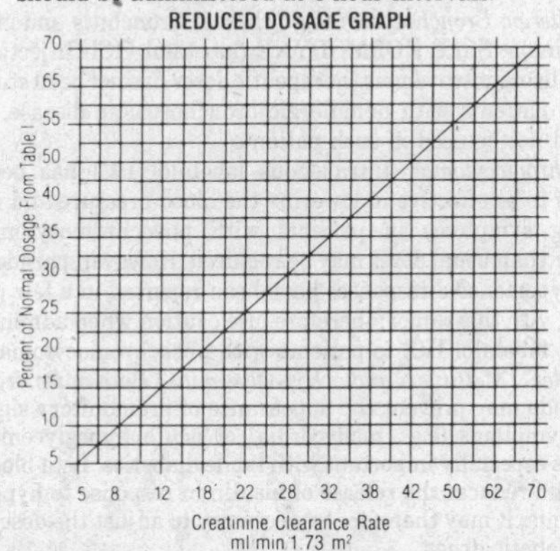

Creatinine clearance can be estimated from serum creatinine levels by the following formula for adult males; multiply by 0.85 for adult females; (Nephron, 1976; 16:31-41):

$$C_{cr} = \frac{(140 - \text{Age})\ (\text{Wt. Kg})}{72 \text{ X } S_{cr}\ (\text{mg}/100 \text{ ml})}$$

The adjusted total daily dose may be administered as one dose at 24-hour intervals, or as 2 or 3 equally divided doses at 12-hour or 8-hour intervals, respectively. Generally, each individual dose should not exceed 3.25 mg/kg. In adults with renal failure who are undergoing hemodialysis, the amount of netilmicin removed from the blood may vary depending upon the dialysis equipment and methods used. (See Clinical Pharmacology.) In adults, a dose of 2.0 mg/kg at the end of each dialysis period is recommended until the results of tests measuring netilmicin serum levels become available. Dosage should then be appropriately adjusted based on these tests.

TABLE I
Dosage Guide for Adults with Normal Renal Function

		For Complicated Urinary Tract Infections, Give 3.0–4.0 mg/kg/day as 1.5–2.0 mg/kg	For Serious Systemic Infections Give 4.0–6.5 mg/kg/day as 1.3–2.2 mg/kg or 2.0–3.25 mg/kg	
Patient's Weight* kg	(lb)	EVERY 12 HOURS mg/dose	EVERY 8 HOURS mg/dose	EVERY 12 HOURS mg/dose
40	(88)	60– 80	52– 88	80–130
45	(99)	68– 90	59– 99	90–146
50	(110)	75–100	65–110	100–163
55	(121)	83–110	72–121	110–179
60	(132)	90–120	78–132	120–195
65	(143)	98–130	85–143	130–211
70	(154)	105–140	91–154	140–228
75	(165)	113–150	98–165	150–244
80	(176)	120–160	104–176	160–260
85	(187)	128–170	111–187	170–276
90	(198)	135–180	117–198	180–293
95	(209)	143–190	124–209	190–309
100	(220)	150–200	130–220	200–325

*The dosage of aminoglycosides in obese patients should be based on an estimate of the lean body mass.
Neonates (less than 6 weeks): 4.0 to 6.5 mg/kg/day given as 2.0 to 3.25 mg/kg every 12 hours.
Infants and Children (6 weeks through 12 years): 5.5 to 8.0 mg/kg/day given either as 1.8 to 2.7 mg/kg every 8 hours, or as 2.7 to 4.0 mg/kg every 12 hours.

ALTERNATE DOSING METHOD FOR PATIENTS WITH NORMAL OR IMPAIRED RENAL FUNCTION

An alternate method of determining dosage regimen (dose and dosing interval) applicable to all ages and all states of renal function (both normal and abnormal) is to employ pharmacokinetic parameters derived from measurements of serum concentrations.

Following the administration of an initial dose of netilmicin and the determination of drug serum concentrations in post-infusion blood samples, the drug's half-life and the patient's elimination rate constant and volume of distribution can be calculated. Desired peak and trough serum levels for a particular patient are then selected by taking into consideration the susceptibility of the causative organism, the severity of infection, and the status of the patient's host-defense mechanisms. The dosage regimen (dose and dosing interval) is then determined using standardized formulae and the appropriate computer program, and the dosage regimen can be adjusted to the nearest practical interval and amount.

ADDITION OF NETILMICIN SULFATE TO VARIOUS INTRAVENOUS PREPARATIONS

In adults, a single dose of netilmicin injection may be diluted in 50 to 200 ml of one of the parenteral solutions listed below. In infants and children, the volume of diluent should be less according to the fluid requirements of the patient. The solution may be infused over a period of one-half to two hours. Tested at concentrations of 2.1 to 3.0 mg/ml, netilmicin sulfate has been shown to be stable in the following large volume parenteral solutions for up to 72 hours when stored in glass containers, both when refrigerated and at room temperature. Use after this time period is not recommended.
[See Table II below].
[See table below].
Parenteral drug products should be inspected visually for particulate matter and discoloration prior to administration, whenever solution and container permit.

TABLE II
LARGE VOLUME PARENTERAL SOLUTIONS IN WHICH NETILMICIN SULFATE IS STABLE

Products/Compositions Tested	**Other Trade Names and Manufacturers**
	(Solutions of Same Composition)
Sterile Water for Injection	
0.9% Sodium Chloride Injection alone or with 5% Dextrose	
5% or 10% Dextrose Injection in Water, or 5% Dextrose in Polysal Injection, or 5% Dextrose with Electrolyte #48 or #75	
Ringer's and Lactated Ringer's, and Lactated Ringer's with 5% Dextrose Injection	
10% Travert with Electrolyte #2 or #3 Injection (Travenol)	Electrolyte #3 (Cooke & Crowley's Solution) with 10% Inverted Sugar Injection (Cutter)
Isolyte E, M, or P with 5% Dextrose Injection	
10% Dextran 40 or 6% Dextran 75 in 5% Dextrose Injection	
Plasma-Lyte 56 or 148 Injection with 5% Dextrose (Travenol)	Normosol-M or R in D5-W (Abbott), Isolyte H or S with 5% Dextrose (McGaw), Polyonic R-148 or M-56 with 5% Dextrose (Cutter)
Plasma-Lyte M Injection 5% Dextrose (Travenol)	Polysal M with 5% Dextrose (Cutter)
Ionosol B in D5-W	
5% Amigen Injection alone or with 5% Dextrose	
Normosol-R	Polyonic R-148 (Cutter), Isolyte S (McGaw), Plasma-Lyte 148 Injection in Water (Travenol)
Polysal (Plain)	
Aminosol 5% Injection	
Fre-Amine II 8.5% Injection	
Plasma-Lyte 148 Injection (approx. pH 7.4) (Travenol)	Normosol-R pH 7.4 (Abbott)
10% Fructose Injection	

HOW SUPPLIED

NETROMYCIN Injection 100 mg/ml is supplied in 1.5 ml vials, box of 10 (NDC 0085-0264-02), and box of 25 (NDC 0085-0264-06); in 15 ml multiple-dose vials, box of 5 (NDC 0085-0264-04). **Store between 2° and 30°C (36° and 86°F).**

ANIMAL PHARMACOLOGY AND/OR ANIMAL TOXICOLOGY

Netilmicin sulfate, administered by the intravenous and intramuscular routes, has been compared to kanamycin, sisomicin, gentamicin, amikacin, and tobramycin in studies ranging in duration from two weeks to three months. Among the aminoglycosides, netilmicin is one of the more potent neuromuscular-blocking agents; however, in six different species, netilmicin sulfate has proven to be the least nephrotoxic and ototoxic of these aminoglycosides, using morphological as well as functional end-points.
In the clinical trials nephrotoxicity and ototoxicity occurred at about the same frequency in netilmicin-treated patients as in those treated with other aminoglycosides.

Schering Biochem Corporation
Manati, Puerto Rico 00701
An Affiliate of Schering Corporation,
Kenilworth, NJ 07033

Revised 11/83

Continued on next page

Information on Schering products appearing on these pages is effective as of September 30, 1986.

Schering—Cont.

NORMODYNE® ℞
[*nŏr'mō-dīn*]
brand of labetalol hydrochloride
Injection

DESCRIPTION

NORMODYNE (labetalol HCl) is an adrenergic receptor blocking agent that has both selective $alpha_1$- and nonselective beta-adrenergic receptor blocking actions in a single substance.
Labetalol HCl is 5-[1-hydroxy-2-[(1-methyl-3-phenylpropyl) amino]ethyl]salicylamide monohydrochloride.
Labetalol HCl has the empirical formula $C_{19}H_{24}N_2O_3$ HCl and a molecular weight of 364.9. It has two asymmetric centers and therefore exists as a molecular complex of two diastereoisomeric pairs.
Labetalol HCl is a white or off-white crystalline powder, soluble in water.
NORMODYNE (labetalol HCl) Injection is a clear, colorless to light yellow aqueous sterile isotonic solution for intravenous injection. It has a pH range of 3.0 to 4.0. Each ml contains 5 mg labetalol HCl, 45 mg anhydrous dextrose, 0.10 mg edetate disodium; 0.80 mg methylparaben and 0.10 mg propylparaben as preservatives; citric acid monohydrate and sodium hydroxide, as necessary, to bring the solution into the pH range.

CLINICAL PHARMACOLOGY

NORMODYNE (labetalol HCl) combines both selective, competitive $alpha_1$-adrenergic blocking and nonselective, competitive beta-adrenergic blocking activity in a single substance. In man, the ratios of alpha- to beta-blockage have been estimated to be approximately 1:3 and 1:7 following oral and intravenous administration, respectively. $Beta_2$-agonist activity has been demonstrated in animals with minimal $beta_1$-agonist (ISA) activity detected. In animals, at doses greater than those required for alpha or beta-adrenergic blockade, a membrane stabilizing effect has been demonstrated.
Pharmacodynamics: The capacity of labetalol HCl to block alpha receptors in man has been demonstrated by attenuation of the pressor effect of phenylephrine and by a significant reduction of the pressor response caused by immersing the hand in ice-cold water ("cold-pressor test"). Labetalol HCl's $beta_1$-receptor blockade in man was demonstrated by a small decrease in the resting heart rate, attenuation of tachycardia produced by isoproterenol or exercise, and by attenuation of the reflex tachycardia to the hypotension produced by amyl nitrite. $Beta_2$-receptor blockade was demonstrated by inhibition of the isoproterenol-induced fall in diastolic blood pressure. Both the alpha- and beta-blocking actions of orally administered labetalol HCl contribute to a decrease in blood pressure in hypertensive patients. Labetalol HCl consistently, in dose related fashion, blunted increases in exercise-induced blood pressure and heart rate, and in their double product. The pulmonary circulation during exercise was not affected by labetalol HCl dosing.
Single oral doses of labetalol HCl administered in patients with coronary artery disease had no significant effect on sinus rate, intraventricular conduction, or QRS duration. The AV conduction time was modestly prolonged in 2 of 7 patients. In another study, intravenous labetalol HCl slightly prolonged AV nodal conduction time and atrial effective refractory period with only small changes in heart rate. The effects on AV nodal refractoriness were inconsistent.
Labetalol HCl produces dose-related falls in blood pressure without reflex tachycardia and without significant reduction in heart rate, presumably through a mixture of its alpha-blocking and beta-blocking effects. Hemodynamic effects are variable with small nonsignificant changes in cardiac output seen in some studies but not others, and small decreases in total peripheral resistance. Elevated plasma renins are reduced.
Doses of labetalol HCl that controlled hypertension did not affect renal function in mild to severe hypertensive patients with normal renal function.
Due to the $alpha_1$-receptor blocking activity of labetalol HCl, blood pressure is lowered more in the standing than in the supine position, and symptoms of postural hypotension can occur. During dosing with intravenous labetalol HCl, the contribution of the postural component should be considered when positioning the patient for treatment, and the patient should not be allowed to move to an erect position unmonitored until their ability to do so is established.
In a clinical pharmacologic study in severe hypertensives, an initial 0.25 mg/kg injection of labetalol HCl administered to patients in the supine position, decreased blood pressure by an average of 11/7 mmHg. Additional injections of 0.5 mg/kg at 15 minute intervals up to a total cumulative dose of 1.75 mg/kg of labetalol HCl caused further dose related decreases in blood pressure. Some patients required cumulative doses of up to 3.25 mg/kg. The maximal effect of each dose level occurred within 5 minutes. Following discontinuation of intravenous treatment with labetalol HCl, the blood pressure rose gradually and progressively, approaching pretreatment baseline values within an average of 16-18 hours in the majority of patients.
Similar results were obtained in the treatment of patients with severe hypertension requiring urgent blood pressure reduction with an initial dose of 20 mg (which corresponds to 0.25 mg/kg for an 80 kg patient) followed by additional doses of either 40 or 80 mg at 10 minute intervals to achieve the desired effect or up to a cumulative dose of 300 mg.
Labetalol HCl administered as a continuous intravenous infusion, with a mean dose of 136 mg (27 to 300 mg) over a period of 2 to 3 hours (mean of 2 hours and 39 minutes) lowered the blood pressure by an average of 60/35 mmHg.
Exacerbation of angina and, in some cases, myocardial infarction and ventricular dysrhythmias have been reported after abrupt discontinuation of therapy with beta-adrenergic blocking agents in patients with coronary artery disease. Abrupt withdrawal of these agents in patients without coronary artery disease has resulted in transient symptoms, including tremulousness, sweating, palpitation, headache, and malaise. Several mechanisms have been proposed to explain these phenomena, among them increased sensitivity to catecholamines because of increased numbers of beta receptors.
Although beta-adrenergic receptor blockade is useful in the treatment of angina and hypertension, there are also situations in which sympathetic stimulation is vital. For example, in patients with severely damaged hearts, adequate ventricular function may depend on sympathetic drive. Beta-adrenergic blockade may worsen AV block by preventing the necessary facilitating effects of sympathetic activity on conduction. $Beta_2$-adrenergic blockade results in passive bronchial constriction by interfering with endogenous adrenergic bronchodilator activity in patients subject to bronchospasm and may also interfere with exogenous bronchodilators in such patients.
Pharmacokinetics and Metabolism Following intravenous infusion, the elimination half-life is about 5.5 hours and the total body clearance is approximately 33 ml/min/kg. The plasma half-life of labetalol following oral administration is about six to eight hours. In patients with decreased hepatic or renal function, the elimination half-life of labetalol is not altered; however, the relative bioavailability in hepatically impaired patients is increased due to decreased "first-pass" metabolism.
The metabolism of labetalol is mainly through conjugation to glucuronide metabolites. These metabolites are present in plasma and are excreted in the urine and, via the bile, into the feces. Approximately 55 to 60% of a dose appears in the urine as conjugates or unchanged labetalol within the first 24 hours of dosing.
Labetalol has been shown to cross the placental barrier in humans. Only negligible amounts of the drug crossed the blood-brain barrier in animal studies. Labetalol is approximately 50% protein bound. Neither hemodialysis nor peritoneal dialysis removes a significant amount of labetalol HCl from the general circulation (<1%).

INDICATIONS AND USAGE

NORMODYNE (labetalol HCl) Injection is indicated for control of blood pressure in severe hypertension.

CONTRAINDICATIONS

NORMODYNE (labetalol HCl) Injection is contraindicated in bronchial asthma, overt cardiac failure, greater than first degree heart block, cardiogenic shock, and severe bradycardia. (See **WARNINGS.**)

WARNINGS

Cardiac Failure: Sympathetic stimulation is a vital component supporting circulatory function in congestive heart failure. Beta blockade carries a potential hazard of further depressing myocardial contractility and precipitating more severe failure. Although beta-blockers should be avoided in overt congestive heart failure, if necessary, labetalol HCl can be used with caution in patients with a history of heart failure who are well-compensated. Congestive heart failure has been observed in patients receiving labetalol HCl. Labetalol HCl does not abolish the inotropic action of digitalis on heart muscle.
In Patients Without a History of Cardiac Failure: In patients with latent cardiac insufficiency, continued depression of the myocardium with beta-blocking agents over a period of time can in some cases lead to cardiac failure. At the first sign or symptom of impending cardiac failure, patients should be fully digitalized and/or be given a diuretic, and the response observed closely. If cardiac failure continues, despite adequate digitalization and diuretic, NORMODYNE (labetalol HCl) therapy should be withdrawn (gradually if possible).
Ischemic Heart Disease: Angina pectoris has not been reported upon labetalol HCl discontinuation. However, following abrupt cessation of therapy with some beta-blocking agents in patients with coronary artery disease, exacerbations of angina pectoris and, in some cases, myocardial infarction have been reported. Therefore, such patients should be cautioned against interruption of therapy without the physician's advice. Even in the absence of overt angina pectoris, when discontinuation of NORMODYNE is planned, the patient should be carefully observed and should be advised to limit physical activity. If angina markedly worsens or acute coronary insufficiency develops, NORMODYNE (labetalol HCl) administration should be reinstituted promptly, at least temporarily, and other measures appropriate for the management of unstable angina should be taken.
Nonallergic Bronchospasm (e.g., chronic bronchitis and emphysema): Since NORMODYNE (labetalol HCl) Injection at the usual intravenous therapeutic doses has not been studied in patients with nonallergic bronchospastic disease, it should not be used in such patients.
Pheochromocytoma: Intravenous labetalol HCl has been shown to be effective in lowering the blood pressure and relieving symptoms in patients with pheochromocytoma; higher than usual doses may be required. However, paradoxical hypertensive responses have been reported in a few patients with this tumor; therefore, use caution when administering labetalol HCl to patients with pheochromocytoma.
Diabetes Mellitus and Hypoglycemia: Beta-adrenergic blockade may prevent the appearance of premonitory signs and symptoms (e.g., tachycardia) of acute hypoglycemia. This is especially important with labile diabetics. Beta-blockade also reduces the release of insulin in response to hyperglycemia; it may therefore be necessary to adjust the dose of antidiabetic drugs.
Major Surgery: The necessity or desirability of withdrawing beta-blocking therapy prior to major surgery is controversial. Protracted severe hypotension and difficulty in restarting or maintaining a heart beat have been reported with beta-blockers. The effect of labetalol HCl's alpha-adrenergic activity has not been evaluated in this setting.
A synergism between labetalol HCl and halothane anesthesia has been shown (see **Drug Interactions**).
Rapid Decreases of Blood Pressure: Caution must be observed when reducing severely elevated blood pressure. Although such findings have not been reported with intravenous labetalol HCl, a number of adverse reactions, including cerebral infarction, optic nerve infarction, angina and ischemic changes in the electrocardiogram, have been reported with other agents when severely elevated blood pressure was reduced over time courses of several hours to as long as one or two days. The desired blood pressure lowering should therefore be achieved over as long a period of time as is compatible with the patient's status.

PRECAUTIONS

General: *Impaired Hepatic Function* may diminish metabolism of NORMODYNE (labetalol HCl) Injection.
Hypotension: Symptomatic postural hypotension (incidence 58%) is likely to occur if patients are tilted or allowed to assume the upright position within 3 hours of receiving NORMODYNE (labetalol HCl) Injection. Therefore, the patient's ability to tolerate an upright position should be established before permitting any ambulation.
Jaundice or Hepatic Dysfunction: On rare occasions, oral labetalol HCl has been associated with jaundice (both hepatic and cholestatic). It is therefore recommended that treatment with labetalol HCl be stopped immediately, should a patient develop jaundice or laboratory evidence of liver injury. Both have been shown to be reversible on stopping therapy.

Information for Patients

The following information is intended to aid in the safe and effective use of this medication. It is not a disclosure of all possible adverse or intended effects. During and immediately following (for up to 3 hours) NORMODYNE Injection, the patient should remain supine. Subsequently, the patient should be advised on how to proceed gradually to become ambulatory, and should be observed at the time of first ambulation.
When the patient is started on NORMODYNE Tablets, following adequate control of blood pressure with NORMODYNE Injection, appropriate directions for titration of dosage should be provided. (See **DOSAGE AND ADMINISTRATION.**)
As with all drugs with beta-blocking activity, certain advice to patients being treated with labetalol HCl is warranted: While no incident of the abrupt withdrawal phenomenon (exacerbation of angina pectoris) has been reported with labetalol HCl, dosing with NORMODYNE Tablets should not be interrupted or discontinued without a physician's advice. Patients being treated with NORMODYNE Tablets should consult a physician at any sign of impending cardiac failure. Also, transient scalp tingling may occur, usually when treatment with NORMODYNE Tablets is initiated (see **ADVERSE REACTIONS**).

Laboratory Tests

Routine laboratory tests are ordinarily not required before or after intravenous labetalol HCl. In patients with concomitant illnesses, such as impaired renal function, appropriate tests should be done to monitor these conditions.

Drug Interactions
Since NORMODYNE (labetalol HCl) Injection may be administered to patients already being treated with other medications, including other antihypertensive agents, careful monitoring of these patients is necessary to detect and treat promptly any undesired effect from concomitant administration.
In one survey, 2.3% of patients taking labetalol HCl orally in combination with tricyclic antidepressants experienced tremor as compared to 0.7% reported to occur with labetalol HCl alone. The contribution of each of the treatments to this adverse reaction is unknown but the possibility of a drug interaction cannot be excluded.
Drugs possessing beta-blocking properties can blunt the bronchodilator effect of beta-receptor agonist drugs in patients with bronchospasm; therefore, doses greater than the normal anti-asthmatic dose of beta-agonist bronchodilator drugs may be required.
Cimetidine has been shown to increase the bioavailability of labetalol HCl administered orally. Since this could be explained either by enhanced absorption or by an alteration of hepatic metabolism of labetalol HCl, special care should be used in establishing the dose required for blood pressure control in such patients.
Synergism has been shown between halothane anesthesia and intravenously administered labetalol HCl. During controlled hypotensive anesthesia using labetalol HCl in association with halothane, high concentrations (3% or above) of halothane should not be used because the degree of hypotension will be increased and because of the possibility of a large reduction in cardiac output and an increase in central venous pressure. The anesthesiologist should be informed when a patient is receiving labetalol HCl.
Labetalol HCl blunts the reflex tachycardia produced by nitroglycerin without preventing its hypotensive effect. If labetalol HCl is used with nitroglycerin in patients with angina pectoris, additional antihypertensive effects may occur.

Drug/Laboratory Test Interactions
The presence of a metabolite of labetalol in the urine may result in falsely increased levels of urinary catecholamines when measured by a nonspecific trihydroxyindole (THI) reaction. In screening patients suspected of having a pheochromocytoma and being treated with labetalol HCl, specific radioenzymatic or high performance liquid chromatography assay techniques should be used to determine levels of catecholamines or their metabolites.

Carcinogenesis, Mutagenesis, Impairment of Fertility
Long-term oral dosing studies with labetalol HCl for 18 months in mice and for 2 years in rats showed no evidence of carcinogenesis. Studies with labetalol HCl, using dominant lethal assays in rats and mice, and exposing microorganisms according to modified Ames tests, showed no evidence of mutagenesis.

Pregnancy Category C
Teratogenic studies have been performed with labetalol in rats and rabbits at oral doses up to approximately 6 and 4 times the maximum recommended human dose (MRHD), respectively. No reproducible evidence of fetal malformations was observed. Increased fetal resorptions were seen in both species at doses approximating the MRHD. There are no adequate and well-controlled studies in pregnant women. Labetalol should be used during pregnancy only if the potential benefit justifies the potential risk to the fetus.

Nonteratogenic Effects
Infants of mothers who were treated with labetalol HCl for hypertension during pregnancy did not appear to be adversely affected by the drug. Oral administration of labetalol to rats during late gestation through weaning at doses of 2 to 4 times the MRHD caused a decrease in neonatal survival.

Labor and Delivery
Labetalol HCl given to pregnant women with hypertension did not appear to affect the usual course of labor and delivery.

Nursing Mothers
Small amounts of labetalol (approximately 0.004% of the maternal dose) are excreted in human milk. Caution should be exercised when NORMODYNE (labetalol HCl) Injection is administered to a nursing woman.

Pediatric Use
Safety and effectiveness in children have not been established.

ADVERSE REACTIONS

NORMODYNE (labetalol HCl) Injection is usually well tolerated. Most adverse effects have been mild and transient and in controlled trials involving 92 patients did not require labetalol HCl withdrawal. Symptomatic postural hypotension (incidence 58%) is likely to occur if patients are tilted or allowed to assume the upright position within 3 hours of receiving NORMODYNE (labetalol HCl) Injection. Moderate hypotension occurred in 1 of 100 patients while supine. Increased sweating was noted in 4 of 100 patients, and flushing occurred in 1 of 100 patients.
The following also were reported with NORMODYNE Injection with the incidence per 100 patients as noted:

Labetalol HCl Daily Dose (mg)	200	300	400	600	800	900	1200	1600	2400
Number of Patients	522	181	606	608	503	117	411	242	175
Dizziness (%)	2	3	3	3	5	1	9	13	16
Fatigue	2	1	4	4	5	3	7	6	10
Nausea	<1	0	1	2	4	0	7	11	19
Vomiting	0	0	<1	<1	<1	0	1	2	3
Dyspepsia	1	0	2	1	1	0	2	2	4
Paresthesias	2	0	2	2	1	1	2	5	5
Nasal Stuffiness	1	1	2	2	2	2	4	5	6
Ejaculation Failure	0	2	1	2	3	0	4	3	5
Impotence	1	1	1	1	2	4	3	4	3
Edema	1	0	1	1	1	0	1	2	2

Cardiovascular System: Ventricular arrhythmia in 1.
Central and Peripheral Nervous Systems: Dizziness in 9; tingling of the scalp/skin 7; hypoesthesia (numbness), and vertigo 1 each.
Gastrointestinal System: Nausea in 13; vomiting 4; dyspepsia and taste distortion, 1 each.
Metabolic Disorders: Transient increases in blood urea nitrogen and serum creatinine levels occurred in 8 of 100 patients; these were associated with drops in blood pressure, generally in patients with prior renal insufficiency.
Psychiatric Disorders: Somnolence/yawning in 3.
Respiratory System: Wheezing in 1.
Skin: Pruritus in 1.
The incidence of adverse reactions depends upon the dose of labetalol HCl. The largest experience is with oral labetalol HCl (see NORMODYNE Tablet Product Information for details). Certain of the side effects increased with increasing oral dose as shown in the table below which depicts the entire U.S. therapeutic trials data base for adverse reactions that are clearly or possibly dose related.
[See table above].
The oculomucocutaneous syndrome associated with the beta-blocker practolol has not been reported with labetalol HCl during investigational use and extensive foreign marketing experience.
Clinical laboratory tests: Among patients dosed with NORMODYNE (labetalol HCl) Tablets, there have been reversible increases of serum transaminases in 4% of patients tested, and more rarely, reversible increases in blood urea.

OVERDOSAGE

Overdosage with NORMODYNE (labetalol HCl) Injection causes excessive hypotension that is posture sensitive and, sometimes, excessive bradycardia. Patients should be placed supine and their legs raised if necessary to improve the blood supply to the brain. If overdosage with labetalol HCl follows oral ingestion, gastric lavage or pharmacologically induced emesis (using syrup of ipecac) may be useful for removal of the drug shortly after ingestion. The following additional measures should be employed if necessary. **Excessive bradycardia**—administer atropine or epinephrine. **Cardiac failure**—administer a digitalis glycoside and a diuretic. Dopamine or dobutamine may also be useful. **Hypotension**—administer vasopressors, eg, norepinephrine. There is pharmacological evidence that norepinephrine may be the drug of choice. **Bronchospasm**—administer epinephrine and/or an aerosolized beta$_2$-agonist. **Seizures**—administer diazepam.
In severe beta-blocker overdose resulting in hypotension and/or bradycardia, glucagon has been shown to be effective when administered in large doses (5 to 10 mg rapidly over 30 seconds, followed by continuous infusion of 5 mg/hr that can be reduced as the patient improves).
Neither hemodialysis nor peritoneal dialysis removes a significant amount of labetalol from the general circulation (<1%).
The oral LD_{50} value of labetalol HCl in the mouse is approximately 600 mg/kg and in the rat is greater than 2 g/kg. The intravenous LD_{50} in these species is 50 to 60 mg/kg.

DOSAGE AND ADMINISTRATION

NORMODYNE (labetalol HCl) Injection is intended for intravenous use in hospitalized patients. DOSAGE MUST BE INDIVIDUALIZED depending upon the severity of hypertension and the response of the patient during dosing.
Patients should always be kept in a supine position during the period of intravenous drug administration. A substantial fall in blood pressure on standing should be expected in these patients. The patient's ability to tolerate an upright position should be established before permitting any ambulation, such as using toilet facilities.
Either of two methods of administration of NORMODYNE Injection may be used: a) repeated intravenous injections, b) slow continuous infusion.
Repeated Intravenous Injection: Initially, NORMODYNE (labetalol HCl) Injection should be given in a dose of 20 mg labetalol HCl (which corresponds to 0.25 mg/kg for an 80 kg patient) by slow intravenous injection over a two-minute period.
Immediately before the injection and at five and ten minutes after injection, supine blood pressure should be measured to evaluate response. Additional injections of 40 mg or 80 mg can be given at ten minute intervals until a desired supine blood pressure is achieved or a total of 300 mg labetalol HCl has been injected. The maximum effect usually occurs within 5 minutes of each injection.
Slow Continuous Infusion: NORMODYNE (labetalol HCl) Injection is prepared for intravenous continuous infusion by diluting the contents with commonly used intravenous fluids (see below). Examples of methods of preparing the infusion solution are:

The contents of two 20 ml vials or ampules (40 ml) are added to 160 ml of a commonly used intravenous fluid such that the resultant 200 ml of solution contains 200 mg of labetalol HCl, 1 mg/ml. The diluted solution should be administered at a rate of 2 ml/min to deliver 2 mg/min.
The contents of one 60 ml vial are added to 240 ml of a commonly used intravenous fluid, such that the resultant 300 ml of solution contains 300 mg of labetalol HCl, 1 mg/ml. The diluted solution should be administered at a rate of 2 ml/min to deliver 2 mg/min.
Alternatively, the contents of two 20 ml vials or ampules (40 ml) of NORMODYNE (labetalol HCl) Injection can be added to 250 ml of a commonly used intravenous fluid. The resultant solution will contain 200 mg of labetalol HCl, approximately 2 mg/3 ml. The diluted solution should be administered at a rate of 3 ml/min to deliver approximately 2 mg/min.

The rate of infusion of the diluted solution may be adjusted according to the blood pressure response, at the discretion of the physician. To facilitate a desired rate of infusion, the diluted solution can be infused using a controlled administration mechanism, e.g., graduated burette or mechanically driven infusion pump.
Since the half life of labetalol is 5 to 8 hours, steady-state blood levels (in the face of a constant rate of infusion) would not be reached during the usual infusion time period. The infusion should be continued until a satisfactory response is obtained and should then be stopped and oral labetalol HCl started (see below). The effective intravenous dose is usually in the range of 50 to 200 mg. A total dose of up to 300 mg may be required in some patients.
Blood Pressure Monitoring: The blood pressure should be monitored during and after completion of the infusion or intravenous injections. Rapid or excessive falls in either systolic or diastolic blood pressure during intravenous treatment should be avoided. In patients with excessive systolic hypertension, the decrease in systolic pressure should be used as an indicator of effectiveness in addition to the response of the diastolic pressure.
Initiation of Dosing with NORMODYNE (labetalol HCl) Tablets: Subsequent oral dosing with NORMODYNE (labetalol HCl) Tablets should begin when it has been established that the supine diastolic blood pressure has begun to rise. The recommended initial dose is 200 mg, followed in 6-12 hours by an additional dose of 200 or 400 mg, depending on the blood pressure response. Thereafter, *inpatient titration with NORMODYNE (labetalol HCl) Tablets* may proceed as follows:

Inpatient Titration Instructions

Regimen	Daily Dose*
200 mg bid	400 mg
400 mg bid	800 mg
800 mg bid	1600 mg
1200 mg bid	2400 mg

*If needed, the total daily dose may be given in three divided doses.

While in the hospital, the dosage of NORMODYNE Tablets may be increased at one day intervals to achieve the desired blood pressure reduction.
For subsequent outpatient titration or maintenance dosing see NORMODYNE Tablets Product Information **DOSAGE AND ADMINISTRATION** for additional recommendations.

Continued on next page

Information on Schering products appearing on these pages is effective as of September 30, 1986.

Schering—Cont.

Compatibility with commonly used intravenous fluids
Parenteral drug products should be inspected visually for particulate matter and discoloration prior to administration, whenever solution and container permit.
NORMODYNE (labetalol HCl) Injection was tested for compatibility with commonly used intravenous fluids at final concentrations of 1.25 mg to 3.75 mg labetalol HCl per ml of the mixture. NORMODYNE Injection was found to be compatible with and stable (for 24 hours refrigerated or at room temperature) in mixtures with the following solutions:
Ringers Injection, USP
Lactated Ringers Injection, USP
5% Dextrose and Ringers Injection
5% Lactated Ringers and 5% Dextrose Injection
5% Dextrose Injection, USP
0.9% Sodium Chloride Injection, USP
5% Dextrose and 0.2% Sodium Chloride Injection, USP
2.5% Dextrose and 0.45% Sodium Chloride Injection, USP
5% Dextrose and 0.9% Sodium Chloride Injection, USP
5% Dextrose and 0.33% Sodium Chloride Injection, USP
NORMODYNE (labetalol HCl) Injection was NOT compatible with 5% Sodium Bicarbonate Injection, USP.

HOW SUPPLIED

NORMODYNE (labetalol HCl) Injection, 5 mg/ml, is supplied in 20 ml (100 mg) ampules, box of 1 (NDC-0085-0362-03); 20 ml (100 mg) (NDC-0085-0362-07) and 60 ml (300 mg) (NDC-0085-0362-05) multi-dose vials, boxes of one.
Store between 2° and 30°C (36° and 86°F). Do not freeze.
Revised 6/86

NORMODYNE® ℞

[*nŏr'mō-dīn*]
brand of labetalol hydrochloride
Tablets

DESCRIPTION

NORMODYNE (labetalol HCl) is an adrenergic receptor blocking agent that has both selective alpha$_1$- and nonselective beta-adrenergic receptor blocking actions in a single substance.
Labetalol HCl is 5-[1-hydroxy-2-[(1-methyl-3-phenylpropyl) amino] ethyl]salicylamide monohydrochloride.
Labetalol HCl has the empirical formula $C_{19}H_{24}N_2O_3$ HCl and a molecular weight of 364.9. It has two asymmetric centers and therefore exists as a molecular complex of two diastereoisomeric pairs.
Labetalol HCl is a white or off-white crystalline powder, soluble in water.
NORMODYNE Tablets contain 100 mg, 200 mg or 300 mg labetalol HCl and are taken orally.
The inactive ingredients for NORMODYNE Tablets, 100 mg, include: corn starch, FD&C Blue No. 2 Al Lake, FD&C Yellow No. 6 Al Lake, hydroxypropyl methylcellulose, lactose, magnesium stearate, methylparaben, PEG, and propylparaben. May also contain: FD&C Blue No. 2 Lake and FD&C Yellow No. 6 Lake.
The inactive ingredients for NORMODYNE Tablets, 200 mg, include: corn starch, hydroxypropyl methylcellulose, lactose, magnesium stearate, methylparaben, PEG, propylparaben, and titanium dioxide.
The inactive ingredients for NORMODYNE Tablets, 300 mg, include: corn starch, FD&C Blue No. 2 Al Lake, hydroxypropyl methylcellulose, lactose, magnesium stearate, methylparaben, PEG, and propylparaben. May also contain: FD&C Blue No. 2 Lake.

CLINICAL PHARMACOLOGY

NORMODYNE (labetalol HCl) combines both selective, competitive alpha$_1$-adrenergic blocking and nonselective, competitive beta-adrenergic blocking activity in a single substance. In man, the ratios of alpha- to beta-blockade have been estimated to be approximately 1:3 and 1:7 following oral and intravenous administration, respectively. Beta$_2$-agonist activity has been demonstrated in animals with minimal beta$_1$-agonist (ISA) activity detected. In animals, at doses greater than those required for alpha or beta-adrenergic blockade, a membrane stabilizing effect has been demonstrated.
Pharmacodynamics: The capacity of labetalol HCl to block alpha receptors in man has been demonstrated by attenuation of the pressor effect of phenylephrine and by a significant reduction of the pressor response caused by immersing the hand in ice-cold water ("cold-pressor test"). Labetalol HCl's beta$_1$-receptor blockade in man was demonstrated by a small decrease in the resting heart rate, attenuation of tachycardia produced by isoproterenol or exercise, and by attenuation of the reflex tachycardia to the hypotension produced by amyl nitrite. Beta$_2$-receptor blockade was demonstrated by inhibition of the isoproterenol-induced fall in diastolic blood pressure. Both the alpha- and beta-blocking actions of orally administered labetalol HCl contribute to a decrease in blood pressure in hypertensive patients. Labetalol HCl consistently, in dose related fashion, blunted increases in exercise-induced blood pressure and heart rate, and in their double product. The pulmonary circulation during exercise was not affected by labetalol HCl dosing.
Single oral doses of labetalol HCl administered in patients with coronary artery disease had no significant effect on sinus rate, intraventricular conduction, or QRS duration. The AV conduction time was modestly prolonged in 2 of 7 patients. In another study, intravenous labetalol HCl slightly prolonged AV nodal conduction time and atrial effective refractory period with only small changes in heart rate. The effects on AV nodal refractoriness were inconsistent.
Labetalol HCl produces dose-related falls in blood pressure without reflex tachycardia and without significant reduction in heart rate, presumably through a mixture of its alpha-blocking and beta-blocking effects. Hemodynamic effects are variable with small nonsignificant changes in cardiac output seen in some studies but not others, and small decreases in total peripheral resistance. Elevated plasma renins are reduced.
Doses of labetalol HCl that controlled hypertension did not affect renal function in mild to severe hypertensive patients with normal renal function.
Due to the alpha$_1$-receptor blocking activity of labetalol HCl, blood pressure is lowered more in the standing than in the supine position, and symptoms of postural hypotension (2%), including rare instances of syncope, can occur. Following oral administration, when postural hypotension has occurred, it has been transient and is uncommon when the recommended starting dose and titration increments are closely followed (See **DOSAGE AND ADMINISTRATION**). Symptomatic postural hypotension is most likely to occur 2 to 4 hours after a dose, especially following the use of large initial doses or upon large changes in dose.
The peak effects of single oral doses of labetalol HCl occur within 2 to 4 hours. The duration of effect depends upon dose, lasting at least 8 hours following single oral doses of 100 mg and more than 12 hours following single oral doses of 300 mg. The maximum, steady-state blood pressure response upon oral, twice-a-day dosing occurs within 24 to 72 hours.
The antihypertensive effect of labetalol has a linear correlation with the logarithm of labetalol plasma concentration, and there is also a linear correlation between the reduction in exercise-induced tachycardia occurring at two hours after oral administration of labetalol HCl and the logarithm of the plasma concentration.
About 70% of the maximum beta-blocking effect is present for five hours after the administration of a single oral dose of 400 mg, with suggestion that about 40% remains at eight hours.
The anti-anginal efficacy of labetalol HCl has not been studied. In 37 patients with hypertension and coronary artery disease, labetalol HCl did not increase the incidence or severity of angina attacks.
Exacerbation of angina and, in some cases, myocardial infarction and ventricular dysrhythmias have been reported after abrupt discontinuation of therapy with beta-adrenergic blocking agents in patients with coronary artery disease. Abrupt withdrawal of these agents in patients without coronary artery disease has resulted in transient symptoms, including tremulousness, sweating, palpitation, headache, and malaise. Several mechanisms have been proposed to explain these phenomena, among them increased sensitivity to catecholamines because of increased numbers of beta receptors.
Although beta-adrenergic receptor blockade is useful in the treatment of angina and hypertension, there are also situations in which sympathetic stimulation is vital. For example, in patients with severely damaged hearts, adequate ventricular function may depend on sympathetic drive. Beta-adrenergic blockade may worsen AV block by preventing the necessary facilitating effects of sympathetic activity on conduction. Beta$_2$-adrenergic blockade results in passive bronchial constriction by interfering with endogenous adrenergic bronchodilator activity in patients subject to bronchospasm and may also interfere with exogenous bronchodilators in such patients.
Pharmacokinetics and Metabolism: Labetalol HCl is completely absorbed from the gastrointestinal tract with peak plasma levels occurring one to two hours after oral administration. The relative bioavailability of labetalol HCl tablets compared to an oral solution is 100%. The absolute bioavailability (fraction of drug reaching systemic circulation) of labetalol when compared to an intravenous infusion is 25%; this is due to extensive "first-pass" metabolism. Despite "first-pass" metabolism there is a linear relationship between oral doses of 100 to 3000 mg and peak plasma levels. The absolute bioavailability of labetalol is increased when administered with food.
The plasma half-life of labetalol following oral administration is about six to eight hours. Steady-state plasma levels of labetalol during repetitive dosing are reached by about the third day of dosing. In patients with decreased hepatic or renal function, the elimination half-life of labetalol is not altered; however, the relative bioavailability in hepatically impaired patients is increased due to decreased "first-pass" metabolism.
The metabolism of labetalol is mainly through conjugation to glucuronide metabolites. These metabolites are present in plasma and are excreted in the urine and, via the bile, into the feces. Approximately 55 to 60% of a dose appears in the urine as conjugates or unchanged labetalol within the first 24 hours of dosing.
Labetalol has been shown to cross the placental barrier in humans. Only negligible amounts of the drug crossed the blood-brain barrier in animal studies. Labetalol is approximately 50% protein bound. Neither hemodialysis nor peritoneal dialysis removes a significant amount of labetalol HCl from the general circulation (<1%).

INDICATIONS AND USAGE

NORMODYNE (labetalol HCl) Tablets are indicated in the management of hypertension. NORMODYNE Tablets may be used alone or in combination with other antihypertensive agents, especially thiazide and loop diuretics.

CONTRAINDICATIONS

NORMODYNE (labetalol HCl) Tablets are contraindicated in bronchial asthma, overt cardiac failure, greater than first degree heart block, cardiogenic shock, and severe bradycardia. (See **WARNINGS.**)

WARNINGS

Cardiac Failure: Sympathetic stimulation is a vital component supporting circulatory function in congestive heart failure. Beta blockade carries a potential hazard of further depressing myocardial contractility and precipitating more severe failure. Although beta-blockers should be avoided in overt congestive heart failure, if necessary, labetalol HCl can be used with caution in patients with a history of heart failure who are well-compensated. Congestive heart failure has been observed in patients receiving labetalol HCl. Labetalol HCl does not abolish the inotropic action of digitalis on heart muscle.
In Patients Without a History of Cardiac Failure: In patients with latent cardiac insufficiency, continued depression of the myocardium with beta-blocking agents over a period of time can, in some cases, lead to cardiac failure. At the first sign or symptom of impending cardiac failure, patients should be fully digitalized and/or be given a diuretic, and the response observed closely. If cardiac failure continues, despite adequate digitalization and diuretic, NORMODYNE (labetalol HCl) therapy should be withdrawn (gradually if possible).
Exacerbation of Ischemic Heart Disease Following Abrupt Withdrawal: Angina pectoris has not been reported upon labetalol HCl discontinuation. However, hypersensitivity to catecholamines has been observed in patients withdrawn from beta-blocker therapy; exacerbation of angina and, in some cases, myocardial infarction have occurred after *abrupt* discontinuation of such therapy. When discontinuing chronically administered NORMODYNE (labetalol HCl), particularly in patients with ischemic heart disease, the dosage should be gradually reduced over a period of one to two weeks and the patient should be carefully monitored. If angina markedly worsens or acute coronary insufficiency develops, NORMODYNE (labetalol HCl) administration should be reinstituted promptly, at least temporarily, and other measures appropriate for the management of unstable angina should be taken. Patients should be warned against interruption or discontinuation of therapy without the physician's advice. Because coronary artery disease is common and may be unrecognized, it may be prudent not to discontinue NORMODYNE (labetalol HCl) therapy abruptly even in patients treated only for hypertension.
Nonallergic Bronchospasm (e.g., chronic bronchitis and emphysema) Patients with bronchospastic disease should, in general, not receive beta-blockers. NORMODYNE may be used with caution, however, in patients who do not respond to, or cannot tolerate, other antihypertensive agents. It is prudent, if NORMODYNE is used, to use the smallest effective dose, so that inhibition of endogenous or exogenous beta-agonists is minimized.
Pheochromocytoma: Labetalol HCl has been shown to be effective in lowering the blood pressure and relieving symptoms in patients with pheochromocytoma. However, paradoxical hypertensive responses have been reported in a few patients with this tumor; therefore, use caution when administering labetalol HCl to patients with pheochromocytoma.
Diabetes Mellitus and Hypoglycemia: Beta-adrenergic blockade may prevent the appearance of premonitory signs and symptoms (e.g., tachycardia) of acute hypoglycemia. This is especially important with labile diabetics. Beta-blockade also reduces the release of insulin in response to hyperglycemia; it may therefore be necessary to adjust the dose of antidiabetic drugs.
Major Surgery: The necessity or desirability of withdrawing beta-blocking therapy prior to major surgery is controversial. Protracted severe hypotension and difficulty in restarting or maintaining a heart beat have been reported with

beta-blockers. The effect of labetalol HCl's alpha-adrenergic activity has not been evaluated in this setting.

A synergism between labetalol HCl and halothane anesthesia has been shown (See **Drug Interactions**).

PRECAUTIONS

General: *Impaired Hepatic Function:* NORMODYNE (labetalol HCl) Tablets should be used with caution in patients with impaired hepatic function since metabolism of the drug may be diminished.

Jaundice or Hepatic Dysfunction: On rare occasions, labetalol HCl has been associated with jaundice (both hepatic and cholestatic). It is therefore recommended that treatment with labetalol HCl be stopped immediately should a patient develop jaundice or laboratory evidence of liver injury. Both have been shown to be reversible on stopping therapy.

Information for Patients

As with all drugs with beta-blocking activity, certain advice to patients being treated with labetalol HCl is warranted. This information is intended to aid in the safe and effective use of this medication. It is not a disclosure of all possible adverse or intended effects. While no incident of the abrupt withdrawal phenomenon (exacerbation of angina pectoris) has been reported with labetalol HCl, dosing with NORMODYNE Tablets should not be interrupted or discontinued without a physician's advice. Patients being treated with NORMODYNE Tablets should consult a physician at any sign of impending cardiac failure. Also, transient scalp tingling may occur, usually when treatment with NORMODYNE Tablets is initiated (See **ADVERSE REACTIONS**).

Laboratory Tests

As with any new drug given over prolonged periods, laboratory parameters should be observed over regular intervals. In patients with concomitant illnesses, such as impaired renal function, appropriate tests should be done to monitor these conditions.

Drug Interactions

In one survey, 2.3% of patients taking labetalol HCl in combination with tricyclic antidepressants experienced tremor as compared to 0.7% reported to occur with labetalol HCl alone. The contribution of each of the treatments to this adverse reaction is unknown but the possibility of a drug interaction cannot be excluded.

Drugs possessing beta-blocking properties can blunt the bronchodilator effect of beta-receptor agonist drugs in patients with bronchospasm; therefore, doses greater than the normal anti-asthmatic dose of beta-agonist bronchodilator drugs may be required.

Cimetidine has been shown to increase the bioavailability of labetalol HCl. Since this could be explained either by enhanced absorption or by an alteration of hepatic metabolism of labetalol HCl, special care should be used in establishing the dose required for blood pressure control in such patients.

Synergism has been shown between halothane anesthesia and intravenously administered labetalol HCl. During controlled hypotensive anesthesia using labetalol HCl in association with halothane, high concentrations (3% or above) of halothane should not be used because the degree of hypotension will be increased and because of the possibility of a large reduction in cardiac output and an increase in central venous pressure. The anesthesiologist should be informed when a patient is receiving labetalol HCl.

Labetalol HCl blunts the reflex tachycardia produced by nitroglycerin without preventing its hypotensive effect. If labetalol HCl is used with nitroglycerin in patients with angina pectoris, additional antihypertensive effects may occur.

Drug/Laboratory Test Interactions

The presence of a metabolite of labetalol in the urine may result in falsely increased levels of urinary catecholamines when measured by a nonspecific trihydroxyindole (THI) reaction. In screening patients suspected of having a pheochromocytoma and being treated with labetalol HCl, specific radioenzymatic or high performance liquid chromatography assay techniques should be used to determine levels of catecholamines or their metabolites.

Carcinogenesis, Mutagenesis, Impairment of Fertility

Long-term oral dosing studies with labetalol HCl for 18 months in mice and for 2 years in rats showed no evidence of carcinogenesis. Studies with labetalol HCl, using dominant lethal assays in rats and mice, and exposing microorganisms according to modified Ames tests, showed no evidence of mutagenesis.

	Labetalol HCl (N=227) %	Placebo (N=98) %	Propranolol (N=84) %	Metoprolol (N=49) %
Body as a whole				
fatigue	5	0	12	12
asthenia	1	1	1	0
headache	2	1	1	2
Gastrointestinal				
nausea	6	1	1	2
vomiting	<1	0	0	0
dyspepsia	3	1	1	0
abdominal pain	0	0	1	2
diarrhea	<1	0	2	0
taste distortion	1	0	0	0
Central and Peripheral Nervous Systems				
dizziness	11	3	4	4
paresthesias	<1	0	0	0
drowsiness	<1	2	2	2
Autonomic Nervous System				
nasal stuffiness	3	0	0	0
ejaculation failure	2	0	0	0
impotence	1	0	1	3
increased sweating	<1	0	0	0
Cardiovascular				
edema	1	0	0	0
postural hypotension	1	0	0	0
bradycardia	0	0	5	12
Respiratory				
dyspnea	2	0	1	2
Skin				
rash	1	0	0	0
Special Senses				
vision abnormality	1	0	0	0
vertigo	2	1	0	0

Pregnancy Category C

Teratogenic studies have been performed with labetalol in rats and rabbits at oral doses up to approximately 6 and 4 times the maximum recommended human dose (MRHD), respectively. No reproducible evidence of fetal malformations was observed. Increased fetal resorptions were seen in both species at doses approximating the MRHD. There are no adequate and well-controlled studies in pregnant women. Labetalol should be used during pregnancy only if the potential benefit justifies the potential risk to the fetus.

Nonteratogenic Effects

Infants of mothers who were treated with labetalol HCl for hypertension during pregnancy did not appear to be adversely affected by the drug. Oral administration of labetalol to rats during late gestation through weaning at doses of 2 to 4 times the MRHD caused a decrease in neonatal survival.

Labor and Delivery

Labetalol HCl given to pregnant women with hypertension did not appear to affect the usual course of labor and delivery.

Nursing Mothers

Small amounts of labetalol (approximately 0.004% of the maternal dose) are excreted in human milk. Caution should be exercised when NORMODYNE Tablets are administered to a nursing woman.

Pediatric Use

Safety and effectiveness in children have not been established.

ADVERSE REACTIONS

Most adverse effects are mild, transient and occur early in the course of treatment. In controlled clinical trials of 3 to 4 months duration, discontinuation of NORMODYNE (labetalol HCl) Tablets due to one or more adverse effect was required in 7% of all patients. In these same trials, beta-blocker control agents led to discontinuation in 8 to 10% of patients, and a centrally acting alpha-agonist in 30% of patients.

The incidence rates of adverse reactions listed in the following table were derived from multicenter controlled clinical trials, comparing labetalol HCl, placebo, metoprolol and propranolol, over treatment periods of 3 and 4 months. Where the frequency of adverse effects for labetalol HCl and placebo is similar, causal relationship is uncertain. The rates are based on adverse reactions considered probably drug-related by the investigator. If all reports are considered, the rates are somewhat higher (e.g., dizziness 20%, nausea 14%, fatigue 11%), but the overall conclusions are unchanged. [See table above].

The adverse effects were reported spontaneously and are representative of the incidence of adverse effects that may be observed in a properly selected hypertensive patient population, i.e., a group excluding patients with bronchospastic disease, overt congestive heart failure, or other contraindications to beta-blocker therapy.

Clinical trials also included studies utilizing daily doses up to 2400 mg in more severely hypertensive patients. Certain of the side effects increased with increasing dose as shown in the table below which depicts the entire U.S. therapeutic trials data base for adverse reactions that are clearly or possibly dose related.

[See table below left].

In addition, a number of other less common adverse events have been reported in clincal trials or the literature:

Cardiovascular: Postural hypotension, including rarely, syncope.

Central and Peripheral Nervous Systems: Paresthesias, most frequently described as scalp tingling. In most cases, it was mild, transient and usually occurred at the beginning of treatment.

Collagen Disorders: Systemic lupus erythematosus; positive antinuclear factor (ANF).

Eyes: Dry eyes.

Immunological System: Antimitochondrial antibodies.

Liver and Biliary System: Cholestasis with or without jaundice.

Musculo-Skeletal System: Muscle cramps; toxic myopathy.

Respiratory System: Bronchospasm.

Skin and Appendages: Rashes of various types, such as generalized maculo-papular; lichenoid; urticarial; bullous lichen planus; psoriaform; facial erythema; Peyronie's disease; reversible alopecia.

Urinary System: Difficulty in micturition, including acute urinary bladder retention.

Following approval for marketing in the United Kingdom, a monitored release survey involving approximately 6,800 patients was conducted for further safety and efficacy evaluation of this product. Results of this survey indicate that the type, severity, and incidence of adverse effects were comparable to those cited above.

Potential Adverse Effects

In addition, other adverse effects not listed above have been reported with other beta-adrenergic blocking agents.

Central Nervous System: Reversible mental depression progressing to catatonia; an acute reversible syndrome characterized by disorientation for time and place, short-term

Continued on next page

Information on Schering products appearing on these pages is effective as of September 30, 1986.

Labetalol HCl Daily Dose (mg)	200	300	400	600	800	900	1200	1600	2400
Number of Patients	522	181	606	608	503	117	411	242	175
Dizziness (%)	2	3	3	3	5	1	9	13	16
Fatigue	2	1	4	4	5	3	7	6	10
Nausea	<1	0	1	2	4	0	7	11	19
Vomiting	0	0	<1	<1	<1	0	1	2	3
Dyspepsia	1	0	2	1	1	0	2	2	4
Paresthesias	2	0	2	2	1	1	2	5	5
Nasal Stuffiness	1	1	2	2	2	2	4	5	6
Ejaculation Failure	0	2	1	2	3	0	4	3	5
Impotence	1	1	1	1	2	4	3	4	3
Edema	1	0	1	1	1	0	1	2	2

Schering—Cont.

memory loss, emotional lability, slightly clouded sensorium, and decreased performance on neuropsychometrics.
Cardiovascular: Intensification of AV block. See **CONTRAINDICATIONS.**
Allergic: Fever combined with aching and sore throat; laryngospasm; respiratory distress.
Hematologic: Agranulocytosis; thrombocytopenic or nonthrombocytopenic purpura.
Gastrointestinal: Mesenteric artery thrombosis; ischemic colitis.
The oculomucocutaneous syndrome associated with the beta-blocker practolol has not been reported with labetalol HCl.
Clinical laboratory tests: There have been reversible increases of serum transaminases in 4% of patients treated with labetalol HCl and tested, and more rarely, reversible increases in blood urea.

OVERDOSAGE

Overdosage with NORMODYNE (labetalol HCl) Tablets causes excessive hypotension that is posture sensitive, and sometimes, excessive bradycardia. Patients should be placed supine and their legs raised if necessary to improve the blood supply to the brain. If overdosage with labetalol HCl follows oral ingestion, gastric lavage or pharmacologically induced emesis (using syrup of ipecac) may be useful for removal of the drug shortly after ingestion. The following additional measures should be employed if necessary: **Excessive bradycardia**—administer atropine or epinephrine. **Cardiac failure**—administer a digitalis glycoside and a diuretic. Deopamine or dobutamine may also be useful. **Hypotension**—administer vasopressors, eg, norepinephrine. There is pharmacological evidence that norepinephrine may be the drug of choice. **Bronchospasm**—administer epinephrine and/or an aerosolized beta$_2$-agonist. **Seizures**—administer diazepam.
In severe beta-blocker overdose resulting in hypotension and/or bradycardia, glucagon has been shown to be effective when administered in large doses (5 to 10 mg rapidly over 30 seconds, followed by continuous infusion of 5 mg/hr that can be reduced as the patient improves).
Neither hemodialysis nor peritoneal dialysis removes a significant amount of labetalol HCl from the general circulation ($<1\%$).
The oral LD_{50} value of labetalol HCl in the mouse is approximately 600 mg/kg and in the rat is greater than 2 g/kg. The intravenous LD_{50} in these species is 50 to 60 mg/kg.

DOSAGE AND ADMINISTRATION

DOSAGE MUST BE INDIVIDUALIZED. The recommended <u>initial</u> dose is 100 mg <u>twice</u> daily whether used alone or added to a diuretic regimen. After 2 or 3 days, using standing blood pressure as an indicator, dosage may be titrated in increments of 100 mg bid every 2 or 3 days. The usual <u>maintenance</u> dosage of labetalol HCl is between 200 and 400 mg <u>twice</u> daily.
Since the full antihypertensive effect of labetalol HCl is usually seen within the first one to three hours of the initial dose or dose increment, the assurance of a lack of an exaggerated hypotensive response can be clinically established in the office setting. The antihypertensive effects of continued dosing can be measured at subsequent visits, approximately 12 hours after a dose, to determine whether further titration is necessary.
Patients with severe hypertension may require from 1200 mg to 2400 mg per day, with or without thiazide diuretics. Should side effects (principally nausea or dizziness) occur with these doses administered bid, the same total daily dose administered tid may improve tolerability and facilitate further titration. Titration increments should not exceed 200 mg bid.
When a diuretic is added, an additive antihypertensive effect can be expected. In some cases this may necessitate a labetalol HCl dosage adjustment. As with most antihypertensive drugs, optimal dosages of NORMODYNE Tablets are usually lower in patients also receiving a diuretic.
When transferring patients from other antihypertensive drugs, NORMODYNE Tablets should be introduced as recommended and the dosage of the existing therapy progressively decreased.

HOW SUPPLIED

NORMODYNE (labetalol HCl) Tablets, <u>100 mg</u>, light-brown, round, scored, film-coated tablets engraved on one side with Schering and product identification numbers 244, and on the other side the number 100 for the strength and "NORMODYNE"; bottles of 100 (NDC-0085-0244-04), 500 (NDC-0085-0244-05), and box of 100 for unit-dose dispensing (NDC-0085-0244-08).
NORMODYNE (labetalol HCl) Tablets, <u>200 mg</u>, white, round, scored, film-coated tablets engraved on one side with Schering and product identification numbers 752, and on the other side the number 200 for the strength and "NORMODYNE"; bottles of 100 (NDC-0085-0752-04), 500 (NDC-0085-0752-05), box of 100 for unit-dose dispensing (NDC-0085-0752-08), and Patient Calendar Package of 56 (4 bottles of 14 tablets) (NDC-0085-0752-03).
NORMODYNE (labetalol HCl) Tablets, <u>300 mg</u>, blue, round, film-coated tablets engraved on one side with Schering and product identification numbers 438, and on the other side the number 300 for the strength and "NORMODYNE"; bottles of 100 (NDC-0085-0438-03), 500 (NDC-0085-0438-05), box of 100 for unit-dose dispensing (NDC-0085-0438-06), and Patient Calendar Package of 56 (4 bottles of 14 tablets) (NDC-0085-0438-02).
NORMODYNE (labetalol HCl) Tablets should be stored between 2° and 30°C (36° and 86°F).
NORMODYNE (labetalol HCl) Tablets in the unit-dose boxes should be protected from excessive moisture.
Revised 6/86

Shown in Product Identification Section, page 428

OPTIMINE® ℞

[*op'tĭ-mēn*]
brand of azatadine maleate, USP
Tablets

DESCRIPTION

OPTIMINE Tablets contain azatadine maleate, an antihistamine having the empirical formula, $C_{20}H_{22}N_2 \cdot 2C_4H_4O_4$, the chemical name, 6,11-Dihydro-11-(1-methyl-4- piperidylidene) -5*H*-benzo[5,6]cyclohepta [1,2-*β*] pyridine maleate (1:2).
The molecular weight of azatadine maleate is 522.54. It is a white to off-white powder and is very soluble in water and soluble in alcohol.
Each OPTIMINE Tablet contains 1 mg azatadine maleate, USP. They also contain: corn starch, lactose, magnesium stearate and povidone.

CLINICAL PHARMACOLOGY

Azatadine maleate is an antihistamine related to cyproheptadine, with antiserotonin, anticholinergic (drying), and sedative effects.
Antihistamines competitively antagonize those pharmacological effects of histamine which are mediated through activation of histamine H_1-receptor sites on effector cells. Histamine-related allergic reactions and tissue injury are blocked or diminished in intensity. Antihistamines antagonize the vasodilator effect of endogenously released histamine, especially in small vessels, and mitigate the effect of histamine which results in increased capillary permeability and edema formation. As consequences of these actions, antihistamines antagonize the physiological manifestations of histamine release in the nose following antigen-antibody interactions, such as congestion related to vascular engorgement, mucosal edema, and profuse, watery secretion, and irritation and sneezing resulting from histamine action on afferent nerve terminals.
Pharmacokinetic studies in normal volunteers dosed orally with radio-labeled azatadine maleate show that the drug is readily absorbed with peak plasma levels at about four hours after dosing. Approximately 50% of the drug is excreted in the urine within five days after administration of a single dose, and no evidence of drug accumulation was seen after daily dosing for 30 days. The elimination half-life of azatadine maleate, based on plasma radioactivity, was approximately 9 hours. Approximately 20% of the drug is excreted unchanged and extensive conjugation of the drug and its metabolites occurs. Azatadine maleate is minimally bound to plasma protein.
While the antihistamines have not been studied for passage through the blood-brain and placental barriers, the occurrence of pharmacologic effects in the central nervous system and in the newborn indicate presence of the drug.

INDICATIONS AND USAGE

OPTIMINE Tablets are indicated for the treatment of perennial and seasonal allergic rhinitis and chronic urticaria.

CONTRAINDICATIONS

Antihistamines *should NOT* be used to treat lower respiratory tract symptoms, including asthma.
Antihistamines, including azatadine maleate, are also contraindicated in patients hypersensitive to this medication and to other antihistamines of similar chemical structure, and in patients receiving monoamine oxidase inhibitor therapy. (See Drug Interactions.)

WARNINGS

Antihistamines should be used with caution in patients with narrow angle glaucoma, stenosing peptic ulcer; pyloroduodenal obstruction; and urinary bladder obstruction due to symptomatic prostatic hypertrophy and narrowing of the bladder neck.
Use with CNS Depressants: Antihistamines have additive effects with alcohol and other CNS depressants (hypnotics, sedatives, tranquilizers, etc.).
Use in Activities Requiring Mental Alertness: Patients should be warned about engaging in activities requiring mental alertness, such as driving a car or operating certain appliances, machinery, etc., until their response to this medication has been determined.
Use in Patients approximately 60 years or older: Antihistamines are more likely to cause dizziness, sedation, and hypotension in patients over 60 years of age.

PRECAUTIONS

General: Azatadine maleate has an atropine-like action and therefore should be used with caution in patients with: a history of bronchial asthma; increased intraocular pressure; hyperthyroidism; cardiovascular disease; hypertension.
Information for Patients: This information is intended to aid in the safe and effective use of this medication. It is not a disclosure of all possible adverse or intended effects.
1. Antihistamines may cause drowsiness.
2. Patients taking antihistamines should not engage in activities requiring mental alertness, such as driving a car or operating machinery, certain appliances, etc., until their response to this medication has been determined.
3. Alcohol or other sedative drugs may enhance the drowsiness caused by antihistamines.
4. Patients should not take this medication if they are receiving a monoamine oxidase (MAO) inhibitor, or if they are receiving oral anticoagulants.
5. This medication should not be given to children less than 12 years of age.

Drug Interactions: MAO inhibitors prolong and intensify the anticholinergic and sedative effects of antihistamines. Additive effects may occur from the concomitant use of antihistamines with tricyclic antidepressants. (See also WARNINGS.) The action of oral anticoagulants may be diminished by antihistamines.
Drug/Laboratory Test Interaction: Antihistamines should be discontinued about four days prior to skin testing procedures since these drugs may prevent or diminish otherwise positive reactions to dermal reactivity indicators.
Carcinogenesis, Mutagenesis, and Impairment of Fertility: Long-term oral dosing studies with azatadine maleate in rats and mice showed no evidence of carcinogenesis. No mutagenic effect was seen in a dominant lethal assay study in mice dosed with azatadine maleate orally and intraperitoneally. There was no impairment of fertility in rats fed azatadine maleate at doses greater than 150 times the recommended human daily dose.
Pregnancy Category B: Reproduction studies have been performed in rats and rabbits at doses up to 188 times and 38 times, respectively, the human dose and have revealed no evidence of impaired fertility or harm to the fetus due to azatadine maleate. There are, however, no adequate and well-controlled studies in pregnant women. Because animal reproduction studies are not always predictive of human response, this drug should be used during pregnancy only if clearly needed. (See **Non-Teratogenic Effects.**)
Non-Teratogenic Effects: Antihistamines should not be used in the third trimester of pregnancy because newborns and premature infants may have severe reactions, such as convulsions, to them.
Nursing Mothers: It is not known whether this drug is excreted in human milk. However, certain antihistamines are known to be excreted in human milk in low concentration. Because of the higher risk of antihistamines for infants generally and for newborns and prematures in particular, a decision should be made whether to discontinue nursing or to discontinue the drug, taking into account the importance of the drug to the mother.
Pediatric Use: Safety and effectiveness in children below the age of 12 years have not been established.

ADVERSE REACTIONS

Slight to moderate drowsiness may occur with azatadine maleate. Other possible side effects common to antihistamines in general include: (the most frequent are underlined).
General: urticaria, drug rash, anaphylactic shock, photosensitivity, excessive perspiration, chills, dryness of mouth, nose, and throat.
Cardiovascular: hypotension, headache, palpitations, tachycardia, extrasystoles.
Hematologic: hemolytic anemia, hypoplastic anemia, thrombocytopenia, agranulocytosis.
Nervous: <u>sedation, sleepiness, dizziness,</u> vertigo, tinnitus, acute labyrinthitis, <u>disturbed coordination,</u> fatigue, confusion, restlessness, excitation, nervousness, tremor, irritability, insomnia, euphoria, paresthesias, blurred vision diplopia, hysteria, neuritis, convulsions.
Gastrointestinal: <u>epigastric distress,</u> anorexia, nausea, vomiting, diarrhea, constipation.
Genitourinary: urinary frequency, difficult urination, urinary retention, early menses.
Respiratory: <u>thickening of bronchial secretions,</u> tightness of chest and wheezing, nasal stuffiness.

DRUG ABUSE AND DEPENDENCE

There is no information to indicate that abuse or dependency occurs with azatadine maleate.
Overdosage: In the event of overdosage, emergency treatment should be started immediately.

Manifestations: Antihistamine overdosage effects may vary from central nervous system depression (sedation, apnea, diminished mental alertness, cardiovascular collapse) to stimulation (insomnia, hallucinations, tremors or convulsions) to death. Other signs and symptoms may be dizziness, tinnitus, ataxia, blurred vision, and hypotension. Stimulation is particularly likely in children, as are atropine-like signs and symptoms (dry mouth; fixed, dilated pupils; flushing; hyperthermia; and gastrointestinal symptoms).

Treatment: The patient should be induced to vomit, even if emesis has occurred spontaneously. Pharmacologic vomiting by the administration of ipecac syrup is a preferred method. However, vomiting should not be induced in patients with impaired consciousness. The action of ipecac is facilitated by physical activity and by the administration of 8 to 12 fluid ounces of water. If emesis does not occur within fifteen minutes, the dose of ipecac should be repeated. Precautions against aspiration must be taken, especially in infants and children. Following emesis, any drug remaining in the stomach may be adsorbed by activated charcoal administered as a slurry with water. If vomiting is unsuccessful or contraindicated, gastric lavage should be performed. Physiologic saline solution is the lavage solution of choice, particularly in children. In adults, tap water can be used; however, as much as possible of the amount administered should be removed before the next instillation. Saline cathartics, such as milk of magnesia, draw water into the bowel by osmosis and, therefore, may be valuable for their action in rapid dilution of bowel content. Dialysis is of little value in antihistamine poisoning. After emergency treatment, the patient should continue to be medically monitored.

Treatment of the signs and symptoms of overdosage is symptomatic and supportive. Stimulants (analeptic agents) should not be used. Vasopressors may be used to treat hypotension. Short acting barbiturates, diazepam, or paraldehyde may be administered to control seizures. Hyperpyrexia, especially in children, may require treatment with tepid water sponge baths or a hypothermic blanket. Apnea is treated with ventilatory support.

DOSAGE AND ADMINISTRATION

DOSAGE SHOULD BE INDIVIDUALIZED ACCORDING TO THE NEEDS AND THE RESPONSE OF THE PATIENT.

OPTIMINE Tablets are not recommended for use in children under 12 years of age.

The usual adult dosage is 1 or 2 mg, twice a day.

HOW SUPPLIED

OPTIMINE Tablets, 1 mg. white, compressed, scored tablets impressed with the Schering trademark and product identification numbers, 282; bottle of 100 (NDC 0085-0282-03).

Store between 2°and 30°C (36°and 86°F).

Revised 12/85

Shown in Product Identification Section, page 428

ORETON® Methyl ℞

[*or 'e-ton*]

brand of methyltestosterone

Tablets, USP

Buccal Tablets, USP

DESCRIPTION

ORETON **Methyl** Tablets and **Buccal** Tablets contain methyltestosterone, USP, a synthetic androgen. Androgens are steroids that develop and maintain primary and secondary male sex characteristics. ORETON **Methyl** Tablets are to be taken orally. ORETON **Methyl Buccal** Tablets are NOT to be swallowed but are to be placed in the lower or upper buccal pouches.

Androgens are derivatives of cyclopentanoperhydrophenanthrene. Endogenous androgens are C-19 steroids with a side chain at C-17, and with two angular methyl groups. Testosterone is the primary endogenous androgen. In their active form, all drugs in the class have a 17-beta-hydroxy group. 17-alpha alkylation (methyltestosterone) increases the pharmacologic activity per unit weight compared to testosterone when given orally.

Methyltestosterone is the 17α-methyl derivative of testosterone, the true testicular hormone. Chemically, methyltestosterone is 17β-Hydroxy-17-methylandrost-4-en-3-one, with the empirical formula $C_{20}H_{30}O_2$, a molecular weight of 302.5.

Methyltestosterone is a white to creamy-white, odorless, slightly hygroscopic powder. It is practically insoluble in water, soluble in alcohol and other organic solvents.

ORETON **Methyl** Tablets contain either 10 mg methyltestosterone, USP and corn starch, lactose and magnesium stearate; or 25 mg of methyltestosterone, USP and corn starch, FD&C Yellow No. 6, lactose and magnesium stearate.

Each ORETON **Methyl Buccal** Tablet contains 10 mg methyltestosterone, USP. They also contain: FD&C Blue No. 2, FD&C Red No. 40, magnesium stearate and PEG.

CLINICAL PHARMACOLOGY

Endogenous androgens are responsible for the normal growth and development of the male sex organs and for maintenance of secondary sex characteristics. These effects include the growth and maturation of prostate, seminal vesicles, penis, and scrotum: the development of male hair distribution, such as beard, pubic, chest, and axillary hair; laryngeal enlargement, vocal chord thickening, alterations in body musculature, and fat distribution. Drugs in this class also cause retention of nitrogen, sodium, potassium, phosphorus, and decreased urinary excretion of calcium. Androgens have been reported to increase protein anabolism and decrease protein catabolism. Nitrogen balance is improved only when there is sufficient intake of calories and protein.

Androgens are responsible for the growth spurt of adolescence and for the eventual termination of linear growth which is brought about by fusion of the epiphyseal growth centers. In children, exogenous androgens accelerate linear growth rates, but may cause a disproportionate advancement in bone maturation. Use over long periods may result in fusion of the epiphyseal growth centers and termination of the growth process. Androgens have been reported to stimulate the production of red blood cells by enhancing the production of erythropoietic stimulating factor.

During exogenous administration of androgens, endogenous testosterone release is inhibited through feedback inhibition of pituitary luteinizing hormone (LH). With large doses of exogenous androgens, spermatogenesis may also be suppressed through feedback inhibition of pituitary follicle stimulating hormone (FSH).

There is a lack of substantial evidence that androgens are effective in fractures, surgery, convalescence, and functional uterine bleeding.

Pharmacokinetics: Testosterone given orally is metabolized by the gut and 44 percent is cleared by the liver in the first pass. Oral doses as high as 400 mg per day are needed to achieve clinically effective blood levels for full replacement therapy. The synthetic androgen (methyltestosterone) is less extensively metabolized by the liver and has a longer half-life. It is more suitable than testosterone for oral administration. Additionally, buccal administration permits the methyltestosterone to be absorbed directly into the systemic venous return so that the unmetabolized hormone is carried directly to the tissues. The buccal tablets have approximately twice the potency of the orally ingested methyltestosterone.

Testosterone in plasma is 98 percent bound to a specific testosterone-estradiol binding globulin, and about one percent is free. Generally, the amount of this sex-hormone binding globulin in the plasma will determine the distribution of testosterone between free and bound forms, and the free testosterone concentration will determine its half-life.

About 90 percent of a dose of testosterone is excreted in the urine as glucuronic and sulfuric acid conjugates of testosterone and its metabolites; about 6 percent of a dose is excreted in the feces, mostly in the unconjugated form. Inactivation of testosterone occurs primarily in the liver. Testosterone is metabolized to various 17-keto steroids through two different pathways. As reported in the literature, the half-life of testosterone varies considerably, ranging from 10 to 100 minutes.

In many tissues the activity of testosterone appears to depend on reduction to dihydrotestosterone, which binds to cytosol receptor proteins. The steroid-receptor complex is transported to the nucleus where it initiates transcription events and cellular changes related to androgen action.

INDICATIONS AND USAGE

In the male: ORETON **Methyl** Tablets and **Methyl Buccal** Tablets are indicated for replacement therapy in conditions associated with a deficiency or absence of endogenous testosterone:

Primary hypogonadism (congenital or acquired)—testicular failure due to cryptorchidism, bilateral torsion, orchitis, vanishing testis syndrome; or orchidectomy.

Hypogonadotropic hypogonadism (congenital or acquired)—idopathic gonadotropin or LHRH deficiency, or pituitary-hypothalamic injury from tumors, trauma, or radiation.

If the above conditions occur prior to puberty, androgen replacement therapy will be needed during the adolescent years for development of secondary sexual characteristics. Prolonged androgen treatment will be required to maintain sexual characteristics in these and other males who develop testosterone deficiency after puberty.

Androgens may be used to stimulate puberty in carefully selected males with clearly delayed puberty. These patients usually have a familial pattern of delayed puberty that is not secondary to a pathological disorder; puberty is expected to occur spontaneously at a relatively late date. Brief treatment with conservative doses may occasionally be justified in these patients if they do not respond to psychological support. The potential adverse effect on bone maturation should be discussed with the patient and parents prior to androgen administration. An X-ray of the hand and wrist to determine bone age should be obtained every 6 months to assess the effect of treatment on the epiphyseal centers. (See WARNINGS.)

In the female: ORETON **Methyl** Tablets and **Methyl Buccal** Tablets may be used secondarily in women with advancing inoperable metastatic (skeletal) mammary cancer who are 1 to 5 years postmenopausal. Primary goals of therapy in these women include ablation of the ovaries. Other methods of counteracting estrogen activity are adrenalectomy, hypophysectomy, and/or antiestrogen therapy. This treatment has also been used in premenopausal women with breast cancer who have benefited from oophorectomy and are considered to have a hormone-responsive tumor. Judgment concerning androgen therapy should be made by an oncologist with expertise in this field.

Androgens, such as methyltestosterone, have been used for the management of postpartum breast pain and engorgement.

CONTRAINDICATIONS

ORETON **Methyl** and **Methyl Buccal** Tablets are contraindicated for use in men with carcinomas of the breast or with known or suspected carcinomas of the prostate, and in women who are or may become pregnant.

When administered to pregnant women, androgens cause virilization of the external genitalia of the female fetus. This virilization includes clitoromegaly, abnormal vaginal development, and fusion of genital folds to form a scrotal-like structure. The degree of masculinization is related to the amount of drug given and to the age of the fetus, and is most likely to occur in the female fetus when the drugs are given in the first trimester. If the patient becomes pregnant while taking these drugs, she should be apprised of the potential hazard to the fetus.

WARNINGS

In patients with breast cancer, androgen therapy may cause hypercalcemia by stimulating osteolysis. In this case, the drugs should be discontinued.

Prolonged use of high doses of androgens has been associated with the development of peliosis hepatis and hepatic neoplasms including hepatocellular carcinoma. (See PRECAUTIONS:—**Carcinogenesis, Mutagenesis, Impairment of Fertility.**) Peliosis hepatis can be a life-threatening or fatal complication.

Cholestatic hepatitis and jaundice occur with 17-alpha-alkylandrogens (such as methyltestosterone) at a relatively low dose. If cholestatic hepatitis with jaundice appears or if liver function tests become abnormal, the androgen should be discontinued and the etiology should be determined. Drug-induced jaundice is reversible when the medication is discontinued.

Geriatric patients treated with androgens may be at an increased risk for the development of prostatic hypertrophy and prostatic carcinoma.

Edema with or without congestive heart failure may be a serious complication in patients with preexisting cardiac, renal, or hepatic disease. In addition to discontinuation of the drug, diuretic therapy may be required.

Gynecomastia frequently develops and occasionally persists in patients being treated for hypogonadism.

Androgen therapy should be used cautiously in healthy males with delayed puberty. The effect on bone maturation should be monitored by assessing bone age of the wrist and hand every 6 months. In children, androgen treatment may accelerate bone maturation without producing compensatory gain in linear growth. This adverse effect may result in compromised adult stature. The younger the child the greater the risk of compromising final mature height.

PRECAUTIONS

General: Women should be observed for signs of virilization (deepening of the voice, hirsutism, acne, clitoromegaly and menstrual irregularities). Discontinuation of drug therapy at the time of evidence of mild virilism is necessary to prevent irreversible virilization. Such virilization is usual following androgen use at high doses. A decision may be made by the patient and the physician that some virilization will be tolerated during treatment for breast carcinoma.

Priapism or excessive sexual stimulation may develop. Males, especially the elderly, may become overstimulated. In treating males for symptoms of climacteric, avoid stimulation to the point of increasing the nervous, mental, and physical activities beyond the patient's cardiovascular capacity.

Oligospermia and reduced ejaculatory volume may occur after prolonged administration or excessive dosage.

Information for the Patients: The physician should instruct patients to report any of the following side effects of androgens:

Adult or Adolescent Males: Too frequent or persistent erections of the penis.

Continued on next page

Schering—Cont.

Women: Hoarseness, acne, changes in menstrual periods, or more hair on the face.
All Patients: Any nausea, vomiting, changes in skin color or ankle swelling.
Any male adolescent patient receiving androgens for delayed puberty should have bone development checked every six months.
Patients should be instructed in the proper taking of ORETON **Methyl Buccal** Tablets. These tablets should **NOT** be swallowed. They should be placed in the space between the gum and cheek and allowed to dissolve, so that the medication enters the body through the lining of the cheek. Avoid eating, drinking, chewing, or smoking while the buccal tablet is in place. The mouth should be rinsed with water after the tablet has dissolved completely.
Laboratory Tests: Women with disseminated breast carcinomas should have frequent determination of urine and serum calcium levels during the course of androgen therapy. (See WARNINGS.)
Because of the hepatoxicity associated with the use of 17-alpha-alkylated androgens, liver function tests should be obtained periodically.
Periodic (every 6 months) X-ray examinations of bone age should be made during treatment of prepubertal males to determine the rate of bone maturation and the effects of androgen therapy on the epiphyseal centers.
Hemoglobin and hematocrit should be checked periodically for polycythemia in patients who are receiving high doses of androgens.
Drug Interactions: Anticoagulants C-17 substituted derivatives of testosterone, such as methandrostenolone, have been reported to decrease the anticoagulant requirements of patients receiving oral anticoagulants. Patients receiving oral anticoagulant therapy require close monitoring especially when androgens are started or stopped.
Oxyphenbutazone Concurrent administration of oxyphenbutazone and androgens may result in elevated serum levels of oxyphenbutazone.
Insulin In diabetic patients the metabolic effects of androgens may decrease blood glucose and insulin requirements.
Drug/Laboratory Test Interferences: Androgens may decrease levels of thyroxine-binding globulin, resulting in decreased total T_4 serum levels and increased resin uptake of T_3 and T_4. Free thyroid hormone levels remain unchanged, however, and there is no clinical evidence of thyroid dysfunction.
Carcinogenesis, Mutagenesis, Impairment of Fertility: *Animal Data:* Testosterone has been tested by subcutaneous injection and implantation in mice and rats. The implant induced cervical-uterine tumors in mice which metastasized in some cases. There is suggestive evidence that injection of testosterone into some strains of female mice increases their susceptibility to hepatoma. Testosterone is also known to increase the number of tumors and decrease the degree of differentiation of chemically induced carcinomas of the liver in rats.
Human Data: There are rare reports of hepatocellular carcinoma in patients receiving long-term therapy with androgens in high doses. Withdrawal of the drugs did not lead to regression of the tumors in all cases.
Geriatric patients treated with androgens may be at an increased risk for the development of prostatic hypertrophy and prostatic carcinoma.
Information on mutagenesis is unknown.
Pregnancy: ***Teratogenic Effects—Pregnancy Category X:*** See CONTRAINDICATIONS.
Nursing Mothers: It is not known whether androgens are excreted in human milk. Because many drugs are excreted in human milk and because of the potential for serious adverse reactions in nursing infants from androgens, a decision should be made whether to discontinue nursing or to discontinue the drug, taking into account the importance of the drug to the mother.
Pediatric Use: Androgen therapy should be used very cautiously in children and only by specialists who are aware of the adverse effects on bone maturation. Skeletal maturation must be monitored every six months by an X-ray of the hand and wrist. (See INDICATIONS AND USAGE, and WARNINGS.)

ADVERSE REACTIONS

Endocrine and Urogenital: ***Female:*** The most common side effects of androgen therapy are amenorrhea and other menstrual irregularities, inhibition of gonadotropin secretion, and virilization, including deepening of the voice and clitoral enlargement. The latter usually is not reversible after androgens are discontinued. When administered to a pregnant woman, androgens cause virilization of external genitalia of the female fetus.
Male: Gynecomastia, and excessive frequency and duration of penile erections. Oligospermia may occur at high dosages. (See CLINICAL PHARMACOLOGY.)
Skin and appendages: Hirsutism, male pattern of baldness, and acne.
Fluid and Electrolyte Disturbances: Retention of sodium, chloride, water, potassium, calcium, and inorganic phosphates.
Gastrointestinal: Nausea, cholestatic jaundice, alterations in liver function tests, rarely hepatocellular neoplasms and peliosis hepatis. (See WARNINGS.)
Hematologic: Suppression of clotting factors, II, V, VII, and X, bleeding in patients on concomitant anticoagulant therapy, and polycythemia.
Nervous System: Increased or decreased libido, headache, anxiety, depression, and generalized paresthesiae.
Metabolic: Increased serum cholesterol.
Miscellaneous: Stomatitis with buccal preparations; rarely anaphylactoid reactions.

OVERDOSAGE

Overdose of medication may be reflected in the occurrence of the signs and symptoms associated with testosterone-anabolic drugs. Nausea and appearance of the early manifestations of edema should be looked for. However, there has been no report of acute overdosage with androgens.

DOSAGE AND ADMINISTRATION

Dosage must be strictly individualized. The suggested dosage for androgens varies depending on the age, sex, and diagnosis of the individual patient. Adjustments and duration of dosage will depend upon the patient's response and the appearance of adverse reactions.
Males: In the androgen-deficient male the following guideline for replacement therapy indicates the usual initial dosages:
[See table below].

	Route	Dose	Frequency
ORETON **Methyl** Tablets	Oral	10–50 mg	Daily
ORETON **Methyl Buccal** Tablets	Buccal	5–25 mg*	Daily

* NOTE: ORETON **Methyl Buccal** Tablets have approximately twice the potency of the orally ingested ORETON **Methyl** Tablets.

Various dosage regimens have been used to induce pubertal changes in hypogonadal males; some experts have advocated lower dosages initially, gradually increasing the dose as puberty progresses, with or without a decrease to maintenance levels. Other experts emphasize that higher dosages are needed to induce pubertal changes and lower dosages can be used for maintenance after puberty. The chronological and skeletal ages must be taken into consideration, both in determining the initial dose and in adjusting the dose.
Dosages used in delayed puberty generally are in the lower ranges of those given above, and are for limited duration, for example, 4 to 6 months.
Females: Women with metastatic breast carcinoma must be followed closely because androgen therapy occasionally appears to accelerate the disease. Thus, many experts prefer to use the shorter acting androgen preparations rather than those with prolonged activity for treating breast carcinoma particularly during the early stages of androgen therapy.
Guideline dosages of androgens for use in the palliative treatment of women with metastatic breast cancer and for the prevention of postpartum breast pain and engorgement are:
[See table above].

	Route	Dose	Frequency
ORETON **Methyl** Tablets			
breast cancer	oral	50–200 mg	daily
postpartum breast pain and engorgement	oral	80 mg	daily (3 to 5 days)
ORETON **Methyl Buccal** Tablets			
breast cancer	buccal	25–100 mg*	daily
postpartum breast pain and engorgement	buccal	40 mg*	daily (3 to 5 days)

* NOTE: ORETON **Methyl Buccal** Tablets have approximately twice the potency of the orally ingested ORETON **Methyl** Tablets.

Administration of Buccal Tablets: ORETON **Methyl Buccal** Tablets should NOT be swallowed, since the hormone is meant to be absorbed through the oral mucous membranes. Place the buccal tablet in the upper or lower buccal pouch between the gum and cheek; let the tablet dissolve completely. Avoid eating, drinking, chewing, or smoking while the buccal tablet is in place. Proper oral hygienic measures (e.g., rinsing mouth with water) are particularly important after the use of buccal tablets.

HOW SUPPLIED

ORETON **Methyl Buccal** Tablets, 10 mg, compressed, lavender-colored, oval tablets impressed with the Schering trademark and product identification letters, BE, or numbers, 970; bottle of 100 (NDC–0085–0970–06).
Store between 2° and 30°C (36° and 86°F).
NOTE: Color of tablets may fade; potency and effectiveness are not impaired.
ORETON **Methyl** Tablets, 10 mg, compressed, white, round tablets impressed with the Schering trademark and product identification letters, JD, or numbers 311; bottle of 100 (NDC– 0085–0311–06).
ORETON **Methyl** Tablets, 25 mg, compressed, peach-colored, round tablets impressed with the Schering trademark and product identification letters, JE, or numbers, 499; bottle of 100 (NDC– 0085–0499–06).
Revised 12/85

Shown in Product Identification Section, page 428

OTOBIOTIC® ℞

[o″to-bi-ah′tik]
brand of polymyxin B sulfate and hydrocortisone
Sterile Otic Solution, USP

DESCRIPTION

OTOBIOTIC Otic Solution is a sterile, antibacterial solution containing an anti-inflammatory agent for use in the external ear. Each ml contains polymyxin B sulfate, USP equivalent to 10,000 units polymyxin B and 5.0 mg hydrocortisone, USP in a propylene glycol, glycerin vehicle which also contains edetate disodium, sodium bisulfite, anhydrous sodium sulfite, and purified water; sulfuric acid used to adjust pH between 3.0 and 5.0.

ACTIONS

Polymyxin B sulfate is effective against *Pseudomonas aeruginosa* and some other gram-negative organisms, including strains of *Escherichia,* that commonly cause otitis externa. The addition of hydrocortisone to the antibiotic affords an anti-inflammatory effect and relief against allergic manifestations and pruritus and reduces the possibility of hypersensitivity and tissue reaction.

INDICATIONS

OTOBIOTIC Otic Solution is indicated for the treatment of superficial bacterial infections of the external auditory canals caused by organisms susceptible to the action of the antibiotic.

CONTRAINDICATIONS

OTOBIOTIC Otic Solution is contraindicated in those individuals who are hypersensitive to corticosteroids, polymyxin or colistin, or to any of its other components, and in infections due to herpes simplex, vaccinia, and zoster-varicella viruses or to fungi.
Perforated tympanic membranes are frequently considered a contraindication to the use of external ear canal medication.

WARNINGS

As with other antibiotic preparations, prolonged treatment with OTOBIOTIC Otic Solution may result in overgrowth of nonsusceptible organisms and fungi.
Infections of the external auditory canals can be of mixed microbial origin and occasionally may be caused by both bacteria and fungi. If the infection is not improved after one week, bacterial and fungal cultures and susceptibility tests should be done to verify the identity of the organism and to determine whether therapy should be changed.
Patients who prefer to warm the medication before using it should be cautioned against heating the solution above body temperature in order to avoid loss of potency.

PRECAUTIONS

If sensitization or irritation occurs, treatment with OTOBIOTIC Otic Solution should be discontinued promptly. Treatment with OTOBIOTIC Otic Solution should not be continued for longer than ten days.
OTOBIOTIC Otic Solution is not for ophthalmic use.

DOSAGE AND ADMINISTRATION

The external auditory canal should be thoroughly cleansed and dried with a sterile cotton applicator before administration of OTOBIOTIC Otic Solution.
For adults, four drops of the solution should be instilled into the affected ear three or four times a day. For infants and children, three drops, instilled into the affected ear three or

four times a day, are suggested because of the smaller capacity of the ear canal.
The patient should lie with the affected ear upward and then the drops should be instilled. This position should be maintained for five minutes to facilitate penetration of the drops into the ear canal. Repeat, if necessary, for the opposite ear.
Note: When placing the dropper in the bottle and during use, do not allow the dropper to touch affected area, fingers, or any other surface. This precaution is necessary to preserve the sterility of the solution.

HOW SUPPLIED

OTOBIOTIC Otic Solution, 15 ml bottle with sterile dropper packaged separately; box of one.
Store between 2° and 30°C (36° and 86°F).

Revised 11/82

PAXIPAM® Ⓒ
[pak'si-pam]
brand of halazepam
Tablets

DESCRIPTION

PAXIPAM Tablets contain halazepam, a benzodiazepine derivative having the chemical name, 7-chloro-1,3-dihydro-5-phenyl-1-(2,2,2-trifluoroethyl)-2*H*-1, 4-benzodiazepin-2-one. Each PAXIPAM Tablet contains 20 mg or 40 mg halazepam. The compound is a white to light cream-colored powder with a molecular weight of 352.8.

CLINICAL PHARMACOLOGY

Central nervous system agents of the 1,4-benzodiazepine class presumably exert their effects by binding at stereo specific receptors at several sites within the central nervous system. Their exact mechanism of action is unknown. Clinically, all benzodiazepines cause a dose-related central nervous system depressant activity varying from mild impairment of task performance to hypnosis.
Halazepam is rapidly and well-absorbed and primarily excreted in the urine. Maximum plasma concentration of halazepam is achieved between one and three hours following oral administration. Studies involving 12 normal subjects indicate the median half-life of elimination of halazepam following a 40 mg dose is approximately 14 hours. The major active plasma metabolite of halazepam is N-desmethyldiazepam. Maximum plasma concentrations of N-desmethyldiazepam usually occur within three to six hours. This metabolite has a half-life of elimination of approximately 50 to 100 hours. Less than one percent of the dose is excreted in the urine as unchanged drug. The major metabolite of halazepam in the urine is a conjugate, 3-hydroxyhalazepam. As with other benzodiazepines, enterohepatic recycling of halazepam and its metabolites may occur in uremic patients.
The degree of plasma protein binding of benzodiazepines is high. Since binding is to serum albumin, the extent of binding is dependent on the albumin concentration. In chronic alcoholics, patients with cirrhosis, and newborns, reduced binding may occur. Protein binding may be greatly reduced in patients with renal insufficiency. Since hepatic biotransformation is the predominant route for the metabolism of benzodiazepines, the disposition of these drugs may be impaired in patients with chronic liver disease. Oral dosing of rats with halazepam for a brief period induced the synthesis of hepatic microsomal drug-metabolizing enzymes. As a result, assuming similar responses in humans, the metabolism of other drugs metabolized in the liver may be increased. The transplacental transfer of halazepam has not been studied. However, other benzodiazepines readily cross the placental barrier. Following administration of halazepam to lactating women, halazepam and its major metabolite, N-desmethyldiazepam, were present in the milk.

INDICATIONS AND USAGE

PAXIPAM Tablets are indicated for the management of anxiety disorders or the short-term relief of the symptoms of anxiety. Anxiety or tension associated with the stress of everyday life usually does not require treatment with an anxiolytic.
The effectiveness of PAXIPAM Tablets for long-term use, that is, more than four months, has not been established. The physician should periodically reassess the usefulness of the drug for the individual patient.

CONTRAINDICATIONS

PAXIPAM Tablets are contraindicated in patients with known sensitivity to this drug or other benzodiazepines. It may be used in patients with open angle glaucoma who are receiving appropriate therapy, but is contraindicated in acute narrow angle glaucoma.

WARNINGS

PAXIPAM Tablets are not of value in the treatment of psychotic patients and should not be employed in lieu of appropriate treatment for psychosis. PAXIPAM Tablets are also not recommended as the primary treatment for major depressive disorders. Because of its depressant CNS effects, patients receiving PAXIPAM Tablets should be cautioned against engaging in hazardous occupations requiring complete mental alertness, such as operating machinery or driving a motor vehicle. For the same reason, patients should be cautioned about the simultaneous ingestion of alcohol and other CNS depressant drugs during treatment with PAXIPAM Tablets.
Benzodiazepines can potentially cause fetal harm when administered to pregnant women. If PAXIPAM Tablets are used during pregnancy, or if the patient becomes pregnant while taking this drug, she should be apprised of the potential hazard to the fetus. Because of experience with other members of the benzodiazepine class, PAXIPAM Tablets are assumed to be capable of causing an increased risk of congenital abnormalities when administered to a pregnant woman during the first trimester. Because use of these drugs is rarely a matter of urgency, their use during the first trimester should almost always be avoided. The possibility that a woman of childbearing potential may be pregnant at the time of institution of therapy should be considered. Patients should be advised that if they become pregnant during therapy or intend to become pregnant, they should communicate with their physicians about the desirability of discontinuing the drug.

PRECAUTIONS

General: If PAXIPAM Tablets are to be combined with other psychotropic agents or anticonvulsant drugs, careful consideration should be given to the pharmacology of the agents to be employed, particularly with compounds which might potentiate the action of benzodiazepines (See Drug Interactions section).
As with other psychotropic medications, the usual precautions with respect to administration of the drug and size of the prescription are indicated for severely depressed patients or those in whom there is reason to expect concealed suicidal ideation or plans.
In elderly and debilitated patients, it is recommended that the dosage be limited to the smallest effective amount to preclude the development of ataxia or oversedation (See DOSAGE AND ADMINISTRATION section). The usual precautions in treating patients with impaired renal or hepatic function should be observed.
Information for Patients: To assure safe and effective use of benzodiazepines, the following information and instructions should be given to the patient:

1. Inform your physician about any alcohol consumption and medicine you are taking now, including drugs you buy without a prescription. Alcohol should generally not be used during treatment with benzodiazepines.
2. Inform your physician if you are planning to become pregnant, if you are pregnant, or if you become pregnant while you are taking this medication.
3. Inform your physician if you are nursing.
4. Until you experience how this medicine affects you, do not drive a car or operate potentially dangerous machinery, etc.
5. If benzodiazepines are used in large doses and/or for an extended period of time, they produce habituation, emotional and physical dependence. Therefore, do not increase the dose even if you think that the drug "does not work anymore."
6. Do not stop taking the drug abruptly without consulting your physician, since withdrawal symptoms can occur.

Laboratory Tests: Laboratory tests are not ordinarily required in otherwise healthy patients.
Drug Interactions: The benzodiazepines, including PAXIPAM Tablets, produce additive CNS depressant effects when co-administered with other psychotropic medications, anticonvulsants, antihistaminics, ethanol, and other drugs which themselves produce CNS depression.
Pharmacokinetic interactions with benzodiazepines have been reported. For example, cimetidine has been reported to reduce diazepam clearance. However, it is not known at this time whether a similar interaction occurs with PAXIPAM Tablets.
Drug/Laboratory Test Interactions: Although interactions between benzodiazepines and commonly employed clinical laboratory tests have occasionally been reported, there is no consistent pattern for a specific drug or specific test.
Carcinogenesis, Mutagenesis, Impairment of Fertility: The results of oral oncogenicity studies in rats and mice treated at doses 5 to 50 times the usual 120 mg daily human dose revealed no evidence of carcinogenicity or other significant pathology. Studies regarding mutagenesis have not been done. Reproduction studies performed in rats have revealed no evidence of impaired fertility.
Pregnancy: Teratogenic Effects: Pregnancy Category D: (See WARNINGS section).
Nonteratogenic Effects: The child born of a mother who is on benzodiazepines may be at some risk for withdrawal symptoms from the drug during the postnatal period. Also, neonatal flaccidity has been reported in children born of mothers who had been receiving benzodiazepines.
Labor and Delivery: PAXIPAM Tablets have no established use in labor or delivery.
Nursing Mothers: Halazepam and its major metabolites are excreted in the milk of lactating postpartum women. Since neonates metabolize benzodiazepines more slowly than adults, and since accumulation of the drug and its metabolites to toxic levels is possible in neonates, the drug should not be given to nursing mothers.
For example, chronic administration of the closely related benzodiazepine, diazepam, to nursing mothers has been reported to cause their infants to become lethargic and lose weight.
Pediatric Use: Safety and effectiveness in children below the age of 18 years have not been established.

ADVERSE REACTIONS

Central Nervous System: The most frequent adverse reactions to PAXIPAM Tablets were CNS disturbances. The most common of these were drowsiness, which occurred in approximately 29 per 100 patients. Other CNS disturbances occurred in approximately 9 per 100 patients (e.g., headache, apathy, psychomotor retardation, disorientation, confusion, euphoria, dysarthria, depression, syncope). Less frequent CNS disturbances were: dizziness, which occurred in approximately 8 per 100 patients; ataxia which occurred in 5 per 100 patients; fatigue, which occurred in approximately 4 per 100 patients; and visual disturbances and paradoxical reaction, which occurred in 1 per 100 patients. Sleep disturbances, changes in libido, and auditory disturbances occurred in fewer than 1 per 100 patients.
Gastrointestinal: Less frequent adverse reactions were: gastrointestinal disturbances (e.g., sense of seasickness, nausea, constipation, increased salivation, difficulty in swallowing, vomiting, gastric disorder) which occurred in approximately 9 per 100 patients; change in appetite, which occurred in approximately 1 per 100 patients; and dry mouth, which occurred in approximately 3 per 100 patients.
Hematologic: Clinically unimportant fluctuations in the white blood and differential counts were reported in less than 5% of 761 patients.
Hepatic: Small to moderate elevations of the following hepatic enzymes were reported; alkaline phosphatase in 20 (2.8%) of 705 patients; SGOT in 35 (5.4%) of 647 patients; SGPT in 3 (<1%) of 336 patients. No serious abnormalities were seen.
The following adverse reactions were reported to occur rarely in those patients treated with PAXIPAM Tablets.
Cardiovascular: Cardiovascular disturbances (e.g., tachycardia, bradycardia, hypotension) were reported to occur in approximately 2 per 100 patients.
Musculoskeletal: Muscular disturbances were reported to occur in approximately 2 per 100 patients.
Other: The following adverse reactions occurred in fewer than 1 per 100 patients: allergic manifestations, genitourinary disturbance, paresthesias, and respiratory disturbance.
Adverse Reactions not reported with the use of PAXIPAM Tablets, but reported with the use of other benzodiazepines are: jaundice, agranulocytosis, edema, slurred speech, minor menstrual irregularities, dystonia, pruritus, incontinence, urinary retention, and diplopia.

DRUG ABUSE AND DEPENDENCE

Physical and Psychological Dependence: Withdrawal symptoms (similar in character to those noted with barbiturates and alcohol) have occurred following abrupt discontinuance of benzodiazepines. These can range from mild dysphoria and insomnia to a major syndrome which may include abdominal and muscle cramps, vomiting, sweating, tremor, and convulsions. These signs and symptoms, especially the more serious ones, are generally more common in those patients who have received excessive doses over an extended period of time. However, withdrawal symptoms have also been reported following abrupt discontinuance of benzodiazepines taken continuously, at therapeutic levels, for several months. Consequently, after extended therapy, abrupt discontinuation should generally be avoided and a gradual tapering in dosage followed.
Patients with a history of seizures or epilepsy, regardless of their concomitant anti-seizure drug therapy, should not be abruptly withdrawn from any CNS depressant agent, including PAXIPAM Tablets. Addiction-prone individuals (such as drug addicts or alcoholics) should be under careful surveillance when receiving halazepam or other psychotropic agents because of the predisposition of such patients to habituation and dependence.
Controlled Substance Class: PAXIPAM is a controlled substance under the Controlled Substance Act and has been assigned by the Drug Enforcement Administration to Schedule IV.

Continued on next page

Information on Schering products appearing on these pages is effective as of September 30, 1986.

Schering—Cont.

OVERDOSAGE

Manifestations of PAXIPAM Tablets overdosage include somnolence, confusion, impaired coordination, diminished reflexes, and coma.

No delayed reactions (e.g., organ toxicity) or clinical laboratory abnormalities have been reported.

General Treatment Of Overdose: Overdosage reports with halazepam are limited. Respiration, pulse, and blood pressure should be monitored, as in all cases of drug overdosage. General supportive measures should be employed, along with immediate gastric lavage. Intravenous fluids should be administered and an adequate airway maintained. Hypotension may be combated by the use of Levophed® (levarterenol) or Aramine® (metaraminol). Dialysis is of limited value. Animal experiments have suggested that forced diuresis or hemodialysis are probably of little value in treating overdosage. As with the management of intentional overdosing with any drug, it should be borne in mind that multiple agents may have been ingested.

DOSAGE AND ADMINISTRATION

Dosage should be individualized for maximum beneficial effect. While the usual daily dosages given below will meet the needs of most patients, there will be some who require higher doses. In such cases, dosage should be increased cautiously to avoid adverse effects.

PAXIPAM Tablets are administered orally in divided doses and the dosage should be individualized according to the severity of symptoms and response of the patient. To facilitate dosing, the tablets are scored. The usual recommended dose is 20 to 40 mg three or four times a day.

The response of the patient to several days of treatment will permit the physician to adjust the dose upward or downward. The optimal dosage usually ranges from 80 to 160 mg daily. In debilitated patients or the elderly (70 years or older), the initial recommended dosage is 20 mg once or twice a day. The dose should be adjusted as needed and tolerated. If side effects occur with the starting dose, the dose should be lowered.

HOW SUPPLIED

PAXIPAM Tablets, 20 mg, orange, compressed, scored tablets impressed with the Schering trademark and product identification numbers, 251; bottles of 100 (NDC-0085-0251-04).

PAXIPAM Tablets, 40 mg, white, compressed, scored tablets impressed with the Schering trademark and product identification numbers, 538; bottles of 100 (NDC-0085-0538-04).

Store between 2° and 30°C (36° and 86°F).

ANIMAL PHARMACOLOGY AND/OR ANIMAL TOXICOLOGY

In animal studies, the antianxiety activity of halazepam was demonstrated by its ability to induce calming effects in normally aggressive species, such as the monkey, and to alleviate suppressed behavior in animals placed in a conflict situation. Halazepam was also shown to block aggressive behavior invoked by stressful stimuli.

Halazepam has relatively little effect on autonomic function and unlike major tranquilizers such as chlorpromazine or haloperidol, it does not cause extrapyramidal side effects. As with other CNS depressants, halazepam at relatively high doses produces transient cardiovascular depressant effects, but no EKG disturbances were seen in dogs.

A battery of tests were performed in monkeys to evaluate the abuse potential of PAXIPAM. Although PAXIPAM did cause physical dependence and positive drug-seeking behavior, these effects were judged to be weaker than those caused by diazepam or chlordiazepoxide in each case. However, the abuse potential of PAXIPAM in man in comparison with that of diazepam or chlordiazepoxide remains to be established.

Revised 9/81

Shown in Product Identification Section, page 428

PERMITIL® ℞

[per'mĭ-til]

brand of fluphenazine hydrochloride

Tablets, USP

Oral Concentrate

DESCRIPTION

PERMITIL products are formulations of fluphenazine hydrochloride, USP, a phenothiazine of the piperazine group. It is available as **Tablets**, 2.5, 5, and 10 mg fluphenazine hydrochloride and as an **Oral Concentrate**, 5 mg fluphenazine hydrochloride per ml and alcohol 1%.

The inactive ingredients for PERMITIL **Tablets** 2.5 mg include: calcium phosphate, corn starch, FD&C Yellow No. 6, lactose, magnesium stearate, and starch.

The inactive ingredients for PERMITIL **Tablets** 5 mg include: calcium phosphate, corn starch, D&C Red No. 33, FD&C Red No. 40, FD&C Yellow No. 6, lactose, magnesium stearate, and starch.

The inactive ingredients for PERMITIL **Tablets** 10 mg include: calcium phosphate, corn starch, D&C Red No. 27 Lake, D&C Red No. 30 Lake, FD&C Yellow No. 6 Lake, lactose, magneisum stearate, and starch.

The inactive ingredients for PERMITIL **Oral Concentrate** include: methylparaben, propylparaben, sodium phosphate, and water.

ACTIONS

Fluphenazine hydrochloride has actions at all levels of the central nervous system, as well as on other organ systems. However, the site and mechanism of action of therapeutic effect are not known.

INDICATIONS

PERMITIL **Tablets** and **Oral Concentrate** are indicated for the management of manifestations of psychotic disorders.

PERMITIL has not been shown effective in the management of behavioral complications in patients with mental retardation.

CONTRAINDICATIONS

PERMITIL is contraindicated in comatose or greatly obtunded patients and in patients receiving large doses of central nervous system depressants (barbiturates, alcohol, narcotics, analgesics, or antihistamines); in the presence of existing blood dyscrasias, bone marrow depression, or liver damage; and in patients who have shown hypersensitivity to PERMITIL products, their components, or related compounds.

PERMITIL is also contraindicated in patients with suspected or established subcortical brain damage, with or without hypothalamic damage, since a hyperthermic reaction with temperatures in excess of 104° F may occur in such patients, sometimes not until 14 to 16 hours after drug administration. Total body ice-packing is recommended for such a reaction; antipyretics may also be useful.

WARNINGS

Tardive dyskinesia, a syndrome consisting of potentially irreversible, involuntary, dyskinetic movements, may develop in patients treated with neuroleptic (antipsychotic) drugs. Although the prevalence of the syndrome appears to be highest among the elderly, especially elderly women, it is impossible to rely upon prevalence estimates to predict, at the inception of neuroleptic treatment, which patients are likely to develop the syndrome. Whether neuroleptic drug products differ in their potential to cause tardive dyskinesia is unknown.

Both the risk of developing the syndrome and the likelihood that it will become irreversible are believed to increase as the duration of treatment and the total cumulative dose of neuroleptic drugs administered to the patient increase. However, the syndrome can develop, although much less commonly, after relatively brief treatment periods at low doses.

There is no known treatment for established cases of tardive dyskinesia, although the syndrome may remit, partially or completely, if neuroleptic treatment is withdrawn. Neuroleptic treatment itself, however, may suppress (or partially suppress) the signs and symptoms of the syndrome, and thereby may possibly mask the underlying disease process. The effect that symptomatic suppression has upon the long-term course of the syndrome is unknown.

Given these considerations, neuroleptics should be prescribed in a manner that is most likely to minimize the occurrence of tardive dyskinesia. Chronic neuroleptic treatment should generally be reserved for patients who suffer from a chronic illness that, 1) is known to respond to neuroleptic drugs, and, 2) for whom alternative, equally effective, but potentially less harmful treatments are not available or appropriate. In patients who do require chronic treatment, the smallest dose and the shortest duration of treatment producing a satisfactory clinical response should be sought. The need for continued treatment should be reassessed periodically.

If signs and symptoms of tardive dyskinesia appear in a patient on neuroleptics, drug discontinuation should be considered. However, some patients may require treatment despite the presence of the syndrome.

(For further information about the description of tardive dyskinesia and its clinical detection, please refer to **Information for Patients** and **ADVERSE REACTIONS.**)

If hypotension develops, epinephrine should not be administered since its action is blocked and partially reversed by fluphenazine hydrochloride. If a vasopressor is needed, norepinephrine may be used. Severe, acute hypotension has occurred with the use of phenothiazines and is particularly likely to occur in patients with mitral insufficiency or pheochromocytoma. Rebound hypertension may occur in pheochromocytoma patients.

PERMITIL can lower the convulsive threshold in susceptible individuals; it should be used with caution in alcohol withdrawal and in patients with convulsive disorders. If the patient is being treated with an anticonvulsant agent, increased dosage of that agent may be required when PERMITIL is used concomitantly.

PERMITIL should be used with caution in patients with psychic depression.

Fluphenazine hydrochloride may impair the mental and/or physical abilities required for the performance of hazardous tasks such as driving a car or operating machinery; therefore, the patient should be warned accordingly.

Usage in Children Safety and effectiveness in children have not been established; therefore, PERMITIL is not recommended for use in children.

Usage in Pregnancy Safe use of fluphenazine hydrochloride during pregnancy and lactation has not been established; therefore, in administering the drug to pregnant patients, nursing mothers, or women who may become pregnant, the possible benefits must be weighed against the possible hazards to mother and child.

PRECAUTIONS

The possibility of suicide in depressed patients remains during treatment and until significant remission occurs. This type of patient should not have access to large quantities of this drug.

As with all phenothiazine compounds, fluphenazine hydrochloride should not be used indiscriminately. Caution should be observed in giving it to patients who have previously exhibited severe adverse reactions to other phenothiazines. Some of the untoward actions of fluphenazine hydrochloride tend to appear more frequently when high doses are used. However, as with other phenothiazine compounds, patients receiving PERMITIL in any dosage should be kept under close supervision.

Neuroleptic drugs elevate prolactin levels; the elevation persists during chronic administration. Tissue culture experiments indicate that approximately one-third of human breast cancers are prolactin dependent *in vitro*, a factor of potential importance if the prescription of these drugs is contemplated in a patient with a previously detected breast cancer. Although disturbances such as galactorrhea, amenorrhea, gynecomastia, and impotence have been reported, the clinical significance of elevated serum prolactin levels is unknown for most patients. An increase in mammary neoplasms has been found in rodents after chronic administration of neuroleptic drugs. Neither clinical studies nor epidemiologic studies conducted to date, however, have shown an association between chronic administration of these drugs and mammary tumorigenesis; the available evidence is considered too limited to be conclusive at this time.

The antiemetic effect of fluphenazine hydrochloride may obscure signs of toxicity due to overdosage of other drugs, or render more difficult the diagnosis of disorders such as brain tumors or intestinal obstruction.

A significant, not otherwise explained, rise in body temperature may suggest individual intolerance to fluphenazine hydrochloride; in which case it should be discontinued.

Patients on large doses of a phenothiazine drug who are undergoing surgery should be watched carefully for possible hypotensive phenomena. Moreover, reduced amounts of anesthetics or central nervous system depressants may be necessary.

Since phenothiazines and central nervous system depressants (opiates, analgesics, antihistamines, barbiturates) can potentiate each other, less than the usual dosage of the added drug is recommended; caution is advised when they are administered concomitantly.

Use with caution in patients who are receiving atropine or related drugs because of additive anticholinergic effects and also in patients who will be exposed to extreme heat or phosphorus insecticides.

The use of alcohol should be avoided since additive effects and hypotension may occur. Patients should be cautioned that their response to alcohol may be increased while they are being treated with PERMITIL. The risk of suicide and the danger of overdose may be increased in patients who use alcohol excessively due to its potentiation of the drug's effect.

Blood counts and hepatic and renal functions should be checked periodically. The appearance of signs of blood dyscrasias requires the discontinuance of the drug and institution of appropriate therapy. If abnormalities in hepatic tests occur, phenothiazine treatment should be discontinued. Renal function in patients on long-term therapy should be monitored: if blood urea nitrogen (BUN) becomes abnormal, treatment with the drug should be discontinued.

The use of phenothiazine derivatives in patients with diminished renal function should be undertaken with caution.

Use with caution in patients suffering from respiratory impairment due to acute pulmonary infections, or in chronic respiratory disorders such as severe asthma or emphysema.

In general, phenothiazines, including fluphenazine hydrochloride, do not produce psychic dependence. Gastritis, nausea and vomiting, dizziness, and tremulousness have been reported following abrupt cessation of high-dose therapy. Reports suggest that these symptoms can be reduced by continuing concomitant antiparkinson agents for several weeks after the phenothiazine is withdrawn.

The possibility of liver damage, corneal and lenticular deposits, and irreversible dyskinesias should be kept in mind when patients are on long-term therapy.

Because photosensitivity has been reported, undue exposure to the sun should be avoided during phenothiazine treatment.

Information for Patients: This information is intended to aid in the safe and effective use of this medication. It is not a disclosure of all possible adverse or intended effects.

Given the likelihood that a substantial proportion of patients exposed chronically to neuroleptics will develop tardive dyskinesia, it is advised that all patients in whom chronic use is contemplated be given, if possible, full information about this risk. The decision to inform patients and/or their guardians must obviously take into account the clinical circumstances and the competency of the patient to understand the information provided.

ADVERSE REACTIONS

Not all of the following adverse reactions have been reported with this specific drug; however, pharmacological similarities among various phenothiazine derivatives require that each be considered. With the piperazine group (of which fluphenazine hydrochloride is an example), the extrapyramidal symptoms are more common, and others (e.g., sedative effects, jaundice, and blood dyscrasias) are less frequently seen.

CNS Effects: *Extrapyramidal reactions:* opisthotonus, trismus, torticollis, retrocollis, aching and numbness of the limbs, motor restlessness, oculogyric crisis, hyperreflexia, dystonia, including protrusion, discoloration, aching and rounding of the tongue, tonic spasm of the masticatory muscles, tight feeling in the throat, slurred speech, dysphagia, akathisia, dyskinesia, parkinsonism, and ataxia. Their incidence and severity usually increase with an increase in dosage, but there is considerable individual variation in the tendency to develop such symptoms. Extrapyramidal symptoms can usually be controlled by the concomitant use of effective antiparkinsonian drugs, such as benztropine mesylate, and/or by reduction in dosage. In some instances, however, these extrapyramidal reactions may persist after discontinuation of treatment with fluphenazine.

Persistent tardive dyskinesia: As with all antipsychotic agents, tardive dyskinesia may appear in some patients on long-term therapy or may appear after drug therapy has been discontinued. Although the risk appears to be greater in elderly patients on high-dose therapy, especially females, it may occur in either sex and in children. The symptoms are persistent and in some patients appear to be irreversible. The syndrome is characterized by rhythmical, involuntary movements of the tongue, face, mouth or jaw (e.g., protrusion of tongue, puffing of cheeks, puckering of mouth, chewing movements). Sometimes these may be accompanied by involuntary movements of the extremities. There is no known effective treatment for tardive dyskinesia; antiparkinsonism agents usually do not alleviate the symptoms of this syndrome. It is suggested that all antipsychotic agents be discontinued if these symptoms appear. Should it be necessary to reinstitute treatment, or increase the dosage of the agent, or switch to a different antipsychotic agent the syndrome may be masked. It has been reported that fine, vermicular movements of the tongue may be an early sign of the syndrome, and if the medication is stopped at that time the syndrome *may not* develop.

Other CNS effects: include cerebral edema; abnormality of cerebrospinal fluid proteins; convulsive seizures, particularly in patients with EEG abnormalities or a history of such disorders; and headaches.

Neuroleptic malignant syndrome has been reported in patients treated with neuroleptic drugs. It is a relatively uncommon, potentially lethal syndrome, characterized by severe extrapyramidal dysfunction, with rigidity and eventual stupor or coma; hyperthermia; and autonomic disturbances, including cardiovascular effects. There is no specific treatment; the neuroleptic drug should be stopped immediately.

Drowsiness may occur, particularly during the first or second week, after which it generally disappears. If troublesome, lower the dosage. Hypnotic effects appear to be minimal, especially in patients who are permitted to remain active.

Adverse behavioral effects include paradoxical exacerbation of psychotic symptoms, catatonic-like states, paranoid reactions, lethargy, paradoxical excitement, restlessness, hyperactivity, nocturnal confusion, bizarre dreams, and insomnia.

Hyperreflexia has been reported in the newborn when a phenothiazine was used during pregnancy.

Autonomic Effects: dry mouth or salivation, nausea, vomiting, diarrhea, anorexia, constipation, obstipation, fecal impaction, urinary retention, frequency or incontinence, bladder paralysis, polyuria, nasal congestion, pallor, myosis, mydriasis, blurred vision, glaucoma, perspiration, hypertension, hypotension, and change in pulse rate occasionally may occur. Significant autonomic effects have been infrequent in patients receiving less than 6 mg fluphenazine hydrochloride daily.

Adynamic ileus occasionally occurs with phenothiazine therapy and if severe, can result in complications and death. It is of particular concern in psychiatric patients who may fail to seek treatment of the condition.

Allergic Effects: urticaria, erythema, eczema, exfoliative dermatitis, pruritus, photosensitivity, asthma, fever, anaphylactoid reactions, laryngeal edema, and angioneurotic edema; contact dermatitis in nursing personnel administering the drug; and in extremely rare instances, individual idiosyncrasy or hypersensitivity to phenothiazines has resulted in cerebral edema, circulatory collapse, and death.

Endocrine Effects: lactation, galactorrhea, moderate breast enlargement in females and gynecomastia in males on large doses, disturbances in the menstrual cycle, amenorrhea, changes in libido, inhibition of ejaculation, syndrome of inappropriate ADH (antidiuretic hormone) secretion, false positive pregnancy tests, hyperglycemia, hypoglycemia, glycosuria.

Cardiovascular Effects: postural hypotension, tachycardia (especially with sudden marked increase in dosage), bradycardia, cardiac arrest, faintness, and dizziness. Occasionally the hypotensive effect may produce a shock-like condition. ECG changes, nonspecific, (quinidine-like effect) usually reversible, have been observed in some patients receiving phenothiazine tranquilizers.

Sudden death has occasionally been reported in patients who have received phenothiazines. In some cases the death was apparently due to cardiac arrest; in others, the cause appeared to be asphyxia due to failure of the cough reflex. In some patients, the cause could not be determined nor could it be established that the death was due to the phenothiazine.

Hematological Effects: agranulocytosis, eosinophilia, leukopenia, hemolytic anemia, thrombocytopenic purpura, and pancytopenia. Most cases of agranulocytosis have occurred between the fourth and tenth weeks of therapy. Patients should be watched closely especially during that period for the sudden appearance of sore throat or signs of infection. If white blood cell and differential cell counts show significant cellular depression, discontinue the drug and start appropriate therapy. However, a slightly lowered white count is not in itself an indication to discontinue the drug.

Other Effects: Special considerations in long-term therapy include pigmentation of the skin, occurring chiefly in the exposed areas; ocular changes consisting of deposition of fine particulate matter in the cornea and lens, progressing in more severe cases to star-shaped lenticular opacities; epithelial keratopathies; and pigmentary retinopathy. Also noted: peripheral edema, reversed epinephrine effect, increase in PBI not attributable to an increase in thyroxine, parotid swelling (rare), hyperpyrexia, systemic lupus erythematosus-like syndrome, increases in appetite and weight, polyphagia, photophobia, and muscle weakness.

Liver damage (biliary stasis) may occur. Jaundice may occur usually between the second and fourth weeks of treatment and is regarded as a hypersensitivity reaction. Incidence is low. The clinical picture resembles infectious hepatitis but with laboratory features of obstructive jaundice. It is usually reversible; however, chronic jaundice has been reported.

DOSAGE AND ADMINISTRATION

In all cases the smallest effective dose should be used. Doses should be initiated at a low level and increased gradually to determine clinical response. Patients who are acutely ill may respond to lower doses than those who are chronically ill. Acutely ill patients may require a rapid increase of dosage. Elderly and debilitated patients and adolescents may respond to low dosages. Outpatients should receive smaller dosages than are given to hospitalized patients who are under close supervision.

Adults: The total daily dose ranges from 0.5 mg to 10 mg and is usually administered in divided doses. In general, a daily dose in excess of 3 mg is rarely necessary. A dose in excess of 20 mg should be used with caution.

Administration of an adequate dose should be continued for sufficiently long periods in order to obtain maximum benefits. After maximum therapeutic response is obtained, dosage may be decreased gradually to the minimal effective maintenance dose.

Geriatric patients: Reduced dosage is usually recommended.

PERMITIL **Oral Concentrate** is a palatable liquid preparation, suitable for administration only with the following diluents: water, saline, Seven-Up, homogenized milk, carbonated orange beverage, and pineapple, apricot, prune, orange, V-8, tomato, and grapefruit juices.

PERMITIL **Oral Concentrate** should not be mixed with beverages containing caffeine (coffee, cola) tannics (tea), or pectinates (apple juice) since physical incompatability may result.

OVERDOSAGE

In the event of overdosage, emergency treatment should be started immediately. All patients suspected of having taken an overdose should be hospitalized as soon as possible.

Manifestations: Overdosage of fluphenazine hydrochloride primarily involves the extrapyramidal mechanism and produces the same side effects described under ADVERSE REACTIONS, but to a more marked degree. It is usually evidenced by stupor or coma; children may have convulsive seizures.

Treatment: Treatment is symptomatic and supportive. There is no specific antidote. The patient should be induced to vomit even if emesis has occurred spontaneously. Pharmacologic vomiting by the administration of ipecac syrup is a preferred method. It should be noted that ipecac has a central mode of action in addition to its local gastric irritant properties, and the central mode of action may be blocked by the antiemetic effect of PERMITIL.

Vomiting should not be induced in patients with impaired consciousness. The action of ipecac is facilitated by physical activity and by the administration of 8 to 12 fluid ounces of water. If emesis does not occur within 15 minutes, the dose of ipecac should be repeated. Precautions against aspiration must be taken, especially in infants and children. Following emesis, any drug remaining in the stomach may be adsorbed by activated charcoal administered as a slurry with water. If vomiting is unsuccessful or contraindicated, gastric lavage should be performed. Isotonic and one-half isotonic saline are the lavage solutions of choice. Saline cathartics, such as milk of magnesia, draw water into the bowel by osmosis and therefore may be valuable for their action in rapid dilution of bowel content.

Standard measures (oxygen, intravenous fluids, corticosteroids) should be used to manage circulatory shock or metabolic acidosis. An open airway and adequate fluid intake should be maintained. Body temperature should be regulated. Hypothermia is expected, but severe hyperthermia may occur and must be treated vigorously. (See CONTRAINDICATIONS.)

An electrocardiogram should be taken and close monitoring of cardiac function instituted if there is any sign of abnormality. Cardiac arthythmias may be treated with neostigmine, pyridostigmine, or propranolol. Digitalis should be considered for cardiac failure. Close monitoring of cardiac function is advisable for not less than five days. Vasopressors such as norepinephrine may be used to treat hypotension, but epinephrine should NOT be used.

Anticonvulsants (an inhalation anesthetic, diazepam or paraldehyde) are recommended for control of convulsions, since fluphenazine hydrochloride increases the central nervous system depressant action, but not the anticonvulsant action of barbiturates.

If acute parkinson-like symptoms result from fluphenazine hydrochloride intoxication, benztropine mesylate or diphenhydramine may be administered.

Central nervous system depression may be treated with nonconvulsant doses of CNS stimulants. Avoid stimulants that may cause convulsions (e.g., picrotoxin and pentylenetetrazol).

Signs of arousal may not occur for 48 hours.

Dialysis is of no value because of low plasma concentrations of the drug.

Since overdosage is often deliberate, patients may attempt suicide by other means during the recovery phase. Deaths by deliberate or accidental overdosage have occurred with this class of drugs.

HOW SUPPLIED

PERMITIL **Tablets,** 2.5 mg, compressed, scored, light orange, oval tablets impressed with the Schering trademark and product identification letters, WDR, or number, 442; bottle of 100 (NDC 0085-0442-04).

PERMITIL **Tablets,** 5 mg, compressed, scored, purple-pink, oval tablets impressed with the Schering trademark and product identification letters WFF, or number, 550; bottle of 100 (NDC 0085-0550-04).

PERMITIL **Tablets,** 10 mg, compressed, scored, light red, oval tablets impressed with the Schering trademark and product identification letters, WFG, or number, 316; bottle of 1000 (NDC 0085-0316-05).

PERMITIL **Oral Concentrate,** 5 mg per ml, a straw-colored, unflavored syrup containing alcohol 1%; bottle of 4 fluid ounces (118 ml), with dropper calibrated both in mg of fluphenazine hydrochloride and in ml of concentrate (NDC 0085-0296-05). **Protect from light and dispense only in amber bottles.**

Store PERMITIL Tablets and Oral Concentrate between 2° and 30°C (36° and 86°F).

Rev. 2/85

Shown in Product Identification Section, page 428

Continued on next page

Information on Schering products appearing on these pages is effective as of September 30, 1986.

Schering—Cont.

POLARAMINE® ℞
[*po-lar 'ah-mēn*]
brand of dexchlorpheniramine maleate
REPETABS® Tablets
Tablets, USP
Syrup, USP

DESCRIPTION

POLARAMINE products contain dexchlorpheniramine maleate, USP, an antihistamine having the formula, $C_{16}H_{19}ClN_2 \cdot C_4H_4O_4$, and a molecular weight of 390.87. Chemically, it is (+)-2-[*p*- Chloro-α-[2-(dimethylamino)ethyl] benzyl] pyridine maleate (1:1).

POLARAMINE **REPETABS** (brand of repeat-action tablets) **Tablets** (4 mg and 6 mg) contain, respectively, 2 or 3 mg dexchlorpheniramine maleate, USP in an outer layer for prompt effect and 2 or 3 mg, respectively, in an inner core for release three to six hours after ingestion.

The inactive ingredients for POLARAMINE **REPETABS** 4 mg include: acacia, butylparaben, calcium phosphate, calcium sulfate, carnauba wax, corn starch, diatomaceous earth, FD&C Red No. 40 Al Lake, FD&C Yellow No. 6 Al Lake, kaolin, lactose, magnesium stearate, neutral soap, oleic acid, potato starch, rosin, stearic acid, sugar, talc, white wax, and zein.

The inactive ingredients for POLARAMINE **REPETABS** 6 mg include: acacia, butylparaben, calcium phosphate, calcium sulfate, carnauba wax, corn starch, diatomaceous earth, FD&C Red No. 40 Al Lake, FD&C Yellow No. 6 Al Lake, kaolin, lactose, magnesium stearate, neutral soap, oleic acid, potato starch, rosin, stearic acid, sugar, talc, white wax, and zein.

POLARAMINE **Tablets** contain 2 mg dexchlorpheniramine maleate, USP. The inactive ingredients include: corn starch, D&C Red No. 27 Al Lake, D&C Red No. 30 Al Lake, FD&C Yellow No. 6 Al Lake, lactose, magnesium stearate, and potato starch.

POLARAMINE **Syrup** contains 2 mg dexchlorpheniramine maleate, USP per 5 ml. The inactive ingredients include: alcohol (6%), FD&C Red No. 40, FD&C Yellow No. 6, flavors, methylparaben, menthol, propylene glycol, propylparaben, sodium citrate, sodium chloride, sorbitol, sugar, and water.

Dexchlorpheniramine maleate is a white, odorless, crystalline powder which in aqueous solution has a pH of between 4 and 5. It is freely soluble in water, soluble in alcohol and in chloroform, but only slightly soluble in benzene or ether.

CLINICAL PHARMACOLOGY

POLARAMINE (dexchlorpheniramine maleate) is an antihistamine with anticholinergic properties. It is capable of producing a slight to moderate sedative effect. Antihistamines appear to compete with histamine for receptor sites on effector cells and are of value clinically in the prevention and relief of many allergic manifestations.

In vitro and *in vivo* assays of the antihistamine potencies of the optically active isomers of chlorpheniramine demonstrate that the predominant activity is in the dextro-isomer. The dextro-isomer is approximately two times more active than the racemic compound. Since dexchlorpheniramine is the dextro-isomer and active moiety of chlorpheniramine, it can be assumed that experience with chlorpheniramine also applies to dexchlorpheniramine.

Chlorpheniramine maleate 4 mg given to fasting human volunteers produced prompt blood levels after oral administration. Peak blood levels were approximately 7 ng/ml at an average time of 3 hours after administration. The half-life of chlorpheniramine maleate ranged from 20 to 24 hours. Following a single dose of tritium-labeled chlorpheniramine maleate to humans, the drug was found to be extensively metabolized whether given orally or by intravenous administration. The drug and metabolites were primarily excreted in the urine, with 19% of the dose appearing in 24 hours and a total of 34% in 48 hours.

Another study in volunteers has demonstrated that a **REPETABS Tablet** containing 12 mg chlorpheniramine maleate gives essentially identical plasma levels of drug as 12 mg of chlorpheniramine given in divided doses.

In a study in normal volunteers, a high flow rate of acidic urine resulted in a high excretion rate of chlorpheniramine maleate. Over a concentration range of 0.28 to 1.24 mcg/ml of plasma, chlorpheniramine maleate was 72 to 69% bound to plasma protein, respectively.

INDICATIONS AND USAGE

POLARAMINE is indicated for the treatment of perennial and seasonal allergic rhinitis; vasomotor rhinitis; allergic conjunctivitis; mild, uncomplicated allergic skin manifestations of urticaria and angioedema; amelioration of allergic reactions to blood or plasma; and dermographism. They are also indicated as therapy for anaphylactic reactions adjunctive to epinephrine and other standard measures after the acute manifestations have been controlled.

CONTRAINDICATIONS

Hypersensitivity to dexchlorpheniramine maleate or other antihistamines of similar chemical structure contraindicates the use of POLARAMINE.

Drug products containing dexchlorpheniramine maleate should not be used in newborn or premature infants because of the possibility of severe reactions such as convulsions.

Antihistamines *should not* be used to treat lower respiratory tract symptoms. Antihistamines are also contraindicated for use in conjunction with monoamine oxidase inhibitor therapy.

WARNINGS

Dexchlorpheniramine, as with all antihistamines, should be used with caution in patients with narrow angle glaucoma, stenosing peptic ulcer, pyloroduodenal obstruction, symptomatic prostatic hypertrophy, and bladder neck obstruction.

Overdoses of antihistamines may cause hallucinations, convulsions, or death, especially in infants and children.

Products containing dexchlorpheniramine maleate have additive effects with alcohol and other CNS depressants (hypnotics, sedatives, tranquilizers, etc.). Patients should not engage in activities requiring mental alertness, such as driving a car or operating machinery.

Antihistamines are more likely to cause dizziness, sedation, and hypotension in elderly patients (approximately 60 years or older).

PRECAUTIONS

General: Dexchlorpheniramine maleate has an atropine-like action and therefore products containing it should be used with caution in patients with: a history of bronchial asthma; increased intraocular pressure; hyperthyroidism; cardiovascular disease; hypertension.

Information for Patients:

1. Dexchlorpheniramine may cause slight to moderate drowsiness.
2. Patients should not engage in activities requiring mental alertness, such as driving or operating machinery.
3. Alcohol or other sedative drugs may enhance the drowsiness caused by antihistamines.
4. Patients should not take POLARAMINE in conjunction with a monoamine oxidase inhibitor or oral anticoagulant.

Drug Interactions: Dexchlorpheniramine maleate may cause severe hypotension when given in conjunction with a monoamine oxidase inhibitor.

Alcohol and other sedative drugs will potentiate the sedative effects of dexchlorpheniramine. (See WARNINGS.)

The action of oral anticoagulants may be inhibited by antihistamines.

Carcinogenesis, Mutagenesis, Impairment of Fertility: Although there have been no oncogenic or mutagenic studies on dexchlorpheniramine, a 103-week oncogenic study in rats on the racemic mixture, chlorpheniramine, did not produce an increase in the incidence of tumors in the drug-treated groups, as compared with the controls.

An Ames mutagenicity test performed on chlorpheniramine and its nitrosation product was negative. An early study in rats with chlorpheniramine maleate revealed a reduction in fertility in female rats at doses approximately 67 times the human dose. More recent studies in rabbits and rats, using more appropriate methodology and doses up to approximately 50 and 85 times the human dose, showed no reduction in fertility in the animals.

Pregnancy Category B: Reproduction studies have been performed in rabbits and rats at doses up to 50 times and 85 times the human dose, respectively, and have revealed no evidence of harm to the fetus due to chlorpheniramine maleate. (See above, "*Impairment of Fertility.*") There are, however, no adequate and well-controlled studies in pregnant women. Because animal reproduction studies are not always predictive of human response, this drug should be used during the first two trimesters of pregnancy only if clearly needed. Dexchlorpheniramine maleate should not be used in the third trimester of pregnancy because newborn and premature infants may have severe reactions to antihistamines. (See CONTRAINDICATIONS.)

Nonteratogenic Effects: Studies of chlorpheniramine maleate done in rats revealed a decrease in the postnatal survival rate of pups of animals dosed with 33 and 67 times the human dose.

Nursing Mothers: It is not known whether this drug is excreted in human milk. Because certain other antihistamines are known to be excreted in human milk, and because dexchlorpheniramine maleate is contraindicated in newborn and premature infants, caution should be exercised when it is administered to a nursing woman.

Pediatric Use: Safety and effectiveness of the 4 and 6 mg **REPETABS Tablets** in children below the ages of 6 and 12 years, respectively, have not been established. Safety and effectiveness of the **Tablets** and **Syrup** in children below the age of 2 years have not been established.

ADVERSE REACTIONS

Slight to moderate drowsiness is the most frequent side effect of dexchlorpheniramine maleate. Other possible side effects of antihistamines include:

General: urticaria, drug rash, anaphylactic shock, photosensitivity, excessive perspiration, chills, dryness of mouth, nose, and throat.

Cardiovascular System: headache, palpitations, tachycardia, extrasystoles, hypotension.

Hematologic System: hemolytic anemia, hypoplastic anemia, thrombocytopenia, agranulocytosis.

Nervous System: sedation, dizziness, vertigo, tinnitus, acute labyrinthitis, disturbed coordination, fatigue, confusion, restlessness, excitation, nervousness, tremor, irritability, insomnia, euphoria, paresthesias, blurred vision, hysteria, neuritis, convulsions.

Gastrointestinal System: epigastric distress, anorexia, nausea, vomiting, diarrhea, constipation.

Genitourinary System: urinary frequency, difficult urination, urinary retention, early menses.

Respiratory System: thickening of bronchial secretions, tightness of chest, wheezing, nasal stuffiness.

OVERDOSAGE

In the event of overdosage, emergency treatment should be started immediately.

Manifestations of antihistamine overdosage may vary from central nervous system depression (sedation, apnea, diminished mental alertness, cardiovascular collapse) to stimulation (insomnia, hallucinations, tremors, or convulsions) to death. Other signs and symptoms may be dizziness, tinnitus, ataxia, blurred vision, and hypotension. Stimulation is particularly likely in children, as are atropine-like signs and symptoms (dry mouth; fixed, dilated pupils; flushing; hyperthermia; and gastrointestinal symptoms).

Treatment—The patient should be induced to vomit, even if emesis has occurred spontaneously. Pharmacologic vomiting by the administration of ipecac syrup is a preferred method. However, vomiting should not be induced in patients with impaired consciousness. The action of ipecac is facilitated by physical activity and by the administration of eight to twelve fluid ounces of water. If emesis does not occur within fifteen minutes, the dose of ipecac should be repeated. Precautions against aspiration must be taken, especially in infants and children. Following emesis, any drug remaining in the stomach may be adsorbed by activated charcoal administered as a slurry with water. If vomiting is unsuccessful or contraindicated, gastric lavage should be performed. Isotonic and one-half isotonic saline are the lavage solutions of choice. Saline cathartics, such as milk of magnesia, draw water into the bowel by osmosis and therefore may be valuable for their action in rapid dilution of bowel content. Dialysis is of little value in antihistamine poisoning. After emergency treatment, the patient should continue to be medically monitored. Treatment of the signs and symptoms of overdosage is symptomatic and supportive. *Stimulants* (analeptic agents) should *not* be used. Vasopressors may be used to treat hypotension. Short-acting barbiturates, diazepam, or paraldehyde may be administered to control seizures. Hyperpyrexia, especially in children, may require treatment with tepid water sponge baths or a hypothermic blanket. Apnea is treated with ventilatory support.

In mice, the oral LD_{50} of dexchlorpheniramine is 258 mg/kg. In humans, the estimated lethal dose of racemic chlorpheniramine is 5 to 10 mg/kg. Thus a dose of 2.5 to 5 mg/kg of dexchlorpheniramine should be similarly regarded.

DOSAGE AND ADMINISTRATION

DOSAGE SHOULD BE INDIVIDUALIZED ACCORDING TO THE NEEDS AND RESPONSE OF THE PATIENT.

POLARAMINE **REPETABS Tablets**—*Adults and children 12 years or older:* one 4 or 6 mg POLARAMINE **REPETABS** Tablet at bedtime or every 8 to 10 hours during the day.

Children 6 to 12 years: one 4 mg **REPETABS** Tablet daily, taken preferably at bedtime.

POLARAMINE **Tablets**—*Adults and children 12 years of age and over:* one tablet every 4 to 6 hours. *Children 6 through 11 years:* one-half tablet every 4 to 6 hours. *Children 2 through 5 years:* one-quarter tablet every 4 to 6 hours.

POLARAMINE **Syrup**—*Adults and children 12 years of age and over:* 1 teaspoonful (2 mg) every 4 to 6 hours. *Children 6 through 11 years:* one-half teaspoonful (1 mg) every 4 to 6 hours. *Children 2 through 5 years:* one-quarter teaspoonful (½ mg) every 4 to 6 hours.

HOW SUPPLIED

POLARAMINE **REPETABS Tablets**, 4 mg, light red, sugar-coated, oval tablets branded in blue-black with the Schering trademark and product identification letters, AGA, or number, 095; bottle of 100.

POLARAMINE **REPETABS Tablets**, 6 mg, bright red, sugar-coated, oval tablets branded in white with the Schering trademark and product identification letters, AGB, or number, 148; bottles of 100 and 1000.

POLARAMANE **Tablets**, 2 mg, red, compressed, oval tablets impressed with the Schering trademark and either product identification letters, AGT, or number, 820; bottle of 100.
POLARAMINE **Syrup**, 2 mg per 5 ml, red-orange-colored, orange-like flavored liquid; 16-fluid ounce (473 ml) bottle.
Store POLARAMINE between 2° and 30°C (36° and 86°F).

Rev. 11/85
Shown in Product Identification Section, page 428

PROVENTIL® Inhaler ℞
[pro-ven 'tĭl]
brand of albuterol
Bronchodilator Aerosol
FOR ORAL INHALATION ONLY

DESCRIPTION

The active component of PROVENTIL Inhaler is albuterol (α^1-[(*tert*-butylamino)methyl] -4- hydroxy- *m* -xylene-α, α'-diol), a relatively selective beta$_2$-adrenergic bronchodilator. Albuterol is the official generic name in the United States. The international generic name for the drug is salbutamol. The molecular weight of albuterol is 239.3, and the empirical formula is $C_{13}H_{21}NO_3$. Albuterol is a white to off-white crystalline solid. It is soluble in ethanol, sparingly soluble in water, and very soluble in chloroform.
PROVENTIL Inhaler is a metered-dose aerosol unit for oral inhalation. It contains a microcrystalline suspension of albuterol in propellants (trichloromonofluoromethane and dichlorodifluoromethane) with oleic acid. Each actuation delivers from the mouthpiece 90 mcg of albuterol. Each canister provides at least 200 inhalations.

CLINICAL PHARMACOLOGY

The prime action of beta-adrenergic drugs is to stimulate adenyl cyclase, the enzyme which catalyzes the formation of cyclic-3′,5′-adenosine monophosphate (cyclic AMP) from adenosine triphosphate (ATP). The cyclic AMP thus formed mediates the cellular responses. By virtue of its relatively selective action on beta$_2$- adrenoceptors, albuterol relaxes smooth muscle of the bronchi, uterus, and vascular supply to skeletal muscle, but may have less cardiac stimulant effects than does isoproterenol.
Albuterol is longer acting than isoproterenol by any route of administration in most patients because it is not a substrate for the cellular uptake processes for catecholamines nor for catechol-*O*-methyl transferase.
Because of its gradual absorption from the bronchi, systemic levels of albuterol are low after inhalation of recommended doses. Studies undertaken with four subjects administered tritiated albuterol, resulted in maximum plasma concentrations occurring within two to four hours. Due to the sensitivity of the assay method, the metabolic rate and half-life of elimination of albuterol in plasma could not be determined. However, urinary excretion provided data indicating that albuterol has an elimination half-life of 3.8 hours. Approximately 72 percent of the inhaled dose is excreted within 24 hours in the urine, and consists of 28 percent of unchanged drug and 44 percent as metabolite.
Results of animal studies show that albuterol does not pass the blood-brain barrier.
The effects of rising doses of albuterol and isoproterenol aerosols were studied in volunteers and asthmatic patients. Results in normal volunteers indicated that albuterol is ½ to ¼ as active as isoproterenol in producing increases in heart rate. In asthmatic patients similar cardiovascular differentiation between the two drugs was also seen.

INDICATIONS AND USAGE

PROVENTIL Inhaler is indicated for the prevention and relief of bronchospasm in patients with reversible obstructive airway disease, and for the prevention of exercise-induced bronchospasm.
In controlled clinical trials the onset of improvement in pulmonary function was within 15 minutes, as determined by both maximal midexpiratory flow rate (MMEF) and FEV$_1$. MMEF measurements also showed that near maximum improvement in pulmonary function generally occurs within 60 to 90 minutes following 2 inhalations of albuterol and that clinically significant improvement generally continues for 3 to 4 hours in most patients. In clinical trials, some patients with asthma showed a therapeutic response (defined by maintaining FEV$_1$ values 15 percent or more above baseline) which was still apparent at 6 hours. Continued effectiveness of albuterol was demonstrated over a 13-week period in these same trials.
In clinical studies, 2 inhalations of albuterol taken approximately 15 minutes prior to exercise, prevented exercise-induced bronchospasm, as demonstrated by the maintenance of FEV$_1$ within 80 percent of baseline values in the majority of patients. One of these studies also evaluated the duration of the prophylactic effect to repeated exercise challenges, which was evident at 4 hours in the majority of patients, and at 6 hours in approximately one third of the patients.

CONTRAINDICATIONS

PROVENTIL Inhaler is contraindicated in patients with a history of hypersensitivity to any of its components.

WARNINGS

As with other adrenergic aerosols, the potential for paradoxical bronchospasm should be kept in mind. If it occurs, the preparation should be discontinued immediately and alternative therapy instituted.
Fatalities have been reported in association with excessive use of inhaled sympathomimetic drugs. The exact cause of death is unknown, but cardiac arrest following the unexpected development of a severe acute asthmatic crisis and subsequent hypoxia is suspected.
The contents of PROVENTIL Inhaler are under pressure. Do not puncture. Do not use or store near heat or open flame. Exposure to temperatures above 120°F may cause bursting. Never throw container into fire or incinerator. Keep out of reach of children.

PRECAUTIONS

Although it has less effect on the cardiovascular system than isoproterenol at recommended dosages, albuterol is a sympathomimetic amine and as such should be used with caution in patients with cardiovascular disorders, including coronary insufficiency and hypertension, in patients with hyperthyroidism or diabetes mellitus, and in patients who are unusually responsive to sympathomimetic amines.
Large doses of intravenous albuterol have been reported to aggravate preexisting diabetes and ketoacidosis. The relevance of this observation to the use of PROVENTIL Inhaler is unknown, since the aerosol dose is much lower than the doses given intravenously.
Although there have been no reports concerning the use of PROVENTIL Inhaler during labor and delivery, it has been reported that high doses of albuterol administered intravenously inhibit uterine contractions. Although this effect is extremely unlikely as a consequence of aerosol use, it should be kept in mind.
Information For Patients: The action of PROVENTIL Inhaler may last up to six hours and therefore it should not be used more frequently than recommended. Increasing the number or frequency of doses without consulting your physician can be dangerous. If recommended dosage does not provide relief of symptoms or symptoms become worse, seek immediate medical attention. While taking PROVENTIL Inhaler, other inhaled medicines should not be used unless prescribed.
See Illustrated Patient Instructions For Use.
Drug Interactions: Other sympathomimetic aerosol bronchodilators should not be used concomitantly with albuterol. If additional adrenergic drugs are to be administered by any route, they should be used with caution to avoid deleterious cardiovascular effects.
Albuterol should be administered with caution to patients being treated with monoamine oxidase inhibitors or tricyclic antidepressants, since the action of albuterol on the vascular system may be potentiated.
Beta-receptor blocking agents and albuterol inhibit the effect of each other.
Carcinogenesis, Mutagenesis, and Impairment of Fertility: In a 2 year study in the rat, albuterol sulfate caused a significant dose-related increase in the incidence of benign leiomyomas of the mesovarium at doses corresponding to 111, 555, and 2,800 times the maximum human inhalational dose. In another study this effect was blocked by the coadministration of propranolol. The relevance of these findings to humans is not known. An 18-month study in mice revealed no evidence of tumorigenicity. Studies with albuterol revealed no evidence of mutagenesis. Reproduction studies in rats revealed no evidence of impaired fertility.
Teratogenic Effects — Pregnancy Category C: Albuterol has been shown to be teratogenic in mice when given in doses corresponding to 14 times the human dose. There are no adequate and well-controlled studies in pregnant women. Albuterol should be used during pregnancy only if the potential benefit justifies the potential risk to the fetus. A reproduction study in CD-1 mice with albuterol (0.025, 0.25, and 2.5 mg/kg, corresponding to 1.4, 14, and 140 times the maximum human inhalational dose) showed cleft palate formation in 5 of 111 (4.5 percent) fetuses at 0.25 mg/kg and in 10 of 108 (9.3 percent) fetuses at 2.5 mg/kg. None were observed at 0.025 mg/kg. Cleft palate also occurred in 22 of 72 (30.5 percent) fetuses treated with 2.5 mg/kg isoproterenol (positive control). A reproduction study in Stride Dutch rabbits revealed cranioschisis in 7 of 19 (37 percent) fetuses at 50 mg/kg, corresponding to 2,800 times the maximum human inhalational dose.
Nursing Mothers: It is not known whether this drug is excreted in human milk. Because of the potential for tumorigenicity shown for albuterol in animal studies, a decision should be made whether to discontinue nursing or to discontinue the drug, taking into account the importance of the drug to the mother.
Pediatric Use: Safety and effectiveness in children below the age of 12 years have not been established.

ADVERSE REACTIONS

The adverse reactions of albuterol are similar in nature to those of other sympathomimetic agents, although the incidence of certain cardiovascular effects is less with albuterol. A 13-week double-blind study compared albuterol and isoproterenol aerosols in 147 asthmatic patients. The results of this study showed that the incidence of cardiovascular effects was: palpitations, less than 10 per 100 with albuterol and less than 15 per 100 with isoproterenol; tachycardia, 10 per 100 with both albuterol and isoproterenol; and increased blood pressure, less than 5 per 100 with both albuterol and isoproterenol. In the same study, both drugs caused tremor or nausea in less than 15 patients per 100; dizziness or heartburn in less than 5 per 100 patients. Nervousness occurred in less than 10 per 100 patients receiving albuterol and in less than 15 per 100 patients receiving isoproterenol. Rare cases of urticaria, angioedema, rash, bronchospasm and oropharyngeal edema have been reported after the use of inhaled albuterol.
In addition, albuterol, like other sympathomimetic agents, can cause adverse reactions such as hypertension, angina, vomiting, vertigo, central nervous system stimulation, insomnia, headache, unusual taste, and drying or irritation of the oropharynx.

OVERDOSAGE

Exaggeration of the effects listed in ADVERSE REACTIONS can occur. Anginal pain and hypertension may result.
As with all sympathomimetic aerosol medications, cardiac arrest and even death may be associated with abuse.
The oral LD$_{50}$ in male and female rats and mice was greater than 2,000 mg/kg. The aerosol LD$_{50}$ could not be determined. Dialysis is not appropriate treatment for overdosage of PROVENTIL Inhaler. The judicious use of a cardioselective beta-receptor blocker, such as metoprolol tartrate, is suggested, bearing in mind the danger of inducing an asthmatic attack.

DOSAGE AND ADMINISTRATION

For treatment of acute episodes of bronchospasm or prevention of asthmatic symptoms, the usual dosage for adults and children 12 years and older is 2 inhalations repeated every 4 to 6 hours; in some patients, 1 inhalation every 4 hours may be sufficient. More frequent administration or a larger number of inhalations is not recommended. For maintenance therapy or prevention of exacerbation of bronchospasm, 2 inhalations, 4 times a day should be sufficient. The use of PROVENTIL Inhaler can be continued as medically indicated to control recurring bouts of bronchospasm. During this time most patients gain optimal benefit from regular use of the inhaler. Safe usage for periods extending over several years has been documented.
If a previously effective dosage regimen fails to provide the usual relief, medical advice should be sought immediately as this is often a sign of seriously worsening asthma which would require reassessment of therapy.
Exercise-Induced Bronchospasm Prevention: The usual dosage for adults and children 12 years and older is 2 inhalations, 15 minutes prior to exercise.
For treatment, see above.

HOW SUPPLIED

PROVENTIL Inhaler, 17.0 g canister; box of one. Each actuation delivers 90 mcg of albuterol from the mouthpiece. It is supplied with an oral adapter and patient's instructions (NDC-0085-0614-02). PROVENTIL Inhaler REFILL canister, 17.0g, with patient's instructions; box of one (NDC-0085-0614-03).
Store between 15° and 30°C (59° and 86°F). Shake well before using.

Revised 2/86
Shown in Product Identification Section, page 428

PROVENTIL® ℞
brand of albuterol sulfate
Syrup

DESCRIPTION

PROVENTIL Syrup contains albuterol sulfate, a relatively selective beta$_2$-adrenergic bronchodilator. Albuterol sulfate has the chemical name α^1-[(*tert*-Butylamino)methyl]-4-hydroxy-*m*-xylene-α,α'-diol sulfate (2:1) (salt).
Albuterol sulfate has a molecular weight of 576.7 and the empirical formula $(C_{13}H_{21}NO_3)_2 \cdot H_2SO_4$. Albuterol sulfate is a white crystalline powder, soluble in water and slightly soluble in ethanol.
The international generic name for albuterol base is salbutamol.

Continued on next page

Information on Schering products appearing on these pages is effective as of September 30, 1986.

Schering—Cont.

PROVENTIL Syrup contains 2 mg of albuterol as 2.4 mg of albuterol sulfate in each teaspoonful (5 ml).
The inactive ingredients for Proventil Syrup include: citric acid, FD&C Yellow No. 6, flavor, hydroxypropyl methylcellulose, saccharin, sodium benzoate, sodium citrate and water.

CLINICAL PHARMACOLOGY

The prime action of beta-adrenergic drugs is to stimulate adenyl cyclase, the enzyme which catalyzes the formation of cyclic-3′,5′-adenosine monophosphate (cyclic AMP) from adenosine triphosphate (ATP). The cyclic AMP thus formed mediates the cellular responses. Based on pharmacologic studies in animals, albuterol appears to exert direct and preferential action on $beta_2$-adrenoceptors including those of the bronchial tree and uterus, and may have less cardiac stimulant effect than isoproterenol, when given in the usual recommended dose.
Albuterol is longer acting than isoproterenol in most patients by any route of administration because it is not a substrate for the cellular uptake processes for catecholamines nor for catechol-*O*-methyl transferase.
After oral administration of 10 ml PROVENTIL Syrup (4 mg albuterol) in normal volunteers, albuterol is rapidly absorbed. Maximum plasma albuterol concentrations of about 18 ng/ml are achieved within 2 hours and the drug is eliminated with a half-life of about 5 hours. In other studies, the analysis of urine samples of patients given 8 mg tritiated albuterol orally showed that 76% of the dose was excreted over 3 days, with the majority of the dose being excreted within the first 24 hours. Sixty percent of this radioactivity was shown to be the metabolite. Feces collected over this period contained 4% of the administered dose.
Animal studies show that albuterol does not pass the blood-brain barrier.

INDICATIONS AND USAGE

PROVENTIL Syrup is indicated for the relief of bronchospasm in adults and in children 2 years of age and older with reversible obstructive airway disease.
In controlled clinical trials in patients with asthma, the onset of improvement in pulmonary function, as measured by maximal midexpiratory flow rate (MMEF) and forced expiratory volume in one second (FEV_1), was within 30 minutes after a dose of PROVENTIL Syrup. Peak improvement of pulmonary function occurred between 2 to 3 hours. In a controlled clinical trial involving 55 children, clinically significant improvement (defined as maintenance of mean values over baseline of 15% or 20% or more in the FEV_1 and MMEF respectively) continued to be recorded up to 6 hours. No decrease in the effectiveness was reported in one uncontrolled study of 32 children who took PROVENTIL Syrup for a 3 month period.

CONTRAINDICATIONS

PROVENTIL Syrup is contraindicated in patients with a history of hypersensitivity to any of its components.

PRECAUTIONS

General: Although albuterol usually has minimal effects on the $beta_1$-adrenoceptors of the cardiovascular system at the recommended dosage, occasionally the usual cardiovascular and CNS stimulatory effects common to all sympathomimetic agents have been seen with patients treated with albuterol necessitating discontinuation. Therefore, albuterol should be used with caution in patients with cardiovascular disorders, including coronary insufficiency and hypertension, in patients with hyperthyroidism or diabetes mellitus, and in patients who are unusually responsive to sympathomimetic amines.
Large doses of intravenous albuterol have been reported to aggravate preexisting diabetes mellitus and ketoacidosis. Additionally, albuterol and other beta-agonists, when given intravenously, may cause a decrease in serum potassium, possibly through intracellular shunting. The decrease is usually transient, not requiring supplementation. The relevance of these observations to the use of PROVENTIL Syrup is unknown.
Information for Patients: The action of PROVENTIL Syrup may last up to six hours and therefore it should not be taken more frequently than recommended. Do not increase the dose or frequency of medication without medical consultation. If symptoms get worse, medical consultation should be sought promptly.
Drug Interactions: The concomitant use of PROVENTIL Syrup and other oral sympathomimetic agents is not recommended since such combined use may lead to deleterious cardiovascular effects. This recommendation does not preclude the judicious use of an aerosol bronchodilator of the adrenergic stimulant type in patients receiving PROVENTIL Syrup. Such concomitant use, however, should be individualized and not given on a routine basis. If regular coadministration is required, then alternative therapy should be considered.
Albuterol should be administered with extreme caution to patients being treated with monoamine oxidase inhibitors or tricyclic antidepressants since the action of albuterol on the vascular system may be potentiated.
Beta-receptor blocking agents and albuterol inhibit the effect of each other.
Carcinogenesis, Mutagenesis, and Impairment of Fertility: Albuterol sulfate, like other agents in its class, caused a significant dose-related increase in the incidence of benign leiomyomas of the mesovarium in a 2-year study in the rat, at doses corresponding to 2, 9, and 46 times the maximum human (child weighing 21 kg) oral dose. In another study this effect was blocked by the coadministration of propranolol. The relevance of these findings to humans is not known. An 18-month study in mice and a lifetime study in hamsters revealed no evidence of tumorigenicity. Studies with albuterol revealed no evidence in mutagenesis. Reproduction studies in rats revealed no evidence of impaired fertility.
Teratogenic Effects—Pregnancy Category C: Albuterol has been shown to be teratogenic in mice when given subcutaneously in doses corresponding to 0.2 times the maximum human (child weighing 21 kg) oral dose. There are no adequate and well-controlled studies in pregnant women. Albuterol should be used during pregnancy only if the potential benefit justifies the potential risk to the fetus. A reproduction study in CD-1 mice with albuterol showed cleft palate formation in 5 of 111 (4.5%) fetuses at 0.25 mg/kg and in 10 of 108 (9.3%) fetuses at 2.5 mg/kg; none was observed at 0.025 mg/kg. Cleft palate also occurred in 22 of 72 (30.5%) fetuses treated with 2.5 mg/kg isoproterenol (positive control). A reproduction study in Stride Dutch rabbits revealed cranioschisis in 7 of 19 (37%) fetuses at 50 mg/kg, corresponding to 46 times the maximum human (child weighing 21 kg) oral dose of albuterol sulfate.
Labor and Delivery: Oral albuterol has been shown to delay preterm labor in some reports. There are presently no well-controlled studies which demonstrate that it will stop preterm labor or prevent labor at term. Therefore, cautious use of PROVENTIL Syrup is required in pregnant patients when given for relief of bronchospasm so as to avoid interference with uterine contractibility. Use in such patients should be restricted to those patients in whom the benefits clearly outweigh the risks.
Nursing Mothers: It is not known whether this drug is excreted in human milk. Because of the potential for tumorigenicity shown for albuterol in animal studies, a decision should be made whether to discontinue nursing or to discontinue the drug, taking into account the importance of the drug to the mother.
Pediatric Use: Safety and effectiveness in children below the age of 2 years have not yet been adequately demonstrated.

ADVERSE REACTIONS

The adverse reactions to albuterol are similar in nature to those of other sympathomimetic agents. The most frequent adverse reactions to PROVENTIL Syrup in adults and older children were tremor, 10 of 100 patients; nervousness and shakiness, each 9 of 100 patients. Other reported adverse reactions were headache, 4 of 100 patients; dizziness and increased appetite, each 3 of 100 patients; hyperactivity and excitement, each 2 of 100 patients; tachycardia, epistaxis, irritable behavior, and sleeplessness, each 1 of 100 patients. The following adverse effects occurred in less than 1 of 100 patients each: muscle spasm; disturbed sleep, epigastric pain; cough; palpitations; stomach ache; irritable behavior; dilated pupils; sweating; chest pain; weakness.
In young children 2 to 6 years of age, some adverse reactions were noted more frequently than in adults and older children. Excitement was noted in approximately 20% of patients and nervousness in 15%. Hyperkinesia occurred in 4% of patients; insomnia, tachycardia, and gastrointestinal symptoms in 2% each. Anorexia, emotional lability, pallor, fatigue, and conjunctivitis were seen in 1%.
In addition, albuterol, like other sympathomimetic agents, can cause adverse reactions such as hypertension, angina, vomiting, vertigo, central nervous system stimulation, unusual taste, and drying or irritation of the oropharynx.
The reactions are generally transient in nature, and it is usually not necessary to discontinue treatment with PROVENTIL Syrup. In selected cases, however, dosage may be reduced temporarily; after the reaction has subsided, dosage should be increased in small increments to the optimal dosage.

OVERDOSAGE

Manifestations of overdosage include anginal pain, hypertension, hypokalemia, and exaggeration of the effects listed in **Adverse Reactions.**
The oral LD_{50} in rats and mice was greater than 2,000 mg/kg. Dialysis is not appropriate treatment for overdosage of PROVENTIL Syrup. The judicious use of a cardioselective beta-receptor blocker, such as metoprolol tartrate, is suggested, bearing in mind the danger of inducing an asthmatic attack.

DOSAGE AND ADMINISTRATION

The following dosages of PROVENTIL Syrup are expressed in terms of albuterol base.
Usual Dose: The usual starting dosage for adults and children over age 14 is 2 mg (1 teaspoonful) or 4 mg (2 teaspoonfuls) three or four times a day.
The usual starting dosage for children 6 to 14 years of age is 2 mg (1 teaspoonful) three or four times a day.
For children 2 to 6 years of age, dosing should be initiated at 0.1 mg/kg of body weight three times a day. This starting dose should not exceed 2 mg (1 teaspoonful) three times a day.
Dosage Adjustment: For adults and children above age 14, dosage above 4 mg four times a day should be used *only* when the patient fails to respond. If a favorable response does not occur, the dosage may be cautiously increased stepwise, but not to exceed 8 mg four times a day.
For children from 6 to 14 years of age who fail to respond to the initial starting dosage of 2 mg four times a day, the dosage may be cautiously increased stepwise, but not to exceed 24 mg per day (given in divided doses).
For children 2 to 6 years of age who do not respond satisfactorily to the initial dosage, the dose may be increased stepwise to 0.2 mg/kg of body weight three times a day, but not to exceed a maximum of 4 mg (2 teaspoonfuls) given three times a day.
For elderly patients and those sensitive to beta-adrenergic stimulation, the initial dose should be restricted to 2 mg three or four times a day and individually adjusted thereafter.

HOW SUPPLIED

PROVENTIL Syrup, a clear orange-yellow liquid with a strawberry flavor, contains 2 mg albuterol as the sulfate per 5 ml, bottles of 16 fluid ounces (NDC 0085-0315-02).
Store between 2° and 30°C (36° and 86°F).
Revised 1/86

PROVENTIL® ℞

[*pro-ven 'til*]
brand of albuterol sulfate
Tablets

DESCRIPTION

PROVENTIL Tablets contain albuterol sulfate, a relatively selective $beta_2$-adrenergic bronchodilator. Albuterol sulfate has the chemical name α^1-[(*tert*-Butylamino) methyl]-4-hydroxy-*m*-xylene-α,α'-diol sulfate (2:1) (salt).
Albuterol sulfate has a molecular weight of 576.7 and the empirical formula $(C_{13}H_{21}NO_3)_2 \cdot H_2SO_4$. Albuterol sulfate is a white crystalline powder, soluble in water and slightly soluble in ethanol.
The international generic name for albuterol base is salbutamol.
Each PROVENTIL Tablet contains 2 or 4 mg of albuterol as 2.4 and 4.8 mg of albuterol sulfate, respectively.
The inactive ingredients for PROVENTIL Tablets 2 and 4 mg include: calcium sulfate, corn starch and magnesium stearate.

CLINICAL PHARMACOLOGY

The prime action of beta-adrenergic drugs is to stimulate adenyl cyclase, the enzyme which catalyzes the formation of cyclic-3′,5′-adenosine monophosphate (cyclic AMP) from adenosine triphosphate (ATP). The cyclic AMP thus formed mediates the cellular responses. Based on pharmacologic studies in animals, albuterol appears to exert direct and preferential action on $beta_2$-adrenoceptors including those of the bronchial tree and uterus, and may have less cardiac stimulant effect than isoproterenol, when given in the usual recommended dose.
Albuterol is longer acting than isoproterenol in most patients by any route of administration because it is not a substrate for the cellular uptake processes for catecholamines nor for catechol-*O*-methyl transferase.
Albuterol is rapidly absorbed after oral administration of 4 mg PROVENTIL Tablets in normal volunteers. Maximum plasma albuterol concentrations of about 18ng/ml are achieved within 2 hours and the drug is eliminated with a half-life of about 5 hours. In other studies, the analysis of urine samples of patients given 8 mg tritiated albuterol orally showed that 76% of the dose was excreted over 3 days, with the majority of the dose being excreted within the first 24 hours. Sixty percent of this radioactivity was shown to be the metabolite. Feces collected over this period contained 4% of the administered dose.
Animal studies show that albuterol does not pass the blood-brain barrier.

INDICATIONS AND USAGE

PROVENTIL Tablets are indicated for the relief of bronchospasm in patients with reversible obstructive airway disease.

In controlled clinical trials in patients with asthma, the onset of improvement in pulmonary function, as measured by maximal midexpiratory flow rate, MMEF, was noted within 30 minutes after a dose of PROVENTIL Tablets with peak improvement occurring between 2 to 3 hours. In controlled clinical trials in which measurements were conducted for 6 hours, significant clinical improvement in pulmonary function (defined as maintaining a 15% or more increase in FEV_1 and a 20% or more increase in MMEF over baseline values) was observed in 60% of patients at 4 hours and in 40% at 6 hours. In other single dose controlled clinical trials, clinically significant improvement was observed in at least 40% of the patients at 8 hours. No decrease in the effectiveness of PROVENTIL Tablets has been reported in patients who received long-term treatment with the drug in uncontrolled studies for periods up to 6 months.

CONTRAINDICATIONS

PROVENTIL Tablets are contraindicated in patients with a history of hypersensitivity to any of its components.

PRECAUTIONS

General: Although albuterol usually has minimal effects on the $beta_1$-adrenoceptors of the cardiovascular system at the recommended dosage, occasionally the usual cardiovascular and CNS stimulatory effects common to all sympathomimetic agents have been seen with patients treated with albuterol necessitating discontinuation. Therefore, albuterol should be used with caution in patients with cardiovascular disorders, including coronary insufficiency and hypertension, in patients with hyperthyroidism or diabetes mellitus, and in patients who are unusually responsive to sympathomimetic amines.

Large doses of intravenous albuterol have been reported to aggravate preexisting diabetes mellitus and ketoacidosis. Additionally, albuterol and other beta agonists, when given intravenously, may cause a decrease in serum potassium, possibly through intracellular shunting. The decrease is usually transient, not requiring supplementation. The relevance of these observations to the use of PROVENTIL Tablets is unknown.

Information for Patients: The action of PROVENTIL Tablets may last for 8 hours or longer and therefore it should not be taken more frequently than recommended. Do not increase the dose or frequency of medication without medical consultation. If symptoms get worse, medical consultation should be sought promptly.

Drug Interactions: The concomitant use of PROVENTIL Tablets and other oral sympathomimetic agents is not recommended since such combined use may lead to deleterious cardiovascular effects. This recommendation does not preclude the judicious use of an aerosol bronchodilator of the adrenergic stimulant type in patients receiving PROVENTIL Tablets. Such concomitant use, however, should be individualized and not given on a routine basis. If regular coadministration is required, then alternative therapy should be considered.

Albuterol should be administered with extreme caution to patients being treated with monoamine oxidase inhibitors or tricyclic antidepressants, since the action of albuterol on the vascular system may be potentiated.

Beta-receptor blocking agents and albuterol inhibit the effect of each other.

Carcinogenesis, Mutagenesis, and Impairment of Fertility: Albuterol sulfate, like other agents in its class, caused a significant dose-related increase in the incidence of benign leiomyomas of the mesovarium in a 2-year study in the rat, at doses corresponding to 3, 16, and 78 times the maximum human oral dose. In another study this effect was blocked by the coadministration of propranolol. The relevance of these findings to humans is not known. An 18-month study in mice and a lifetime study in hamsters revealed no evidence of tumorigenicity. Studies with albuterol revealed no evidence of mutagenesis. Reproduction studies in rats revealed no evidence of impaired fertility.

Teratogenic Effects—Pregnancy Category C: Albuterol has been shown to be teratogenic in mice when given subcutaneously in doses corresponding to 0.4 times the maximum human oral dose. There are no adequate and well-controlled studies in pregnant women. Albuterol should be used during pregnancy only if the potential benefit justifies the potential risk to the fetus. A reproduction study in CD-1 mice with albuterol showed cleft palate formation in 5 of 111 (4.5%) fetuses at 0.25 mg/kg and in 10 of 108 (9.3%) fetuses at 2.5 mg/kg, none were observed at 0.025 mg/kg. Cleft palate also occurred in 22 of 72 (30.5%) fetuses treated with 2.5 mg/kg isoproterenol (positive control). A reproduction study in Stride Dutch rabbits revealed cranioschisis in 7 of 19 (37%) fetuses at 50 mg/kg, corresponding to 78 times the maximum human oral dose of albuterol.

Labor and Delivery: Oral albuterol has been shown to delay preterm labor in some reports. There are presently no well controlled studies which demonstrate that it will stop preterm labor or prevent labor at term. Therefore, cautious use of PROVENTIL Tablets is required in pregnant patients when given for relief of bronchospasm so as to avoid interference with uterine contractibility.

Nursing Mothers: It is not known whether this drug is excreted in human milk. Because of the potential for tumorigenicity shown for albuterol in animal studies, a decision should be made whether to discontinue nursing or to discontinue the drug, taking into account the importance of the drug to the mother.

Pediatric Use: Safety and effectiveness in children below the age of 6 years have not been established.

ADVERSE REACTIONS

The adverse reactions to albuterol are similar in nature to those of other sympathomimetic agents. The most frequent adverse reactions to PROVENTIL Tablets were nervousness and tremor, with each occurring in approximately 20 of 100 patients. Other reported reactions were headache, 7 of 100 patients; tachycardia and palpitations, 5 of 100 patients; muscle cramps, 3 of 100 patients; insomnia, nausea, weakness, and dizziness, each occurred in 2 of 100 patients. Drowsiness, flushing, restlessness, irritability, chest discomfort, and difficulty in micturition each occurred in less than 1 of 100 patients.

In addition, albuterol, like other sympathomimetic agents, can cause adverse reactions such as hypertension, angina, vomiting, vertigo, central nervous system stimulation, unusual taste, and drying or irritation of the oropharynx.

The reactions are generally transient in nature, and it is usually not necessary to discontinue treatment with PROVENTIL Tablets. In selected cases, however, dosage may be reduced temporarily; after the reaction has subsided, dosage should be increased in small increments to the optimal dosage.

OVERDOSAGE

Manifestations of overdosage include anginal pain, hypertension, hypokalemia, and exaggeration of the effects listed in **ADVERSE REACTIONS.**

The oral LD_{50} in rats and mice was greater than 2,000 mg/kg.

Dialysis is not appropriate treatment for overdosage of PROVENTIL Tablets. The judicious use of a cardioselective betareceptor blocker, such as metoprolol tartrate, is suggested, bearing in mind the danger of inducing an asthmatic attack.

DOSAGE AND ADMINISTRATION

The following dosages of PROVENTIL Tablets are expressed in terms of albuterol base.

Usual Dose: The usual starting dosage for children 6 to 12 years of age is 2 mg three or four times a day. The usual starting dosage for adults and children 12 years and over is 2 mg or 4 mg three or four times a day.

Dosage Adjustment: For children from 6 to 12 years of age who fail to respond to the initial starting dosage of 2 mg four times a day, the dosage may be cautiously increased stepwise, but not to exceed 24 mg per day (given in divided doses). For adults and children above age 12, a dosage above 4 mg, four times a day should be used only when the patient fails to respond. If a favorable response does not occur with the 4 mg initial dosage, it should be cautiously increased stepwise up to a maximum of 8 mg four times a day as tolerated.

Elderly Patients and Those Sensitive to Beta-Adrenergic Stimulators: An initial dosage of 2 mg three or four times a day is recommended for elderly patients and for those with a history of unusual sensitivity to beta-adrenergic stimulators. If adequate bronchodilatation is not obtained, dosage may be increased gradually to as much as 8 mg three or four times a day.

The total daily dose should not exceed 32 mg in adults and children 12 years and over.

HOW SUPPLIED

PROVENTIL Tablets, 2 mg albuterol as the sulfate, white, round, compressed tablets, impressed with the product name (PROVENTIL) and the number 2 on one side, and product identification numbers, 252, and scored on the other; bottles of 100 (NDC 0085-0252-02) and 500 (NDC 0085-0252-03).

PROVENTIL Tablets, 4 mg albuterol as the sulfate, white, round, compressed tablets, impressed with the product name (PROVENTIL) and the number 4 on one side, and product identification numbers, 573, and scored on the other; bottles of 100 (NDC 0085-0573-02) and 500 (NDC 0085-0573-03).

Store between 2° and 30°C (36° and 86°F).

Revised 8/85

Shown in Product Identification Section, page 428

Sodium SULAMYD® ℞

[*so'dē-um soo'lah-mĭd*]

brand of sulfacetamide sodium

Ophthalmic Solution, USP 30%—Sterile
Ophthalmic Solution, USP 10%—Sterile
Ophthalmic Ointment, USP 10%—Sterile

DESCRIPTION

Sodium SULAMYD is available in three ophthalmic forms: **Ophthalmic Solution 30%** contains in each ml of sterile aqueous solution 300 mg sulfacetamide sodium, USP, 1.5 mg sodium thiosulfate, with 0.5 mg methylparaben and 0.1 mg propylparaben added as preservatives, and monobasic sodium phosphate as buffer.

Ophthalmic Solution 10% contains in each ml of sterile aqueous solution 100 mg sulfacetamide sodium, USP, 3.1 mg sodium thiosulfate, and 5 mg methylcellulose, with 0.5 mg methylparaben and 0.1 mg propylparaben added as preservatives and monobasic sodium phosphate as buffer.

Ophthalmic Ointment 10% is a sterile ointment, each gram containing 100 mg sulfacetamide sodium, USP, with 0.5 mg methylparaben, 0.1 mg propylparaben and 0.25 mg benzalkonium chloride added as preservatives, and sorbitan monolaurate and water in a bland, unctuous, petrolatum base.

ACTIONS

Sodium SULAMYD exerts a bacteriostatic effect against a wide range of gram-positive and gram-negative microorganisms by restricting, through competition with para-aminobenzoic acid, the synthesis of folic acid which bacteria require for growth.

INDICATIONS

Sodium SULAMYD is indicated for the treatment of conjunctivitis, corneal ulcer, and other superficial ocular infections due to susceptible microorganisms, and as adjunctive treatment in systemic sulfonamide therapy of trachoma.

CONTRAINDICATIONS

Sodium SULAMYD is contraindicated in individuals with known or suspected sensitivity to sulfonamides or to any of the ingredients of the preparations.

PRECAUTIONS

Sodium SULAMYD products are incompatible with silver preparations. Ophthalmic ointments may retard corneal healing. Non-susceptible organisms, including fungi, may proliferate with the use of these preparations. Sulfonamides are inactivated by the para-aminobenzoic acid present in purulent exudates.

Sensitization may recur when a sulfonamide is re-administered irrespective of the route of administration, and cross sensitivity between different sulfonamides may occur. If signs of sensitivity or other untoward reactions occur, discontinue use of the preparation.

ADVERSE REACTIONS

Sulfacetamide sodium may cause local irritation, stinging and burning. While the irritation may be transient, occasionally, use of the medication has to be discontinued.

Although sensitivity reactions to sulfacetamide sodium are rare, an isolated incident of Stevens-Johnson syndrome was reported in a patient who had experienced a previous bullous drug reaction to an orally administered sulfonamide and a single instance of local hypersensitivity was reported which progressed to a fatal syndrome resembling systemic lupus erythematosus.

DOSAGE AND ADMINISTRATION

Sodium SULAMYD Ophthalmic Solution 30%. *For conjunctivitis or corneal ulcer:* instill one drop into lower conjunctival sac every two hours or less frequently according to severity of infection. *For trachoma:* Two drops every two hours; concomitant systemic sulfonamide therapy is indicated.

Sodium SULAMYD Ophthalmic Solution 10%. One or two drops into the lower conjunctival sac every two or three hours during the day and less often at night.

Sodium SULAMYD Ophthalmic Ointment 10%. Apply a small amount four times daily and at bedtime. The ointment may be used adjunctively with either of the solution forms.

HOW SUPPLIED

Sodium SULAMYD Ophthalmic Ointment 10%, 3.5 g tube (NDC 0085-0066-03), box of one. **Store away from heat.**

Sodium SULAMYD Ophthalmic Solution 30%, 15 ml dropper bottle (NDC 0085-0717-06), box of one. **Store between 2° and 30°C (36° and 86°F).**

Sodium SULAMYD Ophthalmic Solution 10%, 5 ml dropper bottle (NDC 0085-0946-03),box of 25; 15 ml dropper bottle (NDC 0085-0946-06), box of one. **Store between 2° and 30°C (36° and 86°F).**

Continued on next page

Information on Schering products appearing on these pages is effective as of September 30, 1986.

Schering—Cont.

On long standing, sulfonamide solutions will darken in color and should be discarded.

Revised 10/84

SOLGANAL® ℞

[sol'gah-nal]

brand of sterile aurothioglucose

Suspension, USP

FOR INTRAMUSCULAR INJECTION ONLY—

NOT FOR INTRAVENOUS USE

WARNINGS

Physicians planning to use SOLGANAL Suspension should thoroughly familiarize themselves with its toxicity and its benefits. The possibility of toxic reactions should always be explained to the patient before starting therapy. Patients should be warned to report promptly any symptom suggesting toxicity. Before **each** injection of SOLGANAL Suspension, the physician should review the results of laboratory work and see the patient to determine the presence or absence of adverse reactions, since some of these can be severe or even fatal.

DESCRIPTION

SOLGANAL is a sterile suspension, for **intramuscular injection only.** SOLGANAL Suspension is an antiarthritic agent which is absorbed gradually following intramuscular injection, producing a therapeutically desired prolonged effect.

Each ml contains 50 mg of aurothioglucose, USP in sterile sesame oil with 2% aluminum monostearate; 1 mg propylparaben is added as preservative. Aurothioglucose contains approximately 50% gold by weight.

The empirical formula for aurothioglucose is $C_6H_{11}AuO_5S$; the molecular weight is 392.18. Chemically it is (1-Thio-D-glucopyranosato) gold.

Aurothioglucose is a nearly odorless, yellow powder which is stable in air. An aqueous solution is unstable on long standing. Aurothioglucose is freely soluble in water but practically insoluble in acetone, in alcohol, in chloroform, and in ether.

CLINICAL PHARMACOLOGY

Although the mechanism of action is not well understood, gold compounds have been reported to decrease synovial inflammation and retard cartilage and bone destruction.

Gold is absorbed from injection sites, reaching peak concentration in blood in four to six hours. Following a single intramuscular injection of 50 mg SOLGANAL Suspension in each of two patients, peak serum levels were about 235 mcg/dl in one patient and 450 mcg/dl in the other. In plasma, 95% is bound to the albumin fraction. Approximately 70% of the gold is eliminated in the urine and approximately 30% in the feces. When a standard weekly treatment schedule is followed, approximately 40% of the administered dose is excreted each week, and the remainder is excreted over a longer period. The biological half-life of gold salts following a single 50 mg dose has been reported to range from 3 to 27 days. Following successive weekly doses, the half-life increases and may be 14 to 40 days after the third dose and up to 168 days after the eleventh weekly dose.

After the initial injection, the serum level of gold rises sharply and declines over the next week. Peak levels with aqueous preparations are higher and decline faster than those with oily preparations. Weekly administration produces a continuous rise in the basal value for several months, after which the serum level becomes relatively stable. After a standard weekly dose, considerable individual variation in the levels of gold has been found. A steady decline in gold levels occurs when the interval between injections is lengthened, and small amounts may be found in the serum for months after discontinuance of therapy. The incidence of toxic reactions is apparently unrelated to the plasma level of gold, but it may be related to the cumulative body content of gold.

Storage of gold in human tissues is dependent upon organ mass as well as upon the concentration of gold. Therefore, tissues having the highest gold levels (weight/weight) do not necessarily contain the greatest total amounts of gold. The major depots, in decreasing order of total gold content, are the bone marrow, liver, skin, and bone, accounting for approximately 85% of body gold. The highest concentrations of gold are found in the lymph nodes, adrenal glands, liver, kidneys, bone marrow, and spleen. Relatively small concentrations are found in articular structures.

Gold passes the blood-brain barrier in hamsters.

Transfer of gold across the human placenta at the twentieth week of pregnancy has been documented. The placenta showed numerous gold deposits and smaller amounts were detected in the fetal liver and kidneys; other tissues provided no evidence of gold deposition.

Gold is excreted into human milk in significant amounts and trace amounts can be demonstrated in the blood of nursing infants. (See PRECAUTIONS, *"Nursing Mothers."*)

INDICATIONS AND USAGE

SOLGANAL Suspension is indicated for the adjunctive treatment of early active rheumatoid arthritis (both of the adult and juvenile types) not adequately controlled by other anti-inflammatory agents and conservative measures. In chronic, advanced cases of rheumatoid arthritis, gold therapy is less valuable.

Antirheumatic measures such as salicylates and other anti-inflammatory drugs (both steroidal and non-steroidal) may be continued after initiation of gold therapy. After improvement commences, these measures may be discontinued slowly as symptoms permit.

See Precautions, "*Laboratory Tests*" **and Dosage and Administration.**

CONTRAINDICATIONS

A history of known hypersensitivity to any component of SOLGANAL Suspension contraindicates its use. Gold therapy is contraindicated in patients with uncontrolled diabetes mellitus, severe debilitation, systemic lupus erythematosus, renal disease, hepatic dysfunction, uncontrolled congestive heart failure, marked hypertension, agranulocytosis, other blood dyscrasias, or hemorrhagic diathesis; or if there is a history of infectious hepatitis. Patients who recently have had radiation, and those who have developed severe toxicity from previous exposure to gold or other heavy metals should not receive SOLGANAL Suspension.

Urticaria, eczema, and colitis are also contraindications.

Gold therapy is usually contraindicated in pregnancy. (See PRECAUTIONS, "*Usage in Pregnancy*".)

Gold salts should not be used with penicillamine (See MANAGEMENT OF ADVERSE REACTIONS) or antimalarials. The safety of coadministration with immunosuppressive agents other than corticosteroids has not been established.

WARNINGS

The following signs should be considered danger signals of gold toxicity, and no additional injection should be given unless further studies reveal some other cause for their presence: rapid reduction of hemoglobin, leukopenia (WBC below 4000/cu mm), eosinophilia above 5%, platelet count below 100,000/cu mm, albuminuria, hematuria, pruritus, dermatitis, stomatitis, jaundice, and petechiae.

Effects that may occur immediately following an injection, or at any time during gold therapy, include: anaphylactic shock, syncope, bradycardia, thickening of the tongue, difficulty in swallowing and breathing, and angioneurotic edema. If such effects are observed, treatment with SOLGANAL Suspension should be discontinued.

Tolerance to gold usually decreases with advancing age. Diabetes mellitus or congestive heart failure should be under control before gold therapy is instituted.

SOLGANAL Suspension should be used with extreme caution in patients with: skin rash, hypersensitivity to other medications, or a history of renal or liver disease.

PRECAUTIONS

General: Before **each** injection, the physician should personally check the patient for adverse reactions and inquiry should be made regarding pruritus, rash, sore mouth, indigestion, and metallic taste. The patient should be observed for at least 15 minutes following each injection. (See also "*Laboratory Tests*".)

Patients with HLA-D locus histocompatibility antigens DRw2 and DRw3 may have a genetic predisposition to develop certain toxic reactions, such as proteinuria, during treatment with gold or D-penicillamine.

SOLGANAL Suspension should be used with caution in patients with compromised cardiovascular or cerebral circulation.

Information for Patients:

1. Promptly report to the physician any unusual symptoms such as pruritus (itching), rash, sore mouth, indigestion, or metallic taste.
2. Increased joint pain may occur for one or two days after an injection and usually subsides after the first few injections.
3. Exposure to sunlight or artificial ultraviolet light should be minimized.
4. Careful oral hygiene is recommended in conjunction with therapy.
5. Patients should be aware of potential hazards if they become pregnant while receiving gold therapy. (See "*Usage in Pregnancy*".)

Laboratory Tests: Before treatment is started, a complete blood count, platelet count, and urinalysis should be done to serve as reference points. Since gold therapy is usually contraindicated in pregnant patients, pregnancy should be ruled out before treatment is started. Throughout the treatment period, urinalysis should be repeated prior to each injection, and complete blood cell and platelet counts should be performed every two weeks. A platelet count is indicated any time that purpura or ecchymosis occurs.

Drug Interactions: Drug interactions have not been reported. (See **Contraindications.**)

Carcinogenesis, Mutagenesis, and Impairment of Fertility: Renal adenomas developed in rats receiving an injectable gold product similar to SOLGANAL Suspension at doses of 2 mg/kg weekly for 46 weeks, followed by 6 mg/kg daily for 47 weeks. These doses were higher and administered more frequently than the recommended human doses. The adenomas were similar histologically to those produced by chronic administration of other gold compounds and heavy metals, such as lead or nickel.

Renal tubular cell neoplasia consisting of renal adenoma and adenocarcinoma were noted in a dose-response relationship in another study in rats using daily intramuscular doses of 3 mg/kg and 6 mg/kg for up to 2 years. These doses were higher and were administered more frequently than the recommended human doses. In this same study, sarcomas at the injection site occurred in some rats but their numbers were not sufficient to demonstrate a dose-response relationship.

No report of renal adenoma or sarcoma at the injection site in man in association with the use of SOLGANAL Suspension has been received.

Gold compounds have not been studied for evaluation of mutagenesis.

Gold sodium thiomalate given subcutaneously did not adversely affect fertility or reproductive performance.

Usage in Pregnancy: Gold therapy is usually contraindicated in pregnant patients. The patient should be warned about the hazards of becoming pregnant while on gold therapy. Rheumatoid arthritis frequently improves when the patient becomes pregnant, thereby eliminating the need for gold therapy. The potential nephrotoxicity of gold should not be superimposed on the increased renal burden which normally occurs in pregnancy and hence, gold therapy should be discontinued upon recognition of pregnancy unless continued use is required in an individual case. The slow excretion of gold and its persistence in body tissues after discontinuation of treatment should be kept in mind when a woman of child-bearing potential being treated with gold plans to become pregnant.

Pregnancy Category C: Gold sodium thiomalate administered subcutaneously, a route not used clinically, has been shown to be teratogenic during the organogenic period in rats and rabbits when given in doses 140 and 175 times, respectively, the usual human dose. Hydrocephalus and microphthalmia were the malformations observed in rats when gold sodium thiomalate was administered at a dose of 25 mg/kg/day from day 6 through day 15 of gestation. In rabbits, limb defects and gastroschisis were the malformations observed when gold sodium thiomalate was administered at doses of 20 to 45 mg/kg/day from day 6 through day 18 of gestation.

Gold compounds administered orally to rabbits from days 6 through 18 of pregnancy resulted in the occurrence of abdominal defects, such as gastroschisis and umbilical hernia; anomalies of the brain, heart, lung, and skeleton; and microphthalmia.

The administration of excessive doses of gold-containing compounds during pregnancy in the above studies was toxic to the mothers and their embryos; the embryotoxic effects probably were secondary to maternal toxicity. Therefore, the significance of these findings in relation to human use is unknown.

There are no adequate and well-controlled studies with SOLGANAL Suspension in pregnant women. Extensive clinical experience with SOLGANAL Suspension has not demonstrated human teratogenicity.

Nursing Mothers: Gold has been demonstated in the milk of lactating mothers. In one patient, a total dose of 135 mg of gold thioglucose was given during the postpartum period. Samples of the maternal milk and urine, and samples of red blood cells and serum of the mother and child were evaluated by atomic absorption spectrophotometry. Trace amounts of gold appeared in the serum and red blood cells of the nursing offspring. It has been postulated that this may be the cause of unexplained rashes, nephritis, hepatitis, and hematologic aberrations in the nursing infants of mothers treated with gold. Because of the potential for serious adverse reactions in nursing infants, a decision should be made whether to discontinue nursing or to discontinue the gold therapy, taking into account the importance of the drug to the mother. The slow excretion of gold and its persistence in the mother after discontinuation of treatment should be kept in mind.

Pediatric Use: Safety and effectiveness in children below the age of six years have not been established.

ADVERSE REACTIONS

Adverse reactions to gold therapy may occur at any time during treatment or many months after therapy has been discontinued. The incidence of toxic reactions is apparently unrelated to the plasma level of gold, but it may be related to the cumulative body content of gold. Higher than conventional dosage schedules may increase the occurrence and severity of toxicity. Severe effects are most common after 300 to 500 mg have been administered.

Cutaneous Reactions: Dermatitis is the most common reaction. Pruritus should be considered a warning signal of an impending cutaneous reaction. Erythema and occasionally the more severe reactions such as papular, vesicular, and exfoliative dermatitis leading to alopecia and shedding of the nails may occur. Chrysiasis (gray-to-blue pigmentation) has been reported, especially on photoexposed areas. Gold dermatitis may be aggravated by exposure to sunlight, or an actinic rash may develop.

Mucous Membrane Reactions: Stomatitis is the second most common adverse reaction. Shallow ulcers on the buccal membranes, on the borders of the tongue and on the palate, diffuse glossitis, or gingivitis may be preceded by the sensation of metallic taste. Careful oral hygiene is recommended. Inflammation of the upper respiratory tract, pharyngitis, gastritis, colitis, tracheitis, and vaginitis have also been reported. Conjunctivitis is rare.

Renal Reactions: Nephrotic syndrome or glomerulitis with hematuria, which is usually relatively mild, subsides completely if recognized early and treatment is discontinued. These reactions become severe and chronic if gold therapy is continued after their onset. Therefore, it is important to perform a urinalysis before each injection and to discontinue treatment promptly if proteinuria or hematuria develops.

Hematologic Reactions: Although rare, blood dyscrasias, including granulocytopenia, agranulocytosis, thrombocytopenia with or without purpura, leukopenia, eosinophilia, panmyelopathy, hemorrhagic diathesis, and hypoplastic and aplastic anemia, have been reported. These reactions may occur separately or in combination.

Nitritoid and Allergic Reactions: These reactions, which may rarely occur with SOLGANAL Suspension and which resemble anaphylactoid effects, include flushing, fainting, dizziness, sweating, malaise, weakness, nausea, and vomiting.

Miscellaneous Reactions: On rare occasions, gastrointestinal symptoms, i.e., nausea, vomiting, colic, anorexia, abdominal cramps, diarrhea, ulcerative enterocolitis, and headache have been reported.

There have been rare reports of iritis and corneal ulcers. Transient, asymptomatic gold deposits in the cornea or conjunctiva may occur.

Other reported reactions include encephalitis, immunological destruction of the synovia, EEG abnormalities, intrahepatic cholestasis, hepatitis with jaundice, toxic hepatitis, acute yellow atrophy, peripheral neuritis, gold bronchitis, pulmonary injury manifested by interstitial pneumonitis or fibrosis, fever, and partial or complete hair loss.

Less common but more severe effects that may occur shortly after an injection or at any time during gold therapy include: anaphylactic shock, syncope, bradycardia, thickening of the tongue, difficulty in swallowing and breathing, and angioneurotic edema. If they are observed, treatment with SOLGANAL Suspension should be discontinued.

Arthralgia may occur for one or two days after an injection and usually subsides after the first few injections. The mechanism of the transient increase in rheumatic symptoms after injection of gold (the so-called nonvasomotor postinjection reaction) is unknown. These reactions are usually mild but occasionally may be so severe that treatment is stopped prematurely.

MANAGEMENT OF ADVERSE REACTIONS

In the event of toxic reactions, gold therapy should be discontinued immediately.

In the presence of mild reactions, it may be sufficient to discontinue the administration of SOLGANAL Suspension for a short period and then to resume treatment with smaller doses.

Dermatitis and pruritus may respond to soothing lotions, other appropriate antipruritic treatment, or topical glucocorticoids.

If dermatitis or stomatitis becomes severe or spreads, systemic glucocorticoid treatment may be indicated. For renal, hematologic, and most other adverse reactions, glucocorticoids may be required in larger doses and for a longer time than for dermatologic reactions. Often this treatment may be required for many months because of the slow elimination of gold from the body.

If severe adverse reactions do not improve with steroid treatment in patients who receive large doses of gold, a chelating agent, such as dimercaprol (BAL), may be used. In one case, it was reported that penicillamine was beneficial in the treatment of gold-induced thrombocytopenia. Adjunctive use of an anabolic steroid with other drugs (i.e., BAL, penicillamine, and corticosteroids) may contribute to recovery of bone marrow deficiency.

In the presence of severe or idiosyncratic reactions, treatment with SOLGANAL Suspension should not be reinstituted.

OVERDOSAGE

Overdosage resulting from too rapid increases in dosing with SOLGANAL Suspension will be manifested by rapid appearance of toxic reactions, particularly those relating to renal damage, such as hematuria, proteinuria, and to hematologic effects, such as thrombocytopenia and granulocytopenia. Other toxic effects, including fever, nausea, vomiting, diarrhea, and various skin disorders such as papulovesicular lesions, urticaria, and exfoliative dermatitis, all attended with severe pruritus, may develop. Treatment consists of prompt discontinuation of the medication, and early administration of dimercaprol. Specific supportive therapy should be given for the renal and hematologic complications. (See also MANAGEMENT OF ADVERSE REACTIONS above).

DOSAGE AND ADMINISTRATION

Adults—The usual dosage schedule for the intramuscular administration of SOLGANAL is as follows: first dose, 10 mg; second and third doses, 25 mg; fourth and subsequent doses, 50 mg. The interval between doses is one week. The 50 mg dose is continued at weekly intervals until 0.8 to 1.0 g SOLGANAL has been given. If the patient has improved and has exhibited no sign of toxicity, the 50 mg dose may be continued many months longer, at three- to four-week intervals. A weekly dose above 50 mg is usually unnecessary and contraindicated; the tendency in gold therapy is toward lower dosage. With this in mind, it may eventually be established that a 25 mg dose is the one of choice. If no improvement has been demonstrated after a total administration of 1.0 g of SOLGANAL Suspension, the necessity for gold therapy should be reevaluated.

Children 6 to 12 years—one-fourth of the adult dose, governed chiefly by body weight, not to exceed 25 mg per dose.

SOLGANAL Suspension should be injected **intramuscularly,** (preferably intragluteally), **never intravenously.** The patient should be lying down and should remain recumbent for approximately 10 minutes after the injection. The vial should be thoroughly shaken in order to suspend all of the active material. Heating the vial to body temperature (by immersion in warm water) will facilitate drawing the suspension into the syringe. An 18-gauge, 1½-inch needle is recommended for depositing the preparation deep into the muscular tissue. For obese patients, an 18-gauge, 2-inch needle may be used. The site usually selected for injection is the upper outer quadrant of the gluteal region.

NOTE: Shake the vial in horizontal position before the dose is withdrawn. Needle and syringe must be dry. The patient should be observed for at least 15 minutes following each injection.

HOW SUPPLIED

SOLGANAL Suspension is available in 10 ml multiple-dose vials containing 5% (50 mg/ml) aurothioglucose; box of one. **Shake well before using. Store between 0° and 30°C (32° and 86°F). Protect from light. Store in carton until contents are used.**

THEOVENT® ℞

[thē-ō-vĕnt]

brand of theophylline anhydrous Long-Acting Capsules

DESCRIPTION

THEOVENT Long-Acting Capsules are a specially formulated preparation of anhydrous theophylline which is gradually released for prolonged effect after oral administration. Each capsule contains either 125 mg or 250 mg of anhydrous theophylline, USP.

Anhydrous theophylline is 1*H*-Purine-2,6-dione, 3,7-dihydro-1,3-dimethyl-, anhydrous.

Anhydrous theophylline is a xanthine compound having the chemical formula, $C_7H_8N_4O_2$, with a molecular weight of 180.17. It is a white, odorless, crystalline powder which is stable in air and has a bitter taste. Theophylline is slightly soluble in water, freely soluble in solutions of alkali hydroxides and in ammonia, while only slightly soluble in alcohol, chloroform, or ether.

CLINICAL PHARMACOLOGY

Theophylline directly relaxes the smooth muscle of the bronchial airways and pulmonary blood vessels, thus acting mainly as a bronchodilator, pulmonary vasodilator, and smooth muscle relaxant. Its bronchodilating action helps relieve wheezing, coughing, and other respiratory symptoms associated with reversible bronchospasm.

Theophylline also possesses other actions typical of the xanthine derivatives: coronary vasodilation; diuretic; and skeletal muscle, cardiac, and cerebral stimulation. Its actions may be mediated through inhibition of phosphodiesterase and a resultant increase in intracellular cyclic AMP. Theophylline also inhibits the release of histamine by mast cells *in vitro* at concentrations higher than those usually attained clinically. *In vitro,* theophylline has been shown to act synergistically with beta agonists that increase intracellular cyclic AMP through the stimulation of adenyl cyclase, but synergism has not been demonstrated in patient studies. More data are needed to determine if theophylline and beta agonists have a clinically important additive effect *in vivo.* Apparently, no development of tolerance occurs with chronic use of theophylline.

Pharmacokinetics: The half-life is shortened by cigarette smoking. Conversely, the half-life is prolonged in patients with alcoholism, reduced hepatic or renal functions, congestive heart failure, and in patients receiving certain macrolide antibiotics, such as troleandomycin or erythromycin, and in patients receiving cimetidine. High fever for prolonged periods, influenza immunization or active infection with influenza may decrease theophylline elimination.

Newborns and neonates have extremely slow clearance rates compared to older infants (over 6 months) and children, and may also have a theophylline half-life of over 24 hours.

Older adults (over age 55) and patients with chronic obstructive pulmonary disease, with or without cor pulmonale or other causes of heart failure, and patients with liver disease may have much lower clearances with a half-life that may exceed 24 hours.

The elimination characteristics of theophylline are as follows:

Patient Population	Theophylline Plasma Clearance Rates (mean ± S.D.)	Average Half-Life (mean ± S.D.)
Children (over 6 months of age)	1.45 ± .58 ml/kg/min	3.7 ± 1.1 hours
Adult non-smokers with uncomplicated asthma	.65 ± .19 ml/kg/min	8.7 ± 2.2 hours

The half-life of theophylline in smokers (of 1 to 2 packs of cigarettes per day) averaged 4 to 5 hours among various studies, much shorter than the half-life in non-smokers, which averaged about 7 to 9 hours. The increase in theophylline clearance caused by smoking is probably the result of induction of drug-metabolizing enzymes that do not readily normalize after cessation of smoking. After cessation of smoking, normalization of theophylline pharmacokinetics may not occur for 3 months to 2 years.

In a single-dose study in 12 normal adult males, a single dose of 500 mg THEOVENT Long-Acting Capsules, administered as 2 capsules each containing 250 mg, given after an 8-hour fast, resulted in a mean peak serum concentration of 7.5 mcg/ml at 4.6 hours after administration. No food was given for four hours after administration of the drug. The relative bioavailability of THEOVENT Long-Acting Capsules was complete compared to that of a standard theophylline syrup.

In a multiple-dose study, 9 asthmatic adults received 500 mg THEOVENT Long-Acting Capsules every 12 hours. Each dose was given either one hour before or one hour after food. Plasma levels in the range of 10 to 20 mcg/ml were achieved by the second day of therapy and were maintained within this range from the second day through the last treatment day (day 4) of the study. On day 4, mean peak serum concentrations were 18.4 mcg/ml; trough concentrations were 9.8 mcg/ml.

The degree of protein binding (55% to 63%) of theophylline at the therapeutic serum concentration has little effect on theophylline distribution.

INDICATIONS AND USAGE

THEOVENT Long-Acting Capsules are indicated for relief and/or prevention of symptoms from asthma and reversible bronchospasm associated with chronic bronchitis and emphysema.

CONTRAINDICATIONS

This product is contraindicated in individuals who have shown hypersensitivity to any of its components, to aminophylline, or to other xanthines, e.g., theobromine or caffeine.

WARNINGS

Status asthmaticus should be considered a medical emergency and is defined as that degree of bronchospasm which is not rapidly responsive to usual doses of conventional bronchodilators. Optimal therapy for such patients frequently requires both additional medication, parenterally administered, and close monitoring, preferably in an intensive care setting.

Although increasing the dose of theophylline may bring about relief, such treatment may be associated with toxicity.

Continued on next page

Information on Schering products appearing on these pages is effective as of September 30, 1986.

Schering—Cont.

The likelihood of such toxicity developing increases significantly when the serum theophylline concentration exceeds 20 mcg/ml. Therefore, determination of serum theophylline levels is recommended to assure maximal benefit without excessive risk.
Serum levels above 20 mcg/ml are rarely found after appropriate administration of the recommended doses. However, in individuals in whom theophylline plasma clearance is reduced for any reason, even conventional doses may result in increased serum levels and potential toxicity. Reduced theophylline clearance has been documented in the following readily identifiable groups: patients with impaired renal or liver function; patients over 55 years of age, particularly males and those with chronic lung disease; those with cardiac failure from any cause; neonates; and those patients taking certain drugs (macrolide antibiotics and cimetidine). Decreased clearance of theophylline may be associated with either influenza immunization or active infection with influenza. In the presence of any of the above factors, it is advisable to monitor theophylline serum levels in all patients. It is especially important that levels be monitored in the subgroups noted. Other circumstances in which it is advisable to monitor serum levels include: unexplained poor control of asthma; occurence of toxic symptoms; addition or removal of other drugs from the therapeutic regimen which affect the metabolism of theophylline; use of unusually high doses.
Although early signs of theophylline toxicity, such as nausea and restlessness, may appear in up to 50% of patients, in some cases more serious signs such as ventricular arrhythmias, convulsions or even death, may be the first signs of toxicity without any previous warning. It is important to discontinue doses which are not tolerated. In situations where therapy is to be resumed, it should be at a lower dosage after all signs of toxicity have disappeared and serum levels have been checked.
Patients with higher than the recommended therapeutic theophylline serum levels are more likely to experience tachycardia than patients whose levels are within the recommended therapeutic range.
Many patients who require theophylline may exhibit tachycardia due to their underlying disease process so that the cause/effect relationship to elevated serum theophylline concentrations may not be appreciated.
Theophylline products may cause dysrhythmia and/or worsen pre-existing arrhythmias and any significant change in rate and/or rhythm warrants monitoring and further investigation.
The occurence of arrhythmias and sudden death (with histological evidence of necrosis of the myocardium) has been recorded in laboratory animals (minipigs, rodents and dogs) when theophylline and beta agonists were administered concomitantly, although not when either was administered alone. The significance of these findings when applied to human usage is currently unknown.

PRECAUTIONS

General: Theophylline should not be administered concurrently with other xanthine medications such as aminophylline and caffeine.
Theophylline half-life is shorter in smokers than in nonsmokers. Therefore, smokers may require larger or more frequent doses. Morphine and curare should be used with caution in patients with airway obstruction as they may suppress respiration and stimulate histamine release. Alternative drugs should be used when possible.
Use theophylline with caution in patients with severe cardiac disease, arrhythmias, acute myocardial injury, congestive heart failure, cor pulmonale, hypertension, severe hypoxemia, hyperthyroidism, liver or renal disease, dehydration, and in the elderly (especially males) and neonates. In particular, great caution should be used in giving theophylline to patients with congestive heart failure. Frequently, such patients have markedly prolonged theophylline serum levels with theophylline persisting in serum for long periods following discontinuation of the drug.
Use theophylline cautiously in patients with a history of peptic ulcer. Theophylline may occasionally act as a local irritant to the G.I. tract although gastrointestinal symptoms are more commonly centrally mediated and associated with serum drug concentrations over 20 mcg/ml.
Information for Patients:
1. This information is intended to aid in the safe and effective use of this medication. It is not a disclosure of all possible adverse or intended effects.
2. Contact a physician immediately if vomiting, nausea, restlessness, convulsions, or irregular heartbeat occurs.
3. Take only the dosage which has been prescribed; especially, do not take a larger dose, or take the drug more frequently, or for a longer time than directed.
4. Do not take other medicines, especially those for asthma or breathing problems, except under advice and supervision of a physician.
5. Avoid drinking large amounts of caffeine-containing beverages, such as tea, coffee (except decaffeinated), cocoa, and cola drinks or eating large amounts of chocolate while taking this medicine, since these products may add to the side effects of theophylline.
6. Inform the physician if symptoms of asthma occur repeatedly, especially near the end of a dosing interval.

Drug Interactions: (See also PRECAUTIONS, *General.*) Toxic synergism with ephedrine has been documented and may occur with some other sympathomimetic bronchodilators. Recent controlled studies suggest that the addition of ephedrine to dosage regimens of theophylline results in an increase in toxic effects, but not in efficacy, when compared to theophylline alone. The concurrent use of theophylline and sympathomimetic drugs is of particular concern in the presence of arrhythmias. The following is a list of other drugs and the effects seen from their interaction with theophylline:

DRUG	EFFECT
lithium carbonate	increased excretion of lithium carbonate
propranolol	antagonism of propranolol
furosemide	increased diuresis
reserpine	tachycardia
cimetidine	increased theophylline blood levels
certain macrolide antibiotics, i.e., troleandomycin, erythromycin	increased theophylline blood levels

Drug-Food Interactions: THEOVENT Long-Acting Capsules have not been adequately studied to determine whether the product's bioavailability is altered when given with food.
Available data suggest that drug administration at the time of food ingestion may influence the absorption characteristics of some or all theophylline controlled-release products resulting in serum values different from those found after administration in the fasting state.
A drug-food effect, if any, would likely have its greatest clinical significance when high theophylline serum levels are being maintained and/or when large single doses (greater than 13 mg/kg or 900 mg) of a controlled-release theophylline product are given. The influence of the type and amount of food on performance of controlled-release theophylline products is under study at this time.
Drug/Laboratory Test Interactions: When plasma levels of theophylline are measured by spectrophotometric methods, coffee, tea, cola beverages, chocolate, and acetaminophen contribute falsely high values.
Carcinogenesis, Mutagenesis, and Impairment of Fertility: Long-term animal studies have not been performed to evaluate the carcinogenic potential, mutagenic potential, or the effect on fertility of xanthine compounds.
Pregnancy Category C: Animal reproduction studies have not been conducted wih theophylline. It is not known whether theophylline can cause fetal harm when administered to a pregnant woman or can affect reproduction capacity. Xanthines should be given to a pregnant woman only if clearly needed.
Nursing Mothers: It has been reported that theophylline distributes readily into breast milk and may cause adverse effects in the infant. Caution must be used if prescribing xanthines to a mother who is nursing, taking into account the risk-benefit of this therapy.
Pediatric Use: Safety and effectiveness of THEOVENT Long-Acting Capsules in children below the age of 6 years have not been established.

ADVERSE REACTIONS

Most adverse reactions are usually due to overdose and include:
Gastrointestinal: hematemesis, nausea, epigastric pain, vomiting, diarrhea.
Central Nervous System: clonic and tonic generalized convulsions, muscle twitching, headaches, irritability, restlessness, insomnia, reflex hyperexcitability.
Cardiovascular: life-threatening ventricular arrhythmias, circulatory failure, extrasystoles, hypotension, tachycardia, palpitations, flushing.
Respiratory: tachypnea.
Renal: albuminuria, increased excretion of renal tubular cells and red blood cells; potentiation of diuresis.
Others: hyperglycemia and inappropriate anti-diuretic hormone syndrome; rash.

OVERDOSAGE

ALTHOUGH EARLY EVIDENCE OF THEOPHYLLINE TOXICITY, SUCH AS NAUSEA AND RESTLESSNESS, IS OFTEN SEEN, IN SOME CASES MORE SERIOUS SIGNS, SUCH AS VENTRICULAR ARRHYTHMIAS OR CONVULSIONS, MAY BE THE FIRST MANIFESTATIONS OF TOXICITY.

Management: Emergency treatment should be started immediately.

A. If overdose is established and seizure has not occurred:
   1. Induce vomiting, even if emesis has occurred spontaneously; the administration of ipecac syrup is the preferred method. Emesis should not be induced in patients with impaired consciousness. The action of ipecac is facilitated by physical activity and the administration of 8 to 12 ounces of water. If emesis does not occur within 15 minutes, the dose of ipecac should be repeated. Precautions against aspiration must be taken, especially in infants and children. If vomiting is unsuccessful or contraindicated, gastric lavage should be performed.
   2. Administer a cathartic (this is particularly important when a sustained-release preparation has been taken).
   3. Administer activated charcoal.

B. If the patient is having a seizure:
   1. Establish an airway.
   2. Administer oxygen.
   3. Treat the seizure with intravenous diazepam 0.1 to 0.3 mg/kg up to 10 mg.
   4. Monitor vital signs, maintain blood pressure, and provide adequate hydration.

C. Post-Seizure Coma:
   1. Maintain airway and oxygenation.
   2. Follow above recommendations to prevent absorption of drug, but perform intubation and lavage instead of inducing emesis. Introduce the cathartic and charcoal via a large bore gastric lavage tube.
   3. Continue to provide full supportive care and adequate hydration while waiting for the drug to be metabolized, which generally occurs rapidly enough that dialysis is not necessary.

D. General:
   Treatment is symptomatic and supportive. *Stimulants (analeptic agents) should not be used.* If atrial arrhythmia occurs during treatment with theophylline, lidocaine should be administered with caution, since both drugs may produce accelerated atrioventricular conduction.
   Intravenous fluids may be required to overcome dehydration, acid-base imbalance, and hypotension; the latter may also be treated with vasopressors. Apnea will require ventilatory support. Hyperpyrexia, especially in children, may be treated with tepid water sponge baths or a hypothermic blanket.

Theophylline is dialyzable; peritoneal and hemodialyses are effective means of removing theophylline and may be useful adjuncts in the management of overdosage. In one case of massive overdose, charcoal hemoperfusion over a 6-hour period rapidly removed theophylline from the serum with notable clinical improvement. Charcoal hemoperfusion should be considered in patients with severe theophylline intoxication as a possible means of preventing irreversible central nervous system damage.
The oral LD_{50} of theophylline is 100 mg/kg in cats and 300 to 400 mg/kg in rabbits.

DOSAGE AND ADMINISTRATION

THEOVENT Long-Acting Capsules have not been adequately studied for the product's bioavailability when administered with food. (See PRECAUTIONS, *Drug-Food Interactions.*) While giving theophylline with food may prevent stomach irritation, the effects of food on the bioavailability of theophylline should be considered.
For most patients, effective use of theophylline, i.e., associated with optimal likelihood of benefit combined with minimal risk of toxicity, is considered to occur when serum levels are maintained between 10 and 20 mcg/ml. Levels above 20 mcg/ml may produce toxicity, and in a small number of patients, toxicity may even be seen with serum levels between 15–20 mcg/ml, particularly during initiation of therapy.
There is considerable variation from patient to patient in the dosage required to achieve and maintain therapeutic and safe levels, primarily due to variable rates of elimination. Therefore, it is essential that dosage be individualized. Titration and monitoring of serum levels should be utilized where available to determine proper dosage. When serum concentration cannot be obtained, restriction of dosage to the amounts and intervals recommended in the guidelines listed below becomes essential. Dosage should be calculated on the basis of lean (ideal) body weight where mg/kg doses are presented. Theophylline does not distribute into fatty tissue.
Dosage guidelines are approximations only and the wide range of theophylline clearance between individuals (particularly those with concomitant disease) makes indiscriminate usage hazardous.
As a practical consideration, it is not always possible to obtain serum level determinations. Under such conditions, restriction of the daily dose (in otherwise healthy adults) to not greater than 13 mg/kg/day (of anhydrous theophylline) in divided doses will result in relatively few patients exceeding serum levels of 20 mcg/ml and the resultant risk of toxicity.

Acute Symptoms: THEOVENT Long-Acting Capsules are not intended for patients experiencing an acute episode of bronchospasm (associated with asthma, chronic bronchitis, or emphysema). Such patients require rapid relief of symptoms and should be treated with an immediate-release or intravenous theophylline preparation (or other bronchodilators) and not with controlled-release products.

Chronic Therapy: It is recommended that the appropriate dosage be established using an immediate-release preparation. Slow clinical titration is generally preferred to help assure acceptance and safety of the medication. Then, if the total 24-hour dose can be given by use of the available strengths of this product, the patients can usually be switched to THEOVENT Long-Acting Capsules giving one-half of the daily dose at 12-hour intervals. However, certain patients, such as the young, smokers, and some nonsmoking adults are likely to metabolize theophylline rapidly and require dosing at 8-hour intervals. Such patients can generally be identified as having trough serum concentrations lower than desired or repeatedly exhibiting symptoms near the end of a dosing interval.

Maximum Dose of Theophylline Where the Serum Concentration is Not Measured:

WARNING: DO NOT ATTEMPT TO MAINTAIN ANY DOSE THAT IS NOT TOLERATED.

Not to exceed the following:	
Age 6–9 years	24 mg/kg/day
Age 9–12 years	20 mg/kg/day
Age 12–16 years	18 mg/kg/day
Age > 16 years	13 mg/kg/day OR 900 mg/day (WHICHEVER IS LESS)

Measurement of Serum Theophylline Concentrations During Chronic Therapy: If the above maximum doses are to be maintained or exceeded, serum theophylline measurement is recommended. The serum sample should be obtained at the time of peak absorption, 1 to 2 hours after administration for immediate-release products and 4 hours after dosing with THEOVENT Long-Acting Capsules. It is important that the patient will have missed no doses during the previous 48 hours and that dosing intervals will have been reasonably typical with no added doses during that period of time. DOSAGE ADJUSTMENT BASED ON SERUM THEOPHYLLINE MEASUREMENTS WHEN THESE INSTRUCTIONS HAVE NOT BEEN FOLLOWED MAY RESULT IN RECOMMENDATIONS THAT PRESENT RISK OF TOXICITY TO THE PATIENT.

Final Adjustment of Dosage:

Dosage adjustment after serum theophylline measurement

If serum theophylline is:		*Directions*
Within normal limits	10 to 20 mcg/ml	Maintain dosage if tolerated. Recheck serum theophylline concentration at 6- to 12-month intervals.*
Too high	20 to 25 mcg/ml	Decrease doses by about 10%. Recheck serum theophylline concentration at 6- to 12-month intervals.*
	25 to 30 mcg/ml	Skip next dose and decrease subsequent doses by about 25%.
	Over 30 mcg/ml	Skip next 2 doses and decrease subsequent doses by 50%. Recheck serum theophylline.
Too low	7.5 to 10 mcg/ml	Increase dose by about 25%.** Recheck serum theophylline concentration at 6- to 12-month intervals.*
	5 to 7.5 mcg/ml	Increase dose by about 25% to the nearest dose increment and recheck serum theophylline for guidance in further dosage adjustment (another increase will probably be needed, but this provides a safety check).

*Finer adjustments in dosage may be needed for some patients.

**Dividing the daily dose into 3 doses administered at 8-hour intervals may be indicated if symptoms occur repeatedly at the end of a dosing interval.

From The Journal of Respiratory Diseases 2(7):16, 1981

Caution should be exercised for younger children who cannot complain of minor side effects. Older adults, those with cor pulmonale, congestive heart failure, and/or liver disease may have unusually low dosage requirements and thus may experience toxicity at the maximal dosage recommended above.

It is important that no patient be maintained on any dosage that is not tolerated. In instructing patients to increase dosage according to the schedule above, they should be instructed not to take a subsequent dose if apparent side effects occur and to resume therapy at a lower dose once adverse effects have disappeared.

HOW SUPPLIED

THEOVENT Long-Acting Capsules, 125 mg, dark green and yellow capsules, branded in blue with Schering and product identification number, 402; bottles of 100 (NDC 0085-0402-01).

THEOVENT Long-Acting Capsules, 250 mg, dark green and clear capsules, branded in blue with Schering and product identification number, 753; bottles of 100 (NDC 0085-0753-01).

Store between 15° and 30°C (59° and 86°F).

Revised 1/85

Shown in Product Identification Section, page 428

TRILAFON® ℞

[*tri 'lah-fon*]

brand of perphenazine, USP

Tablets

REPETABS® Tablets

Concentrate

Injection

DESCRIPTION

TRILAFON products contain perphenazine, USP (4-[3-(2-chlorophenothiazin-10-yl)propyl]-1-piperazineethanol), a piperazinyl phenothiazine having the chemical formula, $C_{21}H_{26}ClN_3OS$. It is available as **Tablets**, 2, 4, 8 and 16 mg; REPETABS (brand of repeat-action tablets) **Tablets**, 4 mg in an outer layer for immediate effect and 4 mg in an inner core for release three to six hours later; **Concentrate**, 16 mg perphenazine per 5 ml and alcohol less than 0.1%; and **Injection**, perphenazine 5 mg per 1 ml.

The inactive ingredients for TRILAFON **Tablets**, 2, 4, 8 and 16 mg. include: acacia, black iron oxide, butylparaben, calcium phosphate, calcium sulfate, carnauba wax, corn starch, gelatin, lactose, magnesium stearate, potato starch, sugar, titanium dioxide, and white wax. May also contain talc.

The inactive ingredients for TRILAFON REPETABS **Tablets** include: acacia, butylparaben, calcium carbonate, calcium sulfate, carnauba wax, corn starch, neutral soap, gelatin, lactose, magnesium stearate, oleic acid, rice starch, rosin, sugar, talc, titanium dioxide, white wax, and zein.

The inactive ingredients for TRILAFON **Concentrate** include: alcohol (less than 0.1%), citric acid, flavors, menthol, sodium phosphate, sorbitol, sugar, and water.

The inactive ingredients for TRILAFON **Injection** include: citric acid, sodium bisulfite, sodium hydroxide, and water.

ACTIONS

Perphenazine has actions at all levels of the central nervous system, particularly the hypothalamus. However, the site and mechanism of action of therapeutic effect are not known.

INDICATIONS

Perphenazine is indicated for use in the management of the manifestations of psychotic disorders; and for the control of severe nausea and vomiting in adults.

TRILAFON has not been shown effective in the management of behavioral complications in patients with mental retardation.

CONTRAINDICATIONS

TRILAFON products are contraindicated in comatose or greatly obtunded patients and in patients receiving large doses of central nervous system depressants (barbiturates, alcohol, narcotics, analgesics, or antihistamines); in the presence of existing blood dyscrasias, bone marrow depression, or liver damage; and in patients who have shown hypersensitivity to TRILAFON products, their components, or related compounds.

TRILAFON products are also contraindicated in patients with suspected or established subcortical brain damage, with or without hypothalamic damage, since a hyperthermic reaction with temperatures in excess of 104°F may occur in such patients, sometimes not until 14 to 16 hours after drug administration. Total body ice-packing is recommended for such a reaction; antipyretics may also be useful.

WARNINGS

Tardive dyskinesia, a syndrome consisting of potentially irreversible, involuntary, dyskinetic movements, may develop in patients treated with neuroleptic (antipsychotic) drugs. Although the prevalence of the syndrome appears to be highest among the elderly, especially elderly women, it is impossible to rely upon prevalence estimates to predict, at the inception of neuroleptic treatment, which patients are likely to develop the syndrome. Whether neuroleptic drug products differ in their potential to cause tardive dyskinesia is unknown.

Both the risk of developing the syndrome and the likelihood that it will become irreversible are believed to increase as the duration of treatment and the total cumulative dose of neuroleptic drugs administered to the patient increase. However, the syndrome can develop, although much less commonly, after relatively brief treatment periods at low doses.

There is no known treatment for established cases of tardive dyskinesia, although the syndrome may remit, partially or completely, if neuroleptic treatment is withdrawn. Neuroleptic treatment itself, however, may suppress (or partially suppress) the signs and symptoms of the syndrome, and thereby may possibly mask the underlying disease process. The effect that symptomatic suppression has upon the long-term course of the syndrome is unknown.

Given these considerations, neuroleptics should be prescribed in a manner that is most likely to minimize the occurrence of tardive dyskinesia. Chronic neuroleptic treatment should generally be reserved for patients who suffer from a chronic illness that, 1) is known to respond to neuroleptic drugs, and 2) for whom alternative, equally effective, but potentially less harmful treatments are not available or appropriate. In patients who do require chronic treatment, the smallest dose and the shortest duration of treatment producing a satisfactory clinical response should be sought. The need for continued treatment should be reassessed periodically.

If signs and symptoms of tardive dyskinesia appear in a patient on neuroleptics, drug discontinuation should be considered. However, some patients may require treatment despite the presence of the syndrome.

(For further information about the description of tardive dyskinesia and its clinical detection, please refer to **Information for Patients** and **Adverse Reactions**.)

If hypotension develops, epinephrine should not be administered since its action is blocked and partially reversed by perphenazine. If a vasopressor is needed, norepinephrine may be used. Severe, acute hypotension has occurred with the use of phenothiazines and is particularly likely to occur in patients with mitral insufficiency or pheochromocytoma. Rebound hypertension may occur in pheochromocytoma patients.

TRILAFON products can lower the convulsive threshold in susceptible individuals; they should be used with caution in alcohol withdrawal and in patients with convulsive disorders. If the patient is being treated with an anticonvulsant agent, increased dosage of that agent may be required when TRILAFON products are used concomitantly.

TRILAFON products should be used with caution in patients with psychic depression.

Perphenazine may impair the mental and/or physical abilities required for the performance of hazardous tasks such as driving a car or operating machinery; therefore, the patient should be warned accordingly.

TRILAFON products are not recommended for children under 12 years of age.

Usage in Pregnancy: Safe use of TRILAFON during pregnancy and lactation has not been established; therefore, in administering the drug to pregnant patients, nursing mothers, or women who may become pregnant, the possible benefits must be weighed against the possible hazards to mother and child.

PRECAUTIONS

The possibility of suicide in depressed patients remains during treatment and until significant remission occurs. This type of patient should not have access to large quantities of this drug.

As with all phenothiazine compounds, perphenazine should not be used indiscriminately. Caution should be observed in giving it to patients who have previously exhibited severe adverse reactions to other phenothiazines. Some of the untoward actions of perphenazine tend to appear more frequently when high doses are used. However, as with other phenothiazine compounds, patients receiving TRILAFON products in any dosage should be kept under close supervision.

Neuroleptic drugs elevate prolactin levels; the elevation persists during chronic administration. Tissue culture experiments indicate that approximately one-third of human breast cancers are prolactin dependent *in vitro*, a factor of potential importance if the prescription of these drugs is contemplated in a patient with a previously detected breast cancer. Although disturbances such as galactorrhea, amenorrhea, gynecomastia, and impotence have been reported, the clinical significance of elevated serum prolactin levels is unknown for most patients. An increase in mammary neoplasms has been found in rodents after chronic administration of neuroleptic drugs. Neither clinical studies nor epide-

Continued on next page

Information on Schering products appearing on these pages is effective as of September 30, 1986.

Schering—Cont.

miologic studies conducted to date, however, have shown an association between chronic administration of these drugs and mammary tumorigenesis, the available evidence is considered too limited to be conclusive at this time.

The antiemetic effect of perphenazine may obscure signs of toxicity due to overdosage of other drugs, or render more difficult the diagnosis of disorders such as brain tumors or intestinal obstruction.

A significant, not otherwise explained, rise in body temperature may suggest individual intolerance to perphenazine, in which case it should be discontinued.

Patients on large doses of a phenothiazine drug who are undergoing surgery should be watched carefully for possible hypotensive phenomena. Moreover, reduced amounts of anesthetics or central nervous system depressants may be necessary.

Since phenothiazines and central nervous system depressants (opiates, analgesics, antihistamines, barbiturates) can potentiate each other, less than the usual dosage of the added drug is recommended, and caution is advised, when they are administered concomitantly.

Use with caution in patients who are receiving atropine or related drugs because of additive anticholinergic effects and also in patients who will be exposed to extreme heat or phosphorus insecticides.

The use of alcohol should be avoided, since additive effects and hypotension may occur. Patients should be cautioned that their response to alcohol may be increased while they are being treated with TRILAFON products. The risk of suicide and the danger of overdose may be increased in patients who use alcohol excessively due to its potentiation of the drug's effect.

Blood counts and hepatic and renal functions should be checked periodically. The appearance of signs of blood dyscrasias requires the discontinuance of the drug and institution of appropriate therapy. If abnormalities in hepatic tests occur, phenothiazine treatment should be discontinued. Renal function in patients on long-term therapy should be monitored; if blood urea nitrogen (BUN) becomes abnormal, treatment with the drug should be discontinued.

The use of phenothiazine derivatives in patients with diminished renal function should be undertaken with caution.

Use with caution in patients suffering from respiratory impairment due to acute pulmonary infections, or in chronic respiratory disorders such as severe asthma or emphysema.

In general, phenothiazines, including perphenazine, do not produce psychic dependence. Gastritis, nausea and vomiting, dizziness, and tremulousness have been reported following abrupt cessation of high-dose therapy. Reports suggest that these symptoms can be reduced by continuing concomitant antiparkinson agents for several weeks after the phenothiazine is withdrawn.

The possibility of liver damage, corneal and lenticular deposits, and irreversible dyskinesias should be kept in mind when patients are on long-term therapy.

Because photosensitivity has been reported, undue exposure to the sun should be avoided during phenothiazine treatment.

Information for Patients: This information is intended to aid in the safe and effective use of this medication. It is not a disclosure of all possible adverse or intended effects.

Given the likelihood that a substantial proportion of patients exposed chronically to neuroleptics will develop tardive dyskinesia, it is advised that all patients in whom chronic use is contemplated be given, if possible, full information about this risk. The decision to inform patients and/or their guardians must obviously take into account the clinical circumstances and the competency of the patient to understand the information provided.

ADVERSE REACTIONS

Not all of the following adverse reactions have been reported with this specific drug; however, pharmacological similarities among various phenothiazine derivatives require that each be considered. In the case of the piperazine group (of which perphenazine is an example) the extrapyramidal symptoms are more common, and others (e.g., sedative effects, jaundice, and blood dyscrasias) are less frequently seen.

CNS Effects: *Extrapyramidal reactions:* opisthotonus, trismus, torticollis, retrocollis, aching and numbness of the limbs, motor restlessness, oculogyric crisis, hyperreflexia, dystonia, including protrusion, discoloration, aching and rounding of the tongue, tonic spasm of the masticatory muscles, tight feeling in the throat, slurred speech, dysphagia, akathisia, dyskinesia, parkinsonism, and ataxia. Their incidence and severity usually increase with an increase in dosage, but there is considerable individual variation in the tendency to develop such symptoms. Extrapyramidal symptoms can usually be controlled by the concomitant use of effective antiparkinsonian drugs, such as benztropine mesylate, and/or by reduction in dosage. In some instances, however, these extrapyramidal reactions may persist after discontinuation of treatment with perphenazine.

Persistent tardive dyskinesia: As with all antipsychotic agents, tardive dyskinesia may appear in some patients on long-term therapy or may appear after drug therapy has been discontinued. Although the risk appears to be greater in elderly patients on high-dose therapy, especially females, it may occur in either sex and in children. The symptoms are persistent and in some patients appear to be irreversible. The syndrome is characterized by rhythmical, involuntary movements of the tongue, face, mouth, or jaw (e.g. protrusion of tongue, puffing of cheeks, puckering of mouth, chewing movements). Sometimes these may be accompanied by involuntary movements of the extremities. There is no known effective treatment for tardive dyskinesia; antiparkinsonism agents usually do not alleviate the symptoms of this syndrome. It is suggested that all antipsychotic agents be discontinued if these symptoms appear. Should it be necessary to reinstitute treatment, or increase the dosage of the agent, or switch to a different antipsychotic agent, the syndrome may be masked. It has been reported that fine, vermicular movements of the tongue may be an early sign of the syndrome, and if the medication is stopped at that time the syndrome may not develop.

Other CNS effects include cerebral edema; abnormality of cerebrospinal fluid proteins; convulsive seizures, particularly in patients with EEG abnormalities or a history of such disorders, and headaches.

Neuroleptic malignant syndrome has been reported in patients treated with neuroleptic drugs. It is a relatively uncommon, potentially lethal syndrome, characterized by severe extrapyramidal dysfunction, with rigidity and eventual stupor or coma; hyperthemia; and autonomic disturbances, including cardiovascular effects. There is no specific treatment; the neuroleptic drug should be stopped immediately.

Drowsiness may occur, particularly during the first or second week, after which it generally disappears. If troublesome, lower the dosage. Hypnotic effects appear to be minimal, especially in patients who are permitted to remain active.

Adverse behavioral effects include paradoxical exacerbation of psychotic symptoms, catatonic-like states, paranoid reactions, lethargy, paradoxical excitement, restlessness, hyperactivity, nocturnal confusion, bizarre dreams, and insomnia.

Hyperreflexia has been reported in the newborn when a phenothiazine was used during pregnancy.

Autonomic Effects: dry mouth or salivation, nausea, vomiting, diarrhea, anorexia, constipation, obstipation, fecal impaction, urinary retention, frequency or incontinence, bladder paralysis, polyuria, nasal congestion, pallor, myosis, mydriasis, blurred vision, glaucoma, perspiration, hypertension, hypotension, and change in pulse rate occasionally may occur. Significant autonomic effects have been infrequent in patients receiving less than 24 mg perphenazine daily.

Adynamic ileus occasionally occurs with phenothiazine therapy and if severe can result in complications and death. It is of particular concern in psychiatric patients, who may fail to seek treatment of this condition.

Allergic Effects: urticaria, erythema, eczema, exfoliative dermatitis, pruritus, photosensitivity, asthma, fever, anaphylactoid reactions, laryngeal edema, and angioneurotic edema; contact dermatitis in nursing personnel administering the drug, and in extremely rare instances, individual idiosyncrasy or hypersensitivity to phenothiazines has resulted in cerebral edema, circulatory collapse, and death.

Endocrine Effects: lactation, galactorrhea, moderate breast enlargement in females and gynecomastia in males on large doses, disturbances in the menstrual cycle, amenorrhea, changes in libido, inhibition of ejaculation, syndrome of inappropriate ADH (antidiuretic hormone) secretion, false positive pregnancy tests, hyperglycemia, hypoglycemia, glycosuria.

Cardiovascular Effects: postural hypotension, tachycardia (especially with sudden marked increase in dosage), bradycardia, cardiac arrest, faintness, and dizziness. Occasionally the hypotensive effect may produce a shock-like condition. ECG changes, nonspecific, (quinidine-like effect) usually reversible, have been observed in some patients receiving phenothiazine tranquilizers.

Sudden death has occasionally been reported in patients who have received phenothiazines. In some cases the death was apparently due to cardiac arrest; in others, the cause appeared to be asphyxia due to failure of the cough reflex. In some patients, the cause could not be determined nor could it be established that the death was due to the phenothiazine.

Hematological Effects: agranulocytosis, eosinophilia, leukopenia, hemolytic anemia, thrombocytopenic purpura, and pancytopenia. Most cases of agranulocytosis have occurred between the fourth and tenth weeks of therapy. Patients should be watched closely especially during that period for the sudden appearance of sore throat or signs of infection. If white blood cell and differential cell counts show significant cellular depression, discontinue the drug and start appropriate therapy. However, a slightly lowered white count is not in itself an indication to discontinue the drug.

Other Effects: Special considerations in long-term therapy include pigmentation of the skin, occurring chiefly in the exposed areas, ocular changes consisting of deposition of fine particulate matter in the cornea and lens, progressing in more severe cases to star-shaped lenticular opacities; epithelial keratopathies; and pigmentary retinopathy. Also noted: peripheral edema, reversed epinephrine effect, increase in PBI not attributable to an increase in thyroxine, parotid swelling (rare), hyperpyrexia, systemic lupus erythematosus-like syndrome, increases in appetite and weight, polyphagia, photophobia, and muscle weakness.

Liver damage (biliary stasis) may occur. Jaundice may occur, usually between the second and fourth weeks of treatment and is regarded as a hypersensitivity reaction. Incidence is low. The clinical picture resembles infectious hepatitis but with laboratory features of obstructive jaundice. It is usually reversible; however, chronic jaundice has been reported.

Side effects with intramuscular TRILAFON **Injection** have been infrequent and transient. Dizziness or significant hypotension after treatment with TRILAFON **Injection** is a rare occurrence.

DOSAGE AND ADMINISTRATION

Dosage must be individualized and adjusted according to the severity of the condition and the response obtained. As with all potent drugs, the best dose is the lowest dose that will produce the desired clinical effect. Since extrapyramidal symptoms increase in frequency and severity with increased dosage, it is important to employ the lowest effective dose. These symptoms have disappeared upon reduction of dosage, withdrawal of the drug or administration of an anti-parkinsonian agent.

Prolonged administration of doses exceeding 24 mg daily should be reserved for hospitalized patients or patients under continued observation for early detection and management of adverse reactions. An antiparkinsonian agent, such as trihexyphenidyl hydrochloride or benztropine mesylate, is valuable in controlling drug-induced, extrapyramidal symptoms.

TRILAFON **Tablets** and REPETABS **Tablets**

Suggested dosages for **Tablets** and REPETABS **Tablets** for various conditions follow:

Moderately disturbed non-hospitalized psychotic patients: **Tablets** 4 to 8 mg t.i.d., or one or two REPETABS **Tablets** b.i.d., initially; reduce as soon as possible to minimum effective dosage.

Hospitalized psychotic patients: **Tablets** 8 to 16 mg b.i.d. to q.i.d. or one to four REPETABS **Tablets** b.i.d.; avoid dosages in excess of 64 mg daily.

Severe nausea and vomiting in adults: **Tablets** 8 to 16 mg daily in divided doses or one REPETABS **Tablet** b.i.d.; 24 mg occasionally may be necessary; early dosage reduction is desirable. Two REPETABS **Tablets** may be administered in acute cases.

TRILAFON **INJECTION**—Intramuscular Administration

The injection is used when rapid effect and prompt control of acute or intractable conditions is required or when oral administration is not feasible. TRILAFON **Injection**, administered by deep intramuscular injection, is well tolerated. The injection should be given with the patient seated or recumbent, and the patient should be observed for a short period after administration.

Therapeutic effect is usually evidenced in 10 minutes and is maximal in 1 to 2 hours. The average duration of effective action is 6 hours, occasionally 12 to 24 hours.

Pediatric dosage has not yet been established. Children over 12 years may receive the lowest limit of adult dosage.

The usual initial dose is 5 mg (1 ml). This may be repeated every 6 hours. Ordinarily, the total daily dosage should not exceed 15 mg in ambulatory patients or 30 mg in hospitalized patients. When required for satisfactory control of symptoms in severe conditions, an initial 10 mg intramuscular dose may be given. Patients should be placed on oral therapy as soon as practicable. Generally, this may be achieved within 24 hours. In some instances, however, patients have been maintained on injectable therapy for several months. It has been established that TRILAFON **Injection** is more potent than TRILAFON **Tablets**. Therefore, equal or higher dosage should be used when the patient is transferred to oral therapy after receiving the injection.

Psychotic conditions: While 5 mg of the **Injection** has a definite tranquilizing effect, it may be necessary to use 10 mg doses to initiate therapy in severely agitated states. Most patients will be controlled and amendable to oral therapy within a maximum of 24 to 48 hours. Acute conditions (hysteria, panic reaction) often respond well to a single dose whereas in chronic conditions, several injections may be required. When transferring patients to oral therapy, it is suggested that increased dosage be employed to maintain adequate clinical control. This should be followed by gradual reduction to the minimal maintenance dose which is effective.

Severe nausea and vomiting in adults: To obtain rapid control of vomiting, administer 5 mg (1 ml); in rare instances it may be necessary to increase the dose to 10 mg, in general, higher doses should be given only to hospitalized patients.

TRILAFON **Injection**—Intravenous Administration

The intravenous administration of TRILAFON **Injection** is seldom required. This route of administration should be used with particular caution and care and only when absolutely necessary to control severe vomiting, intractable hiccoughs, or acute conditions, such as violent retching during surgery. Its use should be limited to recumbent, hospitalized adults in doses not exceeding 5 mg. When employed in this manner, intravenous injection ordinarily should be given as a diluted solution by either fractional injection or a slow drip infusion. In the surgical patient, slow infusion of no more than 5 mg is preferred. When administered in divided doses, TRILAFON **Injection** should be diluted to 0.5 mg/ml (1 ml mixed with 9 ml of physiologic saline solution), and not more than 1 mg per injection given at not less than one-to two-minute intervals. Intravenous injection should be discontinued as soon as symptoms are controlled and should not exceed 5 mg. The possibility of hypotensive and extrapyramidal side effects should be considered and appropriate means for management kept available. Blood pressure and pulse should be monitored continuously during intravenous administration. Pharmacologic and clinical studies indicate that intravenous administration of norepinephrine should be useful in alleviating the hypotensive effect.

TRILAFON **Concentrate**

In hospitalized psychotic patients, the usual dosage range is 8 to 16 mg b.i.d. to q.i.d., depending on the severity of symptoms and individual response. Although a number of investigators have employed higher dosages, a total daily dose of more than 64 mg ordinarily is not required. The **Concentrate** should be diluted only with water, saline, Seven-Up, homogenized milk, carbonated orange drink and pineapple, apricot, prune, orange. V-8, tomato, and grapefruit juices. Trilafon **Concentrate** should not be mixed with beverages containing caffeine (coffee, cola) tannics (tea), or pectinates (apple juice) since physical incompatibility may result. Suggested dilution is approximately two fluid ounces of diluent for each 5 ml (16 mg) teaspoonful of TRILAFON **Concentrate.** For convenience in measuring smaller doses, a graduated dropper marked to measure 8 mg or 4 mg is supplied with each bottle.

OVERDOSAGE

In the event of overdosage, emergency treatment should be started immediately. All patients suspected of having taken an overdose should be hospitalized as soon as possible.

Manifestations: Overdosage of perphenazine primarily involves the extrapyramidal mechanism and produces the same side effects described under ADVERSE REACTIONS, but to a more marked degree. It is usually evidenced by stupor or coma; children may have convulsive seizures.

Treatment: Treatment is symptomatic and supportive. There is no specific antidote. The patient should be induced to vomit even if emesis has occurred spontaneously. Pharmacologic vomiting by the administration of ipecac syrup is a preferred method. It should be noted that ipecac has a central mode of action in addition to its local gastric irritant properties, and the central mode of action may be blocked by the antiemetic effect of TRILAFON products. Vomiting should not be induced in patients with impaired consciousness. The action of ipecac is facilitated by physical activity and by the administration of 8 to 12 fluid ounces of water. If emesis does not occur within 15 minutes, the dose of ipecac should be repeated. Precautions against aspiration must be taken, especially in infants and children. Following emesis, any drug remaining in the stomach may be adsorbed by activated charcoal administered as a slurry with water. If vomiting is unsuccessful or contraindicated, gastric lavage should be performed. Isotonic and one-half isotonic saline are the lavage solutions of choice. Saline cathartics, such as milk of magnesia, draw water into the bowel by osmosis and therefore may be valuable for their action in rapid dilution of bowel content.

Standard measures (oxygen, intravenous fluids, corticosteroids) should be used to manage circulatory shock or metabolic acidosis. An open airway and adequate fluid intake should be maintained. Body temperature should be regulated. Hypothermia is expected, but severe hyperthermia may occur and must be treated vigorously. (See CONTRAINDICATIONS.)

An electrocardiogram should be taken and close monitoring of cardiac function instituted if there is any sign of abnormality. Cardiac arrhythmias may be treated with neostigmine, pyridostigmine, or propranolol. Digitalis should be considered for cadiac failure. Close monitoring of cardiac function is advisable for not less than five days. Vasopressors such as norepinephrine may be used to treat hypotension, but epinephrine should NOT be used.

Anticonvulsants (an inhalation anesthetic, diazepam, or paraldehyde) are recommended for control of convulsions, since perphenazine increases the central nervous system depressant action, but not the anticonvulsant action of barbiturates.

If acute parkinson-like symptoms result from perphenazine intoxication, benztropine mesylate or diphenydramine may be administered.

Central nervous system depression may be treated with nonconvulsant doses of CNS stimulants. Avoid stimulants that may cause convulsions (e.g., picrotoxin and pentylenetetrazol).

Signs of arousal may not occur for 48 hours.

Dialysis is of no value because of low plasma concentrations of the drug.

Since overdosage is often deliberate, patients may attempt suicide by other means during the recovery phase. Deaths by deliberate or accidental overdosage have occurred with this class of drugs.

HOW SUPPLIED

TRILAFON **Tablets** (2 mg): gray, sugar-coated tablets branded in black with the Schering trademark and either product identification letters, ADH, or numbers 705; bottles of 100 (NDC 0085-0705-04) and 500 (NDC 0085-0705-06).

TRILAFON **Tablets** (4 mg): gray, sugar-coated tablets branded in green with the Schering trademark and either product identification letters, ADK, or numbers, 940; bottles of 100 (NDC 0085-0940-05) and 500 (NDC 0085-0940-04).

TRILAFON **Tablets** (8 mg): gray, sugar-coated tablets branded in blue with the Schering trademark and either product identification letters, ADJ, or numbers 313; bottles of 100 (NDC 0085-0313-05) and 500 (NDC 0085-0313-04).

TRILAFON **Tablets** (16 mg): gray, sugar-coated tablets branded in red with the Schering trademark and either product identification letters, ADM, or numbers, 077; bottles of 100 (NDC 0085-0077-05) and 500 (NDC 0085-0077-04).

TRILAFON REPETABS **Tablets** (8 mg): white, sugar-coated tablets branded in gray with the Schering trademark and either product identification letters, ADX, or numbers, 141; bottle of 100 (NDC 0085-0141-06).

TRILAFON **Concentrate**, 16 mg per 5 ml, 4 fluid ounce (118 ml) bottle with graduated dropper (NDC 0085-0363-02). The **Concentrate** is light-sensitive and should be dispensed in amber bottles. **Protect from light. Store in carton until contents are used. Shake well.**

TRILAFON **Injection**, 5 mg per ml, 1-ml ampul for intramuscular or intravenous use, box of 100 (NDC 0085-0012-04). Keep package closed to protect from light. Exposure may cause discoloration. Slight yellowish discoloration will not alter potency or therapeutic efficacy; if markedly discolored, ampul should be discarded. **Protect from light. Store in carton until contents are used.**

Store all TRILAFON Tablets and TRILAFON Concentrate between 2° and 30°C (36° and 86°F).

Revised 7/85

Shown in Product Identification Section, page 428

TRINALIN® ℞

[trin 'a-lin]

brand of azatadine maleate, USP and pseudoephedrine sulfate, USP

Long-Acting Antihistamine/Decongestant REPETABS® Tablets

DESCRIPTION

TRINALIN Long-Acting Antihistamine/Decongestant REPETABS (brand of repeat-action tablets) Tablets contain 1 mg azatadine maleate, USP in the tablet coating and 120 mg pseudoephedrine sulfate, USP, equally distributed between the tablet coating and the barrier-coated core. Following ingestion, the two active components in the coating are quickly liberated; release of the decongestant in the core is delayed for several hours.

Azatadine maleate is an antihistamine having the empirical formula, $C_{20}H_{22}N_2 \cdot 2C_4H_4O_4$, the chemical name, 6,11-Dihydro-11-(1-methyl-4-piperidylidene)-5*H*-benzo[5,6]cyclohepta [1,2-*b*] pyridine maleate (1:2).

The molecular weight of azatadine maleate is 522.54. Azatadine maleate is a white to off-white powder and is very soluble in water and soluble in alcohol.

Pseudoephedrine sulfate, a sympathomimetic amine, is a salt of pseudoephedrine, one of the naturally occurring alkaloids obtained from various species of the plant *Ephedra*. The empirical formula for pseudoephedrine sulfate is $(C_{10}H_{15}NO)_2 \cdot H_2SO_4$; the chemical name is Benzenemethanol, α-[1-(methylamino)ethyl]-, [*S*-(*R**, *R**)]-, sulfate (2:1) (salt).

The molecular weight of pseudoephedrine sulfate is 428.56. It is a white to off-white crystal or powder, very soluble in water, freely soluble in alcohol, and sparingly soluble in chloroform.

The inactive ingredients for TRINALIN REPETABS Tablets are: Acacia, Butylparaben, Calcium Sulfate, Carnauba Wax, Corn Starch, D&C Red No. 30 Al Lake, Neutral Soap, FD&C Yellow No. 6 Al Lake, FD&C Yellow No. 6, Gelatin, Lactose, Magnesium Stearate, Oleic Acid, Povidone, Rosin, Sugar, Talc, White Wax, and Zein.

CLINICAL PHARMACOLOGY

Azatadine maleate is an antihistamine, related to cyproheptadine, with antiserotonin, anticholinergic (drying), and sedative effects. Antihistamines appear to compete with histamine for histamine H_1-receptor sites on effector cells. The antihistamines antagonize those pharmacological effects of histamine which are mediated through activation of H_1-receptor sites and thereby reduce the intensity of allergic reactions and tissue injury response involving histamine release. Antihistamines antagonize the vasodilator effect of endogenously released histamine, especially in small vessels, and mitigate the effect of histamine which results in increased capillary permeability and edema formation. As consequences of these actions, antihistamines antagonize the physiological manifestations of histamine release in the nose following antigen-antibody interaction, such as congestion related to vascular engorgement, mucosal edema, and profuse, watery secretion, and irritation and sneezing resulting from histamine action on afferent nerve terminals.

Pseudoephedrine sulfate (d-isoephedrine sulfate) is an orally effective nasal decongestant which appears to exert its sympathomimetic effect indirectly, predominantly through release of adrenergic mediators from post-ganglionic nerve terminals. In effective recommended oral dosage, pseudoephedrine sulfate produces minimal other sympathomimetic effects, such as pressor activity and CNS stimulation. Use of an orally administered vasoconstrictor for shrinkage of congested nasal mucosa has several advantages: a) it produces a gradual but sustained decongestant effect, causing little, if any "rebound" congestion; b) it facilitates shrinkage of swollen mucosa in upper respiratory areas that are relatively inaccessible to topically applied sprays or drops; c) it relieves nasal obstruction without the additional irritation that may result from local medication.

Pseudoephedrine passes through the blood-brain and placental barriers. While the antihistamines have not been studied systematically for passage through these barriers, the occurrence of pharmacologic effects in the central nervous system and in newborns indicate presence of the drug.

Following administration of the two drugs to normal volunteers in either a single TRINALIN REPETABS Tablet or similar doses in two conventional pseudoephedrine sulfate tablets and a conventional tablet of azatadine maleate, the blood levels of pseudoephedrine and the urinary excretion of azatadine showed that the TRINALIN REPETABS Tablets are bioequivalent to the conventional dosage forms. The apparent elimination half-life of pseudoephedrine in TRINALIN REPETABS Tablets was approximately 6½ hours. The apparent elimination of half-life of azatadine maleate (available from the outer layer of the TRINALIN REPETABS Tablets or from the conventional azatadine maleate tablet) was approximately 12 hours.

INDICATIONS AND USAGE

TRINALIN Long-Acting Antihista.nine/Decongestant REPETABS Tablets are indicated for the relief of the symptoms of upper respiratory mucosal congestion in perennial and allergic rhinitis, and for the relief of nasal congestion and eustachian tube congestion. Analgesics, antibiotics, or both may be administered concurrently, when indicated.

CONTRAINDICATIONS

Antihistamines should not be used to treat lower respiratory tract symptoms, including asthma.

This product is contraindicated in patients with narrow-angle glaucoma or urinary retention, and in patients receiving monoamine oxidase (MAO) inhibitor therapy or within ten days of stopping such treatment. (See Drug Interactions section.) It is also contraindicated in patients with severe hypertension, severe coronary artery disease, hyperthyroidism, and in those who have shown hypersensitivity or idiosyncrasy to its components, to adrenergic agents, or to other drugs of similar chemical structures. Manifestations of patient idiosyncrasy to adrenergic agents include: insomnia, dizziness, weakness, tremor, or arrhythmias.

WARNINGS

TRINALIN REPETABS Tablets should be used with considerable caution in patients with: stenosing peptic ulcer, pyloroduodenal obstruction, urinary bladder obstruction due to symptomatic prostatic hypertrophy, or narrowing of the bladder neck. It should also be administered with caution to patients with cardiovascular disease, including hypertension or ischemic heart disease; increased intraocular pressure (See CONTRAINDICATIONS); diabetes mellitus, or in patients receiving digitalis or oral anticoagulants.

Central nervous system stimulation and convulsions or cardiovascular collapse with accompanying hypotension may be produced by sympathomimetics.

Continued on next page

Information on Schering products appearing on these pages is effective as of September 30, 1986.

Schering—Cont.

Do not exceed recommended dosage.
Use in Activities Requiring Mental Alertness: Patients should be warned about engaging in activities requiring mental alertness, such as driving a car or operating appliances, machinery, etc.
Use in Patients Approximately 60 Years and Older: Antihistamines are more likely to cause dizziness, sedation, and hypotension in patients over 60 years of age. In these patients, sympathomimetics are also more likely to cause adverse reactions, such as confusion, hallucinations, convulsions, CNS depression, and death. For this reason, before considering the use of a repeat-action formulation, the safe use of a short-acting sympathomimetic in that particular patient should be demonstrated.

PRECAUTIONS

General: Because of the atropine-like action of antihistamines, this product should be used with caution in patients with a history of bronchial asthma.
Information for Patients:
1. Products containing antihistamines may cause drowsiness.
2. Patients should not engage in activities requiring mental alertness, such as driving or operating machinery or appliances.
3. Alcohol or other sedative drugs may enhance the drowsiness caused by antihistamines.
4. Patients should not take TRINALIN REPETABS Tablets if they are receiving a monoamine oxidase inhibitor or within 10 days of stopping such treatment, or if they are receiving oral anticoagulants.
5. This medication should not be given to children less than 12 years of age.

Drug Interactions: MAO inhibitors prolong and intensify the effects of antihistamines. Concomitant use of antihistamines with alcohol, tricyclic antidepressants, barbiturates, or other central nervous system depressants may have an additive effect. The action of oral anticoagulants may be inhibited by antihistamines.
When sympathomimetic drugs are given to patients receiving monoamine oxidase inhibitors, hypertensive reactions, including hypertensive crises, may occur. The antihypertensive effects of methyldopa, mecamylamine, reserpine, and veratrum alkaloids may be reduced by sympathomimetics. Beta-adrenergic blocking agents may also interact with sympathomimetics. Increased ectopic pacemaker activity can occur when pseudoephedrine is used concomitantly with digitalis. Antacids increase the rate of absorption of pseudoephedrine, while kaolin decreases it.
Drug/Laboratory Test Interactions: The *in vitro* addition of pseudoephedrine to sera containing the cardiac isoenzyme MB of serum creatine phosphokinase progressively inhibits the activity of the enzyme. The inhibition becomes complete over six hours.
Carcinogenesis, Mutagenesis, and Impairment of Fertility: - There is no animal or laboratory study of the mixture of azatadine maleate and pseudoephedrine sulfate to evaluate carcinogenesis or mutagenesis. Reproduction studies of this mixture in rats showed no evidence of impaired fertility.
Pregnancy Category C: Retarded fetal development and the presence of angulated hyoid wings were seen in the offspring of pregnant rabbits administered TRINALIN at about 12.5 times and 5 times the recommended human dosage, respectively; increased resorption was noted at about 25 times the human dosage. A decreased survival rate at day 21 was seen in rat pups born of mothers given TRINALIN during pregnancy at a dose about 12.5 times the human dosage. There are no adequate and well-controlled studies in pregnant women. TRINALIN REPETABS Tablets should be used during pregnancy only if the potential benefits to the mother justify the potential risks to the infant. (See Nonteratogenic Effects.)
Nonteratogenic Effects: Antihistamines should not be used in the third trimester of pregnancy, because newborns and premature infants may have severe reactions to them such as convulsions.
Nursing Mothers: It is not known whether these drugs are excreted in human milk. However, certain antihistamines and sympathomimetics are known to be excreted in human milk. Because of the higher risks of antihistamines for infants generally and for newborns and prematures in particular, a decision should be made whether to discontinue nursing or to discontinue the drug, taking into account the importance of the drug to the mother.
There is a report of irritability, excessive crying and disturbed sleeping patterns in a nursing infant whose mother had taken a product containing an antihistamine and pseudoephedrine.
Pediatric use: Safety and effectiveness in children below the age of 12 years have not been established.

ADVERSE REACTIONS

The following adverse reactions are associated with antihistamine and sympathomimetic drugs. (Those adverse reactions which occur most frequently with the antihistamines are underlined.)
General: Urticaria, drug rash, anaphylactic shock, photosensitivity, excessive perspiration, chills, dryness of mouth, nose, and throat.
Cardiovascular: Hypertension (see CONTRAINDICATIONS and WARNINGS), hypotension, arrhythmias and cardiovascular collapse, headache, palpitations, extrasystoles, tachycardia, angina.
Hematologic: Hemolytic anemia, hypoplastic anemia, thrombocytopenia, agranulocytosis.
Central Nervous System: Sedation, sleepiness, dizziness, vertigo, tinnitus, acute labyrinthitis, disturbed coordination, fatigue, mydriasis, confusion, restlessness, excitation, nervousness, tension, tremor, irritability, insomnia, euphoria, paresthesias, blurred vision, hysteria, neuritis, convulsions, fear, anxiety, hallucinations, CNS depression, weakness, pallor.
Gastrointestinal: Epigastric distress, anorexia, nausea, vomiting, diarrhea, constipation, abdominal cramps.
Genitourinary: Urinary frequency, urinary retention, dysuria, early menses.
Respiratory: Thickening of bronchial secretions, tightness of chest and wheezing, nasal stuffiness, respiratory difficulty.

DRUG ABUSE AND DEPENDENCE

There is no information to indicate that abuse or dependency occurs with azatadine maleate.
Pseudoephedrine, like other central nervous system stimulants, has been abused. At high doses, subjects commonly experience an elevation of mood, a sense of increased energy and alertness, and decreased appetite. Some individuals become anxious, irritable, and loquacious. In addition to the marked euphoria, the user experiences a sense of markedly enhanced physical strength and mental capacity. With continued use, tolerance develops, the user increases the dose, and toxic signs and symptoms appear. Depression may follow rapid withdrawal.

OVERDOSAGE

In the event of overdosage, emergency treatment should be started immediately.
Manifestations of overdosage may vary from central nervous system depression (sedation, apnea, diminished mental alertness, cyanosis, coma, cardiovascular collapse) to stimulation (insomnia, hallucinations, tremors, or convulsions) to death. Other signs and symptoms may be euphoria, excitement, tachycardia, palpitations, thirst, perspiration, nausea, dizziness, tinnitus, ataxia, blurred vision, and hypertension or hypotension. Stimulation is particularly likely in children, as are atropine-like signs and symptoms (dry mouth; fixed, dilated pupils, flushing; hyperthermia; and gastrointestinal symptoms).
In large doses sympathomimetics may give rise to giddiness, headache, nausea, vomiting, sweating, thirst, tachycardia, precordial pain, palpitations, difficulty in micturition, muscular weakness and tenseness, anxiety, restlessness, and insomnia. Many patients can present a toxic psychosis with delusions and hallucinations. Some may develop cardiac arrhythmias, circulatory collapse, convulsions, coma, and respiratory failure.
The oral LD_{50} of the mixture of the two drugs in mature rats and mice was greater than 1700 mg/kg and 600 mg/kg, respectively.
Treatment—The patient should be induced to vomit, even if emesis has occurred spontaneously. Pharmacologically induced vomiting by the administration of ipecac syrup is a preferred method. However, vomiting should not be induced in patients with impaired consciousness. The action of ipecac is facilitated by physical activity and by the administration of eight to twelve fluid ounces of water. If emesis does not occur within fifteen minutes, the dose of ipecac should be repeated. Precautions against aspiration must be taken, especially in infants and children. Following emesis, any drug remaining in the stomach may be adsorbed by activated charcoal administered as a slurry with water. If vomiting is unsuccessful or contraindicated, gastric lavage should be performed. Isotonic and one-half isotonic saline are the lavage solutions of choice. Saline cathartics, such as milk of magnesia, draw water into the bowel by osmosis and therefore may be valuable for their action in rapid dilution of bowel content. Dialysis is of little value in antihistamine poisoning. After emergency treatment the patient should continue to be medically monitored.
Treatment of the signs and symptoms of overdosage is symptomatic and supportive. Stimulants (analeptic agents) should not be used. Vasopressors may be used to treat hypotension. Short-acting barbiturates, diazepam, or paraldehyde may be administered to control seizures. Hyperpyrexia, especially in children, may require treatment with tepid water sponge baths or a hypothermic blanket. Apnea is treated with ventilatory support.

DOSAGE AND ADMINISTRATION

TRINALIN REPETABS Tablets ARE NOT INTENDED FOR USE IN CHILDREN UNDER 12 YEARS OF AGE. The usual adult dosage is one tablet twice a day.

HOW SUPPLIED

TRINALIN REPETABS Tablets contain 1 mg azatadine maleate and 120 mg pseudoephedrine sulfate. TRINALIN REPETABS Tablets are coral-colored, sugar-coated tablets branded in black with the Schering trademark, or the product name and product identification numbers, 703; bottle of 100 (NDC-0085-0703-04).
Store between 2° and 30°C (36° and 86°F).

Revised 8/85
Shown in Product Identification Section, page 428

VALISONE® ℞

[*val 'ĭ-sōn*]
brand of betamethasone valerate
Cream, USP 0.1%
Ointment, USP 0.1%
Lotion, USP 0.1%
Reduced Strength Cream, USP 0.01%
(potency expressed as betamethasone)
For Dermatologic Use Only
Not for Ophthalmic Use

DESCRIPTION

VALISONE **Cream, Reduced Strength Cream, Ointment** and **Lotion** contain betamethasone valerate, USP, a synthetic adrenocorticoid for dermatologic use. Betamethasone, an analog of prednisolone, has a high degree of corticosteroid activity and a slight degree of mineralocorticosteroid activity. Betamethasone valerate is the 17-valerate ester of betamethasone.
Chemically, betamethasone valerate is 9-Fluoro-11β,17,21-trihydroxy-16β,methylpregna-1, 4-diene-3,20-dione 17-valerate, with the empirical formula $C_{27}H_{37}FO_6$, and a molecular weight of 476.58.
Betamethasone valerate is a white to practically white, odorless crystalline powder, and is practically insoluble in water, freely soluble in acetone and in chloroform, soluble in alcohol, and slightly soluble in benzene and in ether.
Each gram of VALISONE **Cream** 0.1% contains: 1.2 mg betamethasone valerate, USP (equivalent to 1.0 mg betamethasone), in an aqueous hydrophilic emollient cream consisting of mineral oil, white petrolatum, ceteareth-30, cetearyl alcohol, monobasic sodium phosphate, and phosphoric acid; chlorocresol and propylene glycol as preservatives.
Each gram of VALISONE **Ointment** 0.1% contains: 1.2 mg betamethasone valerate, USP (equivalent to 1.0 mg betamethasone), in an ointment base of mineral oil, white petrolatum, and hydrogenated lanolin.
Each gram of VALISONE **Lotion** 0.1% contains: 1.2 mg betamethasone valerate, USP (equivalent to 1.0 mg betamethasone) in a lotion base of isopropyl alcohol (47.5%) and water slightly thickened with carbomer 934P; the pH is adjusted to approximately 4.7 with sodium hydroxide.
Each gram of VALISONE **Reduced Strength Cream** 0.01% contains: 0.12 mg betamethasone valerate, USP (equivalent to 0.1 mg betamethasone), in an aqueous hydrophilic emollient cream consisting of mineral oil, white petrolatum, ceteareth-30, cetearyl alcohol, monobasic sodium phosphate, and phosphoric acid; chlorocresol and propylene glycol as preservatives.

CLINICAL PHARMACOLOGY

The corticosteroids are a class of compounds comprising steroid hormones secreted by the adrenal cortex and their synthetic analogs. In pharmacologic doses corticosteroids are used primarily for their anti-inflammatory and/or immunosuppressive effects.
Topical corticosteroids, such as betamethasone valerate, are effective in the treatment of corticosteroid-responsive dermatoses primarily because of their anti-inflammatory, antipruritic, and vasoconstrictive actions. However, while the physiologic, pharmacologic, and clinical effects of the corticosteroids are well-known, the exact mechanisms of their actions in each disease are uncertain. Betamethasone valerate, a corticosteroid, has been shown to have topical (dermatologic) and systemic pharmacologic and metabolic effects characteristic of this class of drugs.
Pharmacokinetics: The extent of percutaneous absorption of topical corticosteroids is determined by many factors including the vehicle, the integrity of the epidermal barrier, and the use of occlusive dressings.
Topical corticosteroids can be absorbed from normal intact skin. Inflammation and/or other disease processes in the skin increase percutaneous absorption. Occlusive dressings substantially increase the percutaneous absorption of topical corticosteroids. Thus, occlusive dressings may be a valuable therapeutic adjunct for treatment of resistant dermatoses.

Once absorbed through the skin, topical corticosteroids are handled through pharmacokinetic pathways similar to systemically administered corticosteroids. Corticosteroids are bound to plasma proteins in varying degrees. Corticosteroids are metabolized primarily in the liver and are then excreted by the kidneys. Some of the topical corticosteroids and their metabolites are also excreted into the bile.

INDICATIONS AND USAGE

VALISONE **Cream, Reduced Strength Cream, Ointment** and **Lotion** are indicated for relief of the inflammatory and pruritic manifestations of corticosteroid-responsive dermatoses.

CONTRAINDICATIONS

VALISONE **Cream, Reduced Strength Cream, Ointment,** and **Lotion** are contraindicated in patients who are hypersensitive to betamethasone valerate, to other corticosteroids, or to any ingredient in this preparation.

PRECAUTIONS

General: Systemic absorption of topical corticosteroids has produced reversible hypothalamic-pituitary-adrenal (HPA) axis suppression, manifestations of Cushing's syndrome, hyperglycemia, and glucosuria in some patients.

Conditions which augment systemic absorption include the application of the more potent steroids, use over large surface areas, prolonged use, and the addition of occlusive dressings.

Therefore, patients receiving a large dose of a potent topical steroid applied to a large surface area or under an occlusive dressing should be evaluated periodically for evidence of HPA axis suppression by using the urinary free cortisol and ACTH stimulation tests. If HPA axis suppression is noted, an attempt should be made to withdraw the drug, to reduce the frequency of application, or to substitute a less potent steroid.

Recovery of HPA axis function is generally prompt and complete upon discontinuation of the drug. Infrequently, signs and symptoms of steroid withdrawal may occur, requiring supplemental systemic corticosteroids.

Children may absorb proportionally larger amounts of topical corticosteroids and thus be more susceptible to systemic toxicity. (See **PRECAUTIONS-Pediatric Use.**)

If irritation develops, topical corticosteroids should be discontinued and appropriate therapy instituted.

In the presence of dermatological infections, the use of an appropriate antifungal or antibacterial agent should be instituted. If a favorable response does not occur promptly, the corticosteroid should be discontinued until the infection has been adequately controlled.

Information for Patients: Patients using topical corticosteroids should receive the following information and instructions:

1. This medication is to be used as directed by the physician. It is for external use only. Avoid contact with the eyes.
2. Patients should be advised not to use this medication for any disorder other than for which it was prescribed.
3. The treated skin area should not be bandaged or otherwise covered or wrapped as to be occlusive unless directed by the physician.
4. Patients should report any signs of local adverse reactions especially under occlusive dressing.
5. Parents of pediatric patients should be advised not to use tight-fitting diapers or plastic pants on a child being treated in the diaper area, as these garments may constitute occlusive dressings.

Laboratory Tests: The following tests may be helpful in evaluating HPA axis suppression:

Urinary free cortisol test
ACTH stimulation test

Carcinogenesis, Mutagenesis, and Impairment of Fertility: Long-term animal studies have not been performed to evaluate the carcinogenic potential or the effect on fertility of topical corticosteroids.

Studies to determine mutagenicity with prednisolone have revealed negative results.

Pregnancy Category C: Corticosteroids are generally teratogenic in laboratory animals when administered systemically at relatively low dosage levels. The more potent corticosteroids have been shown to be teratogenic after dermal application in laboratory animals. There are no adequate and well-controlled studies in pregnant women on teratogenic effects from topically applied corticosteroids. Therefore, topical corticosteroids should be used during pregnancy only if the potential benefit justifies the potential risk to the fetus. Drugs of this class should not be used extensively on pregnant patients, in large amounts, or for prolonged periods of time.

Nursing Mothers: It is not known whether topical administration of corticosteroids could result in sufficient systemic absorption to produce detectable quantities in breast milk. Systemically administered corticosteroids are secreted into breast milk in quantities not likely to have a deleterious effect on the infant. Nevertheless, caution should be exercised when topical corticosteroids are prescribed for a nursing woman.

Pediatric Use: Pediatric patients may demonstrate greater susceptibility to topical corticosteroid-induced HPA axis suppression and Cushing's syndrome than mature patients because of a larger skin surface area to body weight ratio.

Hypothalamic-pituitary-adrenal (HPA) axis suppression, Cushing's syndrome, and intracranial hypertension, have been reported in children receiving topical corticosteroids. Manifestations of adrenal suppression in children include linear growth retardation, delayed weight gain, low plasma cortisol levels, and absence of response to ACTH stimulation. Manifestations of intracranial hypertension include bulging fontanelles, headaches, and bilateral papilledema.

Administration of topical corticosteroids to children should be limited to the least amount compatible with an effective therapeutic regimen. Chronic corticosteroid therapy may interfere with the growth and development of children.

ADVERSE REACTIONS

The following local adverse reactions have been reported with topical dermatologic corticosteroids, especially under occlusive dressings: burning; itching; irritation; dryness; folliculitis; hypertrichosis; acneiform eruptions; hypopigmentation; perioral dermatitis; allergic contact dermatitis; maceration of the skin; secondary infection; skin atrophy; striae; miliaria.

Systemic absorption of topical corticosteroids has produced reversible hypothalamic-pituitary-adrenal (HPA) axis suppression, manifestations of Cushing's syndrome, hyperglycemia, and glucosuria in some patients.

OVERDOSAGE

Topically applied corticosteroids can be absorbed in sufficient amounts to produce systemic effects (see **PRECAUTIONS.**)

DOSAGE AND ADMINISTRATION

VALISONE **Cream:** Apply a thin film of VALISONE **Cream** 0.1% to the affected skin areas one to three times a day. Dosage once or twice a day is often effective.

VALISONE **Ointment:** Apply a thin film of VALISONE **Ointment** 0.1% to the affected skin areas one to three times a day. Dosage once or twice a day is often effective.

VALISONE **Lotion:** Apply a few drops of VALISONE **Lotion** 0.1% to the affected area and massage lightly until it disappears. Apply twice daily, in the morning and at night. Dosage may be increased in stubborn cases. Following improvement, apply once daily. For the most effective and economical use, apply nozzle very close to affected area and gently squeeze bottle.

VALISONE **Reduced Strength Cream:** Apply a thin film of VALISONE **Reduced Strength Cream** to the affected skin areas one to three times daily. Commonly, treatment twice a day is adequate. In some cases, treatment three times a day is necessary; in others, once a day suffices.

HOW SUPPLIED

VALISONE **Cream** 0.1% is available in 15-gram (NDC 0085-0136-04), 45-gram (NDC 0085-0136-06), and 110-gram (NDC 0085-0136-07) tubes; boxes of one; and a 430-gram jar (NDC 0085-0136-08).

VALISONE **Lotion** 0.1% is available in 20 ml (18.7 g) (NDC 0085-0002-03), and 60 ml (56.2 g) (NDC 0085-0002-05) plastic squeeze bottles; boxes of one. **Protect from light. Store in carton until contents are used.**

VALISONE **Ointment** 0.1% is supplied in 15-gram (NDC 0085-0898-04), and 45-gram (NDC 0085-0898-06) tubes; boxes of one.

VALISONE **Reduced Strength Cream** 0.01% is supplied in 15-gram (NDC 0085-0929-04), and 60-gram (NDC 0085-0929-08) tubes; boxes of one.

Store between 2° and 30°C (36° and 86°F).

Revised 12/85

VANCENASE® Nasal Inhaler ℞

[van 'sen-ās]

brand of beclomethasone dipropionate, USP

For Nasal Inhalation Only

DESCRIPTION

Beclomethasone dipropionate, USP, the active component of VANCENASE Nasal Inhaler, is an anti-inflammatory steroid having the chemical name, 9-Chloro-11β,17,21-trihydroxy-16β-methylpregna-1,4-diene-3,20-dione 17, 21-dipropionate.

Beclomethasone dipropionate is a white to creamy-white odorless powder with a molecular weight of 521.25. It is very slightly soluble in water; very soluble in chloroform; and freely soluble in acetone and in alcohol.

VANCENASE Nasal Inhaler is a metered-dose aerosol unit containing a microcrystalline suspension of beclomethasone dipropionate-trichloromonofluoromethane clathrate in a mixture of propellants (trichloromonofluoromethane and dichlorodifluoromethane) with oleic acid. Each canister contains beclomethasone dipropionate-trichloromonofluoromethane clathrate having a molecular proportion of beclomethasone dipropionate to trichloromonofluoromethane between 3:1 and 3:2. Each actuation delivers from the nasal adapter a quantity of clathrate equivalent to 42 mcg of beclomethasone dipropionate, USP. The contents of one canister provide at least 200 metered doses.

CLINICAL PHARMACOLOGY

Beclomethasone 17,21-dipropionate is a diester of beclomethasone, a synthetic corticosteroid which is chemically related to dexamethasone. Beclomethasone differs from dexamethasone only in having a chlorine at the 9-α position in place of a fluorine. Animal studies showed that beclomethasone dipropionate has potent glucocorticoid and weak mineralocorticoid activity. The mechanisms for the anti-inflammatory action of beclomethasone dipropionate are unknown. The precise mechanism of the aerosolized drug's action in the nose is also unknown. Biopsies of nasal mucosa obtained during clinical studies showed no histopathologic changes when beclomethasone dipropionate was administered intranasally.

The effects of beclomethasone dipropionate on hypothalamic-pituitary-adrenal (HPA) function have been evaluated in adult volunteers, by other routes of administration. Studies are currently being undertaken with beclomethasone dipropionate by the intranasal route, which may demonstrate that there is more or that there is less absorption by this route of administration. There was no suppression of early morning plasma cortisol concentrations when beclomethasone dipropionate was administered in a dose of 1000 mcg/day for one month as an oral aerosol or for three days by intramuscular injection. However, partial suppression of plasma cortisol concentration was observed when beclomethasone dipropionate was administered in doses of 2000 mcg/day either by oral aerosol or intramuscularly. Immediate suppression of plasma cortisol concentrations was observed after single doses of 4000 mcg of beclomethasone dipropionate. Suppression of HPA function (reduction of early morning plasma cortisol levels) has been reported in adult patients who received 1600 mcg daily doses of oral beclomethasone dipropionate for one month. In clinical studies using beclomethasone dipropionate intranasally, there was no evidence of adrenal insufficiency.

Beclomethasone dipropionate is sparingly soluble. When given by nasal inhalation in the form of an aerosolized suspension, the drug is deposited primarily in the nasal passages. A portion of the drug is swallowed. Absorption occurs rapidly from all respiratory and gastrointestinal tissues. There is no evidence of tissue storage of beclomethasone dipropionate or its metabolites. *In vitro* studies, have shown that tissue other than the liver (lung slices) can rapidly metabolize beclomethasone dipropionate to beclomethasone 17-monopropionate and more slowly to free beclomethasone (which has very weak anti-inflammatory activity). However, irrespective of the route of entry, the principal route of excretion of the drug and its metabolites is the feces. In humans, 12% to 15% of an orally administered dose of beclomethasone dipropionate is excreted in the urine as both conjugated and free metabolites of the drug. The half-life of beclomethasone dipropionate in humans is approximately 15 hours.

Studies have shown that the degree of binding to plasma proteins is 87%.

INDICATIONS AND USAGE

VANCENASE Nasal Inhaler is indicated for the relief of the symptoms of seasonal or perennial rhinitis, in those cases poorly responsive to conventional treatment.

VANCENASE is also indicated for the prevention of recurrence of nasal polyps following surgical removal.

Clinical studies in seasonal and perennial rhinitis have shown that improvement is usually apparent within a few days. However, symptomatic relief may not occur in some patients for as long as two weeks. Although systemic effects are minimal at recommended doses, VANCENASE should not be continued beyond three weeks in the absence of significant symptomatic improvement. VANCENASE should not be used in the presence of untreated localized infection involving the nasal mucosa.

Clinical studies have shown that treatment of the symptoms associated with nasal polyps may have to be continued for several weeks or more before a therapeutic result can be fully assessed. Recurrence of symptoms due to polyps can occur after stopping treatment, depending on the severity of the disease.

CONTRAINDICATIONS

Hypersensitivity to any of the ingredients of this preparation contraindicates its use.

Continued on next page

Information on Schering products appearing on these pages is effective as of September 30, 1986.

Schering—Cont.

WARNINGS

The replacement of a systemic corticosteroid with VANCENASE Nasal Inhaler can be accompanied by signs of adrenal insufficiency.

When transferred to VANCENASE Nasal Inhaler, careful attention must be given to patients previously treated for prolonged periods with systemic corticosteroids. This is particularly important in those patients who have associated asthma or other clinical conditions, where too rapid a decrease in systemic corticosteroids may cause a severe exacerbation of their symptoms.

Studies have shown that the combined administration of alternate day prednisone systemic treatment and orally inhaled beclomethasone increased the likelihood of HPA suppression compared to a therapeutic dose of either one alone. Therefore, VANCENASE treatment should be used with caution in patients already on alternate day prednisone regimens for any disease.

PRECAUTIONS

General: During withdrawal from oral steroids, some patients may experience symptoms of withdrawal, e.g., joint and/or muscular pain, lassitude, and depression.

In clinical studies with beclomethasone dipropionate administered intranasally, the development of localized infections of the nose and pharynx with *Candida albicans* has occurred only rarely. When such an infection develops, it may require treatment with appropriate local therapy or discontinuance of treatment with VANCENASE Nasal Inhaler.

Beclomethasone dipropionate is absorbed into the circulation. Use of excessive doses of VANCENASE Nasal Inhaler may suppress HPA function.

VANCENASE should be used with caution, if at all, in patients with active or quiescent tuberculous infections of the respiratory tract, or in untreated fungal, bacterial, systemic viral infections, or ocular herpes simplex.

For VANCENASE to be effective in the treatment of nasal polyps, the aerosol must be able to enter the nose. Therefore, treatment of nasal polyps with VANCENASE should be considered adjunctive therapy to surgical removal and/or the use of other medications which will permit effective penetration of VANCENASE into the nose. Nasal polyps may recur after any form of treatment.

As with any long-term treatment, patients using VANCENASE over several months or longer should be examined periodically for possible changes in the nasal mucosa.

Because of the inhibitory effect of corticosteroids on wound healing, patients who have experienced recent nasal septal ulcers, nasal surgery, or trauma should not use a nasal corticosteroid until healing has occurred.

Although systemic effects have been minimal with recommended doses, this potential increases with excessive doses. Therefore, larger than recommended doses should be avoided.

Information for Patients: Patients should use VANCENASE Nasal Inhaler at regular intervals since its effectiveness depends on its regular use. The patient should take the medication as directed. It is not acutely effective and the prescribed dosage should not be increased. Instead, nasal vasoconstrictors or oral antihistamines may be needed until the effects of VANCENASE Nasal Inhaler are fully manifested. One to two weeks may pass before full relief is obtained. The patient should contact the doctor if symptoms do not improve, or if the condition worsens, or if sneezing or nasal irritation occurs. For the proper use of this unit and to attain maximum improvement, the patient should read and follow the accompanying PATIENT'S INSTRUCTIONS carefully.

Carcinogenesis, Mutagenesis, Impairment of Fertility: Treatment of rats for a total of 95-weeks, 13 weeks by inhalation and 82 weeks by the oral route, resulted in no evidence of carcinogenic activity. Mutagenic studies have not been performed.

Impairment of fertility, as evidenced by inhibition of the estrus cycle in dogs, was observed following treatment by the oral route. No inhibition of the estrus cycle in dogs was seen following treatment with beclomethasone dipropionate by the inhalation route.

Pregnancy Category C: Like other corticoids, parenteral (subcutaneous) beclomethasone dipropionate has been shown to be teratogenic and embryocidal in the mouse and rabbit when given in doses approximately ten times the human dose. In these studies beclomethasone was found to produce fetal resorption, cleft palate, agnathia, microstomia, absence of tongue, delayed ossification, and agenesis of the thymus. No teratogenic or embryocidal effects have been seen in the rat when beclomethasone dipropionate was administered by inhalation at ten times the human dose or orally at 1000 times the human dose. There are no adequate and well-controlled studies in pregnant women. Beclomethasone dipropionate should be used during pregnancy only if the potential benefit justifies the potential risk to the fetus.

Nonteratogenic Effects: Hypoadrenalism may occur in infants born of mothers receiving corticosteroids during pregnancy. Such infants should be carefully observed.

Nursing Mothers: It is not known whether beclomethasone dipropionate is excreted in human milk. Because other corticosteroids are excreted in human milk, caution should be exercised when VANCENASE Nasal Inhaler is administered to nursing women.

Pediatric Use: Safety and effectiveness in children below the age of 12 years have not been established.

ADVERSE REACTIONS

In general, side effects in clinical studies have been primarily associated with the nasal mucous membranes.

Sensations of irritation and burning in the nose (11 per 100 patients) following the use of VANCENASE Nasal Inhaler have been reported. Also, occasional sneezing attacks (10 per 100 patients) have occurred immediately following the use of the intranasal inhaler.

Localized infections of the nose and pharynx with *Candida albicans* have occurred rarely. (See PRECAUTIONS.)

Less than 2 per 100 patients reported transient episodes of bloody discharge from the nose.

Ulceration of the nasal mucosa has been reported rarely.

Extremely rare instances of nasal septum perforation have been reported following the intranasal application of aerosolized corticosteroids. Rare cases of immediate and delayed hypersensitivity reactions, including urticaria, angioedema, rash, and bronchospasm have been reported following the oral and intranasal inhalation of becomethasone.

Systemic corticosteroid side effects were not reported during the controlled clinical trials. If recommended doses are exceeded, however, or if individuals are particularly sensitive, symptoms of hypercorticism, i.e., Cushing's syndrome could occur.

DOSAGE AND ADMINISTRATION

Adults and Children 12 years of age and over: the usual dosage is one inhalation (42 mcg) in each nostril two to four times a day (total dose 168–336 mcg/day). Patients can often be maintained on a maximum dose of one inhalation in each nostril three times a day (252 mcg/day).

The therapeutic effects of corticosteroids, on seasonal or perennial rhinitis or on nasal polyps are not immediate. This should be explained to the patient in advance in order to ensure cooperation and continuation of treatment with the prescribed dosage regimen.

VANCENASE Nasal Inhaler is <u>not</u> recommended for children below 12 years of age.

In the presence of excessive nasal mucus secretion or edema of the nasal mucosa, the drug may fail to reach the site of intended action. In such cases it is advisable to use a nasal vasoconstrictor during the first two to three days of VANCENASE Nasal Inhaler therapy.

Directions for Use: Illustrated PATIENT INSTRUCTIONS for proper use accompany each package of VANCENASE Nasal Inhaler.

CONTENTS UNDER PRESSURE. Do not puncture. Do not use or store near heat or open flame. Exposure to temperatures above 120°F may cause bursting. Never throw container into fire or incinerator. Keep out of reach of children.

OVERDOSAGE

When used at excessive doses, systemic corticosteroid effects such as hypercorticism and adrenal suppression may appear. If such symptoms appear, the dosage should be decreased.

The oral LD_{50} of beclomethasone dipropionate is greater than 1 g/kg in rodents. One canister of VANCENASE Nasal Inhaler contains 8.4 mg of beclomethasone dipropionate, therefore acute overdosage is unlikely.

HOW SUPPLIED

VANCENASE Nasal Inhaler, 16.8 g canister; box of one. Supplied with nasal adapter and PATIENT'S INSTRUCTIONS; (NDC 0085-0041-06).

Store between 2° and 30°C (36° and 86°F).

Revised 1/85

Shown in Product Identification Section, page 428

VANCERIL® Inhaler ℞

[*van 'ser-il*]

brand of beclomethasone dipropionate, USP
FOR ORAL INHALATION ONLY

DESCRIPTION

Beclomethasone dipropionate, USP, the active component of VANCERIL Inhaler, is an anti-inflammatory steroid having the chemical name 9-Chloro-11β,17-21-trihydroxy-16 β-methylpregna-1,4-diene-3, 20-dione 17,21-dipropionate.

VANCERIL Inhaler is a metered-dose aerosol unit containing a microcrystalline suspension of beclomethasone dipropionate-trichloromonofluoromethane clathrate in a mixture of propellants (trichloromonofluoromethane and dichlorodifluoromethane) with oleic acid. Each canister contains beclomethasone dipropionate-trichloromonofluoromethane clathrate having a molecular proportion of beclomethasone dipropionate, USP, to trichloromonofluoromethane between 3:1 and 3:2. Each actuation delivers from the mouthpiece a quantity of clathrate equivalent to 42 mcg. of beclomethasone dipropionate, USP. The contents of one canister provide at least 200 oral inhalations.

CLINICAL PHARMACOLOGY

Beclomethasone 17,21-dipropionate is a diester of beclomethasone, a synthetic corticosteroid which is chemically related to prednisolone. Beclomethasone differs from prednisolone only in having a chlorine at the 9-alpha and a methyl group at the 16-beta position in place of hydrogen. Animal studies showed that beclomethasone dipropionate has potent anti-inflammatory activity. When administered systemically to mice, the anti-inflammatory activity was accompanied by other typical features of glucocorticoid action including thymic involution, liver glycogen deposition, and pituitary-adrenal suppression. However, after systemic administration to rats, the anti-inflammatory action was associated with little or no effect on other tests of glucocorticoid activity.

Beclomethasone dipropionate is sparingly soluble and is poorly mobilized from subcutaneous or intramuscular injection sites. However, systemic absorption occurs after all routes of administration. When given to animals in the form of an aerosolized suspension of the trichloromonofluoromethane clathrate, the drug is deposited in the mouth and nasal passages, the trachea and principal bronchi, and in the lung; a considerable portion of the drug is also swallowed. Absorption occurs rapidly from all respiratory and gastrointestinal tissues, as indicated by the rapid clearance of radioactively labeled drug from local tissues and appearance of tracer in the circulation. There is no evidence of tissue storage of beclomethasone dipropionate or its metabolites. Lung slices can metabolize beclomethasone dipropionate rapidly to beclomethasone 17-monopropionate and more slowly to free beclomethasone (which has very weak anti-inflammatory activity). However, irrespective of the route of administration (injection, oral, or aerosol), the principal route of excretion of the drug and its metabolites is the feces. Less than 10% of the drug and its metabolites is excreted in the urine. In humans, 12% to 15% of an orally administered dose of beclomethasone dipropionate was excreted in the urine as both conjugated and free metabolites of the drug.

The mechanisms responsible for the anti-inflammatory action of beclomethasone dipropionate are unknown. The precise mechanism of the aerosolized drug's action in the lung is also unknown.

INDICATIONS

VANCERIL Inhaler is indicated only for patients who require chronic treatment with corticosteroids for control of the symptoms of bronchial asthma. Such patients would include those already receiving systemic corticosteroids, and selected patients who are inadequately controlled on a nonsteroid regimen and in whom steroid therapy has been withheld because of concern over potential adverse effects.

VANCERIL Inhaler is <u>NOT</u> indicated:

1. For relief of asthma which can be controlled by bronchodilators and other non-steroid medications.
2. In patients who require systemic corticosteroid treatment infrequently.
3. In the treatment of non-asthmatic bronchitis.

CONTRAINDICATIONS

VANCERIL Inhaler is contraindicated in the primary treatment of status asthmaticus or other acute episodes of asthma where intensive measures are required.

Hypersensitivity to any of the ingredients of this preparation contraindicates its use.

WARNINGS

Particular care is needed in patients who are transferred from systemically active corticosteroids to VANCERIL Inhaler because <u>deaths due to adrenal insufficiency have occurred in asthmatic patients during and after transfer from systemic corticosteroids to aerosol beclomethasone dipropionate.</u> After withdrawal from systemic corticosteroids, a number of months are required for recovery of hypothalamic-pituitary-adrenal (HPA) function. During this period of HPA suppression, patients may exhibit signs and symptoms of adrenal insufficiency when exposed to trauma, surgery or infections, particularly gastroenteritis. Although VANCERIL Inhaler may provide control of asthmatic symptoms during these episodes, it does NOT provide the systemic steroid which is necessary for coping with these emergencies.

During periods of stress or a severe asthmatic attack, patients who have been withdrawn from systemic corticosteroids should be instructed to resume systemic steroids (in large doses) immediately and to contact their physician for further instruction. These patients should also be instructed to carry a warning card indicating that they may need supplementary systemic steroids during periods of stress or a severe asthma attack. To assess the risk of adrenal insuffficiency in emergency situations, routine tests of adrenal cortical function, including measurement of early morning resting cortisol levels, should be performed periodically in all patients. An early morning resting cortisol level may be accepted as normal only if it falls at or near the normal mean level.

Localized infections with *Candida albicans* or *Aspergillus niger* have occurred frequently in the mouth and pharynx and occasionally in the larynx. Positive cultures for oral *Candida* may be present in up to 75% of patients. Although the frequency of clinically apparent infection is considerably lower, these infections may require treatment with appropriate antifungal therapy or discontinuance of treatment with VANCERIL Inhaler.

VANCERIL Inhaler is not to be regarded as a bronchodilator and is not indicated for rapid relief of bronchospasm.

Patients should be instructed to contact their physician immediately when episodes of asthma which are not responsive to bronchodilators occur during the course of treatment with VANCERIL. During such episodes, patients may require therapy with systemic corticosteroids.

There is no evidence that control of asthma can be achieved by the administration of VANCERIL in amounts greater than the recommended doses.

Transfer of patients from systemic steroid therapy to VANCERIL Inhaler may unmask allergic conditions previously suppressed by the systemic steroid therapy, e.g., rhinitis, conjunctivitis, and eczema.

PRECAUTIONS

During withdrawal from oral steroids, some patients may experience symptoms of systemically active steroid withdrawal, e.g., joint and/or muscular pain, lassitude and depression, despite maintenance or even improvement of respiratory function (See DOSAGE AND ADMINISTRATION for details).

In responsive patients, beclomethasone dipropionate may permit control of asthmatic symptoms without suppression of HPA function, as discussed below (See CLINICAL STUDIES). Since beclomethasone dipropionate is absorbed into the circulation and can be systemically active, the beneficial effects of VANCERIL Inhaler in minimizing or preventing HPA dysfunction may be expected only when recommended dosages are not exceeded.

The long-term effects of beclomethasone dipropionate in human subjects are still unknown. In particular, the local effects of the agent on developmental or immunologic processes in the mouth, pharynx, trachea, and lung are unknown. There is also no information about the possible long-term systemic effects of the agent.

The potential effects of VANCERIL on acute, recurrent, or chronic pulmonary infections, including active or quiescent tuberculosis, are not known. Similarly, the potential effects of long-term administration of the drug on lung or other tissues are unknown.

Pulmonary infiltrates with eosinophilia may occur in patients on VANCERIL Inhaler therapy. Although it is possible that in some patients this state may become manifest because of systemic steroid withdrawal when inhalational steroids are administered, a causative role for beclomethasone dipropionate and/or its vehicle cannot be ruled out.

Use in Pregnancy: Glucocorticoids are known teratogens in rodent species and beclomethasone dipropionate is no exception.

Teratology studies were done in rats, mice, and rabbits treated with subcutaneous beclomethasone dipropionate. Beclomethasone dipropionate was found to produce fetal resorptions, cleft palate, agnathia, microstomia, absence of tongue, delayed ossification and partial agenesis of the thymus. Well-controlled trials relating to fetal risk in humans are not available. Glucocorticoids are secreted in human milk. It is not known whether beclomethasone dipropionate would be secreted in human milk but it is safe to assume that it is likely. The use of beclomethasone dipropionate in pregnancy, nursing mothers, or women of childbearing potential requires that the possible benefits of the drug be weighed against the potential hazards to the mother, embryo, or fetus. Infants born of mothers who have received substantial doses of corticosteroids during pregnancy should be carefully observed for hypoadrenalism.

ADVERSE REACTIONS

Deaths due to adrenal insufficiency have occurred in asthmatic patients during and after transfer from systemic corticosteroids to aerosol beclomethasone dipropionate (See WARNINGS).

Suppression of HPA function (reduction of early morning plasma cortisol levels) has been reported in adult patients who received 1600 mcg. daily doses of VANCERIL for one month. A few patients on VANCERIL have complained of hoarseness or dry mouth.

Rare cases of immediate and delayed hypersensitivity reactions, including urticaria, angioedema, rash and bronchospasm have been reported following the oral and intranasal inhalation of beclomethasone.

DOSAGE AND ADMINISTRATION

Adults: The usual dosage is two inhalations (84 mcg.) given three or four times a day. In patients with severe asthma, it is advisable to start with 12 to 16 inhalations a day and adjust the dosage downward according to the response of the patient. The maximal daily intake should not exceed 20 inhalations, 840 mcg. (0.84 mg.), in adults.

Children 6 to 12 years of age: The usual dosage is one or two inhalations (42 to 84 mcg.) given three or four times a day according to the response of the patient. The maximal daily intake should not exceed ten inhalations, 420 mcg. (0.42 mg.), in children 6 to 12 years of age. Insufficient clinical data exist with respect to the administration of VANCERIL Inhaler in children below the age of 6.

Rinsing the mouth after inhalation is advised.

Patients receiving bronchodilators by inhalation should be advised to use the bronchodilator before VANCERIL Inhaler in order to enhance penetration of beclomethasone dipropionate into the bronchial tree. After use of an aerosol bronchodilator, several minutes should elapse before use of the VANCERIL Inhaler to reduce the potential toxicity from the inhaled fluorocarbon propellants in the two aerosols.

Different considerations must be given to the following groups of patients in order to obtain the full therapeutic benefit of VANCERIL Inhaler.

Patients not receiving systemic steroids: The use of VANCERIL Inhaler is straightforward in patients who are inadequately controlled with non-steroid medications but in whom systemic steroid therapy has been withheld because of concern over potential adverse reactions. In patients who respond to VANCERIL, an improvement in pulmonary function is usually apparent within one to four weeks after the start of VANCERIL Inhaler.

Patients receiving systemic steroids: In those patients dependent on systemic steroids, transfer to VANCERIL and subsequent management may be more difficult because recovery from impaired adrenal function is usually slow. Such suppression has been known to last for up to 12 months. Clinical studies, however, have demonstrated that VANCERIL may be effective in the management of these asthmatic patients and may permit replacement or significant reduction in the dosage of systemic corticosteroids.

The patient's asthma should be reasonably stable before treatment with VANCERIL Inhaler is started. Initially, the aerosol should be used concurrently with the patient's usual maintenance dose of systemic steroid. After approximately one week, gradual withdrawal of the systemic steroid is started by reducing the daily or alternate daily dose. The next reduction is made after an interval of one or two weeks, depending on the response of the patient. Generally, these decrements should not exceed 2.5 mg. of prednisone or its equivalent. A slow rate of withdrawal cannot be overemphasized. During withdrawal, some patients may experience symptoms of systemically active steroid withdrawal, e.g., joint and/or muscular pain, lassitude and depression, despite maintenance or even improvement of respiratory function. Such patients should be encouraged to continue with the Inhaler but should be watched carefully for objective signs of adrenal insufficiency, such as hypotension and weight loss. If evidence of adrenal insufficiency occurs, the systemic steroid dose should be boosted temporarily and thereafter further withdrawal should continue more slowly. During periods of stress or a severe asthma attack, transfer patients will require supplementary treatment with systemic steroids. Exacerbations of asthma which occur during the course of treatment with VANCERIL Inhaler should be treated with a short course of systemic steroid which is gradually tapered as these symptoms subside. There is no evidence that control of asthma can be achieved by administration of VANCERIL in amounts greater than the recommended doses.

Directions for Use: Illustrated patient instructions for proper use accompany each package of VANCERIL Inhaler. CONTENTS UNDER PRESSURE. Do not puncture. Do not use or store near heat or open flame. Exposure to temperatures above 120°F. may cause bursting. Never throw container into fire or incinerator. Keep out of reach of children.

HOW SUPPLIED

VANCERIL Inhaler 16.8 g canister supplied with an oral adapter and patient's instructions; box of one. (NDC-0085-0736-04).

Store between 2° and 30°C (36° and 86°F).

ANIMAL PHARMACOLOGY AND TOXICOLOGY

Studies in a number of animal species including rats, rabbits, and dogs have shown no unusual toxicity during acute experiments. However, the effects of beclomethasone dipropionate in producing signs of glucocorticoid excess during chronic administration by various routes were dose related.

CLINICAL STUDIES

The effects of beclomethasone dipropionate on hypothalamic-pituitary-adrenal (HPA) function have been evaluated in adult volunteers. There was no suppression of early morning plasma cortisol concentrations when beclomethasone dipropionate was administered in a dose of 1000 mcg./day for one month as an aerosol or for three days by intramuscular injection. However, partial suppression of plasma cortisol concentration was observed when beclomethasone dipropionate was administered in doses of 2000 mcg./day either intramuscularly or by aerosol. Immediate suppression of plasma cortisol concentrations was observed after single doses of 4000 mcg. of beclomethasone dipropionate.

In one study, the effects of beclomethasone dipropionate on HPA function were examined in patients with asthma. There was no change in basal early morning plasma cortisol concentrations or in the cortisol responses to tetracosactrin (ACTH 1:24) stimulation after daily administration of 400, 800 or 1200 mcg. of beclomethasone dipropionate for 28 days. After daily administration of 1600 mcg. each day for 28 days, there was a slight reduction in basal cortisol concentrations and a statistically significant ($p < .01$) reduction in plasma cortisol responses to tetracosactrin stimulation. The effects of a more prolonged period of beclomethasone dipropionate administration on HPA function have not been evaluated. However, a number of investigators have noted that when systemic corticosteroid therapy in asthmatic subjects can be replaced with recommended doses of beclomethasone dipropionate, there is gradual recovery of endogenous cortisol concentrations to the normal range. There is still no documented evidence of recovery from other adverse systemic corticosteroid-induced reactions during prolonged therapy of patients with beclomethasone dipropionate.

Clinical experience has shown that some patients with bronchial asthma who require corticosteroid therapy for control of symptoms can be partially or completely withdrawn from systemic corticosteroid if therapy with beclomethasone dipropionate aerosol is substituted. Beclomethasone dipropionate aerosol is not effective for all patients with bronchial asthma or at all stages of the disease in a given patient.

The early clinical experience has revealed several new problems which may be associated with the use of beclomethasone dipropionate by inhalation for treatment of patients with bronchial asthma:

1. There is a risk of adrenal insufficiency when patients are transferred from systemic corticosteroids to aerosol beclomethasone dipropionate. Although the aerosol may provide adequate control of asthma during the transfer period, it does not provide the systemic steroid which is needed during acute stress situations. Deaths due to adrenal insufficiency have occurred in asthmatic patients during and after transfer from systemic corticosteroids to aerosol beclomethasone dipropionate. (See WARNINGS.)
2. Transfer of patients from systemic steroid therapy to beclomethasone dipropionate aerosol may unmask allergic conditions which were previously controlled by the systemic steroid therapy, e.g., rhinitis, conjunctivitis, and eczema.
3. Localized infections with *Candida albicans* or *Aspergillus niger* have occurred frequently in the mouth and pharynx and occasionally in the larynx. It has been reported that up to 75% of the patients who receive prolonged treatment with beclomethasone dipropionate have positive oral cultures for *Candida albicans.* The incidence of clinically apparent infection is considerably lower but may require therapy with appropriate antifungal agents or discontinuation of treatment with beclomethasone dipropionate aerosol.

The long-term effects of beclomethasone dipropionate in human subjects are still unknown. In particular, the local effects of the agent on developmental or immunologic processes in the mouth, pharynx, trachea and lung are unknown. There is also no information about the possible long-term systemic effects of the agent. The possible relevance of the data in animal studies to results in human subjects cannot be evaluated.

Revised 9/85

Shown in Product Identification Section, page 428

Information on Schering products appearing on these pages is effective as of September 30, 1986.

Products are cross-indexed by generic and chemical names in the **YELLOW SECTION**

Schmid Laboratories, Inc.
ROUTE 46 WEST
LITTLE FALLS, NJ 07424-0415

KORO-FLEX® ℞
ARCING SPRING DIAPHRAGM

DESCRIPTION
The KORO-FLEX (R) ARCING SPRING DIAPHRAGM is made of natural, dipped, latex rubber. The improved contouring spring is actually 5 (five) springs in one.

ACTION
When compressed, it assumes a half moon shape which facilitates introduction beyond the cervix for simple, correct placement. When properly fitted, it will help to prevent sperm from entering the cervical canal. It also holds the spermicide in place.

INDICATIONS
KORO-FLEX Diaphragms, when used in conjunction with an appropriate spermicide such as KOROMEX (R) CONTRACEPTIVE CRYSTAL CLEAR GEL, KOROMEX (R) CONTRACEPTIVE JELLY or KOROMEX (R) CONTRACEPTIVE CREAM, are indicated for the prevention of pregnancy in women who choose diaphragms as their method of contraception.

PRECAUTIONS
While there has been no established link between the use of a diaphragm and Toxic Shock Syndrome (TSS), a few women wearing diaphragms have developed symptoms of the condition. In many of these situations, the women wore the diaphragm for more than 24 hours. It shall be recommended, therefore, that the diaphragm not be worn continuously for more than 24 hours.
Symptoms of TSS include sudden high fever (generally 102°F or over), vomiting, diarrhea, dizziness, fainting, or near fainting when standing up and a rash that resembles sunburn. Other signs of TSS may include sore throat, weakness, aching of muscles and joints, and redness of the eyes. If the patient experiences a high fever and one or more other TSS symtoms, she should be instructed to remove the diaphragm and contact her physician immediately.

INSTRUCTIONS
To be effective, the diaphragm should always be used with contraceptive gel, jelly or cream. This must be spread around the inner surface of the diaphragm as well as on the rim. Proper placement of the diaphragm is essential.
The diaphragm may be inserted up to 6 (six) hours before intercourse. If more than 6 (six) hours has elapsed after insertion of the diaphragm or for each repeated intercourse, an additional applicatorful of contraceptive gel, jelly, or cream must be used. The diaphragm SHOULD NOT be removed for this additional application.
The diaphragm must be left in place for at least 6 (six) hours after the last intercourse. Douching is not necessary. However, if recommended, the woman must wait for a full 6 (six) hours after the last intercourse. The diaphragm should not be left in place for more than 24 hours.

HOW SUPPLIED
KORO-FLEX ARCING SPRING DIAPHRAGMS are available in two convenient packages: KORO-FLEX ARCING SPRING DIAPHRAGM KIT (stock #136), contains trial sizes of KOROMEX CONTRACEPTIVE CRYSTAL CLEAR GEL, KOROMEX CONTRACEPTIVE JELLY, KOROMEX CONTRACEPTIVE CREAM, and a white plastic case. Available in sizes 60 mm–95 mm in 5 mm gradations.
KORO-FLEX ARCING SPRING DIAPHRAGM SET (stock #536), contains a regular tube of KOROMEX CONTRACEPTIVE CRYSTAL CLEAR GEL, trial sizes of KOROMEX CONTRACEPTIVE JELLY and KOROMEX CONTRACEPTIVE CREAM, a gel/jelly/cream applicator, white plastic case, and a convenient zippered pouch. Available in sizes 60 mm–95 mm in 5 mm gradations.

KOROMEX® ℞
COIL SPRING DIAPHRAGM

DESCRIPTION
The KOROMEX COIL SPRING DIAPHRAGM is made of natural, dipped, latex rubber. The plated spring is tension-controlled.

ACTION
When properly fitted, it will help to prevent sperm from entering the cervical canal. It also holds the spermicide in place.

INDICATIONS
KORMEX Diaphragms, when used in conjunction with an appropriate spermicide such as KOROMEX (R) CONTRACEPTIVE CRYSTAL CLEAR GEL, KOROMEX (R) CONTRACEPTIVE JELLY or KOROMEX (R) CONTRACEPTIVE CREAM, are indicated for the prevention of pregnancy in women who choose diaphragms as their method of contraception.

PRECAUTIONS
While there has been no established link between use of a diaphragm and Toxic Shock Syndrome (TSS), a few women wearing diaphragms have developed symptoms of the condition. In many of these situations, the women wore the diaphragm for more than 24 hours. It should be recommended therefore, that the diaphragm not be worn continuously for more than 24 hours.
Symptoms of TSS include sudden high fever (generally 102°F or over), vomiting, diarrhea, dizziness, fainting, or near fainting when standing up, and a rash that resembles sunburn. Other signs of TSS may include: sore throat, weakness, aching of muscles and joints, and redness of the eyes. If the patient experiences a high fever and one or more other TSS symptoms, she should be instructed to remove the diaphragm and contact her physician immediately.

INSTRUCTIONS
To be effective, the diaphragm should always be used with a contraceptive gel, jelly, or cream. This must be spread around the inner surface of the diaphragm as well as on the rim. Proper placement of the diaphragm is essential.
The diaphragm may be inserted up to 6 (six) hours before intercourse. If more than 6 (six) hours has elapsed after insertion of the diaphragm or for each repeated intercourse, an additional applicatorful of contraceptive gel, jelly, or cream must be used. The diaphragm SHOULD NOT be removed for this additional application.
The diaphragm must be left in place for at least 6 (six) hours after the last intercourse. Douching is not necessary. However, if recommended, the woman must wait a full 6 (six) hours after the last intercourse. The diaphragm should not be left in place for more than 24 hours.

HOW SUPPLIED
KORMEX COIL SPRING DIAPHRAGMS are available in two convenient packages: KOROMEX COIL SPRING DIAPHRAGM KIT (stock #131), contains trial sizes of KOROMEX CONTRACEPTIVE CRYSTAL CLEAR GEL, KOROMEX CONTRACEPTIVE JELLY, KOROMEX CONTRACEPTIVE CREAM, and a white plastic case. Available in sizes 50 mm–95 mm in 5 mm gradations.
KOROMEX COIL SPRING DIAPHRAGM COMPACT SET (Stock #541), contains a regular tube of KOROMEX CONTRACEPTIVE CRYSTAL CLEAR GEL, trial sizes of KOROMEX CONTRACEPTIVE JELLY and KOROMEX CONTRACEPTIVE CREAM, a diaphragm introducer, a gel/jelly/cream applicator, white plastic case, and a convenient zippered pouch. Available in sizes 60 mm–95 mm in 5 mm gradations.

VAGISEC PLUS® SUPPOSITORIES ℞
[*vaj 'ĕ-sĕk"*]
VAGISEC® MEDICATED DOUCHE LIQUID CONCENTRATE

DESCRIPTION
VAGISEC PLUS SUPPOSITORIES contain a combination of trichomonacidal and bactericidal agents and provide continued medication by gradual liquefaction. Each vaginal suppository contains the following ingredients:

9-aminoacridine HCl	6.00 mg.
Polyoxyethylene nonyl phenol	5.25 mg.
Sodium edetate	0.66 mg.
Sodium dioctyl sulfosuccinate	0.07 mg.

in a polyethylene glycol base containing glycerin and citric acid.
VAGISEC MEDICATED DOUCHE LIQUID CONCENTRATE contains a combination of polyoxyethylene nonyl phenol, sodium edetate, and sodium dioctyl sulfosuccinate, a complex proven to be effective trichomonacide when used as a vaginal douche (Vagisec Liquid).

CLINICAL PHARMACOLOGY
9-aminoacridine is a broad-spectrum anti-infective of extensive medical acceptance for the topical treatment of bacterial infections. The combination of polyoxyethylene nonyl phenol, sodium edetate, and sodium dioctyl sulfosuccinate is a trichomonacide which when in solution and diluted disintegrates the flagellates through marked changes in surface tension.

INDICATIONS AND USAGE
The Vagisec Liquid/Suppository regimen is indicated for the specific treatment, in adults, of vaginitis, as evidenced by pruritus, malodorous leukorrhea, erythema of the vaginal mucosa, dyspareunia, caused by Trichomonas vaginalis and mixed vaginal infections complicated by a bacterial moiety. The presence of trichomonads can be established by a hanging drop mount preparation of the discharge from the posterior fornix and confirmed by cultures grown on STS medium; the atypical bacterial moiety can be identified by examination of gram-stained preparations of smeared vaginal secretions.

CONTRAINDICATIONS
Douching is not recommended during pregnancy. VAGISEC Medicated Douche and VAGISEC PLUS Suppositories are spermicidal and should not be used when the patient is trying to conceive.

PRECAUTIONS
General: The full course of therapy must be completed to eliminate the infecting micro-organisms from the vagina. It is generally desirable to continue treatment through the menses in order to guard against potential flare-ups since the presence of blood favors the rapid growth of Trichomonas. Recurrence of vaginitis often indicates extravaginal foci or infection in cervical, vestibular and urethral glands, etc. or reinfection by the sexual partner.
Information for Patients: During treatment, patient should refrain from intercourse, or the partner should wear a prophylactic. To prevent flare-ups after completion of therapy and for continued vaginal cleanliness, the patient is advised to continue with VAGISEC Liquid as a regular douche, but no more than twice weekly unless otherwise directed by physician.
Laboratory Tests: No patient should be considered cured until cultures on STS medium and gram-stained preparations of smeared vaginal secretions, taken at monthly intervals for 3 months following treatment, show absence of trichomonads and a return to the normal vaginal bacterial flora.

ADVERSE REACTIONS
No significant adverse reactions have been reported to date for Vagisec Plus Suppositories or Vagisec Liquid. Any minor irritation is generally relieved by discontinuance of douche for 24 hours.

OVERDOSAGE
Antidote: Copious use of water. The dilute Vagisec solution is non-toxic.

DOSAGE & ADMINISTRATION
Office Treatment (Adult): For the treatment of vaginal trichomoniasis and mixed vaginal infections, best results are obtained by scrubbing the vagina with VAGISEC Liquid, diluted 1:100 by the physician in the office: 3 scrubs the first week, 2 the second. A suppository is inserted after each office scrub in the Liquid/Suppository regimen. Patient should be instructed to continue treatment at home. *Home Treatment:* The combination douche and suppositories (Liquid/Suppository regimen) is recommended for home use. The usual daily home treatment is VAGISEC Medicated Douche in the morning, followed by a VAGISEC PLUS Suppository inserted deep in the vagina, using tip of finger, and a second suppository inserted in like manner at bedtime for a period of 14 days. Treatment should be omitted the night and morning preceding an office visit. In chronic or stubborn cases, therapy may be repeated with no interval between courses. The Liquid/Suppository regimen may be continued throughout the menstrual cycle. It is advisable to continue treatment through two menstrual periods. Patients should be reexamined 3 days after home treatment has been discontinued. The full course of therapy must be completed to eliminate the infecting micro-organisms from the vagina. No patient should be considered cured until vaginal smears or cultures, taken at monthly intervals for 3 months following treatment, show absence of trichomonads and a return to the normal vaginal flora.

HOW SUPPLIED
VAGISEC PLUS® SUPPOSITORIES—box of 28 plastic-wrapped 3 gram suppositories. VAGISEC® MEDICATED DOUCHE LIQUID CONCENTRATE—4 oz. plastic bottle with instructions for dilution and douching.

CAUTION
Federal law prohibits dispensing VAGISEC PLUS Suppositories without prescription.

IDENTIFICATION PROBLEM?
Consult PDR's
Product Identification Section
where you'll find over 1200
products pictured actual size
and in full color.

Sclavo Inc.
5 MANSARD COURT
WAYNE, NJ 07470

COMPLETE INFORMATION FOR THE BELOW LISTED PRODUCTS IS FURNISHED IN THE PACKAGING.

ANTIRABIES SERUM (equine) USP ℞
CHOLERA VACCINE, USP ℞
DIPHTHERIA ANTITOXIN (equine) USP ℞
DIPHTHERIA TOXOID, USP ℞
DIPHTHERIA AND TETANUS TOXOIDS ADSORBED, USP (For Pediatric Use) ℞
SclavoTest®-PPD Tuberculin Purified Protein Derivative (PPD) Multiple Puncture Device
For product information, consult Diagnostic Product Information Section.
TETANUS ANTITOXIN (equine) USP ℞
TETANUS TOXOID, ADSORBED, USP ℞
TETANUS AND DIPHTHERIA TOXOIDS ADSORBED, USP For Adult Use ℞

EDUCATIONAL MATERIAL

SclavoTest Brochure Free on Request to Physicians
"Tuberculin Skin Testing: Mantoux or Multiple Puncture Device" Paper by J. J. Piecoro, Jr., Pharm D, H. David Wilson, M.D. and Irene G. Melvin, M.S. Available on request to physicians free.

Scot-Tussin Pharmacal Co., Inc.
50 CLEMENCE STREET
CRANSTON, RI 02920-0217

S–T FORTE™ SUGAR-FREE S–T FORTE™ Syrup Ⓒ-III

Complete prescribing information is furnished in the packaging.

COMPOSITION
Each 5 ml (1 teaspoonful) contains:
Hydrocodone Bitartrate, USP .... 2.5 mg
(**Warning:** May be habit forming)
Phenylephrine HCl, USP .... 5 mg
Phenylpropanolamine HCl, USP .... 5 mg
Pheniramine Maleate, USP .... 13.33 mg
Guaifenesin, USP .... 80 mg
Alcohol 5 per cent by vol.

HOW SUPPLIED
Syrup: Pints (NDC 0372-0004-16); Gallons (NDC 0372-0004-28).
Sugar-Free: Pints (NDC 0372-0005-16); Gallons (NDC 0372-0005-28).

SCOT-TUSSIN® SUGAR-FREE; ALCOHOL-FREE; DM COUGH & COLD MEDICINE — OTC

COMPOSITION
Each 5 ml (1 teaspoonful) contains:
Dextromethorphan HBr., USP .... 15 mg.
Chlorpheniramine Maleate, USP .... 2 mg.

HOW SUPPLIED
Bottles of 4 fl. oz. (NDC 0372-0036-04)

SCOT-TUSSIN® SUGAR-FREE; DECONGESTANT-FREE EXPECTORANT DYE-FREE & SODIUM-FREE COUGH FORMULA — OTC

COMPOSITION
Each 5 ml (1 teaspoonful) contains:
Guaifenesin, USP .... 200 mg
Alcohol 3.5 per cent

HOW SUPPLIED
Bottles of 4 fl. oz. (NDC 0372-0006-04).

TUSSIREX™ SUGAR-FREE; ALCOHOL-FREE NATURAL COLORING TUSSIREX™ "DYE-FREE" Syrup Ⓒ-V

Complete prescribing information is furnished in the packaging.

COMPOSITION
Each 5 ml (1 teaspoonful) contains:
Codeine Phosphate, USP .... 10 mg
(**Warning:** May be habit forming)
Pheniramine Maleate, USP .... 13.33 mg
Phenylephrine HCl., USP .... 4.17 mg
Sodium Citrate, USP .... 83.33 mg
Sodium Salicylate, USP .... 83.33 mg
Caffeine Citrate, USP .... 25 mg

HOW SUPPLIED
Both Tussirex™ Sugar-Free (yellow, lemon flavor), and Tussirex™ Syrup "Dye-Free" are available in pint (sugar-free NDC 0372-0018-16; syrup NDC 0372-0017-16), and gallon (sugar-free NDC 0372-0018-28; syrup NDC 0372-0017-28) bottles.

Searle Pharmaceuticals Inc.
BOX 5110
CHICAGO, IL 60680

Searle & Co.*
SAN JUAN, PUERTO RICO 00936

Alphabetic Product Listing*
Product, ID#, (NDC†), Form, Strength

*Aldactazide, 1011, Tablet, 25 mg/25 mg
*Aldactazide, 1021, Tablet, 50 mg/50 mg
*Aldactone, 1001, Tablet, 25 mg
*Aldactone, 1041, Tablet, 50 mg
*Aldactone, 1031, Tablet, 100 mg
Aminophyllin Injection, 1213, Ampul, 250 mg/10 ml
Aminophyllin Injection, 1223, Ampul, 500 mg/20 ml
*Aminophyllin, 1231, Tablet, 100 mg
*Aminophyllin, 1251, Tablet, 200 mg
*Anavar, 1401, Tablet, 2.5 mg
*Banthīne, 1501, Tablet, 50 mg
Calan, 1853, Ampul, 5 mg/2 ml
Calan, 1958, Syringe, I.V., 5 mg/2 ml
Calan, 1968, Syringe, I.V., 10 mg/4 ml
*Calan, 1851, Tablet, 80 mg
*Calan, 1861, Tablet, 120 mg
Calan, 1864, Vial, I.V., 5 mg/2 ml
Calan, 1874, Vial, I.V., 10 mg/4 ml
Chlorthalidone, 531, Tablet, 25 mg
Chlorthalidone, 541, Tablet, 50 mg
Cu-7 (Product Information only)
*Demulen 1/35-21, Compack, 151, Tablet, 1 mg/35 mcg
*Demulen 1/35-21, Refill, 151, Tablet, 1 mg/35 mcg
*Demulen 1/35-28, Compack, 151 (0161), Tablet, 1 mg/35 mcg
*Demulen 1/35-28, Refill, 151 (0161), Tablet, 1 mg/35 mcg
*Demulen 1/50-21, Compack, 71, Tablet, 1 mg/50 mcg
*Demulen 1/50-21, Refill, 71, Tablet, 1 mg/50 mcg
*Demulen 1/50-28, Compack, 71 (0081), Tablet, 1 mg/50 mcg
*Demulen 1/50-28, Refill, 71 (0081), Tablet, 1 mg/50 mcg
Diulo, 501, Tablet, 2½ mg
Diulo, 511, Tablet, 5 mg
Diulo, 521, Tablet, 10 mg
Dramamine Injection, 1703, Ampul, 50 mg/1 ml
Dramamine Injection, 1724, Vial, 250 mg/5 ml
Dramamine, 1736, Liquid, 12.5 mg/4 ml, 16 oz
Dramamine, 1701, Tablet, 50 mg (1,000s)
Dramamine, 1701, Unit Dose, Tablet, 50 mg, 100s
*Enovid, 51, Tablet, 5 mg/75 mcg
*Enovid, 101, Tablet, 10 mg (9.85 mg/0.15 mg)
*Enovid-E 21, Compack, 131, Tablet, 2.5 mg/0.1 mg
*Enovid-E 21, Refill, 131, Tablet, 2.5 mg/0.1 mg
*Flagyl, 1831, Tablet, 250 mg
*Flagyl, 500 (1821), Tablet, 500 mg
Flagyl I.V., 1804, Vial (partial fill, lyoph. pwd.), 500 mg
Flagyl I.V. RTU, 1844, Vial, 500 mg/100 ml
Flagyl I.V. RTU, 1847, Plastic Container, 500 mg/100 ml
Furosemide, 571, Tablet, 20 mg
Furosemide, 581, Tablet, 40 mg
Haloperidol, 896, Oral Solution, 2 mg/ml
Haloperidol, 831, Tablet, 0.5 mg
Haloperidol, 841, Tablet, 1 mg
Haloperidol, 851, Tablet, 2 mg
Haloperidol, 861, Tablet, 5 mg
Haloperidol, 871, Tablet, 10 mg
*Lomotil Ⓒ, 61, Tablet, 2.5 mg/0.025 mg
*Lomotil Ⓒ, Liquid, 66, 2.5 mg/0.025 mg per 5 ml
Nitrodisc, 2058, 5 mg/24 hr
Nitrodisc, 2078, 7.5 mg/24 hr
Nitrodisc, 2068, 10 mg/24 hr
*Norpace, 2752, Capsule, 100 mg
*Norpace, 2762, Capsule, 150 mg
*Norpace CR, 2732, Capsule, 100 mg
*Norpace CR, 2742, Capsule, 150 mg
*Ovulen-21, Compack, 401, Tablet, 1 mg/0.1 mg
*Ovulen-21, Refill, 401, Tablet, 1 mg/0.1 mg
*Ovulen-28, Compack, 401 (0421), Tablet, 1 mg/0.1 mg
*Ovulen-28, Refill, 401 (0421), Tablet, 1 mg/0.1 mg
*Pro-Banthīne, 601, Tablet, 15 mg
*Pro-Banthīne, Unit Dose, 601, Tablet, 15 mg
*Pro-Banthīne, 611, Tablet, 7½ mg
Tatum-T (Product Information only)
*Theo-24, 2832, Capsule, 100 mg
*Theo-24, 2842, Capsule, 200 mg
*Theo-24, 2852, Capsule, 300 mg

* Products of Searle & Co.

† When the product ID# is not the same as the NDC#, the NDC# appears in parentheses.

Products without reference marks are Searle Pharmaceuticals Inc. products. Products with asterisks are Searle & Co. products.

Various educational materials are available for physicians, pharmacists, nurses, physicians' assistants, and patients (through the physician). Please ask your Searle representative for information about these materials.

Searle Pharmaceuticals Inc.
BOX 5110
CHICAGO, IL 60680

AMINOPHYLLIN INJECTION™ ℞
[*ă-mĭ-noph 'yl-lĭn*]
(aminophylline injection USP)

DESCRIPTION
Aminophyllin Injection is a sterile solution of theophylline in water for injection prepared with the aid of ethylenediamine. Aminophyllin Injection contains anhydrous theophylline USP 19.7 mg/ml and ethylenediamine USP 3.6 mg/ml (equivalent to aminophylline dihydrate 25 mg/ml) in water for injection.
Aminophylline is a 2:1 complex of theophylline ($C_7H_8N_4O_2$), a bronchodilator, and ethylenediamine ($C_2H_8N_2$).
Aminophylline is white or slightly yellowish granules or powder, having a slight ammoniacal odor and a bitter taste.

CLINICAL PHARMACOLOGY
Theophylline directly relaxes the smooth muscle of the bronchial airways and pulmonary blood vessels, thus acting mainly as a bronchodilator and smooth muscle relaxant. The drug also possesses other actions typical of the xanthine derivatives: coronary vasodilation, cardiac stimulation, diuresis, cerebral stimulation, and skeletal muscle stimulation. The actions of theophylline may be mediated through inhibition of phosphodiesterase and a resultant increase in intracellular cyclic AMP. *In vitro,* theophylline inhibits the release of histamine by mast cells at concentrations generally higher than attained *in vivo. In vitro,* theophylline has been shown to act synergistically with beta agonists that increase intracellular cyclic AMP through the stimulation of adenyl cyclase. More data are needed to determine if theophylline and beta agonists have a clinically important additive effect *in vivo.*

Pharmacokinetics:

Theophylline Elimination Characteristics

	Theophylline Clearance Rates (mean ± S.D.)	Half-life Average (mean ± S.D.)
Children (over 6 months of age)	1.45 ± 0.58 ml/kg/min	3.7 ± 1.1 hr
Adult nonsmokers with uncomplicated asthma	0.65 ± 0.19 ml/kg/min	8.7 ± 2.2 hr

The half-life of theophylline is prolonged in patients with alcoholism, reduced hepatic or renal function, or congestive heart failure, and in patients receiving cimetidine or macro-

Continued on next page

Searle Pharm.—Cont.

lide antibiotics such as troleandomycin and erythromycin. High fever for prolonged periods may reduce the rate of theophylline elimination.

Newborn infants have extremely slow theophylline clearance rates. The theophylline half-life in newborn infants may exceed 24 hours. Not until the age of 3 to 6 months do clearance rates approach those seen in older children.

Patients over age 55 and patients with chronic obstructive pulmonary disease, cardiac failure, or liver insufficiency may have much slower clearance rates with half-lives that exceed 24 hours.

The average half-life of theophylline in smokers (1 to 2 packs/day) is 4 to 5 hours; the average half-life in nonsmokers is 7 to 10 hours. The increase in theophylline clearance caused by smoking is probably the result of induction of drug-metabolizing enzymes. The effect of smoking on theophylline pharmacokinetics may persist for 3 months to 2 years after smoking is discontinued.

Tolerance does not appear to develop during long-term use of theophylline.

INDICATIONS AND USAGE

Aminophyllin Injection is indicated for relief of acute bronchial asthma and for reversible bronchospasm associated with chronic bronchitis and emphysema.

CONTRAINDICATIONS

Patients with a history of hypersensitivity to aminophylline or its components (theophylline or ethylenediamine) should not be treated with Aminophyllin Injection (aminophylline).

WARNINGS

Status asthmaticus is a medical emergency. Optimal therapy frequently requires additional medication including corticosteroids when the patient is not rapidly responsive to bronchodilators.

Excessive theophylline doses may be associated with toxicity. The determination of theophylline serum levels is recommended to assure maximal benefit without excessive risk. Incidence of toxicity increases at theophylline serum levels greater than 20 mcg/ml.

Morphine and curare should be used with caution in patients with airflow obstruction because they stimulate histamine release and can induce asthmatic attacks. They may also suppress respiration leading to respiratory failure. Alternative drugs should be chosen whenever possible.

There is an excellent correlation between high serum levels of theophylline resulting from conventional doses and associated clinical manifestations of toxicity in (1) patients with lowered body plasma clearances (due to transient cardiac decompensation), (2) patients with liver dysfunction or chronic obstructive lung disease, (3) patients who are older than 55 years of age, particularly males.

Decreased clearance of theophylline may be associated with either influenza immunization or active influenza, and with other viral infections.

Less serious signs of theophylline toxicity such as nausea and restlessness may appear in up to 50% of patients. However, serious side effects such as ventricular arrhythmias and convulsions may appear as the first signs of toxicity.

Many patients who have high theophylline serum levels exhibit tachycardia. Theophylline products may cause arrhythmias or worsen preexisting arrhythmias. Halothane anesthesia in the presence of aminophylline may produce sinus tachycardia or ventricular arrhythmias.

Aminophylline injection should not be injected rapidly (no more than 25 mg/min) or through a central venous catheter. Intravenous doses given too rapidly or excessive doses given by any route of administration may be expected to be toxic, causing gastrointestinal, central nervous system, cardiovascular, and/or respiratory symptoms (see *OVERDOSAGE*).

Some children may be unusually sensitive to aminophylline. Toxic synergism with ephedrine or other sympathomimetic drugs may occur.

Caution should be used when aminophylline is given to patients with impaired liver function. Serum levels in such patients may persist longer than expected.

In minipigs, rodents, and dogs, arrhythmia and sudden death (with histological evidence of myocardial necrosis) have been observed when theophylline and beta agonists were administered concomitantly but not when either was administered alone. The significance of these findings for human use is unknown.

PRECAUTIONS

General: Mean half-life in smokers is shorter than in nonsmokers; therefore smokers may require larger doses of aminophylline. Aminophylline should not be administered concomitantly with other xanthine medications. Use with caution in patients with severe cardiac disease, severe hypoxemia, hypertension, hyperthyroidism, acute myocardial [illegible] cor pulmonale, congestive heart failure, or hepatic [illegible] and in the elderly (especially males) and in neo-

Particular caution should be used in giving aminophylline to patients in congestive heart failure. Frequently, such patients have markedly prolonged theophylline serum levels with theophylline persisting in serum for long periods following discontinuation of the drug.

Convulsions may occur in patients with aminophylline overdosage with serum levels of 30 mcg/ml or higher. Aminophylline may lower the seizure threshold.

Methylxanthines are known to increase gastric acidity. Therefore, aminophylline should be used cautiously in patients with a history of peptic ulcer since the disease may be exacerbated. Theophylline may occasionally act as a local irritant to the gastrointestinal tract, although gastrointestinal symptoms are more commonly mediated through the central nervous system and are usually associated with serum drug concentrations over 20 mcg/ml.

Laboratory tests: The determination of serum theophylline levels is highly recommended.

Drug interactions: Elevated serum levels of theophylline may occur in patients treated concomitantly with theophylline preparations and cimetidine, troleandomycin, erythromycin, allopurinol, or oral contraceptive steroids. Therefore, such patients should be watched carefully for signs of theophylline toxicity and the dose of aminophylline decreased if necessary. If ephedrine or other sympathomimetic drugs are given concomitantly with aminophylline, toxic synergism may occur. Co-medication with phenobarbital, phenytoin, or rifampin may increase theophylline clearance, and an increase of the aminophylline dose may be required.

Interaction	Effect
With lithium carbonate	Increased excretion of lithium carbonate
With propranolol	Antagonism of propranolol effect
With cimetidine	Increased theophylline serum levels
With troleandomycin or erythromycin	Increased theophylline serum levels
With intravenous isoproterenol	Decreased theophylline serum levels

Drug/Laboratory test interactions: Consumption of coffee, tea, cola beverages, chocolate, or acetaminophen contributes to falsely high serum theophylline levels when theophylline is measured spectrophotometrically without previous isolation by chromatography.

Mutagenesis: Theophylline has been shown to be mutagenic in *Escherichia coli* and other lower organisms (*Euglena gracillis* and *Ophiostoma multiannulatum*) and to produce chromosome breaks in cultured mouse cells and cultured human lymphocytes. The drug had no mutagenic activity *in vivo* in a dominant lethal test using mice.

Use in pregnancy: Limited animal studies have shown teratogenic activity of theophylline in mice and rats. Safe use in pregnancy has not been established relative to possible adverse effects on fetal development, but neither have adverse effects on fetal development been established. This is true for most antiasthmatic medications. Use of aminophylline in pregnant women should be balanced against the risk of uncontrolled asthma.

Nursing mothers: Theophylline is excreted in breast milk and may cause adverse effects in the infant. Caution must be used when prescribing aminophylline to a nursing mother, taking into account the risk/benefit of this therapy.

Pediatric use: Due to the marked variation in theophylline metabolism in infants, this drug is not recommended for infants under 6 months of age.

ADVERSE REACTIONS

The most consistent adverse reactions are usually due to overdose and are:

1. Gastrointestinal: nausea, vomiting, epigastric pain, hematemesis, diarrhea.
2. Central nervous system: headaches, irritability, restlessness, insomnia, reflex hyperexcitability, muscle twitching, clonic and tonic generalized convulsions, coma.
3. Cardiovascular: palpitation, tachycardia, extrasystoles, flushing, hypotension, circulatory failure, ventricular arrhythmias.
4. Respiratory: tachypnea.
5. Renal: albuminuria, microhematuria, potentiation of diuresis.
6. Others: hyperglycemia and inappropriate ADH (antidiuretic hormone) syndrome; rash (ethylenediamine).

OVERDOSAGE

Management of Toxic Symptoms:

1. Discontinue drug immediately.
2. There is no known specific antidote.
3. Treatment is supportive and symptomatic.
4. Avoid administration of sympathomimetic drugs.
5. Theophylline is dialyzable; charcoal hemoperfusion should be considered in severe theophylline toxic reactions.
6. Administer intravenous fluids, oxygen, and other supportive measures to prevent hypotension, correct dehydration and acid-base imbalance.
7. For hyperthermia, use a cooling blanket or give sponge baths as necessary.
8. Maintain patent airway and use artificial respiration (mechanical ventilation) in case of respiratory depression.
9. Control convulsions with appropriate parenteral medication(s) such as short-acting barbiturates, diazepam (0.1 to 0.3 mg/kg up to a total dose of 10 mg), or phenytoin.
10. Monitor theophylline serum levels until below 20 mcg/ml.

DOSAGE AND ADMINISTRATION

Therapeutic theophylline serum levels associated with optimal likelihood for benefit and minimal risk of toxicity are considered to be between 10 and 20 mcg/ml. Levels above 20 mcg/ml may produce toxic effects. There is great variation from patient to patient in dosage needed in order to achieve a therapeutic serum level because of variable rates of elimination. Because of this wide interpatient variation, and the relatively narrow therapeutic serum level range, dosage must be individualized. Monitoring of theophylline serum levels is highly recommended. Continuous cardiac monitoring may offer additional safety. Patients should be closely monitored for signs of toxicity. Dosage should be temporarily discontinued and resumed later at a lower dose if any signs of theophylline toxicity are present.

Dosage should be calculated on the basis of lean (ideal) body weight where mg/kg doses are stated. Theophylline does not distribute into fatty tissue.

Due to the marked variation in theophylline metabolism in infants, this drug is not recommended for infants under 6 months of age.

Aminophylline Dosage for Patient Population:

A. Not currently receiving theophylline products:

Group	Loading Dose* (mg/kg)	Maintenance Dose for Next 12 Hours (mg/kg/hr)	Maintenance Dose Beyond 12 Hours (mg/kg/hr)
1. Children 6 months to 9 years	6 (5)†	1.2 (1.0)†	1.0 (0.8)†
2. Children age 9 to 16 and young adult smokers	6 (5)	1.0 (0.8)	0.8 (0.65)
3. Otherwise healthy nonsmoking adults	6 (5)	0.7 (0.6)	0.5 (0.4)
4. Older patients and patients with cor pulmonale	6 (5)	0.6 (0.5)	0.3 (0.24)
5. Patients with congestive heart failure, liver disease	6 (5)	0.5 (0.4)	0.1–0.2 (0.08–0.16)

* Administer slowly, no faster than 25 mg/min.

† Equivalent anhydrous theophylline indicated in parentheses.

B. Currently receiving theophylline products: Determine, where possible, the time, amount, route of administration, and form of the patient's last dose.

The loading dose for theophylline is based on the principle that each 0.5 mg/kg of theophylline administered as a loading dose will result in a 1 mcg/ml increase in serum theophylline concentration. Ideally, the loading dose should be deferred if serum theophylline concentration can be rapidly obtained. If this is not possible, the clinician must exercise judgment in selecting a dose based on the potential for benefit and risk. When there is sufficient respiratory distress to warrant a small risk, 2.5 mg/kg of anhydrous theophylline (3.1 mg/kg of intravenous aminophylline) is likely to increase the serum concentration when administered as a loading dose in rapidly absorbed form by approximately 5 mcg/ml. If the patient is not already experiencing theophylline toxicity, this is unlikely to result in dangerous adverse effects.

Subsequent to the decision regarding modification of the loading dose in this group of patients, the maintenance dosage recommendations are the same as those described above.

Aminophyllin Injection in intravenous ampuls of 10 ml (250 mg) or 20 ml (500 mg) can either be injected very slowly by syringe or, more conveniently, may be infused in a small quantity (usually 100 or 200 ml) of 5% dextrose injection or 0.9% sodium chloride injection. This solution is sometimes given "piggyback" through an I.V. system already in place. Do not exceed the rate of 25 mg/min.

Thereafter, maintenance therapy can be administered by a large volume infusion to deliver the desired amount of drug each hour. Aminophylline is compatible with most commonly used I.V. solutions.

Oral therapy should be substituted for intravenous aminophylline as soon as adequate improvement is achieved.

Parenteral drug products should be inspected visually for particulate matter and discoloration prior to administration, whenever solution and container permit. Use only if solution is clear and no crystals are present.

INTRAVENOUS ADMIXTURE INCOMPATIBILITY: Although there have been reports of aminophylline precipitating in acidic media, these reports do not apply to the dilute solutions found in intravenous infusions. Aminophyllin Injection (aminophylline) should not be mixed in a syringe with other drugs but should be added separately to the intravenous solution.

When an intravenous solution containing aminophylline is given "piggyback," the intravenous system already in place should be turned off while the aminophylline is infused if there is a potential problem with admixture incompatibility.

The following may be incompatible when mixed with aminophylline in intravenous fluids: anileridine HCl, ascorbic acid, chlorpromazine, codeine phosphate, dimenhydrinate, dobutamine HCl, epinephrine HCl, erythromycin gluceptate, hydralazine HCl, insulin, levorphanol tartrate, meperidine HCl, methadone HCl, methicillin sodium, morphine sulfate, norepinephrine bitartrate, oxytetracycline HCl, penicillin G potassium, phenobarbital sodium, phenytoin sodium, prochlorperazine maleate, promazine HCl, promethazine HCl, tetracycline HCl, vancomycin HCl, vitamin B complex with C.

HOW SUPPLIED

Aminophyllin Injection is available in 10-ml (250 mg) or 20-ml (500 mg) ampuls, aqueous solution, USP; cartons of 25 and boxes of 100.

Store below 86°F (30°C) and protect from light and from freezing.

Tablets Shown in Product Identification Section, page 429

CALAN® ℞

[cal'an]
(verapamil hydrochloride)
For Intravenous Injection

DESCRIPTION

Calan (verapamil HCl) is a calcium antagonist or slow-channel inhibitor available as a sterile solution for intravenous injection in 5-mg (2 ml) ampuls, 5-mg (2 ml) and 10-mg (4 ml) syringes, and 5-mg (2 ml) and 10-mg (4 ml) vials. Each form contains verapamil HCl 2.5 mg/ml and sodium chloride 8.5 mg/ml in water for injection. Hydrochloric acid and/or sodium hydroxide is used for pH adjustment. The pH of the solution is between 4.1 and 6.0.

The structural formula of verapamil HCl is given below:

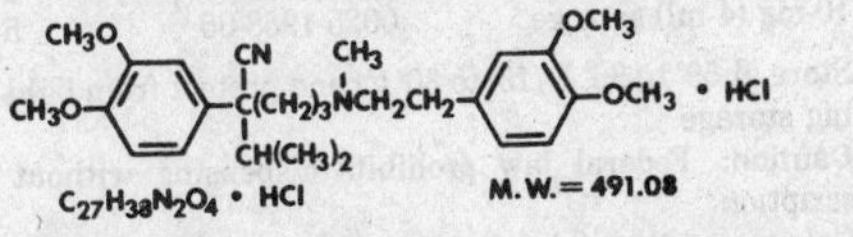

$C_{27}H_{38}N_2O_4 \cdot HCl$ M.W. = 491.08

Benzeneacetonitrile, α-[3-[[2-(3,4-dimethoxyphenyl) ethyl] methylamino] propyl]-3, 4-dimethoxy-α- (1-methylethyl) hydrochloride

Verapamil HCl is an almost white, crystalline powder, practically free of odor, with a bitter taste. It is soluble in water, chloroform, and methanol. Verapamil HCl is not chemically related to other antiarrhythmic drugs.

CLINICAL PHARMACOLOGY

Mechanism of action: Calan (verapamil HCl) inhibits the calcium ion (and possibly sodium ion) influx through slow channels into conductile and contractile myocardial cells and vascular smooth muscle cells. The antiarrhythmic effect of Calan appears to be due to its effect on the slow channel in cells of the cardiac conductile system.

Electrical activity through the SA and AV nodes depends, to a significant degree, upon calcium influx through the slow channel. By inhibiting this influx, Calan slows AV conduction and prolongs the effective refractory period within the AV node in a rate-related manner. This effect results in a reduction of the ventricular rate in patients with atrial flutter and/or atrial fibrillation and a rapid ventricular response. By interrupting reentry at the AV node, Calan can restore normal sinus rhythm in patients with paroxysmal supraventricular tachycardias (PSVT), including Wolff-Parkinson-White (WPW) syndrome. Calan has no effect on conduction across accessory bypass tracts. Calan does not alter the normal atrial action potential or intraventricular conduction time but depresses amplitude, velocity of depolarization, and conduction in depressed atrial fibers.

In the isolated rabbit heart, concentrations of Calan that markedly affect SA nodal fibers or fibers in the upper and middle regions of the AV node have very little effect on fibers in the lower AV node (NH region) and no effect on atrial action potentials or His bundle fibers.

Calan does not induce peripheral arterial spasm.

Calan has a local anesthetic action that is 1.6 times that of procaine on an equimolar basis. It is not known whether this action is important at the doses used in man.

Calan does not alter total serum calcium levels.

Hemodynamics: Calan (verapamil HCl) reduces afterload and myocardial contractility. In most patients, including those with organic cardiac disease, the negative inotropic action of Calan is countered by reduction of afterload, and cardiac index is usually not reduced, but in patients with moderately severe to severe cardiac dysfunction (pulmonary wedge pressure above 20 mm Hg, ejection fraction less than 30%), acute worsening of heart failure may be seen. Peak therapeutic effects occur within 3 to 5 minutes after a bolus injection. The commonly used intravenous doses of 5-10 mg Calan produce transient, usually asymptomatic, reduction in normal systemic arterial pressure, systemic vascular resistance and contractility; left ventricular filling pressure is slightly increased.

Pharmacokinetics: Intravenously administered Calan (verapamil HCl) has been shown to be rapidly metabolized. Following intravenous infusion in man, verapamil is eliminated bi-exponentially, with a rapid early distribution phase (half-life about 4 minutes) and a slower terminal elimination phase (half-life 2-5 hours). In healthy men, orally administered Calan undergoes extensive metabolism in the liver, with 12 metabolites having been identified, most in only trace amounts. The major metabolites have been identified as various N- and O-dealkylated products of Calan. Approximately 70% of an administered dose is excreted in the urine and 16% or more in the feces within 5 days. About 3% to 4% is excreted as unchanged drug.

INDICATIONS AND USAGE

Calan (verapamil HCl) is indicated for the treatment of supraventricular tachyarrhythmias, including:

- Rapid conversion to sinus rhythm of paroxysmal supraventricular tachycardias, including those associated with accessory bypass tracts (Wolff-Parkinson-White [WPW] and Lown-Ganong-Levine [LGL] syndromes). When clinically advisable, appropriate vagal maneuvers (eg, Valsalva maneuver) should be attempted prior to Calan administration.
- Temporary control of rapid ventricular rate in atrial flutter or atrial fibrillation, **except** when the atrial flutter and/or atrial fibrillation are associated with accessory bypass tracts (Wolff-Parkinson-White [WPW] and Lown-Ganong-Levine [LGL] syndromes).

In controlled studies in the U.S., about 60% of patients with supraventricular tachycardia converted to normal sinus rhythm within 10 minutes after intravenous verapamil HCl. Uncontrolled studies reported in the world literature describe a conversion rate of about 80%. About 70% of patients with atrial flutter and/or fibrillation with a fast ventricular rate respond with a decrease in heart rate of at least 20%. Conversion of atrial flutter or fibrillation to sinus rhythm is uncommon (about 10%) after verapamil HCl and may reflect the spontaneous conversion rate, since the conversion rate after placebo was similar. The effect of a single injection lasts for 30–60 minutes when conversion to sinus rhythm does not occur.

Because a small fraction (< 1.0%) of patients treated with verapamil HCl respond with life-threatening adverse responses (rapid ventricular rate in atrial flutter/fibrillation with an accessory bypass tract, marked hypotension, or extreme bradycardia/asystole—see *Contraindictions* and *Warnings*), the initial use of intravenous verapamil HCl should, if possible, be in a treatment setting with monitoring and resuscitation facilities, including DC-cardioversion capability (see *Suggested Treatment of Acute Cardiovascular Adverse Reactions*). As a familiarity with the patient's response is gained, an office setting may be acceptable.

Cardioversion has been used safely and effectively after intraveneous Calan.

CONTRAINDICATIONS

Intravenous verapamil HCl is contraindicated in:

1. Severe hypotension or cardiogenic shock
2. Second- or third-degree AV block (except in patients with a functioning artificial ventricular pacemaker).
3. Sick sinus syndrome (except in patients with a functioning artificial ventricular pacemaker)
4. Severe congestive heart failure (unless secondary to a supraventricular tachycardia amenable to verapamil therapy)
5. Patients receiving **intravenous** beta-adrenergic blocking drugs (eg, propranolol). **Intravenous** verapamil and **intravenous** beta-adrenergic blocking drugs should not be administered in close proximity to each other (within a few hours), since both may have a depressant effect on myocardial contractility and AV conduction.
6. Patients with atrial flutter or atrial fibrillation and an accessory bypass tract (eg. Wolff-Parkinson-White, Lown-Ganong-Levine syndromes). These patients are at risk to develop ventricular tachyarrhythmia including ventricular fibrillation if verapamil is administered.
7. Ventricular tachycardia. Administration of intravenous verapamil to patients with wide-complex ventricular tachycardia (QRS ≥ 0.12 sec) can result in marked hemodynamic deterioration and ventricular fibrillation. Proper pretherapy diagnosis and differentiation from wide-complex supraventricular tachycardia is imperative in the emergency room setting.
8. Known hypersensitivity to verapamil HCl

WARNINGS

CALAN SHOULD BE GIVEN AS A SLOW INTRAVENOUS INJECTION OVER AT LEAST A TWO-MINUTE PERIOD OF TIME. (See *Dosage and Administration.*)

Hypotension: Intravenous verapamil often produces a decrease in blood pressure below baseline levels that is usually transient and asymptomatic but may result in dizziness. Systolic pressure less than 90 mm Hg and/or diastolic pressure less than 60 mm Hg was seen in 5%–10% of patients in controlled U.S. trials in supraventricular tachycardia and in about 10% of the patients with atrial flutter/fibrillation. The incidence of symptomatic hypotension observed in studies conducted in the U.S. was approximately 1.5%. Three of the five symptomatic patients required pharmacologic treatment (norepinephrine bitartrate IV, metaraminol bitartrate IV, or 10% calcium gluconate IV). All recovered without sequelae.

Extreme bradycardia/asystole: Verapamil affects the AV and SA nodes and rarely may produce second- or third-degree AV block, bradycardia, and, in extreme cases, asystole. This is more likely to occur in patients with a sick sinus syndrome (SA nodal disease), which is more common in older patients. Bradycardia associated with sick sinus syndrome was reported in 0.3% of the patients treated in controlled double-blind trials in the U.S. The total incidence of bradycardia (ventricular rate less than 60 beats/min) was 1.2% in these studies. Asystole in patients other than those with sick sinus syndrome is usually of short duration (few seconds or less), with spontaneous return to AV nodal or normal sinus rhythm. If this does not occur promptly, appropriate treatment should be initiated immediately. (See *Adverse Reactions* including suggested treatment of adverse reactions.)

Heart failure: When heart failure is not severe or rate related, it should be controlled with digitalis glycosides and diuretics, as appropriate, before Calan is used.

In patients with moderately severe to severe cardiac dysfunction (pulmonary wedge pressure above 20 mm Hg, ejection fraction less than 30%), acute worsening of heart failure may be seen.

Concomitant antiarrhythmic therapy

Digitalis: Intravenous verapamil has been used concomitantly with digitalis preparations without the occurrence of serious adverse effects. However, since both drugs slow AV conduction, patients should be monitored for AV block or excessive bradycardia.

Procainamide: Intravenous verapamil has been administered to a small number of patients receiving oral procainamide without the occurrence of serious adverse effects.

Quinidine: Intravenous verapamil has been administered to a small number of patients receiving oral quinidine without the occurrence of serious adverse effects. However, a few cases of hypotension have been reported in patients taking oral quinidine who received intravenous verapamil. Caution should therefore be used when employing this combination of drugs.

Beta-adrenergic blocking drugs: Intravenous verapamil has been administered to patients receiving **oral** beta blockers without the development of serious adverse effects. However, since both drugs may depress myocardial contractility or AV conduction, the possibility of detrimental interactions should be considered. The concomitant administration of **intravenous** beta blockers and **intravenous** verapamil has resulted in serious adverse reactions (see *Contraindications*), especially in patients with severe cardiomyopathy, congestive heart failure, or recent myocardial infarction.

Disopyramide: Until data on possible interactions between verapamil and disopyramide are obtained, disopyramide should not be administered within 48 hours before or 24 hours after verapamil administration.

Heart block: Calan prolongs AV conduction time. While high-degree AV block has not been observed in controlled clinical trials in the U.S., a low percentage (less than 0.5%) has been reported in the world literature. Development of second- or third-degree AV block or unifascicular, bifascicular, or trifascicular bundle branch block requires reduction in subsequent doses or discontinuation of verapamil and institution of appropriate therapy, if needed. (See *Adverse Reactions* and *Concomitant antiarrhythmic therapy.*)

Hepatic and renal failure: Significant hepatic and renal failure should not increase the effects of a single intravenous dose of Calan but may prolong its duration. Repeated injections of intravenous Calan in such patients may lead to accumulation and an excessive pharmacologic effect of the drug. There is no experience to guide use of multiple doses in such patients, and this generally should be avoided. If repeated injections are essential, blood pressure and PR interval should be closely monitored and smaller repeat doses should be utilized. Data on the clearance of verapamil by dialysis are not yet available.

Continued on next page

Searle Pharm.—Cont.

Premature ventricular contractions: During conversion to normal sinus rhythm or marked reduction in ventricular rate, a few benign complexes of unusual appearance (sometimes resembling premature ventricular contractions) may be seen after treatment with verapamil. Similar complexes are seen during spontaneous conversion of supraventricular tachycardia and after DC-cardioversion or other pharmacologic therapy. These complexes appear to have no clinical significance.

Duchenne's muscular dystrophy: Intravenous verapamil can precipitate respiratory muscle failure in these patients and should, therefore, be used with caution.

Increased intracranial pressure: Intravenous verapamil has been seen to increase intracranial pressure in patients with supratentorial tumors at the time of anesthesia induction. Caution should be taken and appropriate monitoring performed.

PRECAUTIONS

Drug interactions: (See *Warnings: Concomitant antiarrhythmic therapy.*) Intravenous verapamil has been used concomitantly with other cardioactive drugs (eg, digitalis) without evidence of serious negative drug interactions. In rare instances, including when patients with severe cardiomyopathy, congestive heart failure, or recent myocardial infarction were given **intravenous** beta-adrenergic blocking agents or disopyramide concomitantly with intravenous verapamil, serious adverse effects have occurred. Concomitant use of verapamil with agents that decrease adrenergic function may result in an exaggerated hypotensive response. Animal studies suggest concomitant use of intravenous verapamil and intravenous dantrolene sodium may result in cardiovascular collapse. The clinical relevance of these findings is unknown. Cimetidine has no effect on intravenous Calan kinetics. As verapamil is highly bound to plasma proteins, it should be administered with caution to patients receiving other highly protein-bound drugs.

Animal experiments have shown that inhalation anesthetics depress cardiovascular activity by decreasing the inward movement of calcium ions. When used concomitantly, inhalation anesthetics and calcium antagonists, such as verapamil, should each be titrated carefully to avoid excessive cardiovascular depression.

Clinical data and animal studies suggest that verapamil may potentiate the activity of neuromuscular blocking agents (curare-like and depolarizing). It may be necessary to decrease the dose of verapamil and/or the dose of the neuromuscular blocking agent when the drugs are used concomitantly.

Pregnancy: Pregnancy Category C. Reproduction studies have been performed in rabbits and rats at **oral** verapamil doses up to 1.5 (15 mg/kg/day) and 6 (60 mg/kg/day) times the human oral daily dose, respectively, and have revealed no evidence of teratogenicity. In the rat, however, this multiple of the human dose was embryocidal and retarded fetal growth and development, probably because of adverse maternal effects reflected in reduced weight gains of the dams. This oral dose has also been shown to cause hypotension in rats. There are, however, no adequate and well-controlled studies in pregnant women. Because animal reproduction studies are not always predictive of human response, this drug should be used during pregnancy only if clearly needed.

Labor and delivery: There have been few controlled studies to determine whether the use of verapamil during labor or delivery has immediate or delayed adverse effects on the fetus, or whether it prolongs the duration of labor or increases the need for forceps delivery or other obstetric intervention. Such adverse experiences have not been reported in the literature, despite a long history of use of intravenous Calan in Europe in the treatment of cardiac side effects of beta-adrenergic agonist agents used to treat premature labor.

Nursing mothers: Verapamil crosses the placental barrier and can be detected in umbilical vein blood at delivery. Also, verapamil is excreted in human milk. Because of the potential for serious adverse reactions in nursing infants from verapamil, nursing should be discontinued while verapamil is administered.

Pediatric use: Controlled studies with verapamil have not been conducted in pediatric patients, but uncontrolled experience with intravenous administration in more than 250 patients, about half under 12 months of age and about 25% newborn, indicates that results of treatment are similar to those in adults. However, in rare instances, severe hemodynamic side effects have occurred following the intravenous administration of verapamil in neonates and infants. Caution should therefore be used when administering verapamil to this group of pediatric patients. The most commonly used single doses in patients up to 12 months of age have ranged from 0.1 to 0.2 mg/kg of body weight, while in patients aged 1 to 15 years, the most commonly used single doses ranged from 0.1 to 0.3 mg/kg of body weight. Most of the patients received the lower dose of 0.1 mg/kg once, but in some cases, the dose was repeated once or twice every 10 to 30 minutes.

ADVERSE REACTIONS

The following reactions were reported with intravenous verapamil use in controlled U.S. clinical trials involving 324 patients:

Cardiovascular: Symptomatic hypotension (1.5%); bradycardia (1.2%); severe tachycardia (1.0%). The worldwide experience in open clinical trials in more than 7,900 patients was similar.

Central nervous system effects: Dizziness (1.2%); headache (1.2%). Although rare, cases of seizures during verapamil injection have been reported.

Gastrointestinal: Nausea (0.9%); abdominal discomfort (0.6%).

In rare cases of hypersensitivity, broncho/laryngeal spasm accompanied by itch and urticaria has been reported.

The following reactions were reported in a few patients: emotional depression, rotary nystagmus, sleepiness, vertigo, muscle fatigue, or diaphoresis.

Suggested Treatment of Acute Cardiovascular Adverse Reactions*

The frequency of these adverse reactions was quite low, and experience with their treatment has been limited.

[See table below].

OVERDOSAGE

Treatment of overdosage should be supportive and individualized. Beta-adrenergic stimulation and/or parenteral administration of calcium solutions (calcium chloride) have been effectively used in treatment of deliberate overdosage with oral verapamil. Clinically significant hypotensive reactions or high-degree AV block should be treated with vasopressor agents or cardiac pacing, respectively. Asystole should be handled by the usual measures including isoproterenol hydrochloride, other vasopressor agents, or cardiopulmonary resuscitation (see *Suggested Treatment of Acute Cardiovascular Adverse Reactions*).

DOSAGE AND ADMINISTRATION

For intravenous use only. CALAN SHOULD BE GIVEN AS A SLOW INTRAVENOUS INJECTION OVER AT LEAST A TWO-MINUTE PERIOD OF TIME UNDER CONTINUOUS ECG AND BLOOD PRESSURE MONITORING. The recommended intravenous doses of Calan (verapamil HCl) are as follows:

Adult:

Initial dose—5–10 mg (0.075–0.15 mg/kg body weight) given as an intravenous bolus.

Repeat dose—10 mg (0.15 mg/kg body weight) 30 minutes after the first dose if the initial response is not adequate.

Older Patients—The dose should be administered over at least 3 minutes to minimize the risk of untoward drug effects.

Pediatric:

Initial dose

0–1 year: 0.1–0.2 mg/kg body weight (usual single dose range: 0.75–2 mg) should be administered as an intravenous bolus.

1–15 years: 0.1–0.3 mg/kg body weight (usual single dose range: 2–5 mg) should be administered as an intravenous bolus. *Do not exceed 5 mg.*

Repeat dose

0–1 year: 0.1–0.2 mg/kg body weight (usual single dose range: 0.75–2 mg) 30 minutes after the first dose if the initial response is not adequate.

1–15 years: 0.1–0.3 mg/kg body weight (usual single dose range: 2–5 mg) 30 minutes after the first dose if the initial response is not adequate. *Do not exceed 10 mg as a single dose.*

Note: Parenteral drug products should be inspected visually for particulate matter and discoloration prior to administration, whenever solution and container permit. Use only if solution is clear and vial seal is intact. Unused amount of solution should be discarded immediately following withdrawal of any portion of contents.

For stability reasons this product is not recommended for dilution with Sodium Lactate Injection USP in polyvinyl chloride bags. Admixing intravenous Calan with albumin, amphotericin B, hydralazine HCl, and trimethoprim with sulfamethoxazole should be avoided. Calan will precipitate in any solution with a pH above 6.0.

HOW SUPPLIED

All forms are individually packaged.

Size	NDC Number	Carton Size
5-mg (2 ml) ampul	0025-1853-10	10
5-mg (2 ml) vial	0025-1864-05	5
10-mg (4 ml) vial	0025-1874-05	5
5-mg (2 ml) syringe	0025-1958-05	5
10-mg (4 ml) syringe	0025-1968-05	5

Store at 59° to 86° F (15° to 30° C) and protect from light during storage.

Caution: Federal law prohibits dispensing without prescription.

Calan ampuls, vials, and syringes are manufactured for Searle Pharmaceuticals Inc.

Shown in Product Identification Section, page 429

Adverse Reaction	Proven Effective Treatment	Supportive Treatment
1. Symptomatic hypotension requiring treatment	Dopamine HCl IV Calcium chloride IV Norepinephrine bitartrate IV Metaraminol bitartrate IV Isoproterenol HCl IV	Intravenous fluids Trendelenburg position
2. Bradycardia, AV block, Asystole	Isoproterenol HCl IV Calcium chloride IV Norepinephrine bitartrate IV Atropine sulfate IV Cardiac pacing	Intravenous fluids (slow drip)
3. Rapid ventricular rate (due to antegrade conduction in flutter/fibrillation with WPW or LGL syndromes)	DC-cardioversion (high energy may be required) Procainamide IV Lidocaine HCl IV	Intravenous fluids (slow drip)

*Treatment and dosage should depend on the severity of the clinical situation and the judgment and experience of the physician.

CU-7® ℞

[cē′ū-sev″en]

(intrauterine copper contraceptive)

DESCRIPTION

The plastic component of the Cu-7 is composed of pharmaceutical grade polypropylene homopolymer with barium sulfate added to render it radiopaque. Its shape approximates the number 7. It is substantially smaller than previously available intrauterine devices; the vertical dimension measures 36 mm and the horizontal, 26 mm.

Coiled around the vertical limb is 89 mg of copper wire providing approximately 200 mm^2 of exposed copper surface area. A retrieval thread is fastened to the free end of the vertical limb of the Cu-7.

The Cu-7 is supplied with a simple tubular plastic inserter. All components are sterile.

[The following sections apply to both Cu-7 and Tatum-T.]

CLINICAL PHARMACOLOGY

Available data indicate that the contraceptive effectiveness of the Cu-7 or Tatum-T is enhanced by a minute quantity of copper released continuously from the coiled copper into the uterine cavity.

The exact mechanism by which metallic copper enhances the contraceptive effect of an IUD has not been conclusively demonstrated. Various hypotheses have been advanced, the most common being that copper placed in the uterus interferes with enzymatic or other processes that regulate blastocyst implantation.

Animal studies suggest that copper may play an additional role by reduction of sperm transport within the uterine environment.

INDICATION AND USAGE

The Cu-7 or Tatum-T is indicated for contraception.

CONTRAINDICATIONS

The Cu-7 or Tatum-T should not be inserted when any of the following conditions exist: pregnancy or suspicion of pregnancy; abnormalities of the uterus resulting in distortion of the uterine cavity; acute pelvic inflammatory disease, a history of repeated or recent pelvic inflammatory disease, or a history of severe pelvic inflammatory disease; genital actinomycosis; postpartum endometritis or infected abortion in the past three months; known or suspected uterine or cervical disease such as hyperplasia or carcinoma including unresolved, abnormal Pap test; vaginal bleeding of unknown etiology; untreated acute cervicitis until infection is controlled; diagnosed Wilson's disease; known or suspected allergy to copper; previous ectopic pregnancy; significant anemia; and valvular heart disease, leukemia, or use of chronic corticosteroid therapy because of the increased susceptibility to infection with certain microorganisms which may possibly be introduced at the time of an IUD insertion.

WARNINGS

1. *Pregnancy:* (a) *Long-term effects.* The long-term effects on the offspring of the presence of copper in the uterus when pregnancy occurs with the Cu-7 or Tatum-T are unknown.
(b) *Septic abortion.* Reports have indicated an increased incidence of septic abortion associated in some instances with septicemia, septic shock and death in patients becoming pregnant with an IUD in place. Most of these reports have been associated with the mid-trimester of pregnancy. In some cases, the initial symptoms have been insidious and not easily recognized. If pregnancy should occur with a Cu-7 or Tatum-T in situ, the Cu-7 or Tatum-T should be removed if the thread is visible or, if removal proves to be or would be difficult, interruption of the pregnancy should be considered and offered to the patient as an option, bearing in mind that the risks associated with an elective abortion increase with gestational age.
(c) *Continuation of pregnancy.* If the patient chooses to continue the pregnancy and the Cu-7 or Tatum-T remains in situ, she must be warned of the increased risk of spontaneous abortion and the increased risk of sepsis, including death. The patient must be closely observed and she must be advised to report immediately all abnormal symptoms, such as flu-like syndrome, fever, abdominal cramping and pain, bleeding, or vaginal discharge, because generalized symptoms of septicemia may be insidious.
2. *Ectopic pregnancy:* (a) A pregnancy which occurs with an IUD in situ is more likely to be ectopic than a pregnancy occurring without an IUD. Therefore, patients who become pregnant while using a Cu-7 or Tatum-T should be carefully evaluated for the possibility of an ectopic pregnancy.
(b) Special attention should be directed to patients with delayed menses, slight metrorrhagia and/or unilateral pelvic pain, and to those patients who wish to interrupt a pregnancy occurring in the presence of a Cu-7 or Tatum-T, to determine whether ectopic pregnancy has occurred.
3. *Pelvic infection:* An increased risk of pelvic inflammatory disease associated with the use of IUDs has been reported. While unconfirmed, this risk appears to be greatest for young women who are nulliparous and/or who have a multiplicity of sexual partners. Salpingitis can result in tubal damage and occlusion, thereby threatening future fertility. Therefore, it is recommended that patients be taught to look for symptoms of pelvic inflammatory disease. The decision to use an IUD in a particular case must be made by the physician and patient with the consideration of a possible deleterious effect on future fertility. This consideration is especially important for women who may wish to have children at a later date, particularly nulliparous women.
Pelvic infection may occur with a Cu-7 or Tatum-T in situ and at times result in the development of tubo-ovarian abscesses or general peritonitis. The symptoms of pelvic infection include: new development of menstrual disorders (prolonged or heavy bleeding), abnormal vaginal discharge, abdominal or pelvic pain, dyspareunia, fever. The symptoms are especially significant if they occur following the first two or three cycles after insertion. Appropriate aerobic and anaerobic bacteriologic studies and tests for *Chlamydia trachomatis* should be done and antibiotic therapy initiated promptly. If the infection does not show marked clinical improvement within 24 to 48 hours, the Cu-7 or Tatum-T should be removed and the continuing treatment reassessed on the basis of the results of culture and sensitivity tests. Genital actinomycosis has been associated primarily with long-term IUD use. It has been reported with the use of copper-bearing IUDs as well. Treatment requires prompt removal of the IUD and appropriate antibiotic therapy.
4. *Embedment:* Partial penetration or lodging of the Cu-7 or Tatum-T in the endometrium or myometrium can result in a difficult removal. This may occur more frequently in smaller uteri. (See removal instructions.)
5. *Perforation:* Partial or total perforation of the uterine wall or cervix may occur with the use of the Cu-7 or Tatum-T, usually during insertions into patients sooner than two months after abortion or delivery, or in uterine cavities too small for the Cu-7 or Tatum-T. An increased risk of perforation has been reported to occur when an IUD is inserted into lactating women compared to nonlactating parous women. The possibility of perforation must be kept in mind during insertion and at the time of any subsequent examination. If perforation occurs, investigation by appropriate means, including laparotomy or laparoscopy, should be carried out as soon as medically feasible, and the Cu-7 or Tatum-T located and removed from any site other than its correct position in the endometrial cavity. Abdominal adhesions, intestinal penetration, intestinal obstruction, and local inflammatory reaction with abscess formation and erosion of adjacent viscera may result if the Cu-7 or Tatum-T is left in the peritoneal cavity. Perforation by IUDs into urinary bladder, small or large bowel, or appendix has been reported.
6. *Medical diathermy:* The use of medical diathermy (shortwave and microwave) in a patient with a metal-containing IUD may cause heat injury to the surrounding tissue. Therefore, medical diathermy to the abdominal and sacral areas should not be used on patients using a Cu-7 or Tatum-T.
7. *Effects of copper:* Additional amounts of copper available to the body from the Cu-7 or Tatum-T may precipitate symptoms in women with undiagnosed Wilson's disease. The incidence of Wilson's disease is 1 in 200,000.
Malonaldehyde (MA) is a normal trace by-product of both prostaglandin biosynthesis and the oxidative breakdown of body fat, and occurs naturally in the human body. MA and related fat breakdown products have been reported to be mutagenic in a variety of test systems, and systemically carcinogenic when applied to the skin of mice at higher than naturally occurring levels. A study has reported that levels of MA were detected in the cervical mucus of women using copper-bearing IUDs, but not in controls. The author stated that increased levels of MA within the uterus represent an increased risk of carcinogenesis. The concentrations of MA reported to be mutagenic in bacterial or cell culture systems or carcinogenic in mice are higher than the concentration of MA observed in the cervical mucus of women using copper-bearing IUDs.

PRECAUTIONS

1. *Patient counseling.* Prior to the insertion the physician, nurse, or other trained health professional must provide the patient with the Patient Brochure. The patient should be given the opportunity to read the brochure and discuss fully any questions she may have concerning the Cu-7 or Tatum-T as well as other methods of contraception.
2. *Patient evaluation and clinical considerations.* (a) A complete medical history should be obtained to determine conditions that might influence the selection of an IUD. A physical examination should include a pelvic examination, Pap test, chlamydia test, gonorrhea culture, and, if indicated, appropriate tests for other forms of genital disease including genital actinomycosis, which usually can be detected by the Pap test. The physician should determine that the patient is not pregnant.
(b) The uterus should be carefully sounded prior to the insertion to determine the degree of patency of the endocervical canal and the internal os, and the direction and depth of the uterine cavity. Exercise care to avoid perforation with the sound. DO NOT USE THE Cu-7 OR Tatum-T INSERTION INSTRUMENT AS A SOUND. In occasional cases, severe cervical stenosis may be encountered. Do not use excessive force to overcome this resistance.
(c) The uterus usually sounds to a depth of 6 cm to 8 cm. Insertion of a Cu-7 or Tatum-T into a uterine cavity measuring less than 6.5 cm by sounding may increase the incidence of pain, bleeding, partial or complete expulsion, perforation, and possibly pregnancy.
(d) To reduce the possibility of insertion in the presence of an existing undetermined pregnancy, the optimal time for insertion is the latter part of the menstrual flow or one or two days thereafter. The Cu-7 or Tatum-T should not be inserted post partum or post abortion until involution of the uterus is complete. The incidence of perforation and expulsion is greater if involution is not complete.
It is, however, necessary to place the Cu-7 or Tatum-T as high as possible within the uterine cavity to help avoid partial or complete expulsion that could result in pregnancy.
Since the Cu-7 or Tatum-T represents a different design in intrauterine contraception, physicians are cautioned that it is imperative for them to become thoroughly familiar with the instructions for use before attempting placement of the Cu-7 or Tatum-T.
(e) IUDs should be used with caution in those patients who have an anemia or a history of menorrhagia or hypermenorrhea. Patients experiencing menorrhagia and/or metrorrhagia following IUD insertion may be at risk for the development of hypochromic microcytic anemia. Also, IUDs should be used with caution in patients receiving anticoagulants or having a coagulopathy.
(f) Syncope, bradycardia or other neurovascular episodes may occur during insertion or removal of IUDs, especially in patients with a previous disposition to these conditions.
(g) Patients with valvular or congenital heart disease are more prone to develop subacute bacterial endocarditis than patients who do not have valvular or congenital heart disease. Use of an IUD in these patients may represent a potential source of septic emboli. See *Contraindications.*
(h) Use of an IUD in those patients with acute cervicitis should be postponed until proper treatment has cleared up the infection.
(i) Since the Cu-7 or Tatum-T may be partially or completely expelled, patients should be reexamined and evaluated shortly after the first postinsertion menses, but definitely within three months after insertion. Thereafter annual examination with appropriate medical and laboratory evaluation, and a Pap test, including examination for *Actinomyces* organisms, should be carried out. The Cu-7 or Tatum-T should be replaced every three years.
(j) The patient should be told that some bleeding or cramping may occur during the first few weeks after insertion, but if these symptoms continue or are severe she should report them to her physician. She should be instructed on how to check after each menstrual period to make certain that the thread still protrudes from the cervix and cautioned that there is no contraceptive protection if the Cu-7 or Tatum-T has been expelled. She should also be cautioned not to dislodge the Cu-7 or Tatum-T by pulling on the thread. If a partial expulsion occurs, removal is indicated and a new Cu-7 or Tatum-T may be inserted. The patient should be told to return within three years for removal of the Cu-7 or Tatum-T and for replacement if desired.
(k) A copper-induced urticarial allergic skin reaction may develop in women using a copper-containing IUD. If symptoms of such an allergic response occur, the patient should be instructed to tell the consulting physician that a copper-containing device is being used.
(l) The Cu-7 or Tatum-T should be removed for the following medical reasons: menorrhagia and/or metrorrhagia producing significant anemia; uncontrolled pelvic infection; genital actinomycosis; intractable pain often aggravated by intercourse, dyspareunia; pregnancy, if the thread is visible; endometrial or cervical malignancy; uterine or cervical perforation; or any indication of partial expulsion.
(m) If the retrieval thread cannot be visualized it may have retracted into the uterus or have been broken off, or the Cu-7 or Tatum-T may have been expelled. Localization usually can be made by feeling with a probe; if not, contact hysteroscopy, x-ray, or sonography can be used. When the physician elects to recover a Cu-7 or Tatum-T with the thread not visible, the removal instructions should be considered.
(n) If any patient with a Cu-7 or Tatum-T suddenly develops overt clinical hepatitis or abnormal liver function tests, appropriate diagnostic procedures should be initiated.
(o) It has been reported that IUDs may be less effective in insulin-dependent diabetics.

ADVERSE REACTIONS

Perforations of uterus and cervix have occurred. Perforation into the abdomen has been followed by abdominal adhesions, intestinal penetration, intestinal obstruction, local inflammatory reaction with abscess formation and erosion of adjacent viscera. Perforation of the urinary bladder by IUDs has occurred. Pregnancy has occurred with the Cu-7 or Tatum-T in situ and when the Cu-7 or Tatum-T has been partially or completely expelled.
The incidence of spontaneous abortion, when conception occurs with intrauterine devices in situ, appears to be increased over that in unprotected women. Insertion cramping, usually of no more than a few seconds' duration, may occur; however, some women may experience residual cramping for several hours or even days. Intermenstrual spotting or bleeding, or prolonged or increased menstrual flow may occur.
Pelvic infection including salpingitis with tubal damage or occlusion has been reported. This may result in future infertility. Complete or partial expulsion of the Cu-7 or Tatum-T may sometimes occur, particularly in those patients with uteri measuring less than 6.5 cm by sounding. Urticarial allergic skin reaction may occur. The following complaints have also been reported with IUDs although their relation to the Cu-7 or Tatum-T has not been established: amenorrhea or delayed menses, backaches, cervical erosion, cystic masses in the pelvis, vaginitis, leg pain or soreness, erythema nodosum, weight loss or gain, nervousness, dyspareunia, cystitis, endometritis, septic abortion, mycotic chorioamnionitis, septicemia, leukorrhea, ectopic pregnancy, difficult removal, uterine embedment, anemia, pain, neurovascular episodes including bradycardia and syncope secondary to insertion, dysmenorrhea, and fragmentation of the IUD.

[*The following sections do not apply to Tatum-T. See* **Directions for Use, Clinical Studies, Procedure for Insertion, and Removal of the Tatum-T** *under that product's heading.*]

Continued on next pa

Searle Pharm.—Cont.

DIRECTIONS FOR USE

The Cu-7 is to be placed within the uterine cavity. See the *Procedure for Insertion* that follows, which describes two insertion techniques.

The small diameter of the Cu-7 inserter tube facilitates easy insertion in nulligravidous and nulliparous, as well as parous, women. The optimal time of insertion is during the latter part of the menstrual flow or one or two days thereafter. The cervical canal is relatively more patent at this time, and there is little chance that the patient may be pregnant.

Present information indicates that efficacy is retained for 36 months. There is no evidence that contraceptive efficacy decreases with time up to three years of use, but unless new data support a longer period of efficacy and safety, the Cu-7 must be removed within 36 months from the date of insertion and a new one inserted if desired. If partial expulsion occurs, removal is indicated, and a new Cu-7 may be inserted. Removal of the Cu-7 may also be indicated in the event of heavy or persistent bleeding.

The physician should become thoroughly familiar with the instructions for use before attempting insertion or removal of the Cu-7.

CLINICAL STUDIES

Different event rates have been reported with the use of different intrauterine contraceptives. Inasmuch as these rates are usually derived from separate studies conducted by different investigators in several population groups, a comparison cannot be made with precision. Even in different studies with the same contraceptive, considerably different rates are likely to be obtained because of differing characteristics of the study population. Furthermore, event rates per unit of time tend to be lower as clinical experience is expanded, possibly due to retention in the clinical study of those patients who accept the treatment regimen, not having discontinued due to adverse reactions or pregnancy, so that those remaining in the study were those less susceptible. In clinical trials of the Cu-7 conducted by Searle, use effectiveness was determined as follows for parous and nulliparous women, as tabulated by the life table method. (Rates are expressed as cumulative events per 100 women through 12, 24, and 36 months of use.)

This experience encompasses 373,948 woman-months of use, including 12 months for 11,288 women, 24 months for 7,518, and 36 months for 3,371.

Cumulative rates were:

[See table below].

Procedure for Insertion

The Cu-7 may be inserted easily at any time during the menstrual cycle. It is *not* necessary to delay insertion until a menstrual flow is in progress; however, the possibility of existing undetermined pregnancy is lessened if insertion is made during or shortly following a menstrual period.

The cervix should be cleansed with antiseptic solution and its anterior lip grasped with a tenaculum prior to sounding the uterus and insertion of the Cu-7. Insertion of the Cu-7 into a severely anteverted or severely retroverted uterus may be difficult unless sufficient tension is applied to the tenaculum. Determination of the depth and direction of the uterine cavity should be made with a sound prior to insertion.

An aseptic technique should be employed. Sterile gloves are recommended; however, the sterile sheath covering the Cu-7 in the package may be used to avoid handling any part of the copper figure seven or the tube which will enter the cervical canal.

To load the Cu-7 into the tube, fold the transverse arm against the copper-clad stem and push it into the tube until only the mushroom tip protrudes. Center the dot (thread knot) on the stem of the plastic carrier with the long axis (horizontal plane) of the cervical stop.

CAUTION

DO NOT leave the Cu-7 folded in the tube longer than two minutes or the plastic will lose its "memory"; it will then fail to resume its original configuration within the uterus and thus invite loss of effectiveness and early expulsion.

DO NOT remove the thread-retaining clip from the insertion rod until after insertion has been made and you are ready to deposit the Cu-7 within the uterine cavity.

DO NOT force the insertion. It is generally believed that most perforations occur at the time of insertion, although the perforation may not be detected until some time later. The position of the uterus should be determined during the pre-insertion examination. Great care must be exercised during the pre-insertion sounding and subsequent insertion.

Note: If the uterine cavity measures under 6.5 cm, the incidence of pain, bleeding, partial or complete expulsion, perforation, and possibly pregnancy increases. Insertion is not recommended into a uterus that sounds under 5.5 cm.

Release Technique

Note: After sounding, the cervical stop should be set at the depth measured on the sound. *See Figure 1.* Load the Cu-7 into the tube and immediately begin the insertion. DO NOT leave the Cu-7 in the tube longer than 2 minutes.

1. Apply tension with the tenaculum and gently insert the loaded instrument through the cervical canal, *see Figure 2*, to the fundus, *see Figure 3*, at which time the cervical stop should be at the cervix. Pinch the thread-retaining clip to the tube-stop during insertion to prevent the tube from crimping. The end of the rod should be touching the end of the Cu-7 at all times. Keep the cervical stop in the horizontal plane until it reaches the cervix. DO NOT FORCE.

2. Hold the rod firmly with the cervical stop at the cervix and free the thread by pressing the thread-retaining clip from the rod. Release the Cu-7 into the uterine cavity by *withdrawing* the tube to ½ inch from the handle. (DO NOT PUSH ON THE HANDLE; perforation could result.) *See Figure 4.*

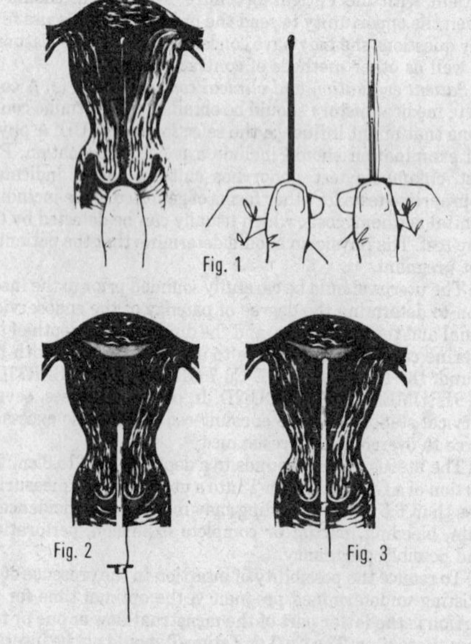

Fig. 1

Fig. 2

Fig. 3

3. Hold the tube still (do not withdraw further) and gently push the rod all of the way into the tube to correctly seat the Cu-7 entirely within the uterine cavity. *See Figure 5.*

4. Withdraw the insertion instrument and cut the thread at least 2 in (5 cm) from the external os. DO NOT PULL OUT EXCESS THREAD BEFORE CUTTING. *See Figure 6.*

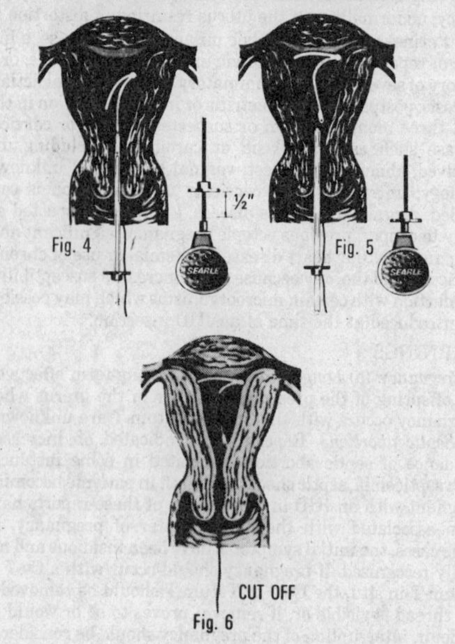

Fig. 4

Fig. 5

Fig. 6

Push-In Technique

Note: The cervical stop has been preset on the tube at 34 mm from the proximal end. *See Figure 1.* This will allow proper placement of the Cu-7 in a uterus which sounds to 2¾ in (7.0 cm) using *this* insertion technique only. (Since the cervical stop may have moved during shipment, this measurement should be verified.) If the uterus sounds to a depth greater than 2¾ in (7.0 cm), the cervical stop should be moved farther from the end of the tube by that many inches (centimeters). If the uterus sounds to a depth less than 2¾ in (7.0 cm), the cervical stop should be moved that much closer to the end of the tube.

1. Apply tension with the tenaculum and gently insert the loaded instrument through the cervical canal to the cervical stop, *see Figure 2.* Pinch the thread-retaining clip to the tube-stop during insertion to prevent the tube from crimping. The end of the rod should be touching the end of the Cu-7 at all times. Keep the cervical stop in the horizontal plane until it reaches the cervix. DO NOT FORCE.

2. Hold the tube firmly; remove the thread-retaining clip by pressing it off the rod and gently push the rod, *see Figure 3,* all the way into the tube to correctly seat the Cu-7 entirely within the uterine cavity. *See Figure 4.*

3. Withdraw the insertion instrument and cut the thread at least 2 in (5 cm) from the external os. DO NOT PULL OUT EXCESS THREAD BEFORE CUTTING. *See Figure 5.*

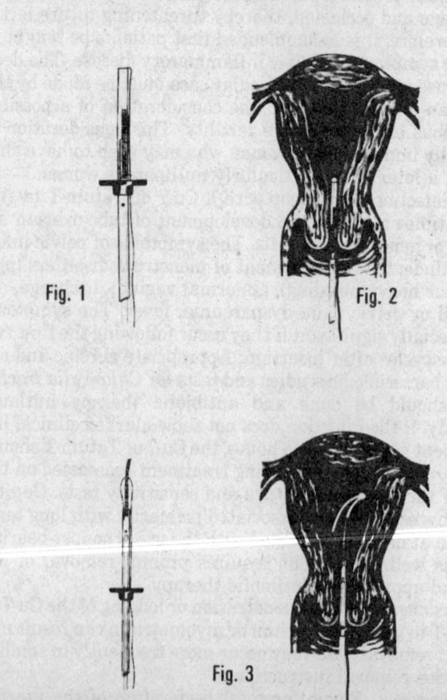

Fig. 1

Fig. 2

Fig. 3

	12 Months		24 Months		36 Months	
	Parous	Nulliparous	Parous	Nulliparous	Parous	Nulliparous
Pregnancy	1.9	1.7	3.0	2.6	3.5	3.1
Expulsion	5.6	7.8	6.7	9.0	7.2	9.4
Medical removal	10.9	13.7	18.3	20.9	24.8	28.7
Continuation	69.8	65.9	45.7	45.8	21.6	17.8

After elective removal of the Cu-7 for desire to become pregnant, 60% of the women conceived within three months and 75% had conceived within one year of removal.

Cu-7® Insertion Instrument

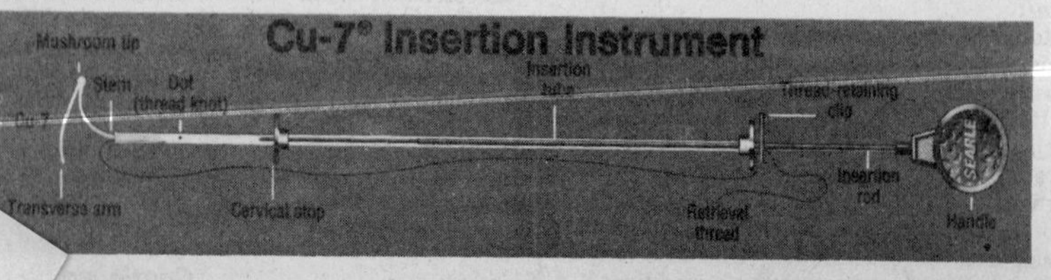

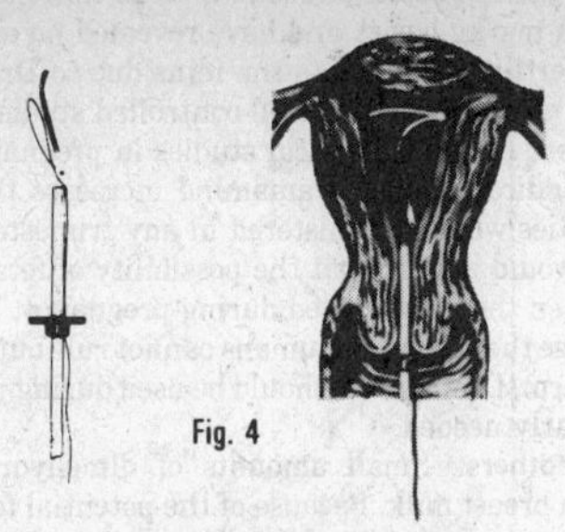

Fig. 4

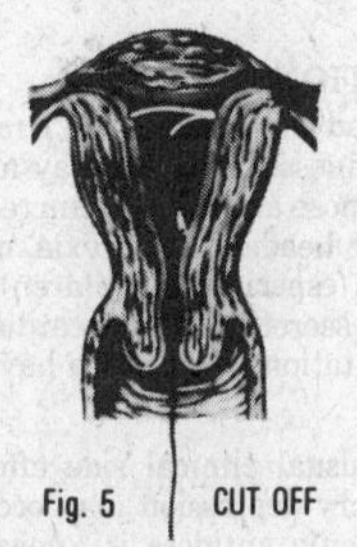

Fig. 5 CUT OFF

Removal of the Cu-7

ROUTINE REMOVAL—THREAD VISIBLE:

1. DO NOT exert a sudden pull or jerk on the retrieval thread. Exert a firm, steady pull on the thread. A jerk may cause the thread to break.

2. A ring (sponge) forceps, with its smooth edges and minimal crushing force, is a good instrument with which to grasp the thread.

3. Other instruments may be used, but care must be exerted to avoid crushing or cutting the thread.

4. Avoid winding or angulating the thread about the jaws of the withdrawal instrument.

5. Utilize the minimum force needed to remove the Cu-7.

6. Should resistance be encountered, dislodge the Cu-7 by the aseptic use of a slim instrument (eg, uterine dressing forceps) before making further removal attempts.

THREAD NOT VISIBLE: If the Cu-7 is in the uterus and the thread is not visible, the following procedures should be considered when you elect to recover it:

1. Aseptic use of a slim instrument (eg, uterine dressing forceps) or contact hysteroscopy will frequently permit removal in the office.

2. Hysteroscopy under hospital conditions may be required.

3. D & C and also suction aspiration have been used as alternative measures.

NOTE: If intrauterine manipulative procedures are required, allow an appropriate healing period before inserting a new Cu-7.

DIULO™ ℞

[dī'ū-lō]
(metolazone)

DESCRIPTION

Each Diulo tablet contains 2½, 5, or 10 mg of metolazone, a diuretic/saluretic/antihypertensive drug. Metolazone has the molecular formula $C_{16}H_{16}ClN_3O_3S$. The structural formula of the metolazone molecule is

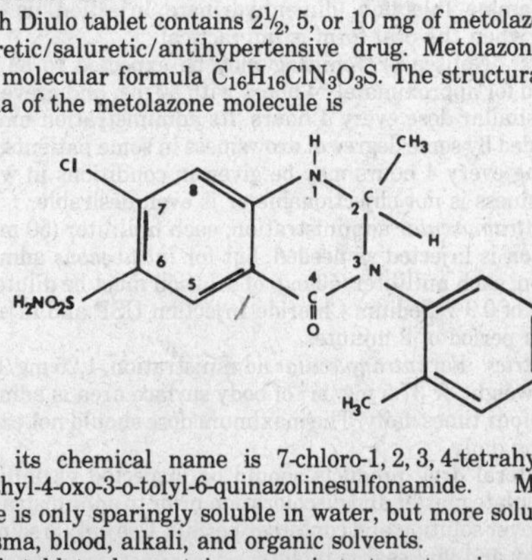

and its chemical name is 7-chloro-1, 2, 3, 4-tetrahydro-2-methyl-4-oxo-3-o-tolyl-6-quinazolinesulfonamide. Metolazone is only sparingly soluble in water, but more soluble in plasma, blood, alkali, and organic solvents.

Diulo tablets also contain magnesium stearate, microcrystalline cellulose, and dye: 2½ mg—D&C Red No. 33; 5 mg—FD&C Blue No. 2; 10 mg—D&C Yellow No. 10 and FD&C Yellow No. 6.

ACTIONS

Diulo (metolazone) is a diuretic/saluretic/antihypertensive drug whose action results in an interference with the renal tubular mechanism of electrolyte reabsorption. The mechanism of this action is unknown. Diulo acts primarily to inhibit sodium reabsorption at the cortical diluting site and in the proximal convoluted tubule. Sodium and chloride ions are excreted in approximately equivalent amounts. The increased delivery of sodium to the distal-tubular exchange site may result in increased potassium excretion.

Drug Interaction Studies: In animals pretreated with metolazone, the drug did not alter the characteristic effect of heparin on clotting time nor protamine antagonism; dicumarol on prothrombin time nor Vitamin K antagonism; the response of guanethidine, reserpine and hydralazine to cardiovascular parameters nor the pressor response of the subsequent dose of norepinephrine.

Metolazone and furosemide, administered concurrently have produced marked diuresis in some patients whose edema or ascites was refractory to treatment with maximum recommended doses of these or other diuretics administered alone. The mechanism of this interaction is not known.

In clinical usage, metolazone does not inhibit carbonic anhydrase. Its proximal action has been evidenced in humans by increased excretion of phosphate and magnesium ions, by markedly increased fractional excretion of sodium in patients with severely compromised glomerular filtration, and in animals by the results of micropuncture studies. Decrease in calcium ion excretion has not been noted.

At maximum therapeutic dosage Diulo is approximately equal to thiazide diuretics in its diuretic potency. However, Diulo may produce diuresis in patients with glomerular filtration rates below 20 ml/min.

When Diulo is given, diuresis and saluresis usually begin within one hour and persist for 12 to 24 hours depending on dosage. Maximum effect occurs about two hours after administration. At the higher recommended dosages, effect may be prolonged beyond 24 hours. *A single daily dose is recommended.* For most patients the duration of effect can be varied by adjusting the daily dose.

The prolonged duration of action of Diulo is attributed to protein binding and enterohepatic recycling. A small amount of Diulo is metabolized and the fraction so changed is nontoxic. The primary route of excretion is renal.

The mechanism whereby diuretics function in the control of hypertension is unknown; both renal and extrarenal actions may be involved. An antihypertensive effect may be seen as early as three to four days after Diulo has been started. Administration for three to four weeks, however, is usually required for optimum antihypertensive effect.

INDICATIONS AND USAGE

Diulo (metolazone) is indicated in the management of hypertension either as the sole therapeutic agent or to enhance the effectiveness of other antihypertensive drugs in the more severe forms of hypertension.

Diulo (metolazone) is indicated for the treatment of salt and water retention including

— edema accompanying congestive heart failure
— edema accompanying renal diseases, including the nephrotic syndrome, and states of diminished renal function.

Usage in Pregnancy

The routine use of diuretics in an otherwise healthy woman is inappropriate and exposes mother and fetus to unnecessary hazard. Diuretics do not prevent development of toxemia of pregnancy, and there is no satisfactory evidence that they are useful in the treatment of developed toxemia.

Edema during pregnancy may arise from pathological causes or from the physiologic and mechanical consequences of pregnancy. Diulo is indicated in pregnancy when edema is due to pathologic causes, just as it is in the absence of pregnancy (however, see *Precautions,* below). Dependent edema in pregnancy, resulting from restriction of venous return by the expanded uterus, is properly treated through elevation of the lower extremities and use of support hose; use of diuretics to lower intravascular volume in this case is illogical and unnecessary. There is hypervolemia during normal pregnancy which is harmful to neither the fetus nor the mother (in the absence of cardiovascular disease), but which is associated with edema, including generalized edema, in the majority of pregnant women. If this edema produces discomfort, increased recumbency will often provide relief. In rare instances, this edema may cause extreme discomfort which is not relieved by rest. In these cases, a short course of diuretics may provide relief and may be appropriate.

CONTRAINDICATIONS

Anuria.

Hepatic coma or pre-coma; known allergy or hypersensitivity to metolazone.

WARNINGS

Rarely, the rapid onset of severe hyponatremia and/or hypokalemia has been reported following initial doses of thiazide or non-thiazide diuretics. When symptoms consistent with severe electrolyte imbalance appear rapidly, Diulo should be discontinued and supportive means should be initiated immediately. Appropriateness of diuretic therapy should be carefully reevaluated.

While not reported to date, cross-allergy theoretically may occur when metolazone is given to patients known to be allergic to sulfonamide-derived drugs, thiazides, or quinethazone.

Hypokalemia may occur, with consequent weakness, cramps, and cardiac dysrhythmias. Hypokalemia is a particular hazard in digitalized patients; dangerous or fatal arrhythmias may be precipitated.

Azotemia and hyperuricemia may be noted or precipitated during the administration of metolazone. Infrequently, gouty attacks have been reported in persons with history of gout.

If azotemia and oliguria worsen during treatment of patients with severe renal disease, Diulo should be discontinued.

Until additional data have been obtained, Diulo is not recommended for patients in the pediatric age group.

Unusually large or prolonged effects on volume and electrolytes may result when metolazone and furosemide are administered concurrently. It is recommended that concurrent administration of these diuretics for treatment of resistant edema be started under hospital conditions in order to provide for adequate monitoring.

When Diulo is used with other antihypertensive drugs, particular care must be taken, especially during initial therapy. Dosage of other antihypertensive agents, especially the ganglionic blockers, should be reduced.

Diulo may be given with a potassium-sparing diuretic when indicated. In this circumstance, diuresis may be potentiated and dosages should be reduced. Potassium retention and hyperkalemia may result; the serum potassium should be determined frequently. Potassium supplementation is contraindicated when a potassium-sparing diuretic is given.

PRECAUTIONS

Periodic determination of serum electrolytes to detect possible electrolyte imbalance should be performed at appropriate intervals. Blood urea nitrogen, uric acid, and glucose levels should be assessed at intervals during diuretic therapy.

All patients receiving Diulo (metolazone) therapy should be observed for clinical signs of fluid and/or electrolyte imbalance; namely, hyponatremia, hypochloremic alkalosis, and hypokalemia. Serum and urine electrolyte determinations are particularly important when the patient is vomiting excessively or receiving parenteral fluids. Medication such as digitalis may also influence serum electrolytes. Warning signs, irrespective of cause, are: dryness of mouth, thirst, weakness, lethargy, drowsiness, restlessness, muscle pains or cramps, muscular fatigue, hypotension, oliguria, tachycardia, and gastrointestinal disturbances such as nausea and vomiting.

The serum potassium should be determined at regular intervals, and potassium supplementation instituted whenever indicated. Hypokalemia will be more common in association with intensive or prolonged diuretic therapy, with concomitant steroid or ACTH therapy, and with inadequate electrolyte intake.

While not reported to date for metolazone, related diuretics have increased responsiveness to tubocurarine and decreased arterial responsiveness to norepinephrine. Accordingly, it may be advisable to discontinue Diulo three days before elective surgery.

Caution should be observed when administering Diulo to hyperuricemic or gouty patients. Diulo exerts minimal effects on glucose metabolism; insulin requirements may be affected in diabetics, and hyperglycemia and glycosuria may occur in patients with latent diabetes.

Chloride deficit and hypochloremic alkalosis may occur. In patients with severe edema accompanying cardiac failure or renal disease, a low-salt syndrome may be produced; hot weather and a low-salt diet will contribute.

Caution should be observed when administering Diulo to patients with severely impaired renal function. As most of the drug is excreted by the renal route, cumulative effects may be seen in this circumstance.

Orthostatic hypotension may occur; this may be potentiated by alcohol, barbiturates, narcotics, or concurrent therapy with other antihypertensive drugs.

While not reported for metolazone, use of other diuretics has been associated on rare occasions with pathological changes in the parathyroid glands and with hypercalcemia. This possibility should be kept in mind with clinical use of Diulo.

Usage in Pregnancy

Diulo crosses the placental barrier and appears in cord blood. The use of Diulo in pregnant women requires that the anticipated benefit be weighed against possible hazards to the fetus. These hazards include fetal or neonatal jaundice, thrombocytopenia, and possibly other adverse reactions whic' have occurred in the adult.

Continued on next p

Searle Pharm.—Cont.

Nursing Mothers
Metolazone appears in breast milk. If use of the drug is deemed essential, the patient should stop nursing.

ADVERSE REACTIONS

Adverse reactions encountered during therapy with potent medications should be considered in two groups: those that represent extensions of the expected pharmacologic actions of the drug, and those which are pharmacologically unexpected, idiosyncratic, specially toxic, due to allergy or hypersensitivity, or due to unexplained causes.
For Diulo (metolazone), adverse reactions constituting extensions of the expected pharmacologic actions of this potent diuretic/saluretic/antihypertensive drug may include:
Gastrointestinal reactions: constipation.
Central nervous system reactions: syncope, dizziness, drowsiness.
Cardiovascular reactions: orthostatic hypotension, excessive volume depletion, hemoconcentration, venous thrombosis.
Other reactions: dryness of the mouth, symptomatic and asymptomatic hypokalemia, hyponatremia, hypochloremia; hypochloremic alkalosis, hypophosphatemia, hyperuricemia, hyperglycemia, glycosuria, increase in BUN or creatinine, fatigue, muscle cramps or spasm, weakness, restlessness sometimes resulting in insomnia.
In the second classification, adverse reactions to Diulo may include:
Gastrointestinal reactions: nausea, vomiting, anorexia, diarrhea, abdominal bloating, epigastric distress, intrahepatic cholestatic jaundice, hepatitis.
Central nervous system reactions: vertigo, headache, paresthesias.
Hematologic reactions: leukopenia, aplastic anemia.
Dermatologic-hypersensitivity reactions: urticaria and other skin rashes, purpura, necrotizing angiitis (cutaneous vasculitis).
Cardiovascular reactions: palpitation, chest pain.
Other reactions: chills, acute gouty attacks, transient blurred vision.
Adverse reactions which have occurred with other diuretics include: pancreatitis, xanthopsia, agranulocytosis, thrombocytopenia, and photosensitivity. These reactions should be considered as possible occurrences with clinical usage of Diulo.
Whenever adverse reactions are moderate or severe, Diulo dosage should be reduced or therapy withdrawn.

DOSAGE AND ADMINISTRATION

Therapy should be individualized according to patient response. Programs of therapy with Diulo (metolazone) should be titrated to gain a maximal initial therapeutic response, and to determine the minimal dose possible to maintain that therapeutic response.
Diulo is a potent drug with a prolonged, 12- to 24-hour duration of action. When an initially-desired therapeutic effect has been obtained, it is ordinarily advisable to reduce the dosage of Diulo to a lower maintenance level. The time interval required for the initial higher-dosage regimen may vary from days in edematous states to three or four weeks in the treatment of elevated blood pressure.
The daily dosage depends on the severity of each patient's condition, sodium intake, and responsiveness. Therefore, dosage adjustment is usually necessary during the course of therapy. A decision to reduce the daily dosage of Diulo from a higher induction level to a lower maintenance level should be based on the results of thorough clinical and laboratory evaluations. If antihypertensive drugs or diuretics are given concurrently with Diulo, careful dosage adjustment may be necessary.

Usual Dosage
Suitable initial dosages will usually fall in the ranges given:
Edema of cardiac failure:
Diulo 5–10 mg, once daily
Edema of renal disease:
Diulo 5–20 mg, once daily
Mild to moderate essential hypertension:
Diulo 2½–5 mg, once daily
For patients with congestive cardiac failure who tend to experience paroxysmal nocturnal dyspnea, it is usually advisable to employ a dosage near the upper end of the range, to ensure prolongation of diuresis and saluresis for a full 24-hour period.

HOW SUPPLIED

Diulo (metolazone) is supplied as tablets containing 2½, [illegible] and 10 mg of metolazone.
[illegible]lo 2½-mg tablets are round, pink tablets with [illegible] debossed on one side and 501 on the other side.
[illegible] tablets are round, blue tablets with SEARLE [illegible] side and 511 on the other side.
[illegible]blets are round, yellow tablets with [illegible]d on one side and 521 on the other side.

Diulo 2½ mg, 5 mg, and 10 mg are available in bottles of 100 tablets.
Shown in Product Identification Section, page 429

DRAMAMINE® Liquid
[dram 'uh-meen]
(dimenhydrinate syrup USP)
DRAMAMINE® Tablets
DRAMAMINE INJECTION™ ℞
(dimenhydrinate injection USP)

DESCRIPTION

Dimenhydrinate, an antinauseant/antiemetic, is the 8-chlorotheophylline (8-chloro-3,7-dihydro-1,3-dimethyl-1H-purine-2,6-dione) salt of diphenhydramine (2-diphenylmethoxy-N,N-dimethylethanamine). The structural formula of dimenhydrinate is

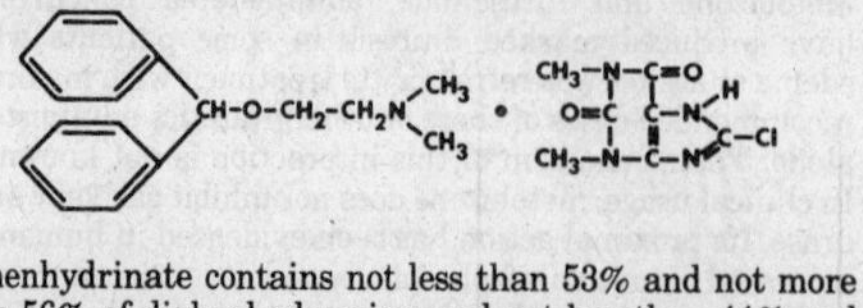

Dimenhydrinate contains not less than 53% and not more than 56% of diphenhydramine, and not less than 44% and not more than 47% of 8-chlorotheophylline, calculated on the dried basis.
Dramamine Injection ampuls and vials contain a sterile solution of dimenhydrinate 50 mg/ml in benzyl alcohol 5%, propylene glycol 50%, and water for injection.
Inactive ingredients of Dramamine tablets include acacia, carboxymethylcellulose sodium, corn starch, magnesium stearate, and sodium sulfate. Inactive ingredients of Dramamine liquid include cherry flavor, coloring, ethyl alcohol 5%, glycerin, methylparaben, sucrose, and water.

CLINICAL PHARMACOLOGY

While the precise mode of action of dimenhydrinate is not known, it has a depressant action on hyperstimulated labyrinthine function.

INDICATIONS AND USAGE

Dramamine is indicated for the prevention and treatment of the nausea, vomiting, or vertigo of motion sickness.

CONTRAINDICATIONS

Neonates and patients with a history of hypersensitivity to dimenhydrinate or its components (diphenhydramine or 8-chlorotheophylline) should not be treated with Dramamine Injection.

WARNINGS

Caution should be used when Dramamine is taken in conjunction with certain antibiotics that may cause ototoxicity, since Dramamine is capable of masking ototoxic symptoms and an irreversible state may be reached. As with any drug, pregnant or nursing women should seek the advice of a health professional before using this product.
This drug may impair the mental and/or physical abilities required for the performance of potentially hazardous tasks, such as driving a vehicle or operating machinery. The concomitant use of alcohol or other central nervous system depressants may have an additive effect. Therefore, patients should be warned accordingly.
Dimenhydrinate should be used with caution in patients having conditions which might be aggravated by anticholinergic therapy (ie, prostatic hypertrophy, stenosing peptic ulcer, pyloroduodenal obstruction, bladder neck obstruction, narrow-angle glaucoma, bronchial asthma, or cardiac arrhythmias).
This preparation should not be injected intra-arterially.
Usage in Children: For infants and children especially, antihistamines in overdosage may cause hallucinations, convulsions, or death.
As in adults, antihistamines may diminish mental alertness in children. In the young child, particularly, they may produce excitation.

PRECAUTIONS

General: Drowsiness may be experienced by some patients, especially with high dosage. This condition frequently is not undesirable in conditions for which the drug is used.
Information for Patients: Because of the potential for drowsiness, patients taking Dramamine should be cautioned against operating automobiles or dangerous machinery. See *Warnings.*
Carcinogenesis, mutagenesis, impairment of fertility: Mutagenicity screening tests performed with dimenhydrinate, diphenhydramine, and 8-chlorotheophylline produced positive results in the bacterial systems and negative results in the mammalian systems. There are no human data that indicate Dramamine is a carcinogen or mutagen or that it impairs fertility.
Pregnancy: Pregnancy Category B. Reproduction studies have been performed in rats at doses up to 20 times the human dose, and in rabbits at doses up to 25 times the human dose (on an mg/kg basis), and have revealed no evidence of impaired fertility or harm to the fetus due to Dramamine. There are no adequate and well-controlled studies in pregnant women. However, clinical studies in pregnant women have not indicated that Dramamine increases the risk of abnormalities when administered in any trimester of pregnancy. It would appear that the possibility of fetal harm is remote when the drug is used during pregnancy. Nevertheless, because the studies in humans cannot rule out the possibility of harm, Dramamine should be used during pregnancy only if clearly needed.
Nursing mothers: Small amounts of dimehydrinate are excreted in breast milk. Because of the potential for adverse reactions in nursing infants from dimenhydrinate, a decision should be made whether to discontinue nursing or to discontinue the drug, taking into account the importance of the drug to the mother.

ADVERSE REACTIONS

The most frequent adverse reaction to Dramamine (dimenhydrinate) is drowsiness. Dizziness may also occur. Symptoms of dry mouth, nose and throat, blurred vision, difficult or painful urination, headache, anorexia, nervousness, restlessness or insomnia (especially in children), skin rash, thickening of bronchial secretions, tachycardia, epigastric distress, lassitude, excitation, and nausea have been reported.

OVERDOSAGE

Drowsiness is the usual clinical side effect. Convulsions, coma, and respiratory depression may occur with massive overdosage. No specific antidote is known. If respiratory depression occurs, mechanically assisted respiration should be initiated and oxygen administered. Convulsions should be treated with appropriate doses of diazepam. Phenobarbital (5 to 6 mg/kg) may be given to control convulsions in children.
The oral LD_{50} in mice and rats is 203 mg/kg and 1320 mg/kg, respectively. The intraperitoneal LD_{50} in mice is 149 mg/kg.

DOSAGE AND ADMINISTRATION

Dramamine Tablets: To prevent motion sickness, the first dose should be taken ½ to 1 hour before starting the activity. Additional medication depends on travel conditions.
Dosage: Adults: Nausea or vomiting may be expected to be controlled for approximately 4 hours with 50 mg of Dramamine, and prevented by a similar dose every 4 hours. Its administration may be attended by some degree of drowsiness in some patients, and 100 mg every 4 hours may be given in conditions in which drowsiness is not objectionable or is even desirable. The usual adult dosage is 1 to 2 tablets every 4 to 6 hours, not to exceed 8 tablets in 24 hours. *Children 6 to 12 years:* ½ to 1 tablet every 6 to 8 hours, not to exceed 3 tablets in 24 hours. *Children 2 to 6 years:* Up to ½ tablet every 6 to 8 hours, not to exceed 1½ tablets in 24 hours. Children may also be given Dramamine (dimenhydrinate) cherry-flavored liquid in accordance with directions for use. Not for frequent or prolonged use except on advice of a physician. Do not exceed recommended dosage.
Dramamine Liquid: To prevent motion sickness, the first dose should be taken ½ to 1 hour before starting the activity. Additional medication depends on travel conditions.
Dosage: Adults: 4 to 8 teaspoonfuls (4 ml per teaspoonful) every 4 to 6 hours, not to exceed 32 teaspoonfuls in 24 hours. *Children 6 to 12 years:* 2 to 4 teaspoonfuls (4 ml per teaspoonful) every 6 to 8 hours, not to exceed 12 teaspoonfuls in 24 hours. *Children 2 to 6 years:* 1 to 2 teaspoonfuls every 6 to 8 hours, not to exceed 6 teaspoonfuls in 24 hours. *Children under 2 years:* Only on advice of a physician.
Not for frequent or prolonged use except on advice of a physician. Do not exceed recommended dosage. Use of a measuring device is recommended for all liquid medication.
Dramamine Injection (dimenhydrinate injection) is indicated when the oral form is impractical.
Adults: Nausea or vomiting may be expected to be controlled for approximately 4 hours with 50 mg, and prevented by a similar dose every 4 hours. Its administration may be attended by some degree of drowsiness in some patients, and 100 mg every 4 hours may be given in conditions in which drowsiness is not objectionable or is even desirable.
For *intramuscular* administration, each milliliter (50 mg) of solution is injected as needed, but for *intravenous* administration, each milliliter (50 mg) of solution must be diluted in 10 ml of 0.9% Sodium Chloride Injection USP and injected over a period of 2 minutes.
Pediatric: For *intramuscular* administration, 1.25 mg/kg of body weight or 37.5 mg/m^2 of body surface area is administered four times daily. The maximum dose should not exceed 300 mg daily.
Parenteral drug products should be inspected visually for particulate matter and discoloration prior to administration, whenever solution and container permit. Use only if solution is clear and vial seal is intact.

HOW SUPPLIED

Dramamine (dimenhydrinate) is supplied in the following dosage forms and package sizes:

For oral use—**tablets**, scored, white, 50 mg, with SEARLE debossed on one side and 1701 on the other side; bottles of 1,000, and cartons of 100 single-dose individually blister-sealed tablets; **liquid**, 12.5 mg/ 4 ml, ethyl alcohol 5%, bottles of 16 fl oz.

Dramamine Injection (dimenhydrinate) is supplied in 1-ml ampuls, each containing 50 mg of dimenhydrinate, in cartons of 5, 25, and 100, and in 5-ml (50 mg/ml, 250 mg total) vials in cartons of 5 and 25.

Dramamine Tablets are manufactured for Searle Pharmaceuticals Inc. by Searle & Co. Dramamine ampuls and vials are manufactured for Searle Pharmaceuticals Inc.

[Please note: Other sizes of Dramamine Tablets and Liquid are also shown under Procter & Gamble in the PDR For Nonprescription Drugs.]

Tablets are shown in Product Identification Section, page 429

FLAGYL I.V.™ ℞
[flaj'yl]
(metronidazole hydrochloride)
Single-Dose, 500 mg, glass vials (lyophilized powder)
NSN 6505-01-153-4364 (VA)

FLAGYL I.V.™ RTU® ℞
(metronidazole) Ready-to-Use
Single-Dose, 500 mg/100 ml, RTU glass vials
NSN 6505-01-123-2457 (VA)
Single-Dose, 500 mg/100 ml, RTU plastic containers
NSN 6505-01-139-4931 (VA)
Sterile
For Intravenous Infusion Only

WARNING

Metronidazole has been shown to be carcinogenic in mice and rats (see *Warnings*). Its use, therefore, should be reserved for the conditions described in the *Indications and Usage* section below.

DESCRIPTION

Flagyl I.V., sterile (metronidazole hydrochloride), and Flagyl I.V. RTU, sterile (metronidazole), are parenteral dosage forms of the synthetic antibacterial agents 1-(β-hydroxyethyl)-2-methyl-5-nitroimidazole hydrochloride and 1-(β-hydroxyethyl)-2-methyl-5-nitroimidazole, respectively.

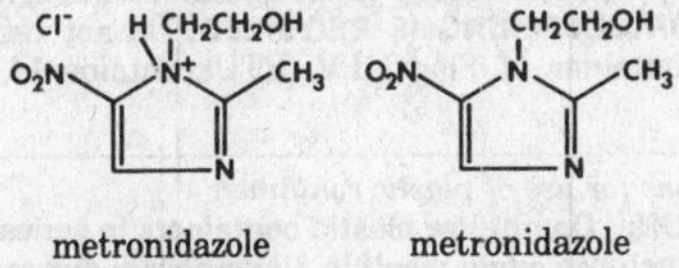

metronidazole hydrochloride   metronidazole

Each single-dose vial of lyophilized Flagyl I.V. contains sterile, nonpyrogenic metronidazole hydrochloride, equivalent to 500 mg metronidazole, and 415 mg mannitol.

Each Flagyl I.V. RTU 100-ml single-dose glass vial or plastic container contains a sterile, nonpyrogenic, isotonic, buffered solution of 500 mg metronidazole, 47.6 mg sodium phosphate, 22.9 mg citric acid, and 790 mg sodium chloride in Water for Injection USP. Flagyl I.V. RTU has a tonicity of 310 mOsm/L and a pH of 5 to 7. Each container contains 14 mEq of sodium.

The plastic container is fabricated from a specially formulated polyvinyl chloride plastic. Water can permeate from inside the container into the overwrap in amounts insufficient to affect the solution significantly. Solutions in contact with the plastic container can leach out certain of its chemical components in very small amounts within the expiration period, eg, di 2-ethylhexyl phthalate (DEHP), up to 5 parts per million. However, the safety of the plastic has been confirmed in tests in animals according to USP biological tests for plastic containers as well as by tissue culture toxicity studies.

CLINICAL PHARMACOLOGY

Metronidazole is a synthetic antibacterial compound. Disposition of metronidazole in the body is similar for both oral and intravenous dosage forms, with an average elimination half-life in healthy humans of eight hours.

The major route of elimination of metronidazole and its metabolites is via the urine (60–80% of the dose), with fecal excretion accounting for 6–15% of the dose. The metabolites that appear in the urine result primarily from side-chain oxidation [1-(β-hydroxyethyl) -2- hydroxymethyl-5-nitroimidazole and 2-methyl-5-nitroimidazole-1-yl-acetic acid] and glucuronide conjugation, with unchanged metronidazole accounting for approximately 20% of the total. Renal clearance of metronidazole is approximately 10 ml/ min/1.73m.[2]

Metronidazole is the major component appearing in the plasma, with lesser quantities of the 2-hydroxymethyl metabolite also being present. Less than 20% of the circulating metronidazole is bound to plasma proteins. Both the parent compound and the metabolite possess *in vitro* bactericidal activity against most strains of anaerobic bacteria.

Metronidazole appears in cerebrospinal fluid, saliva, and breast milk in concentrations similar to those found in plasma. Bactericidal concentrations of metronidazole have also been detected in pus from hepatic abscesses.

Plasma concentrations of metronidazole are proportional to the administered dose. An eight-hour intravenous infusion of 100–4,000 mg of metronidazole in normal subjects showed a linear relationship between dose and peak plasma concentration.

In patients treated with Flagyl I.V., using a dosage regimen of 15 mg/kg loading dose followed six hours later by 7.5 mg/kg every six hours, peak steady-state plasma concentrations of metronidazole averaged 25 mcg/ml with trough (minimum) concentrations averaging 18 mcg/ml.

Decreased renal function does not alter the single-dose pharmacokinetics of metronidazole. However, plasma clearance of metronidazole is decreased in patients with decreased liver function.

In one study newborn infants appeared to demonstrate diminished capacity to eliminate metronidazole. The elimination half-life, measured during the first three days of life, was inversely related to gestational age. In infants whose gestational ages were between 28 and 40 weeks, the corresponding elimination half-lives ranged from 109 to 22.5 hours.

Microbiology: Metronidazole is active *in vitro* against most obligate anaerobes, but does not appear to possess any clinically relevant activity against facultative anaerobes or obligate aerobes. Against susceptible organisms, metronidazole is generally bactericidal at concentrations equal to or slightly higher than the minimal inhibitory concentrations. Metronidazole has been shown to have *in vitro* and clinical activity against the following organisms:

Anaerobic gram-negative bacilli, including:
Bacteroides species, including the *Bacteroides fragilis* group (*B. fragilis, B. distasonis, B. ovatus, B. thetaiotaomicron, B. vulgatus*)
Fusobacterium species.

Anaerobic gram-positive bacilli, including:
Clostridium species and susceptible strains of *Eubacterium*

Anaerobic gram-positive cocci, including:
Peptococcus species
Peptostreptococcus species

Susceptibility Tests: Bacteriologic studies should be performed to determine the causative organisms and their susceptibility to metronidazole; however, the rapid, routine susceptibility testing of individual isolates of anaerobic bacteria is not always practical, and therapy may be started while awaiting these results.

Quantitative methods give the most accurate estimates of susceptibility to antibacterial drugs. A standardized agar dilution method and a broth microdilution method are recommended.[1]

Control strains are recommended for standardized susceptibility testing. Each time the test is performed, one or more of the following strains should be included: *Clostridium perfringens* ATCC 13124, *Bacteroides fragilis* ATCC 25285, and *Bacteroides thetaiotaomicron* ATCC 29741. The mode metronidazole MICs for those three strains are reported to be 0.25, 0.25, and 0.5 mcg/ml, respectively.

A clinical laboratory test is considered under acceptable control if the results of the control strains are within one doubling dilution of the mode MICs reported for metronidazole.

A bacterial isolate may be considered susceptible if the MIC value for metronidazole is not more than 16 mcg/ml. An organism is considered resistant if the MIC is greater than 16 mcg/ml. A report of "resistant" from the laboratory indicates that the infecting organism is not likely to respond to therapy.

INDICATIONS AND USAGE

Treatment of Anaerobic Infections

Flagyl I.V. (metronidazole hydrochloride) and Flagyl I.V. RTU (metronidazole) are indicated in the treatment of serious infections caused by susceptible anaerobic bacteria. Indicated surgical procedures should be performed in conjunction with Flagyl I.V. or Flagyl I.V. RTU therapy. In a mixed aerobic and anaerobic infection, antibiotics appropriate for the treatment of the aerobic infection should be used in addition to Flagyl I.V. or Flagyl I.V. RTU.

Flagyl I.V. and Flagyl I.V. RTU are effective in *Bacteroides fragilis* infections resistant to clindamycin, chloramphenicol, and penicillin.

INTRA-ABDOMINAL INFECTIONS, including peritonitis, intra-abdominal abscess, and liver abscess, caused by *Bacteroides* species including the *B. fragilis* group (*B. fragilis, B. distasonis, B. ovatus, B. thetaiotaomicron, B. vulgatus*), *Clostridium* species, *Eubacterium* species, *Peptococcus* species, and *Peptostreptococcus* species.

SKIN AND SKIN STRUCTURE INFECTIONS caused by *Bacteroides* species including the *B. fragilis* group, *Clostridium* species, *Peptococcus* species, *Peptostreptococcus* species, and *Fusobacterium* species.

GYNECOLOGIC INFECTIONS, including endometritis, endomyometritis, tubo-ovarian abscess, and postsurgical vaginal cuff infection, caused by *Bacteroides* species including the *B. fragilis* group, *Clostridium* species, *Peptococcus* species, and *Peptostreptococcus* species.

BACTERIAL SEPTICEMIA caused by *Bacteroides* species including the *B. fragilis* group, and *Clostridium* species.

BONE AND JOINT INFECTIONS, as adjunctive therapy, caused by *Bacteroides* species including the *B. fragilis* group.

CENTRAL NERVOUS SYSTEM (CNS) INFECTIONS, including meningitis and brain abscess, caused by *Bacteroides* species including the *B. fragilis* group.

LOWER RESPIRATORY TRACT INFECTIONS, including pneumonia, empyema, and lung abscess, caused by *Bacteroides* species including the *B. fragilis* group.

ENDOCARDITIS caused by *Bacteroides* species including the *B. fragilis* group.

Prophylaxis

The prophylactic administration of Flagyl I.V. or Flagyl I.V. RTU preoperatively, intraoperatively, and postoperatively may reduce the incidence of postoperative infection in patients undergoing elective colorectal surgery which is classified as contaminated or potentially contaminated.

Prophylactic use of Flagyl I.V. or Flagyl I.V. RTU should be discontinued within 12 hours after surgery. If there are signs of infection, specimens for cultures should be obtained for the identification of the causative organisms(s) so that appropriate therapy may be given (see *Dosage and Administration*).

CONTRAINDICATIONS

Flagyl I.V. and Flagyl I.V. RTU are contraindicated in patients with a prior history of hypersensitivity to metronidazole or other nitroimidazole derivatives.

WARNINGS

Convulsive Seizures and Peripheral Neuropathy: Convulsive seizures and peripheral neuropathy, the latter characterized mainly by numbness or paresthesia of an extremity, have been reported in patients treated with metronidazole. The appearance of abnormal neurologic signs demands the prompt evaluation of the benefit/risk ratio of the continuation of therapy.

Tumorigenicity in Rodents: Metronidazole has shown evidence of carcinogenic activity in studies involving chronic, oral administration in mice and rats, but similar studies in the hamster gave negative results. Also, metronidazole has shown mutagenic activity in a number of *in vitro* assay systems, but studies in mammals *(in vivo)* failed to demonstrate a potential for genetic damage.

PRECAUTIONS

General: Patients with severe hepatic disease metabolize metronidazole slowly, with resultant accumulation of metronidazole and its metabolites in the plasma. Accordingly, for such patients, doses below those usually recommended should be administered cautiously.

Administration of solutions containing sodium ions may result in sodium retention. Care should be taken when administering Flagyl I.V. RTU to patients receiving corticosteroids or to patients predisposed to edema.

Known or previously unrecognized candidiasis may present more prominent symptoms during therapy with Flagyl I.V. (metronidazole hydrochloride) or Flagyl I.V. RTU (metronidazole) and requires treatment with a candicidal agent.

Laboratory Tests: Metronidazole is a nitroimidazole, and Flagyl I.V. or Flagyl I.V. RTU should be used with care in patients with evidence of or history of blood dyscrasia. A mild leukopenia has been observed during its administration; however, no persistent hematologic abnormalities attributable to metronidazole have been observed in clinical studies. Total and differential leukocyte counts are recommended before and after therapy.

Drug Interactions: Metronidazole has been reported to potentiate the anticoagulant effect of warfarin and other oral coumarin anticoagulants, resulting in a prolongation of prothrombin time. This possible drug interaction should be considered when Flagyl I.V. or Flagyl I.V. RTU is prescribed for patients on this type of anticoagulant therapy.

The simultaneous administration of drugs that induce microsomal liver enzymes, such as phenytoin or phenobarbital, may accelerate the elimination of metronidazole, resulting in reduced plasma levels; impaired clearance of phenytoin has also been reported.

The simultaneous administration of drugs that decrease microsomal liver enzyme activity, such as cimetidine, may prolong the half-life and decrease plasma clearance of metronidazole.

Alcoholic beverages should not be consumed during metronidazole therapy because abdominal cramps, nausea, vomiting, headaches, and flushing may occur.

Continued on next pa[ge]

Searle Pharm.—Cont.

Drug/Laboratory Test Interactions: Metronidazole may interfere with certain types of determinations of serum chemistry values, such as aspartate aminotransferase (AST, SGOT), alanine aminotransferase (ALT, SGPT), lactate dehydrogenase (LDH), triglycerides, and hexokinase glucose. Values of zero may be observed. All of the assays in which interference has been reported involve enzymatic coupling of the assay to oxidation-reduction of nicotine adenine dinucleotide ($NAD^+ \rightleftarrows NADH$). Interference is due to the similarity in absorbance peaks of NADH (340 nm) and metronidazole (322 nm) at pH 7.

Carcinogenesis: See *Warnings.*

Pregnancy: Teratogenic Effects—Pregnancy Category B. Metronidazole crosses the placental barrier and enters the fetal circulation rapidly. Reproduction studies have been performed in rats at doses up to five times the human dose and have revealed no evidence of impaired fertility or harm to the fetus due to metronidazole. Metronidazole administered intraperitoneally to pregnant mice at approximately the human dose caused fetotoxicity; administered orally to pregnant mice, no fetotoxicity was observed. There are, however, no adequate and well-controlled studies in pregnant women. Because animal reproduction studies are not always predictive of human response, and because metronidazole is a carcinogen in rodents, these drugs should be used during pregnancy only if clearly needed.

Nursing Mothers: Because of the potential for tumorigenicity shown for metronidazole in mouse and rat studies, a decision should be made whether to discontinue nursing or to discontinue the drug, taking into account the importance of the drug to the mother. Metronidazole is secreted in breast milk in concentrations similar to those found in plasma.

Pediatric Use: Safety and effectiveness in children have not been established.

ADVERSE REACTIONS

Two serious adverse reactions reported in patients treated with Flagyl I.V. or Flagyl I.V. RTU have been convulsive seizures and peripheral neuropathy, the latter characterized mainly by numbness or paresthesia of an extremity. Since persistent peripheral neuropathy has been reported in some patients receiving prolonged oral administration of Flagyl® (metronidazole), patients should be observed carefully if neurologic symptoms occur and a prompt evaluation made of the benefit/risk ratio of the continuation of therapy.

The following reactions have also been reported during treatment with Flagyl I.V. (metronidazole hydrochloride) or Flagyl I.V. RTU (metronidazole):

- Gastrointestinal: Nausea, vomiting, abdominal discomfort, diarrhea, and an unpleasant metallic taste.
- Hematopoietic: Reversible neutropenia (leukopenia).
- Dermatologic: Erythematous rash and pruritus.
- Central Nervous System: Headache, dizziness, syncope, ataxia, and confusion.
- Local Reactions: Thrombophlebitis after intravenous infusion. This reaction can be minimized or avoided by avoiding prolonged use of indwelling intravenous catheters.
- Other: Fever. Instances of a darkened urine have also been reported, and this manifestation has been the subject of a special investigation. Although the pigment which is probably responsible for this phenomenon has not been positively identified, it is almost certainly a metabolite of metronidazole and seems to have no clinical significance.

The following adverse reactions have been reported during treatment with oral Flagyl (metronidazole):

- Gastrointestinal: Nausea, sometimes accompanied by headache, anorexia and occasionally vomiting; diarrhea, epigastric distress, abdominal cramping, and constipation.
- Mouth: A sharp, unpleasant metallic taste is not unusual. Furry tongue, glossitis, and stomatitis have occurred; these may be associated with a sudden overgrowth of *Candida* which may occur during effective therapy.
- Hematopoietic: Reversible neutropenia (leukopenia); rarely, reversible thrombocytopenia.
- Cardiovascular: Flattening of the T-wave may be seen in electrocardiographic tracings.
- Central Nervous System: Convulsive seizures, peripheral neuropathy, dizziness, vertigo, incoordination, ataxia, confusion, irritability, depression, weakness, and insomnia.
- Hypersensitivity: Urticaria, erythematous rash, flushing, nasal congestion, dryness of mouth (or vagina or vulva), and fever.
- Renal: Dysuria, cystitis, polyuria, incontinence, a sense of pelvic pressure, and darkened urine.
- [illegible] Proliferation of *Candida* in the vagina, dyspareu[illegible]ease of libido, proctitis, and fleeting joint pains [illegible] resembling "serum sickness." If patients [illegible]etronidazole drink alcoholic beverages, they [illegible]ience abdominal distress, nausea, vomiting, flushing, or headache. A modification of the taste of alcoholic beverages has also been reported.

Crohn's disease patients are known to have an increased incidence of gastrointestinal and certain extraintestinal cancers. There have been some reports in the medical literature of breast and colon cancer in Crohn's disease patients who have been treated with metronidazole at high doses for extended periods of time. A cause and effect relationship has not been established. Crohn's disease is not an approved indication for Flagyl I.V. or Flagyl I.V. RTU.

OVERDOSAGE

Use of dosages of Flagyl I.V. (metronidazole hydrochloride) higher than those recommended has been reported. These include the use of 27 mg/kg three times a day for 20 days, and the use of 75 mg/kg as a single loading dose followed by 7.5 mg/kg maintenance doses. No adverse reactions were reported in either of the two cases.

Single oral doses of metronidazole, up to 15 g, have been reported in suicide attempts and accidental overdoses. Symptoms reported include nausea, vomiting, and ataxia.

Oral metronidazole has been studied as a radiation sensitizer in the treatment of malignant tumors. Neurotoxic effects, including seizures and peripheral neuropathy, have been reported after 5 to 7 days of doses of 6 to 10.4 g every other day.

Treatment: There is no specific antidote for overdose; therefore, management of the patient should consist of symptomatic and supportive therapy.

DOSAGE AND ADMINISTRATION

Treatment of Anaerobic Infections

The recommended dosage schedule for *adults* is:

Loading dose:

15 mg/kg infused over one hour (approximately 1 g for a 70-kg adult).

Maintenance Dose:

7.5 mg/kg infused over one hour every six hours (approximately 500 mg for a 70-kg adult). The first maintenance dose should be instituted six hours following the initiation of the loading dose.

Parenteral therapy may be changed to oral Flagyl (metronidazole) when conditions warrant, based upon the severity of the disease and the response of the patient to Flagyl I.V. or Flagyl I.V. RTU (metronidazole) treatment. The usual adult oral dosage is 7.5 mg/kg every six hours.

A maximum of 4 g should not be exceeded during a 24-hour period.

Patients with severe hepatic disease metabolize metronidazole slowly, with resultant accumulation of metronidazole and its metabolites in the plasma. Accordingly, for such patients, doses below those usually recommended should be administered cautiously. Close monitoring of plasma metronidazole levels[2] and toxicity is recommended.

In patients receiving Flagyl I.V. or Flagyl I.V. RTU in whom gastric secretions are continuously removed by nasogastric aspiration, sufficient metronidazole may be removed in the aspirate to cause a reduction in serum levels.

The dose of Flagyl I.V. or Flagyl I.V. RTU should not be specifically reduced in anuric patients since accumulated metabolites may be rapidly removed by dialysis.

The usual duration of therapy is 7 to 10 days; however, infections of the bone and joint, lower respiratory tract, and endocardium may require longer treatment.

Prophylaxis

For surgical prophylactic use, to prevent postoperative infection in contaminated or potentially contaminated colorectal surgery, the recommended dosage schedule for adults is:

a. 15 mg/kg infused over 30 to 60 minutes and completed approximately one hour before surgery; followed by
b. 7.5 mg/kg infused over 30 to 60 minutes at 6 and 12 hours after the initial dose.

It is important that (1) administration of the initial preoperative dose be completed approximately one hour before surgery so that adequate drug levels are present in the serum and tissues at the time of initial incision, and (2) Flagyl I.V. or Flagyl I.V. RTU be administered, if necessary, at 6-hour intervals to maintain effective drug levels. Prophylactic use of Flagyl I.V. or Flagyl I.V. RTU should be limited to the day of surgery only, following the above guidelines.

CAUTION: Flagyl I.V. (metronidazole hydrochloride) or Flagyl I.V. RTU (metronidazole) is to be administered by slow intravenous drip infusion only, either as a continuous or intermittent infusion. I.V. admixtures containing metronidazole and other drugs should be avoided. Additives should not be introduced into the Flagyl I.V. RTU solution. If used with a primary intravenous fluid system, the primary solution should be discontinued during metronidazole infusion. DO NOT USE EQUIPMENT CONTAINING ALUMINUM (EG, NEEDLES, CANNULAE) THAT WOULD COME IN CONTACT WITH THE DRUG SOLUTION.

FLAGYL I.V.

Flagyl I.V. <u>cannot</u> be given by direct intravenous injection (I.V. bolus) because of the low pH (0.5 to 2.0) of the reconstituted product. FLAGYL I.V. MUST BE FURTHER DILUTED AND NEUTRALIZED FOR I.V. INFUSION.

Flagyl I.V. is prepared for use in two steps:

NOTE: ORDER OF MIXING IS IMPORTANT

A. Reconstitution.
B. Dilution in intravenous solution followed by pH neutralization with sodium bicarbonate injection into the dilution.

Reconstitution: To prepare the solution, add 4.4 ml of one of the following diluents and mix thoroughly: Sterile Water for Injection, USP; Bacteriostatic Water for Injection, USP; 0.9% Sodium Chloride Injection, USP; or Bacteriostatic 0.9% Sodium Chloride Injection, USP. The resultant approximate withdrawal volume is 5.0 ml with an approximate concentration of 100 mg/ml.

The pH of the reconstituted product will be in the range of 0.5 to 2.0. Reconstituted Flagyl I.V. is clear, and pale yellow to yellow-green in color.

Dilution in Intravenous Solutions: Properly reconstituted Flagyl I.V. may be added to a glass or plastic I.V. container not to exceed a concentration of 8 mg/ml. Any of the following intravenous solutions may be used: 0.9% Sodium Chloride Injection, USP; 5% Dextrose Injection, USP; or Lactated Ringer's Injection, USP.

NEUTRALIZATION IS REQUIRED PRIOR TO ADMINISTRATION

The final product should be mixed thoroughly and used within 24 hours.

Neutralization For Intravenous Infusion: Neutralize the intravenous solution containing Flagyl I.V. with approximately 5 mEq of sodium bicarbonate injection for each 500 mg of Flagyl I.V. used. Mix thoroughly. The pH of the neutralized intravenous solution will be approximately 6.0 to 7.0. Carbon dioxide gas will be generated with neutralization. It may be necessary to relieve gas pressure within the container.

Note: When the contents of one vial (500 mg) are diluted and neutralized to 100 ml, the resultant concentration is 5 mg/ml. Do not exceed an 8 mg/ml concentration of Flagyl I.V. in the neutralized intravenous solution, since neutralization will decrease the aqueous solubility and precipitation may occur. DO NOT REFRIGERATE NEUTRALIZED SOLUTIONS; otherwise, precipitation may occur.

Storage and Stability: Reconstituted vials of Flagyl I.V. are chemically stable for 96 hours when stored below 86°F (30°C) in room light.

Use diluted and neutralized intravenous solutions containing Flagyl I.V. within 24 hours of mixing.

FLAGYL I.V. RTU

Flagyl I.V. RTU is a ready-to-use isotonic solution. **NO DILUTION OR BUFFERING IS REQUIRED.** Do not refrigerate. Each container of Flagyl I.V. RTU contains 14 mEq of sodium.

Directions for use of plastic container:

CAUTION: Do not use plastic containers in series connections. Such use could result in air embolism due to residual air (approximately 15 ml) being drawn from the primary container before administration of the fluid from the secondary container is complete.

To open. Tear overwrap down side at slit and remove solution container. Some opacity of the plastic due to moisture absorption during the sterilization process may be observed. This is normal and does not affect the solution quality or safety. The opacity will diminish gradually. Check for minute leaks by squeezing inner bag firmly. If leaks are found discard solution as sterility may be impaired.

Preparation for administration:

1. Suspend container from eyelet support.
2. Remove plastic protector from outlet port at bottom of container.
3. Attach administration set. Refer to complete directions accompanying set.

Parenteral drug products should be inspected visually for particulate matter and discoloration prior to administration, whenever solution and container permit. Do not use if cloudy or precipitated or if the seal is not intact.

Use sterile equipment. It is recommended that the intravenous administration apparatus be replaced at least once every 24 hours.

HOW SUPPLIED

FLAGYL I.V.

Flagyl I.V., sterile (metronidazole hydrochloride), is supplied in single-dose lyophilized vials each containing 500 mg metronidazole equivalent, individually packaged in cartons of 10 vials.

Flagyl I.V., prior to reconstitution, should be stored below 86°F (30°C) and protected from light.

FLAGYL I.V. RTU

In plastic container: Flagyl I.V. RTU, sterile (metronidazole), is supplied in 100-ml single-dose containers, each containing an isotonic, buffered solution of 500 mg metronidazole, individually packaged in boxes of 24.

In glass: Flagyl I.V. RTU, sterile (metronidazole), is supplied in 100-ml single-dose vials, each containing an isotonic,

buffered solution of 500 mg metronidazole, individually packaged in cartons of 6 vials.
Flagyl I.V. RTU should be stored at controlled room temperature, 59° to 86° F (15° to 30°C), and protected from light during storage.

---

1. Proposed standard: PSM-11—Proposed Reference Dilution Procedure for Antimicrobic Susceptibility Testing of Anaerobic Bacteria, National Committee for Clinical Laboratory Standards, and Sutter, et al.: Collaborative Evaluation of a Proposed Reference Dilution Method of Susceptibility Testing of Anaerobic Bacteria, Antimicrob. Agents Chemother. *16:* 495–502 (Oct.) 1979; and Tally, et al: *In Vitro* Activity of Thienamycin, Antimicrob. Agents Chemother. *14:* 436–438 (Sept.) 1978.
2. Ralph, E.D., and Kirby, W.M.M.: Bioassay of Metronidazole With Either Anaerobic or Aerobic Incubation, J. Infect. Dis. *132:* 587–591 (Nov.) 1975; or Gulaid, et al.: Determination of Metronidazole and Its Major Metabolites in Biological Fluids by High Pressure Liquid Chromatography, Br. J. Clin. Pharmacol. *6:* 430–432, 1978.

Shown in Product Identification Section, page 429

NITRODISC® ℞

[*nī 'trō 'disc*]
(nitroglycerin transdermal system)
5 mg/24 hr; 7.5 mg/24 hr; 10 mg/24 hr

DESCRIPTION

Nitrodisc incorporates a patented Microseal Drug Delivery™ system consisting of a solid, nitroglycerin-impregnated polymer bonded to a flexible, nonsensitizing adhesive bandage. It is designed to be applied topically. Nitrodisc provides constant and controlled drug delivery over a uniform skin surface area for 24 hours.
Nitrodisc is available in three strengths which release 5 mg, 7.5 mg, or 10 mg of nitroglycerin during a 24-hour period. The 5 mg/24 hr system contains 16 mg of nitroglycerin over an 8 cm^2 releasing surface. The 7.5 mg/24 hr system contains 24 mg of nitroglycerin over a 12 cm^2 releasing surface. The 10 mg/24 hr system contains 32 mg of nitroglycerin over a 16 cm^2 releasing surface (see *How Supplied* section).
Inactive ingredients are lactose, polyethylene glycol, water, silicone rubber, plasticizers, aluminum foil laminate, polyethylene foam, and acrylic adhesive.

CLINICAL PHARMACOLOGY

When Nitrodisc is applied to the skin, nitroglycerin is absorbed continuously through the skin into the systemic circulation. This results in active drug reaching the target organs (heart and peripheral vasculature) before being inactivated by the liver. Nitroglycerin is a smooth muscle relaxant with vascular effects manifested predominantly by venous dilation and pooling. The major beneficial effect of nitroglycerin in angina pectoris is due to a reduction in myocardial oxygen consumption secondary to vascular smooth muscle relaxation and consequent reduced cardiac preload and afterload. In addition, a direct effect of nitroglycerin on the coronary vessels is recognized as well.
In normal volunteers, transdermal absorption of nitroglycerin from Nitrodisc occurred in a continuous and well-controlled manner for a minimum of 24 hours. Detectable plasma levels were attained within 1 hour after the application of the disc and remained at a similar level for 24 hours. Precise definition of "therapeutic plasma level" is not known at this time. Plasma levels of nitroglycerin were still detectable 30 minutes after removal of the system.
The amount of nitroglycerin released (5 mg/24 hr, 7.5 mg/24 hr, or 10 mg/24 hr) represents the mean release rate of nitroglycerin from the disc as determined from healthy volunteers and, hence, the amount potentially available for absorption through the skin. Absorption will vary among individuals.

INDICATIONS AND USAGE

Nitrodisc has been conditionally approved by the FDA for the prevention and treatment of angina pectoris due to coronary artery disease. The conditional approval reflects a determination that the drug may be marketed while further investigation of its effectiveness is undertaken. A final evaluation of the effectiveness of the product will be announced by the FDA.

CONTRAINDICATIONS

Nitrodisc (nitroglycerin) is contraindicated in patients known to be intolerant of organic nitrate drugs and in patients with marked anemia.

WARNINGS

In patients with acute myocardial infarction or congestive heart failure, Nitrodisc should be used under careful clinical and/or hemodynamic monitoring.
In terminating treatment of patients with angina, both the dosage and frequency of application must be gradually reduced over a period of 4 to 6 weeks to prevent potential withdrawal reactions, which are characteristic of all vasodilators in the nitrate class.

PRECAUTIONS

Symptoms of hypotension, such as faintness, weakness, or dizziness, particularly orthostatic hypotension, may be due to overdosage. When these symptoms occur, the dosage should be reduced or use of the product discontinued.
Nitrodisc is not intended for immediate relief of anginal attacks. For this purpose, occasional use of sublingual preparations may be necessary.
Pregnancy: Pregnancy Category C. Animal reproduction studies have not been conducted with Nitrodisc. It is also not known whether nitroglycerin can cause fetal harm when administered to a pregnant woman or can affect reproduction capacity. Nitroglycerin should be given to a pregnant woman only if clearly needed.
Nursing mothers: It is not known whether nitroglycerin is excreted in human milk. Because many drugs are excreted in human milk, caution should be exercised when Nitrodisc is administered to a nursing woman.

ADVERSE REACTIONS

Transient headache is the most common side effect, especially when higher doses of the drug are used. These headaches should be treated with mild analgesics while Nitrodisc therapy is continued. When such headaches are unresponsive to treatment, the nitroglycerin dosage should be reduced or use of the product discontinued.
Adverse reactions reported less frequently include hypotension, increased heart rate, faintness, flushing, dizziness, nausea, vomiting, and dermatitis. With the exception of dermatitis, these symptoms are attributable to the known pharmacologic effects of nitroglycerin, but may be symptoms of overdosage. When they persist, Nitrodisc (nitroglycerin) dose should be reduced or use of the product discontinued.

DOSAGE AND ADMINISTRATION

Nitrodisc should be applied once each day. To use Nitrodisc, follow the instructions on the package. Nitrodisc should be applied to an intact skin site free of hair and not subject to excessive movement. It should not be applied to the distal parts of the extremities. A suitable area should be shaved free of hair, if necessary. The application site should be changed slightly each time to avoid undue skin irritation. A new Nitrodisc should be applied if the product loosens.
The optimal dosage regimen should be selected based upon the clinical response, the side effects, and the effects of therapy upon blood pressure and heart rate. It is recommended that therapy be initiated with Nitrodisc 5 mg/24 hr and that Nitrodisc 7.5 mg/24 hr or Nitrodisc 10 mg/24 hr be utilized when a greater response is desired. In the event that higher doses are necessary, multiple discs may be applied.
Patient Instructions for Application: These are provided with the product.

HOW SUPPLIED

Nitrodisc	5 mg/ 24 hr	7.5 mg/ 24 hr	10 mg/ 24 hr
Drug released per 24 hours	5 mg	7.5 mg	10 mg
Total drug content	16 mg	24 mg	32 mg
Drug releasing surface	8 cm^2	12 cm^2	16 cm^2

Nitrodisc (nitroglycerin transdermal system) is supplied in cartons of 30 discs and in cartons of 30 and 100 discs (labeled for institutional use). Store at a controlled room temperature of 59°–86°F (15°–30°C). **Do not refrigerate.** Extremes of temperature and/or humidity should be avoided.

Shown in Product Identification Section, page 429

	12 Months		24 Months		36 Months	
	Parous	Nulliparous	Parous	Nulliparous	Parous	Nulliparous
Pregnancy	3.0	2.1	4.9	4.5	6.0	5.8
Expulsion	7.8	8.0	9.8	9.6	10.8	10.9
Medical removal	10.9	13.9	18.2	21.9	23.3	26.9
Continuation	73.4	71.4	55.0	53.9	41.9	40.1

It has been reported that the return of fertility (cumulative gross rate) after elective removal of the Tatum-T in women desiring pregnancy was 87% at one year after removal.

Tatum-T Placement Instrument

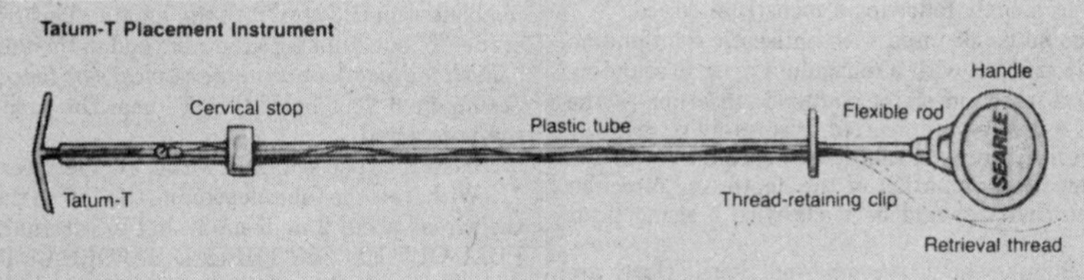

TATUM-T® ℞

[*tā 'tum-tē"*]
(intrauterine copper contraceptive)

DESCRIPTION

The plastic component of the Tatum-T (intrauterine copper contraceptive) is composed of polyethylene with barium sulfate added to render it radiopaque. Its shape approximates the letter T. The vertical dimension measures 36 mm and the horizontal, 32 mm.
Coiled around the vertical limb is 120 mg of copper wire providing approximately 210 mm^2 of exposed copper surface area. A retrieval thread is fastened to the free end of the vertical limb of the Tatum-T.
The Tatum-T is supplied with a simple tubular plastic inserter. All components are sterile.

For **Clinical Pharmacology, Indications and Usage, Contraindications, Warnings, Precautions,** and **Adverse Reactions,** *see Cu-7 (intrauterine copper contraceptive) under this manufacturer.*

DIRECTIONS FOR USE

The Tatum-T is to be placed within the uterine cavity. See the *Procedure for Insertion* for the insertion technique.
The optimal time of insertion is during the latter part of the menstrual flow or one or two days thereafter. The cervical canal is relatively more patent at this time, and there is little chance that the patient may be pregnant.
Present information indicates that efficacy is retained for 36 months. There is no evidence that contraceptive efficacy decreases with time up to three years of use, but unless new data support a longer period of efficacy and safety, the Tatum-T must be removed within 36 months from the date of insertion and a new one inserted if desired. If partial expulsion occurs, removal is indicated, and a new Tatum-T may be inserted. Removal of the Tatum-T may also be indicated in the event of heavy or persistent bleeding.
The physician should become thoroughly familiar with the instructions for use before attempting insertion or removal of the Tatum-T.

CLINICAL STUDIES

Different event rates have been reported with the use of different intrauterine contraceptives. Inasmuch as these rates are usually derived from separate studies conducted by different investigators in several population groups, a comparison cannot be made with precision. Even in different studies with the same contraceptive, considerably different rates are likely to be obtained because of differing characteristics of the study population. Furthermore, event rates per unit of time tend to be lower as clinical experience is expanded, possibly due to retention in the clinical study of those patients who accept the treatment regimen, not having discontinued due to adverse reactions or pregnancy, so that those remaining in the study were those less susceptible. In clinical trials of the Tatum-T conducted in the United States and Canada, use effectiveness was determined as follows for parous and nulliparous women, as tabulated by the life table method. (Rates are expressed as cumulative events per 100 women through 12, 24, and 36 months of use.)
This experience encompasses 236,060 woman-months of use, including 12 months for 8,232 women, 24 months for 4,247, and 36 months for 1,408.
Cumulative rates were:
[See table above].

Procedure for Insertion

Physicians are cautioned that it is imperative that they become thoroughly familiar with the instructions for insertion before attempting placement of the "T." The insertion technique is different in several respects from that employed with other intrauterine contraceptives currently available;

Continued on next page

Searle Pharm.—Cont.

particular attention should be paid to the illustrations and instructions.

The Tatum-T may be inserted easily at any time during the menstrual cycle. It is *not* necessary to delay insertion until a menstrual flow is in progress; however, the possibility of existing undetermined pregnancy is lessened if insertion is made during or shortly following a menstrual period.

The cervix should be cleansed with antiseptic solution and its anterior lip grasped with a tenaculum prior to sounding the uterus and insertion of the Tatum-T. Insertion of the Tatum-T into a severely anteverted or severely retroverted uterus may be difficult unless sufficient tension is applied to the tenaculum. Determination of the depth and direction of the uterine cavity should be made with a sound prior to insertion.

An aseptic technique should be employed. Sterile gloves are recommended; however, the package itself may be used to set the cervical stop and to load the "T" into the insertion tube. A small loading device is contained within the package to facilitate this step. Exercise care to avoid contaminating the "T" or that part of the tube which will enter the cervical canal.

CAUTION

DO NOT load the "T" into the tube until after the cervical stop on the tube has been set to the sounded depth nor leave it loaded longer than 2 minutes. The plastic of the Tatum-T is soft and it will lose its "memory"; it will then fail to return to its "T" configuration within the uterus and thus invite loss of effectiveness and early expulsion.

DO NOT push the "T" into the tube so that less than 1/4 in of the frame protrudes; placement may be improper; the arms may be damaged. If more than 1/4 in protrudes, the risk of perforation is increased.

DO NOT remove the thread-retaining clip from the insertion rod until after insertion has been made and you are ready to deposit the Tatum-T within the uterine cavity. The thread-retaining clip on the rod prevents the "T" and/or rod from falling to a non-sterile surface. When held against the end of the tube during the loading procedure, it helps to keep the "T" from being pushed too far into the tube and prevents premature ejection of the "T" during the insertion procedure.

DO NOT force the insertion. It is generally believed that most perforations occur at the time of insertion, although the perforation may not be detected until some time later. The position of the uterus should be determined during the pre-insertion examination. Great care must be exercised during the pre-insertion sounding and subsequent insertion.

Note: If the uterine cavity measures under 6.5 cm, the incidence of pain, bleeding, partial or complete expulsion, perforation, and possibly pregnancy, increases. Insertion is not recommended into a uterus that sounds under 6.0 cm.

1. Sterile gloves are recommended for the insertion procedure. If sterile gloves are used, the instrument may be removed from the package when setting the cervical stop and loading it into the insertion tube. If sterile gloves are not used then the package containing the "T" should be used for these procedures. (The package should be torn open just over halfway.)
2. After sounding, adjust the 1/4-in-thick blue cervical stop on the tube. The edge closer to the handle must be set at the sounded depth of the uterus, *see Figure 1,* because the "T" protrudes 1/4 in from the end of the tube. If the package is being used to set the cervical stop, do not put the sound inside the package since it could contaminate the "T".
3. The plastic loading device affixed to the cardboard backing near the "T" will help facilitate loading the "T" into the tube. NOTE: It is easier to load the "T" when the sides of the loading device are not squeezed together. For this reason it is best to hold the cardboard backing and not the device. Free the insertion instrument from the cardboard mount. Holding the insertion instrument midway between the cervical stop and the handle, push the insertion rod and tube so that the arms of the "T" slide into the cul-de-sac of the loading device. *See Figure 2.* The arms of the "T" are now folded against the tube. Retract the tube and rod together until the tube clears the arms of the "T". Again push the insertion instrument towards the loading device, trapping the arms of the "T" in the tube until 1/4 in (~0.6 cm) of the folded "T" protrudes and the end of the rod just touches the stem of the "T". *See Figure 3.* To release the "T" from the loading device, rotate the insertion instrument 90° and slide the inserter out. If the package is being used to maintain sterility, the insertion instrument should not be completely removed from the package until the cervical stop has been aligned. Align the folded arms of the "T" with the wings of the cervical stop. After the cervical stop has been aligned, open the package the rest of the way.
4. Immediately apply gentle traction on the uterus with a tenaculum and insert the Tatum-T through the cervical canal up to the fundus. *See Figure 4.* Maintain or align the cervical stop at the cervix in a horizontal plane.
5. Press the thread-retaining clip back toward the handle to free the thread. Hold the rod firmly, but without undue pressure against the stem of the "T," and withdraw the tube to about 1/2 in (1.3 cm) from the handle. This frees the arms of the "T" but still keeps the stem end in the tube. *See Figure 5. Push the tube back until the cervical stop touches the cervix. See Figure 6.* This holds the "T" near the fundus while the rod is removed.
6. Hold the tube still and withdraw the insertion rod.
7. Withdraw the tube, depositing the "T" in the uterus. Cut the thread about 2 in (5 cm) from the external os. DO NOT PULL OUT EXCESS THREAD BEFORE CUTTING.

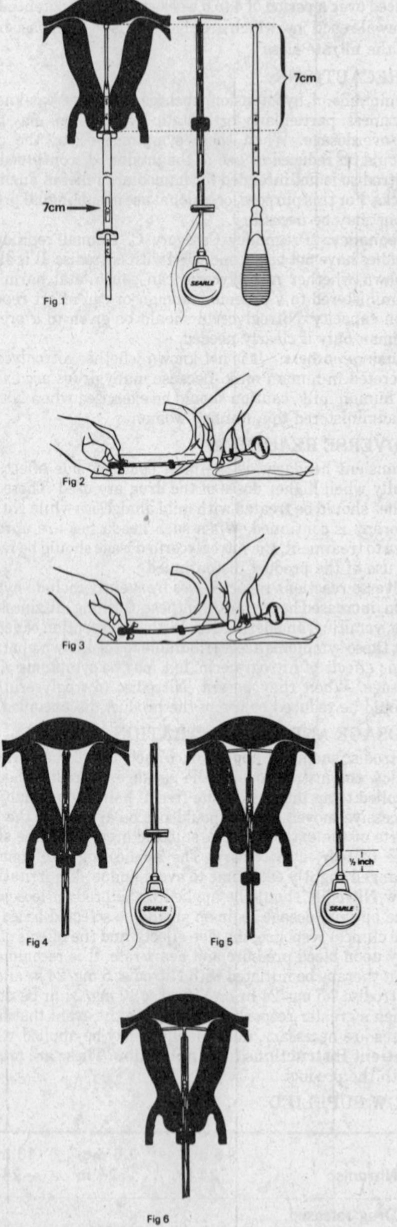

Removal of the Tatum-T

ROUTINE REMOVAL—THREAD VISIBLE:

1. DO NOT exert a sudden pull or jerk on the retrieval thread. Exert a firm, steady pull on the thread. A jerk may cause the thread to break.

2. A ring (sponge) forceps, with its smooth edges and minimal crushing force, is a good instrument with which to grasp the thread.

3. Other instruments may be used, but care must be exerted to avoid crushing or cutting the thread.

4. Avoid winding or angulating the thread about the jaws of the withdrawal instrument.

5. Utilize the minimum force needed to remove the Tatum-T.

6. Should resistance be encountered, dislodge the Tatum-T with a probe or uterine sound before making further removal attempts.

THREAD NOT VISIBLE: If the Tatum-T is in the uterus and the thread is not visible, the following procedures should be considered when you elect to recover it:

1. Aseptic use of a slim instrument (eg, uterine dressing forceps) or contact hysteroscopy will frequently permit removal in the office.

2. Hysteroscopy under hospital conditions may be required.

3. D & C and also suction aspiration have been used as alternative measures.

NOTE: If intrauterine manipulative procedures are required, allow an appropriate healing period before inserting a new Tatum-T.

The preceding prescribing information for Searle Pharmaceuticals Inc. was current on September 1, 1986.

Searle & Co.
SAN JUAN, PUERTO RICO 00936

ALDACTAZIDE® ℞
[al-dac 'tuh "zīde]
(spironolactone with hydrochlorothiazide)

WARNING

Spironolactone, an ingredient of Aldactazide, has been shown to be a tumorigen in chronic toxicity studies in rats (see *Warnings*). Aldactazide should be used only in those conditions described under *Indications and Usage.* Unnecessary use of this drug should be avoided.

Fixed-dose combination drugs are not indicated for initial therapy of edema or hypertension. Edema or hypertension requires therapy titrated to the individual patient. If the fixed combination represents the dosage so determined, its use may be more convenient in patient management. The treatment of hypertension and edema is not static, but must be reevaluated as conditions in each patient warrant.

DESCRIPTION

Aldactazide oral tablets contain:

spironolactone	25 mg
hydrochlorothiazide	25 mg
or	
spironolactone	50 mg
hydrochlorothiazide	50 mg

Spironolactone (Aldactone®), an aldosterone antagonist, is 17-hydroxy-7α-mercapto-3-oxo-17α-pregn-4-ene-21-carboxylic acid γ-lactone acetate and has the following structural formula:

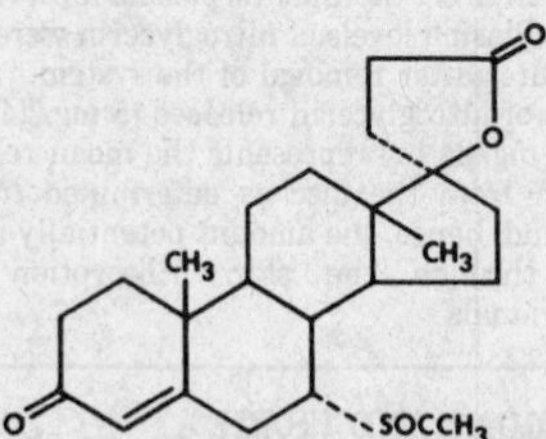

Spironolactone is practically insoluble in water, soluble in alcohol, and freely soluble in benzene and in chloroform. Hydrochlorothiazide, a diuretic and antihypertensive, is 6-chloro-3, 4-dihydro-2H-1,2,4-benzothiadiazine-7-sulfonamide 1,1-dioxide and has the following structural formula:

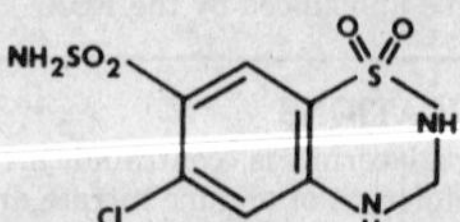

Hydrochlorothiazide is slightly soluble in water and freely soluble in sodium hydroxide solution.

Inactive ingredients include calcium sulfate, corn starch, flavor, hydroxypropyl cellulose, hydroxypropyl methylcellulose, iron oxide, magnesium stearate, polyethylene glycol, povidone, and titanium dioxide.

CLINICAL PHARMACOLOGY

Aldactazide is a combination of two diuretic agents with different but complementary mechanisms and sites of action, thereby providing additive diuretic and antihypertensive effects. Additionally, the spironolactone component helps to minimize the potassium loss characteristically induced by the thiazide component.

The diuretic effect of spironolactone is mediated through its action as a specific pharmacologic antagonist of aldosterone, primarily by competitive binding of receptors at the aldosterone-dependent sodium-potassium exchange site in the distal convoluted renal tubule. Hydrochlorothiazide promotes the excretion of sodium and water primarily by inhibiting their reabsorption in the cortical diluting segment of the renal tubule.

Aldactazide is effective in significantly lowering the systolic and diastolic blood pressure in many patients with essential hypertension, even when aldosterone secretion is within normal limits.

Both spironolactone and hydrochlorothiazide reduce exchangeable sodium, plasma volume, body weight, and blood pressure. The diuretic and antihypertensive effects of the individual components are potentiated when spironolactone and hydrochlorothiazide are given concurrently.

In the human, the bioavailability of both spironolactone and hydrochlorothiazide from orally administered Aldactazide 25 mg/25 mg uncoated tablets and Aldactazide film-coated tablets has been evaluated in hypertensive subjects. Equivalent doses of the film-coated tablets, which contain microcrystalline spironolactone, showed 20% to 25% higher bioavailability of spironolactone compared to the uncoated Aldactazide tablets. Hydrochlorothiazide bioavailability was similar in the film-coated and uncoated tablets.

Spironolactone is rapidly and extensively metabolized. The primary metabolite is canrenone, which attains peak serum levels at two to four hours following single oral administration. Canrenone plasma concentrations decline in two distinct phases, being rapid in the first 12 hours and slower from 12 to 96 hours. The log-linear phase half-life of canrenone, following multiple doses of Aldactone (spironolactone), is between 13 and 24 hours. Both spironolactone and canrenone are more than 90% bound to plasma proteins. The metabolites of spironolactone are excreted primarily in urine, but also in bile.

Hydrochlorothiazide is rapidly absorbed following oral administration. Onset of action is observed within one hour and persists for 6 to 12 hours. Plasma concentrations attain peak levels at one to two hours and decline with a half-life of four to five hours. Hydrochlorothiazide undergoes only slight metabolic alteration and is excreted in urine. It is distributed throughout the extracellular space, with essentially no tissue accumulation except in the kidney.

INDICATIONS AND USAGE

Spironolactone, an ingredient of Aldactazide, has been shown to be a tumorigen in chronic toxicity studies in rats (see *Warnings* section). Aldactazide should be used only in those conditions described below. Unnecessary use of this drug should be avoided.

Aldactazide is indicated for:

Edematous conditions for patients with:

Congestive heart failure: For the management of edema and sodium retention when the patient is only partially responsive to, or is intolerant of, other therapeutic measures. The treatment of diuretic-induced hypokalemia in patients with congestive heart failure when other measures are considered inappropriate. The treatment of patients with congestive heart failure taking digitalis when other therapies are considered inadequate or inappropriate.

Cirrhosis of the liver accompanied by edema and/or ascites: Aldosterone levels may be exceptionally high in this condition. Aldactazide is indicated for maintenance therapy together with bed rest and the restriction of fluid and sodium.

The nephrotic syndrome: For nephrotic patients when treatment of the underlying disease, restriction of fluid and sodium intake, and the use of other diuretics do not provide an adequate response.

Essential hypertension

For patients with essential hypertension in whom other measures are considered inadequate or inappropriate. In hypertensive patients for the treatment of a diuretic-induced hypokalemia when other measures are considered inappropriate.

Usage in Pregnancy. The routine use of diuretics in an otherwise healthy woman is inappropriate and exposes mother and fetus to unnecessary hazard. Diuretics do not prevent development of toxemia of pregnancy, and there is no satisfactory evidence that they are useful in the treatment of developing toxemia.

Edema during pregnancy may arise from pathologic causes or from the physiologic and mechanical consequences of pregnancy. Aldactazide is indicated in pregnancy when edema is due to pathologic causes just as it is in the absence of pregnancy (however, see *Warnings* section). Dependent edema in pregnancy, resulting from restriction of venous return by the expanded uterus, is properly treated through elevation of the lower extremities and use of support hose; use of diuretics to lower intravascular volume in this case is unsupported and unnecessary. There is hypervolemia during normal pregnancy which is harmful to neither the fetus nor the mother (in the absence of cardiovascular disease), but which is associated with edema, including generalized edema, in the majority of pregnant women. If this edema produces discomfort, increased recumbency will often provide relief. In rare instances, this edema may cause extreme discomfort which is not relieved by rest. In these cases, a short course of diuretics may provide relief and may be appropriate.

CONTRAINDICATIONS

Aldactazide is contraindicated in patients with anuria, acute renal insufficiency, significant impairment of renal function, or hyperkalemia, and in patients who are allergic to thiazide diuretics or to other sulfonamide-derived drugs. Aldactazide may also be contraindicated in acute or severe hepatic failure.

WARNINGS

Potassium supplementation, either in the form of medication or as a diet rich in potassium, should not ordinarily be given in association with Aldactazide therapy. Excessive potassium intake may cause hyperkalemia in patients receiving Aldactazide (see *Precautions* section). Aldactazide should not be administered concurrently with other potassium-sparing diuretics.

Sulfonamide derivatives, including thiazides, have been reported to exacerbate or activate systemic lupus erythematosus.

Spironolactone has been shown to be a tumorigen in chronic toxicity studies performed in rats, with its proliferative effects manifested on endocrine organs and the liver. In one study using 25, 75, and 250 times the usual daily human dose (2 mg/kg) there was a statistically significant dose-related increase in benign adenomas of the thyroid and testes. In female rats there was a statistically significant increase in malignant mammary tumors at the mid-dose only. In male rats there was a dose-related increase in proliferative changes in the liver. At the highest dosage level (500 mg/kg), the range of effects included hepatocytomegaly, hyperplastic nodules, and hepatocellular carcinoma; the last was not statistically significant at a value of $p = 0.05$. A dose-related (above 20 mg/kg/day) incidence of myelocytic leukemia was observed in rats fed daily doses of potassium canrenoate for a period of one year. In long-term (two-year) oral carcinogenicity studies of potassium canrenoate in the rat, myelocytic leukemia and hepatic, thyroid, testicular, and mammary tumors were observed. Potassium canrenoate did not produce a mutagenic effect in tests using bacteria or yeast. It did produce a postive mutagenic effect in several *in vitro* tests in mammalian cells following metabolism activation. In an *in vivo* mammalian system potassium canrenoate was not mutagenic. Canrenone and canrenoic acid are the major metabolites of potassium canrenoate. Spironolactone is also metabolized to canrenone. An increased incidence of leukemia was not observed in chronic rat toxicity studies conducted with spironolactone at doses up to 500 mg/kg/day.

PRECAUTIONS

Patients receiving Aldactazide therapy should be carefully evaluated for possible disturbances of fluid and electrolyte balance. Hyperkalemia may occur in patients with impaired renal function or excessive potassium intake and can cause cardiac irregularities which may be fatal. Consequently, no potassium supplement should ordinarily be given with Aldactazide. Hyperkalemia can be treated promptly by the rapid intravenous administration of glucose (20% to 50%) and regular insulin, using 0.25 to 0.5 units of insulin per gram of glucose. This is a temporary measure to be repeated as required. Aldactazide should be discontinued and potassium intake (including dietary potassium) restricted.

Hypokalemia may develop as a result of profound diuresis, particularly when Aldactazide is used concomitantly with loop diuretics, glucocorticoids, or ACTH. Hypokalemia may exaggerate the effects of digitalis therapy. Potassium depletion may induce signs of digitalis intoxication at previously tolerated dosage levels.

Warning signs of possible fluid and electrolyte imbalance include dryness of the mouth, thirst, weakness, lethargy, drowsiness, restlessness, muscle pains or cramps, muscular fatigue, hypotension, oliguria, tachycardia, and gastrointestinal symptoms.

Aldactazide therapy may cause a transient elevation of BUN. This appears to represent a concentration phenomenon rather than renal toxicity, since the BUN returns to normal after Aldactazide is discontinued. Progressive elevation of BUN is suggestive of the presence of preexisting renal impairment.

Reversible hyperchloremic metabolic acidosis, usually in association with hyperkalemia, has been reported to occur in some patients with decompensated hepatic cirrhosis, even in the presence of normal renal function.

Dilutional hyponatremia, manifested by dryness of the mouth, thirst, lethargy, and drowsiness, and confirmed by a low serum sodium level, may be induced, especially when Aldactazide is administered in combination with other diuretics. A true low-salt syndrome may rarely develop with Aldactazide therapy and may be manifested by increasing mental confusion similar to that observed with hepatic coma. This syndrome is differentiated from dilutional hyponatremia in that it does not occur with obvious fluid retention. Its treatment requires that diuretic therapy be discontinued and sodium administered.

Gynecomastia may develop in association with the use of spironolactone, and physicians should be alert to its possible onset. The development of gynecomastia appears to be related to both dosage level and duration of therapy and is normally reversible when Aldactazide is discontinued. In rare instances some breast enlargement may persist.

Thiazides have been demonstrated to alter the metabolism of uric acid and carbohydrates, with possible development of hyperuricemia, gout, and decreased glucose tolerance. Thiazides may temporarily exaggerate abnormalities of glucose metabolism in diabetic patients or cause abnormalities to appear in patients with latent diabetes.

The antihypertensive effects of hydrochlorothiazide may be enhanced in patients who have undergone sympathectomy.

Pathologic changes in the parathyroid gland with hypercalcemia and hypophosphatemia have been observed in patients on prolonged thiazide therapy. Thiazides may also decrease serum PBI levels without evidence of alteration of thyroid function.

Both spironolactone and hydrochlorothiazide reduce the vascular responsiveness to norepinephrine. Therefore, caution should be exercised in the management of patients subjected to regional or general anesthesia while they are being treated with Aldactazide. Thiazides may also increase the responsiveness to tubocurarine.

Spironolactone has been shown to increase the half-life of digoxin. This may result in increased serum digoxin levels and subsequent digitalis toxicity. It may be necessary to reduce the maintenance and digitalization doses when spironolactone is administered, and the patient should be carefully monitored to avoid over- or underdigitalization.

Several reports of possible interference with digoxin radioimmunoassays by spironolactone, or its metabolites, have appeared in the literature. Neither the extent nor the potential clinical significance of its interference (which may be assay-specific) has been fully established.

Usage in Pregnancy. Spironolactone or its metabolites may, and hydrochlorothiazide does, cross the placental barrier. Therefore, the use of Aldactazide in pregnant women requires that the anticipated benefit be weighed against possible hazards to the fetus. These hazards include fetal or neonatal jaundice, thrombocytopenia, and possible other adverse reactions which have been reported in the adult.

Nursing Mothers. Canrenone, a metabolite of spironolactone, and hydrochlorothiazide appear in breast milk. If use of these drugs is deemed essential, an alternative method of infant feeding should be instituted.

ADVERSE REACTIONS

Gynecomastia is observed not infrequently. A few cases of agranulocytosis have been reported in patients taking spironolactone. Other adverse reactions that have been reported in association with the use of spironolactone are: gastrointestinal symptoms including cramping and diarrhea, drowsiness, lethargy, headache, maculopapular or erythematous cutaneous eruptions, urticaria, mental confusion, drug fever, ataxia, inability to achieve or maintain erection, irregular menses or amenorrhea, postmenopausal bleeding, hirsutism, and deepening of the voice. Carcinoma of the breast has been reported in patients taking spironolactone, but a cause and effect relationship has not been established.

Adverse reactions reported in association with the use of thiazides include: gastrointestinal symptoms (anorexia, nausea, vomiting, diarrhea, abdominal cramps), purpura, thrombocytopenia, leukopenia, agranulocytosis, dermatologic symptoms (cutaneous eruptions, pruritus, erythema multiforme), paresthesia, acute pancreatitis, jaundice, dizziness, vertigo, headache, xanthopsia, photosensitivity, necrotizing angiitis, aplastic anemia, orthostatic hypotension, muscle spasm, weakness, and restlessness.

Adverse reactions are usually reversible upon discontinuation of Aldactazide.

DOSAGE AND ADMINISTRATION

Optimal dosage should be established by individual titration of the components (see Box Warning).

Edema in adults (*congestive heart failure, hepatic cirrhosis, or nephrotic syndrome*). The usual maintenance dose of Aldactazide is 100 mg each of spironolactone and hydrochlorothiazide daily, administered in a single dose or in divided doses, but may range from 25 mg to 200 mg of each component daily depending on the response to the initial titration. In some

Continued on next page

Searle & Co.—Cont.

instances it may be desirable to administer separate tablets of either Aldactone (spironolactone) or hydrochlorothiazide in addition to Aldactazide in order to provide optimal individual therapy.
The onset of diuresis with Aldactazide occurs promptly and, due to prolonged effect of the spironolactone component, persists for two to three days after Aldactazide is discontinued.
Edema in children. The usual daily maintenance dose of Aldactazide should be that which provides 0.75 to 1.5 mg of spironolactone per pound of body weight (1.65 to 3.3 mg/kg).
Essential hypertension. Although the dosage will vary depending on the results of titration of the individual ingredients, many patients will be found to have an optimal response to 50 mg to 100 mg each of spironolactone and hydrochlorothiazide daily, given in a single dose or in divided doses.
Concurrent potassium supplementation is not recommended when Aldactazide is used in the long-term management of hypertension or in the treatment of most edematous conditions, since the spironolactone content of Aldactazide is usually sufficient to minimize loss induced by the hydrochlorothiazide component.

HOW SUPPLIED

Aldactazide tablets containing 25 mg of spironolactone (Aldactone) and 25 mg of hydrochlorothiazide are round, tan, film coated, with SEARLE and 1011 debossed on one side and ALDACTAZIDE and 25 on the other side; bottles of 100, 500, 1,000, and 2,500, and cartons of 100 unit-dose individually blister-sealed tablets.
Aldactazide tablets containing 50 mg of spironolactone (Aldactone) and 50 mg of hydrochlorothiazide are oblong, tan, scored, film coated, with SEARLE and 1021 debossed on the scored side and ALDACTAZIDE and 50 on the other side; bottles of 100 and cartons of 100 unit-dose individually blister-sealed tablets.

Shown in Product Identification Section, page 429

ALDACTONE® ℞

[al-dac 'tone]
(spironolactone)

> **Warning**
> Spironolactone has been shown to be a tumorigen in chronic toxicity studies in rats (see *Warnings*). Aldactone should be used only in those conditions described under *Indications and Usage*. Unnecessary use of this drug should be avoided.

DESCRIPTION

Aldactone oral tablets contain 25 mg, 50 mg, or 100 mg of the aldosterone antagonist spironolactone, 17- hydroxy-7α -mercapto-3-oxo-17α -pregn-4-ene-21-carboxylic acid γ-lactone acetate, which has the following structural formula:

Spironolactone is practically insoluble in water, soluble in alcohol, and freely soluble in benzene and in chloroform.
Inactive ingredients include calcium sulfate, corn starch, flavor, hydroxypropyl cellulose, hydroxypropyl methylcellulose, iron oxide, magnesium stearate, polyethylene glycol, povidone, and titanium dioxide.

CLINICAL PHARMACOLOGY

Aldactone (spironolactone) is a specific pharmacologic antagonist of aldosterone, acting primarily through competitive binding of receptors at the aldosterone-dependent sodium-potassium exchange site in the distal convoluted renal tubule. Aldactone causes increased amounts of sodium and water to be excreted, while potassium is retained. Aldactone acts both as a diuretic and as an antihypertensive drug by this mechanism. It may be given alone or with other diuretic agents which act more proximally in the renal tubule.
Increased levels of the mineralocorticoid, aldosterone, are present in primary and secondary hyperaldosteronism. Edematous states in which secondary aldosteronism is usually involved include congestive heart failure, hepatic cirrhosis, and the nephrotic syndrome. By competing with aldosterone for receptor sites, Aldactone provides effective therapy for the edema and ascites in those conditions. Aldactone counteracts secondary aldosteronism induced by the volume depletion and associated sodium loss caused by active diuretic therapy.
Aldactone is effective in lowering the systolic and diastolic blood pressure in patients with primary hyperaldosteronism. It is also effective in most cases of essential hypertension, despite the fact that aldosterone secretion may be within normal limits in benign essential hypertension.
Through its action in antagonizing the effect of aldosterone, Aldactone inhibits the exchange of sodium for potassium in the distal renal tubule and helps to prevent potassium loss.
Aldactone has not been demonstrated to elevate serum uric acid, to precipitate gout, or to alter carbohydrate metabolism.
In the human, the bioavailability of spironolactone from orally administered Aldactone 25-mg and 100-mg film-coated tablets, which contain microcrystalline spironolactone, has been evaluated in hypertensive subjects. Equivalent doses showed 35% and 20% higher bioavailability of spironolactone from the 25-mg and 100-mg film-coated tablets, respectively, compared to the 25-mg uncoated Aldactone tablets.
Spironolactone is rapidly and extensively metabolized. The primary metabolite is canrenone, which attains peak serum levels at two to four hours following single oral administration. In the dose range of 25 mg to 200 mg, an approximately linear relationship exists between a single dose of spironolactone and plasma levels of canrenone. Plasma concentrations of canrenone decline in two distinct phases, the first phase lasting from 3 to 12 hours, being more rapid than the second phase lasting from 12 to 96 hours. Canrenone clearance data, following multiple doses of spironolactone, indicate that accumulation of canrenone in the body with 100 mg once a day would be lower than with 25 mg four times a day. Both spironolactone and canrenone are more than 90% bound to plasma proteins. The metabolites of spironolactone are excreted primarily in urine, but also in bile.

INDICATIONS AND USAGE

Aldactone (spironolactone) is indicated in the management of:

Primary hyperaldosteronism for:
- Establishing the diagnosis of primary hyperaldosteronism by therapeutic trial.
- Short-term preoperative treatment of patients with primary hyperaldosteronism.
- Long-term maintenance therapy for patients with discrete aldosterone-producing adrenal adenomas who are judged to be poor operative risks or who decline surgery.
- Long-term maintenance therapy for patients with bilateral micro- or macronodular adrenal hyperplasia (idiopathic hyperaldosteronism).

Edematous conditions for patients with:
- **Congestive heart failure:** For the management of edema and sodium retention when the patient is only partially responsive to, or is intolerant of, other therapeutic measures. Aldactone is also indicated for patients with congestive heart failure taking digitalis when other therapies are considered inappropriate.
- **Cirrhosis of the liver accompanied by edema and/or ascites:** Aldosterone levels may be exceptionally high in this condition. Aldactone is indicated for maintenance therapy together with bed rest and the restriction of fluid and sodium.
- **The nephrotic syndrome:** For nephrotic patients when treatment of the underlying disease, restriction of fluid and sodium intake, and the use of other diuretics do not provide an adequate response.

Essential hypertension
Usually in combination with other drugs, Aldactone is indicated for patients who cannot be treated adequately with other agents or for whom other agents are considered inappropriate.

Hypokalemia
For the treatment of patients with hypokalemia when other measures are considered inappropriate or inadequate. Aldactone is also indicated for the prophylaxis of hypokalemia in patients taking digitalis when other measures are considered inadequate or inappropriate.

Usage in Pregnancy. The routine use of diuretics in an otherwise healthy woman is inappropriate and exposes mother and fetus to unnecessary hazard. Diuretics do not prevent development of toxemia of pregnancy, and there is no satisfactory evidence that they are useful in the treatment of developing toxemia.
Edema during pregnancy may arise from pathologic causes or from the physiologic and mechanical consequences of pregnancy.
Aldactone is indicated in pregnancy when edema is due to pathologic causes just as it is in the absence of pregnancy (however, see *Warnings* section). Dependent edema in pregnancy, resulting from restriction of venous return by the expanded uterus, is properly treated through elevation of the lower extremities and use of support hose; use of diuretics to lower intravascular volume in this case is unsupported and unnecessary. There is hypervolemia during normal pregnancy which is harmful to neither the fetus nor the mother (in the absence of cardiovascular disease), but which is associated with edema, including generalized edema, in the majority of pregnant women. If this edema produces discomfort, increased recumbency will often provide relief. In rare instances, this edema may cause extreme discomfort which is not relieved by rest. In these cases, a short course of diuretics may provide relief and may be appropriate.

CONTRAINDICATIONS

Aldactone is contraindicated for patients with anuria, acute renal insufficiency, significant impairment of renal function, or hyperkalemia.

WARNINGS

Potassium supplementation, either in the form of medication or as a diet rich in potassium, should not ordinarily be given in association with Aldactone therapy. Excessive potassium intake may cause hyperkalemia in patients receiving Aldactone (see *Precautions* section). Aldactone should not be administered concurrently with other potassium-sparing diuretics.
Spironolactone has been shown to be a tumorigen in chronic toxicity studies performed in rats, with its proliferative effects manifested on endocrine organs and the liver. In one study using 25, 75, and 250 times the usual daily human dose (2 mg/kg) there was a statistically significant dose-related increase in benign adenomas of the thyroid and testes. In female rats there was a statistically significant increase in malignant mammary tumors at the mid-dose only. In male rats there was a dose-related increase in proliferative changes in the liver. At the highest dosage level (500 mg/kg) the range of effects included hepatocytomegaly, hyperplastic nodules, and hepatocellular carcinoma; the last was not statistically significant at a value of $p = 0.05$. A dose-related (above 20 mg/kg/day) incidence of myelocytic leukemia was observed in rats fed daily doses of potassium canrenoate for a period of one year. In long-term (two-year) oral carcinogenicity studies of potassium canrenoate in the rat, myelocytic leukemia and hepatic, thyroid, testicular, and mammary tumors were observed. Potassium canrenoate did not produce a mutagenic effect in tests using bacteria or yeast. It did produce a positive mutagenic effect in several *in vitro* tests in mammalian cells following metabolism activation. In an *in vivo* mammalian system potassium canrenoate was not mutagenic. Canrenone and canrenoic acid are the major metabolites of potassium canrenoate. Spironolactone is also metabolized to canrenone. An increased incidence of leukemia was not observed in chronic rat toxicity studies conducted with spironolactone at doses up to 500 mg/kg/day.

PRECAUTIONS

General: Because of the diuretic action of Aldactone (spironolactone), patients should be carefully evaluated for possible disturbances of fluid and electrolyte balance. Hyperkalemia may occur in patients with impaired renal function or excessive potassium intake and can cause cardiac irregularities which may be fatal. Consequently, no potassium supplement should ordinarily be given with Aldactone. Hyperkalemia can be treated promptly by the rapid intravenous administration of glucose (20% to 50%) and regular insulin, using 0.25 to 0.5 units of insulin per gram of glucose. This is a temporary measure to be repeated as required. Aldactone should be discontinued and potassium intake (including dietary potassium) restricted.
Reversible hyperchloremic metabolic acidosis, usually in association with hyperkalemia, has been reported to occur in some patients with decompensated hepatic cirrhosis, even in the presence of normal renal function.
Hyponatremia, manifested by dryness of the mouth, thirst, lethargy, and drowsiness, and confirmed by a low serum sodium level, may be caused or aggravated, especially when Aldactone is administered in combination with other diuretics.
Gynecomastia may develop in association with the use of spironolactone, and physicians should be alert to its possible onset. The development of gynecomastia appears to be related to both dosage level and duration of therapy and is normally reversible when Aldactone is discontinued. In rare instances some breast enlargement may persist.
Aldactone therapy may cause a transient elevation of BUN, especially in patients with preexisting renal impairment. Aldactone may cause mild acidosis.
Drug interactions: When used in combination with other diuretics or antihypertensive agents Aldactone potentiates their effects. Therefore, the dosage of such drugs, particularly the ganglionic blocking agents, should be reduced by at least 50% when Aldactone is added to the regimen.
Spironolactone reduces the vascular responsiveness to norepinephrine. Therefore, caution should be exercised in the management of patients subjected to regional or general anesthesia while they are being treated with Aldactone.
Spironolactone has been shown to increase the half-life of digoxin. This may result in increased serum digoxin levels and subsequent digitalis toxicity. It may be necessary to reduce the maintenance and digitalization doses when spirono-

lactone is administered, and the patient should be carefully monitored to avoid over- or underdigitalization.

Drug/Laboratory test interactions: Several reports of possible interference with digoxin radioimmunoassays by spironolactone, or its metabolites, have appeared in the literature. Neither the extent nor the potential clinical significance of its interference (which may be assay-specific) has been fully established.

Usage in pregnancy: Spironolactone or its metabolites may cross the placental barrier. Therefore, the use of Aldactone in pregnant women requires that the anticipated benefit be weighed against possible hazard to the fetus.

Nursing mothers: Canrenone, a metabolite of spironolactone, appears in breast milk. If use of the drug is deemed essential, an alternative method of infant feeding should be instituted.

ADVERSE REACTIONS

Gynecomastia is observed not infrequently. A few cases of agranulocytosis have been reported in patients taking spironolactone. Other adverse reactions that have been reported in association with Aldactone are: gastrointestinal symptoms including cramping and diarrhea, drowsiness, lethargy, headache, maculopapular or erythematous cutaneous eruptions, urticaria, mental confusion, drug fever, ataxia, inability to achieve or maintain erection, irregular menses or amenorrhea, postmenopausal bleeding, hirsutism, and deepening of the voice. Carcinoma of the breast has been reported in patients taking spironolactone, but a cause and effect relationship has not been established.

Adverse reactions are usually reversible upon discontinuation of the drug.

DOSAGE AND ADMINISTRATION

Primary hyperaldosteronism. Aldactone may be employed as an initial diagnostic measure to provide presumptive evidence of primary hyperaldosteronism while patients are on normal diets.

Long test: Aldactone (spironolactone) is administered at a daily dosage of 400 mg for three to four weeks. Correction of hypokalemia and of hypertension provides presumptive evidence for the diagnosis of primary hyperaldosteronism.

Short test: Aldactone is administered at a daily dosage of 400 mg for four days. If serum potassium increases during Aldactone administration but drops when Aldactone is discontinued, a presumptive diagnosis of primary hyperaldosteronism should be considered.

After the diagnosis of hyperaldosteronism has been established by more definitive testing procedures, Aldactone may be administered in doses of 100 to 400 mg daily in preparation for surgery. For patients who are considered unsuitable for surgery, Aldactone may be employed for long-term maintenance therapy at the lowest effective dosage determined for the individual patient.

Edema in adults (*congestive heart failure, hepatic cirrhosis, or nephrotic syndrome*). An initial daily dosage of 100 mg of Aldactone administered in either single or divided doses is recommended, but may range from 25 to 200 mg daily. When given as the sole agent for diuresis, Aldactone should be continued for at least five days at the initial dosage level, after which it may be adjusted to the optimal therapeutic or maintenance level administered in either single or divided daily doses. If, after five days, an adequate diuretic response to Aldactone has not occurred, a second diuretic which acts more proximally in the renal tubule may be added to the regimen. Because of the additive effect of Aldactone when administered concurrently with such diuretics, an enhanced diuresis usually begins on the first day of combined treatment; combined therapy is indicated when more rapid diuresis is desired. The dosage of Aldactone should remain unchanged when other diuretic therapy is added.

Edema in children. The initial daily dosage should provide approximately 1.5 mg of Aldactone per pound of body weight (3.3 mg/kg) administered in either single or divided doses.

Essential hypertension. For adults, an initial daily dosage of 50 to 100 mg of Aldactone administered in either single or divided doses is recommended. Aldactone may also be given with diuretics which act more proximally in the renal tubule or with other antihypertensive agents. Treatment with Aldactone should be continued for at least two weeks, since the maximum response may not occur before this time. Subsequently, dosage should be adjusted according to the response of the patient.

Hypokalemia. Aldactone in a dosage ranging from 25 mg to 100 mg daily is useful in treating a diuretic-induced hypokalemia, when oral potassium supplements or other potassium-sparing regimens are considered inappropriate.

HOW SUPPLIED

Aldactone 25-mg tablets are round, light yellow, film coated, with SEARLE and 1001 debossed on one side and ALDACTONE and 25 on the other side; bottles of 100, 500, 1,000, and 2,500, and cartons of 100 unit-dose individually blister-sealed tablets.

Aldactone 50-mg tablets are oval, light orange, scored, film coated, with SEARLE and 1041 debossed on the scored side and ALDACTONE and 50 on the other side; bottles of 100 and cartons of 100 unit-dose individually blister-sealed tablets.

Aldactone 100-mg tablets are round, peach colored, scored, film coated, with SEARLE and 1031 debossed on the scored side and ALDACTONE and 100 on the other side; bottles of 100 and cartons of 100 unit-dose individually blister-sealed tablets.

Shown in Product Identification Section, page 429

AMINOPHYLLIN™ Tablets ℞

[*ă-mĭ-nŏph 'yl-lĭn*]
(aminophylline)

DESCRIPTION

Each tablet contains 100 mg or 200 mg of aminophylline USP calculated as the dihydrate, which is equivalent to 79 mg and 158 mg of anhydrous theophylline, respectively. Aminophylline USP (anhydrous) is a soluble complex containing approximately 85% anhydrous theophylline and 15% ethylenediamine. Aminophylline is white or slightly yellowish granules or powder, having a slight ammoniacal odor and a bitter taste.

Inactive ingredients of Aminophyllin 100-mg tablets include acacia, corn starch, magnesium stearate, potassium phosphate, sodium sulfate, and sodium sulfite. Inactive ingredients of Aminophyllin 200-mg tablets include corn starch, magnesium stearate, potassium phosphate, sodium sulfite, and talc.

ACTIONS

Aminophylline directly relaxes the smooth muscle of the bronchial airways and pulmonary blood vessels, thus acting mainly as a bronchodilator, pulmonary vasodilator, and smooth muscle relaxant. The drug also possesses other actions typical of the xanthine derivatives: coronary vasodilator, diuretic, cardiac stimulant, cerebral stimulant, and skeletal muscle stimulant.

INDICATIONS AND USAGE

Aminophyllin Tablets are indicated for the relief and/or prevention of symptoms from asthma and reversible bronchospasm associated with chronic bronchitis and emphysema.

CONTRAINDICATIONS

Aminophylline should not be administered to patients with active peptic ulcer disease, since it may increase the volume and acidity of gastric secretions.

Patients with a history of hypersensitivity to aminophylline or theophylline should not be treated with the drug.

Aminophylline should not be administered with other xanthine preparations.

WARNINGS

Excessive doses may be expected to be toxic. Some children may be unusually sensitive to aminophylline. Toxic synergism with ephedrine and other sympathomimetic bronchodilator drugs may occur. Halothane anesthesia in the presence of aminophylline may produce sinus tachycardia or ventricular arrhythmias.

Usage in Pregnancy. Safe use in pregnancy has not been established relative to possible adverse effects on fetal development. Therefore, aminophylline should not be used in pregnant women unless, in the judgment of the physician, the potential benefits outweigh the possible hazards.

PRECAUTIONS

Use with caution in patients with severe cardiac disease, hypertension, hyperthyroidism, acute myocardial injury, cor pulmonale, severe hypoxemia, hepatic impairment, or alcoholism, and in the elderly (especially males) and in neonates. Particular caution in dose administration must be exercised in patients with a history of peptic ulcer since the condition may be exacerbated. Chronic oral administration in high doses may be associated with gastrointestinal irritation.

Caution should be used in giving aminophylline to patients in congestive heart failure. Serum levels in such patients have persisted for long periods following discontinuation of the drug.

Theophylline half-life is shorter in smokers than nonsmokers; therefore, smokers may require larger or more frequent doses.

Aminophylline may lower the seizure threshold.

Elevated serum levels of theophylline may occur in patients treated concomitantly with aminophylline and cimetidine, troleandomycin, erythromycin, allopurinol, or oral contraceptive steroids. The addition of ephedrine or other sympathomimetic drugs to regimens of aminophylline increases the toxicity potential and may result in symptoms of overdosage, due to the additive pharmacological effects of these compounds. Co-medication with phenobarbital, phenytoin, or rifampin may increase theophylline clearance and an increase of the aminophylline dose may be required. The excretion of lithium carbonate is increased in patients receiving aminophylline. Aminophylline may antagonize the effects of propranolol.

Consumption of coffee, tea, cola beverages, chocolate, or acetaminophen contributes to falsely high serum theophylline levels when theophylline is measured spectrophotometrically without previous isolation by chromatography.

Mutagenesis: Theophylline has been shown to be mutagenic in *Escherichia coli* and other lower organisms (*Euglena gracilis* and *Ophiostoma multiannulatum*) and to produce chromosome breaks in cultured mouse cells and cultured human lymphocytes. The drug had no mutagenic activity *in vivo* in a dominant lethal test using mice.

Limited animal studies have shown teratogenic activity of theophylline in mice and rats.

Theophylline is excreted in breast milk and may cause adverse effects in the infant. Caution must be used when prescribing aminophylline to a nursing mother, taking into account the risk/benefit of this therapy.

Due to the marked variation in theophylline metabolism in infants under 6 months of age, aminophylline is not recommended for this age group.

ADVERSE REACTIONS

The most consistent adverse reactions observed with *therapeutic* amounts of aminophylline are:

1. Gastrointestinal: Nausea, vomiting, anorexia, bitter aftertaste, dyspepsia, heavy feeling in the stomach, and gastrointestinal distress.
2. Central nervous system: Dizziness, vertigo, lightheadedness, headache, nervousness, insomnia, and agitation.
3. Cardiovascular: Palpitation, tachycardia, flushing, and extrasystoles.
4. Respiratory: Increase in respiratory rate.
5. Dermatologic: Urticaria.

OVERDOSAGE

The most consistent reactions observed with *toxic* overdoses of aminophylline are:

1. Gastrointestinal: Nausea, vomiting, epigastric pain, hematemesis, and diarrhea.
2. Central nervous system: In addition to those cited above, the patient may exhibit hyperreflexia, fasciculations, and clonic and tonic convulsions. These are especially prone to occur in cases of overdosage in infants and small children.
3. Cardiovascular: In addition to those outlined above, marked hypotension and circulatory failure may be manifest.
4. Respiratory: Tachypnea and respiratory arrest may occur.
5. Renal: Albuminuria and microhematuria may occur. Increased excretion of renal tubular cells has been observed.
6. General systemic effects: Syncope, collapse, fever, and dehydration.

Management of Toxic Symptoms:

1. Discontinue drug immediately.
2. There is no known specific antidote.
3. Gastric lavage.
4. Emetic medication may be of value.
5. Avoid administration of sympathomimetic drugs.
6. Intravenous fluids, oxygen, and other supportive measures to prevent hypotension and overcome dehydration.
7. Central nervous system stimulation and seizures may respond to short-acting barbiturates.
8. Monitor serum levels until below 20 mcg/ml.

DOSAGE AND ADMINISTRATION

The oral dose for adults should be adjusted according to the need and response of the patient. Usually a daily dose in the range of 600 to 1600 mg, administered in 3 or 4 divided doses, will provide the desired therapeutic effect. Similarly, the dose for children should be adjusted according to the response. An oral dose of 12 mg/kg/24 hours, administered in four divided doses, will usually provide the desired therapeutic effect in children.

Therapeutic serum levels are considered to be between 10 mcg/ml and 20 mcg/ml. Levels above 20 mcg/ml may produce toxic effects. There is great variation from patient to patient in dosage needed to achieve a therapeutic serum level and in the duration of action of oral aminophylline. Because of these wide variations and the relatively narrow therapeutic serum-level range, dosage must be individualized with monitoring of theophylline serum levels, particularly when prolonged use is planned.

HOW SUPPLIED

Aminophyllin Tablets are supplied as:

Round, white, scored tablets with 1231 debossed on the scored side and SEARLE on the other side, each tablet containing 100 mg of aminophylline; bottles of 100 and 1,000, and cartons of 100 unit-dose individually blister-sealed tablets.

Continued on next page

Searle & Co.—Cont.

Oval, white, scored tablets with 1251 debossed on the scored side and SEARLE on the other side, each tablet containing 200 mg of aminophylline; bottles of 100 and 1,000, and cartons of 100 unit-dose individually blister-sealed tablets.

Shown in Product Identification Section, page 429

ANAVAR® ℞
[an 'uh-var]
(oxandrolone)

DESCRIPTION

Anavar oral tablets contain 2.5 mg of the anabolic steroid oxandrolone, a synthetic derivative of testosterone. Oxandrolone is 17β-hydroxy-17α -methyl -2- oxa-5α -androstan - 3- one with the following structural formula:

Inactive ingredients include corn starch, lactose, magnesium stearate, and methylcellulose.

CLINICAL PHARMACOLOGY

Anavar is used primarily for its protein anabolic effect and its catabolism-inhibiting effect on tissue. Nitrogen balance is improved by anabolic agents, but only when the intake of calories and protein is sufficient. It has not been established whether this positive nitrogen balance indicates a primary benefit in the utilization of protein-building dietary substances. Some clinical effects and adverse reactions reported demonstrate the androgenic properties of drugs of this class. Complete dissociation of anabolic from androgenic effects has not been achieved. The actions of anabolic steroids are therefore similar to those of male sex hormones with the possibility that serious disturbances of growth and sexual development may be caused if given to young children.

Use of androgens in children over long periods of time may result in fusion of the epiphyseal growth centers.

Anabolic steroids have been reported to increase low-density lipoproteins and decrease high-density lipoproteins. Serum lipid determination should be done periodically.

During exogenous administration of anabolic androgens, endogenous testosterone release is inhibited through inhibition of pituitary luteinizing hormone (LH). At large doses spermatogenesis may be suppressed through feedback inhibition of pituitary follicle-stimulating hormone (FSH).

INDICATIONS AND USAGE

Anavar is indicated as adjunctive therapy to promote weight gain after weight loss following extensive surgery, chronic infections, or severe trauma, and in some patients who without definite pathophysiologic reasons fail to gain or to maintain normal weight, to offset the protein catabolism associated with prolonged administration of corticosteroids, and for the relief of the bone pain frequently accompanying osteoporosis. (See *Dosage and Administration.*)

CONTRAINDICATIONS

1. Carcinoma of the prostate or male breast.
2. Carcinoma of the breast in some women.
3. Nephrosis or the nephrotic phase of nephritis.
4. Pregnancy, because of possible masculinization of the fetus. Anavar has been shown to cause embryotoxicity, fetotoxicity, infertility, and masculinization of female animal offspring when given in doses 9 times the human dose. No *in vitro* mutagenicity tests have been conducted.
5. Hypercalcemia.

WARNINGS

ANABOLIC STEROIDS DO NOT ENHANCE ATHLETIC ABILITY.

Geriatric patients treated with anabolic/androgenic steroids may be at an increased risk for the development of prostatic hypertrophy and prostatic carcinoma.

There have been rare reports of hepatocellular neoplasms, including carcinoma, and peliosis hepatis in association with anabolic/androgenic steroid therapy.

Cholestatic hepatitis and jaundice may occur with 17-alpha-alkylated androgens at a relatively low dose. If cholestatic hepatitis with jaundice appears or if liver function tests become abnormal, Anavar should be discontinued and the etiology should be determined. Drug-induced jaundice is reversible when the medication is discontinued.

Hypercalcemia may develop both spontaneously and as a result of hormonal therapy in women with disseminated breast carcinoma. Anavar therapy should be discontinued if hypercalcemia occurs.

Edema with or without congestive heart failure may be a serious complication in patients with preexisting cardiac, renal, or hepatic disease. Therapy with Anavar may increase the edema.

In children, androgen therapy may accelerate bone maturation without producing compensatory gain in linear growth. The effect on bone maturation should be monitored. (See *Precautions/Laboratory tests.*)

PRECAUTIONS

General: Women should be observed for signs of virilization (deepening of the voice, hirsutism, acne, clitoromegaly, and menstrual irregularities). Discontinuation of drug therapy at the time of evidence of mild virilism is necessary to prevent irreversible virilization.

Suppression of clotting factors II, V, VII, and X has been observed.

Information for patients: The physician should instruct patients to report any of the following side effects of androgens:

Prepubertal males: Too frequent or persistent erections of the penis.

Females: Hoarseness, acne, changes in menstrual periods, or more facial hair.

All patients: Nausea, vomiting, changes in skin color, or ankle swelling.

Laboratory tests:

1. Women with disseminated breast carcinoma should have frequent determination of urine and serum calcium levels during the course of therapy (see *Warnings*).
2. Because of the hepatotoxicity associated with the use of 17-alpha-alkylated androgens, liver function tests should be obtained periodically.
3. Periodic (every 6 months) x-ray examinations of bone age should be made during treatment of prepubertal males to determine the rate of bone maturation and the effects of androgen therapy on the epiphyseal centers.
4. Serum lipid determinations should be done periodically as anabolic/androgenic steroids have been reported to increase low-density lipoproteins and decrease high-density lipoproteins.
5. Serum cholesterol levels may increase during therapy. Therefore, caution is required when administering these agents to patients with a history of myocardial infarction or coronary artery disease. Serial determinations of serum cholesterol should be made and therapy adjusted accordingly.

Drug interactions

Anticoagulants: C-17 substituted derivatives of testosterone have been reported to decrease the anticoagulant requirements of patients receiving oral anticoagulants. Patients receiving oral anticoagulant therapy require close monitoring, especially when androgens are started or stopped.

Insulin: In diabetic patients the metabolic effects of androgens may decrease blood glucose and insulin requirements.

Oral hypoglycemic agents: Anavar may inhibit the metabolism of oral hypoglycemic agents.

Adrenal steroids or ACTH: In patients with edema, concomitant administration with adrenal steroids or ACTH may increase the edema.

Drug/Laboratory test interactions: If thyroid function tests are performed, the physician should be aware that androgens may decrease levels of thyroxine-binding globulin, resulting in decreased total T_4 serum levels and increased resin uptake of T_3 and T_4. In addition, a decrease in PBI and radioactive iodine uptake may occur.

Alterations in the metyrapone test have occurred.

Carcinogenesis, mutagenesis, impairment of fertility

Animal data: In two-year chronic oral rat studies, a dose-related reduction of spermatogenesis and decreased organ weights (testes, prostate, seminal vesicles, ovaries, uterus, adrenals, and pituitary) were shown. Anavar has not been tested in laboratory animals for carcinogenic or mutagenic effects.

Human data: There are rare reports of hepatocellular carcinoma in patients receiving long-term therapy with anabolic/androgenic steroids in high doses. Withdrawal of the drugs did not lead to regression of the tumors in all cases. Geriatric patients treated with androgens may be at an increased risk for the development of prostatic hypertrophy and prostatic carcinoma.

Pregnancy: Teratogenic effects; Pregnancy Category X. See *Contraindications.*

Nursing mothers: It is not known whether anabolic steroids are excreted in human milk. Because of the potential for serious adverse reactions in nursing infants from Anavar, a decision should be made whether to discontinue nursing or to discontinue the drug, taking into account the importance of the drug to the mother.

Pediatric use: Anabolic/androgenic steroid therapy should be used very cautiously in children and only by specialists who are aware of the effects on bone maturation. Skeletal maturation should be monitored every six months by an x-ray of hand and wrist. (See *Warnings.*)

ADVERSE REACTIONS

The following adverse reactions have been associated with use of anabolic steroids:

Endocrine: Masculinization of the fetus, increased or decreased libido, inhibition of gonadotropin secretion, and premature closure of epiphyses in children.

In *males:*

Prepubertal

Phallic enlargement

Increased frequency or persistence of erections

Postpubertal

Inhibition of testicular function and oligospermia

Gynecomastia

In *females:*

Hirsutism, male-pattern baldness, deepening of the voice, and clitoral enlargement. (These changes are usually irreversible even after prompt discontinuance of therapy and are not prevented by concomitant use of estrogens.)

Menstrual irregularities

When administered to a pregnant woman, anabolic/androgenic steroids cause virilization of external genitalia of the female fetus.

Gastrointestinal: Nausea, abdominal fullness, loss of appetite, vomiting, and burning of the tongue.

Dermatologic: Acne (especially in females and prepubertal males).

Hepatic: Cholestatic jaundice, alterations in liver function tests and, rarely, hepatocellular neoplasms and peliosis hepatis (see *Warnings*).

General: Bleeding in patients on concomitant anticoagulant therapy.

Fluid and electrolyte disturbances: Retention of sodium, chloride, water, potassium, calcium, and inorganic phosphate.

Metabolism: Increased serum cholesterol.

OVERDOSAGE

No symptoms or signs associated with overdosage have been reported. It is possible that sodium and water retention may occur.

The oral LD_{50} of oxandrolone in mice and dogs is greater than 5,000 mg/kg. No specific antidote is known, but gastric lavage may be used.

DOSAGE AND ADMINISTRATION

Therapy with anabolic steroids is adjunctive to and not a replacement for conventional therapy. The duration of therapy with Anavar (oxandrolone) will depend on the response of the patient and the possible appearance of adverse reactions. Therapy should be intermittent.

Adults. The *usual adult dosage* of Anavar is one 2.5-mg tablet two to four times daily. However, the response of individuals to anabolic steroids varies, and a daily dosage of as little as 2.5 mg or as much as 20 mg may be required to achieve the desired response. A course of therapy of two to four weeks is usually adequate. This may be repeated intermittently as indicated.

Children. For children the *total daily dosage* of Anavar is 0.25 mg per kilogram or 0.12 mg per pound of body weight. This may be repeated intermittently as indicated.

HOW SUPPLIED

Anavar 2.5-mg tablets are oval, white, and scored, with 1401 debossed on the scored side and SEARLE on the other side; bottles of 100.

Federal law prohibits dispensing without prescription.

Shown in Product Identification Section, page 429

CALAN® Tablets ℞
[cal 'an]
(verapamil hydrochloride)

DESCRIPTION

Calan (verapamil HCl) is a calcium ion influx inhibitor (slow-channel blocker or calcium ion antagonist) available for oral administration in film-coated tablets containing 80 mg or 120 mg of verapamil hydrochloride.

The structural formula of verapamil HCl is

$C_{27}H_{38}N_2O_4 \cdot HCl$ M.W. = 491.08

Benzeneacetonitrile, α-[3-[[2-(3, 4-dimethoxyphenyl) ethyl] methylamino]propyl]-3,4-dimethoxy-α-(1-methylethyl) hydrochloride.

Verapamil HCl is an almost white, crystalline powder, practically free of odor, with a bitter taste. It is soluble in water, chloroform, and methanol. Verapamil HCl is not chemically related to other cardioactive drugs.

Inactive ingredients include cellulose, corn starch, gelatin, hydroxypropyl cellulose, hydroxypropyl methylcellulose, iron oxide, lactose, magnesium stearate, polyethylene glycol, talc, and titanium dioxide.

CLINICAL PHARMACOLOGY

Calan is a calcium ion influx inhibitor (slow-channel blocker or calcium ion antagonist) that exerts its pharmacologic effects by modulating the influx of ionic calcium across the cell membrane of the arterial smooth muscle as well as in conductile and contractile myocardial cells.

Mechanism of action: The precise mechanism of action of Calan as an antianginal agent remains to be fully determined, but includes the following two mechanisms:

1. *Relaxation and prevention of coronary artery spasm:* Calan dilates the main coronary arteries and coronary arterioles, both in normal and ischemic regions, and is a potent inhibitor of coronary artery spasm, whether spontaneous or ergonovine-induced. This property increases myocardial oxygen delivery in patients with coronary artery spasm and is responsible for the effectiveness of Calan in vasospastic (Prinzmetal's or variant) as well as unstable angina at rest. Whether this effect plays any role in classical effort angina is not clear, but studies of exercise tolerance have not shown an increase in the maximum exercise rate–pressure product, a widely accepted measure of oxygen utilization. This suggests that, in general, relief of spasm or dilation of coronary arteries is not an important factor in classical angina.
2. *Reduction of oxygen utilization:* Calan regularly reduces arterial pressure at rest and at a given level of exercise by dilating peripheral arterioles and reducing the total peripheral resistance (afterload) against which the heart works. This unloading of the heart reduces myocardial energy consumption and oxygen requirements and probably accounts for the effectiveness of Calan in chronic stable effort angina.

Electrical activity through the SA and AV nodes depends, to a significant degree, on calcium influx through the slow channel. By inhibiting this influx, Calan slows AV conduction and prolongs the effective refractory period within the AV node in a rate-related manner. It can interfere with sinus node impulse generation and induce sinus arrest in patients with sick sinus syndrome; it also can induce atrioventricular block, although this has been seen rarely in clinical use. Calan may shorten the antegrade effective refractory period of the accessory bypass tracts. Calan does not alter the normal atrial action potential or intraventricular conduction time, but depresses amplitude, velocity of depolarization, and conduction in depressed atrial fibers.

Calan (verapamil HCl) has a local anesthetic action that is 1.6 times that of procaine on an equimolar basis. It is not known whether this action is important at the doses used in man.

Calan does not alter total serum calcium levels.

Pharmacokinetics and metabolism: More than 90% of the orally administered dose of Calan is absorbed. Because of rapid biotransformation of verapamil during its first pass through the portal circulation, absolute bioavailability ranges from 20% to 35%. Peak plasma concentrations are reached between 1 and 2 hours after oral administration. Chronic oral administration of 120 mg of verapamil every 6 hours resulted in plasma levels of verapamil ranging from 125 to 400 ng/ml, with higher values reported occasionally. A close relationship exists between verapamil plasma concentration and prolongation of the PR interval. The mean elimination half-life in single-dose studies ranged from 2.8 to 7.4 hours. In these same studies, after repetitive dosing, the half-life increased to a range from 4.5 to 12.0 hours (after less than 10 consecutive doses given 6 hours apart). Half-life may increase during titration due to saturation of hepatic enzyme systems as plasma verapamil levels rise.

Verapamil is highly bound to plasma proteins. In healthy men, orally administered Calan undergoes extensive metabolism in the liver. Twelve metabolites have been identified in plasma; all except norverapamil are present in trace amounts only. Norverapamil can reach steady-state plasma concentrations approximately equal to those of verapamil itself. The major metabolites of verapamil have been identified as various N- and O-dealkylated products of verapamil. Approximately 70% of an administered dose is excreted as metabolites in the urine and 16% or more in the feces within 5 days. About 3% to 4% is excreted in the urine as unchanged drug. Approximately 90% is bound to plasma proteins. In patients with hepatic insufficiency, metabolism is delayed and elimination half-life prolonged up to 14 to 16 hours (see *Precautions*); the volume of distribution is increased and plasma clearance reduced to about 30% of normal. Verapamil clearance values suggest that patients with liver dysfunction may attain therapeutic verapamil plasma concentrations with one third of the oral daily dose required for patients with normal liver function.

Hemodynamics and myocardial metabolism: In animals and man, Calan (verapamil HCl) reduces afterload and myocardial contractility. In most patients, including those with organic cardiac disease, the negative inotropic action of Calan is countered by reduction of afterload, and cardiac index is usually not reduced. However, in patients with severe left ventricular dysfunction (eg, pulmonary wedge pressure above 20 mm Hg or ejection fraction less than 30%), or in patients taking beta-adrenergic blocking agents or other cardiodepressant drugs, deterioration of ventricular function may occur (see *Drug interactions*).

Pulmonary function: Calan does not induce bronchoconstriction and, hence, does not impair ventilatory function.

INDICATIONS AND USAGE

Calan tablets are indicated for the treatment of angina pectoris, including:

1. Angina at rest, including:
   - Vasospastic (Prinzmetal's variant) angina
   - Unstable (crescendo, preinfarction) angina
2. Chronic stable angina (classic effort-associated angina)

CONTRAINDICATIONS

Verapamil HCl tablets are contraindicated in:

1. Severe left ventricular dysfunction (see *Warnings*)
2. Hypotension (systolic pressure less than 90 mm Hg) or cardiogenic shock
3. Sick sinus syndrome (except in patients with a functioning artificial ventricular pacemaker)
4. Second- or third-degree AV block
5. Patients with atrial flutter or atrial fibrillation and an accessory bypass tract (eg, Wolff-Parkinson-White, Lown-Ganong-Levine syndromes). (See *Warnings*.)

WARNINGS

Heart failure: Verapamil has a negative inotropic effect, which in most patients is compensated by its afterload reduction (decreased peripheral vascular resistance) properties without a net impairment of ventricular performance. In clinical studies involving 1,166 patients, 11 (0.9%) developed congestive heart failure or pulmonary edema. Congestive heart failure/pulmonary edema led to discontinuation or reduction of dosage of verapamil in 6 patients (0.5%). Verapamil should be avoided in patients with severe left ventricular dysfunction (eg, ejection fraction less than 30%) or moderate to severe symptoms of cardiac failure and in patients with any degree of ventricular dysfunction if they are receiving a beta-blocker (see *Drug interactions*). Patients with milder ventricular dysfunction should, if possible, be controlled with optimum doses of digitalis and/or diuretics before verapamil treatment. **(Note interactions with digoxin under *Precautions*.)**

Hypotension: Occasionally, the pharmacologic action of verapamil may produce a decrease in blood pressure below normal levels, which may result in dizziness or symptomatic hypotension. Hypotension is usually asymptomatic, orthostatic, mild, and can be controlled by a decrease in the Calan (verapamil HCl) dose. The incidence of hypotension observed in 1,166 patients enrolled in clinical trials was 2.9%.

Elevated liver enzymes: Elevations of transaminases with and without concomitant elevations in alkaline phosphatase and bilirubin have been reported. Such elevations have sometimes been transient and may disappear even in the face of continued verapamil treatment. However, four cases of hepatocellular injury produced by verapamil have been proven by rechallenge; two of these four cases had clinical symptoms of malaise, fever, and/or right upper quadrant pain, in addition to elevation of SGOT, SGPT, and alkaline phosphatase. Periodic monitoring of liver function in patients receiving verapamil is therefore prudent.

Accessory bypass tract (Wolff-Parkinson-White or Lown-Ganong-Levine): Some patients with paroxysmal and/or chronic atrial fibrillation or atrial flutter and a coexisting accessory AV pathway have been shown to develop increased antegrade conduction across the accessory pathway bypassing the AV node, producing a very rapid ventricular response or ventricular fibrillation after receiving intravenous verapamil (or digitalis). Although a risk of this occurring with oral verapamil has not been established, such patients receiving oral verapamil may be at risk and its use in these patients is contraindicated (see *Contraindications*).

Atrioventricular block: The effect of verapamil on AV conduction and the SA node leads to first-degree AV block and transient bradycardia, sometimes accompanied by nodal escape rhythms, fairly commonly during the peaks of serum concentration. Higher degrees of AV block, however, were infrequently observed (0.8%). Marked first-degree block or progressive development to second- or third-degree AV block requires a reduction in dosage or, in rare instances, discontinuation of verapamil HCl and institution of appropriate therapy, depending on the clinical situation.

Patients with hypertrophic cardiomyopathy (IHSS): In 120 patients with hypertrophic cardiomyopathy (most of them refractory or intolerant to propranolol) who received therapy with verapamil at doses up to 720 mg/day, a variety of serious adverse effects was seen. Three patients died in pulmonary edema; all had a past history of severe left ventricular outflow obstruction and left ventricular dysfunction. Eight other patients had pulmonary edema and/or severe hypotension; abnormally high (greater than 20 mm Hg) pulmonary wedge pressure and a marked left ventricular outflow obstruction were present in most of these patients. Concomitant administration of quinidine preceded the severe hypotension in 3 of the 8 patients (2 of whom developed pulmonary edema). Sinus bradycardia occurred in 11% of the patients, second-degree AV block in 4%, and sinus arrest in 2%. It must be appreciated that this group of patients had a serious disease with a high mortality rate. Most adverse effects responded well to dose reduction, and only rarely did verapamil use have to be discontinued.

PRECAUTIONS

General

Use in patients with impaired hepatic function: Since verapamil is highly metabolized by the liver, it should be administered cautiously to patients with impaired hepatic function. Severe liver dysfunction prolongs the elimination half-life of verapamil to about 14 to 16 hours; hence, approximately 30% of the dose given to patients with normal liver function should be administered to these patients. Careful monitoring for abnormal prolongation of the PR interval or other signs of excessive pharmacologic effects (see *Overdosage*) should be carried out.

Use in patients with attenuated (decreased) neuromuscular transmission: It has been reported that verapamil decreases neuromuscular transmission in patients with Duchenne's muscular dystrophy, and that verapamil prolongs recovery from the neuromuscular blocking agent vecuronium. It may be necessary to decrease the dosage of verapamil when it is administered to patients with attenuated neuromuscular transmission.

Use in patients with impaired renal function: About 70% of an administered dose of verapamil is excreted as metabolites in the urine. Until further data are available, verapamil should be administered cautiously to patients with impaired renal function. These patients should be carefully monitored for abnormal prolongation of the PR interval or other signs of overdosage (see *Overdosage*).

Drug interactions

Beta-blockers: Controlled studies in small numbers of patients suggest that the concomitant use of Calan (verapamil HCl) and beta-blocking agents may be beneficial in patients with chronic stable angina, but available information is not sufficient to predict with confidence the effects of concurrent treatment, especially in patients with left ventricular dysfunction or cardiac conduction abnormalities.

The combination can have adverse effects on cardiac function. In one study involving 15 patients treated with high doses of propranolol (median dose, 480 mg/day; range, 160 to 1,280 mg/day) for severe angina, with preserved left ventricular function (ejection fraction greater than 35%), the hemodynamic effects of additional therapy with verapamil HCl were assessed using invasive methods. The addition of verapamil to high-dose beta-blockers induced modest negative inotropic and chronotropic effects that were not severe enough to limit short-term (48 hours) combination therapy in this study. These modest cardiodepressant effects persisted for greater than 6 but less than 30 hours after abrupt withdrawal of beta-blockers and were closely related to plasma levels of propranolol. The primary verapamil/beta-blocker interaction in this study appeared to be hemodynamic rather than electrophysiologic.

In 3 other studies involving 51 patients, verapamil did not induce negative inotropic or chronotropic effects in patients with preserved left ventricular function receiving low or moderate doses of propranolol (less than or equal to 320 mg/day). Because of the still limited experience with combination therapy, verapamil should be used alone, if possible. If combined therapy is used, close surveillance of vital signs and clinical status should be carried out and the need for concomitant treatment with propranolol reassessed periodically. Combined therapy should usually be avoided in patients with atrioventricular conduction abnormalities and those with depressed left ventricular function.

Digitalis: Chronic verapamil treatment increases serum digoxin levels by 50% to 70% during the first week of therapy, and this can result in digitalis toxicity. Maintenance and digitalization doses should be reduced when verapamil is administered, and the patient should be carefully monitored to avoid over- or underdigitalization. Whenever overdigitalization is suspected, the daily dose of digoxin should be reduced or temporarily discontinued. On discontinuation of Calan (verapamil HCl) use, the patient should be monitored to avoid underdigitalization.

Antihypertensive agents: Verapamil administered concomitantly with oral antihypertensive agents (eg, vasodilators, diuretics) may have an additive effect on lowering blood pressure. Patients receiving these combinations should be appropriately monitored. In patients who have recently received drugs such as methyldopa, which attenuate alpha-adrenergic response, combined therapy of verapamil and propranolol should probably be avoided (severe hypotension may occur).

Disopyramide: Until data on possible interactions between verapamil and disopyramide are obtained, disopyramide should not be administered within 48 hours before or 24 hours after verapamil administration.

Continued on next page

Searle & Co.—Cont.

Quinidine: In a small number of patients with hypertrophic cardiomyopathy (IHSS), concomitant use of verapamil and quinidine resulted in significant hypotension. Until further data are obtained, combined therapy of verapamil and quinidine in patients with hypertrophic cardiomyopathy should probably be avoided.

Nitrates: Verapamil has been given concomitantly with short- and long-acting nitrates without any undesirable drug interactions. The pharmacologic profile of both drugs and the clinical experience suggest beneficial interactions.

Inhalation anesthetics: Animal experiments have shown that inhalation anesthetics depress cardiovascular activity by decreasing the inward movement of calcium ions. When used concomitantly, inhalation anesthetics and calcium antagonists, such as verapamil, should each be titrated carefully to avoid excessive cardiovascular depression.

Neuromuscular blocking agents: Clinical data and animal studies suggest that verapamil may potentiate the activity of neuromuscular blocking agents (curare-like and depolarizing). It may be necessary to decrease the dose of verapamil and/or the dose of the neuromuscular blocking agent when the drugs are used concomitantly.

Carbamazepine: The concomitant oral administration of verapamil and carbamazepine may produce increased plasma concentrations of free carbamazepine due to a decreased rate of carbamazepine metabolism. This may produce carbamazepine side effects such as diplopia, headache, ataxia, or dizziness.

Carcinogenesis, mutagenesis, impairment of fertility: Adequate animal carcinogenicity studies have not been performed with verapamil. An 18-month toxicity study in rats, at a low multiple (6-fold) of the maximum recommended human dose, and not the maximum tolerated dose, did not suggest a tumorigenic potential. A 2-year carcinogenicity study will be carried out in rats.

Verapamil was not mutagenic in the Ames test in 5 test strains at 3 mg per plate with or without metabolic activation.

Studies in female rats at daily dietary doses up to 5.5 times (55 mg/kg/day) the maximum recommended human dose did not show impaired fertility. Effects on male fertility have not been determined.

Pregnancy: Pregnancy Category C. Reproduction studies have been performed in rabbits and rats at oral doses up to 1.5 (15 mg/kg/day) and 6 (60 mg/kg/day) times the human oral daily dose, respectively, and have revealed no evidence of teratogenicity. In the rat, however, this multiple of the human dose was embryocidal and retarded fetal growth and development, probably because of adverse maternal effects reflected in reduced weight gains of the dams. This oral dose has also been shown to cause hypotension in rats. There are no adequate and well-controlled studies in pregnant women. Because animal reproduction studies are not always predictive of human response, this drug should be used during pregnancy only if clearly needed.

Labor and delivery: It is not known whether the use of verapamil during labor or delivery has immediate or delayed adverse effects on the fetus, or whether it prolongs the duration of labor or increases the need for forceps delivery or other obstetric intervention. Such adverse experiences have not been reported in the literature, despite a long history of use of verapamil in Europe in the treatment of cardiac side effects of beta-adrenergic agonist agents used to treat premature labor.

Nursing mothers: Verapamil is excreted in human milk. Because of the potential for adverse reactions in nursing infants from verapamil, nursing should be discontinued while verapamil is administered.

Animal pharmacology and/or animal toxicology: Chronic animal toxicology studies indicate that verapamil causes lenticular and/or suture line changes at 30 mg/kg/day or greater, and frank cataracts at 62.5 mg/kg/day or greater in the beagle dog but not in the rat. These effects are thought to be species specific. Development of cataracts due to verapamil has not been reported in man.

ADVERSE REACTIONS

Serious adverse reactions are rare when Calan (verapamil HCl) therapy is initiated with upward dose titration within the recommended single and total daily dose. The following reactions to orally administered verapamil were reported from clinical studies involving 1,166 patients with angina or arrhythmia.

Adverse reactions occurred at a similar rate in controlled clinical trials and uncontrolled clinical experience.

Cardiovascular: Hypotension (2.9%), peripheral edema (1.7%), AV block: third-degree (0.8%), bradycardia: HR <50/min (1.1%), CHF or pulmonary edema (0.9%).

Central nervous system: Dizziness (3.6%), headache (1.8%), fatigue (1.1%).

Gastrointestinal: Constipation (6.3%), nausea (1.6%); elevations of liver enzymes have been reported (see *Warnings*).

The following reactions, reported in less than 0.5% of patients, occurred under circumstances where a causal relationship is not certain, and are therefore mentioned to alert the physician to a possible relationship: confusion, paresthesia, insomnia, somnolence, equilibrium disorders, blurred vision, syncope, muscle cramps, shakiness, claudication, hair loss, macular eruptions, spotty menstruation, ecchymosis, bruising, impotence, gynecomastia, and psychotic symptoms. In addition, more serious adverse events were observed, not readily distinguishable from the natural history of the disease in these patients. Of the 1,166 patients evaluated, 16 (1.4%) had myocardial infarctions. Nine of these 16 patients had myocardial infarctions while being treated for unstable angina, 4 of these were receiving placebo, the remaining 5 received verapamil.

The daily dose of verapamil was reduced in 6.3% and discontinued in 5.5% of the 1,166 patients. In general, the highest incidence of adverse reactions was seen in the dose-titration periods in all the studies.

Treatment of acute cardiovascular adverse reactions: The frequency of cardiovascular adverse reactions that require therapy is rare; hence, experience with their treatment is limited. Whenever severe hypotension or complete AV block occur following oral administration of verapamil, the appropriate emergency measures should be applied immediately; eg, intravenously administered isoproterenol HCl, norepinephrine bitartrate, atropine sulfate (all in the usual doses), or calcium gluconate (10% solution). In patients with hypertrophic cardiomyopathy (IHSS), alpha-adrenergic agents (phenylephrine HCl, metaraminol bitartrate, or methoxamine HCl) should be used to maintain blood pressure, and isoproterenol and norepinephrine should be avoided. If further support is necessary, dopamine HCl or dobutamine HCl may be administered. Actual treatment and dosage should depend on the severity of the clinical situation and the judgment and experience of the treating physician.

OVERDOSAGE

Treatment of overdosage should be supportive. Beta-adrenergic stimulation or parenteral administration of calcium solutions may increase calcium ion flux across the slow channel, and have been used effectively in treatment of deliberate overdosage with verapamil. Clinically significant hypotensive reactions or fixed high-degree AV block should be treated with vasopressor agents or cardiac pacing, respectively. Asystole should be handled by the usual measures, including cardiopulmonary resuscitation.

DOSAGE AND ADMINISTRATION

The dose of verapamil must be individualized by titration. Calan (verapamil HCl) is available in 80-mg and 120-mg tablets. The usual initial dose is 80 mg every 6 to 8 hours. Dosage may be increased at daily (eg, patients with unstable angina) or weekly intervals until optimum clinical response is obtained. In general, maximum effects of any given dosage would be apparent during the first 24 to 48 hours of therapy, but note that between 24 and 48 hours, the half-life of verapamil increases; therefore, the maximum response may be delayed. The total daily dose ranges from 240 to 480 mg. The optimum daily dose for most patients ranges from 320 to 480 mg. The usefulness and safety of dosages exceeding 480 mg/day in angina pectoris have not been established.

HOW SUPPLIED

Calan 80-mg tablets are oval, peach colored, scored, film coated, with CALAN debossed on one side and 80 on the other, supplied as:

NDC Number	Size
0014-1851-31	bottle of 100
0014-1851-51	bottle of 500
0014-1851-52	bottle of 1,000
0014-1851-34	carton of 100 unit dose

Calan 120-mg tablets are oval, brown, scored, film coated, with CALAN 120 debossed on one side, supplied as:

NDC Number	Size
0014-1861-31	bottle of 100
0014-1861-51	bottle of 500
0014-1861-52	bottle of 1,000
0014-1861-34	carton of 100 unit dose

Store at 59° to 86°F (15° to 30°C).

Shown in Product Identification Section, page 429

SEARLE ORAL CONTRACEPTIVES

DEMULEN 1/35™–21 ℞
DEMULEN 1/35™–28 ℞
DEMULEN 1/50™–21 ℞
DEMULEN 1/50™–28 ℞
[dem 'ū-len]
(ethynodiol diacetate with ethinyl estradiol)

OVULEN-21® ℞
OVULEN-28® ℞
[ov 'ū-len]
(ethynodiol diacetate with mestranol)

ENOVID-E® 21 ℞
ENOVID® 5 mg ℞
ENOVID® 10 mg ℞
[ē-nov 'id]
(norethynodrel with mestranol)

DESCRIPTION

Demulen 1/35™-21 and Demulen 1/35™-28. Each white tablet contains 1 mg of ethynodiol diacetate and 35 mcg of ethinyl estradiol, and the inactive ingredients include calcium acetate, calcium phosphate, corn starch, hydrogenated castor oil, and povidone. Each blue tablet in the Demulen 1/35™-28 package is a placebo containing no active ingredients, and the inactive ingredients include calcium sulfate, corn starch, FD&C Blue No. 1 Lake, magnesium stearate, and sucrose.

Demulen 1/50™-21 and Demulen 1/50™-28. Each white tablet contains 1 mg of ethynodiol diacetate and 50 mcg of ethinyl estradiol, and the inactive ingredients include calcium acetate, calcium phosphate, corn starch, hydrogenated castor oil, and povidone. Each pink tablet in the Demulen 1/50™-28 package is a placebo containing no active ingredients, and the inactive ingredients include calcium sulfate, corn starch, FD&C Red No. 3, FD&C Yellow No. 6, magnesium stearate, and sucrose.

Ovulen-21 and Ovulen-28. Each white tablet contains 1 mg of ethynodiol diacetate and 0.1 mg of mestranol, and the inactive ingredients include calcium acetate, calcium phosphate, corn starch, hydrogenated castor oil, and povidone. Each pink tablet in the Ovulen-28 package is a placebo containing no active ingredients, and the inactive ingredients include calcium sulfate, corn starch, FD&C Red No. 3, FD&C Yellow No. 6, magnesium stearate, and sucrose.

Enovid-E 21. Each tablet contains 2.5 mg of norethynodrel and 0.1 mg of mestranol. Inactive ingredients include acacia, corn starch, FD&C Red No. 3, FD&C Yellow No. 6, magnesium stearate, sodium phosphate, sodium sulfate, and sucrose.

Enovid 5 mg. Each tablet contains 5 mg of norethynodrel and 75 mcg of mestranol. Inactive ingredients include acacia, corn starch, FD&C Red No. 3, FD&C Yellow No. 6, magnesium stearate, sodium phosphate, sodium sulfate, and sucrose.

Enovid 10 mg. Each tablet contains 9.85 mg of norethynodrel and 0.15 mg of mestranol. Inactive ingredients include acacia, corn starch, FD&C Red No. 40, FD&C Yellow No. 6, magnesium stearate, and sodium sulfate.

The chemical name for norethynodrel is 17α-ethynyl-17-hydroxy-5(10)-estren-3-one, for mestranol it is 3-methoxy-19-nor-17α-pregna-1,3,5(10)-trien-20-yn-17-ol, for ethynodiol diacetate it is 19-nor-17α-pregn-4-en-20-yne-3β,17-diol diacetate, and for ethinyl estradiol it is 19-nor-17α-pregna-1, 3, 5(10)-trien-20-yne-3,17-diol. Their structural formulas are as follows:

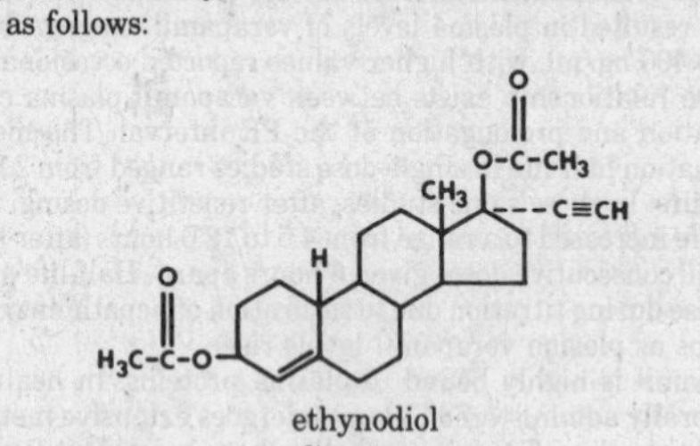

ethynodiol diacetate

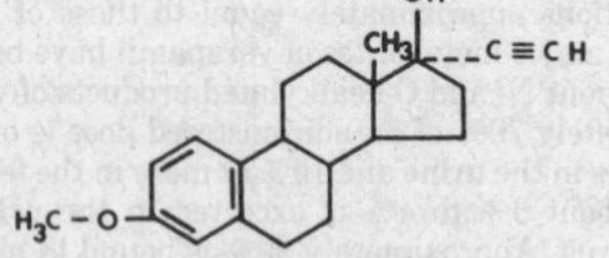

mestranol

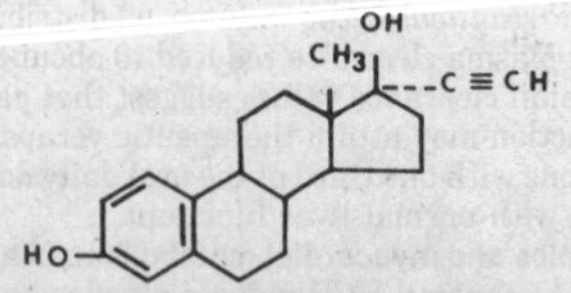

ethinyl estradiol

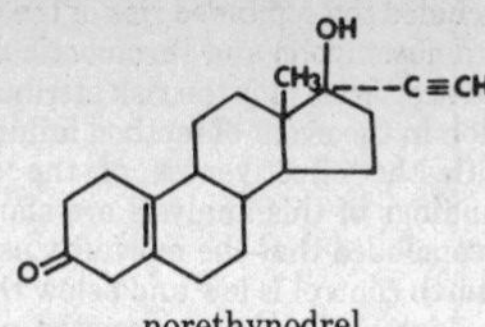

norethynodrel

Therapeutic Class: Oral contraceptive (except for Enovid 10 mg). Estrogen-progestogen combination (Enovid 5 mg and 10 mg only).

CLINICAL PHARMACOLOGY

Combination oral contraceptives act primarily through the mechanism of gonadotropin suppression due to the estrogenic and progestational activity of their components. Although the primary mechanism of action is inhibition of ovulation, alterations in the genital tract, including changes in the cervical mucus (which reduce sperm penetration) and the endometrium (which reduce the likelihood of implantation) may also contribute to contraceptive effectiveness.

Enovid 5 mg or Enovid 10 mg, when used for the treatment of endometriosis, may be administered to induce changes in areas of endometriosis similar to those that occur during pregnancy. In many instances when Enovid 5 mg or Enovid 10 mg is taken continuously the areas of endometriosis develop a decidua-like response followed by necrosis, which may result in destruction of the abnormally located tissue and resolution of the lesions.

INDICATIONS AND USAGE

Demulen 1/35, Demulen 1/50, Ovulen, Enovid-E, and Enovid 5 mg are indicated for the prevention of pregnancy in women who elect to use oral contraceptives as a method of contraception.

Enovid 5 mg and Enovid 10 mg are indicated for the treatment of endometriosis, for the treatment of hypermenorrhea, and for the production of cyclic withdrawal bleeding.

NOTE: The contraindication, warning, precaution, and adverse reaction information in this monograph also applies when Enovid 5 mg is prescribed for indications other than contraception or when Enovid 10 mg is prescribed.

Oral contraceptives are highly effective. The pregnancy rate in women using conventional combination oral contraceptives (containing 35 mcg or more of ethinyl estradiol or 50 mcg or more of mestranol) is generally reported to be less than 1 pregnancy per 100 woman-years of use. Slightly higher rates (somewhat more than 1 pregnancy per 100 woman-years of use) are reported for some combination products containing 35 mcg or less of ethinyl estradiol, and rates on the order of 3 pregnancies per 100 woman-years are reported for the progestogen-only oral contraceptives.

These rates are derived from separate studies conducted by different investigators in several population groups; therefore, a precise comparison cannot be made. Furthermore, pregnancy rates tend to be lower as clinical studies are continued, possibly due to selective retention in the longer studies of those patients who accept the treatment regimen and do not discontinue as a result of adverse reactions, pregnancy, or other reasons. In Table 1 ranges of pregnancy rates as reported in the literature[1] are shown for other means of contraception. The efficacy of these means of contraception, except for the IUD, depends upon the degree of adherence to the method.

In clinical trials with Ovulen, 5,938 patients completed 83,463 cycles, and a total of 8 pregnancies were reported. This represents a pregnancy rate of 0.12 per 100 woman-years.

In clinical trials with Enovid-E, 1,657 patients completed 28,400 cycles, and a total of 8 pregnancies were reported. This represents a pregnancy rate of 0.34 per 100 woman-years.

In clinical trials with Demulen 1/50, 2,256 patients completed 30,409 cycles, and a total of 30 pregnancies were reported. This represents a pregnancy rate of 1.18 per 100 woman-years.

In clinical trials with Demulen 1/35, 1,231 patients completed 14,641 cycles, and a total of 15 pregnancies were reported. This represents a pregnancy rate of 1.23 per 100 woman-years.

In clinical trials with Demulen 1/35, the incidence of delayed or breakthrough bleeding was 44% at cycle 6. However, only 9.9% of the patients dropped out of the study due to bleeding.

Table 1
Pregnancies per 100 Woman-Years

Method	*Range*
IUD	<1 to 6
Diaphragm with spermicidal cream or gel	2 to 20
Condom	3 to 36
Spermicidal aerosol foams	2 to 29
Spermicidal gels and creams	4 to 36
Periodic abstinence (rhythm), all types	<1 to 47
1. Calendar method	14 to 47
2. Temperature method	1 to 20
3. Temperature method (intercourse only in postovulatory phase)	<1 to 7
4. Mucus method	1 to 25
No contraception	60 to 80

Dose-related Risk of Thromboembolism From Oral Contraceptives: Studies have shown a positive association between the dose of estrogens in oral contraceptives and the risk of thromboembolism[2,96,97] (see *Warning* No. 1). For this reason, it is prudent and in keeping with good principles of therapeutics to minimize exposure to estrogen. The oral contraceptive product prescribed for any given patient should be that product which contains the least amount of estrogen that is compatible with an acceptable pregnancy rate and patient acceptance. It is recommended that new users of oral contraceptives be started on preparations containing 50 mcg or less of estrogen.

CONTRAINDICATIONS

Oral contraceptives should not be used in women with any of the following conditions:

1. Thrombophlebitis or thromboembolic disorders.
2. A past history of deep vein thrombophlebitis or thromboembolic disorders.
3. Cerebral vascular disease, myocardial infarction or coronary artery disease, or a past history of these conditions.
4. Known or suspected carcinoma of the breast.
5. Known or suspected estrogen-dependent neoplasia.
6. Undiagnosed abnormal genital bleeding.
7. Known or suspected pregnancy (see *Warning* No. 5).
8. Past or present, benign or malignant liver tumors among women who developed these tumors during the use of oral contraceptives or other estrogen-containing products (see *Warning* No. 4).

WARNINGS

Cigarette-smoking increases the risk of serious cardiovascular side effects from oral contraceptive use. This risk increases with age and with heavy smoking (15 or more cigarettes per day) and is quite marked in women over 35 years of age. Women who use oral contraceptives should be strongly advised not to smoke.

The use of oral contraceptives is associated with increased risk of several serious conditions including venous and arterial thromboembolism, thrombotic and hemorrhagic stroke, myocardial infarction, visual disorders, hepatic tumors, gallbladder disease, hypertension, and fetal abnormalities. Practitioners prescribing oral contraceptives should be familiar with the following information relating to these and other risks.

1. *Thromboembolic Disorders and Other Vascular Problems.* An increased risk of thromboembolic and thrombotic disease associated with the use of oral contraceptives is well established. One study in Great Britain[3] demonstrated an increased relative risk for fatal venous thromboembolism; several British[4,5,14,22,92,156] and U.S.[6-8,23,98-101,126] studies demonstrated an increased relative risk for nonfatal venous thromboembolism. U.S. studies[6,9,10,99,101-103] demonstrated an increased relative risk for stroke, which had not been shown in prior British studies.[3-5] In these studies it was estimated that users of oral contraceptives were 1.9 to 11 times more likely than nonusers to manifest these diseases without evident cause (Table 2). In a British study of idiopathic deep vein thrombosis and pulmonary embolism, the projected annual hospitalization rates for women aged 16–40 were 47 per 100,000 users and 5 for nonusers.[77] In one British mortality study,[3] overall excess mortality due to pulmonary embolism or stroke was on the order of 1.3 to 3.4 deaths annually per 100,000 users and increased with age.

Cerebrovascular Disorders: In a collaborative U.S. study[9,10] of cerebrovascular disorders in women with and without predisposing causes, it was estimated that the risk of hemorrhagic stroke was 2.0 times greater in users than in nonusers, and the risk of thrombotic stroke was 4.0[10] to 9.5[9] times greater in users than in nonusers (Table 2). Analysis of mortality trends in 21 countries indicates that, since oral contraceptives first became available, changes in mortality from nonrheumatic heart disease and hypertension, cerebrovascular disease, and all nonrheumatic cardiovascular disease among women aged 15 to 44 years have been associated with changes in the prevalence of oral contraceptive use in each country.[11]

Table 2. *Summary of Relative Risks of Thromboembolic Disorders and Other Vascular Problems in Oral Contraceptive Users Compared with Nonusers.*

Disorders	*Relative Risk*
Idiopathic thromboembolic disease	2 to 11 times greater
Postsurgery thromboembolic complications	4 to 7 times greater
Thrombotic stroke	4 to 9.5 times greater
Hemorrhagic stroke	2.0 to 2.3 times greater
Myocardial infarction	2 to 12 times greater

In May 1974 the Royal College of General Practitioners[12] issued an interim report of its continuing large-scale prospective study comparing a user group with a nonuser group. It stated: "A statistically significant higher rate of reporting of cerebrovascular accidents in Takers is evident, but the numbers are too small to justify an estimation of the degree of risk." A 1981 analysis of data from this study was reported[13] to show a 4-fold increased mortality from circulatory diseases, mainly from myocardial infarction and hemorrhagic stroke, in users. The excess mortality was associated with age and smoking in users. A 1983 analysis[138] of arterial diseases reported a significantly increased incidence of cerebrovascular disease among current oral contraceptive users. Risk appeared to increase with duration of use up to 8 years. Categories with a significantly increased incidence included cerebral thrombosis or embolism, and transient ischemic attacks, but not hemorrhagic strokes. Incidence of peripheral arterial thromboembolism, Raynaud's disease, and acute myocardial infarction was increased in current users. Women aged 30 years and older had appreciably higher rates of arterial disease than did younger women. Smoking increased the risk for older women in each usage group, the greatest risk being in current users aged 35 years and older who smoked. Expressed as the percentage of women diagnosed as having an arterial disease who died of that disease, the case-fatality rates were 2 to 3 times greater for users who smoked than for women in the other groups.

In October 1976 an interim report was issued on the long-term follow-up study of the British Family Planning Association.[14] There was a highly significant association between oral contraceptive use and stroke, although total numbers were small in this study also. The increase in risk of venous thrombosis and pulmonary embolism among users was about 4-fold and was statistically highly significant. In later reports[15] it was noted that mortality from nonrheumatic heart disease was greater in women who had ever used oral contraceptives. A 1984 report[147] on stroke found pill use to be a significant risk factor for nonhemorrhagic stroke, but not for subarachnoid hemorrhage. Smoking and hypertension were significant risk factors only for the latter.

In the Walnut Creek prospective study,[99,101,102] the risk of subarachnoid hemorrhage was associated with heavy smoking, age, and use of the pill.

Myocardial Infarction: An increased risk of myocardial infarction associated with the use of oral contraceptives has been reported in Great Britain,[16-19,136,138] confirming a previously suspected association.[3] The morbidity study[16,17] found that the greater the number of underlying risk factors for coronary artery disease (cigarette-smoking, hypertension, hypercholesterolemia, obesity, diabetes, history of preeclamptic toxemia), the higher the risk of developing myocardial infarction, regardless of whether the patient was an oral contraceptive user or not. Oral contraceptives were considered an additional risk factor.

The annual excess rate of fatal myocardial infarction in British oral contraceptive users was estimated to be approximately 3.5 cases per 100,000 women users in the 30- to 39-year age group and 20 per 100,000 women users in the 40- to 44-year age group.[19] (These estimates are based on British vital statistics, which show acute myocardial infarction death rates 2 to 3 times less than in the U.S. for women in these age groups. In an attempt to extrapolate these figures to U.S. women, it was estimated that the annual excess rates in users are 25.7 cases per 100,000 for women aged 30–39 with predisposing conditions versus 1.5 cases without; corresponding estimates for women aged 40–44 were 86.2 versus 5.1.[78]) The annual excess rate of hospitalization for nonfatal myocardial infarction in married British oral contraceptive users was estimated to be approximately 3.5 per 100,000 women users in the 30- to 39-year age group and 47 per 100,000 women users in the 40- to 44-year age group.[16]

Smoking is considered a major predisposing condition to myocardial infarction. In terms of relative risk, it has been estimated[20] that oral contraceptive users who do not smoke are about twice as likely to have a fatal myocardial infarction as nonusers who do not smoke. Oral contraceptive users who are also smokers have about a 5-fold increased risk of fatal infarction compared to users who do not smoke, but about a 10- to 12-fold increased risk compared to nonusers who do not smoke. Furthermore, the amount of smoking is also an important factor. In determining the importance of these relative risks, however, the baseline rates for various age groups, as shown in Table 3, must be given serious consideration. The importance of other predisposing conditions mentioned above in determining relative and absolute risks

Continued on next page

Searle & Co.—Cont.

has not been quantified; it is likely that the same synergistic action exists, but perhaps to a lesser extent.
Similar findings relating nonfatal and fatal myocardial infarction, oral contraceptives, smoking, and age were subsequently published in the U.S.[91,99,104–108,152] and by the Royal College of General Practitioners in Great Britain. [13,138]

Table 3. *Estimated Annual Mortality Rate per 100,000 Women from Myocardial Infarction by Use of Oral Contraceptives, Smoking Habits, and Age in Years*[20]

	Myocardial infarction			
	Women aged 30–39		Women aged 40–44	
Smoking habits	Users	Non-users	Users	Non-users
All smokers	10.2	2.6	62.0	15.9
Heavy*	13.0	5.1	78.7	31.3
Light	4.7	0.9	28.6	5.7
Nonsmokers	1.8	1.2	10.7	7.4
Smokers and nonsmokers	5.4	1.9	32.8	11.7

*15 or more cigarettes per day

Risk of Dose: Reports of thromboembolism following the use of oral contraceptives containing 50 mcg or more of estrogen received by drug safety committees in Great Britain, Sweden, and Denmark were compared with the distribution expected from market research estimates of sales.[2] A positive correlation was found between the dose of estrogen and the reporting of thromboembolism, including coronary thrombosis, in excess of that predicted by sales estimates. Preparations containing 100 mcg or more of estrogen were associated with a higher risk of thromboembolism than those containing 50 to 80 mcg of estrogen. The authors' analysis did suggest, however, that the quantity of estrogen may not be the sole factor involved. Any influence on the part of the progestogens was not considered, which may have been responsible for certain discrepancies in the data. No significant differences were detected between preparations containing the same dose of estrogen nor between the two estrogens ethinyl estradiol and mestranol. A subsequent study of a similar nature in Great Britain found a positive association between the dose of progestogen or estrogen and certain thromboembolic conditions, [96] which is consistent with findings of the Royal College study. [12,92,135] Swedish authorities noted decreased reporting of thromboembolic episodes when higher estrogen preparations were no longer prescribed.[97] Careful epidemiologic studies to determine the degree of thromboembolic risk associated with progestogen-only oral contraceptives have not been performed. Cases of thromboembolic disease have been reported in women using these products, and they should not be presumed to be free of excess risk.
The relative risk of oral contraceptive use one month prior to hospitalization for various types of thromboembolism was calculated in a U.S. retrospective case-control study.[8] If no account is taken of the relative estrogenic potency of different estrogens and if any possible influence of the different progestogenic components is ignored, the products employed may be divided into those containing less than 100 mcg and those containing 100 mcg or more of estrogen. For all cases combined, the larger-dose category was associated with only a slightly higher relative risk; for the idiopathic subgroup, the relative risk was approximately doubled with the larger estrogen content, but the confidence limits overlapped considerably and the differences, therefore, were not statistically significant. Apparently there was less of an increased relative risk for the subgroup with predispositions to thromboembolism.[98]
In the British Family Planning Association study,[147] no nonhemorrhagic strokes occurred during 9,100 woman-years of current use of pills containing less than 50 mcg of estrogen, in contrast to 13 observed during 39,400 woman-years of current use of pills with higher doses.
The risk of thromboembolic and thrombotic disorders, both in users and in nonusers of oral contraceptives, increases with age. Oral contraceptives have been considered an independent risk factor for these events.
Persistence of Risk: A 1977 analysis[13a] of the mortality data from the prospective study of the Royal College of General Practitioners (RCGP) suggested that the risk of circulatory disease increases with the duration of oral contraceptive use and may persist after discontinuation. The ratio of the mortality rate from circulatory disease in former users to that in controls was 4.3 to 1 ($P < 0.01$), and was still 3.7 to 1 even after excluding the two deaths from malignant hypertension, where use was stopped because of the onset of hypertension. For the category of fatal subarachnoid hemorrhage, the rate ratio comparing former users to controls was also statistically significant.
In 1981, a new analysis of the RCGP mortality data[13] showed significantly increased risk ratios in former users for the categories of all nonrheumatic heart disease plus hypertension (4.6 to 1), cerebrovascular disease (3.6 to 1), as well as the subcategory of subarachnoid hemorrhage (4.5 to 1). Overall, the incidence of fatal circulatory disease for former users was 4.3 times that of the controls.
A 1983 analysis of the incidence of arterial disease in the RCGP study[138] showed that the incidence of all cerebrovascular disease, fatal and nonfatal, was significantly greater in former users than in controls (risk ratio = 2.6) and remained elevated for at least 6 years after discontinuation of oral contraceptives. Former users had significantly increased rates for cerebral thrombosis (4 vs 0), transient ischemic attacks (8.7 to 1), and "other" cerebrovascular disease (3.8 to 1).
In the Walnut Creek prospective study,[102] former use of oral contraceptives was significantly associated with increased risk of subarachnoid hemorrhage, the relative risk being 5.3.
In a U.S. hospital-based, case-control study,[137] when the duration of oral contraceptive use was considered, the data suggested that the rate of myocardial infarction is increased approximately 2- to 3-fold in older women who had used oral contraceptives for more than 10 years before discontinuation. The excess risk associated with long-term use was evident in subjects who had stopped less than 5 years previously, as well as in those who had stopped 5 to 9 years previously. Whether the excess risk persisted for more than 10 years after discontinuation could not be assessed because of a paucity of data.
In summary, persistence of risk after discontinuation of oral contraceptives has been reported for circulatory disease in general,[13,13a] for nonrheumatic heart disease,[13,137] and for cerebrovascular disease,[13,138] including subarachnoid hemorrhage,[13,13a,102] cerebral thrombosis,[138] and transient ischemic attacks.[138]
Estimate of Excess Mortality from Circulatory Diseases: A large prospective study[13] carried out in the U.K. provided estimates of the mortality rate per 100,000 women per year from diseases of the circulatory system for users and nonusers of oral contraceptives according to age, smoking habits, and duration of use. The overall annual excess death rate from circulatory diseases for oral contraceptive users was estimated at 23 per 100,000 for women of all ages. The rates for nonsmokers and smokers, respectively, were: ages 25–34, 2 and 10 per 100,000; ages 35–44, 15 and 48 per 100,000; and ages 45 and older, 41 and 179 per 100,000. The risk was statistically significant only in cigarette-smokers over age 34. The majority of deaths were due to subarachnoid hemorrhage or ischemic heart disease. Relative risk for women who had ever used oral contraceptives rose with increasing parity, a new observation that needs confirmation.
The available data from a variety of sources have been analyzed[21] to estimate the risk of death associated with various methods of contraception. The estimates of risk of death for each method included the combined risk of the contraceptive method (eg, thromboembolic and thrombotic disease in the case of oral contraceptives) plus the risk attributable to pregnancy or abortion in the event of method failure. This latter risk varies with the effectiveness of the contraceptive method. The findings of this analysis are shown in Figure 1.[21] The study concluded that the mortality associated with all methods of birth control is low and below that associated with childbirth, except for that associated with oral contraceptives in women over 40 who smoke. (The rates given for pill only/smokers for each age group are for smokers as a class. For "heavy" smokers [more than 15 cigarettes a day], the rates given would be about double; for "light" smokers [less than 15 cigarettes a day], about 50 percent.[20]) The mortality associated with oral contraceptive use in nonsmokers over 40 is higher than with any other method of contraception in that age group. The lowest mortality is associated with the condom or diaphragm backed up by early legal abortion.

Figure 1 Estimated annual number of deaths associated with control of fertility and no control per 100 000 nonsterile women by regimen of control and age of woman

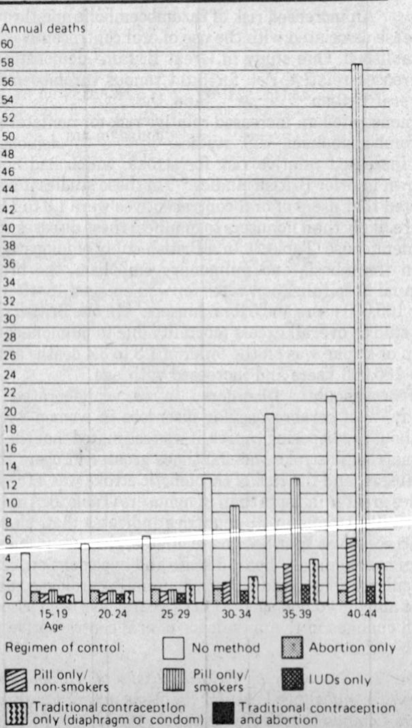

The risk of thromboembolic and thrombotic disease associated with oral contraceptives increases with age after approximately age 30 and, for myocardial infarction, is further increased by hypertension, hypercholesterolemia, obesity, diabetes, or history of preeclamptic toxemia, and especially by cigarette-smoking.[20,78,79]
Based on the data currently available, the following table gives a gross estimate of the risk of death from circulatory disorders associated with the use of oral contraceptives:

Table 4. *Smoking Habits and Other Predisposing Conditions—Risk Associated with Use of Oral Contraceptives*

Age	Below 30	30–39	40+
Heavy smokers	C	B	A
Light smokers	D	C	B
Nonsmokers (no predisposing conditions)	D	C,D	C
Nonsmokers (other predisposing conditions)	C	C,B	B,A

A—Use associated with very high risk.
B—Use associated with high risk.
C—Use associated with moderate risk.
D—Use associated with low risk.

The physician and patient should be alert to the earliest manifestations of thromboembolic and thrombotic disorders (eg, thrombophlebitis, pulmonary embolism, cerebrovascular insufficiency, coronary artery disease or myocardial infarction, retinal thrombosis, and mesenteric thrombosis). Should any of these occur or be suspected, the drug should be discontinued immediately.
A 4- to 7-fold increased risk of postsurgery thromboembolic complications has also been reported in oral contraceptive users.[22,23] If feasible, oral contraceptives should be discontinued at least 4 weeks before elective surgery or during periods of prolonged immobilization. The decision as to when to resume oral contraception following major surgery or bed rest should balance the recognized risks of postsurgery thromboembolic complications with the need to reinstate contraceptive practices.
The Royal College of General Practitioners in a large prospective study reported a higher incidence of superficial and deep vein thrombosis in users, the former being correlated with the progestogen dose. The RCGP data suggest that the presence of varicose veins substantially increases the risk of superficial venous thrombosis of the leg, the risk depending upon the severity of the varicosities. The evidence suggests that the presence of varicose veins has little effect on the development of deep vein thrombosis in the leg.[92] Other prospective studies have also reported a higher incidence of venous thrombosis in users.[14,99–101,109]
2. *Ocular Lesions.* There have been reports of neuro-ocular lesions such as optic neuritis or retinal thrombosis associated with the use of oral contraceptives. Discontinue medication if there is unexplained, gradual or sudden, partial or complete loss of vision; proptosis or diplopia; papilledema; or any evidence of retinal vascular lesions. Appropriate diagnostic and therapeutic measures should be instituted.
3. *Carcinoma.* Long-term continuous administration of either natural or synthetic estrogens in certain animal species increases the frequency of certain carcinomas, and/or nonmalignant neoplasms, such as those of the breast, uterus, cervix, vagina, ovary, liver, and pituitary. Certain synthetic progestogens, none currently contained in oral contraceptives, have been noted to increase the incidence of mammary nodules, benign and malignant, in dogs.
There is now evidence that estrogens increase the risk of carcinoma of the endometrium in humans. In several independent, retrospective case-control studies,[24–28,80,93] an increased relative risk (2.2 to 13.9 times) was reported, associ-

ating endometrial carcinoma with the prolonged use of estrogens in postmenopausal women who took estrogen replacement medication to relieve menopausal symptoms. This risk was independent of the other known risk factors for endometrial cancer and appeared to depend both on duration of treatment[24,27,28] and on estrogen dose.[26–28] These findings are supported by the observation that incidence rates of endometrial cancer have increased sharply since 1969 in 8 different areas of the U.S. with population-based cancer-reporting systems, an increase which may be related to the rapidly expanding use of estrogens during the past decade.[29] There is no evidence at present that "natural" estrogens are more or less hazardous than "synthetic" estrogens at equiestrogenic doses.

One publication[30] reported on the first 30 cases submitted by physicians to a registry of cases of adenocarcinoma of the endometrium in women under 40 on oral contraceptives. Of the adenocarcinomas found in women without predisposing risk factors for adenocarcinoma of the endometrium (eg, irregular bleeding at the time oral contraceptives were first given, polycystic ovaries), nearly all occurred in women who had used a sequential oral contraceptive. These products are no longer marketed. No statistical association has been reported suggesting an increased risk of endometrial cancer in users of conventional combination or progestogen-only oral contraceptives, although individual cases have been reported.

Several studies[7,31–35,99,121,122] have shown no increased risk of breast cancer to women taking oral contraceptives or estrogens. In one study,[36,37] however, while no overall increased risk of breast cancer was noted in women treated with oral contraceptives, a greater risk was suggested for the subgroups of oral contraceptive users with documented benign breast disease and for long-term (2–4 years) users. Another study[123,142] reported increased risk of breast cancer in women who had used the pill for more than 4 years before their first full-term pregnancy. One other study[38] indicated an increasing risk of breast cancer in women taking menopausal estrogens, which increased with duration of follow-up. Several other studies have also shown oral contraceptives[127–129,133,140,141,144,146,148] or estrogens[130,145] to be associated with breast cancer, particularly in connection with other risk factors[127–129] (eg, family history, previous breast biopsy, late age of first delivery) and long duration of use.[127,128,130,146] A reduced occurrence of benign breast tumors in users of oral contraceptives has been well documented.[7,12,14,31,36,39,40,86,99]

Some epidemiologic studies[41,81–84,99,109,120,143,149,150] have suggested an increased risk of cervical dysplasia, erosion, and carcinoma in long-term pill users; however, cause and effect has not been established. There have been other reports of microglandular dysplasia of the cervix in users.

In summary, there is at present no consistent evidence from human studies of an increased risk of cancer associated with oral contraceptives.[42] Close clinical surveillance of all women taking oral contraceptives is, nevertheless, essential. In all cases of undiagnosed persistent or recurrent abnormal vaginal bleeding, nonfunctional causes should be borne in mind and appropriate diagnostic measures should be taken to rule out malignancy. Women who have a strong family history of breast cancer or who have breast nodules, fibrocystic disease, recurrent cystic mastitis, abnormal mammograms, or cervical dysplasia should be monitored with particular care if they elect to use oral contraceptives.

4. *Hepatic Lesions (adenomas, hepatomas, hamartomas, regenerating nodules, focal nodular hyperplasia, hemangiomas, peliosis hepatis, sinusoidal dilatation, hepatocellular carcinoma, etc).* Benign hepatic adenomas and other hepatic lesions have been associated with the use of oral contraceptives.[43,45,46,85] One study[46] reported that oral contraceptive formulations with high "hormonal potency" were associated with a higher risk than lower-potency formulations, as was age over 30 years. Although benign, these hepatic lesions may rupture and may cause death through intra-abdominal hemorrhage. This has been reported in short-term as well as long-term users of oral contraceptives. Two studies related risk with duration of use of the contraceptive, the risk being much greater after 4 or more years of oral contraceptive use.[45,46] Long-term users of oral contraceptives have an estimated annual incidence of hepatocellular adenoma of 3 to 4 per 100,000.[46] While such hepatic lesions are rare, they should be considered in women presenting with abdominal pain and tenderness, abdominal mass, or shock. Patients with liver tumors have demonstrated variable clinical features, which may make preoperative diagnosis difficult. About one quarter of the cases presented because of abdominal masses; up to one half had signs and symptoms of acute intraperitoneal hemorrhage. Routine radiologic and laboratory studies may not be helpful. Liver scans may clearly show a focal defect. Hepatic arteriography or computed tomography may be useful procedures in diagnosing primary liver neoplasms.

Cases of hepatocellular carcinoma have been reported in women taking oral contraceptives. The relationship of these drugs to this type of malignancy is not known at this time, although epidemiologic studies[157–159] have estimated a relative risk as high as 7 to 20 for users for 8 or more years as compared to nonusers.[158,159]

Oral contraceptives are contraindicated if there are past or present, benign or malignant liver tumors among women who developed these tumors during the use of oral contraceptives or other estrogen-containing products.

5. *Use In or Immediately Preceding Pregnancy, Birth Defects in Offspring, and Malignancy in Offspring.* The use of female sex hormones, both estrogens and progestogens, during early pregnancy may seriously damage the offspring. It has been reported that females exposed in utero to diethylstilbestrol and other nonsteroidal estrogens have an increased risk of developing in later life a form of vaginal or cervical cancer that is ordinarily extremely rare.[47,48] This risk has been estimated to be on the order of 1 in 1,000 exposures or less.[49,50] The excess incidence for dysplasia and carcinoma in situ has been estimated at 7.8 cases per 1,000 woman-years.[154] Although there is no evidence at the present time that oral contraceptives further enhance the risk of developing this type of malignancy, such patients should be monitored with particular care if they elect to use oral contraceptives instead of other methods of contraception. Furthermore, a high percentage of such exposed women (from 30% to 90%) have been found to have adenosis (epithelial changes) of the vagina and cervix.[51–55] Although these changes are histologically benign, it is not known whether this condition is a precursor of malignancy. DES-exposed daughters appear to have an increased risk of unfavorable outcome of pregnancy.[110–112] DES-exposed male children may develop abnormalities of the urogenital tract[56–58,131] and sperm.[131] Although similar data are not available for the use of other estrogens, it cannot be presumed that they would not induce similar changes.

Several reports suggest an association between fetal exposure to female sex hormones, including oral contraceptives, and congenital anomalies,[59–64,94,113–116] including multiple congenital anomalies described by the acronym VACTERL, for vertebral, anal, cardiac, tracheoesophageal, renal, and limb defects.[61,62,113] There appears to be a preferential expression of these defects by exposed male offspring.[63,65,115,121] In one case-control study[63] it was estimated that there was a 4.7-fold increased risk of limb-reduction defects in infants exposed in utero to sex hormones (oral contraceptives, hormonal withdrawal tests for pregnancy, or attempted treatment for threatened abortion). Some of these exposures were very short and involved only a few days of treatment. The data suggest that the risk of limb-reduction defects in exposed fetuses is somewhat less than 1 in 1,000 live births. In a large prospective study,[64] cardiovascular defects in children born to women who received female hormones, including oral contraceptives, during early pregnancy occurred at a rate of 18.2 per 1,000 births, compared to 7.8 per 1,000 for children not so exposed in utero. These results are statistically significant. The incidence of twin births may be increased for women who conceive shortly after discontinuing use of the pill.[14,63,117,118,124]

In the past, female sex hormones have been used during pregnancy in an attempt to treat threatened or habitual abortion. There is considerable evidence that estrogens are ineffective for these indications, and there is no evidence from well-controlled studies that progestogens are effective for these uses.

There is some evidence that triploidy and possibly other types of polyploidy are increased among abortuses from women who become pregnant soon after stopping oral contraceptives.[66] Embryos with these anomalies are virtually always aborted spontaneously. Whether there is an overall increase in spontaneous abortion of pregnancies conceived soon after stopping the oral contraceptives is unknown. A highly significant ($P < 0.001$) increase of lymphocytic chromosome aberrations in oral contraceptive users has been reported.[160]

The safety of this product in pregnancy has not been demonstrated. Pregnancy should be ruled out before initiating or continuing the contraceptive regimen. Pregnancy should always be considered if withdrawal bleeding does not occur. It is recommended that for any patient who has missed 2 consecutive periods, pregnancy should be ruled out before continuing the contraceptive regimen. If the patient has not adhered to the prescribed schedule, the possibility of pregnancy should be considered at the time of the first missed period, and further use of oral contraceptives should be withheld until pregnancy has been ruled out. If pregnancy is confirmed, the patient should be apprised of the potential risks to the fetus, and the advisability of continuation of the pregnancy should be discussed in the light of these risks.

It is recommended that women who discontinue oral contraceptives with the intent of becoming pregnant use an alternative form of contraception for a period of time before attempting to conceive. Many clinicians recommend 3 months, although no precise information is available on which to base this recommendation.

The administration of progestogen-only or progestogen-estrogen combinations to induce withdrawal bleeding should not be used as a test of pregnancy.

6. *Gallbladder Disease.* Reports of studies[7,8,12,14,33] indicate an increased risk for surgically confirmed gallbladder disease in users of oral contraceptives or estrogens. In one study,[12] an increased risk appeared after 2 years of use and doubled after 4 or 5 years of use. In one of the other studies[7] an increased risk was apparent between 6 and 12 months of use.

7. *Carbohydrate and Lipid Metabolism.* A decrease in glucose tolerance has been observed in a significant percentage of patients on oral contraceptives. For this reason, prediabetic and diabetic patients should be carefully observed while receiving oral contraceptives. An increase in triglycerides and total phospholipids has been observed in patients receiving oral contraceptives.[67] The clinical significance of this finding remains to be defined.

8. *Elevated Blood Pressure.* An increase in blood pressure has been reported in patients receiving oral contraceptives.[12,69,109] There is evidence that the degree of hypertension may correlate directly with increasing dosage of progestogen.[86] In some women, hypertension may occur within a few months of beginning oral contraceptive use. The prevalence of hypertension in users is low in the first year of use, and may be no higher than that in a comparable group of nonusers. The prevalence in users increases, however, with longer exposure and, in the fifth year of use, is $2\frac{1}{2}$ to 3 times the reported prevalence in the first year. Age is also strongly correlated with the development of hypertension in oral contraceptive users.

Women with a history of elevated blood pressure (hypertension), preexisting renal disease, a history of toxemia or elevated blood pressure during pregnancy, a familial tendency to hypertension or its consequences, or a history of excessive weight gain or fluid retention during the menstrual cycle may be more likely to develop elevation of blood pressure when given oral contraceptives and, therefore, should be monitored closely.[68] Even though elevated blood pressure may remain within the "normal" range, the clinical implications of elevations should not be ignored and close surveillance is indicated, particularly for women with other risk factors for cardiovascular disease or stroke.[69] High blood pressure may or may not persist after discontinuation of the oral contraceptive.

9. *Headache.* The onset or exacerbation of migraine or development of headache of a new pattern which is recurrent, persistent, or severe, requires discontinuation of oral contraceptives and evaluation of the cause.

10. *Bleeding Irregularities.* Breakthrough bleeding, spotting, and amenorrhea are frequent reasons for discontinuance of oral contraceptives. In breakthrough bleeding, as in all cases of irregular vaginal bleeding, nonfunctional causes should be borne in mind. In patients with undiagnosed persistent or recurrent abnormal vaginal bleeding, adequate diagnostic measures are indicated to rule out pregnancy or malignancy. If a pathologic basis has been excluded, passage of time or a change to another formulation may correct the bleeding problem. A change to an oral contraceptive with a higher estrogen content, while potentially useful in minimizing menstrual irregularity, should be made only when considered necessary since this may increase the risk of thromboembolic disease.

Women with a past history of oligomenorrhea or secondary amenorrhea or young women who have not established regular cycles may have a tendency to remain anovulatory or to become amenorrheic after discontinuation of oral contraceptives. Women with these preexisting problems should be informed of these possibilities and encouraged to use other contraceptive methods. Post-use anovulation, possibly prolonged, may also occur in women without previous irregularities. A higher incidence of galactorrhea and of pituitary tumors (eg, adenomas) has been associated with amenorrhea in former users compared with nonusers.[87] One study[70] reported a 16-fold increased prevalence of pituitary prolactin-secreting tumors among patients with postpill amenorrhea when galactorrhea was present. A case-control study[44] reported an increased risk of galactorrhea following discontinuation of oral contraceptives by women who did not have pituitary tumors.

11. *Ectopic Pregnancy.* Contraceptive failure may result in either ectopic or intrauterine pregnancy. In failures with combination-type oral contraceptives, the ratio of ectopic to intrauterine pregnancies is no higher than in women who are not receiving oral contraceptives.

12. *Breast Feeding.* Oral contraceptives given in the postpartum period may interfere with lactation. There may be a decrease in the quantity and quality of the breast milk. Furthermore, a small fraction of the hormonal agents in oral contraceptives has been identified in the milk of mothers receiving these drugs.[71,88,89] The effects, if any, on the breast-fed child have not been determined. If feasible, the use of oral contraceptives should be deferred until the infant has been weaned.

13. *Infertility.* There is evidence of fertility impairment in women discontinuing oral contraceptives in comparison

Continued on next page

Searle & Co.—Cont.

with those discontinuing other methods.[14,90,132,155] While the impairment diminishes with time, there is still an appreciable difference in the results in nulliparous women aged 25 to 29 at 30 months after discontinuation of birth control; the difference is negligible after 48 months. However, among nulliparas aged 30–34, the impairment persists up to 72 months and appears more severe for users for 2 or more years. For parous women aged 25 to 34 the difference is no longer apparent 30 months after cessation of contraception.

PRECAUTIONS

General. 1. A complete medical and family history should be taken and a thorough physical examination should be performed prior to the initiation of oral contraceptives. The pretreatment and periodic physical examinations should include special reference to blood pressure, breasts, abdomen, and pelvic organs, including a Pap smear and relevant laboratory tests. As a general rule, oral contraceptives should not be prescribed for longer than one year without the performance of another physical examination (see *Warnings*).

2. Preexisting uterine leiomyomata may increase in size during oral contraceptive use.

3. Oral contraceptives appear to be associated with an increased incidence of mental depression. Therefore, patients with a history of depression should be carefully observed and the drug discontinued if depression recurs to a serious degree. Patients becoming significantly depressed while taking oral contraceptives should stop the medication and use an alternative method of contraception in an attempt to determine whether the symptom is drug related.

4. Oral contraceptives may cause some degree of fluid retention. They should be prescribed with caution, and only with careful monitoring, in patients with conditions which might be aggravated by fluid retention, such as convulsive disorders, migraine syndrome, asthma, or cardiac, hepatic, or renal dysfunction.

5. Patients with a past history of jaundice during pregnancy have an increased risk of recurrence of jaundice and should be carefully observed while receiving oral contraceptives. If jaundice develops in any patient receiving such drugs, the medication should be discontinued while the cause is investigated. Cholestatic jaundice has been reported after combined treatment with oral contraceptives and troleandomycin. Hepatotoxicity following a combination of oral contraceptives and cyclosporine has also been reported.

6. Steroid hormones may be poorly metabolized in patients with impaired liver function and should be administered with caution in such patients.

7. Oral contraceptive users may have disturbances in normal tryptophan metabolism, which may result in a relative pyridoxine deficiency. The clinical significance of this is unknown, although megaloblastic anemia has been reported.

8. Serum folate levels may be depressed by oral contraceptive therapy. Since the pregnant woman is predisposed to folate deficiency and the incidence of folate deficiency increases with lengthening gestation, it is possible that if a woman becomes pregnant shortly after stopping oral contraceptives, she may have a greater chance of developing folate deficiency and complications attributable to this deficiency.

9. The pathologist should be advised of oral contraceptive therapy when relevant specimens are submitted.

10. Certain endocrine and liver function tests may be affected by estrogen-containing oral contraceptives. Therefore, it is recommended that any abnormal tests be repeated after the drug has been withdrawn for two months. The following alterations in laboratory results have been observed with the use of oral contraceptives:

a. Hepatic function: Increased sulfobromophthalein retention and other abnormalities in tests of liver function.
b. Coagulation tests: Increased prothrombin and coagulation factors VII, VIII, IX, and X; decreased antithrombin III; increased platelet aggregability.
c. Thyroid function: Increased thyroid-binding globulin (TBG) leading to increased circulating total thyroid hormone, as measured by protein-bound iodine (PBI) or T^4 by column or radioimmunoassay. Free T^3 resin uptake is decreased, reflecting the elevated TBG; free T^4 concentration is unaltered.
d. Decreased pregnanediol excretion.
e. Reduced response to metyrapone test.
f. Increased blood transcortin and corticosteroid levels.
g. Increased blood triglyceride and phospholipid concentrations.
h. Reduced serum folate concentration.
i. Impaired glucose tolerance.
j. Altered plasma levels of trace minerals (eg, increased ceruloplasmin).

11. The influence of prolonged oral contraceptive therapy on pituitary, ovarian, adrenal, hepatic, or uterine function, or on the immune response, has not been established.

12. Treatment with oral contraceptives may mask the onset of the climacteric. (See *Warnings* section regarding risks in this age group.)

13. The prevalence of cervical *Chlamydia trachomatis* in oral contraceptive users is increased several-fold. It should not be assumed that oral contraceptives afford protection against pelvic inflammatory disease from *Chlamydia*.[151]

Information for the Patient. See patient labeling printed at end.

Drug Interactions. Oral contraceptives may be rendered less effective and increased incidence of breakthrough bleeding may occur by virtue of drug interaction with rifampin, isoniazid, ampicillin, neomycin, penicillin V, tetracycline, chloramphenicol, sulfonamides, nitrofurantoin, griseofulvin, barbiturates, phenytoin, primidone, phenylbutazone, analgesics, tranquilizers, and antimigraine preparations.[72–74,95,125,153] Oral contraceptives may alter the effectiveness of other types of drugs, such as oral anticoagulants, anticonvulsants, tranquilizers (eg, diazepam), tricyclic antidepressants, antihypertensive agents (eg, guanethidine), theophylline, caffeine, vitamins, hypoglycemic agents, clofibrate, glucocorticoids, and acetaminophen.[72,119,134,139,153] (See *Precaution* No. 5).

Carcinogenesis. See *Warnings* No. 3 and 4 for information on the carcinogenic potential of oral contraceptives.

Pregnancy. Pregnancy category X. See *Contraindication* No. 7 and *Warning* No. 5.

Nursing Mothers. See *Warning* No. 12.

ADVERSE REACTIONS

An increased risk of the following serious adverse reactions has been associated with the use of oral contraceptives (see *Warnings*):

- Thrombophlebitis and thrombosis
- Pulmonary embolism
- Arterial thromboembolism
- Raynaud's disease
- Myocardial infarction and coronary thrombosis
- Cerebral thrombosis
- Cerebral hemorrhage
- Hypertension
- Gallbladder disease
- Budd-Chiari syndrome
- Benign adenomas and other hepatic lesions, with or without intra-abdominal bleeding
- Hepatocellular carcinoma
- Congenital anomalies

There is evidence of an association between the following conditions and the use of oral contraceptives, although confirmatory studies have not been done:

- Mesenteric thrombosis
- Neuro-ocular lesions, (eg, retinal thrombosis and optic neuritis)

The following adverse reactions have been reported in patients receiving oral contraceptives and are believed to be drug related:

- Nausea and vomiting
  (Usually the most common adverse reactions, occurring in approximately 10% or fewer patients during the first cycle. Other reactions, as a general rule, are seen much less frequently or only occasionally.)
- Gastrointestinal symptoms (eg, abdominal cramps and bloating)
- Breakthrough bleeding
- Spotting
- Change in menstrual flow
- Dysmenorrhea
- Amenorrhea during and after use
- Infertility after discontinuation
- Edema
- Chloasma or melasma, which may persist when the drug is discontinued
- Breast changes: tenderness, enlargement, and secretion
- Change in weight (increase or decrease)
- Change in cervical erosion and secretion
- Endocervical hyperplasia
- Possible diminution in lactation when given immediately post partum
- Cholestatic jaundice
- Migraine
- Increase in size of uterine leiomyomata
- Rash (allergic)
- Mental depression
- Reduced tolerance to carbohydrates
- Vaginal candidiasis
- Change in corneal curvature (steepening)
- Intolerance to contact lenses

The following adverse reactions or conditions have been reported in users of oral contraceptives, and the association has been neither confirmed nor refuted:

- Premenstrual-like syndrome
- Cataracts
- Changes in libido
- Chorea
- Changes in appetite
- Cystitis-like syndrome
- Headache
- Paresthesia
- Nervousness
- Dizziness
- Auditory disturbances
- Rhinitis
- Fatigue
- Backache
- Hirsutism
- Loss of scalp hair
- Erythema multiforme
- Erythema nodosum
- Hemorrhagic eruption
- Herpes gestationis
- Hemolytic uremic syndrome
- Malignant hypertension
- Itching
- Vaginitis
- Porphyria
- Impaired renal function
- Acute renal failure, sometimes irreversible
- Premature ventricular contractions
- Pulmonary hypertension
- Thrombotic thrombocytopenia purpura
- Anemia
- Pancreatitis
- Hepatitis
- Colitis
- Crohn's disease
- Gingivitis
- Dry socket
- Lupus erythematosus
- Rheumatoid arthritis
- Pituitary tumors (eg, adenoma) with amenorrhea and/or galactorrhea after OC use
- Malignant melanoma
- Endometrial, cervical, and breast carcinoma (see *Warning* No. 3)

ACUTE OVERDOSAGE

Serious ill effects have not been reported following the acute ingestion of large doses of oral contraceptives by young children.[75,76] Overdosage may cause nausea, and withdrawal bleeding might occur in females.

DOSAGE AND ADMINISTRATION

Contraception: Demulen 1/35™-21, Demulen 1/35™-28, Demulen 1/50™-21, Demulen 1/50™-28, Ovulen-21, Ovulen-28, Enovid-E 21, and Enovid 5 mg.

To achieve maximum contraceptive effectiveness, oral contraceptives must be taken exactly as directed and at intervals of 24 hours.

IMPORTANT: The patient should be instructed to use an additional method of protection until after the first week of administration *in the initial cycle.* The possibility of ovulation and conception prior to initiation of use should be considered.

Enovid 5 mg 20-Tablet Dosage Schedule: The patient should take one tablet daily for twenty consecutive days beginning each 20-tablet course on day 5 of her menstrual cycle or eight days after taking the last pill from the previous cycle, whichever occurs first. The first day of menstruation is counted as day 1.

Demulen 1/35™-21, Demulen 1/35™-28, Demulen 1/50™-21, Demulen 1/50™-28, Ovulen-21, Ovulen-28, and Enovid-E 21 Dosage Schedules: The Demulen 1/35™-21, Demulen 1/50™-21, Ovulen-21, and Enovid-E 21 Compack® tablet dispensers contain 21 tablets arranged in three numbered rows of 7 tablets each.

The Demulen 1/35™-28, Demulen 1/50™-28, and Ovulen-28 tablet dispensers contain 21 white active tablets arranged in three numbered rows of 7 tablets each, followed by a fourth row of 7 pink (blue for Demulen 1/35™-28) placebo tablets.

Days of the week are printed above the tablets, starting with Sunday on the left.

Two dosage schedules are described, one of which may be more convenient or suitable than the other for an individual patient.

Schedule #1: Sunday Start: The patient begins taking Demulen 1/35™-21, Demulen 1/35™-28, Demulen 1/50™-21, Demulen 1/50™-28, Ovulen-21, Ovulen-28, or Enovid-E 21, from the first row of her package, one tablet daily, starting on the first Sunday after the onset of menstruation. If the patient's period begins on a Sunday she takes her first tablet that very same day. The 21st tablet or the 28th tablet, depending on whether the patient is taking the 21- or 28-tablet course, will then be taken on a Saturday.

Subsequent Cycles:

21-tablet course—The patient begins a new 21-tablet course on the eighth day, Sunday, after taking her last tablet. All subsequent cycles will also begin on Sunday, one tablet being taken each day for three weeks followed by a week of no pill-taking.

28-tablet course—The patient begins a new 28-tablet course on the next day, Sunday, and all subsequent cycles will also begin on Sunday, one tablet being taken each and every day.

With a Sunday-start schedule, a woman whose period begins on the day of or one to four days before taking the first tablet should expect a diminution of flow and fewer menstrual days. The initial cycle will likely be shortened by from one to five days. Thereafter, cycles should be about 28 days in length.

Schedule #2: Day 5 Start: The patient begins taking Demulen 1/35™-21, Demulen 1/50™-21, Ovulen-21, or Enovid-E 21 from the first row of her package, one tablet daily, starting with the pill day which corresponds to day 5 of her menstrual cycle; the first day of menstruation is counted as day 1. After the last (Saturday) tablet in row #3 has been taken, if any remain in the first row, the patient completes her 21-tablet schedule starting with Sunday in row #1.

Subsequent Cycles: The patient begins a new 21-tablet course on the eighth day after taking her last tablet, again starting the same day of the week on which she began her first course. All subsequent cycles will also begin on that same day, one tablet being taken each day for three weeks followed by a week of no pill-taking.

Postpartum Administration. Ovulen-21 and Ovulen-28 oral contraceptives may be prescribed at the first postpartum examination regardless of whether or not the patient has experienced spontaneous menstruation. In non-nursing mothers, administration may be initiated immediately after delivery if desired or on the first Sunday after delivery. If preferred the tablets may be started on the day the patient leaves the hospital. (For nursing mothers, see *Warning* No. 12.) Increased risk of thromboembolism during the postpartum period must be considered. (See *Contraindications, Warnings,* and *Precautions.*)

Hypermenorrhea; Production of Cyclic Withdrawal Bleeding: Enovid 5 mg or 10 mg only. Most patients with hypermenorrhea may be expected to respond to Enovid 5-mg or 10-mg therapy within 24 to 48 hours. Regular withdrawal bleeding may then be induced by cyclic administration. Vaginal bleeding at times other than the regular menstrual period requires that a diagnosis be established prior to beginning therapy.

For emergency control of severe bleeding in patients with hypermenorrhea give 20 to 30 mg of Enovid daily until the bleeding is controlled, then reduce the daily dose to 10 mg and continue through day 24 of the cycle. Then discontinue Enovid and withdrawal flow usually will begin approximately two to three days later.

Cyclic withdrawal bleeding may be produced after treatment in this initial cycle by giving the patient 5 to 10 mg of Enovid 5 mg or 10 mg daily from day 5 through day 24 of the next two or three cycles. A new course of Enovid therapy should be started on day 5 of her menstrual cycle or eight days after the last pill from the previous cycle, whichever occurs first. The first day of menstruation is counted as day 1.

Endometriosis: Enovid 5 mg or 10 mg only. A daily dose of Enovid should be given for six to nine months or longer on the following schedule: 5 or 10 mg should be given for two weeks beginning on day 5 of a menstrual cycle. This daily dose should be given continuously (without cyclic interruption) and increased 5 or 10 mg at two-week intervals until the patient is receiving 20 mg daily. This dose of 20 mg should be continued for six to nine months and further increased (up to 40 mg daily) if breakthrough bleeding occurs.

Therapy may be discontinued after six months if the disease is mild and the lesions are no longer palpable. If the disorder is more severe continue treatment for nine months or longer. When surgery is contemplated, prior administration of Enovid may facilitate the surgical procedure. (See *Warning* No. 1 concerning discontinuation prior to elective surgery.)

Special Notes: *Spotting or Breakthrough Bleeding.* If spotting (bleeding insufficient to require a pad) or breakthrough bleeding (heavier bleeding similar to a menstrual flow) occurs when these products are used for contraception the patient should continue taking her tablets as directed. The incidence of spotting or breakthrough bleeding is minimal, most frequently occurring in the first cycle. Ordinarily spotting or breakthrough bleeding will stop within a week. Usually the patient will begin to cycle regularly within two or three courses of tablet-taking. If breakthrough bleeding occurs while the patient is taking Enovid for hypermenorrhea she should immediately increase the daily dosage by 5 or 10 mg until bleeding has been controlled for three days, after which the original dosage usually may be resumed. In the event of spotting or breakthrough bleeding organic causes should be borne in mind. (See *Warning* No. 10.)

Missed Menstrual Periods. Withdrawal flow will normally occur two or three days after the last active tablet is taken. Failure of withdrawal bleeding ordinarily does not mean that the patient is pregnant, providing the dosage schedule has been correctly followed. (See *Warning* No. 5.)

If the patient has *not* adhered to the prescribed dosage regimen, the possibility of pregnancy should be considered after the first missed period, and oral contraceptives should be withheld until pregnancy has been ruled out.

If the patient has adhered to the prescribed regimen and misses two consecutive periods, pregnancy should be ruled out before continuing the contraceptive regimen.

The first intermenstrual interval after discontinuing the tablets is usually prolonged; consequently, a patient for whom a 28-day cycle is usual might not begin to menstruate for 35 days or longer. Ovulation in such prolonged cycles will occur correspondingly later in the cycle. Posttreatment cycles after the first one, however, are usually typical for the individual woman prior to taking tablets. (See *Warnings* No. 10 and 11.)

Missed Tablets (Contraception). If a woman misses taking one active tablet the missed tablet should be taken as soon as it is remembered. In addition, the next tablet should be taken at the usual time. If two consecutive active tablets are missed the dosage should be doubled for the next two days. The regular schedule should then be resumed, but an additional method of protection is recommended for the remainder of the cycle.

While there is little likelihood of ovulation if only one active tablet is missed, the possibility of spotting or breakthrough bleeding is increased and should be expected if two or more successive active tablets are missed. However, the possibility of ovulation increases with each successive day that scheduled active tablets are missed.

If one or more placebo tablets of Demulen 1/35™ -28, Demulen 1/50™-28, or Ovulen-28 are missed, the Demulen 1/35™-28, Demulen 1/50™-28, or Ovulen-28 schedule should be resumed on the following Sunday (the eighth day after the last white tablet was taken). Omission of placebo tablets in the 28-tablet courses does not increase the possibility of conception provided that this schedule is followed.

HOW SUPPLIED

Demulen 1/35: Each white Demulen 1/35 tablet is round in shape, with a debossed SEARLE on one side and 151 and design on the other side, and contains 1 mg of ethynodiol diacetate and 35 mcg of ethinyl estradiol.

Demulen 1/35™-21 is packaged in cartons of 6 and 24 Compack tablet dispensers of 21 tablets each, and in cartons of 12 Compack refills of 21 tablets each.

Demulen 1/35™-28 is packaged in cartons of 6 and 24 Compack tablet dispensers and in cartons of 12 Compack refills. Each Compack and refill contains 21 white Demulen 1/35 tablets and 7 blue placebo tablets. (Placebo tablets have a debossed SEARLE on one side and a "P" on the other side.)

Demulen: 1/50: Each white Demulen 1/50 tablet is round in shape, with a debossed SEARLE on one side and 71 on the other side, and contains 1 mg of ethynodiol diacetate and 50 mcg of ethinyl estradiol.

Demulen 1/50™-21 is packaged in cartons of 6 and 24 Compack tablet dispensers of 21 tablets each, and in cartons of 12 Compack refills of 21 tablets each.

Demulen 1/50™-28 is packaged in cartons of 6 and 24 Compack tablet dispensers and in cartons of 12 Compack refills. Each Compack and refill contains 21 white Demulen 1/50 tablets and 7 pink placebo tablets. (Placebo tablets have a debossed SEARLE on one side and a "P" on the other side.)

Ovulen: Each white Ovulen tablet is pentagonal in shape, with a debossed SEARLE on one side and 401 on the other side, and contains 1 mg of ethynodiol diacetate and 0.1 mg of mestranol.

Ovulen-21 is packaged in cartons of 6 and 24 Compack tablet dispensers of 21 tablets each, and in cartons of 12 Compack refills of 21 tablets each.

Ovulen-28 is packaged in cartons of 6 Compack tablet dispensers and in cartons of 12 Compack refills. Each Compack and refill contains 21 white Ovulen tablets and 7 pink placebo tablets. (Placebo tablets have a debossed SEARLE on one side and a "P" on the other side.)

Enovid-E: Each Enovid-E tablet is pale pink, round in shape, with a debossed SEARLE E on one side and 131 on the other side, and contains 2.5 mg of norethynodrel and 0.1 mg of mestranol.

Enovid-E 21 is packaged in cartons of 6 Compack tablet dispensers of 21 tablets each, and in cartons of 12 Compack refills of 21 tablets each.

Enovid 5 mg: Each Enovid 5 mg tablet is pink, round in shape, with a debossed SEARLE 5 on one side and 51 on the other side, and contains 5 mg of norethynodrel and 75 mcg of mestranol. Enovid 5 mg is packaged in bottles of 100 tablets each.

Enovid 10 mg: Each Enovid 10 mg tablet is coral colored, round in shape, with a debossed SEARLE 10 on one side and 101 on the other side, and contains 9.85 mg of norethynodrel and 0.15 mg of mestranol. Enovid 10 mg is packaged in bottles of 50 tablets each.

REFERENCES

1. Population Reports, Series H, No. 2 (May) 1974; Series I, No. 1 (June) 1974; Series B, No. 3 (May) 1979; Series H, No. 3 (Jan.) 1975; Series H, No. 4 (Jan.) 1976; Population Information Program, Geo. Washington U. Medical Center, Washington, D.C. **2.** Inman, W. H. W., et al.: Br. Med. J. *2*:203 (April 25) 1970. **3.** Inman, W. H. W., et al.: Br. Med. J. *2*:193 (April 27) 1968. **4.** Royal College of General Practitioners: J. Coll. Gen. Pract. *13*:267 (May) 1967. **5.** Vessey, M. P., et al.: Br. Med. J. *2*:651 (June 14) 1969. **6.** Sartwell, P. E., et al.: Am. J. Epidemiol. *90*:365 (Nov.) 1969. **7.** Boston Collaborative Drug Surveillance Programme: Lancet *1*:1399 (June 23) 1973. **8.** Stolley, P.D., et al.: Am. J. Epidemiol. *102*:197 (Sept.) 1975. **9.** Collaborative Group for the Study of Stroke in Young Women: N. Engl. J. Med. *288*:871 (April 26) 1973.

10. Collaborative Group for the Study of Stroke in Young Women: J.A.M.A. *231*:718 (Feb. 17) 1975. **11.** Beral, V.: Lancet *2*:1047 (Nov. 13) 1976. **12.** Royal College of General Practitioners: Oral Contraceptives and Health, New York, Pitman Publ. Corp., May 1974. **13.** Layde, P., et al.: Lancet *1*:541 (March 7) 1981. **13a.** Beral, V., et al.: Lancet *2*:727 (Oct. 8) 1977. **14.** Vessey, M., et al.: J. Biosoc. Sci. *8*:373 (Oct.) 1976. **15.** Vessey, M., et al.: Lancet *2*:731 (Oct. 8) 1977; *1*:549 (March 7) 1981. **16.** Mann, J. I., et al.: Br. Med. J. *2*:241 (May 3) 1975. **17.** Mann, J. I., et al.: Br. Med. J. *3*:631 (Sept. 13) 1975. **18.** Mann, J. I., et al.: Br. Med. J. *2*:245 (May 3) 1975. **19.** Mann, J. I., et al.: Br. Med. J. *2*:445 (Aug. 21) 1976.

20. Jain, A. K.: Stud. Fam. Plann. *8*:50 (March) 1977. **21.** Tietze, C.: Fam. Plann. Perspect. *9*:74 (March-April) 1977. **22.** Vessey, M. P., et al.: Br. Med. J. *3*:123 (July 18) 1970. **23.** Greene, G. R., et al.: Am. J. Public Health *62*:680 (May) 1972. **24.** Ziel, H. K., et al.: N. Engl. J. Med. *293*:1167 (Dec. 4) 1975. **25.** Smith, D. C., et al.: N. Engl. J. Med. *293*:1164 (Dec. 4) 1975. **26.** Mack, T. M., et al.: N. Engl. J. Med. *294*:1262 (June 3) 1976. **27.** Gray, L. A., et al.: Obstet. Gynecol. *49*:385 (April) 1977. **28.** McDonald, T. W., et al.: Am. J. Obstet. Gynecol. *127*:572 (March 15) 1977. **29.** Weiss, N. S., et al.: N. Engl. J. Med. *294*:1259 (June 3) 1976.

30. Silverberg, S. G., et al.: Cancer *39*:592 (Feb.) 1977. **31.** Vessey, M. P., et al.: Br. Med. J. *3*:719 (Sept. 23) 1972. **32.** Vessey, M. P., et al.: Lancet *1*:941 (April 26) 1975. **33.** Boston Collaborative Drug Surveillance Program: N. Engl. J. Med. *290*:15 (Jan. 3) 1974. **34.** Arthes, F. G., et al.: Cancer *28*:1391 (Dec.) 1971. **35.** Casagrande, J., et al.: J. Natl. Cancer Inst. *56*:839 (April) 1976. **36.** Fasal, E., et al.: J. Natl. Cancer Inst. *55*:767 (Oct.) 1975. **37.** Paffenbarger, R. S., et al.: Cancer *49*:1887 (April Suppl.) 1977. **38.** Hoover, R., et al.: N. Engl. J. Med. *295*:401 (Aug. 19) 1976. **39.** Kelsey, J. L., et al.: Am. J. Epidemiol. *107*:236 (March) 1978.

40. Ory, H., et al.: N. Engl. J. Med. *294*:419 (Feb. 19) 1976. **41.** Stern, E., et al.: Science *196*:1460 (June 24) 1977. **42.** Population Reports, Series A, No. 4 (May) 1977: Population Information Program, Geo. Washington U. Medical Center, Washington, D.C. **43.** Baum, J. K., et al.: Lancet *2*:926 (Oct. 27) 1973. **44.** Taler, S.J., et al.: Obstet. Gynecol. *65*:665 (May) 1985. **45.** Edmondson, H. A., et al.: N. Engl. J. Med. *294*:470 (Feb. 26) 1976. **46.** Rooks, J. B., et al.: J.A.M.A. *242*: 644 (Aug. 17) 1979. **47.** Herbst, A. L., et al.: N. Engl. J. Med. *284*:878 (April 22) 1971. **48.** Greenwald, P., et al.: N. Engl. J. Med. *285*:390 (Aug. 12) 1971. **49.** Lanier, A. P., et al.: Mayo Clin. Proc. *48*:793 (Nov.) 1973.

50. Herbst, A. L., et al.: Am. J. Obstet. Gynecol. *128*:43 (May 1) 1977. **51.** Herbst, A. L., et al.: Obstet. Gynecol. *40*:287 (Sept.) 1972. **52.** Herbst, A. L., et al.: Am. J. Obstet. Gynecol. *118*:607 (March 1) 1974. **53.** Herbst, A. L., et al.: N. Engl. J. Med. *292*:334 (Feb. 13) 1975. **54.** Stafl, A., et al.: Obstet. Gynecol. *43*:118 (Jan.) 1974. **55.** Sherman, A. I., et al.: Obstet. Gynecol. *44*:531 (Oct.) 1974. **56.** Bibbo, M., et al.: J. Reprod. Med. *15*:29 (July) 1975. **57.** Gill, W., et al.: J. Reprod. Med. *16*:147 (April) 1976. **58.** Henderson, B., et al.: Pediatrics *58*:505 (Oct.) 1976. **59.** Gal, I., et al.: Nature *240*:241 (Nov. 24) 1972.

60. Levy, E. P., et al.: Lancet *1*:611 (March 17) 1973. **61.** Nora, J. J., et al.: Lancet *1*:941 (April 28) 1973. **62.** Nora, A. H., et al.: Arch. Environ. Health *30*:17 (Jan.) 1975; Adv. Plann. Parent. *12*:156, 1978. **63.** Janerich, D. T., et al.: N. Engl. J. Med. *291*:697 (Oct. 3) 1974. **64.** Heinonen, O. P., et al.: N. Engl. J. Med. *296*:67 (Jan. 13) 1977. **65.** Nora, J. J., et al.: N. Engl. J. Med. *291*:731 (Oct. 3) 1974. **66.** Carr, D. H.: Can. Med. Assoc. J. *103*:343 (Aug. 15 & 29) 1970. **67.** Wynn, V., et al.: Lancet *2*:720 (Oct. 1) 1966. **68.** Laragh, J. H.: Am. J. Obstet. Gynecol. *126*:141 (Sept.) 1976. **69.** Fisch, I. R., et al.: J.A.M.A. *237*:2499 (June 6) 1977.

70. Van Campenhout, J., et al.: Fertil. Steril. *28*:728 (July) 1977. **71.** Laumas, K. R., et al.: Am. J. Obstet. Gynecol. *98*:411 (June 1) 1967. **72.** Stockley, I.: Pharmaceut. J. *216*:140 (Feb. 14) 1976. **73.** Hempel, E., et al.: Drugs *12*:442 (Dec.) 1976. **74.** Bessot, J.-C., et al.: Nouv. Presse Med. *6*:1568 (April 30) 1977. **75.** Francis, W. G., et al.: Can. Med. Assoc. J. *92*:191 (Jan. 23) 1965. **76.** Verhulst, H. L., et al.: J. Clin. Pharmacol. 7:9 (Jan.-Feb.) 1967. **77.** Vessey, M. P., et al.: Br. Med. J. *2*:199 (April 27) 1968. **78.** Ory, H. W.: J.A.M.A. *237*:2619 (June 13) 1977. **79.** Jain, A. K.: Am. J. Obstet. Gynecol. *126*:301 (Oct. 1) 1976.

80. Ziel, H. K., et al.: Am. J. Obstet. Gynecol. *124*:735 (April 1) 1976. **81.** Peritz, E., et al.: Am. J. Epidemiol. *106*:462 (Dec.) 1977. **82.** Ory, H. W., et al.: in Garattini, S., and Berendes, H. (eds.), Pharmacology of Steroid Contraceptive Drugs, Raven Press, N.Y., 1977. **83.** Goldacre, M. J., et al.: Br. Med. J. *1*:748 (March 25) 1978. **84.** Meisels, A., et al.: Cancer *40*:3076 (Dec.) 1977. **85.** Klatskin, G.: Gastroenterology *73*:386 (Aug.) 1977.

Continued on next page

Searle & Co.—Cont.

86. Kay, C. R.: Lancet *1*:624 (March 19) 1977. **87.** March, C. M., et al.: Fertil. Steril. *28*:346 (March) 1977. **88.** Saxena, B. N., et al.: Contraception *16*:605 (Dec.) 1977. **89.** Nilsson, S., et al.: Contraception *17*:131 (Feb.) 1978.
90. Vessey, M. P., et al.: Br. Med. J. *1*:265 (Feb. 4) 1978. **91.** Jick, H., et al.: J.A.M.A. *239*:1403, 1407 (April 3) 1978. **92.** Kay, C. R.: J. R. Coll. Gen. Pract. *28*:393 (July) 1978. **93.** Hoogerland, D. L., et al.: Gynecol. Oncol. *6*:451 (Oct.) 1978. **94.** Lorber, C. A., et al.: Fertil. Steril. *31*:21 (Jan.) 1979. **95.** Bacon, J. F., et al.: Br. Med. J. *280*:293 (Feb. 2) 1980. **96.** Meade, T. W., et al.: Br. Med. J. *280*:1157 (May 10) 1980. **97.** Böttiger, L. E., et al.: Lancet *1*:1097 (May 24) 1980. **98.** Maguire, M. G., et al.: Am. J. Epidemiol. *110*:188 (Aug.) 1979. **99.** Ramcharan, S., et al.: The Walnut Creek Contraceptive Drug Study, Vol. 3, U.S. Govt. Ptg. Off., 1981; J. Reprod. Med. *25*:346 (Dec.) 1980.
100. Petitti, D. B., et al.: Am. J. Epidemiol. *108*:480 (Dec.) 1978. **101.** Petitti, D. B., et al.: J.A.M.A. *242*:1150 (Sept. 14) 1979. **102.** Petitti, D. B., et al.: Lancet *2*:234 (July 29) 1978. **103.** Jick, H., et al.: Ann. Int. Med. *88*:58 (July) 1978. **104.** Jick, H., et al.: J.A.M.A. *240*:2548 (Dec. 1) 1978. **105.** Shapiro, S., et al.: Lancet *1*:743 (April 7) 1979. **106.** Rosenberg, L., et al.: Am. J. Epidemiol. *111*:59 (Jan.) 1980. **107.** Kreuger, D. E., et al.: Am. J. Epidemiol. *111*:655 (June) 1980. **108.** Arthes, F. G., et al.: Chest *70*:574 (Nov.) 1976. **109.** Hoover, R., et al.: Am. J. Public Health *18*:335 (April) 1978.
110. Herbst, A. L., et al.: J. Reprod. Med. *24*:62 (Feb.) 1980. **111.** Barnes, A. B., et al.: N. Engl. J. Med. *302*:609 (March 13) 1980. **112:** Cousins, L., et al.: Obstet. Gynecol. *56*:70 (July) 1980. **113.** Nora, J. J., et al.: J.A.M.A. *240*:837 (Sept. 1) 1978. **114.** Aarskog, D.: N. Engl. J. Med. *300*:75 (Jan. 11) 1979. **115.** Janerich, D. T., et al.: Am. J. Epidemiol. *112*:73 (July) 1980. **116.** Kasan, P. N., et al.: Br. J. Obstet. Gynaecol. *87*:545 (July) 1980. **117.** Rothman, K. J.: N. Engl. J. Med. *297*:468 (Sept. 1) 1977. **118.** Bracken, M. B.: Am. J. Obstet. Gynecol. *133*:432 (Feb. 15) 1979. **119.** De Teresa, E., et al.: Br. Med. J. *2*:1260 (Nov. 17) 1979.
120. Swan, S., et al.: Am. J. Obstet. Gynecol. *139*:52 (Jan. 1) 1981. **121.** Kay, C. R.: Br. Med. J. *282*:2089 (June 27) 1981. **122.** Vessey, M. P., et al.: Br. Med. J. *282*:2093 (June 27) 1981. **123.** Pike, M. C., et al.: Br. J. Cancer *43*:72 (Jan.) 1981. **124.** Harlap, S., et al.: Obstet. Gynecol. *55*:447 (April) 1980. **125.** Back, D. J., et al.: Drugs *21*:46 (Jan.) 1981. **126.** Porter, J. B., et al.: Obstet. Gynecol. *59*:229 (March) 1982. **127.** Lees, A.W., et al.: Int. J. Cancer *22*:700, 1978. **128.** Brinton, L. A., et al.: J. Natl. Cancer Inst. (JNCI) *62*:37 (Jan.) 1979. **129.** Black, M. M.: Pathol. Res. Pract. *166*:491. 1980; Cancer *46*:2747 (Dec.) 1980; Cancer *51*: 2147 (June 1) 1983.
130. Hoover, R., et al.: JNCI *67*:815 (Oct.) 1981. **131.** Gill, W. B., et al.: J. Urol. *122*:36 (July) 1979. **132.** Linn, S., et al.: J.A.M.A. *247*:629 (Feb. 5) 1982. **133.** Clavel, F., et al.: Bull. Cancer (Paris) *68*:449 (Dec.) 1981. **134.** Abernethy, D. R., et al.: N. Engl. J. Med. *306*:791 (April 1) 1982. **135.** Kay, C. R.: Am. J. Obstet. Gynecol. *142*:762 (March 15) 1982. **136.** Adam, S. A., et al.: Br. J. Obstet. Gynaecol. *88*:838 (Aug.) 1981. **137.** Slone, D., et al.: N. Engl. J. Med. *305*:420 (Aug. 20) 1981. **138.** Layde, P.M., et al.: J.R. Coll. Gen. Pract. *33*:75 (Feb.) 1983. **139.** Abernethy, D. R., et al.: Obstet. Gynecol. *60*:338 (Sept.) 1982.
140. Brinton, L.A., et al.: Int. J. Epidemiol. *11*:316, 1982. **141.** Harris, N.V., et al.: Am. J. Epidemiol. *116*: 643 (Oct.) 1982. **142.** Pike, M.C., et al.: Lancet *2*:926 (Oct. 22) 1983. **143.** Vessey, M.P., et al.: Lancet *2*:930 (Oct. 22) 1983. **144.** Jick, H., et al.: Am. J. Epidemiol. *112*:577 (Nov.) 1980. **145.** Jick, H., et al.: Am. J. Epidemiol. *112*:586 (Nov.) 1980. **146.** McPherson, K., et al.: Lancet *2*:1414 (Dec. 17) 1983. **147.** Vessey, M.P., et al.: Br. Med. J. *289*:530 (Sept. 1) 1984. **148.** Olsson, H., et al.: Lancet *1*:748 (March 30) 1985. **149.** Thomas, D.B., et al.: Br. Med. J. *290*:961 (March 30) 1985.
150. Dallenbach-Hellweg, G.: Path. Res. Pract. *179*:38, 1984. **151.** Washington, A.E., et al.: J.A.M.A. *253*:2246 (April 19) 1985. **152.** Rosenberg, L., et al.: J.A.M.A. *253*:2965 (May 24/31) 1985. **153.** Baciewicz, A.M.: Therap. Drug Monitor. *7*:26 (March) 1985. **154.** Robboy, S.J., et al.: J.A.M.A. *252*:2979 (Dec. 7) 1984. **155.** Vessey, M.P., et al.: Br. J. Fam. Plan. *11*:120 (Jan.) 1986. **156.** Vessey, M.P., et al.: Br. Med. J. *292*:526 (Feb. 22) 1986. **157.** Henderson, B.E., et al.: Br. J. Cancer *48*:437 (July) 1983. **158.** Neuberger, J., et al.: Br. Med. J. *292*:1355 (May 24) 1986. **159.** Forman, D., et al.: Br. Med. J. *292*:1357 (May 24) 1986.
160. Pinto, M.R.: Mutat. Res. *169*:149 (March) 1986.

Brief Summary of Patient Labeling

Cigarette-smoking increases the risk of serious adverse effects on the heart and blood vessels from oral contraceptive use. This risk increases with age and with heavy smoking (15 or more cigarettes per day) and is quite marked in women over 35 years of age. Women who use oral contraceptives should not smoke.

In the detailed leaflet, "What You Should Know About Oral Contraceptives," which you have received, the risks and benefits of oral contraceptives are discussed in much more detail. This leaflet also provides information on other forms of contraception. Please take time to read it carefully for it may have been recently revised.

If you have any questions or problems regarding this information, contact your doctor.

Oral contraceptives taken as directed are about 99% effective in preventing pregnancy. (The mini-pill, however, is somewhat less effective.) Forgetting to take your pills increases the chance of pregnancy.

Women who have or have had clotting disorders, cancer of the breast or sex organs, unexplained vaginal bleeding, stroke, heart attack, chest pains on exertion (angina pectoris), liver tumors associated with the use of the pill or with other estrogen-containing products, or who suspect they may be pregnant should not use oral contraceptives.

Most side effects of the pill are not serious. The most common side effects are nausea, vomiting, bleeding between menstrual periods, weight gain, and breast tenderness. However, proper use of oral contraceptives requires that they be taken under your doctor's continuing supervision, because they can be associated with serious side effects which may be fatal. Fortunately, these are very uncommon, but the risks may persist after use of the pill is discontinued. The serious side effects are:

1. Blood clots in the legs, arms, lungs, brain, heart, eyes, abdomen, or elsewhere in the body.
2. Bleeding in the brain (hemorrhage) as a result of bursting of a blood vessel.
3. Disorders of vision.
4. Liver tumors, which may rupture and cause severe bleeding.
5. Birth defects if the pill is taken during pregnancy.
6. High blood pressure.
7. Gallbladder disease.

The symptoms associated with these serious side effects are discussed in the detailed leaflet given you with your supply of pills. Notify your doctor if you notice any unusual physical disturbance while taking the pill.

Breast cancer and other cancers have developed in certain animals when given the estrogens in oral contraceptives for long periods. These findings suggest that oral contraceptives may also cause cancer in humans. However, studies to date in women taking currently marketed oral contraceptives have not confirmed that oral contraceptives cause cancer in humans.

Caution: Oral contraceptives are of no value in the prevention or treatment of venereal disease.

Various drugs, such as antibiotics, may also decrease the effectiveness of oral contraceptives.

Detailed Patient Labeling: What You Should Know About Oral Contraceptives

Oral contraceptives (the pill) are the most effective way (except for sterilization) to prevent pregnancy if you follow the directions for their use and are careful not to skip doses or take them irregularly. They are also convenient and, for most women, free of serious or unpleasant side effects. Oral contraceptives must always be taken under the continuing supervision of a doctor.

It is important that any woman who considers using an oral contraceptive understands the risks involved. Although the oral contraceptives have important advantages over other methods of contraception, they have certain risks that no other method has. Only you can decide whether the advantages are worth these risks. This leaflet will tell you about the most important risks. It will explain how you can help your doctor prescribe the pill as safely as possible by telling him/her about yourself and being alert for the earliest signs of trouble. And it will tell you how to use the pill properly, so that it will be as effective as possible. THERE IS MORE DETAILED INFORMATION AVAILABLE IN THE LEAFLET PREPARED FOR DOCTORS. Your pharmacist can show you a copy; you may need your doctor's help in understanding parts of it.

Enovid 5 mg or 10 mg can be prescribed as a treatment for endometriosis and as a treatment for hypermenorrhea and regulating periods. If you are taking Enovid 5 mg or 10 mg for one of these other conditions besides contraception the warning information in this detailed leaflet also applies, so please read this leaflet.

Caution: Oral contraceptives are of no value in the prevention or treatment of venereal disease.

Cigarette-smoking increases the risk of serious adverse effects on the heart and blood vessels from oral contraceptive use. This risk increases with age and with heavy smoking (15 or more cigarettes per day) and is quite marked in women over 35 years of age. Women who use oral contraceptives should not smoke.

Who Should Not Use Oral Contraceptives:
You should not use oral contraceptives:

A. If you have any of the following conditions:
   1. Blood clots in the legs, lungs, eyes, or elsewhere in the body.
   2. Chest pains on exertion (angina pectoris).
   3. Known or suspected cancer of the breast or sex organs, such as the womb (uterus), vagina, or cervix.
   4. Unusual vaginal bleeding that has not been diagnosed by your doctor.
   5. Known or suspected pregnancy (one or more menstrual periods missed).
B. If you have had any of the following conditions:
   1. Heart attack or stroke (clots or bleeding in the brain).
   2. Blood clots in the legs, lungs, eyes, or elsewhere in the body.
   3. Liver tumor associated with use of the pill or other estrogen-containing products.
C. If you have scanty or irregular periods or are a young woman without a regular cycle, you should use another method of contraception because, if you use the pill, you may have difficulty becoming pregnant or may fail to have menstrual periods after discontinuing the pill.

Deciding to Use Oral Contraceptives. If you do not have any of the conditions listed above and are thinking about using oral contraceptives, to help you decide, you need information about the advantages and risks of oral contraceptives and of other contraceptive methods as well. This leaflet describes the advantages and risks of oral contraceptives. Except for sterilization, the intrauterine device (IUD), and abortion, which have their own specific risks, the only risks of other methods of contraception are those due to pregnancy should the method fail. Your doctor can answer questions you may have with respect to other methods of contraception, and further questions you may have on oral contraceptives after reading this leaflet.

1. *What Oral Contraceptives Are and How They Work.*
Oral contraceptives are of two types. The most common, often simply called "the pill," is a *combination* of an estrogen and a progestogen, the two kinds of female hormones. The amount of estrogen and progestogen can vary, but the amount of estrogen is more important because both the effectiveness and some of the dangers of oral contraceptives have been related to the amount of estrogen. This combination oral contraceptive works principally by preventing release of an egg from the ovary during the cycle in which the pills are taken. When the amount of estrogen is 50 micrograms or more, and the pill is taken as directed, oral contraceptives are more than 99% effective (that is, there would be less than 1 pregnancy in 100 women using the pill for one year). Pills that contain 20 to 35 micrograms of estrogen vary slightly in effectiveness, ranging from 98% to more than 99% effective.
The second type of oral contraceptive, often called the mini-pill, contains only a progestogen. It works in part by preventing release of an egg from the ovary, but also by keeping sperm from reaching the egg and by making the womb (uterus) less receptive to any fertilized egg that reaches it. The mini-pill is less effective than the combination oral contraceptive, about 97% effective. In addition, the mini-pill has a tendency to cause irregular bleeding, which may be quite inconvenient, or cessation of bleeding entirely. The mini-pill is used despite its lower effectiveness in the hope that it will prove not to have some of the serious side effects of the estrogen-containing pill, but it is not yet certain that the mini-pill does in fact have fewer serious side effects. The following discussion, while based mainly on information about the combination pills, should be considered to apply as well to the mini-pill.

2. *Other Nonsurgical Ways to Prevent Pregnancy.*
As this leaflet will explain, oral contraceptives have several serious risks. Other methods of contraception have lesser risks or none at all. They are also less effective than oral contraceptives, but, used properly, may be effective enough for many women. The following table gives reported pregnancy rates (the number of women out of 100 who would become pregnant in one year) for these methods:

Pregnancies per 100 Women per Year

Method	*Range*
Intrauterine device (IUD)	less than 1 to 6
Diaphragm with spermicidal cream or jelly	2 to 20
Condom (rubber)	3 to 36
Spermicidal aerosol foams	2 to 29
Spermicidal jellies or creams	4 to 36
Periodic abstinence (rhythm), all types	less than 1 to 47
1. Calendar method	14 to 47
2. Temperature method	1 to 20
3. Temperature method (intercourse only in postovulatory phase)	less than 1 to 7
4. Mucus method	1 to 25
No contraception	60 to 80

These figures (except for the IUD) vary widely because people differ in how well they use each method. Very faithful users of the various methods obtain the best results, except for users of the periodic abstinence (rhythm) calendar method. Effective use of these methods, except for the IUD, requires somewhat more effort than simply taking a single pill every day, but it is an effort that many couples undertake successfully. Your doctor can tell you a great deal more about these methods of contraception and their effectiveness.

3. *The Dangers of Oral Contraceptives.*

a. *Circulatory disorders (blood clots, strokes, and heart attacks).* Blood clots occasionally form in the blood vessels of the body and, though rare, are the most common of the serious side effects of oral contraceptives. Clotting can result in a stroke (a clot in the brain), a heart attack (a clot in a blood vessel of the heart), or a pulmonary embolus (a clot that forms in the legs or abdominal region, then breaks off and travels to the lungs), or loss of a limb (a clot in a blood vessel in, or leading to, an arm or leg). Clots can also form in the blood vessels of the intestines or liver. Any of these events can be fatal (lead to death). Clots also occur rarely in the blood vessels of the eye, resulting in blindness or impairment of vision in that eye. There is some evidence that the risk of clotting may increase with higher estrogen doses. It is therefore important for your doctor to keep the dose of estrogen as low as possible, so long as the oral contraceptive used has an acceptable pregnancy rate and doesn't cause unacceptable changes in the menstrual pattern. Higher doses of progestogen have also been suggested as increasing the risk of clotting. Furthermore, cigarette-smoking by oral contraceptive users increases the risk of serious adverse effects on the heart and blood vessels. This risk increases with age and with heavy smoking (15 or more cigarettes per day) and begins to become quite marked in women over 35 years of age. For this reason, women who use oral contraceptives should not smoke.

The risk of abnormal clotting increases with age both in users and in nonusers of oral contraceptives, but the increased risk with the oral contraceptives appears to be present at all ages.

The risks of circulatory disorders may persist or continue after the pill is stopped. This has been reported for circulatory disorders in general, for heart disease or heart attacks, and for strokes caused either by a bursting blood vessel in the brain or by blood clots in the brain.

For oral contraceptive users in general, it has been estimated that in women between the ages of 25 and 34 the risk of death due to circulatory disorders in nonsmokers is about 1 in 23,000 per year. In contrast, for nonusers of the pill the risk is about 1 in 37,000 per year. Estimates of the risk of death due to circulatory disorders can be made, depending upon the woman's age, whether or not she uses oral contraceptives, and whether or not she smokes cigarettes. In the age group 25–34 years, women who use the pill have a risk of 1 in 7,000 (for smokers) to 1 in 23,000 (for nonsmokers) per year. This may be compared to the corresponding risk in women who have not used the pill: 1 in 24,000 (for smokers) to 1 in 37,000 (for nonsmokers) per year. The risks are greater in older women; thus, in the age group 35–44 years, women who use the pill have a risk of 1 in 1,600 (for smokers) to 1 in 4,700 (for nonsmokers) per year. The corresponding risk for women who have not used the pill is 1 in 6,600 (for smokers) to 1 in 16,000 (for nonsmokers) per year.

For women aged 16 to 40 it is estimated that about 1 in 2,000 using oral contraceptives will be hospitalized each year because of abnormal clotting in the veins or lungs. Among nonusers of the same age, about 1 in 20,000 would be hospitalized each year for these disorders.

Disease of the arteries characterized by paleness, numbness, or tingling in the fingers or toes has been reported to be more common in pill users.

Strokes are caused by a bursting blood vessel in the brain (hemorrhage) or a loss of blood circulation to the brain due to blood clots. When they occur, paralysis of all or part of the body may result; death can result. The risk of strokes due to clots or hemorrhages in the brain has been reported to be increased in pill users when compared with nonusers.

It has been estimated that pill users are twice as likely as nonusers to have a stroke due to a bursting blood vessel in the brain. It has further been estimated that pill users are 4 to 10 times as likely as nonusers to have a stroke due to clotting in a blood vessel in or leading to the brain.

It has been reported that women using the pill may have a greater risk of heart attack than nonusers. Even without the pill the risk of having a heart attack increases with age and is also increased by additional risk factors such as high blood pressure, high blood cholesterol, obesity, diabetes, cigarette-smoking, or the occurrence during pregnancy of high blood pressure, swelling of the legs, or protein in the urine. Without any risk factors present, the use of oral contraceptives alone may double the risk of heart attack. However, the combination of cigarette-smoking, especially heavy smoking, and oral contraceptive use greatly increases the risk of heart attack. Oral contraceptive users who smoke are about five times more likely to have a heart attack than users who do not smoke, and about ten times more likely to have a heart attack than nonusers who do not smoke. It has been estimated that users between the ages of 30 and 39 who smoke have about a 1 in 10,000 chance each year of having a fatal heart attack compared to about a 1 in 50,000 chance in users who do not smoke, and about a 1 in 100,000 chance in nonusers who do not smoke. In the age group 40 to 44, the risk is about 1 in 1,700 per year for users who smoke compared to about 1 in 10,000 for users who do not smoke, and to about 1 in 14,000 per year for nonusers who do not smoke. Heavy smoking (about 15 cigarettes or more a day) further increases the risk. If you do not smoke and have none of the other heart attack risk factors described above, you will have a smaller risk than listed. If you have several heart attack risk factors, the risk may be considerably greater than listed. The above are average figures for Great Britain; comparable estimates for the U.S. have been higher.

Oral contraceptives should never be used at any age by women who have had a stroke, a heart attack, or chest pains on exertion (angina pectoris), or who have had blood clots in the legs, lungs, or elsewhere.

Anyone using the pill who has severe leg or chest pains, coughs up blood, has difficulty in breathing, severe headache or vomiting, dizziness or fainting, disturbances of vision or speech, weakness, numbness, or pain in an arm or leg should call her doctor immediately and stop taking the pill, and use another method of contraception.

b. *Formation of tumors.* When certain animals are given the female sex hormone estrogen (which is an ingredient in oral contraceptives) continuously for long periods, cancers may develop in organs such as the breast, cervix, vagina, liver, womb, ovary, and pituitary.

These findings suggest that oral contraceptives may cause cancer in humans. However, studies to date in women taking currently marketed oral contraceptives have not confirmed that oral contraceptives cause cancer in humans, but it remains possible they will be discovered in the future to do so. Several studies have found no increase in breast cancer in users, although it has been suggested that oral contraceptives might cause an increase in breast cancer in women who already have benign (noncancerous) breast disease (for example, cysts), in long-term (2–4 years) users, or in the presence of other risk factors (such as a family history of breast cancer, a previous breast biopsy, or delay in having the first child).

Women with a family history of breast cancer or who have breast nodules (lumps), fibrocystic disease (breast cysts), or abnormal mammograms (x-ray pictures of the breasts), or who were exposed to the estrogen diethylstilbestrol (DES) during their mother's pregnancy, or who have abnormal Pap smears should be followed very closely by their doctors if they choose to use oral contraceptives instead of another method of contraception. Many studies have shown that women taking oral contraceptives have less risk of getting benign (noncancerous) breast disease than those who have not used oral contraceptives. There is strong evidence that estrogens (one component of combination-type oral contraceptives), when given for periods of more than one year to women after the menopause (change-of-life), increase the risk of cancer of the womb (uterus). There is also some evidence that the sequential oral contraceptive, a kind of oral contraceptive that is no longer sold, may increase the risk of cancer of the womb. There is no evidence, however, that the oral contraceptives now available increase the risk of this type of cancer, although some individual cases have been reported. Cancer of the cervix may develop more readily in long-term users of the pill, particularly if they have had preexisting abnormal Pap smears. Cervical erosion and cell abnormalities, as well as chlamydial infections, have been reported to be more frequent in pill users.

Very rarely, oral contraceptive users may have a noncancerous tumor of the liver. These tumors do not spread, but they may rupture and cause internal bleeding, which may be fatal. This has been reported in short-term as well as long-term users, although increasing duration of use increases the risk. Long-term users have an estimated annual incidence of 3 to 4 per 100,000. One study reported that oral contraceptive products with a high "hormonal potency" were associated with a higher risk than lower-potency products, as was age over 30 years. Cases of cancer of the liver have been reported in women using oral contraceptives also. Users for 8 or more years were estimated to be 7 to 20 times more likely to develop this cancer than were nonusers.

A type of skin cancer that has been linked to exposure to sunlight (malignant melanoma) has been reported to be more frequent among pill users. It was not possible to determine what the effect was of greater exposure to sunlight in users.

c. *Dangers to a developing baby if oral contraceptives are used in or immediately preceding pregnancy.* Oral contraceptives should not be taken by pregnant women because they may damage the developing baby. There is an increased risk to the baby of abnormalities of such parts of the body as the backbone, anus, heart, windpipe, esophagus, kidneys, arms, and legs. In addition, the developing female child whose mother has received DES, a synthetic estrogen, during pregnancy has a risk of getting cancer of the vagina or cervix in her teens or young adulthood. This risk is estimated to be about 1 in 1,000 exposures or less. DES-exposed daughters appear to have an increased risk of unfavorable outcome of pregnancy. Abnormalities of the urinary and sex organs and sperm have been reported in DES-exposed male babies as well. It is possible that other estrogens, such as the estrogens in oral contraceptives, could have the same effect in the baby if the mother takes them during pregnancy.

Occasionally women who are taking the pill miss periods. It has been reported to occur as frequently as several times each year in some women, depending on various factors such as age and prior history. (Your doctor is the best source of information about this.) The pill should not be used when you are pregnant or suspect you may be pregnant. Very rarely, women who are using the pill as directed become pregnant. The likelihood of becoming pregnant is higher if you occasionally miss one or two pills. Therefore, if you miss a period you should consult your physician before continuing to take the pill. If you miss a period, especially if you have not taken the pill regularly, you should use an alternative method of contraception until pregnancy has been ruled out; if you have missed more than one pill at any time, you should immediately start using an additional method of contraception and complete your pill cycle.

You should not attempt to become pregnant for at least three months after discontinuing oral contraceptives. Use another method of contraception during this period of time. The reason for this is that during this period there may be an increased risk of miscarriage and deformity to the baby, or an increased chance of having twins. Whether there is an overall increase in miscarriage in women who become pregnant soon after stopping the pill as compared with women who did not use the pill is not known, but it is possible that there may be.

If, however, you do become pregnant soon after stopping oral contraceptives, and do not have a miscarriage, there is no evidence that the baby has an increased risk of being abnormal.

d. *Gallbladder disease.* Women who use oral contraceptives have a greater risk than nonusers of having gallbladder disease requiring surgery. The increased risk may first appear within one year of use and may double after 4 or 5 years of use.

e. *Other side effects of oral contraceptives.* Some women using oral contraceptives experience unpleasant side effects from the pill which are not dangerous and are not likely to damage their health. Some of these side effects are similar to symptoms women experience in early pregnancy and may be temporary. Your breasts may feel tender, be enlarged, or have a discharge; nausea and vomiting or other stomach or intestinal problems may occur; you may gain or lose weight, and your ankles may swell. A spotty darkening of the skin, particularly of the face, is possible and may persist after the drug is discontinued. An allergic or other type of rash or vaginal yeast infection might occur. You may notice unexpected vaginal bleeding, change in discharge, or changes in your menstrual period. Irregular bleeding is frequently seen when the mini-pill or the combination oral contraceptives containing less than 50 micrograms of estrogen are used. These should all be reported to your doctor.

Other side effects include worsening of migraine, asthma, convulsive disorders (such as epilepsy), and kidney, liver, or heart disease because of a tendency for water to be retained in the body when oral contraceptives are used. Other side effects are painful periods; growth of preexisting fibroid tumors of the womb; mental depression; and liver problems with jaundice (yellowing of the whites of the eyes or of the skin). Your doctor may find that levels of sugar and fatty substances in your blood are elevated; the long-term effects of these changes are not known. Some women develop high blood pressure while taking oral contraceptives, which ordinarily, but not always, returns to the original levels when the oral contraceptive is stopped. The degree of blood pressure rise may be related to the amount of progestogen in the pill. Women with a history of increased blood pressure, kidney disease, or toxemia during pregnancy (increased blood pressure, swelling of the legs, protein in the urine, or convulsions), or a family tendency to high blood pressure or its consequences (stroke, heart disease, kidney disease, blood vessel problems), or a history of excessive weight gain or swelling of the legs during their menstrual cycle, may be more likely to develop increased blood pressure when given oral contraceptives; therefore, they should have their blood pressure taken frequently. High blood pressure predisposes one to stroke, heart attacks, kidney disease, and other diseases of the blood vessels. The effect of prolonged use of oral contraceptives on several of your organs (pituitary, liver, ovaries, womb, and adrenals) or immune system is not known at this time.

Continued on next page

Searle & Co.—Cont.

Increased damage to the chromosomes of white blood cells has been reported in pill users. The significance for cancer or birth defects is unknown.

Other conditions, although not proved to be caused by oral contraceptives, are occasionally reported. These include more frequent urination and some discomfort when urinating, kidney disease, nervousness, dizziness, hearing problems, inflammation of the nasal passages, loss of scalp hair, an increase in body hair, an increase or decrease in sex drive, appetite changes, gum disease, dry socket, cataracts, a need for a change in contact lens prescription or inability to use contact lenses, tiredness, backache, vaginal infections, itching, anemia, blood cell breakdown with kidney failure, headache, symptoms similar to those you get before a period; breast, womb, cervical, and liver cancer; inflammation of the pancreas, liver, or large or small intestine; chorea (spasmodic movements), burning or prickly sensation, rheumatoid arthritis, pulmonary hypertension, abnormal heart rhythm, and a bruising disease caused by decreased blood platelets (TTP).

After you stop using oral contraceptives, there may be a delay before you are able to become pregnant or before you resume having menstrual periods. This is especially true of women who had irregular menstrual cycles prior to the use of oral contraceptives.

One study showed that this delay in becoming pregnant can persist up to 72 months after stopping the pill if you have never had children and are over 30 years old. The delay appears to be more severe if the pill has been used for 2 years or more by such women. For women who have had children, the delay can persist to 30 months, regardless of age. For women who have not had children and who are less than 30, the delay may persist to 48 months. Very rarely there may be secretions from the breast associated with the absence of periods, which might be due to a noncancerous tumor of the pituitary gland requiring surgery. This may occur more frequently in former users of the pill than in nonusers. As discussed previously, you should wait at least three months after stopping the pill before you try to become pregnant. During the first three months after stopping oral contraceptives, use another form of contraception. You should consult your doctor before resuming use of oral contraceptives after childbirth, especially if you plan to nurse your baby. Drugs in oral contraceptives are known to appear in the milk, and the long-range effect on babies is not known at this time. Furthermore, oral contraceptives may cause a decrease in your milk supply as well as in the quality of the milk.

4. *Comparison of the Risks of Oral Contraceptives and Other Contraceptive Methods.*

The many studies on the risks and effectiveness of oral contraceptives and other methods of contraception have been analyzed to estimate the risk of death associated with various methods of contraception. This risk has two parts: (a) the risk of the method itself (for example, the risk that oral contraceptives might cause death due to abnormal blood clotting), and (b) the risk of death due to pregnancy or abortion in the event the method should fail. The results of this analysis are shown in the following bar graph. The height of the bars indicates the number of deaths per 100,000 women each year. There are six sets of bars, each set referring to a specific age group of women. Within each set of bars, there is a single bar for each of the different contraceptive methods.

For oral contraceptives, there are two bars—one for smokers and the other for nonsmokers. The analysis is based on present knowledge and new information could, of course, alter it. The analysis shows that the risk of death from all methods of birth control is low and below that associated with the risks of childbirth, *except for oral contraceptives in women over 40 who smoke.* The risk of death associated with pill use in nonsmokers over 40 is higher than with any other method of contraception in that age group. It shows that the lowest risk of death is associated with the condom or diaphragm (traditional contraception) backed up by early legal abortion in case of failure of the condom or diaphragm to prevent pregnancy. Also, at any age, the risk of death (due to unexpected pregnancy) from use of traditional contraception, even without a backup of abortion, is generally the same as, or less than, that from use of oral contraceptives.

How to Use Oral Contraceptives as Safely and Effectively as Possible, Once You Have Decided to Use Them:

1. *What to Tell Your Doctor.* You can make use of the pill as safe as possible, by telling your doctor if you have any of the following:

a. Conditions that mean you should not use oral contraceptives:

If you *now* have any of the following:

1. Blood clots in the legs, lungs, eyes, or elsewhere in the body.
2. Chest pains on exertion (angina pectoris).
3. Known or suspected cancer of the breast or sex organs, such as the womb (uterus), vagina, or cervix.
4. Unusual vaginal bleeding that has not been diagnosed by your doctor.

Figure 1 Estimated annual number of deaths associated with control of fertility and no control per 100 000 nonsterile women by regimen of control and age of woman

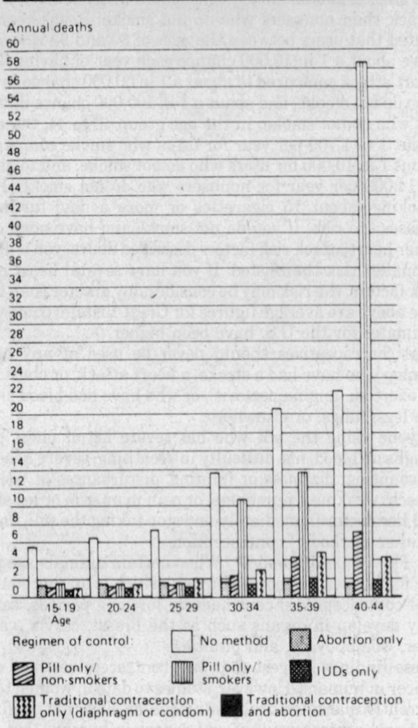

5. Known or suspected pregnancy (one or more menstrual periods missed).

If you have *ever* had any of the following:

1. Heart attack or stroke (clots or bleeding in the brain).
2. Blood clots in the legs, lungs, eyes, or elsewhere in the body.
3. Liver tumor associated with use of the pill or other estrogen-containing products.

b. Inform your doctor of the following conditions since s/he will want to watch them closely or they might cause him/her to suggest another method of contraception:

A family history of breast cancer

Breast nodules (lumps), fibrocystic disease (breast cysts), abnormal mammograms (x-ray pictures of the breasts), or abnormal Pap smears

Diabetes

High blood pressure

High blood cholesterol

Cigarette-smoking

Migraine

Heart or kidney disease

Asthma

Problems during a prior pregnancy

Epilepsy

Mental depression

Fibroid tumors of the womb

History of jaundice (yellowing of the whites of the eyes or of the skin)

Gallbladder disease

Varicose veins

Tuberculosis

Plans for elective surgery

Previous problems with your periods (irregularities)

Use of any of the following kinds of drugs, which might interact with the pill: antibiotics (such as rifampin, ampicillin, and tetracycline), sulfa drugs, drugs for epilepsy or migraine, painkillers, tranquilizers, sedatives or sleeping pills, blood-thinning drugs, cortisone-like drugs, vitamins, drugs being used for the treatment of depression, high blood pressure, high blood sugar (diabetes), elevated blood lipids, or asthma

c. Once you are using oral contraceptives, you should be alert for signs of a serious adverse effect and call your doctor immediately if any of these occur:

Sharp pain in the chest, coughing up of blood, or sudden shortness of breath (indicating possible clots in the lungs).

Pain in the calf (possible clot in the leg).

Crushing chest pain or heaviness (indicating possible heart attack).

Sudden severe headache or vomiting, dizziness or fainting, disturbance of vision or speech, or weakness or numbness in an arm or leg (indicating a possible stroke).

Sudden partial or complete loss of vision (indicating a possible clot in the blood vessels of the eye).

Abnormal vaginal bleeding.

Breast discharge or lumps (you should ask your doctor to show you how to examine your own breasts).

Severe and/or persistent pain or a mass in the abdomen (indicating a possible tumor of the liver, which might have ruptured).

Severe depression.

Yellowing of the whites of the eyes or of the skin (jaundice).

Unusual swelling.

Other unusual conditions.

2. *How to Take the Pill So That It Is Most Effective. Dosage Schedules.* See later sections in this leaflet concerning spotting, breakthrough bleeding, forgotten pills, and missed menstruation.

When you first begin to use the pill, you should use an additional method of protection until you have taken your first seven pills.

To remove a pill, press down on it. The pill will drop through a hole in the bottom of the Compack®.

The "20-pill" Schedule. Enovid® 5 mg may be prescribed on the 20-pill schedule.

Take a pill each day for 20 consecutive days, beginning each pill cycle on day 5 after your period starts, just as you did during the first pill cycle, or on the eighth day after having taken the last pill, whichever occurs first. Count the day you start to menstruate as day 1.

Continue this 20-pill schedule, cycle after cycle, regardless of whether your flow has or has not ceased when you start or whether you happen to spot or experience unexpected (breakthrough) bleeding during a cycle.

You will probably have your periods about every 27 days.

The Two "three weeks on—one week off" Schedules. Your Demulen 1/35™-21, Demulen 1/50™ -21, Ovulen 21, or Enovid-E 21 Compack contains 21 tablets arranged in three numbered rows with the days of the week printed above them.

Day-5 Schedule. If you are to begin on day 5, count the day you start to menstruate as day 1 and determine which day to start. Start in row #1 with the pill under the day which corresponds to day 5 after your flow began. Continue to take one pill each day on consecutive days of the week.

After the last (Saturday) pill in row #3 has been taken, if any remain in the first row, complete your 21-pill schedule by taking one pill daily starting with Sunday in row #1. Then stop for one week before starting to take the pills again. Begin your next pill cycle on the same day of the week that you began the first cycle.

Sunday Schedule. Start taking the pills on the first Sunday after your period begins unless your period begins on Sunday. If your period begins on Sunday start taking the pill that very same day.

Begin in row #1 and take your pills, one each day on consecutive days, for three weeks (21 days), then stop taking them for one week (7 days) before starting to take the pills again on Sunday.

Whether you begin on "day 5" or on Sunday, continue taking your pills as directed, month after month, regardless of whether your flow has or has not ceased or whether you may have experienced spotting or unexpected (breakthrough) bleeding during your pill cycle. You will probably have your period about every 28 days.

The "Pill-a-day" Schedule. Your Demulen 1/35™-28, Demulen 1/50™-28, or Ovulen-28 Compack contains 28 pills arranged in four numbered rows of seven pills each with the days of the week printed above them.

You must take your pills in order, one pill each day. Begin with the Sunday pill in row #1.

1—Start taking the pills on the first Sunday after your period begins unless your period begins on Sunday. *If your period begins on Sunday start taking the pills that very same day.*

2—Continue to take one pill each day on consecutive days of the week.

3—After the Saturday pill in row #1 has been taken begin taking pills in row #2, and so on, until the Saturday pill in row #4 has been taken.

4—Replace the Refill in your Compack at once, and begin a new pill cycle the next day, starting with the Sunday pill in row #1.

You will probably have your period about every 28 days, while you are taking the pink (blue for Demulen 1/35™-28) pills.

Continue your pill-a-day schedule, month after month, regardless of whether your flow ceases while you are taking the colored pills, or whether you experience spotting or unexpected (breakthrough) bleeding during a cycle.

Take your pill faithfully every "pill day"!

It is important that you take a pill without fail every pill day at intervals of 24 hours, for two reasons. First, your ovaries may release an egg and therefore you may become pregnant if you do not take your pills regularly. Second, you may spot or start to flow between your periods. This may be inconvenient.

Take your pill at the same time every day!
You are probably wondering why the same time of day is important. By taking your pill at the same time every day it becomes a good habit, and you are much less likely to forget. You may wish to keep your pills in the medicine cabinet near your toothbrush as a reminder to take them when you brush your teeth at night. The best time to take your daily pill may be either with your evening meal or at bedtime. You may find it helpful to associate your pill-taking with something else you do every day at a particular time.
Another very important reason for you to take your pills as "regular as clockwork" is that you are protected best when you take one every 24 hours; they are made to work that way. Just remember that once every day is not the same as once every 24 hours. Here is why: Suppose you were to take your Monday pill in the morning when you get up, and then not take your Tuesday pill till the evening before you go to bed. True, you will have taken a pill each day, on Monday and on Tuesday—but the time between pill-taking will probably have been more than 36 hours, or more than 1½ days! You might spot. Chances are you would still be protected and would not get pregnant, but why risk it when it is so easy to guarantee yourself maximal protection by taking your pill faithfully every pill day and at the same time every pill day?
In summary, you should take the pills exactly as directed and at intervals of 24 hours in order to achieve maximum contraceptive effectiveness.
Spotting. This is a slight staining between your menstrual periods which may not even require a pad. Some women spot even though they take their pills exactly as directed. Many women spot although they have never taken the pills. Spotting does not mean that your ovaries are releasing an egg. Spotting may be the result of irregular pill-taking. Getting back on schedule will usually stop it.
If you should spot while taking the pills you should not be alarmed because spotting usually stops by itself within a few days. It seldom occurs after the first pill cycle. Consult your doctor if spotting persists for more than a few days or if it occurs after the second cycle.
Unexpected (Breakthrough) Bleeding. Unexpected (breakthrough) bleeding does not mean your ovaries have released an egg. It seldom occurs, but when it does happen it is most common in the first pill cycle. It is a flow much like a regular period, requiring the use of a pad or tampon.
If you experience breakthrough bleeding use a pad or tampon and continue with your schedule. Usually your periods will become regular within a few cycles. Breakthrough bleeding will seldom bother you again.
Consult your doctor if breakthrough bleeding does not stop within a week or if it occurs after the second cycle.
Forgotten Pills. There is little likelihood of your getting pregnant if only one active pill is missed; however, the possibility increases with each successive day that the scheduled active pills are missed. If you forget to take a pill one day, take two the next day—the one you forgot as soon as you remember and your regular pill at your usual time.
If you forget your pills (except the inactive colored pills in Demulen 1/35™-28, Demulen 1/50™-28, or Ovulen-28) on two consecutive days, do not be surprised if you spot or start to flow. You should take two pills each day for the next two days, and use an additional method of protection for the remainder of the cycle.
If you are using Demulen 1/35™-28, Demulen 1/50™-28, or Ovulen-28 and forget to take one or more colored pills, begin a new cycle on the next Sunday; use a new package and start taking the white pills. Missing the colored pills does not increase your chances of getting pregnant providing the white pill schedule has been followed.
Missed Menstruation. At times there may be no menstrual period after a cycle of pills. Therefore, if you miss one menstrual period but have taken the pills *exactly as you were supposed to*, continue as usual into the next cycle. You may wish to call your doctor. If you have not taken the pills correctly and miss a menstrual period, *you may be pregnant* and should stop taking oral contraceptives until your doctor determines whether or not you are pregnant. Until you can get to your doctor, use another form of contraception. If two consecutive menstrual periods are missed, you should stop taking the pills until it is determined whether you are pregnant. If you do become pregnant while using oral contraceptives, you should discuss the risks to the developing baby with your doctor.
3. *Periodic Examinations.* Your doctor will take a complete medical and family history before prescribing oral contraceptives. At that time and about once a year thereafter, s/he will generally examine your blood pressure, breasts, abdomen, and internal female organs (including a Pap smear test for cancer of the cervix) and perform certain laboratory tests. Certain health problems or conditions in your medical or family history may require that your doctor see you more frequently while you are taking the pill.
4. *Using Enovid for Purposes Other Than Contraception.* Since dosage schedules for these uses must be individualized for each patient, please follow the directions of your doctor.

SUMMARY

Oral contraceptives are the most effective method, except sterilization, for preventing pregnancy. Other methods, when used conscientiously, are also very effective and have fewer risks. The serious side effects of oral contraceptives are uncommon, but the risk of experiencing them may persist after discontinuing the pill. The pill is a very convenient method for preventing pregnancy.
Women who use oral contraceptives should not smoke.
If you have certain conditions or have had these conditions in the past, you should not use oral contraceptives because of increased risk. These conditions are listed in this leaflet. If you do not have these conditions, and decide to use the pill, please read this leaflet carefully so that you can use the pill safely and effectively. Be certain to read new revisions of this leaflet.
Based on your doctor's assessment of your medical needs, this drug has been prescribed for you. Do not give it to anyone else.
See your doctor regularly, ask any questions you may have about the use of the pill, and report any special problems that may arise.

These products are shown in the Product Identification Section, page 429

ENOVID-E® 21 ℞

[*ē-nov 'id-ē*]
(norethynodrel with mestranol)

See Demulen products under Searle & Co. for Enovid-E 21 prescribing information.
Shown in Product Identification Section, page 429

ENOVID® 5 mg ℞
ENOVID® 10 mg ℞

[*ē-nov 'id*]
(norethynodrel with mestranol)

See Demulen products under Searle & Co. for Enovid 5 mg and Enovid 10 mg prescribing information.
Shown in Product Identification Section, page 429

FLAGYL® Tablets ℞

[*flaj 'yl*]
(metronidazole)

> **WARNING**
> Metronidazole has been shown to be carcinogenic in mice and rats (see *Warnings*). Unnecessary use of the drug should be avoided. Its use should be reserved for the conditions described in the *Indications and Usage* section below.

DESCRIPTION

Flagyl (metronidazole) is an oral synthetic antiprotozoal and antibacterial agent, 1-(β-hydroxyethyl)-2-methyl-5-nitroimidazole, which has the following structural formula:

CH_2CH_2OH O_2N N CH_3 N

Inactive ingredients include cellulose, FD&C Blue No. 2 Lake, hydroxypropyl cellulose, hydroxypropyl methylcellulose, polyethylene glycol, stearic acid, and titanium dioxide.

CLINICAL PHARMACOLOGY

Disposition of metronidazole in the body is similar for both oral and intravenous dosage forms, with an average elimination half-life in healthy humans of eight hours.
The major route of elimination of metronidazole and its metabolites is via the urine (60–80% of the dose), with fecal excretion accounting for 6–15% of the dose. The metabolites that appear in the urine result primarily from side-chain oxidation [1-(β-hydroxyethyl)- 2-hydroxymethyl-5-nitroimidazole and 2-methyl-5-nitroimidazole-1-yl-acetic acid] and glucuronide conjugation, with unchanged metronidazole accounting for approximately 20% of the total. Renal clearance of metronidazole is approximately 10 ml/min/1.73 m^2.
Metronidazole is the major component appearing in the plasma, with lesser quantities of the 2-hydroxymethyl metabolite also being present. Less than 20% of the circulating metronidazole is bound to plasma proteins. Both the parent compound and the metabolite possess *in vitro* bactericidal activity against most strains of anaerobic bacteria and *in vitro* trichomonacidal activity.
Metronidazole appears in cerebrospinal fluid, saliva, and breast milk in concentrations similar to those found in plasma. Bactericidal concentrations of metronidazole have also been detected in pus from hepatic abscesses.
Following oral administration metronidazole is well absorbed, with peak plasma concentrations occurring between one and two hours after administration. Plasma concentrations of metronidazole are proportional to the administered dose. Oral administration of 250 mg, 500 mg, or 2,000 mg produced peak plasma concentrations of 6 mcg/ml, 12 mcg/ml, and 40 mcg/ml, respectively. Studies reveal no significant bioavailability differences between males and females; however, because of weight differences, the resulting plasma levels in males are generally lower.
Decreased renal function does not alter the single-dose pharmacokinetics of metronidazole. However, plasma clearance of metronidazole is decreased in patients with decreased liver function.
Microbiology: *Trichomonas vaginalis, Entamoeba histolytica.* Flagyl (metronidazole) possesses direct trichomonacidal and amebacidal activity against *T. vaginalis* and *E. histolytica.* The *in vitro* minimal inhibitory concentration (MIC) for most strains of these organisms is 1 mcg/ml or less.
Anaerobic Bacteria. Metronidazole is active *in vitro* against most obligate anaerobes, but does not appear to possess any clinically relevant activity against facultative anaerobes or obligate aerobes. Against susceptible organisms, metronidazole is generally bactericidal at concentrations equal to or slightly higher than the minimal inhibitory concentrations. Metronidazole has been shown to have *in vitro* and clinical activity against the following organisms:

Anaerobic gram-negative bacilli, including:
- *Bacteroides* species including the *Bacteroides fragilis* group (*B. fragilis, B. distasonis, B. ovatus, B. thetaiotaomicron, B. vulgatus)*
- *Fusobacterium* species

Anaerobic gram-positive bacilli, including:
- *Clostridium* species and susceptible strains of *Eubacterium*

Anaerobic gram-positive cocci, including:
- *Peptococcus* species
- *Peptostreptococcus* species

Susceptibility Tests: Bacteriologic studies should be performed to determine the causative organisms and their susceptibility to metronidazole; however, the rapid, routine susceptibility testing of individual isolates of anaerobic bacteria is not always practical, and therapy may be started while awaiting these results.
Quantitative methods give the most precise estimates of susceptibility to antibacterial drugs. A standardized agar dilution method and a broth microdilution method are recommended.[1]
Control strains are recommended for standardized susceptibility testing. Each time the test is performed, one or more of the following strains should be included: *Clostridium perfringens* ATCC 13124, *Bacteroides fragilis* ATCC 25285, and *Bacteroides thetaiotaomicron* ATCC 29741. The mode metronidazole MICs for those three strains are reported to be 0.25, 0.25, and 0.5 mcg/ml, respectively.
A clinical laboratory is considered under acceptable control if the results of the control strains are within one doubling dilution of the mode MICs reported for metronidazole.
A bacterial isolate may be considered susceptible if the MIC value for metronidazole is not more than 16 mcg/ml. An organism is considered resistant if the MIC is greater than 16 mcg/ml. A report of "resistant" from the laboratory indicates that the infecting organism is not likely to respond to therapy.

INDICATIONS AND USAGE

Symptomatic Trichomoniasis. Flagyl is indicated for the treatment of symptomatic trichomoniasis in females and males when the presence of the trichomonad has been confirmed by appropriate laboratory procedures (wet smears and/or cultures).
Asymptomatic Trichomoniasis. Flagyl is indicated in the treatment of asymptomatic females when the organism is associated with endocervicitis, cervicitis, or cervical erosion. Since there is evidence that presence of the trichomonad can interfere with accurate assessment of abnormal cytological smears, additional smears should be performed after eradication of the parasite.
Treatment of Asymptomatic Consorts. *T. vaginalis* infection is a venereal disease. Therefore, asymptomatic sexual partners of treated patients should be treated simultaneously if the organism has been found to be present, in order to prevent reinfection of the partner. The decision as to whether to treat an asymptomatic male partner who has a negative culture or one for whom no culture has been attempted is an individual one. In making this decision, it should be noted that there is evidence that a woman may become reinfected if her consort is not treated. Also, since there can be considerable difficulty in isolating the organism from the asymptomatic male carrier, negative smears and cultures cannot be relied upon in this regard. In any event, the consort should be treated with Flagyl in cases of reinfection.

Continued on next page

Searle & Co.—Cont.

Amebiasis. Flagyl is indicated in the treatment of acute intestinal amebiasis (amebic dysentery) and amebic liver abscess.

In amebic liver abscess, Flagyl therapy does not obviate the need for aspiration or drainage of pus.

Anaerobic Bacterial Infections. Flagyl is indicated in the treatment of serious infections caused by susceptible anaerobic bacteria. Indicated surgical procedures should be performed in conjunction with Flagyl therapy. In a mixed aerobic and anaerobic infection, antibiotics appropriate for the treatment of the aerobic infection should be used in addition to Flagyl.

In the treatment of most serious anaerobic infections, Flagyl I.V.™ (metronidazole hydrochloride) or Flagyl I.V.™ RTU® (metronidazole) is usually administered initially. This may be followed by oral therapy with Flagyl (metronidazole) at the discretion of the physician.

INTRA-ABDOMINAL INFECTIONS, including peritonitis, intra-abdominal abscess, and liver abscess, caused by *Bacteroides* species including the *B. fragilis* group (*B. fragilis, B. distasonis, B. ovatus, B. thetaiotaomicron, B. vulgatus), Clostridium* species, *Eubacterium* species, *Peptococcus* species, and *Peptostreptococcus* species.

SKIN AND SKIN STRUCTURE INFECTIONS caused by *Bacteroides* species including the *B. fragilis* group, *Clostridium* species, *Peptococcus* species, *Peptostreptococcus* species, and *Fusobacterium* species.

GYNECOLOGIC INFECTIONS, including endometritis, endomyometritis, tubo-ovarian abscess, and postsurgical vaginal cuff infection, caused by *Bacteroides* species including the *B. fragilis* group, *Clostridium* species, *Peptococcus* species, and *Peptostreptococcus* species.

BACTERIAL SEPTICEMIA caused by *Bacteroides* species including the *B. fragilis* group, and *Clostridium* species.

BONE AND JOINT INFECTIONS, as adjunctive therapy, caused by *Bacteroides* species including the *B. fragilis* group.

CENTRAL NERVOUS SYSTEM (CNS) INFECTIONS, including meningitis and brain abscess, caused by *Bacteroides* species including the *B. fragilis* group.

LOWER RESPIRATORY TRACT INFECTIONS, including pneumonia, empyema, and lung abscess, caused by *Bacteroides* species including the *B. fragilis* group.

ENDOCARDITIS caused by *Bacteroides* species including the *B. fragilis* group.

CONTRAINDICATIONS

Flagyl is contraindicated in patients with a prior history of hypersensitivity to metronidazole or other nitroimidazole derivatives.

In patients with trichomoniasis, Flagyl is contraindicated during the first trimester of pregnancy. (See *Warnings.*)

WARNINGS

Convulsive Seizures and Peripheral Neuropathy: Convulsive seizures and peripheral neuropathy, the latter characterized mainly by numbness or paresthesia of an extremity, have been reported in patients treated with metronidazole. The appearance of abnormal neurologic signs demands the prompt discontinuation of Flagyl therapy. Flagyl should be administered with caution to patients with central nervous system diseases.

Tumorigenicity Studies in Rodents: Metronidazole has shown evidence of carcinogenic activity in a number of studies involving chronic, oral administration in mice and rats. Prominent among the effects in the mouse was the promotion of pulmonary tumorigenesis. This has been observed in all six reported studies in that species, including one study in which the animals were dosed on an intermittent schedule (administration during every fourth week only). At very high dose levels (approx. 500 mg/kg/day) there was a statistically significant increase in the incidence of malignant liver tumors in males. Also, the published results of one of the mouse studies indicate an increase in the incidence of malignant lymphomas as well as pulmonary neoplasms associated with lifetime feeding of the drug. All these effects are statistically significant.

Several long-term, oral-dosing studies in the rat have been completed. There were statistically significant increases in the incidence of various neoplasms, particularly in mammary and hepatic tumors, among female rats administered metronidazole over those noted in the concurrent female control groups.

Two lifetime tumorigenicity studies in hamsters have been performed and reported to be negative.

Mutagenicity Studies: Although metronidazole has shown mutagenic activity in a number of *in vitro* assay systems, studies in mammals (*in vivo*) have failed to demonstrate a potential for genetic damage.

PRECAUTIONS

General: Patients with severe hepatic disease metabolize metronidazole slowly, with resultant accumulation of metronidazole and its metabolites in the plasma. Accordingly, for such patients, doses below those usually recommended should be administered cautiously.

Known or previously unrecognized candidiasis may present more prominent symptoms during therapy with Flagyl and requires treatment with a candicidal agent.

Information for Patients: Alcoholic beverages should be avoided while taking Flagyl and for at least one day afterward. See *Drug Interactions.*

Laboratory Tests: Flagyl (metronidazole) is a nitroimidazole and should be used with care in patients with evidence of or history of blood dyscrasia. A mild leukopenia has been observed during its administration; however, no persistent hematologic abnormalities attributable to metronidazole have been observed in clinical studies. Total and differential leukocyte counts are recommended before and after therapy for trichomoniasis and amebiasis, especially if a second course of therapy is necessary, and before and after therapy for anaerobic infection.

Drug Interactions: Metronidazole has been reported to potentiate the anticoagulant effect of warfarin and other oral coumarin anticoagulants, resulting in a prolongation of prothrombin time. This possible drug interaction should be considered when Flagyl is prescribed for patients on this type of anticoagulant therapy.

The simultaneous administration of drugs that induce microsomal liver enzymes, such as phenytoin or phenobarbital, may accelerate the elimination of metronidazole, resulting in reduced plasma levels; impaired clearance of phenytoin has also been reported.

The simultaneous administration of drugs that decrease microsomal liver enzyme activity, such as cimetidine, may prolong the half-life and decrease plasma clearance of metronidazole.

Alcoholic beverages should not be consumed during Flagyl therapy and for at least one day afterward because abdominal cramps, nausea, vomiting, headaches, and flushing may occur.

Drug/Laboratory Test Interactions: Metronidazole may interfere with certain types of determinations of serum chemistry values, such as aspartate aminotransferase (AST, SGOT), alanine aminotransferase (ALT, SGPT), lactate dehydrogenase (LDH), triglycerides, and hexokinase glucose. Values of zero may be observed. All of the assays in which interference has been reported involve enzymatic coupling of the assay to oxidation-reduction of nicotine adenine dinucleotide ($NAD^+ \rightleftharpoons NADH$).

Interference is due to the similarity in absorbance peaks of NADH (340 nm) and metronidazole (322 nm) at pH 7.

Carcinogenesis: See *Warnings.*

Pregnancy: Teratogenic Effects—Pregnancy Category B. Metronidazole crosses the placental barrier and enters the fetal circulation rapidly. Reproduction studies have been performed in rats at doses up to five times the human dose and have revealed no evidence of impaired fertility or harm to the fetus due to metronidazole. Metronidazole administered intraperitoneally to pregnant mice at approximately the human dose caused fetotoxicity; administered orally to pregnant mice, no fetotoxicity was observed. There are, however, no adequate and well-controlled studies in pregnant women. Because animal reproduction studies are not always predictive of human response, and because metronidazole is a carcinogen in rodents, this drug should be used during pregnancy only if clearly needed (see *Contraindications*).

Use of Flagyl for trichomoniasis in the second and third trimesters should be restricted to those in whom local palliative treatment has been inadequate to control symptoms.

Nursing Mothers: Because of the potential for tumorigenicity shown for metronidazole in mouse and rat studies, a decision should be made whether to discontinue nursing or to discontinue the drug, taking into account the importance of the drug to the mother. Metronidazole is secreted in breast milk in concentrations similar to those found in plasma.

Pediatric Use: Safety and effectiveness in children have not been established, except for the treatment of amebiasis.

ADVERSE REACTIONS

Two serious adverse reactions reported in patients treated with Flagyl (metronidazole) have been convulsive seizures and peripheral neuropathy, the latter characterized mainly by numbness or paresthesia of an extremity. Since persistent peripheral neuropathy has been reported in some patients receiving prolonged administration of Flagyl, patients should be specifically warned about these reactions and should be told to stop the drug and report immediately to their physicians if any neurologic symptoms occur.

The most common adverse reactions reported have been referable to the gastrointestinal tract, particularly nausea reported by about 12% of patients, sometimes accompanied by headache, anorexia, and occasionally vomiting; diarrhea; epigastric distress; and abdominal cramping. Constipation has also been reported.

The following reactions have also been reported during treatment with Flagyl (metronidazole):

Mouth: A sharp, unpleasant metallic taste is not unusual. Furry tongue, glossitis, and stomatitis have occurred; these may be associated with a sudden overgrowth of *Candida* which may occur during effective therapy.

Hematopoietic: Reversible neutropenia (leukopenia).

Cardiovascular: Flattening of the T-wave may be seen in electrocardiographic tracings.

Central Nervous System: Convulsive seizures, peripheral neuropathy, dizziness, vertigo, incoordination, ataxia, confusion, irritability, depression, weakness, and insomnia.

Hypersensitivity: Urticaria, erythematous rash, flushing, nasal congestion, dryness of mouth (or vagina or vulva), and fever.

Renal: Dysuria, cystitis, polyuria, incontinence, and a sense of pelvic pressure. Instances of darkened urine have been reported by approximately one patient in 100,000. Although the pigment which is probably responsible for this phenomenon has not been positively identified, it is almost certainly a metabolite of metronidazole and seems to have no clinical significance.

Other: Proliferation of *Candida* in the vagina, dyspareunia, decrease of libido, proctitis, and fleeting joint pains sometimes resembling "serum sickness." If patients receiving Flagyl drink alcoholic beverages, they may experience abdominal distress, nausea, vomiting, flushing, or headache. A modification of the taste of alcoholic beverages has also been reported.

Crohn's disease patients are known to have an increased incidence of gastrointestinal and certain extraintestinal cancers. There have been some reports in the medical literature of breast and colon cancer in Crohn's disease patients who have been treated with metronidazole at high doses for extended periods of time. A cause and effect relationship has not been established. Crohn's disease is not an approved indication for Flagyl.

OVERDOSAGE

Single oral doses of metronidazole, up to 15 g, have been reported in suicide attempts and accidental overdoses. Symptoms reported include nausea, vomiting, and ataxia.

Oral metronidazole has been studied as a radiation sensitizer in the treatment of malignant tumors. Neurotoxic effects, including seizures and peripheral neuropathy, have been reported after 5 to 7 days of doses of 6 to 10.4 g every other day.

Treatment: There is no specific antidote for Flagyl overdose; therefore, management of the patient should consist of symptomatic and supportive therapy.

DOSAGE AND ADMINISTRATION

Trichomoniasis:

In the Female:

One-day treatment—two grams of Flagyl, given either as a single dose or in two divided doses of one gram each given in the same day.

Seven-day course of treatment—250 mg three times daily for seven consecutive days. There is some indication from controlled comparative studies that cure rates as determined by vaginal smears, signs and symptoms, may be higher after a seven-day course of treatment than after a one-day treatment regimen.

The dosage regimen should be individualized. Single-dose treatment can assure compliance, especially if administered under supervision, in those patients who cannot be relied on to continue the seven-day regimen. A seven-day course of treatment may minimize reinfection of the female long enough to treat sexual contacts. Further, some patients may tolerate one course of therapy better than the other.

Pregnant patients should not be treated during the first trimester with either regimen. If treated during the second or third trimester, the one-day course of therapy should not be used, as it results in higher serum levels which reach the fetal circulation. (See *Contraindications* and *Precautions.*)

When repeat courses of the drug are required, it is recommended that an interval of four to six weeks elapse between courses and that the presence of the trichomonad be reconfirmed by appropriate laboratory measures. Total and differential leukocyte counts should be made before and after re-treatment.

In the Male: Treatment should be individualized as for the female.

Amebiasis:

Adults:

For acute intestinal amebiasis (acute amebic dysentery): 750 mg orally three times daily for 5 to 10 days.

For amebic liver abscess: 500 mg or 750 mg orally three times daily for 5 to 10 days.

Children: 35 to 50 mg/kg/24 hours, divided into three doses, orally for 10 days.

Anaerobic Bacterial Infections: In the treatment of most serious anaerobic infections, Flagyl I.V.™ (metronidazole hydrochloride) or Flagyl I.V.™RTU® (metronidazole) is usually administered initially.

The usual adult *oral* dosage is 7.5 mg/kg every six hours (approx. 500 mg for a 70-kg adult). A maximum of 4 g should not be exceeded during a 24-hour period.

The usual duration of therapy is 7 to 10 days; however, infections of the bone and joint, lower respiratory tract, and endocardium may require longer treatment.

Patients with severe hepatic disease metabolize metronidazole slowly, with resultant accumulation of metronidazole and its metabolites in the plasma. Accordingly, for such patients, doses below those usually recommended should be administered cautiously. Close monitoring of plasma metronidazole levels[2] and toxicity is recommended.

The dose of Flagyl should not be specifically reduced in anuric patients since accumulated metabolites may be rapidly removed by dialysis.

HOW SUPPLIED

Flagyl 250-mg tablets are round, blue, film coated, with SEARLE and 1831 debossed on one side and FLAGYL and 250 on the other side; bottles of 50, 100, 250, 1,000, and 2,500, and cartons of 100 unit-dose individually blister-sealed tablets.

Flagyl 500-mg tablets are oblong, blue, film coated, with FLAGYL debossed on one side and 500 on the other side; bottles of 50, 100, and 500, and cartons of 100 unit-dose individually blister-sealed tablets.

Storage and Stability: Store below 86°F (30°C) and protect from light.

1. Proposed standard: PSM-11—Proposed Reference Dilution Procedure for Antimicrobic Susceptibility Testing of Anaerobic Bacteria, National Committee for Clinical Laboratory Standards, and Sutter, et al.: Collaborative Evaluation of a Proposed Reference Dilution Method of Susceptibility Testing of Anaerobic Bacteria, Antimicrob. Agents Chemother. *16:* 495–502 (Oct.) 1979; and Tally, et al.: *In Vitro* Activity of Thienamycin, Antimicrob. Agents Chemother. *14:* 436–438 (Sept.) 1978.

2. Ralph, E.D., and Kirby, W.M.M.: Bioassay of Metronidazole With Either Anaerobic or Aerobic Incubation, J. Infect. Dis. *132:* 587–591 (Nov.) 1975; or Gulaid, et al.: Determination of Metronidazole and Its Major Metabolites in Biological Fluids by High Pressure Liquid Chromatography, Br. J. Clin. Pharmacol. *6:* 430–432, 1978.

Shown in Product Identification Section, page 429

LOMOTIL® Liquid Ⓒ
LOMOTIL® Tablets Ⓒ
[*lō-mō'til*]
(diphenoxylate hydrochloride with atropine sulfate)

DESCRIPTION

Each Lomotil tablet and each 5 ml of Lomotil liquid for oral use contains:

diphenoxylate hydrochloride .... 2.5 mg
(Warning—May be habit forming.)
atropine sulfate .... 0.025 mg

Diphenoxylate hydrochloride, an antidiarrheal, is ethyl 1-(3-cyano-3,3-diphenylpropyl)-4-phenylisonipecotate monohydrochloride and has the following structural formula:

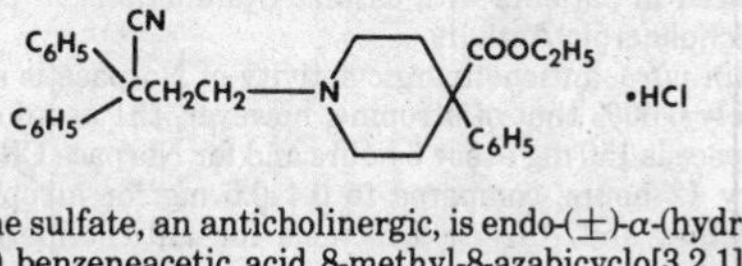

Atropine sulfate, an anticholinergic, is endo-(±)-α-(hydroxymethyl) benzeneacetic acid 8-methyl-8-azabicyclo[3.2.1] oct-3-yl ester sulfate (2:1) (salt) monohydrate and has the following structural formula:

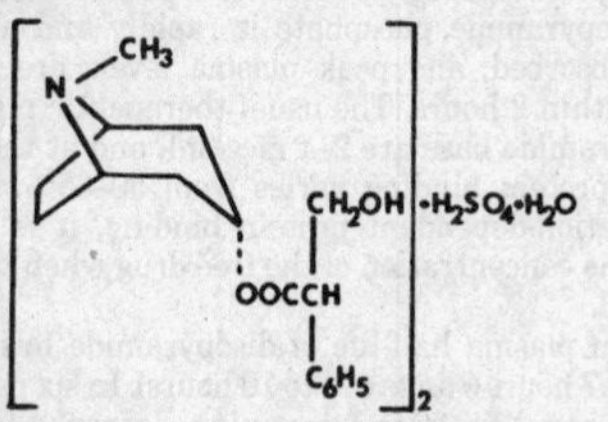

Inactive ingredients of Lomotil tablets include acacia, corn starch, magnesium stearate, sorbitol, sucrose, and talc. Inactive ingredients of Lomotil liquid include cherry flavor, citric acid, ethyl alcohol 15%, FD&C Yellow No. 6, glycerin, sodium phosphate, sorbitol, and water.

IMPORTANT INFORMATION

Lomotil is classified as a Schedule V controlled substance by federal law. Diphenoxylate hydrochloride is chemically related to the narcotic meperidine. Therefore, in case of overdosage, treatment is similar to that for meperidine or morphine intoxication, in which prolonged and careful monitoring is essential. Respiratory depression may be evidenced as late as 30 hours after ingestion and may recur in spite of an initial response to narcotic antagonists. A subtherapeutic amount of atropine sulfate is present to discourage deliberate overdosage. LOMOTIL IS *NOT* AN INNOCUOUS DRUG AND DOSAGE RECOMMENDATIONS SHOULD BE STRICTLY ADHERED TO, ESPECIALLY IN CHILDREN. KEEP THIS AND ALL MEDICATIONS OUT OF REACH OF CHILDREN.

CLINICAL PHARMACOLOGY

Diphenoxylate is rapidly and extensively metabolized in man by ester hydrolysis to diphenoxylic acid (difenoxine), which is biologically active and the major metabolite in the blood. After a 5-mg oral dose of carbon-14 labeled diphenoxylate hydrochloride in ethanolic solution was given to three healthy volunteers, an average of 14% of the drug plus its metabolites was excreted in the urine and 49% in the feces over a four-day period. Urinary excretion of the unmetabolized drug constituted less than 1% of the dose, and diphenoxylic acid plus its glucuronide conjugate constituted about 6% of the dose. In a 16-subject crossover bioavailability study, a linear relationship in the dose range of 2.5 to 10 mg was found between the dose of diphenoxylate hydrochloride (given as Lomotil liquid) and the peak plasma concentration, the area under the plasma concentration-time curve, and the amount of diphenoxylic acid excreted in the urine. In the same study the bioavailability of the tablet compared with an equal dose of the liquid was approximately 90%. The average peak plasma concentration of diphenoxylic acid following ingestion of four 2.5-mg tablets was 163 ng/ml at about 2 hours, and the elimination half-life of diphenoxylic acid was approximately 12 to 14 hours.

In dogs, diphenoxylate hydrochloride has a direct effect on circular smooth muscle of the bowel that conceivably results in segmentation and prolongation of gastrointestinal transit time. The clinical antidiarrheal action of diphenoxylate hydrochloride may thus be a consequence of enhanced segmentation that allows increased contact of the intraluminal contents with the intestinal mucosa.

INDICATIONS AND USAGE

Lomotil is effective as adjunctive therapy in the management of diarrhea.

CONTRAINDICATIONS

Lomotil is contraindicated in patients with

1. Known hypersensitivity to diphenoxylate or atropine.
2. Obstructive jaundice.
3. Diarrhea associated with pseudomembranous enterocolitis.

WARNINGS

LOMOTIL IS *NOT* AN INNOCUOUS DRUG AND DOSAGE RECOMMENDATIONS SHOULD BE STRICTLY ADHERED TO, ESPECIALLY IN CHILDREN. LOMOTIL IS NOT RECOMMENDED FOR CHILDREN UNDER 2 YEARS OF AGE. OVERDOSAGE MAY RESULT IN SEVERE RESPIRATORY DEPRESSION AND COMA, POSSIBLY LEADING TO PERMANENT BRAIN DAMAGE OR DEATH (SEE *OVERDOSAGE*). THEREFORE, KEEP THIS MEDICATION OUT OF THE REACH OF CHILDREN.

THE USE OF LOMOTIL SHOULD BE ACCOMPANIED BY APPROPRIATE FLUID AND ELECTROLYTE THERAPY, WHEN INDICATED. IF SEVERE DEHYDRATION OR ELECTROLYTE IMBALANCE IS PRESENT, LOMOTIL SHOULD BE WITHHELD UNTIL APPROPRIATE CORRECTIVE THERAPY HAS BEEN INITIATED. DRUG-INDUCED INHIBITION OF PERISTALSIS MAY RESULT IN FLUID RETENTION IN THE INTESTINE, WHICH MAY FURTHER AGGRAVATE DEHYDRATION AND ELECTROLYTE IMBALANCE.

LOMOTIL SHOULD BE USED WITH SPECIAL CAUTION IN YOUNG CHILDREN BECAUSE THIS AGE GROUP MAY BE PREDISPOSED TO DELAYED DIPHENOXYLATE TOXICITY AND BECAUSE OF THE GREATER VARIABILITY OF RESPONSE IN THIS AGE GROUP.

Antiperistaltic agents may prolong and/or worsen diarrhea associated with organisms that penetrate the intestinal mucosa (toxigenic *E. coli, Salmonella, Shigella*), and pseudomembranous enterocolitis associated with broad-spectrum antibiotics. Antiperistaltic agents should not be used in these conditions.

In some patients with acute ulcerative colitis, agents that inhibit intestinal motility or prolong intestinal transit time have been reported to induce toxic megacolon. Consequently, patients with acute ulcerative colitis should be carefully observed and Lomotil therapy should be discontinued promptly if abdominal distention occurs or if other untoward symptoms develop.

Since the chemical structure of diphenoxylate hydrochloride is similar to that of meperidine hydrochloride, the concurrent use of Lomotil with monoamine oxidase (MAO) inhibitors may, in theory, precipitate hypertensive crisis.

Lomotil should be used with extreme caution in patients with advanced hepatorenal disease and in all patients with abnormal liver function since hepatic coma may be precipitated.

Diphenoxylate hydrochloride may potentiate the action of barbiturates, tranquilizers, and alcohol. Therefore, the patient should be closely observed when any of these are used concomitantly.

PRECAUTIONS

General: Since a subtherapeutic dose of atropine has been added to the diphenoxylate hydrochloride, consideration should be given to the precautions relating to the use of atropine. In children, Lomotil should be used with caution since signs of atropinism may occur even with recommended doses, particularly in patients with Down's syndrome.

Information for patients: INFORM THE PATIENT (PARENT OR GUARDIAN) NOT TO EXCEED THE RECOMMENDED DOSAGE AND TO KEEP LOMOTIL OUT OF THE REACH OF CHILDREN AND IN A CHILD-RESISTANT CONTAINER. INFORM THE PATIENT OF THE CONSEQUENCES OF OVERDOSAGE, INCLUDING SEVERE RESPIRATORY DEPRESSION AND COMA, POSSIBLY LEADING TO PERMANENT BRAIN DAMAGE OR DEATH. Lomotil may produce drowsiness or dizziness. The patient should be cautioned regarding activities requiring mental alertness, such as driving or operating dangerous machinery. Potentiation of the action of alcohol, barbiturates, and tranquilizers with concomitant use of Lomotil should be explained to the patient. The physician should also provide the patient with other information in this labeling, as appropriate.

Drug interactions: Known drug interactions include barbiturates, tranquilizers, and alcohol. Lomotil may interact with MAO inhibitors (see *Warnings*).

In studies with male rats, diphenoxylate hydrochloride was found to inhibit the hepatic microsomal enzyme system at a dose of 2 mg/kg/day. Therefore, diphenoxylate has the potential to prolong the biological half-lives of drugs for which the rate of elimination is dependent on the microsomal drug metabolizing enzyme system.

Carcinogenesis, mutagenesis, impairment of fertility: No long-term study in animals has been performed to evaluate carcinogenic potential. Diphenoxylate hydrochloride was administered to male and female rats in their diets to provide dose levels of 4 and 20 mg/kg/day throughout a three-litter reproduction study. At 50 times the human dose (20 mg/kg/day), female weight gain was reduced and there was a marked effect on fertility as only 4 of 27 females became pregnant in three test breedings. The relevance of this finding to usage of Lomotil in humans is unknown.

Pregnancy: Pregnancy Category C. Diphenoxylate hydrochloride has been shown to have an effect on fertility in rats when given in doses 50 times the human dose (see above discussion). Other findings in this study include a decrease in maternal weight gain of 30% at 20 mg/kg/day and of 10% at 4 mg/kg/day. At 10 times the human dose (4 mg/kg/day), average litter size was slightly reduced.

Teratology studies were conducted in rats, rabbits, and mice with diphenoxylate hydrochloride at oral doses of 0.4 to 20 mg/kg/day. Due to experimental design and small numbers of litters, embryotoxic, fetotoxic, or teratogenic effects cannot be adequately assessed. However, examination of the available fetuses did not reveal any indication of teratogenicity.

There are no adequate and well-controlled studies in pregnant women. Lomotil should be used during pregnancy only if the anticipated benefit justifies the potential risk to the fetus.

Nursing mothers: Caution should be exercised when Lomotil is administered to a nursing woman, since the physicochemical characteristics of the major metabolite, diphenoxylic acid, are such that it may be excreted in breast milk and since it is known that atropine is excreted in breast milk.

Pediatric use: Lomotil may be used as an adjunct to the treatment of diarrhea but should be accompanied by appropriate fluid and electrolyte therapy, if needed. LOMOTIL IS NOT RECOMMENDED FOR CHILDREN UNDER 2 YEARS OF AGE. Lomotil should be used with special caution in young children because of the greater variability of response in this age group. See *Warnings* and *Dosage and Administration*. In case of accidental ingestion by children, see *Overdosage* for recommended treatment.

ADVERSE REACTIONS

At *therapeutic* doses, the following have been reported; they are listed in decreasing order of severity, but not of frequency:

Nervous system: numbness of extremities, euphoria, depression, malaise/lethargy, confusion, sedation/drowsiness, dizziness, restlessness, headache.

Allergic: anaphylaxis, angioneurotic edema, urticaria, swelling of the gums, pruritus.

Gastrointestinal system: toxic megacolon, paralytic ileus, pancreatitis, vomiting, nausea, anorexia, abdominal discomfort.

The following atropine sulfate effects are listed in decreasing order of severity, but not of frequency: hyperthermia, tachy-

Continued on next page

Searle & Co.—Cont.

cardia, urinary retention, flushing, dryness of the skin and mucous membranes. These effects may occur especially in children.

THIS MEDICATION SHOULD BE KEPT IN A CHILD-RESISTANT CONTAINER AND OUT OF THE REACH OF CHILDREN SINCE AN OVERDOSAGE MAY RESULT IN SEVERE RESPIRATORY DEPRESSION AND COMA, POSSIBLY LEADING TO PERMANENT BRAIN DAMAGE OR DEATH.

DRUG ABUSE AND DEPENDENCE

Controlled substance: Lomotil is classified as a Schedule V controlled substance by federal regulation. Diphenoxylate hydrochloride is chemically related to the narcotic analgesic meperidine.

Drug abuse and dependence: In doses used for the treatment of diarrhea, whether acute or chronic, diphenoxylate has not produced addiction.

Diphenoxylate hydrochloride is devoid of morphine-like subjective effects at therapeutic doses. At high doses it exhibits codeine-like subjective effects. The dose which produces antidiarrheal action is widely separated from the dose which causes central nervous system effects. The insolubility of diphenoxylate hydrochloride in commonly available aqueous media precludes intravenous self-administration. A dose of 100 to 300 mg/day, which is equivalent to 40 to 120 tablets, administered to humans for 40 to 70 days, produced opiate withdrawal symptoms. Since addiction to diphenoxylate hydrochloride is possible at high doses, the recommended dosage should not be exceeded.

OVERDOSAGE

RECOMMENDED DOSAGE SCHEDULES SHOULD BE STRICTLY FOLLOWED. THIS MEDICATION SHOULD BE KEPT IN A CHILD-RESISTANT CONTAINER AND OUT OF THE REACH OF CHILDREN, SINCE AN OVERDOSAGE MAY RESULT IN SEVERE, EVEN FATAL, RESPIRATORY DEPRESSION.

Diagnosis: Initial signs of overdosage may include dryness of the skin and mucous membranes, mydriasis, restlessness, flushing, hyperthermia, and tachycardia followed by lethargy or coma, hypotonic reflexes, nystagmus, pinpoint pupils, and respiratory depression. Respiratory depression may be evidenced as late as 30 hours after ingestion and may recur in spite of an initial response to narcotic antagonists.

TREAT ALL POSSIBLE LOMOTIL OVERDOSAGES AS SERIOUS AND MAINTAIN MEDICAL OBSERVATION FOR AT LEAST 48 HOURS, PREFERABLY UNDER CONTINUOUS HOSPITAL CARE.

Treatment: In the event of overdose, induction of vomiting, gastric lavage, establishment of a patent airway, and possibly mechanically assisted respiration are advised. *In vitro* and animal studies indicate that activated charcoal may significantly decrease the bioavailability of diphenoxylate. In non-comatose patients, a slurry of 100 g of activated charcoal can be administered immediately after the induction of vomiting or gastric lavage.

A pure narcotic antagonist (eg, naloxone) should be used in the treatment of respiratory depression caused by Lomotil. When a narcotic antagonist is administered intravenously, the onset of action is generally apparent within two minutes. It may also be administered subcutaneously or intramuscularly, providing a slightly less rapid onset of action but a more prolonged effect.

To counteract respiratory depression caused by Lomotil overdosage, the following dosage schedule for the narcotic antagonist naloxone hydrochloride should be followed:

Adult dosage: The usual initial adult dose of naloxone hydrochloride is 0.4 mg (1 ml) administered intravenously. If respiratory function does not adequately improve after the initial dose, the same I.V. dose may be repeated at two- to three-minute intervals.

Children: The usual initial dose of naloxone hydrochloride for children is 0.01 mg/kg of body weight administered intravenously and repeated at two- to three-minute intervals if necessary.

Following initial improvement of respiratory function, repeated doses of naloxone hydrochloride may be required to counteract recurrent respiratory depression. Supplemental intramuscular doses of naloxone hydrochloride may be utilized to produce a longer-lasting effect.

Since the duration of action of diphenoxylate hydrochloride is longer than that of naloxone hydrochloride, improvement of respiration following administration may be followed by recurrent respiratory depression. Consequently, continuous observation is necessary until the effect of diphenoxylate hydrochloride on respiration has passed. This effect may persist for many hours. The period of observation should extend over at least 48 hours, preferably under continuous hospital care. Although signs of overdosage and respiratory depression may not be evident soon after ingestion of diphenoxylate hydrochloride, respiratory depression may occur from 12 to 30 hours later.

DOSAGE AND ADMINISTRATION

DO NOT EXCEED RECOMMENDED DOSAGE.

Adults: The recommended initial dosage is two Lomotil tablets four times daily or 10 ml (two regular teaspoonfuls) of Lomotil liquid four times daily (20 mg per day). Most patients will require this dosage until initial control has been achieved, after which the dosage may be reduced to meet individual requirements. Control may often be maintained with as little as 5 mg (two tablets or 10 ml of liquid) daily. Clinical improvement of acute diarrhea is usually observed within 48 hours. If clinical improvement of chronic diarrhea after treatment with a maximum daily dose of 20 mg of diphenoxylate hydrochloride is not observed within 10 days, symptoms are unlikely to be controlled by further administration.

Children: Lomotil is not recommended in children under 2 years of age and should be used with special caution in young children (see Warnings *and* Precautions*). The nutritional status and degree of dehydration must be considered. In children under 13 years of age, use Lomotil liquid. Do not use Lomotil tablets for this age group.*

Only the plastic dropper should be used when measuring Lomotil liquid for administration to children.

Dosage schedule for children: The recommended initial total daily dosage of Lomotil liquid for children is 0.3 to 0.4 mg/kg, administered in four divided doses. The following table provides an *approximate* initial daily dosage recommendation for children.

Age (years)	Approximate weight (kg)	(lb)	Dosage in ml (four times daily)
2	11–14	24–31	1.5–3.0
3	12–16	26–35	2.0–3.0
4	14–20	31–44	2.0–4.0
5	16–23	35–51	2.5–4.5
6–8	17–32	38–71	2.5–5.0
9–12	23–55	51–121	3.5–5.0

These pediatric schedules are the best approximation of an average dose recommendation which may be adjusted downward according to the overall nutritional status and degree of dehydration encountered in the sick child. Reduction of dosage may be made as soon as initial control of symptoms has been achieved. Maintenance dosage may be as low as one-fourth of the initial daily dosage. If no response occurs within 48 hours, Lomotil is unlikely to be effective.

KEEP THIS AND ALL MEDICATIONS OUT OF THE REACH OF CHILDREN.

HOW SUPPLIED

Tablets—round, white, with SEARLE debossed on one side and 61 on the other side and containing 2.5 mg of diphenoxylate hydrochloride and 0.025 mg of atropine sulfate, supplied as:

NDC Number	Size
0014-0061-31	bottle of 100
0014-0061-51	bottle of 500
0014-0061-52	bottle of 1,000
0014-0061-55	bottle of 2,500
0014-0061-34	carton of 100 unit dose

Liquid—containing 2.5 mg of diphenoxylate hydrochloride and 0.025 mg of atropine sulfate per 5 ml; bottles of 2 fl oz (NDC Number 0014-0066-02).

A plastic dropper calibrated in increments of ½ ml (¼ mg) with a capacity of 2 ml (1 mg) accompanies each 2-oz bottle of Lomotil liquid. Only this plastic dropper should be used when measuring Lomotil liquid for administration to children.

Shown in Product Identification Section, page 429

NORPACE® Capsules ℞
[*nor 'pāce*]
(disopyramide phosphate)
100 mg-NSN 6505-01-220-6314 (VA)
150 mg-NSN 6505-01-220-6313 (VA)
(bottles of 120 capsules)

NORPACE® CR Capsules ℞
(disopyramide phosphate)
Controlled-Release
100 mg-NSN 6505-01-158-2170 (VA)
150 mg-NSN 6505-01-158-6361 (VA)
(bottles of 100 capsules)

DESCRIPTION

Norpace (disopyramide phosphate) is an antiarrhythmic drug available for oral administration in immediate-release and controlled-release capsules containing 100 mg or 150 mg of disopyramide base, present as the phosphate. The base content of the phosphate salt is 77.6%. The structural formula of Norpace is:

[See Chemical Formula at top of next column].

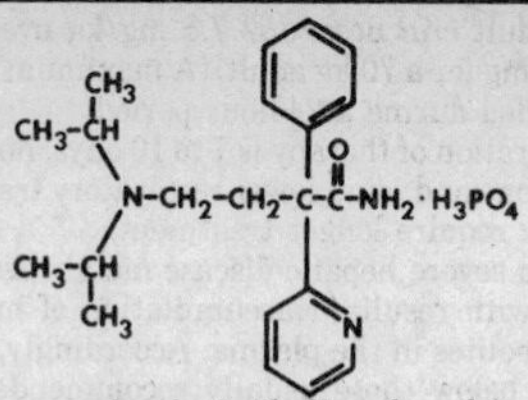

α-[2-(diisopropylamino) ethyl]-α-phenyl-2-pyridine-acetamide phosphate

Norpace is freely soluble in water, and the free base (pKa 10.4) has an aqueous solubility of 1 mg/ml. The chloroform: water partition coefficient of the base is 3.1 at pH 7.2.

Norpace is a racemic mixture of *d*- and *l*-isomers. This drug is not chemically related to other antiarrhythmic drugs.

Norpace CR (controlled-release) capsules are designed to afford a gradual and consistent release of disopyramide. Thus, for maintenance therapy, Norpace CR provides the benefit of less frequent dosing (every 12 hours) as compared with the every-6-hour dosage schedule of immediate-release Norpace capsules.

Inactive ingredients of Norpace include corn starch, edible ink, FD&C Red No. 3, FD&C Yellow No. 6, gelatin, lactose, talc, and titanium dioxide; the 150-mg capsule also contains FD&C Blue No. 1.

Inactive ingredients of Norpace CR include corn starch, D&C Yellow No. 10, edible ink, ethylcellulose, FD&C Blue No. 1, gelatin, shellac, sucrose, talc, and titanium dioxide; the 150-mg capsule also contains FD&C Red No. 3 and FD&C Yellow No. 6.

CLINICAL PHARMACOLOGY

Mechanisms of Action

Norpace (disopyramide phosphate) is a Type 1 antiarrhythmic drug (ie, similar to procainamide and quinidine). *In animal studies* Norpace decreases the rate of diastolic depolarization (phase 4) in cells with augmented automaticity, decreases the upstroke velocity (phase 0) and increases the action potential duration of normal cardiac cells, decreases the disparity in refractoriness between infarcted and adjacent normally perfused myocardium, and has no effect on alpha- or beta-adrenergic receptors.

Electrophysiology

In man, Norpace at therapeutic plasma levels shortens the sinus node recovery time, lengthens the effective refractory period of the atrium, and has a minimal effect on the effective refractory period of the AV node. Little effect has been shown on AV-nodal and His-Purkinje conduction times or QRS duration. However, prolongation of conduction in accessory pathways occurs.

Hemodynamics

At recommended oral doses, Norpace rarely produces significant alterations of blood pressure in patients without congestive heart failure (see *Warnings*). With intravenous Norpace, either increases in systolic/diastolic or decreases in systolic blood pressure have been reported, depending on the infusion rate and the patient population. Intravenous Norpace may cause cardiac depression with an approximate mean 10% reduction of cardiac output, which is more pronounced in patients with cardiac dysfunction.

Anticholinergic Activity

The *in vitro* anticholinergic activity of Norpace is approximately 0.06% that of atropine; however, the usual dose for Norpace is 150 mg every 6 hours and for Norpace CR 300 mg every 12 hours, compared to 0.4–0.6 mg for atropine (see *Warnings* and *Adverse Reactions* for anticholinergic side effects).

Pharmacokinetics

Following oral administration of immediate-release Norpace, disopyramide phosphate is rapidly and almost completely absorbed, and peak plasma levels are usually attained within 2 hours. The usual therapeutic plasma levels of disopyramide base are 2–4 mcg/ml, and at these concentrations protein binding varies from 50–65%. Because of concentration-dependent protein binding, it is difficult to predict the concentration of the free drug when total drug is measured.

The mean plasma half-life of disopyramide in healthy humans is 6.7 hours (range of 4 to 10 hours). In six patients with impaired renal function (creatinine clearance less than 40 ml/min), disopyramide half-life values were 8 to 18 hours.

After the oral administration of 200 mg of disopyramide to 10 cardiac patients with borderline to moderate heart failure, the time to peak serum concentration of 2.3 ± 1.5 hours (mean ± SD) was increased, and the mean peak serum concentration of 4.8 ± 1.6 mcg/ml was higher than in healthy volunteers. After intravenous administration in these same patients, the mean elimination half-life was 9.7 ± 4.2 hours (range in healthy volunteers of 4.4 to 7.8 hours). In a second study of the oral administration of disopyramide to 7 patients with heart disease, including left ventricular dysfunction, the mean plasma half-life was slightly prolonged to 7.8 ± 1.9 hours (range of 5 to 9.5 hours).

In healthy men about 50% of a given dose of disopyramide is excreted in the urine as the unchanged drug, about 20% as the mono-N-dealkylated metabolite, and 10% as the other metabolites. The plasma concentration of the major metabolite is approximately one tenth that of disopyramide. Altering the urinary pH in man does not affect the plasma half-life of disopyramide.

In a crossover study in healthy subjects, the bioavailability of disopyramide from Norpace CR capsules was similar to that from the immediate-release capsules. With a single 300-mg oral dose, peak disopyramide plasma concentrations of 3.23 ± 0.75 mcg/ml (mean ± SD) at 2.5 ± 2.3 hours were obtained with two 150-mg immediate-release capsules and 2.22 ± 0.47 mcg/ml at 4.9 ± 1.4 hours with two 150-mg Norpace CR capsules. The elimination half-life of disopyramide was 8.31 ± 1.83 hours with the immediate-release capsules and 11.65 ± 4.72 hours with Norpace CR capsules. The amount of disopyramide and mono-N-dealkylated metabolite excreted in the urine in 48 hours was 128 and 48 mg, respectively, with the immediate-release capsules, and 112 and 33 mg, respectively, with Norpace CR capsules. The differences in the urinary excretion of either constituent were not statistically significant.

Following multiple doses, steady-state plasma levels of between 2 and 4 mcg/ml were attained following either 150 mg every-6-hour dosing with immediate-release capsules or 300 mg every-12-hour dosing with Norpace CR capsules.

INDICATIONS AND USAGE

Norpace or Norpace CR should be prescribed only after appropriate electrocardiographic assessment.

Norpace and Norpace CR are indicated for suppression and prevention of recurrence of the following cardiac arrhythmias when they occur singly or in combination:

1. Unifocal premature (ectopic) ventricular contractions.
2. Premature (ectopic) ventricular contractions of multifocal origin.
3. Paired premature ventricular contractions (couplets).
4. Episodes of ventricular tachycardia (persistent ventricular tachycardia is ordinarily treated with DC-cardioversion).

In controlled trials of ambulatory patients, 150 mg of Norpace every 6 hours was as effective as 325 mg of quinidine every 6 hours in reducing the frequency of ventricular ectopic activity. Norpace was equally effective in digitalized and nondigitalized patients. Norpace is also equally effective in the treatment of primary cardiac arrhythmias and those which occur in association with organic heart disease, including coronary artery disease.

Oral disopyramide phosphate has not been adequately studied in patients with acute myocardial infarction or in patients with persistent ventricular tachycardia or atrial arrhythmias.

Norpace CR should not be used initially if rapid establishment of disopyramide plasma levels is desired.

Type 1 antiarrhythmic drugs are usually not effective in treating arrhythmias secondary to digitalis intoxication and, therefore, Norpace or Norpace CR is not indicated for such cases.

The value of antiarrhythmic drugs in preventing sudden death in patients with serious ventricular ectopic activity has not been established.

CONTRAINDICATIONS

Norpace and Norpace CR are contraindicated in the presence of cardiogenic shock, preexisting second- or third-degree AV block (if no pacemaker is present), congenital Q-T prolongation, or known hypersensitivity to the drug.

WARNINGS

Negative Inotropic Properties:

Heart Failure/Hypotension

Norpace or Norpace CR may cause or worsen congestive heart failure or produce severe hypotension as a consequence of its negative inotropic properties. Hypotension has been observed primarily in patients with primary cardiomyopathy or inadequately compensated congestive heart failure. Norpace or Norpace CR should not be used in patients with uncompensated or marginally compensated congestive heart failure or hypotension unless the congestive heart failure or hypotension is secondary to cardiac arrhythmia. Patients with a history of heart failure may be treated with Norpace or Norpace CR, but careful attention must be given to the maintenance of cardiac function, including optimal digitalization. If hypotension occurs or congestive heart failure worsens, Norpace or Norpace CR should be discontinued and, if necessary, restarted at a lower dosage only after adequate cardiac compensation has been established.

QRS Widening

Although it is unusual, significant widening (greater than 25%) of the QRS complex may occur during Norpace or Norpace CR administration; in such cases Norpace or Norpace CR should be discontinued.

Q-T Prolongation

As with other Type 1 antiarrhythmic drugs, prolongation of the Q-T interval (corrected) and worsening of the arrhythmia, including ventricular tachycardia and ventricular fibrillation, may occur. Patients who have evidenced prolongation of the Q-T interval in response to quinidine may be at particular risk. If a Q-T prolongation of greater than 25% is observed and if ectopy continues, the patient should be monitored closely, and consideration be given to discontinuing Norpace or Norpace CR.

Hypoglycemia

In rare instances significant lowering of blood glucose values has been reported during Norpace administration. The physician should be alert to this possibility, especially in patients with congestive heart failure, chronic malnutrition, hepatic, renal, or other diseases, or drugs (eg, beta adrenoceptor blockers, alcohol) which could compromise preservation of the normal glucoregulatory mechanisms in the absence of food. In these patients the blood glucose levels should be carefully followed.

Concomitant Antiarrhythmic Therapy

The concomitant use of Norpace or Norpace CR with other Type 1 antiarrhythmic agents (such as quinidine or procainamide) and/or propranolol should be reserved for patients with life-threatening arrhythmias who are demonstrably unresponsive to single-agent antiarrhythmic therapy. Such use may produce serious negative inotropic effects, or may excessively prolong conduction. This should be considered particularly in patients with any degree of cardiac decompensation or those with a prior history thereof. Patients receiving more than one antiarrhythmic drug must be carefully monitored.

Heart Block

If first-degree heart block develops in a patient receiving Norpace or Norpace CR, the dosage should be reduced. If the block persists despite reduction of dosage, continuation of the drug must depend upon weighing the benefit being obtained against the risk of higher degrees of heart block. Development of second- or third-degree AV block or unifascicular, bifascicular, or trifascicular block requires discontinuation of Norpace or Norpace CR therapy, unless the ventricular rate is adequately controlled by a temporary or implanted ventricular pacemaker.

Anticholinergic Activity

Because of its anticholinergic activity, disopyramide phosphate should not be used in patients with glaucoma, myasthenia gravis, or urinary retention unless adequate overriding measures are taken; these consist of the topical application of potent miotics (eg, pilocarpine) for patients with glaucoma, and catheter drainage or operative relief for patients with urinary retention. Urinary retention may occur in patients of either sex as a consequence of Norpace or Norpace CR administration, but males with benign prostatic hypertrophy are at particular risk. In patients with a family history of glaucoma, intraocular pressure should be measured before initiating Norpace or Norpace CR therapy. Disopyramide phosphate should be used with special care in patients with myasthenia gravis since its anticholinergic properties could precipitate a myasthenic crisis in such patients.

PRECAUTIONS

General

Atrial Tachyarrhythmias

Patients with atrial flutter or fibrillation should be digitalized prior to Norpace or Norpace CR administration to ensure that drug-induced enhancement of AV conduction does not result in an increase of ventricular rate beyond physiologically acceptable limits.

Conduction Abnormalities

Care should be taken when prescribing Norpace or Norpace CR for patients with sick sinus syndrome (bradycardia-tachycardia syndrome), Wolff-Parkinson-White syndrome (WPW), or bundle branch block. The effect of disopyramide phosphate in these conditions is uncertain at present.

Cardiomyopathy

Patients with myocarditis or other cardiomyopathy may develop significant hypotension in response to the usual dosage of disopyramide phosphate, probably due to cardiodepressant mechanisms. Therefore, a loading dose of Norpace should not be given to such patients, and initial dosage and subsequent dosage adjustments should be made under close supervision (see *Dosage and Administration*).

Renal Impairment

More than 50% of disopyramide is excreted in the urine unchanged. Therefore Norpace dosage should be reduced in patients with impaired renal function (see *Dosage and Administration*). The electrocardiogram should be carefully monitored for prolongation of PR interval, evidence of QRS widening, or other signs of overdosage (see *Overdosage*).

Norpace CR is not recommended for patients with severe renal insufficiency (creatinine clearance 40 ml/min or less).

Hepatic Impairment

Hepatic impairment also causes an increase in the plasma half-life of disopyramide. Dosage should be reduced for patients with such impairment. The electrocardiogram should be carefully monitored for signs of overdosage (see *Overdosage*).

Patients with cardiac dysfunction have a higher potential for hepatic impairment; this should be considered when administering Norpace or Norpace CR.

Potassium Imbalance

Antiarrhythmic drugs may be ineffective in patients with hypokalemia, and their toxic effects may be enhanced in patients with hyperkalemia. Therefore, potassium abnormalities should be corrected before starting Norpace or Norpace CR therapy.

Drug Interactions

If phenytoin or other hepatic enzyme inducers are taken concurrently with Norpace or Norpace CR, lower plasma levels of disopyramide may occur. Monitoring of disopyramide plasma levels is recommended in such concurrent use to avoid ineffective therapy. Other antiarrhythmic drugs (eg, quinidine, procainamide, lidocaine, propranolol) have occasionally been used concurrently with Norpace. Excessive widening of the QRS complex and/or prolongation of the Q-T interval may occur in these situations (see *Warnings*). In healthy subjects, no significant drug-drug interaction was observed when Norpace was coadministered with either propranolol or diazepam. Concomitant administration of Norpace and quinidine resulted in slight increases in plasma disopyramide levels and slight decreases in plasma quinidine levels. Norpace does not increase serum digoxin levels.

Carcinogenesis, Mutagenesis, Impairment of Fertility

Eighteen months of Norpace administration to rats, at oral doses up to 400 mg/kg/day (about 30 times the usual daily human dose of 600 mg/day, assuming a patient weight of at least 50 kg), revealed no evidence of carcinogenic potential. An evaluation of mutagenic potential by Ames test was negative. Norpace, at doses up to 250 mg/kg/day, did not adversely affect fertility of rats.

Pregnancy

Teratogenic Effects: Pregnancy Category C. Norpace was associated with decreased numbers of implantation sites and decreased growth and survival of pups when administered to pregnant rats at 250 mg/kg/day (20 or more times the usual daily human dose of 12 mg/kg, assuming a patient weight of at least 50 kg), a level at which weight gain and food consumption of dams were also reduced. Increased resorption rates were reported in rabbits at 60 mg/kg/day (5 or more times the usual daily human dose). Effects on implantation, pup growth and survival were not evaluated in rabbits. There are no adequate and well-controlled studies in pregnant women. Norpace or Norpace CR should be used during pregnancy only if the potential benefit justifies the potential risk to the fetus.

Nonteratogenic Effects: **Norpace has been reported to stimulate contractions of the pregnant uterus.** Disopyramide has been found in human fetal blood.

Labor and Delivery

It is not known whether the use of Norpace or Norpace CR during labor or delivery has immediate or delayed adverse effects on the fetus, or whether it prolongs the duration of labor or increases the need for forceps delivery or other obstetric intervention.

Nursing Mothers

Studies in rats have shown that the concentration of disopyramide and its metabolites is between one and three times greater in milk than it is in plasma. Following oral administration, disopyramide has been detected in human milk at a concentration not exceeding that in plasma. Because of the potential for serious adverse reactions in nursing infants from Norpace or Norpace CR, a decision should be made whether to discontinue nursing or to discontinue the drug, taking into account the importance of the drug to the mother.

ADVERSE REACTIONS

The adverse reactions which were reported in Norpace clinical trials encompass observations in 1,500 patients, including 90 patients studied for at least 4 years. The most serious adverse reactions are hypotension and congestive heart failure. The most common adverse reactions, which are dose dependent, are associated with the anticholinergic properties of the drug. These may be transitory, but may be persistent or can be severe. Urinary retention is the most serious anticholinergic effect.

The following reactions were reported in 10–40% of patients:
- Anticholinergic: dry mouth (32%), urinary hesitancy (14%), constipation (11%)

The following reactions were reported in 3–9% of patients:
- Anticholinergic: blurred vision, dry nose/eyes/ throat
- Genitourinary: urinary retention, urinary frequency and urgency
- Gastrointestinal: nausea, pain/bloating/gas
- General: dizziness, general fatigue/muscle weakness, headache, malaise, aches/pains

The following reactions were reported in 1–3% of patients:
- Genitourinary: impotence

Continued on next page

Searle & Co.—Cont.

Cardiovascular: hypotension with or without congestive heart failure, increased congestive heart failure (see *Warnings*), cardiac conduction disturbances (see *Warnings*), edema/ weight gain, shortness of breath, syncope, chest pain
Gastrointestinal: anorexia, diarrhea, vomiting
Dermatologic: generalized rash/dermatoses, itching
Central nervous system: nervousness
Other: hypokalemia, elevated cholesterol/triglycerides

The following reactions were reported in less than 1%:

Depression, insomnia, dysuria, numbness/tingling, elevated liver enzymes, AV block, elevated BUN, elevated creatinine, decreased hemoglobin/hematocrit

Hypoglycemia has been reported in association with Norpace administration (see *Warnings*).

Infrequent occurrences of reversible cholestatic jaundice, fever, and respiratory difficulty have been reported in association with disopyramide therapy, as have rare instances of thrombocytopenia, reversible agranulocytosis, and gynecomastia. Rarely, acute psychosis has been reported following Norpace therapy, with prompt return to normal mental status when therapy was stopped. The physician should be aware of these possible reactions and should discontinue Norpace or Norpace CR therapy promptly if they occur.

OVERDOSAGE

Symptoms

Deliberate or accidental overdose of oral disopyramide may be followed by apnea, loss of consciousness, cardiac arrhythmias, and loss of spontaneous respiration. Death has occurred following overdose.

Toxic plasma levels of disopyramide produce excessive widening of the QRS complex and Q-T interval, worsening of congestive heart failure, hypotension, varying kinds and degrees of conduction disturbance, bradycardia, and finally asystole. Obvious anticholinergic effects are also observed.

The approximate oral LD_{50} of disopyramide phosphate is 580 and 700 mg/kg for rats and mice, respectively.

Treatment

Experience indicates that prompt and vigorous treatment of overdosage is necessary even in the absence of symptoms. Such treatment may be lifesaving. No specific antidote for disopyramide phosphate has been identified. Treatment should be symptomatic and may include induction of emesis or gastric lavage, administration of a cathartic followed by activated charcoal by mouth or stomach tube, intravenous administration of isoproterenol and dopamine, insertion of an intra-aortic balloon for counterpulsation, and mechanically assisted ventilation. Hemodialysis or, preferably, hemoperfusion with charcoal may be employed to lower serum concentration of the drug.

The electrocardiogram should be monitored, and supportive therapy with cardiac glycosides and diuretics should be given as required.

If progressive AV block should develop, endocardial pacing should be implemented. In case of any impaired renal function, measures to increase the glomerular filtration rate may reduce the toxicity (disopyramide is excreted primarily by the kidney).

The anticholinergic effects can be reversed with neostigmine at the discretion of the physician.

Altering the urinary pH in humans does not affect the plasma half-life or the amount of disopyramide excreted in the urine.

DOSAGE AND ADMINISTRATION

The dosage of Norpace or Norpace CR must be individualized for each patient on the basis of response and tolerance. The usual adult dosage of Norpace or Norpace CR is 400 to 800 mg per day given in divided doses. The recommended dosage for most adults is 600 mg/day given in divided doses (either 150 mg every 6 hours for immediate-release Norpace or 300 mg every 12 hours for Norpace CR). For patients whose body weight is less than 110 pounds (50 kg), the recommended dosage is 400 mg/day given in divided doses (either 100 mg every 6 hours for immediate-release Norpace or 200 mg every 12 hours for Norpace CR).

For patients with cardiomyopathy or possible cardiac decompensation, a loading dose, as discussed below, should not be given and initial dosage should be limited to 100 mg of immediate-release Norpace every 6 to 8 hours. Subsequent dosage adjustments should be made gradually, with close monitoring for the possible development of hypotension and/ or congestive heart failure (see *Warnings*).

For patients with moderate renal insufficiency (creatinine clearance greater than 40 ml/min) or hepatic insufficiency, the recommended dosage is 400 mg/day given in divided doses (either 100 mg every 6 hours for immediate-release Norpace or 200 mg every 12 hours for Norpace CR).

For patients with severe renal insufficiency (C_{cr} 40 ml/min or less) the recommended dosage regimen of immediate-release Norpace is 100 mg at intervals shown in the table below, with or without an initial loading dose of 150 mg.

IMMEDIATE-RELEASE NORPACE DOSAGE INTERVAL FOR PATIENTS WITH RENAL INSUFFICIENCY

Creatinine clearance (ml/min)	40–30	30–15	less than 15
Approximate maintenance-dosing interval	q 8 hr	q 12 hr	q 24 hr

The above dosing schedules are for Norpace immediate-release capsules; Norpace CR is not recommended for patients with severe renal insufficiency.

For patients in whom rapid control of ventricular arrhythmia is essential, an initial loading dose of 300 mg of immediate-release Norpace (200 mg for patients whose body weight is less than 110 pounds) is recommended, followed by the appropriate maintenance dosage. Therapeutic effects are usually attained 30 minutes to 3 hours after administration of a 300-mg loading dose. If there is no response or evidence of toxicity within 6 hours of the loading dose, 200 mg of immediate-release Norpace every 6 hours may be prescribed instead of the usual 150 mg. If there is no response to this dosage within 48 hours, either Norpace should then be discontinued or the physician should consider hospitalizing the patient for careful monitoring while subsequent immediate-release Norpace doses of 250 mg or 300 mg every 6 hours are given. A limited number of patients with severe refractory ventricular tachycardia have tolerated daily doses of Norpace up to 1600 mg per day (400 mg every 6 hours) resulting in disopyramide plasma levels up to 9 mcg/ml. If such treatment is warranted, it is essential that patients be hospitalized for close evaluation and continuous monitoring.

Norpace CR should not be used initially if rapid establishment of disopyramide plasma levels is desired.

Transferring to Norpace or Norpace CR

The following dosage schedule based on theoretical considerations rather than experimental data is suggested for transferring patients with normal renal function from either quinidine sulfate or procainamide therapy (Type 1 antiarrhythmic agents) to Norpace or Norpace CR therapy:

Norpace or Norpace CR should be started using the regular maintenance schedule **without a loading dose** 6–12 hours after the last dose of quinidine sulfate or 3–6 hours after the last dose of procainamide.

In patients in whom withdrawal of quinidine sulfate or procainamide is likely to produce life-threatening arrhythmias, the physician should consider hospitalization of the patient.

When transferring a patient from immediate-release Norpace to Norpace CR, the maintenance schedule of Norpace CR may be started 6 hours after the last dose of immediate-release Norpace.

Pediatric Dosage

Controlled clinical studies have not been conducted in pediatric patients; however, the following suggested dosage table is based on published clinical experience.

Total daily dosage should be divided and equal doses administered orally every 6 hours or at intervals according to individual patient needs. Disopyramide plasma levels and therapeutic response must be monitored closely. Patients should be hospitalized during the initial treatment period, and dose titration should start at the lower end of the ranges provided below.

SUGGESTED TOTAL DAILY DOSAGE*

Age (years)	Disopyramide (mg/kg body weight/day)
Under 1	10 to 30
1 to 4	10 to 20
4 to 12	10 to 15
12 to 18	6 to 15

* Dosage is expressed in milligrams of disopyramide base. Since Norpace (disopyramide phosphate) 100-mg capsules contain 100 mg of disopyramide base, the pharmacist can readily prepare a 1-mg/ml to 10-mg/ml liquid suspension by adding the entire contents of Norpace capsules to cherry syrup, NF. The resulting suspension, when refrigerated, is stable for one month and should be thoroughly shaken before the measurement of each dose. The suspension should be dispensed in an amber glass bottle with a child-resistant closure.
Norpace CR capsules should not be used to prepare the above suspension.

HOW SUPPLIED

Norpace (disopyramide phosphate) is supplied in hard gelatin capsules containing either 100 mg or 150 mg of disopyramide base, present as the phosphate.

Norpace 100-mg capsules are white and orange, with markings SEARLE, 2752, NORPACE, and 100 MG.

NDC Number	Size
0014-2752-31	bottle of 100
0014-2752-51	bottle of 500
0014-2752-52	bottle of 1,000
0014-2752-34	carton of 100 unit dose

Norpace 150-mg capsules are brown and orange, with markings SEARLE, 2762, NORPACE, and 150 MG.

NDC Number	Size
0014-2762-31	bottle of 100
0014-2762-51	bottle of 500
0014-2762-52	bottle of 1,000
0014-2762-34	carton of 100 unit dose

Norpace CR (disopyramide phosphate) Controlled-Release is supplied as specially prepared controlled-release beads in hard gelatin capsules containing either 100 mg or 150 mg of disopyramide base, present as the phosphate.

Norpace CR 100-mg capsules are white and light green, with markings SEARLE, 2732, NORPACE CR, and 100 mg.

NDC Number	Size
0014-2732-31	bottle of 100
0014-2732-51	bottle of 500
0014-2732-34	carton of 100 unit dose

Norpace CR 150-mg capsules are brown and light green, with markings SEARLE, 2742, NORPACE CR, and 150 mg.

NDC Number	Size
0014-2742-31	bottle of 100
0014-2742-51	bottle of 500
0014-2742-34	carton of 100 unit dose

Store below 86°F (30°C).

Caution: Federal law prohibits dispensing without prescription.

Certain manufacturing operations for Norpace CR have been performed by G. D. Searle & Co. LTD., Morpeth, England.

Shown in Product Identification Section, page 429

OVULEN-21® ℞
OVULEN-28® ℞

[*ov 'ū-len*]
(ethynodiol diacetate with mestranol)

See Demulen products under Searle & Co. for Ovulen prescribing information.

Shown in Product Identification Section, page 429

PRO-BANTHĪNE® Tablets ℞

[*prō-ban 'thīne*]
(propantheline bromide USP)

DESCRIPTION

Pro-Banthīne oral tablets contain 15 mg or $7\frac{1}{2}$ mg of the anticholinergic propantheline bromide, (2-hydroxyethyl)-diisopropylmethylammonium bromide xanthene-9-carboxylate.

The structural formula of Pro-Banthīne is

$$\left[\text{COOCH}_2\text{CH}_2\overset{+}{\text{N}}[\text{CH(CH}_3)_2]_2 \; (\text{CH}_3) \right] Br^-$$

Inactive ingredients include calcium carbonate, corn starch, edible ink, flavor, lactose, magnesium carbonate, magnesium stearate, sucrose, talc, titanium dioxide, and waxes. The 15-mg tablet also contains coloring agents.

CLINICAL PHARMACOLOGY

Pro-Banthīne inhibits gastrointestinal motility and diminishes gastric acid secretion. The drug also inhibits the action of acetylcholine at the postganglionic nerve endings of the parasympathetic nervous system.

Propantheline bromide is extensively metabolized in man primarily by hydrolysis to the inactive materials xanthene-9-carboxylic acid and (2-hydroxyethyl) diisopropylmethylammonium bromide. After a single 30-mg oral dose given as two 15-mg tablets the mean peak plasma concentration of propantheline was 21 ng/ml at one hour in six healthy subjects.

The plasma elimination half-life of propantheline is about 1.6 hours. Approximately 70% of the dose is excreted in the urine, mostly as metabolites. The urinary excretion of propantheline is about 3% after oral tablet administration.

INDICATIONS AND USAGE

Pro-Banthīne is effective as adjunctive therapy in the treatment of peptic ulcer.

CONTRAINDICATIONS

Pro-Banthīne (propantheline bromide) is contraindicated in patients with:

1. Glaucoma, since mydriasis is to be avoided.
2. Obstructive disease of the gastrointestinal tract (pyloroduodenal stenosis, achalasia, paralytic ileus, etc).
3. Obstructive uropathy (eg, bladder-neck obstruction due to prostatic hypertrophy).
4. Intestinal atony of elderly or debilitated patients.
5. Severe ulcerative colitis or toxic megacolon complicating ulcerative colitis.
6. Unstable cardiovascular adjustment in acute hemorrhage.
7. Myasthenia gravis.

WARNINGS

In the presence of a high environmental temperature, heat prostration (fever and heat stroke due to decreased sweating) can occur with the use of Pro-Banthīne.

Diarrhea may be an early symptom of incomplete intestinal obstruction, especially in patients with ileostomy or colostomy. In this instance treatment with Pro-Banthīne would be inappropriate and possibly harmful.

With overdosage, a curare-like action may occur (ie, neuromuscular blockade leading to muscular weakness and possible paralysis).

Pro-Banthīne may cause increased heart rate and, therefore, should be used with caution in patients with heart disease.

PRECAUTIONS

General: Pro-Banthīne (propantheline bromide) should be used with caution in the elderly and in all patients with autonomic neuropathy, hepatic or renal disease, hyperthyroidism, coronary heart disease, congestive heart failure, cardiac tachyarrhythmias, hypertension, or hiatal hernia associated with reflux esophagitis, since anticholinergics may aggravate this condition.

In patients with ulcerative colitis, large doses of Pro-Banthīne may suppress intestinal motility to the point of producing paralytic ileus and, for this reason, may precipitate or aggravate toxic megacolon, a serious complication of the disease.

Information for patients: Pro-Banthīne may produce drowsiness or blurred vision. The patient should be cautioned regarding activities requiring mental alertness, such as operating a motor vehicle or other machinery or performing hazardous work, while taking this drug.

Drug interactions: Anticholinergics may delay absorption of other medication given concomitantly.

Excessive cholinergic blockade may occur if Pro-Banthīne is given concomitantly with belladonna alkaloids, synthetic or semisynthetic anticholinergic agents, narcotic analgesics such as meperidine, Type 1 antiarrhythmic drugs (eg, disopyramide, procainamide, or quinidine), antihistamines, phenothiazines, tricyclic antidepressants, or other psychoactive drugs. Pro-Banthīne may also potentiate the sedative effect of phenothiazines. Increased intraocular pressure may result from concurrent administration of anticholinergics and corticosteroids.

Concurrent use of Pro-Banthīne with slow-dissolving tablets of digoxin may cause increased serum digoxin levels. This interaction can be avoided by using only those digoxin tablets that rapidly dissolve by USP standards.

Carcinogenesis, mutagenesis, impairment of fertility: No long-term fertility, carcinogenicity, or mutagenicity studies have been done with Pro-Banthīne.

Pregnancy. Pregnancy Category C. Animal reproduction studies have not been conducted with Pro-Banthīne. It is also not known whether Pro-Banthīne can cause fetal harm when administered to a pregnant woman or can affect reproduction capacity. Pro-Banthīne should be given to a pregnant woman only if clearly needed.

Nursing mothers: It is not known whether this drug is excreted in human milk. Because many drugs are excreted in human milk, caution should be exercised when Pro-Banthīne is administered to a nursing woman. Suppression of lactation may occur with anticholinergic drugs.

Pediatric use: Safety and effectiveness in children have not been established.

ADVERSE REACTIONS

Varying degrees of drying of salivary secretions may occur as well as decreased sweating. Ophthalmic side effects include blurred vision, mydriasis, cycloplegia, and increased ocular tension. Other reported adverse reactions include urinary hesitancy and retention, tachycardia, palpitations, loss of the sense of taste, headache, nervousness, mental confusion, drowsiness, weakness, dizziness, insomnia, nausea, vomiting, constipation, bloated feeling, impotence, suppression of lactation, and allergic reactions or drug idiosyncracies, including anaphylaxis, urticaria, and other dermal manifestations.

OVERDOSAGE

The symptoms of overdosage with Pro-Banthīne progress from an intensification of the usual side effects to CNS disturbances (from restlessness and excitement to psychotic behavior), circulatory changes (flushing, fall in blood pressure, circulatory failure), respiratory failure, paralysis, and coma.

Measures to be taken are (1) immediate induction of emesis or lavage of the stomach, (2) injection of physostigmine 0.5 to 2 mg intravenously, repeated as necessary up to a total of 5 mg, and (3) monitoring of vital signs and managing as necessary.

Fever may be treated symptomatically (cooling blanket or alcohol sponging). Excitement of a degree which demands attention may be managed with thiopental sodium 2% solution given slowly intravenously or diazepam, 5 to 10 mg intravenously or 10 mg intramuscularly. In the event of progression of the curare-like effect to paralysis of the respiratory muscles, mechanical respiration should be instituted and maintained until effective respiratory action returns.

DOSAGE AND ADMINISTRATION

The usual initial adult dosage of Pro-Banthīne tablets is 15 mg taken 30 minutes before each meal and 30 mg at bedtime (a total of 75 mg daily). Subsequent dosage adjustment should be made according to the patient's individual response and tolerance. The administration of one 7½-mg tablet three times a day is convenient for patients with mild manifestations, for geriatric patients, and for those of small stature.

HOW SUPPLIED

Pro-Banthīne 15-mg tablets are round, peach colored, sugar coated, with SEARLE imprinted on one side and 601 on the other side; bottles of 100 and 500, and cartons containing 100 unit-dose, individually blister-sealed tablets.

Pro-Banthīne 7½-mg tablets are round, white, sugar coated, with SEARLE imprinted on one side and 611 on the other side; bottles of 100.

Shown in Product Identification Section, page 429

THEO-24® ℞

[thē'ō-24]

(theophylline anhydrous)

DESCRIPTION

Theo-24 oral capsules contain 100 mg, 200 mg, or 300 mg of anhydrous theophylline, a bronchodilator, in a controlled-release formulation which allows a 24-hour dosing interval for appropriate patients.

The structural formula of theophylline, 3,7-dihydro-1,3-dimethyl-1*H*-purine-2,6-dione, is:

Theophylline is a white, odorless, crystalline powder having a bitter taste.

Inactive ingredients are edible ink, ethylcellulose, gelatin, shellac, silicon dioxide, starch, sucrose, talc, titanium dioxide, and coloring agents: 100-mg—includes FD&C Yellow No. 6; 200-mg—FD&C Red No. 3 and other colors; 300-mg—FD&C Blue No. 1 and other colors.

CLINICAL PHARMACOLOGY

Theophylline directly relaxes the smooth muscle of the bronchial airways and pulmonary blood vessels, thus acting mainly as a bronchodilator and smooth muscle relaxant. The drug also possesses other actions typical of the xanthine derivatives: coronary vasodilation, cardiac stimulation, diuresis, cerebral stimulation, and skeletal muscle stimulation. The actions of theophylline may be mediated through inhibition of phosphodiesterase and a resultant increase in intracellular cyclic AMP. *In vitro,* theophylline also has been shown to act synergistically with beta agonists that increase intracellular cyclic AMP through the stimulation of adenyl cyclase. More data are needed to determine if theophylline and beta agonists have a clinically important additive effect *in vivo.*

Pharmacokinetics:

Theophylline Elimination Characteristics

	Theophylline Clearance Rates (mean ± S.D.)	Half-Life Average (mean ± S.D.)
Children (over 6 months of age)	1.45 ± 0.58 ml/kg/min	3.7 ± 1.1 hr
Adult nonsmokers with uncomplicated asthma	0.65 ± 0.19 ml/kg/min	8.7 ± 2.2 hr

The half-life of theophylline is prolonged in patients with alcoholism, reduced hepatic or renal function, or congestive heart failure, and in patients receiving cimetidine or macrolide antibiotics such as troleandomycin and erythromycin. High fever for prolonged periods may reduce the rate of theophylline elimination.

Newborn infants have extremely slow theophylline clearance rates. The theophylline half-life in newborn infants may exceed 24 hours. Not until the age of 6 months do clearance rates approach those seen in older children.

Patients over age 55 and patients with chronic obstructive pulmonary disease, cardiac failure, or liver insufficiency may have much slower clearance rates with half-lives that exceed 24 hours.

The average half-life of theophylline in smokers (1 to 2 packs/day) is 4 to 5 hours; the average half-life in nonsmokers is 7 to 10 hours. The increase in theophylline clearance caused by smoking is probably the result of induction of drug-metabolizing enzymes. The effect of smoking on theophylline pharmacokinetics may persist for 3 months to 2 years after smoking is discontinued.

Tolerance does not appear to develop during long-term use of theophylline.

Theo-24 capsules contain hundreds of coated beads of theophylline. Each bead is an individual controlled-release delivery system. After dissolution of the capsules these beads are released and distributed in the gastrointestinal tract, thus minimizing the probability of high local concentrations of theophylline at any particular site.

Following the single-dose administration (8 mg/kg) of Theo-24 to 20 normal subjects who had fasted overnight and 2 hours after morning dosing, peak serum theophylline concentrations of 4.8 ± 1.5 (S.D.) mcg/ml were obtained at 13.3 ±4.7 (S.D.) hours. The fraction of the amount of the dose absorbed was approximately 13% at 3 hours, 31% at 6 hours, 55% at 12 hours, 70% at 16 hours, and 88% at 24 hours. The extent of theophylline bioavailability from Theo-24 was comparable to the most widely used 12-hour controlled-release product when both products were administered every 12 hours.

In a 6-day multiple-dose study involving 18 subjects (with theophylline clearance rates between 0.57 and 1.02 ml/kg/min) who had fasted overnight and 2 hours after morning dosing, Theo-24 given once daily in a dose of 1500 mg produced serum theophylline levels that ranged between 5.7 mcg/ml and 22 mcg/ml. The mean minimum and maximum values were 11.6 mcg/ml and 18.1 mcg/ml, respectively, with an average peak-trough difference of 6.5 mcg/ml. A 24-hour single-dose study demonstrated an approximately proportional increase in serum levels as the dose was increased from 600 to 1500 mg.

Taking Theo-24 with a high-fat-content meal may result in a significant increase in peak serum level and in the extent of absorption of theophylline as compared to administration in the fasted state (see *Precautions: Drug/Food interactions*).

INDICATIONS AND USAGE

Theo-24 is indicated for the relief and/or prevention of symptoms of asthma and for reversible bronchospasm associated with chronic bronchitis and emphysema.

CONTRAINDICATIONS

Theo-24 (theophylline anhydrous) is contraindicated in patients who have shown hypersensitivity to theophylline.

WARNINGS

Status asthmaticus is a medical emergency and is defined as that degree of bronchospasm not rapidly responsive to recommended doses of usual bronchodilators. Oral theophylline alone is not appropriate treatment for status asthmaticus. Patients with status asthmaticus require *medication administered parenterally* and *close monitoring,* preferably in an intensive-care setting.

Optimum therapeutic response occurs in many patients when the serum theophylline concentration is 10 to 20 mcg/ml. In other patients satisfactory results (as determined by both relief of symptoms and improvement in pulmonary function) may be obtained at lower levels. In still others, adequate response may require higher levels. The physician should adjust the desired serum concentration range to the patients' requirements, keeping in mind that *an increased probability of toxicity exists when levels exceed 20 mcg/ml.* Therefore, in order to assure maximum benefit without excessive risk, measurement of serum levels is highly recommended.

Serum levels above 20 mcg/ml are rarely found after appropriate administration of the recommended doses. However, in individuals in whom theophylline plasma clearance is reduced *for any reason,* even conventional doses may result in increased serum levels with subsequent toxicity. Reduced theophylline clearance has been documented in the following readily identifiable groups:

1. Patients with impaired renal or liver function.
2. Patients over 55 years of age, particularly males and those with chronic lung disease.

Continued on next page

Searle & Co.—Cont.

3. Patients with cardiac failure from any cause.
4. Neonates.
5. Patients taking certain drugs (macrolide antibiotics, cimetidine, or oral contraceptives).

Decreased clearance of theophylline may be associated with either influenza immunization or active influenza, and with other viral infections. Reduction of dosage and measurement of serum theophylline levels are especially appropriate in the above individuals.

Although the effects of theophylline are dose related, *serious toxicity is not reliably preceded by less severe side effects.* Ventricular arrhythmias, convulsions, or even death may appear as the first sign of toxicity without previous warning. Less serious signs of theophylline toxicity (ie, nausea and restlessness) may occur frequently when initiating therapy, but are usually transient; when such signs are persistent during maintenance therapy, they are often associated with serum concentrations above 20 mcg/ml.

Patients who require theophylline may exhibit tachycardia due to the underlying disease process so that the cause/effect relationship to elevated serum theophylline concentrations will not be recognized.

Theophylline products may cause arrhythmias or worsen preexisting arrhythmias. Any significant change in cardiac rate and/or rhythm warrants monitoring and further investigation. Halothane anesthesia in the presence of theophylline may produce sinus tachycardia or ventricular arrhythmias.

In minipigs, rodents, and dogs, arrhythmia and sudden death (with histological evidence of myocardial necrosis) have been observed when theophylline and beta agonists were administered concomitantly but not when either was administered alone. The significance of these findings for human use is unknown.

PRECAUTIONS

General: Use with caution in patients with severe cardiac disease, hypertension, acute myocardial injury, congestive heart failure, cor pulmonale, severe hypoxemia, hyperthyroidism, hepatic impairment, or alcoholism, and in the elderly (especially males) and in neonates. Particular caution should be used in administering theophylline to patients with congestive heart failure. Reduced theophylline clearance in these patients may cause serum theophylline levels to persist long after the drug is discontinued.

Individuals who are rapid metabolizers of theophylline (such as the young, smokers, and some nonsmoking adults) may not be suitable candidates for once-a-day dosing. Dividing the daily dose into two doses may be indicated if symptoms of bronchospasm occur repeatedly, especially near the end of a 24-hour dosing interval, or if the patient exhibits wider peak-trough differences than desired.

Convulsions may occur in patients with theophylline overdosage when serum theophylline concentrations exceed 30 mcg/ml. Theophylline may lower the seizure threshold.

Theophylline should not be administered concomitantly with other xanthine medications.

Methylxanthines are known to increase gastric acidity. Therefore, theophylline should be used cautiously in patients with a history of peptic ulcer since the disease may be exacerbated. Theophylline may occasionally act as a local irritant to the gastrointestinal tract, although gastrointestinal symptoms are more commonly mediated through the central nervous system and are usually associated with serum drug concentrations over 20 mcg/ml.

Information for patients: Patients should be instructed to take this medication in the morning, at approximately the same time each day, and to not exceed the prescribed dose. Patients who require a relatively high dose of theophylline (ie, a dose equal to or greater than 900 mg or 13 mg/kg, whichever is less) should be informed of important considerations relating to time of drug administration and meal content (see *Precautions: Drug/Food interactions;* and *Dosage and Administration).*

As with any controlled-release theophylline product the patient should alert the physician if symptoms occur repeatedly, especially near the end of a dosing interval.

Laboratory tests: The determination of serum theophylline levels is highly recommended.

Drug interactions:

Drug/Drug interactions: Elevated serum levels of theophylline may occur in patients treated concomitantly with theophylline and cimetidine, ranitidine, troleandomycin, erythromycin, allopurinol, or oral contraceptive steroids. Therefore, such patients should be watched carefully for signs of theophylline toxicity and the dose of theophylline decreased if necessary. Increased toxicity may occur when ephedrine or other sympathomimetic drugs are given concomitantly with theophylline. Co-medication with phenobarbital, phenytoin, or rifampin may increase theophylline clearance and an increase of the theophylline dose may be required. The excretion of lithium carbonate is increased in patients receiving aminophylline (theophylline with ethylenediamine). Aminophylline may antagonize the effects of propranolol.

Drug/Food interactions: *Taking Theo-24 less than one hour before a high-fat-content meal, such as 8 oz whole milk, 2 fried eggs, 2 bacon strips, 2 oz hashed brown potatoes, and 2 slices of buttered toast (about 985 calories, including approximately 71 g of fat) may result in a significant increase in peak serum level and in the extent of absorption of theophylline as compared to administration in the fasted state. In some cases (especially with doses of 900 mg or more taken less than one hour before a high-fat-content meal) serum theophylline levels may exceed the 20 mcg/ml level, above which theophylline toxicity is more likely to occur.*

Drug/Laboratory test interactions: Consumption of coffee, tea, cola beverages, chocolate, or acetaminophen contributes to falsely high serum theophylline levels when theophylline is measured spectrophotometrically without previous isolation by chromatography.

Carcinogenesis, mutagenesis, and impairment of fertility: Theophylline has been shown to be mutagenic in *Escherichia coli* and other lower organisms (*Euglena gracilis* and *Ophiostoma multiannulatum*) and to produce chromosome breaks in cultured mouse cells and cultured human lymphocytes. The drug had no mutagenic activity *in vivo* in a dominant lethal test using mice. Long-term animal studies have not been performed with theophylline to evaluate carcinogenic potential, mutagenic potential, or effect on fertility.

Pregnancy: Pregnancy Category C. Limited animal studies have shown teratogenic activity of theophylline in mice and rats. It is not known whether theophylline can cause fetal harm when administered to a pregnant woman or can affect reproductive capacity. Xanthines should be given to a pregnant woman only if clearly needed.

Nursing mothers: Theophylline is excreted in breast milk and may cause adverse effects in the infant. Caution must be used when prescribing theophylline to a nursing mother, taking into account the risk/benefit of this therapy.

Pediatric use: Safety and effectiveness in children under 12 years of age have not been established with this product.

ADVERSE REACTIONS

The most consistent adverse reactions are usually due to overdose and are:

1. Gastrointestinal: nausea, vomiting, epigastric pain, hematemesis, diarrhea.
2. Central nervous system: headaches, irritability, restlessness, insomnia, reflex hyperexcitability, muscle twitching, clonic and tonic generalized convulsions, coma.
3. Cardiovascular: palpitation, tachycardia, extrasystoles, flushing, hypotension, circulatory failure, ventricular arrhythmias.
4. Respiratory: tachypnea.
5. Renal: albuminuria, microhematuria, potentiation of diuresis.
6. Other: hyperglycemia and inappropriate ADH (antidiuretic hormone) syndrome, rash.

OVERDOSAGE

Management: If overdose following oral administration is suspected and a seizure has not occurred:

A. Induce vomiting or perform gastric lavage.
B. Administer activated charcoal.
C. Administer a cathartic, particularly if a controlled-release preparation has been taken.

If patient is having a seizure:

A. Establish an airway.
B. Administer oxygen.
C. Treat the seizure with intravenous diazepam, 0.1 to 0.3 mg/kg up to a total dose of 10 mg.
D. Monitor vital signs, maintain blood pressure, and provide adequate hydration.

If patient is in post-seizure coma:

A. Maintain airway and oxygenation.
B. Gastric lavage must be performed and a cathartic and activated charcoal introduced via a large-bore tube.
C. Continue to provide full supportive care and adequate hydration while waiting for drug to be metabolized. The drug is metabolized rapidly enough by most patients so that dialysis is usually not needed. If serum levels exceed 50 mcg/ml, charcoal hemoperfusion may be indicated.

DOSAGE AND ADMINISTRATION

Patients who require a relatively high dose of theophylline (ie, a dose equal to or greater than 900 mg or 13 mg/kg, whichever is less) should not take Theo-24 less than one hour before a high-fat-content meal since this may result in a significant increase in peak serum level and in the extent of absorption of theophylline as compared to administration in the fasted state (see *Precautions: Drug/Food interactions*).

Effective use of theophylline (ie, the concentration of drug in the serum associated with optimal benefit and minimal risk of toxicity) is considered to occur when the theophylline concentration is maintained from 10 to 20 mcg/ml. The early studies from which these levels were derived were carried out in patients immediately or shortly after recovery from acute exacerbations of their disease (some hospitalized with status asthmaticus).

Although the 20 mcg/ml level remains appropriate as a critical value (above which toxicity is more likely to occur) for safety purposes, additional data are now available which indicate that the serum theophylline concentrations required to produce maximum physiologic benefit may, in fact, fluctuate with the degree of bronchospasm present and are variable. Therefore, the physician should individualize the range appropriate to the patient's requirements, based on both symptomatic response and improvement in pulmonary function. It should be stressed that serum theophylline concentrations maintained at the upper level of the 10 to 20 mcg/ml range may be associated with potential toxicity when factors known to reduce theophylline clearance are operative. (See *Precautions,* including *Drug interactions.*)

Theo-24, like other controlled-release theophylline products, is intended for patients with relatively continuous or recurring symptoms who have a need to maintain therapeutic serum levels of theophylline. It is not intended for patients experiencing an acute episode of bronchospasm (associated with asthma, chronic bronchitis, or emphysema). Such patients require *rapid* relief of symptoms and should be treated with an immediate-release or intravenous theophylline preparation (or other bronchodilators) and not with controlled-release products.

Patients who metabolize theophylline at a normal or slow rate are reasonable candidates for once-daily dosing with Theo-24. Patients who metabolize theophylline rapidly (eg, the young, smokers, and some nonsmoking adults) and who have symptoms repeatedly at the end of a dosing interval, will require either increased doses given once a day, or preferably, are likely to be better controlled by a schedule of twice-daily dosing. Those patients who require increased daily doses are more likely to experience relatively wide peak-trough differences and may be candidates for twice-a-day dosing with Theo-24.

Patients should be instructed to take this medication each morning at approximately the same time and not to exceed the prescribed dose.

Recent studies suggest that dosing of controlled-release theophylline products at night (after the evening meal) results in serum concentrations of theophylline which are not identical to those recorded during waking hours and may be characterized by early trough and delayed peak levels. This appears to occur whether the drug is given as an immediate-release, controlled-release, *or* intravenous product. To avoid this phenomenon when two doses per day are prescribed, it is recommended that the second dose be given 10 to 12 hours after the morning dose and before the evening meal.

Food and posture, along with changes associated with circadian rhythm, may influence the rate of absorption and/or clearance rates of theophylline from controlled-release dosage forms administered at night. The exact relationship of these and other factors to nighttime serum concentrations and the clinical significance of such findings require additional study. Therefore, it is not recommended that Theo-24 (when used as a once-a-day product) be administered at night.

Since there is a wide variation from patient to patient in the total dose of theophylline required to attain the desired level in the serum, it is essential that the dose be titrated and that serum levels be monitored before and after *transfer* to any sustained-release product.

When serum levels are not measured, the initial dosage should be restricted to the amount recommended below (see *Initiation of Therapy*).

As a practical consideration, it is not always possible to obtain serum level determinations. Under such conditions, restriction of the daily dose (in otherwise healthy adults) to not greater than 13 mg/kg/day (or 900 mg, whichever is lower) will result in relatively few patients exceeding serum levels of 20 mcg/ml, thereby reducing the risk of developing toxicity.

Dosage Guidelines

WARNING: DO NOT ATTEMPT TO MAINTAIN ANY DOSE THAT IS NOT TOLERATED. Dosage guidelines are approximations only, and the wide range of clearance of theophylline among individuals (particularly those with concomitant disease) makes indiscriminate usage hazardous.

Because a high-fat-content meal may significantly increase the peak level and extent of absorption of theophylline from Theo-24, patients receiving large single doses (ie, equal to or greater than 900 mg or 13 mg/kg, whichever is less) should be instructed to avoid eating a high-fat-content morning meal or to take their medication at least one hour before eating. If the physician cannot be assured that the patient will follow this regimen, then the patient should be placed on a twice-daily dosing regimen.

For patients receiving lower once-daily single doses (less than 900 mg), very high peak levels are less likely to occur when Theo-24 (theophylline anhydrous) is taken with food. With close monitoring, patients less certain to observe the fasting requirements could be treated with once-daily dosing.

It is recommended that dosing be considered in three stages: (I) initiation of therapy with Theo-24, (II) titration and adjustment, and (III) chronic maintenance.

I. Initiation of Therapy with Theo-24:

A. *Transfer of patients* already on established daily doses of theophylline (whether stabilized on immediate- or controlled-release products) can be accomplished by administering the total daily dosage as a single dose given in the morning (eg, 300 mg of an immediate-release product given t.i.d. should be given as 900 mg of Theo-24). The initial transfer should not be made at doses exceeding 900 mg/day or 13 mg/kg/day, whichever is less. Subsequent dose titration should be done on the basis of serum levels and with appropriate attention to the time of drug administration and meal content as noted above.

It must be recognized that the peak and trough serum theophylline levels produced by once-daily dosing may vary (usually wider peak-trough differences) from those produced by the previous product and/or dosage regimen.

B. *For initiation of therapy with Theo-24* in patients who are not currently taking a theophylline product, the total daily dose, administered in the morning, must be established in accordance with the following guidelines:

Body Weight	Daily Dose
Children	
30 to 35 kg	300 mg
35 kg and above	400 mg
Adults	400 mg

Theophylline does not distribute into fatty tissue. Therefore, dosage should be calculated on the basis of lean (ideal) body weight where mg/kg doses are presented.

If appropriate serum theophylline concentrations or adequate improvement in pulmonary function is not obtained after 3 days, the instructions in Part II (below) should be followed.

II. Titration and Adjustment of Dose:

This phase of adjustment should be implemented either by the use of serum concentration measurements or by empirical principles when serum level determinations are not available.

A. *If serum levels can be measured:*

After 3 days' therapy with Theo-24, serum levels should be determined for peak concentration (sample obtained 12 hours after the morning dose) and trough concentration (24 hours after the morning dose). It is important that the patient has not missed or added any dose during the 72-hour period and that dosing intervals have been reasonably consistent. DOSE ADJUSTMENT BASED ON MEASUREMENTS WHEN THESE INSTRUCTIONS HAVE NOT BEEN FOLLOWED MAY RESULT IN TOXICITY.

Based on the results of the peak-trough values obtained, *three possibilities* exist:

1. The values of serum theophylline concentration fall within the desired range. If this result is obtained, the dosage should be maintained if it is tolerated.
2. If the serum theophylline concentration is too high, the dosage should be reduced as follows:
   a. If the values are between 20 and 25 mcg/ml, the daily dose may be reduced by about 10% and serum theophylline levels should be rechecked after 3 days.
   b. If the values are between 25 and 30 mcg/ml, the next dose should be skipped and the daily dose reduced by about 25%. The serum concentration should be rechecked after 3 days.
   c. If the values are over 30 mcg/ml, the next dose should be skipped and the daily dose reduced by 50%. The serum concentration should be rechecked after 3 days.
3. If the serum theophylline concentration is too low, the dosage should be increased at 3-day intervals by 100 mg or 200 mg (or 25% of the current dose), depending upon the desired goal. The serum concentration may be rechecked at appropriate intervals, but at least at the end of this adjustment period.

B. *If serum levels cannot be measured:*

1. If the clinical response is satisfactory then the total daily dose should be maintained.
2. If the response is unsatisfactory (due to persistence of symptoms or minimal improvement in measured function) after 3 days, then the dose may be increased by 100-mg increments. Reevaluation should be undertaken every 3 days.
3. If the response is still unsatisfactory and there are no adverse reactions, the dose may be cautiously adjusted upward in increments of 100 mg/day at 3- to 5-day intervals up to 900 mg (or 13 mg/kg/day, whichever is less).
4. If a response is accompanied by adverse reactions, then the next dose should be withheld or reduced by 25% depending on the severity of the reactions.

III. Chronic Maintenance

After the dose is established theophylline serum concentrations usually remain stable. However, as noted elsewhere (see *Precautions* and *Warnings*), certain exogenous and endogenous factors alter theophylline elimination (including concomitant disease and drug interactions) which require drug monitoring and adjustments in total daily dose requirements while such factors are operative.

Older adults, those with cor pulmonale, congestive heart failure, and/or liver disease may have unusually low dosage requirements and thus may experience toxicity at the minimal dosage recommended above.

If the patient's condition is otherwise clinically stable and none of the recognized factors which alter elimination are present, measurement of serum levels need be repeated only every 6 to 12 months.

HOW SUPPLIED

Theo-24 (theophylline anhydrous) is supplied in controlled-release capsules containing 100, 200, or 300 mg of anhydrous theophylline.

Theo-24 100-mg capsules are gold and clear, with markings Theo-24, 100 mg, SEARLE, and 2832.

Theo-24 200-mg capsules are orange and clear, with markings Theo-24, 200 mg, SEARLE, and 2842.

Theo-24 300-mg capsules are red and clear, with markings Theo-24, 300 mg, SEARLE, and 2852.

Available in bottles of 100, 500 (except 100 mg), and cartons of 100 unit-dose individually blister-sealed capsules.

Shown in Product Identification Section, page 429

The preceding prescribing information for Searle & Co. products was current on September 1, 1986.

SERES Laboratories, Inc.

3331 INDUSTRIAL DRIVE
BOX 470
SANTA ROSA, CA 95402

CANTHARONE® ℞

[kan'tha-rone]
(cantharidin collodion)
For External Use Only

DESCRIPTION

CANTHARONE, cantharidin collodion, is a topical liquid containing 0.7% cantharidin, acetone, pyroxylin, castor oil and camphor.

HOW SUPPLIED

7.5 mL bottles (NDC 50694-096-01). Close tightly immediately after use. Keep away from heat.
Revised July, 1985
Direct inquiries to Kathryn MacLeod, Ph.D.

CANTHARONE® PLUS ℞

[kan'tha rone PLUS]
For External Use Only

DESCRIPTION

CANTHARONE PLUS is a topical liquid containing 30% salicylic acid, 5% podophyllin, 1% cantharidin, octylphenyl-polyethylene glycol, cellosolve, ethocel, pyroxylin, castor oil and acetone.

HOW SUPPLIED

7.5 mL bottles (NDC 50694-097-01). Close tightly immediately after use. Keep away from heat. Do not refrigerate.
Revised July, 1985
Direct inquiries to Kathryn MacLeod, Ph.D.

NIGHT CAST™ Formula R

(Medicated Acne Mask)

DESCRIPTION

Contains 4% sulfur, 1.5% salicylic acid and 33% alcohol in a non-comedogenic vehicle.

HOW SUPPLIED

4 fl. oz. in a plastic dispenser bottle.
(NDC 50694-201-04) Revised July 1986
Direct inquiries to Kathryn MacLeod, Ph.D.

NIGHT CAST™ Formula S

(Medicated Acne Mask)

DESCRIPTION

Contains 8% sulfur, 2% resorcinol and 31% alcohol in a non-comedogenic vehicle.

HOW SUPPLIED

4 fl. oz. in a plastic dispenser bottle.
(NDC 50694-202-04) Revised July 1986
Direct inquiries to Kathryn MacLeod, Ph.D.

Serono Laboratories, Inc.

280 POND STREET
RANDOLPH, MA 02368

Serono Laboratories, Inc. will be pleased to answer inquiries about the following products:

PERGONAL® ℞

[per'go-nal]
(menotropins for injection, USP)
For Intramuscular Injection

PRODUCT OVERVIEW

KEY FACTS

Pergonal® is a purified, lyophilized preparation of gonadotropins, and contains equal amounts of follice stimulating hormone and luteinizing hormone. Pergonal® is administered by intramuscular injection immediately after reconstitution with Sodium Chloride for Injection, USP.

MAJOR USES

Women: Pergonal® is used to stimulate follicular development in hypogonadotropic anovulatory women who do not have primary ovarian failure.

Men: Pergonal® is used concomitantly with Profasi® HP (hCG) to stimulate spermatogenesis in men with infertility due to primary or secondary hypogonadotropic hypogonadism.

SAFETY INFORMATION

Pergonal® is contraindicated in individuals who have previously demonstrated hypersensitivity to the drug. In rare instances, women may experience excessive ovarian enlargement, ascites, and pleural effusion requiring hospitalization. The risk can be minimized through careful patient monitoring. Multiple births, 90% of which are twins, have been reported in 20% of pregnancies resulting from Pergonal® therapy.

PRESCRIBING INFORMATION

PERGONAL® ℞

[per'go-nal]
(menotropins for injection, USP)

DESCRIPTION

Pergonal® (Menotropins for Injection, USP) is a purified preparation of gonadotropins extracted from the urine of postmenopausal women. Each ampule of Pergonal® contains 75 IU or 150 IU of follicle-stimulating hormone (FSH) activity and 75 IU or 150 IU of luteinizing hormone (LH) activity, respectively, plus 10 mg lactose in a sterile, lyophilized form. Pergonal® is administered by intramuscular injection.

Pergonal® is biologically standardized for FSH and LH (ICSH) gonadotropin activities in terms of the Second International Reference Preparation for Human Menopausal Gonadotropins established in September, 1964 by the Expert Committee on Biological Standards of the World Health Organization.

Both FSH and LH are glycoproteins that are acidic and water soluble. Therapeutic class: Infertility.

CLINICAL PHARMACOLOGY

Women:

Pergonal® administered for seven to twelve days produces ovarian follicular growth in women who do not have primary ovarian failure. Treatment with Pergonal® in most instances results only in follicular growth and maturation. In order to effect ovulation, human chorionic gonadotropin (hCG) must be given following the administration of Pergonal® when clinical assessment of the patient indicates that sufficient follicular maturation has occurred.

Men:

Pergonal® administered concomitantly with human chorionic gonadotropin (hCG) for at least three months induces spermatogenesis in men with primary or secondary pituitary hypofunction who have achieved adequate masculinization with prior hCG therapy.

Continued on next page

Serono—Cont.

INDICATIONS AND USAGE

Women:

Pergonal® and hCG given in a sequential manner are indicated for the induction of ovulation and pregnancy in the anovulatory infertile patient, in whom the cause of anovulation is functional and is not due to primary ovarian failure.

Men:

Pergonal® with concomitant hCG is indicated for the stimulation of spermatogenesis in men who have primary or secondary hypogonadotropic hypogonadism.

Pergonal® with concomitant hCG has proven effective in inducing spermatogenesis in men with primary hypogonadotropic hypogonadism due to a congenital factor or prepubertal hypophysectomy and in men with secondary hypogonadotropic hypogonadism due to hypophysectomy, craniopharyngioma, cerebral aneurysm or chromophobe adenoma.

SELECTION OF PATIENTS

Women:

1. Before treatement with Pergonal® is instituted, a thorough gynecologic and endocrinologic evaluation must be performed. This should include a hysterosalpingogram (to rule out uterine and tubal pathology) and documentation of anovulation by means of basal body temperature, serial vaginal smears, examination of cervical mucus, determination of urinary pregnanediol and endometrial biopsy.
2. Primary ovarian failure should be excluded by the determination of gonadotropin levels.
3. Careful examination should be made to rule out the presence of an early pregnancy.
4. Patients in late reproductive life have a greater predilection to endometrial carcinoma as well as a higher incidence of anovulatory disorders. Cervical dilation and curettage should always be done for diagnosis before starting Pergonal® therapy in such patients.
5. Evaluation of the husband's fertility potential should be included in the workup.

Men:

Patient selection should be made based on a documented lack of pituitary function. Prior to hormonal therapy, these patients will have low testosterone levels and low or absent gonadotropin levels. Patients with primary hypogonadotropic hypogonadism will have a sub-normal development of masculinization, and those with secondary hypogonadotropic hypogonadism will have decreased masculinization.

CONTRAINDICATIONS

Women:

Pergonal® is contraindicated in women who have:

1. A high gonadotropin level indicating primary ovarian failure.
2. Overt thyroid and adrenal dysfunction.
3. An organic intracranial lesion such as a pituitary tumor.
4. The presence of any cause of infertility other than anovulation, as stated in the indications.
5. Abnormal bleeding of undetermined origin.
6. Ovarian cysts or enlargement not due to polycystic ovary syndrome.
7. Pergonal® is contraindicated in women who are pregnant and may cause fetal harm when administered to a pregnant woman. There are no human data on the effects of Pergonal® when administered during pregnancy. If this drug is inadvertently used during pregnancy, the patient should be apprised of the potential hazard to the fetus.

Men:

Pergonal® is contraindicated in men who have:

1. Normal gonadotropin levels indicating normal pituitary function.
2. Elevated gonadotropin levels indicating primary testicular failure.
3. Infertility disorders other than hypogonadotropic hypogonadism.

WARNINGS

Pergonal® is a drug that should only be used by physicians who are thoroughly familiar with infertility problems. It is a potent gonadotropic substance capable of causing mild to severe adverse reactions in women. In female patients it must be used with a great deal of care.

Overstimulation of the Ovary During Pergonal® Therapy: In order to minimize the hazard associated with the occasional abnormal ovarian enlargement associated with Pergonal®-hCG therapy, the lowest dose consistent with expectation of good results should be used. Careful monitoring of ovarian response can further minimize the risk of overstimulation.

Mild to moderate uncomplicated ovarian enlargement which may be accompanied by abdominal distension and/or abdominal pain occurs in approximately 20% of those treated with Pergonal® and hCG, and generally regresses without treatment within two or three weeks.

The hyperstimulation syndrome characterized by sudden ovarian enlargement accompanied by ascites with or without pain and/or pleural effusion occurs in approximately 0.4% of patients when the recommended dose is administered and in 1.3% of patients when higher than recommended doses are included.

If hyperstimulation occurs, treatment should be stopped and the patient hospitalized. The hyperstimulation syndrome develops rapidly over a period of three to four days and generally occurs during the two week period immediately following treatment. The phenomenon of hemoconcentration associated with fluid loss into the abdominal cavity has been seen to occur and should be thoroughly assessed in the following manner: 1) fluid intake and output, 2) weight, 3) hematocrit, 4) serum and urinary electrolytes, and 5) urine specific gravity. These determinations are to be performed daily or more often if the need arises. Treatment is primarily symptomatic and would consist of bed rest, fluid and electrolyte replacement and analgesics if needed. The ascitic fluid should never be removed because of the potential danger of injury to the ovary.

Hemoperitoneum may occur from ruptured ovarian cysts. This is usually the result of pelvic examination. If this does occur, and if bleeding becomes such that surgery is required, the conservative approach with partial resection of the enlarged ovary or ovaries is generally adequate.

Intercourse should be prohibited in those patients in whom significant ovarian enlargement occurs after ovulation because of the danger of hemoperitoneum resulting from ruptured ovarian cycsts.

Arterial Thromboembolism:

Arterial thromboembolism following Pergonal® and hCG therapy has been reported in four patients, two of whom died.

Multiple Births:

Of the pregnancies following therapy with Pergonal® and hCG, 80% have resulted in single births and 20% in multiple births, most of which have been twins. Fifteen percent of the total pregnancies resulted in twins, of which 93% were viable (78 surviving infants from 43 sets of twins). Five percent of the total pregnancies have resulted in three or more conceptuses, of which 20% were viable (nine surviving infants from three sets of triplets, four surviving infants from four sets of quadruplets, and no surviving infants from four sets of quintuplets). The patient and her husband should be advised of the frequency and potential hazards of multiple pregnancy before starting treatment.

PRECAUTIONS

General: Careful attention should be given to diagnosis in the selection of candidates for Pergonal® therapy (see "Indications and Usage—Selection of Patients").

Information for Patients: Prior to therapy with Pergonal®, patients should be informed of the duration of treatment and the monitoring of their condition that will be required. Possible adverse reactions (see "Adverse Reactions" section) and the risk of multiple births should also be discussed.

Laboratory Tests:

Women:

Treatment for Induction of Ovulation

In most instances, treatment with Pergonal® results only in follicular growth and maturation. In order to effect ovulation, hCG must be given following the administration of Pergonal® when clinical assessment of the patient indicates that sufficient follicular maturation has occurred. This is indirectly estimated by the estrogenic effect upon the target organs. These indices of estrogenic activity include:

a) Changes in the vaginal smear;
b) Appearance and volume of the cervical mucus;
c) Spinnbarkeit; and
d) Ferning of the cervical mucus.

A combination of the above clinical indices, along with serum or urinary estrogen determinations and ultrasonography, provides an acceptable means for monitoring the growth and development of follicles, timing the hCG administration, as well as minimizing the risk of hyperstimulation.

The clinical confirmation of ovulation, with the exception of pregnancy, is obtained by indirect indices of progesterone production. The indices most generally used are as follows:

a) A rise in basal body temperature;
b) Change of the cervical mucus from a "fern" pattern to a "cellular"pattern;
c) Vaginal cytology characteristic of the luteal phase of the menstrual cycle;
d) Increase in urinary pregnanediol; and
e) Menstruation following the shift in basal body temperature.

Because of the subjectivity of the various tests for the determination of follicular maturation and ovulation, it cannot be over-emphasized that the physician should choose tests with which he/she is thoroughly familiar.

Drug Interactions: No clinically signficant drug/drug or drug/food adverse interactions have been reported during Pergonal® therapy.

Carcinogenesis and Mutagenesis: Long-term toxicity studies in animals have not been performed to evaluate the carcinogenic potential of Pergonal®.

Pregnancy: Pregnancy Category X. See "Contraindications" section.

Nursing Mothers: It is not known whether this drug is excreted in human milk. Because many drugs are excreted in human milk, caution should be exercised if Pergonal® is administered to a nursing woman.

ADVERSE REACTIONS

Women:

1. Arterial Thromboembolism (see "Warnings"above)
2. Hyperstimulation Syndrome
3. Hemoperitoneum
4. Abnormal Ovarian Enlargement
5. Ectopic Pregnancy
6. Sensitivity to Pergonal®
   Occasional febrile reactions after the administration of Pergonal® have occurred. It is not clear whether or not these were pyrogenic responses or possible allergic reactions.
7. Pain, rash, swelling and/or irritation at the site of injection
8. Defects at Birth
   From 287 completed pregnancies following Pergonal®-hCG therapy five incidents of birth defects have been reported (1.7%). One infant had multiple congenital anomalies consisting of imperforate anus, aplasia of the sigmoid colon, third degree hypospadias, cecovesicle fistula, bifid scrotum, meningocele, bilateral internal tibial torsion, and right metatarsus adductus. Another infant was born with an imperforate anus and possible congenital heart lesions; another had a supernumerary digit; another was born with hypospadias and exstrophy of the bladder; and the fifth child had Down's syndrome. None of the investigators felt that these defects were drug-related. Subsequently one report of an infant death due to hydrocephalus and cardiac anomalies has been received.

Men:

1. Gynecomastia may occur occasionally during Pergonal®-hCG therapy. This is a known effect of hCG treatment.
2. Erythrocytosis (hct 50%, hgb 17.8 g%) was recorded in one patient.

DRUG ABUSE AND DEPENDENCE

There have been no reports of abuse or dependence with Pergonal®.

OVERDOSAGE

Aside from possible ovarian hyperstimulation (see "Warnings"), little is known concerning the consequences of acute overdosage with Pergonal®.

DOSAGE AND ADMINISTRATION

Women:

1. Dosage:

The dose of Pergonal® to produce maturation of the follicle must be individualized for each patient. It is recommended that the initial dose to any patient should be 75 IU of FSH/LH per day, **ADMINISTERED INTRAMUSCULARLY**, for seven to twelve days followed by hCG, 5,000 U to 10,000 U, one day after the last dose of Pergonal®. The hyperstimulation syndrome has not occurred with administration of 75 IU of FSH/LH per day for up to twelve days. Administration of Pergonal®should not exceed 12 days in a single course of therapy. The patient should be treated until indices of estrogenic activity, as indicated under "Precautions" above, are equivalent to or greater than those of the normal individual. If serum or urinary estradiol determinations or ultrasonographic visualizations are available, they may be useful as a guide to therapy. If the ovaries are abnormally enlarged on the last day of Pergonal® therapy, hCG should not be administered in this course of therapy; this will reduce the chances of development of the hyperstimulation syndrome. If there is evidence of ovulation but no pregnancy, repeat this dosage regime for at least two more courses before increasing the dose of Pergonal® to 150 IU of FSH/LH per day for seven to twelve days. As before, this dose should be followed by 5,000 U to 10,000 U of hCG one day after the last dose of Pergonal®. A Pergonal® dose of 150 IU of FSH/LH per day has proven to be the most effective dose. If evidence of ovulation is present, but pregnancy does not ensue, repeat the same dose for two more courses. Doses larger than this are not routinely recommended.

During treatment with both Pergonal® and hCG and during a two-week post-treatment period, patients should be examined at least every other day for signs of excessive ovarian stimulation. It is recommended that Pergonal® administration be stopped if the ovaries become abnormally enlarged or abdominal pain occurs. Most of the ovarian hyperstimulation occurs after treatment has been discontinued and reaches its maximum at about seven to ten days post-ovulation. Patients should be followed for at least two weeks after hCG administration.

The couple should be encouraged to have intercourse daily, beginning on the day prior to the administration of hCG until ovulation becomes apparent from the indices employed for the determination of progestational activity.

Care should be taken to insure insemination. In the light of the foregoing indices and parameters mentioned, it should become obvious that, unless a physician is willing to devote considerable time to these patients and be familiar with and conduct the necessary laboratory studies, he/she should not use Pergonal®.

2. Administration:

Dissolve the contents of one ampule of Pergonal® in one to two ml of sterile saline and **ADMINISTER INTRAMUSCULARLY** immediately. Any unused reconstituted material should be discarded.

Men:

1. Dosage:

Prior to concomitant therapy with Pergonal® and hCG, pretreatment with hCG alone (5,000 U three times a week) is required. Treatment should continue for a period sufficient to achieve serum testosterone levels within the normal range and masculinization as judged by the appearance of secondary sex characteristics. Such pretreatment may require four to six months, then the recommended dose of Pergonal® is 75 IU FSH/LH **ADMINISTERED INTRAMUSCULARLY**, three times a week and the recommended dose of hCG is 2,000 U twice a week. Therapy should be carried on for a minimum of four more months to insure detecting spermatozoa in the ejaculate, as it takes 74± 4 days in the human male for germ cells to reach the spermatozoa stage.

If the patient has not responded with evidence of increased spermatogenesis at the end of four months of therapy, treatment may continue with 75 IU FSH/LH three times a week, or the dose can be increased to 150 IU FSH/LH three times a week, with the hCG dose unchanged.

2. Administration:

Dissolve the contents of one ampule of Pergonal® in one to two ml of sterile saline and **ADMINISTER INTRAMUSCULARLY** immediately. Any unused reconstituted material should be discarded.

HOW SUPPLIED

Pergonal® is supplied in a sterile lyophilized form in snap-top ampules containing 75 IU or 150 IU FSH/LH activity.

The following package combinations are available:

—1 ampule 75 IU Pergonal® and 1 ampule 2 ml Sodium Chloride Injection (USP), NDC 44087-0571-7.

—10 ampules 75 IU Pergonal® and 10 ampules 2 ml Sodium Chloride Injection (USP), NDC 44087-5075-3.

—1 ampule 150 IU Pergonal® and 1 ampule 2 ml Sodium Chloride Injection (USP), NDC 44087-5150-1.

By biological assay, one IU of LH for the Second International Reference Preparation (2nd-IRP) for hMG is biologically equivalent to approximately ½ IU of hCG.

Lyophilized powder may be stored refrigerated or at room temperature (3–30°C/37–86°F). Use immediately after reconstitution. Discard unused material.

CLINICAL STUDIES

Women:

The results of the clinical experience and effectiveness of the administration of Pergonal® to 1,286 patients in 3.002 courses of therapy are summarized below. The values include patients who were treated with other than the recommended dosage regime. The values for the presently recommended dosage regime are essentially the same, except for the fact that the hyperstimulation syndrome has not occurred with administration of 75 IU of Pergonal® per day for nine to twelve days and the incidence of the hyperstimulation syndrome with administration of 150 IU of Pergonal® per day for nine to twelve days has not exceeded 0.4%.

	%
Patients ovulating	75
Patients pregnant	25
Patients aborting	25*
Multiple pregnancies	20†
Twins	15†
Three or more conceptuses	5†
Fetal abnormalities	1.7†
Hyperstimulation syndrome	1.3

* Based on total pregnancies

† Based on total deliveries

Results by diagnosis group are summarized below. (These values include patients who were treated with other than the present recommended dosage regime):

[See table above right].

Men:

Clinical results of the treatment of men with primary or secondary hypogonadotropic hypogonadism are as follows:

In the Serono Cooperative study, with an adequate treatment period of 3 to 8 months, 60 of 70 men with primary hypogonadotropic hypogonadism and 8 of 11 men with secondary hypogonadotropic hypogonadism responded with mean increases in their sperm counts from less than 5 to 24 million spermatozoa per milliliter of ejaculate. Forty-one wives of 54 men with primary hypogonadotropic hypogonadism desiring offspring and 7 wives of men with secondary hypogonadotropic hypogonadism conceived. Patients treated with Pergonal® and hCG for less than 3 months or with Pergonal® alone did not respond to therapy.

	% Pts. Ovul	% Pts. Preg.	% Abort	% Multi Preg.	% Twins	% 3 or More Conceptuses	% Hyper-stim. Syndr.
Primary Amenorrhea	62	22	14	25	25	0	0
Secondary Amenorrhea	61	28	24	28	18	10	1.9
Secondary Amen. with Galactorrhea	77	42	21	41	31	10	1.2
Polycystic Ovaries	76	26	39	17	17	0	1.1
Anovulatory Cycles	77	24	15	14	9	5	2.0
Miscellaneous	83	20	36	2	2	0	0.1

A world-wide data search revealed that of 160 recorded pregnancies as the result of use of Pergonal®-hCG in men, there were 7 spontaneous abortions, one ectopic pregnancy and 3 congenital anomalies at birth (esophageal atresia in a female infant which was later corrected by surgery, unilateral cryptorchidism, inguinal hernia).

Caution: Federal law prohibits dispensing without prescription.

Manufactured for:
SERONO LABORATORIES, INC.
Randolph, MA 02368
by: Laboratories Serono, SA
Aubonne, Switzerland

Revised: 3/86

Date of Printing: 4/86

PROFASI® HP ℞

[pro 'fah-se]

(human chorionic gonadotropin, USP)

FOR INTRAMUSCULAR USE ONLY

PRODUCT OVERVIEW

KEY FACTS

Profasi® HP is a lyophilized preparation of human chorionic gonadotropin. It is administered by intramuscular injection after reconstitution with Bacteriostatic Water for Injection, USP.

MAJOR USES

Women: Profasi® HP is used to induce ovulation in women who have been appropriately treated with Pergonal®.

Men: Profasi® HP is used to treat hypogonadotropic males, or to treat prepubertal cryptorchidism not due to anatomical obstruction.

SAFETY INFORMATION

Profasi® HP should not be administered to patients who have previously demonstrated hypersensitivity to human chorionic gonadotropin. Women who have experienced excessive ovarian enlargement and overstimulation while undergoing Pergonal® treatment should not be given hCG. When treating prepubertal cryptorchidism, therapy should be discontinued if signs of precocious puberty occur.

PRESCRIBING INFORMATION

PROFASI® HP ℞

[pro 'fah-se]

(human chorionic gonadotropin, USP)

FOR INTRAMUSCULAR USE ONLY

DESCRIPTION

Human chorionic gonadotropin (HCG), a polypeptide hormone produced by the human placenta, is composed of an alpha and a beta sub-unit. The alpha sub-unit is essentially identical to the alpha sub-units of the human pituitary gonadotropins, luteinizing hormone (LH) and follicle-stimulating hormone (FSH), as well as to the alpha sub-unit of human thyroid-stimulating hormone (TSH). The beta sub-units of these hormones differ in amino acid sequence.

Chorionic Gonadotropin is a water soluble glycoprotein derived from human pregnancy urine. The sterile lyophilized powder is stable. When reconstituted the solution should be refrigerated and should be used within 60 days.

Each vial when reconstituted will contain:

Chorionic Gonadotropin: 5,000 USP Units or 10,000 USP Units; Mannitol: 100 mg with Dibasic Sodium Phosphate and Monobasic Sodium Phosphate to adjust pH.

In addition, when reconstituted with the diluent provided (Bacteriostatic Water for Injection, USP containing 0.9% v/v Benzyl Alcohol) each serum vial will contain Benzyl Alcohol 0.9%.

CLINICAL PHARMACOLOGY

The action of HCG is virtually identical to that of pituitary LH, although HCG appears to have a small degree of FSH activity as well. It stimulates production of gonadal steroid hormones by stimulating the interstitial cells (Leydig cells) of the testis to produce androgens and the corpus luteum of the ovary to produce progesterone. Androgen stimulation in the male leads to the development of secondary sex characteristics and may stimulate testicular descent when no anatomical impediment to descent is present. This descent is usually reversible when HCG is discontinued. During the normal menstrual cycle, LH participates with FSH in the development and maturation of the normal ovarian follicle, and the mid-cycle LH surge triggers ovulation. HCG can substitute for LH in this function.

During a normal pregnancy, HCG secreted by the placenta maintains the corpus luteum after LH secretion decreases, supporting continued secretion of estrogen and progesterone and preventing menstruation. HCG HAS NO KNOWN EFFECT ON FAT MOBILIZATION, APPETITE OR SENSE OF HUNGER, OR BODY FAT DISTRIBUTION.

INDICATIONS AND USAGE

HCG HAS NOT BEEN DEMONSTRATED TO BE EFFECTIVE ADJUNCTIVE THERAPY IN THE TREATMENT OF OBESITY. THERE IS NO SUBSTANTIAL EVIDENCE THAT IT INCREASES WEIGHT LOSS BEYOND THAT RESULTING FROM CALORIC RESTRICTION, THAT IT CAUSES A MORE ATTRACTIVE OR "NORMAL" DISTRIBUTION OF FAT, OR THAT IT DECREASES THE HUNGER AND DISCOMFORT ASSOCIATED WITH CALORIE-RESTRICTED DIETS.

1. Prepubertal cryptorchidism not due to anatomical obstruction. In general, HCG is thought to induce testicular descent in situations when descent would have occurred at puberty. HCG thus may help predict whether or not orchiopexy will be needed in the future. Although, in some cases, descent following HCG administration is permanent, in most cases, the response is temporary. Therapy is usually instituted between the ages of 4 and 9.
2. Selected cases of hypogonadotropic hypogonadism (hypogonadism secondary to a pituitary deficiency) in males.
3. Induction of ovulation and pregnancy in the anovulatory, infertile woman in whom the cause of anovulation is secondary and not due to primary ovarian failure, and who has been appropriately pre-treated with human menotropins.

CONTRAINDICATIONS

Precocious puberty, prostatic carcinoma or other androgen-dependent neoplasm, prior allergic reaction to HCG.

WARNINGS

HCG should be used in conjunction with human menopausal gonadotropins only by physicians experienced with infertility problems who are familiar with the criteria for patient selection, contraindications, warnings, precautions, and adverse reactions described in the package insert for menotropins. The principal serious adverse reactions during this use are: (1) Ovarian hyperstimulation, a syndrome of sudden ovarian enlargement, ascites with or without pain, and/or pleural effusion, (2) Rupture of ovarian cysts with resultant hemoperitoneum, (3) Multiple births, and (4) Arterial thromboembolism.

PRECAUTIONS

1. Induction of androgen secretion by HCG may induce precocious puberty in patients treated for cryptorchidism. Therapy should be discontinued if signs of precocious puberty occur.
2. Since androgens may cause fluid retention, HCG should be used with caution in patients with cardiac or renal disease, epilepsy, migraine, or asthma.

ADVERSE REACTIONS

Headache, irritability, restlessness, depression, fatigue, edema, precocious puberty, gynecomastia, pain at the site of injection.

DOSAGE AND ADMINISTRATION

(Intramuscular Use Only): The dosage regimen employed in any particular case will depend upon the indication for use,

Continued on next page

Serono—Cont.

the age and weight of the patient, and the physician's preference. The following regimens have been advocated by various authorities.

Prepubertal cryptorchidism not due to anatomical obstruction:

1. 4,000 USP Units three times weekly for three weeks.
2. 5,000 USP Units every second day for four injections.
3. 15 injections of 500 to 1,000 USP Units over a period of six weeks.
4. 500 USP Units three times weekly for four to six weeks. If this course of treatment is not successful, another is begun one month later, giving 1,000 USP Units per injection.

Selected cases of hypogonadotropic hypogonadism in males:

1. 500 to 1,000 USP Units three times a week for three weeks, followed by the same dose twice a week for three weeks.
2. 4,000 USP Units three times weekly for six to nine months, following which the dosage may be reduced to 2,000 USP Units three times weekly for an additional three months.

Induction of ovulation and pregnancy in the anovulatory, unfertile woman in whom the cause of anovulation is secondary and not due to primary ovarian failure and who has been appropriately pre-treated with human menotropins (see prescribing information for menotropins for dosage and administration for that drug product):

5,000 to 10,000 USP Units one day following the last dose of menotropins (a dosage of 10,000 USP Units is recommended in the labeling for menotropins).

HOW SUPPLIED

Regular 10 ml lyophilized multiple dose vial

5,000 USP Units per Vial—NDC 44087-8005-3

10,000 USP Units per Vial—NDC 44087-8010-3 with 10 ml vial Bacteriostatic Water for Injection, USP (containing Benzyl Alcohol 0.9% v/v).

CAUTION

Federal law prohibits dispensing without prescription.

DIRECTIONS FOR RECONSTITUTION

TWO-VIAL PACKAGE: Withdraw sterile air from lyophilized vial and inject into diluent vial. Remove 10 ml from diluent and add to lyophilized vial; agitate gently until solution is complete.

SEROPHENE® ℞

[se ″ro-fēn]

(clomiphene citrate tablets, U.S.P.)

PRODUCT OVERVIEW

KEY FACTS

Serophene® is an orally administered, nonsteroidal compound with some estrogenic activity. The exact mechanism of action is unknown, although it appears to involve the pituitary by stimulating release of pituitary gonadotropins to mediate ovulation.

MAJOR USES

Serophene® is effective in inducing ovulation in infertile women with physiological indications of normal estrogen production. Reduced estrogen levels, while less favorable, do not prevent successful therapy.

SAFETY INFORMATION

Serophene® is contraindicated in patients who have previously experienced hypersensitivity to clomiphene citrate. Visual disturbances, vasomotor flushes, and ovarian enlargement occasionally occur. Because the teratogenic potential of clomiphene citrate is unknown, it should not be administered during pregnancy. Multiple births occur in appoximately 10% of pregnancies resulting from clomiphene citrate therapy; 99% of these are twins.

PRESCRIBING INFORMATION

SEROPHENE® ℞

[se ″ro-fēn]

(clomiphene citrate tablets, U.S.P.)

DESCRIPTION

Each scored white tablet contains:

Clomiphene Citrate USP 50 mg. Clomiphene citrate is designated chemically as 2-[p-(2-chloro-1,2-diphenylvinyl) phenoxy] triethylamine dihydrogen citrate and is represented structurally as:

$$(C_2H_5)_2NCH_2CH_2O\text{-}C_6H_4\text{-}C(C_6H_5){=}CCl\text{-}C_6H_5 \cdot C_6H_8O_7$$

clomiphene citrate USP (Serophene)

As shown, one molecule of citric acid is chemically bound with one molecule of the organic base, clomiphene.

Clomiphene citrate is a chemical analog of other triarylethylene compounds such as chlorotrianisene and the cholesterol inhibitor, triparanol.

ACTIONS

Clomiphene citrate, an orally-administered, non-steroidal agent, may induce ovulation in selected anovulatory women. It is a drug of considerable pharmacologic potency. Careful evaluation and selection of the patient and close attention to the timing of the dose is mandatory prior to treatment with clomiphene citrate. Conservative selection and management of the patient contribute to successful therapy of anovulation. Clomiphene citrate induces ovulation in most selected anovulatory patients. The various criteria for ovulation include: an ovulation peak of estrogen excretion followed by a biphasic basal body temperature curve; urinary excretion of pregnanediol at post-ovulatory levels and, endometrial histologic findings characteristic of the luteal phase.

A review of eleven publications appearing between 1964 and 1978 showed that pregnancy occurred in 35% of 5154 patients with ovulatory dysfunction who received clomiphene citrate.

[See table below].

Clomiphene citrate therapy appears to mediate ovulation through increased output of pituitary gonadotropins. These stimulate the maturation and endocrine activity of the ovarian follicle which is followed by the development and function of the corpus luteum. Increased urinary excretion of gonadotropins and estrogen suggest involvement of the pituitary.

Studies with ^{14}C labeled clomiphene citrate have shown that it is readily absorbed orally in humans, and is excreted principally in the feces. An average of 51% of the administered dose was excreted after 5 days. After intravenous administration 37% was excreted in 5 days. The appearance of ^{14}C in the feces six weeks after administration suggests that the remaining drug and/or metabolites are slowly excreted from a sequestered enterohepatic recirculation pool.

INDICATIONS

Clomiphene citrate is indicated for the treatment of ovulatory failure in patients desiring pregnancy, and whose husbands are fertile and potent. Impediments to this goal must be excluded or adequately treated before beginning therapy.

Administration of clomiphene citrate is indicated only in patients with demonstrated ovulatory dysfunction and in whom the following conditions apply:

1. Normal liver function.
2. Physiologic indications of normal endogenous estrogen (as estimated from vaginal smears, endometrial biopsy, assay of urinary estrogen, or from bleeding in response to progesterone). Reduced estrogen levels, while less favorable, do not prevent successful therapy.
3. Clomiphene citrate therapy is not effective for those patients with primary pituitary or ovarian failure. It cannot substitute for appropriate therapy of other disturbances leading to ovulatory dysfunction, e.g., diseases of the thyroid or adrenals.
4. Particularly careful evaluation prior to clomiphene citrate therapy should be done in patients with abnormal uterine bleeding. It is most important that neoplastic lesions are detected.

CONTRAINDICATIONS

Pregnancy

Although no direct effect of clomiphene citrate therapy on the human fetus has been seen, clomiphene citrate should not be administered in cases of suspected pregnancy as such effects have been reported in animals. To prevent inadvertent clomiphene citrate administration during early pregnancy, the basal body temperature should be recorded throughout all treatment cycles, and therapy should be discontinued if pregnancy is suspected. If the basal body temperature following clomiphene citrate is biphasic and is not followed by menses, the possibility of an ovarian cyst and/or pregnancy should be excluded. Until the correct diagnosis has been determined, the next course of therapy should be delayed.

Liver Disease

Patients with liver disease or a history of liver dysfunction should not receive clomiphene citrate therapy.

Abnormal Uterine Bleeding

Clomiphene citrate is contraindicated in patients with abnormal uterine bleeding.

WARNINGS

Visual Symptoms

Patients should be warned that blurring and/or other visual symptoms may occur occasionally with clomiphene citrate therapy. These may make activities such as driving or operating machinery more hazardous than usual, particularly under conditions of variable lighting. While their significance is not yet understood (see ADVERSE REACTIONS), patients having any visual symptoms, should discontinue treatment and have a complete ophthalmologic evaluation.

PRECAUTIONS

Diagnosis Prior to Clomiphene Citrate Therapy

Careful evaluation should be given to candidates for clomiphene citrate therapy. A complete pelvic examination should be performed prior to treatment and repeated before each subsequent course. Clomiphene citrate should not be given to patients with an ovarian cyst, as further ovarian enlargement may result.

Since the incidence of endometrial carcinoma and of ovulatory disorders increases with age, endometrial biopsy should always exclude the former as causative in such patients. If abnormal uterine bleeding is present, full diagnostic measures are necessary.

Ovarian Overstimulation During Treatment with Clomiphene Citrate

To minimize the hazard associated with the occasional abnormal ovarian enlargement during clomiphene citrate therapy (see ADVERSE REACTIONS), the lowest dose producing good results should be chosen. Some patients with polycystic ovary syndrome are unusually sensitive to gonadotropin and may have an exaggerated response to usual doses of clomiphene citrate. Maximal enlargement of the ovary, whether abnormal or physiologic, does not occur until several days after discontinuation of clomiphene citrate. The patient complaining of pelvic pains after receiving clomiphene citrate should be examined carefully. If enlargement of the ovary occurs, clomiphene citrate therapy should be withheld until the ovaries have returned to pretreatment size, and the dosage or duration of the next course should be reduced. The ovarian enlargement and cyst formation following clomiphene citrate therapy regress spontaneously within a few days or weeks after discontinuing treatment. Therefore, unless a strong indication for laparotomy exists, such cystic enlargement always should be managed conservatively.

Multiple Pregnancy

In the reviewed publications, the incidence of multiple pregnancies was increased during those cycles in which clomiphene citrate was given. Among the 1803 pregnancies on which the outcome was reported, 90% were single and 10% twins. Less than 1% of the reported deliveries resulted in triplets or more.

Of these multiple pregnancies, 96-99% resulted in the births of live infants. The patient and her husband should be advised of the frequency and potential hazards of multiple pregnancy before starting treatment.

ADVERSE REACTIONS

Symptoms

Side effects are not prominent at the recommended dosage of clomiphene citrate and infrequently interfere with treatment. Side effects tend to occur more frequently at higher doses and in the longer treatment courses used in some early studies. The more common side effects and the percent of patients experiencing them include vasomotor flushes (11%), abdominal discomfort (7.4%), abnormal uterine bleeding (0.5%), ovarian enlargement (14%), breast tenderness (2.1%), and visual symptoms (1.6%). The vasomotor symptoms resemble menopausal "hot flushes", and are not usually severe. They promptly disappear after treatment is discontinued. Abdominal discomfort may resemble ovulatory

Serophene

PREGNANCIES FOLLOWING CLOMIPHENE CITRATE U.S.P.[a]

			(Range)
Number of Patients	=	5154	
Percent of Patients Ovulating[b]	=	75	(50-94)%
Percent of Ovulatory Cycles	=	53	(33-69)%
Percent of Patients Pregnant	=	35	(11-52)%
Percent Patients Pregnant / Percent Patients Ovulating	=	46	(22-61)%
Percent Live Births	=	86	(74-99.8)%
Percent Abortions	=	14	(0.2-26)%
Percent of Single Births	=	90	(67-100)%
Percent Surviving	=	99	(98.2-100)%
Percent of Multiple Births	=	10	(0-33)%
Percent Surviving	=	96	(82-100)%

a) includes patients receiving other than recommended dosage regimen.

b) average from studies

(mittelschmerz) or premenstrual phenomena, or that due to ovarian enlargement. In addition, nausea and vomiting (2.1%), nervousness and insomnia (1.9%), headache (1%), dizziness and lightheadedness (1%), increased urination (0.9%), depression and fatigue (0.8%), urticaria and allergic dermatitis (0.6%), weight gain (0.4%), and reversible hair loss (0.3%) have been reported.

When clomiphene citrate is administered at the recommended dose, abnormal ovarian enlargement (see PRECAUTIONS) is infrequent, although the usual cyclic variation in ovarian size may be exaggerated. Similarly, mid-cycle ovarian pain (mittelschmerz) may be accentuated. With prolonged or higher dosage, ovarian enlargement and cyst formation (usually luteal) may occur more often and the luteal phase of the cycle may be prolonged. Patients with polycystic ovary disease may be unusually sensitive to clomiphene therapy. Rare occurrences of massive ovarian enlargement have been reported, for example, in a patient with polycystic ovary syndrome whose clomiphene citrate therapy consisted of 100 mg daily for 14 days. Since abnormal ovarian enlargement usually regresses spontaneously, most of these patients should be treated conservatively.

The incidence of visual symptoms (see WARNINGS for further recommendations), usually described as "blurring" or spots or flashes (scintillating scotomata), correlates with increasing total dose. The symptoms disappear within a few days or weeks after clomiphene citrate is discontinued. This may be due to intensification and/or prolongation of afterimages. Symptoms often appear first, or are accentuated, upon exposure to a more brightly lit environment. While measured visual acuity has not generally been affected, in one patient taking 200 mg daily, visual blurring developed on the seventh day of treatment, and progressed to severe diminution of visual acuity by the tenth day. No other abnormality was coincident, and the visual acuity was normal by the third day after treatment was stopped. Ophthalmologically definable scotomata and electroretinographic retinal function changes have also been reported.

BSP Laboratory Studies

Greater than 5% retention of sulfobromophthalein (BSP) has been reported in approximately 10 to 20% of patients in whom it was measured. Retention was usually minimal but was elevated during prolonged clomiphene citrate administration or with apparently unrelated liver disease. In some patients, pre-existing BSP retention decreased even though clomiphene citrate therapy was continued. Other liver function tests were usually normal.

Other Laboratory Studies

Clomiphene citrate has not been reported to cause a significant abnormality in hematologic or renal tests, in protein bound iodine, or in serum cholesterol levels.

Birth Defects

Of 1803 births following clomiphene citrate administration, 45 infants with birth defects were reported for a cumulative rate of 2.5%.

Six cases of Down's Syndrome, one neonatal death with multiple malformations and one case each of the following were reported: extropia, club foot, tibial torsion, blocked tear duct and hemangioma. The other congenital abnormalities were not described. The investigators did not report that these were presumed to be due to therapy. The cumulative rate of congenital abnormalities does not exceed that reported in the general population.

DOSAGE AND ADMINISTRATION

General Considerations

Physicians experienced in managing gynecologic or endocrine disorders should supervise the work-up and treatment of candidate patients for clomiphene citrate therapy. Patients should be chosen for clomiphene citrate therapy only after careful diagnostic evaluation (see INDICATIONS). The plan of therapy should be outlined in advance. Impediments to achieving the goal of therapy must be excluded or adequately treated before beginning clomiphene citrate.

In determining a starting dose schedule, efficacy must be balanced against potential side effects. For example, the available data so far suggests that ovulation and pregnancy are slightly more attainable with 100 mg/day for 5 days than with 50 mg/day for 5 days. As the dosage is increased, however, ovarian overstimulation and other side effects may be expected to increase. Although the data do not yet establish a relationship between dose level and multiple births, it is reasonable that such a correlation exists on pharmacologic grounds.

For these reasons, treatment of the usual patient should initiate with a 50 mg daily dose for 5 days. The dose may be increased only in those patients who do not respond to the first course (see Recommended Dosage). Special treatment with lower dosage over shorter duration is particularly recommended if unusual sensitivity to pituitary gonadotropin is suspected, including patients with polycystic ovary syndrome (see PRECAUTIONS).

Recommended Dosage

The recommended dosage for the first course of clomiphene citrate is 50 mg (1 tablet) daily for 5 days. Therapy may be started at any time if the patient has had no recent uterine bleeding. If progestin-induced bleeding is intended, or if spontaneous uterine bleeding occurs prior to therapy, the regimen of 50 mg daily for 5 days should be started on or about the fifth day of the cycle. When ovulation occurs at this dosage, there is no advantage to increasing the dose in subsequent cycles of treatment.

If ovulation does not appear to have occurred after the first course of therapy, a second course of 100 mg daily (two 50 mg tablets given as a single daily dose) for 5 days may be started. This course may begin as early as 30 days after the previous one. Increasing the dosage or duration of therapy beyond 100 mg/day for 5 days should not be undertaken.

The majority of patients who respond do so during the first course of therapy, and 3 courses constitute an adequate therapeutic trial. If ovulatory menses do not occur, the diagnosis should be re-evaluated. Treatment beyond this is not recommended in the patient who does not exhibit evidence of ovulation.

Pregnancy

Properly timed coitus is very important for good results. For regularity of cyclic ovulatory response it is also important that each course of clomiphene citrate be started on or about the fifth day of the cycle, once ovulation has been established. As with other therapeutic modalities, Serophene® therapy follows the rule of diminishing returns, such that likelihood of conception diminishes with each succeeding course of therapy. If pregnancy has not been achieved after 3 ovulatory responses to Serophene, further treatment is not generally recommended. Before starting treatment patients should be advised of the possibility and potential hazards of multiple pregnancy if conception occurs following clomiphene citrate therapy.

Long-Term Cyclic Therapy—Not Recommended

Since the relative safety of long-term cyclic therapy has not yet been conclusively demonstrated, and since the majority of patients will ovulate following 3 courses, long-term cyclic therapy is not recommended.

HOW SUPPLIED

Serophene is available as 50 mg scored white tablets in the following package combinations:

• 1 carton 10 tablets, NDC 44087-8090-6

Each carton contains 2 strips of 5 tablets each.

• 1 carton 30 tablets, NDC 44087-8090-1

Each carton contains 3 strips of 10 tablets, each in a 2 × 5 arrangement.

Protect from light, moisture, and excessive heat. Dispense in well-closed, light resistant container as defined in the USP, with child resistant closure.

PRDUCT INFORMATION

AVAILABLE ONLY ON PRESCRIPTION.

For additional information, please contact:
Serono Laboratories, Inc.
Medical Information Services
280 Pond Street
Randolph, MA 02368
800-225-5185 (Toll free, outside MA)
617-963-8154 (Inside MA)

Sigma-Tau, Inc.
723 NORTH BEERS STREET
HOLMDEL, NJ 07733

CARNITOR® ℞
[kar'nĭ-tor]
(L-carnitine)

DESCRIPTION

L-carnitine is L-beta–hydroxy–gamma–trimethylamino butyric acid (inner salt). It is a white powder with a melting point of 196–197°C and is readily soluble in water. The L-isomer of carnitine is the biologically active form

$$CH_3-\overset{\displaystyle CH_3}{\underset{\displaystyle CH_3}{N^+}}-CH_2-\underset{\displaystyle OH}{CH}-CH_2-COO^-$$

CLINICAL PHARMACOLOGY

L-carnitine is essential for the transport of long chain fatty acids across the inner mitochondrial membrane into the mitochondrial matrix where they undergo β–oxidation.

INDICATIONS AND USAGE

L-carnitine is indicated in the treatment of primary systemic carnitine deficiency.

CONTRAINDICATIONS

None known.

WARNINGS

None.

PRECAUTIONS

Mutagenicity tests have been performed in **Salmonella typhimurium, Saccharomyces cerevisiae,** and **Schizosaccharomyces pombe** that do not indicate that L-carnitine is mutagenic. Long-term animal studies have not been conducted to evaluate the carcinogenicity of the compound.

Pregnancy Category B. Reproductive studies have been performed in rats and rabbits using parenteral administration at doses equivalent on a mg/kg basis to the suggested oral adult dosage and have revealed no harm to the fetus due to L-carnitine. There are, however, no adequate and well-controlled studies in pregnant women. Because animal reproduction studies are not always predictive of human response, this drug should be used during pregnancy only if clearly needed.

ADVERSE REACTIONS

The most frequent type of adverse reaction occurring during treatment with L-carnitine is gastrointestinal.

In clinical studies, 41% of patients reported one or more gastrointestinal complaints which tended to be transient.

Typical complaints included nausea, diarrhea, and abdominal distress. Patient odor was the next most frequent adverse effect which had an incidence of 11%. Decreasing the dosage often diminishes or eliminates drug-related patient body odor or gastrointestinal symptoms when present.

DOSAGE AND ADMINISTRATION

Adults: The recommended oral dosage for adults is 990 mg two or three times a day, depending on clinical response.

Infants and children: The recommended oral dosage for infants and children is between 50 and 100 mg/kg/day in divided doses, with a maximum of 3 grams/day. The exact dosage will depend on clinical response.

BIOAVAILABILITY

The bioavailability/pharmacokinetics of L-carnitine tablets have not been determined in well controlled studies.

HOW SUPPLIED

L-carnitine is supplied as 330 mg, individually foil wrapped tablets in boxes of 90. Store at room temperature.

Enteral liquid, 10 ml unit dose containing 1.0 g of L-carnitine in aluminium foil container. Unit dose containers are provided in plastic trays, ten units per tray. Trays are packed 10 or 16 per case. Store upright at room temperature. Avoid freezing or excessive heat.

SmithKline Consumer Products
A SmithKline Beckman Company
P.O. BOX 8082
PHILADELPHIA, PA 19101

ECOTRIN®
Analgesics: Aspirin
Antiarthritic

DESCRIPTION

'Ecotrin' is enteric-coated aspirin (acetylsalicylic acid) available in tablet and capsule forms. Both forms are available in 325 mg. and 500 mg. dosage units.

In the tablet form, the enteric coating covers a core of aspirin. The enteric coating is designed to resist disintegration in the stomach, but to dissolve in the more alkaline environment of the duodenum. Inactive Ingredients (listed for individuals with specific allergies): Cellulose, Cellulose Acetate Phthalate, D&C Yellow 10, Diethyl Phthalate, FD&C Yellow 6, Silicon Dioxide, Sodium Starch Glycolate, Starch, Stearic Acid, Titanium Dioxide, and trace amounts of other inactive ingredients.

In the capsule form, hundreds of aspirin granules, each with an enteric coating, are contained within a gelatin capsule. The granules are released in the stomach as the capsule dissolves, but resist disintegration until they pass into the duodenum. Inactive Ingredients (listed for individuals with specific allergies): Benzyl Alcohol, Cellulose Acetate Phthalate, Cetyl Alcohol, Cetylpyridinium Chloride, FD&C Red 3, Yellow 6, Gelatin, Sodium Lauryl Sulfate, Talc, and other ingredients.

INDICATIONS

'Ecotrin' is indicated for conditions requiring chronic or long-term aspirin therapy. The enteric coating is resistant to disintegration in the acid environment of the stomach, but does dissolve in the neutral-to-basic environment of the duodenum. Such action tends to protect the stomach from injury

Continued on next page

SmithKline Consumer—Cont.

that may result from ingestion of plain, i.e., non-enteric coated, aspirin (see SAFETY).
'Ecotrin' may also be recommended for the antiplatelet indications of aspirin. For additional information, see the ANTIPLATELET EFFECT section.

DOSAGE

The OTC maximum dosage for aspirin is 4000 mg. per day in divided doses, i.e., 2–325 mg. tablets or capsules, q4h, or 3–325 mg. tablets or capsules, or 2–500 mg. tablets or capsules, q6h.
Under a physician's direction, the dosage can be increased or otherwise modified as appropriate to the clinical situation. However, the physician should be attentive to plasma salicylate levels. The physician may also want to caution the patient to be alert to the development of tinnitus as an indicator of elevated salicylate levels. It should be noted that patients with a high frequency hearing loss that often occurs in older individuals may have difficulty perceiving the tinnitus and so it may not be a reliable indicator in such individuals.

BIOAVAILABILITY

The bioavailability of aspirin from 'Ecotrin' has been demonstrated in a number of salicylate excretion studies. The studies show levels of salicylate (and metabolites) in urine excreted over 48 hours for 'Ecotrin' do not differ statistically from plain, i.e., non-enteric coated, aspirin.
Plasma studies, in which both tablet and capsule forms of 'Ecotrin' have been compared with plain aspirin in steady-state studies over eight days, also demonstrate that the enteric-coated forms provide plasma salicylate levels not statistically different from plain aspirin.
Information regarding salicylate levels over a range of doses was generated in a study in which 24 healthy volunteers (12 male and 12 female) took daily (divided) doses of either 2600 mg., 3900 mg., or 5200 mg. of 'Ecotrin'. Plasma salicylate levels generally acknowledged to be anti-inflammatory (15 mg./dL.) were attained at daily doses of 5200 mg., on Day 2 by females and Day 3 by males. At 3900 mg., anti-inflammatory levels were attained at Day 3 by females and Day 4 by males.
Dissolution of the enteric coating occurs at a neutral-to-basic pH and is therefore dependent on gastric emptying into the duodenum. With continued dosing, appropriate plasma levels are maintained.

SAFETY

The safety of both 'Ecotrin' tablets and capsules has been demonstrated in a number of clinical studies comparing endoscopic findings from 'Ecotrin', plain aspirin, as well as plain buffered and "arthritis-strength" buffered preparations. In these studies, all forms of aspirin were dosed to the OTC maximum (3900–4000 mg. per day) for 14 days. The normal healthy volunteers participating in these studies were gastroscoped before and after the 14-day courses of treatment, and 14-day drug-free periods followed active drug. Compared to all the other preparations, there was statistically significantly less gastric damage during the 'Ecotrin' courses. There was also statistically less duodenal damage when compared with the plain, i.e., non-enteric coated, aspirin.
Details of studies demonstrating the safety and bioavailability of 'Ecotrin' are available to health care professionals. Write: Medical Affairs Department, SmithKline Consumer Products, P.O. Box 8082, Philadelphia, PA 19101.

WARNING

Consumer Warning: Children and teenagers should not use this medicine for chicken pox or flu symptoms before a doctor is consulted about Reye syndrome, a rare but serious illness. If pain persists for more than 10 days, or if redness is present, or in arthritic or rheumatic conditions affecting children under 12, consult a physician immediately. Discontinue use if dizziness, ringing in ears, or impaired hearing occurs. If you experience persistent or unexplained stomach upset, consult a physician. Keep this and all drugs out of children's reach. In case of accidental overdose, seek professional assistance or contact a poison control center immediately. As with any medicine, if you are pregnant or nursing a baby, seek the advice of a health professional before using this product. Store at controlled room temperature (59°–86°F.).
Professional Warning: There have been occasional reports in the literature concerning individuals with impaired gastric emptying in whom there may be retention of one or more 'Ecotrin' tablets over time. This phenomenon may occur as a result of outlet obstruction from ulcer disease alone or combined with hypotonic gastric peristalsis. Because of the integrity of the enteric coating in an acidic environment, these tablets may accumulate and form a bezoar in the stomach. Individuals with this condition may present with complaints of early satiety or of vague upper abdominal distress. Diagnosis may be made by endoscopy or by abdominal films which show opacities suggestive of a mass of small tablets. Management may vary according to the condition of the patient. Options include: gastrotomy and alternating slightly basic and neutral lavage (*Ref.: Baum, J.: Enteric-Coated Aspirin and the Problem of Gastric Retention. J. Rheum., 1984:11, 250-1.*). While there has been no clinical experience, it has been suggested that such individuals may also be treated with parenteral cimetidine (to reduce acid secretion) and then given sips of slightly basic liquids. Progess may be followed with plasma salicylate levels or via recognition of tinnitus by the patient.
It should be kept in mind that individuals with a history of partial or complete gastrectomy may produce reduced amounts of acid and therefore have an elevated gastric pH. Under these circumstances, the benefits offered by the acid-resistant enteric coating may not exist.

ANTIPLATELET EFFECT

FDA has approved the professional labeling of aspirin to reduce the risk of death and/or nonfatal myocardial infarction (MI) in patients with a previous infarction or unstable angina pectoris. Previously, wording was added to the professional labeling of aspirin indicating its use in reducing the risk of transient ischemic attacks in men.
Labeling for both indications follows:

Aspirin for Myocardial Infarction

Indication: Aspirin is indicated to reduce the risk of death and/or nonfatal myocardial infarction in patients with a previous infarction or unstable angina pectoris.
Clinical Trials: The indication is supported by the results of six, large, randomized multicenter, placebo-controlled studies involving 10,816 predominantly male, post-myocardial infarction (MI) patients and one randomized placebo-controlled study of 1,266 men with unstable angina.[1–7] Therapy with aspirin was begun at intervals after the onset of acute MI varying from less than three days to more than five years and continued for periods of from less than one year to four years. In the unstable angina study, treatment was started within one month after the onset of unstable angina and continued for 12 weeks, and patients with complicating conditions such as congestive heart failure were not included in the study.
Aspirin therapy in MI patients was associated with about a 20 percent reduction in the risk of subsequent death and/or nonfatal reinfarction, a median absolute decrease of 3 percent from the 12 to 22 percent event rates in the placebo groups. In aspirin-treated unstable angina patients, the reduction in risk was about 50 percent, a reduction in event rate in the placebo group over the 12 weeks of the study.
Daily dosage of aspirin in the post-myocardial infarction studies was 300 mg. in one study and 900 to 1500 mg. in five studies. A dose of 325 mg. was used in the study of unstable angina.

ADVERSE REACTIONS

Gastrointestinal Reactions: Doses of 1000 mg. per day of aspirin caused gastrointestinal symptoms and bleeding that in some cases were clinically significant. In the largest post-infarction study (the Aspirin Myocardial Infarction Study [AMIS] with 4,500 people), the percentage incidences of gastrointestinal symptoms of a standard, solid-tablet formulation and placebo-treated subjects, respectively, were: stomach pain (14.5%; 4.4%); heartburn (11.9%; 4.8%); nausea and/or vomiting (7.6%; 2.1%); hospitalization for gastrointestinal disorder (4.9%; 3.5%). In the AMIS and other trials, aspirin-treated patients had increased rates of gross gastrointestinal bleeding. Symptoms and signs of gastrointestinal irritation were not significantly increased in subjects treated for unstable angina with buffered aspirin in solution.
Cardiovascular and Biochemical: In the AMIS trial, the dosage of 1000 mg. per day of aspirin was associated with small increases in systolic blood pressure (BP) (average 1.5 to 2.1 mmHg) and diastolic BP (0.5 to 0.6 mmHg), depending upon whether maximal or last available readings were used. Blood urea nitrogen and uric acid levels were also increased, but by less than 1.0 mg.%. Subjects with marked hypertension or renal insufficiency had been excluded from the trial so that the clinical importance of these observations for such subjects or for any subjects treated over more prolonged periods is not known. It is recommended that patients placed on long-term aspirin treatment, even at doses of 300 mg. per day, be seen at regular intervals to assess changes in these measurements.
Sodium in Buffered Aspirin for Solution Formulations: One tablet daily of buffered aspirin in solution adds 553 mg. of sodium to that in the diet and may not be tolerated by patients with active sodium-retaining states such as congestive heart or renal failure. This amount of sodium adds about 30 percent to the 70 to 90 meq. intake suggested as appropriate for dietary hypertension in the 1984 Report of the Joint National Committee on Detection, Evaluation, and Treatment of High Blood Pressure.[8]
Dosage and Administration: Although most of the studies used dosages exceeding 300 mg. daily, two trials used only 300 mg. and pharmacologic data indicate that this dose inhibits platelet function fully. Therefore, 300 mg. or a conventional 325 mg. aspirin dose daily is a reasonable, routine dose that would minimize gastrointestinal adverse reactions. This use of aspirin applies to both solid, oral dosage forms (buffered and plain aspirin) and buffered aspirin in solution.

References:

1. Elwood, P.C., et al.: A Randomized Controlled Trial of Acetylsalicylic Acid in the Secondary Prevention of Mortality from Myocardial Infarction, *Br. Med. J.* 1:436–440, 1974.
2. The Coronary Drug Project Research Group: Aspirin in Coronary Heart Disease, *J. Chronic Dis.* 29:625–642, 1976.
3. Breddin, K., et al.: Secondary Prevention of Myocardial Infarction: A Comparison of Acetylsalicylic Acid, Phenprocoumon or Placebo, *Homeostasis* 470:263–268, 1979.
4. Aspirin Myocardial Infarction Study Research Group: A Randomized Controlled Trial of Aspirin in Persons Recovered from Myocardial Infarction, *J.A.M.A.* 243:661–669, 1980.
5. Elwood, P.C., and Sweetnam, P.M.: Aspirin and Secondary Mortality After Myocardial Infarction, *Lancet* pp. 1313–1315, Dec. 22–29, 1979.
6. The Persantine-Aspirin Reinfarction Study Research Group, Persantine and Aspirin in Coronary Heart Disease, *Circulation* 62:449–469, 1980.
7. Lewis, H.D., et al.: Protective Effects of Aspirin Against Acute Myocardial Infarction and Death in Men with Unstable Angina, Results of a Veterans Administration Cooperative Study, *N. Engl. J. Med.* 309:396–403, 1983.
8. 1984 Report of the Joint National Committee on Detection, Evaluation, and Treatment of High Blood Pressure, U.S. Department of Health and Human Services and U.S. Public Health Service, National Institutes of Health. NIH Pub. No. 84-1088.

For Recurrent TIAs in Men

There is evidence that aspirin is safe and effective for reducing the risk of recurrent transient ischemic attacks (TIAs) or stroke in men who have transient ischemia of the brain due to fibrin emboli. There is no evidence that aspirin is effective in reducing TIAs in women, or is of benefit in the treatment of completed strokes in men or women.
Patients presenting with signs and/or symptoms of TIAs should have a complete medical and neurologic evaluation. Consideration should be given to other disorders which may resemble TIAs. It is important to evaluate and treat, if appropriate, diseases associated with TIAs and stroke, such as hypertension and diabetes.
Dosage: The recommended dosage for this new indication is 1300 mg./day (650 mg. b.i.d. or 325 mg. q.i.d.).

SUPPLIED

'Ecotrin' Tablets
325 mg. in bottles of 36, 100, 250 and 1000.
500 mg. in bottles of 24, 60 and 150.
'Ecotrin' Capsules
325 mg. in bottles of 70.
500 mg. in bottles of 50.
TAMPER-RESISTANT PACKAGE FEATURE: BOTTLE HAS IMPRINTED SEAL UNDER CAP; DO NOT USE IF BROKEN.

FEOSOL® CAPSULES
Hematinic

DESCRIPTION

'Feosol' Capsules provide the body with ferrous sulfate—iron in its most efficient form—for simple iron deficiency and iron-deficiency anemia. The special targeted-release capsule formulation—ferrous sulfate in pellets—reduces stomach upset, a common problem with iron.

FORMULA

Each capsule contains 159 mg. of dried ferrous sulfate USP (50 mg. of elemental iron), equivalent to 250 mg. of ferrous sulfate USP. Inactive Ingredients: Benzyl Alcohol, Cetylpyridinium Chloride, D&C Red No. 33, D&C Yellow No. 10, FD&C Blue No. 1 Aluminum Lake, FD&C Red No. 40 Aluminum Lake, FD&C Red No. 3 Aluminum Lake, Gelatin, Glyceryl Distearate, Glyceryl Monostearate, Iron Oxide, Polyethylene Glycol 8000, Povidone, Shellac, Sodium Lauryl Sulfate, Starch, Sucrose, Titanium Dioxide, White Wax.

DOSAGE

Adults: 1 or 2 capsules as directed by a physician. Children: As directed by a physician.
TAMPER-RESISTANT PACKAGE FEATURE
EACH CAPSULE IN SEALED UNIT; DO NOT USE IF BROKEN (30's). BOTTLE HAS IMPRINTED SEAL UNDER CAP; DO NOT USE IF BROKEN (100's and 500's).

WARNING

Do not exceed recommended dosage. The treatment of any anemic condition should be under the advice and supervision of a physician. Iron-containing medication may occasionally cause constipation or diarrhea. Since oral iron products interfere with absorption of oral tetracycline antibiotics, these products should not be taken within two hours of each other. Keep this and all drugs out of the reach of children. In case of

accidental overdose, seek professional assistance or contact a poison control center immediately. As with any drug, if you are pregnant or nursing a baby, seek the advice of a health professional before using this product.
Store at controlled room temperature (59°–86°F.).

HOW SUPPLIED

Packages of 30, bottles of 100 and 500 capsules; in Single Unit Packages of 100 capsules (intended for institutional use only).
Also available in Tablets and Elixir.

FEOSOL® ELIXIR
Hematinic

DESCRIPTION

'Feosol' Elixir, an unusually palatable iron elixir, provides the body with ferrous sulfate—iron in its most efficient form. The standard elixir for simple iron deficiency and iron-deficiency anemia when the need for such therapy has been determined by a physician. Each 5 ml. (1 teaspoonful) contains ferrous sulfate, USP, 220 mg. (44 mg. of elemental iron); alcohol, 5%.

Inactive Ingredients (listed for individuals with specific allergies): Citric Acid, FD&C Yellow 6, Flavors, Glucose, Saccharin Sodium, Sucrose, Purified Water.

USUAL DOSAGE

Adults—1 to 2 teaspoonful three times daily preferably between meals. Children—½ to 1 teaspoonful three times daily preferably between meals. Infants—as directed by physician. Mix with water or fruit juice to avoid temporary staining of teeth; do not mix with milk or wine-based vehicles.

TAMPER-RESISTANT PACKAGE FEATURE: IMPRINTED SEAL AROUND BOTTLE CAP; DO NOT USE IF BROKEN.

WARNING

The treatment of any anemic condition should be under the advice and supervision of a physician. Since oral iron products interfere with absorption of oral tetracycline antibiotics, these products should not be taken within two hours of each other. Occasional gastrointestinal discomfort (such as nausea) may be minimized by taking with meals and by beginning with one teaspoonful the first day, two the second, etc. until the recommended dosage is reached. Iron-containing medication may occasionally cause constipation or diarrhea, and liquids may cause temporary staining of the teeth (this is less likely when diluted). Keep this and all drugs out of reach of children. In case of accidental overdose, seek professional assistance or contact a poison control center immediately. As with any drug, if you are pregnant or nursing a baby, seek the advice of a health professional before using this product.
Store at controlled room temperature (59°–86°F.).

HOW SUPPLIED

A clear orange liquid in 16 fl. oz. bottles.

ALSO AVAILABLE

'Feosol' Tablets, 'Feosol' Capsules.

FEOSOL® TABLETS
Hematinic

PRODUCT INFORMATION

'Feosol' Tablets provide the body with ferrous sulfate, iron in its most efficient form, for iron deficiency and iron-deficiency anemia when the need for such therapy has been determined by a physician. The distinctive triangular-shaped tablet has a coating to prevent oxidation and improve palatability.

FORMULA

Active Ingredient: Each tablet contains 200 mg. of dried ferrous sulfate USP (65 mg. of elemental iron), equivalent to 325 mg. (5 grains) of ferrous sulfate USP. Inactive Ingredients (listed for individuals with specific allergies): Calcium Sulfate, D&C Yellow 10, FD&C Blue 2, Glucose, Hydroxypropyl Methylcellulose, Mineral Oil, Polyethylene Glycol, Sodium Lauryl Sulfate, Starch, Stearic Acid, Talc, and trace amounts of other inactive ingredients.

USUAL DOSAGE

Adults—one tablet 3 to 4 times daily, after meals and upon retiring. Children 6 to 12 years—one tablet three times a day after meals. Children under 6 years and infants—use 'Feosol' Elixir.

TAMPER-RESISTANT PACKAGE FEATURE: BOTTLE HAS IMPRINTED SEAL UNDER CAP; DO NOT USE IF BROKEN.

WARNINGS

Do not exceed recommended dosage. The treatment of any anemic condition should be under the advice and supervision of a physician. Since oral iron products interfere with absorption of oral tetracycline antibiotics, these products should not be taken within two hours of each other. Occasional gastrointestinal discomfort (such as nausea) may be minimized by taking with meals and by beginning with one tablet the first day, two the second, etc. until the recommended dosage is reached. Iron-containing medication may occasionally cause constipation or diarrhea. Keep this and all drugs out of reach of children. In case of accidental overdose, seek professional assistance or contact a poison control center immediately. As with any drug, if you are pregnant or nursing a baby, seek the advice of a health professional before using this product.
Store at controlled room temperature (59°–86°F.).

HOW SUPPLIED

Bottles of 100 or 1000 tablets; in Single Unit Packages of 100 tablets (intended for institutional use only).
Also available in Capsules and Elixir.

FEOSOL PLUS®
Hematinic: Iron plus vitamins

DESCRIPTION

For use in iron deficiency and iron-deficiency anemia where additional vitamins are indicated.

FORMULA

Each 'Feosol Plus' capsule contains:

Dried ferrous sulfate	200 mg.
(equivalent to 325 mg. ferrous sulfate USP: 65 mg. of elemental iron)	
Folic acid	0.2 mg.
Ascorbic acid (Vitamin C)	50 mg.
Thiamine HCl (Vitamin B_1)	2 mg.
Riboflavin (Vitamin B_2)	2 mg.
Pyridoxine HCl (Vitamin B_6)	2 mg.
Vitamin B_{12} (activity equivalent)	5 mcg.
(derived from streptomyces fermentation)	
Nicotinic acid (niacin)	20 mg.

Inactive Ingredients (listed for individuals with specific allergies): Benzyl Alcohol, Cetylpyridinium Chloride, D&C Red 33, Yellow 10, FD&C Green 3, Gelatin, Mineral Oil, Sodium Lauryl Sulfate, Starch, and trace amounts of other inactive ingredients.

USUAL DOSAGE

Adults and children (over 3 years): One capsule twice daily or as directed by physician.

TAMPER-RESISTANT PACKAGE FEATURE: BOTTLE HAS IMPRINTED SEAL UNDER CAP; DO NOT USE IF BROKEN.

WARNING

The treatment of any anemic condition should be under the advice and supervision of a physician. Since oral iron products tend to interfere with absorption of oral tetracycline antibiotics, these products should not be taken within two hours of each other. Keep this and all drugs out of reach of children. In case of accidental overdose, seek professional assistance or contact a poison control center immediately. Iron-containing medication may occasionally cause constipation or diarrhea. As with any drug, if you are pregnant or nursing a baby, seek the advice of a health professional before using this product.

HOW SUPPLIED

Bottles of 100 capsules.

TELDRIN®
Chlorpheniramine maleate
Timed-Release Allergy Capsules

Antihistamine

FORMULA

Active Ingredient: Each capsule contains Chlorpheniramine Maleate, 12 mg. Inactive Ingredients (listed for individuals with specific allergies): Benzyl Alcohol, Cetylpyridinium Chloride, D&C Red 33, Ethylcellulose, FD&C Green 3, Red 3, Red 40, Yellow 6, Gelatin, Hydrogenated Castor Oil, Silicon Dioxide, Sodium Lauryl Sulfate, Starch, Sucrose, and trace amounts of other inactive ingredients.

DESCRIPTION

Each 'Teldrin' Timed-Release capsule contains chlorpheniramine maleate, Maximum Strength 12 mg., so formulated that a portion of the antihistamine dose is released initially, and the remaining medication is released gradually over a prolonged period.

INDICATIONS FOR USE

Hay fever and allergies are caused by grass and tree pollen, dust and pollution. 'Teldrin' provides up to 12 hours of relief from hay fever/upper respiratory allergy symptoms; sneezing; runny nose; itchy, watery eyes.

DOSAGE

Adults and children over 12 years of age: Just one capsule in the morning, and one in the evening. Do not give to children under 12 without the advice and consent of a physician. Not to exceed 24 mg. (2 capsules of 12 mg.) in 24 hours.

TAMPER-RESISTANT PACKAGE FEATURES

- The carton is protected by a clear overwrap printed with "safety sealed"; do not use if overwrap is missing or broken.
- Each capsule is encased in a plastic cell with a foil back; do not use if the cell or foil is broken.
- Each 'TELDRIN' capsule is protected by a green PERMA-SEAL™ band which bonds the two capsule halves together; do not use if capsule or band is broken.
- A package insert is provided for information on tamper-resistant packaging.

WARNING

Do not take this product if you have asthma, glaucoma, or difficulty in urination due to enlargement of the prostate gland, except under the advice and supervision of a physician. Do not drive or operate heavy machinery as this preparation may cause drowsiness. Avoid alcoholic beverages while taking this product. May cause excitability, especially in children. Keep this and all drugs out of the reach of children. In case of accidental overdose, seek professional assistance or contact a poison control center immediately. As with any drug, if you are pregnant or nursing a baby, seek the advice of a health professional before using this product.
Store at controlled room temperature (59°–86°F.).

HOW SUPPLIED

Packages of 12, 24 and 48 capsules.

Smith Kline &French Laboratories
Division of SmithKline Beckman Corporation
1500 SPRING GARDEN ST.
P.O. BOX 7929
PHILADELPHIA, PA 19101

SK&F Co.
Carolina, P.R. 00630
Subsidiary of SmithKline Beckman Corporation

SK&F Lab Co.
Carolina, P.R. 00630
Subsidiary of SmithKline Beckman Corporation

SK&F PRODUCT CODE INDEX

Code	Product, Form and Strength
C44	'Compazine' *Spansule* capsules 10 mg.
C46	'Compazine' *Spansule* capsules 15 mg.
C47	'Compazine' *Spansule* capsules 30 mg.
C60	'Compazine' Suppositories 2 ½ mg.
C61	'Compazine' Suppositories 5 mg.
C62	'Compazine' Suppositories 25 mg.
C66	'Compazine' Tablets 5 mg.
C67	'Compazine' Tablets 10 mg.
C69	'Compazine' Tablets 25 mg.
D14	'Cytomel' Tablets 5 mcg.
D16	'Cytomel' Tablets 25 mcg.
D17	'Cytomel' Tablets 50 mcg.
D62	'Darbid' Tablets 5 mg.
E12	'Dexedrine' *Spansule* capsules 5 mg.
E13	'Dexedrine' *Spansule* capsules 10 mg.
E14	'Dexedrine' *Spansule* capsules 15 mg.
E19	'Dexedrine' Tablets 5 mg.
E33	'Dibenzyline' Capsules 10 mg.
J09	'Eskalith' Tablets 300 mg.
J10	'Eskalith' Controlled Release Tablets 450 mg.
120	'SK-Amitriptyline HCl' Tablets 10 mg.
121	'SK-Amitriptyline HCl' Tablets 25 mg.
124	'SK-Amitriptyline HCl' Tablets 75 mg.
131	'SK-Amitriptyline HCl' Tablets 100 mg.
101	'SK-Ampicillin' Capsules 250 mg.
102	'SK-Ampicillin' Capsules 500 mg.
494	'SK-APAP' with CODEINE Tablets 300 mg./15 mg.
496	'SK-APAP' with CODEINE Tablets 300 mg./30 mg.
497	'SK-APAP' with CODEINE Tablets 300 mg./60 mg.
133	'SK-Bamate' Tablets 200 mg.

Continued on next page

Smith Kline & French—Cont.

134 'SK-Bamate' Tablets 400 mg.
420 'SK-Chlorothiazide' Tablets 500 mg.
423 'SK-Diphenoxylate' Tablets 2.5 mg./0.025 mg.
379 'SK-Dipyridamole' Tablets 25 mg.
380 'SK-Dipyridamole' Tablets 50 mg.
381 'SK-Dipyridamole' Tablets 75 mg.
367 'SK-Erythromycin' Tablets 250 mg.
369 'SK-Erythromycin' Tablets 500 mg.
340 'SK-Furosemide' Tablets 20 mg.
341 'SK-Furosemide' Tablets 40 mg.
441 'SK-Lygen' Capsules 5 mg.
442 'SK-Lygen' Capsules 10 mg.
443 'SK-Lygen' Capsules 25 mg.
319 'SK-Oxycodone' with Aspirin Tablets
320 'SK-Oxycodone' with Acetaminophen Tablets
111 'SK-Penicillin G' Tablets 400,000 units
116 'SK-Penicillin VK' Tablets 250 mg.
117 'SK-Penicillin VK' Tablets 500 mg.
321 'SK-Pramine' Tablets 10 mg.
322 'SK-Pramine' Tablets 25 mg.
323 'SK-Pramine' Tablets 50 mg.
339 'SK-Prednisone' Tablets 5 mg.
499 'SK-Probenecid' Tablets 500 mg.
171 'SK-Quinidine Sulfate' Tablets 200 mg.
463 'SK-65' Capsules 65 mg.
468 'SK-65 Compound' Capsules
474 'SK-65 APAP' Tablets
126 'SK-Tetracycline HCl' Capsules 250 mg.
127 'SK-Tetracycline HCl' Capsules 500 mg.
409 'SK-Tolbutamide' Tablets 500 mg.
S03 *'Stelazine' Tablets 1 mg.
S04 *'Stelazine' Tablets 2 mg.
S06 *'Stelazine' Tablets 5 mg.
S07 *'Stelazine' Tablets 10 mg.
T63 'Thorazine' *Spansule* capsules 30 mg.
T64 'Thorazine' *Spansule* capsules 75 mg.
T66 'Thorazine' *Spansule* capsules 150 mg.
T67 'Thorazine' *Spansule* capsules 200 mg.
T69 'Thorazine' *Spansule* capsules 300 mg.
T70 'Thorazine' Suppositories 25 mg.
T71 'Thorazine' Suppositories 100 mg.
T73 'Thorazine' Tablets 10 mg.
T74 'Thorazine' Tablets 25 mg.
T76 'Thorazine' Tablets 50 mg.
T77 'Thorazine' Tablets 100 mg.
T79 'Thorazine' Tablets 200 mg.

*A product of SK&F Co., Carolina, P.R. 00630, Subsidiary of SmithKline Beckman Corporation, Philadelphia, Pa.

ANCEF® ℞
[an-sef']
(brand of sterile cefazolin sodium and cefazolin sodium injection)

PRODUCT OVERVIEW

KEY FACTS

'Ancef' is a semi-synthetic cephalosporin for parenteral administration. 'Ancef' has proven to be active against a number of gram-positive and gram-negative organisms *in vitro* and in clinical infections.

MAJOR USES

'Ancef' is indicated in the treatment of serious infections due to susceptible organisms listed below in the full prescribing information. These include infections of the urinary tract, respiratory tract, skin and skin structure, biliary tract, bone and joint and genital infections, as well as septicemia and endocarditis. 'Ancef' is also indicated for perioperative prophylaxis in patients undergoing surgical procedures classified as contaminated or potentially contaminated.

SAFETY INFORMATION

'Ancef' is contraindicated in patients with known allergy to cefazolin or other cephalosporins. Careful inquiry should be made concerning previous hypersensitivity to cephalosporins and penicillin. 'Ancef' should be administered cautiously to penicillin-sensitive patients. Serious acute hypersensitivity reactions may require epinephrine and other emergency measures. Because pseudomembranous colitis has been reported with the use of cephalosporins, it is important to consider its diagnosis in patients who develop diarrhea in association with antibiotic use.

PRESCRIBING INFORMATION

ANCEF® ℞
[an-sef']
(brand of sterile cefazolin sodium and cefazolin sodium injection)

DESCRIPTION

Ancef (sterile cefazolin sodium, SK&F) is a semi-synthetic cephalosporin for parenteral administration. It is the sodium salt of 3- {[(5-methyl-1, 3, 4-thiadiazol-2-yl) thio]-methyl}-8-oxo-7- [2-(1H-tetrazol -1- yl) acetamido] -5- thia-1-azabicyclo [4.2.0] oct-2-ene-2-carboxylic acid.

The sodium content is 46 mg. per gram of cefazolin.

'Ancef' in lyophilized form is supplied in vials equivalent to 250 mg., 500 mg. or 1 gram of cefazolin, in "Piggyback" Vials for intravenous admixture equivalent to 500 mg. or 1 gram of cefazolin; and in Pharmacy Bulk Vials equivalent to 5 grams or 10 grams of cefazolin.

'Ancef' is also supplied as a frozen, sterile, nonpyrogenic solution of cefazolin sodium in an iso-osmotic diluent in plastic containers. After thawing, the solution is intended for intravenous use.

The plastic container is fabricated from specially formulated polyvinyl chloride. Solutions in contact with the plastic container can leach out certain of its chemical components in very small amounts within the expiration period, e.g., di 2-ethylhexyl phthalate (DEHP), up to 5 parts per million. However, the safety of the plastic has been confirmed in tests in animals according to the USP biological tests for plastic containers as well as by tissue culture toxicity studies.

CLINICAL PHARMACOLOGY

Human Pharmacology: After intramuscular administration of 'Ancef' to normal volunteers, the mean serum concentrations were 37 mcg./ml. at one hour and 3 mcg./ml. at eight hours following a 500 mg. dose, and 64 mcg./ml. at one hour and 7 mcg./ml. at eight hours following a 1 gram dose.

Studies have shown that following intravenous administration of 'Ancef' to normal volunteers, mean serum concentrations peaked at approximately 185 mcg./ml. and were approximately 4 mcg./ml. at eight hours for a 1 gram dose.

The serum half-life for 'Ancef' is approximately 1.8 hours following I.V. administration and approximately 2.0 hours following I.M. administration.

In a study (using normal volunteers) of constant intravenous infusion with dosages of 3.5 mg./kg. for one hour (approximately 250 mg.) and 1.5 mg./kg. the next two hours (approximately 100 mg.), 'Ancef' produced a steady serum level at the third hour of approximately 28 μg./ml.

Studies in patients hospitalized with infections indicate that Ancef (sterile cefazolin sodium, SK&F) produces mean peak serum levels approximately equivalent to those seen in normal volunteers.

Bile levels in patients without obstructive biliary disease can reach or exceed serum levels by up to five times; however, in patients with obstructive biliary disease, bile levels of 'Ancef' are considerably lower than serum levels (< 1.0 μg./ml.).

In synovial fluid, the 'Ancef' level becomes comparable to that reached in serum at about four hours after drug administration.

Studies of cord blood show prompt transfer of 'Ancef' across the placenta. 'Ancef' is present in very low concentrations in the milk of nursing mothers.

'Ancef' is excreted unchanged in the urine. In the first six hours approximately 60% of the drug is excreted in the urine and this increases to 70%–80% within 24 hours. 'Ancef' achieves peak urine concentrations of approximately 2400 μg./ml. and 4000 μg./ml. respectively following 500 mg. and 1 gram intramuscular doses.

In patients undergoing peritoneal dialysis (2 l./hr.), 'Ancef' produced mean serum levels of approximately 10 and 30 μg./ml. after 24 hours' instillation of a dialyzing solution containing 50 mg./l. and 150 mg./l., respectively. Mean peak levels were 29 μg./ml. (range 13–44 μg./ml.) with 50 mg./l. (three patients), and 72 μg./ml. (range 26–142 μg./ml.) with 150 mg./l. (six patients). Intraperitoneal administration of 'Ancef' is usually well tolerated.

Controlled studies on adult normal volunteers, receiving 1 gram 4 times a day for 10 days, monitoring CBC, SGOT, SGPT, bilirubin, alkaline phosphatase, BUN, creatinine, and urinalysis, indicated no clinically significant changes attributed to 'Ancef'.

Microbiology: *In vitro* tests demonstrate that the bactericidal action of cephalosporins results from inhibition of cell wall synthesis. Ancef (sterile cefazolin sodium, SK&F) is active against the following organisms *in vitro* and in clinical infections:

Staphylococcus aureus (including penicillinase-producing strains)
Staphylococcus epidermidis
Methicillin-resistant staphylococci are uniformly resistant to cefazolin
Group A beta-hemolytic streptococci and other strains of streptococci (many strains of enterococci are resistant)
Streptococcus pneumoniae (formerly *D. pneumoniae)*
Escherichia coli
Proteus mirabilis
Klebsiella species
Enterobacter aerogenes
Hemophilus influenzae

Most strains of indole positive Proteus (*Proteus vulgaris*), *Enterobacter cloacae, Morganella morganii,* and *Providencia rettgeri* are resistant. *Serratia, Pseudomonas, Mima, Herellea* species are almost uniformly resistant to cefazolin.

Disk Susceptibility Tests

Disk diffusion technique—Quantitative methods that require measurement of zone diameters give the most precise estimates of antibiotic susceptibility. One such procedure[1] has been recommended for use with disks to test susceptibility to cefazolin.

Reports from a laboratory using the standardized single-disk susceptibility test[1] with a 30 mcg. cefazolin disk should be interpreted according to the following criteria:

Susceptible organisms produce zones of 18 mm. or greater, indicating that the tested organism is likely to respond to therapy.

Organisms of intermediate susceptibility produce zones 15 to 17 mm., indicating that the tested organism would be susceptible if high dosage is used or if the infection is confined to tissues and fluids (e.g., urine), in which high antibiotic levels are attained.

Resistant organisms produce zones of 14 mm. or less, indicating that other therapy should be selected.

For gram-positive isolates, a zone of 18 mm. is indicative of a cefazolin-susceptible organism when tested with either the cephalosporin-class disk (30 mcg. cephalothin) or the cefazolin disk (30 mcg. cefazolin).

Gram-negative organisms should be tested with the cefazolin disk (using the above criteria), since cefazolin has been shown by *in vitro* tests to have activity against certain strains of *Enterobacteriaceae* found resistant when tested with the cephalothin disk. Gram-negative organisms having zones of less than 18 mm. around the cephalothin disk may be susceptible to cefazolin.

Standardized procedures require use of control organisms. The 30 mcg. cefazolin disk should give zone diameter between 23 and 29 mm. for *E. coli* ATCC 25922 and between 29 and 35 mm. for *S. aureus* ATCC 25923.

The cefazolin disk should not be used for testing susceptibility to other cephalosporins.

Dilution techniques—A bacterial isolate may be considered susceptible if the minimal inhibitory concentration (MIC) for cefazolin is not more than 16 mcg. per ml. Organisms are considered resistant if the MIC is equal to or greater than 64 mcg. per ml.

The range of MIC's for the control strains are as follows:
S. aureus ATCC 25923, 0.25-1.0 mcg./ml.
E. coli ATCC 25922, 1.0-4.0 mcg./ml.

INDICATIONS AND USAGE

Ancef (sterile cefazolin sodium, SK&F) is indicated in the treatment of the following serious infections due to susceptible organisms:

RESPIRATORY TRACT INFECTIONS due to *Streptococcus pneumoniae* (formerly *D. pneumoniae*), *Klebsiella* species, *Hemophilus influenzae, Staphylococcus aureus* (penicillin-sensitive and penicillin-resistant), and group A beta-hemolytic streptococci.

Injectable benzathine penicillin is considered to be the drug of choice in treatment and prevention of streptococcal infections, including the prophylaxis of rheumatic fever.

'Ancef' is effective in the eradication of streptococci from the nasopharynx; however, data establishing the efficacy of 'Ancef' in the subsequent prevention of rheumatic fever are not available at present.

URINARY TRACT INFECTIONS due to *Escherichia coli, Proteus mirabilis, Klebsiella* species, and some strains of enterobacter and enterococci.

SKIN AND SKIN STRUCTURE INFECTIONS due to *Staphylococcus aureus* (penicillin-sensitive and penicillin-resistant), group A beta-hemolytic streptococci and other strains of streptococci.

BILIARY TRACT INFECTIONS due to *Escherichia coli,* various strains of streptococci, *Proteus mirabilis, Klebsiella* species and *Staphylococcus aureus.*

BONE AND JOINT INFECTIONS due to *Staphylococcus aureus.*

GENITAL INFECTIONS (i.e., prostatitis, epididymitis) due to *Escherichia coli, Proteus mirabilis, Klebsiella* species, and some strains of enterococci.

SEPTICEMIA due to *Streptococcus pneumoniae* (formerly *D. pneumoniae*), *Staphylococcus aureus* (penicillin-sensitive and penicillin-resistant), *Proteus mirabilis, Escherichia coli,* and *Klebsiella* species.

ENDOCARDITIS due to *Staphylococcus aureus* (penicillin-sensitive and penicillin-resistant) and group A beta-hemolytic streptococci.

Appropriate culture and susceptibility studies should be performed to determine susceptibility of the causative organism to 'Ancef'.

PERIOPERATIVE PROPHYLAXIS: The prophylactic administration of 'Ancef' preoperatively, intraoperatively, and postoperatively may reduce the incidence of certain postoperative infections in patients undergoing surgical procedures which are classified as contaminated or potentially contaminated (e.g., vaginal hysterectomy, and cholecystectomy in high-risk patients such as those over 70 years of age, with acute cholecystitis, obstructive jaundice, or common duct bile stones).

The perioperative use of 'Ancef' may also be effective in surgical patients in whom infection at the operative site would present a serious risk (e.g., during open-heart surgery and prosthetic arthroplasty).

The prophylactic administration of 'Ancef' should usually be discontinued within a 24-hour period after the surgical procedure. In surgery where the occurrence of infection may be particularly devastating (e.g., open-heart surgery and prosthetic arthroplasty), the prophylactic administration of 'Ancef' may be continued for 3 to 5 days following the completion of surgery.

If there are signs of infection, specimens for cultures should be obtained for the identification of the causative organism so that appropriate therapy may be instituted.

(See Dosage and Administration.)

CONTRAINDICATIONS

ANCEF (STERILE CEFAZOLIN SODIUM, SK&F) IS CONTRAINDICATED IN PATIENTS WITH KNOWN ALLERGY TO THE CEPHALOSPORIN GROUP OF ANTIBIOTICS.

WARNINGS

BEFORE CEFAZOLIN THERAPY IS INSTITUTED, CAREFUL INQUIRY SHOULD BE MADE CONCERNING PREVIOUS HYPERSENSITIVITY REACTIONS TO CEPHALOSPORINS AND PENICILLIN. CEPHALOSPORIN C DERIVATIVES SHOULD BE GIVEN CAUTIOUSLY IN PENICILLIN-SENSITIVE PATIENTS.

SERIOUS ACUTE HYPERSENSITIVITY REACTIONS MAY REQUIRE EPINEPHRINE AND OTHER EMERGENCY MEASURES.

There is some clinical and laboratory evidence of partial cross-allergenicity of the penicillins and the cephalosporins. Patients have been reported to have had severe reactions (including anaphylaxis) to both drugs.

Any patient who has demonstrated some form of allergy, particularly to drugs, should receive antibiotics cautiously. No exception should be made with regard to 'Ancef'.

Pseudomembranous colitis has been reported with the use of cephalosporins (and other broad-spectrum antibiotics); therefore, it is important to consider its diagnosis in patients who develop diarrhea in association with antibiotic use.

Treatment with broad-spectrum antibiotics alters normal flora of the colon and may permit overgrowth of clostridia. Studies indicate a toxin produced by *Clostridium difficile* is one primary cause of antibiotic-associated colitis. Cholestyramine and colestipol resins have been shown to bind the toxin *in vitro*.

Mild cases of colitis may respond to drug discontinuance alone.

Moderate to severe cases should be managed with fluid, electrolyte and protein supplementation as indicated.

When the colitis is not relieved by drug discontinuance or when it is severe, oral vancomycin is the treatment of choice for antibiotic-associated pseudomembranous colitis produced by *C. difficile*. Other causes of colitis should also be considered.

PRECAUTIONS

General—Prolonged use of Ancef (sterile cefazolin sodium, SK&F) may result in the overgrowth of nonsusceptible organisms. Careful clinical observation of the patient is essential.

When 'Ancef' is administered to patients with low urinary output because of impaired renal function, lower daily dosage is required (see Dosage and Administration).

'Ancef', as with all cephalosporins, should be prescribed with caution in individuals with a history of gastrointestinal disease, particularly colitis.

Drug Interactions—Probenecid may decrease renal tubular secretion of cephalosporins when used concurrently, resulting in increased and more prolonged cephalosporin blood levels.

Drug/Laboratory Test Interactions—A false positive reaction for glucose in the urine may occur with Benedict's solution, Fehling's solution, or with Clinitest® tablets, but not with enzyme-based tests such as Clinistix® and Tes-Tape®. Positive direct and indirect antiglobulin (Coombs) tests have occurred; these may also occur in neonates whose mothers received cephalosporins before delivery.

Carcinogenesis/Mutagenesis — Mutagenicity studies and long-term studies in animals to determine the carcinogenic potential of Ancef (sterile cefazolin sodium, SK&F) have not been performed.

Pregnancy — Teratogenic Effects — Pregnancy Category B. Reproduction studies have been performed in rats, mice and rabbits at doses up to 25 times the human dose and have revealed no evidence of impaired fertility or harm to the fetus due to 'Ancef'. There are, however, no adequate and well-controlled studies in pregnant women. Because animal reproduction studies are not always predictive of human response, this drug should be used during pregnancy only if clearly needed.

Labor and Delivery—When cefazolin has been administered prior to caesarean section, drug levels in cord blood have been approximately one quarter to one third of maternal drug levels. The drug appears to have no adverse effect on the fetus.

Nursing Mothers—'Ancef' is present in very low concentrations in the milk of nursing mothers. Caution should be exercised when 'Ancef' is administered to a nursing woman.

Pediatric Use—Safety and effectiveness for use in prematures and infants under one month of age have not been established. See Dosage and Administration for recommended dosage in children over one month.

ADVERSE REACTIONS

The following reactions have been reported:

Gastrointestinal: Diarrhea, oral candidiasis (oral thrush), vomiting, nausea, stomach cramps, anorexia. Symptoms of pseudomembranous colitis can appear during antibiotic treatment. Nausea and vomiting have been reported rarely.

Allergic: Anaphylaxis, eosinophilia, itching, drug fever, skin rash.

Hematologic: Neutropenia, leukopenia, thrombocythemia.

Hepatic and Renal: Transient rise in SGOT, SGPT, BUN and alkaline phosphatase levels has been observed without clinical evidence of renal or hepatic impairment.

Local Reactions: Rare instances of phlebitis have been reported at site of injection. Pain at the site of injection after intramuscular administration has occurred infrequently. Some induration has occurred.

Other Reactions: Genital and anal pruritus (including vulvar pruritus, genital moniliasis, and vaginitis).

DOSAGE AND ADMINISTRATION

Usual Adult Dosage

Type of Infection	Dose	Frequency
Moderate to severe infections	500 mg. to 1 gram	every 6 to 8 hrs.
Mild infections caused by susceptible gram + cocci	250 mg. to 500 mg.	every 8 hours
Acute, uncomplicated urinary tract infections	1 gram	every 12 hours
Pneumococcal pneumonia	500 mg.	every 12 hours
Severe, life-threatening infections (e.g., endocarditis, septicemia)*	1 gram to 1.5 grams	every 6 hours

* In rare instances, doses of up to 12 grams of 'Ancef' per day have been used.

Perioperative Prophylactic Use

To prevent postoperative infection in contaminated or potentially contaminated surgery, recommended doses are:

a. 1 gram I.V. or I.M. administered ½ hour to 1 hour prior to the start of surgery.
b. For lengthy operative procedures (e.g., 2 hours or more), 500 mg. to 1 gram I.V. or I.M. during surgery (administration modified depending on the duration of the operative procedure).
c. 500 mg. to 1 gram I.V. or I.M. every 6 to 8 hours for 24 hours postoperatively.

It is important that (1) the preoperative dose be given just (½ to 1 hour) prior to the start of surgery so that adequate antibiotic levels are present in the serum and tissues at the time of initial surgical incision; and (2) 'Ancef' be administered, if necessary, at appropriate intervals during surgery to provide sufficient levels of the antibiotic at the anticipated moments of greatest exposure to infective organisms.

In surgery where the occurrence of infection may be particularly devastating (e.g., open-heart surgery and prosthetic arthroplasty), the prophylactic administration of Ancef (sterile cefazolin sodium, SK&F) may be continued for 3 to 5 days following the completion of surgery.

Dosage Adjustment for Patients with Reduced Renal Function

'Ancef' may be used in patients with reduced renal function with the following dosage adjustments: Patients with a creatinine clearance of 55 ml./min. or greater or a serum creatinine of 1.5 mg. % or less can be given full doses. Patients with creatinine clearance rates of 35 to 54 ml./min. or serum creatinine of 1.6 to 3.0 mg. % can also be given full doses but dosage should be restricted to at least 8 hour intervals. Patients with creatinine clearance rates of 11 to 34 ml./min. or serum creatinine of 3.1 to 4.5 mg. % should be given ½ the usual dose every 12 hours. Patients with creatinine clearance rates of 10 ml./min. or less or serum creatinine of 4.6 mg. % or greater should be given ½ the usual dose every 18 to 24 hours. All reduced dosage recommendations apply after an initial loading dose appropriate to the severity of the infection. Patients undergoing peritoneal dialysis: See Human Pharmacology.

Pediatric Dosage

In children, a total daily dosage of 25 to 50 mg. per kg. (approximately 10 to 20 mg. per pound) of body weight, divided into three or four equal doses, is effective for most mild to moderately severe infections. Total daily dosage may be increased to 100 mg. per kg. (45 mg. per pound) of body weight for severe infections. Since safety for use in premature infants and in infants under one month has not been established, the use of Ancef (sterile cefazolin sodium, SK&F) in these patients is not recommended.

Pediatric Dosage Guide

Weight		25 mg./kg./Day Divided into 3 Doses		25 mg./kg./Day Divided into 4 Doses	
Lbs.	Kg.	Approximate Single Dose mg./q8h	Vol. (ml.) needed with dilution of 125 mg./ml.	Approximate Single Dose mg./q6h	Vol. (ml.) needed with dilution of 125 mg./ml.
10	4.5	40 mg.	0.35 ml.	30 mg.	0.25 ml.
20	9.0	75 mg.	0.60 ml.	55 mg.	0.45 ml.
30	13.6	115 mg.	0.90 ml.	85 mg.	0.70 ml.
40	18.1	150 mg.	1.20 ml.	115 mg.	0.90 ml.
50	22.7	190 mg.	1.50 ml.	140 mg.	1.10 ml.

Weight		50 mg./kg./Day Divided into 3 Doses		50 mg./kg./Day Divided into 4 Doses	
Lbs.	Kg.	Approximate Single Dose mg./q8h	Vol. (ml.) needed with dilution of 225 mg./ml.	Approximate Single Dose mg./q6h	Vol. (ml.) needed with dilution of 225 mg./ml.
10	4.5	75 mg.	0.35 ml.	55 mg.	0.25 ml.
20	9.0	150 mg.	0.70 ml.	110 mg.	0.50 ml.
30	13.6	225 mg.	1.00 ml.	170 mg.	0.75 ml.
40	18.1	300 mg.	1.35 ml.	225 mg.	1.00 ml.
50	22.7	375 mg.	1.70 ml.	285 mg.	1.25 ml.

In children with mild to moderate renal impairment (creatinine clearance of 70 to 40 ml./min.), 60 percent of the normal daily dose given in equally divided doses every 12 hours should be sufficient. In patients with moderate impairment (creatinine clearance of 40 to 20 ml./min.), 25 percent of the normal daily dose given in equally divided doses every 12 hours should be adequate. Children with severe renal impairment (creatinine clearance of 20 to 5 ml./min.) may be given 10 percent of the normal daily dose every 24 hours. All dosage recommendations apply after an initial loading dose.

RECONSTITUTION

Preparation of Parenteral Solution

Parenteral drug products should be SHAKEN WELL when reconstituted, and inspected visually for particulate matter prior to administration. If particulate matter is evident in reconstituted fluids, the drug solutions should be discarded. When reconstituted or diluted according to the instructions below, Ancef (sterile cefazolin sodium, SK&F) is stable for 24 hours at room temperature or for 96 hours if stored under refrigeration. Reconstituted solutions may range in color from pale yellow to yellow without a change in potency.

Single-Dose Vials

For I.M. injection, I.V. direct (bolus) injection, or I.V. infusion, reconstitute with Sterile Water for Injection according to the following table. SHAKE WELL.

Vial Size	Amount of Diluent	Approximate Concentration	Approximate Available Volume
250 mg.	2.0 ml.	125 mg./ml.	2.0 ml.
500 mg.	2.0 ml.	225 mg./ml.	2.2 ml.
1 gram	2.5 ml.	330 mg./ml.	3.0 ml.

Pharmacy Bulk Vials

Add Sterile Water for Injection, Bacteriostatic Water for Injection, or Sodium Chloride Injection according to the table below. SHAKE WELL.

Continued on next page

Smith Kline & French—Cont.

Vial Size	Amount of Diluent	Approximate Concentration	Approximate Available Volume
5 grams	23 ml.	1 gram/5 ml.	26 ml.
	48 ml.	1 gram/10 ml.	51 ml.
10 grams	45 ml.	1 gram/5 ml.	51 ml.
	96 ml.	1 gram/10 ml.	102 ml.

"Piggyback" Vials

Reconstitute with 50 to 100 ml. of Sodium Chloride Injection or other I.V. solution listed under ADMINISTRATION. When adding diluent to vial, allow air to escape by using a small vent needle or by pumping the syringe. SHAKE WELL. Administer with primary I.V. fluids, as a single dose.

ADMINISTRATION

Intramuscular Administration—Reconstitute vials with Sterile Water for Injection according to the dilution table above. Shake well until dissolved. 'Ancef' should be injected into a large muscle mass. Pain on injection is infrequent with 'Ancef'.

Intravenous Administration—Direct (bolus) injection: Following reconstitution according to the above table, further dilute vials with approximately 5 ml. Sterile Water for Injection. Inject the solution slowly over 3 to 5 minutes, directly or through tubing for patients receiving parenteral fluids (see list below).

Intermittent or continuous infusion: Dilute reconstituted 'Ancef' in 50 to 100 ml. of one of the following solutions:

Sodium Chloride Injection
5% or 10% Dextrose Injection
5% Dextrose in Lactated Ringer's Injection
5% Dextrose and 0.9% Sodium Chloride Injection (also may be used with 5% Dextrose and 0.45% or 0.2% Sodium Chloride Injection)
Lactated Ringer's Injection
Invert Sugar 5% or 10% in Sterile Water for Injection
Ringer's Injection
5% Sodium Bicarbonate in Sterile Water for Injection

DIRECTIONS FOR USE OF ANCEF (CEFAZOLIN SODIUM INJECTION, SK&F) PLASTIC CONTAINERS

'Ancef' supplied as a frozen, sterile, nonpyrogenic solution in plastic containers is to be administered either as a continuous or intermittent infusion.

Thaw container at room temperature. After thawing, check for minute leaks by squeezing bag firmly. If leaks are found, discard solution as sterility may be impaired. Additives should not be introduced into this solution. Do not use if the solution is cloudy or precipitated or if the seal is not intact. After thawing, the solution is stable for 24 hours at room temperature and 10 days if stored under refrigeration (5°C). DO NOT REFREEZE.

Use sterile equipment. It is recommended that the intravenous administration apparatus be replaced at least once every 48 hours.

CAUTION: Do not use plastic containers in series connections. Such use could result in air embolism due to residual air being drawn from the primary container before administration of the fluid from the secondary container is complete.

Preparation for administration:

1. Suspend container from eyelet support.
2. Remove plastic protector from outlet port at bottom of container.
3. Attach administration set. Refer to complete directions accompanying set.

HOW SUPPLIED

Ancef (sterile cefazolin sodium, SK&F)—supplied in vials equivalent to 250 mg., 500 mg. or 1 gram of cefazolin; in "Piggyback" Vials for intravenous admixture equivalent to 500 mg. or 1 gram of cefazolin; and in Pharmacy Bulk Vials equivalent to 5 grams or 10 grams of cefazolin.

Ancef (cefazolin sodium injection, SK&F) as a frozen, sterile, nonpyrogenic solution in plastic containers—supplied in 50 ml. single-dose containers equivalent to 500 mg. or 1 gram of cefazolin in 5% Dextrose (D5W). Do not store above −20°C.

'Ancef' supplied as a frozen, sterile, nonpyrogenic solution in plastic containers is manufactured for Smith Kline &French Laboratories by Travenol Laboratories, Inc., Deerfield, IL 60015.

Military—Vial, 10 gram, 100 ml., 6505-01-184-1574; 5 gram, 100 ml., 10's, 6505-01-058-2046; 1 gram, 6505-01-010-0832; 500 mg., 6505-01-010-0833.

Veterans Administration—500 mg., 6505-01-010-0833; 1 gram, 6505-01-010-0832; 10 gram, 6505-01-008-3408.

1 Bauer, A.W.; Kirby, W.M.M.; Sherris, J.C., and Turck, M.: Antibiotic Testing by a Standardized Single Disc Method, Am. J. Clin. Path. 45:493, 1966. Standardized Disc Susceptibility Test, Federal Register 39:19182-19184, 1974.

AF:L38

Shown in Product Identification Section, page 430

ANSPOR® ℞

[*an-spore'*]

(brand of cephradine)
Capsules, 250 mg. and 500 mg.
and
for Oral Suspension, 125 mg./5 ml. and 250 mg./5 ml.

('Anspor' is manufactured for Smith Kline &French Laboratories, Division of SmithKline Beckman Corporation, Philadelphia, Pa., by Squibb Manufacturing, Inc., Humacao, P.R., Subsidiary of E.R. Squibb & Sons, Inc.)

DESCRIPTION

Cephradine is a semisynthetic cephalosporin antibiotic chemically designated as (6*R*, 7*R*)-7-[(*R*)-2-amino-2-(1, 4-cyclohexadien-1-y1)acetamido]-3-methyl-8-oxo-5-thia-1-azabicyclo[4.2.0]oct-2-ene-2-carboxylic acid.

Capsules—Each Anspor (cephradine, SK&F) capsule contains cephradine as follows: 250 mg.—opaque orange cap and opaque white body imprinted with the product name ANSPOR, SKF and 250; 500 mg.—opaque orange cap and body imprinted with the product name ANSPOR, SKF and 500. Inactive ingredients consist of FD&C Red No. 3, FD&C Yellow No. 6, gelatin, lactose, magnesium stearate, talc, titanium dioxide and trace amounts of other inactive ingredients.

For Oral Suspension—When reconstituted as directed, the fruit-flavored suspension contains cephradine as follows: 125 mg./5 ml. (yellow-orange) or 250 mg./5 ml. (red). Inactive ingredients consist of citric acid, FD&C Red No. 40 (250 mg./5 ml. strength), FD&C Yellow No. 6 (125 mg./5 ml. strength), flavors, guar gum, methylcellulose, sodium citrate and sucrose.

CLINICAL PHARMACOLOGY

Human Pharmacology: Anspor (cephradine, SK&F) is acid stable. It is rapidly absorbed after oral administration in the fasting state. Following doses of 250 mg. and 500 mg. in normal adult volunteers, average peak serum levels within one hour were approximately 9 and 16.5 mcg. per ml. respectively. The presence of food in the gastrointestinal tract delays the absorption but does not affect the total amount of cephradine absorbed. Over 90 percent of the drug is excreted unchanged in the urine within 6 hours. Peak urine concentrations are approximately 1600 mcg. per ml. following a 250 mg. dose and 3200 mcg. per ml. following a 500 mg. dose.

Microbiology: *In vitro* tests demonstrate that the cephalosporins are bactericidal because of their inhibition of cell-wall synthesis. Cephradine is active against the following organisms *in vitro* and in clinical infections:

Beta-hemolytic streptococci
Staphylococci, including coagulase-positive, coagulase-negative, and penicillinase-producing strains
Streptococcus pneumoniae (formerly *D. pneumoniae*)
Escherichia coli
Proteus mirabilis
Klebsiella sp.
Hemophilus influenzae

Note—Some strains of enterococci *(Streptococcus faecalis)* are resistant to cephradine. It is not active against most strains of *Enterobacter* sp., *Pr. morganii*, and *Pr. vulgaris*. It has no activity against *Pseudomonas* or *Herellea* species. When tested by *in vitro* methods, staphylococci exhibit cross-resistance between cephradine and methicillin-type antibiotics.

Disc Susceptibility Tests: Quantitative methods that require measurement of zone diameters give the most precise estimates of antibiotic susceptibility. One recommended procedure (21 CFR § 460.1) uses cephalosporin class discs for testing susceptibility; interpretations correlate zone diameters of this disc test with MIC values for cephradine. With this procedure, a report from the laboratory of "resistant" indicates that the infecting organism is not likely to respond to therapy. A report of "intermediate susceptibility" suggests that the organism would be susceptible if the infection is confined to the urinary tract, as high antibiotic levels can be obtained in the urine, or if high dosage is used in other types of infection.

INDICATIONS AND USAGE

Anspor (cephradine, SK&F) Capsules and 'Anspor' for Oral Suspension are indicated in the treatment of the following infections when caused by susceptible strains of designated microorganisms:

Infections of the respiratory tract (e.g., tonsillitis, pharyngitis, and lobar pneumonia) caused by group A beta-hemolytic streptococci and *Streptococcus pneumoniae* (formerly *D. pneumoniae*).

(Penicillin is the usual drug of choice in the treatment and prevention of streptococcal infections, including the prophylaxis of rheumatic fever. 'Anspor' is generally effective in the eradication of streptococci from the nasopharynx; substantial data establishing the efficacy of 'Anspor' in the subsequent prevention of rheumatic fever are not available at present.)

Otitis media caused by group A beta-hemolytic streptococci, *Streptococcus pneumoniae* (formerly *D. pneumoniae*), *Hemophilus influenzae* and staphylococci.

Skin and skin structure infections caused by staphylococci (penicillin-susceptible and penicillin-resistant) and beta-hemolytic streptococci.

Infections of the urinary tract, including prostatitis, caused by *Escherichia coli*, *Pr. mirabilis*, and *Klebsiella* sp.

Note—Culture and susceptibility tests should be initiated prior to and during therapy. Renal function studies should be performed when indicated.

CONTRAINDICATIONS

Cephradine is contraindicated in patients with known hypersensitivity to the cephalosporin group of antibiotics.

WARNINGS

BEFORE CEPHRADINE THERAPY IS INSTITUTED, CAREFUL INQUIRY SHOULD BE MADE CONCERNING PREVIOUS HYPERSENSITIVITY REACTIONS TO CEPHALOSPORINS AND PENICILLIN. CEPHALOSPORIN C DERIVATIVES SHOULD BE GIVEN CAUTIOUSLY IN PENICILLIN-SENSITIVE PATIENTS.

SERIOUS ACUTE HYPERSENSITIVITY REACTIONS MAY REQUIRE EPINEPHRINE AND OTHER EMERGENCY MEASURES.

There is some clinical and laboratory evidence of partial cross-allergenicity of the penicillins and the cephalosporins. Patients have been reported to have had severe reactions (including anaphylaxis) to both drugs.

Any patient who has demonstrated some form of allergy, particularly to drugs, should receive antibiotics cautiously. No exception should be made with regard to Anspor (cephradine, SK&F).

Pseudomembranous colitis has been reported with the use of cephalosporins (and other broad-spectrum antibiotics); therefore, it is important to consider its diagnosis in patients who develop diarrhea in association with antibiotic use.

Treatment with broad-spectrum antibiotics alters normal flora of the colon and may permit overgrowth of clostridia. Studies indicate a toxin produced by *Clostridium difficile* is one primary cause of antibiotic-associated colitis. Cholestyramine and colestipol resins have been shown to bind the toxin *in vitro*.

Mild cases of colitis may respond to drug discontinuance alone.

Moderate to severe cases should be managed with fluid, electrolyte and protein supplementation as indicated.

When the colitis is not relieved by drug discontinuance or when it is severe, oral vancomycin is the treatment of choice for antibiotic-associated pseudomembranous colitis produced by *C. difficile*. Other causes of colitis should also be considered.

PRECAUTIONS

General—Patients should be followed carefully so that any side effects or unusual manifestations of drug idiosyncrasy may be detected. If a hypersensitivity reaction occurs, the drug should be discontinued and the patient treated with the usual agents, e.g., pressor amines, antihistamines, or corticosteroids.

Administer cephradine with caution in the presence of markedly impaired renal function. In patients with known or suspected renal impairment, careful clinical observation and appropriate laboratory studies should be made prior to and during therapy as cephradine accumulates in the serum and tissues. See DOSAGE AND ADMINISTRATION section for information on treatment of patients with impaired renal function.

Prolonged use of antibiotics may promote the overgrowth of nonsusceptible organisms. Should superinfection occur during therapy, appropriate measures should be taken.

Anspor (cephradine, SK&F), as with all cephalosporins, should be prescribed with caution in individuals with a history of gastrointestinal disease, particularly colitis.

Information for Patients—Cephradine may be taken without regard to meals, unless gastrointestinal irritation occurs.

Diabetic patients receiving 'Anspor' should be cautioned to check with physicians before changing diet or dosage of diabetes medication. A false positive reaction for glucose in the urine may occur with Benedict's solution, Fehling's solution, or with Clinitest® tablets, but not with enzyme-based tests such as Clinistix® and Tes-Tape®.

Laboratory Tests—In chronic urinary tract infections, frequent bacteriologic tests are necessary during drug therapy and may be necessary for several months afterwards.

Drug Interactions—Probenecid may decrease renal tubular secretion of cephalosporins when used concurrently, resulting in increased and more prolonged cephalosporin blood levels.

Drug/Laboratory Test Interactions—After treatment with cephradine, a false positive reaction for glucose in the urine may occur with Benedict's solution, Fehling's solution, or with Clinitest® tablets, but not with enzyme-based tests such as Clinistix® and Tes-Tape®.

A false positive direct Coombs test has been reported after treatment with other cephalosporins; therefore, it should be recognized that a positive Coombs test may be due to the drug.

Carcinogenesis/Mutagenesis — Mutagenicity studies and long-term studies in animals to determine the carcinogenic potential of Anspor (cephradine, SK&F) have not been performed.

Pregnancy—*Teratogenic Effects*—Pregnancy Category B. Reproduction studies have been performed in mice and rats receiving doses up to four times the maximum human dose and have revealed no evidence of impaired fertility or harm to the fetus due to cephradine. There are, however, no adequate and well-controlled studies in pregnant women. Because animal reproduction studies are not always predictive of human response, this drug should be used during pregnancy only if clearly needed.

Nursing Mothers—Cephradine is present in very low concentrations in the milk of nursing mothers. Caution should be exercised when cephradine is administered to a nursing woman.

Pediatric Use—Safety and effectiveness for use in infants under nine months of age have not been established. See DOSAGE AND ADMINISTRATION section for recommended dosage in children over nine months.

ADVERSE REACTIONS

As with other cephalosporins, untoward reactions are limited essentially to gastrointestinal disturbances and to hypersensitivity phenomena. The latter are more likely to occur in individuals who have previously demonstrated hypersensitivity and those with a history of allergy, asthma, hay fever, or urticaria.

The following adverse reactions have been reported following the use of cephradine:

Gastrointestinal: Diarrhea or loose stools, vomiting, glossitis, nausea, abdominal pain and heartburn.

Symptoms of pseudomembranous colitis can appear during antibiotic treatment.

Nausea and vomiting have been reported rarely.

Allergic: Anaphylaxis, mild urticaria or skin rash, pruritus, joint pains.

Hematologic: Mild, transient eosinophilia, leukopenia and neutropenia.

Liver: Transient mild rise of SGOT, SGPT, and total bilirubin has been observed with no evidence of hepatocellular damage.

Renal: Transitory rises in BUN have been observed in some patients treated with cephalosporins; their frequency increases in patients over 50 years old. In adults for whom serum creatinine determinations were performed, the rise in BUN was not accompanied by a rise in serum creatinine.

Other: Dizziness and tightness in the chest and candidal vaginitis.

DOSAGE AND ADMINISTRATION

Anspor (cephradine, SK&F) may be given without regard to meals.

Adults: For skin and soft-tissue and respiratory tract infections (other than lobar pneumonia), the usual dose is 250 mg. every 6 hours or 500 mg. every 12 hours. For acute infections of the urinary tract, including prostatitis, and pneumococcal lobar pneumonia, the usual dose is 500 mg. every 6 hours or 1 gram every 12 hours. Severe or chronic infections may require larger doses.

Children: No adequate information is available on the efficacy of b.i.d. regimens in children under nine months of age. The usual dose in children over nine months of age is 25 to 50 mg./kg./day administered in equally divided doses every 6 or 12 hours. For otitis media due to *H. influenzae*, doses are from 75 to 100 mg./kg./day administered in equally divided doses every 6 or 12 hours. Doses for children should not exceed doses recommended for adults. The maximum dose should not exceed 4 grams per day.

All patients, regardless of age and weight: Larger doses (up to 1 gram, q.i.d.) may be given for severe or chronic infections.

As with antibiotic therapy generally, therapy should be continued for a minimum of 48 to 72 hours after the patient becomes asymptomatic or evidence of bacterial eradication has been obtained. In infections caused by group A beta-hemolytic streptococci, a minimum of 10 days of treatment is recommended to guard against the risk of rheumatic fever or glomerulonephritis. In the treatment of chronic urinary tract infection, frequent bacteriologic and clinical appraisal is necessary during therapy and may be necessary for several months afterwards. Persistent infections may require treatment for several weeks. Prolonged intensive therapy is recommended for prostatitis. Doses smaller than those indicated are not recommended.

Patients with Impaired Renal Function

Not on Dialysis: The following initial dosage schedule is suggested as a guideline based on creatinine clearance. Further modification in the dosage schedule may be required because of individual variations in absorption.

Creatinine Clearance	Dose	Time Interval
>20 ml./min.	500 mg.	6 hours
5–20 ml./min.	250 mg.	6 hours
<5 ml./min.	250 mg.	12 hours

On Chronic, Intermittent Hemodialysis:

250 mg. Start
250 mg. at 12 hours
250 mg. 36–48 hours (after start)

Children may require dosage modification proportional to their weight and severity of infection.

HOW SUPPLIED

Anspor (cephradine, SK&F) Capsules: 250 mg. in bottles of 100 and in Single Unit Packages of 100 (intended for institutional use only); 500 mg. in bottles of 20 and 100 and in Single Unit Packages of 100 (intended for institutional use only). 'Anspor' for Oral Suspension after reconstitution provides 125 mg. or 250 mg. of cephradine per 5 ml. (one teaspoonful) in 100 ml. bottles.

NOTES ON STABILITY

Anspor (cephradine, SK&F) Capsules—Do not store above 86°F.; keep bottle tightly closed. 'Anspor' for Oral Suspension—Prior to reconstitution, do not store above 86°F. After reconstitution, suspensions retain their potency for seven days at room temperature and for 14 days if refrigerated.

Shown in Product Identification Section, page 430

AN:L14

CEFIZOX® ℞
[sef'eh-zocks]
(brand of sterile ceftizoxime sodium)

PRODUCT OVERVIEW

KEY FACTS

'Cefizox' is a sterile, semisynthetic cephalosporin antibiotic for parenteral (I.V., I.M.) administration. 'Cefizox' is highly resistant to a broad spectrum of beta-lactamases, and is active against a wide range of both aerobic and anaerobic gram-positive and gram-negative organisms.

MAJOR USES

'Cefizox' is indicated in the treatment of infections due to susceptible microorganisms listed below in the full prescribing information. In particular, because of its mixed aerobic/anaerobic coverage, 'Cefizox' has proven to be useful for treating intra-abdominal infections.

SAFETY INFORMATION

'Cefizox' is contraindicated in patients who have shown hypersensitivity to ceftizoxime or the cephalosporin group of antibiotics. Careful inquiry should be made concerning previous hypersensitivity reactions to drug. 'Cefizox' should be administered with caution to penicillin-sensitive patients. Serious acute hypersensitivity reactions may require epinephrine and other emergency measures. Because pseudomembranous colitis has been reported with the use of cephalosporins, it is important to consider its diagnosis in patients who develop diarrhea in association with antibiotic use.

PRESCRIBING INFORMATION

CEFIZOX® ℞
[sef'eh-zocks]
(brand of sterile ceftizoxime sodium and ceftizoxime sodium injection)

DESCRIPTION

Cefizox (sterile ceftizoxime sodium, FSK) is a sterile, semisynthetic, broad-spectrum, beta-lactamase resistant cephalosporin antibiotic for parenteral (I.V., I.M.) administration. It is the sodium salt of [6R-[6α, 7 β(Z)]]-7-[[(2,3-dihydro-2-imino-4-thiazolyl) (methoxyimino) acetyl] amino]-8-oxo-5-thia-1-azabicyclo [4.2.0] oct-2- ene-2-carboxylic acid. Its sodium content is approximately 60 mg. (2.6 mEq.) per gram of ceftizoxime activity.

Sterile ceftizoxime sodium is a white to pale yellow crystalline powder.

'Cefizox' is supplied in vials equivalent to 1 gram or 2 grams of ceftizoxime, and in "Piggyback" Vials for intravenous admixture equivalent to 1 gram or 2 grams of ceftizoxime. 'Cefizox', equivalent to 1 gram or 2 grams of ceftizoxime, is also supplied as a frozen, sterile, nonpyrogenic solution of ceftizoxime sodium in an iso-osmotic diluent in plastic containers. After thawing, the solution is intended for intravenous use.

The plastic container is fabricated from specially formulated polyvinyl chloride. Solutions in contact with the plastic container can leach out certain of its chemical components in very small amounts within the expiration period, e.g., di 2-ethylhexyl phthalate (DEHP), up to 5 parts per million. However, the safety of the plastic has been confirmed in tests in animals according to the USP biological tests for plastic containers as well as by tissue culture toxicity studies.

CLINICAL PHARMACOLOGY

The table below demonstrates the serum levels and duration of Cefizox (sterile ceftizoxime sodium, FSK) following intramuscular administration of 500 mg. and 1.0 gram doses respectively to normal volunteers.

[See table above].

Serum Concentrations After Intramuscular Administration
Serum Concentration (mcg./ml.)

Dose	½ hr.	1 hr.	2 hrs.	4 hrs.	6 hrs.	8 hrs.
500 mg.	13.3	13.7	9.2	4.8	1.9	0.7
1.0 gram	36.0	39.0	31.0	15.0	6.0	3.0

Following intravenous administration of 1.0, 2.0 and 3.0 gram doses of 'Cefizox' to normal volunteers, the following serum levels were obtained:

[See table below].

ND = Not Done

Serum Concentrations After Intravenous Administration
Serum Concentration (mcg./ml.)

Dose	5 mins.	10 mins.	30 mins.	1 hr.	2 hrs.	4 hrs.	8 hrs.
1.0 gram	ND	ND	60.5	38.9	21.5	8.4	1.4
2.0 grams	131.8	110.9	77.5	53.6	33.1	12.1	2.0
3.0 grams	221.1	174.0	112.7	83.9	47.4	26.2	4.8

A serum half-life of approximately 1.7 hours was observed after intravenous or intramuscular administration.

'Cefizox' is 30% protein bound.

'Cefizox' is not metabolized, and is excreted virtually unchanged by the kidneys in 24 hours. This provides a high urinary concentration. Concentrations greater than 6,000 mcg./ml. have been achieved in the urine by 2 hours after a 1 gram dose of 'Cefizox' intravenously. Probenecid slows tubular secretion and produces even higher serum levels, increasing the duration of measurable serum concentrations.

'Cefizox' achieves therapeutic levels in various body fluids, e.g., cerebrospinal fluid (in patients with inflamed meninges), bile, surgical wound fluid, pleural fluid, aqueous humor, ascitic fluid, peritoneal fluid, prostatic fluid and saliva, and the following body tissues: heart, gallbladder, bone, biliary, peritoneal, prostatic and uterine.

In clinical experience to date, no disulfiram-like reactions have been reported with Cefizox (sterile ceftizoxime sodium, FSK).

Microbiology

The bactericidal action of 'Cefizox' results from inhibition of cell-wall synthesis. 'Cefizox' is highly resistant to a broad spectrum of beta-lactamases (penicillinase and cephalosporinase), including Richmond types I, II, III, TEM, and IV, produced by both aerobic and anaerobic gram-positive and gram-negative organisms. 'Cefizox' is active against a wide range of gram-positive and gram-negative organisms, and is usually active against the following organisms *in vitro* and in clinical situations (see Indications and Usage):

Gram-Positive Aerobes:

Staphylococcus sp. including penicillinase and nonpenicillinase producing *S. aureus* and *S. epidermidis.* Note: Methicillin-resistant staphylococci are resistant to cephalosporins, including ceftizoxime.

Streptococcus sp. including *S. pneumoniae* (formerly *D. pneumoniae*) and *S. pyogenes.*

Note: 'Cefizox' is usually inactive *in vitro* against most strains of enterococci, eg, *S. faecalis.*

Gram-Negative Aerobes:

Klebsiella sp. including *K. pneumoniae*
Escherichia coli
Enterobacter sp.
Pseudomonas sp. including *Ps. aeruginosa*

Continued on next page

Smith Kline & French—Cont.

Proteus mirabilis
Proteus vulgaris
Morganella morganii (formerly *Proteus morganii*) and
Providencia rettgeri (formerly *Proteus rettgeri*)
Serratia sp. including *S. marcescens*
Haemophilus sp. including ampicillin-resistant strains of *H. influenzae*
Neisseria gonorrhoeae

Anaerobes:
Bacteroides sp. including *B. fragilis*
Anaerobic cocci including *Peptococcus* sp. *Peptostreptococcus* sp.

'Cefizox' is usually active against strains of *Acinetobacter* sp. Cefizox (sterile ceftizoxime sodium, FSK) is usually active against the following organisms *in vitro*, but the clinical significance of these data has not been established:

Gram-Positive Aerobes:
Corynebacterium diphtheriae

Gram-Negative Aerobes:
Shigella sp.
Providencia stuartii
Salmonella sp.
Aeromonas hydrophila
Yersinia enterocolitica
Moraxella sp.
Pasteurella multocida
Neisseria meningitidis
Citrobacter sp.

Anaerobes:
Actinomyces sp.
Veillonella sp.
Eubacterium sp.
Clostridium sp. (Note: Most strains of *C. difficile* are resistant.)
Fusobacterium sp.
Bifidobacterium sp.
Propionibacterium sp.

Susceptibility Testing
Quantitative methods that require measurement of zone diameters give the most precise estimate of antibiotic susceptibility. One such procedure* has been recommended for use with disks to test susceptibility to ceftizoxime.

Reports from the laboratory giving results of the standard single-disk susceptibility test with a 30 mcg. ceftizoxime disk should be interpreted according to the following criteria (with the exception of *Ps. aeruginosa*):

Susceptible organisms produce zones of 20 mm. or greater, indicating that the test organism is likely to respond to therapy.

Organisms that produce zones of 15 to 19 mm. are expected to be susceptible if high dosage is used or if the infection is confined to tissues and fluids (e.g., urine) in which high antibiotic levels are attained.

Resistant organisms produce zones of 14 mm. or less, indicating that other therapy should be selected.

Organisms should be tested with the 'Cefizox' disk, since 'Cefizox' has been shown by *in vitro* tests to be active against certain strains found resistant when other beta-lactam disks are used.

Susceptibility Testing for Pseudomonas in Urinary Tract Infections
Most strains of *Ps. aeruginosa* are moderately susceptible to Cefizox (sterile ceftizoxime sodium, FSK). 'Cefizox' achieves high levels in the urine (greater than 6,000 mcg./ml. at 2 hours with 1 gram I.V.) and therefore the following zone sizes should be used when testing 'Cefizox' for treatment of urinary tract infections caused by *Ps. aeruginosa:*

Susceptible organisms produce zones of 20 mm. or greater, indicating that the test organism is likely to respond to therapy.

Organisms that produce zones of 11 to 19 mm. are expected to be susceptible when the infection is confined to the urinary tract in which high antibiotic levels are attained.

Resistant organisms produce zones of 10 mm. or less, indicating that other therapy should be selected.

A bacterial isolate may be considered susceptible if the MIC value for 'Cefizox' is equal to or less than 16 mcg./ml. Organisms are considered moderately susceptible if the MIC is greater than 16 mcg./ml. but less than 64 mcg./ml. Organisms are considered resistant if the MIC is 64 mcg./ml. or greater. For most organisms the MBC value for 'Cefizox' is the same as the MIC value.

The standardized quality control procedure requires use of control organisms. The 30 mcg. ceftizoxime disk should give the zone diameters listed below for the quality control strains.

Organism	ATCC	Zone Size Range
E. coli	25922	30–36 mm.
S. aureus	25923	27–35 mm.
Ps. aeruginosa	27853	12–17 mm.

INDICATIONS AND USAGE
Cefizox (sterile ceftizoxime sodium, FSK) is indicated in the treatment of infections due to susceptible strains of the microorganisms listed below:

LOWER RESPIRATORY TRACT INFECTIONS caused by *Streptococcus* sp. including *S. pneumoniae* (formerly *D. pneumoniae*), but excluding enterococci; *Klebsiella* sp.; *Proteus mirabilis; Escherichia coli; Haemophilus influenzae* including ampicillin-resistant strains; *Staphylococcus aureus* (penicillinase and nonpenicillinase producing); *Serratia* sp.; *Enterobacter* sp.; and *Bacteroides* sp.

URINARY TRACT INFECTIONS caused by *Staphylococcus aureus* (penicillinase and nonpenicillinase producing); *Escherichia coli; Pseudomonas* sp. including *Ps. aeruginosa; Proteus mirabilis; P. vulgaris; Providencia rettgeri* (formerly *Proteus rettgeri*) and *Morganella morganii* (formerly *Proteus morganii*); *Klebsiella* sp.; *Serratia* sp. including *S. marcescens; Enterobacter* sp.

GONORRHEA. Uncomplicated cervical and urethral gonorrhea caused by *Neisseria gonorrhoeae.*

INTRA-ABDOMINAL INFECTIONS caused by *Escherichia coli; Staphylococcus epidermidis; Streptococcus* sp. (excluding enterococci); *Enterobacter* sp.; *Klebsiella* sp.; *Bacteroides* sp. including *B. fragilis;* and anaerobic cocci, including *Peptococcus* sp. and *Peptostreptococcus* sp.

SEPTICEMIA caused by *Streptococcus* sp. including *S. pneumoniae* (formerly *D. pneumoniae*), but excluding enterococci; *Staphylococcus aureus* (penicillinase and nonpenicillinase producing); *Escherichia coli; Bacteroides* sp. including *B. fragilis; Klebsiella* sp.; and *Serratia* sp.

SKIN AND SKIN STRUCTURE INFECTIONS caused by *Staphylococcus aureus* (penicillinase and nonpenicillinase producing); *Staphylococcus epidermidis; Escherichia coli; Klebsiella* sp.; *Streptococcus* sp. including *Streptococcus pyogenes* (group A beta-hemolytic), but excluding enterococci; *Proteus mirabilis; Serratia* sp.; *Enterobacter* sp.; *Bacteroides* sp. including *B. fragilis;* and anaerobic cocci, including *Peptococcus* sp. and *Peptostreptococcus* sp.

BONE AND JOINT INFECTIONS caused by *Staphylococcus aureus* (penicillinase and nonpenicillinase producing); *Streptococcus* sp. (excluding enterococci); *Proteus mirabilis; Bacteroides* sp.; and anaerobic cocci, including *Peptococcus* sp. and *Peptostreptococcus* sp.

MENINGITIS caused by *Haemophilus influenzae.* 'Cefizox' has also been used successfully in the treatment of a limited number of pediatric and adult cases of meningitis caused by *Streptococcus pneumoniae.*

'Cefizox' has been effective in the treatment of seriously ill, compromised patients, including those who were debilitated, immunosuppressed or neutropenic.

Infections caused by aerobic gram-negative and by mixtures of organisms resistant to other cephalosporins, aminoglycosides, or penicillins have responded to treatment with 'Cefizox'.

Because of the serious nature of some urinary tract infections due to *Ps. aeruginosa* and because many strains of *Pseudomonas* species are only moderately susceptible to 'Cefizox', higher dosage is recommended. Other therapy should be instituted if the response is not prompt.

Susceptibility studies on specimens obtained prior to therapy should be used to determine the response of causative organisms to 'Cefizox'. Therapy with 'Cefizox' may be initiated pending results of the studies; however, treatment should be adjusted according to study findings. In serious infections 'Cefizox' has been used concomitantly with aminoglycosides (see Precautions). Before using 'Cefizox' concomitantly with other antibiotics, the prescribing information for those agents should be reviewed for contraindications, warnings, precautions and adverse reactions. Renal function should be carefully monitored.

CONTRAINDICATIONS
Cefizox (sterile ceftizoxime sodium, FSK) is contraindicated in patients who have known allergy to the drug.

WARNINGS
BEFORE THERAPY WITH CEFIZOX (STERILE CEFTIZOXIME SODIUM, FSK) IS INSTITUTED, CAREFUL INQUIRY SHOULD BE MADE TO DETERMINE WHETHER THE PATIENT HAS HAD PREVIOUS HYPERSENSITIVITY REACTIONS TO CEPHALOSPORINS, PENICILLINS, OR OTHER DRUGS. THIS PRODUCT SHOULD BE GIVEN CAUTIOUSLY TO PENICILLIN-SENSITIVE PATIENTS. ANTIBIOTICS SHOULD BE ADMINISTERED WITH CAUTION TO ANY PATIENT WHO HAS DEMONSTRATED SOME FORM OF ALLERGY, PARTICULARLY TO DRUGS. SERIOUS ACUTE HYPERSENSITIVITY REACTIONS MAY REQUIRE EPINEPHRINE AND OTHER EMERGENCY MEASURES.

***Pseudomembranous colitis* has been reported with the use of cephalosporins (and other broad-spectrum antibiotics); therefore, it is important to consider its diagnosis in patients who developed diarrhea in association with antibiotic use.**
Treatment with broad-spectrum antibiotics alters normal flora of the colon and may permit overgrowth of *Clostridia.* Studies indicate a toxin produced by *Clostridium difficile* is one primary cause of antibiotic-associated colitis. Cholestyramine and colestipol resins have been shown to bind the toxin *in vitro.*

Mild cases of colitis may respond to drug discontinuance alone.

Moderate to severe cases should be managed with fluid, electrolyte and protein supplementation as indicated.

When the colitis is not relieved by drug discontinuance or when it is severe, oral vancomycin is the treatment of choice for antibiotic-associated pseudomembranous colitis produced by *C. difficile.* Other causes of colitis should also be considered.

PRECAUTIONS
General: As with all broad-spectrum antibiotics, Cefizox (sterile ceftizoxime sodium, FSK) should be prescribed with caution in individuals with a history of gastrointestinal disease, particularly colitis.

Although 'Cefizox' has not been shown to produce an alteration in renal function, renal status should be evaluated, especially in seriously ill patients receiving maximum dose therapy. As with any antibiotic, prolonged use may result in overgrowth of nonsusceptible organisms. Careful observation is essential; appropriate measures should be taken if superinfection occurs.

Drug Interactions: Although the occurrence has not been reported with 'Cefizox', nephrotoxicity has been reported following concomitant administration of other cephalosporins and aminoglycosides.

Pregnancy: (Category B.) Reproduction studies have been performed in rats and rabbits and have revealed no evidence of impaired fertility or harm to the fetus due to 'Cefizox'. There are, however, no adequate and well-controlled studies in pregnant women. Because animal reproduction studies are not always predictive of human response, this drug should be used during pregnancy only if clearly needed.

Labor and Delivery: Safety of 'Cefizox' use during labor and delivery has not been established.

Nursing Mothers: 'Cefizox' is excreted in human milk in low concentrations. Caution should be exercised when 'Cefizox' is administered to a nursing woman.

Infants and Children: Safety and efficacy in infants from birth to six months of age have not been established. In children six months of age and older, treatment with 'Cefizox' has been associated with transient elevated levels of eosinophils, SGOT, SGPT and CPK (creatine phosphokinase). The CPK elevation may be related to I.M. administration.

ADVERSE REACTIONS
Ceftizoxime is generally well tolerated. The *most* frequent adverse reactions (*greater than* 1% but less than 5%) are:
Hypersensitivity—Rash, pruritus, fever.
Hepatic—Transient elevation in SGOT, SGPT and alkaline phosphatase.
Hematologic—Transient eosinophilia, thrombocytosis. Some individuals have developed a positive Coombs test.
Local—Injection site—Burning, cellulitis, phlebitis with I.V. administration, pain, induration, tenderness, paresthesia.
The *less* frequent adverse reactions (*less than* 1%) are:
Hypersensitivity—Numbness has been reported rarely.
Hepatic—Elevation of bilirubin has been reported rarely.
Renal—Transient elevations of BUN and creatinine have been occasionally observed with ceftizoxime.
Hematologic—Anemia, leukopenia, neutropenia and thrombocytopenia have been reported rarely.
Genitourinary—Vaginitis has rarely occurred.
Gastrointestinal—Diarrhea; nausea and vomiting have been reported occasionally.
Symptoms of pseudomembranous colitis can appear during or after antibiotic treatment. (See Warnings section.)

DOSAGE AND ADMINISTRATION
The usual adult dosage is 1 or 2 grams of Cefizox (sterile ceftizoxime sodium, FSK) every 8 to 12 hours. Proper dosage and route of administration should be determined by the condition of the patient, severity of the infection and susceptibility of the causative organisms.
[See table on top next page].

Because of the serious nature of urinary tract infections due to *Ps. aeruginosa* and because many strains of *Pseudomonas* species are only moderately susceptible to 'Cefizox', higher dosage is recommended. Other therapy should be instituted if the response is not prompt.

A single, 1 gram I.M. dose is the usual dose for treatment of uncomplicated gonorrhea.

The intravenous route may be preferable for patients with bacterial septicemia, localized parenchymal abscesses (such as intra-abdominal abscess), peritonitis, or other severe or life-threatening infections.

In those with normal renal function, the intravenous dosage for such infections is 2 to 12 grams of Cefizox (sterile ceftizoxime sodium, FSK) daily. In conditions such as bacterial septicemia, 6 to 12 grams/day may be given initially by the intravenous route for several days, and the dosage may then be gradually reduced according to clinical response and laboratory findings.

Pediatric Dosage Schedule

	Unit Dose	Frequency
Children 6 months and older	50 mg./kg.	q6-8h

Dosage may be increased to a total daily dose of 200 mg./kg. (not to exceed the maximum adult dose for serious infection).

Impaired Renal Function

Modification of 'Cefizox' dosage is necessary in patients with impaired renal function. Following an initial loading dose of 500 mg.–1.0 gram I.M. or I.V., the maintenance dosing schedule shown below should be followed. Further dosing should be determined by therapeutic monitoring, severity of the infection and susceptibility of the causative organisms.

When only the serum creatinine level is available, creatinine clearance may be calculated from the following formula. The serum creatinine level should represent current renal function at the steady state.

$$\text{Males}\quad Clcr = \frac{\text{Weight (kg.)} \times (140-\text{age})}{72 \times \text{serum creatinine (mg./100 ml.)}}$$

Females 0.85 of the above values

In patients undergoing hemodialysis no additional supplemental dosing is required following hemodialysis; however, dosing should be timed so that the patient receives the dose (according to the table below) at the end of the dialysis.

Dosage in Adults with Reduced Renal Function

Creatinine Clearance ml./min.	Renal Function	Less Severe Infections	Life-Threatening Infections
79–50	Mild impairment	500 mg. q8h	0.75 gram–1.5 grams q8h
49–5	Moderate to severe impairment	250 mg.–500 mg. q12h	0.5 gram–1.0 gram q12h
4–0	Dialysis patients	500 mg. q48h or 250 mg. q24h	0.5 gram–1.0 gram q48h or 0.5 gram q24h

Preparation of Parenteral Solution

RECONSTITUTION

I.M. Administration: Reconstitute with Sterile Water for Injection. SHAKE WELL.

Vial Size	Diluent to Be Added	Approx. Avail. Vol.	Approx. Avg. Concentration
1 gram	3.0 ml.	3.7 ml.	270 mg./ml.
2 grams*	6.0 ml.	7.4 ml.	270 mg./ml.

*When administering 2 gram I.M. doses, the dose should be divided and given in different large muscle masses.

I.V. Administration: Reconstitute with Sterile Water for Injection. SHAKE WELL.

Vial Size	Diluent to Be Added	Approx. Avail. Vol.	Approx. Avg. Concentration
1 gram	10 ml.	10.7 ml.	95 mg./ml.
2 grams	20 ml.	21.4 ml.	95 mg./ml.

These solutions of Cefizox (sterile ceftizoxime sodium, FSK) are stable 24 hours at room temperature or 96 hours if refrigerated (5°C.).

Parenteral drug products should be inspected visually for particulate matter prior to administration. If particulate matter is evident in reconstituted fluids, then the drug solution should be discarded. Reconstituted solutions may range from yellow to amber without changes in potency.

"Piggyback" Vials: Reconstitute with 50 to 100 ml. of Sodium Chloride Injection or any other I.V. solution listed below. SHAKE WELL.

Administer with primary I.V. fluids, as a single dose. These solutions of 'Cefizox' are stable 24 hours at room temperature or 96 hours if refrigerated (5°C.).

A solution of 1 gram 'Cefizox' in 13 ml. Sterile Water for Injection is isotonic.

I.M. Injection: Inject well within the body of a relatively large muscle. Aspiration is necessary to avoid inadvertent injection into a blood vessel. When administering 2 gram I.M. doses, the dose should be divided and given in different large muscle masses.

I.V. Administration: Direct (bolus) injection, slowly over 3 to 5 minutes, directly or through tubing for patients receiving parenteral fluids (see list below). Intermittent or continuous infusion, dilute reconstituted 'Cefizox' in 50 to 100 ml. of one of the following solutions:

Sodium Chloride Injection
5% or 10% Dextrose Injection
5% Dextrose and 0.9%, 0.45%, or 0.2% Sodium Chloride Injection
Ringer's Injection
Lactated Ringer's Injection
Invert Sugar 10% in Sterile Water for Injection
5% Sodium Bicarbonate in Sterile Water for Injection
5% Dextrose in Lactated Ringer's Injection (only when reconstituted with 4% Sodium Bicarbonate Injection)

In these fluids 'Cefizox' is stable 24 hours at room temperature or 96 hours if refrigerated (5°C.).

General Guidelines for Dosage of 'Cefizox'

Type of Infection	Daily Dose (Grams)	Frequency and Route
Uncomplicated Urinary Tract	1	500 mg. q12h I.M. or I.V.
Other Sites	2–3	1 gram q8–12h I.M. or I.V.
Severe or Refractory	3–6	1 gram q8h I.M. or I.V. 2 grams q8–12h I.M.* or I.V.
Life-Threatening†	9–12	3–4 grams q8h I.V.

*When administering 2 gram I.M. doses, the dose should be divided and given in different large muscle masses.
† In life-threatening infections dosages up to 2 grams every 4 hours have been given.

DIRECTIONS FOR USE OF CEFIZOX (CEFTIZOXIME SODIUM INJECTION, FSK) PLASTIC CONTAINERS

'Cefizox' supplied as a frozen, sterile, nonpyrogenic solution in plastic containers is to be administered either as a continuous or intermittent infusion.

Thaw container at room temperature. After thawing, check for minute leaks by squeezing bag firmly. If leaks are found, discard solution as sterility may be impaired. Additives should not be introduced into this solution. Do not use if the solution is cloudy or precipitated or if the seal is not intact. After thawing, the solution is stable for 24 hours at room temperature or 10 days if stored under refrigeration (5°C.). DO NOT REFREEZE.

Use sterile equipment. It is recommended that the intravenous administration apparatus be replaced at least once every 48 hours.

CAUTION: Do not use plastic containers in series connections. Such use could result in air embolism due to residual air being drawn from the primary container before administration of the fluid from the secondary container is complete.

Preparation for administration:

1. Suspend container from eyelet support.
2. Remove plastic protector from outlet port at bottom of container.
3. Attach administration set. Refer to complete directions accompanying set.

HOW SUPPLIED

Cefizox (sterile ceftizoxime sodium, FSK)—supplied in vials equivalent to 1 gram or 2 grams of ceftizoxime; in "Piggyback" Vials for I.V. admixture equivalent to 1 gram or 2 grams of ceftizoxime.

Note: Unreconstituted Cefizox (sterile ceftizoxime sodium, FSK) should be protected from excessive light, and stored at controlled room temperature (59°–86°F.) in the original package until used.

Cefizox (ceftizoxime sodium injection, FSK) as a frozen, sterile, nonpyrogenic solution in plastic containers—supplied in 50 ml. single-dose containers equivalent to 1 gram or 2 grams of ceftizoxime in 5% Dextrose (D5W). Do not store above −20°C.

'Cefizox' supplied as a frozen, sterile, nonpyrogenic solution in plastic containers is manufactured for Fujisawa SmithKline Corporation by Travenol Laboratories, Inc., Deerfield, IL 60015.

* Am. J. Clin. Pathol. 45:493, 1966; Federal Register 39:19182–19184, 1974.

CF:L14

Shown in Product Identification Section, page 430

COMPAZINE® ℞

[komp 'ah-zeen]
(brand of prochlorperazine)

PRODUCT OVERVIEW

KEY FACTS

'Compazine' is a phenothiazine derivative of the piperazine group, available in 13 dosage forms and strengths for oral, rectal or parenteral administration. The Spansule® sustained release capsule dosage form provides an equivalent milligram dose of tablets given in divided doses.

MAJOR USES

'Compazine' is indicated for control of severe nausea and vomiting. 'Compazine' is also indicated in the management of the manifestations of psychotic disorders, as well as the short-term treatment of generalized non-psychotic anxiety, where it is considered second-line therapy.

SAFETY INFORMATION

'Compazine' is contraindicated in comatose states, pediatric surgery, children under 2 years of age or under 20 pounds, and in the presence of large amounts of CNS depressants. 'Compazine'-induced EPS may be confused with the CNS signs of Reye's syndrome or other encephalopathy. Avoid using in children and adolescents whose signs and symptoms suggest Reye's syndrome. Use 'Compazine' in children with acute illnesses or dehydration only under close supervision, since they appear much more susceptible to EPS, particularly dystonias, than adults. Pregnant patients, patients with bone marrow depression or with previous hypersensitivity reactions to a phenothiazine should not receive 'Compazine' unless the potential benefits outweigh possible hazards.

PRESCRIBING INFORMATION

COMPAZINE® ℞

[komp 'ah-zeen]
(brand of prochlorperazine)

DESCRIPTION

Tablets—Each round, yellow-green, coated tablet contains prochlorperazine maleate equivalent to prochlorperazine as follows: 5 mg. imprinted SKF and C66; 10 mg. imprinted SKF and C67; 25 mg. imprinted SKF and C69. Inactive ingredients consist of acacia, calcium sulfate, D&C Green No. 5, D&C Yellow No. 10, FD&C Blue No. 1, FD&C Yellow No. 6, gelatin, mineral oil, starch, stearic acid, sucrose, talc and trace amounts of other inactive ingredients.

Spansule® sustained release capsules—Each 'Compazine' *Spansule* capsule is so prepared that an initial dose is released promptly and the remaining medication is released gradually over a prolonged period.

Each capsule, with black cap and natural body, contains prochlorperazine maleate equivalent to prochlorperazine as follows: 10 mg. imprinted SKF and C44; 15 mg. imprinted SKF and C46; 30 mg. imprinted SKF and C47. Inactive ingredients consist of benzyl alcohol, cetylpyridinium chloride, D&C Green No. 5, D&C Yellow No. 10, FD&C Blue No. 1, FD&C Red No. 40, FD&C Yellow No. 6, gelatin, glyceryl monostearate, sodium lauryl sulfate, starch, sucrose, wax and trace amounts of other inactive ingredients.

Ampuls, 2 ml. (5 mg./ml.)—Each ml. contains, in aqueous solution, 5 mg. prochlorperazine as the edisylate, 1 mg. sodium sulfite, 1 mg. sodium bisulfite, 8 mg. sodium phosphate and 12 mg. sodium biphosphate.

Multiple-dose Vials, 10 ml. (5 mg./ml.)—Each ml. contains, in aqueous solution, 5 mg. prochlorperazine as the edisylate, 5 mg. sodium biphosphate, 12 mg. sodium tartrate, 0.9 mg. sodium saccharin, and 0.75% benzyl alcohol as preservative.

Disposable Syringes, 2 ml. (5 mg./ml.)—Each ml. contains, in aqueous solution, 5 mg. prochlorperazine as the edisylate, 5 mg. sodium biphosphate, 12 mg. sodium tartrate, 0.9 mg. sodium saccharin, and 0.75% benzyl alcohol as preservative.

Suppositories—Each suppository contains $2\frac{1}{2}$ mg., 5 mg., or 25 mg. of prochlorperazine; with glycerin, glyceryl monopalmitate, glyceryl monostearate, hydrogenated cocoanut oil fatty acids and hydrogenated palm kernel oil fatty acids.

Syrup—Each 5 ml. (one teaspoonful) of clear, yellow-orange, fruit-flavored liquid contains 5 mg. of prochlorperazine as the edisylate. Inactive ingredients consist of FD&C Yellow No. 6, flavors, polyoxyethylene polyoxypropylene glycol, sodium benzoate, sodium citrate, sucrose and water.

INDICATIONS

For control of severe nausea and vomiting.
For management of the manifestations of psychotic disorders.

Continued on next page

Smith Kline & French—Cont.

Compazine (prochlorperazine, SK&F) is effective for the short-term treatment of generalized non-psychotic anxiety. However, 'Compazine' is not the first drug to be used in therapy for most patients with non-psychotic anxiety, because certain risks associated with its use are not shared by common alternative treatments (e.g., benzodiazepines).

When used in the treatment of non-psychotic anxiety, 'Compazine' should not be administered at doses of more than 20 mg. per day or for longer than 12 weeks, because the use of 'Compazine' at higher doses or for longer intervals may cause persistent tardive dyskinesia that may prove irreversible. (See Warnings section.)

The effectiveness of 'Compazine' as treatment for non-psychotic anxiety was established in four-week clinical studies of outpatients with generalized anxiety disorder. This evidence does not predict that 'Compazine' will be useful in patients with other non-psychotic conditions in which anxiety, or signs that mimic anxiety, are found (e.g., physical illness, organic mental conditions, agitated depression, character pathologies, etc.).

'Compazine' has not been shown effective in the management of behavioral complications in patients with mental retardation.

CONTRAINDICATIONS

Do not use in comatose states or in the presence of large amounts of central nervous system depressants (alcohol, barbiturates, narcotics, etc.).

Do not use in pediatric surgery.

Do not use in children under 2 years of age or under 20 lbs.

Do not use in children for conditions for which dosage has not been established.

WARNINGS

The extrapyramidal symptoms which can occur secondary to Compazine (prochlorperazine, SK&F) may be confused with the central nervous system signs of an undiagnosed primary disease responsible for the vomiting, e.g., Reye's syndrome or other encephalopathy. The use of 'Compazine' and other potential hepatotoxins should be avoided in children and adolescents whose signs and symptoms suggest Reye's syndrome.

Tardive Dyskinesia: Tardive dyskinesia, a syndrome consisting of potentially irreversible, involuntary, dyskinetic movements, may develop in patients treated with neuroleptic (antipsychotic) drugs. Although the prevalence of the syndrome appears to be highest among the elderly, especially elderly women, it is impossible to rely upon prevalence estimates to predict, at the inception of neuroleptic treatment, which patients are likely to develop the syndrome. Whether neuroleptic drug products differ in their potential to cause tardive dyskinesia is unknown.

Both the risk of developing the syndrome and the likelihood that it will become irreversible are believed to increase as the duration of treatment and the total cumulative dose of neuroleptic drugs administered to the patient increase. However, the syndrome can develop, although much less commonly, after relatively brief treatment periods at low doses.

There is no known treatment for established cases of tardive dyskinesia, although the syndrome may remit, partially or completely, if neuroleptic treatment is withdrawn. Neuroleptic treatment itself, however, may suppress (or partially suppress) the signs and symptoms of the syndrome and thereby may possibly mask the underlying disease process. The effect that symptomatic suppression has upon the long-term course of the syndrome is unknown.

Given these considerations, neuroleptics should be prescribed in a manner that is most likely to minimize the occurrence of tardive dyskinesia. Chronic neuroleptic treatment should generally be reserved for patients who suffer from a chronic illness that, 1) is known to respond to neuroleptic drugs, and, 2) for whom alternative, equally effective, but potentially less harmful treatments are *not* available or appropriate. In patients who do require chronic treatment, the smallest dose and the shortest duration of treatment producing a satisfactory clinical response should be sought. The need for continued treatment should be reassessed periodically.

If signs and symptoms of tardive dyskinesia appear in a patient on neuroleptics, drug discontinuation should be considered. However, some patients may require treatment despite the presence of the syndrome.

For further information about the description of tardive dyskinesia and its clinical detection, please refer to the sections on Precautions and Adverse Reactions.

Patients with bone marrow depression or who have previously demonstrated a hypersensitivity reaction (e.g., blood dyscrasias, jaundice) with a phenothiazine should not receive any phenothiazine, including 'Compazine', unless in the judgment of the physician the potential benefits of treatment outweigh the possible hazards.

Compazine (prochlorperazine, SK&F) may impair mental and/or physical abilities, especially during the first few days of therapy. Therefore, caution patients about activities requiring alertness (e.g., operating vehicles or machinery).

Phenothiazines may intensify or prolong the action of central nervous system depressants (e.g., alcohol, anesthetics, narcotics).

Usage in Pregnancy: Safety for the use of 'Compazine' during pregnancy has not been established. Therefore, 'Compazine' is not recommended for use in pregnant patients except in cases of severe nausea and vomiting that are so serious and intractable that, in the judgment of the physician, drug intervention is required and potential benefits outweigh possible hazards.

There have been reported instances of prolonged jaundice, extrapyramidal signs, hyperreflexia or hyporeflexia in newborn infants whose mothers received phenothiazines.

Nursing Mothers: There is evidence that phenothiazines are excreted in the breast milk of nursing mothers.

PRECAUTIONS

The antiemetic action of 'Compazine' may mask the signs and symptoms of overdosage of other drugs and may obscure the diagnosis and treatment of other conditions such as intestinal obstruction, brain tumor and Reye's syndrome (See Warnings).

When 'Compazine' is used with cancer chemotherapeutic drugs, vomiting as a sign of the toxicity of these agents may be obscured by the antiemetic effect of 'Compazine'.

Because hypotension may occur, large doses and parenteral administration should be used cautiously in patients with impaired cardiovascular systems. To minimize the occurrence of hypotension after injection, keep patient lying down and observe for at least ½ hour. If hypotension occurs after parenteral or oral dosing, place patient in head-low position with legs raised. If a vasoconstrictor is required, Levophed®* and Neo-Synephrine®† are suitable. Other pressor agents, including epinephrine, should not be used because they may cause a paradoxical further lowering of blood pressure.

Aspiration of vomitus has occurred in a few post-surgical patients who have received 'Compazine' as an antiemetic. Although no causal relationship has been established, this possibility should be borne in mind during surgical aftercare.

Deep sleep, from which patients can be aroused, and coma have been reported, usually with overdosage.

Neuroleptic drugs elevate prolactin levels; the elevation persists during chronic administration. Tissue culture experiments indicate that approximately one-third of human breast cancers are prolactin-dependent *in vitro*, a factor of potential importance if the prescribing of these drugs is contemplated in a patient with a previously detected breast cancer. Although disturbances such as galactorrhea, amenorrhea, gynecomastia and impotence have been reported, the clinical significance of elevated serum prolactin levels is unknown for most patients. An increase in mammary neoplasms has been found in rodents after chronic administration of neuroleptic drugs. Neither clinical nor epidemiologic studies conducted to date, however, have shown an association between chronic administration of these drugs and mammary tumorigenesis; the available evidence is considered too limited to be conclusive at this time.

As with all drugs which exert an anticholinergic effect, and/or cause mydriasis, prochlorperazine should be used with caution in patients with glaucoma.

Because phenothiazines may interfere with thermoregulatory mechanisms, use with caution in persons who will be exposed to extreme heat.

Phenothiazines can diminish the effect of oral anticoagulants.

Phenothiazines can produce alpha-adrenergic blockade.

Thiazide diuretics may accentuate the orthostatic hypotension that may occur with phenothiazines.

Antihypertensive effects of guanethidine and related compounds may be counteracted when phenothiazines are used concomitantly.

Concomitant administration of propranolol with phenothiazines results in increased plasma levels of both drugs.

Phenothiazines may lower the convulsive threshold; dosage adjustments of anticonvulsants may be necessary. Potentiation of anticonvulsant effects does not occur. However, it has been reported that phenothiazines may interfere with the metabolism of Dilantin®‡ and thus precipitate Dilantin‡ toxicity.

The presence of phenothiazines may produce false positive phenylketonuria (PKU) test results.

Long-Term Therapy: Given the likelihood that some patients exposed chronically to neuroleptics will develop tardive dyskinesia, it is advised that all patients in whom chronic use is contemplated be given, if possible, full information about this risk. The decision to inform patients and/or their guardians must obviously take into account the clinical circumstances and the competency of the patient to understand the information provided.

To lessen the likelihood of adverse reactions related to cumulative drug effect, patients with a history of long-term therapy with Compazine (prochlorperazine, SK&F) and/or other neuroleptics should be evaluated periodically to decide whether the maintenance dosage could be lowered or drug therapy discontinued.

Children with acute illnesses (e.g., chickenpox, C.N.S. infections, measles, gastroenteritis) or dehydration seem to be much more susceptible to neuromuscular reactions, particularly dystonias, than are adults. In such patients, the drug should be used only under close supervision.

Drugs which lower the seizure threshold, including phenothiazine derivatives, should not be used with Amipaque®§. As with other phenothiazine derivatives, Compazine (prochlorperazine, SK&F) should be discontinued at least 48 hours before myelography, should not be resumed for at least 24 hours postprocedure, and should not be used for the control of nausea and vomiting occurring either prior to myelography with Amipaque§, or postprocedure.

ADVERSE REACTIONS

Drowsiness, dizziness, amenorrhea, blurred vision, skin reactions and hypotension may occur.

Cholestatic jaundice has occurred. If fever with grippe-like symptoms occurs, appropriate liver studies should be conducted. If tests indicate an abnormality, stop treatment. There have been a few observations of fatty changes in the livers of patients who have died while receiving the drug. No causal relationship has been established.

Leukopenia and agranulocytosis have occurred. Warn patients to report the sudden appearance of sore throat or other signs of infection. If white blood cell and differential counts indicate leukocyte depression, stop treatment and start antibiotic and other suitable therapy.

Neuromuscular (Extrapyramidal) Reactions

These symptoms are seen in a significant number of hospitalized mental patients. They may be characterized by motor restlessness, be of the dystonic type, or they may resemble parkinsonism.

Depending on the severity of symptoms, dosage should be reduced or discontinued. If therapy is reinstituted, it should be at a lower dosage. Should these symptoms occur in children or pregnant patients, the drug should be stopped and not reinstituted. In most cases barbiturates by suitable route of administration will suffice. (Or, injectable Benadryl®‖ may be useful.) In more severe cases, the administration of an anti-parkinsonism agent, except levodopa, usually produces rapid reversal of symptoms. Suitable supportive measures such as maintaining a clear airway and adequate hydration should be employed.

Motor Restlessness: Symptoms may include agitation or jitteriness and sometimes insomnia. These symptoms often disappear spontaneously. At times these symptoms may be similar to the original neurotic or psychotic symptoms. Dosage should not be increased until these side effects have subsided.

If this phase becomes too troublesome, the symptoms can usually be controlled by a reduction of dosage or concomitant administration of a barbiturate.

Dystonias: Symptoms may include: spasm of the neck muscles, sometimes progressing to torticollis; extensor rigidity of back muscles, sometimes progressing to opisthotonos; carpopedal spasm, trismus, swallowing difficulty, oculogyric crisis and protrusion of the tongue.

These usually subside within a few hours, and almost always within 24 to 48 hours, after the drug has been discontinued.

In mild cases, reassurance or a barbiturate is often sufficient. *In moderate cases,* barbiturates will usually bring rapid relief. *In more severe adult cases,* the administration of an anti-parkinsonism agent, except levodopa, usually produces rapid reversal of symptoms. *In children,* reassurance and barbiturates will usually control symptoms. (Or, injectable Benadryl‖ may be useful. Note: See Benadryl‖ prescribing information for appropriate *children's* dosage.) If appropriate treatment with anti-parkinsonism agents or Benadryl‖ fails to reverse the signs and symptoms, the diagnosis should be reevaluated.

Pseudo-parkinsonism: Symptoms may include: mask-like facies; drooling; tremors; pillrolling motion; cogwheel rigidity; and shuffling gait. Reassurance and sedation are important. In most cases these symptoms are readily controlled when an anti-parkinsonism agent is administered concomitantly. Anti-parkinsonism agents should be used only when required. Generally, therapy of a few weeks to two or three months will suffice. After this time patients should be evaluated to determine their need for continued treatment. (Note: Levodopa has not been found effective in pseudo-parkinsonism.) Occasionally it is necessary to lower the dosage of Compazine (prochlorperazine, SK&F) or to discontinue the drug.

Tardive Dyskinesia: As with all antipsychotic agents, tardive dyskinesia may appear in some patients on long-term therapy or may appear after drug therapy has been discontinued. The syndrome can also develop, although much less frequently, after relatively brief treatment periods at low doses. This syndrome appears in all age groups. Although its prevalence appears to be highest among elderly patients, especially elderly women, it is impossible to rely upon prevalence estimates to predict at the inception of neuroleptic treatment which patients are likely to develop the syndrome. The symptoms are persistent and in some patients appear to be irreversible. The syndrome is characterized by rhythmical involuntary movements of the tongue, face, mouth or jaw (e.g., protrusion of tongue, puffing of cheeks, puckering of mouth, chewing movements). Sometimes these may be accompanied by involuntary movements of extremities. In rare instances, these involuntary movements of the extremities are the only manifestations of tardive dyskinesia. A variant of tardive dyskinesia, tardive dystonia, has also been described.

There is no known effective treatment for tardive dyskinesia; anti-parkinsonism agents do not alleviate the symptoms of this syndrome. It is suggested that all antipsychotic agents be discontinued if these symptoms appear. Should it be necessary to reinstitute treatment, or increase the dosage of the agent, or switch to a different antipsychotic agent, the syndrome may be masked.

It has been reported that fine vermicular movements of the tongue may be an early sign of the syndrome and if the medication is stopped at that time the syndrome may not develop.

Contact Dermatitis: Avoid getting the Injection solution on hands or clothing because of the possibility of contact dermatitis.

Adverse Reactions Reported with Compazine (prochlorperazine, SK&F) or Other Phenothiazine Derivatives: Adverse reactions with different phenothiazines vary in type, frequency, and mechanism of occurrence, i.e., some are dose-related, while others involve individual patient sensitivity. Some adverse reactions may be more likely to occur, or occur with greater intensity, in patients with special medical problems, e.g., patients with mitral insufficiency or pheochromocytoma have experienced severe hypotension following recommended doses of certain phenothiazines.

Not all of the following adverse reactions have been observed with every phenothiazine derivative, but they have been reported with one or more and should be borne in mind when drugs of this class are administered: extrapyramidal symptoms (opisthotonos, oculogyric crisis, hyperreflexia, dystonia, akathisia, dyskinesia, parkinsonism) some of which have lasted months and even years—particularly in elderly patients with previous brain damage; grand mal and petit mal convulsions, particularly in patients with EEG abnormalities or history of such disorders; altered cerebrospinal fluid proteins; cerebral edema; intensification and prolongation of the action of central nervous system depressants (opiates, analgesics, antihistamines, barbiturates, alcohol), atropine, heat, organophosphorus insecticides; autonomic reactions (dryness of mouth, nasal congestion, headache, nausea, constipation, obstipation, adynamic ileus, ejaculatory disorders /impotence, priapism, atonic colon, urinary retention, miosis and mydriasis); reactivation of psychotic processes, catatonic-like states; hypotension (sometimes fatal); cardiac arrest; blood dyscrasias (pancytopenia, thrombocytopenic purpura, leukopenia, agranulocytosis, eosinophilia, hemolytic anemia, aplastic anemia); liver damage (jaundice, biliary stasis); endocrine disturbances (hyperglycemia, hypoglycemia, glycosuria, lactation, galactorrhea, gynecomastia, menstrual irregularities, false positive pregnancy tests); skin disorders (photosensitivity, itching, erythema, urticaria, eczema up to exfoliative dermatitis); other allergic reactions (asthma, laryngeal edema, angioneurotic edema, anaphylactoid reactions); peripheral edema; reversed epinephrine effect; hyperpyrexia; mild fever after large I.M. doses; increased appetite; increased weight; a systemic lupus erythematosus-like syndrome; pigmentary retinopathy; with prolonged administration of substantial doses, skin pigmentation, epithelial keratopathy, and lenticular and corneal deposits.

EKG changes—particularly nonspecific, usually reversible Q and T wave distortions—have been observed in some patients receiving phenothiazine tranquilizers.

Although phenothiazines cause neither psychic nor physical dependence, sudden discontinuance in long-term psychiatric patients may cause temporary symptoms, e.g., nausea and vomiting, dizziness, tremulousness.

Rare occurrences of neuroleptic malignant syndrome have been reported in patients receiving neuroleptic drugs. This syndrome is comprised of the symptom complex of hyperthermia, altered consciousness, muscular rigidity and autonomic dysfunction and is potentially fatal.

Note: There have been occasional reports of sudden death in patients receiving phenothiazines. In some cases, the cause appeared to be cardiac arrest or asphyxia due to failure of the cough reflex.

DOSAGE AND ADMINISTRATION

Notes on Injection: *Stability*—This solution should be protected from light. Slight yellowish discoloration will not alter potency. If markedly discolored, solution should be discarded.

Compatibility—It is recommended that Compazine (prochlorperazine, SK&F) Injection not be mixed with other agents in the syringe. Do not dilute the contents of 'Compazine' ampuls with any diluent that contains parabens as a preservative.

DOSAGE AND ADMINISTRATION—ADULTS

(For children's dosage and administration, see below.) Dosage should be increased more gradually in debilitated or emaciated patients.

Elderly Patients: In general, dosages in the lower range are sufficient for most elderly patients. Since they appear to be more susceptible to hypotension and neuromuscular reactions, such patients should be observed closely. Dosage should be tailored to the individual, response carefully monitored, and dosage adjusted accordingly. Dosage should be increased more gradually in elderly patients.

1. To Control Severe Nausea and Vomiting: Adjust dosage to the response of the individual. Begin with the lowest recommended dosage.

Oral Dosage: Usually 5 or 10 mg. 3 or 4 times daily; by 'Spansule' capsule, usually one 15 mg. capsule on arising or one 10 mg. capsule q12h.

Rectal Dosage: 25 mg. twice daily.

I.M. Dosage: Initially 5 to 10 mg. (1–2 ml.) injected *deeply* into the upper outer quadrant of the buttock. If necessary, repeat every 3 or 4 hours. Total I.M. dosage should not exceed 40 mg. per day.

Subcutaneous administration is not advisable because of local irritation.

2. Adult Surgery (for severe nausea and vomiting): Total parenteral dosage should not exceed 40 mg. per day. Hypotension is a possibility if the drug is given by I.V. injection or infusion.

I.M. Dosage: 5 to 10 mg. (1–2 ml.) 1 to 2 hours before induction of anesthesia (repeat once in 30 minutes, if necessary), or to control acute symptoms during and after surgery (repeat once if necessary).

I.V. Injection: 5 to 10 mg. (1–2 ml.) 15 to 30 minutes before induction of anesthesia, or to control acute symptoms during or after surgery. Repeat once if necessary. Compazine (prochlorperazine, SK&F) may be administered either undiluted or diluted in isotonic solution, but a single dose of the drug should not exceed 10 mg. The rate of administration should not exceed 5 mg./ml./min. When administered I.V., do not use bolus injection.

I.V. Infusion: 20 mg. (4 ml.) per liter of isotonic solution. Do not dilute in less than one liter of isotonic solution. Add to I.V. infusion 15 to 30 minutes before induction.

3. In Adult Psychiatric Disorders: Adjust dosage to the response of the individual and according to the severity of the condition. Begin with the lowest recommended dose. Although response ordinarily is seen within a day or two, longer treatment is usually required before maximal improvement is seen.

Oral Dosage: *Non-Psychotic Anxiety*—Usual dosage is 5 mg. 3 or 4 times daily; by 'Spansule' capsule, usually one 15 mg. capsule on arising or one 10 mg. capsule q12h. Do not administer in doses of more than 20 mg. per day or for longer than 12 weeks.

Psychotic Disorders —In relatively mild conditions, as seen in private psychiatric practice or in outpatient clinics, dosage is 5 or 10 mg. 3 or 4 times daily.

In moderate to severe conditions, for hospitalized or adequately supervised patients, usual starting dosage is 10 mg. 3 or 4 times daily. Increase dosage gradually until symptoms are controlled or side effects become bothersome. When dosage is increased by small increments every 2 or 3 days, side effects either do not occur or are easily controlled. Some patients respond satisfactorily on 50 to 75 mg. daily.

In more severe disturbances, optimum dosage is usually 100 to 150 mg. daily.

I.M. Dosage: For immediate control of severely disturbed adults, inject an initial dose of 10 to 20 mg. (2–4 ml.) *deeply* into the upper outer quadrant of the buttock. Many patients respond shortly after the first injection. If necessary, however, repeat the initial dose every 2 to 4 hours (or, in resistant cases, every hour) to gain control of the patient. More than 3 or 4 doses are seldom necessary. After control is achieved, switch patient to an oral form of the drug at the same dosage level or higher. If, in rare cases, parenteral therapy is needed for a prolonged period, give 10 to 20 mg. (2–4 ml.) every 4 to 6 hours. Pain and irritation at the site of injection have seldom occurred.

Subcutaneous administration is not advisable because of local irritation.

DOSAGE AND ADMINISTRATION—CHILDREN

Do not use in pediatric surgery.

Children seem more prone to develop extrapyramidal reactions, even on moderate doses. Therefore, use lowest effective dosage. Tell parents not to exceed prescribed dosage, since the possibility of adverse reactions increases as dosage rises. Occasionally the patient may react to the drug with signs of restlessness and excitement; if this occurs, do not administer additional doses. Take particular precaution in administering the drug to children with acute illnesses or dehydration (see under Dystonias).

When writing a prescription for the 2½ mg. size suppository, write "2½," not "2.5"; this will help avoid confusion with the 25 mg. adult size.

1. Severe Nausea and Vomiting in Children: Compazine (prochlorperazine, SK&F) should not be used in children under 20 pounds in weight or two years of age. It should not be used in conditions for which children's dosages have not been established. Dosage and frequency of administration should be adjusted according to the severity of the symptoms and the response of the patient. The duration of activity following intramuscular administration may last up to 12 hours. Subsequent doses may be given by the same route if necessary.

Oral or Rectal Dosage: More than one day's therapy is seldom necessary.

Weight	Usual Dosage	Not to Exceed
under 20 lbs.	not recommended	
20-29 lbs.	2½ mg. 1 or 2 times a day	7.5 mg. per day
30-39 lbs.	2½ mg. 2 or 3 times a day	10 mg. per day
40-85 lbs.	2½ mg. 3 times a day or 5 mg. 2 times a day	15 mg. per day

I.M. Dosage: Calculate each dose on the basis of 0.06 mg. of the drug per lb. of body weight; give by deep I.M. injection. Control is usually obtained with one dose.

2. In Psychotic Children:

Oral or Rectal Dosage: For children 2 to 12 years, starting dosage is 2½ mg. 2 or 3 times daily. Do not give more than 10 mg. the first day. Then increase dosage according to patient's response.

FOR AGES 2–5, total daily dosage usually does not exceed 20 mg.

FOR AGES 6–12, total daily dosage usually does not exceed 25 mg.

I.M. Dosage: For ages under 12, calculate each dose on the basis of 0.06 mg. of Compazine (prochlorperazine, SK&F) per lb. of body weight; give by deep I.M. injection. Control is usually obtained with one dose. After control is achieved, switch the patient to an oral form of the drug at the same dosage level or higher.

OVERDOSAGE

(See also Adverse Reactions.)

Symptoms—Primarily involvement of the extrapyramidal mechanism producing some of the dystonic reactions described above.

Symptoms of central nervous system depression to the point of somnolence or coma. Agitation and restlessness may also occur. Other possible manifestations include convulsions, EKG changes and cardiac arrhythmias, fever, and autonomic reactions such as hypotension, dry mouth and ileus.

TREATMENT—It is important to determine other medications taken by the patient since multiple dose therapy is common in overdosage situations. Treatment is essentially symptomatic and supportive. Early gastric lavage is helpful. Keep patient under observation and maintain an open airway, since involvement of the extrapyramidal mechanism may produce dysphagia and respiratory difficulty in severe overdosage. **Do not attempt to induce emesis because a dystonic reaction of the head or neck may develop that could result in aspiration of vomitus.** Extrapyramidal symptoms may be treated with anti-parkinsonism drugs, barbiturates, or Benadryl[ll]. See prescribing information for these products. Care should be taken to avoid increasing respiratory depression.

If administration of a stimulant is desirable, amphetamine, dextroamphetamine, or caffeine with sodium benzoate is recommended. Stimulants that may cause convulsions (e.g., picrotoxin or pentylenetetrazol) should be avoided.

If hypotension occurs, the standard measures for managing circulatory shock should be initiated. If it is desirable to administer a vasoconstrictor, Levophed* and Neo-Synephrine† are most suitable. Other pressor agents, including epinephrine, are not recommended because phenothiazine derivatives may reverse the usual elevating action of these agents and cause a further lowering of blood pressure.

Limited experience indicates that phenothiazines are *not* dialyzable.

Special note on 'Spansule' capsules—Since much of the 'Spansule' capsule medication is coated for gradual release, therapy directed at reversing the effects of the ingested drug and at supporting the patient should be continued for as long as overdosage symptoms remain. Saline cathartics are useful for hastening evacuation of pellets that have not already released medication.

HOW SUPPLIED

Tablets—5 and 10 mg., in bottles of 100 and 1000; in Single Unit Packages of 100 (intended for institutional use only).

Continued on next page

Smith Kline & French—Cont.

For use in severe neuropsychiatric conditions, 25 mg., in bottles of 100 and 1000.
'Spansule' capsules—10, 15 and 30 mg., in bottles of 50 and 500; in Single Unit Packages of 100 (intended for institutional use only).
Ampuls—2 ml. (5 mg./ml.), in boxes of 10 and 100.
Multiple-dose Vials—10 ml. (5 mg./ml.), in boxes of 1, 20 and 100.
Disposable Syringes—2 ml. (5 mg./ml.), in individual cartons.
Suppositories—2½ mg. (for young children), 5 mg. (for older children) and 25 mg. (for adults), in boxes of 12.
Syrup—5 mg./5 ml. (1 teaspoonful) in 4 fl. oz. bottles.
Veterans Administration—Injection, 10 ml., 100's, 6505-00-684-9630A; 'Spansule' Capsules, 15 mg., 500's, 6505-00-014-1188.
Military—Injection, 2 ml., 100's, 6505-00-656-1610; Suppositories, 2½ mg., 12's, 6505-00-133-5213; 25 mg., 12's, 6505-00-133-5214; Tablets, 5 mg., S.U.P. 100's 6505-00-118-2563.

---

* Norepinephrine bitartrate, Winthrop-Breon Laboratories.
† Phenylephrine hydrochloride, Winthrop-Breon Laboratories.
‡ Phenytoin, Parke-Davis.
§ Metrizamide, Winthrop-Breon Laboratories.
ǁ Diphenhydramine hydrochloride, Parke-Davis.

CZ:L69

Shown in Product Identification Section, page 430

CYTOMEL® ℞
[sigh "toe 'mel]
brand of liothyronine sodium
Tablets

DESCRIPTION

Thyroid hormone drugs are natural or synthetic preparations containing tetraiodothyronine (T_4, levothyroxine) sodium or triiodothyronine (T_3, liothyronine) sodium or both. T_4 and T_3 are produced in the human thyroid gland by the iodination and coupling of the amino acid tyrosine. T_4 contains four iodine atoms and is formed by the coupling of two molecules of diiodotyrosine (DIT). T_3 contains three atoms of iodine and is formed by the coupling of one molecule of DIT with one molecule of monoiodotyrosine (MIT). Both hormones are stored in the thyroid colloid as thyroglobulin.
Thyroid hormone preparations belong to two categories: (1) natural hormonal preparations derived from animal thyroid, and (2) synthetic preparations. Natural preparations include desiccated thyroid and thyroglobulin. Desiccated thyroid is derived from domesticated animals that are used for food by man (either beef or hog thyroid), and thyroglobulin is derived from thyroid glands of the hog. The United States Pharmacopeia (USP) has standardized the total iodine content of natural preparations. Thyroid USP contains not less than (NLT) 0.17 percent and not more than (NMT) 0.23 percent iodine, and thyroglobulin contains not less than (NLT) 0.7 percent of organically bound iodine. Iodine content is only an indirect indicator of true hormonal biologic activity.
Cytomel (liothyronine sodium, SK&F) Tablets contain liothyronine (L-triiodothyronine or LT_3), a synthetic form of a natural thyroid hormone, and is available as the sodium salt.
Twenty-five mcg. of liothyronine is equivalent to approximately 1 grain of desiccated thyroid or thyroglobulin and 0.1 mg. of L-thyroxine.
Each round, white Cytomel (liothyronine sodium, SK&F) tablet contains liothyronine sodium equivalent to liothyronine as follows: 5 mcg. debossed SKF and D14; 25 mcg. scored and debossed SKF and D16; 50 mcg. scored and debossed SKF and D17. Inactive ingredients consist of calcium sulfate, gelatin, starch, stearic acid, sucrose and talc.

CLINICAL PHARMACOLOGY

The mechanisms by which thyroid hormones exert their physiologic action are not well understood. These hormones enhance oxygen consumption by most tissues of the body, increase the basal metabolic rate and the metabolism of carbohydrates, lipids and proteins. Thus, they exert a profound influence on every organ system in the body and are of particular importance in the development of the central nervous system.

Pharmacokinetics
Since liothyronine sodium (T_3) is not firmly bound to serum protein, it is readily available to body tissues. The onset of activity of liothyronine sodium is rapid, occurring within a few hours. Maximum pharmacologic response occurs within two or three days, providing early clinical response. The biological half-life is about 2-½ days.
T_3 is almost totally absorbed, 95 percent in four hours. The hormones contained in the natural preparations are absorbed in a manner similar to the synthetic hormones.
Liothyronine sodium has a rapid cutoff of activity which permits quick dosage adjustment and facilitates control of the effects of overdosage, should they occur.
The higher affinity of levothyroxine (T_4) for both thyroid-binding globulin and thyroid-binding prealbumin as compared to triiodothyronine (T_3) partially explains the higher serum levels and longer half-life of the former hormone. Both protein-bound hormones exist in reverse equilibrium with minute amounts of free hormone, the latter accounting for the metabolic activity.

INDICATIONS AND USAGE

Thyroid hormone drugs are indicated:
1. As replacement or supplemental therapy in patients with hypothyroidism of any etiology, except transient hypothyroidism during the recovery phase of subacute thyroiditis. This category includes cretinism, myxedema and ordinary hypothyroidism in patients of any age (children, adults, the elderly), or state (including pregnancy); primary hypothyroidism resulting from functional deficiency, primary atrophy, partial or total absence of thyroid gland, or the effects of surgery, radiation, or drugs, with or without the presence of goiter; and secondary (pituitary) or tertiary (hypothalamic) hypothyroidism (See WARNINGS).
2. As pituitary thyroid-stimulating hormone (TSH) suppressants, in the treatment or prevention of various types of euthyroid goiters, including thyroid nodules, subacute or chronic lymphocytic thyroiditis (Hashimoto's) and multinodular goiter.
3. As diagnostic agents in suppression tests to differentiate suspected mild hyperthyroidism or thyroid gland autonomy.

Cytomel (liothyronine sodium, SK&F) Tablets can be used in patients allergic to desiccated thyroid or thyroid extract derived from pork or beef.

CONTRAINDICATIONS

Thyroid hormone preparations are generally contraindicated in patients with diagnosed but as yet uncorrected adrenal cortical insufficiency, untreated thyrotoxicosis and apparent hypersensitivity to any of their active or extraneous constituents. There is no well-documented evidence from the literature, however, of true allergic or idiosyncratic reactions to thyroid hormone.

WARNINGS

> Drugs with thyroid hormone activity, alone or together with other therapeutic agents, have been used for the treatment of obesity. In euthyroid patients, doses within the range of daily hormonal requirements are ineffective for weight reduction. Larger doses may produce serious or even life-threatening manifestations of toxicity, particularly when given in association with sympathomimetic amines such as those used for their anorectic effects.

The use of thyroid hormones in the therapy of obesity, alone or combined with other drugs, is unjustified and has been shown to be ineffective. Neither is their use justified for the treatment of male or female infertility unless this condition is accompanied by hypothyroidism.
Thyroid hormones should be used with great caution in a number of circumstances where the integrity of the cardiovascular system, particularly the coronary arteries, is suspected. These include patients with angina pectoris or the elderly, in whom there is a greater likelihood of occult cardiac disease. In these patients, liothyronine sodium therapy should be initiated with low doses, with due consideration for its relatively rapid onset of action. Starting dosage of Cytomel (liothyronine sodium, SK&F) Tablets is 5 mcg. daily, and should be increased by no more than 5 mcg. increments at two-week intervals. When, in such patients, a euthyroid state can only be reached at the expense of an aggravation of the cardiovascular disease, thyroid hormone dosage should be reduced.
Morphologic hypogonadism and nephrosis should be ruled out before the drug is administered. If hypopituitarism is present, the adrenal deficiency must be corrected prior to starting the drug.
Myxedematous patients are very sensitive to thyroid; dosage should be started at a very low level and increased gradually.
Severe and prolonged hypothyroidism can lead to a decreased level of adrenocortical activity commensurate with the lowered metabolic state. When thyroid-replacement therapy is administered, the metabolism increases at a greater rate than adrenocortical activity. This can precipitate adrenocortical insufficiency. Therefore, in severe and prolonged hypothyroidism, supplemental adrenocortical steroids may be necessary.
In rare instances the administration of thyroid hormone may precipitate a hyperthyroid state or may aggravate existing hyperthyroidism.

PRECAUTIONS

General—Thyroid hormone therapy in patients with concomitant diabetes mellitus or insipidus or adrenal cortical insufficiency aggravates the intensity of their symptoms. Appropriate adjustments of the various therapeutic measures directed at these concomitant endocrine diseases are required.
The therapy of myxedema coma requires simultaneous administration of glucocorticoids.
Hypothyroidism decreases and hyperthyroidism increases the sensitivity to oral anticoagulants. Prothrombin time should be closely monitored in thyroid-treated patients on oral anticoagulants and dosage of the latter agents adjusted on the basis of frequent prothrombin time determinations.
In infants, excessive doses of thyroid hormone preparations may produce craniosynostosis.

Information for the Patient—Patients on thyroid hormone preparations and parents of children on thyroid therapy should be informed that:
1. Replacement therapy is to be taken essentially for life, with the exception of cases of transient hypothyroidism, usually associated with thyroiditis, and in those patients receiving a therapeutic trial of the drug.
2. They should immediately report during the course of therapy any signs or symptoms of thyroid hormone toxicity, e.g., chest pain, increased pulse rate, palpitations, excessive sweating, heat intolerance, nervousness, or any other unusual event.
3. In case of concomitant diabetes mellitus, the daily dosage of antidiabetic medication may need readjustment as thyroid hormone replacement is achieved. If thyroid medication is stopped, a downward readjustment of the dosage of insulin or oral hypoglycemic agent may be necessary to avoid hypoglycemia. At all times, close monitoring of urinary glucose levels is mandatory in such patients.
4. In case of concomitant oral anticoagulant therapy, the prothrombin time should be measured frequently to determine if the dosage of oral anticoagulants is to be readjusted.
5. Partial loss of hair may be experienced by children in the first few months of thyroid therapy, but this is usually a transient phenomenon and later recovery is usually the rule.

Laboratory Tests—Treatment of patients with thyroid hormones requires the periodic assessment of thyroid status by means of appropriate laboratory tests besides the full clinical evaluation. The TSH suppression test can be used to test the effectiveness of any thyroid preparation, bearing in mind the relative insensitivity of the infant pituitary to the negative feedback effect of thyroid hormones. Serum T_4 levels can be used to test the effectiveness of all thyroid medications except products containing liothyronine sodium. When the total serum T_4 is low but TSH is normal, a test specific to assess unbound (free) T_4 levels is warranted. Specific measurements of T_4 and T_3 by competitive protein binding or radioimmunoassay are not influenced by blood levels of organic or inorganic iodine and have essentially replaced older tests of thyroid hormone measurements, i.e., PBI, BEI and T_4 by column.

Drug Interactions
Oral Anticoagulants—Thyroid hormones appear to increase catabolism of vitamin K-dependent clotting factors. If oral anticoagulants are also being given, compensatory increases in clotting factor synthesis are impaired. Patients stabilized on oral anticoagulants who are found to require thyroid replacement therapy should be watched very closely when thyroid is started. If a patient is truly hypothyroid, it is likely that a reduction in anticoagulant dosage will be required. No special precautions appear to be necessary when oral anticoagulant therapy is begun in a patient already stabilized on maintenance thyroid replacement therapy.
Insulin or Oral Hypoglycemics—Initiating thyroid replacement therapy may cause increases in insulin or oral hypoglycemic requirements. The effects seen are poorly understood and depend upon a variety of factors such as dose and type of thyroid preparations and endocrine status of the patient. Patients receiving insulin or oral hypoglycemics should be closely watched during initiation of thyroid replacement therapy.
Cholestyramine—Cholestyramine binds both T_4 and T_3 in the intestine, thus impairing absorption of these thyroid hormones. *In vitro* studies indicate that the binding is not easily removed. Therefore, four to five hours should elapse between administration of cholestyramine and thyroid hormones.
Estrogen, Oral Contraceptives—Estrogens tend to increase serum thyroxine-binding globulin (TBg). In a patient with a nonfunctioning thyroid gland who is receiving thyroid replacement therapy, free levothyroxine may be decreased when estrogens are started thus increasing thyroid requirements. However, if the patient's thyroid gland has sufficient function, the decreased free thyroxine will result in a compensatory increase in thyroxine output by the thyroid. Therefore, patients without a functioning thyroid gland who are on thyroid replacement therapy may need to increase their thyroid dose if estrogens or estrogen-containing oral contraceptives are given.
Tricyclic Antidepressants—Use of thyroid products with imipramine and other tricyclic antidepressants may in-

crease receptor sensitivity and enhance antidepressant activity; transient cardiac arrhythmias have been observed. Thyroid hormone activity may also be enhanced.

Digitalis—Thyroid preparations may potentiate the toxic effects of digitalis. Thyroid hormonal replacement increases metabolic rate, which requires an increase in digitalis dosage.

Ketamine—When administered to patients on a thyroid preparation, this parenteral anesthetic may cause hypertension and tachycardia. Use with caution and be prepared to treat hypertension, if necessary.

Levarterenol—Thyroxine increases the adrenergic effect of catecholamines such as epinephrine and norepinephrine. Therefore, injection of these agents into patients receiving thyroid preparations increases the risk of precipitating coronary insufficiency, especially in patients with coronary artery disease. Careful observation is required.

Drug/Laboratory Test Interactions—The following drugs or moieties are known to interfere with laboratory tests performed in patients on thyroid hormone therapy: androgens, corticosteroids, estrogens, oral contraceptives containing estrogens, iodine-containing preparations and the numerous preparations containing salicylates.

1. Changes in TBg concentration should be taken into consideration in the interpretation of T_4 and T_3 values. In such cases, the unbound (free) hormone should be measured. Pregnancy, estrogens and estrogen-containing oral contraceptives increase TBg concentrations. TBg may also be increased during infectious hepatitis. Decreases in TBg concentrations are observed in nephrosis, acromegaly and after androgen or corticosteroid therapy. Familial hyper- or hypo-thyroxine-binding-globulinemias have been described. The incidence of TBg deficiency approximates 1 in 9000. The binding of thyroxine by thyroxine-binding prealbumin (TBPA) is inhibited by salicylates.
2. Medicinal or dietary iodine interferes with all *in vivo* tests of radioiodine uptake, producing low uptakes which may not be reflective of a true decrease in hormone synthesis.
3. The persistence of clinical and laboratory evidence of hypothyroidism in spite of adequate dosage replacement indicates either poor patient compliance, poor absorption, excessive fecal loss, or inactivity of the preparation. Intracellular resistance to thyroid hormone is quite rare.

Carcinogenesis, Mutagenesis and Impairment of Fertility—A reportedly apparent association between prolonged thyroid therapy and breast cancer has not been confirmed and patients on thyroid for established indications should not discontinue therapy. No confirmatory long-term studies in animals have been performed to evaluate carcinogenic potential, mutagenicity, or impairment of fertility in either males or females.

Pregnancy—Category A. Thyroid hormones do not readily cross the placental barrier. The clinical experience to date does not indicate any adverse effect on fetuses when thyroid hormones are administered to pregnant women. On the basis of current knowledge, thyroid replacement therapy to hypothyroid women should not be discontinued during pregnancy.

Nursing Mothers—Minimal amounts of thyroid hormones are excreted in human milk. Thyroid is not associated with serious adverse reactions and does not have a known tumorigenic potential. However, caution should be exercised when thyroid is administered to a nursing woman.

Pediatric Use—Pregnant mothers provide little or no thyroid hormone to the fetus. The incidence of congenital hypothyroidism is relatively high (1:4000) and the hypothyroid fetus would not derive any benefit from the small amounts of hormone crossing the placental barrier. Routine determinations of serum T_4 and/or TSH is strongly advised in neonates in view of the deleterious effects of thyroid deficiency on growth and development.

Treatment should be initiated immediately upon diagnosis and maintained for life, unless transient hypothyroidism is suspected, in which case, therapy may be interrupted for two to eight weeks after the age of three years to reassess the condition. Cessation of therapy is justified in patients who have maintained a normal TSH during those two to eight weeks.

ADVERSE REACTIONS

Adverse reactions, other than those indicative of hyperthyroidism because of therapeutic overdosage, either initially or during the maintenance period are rare (See OVERDOSAGE).

In rare instances, allergic skin reactions have been reported with Cytomel (liothyronine sodium, SK&F) Tablets.

OVERDOSAGE

Signs and Symptoms—Headache, irritability, nervousness, sweating, tachycardia, increased bowel motility and menstrual irregularities. Angina pectoris or congestive heart failure may be induced or aggravated. Shock may also develop. Massive overdosage may result in symptoms resembling thyroid storm. Chronic excessive dosage will produce the signs and symptoms of hyperthyroidism.

Treatment of Overdosage—Dosage should be reduced or therapy temporarily discontinued if signs and symptoms of overdosage appear. Treatment may be reinstituted at a lower dosage. In normal individuals, normal hypothalamic-pituitary-thyroid axis function is restored in six to eight weeks after thyroid suppression.

Treatment of acute massive thyroid hormone overdosage is aimed at reducing gastrointestinal absorption of the drugs and counteracting central and peripheral effects, mainly those of increased sympathetic activity. Vomiting may be induced initially if further gastrointestinal absorption can reasonably be prevented and barring contraindications such as coma, convulsions, or loss of the gagging reflex. Treatment is symptomatic and supportive. Oxygen may be administered and ventilation maintained. Cardiac glycosides may be indicated if congestive heart failure develops. Measures to control fever, hypoglycemia, or fluid loss should be instituted if needed. Antiadrenergic agents, particularly propranolol, have been used advantageously in the treatment of increased sympathetic activity. Propranolol may be administered intravenously at a dosage of 1 to 3 mg. over a 10-minute period or orally, 80 to 160 mg./day, especially when no contraindications exist for its use.

DOSAGE AND ADMINISTRATION

The dosage of thyroid hormones is determined by the indication and must in every case be individualized according to patient response and laboratory findings.

Thyroid hormones are given orally. In acute, emergency conditions, injectable levothyroxine sodium may be given intravenously when oral administration is not feasible or desirable, as in the treatment of myxedema coma or during total parenteral nutrition. Injectable liothyronine sodium is also available from Smith Kline &French Laboratories upon request, under investigational status, for the treatment of myxedema coma. Intramuscular administration of these two preparations is not advisable because of reported poor absorption.

With Cytomel (liothyronine sodium, SK&F) Tablets once-a-day dosage is recommended; although liothyronine sodium has a rapid cutoff, its metabolic effects persist for a few days following discontinuance.

Mild Hypothyroidism: Recommended starting dosage is 25 mcg. daily. Daily dosage then may be increased by 12.5 or 25 mcg. every one or two weeks. Usual maintenance dose is 25-75 mcg. daily. Smaller doses may be fully effective in some patients, while dosage of 100 mcg. daily may be required in others.

The rapid onset and dissipation of action of liothyronine sodium (T_3), as compared with levothyroxine sodium (T_4), has led some clinicians to prefer its use in patients who might be more susceptible to the untoward effects of thyroid medication. However, the wide swings in serum T_3 levels that follow its administration and the possibility of more pronounced cardiovascular side effects tend to counterbalance the stated advantages.

Cytomel (liothyronine sodium, SK&F) Tablets may be used in preference to levothyroxine (T_4) during radioisotope scanning procedures, since induction of hypothyroidism in those cases is more abrupt and can be of shorter duration. It may also be preferred when impairment of peripheral conversion of T_4 and T_3 is suspected.

Myxedema: Recommended starting dosage is 5 mcg. daily. This may be increased by 5 to 10 mcg. daily every one or two weeks. When 25 mcg. daily is reached, dosage may often be increased by 12.5 or 25 mcg. every one or two weeks. Usual maintenance dose is 50 to 100 mcg. daily.

Myxedema Coma: Myxedema coma is usually precipitated in the hypothyroid patient of long standing by intercurrent illness or drugs such as sedatives and anesthetics and should be considered a medical emergency. A 'Cytomel' Injection Kit for the emergency treatment of myxedema coma is available from Smith Kline &French Laboratories upon request, under investigational status. Instructions which accompany this kit provide information on administration.

Congenital Hypothyroidism: Recommended starting dosage is 5 mcg. daily, with a 5 mcg. increment every three to four days until the desired response is achieved. Infants a few months old may require only 20 mcg. daily for maintenance. At one year, 50 mcg. daily may be required. Above three years, full adult dosage may be necessary (See PRECAUTIONS, Pediatric Use).

Simple (non-toxic) Goiter: Recommended starting dosage is 5 mcg. daily. This dosage may be increased by 5 to 10 mcg. daily every one or two weeks. When 25 mcg. daily is reached, dosage may be increased every week or two by 12.5 or 25 mcg. Usual maintenance dosage is 75 mcg. daily.

In the elderly or in children, therapy should be started with 5 mcg. daily and increased only by 5 mcg. increments at the recommended intervals.

When switching a patient to Cytomel (liothyronine sodium, SK&F) Tablets from thyroid, L-thyroxine or thyroglobulin, discontinue the other medication, initiate 'Cytomel' at a low dosage, and increase gradually according to the patient's response. When selecting a starting dosage, bear in mind that this drug has a rapid onset of action, and that residual effects of the other thyroid preparation may persist for the first several weeks of therapy.

Thyroid Suppression Therapy: Administration of thyroid hormone in doses higher than those produced physiologically by the gland results in suppression of the production of endogenous hormone. This is the basis for the thyroid suppression test and is used as an aid in the diagnosis of patients with signs of mild hyperthyroidism in whom baseline laboratory tests appear normal or to demonstrate thyroid gland autonomy in patients with Graves' ophthalmopathy. ^{131}I uptake is determined before and after the administration of the exogenous hormone. A 50 percent or greater suppression of uptake indicates a normal thyroid-pituitary axis and thus rules out thyroid gland autonomy.

Cytomel (liothyronine sodium, SK&F) Tablets are given in doses of 75-100 mcg./day for seven days, and radioactive iodine uptake is determined before and after administration of the hormone. If thyroid function is under normal control, the radioiodine uptake will drop significantly after treatment. Cytomel (liothyronine sodium, SK&F) Tablets should be administered cautiously to patients in whom there is a strong suspicion of thyroid gland autonomy, in view of the fact that the exogenous hormone effects will be additive to the endogenous source.

HOW SUPPLIED

Cytomel (liothyronine sodium, SK&F) tablets: 5 mcg. in bottles of 100; 25 mcg. in bottles of 100 and 1000; and 50 mcg. in bottles of 100.

CY:L30

Shown in Product Identification Section, page 430

DARBID® TABLETS, 5 mg. ℞

[*dahr'bid*]

(brand of isopropamide iodide)

DESCRIPTION

Darbid (brand of isopropamide iodide) is available as a tablet for oral administration. Each round, pink, coated tablet is imprinted SKF and D62 and contains isopropamide iodide equivalent to 5 mg. of isopropamide. Inactive ingredients consist of acacia, calcium sulfate, FD&C Red No. 3, FD&C Yellow No. 6, gelatin, iron oxide, mineral oil, starch, stearic acid, sucrose, talc, titanium dioxide and trace amounts of other inactive ingredients.

Chemically, Darbid (isopropamide iodide, SK&F) is (3-carbamoyl-3, 3-diphenylpropyl) diisopropylmethyl ammonium iodide.

ACTIONS

Isopropamide iodide is a synthetic anticholinergic that produces 10- to 12-hour gastric acid antisecretory effect and gastrointestinal antispasmodic response in man.

INDICATIONS

'Darbid' is effective as adjunctive therapy in the treatment of peptic ulcer.

'DARBID' HAS NOT BEEN SHOWN TO BE EFFECTIVE AS SOLE THERAPY IN CONTRIBUTING TO THE HEALING OF PEPTIC ULCER, DECREASING THE RATE OF RECURRENCE OR PREVENTING COMPLICATIONS.

To be effective, dosage must be titrated to the individual patient's needs.

CONTRAINDICATIONS

Glaucoma; obstructive uropathy (e.g., bladder neck obstruction due to prostatic hypertrophy); obstructive disease of the gastrointestinal tract (as in achalasia, pyloroduodenal stenosis, etc.); obstructive or paralytic ileus, intestinal atony of the elderly or debilitated patient; unstable cardiovascular status in acute hemorrhage; severe ulcerative colitis; toxic megacolon complicating ulcerative colitis; myasthenia gravis.

WARNINGS

In the presence of a high environmental temperature, heat prostration (fever and heat stroke due to decreased sweating) can occur.

In patients with diarrhea due to incomplete intestinal obstruction (especially those with ileostomy or colostomy), treatment with Darbid (isopropamide iodide, SK&F) would be inappropriate and possibly harmful.

'Darbid' may produce drowsiness or blurred vision. In this event, the patient should be warned not to engage in activities requiring mental alertness such as operating a motor vehicle or other machinery or perform hazardous work while taking this drug.

Usage in Pregnancy: In pregnancy, lactation, and in women who may bear children, the potential benefits of the drug must be weighed against possible hazards.

PRECAUTIONS

Use cautiously in elderly patients.

Since the iodine in isopropamide iodide may alter PBI test results and will suppress I^{131} uptake, it is suggested that

Continued on next page

Smith Kline & French—Cont.

therapy be discontinued one week prior to these tests. Also, iodine skin rash may occur rarely.
Use with caution in patients with:
Autonomic neuropathy.
Hepatic or renal disease.
Ulcerative colitis (large doses may suppress intestinal motility to the point of producing paralytic ileus, and the use of this drug may precipitate or aggravate the serious complication of toxic megacolon).
Hyperthyroidism, coronary heart disease, congestive heart failure, cardiac arrhythmia, hypertension and nonobstructing prostatic hypertrophy.
Hiatal hernia associated with reflux esophagitis (anticholinergic drugs may aggravate this condition).
It should be noted that the use of anticholinergic drugs in the treatment of gastric ulcer may produce a delay in gastric emptying time (antral stasis) and, thus, complicate therapy.
Do not rely on the use of the drug in the presence of complication of biliary tract disease.
Investigate any tachycardia before giving anticholinergic (atropine-like) drugs, since they may increase the heart rate.
With overdosage, a curare-like action may occur.

ADVERSE REACTIONS

Anticholinergics produce certain pharmacological effects which may be desirable or undesirable, depending upon the individual patient's response. The physician must delineate these.
Adverse reactions which have occurred with Darbid (isopropamide iodide, SK&F) include: xerostomia (dry mouth); urinary hesitancy and retention; blurred vision; tachycardia; palpitations; mydriasis (dilatation of the pupils); cycloplegia; constipation; bloated feeling; nausea; dysphagia; fever; and nasal congestion.
Other adverse reactions possible with anticholinergics include: increased ocular tension; loss of taste; headaches; nervousness; drowsiness; weakness; dizziness; insomnia; vomiting; impotence; suppression of lactation; severe allergic reaction or drug idiosyncrasies including anaphylaxis; urticaria and other dermal manifestations; some degree of mental confusion and/or excitement, especially in elderly persons.
Decreased sweating may occur. It should be noted that adrenergic innervation of the eccrine sweat glands on the palms and soles makes complete control of sweating impossible. An end point of complete anhidrosis cannot occur because large doses of drug would be required, and this would produce severe side effects from parasympathetic paralysis.

DOSAGE AND ADMINISTRATION

Not for use in children under 12. Adults and children over 12—Usual starting dose is one 5 mg. tablet b.i.d. (every 12 hours). Patients with severe symptoms may require two 5 mg. tablets b.i.d., or more. Dosage should be individualized and titrated to the patient's need for greatest therapeutic effect.

OVERDOSAGE

Involves the cardiovascular, respiratory, gastrointestinal, central and peripheral nervous systems. SYMPTOMS—May include dryness of mouth, dysphagia, thirst, blurred vision, dilated pupils, photophobia, fever, rapid pulse and respiration, disorientation. Depression and circulatory collapse may result from severe overdosage. TREATMENT—Gastric lavage, repeated several times.
Respiratory depression should be promptly treated by the use of oxygen and stimulants. If marked excitement is present, one of the short-acting barbiturates, chloral hydrate, or gas anesthesia may be used. Otherwise do not administer sedation. Hyperpyrexia may be treated with physical cooling measures. Force fluids by mouth or, if necessary, by intravenous administration.
While pilocarpine or similar drugs are sometimes recommended for the relief of dry mouth, many authorities feel that these drugs are not indicated, since they relieve the minor peripheral effect but do not influence the more serious central effects and, thus, may merely mask signs of drug activity. If photophobia occurs, the patient should be kept in a darkened room.

HOW SUPPLIED

Tablets, 5 mg., in bottles of 50.

DB:L16

Shown in Product Identification Section, page 430

DEXEDRINE® Ⓒ II

[*dex 'eh-dreen*]
(brand of dextroamphetamine sulfate)
SPANSULE® CAPSULES, TABLETS and ELIXIR

WARNING

AMPHETAMINES HAVE A HIGH POTENTIAL FOR ABUSE. THEY SHOULD THUS BE TRIED ONLY IN WEIGHT REDUCTION PROGRAMS FOR PATIENTS IN WHOM ALTERNATIVE THERAPY HAS BEEN INEFFECTIVE. ADMINISTRATION OF AMPHETAMINES FOR PROLONGED PERIODS OF TIME IN OBESITY MAY LEAD TO DRUG DEPENDENCE AND MUST BE AVOIDED. PARTICULAR ATTENTION SHOULD BE PAID TO THE POSSIBILITY OF SUBJECTS OBTAINING AMPHETAMINES FOR NON-THERAPEUTIC USE OR DISTRIBUTION TO OTHERS, AND THE DRUGS SHOULD BE PRESCRIBED OR DISPENSED SPARINGLY.

DESCRIPTION

Dexedrine (dextroamphetamine sulfate, SK&F) is the dextro isomer of the compound *d,l*-amphetamine sulfate, a sympathomimetic amine of the amphetamine group. Chemically, dextroamphetamine is *d*-alpha-methylphenethylamine, and is present in all forms of 'Dexedrine' as the neutral sulfate.
Spansule® capsules
Each 'Spansule' sustained release capsule is so prepared that an initial dose is released promptly and the remaining medication is released gradually over a prolonged period.
Each capsule, with brown cap and natural body, contains dextroamphetamine sulfate as follows: 5 mg. imprinted SKF and E12; 10 mg. imprinted SKF and E13, 15 mg. imprinted SKF and E14. Inactive ingredients consist of acacia, benzyl alcohol, calcium sulfate, cetylpyridinium chloride, FD&C Blue No. 1, FD&C Red No. 40, FD&C Yellow No. 5 (tartrazine), FD&C Yellow No. 6, gelatin, glyceryl distearate, glyceryl monostearate, sodium lauryl sulfate, starch, sucrose, wax and trace amounts of other inactive ingredients.
Tablets
Each triangular, orange, scored tablet is debossed SKF and E19 and contains dextroamphetamine sulfate, 5 mg. Inactive ingredients consist of calcium sulfate, FD&C Yellow No. 5 (tartrazine), FD&C Yellow No. 6, gelatin, lactose, mineral oil, starch, stearic acid, sucrose, talc and trace amounts of other inactive ingredients.
Elixir
Each 5 ml. (one teaspoonful) of clear, orange-colored, orange-flavored liquid contains dextroamphetamine sulfate, 5 mg., and alcohol, 10%. Inactive ingredients consist of benzoic acid, citric acid, FD&C Yellow No. 5 (tartrazine), FD&C Yellow No. 6, flavor, sucrose, water and wine.

CLINICAL PHARMACOLOGY

Amphetamines are non-catecholamine, sympathomimetic amines with CNS stimulant activity. Peripheral actions include elevations of systolic and diastolic blood pressures and weak bronchodilator and respiratory stimulant action.
There is neither specific evidence which clearly establishes the mechanism whereby amphetamines produce mental and behavioral effects in children, nor conclusive evidence regarding how these effects relate to the condition of the central nervous system.
Drugs of this class used in obesity are commonly known as "anorectics" or "anorexigenics." It has not been established, however, that the action of such drugs in treating obesity is primarily one of appetite suppression. Other central nervous system actions, or metabolic effects, may be involved, for example.
Adult obese subjects instructed in dietary management and treated with "anorectic" drugs lose more weight on the average than those treated with placebo and diet, as determined in relatively short-term clinical trials.
The magnitude of increased weight loss of drug-treated patients over placebo-treated patients is only a fraction of a pound a week. The rate of weight loss is greatest in the first weeks of therapy for both drug and placebo subjects and tends to decrease in succeeding weeks. The origins of the increased weight loss due to the various possible drug effects are not established. The amount of weight loss associated with the use of an "anorectic" drug varies from trial to trial, and the increased weight loss appears to be related in part to variables other than the drug prescribed, such as the physician-investigator, the population treated, and the diet prescribed. Studies do not permit conclusions as to the relative importance of the drug and nondrug factors on weight loss.
The natural history of obesity is measured in years, whereas the studies cited are restricted to a few weeks' duration; thus, the total impact of drug-induced weight loss over that of diet alone must be considered clinically limited.
Dexedrine (dextroamphetamine sulfate, SK&F) *Spansule* capsules are formulated to release the active drug substance *in vivo* in a more gradual fashion than the standard formulation, as demonstrated by blood levels. The formulation has not been shown superior in effectiveness over the same dosage of the standard, noncontrolled-release formulations given in divided doses.
Pharmacokinetics
Elixir—Ingestion of 10 mg. of dextroamphetamine sulfate in elixir form by healthy volunteers produced an average peak dextroamphetamine blood level of 33.2 ng./ml. The half-life was 11.75 hours. The average urinary recovery was 38% in 48 hours.
Tablet—The single ingestion of two 5 mg. tablets by healthy volunteers produced an average peak dextroamphetamine blood level of 29.2 ng./ml. at 2 hours post-administration. The average half-life was 10.25 hours. The average urinary recovery was 45% in 48 hours.
'Spansule' capsule—Ingestion of a 'Spansule' capsule containing 15 mg. radiolabeled dextroamphetamine sulfate by healthy volunteers produced a peak blood level of radioactivity, on the average, at 8-10 hours post-administration with peak urinary recovery seen at 12–24 hours.

INDICATIONS AND USAGE

Dexedrine (dextroamphetamine sulfate, SK&F) is indicated:
1. In Narcolepsy.
2. In Attention Deficit Disorder with Hyperactivity, as an integral part of a total treatment program which typically includes other remedial measures (psychological, educational, social) for a stabilizing effect in children with a behavioral syndrome characterized by the following group of developmentally inappropriate symptoms: moderate to severe distractibility, short attention span, hyperactivity, emotional lability, and impulsivity. The diagnosis of this syndrome should not be made with finality when these symptoms are only of comparatively recent origin. Nonlocalizing (soft) neurological signs, learning disability, and abnormal EEG may or may not be present, and a diagnosis of central nervous system dysfunction may or may not be warranted.
3. In Exogenous Obesity, as a short-term (a few weeks) adjunct in a regimen of weight reduction based on caloric restriction, for patients refractory to alternative therapy, e.g., repeated diets, group programs, and other drugs. The limited usefulness of amphetamines (see CLINICAL PHARMACOLOGY) should be weighed against possible risks inherent in use of the drug, such as those described below.

CONTRAINDICATIONS

Advanced arteriosclerosis, symptomatic cardiovascular disease, moderate to severe hypertension, hyperthyroidism, known hypersensitivity or idiosyncrasy to the sympathomimetic amines, glaucoma.
Agitated states.
Patients with a history of drug abuse.
During or within 14 days following the administration of monoamine oxidase inhibitors (hypertensive crises may result).

WARNING

When tolerance to the "anorectic" effect develops, the recommended dose should not be exceeded in an attempt to increase the effect; rather, the drug should be discontinued.

PRECAUTIONS

General: Caution is to be exercised in prescribing amphetamines for patients with even mild hypertension.
The least amount feasible should be prescribed or dispensed at one time in order to minimize the possibility of overdosage.
These products contain FD&C Yellow No. 5 (tartrazine), which may cause allergic-type reactions (including bronchial asthma) in certain susceptible individuals. Although the overall incidence of FD&C Yellow No. 5 (tartrazine) sensitivity in the general population is low, it is frequently seen in patients who also have aspirin hypersensitivity.
Information for Patients: Amphetamines may impair the ability of the patient to engage in potentially hazardous activities such as operating machinery or vehicles; the patient should therefore be cautioned accordingly.
Drug Interactions
Acidifying agents—Gastrointestinal acidifying agents (guanethidine, reserpine, glutamic acid HCl, ascorbic acid, fruit juices, etc.) lower absorption of amphetamines. Urinary acidifying agents (ammonium chloride, sodium acid phosphate, etc.) increase the concentration of the ionized species of the amphetamine molecule, thereby increasing urinary excretion. Both groups of agents lower blood levels and efficacy of amphetamines.
Adrenergic blockers—Adrenergic blockers are inhibited by amphetamines.
Alkalinizing agents—Gastrointestinal alkalinizing agents (sodium bicarbonate, etc.) increase absorption of amphetamines. Urinary alkalinizing agents (acetazolamide, some thiazides) increase the concentration of the non-ionized species of the amphetamine molecule, thereby decreasing uri-

nary excretion. Both groups of agents increase blood levels and therefore potentiate the actions of amphetamines.
Antidepressants, tricyclic—Amphetamines may enhance the activity of tricyclic or sympathomimetic agents; d-amphetamine with desipramine or protriptyline and possibly other tricyclics cause striking and sustained increases in the concentration of d-amphetamine in the brain; cardiovascular effects can be potentiated.
MAO inhibitors—MAOI antidepressants, as well as a metabolite of furazolidone, slow amphetamine metabolism. This slowing potentiates amphetamines, increasing their effect on the release of norepinephrine and other monoamines from adrenergic nerve endings; this can cause headaches and other signs of hypertensive crisis. A variety of neurological toxic effects and malignant hyperpyrexia can occur, sometimes with fatal results.
Antihistamines—Amphetamines may counteract the sedative effect of antihistamines.
Antihypertensives—Amphetamines may antagonize the hypotensive effects of antihypertensives.
Chlorpromazine—Chlorpromazine blocks dopamine and norepinephrine reuptake, thus inhibiting the central stimulant effects of amphetamines, and can be used to treat amphetamine poisoning.
Ethosuximide—Amphetamines may delay intestinal absorption of ethosuximide.
Haloperidol—Haloperidol blocks dopamine and norepinephrine reuptake, thus inhibiting the central stimulant effects of amphetamines.
Lithium carbonate—The antiobesity and stimulatory effects of amphetamines may be inhibited by lithium carbonate.
Meperidine—Amphetamines potentiate the analgesic effect of meperidine.
Methenamine therapy—Urinary excretion of amphetamines is increased, and efficacy is reduced, by acidifying agents used in methenamine therapy.
Norepinephrine—Amphetamines enhance the adrenergic effect of norepinephrine.
Phenobarbital—Amphetamines may delay intestinal absorption of phenobarbital; co-administration of phenobarbital may produce a synergistic anticonvulsant action.
Phenytoin—Amphetamines may delay intestinal absorption of phenytoin; co-administration of phenytoin may produce a synergistic anticonvulsant action.
Propoxyphene—In cases of propoxyphene overdosage, amphetamine CNS stimulation is potentiated and fatal convulsions can occur.
Veratrum alkaloids—Amphetamines inhibit the hypotensive effect of veratrum alkaloids.

Drug/Laboratory Test Interactions

- Amphetamines can cause a significant elevation in plasma corticosteroid levels. This increase is greatest in the evening.
- Amphetamines may interfere with urinary steroid determinations.

Carcinogenesis/Mutagenesis: Mutagenicity studies and long-term studies in animals to determine the carcinogenic potential of Dexedrine (dextroamphetamine sulfate, SK&F) have not been performed.

Pregnancy—Teratogenic Effects: Pregnancy Category C. 'Dexedrine' has been shown to have embryotoxic and teratogenic effects when administered to A/Jax mice and C57BL mice in doses approximately 41 times the maximum human dose. Embryotoxic effects were not seen in New Zealand white rabbits given the drug in doses 7 times the human dose nor in rats given 12.5 times the maximum human dose. There are no adequate and well-controlled studies in pregnant women. 'Dexedrine' should be used during pregnancy only if the potential benefit justifies the potential risk to the fetus.

Nonteratogenic Effects: Infants born to mothers dependent on amphetamines have an increased risk of premature delivery and low birth weight. Also, these infants may experience symptoms of withdrawal as demonstrated by dysphoria, including agitation, and significant lassitude.

Nursing Mothers: It is not known whether this drug is excreted in breast milk; efforts to measure amphetamines in breast milk have been unsuccessful. Because many drugs are excreted in human milk, caution should be exercised when 'Dexedrine' is administered to a nursing woman.

Pediatric Use: Long-term effects of amphetamines in children have not been well established.
Amphetamines are not recommended for use as anorectic agents in children under 12 years of age, or in children under 3 years of age with Attention Deficit Disorder with Hyperactivity described under INDICATIONS AND USAGE.
Clinical experience suggests that in psychotic children, administration of amphetamines may exacerbate symptoms of behavior disturbance and thought disorder.
Amphetamines have been reported to exacerbate motor and phonic tics and Tourette's syndrome. Therefore, clinical evaluation for tics and Tourette's syndrome in children and their families should precede use of stimulant medications.
Data are inadequate to determine whether chronic administration of amphetamines may be associated with growth inhibition; therefore, growth should be monitored during treatment.
Drug treatment is not indicated in all cases of Attention Deficit Disorder with Hyperactivity and should be considered only in light of the complete history and evaluation of the child. The decision to prescribe amphetamines should depend on the physician's assessment of the chronicity and severity of the child's symptoms and their appropriateness for his/her age. Prescription should not depend solely on the presence of one or more of the behavioral characteristics.
When these symptoms are associated with acute stress reactions, treatment with amphetamines is usually not indicated.

ADVERSE REACTIONS

Cardiovascular: Palpitations, tachycardia, elevation of blood pressure.

Central Nervous System: Psychotic episodes at recommended doses (rare), overstimulation, restlessness, dizziness, insomnia, euphoria, dyskinesia, dysphoria, tremor, headache, exacerbation of motor and phonic tics and Tourette's syndrome.

Gastrointestinal: Dryness of the mouth, unpleasant taste, diarrhea, constipation, other gastrointestinal disturbances. Anorexia and weight loss may occur as undesirable effects when amphetamines are used for other than the anorectic effect.

Allergic: Urticaria.

Endocrine: Impotence, changes in libido.

DRUG ABUSE AND DEPENDENCE

Dextroamphetamine sulfate is a Schedule II controlled substance.
Amphetamines have been extensively abused. Tolerance, extreme psychological dependence, and severe social disability have occurred. There are reports of patients who have increased the dosage to many times that recommended. Abrupt cessation following prolonged high dosage administration results in extreme fatigue and mental depression; changes are also noted on the sleep EEG.
Manifestations of chronic intoxication with amphetamines include severe dermatoses, marked insomnia, irritability, hyperactivity, and personality changes. The most severe manifestation of chronic intoxication is psychosis, often clinically indistinguishable from schizophrenia. This is rare with oral amphetamines.

OVERDOSAGE

Individual patient response to amphetamines varies widely. While toxic symptoms occasionally occur as an idiosyncrasy at doses as low as 2 mg., they are rare with doses of less than 15 mg.; 30 mg. can produce severe reactions, yet doses of 400 to 500 mg. are not necessarily fatal.
In rats, the oral LD_{50} of dextroamphetamine sulfate is 96.8 mg./kg.
SYMPTOMS—Manifestations of acute overdosage with amphetamines include restlessness, tremor, hyperreflexia, rapid respiration, confusion, assaultiveness, hallucinations, panic states.
Fatigue and depression usually follow the central stimulation.
Cardiovascular effects include arrhythmias, hypertension or hypotension and circulatory collapse. Gastrointestinal symptoms include nausea, vomiting, diarrhea, and abdominal cramps. Fatal poisoning is usually preceded by convulsions and coma.
TREATMENT—Management of acute amphetamine intoxication is largely symptomatic and includes gastric lavage and sedation with a barbiturate. Experience with hemodialysis or peritoneal dialysis is inadequate to permit recommendation in this regard. Acidification of the urine increases amphetamine excretion. If acute, severe hypertension complicates amphetamine overdosage, administration of intravenous phentolamine (Regitine®, CIBA) has been suggested. However, a gradual drop in blood pressure will usually result when sufficient sedation has been achieved.
Chlorpromazine antagonizes the central stimulant effects of amphetamines and can be used to treat amphetamine intoxication.
Since much of the 'Spansule' capsule medication is coated for gradual release, therapy directed at reversing the effects of the ingested drug and at supporting the patient should be continued for as long as overdosage symptoms remain. Saline cathartics are useful for hastening the evacuation of pellets that have not already released medication.

DOSAGE AND ADMINISTRATION

Regardless of indication, amphetamines should be administered at the lowest effective dosage and dosage should be individually adjusted. Late evening doses—particularly with the 'Spansule' capsule form—should be avoided because of the resulting insomnia.

Narcolepsy: Usual dose 5 to 60 milligrams per day in divided doses, depending on the individual patient response.
Narcolepsy seldom occurs in children under 12 years of age; however, when it does, Dexedrine (dextroamphetamine sulfate, SK&F) may be used. The suggested initial dose for patients aged 6–12 is 5 mg. daily; daily dose may be raised in increments of 5 mg. at weekly intervals until optimal response is obtained. In patients 12 years of age and older, start with 10 mg. daily; daily dosage may be raised in increments of 10 mg. at weekly intervals until optimal response is obtained. If bothersome adverse reactions appear (e.g., insomnia or anorexia), dosage should be reduced. 'Spansule' capsules may be used for once-a-day dosage wherever appropriate. With tablets or elixir, give first dose on awakening; additional doses (1 or 2) at intervals of 4 to 6 hours.

Attention Deficit Disorder with Hyperactivity: Not recommended for children under 3 years of age.

In children from 3 to 5 years of age, start with 2.5 mg. daily, by tablet or elixir; daily dosage may be raised in increments of 2.5 mg. at weekly intervals until optimal response is obtained.

In children 6 years of age and older, start with 5 mg. once or twice daily; daily dosage may be raised in increments of 5 mg. at weekly intervals until optimal response is obtained. Only in rare cases will it be necessary to exceed a total of 40 milligrams per day.
'Spansule' capsules may be used for once-a-day dosage wherever appropriate.
With tablets or elixir, give first dose on awakening; additional doses (1 or 2) at intervals of 4 to 6 hours.
Where possible, drug administration should be interrupted occasionally to determine if there is a recurrence of behavioral symptoms sufficient to require continued therapy.

Exogenous Obesity: Usual dosage is one 10 or 15 mg. 'Spansule' capsule daily, taken in the morning, or up to 30 mg. daily by tablets or elixir, taken in divided doses of 5 to 10 mg. 30 to 60 minutes before meals. Not recommended for this use in children under 12 years of age.

HOW SUPPLIED

'Spansule' capsules available: 5 mg., in bottles of 50; 10 mg. and 15 mg., in bottles of 50 and 500.
Tablets, 5 mg., available in bottles of 100 and 1000.
Elixir, 5 mg./5 ml., available in 16 fl. oz. (473 ml.) bottles.
DX:L35

Shown in Product Identification Section, page 430

DIBENZYLINE® Capsules ℞

[di-benz 'eh-leen]
(brand of phenoxybenzamine hydrochloride)

DESCRIPTION

Each 'DIBENZYLINE' capsule, with red cap and red body, is imprinted SKF and E33 and contains phenoxybenzamine hydrochloride, 10 mg. Inactive ingredients consist of benzyl alcohol, cetylpyridinium chloride, D&C Red No. 33, FD&C Red No. 3, FD&C Yellow No. 6, gelatin, lactose, sodium lauryl sulfate and trace amounts of other inactive ingredients.
'Dibenzyline' is N-(2-Chloroethyl)-N-(1-methyl-2-phenoxyethyl) benzylamine hydrochloride.
Phenoxybenzamine hydrochloride is a colorless, crystalline powder with a molecular weight of 340.3 which melts between 136° and 141°C. It is soluble in water, alcohol and chloroform; insoluble in ether.

ACTIONS

Dibenzyline (phenoxybenzamine hydrochloride, SK&F) is a long-acting, adrenergic, α-receptor blocking agent which can produce and maintain "chemical sympathectomy" by oral administration. It increases blood flow to the skin, mucosa and abdominal viscera, and lowers both supine and erect blood pressures. It has no effect on the parasympathetic system.

INDICATION

Pheochromocytoma, to control episodes of hypertension and sweating. If tachycardia is excessive, it may be necessary to use a beta-blocking agent concomitantly.

CONTRAINDICATIONS

Conditions where a fall in blood pressure may be undesirable.

WARNING

'Dibenzyline'-induced *alpha*-adrenergic blockade leaves *beta*-adrenergic receptors unopposed. Compounds that stimulate both types of receptors may therefore produce an exaggerated hypotensive response and tachycardia.

PRECAUTIONS

Phenoxybenzamine hydrochloride has shown *in vitro* mutagenic activity in the Ames test and in the mouse lymphoma assay; it has not shown mutagenic activity in the micronucleus test in mice. In rats and mice repeated intraperitoneal administration of phenoxybenzamine hydrochloride resulted in peritoneal sarcomas. Chronic oral dosing in rats has produced malignant tumors of the gastrointestinal tract.
The clinical significance of such test results is not established. Nevertheless, these results should be given consideration in determining the benefit-risk ratio as it applies to the individual patient.

Continued on next page

Smith Kline & French—Cont.

Administer with caution in patients with marked cerebral or coronary arteriosclerosis or renal damage. Adrenergic blocking effect may aggravate symptoms of respiratory infections.

ADVERSE REACTIONS

Nasal congestion, miosis, postural hypotension, tachycardia and inhibition of ejaculation may occur. These so-called "side effects" are actually evidence of adrenergic blockade and vary according to the degree of blockade. Furthermore, they tend to decrease as therapy is continued. Gastrointestinal irritation, drowsiness and fatigue have also been reported.

DOSAGE AND ADMINISTRATION

The dosage should be adjusted to fit the needs of each patient. Small initial doses should be *slowly* increased until the desired effect is obtained or the side effects from blockade become troublesome. *After each increase, the patient should be observed on that level before instituting another increase.* The dosage should be carried to a point where symptomatic relief and/or objective improvement are obtained, but not so high that the side effects from blockade become troublesome. Initially, 10 mg. of Dibenzyline (phenoxybenzamine hydrochloride, SK&F) twice a day. Dosage should be increased every other day, usually to 20 to 40 mg. two or three times a day, until an optimal dosage is obtained, as judged by blood pressure control.

OVERDOSAGE

SYMPTOMS—These are largely the result of block of the sympathetic nervous system and of the circulating epinephrine. They may include postural hypotension resulting in dizziness or fainting; tachycardia, particularly postural; vomiting; lethargy; shock. TREATMENT—When symptoms and signs of overdosage exist, discontinue the drug. Treatment of circulatory failure, if present, is a prime consideration. In cases of mild overdosage, recumbent position with legs elevated usually restores cerebral circulation. In the more severe cases, the usual measures to combat shock should be instituted. Usual pressor agents are *not* effective. Epinephrine is contraindicated because it stimulates both α and β receptors; since α receptors are blocked, the net effect of epinephrine administration is vasodilation and a further drop in blood pressure (epinephrine reversal).
The patient may have to be kept flat for 24 hours or more in the case of overdose, as the effect of the drug is prolonged. Leg bandages and an abdominal binder may shorten the period of disability.
I.V. infusion of levarterenol bitartrate* may be used to combat severe hypotensive reactions, because it stimulates α receptors primarily. Although Dibenzyline (phenoxybenzamine hydrochloride, SK&F) is an α adrenergic blocking agent, a sufficient dose of levarterenol bitartrate will overcome this effect.

HOW SUPPLIED

Dibenzyline (phenoxybenzamine hydrochloride, SK&F) capsules, 10 mg., in bottles of 100.

*Available as Levophed® Bitartrate (brand of levarterenol bitartrate) from Winthrop Laboratories.

DI:L22

Shown in Product Identification Section, page 430

DYAZIDE® Capsules ℞

[dye-uh-zide']

('Dyazide' is a product of SK&F Co., Carolina, P.R. 00630, Subsidiary of SmithKline Beckman Corporation, Philadelphia, Pa.)

> **WARNING**
> This fixed combination drug is not indicated for initial therapy of edema or hypertension. Edema or hypertension requires therapy titrated to the individual patient. If the fixed combination represents the dosage so determined, its use may be more convenient in patient management. The treatment of hypertension and edema is not static, but must be reevaluated as conditions in each patient warrant.

DESCRIPTION

Hydrochlorothiazide is 6-chloro-3, 4-dihydro-2*H*-1, 2, 4-benzothiadiazine-7-sulfonamide 1,1 -dioxide.
Triamterene is 2, 4, 7-triamino-6-phenylpteridine.
Hydrochlorothiazide is slightly soluble in water. It is soluble in dilute ammonia, dilute aqueous sodium hydroxide, and dimethylformamide. It is sparingly soluble in methanol.
At 50°C., triamterene is practically insoluble in water (less than 0.1%). It is soluble in formic acid, sparingly soluble in methoxyethanol, and very slightly soluble in alcohol.
Each 'Dyazide' capsule, with opaque red cap and opaque white body, contains hydrochlorothiazide 25 mg., and the potassium-sparing agent triamterene 50 mg., and is imprinted with the product name DYAZIDE and SKF. Inactive ingredients consist of benzyl alcohol, cetylpyridinium chloride, D&C Red No. 33, FD&C Yellow No. 6, gelatin, lactose, magnesium stearate, povidone, sodium lauryl sulfate, titanium dioxide and trace amounts of other inactive ingredients.

ACTION

'Dyazide' is a diuretic/antihypertensive drug product that combines the natriuretic, hydrochlorothiazide, and the potassium-sparing natriuretic, triamterene, each of which complements the action of the other. The hydrochlorothiazide component blocks the reabsorption of sodium and chloride ions, and thereby increases the quantity of sodium traversing the distal tubule and the volume of water excreted. A portion of the additional sodium presented to the distal tubule is exchanged there for potassium and hydrogen ions. With continued use of hydrochlorothiazide and depletion of sodium, compensatory mechanisms tend to increase this exchange and may produce excessive loss of potassium, hydrogen and chloride ions. Hydrochlorothiazide also decreases the excretion of calcium and uric acid, may increase the excretion of iodide and may reduce glomerular filtration rate. The exact mechanism of the antihypertensive effect of hydrochlorothiazide is not known.
The triamterene component of 'Dyazide' exerts its diuretic effect on the distal renal tubule to inhibit the reabsorption of sodium in exchange for potassium and hydrogen ions. Its natriuretic activity is limited by the amount of sodium reaching its site of action. Although it blocks the increase in this exchange that is stimulated by mineralocorticoids (chiefly aldosterone) it is not a competitive antagonist of aldosterone and its activity can be demonstrated in adrenalectomized rats and patients with Addison's disease. As a result the dose of triamterene required is not proportionally related to the level of mineralocorticoid activity, but is dictated by the response of the individual patient, and the kaliuretic effect of concomitantly administered drugs. By inhibiting the distal tubular exchange mechanism, triamterene maintains or increases the sodium excretion and reduces the excess loss of potassium, hydrogen, and chloride ions induced by hydrochlorothiazide. As with hydrochlorothiazide, triamterene may reduce glomerular filtration and renal plasma flow. Via this mechanism it may reduce uric acid excretion although it has no tubular effect on uric acid reabsorption or secretion. Triamterene does not affect calcium excretion. No predictable antihypertensive effect has been demonstrated for triamterene.
Duration of diuretic activity and effective dosage range of the hydrochlorothiazide and triamterene components of 'Dyazide' are similar. Onset of diuresis with 'Dyazide' takes place within one hour, peaks at two-three hours and tapers off during the subsequent seven to nine hours.

INDICATIONS

This combination drug finds its usefulness primarily in the treatment of edema. Any usefulness of triamterene when used with a thiazide in hypertension will derive from its potassium-sparing effect. Either its main diuretic effect or potassium-sparing effect when used with a thiazide drug should be determined by individual titration. (See box warning.)
When the fixed combination represents the dosage determined by titration, 'Dyazide' is indicated as adjunctive therapy in edema associated with congestive heart failure, hepatic cirrhosis and the nephrotic syndrome. It is also indicated in corticosteroid and estrogen induced edema and idiopathic edema.
When the potassium-sparing action of its triamterene component is warranted and the fixed combination represents the dosage determined by titration, 'Dyazide' is indicated in the management of hypertension as determined by individual dosage titration of all agents employed. (See box warning.)
Usage in Pregnancy. The routine use of diuretics in an otherwise healthy woman is inappropriate and exposes mother and fetus to unnecessary hazard. Diuretics do not prevent development of toxemia of pregnancy, and there is no satisfactory evidence that they are useful in the treatment of developed toxemia.
Edema during pregnancy may arise from pathological causes or from the physiologic and mechanical consequences of pregnancy. Diuretics are indicated in pregnancy when edema is due to pathologic causes, just as they are in the absence of pregnancy (however, see Warnings, below). Dependent edema in pregnancy, resulting from restriction of venous return by the expanded uterus, is properly treated through elevation of the lower extremities and use of support hose; use of diuretics to lower intravascular volume in this case is illogical and unnecessary. There is hypervolemia during normal pregnancy which is harmful to neither the fetus nor the mother (in the absence of cardiovascular disease), but which is associated with edema, including generalized edema, in the majority of pregnant women. If this edema produces discomfort, increased recumbency will often provide relief. In rare instances, this edema may cause extreme discomfort which is not relieved by rest. In these cases, a short course of diuretics may provide relief and may be appropriate.

CONTRAINDICATIONS

'Dyazide' should not be given to patients receiving other potassium-sparing agents such as spironolactone or amiloride. Two deaths have been reported in patients receiving concomitant spironolactone and triamterene or 'Dyazide'. In one case dosage recommendations were exceeded; in the other serum electrolytes were not properly monitored.
'Dyazide' is contraindicated for further use in patients who exhibit anuria or progressive renal dysfunction, including increasing oliguria and increasing azotemia or in patients who develop hyperkalemia while on the drug.
'Dyazide' should not be used in patients with pre-existing elevated serum potassium, as is sometimes seen in patients with impaired renal function. Increasing hepatic dysfunction in patients on 'Dyazide' contraindicates further use of the preparation. Hypersensitivity to either drug in the preparation or to other sulfonamide-derived drugs is a contraindication.

WARNINGS

Patients should not be placed on dietary potassium supplements, potassium salts, or potassium-containing salt substitutes in conjunction with 'Dyazide' unless they develop hypokalemia or their dietary intake of potassium is markedly impaired. Because of the potassium conserving effect of triamterene, hypokalemia is an uncommon occurrence with the use of 'Dyazide'.
If the need for supplementary potassium is demonstrated by repeated low serum potassium determinations a form other than potassium tablets should be used since these have been implicated in the development of nonspecific small bowel lesions consisting of stenosis with or without ulceration.
Abnormal elevation of serum potassium, though uncommon, is potentially the most severe electrolyte disturbance with 'Dyazide' therapy. Hyperkalemia has been reported and in some cases has been associated with cardiac irregularities. Hyperkalemia is more likely to occur in patients who are severely ill, with relatively small urine volumes (less than one liter per day), or in elderly or diabetic patients with confirmed or suspected renal insufficiency. Acute transient hyperkalemia has been observed during intravenous glucose tolerance testing of diabetics dosed with the triamterene component of 'Dyazide'. Fatalities due to hyperkalemia have been reported, accordingly no potassium supplements should ordinarily be given with 'Dyazide' therapy, and periodic determinations of serum potassium should be made. If hyperkalemia develops, withdraw 'Dyazide', substitute a thiazide alone, and restrict potassium intake.
If hyperkalemia is present or suspected, an electrocardiogram should be obtained. If the ECG shows no widening of the QRS or arrhythmia in the presence of hyperkalemia, it is usually sufficient to discontinue 'Dyazide' and any potassium supplementation and substitute a thiazide alone. Sodium polystyrene sulfonate (Kayexalate®, Winthrop) may be administered to enhance the excretion of excess potassium. **The presence of a widened QRS complex or arrhythmia in association with hyperkalemia requires prompt additional therapy.** For tachyarrhythmia, infuse 44 mEq. of sodium bicarbonate or 10 ml. of 10% calcium gluconate or calcium chloride over several minutes. For asystole, bradycardia or A-V block transvenous pacing is also recommended.
The effect of calcium and sodium bicarbonate is transient and repeated administration may be required. When indicated by the clinical situation, excess K^+ may be removed by dialysis or oral or rectal administration of Kayexalate®. Infusion of glucose and insulin has also been used to treat hyperkalemia.
Sensitivity reactions may occur in patients with or without a history of allergy or bronchial asthma.
The possibility of exacerbation or activation of systemic lupus erythematosus has been reported with thiazide diuretics.
Usage in Pregnancy. Thiazides cross the placental barrier and appear in cord blood. The use of thiazides in pregnant women requires that the anticipated benefit be weighed against possible hazards to the fetus. These hazards include fetal or neonatal jaundice, thrombocytopenia, and possibly other adverse reactions which have occurred in the adult.
Nursing Mothers. Thiazides appear and triamterene may appear in breast milk. If use of the drug product is deemed essential, the patient should stop nursing.

Usage in Children

Adequate information on the use of 'Dyazide' in children is not available.

PRECAUTIONS

The bioavailability of the hydrochlorothiazide component of 'Dyazide' is about 50% of the bioavailability of the single entity. Theoretically, a patient transferred from the single entities triamterene and hydrochlorothiazide may show an increase in blood pressure or fluid retention. Similarly, it is

also possible that the lesser hydrochlorothiazide bioavailability could lead to increased serum potassium levels. However, extensive clinical experience with 'Dyazide' suggests that these conditions have not been commonly observed in clinical practice.
Electrolyte imbalance, often encountered in such conditions as heart failure, renal disease, or cirrhosis of the liver, may also be aggravated by diuretics, and should be considered during 'Dyazide' therapy when using high doses for prolonged periods or in patients on a salt-restricted diet. Serum determinations of electrolytes should be performed, and are particularly important if the patient is vomiting excessively or receiving fluids parenterally. Possible fluid and electrolyte imbalance may be indicated by such warning signs as: dry mouth, thirst, weakness, lethargy, drowsiness, restlessness, muscle pain or cramps, muscular fatigue, hypotension, oliguria, tachycardia, and gastrointestinal symptoms.
Because of the potassium-sparing characteristic of triamterene, hypokalemia is uncommon with 'Dyazide' but may occur in some cases when the triamterene component is unable to completely compensate for the potassium-wasting effect of the hydrochlorothiazide component or the disease. The myocardial effects of digitalis may be exaggerated in patients with hypokalemia. In these patients signs of digitalis intoxication may be produced by previously tolerated doses of digitalis.
Hypokalemia is uncommon with 'Dyazide' but should it develop, corrective measures should be taken such as potassium supplementation or increased dietary intake of potassium-rich foods. Institute such measures cautiously with frequent determinations of serum potassium levels. Discontinue corrective measures immediately if laboratory determinations reveal an abnormal elevation of serum potassium. Discontinue 'Dyazide' and substitute a thiazide diuretic alone until potassium levels return to normal.
Although any chloride deficit is generally mild and usually does not require specific treatment except under extraordinary circumstances (as in liver disease or renal disease), chloride replacement may be required in the treatment of metabolic alkalosis. Dilutional hyponatremia may occur in edematous patients in hot weather; appropriate therapy is water restriction, rather than administration of salt, except in rare instances when the hyponatremia is life threatening. In actual salt depletion, appropriate replacement is the therapy of choice.
'Dyazide' may produce an elevated blood urea nitrogen level, creatinine level, or both. This apparently is secondary to a reversible reduction of glomerular filtration rate or a depletion of intravascular fluid volume (prerenal azotemia) rather than renal toxicity; levels return to normal when 'Dyazide' is discontinued. Elevated levels are seldom seen with every-other-day therapy. If azotemia increases, discontinue 'Dyazide'. Cumulative effects of the drug may develop in patients with impaired renal function. Periodic BUN or serum creatinine determinations should be made, especially in elderly patients and in patients with suspected or confirmed renal insufficiency.
Triamterene has been found in renal stones in association with the other usual calculus components. Therefore, 'Dyazide' should be used with caution in patients with histories of stone formation.
A possible interaction resulting in acute renal failure has been reported in a few patients on 'Dyazide' when treated with indomethacin, a nonsteroidal anti-inflammatory agent. Caution is advised in administering nonsteroidal anti-inflammatory agents with 'Dyazide'.
Potassium-sparing agents should be used with caution in conjunction with angiotensin-converting enzyme (ACE) inhibitors due to an increased risk of hyperkalemia.
Thiazides should be used with caution in patients with impaired hepatic function. They can precipitate hepatic coma in patients with severe liver disease. Potassium depletion induced by the thiazide may be important in this connection. Administer 'Dyazide' cautiously and be alert for such early signs of impending coma as confusion, drowsiness and tremor; if mental confusion increases discontinue 'Dyazide' for a few days. Attention must be given to other factors that may precipitate hepatic coma, such as blood in the gastrointestinal tract or preexisting potassium depletion.
Patients should be observed regularly for the possible occurrence of blood dyscrasias, liver damage, or other idiosyncratic reactions. There have been reports of blood dyscrasias in patients receiving triamterene. Leukopenia, thrombocytopenia, agranulocytosis, and aplastic and hemolytic anemia have been reported with the thiazides. Cirrhotics with splenomegaly may have marked variations in their blood pictures—including thrombocyte and leukocyte levels—which are not related to drug therapy. Since the triamterene component of 'Dyazide' is a weak folic acid antagonist, it may contribute to the appearance of megaloblastosis in cases where folic acid stores are depleted. Periodic blood studies in these patients are recommended.
The antihypertensive effects of 'Dyazide' may be enhanced in the post-sympathectomy patient.
Diabetes mellitus which has been latent may become manifest during thiazide administration.
Thiazides may cause hyperglycemia and glycosuria, and alter insulin requirements in diabetes. 'Dyazide' may have similar effects; concurrent use with chlorpropamide may increase the risk of severe hyponatremia. Hyperuricemia may be observed, with possible occurrence of gout. Triamterene may cause a decreasing alkali reserve with the possibility of metabolic acidosis.
Thiazides may add to or potentiate the action of other antihypertensive drugs. See Dosage and Administration for concomitant use with other antihypertensive drugs.
Thiazides have been shown to decrease arterial responsiveness to norepinephrine (an effect attributed to loss of sodium). This diminution is not sufficient to preclude effectiveness of the pressor agent for therapeutic use. Thiazides have also been shown to increase the paralyzing effect of nondepolarizing muscle relaxants such as tubocurarine (an effect attributed to potassium loss); consequently caution should be observed in patients undergoing surgery.
Thiazides may decrease serum PBI levels without signs of thyroid disturbance.
Calcium excretion is decreased by thiazides. Pathologic changes in the parathyroid glands with hypercalcemia and hypophosphatemia have been observed in a few patients on prolonged thiazide therapy. The common complications of hyperparathyroidism such as renal lithiasis, bone resorption, and peptic ulceration have not been seen. Thiazides should be discontinued before carrying out tests for parathyroid function.
Triamterene and quinidine have similar fluorescence spectra; thus, 'Dyazide' will interfere with the fluorescent measurement of quinidine.
Lithium generally should not be given with diuretics because they reduce its renal clearance and increase the risk of lithium toxicity. Read circulars for lithium preparations before use of such concomitant therapy with 'Dyazide'.
Concurrent use of hydrochlorothiazide with amphotericin B or corticosteroids or corticotropin (ACTH) may intensify electrolyte imbalance, particularly hypokalemia, although the presence of triamterene minimizes the hypokalemic effects.
The effects of oral anticoagulants may be decreased when used concurrently with hydrochlorothiazide; dosage adjustments may be necessary.

ADVERSE REACTIONS

Side effects observed in association with the use of 'Dyazide' include: muscle cramps, weakness, dizziness, headache and dry mouth; anaphylaxis, rash, urticaria, photosensitivity, purpura and other dermatological conditions; nausea and vomiting, diarrhea, constipation, and other gastrointestinal disturbances (such nausea can usually be prevented by giving the drug after meals). It should be noted that symptoms of nausea and vomiting can also be indicative of electrolyte imbalance (see Precautions). Postural hypotension (may be aggravated by alcohol, barbiturates, or narcotics). Impotence has been reported in a few patients on 'Dyazide', although a causal relationship has not been established.
Triamterene has been found in renal stones in association with the other usual calculus components (see Precautions).
Thiazides alone have been known to cause necrotizing vasculitis, paresthesias, icterus, pancreatitis, xanthopsia, and respiratory distress including pneumonitis and pulmonary edema, transient blurred vision, sialadenitis, and vertigo. Rare incidents of acute interstitial nephritis have been reported with the use of 'Dyazide'.
Newborn, whose mothers had received thiazides during pregnancy, in rare instances have developed thrombocytopenia or pancreatitis.

DOSAGE AND ADMINISTRATION

As determined by individual titration. (See box warning.)

Adults:

The usual dose is one or two capsules twice daily after meals. Some patients may be maintained on one capsule daily or every other day. Maximum daily dose should not exceed four capsules, and at this dosage, the incidence of side effects may increase.
Since 'Dyazide' has an antihypertensive effect, hypotensive drugs used concomitantly should be added at reduced dosage—at least one half the usual dosage—particularly if it is a ganglionic or peripheral adrenergic blocking agent. Adjust dosage as indicated.

Children:

Adequate information on the use of 'Dyazide' in children is not available.
Note: Potassium supplementation used concurrently with other diuretics should be discontinued when titrating with triamterene. They should not be reinstituted when the patient is placed on 'Dyazide' unless the triamterene component does not completely compensate for the potassium loss.

OVERDOSAGE

Electrolyte imbalance is the major concern (See Warnings section). Symptoms reported include: polyuria, nausea, vomiting, weakness, lassitude, fever, flushed face, and hyperactive deep tendon reflexes. If hypotension occurs, it may be treated with pressor agents such as levarterenol to maintain blood pressure. Carefully evaluate the electrolyte pattern and fluid balance. Induce immediate evacuation of the stomach through emesis or gastric lavage. There is no specific antidote.
Although triamterene is largely protein-bound (approximately 67%), there may be some benefit to dialysis in cases of overdosage.

HOW SUPPLIED

Capsules containing 25 mg. hydrochlorothiazide and 50 mg. triamterene, in bottles of 1000 capsules; in Single Unit Packages (unit-dose) of 100 (intended for institutional use only); in Patient-Pak™ unit-of-use bottles of 100.
Military—Capsules, 1000's, 6505-00-901-0043; 100's, 6505-00-901-0024; 100's (SUP), 6505-00-524-7060.
Veterans Administration—Capsules, 100's, 6505-00-901-0024A; 1000's, 6505-00-901-0043A; 100's (SUP), 6505-00-524-7060A.

DZ:L42

Shown in Product Identification Section, page 430

DYRENIUM® ℞

[di-ren 'ee-um]
(brand of triamterene)

('Dyrenium' is a product of SK&F Co., Carolina, P.R. 00630, Subsidiary of SmithKline Beckman Corporation, Philadelphia, Pa.)

DESCRIPTION

Dyrenium (triamterene, SK&F CO.) is a potassium-conserving diuretic.
Triamterene is 2,4,7-triamino-6-phenylpteridine. Its molecular weight is 253.27. At 50°C., triamterene is slightly soluble in water. It is soluble in dilute ammonia, dilute aqueous sodium hydroxide and dimethylformamide. It is sparingly soluble in methanol.
Each capsule, with opaque red cap and body, contains triamterene, 50 or 100 mg., and is imprinted with the product name DYRENIUM, strength (50 or 100) and SKF. Inactive ingredients consist of benzyl alcohol, cetylpyridinium chloride, D&C Red No. 33, FD&C Yellow No. 6, gelatin, lactose, magnesium stearate, povidone, sodium lauryl sulfate, titanium dioxide and trace amounts of other inactive ingredients.

CLINICAL PHARMACOLOGY

Triamterene has a unique mode of action; it inhibits the reabsorption of sodium ions in exchange for potassium and hydrogen ions at that segment of the distal tubule under the control of adrenal mineralocorticoids (especially aldosterone). This activity is not directly related to aldosterone secretion or antagonism; it is a result of a direct effect on the renal tubule.
The fraction of filtered sodium reaching this distal tubular exchange site is relatively small, and the amount which is exchanged depends on the level of mineralocorticoid activity. Thus, the degree of natriuresis and diuresis produced by inhibition of the exchange mechanism is necessarily limited. Increasing the amount of available sodium and the level of mineralocorticoid activity by the use of more proximally acting diuretics will increase the degree of diuresis and potassium conservation.
Triamterene occasionally causes increases in serum potassium which can result in hyperkalemia. It does not produce alkalosis because it does not cause excessive excretion of titratable acid and ammonium.
Triamterene has been shown to cross the placental barrier and appear in the cord blood of animals.

Pharmacokinetics

Onset of action is two to four hours after ingestion. In normal volunteers the mean peak serum levels were 30 ng./ml. at three hours. The average percent of drug recovered in the urine (0–48 hours) was 21%. Triamterene is primarily metabolized to the sulfate conjugate of hydroxytriamterene. Both the plasma and urine levels of this metabolite greatly exceed triamterene levels. Triamterene is rapidly absorbed, with somewhat less than 50% of the oral dose reaching the urine. Most patients will respond to Dyrenium (triamterene, SK&F CO.) during the first day of treatment. Maximum therapeutic effect, however, may not be seen for several days. Duration of diuresis depends on several factors, especially renal function, but it generally tapers off seven to nine hours after administration.

INDICATIONS AND USAGE

Dyrenium (triamterene, SK&F CO.) is indicated in the treatment of edema associated with congestive heart failure, cirrhosis of the liver, and the nephrotic syndrome; also in steroid-induced edema, idiopathic edema, and edema due to secondary hyperaldosteronism.
'Dyrenium' may be used alone or with other diuretics either for its added diuretic effect or its potassium-conserving potential. It also promotes increased diuresis when patients

Continued on next page

Smith Kline & French—Cont.

prove resistant or only partially responsive to thiazides or other diuretics because of secondary hyperaldosteronism.

Usage in Pregnancy. The routine use of diuretics in an otherwise healthy woman is inappropriate and exposes mother and fetus to unnecessary hazard. Diuretics do not prevent development of toxemia of pregnancy, and there is no satisfactory evidence that they are useful in the treatment of developed toxemia.

Edema during pregnancy may arise from pathological causes or from the physiologic and mechanical consequences of pregnancy. Diuretics are indicated in pregnancy when edema is due to pathologic causes, just as they are in the absence of pregnancy (however, see Precautions below). Dependent edema in pregnancy, resulting from restriction of venous return by the expanded uterus, is properly treated through elevation of the lower extremities and use of support hose; use of diuretics to lower intravascular volume in this case is illogical and unnecessary. There is hypervolemia during normal pregnancy which is harmful to neither the fetus nor the mother (in the absence of cardiovascular disease), but which is associated with edema, including generalized edema, in the majority of pregnant women. If this edema produces discomfort, increased recumbency will often provide relief. In rare instances, this edema may cause extreme discomfort which is not relieved by rest. In these cases, a short course of diuretics may provide relief and may be appropriate.

CONTRAINDICATIONS

Anuria. Severe or progressive kidney disease or dysfunction with the possible exception of nephrosis. Severe hepatic disease. Hypersensitivity to the drug.

Dyrenium (triamterene, SK&F CO.) should not be used in patients with preexisting elevated serum potassium, as is sometimes seen in patients with impaired renal function or azotemia, or in patients who develop hyperkalemia while on the drug. Patients should not be placed on dietary potassium supplements, potassium salts, or potassium-containing salt substitutes in conjunction with 'Dyrenium'.

'Dyrenium' should not be given to patients receiving other potassium-conserving agents such as spironolactone, amiloride hydrochloride, or other formulations containing triamterene. Two deaths have been reported in patients receiving concomitant spironolactone and 'Dyrenium' or Dyazide®. Although dosage recommendations were exceeded in one case and in the other serum electrolytes were not properly monitored, these two drugs should not be given concomitantly.

WARNINGS

There have been isolated reports of hypersensitivity reactions; therefore, patients should be observed regularly for the possible occurrence of blood dyscrasias, liver damage, or other idiosyncratic reactions.

Periodic BUN and serum potassium determinations should be made to check kidney function, especially in patients with suspected or confirmed renal insufficiency. It is particularly important to make serum potassium determinations in elderly or diabetic patients receiving the drug; these patients should be observed carefully for possible serum potassium increases.

If hyperkalemia is present or suspected, an electrocardiogram should be obtained. If the ECG shows no widening of the QRS or arrhythmia in the presence of hyperkalemia, it is usually sufficient to discontinue Dyrenium (triamterene, SK&F CO.) and any potassium supplementation and substitute a thiazide alone. Sodium polystyrene sulfonate (Kayexalate®, Winthrop) may be administered to enhance the excretion of excess potassium. **The presence of a widened QRS complex or arrhythmia in association with hyperkalemia requires prompt additional therapy.** For tachyarrhythmia, infuse 44 mEq. of sodium bicarbonate or 10 ml. of 10% calcium gluconate or calcium chloride over several minutes. For asystole, bradycardia, or A-V block transvenous pacing is also recommended.

The effect of calcium and sodium bicarbonate is transient and repeated administration may be required. When indicated by the clinical situation, excess K^+ may be removed by dialysis or oral or rectal administration of Kayexalate®. Infusion of glucose and insulin has also been used to treat hyperkalemia.

PRECAUTIONS

General

Dyrenium (triamterene, SK&F CO.) tends to conserve potassium rather than to promote the excretion as do many diuretics and, occasionally, can cause increases in serum potassium which, in some instances, can result in hyperkalemia. In rare instances, hyperkalemia has been associated with cardiac irregularities.

Electrolyte imbalance often encountered in such diseases as congestive heart failure, renal disease, or cirrhosis may be aggravated or caused independently by any effective diuretic agent including 'Dyrenium'. The use of full doses of a diuretic when salt intake is restricted can result in a low-salt syndrome.

Triamterene can cause mild nitrogen retention which is reversible upon withdrawal of the drug and is seldom observed with intermittent (every-other-day) therapy.

Triamterene may cause a decreasing alkali reserve with the possibility of metabolic acidosis.

By the very nature of their illness, cirrhotics with splenomegaly sometimes have marked variations in their blood pictures. Since triamterene is a weak folic acid antagonist, it may contribute to the appearance of megaloblastosis in cases where folic acid stores have been depleted. Therefore, periodic blood studies in these patients are recommended. They should also be observed for exacerbations of underlying liver disease.

Triamterene has elevated uric acid, especially in persons predisposed to gouty arthritis.

Triamterene has been reported in renal stones in association with other calculus components. 'Dyrenium' should be used with caution in patients with histories of renal stones.

Information for Patients

To help avoid stomach upset, it is recommended that the drug be taken after meals.

If a single daily dose is prescribed, it may be preferable to take it in the morning to minimize the effect of increased frequency of urination on nighttime sleep.

If a dose is missed, the patient should not take more than the prescribed dose at the next dosing interval.

Laboratory Tests

Hyperkalemia will rarely occur in patients with adequate urinary output, but it is a possibility if large doses are used for considerable periods of time. If hyperkalemia is observed, Dyrenium (triamterene, SK&F CO.) should be withdrawn. The normal adult range of serum potassium is 3.5 to 5.0 mEq. per liter with 4.5 mEq. often being used for a reference point. Potassium levels persistently above 6 mEq. per liter require careful observation and treatment. Normal potassium levels tend to be higher in neonates (7.7 mEq. per liter) than in adults.

Serum potassium levels do not necessarily indicate true body potassium concentration. A rise in plasma pH may cause a decrease in plasma potassium concentration and an increase in the intracellular potassium concentration. Because 'Dyrenium' conserves potassium, it has been theorized that in patients who have received intensive therapy or been given the drug for prolonged periods, a rebound kaliuresis could occur upon abrupt withdrawal. In such patients withdrawal of 'Dyrenium' should be gradual.

Drug Interactions

Caution should be used when lithium and diuretics are used concomitantly because diuretic-induced sodium loss may reduce the renal clearance of lithium and increase serum lithium levels with risk of lithium toxicity. Patients receiving such combined therapy should have serum lithium levels monitored closely and the lithium dosage adjusted if necessary.

A possible interaction resulting in acute renal failure has been reported in a few subjects when indomethacin, a nonsteroidal anti-inflammatory agent, was given with triamterene. Caution is advised in administering nonsteroidal anti-inflammatory agents with triamterene.

The effects of the following drugs may be potentiated when given together with triamterene: antihypertensive medication, other diuretics, preanesthetic and anesthetic agents, skeletal muscle relaxants (nondepolarizing).

The following agents, given together with triamterene, may promote serum potassium accumulation and possibly result in hyperkalemia because of the potassium-sparing nature of triamterene, especially in patients with renal insufficiency: blood from blood bank (may contain up to 30 mEq. of potassium per liter of plasma or up to 65 mEq. per liter of whole blood when stored for more than 10 days); low-salt milk (may contain up to 60 mEq. of potassium per liter); potassium-containing medications (such as parenteral penicillin G potassium); salt substitutes (most contain substantial amounts of potassium).

Dyrenium (triamterene, SK&F CO.) may raise blood glucose levels; for adult-onset diabetes, dosage adjustments of hypoglycemic agents may be necessary during and after therapy; concurrent use with chlorpropamide may increase the risk of severe hyponatremia.

Drug/Laboratory Test Interactions

Triamterene and quinidine have similar fluorescence spectra; thus, triamterene will interfere with the fluorescent measurement of quinidine.

Carcinogenesis, Mutagenesis, Impairment of Fertility

Long-term studies to determine the carcinogenic potential of triamterene are not available. Studies to determine the mutagenic potential of triamterene are not available. Reproductive studies have been performed in rats at doses up to 30 times the human dose and have revealed no evidence of impaired fertility.

Pregnancy

Teratogenic Effects: Pregnancy Category B. Reproduction studies have been performed in rats at doses up to 30 times the human dose and have revealed no evidence of impaired fertility or harm to the fetus due to triamterene. There are, however, no adequate and well-controlled studies in pregnant women. Because animal reproductive studies are not always predictive of human reponse, this drug should be used during pregnancy only if clearly needed.

Nonteratogenic Effects: Triamterene has been shown to cross the placental barrier and appear in the cord blood of animals; this may occur in humans. The use of 'Dyrenium' in pregnant women requires that the anticipated benefit be weighed against possible hazards to the fetus. These possible hazards include adverse reactions which have occurred in the adult.

Nursing Mothers: Triamterene appears in animal milk; this may occur in humans. If use of the drug is deemed essential, the patient should stop nursing.

Pediatric Use: Safety and effectiveness in children have not been established.

ADVERSE REACTIONS

Adverse effects are listed in decreasing order of frequency; however, the most serious adverse effects are listed first regardless of frequency. All adverse effects occur rarely (that is, one in 1000, or less).

Hypersensitivity: anaphylaxis, rash, photosensitivity.
Metabolic: hyperkalemia, hypokalemia.
Renal: azotemia, elevated BUN and creatinine, renal stones, acute interstitial nephritis (rare).
Gastrointestinal: jaundice and/or liver enzyme abnormalities, nausea and vomiting, diarrhea.
Hematologic: thrombocytopenia, megaloblastic anemia.
Central Nervous System: weakness, fatigue, dizziness, headache, dry mouth.

OVERDOSAGE

In the event of overdosage it can be theorized that electrolyte imbalance would be the major concern, with particular attention to possible hyperkalemia. Other symptoms that might be seen would be nausea and vomiting, other g.i. disturbances, and weakness. It is conceivable that some hypotension could occur. As with an overdose of any drug, immediate evacuation of the stomach should be induced through emesis and gastric lavage. Careful evaluation of the electrolyte pattern and fluid balance should be made. There is no specific antidote.

The oral LD_{50} in mice is 380 mg./kg. The amount of drug in a single dose ordinarily associated with symptoms of overdose or likely to be life-threatening is not known.

Although triamterene is 67% protein-bound, there may be some benefit to dialysis in cases of overdosage.

DOSAGE AND ADMINISTRATION

Adult Dosage

Dosage should be titrated to the needs of the individual patient. When used alone, the usual starting dose is 100 mg. twice daily after meals. When combined with another diuretic or antihypertensive agent, the total daily dosage of each agent should usually be lowered initially and then adjusted to the patient's needs. The total daily dosage should not exceed 300 mg. Please refer to Precautions—General.

When Dyrenium (triamterene, SK&F CO.) is added to other diuretic therapy or when patients are switched to 'Dyrenium' from other diuretics, all potassium supplementation should be discontinued.

HOW SUPPLIED

Capsules: 50 mg. in bottles of 100 and in Single Unit Packages of 100 (intended for institutional use only); 100 mg. in bottles of 100 and 1000 and in Single Unit Packages of 100 (intended for institutional use only).

DY:L31

Shown in Product Identification Section, page 430

ESKALITH® ℞

[ess-kah 'lith]
(brand of lithium carbonate)
Capsules, 300 mg.
Tablets, 300 mg.

ESKALITH CR® ℞

(brand of lithium carbonate)
Controlled Release Tablets, 450 mg.

WARNING

Lithium toxicity is closely related to serum lithium levels, and can occur at doses close to therapeutic levels. Facilities for prompt and accurate serum lithium determinations should be available before initiating therapy (see DOSAGE AND ADMINISTRATION).

DESCRIPTION

'Eskalith' contains lithium carbonate, a white, light alkaline powder with molecular formula Li_2CO_3 and molecular weight 73.89. Lithium is an element of the alkali-metal group with atomic number 3, atomic weight 6.94 and an emission line at 671 nm on the flame photometer.

'Eskalith' Capsules: Each capsule, with opaque gray cap and opaque yellow body, is imprinted with the product name ESKALITH and SKF and contains lithium carbonate, 300 mg. Inactive ingredients consist of benzyl alcohol, cetylpyridinium chloride, D&C Yellow No. 10, FD&C Green No. 3, FD&C Red No. 40, FD&C Yellow No. 6, gelatin, lactose, magnesium stearate, povidone, sodium lauryl sulfate, titanium dioxide and trace amounts of other inactive ingredients.
'Eskalith' Tablets: Each round, gray, scored tablet is debossed SKF and J09 and contains lithium carbonate, 300 mg. Inactive ingredients consist of cellulose, iron oxide, lactose, magnesium stearate and sodium lauryl sulfate.
'Eskalith CR' Controlled Release Tablets: Each round, buff, scored tablet is debossed SKF and J10 and contains lithium carbonate, 450 mg. Inactive ingredients consist of alginic acid, gelatin, iron oxide, magnesium stearate and sodium starch glycolate.
'Eskalith CR' tablets 450 mg. are designed to release a portion of the dose initially and the remainder gradually; the release pattern of the controlled release tablets reduces the variability in lithium blood levels seen with the immediate release dosage forms.

ACTIONS

Preclinical studies have shown that lithium alters sodium transport in nerve and muscle cells and effects a shift toward intraneuronal metabolism of catecholamines, but the specific biochemical mechanism of lithium action in mania is unknown.

INDICATIONS

Eskalith (lithium carbonate, SK&F) is indicated in the treatment of manic episodes of manic-depressive illness. Maintenance therapy prevents or diminishes the intensity of subsequent episodes in those manic-depressive patients with a history of mania.
Typical symptoms of mania include pressure of speech, motor hyperactivity, reduced need for sleep, flight of ideas, grandiosity, elation, poor judgment, aggressiveness, and possibly hostility. When given to a patient experiencing a manic episode, 'Eskalith' may produce a normalization of symptomatology within 1 to 3 weeks.

WARNINGS

Lithium should generally not be given to patients with significant renal or cardiovascular disease, severe debilitation or dehydration, or sodium depletion, since the risk of lithium toxicity is very high in such patients. If the psychiatric indication is life-threatening, and if such a patient fails to respond to other measures, lithium treatment may be undertaken with extreme caution, including daily serum lithium determinations and adjustment to the usually low doses ordinarily tolerated by these individuals. In such instances, hospitalization is a necessity.
Chronic lithium therapy may be associated with diminution of renal concentrating ability, occasionally presenting as nephrogenic diabetes insipidus, with polyuria and polydipsia. Such patients should be carefully managed to avoid dehydration with resulting lithium retention and toxicity. This condition is usually reversible when lithium is discontinued.
Morphologic changes with glomerular and interstitial fibrosis and nephron atrophy have been reported in patients on chronic lithium therapy. Morphologic changes have also been seen in manic-depressive patients never exposed to lithium. The relationship between renal functional and morphologic changes and their association with lithium therapy have not been established.
When kidney function is assessed, for baseline data prior to starting lithium therapy or thereafter, routine urinalysis and other tests may be used to evaluate tubular function (e.g., urine specific gravity or osmolality following a period of water deprivation, or 24-hour urine volume) and glomerular function (e.g., serum creatinine or creatinine clearance). During lithium therapy, progressive or sudden changes in renal function, even within the normal range, indicate the need for reevaluation of treatment.
An encephalopathic syndrome (characterized by weakness, lethargy, fever, tremulousness and confusion, extrapyramidal symptoms, leukocytosis, elevated serum enzymes, BUN and FBS) followed by irreversible brain damage has occurred in a few patients treated with lithium plus haloperidol. A causal relationship between these events and the concomitant administration of lithium and haloperidol has not been established; however, patients receiving such combined therapy should be monitored closely for early evidence of neurologic toxicity and treatment discontinued promptly if such signs appear. The possibility of similar adverse interactions with other antipsychotic medication exists.
Lithium toxicity is closely related to serum lithium levels, and can occur at doses close to therapeutic levels (see DOSAGE AND ADMINISTRATION).
Outpatients and their families should be warned that the patient must discontinue lithium carbonate therapy and contact his physician if such clinical signs of lithium toxicity as diarrhea, vomiting, tremor, mild ataxia, drowsiness, or muscular weakness occur.
Lithium carbonate may impair mental and/or physical abilities. Caution patients about activities requiring alertness (e.g., operating vehicles or machinery).
Lithium may prolong the effects of neuromuscular blocking agents. Therefore, neuromuscular blocking agents should be given with caution to patients receiving lithium.
Usage in Pregnancy: Adverse effects on implantation in rats, embryo viability in mice, and metabolism *in vitro* of rat testes and human spermatozoa have been attributed to lithium, as have teratogenicity in submammalian species and cleft palates in mice.
In humans, lithium carbonate may cause fetal harm when administered to a pregnant woman. Data from lithium birth registries suggest an increase in cardiac and other anomalies, especially Ebstein's anomaly. If this drug is used during pregnancy, or if a patient becomes pregnant while taking this drug, the patient should be apprised of the potential hazard to the fetus.
Usage in Nursing Mothers: Lithium is excreted in human milk. Nursing should not be undertaken during lithium therapy except in rare and unusual circumstances where, in the view of the physician, the potential benefits to the mother outweigh possible hazards to the child.
Usage in Children: Since information regarding the safety and effectiveness of lithium carbonate in children under 12 years of age is not available, its use in such patients is not recommended at this time.

PRECAUTIONS

The ability to tolerate lithium is greater during the acute manic phase and decreases when manic symptoms subside (see DOSAGE AND ADMINISTRATION).
Caution should be used when lithium and diuretics are used concomitantly because diuretic-induced sodium loss may reduce the renal clearance of lithium and increase serum lithium levels with risk of lithium toxicity. Patients receiving such combined therapy should have serum lithium levels monitored closely and the lithium dosage adjusted if necessary.
The distribution space of lithium approximates that of total body water. Lithium is primarily excreted in urine with insignificant excretion in feces. Renal excretion of lithium is proportional to its plasma concentration. The half-life of elimination of lithium is approximately 24 hours. Lithium decreases sodium reabsorption by the renal tubules which could lead to sodium depletion. Therefore, it is essential for the patient to maintain a normal diet, including salt, and an adequate fluid intake (2500–3000 ml.) at least during the initial stabilization period. Decreased tolerance to lithium has been reported to ensue from protracted sweating or diarrhea and, if such occur, supplemental fluid and salt should be administered under careful medical supervision and lithium intake reduced or suspended until the condition is resolved.
In addition to sweating and diarrhea, concomitant infection with elevated temperatures may also necessitate a temporary reduction or cessation of medication.
Previously existing underlying thyroid disorders do not necessarily constitute a contraindication to lithium treatment; where hypothyroidism exists, careful monitoring of thyroid function during lithium stabilization and maintenance allows for correction of changing thyroid parameters, if any; where hypothyroidism occurs during lithium stabilization and maintenance, supplemental thyroid treatment may be used.
Indomethacin has been reported to increase steady state plasma lithium levels from 30 to 59 percent. There is also some evidence that other nonsteroidal anti-inflammatory agents may have a similar effect. When such combinations are used, increased plasma lithium level monitoring is recommended.

ADVERSE REACTIONS

Adverse reactions are seldom encountered at serum lithium levels below 1.5 mEq./l., except in the occasional patient unusually sensitive to lithium. Mild to moderate toxic reactions may occur at levels from 1.5 to 2.5 mEq./l., and moderate to severe reactions may be seen at levels from 2.0 to 2.5 mEq./l., depending upon the individual response to the drug.
Fine hand tremor, polyuria, and mild thirst may occur during initial therapy for the acute manic phase, and may persist throughout treatment. Transient and mild nausea and general discomfort may also appear during the first few days of lithium administration.
These side effects are an inconvenience rather than a disabling condition, and usually subside with continued treatment or a temporary reduction or cessation of dosage. If persistent, a cessation of dosage is indicated.
Diarrhea, vomiting, drowsiness, muscular weakness, and lack of coordination may be early signs of lithium intoxication, and can occur at lithium levels below 2.0 mEq./l. At higher levels, ataxia, giddiness, tinnitus, blurred vision, and a large output of dilute urine may be seen. Serum lithium levels above 3.0 mEq./l. may produce a complex clinical picture, involving multiple organs and organ systems. Serum lithium levels should not be permitted to exceed 2.0 mEq./l. during the acute treatment phase.
The following reactions have been reported and appear to be related to serum lithium levels, including levels within the therapeutic range: **Neuromuscular/Central Nervous System**—tremor, muscle hyperirritability (fasciculations, twitching, clonic movements of whole limbs), hypertonicity, ataxia, choreo-athetotic movements, hyperactive deep tendon reflex, extrapyramidal symptoms, blackout spells, epileptiform seizures, slurred speech, dizziness, vertigo, incontinence of urine or feces, somnolence, psychomotor retardation, restlessness, confusion, stupor, coma, tongue movements, tics, tinnitus, hallucinations, poor memory, slowed intellectual functioning, startled response, worsening of organic brain syndromes; **Cardiovascular**—cardiac arrhythmia, hypotension, peripheral circulatory collapse, bradycardia, sinus node dysfunction with severe bradycardia (which may result in syncope); **Gastrointestinal**—anorexia, nausea, vomiting, diarrhea, gastritis, salivary gland swelling, abdominal pain, excessive salivation, flatulence, indigestion; **Genitourinary**—albuminuria, oliguria, polyuria with thirst, sometimes resembling diabetes insipidus, glycosuria, decreased creatinine clearance; **Dermatologic**—drying and thinning of hair, alopecia, anesthesia of skin, chronic folliculitis, xerosis cutis, psoriasis or its exacerbation, generalized pruritus with or without rash, cutaneous ulcers, angioedema; **Autonomic**—blurred vision, dry mouth, impotence/sexual dysfunction; **Thyroid Abnormalities**—euthyroid goiter and/or hypothyroidism (including myxedema) accompanied by lower T_3 and T_4. I^{131} uptake may be elevated. (See Precautions.) Paradoxically, rare cases of hyperthyroidism have been reported; **EEG Changes**—diffuse slowing, widening of the frequency spectrum, potentiation and disorganization of background rhythm; **EKG Changes**—reversible flattening, isoelectricity or inversion of T-waves; **Miscellaneous**—fatigue, lethargy, transient scotomata, dehydration, weight loss, leukocytosis, headache, transient hyperglycemia, hypercalcemia, hyperparathyroidism, excessive weight gain, edematous swelling of ankles or wrists, metallic taste, dysgeusia/taste distortion, salty taste, swollen lips, tightness in chest, swollen and/or painful joints, fever, polyarthralgia, dental caries.
A few reports have been received of the development of painful discoloration of fingers and toes and coldness of the extremities within one day of the starting of treatment with lithium. The mechanism through which these symptoms (resembling Raynaud's syndrome) developed is not known. Recovery followed discontinuance.
Cases of pseudotumor cerebri (increased intracranial pressure and papilledema) have been reported with lithium use. If undetected, this condition may result in enlargement of the blind spot, constriction of visual fields and eventual blindness due to optic atrophy.
Lithium should be discontinued, if clinically possible, if this syndrome occurs.

DOSAGE AND ADMINISTRATION

Immediate release capsules and tablets are usually given t.i.d. or q.i.d. Doses of controlled release tablets are usually given b.i.d. (approximately 12-hour intervals). When initiating therapy with immediate release or controlled release lithium, dosage must be individualized according to serum levels and clinical response.
When switching a patient from immediate release capsules or tablets to the Eskalith CR (lithium carbonate, SK&F) Controlled Release Tablets, give the same total daily dose when possible. Most patients on maintenance therapy are stabilized on 900 mg. daily, e.g., 450 mg. 'Eskalith CR' b.i.d. When the previous dosage of immediate release lithium is not a multiple of 450 mg., for example, 1500 mg., initiate 'Eskalith CR' dosage at the multiple of 450 mg. nearest to, but *below*, the original daily dose, i.e., 1350 mg. When the two doses are unequal, give the larger dose in the evening. In the above example, with a total daily dosage of 1350 mg., generally 450 mg. 'Eskalith CR' should be given in the morning and 900 mg. 'Eskalith CR' in the evening. If desired, the total daily dosage of 1350 mg. can be given in three equal 450 mg. 'Eskalith CR' doses. These patients should be monitored at 1–2 week intervals, and dosage adjusted if necessary, until stable and satisfactory serum levels and clinical state are achieved.
When patients require closer titration than that available with 'Eskalith CR' doses in increments of 450 mg., immediate release capsules or tablets should be used.
Acute Mania—Optimal patient response to Eskalith (lithium carbonate, SK&F) can usually be established and maintained with 1800 mg. per day in divided doses. Such doses will normally produce the desired serum lithium level ranging between 1.0 and 1.5 mEq./l.
Dosage must be individualized according to serum levels and clinical response. Regular monitoring of the patient's clinical state and serum lithium levels is necessary. Serum levels should be determined twice per week during the acute phase, and until the serum level and clinical condition of the patient have been stabilized.
Long-Term Control—The desirable serum lithium levels are 0.6 to 1.2 mEq./l. Dosage will vary from one individual to

Continued on next page

Smith Kline & French—Cont.

another, but usually 900 mg. to 1200 mg. per day in divided doses will maintain this level. Serum lithium levels in uncomplicated cases receiving maintenance therapy during remission should be monitored at least every two months.
Patients abnormally sensitive to lithium may exhibit toxic signs at serum levels of 1.0 to 1.5 mEq./l. Elderly patients often respond to reduced dosage, and may exhibit signs of toxicity at serum levels ordinarily tolerated by other patients.
N.B.: Blood samples for serum lithium determinations should be drawn immediately prior to the next dose when lithium concentrations are relatively stable (i.e., 8–12 hours after the previous dose). Total reliance must not be placed on serum levels alone. Accurate patient evaluation requires both clinical and laboratory analysis.

OVERDOSAGE

The toxic levels for lithium are close to the therapeutic levels. It is therefore important that patients and their families be cautioned to watch for early toxic symptoms and to discontinue the drug and inform the physician should they occur. Toxic symptoms are listed in detail under ADVERSE REACTIONS.

Treatment

No specific antidote for lithium poisoning is known. Early symptoms of lithium toxicity can usually be treated by reduction or cessation of dosage of the drug and resumption of the treatment at a lower dose after 24 to 48 hours. In severe cases of lithium poisoning, the first and foremost goal of treatment consists of elimination of this ion from the patient. Treatment is essentially the same as that used in barbiturate poisoning: 1) gastric lavage, 2) correction of fluid and electrolyte imbalance, and 3) regulation of kidney function. Urea, mannitol, and aminophylline all produce significant increases in lithium excretion. Hemodialysis is an effective and rapid means of removing the ion from the severely toxic patient. Infection prophylaxis, regular chest X-rays, and preservation of adequate respiration are essential.

HOW SUPPLIED

Capsules containing 300 mg. lithium carbonate per capsule, in bottles of 100 and 500.
Tablets containing 300 mg. lithium carbonate per tablet, in bottles of 100.
Controlled Release Tablets containing 450 mg. lithium carbonate per tablet, in bottles of 100.

EL:L31

Shown in Product Identification Section, page 430

HISPRIL® ℞

[hiss 'prill]
(brand of diphenylpyraline hydrochloride)
SPANSULE® CAPSULES 5 mg.

DESCRIPTION

Hispril®, brand of diphenylpyraline HCl, is an antihistamine.
Each 'Spansule' capsule contains diphenylpyraline hydrochloride, 5 mg., so prepared that an initial dose is released promptly and the remaining medication is released gradually over a prolonged period.

ACTIONS

Diphenylpyraline hydrochloride is an antihistamine with anticholinergic (drying) and sedative side effects. Antihistamines appear to compete with histamine for cell receptor sites on effector cells.

INDICATIONS

For the symptomatic treatment of perennial and seasonal allergic rhinitis; vasomotor rhinitis; allergic conjunctivitis due to inhalant allergens and foods; mild, uncomplicated allergic skin manifestations of urticaria and angioedema; amelioration of allergic reactions to blood or plasma; dermographism; and as therapy for anaphylactic reactions adjunctive to epinephrine and other standard measures after the acute manifestations have been controlled.

CONTRAINDICATIONS

Use in Newborn or Premature Infants—This drug should *not* be used in newborn or premature infants.
Use in Nursing Mothers—Because of the higher risk of antihistamines for infants generally and for newborns and prematures in particular, antihistamine therapy is contraindicated in nursing mothers.
Use in Lower Respiratory Disease—Antihistamines *should NOT* be used to treat lower respiratory tract symptoms including asthma.
Antihistamines are also contraindicated in the following conditions:

Hypersensitivity to diphenylpyraline hydrochloride and other antihistamines of similar chemical structure
Monoamine oxidase inhibitor therapy (See Drug Interactions section)

WARNINGS

Antihistamines should be used with considerable caution in patients with:

Narrow angle glaucoma
Stenosing peptic ulcer
Pyloroduodenal obstruction
Symptomatic prostatic hypertrophy
Bladder neck obstruction

Use in Children—In infants and children, especially, antihistamines in *overdosage* may cause hallucinations, convulsions, or death.
As in adults, antihistamines may diminish mental alertness in children. In the young child, particularly, they may produce excitation.
Use in Pregnancy—Experience with this drug in pregnant women is inadequate to determine whether there exists a potential for harm to the developing fetus.
Use with CNS Depressants—Diphenylpyraline hydrochloride has additive effects with alcohol and other CNS depressants (hypnotics, sedatives, tranquilizers, etc.).
Use in Activities Requiring Mental Alertness—Patients should be warned about engaging in activities requiring mental alertness as driving a car or operating appliances, machinery, etc.
Use in the Elderly (approximately 60 years or older)—Antihistamines are more likely to cause dizziness, sedation, and hypotension in the elderly than in younger patients.

PRECAUTIONS

Diphenylpyraline hydrochloride has an atropine-like action and, therefore, should be used with caution in patients with:

History of bronchial asthma
Increased intraocular pressure
Hyperthyroidism
Cardiovascular disease
Hypertension

Drug Interactions—MAO inhibitors prolong and intensify the anticholinergic (drying) effects of antihistamines.

ADVERSE REACTIONS

The most frequent adverse reactions are underlined:

1. **General:** Urticaria, drug rash, anaphylactic shock, photosensitivity, excessive perspiration, chills, dryness of mouth, nose, and throat.
2. **Cardiovascular System:** Hypotension, headache, palpitations, tachycardia, extrasystoles.
3. **Hematologic System:** Hemolytic anemia, thrombocytopenia, agranulocytosis.
4. **Nervous System:** <u>Sedation,</u> <u>sleepiness,</u> <u>dizziness,</u> <u>disturbed</u> <u>coordination,</u> fatigue, confusion, restlessness, excitation, nervousness, tremor, irritability, insomnia, euphoria, paresthesias, blurred vision, diplopia, vertigo, tinnitus, acute labyrinthitis, hysteria, neuritis, convulsions.
5. **G.I. System:** <u>Epigastric</u> <u>distress,</u> anorexia, nausea, vomiting, diarrhea, constipation.
6. **G.U. System:** Urinary frequency, difficult urination, urinary retention, early menses.
7. **Respiratory System:** <u>Thickening</u> <u>of</u> <u>bronchial</u> <u>secretions,</u> tightness of chest and wheezing, nasal stuffiness.

OVERDOSAGE

Antihistamine overdosage reactions may vary from central nervous system depression to stimulation. Stimulation is particularly likely in children. Atropine-like signs and symptoms—dry mouth; fixed, dilated pupils; flushing; and gastrointestinal symptoms may also occur. Marked cerebral irritation, resulting in jerking of muscles and possible convulsions, may be followed by deep stupor.
If vomiting has not occurred spontaneously the patient should be induced to vomit. This is best done by having him drink a glass of water or milk after which he should be made to gag. Precautions against aspiration must be taken, especially in infants and children.
If vomiting is unsuccessful gastric lavage is indicated within 3 hours after ingestion and even later if large amounts of milk or cream were given beforehand. Isotonic and ½ isotonic saline is the lavage solution of choice.
Saline cathartics, as milk of magnesia, by osmosis draw water into the bowel and therefore are valuable for their action in rapid dilution of bowel content.
Do not treat CNS depression with analeptics which might precipitate convulsions. Use only short-acting depressants to treat convulsions.
Stimulants should *not* be used.
If a vasoconstrictor is required for hypotension, levarterenol bitartrate, USP, may be used. Other pressor agents, including epinephrine, should not be used as they may cause a paradoxical further lowering of blood pressure.
Special note on 'Spansule' capsules—Since much of the 'Spansule' capsule medication is coated for gradual release, therapy directed at reversing the effects of the ingested drug and at supporting the patient should be continued for as long as overdosage symptoms remain. Saline cathartics are useful for hastening evacuation of pellets that have not already released medication.

DOSAGE AND ADMINISTRATION

DOSAGE SHOULD BE INDIVIDUALIZED ACCORDING TO THE NEEDS AND THE RESPONSE OF THE PATIENT.
Adults—One capsule (5 mg.), q12h.
Older Children (6–12 years)—One 5 mg. capsule daily is usually sufficient. The physician should bear in mind that in children a higher incidence and a greater degree of antihistaminic side effects may be encountered. Do not use in children under 6 years.

HOW SUPPLIED

Bottles of 50 capsules.

HI:L18

Shown in Product Identification Section, page 430

MONOCID® ℞

[mon 'oh-sid]
brand of sterile cefonicid sodium

PRODUCT OVERVIEW

KEY FACTS

'Monocid' is a sterile, lyophilized, semisynthetic, broad-spectrum cephalosporin antibiotic for parenteral (I.V., I.M.) administration. The 4.5 hour serum half-life of 'Monocid', combined with therapeutic serum and tissue levels, allows dosing once daily (every 24 hours).

MAJOR USES

'Monocid' is indicated in the treatment of infections due to susceptible strains of the microorganisms listed below in the full prescribing information. In particular, 'Monocid' has been proven to be clinically effective in lower respiratory tract infections, including ampicillin-sensitive and ampicillin-resistant *H. influenzae*, and as single-dose prophylaxis in surgical procedures classified as contaminated or potentially contaminated.

SAFETY INFORMATION

'Monocid' is contraindicated in patients who have shown hypersensitivity to cefonicid, penicillin, or the cephalosporin group of antibiotics. Careful inquiry should be made concerning previous hypersensitivity reactions to drugs. 'Monocid' should be administered with caution to penicillin-sensitive patients. Serious acute hypersensitivity reactions may require epinephrine and other emergency measures. Because pseudomembranous colitis has been reported with the use of cephalosporins, it is important to consider its diagnosis in patients who develop diarrhea in association with antibiotic use.

PRESCRIBING INFORMATION

MONOCID® ℞

[mon 'oh-sid]
brand of sterile cefonicid sodium
(lyophilized)

DESCRIPTION

Monocid (sterile cefonicid sodium, SK&F), a sterile, lyophilized, semisynthetic, broad-spectrum cephalosporin antibiotic for intravenous and intramuscular administration, is 5-Thia-1-azabicyclo [4.2.0] oct-2-ene-2-carboxylic acid, 7-[(hydroxyphenylacetyl)-amino]-8-oxo-3-[[[1-(sulfomethyl)-1*H*-tetrazol-5-yl]thio] methyl]-disodium salt, [6*R*-[6α, 7β(*R* *)]]. Cefonicid sodium contains 85 mg. (3.7 mEq.) sodium per gram of cefonicid activity.

CLINICAL PHARMACOLOGY

Human Pharmacology

The table below demonstrates the levels and duration of Monocid (sterile cefonicid sodium, SK&F) in serum following intravenous and intramuscular administration of 1 gram to normal volunteers.
[See table left].

Serum Concentrations After 1 Gram Administration (mcg./ml.)

Interval	5 min.	15 min.	30 min.	1 hr.	2 hr.	4 hr.	6 hr.	8 hr.	10 hr.	12 hr.	24 hr.
I.V.	221.3	176.4	147.6	124.2	88.9	61.4	40.0	29.3	20.6	15.2	2.6
I.M.	13.5	45.9	73.1	98.6	97.1	77.8	54.9	38.5	28.9	20.6	4.5

Serum half-life is approximately 4.5 hours with intravenous and intramuscular administration. 'Monocid' is highly (greater than 90%) and reversibly protein bound.
'Monocid' is not metabolized; 99% is excreted unchanged in the urine in 24 hours. A 500 mg. I.M. dose provides a high

(384 mcg./ml.) urinary concentration at 6–8 hours. Probenecid, given concurrently with 'Monocid', slows renal excretion, produces higher peak serum levels and significantly increases the serum half-life of the drug (8.2 hours).
'Monocid' reaches therapeutic levels in the following tissues and fluids:
[See table right].
Note: Although 'Monocid' reaches therapeutic levels in bile, those levels are lower than those seen with other cephalosporins, and amounts of 'Monocid' released into the gastrointestinal tract are minute. This small amount of 'Monocid' in the gastrointestinal tract is thought to be the reason for the low incidence of gastrointestinal reactions following therapy with 'Monocid'.
No disulfiram-like reactions were reported in a crossover study conducted in healthy volunteers receiving 'Monocid' and alcohol.

Microbiology

The bactericidal action of Monocid (sterile cefonicid sodium, SK&F) results from inhibition of cell-wall synthesis. 'Monocid' is highly resistant to beta-lactamases produced by *Staphylococcus aureus, Hemophilus influenzae, Neisseria gonorrhoeae* and Richmond type I beta-lactamases. 'Monocid' is resistant to degradation by beta-lactamases from certain members of *Enterobacteriaceae*. Active against a wide range of gram-positive and gram-negative organisms, 'Monocid' is usually active against the following organisms *in vitro* and in clinical situations:
Gram-Positive Aerobes: *Staphylococcus aureus* (beta-lactamase producing and non-beta-lactamase producing) and *S. epidermidis* (Note: Methicillin-resistant staphylococci are resistant to cephalosporins, including cefonicid.); *Streptococcus pneumoniae, S. pyogenes* (Group A beta-hemolytic *Streptococcus*), and *S. agalactiae* (Group B *Streptococcus*).
Gram-Negative Aerobes: *Escherichia coli; Klebsiella pneumoniae; Proteus mirabilis* (indole-negative *Proteus*); and *Hemophilus influenzae* (ampicillin-sensitive and -resistant).
In addition to the preceding, 'Monocid' is usually active against the following organisms *in vitro*, but the clinical significance of these data has not been established:
Gram-Negative Aerobes: *Klebsiella oxytoca; Providencia rettgerii* (formerly *Proteus rettgerii*); *Enterobacter aerogenes; Neisseria gonorrhoeae* (penicillin-sensitive and -resistant); *Citrobacter freundii* and *C. diversus.*
Gram-Positive Anaerobes: *Clostridium perfringens: Peptostreptococcus anaerobius; Peptococcus magnus; P. prevotii;* and *Propionibacterium acnes.*
Gram-Negative Anaerobes: *Fusobacterium nucleatum.*
'Monocid' is usually inactive *in vitro* against most strains of *Pseudomonas, Serratia, Enterococcus* and *Acinetobacter.* Most strains of *B. fragilis* are resistant.

Susceptibility Testing

Results from standardized single-disk susceptibility tests using a 30 mcg. 'Monocid' disk should be interpreted according to the following criteria:

Zones of 18 mm. or greater indicate that the tested organism is susceptible to 'Monocid' and is likely to respond to therapy.

Zones from 15 to 17 mm. indicate that the tested organism is of intermediate (moderate) susceptibility, and is likely to respond to therapy if a higher dosage is used or if the infection is confined to tissues and fluids in which high antibiotic levels are attained.

Zones of 14 mm. or less indicate that the organism is resistant.

Only the 'Monocid' disk should be used to determine susceptibility, since *in vitro* tests show that 'Monocid' has activity against certain strains not susceptible to other cephalosporins. The 'Monocid' disk should not be used for testing susceptibility to other cephalosporins.
A bacterial isolate may be considered susceptible if the MIC value for 'Monocid' is equal to or less than 8 mcg./ml. in accordance with NCCLS* guidelines. Organisms are considered resistant if the MIC is equal to or greater than 32 mcg./ml. For most organisms the MBC value for 'Monocid' is the same as the MIC value.
* National Committee for Clinical Laboratory Standards
The standardized quality control procedure requires use of control organisms. The 30 mcg. 'Monocid' disk should give the zone diameters listed below for the quality control strains.

Organism	ATCC	Zone Size Range
E. coli	25922	25–29 mm.
S. aureus	25923	22–28 mm.

INDICATIONS AND USAGE

Monocid (sterile cefonicid sodium, SK&F) is indicated in the treatment of infections due to susceptible strains of the microorganisms listed below:
LOWER RESPIRATORY TRACT INFECTIONS, due to *Streptococcus pneumoniae* (formerly *D. pneumoniae*); *Klebsiella pneumoniae; Escherichia coli;* and *Hemophilus influenzae* (ampicillin-resistant and ampicillin-sensitive).
URINARY TRACT INFECTIONS, due to *Escherichia coli; Proteus mirabilis* (indole-negative *Proteus*); and *Klebsiella pneumoniae.*

Tissue and Body Fluid Levels

Tissue or Body Fluid	Dosage and Route (No. of Patients Sampled)	Time of Sampling After Dose	Average Tissue or Fluid Levels (mcg./g. or/ml.)
Bone	1 g. I.M. (7)	60–90 min.	6.8
	1 g. I.V. (10)	44–99 min.	14.0
Gallbladder	1 g. I.M. (10)	60–70 min.	15.5
Bile	1 g. I.M. (10)	60–70 min.	7.5
Prostate	1 g. I.M. (10)	50–115 min.	13.0
Uterine Tissue	1 g. I.M. (6)	60–90 min.	17.5
Wound Fluid	1 g. I.M. (10)	60–75 min.	37.7
Purulent Wound	1 g. I.M. (9)	60 min.	11.5
Adipose Tissue	1 g. I.M. (5)	60 min.	4.0
Atrial Appendage	1 g. I.M. (7)	77–170 min.	7.5
	2 g. I.M. (7)	105–170 min.	8.7
	15 mg./kg. I.V. (10)	53–160 min.	15.4

SKIN AND SKIN STRUCTURE INFECTIONS, due to *Staphylococcus aureus* and *S. epidermidis; Streptococcus pyogenes* (Group A *Streptococcus*) and *S. agalactiae* (Group B *Streptococcus*).
SEPTICEMIA, due to *Streptococcus pneumoniae* (formerly *D. pneumoniae*) and *Escherichia coli.*
BONE AND JOINT INFECTIONS, due to *Staphylococcus aureus.*
SURGICAL PROPHYLAXIS
Administration of a single 1 gram dose of 'Monocid' before surgery may reduce the incidence of postoperative infections in patients undergoing surgical procedures classified as contaminated or potentially contaminated (e.g., colorectal surgery, vaginal hysterectomy, or cholecystectomy in high-risk patients), or in patients in whom infection at the operative site would present a serious risk (e.g., prosthetic arthroplasty, open heart surgery). Although cefonicid has been shown to be as effective as cefazolin in prevention of infection following coronary artery bypass surgery, no placebo-controlled trials have been conducted to evaluate any cephalosporin antibiotic in the prevention of infection following coronary artery bypass surgery or prosthetic heart valve replacement.
In cesarean section, the use of 'Monocid' (after the umbilical cord has been clamped) may reduce the incidence of certain postoperative infections.
When administered one hour prior to surgical procedures for which it is indicated, a single 1 gram dose of 'Monocid' provides protection from most infections due to susceptible organisms throughout the course of the procedure and for approximately 24 hours after administration. Intraoperative and postoperative administration of 'Monocid' is not necessary. Daily doses of 'Monocid' may be administered for two additional days in patients undergoing prosthetic arthroplasty or open heart surgery.
If there are signs of infection, the causative organisms should be identified and appropriate therapy determined through susceptibility testing.
Studies on specimens obtained prior to therapy should be used to determine the susceptibility of the causative organisms to 'Monocid'. Therapy with 'Monocid' may be initiated pending results of the studies; however, treatment should be adjusted according to study findings.
Before using 'Monocid' concomitantly with other antibiotics, the prescribing information for those agents should be reviewed for contraindications, warnings, precautions and adverse reactions. Renal function should be carefully monitored.

CONTRAINDICATIONS

Monocid (sterile cefonicid sodium, SK&F) is contraindicated in persons who have shown hypersensitivity to cephalosporin antibiotics.

WARNINGS

BEFORE THERAPY WITH MONOCID (STERILE CEFONICID SODIUM, SK&F) IS INSTITUTED, CAREFUL INQUIRY SHOULD BE MADE TO DETERMINE WHETHER THE PATIENT HAS HAD PREVIOUS HYPERSENSITIVITY REACTIONS TO CEPHALOSPORINS, PENICILLINS, OR OTHER DRUGS. THIS PRODUCT SHOULD BE GIVEN CAUTIOUSLY TO PENICILLIN-SENSITIVE PATIENTS. ANTIBIOTICS SHOULD BE ADMINISTERED WITH CAUTION TO ANY PATIENT WHO HAS DEMONSTRATED SOME FORM OF ALLERGY, PARTICULARLY TO DRUGS. SERIOUS ACUTE HYPERSENSITIVITY REACTIONS MAY REQUIRE EPINEPHRINE AND OTHER EMERGENCY MEASURES.
Pseudomembranous colitis has been reported with the use of cephalosporins (and other broad-spectrum antibiotics); therefore, it is important to consider that diagnosis in patients who develop diarrhea in association with antibiotic use.
Treatment with broad-spectrum antibiotics alters normal flora of the colon and may permit overgrowth of Clostridia. Studies indicate a toxin produced by *Clostridium difficile* is one primary cause of antibiotic-associated colitis. Cholestyramine and colestipol resins have been shown to bind the toxin *in vitro.*
Mild cases of colitis may respond to drug discontinuance alone.
Moderate to severe cases should be managed with fluid, electrolyte and protein supplementation as indicated.
When the colitis is not relieved by drug discontinuance and when it is severe, oral vancomycin is the treatment of choice for antibiotic-associated pseudomembranous colitis produced by *C. difficile.* Other causes of colitis should also be considered.

PRECAUTIONS

General: With any antibiotic, prolonged use may result in overgrowth of nonsusceptible organisms. Careful observation is essential, and appropriate measures should be taken if superinfection occurs.
Drug Interactions: Nephrotoxicity has been reported following concomitant administration of other cephalosporins and aminoglycosides.
Pregnancy: (Category B.) Reproduction studies have been performed in mice, rabbits and rats at doses up to an equivalent of 40 times the usual adult human dose and have revealed no evidence of impaired fertility or harm to the fetus due to Monocid (sterile cefonicid sodium, SK&F). There are, however, no adequate and well-controlled studies in pregnant women. Because animal reproduction studies are not always predictive of human response, this drug should be used in pregnancy only if clearly needed.
Labor and Delivery: In cesarean section, 'Monocid' should be administered only after the umbilical cord has been clamped.
Nursing Mothers: 'Monocid' is excreted in human milk in low concentrations. Caution should be exercised when 'Monocid' is administered to a nursing woman.
Pediatric Use: Safety and effectiveness in children have not been established.
Beta-lactam antibiotics with methyl-thio-tetrazole side chains have been shown to cause testicular atrophy in prepubertal rats, which persisted into adulthood and resulted in decreased spermatogenesis and decreased fertility. Cefonicid, which contains a methylsulfonic-thio-tetrazole moiety, has no adverse effect on the male reproductive system of prepubertal, juvenile or adult rats when given under identical conditions.

ADVERSE REACTIONS

Monocid (sterile cefonicid sodium, SK&F) is generally well tolerated and adverse reactions have occurred infrequently. The most common adverse reaction has been pain on I.M. injection. On-therapy conditions occurring in greater than 1% of 'Monocid'-treated patients were:

Injection Site Phenomena (5.7%): Pain and/or discomfort on injection; less often, burning, phlebitis at I.V. site.
Increased Platelets (1.7%).
Increased Eosinophils (2.9%).
Liver Function Test Alterations (1.6%): Increased alkaline phosphatase, increased SGOT, increased SGPT, increased GGTP, increased LDH.

Less frequent on-therapy conditions occurring in less than 1% of 'Monocid'-treated patients were:

Hypersensitivity Reactions: Fever, rash, pruritus, erythema, myalgia and anaphylactoid-type reactions have been reported.
Hematology: Decreased WBC, neutropenia, thrombocytopenia, positive Coombs' test.
Diarrhea.

DOSAGE AND ADMINISTRATION

General

The usual adult dosage is 1 gram of Monocid (sterile cefonicid sodium, SK&F) given once every 24 hours, intravenously or by deep intramuscular injection. Doses in excess of 1 gram daily are rarely necessary; however, in exceptional cases dosage of up to 2 grams given once daily have been well tolerated. When administering 2 gram I.M. doses once daily, one-

Continued on next page

Smith Kline & French—Cont.

half the dose should be administered in different large muscle masses.

Surgical Prophylaxis

When administered one hour prior to appropriate surgical procedures (see INDICATIONS AND USAGE), a 1 gram dose of 'Monocid' provides protection from most infections due to susceptible organisms throughout the course of the procedure and for approximately 24 hours after administration. Intraoperative and postoperative administration of 'Monocid' is not necessary. Daily doses of 'Monocid' may be administered for two additional days in patients undergoing prosthetic arthroplasty or open heart surgery.
In cesarean section 'Monocid' should be administered only after the umbilical cord has been clamped.

General Guidelines for Dosage of 'Monocid', I.V. or I.M.

Type of Infection	Daily Dose (grams)	Frequency
Uncomplicated Urinary Tract	0.5	once every 24 hours
Mild to Moderate	1	once every 24 hours
Severe or Life-Threatening	2*	once every 24 hours
Surgical Prophylaxis	1	1 hour preoperatively

* When administering 2 gram I.M. doses once daily, one-half the dose should be administered in different large muscle masses.

Impaired Renal Function

Modification of Monocid (sterile cefonicid sodium, SK&F) dosage is necessary in patients with impaired renal function. Following an initial loading dosage of 7.5 mg./kg. I.M. or I.V., the maintenance dosing schedule shown below should be followed. Further dosing should be determined by therapeutic monitoring, severity of the infection and susceptibility of the causative organism.
[See table below].
Note: It is not necessary to administer additional dosage following dialysis.

Preparation of Parenteral Solution

Parenteral drug products should be SHAKEN WELL when reconstituted, and inspected visually for particulate matter prior to administration. If particulate matter is evident in reconstituted fluids, the drug solutions should be discarded.
RECONSTITUTION

Single-Dose Vials

For I.M. injection, I.V. direct (bolus) injection, or I.V. infusion, reconstitute with Sterile Water for Injection according to the following table. SHAKE WELL.

Vial Size	Diluent to Be Added	Approx. Avail. Volume	Approx. Avg. Concentration
500 mg.	2.0 ml.	2.2 ml.	220 mg./ml.
1 gram	2.5 ml.	3.1 ml.	325 mg./ml.

These solutions of Monocid (sterile cefonicid sodium, SK&F) are stable 24 hours at room temperature or 72 hours if refrigerated (5°C.). Slight yellowing does not affect potency.
For I.V. infusion, dilute reconstituted solution in 50 to 100 ml. of the parenteral fluids listed under ADMINISTRATION.

Pharmacy Bulk Vials (10 grams)

For I.M. injection, I.V. direct (bolus) injection or I.V. infusion, reconstitute with Sterile Water for Injection, Bacteriostatic Water for Injection, or Sodium Chloride Injection according to the following table:

Amount of Diluent	Approx. Concentration	Approx. Avail. Volume
25 ml.	1 gram/3 ml.	31 ml.
45 ml.	1 gram/5 ml.	51 ml.

These solutions of 'Monocid' are stable 24 hours at room temperature or 72 hours if refrigerated (5°C.). Slight yellowing does not affect potency.
For I.V. infusion add to parenteral fluids listed under ADMINISTRATION.

"Piggyback" Vials

Reconstitute with 50 to 100 ml. of Sodium Chloride Injection or other I.V. solution listed under ADMINISTRATION. Administer with primary I.V. fluids, as a single dose. These solutions of 'Monocid' are stable 24 hours at room temperature or 72 hours if refrigerated (5°C.). Slight yellowing does not affect potency.
A solution of 1 gram of 'Monocid' in 18 ml. of Sterile Water for Injection is isotonic.

ADMINISTRATION

I.M. Injection: Inject well within the body of a relatively large muscle. Aspiration is necessary to avoid inadvertent injection into a blood vessel. When administering 2 gram I.M. doses once daily, one-half the dose should be given in different large muscle masses.

I.V. Administration: For direct (bolus) injection, administer reconstituted 'Monocid' slowly over 3 to 5 minutes, directly or through tubing for patients receiving parenteral fluids (see list below). For infusion, dilute reconstituted 'Monocid' in 50 to 100 ml. of one of the following solutions:

0.9% Sodium Chloride Injection, USP
5% Dextrose Injection, USP
5% Dextrose and 0.9% Sodium Chloride Injection, USP
5% Dextrose and 0.45% Sodium Chloride Injection, USP
5% Dextrose and 0.2% Sodium Chloride Injection, USP
10% Dextrose Injection, USP
Ringer's Injection, USP
Lactated Ringer's Injection, USP
5% Dextrose and Lactated Ringer's Injection
10% Invert Sugar in Sterile Water for Injection
5% Dextrose and 0.15% Potassium Chloride Injection
Sodium Lactate Injection, USP

In these fluids 'Monocid' is stable 24 hours at room temperature or 72 hours if refrigerated (5°C.). Slight yellowing does not affect potency.

HOW SUPPLIED

Monocid (sterile cefonicid sodium, SK&F) is supplied in vials equivalent to 500 mg. and 1 gram of cefonicid; in "Piggyback" Vials for I.V. admixture equivalent to 1 gram of cefonicid; and in Pharmacy Bulk Vials equivalent to 10 grams of cefonicid.

MC:L15

Shown in Product Identification Section, page 430

Dosage of 'Monocid' in Adults with Reduced Renal Function

(Monitor renal function and adjust accordingly.)

Creatinine Clearance (ml./min. per 1.73 M^2)	Dosage Regimen: Mild to Moderate Infections	Dosage Regimen: Severe Infections
79–60	10 mg./kg. (every 24 hours)	25 mg./kg. (every 24 hours)
59–40	8 mg./kg. (every 24 hours)	20 mg./kg. (every 24 hours)
39–20	4 mg./kg. (every 24 hours)	15 mg./kg. (every 24 hours)
19–10	4 mg./kg. (every 48 hours)	15 mg./kg. (every 48 hours)
9–5	4 mg./kg. (every 3 to 5 days)	15 mg./kg. (every 3 to 5 days)
<5	3 mg./kg. (every 3 to 5 days)	4 mg./kg. (every 3 to 5 days)

ORNADE® SPANSULE® CAPSULES ℞

[or 'naid]

PRODUCT OVERVIEW

KEY FACTS

Ornade® Spansule® capsules contain phenylpropanolamine HCl, a decongestant that provides vasoconstriction similar to that of ephedrine but with less CNS stimulation, and chlorpheniramine maleate, an antihistamine.
Spansule® capsules are prepared so that an initial dose is released promptly and the remaining dose is released gradually over a prolonged period of time, thus permitting b.i.d. dosing.

MAJOR USE

Ornade® Spansule® capsules are for symptomatic relief of nasal congestion, runny nose, sneezing, itchy nose or throat, and itchy and watery eyes due, for example, to the common cold or allergic rhinitis.

SAFETY INFORMATION

Ornade® Spansule® capsules are contraindicated in patients with: hypersensitivity to either phenylpropanolamine HCl or chlorpheniramine maleate; severe hypertension; coronary artery disease; stenosing peptic ulcer; pyloroduodenal or bladder neck obstruction; concurrent MAO inhibitor therapy. They should not be used to treat lower respiratory tract conditions including asthma. They should not be used in nursing mothers, or in newborn or premature infants or in children under 12. Further, patients should be cautioned about activities requiring alertness and about the possible additive effects of alcohol and other CNS depressants.

PRESCRIBING INFORMATION

ORNADE® SPANSULE® CAPSULES ℞

[or 'naid]

DESCRIPTION

Each 'Ornade' *Spansule* capsule, with opaque red cap and natural body, is imprinted with the product name ORNADE and SKF and contains phenylpropanolamine hydrochloride, 75 mg. and chlorpheniramine maleate, 12 mg. Inactive ingredients consist of benzyl alcohol, cetylpyridinium chloride, FD&C Blue No. 1, FD&C Red No. 3, FD&C Yellow No. 6, gelatin, glyceryl distearate, iron oxide, polyethylene glycol, povidone, silicon dioxide, sodium lauryl sulfate, starch, sucrose, titanium dioxide, wax and trace amounts of other inactive ingredients.
Each 'Ornade' *Spansule* capsule is so prepared that an initial dose is released promptly and the remaining medication is released gradually over a prolonged period.
A single capsule dose produces blood levels comparable to those produced by administration of three 25 mg. doses of phenylpropanolamine hydrochloride and three 4 mg. doses of chlorpheniramine maleate in conventional release form given at four-hour intervals.

ACTIONS

Phenylpropanolamine hydrochloride is a decongestant that provides vasoconstriction similar to that of ephedrine, but with less CNS stimulation.
Chlorpheniramine maleate is an antihistamine with anticholinergic (drying) and sedative side effects. Antihistamines appear to compete with histamines for H_1 cell receptor sites on effector cells.

INDICATIONS

For symptomatic relief of nasal congestion, runny nose, sneezing, itchy nose or throat, and itchy and watery eyes as may occur with the common cold or in allergic rhinitis (e.g., hay fever).
N.B.: A final determination has not been made on the effectiveness of this drug combination in accordance with efficacy requirements of the 1962 Amendments to the Food, Drug and Cosmetic Act.

CONTRAINDICATIONS

Hypersensitivity to either ingredient; severe hypertension; coronary artery disease; stenosing peptic ulcer; pyloroduodenal or bladder neck obstruction.
'Ornade' *Spansule* capsules should NOT be used to treat lower respiratory tract conditions, including asthma.
As with any product containing a sympathomimetic, 'Ornade' *Spansule* capsules should NOT be used in patients taking MAO inhibitors.
Because of the higher risk of antihistamine side effects in infants generally, and for newborns and prematures in particular, antihistamine therapy is contraindicated in nursing mothers. This drug product should NOT be used in newborn or premature infants.

WARNINGS

Caution patients about activities requiring alertness (e.g., operating vehicles or machinery). Patients should also be warned about the possible additive effects of alcohol and other CNS depressants (hypnotics, sedatives, tranquilizers, etc.).

PRECAUTIONS

Use with caution in patients with narrow-angle glaucoma, hypertension, cardiovascular disease, prostatic hypertrophy, hyperthyroidism, or diabetes. Patients taking this medication should be cautioned not to take simultaneously other products containing phenylpropanolamine HCl or amphetamines.

Use in Children: In infants and children, antihistamines in *overdosage* may cause hallucinations, convulsions, or death. As in adults, antihistamines may diminish mental alertness in children. In the young child, particularly, they may produce excitation.

Use in Pregnancy: Experience with this drug in pregnant women is inadequate to determine whether there exists a potential for harm to the developing fetus. Therefore, 'Ornade' *Spansule* capsules should be used in pregnant women only when clearly needed in the judgment of the physician.

Use in the Elderly (approximately 60 years or older): The risk of dizziness, sedation, and hypotension is greater in the elderly patient.

ADVERSE REACTIONS

General: excessive dryness of nose, throat, or mouth; headache; rash; weakness.

Cardiovascular System: angina pain; palpitations; hypertension; hypotension.

Hematologic: thrombocytopenia; leukopenia; hemolytic anemia; agranulocytosis.

Nervous System: drowsiness; nervousness or insomnia; dizziness; irritability; incoordination; tremor; convulsions; visual disturbances.

GI System: nausea; vomiting; epigastric distress; diarrhea; abdominal pain; anorexia; constipation.

GU System: difficulty in urination; dysuria.

Respiratory System: tightness of chest.

DOSAGE AND ADMINISTRATION

Adults and children over 12 years of age—one capsule every 12 hours.

'Ornade' *Spansule* capsules should not be used in children under 12.

OVERDOSAGE

Symptoms may vary from central nervous system depression to stimulation. Also, atropine-like signs and symptoms (dry mouth; fixed, dilated pupils; flushing, etc.) as well as gastrointestinal symptoms may occur. Marked cerebral irritation resulting in jerking of muscles and possible convulsions may be followed by deep stupor and respiratory failure. Acute hypertension or cardiovascular collapse with accompanying hypotension may occur.

Treatment of Overdosage: Immediate evacuation of the stomach should be induced by emesis and gastric lavage. Since much of the 'Spansule' capsule medication is coated for gradual release, saline cathartics should be administered to hasten evacuation of pellets that have not already released medication.

Respiratory depression should be treated promptly with oxygen. Do not treat respiratory or CNS depression with analeptics that might precipitate convulsions; if convulsions or marked CNS excitement occurs, only short-acting barbiturates or chloral hydrate should be used.

SUPPLIED

'Spansule' capsules (brand of sustained release capsules) containing phenylpropanolamine hydrochloride 75 mg. and chlorpheniramine maleate 12 mg., in bottles of 50 and 500, and in Single Unit Packages of 100 (intended for institutional use only).

Military—Capsules, 500's, 6505-01-108-9574.

Veterans Administration—Capsules, 500's, 6505-01-108-9574A.

Shown in Product Identification Section, page 430

OR:L33

PAREDRINE® 1% ℞

[pah-red 'drin]

(brand of hydroxyamphetamine hydrobromide)

with BORIC ACID, OPHTHALMIC SOLUTION

DESCRIPTION

Hydroxyamphetamine hydrobromide, 1%, in distilled water. Made tear-isotonic with 2% boric acid, and preserved with thimerosal, 1:50,000.

ACTION

Dilates the pupil; probably by stimulating the dilator muscles of the iris.

INDICATION

To dilate the pupil; produces a pupillary dilatation which lasts for a few hours.

CONTRAINDICATION

Narrow-angle glaucoma.

PRECAUTIONS

Use with caution in patients with hypertension, hyperthyroidism and diabetes.

ADVERSE REACTIONS

With widely dilated pupils there will likely be increased intraocular pressure, photophobia and blurring of vision.

DOSAGE AND ADMINISTRATION

Instil 1 or 2 drops into the conjunctival sac.

OVERDOSAGE

Symptoms—Dilatation of pupils. *Treatment*—Dilute pilocarpine (1%) may be administered if desired. Instil one drop at intervals. Repeat as necessary. **Accidental ingestion**—Symptoms—These may include marked rise in blood pressure, palpitation, cardiac arrhythmias, substernal discomfort, headache, sweating, nausea, vomiting and gastrointestinal irritation. *Treatment*—Sedation is indicated. Further treatment is symptomatic. Shock, if present, should be treated promptly. If hypertension is prominent, measures should be taken to lower blood pressure.

HOW SUPPLIED

½ fl. oz. (15 ml.) bottles.

PHO:L27

PARNATE® ℞

[pahr 'naight]

(brand of tranylcypromine sulfate)

Before prescribing, the physician should be familiar with the entire contents of this prescribing information.

DESCRIPTION

Chemically, tranylcypromine sulfate is (±)-*trans*-2-phenylcyclopropylamine sulfate (2:1).

Each round, rose-red, coated tablet is imprinted with the product name PARNATE and SKF and contains tranylcypromine sulfate equivalent to 10 mg. of tranylcypromine.

Inactive ingredients consist of acacia, calcium sulfate, cellulose, ethylcellulose, FD&C Red No. 3, gelatin, iron oxide, magnesium stearate, starch, sucrose and trace amounts of other inactive ingredients.

ACTION

Tranylcypromine is a non-hydrazine monoamine oxidase inhibitor with a rapid onset of activity. It increases the concentration of epinephrine, norepinephrine, and serotonin in storage sites throughout the nervous system, and in theory, this increased concentration of monoamines in the brainstem is the basis for its antidepressant activity. When tranylcypromine is withdrawn, monoamine oxidase activity is recovered in 3 to 5 days, although the drug is excreted in 24 hours.

INDICATIONS

For the treatment of Major Depressive Episode Without Melancholia.

Parnate (tranylcypromine sulfate, SK&F) should be used in adult patients who can be closely supervised. It should rarely be the first antidepressant drug given. Rather, the drug is suited for patients who have failed to respond to the drugs more commonly administered for depression.

The effectiveness of 'Parnate' has been established in adult outpatients, most of whom had a depressive illness which would correspond to a diagnosis of Major Depressive Episode Without Melancholia. As described in the American Psychiatric Association's Diagnostic and Statistical Manual, third edition (DSM III), Major Depressive Episode implies a prominent and relatively persistent (nearly every day for at least two weeks) depressed or dysphoric mood that usually interferes with daily functioning and includes at least four of the following eight symptoms: change in appetite, change in sleep, psychomotor agitation or retardation, loss of interest in usual activities or decrease in sexual drive, increased fatigability, feelings of guilt or worthlessness, slowed thinking or impaired concentration, and suicidal ideation or attempts.

The effectiveness of 'Parnate' in patients who meet the criteria for Major Depressive Episode with Melancholia (endogenous features) has not been established.

SUMMARY OF CONTRAINDICATIONS

Parnate (tranylcypromine sulfate, SK&F) should not be administered in combination with any of the following: MAO inhibitors or dibenzazepine derivatives; sympathomimetics (including amphetamines); some central nervous system depressants (including narcotics and alcohol); antihypertensive, diuretic, antihistaminic, sedative or anesthetic drugs; cheese or other foods with a high tyramine content; or excessive quantities of caffeine.

Parnate (tranylcypromine sulfate, SK&F) should not be administered to any patient beyond 60 years of age or with a confirmed or suspected cerebrovascular defect or to any patient with cardiovascular disease, hypertension or history of headache.

(For complete discussion of contraindications and warnings, see below.)

CONTRAINDICATIONS

Parnate (tranylcypromine sulfate, SK&F) is contraindicated:

1. In patients with cerebrovascular defects or cardiovascular disorders

'Parnate' should not be administered to any patient with a confirmed or suspected cerebrovascular defect or to any patient with cardiovascular disease or hypertension. The drug should also be withheld from individuals beyond the age of 60 because of the possibility of existing cerebral sclerosis with damaged vessels.

2. In the presence of pheochromocytoma

'Parnate' should not be used in the presence of pheochromocytoma since such tumors secrete pressor substances.

3. In combination with MAO inhibitors or with dibenzazepine-related entities

Parnate (tranylcypromine sulfate, SK&F) should not be administered together or in rapid succession with other MAO inhibitors or with dibenzazepine-related entities. Hypertensive crises or severe convulsive seizures may occur in patients receiving such combinations.

In patients being transferred to 'Parnate' from another MAO inhibitor or from a dibenzazepine-related entity, allow a medication-free interval of at least a week, then initiate 'Parnate' using half the normal starting dosage for at least the first week of therapy. Similarly, at least a week should elapse between the discontinuance of 'Parnate' and the administration of another MAO inhibitor or a dibenzazepine-related entity, or the readministration of 'Parnate'.

Other MAO Inhibitors

Generic Name	Trademark
Furazolidone	Furoxone® (Norwich Eaton)
Isocarboxazid	Marplan® (Roche Laboratories)
Pargyline HCl	Eutonyl® (Abbott Laboratories)
Pargyline HCl and methyclothiazide	Eutron® (Abbott Laboratories)
Phenelzine sulfate	Nardil® (Parke-Davis)
Procarbazine HCl	Matulane® (Roche Laboratories)

Dibenzazepine-Related and Other Tricyclics

Generic Name	Trademark
Amitriptyline HCl	Amitril® (Parke-Davis)
	Elavil® (Merck Sharp & Dohme)
	Endep® (Roche Products)
	SK-Amitriptyline HCl™ (Smith Kline &French)
Perphenazine and amitriptyline HCl	Etrafon® (Schering)
	Triavil® (Merck Sharp & Dohme)
Desipramine HCl	Norpramin® (Merrell Dow)
	Pertofrane® (USV Laboratories)
Imipramine HCl	Janimine® (Abbott Laboratories)
	SK-Pramine™ (Smith Kline &French)
	Tofranil® (Geigy Pharmaceuticals)
Nortriptyline HCl	Aventyl® (Eli Lilly & Co.)
	Pamelor® (Sandoz)
Protriptyline HCl	Vivactil® (Merck Sharp & Dohme)
Doxepin HCl	Adapin® (Pennwalt)
	Sinequan® (Roerig)
Carbamazepine	Tegretol® (Geigy Pharmaceuticals)
Cyclobenzaprine HCl	Flexeril® (Merck Sharp & Dohme)
Amoxapine	Asendin® (Lederle)
Maprotiline HCl	Ludiomil® (CIBA)
Trimipramine maleate	Surmontil® (Wyeth Laboratories)

4. In combination with sympathomimetics

Parnate (tranylcypromine sulfate, SK&F) should not be administered in combination with sympathomimetics, including amphetamines, and over-the-counter drugs such as cold, hay fever or weight-reducing preparations that contain vasoconstrictors.

During 'Parnate' therapy, it appears that certain patients are particularly vulnerable to the effects of sympathomimetics when the activity of certain enzymes is inhibited. Use of sympathomimetics and compounds such as methyldopa, dopamine, levodopa and tryptophane with 'Parnate' may precipitate hypertension, headache, and related symptoms. In addition, use with tryptophane may precipitate disorien-

Continued on next page

Smith Kline & French—Cont.

tation, memory impairment, and other neuroleptic and behavioral signs.

5. In combination with meperidine
Do not use meperidine concomitantly with MAO inhibitors or within two or three weeks following MAOI therapy. Serious reactions have been precipitated with concomitant use, including coma, severe hypertension or hypotension, severe respiratory depression, convulsions, malignant hyperpyrexia, excitation, peripheral vascular collapse and death. It is thought that these reactions may be mediated by accumulation of 5-HT (serotonin) consequent to MAO inhibition.

6. In combination with cheese or other foods with a high tyramine content
Hypertensive crises have sometimes occurred during 'Parnate' therapy after ingestion of foods with a high tyramine content. In general, the patient should avoid protein foods in which aging or protein breakdown is used to increase flavor. In particular, patients should be instructed not to take foods such as cheese (particularly strong or aged varieties), sour cream, Chianti wine, sherry, beer, pickled herring, liver, canned figs, raisins, bananas or avocados (particularly if overripe), chocolate, soy sauce, the pods of broad beans (fava beans), yeast extracts, or meat prepared with tenderizers.

7. In patients undergoing elective surgery
Patients taking 'Parnate' should not undergo elective surgery requiring general anesthesia. Also, they should not be given cocaine or local anesthesia containing sympathomimetic vasoconstrictors. The possible combined hypotensive effects of 'Parnate' and spinal anesthesia should be kept in mind. 'Parnate' should be discontinued at least 10 days prior to elective surgery.

ADDITIONAL CONTRAINDICATIONS

In general, the physician should bear in mind the possibility of a lowered margin of safety when Parnate (tranylcypromine sulfate, SK&F) is administered in combination with potent drugs.

1. 'Parnate' should not be used in combination with some central nervous system depressants such as narcotics and alcohol, or with hypotensive agents. A marked potentiating effect on these classes of drugs has been reported.
2. Anti-parkinsonism drugs should be used with caution in patients receiving 'Parnate' since severe reactions have been reported.
3. 'Parnate' should not be used in patients with a history of liver disease or in those with abnormal liver function tests.
4. Excessive use of caffeine in any form should be avoided in patients receiving 'Parnate'.

WARNING TO PHYSICIANS

Parnate (tranylcypromine sulfate, SK&F) is a potent agent with the capability of producing serious side effects. 'Parnate' is not recommended in those depressive reactions where other antidepressant drugs may be effective. **It should be reserved for patients who can be closely supervised and who have not responded satisfactorily to the drugs more commonly administered for depression.**

Before prescribing, the physician should be completely familiar with the full material on dosage, side effects, and contraindications on these pages, with the principles of MAO inhibitor therapy and the side effects of this class of drugs. Also, the physician should be familiar with the symptomatology of mental depressions and alternate methods of treatment to aid in the careful selection of patients for 'Parnate' therapy. In depressed patients, the possibility of suicide should always be considered and adequate precautions taken.

Pregnancy Warning: Use of any drug in pregnancy, during lactation, or in women of childbearing age requires that the potential benefits of the drug be weighed against its possible hazards to mother and child. Animal reproductive studies show that 'Parnate' passes through the placental barrier into the fetus of the rat. Also, it passes into milk of the lactating dog. The absence of a harmful action of 'Parnate' on fertility or on postnatal development by either prenatal treatment or from the milk of treated animals has not been demonstrated.

WARNING TO THE PATIENT

Patients should be instructed to report promptly the occurrence of headache or other unusual symptoms.

Patients should be warned against eating the foods listed in Section 6 under Contraindications while on Parnate (tranylcypromine sulfate, SK&F) therapy. Also, they should be told not to drink alcoholic beverages.

Patients should be warned against self-medication with proprietary (over-the-counter) drugs such as cold, hay fever or weight-reducing preparations that contain pressor agents. They should be advised not to consume excessive amounts of caffeine in any form.

WARNINGS

HYPERTENSIVE CRISES: The most important reaction associated with Parnate (tranylcypromine sulfate, SK&F) is the occurrence of hypertensive crises which have sometimes been fatal.

These crises are characterized by some or all of the following symptoms: occipital headache which may radiate frontally, palpitation, neck stiffness or soreness, nausea or vomiting, sweating (sometimes with fever and sometimes with cold, clammy skin) and photophobia. Either tachycardia or bradycardia may be present, and associated constricting chest pain and dilated pupils may occur. **Intracranial bleeding, sometimes fatal in outcome, has been reported in association with the paradoxical increase in blood pressure.**

In all patients taking 'Parnate' blood pressure should be followed closely to detect evidence of any pressor response. It is emphasized that full reliance should not be placed on blood pressure readings, but that the patient should also be observed frequently.

Therapy should be discontinued immediately upon the occurrence of palpitation or frequent headaches during 'Parnate' therapy. These signs may be prodromal of a hypertensive crisis.

Important: Recommended treatment in hypertensive crises

If a hypertensive crisis occurs, Parnate (tranylcypromine sulfate, SK&F) should be discontinued and therapy to lower blood pressure should be instituted immediately. Headache tends to abate as blood pressure is lowered. On the basis of present evidence, phentolamine (available as Regitine®*) is recommended. (The dosage reported for phentolamine is 5 mg. i.v.) Care should be taken to administer this drug slowly in order to avoid producing an excessive hypotensive effect. Fever should be managed by means of external cooling. Other symptomatic and supportive measures may be desirable in particular cases. Do not use parenteral reserpine.

PRECAUTIONS

Hypotension—Hypotension has been observed during Parnate (tranylcypromine sulfate, SK&F) therapy. Symptoms of postural hypotension are seen most commonly but not exclusively in patients with pre-existent hypertension; blood pressure usually returns rapidly to pretreatment levels upon discontinuation of the drug. At doses above 30 mg. daily, postural hypotension is a major side effect and may result in syncope. Dosage increases should be made more gradually in patients showing a tendency toward hypotension at the beginning of therapy. Postural hypotension may be relieved by having the patient lie down until blood pressure returns to normal.

Also, when 'Parnate' is combined with those phenothiazine derivatives or other compounds known to cause hypotension, the possibility of additive hypotensive effects should be considered.

OTHER PRECAUTIONS

There have been reports of drug dependency in patients using doses of tranylcypromine significantly in excess of the therapeutic range. Some of these patients had a history of previous substance abuse. The following withdrawal symptoms have been reported: restlessness, anxiety, depression, confusion, hallucinations, headache, weakness and diarrhea.

Drugs which lower the seizure threshold, including MAO inhibitors, should not be used with Amipaque®†. As with other MAO inhibitors, Parnate (tranylcypromine sulfate, SK&F) should be discontinued at least 48 hours before myelography and should not be resumed for at least 24 hours postprocedure.

In depressed patients, the possibility of suicide should always be considered and adequate precautions taken. Exclusive reliance on drug therapy to prevent suicidal attempts is unwarranted, as there may be a delay in the onset of therapeutic effect or an increase in anxiety and agitation. Also, of course, some patients fail to respond to drug therapy or may respond only temporarily.

MAO inhibitors may have the capacity to suppress anginal pain that would otherwise serve as a warning of myocardial ischemia. The usual precautions should be observed in patients with impaired renal function since there is a possibility of accumulative effects in such patients.

Although excretion of 'Parnate' is rapid, inhibition of MAO may persist up to 10 days following discontinuation.

Because the influence of 'Parnate' on the convulsive threshold is variable in animal experiments, suitable precautions should be taken if epileptic patients are treated.

Some MAO inhibitors have contributed to hypoglycemic episodes in diabetic patients receiving insulin or oral hypoglycemic agents. Therefore, 'Parnate' should be used with caution in diabetics using these drugs.

'Parnate' may aggravate coexisting symptoms in depression, such as anxiety and agitation.

Use 'Parnate' with caution in hyperthyroid patients because of their increased sensitivity to pressor amines.

'Parnate' should be administered with caution to patients receiving Antabuse®‡. In a single study, rats given high intraperitoneal doses of *d* or *l* isomers of tranylcypromine sulfate plus disulfiram experienced severe toxicity including convulsions and death. Additional studies in rats given high oral doses of racemic tranylcypromine sulfate ('Parnate') and disulfiram produced no adverse interaction.

ADVERSE REACTIONS

Overstimulation which may include increased anxiety, agitation and manic symptoms is usually evidence of excessive therapeutic action. Dosage should be reduced, or a phenothiazine tranquilizer should be administered concomitantly.

Patients may experience restlessness or insomnia; may notice some weakness, drowsiness, episodes of dizziness, or dry mouth; or may report nausea, diarrhea, abdominal pain, or constipation. Most of these effects can be relieved by lowering the dosage or by giving suitable concomitant medication.

Tachycardia, significant anorexia, edema, palpitation, blurred vision, chills, and impotence have each been reported.

Headaches without blood pressure elevation have occurred.

Rare instances of hepatitis and skin rash have been reported.

Impaired water excretion compatible with the syndrome of inappropriate secretion of antidiuretic hormone (SIADH) has been reported.

Tinnitus, muscle spasm and tremors, paresthesia and urinary retention have been reported so rarely that the role of Parnate (tranylcypromine sulfate, SK&F) cannot be established.

Blood toxicity has not been reported.

DOSAGE AND ADMINISTRATION

Dosage should be adjusted to the requirements of the individual patient. Improvement should be seen within 48 hours to three weeks after starting therapy.

The usual effective dosage is 30 mg. per day, usually given in divided doses. If there are no signs of improvement after a reasonable period (up to two weeks), then the dosage may be increased in 10 mg. per day increments at intervals of one to three weeks; the dosage range may be extended to a maximum of 60 mg. per day from the usual 30 mg. per day.

Withdrawal from Parnate (tranylcypromine sulfate, SK&F) should be gradual.

OVERDOSAGE

Symptoms: The characteristic symptoms that may be caused by overdosage are usually those described on the preceding pages.

However, an intensification of these symptoms and sometimes severe additional manifestations may be seen, depending on the degree of overdosage and on individual susceptibility. Some patients exhibit insomnia, restlessness and anxiety, progressing in severe cases to agitation, mental confusion and incoherence. Hypotension, dizziness, weakness and drowsiness may occur, progressing in severe cases to extreme dizziness and shock. A few patients have displayed hypertension with severe headache and other symptoms. Rare instances have been reported in which hypertension was accompanied by twitching or myoclonic fibrillation of skeletal muscles with hyperpyrexia, sometimes progressing to generalized rigidity and coma.

Treatment: Gastric lavage is helpful if performed early. Treatment should normally consist of general supportive measures, close observation of vital signs and steps to counteract specific symptoms as they occur, since MAO inhibition may persist. The management of hypertensive crises is described under Hypertensive Crises.

External cooling is recommended if hyperpyrexia occurs. Barbiturates have been reported to help relieve myoclonic reactions, but frequency of administration should be controlled carefully because Parnate (tranylcypromine sulfate, SK&F) may prolong barbiturate activity. When hypotension requires treatment, the standard measures for managing circulatory shock should be initiated. If pressor agents are used, the rate of infusion should be regulated by careful observation of the patient because an exaggerated pressor response sometimes occurs in the presence of MAO inhibition.

Remember that the toxic effect of 'Parnate' may be delayed or prolonged following the last dose of the drug. Therefore, the patient should be closely observed for at least a week.

HOW SUPPLIED

Tablets, containing tranylcypromine sulfate equivalent to 10 mg. of tranylcypromine, in bottles of 100 and 1000.

---

* Phentolamine mesylate, U.S.P., CIBA.
† Metrizamide, Winthrop-Breon Laboratories.
‡Disulfiram, Ayerst Laboratories.

PT:L48

Shown in Product Identification Section, page 430

RIDAURA® ℞
[ri-door'ah]
(brand of auranofin)
Capsules

PRODUCT OVERVIEW

KEY FACTS

Ridaura (auranofin, SK&F) is an oral form (3 mg. capsules) of gold therapy for adult rheumatoid arthritis. 'Ridaura' may modify disease activity as manifested by synovitis and associated symptoms, and reflected by laboratory parameters such as ESR. Gold therapy cannot reverse structural damage to joint cartilage and bone caused by previous disease. The greatest potential benefit occurs in patients with active synovitis, particularly in its early stage.

MAJOR USES

'Ridaura' is indicated in the management of adults with active classical or definite rheumatoid arthritis (ARA criteria) who have had an insufficient therapeutic response to, or are intolerant of, an adequate trial of full doses of one or more nonsteroidal anti-inflammatory drugs. 'Ridaura' should be added to a comprehensive baseline program for rheumatoid arthritis patients, including NSAIDS and non-drug therapies.

SAFETY INFORMATION

See complete list of CONTRAINDICATIONS, WARNINGS, PRECAUTIONS and ADVERSE REACTIONS below.

PRESCRIBING INFORMATION

RIDAURA® ℞
[ri-door'ah]
(brand of auranofin)
Capsules

> Ridaura (auranofin, SK&F) contains gold and, like other gold-containing drugs, can cause gold toxicity, signs of which include: fall in hemoglobin, leukopenia below 4,000 WBC/cu mm, granulocytes below 1,500/cu mm, decrease in platelets below 150,000/cu mm, proteinuria, hematuria, pruritus, rash, stomatitis or persistent diarrhea. Therefore, the results of recommended laboratory work (See PRECAUTIONS) should be reviewed before writing each 'Ridaura' prescription. Like other gold preparations, 'Ridaura' is only indicated for use in selected patients with active rheumatoid arthritis. Physicians planning to use 'Ridaura' should be experienced with chrysotherapy and should thoroughly familiarize themselves with the toxicity and benefits of 'Ridaura'.
> In addition, the following precautions should be routinely employed:
> 1. The possibility of adverse reactions should be explained to patients before starting therapy.
> 2. Patients should be advised to report promptly any symptoms suggesting toxicity. (See PRECAUTIONS —Information for Patients.)

DESCRIPTION

Ridaura (auranofin, SK&F) is available in oral form as capsules containing 3 mg. auranofin.
Auranofin is (2,3,4,6-tetra-O-acetyl-1-thio-β-D-glucopyranosato-S-) (triethylphosphine) gold.
Auranofin contains 29% gold and has the following chemical structure:

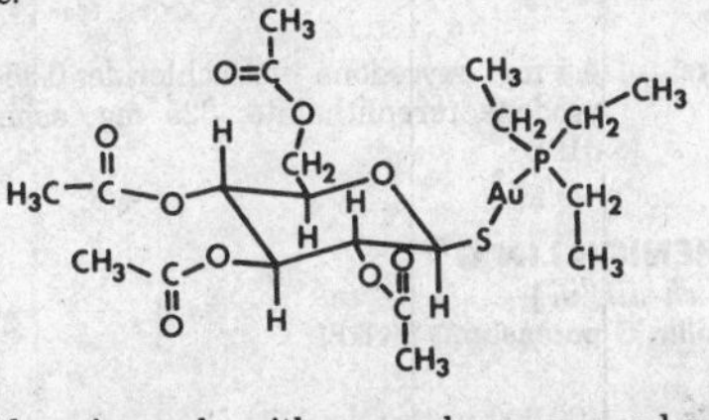

Each 'Ridaura' capsule, with opaque brown cap and opaque tan body, contains auranofin, 3 mg., and is imprinted with the product name RIDAURA and SKF. Inactive ingredients consist of benzyl alcohol, cellulose, cetylpyridinium chloride, D&C Red No. 33, FD&C Blue No. 1, FD&C Red No. 40, FD&C Yellow No. 6, gelatin, lactose, magnesium stearate, povidone, sodium lauryl sulfate, sodium starch glycolate, starch, titanium dioxide and trace amounts of other inactive ingredients.

CLINICAL PHARMACOLOGY

The mechanism of action of Ridaura (auranofin, SK&F) is not understood. In patients with adult rheumatoid arthritis, 'Ridaura' may modify disease activity as manifested by synovitis and associated symptoms, and reflected by laboratory parameters such as ESR. There is no substantial evidence, however, that gold-containing compounds induce remission of rheumatoid arthritis.

Pharmacokinetics: Pharmacokinetic studies were performed in rheumatoid arthritis patients, not in normal volunteers. Auranofin is rapidly metabolized and intact auranofin has never been detected in the blood. Thus, studies of the pharmacokinetics of auranofin have involved measurement of gold concentrations. Approximately 25% of the gold in auranofin is absorbed.
The mean terminal plasma half-life of auranofin gold at steady state was 26 days (range 21 to 31 days; n=5). The mean terminal body half-life was 80 days (range 42 to 128; n=5). Approximately 60% of the absorbed gold (15% of the administered dose) from a single dose of auranofin is excreted in urine; the remainder is excreted in the feces.
In clinical studies, steady state blood-gold concentrations are achieved in about three months. In patients on 6 mg. auranofin/day, mean steady state blood-gold concentrations were 0.68 ± 0.45 mcg./ml. (n=63 patients). In blood, approximately 40% of auranofin gold is associated with red cells, and 60% associated with serum proteins. In contrast, 99% of injectable gold is associated with serum proteins.
Mean blood-gold concentrations are proportional to dose; however, no correlation between blood-gold concentrations and safety or efficacy has been established.

INDICATIONS AND USAGE

Ridaura (auranofin, SK&F) is indicated in the management of adults with active classical or definite rheumatoid arthritis (ARA criteria) who have had an insufficient therapeutic response to, or are intolerant of, an adequate trial of full doses of one or more nonsteroidal anti-inflammatory drugs. 'Ridaura' should be added to a comprehensive baseline program, including non-drug therapies.
Unlike anti-inflammatory drugs, 'Ridaura' does not produce an immediate response. Therapeutic effects may be seen after three to four months of treatment, although improvement has not been seen in some patients before six months.
When cartilage and bone damage has already occurred, gold cannot reverse structural damage to joints caused by previous disease. The greatest potential benefit occurs in patients with active synovitis, particularly in its early stage.
In controlled clinical trials comparing 'Ridaura' with injectable gold, 'Ridaura' was associated with fewer dropouts due to adverse reactions, while injectable gold was associated with fewer dropouts for inadequate or poor therapeutic effect. Physicians should consider these findings when deciding on the use of 'Ridaura' in patients who are candidates for chrysotherapy.

CONTRAINDICATIONS

Ridaura (auranofin, SK&F) is contraindicated in patients with a history of any of the following gold-induced disorders: anaphylactic reactions, necrotizing enterocolitis, pulmonary fibrosis, exfoliative dermatitis, bone marrow aplasia or other severe hematologic disorders.

WARNINGS

Danger signs of possible gold toxicity include fall in hemoglobin, leukopenia below 4,000 WBC/cu mm, granulocytes below 1,500/cu mm, decrease in platelets below 150,000/cu mm, proteinuria, hematuria, pruritus, rash, stomatitis or persistent diarrhea.
Thrombocytopenia has occurred in 1–3% of patients (See ADVERSE REACTIONS) treated with Ridaura (auranofin, SK&F), some of whom developed bleeding. The thrombocytopenia usually appears to be peripheral in origin and is usually reversible upon withdrawal of 'Ridaura'. Its onset bears no relationship to the duration of 'Ridaura' therapy and its course may be rapid. While patients' platelet counts should normally be monitored at least monthly (See PRECAUTIONS—Laboratory Tests), the occurrence of a precipitous decline in platelets or a platelet count less than 100,000/cu mm or signs and symptoms (e.g., purpura, ecchymoses or petechiae) suggestive of thrombocytopenia indicates a need to immediately withdraw 'Ridaura' and other therapies with the potential to cause thrombocytopenia, and to obtain additional platelet counts. No additional 'Ridaura' should be given unless the thrombocytopenia resolves and further studies show it was not due to gold therapy.
Proteinuria has developed in 3–9% of patients (See ADVERSE REACTIONS) treated with 'Ridaura'. If clinically significant proteinuria or microscopic hematuria is found (See PRECAUTIONS—Laboratory Tests), 'Ridaura' and other therapies with the potential to cause proteinuria or microscopic hematuria should be stopped immediately.

PRECAUTIONS

General: The safety of concomitant use of Ridaura (auranofin, SK&F) with injectable gold, hydroxychloroquine, penicillamine, immunosuppressive agents (e.g., cyclophosphamide, azathioprine, or methotrexate) or high doses of corticosteroids has not been established.
Medical problems that might affect the signs or symptoms used to detect 'Ridaura' toxicity should be under control before starting Ridaura (auranofin, SK&F).
The potential benefits of using 'Ridaura' in patients with progressive renal disease, significant hepatocellular disease, inflammatory bowel disease, skin rash or history of bone marrow depression should be weighed against 1) the potential risks of gold toxicity on organ systems previously compromised or with decreased reserve, and 2) the difficulty in quickly detecting and correctly attributing the toxic effect.
The following adverse reactions have been reported with the use of gold preparations and require modification of 'Ridaura' treatment or additional monitoring. See ADVERSE REACTIONS for the approximate incidence of those reactions specifically reported with 'Ridaura'.
Gastrointestinal Reactions: Gastrointestinal reactions reported with gold therapy include diarrhea/loose stools, nausea, vomiting, anorexia and abdominal cramps. The most common reaction to 'Ridaura' is diarrhea/loose stools reported in approximately 50% of the patients. This is generally manageable by reducing the dosage (e.g., from 6 mg. daily to 3 mg.) and in only 6% of the patients is it necessary to discontinue 'Ridaura' permanently.
Ulcerative enterocolitis is a rare serious gold reaction. Therefore, patients with gastrointestinal symptoms should be monitored for the appearance of gastrointestinal bleeding.
Cutaneous Reactions: Dermatitis is the most common reaction to injectable gold therapy and the second most common reaction to 'Ridaura'. *Any eruption, especially if pruritic, that develops during treatment should be considered a gold reaction until proven otherwise.* Pruritus often exists before dermatitis becomes apparent, and therefore should be considered to be a warning signal of a cutaneous reaction. Gold dermatitis may be aggravated by exposure to sunlight or an actinic rash may develop. The most serious form of cutaneous reaction reported with injectable gold is generalized exfoliative dermatitis.
Mucous Membrane Reactions: Stomatitis, another common gold reaction, may be manifested by shallow ulcers on the buccal membranes, on the borders of the tongue, and on the palate or in the pharynx. Stomatitis may occur as the only adverse reaction or with a dermatitis. Sometimes diffuse glossitis or gingivitis develops. A metallic taste may precede these oral mucous membrane reactions and should be considered a warning signal.
Renal Reactions: Gold can produce a nephrotic syndrome or glomerulitis with proteinuria and hematuria. These renal reactions are usually relatively mild and subside completely if recognized early and treatment is discontinued. They may become severe and chronic if treatment is continued after the onset of the reaction. *Therefore it is important to perform urinalyses regularly* and to discontinue treatment promptly if proteinuria or hematuria develops.
Hematologic Reactions: Blood dyscrasias including leukopenia, granulocytopenia and thrombocytopenia have all been reported as reactions to injectable gold and 'Ridaura'. These reactions may occur separately or in combination at anytime during treatment. Because they have potentially serious consequences, *blood dyscrasias should be constantly watched for through regular monitoring (at least monthly) of the formed elements of the blood throughout treatment.*
Miscellaneous Reactions: Rare reactions attributed to gold include cholestatic jaundice; gold bronchitis and interstitial pneumonitis and fibrosis; peripheral neuropathy; partial or complete hair loss; fever.
Information for Patients: Patients should be advised of the possibility of toxicity from 'Ridaura' and of the signs and symptoms that they should report promptly. (Patient information sheets are available.)
Women of childbearing potential should be warned of the potential risks of 'Ridaura' therapy during pregnancy (See PRECAUTIONS—Pregnancy).
Laboratory Tests: CBC with differential, platelet count, urinalysis, and renal and liver function tests should be performed prior to Ridaura (auranofin, SK&F) therapy to establish a baseline and to identify any preexisting conditions.
CBC with differential, platelet count and urinalysis should then be monitored at least monthly; other parameters should be monitored as appropriate.
Drug Interactions: In a single patient-report, there is the suggestion that concurrent administration of 'Ridaura' and phenytoin may have increased phenytoin blood levels.
Carcinogenesis/Mutagenesis: In a 24-month study in rats, animals treated with auranofin at 0.4, 1.0 or 2.5 mg./kg./day orally (3, 8 or 21 times the human dose) or gold sodium thiomalate at 2 or 6 mg./kg. injected twice weekly (4 or 12 times the human dose) were compared to untreated control animals.
There was a significant increase in the frequency of renal tubular cell karyomegaly and cytomegaly and renal adenoma in the animals treated with 1.0 or 2.5 mg./kg./day of auranofin and 2 or 6 mg./kg. twice weekly of gold sodium thiomalate. Malignant renal epithelial tumors were seen in the 1.0 mg./kg./day and the 2.5 mg./kg./day auranofin and in the 6 mg./kg. twice weekly gold sodium thiomalate-treated animals.
In a 12-month study, rats treated with auranofin at 23 mg./kg./day (192 times the human dose) developed tumors of

Continued on next page

Smith Kline & French—Cont.

the renal tubular epithelium, whereas those treated with 3.6 mg./kg./day (30 times the human dose) did not.

In an 18-month study in mice given oral auranofin at doses of 1, 3 and 9 mg./kg./day (8, 24 and 72 times the human dose), there was no statistically significant increase above controls in the instances of tumors.

In the mouse lymphoma forward mutation assay, auranofin at high concentrations (313 to 700 ng./ml.) induced increases in the mutation frequencies in the presence of a rat liver microsomal preparation. Auranofin produced no mutation effects in the Ames test (Salmonella), in the *in vitro* assay (Forward and Reverse Mutation Inducement Assay with Saccharomyces), in the *in vitro* transformation of BALB/T3 cell mouse assay or in the Dominant Lethal Assay.

Pregnancy: Teratogenic Effects—Pregnancy Category C. Use of Ridaura (auranofin, SK&F) by pregnant women is not recommended. Furthermore, women of childbearing potential should be warned of the potential risks of 'Ridaura' therapy during pregnancy. (See below.)

Pregnant rabbits given auranofin at doses of 0.5, 3 or 6 mg./kg./day (4.2 to 50 times the human dose) had impaired food intake, decreased maternal weights, decreased fetal weights and an increase above controls in the incidence of resorptions, abortions and congenital abnormalities, mainly abdominal defects such as gastroschisis and umbilical hernia.

Pregnant rats given auranofin at a dose of 5 mg./kg./day (42 times the human dose) had an increase above controls in the incidence of resorptions and a decrease in litter size and weight linked to maternal toxicity. No such effects were found in rats given 2.5 mg./kg./day (21 times the human dose).

Pregnant mice given auranofin at a dose of 5 mg./kg./day (42 times the human dose) had no teratogenic effects.

There are no adequate and well-controlled 'Ridaura' studies in pregnant women.

Nursing Mothers: Nursing during 'Ridaura' therapy is not recommended. Following auranofin administration to rats and mice, gold is excreted in milk. Following the administration of injectable gold, gold appears in the milk of nursing women; human data on auranofin are not available.

Pediatric Use: Ridaura (auranofin, SK&F) is not recommended for use in children because its safety and effectiveness have not been established.

ADVERSE REACTIONS

The adverse reactions incidences listed below are based on observations of 4,784 'Ridaura'-treated patients (2,474 U.S., 2,310 foreign), of whom 2,729 were treated more than one year and 573 for more than three years. The highest incidence is during the first six months of treatment; however, reactions can occur after many months of therapy. With rare exceptions, all patients were on concomitant nonsteroidal anti-inflammatory therapy; some of them were also taking low dosages of corticosteroids.

Reactions occurring in more than 1% of 'Ridaura'-treated patients

Gastrointestinal: loose stools or diarrhea (47%); abdominal pain (14%); nausea with or without vomiting (10%); constipation; anorexia*; flatulence*; dyspepsia*; dysgeusia.

Dermatological: rash (24%); pruritus (17%); hair loss; urticaria.

Mucous Membrane: stomatitis (13%); conjunctivitis*; glossitis.

Hematological: anemia; leukopenia; thrombocytopenia; eosinophilia.

Renal: proteinuria*; hematuria.

Hepatic: elevated liver enzymes.

Reactions occurring in less than 1% of 'Ridaura'-treated patients

Gastrointestinal: dysphagia; gastrointestinal bleeding†; melena†; positive stool for occult blood†; ulcerative enterocolitis.

Dermatological: angioedema.

Mucous Membrane: gingivitis†.

Hematological: neutropenia†; agranulocytosis.

Hepatic: jaundice.

Respiratory: interstitial pneumonitis.

Neurological: peripheral neuropathy.

Reactions reported with injectable gold preparations, but not with Ridaura (auranofin, SK&F) (based on 4,784 patients in clinical trials and on postmarketing experience)

Cutaneous Reactions: generalized exfoliative dermatitis.

Hematologic Reactions: pancytopenia, aplastic anemia.

Nitritoid, Anaphylactoid and Anaphylactic Reactions: Reactions of the "nitritoid type" which may resemble anaphylactic reactions.

Incidence of Adverse Reactions for Specific Categories—18 Comparative Trials

	'Ridaura' (445 patients)	Injectable Gold (445 patients)
Proteinuria	0.9%	5.4%
Rash	26 %	39 %
Diarrhea	42.5%	13 %
Stomatitis	13 %	18 %
Anemia	3.1%	2.7%
Leukopenia	1.3%	2.2%
Thrombocytopenia	0.9%	2.2%
Elevated liver function tests	1.9%	1.7%
Pulmonary	0.2%	0.2%

OVERDOSAGE

The acute oral LD_{50} for auranofin is 310 mg./kg. in adult mice and 265 mg./kg. in adult rats. The minimum lethal dose in rats is 30 mg./kg.

In case of acute overdosage, immediate induction of emesis or gastric lavage and appropriate supportive therapy are recommended.

'Ridaura' overdosage experience is limited. A 50-year-old female, previously on 6 mg. 'Ridaura' daily, took 27 mg. (9 capsules) daily for 10 days and developed an encephalopathy and peripheral neuropathy. 'Ridaura' was discontinued and she eventually recovered.

There has been no experience with treating 'Ridaura' overdosage with modalities such as chelating agents. However, they have been used with injectable gold and may be considered for 'Ridaura' overdosage.

DOSAGE AND ADMINISTRATION

Usual Adult Dosage: The usual adult dosage of Ridaura (auranofin, SK&F) is 6 mg. daily, given either as 3 mg. twice daily or 6 mg. once daily. Initiation of therapy at dosages exceeding 6 mg. daily is not recommended because it is associated with an increased incidence of diarrhea. If response is inadequate after six months, an increase to 9 mg. (3 mg. three times daily) may be tolerated. If response remains inadequate after a three-month trial of 9 mg. daily, 'Ridaura' therapy should be discontinued. Safety at dosages exceeding 9 mg. daily has not been studied.

Transferring from Injectable Gold: In controlled clinical studies, patients on injectable gold have been transferred to Ridaura (auranofin, SK&F) by discontinuing the injectable agent and starting oral therapy with 'Ridaura', 6 mg. daily. When patients are transferred to 'Ridaura', they should be informed of its adverse reaction profile, in particular the gastrointestinal reactions. (See PRECAUTIONS—Information for Patients.) At six months, control of disease activity of patients transferred to 'Ridaura' and those maintained on the injectable agent was not different. Data beyond six months are not available.

HOW SUPPLIED

Capsules, containing 3 mg. auranofin, in bottles of 60.

STORAGE AND HANDLING

Store at controlled room temperature.

RI:L23

Shown in Product Identification Section, page 430

SK-LINE®

SK-AMITRIPTYLINE HCI™ ℞
[*am'eh-trip"teh'leen*]
(amitriptyline hydrochloride, SK&F)

Tablets: 10 mg. (No. 120), 25 mg. (No. 121), 75 mg. (No. 124), 100 mg. (No. 131).

SK-AMPICILLIN® ℞
[*amp'eh-sill'in*]
(ampicillin, SK&F)

Capsules: 250 mg. (No. 101), 500 mg. (No. 102).
For Oral Suspension: 125 mg./5 ml. (No. 103), 250 mg./5 ml. (No. 104), 100 mg./ml. (No. 109).

SK-AMPICILLIN-N® ℞
[*amp'eh-sill'in*]
(sterile ampicillin sodium, SK&F)

Injection: 500 mg. (No. 106).

SK-APAP™ with CODEINE Ⓒ-III
[*ay'pap*]
(acetaminophen, codeine phosphate)

Tablets: 300 mg./15 mg. (No. 494), 300 mg./30 mg. (No. 496), 300 mg./60 mg. (No. 497).

SK-BAMATE™ Ⓒ-IV
[*bam'ate*]
(meprobamate, SK&F)

Tablets: 200 mg. (No. 133), 400 mg. (No. 134).

SK-CHLOROTHIAZIDE™ ℞
[*klor'oh-thigh'ah-zide*]
(chlorothiazide, SK&F)

Tablets: 500 mg. (No. 420).

SK-DIPHENOXYLATE™ Ⓒ-V
[*di'fen-ox"il-ate*]
(diphenoxylate HCl, atropine sulfate, SK&F)

Tablets: 2.5 mg./0.025 mg. (No. 423).

SK-DIPYRIDAMOLE™ ℞
[*die-pie-rid'ah-mole*]
(dipyridamole, SK&F)

Tablets: 25 mg. (No. 379), 50 mg. (No. 380), 75 mg. (No. 381).

SK-ERYTHROMYCIN™ ℞
[*ĕ-rith"ro-mi'sin*]
(erythromycin stearate, SK&F)

Tablets: 250 mg. (No. 367), 500 mg. (No. 369).

SK-FUROSEMIDE™ ℞
[*few-row"seh-mide'*]
(furosemide, SK&F)

Tablets: 20 mg. (No. 340), 40 mg. (No. 341).

SK-LYGEN® Ⓒ-IV
[*lye'gen*]
(chlordiazepoxide hydrochloride, SK&F)

Capsules: 5 mg. (No. 441), 10 mg. (No. 442), 25 mg. (No. 443).

SK-OXYCODONE™ with ACETAMINOPHEN Ⓒ-II
[*ox-e'co-doan*]

Tablets: 5 mg. oxycodone hydrochloride; 325 mg. acetaminophen (No. 320).

SK-OXYCODONE™ with ASPIRIN Ⓒ-II
[*ox-e'co-doan*]

Tablets: 4.5 mg. oxycodone hydrochloride; 0.38 mg. oxycodone terephthalate; 325 mg. aspirin (No. 319).

SK-PENICILLIN G™ ℞
[*penn'eh-sill"in*]
(penicillin G potassium, SK&F)

Tablets: 400,000 units (No. 111).

SK-PENICILLIN VK™ ℞
[*pen'eh-sill"in*]
(penicillin V potassium, SK&F)

Tablets: 250 mg. (No. 116), 500 mg. (No. 117).
For Oral Solution: 125 mg./5 ml. (No. 118), 250 mg./5 ml. (No. 119).

SK-POTASSIUM CHLORIDE™ ℞
[*po-tas'e-um klo'rīd*]
(potassium chloride, SK&F)

Oral Solution: 10% solution (No. 456), 20% solution, (No. 457).

---

* Reactions marked with an asterisk occurred in 3–9% of the patients. The other reactions listed occurred in 1–3%.

† Reactions marked with a dagger occurred in 0.1–1% of the patients. The other reactions listed occurred in less than 0.1%.

SK-PRAMINE™ ℞
[pram 'een]
(imipramine hydrochloride, SK&F)

Tablets: 10 mg. (No. 321), 25 mg. (No. 322), 50 mg. (No. 323).

SK-PREDNISONE™ ℞
[pred-neh 'soan]
(prednisone, SK&F)

Tablets: 5 mg. (No. 339).

SK-QUINIDINE SULFATE™ ℞
[kwin 'eh-deen sul-fate]
(quinidine sulfate, SK&F)

Tablets: 200 mg. (No. 171).

SK-65® Ⓒ
(propoxyphene hydrochloride, SK&F)

Capsules: 65 mg. (No. 463).

SK-65 APAP® Ⓒ
[ay 'pap]

Each tablet: 65 mg. propoxyphene HCl, 650 mg. acetaminophen (No. 474).

SK-65® COMPOUND Ⓒ

Each capsule: 65 mg. propoxyphene HCl, 389 mg. aspirin, 32.4 mg. caffeine (No. 468).

SK-TERPIN HYDRATE and CODEINE ™ Ⓒ
[ter 'pin hi 'drate]
(terpin hydrate and codeine, SK&F)

Elixir: 85 mg./10 mg./5 ml. (No. 354).

SK-TETRACYCLINE HCl™ CAPSULES ℞
[tet-rah-sigh 'clean]
(tetracycline hydrochloride, SK&F)

250 mg. (No. 126), 500 mg. (No. 127).

SK-TOLBUTAMIDE™ ℞
[toll-bu 'tah-mide]
(brand of tolbutamide)

Tablets: 500 mg. (No. 409).

STELAZINE® ℞
[stel 'ah-zeen]
(brand of trifluoperazine hydrochloride)

('Stelazine' is a product of SK&F Co., Carolina, P.R. 00630, Subsidiary of SmithKline Beckman Corporation, Philadelphia, Pa.)

DESCRIPTION

Tablets: Modified Formulation—Each round, blue, film-coated tablet contains trifluoperazine hydrochloride equivalent to trifluoperazine as follows: 1 mg. imprinted SKF and S03; 2 mg. imprinted SKF and S04; 5 mg. imprinted SKF and S06; 10 mg. imprinted SKF and S07. Inactive ingredients consist of cellulose, croscarmellose sodium, FD&C Blue No. 2, FD&C Yellow No. 6, gelatin, lactose, magnesium stearate, talc, titanium dioxide and trace amounts of other inactive ingredients.

NOTE: Stelazine (trifluoperazine HCl, SK&F) tablets have been changed from blue, sugar-coated tablets to blue, film-coated tablets. The film-coated tablets differ in size from the corresponding sugar-coated tablets, but the drug content remains unchanged.

Multiple-dose Vials, 10 ml. (2 mg./ml.)—Each ml. contains, in aqueous solution, trifluoperazine, 2 mg., as the hydrochloride; sodium tartrate, 4.75 mg.; sodium biphosphate, 11.6 mg.; sodium saccharin, 0.3 mg.; benzyl alcohol, 0.75%, as preservative.

Concentrate (intended for institutional use only)—Each ml. of clear, yellow, banana-vanilla flavored liquid contains 10 mg. of trifluoperazine as the hydrochloride. Inactive ingredients consist of D&C Yellow No. 10, FD&C Yellow No. 6, flavor, sodium benzoate, sodium bisulfite, sucrose and water.

N.B.: The Concentrate is for use in severe neuropsychiatric conditions when oral medication is preferred and other oral forms are considered impractical.

INDICATIONS

For the management of the manifestations of psychotic disorders.

Stelazine (trifluoperazine HCl, SK&F) is effective for the short-term treatment of generalized non-psychotic anxiety. However, 'Stelazine' is not the first drug to be used in therapy for most patients with non-psychotic anxiety because certain risks associated with its use are not shared by common alternative treatments (i.e., benzodiazepines).

When used in the treatment of non-psychotic anxiety, 'Stelazine' should not be administered at doses of more than 6 mg. per day or for longer than 12 weeks because the use of 'Stelazine' at higher doses or for longer intervals may cause persistent tardive dyskinesia that may prove irreversible (see Warnings section).

The effectiveness of 'Stelazine' as a treatment for non-psychotic anxiety was established in a four-week clinical multicenter study of outpatients with generalized anxiety disorder (DSM-III). This evidence does not predict that 'Stelazine' will be useful in patients with other non-psychotic conditions in which anxiety, or signs that mimic anxiety, are found (i.e., physical illness, organic mental conditions, agitated depression, character pathologies, etc.).

'Stelazine' has not been shown effective in the management of behavioral complications in patients with mental retardation.

CONTRAINDICATIONS

Comatose or greatly depressed states due to central nervous system depressants, and in cases of existing blood dyscrasias, bone marrow depression and pre-existing liver damage.

WARNINGS

Tardive Dyskinesia: Tardive dyskinesia, a syndrome consisting of potentially irreversible, involuntary, dyskinetic movements, may develop in patients treated with neuroleptic (antipsychotic) drugs. Although the prevalence of the syndrome appears to be highest among the elderly, especially elderly women, it is impossible to rely upon prevalence estimates to predict, at the inception of neuroleptic treatment, which patients are likely to develop the syndrome. Whether neuroleptic drug products differ in their potential to cause tardive dyskinesia is unknown.

Both the risk of developing the syndrome and the likelihood that it will become irreversible are believed to increase as the duration of treatment and the total cumulative dose of neuroleptic drugs administered to the patient increase. However, the syndrome can develop, although much less commonly, after relatively brief treatment periods at low doses.

There is no known treatment for established cases of tardive dyskinesia, although the syndrome may remit, partially or completely, if neuroleptic treatment is withdrawn. Neuroleptic treatment itself, however, may suppress (or partially suppress) the signs and symptoms of the syndrome and thereby may possibly mask the underlying disease process. The effect that symptomatic suppression has upon the long-term course of the syndrome is unknown.

Given these considerations, neuroleptics should be prescribed in a manner that is most likely to minimize the occurrence of tardive dyskinesia. Chronic neuroleptic treatment should generally be reserved for patients who suffer from a chronic illness that 1) is known to respond to neuroleptic drugs, and, 2) for whom alternative, equally effective, but potentially less harmful treatments are *not* available or appropriate. In patients who do require chronic treatment, the smallest dose and the shortest duration of treatment producing a satisfactory clinical response should be sought. The need for continued treatment should be reassessed periodically.

If signs and symptoms of tardive dyskinesia appear in a patient on neuroleptics, drug discontinuation should be considered. However, some patients may require treatment despite the presence of the syndrome.

For further information about the description of tardive dyskinesia and its clinical detection, please refer to the sections on Precautions and Adverse Reactions.

Patients who have demonstrated a hypersensitivity reaction (e.g., blood dyscrasias, jaundice) with a phenothiazine should not be re-exposed to any phenothiazine, including Stelazine (trifluoperazine HCl, SK&F), unless in the judgment of the physician the potential benefits of treatment outweigh the possible hazard.

'Stelazine' may impair mental and/or physical abilities, especially during the first few days of therapy. Therefore, caution patients about activities requiring alertness (e.g., operating vehicles or machinery).

If agents such as sedatives, narcotics, anesthetics, tranquilizers, or alcohol are used either simultaneously or successively with the drug, the possibility of an undesirable additive depressant effect should be considered.

Usage in Pregnancy: Safety for the use of 'Stelazine' during pregnancy has not been established. Therefore, it is not recommended that the drug be given to pregnant patients except when, in the judgment of the physician, it is essential. The potential benefits should clearly outweigh possible hazards. There are reported instances of prolonged jaundice, extrapyramidal signs, hyperreflexia or hyporeflexia in newborn infants whose mothers received phenothiazines.

Reproductive studies in rats given over 600 times the human dose showed an increased incidence of malformations above controls and reduced litter size and weight linked to maternal toxicity. These effects were not observed at half this dosage. No adverse effect on fetal development was observed in rabbits given 700 times the human dose nor in monkeys given 25 times the human dose.

Nursing Mothers: There is evidence that phenothiazines are excreted in the breast milk of nursing mothers.

PRECAUTIONS

Given the likelihood that some patients exposed chronically to neuroleptics will develop tardive dyskinesia, it is advised that all patients in whom chronic use is contemplated be given, if possible, full information about this risk. The decision to inform patients and/or their guardians must obviously take into account the clinical circumstances and the competency of the patient to understand the information provided.

Thrombocytopenia and anemia have been reported in patients receiving the drug. Agranulocytosis and pancytopenia have also been reported—warn patients to report the sudden appearance of sore throat or other signs of infection. If white blood cell and differential counts indicate cellular depression, stop treatment and start antibiotic and other suitable therapy.

Jaundice of the cholestatic type of hepatitis or liver damage has been reported. If fever with grippe-like symptoms occurs, appropriate liver studies should be conducted. If tests indicate an abnormality, stop treatment.

One result of therapy may be an increase in mental and physical activity. For example, a few patients with angina pectoris have complained of increased pain while taking the drug. Therefore, angina patients should be observed carefully and, if an unfavorable response is noted, the drug should be withdrawn.

Because hypotension has occurred, large doses and parenteral administration should be avoided in patients with impaired cardiovascular systems. To minimize the occurrence of hypotension after injection, keep patient lying down and observe for at least ½ hour. If hypotension occurs from parenteral or oral dosing, place patient in head-low position with legs raised. If a vasoconstrictor is required, Levophed®* and Neo-Synephrine®† are suitable. Other pressor agents, including epinephrine, should not be used as they may cause a paradoxical further lowering of blood pressure.

Since certain phenothiazines have been reported to produce retinopathy, the drug should be discontinued if ophthalmoscopic examination or visual field studies should demonstrate retinal changes.

An antiemetic action of Stelazine (trifluoperazine HCl, SK&F) may mask the signs and symptoms of toxicity or overdosage of other drugs and may obscure the diagnosis and treatment of other conditions such as intestinal obstruction, brain tumor and Reye's syndrome.

With prolonged administration at high dosages, the possibility of cumulative effects, with sudden onset of severe central nervous system or vasomotor symptoms, should be kept in mind.

Neuroleptic drugs elevate prolactin levels; the elevation persists during chronic administration. Tissue culture experiments indicate that approximately one-third of human breast cancers are prolactin-dependent in vitro, a factor of potential importance if the prescribing of these drugs is contemplated in a patient with a previously detected breast cancer. Although disturbances such as galactorrhea, amenorrhea, gynecomastia and impotence have been reported, the clinical significance of elevated serum prolactin levels is unknown for most patients. An increase in mammary neoplasms has been found in rodents after chronic administration of neuroleptic drugs. Neither clinical nor epidemiologic studies conducted to date, however, have shown an association between chronic administration of these drugs and mammary tumorigenesis; the available evidence is considered too limited to be conclusive at this time.

Because phenothiazines may interfere with thermoregulatory mechanisms, use with caution in persons who will be exposed to extreme heat.

As with all drugs which exert an anticholinergic effect, and/or cause mydriasis, trifluoperazine should be used with caution in patients with glaucoma.

Phenothiazines may diminish the effect of oral anticoagulants.

Phenothiazines can produce alpha-adrenergic blockade.

Concomitant administration of propranolol with phenothiazines results in increased plasma levels of both drugs.

Antihypertensive effects of guanethidine and related compounds may be counteracted when phenothiazines are used concurrently.

Thiazide diuretics may accentuate the orthostatic hypotension that may occur with phenothiazines.

Continued on next page

Smith Kline & French—Cont.

Phenothiazines may lower the convulsive threshold; dosage adjustments of anticonvulsants may be necessary. Potentiation of anticonvulsant effects does not occur. However, it has been reported that phenothiazines may intefere with the metabolism of Dilantin®‡ and thus precipitate Dilantin‡ toxicity.

Drugs which lower the seizure threshold, including phenothiazine derivatives, should not be used with Amipaque®§.

As with other phenothiazine derivatives, 'Stelazine' should be discontinued at least 48 hours before myelography, should not be resumed for at least 24 hours postprocedure, and should not be used for the control of nausea and vomiting occurring either prior to myelography or postprocedure with Amipaque§.

The presence of phenothiazines may produce false positive phenylketonuria (PKU) test results.

Long-Term Therapy: To lessen the likelihood of adverse reactions related to cumulative drug effect, patients with a history of long-term therapy with Stelazine (trifluoperazine HCl, SK&F) and/or other neuroleptics should be evaluated periodically to decide whether the maintenance dosage could be lowered or drug therapy discontinued.

ADVERSE REACTIONS

Drowsiness, dizziness, skin reactions, rash, dry mouth, insomnia, amenorrhea, fatigue, muscular weakness, anorexia, lactation, blurred vision and neuromuscular (extrapyramidal) reactions.

Neuromuscular (Extrapyramidal) Reactions

These symptoms are seen in a significant number of hospitalized mental patients. They may be characterized by motor restlessness, be of the dystonic type, or they may resemble parkinsonism.

Depending on the severity of symptoms, dosage should be reduced or discontinued. If therapy is reinstituted, it should be at a lower dosage. Should these symptoms occur in children or pregnant patients, the drug should be stopped and not reinstituted. In most cases barbiturates by suitable route of administration will suffice. (Or, injectable Benadryl®[ll] may be useful.) In more severe cases, the administration of an anti-parkinsonism agent, except levodopa, usually produces rapid reversal of symptoms. Suitable supportive measures such as maintaining a clear airway and adequate hydration should be employed.

Motor Restlessness: Symptoms may include agitation or jitteriness and sometimes insomnia. These symptoms often disappear spontaneously. At times these symptoms may be similar to the original neurotic or psychotic symptoms. Dosage should not be increased until these side effects have subsided.

If this phase becomes too troublesome, the symptoms can usually be controlled by a reduction of dosage or concomitant administration of a barbiturate.

Dystonias: Symptoms may include: spasm of the neck muscles, sometimes progressing to torticollis; extensor rigidity of back muscles, sometimes progressing to opisthotonos; carpopedal spasm, trismus, swallowing difficulty, oculogyric crisis and protrusion of the tongue.

These usually subside within a few hours, and almost always within 24 to 48 hours, after the drug has been discontinued.

In mild cases, reassurance or a barbiturate is often sufficient. *In moderate cases,* barbiturates will usually bring rapid relief. *In more severe adult cases,* the administration of an anti-parkinsonism agent, except levodopa, usually produces rapid reversal of symptoms. Also, intravenous caffeine with sodium benzoate seems to be effective. *In children,* reassurance and barbiturates will usually control symptoms. (Or, injectable Benadryl[ll] may be useful.) Note: See Benadryl[ll] prescribing information for appropriate children's dosage. If appropriate treatment with anti-parkinsonism agents or Benadryl[ll] fails to reverse the signs and symptoms, the diagnosis should be reevaluated.

Pseudo-parkinsonism: Symptoms may include: mask-like facies; drooling; tremors; pillrolling motion; cogwheel rigidity; and shuffling gait. Reassurance and sedation are important. In most cases these symptoms are readily controlled when an anti-parkinsonism agent is administered concomitantly. Anti-parkinsonism agents should be used only when required. Generally, therapy of a few weeks to two or three months will suffice. After this time patients should be evaluated to determine their need for continued treatment. (Note: Levodopa has not been found effective in pseudo-parkinsonism.) Occasionally it is necessary to lower the dosage of Stelazine (trifluoperazine HCl, SK&F) or to discontinue the drug.

Tardive Dyskinesia: As with all antipsychotic agents, tardive dyskinesia may appear in some patients on long-term therapy or may appear after drug therapy has been discontinued. The syndrome can also develop, although much less frequently, after relatively brief treatment periods at low doses. This syndrome appears in all age groups. Although its prevalence appears to be highest among elderly patients, especially elderly women, it is impossible to rely upon prevalence estimates to predict at the inception of neuroleptic treatment which patients are likely to develop the syndrome. The symptoms are persistent and in some patients appear to be irreversible. The syndrome is characterized by rhythmical involuntary movements of the tongue, face, mouth or jaw (e.g., protrusion of tongue, puffing of cheeks, puckering of mouth, chewing movements). Sometimes these may be accompanied by involuntary movements of extremities. In rare instances, these involuntary movements of the extremities are the only manifestations of tardive dyskinesia. A variant of tardive dyskinesia, tardive dystonia, has also been described.

There is no known effective treatment for tardive dyskinesia; anti-parkinsonism agents do not alleviate the symptoms of this syndrome. If clinically feasible, it is suggested that all antipsychotic agents be discontinued if these symptoms appear. Should it be necessary to reinstitute treatment, or increase the dosage of the agent, or switch to a different antipsychotic agent, the syndrome may be masked.

It has been reported that fine vermicular movements of the tongue may be an early sign of the syndrome and if the medication is stopped at that time the syndrome may not develop.

Adverse Reactions Reported with Stelazine (trifluoperazine HCl, SK&F) or Other Phenothiazine Derivatives: Adverse effects with different phenothiazines vary in type, frequency, and mechanism of occurrence, i.e., some are dose-related, while others involve individual patient sensitivity. Some adverse effects may be more likely to occur, or occur with greater intensity, in patients with special medical problems, e.g., patients with mitral insufficiency or pheochromocytoma have experienced severe hypotension following recommended doses of certain phenothiazines.

Not all of the following adverse reactions have been observed with every phenothiazine derivative, but they have been reported with one or more and should be borne in mind when drugs of this class are administered: extrapyramidal symptoms (opisthotonos, oculogyric crisis, hyperreflexia, dystonia, akathisia, dyskinesia, parkinsonism) some of which have lasted months and even years—particularly in elderly patients with previous brain damage; grand mal and petit mal convulsions, particularly in patients with EEG abnormalities or history of such disorders; altered cerebrospinal fluid proteins; cerebral edema; intensification and prolongation of the action of central nervous system depressants (opiates, analgesics, antihistamines, barbiturates, alcohol), atropine, heat, organophosphorus insecticides; autonomic reactions (dryness of mouth, nasal congestion, headache, nausea, constipation, obstipation, adynamic ileus, ejaculatory disorders/impotence, priapism, atonic colon, urinary retention, miosis and mydriasis); reactivation of psychotic processes, catatonic-like states; hypotension (sometimes fatal); cardiac arrest; blood dyscrasias (pancytopenia, thrombocytopenic purpura, leukopenia, agranulocytosis, eosinophilia, hemolytic anemia, aplastic anemia); liver damage (jaundice, biliary stasis); endocrine disturbances (hyperglycemia, hypoglycemia, glycosuria, lactation, galactorrhea, gynecomastia, menstrual irregularities, false positive pregnancy tests); skin disorders (photosensitivity, itching, erythema, urticaria, eczema up to exfoliative dermatitis); other allergic reactions (asthma, laryngeal edema, angioneurotic edema, anaphylactoid reactions); peripheral edema; reversed epinephrine effect; hyperpyrexia; mild fever after large I.M. doses; increased appetite; increased weight; a systemic lupus erythematosus-like syndrome; pigmentary retinopathy; with prolonged administration of substantial doses, skin pigmentation, epithelial keratopathy, and lenticular and corneal deposits.

EKG changes—particularly nonspecific, usually reversible Q and T wave distortions—have been observed in some patients receiving phenothiazine tranquilizers. Although phenothiazines cause neither psychic nor physical dependence, sudden discontinuance in long-term psychiatric patients may cause temporary symptoms, e.g., nausea and vomiting, dizziness, tremulousness.

Rare occurrences of neuroleptic malignant syndrome (NMS) have been reported in patients receiving neuroleptic drugs. This syndrome is comprised of the symptom complex of hyperthermia, altered consciousness, muscular rigidity and autonomic dysfunction and is potentially fatal.

Note: There have been occasional reports of sudden death in patients receiving phenothiazines. In some cases, the cause appeared to be cardiac arrest or asphyxia due to failure of the cough reflex.

DOSAGE AND ADMINISTRATION—ADULTS

Dosage should be adjusted to the needs of the individual. The lowest effective dosage should always be used. Dosage should be increased more gradually in debilitated or emaciated patients. When maximum response is achieved, dosage may be reduced gradually to a maintenance level. Because of the inherent long action of the drug, patients may be controlled on convenient b.i.d. administration; some patients may be maintained on once-a-day administration.

When Stelazine (trifluoperazine HCl, SK&F) is administered by intramuscular injection, equivalent oral dosage may be substituted once symptoms have been controlled.

Note: Although there is little likelihood of contact dermatitis due to the drug, persons with known sensitivity to phenothiazine drugs should avoid direct contact.

Elderly Patients: In general, dosages in the lower range are sufficient for most elderly patients. Since they appear to be more susceptible to hypotension and neuromuscular reactions, such patients should be observed closely. Dosage should be tailored to the individual, response carefully monitored, and dosage adjusted accordingly. Dosage should be increased more gradually in elderly patients.

Non-psychotic Anxiety

Usual dosage is 1 or 2 mg. twice daily. Do not administer at doses of more than 6 mg. per day or for longer than 12 weeks.

Psychotic Disorders

Oral: Usual starting dosage is 2 mg. to 5 mg. b.i.d. (Small or emaciated patients should always be started on the lower dosage.)

Most patients will show optimum response on 15 mg. or 20 mg. daily, although a few may require 40 mg. a day or more. Optimum therapeutic dosage levels should be reached within two or three weeks.

When the Concentrate dosage form is to be used, it should be added to 60 ml. (2 fl. oz.) or more of diluent *just prior to administration* to insure palatability and stability. Vehicles suggested for dilution are: tomato or fruit juice, milk, simple syrup, orange syrup, carbonated beverages, coffee, tea, or water. Semisolid foods (soup, puddings, etc.) may also be used.

Intramuscular (for prompt control of severe symptoms): Usual dosage is 1 mg. to 2 mg. (½-1 ml.) by deep intramuscular injection q4-6h, p.r.n. More than 6 mg. within 24 hours is rarely necessary.

Only in very exceptional cases should intramuscular dosage exceed 10 mg. within 24 hours. Injections should not be given at intervals of less than 4 hours because of a possible cumulative effect.

Note: Stelazine (trifluoperazine HCl, SK&F) Injection has been usually well tolerated and there is little, if any, pain and irritation at the site of injection.

The Injection should be protected from light. Exposure may cause discoloration. Slight yellowish discoloration will not alter potency or efficacy. If markedly discolored, the solution should be discarded.

DOSAGE AND ADMINISTRATION—PSYCHOTIC CHILDREN

Dosage should be adjusted to the weight of the child and severity of the symptoms. These dosages are for children, ages 6 to 12, who are hospitalized or under close supervision.

Oral: The starting dosage is 1 mg. administered once a day or b.i.d. Dosage may be increased gradually until symptoms are controlled or until side effects become troublesome.

While it is usually not necessary to exceed dosages of 15 mg. daily, some older children with severe symptoms may require higher dosages.

Intramuscular: There has been little experience with the use of Stelazine (trifluoperazine HCl, SK&F) Injection in children. However, if it is necessary to achieve rapid control of severe symptoms, 1 mg. (½ ml.) of the drug may be administered intramuscularly once or twice a day.

OVERDOSAGE

(See also under Adverse Reactions.)

Symptoms—Primarily involvement of the extrapyramidal mechanism producing some of the dystonic reactions described above. Symptoms of central nervous system depression to the point of somnolence or coma. Agitation and restlessness may also occur. Other possible manifestations include convulsions, EKG changes and cardiac arrhythmias, fever, and autonomic reactions such as hypotension, dry mouth and ileus.

Treatment—It is important to determine other medications taken by the patient since multiple dose therapy is common in overdosage situations. Treatment is essentially symptomatic and supportive. Early gastric lavage is helpful. Keep patient under observation and maintain an open airway, since involvement of the extrapyramidal mechanism may produce dysphagia and respiratory difficulty in severe overdosage. **Do not attempt to induce emesis because a dystonic reaction of the head or neck may develop that could result in aspiration of vomitus.** Extrapyramidal symptoms may be treated with anti-parkinsonism drugs, barbiturates, or Benadryl[ll]. See prescribing information for these products. Care should be taken to avoid increasing respiratory depression. If administration of a stimulant is desirable, amphetamine, dextroamphetamine, or caffeine with sodium benzoate is recommended. Stimulants that may cause convulsions (e.g., picrotoxin or pentylenetetrazol) should be avoided.

If hypotension occurs, the standard measures for managing circulatory shock should be initiated. If it is desirable to administer a vasoconstrictor, Levophed* and Neo-Synephrine† are most suitable. Other pressor agents, including epinephrine, are not recommended because phenothiazine derivatives may reverse the usual elevating action of these agents and cause a further lowering of blood pressure.

Limited experience indicates that phenothiazines are *not* dialyzable.

HOW SUPPLIED

Tablets, 1 mg. and 2 mg., in bottles of 100 and 1000; in Single Unit Packages of 100 (intended for institutional use only).
For psychiatric patients who are hospitalized or under close supervision:
Tablets, 5 mg. and 10 mg., in bottles of 100 and 1000; in Single Unit Packages of 100 (intended for institutional use only).
Multiple-dose Vials, 10 ml. (2 mg./ml.), in boxes of 1 and 20.
Concentrate (intended for institutional use only)—10 mg./ml., in 2 fl. oz. bottles and in cartons of 12 bottles. Each bottle is packaged with a graduated dropper.
The Concentrate form is light-sensitive. For this reason, it should be protected from light and dispensed in amber bottles. *Refrigeration is not required.*
Military—Tablets, 2 mg., S.U.P. 100's, 6505-00-132-0143; 5 mg., S.U.P. 100's, 6505-00-132-0144; 10 mg., S.U.P. 100's, 6505-00-132-0188.

* Norepinephrine bitartrate, Winthrop-Breon Laboratories.
† Phenylephrine hydrochloride, Winthrop-Breon Laboratories.
‡ Phenytoin, Parke-Davis.
§ Metrizamide, Winthrop-Breon Laboratories.
‖ Diphenhydramine hydrochloride, Parke-Davis.

SZ:L59

Shown in Product Identification Section, page 430

TAGAMET® ℞

[tag'ah-met]
(brand of cimetidine tablets cimetidine hydrochloride liquid and cimetidine hydrochloride injection)

('Tagamet' is a product of SK&F Lab Co., Carolina, P.R. 00630, Subsidiary of SmithKline Beckman Corporation, Philadelphia, Pa.)

DESCRIPTION

'Tagamet' (brand of cimetidine) is a histamine H_2 receptor antagonist. Chemically it is *N″*-cyano-N-methyl-*N′*-[2-[[(5-methyl-1H-imidazol-4-yl) methyl] thio]-ethyl]-guanidine.
The empirical formula for cimetidine is $C_{10}H_{16}N_6S$ and for cimetidine hydrochloride, $C_{10}H_{16}N_6SHCl$; these represent molecular weights of 252.34 and 288.80, respectively.
Cimetidine contains an imidazole ring, and is chemically related to histamine.
(The liquid and injection dosage forms contain cimetidine as the hydrochloride.)
Cimetidine has a bitter taste and characteristic odor.
Tablets: Each light green, film-coated tablet contains cimetidine as follows: 200 mg.—round, imprinted with the product name TAGAMET, SKF and 200; 300 mg.—round, imprinted with the product name TAGAMET, SKF and 300; 400 mg.—capsule-shaped, imprinted with the product name TAGAMET, SKF and 400; 800 mg.—oval Tiltab™ tablets, imprinted with the product name TAGAMET, SKF and 800. Inactive ingredients consist of cellulose, D&C Yellow No. 10, FD&C Blue No. 2, FD&C Yellow No. 6, hydroxypropyl methylcellulose, iron oxides, magnesium stearate, povidone, propylene glycol, sodium lauryl sulfate, sodium starch glycolate, starch, titanium dioxide and trace amounts of other inactive ingredients.
Liquid: Each 5 ml. (one teaspoonful) of clear, light orange, mint-peach flavored liquid contains cimetidine hydrochloride equivalent to cimetidine, 300 mg.; alcohol, 2.8%. Inactive ingredients consist of FD&C Yellow No. 6, flavors, methylparaben, polyoxyethylene polyoxypropylene glycol, propylene glycol, propylparaben, saccharin sodium, sodium chloride, sodium phosphate, sorbitol and water.
Vials: Each 2 ml. contains, in aqueous solution, cimetidine hydrochloride equivalent to cimetidine, 300 mg.; phenol, 10 mg.
Multiple-dose Vials: 8 ml. (300 mg./2 ml.): Each 2 ml. contains, in aqueous solution, cimetidine hydrochloride equivalent to cimetidine, 300 mg.; phenol, 10 mg.
Single-dose Prefilled Disposable Syringes: Each 2 ml. contains, in aqueous solution, cimetidine hydrochloride equivalent to cimetidine, 300 mg.; phenol, 10 mg.
Single-dose Premixed Plastic Containers: Each 50 ml. contains cimetidine hydrochloride equivalent to 300 mg. cimetidine and 0.45 grams sodium chloride.
The plastic container is fabricated from specially formulated polyvinyl chloride. The amount of water that can permeate from inside the container into the overwrap is insufficient to affect the solution significantly. Solutions in contact with the plastic container can leach out certain of its chemical components in very small amounts within the expiration period, e.g., di 2-ethylhexyl phthalate (DEHP), up to 5 parts per million. However, the safety of the plastic has been confirmed in tests in animals according to the USP biological tests for plastic containers as well as by tissue culture toxicity studies.

CLINICAL PHARMACOLOGY

'Tagamet' (brand of cimetidine) competitively inhibits the action of histamine at the histamine H_2 receptors of the parietal cells and thus is a histamine H_2-receptor antagonist.
'Tagamet' is not an anticholinergic agent. Studies have shown that 'Tagamet' inhibits both daytime and nocturnal basal gastric acid secretion. 'Tagamet' also inhibits gastric acid secretion stimulated by food, histamine, pentagastrin, caffeine and insulin.

Antisecretory Activity

1) **Acid Secretion:** *Nocturnal:* 'Tagamet' 800 mg. at bedtime reduces mean hourly H^+ activity by greater than 85% over an eight-hour period in duodenal ulcer patients, with no effect on daytime acid secretion. 'Tagamet' 1600 mg. h.s. produces 100% inhibition of mean hourly H^+ activity over an eight-hour period in duodenal ulcer patients, but also reduces H^+ activity by 35% for an additional five hours into the following morning. 'Tagamet' 400 mg. b.i.d. and 300 mg. q.i.d. decrease nocturnal acid suppression in a dose-related manner, i.e., 47%–83% over a six- to eight-hour period and 54% over a nine-hour period, respectively.
Food Stimulated: During the first hour after a standard experimental meal, oral 'Tagamet' 300 mg. inhibited gastric acid secretion in duodenal ulcer patients by at least 50%. During the subsequent two hours 'Tagamet' inhibited gastric acid secretion by at least 75%.
The effect of a 300 mg. breakfast dose of 'Tagamet' continued for at least four hours and there was partial suppression of the rise in gastric acid secretion following the luncheon meal in duodenal ulcer patients. This suppression of gastric acid output was enhanced and could be maintained by another 300 mg. dose of 'Tagamet' given with lunch.
In another study, 'Tagamet' 300 mg. given with the meal increased gastric pH as compared with placebo.

	Mean Gastric pH	
	'Tagamet'	Placebo
1 hour	3.5	2.6
2 hours	3.1	1.6
3 hours	3.8	1.9
4 hours	6.1	2.2

24-Hour Mean H^+ Activity: 'Tagamet' 800 mg. h.s., 400 mg. b.i.d. and 300 mg. q.i.d. all provide a similar, moderate (less than 60%) level of 24-hour acid suppression. However, the 800 mg. h.s. regimen exerts its entire effect on nocturnal acid, and does not affect daytime gastric physiology.
Chemically Stimulated: Oral 'Tagamet' (brand of cimetidine) significantly inhibited gastric acid secretion stimulated by betazole (an isomer of histamine), pentagastrin, caffeine and insulin as follows:

Stimulant	Stimulant Dose	'Tagamet'	% Inhibition
Betazole	1.5mg/kg (sc)	300mg (po)	85% at 2½ hours
Pentagastrin	6mcg/kg/hr (iv)	100mg/hr (iv)	60% at 1 hour
Caffeine	5mg/kg/hr (iv)	300mg (po)	100% at 1 hour
Insulin	0.03 units/kg/hr (iv)	100mg/hr (iv)	82% at 1 hour

When food and betazole were used to stimulate secretion, inhibition of hydrogen ion concentration usually ranged from 45–75% and the inhibition of volume ranged from 30–65%.
2) **Pepsin:** Oral 'Tagamet' 300 mg. reduced total pepsin output as a result of the decrease in volume of gastric juice.
3) **Intrinsic Factor:** Intrinsic factor secretion was studied with betazole as a stimulant. Oral 'Tagamet' 300 mg. inhibited the rise in intrinsic factor concentration produced by betazole, but some intrinsic factor was secreted at all times.

Other

Lower Esophageal Sphincter Pressure and Gastric Emptying

'Tagamet' has no effect on lower esophageal sphincter (LES) pressure or the rate of gastric emptying.

Pharmacokinetics

'Tagamet' is rapidly absorbed after oral administration and peak levels occur in 45–90 minutes. The half-life of 'Tagamet' is approximately 2 hours. Both oral and parenteral (IV or IM) administration provide comparable periods of therapeutically effective blood levels; blood concentrations remain above that required to provide 80% inhibition of basal gastric acid secretion for 4–5 hours following a dose of 300 mg.
The principal route of excretion of 'Tagamet' is the urine. Following parenteral administration, most of the drug is excreted as the parent compound; following oral administration, the drug is more extensively metabolized, the sulfoxide being the major metabolite. Following a single oral dose, 48% of the drug is recovered from the urine after 24 hours as the parent compound. Following IV or IM administration, approximately 75% of the drug is recovered from the urine after 24 hours as the parent compound.

CLINICAL TRIALS

Duodenal Ulcer

'Tagamet' (brand of cimetidine) has been shown to be effective in the treatment of active duodenal ulcer and, at reduced dosage, in maintenance therapy following healing of active ulcers.
Active Duodenal Ulcer: 'Tagamet' accelerates the rate of duodenal ulcer healing. Healing rates reported in U.S. and foreign controlled trials with 'Tagamet' are summarized below, beginning with the regimen providing the lowest nocturnal dose.

Duodenal Ulcer Healing Rates with Various 'Tagamet' Dosage Regimens*

Regimen	300 mg. q.i.d.	400 mg. b.i.d.	800 mg. h.s.	1600 mg. h.s.
week 4	68%	73%	80%	86%
week 6	80%	80%	89%	—
week 8	—	92%	94%	—

*Averages from controlled clinical trials.

A U.S., double-blind, placebo-controlled, dose-ranging study demonstrated that all once-daily at bedtime (h.s.) 'Tagamet' regimens were superior to placebo in ulcer healing and that 'Tagamet' 800 mg. h.s. healed 75% of patients at four weeks. The healing rate with 800 mg. h.s. was significantly superior to 400 mg. h.s. (66%) and not significantly different from 1600 mg. h.s. (81%).
In the U.S. dose-ranging trial, over 80% of patients receiving 'Tagamet' 800 mg. h.s. experienced nocturnal pain relief after one day. Relief from daytime pain was reported in approximately 70% of patients after two days. As with ulcer healing, the 800 mg. h.s. dose was superior to 400 mg. h.s. and not different from 1600 mg. h.s.
In foreign, double-blind studies with 'Tagamet' 800 mg. h.s., 79–85% of patients were healed at four weeks.
While short-term treatment with 'Tagamet' (brand of cimetidine) can result in complete healing of the duodenal ulcer, acute therapy will not prevent ulcer recurrence after 'Tagamet' has been discontinued. Some follow-up studies have reported that the rate of recurrence once therapy was discontinued was slightly higher for patients healed on 'Tagamet' than for patients healed on other forms of therapy; however, the 'Tagamet'-treated patients generally had more severe disease.
Maintenance Therapy in Duodenal Ulcer: Treatment with a reduced dose of 'Tagamet' has been proven effective as maintenance therapy following healing of active duodenal ulcers.
In numerous placebo-controlled studies conducted worldwide, the percent of patients with observed ulcers at the end of one year's therapy with 'Tagamet' 400 mg. h.s. was significantly lower (10%–45%) than in patients receiving placebo (44%–70%). Thus, from 55% to 90% of patients were maintained free of observed ulcers at the end of one year with 'Tagamet' 400 mg. h.s.
Factors such as smoking, duration and severity of disease, gender, and genetic traits may contribute to variations in actual percentages.
Trials of other anti-ulcer therapy, whether placebo-controlled, positive-controlled or open, have demonstrated a range of results similar to that seen with 'Tagamet'.

Active Benign Gastric Ulcer

'Tagamet' has been shown to be effective in the short-term treatment of active benign gastric ulcer.
In a multicenter, double-blind U.S. study, patients with endoscopically confirmed benign gastric ulcer were treated with 'Tagamet' 300 mg. four times a day or with placebo for six weeks. Patients were limited to those with ulcers ranging from 0.5–2.5 cm. in size. Endoscopically confirmed healing at six weeks was seen in significantly* more 'Tagamet'-treated patients than in patients receiving placebo, as shown below:

	'Tagamet'	Placebo
week 2	14/63 (22%)	7/63 (11%)
total at week 6	43/65 (66%)*	30/67 (45%)

*$p < 0.05$

Similarly, in worldwide double-blind clinical studies, endoscopically evaluated benign gastric ulcer healing rates were consistently higher with 'Tagamet' than with placebo.

Pathological Hypersecretory Conditions (such as Zollinger-Ellison Syndrome)

'Tagamet' significantly inhibited gastric acid secretion and reduced occurrence of diarrhea, anorexia and pain in patients with pathological hypersecretion associated with Zollinger-Ellison Syndrome, systemic mastocytosis and

Continued on next page

Smith Kline & French—Cont.

multiple endocrine adenomas. Use of 'Tagamet' was also followed by healing of intractable ulcers.

INDICATIONS

'Tagamet' (brand of cimetidine) is indicated in:

(1) **Short-term treatment of active duodenal ulcer.** Most patients heal within 4 weeks and there is rarely reason to use 'Tagamet' at full dosage for longer than 6–8 weeks (see Dosage and Administration–Duodenal Ulcer). Concomitant antacids should be given as needed for relief of pain. However, simultaneous administration of 'Tagamet' and antacids is not recommended, since antacids have been reported to interfere with the absorption of 'Tagamet'.

(2) **Maintenance therapy for duodenal ulcer patients at reduced dosage after healing of active ulcer.** Patients have been maintained on continued treatment with 'Tagamet' 400 mg. h.s. for periods of up to five years.

(3) **Short-term treatment of active benign gastric ulcer.** There is no information concerning usefulness of treatment periods of longer than 8 weeks.

(4) **The treatment of pathological hypersecretory conditions** (i.e., Zollinger-Ellison Syndrome, systemic mastocytosis, multiple endocrine adenomas).

CONTRAINDICATIONS

There are no known contraindications to the use of 'Tagamet' (brand of cimetidine). However, the physician should refer to the Precautions section regarding usage in pregnant, nursing, or pediatric patients.

PRECAUTIONS

'Tagamet' (brand of cimetidine) has demonstrated a weak antiandrogenic effect. In animal studies this was manifested as reduced prostate and seminal vesicle weights. However, there was no impairment of mating performance or fertility, nor any harm to the fetus in these animals at doses 9 to 56 times the full therapeutic dose of 'Tagamet', as compared with controls. The cases of gynecomastia seen in patients treated for one month or longer may be related to this effect.
In human studies, 'Tagamet' has been shown to have no effect on spermatogenesis, sperm count, motility, morphology or *in vitro* fertilizing capacity.
In a 24-month toxicity study conducted in rats, at dose levels of 150, 378 and 950 mg./kg./day (approximately 9 to 56 times the recommended human dose), there was a small increase in the incidence of benign Leydig cell tumors in each dose group; when the combined drug-treated groups and control groups were compared, this increase reached statistical significance. In a subsequent 24-month study, there were no differences between the rats receiving 150 mg./kg./day and the untreated controls. However, a statistically significant increase in benign Leydig cell tumor incidence was seen in the rats that received 378 and 950 mg./kg./day. These tumors were common in control groups as well as treated groups and the difference became apparent only in aged rats.
Rare instances of cardiac arrhythmias and hypotension have been reported following the rapid administration of 'Tagamet' HCl (brand of cimetidine hydrochloride) Injection by intravenous bolus.
Symptomatic response to 'Tagamet' therapy does not preclude the presence of a gastric malignancy. There have been rare reports of transient healing of gastric ulcers despite subsequently documented malignancy.
Reversible confusional states (see Adverse Reactions) have been observed on occasion, predominantly, but not exclusively, in severely ill patients. Advancing age (50 or more years) and preexisting liver and/or renal disease appear to be contributing factors. In some patients these confusional states have been mild and have not required discontinuation of 'Tagamet' therapy. In cases where discontinuation was judged necessary, the condition usually cleared within 3-4 days of drug withdrawal.
Drug Interactions: 'Tagamet', apparently through an effect on certain microsomal enzyme systems, has been reported to reduce the hepatic metabolism of warfarin-type anticoagulants, phenytoin, propranolol, chlordiazepoxide, diazepam, lidocaine, theophylline and metronidazole, thereby delaying elimination and increasing blood levels of these drugs.
Clinically significant effects have been reported with the warfarin anticoagulants; therefore, close monitoring of prothrombin time is recommended, and adjustment of the anticoagulant dose may be necessary when 'Tagamet' is administered concomitantly. Interaction with phenytoin, lidocaine and theophylline has also been reported to produce adverse clinical effects.
However, a crossover study in healthy subjects receiving either 'Tagamet' 300 mg. q.i.d. or 800 mg. h.s. concomitantly with a 300 mg. b.i.d. dosage of theophylline (Theo-Dur®), demonstrated less alteration in steady-state theophylline peak serum levels with the 800 mg. h.s. regimen, particularly in subjects aged 54 years and older. Data beyond ten days are not available. (Note: All patients receiving theophylline should be monitored appropriately, regardless of concomitant drug therapy.)
Dosage of the drugs mentioned above and other similarly metabolized drugs, particularly those of low therapeutic ratio or in patients with renal and/or hepatic impairment, may require adjustment when starting or stopping concomitantly administered 'Tagamet' to maintain optimum therapeutic blood levels.
Additional clinical experience may reveal other drugs affected by the concomitant administration of 'Tagamet'.
Usage in Pregnancy: There has been no experience to date with the use of 'Tagamet' in pregnant patients. However, animal studies have demonstrated that 'Tagamet' crosses the placental barrier. Teratology studies (100–950 mg./kg./day) have shown no effects attributable to 'Tagamet' on litter parameters or early development of the young. 'Tagamet' should not be used in pregnant patients or women of childbearing potential unless, in the judgment of the physician, the anticipated benefits outweigh the potential risks.
Nursing Mothers: Cimetidine is secreted in human milk and, as a general rule, nursing should not be undertaken while a patient is on a drug.
Pediatric Use: Clinical experience in children is limited. Therefore, 'Tagamet' therapy cannot be recommended for children under 16, unless, in the judgment of the physician, anticipated benefits outweigh the potential risks. In very limited experience, doses of 20–40 mg./kg. per day have been used.

ADVERSE REACTIONS

Mild and transient diarrhea, dizziness, somnolence and rash have been reported in a small number of patients, e.g., approximately 1 in 100, during treatment with 'Tagamet' (brand of cimetidine). A few cases of headache, ranging from mild to severe, have been reported; these cleared on withdrawal of the drug.
There have been rare reports of reversible arthralgia and myalgia; exacerbation of joint symptoms in patients with preexisting arthritis has also been reported. Such symptoms have usually been alleviated by a reduction in 'Tagamet' (brand of cimetidine) dosage. A few cases of polymyositis have been reported, but no causal relationship has been established.
Reversible confusional states, e.g., mental confusion, agitation, psychosis, depression, anxiety, hallucinations, disorientation, have been reported predominantly, but not exclusively, in severely ill patients. They have usually developed within 2-3 days of initiation of 'Tagamet' therapy and have cleared within 3-4 days of discontinuation of the drug.
Gynecomastia has been reported in patients treated for one month or longer. In patients being treated for pathological hypersecretory states, this occurred in about 4 percent of cases while in all others the incidence was 0.3% to 1% in various studies. No evidence of induced endocrine dysfunction was found, and the condition remained unchanged or returned toward normal with continuing 'Tagamet' (brand of cimetidine) treatment.
Reversible impotence has been reported in patients with pathological hypersecretory disorders, e.g., Zollinger-Ellison Syndrome, receiving 'Tagamet', particularly in high doses, for at least 12 months (range 12–79 months, mean 38 months). However, in large-scale surveillance studies at regular dosage, the incidence has not exceeded that commonly reported in the general population.
Reversible alopecia has been reported very rarely.
Decreased white blood cell counts in 'Tagamet'-treated patients (approximately 1 per 100,000 patients), including agranulocytosis (approximately 3 per million patients), have been reported, including a few reports of recurrence on rechallenge. Most of these reports were in patients who had serious concomitant illnesses and received drugs and/or treatment known to produce neutropenia. Thrombocytopenia (approximately 3 per million patients) and a few cases of aplastic anemia have also been reported.
Regularly observed small increases in plasma creatinine and some increases in serum transaminase have been reported. These did not progress with continued therapy and disappeared at the end of therapy.
Rare cases of fever, interstitial nephritis, urinary retention, pancreatitis and allergic reactions, including hypersensitivity vasculitis, which cleared on withdrawal of the drug, have been reported. Adverse hepatic effects have been reported rarely. These were reversible and cholestatic or mixed cholestatic-hepatocellular in nature. Because of the predominance of cholestatic features, severe parenchymal injury is considered highly unlikely.
There has been reported a single case of biopsy-proven periportal hepatic fibrosis in a patient receiving 'Tagamet'.

DOSAGE AND ADMINISTRATION

Duodenal Ulcer

Active Duodenal Ulcer: Clinical studies have indicated that suppression of nocturnal acid is the most important factor in duodenal ulcer healing (see Clinical Pharmacology—Acid Secretion). This is supported by recent clinical trials (see Clinical Trials—Active Duodenal Ulcer). Therefore, there is no apparent rationale, except for familiarity with use, for treating with anything other than a once-daily at bedtime dosage regimen (h.s.).
In a U.S. dose-ranging study of 400 mg. h.s., 800 mg. h.s. and 1600 mg. h.s., a continuous dose response relationship for ulcer healing was demonstrated.
However, 800 mg. h.s. is the dose of choice for most patients, as it provides a high healing rate (the difference between 800 mg. h.s. and 1600 mg. h.s. being small), maximal pain relief, a decreased potential for drug interactions (see Precautions—Drug Interactions) and maximal patient convenience. Patients unhealed at four weeks, or those with persistent symptoms, have been shown to benefit from two to four weeks of continued therapy.
It has been shown that patients who both have an endoscopically demonstrated ulcer larger than 1.0 cm. and are also heavy smokers (i.e., smoke one pack of cigarettes or more per day) are more difficult to heal. There is some evidence which suggests that more rapid healing can be achieved in this subpopulation with 'Tagamet' 1600 mg. at bedtime. While early pain relief with either 800 mg. h.s. or 1600 mg. h.s. is equivalent in all patients, 1600 mg. h.s. provides an appropriate alternative when it is important to ensure healing within four weeks for this subpopulation. Alternatively, approximately 94% of all patients will also heal in eight weeks with 'Tagamet' 800 mg. h.s.
Other 'Tagamet' regimens in the U.S. which have been shown to be effective are: 300 mg. four times daily, with meals and at bedtime, the original regimen with which U.S. physicians have the most experience, and 400 mg. twice daily, in the morning and at bedtime (see Clinical Trials—Active Duodenal Ulcer).
Concomitant antacids should be given as needed for relief of pain. However, simultaneous administration of 'Tagamet' and antacids is not recommended, since antacids have been reported to interfere with the absorption of 'Tagamet' (brand of cimetidine).
While healing with 'Tagamet' often occurs during the first week or two, treatment should be continued for 4–6 weeks unless healing has been demonstrated by endoscopic examination.

Maintenance Therapy for Duodenal Ulcer: In those patients requiring maintenance therapy, the recommended adult oral dose is 400 mg. at bedtime.

Active Benign Gastric Ulcer

The recommended adult oral dosage for short-term treatment of active benign gastric ulcer is 300 mg. four times a day with meals and at bedtime. Controlled clinical studies were limited to six weeks of treatment (see Clinical Trials). Symptomatic response to 'Tagamet' does not preclude the presence of a gastric malignancy. It is important to follow gastric ulcer patients to assure rapid progress to complete healing.

Pathological Hypersecretory Conditions (such as Zollinger-Ellison Syndrome)

Recommended adult oral dosage: 300 mg. four times a day with meals and at bedtime. In some patients it may be necessary to administer 'Tagamet' 300 mg. doses more frequently. Doses should be adjusted to individual patient needs, but should not usually exceed 2400 mg. per day and should continue as long as clinically indicated.

Parenteral Administration

In hospitalized patients with pathological hypersecretory conditions or intractable ulcers, or in patients who are unable to take oral medication, 'Tagamet' may be administered parenterally.
All parenteral drug products should be inspected visually for particulate matter and discoloration prior to administration.

Recommendations for parenteral administration:

Intramuscular injection: 300 mg. q 6–8 hours (no dilution necessary). Transient pain at the site of injection has been reported.

Intravenous injection: 300 mg. q 6–8 hours. Dilute 'Tagamet' HCl (brand of cimetidine hydrochloride) Injection, 300 mg., in Sodium Chloride Injection (0.9%) or another compatible i.v. solution (see Stability of 'Tagamet' HCl Injection) to a total volume of 20 ml. and inject over a period of not less than 2 minutes (see Precautions).

Intermittent intravenous infusion: 300 mg. q 6–8 hours. Dilute 'Tagamet' HCl Injection, 300 mg., in at least 50 ml. of Dextrose Injection (5%) or another compatible i.v. solution (see Stability of 'Tagamet' HCl Injection), or use premixed 'Tagamet' HCl Injection 300 mg. in 0.9% Sodium Chloride in 50 ml. plastic containers. Infuse over 15–20 minutes.

DIRECTIONS FOR USE OF 'TAGAMET' HCl (brand of cimetidine hydrochloride) INJECTION IN PLASTIC CONTAINERS

To open: Tear overwrap down side at slit and remove solution containers.
Some opacity of the plastic due to moisture absorption during the sterilization process may be observed. This is normal and does not affect solution quality or safety. The opacity will diminish gradually.

Do not add other drugs to premixed 'Tagamet' HCl Injection in plastic containers.

CAUTION: Check for minute leaks by squeezing inner bag firmly. If leaks are found, discard solution as sterility may be impaired. Additives should not be introduced into this solution. Do not use if the solution is cloudy or precipitated or if the seal is not intact.

Do not use plastic containers in series connections. Such use could result in air embolism due to residual air being drawn from the primary container before administration of the fluid from the secondary container is complete.

Use sterile equipment.

Preparation for administration:

1. Suspend container from eyelet support.
2. Remove plastic protector from outlet port at bottom of container.
3. Attach administration set. Refer to complete directions accompanying set.

In some patients it may be necessary to increase dosage. When this is necessary, the increases should be made by more frequent administration of a 300 mg. dose but should not exceed 2400 mg. per day.

Dosage Adjustment for Patients with Impaired Renal Function

Patients with severely impaired renal function have been treated with 'Tagamet'. However, such usage has been very limited. On the basis of this experience the recommended dosage is 300 mg. q 12 hours orally or by intravenous injection. Should the patient's condition require, the frequency of dosing may be increased to q 8 hours or even further with caution. In severe renal failure accumulation may occur and the lowest frequency of dosing compatible with an adequate patient response should be used. When liver impairment is also present, further reductions in dosage may be necessary. Hemodialysis reduces the level of circulating 'Tagamet'. Ideally, the dosage schedule should be adjusted so that the timing of a scheduled dose coincides with the end of hemodialysis.

Stability of 'Tagamet' HCl Injection

When added to or diluted with most commonly used intravenous solutions, e.g., Sodium Chloride Injection (0.9%), Dextrose Injection (5% or 10%), Lactated Ringer's Solution, 5% Sodium Bicarbonate Injection, 'Tagamet' HCl (brand of cimetidine hydrochloride) Injection should not be used after more than 48 hours of storage at room temperature.

'Tagamet' HCl Injection premixed in plastic containers is stable through the labeled expiration date when stored under the recommended conditions.

OVERDOSAGE

The usual measures to remove unabsorbed material from the gastrointestinal tract, clinical monitoring and supportive therapy should be employed. Studies in animals indicate that toxic doses are associated with respiratory failure and tachycardia which may be controlled by assisted respiration and the administration of a beta-blocker.

Human experience with gross overdosage is limited. However, in the few cases which have been reported, doses up to 10 grams have not been associated with any untoward effects.

HOW SUPPLIED

Tablets: 200 mg. tablets in bottles of 100; 300 mg. tablets in bottles of 100 and Single Unit Packages of 100 (intended for institutional use only); 400 mg. tablets in bottles of 60 and Single Unit Packages of 100 (intended for institutional use only), and 800 mg. Tiltab™ tablets in bottles of 30.

Liquid: 300 mg./5 ml., in 8 fl. oz. (237 ml.) amber glass bottles and in single-dose units (300 mg./5 ml.), in packages of 10 (intended for institutional use only).

Injection:

Vials: 300 mg./2 ml. in single-dose vials, in packages of 10 and 30, and in 8 ml. multiple-dose vials, in packages of 10 and 25. **Prefilled Syringes:** 300 mg./2 ml. in single-dose prefilled disposable syringes. **Plastic Containers:** 300 mg. in 50 ml. of 0.9% Sodium Chloride in single-dose plastic containers, in packages of 4 units.

Exposure of the premixed product to excessive heat should be avoided. It is recommended the product be stored at controlled room temperature. Brief exposure up to 40°C does not adversely affect the premixed product.

'Tagamet' HCl (brand of cimetidine hydrochloride) Injection premixed in single-dose plastic containers is manufactured for SK&F Lab Co. by Travenol Laboratories, Inc., Deerfield, IL 60015.

Military—Tablets, 200 mg., 100's, 6505-01-103-6335; 300 mg., SUP, 100's, 6505-01-050-3546, and 300 mg., 100's, 6505-01-050-3547; 400 mg., 60's, 6505-01-176-0712; Injection, 2 ml., 10's, 6505-01-051-4698; 8 ml., 10's, 6505-01-069-1661; Liquid, 300 mg., 8 oz., 6505-01-119-0616.

Veterans Administration—Tablets, 200 mg., 100's, 6505-01-103-6335A; 300 mg., 100's, 6505-01-050-3547A; 300 mg., SUP, 100's, 6505-01-050-3546A; 400 mg., 60's, 6505-01-176-0712; Liquid, 300 mg., 8 oz., 6505-01-119-0616A; Injection, 2 ml., 10's, 6505-01-051-4698B; 8 ml., 10's, 6505-01-069-1661B.

TG:L69

Shown in Product Identification Section, page 431

Table 2. Ceftazidime Concentrations in Body Tissues and Fluids

Tissue or Fluid	Dose/ Route	No. Patients	Time of Sample Post-Dose	Average Tissue or Fluid Level (mcg./ml.)
Urine	500 mg. I.M.	6	0–2 hours	2,100
	2 g. I.V.	6	0–2 hours	12,000
Bile	2 g. I.V.	3	90 min.	36.4
Synovial fluid	2 g. I.V.	13	2 hours	25.6
Peritoneal fluid	2 g. I.V.	8	2 hours	48.6
Sputum	1 g. I.V.	8	1 hour	9
Cerebrospinal fluid	2 g. q8h I.V.	5	120 min.	9.8
(inflamed meninges)	2 g. q8h I.V.	6	180 min.	9.4
Aqueous humor	2 g. I.V.	13	1–3 hours	11
Blister fluid	1 g. I.V.	7	2–3 hours	19.7
Lymphatic fluid	1 g. I.V.	7	2–3 hours	23.4
Bone	2 g. I.V.	8	0.67 hour	31.1
Heart muscle	2 g. I.V.	35	30–280 min.	12.7
Skin	2 g. I.V.	22	30–180 min.	6.6
Skeletal muscle	2 g. I.V.	35	30–280 min.	9.4
Myometrium	2 g. I.V.	31	1–2 hours	18.7

TAZICEF™ ℞

[*taz'i-sef*]

(brand of ceftazidime for injection)

PRODUCT OVERVIEW

KEY FACTS

'Tazicef' is a new cephalosporin with enhanced antipseudomonal activity. A wide range of gram-negative organisms, including strains resistant to gentamicin and other aminoglycosides, are susceptible to ceftazidime *in vitro*. Ceftazidime has also been shown to be active against gram-positive organisms. Ceftazidime achieves therapeutic levels in serum which allow for q8-12h dosing.

MAJOR USES

'Tazicef' is indicated for the treatment of patients with infections caused by susceptible strains of the designated organisms in the diseases listed in the full prescribing information below. In particular, ceftazidime has been proven to be clinically effective against *Pseudomonas* in skin and skin structure infections, respiratory tract infections, urinary tract infections, and, concomitantly with an anti-gram-negative agent, in infections in neutropenic patients.

SAFETY INFORMATION

'Tazicef' is contraindicated in patients who have shown hypersensitivity to ceftazidime or the cephalosporin group of antibiotics. Careful inquiry should be made concerning previous hypersensitivity reactions to drugs. 'Tazicef' should be administered with caution to penicillin-sensitive patients. Serious acute hypersensitivity reactions may require epinephrine and other emergency measures. Because pseudomembranous colitis has been reported with the use of cephalosporins, it is important to consider its diagnosis in patients who develop diarrhea in association with antibiotic use.

PRESCRIBING INFORMATION

TAZICEF™ ℞

[*taz'i-sef*]

(brand of ceftazidime for injection)

For Intravenous or Intramuscular Use

('Tazicef' is manufactured for Smith Kline &French Laboratories, Division of SmithKline Beckman Corporation, Philadelphia, Pa. by Merck & Co., Rahway, N.J.)

DESCRIPTION

Ceftazidime is a semisynthetic, broad-spectrum, beta-lactam antibiotic for parenteral administration. It is the pentahydrate of Pyridinium, 1-[[7-[[(2-amino-4-thiazolyl)[(1-carboxy-1-methylethoxy) imino]acetyl]amino]-2-carboxy-8-oxo-5-thia-1-azabicyclo (4.2.0.)oct-2-en-3-yl] methyl]-,hydroxide,inner salt, [6R-[6α,7β(Z)]].

Tazicef (ceftazidime for injection, SK&F) is a sterile, dry, powdered mixture of ceftazidime pentahydrate and sodium carbonate. The sodium carbonate at a concentration of 118 mg./g. of ceftazidime activity has been admixed to facilitate dissolution. The total sodium content of the mixture is approximately 54 mg. (2.3 mEq.)/g. of ceftazidime activity. Solutions of 'Tazicef' range in color from light yellow to amber, depending upon the diluent and volume used. The pH of freshly reconstituted solutions usually ranges from 5.0 to 8.0.

CLINICAL PHARMACOLOGY

After intravenous administration of 500 mg. and 1 g. doses of ceftazidime over five minutes to normal adult male volunteers, mean peak serum concentrations of 45 mcg./ml. and 90 mcg./ml., respectively, were achieved. After intravenous infusion of 500 mg., 1 g. and 2 g. doses of ceftazidime over 20 to 30 minutes to normal adult male volunteers, mean peak serum concentrations of 42 mcg./ml., 69 mcg./ml. and 170 mcg./ml., respectively, were achieved. The average serum concentrations following intravenous infusion of 500 mg., 1 g. and 2 g. doses to these volunteers over an eight-hour interval are given in Table 1.

Table 1

Ceftazidime I.V. Dosage	Serum Concentrations (mcg./ml.)				
	0.5 hr.	1 hr.	2 hr.	4 hr.	8 hr.
500 mg.	42	25	12	6	2
1 g.	60	39	23	11	3
2 g.	129	75	42	13	5

The absorption and elimination of ceftazidime were directly proportional to the size of the dose. The half-life following intravenous administration was approximately 1.9 hours. Less than 10% of ceftazidime was protein bound. The degree of protein binding was independent of concentration. There was no evidence of accumulation of ceftazidime in the serum in individuals with normal renal function following multiple intravenous doses of 1 g. and 2 g. every eight hours for ten days.

Following intramuscular administration of 500 mg. and 1 g. doses of ceftazidime to normal adult volunteers, the mean peak serum concentrations were 17 mcg./ml. and 39 mcg./ml., respectively, at approximately one hour. Serum concentrations remained above 4 mcg./ml. for six and eight hours after the intramuscular administration of 500 mg. and 1 g. doses, respectively. The half-life of ceftazidime in these volunteers was approximately two hours.

The presence of hepatic dysfunction had no effect on the pharmacokinetics of ceftazidime in individuals administered 2 g. intravenously every eight hours for five days. Therefore, a dosage adjustment from the normal recommended dosage is not required for patients with hepatic dysfunction, provided renal function is not impaired.

Approximately 80%–90% of an intramuscular or intravenous dose of ceftazidime is excreted unchanged by the kidneys over a 24-hour period. After the intravenous administration of single 500 mg. or 1 g. doses, approximately 50% of the dose appeared in the urine in the first two hours. An additional 20% was excreted between two and four hours after dosing, and approximately another 12% of the dose appeared in the urine between four and eight hours later. The elimination of ceftazidime by the kidneys resulted in high therapeutic concentrations in the urine.

The mean renal clearance of ceftazidime was approximately 100 ml./min. The calculated plasma clearance of approximately 115 ml./min. indicated nearly complete elimination of ceftazidime by the renal route. Administration of probenecid prior to dosing had no effect on the elimination kinetics of ceftazidime. This suggests that ceftazidime is eliminated by glomerular filtration and is not actively secreted by renal tubular mechanisms.

Since ceftazidime is eliminated almost solely by the kidneys, its serum half-life is significantly prolonged in patients with impaired renal function. Consequently, dosage adjustments in such patients as described in the DOSAGE AND ADMINISTRATION section are suggested.

Therapeutic concentrations of ceftazidime are achieved in the following body tissues and fluid.

[See table above].

Microbiology

Ceftazidime is bactericidal in action, exerting its effect by inhibition of enzymes responsible for cell-wall synthesis. A wide range of gram-negative organisms is susceptible to cef-

Continued on next page

Smith Kline & French—Cont.

tazidime *in vitro,* including strains resistant to gentamicin and other aminoglycosides. In addition, ceftazidime has been shown to be active against gram-positive organisms. It is highly stable to most clinically important beta-lactamases, plasmid or chromosomal, which are produced by both gram-negative and gram-positive organisms, and consequently is active against many strains resistant to ampicillin and other cephalosporins.

Ceftazidime has been shown to be active against the following organisms both *in vitro* and in clinical infections (see INDICATIONS AND USAGE).

Aerobes, Gram-Negative: *Pseudomonas* species (including *Pseudomonas aeruginosa*); *Klebsiella* species (including *Klebsiella pneumoniae*); *Proteus mirabilis; Proteus vulgaris; Escherichia coli; Enterobacter* species, including *Enterobacter cloacae* and *Enterobacter aerogenes; Citrobacter* species, including *Citrobacter freundii* and *Citrobacter diversus; Serratia* species; *Haemophilus influenzae,* including ampicillin-resistant strains; and *Neisseria meningitidis.*

Aerobes, Gram-Positive: *Staphylococcus aureus,* including penicillinase- and non-penicillinase-producing strains; *Streptococcus pyogenes* (group A beta-hemolytic streptococci); *Streptococcus agalactiae* (group B streptococci); and *Streptococcus pneumoniae.*

Anaerobes: *Bacteroides* species (NOTE: Many strains of *Bacteroides fragilis* are resistant).

Ceftazidime has also been shown to demonstrate *in vitro* activity against the following microorganisms, although its clinical significance is not known: *Staphylococcus epidermidis; Morganella morganii* (formerly *Proteus morganii*); *Providencia* species (including *Providencia rettgeri,* formerly *Proteus rettgeri*); *Acinetobacter* species; *Salmonella* species; *Clostridium* species (not including *Clostridium difficile*); *Peptococcus* species; *Peptostreptococcus* species; *Neisseria gonorrhoeae; Haemophilus parainfluenzae; Yersinia enterocolitica;* and *Shigella* species.

Ceftazidime and the aminoglycosides have been shown to be synergistic *in vitro* against *P. aeruginosa* and the *Enterobacteriaceae.* Ceftazidime and carbenicillin have also been shown to be synergistic *in vitro* against *P. aeruginosa.*

Ceftazidime is not active *in vitro* against: methicillin-resistant staphylococci; *Streptococcus faecalis* and many other enterococci; *Listeria monocytogenes; Campylobacter* species; or *Clostridium difficile.*

Susceptibility Tests

Quantitative methods that require measurement of zone diameters give the most precise estimate of antibiotic susceptibility. One such procedure[1–3] has been recommended for use with disks to test susceptibility to ceftazidime.

Reports from the laboratory giving results of the standard single-disk susceptibility test with a 30 mcg. ceftazidime disk should be interpreted according to the following criteria:

Susceptible organisms produce zones of 18 mm. or greater, indicating that the test organism is likely to respond to therapy.

Organisms that produce zones of 15 mm. to 17 mm. are expected to be susceptible if high dosage is used or if the infection is confined to tissues and fluids (e.g., urine) in which high antibiotic levels are attained.

Resistant organisms produce zones of 14 mm. or less, indicating that other therapy should be selected.

Organisms should be tested with the ceftazidime disk, since ceftazidime has been shown by *in vitro* tests to be active against certain strains found resistant when other beta-lactam disks are used.

Standardized procedures require the use of laboratory control organisms. The 30 mcg. ceftazidime disk should give zone diameters between 25 mm. and 32 mm. for *E. coli* ATCC 25922. For *P. aeruginosa* ATCC 27853, the zone diameters should be between 22 mm. and 29 mm. For *S. aureus* ATCC 25923, the zone diameters should be between 16 mm. and 20 mm.

In other susceptibility testing procedures, e.g., ICS agar dilution or the equivalent, a bacterial isolate may be considered susceptible if the MIC value for ceftazidime is not more than 16 mcg./ml. Organisms are considered resistant to ceftazidime if the MIC is equal to or greater than 64 mcg./ml. Organisms having an MIC value of less than 64 mcg./ml. but greater than 16 mcg./ml. are expected to be susceptible if high dosage is used or if the infection is confined to tissues and fluids (e.g., urine) in which high antibiotic levels are attained.

As with standard diffusion methods, dilution procedures require the use of laboratory control organisms. Standard ceftazidime powder should give MIC values in the range of 4 mcg./ml. and 16 mcg./ml. for *S. aureus* ATCC 25923. For *E. coli* ATCC 25922, the MIC range should be between 0.125 mcg./ml. and 0.5 mcg./ml. For *P. aeruginosa* ATCC 27853, the MIC range should be between 0.5 mcg./ml. and 2 mcg./ml.

INDICATIONS AND USAGE

Tazicef (ceftazidime for injection, SK&F) is indicated for the treatment of patients with infections caused by susceptible strains of the designated organisms in the diseases listed below:

LOWER RESPIRATORY TRACT INFECTIONS, including pneumonia, caused by *P. aeruginosa* and other *Pseudomonas* species; *H. influenzae,* including ampicillin-resistant strains; *Klebsiella* species; *Enterobacter* species, *P. mirabilis; E. coli; Serratia* species; *Citrobacter* species; *S. pneumoniae;* and *S. aureus* (methicillin-susceptible strains).

SKIN AND SKIN STRUCTURE INFECTIONS, caused by *P. aeruginosa, Klebsiella* species; *E. coli; Proteus* species including *P. mirabilis* and indole-positive *Proteus, Enterobacter* species; *Serratia* species; *S. aureus* (methicillin-susceptible strains) and *S. pyogenes* (group A beta-hemolytic streptococci).

URINARY TRACT INFECTIONS, both complicated and uncomplicated, caused by *P. aeruginosa; Enterobacter* species; *Proteus* species, including *P. mirabilis* and indole-positive *Proteus; Klebsiella* species and *E. coli.*

BACTERIAL SEPTICEMIA, caused by *P. aeruginosa, Klebsiella* species; *H. influenzae; E. coli, Serratia* species, *S. pneumoniae* and *S. aureus* (methicillin-susceptible strains).

BONE AND JOINT INFECTIONS, caused by *P. aeruginosa; Klebsiella* species; *Enterobacter* species; and *S. aureus* (methicillin-susceptible strains).

GYNECOLOGICAL INFECTIONS, including endometritis, pelvic cellulitis and other infections of the female genital tract caused by *E. coli.*

INTRA-ABDOMINAL INFECTIONS, including peritonitis caused by *E. coli, Klebsiella* species; *S. aureus* (methicillin-susceptible strains), and polymicrobial infections caused by aerobic and anaerobic organisms, and *Bacteroides* species (many strains of *B. fragilis* are resistant).

CENTRAL NERVOUS SYSTEM INFECTIONS, including meningitis caused by *H. influenzae* and *Neisseria meningitidis.* Ceftazidime has also been used successfully in a limited number of cases of meningitis due to *P. aeruginosa* and *S. pneumoniae.*

Specimens for bacterial cultures should be obtained prior to therapy in order to isolate and identify causative organisms and to determine their susceptibility to ceftazidime. Therapy may be instituted before results of susceptibility studies are known; however, once these results become available, the antibiotic treatment should be adjusted accordingly.

Tazicef (ceftazidime for injection, SK&F) may be used alone in cases of confirmed or suspected sepsis. Ceftazidime has been used successfully in clinical trials as empiric therapy in cases where various concomitant therapies with other antibiotics have been used.

'Tazicef' may also be used concomitantly with other antibiotics, such as aminoglycosides, vancomycin and clindamycin, in severe and life-threatening infections and in the immunocompromised patient. When such concomitant treatment is appropriate, prescribing information in the labeling for the other antibiotics should be followed. The dose depends on the severity of the infection and the patient's condition.

CONTRAINDICATIONS

'Tazicef' is contraindicated in patients who have shown hypersensitivity to ceftazidime or the cephalosporin group of antibiotics.

WARNINGS

BEFORE THERAPY WITH 'TAZICEF' IS INSTITUTED, CAREFUL INQUIRY SHOULD BE MADE TO DETERMINE WHETHER THE PATIENT HAS HAD PREVIOUS HYPERSENSITIVITY REACTIONS TO CEFTAZIDIME, CEPHALOSPORINS, PENICILLINS, OR OTHER DRUGS. ANTIBIOTICS SHOULD BE ADMINISTERED WITH CAUTION TO ANY PATIENT WHO HAS DEMONSTRATED SOME FORM OF ALLERGY, PARTICULARLY TO DRUGS. THIS PRODUCT SHOULD BE GIVEN WITH CAUTION TO PATIENTS WITH TYPE 1 HYPERSENSITIVITY REACTIONS TO PENICILLIN. IF AN ALLERGIC REACTION TO 'TAZICEF' OCCURS, DISCONTINUE TREATMENT WITH THE DRUG. SERIOUS ACUTE HYPERSENSITIVITY REACTIONS MAY REQUIRE EPINEPHRINE AND OTHER EMERGENCY MEASURES.

Pseudomembranous colitis has been reported with the use of cephalosporins (and other broad-spectrum antibiotics); therefore, it is important to consider its diagnosis in patients who develop diarrhea in association with antibiotic use.

Treatment with broad-spectrum antibiotics alters normal flora of the colon and may permit overgrowth of clostridia. Studies indicate a toxin produced by *C. difficile* is one primary cause of antibiotic-associated colitis.

Mild cases of colitis may respond to drug discontinuance alone. Moderate to severe cases should be managed with fluid, electrolyte and protein supplementation as indicated. When the colitis is not relieved by drug discontinuance or when it is severe, oral vancomycin is the treatment of choice for antibiotic-associated pseudomembranous colitis produced by *C. difficile.* Other causes of colitis should also be considered.

PRECAUTIONS

Ceftazidime has not been shown to be nephrotoxic; however, because high and prolonged serum antibiotic concentrations can occur from usual doses in patients with transient or persistent reduction of urinary output because of renal insufficiency, the total daily dosage should be reduced when ceftazidime is administered to such patients (see DOSAGE AND ADMINISTRATION). Continued dosage should be determined by degree of renal impairment, severity of infection and susceptibility of the causative organisms.

As with other antibiotics, prolonged use of Tazicef (ceftazidime for injection, SK&F) may result in overgrowth of nonsusceptible organisms. Repeated evaluation of the patient's condition is essential. If superinfection occurs during therapy, appropriate measures should be taken.

'Tazicef' should be prescribed with caution in individuals with a history of gastrointestinal disease, particularly colitis.

Drug Interactions: Nephrotoxicity has been reported following concomitant administration of cephalosporins with aminoglycoside antibiotics or potent diuretics, such as furosemide. Renal function should be carefully monitored, especially if higher dosages of the aminoglycosides are to be administered or if therapy is prolonged, because of the potential nephrotoxicity and ototoxicity of aminoglycoside antibiotics. Nephrotoxicity and ototoxicity were not noted when ceftazidime was given alone in clinical trials.

Carcinogenesis, Mutagenesis, Impairment of Fertility: Long-term studies in animals have not been performed to evaluate carcinogenic potential. However, a mouse micronucleus test and an Ames test were both negative for mutagenic effects.

Usage in Pregnancy: Pregnancy Category B. Reproduction studies have been performed in mice and rats at doses up to 40 times the human dose and have revealed no evidence of impaired fertility or harm to the fetus due to ceftazidime. There are, however, no adequate and well-controlled studies in pregnant women. Because animal reproduction studies are not always predictive of human response, this drug should be used during pregnancy only if clearly needed.

Nursing Mothers: Ceftazidime is excreted in human milk in low concentrations. Caution should be exercised when 'Tazicef' is administered to a nursing woman.

ADVERSE REACTIONS

Ceftazidime is generally well tolerated. The incidence of adverse reactions associated with the administration of ceftazidime was low in clinical trials. The most common were local reactions following intravenous injection, and allergic and gastrointestinal reactions. Other adverse reactions were encountered infrequently. No disulfiram-like reactions were reported. The following adverse effects from premarketing clinical trials were considered to be either related to ceftazidime therapy or were of uncertain etiology.

Local Effects, reported in less than 2% of patients, were phlebitis and inflammation at the site of injection (1 in 69 patients).

Hypersensitivity Reactions, reported in 2% of patients, were pruritus, rash and fever. Immediate hypersensitivity reactions occurred in 1 in 285 patients.

Gastrointestinal Symptoms, reported in less than 2% of patients, were diarrhea (1 in 78), nausea (1 in 156), vomiting (1 in 500) and abdominal pain (1 in 416).

Symptoms of pseudomembranous colitis can appear during or after antibiotic treatment (See WARNINGS section).

Less Frequent Adverse Events (less than 1%) were candidiasis and vaginitis; central nervous system events which included headache, dizziness and paresthesia.

Laboratory Test Changes noted during ceftazidime clinical trials were transient and included: eosinophilia (1 in 13), positive Coombs' test without hemolysis (1 in 23), thrombocytosis (1 in 45), and slight elevations in one or more of the hepatic enzymes, SGOT (1 in 16), SGPT (1 in 15), LDH (1 in 18) and alkaline phosphatase (1 in 23). As with some other cephalosporins, transient elevations of blood urea, blood urea nitrogen and/or serum creatinine were observed occasionally. Transient leukopenia, neutropenia, thrombocytopenia and lymphocytosis were seen very rarely.

DOSAGE AND ADMINISTRATION

Dosage: The usual adult dosage is 1 g. administered intravenously or intramuscularly every eight or 12 hours. The dosage and route should be determined by the susceptibility of the causative organisms, the severity of infection and the condition and renal function of the patient.

The guidelines for dosage of 'Tazicef' are listed in Table 3. The following dosage schedule is recommended.

[See table on top next page].

Impaired Hepatic Function: No adjustment in dosage is required for patients with hepatic dysfunction.

Impaired Renal Function: Ceftazidime is excreted by the kidneys, almost exclusively by glomerular filtration. Therefore, in patients with impaired renal function (GFR <50 ml./min.), it is recommended that the dosage of ceftazidime be reduced to compensate for its slower excretion. In patients with suspected renal insufficiency, an initial loading dose of

1 g. of ceftazidime may be given. An estimate of GFR should be made to determine the appropriate maintenance dose. The recommended dosage is presented in Table 4.

Table 4. Recommended Maintenance Doses of Tazicef (ceftazidime for injection, SK&F) in Renal Insufficiency

Creatinine Clearance (ml./min.)	Recommended Unit Dose of Ceftazidime	Frequency of Dosing
50–31	1 g.	q12h
30–16	1 g.	q24h
15–6	500 mg.	q24h
<5	500 mg.	q48h

When only serum creatinine is available, the following formula (Cockcroft's equation)[4] may be used to estimate creatinine clearance. The serum creatinine should represent a steady state of renal function:

Males:

$$\text{Creatinine clearance (ml./min.)} = \frac{\text{Weight (kg.)} \times (140 - \text{age})}{72 \times \text{serum creatinine (mg./dl.)}}$$

Females:

0.85 × above value

In patients with severe infections who would normally receive 6 g. of ceftazidime daily were it not for renal insufficiency, the unit dose given in the table above may be increased by 50% or the dosing frequency increased appropriately. Further dosing should be determined by therapeutic monitoring, severity of the infection and susceptibility of the causative organism.

In children as for adults, the creatinine clearance should be adjusted for body surface area or lean body mass and the dosing frequency reduced in cases of renal insufficiency.

In patients undergoing hemodialysis, a loading dose of 1 g. is recommended, followed by 1 g. after each hemodialysis period.

Tazicef (ceftazidime for injection, SK&F) can also be used in patients undergoing intra-peritoneal dialysis (IPD) and continuous ambulatory peritoneal dialysis (CAPD). In such patients, a loading dose of 'Tazicef' 1 g. may be given, followed by 500 mg. every 24 hours. In addition to intravenous use, 'Tazicef' can be incorporated in the dialysis fluid at a concentration of 250 mg. for 2 liters of dialysis fluid.

NOTE: Generally, 'Tazicef' should be continued for two days after the signs and symptoms of infection have disappeared, but in complicated infections longer therapy may be required.

RECONSTITUTION

Single Dose Vials:

For I.M. injection, I.V. direct (bolus) injection, or I.V. infusion, reconstitute with Sterile Water for Injection according to the following table. The vacuum may assist entry of the diluent. SHAKE WELL.

Table 5

Vial Size	Diluent to Be Added	Approx. Avail. Volume	Approx. Avg. Concentration
Intramuscular or Intravenous Direct (bolus) Injection			
1 gram	3.0 ml.	3.6 ml.	280 mg./ml.
Intravenous Infusion			
1 gram	10 ml.	10.6 ml.	95 mg./ml.
2 gram	10 ml.	11.2 ml.	180 mg./ml.

Withdraw the total volume of solution into the syringe (the pressure in the vial may aid withdrawal). The withdrawn solution may contain some bubbles of carbon dioxide.

NOTE: As with the administration of all parenteral products, accumulated gases should be expressed from the syringe immediately before injection of 'Tazicef'.

These solutions of 'Tazicef' are stable for 18 hours at room temperature or seven days if refrigerated (5°C.). Slight yellowing does not affect potency.

For I.V. infusion, dilute reconstituted solution in 50 to 100 ml. of one of the parenteral fluids listed under COMPATIBILITY AND STABILITY.

"Piggyback" Vials:

For I.V. infusion, reconstitute with 10 ml. of Sodium Chloride Injection according to the following table. The vacuum may assist entry of the diluent. SHAKE WELL.

Table 6

Vial Size	Diluent to Be Added	Approx. Avail. Volume	Approx. Avg. Concentration
1 gram	100 ml.*	100 ml.	10 mg./ml.
2 gram	100 ml.*	100 ml.	20 mg./ml.

* Addition should be in two stages.

Insert a gas relief needle through the vial closure to relieve the internal pressure. With the gas relief needle in position, add the remaining 90 ml. of Sodium Chloride Injection. Remove the gas relief needle and syringe needle; shake the vial and set up for infusion in the normal way.

NOTE: To preserve product sterility, it is important that a gas relief needle is not inserted through the vial closure before the product has dissolved.

These solutions of Tazicef (ceftazidime for injection, SK&F) are stable for 18 hours at room temperature or seven days if refrigerated (5°C.). Slight yellowing does not affect potency.

Administration: 'Tazicef' may be given intravenously or by deep intramuscular injection into a large muscle mass such as the upper outer quadrant of the gluteus maximus or lateral part of the thigh.

Intramuscular Administration: For intramuscular administration, 'Tazicef' should be reconstituted with Sterile Water for Injection. Refer to Table 5.

Intravenous Administration: The I.V. route is preferable for patients with bacterial septicemia, bacterial meningitis, peritonitis, or other severe or life-threatening infections, or for patients who may be poor risks because of lowered resistance resulting from such debilitating conditions as malnutrition, trauma, surgery, diabetes, heart failure or malignancy, particularly if shock is present or pending.

For direct intermittent intravenous administration, reconstitute 'Tazicef' as directed in Table 5 with Sterile Water for Injection. Slowly inject directly into the vein over a period of three to five minutes or give through the tubing of an administration set while the patient is also receiving one of the compatible intravenous fluids (See COMPATIBILITY AND STABILITY).

For intravenous infusion, reconstitute the 1 or 2 g. piggyback vial with 100 ml. of Sodium Chloride Injection or one of the compatible intravenous fluids listed under the COMPATIBILITY AND STABILITY section. Alternatively, reconstitute the 1 g. or 2 g. vial and add an appropriate quantity of the resulting solution to an I.V. container with one of the compatible intravenous fluids.

Intermittent intravenous infusion with a Y-type administration set can be accomplished with compatible solutions. However, during infusion of a solution containing 'Tazicef' it is advisable to discontinue the other solution.

All vials of 'Tazicef' as supplied are under reduced pressure. When 'Tazicef' is dissolved, carbon dioxide is released and a positive pressure develops. See RECONSTITUTION.

Solutions of 'Tazicef', like those of most beta-lactam antibiotics, should not be added to solutions of aminoglycoside antibiotics because of potential interaction.

However, if concurrent therapy with 'Tazicef' and an aminoglycoside is indicated, each of these antibiotics can be administered separately to the same patient.

COMPATIBILITY AND STABILITY

Intramuscular: 'Tazicef', when reconstituted as directed with Sterile Water for Injection, maintains satisfactory potency for 18 hours at room temperature or for seven days under refrigeration (5°C.). Solutions in Sterile Water for Injection that are frozen immediately after reconstitution in the original container are stable for three months when stored at −20°C. Once thawed, solutions should not be refrozen. Thawed solutions may be stored for up to eight hours at room temperature or for four days in a refrigerator (5°C.).

Intravenous: Tazicef (ceftazidime for injection, SK&F), when reconstituted as directed with Sterile Water for Injection, maintains satisfactory potency for 18 hours at room temperature or for seven days under refrigeration (5°C.). Solutions in Sterile Water for Injection in the original container or in 0.9% Sodium Chloride Injection in Viaflex® small volume containers that are frozen immediately after reconstitution are stable for three months when stored at −20°C. For larger volumes where it may be necessary to warm the frozen product (to a maximum of 40°C.), care should be taken to avoid heating after thawing is complete. Once thawed, solutions should not be refrozen. Thawed solutions may be stored for up to eight hours at room temperature or for four days in a refrigerator (5°C.).

'Tazicef' is compatible with the more commonly used intravenous infusion fluids. Solutions at concentrations between 1 mg./ml. and 40 mg./ml. in the following infusion fluids may be stored for up to 18 hours at room temperature or seven days if refrigerated: 0.9% Sodium Chloride Injection; Ringer's Injection USP; Lactated Ringer's Injection USP; 5% Dextrose Injection; 5% Dextrose and 0.225% Sodium Chloride Injection; 5% Dextrose and 0.45% Sodium Chloride Injection; 5% Dextrose and 0.9% Sodium Chloride Injection; 10% Dextrose Injection.

'Tazicef' is less stable in Sodium Bicarbonate Injection than in other intravenous fluids. It is not recommended as a diluent. Solutions of 'Tazicef' in 5% Dextrose and 0.9% Sodium Chloride Injection are stable for at least six hours at room temperature in plastic tubing, drip chambers and volume control devices of common intravenous infusion sets.

Ceftazidime at a concentration of 20 mg./ml. has been found compatible for 18 hours at room temperature or seven days under refrigeration in Sterile Water for Injection when admixed with: cefazolin sodium (Ancef®) 330 mg./ml.; heparin 1000 units/ml.; and cimetidine HCl (Tagamet® HCl) 150 mg./ml.

Ceftazidime at a concentration of 20 mg./ml. has been found compatible for 18 hours at room temperature or seven days under refrigeration in 5% Dextrose Injection when admixed with Potassium Chloride 40 mEq/l.

Note: Parenteral drug products should be inspected visually for particulate matter prior to administration wherever solution and container permit.

As with other cephalosporins, 'Tazicef' powder as well as solutions tend to darken depending on storage conditions; within the stated recommendations, however, product potency is not adversely affected.

HOW SUPPLIED

Tazicef (ceftazidime for injection, SK&F) is supplied in vials equivalent to 1 gram and 2 grams of ceftazidime; in "Piggyback" Vials for I.V. admixture equivalent to 1 gram and 2 grams of ceftazidime.

REFERENCES

1. Bauer, A.W.; Kirby, W.M.M., and Sherris, J.C., et al.: Antibiotic susceptibility testing by a standardized single disc method, Am. J. Clin. Pathol. 45:493, 1966. 2. National Committee for Clinical Laboratory Standards, Approved Standard: Performance Standards for Antimicrobial Disc Susceptibility Tests (M2-A3), December, 1984. 3. Standardized disc susceptibility test, Federal Register 39:19182–19184, 1974. 4. Cockcroft, D.W., and Gault, M.H.: Prediction of creatinine clearance from serum creatinine, Nephron 16:31–41, 1976.

TF:L2

Shown in Product Identification Section, page 431

Continued on next page

Table 3. Recommended Dosage Schedule

	Dose	Frequency
Adults		
Usual recommended dose	1 g. I.V. or I.M.	q8–12h
Uncomplicated urinary tract infections	250 mg. I.V. or I.M.	q12h
Bone and joint infections	2 g. I.V.	q12h
Complicated urinary tract infections	500 mg. I.V. or I.M.	q8–12h
Uncomplicated pneumonia; mild skin and skin structure infections	500 mg.–1 g. I.V. or I.M.	q8h
Serious gynecological and intra-abdominal infections	2 g. I.V.	q8h
Meningitis	2 g. I.V.	q8h
Very severe life-threatening infections, especially in immunocompromised patients	2 g. I.V.	q8h
Pseudomonal lung infections in patients with cystic fibrosis with normal renal function*	30–50 mg./kg. I.V. to a maximum of 6 g./day	q8h
Neonates (0–4 weeks)	30 mg./kg. I.V.	q12h
Infants and children (1 month–12 years)	30–50 mg./kg. I.V. to a maximum of 6 g./day†	q8h

* Although clinical improvement has been shown, bacteriological cures cannot be expected in patients with chronic respiratory disease and cystic fibrosis.

† The higher dose should be reserved for immunocompromised children or children with cystic fibrosis or meningitis.

Smith Kline & French—Cont.

THORAZINE® ℞
[*thor'ah-zeen*]
(brand of chlorpromazine)

DESCRIPTION

Thorazine (chlorpromazine, SK&F) is 10 - (3 - dimethylaminopropyl) -2-chlorphenothiazine, a dimethylamine derivative of phenothiazine. It is present in oral and injectable forms as the hydrochloride salt, and in the suppositories as the base.

Tablets—Each round, orange, coated tablet contains chlorpromazine hydrochloride as follows: 10 mg. imprinted SKF and T73; 25 mg. imprinted SKF and T74; 50 mg. imprinted SKF and T76; 100 mg. imprinted SKF and T77; 200 mg. imprinted SKF and T79. Inactive ingredients consist of benzoic acid, croscarmellose sodium, D&C Yellow No. 10, FD&C Blue No. 2, FD&C Yellow No. 6, gelatin, hydroxypropyl methylcellulose, lactose, magnesium stearate, methylparaben, polyethylene glycol, propylparaben, talc, titanium dioxide and trace amounts of other inactive ingredients.

Spansule® sustained release capsules—Each 'Thorazine' *Spansule* capsule is so prepared that an initial dose is released promptly and the remaining medication is released gradually over a prolonged period.

Each capsule, with opaque orange cap and natural body, contains chlorpromazine hydrochloride as follows: 30 mg. imprinted SKF and T63; 75 mg. imprinted SKF and T64; 150 mg. imprinted SKF and T66; 200 mg. imprinted SKF and T67; 300 mg. imprinted SKF and T69. Inactive ingredients consist of benzyl alcohol, calcium sulfate, cetylpyridinium chloride, FD&C Yellow No. 6, gelatin, glyceryl distearate, glyceryl monostearate, iron oxide, povidone, silicon dioxide, sodium lauryl sulfate, starch, sucrose, titanium dioxide, wax and trace amounts of other inactive ingredients.

Ampuls—Each ml. contains, in aqueous solution, chlorpromazine hydrochloride, 25 mg.; ascorbic acid, 2 mg.; sodium bisulfite, 1 mg.; sodium chloride, 6 mg.; sodium sulfite, 1 mg.

Multiple-dose Vials—Each ml. contains, in aqueous solution, chlorpromazine hydrochloride, 25 mg.; ascorbic acid, 2 mg.; sodium bisulfite, 1 mg.; sodium chloride, 1 mg.; sodium sulfite, 1 mg.; benzyl alcohol, 2%, as a preservative.

Syrup—Each 5 ml. (one teaspoonful) of clear, orange-custard flavored liquid contains chlorpromazine hydrochloride, 10 mg. Inactive ingredients consist of citric acid, flavors, sodium benzoate, sucrose and water.

Suppositories—Each suppository contains chlorpromazine, 25 or 100 mg., glycerin, glyceryl monopalmitate, glyceryl monostearate, hydrogenated coconut oil fatty acids, and hydrogenated kernel oil fatty acids.

Concentrate—Each ml. of clear, custard flavored liquid contains chlorpromazine hydrochloride, 30 or 100 mg. Inactive ingredients consist of calcium disodium edetate, citric acid, flavors, hydroxypropyl methylcellulose, propylene glycol, saccharin sodium, sodium benzoate, water and trace amounts of other inactive ingredients.

ACTIONS

The precise mechanism whereby the therapeutic effects of chlorpromazine are produced is not known. The principal pharmacological actions are psychotropic. It also exerts sedative and antiemetic activity. Chlorpromazine has actions at all levels of the central nervous system— primarily at subcortical levels—as well as on multiple organ systems. Chlorpromazine has strong antiadrenergic and weaker peripheral anticholinergic activity; ganglionic blocking action is relatively slight. It also possesses slight antihistaminic and antiserotonin activity.

INDICATIONS

For the management of manifestations of psychotic disorders.
To control nausea and vomiting.
For relief of restlessness and apprehension before surgery.
For acute intermittent porphyria.
As an adjunct in the treatment of tetanus.
To control the manifestations of the manic type of manic-depressive illness.
For relief of intractable hiccups.
For the treatment of severe behavioral problems in children marked by combativeness and/or explosive hyperexcitable behavior (out of proportion to immediate provocations), and in the short-term treatment of hyperactive children who show excessive motor activity with accompanying conduct disorders consisting of some or all of the following symptoms: impulsivity, difficulty sustaining attention, aggressivity, mood lability and poor frustration tolerance.

> Thorazine (chlorpromazine, SK&F) is considered possibly effective in the treatment of non-psychotic anxiety. However, 'Thorazine' is not the first drug to be used in therapy for most patients with non-psychotic anxiety because certain risks associated with its use are not shared by common alternative treatments (e.g., benzodiazepines).
> When used in the treatment of non-psychotic anxiety, 'Thorazine' should not be administered in doses of more than 100 mg. per day or for longer than 12 weeks because the use of 'Thorazine' at higher doses or for longer intervals may cause persistent tardive dyskinesia that may prove irreversible. (See Warnings section.)
> Final classification by the FDA of the non-psychotic anxiety indication requires further investigation.

CONTRAINDICATIONS

Do not use in comatose states or in the presence of large amounts of central nervous system depressants (alcohol, barbiturates, narcotics, etc.).

WARNINGS

The extrapyramidal symptoms which can occur secondary to 'Thorazine' may be confused with the central nervous system signs of an undiagnosed primary disease responsible for the vomiting, e.g., Reye's syndrome or other encephalopathy. The use of 'Thorazine' and other potential hepatotoxins should be avoided in children and adolescents whose signs and symptoms suggest Reye's syndrome.

Tardive Dyskinesia: Tardive dyskinesia, a syndrome consisting of potentially irreversible, involuntary, dyskinetic movements, may develop in patients treated with neuroleptic (antipsychotic) drugs. Although the prevalence of the syndrome appears to be highest among the elderly, especially elderly women, it is impossible to rely upon prevalence estimates to predict, at the inception of neuroleptic treatment, which patients are likely to develop the syndrome. Whether neuroleptic drug products differ in their potential to cause tardive dyskinesia is unknown.

Both the risk of developing the syndrome and the likelihood that it will become irreversible are believed to increase as the duration of treatment and the total cumulative dose of neuroleptic drugs administered to the patient increase. However, the syndrome can develop, although much less commonly, after relatively brief treatment periods at low doses.

There is no known treatment for established cases of tardive dyskinesia, although the syndrome may remit, partially or completely, if neuroleptic treatment is withdrawn. Neuroleptic treatment itself, however, may suppress (or partially suppress) the signs and symptoms of the syndrome and thereby may possibly mask the underlying disease process. The effect that symptomatic suppression has upon the long-term course of the syndrome is unknown.

Given these considerations, neuroleptics should be prescribed in a manner that is most likely to minimize the occurrence of tardive dyskinesia. Chronic neuroleptic treatment should generally be reserved for patients who suffer from a chronic illness that, 1) is known to respond to neuroleptic drugs, and, 2) for whom alternative, equally effective, but potentially less harmful treatments are *not* available or appropriate. In patients who do require chronic treatment, the smallest dose and the shortest duration of treatment producing a satisfactory clinical response should be sought. The need for continued treatment should be reassessed periodically.

If signs and symptoms of tardive dyskinesia appear in a patient on neuroleptics, drug discontinuation should be considered. However, some patients may require treatment despite the presence of the syndrome.

For further information about the description of tardive dyskinesia and its clinical detection, please refer to the sections on Precautions and Adverse Reactions.

Patients with bone marrow depression or who have previously demonstrated a hypersensitivity reaction (e.g., blood dyscrasias, jaundice) with a phenothiazine should not receive any phenothiazine, including 'Thorazine', unless in the judgment of the physician the potential benefits of treatment outweigh the possible hazard.

'Thorazine' may impair mental and/or physical abilities, especially during the first few days of therapy. Therefore, caution patients about activities requiring alertness (e.g., operating vehicles or machinery).

The use of alcohol with this drug should be avoided due to possible additive effects and hypotension.

'Thorazine' may counteract the antihypertensive effect of guanethidine and related compounds.

Usage in Pregnancy: Safety for the use of Thorazine (chlorpromazine, SK&F) during pregnancy has not been established. Therefore, it is not recommended that the drug be given to pregnant patients except when, in the judgment of the physician, it is essential. The potential benefits should clearly outweigh possible hazards. There are reported instances of prolonged jaundice, extrapyramidal signs, hyperreflexia or hyporeflexia in newborn infants whose mothers received phenothiazines.

Reproductive studies in rodents have demonstrated potential for embryotoxicity, increased neonatal mortality and nursing transfer of the drug. Tests in the offspring of the drug-treated rodents demonstrate decreased performance. The possibility of permanent neurological damage cannot be excluded.

Nursing Mothers: There is evidence that chlorpromazine is excreted in the breast milk of nursing mothers.

PRECAUTIONS

Given the likelihood that some patients exposed chronically to neuroleptics will develop tardive dyskinesia, it is advised that all patients in whom chronic use is contemplated be given, if possible, full information about this risk. The decision to inform patients and/or their guardians must obviously take into account the clinical circumstances and the competency of the patient to understand the information provided.

Thorazine (chlorpromazine, SK&F) should be administered cautiously to persons with cardiovascular or liver disease. There is evidence that patients with a history of hepatic encephalopathy due to cirrhosis have increased sensitivity to the C.N.S. effects of 'Thorazine' (i.e., impaired cerebration and abnormal slowing of the EEG).

Because of its C.N.S. depressant effect, 'Thorazine' should be used with caution in patients with chronic respiratory disorders such as severe asthma, emphysema and acute respiratory infections, particularly in children.

Because 'Thorazine' can suppress the cough reflex, aspiration of vomitus is possible.

Thorazine (chlorpromazine, SK&F) prolongs and intensifies the action of C.N.S. depressants such as anesthetics, barbiturates and narcotics. When 'Thorazine' is administered concomitantly, about ¼ to ½ the usual dosage of such agents is required. When 'Thorazine' is not being administered to reduce requirements of C.N.S. depressants, it is best to stop such depressants before starting 'Thorazine' treatment. These agents may subsequently be reinstated at low doses and increased as needed.

Note: 'Thorazine' does *not* intensify the anticonvulsant action of barbiturates. Therefore, dosage of anticonvulsants, including barbiturates, should *not* be reduced if 'Thorazine' is started. Instead, start 'Thorazine' at low doses and increase as needed.

Use with caution in persons who will be exposed to extreme heat, organophosphorus insecticides, and in persons receiving atropine or related drugs.

'Thorazine' tablets have recently been reformulated to remove FD&C Yellow No. 5 (tartrazine).

However, until the transition process is complete, some lots of 'Thorazine' tablets containing FD&C Yellow No. 5 (tartrazine) will still be in stock. FD&C Yellow No. 5 (tartrazine) may cause allergic-type reactions (including bronchial asthma) in certain susceptible individuals. Although the overall incidence of FD&C Yellow No. 5 (tartrazine) sensitivity in the general population is low, it is frequently seen in patients who also have aspirin sensitivity.

For specific information, contact Smith Kline &French Laboratories (outside Pa., call toll-free: 1-800-523-4835, ext. 5231; in Pa., call collect: 215-751-5231).

Neuroleptic drugs elevate prolactin levels; the elevation persists during chronic administration. Tissue culture experiments indicate that approximately one-third of human breast cancers are prolactin-dependent in vitro, a factor of potential importance if the prescribing of these drugs is contemplated in a patient with a previously detected breast cancer. Although disturbances such as galactorrhea, amenorrhea, gynecomastia and impotence have been reported, the clinical significance of elevated serum prolactin levels is unknown for most patients. An increase in mammary neoplasms has been found in rodents after chronic administration of neuroleptic drugs. Neither clinical nor epidemiologic studies conducted to date, however, have shown an association between chronic administration of these drugs and mammary tumorigenesis; the available evidence is considered too limited to be conclusive at this time.

As with all drugs which exert an anticholinergic effect, and/or cause mydriasis, chlorpromazine should be used with caution in patients with glaucoma.

Chlorpromazine diminishes the effect of oral anticoagulants.

Phenothiazines can produce alpha-adrenergic blockade.

Chlorpromazine may lower the convulsive threshold; dosage adjustments of anticonvulsants may be necessary. Potentiation of anticonvulsant effects does not occur. However, it has been reported that chlorpromazine may interfere with the metabolism of Dilantin®* and thus precipitate Dilantin* toxicity.

Concomitant administration with propranolol results in increased plasma levels of both drugs.

Thiazide diuretics may accentuate the orthostatic hypotension that may occur with phenothiazines.

The presence of phenothiazines may produce false positive phenylketonuria (PKU) test results.

Drugs which lower the seizure threshold, including phenothiazine derivatives, should not be used with Amipaque®†.

As with other phenothiazine derivatives, 'Thorazine' should be discontinued at least 48 hours before myelography, should not be resumed for at least 24 hours postprocedure, and should not be used for the control of nausea and vomiting occurring either prior to myelography or postprocedure with Amipaque†.

Long-Term Therapy: To lessen the likelihood of adverse reactions related to cumulative drug effect, patients with a history of long-term therapy with 'Thorazine' and/or other neuroleptics should be evaluated periodically to decide whether the maintenance dosage could be lowered or drug therapy discontinued.

Antiemetic Effect: The antiemetic action of 'Thorazine' may mask the signs and symptoms of overdosage of other drugs and may obscure the diagnosis and treatment of other conditions such as intestinal obstruction, brain tumor and Reye's syndrome. (See Warnings.)

When 'Thorazine' is used with cancer chemotherapeutic drugs, vomiting as a sign of the toxicity of these agents may be obscured by the antiemetic effect of 'Thorazine'.

Abrupt Withdrawal: Like other phenothiazines, Thorazine (chlorpromazine, SK&F) is not known to cause psychic dependence and does not produce tolerance or addiction. There may be, however, following abrupt withdrawal of high-dose therapy, some symptoms resembling those of physical dependence such as gastritis, nausea and vomiting, dizziness and tremulousness. These symptoms can usually be avoided or reduced by gradual reduction of the dosage or by continuing concomitant anti-parkinsonism agents for several weeks after 'Thorazine' is withdrawn.

ADVERSE REACTIONS

Note: Some adverse effects of 'Thorazine' may be more likely to occur, or occur with greater intensity, in patients with special medical problems, e.g., patients with mitral insufficiency or pheochromocytoma have experienced severe hypotension following recommended doses.

Drowsiness, usually mild to moderate, may occur, particularly during the first or second week, after which it generally disappears. If troublesome, dosage may be lowered.

Jaundice: Overall incidence has been low, regardless of indication or dosage. Most investigators conclude it is a sensitivity reaction. Most cases occur between the second and fourth weeks of therapy. The clinical picture resembles infectious hepatitis, with laboratory features of obstructive jaundice, rather than those of parenchymal damage. It is usually promptly reversible on withdrawal of the medication; however, chronic jaundice has been reported.

There is no conclusive evidence that preexisting liver disease makes patients more susceptible to jaundice. Alcoholics with cirrhosis have been successfully treated with Thorazine (chlorpromazine, SK&F) without complications. Nevertheless, the medication should be used cautiously in patients with liver disease. Patients who have experienced jaundice with a phenothiazine should not, if possible, be reexposed to 'Thorazine' or other phenothiazines.

If fever with grippe-like symptoms occurs, appropriate liver studies should be conducted. If tests indicate an abnormality, stop treatment.

Liver function tests in jaundice induced by the drug may mimic extrahepatic obstruction; withhold exploratory laparotomy until extrahepatic obstruction is confirmed.

Hematological Disorders, including agranulocytosis, eosinophilia, leukopenia, hemolytic anemia, aplastic anemia, thrombocytopenic purpura and pancytopenia have been reported.

Agranulocytosis—Warn patients to report the sudden appearance of sore throat or other signs of infection. If white blood cell and differential counts indicate cellular depression, stop treatment and start antibiotic and other suitable therapy.

Most cases have occurred between the 4th and 10th weeks of therapy; patients should be watched closely during that period.

Moderate suppression of white blood cells is not an indication for stopping treatment unless accompanied by the symptoms described above.

Cardiovascular:

Hypotensive Effects—Postural hypotension, simple tachycardia, momentary fainting and dizziness may occur after the first injection; occasionally after subsequent injections; rarely, after the first oral dose. Usually recovery is spontaneous and symptoms disappear within ½ to 2 hours. Occasionally, these effects may be more severe and prolonged, producing a shock-like condition.

To minimize hypotension after injection, keep patient lying down and observe for at least ½ hour. To control hypotension, place patient in head-low position with legs raised. If a vasoconstrictor is required, Levophed®‡ and Neo-Synephrine®§ are the most suitable. Other pressor agents, including epinephrine, should not be used as they may cause a paradoxical further lowering of blood pressure.

EKG Changes—particularly nonspecific, usually reversible Q and T wave distortions—have been observed in some patients receiving phenothiazine tranquilizers, including Thorazine (chlorpromazine, SK&F).

Note: Sudden death, apparently due to cardiac arrest, has been reported.

C.N.S. Reactions:

Neuromuscular (Extrapyramidal) Reactions— Neuromuscular reactions include dystonias, motor restlessness, pseudoparkinsonism and tardive dyskinesia, and appear to be dose-related. They are discussed in the following paragraphs:

Dystonias: Symptoms may include spasm of the neck muscles, sometimes progressing to acute, reversible torticollis; extensor rigidity of back muscles, sometimes progressing to opisthotonos; carpopedal spasm, trismus, swallowing difficulty, oculogyric crisis and protrusion of the tongue.

These usually subside within a few hours, and almost always within 24 to 48 hours after the drug has been discontinued.

In mild cases, reassurance or a barbiturate is often sufficient. *In moderate cases,* barbiturates will usually bring rapid relief. *In more severe adult cases,* the administration of an anti-parkinsonism agent, except levodopa, usually produces rapid reversal of symptoms. *In children,* reassurance and barbiturates will usually control symptoms. (Or, parenteral Benadryl®[ll] may be useful. See Benadryl[ll] prescribing information for appropriate children's dosage.) If appropriate treatment with anti-parkinsonism agents or Benadryl[ll] fails to reverse the signs and symptoms, the diagnosis should be reevaluated.

Suitable supportive measures such as maintaining a clear airway and adequate hydration should be employed when needed. If therapy is reinstituted, it should be at a lower dosage. Should these symptoms occur in children or pregnant patients, the drug should not be reinstituted.

Motor Restlessness: Symptoms may include agitation or jitteriness and sometimes insomnia. These symptoms often disappear spontaneously. At times these symptoms may be similar to the original neurotic or psychotic symptoms. Dosage should not be increased until these side effects have subsided.

If these symptoms become too troublesome, they can usually be controlled by a reduction of dosage or concomitant administration of a barbiturate.

Pseudo-parkinsonism: Symptoms may include: mask-like facies, drooling, tremors, pillrolling motion, cogwheel rigidity and shuffling gait. In most cases these symptoms are readily controlled when an anti-parkinsonism agent is administered concomitantly. Anti-parkinsonism agents should be used only when required. Generally, therapy of a few weeks to two or three months will suffice. After this time patients should be evaluated to determine their need for continued treatment. (Note: Levodopa has not been found effective in neuroleptic-induced pseudo-parkinsonism.) Occasionally it is necessary to lower the dosage of Thorazine (chlorpromazine, SK&F) or to discontinue the drug.

Tardive Dyskinesia: As with all antipsychotic agents, tardive dyskinesia may appear in some patients on long-term therapy or may appear after drug therapy has been discontinued. The syndrome can also develop, although much less frequently, after relatively brief treatment periods at low doses. This syndrome appears in all age groups. Although its prevalence appears to be highest among elderly patients, especially elderly women, it is impossible to rely upon prevalence estimates to predict at the inception of neuroleptic treatment which patients are likely to develop the syndrome. The symptoms are persistent and in some patients appear to be irreversible. The syndrome is characterized by rhythmical involuntary movements of the tongue, face, mouth or jaw (e.g., protrusion of tongue, puffing of cheeks, puckering of mouth, chewing movements). Sometimes these may be accompanied by involuntary movements of extremities. In rare instances, these involuntary movements of the extremities are the only manifestations of tardive dyskinesia. A variant of tardive dyskinesia, tardive dystonia, has also been described.

There is no known effective treatment for tardive dyskinesia; anti-parkinsonism agents do not alleviate the symptoms of this syndrome. If clinically feasible, it is suggested that all antipsychotic agents be discontinued if these symptoms appear. Should it be necessary to reinstitute treatment, or increase the dosage of the agent, or switch to a different antipsychotic agent, the syndrome may be masked.

It has been reported that fine vermicular movements of the tongue may be an early sign of the syndrome and if the medication is stopped at that time the syndrome may not develop.

Adverse Behavioral Effects—Psychotic symptoms and catatonic-like states have been reported rarely.

Other C.N.S. Effects—Cerebral edema has been reported.

Convulsive seizures *(petit mal* and *grand mal)* have been reported, particularly in patients with EEG abnormalities or history of such disorders.

Abnormality of the cerebrospinal fluid proteins has also been reported.

Allergic Reactions of a mild urticarial type or photosensitivity are seen. Avoid undue exposure to sun. More severe reactions, including exfoliative dermatitis, have been reported occasionally.

Contact dermatitis has been reported in nursing personnel; accordingly, the use of rubber gloves when administering 'Thorazine' liquid or injectable is recommended.

In addition, asthma, laryngeal edema, angioneurotic edema and anaphylactoid reactions have been reported.

Endocrine Disorders: Lactation and moderate breast engorgement may occur in females on large doses. If persistent, lower dosage or withdraw drug. False-positive pregnancy tests have been reported, but are less likely to occur when a serum test is used. Amenorrhea and gynecomastia have also been reported. Hyperglycemia, hypoglycemia and glycosuria have been reported.

Autonomic Reactions: Occasional dry mouth; nasal congestion; nausea; obstipation; constipation; adynamic ileus; urinary retention; priapism; miosis and mydriasis, atonic colon, ejaculatory disorders/impotence.

Special Considerations in Long-Term Therapy: Skin pigmentation and ocular changes have occurred in some patients taking substantial doses of Thorazine (chlorpromazine, SK&F) for prolonged periods.

Skin Pigmentation—Rare instances of skin pigmentation have been observed in hospitalized mental patients, primarily females who have received the drug usually for three years or more in dosages ranging from 500 mg. to 1500 mg. daily. The pigmentary changes, restricted to exposed areas of the body, range from an almost imperceptible darkening of the skin to a slate gray color, sometimes with a violet hue. Histological examination reveals a pigment, chiefly in the dermis, which is probably a melanin-like complex. The pigmentation may fade following discontinuance of the drug.

Ocular Changes—Ocular changes have occurred more frequently than skin pigmentation and have been observed both in pigmented and nonpigmented patients receiving Thorazine (chlorpromazine, SK&F) usually for two years or more in dosages of 300 mg. daily and higher. Eye changes are characterized by deposition of fine particulate matter in the lens and cornea. In more advanced cases, star-shaped opacities have also been observed in the anterior portion of the lens. The nature of the eye deposits has not yet been determined. A small number of patients with more severe ocular changes have had some visual impairment. In addition to these corneal and lenticular changes, epithelial keratopathy and pigmentary retinopathy have been reported. Reports suggest that the eye lesions may regress after withdrawal of the drug.

Since the occurrence of eye changes seems to be related to dosage levels and/or duration of therapy, it is suggested that long-term patients on moderate to high dosage levels have periodic ocular examinations.

Etiology—The etiology of both of these reactions is not clear, but exposure to light, along with dosage/duration of therapy, appears to be the most significant factor. If either of these reactions is observed, the physician should weigh the benefits of continued therapy against the possible risks and, on the merits of the individual case, determine whether or not to continue present therapy, lower the dosage, or withdraw the drug.

Other Adverse Reactions: Mild fever may occur after large I.M. doses. Hyperpyrexia has been reported. Increases in appetite and weight sometimes occur. Peripheral edema and a systemic lupus erythematosus-like syndrome have been reported.

Rare occurrences of neuroleptic malignant syndrome (NMS) have been reported in patients receiving neuroleptic drugs. This syndrome is comprised of the symptom complex of hyperthermia, altered consciousness, muscular rigidity and autonomic dysfunction and is potentially fatal.

Note: There have been occasional reports of sudden death in patients receiving phenothiazines. In some cases, the cause appeared to be cardiac arrest or asphyxia due to failure of the cough reflex.

DOSAGE AND ADMINISTRATION

Adjust dosage to individual and the severity of his condition, recognizing that the milligram for milligram potency relationship among all dosage forms has not been precisely established clinically. It is important to increase dosage until symptoms are controlled. Dosage should be increased more gradually in debilitated or emaciated patients. In continued therapy, gradually reduce dosage to the lowest effective maintenance level, after symptoms have been controlled for a reasonable period.

In general, dosage recommendations for other oral forms of the drug may be applied to Spansule® brand sustained release capsules on the basis of total daily dosage in milligrams.

The 100 mg. and 200 mg. tablets and the 300 mg. 'Spansule' capsules are for use in severe neuropsychiatric conditions.

Increase parenteral dosage only if hypotension has not occurred. Before using I.M., see Important Notes on Injection.

Elderly Patients: In general, dosages in the lower range are sufficient for most elderly patients. Since they appear to be more susceptible to hypotension and neuromuscular reactions, such patients should be observed closely. Dosage should be tailored to the individual, response carefully monitored, and dosage adjusted accordingly. Dosage should be increased more gradually in elderly patients.

Continued on next page

Smith Kline & French—Cont.

General Medicine:

Adults: EXCESSIVE ANXIETY, TENSION AND AGITATION—*Oral:* 10 mg. t.i.d. or q.i.d., or 25 mg. b.i.d. or t.i.d. MORE SEVERE CASES—*Oral:* 25 mg. t.i.d. After 1 or 2 days, daily dosage may be increased by 20 to 50 mg. semiweekly, until patient becomes calm and cooperative. (Maximum improvement may not be seen for weeks or even months.) Continue optimum dosage for 2 weeks; then gradually reduce to maintenance level. Daily dosage of 200 mg. is not unusual. Some patients require higher dosages (e.g., 800 mg. daily is not uncommon in discharged mental patients).
TREATMENT OF NON-PSYCHOTIC ANXIETY—Do not administer in doses of more than 100 mg. per day or for longer than 12 weeks.
PROMPT CONTROL OF SEVERE SYMPTOMS —*I.M.:* 25 mg. (1 ml.). If necessary, repeat in 1 hour. Subsequent doses should be oral, 25 to 50 mg. t.i.d.
NAUSEA AND VOMITING—*Oral:* 10 to 25 mg. q4-6h, p.r.n., increased, if necessary. *I.M.:* 25 mg. (1 ml.). If no hypotension occurs, give 25 to 50 mg. q3-4h, p.r.n., until vomiting stops. Then switch to oral dosage. *Rectal:* One 100 mg. suppository q6-8h, p.r.n. In some patients, half this dose will do.
INTRACTABLE HICCUPS—*Oral:* 25 to 50 mg. t.i.d. or q.i.d. If symptoms persist for 2-3 days, give 25 to 50 mg. (1-2 ml.) I.M. Should symptoms persist, use *slow* I.V. infusion with patient flat in bed: 25 to 50 mg. (1-2 ml.) in 500 to 1,000 ml. of saline. Follow blood pressure closely.
ACUTE INTERMITTENT PORPHYRIA—*Oral:* 25 to 50 mg. t.i.d. or q.i.d. Can usually be discontinued after several weeks, but maintenance therapy may be necessary for some patients. *I.M.:* 25 mg. (1 ml.) t.i.d. or q.i.d. until patient can take oral therapy.
TETANUS—*I.M.:* 25 to 50 mg. (1-2 ml.) given 3 or 4 times daily, usually in conjunction with barbiturates. Total doses and frequency of administration must be determined by the patient's response, starting with low doses and increasing gradually. *I.V.:* 25 to 50 mg. (1-2 ml.). Dilute to at least 1 mg. per ml. and administer at a rate of 1 mg. per minute.

Children: NAUSEA AND VOMITING—Thorazine (chlorpromazine, SK&F) should generally not be used in children under 6 months of age. It should not be used in conditions for which children's dosages have not been established. Dosage and frequency of administration should be adjusted according to the severity of the symptoms and response of the patient. The duration of activity following intramuscular administration may last up to 12 hours. Subsequent doses may be given by the same route if necessary. *Oral:* ¼ mg./lb. body weight q4-6h (e.g., 40 lb. child—10 mg. q4-6h). *Rectal:* ½ mg./lb. body weight q6-8h, p.r.n. (e.g., 20-30 lb. child—half of a 25 mg. suppository q6-8h). *I.M.:* ¼ mg./lb. body weight q6-8h, p.r.n. *Maximum I.M. Dosage:* Children up to 5 yrs. (or 50 lbs.), not over 40 mg./day; 5-12 yrs. (or 50-100 lbs.), not over 75 mg./day except in severe cases. (For mental and emotional disorders, see Psychiatry, below.)
TETANUS—*I.M.* or *I.V.:* ¼ mg./lb. body weight q6-8h. When given I.V., dilute to at least 1 mg./ml. and administer at rate of 1 mg. per 2 minutes. In children up to 50 lbs., do not exceed 40 mg. daily; 50 to 100 lbs., do not exceed 75 mg., except in severe cases.

Surgery:

Adults: PREOPERATIVE—*Oral:* 25 to 50 mg., 2 to 3 hours before the operation. *I.M.:* 12.5 to 25 mg. (0.5-1 ml.), 1 to 2 hours before operation. DURING SURGERY—Administer only to control acute nausea and vomiting. *I.M.:* 12.5 mg. (0.5 ml.). Repeat in ½ hour if necessary and if no hypotension occurs. *I.V.:* 2 mg. per fractional injection, at 2-minute intervals. Do not exceed 25 mg. Dilute to 1 mg./ml., i.e., 1 ml. (25 mg.) mixed with 24 ml. of saline. POSTOPERATIVE —*Oral:* 10 to 25 mg. q4-6h, p.r.n. *I.M.:* 12.5 to 25 mg. (0.5-1 ml.). Repeat in 1 hour if necessary and if no hypotension occurs.

Children: Thorazine (chlorpromazine, SK&F) should generally not be used in children under 6 months of age except where potentially lifesaving. It should not be used in conditions for which specific children's dosages have not been established. PREOPERATIVE—¼ mg./lb. body weight, either *orally* 2 to 3 hours before operation, or *I.M.* 1 to 2 hours before. DURING SURGERY—*I.M.:* ⅛ mg./lb. body weight. Repeat in ½ hour if necessary and if no hypotension occurs. *I.V.:* 1 mg. per fractional injection at 2-minute intervals and not exceeding recommended I.M. dosage. Always dilute to 1 mg./ml., i.e., 1 ml. (25 mg.) mixed with 24 ml. of saline. POSTOPERATIVE—¼ mg./lb. body weight, either *orally* q4-6h, p.r.n., or *I.M.* Repeat in 1 hour if necessary and if no hypotension occurs.

Psychiatry:

Increase dosage gradually until symptoms are controlled. Maximum improvement may not be seen for weeks or even months. Continue optimum dosage for 2 weeks; then gradually reduce dosage to the lowest effective maintenance level.

Adults: OFFICE PATIENTS OR OUTPATIENTS —*Oral:* 10 mg. t.i.d. or q.i.d., or 25 mg. b.i.d. or t.i.d. MORE SEVERE CASES—*Oral:* 25 mg. t.i.d. After 1 or 2 days, daily dosage may be increased by 20-50 mg. at semiweekly intervals until patient becomes calm and cooperative. TREATMENT OF NON-PSYCHOTIC ANXIETY—Do not administer in doses of more than 100 mg. per day or for longer than 12 weeks.
PROMPT CONTROL OF SEVERE SYMPTOMS—*I.M.:* 25 mg. (1 ml.). If necessary, repeat in 1 hour. Subsequent doses should be oral, 25-50 mg. t.i.d.
HOSPITALIZED PATIENTS: ACUTELY AGITATED, MANIC, OR DISTURBED—*I.M.:* 25 mg. (1 ml.). If necessary, give additional 25 to 50 mg. injection in 1 hour. Increase subsequent I.M. doses gradually over several days—up to 400 mg. q4-6h in exceptionally severe cases—until patient is controlled. Usually patient becomes quiet and cooperative within 24 to 48 hours and oral doses may be substituted and increased until the patient is calm. 500 mg. a day is generally sufficient. While gradual increases to 2,000 mg. a day or more may be necessary, there is usually little therapeutic gain to be achieved by exceeding 1,000 mg. a day for extended periods. In general, dosage levels should be lower in the elderly, the emaciated and the debilitated. LESS ACUTELY AGITATED PATIENTS—*Oral:* 25 mg. t.i.d. Increase gradually until effective dose is reached—usually 400 mg. daily.

Children: OFFICE PATIENTS OR OUTPATIENTS—Select route of administration according to severity of patient's condition and increase dosage gradually as required. *Oral:* ¼ mg./lb. body weight q4-6h, p.r.n. (e.g., for 40 lb. child—10 mg. q4-6h). *Rectal:* ½ mg./lb. body weight q6-8h, p.r.n. (e.g., for 20-30 lb. child—half a 25 mg. suppository q6-8h). *I.M.:* ¼ mg./lb. body weight q6-8h, p.r.n.
HOSPITALIZED PATIENTS—As with outpatients, start with low doses and increase dosage gradually. In severe behavior disorders or psychotic conditions, higher dosages (50-100 mg. daily, and in older children, 200 mg. daily or more) may be necessary. There is little evidence that behavior improvement in severely disturbed mentally retarded patients is further enhanced by doses beyond 500 mg. per day. *Maximum I.M. Dosage:* Children up to 5 years (or 50 lbs.), not over 40 mg./day; 5-12 years (or 50-100 lbs.), not over 75 mg./day except in unmanageable cases.

IMPORTANT NOTES ON INJECTION

Inject slowly, deep into upper outer quadrant of buttock.
Because of possible hypotensive effects, reserve parenteral administration for bedfast patients or for acute ambulatory cases, and keep patient lying down for at least ½ hour after injection. If irritation is a problem, dilute Injection with saline or 2% procaine; mixing with other agents in the syringe is not recommended. Subcutaneous injection is not advised. Avoid injecting undiluted Thorazine (chlorpromazine, SK&F) into vein. I.V. route is only for severe hiccups, surgery and tetanus.
Because of the possibility of contact dermatitis, avoid getting solution on hands or clothing. Protect from light, or discoloration may occur. Slight yellowing will not alter potency. Discard if markedly discolored.

Note on Concentrate: When the Concentrate is to be used, add the desired dosage of Concentrate to 60 ml. (2 fl. oz.) or more of diluent *just prior to administration.* This will insure palatability and stability. Vehicles suggested for dilution are: tomato or fruit juice, milk, simple syrup, orange syrup, carbonated beverages, coffee, tea, or water. Semisolid foods (soups, puddings, etc.) may also be used. The Concentrate is light sensitive; it should be protected from light and dispensed in amber glass bottles. *Refrigeration is not required.*

OVERDOSAGE

(See also Adverse Reactions.)
SYMPTOMS—Primarily symptoms of central nervous system depression to the point of somnolence or coma. Hypotension and extrapyramidal symptoms.
Other possible manifestations include agitation and restlessness, convulsions, fever, autonomic reactions such as dry mouth and ileus, EKG changes and cardiac arrhythmias.
TREATMENT—It is important to determine other medications taken by the patient since multiple dose therapy is common in overdosage situations. Treatment is essentially symptomatic and supportive. Early gastric lavage is helpful. Keep patient under observation and maintain an open airway, since involvement of the extrapyramidal mechanism may produce dysphagia and respiratory difficulty in severe overdosage. **Do not attempt to induce emesis because a dystonic reaction of the head or neck may develop that could result in aspiration of vomitus.** Extrapyramidal symptoms may be treated with anti-parkinsonism drugs, barbiturates, or Benadryl[||]. See prescribing information for these products. Care should be taken to avoid increasing respiratory depression.
If administration of a stimulant is desirable, amphetamine, dextroamphetamine, or caffeine with sodium benzoate is recommended. Stimulants that may cause convulsions (e.g., picrotoxin or pentylenetetrazol) should be avoided.
If hypotension occurs, the standard measures for managing circulatory shock should be initiated. If it is desirable to administer a vasoconstrictor, Levophed‡ and Neo-Synephrine§ are most suitable. Other pressor agents, including epinephrine, are not recommended because phenothiazine derivatives may reverse the usual elevating action of these agents and cause a further lowering of blood pressure.
Limited experience indicates that phenothiazines are *not* dialyzable.
Special note on 'Spansule' capsules—Since much of the 'Spansule' capsule medication is coated for gradual release, therapy directed at reversing the effects of the ingested drug and at supporting the patient should be continued for as long as overdosage symptoms remain. Saline cathartics are useful for hastening evacuation of pellets that have not already released medication.

HOW SUPPLIED

Tablets: 10 mg., 25 mg. or 50 mg., in bottles of 100 and 1000; in Single Unit Packages of 100 (intended for institutional use only). For use in severe neuropsychiatric conditions, 100 mg. and 200 mg., in bottles of 100 and 1000; in Single Unit Packages of 100 (intended for institutional use only).
Spansule® brand of sustained release capsules: 30 mg., 75 mg., 150 mg. or 200 mg., in bottles of 50 and 500; in Single Unit Packages of 100 (intended for institutional use only). For use in severe neuropsychiatric conditions, 300 mg., in bottles of 50; in Single Unit Packages of 100 (intended for institutional use only).
Ampuls: 1 ml. and 2 ml. (25 mg./ml.), in boxes of 10, 100 and 500.
Multiple-dose Vials: 10 ml. (25 mg./ml.), in boxes of 1, 20 and 100.
Syrup: 10 mg./5 ml. in 4 fl. oz. bottles.
Suppositories: 25 mg. or 100 mg., in boxes of 12.
Concentrate (intended for institutional use only): *30 mg./ml.* in 4 fl. oz. bottles, in cartons of 36 bottles, and in 1 gallon bottles. *100 mg./ml.* in 8 fl. oz. bottles, in cartons of 12.
Veterans Administration—Tablets, 100 mg., 90's, unit of use, 6505-01-074-0980A and 120's, 6505-01-074-0981A; Tablets, 200 mg., 90's, unit of use, 6505-01-074-7738A and 120's, 6505-01-075-1765A; 'Spansule' Capsules, 150 mg., 500's, 6505-00-022-1324; Injection, 2 ml., 100's, 6505-00-619-8639A.
Military—Tablets, 25 mg., S.U.P., 100's, 6505-00-118-2529; Tablets, 100 mg., S.U.P., 100's, 6505-00-132-0372.

* Phenytoin, Parke-Davis.
† Metrizamide, Winthrop-Breon Laboratories.
‡ Norepinephrine, Winthrop-Breon Laboratories.
§ Phenylephrine hydrochloride, Winthrop-Breon Laboratories.
|| Diphenhydramine hydrochloride, Parke-Davis.

Shown in Product Identification Section, page 431

TZ:L67

TUSS-ORNADE® ℞

[tuss 'or-naid']
LIQUID

DESCRIPTION

Each 5 ml. (one teaspoonful) of clear, fruit-flavored 'Tuss-Ornade' Liquid contains caramiphen edisylate, 6.7 mg.; phenylpropanolamine hydrochloride, 12.5 mg.; and alcohol, 5.0%. Inactive ingredients consist of citric acid, flavors, glycerin, menthol, methylparaben, propylparaben, sodium citrate, sorbitol and water.

ACTIONS

The 'Tuss-Ornade' formula contains caramiphen edisylate, a synthetic, non-narcotic cough suppressant, and phenylpropanolamine hydrochloride, a vasoconstrictor with decongestant action on nasal and upper respiratory tract mucosal membranes.

INDICATIONS

For the symptomatic relief of coughs and nasal congestion associated with common colds.
N.B.: A final determination has not been made on the effectiveness of this drug combination in accordance with efficacy requirements of the 1962 Amendments to the Food, Drug and Cosmetic Act.

CONTRAINDICATIONS

Hypersensitivity to either of the components; concurrent MAO inhibitor therapy; severe hypertension; bronchial asthma; coronary artery disease.
Do not use 'Tuss-Ornade' Liquid in children under 15 pounds or in children less than six months of age.

WARNINGS

Caution patients about activities requiring alertness (e.g., operating vehicles or machinery). Patients should also be warned about the possible additive effects of alcohol and other CNS depressants.

PRECAUTIONS

Use with caution in patients with cardiovascular disease, glaucoma, prostatic hypertrophy, thyroid disease or diabetes. Use with caution in patients in whom productive cough is desirable to clear excessive secretions from the bronchial tree. Patients taking this medication should be cautioned not to take simultaneously other products containing phenylpropanolamine HCl or amphetamines.

Usage in Pregnancy: Safe use in pregnancy has not been established. This drug should not be used in pregnancy, nursing mothers, or women of childbearing potential unless, in the judgment of the physician, the anticipated benefits outweigh the potential risks.

ADVERSE REACTIONS

Adverse effects associated with products containing a centrally acting antitussive or sympathomimetic amine may occur and include: nausea, gastrointestinal upset, diarrhea, constipation, dizziness, drowsiness, nervousness, insomnia, anorexia, weakness, tightness of chest, angina pain, irritability, palpitations, headache, incoordination, tremor, difficulty in urination, dysuria, hypertension, hypotension, visual disturbances.

DOSAGE AND ADMINISTRATION

Adults and children over 12 years—2 teaspoonfuls every 4 hours; do not exceed 12 teaspoonfuls in 24 hours. Children 6 to 12 years—1 teaspoonful every 4 hours; do not exceed 6 teaspoonfuls in 24 hours. Children 2 to 6 years—½ teaspoonful every 4 hours; do not exceed 3 teaspoonfuls in 24 hours. Data are not available on which to base dosage recommendations for children under 2 years of age. **Do not use in children under 15 pounds or less than 6 months old.**

OVERDOSAGE

Symptoms—May include dryness of mouth, dysphagia, thirst, blurred vision, dilated pupils, photophobia, fever, rapid pulse and respiration, disorientation, dizziness, nausea, fainting, tachycardia, and either excitation or depression of the central nervous system.

Treatment—Immediate evacuation of the stomach should be induced by emesis and gastric lavage, repeated as necessary. Respiratory depression should be treated promptly with oxygen and respiratory stimulants. Do not treat respiratory or CNS depression with analeptics that might precipitate convulsions. If marked excitement occurs, a short-acting barbiturate or chloral hydrate may be used.

SUPPLIED

Liquid containing caramiphen edisylate 6.7 mg.; phenylpropanolamine hydrochloride 12.5 mg.; and alcohol 5.0% per 5 ml. (one teaspoonful), in 16 fl. oz. bottles.

TOL:L15

TUSS-ORNADE® ℞

[tuss 'or-naid ']

SPANSULE® CAPSULES

PRODUCT OVERVIEW

KEY FACTS

Tuss-Ornade® Spansule® capsules contain caramiphen edisylate, a non-narcotic cough suppressant, and phenylpropanolamine HCl, a decongestant that provides vasoconstriction similar to that of ephedrine but with less CNS stimulation. Spansule® capsules are prepared so that an initial dose is released promptly and the remaining medication is released gradually over a prolonged period of time, thus permitting b.i.d. dosing.

MAJOR USE

Tuss-Ornade® Spansule® capsules are for symptomatic relief of coughs and nasal congestion associated with the common cold.

SAFETY INFORMATION

Tuss-Ornade® Spansule® capsules are contraindicated in patients with: hypersensitivity to either caramiphen edisylate or phenylpropanolamine HCl; concurrent MAO inhibitor therapy; severe hypertension; bronchial asthma; coronary artery disease. They should not be used in children under the age of 12 years. Further, patients should be cautioned about activities requiring alertness and about the possible additive effects of alcohol and other CNS depressants.

PRESCRIBING INFORMATION

TUSS-ORNADE® ℞

[tuss 'or-naid ']

SPANSULE® CAPSULES

DESCRIPTION

Each 'Tuss-Ornade' *Spansule* capsule, with opaque light blue cap and natural body, is imprinted with the product name TUSS-ORNADE and SKF and contains caramiphen edisylate, 40 mg. and phenylpropanolamine hydrochloride,75 mg. Inactive ingredients consist of benzyl alcohol, cetylpyridinium chloride, D&C Red No. 33, FD&C Blue No. 1, FD&C Red No. 3, FD&C Yellow No. 6, gelatin, glyceryl distearate, polyethylene glycol, povidone, silicon dioxide, sodium lauryl sulfate, starch, sucrose, titanium dioxide, wax and trace amounts of other inactive ingredients.

Each 'Tuss-Ornade' *Spansule* capsule is so prepared that an initial dose is released promptly and the remaining medication is released gradually over a prolonged period.

ACTIONS

The 'Tuss-Ornade' formula contains caramiphen edisylate, a synthetic, non-narcotic cough suppressant, and phenylpropanolamine hydrochloride, a vasoconstrictor with decongestant action on nasal and upper respiratory tract mucosal membranes.

Pharmacokinetics: At steady-state conditions, the following peak levels are reached after the oral administration of a 'Spansule' capsule: 24 ng./ml. caramiphen in 4.6 hours; 200 ng./ml. phenylpropanolamine in 5.5 hours; the half-lives are approximately 11 and 8 hours, respectively.

INDICATIONS

For the symptomatic relief of coughs and nasal congestion associated with common colds.

N.B.: A final determination has not been made on the effectiveness of this drug combination in accordance with efficacy requirements of the 1962 Amendments to the Food, Drug and Cosmetic Act.

CONTRAINDICATIONS

Hypersensitivity to either of the components; concurrent MAO inhibitor therapy; severe hypertension; bronchial asthma; coronary artery disease.

Do not use 'Tuss-Ornade' *Spansule* capsules in children under 12 years of age.

WARNINGS

Caution patients about activities requiring alertness (e.g., operating vehicles or machinery). Patients should also be warned about the possible additive effects of alcohol and other CNS depressants.

PRECAUTIONS

Use with caution in persons with cardiovascular disease, glaucoma, prostatic hypertrophy, thyroid disease or diabetes. Use with caution in patients in whom productive cough is desirable to clear excessive secretions from the bronchial tree. Patients taking this medication should be cautioned not to take simultaneously other products containing phenylpropanolamine HCl or amphetamines.

Usage in Pregnancy: Safe use in pregnancy has not been established. This drug should not be used in pregnancy, nursing mothers, or women of childbearing potential unless, in the judgment of the physician, the anticipated benefits outweigh the potential risks.

ADVERSE REACTIONS

Adverse effects associated with products containing a centrally acting antitussive or sympathomimetic amine may occur and include: nausea, gastrointestinal upset, diarrhea, constipation, dizziness, drowsiness, nervousness, insomnia, anorexia, weakness, tightness of chest, angina pain, irritability, palpitation, headache, incoordination, tremor, difficulty in urination, dysuria, hypertension, hypotension, visual disturbances.

DOSAGE AND ADMINISTRATION

'Tuss-Ornade' *Spansule* capsules: Adults and children over 12 years of age—one 'Tuss-Ornade' *Spansule* capsule every 12 hours. **Do not use in children under 12 years of age.**

OVERDOSAGE

Symptoms—May include dryness of mouth, dysphagia, thirst, blurred vision, dilated pupils, photophobia, fever, rapid pulse and respiration, disorientation, dizziness, nausea, fainting, tachycardia, and either excitation or depression of the central nervous system.

Treatment—Immediate evacuation of the stomach should be induced by emesis and gastric lavage, repeated as necessary. Respiratory depression should be treated promptly with oxygen and respiratory stimulants. Do not treat respiratory or CNS depression with analeptics that might precipitate convulsions. If marked excitement occurs, a short-acting barbiturate or chloral hydrate may be used.

Since much of the 'Spansule' capsule medication is coated for gradual release, saline cathartics should be administered to hasten evacuation of pellets that have not already released medication.

SUPPLIED

'Spansule' capsules (brand of sustained release capsules) containing caramiphen edisylate 40 mg. and phenylpropanolamine hydrochloride 75 mg., in bottles of 50 and 500.

TO:L31

Shown in Product Identification Section, page 431

URISPAS® ℞

[yore 'eh-spaz]

(brand of flavoxate HCl)

100 mg. tablets

Urinary tract spasmolytic

DESCRIPTION

Urispas (flavoxate HCl, SK&F) tablets contain flavoxate hydrochloride, a synthetic urinary tract spasmolytic.

Chemically, flavoxate hydrochloride is 2-piperidinoethyl 3-methyl-4- oxo-2-phenyl-4H-1-benzopyran -8- carboxylate hydrochloride. The empirical formula of flavoxate hydrochloride is $C_{24}H_{25}NO_4 \cdot HCl$. The molecular weight is 427.94.

'Urispas' is supplied in tablets for oral administration. Each round, white, film-coated 'Urispas' tablet is debossed SKF and V90 and contains flavoxate hydrochloride, 100 mg. Inactive ingredients consist of calcium phosphate, castor oil, cellulose acetate phthalate, magnesium stearate, polyethylene glycol, starch and talc.

CLINICAL PHARMACOLOGY

Flavoxate hydrochloride counteracts smooth muscle spasm of the urinary tract and exerts its effect directly on the muscle.

In a single study of 11 normal male subjects, the time to onset of action was 55 minutes. The peak effect was observed at 112 minutes. 57% of the flavoxate HCl was excreted in the urine within 24 hours.

INDICATIONS AND USAGE

Urispas (flavoxate HCl, SK&F) is indicated for symptomatic relief of dysuria, urgency, nocturia, suprapubic pain, frequency and incontinence as may occur in cystitis, prostatitis, urethritis, urethrocystitis/urethrotrigonitis. 'Urispas' is not indicated for definitive treatment, but is compatible with drugs used for the treatment of urinary tract infections.

CONTRAINDICATIONS

Urispas (flavoxate HCl, SK&F) is contraindicated in patients who have any of the following obstructive conditions: pyloric or duodenal obstruction, obstructive intestinal lesions or ileus, achalasia, gastrointestinal hemorrhage, and obstructive uropathies of the lower urinary tract.

WARNINGS

Urispas (flavoxate HCl, SK&F) should be given cautiously in patients with suspected glaucoma.

PRECAUTIONS

Information for Patients: Patients should be informed that if drowsiness and blurred vision occur, they should not operate a motor vehicle or machinery or participate in activities where alertness is required.

Carcinogenesis, Mutagenesis, Impairment of Fertility: Mutagenicity studies and long-term studies in animals to determine the carcinogenic potential of Urispas (flavoxate HCl, SK&F) have not been performed.

Pregnancy: Teratogenic Effects—Pregnancy Category B. Reproduction studies have been performed in rats and rabbits at doses up to 34 times the human dose and revealed no evidence of impaired fertility or harm to the fetus due to flavoxate HCl. There are, however, no well-controlled studies in pregnant women. Because animal reproduction studies are not always predictive of human response, this drug should be used during pregnancy only if clearly needed.

Nursing Mothers: It is not known whether this drug is excreted in human milk. Because many drugs are excreted in human milk, caution should be exercised when 'Urispas' is administered to a nursing woman.

Pediatric Use: Safety and effectiveness in children below the age of 12 years have not been established.

ADVERSE REACTIONS

The following adverse reactions have been observed, but there are not enough data to support an estimate of their frequency.

Gastrointestinal: Nausea, vomiting, dry mouth.

CNS: Vertigo, headache, mental confusion, especially in the elderly, drowsiness, nervousness.

Hematologic: Leukopenia (one case which was reversible upon discontinuation of the drug).

Cardiovascular: Tachycardia and palpitation.

Allergic: Urticaria and other dermatoses, eosinophilia and hyperpyrexia.

Ophthalmic: Increased ocular tension, blurred vision, disturbance in eye accommodation.

Renal: Dysuria.

OVERDOSAGE

The oral LD_{50} for flavoxate HCl in rats is 4273 mg./kg. The oral LD_{50} for flavoxate HCl in mice is 1837 mg./kg.

It is not known whether flavoxate HCl is dialyzable.

DOSAGE AND ADMINISTRATION

Adults and children over 12 years of age: One or two 100 mg. tablets three or four times a day. With improvement of

Continued on next page

Smith Kline & French—Cont.

symptoms, the dose may be reduced. This drug cannot be recommended for infants and children under 12 years of age because safety and efficacy have not been demonstrated in this age group.

HOW SUPPLIED

Urispas (flavoxate HCl, SK&F) tablets, 100 mg., in bottles of 100 and in Single Unit Packages of 100 (intended for institutional use only).

UR:L13

Shown in Product Identification Section, page 431

VONTROL® ℞

[vohn 'trole]

(brand of diphenidol)

'Vontrol' may cause hallucinations, disorientation, or confusion. For this reason, its use is limited to patients who are hospitalized or under comparable, continuous, close, professional supervision. Even then, the physician should carefully weigh the benefits against the possible risks and give due consideration to alternate therapeutic measures.

DESCRIPTION

Diphenidol, α, α-diphenyl-1-piperidinebutanol, is a compound not related to the antihistamines, phenothiazines, barbiturates, or other agents with antivertigo or antiemetic action.

Each round, orange 'Vontrol' tablet is debossed SKF and 25 and contains diphenidol hydrochloride equivalent to diphenidol, 25 mg. Inactive ingredients consist of acacia, calcium sulfate, cellulose, FD&C Yellow No. 5 (tartrazine), FD&C Yellow No. 6, magnesium stearate and starch.

ACTIONS

'Vontrol' (diphenidol, SK&F) apparently exerts a specific antivertigo effect on the vestibular apparatus to control vertigo and inhibits the chemoreceptor trigger zone to control nausea and vomiting.

INDICATIONS (SEE WARNINGS)

1) VERTIGO—'Vontrol' is indicated in peripheral (labyrinthine) vertigo and associated nausea and vomiting, as seen in such conditions as: Meniere's disease, middle- and inner-ear surgery (labyrinthitis).
2) NAUSEA AND VOMITING—'Vontrol' is indicated in the control of nausea and vomiting, as seen in such conditions as: postoperative states, malignant neoplasms and labyrinthine disturbances.

CONTRAINDICATIONS

Known hypersensitivity to the drug is a contraindication. Anuria is a contraindication. (Since approximately 90% of the drug is excreted in the urine, renal shutdown could cause systemic accumulation.)

WARNINGS

'Vontrol' (diphenidol, SK&F) may cause hallucinations, disorientation or confusion. For this reason, its use is limited to patients who are hospitalized or under comparable, continuous, close, professional supervision. Even then, the physician should carefully weigh the benefits against the possible risks and give due consideration to alternate therapeutic measures.

The incidence of auditory and visual hallucinations, disorientation and confusion appears to be less than ½% or approximately one in 350 patients. The reaction has usually occurred within three days of starting the drug in recommended dosage and has subsided spontaneously usually within three days after discontinuation of the drug. Patients on 'Vontrol' should be observed closely and in the event of such a reaction the drug should be stopped.

Usage in Pregnancy: Use of any drug in pregnancy, lactation or in women of childbearing age requires that the potential benefits of the drug be weighed against its possible hazards to the mother and child.

In animal teratogenesis and reproduction studies of 'Vontrol' (diphenidol, SK&F), there were no significant differences between drug-treated groups and untreated control groups, except as noted under animal Reproduction Studies (see "Pharmacology [animal]").

In 936 patients who received 'Vontrol' during pregnancy, the incidences of normal and abnormal birth were comparable to those reported in the literature for the average population of pregnant patients. And in no instance was there any evidence that 'Vontrol' played a part in birth abnormality (see "In Pregnancy").

'Vontrol' is not indicated for use in nausea and vomiting of pregnancy, since the therapeutic value and safety in this indication have not yet been determined.

PRECAUTIONS

The antiemetic action of 'Vontrol' (diphenidol, SK&F) may mask signs of overdose of drugs (e.g., digitalis) or may obscure diagnosis of conditions such as intestinal obstruction and brain tumor.

Although there have been no reports of blood dyscrasias with 'Vontrol', patients should be observed regularly for any idiosyncratic reactions.

'Vontrol' has a weak peripheral anticholinergic effect and should be used with care in patients with glaucoma, obstructive lesions of the gastrointestinal and genitourinary tracts, such as stenosing peptic ulcer, prostatic hypertrophy, pyloric and duodenal obstruction, and organic cardiospasm.

'Vontrol' Tablets contain FD&C Yellow No. 5 (tartrazine) which may cause allergic-type reactions (including bronchial asthma) in certain susceptible individuals. Although the overall incidence of FD&C Yellow No. 5 (tartrazine) sensitivity in the general population is low, it is frequently seen in patients who also have aspirin hypersensitivity.

Usage in Children

'Vontrol' is not recommended for use in children under 50 pounds. (See Dosage and Administration—Children.)

ADVERSE REACTIONS

Auditory and visual hallucinations, disorientation and confusion have been reported. Drowsiness, overstimulation, depression, sleep disturbance, dry mouth, g.i. irritation (nausea and indigestion), or blurred vision may occur.

Rarely, slight dizziness, skin rash, malaise, headache, or heartburn may occur. Mild jaundice of questionable relationship to the use of 'Vontrol' (diphenidol, SK&F) has been reported. Slight, transient lowering of blood pressure has been reported in a few patients.

(See laboratory studies under "Pharmacology [human]".)

DOSAGE AND ADMINISTRATION (SEE WARNINGS)

ADULTS—FOR VERTIGO OR NAUSEA AND VOMITING: The usual dose is one tablet (25 mg.) every four hours as needed. Some patients may require two tablets (50 mg.).

CHILDREN—FOR NAUSEA AND VOMITING: These recommendations are for nausea and vomiting only. There has been no experience with 'Vontrol' in vertigo in children. Unit doses in children are best calculated by body weight: usually 0.4 mg./lb.

Children's doses usually should not be given more often than every four hours. However, if symptoms persist after the first dose, administration may be repeated after one hour. Thereafter, doses may be given every four hours as needed. The total dose in 24 hours should not exceed 2.5 mg./lb.

NOTE: The drug is not recommended for use in children under 50 pounds. The dosage for children 50 to 100 pounds is one tablet (25 mg.).

OVERDOSAGE

In the event of overdosage, the patient should be managed according to his symptoms. Treatment is essentially supportive, with maintenance of blood pressure and respiration, plus careful observation. Early gastric lavage may be indicated depending on the amount of overdose and nature of symptoms.

HOW SUPPLIED

Tablets containing 25 mg. diphenidol, as the hydrochloride, in bottles of 100.

PHARMACOLOGY (animal): 'Vontrol' (diphenidol, SK&F) exerts its antiemetic effect primarily by inhibiting the chemoreceptor trigger zone, as evidenced by its activity in blocking emesis induced by apomorphine in dogs. In this regard 'Vontrol', as the hydrochloride salt, has a potency equal to the potent phenothiazine antiemetic, chlorpromazine hydrochloride. In animals 'Vontrol' has only weak parasympatholytic activity and no significant sedative, tranquilizing or antihistaminic action or effects on blood pressure, heart rate, respiration or the electrocardiogram.

Subacute and chronic toxicity studies in rats and dogs, in which large doses of 'Vontrol', as the hydrochloride salt, were administered orally and intramuscularly for periods up to one year, revealed no significant effects on hematology, liver function, kidney function or blood glucose determinations. Histological examination of the animals' tissues did not reveal any significant lesions attributable to administration of 'Vontrol'.

Reproduction Studies: Teratogenesis and reproduction studies were carried out in rats and rabbits. In rats, 'Vontrol' (diphenidol, SK&F), as the hydrochloride salt, was fed daily to male and female animals in doses of 20 mg./kg. and 40 mg./kg. (approximately three and six times the maximum recommended daily dose in adult humans) for 60 days before mating, and during mating, gestation and lactation for each of two litters. There were no significant differences between drug-treated and untreated control groups with regard to conception rate, litter size, live birth or viability in either of the two litters. There was no congenital anomaly among the offspring. In rabbits, 'Vontrol', as the hydrochloride salt, was fed in the diets in doses of 5 mg./kg. or 75 mg./kg. (approximately equal to, and 12 times as much as, the maximum recommended daily dose in adult humans) from the first day of gestation through the 26th or 27th day of gestation, when the young were delivered by Cesarean section. There were no significant differences between drug-treated and control groups with regard to number and weight of fetuses, numbers of resorption sites or viable fetuses. There was also no statistically significant difference between drug-treated and control groups with regard to the total percentage of underdeveloped fetuses. However, when data were calculated on the basis of a ratio between underdeveloped fetuses and number of pregnant does, an adverse dose-related effect was observed in the high-dose test group.

PHARMACOLOGY (human): Three double-blind controlled studies comparing 'Vontrol' (diphenidol, SK&F) to placebo were carried out: one in 32 male volunteers over a four-week period; one in 45 volunteers of whom 15 were studied for 12 weeks and 17 for 24 weeks; and one in 48 volunteers of whom 36 were studied for 12 weeks.

In the first study 'Vontrol', as the hydrochloride salt, was given orally in daily doses that were started at 75 mg. during the first week and graduated up to 200 mg. by the fourth week. In the second study, one group received 'Vontrol' orally, as the hydrochloride salt, titrated up to 500 mg. daily, then down to 200 mg. daily; another group received a maximum of 200 mg. daily. In the third study, patients received oral doses of 200 mg. to 300 mg. of 'Vontrol' daily, as the hydrochloride or pamoate salts.

The studies included these laboratory determinations: complete blood counts (including hemoglobin and hematocrit determinations), urinalyses (including microscopic examination), serum alkaline phosphatase, serum bilirubin, and bromsulphalein retention. The studies also included records of weight and blood pressure and, in one, electrocardiograms.

In two of these studies, clinical laboratory changes were seen among volunteers in both treated and control groups. The changes included: extrasystoles, white cells in the urine, increase in prothrombin time, rise in hematocrit, rise in leucocytes, rise in eosinophils, and rise or reduction in neutrophils. At no time in any study did changes in the treated group differ significantly from those in the control group.

'Vontrol', as the hydrochloride salt, was given orally to 17 children (aged five to 15). Total daily doses ranged from 90 to 240 mg. Complete blood counts and, in some patients, urinalyses were done before treatment and after approximately four days of treatment. There was no significant difference between pre- and post-treatment laboratory determinations in any child. No side effects were seen.

EXCRETION: Following oral administration of 'Vontrol' (diphenidol, SK&F) to dogs, as the hydrochloride or pamoate salts, and to humans, as the hydrochloride salt, peak blood concentration of the drug generally occurs in one and a half to three hours. In dogs and rats, virtually all of an oral dose of C^{14}-labeled 'Vontrol' is excreted in the urine and feces within three to four days, as determined by radioactivity counts. Approximately the same percentage of an administered dose appeared in the urine of dogs following either oral administration of the hydrochloride salt or rectal administration of the free base.

IN PREGNANCY: Investigators kept follow-up records on 936 patients who had received 'Vontrol' (diphenidol, SK&F) at some time during pregnancy, primarily during the first trimester.

Of the 936 women, 864 (92%) had normal births of normal infants.

Seventy-two (8%) of the women experienced some birth abnormality. Of the 72, six patients had premature but otherwise normal infants, 40 patients aborted, 10 had stillbirths, and 16 had infants with miscellaneous defects. These included hernias, congenital heart defects, hydrocephalus, internal strabismus, anencephalus, enlarged thyroid, and hypospadia.

These incidences of abnormal birth are lower than those generally reported in the literature for the average population of pregnant patients. And in no instance was there any evidence that the administration of 'Vontrol' played a part in birth abnormality.

VN:L15

Shown in Product Identification Section, page 431

EDUCATIONAL MATERIAL

BOOKLETS

"Essentials of Immune Response, Inflammation and the Pathogenesis of Rheumatoid Arthritis," a 63-page booklet (6½" × 8½"). Reviews current thinking on the pathogenesis of rheumatoid arthritis and, briefly, the basic terminology and principles of immunology and inflammation. Free to physicians and allied health personnel.

"Essentials of a Differential Diagnosis of Rheumatoid Arthritis," a 66-page booklet (6½" × 8½"). Provides a logical stepwise approach to rheumatoid arthritis diagnosis. Free to physicians and allied health personnel.

"Essentials of Managing Rheumatoid Arthritis," a 54-page booklet (6½" × 8½"). Examines the drug and nondrug therapies used to manage rheumatoid arthritis. Free to physicians and allied health personnel.

PATIENT I.D. CARDS

"I am taking Eskalith®/ Eskalith CR® (brand of lithium carbonate)." Packet of 10 wallet-size (2½" × 3½") cards. Provides information to emergency room or other medical personnel about the patient and attending physician and about possible drug-related side effects and their management. Free to physicians.

"I am taking Stelazine® (brand of trifluoperazine hydrochloride)." Packet of 10 wallet-size (2½" × 3½") fold-out cards. Provides information to emergency room or other medical personnel about the patient and attending physician and about possible drug-related side effects and their management. Free to physicians.

"I am taking Parnate® (brand of tranylcypromine sulfate)." Packet of 10 wallet-size (2½" × 3½") cards. Provides information to emergency room or other medical personnel about the patient and attending physician and about possible drug-related side effects and their management. Free to physicians.

PATIENT INFORMATION

Patient information on Dyazide® (triamterene and hydrochlorothiazide). Pad (8½" × 11") of 50 sheets. Provides basic information about high blood pressure and 'Dyazide', including special considerations about diet, possible drug interactions, and side effects. Free to physicians. Patient I.D. Card.

Instruction sheets for patients on Parnate® (brand of tranylcypromine sulfate). Pad (4¼" × 8") of 24 sheets. Serves as a reminder of principal instructions about 'Parnate' therapy, e.g.: the importance of following dosage instructions exactly; the need for consulting before taking any other drugs; what foods and beverages must be avoided; what symptoms should be reported promptly. A carbon copy is provided for the physician's records. Free to physicians.

Instructions for patients on Ridaura® (brand of auranofin). Pad (5" × 8") of 15 sheets. Serves as a reminder of the main instructions about 'Ridaura' therapy, including time to onset of response, what symptoms to report promptly, and the need for regular laboratory monitoring. Free to physicians and pharmacists.

Smith Laboratories, Inc.

2215 SANDERS ROAD
NORTHBROOK, IL 60062

CHYMODIACTIN® ℞

[ki″mō-dī-ac′tin]
(chymopapain for injection)
with Diluent

WARNINGS

Chymodiactin® should only be used in a hospital setting by physicians experienced and trained in the diagnosis of lumbar disc disease and all standard treatment modalities, including surgery. Additionally, these physicians and their support personnel should be competent in the diagnosis and management of all potential complications from the use of Chymodiactin.

Anaphylaxis, which can be fatal, has occurred in approximately 0.5% of patients receiving Chymodiactin (0.4% for patients under local anesthesia v. 0.5% for patients under general anesthesia).

Paraplegia/paraparesis, central nervous system hemorrhage, and other serious neurologic adverse events have been observed soon (within hours or days) after chymopapain injection at a rate of about 1 in 2,000. Acute transverse myelitis/acute transverse myelopathy has been observed 2–3 weeks following chymopapain injection at a rate of about 1 in 18,000, which is significantly higher than the incidence reported in the medical literature. A cause and effect relationship between these neurologic events and chymopapain when properly injected has not been established.

Chymopapain is extremely toxic when injected intrathecally, as are some radiopaque contrast media used for discography. Therefore, great care must be taken to assure that the dura is not penetrated and that chymopapain, or contrast medium if used, does not enter the subarachnoid space. If there is any question regarding needle tip location within the nucleus of the disc or if contrast medium is used and it extravasates into the subarachnoid space, the procedure should be abandoned and chymopapain should not be injected.

Discography at the time of chemonucleolysis is not recommended unless it is determined that the benefits outweigh the risks. Chemonucleolysis should be limited to the disc producing the patient's signs and symptoms and should be performed using supplemented local anesthesia whenever possible.

DESCRIPTION

Chymodiactin is a proteolytic enzyme in the form of a sterile, nonpyrogenic, lyophilized powder. The unit of chymopapain activity is the picoKatal (pKat). The enzyme forms, under the conditions of the assay, 1 picomole of p-nitroaniline per second from DL-benzoyl arginine-p-nitroanilide (BAPNA) substrate. In general, 1 mg of chymopapain contains approximately 500 pKat units.

Chymodiactin is available in 2 ml and 5 ml vial sizes, and is accompanied by a vial of Sterile Water for Injection, USP, which is to be used as diluent. The 2 ml vial, which is to be reconstituted with 2 ml of diluent, contains 4,000 pKat units of Chymodiactin and 1.4 mg of sodium L-cysteinate hydrochloride. The 5 ml vial, which is to be reconstituted with 5 ml of diluent, contains 10,000 pKat units of Chymodiactin and 3.6 mg of sodium L-cysteinate hydrochloride. The concentration of the solution in a reconstituted vial is 2,000 pKat units of active drug per ml. The vial contains no preservatives.

The proteolytic enzyme chymopapain is derived from the crude latex of *Carica papaya*. Sodium L-cysteinate hydrochloride is added as a reducing agent for this sulphur containing enzyme to maintain the sulphur in the sulphydryl form. The pH of the reconstituted drug is 5.5 to 6.5.

CLINICAL PHARMACOLOGY

Chymodiactin is injected into the herniated nucleus pulposus of the lumbar intervertebral disc resulting in rapid hydrolysis of the noncollagenous polypeptides or proteins that maintain the tertiary structure of the chondromucoprotein of the nucleus pulposus. By causing degradation of the chondromucoprotein, the intradiscal osmotic activity is lessened, thereby decreasing fluid absorption and reducing intradiscal pressure. The foregoing mechanism of action is based on animal *in vitro* and *in vivo* data. Although the mechanism of action in the human has not been established directly, operative findings in patients who have had surgery following injection have usually revealed the nucleus pulposus to be absent from its former site. A temporary increase in urinary mucopolysaccharide occurs in man following intradiscal injection of chymopapain. After intradiscal injection of chymopapain in humans it appears that the inhibitory activity of the alpha$_2$-macroglobulin prevents expression of any significant proteolytic activity outside the disc.

As Chymodiactin is injected directly into the herniated lumbar intervertebral disc, absorption, distribution, and metabolism are not necessary for it to achieve its intended purpose. Pharmacological activity has been demonstrated by direct observation both *in vivo* and *in vitro* in animals, *in vitro* in human disc tissue, and pharmacokinetically in the human by observation of increases in urinary excretion of substances known to be in high concentration in the disc.

After injection into the central portion of human lumbar intervertebral discs (*in vivo*) there is an increase in the urinary concentration of glycosaminoglycans of the type known to occur in human intervertebral discs; and chymopapain or its immunologically reactive fragments (CIP) are also detectable by radioimmunoassay in plasma at 30 minutes and are declining at 24 hours. Small amounts of CIP are also detected in the urine. These findings indicate that, after intradiscal injection of chymopapain, CIP diffuses rapidly into plasma. Due to the inhibitory activity of the plasma alpha$_2$-macroglobulin and the low concentration of CIP, it is unlikely that any proteolytic activity is expressed outside the disc.

In a randomized, double-blind comparison of drug and placebo, approximately 75% of patients responded successfully to drug, compared to approximately 45% for placebo, using the randomization code-break as the criterion for efficacy. When the placebo failures were then treated with drug, 90% of them responded with partial or total relief of their symptoms. In a multicenter, open-label study involving approximately 1,500 patients, therapeutic results were also favorable, with success rates ranging from 80% to 89% depending on the criteria used to determine outcome.

INDICATIONS AND USAGE

Chymodiactin intradiscal injection is indicated for the treatment of patients with documented herniated lumbar intervertebral discs whose symptoms and signs, particularly sciatica, have not responded to an adequate period or periods of conservative therapy. Chymodiactin has not been studied in the treatment of herniated discs in areas other than the lumbar spine.

Chymodiactin should only be used by physicians who routinely care for the patients, described above, who are qualified by training and experience to perform laminectomy, discectomy, or other spinal procedures, and who have received specialized training in chemonucleolysis. The appropriate use of Chymodiactin in chemonucleolysis requires precise diagnosis, and the ability to employ skillfully all appropriate diagnostic and treatment modalities necessary, including surgical intervention other than chemonucleolysis (laminectomy/discectomy) and all aspects of pre- and postoperative patient management. Proper selection of patients for whom chemonucleolysis is applicable requires extensive training and experience in the diagnosis and management of all spinal disorders, since there are circumstances in which nerve root compression resulting from conditions other than a herniated disc can produce similar signs and symptoms.

Chymodiactin should be used only in hospitals. Support personnel, as well as physicians, should be qualified in the diagnosis and management of all potential complications of the use of Chymodiactin.

CONTRAINDICATIONS

Chymodiactin is contraindicated in patients with a known sensitivity to chymopapain, papaya or papaya derivatives such as certain papain-containing contact lens cleaners and meat tenderizer preparations. Other contraindications are severe spondylolisthesis; significant spinal stenosis; severe, progressing paralysis as indicated by rapidly progressing neurologic dysfunction; and evidence of spinal cord tumor or other lesions producing spinal motor or sensory dysfunction (e.g. cauda equina lesion).

Chymopapain is a foreign protein and its injection has the potential for generating an immunologic response. Therefore, the use of Chymodiactin is contraindicated in patients who have previously been injected with any form of chymopapain.

Chymodiactin has not been studied in regions of the spine other than the lumbar area; therefore, its use is contraindicated in any spinal region other than the lumbar area.

WARNINGS

(1) Anaphylaxis of a severe to mild nature has been observed after injection of Chymodiactin in about 0.5% of patients and may be life threatening if not treated promptly and correctly. *At least one open intravenous line must always be in place to permit rapid and adequate management of such an occurrence.* The reaction can be immediate or delayed up to two hours after injection and can last for minutes to several hours or longer. The patient may present with almost immediate hypotension and/or bronchospasm, the former being more common. These may proceed to laryngeal edema, cardiac arrhythmia, cardiac arrest, coma, and death. Speed in diagnosis and treatment is of the essence since the clinical signs, severity, progression, and duration of an anaphylactic reaction are highly unpredictable. The patient must also be observed for the development of other signs of allergic response, such as erythema, pilomotor erection, rash, pruritic urticaria, conjunctivitis, vasomotor rhinitis, angioedema, or various gastrointestinal disturbances.

Data obtained from postmarketing surveillance of over 71,000 patients demonstrate the incidence of anaphylaxis secondary to Chymodiactin injection varies by gender and type of anesthesia:

	Local	General	Overall
Male	0.3%	0.3%	0.3%
Female	0.6%	0.9%	0.8%
Overall	0.4%	0.5%	0.5%

The anaphylaxis rate is statistically significantly higher for females (0.8% v. 0.3% for males) and for patients who received general anesthesia (0.5% v. 0.4% for local anesthesia). In the population where race has been reported the incidence is statiscally significantly higher in black females.

Clinical judgment, speed of therapy, and choice of agents all enter into the treatment of anaphylaxis. *Epinephrine is the definitive therapeutic agent in the immediate treatment of anaphylaxis. Substitution of other agents such as steroids should be reserved for cases where epinephrine is not appropriate.*

(2) Paraplegia/paraparesis, (e.g. as are seen in the cauda equina syndrome), other serious neurologic adverse events, and subarachnoid and intracerebral hemorrhage, and seizures have been observed soon (within hours or days) after chymopapain injection at a rate of about 1 in 2,000. Causal relationships to the drug when properly injected have not been established. Needle trauma and/or injection of chymopapain and contrast media into the spinal fluid may be causes in some of these reported cases. Other less severe neurologic reactions have included burning sacral, leg pain, hypalgesia, leg weakness, foot drop, cramping in both calves, pain in the opposite leg, paresthesia, tingling in legs, and numbness of legs/toes.

Acute transverse myelitis/acute transverse myelopathy has been reported in association with the injection of chymopapain at a rate of about 1 in 18,000. Although cause and effect relationship to the injection of chymopapain itself has not been established, the reported rate is significantly higher than the incidence reported in the medical literature. These patients are characterized clinically by the delayed (2–3 weeks) onset of paraplegia or paraparesis without prior signs or symptoms.

Regarding serious neurologic adverse events, the following should be noted:

Continued on next page

Smith—Cont.

(a) In nearly all of the cases of serious neurologic adverse events, discography was performed as part of the procedure. As noted above, the injection of contrast agent and chymopapain into the spinal fluid may be a cause in some of the reported cases. Additionally, several of the patients experiencing neurologic adverse events who did not have discography performed prior to the procedure experienced only transient problems. Based on this information and the results of a study in baboons (see **Animal Pharmacology and Toxicology**), *it is recommended that discography not be performed as part of the chemonucleolysis procedure unless, in the judgment of the surgeon, the benefits outweigh the risks for a particular patient.* A water or saline acceptance test may be used as an alternative to discography to indicate that the disc is abnormal and to attempt reproduction of sciatic pain in the patient receiving local anesthesia.

(b) Patients receiving injections at two or more disc spaces appear to be at increased risk of serious neurologic adverse events. Therefore, *chemonucleolysis should be limited to the one disc producing the patient's symptoms unless definitive signs, symptoms, and diagnostic procedures indicate that more than one disc is at fault.*

(c) Nearly all of the patients who experienced a serious neurologic adverse event had the procedure performed under general anesthesia. Local anesthesia provides an awake patient, more likely to experience pain and complain if the needle impinges on nerve tissue. Also, it is unlikely that a patient under local anesthesia will tolerate an excessive number of attempts to place the needle. Although the final choice of anesthetic rests with the patient's physician. *it is recommended that local or supplemented local anesthesia be used for chemonucleolysis whenever possible.*

(d) Patients who have had prior surgery of the lumbar spine appear to be at increased risk of experiencing a serious neurologic adverse event. Therefore, it is recommended that such patients be selected for chemonucleolysis only after careful consideration of the risk/benefit ratio.

(e) A number of patients with a history of hypertension, known or suspected cerebrovascular anomaly, previous cerebrovascular accident, or a strong family history of cerebrovascular accident have experienced extensive, severe, or fatal central nervous system hemorrhage following chemonucleolysis.

(3) *The drug is extremely toxic when injected intrathecally in animals. Therefore, great caution must be exercised in assuring that Chymodiactin is not injected intrathecally. The transdural or posterior approach for needle placement must be avoided.*

(4) Certain radiopaque contrast media used for discography are neurotoxic when injected intrathecally. The toxicity of these materials may be enhanced by intrathecal bleeding. If Chymodiactin is inadvertently administered intrathecally, disruption of the capillaries may occur resulting in intrathecal bleeding.

PRECAUTIONS

Patient Selection:

(1) A careful history should be obtained to determine if the patient has multiple allergies, especially a known allergy to papaya or payaya derivatives or iodine. Absorbable iodine should not be used during myelography (or discography, if performed—see **Warnings**) in patients allergic to iodine.
The use of a preoperative screening test for chymopapain-specific IgE antibody should be considered to identify patients at risk for anaphylaxis.

(2) A number of patients with a history of prior surgery of the lumbar spine, hypertension, known or suspected cerebrovascular anomaly, previous cerebrovascular accident, or strong family history of cerebrovascular accident have experienced a serious neurologic adverse event following chemonucleolysis. (See **Warnings.**)

(3) Females, particularly black females, are more likely to develop anaphylactic reactions secondary to Chymodiactin. (See **Warnings.**)

(4) In case of anaphylaxis, beta-blocker therapy may block the action of epinephrine.

Pretreatment:

(1) It is recommended that patients be pretreated prior to the injection of Chymodiactin with histamine receptor (H_1 and H_2) antagonists to lessen the severity of an anaphylactic reaction. One regimen that has been widely used is cimetidine 300 mg orally every 6 hours and diphenhydramine 50 mg orally every 6 hours for 24 hours prior to chemonucleolysis.

(2) Because of the abrupt decrease in intravascular volume during anaphylaxis, patients should be well hydrated by oral or intravenous fluids prior to chemonucleolysis. At least one open intravenous line must always be in place to permit rapid and adequate management of such an occurence.

Procedure:

(1) The choice of anesthetic for a specific patient should be made by the attending surgeon and anesthesiologist; however, local or supplemented local anesthetic is recommended whenever possible.
The advantages of local or supplemented local anesthesia are thought to be: a lower anaphylaxis rate (0.4%); possible ease of recognition of impending anaphylaxis because earliest symptoms can be reported by an awake patient; possible correlation of sciatic pain with a specific disc because the patient is awake; and possible decreased risk of experiencing a serious neurologic adverse event secondary to difficult needle placement. (See **Warnings.**)
The advantages of general anesthesia are thought to be: ease of airway management if anaphylaxis should develop; more precise patient positioning for injection; and less patient discomfort. A disadvantage of general anesthesia is a higher rate of anaphylaxis (0.5%). If halothane anesthesia is used, it should be noted that if epinephrine HCl is required for treatment of an anaphylactic reaction, there is a potential arrhythmogenic interaction of the two drugs.

(2) Needle placement for the intradiscal administration of Chymodiactin should be made by physicians experienced in needle placement via the lateral approach to avoid puncture of the dura mater. Clinical trials have not been conducted using the posterior approach for needle placement and serious neurologic toxicity has been reported using a posterior transdural approach; therefore, this method of needle placement must be avoided. Prior to injection of Chymodiactin, visualization of the needle tip position in the disc must be confirmed using x-ray image intensifier for both the anteroposterior and lateral views. *If high quality x-ray equipment including an image intensifier is not available, chemonucleolysis should not be performed.*

(3) If discography is deemed essential at the time of the chemonucleolysis procedure (see **Warnings**), at least 15 minutes should elapse after the administration of radiopaque contrast medium to be sure there has been no reaction from the contrast agent.

(4) For 3 minutes prior to Chymodiactin injection, 100% O_2 may be administered to the patient by the anesthesiologist to maximize oxygenation in case of anaphylaxis.

(5) A test dose injection of 0.2 ml of Chymodiactin followed by a 10–15 minute wait is recommended prior to the injection of the full therapeutic dose. The purpose of the test dose is to help identify those patients who are most sensitive to chymopapain, and patients who develop signs and/or symptoms of anaphylaxis following the test dose must not receive the therapeutic dose. However, some patients have been reported who failed to react to the test dose, but developed anaphylaxis to the therapeutic dose, suggesting that sensitivity to Chymodiactin may be dose related.

Patient Instructions:

(1) Patients should be instructed that after injection they may experience back pain or involuntary muscle spasm in the lower area of the back for several days. This is not uncommon nor is a residual stiffness or soreness of the low back which may persist for several months.

(2) Patients should be instructed to anticipate the possibility of any of the following delayed allergic reactions which may occur as late as 15 days after injection: rash of any type, urticaria, or itching. If any of these occur, patients should contact their physician.

Pregnancy: Pregnancy Category C. Animal reproduction studies have not been conducted with Chymodiactin. It is also not known whether Chymodiactin can cause fetal harm when administered to a pregnant woman or can affect reproduction capacity. Chymodiactin should be given to a pregnant woman only if clearly needed.

Pediatric Use: Safety and effectiveness of Chymodiactin has not been studied in pediatric patients; therefore, the drug should not be used in children.

ADVERSE REACTIONS

Based on postmarketing surveillance reports, the overall frequency of anaphylaxis is 0.5% or about 1 in 200 patients. The frequency in females is approximately 0.8%, in males approximately 0.3%. The frequency when general anesthesia is employed is 0.5%, when local anesthesia is employed, 0.4%. These differences are statistically significant.
Fatalities have been reported following injection of Chymodiactin. Some of these fatalities, such as those due to anaphylaxis or complications of anaphylaxis, disc space infection, or central nervous system hemorrhage, may be associated with either the drug or the procedure. Others appear to be coincidental. The overall mortality rate following Chymodiactin injection is approximately 1 in 5,000 patients (0.02%). For purposes of comparison, mortality associated with laminectomy has been reported to range from 0.02% to 0.1%.
Paraplegia/paraparesis, (e.g as are seen in the cauda equina syndrome), other serious neurologic adverse events, and subarachnoid and intracerebral hemorrhage, and seizures have been observed soon (within hours or days) after chymopapain injection at a rate of about 1 in 2,000. Causal relationships to the drug when properly injected have not been established. Needle trauma and/or injection of chymopapain and contrast media into the spinal fluid may be causes in some of these reported cases. Other less severe neurologic reactions have included burning sacral, leg pain, hypalgesia, leg weakness, foot drop, cramping in both calves, pain in the opposite leg, paresthesia, tingling in legs, and numbness of legs/toes.
Acute transverse myelitis/acute transverse myelopathy has been reported in association with the injection of chymopapain at a rate of about 1 in 18,000. Although cause and effect relationship to the injection of chymopapain itself has not been established, the reported rate is significantly higher than the incidence reported in the medical literature. These patients are characterized clinically by the delayed (2–3 weeks) onset of paraplegia or paraparesis without prior signs or symptoms.
Discitis, both bacterial and aseptic, has been reported.
Less severe, but more frequent adverse reactions include back pain/stiffness/soreness in approximately 50% of treated patients and/or back spasm in approximately 30%.
Less frequent adverse reactions, occurring in less than 1% of patients studied include rash, itching, urticaria, nausea, paralytic ileus, urinary retention, headache, and dizziness.

DRUG ABUSE AND DEPENDENCE

Chymodiactin injection does not lend itself to drug abuse and dependence.

OVERDOSAGE

Overdosage has not occurred in the clinical trials of Chymodiactin.

DOSAGE AND ADMINISTRATION

Each 2 ml vial of Chymodiactin contains 4,000 pKat units of enzyme and should be reconstituted with 2.0 ml Sterile Water for Injection, USP. Each 5 ml vial of Chymodiactin contains 10,000 pKat units of the enzyme and should be reconstituted with 5.0 ml Sterile Water for Injection, USP. The concentration of solution in the reconstituted vial is 2,000 pKat units of Chymodiactin per ml. Recommended dosage is 2,000 to 4,000 pKat units per disc, usually 3,000 pKat units per disc, or a volume of injection of 1 to 2 ml, usually 1.5 ml per disc. If more than one disc is to be injected (see **Warnings**), an individual patient should not receive more than 8,000 pKat units.
A 5 ml vial of Sterile Water for Injection, USP is supplied with each vial of Chymodiactin. *This is the only diluent which should be used to reconstitute the drug. Bacteriostatic Water for Injection, USP, must not be used* because it may inactivate the enzyme.
Alcohol should be used to cleanse the vial stopper prior to insertion of needles into the vial. However, since residual alcohol may inactivate the enzyme, it should be allowed to air dry before continuing with the reconstitution process.
Parenteral drug products should be inspected visually for particulate matter and discoloration prior to administration.
Care should be exercised in the selection of proper size and use of needles inserted into the vials in the reconstitution process to reduce the possibility of coring the stopper. The manufacturing process results in a residual vacuum in the vial; therefore, the use of automatic filling syringes is not recommended.
The drug must be used within two hours of its reconstitution with Sterile Water for Injection, USP. Unused drug must be promptly discarded and not stored for future use.
Chymodiactin is limited to use under the professional supervision of a physician licensed by law to administer it, with the following additional considerations:

The appropriate use of Chymodiactin in chemonucleolysis, as pointed out in the **Indications and Usage** section of the labeling, requires precise diagnosis, and the ability to employ skillfully all acceptable diagnostic and treatment modalities as necessary, including surgical intervention other than chemonucleolysis, *e.g.*, laminectomy, including all aspects of pre- and postoperative patient care.

The proper selection of patients for whom chemonucleolysis is applicable is of the utmost importance and requires extensive training and experience in the diagnosis and management of all spinal disorders and diseases, since there are circumstances in which nerve root compression resulting from conditions other than the herniated disc can produce similar signs and symptoms.

The use of Chymodiactin, therefore, should be limited to physicians who are trained not only in chemonucleolysis but who are qualified by training and experience to care routinely for such patients in other ways.

Chymodiactin should be used only in a hospital setting with the assistance of trained personnel, and in such a manner as to assure immediate and proper management of all potential complications.

HOW SUPPLIED
Chymodiactin is supplied as a sterile, nonpyrogenic, lyophilized powder in single vials containing either 4,000 or 10,000 pKat units of enzymatic activity. Each vial of Chymodiactin is accompanied with a 5 ml vial of Sterile Water for Injection, USP, which is to be used as diluent.
Caution: Although a 5 ml vial of Sterile Water for Injection, USP, is supplied with both vial sizes, *only 2 ml of diluent is to be used when reconstituting the 4,000 pKat unit vial.*
Chymodiactin can be shipped unrefrigerated; however, it should be stored refrigerated (36° to 46°F or 2° to 8°C) until reconstituted for use.
Animal Pharmacology and Toxicology: Injection of Chymodiactin into the lumbar intervertebral disc of mature beagle dogs revealed narrowing of the intervertebral space noted on radiographs obtained at 48 hours and at 14 days. In dogs sacrificed at 14 days following injection, cavitation of the nucleus pulposus was observed, but the end plates were unaffected.
Chymopapain has previously been shown to dissolve the nucleus pulposus of dogs and rabbits at doses as low as 100 pKat units/disc and 50 pKat units/disc, respectively. Doses of 3,000 pKat units/disc cause thinning of only the inner portion of the annulus in rabbits but do not penetrate the entire structure, while doses as high as 24,000 pKat units/disc in dogs resulted in no apparent significant change in the peripheral portion of the annulus. *In vitro* studies demonstrated that chymopapain solubilized the mucopolysaccharide protein complex of human nucleus pulposus, but did not attack the collagen of this structure.
When chymopapain is injected into dogs, doses up to 100 times greater than that required to remove the nucleus pulposus were well tolerated when injected intravenously, intradiscally, and epidurally. The drug is extremely toxic when injected intrathecally; the approximate LD_{50} is 15 pKat units/kg in rabbits, 150 pKat units/kg in dogs and 200 pKat units/kg in baboons. Therefore, great caution must be exercised in assuring that Chymodiactin is not injected intrathecally.
In baboons the serial injection into the spinal fluid of contrast agents (Renografin®, Conray or Amipaque®) followed by Chymodiactin 15 minutes later produced serious neurotoxicity, including weakness, paralysis and death. When administered singly at the same doses, Conray, Amipaque, and Chymodiactin were not toxic; Renografin was less toxic singly than in combination with Chymodiactin. This information supports the clinical observation that the documented entry of contrast agent and presumed entry of chymopapain into the spinal fluid can produce serious neurotoxicity including paraplegia and central nervous system hemorrhage.

Smith Laboratories, Inc.
Northbrook, Illinois 60062
July 1986 SL-9050-R2

Solgar Vitamin Company, Inc.
410 OCEAN AVENUE
LYNBROOK, NY 11563

STRESS FORMULA
B–COMPLEX WITH C

Provides dietary supplementation for Vitamin C and B-Complex.

SUPPLIED
Bottles of 100, 250 and 500 tablets.

BETA CAROTENE CAPSULES (Natural)
(PROVITAMIN A)

Each capsule provides: Natural Beta Carotene (Provitamin A) sufficient to convert to 11,000 IU of Vitamin A.

SUPPLIED
Bottles of 50 and 100 capsules.

BIOTIN TABLETS
300 mcg, 600 mcg (VITAMIN H)

SUPPLIED
Bottles of 100 and 250 tablets.

CALCIUM 600
From Oyster Shells

Two tablets provide 1200 mg of calcium (calcium carbonate) with 400 IU of vitamin D.

SUPPLIED
Bottles of 60 and 120 tablets.

CHEWS–EZE TABLETS
NATURAL CHILDREN'S CHEWABLE VITAMIN SUPPLEMENT WITH BEE POLLEN AND ORANGE JUICE CRYSTALS.
SALT AND STARCH FREE
• VEGETARIAN FORMULA

Provides essential multi-vitamins for children under 4 years of age. Chew or allow to dissolve in the mouth. May be crushed and sprinkled over cereal or dissolved in milk or other liquids.
Each Tablet Provides:

Vitamin A	5000 IU
Vitamin D	400 IU
Vitamin B-1	3 mg
Vitamin B-2	6 mg
Niacinamide	1.71 mg
Vitamin C	100 mg
Vitamin B-12	5 mcg
Vitamin E	5 IU

SUPPLIED
Bottles of 30, 90, 180 tablets.

CHOLINE/INOSITOL TABLETS
250/250 mg

A dietary supplement containing Choline and Inositol, members of the B-Complex family.

SUPPLIED
Bottles of 100 and 250 tablets.

FORMULA B–50 CAPSULES
HIGH POTENCY B-COMPLEX FORMULA

A balanced proportion of all the recognized B-Complex factors.
Each Capsule Provides:

Vitamin B-1	50 mg
Vitamin B-2	50 mg
Vitamin B-6	50 mg
Vitamin B-12	50 mcg
Niacinamide	50 mg
Folic Acid	400 mcg
Pantothenic Acid	50 mg
Para Aminobenzoic Acid	50 mg
Choline Bitartrate	50 mg
Inositol	50 mg
Biotin	50 mcg

SUPPLIED
Bottles of 50, 100 and 250 capsules.

FORMULA VM–75 MULTIVITAMIN & MINERAL TABLETS
EXTRA HIGH POTENCY— BALANCED B-COMPLEX WITH CHELATED MINERALS

Each Tablet Daily Provides:

Vitamin C (with Rose Hips)	250 mg
Vitamin E (d-Alpha Tocopherol)	150 IU
Vitamin A (Palmitate and Beta-Carotene)	25,000 IU
Vitamin D	1,000 IU
Vitamin B-1 (Thiamine)	75 mg
Vitamin B-2 (Riboflavin)	75 mg
Vitamin B-6 (Pyridoxine)	75 mg
Vitamin B-12	75 mcg
Niacinamide	75 mg
Choline Bitartrate	75 mg
Inositol	75 mg
Para Aminobenzoic Acid	75 mg
Pantothenic Acid	75 mg
Biotin	75 mcg
Folic Acid	400 mcg
Rutin	25 mg
Citrus Bioflavonoid Complex	25 mg
Hesperidin Complex	5 mg
Betaine HCl	25 mg
Glutamic Acid	25 mg
Iodine (Kelp)	150 mcg
Calcium Amino Acid Chelate	50 mg
Potassium Amino Acid Complex	10 mg
Iron Amino Acid Chelate	10 mg
Magnesium Amino Acid Chelate	7.2 mg
Manganese Amino Acid Chelate	6.1 mg
Zinc Amino Acid Chelate	15 mg
Selenium (L-selenomethionine)	10 mcg

SUPPLIED
Bottles of 30, 60, 90 and 180 tablets.

HY–C TABLETS
HIGH POTENCY VITAMIN C SUPPLEMENT

Vitamin C with Rose Hips and Citrus Bioflavonoid Complex. Rutin and Hesperidin Complex.
Each Tablet Contains:

Vitamin C	600 mg
Citrus Bioflavonoid Complex	100 mg
Rutin	50 mg
Hesperidin Complex	25 mg

SUPPLIED
Bottles of 50, 100, 250, 500 and 1000 tablets.

LIVER TABLETS
11 GRAINS

Natural Desiccated and Defatted Argentinian Liver fortified with Vitamin B-12 and Red Bone Marrow. Provides the naturally occurring B-Complex Factors and Amino Acids found in Dried Beef Liver.

SUPPLIED
Bottles of 100, 250, 500 and 1000 tablets.

L–TRYPTOPHAN CAPSULES
(Free-form)
500 mg

SUPPLIED
Bottles of 30, 60 and 90 capsules.

VITAMIN B–1 TABLETS (Thiamine)
25 mg, 50 mg, 100 mg and 500 mg

SUPPLIED
Bottles of 100, 250 and 500 tablets.

VITAMIN B–2 TABLETS (Riboflavin)
10 mg, 25 mg, 50 mg and 100 mg

SUPPLIED
Bottles of 100, 250 and 500 tablets.

VITAMIN B–6 TABLETS (Pyridoxine)
25 mg, 50 mg, 100 mg and 500 mg

SUPPLIED
Bottles of 100, 250 and 500 tablets.

VITAMIN B–12 TABLETS
50 mcg, 100 mcg, 250 mcg, 500 mcg and 1000 mcg

SUPPLIED
Bottles of 100, 250 and 500 tablets.

VITAMIN C TABLETS OR CAPSULES (Ascorbic Acid)
500 mg

SUPPLIED
Bottles of 100, 250 and 500 tablets or capsules.

VITAMIN E CAPSULES (Natural)
100 IU, 200 IU, 400 IU and 1000 IU
D-ALPHA TOCOPHEROL plus MIXED TOCOPHEROLS

SUPPLIED
Bottles of 50, 100, 250, 500 and 1000 capsules.

ZINC "50" TABLETS

Each Tablet Provides:

Zinc Gluconate (Organically Complexed)	409 mg
providing elemental Zinc	50 mg

SUPPLIED
Bottles of 100, 250 and 500 tablets.

E. R. Squibb & Sons, Inc.
GENERAL OFFICES
P.O. BOX 4000
PRINCETON, NJ 08540

For listing of standard and purified insulins, see Squibb-Novo, Inc.

UNILOG®
(Tablet and Capsule Identification Code)
NUMERICAL INDEX

Unilog Number | **Product**

F16 Principen with Probenecid
(Ampicillin-Probenecid Capsules)
113 Velosef '250' Capsules
(Cephradine Capsules USP) 250 mg
114 Velosef '500' Capsules
(Cephradine Capsules USP) 500 mg
160 Ethril '250'
(Erythromycin Stearate Tablets USP) 250 mg
161 Ethril '500'
(Erythromycin Stearate Tablets USP) 500 mg
164 Pentids Tablets
(Penicillin G Potassium Tablets USP) 200,000 u.
165 Pentids '400' Tablets
(Penicillin G Potassium Tablets USP) 400,000 u.
168 Pentids '800' Tablets
(Penicillin G Potassium Tablets USP) 800,000 u.
196 Vitamin C Tablets 250 mg
197 Vitamin C Tablets 500 mg
201 Aspirin Tablets USP, 5 gr. (324 mg)
230 Trimox '250' Capsules
(Amoxicillin Capsules USP) 250 mg
231 Trimox '500' Capsules
(Amoxicillin Capsules USP) 500 mg
338 Capozide (Captopril-Hydrochlorothiazide Tablets) 25 mg–15 mg
349 Capozide (Captopril-Hydrochlorothiazide Tablets) 25 mg–25 mg
355 Valadol Tablets
(Acetaminophen Tablets USP) 325 mg (5 gr.)
384 Capozide (Captopril-Hydrochlorothiazide Tablets) 50 mg–15 mg
390 Capozide (Captopril-Hydrochlorothiazide Tablets) 50 mg–25 mg
429 Florinef Acetate
(Fludrocortisone Acetate Tablets USP) 0.1 mg
450 Capoten (Captopril Tablets) 12.5 mg
452 Capoten (Captopril Tablets) 25 mg
455 Oragrafin Sodium Capsules
(Ipodate Sodium Capsules USP) 500 mg
457 Mycostatin Vaginal Tablets
(Nystatin Vaginal Tablets USP) 100,000 u.
478 Engran-HP Tablets
(Multi-Vitamin and Multi-Mineral Supplement)
482 Capoten (Captopril Tablets) 50 mg
485 Capoten (Captopril Tablets) 100 mg
512 Kenacort
(Triamcinolone Tablets USP) 4 mg
518 Kenacort
(Triamcinolone Tablets USP) 8 mg
535 Theragran Hematinic
(Therapeutic Formula Vitamin Tablets with Hematinics)
537 Niacin Tablets USP, 500 mg
549 Iron and Vitamin C Tablets
573 Ora-Testryl
(Fluoxymesterone Tablets USP) 5 mg
580 Mycostatin Oral Tablets
(Nystatin Tablets USP) 500,000 u.
603 Sumycin '500' Tablets
(Tetracycline Hydrochloride Tablets USP) 500 mg
610 Niacin Tablets USP, 25 mg
611 Niacin Tablets USP, 50 mg
612 Niacin Tablets USP, 100 mg
623 Noctec Capsules
(Chloral Hydrate Capsules USP) 250 mg ($3\frac{3}{4}$ grains)
626 Noctec Capsules
(Chloral Hydrate Capsules USP) 500 mg ($7\frac{1}{2}$ grains)
637 Nydrazid Tablets
(Isoniazid Tablets USP) 100 mg
648 Veetids '500' Tablets
(Penicillin V Potassium Tablets USP) 500 mg (800,000 u.)
655 Sumycin '250' Capsules
(Tetracycline Hydrochloride Capsules USP) 250 mg
663 Sumycin '250' Tablets
(Tetracycline Hydrochloride Tablets USP) 250 mg
684 Veetids '250' Tablets
(Penicillin V Potassium Tablets USP) 250 mg (400,000 u.)
690 Teslac Tablets
(Testolactone Tablets USP) 50 mg
763 Sumycin '500' Capsules
(Tetracycline Hydrochloride Capsules USP) 500 mg
779 Mysteclin-F Capsules
(Tetracycline - Amphotericin B Capsules) 250 mg c̄ 50 mg
830 Hydrea Capsules
(Hydroxyurea Capsules USP) 500 mg
872 Comoxol Tablets
(Sulfamethoxazole and Trimethoprim Tablets USP)
400 mg—80 mg
873 Comoxol Tablets
(Sulfamethoxazole and Trimethoprim Tablets USP)
800 mg—160 mg
876 Trigesic Tablets
(Analgesic Compound)
883 Vivox Capsules
(Doxycycline Hyclate Capsules USP) 50 mg
884 Vivox Capsules
(Doxycycline Hyclate Capsules USP) 100 mg
887 Terfonyl Tablets
(Trisulfapyrimidines Tablets USP) 500 mg
897 Vivox Tablets
(Doxycycline Hyclate Tablets USP) 100 mg
915 Vitamin B_1 Tablets 50 mg
916 Vitamin B_1 Tablets USP 100 mg
971 Principen '250' Capsules
(Ampicillin Capsules USP) 250 mg
974 Principen '500' Capsules
(Ampicillin Capsules USP) 500 mg

CAPOTEN® TABLETS ℞
[kap'o-ten"]
Captopril Tablets

DESCRIPTION

CAPOTEN (captopril) is the first of a new class of antihypertensive agents, a specific competitive inhibitor of angiotensin I-converting enzyme (ACE), the enzyme responsible for the conversion of angiotensin I to angiotensin II. Captopril is also effective in the management of heart failure.

CAPOTEN (captopril) is designated chemically as 1-[(2S)-3-mercapto-2-methylpropionyl]-L-proline (MW 217.29).

Captopril is a white to off-white crystalline powder that may have a slight sulfurous odor; it is soluble in water (approx. 160 mg/mL), methanol, and ethanol and sparingly soluble in chloroform and ethyl acetate.

CAPOTEN (captopril) is available in potencies of 12.5 mg, 25 mg, 50 mg, and 100 mg as scored tablets for oral administration. Inactive ingredients: cellulose, corn starch, lactose, and stearic acid.

CLINICAL PHARMACOLOGY

Mechanism of Action—The mechanism of action of CAPOTEN (captopril) has not yet been fully elucidated. Its beneficial effects in hypertension and heart failure appear to result primarily from suppression of the renin-angiotensin-aldosterone system. However, there is no consistent correlation between renin levels and response to the drug. Renin, an enzyme synthesized by the kidneys, is released into the circulation where it acts on a plasma globulin substrate to produce angiotensin I, a relatively inactive decapeptide. Angiotensin I is then converted by angiotensin converting enzyme (ACE) to angiotensin II, a potent endogenous vasoconstrictor substance. Angiotensin II also stimulates aldosterone secretion from the adrenal cortex, thereby contributing to sodium and fluid retention.

CAPOTEN (captopril) prevents the conversion of angiotensin I to angiotensin II by inhibition of ACE, a peptidyldipeptide carboxy hydrolase. This inhibition has been demonstrated in both healthy human subjects and in animals by showing that the elevation of blood pressure caused by exogenously administered angiotensin I was attenuated or abolished by captopril. In animal studies, captopril did not alter the pressor responses to a number of other agents, including angiotensin II and norepinephrine, indicating specificity of action.

ACE is identical to "bradykininase," and CAPOTEN (captopril) may also interfere with the degradation of the vasodepressor peptide, bradykinin. Increased concentrations of bradykinin or prostaglandin E_2 may also have a role in the therapeutic effect of CAPOTEN.

Inhibition of ACE results in decreased plasma angiotensin II and increased plasma renin activity (PRA), the latter resulting from loss of negative feedback on renin release caused by reduction in angiotensin II. The reduction of angiotensin II leads to decreased aldosterone secretion, and, as a result, small increases in serum potassium may occur along with sodium and fluid loss.

The antihypertensive effects persist for a longer period of time than does demonstrable inhibition of circulating ACE. It is not known whether the ACE present in vascular endothelium is inhibited longer than the ACE in circulating blood.

Pharmacokinetics—After oral administration of therapeutic doses of CAPOTEN (captopril), rapid absorption occurs with peak blood levels at about one hour. The presence of food in the gastrointestinal tract reduces absorption by about 30 to 40 percent; captopril therefore should be given one hour before meals. Based on carbon-14 labeling, average minimal absorption is approximately 75 percent. In a 24-hour period, over 95 percent of the absorbed dose is eliminated in the urine; 40 to 50 percent is unchanged drug; most of the remainder is the disulfide dimer of captopril and captopril-cysteine disulfide.

Approximately 25 to 30 percent of the circulating drug is bound to plasma proteins. The apparent elimination half-life for total radioactivity in blood is probably less than 3 hours. An accurate determination of half-life of unchanged captopril is not, at present, possible, but it is probably less than 2 hours. In patients with renal impairment, however, retention of captopril occurs (see DOSAGE AND ADMINISTRATION).

Pharmacodynamics—Administration of CAPOTEN (captopril) results in a reduction of peripheral arterial resistance in hypertensive patients with either no change, or an increase, in cardiac output. There is an increase in renal blood flow following administration of CAPOTEN (captopril) and glomerular filtration rate is usually unchanged.

Reductions of blood pressure are usually maximal 60 to 90 minutes after oral administration of an individual dose of CAPOTEN (captopril). The duration of effect is dose related. The reduction in blood pressure may be progressive, so to achieve maximal therapeutic effects, several weeks of therapy may be required. The blood pressure lowering effects of captopril and thiazide-type diuretics are additive. In contrast, captopril and beta-blockers have a less than additive effect.

Blood pressure is lowered to about the same extent in both standing and supine positions. Orthostatic effects and tachycardia are infrequent but may occur in volume-depleted patients. Abrupt withdrawal of CAPOTEN has not been associated with a rapid increase in blood pressure.

In patients with heart failure, significantly decreased peripheral (systemic vascular) resistance and blood pressure (afterload), reduced pulmonary capillary wedge pressure (preload) and pulmonary vascular resistance, increased cardiac output, and increased exercise tolerance time (ETT) have been demonstrated. These hemodynamic and clinical effects occur after the first dose and appear to persist for the duration of therapy. Placebo controlled studies of 12 weeks duration show no tolerance to beneficial effects on ETT; open studies, with exposure up to 18 months in some cases, also indicate that ETT benefit is maintained. Clinical improvement has been observed in some patients where acute hemodynamic effects were minimal.

Studies in rats and cats indicate that CAPOTEN (captopril) does not cross the blood-brain barrier to any significant extent.

INDICATIONS AND USAGE

Hypertension: CAPOTEN (captopril) is indicated for the treatment of hypertension.

In using CAPOTEN, consideration should be given to the risk of neutropenia/agranulocytosis (see WARNINGS).

CAPOTEN may be used as initial therapy for patients with normal renal function, in whom the risk is relatively low. In patients with impaired renal function, particularly those with collagen vascular disease, captopril should be reserved for hypertensives who have either developed unacceptable side effects on other drugs, or have failed to respond satisfactorily to drug combinations.

CAPOTEN is effective alone and in combination with other antihypertensive agents, especially thiazide-type diuretics. The blood pressure lowering effects of captopril and thiazides are approximately additive.

Heart Failure: CAPOTEN (captopril) is indicated in patients with heart failure who have not responded adequately to or cannot be controlled by conventional diuretic and digitalis therapy. CAPOTEN is to be used with diuretics and digitalis.

WARNINGS

Neutropenia/Agranulocytosis—Neutropenia ($<1000/mm^3$) with myeloid hypoplasia has resulted from use of captopril. About half of the neutropenic patients developed systemic or oral cavity infections or other features of the syndrome of agranulocytosis.

The risk of neutropenia is dependent on the clinical status of the patient:

In clinical trials in patients with hypertension who have normal renal function (serum creatinine less than 1.6

mg/dL and no collagen vascular disease), neutropenia has been seen in one patient out of over 8,600 exposed.

In patients with some degree of renal failure (serum creatinine at least 1.6 mg/dL) but no collagen vascular disease, the risk of neutropenia in clinical trials was about 1 per 500, a frequency over 15 times that for uncomplicated hypertension. Daily doses of captopril were relatively high in these patients, particularly in view of their diminished renal function. In foreign marketing experience in patients with renal failure, use of allopurinol concomitantly with captopril has been associated with neutropenia but this association has not appeared in U.S. reports.

In patients with collagen vascular diseases (e.g., systemic lupus erythematosus, scleroderma) and impaired renal function, neutropenia occurred in 3.7 percent of patients in clinical trials.

While none of the over 750 patients in formal clinical trials of heart failure developed neutropenia, it has occurred during the subsequent clinical experience. About half of the reported cases had serum creatinine > 1.6 mg/dL and more than 75 percent were in patients also receiving procainamide. In heart failure, it appears that the same risk factors for neutropenia are present.

The neutropenia has usually been detected within three months after captopril was started. Bone marrow examinations in patients with neutropenia consistently showed myeloid hypoplasia, frequently accompanied by erythroid hypoplasia and decreased numbers of megakaryocytes (e.g., hypoplastic bone marrow and pancytopenia); anemia and thrombocytopenia were sometimes seen.

In general, neutrophils returned to normal in about two weeks after captopril was discontinued, and serious infections were limited to clinically complex patients. About 13 percent of the cases of neutropenia have ended fatally, but almost all fatalities were in patients with serious illness, having collagen vascular disease, renal failure, heart failure or immunosuppressant therapy, or a combination of these complicating factors.

Evaluation of the hypertensive or heart failure patient should always include assessment of renal function.

If captopril is used in patients with impaired renal function, white blood cell and differential counts should be evaluated prior to starting treatment and at approximately two-week intervals for about three months, then periodically.

In patients with collagen vascular disease or who are exposed to other drugs known to affect the white cells or immune response, particularly when there is impaired renal function, captopril should be used only after an assessment of benefit and risk, and then with caution.

All patients treated with captopril should be told to report any signs of infection (e.g., sore throat, fever). If infection is suspected, white cell counts should be performed without delay.

Since discontinuation of captopril and other drugs has generally led to prompt return of the white count to normal, upon confirmation of neutropenia (neutrophil count < $1000/mm^3$) the physician should withdraw captopril and closely follow the patient's course.

Proteinuria—Total urinary proteins greater than 1 g per day were seen in about 0.7 percent of patients receiving captopril. About 90 percent of affected patients had evidence of prior renal disease or received relatively high doses of captopril (in excess of 150 mg/day), or both. The nephrotic syndrome occurred in about one-fifth of proteinuric patients. In most cases, proteinuria subsided or cleared within six months whether or not captopril was continued. Parameters of renal function, such as BUN and creatinine, were seldom altered in the patients with proteinuria.

Since most cases of proteinuria occurred by the eighth month of therapy with captopril, patients with prior renal disease or those receiving captopril at doses greater than 150 mg per day, should have urinary protein estimations (dip-stick on first morning urine) prior to treatment, and periodically thereafter.

Hypotension—Excessive hypotension was rarely seen in hypertensive patients but is a possible consequence of captopril use in severely salt/volume depleted persons such as those treated vigorously with diuretics, for example, patients with severe congestive heart failure (see PRECAUTIONS [Drug Interactions]).

In heart failure, where the blood pressure was either normal or low, transient decreases in mean blood pressure greater than 20 percent were recorded in about half of the patients. This transient hypotension may occur after any of the first several doses and is usually well tolerated, producing either no symptoms or brief mild lightheadedness, although in rare instances it has been associated with arrhythmia or conduction defects. Hypotension was the reason for discontinuation of drug in 3.6 percent of patients with heart failure.

BECAUSE OF THE POTENTIAL FALL IN BLOOD PRESSURE IN THESE PATIENTS, THERAPY SHOULD BE STARTED UNDER VERY CLOSE MEDICAL SUPERVISION. A starting dose of 6.25 or 12.5 mg tid may minimize the hypotensive effect. Patients should be followed closely for the first two weeks of treatment and whenever the dose of captopril and/or diuretic is increased.

Hypotension is not *per se* a reason to discontinue captopril. Some decrease of systemic blood pressure is a common and desirable observation upon initiation of CAPOTEN (captopril) treatment in heart failure. The magnitude of the decrease is greatest early in the course of treatment; this effect stabilizes within a week or two, and generally returns to pretreatment levels, without a decrease in therapeutic efficacy, within two months.

PRECAUTIONS

General—*Impaired Renal Function*—Hypertension—Some patients with renal disease, particularly those with severe renal artery stenosis, have developed increases in BUN and serum creatinine after reduction of blood pressure with captopril. Captopril dosage reduction and/or discontinuation of diuretic may be required. For some of these patients, it may not be possible to normalize blood pressure and maintain adequate renal perfusion.

Heart Failure—About 20 percent of patients develop stable elevations of BUN and serum creatinine greater than 20 percent above normal or baseline upon long-term treatment with captopril. Less than 5 percent of patients, generally those with severe preexisting renal disease, required discontinuaton of treatment due to progressively increasing creatinine; subsequent improvement probably depends upon the severity of the underlying renal disease.

See CLINICAL PHARMACOLOGY, DOSAGE AND ADMINISTRATION, ADVERSE REACTIONS [Altered Laboratory Findings].

Valvular Stenosis: There is concern, on theoretical grounds, that patients with aortic stenosis might be at particular risk of decreased coronary perfusion when treated with vasodilators because they do not develop as much after-load reduction as others.

Surgery/Anesthesia: In patients undergoing major surgery or during anesthesia with agents that produce hypotension, captopril will block angiotensin II formation secondary to compensatory renin release. If hypotension occurs and is considered to be due to this mechanism, it can be corrected by volume expansion.

Information for Patients—Patients should be told to report promptly any indication of infection (e.g., sore throat, fever), which may be a sign of neutropenia, or of progressive edema which might be related to proteinuria and nephrotic syndrome.

All patients should be cautioned that excessive perspiration and dehydration may lead to an excessive fall in blood pressure because of reduction in fluid volume. Other causes of volume depletion such as vomiting or diarrhea may also lead to a fall in blood pressure; patients should be advised to consult with the physician.

Patients should be warned against interruption or discontinuation of medication unless instructed by the physician.

Heart failure patients on captopril therapy should be cautioned against rapid increases in physical activity.

Patients should be informed that CAPOTEN (captopril) should be taken one hour before meals (see DOSAGE AND ADMINISTRATION).

Drug Interactions—*Hypotension—Patients on Diuretic Therapy:* Patients on diuretics and especially those in whom diuretic therapy was recently instituted, as well as those on severe dietary salt restriction or dialysis, may occasionally experience a precipitous reduction of blood pressure usually within the first hour after receiving the initial dose of captopril.

The possibility of hypotensive effects with captopril can be minimized by either discontinuing the diuretic or increasing the salt intake approximately one week prior to initiation of treatment with CAPOTEN (captopril) or initiating therapy with small doses (6.25 or 12.5 mg). Alternatively, provide medical supervision for at least one hour after the initial dose. If hypotension occurs, the patient should be placed in a supine position and, if necessary, receive an intravenous infusion of normal saline. This transient hypotensive response is not a contraindication to further doses which can be given without difficulty once the blood pressure has increased after volume expansion.

Agents Having Vasodilator Activity: Data on the effect of concomitant use of other vasodilators in patients receiving CAPOTEN (captopril) for heart failure are not available; therefore, nitroglycerin or other nitrates (as used for management of angina) or other drugs having vasodilator activity should, if possible, be discontinued before starting CAPOTEN. If resumed during CAPOTEN therapy, such agents should be administered cautiously, and perhaps at lower dosage.

Agents Causing Renin Release: Captopril's effect will be augmented by antihypertensive agents that cause renin release. For example, diuretics (e.g., thiazides) may activate the renin-angiotensin-aldosterone system.

Agents Affecting Sympathetic Activity: The sympathetic nervous system may be especially important in supporting blood pressure in patients receiving captopril alone or with diuretics. Therefore, agents affecting sympathetic activity (e.g., ganglionic blocking agents or adrenergic neuron blocking agents) should be used with caution. Beta-adrenergic blocking drugs add some further antihypertensive effect to captopril, but the overall response is less than additive.

Agents Increasing Serum Potassium: Since captopril decreases aldosterone production, elevation of serum potassium may occur. Potassium-sparing diuretics such as spironolactone, triamterene, or amiloride, or potassium supplements should be given only for documented hypokalemia, and then with caution, since they may lead to a significant increase of serum potassium. Salt substitutes containing potassium should also be used with caution.

Inhibitors Of Endogenous Prostaglandin Synthesis: It has been reported that indomethacin may reduce the antihypertensive effect of captopril, especially in cases of low renin hypertension. Other nonsteroidal anti-inflammatory agents (e.g., aspirin) may also have this effect.

Drug/Laboratory Test Interaction—Captopril may cause a false-positive urine test for acetone.

Carcinogenesis, Mutagenesis and Impairment of Fertility—Two-year studies with doses of 50 to 1350 mg/kg/day in mice and rats failed to show any evidence of carcinogenic potential.

Studies in rats have revealed no impairment of fertility.

Animal Toxicology—Chronic oral toxicity studies were conducted in rats (2 years), dogs (47 weeks; 1 year), mice (2 years), and monkeys (1 year). Significant drug related toxicity included effects on hematopoiesis, renal toxicity, erosion/ulceration of the stomach, and variation of retinal blood vessels.

Reductions in hemoglobin and/or hematocrit values were seen in mice, rats, and monkeys at doses 50 to 150 times the maximum recommended human dose (MRHD). Anemia, leukopenia, thrombocytopenia, and bone marrow suppression occurred in dogs at doses 8 to 30 times MRHD. The reductions in hemoglobin and hematocrit values in rats and mice were only significant at 1 year and returned to normal with continued dosing by the end of the study. Marked anemia was seen at all dose levels (8 to 30 times MRHD) in dogs, whereas moderate to marked leukopenia was noted only at 15 and 30 times MRHD and thrombocytopenia at 30 times MRHD. The anemia could be reversed upon discontinuation of dosing. Bone marrow suppression occurred to a varying degree, being associated only with dogs that died or were sacrificed in a moribund condition in the 1 year study. However, in the 47-week study at a dose 30 times MRHD, bone marrow suppression was found to be reversible upon continued drug administration.

Captopril caused hyperplasia of the juxtaglomerular apparatus of the kidneys at doses 7 to 200 times the MRHD in rats and mice, at 20 to 60 times MRHD in monkeys, and at 30 times the MRHD in dogs.

Gastric erosions/ulcerations were increased in incidence at 20 and 200 times MRHD in male rats and at 30 to 65 times MRHD in dogs and monkeys, respectively. Rabbits developed gastric and intestinal ulcers when given oral doses approximately 30 times MRHD for only 5 to 7 days.

In the two-year rat study, irreversible and progressive variations in the caliber of retinal vessels (focal sacculations and constrictions) occurred at all dose levels (7 to 200 times MRHD) in a dose-related fashion. The effect was first observed in the 88th week of dosing, with a progressively increased incidence thereafter, even after cessation of dosing.

Pregnancy: Category C—Captopril was embryocidal in rabbits when given in doses about 2 to 70 times (on a mg/kg basis) the maximum recommended human dose, and low incidences of craniofacial malformations were seen. These effects in rabbits were most probably due to the particularly marked decrease in blood pressure caused by the drug in this species.

Captopril given to pregnant rats at 400 times the recommended human dose continuously during gestation and lactation caused a reduction in neonatal survival.

No teratogenic effects (malformations) have been observed after large doses of captopril in hamsters and rats.

Captopril crosses the human placenta.

There are no adequate and well-controlled studies in pregnant women. Captopril should be used during pregnancy, or for patients likely to become pregnant, only if the potential benefit justifies a potential risk to the fetus.

Nursing Mothers—Concentrations of captopril in human milk are approximately one percent of those in maternal blood. The effect of low levels of captopril on the nursing infant has not been determined. Caution should be exercised when captopril is administered to a nursing woman, and, in general, nursing should be interrupted.

Pediatric Use—Safety and effectiveness in children have not been established although there is limited experience with the use of captopril in children from 2 months to 15 years of age with secondary hypertension and varying degrees of renal insufficiency. Dosage, on a weight basis, was comparable to that used in adults. CAPOTEN (captopril) should be used in children only if other measures for controlling blood pressure have not been effective.

Continued on next page

Squibb—Cont.

ADVERSE REACTIONS

Reported incidences are based on clinical trials involving approximately 7000 patients.

Renal—About one of 100 patients developed proteinuria (see WARNINGS).

Each of the following has been reported in approximately 1 to 2 of 1000 patients and are of uncertain relationship to drug use: renal insufficiency, renal failure, polyuria, oliguria, and urinary frequency.

Hematologic—Neutropenia/agranulocytosis has occurred (see WARNINGS). Cases of anemia, thrombocytopenia, and pancytopenia have been reported.

Dermatologic—Rash, often with pruritus, and sometimes with fever, arthralgia, and eosinophilia, occurred in about 4 to 7 (depending on renal status and dose) of 100 patients, usually during the first four weeks of therapy. It is usually maculopapular, and rarely urticarial. The rash is usually mild and disappears within a few days of dosage reduction, short-term treatment with an antihistaminic agent, and/or discontinuing therapy; remission may occur even if captopril is continued. Pruritus, without rash, occurs in about 2 of 100 patients. Between 7 and 10 percent of patients with skin rash have shown an eosinophilia and/or positive ANA titers. A reversible associated pemphigoid-like lesion, and photosensitivity, have also been reported.

Angioedema of the face, mucous membranes of the mouth, or of the extremities has been observed in approximately 1 of 1000 patients and is reversible on discontinuance of captopril therapy. One case of laryngeal edema has been reported.

Flushing or pallor has been reported in 2 to 5 of 1000 patients.

Cardiovascular—Hypotension may occur; see WARNINGS and PRECAUTIONS [Drug Interactions] for discussion of hypotension on initiation of captopril therapy.

Tachycardia, chest pain, and palpitations have each been observed in approximately 1 of 100 patients.

Angina pectoris, myocardial infarction, Raynaud's syndrome, and congestive heart failure have each occurred in 2 to 3 of 1000 patients.

Dysgeusia—Approximately 2 to 4 (depending on renal status and dose) of 100 patients developed a diminution or loss of taste perception. Taste impairment is reversible and usually self-limited (2 to 3 months) even with continued drug administration. Weight loss may be associated with the loss of taste.

The following have been reported in about 0.5 to 2 percent of patients but did not appear at increased frequency compared to placebo or other treatments used in controlled trials; gastric irritation, abdominal pain, nausea, vomiting, diarrhea, anorexia, constipation, aphthous ulcers, peptic ulcer, dizziness, headache, malaise, fatigue, insomnia, dry mouth, dyspnea, cough, alopecia, paresthesias.

Altered Laboratory Findings—Elevations of liver enzymes have been noted in a few patients but no causal relationship to captopril use has been established. Rare cases of cholestatic jaundice, and of hepatocellular injury with or without secondary cholestasis, have been reported in association with captopril administration.

A transient elevation of BUN and serum creatinine may occur, especially in patients who are volume-depleted or who have renovascular hypertension. In instances of rapid reduction of longstanding or severely elevated blood pressure, the glomerular filtration rate may decrease transiently, also resulting in transient rises in serum creatinine and BUN.

Small increases in the serum potassium concentration frequently occur, especially in patients with renal impairment (see PRECAUTIONS).

OVERDOSAGE

Correction of hypotension would be of primary concern. Volume expansion with an intravenous infusion of normal saline is the treatment of choice for restoration of blood pressure.

Captopril may be removed from the general circulation by hemodialysis.

DOSAGE AND ADMINISTRATION

CAPOTEN (captopril) should be taken one hour before meals. Dosage must be individualized.

Hypertension—Initiation of therapy requires consideration of recent antihypertensive drug treatment, the extent of blood pressure elevation, salt restriction, and other clinical circumstances. If possible, discontinue the patient's previous antihypertensive drug regimen for one week before starting CAPOTEN.

The initial dose of CAPOTEN (captopril) is 25 mg bid or tid. If satisfactory reduction of blood pressure has not been achieved after one or two weeks, the dose may be increased to 50 mg bid or tid. Concomitant sodium restriction may be beneficial when CAPOTEN is used alone.

The dose of CAPOTEN in hypertension usually does not exceed 50 mg tid. Therefore, if the blood pressure has not been satisfactorily controlled after one to two weeks at this dose (and the patient is not already receiving a diuretic), a modest dose of a thiazide-type diuretic (e.g., hydrochlorothiazide, 25 mg daily) should be added. The diuretic dose may be increased at one- to two-week intervals until its highest usual antihypertensive dose is reached.

If CAPOTEN (captopril) is being started in a patient already receiving a diuretic, CAPOTEN therapy should be initiated under close medical supervision (see WARNINGS and PRECAUTIONS [Drug Interactions] regarding hypotension), with dosage and titration of CAPOTEN as noted above.

If further blood pressure reduction is required, the dose of CAPOTEN may be increased to 100 mg bid or tid and then, if necessary, to 150 mg bid or tid (while continuing the diuretic). The usual dose range is 25 to 150 mg bid or tid. A maximum daily dose of 450 mg CAPOTEN should not be exceeded.

For patients with severe hypertension (e.g., accelerated or malignant hypertension), when temporary discontinuation of current antihypertensive therapy is not practical or desirable, or when prompt titration to more normotensive blood pressure levels is indicated, diuretic should be continued but other current antihypertensive medication stopped and CAPOTEN dosage promptly initiated at 25 mg bid or tid, under close medical supervision.

When necessitated by the patient's clinical condition, the daily dose of CAPOTEN may be increased every 24 hours or less under continuous medical supervision until a satisfactory blood pressure response is obtained or the maximum dose of CAPOTEN (captopril) is reached. In this regimen, addition of a more potent diuretic, e.g., furosemide, may also be indicated.

Beta-blockers may also be used in conjunction with CAPOTEN therapy (see PRECAUTIONS [Drug Interactions]), but the effects of the two drugs are less than additive.

Heart Failure—Initiation of therapy requires consideration of recent diuretic therapy and the possibility of severe salt/volume depletion. In patients with either normal or low blood pressure, who have been vigorously treated with diuretics and who may be hyponatremic and/or hypovolemic, a starting dose of 6.25 or 12.5 mg tid may minimize the magnitude or duration of the hypotensive effect (see WARNINGS, [Hypotension]); for these patients, titration to the usual daily dosage can then occur within the next several days.

For most patients the usual initial daily dosage is 25 mg tid. After a dose of 50 mg tid is reached, further increases in dosage should be delayed, where possible, for at least two weeks to determine if a satisfactory response occurs. Most patients studied have had a satisfactory clinical improvement at 50 or 100 mg tid. A maximum daily dose of 450 mg of CAPOTEN (captopril) should not be exceeded.

CAPOTEN is to be used in conjunction with a diuretic and digitalis. CAPOTEN therapy must be initiated under very close medical supervision.

Dosage Adjustment in Renal Impairment—Because CAPOTEN (captopril) is excreted primarily by the kidneys, excretion rates are reduced in patients with impaired renal function. These patients will take longer to reach steady-state captopril levels and will reach higher steady-state levels for a given daily dose than patients with normal renal function. Therefore, these patients may respond to smaller or less frequent doses.

Accordingly, for patients with significant renal impairment, initial daily dosage of CAPOTEN (captopril) should be reduced, and smaller increments utilized for titration, which should be quite slow (one- to two-week intervals). After the desired therapeutic effect has been achieved, the dose should be slowly back-titrated to determine the minimal effective dose. When concomitant diuretic therapy is required, a loop diuretic (e.g., furosemide), rather than a thiazide diuretic, is preferred in patients with severe renal impairment.

HOW SUPPLIED

12.5 mg tablets in bottles of 100, **25 mg tablets** in bottles of 100 and 1000, **50 mg tablets** in bottles of 100, and **100 mg tablets** in bottles of 100. Bottles contain a desiccant-charcoal canister.

Unimatic® unit-dose packs containing 100 tablets are also available for each potency: **12.5 mg, 25 mg, 50 mg,** and **100 mg.**

The **12.5 mg tablet** is a flat oval with a partial bisect bar; the **25 mg tablet** is a biconvex rounded square with a quadrisect bar; the **50 and 100 mg tablets** are biconvex ovals with a bisect bar.

All captopril tablets are white and may exhibit a slight sulfurous odor. Tablet identification numbers: 12.5 mg, **450;** 25 mg, **452;** 50 mg, **482;** and 100 mg, **485.**

Storage—Do not store above 86°F. Keep bottles tightly closed (protect from moisture).

(J3-658D)

Shown in Product Identification Section, page 431

CAPOZIDE® 25/15 ℞
CAPOZIDE® 25/25 ℞
CAPOZIDE® 50/15 ℞
CAPOZIDE® 50/25 ℞

[*kap'o-zīd"*]

Captopril-Hydrochlorothiazide Tablets

DESCRIPTION

CAPOZIDE (Captopril-Hydrochlorothiazide Tablets) for oral administration combines two antihypertensive agents: CAPOTEN® (captopril) and hydrochlorothiazide. Captopril, the first of a new class of antihypertensive agents, is a specific competitive inhibitor of angiotensin I-converting enzyme (ACE), the enzyme responsible for the conversion of angiotensin I to angiotensin II. Hydrochlorothiazide is a benzothiadiazide (thiazide) diuretic-antihypertensive. CAPOZIDE tablets are available in four combinations of captopril with hydrochlorothiazide: 25 mg with 15 mg, 25 mg with 25 mg, 50 mg with 15 mg, and 50 mg with 25 mg. Inactive ingredients: cellulose, colorant (FD&C Yellow No. 6), lactose, magnesium stearate, pregelatinized starch, and stearic acid.

Captopril is designated chemically as 1-[(2S)-3-mercapto-2-methylpropionyl]-L-proline; hydrochlorothiazide is 6-Chloro-3, 4-dihydro-2*H*-1, 2, 4-benzothiadiazine-7- sulfonamide 1,1-dioxide.

Captopril is a white to off-white crystalline powder that may have a slight sulfurous odor; it is soluble in water (approx. 160 mg/mL), methanol, and ethanol and sparingly soluble in chloroform and ethyl acetate.

Hydrochlorothiazide is a white crystalline powder slightly soluble in water but freely soluble in sodium hydroxide solution.

CLINICAL PHARMACOLOGY

Captopril—Mechanism of Action—The mechanism of action of captopril has not yet been fully elucidated. Its beneficial effects in hypertension and heart failure appear to result primarily from suppression of the renin-angiotensin-aldosterone system. However, there is no consistent correlation between renin levels and response to the drug. Renin, an enzyme synthesized by the kidneys, is released into the circulation where it acts on a plasma globulin substrate to produce angiotensin I, a relatively inactive decapeptide. Angiotensin I is then converted by angiotensin converting enzyme (ACE) to angiotensin II, a potent endogenous vasoconstrictor substance. Angiotensin II also stimulates aldosterone secretion from the adrenal cortex, thereby contributing to sodium and fluid retention.

Captopril prevents the conversion of angiotensin I to angiotensin II by inhibition of ACE, a peptidyldipeptide carboxy hydrolase. This inhibition has been demonstrated in both healthy human subjects and in animals by showing that the elevation of blood pressure caused by exogenously administered angiotensin I was attenuated or abolished by captopril. In animal studies, captopril did not alter the pressor responses to a number of other agents, including angiotensin II and norepinephrine, indicating specificity of action.

ACE is identical to "bradykininase" and captopril may also interfere with the degradation of the vasodepressor peptide, bradykinin. Increased concentrations of bradykinin or prostaglandin E_2 may also have a role in the therapeutic effect of captopril.

Inhibition of ACE results in decreased plasma angiotensin II and increased plasma renin activity (PRA), the latter resulting from loss of negative feedback on renin release caused by reduction in angiotensin II. The reduction of angiotensin II leads to decreased aldosterone secretion, and, as a result, small increases in serum potassium may occur along with sodium and fluid loss.

The antihypertensive effects persist for a longer period of time than does demonstrable inhibition of circulating ACE. It is not known whether the ACE present in vascular endothelium is inhibited longer than the ACE in circulating blood.

Pharmacokinetics—After oral administration of therapeutic doses of captopril, rapid absorption occurs with peak blood levels at about one hour. The presence of food in the gastrointestinal tract reduces absorption by about 30 to 40 percent; captopril therefore should be given one hour before meals. Based on carbon-14 labeling, average minimal absorption is approximately 75 percent. In a 24-hour period, over 95 percent of the absorbed dose is eliminated in the urine; 40 to 50 percent is unchanged drug; most of the remainder is the disulfide dimer of captopril and captopril-cysteine disulfide.

Approximately 25 to 30 percent of the circulating drug is bound to plasma proteins. The apparent elimination half-life for total radioactivity in blood is probably less than three hours. An accurate determination of half-life of unchanged captopril is not, at present, possible, but it is probably less than two hours. In patients with renal impairment, however, retention of captopril occurs (see DOSAGE AND ADMINISTRATION).

Pharmacodynamics—Administration of captopril results in a reduction of peripheral arterial resistance in hypertensive patients with either no change, or an increase, in cardiac output. There is an increase in renal blood flow following administration of captopril and glomerular filtration rate is usually unchanged. In patients with heart failure, significantly decreased peripheral (systemic vascular) resistance and blood pressure (afterload), reduced pulmonary capillary wedge pressure (preload) and pulmonary vascular resistance, increased cardiac output, and increased exercise tolerance time (ETT) have been demonstrated.

Reductions of blood pressure are usually maximal 60 to 90 minutes after oral administration of an individual dose of captopril. The duration of effect is dose related. The reduction in blood pressure may be progressive, so to achieve maximal therapeutic effects, several weeks of therapy may be required. The blood pressure lowering effects of captopril and thiazide-type diuretics are additive. In contrast, captopril and beta-blockers have a less than additive effect.

Blood pressure is lowered to about the same extent in both standing and supine positions. Orthostatic effects and tachycardia are infrequent but may occur in volume-depleted patients. Abrupt withdrawal of captopril has not been associated with a rapid increase in blood pressure.

Studies in rats and cats indicate that captopril does not cross the blood-brain barrier to any significant extent.

Hydrochlorothiazide—Thiazides affect the renal tubular mechanism of electrolyte reabsorption. At maximal therapeutic dosage all thiazides are approximately equal in their diuretic potency.

Thiazides increase excretion of sodium and chloride in approximately equivalent amounts. Natriuresis causes a secondary loss of potassium and bicarbonate.

The mechanism of the antihypertensive effect of thiazides is unknown. Thiazides do not affect normal blood pressure.

The mean plasma half-life of hydrochlorothiazide in fasted individuals has been reported to be approximately 2.5 hours. Onset of diuresis occurs in two hours and the peak effect at about four hours. Its action persists for approximately six to twelve hours. Hydrochlorothiazide is eliminated rapidly by the kidney.

INDICATIONS AND USAGE

CAPOZIDE (Captopril-Hydrochlorothiazide Tablets) is indicated for the treatment of hypertension. The blood pressure lowering effects of captopril and thiazides are approximately additive.

This fixed combination drug is not indicated for initial therapy of hypertension. If the fixed combination represents the dose titrated to the individual patient's needs, it may be more convenient than the separate components.

In using CAPOZIDE, consideration should be given to the risk of neutropenia/agranulocytosis (see WARNINGS).

CAPOZIDE may be used for patients with normal renal function, in whom the risk is relatively low. In patients with impaired renal function, particularly those with collagen vascular disease, CAPOZIDE should be reserved for hypertensives who have either developed unacceptable side effects on other drugs, or have failed to respond satisfactorily to other drug combinations.

CONTRAINDICATIONS

Hydrochlorothiazide—Hydrochlorothiazide is contraindicated in anuria. It is also contraindicated in patients who have previously demonstrated hypersensitivity to hydrochlorothiazide or other sulfonamide-derived drugs.

WARNINGS

Captopril—Neutropenia/Agranulocytosis—Neutropenia ($<1000/mm^3$) with myeloid hypoplasia has resulted from use of captopril. About half of the neutropenic patients developed systemic or oral cavity infections or other features of the syndrome of agranulocytosis.

The risk of neutropenia is dependent on the clinical status of the patient:

In clinical trials in patients with hypertension who have normal renal functions (serum creatinine less than 1.6 mg/dL and no collagen vascular disease), neutropenia has been seen in one patient out of over 8,600 exposed.

In patients with some degree of renal failure (serum creatinine at least 1.6 mg/dL) but no collagen vascular disease, the risk of neutropenia in clinical trials was about 1 per 500, a frequency over 15 times that for uncomplicated hypertension. Daily doses of captopril were relatively high in these patients, particularly in view of their diminished renal function. In foreign marketing experience in patients with renal failure, use of allopurinol concomitantly with captopril has been associated with neutropenia but this association has not appeared in U.S. reports.

In patients with collagen vascular diseases (e.g., systemic lupus erythematosus, scleroderma) and impaired renal function, neutropenia occurred in 3.7 percent of patients in clinical trials.

While none of the over 750 patients in formal clinical trials of heart failure developed neutropenia, it has occurred during the subsequent clinical experience. About half of the reported cases had serum creatinine ≥ 1.6 mg/dL and more than 75 percent were in patients also receiving procainamide. In heart failure, it appears that the same risk factors for neutropenia are present.

The neutropenia has usually been detected within three months after captopril was started. Bone marrow examinations in patients with neutropenia consistently showed myeloid hypoplasia, frequently accompanied by erythroid hypoplasia and decreased numbers of megakaryocytes (e.g., hypoplastic bone marrow and pancytopenia); anemia and thrombocytopenia were sometimes seen.

In general, neutrophils returned to normal in about two weeks after captopril was discontinued, and serious infections were limited to clinically complex patients. About 13 percent of the cases of neutropenia have ended fatally, but almost all fatalities were in patients with serious illness, having collagen vascular disease, renal failure, heart failure or immunosuppressant therapy, or a combination of these complicating factors.

Evaluation of the hypertensive or heart failure patient should always include assessment of renal function.

If captopril is used in patients with impaired renal function, white blood cell and differential counts should be evaluated prior to starting treatment and at approximately two-week intervals for about three months, then periodically.

In patients with collagen vascular disease or who are exposed to other drugs known to affect the white cells or immune response, particularly when there is impaired renal function, captopril should be used only after an assessment of benefit and risk, and then with caution.

All patients treated with captopril should be told to report any signs of infection (e.g., sore throat, fever). If infection is suspected, white cell counts should be performed without delay.

Since discontinuation of captopril and other drugs has generally led to prompt return of the white count to normal, upon confirmation of neutropenia (neutrophil count $<1000/mm^3$) the physician should withdraw captopril and closely follow the patient's course.

Proteinuria—Total urinary proteins greater than 1 g per day were seen in about 0.7 percent of patients receiving captopril. About 90 percent of affected patients had evidence of prior renal disease or received relatively high doses of captopril (in excess of 150 mg/day), or both. The nephrotic syndrome occurred in about one-fifth of proteinuric patients. In most cases, proteinuria subsided or cleared within six months whether or not captopril was continued. Parameters of renal function, such as BUN and creatinine, were seldom altered in the patients with proteinuria.

Since most cases of proteinuria occurred by the eighth month of therapy with captopril, patients with prior renal disease or those receiving captopril at doses greater than 150 mg per day, should have urinary protein estimations (dipstick on first morning urine) prior to treatment, and periodically thereafter.

Hypotension—Excessive hypotension was rarely seen in hypertensive patients but is a possible consequence of captopril use in severely salt/volume depleted persons such as those treated vigorously with diuretics, for example, patients with severe congestive heart failure (see PRECAUTIONS [Drug Interactions]).

Hydrochlorothiazide—Thiazides should be used with caution in severe renal disease. In patients with renal disease, thiazides may precipitate azotemia. Cumulative effects of the drug may develop in patients with impaired renal function.

Thiazides should be used with caution in patients with impaired hepatic function or progressive liver disease, since minor alterations of fluid and electrolyte balance may precipitate hepatic coma.

Sensitivity reactions may occur in patients with or without a history of allergy or bronchial asthma.

The possibility of exacerbation or activation of systemic lupus erythematosus has been reported.

PRECAUTIONS

General—Captopril—*Impaired Renal Function*—Some patients with renal disease, particularly those with severe renal artery stenosis, have developed increases in BUN and serum creatinine after reduction of blood pressure with captopril. Captopril dosage reduction and/or discontinuation of diuretic may be required. For some of these patients, it may not be possible to normalize blood pressure and maintain adequate renal perfusion (see CLINICAL PHARMACOLOGY, DOSAGE AND ADMINISTRATION, ADVERSE REACTIONS [Altered Laboratory Findings]).

Surgery/Anesthesia—In patients undergoing major surgery or during anesthesia with agents that produce hypotension, captopril will block angiotensin II formation secondary to compensatory renin release. If hypotension occurs and is considered to be due to this mechanism, it can be corrected by volume expansion.

Hydrochlorothiazide—All patients receiving thiazide therapy should be observed for clinical signs of fluid or electrolyte imbalance; namely hyponatremia, hypochloremic alkalosis, and hypokalemia. Serum and urine electrolyte determinations are particularly important when the patient is vomiting excessively or receiving parenteral fluids. Warning signs, irrespective of cause include dryness of mouth, thirst, weakness, lethargy, drowsiness, restlessness, muscle pains or cramps, muscular fatigue, hypotension, oliguria, tachycardia, and gastrointestinal disturbances such as nausea and vomiting.

Hypokalemia may develop, especially with brisk diuresis, when severe cirrhosis is present. Interference with adequate oral electrolyte intake will also contribute to hypokalemia. Hypokalemia can sensitize or exaggerate the response of the heart to the toxic effects of digitalis (e.g., increased ventricular irritability). Because captopril reduces the production of aldosterone, concomitant therapy with captopril reduces the diuretic-induced hypokalemia. Fewer patients may require potassium supplements and/or foods with a high potassium content (see Drug Interactions, Agents Increasing Serum Potassium).

Any chloride deficit is generally mild and usually does not require specific treatment except under extraordinary circumstances (as in liver disease or renal disease). Dilutional hyponatremia may occur in edematous patients in hot weather; appropriate therapy is water restriction, rather than administration of salt except in rare instances when the hyponatremia is life-threatening. In actual salt depletion, appropriate replacement is the therapy of choice.

Hyperuricemia may occur or frank gout may be precipitated in certain patients receiving thiazide therapy.

Diabetes mellitus which has been latent may become manifest during thiazide administration.

The antihypertensive effects of the drug may be enhanced in the postsympathectomy patient.

If progressive renal impairment becomes evident, as indicated by rising nonprotein nitrogen or blood urea nitrogen, a careful reappraisal of therapy is necessary with consideration given to withholding or discontinuing diuretic therapy.

Thiazides may decrease serum PBI levels without signs of thyroid disturbance.

Calcium excretion is decreased by thiazides. Pathologic changes in the parathyroid gland with hypercalcemia and hypophosphatemia have been observed in a few patients on prolonged thiazide therapy. The common complications of hyperparathyroidism have not been seen.

Information for Patients—Patients should be told to report promptly any indication of infection (e.g., sore throat, fever), which may be a sign of neutropenia, or of progressive edema which might be related to proteinuria and nephrotic syndrome.

All patients should be cautioned that excessive perspiration and dehydration may lead to an excessive fall in blood pressure because of reduction in fluid volume. Other causes of volume depletion such as vomiting or diarrhea may also lead to a fall in blood pressure; patients should be advised to consult with the physician.

Patients should be warned against interruption or discontinuation of medication unless instructed by the physician.

Heart failure patients on captopril therapy should be cautioned against rapid increases in physical activity.

Patients should be informed that CAPOZIDE (Captopril-Hydrochlorothiazide Tablets) should be taken one hour before meals (see DOSAGE AND ADMINISTRATION).

Laboratory Tests—Serum and urine electrolyte levels should be regularly monitored (see WARNINGS [Captopril and Hydrochlorothiazide], also PRECAUTIONS [General, Hydrochlorothiazide]).

Drug Interactions—Captopril—

Hypotension—Patients on Diuretic Therapy: Patients on diuretics and especially those in whom diuretic therapy was recently instituted, as well as those on severe dietary salt restrictions or dialysis, may occasionally experience a precipitous reduction of blood pressure usually within the first hour after receiving the initial dose of captopril.

The possibility of hypotensive effects with captopril can be minimized by either discontinuing the diuretic or increasing the salt intake approximately one week prior to initiation of treatment with captopril or initiating therapy with small doses (6.25 or 12.5 mg). Alternatively, provide medical supervision for at least one hour after the initial dose. If hypotension occurs, the patient should be placed in a supine position and, if necessary, receive an intravenous infusion of normal saline. This transient hypotensive response is not a contraindication to further doses which can be given without difficulty once the blood pressure has increased after volume expansion.

Agents Having Vasodilator Activity: Data on the effect of concomitant use of other vasodilators in patients receiving captopril for heart failure are not available; therefore, nitroglycerin or other nitrates (as used for management of angina) or other drugs having vasodilator activity should, if possible, be discontinued before starting captopril. If resumed during captopril therapy, such agents should be administered cautiously, and perhaps at lower dosage.

Agents Causing Renin Release: Captopril's effect will be augmented by antihypertensive agents that cause renin release. For example, diuretics (e.g., thiazides) may activate the renin-angiotensin-aldosterone system.

Agents Affecting Sympathetic Activity: The sympathetic nervous system may be especially important in supporting

Continued on next page

Squibb—Cont.

blood pressure in patients receiving captopril alone or with diuretics. Therefore, agents affecting sympathetic activity (e.g., ganglionic blocking agents or adrenergic neuron blocking agents) should be used with caution. Beta-adrenergic blocking drugs add some further antihypertensive effect to captopril, but the overall response is less than additive.

Agents Increasing Serum Potassium: Since captopril decreases aldosterone production, elevation of serum potassium may occur. Potassium-sparing diuretics such as spironolactone, triamterene, or amiloride, or potassium supplements, should be given only for documented hypokalemia, and then with caution, since they may lead to a significant increase of serum potassium. Salt substitutes containing potassium should also be used with caution.

Inhibitors Of Endogenous Prostaglandin Synthesis: It has been reported that indomethacin may reduce the antihypertensive effect of captopril, expecially in cases of low renin hypertension. Other nonsteroidal anti-inflammatory agents (e.g., aspirin) may also have this effect.

Hydrochlorothiazide—When administered concurrently the following drugs may interact with thiazide diuretics:

Alcohol, barbiturates, or narcotics—potentiation of orthostatic hypotension may occur.

Antidiabetic drugs (oral agents and insulin)—hyperglycemia induced by thiazides may require dosage adjustment of the antidiabetic drug.

Other antihypertensive drugs—additive effect or potentiation. Potentiation occurs with ganglionic or peripheral adrenergic blocking drugs.

Corticosteroids, ACTH—intensified electrolyte depletion, particularly hypokalemia.

Preanesthetic and anesthetic agents—effects of preanesthetic and anesthetic agents may be potentiated; adjust dosage of these agents accordingly.

Pressor amines (e.g., norepinephrine)—possible decreased response to pressor amines but not sufficient to preclude their use.

Skeletal muscle relaxants, nondepolarizing (e.g., tubocurarine)—possible increased responsiveness to the muscle relaxant.

Lithium—should not generallly be given with diuretics; diuretic agents reduce the renal clearance of lithium and add a high risk of lithium toxicity. Refer to the package insert for lithium preparations before use of such preparations with CAPOZIDE. (Captopril-Hydrochlorothiazide Tablets).

Drug/Laboratory Test Interactions—Captopril—Captopril may cause a false-positive urine test for acetone.

Hydrochlorothiazide—Thiazides should be discontinued before carrying out tests for parathyroid function (see PRECAUTIONS [General, Hydrochlorothiazide]).

Carcinogenesis, Mutagenesis, Impairment of Fertility—Captopril—Two-year studies with doses of 50 to 1350 mg/kg/day in mice and rats failed to show any evidence of carcinogenic potential.

Studies in rats have revealed no impairment of fertility.

Animal Toxicology—Chronic oral toxicity studies were conducted in rats (2 years), dogs (47 weeks; 1 year), mice (2 years), and monkeys (1 year). Significant drug-related toxicity included effects on hematopoiesis, renal toxicity, erosion/ulceration of the stomach, and variation of retinal blood vessels.

Reductions in hemoglobin and/or hematocrit values were seen in mice, rats, and monkeys at doses 50 to 150 times the maximum recommended human dose (MRHD). Anemia, leukopenia, thrombocytopenia, and bone marrow suppression occurred in dogs at doses 8 to 30 times MRHD. The reductions in hemoglobin and hematocrit values in rats and mice were only significant at 1 year and returned to normal with continued dosing by the end of the study. Marked anemia was seen at all dose levels (8 to 30 times MRHD) in dogs, whereas moderate to marked leukopenia was noted only at 15 and 30 times MRHD and thrombocytopenia at 30 times MRHD. The anemia could be reversed upon discontinuation of dosing. Bone marrow suppression occurred to a varying degree, being associated only with dogs that died or were sacrificed in a moribund condition in the 1-year study. However, in the 47-week study at a dose 30 times MRHD, bone marrow suppression was found to be reversible upon continued drug administration.

Captopril caused hyperplasia of the juxtaglomerular apparatus of the kidneys at doses 7 to 200 times the MRHD in rats and mice, at 20 to 60 times MRHD in monkeys, and at 30 times the MRHD in dogs.

Gastric erosions/ulcerations were increased in incidence at 20 and 200 times MRHD in male rats and at 30 and 65 times MRHD in dogs and monkeys, respectively. Rabbits developed gastric and intestinal ulcers when given oral doses approximately 30 times MRHD for only five to seven days.

In the two-year rat study, irreversible and progressive variations in the caliber of retinal vessels (focal sacculations and constrictions) occurred at all dose levels (7 to 200 times MRHD) in a dose-related fashion. The effect was first observed in the 88th week of dosing, with a progressively increased incidence thereafter, even after cessation of dosing.

Hydrochlorothiazide—Long-term studies in animals have not been performed to evaluate carcinogenic potential, mutagenesis, or whether this drug affects fertility in males or females.

Pregnancy—Category C—Captopril—Captopril was embryocidal in rabbits when given in doses about 2 to 70 times (on a mg/kg basis) the maximum recommended human dose, and low incidences of craniofacial malformations were seen. These effects in rabbits were most probably due to the particularly marked decrease in blood pressure caused by the drug in this species.

Captopril given to pregnant rats at 400 times the recommended human dose continuously during gestation and lactation caused a reduction in neonatal survival.

No teratogenic effects (malformations) have been observed after large doses of captopril in hamsters and rats.

Captopril crosses the human placenta.

Hydrochlorothiazide—Teratology studies have been performed in pregnant rats using captopril and hydrochlorothiazide individually and in combination; each agent was administered in doses up to 1350 mg/kg (400 times the maximum recommended human dose for hydrochlorothiazide). No evidence of embryotoxicity, fetotoxicity, or teratogenicity was found in any group.

There are no adequate and well-controlled studies with captopril and hydrochlorothiazide in pregnant women. Because animal reproduction studies are not always predictive of human response, CAPOZIDE should be used during pregnancy, or for patients likely to become pregnant, only if the potential benefit justifies a potential risk to the fetus.

Pregnancy — Nonteratogenic Effects — Hydrochlorothiazide—Thiazides cross the placental barrier and appear in cord blood. The use of thiazides in pregnant women requires that the anticipated benefit be weighed against possible hazards to the fetus. These hazards include fetal or neonatal jaundice, thrombocytopenia, and possibly other adverse reactions which have occurred in the adult.

Nursing Mothers—Both captopril and hydrochlorothiazide are excreted in human milk. Because of the potential for serious adverse reactions in nursing infants from both drugs, a decision should be made whether to discontinue nursing or to discontinue therapy taking into account the importance of CAPOZIDE (Captopril-Hydrochlorothiazide Tablets) to the mother.

Pediatric Use—Safety and effectiveness in children have not been established although there is limited experience with the use of captopril in children from 2 months to 15 years of age with secondary hypertension and varying degrees of renal insufficiency. Dosage, on a weight basis, was comparable to that used in adults. CAPOZIDE (Captopril-Hydrochlorothiazide Tablets) should be used in children only if other measures for controlling blood pressure have not been effective.

ADVERSE REACTIONS

Captopril—Reported incidences are based on clinical trials involving approximately 7000 patients.

Renal—About one of 100 patients developed proteinuria (see WARNINGS).

Each of the following has been reported in approximately 1 to 2 of 1000 patients and is of uncertain relationship to drug use: renal insufficiency, renal failure, polyuria, oliguria, and urinary frequency.

Hematologic—Neutropenia/agranulocytosis has occurred (see WARNINGS). Cases of anemia, thrombocytopenia, and pancytopenia have been reported.

Dermatologic—Rash, often with pruritus, and sometimes with fever, arthralgia, and eosinophilia, occurred in about 4 to 7 (depending on renal status and dose) of 100 patients, usually during the first four weeks of therapy. It is usually maculopapular, and rarely urticarial. The rash is usually mild and disappears within a few days of dosage reduction, short-term treatment with an antihistaminic agent, and/or discontinuing therapy; remission may occur even if captopril is continued. Pruritus, without rash, occurs in about 2 of 100 patients. Between 7 and 10 percent of patients with skin rash have shown and eosinophilia and/or positive ANA titers. A reversible associated pemphigoid-like lesion, and photosensitivity, have also been reported.

Angioedema of the face, mucous membranes of the mouth, or of the extremities has been observed in approximately 1 of 1000 patients and is reversible on discontinuance of captopril therapy. One case of laryngeal edema has been reported.

Flushing or pallor has been reported in 2 to 5 of 1000 patients.

Cardiovascular—Hypotension may occur; see WARNINGS and PRECAUTIONS (Drug Interactions) for discussion of hypotension on initiation of captopril therapy.

Tachycardia, chest pain, and palpitations have each been observed in approximately 1 of 100 patients.

Angina pectoris, myocardial infarction, Raynaud's syndrome, and congestive heart failure have each occurred in 2 to 3 of 1000 patients.

Dysgeusia—Approximately 2 to 4 (depending on renal status and dose) of 100 patients developed a diminution or loss of taste perception. Taste impairment is reversible and usually self-limited (2 to 3 months) even with continued drug administration. Weight loss may be associated with the loss of taste.

The following have been reported in about 0.5 to 2 percent of patients but did not appear at increased frequency compared to placebo or other treatments used in controlled trials: gastric irritation, abdominal pain, nausea, vomiting, diarrhea, anorexia, constipation, aphthous ulcers, peptic ulcer, dizziness, headache, malaise, fatigue, insomnia, dry mouth, dyspnea, cough, alopecia, paresthesias.

Hydrochlorothiazide—*Gastrointestinal System*—anorexia, gastric irritation, nausea, vomiting, cramping, diarrhea, constipation, jaundice (intrahepatic cholestatic jaundice), pancreatitis, and sialadenitis.

Central Nervous System—dizziness, vertigo, paresthesias, headache, and xanthopsia.

Hematologic—Leukopenia, agranulocytosis, thrombocytopenia, aplastic anemia, and hemolytic anemia.

Cardiovascular—orthostatic hypotension.

Hypersensitivity—purpura, photosensitivity, rash, urticaria, necrotizing angiitis (vasculitis; cutaneous vasculitis), fever, respiratory distress including pneumonitis, and anaphylactic reactions.

Other—hyperglycemia, glycosuria, hyperuricemia, muscle spasm, weakness, restlessness, and transient blurred vision. Whenever adverse reactions are moderate or severe, thiazide dosage should be reduced or therapy withdrawn.

Altered Laboratory Findings—Elevations of liver enzymes have been noted in a few patients but no causal relationship to captopril use has been established. Rare cases of cholestatic jaundice and of hepatocellular injury with or without secondary cholestasis have been reported in association with captopril administration.

A transient elevation of BUN and serum creatinine may occur, especially in patients who are volume-depleted or who have renovascular hypertension. In instances of rapid reduction of longstanding or severely elevated blood pressure, the glomerular filtration rate may decrease transiently, also resulting in transient rises in serum creatinine and BUN.

Small increases in the serum potassium concentration frequently occur, especially in patients with renal impairment (see PRECAUTIONS).

OVERDOSAGE

Captopril—Correction of hypotension would be of primary concern. Volume expansion with an intravenous infusion of normal saline is the treatment of choice for restoration of blood pressure.

Captopril may be removed from the general circulation by hemodialysis.

Hydrochlorothiazide—In addition to the expected diuresis, overdosage of thiazides may produce varying degrees of lethargy which may progress to coma within a few hours, with minimal depression of respiration and cardiovascular function and without evidence of serum electrolyte changes or dehydration. The mechanism of thiazide-induced CNS depression is unknown. Gastrointestinal irritation and hypermotility may occur. Transitory increase in BUN has been reported, and serum electrolyte changes may occur, especially in patients with impaired renal function.

In addition to gastric lavage and supportive therapy for stupor or coma, symptomatic treatment of gastrointestinal effects may be needed. The degree to which hydrochlorothiazide is removed by hemodialysis has not been clearly established. Measures as required to maintain hydration, electrolyte balance, respiration, and cardiovascular and renal function should be instituted.

DOSAGE AND ADMINISTRATION

DOSAGE MUST BE INDIVIDUALIZED (SEE INDICATIONS AND USAGE).

CAPOZIDE (Captopril-Hydrochlorothiazide Tablets) should be taken one hour before meals.

The usual initial dose of captopril is 25 mg bid or tid. Hydrochlorothiazide is usually given at a total daily dose of 25 to 100 mg.

The approximate daily dose of captopril and hydrochlorothiazide, as determined by titration of the individual components (see INDICATIONS AND USAGE), may be administered by utilizing an appropriate potency of CAPOZIDE bid. For example, CAPOZIDE may be administered beginning with the 25 mg/15 mg combination tablet bid. Increased captopril dosage may be obtained by utilizing the 50 mg/15 mg combination tablet bid or increased hydrochlorothiazide dosage may be obtained by utilizing the 25 mg/25 mg combination tablet bid. CAPOZIDE 25 mg/15 mg and 50 mg/15 mg tablets may also be utilized in tid dosage regimens to provide higher daily dosages.

If additional control beyond that provided by the 50 mg/15 mg tid CAPOZIDE dose is indicated, it is recommended that other antihypertensive agents be added to the regimen.

A maximum daily dose of 450 mg captopril should not be exceeded.

Beta-blockers may be used in conjunction with CAPOZIDE therapy (see PRECAUTIONS [Drug Interactions]), but the effects are less than additive. Other agents may be added gradually beginning with 50 percent of the usual recommended starting dose to avoid an excessive fall in blood pressure.

For patients with severe hypertension (e.g., accelerated or malignant hypertension), the dosage increments may be made more frequently than every two weeks with the patient under continuous medical supervision until a satisfactory blood pressure response is obtained or the maximal dose of captopril is reached.

Dosage Adjustment in Renal Impairment—Because captopril and hydrochlorothiazide are excreted primarily by the kidneys, excretion rates are reduced in patients with impaired renal function. These patients will take longer to reach steady-state captopril levels and will reach higher steady-state levels for a given daily dose than patients with normal renal function. Therefore, these patients may respond to smaller or less frequent doses of CAPOZIDE.

After the desired therapeutic effect has been achieved, the dose intervals should be increased or the total daily dose reduced until the minimal effective dose is achieved. When concomitant diuretic therapy is required in patients with severe renal impairment, a loop diuretic (e.g., furosemide), rather than a thiazide diuretic is preferred for use with captopril; therefore, for patients with severe renal dysfunction the captopril-hydrochlorothiazide combination tablet is not usually recommended.

HOW SUPPLIED

CAPOZIDE (Captopril-Hydrochlorothiazide Tablets)

25 mg captopril combined with 15 mg hydrochlorothiazide in bottles of 100. Tablets are white with distinct orange mottling; they are biconvex rounded squares with quadrisect bars. Tablet identification no. **338.**

25 mg captopril combined with 25 mg hydrochlorothiazide in bottles of 100. Tablets are peach-colored and may show slight mottling; they are biconvex rounded squares with quadrisect bars. Tablet identification no. **349.**

50 mg. captopril combined with 15 mg hydrochlorothiazide in bottles of 100. Tablets are white with distinct orange mottling; they are biconvex ovals with a bisect bar. Tablet identification no. **384.**

50 mg captopril combined with 25 mg hydrochlorothiazide in bottles of 100. Tablets are peach-colored and may show slight mottling; they are biconvex ovals with a bisect bar. Tablet identification no. **390.**

Storage: Keep bottles tightly closed (protect from moisture); do not store above 86°F.

(J4-005C)

Shown in Product Identification Section, page 431

COMOXOL™ 400/80 ℞
COMOXOL™ 800/160

[*kō-mox 'ol*]

Sulfamethoxazole and Trimethoprim Tablets USP

DESCRIPTION

Sulfamethoxazole and Trimethoprim is a synthetic antibacterial combination product available in tablets, each containing 400 mg sulfamethoxazole and 80 mg trimethoprim, and in double strength (DS) tablets, each containing 800 mg sulfamethoxazole and 160 mg trimethoprim. Inactive ingredients: magnesium stearate, sodium starch glycolate, and starch (corn).

Sulfamethoxazole is N′-(5-methyl-3-isoxazolyl) sulfanilamide. It is a white to off-white, practically odorless, crystalline powder. It is practically insoluble in water, in ether, and in chloroform; freely soluble in acetone and in dilute solutions of sodium hydroxide; and sparingly soluble in alcohol.

Trimethoprim is 2,4-diamino-5-(3,4,5-trimethoxybenzyl) pyrimidine. It is white to cream colored, odorless crystals or crystalline powder. It is very soluble in water; soluble in benzyl alcohol; sparingly soluble in chloroform and in methanol; slightly soluble in alcohol and in acetone; and practically insoluble in ether and in carbon tetrachloride.

CLINICAL PHARMACOLOGY

Sulfamethoxazole and Trimethoprim are rapidly absorbed following oral administration. Both sulfamethoxazole and trimethoprim exist in the blood as unbound, protein-bound and metabolized forms; sulfamethoxazole also exists as the conjugated form. The metabolism of sulfamethoxazole occurs predominantly by N_4-acetylation, although the glucuronide conjugate has been identified. The principal metabolites of trimethoprim are the 1- and 3-oxides and the 3′- and 4′-hydroxy derivatives. The free forms of sulfamethoxazole and trimethoprim are considered to be the therapeutically active forms. Approximately 44 percent of trimethoprim and 70 percent of sulfamethoxazole are bound to plasma proteins. The presence of 10 mg percent sulfamethoxazole in plasma decreases the protein binding of trimethoprim by an insignificant degree; trimethoprim does not influence the protein binding of sulfamethoxazole.

REPRESENTATIVE MINIMUM INHIBITORY CONCENTRATION VALUES FOR SULFAMETHOXAZOLE AND TRIMETHOPRIM SUSCEPTIBLE ORGANISMS (MIC-μg/mL)

Bacteria	TMP alone	SMX-alone	TMP/SMX (1:19) TMP	SMX
Escherichia coli	0.05–1.5	1.0–245	0.05–0.5	0.95–9.5
Proteus species				
indole positive	0.5–5.0	7.35–300	0.05–1.5	0.95–28.5
Morganella morganii	0.5–5.0	7.35–300	0.05–1.5	0.95–28.5
Proteus mirabilis	0.5–1.5	7.35–30	0.05–0.15	0.95–2.85
Klebsiella species	0.15–5.0	2.45–245	0.05–1.5	0.95–28.5
Enterobacter species	0.15–5.0	2.45–245	0.05–1.5	0.95–28.5
Haemophilus influenzae	0.15–1.5	2.85–95	0.015–1.15	0.285–2.85
Streptococcus pneumoniae	0.15–1.5	7.35–24.5	0.05–0.15	0.95–2.85
Shigella flexneri†	<0.01–0.04	<0.16–>320	<0.002–0.03	0.04–0.625
Shigella sonnei†	0.02–0.08	0.625–>320	0.004–0.06	0.08–1.25

TMP = Trimethoprim SMX = Sulfamethoxazole

†Rudoy RC, Nelson JD, Haitalin KC, *Antimicrobial Agents and Chemotherapy* 5:439–43, 1974.

Peak blood levels for the individual components occur 1 to 4 hours after oral administration. The mean serum half-lives of sulfamethoxazole and trimethoprim, 10 and 8 to 10 hours, respectively. However, patients with severely impaired renal function exhibit an increase in the half-lives of both components, requiring dosage regimen adjustment (see DOSAGE AND ADMINISTRATION section). Detectable amounts of sulfamethoxazole and trimethoprim are present in the blood 24 hours after drug administration. During administration of 800 mg sulfamethoxazole and 160 mg trimethoprim b.i.d., the mean steady state plasma concentration of trimethoprim was 1.72 μg/mL. The steady state minimal plasma levels of free and total sulfamethoxazole were 57.4 μg/mL and 68.0 μg/mL, respectively. These steady state levels were achieved after three days of drug administration.[1]

Excretion of sulfamethoxazole and trimethoprim is primarily by the kidneys through both glomerular filtration and tubular secretion. Urine concentrations of both sulfamethoxazole and trimethoprim are considerably higher than are the concentrations in the blood. The average percentage of the dose recovered in urine from 0 to 72 hours after a single oral dose is 84.5 percent for total sulfonamide and 66.8 percent for free trimethoprim. Thirty percent of the total sulfonamide is excreted as free sulfamethoxazole, with the remaining as N_4-acetylated metabolite.[2] When administered together as sulfamethoxazole and trimethoprim, neither sulfamethoxazole nor trimethoprim affects the urinary excretion pattern of the other.

Both sulfamethoxazole and trimethoprim distribute to sputum, vaginal fluid, and middle ear fluid; trimethoprim also distributes to bronchial secretion, and both pass the placental barrier and are excreted in breast milk.

Microbiology—Sulfamethoxazole inhibits bacterial synthesis of dihydrofolic acid by competing with para-aminobenzoic acid (PABA). Trimethoprim blocks the production of tetrahydrofolic acid from dihydrofolic acid by binding to and reversibly inhibiting the required enzyme, dihydrofolate reductase. Thus, sulfamethoxazole and trimethoprim block two consecutive steps in the biosynthesis of nucleic acids and proteins essential to many bacteria.

In vitro studies have shown that bacterial resistance develops more slowly with sulfamethoxazole and trimethoprim than with sulfamethoxazole or trimethoprim alone.

In vitro serial dilution tests have shown that the spectrum of antibacterial activity of sulfamethoxazole and trimethoprim includes the common urinary tract pathogens with the exception of *Pseudomonas aeruginosa*. The following organisms are usually susceptible: *Escherichia coli, Klebsiella species, Enterobacter species, Morganella morganii, Proteus mirabilis* and indole-positive *Proteus* species including *Proteus vulgaris.*

The usual spectrum of antimicrobial activity of sulfamethoxazole and trimethoprim includes the bacterial pathogens isolated from middle ear exudate and from bronchial secretions: *Haemophilus influenzae,* including ampicillin-resistant strains, and *Streptococcus pneumoniae. Shigella flexneri* and *Shigella sonnei* are also usually susceptible.

[See table above].

The recommended quantitative disc susceptibility method may be used for estimating the susceptibility of bacteria to sulfamethoxazole and trimethoprim.[3,4] With this procedure, a report from the laboratory of "Susceptible to sulfamethoxazole-trimethoprim" indicates that the infection is likely to respond to therapy with sulfamethoxazole and trimethoprim. If the infection is confined to the urine, a report of "Intermediate susceptibility to trimethoprim and sulfamethoxazole" also indicates that the infection is likely to respond. A report of "Resistant to trimethoprim and sulfamethoxazole" indicates that the infection is unlikely to respond to therapy with sulfamethoxazole and trimethoprim.

INDICATIONS AND USAGE

Urinary Tract Infections—For the treatment of urinary tract infections due to susceptible strains of the following organisms: *Escherichia coli, Klebsiella* species, *Enterobacter,* species, *Proteus morganii, Proteus Mirabilis,* and *Proteus vulgaris.* It is recommended that initial episodes of uncomplicated urinary tract infections be treated with a single effective antibacterial agent rather than the combination.

Acute Otitis Media—For the treatment of acute otitis media in children due to susceptible strains of *Streptococcus pneumoniae or Haemophilusus influenzae* when in the judgment of the physician sulfamethoxazole and trimethoprim offer some advantage over the use of other antimicrobial agents. To date, there are limited data on the safety of repeated use of sulfamethoxazole and trimethoprim in children under two years of age. Sulfamethoxazole and trimethoprim are not indicated for prophylactic or prolonged administration in otitis media at any age.

Acute Exacerbations of Chronic Bronchitis in Adults—For the treatment of acute exacerbations of chronic bronchitis due to susceptible strains of *Streptococcus pneumoniae* or *Haemophilus influenzae* when, in the judgment of the physician, sulfamethoxazole and trimethoprim offer some advantage over the use of a single antimicrobial agent.

Shigellosis—For the treatment of enteritis caused by susceptible strains of *Shigella flexneri* and *Shigella sonnei* when antibacterial therapy is indicated.

Pneumocystis carinii Pneumonitis—For the treatment of documented *Pneumocystis carinii* pneumonitis.

CONTRAINDICATIONS

Hypersensitivity to trimethoprim or sulfonamides. Patients with documented megaloblastic anemia due to folate deficiency.

Pregnancy at term and during the nursing period, because sulfonamides pass the placenta and are excreted in the milk and may cause kernicterus. Infants less than two months of age.

WARNINGS

FATALITIES ASSOCIATED WITH THE ADMINISTRATION OF SULFONAMIDES, ALTHOUGH RARE, HAVE OCCURRED DUE TO SEVERE REACTIONS, INCLUDING STEVENS-JOHNSON SYNDROME, TOXIC EPIDERMAL NECROLYSIS, FULMINANT HEPATIC NECROSIS, AGRANULOCYTOSIS, APLASTIC ANEMIA AND OTHER BLOOD DYSCRASIAS.

SULFAMETHOXAZOLE AND TRIMETHOPRIM SHOULD BE DISCONTINUED AT THE FIRST APPEARANCE OF SKIN RASH OR ANY SIGN OF ADVERSE REACTION. Clinical signs, such as rash, sore throat, fever, pallor, purpura or jaundice may be early indications of serious reactions. In rare instances a skin rash may be followed by more severe reactions, such as Stevens-Johnson syndrome, toxic epidermal necrolysis, hepatic necrosis or serious blood disorder. Complete blood counts should be done frequently in patients receiving sulfonamides.

SULFAMETHOXAZOLE AND TRIMETHOPRIM SHOULD NOT BE USED IN THE TREATMENT OF STREPTOCOCCAL PHARYNGITIS. Clinical studies have documented that patients with Group A, β-hemolytic streptococcal tonsillopharyngitis have a greater incidence of bacteriologic failure when treated with sulfamethoxazole and trimethoprim than do those patients treated with penicillin, as evidenced by failure to eradicate this organism from the tonsillopharyngeal area.

PRECAUTIONS

General—Sulfamethoxazole and trimethoprim should be given with caution to patients with impaired renal or hepatic function, to those with possible folate deficiency and to those with severe allergy or bronchial asthma. In glucose-6-phosphate dehydrogenase-deficient individuals, hemolysis may occur. This reaction is frequently dose-related.

Information for Patients—Patients should be instructed to maintain an adequate fluid intake in order to prevent crystalluria and stone formation.

Continued on next page

Squibb—Cont.

Laboratory Tests—Complete blood counts should be done frequently in patients receiving sulfamethoxazole and trimethoprim: if a significant reduction in the count of any formed blood element is noted, sulfamethoxazole and trimethoprim should be discontinued. Urinalysis with careful microscopic examination and renal function tests should be performed during therapy, particularly for those patients with impaired renal function.

Drug Interactions—In elderly patients concurrently receiving certain diuretics, primarily thiazides, an increased incidence of thrombocytopenia with purpura has been reported. It has been reported that sulfamethoxazole and trimethoprim may prolong the prothrombin time in patients who are receiving the anticoagulant warfarin. This interaction should be kept in mind when sulfamethoxazole and trimethoprim are given to patients already on anticoagulant therapy, and the coagulation time should be reassessed.

Sulfamethoxazole and trimethoprim may inhibit the hepatic metabolism of phenytoin. Sulfamethoxazole and trimethoprim, given at a common clinical dosage, increased the phenytoin half-life by 39 percent and decreased the phenytoin metabolic clearance rate by 27 percent. When administering these drugs concurrently, one should be alert for possible excessive phenytoin effect. Sulfonamides can also displace methotrexate from plasma protein binding sites, thus increasing methotrexate concentrations.

Drug/Laboratory Test Interactions—Sulfamethoxazole and trimethoprim, specifically the trimethoprim component, can interfere with a serum methotrexate assay as determined by the competitive binding protein technique (CBPA) when a bacterial dihydrofolate reductase is used as the binding protein. No interference occurs, however, if methotrexate is measured by a radioimmunoassay (RIA).

Carcinogenesis, Mutagenesis, Impairment of Fertility: Carcinogenesis—Long-term studies in animals to evaluate carcinogenic potential have not been conducted with sulfamethoxazole and trimethoprim. **Mutagenesis**—Bacterial mutagenic studies have not been performed with sulfamethoxazole and trimethoprim in combination. Trimethoprim was demonstrated to be nonmutagenic in the Ames assay. No chromosomal damage was observed in human leukocytes cultured *in vitro* with sulfamethoxazole and trimethoprim alone or in combination; the concentrations used exceeded blood levels of these compounds following therapy with sulfamethoxazole and trimethoprim. Observations of leukocytes obtained from patients treated with sulfamethoxazole and trimethoprim revealed no chromosomal abnormalities.

Impairment of Fertility—No adverse effects on fertility or general reproductive performance were observed in rats given oral dosages as high as 350 mg/kg/day sulfamethoxazole plus 70 mg/kg/day trimethoprim.

Pregnancy, Teratogenic Effects: Pregnancy Category C: In rats, oral doses of 533 mg/kg sulfamethoxazole or 200 mg/kg trimethoprim produced teratological effects manifested mainly as cleft palates. The highest dose which did not cause cleft palates in rats was 512 mg/kg of sulfamethoxazole or 192 mg/kg trimethoprim when administered separately. In two studies in rats, no teratology was observed when 512mg/kg of sulfamethoxazole was used in combination with 128 mg/kg of trimethoprim. In one study, however, cleft palates were observed in one litter out of 9 when 355 mg/kg of sulfamethoxazole was used in combination with 88 mg/kg of trimethoprim.

In some rabbit studies, an overall increase in fetal loss (dead and resorbed and malformed conceptuses) was associated with doses of trimethoprim six times the human therapeutic dose.

While there are no large, well-controlled studies on the use of sulfamethoxazole and trimethoprim in pregnant women, Brumfitt and Pursell,[5] in a retrospective study, reported the outcome of 186 pregnancies during which the mother received either placebo or sulfamethoxazole and trimethoprim. The incidence of congenital abnormalities was 4.5 percent (3 of 66) in those who received placebo and 3.3 percent (4 of 120) in those receiving trimethoprim and sulfamethoxazole. There were no abnormalities in the 10 children whose mothers received the drug during the first trimester. In a separate survey, Brumfitt and Pursell also found no congenital abnormalities in 35 children whose mothers had received oral sulfamethoxazole and trimethoprim at the time of conception or shortly thereafter.

Because sulfamethoxazole and trimethoprim may interfere with folic acid metabolism, sulfamethoxazole and trimethoprim should be used during pregnancy only if the potential benefit justifies the potential risk to the fetus.

Pregnancy, Nonteratogenic Effects: See CONTRAINDICATIONS section.

Nursing Mothers: See CONTRAINDICATIONS section.

Pediatric Use: Sulfamethoxazole and trimethoprim are not recommended for infants younger than two months of age (see INDICATIONS AND USAGE and CONTRAINDICATIONS sections).

ADVERSE REACTIONS

The most common adverse effects are gastrointestinal disturbances (nausea, vomiting, anorexia) and allergic skin reactions (such as rash and urticaria). FATALITIES ASSOCIATED WITH THE ADMINISTRATION OF SULFONAMIDES, ALTHOUGH RARE, HAVE OCCURRED DUE TO SEVERE REACTIONS, INCLUDING STEVENS-JOHNSON SYNDROME, TOXIC EPIDERMAL NECROLYSIS, FULMINANT HEPATIC NECROSIS, AGRANULOCYTOSIS, APLASTIC ANEMIA AND OTHER BLOOD DYSCRASIAS (SEE WARNINGS SECTION).

Hematologic: Agranulocytosis, aplastic anemia, thrombocytopenia, leukopenia, neutropenia, hemolytic anemia, megaloblastic anemia, hypoprothrombinemia, methemoglobinemia, eosinophilia.

Allergic reactions: Stevens-Johnson syndrome, toxic epidermal necrolysis, anaphylaxis, allergic myocarditis, erythema multiforme, exofoliative dermatitis, angioedema, Henoch-Schonlein purpura, serum sickness-like syndrome, generalized allergic reactions, generalized skin eruptions, photosensitivity, conjunctival and scleral injection, pruritus, urticaria and rash. In addition, periarteritis nodosa and systemic lupus erythematosus have been reported.

Gastrointestinal: Hepatitis including cholestatic jaundice and hepatic and hepatic necrosis, elevation of serum transaminase and bilirubin, pseudomembranous, enterocolitis, pancreatitis, stomatitis, glossitis, nausea, emesis, abdominal pain, diarrhea, anorexia.

Genitourinary: Renal failure, interstitial nephritis, BUN and serum creatinine elevation, toxic nephrosis with oliguria and anuria, and crystalluria.

Neurologic: Convulsions, peripheral neuritis, ataxia, vertigo, tinnitus, headache.

Psychiatric: Hallucinations, depression, apathy, nervousness.

Endocrine: The sulfonamides bear certain chemical similarities to some goitrogens, diuretics (acetazolamide and the thiazides) and oral hypoglycemic agents. Cross-sensitivity may exist with these agents. Diuresis and hypoglycemia have occurred rarely in patients receiving sulfonamides.

Musculoskeletal: Arthralgia and myalgia.

Miscellaneous: Weakness, fatigue, insomnia.

OVERDOSAGE

Acute—The amount of a single dose of sulfamethoxazole and trimethoprim that is either associated with symptoms of overdosage or is likely to be life-threatening has not been reported. Signs and symptoms of overdosage reported with sulfonamides include anorexia, colic, nausea, vomiting, dizziness, headache, drowsiness and unconsciousness. Pyrexia, hematuria and crystalluria may be noted. Blood dyscrasias and jaundice are potential late manifestations of overdosage. Signs of acute overdosage with trimethoprim include nausea, vomiting, dizziness, headache, mental depression, confusion and bone marrow depression.

General principles of treatment include the institution of gastric lavage or emesis; forcing oral fluids; and the administration of intravenous fluids if urine output is low and renal function is normal. Acidification of the urine will increase renal elimination of trimethoprim. The patient should be monitored with blood counts and appropriate blood chemistries, including electrolytes. If a significant blood dyscrasia or jaundice occurs, specific therapy should be instituted for these complications. Peritoneal dialysis is not effective and hemodialysis is only moderately effective in eliminating trimethoprim and sulfamethoxazole.

Chronic—Use of sulfamethoxazole and trimethoprim at high doses and/or for extended periods of time may cause bone marrow depression manifested as thrombocytopenia, leukopenia and/or megaloblastic anemia. If signs of bone marrow depression occur, the patient should be given leucovorin 5 to 15 mg daily until normal hematopoiesis is restored.

DOSAGE AND ADMINISTRATION

Not recommended for use in infants less than two months of age.

Urinary Tract Infections and Shigellosis in Adults and Children, and Acute Otitis Media in Children—

Adults: The usual adult dosage in the treatment of urinary tract infections is one sulfamethoxazole and trimethoprim DS (double strength) tablet, or two sulfamethoxazole and trimethoprim tablets, every 12 hours for 10 to 14 days. An identical daily dosage is used for 5 days in the treatment of shigellosis.

Children: The recommended dose for children with urinary tract infections or acute otitis media is 40 mg/kg sulfamethoazole and 8 mg/kg trimethoprim per 24 hours, given in two divided doses every 12 hours for 10 days. An identical daily dosage is used for 5 days in the treatment of shigellosis. The following table is a guideline for the attainment of this dosage.

Children two months of age or older:

Weight lb	Weight kg	Dose—every 12 hours Tablets
44	20	1
66	30	1½
88	40	2 (or 1 DS tablet)

For patients with impaired renal function: When renal function is impaired, a reduced dosage should be employed using the following table:

Creatinine Clearance (mL/min)	Recommended Dosage Regimen
above 30	standard regimen
15–30	½ the usual regimen
below 15	use not recommended

Acute Exacerbations of Chronic Bronchitis in Adults—The usual adult dosage in the treatment of acute exacerbations of chronic bronchitis is one sulfamethoxazole and trimethoprim DS (double strength) tablet, or two sufamethoxazole and trimethoprim tablets every 12 hours for 14 days.

***Pneumocystis carinii* Pneumonitis**—The recommended dosage for patients with *Pneumocystis carinii* pneumonitis is 100 mg/kg sulfamethoxazole and 20 mg/kg trimethoprim per 24 hours given in equally divided doses every 6 hours for 14 days. The following table is a guideline for attainment of this dosage in children.

Weight lb	Weight kg	Dose—every 6 hours Tablets
35	16	1
53	24	1½
70	32	2 (or 1 DS tablet)

HOW SUPPLIED

COMOXOL (Sulfamethoxazole and Trimethoprim Tablets USP)

COMOXOL 400/80

Sulfamethoxazole 400 mg and trimethoprim 80 mg per tablet. White, round-shaped tablets in bottles of 100 and 500. Imprinted: upper side, SQUIBB; lower side, **872.**

COMOXOL 800/160, Double Strength

Sulfamethoxazole 800 mg and trimethoprim 160 mg per tablet. White, capsule-shaped tablets in bottles of 100 and 500. Imprinted: upper side, SQUIBB; lower side, **873.**

Storage: Store at controlled room temperature 15°–30° C (59°–86° F). Dispense in well-closed, light-resistant, child-proof containers.

REFERENCES

1. Kremers P, Duvivier J, Heusghem C: Pharmacokinetic Studies of Co-Trimoxazole in Man after Single and Repeated Doses. J Clin Pharmacol 14:112–117, 1974.
2. Kaplan SA, et al: Pharmacokinetic Profile of Trimethoprim-Sulfamethoxazole in Man. J Infect Dis 128:S547–S554, November 1973.
3. Federal Register, 37:20527–20529, 1972.
4. Bauer AW, Kirby WMM, Sherris JC, Turck M: Antibiotic Susceptibility Testing by Standardized Single Disk Method. Am J Clin Path 45:493–496, April 1966.
5. Brumfitt W and Pursell R: Trimethoprim/Sulfamethoxazole in the Treatment of Bacteriuria in Women. J Infect Dis 128 (Suppl):S657–S663, November 1973.

(J4-007B)

Shown in Product Identification Section, page 431

CRYSTICILLIN® 300 A.S. ℞
CRYSTICILLIN® 600 A.S. ℞

[*kris "ti-sil 'in*]

(Sterile Penicillin G Procaine Suspension USP)

DESCRIPTION

Crysticillin 300 A.S. and Crysticillin 600 A.S. are aqueous suspensions providing 300,000 u per mL and 600,000 u per 1.2 mL (500,000 u/mL) penicillin G procaine, respectively. The vials providing 300,000 u per mL also contain 0.13% methylparaben, 0.02% propylparaben, and 0.25% phenol as preservatives; 0.5% lecithin; 0.5% povidone; 1% sodium citrate; not more than 0.01% sodium formaldehyde sulfoxylate; and 0.075% carboxymethylcellulose sodium. The vials providing 600,000 u per 1.2 mL also contain 0.13% methylparaben, 0.02% propylparaben, and 0.18% phenol as preservatives; 0.3% povidone; 1% sodium citrate; 0.05% sodium carboxymethylcellulose; not more than 0.03% sodium formaldehyde sulfoxylate; and 2.3% lecithin.

CLINICAL PHARMACOLOGY

Penicillin G is bactericidal against penicillin-susceptible microorganisms during the stage of active multiplication. It acts by inhibiting biosynthesis of cell-wall mucopeptide. It is not active against the penicillinase-producing bacteria, which include many strains of staphylococci. Penicillin G is highly active *in vitro* against staphylococci (except penicillinase-producing strains), streptococci (groups A, C, G, H, L, and M), and pneumococci. Other organisms susceptible *in vitro* to penicillin G are *Neisseria gonorrhoeae, Corynebacterium diphtheriae, Bacillus anthracis,* Clostridia, *Actinomyces bovis, Streptobacillus moniliformis, Listeria monocytogenes,* and Leptospira; *Treponema pallidum* is extremely susceptible.

Susceptibility plate testing: If the Kirby-Bauer method of disc susceptibility is used, a 10 u penicillin disc should give a zone greater than 28 mm when tested against a penicillin-susceptible bacterial strain.

Penicillin G procaine is an equimolar compound of procaine and penicillin G administered intramuscularly as a suspension. It dissolves slowly at the site of injection, giving a plateau type of blood level at about four hours which falls slowly during the next 15 to 20 hours.

Approximately 60 percent of penicillin G is bound to serum protein. The drug is distributed throughout the body tissues in widely varying amounts. Highest levels are found in the kidneys with lesser amounts in the liver, skin, and intestines. Penicillin G penetrates into all other tissues to a lesser degree with a very small level found in the cerebrospinal fluid. The drug is excreted rapidly by tubular excretion in patients with normal kidney function. In neonates and young infants, and in individuals with impaired kidney function, excretion is considerably delayed. Approximately 60 to 90 percent of a dose of parenteral penicillin G is excreted in the urine within 24 to 36 hours.

INDICATIONS AND USAGE

Crysticillin 300 A.S. and Crysticillin 600 A.S. (Sterile Penicillin G Procaine Suspension USP) are indicated in the treatment of moderately severe infections due to penicillin G-susceptible microorganisms. Therapy should be guided by bacteriological studies, including susceptibility tests, and by clinical response. Note: severe pneumonia, empyema, bacteremia, pericarditis, meningitis, peritonitis, and septic arthritis are better treated with aqueous penicillin G during the acute stage; when high, sustained serum levels are required, aqueous penicillin G, either IM or IV should be used.

The following infections will usually respond to adequate dosage:

Streptococcal infections Group A without bacteremia—Moderately severe to severe infections of the upper respiratory tract, skin and skin structures infections, scarlet fever, and erysipelas. Note: streptococci in groups A, C, G, H, L, and M are very susceptible to penicillin G. Other groups, including group D (enterococcus) are resistant. Aqueous penicillin is recommended for streptococcal infections with bacteremia.

Pneumococcal infections—Moderately severe infections of the respiratory tract.

Staphylococcal infections—penicillin G susceptible—Moderately severe infections of the skin and skin structures. Note: reports indicate an increasing number of strains of staphylococci resistant to penicillin G, emphasizing the need for culture and susceptibility studies in treating suspected staphylococcal infections. Indicated surgical procedures should be performed.

Vincent's gingivitis and pharyngitis (fusospirochetosis)—Moderately severe infections of the oropharynx. Note: necessary dental care should be accomplished in infections involving the gum tissue.

Syphilis (*T. pallidum*)—All stages; **Gonorrheal infections** (acute and chronic—without bacteremia)—With adequate recommended doses; **Treponema**—Yaws, Bejel, Pinta; **Diphtheria**—as an adjunct to antitoxin for the prevention of the carrier state; **Anthrax; Rat-bite fever** (*S. moniliformis* and *S. minus*); **Erysipeloid.**

Subacute bacterial endocarditis (group A streptococcus)—Only in extremely susceptible infections.

CONTRAINDICATIONS

Contraindicated in patients with a history of hypersensitivity to procaine or any penicillin.

WARNINGS

Serious and occasional fatal hypersensitivity (anaphylactoid) reactions have been reported in patients on penicillin therapy. Although anaphylaxis is more frequent following parenteral administration, it has occurred in patients on oral penicillins. These reactions are more apt to occur in individuals with a history of sensitivity to multiple allergens.

There have been well-documented reports of individuals with a history of penicillin hypersensitivity who have experienced severe hypersensitivity reactions when treated with cephalosporins. Before therapy with a penicillin, careful inquiry should be made concerning previous hypersensitivity reactions to penicillins, cephalosporins, and other allergens. If an allergic reaction occurs, the drug should be discontinued and the patient treated with the usual agents, e.g., pressor amines, antihistamines, and corticosteroids. Serious anaphylactoid reactions are not controlled by antihistamines alone, and require such emergency measures as the immediate use of epinephrine, aminophylline, oxygen, and intravenous corticosteroids.

Immediate toxic reactions to procaine may occur in some individuals, particularly when a large single dose is administered in the treatment of gonorrhea (4.8 million u). These reactions may be manifested by mental disturbances including anxiety, confusion, agitation, depression, weakness, seizures, hallucinations, combativeness, and expressed "fear of impending death." The reactions noted in carefully controlled studies occurred in approximately one in 500 patients treated for gonorrhea. Reactions are transient, lasting from 15 to 30 minutes.

PRECAUTIONS

Penicillin should be used with caution in individuals with histories of significant allergies and/or asthma.

A small percentage of patients are sensitive to procaine. If there is a history of sensitivity, make the usual test: inject intradermally 0.1 mL of a 1 to 2% procaine hydrochloride solution. Development of an erythema, wheal, flare or eruption indicates procaine sensitivity. Sensitivity should be treated by the usual methods, and procaine penicillin preparations should not be used. Antihistamines appear beneficial in the treatment of procaine reactions.

The use of antibiotics may result in overgrowth of nonsusceptible organisms. Constant observation of the patient is essential. If new infections due to bacteria or fungi appear during therapy, the drug should be discontinued and appropriate measures taken. Whenever allergic reactions occur, penicillin should be withdrawn unless, in the opinion of the physician, the condition being treated is life-threatening and amenable only to penicillin therapy.

Care should be taken to avoid accidental intravenous administration.

In prolonged therapy with penicillin, and particularly with high dosage schedules, periodic evaluation of the renal and hematopoietic systems is recommended.

In streptococcal infections, therapy must be sufficient to eliminate the organism (10 days minimum); otherwise the sequelae of streptococcal disease may occur. Cultures should be taken following the completion of treatment to determine whether streptococci have been eradicated.

In suspected staphylococcal infections, proper laboratory studies, including susceptibility tests, should be performed.

When treating gonococcal infections in which primary or secondary syphilis may be suspected, proper diagnostic procedures, including darkfield examinations, should be done. In all cases in which concomitant syphilis is suspected, monthly serological tests should be made for at least four months. All cases of penicillin-treated syphilis should receive clinical and serological examinations every six months for at least two or three years.

ADVERSE REACTIONS

Penicillin is a substance of low toxicity, but does possess a significant index of sensitization. The hypersensitivity reactions reported are skin rashes ranging from maculopapular eruptions to exfoliative dermatitis; urticaria; and serum sickness-like reactions including chills, fever, edema, arthralgia, and prostration. Hemolytic anemia, leukopenia, thrombocytopenia, neuropathy, and nephropathy are infrequent reactions and are usually associated with high doses of parenteral penicillin. Severe and often fatal anaphylaxis has been reported; these reactions require emergency measures (see WARNINGS). As with other treatments for syphilis, the Jarisch-Herxheimer reaction has been reported.

Procaine toxicity manifestations have been reported (see WARNINGS). Procaine hypersensitivity reactions have not been reported with this drug.

DOSAGE AND ADMINISTRATION

For intramuscular use only

The product is ready for immediate injection after vigorous shaking of the vial to insure a uniform suspension.

Injection is made rapidly by the intramuscular route. The preferred site is the upper outer quadrant of the gluteal area. Injections are easier to make and there is less likelihood of needle blockage if a small bore syringe is used; use a 20-gauge needle. Avoid using a syringe with a loosely-fitting plunger as crystals may creep between the walls and cause it to "freeze". Remove the needle and plunger from the syringe soon after injection to prevent "freezing" of the remaining crystals.

The usual dosage recommendation is as follows:

Streptococcal infections (Group A)—moderately severe to severe tonsillitis, erysipelas, scarlet fever, infections of the upper respiratory tract, and skin and skin structures infections: 600,000 to 1,200,000 u daily for a minimum of 10 days.

Pneumococcal infections (uncomplicated)— moderately severe: 600,000 to 1,200,000 u daily.

Staphylococcal infections—moderately severe to severe: 600,000 to 1,200,000 u daily.

Vincent's gingivitis and pharyngitis (fusospirochetosis): 600,000 to 1,200,000 u daily.

Syphilis—*Primary, secondary and latent* with a negative spinal fluid in adults and children over 12 years of age: 600,000 u daily for eight days—total 4,800,000 u; *Late* (tertiary, neurosyphilis and latent syphilis with positive or no spinal fluid examination): 600,000 u daily for 10 to 15 days—total 6 to 9 million u; *Congenital* (under 32 kg [70 lb] body weight): 10,000 u/kg/day for 10 days.

Gonorrheal infections (uncomplicated): 4.8 million u divided into at least two doses at one visit for males and females; one gram of oral probenecid is given 30 minutes before the injections. Follow-up cultures should be obtained from the original site(s) of infection 7 to 14 days after therapy. In women, it is also desirable to obtain culture test-of-cure from both the endocervical and anal canals. Note: gonorrheal endocarditis should be treated intensively with aqueous penicillin G.

Yaws, Bejel, and Pinta—treat same as syphilis in corresponding stage of disease.

Diphtheria—*adjunctive therapy with antitoxin:* 300,000 to 600,000 u daily; **Anthrax**—cutaneous: 600,000 to 1,200,000 u daily; **Rat-bite fever** (*S. moniliformis* and *S. minus*) and **Erysipeloid**: 600,000 to 1,200,000 u daily.

Bacterial endocarditis (group A streptococcus) —only in extremely susceptible infections: 600,000 to 1,200,000 u daily.

HOW SUPPLIED

Crysticillin 300 A.S. (Sterile Penicillin G Procaine Suspension USP) is available in 10 mL vials; Crysticillin 600 A.S. is available in 12 mL vials.

Storage: Store below 15° C. (59° F.); avoid freezing.

(J2-661D/662D)

ETHRIL® '250' ℞
ETHRIL® '500' ℞

Erythromycin Stearate Tablets USP

DESCRIPTION

Erythromycin is produced by a strain of *Streptomyces erythreus* and belongs to the macrolide group of antibiotics. It is basic and readily forms salts with acids. The base, the stearate salt, and the esters are poorly soluble in water and are suitable for oral administration

Ethril '250' and Ethril '500' tablets (Erythromycin Stearate Tablets) are available for oral administration as FILMLOK tablets providing erythromycin stearate equivalent to 250 mg and 500 mg erythromycin, respectively. Inactive ingredients: calcium stearate, cellulose, colorants [FD&C Yellow No. 5 (tartrazine) in the 500 mg tablets only; FD&C Red No. 3], flavor, polacrilin potassium, povidone, sodium citrate, and other ingredients.

CLINICAL PHARMACOLOGY

Erythromycin is a protein-synthesis inhibitor—without, itself, affecting nucleic acid synthesis. Resistance to erythromycin by some strains of *Hemophilus influenzae* and staphylococci has been demonstrated. Culture and susceptibility testing should be done. If the Kirby-Bauer method of disc susceptibility is used, a 15 mcg erythromycin disc should give a zone diameter of at least 18 mm when tested against an erythromycin-susceptible organism.

Orally administered erythromycin is readily absorbed by most patients, especially on an empty stomach, but patient variation has been observed.

After absorption, erythromycin diffuses readily into most body fluids. In the absence of meningeal inflammation, low concentrations are normally achieved in the spinal fluid, but passage of the drug across the blood-brain barrier increases in meningitis. In the presence of normal hepatic function, erythromycin is concentrated in the liver and excreted in the bile; the effect of hepatic dysfunction on excretion of erythromycin by the liver into the bile is not known. After oral administration, less than 5 percent of the activity of the administered dose can be recovered in the urine.

Erythromycin crosses the placental barrier, but fetal plasma levels are low.

INDICATIONS AND USAGE

Streptococcus pyogenes (Group A beta-hemolytic streptococci): Upper and lower respiratory tract, skin, and skin structures infections of mild to moderate severity.

Sterile Penicillin G Benzathine Suspension USP is considered by the American Heart Association to be the drug of choice in the treatment and prevention of streptococcal pharyngitis and in long-term prophylaxis of rheumatic fever. When oral medication is preferred for the treatment of streptococcal pharyngitis, penicillin G. V. or erythromycin are alternate drugs of choice. When oral medication is given, the importance of strict adherence to the prescribed dosage regimen by the patient must be stressed. A therapeutic dose should be administered for at least 10 days.

Prevention of bacterial endocarditis: Although no controlled efficacy trials have been conducted, oral erythromycin has been suggested by the American Heart Association and the American Dental Association for use in a regimen for prophylaxis against bacterial endocarditis in patients hypersensitive to penicillin who have congenital heart disease or rheumatic or other acquired valvular heart disease when they undergo dental procedures and surgical procedures of

Continued on next page

Squibb—Cont.

the upper respiratory tract.[1] Erythromycin is not suitable prior to genitourinary or gastrointestinal tract surgery. **NOTE: When selecting antibiotics for the prevention of bacterial endocarditis the physician or dentist should read the full joint statement of the American Heart Association and the American Dental Association.[1] Staphylococcus aureus:** Acute infections of skin and skin structures of mild to moderate severity. Resistance may develop during treatment.[1] **Streptococcus pneumoniae** (formerly *Diplococcus pneumoniae*): Upper respiratory tract infections (e.g., otitis media, pharyngitis) and lower respiratory tract infections (e.g., pneumonia) of mild to moderate degree. **Mycoplasma pneumoniae** (Eaton agent, PPLO): In the treatment of primary atypical pneumonia, when due to this organism. **Hemophilus influenzae:** Upper respiratory tract infections of mild to moderate severity when used concomitantly with adequate doses of sulfonamides. Not all strains of this organism are susceptible at the erythromycin concentrations ordinarily achieved (see appropriate sulfonamide labeling for prescribing information). **Treponema pallidum:** Erythromycin is an alternate choice of treatment for primary syphilis in patients allergic to the penicillins. Patients who are suspected of having syphilis should have a microscopic examination for *T. pallidum* (by immunofluorescence or darkfield) before receiving erythromycin and monthly tests for a minimum of four months. In the treatment of primary syphilis, spinal fluid examinations should be done before treatment and as part of follow-up after therapy. **Corynebacterium diphtheriae** and **C. minutissimum:** As an adjunct to antitoxin, to prevent establishment of carriers and to eradicate the organism in carriers. In the treatment of erythrasma. **Entamoeba histolytica:** In the treatment of intestinal amebiasis only. Extraenteric amebiasis requires treatment with other agents. **Listeria monocytogenes:** Infections due to this organism. **Neisseria gonorrhoeae:** Erythromycin lactobionate for injection in conjunction with erythromycin stearate orally, as an alternative drug in the treatment of acute pelvic inflammatory disease caused by *N. gonorrhoeae* in female patients with a history of sensitivity to penicillin. Before treatment of gonorrhea, patients who are suspected of having syphilis should have a microscopic examination for *T. pallidum* (by immunofluorescence or darkfield) before receiving erythromycin and monthly tests for a minimum of four months. **Legionnaires' disease:** Although no controlled clinical efficacy studies have been conducted, *in vitro* and limited preliminary clinical data suggest that erythromycin may be effective in treating Legionnaires' disease. **Chlamydia trachomatis:** Erythromycins are indicated for treatment of urogenital infections during pregnancy caused by *Chlamydia trachomatis.* When tetracyclines are contraindicated or not tolerated, erythromycin is indicated for the treatment of uncomplicated urethreal, endocervical, or rectal infections in adults due to *Chlamydia trachomatis.*

CONTRINDICATIONS

Erythromycin is contraindicated in patients with known hypersensitivity to this antibiotic.

WARNING

Usage In Pregnancy: Safety for use in pregnancy has not been established.

PRECAUTIONS

Erythromycin is principally excreted by the liver. Caution should be exercised in administering the antibiotic to patients with impaired hepatic function. There have been reports of hepatic dysfunction, with or without jaundice, occurring in patients receiving oral erythromycin products.

Recent data from studies of erythromycin reveal that its use in patients who are receiving high doses of theophylline may be associated with an increase of serum theophylline levels and potential theophylline toxicity. In case of theophylline toxicity and/or elevated serum theophylline levels, the dose of theophylline should be reduced while the patient is receiving concomitant erythromycin therapy.

Surgical procedures should be performed when indicated.

Ethril '500' (Erythromycin Stearate Tablets USP) contain FD&C Yellow No. 5 (tartrazine) which may cause allergic-type reactions (including bronchial asthma) in certain susceptible individuals. Although the overall incidence of FD&C Yellow No. 5 (tartrazine) sensitivity in the general population is low, it is frequently seen in patients who also have aspirin hypersensitivity.

ADVERSE REACTIONS

The most frequent side effects of erythromycin preparations are gastrointestinal, such as abdominal cramping and discomfort; these are dose related. Nausea, vomiting, and diarrhea occur infrequently with usual oral doses.

During prolonged or repeated therapy, there is a possibility of overgrowth of nonsusceptible bacteria or fungi. If such infections occur, the drug should be discontinued and appropriate therapy instituted.

Mild allergic reactions such as urticaria and other skin rashes have occurred. Serious allergic reactions, including anaphylaxis, have been reported.

There have been isolated reports of reversible hearing loss occurring chiefly in patients with renal insufficiency and in patients receiving high doses of erythromycin.

DOSAGE AND ADMINISTRATION

Optimum blood levels are obtained when doses are given on an empty stomach.

Adults: The usual dose is 250 mg every six hours. Dosage may be increased up to 4 or more grams per day according to the severity of the infection.

Children: Age, weight, and severity of the infection are important factors in determining the proper dosage. The usual dosage, in divided doses, is 30 to 50 mg/kg/day. For more severe infections this dose may be doubled.

If dosage is desired on a twice-a-day schedule in either adults or children, one half of the total daily dose may be given every 12 hours, one hour before meals.

In the treatment of streptococcal infections, a therapeutic dosage of erythromycin should be administered for at least 10 days. In continuous *prophylaxis* of streptococcal infections in persons with a history of rheumatic heart disease, the dose is 250 mg twice a day.

For prophylaxis against bacterial endocarditis[1] in patients with congenital heart disease or rheumatic or other acquired valvular heart disease when undergoing dental procedures or surgical procedures of the upper respiratory tract, give 1 g (20 mg/kg for children) orally one hour before the procedure, and then 500 mg (10 mg/kg for children) orally six hours later. Children's total doses should not exceed the maximum adult dosages.

For treatment of primary syphilis, the dose is 30 to 40 g given in divided doses over a period of 10 to 15 days.

For treatment of acute pelvic inflammatory disease caused by *N. gonorrhoeae*, 500 mg erythromycin lactobionate for injection every six hours for three days, followed by one Ethril '250' every six hours for seven days.

For dysenteric amebiasis, the dose for adults is 250 mg four times daily for 10 to 14 days; for children, the dose is 30 to 50 mg/kg/day in divided doses for 10 to 14 days.

For treatment of Legionnaires' disease: Although optimal doses have not been established, doses utilized in reported clinical data were 1 to 4 grams erythromycin stearate or base daily in divided does.

Urogenital infections during pregnancy due to Chlamydia trachomatis: Although the optimal dose and duration of therapy have not been established, the suggested treatment is erythromycin 500 mg, by mouth, four times a day on an empty stomach for at least seven days. For women who cannot tolerate this regimen, a decreased dose of 250 mg, by mouth, four times a day should be used for at least 14 days.[2]

For adults with uncomplicated urethral, endocervical, or rectal infections caused by Chlamydia trachomatic in whom tetracyclines are contraindicated or not tolerated: 500 mg, by mouth, four times a day for at least seven days.[2]

HOW SUPPLIED

Ethril '250' and Ethril '500' (Erythromycin Stearate Tablets USP) are avaialable for oral administration as FILMLOK®* tablets providing erythromycin stearate equivalent to 250 mg and 500 mg erythromycin, respectively.

Storage: Store at room temperature; avoid excessive heat. Keep from light to prevent discoloration.

REFERENCES

1. American Heart Association: Prevention of bacterial endocarditis. Circulation 70: 1123A–1127A, 1984.
2. CDC Sexually Transmitted Diseases Treatment Guidelines 1982.

* FILMLOK is a Squibb trademark for veneer-coated tablets.
(J2–594H)

FUNGIZONE® ℞

[fun'ji-zōn]
(Amphotericin B)
CREAM/LOTION/OINTMENT

DESCRIPTION

Fungizone Cream (Amphotericin B Cream USP) contains the antifungal antibiotic Amphotericin B USP at a concentration of 3% (30 mg/gram) in a pleasantly tinted aqueous vehicle, which also contains titanium dioxide, thimerosal, propylene glycol, cetearyl alcohol (and) ceteareth-20, white petrolatum, methylparaben, propylparaben, sorbitol solution, glyceryl monostearate, polyethylene glycol monostearate, simethicone, and sorbic acid.

Fungizone Lotion (Amphotericin B Lotion USP) contains the antifungal antibiotic Amphotericin B USP at a concentration of 3% (30 mg/mL) in a tinted aqueous lotion vehicle, which is pleasantly scented, and also contains thimerosal, titanium dioxide, guar gum, propylene glycol, cetyl alcohol, stearyl alcohol, sorbitan monopalmitate, polysorbate 20, glyceryl monostearate, polyethylene glycol monostearate, simethicone, sorbic acid, methylparaben, and propylparaben.

Fungizone Ointment (Amphotericin B Ointment USP) contains the antifungal antibiotic Amphotericin B USP at a concentration of 3% (30 mg/gram) in a tinted form of Plastibase® (Plasticized Hydrocarbon Gel), a polyethylene and mineral oil gel base with titanium dioxide.

CLINICAL PHARMACOLOGY

Amphotericin B is an antibiotic with antifungal activity which is produced by a strain of *Streptomyces nodosus.* It has been shown to exhibit greater *in vitro* activity than nystatin against *Candida* (Monilia) *albicans.* In clinical studies involving cutaneous and mucocutaneous candidal infections, results with topical preparations of amphotericin B were comparable to those obtained with nystatin in similar formulations.

Although amphotericin B exhibits some *in vitro* activity against the superficial dermatophytes (ringworm organisms), it has not demonstrated an effectiveness *in vivo* on topical application. Amphotericin B has no significant effect either *in vitro* or clinically against gram-positive or gram-negative bacteria, or viruses.

INDICATIONS AND USAGE

Fungizone (Amphotericin B) topical preparations are indicated in the treatment of cutaneous and mucocutaneous mycotic infections caused by Candida (Monilia) species.

CONTRAINDICATIONS

The preparations are contraindicated in patients with a history of hypersensitivity to any of their components.

PRECAUTIONS

Should a reaction of hypersensitivity occur the drug should be immediately withdrawn and appropriate measures taken.

ADVERSE REACTIONS

Fungizone Cream (Amphotericin B Cream USP)—No evidence of any systemic toxicity or side effects has been observed during or following the use of the Cream. The preparation is usually well tolerated by all age groups. It is not a primary irritant and apparently has only a slight sensitizing potential. It may have a "drying" effect on some skin, and local irritation characterized by erythema, pruritus, or a burning sensation sometimes occurs, particularly in intertriginous areas.

Fungizone Lotion (Amphotericin B Lotion USP)—No evidence of any systemic toxicity or side effects has been observed during or following even prolonged, intensive and extensive application of the Lotion. The preparation is extremely well tolerated by all age groups, including infants, even when therapy must be continued for many months. It is not a primary irritant and apparently has only a slight sensitizing potential. Local intolerance, which seldom occurs, has included increased pruritus with or without other subjective or objective evidence of local irritation, or exacerbation of preexisting candidal lesions. Allergic contact dermatitis is rare.

Fungizone Ointment (Amphotericin B Ointment USP)—No evidence of any systemic toxicity or side effects has been observed during or following even prolonged, intensive and extensive application of the Ointment. The preparation is usually well tolerated by all age groups. It is not a primary irritant and apparently has only a slight sensitizing potential. However, it is well to remember that any oleaginous ointment vehicle may occasionally irritate when applied to moist, intertriginous areas.

DOSAGE AND ADMINISTRATION

Fungizone (Amphotericin B) Cream, Lotion, or Ointment should be applied liberally to the candidal lesions two to four times daily. Duration of therapy depends on individual patient response. Intertriginous lesions usually respond within a few days, and treatment may be completed in one to three weeks. Similarly, candidiasis of the diaper area, perleche, and glabrous skin lesions usually clear in one to two weeks. Interdigital (erosio) lesions may require two to four weeks of intensive therapy; paronychias also require relatively prolonged therapy, and those onychomycoses which respond may require several months or more of treatment. (Relapses are frequently encountered in the last three clinical conditions.)

NOTE: When rubbed into the lesion, the Cream discolors the skin minimally. The Lotion and Ointment do not stain the skin when thoroughly rubbed into the lesion although nail lesions may be stained. The patient should be informed that any discoloration of fabrics from the Cream may be removed by hand-washing the fabric with soap and warm water, that any discoloration of fabrics from the Lotion is readily removed with soap and warm water, or that any discoloration of fabrics from the Ointment may be removed by applying a standard cleaning fluid.

HOW SUPPLIED

Fungizone Cream (Amphotericin B Cream USP) is supplied in tubes of 20 grams.

Fungizone Lotion (Amphotericin B Lotion USP) is supplied in 30 mL plastic squeeze bottles (Military Depot Item, NSN 6505-00-890-1486).

Fungizone Ointment (Amphotericin B Ointment USP) is supplied in tubes of 20 grams.

Storage: Store the Cream and Lotion at room temperature; avoid freezing. Store the Ointment at room temperature.
(J2-224E/J3-521/J2-151D)

FUNGIZONE® INTRAVENOUS ℞

[fun'ji-zōn]
(Amphotericin B for Injection USP)

WARNING
This drug should be used *primarily* for treatment of patients with progressive and potentially fatal fungal infections; it should not be used to treat the common clinically inapparent forms of fungal disease which show only positive skin or serologic tests.

DESCRIPTION

Fungizone Intravenous (Amphotericin B for Injection USP) is an antifungal antibiotic derived from a strain of *Streptomyces nodosus.* Crystalline amphotericin B is insoluble in water; therefore, the antibiotic is "solubilized" by the addition of sodium desoxycholate to form a mixture which provides a colloidal dispersion for parenteral administration.

ACTIONS

Microbiology

Amphotericin B shows a high order of *in vitro* activity against many species of fungi. *Histoplasma capsulatum, Coccidiodes immitis, Candida* species, *Blastomyces dermatitidis, Rhodotorula, Cryptococcus neoformans, Sporotrichum schenckii, Mucor mucedo,* and *Aspergillus fumigatus* are all inhibited by concentrations of amphotericin B ranging from 0.03 to 1.0 mcg/mL *in vitro.* The antibiotic is without effect on bacteria, rickettsiae, and viruses.

Clinical Pharmacology

Amphotericin B is fungistatic or fungicidal depending on the concentration obtained in body fluids and the susceptibility of the fungus. The drug probably acts by binding to sterols in the fungus cell membrane with a resultant change in membrane permeability which allows leakage of a variety of small molecules. Mammalian cell membranes also contain sterols and it has been suggested that the damage to human cells and fungal cells may share common mechanisms.

An initial intravenous infusion of 1 to 5 mg of amphotericin B per day, gradually increased to 0.65 mg/kg daily, produces peak plasma concentrations of approximately 2 to 4 mcg/mL which can persist between doses since the plasma half-life of amphotericin B is about 24 hours. (For recommended dosages, see the DOSAGE AND ADMINISTRATION section.) It has been reported that amphotericin B is highly bound (>90%) to plasma proteins and is poorly dialyzable.

Amphotericin B is excreted very slowly by the kidneys with two to five percent of a given dose being excreted in biologically active form. After treatment is discontinued, the drug can be detected in the urine for at least seven weeks. The cumulative urinary output over a seven-day period amounts to approximately 40 percent of the amount of drug infused. Details of tissue distribution and possible metabolic pathways are not known.

INDICATIONS

Fungizone Intravenous should be administered primarily to patients with progressive, potentially fatal infections. This potent drug should not be used to treat the common inapparent forms of fungal disease which show only positive skin or serologic tests.

Fungizone Intravenous (Amphotericin B for Injection USP) is specifically intended to treat cryptococcosis (torulosis); North American blastomycosis; the disseminated forms of moniliasis, coccidioidomycosis, and histoplasmosis; mucormycosis (phycomycosis) caused by species of the genera *Mucor, Rhizopus, Absidia, Entomophthora,* and *Basidiobolus;* sporotrichosis (*Sporothrix schenckii* [formerly *Sporotrichum schenckii*]); aspergillosis (*Aspergillus fumigatus*).

Amphotericin B may be helpful in the treatment of American mucocutaneous leishmaniasis, but is not the drug of choice in primary therapy.

CONTRAINDICATIONS

This product is contraindicated in those patients who have shown hypersensitivity to it unless, in the opinion of the physician, the condition requiring treatment is life-threatening and amenable only to amphotericin B therapy.

WARNINGS

Amphotericin B is frequently the only effective treatment available for potentially fatal fungal disease. In each case, its possible life-saving benefit must be balanced against its untoward and dangerous side effects.

Usage in Pregnancy: Safety for use in pregnancy has not been established; therefore, it should be used during pregnancy only if the possible benefits to be derived outweigh the potential risks involved.

PRECAUTIONS

Prolonged therapy with amphotericin B is usually necessary. Unpleasant reactions are quite common when the drug is given parenterally at therapeutic dosage levels. **Some of these reactions are potentially dangerous.** Hence, amphotericin B should be used parenterally only in hospitalized patients or those under close clinical observation by medically trained personnel and should be reserved for those patients in whom a diagnosis of the progressive, potentially fatal forms of susceptible mycotic infections has been firmly established, preferably by positive culture or histologic study.

Corticosteroids should not be administered concomitantly unless they are necessary to control drug reactions. Other nephrotoxic antibiotics and antineoplastic agents such as nitrogen mustard should not be given concomitantly except with great caution.

Laboratory facilities must be available to perform blood urea nitrogen and serum creatinine or endogenous creatinine clearance tests. These determinations should be made at least weekly during therapy. If the BUN exceeds 40 mg per 100 mL or the serum creatinine exceeds 3.0 mg per 100 mL the drug should be discontinued or the dosage markedly reduced until renal function is improved. Weekly hemograms and serum potassium determinations are also advisable. Low serum magnesium levels have also been noted during treatment with amphotericin B. Therapy should be discontinued if liver function test results (elevated bromsulphalein, alkaline phosphatase and bilirubin) are abnormal.

Whenever medication is interrupted for a period longer than seven days, therapy should be resumed by starting with the lowest dosage level, e.g., 0.25 mg/kg of body weight, and increased gradually as outlined under DOSAGE AND ADMINISTRATION.

ADVERSE REACTIONS

While some few patients may tolerate full intravenous doses of amphotericin B without difficulty, most will exhibit some intolerance, often at less than the full therapeutic dosage. They may be made less severe by giving aspirin, antihistamines, and antiemetics. Administration of the drug on alternate days may decrease anorexia and phlebitis. Intravenous administration of small doses of adrenal corticosteroids just prior to or during the amphotericin B infusion may decrease febrile reactions. The dosage and duration of such corticosteroid therapy should be kept to a minimum. Adding a small amount of heparin to the infusion may lessen the incidence of thrombophlebitis. Extravasation may cause chemical irritation.

The adverse reactions that are most commonly observed are: fever (sometimes with shaking chills); headache; anorexia; weight loss; nausea and vomiting; malaise; dyspepsia; diarrhea; generalized pain including muscle and joint pains, cramping epigastric pain, and local venous pain at the injection site with phlebitis and thrombophlebitis; and normochromic, normocytic anemia. Abnormal renal function including hypokalemia, azotemia, hyposthenuria, renal tubular acidosis and nephrocalcinosis is also commonly observed, and usually improves upon interruption of therapy; however, some permanent impairment often occurs, especially in those patients receiving large amounts (over 5 g) of amphotericin B. Supplemental alkali medication may decrease renal tubular acidosis complications.

The following adverse reactions occur less frequently or rarely: anuria; oliguria; cardiovascular toxicity including arrhythmias, ventricular fibrillation, cardiac arrest, hypertension, and hypotension; coagulation defects; thrombocytopenia; leukopenia; agranulocytosis; eosinophilia; leukocytosis; melena or hemorrhagic gastroenteritis; maculopapular rash; hearing loss; tinnitus; transient vertigo; blurred vision or diplopia; peripheral neuropathy; convulsions and other neurologic symptoms; pruritus (without rash); anaphylactoid reactions; acute liver failure; and flushing.

DOSAGE AND ADMINISTRATION

Fungizone Intravenous (Amphotericin B for Injection USP) should be administered by *slow* intravenous infusion. Intravenous infusion should be given over a period of approximately six hours observing the usual precautions for intravenous therapy. The recommended concentration for intravenous infusion is 0.1 mg/mL (1 mg/10 mL).

Dosage must be adjusted to the specific requirements of each patient since tolerance to amphotericin B varies individually. Therapy is usually instituted with a daily dose of 0.25 mg/kg of body weight and **gradually** increased as tolerance permits. There are insufficient data presently available to define total dosage requirements and duration of treatment necessary for eradication of mycoses such as phycomycosis. The optimal dose is unknown. Total daily dosage may range up to 1.0 mg/kg of body weight or alternate day dosages ranging up to 1.5 mg/kg Several months of therapy are usually necessary; a shorter period of therapy may produce an inadequate response and lead to relapse.

CAUTION

Under no circumstances should a total daily dosage of 1.5 mg/kg be exceeded.

Therapy with intravenous amphotericin B for sporotrichosis has ranged up to nine months. The usual dose per injection is 20 mg.

Aspergillosis has been treated with amphotericin B intravenously for a period up to 11 months with a total dose up to 3.6 g.

Rhinocerebral phycomycosis, a fulminating disease, generally occurs in association with diabetic ketoacidosis. It is, therefore, imperative that rapid restoration of diabetic control be instituted before successful treatment with Fungizone Intravenous (Amphotericin B for Injection USP) can be accomplished. In contradistinction, pulmonary phycomycosis, which is more common in association with hematologic malignancies, is often an incidental finding at autopsy. A cumulative dose of at least 3 g of amphotericin B is recommended. Although a total dose of 3 to 4 g will infrequently cause lasting renal impairment, this would seem a reasonable minimum where there is clinical evidence of invasion of the deep tissues; since rhinocerebral phycomycosis usually follows a rapidly fatal course, the therapeutic approach must necessarily be more aggressive than that used in more indolent mycoses.

PREPARATION OF SOLUTIONS

Reconstitute as follows: An initial concentrate of 5 mg amphotericin B per mL is first prepared by rapidly expressing 10 mL Sterile Water for Injection USP *without a bacteriostatic agent* directly into the lyophilized cake, using a sterile needle (minimum diameter: 20 gauge) and syringe. Shake the vial immediately until the colloidal solution is clear. The infusion solution, providing 0.1 mg amphotericin B per mL, is then obtained by further dilution (1:50) with 5% Dextrose Injection USP *of pH above 4.2.* The pH of each container of Dextrose Injection should be ascertained before use. Commercial Dextrose Injection usually has a pH above 4.2; however, if it is below 4.2, then 1 or 2 mL of buffer should be added to the Dextrose Injection before it is used to dilute the concentrated solution of amphotericin B. The recommended buffer has the following composition:

Dibasic sodium phosphate (anhydrous)	1.59 g
Monobasic sodium phosphate (anhydrous)	0.96 g
Water for Injection USP	qs 100.0 mL

The buffer should be sterilized before it is added to the Dextrose Injection, either by filtration through a bacterial retentive stone, mat, or membrane, or by autoclaving for 30 minutes at 15 lb pressure (121° C.).

CAUTION

Aseptic technique must be strictly observed in all handling, since no preservative or bacteriostatic agent is present in the antibiotic or in the materials used to prepare it for administration. **All entries into the vial or into the diluents must be made with a sterile needle. Do not reconstitute with saline solutions. The use of any diluent other than the ones recommended or the presence of a bacteriostatic agent** (e.g., benzyl alcohol) **in the diluent may cause precipitation of the antibiotic. Do not use the initial concentrate or the infusion solution if there is any evidence of precipitation or foreign matter in either one.**

An in-line membrane filter may be used for intravenous infusion of amphotericin B; **however, the mean pore diameter of the filter should not be less than 1.0 micron in order to assure passage of the antibiotic dispersion.**

HOW SUPPLIED

Fungizone Intravenous is supplied in vials as a sterile lyophilized cake (which may partially reduce to powder following manufacture) providing 50 mg amphotericin B and 41 mg sodium desoxycholate with 20.2 mg sodium phosphates as a buffer. At the time of manufacture, the air in the container is replaced by nitrogen. [Military Depot Item: NSN 6505-01-084-9453.]

Storage: Prior to reconstitution, Fungizone Intravenous (Amphotericin B for injection USP) should be stored in the refrigerator, protected against exposure to light. The concentrate (5 mg amphotericin B per mL after reconstitution with 10 mL Sterile Water for Injection USP) may be stored in the dark, at room temperature for 24 hours, or at refrigerator temperatures for one week with minimal loss of potency and clarity. Any unused material should then be discarded. Solutions prepared for intravenous infusion (0.1 mg or less amphotericin B per mL) should be used promptly after preparation and should be protected from light during administration.
(J3-640)

Continued on next page

Squibb—Cont.

HYDREA® ℞
[hī″drē′ah]
(Hydroxyurea Capsules USP)

DESCRIPTION

Hydrea (Hydroxyurea Capsules USP) is an antineoplastic agent, available for oral use as capsules providing 500 mg hydroxyurea.
Inactive ingredients: citric acid, colorants (D&C Yellow No. 10; FD&C Blue No. 1 and Red No. 3), gelatin, lactose, magnesium stearate, sodium phosphate, and titanium dioxide. Hydroxyurea occurs as an essentially tasteless, white crystalline powder.

ACTIONS

Mechanism of Action
The precise mechanism by which hydroxyurea produces its cytotoxic effects cannot, at present, be described. However, the reports of various studies in tissue culture in rats and man lend support to the hypothesis that hydroxyurea causes an immediate inhibition of DNA synthesis without interfering with the synthesis of ribonucleic acid or of protein. This hypothesis explains why, under certain conditions, hydroxyurea may induce teratogenic effects.
Three mechanisms of action have been postulated for the increased effectiveness of concomitant use of hydroxyurea therapy with irradiation on squamous cell (epidermoid) carcinomas of the head and neck. *In vitro* studies utilizing Chinese hamster cells suggest that hydroxyurea (1) is lethal to normally radioresistant S-stage cells, and (2) holds other cells of the cell cycle in the G1 or pre-DNA synthesis stage where they are most susceptible to the effects of irradiation. The third mechanism of action has been theorized on the basis of *in vitro* studies of HeLa cells: it appears that hydroxyurea, by inhibition of DNA synthesis, hinders the normal repair process of cells damaged but not killed by irradiation, thereby decreasing their survival rate; RNA and protein syntheses have shown no alteration.
Absorption, Metabolism, Fate and Excretion
After oral administration in man, hydroxyurea is readily absorbed from the gastrointestinal tract. The drug reaches peak serum concentrations within 2 hours; by 24 hours the concentration in the serum is essentially zero. Approximately 80 percent of an oral or intravenous dose of 7 to 30 mg/kg may be recovered in the urine within 12 hours.
Animal Pharmacology and Toxicology
The oral LD_{50} of hydroxyurea is 7330 mg/kg in mice and 5780 mg/kg in rats, given as a single dose.
In subacute and chronic toxicity studies in the rat, the most consistent pathological findings were an apparent dose-related mild to moderate bone marrow hypoplasia as well as pulmonary congestion and mottling of the lungs. At the highest dosage levels (1260 mg/kg/day for 37 days then 2520 mg/kg/day for 40 days), testicular atrophy with absence of spermatogenesis occurred; in several animals, hepatic cell damage with fatty metamorphosis was noted. In the dog, mild to marked bone marrow depression was a consistent finding except at the lower dosage levels. Additionally, at the higher dose levels (140 to 420 mg or 140 to 1260 mg/kg/week given 3 or 7 days weekly for 12 weeks), growth retardation, slightly increased blood glucose values, and hemosiderosis of the liver or spleen were found; reversible spermatogenic arrest was noted. In the monkey, bone marrow depression, lymphoid atrophy of the spleen, and degenerative changes in the epithelium of the small and large intestines were found. At the higher, often lethal, doses (400 to 800 mg/kg/day for 7 to 15 days), hemorrhage and congestion were found in the lungs, brain and urinary tract. Cardiovascular effects (changes in heart rate, blood pressure, orthostatic hypotension, EKG changes) and hematological changes (slight hemolysis, slight methemoglobinemia) were observed in some species of laboratory animals at doses exceeding clinical levels.

INDICATIONS AND USAGE

Significant tumor response to Hydrea (Hydroxyurea Capsules USP) has been demonstrated in melanoma, resistant chronic myelocytic leukemia, and recurrent, metastatic, or inoperable carcinoma of the ovary.
Hydrea used concomitantly with irradiation therapy is intended for use in the local control of primary squamous cell (epidermoid) carcinomas of the head and neck, excluding the lip.

CONTRAINDICATIONS

Hydroxyurea is contraindicated in patients with marked bone marrow depression, i.e., leukopenia (less than 2500 WBC) or thrombocytopenia (less than 100,000), or severe anemia.

WARNINGS

Treatment with hydroxyurea should not be initiated if bone marrow function is markedly depressed (—see CONTRAINDICATIONS). Bone marrow suppression may occur, and leukopenia is generally its first and most common manifestation. Thrombocytopenia and anemia occur less often, and are seldom seen without a preceding leukopenia. However, the recovery from myelosuppression is rapid when therapy is interrupted. It should be borne in mind that bone marrow depression is more likely in patients who have previously received radiotherapy or cytotoxic cancer chemotherapeutic agents; hydroxyurea should be used cautiously in such patients.
Patients who have received irradiation therapy in the past may have an exacerbation of postirradiation erythema.
Severe anemia must be corrected with whole blood replacement before initiating therapy with hydroxyurea.
Erythrocytic abnormalities: megaloblastic erythropoiesis, which is self-limiting, is often seen early in the course of hydroxyurea therapy. The morphologic change resembles pernicious anemia, but is not related to vitamin B_{12} or folic acid deficiency. Hydroxyurea may also delay plasma iron clearance and reduce the rate of iron utilization by erythrocytes, but it does not appear to alter the red blood cell survival time.
Hydroxyurea should be used with caution in patients with marked renal dysfunction.
Elderly patients may be more sensitive to the effects of hydroxyurea, and may require a lower dose regimen.
Usage in Pregnancy—Drugs which affect DNA synthesis, such as hydroxyurea, may be potential mutagenic agents. The physician should carefully consider this possibility before administering this drug to male or female patients who may contemplate conception.
Hydrea (Hydroxyurea Capsules USP) is a known teratogenic agent in animals. Therefore, hydroxyurea should not be used in women who are or may become pregnant unless in the judgment of the physician the potential benefits outweigh the possible hazards.

PRECAUTIONS

Therapy with hydroxyurea requires close supervision. The complete status of the blood, including bone marrow examination, if indicated, as well as kidney function and liver function should be determined prior to, and repeatedly during, treatment. The determination of the hemoglobin level, total leukocyte counts, and platelet counts should be performed at least once a week throughout the course of hydroxyurea therapy. If the white blood cell count decreases to less than 2500/mm^3, or the platelet count to less than 100,000/mm^3, therapy should be interrupted until the values rise significantly toward normal levels. Anemia, if it occurs, should be managed with whole blood replacement, without interrupting hydroxyurea therapy.

ADVERSE REACTIONS

Adverse reactions have been primarily bone marrow depression (leukopenia, anemia, and occasionally thrombocytopenia), and less frequently gastrointestinal symptoms (stomatitis, anorexia, nausea, vomiting, diarrhea, and constipation), and dermatological reactions such as maculopapular rash and facial erythema. Dysuria and alopecia occur very rarely. Large doses may produce moderate drowsiness. Neurological disturbances have occurred extremely rarely and were limited to headache, dizziness, disorientation, hallucinations, and convulsions. Hydroxyurea occasionally may cause temporary impairment of renal tubular function accompanied by elevations in serum uric acid, BUN, and creatinine levels. Abnormal BSP retention has been reported. Fever, chills, malaise, and elevation of hepatic enzymes have also been reported.
Adverse reactions observed with combined hydroxyurea and irradiation therapy are similar to those reported with the use of hydroxyurea alone. These effects primarily include bone marrow depression (anemia and leukopenia), and gastric irritation. Almost all patients receiving an adequate course of combined hydroxyurea and irradiation therapy will demonstrate concurrent leukopenia. Platelet depression (less than 100,000 cells/mm^3) has occurred rarely and only in the presence of marked leukopenia. Gastric distress has also been reported with irradiation alone and in combination with hydroxyurea therapy.
It should be borne in mind that therapeutic doses of irradiation alone produce the same adverse reactions as hydroxyurea; combined therapy may cause an increase in the incidence and severity of these side effects.
Although inflammation of the mucous membranes at the irradiated site (mucositis) is attributed to irradiation alone, some investigators believe that the more severe cases are due to combination therapy.

DOSAGE AND ADMINISTRATION

Because of the rarity of melanoma, resistant chronic myelocytic leukemia, carcinoma of the ovary, and carcinomas of the head and neck in children, dosage regimens have not been established.
All dosage should be based on the patient's actual or ideal weight, whichever is less.
NOTE: If the patient prefers, or is unable to swallow capsules, the contents of the capsules may be emptied into a glass of water and taken immediately. Some inert material used as a vehicle in the capsule may not dissolve, and may float on the surface.

Solid Tumors

Intermittent Therapy: 80 mg/kg administered orally as *single* dose every *third* day
Continuous Therapy: 20 to 30 mg/kg administered orally as a *single* dose *daily*
The intermittent dosage schedule offers the advantage of reduced toxicity since patients on this dosage regimen have rarely required complete discontinuance of therapy because of toxicity.
Concomitant Therapy with Irradiation (*Carcinoma of the head and neck*)—80 mg/kg administered orally as a *single* dose every *third* day.
Administration of Hydrea (Hydroxyurea Capsules USP) should be begun at least seven days before initiation of irradiation and continued during radiotherapy as well as indefinitely afterwards provided that the patient may be kept under adequate observation and evidences no unusual or severe reactions.
Irradiation should be given at the maximum dose considered appropriate for the particular therapeutic situation; adjustment of irradiation dosage is not usually necessary when Hydrea is used concomitantly.

Resistant Chronic Myelocytic Leukemia

Until the intermittent therapy regimen has been evaluated, CONTINUOUS therapy (20 to 30 mg/kg administered orally as a *single* dose *daily*) is recommended.

An adequate trial period for determining the antineoplastic effectiveness of Hydrea is six weeks of therapy. When there is regression in tumor size or arrest in tumor growth, therapy should be continued indefinitely. Therapy should be interrupted if the white blood cell count drops below 2500/mm^3, or the platelet count below 100,000/mm^3. In these cases, the counts should be rechecked after three days, and therapy resumed when the counts rise significantly toward normal values. Since the hematopoietic rebound is prompt, it is usually necessary to omit only a few doses. If prompt rebound has not occurred during combined hydroxyurea and irradiation therapy, irradiation may also be interrupted. However, the need for postponement of irradiation has been rare; radiotherapy has usually been continued using the recommended dosage and technique. Anemia, if it occurs, should be corrected with whole blood replacement, without interrupting hydroxyurea therapy. Because hematopoiesis may be compromised by extensive irradiation or by other antineoplastic agents, it is recommended that Hydrea be administered cautiously to patients who have recently received extensive radiation therapy or chemotherapy with other cytotoxic drugs.
Pain or discomfort from inflammation of the mucous membranes at the irradiated site (mucositis) is usually controlled by measures such as topical anesthetics and orally administered analgesics. If the reaction is severe, hydroxyurea therapy may be temporarily interrupted; if it is extremely severe, irradiation dosage may, in addition, be temporarily postponed. However, it has rarely been necessary to terminate these therapies.
Severe gastric distress, such as nausea, vomiting, and anorexia resulting from combined therapy may usually be controlled by temporary interruption of Hydrea (Hydroxyurea Capsules USP) administration; rarely has the additional interruption of irradiation been necessary.

HOW SUPPLIED

Bottles of 100.
Storage: Store at room temperature; avoid excessive heat; keep bottle tightly closed. Dispense in tight containers.
(J4-072)

Shown in Product Identification Section, page 431

KENALOG® ℞
[ken′ah-log]
Triamcinolone Acetonide USP
CREAM/LOTION/OINTMENT/SPRAY

DESCRIPTION

The topical corticosteroids constitute a class of primary synthetic steroids used as anti-inflammatory and antipruritic agents. The steroids in this class include triamcinolone acetonide. Triamcinolone acetonide is designated chemically as 9-Fluoro-11β, 16α, 17, 21,-tetrahydroxypregna-1,4-diene-3, 20-dione cyclic 16, 17-acetal with acetone.
Each gram of 0.025%, 0.1%, and 0.5% Kenalog Cream (Triamcinolone Acetonide Cream) provides 0.25 mg, 1 mg, or 5 mg triamcinolone acetonide, respectively, in a vanishing cream base containing propylene glycol, cetearyl alcohol (and) ceteareth-20, white petrolatum, sorbitol solution, glyceryl monostearate, polyethylene glycol monostearate, simethicone, sorbic acid, and purified water.
Each mL of 0.025% and 0.1% Kenalog Lotion (Triamcinolone Acetonide Lotion) provides 0.25 mg and 1 mg triamcino-

lone acetonide, respectively, in a lotion base containing propylene glycol, cetyl alcohol, stearyl alcohol, sorbitan monopalmitate, polysorbate 20, simethicone, and purified water.
Each gram of 0.025%, 0.1%, and 0.5% Kenalog Ointment (Triamcinolone Acetonide Ointment) provides 0.25 mg, 1 mg, or 5 mg triamcinolone acetonide, respectively, in Plastibase® (Plasticized Hydrocarbon Gel), a polyethylene and mineral oil gel base.
Kenalog Spray (Triamcinolone Acetonide Topical Aerosol) is **for dermatologic use only.** A two-second application, which covers an area approximately the size of the hand, delivers an amount of triamcinolone acetonide not exceeding 0.2 mg. After spraying, the nonvolatile vehicle remaining on the skin contains approximately 0.2% triamcinolone acetonide. Each gram of spray provides 0.147 mg triamcinolone acetonide in a vehicle of isopropyl palmitate, dehydrated alcolol (10.3%), and isobutane propellant.

CLINICAL PHARMACOLOGY

Topical corticosteroids share anti-inflammatory, antipruritic and vasoconstrictive actions.
The mechanism of anti-inflammatory activity of the topical corticosteroids is unclear. Various laboratory methods, including vasoconstrictor assays, are used to compare and predict potencies and/or clinical efficacies of the topical corticosteroids. There is some evidence to suggest that a recognizable correlation exists between vasoconstrictor potency and therapeutic efficacy in man.
Pharmacokinetics—The extent of percutaneous absorption of topical corticosteroids is determined by many factors including the vehicle, the integrity of the epidermal barrier, and the use of occlusive dressings.
Topical corticosteroids can be absorbed from normal intact skin. Inflammation and/or other disease processes in the skin increase percutaneous absorption. Occlusive dressings substantially increase the percutaneous absorption of topical corticosteroids. Thus, occlusive dressings may be a valuable therapeutic adjunct for treatment of resistant dermatoses (see DOSAGE AND ADMINISTRATION).
Once absorbed through the skin, topical corticosteroids are handled through pharmacokinetic pathways similar to systemically administered corticosteroids. Corticosteroids are bound to plasma proteins in varying degrees. Corticosteroids are metabolized primarily in the liver and are then excreted by the kidneys. Some of the topical corticosteroids and their metabolites are also excreted into the bile.

INDICATIONS AND USAGE

Kenalog (Triamcinolone Acetonide) Creams, Lotions, Ointments, and Spray are indicated for relief of the inflammatory and pruritic manifestations of corticosteroid-responsive dermatoses.

CONTRAINDICATIONS

Topical corticosteroids are contraindicated in those patients with a history of hypersensitivity to any of the components of the preparations.

PRECAUTIONS

General—Systemic absorption of topical corticosteroids has produced reversible hypothalamic-pituitary-adrenal (HPA) axis suppression, manifestations of Cushing's syndrome, hyperglycemia, and glycosuria in some patients.
Conditions which augment systemic absorption include the application of the more potent steroids, use over large surface areas, prolonged use, and the addition of occlusive dressings.
Therefore, patients receiving a large dose of any potent topical steroid applied to a large surface area or under an occlusive dressing should be evaluated periodically for evidence of HPA axis suppression by using the urinary free cortisol and ACTH stimulation tests, and for impairment of thermal homeostasis. If HPA axis suppression or elevation of the body temperature occurs, an attempt should be made to withdraw the drug, to reduce the frequency of application, substitute a less potent steroid, or use a sequential approach when utilizing the occlusive technique.
Recovery of HPA axis function and thermal homeostasis are generally prompt and complete upon discontinuation of the drug. Infrequently, signs and symptoms of steroid withdrawal may occur, requiring supplemental systemic corticosteroids. Occasionally, a patient may develop a sensitivity reaction to a particular occlusive dressing material or adhesive and a substitute material may be necessary.
Children may absorb proportionally larger amounts of topical corticosteroids and thus be more susceptible to systemic toxicity (see PRECAUTIONS, Pediatric Use).
If irritation develops, topical corticosteroids should be discontinued and appropriate therapy instituted.
In the presence of dermatological infections, the use of an appropriate antifungal or antibacterial agent should be instituted. If a favorable response does not occur promptly, the corticosteroid should be discontinued until the infection has been adequately controlled.
These preparations are not for ophthalmic use.
Information for the Patient: Patients using topical corticosteroids should receive the following information and instructions:

1. This medication is to be used as directed by the physician. It is for external use only. Avoid contact with the eyes.
2. Patients should be advised not to use this medication for any disorder other than for which it was prescribed.
3. The treated skin area should not be bandaged or otherwise covered or wrapped as to be occlusive unless directed by the physician.
4. Patients should report any signs of local adverse reactions especially under occlusive dressing.
5. Parents of pediatric patients should be advised not to use tight-fitting diapers or plastic pants on a child being treated in the diaper area, as these garments may constitute occlusive dressings.

Laboratory Tests—A urinary free cortisol test and ACTH stimulation test may be helpful in evaluating HPA axis suppression.
Carcinogenesis, Mutagenesis, and Impairment of Fertility—Long-term animal studies have not been performed to evaluate the carcinogenic potential or the effect on fertility of topical corticosteroids.
Studies to determine mutagenicity with prednisolone and hydrocortisone showed negative results.
Pregnancy: Teratogenic Effects—Category C. Corticosteroids are generally teratogenic in laboratory animals when administered systemically at relatively low dosage levels. The more potent corticosteroids have been shown to be teratogenic after dermal application in laboratory animals. There are no adequate and well-controlled studies in pregnant women on teratogenic effects from topically applied corticosteroids. Therefore, topical corticosteroids should be used during pregnancy only if the potential benefit justifies the potential risk to the fetus. Drugs of this class should not be used extensively on pregnant patients, in large amounts, or for prolonged periods of time.
Nursing Mothers—It is not known whether topical administration of corticosteroids could result in sufficient systemic absorption to produce detectable quantities in breast milk. Systemically administered corticosteroids are secreted into breast milk in quantities **not** likely to have a deleterious effect on the infant. Nevertheless, caution should be exercised when topical corticosteroids are administered to a nursing woman.
Pediatric Use—Pediatric patients may demonstrate greater susceptibility to topical corticosteroid-induced HPA axis suppression and Cushing's syndrome than mature patients because of a larger skin surface area to body weight ratio.
HPA axis suppression, Cushing's syndrome, and intracranial hypertension have been reported in children receiving topical corticosteroids. Manifestations of adrenal suppression in children include linear growth retardation, delayed weight gain, low plasma cortisol levels, and absence of response to ACTH stimulation. Manifestations of intracranial hypertension include bulging fontanelles, headaches, and bilateral papilledema.
Administration of topical corticosteroids to children should be limited to the least amount compatible with an effective therapeutic regimen. Chronic corticosteroid therapy may interfere with the growth and development of children.

ADVERSE REACTIONS

The following local adverse reactions are reported infrequently with topical corticosteroids, but may occur more frequently with the use of occlusive dressings (reactions are listed in an approximate decreasing order of occurrence): burning, itching, irritation, dryness, folliculitis, hypertrichosis, acneiform eruptions, hypopigmentation, perioral dermatitis, allergic contact dermatitis, maceration of the skin, secondary infection, skin atrophy, striae, and miliaria.

OVERDOSAGE

Topically applied corticosteroids can be absorbed in sufficient amounts to produce systemic effects (see PRECAUTIONS, General).

DOSAGE AND ADMINISTRATION

Kenalog Cream (Triamcinolone Acetonide Cream) 0.025%: Apply to the affected area two to four times daily. Rub in gently.
Kenalog Cream (Triamcinolone Acetonide Cream) 0.1% or 0.5%: Apply, as appropriate, to the affected area two to three times daily. Rub in gently.
Kenalog Lotion (Triamcinolone Acetonide Lotion) 0.025%: Apply to the affected area two to four times daily. Rub in gently.
Kenalog Lotion (Triamcinolone Acetonide Lotion) 0.1%): Apply to the affected area two to three times daily. Rub in gently.
Kenalog Ointment (Triamcinolone Acetonide Ointment) 0.025%: Apply a thin film to the affected area two to four times daily.
Kenalog Ointment (Triamcinolone Acetonide Ointment) 0.1% or 0.5%: Apply a thin film, as appropriate, to the affected area two to three times daily.
Kenalog Spray (Triamcinolone Acetonide Topical Aerosol): Directions for use of the spray can are provided on the label. The preparation may be applied to any area of the body, but when it is sprayed about the face, care should be taken to see that the eyes are covered, and that inhalation of the spray is avoided. Three or four applications daily are generally adequate.
Occlusive Dressing Technique—Kenalog Cream (Triamcinolone Acetonide Cream) 0.025%, 0.1%, and 0.5% and Kenalog Lotion (Triamcinolone Acetonide Lotion) 0.025% and 0.1%: Occlusive dressings may be used for the management of psoriasis or other recalcitrant conditions. Gently rub a small amount of the preparation into the lesion until it disappears. Reapply the preparation leaving a thin coating on the lesion, cover with a pliable nonporous film, and seal the edges. If needed, additional moisture may be provided by covering the lesion with a dampened clean cotton cloth before the nonporous film is applied or by briefly wetting the affected area with water immediately prior to applying the medication. The frequency of changing dressings is best determined on an individual basis. It may be convenient to apply the preparation under an occlusive dressing in the evening and to remove the dressing in the morning (i.e., 12-hour occlusion). When utilizing the 12-hour occlusion regimen, additional preparation should be applied, without occlusion, during the day. Reapplication is essential at each dressing change.
If an infection develops, the use of occlusive dressings should be discontinued and appropriate antimicrobial therapy instituted.
Kenalog Ointment (Triamcinolone Acetonide Ointment) 0.025%, 0.1% and 0.5% and Kenalog Spray (Triamcinolone Acetonide Topical Aerosol): Occlusive dressings may be used for the management of psoriasis or other recalcitrant conditions. Apply a thin coating of the preparation onto the lesion, cover with a pliable nonporous film, and seal the edges. If needed, additional moisture may be provided by covering the lesion with a dampened clean cotton cloth before the nonporous film is applied or by briefly wetting the affected area with water immediately prior to applying the medication. The frequency of changing dressings is best determined on an individual basis. It may be convenient to apply the preparation under an occlusive dressing in the evening and to remove the dressing in the morning (i.e., 12-hour occlusion). When utilizing the 12-hour occlusion regimen, additional preparation should be applied, without occlusion, during the day. Reapplication is essential at each dressing change.
If an infection develops, the use of occlusive dressings should be discontinued and appropriate antimicrobial therapy instituted.

HOW SUPPLIED

The 0.025% Cream and Ointment are supplied in 15 g, 60 g and 80 g tubes, and 240 g (8 oz) jars. The 0.1% Cream and Ointment are supplied in 15 g, 60 g, and 80 g tubes and in 240 g (8 oz) jars. The 0.5% Cream and Ointment are supplied in 20 g tubes. The 0.1% and 0.025% Creams and 0.1% Ointment are also supplied in 5.25 lb jars. The 0.025% Lotion is supplied in 60 mL plastic squeeze bottles. The 0.1% Lotion is supplied in 15 mL and 60 mL plastic squeeze bottles. [60 mL bottle, V.A. Depot Item NSN 6505-00-282-5118A]. The Spray is supplied in 23 g and 63 g aerosol cans (each can is supplied with a spray tube applicator). [63 g cans, Military Depot Item, NSN 6505-01-066-1325].
Storage
Store the creams and lotions at room temperature; avoid freezing Store the ointments at room temperature. Store the spray at room temperature; avoid excessive heat.
(J3-555C/528E/557D/232G)

KENALOG®-40 INJECTION ℞

[*ken 'ah-log"*]
(Sterile Triamcinolone Acetonide Suspension USP)
NOT FOR INTRAVENOUS OR INTRADERMAL USE

DESCRIPTION

Kenalog-40 Injection (Sterile Triamcinolone Acetonide Suspension USP) provides a synthetic corticosteroid with marked anti-inflammatory action. Each mL of the sterile, aqueous suspension provides 40 mg of triamcinolone acetonide, with sodium chloride for isotonicity, 0.9% (w/v) benzyl alcohol as a preservative, 0.75% [carboxymethylcellulose sodium, and 0.04% polysorbate 80. Sodium hydroxide or hydrochloric acid may be present to adjust pH to 5.0 to 7.5. At the time of manufacture, the air in the container is replaced by nitrogen.

Continued on next page

Squibb—Cont.

ACTIONS

Naturally occurring glucocorticoids (hydrocortisone), which also have salt-retaining properties, are used as replacement therapy in adrenocortical deficiency states. Their synthetic analogs are primarily used for their potent anti-inflammatory effects in disorders of many organ systems.
Glucocorticoids cause profound and varied metabolic effects. In addition, they modify the body's immune responses to diverse stimuli.
Kenalog-40 Injection has an extended duration of effect which may be permanent, or sustained over a period of several weeks. Studies indicate that following a single intramuscular dose of 60 to 100 mg of triamcinolone acetonide, adrenal suppression occurs within 24 to 48 hours and then gradually returns to normal, usually in 30 to 40 days. This finding correlates closely with the extended duration of therapeutic action achieved with the drug.

INDICATIONS

Intramuscular

Where oral therapy is not feasible or is temporarily undesirable in the judgment of the physician, Kenalog-40 Injection (Sterile Triamcinolone Acetonide Suspension USP) is indicated for intramuscular use as follows:

1. *Endocrine disorders*—Nonsuppurative thyroiditis.
2. *Rheumatic disorders*—As adjunctive therapy for short-term administration (to tide the patient over an acute episode or exacerbation) in: posttraumatic osteoarthritis; synovitis of osteoarthritis; rheumatoid arthritis; acute and subacute bursitis; epicondylitis; acute nonspecific tenosynovitis; acute gouty arthritis; psoriatic arthritis; ankylosing spondylitis; juvenile rheumatoid arthritis.
3. *Collagen diseases*—During an exacerbation or as maintenance therapy in selected cases of: systemic lupus erythematosus; acute rheumatic carditis.
4. *Dermatologic diseases*—Pemphigus; severe erythema multiforme (Stevens-Johnson syndrome); exfoliative dermatitis; bullous dermatitis herpetiformis; severe seborrheic dermatitis; severe psoriasis.
5. *Allergic states*—Control of severe or incapacitating allergic conditions intractable to adequate trials of conventional treatment in: bronchial asthma; contact dermatitis; atopic dermatitis; seasonal or perennial allergic rhinitis.
6. *Ophthalmic diseases*—Severe chronic allergic and inflammatory processes involving the eye, such as: herpes zoster ophthalmicus; iritis; irridocyclitis; chorioretinitis; diffuse posterior uveitis and choroiditis; optic neuritis; sympathetic ophthalmia; anterior segment inflammation.
7. *Gastrointestinal diseases*—To tide the patient over a critical period of disease in: ulcerative colitis (systemic therapy); regional enteritis (systemic therapy).
8. *Respiratory diseases*—Symptomatic sarcoidosis; berylliosis; aspiration pneumonitis.
9. *Hematologic disorders*—Acquired (autoimmune) hemolytic anemia.
10. *Neoplastic diseases*—For palliative management of: leukemias and lymphomas in adults; acute leukemia of childhood.
11. *Edematous state*—To induce diuresis or remission of proteinuria in the nephrotic syndrome, without uremia, of the idiopathic type or that due to lupus erythematosus.

Intra-Articular

Kenalog-40 Injection (Sterile Triamcinolone Acetonide Suspension USP) is indicated for intra-articular or intrabursal administration, and for injections into tendon sheaths, as adjunctive therapy for short-term administration (to tide the patient over an acute episode or exacerbation) in: synovitis of osteoarthritis; rheumatoid arthritis; acute and subacute bursitis; acute gouty arthritis; epicondylitis; acute nonspecific tenosynovitis; posttraumatic osteoarthritis.

CONTRAINDICATIONS

Corticosteroids are contraindicated in patients with systemic fungal infections. Intramuscular corticosteroid preparations are contraindicated for idiopathic thrombocytopenic purpura.

WARNINGS

Because it is a suspension, the preparation should **not** be administered intravenously. Strict aseptic technique is mandatory. This preparation is not recommended for children under six years of age.
Adequate studies to demonstrate the safety of administration of Kenalog-40 Injection (Sterile Triamcinolone Acetonide Suspension USP) by intraturbinal, subconjunctival, subtenon and retrobulbar injections have not been performed. Several instances of blindness have been reported following injection of corticosteroid suspensions into the nasal turbinates and also following the intralesional injection about the head.
When patients who are receiving corticosteroid therapy are subjected to unusual stress, increased dosage of rapidly acting corticosteroids is indicated before, during, and after the stressful situation.
Corticosteroids may mask some signs of infection, and new infections may appear during their use. There may be decreased resistance and inability to localize infection when corticosteroids are used. If an infection occurs during corticosteroid therapy, it should be promptly controlled by suitable antimicrobial therapy (see PRECAUTIONS).
Prolonged use of corticosteroids may produce posterior subcapsular cataracts, glaucoma with possible damage to the optic nerves, and may enhance the establishment of secondary ocular infections due to fungi or viruses.
Average and large doses of hydrocortisone or cortisone can cause elevation of blood pressure, salt and water retention, and increased excretion of potassium. These effects are less likely to occur with the synthetic derivatives except when they are used in large doses; dietary salt restriction and potassium supplementation may be necessary (see PRECAUTIONS). All corticosteroids increase calcium excretion.
Patients should not be vaccinated against smallpox while on corticosteroid therapy. Other immunization procedures should not be undertaken in patients who are on corticosteroids, especially on high dose, because of possible hazards of neurological complications and a lack of antibody response.
The use of corticosteroids in patients with active tuberculosis should be restricted to those cases of fulminating or disseminated tuberculosis in which the corticosteroid is used for the management of the disease in conjunction with an appropriate antituberculous regimen. If corticosteroids are indicated in patients with latent tuberculosis or tuberculin reactivity, close observation is necessary since reactivation of the disease may occur. During prolonged corticosteroid therapy, these patients should receive chemoprophylaxis.
Because rare instances of anaphylactoid reactions have occurred in patients receiving parenteral corticosteroid therapy, appropriate precautionary measures should be taken prior to administration, especially when the patient has a history of allergy to any drug.
Unless a **deep** intramuscular injection is given, local atrophy is likely to occur. (For recommendations on injection techniques, see DOSAGE AND ADMINISTRATION.) Due to the significantly higher incidence of local atrophy when the material is injected into the deltoid area, this injection site should be avoided in favor of the gluteal area. Only very unusual circumstances would warrant injection into the deltoid area.
Usage in Pregnancy: Since adequate human reproduction studies have not been done with corticosteroids, the use of these drugs in pregnancy, nursing mothers, or women of child-bearing potential requires that the possible benefits of the drug be weighed against the potential hazards to the mother and the embryo, fetus, or nursing infant. Infants born of mothers who have received substantial doses of corticosteroids during pregnancy should be carefully observed for signs of hypoadrenalism.

PRECAUTIONS

Drug-induced secondary adrenocortical insufficiency may be minimized by a gradual reduction of dosage. This type of relative insufficiency may persist for months after discontinuation of therapy; therefore, in any situation of stress (such as trauma, surgery, or severe illness) occurring during that period, hormone therapy should be reinstituted. Since mineralocorticoid secretion may be impaired, salt and/or a mineralocorticoid should be administered concurrently.
There is an enhanced corticosteroid effect in patients with hypothyroidism and in those with cirrhosis.
Corticosteroids should be used cautiously in patients with ocular herpes simplex because of possible corneal perforation.
The lowest possible dose of corticosteroid should be used to control the condition being treated. A gradual reduction in dosage should be made when possible.
Psychic derangements may appear when corticosteroids are used. These may range from euphoria, insomnia, mood swings, personality changes and severe depression to frank psychotic manifestations. Existing emotional instability or psychotic tendencies may also be aggravated by corticosteroids.
Aspirin should be used cautiously in conjunction with corticosteroids in patients with hypoprothrombinemia.
Corticosteroids should be used with caution in patients with nonspecific ulcerative colitis if there is a probability of impending perforation, abscess, or other pyogenic infection. Corticosteroids should also be used cautiously in patients with diverticulitis, fresh intestinal anastomoses, active or latent peptic ulcer, renal insufficiency, hypertension, osteoporosis, acute glomerulonephritis, vaccinia, varicella, exanthema, Cushing's syndrome, antibiotic resistant infections, diabetes mellitus, congestive heart failure, chronic nephritis, thromboembolitic tendencies, thrombophlebitis, convulsive disorders, metastatic carcinoma, and myasthenia gravis.
Growth and development of infants and children on prolonged corticosteroid therapy should be carefully observed.
Although therapy with Kenalog-40 Injection (Sterile Triamcinolone Acetonide Suspension USP) will ameliorate symptoms, it is in no sense a cure and the hormone has no effect on the cause of the inflammation. Therefore, this method of treatment does not obviate the need for the conventional measures usually employed.
Intra-articular injection of a corticosteroid may produce systemic as well as local effects. The inadvertent injection of the suspension into the soft tissues surrounding a joint is not harmful, but may lead to the occurrence of systemic effects, and is the most common cause of failure to achieve the desired local results.
Following intra-articular steroid therapy, patients should be specifically warned to avoid overuse of joints in which symptomatic benefit has been obtained. Negligence in this matter may permit an increase in joint deterioration that will more than offset the beneficial effects of the steroid. To detect deterioration, follow-up x-ray examination is suggested in selected cases.
Overdistention of the joint capsule and deposition of steroid along the needle track should be avoided in intra-articular injection since this may lead to subcutaneous atrophy.
Corticosteroids should not be injected into unstable joints.
Repeated intra-articular injection may in some cases result in instability of the joint. In selected cases, particularly when repeated injections are given, x-ray follow-up is suggested.
An increase in joint discomfort has seldom occurred. A marked increase in pain accompanied by local swelling, further restriction of joint motion, fever, and malaise are suggestive of a septic arthritis. If these complications should appear, and the diagnosis of septic arthritis is confirmed, administration of triamcinolone acetonide should be stopped, and antimicrobial therapy should be instituted immediately and continued for 7 to 10 days after all evidence of infection has disappeared. Appropriate examination of any joint fluid present is necessary to exclude a septic process.
Local injection of a steroid into a previously infected joint is to be avoided.
Kenalog-40 Injection (Sterile Triamcinolone Acetonide Suspension USP) should be administered only with full knowledge of characteristic activity of, and varied responses to, adrenocortical hormones. Like other potent corticosteroids, triamcinolone acetonide should be used under close clinical supervision. Triamcinolone acetonide can cause elevation of blood pressure, salt and water retention, and increased potassium and calcium excretion necessitating dietary salt restriction and potassium supplementation. Edema may occur in the presence of renal disease with a fixed or decreased glomerular filtration rate.
During prolonged therapy, **a liberal protein intake is essential** for counteracting the tendency to gradual weight loss sometimes associated with negative nitrogen balance, wasting and weakness of skeletal muscles.
When local or systemic microbial infections are present, therapy with triamcinolone acetonide is not recommended, but may be employed with caution and only in conjunction with appropriate antibiotic or chemotherapeutic medication. Triamcinolone acetonide may mask signs of infection and enhance dissemination of the infecting organism. Hence, all patients receiving triamcinolone acetonide should be watched for evidence of intercurrent infection. Should infection occur, vigorous, appropriate anti-infective therapy should be initiated. If possible, abrupt cessation of steroids should be avoided because of the danger of superimposing adrenocortical insufficiency on the infectious process.
Menstrual irregularities may occur, and this possibility should be mentioned to female patients past menarche.
In peptic ulcer, recurrence may be asymptomatic until perforation or hemorrhage occurs. Long-term adrenocorticoid therapy may evoke hyperacidity or peptic ulcer; therefore, as a prophylactic measure, an ulcer regimen and the administration of an antacid are highly recommended. X-rays should be taken in peptic ulcer patients complaining of gastric distress, or when therapy is prolonged. Whether or not changes are observed, an ulcer regimen is recommended.
As with other corticosteroids, the possibility of other severe reactions should be considered. If such reactions should occur, appropriate corrective measures should be instituted and use of the drug discontinued.
Continued supervision of the patient after termination of triamcinolone acetonide therapy is essential, since there may be a sudden reappearance of severe manifestations of the disease for which the patient was treated.

ADVERSE REACTIONS

Following Administration by Any Route — Patients should be watched closely for the following adverse reactions which may be associated with any corticosteroid therapy:
Fluid and electrolyte disturbances — sodium retention, fluid retention, congestive heart failure in susceptible patients, potassium loss, cardiac arrhythmias or ECG changes due to potassium deficiency, hypokalemic alkalosis, and hypertension.
Musculoskeletal — muscle weakness, fatigue, steroid myopathy, loss of muscle mass, osteoporosis, vertebral compression

fractures, delayed healing of fractures, aseptic necrosis of femoral and humeral heads, pathologic fractures of long bones, and spontaneous fractures.
Gastrointestinal — peptic ulcer with possible subsequent perforation and hemorrhage, pancreatitis, abdominal distention, and ulcerative esophagitis.
Dermatologic — impaired wound healing, thin fragile skin, petechiae and ecchymoses, facial erythema, increased sweating, purpura, striae, hirsutism, acneiform eruptions, lupus erythematosus-like lesions and suppressed reactions to skin tests.
Neurological — convulsions, increased intracranial pressure with papilledema (pseudo-tumor cerebri) usually after treatment, vertigo, headache, neuritis or paresthesias, and aggravation of preexisting psychiatric conditions.
Endocrine — menstrual irregularities; development of the cushingoid state; suppression of growth in children; secondary adrenocortical and pituitary unresponsiveness, particularly in times of stress (e.g., trauma, surgery, or illness); decreased carbohydrate tolerance; manifestations of latent diabetes mellitus and increased requirements for insulin or oral hypoglycemic agents in diabetics.
Ophthalmic — posterior subcapsular cataracts, increased intraocular pressure, glaucoma, and exophthalmos.
Metabolic — hyperglycemia, glycosuria, and negative nitrogen balance due to protein catabolism.
Others — necrotizing angiitis, thrombophlebitis, thromboembolism, aggravation or masking of infections, insomnia, syncopal episodes, and anaphylactoid reactions.
Following Intramuscular Administration — Severe pain has been reported in a few cases. Sterile abscess formation, subcutaneous and cutaneous atrophy, hyperpigmentation and hypopigmentation and charcot-like arthropathy have also occurred.
Following Intra-Articular Administration — Undesirable reactions have included postinjection flare, transient pain, occasional irritation at the injection site, sterile abscess formation, hyperpigmentation and hypopigmentation, charcot-like arthropathy and occasional brief increase in joint discomfort.

DOSAGE AND ADMINISTRATION

General

The initial dose of Kenalog-40 Injection (Sterile Triamcinolone Acetonide Suspension USP) may vary from 2.5 to 60 mg per day depending on the specific disease entity being treated (see **Dosage** section below). In situations of less severity, lower doses will generally suffice while in selected patients higher initial doses may be required. Usually the parenteral dosage ranges are one-third to one-half the oral dose given every 12 hours. However, in certain overwhelming, acute, life-threatening situations, administration of dosages exceeding the usual dosages may be justified and may be in multiples of the oral dosages.
The initial dosage should be maintained or adjusted until a satisfactory response is noted. If after a reasonable period of time there is a lack of satisfactory clinical response, Kenalog-40 Injection should be discontinued and the patient transferred to other appropriate therapy. **IT SHOULD BE EMPHASIZED THAT DOSAGE REQUIREMENTS ARE VARIABLE AND MUST BE INDIVIDUALIZED ON THE BASIS OF THE DISEASE UNDER TREATMENT AND THE RESPONSE OF THE PATIENT.** After a favorable response is noted, the proper maintenance dosage should be determined by decreasing the initial drug dosage in small increments at appropriate time intervals until the lowest dosage which will maintain an adequate clinical response is reached. It should be kept in mind that constant monitoring is needed in regard to drug dosage. Included in the situations which may make dosage adjustments necessary are changes in clinical status secondary to remissions or exacerbations in the disease process, the patient's individual drug responsiveness, and the effect of patient exposure to stressful situations not directly related to the disease entity under treatment; in this latter situation it may be necessary to increase the dosage of Kenalog-40 Injection for a period of time consistent with the patient's condition. If after long-term therapy the drug is to be stopped, it is recommended that it be withdrawn gradually rather than abruptly.

Dosage

Systemic: Although Kenalog-40 Injection (Sterile Triamcinolone Acetonide Suspension USP) may be administered intramuscularly for initial therapy, most physicians prefer to adjust the dose orally until adequate control is attained. Intramuscular administration provides a sustained or depot action which can be used to supplement or replace initial oral therapy. With intramuscular therapy, greater supervision of the amount of steroid used is made possible in the patient who is inconsistent in following an oral dosage schedule. In maintenance therapy, the patient-to-patient response is not uniform and, therefore, the dose must be individualized for optimal control.
For **adults and children over 12 years of age,** the suggested initial dose is 60 mg, **injected deeply into the gluteal muscle.** Subcutaneous fat atrophy may occur if care is not taken to inject the preparation intramuscularly. Dosage is usually adjusted within the range of 40 to 80 mg, depending upon patient response and duration of relief. However, some patients may be well controlled on dosages as low as 20 mg or less. Patients with hay fever or pollen asthma who are not responding to pollen administration and other conventional therapy may obtain a remission of symptoms lasting throughout the pollen season after one injection of 40 to 100 mg.
For **children from 6 to 12 years of age,** the suggested initial dose is 40 mg, although dosage depends more on the severity of symptoms than on age or weight. There is insufficient clinical experience with Kenalog-40 Injection to recommend its use in children under six years of age.
Local: For intra-articular or intrabursal administration and for injection into tendon sheaths, the initial dose of Kenalog-40 Injection (Sterile Triamcinolone Acetonide Suspension USP) may vary from 2.5 to 5 mg for smaller joints and from 5 to 15 mg for larger joints depending on the specific disease entity being treated. (A more dilute form of Sterile Triamcinolone Acetonide Suspension USP is available—see ALSO AVAILABLE.) For adults, doses up to 10 mg for smaller areas and up to 40 mg for larger areas have usually been sufficient to alleviate symptoms. Single injections into several joints for multiple locus involvement, up to a total of 80 mg, have been given without undue reactions. A single local injection of triamcinolone acetonide is frequently sufficient, but several injections may be needed for adequate relief of symptoms. The lower dosages in the initial dosage range of triamcinolone acetonide may produce the desired effect when the corticosteroid is administered to provide a localized concentration. The site of the injection and the volume of the injection should be carefully considered when triamcinolone acetonide is administered for this purpose.

Administration

General: Shake the vial before use to insure a uniform suspension. Prior to withdrawal, inspect suspension for clumping or granular appearance (agglomeration). An agglomerated product results from exposure to freezing temperatures and should not be used. After withdrawal, inject without delay to prevent settling in the syringe. Careful technique should be employed to avoid the possibility of entering a blood vessel or introducing infection.
Routine laboratory studies, such as urinalysis, two-hour postprandial blood sugar, determination of blood pressure and body weight and a chest x-ray should be made at regular intervals during prolonged therapy. Upper GI x-rays are desirable in patients with an ulcer history or significant dyspepsia.
Systemic: For systemic therapy, injection should be made **deeply into the gluteal muscle** to insure intramuscular delivery (see WARNINGS). For adults, a minimum needle length of 1 ½ inches is recommended. In obese patients, a longer needle may be required. Use alternate sites for subsequent injections.
Local: For treatment of joints, the usual intra-articular injection technique, as described in standard textbooks, should be followed. If an excessive amount of synovial fluid is present in the joint, some, but not all, should be aspirated to aid in the relief of pain and to prevent undue dilution of the corticosteroid.
With intra-articular or intrabursal administration, and with injection of the drug into tendon sheaths, the use of a local anesthetic may often be desirable. When a local anesthetic is used, its package insert should be read with care and all the precautions connected with its use should be observed. It should be injected into the surrounding soft tissues prior to the injection of the corticosteroid. A small amount of the anesthetic solution may be instilled into the joint. Care should be taken with intra-articular and intrabursal injections (particularly in the deltoid region) and with injection into tendon sheaths to avoid injecting the suspension into the tissues surrounding the site since this may lead to tissue atrophy.
In treating acute nonspecific tenosynovitis, care should be taken to insure that the injection of the corticosteroid is made into the tendon sheath rather than the tendon substance. Epicondylitis (tennis elbow) may be treated by infiltrating the preparation into the area of greatest tenderness.

HOW SUPPLIED

In vials of 1, 5, and 10 mL [5 mL vial—Military Depot Item, NSN 6505-00-885-6216 and V.A. Depot Item, NSN6505-00-885-6216A].
Also Available: Kenalog-10 Injection (Sterile Triamcinolone Acetonide Suspension USP) providing 10 mg triamcinolone acetonide per mL, with sodium chloride for isotonicity, 0.9% (w/v) benzyl alcohol as a preservative, 0.75% sodium carboxymethylcellulose, and 0.04% polysorbate 80. See package insert for full information.
Storage: Store at room temperature; avoid freezing. Protect from light.
(J3-064F)

KENALOG® -10 INJECTION ℞

[ken 'ah-log"]
(Sterile Triamcinolone Acetonide Suspension USP)
For Intra-articular, Intrabursal or Intradermal Use
NOT FOR INTRAVENOUS OR INTRAMUSCULAR USE

DESCRIPTION

Kenalog-10 Injection (Sterile Triamcinolone Acetonide Suspension USP) provides triamcinolone acetonide, a synthetic corticosteroid with marked anti-inflammatory action, in a sterile aqueous suspension suitable for intradermal, intra-articular, and intrabursal injection and for injection into tendon sheaths. This preparation is NOT suitable for intravenous or intramuscular use. Each mL of the sterile aqueous suspension provides 10 mg triamcinolone acetonide, with sodium chloride for isotonicity, 0.9% (w/v) benzyl alcohol as a preservative, 0.75% carboxymethylcellulose sodium, and 0.04% polysorbate 80; sodium hydroxide or hydrochloric acid may have been added to adjust pH between 5.0 and 7.5. At the time of manufacture, the air in the container is replaced by nitrogen.
The chemical name for triamcinolone acetonide is 9-fluoro-11β, 16α, 17, 21-tetrahydroxypregna-1,4-diene-3,20-dione cyclic 16, 17-acetal with acetone.

CLINICAL PHARMACOLOGY

Naturally occurring glucocorticoids (hydrocortisone), which also have salt-retaining properties, are used as replacement therapy in adrenocortical deficiency states. Their synthetic analogs are primarily used for their potent anti-inflammatory effects in disorders of many organ systems.
Glucocorticoids cause profound and varied metabolic effects. In addition, they modify the body's immune responses to diverse stimuli.

INDICATIONS AND USAGE

Intra-Articular:

Kenalog-10 Injection (Sterile Triamcinolone Acetonide Suspension USP) is indicated for intra-articular or intrabursal administration, and for injections into tendon sheaths, as adjunctive therapy for short-term administration (to tide the patient over an acute episode or exacerbation) in: synovitis of osteoarthritis, rheumatoid arthritis, acute and subacute bursitis, acute gouty arthritis, epicondylitis, acute nonspecific tenosynovitis, and post-traumatic osteoarthritis.

Intradermal:

Intralesional administration of Kenalog-10 Injection is indicated for the treatment of keloids, discoid lupus erythematosus, necrobiosis lipoidica diabeticorum, alopecia areata, and localized hypertrophic, infiltrated, inflammatory lesions of: lichen planus, psoriatic plaques, granuloma annulare, and lichen simplex chronicus (neurodermatitis). Kenalog-10 Injection also may be useful in cystic tumors of an aponeurosis or tendon (ganglia).

CONTRAINDICATIONS

Corticosteroids are contraindicated in patients with systemic fungal infections.

WARNINGS

Because it is a suspension, the preparation should *not* be administered intravenously. Strict aseptic technique is mandatory.
When patients who are receiving corticosteroid therapy are subjected to unusual stress, increased dosage of rapidly acting corticosteroids is indicated before, during, and after the stressful situation. Kenalog-10 Injection (Sterile Triamcinolone Acetonide Suspension USP), as a long-acting preparation, is *not* suitable for use in acute stress situations.
Corticosteroids may mask some signs of infection, and new infections may appear during their use. There may be decreased resistance and inability to localize infection when corticosteroids are used. If an infection occurs during corticosteroid therapy, it should be promptly controlled by suitable antimicrobial therapy (see PRECAUTIONS).
Prolonged use of corticosteroids may produce posterior subcapsular cataracts, glaucoma with possible damage to the optic nerves, and may enhance the establishment of secondary ocular infections due to fungi or viruses.
Average and large doses of hydrocortisone or cortisone can cause elevation of blood pressure, salt and water retention, and increased excretion of potassium. These effects are less likely to occur with the synthetic derivatives except when they are used in large doses; dietary salt restriction and potassium supplementation may be necessary (see PRECAUTIONS). All corticosteroids increase calcium excretion.
Patients should not be vaccinated against smallpox while on corticosteroid therapy. Other immunization procedures should not be undertaken in patients who are on corticosteroids, especially on high dose, because of possible hazards of neurological complications and a lack of antibody response.

Continued on next page

Squibb—Cont.

The use of triamcinolone acetonide in patients with active tuberculosis should be restricted to those cases of fulminating or disseminated tuberculosis in which the corticosteroid is used for the management of the disease in conjunction with an appropriate antituberculous regimen. If corticosteroids are indicated in patients with latent tuberculosis or tuberculin reactivity, close observation is necessary since reactivation of the disease may occur. During prolonged corticosteroid therapy these patients should receive chemoprophylaxis.
Because rare instances of anaphylactoid reactions have occurred in patients receiving parenteral corticosteroid therapy, appropriate precautionary measures should be taken prior to administration, especially when the patient has a history of allergy to any drug.
Safety of use of Kenalog-10 Injection (Sterile Triamcinolone Acetonide Suspension USP) by intraturbinal, subconjunctival, subtenons, and retrobulbar injection has not been established.
Usage in Pregnancy — Since adequate human reproduction studies have not been done with corticosteroids, the use of these drugs in pregnancy, nursing mothers, or women of child-bearing potential requires that the possible benefits of the drug be weighed against the potential hazards to the mother and the embryo, fetus, or nursing infant. Infants born of mothers who have received substantial doses of corticosteroids during pregnancy should be carefully observed for signs of hypoadrenalism.

PRECAUTIONS

Drug-induced secondary adrenocortical insufficiency may be minimized by a gradual reduction of dosage. This type of relative insufficiency may persist for months after discontinuation of therapy; therefore, in any situation of stress (such as trauma, surgery, or severe illness) occurring during that period, hormone therapy should be reinstituted. Since mineralocorticoid secretion may be impaired, salt and/or a mineralocorticoid should be administered concurrently.
There is enhanced corticosteroid effect in patients with hypothyroidism and in those with cirrhosis.
Corticosteroids should be used cautiously in patients with ocular herpes simplex because of possible corneal perforation.
The lowest possible dose of corticosteroid should be used to control the condition being treated. A gradual reduction in dosage should be made when possible.
Psychic derangements may appear when corticosteroids are used. These may range from euphoria, insomnia, mood swings, personality changes, and severe depression, to frank psychotic manifestations. Existing emotional instability or psychotic tendencies may also be aggravated by corticosteroids.
Aspirin should be used cautiously in conjunction with corticosteroids in patients with hypoprothrombinemia.
Corticosteroids should be used with caution in patients with nonspecific ulcerative colitis if there is a probability of impending perforation, abscess, or other pyogenic infection. Corticosteroids should also be used cautiously in patients with diverticulitis, fresh intestinal anastomoses, active or latent peptic ulcer, renal insufficiency, hypertension, osteoporosis, and myasthenia gravis.
Growth and development of infants and children on prolonged corticosteroid therapy should be carefully observed.
Although therapy with Kenalog-10 Injection (Sterile Triamcinolone Acetonide Suspension USP) may ameliorate symptoms, it is in no sense a cure and the hormone has no effect on the cause of the inflammation. Therefore, this method of treatment does not obviate the need for the conventional measures usually employed.
Intra-articular injection of a corticosteroid may produce systemic as well as local effects. The inadvertent injection of the suspension into the soft tissues surrounding a joint is not harmful, but is the most common cause of failure to achieve the desired local results.
Following intra-articular steroid therapy, patients should be specifically warned to avoid overuse of joints in which symptomatic benefit has been obtained. Negligence in this matter may permit an increase in joint deterioration that will more than offset the beneficial effects of the steroid. To detect deterioration follow-up x-ray examination is suggested in selected cases.
Overdistention of the joint capsule and deposition of steroid along the needle track should be avoided in intra-articular injection since this may lead to subcutaneous atrophy.
Corticosteroids should not be injected into unstable joints. Repeated intra-articular injection may in some cases result in instability of the joint. In selected cases, particularly when repeated injections are given, x-ray follow-up is suggested.
An increase in joint discomfort has seldom occurred. A marked increase in pain accompanied by local swelling, further restriction of joint motion, fever, and malaise are suggestive of a septic arthritis. If these complications should appear, and the diagnosis of septic arthritis is confirmed, administration of triamcinolone acetonide should be stopped, and antimicrobial therapy should be instituted immediately and continued for 7 to 10 days after all evidence of infection has disappeared. Appropriate examination of any joint fluid present is necessary to exclude a septic process. Local injection of a steroid into a previously infected joint is to be avoided.
Kenalog-10 Injection (Sterile Triamcinolone Acetonide Suspension USP) should be administered only with full knowledge of characteristic activity of, and varied responses to, adrenocortical hormones. Like other potent corticosteroids, triamcinolone acetonide should be used under close clinical supervision. Triamcinolone acetonide can cause elevation of blood pressure, salt and water retention, and increased potassium and calcium excretion necessitating dietary salt restriction and potassium supplementation. Edema may occur in the presence of renal disease with a fixed or decreased glomerular filtration rate.
During prolonged therapy, *a liberal protein intake is essential* for counteracting the tendency to gradual weight loss sometimes associated with negative nitrogen balance, wasting and weakness of skeletal muscles.
When local or systemic microbial infections are present, therapy with triamcinolone acetonide is not recommended, but may be employed with caution and only in conjunction with appropriate antibiotic or chemotherapeutic medication. Triamcinolone acetonide may mask signs of infection and enhance dissemination of the infecting organism. Hence, all patients receiving triamcinolone acetonide should be watched for evidence of intercurrent infection. Should infection occur, vigorous, appropriate anti-infective therapy should be initiated. If possible, abrupt cessation of steroids should be avoided because of the danger of superimposing adrenocortical insufficiency on the infectious process.
Menstrual irregularities may occur, and this possibility should be mentioned to female patients past menarche.
In peptic ulcer, recurrence may be asymptomatic until perforation or hemorrhage occurs. X-rays should be taken in peptic ulcer patients complaining of gastric distress, or when therapy is prolonged. Whether or not changes are observed, an ulcer regimen is recommended.
As with other corticosteroids, the possibility of other severe reactions should be considered. If such reactions should occur, appropriate corrective measures should be instituted and use of the drug discontinued.
Continued supervision of the patient after termination of triamcinolone acetonide therapy is essential, since there may be a sudden reappearance of severe manifestations of the disease for which the patient was treated.

ADVERSE REACTIONS

Undesirable reactions following intra-articular administration of the preparation have included postinjection flare, transient pain, occasional local irritation at the injection site, sterile abscesses, hyper- and hypopigmentation, charcot-like arthropathy, and occasional brief increase in joint discomfort; following intradermal administration, rare instances of blindness associated with intralesional therapy around the face and head, transient local discomfort, sterile abscesses, hyper- and hypopigmentation, and subcutaneous and cutaneous atrophy (which usually disappears, unless the basic disease process is itself atrophic) have occurred.
Since systemic absorption may occasionally occur with intra-articular or other local administration, patients should be watched closely for the following adverse reactions which may be associated with any corticosteroid therapy:
Fluid and electrolyte disturbances—sodium retention, fluid retention, congestive heart failure in susceptible patients, potassium loss, cardiac arrythmias or ECG changes due to potassium deficiency, hypokalemic alkalosis, and hypertension.
Musculoskeletal—muscle weakness, fatigue, steroid myopathy, loss of muscle mass, osteoporosis, vertebral compression fractures, delayed healing of fractures, aseptic necrosis of femoral and humeral heads, pathologic fractures of long bones, and spontaneous fractures.
Gastrointenstinal—peptic ulcer with possible subsequent perforation and hemorrhage, pancreatitis, abdominal distention, and ulcerative esophagitis.
Dermatologic—impaired wound healing, thin fragile skin, petechiae and ecchymoses, facial erythema, increased sweating, purpura, striae, hirsutism, acneiform eruptions, lupus erythematosus-like lesions and suppressed reactions to skin tests.
Neurological—convulsions, increased intracranial pressure with papilledema (pseudo-tumor cerebri) usually after treatment, vertigo, headache, neuritis or paresthesias, and aggravation of pre-existing psychiatric conditions.
Endocrine—menstrual irregularities; development of the cushingoid state; suppression of growth in children; secondary adrenocortical and pituitary unresponsiveness, particularly in times of stress (e.g., trauma, surgery, or illness); decreased carbohydrate tolerance; manifestations of latent diabetes mellitus; and increased requirements for insulin or oral hypoglycemic agents in diabetics.
Ophthalmic—posterior subcapsular cataracts, increased intraocular pressure, glaucoma, and exophthalmos.
Metabolic—hyperglycemia, glycosuria, and negative nitrogen balance due to protein catabolism.
Others—necrotizing angiitis, thrombophlebitis, thromboembolism, aggravation or masking of infections, insomnia, syncopal episodes, and anaphylactoid reactions.

DOSAGE AND ADMINISTRATION

Dosage: The initial dose of Kenalog-10 Injection (Sterile Triamcinolone Acetonide Suspension USP) for intra-articular or intrabursal administration and for injection into tendon sheaths may vary from 2.5 mg to 5 mg for smaller joints and from 5 to 15 mg for larger joints depending on the specific disease entity being treated. Single injections into several joints for multiple locus involvement, up to a total of 20 mg or more, have been given without incident. For intradermal administration, the initial dose of triamcinolone acetonide will vary depending upon the specific disease entity being treated but should be limited to 1.0 mg (0.1 mL) per injection site, since larger volumes are more likely to produce cutaneous atrophy. Multiple sites (separated by one centimeter or more) may be so injected, keeping in mind that the greater the *total* volume employed the more corticosteroid becomes available for possible systemic absorption and subsequent corticosteroid effects. Such injections may be repeated, if necessary, at weekly or less frequent intervals.
The lower dosages in the initial dosage range of triamcinolone acetonide may produce the desired effect when the corticosteroid is administered to provide a localized concentration. The site of the injection and the volume of the injection should be carefully considered when triamcinolone acetonide is administered for this purpose. The inital dosage should be maintained or adjusted until a satisfactory response is noted. If after a reasonable period of time there is a lack of satisfactory clinical response, Kenalog-10 Injection should be discontinued and the patient transferred to other appropriate therapy. IT SHOULD BE EMPHASIZED THAT DOSAGE REQUIREMENTS ARE VARIABLE AND MUST BE INDIVIDUALIZED ON THE BASIS OF THE DISEASE UNDER TREATMENT AND THE RESPONSE OF THE PATIENT. After a favorable response is noted, the proper maintenance dosage should be determined by decreasing the initial drug dosage in small increments at appropriate time intervals until the lowest dosage which will maintain an adequate clinical response is reached. It should be kept in mind that constant monitoring is needed in regard to drug dosage. Included in the situations which may make dosage adjustments necessary are changes in clinical status secondary to remissions or exacerbations in the disease process, the patient's individual drug responsiveness, and the effect of patient exposure to stressful situations not directly related to the disease entity under treatment; in this latter situation it may be necessary to increase the dosage of Kenalog-10 Injection (Sterile Triamcinolone Acetonide Suspension USP) for a period of time consistent with the patient's condition. If the drug is to be stopped after long-term therapy, it is recommended that it be withdrawn gradually rather than abruptly.
Administration: Shake the vial before use to insure a uniform suspension. Prior to withdrawal, inspect suspension for clumping or granular appearance (agglomeration). An agglomerated product results from exposure to freezing temperatures and should not be used. After withdrawal, inject without delay to prevent settling in the syringe. Careful technique should be employed to avoid the possibility of entering a blood vessel or introducing infection.
Routine laboratory studies, such as urinalysis, two-hour post-prandial blood sugar, determination of blood pressure and body weight, and a chest x-ray should be made at regular intervals during prolonged therapy. Upper GI x-rays are desirable in patients with an ulcer history or significant dyspepsia.
For treatment of joints, the usual intra-articular injection technique, as described in standard textbooks, should be followed. If an excessive amount of synovial fluid is present in the joint, some, but not all, should be aspirated to aid in the relief of pain and to prevent undue dilution of the steroid.
With intra-articular or intrabursal administration, and with injection of Kenalog-10 Injection into tendon sheaths, the use of a local anesthetic may often be desirable. When a local anesthetic is used, its package insert should be read with care and all the precautions connected with its use should be observed. It should be injected into the surrounding soft tissue prior to the injection of the corticosteroid. A small amount of the anesthetic solution may be instilled into the joint.
In treating acute nonspecific tenosynovitis, care should be taken to insure that the injection of Kenalog-10 Injection is made into the tendon sheath rather than the tendon substance. Epicondylitis (tennis elbow) may be treated by infiltrating the preparation into the area of greatest tenderness.
For treatment of dermal lesions, Kenalog-10 Injection is injected directly into the lesion, i.e., intradermally or sometimes subcutaneously. For accuracy of dosage measurement and ease of administration, it is preferable to employ a tuber-

culin syringe and a small bore needle (23 to 25 gauge). Ethyl chloride spray may be used to alleviate the discomfort of the injection.

HOW SUPPLIED

Kenalog-10 Injection (Sterile Triamcinolone Acetonide Suspension USP) is supplied in 5 mL multiple-dose vials providing 10 mg triamcinolone acetonide per ml. [Military Depot Item, NSN 6505-00-065-6772].

Storage: Store at room temperature; avoid freezing; protect from light.

(J3-526A)

KENALOG® IN ORABASE® ℞

[*ken'ah-log" in or'a-bās"*]

(Triamcinolone Acetonide Dental Paste USP)

DESCRIPTION

Each gram of Kenalog in Orabase provides 1 mg. (0.1%) triamcinolone acetonide in emollient dental paste containing gelatin, pectin, and carboxymethylcellulose sodium in Plastibase® (Plasticized Hydrocarbon Gel), a polyethylene and mineral oil gel base.

ACTIONS

Triamcinolone acetonide is a synthetic corticosteroid which possesses anti-inflammatory, antipruritic, and antiallergic action. The emollient dental paste acts as an adhesive vehicle for applying the active medication to the oral tissues. The vehicle provides a protective covering which may serve to temporarily reduce the pain associated with oral irritation.

INDICATIONS

Kenalog in Orabase (Triamcinolone Acetonide Dental Paste USP) is indicated for adjunctive treatment and for the temporary relief of symptoms associated with oral inflammatory lesions and ulcerative lesions resulting from trauma.

CONTRAINDICATIONS

This preparation is contraindicated in patients with a history of hypersensitivity to any of its components.

Because it contains a corticosteroid, the preparation is contraindicated in the presence of fungal, viral, or bacterial infections of the mouth or throat.

WARNING

Usage in Pregnancy—Safe use of this preparation during pregnancy has not been established with respect to possible adverse reactions upon fetal development; therefore, it should not be used in women of child-bearing potential and particularly during early pregnancy unless, in the judgment of the physician or dentist, the potential benefits outweigh the possible hazards.

PRECAUTIONS

Patients with tuberculosis, peptic ulcer or diabetes mellitus should not be treated with any corticosteroid preparation without the advice of the patient's physician.

It should be borne in mind that the normal defensive responses of the oral tissues are depressed in patients receiving topical corticosteroid therapy. Virulent strains of oral microorganisms may multiply without producing the usual warning symptoms of oral infections.

The small amount of steroid released when the preparation is used as recommended makes systemic effects very unlikely; however, they are a possibility when topical corticosteroid preparations are used over a long period of time.

If local irritation or sensitization should develop, the preparation should be discontinued and appropriate therapy instituted.

If significant regeneration or repair of oral tissues has not occurred in seven days, additional investigation into the etiology of the oral lesion is advised.

ADVERSE REACTIONS

Prolonged administration may elicit the adverse reactions known to occur with systemic steroid preparations; for example, adrenal suppression, alteration of glucose metabolism, protein catabolism, peptic ulcer activations, and others. These are usually reversible and disappear when the hormone is discontinued.

DOSAGE AND ADMINISTRATION

Press a small dab (about one-quarter of an inch) to the lesion until a thin film develops. A larger quantity may be required for coverage of some lesions. For optimal results use only enough to coat the lesion with a thin film. Do not rub in. Attempting to spread this preparation may result in a granular, gritty sensation and cause it to crumble. After application, however, a smooth, slippery film develops.

The preparation should be applied at bedtime to permit steroid contact with the lesion throughout the night. Depending on the severity of symptoms, it may be necessary to apply the preparation two or three times a day, preferably after meals. If significant repair or regeneration has not occurred in seven days, further investigation is advisable.

HOW SUPPLIED

5 gram tubes (Military Depot Item, NSN 6505-00-926-8913).

Storage: Store at room temperature; keep tube tightly closed.

(J2-482F)

MYCOLOG®-II ℞

[*mīk'ō-log"*]

Nystatin and Triamcinolone Acetonide Cream and Ointment
For Dermatologic Use Only; Not for Ophthalmic Use

DESCRIPTION

MYCOLOG-II Cream and Ointment (Nystatin and Triamcinolone Acetonide Cream and Ointment) for dermatologic use contains the antifungal agent nystatin and the synthetic corticosteroid triamcinolone acetonide.

Nystatin is a polyene antimycotic obtained from *Streptomyces noursei*. It is a yellow to light tan powder with a cereal-like odor, very slightly soluble in water, and slightly to sparingly soluble in alcohol.

Triamcinolone acetonide is designated chemically as 9-fluoro-11β,16α,17,21-tetrahydroxypregna-1,4-diene-3,20-dione cyclic 16,17-acetal with acetone. The white to cream crystalline powder has a slight odor, is practically insoluble in water, and very soluble in alcohol.

MYCOLOG-II Cream (Nystatin and Triamcinolone Acetonide Cream) is a soft, smooth, cream having a light yellow to buff color. Each gram provides 100,000 units nystatin and 1.0 mg triamcinolone acetonide in an aqueous perfumed vanishing cream base with aluminum hydroxide concentrated wet gel, titanium dioxide, glyceryl monostearate, polyethylene glycol monostearate, simethicone, sorbic acid, propylene glycol, white petrolatum, cetearyl alcohol (and) ceteareth-20, and sorbitol solution.

MYCOLOG-II Ointment (Nystatin and Triamcinolone Acetonide Ointment) provides, in each gram, 100,000 units nystatin and 1 mg triamcinolone acetonide in a protective ointment base, Plastibase® (Plasticized Hydrocarbon Gel), a polyethylene and mineral oil gel base.

These preparations are for dermatologic use only; not for ophthalmic use.

CLINICAL PHARMACOLOGY

Nystatin—Nystatin exerts its antifungal activity against a variety of pathogenic and nonpathogenic yeasts and fungi by binding to sterols in the cell membrane. The binding process renders the cell membrane incapable of functioning as a selective barrier. Nystatin provides specific anticandidal activity to *Candida* (Monilia) *albicans* and other *Candida* species, but is not active against bacteria, protozoa, trichomonads, or viruses.

Nystatin is not absorbed from intact skin or mucous membranes.

Triamcinolone Acetonide—Triamcinolone acetonide is primarily effective because of its anti-inflammatory, antipruritic and vasoconstrictive actions, characteristic of the topical corticosteroid class of drugs. The pharmacologic effects of the topical corticosteroids are well-known; however, the mechanisms of their dermatologic actions are unclear. Various laboratory methods, including vasoconstrictor assays, are used to compare and predict potencies and/or clinical efficacies of the topical corticosteroids. There is some evidence to suggest that a recognizable correlation exists between vasoconstrictor potency and therapeutic efficacy in man.

Pharmacokinetics—The extent of percutaneous absorption of topical corticosteroids is determined by many factors including the vehicle, the integrity of the epidermal barrier, and the use of occlusive dressings (see DOSAGE AND ADMINISTRATION).

Topical corticosteroids can be absorbed from normal intact skin. Inflammation and/or other disease processes in the skin increase percutaneous absorption. Occlusive dressings substantially increase the percutaneous absorption of topical corticosteroids (see DOSAGE AND ADMINISTRATION). Once absorbed through the skin, topical corticosteroids are handled through pharmacokinetic pathways similar to systemically administered corticosteroids. Corticosteroids are bound to plasma proteins in varying degrees. Corticosteroids are metabolized primarily in the liver and are then excreted by the kidneys. Some of the topical corticosteroids and their metabolites are also excreted into the bile.

Nystatin and Triamcinolone Acetonide—During clinical studies of mild to severe manifestations of cutaneous candidiasis, patients treated with nystatin and triamcinolone acetonide showed a faster and more pronounced clearing of erythema and pruritus than patients treated with nystatin or triamcinolone acetonide alone.

INDICATIONS AND USAGE

MYCOLOG-II Cream and Ointment (Nystatin and Triamcinolone Acetonide Cream and Ointment) are indicated for the treatment of cutaneous candidiasis; it has been demonstrated that the nystatin-steroid combination provides greater benefit than the nystatin component alone during the first few days of treatment.

CONTRAINDICATIONS

This preparation is contraindicated in those patients with a history of hypersensitivity to any of its components.

PRECAUTIONS

General—Systemic absorption of topical corticosteroids has produced reversible hypothalamic-pituitary-adrenal (HPA) axis suppression, manifestations of Cushing's syndrome, hyperglycemia, and glucosuria in some patients.

Conditions that augment systemic absorption include application of the more potent steroids, use over large surface areas, prolonged use, and the addition of occlusive dressings (see DOSAGE AND ADMINISTRATION).

Therefore, patients receiving a large dose of any potent topical steroid applied to a large surface area should be evaluated periodically for evidence of HPA axis suppression by using the urinary free cortisol and ACTH stimulation tests, and for impairment of thermal homeostasis. If HPA axis suppression or elevation of the body temperature occurs, an attempt should be made to withdraw the drug, to reduce the frequency of application, or to substitute a less potent steroid.

Recovery of HPA axis function and thermal homeostasis are generally prompt and complete upon discontinuation of the drug. Infrequently, signs and symptoms of steroid withdrawal may occur, requiring supplemental systemic corticosteroids.

Children may absorb proportionally larger amounts of topical corticosteroids and thus be more susceptible to systemic toxicity (see PRECAUTIONS, Pediatric Use).

If irritation or hypersensitivity develops with the combination nystatin and triamcinolone acetonide, treatment should be discontinued and appropriate therapy instituted.

Information for the Patient—Patients using this medication should receive the following information and instructions:

1. This medication is to be used as directed by the physician. It is for external use only. Avoid contact with the eyes.
2. Patients should be advised not to use this medication for any disorder other than for which it was prescribed.
3. The treated skin area should not be bandaged or otherwise covered or wrapped as to be occluded (see DOSAGE AND ADMINISTRATION).
4. Patients should report any signs of local adverse reactions.
5. When using this medication in the inguinal area, patients should be advised to apply the cream or ointment sparingly and to wear loose fitting clothing.
6. Parents of pediatric patients should be advised not to use tight-fitting diapers or plastic pants on a child being treated in the diaper area, as these garments may constitute occlusive dressings.
7. Patients should be advised on preventive measures to avoid reinfection.

Laboratory Tests—If there is a lack of therapeutic response, appropriate microbiological studies (e.g., KOH smears and/or cultures) should be repeated to confirm the diagnosis and rule out other pathogens, before instituting another course of therapy.

A urinary free cortisol test and ACTH stimulation test may be helpful in evaluating hypothalamic-pituitary-adrenal (HPA) axis suppression due to corticosteroid.

Carcinogenesis, Mutagenesis, and Impairment of Fertility—Long-term animal studies have not been performed to evaluate carcinogenic or mutagenic potential, or possible impairment of fertility in males or females.

Pregnancy Category C—There are no teratogenic studies with combined nystatin and triamcinolone acetonide. Corticosteroids are generally teratogenic in laboratory animals when administered systemically at relatively low dosage levels. The more potent corticosteroids have been shown to be teratogenic after dermal application in laboratory animals. Therefore, any topical corticosteroid preparation should be used during pregnancy only if the potential benefit justifies the potential risk to the fetus.

Topical preparations containing corticosteroids should not be used extensively on pregnant patients, in large amounts, or for prolonged periods of time.

Nursing Mothers—It is not known whether any component of this preparation is excreted in human milk. Because many drugs are excreted in human milk, caution should be exercised during use of this preparation by a nursing woman.

Pediatric Use—In clinical studies of a limited number of pediatric patients ranging in age from two months through 12 years, nystatin-triamcinolone cream formulation cleared or significantly ameliorated the disease state in most patients.

Pediatric patients may demonstrate greater susceptibility to topical corticosteroid-induced hypothalamic-pituitary-adrenal (HPA) axis suppression and Cushing's syndrome than mature patients because of a larger skin surface area to body weight ratio.

HPA axis suppression, Cushing's syndrome, and intracranial hypertension have been reported in children receiving

Continued on next page

Squibb—Cont.

topical corticosteroids. Manifestations of adrenal suppression in children include linear growth retardation, delayed weight gain, low plasma cortisol levels, and absence of response to ACTH stimulation. Manifestations of intracranial hypertension include bulging frontanelles, headaches, and bilateral papilledema.
Administration of topical corticosteroids to children should be limited to the least amount compatible with an effective therapeutic regimen. Chronic corticosteroid therapy may interfere with the growth and development of children.

ADVERSE REACTIONS
A single case (approximately one percent of patients studied) of acneform eruption occurred with use of combined nystatin and triamcinolone acetonide in clinical studies.
Nystatin is virtually nontoxic and nonsensitizing and is well tolerated by all age groups, even during prolonged use. Rarely, irritation may occur.
The following local adverse reactions are reported infrequently with topical corticosteroids (reactions are listed in an approximate decreasing order of occurrence): burning, itching, irritation, dryness, folliculitis, hypertrichosis, acneform eruptions, hypopigmentation, perioral dermatitis, allergic contact dermatitis, maceration of the skin, secondary infection, skin atrophy, striae, and miliaria.

OVERDOSAGE
Topically applied corticosteroids can be absorbed in sufficient amounts to produce systemic effects (see PRECAUTIONS, General); however, acute overdosage and serious adverse effects with dermatologic use are unlikely.

DOSAGE AND ADMINISTRATION
MYCOLOG-II Cream (Nystatin and Triamcinolone Acetonide Cream) is usually applied to the affected areas twice daily in the morning and evening by gently and thoroughly massaging the preparation into the skin. The cream should be discontinued if symptoms persist after 25 days of therapy. (See PRECAUTIONS, Laboratory Tests.)
MYCOLOG-II Cream should *not* be used with occlusive dressings.
A thin film of Mycolog-II Ointment (Nystatin and Triamcinolone Acetonide Ointment) is usually applied to the affected areas twice daily in the morning and evening.
The preparation should be discontinued if symptoms persist after 25 days of therapy (see PRECAUTIONS, Laboratory Tests).
MYCOLOG-II Ointment should *not* be used with occlusive dressings.

HOW SUPPLIED
MYCOLOG-II Cream (Nystatin and Triamcinolone Acetonide Cream) is supplied in 15 g, 30 g, and 60 g tubes and 120 g jars.
MYCOLOG-II Ointment (Nystatin and Triamcinolone Acetonide Ointment) is supplied in 15 g, 30 g, and 60 g tubes and 120 g jars.
Storage: Store at room temperature; avoid freezing cream.
(J4-019/J4-024)

MYCOSTATIN® CREAM ℞
[*mīk 'ō-stat "in*]
(Nystatin Cream)
MYCOSTATIN OINTMENT ℞
(Nystatin Ointment USP)
MYCOSTATIN TOPICAL POWDER ℞
(Nystatin Topical Powder)

DESCRIPTION
Mycostatin Cream (Nystatin Cream) contains the antifungal antibiotic Nystatin USP at a concentration of 100,000 units per gram in an aqueous, perfumed vanishing cream base containing aluminum hydroxide concentrated wet gel, titanium dioxide, propylene glycol, cetearyl alcohol (and) ceteareth-20, white petrolatum, sorbitol solution, glyceryl monostearate, polyethylene glycol monostearate, sorbic acid and simethicone.
Mycostatin Ointment (Nystatin Ointment USP) provides 100,000 units Nystatin USP per gram in Plastibase® (Plasticized Hydrocarbon Gel), a polyethylene and mineral oil gel base.
Mycostatin Topical Powder (Nystatin Topical Powder) provides, in each gram, 100,000 units Nystatin USP dispersed in Talc USP.

CLINICAL PHARMACOLOGY
Nystatin is an antifungal antibiotic which is both fungistatic and fungicidal *in vitro* against a wide variety of yeasts and yeast-like fungi. It probably acts by binding to sterols in the cell membrane of the fungus with a resultant change in membrane permeability allowing leakage of intracellular components. Nystatin is a polyene antibiotic of undetermined structural formula that is obtained from *Streptomyces noursei*, and is the first well tolerated antifungal antibiotic of dependable efficacy for the treatment of cutaneous, oral and intestinal infections caused by *Candida* (Monilia) *albicans* and other Candida species. It exhibits no appreciable activity against bacteria.
Nystatin provides specific therapy for all localized forms of candidiasis. Symptomatic relief is rapid, often occurring within 24 to 72 hours after the initiation of treatment. Cure is effected both clinically and mycologically in most cases of localized candidiasis.

INDICATIONS AND USAGE
Mycostatin topical preparations are indicated in the treatment of cutaneous or mucocutaneous mycotic infections caused by *Candida* (Monilia) *albicans* and other Candida species.

CONTRAINDICATIONS
Mycostatin topical preparations are contraindicated in patients with a history of hypersensitivity to any of their components.

PRECAUTIONS
Should a reaction of hypersensitivity occur the drug should be immediately withdrawn and appropriate measures taken.

ADVERSE REACTIONS
Nystatin is virtually nontoxic and nonsensitizing and is well tolerated by all age groups including debilitated infants, even on prolonged administration. If irritation on topical application should occur, discontinue medication.

DOSAGE AND ADMINISTRATION
The cream and the ointment should be applied liberally to affected areas twice daily or as indicated until healing is complete. The powder should be applied to candidal lesions two or three times daily until lesions have healed. For fungal infection of the feet caused by Candida species, the powder should be dusted freely on the feet as well as in shoes and socks. The cream is usually preferred to the ointment in candidiasis involving intertriginous areas; very moist lesions, however, are best treated with the topical dusting powder. The preparations do not stain skin or mucous membranes and they provide a simple, convenient means of treatment.

HOW SUPPLIED
Mycostatin Cream (Nystatin Cream) is supplied in tubes of 15 g and 30 g.
Mycostatin Ointment (Nystatin Ointment USP) is supplied in tubes of 15 g and 30 g.
Mycostatin Topical Powder (Nystatin Topical Powder) is supplied in plastic squeeze bottles of 15 g (½ oz) [Military Depot Item, NSN 6505-00-890-1218].
Storage: Store the cream at room temperature; avoid freezing. Store the ointment at room temperature. Store the topical powder at room temperature; avoid excessive heat; keep bottle tightly closed.
(J3-331B)

MYCOSTATIN® ORAL SUSPENSION ℞
[*mīk 'ō-stat "in*]
(Nystatin Oral Suspension USP)

DESCRIPTION
Nystatin is an antifungal antibiotic which is both fungistatic and fungicidal *in vitro* against a wide variety of yeasts and yeast-like fungi. It is a polyene antibiotic of undetermined structural formula that is obtained from *Streptomyces noursei.* Mycostatin Oral Suspension is provided for oral administration containing 100,000 units nystatin per mL. Inactive ingredients: alcohol (not > 1% v/v), carboxymethylcellulose sodium, flavors, glycerin, methylparaben, propylparaben, saccharin sodium, sodium phosphate, sucrose (50% w/v), and purified water.

CLINICAL PHARMACOLOGY
Nystatin probably acts by binding to sterols in the cell membrane of the fungus with a resultant change in membrane permeability allowing leakage of intracellular components. It exhibits no appreciable activity against bacteria or trichomonads.
Following oral administration, nystatin is sparingly absorbed with no detectable blood levels when given in the recommended doses. Most of the orally administered nystatin is passed unchanged in the stool.

INDICATIONS AND USAGE
Mycostatin Oral Suspension is indicated for the treatment of candidiasis in the oral cavity.

CONTRAINDICATION
The preparation is contraindicated in patients with a history of hypersensitivity to any of its components.

PRECAUTIONS
Usage in Pregnancy—No adverse effects or complications have been attributed to nystatin in infants born to women treated with nystatin.

ADVERSE REACTIONS
Nystatin is virtually nontoxic and nonsensitizing and is well tolerated by all age groups including debilitated infants, even on prolonged administration. Large oral doses have occasionally produced diarrhea, gastrointestinal distress, nausea, and vomiting.

DOSAGE AND ADMINISTRATION
INFANTS—2 mL (200,000 units nystatin) four times daily (1 mL in each side of mouth).
NOTE: Limited clinical studies in premature and low birth weight infants indicate that 1 mL four times daily is effective.
CHILDREN AND ADULTS—4-6 mL (400,000 to 600,000 units nystatin) four times daily (one-half of dose in each side of mouth). The preparation should be retained in the mouth as long as possible before swallowing.
Continue treatment for at least 48 hours after perioral symptoms have disappeared and cultures returned to normal.

HOW SUPPLIED
Mycostatin Oral Suspension (Nystatin Oral Suspension USP) is available as a pleasant-tasting, ready-to-use suspension containing 100,000 units nystatin per mL in 60 mL bottles (each supplied with a calibrated dropper) [NSN 6505-00-216-5051] 473 mL bottles, and UNIMATIC® bottles containing a single 5 mL dose.
Storage: Store at room temperature; avoid freezing.
(J3-208J)

MYCOSTATIN® ORAL TABLETS ℞
[*mīk 'ō-stat "in*]
(Nystatin Tablets USP)

DESCRIPTION
Nystatin is an antifungal antibiotic which is both fungistatic and fungicidal *in vitro* against a wide variety of yeasts and yeast-like fungi. It is a polyene antibiotic of undetermined structural formula that is obtained from *Streptomyces noursei.* Mycostatin Oral Tablets are provided for oral administration as coated tablets containing 500,000 units nystatin. Inactive ingredients: cellulose, colorants (FD&C Blue No. 2, Red No. 3, and Yellow No. 6), cornstarch, flavor, lactose, magnesium stearate, povidone, stearic acid and other ingredients.

CLINICAL PHARMACOLOGY
Nystatin probably acts by binding to sterols in the cell membrane of the fungus with a resultant change in membrane permeability allowing leakage of intracellular components. It exhibits no appreciable activity against bacteria or trichomonads.
Following oral administration, nystatin is sparingly absorbed with no detectable blood levels when given in the recommended doses. Most of the orally administered nystatin is passed unchanged in the stool.

INDICATIONS AND USAGE
Mycostatin Oral Tablets (Nystatin Tablets USP) are intended for the treatment of intestinal candidiasis.

CONTRAINDICATIONS
Mycostatin Oral Tablets are contraindicated in patients with a history of hypersensitivity to any of their components.

PRECAUTIONS
Usage in Pregnancy—No adverse effects or complications have been attributed to nystatin in infants born to women treated with nystatin.

ADVERSE REACTIONS
Nystatin is virtually nontoxic and nonsensitizing and is well tolerated by all age groups including debilitated infants, even on prolonged administration. Large oral doses have occasionally produced diarrhea, gastrointestinal distress, nausea and vomiting.

DOSAGE AND ADMINISTRATION
The usual therapeutic dosage is one to two tablets (500,000 to 1,000,000 units nystatin) three times daily. Treatment should generally be continued for at least 48 hours after clinical cure to prevent relapse.

HOW SUPPLIED
Mycostatin Oral Tablets (Nystatin Tablets USP) are available for oral administration as FILMLOK® tablets providing 500,000 units nystatin per tablet in bottles of 100 and UNIMATIC® cartons of 100. (Filmlok is a Squibb trademark for veneer-coated tablets.) [Bottles of 100, Military Depot Item, NSN6505-00-118-1949.]
Storage: Store at room temperature; avoid excessive heat. Dispense in tight, light-resistant containers.
(J3-513B)
Shown in Product Identification Section, page 431

MYCOSTATIN® VAGINAL TABLETS ℞
[*mīk'ō-stat"in*]
(Nystatin Vaginal Tablets USP)

DESCRIPTION

Nystatin is an antimycotic polyene antibiotic obtained from *Streptomyces noursei.*
Mycostatin Vaginal Tablets (Nystatin Vaginal Tablets USP) are available as diamond-shaped compressed tablets for intravaginal administration, providing 100,000 units of nystatin dispersed in lactose with ethyl cellulose, stearic acid, and starch.

CLINICAL PHARMACOLOGY

Nystatin is both fungistatic and fungicidal *in vitro* against a wide variety of yeasts and yeast-like fungi. Nystatin acts by binding to sterols in the cell membrane of sensitive fungi with a resultant change in membrane permeability allowing leakage of intracellular components. Nystatin exhibits no appreciable activity against bacteria, protozoa, trichomonads, or viruses.
Nystatin is not absorbed from intact skin or mucous membranes.

INDICATIONS AND USAGE

Mycostatin Vaginal Tablets (Nystatin Vaginal Tablets USP) are effective for the local treatment of vulvovaginal candidiasis (moniliasis). The diagnosis should be confirmed, prior to therapy, by KOH smears and/or cultures. Other pathogens commonly associated with vulvovaginitis (Trichomonas and *Haemophilus vaginalis*) do not respond to nystatin and should be ruled out by appropriate laboratory methods.

CONTRAINDICATIONS

This preparation is contraindicated in patients with a history of hypersensitivity to any of its components.

PRECAUTIONS

General: Discontinue treatment if sensitization or irritation is reported during use.
Information for Patients: The patient should be informed of symptoms of sensitization or irritation and told to report them promptly.
The patient should be warned against interruption or discontinuation of medication even during menstruation and even though symptomatic relief may occur within a few days.
The patient should be advised that adjunctive measures such as therapeutic douches are unnecessary and sometimes inadvisable, but cleansing douches may be used by nonpregnant women, if desired, for esthetic purposes.
Laboratory Tests: If there is a lack of response to Mycostatin Vaginal Tablets (Nystatin Vaginal Tablets USP), appropriate microbiological studies should be repeated to confirm the diagnosis and rule out other pathogens, before instituting another course of antimycotic therapy (see INDICATIONS AND USAGE).
Carcinogenesis, Mutagenesis, Impairment of Fertility: Long-term studies in animals have not been performed to evaluate carcinogenic potential, mutagenesis, or whether this medication affects fertility in females.
Pregnancy: Teratogenic Effects: Category A. There have been no reports that use of nystatin vaginal tablets by pregnant women increases the risk of fetal abnormalities or affects later growth, development, and functional maturation of the child. Nevertheless, because the possibility of harm cannot be ruled out, nystatin vaginal tablets should be used during pregnancy only if the physician considers it essential to the welfare of the patient.
Animal reproduction studies have not been conducted with nystatin vaginal tablets.
Pediatric Use: Safety and effectiveness in children have not been established.

ADVERSE REACTIONS

Nystatin is virtually nontoxic and nonsensitizing and is well tolerated by all age groups, even on prolonged administration. Rarely, irritation or sensitization may occur (see PRECAUTIONS).

DOSAGE AND ADMINISTRATION

The usual dosage is one tablet (100,000 units nystatin) daily for two weeks. The tablets should be deposited high in the vagina by means of the applicator. "Instructions for the Patient" are enclosed in each package.

HOW SUPPLIED

Mycostatin Vaginal Tablets (Nystatin Vaginal Tablets USP) are available in packages of 15 (NSN 6505-00-616-9128) and 30 individually foil wrapped tablets with applicator and in UNIMATIC® cartons of 50 unit-dose packs per carton—each celloprotected unit-dose pack contains one individually foil wrapped tablet, one applicator, and one "Instructions for the Patient" leaflet.
Storage: Store in refrigerator below 15° C (59° F).
(J3-635)

Shown in Product Identification Section, page 431

MYSTECLIN–F® CAPSULES ℞
[*mī-stek'lin-ef*]
(Tetracycline and Amphotericin B Capsules USP)
MYSTECLIN–F® SYRUP ℞
(Tetracycline and Amphotericin B Oral Suspension USP)

> Recently, a panel of the National Academy of Sciences—National Research Council has stated that in its informed judgment Mysteclin-F is ineffective as a fixed combination. Further, it stated, "The Panel is not aware of evidence of proved efficacy of this combination in the prevention of disease due to monilial organisms, although suppression of growth of monilia may be accomplished. It should be noted that the apparent reduction of organisms in the feces may be an artifact due to residual antibiotic activity and thus may not reflect the true state in the patient. It is preferable, in the Panel's opinion, to prescribe antifungal drugs when clinically indicated, rather than to use them indiscriminately as 'prophylaxis' against an uncommon clinical entity seen during therapy with tetracyclines and other antibiotics."

DESCRIPTION

Mysteclin-F Capsules (Tetracycline and Amphotericin B Capsules) contain tetracycline equivalent to 250 mg tetracycline hydrochloride with 50 mg amphotericin B. Inactive ingredients: colorants (D&C Red No. 33 and Yellow No. 10; FD&C Blue No. 1 and Red No. 3), gelatin, lactose, magnesium stearate, mineral oil, potassium metaphosphate, and titanium dioxide. Mysteclin-F Syrup (Tetracycline and Amphotericin B Oral Suspension) is a fruit-flavored syrup containing, in each 5 mL teaspoonful, tetracycline equivalent to 125 mg tetracycline hydrochloride and 25 mg amphotericin B. Inactive ingredients: citric acid, colorates (D&C Red No. 22 and Yellow No. 10), flavors, polysorbate 40, potassium citrate, potassium metaphosphate, saccharin sodium, sodium benzoate, sodium metabisulfite, sorbitol solution, sucrose tragacanth, and purified water.

CLINICAL PHARMACOLOGY

Mysteclin-F (Tetracycline—Amphotericin B) Capsules and Syrup have been designed to provide simultaneous antimicrobial therapy and anticandidal prophylaxis, a concept first developed by Squibb.
The preparations, which contain the broad spectrum antibiotic tetracycline, well known for its pronounced antimicrobial effect against a wide range of pathogenic organisms, produce exceptionally high initial tetracycline blood levels as well as excellent diffusion to tissues and body fluids.
Furthermore, these preparations also contain **prophylactic** amounts of the antifungal antibiotic, amphotericin B. This antibiotic, first isolated and described by the Squibb Institute for Medical Research, is substantially more active *in vitro* against *Candida* strains than nystatin[1,2,5], and has been widely used by the intravenous route in the treatment of many deep-seated mycotic infections.
Given orally, amphotericin B is extremely well tolerated[3–6] and is virtually nontoxic in prophylactic doses. Although poorly absorbed from the gut, amphotericin B has a high degree of activity against *Candida* species in the intestinal tract and prevents the overgrowth of these organisms commonly associated with broad spectrum antibiotic therapy (amphotericin B has no antibacterial activity). By suppressing overgrowth of *Candida* in the gastrointestinal tract, thereby minimizing a possible reservoir of this organism, Mysteclin-F (Tetracycline—Amphotericin B) provides added protection for the patient against troublesome, or even serious, candidal superinfections, e.g., intestinal (diarrheal), anogenital, vulvovaginal, mucocutaneous candidiasis.
Note: Microorganisms that have become insensitive to one tetracycline invariably exhibit cross-resistance to other tetracyclines. In addition, gram-negative bacilli made tetracycline resistant may also show cross-resistance to chloramphenicol.

INDICATIONS AND USAGE

Candidal overgrowth occurs in a large number of patients taking broad spectrum antibiotics. Although it is impossible to predict exactly which patient will develop candidal complications and which will not, certain types of patients are known to be particularly susceptible to candidiasis. Among these are elderly or debilitated patients; patients on high or prolonged antibiotic dosage; diabetics; infants; patients on corticoid therapy; patients who have developed candidiasis on previous broad spectrum therapy; women, particularly during pregnancy. Because the danger of candidal complications is greatest in these patients, they are potential candidates for therapy with Mysteclin-F.
Mysteclin-F (Tetracycline and Amphotericin B) Capsules and Syrup are indicated for the many common infections, including those of the respiratory, gastrointestinal and genitourinary systems, which are amenable to tetracycline therapy. Infections caused by gram-positive and gram-negative bacteria, spirochetes, viruses of the lymphogranuloma-psittacosis-trachoma group, rickettsiae and *Endamoeba histolytica* can be expected to respond. Because of the wide range of antimicrobial activity, the preparations are particularly useful in the treatment of mixed infections due to susceptible organisms.
Mysteclin-F (Tetracycline and Amphotericin B) Capsules and Syrup are also a useful part of the armamentarium in the management of chronic cases of acne vulgaris which, in the judgment of the clinician, require long-term treatment. The cystic and pustular forms of this condition respond most satisfactorily to tetracycline therapy; the papular form may also show improvement in some individuals. Because long-term maintenance therapy with tetracycline is involved, the presence of amphotericin B in the product is a particular advantage, helping to guard against the risk of candidal overgrowth.
Note: A number of strains of staphylococci and streptococci have shown resistance to tetracyclines. A few strains of pneumococci, *E. coli* and shigellae also have been reported as resistant. Indicated laboratory studies, including sensitivity tests, should be performed.

CONTRAINDICATIONS

These products should not be used in persons with a history of hypersensitivity to any of their components.

WARNINGS

THE USE OF DRUGS OF THE TETRACYCLINE CLASS DURING TOOTH DEVELOPMENT (LAST HALF OF PREGNANCY, INFANCY, AND CHILDHOOD TO AGE OF EIGHT YEARS) MAY CAUSE PERMANENT DISCOLORATION OF THE TEETH (YELLOW-GRAY-BROWN). This reaction is more common during long-term use of the drugs but has been observed following repeated short-term courses. Enamel hypoplasia has also been reported. TETRACYCLINE DRUGS, THEREFORE, SHOULD NOT BE USED IN THIS AGE GROUP UNLESS OTHER DRUGS ARE NOT LIKELY TO BE EFFECTIVE OR ARE CONTRAINDICATED.
If renal impairment exists, even usual oral or parenteral doses may lead to excessive systemic accumulation of the drug and possible liver toxicity. Under such conditions, lower-than-usual doses are indicated and if therapy is prolonged, tetracycline serum level determinations may be advisable.
Certain hypersensitive individuals may develop a photodynamic reaction precipitated by exposure to direct sunlight during the use of this drug. This reaction is usually of the photoallergic type which may also be produced by other tetracycline derivatives. Individuals with a history of photosensitivity reactions should be instructed to avoid exposure to direct sunlight while under treatment with this or other tetracycline drugs and treatment should be discontinued at first evidence of skin discomfort.
NOTE: Photosensitization reactions have occurred most frequently with demethylchlortetracycline, less with chlortetracycline and very rarely with oxytetracycline and tetracycline.

PRECAUTIONS

As with any antibiotic preparation, prolonged use may result in overgrowth of nonsusceptible organisms. Constant observation of the patient is essential. Should superinfection occur, the preparation should be discontinued and/or appropriate therapy instituted. *Note:* Superinfection of the bowel by staphylococci may be life threatening.
Tetracycline may form a stable calcium complex in any bone forming tissue with no serious harmful effects reported thus far in humans. However, use of tetracycline during tooth development (i.e., latter half of gestation, neonatal period and early childhood) may cause discoloration of the teeth (i.e., yellow-gray-brownish). This effect occurs mostly during long-term use of the drug but it has also been observed in usual short treatment courses.
During long-term therapy, periodic assessment of organ system function, including renal, hepatic, and hematopoietic systems, should be made.
Increased intracranial pressure with bulging fontanels has been observed in infants taking therapeutic doses of tetracycline. Occurrence has been rare and all signs and symptoms have disappeared rapidly upon cessation of treatment.
Since sensitivity reactions are more likely to occur in persons with a history of allergy, asthma, hay fever, or urticaria, the preparation should be used with caution in such individuals. Cross-sensitization among the various tetracyclines is extremely common.
In the treatment of gonorrhea, patients with a suspected lesion of syphilis should have darkfield examinations before receiving tetracycline and monthly serologic tests for a minimum of three months.
The use of tetracycline in staphylococcal infections does not preclude the need for indicated surgical procedures.

Continued on next page

Squibb—Cont.

ADVERSE REACTIONS

Oral administration of amphotericin B is usually well tolerated.

The following adverse reactions have been reported with tetracycline preparations:

Gastrointestinal irritation (anorexia, epigastric distress, nausea, vomiting) as well as bulky loose stools, and diarrhea may occur. Glossitis, stomatitis, enterocolitis, proctitis, and pruritus ani may occur in some patients. Black hairy tongue, sore throat, dysphagia, and hoarseness have also been reported. However, tetracycline is generally well tolerated, undesirable gastrointestinal side effects occurring significantly less frequently than with the two analogues, oxytetracycline and chlortetracycline.

Tetracyclines may also cause maculopapular and erythematous skin rashes. A rare case of exfoliative dermatitis has been reported. Photosensitivity, manifested by an exaggerated sunburn reaction has been observed in some individuals (see *Warnings*). Onycholysis and discoloration of the nails have been reported rarely.

Rise in BUN has been reported and is apparently dose related. Urinary loss of nitrogen has been observed in some patients receiving tetracyclines and may result in negative nitrogen balance. Increased excretion of sodium has also been reported. The development of peptic ulcers and bleeding has been observed in uremic patients receiving tetracyclines.

Hypersensitivity reactions may include urticaria, serum sickness-like reactions (fever, rash, arthralgia), angioneurotic edema, and anaphylactoid shock. If allergic reactions occur, or if an individual idiosyncrasy appears, tetracycline therapy should be discontinued.

Increased intracranial pressure with bulging fontanels has been reported in infants following full therapeutic doses of tetracycline. This symptom disappears rapidly when administration of tetracycline is discontinued (see *Precautions*).

The use of tetracycline during the mineralization phase of tooth development (latter half of gestation, neonatal period, and early childhood) may cause discoloration of the teeth (yellow-gray-brownish) which may sometimes be accompanied by enamel hypoplasia (see *Warnings*).

Anemia, thrombocytopenic purpura, neutropenia, and eosinophilia have been reported. Tetracyclines may delay blood coagulation.

Hepatic cholestasis has been reported rarely, and is usually associated with high dosage levels of tetracycline.

DOSAGE AND ADMINISTRATION

Dosage should be based on the tetracycline content. **Adults:** For the many common infections amenable to tetracycline therapy, adults should receive a minimum of 250 mg four times daily. Higher dosages, such as 500 mg four times daily, may be required for severe infections or for those infections which do not respond to the smaller dose. **For children above eight years of age:** In general, the pediatric dosage should supply 10 to 20 mg tetracycline per pound of body weight each day, in divided doses, depending on the type and severity of the infection.

Representative pediatric dosages of Mysteclin-F Syrup (Tetracycline and Amphotericin B Oral Suspension USP) are as follows: 20 lbs: ½ teaspoonful qid; 40 lbs: 1 teaspoonful qid; 60 lbs: 1½ teaspoonfuls qid; 80 lbs: 2 teaspoonfuls qid.

Oral forms of tetracycline should be given one hour before or two hours following meals. Pediatric dosage forms (oral) should not be given with milk formulas or other calcium containing food, and should be given at least one hour prior to feeding.

Treatment of most common infections should continue for 24 to 48 hours after symptoms and fever subside. However, if the capsules or syrup are used in the treatment of streptococcal infections due to susceptible organisms, therapy should be continued for a full 10 days to guard against the risk of rheumatic fever or glomerulonephritis. Higher dosage and even more prolonged therapy is necessary for subacute bacterial endocarditis and may be required in certain staphylococcal infections.

In chronic cases of acne vulgaris which, in the judgment of the clinician, require long-term treatment, the recommended initial dosage of the capsules or syrup is 1 gram daily in divided doses. When improvement is noted, usually within one week, dosage should be gradually reduced to maintenance levels ranging from 125 to 500 mg daily. In some patients it may be possible to maintain adequate remission of lesions with alternate-day or intermittent therapy. Tetracycline therapy of acne vulgaris should augment the other standard measures known to be of value.

HOW SUPPLIED

Mysteclin-F Capsules (Tetracycline and Amphotericin B Capsules USP) contain tetracycline equivalent to 250 mg tetracyline hydrochloride with 50 mg amohotericin B supplied in bottles of 16 and 100.

Unimatic® unit-dose packs containing 100 tablets are also available. Mysteclin-F Syrup (Tetracycline and Amphotericin B Oral Suspension USP) contains, in each 5 mL teaspoonful, tetracycline equivalent to 125 mg tetracycline hydrochloride and 25 mg amphotericin B in 240 mL bottles.

Storage: Store the capsules at room temperature; avoid excessive heat; keep tightly closed. Dispense in tight containers. Store the syrup below 30°C. (86°F.); protect from light; keep tightly closed. Dispense in tight light-resistant containers.

REFERENCES

1. Lechevalier H: Antibiotics Annual 1959-1960, New York, Antibiotica, Inc., 1960, p. 614
2. Quinn LY, Wilbur RE, Catron DV: *Antibiotics & Chemother* 10:95 1960
3. Reiss, F, *In* Muschenheim C, Robitzek EH, Vandow JE, Reiss F: *New York J Med* 59:4187 (4209) 1959
4. Halde C, Wright ET, Pollard WH, II, Newcomer VD, Sternberg TH: Antibiotics Annual 1956–1957, New York, Medical Encyclopedia, Inc., 1957, p. 123
5. Stough AR, Groel JT, Kroeger WH: *Antibiotic Med* 6:653 1959
6. Kozinn PJ, Burchall JJ, Taschdjian CL: Presented at the 7th Annual Symposium on Antibiotics, Washington, D.C., Nov. 4–6, 1959.

(J2-049C/596C)

PENICILLIN G POTASSIUM FOR INJECTION USP ℞

DESCRIPTION

Penicillin G Potassium for Injection USP is crystalline penicillin G potassium as a sterile powder. The preparation contains approximately 27 mg citrate buffer (composed of sodium citrate and not more than 0.94 mg citric acid) with approximately 1.7 mEq potassium and 0.3 mEq sodium per million units of penicillin.

CLINICAL PHARMACOLOGY

Penicillin G is bactericidal against penicillin-susceptible microorganisms during the stage of active multiplication. It acts by inhibiting biosynthesis of cell-wall mucopeptide. It is not active against the penicillinase-producing bacteria, which include many strains of staphylococci. Penicillin G is highly active *in vitro* against staphylococci (except penicillinase-producing strains), streptococci (groups A, C, G, H, L, and M) and pneumococci. Other organisms sensitive *in vitro* to penicillin G are *Neisseria gonorrhoeae, Corynebacterium diphtheriae, Bacillus anthracis,* Clostridia, *Actinomyces bovis, Streptobacillus moniliformis, Listeria monocytogenes,* and *Leptospira; Treponema pallidum* is extremely susceptible. Some species of gram-negative bacilli are susceptible to moderate to high concentrations of penicillin G obtained with intravenous administration. These include most strains of *Escherichia coli;* all strains of *Proteus mirabilis, Salmonella,* and *Shigella;* and some strains of *Enterobacter aerogenes* (formerly *Aerobacter aerogenes*) and *Alcaligenes faecalis.*

Susceptibility plate testing: If the Kirby-Bauer method of disc susceptibility is used, a 10 u. penicillin disc should give a zone greater than 28 mm. when tested against a penicillin-susceptible bacterial strain.

Aqueous penicillin G is rapidly absorbed following both intramuscular and subcutaneous injection. Approximately 60 percent of the total dose of 300,000 u. is excreted in the urine within this five-hour period. Therefore, high and frequent doses are required to maintain the elevated serum levels desirable in treating certain severe infections in individuals with normal kidney function. In neonates and young infants, and in individuals with impaired kidney function, excretion is considerably delayed.

INDICATIONS AND USAGE

Penicillin G Potassium for Injection USP is indicated in the treatment of severe infections caused by penicillin G-susceptible microorganisms when rapid and high penicillinemia is required. Therapy should be guided by bacteriological studies, including susceptibility tests, and by clinical response.

The following infections will usually respond to adequate dosage:

Streptococcal infections. Note: streptococci in groups A, C, G, H, L, and M are very susceptible to penicillin G. Some group D organisms are susceptible to the high serum levels obtained with aqueous penicillin G. Aqueous penicillin G potassium is the penicillin dosage form of choice for bacteremia, empyema, severe pneumonia, pericarditis, endocarditis, meningitis, and other severe infections caused by susceptible strains of the gram-positive species listed above.

Pneumococcal infections; Staphylococcal infections—penicillin G-susceptible; **Anthrax; Actinomycosis; Clostridial infections** (including tetanus); **Diphtheria** (to prevent the carrier state); **Erysipeloid endocarditis** *(Erysipelothrix insidiosa);* **Vincent's gingivitis and pharyngitis** (fusospirochetosis)—Severe infections of the oropharynx (Note: necessary dental care should be accomplished in infections involving gum tissue.) and **lower respiratory tract and genital area infections** due to *F. fusiformisaris* spirochetes; **Gram-negative bacillary infections** (bacteremias)—*(E. coli, E. aerogenes, A. faecalis,* Salmonella, Shigella and *P. mirabilis);* **Listeria infections** *(L. monocytogenes);* **Meningitis and endocarditis; Pasteurella infections** *(P. multocida): Bacteremia* and *meningitis;* **Rat-bite fever** *(S. minus or S. moniliformis);* **Gonorrheal endocarditis and arthritis** *(N. gonorrhoeae);* **Syphilis** *(T. pallidum)* including congenital syphilis; **Meningococcic meningitis.**

Prevention of bacterial endocarditis *(Patients unable to take oral antibiotics)*—Although no controlled clinical efficacy studies have been conducted, aqueous crystalline penicillin G for injection (**except** penicillin G procaine suspension) has been suggested by the American Heart Association and the American Dental Association for prophylaxis against bacterial endocarditis in patients with congenital heart disease or rheumatic or other acquired valvular heart disease when they undergo dental procedures and surgical procedures of the upper respiratory tract.[1] Since it may happen that *alpha* hemolytic streptococci relatively resistant to penicillin may be found when patients are receiving continuous oral penicillin for secondary prevention of rheumatic fever, prophylactic agents other than penicillin may be chosen for these patients and prescribed in addition to their continuous rheumatic fever prophylactic regimen. **NOTE: When selecting antibiotics for the prevention of bacterial endocarditis the physician or dentist should read the full joint statement of the American Heart Association and the American Dental Association.**

CONTRAINDICATIONS

Contraindicated in patients with a history of hypersensitivity to any penicillin.

WARNINGS

Serious and occasional fatal hypersensitivity (anaphylactoid) reactions have been reported in patients on penicillin therapy. Although anaphylaxis is more frequent following parenteral administration, it has occurred in patients on oral penicillins. These reactions are more apt to occur in individuals with a history of sensitivity to multiple allergens.

There have been well-documented reports of individuals with a history of penicillin hypersensitivity who have experienced severe hypersensitivity reactions when treated with cephalosporins. Before therapy with a penicillin, careful inquiry should be made concerning previous hypersensitivity reactions to penicillins, cephalosporins, and other allergens. If an allergic reaction occurs, the drug should be discontinued and the patient treated with the usual agents, e.g., pressor amines, antihistamines, and corticosteroids. Serious anaphylactoid reactions are not controlled by antihistamines alone, and require such emergency measures as the immediate use of epinephrine, aminophylline, oxygen, and intravenous corticosteroids.

PRECAUTIONS

Penicillin should be used with caution in individuals with histories of significant allergies and/or asthma.

In prolonged therapy with penicillin and particularly with high dosage schedules, periodic evaluation of the renal and hematopoietic systems is recommended.

In streptococcal infections, therapy must be sufficient to eliminate the organism (ten days minimum); otherwise the sequelae of streptococcal disease may occur. Cultures should be taken following the completion of treatment to determine whether streptococci have been eradicated.

In high doses (above 10 million u), intravenous aqueous penicillin G potassium should be administered slowly because of the adverse effects of electrolyte imbalance from the potassium content of the penicillin. The patient's renal, cardiac and vascular status should be evaluated and if impairment of function is suspected or known to exist, a reduction in the total dosage should be considered. Frequent evaluation of electrolyte balance, and renal and hematopoietic function is recommended during therapy when high doses of intravenous aqueous penicillin G potassium are used.

Prolonged use of antibiotics may promote overgrowth of nonsusceptible organisms, including fungi. Should superinfection occur, appropriate measures should be taken. Indwelling intravenous catheters encourage superinfections and should be avoided whenever possible.

Therapy of susceptible infections should be accompanied by any indicated surgical procedures. In suspected staphylococcal infections, proper laboratory studies, including susceptibility tests should be performed.

When treating gonococcal infections in which primary or secondary syphilis may be suspected, proper diagnostic procedures, including darkfield examinations, should be done. In all cases in which concomitant syphilis is suspected, monthly serological tests should be made for at least four months. All cases of penicillin-treated syphilis should receive clinical and serological examinations every six months for at least two or three years.

Any entry into the container to effect solution of the powder or withdrawal of contents must be accomplished with strict aseptic technique and sterile equipment.

ADVERSE REACTIONS

Penicillin is a substance of low toxicity but does possess a significant index of sensitization.

The hypersensitivity reactions reported are skin rashes ranging from maculopapular eruptions to exfoliative dermatitis; urticaria; and serum sickness-like reactions including chills, fever, edema, arthralgia, and prostration. Severe and occasionally fatal anaphylaxis has occurred (see WARNINGS).

Hemolytic anemia, leukopenia, thrombocytopenia, neuropathy, and nephropathy are rarely observed adverse reactions and are usually associated with high intravenous dosage. Urticaria, other skin rashes, and serum sickness-like reactions may be controlled by antihistamines and, if necessary, corticosteroids. Whenever such reactions occur, penicillin should be discontinued unless, in the opinion of the physician, the condition being treated is life-threatening and amenable only to penicillin therapy. Patients given continuous intravenous therapy with penicillin G potassium in high dosage (10 million to 100 million u daily) may suffer severe or even fatal potassium poisoning, particularly if renal insufficiency is present. Hyperreflexia, convulsions and coma may be indicative of this syndrome.

The Jarisch-Herxheimer reaction has been reported in patients treated for syphilis.

DOSAGE AND ADMINISTRATION

Penicillin G Potassium for Injection USP may be given intramuscularly or by continuous intravenous drip.

The 10,000,000 and 20,000,000 u preparations of Penicillin G Potassium for Injection USP should be administered by intravenous infusion only.

The usual dose recommendation is as follows:

Severe infections due to susceptible strains of streptococci, pneumococci, and staphylococci; bacteremia, pneumonia, endocarditis, pericarditis, empyema, meningitis and other severe infections: a minimum of 5 million u daily.

Anthrax: a minimum of 5 million u/day in divided doses until cure is effected; **Actinomycosis:** 1 to 6 million u/day for cervicofacial cases; 10 to 20 million u/day for thoracic and abdominal disease; **Clostridial infections** (as adjunctive therapy to antitoxin): 20 million u/day; **Diphtheria**—adjunctive therapy to antitoxin for prevention of the carrier state: 300,000 to 400,000 u/day in divided doses for 10 to 12 days; **Erysipeloid:** *Endocarditis:* 2 to 20 million u/day for four to six weeks; **Fusospirochetal infections** (fusospirochetosis)—severe infections of the oropharynx, lower respiratory tract and genital area: 5 to 10 million u/day; **Gram-negative bacillary infections** *(E. coli, E. aerogenes, A. faecalis,* Salmonella, Shigella, and *P. mirabilis); Bacteremia:* 20 to 80 million u/day; **Listeria infections** *(L. monocytogenes): Neonates:* 500,000 to 1 million u/day; *Adults with meningitis:* 15 to 20 million u/day for two weeks; *Adults with endocarditis:* 15 to 20 million u/ day for four weeks; **Pasteurella infections** *(P. multocida):* Bacteremia and *meningitis:* 4 to 6 million u/day for two weeks; **Rat-bite fever** *(S. minus* or *S. moniliformis):* 12 to 15 million u/day for three to four weeks.

Gonorrheal endocarditis and arthritis: a minimum of 5 million u daily.

Syphilis—aqueous penicillin G potassium may be used in the treatment of acquired and congenital syphilis but, because of the necessity of frequent dosage, hospitalization is recommended. Dosage and duration of therapy is determined by the age of the patient and the stage of the disease.

Meningococcic meningitis: 1 to 2 million u IM every two hours or continuous IV drip of 20 to 30 million u/day.

Prevention of bacterial endocarditis *Patients unable to take oral antibiotics)*—For prophylaxis against bacterial endocarditis[1] in patients with congenital heart disease or rheumatic or other acquired valvular heart disease when undergoing dental procedures or surgical procedures of the upper respiratory tract, administer 2 million u (50,000 u/kg for children) aqueous penicillin G, **except** penicillin G procaine suspension, intravenously or intramuscularly 30 to 60 minutes before the procedure and 1 million u (25,000 u/kg for children) six hours later. Doses for children should not exceed recommendations for adults for a single dose or for a 24-hour period.

Preparation of Solutions: Solutions of penicillin should be prepared as follows: Loosen powder. Hold vial horizontally and rotate it while *slowly* directing the stream of diluent against the wall of the vial. Shake vial vigorously after all the diluent has been added. Depending on the route of administration, use Sterile Water for Injection USP, isotonic Sodium Chloride Injection USP, or Dextrose Injection USP. NOTE: Penicillins are rapidly inactivated in the presence of carbohydrate solutions at alkaline pH.

RECONSTITUTION: 1,000,000 u vial—add 9.6 mL, 4.6 mL, or 3.6 mL diluent to provide 100,000 u, 200,000 u, or 250,000 u per mL, respectively: 5,000,000 u vial — add 23 mL, 18 mL, 8 mL, or 3 mL diluent to provide 200,000 u, 250,000 u, 500,000 u, or 1,000,000 u per mL, respectively. For *IV infusion only:* 10,000,000 u vial—add 15.5 mL or 5.4 mL diluent to provide 500,000 u or 1,000,000 u per mL, respectively: 20,000,000 u vial—add 31.6 mL diluent to provide 500,000 u per mL.

HOW SUPPLIED

Penicillin G Potassium for Injection USP is available in vials providing 1, 5, 10 and 20 million u of crystalline penicillin G potassium.

Storage: The dry powder is relatively stable and may be stored at room temperature without significant loss of potency. Sterile solutions may be kept in the refrigerator one week without significant loss of potency. Solutions prepared for intravenous infusion are stable at room temperature for at least 24 hours.

REFERENCE

1. American Heart Association: Prevention of bacterial endocarditis. Circulation 70: 1123A-1127A, 1984

For information contact:
Squibb-Marsam, Inc., Cherry Hill, N.J. 08034
(J4-086A)

PENICILLIN G SODIUM FOR INJECTION USP ℞

DESCRIPTION

Penicillin G Sodium for Injection is crystalline penicillin G sodium as a sterile powder. The preparation contains approximately 28 mg citrate buffer (composed of sodium citrate and not more than 0.92 mg citric acid) and 2.0 mEq sodium per million units of penicillin.

CLINICAL PHARMACOLOGY

Penicillin G is bactericidal against penicillin-susceptible microorganisms during the stage of active multiplication. It acts by inhibiting biosynthesis of cell-wall mucopeptide. It is not active against the penicillinase-producing bacteria, which include many strains of staphylococci. Penicillin G is highly active *in vitro* against staphylococci (except penicillinase-producing strains), streptococci (groups A, C, G, H, L, and M) and pneumococci. Other organisms susceptible *in vitro* to penicillin G are *Neisseria gonorrhoeae, Corynebacterium diphtheriae, Bacillus anthracis,* Clostridia, *Actinomyces bovis, Streptobadcillus moniliformis, Literia monocytogenes,* and Leptospira; *Treponema pallidum* is extremely susceptible. Some species of gram-negative bacilli are susceptible to moderate to high concentrations of penicillin G obtained with intravenous administration. These include most strains of *Escherichia coli;* all strains of *Proteus mirabilis,* Salmonella, and Shigella; and some strains of *Enterobacter aerogenes* (formerly *Aerobacter aerogenes*) and *Alcaligenes faecalis.*

Susceptibility plate testing: If the Kirby-Bauer method of disc susceptibility is used, a 10 u penicillin disc should give a zone greater than 28 mm when tested against a penicillin-susceptible bacterial strain.

Aqueous penicillin G is rapidly absorbed following both intramuscular and subcutaneous injection. Approximately 60 percent of the total dose of 300,000 u is excreted in the urine within this five-hour period. Therefore, high and frequent doses are required to maintain the elevated serum levels desirable in treating certain severe infections in individuals with normal kidney function. In neonates and young infants and in individuals with impaired kidney function, excretion is considerably delayed.

INDICATIONS AND USAGE

Penicillin G Sodium for Injection is indicated in the treatment of severe infections caused by penicillin G-susceptible microorganisms when rapid and high penicillinemia is required. Therapy should be guided by bacteriological studies, including susceptibility tests, and by clinical response.

The following infections will usually respond to adequate dosage:

Streptococcal infections. Note: streptococci in groups A, C, G, H, L, and M are very susceptible to penicillin G. Some group D organisms are susceptible to the high serum levels obtained with aqueous penicillin G. Aqueous penicillin G sodium is the penicillin dosage form of choice for bacteremia, empyema, severe pneumonia, pericarditis, endocarditis, meningitis, and other severe infections caused by susceptible strains of the gram-positive species listed above.

Pneumococcal infections; Staphylococcal infections—penicillin G-susceptible; **Anthrax; Actinomycosis; Clostridial infections** (including tetanus); **Diphtheria** (to prevent the carrier state); **Erysipeloid endocarditis** (*Erysipelothrix insidiosa*); **Vincent's gingivitis and pharyngitis** (fusospirochetosis)—Severe infections of the oropharynx (Note: necessary dental care should be accomplished in infections involving gum tissue.) and **lower respiratory tract and genital area infections** due to *F. fusiformisans* spirochetes; **Gram-negative bacillary infections** (bacteremias)—*(E. coli, E. aerogenes, A. faecalis,* salmonella, Shigella and *P. mirabilis*); **Listeria infections** (*L. monocytogenes*); **Meningitis and endocarditis; Pasteurella infections** (*P. multocida*)- *Bacteremia* and *meningitis;* **Rat-bite fever** (*S. minus* or *S. moniliformis*); **Gonorrheal endocarditis and arthritis** (*N. gonorrhoeae*); **Syphilis** (*T. pallidum*) including congenital syphilis; **Miningococcic meningitis.**

Prevention of bacterial endocarditis (*Patients unable to take oral antibiotics*) Although no controlled clinical efficacy studies have been conducted, aqueous crystalline penicillin G for injection (**except penicillin G procaine suspension**) has been suggested by the American Heart Association and the American Dental Association for prophylaxis against bacterial endocarditis in patients with congenital heart disease or rheumatic or other acquired valvular heart disease when they undergo dental procedures and surgical procedures of the upper respiratory tract.[1] Since it may happen that *alpha* hemolytic streptococci relatively resistant to penicillin may be found when patients are receiving continuous oral penicillin for secondary prevention of rheumatic fever, prophylactic agents other than penicillin may be chosen for these patients and prescribed in addition to their continuous rheumatic fever prophylactic regimen. **NOTE: When selecting antibiotics for the prevention of bacterial endocarditis the physician or dentist should read the full joint statement of the American Heart Association and the American Dental Association.[1]**

CONTRAINDICATIONS

Contraindicated in patients with a history of hypersensitivity to any penicillin.

WARNINGS

Serious and occasional fatal hypersensitivity (anaphylactoid reactions have been reported in patients on penicillin therapy. Although anaphylaxis is more frequent following parenteral administration, it has occurred in patients on oral penicillins. These reactions are more apt to occur in individuals with a history of sensitivity to multiple allergens.

There have been well-documented reports of individuals with a history of penicillin hypersensitivity who have experienced severe hypersensitivity reactions when treated with caphalosporins. Before therapy with a penicillin, careful inquiry should be made concerning previous hypersensitivity reactions to penicillins, cephalosporins, and other allergens. If an allergic reaction occurs, the drug should be discontinued and the patient treated with the usual agents, e.g., pressor amines, antihistamines, and corticosteroids. Serious anaphylactoid reactions are not controlled by antihistamines alone, and require such emergency measures as the immediate use of epinephrine, aminophylline, oxygen, and intravenous corticosteroids.

PRECAUTIONS

Penicillin should be used with caution in individuals with histories of significant allergies and/or asthma.

In prolonged therapy with penicillin and particularly with high dosage schedules, periodic evaluation of the renal and hematopoietic systems is recommended.

In streptococcal infections, therapy must be sufficient to eliminate the organism (10 days minimum); otherwise the sequelae of streptococcal disease may occur. Cultures should be taken following the completion of treatment to determine whether streptococci have been eradicated.

In high doses (above 10 million u), intravenous aqueous penicillin G sodium should be administered slowly because of the adverse effects of electrolyte imbalance from the sodium content of the penicillin. The patient's renal, cardiac and vascular status should be evaluated and if impairment of function is suspected or known to exist, a reduction in the total dosage should be considered. Frequent evaluation of electrolyte balance, and renal and hematopoietic function is recommended during therapy when high doses of intravenous aqueous penicillin G sodium are used.

Prolonged use of antibiotics may promote overgrowth of nonsusceptible organisms, including fungi. Should superinfection occur, appropriate measures should be taken. Indwelling intravenous catheters encourage superinfections and should be avoided whenever possible.

Therapy of susceptible infections should be accompanied by any indicated surgical procedures. In suspected staphylococcal infections, proper laboratory studies, including susceptibility tests, should be performed.

When treating gonococcal infections in which primary or secondary syphilis may be suspected, proper diagnostic procedures, including darkfield examinations, should be done. In all cases in which concomitant syphilis is suspected, monthly serological tests should be made for at least four months. All cases of penicillin-treated syphilis should receive clinical and serological examinations every six months for at least two or three years.

Any entry into the container to effect solution of the powder or withdrawal must be accomplished with strict aseptic technique and sterile equipment.

ADVERSE REACTIONS

Penicillin is a substance of low toxicity but does possess a significant index of sensitization.

The hypersensitivity reactions reported are skin rashes ranging from maculopapular eruptions to exfoliative derma-

Continued on next page

Squibb—Cont.

titis; urticaria; and serum sickness-like reactions including chills, fever, edema, arthralgia, and prostration. Severe and occasionally fatal anaphylaxis has occurred (se WARNINGS).
Hemolytic anemia, leukopenia, thrombocytopenia, neuropathy, and nephropathy are rarely observed adverse reactions and are usually associated with high intravenous dosage. Urticaria, other skin rashes, and serum sickness-like reactions may be controlled by antihistamines and, if necessary, corticosteroids. Whenever such reactions occur, penicillin should be discontinued unless, in the opinion of the physician, the condition being treated is life-threatening and amenable only to penicillin therapy. High dosage of penicillin G sodium may result in congestive heart failure due to high sodium intake.
The Harisch-Herxheimer reaction has been reported in patients treated for syphilis.

DOSAGE AND ADMINISTRATION

Penicillin G Sodium for Injection may be given intramuscularly or by continuous intravenous drip.
The usual dosage recommendation is as follows:
Severe infections due to susceptible strains of streptococci, pneumococci, and staphylococci; bacteremia, pneumonia, endocarditis, pericarditis, empyema, meningitis and other severe infectons: a minimum of 5 million u daily.
Anthrax: a minimum of 5 million u/day in divided doses until cure is effected; **Actinomycosis:** 1 to 6 million u/day for cervicofacial cases; 10 to 20 million u/day for thoracic and abdominal disease; **Clostridial infections** (as adjunctive therapy to antitoxin): 20 million u/day; **Diphtheria** —adjunctive therapy to antitoxin for prevention of the carrier state: 300,000 to 400,000 u/day in divided doses for 10 to 12 days; **Erysipeloid:** *Endocarditis:* 2 to 20 million u/day for four to six weeks; **Fusospirochetal infections** (fusospirochetosis) —severe infections of the oropharynx, lower respiratory tract and genital area: 5 to 10 million u/day; **Gram-negative bacillary infections** (*E. coli, E. aerogenes, A. faecalis,* Salmonella, Shigella, and *P. mirabilis*); *Bacteremia:* 20 to 80 million u/day; **Listeria infections** (*L. monocytogenes*); *Neonates:* 500,000 to 1 million u/day; *Adults with meningitis:* 15 to 20 million u/day for two weeks; *Adults with endocarditis:* 15 to 20 million u/day for four weeks; **Pasteurella infections** (*P. multocida*): *Bacteremia and meningitis:* 4 to 6 million u/day for two weeks; **Rat-bite fever** (*S. minus* or *S. moniliformis*): 12 to 15 million u/day for three to four weeks.
Gonorrheal endocarditis and arthritis: a minimum of 5 million u daily.
Syphilis —aqueous penicillin G sodium may be used in the treatment of acquired and congenital syphilis but, because of the necessity of frequent dosage, hospitalization is recommended. Dosage and duration of therapy is determined by the age of the patient and the stage of the disease.
Meningococcic meningitis: 1 to 2 million u IM every two hours or continuous IV drip of 20 to 30 million u/day.
Prevention of bacterial endocarditis (*Patients unable to take oral antibiotics*)—For prophylaxis against bacterial endocarditis[1] in patients with congenital heart disease or rheumatic or other acquired valvular heart disease when undergoing dental procedures or surgical procedures of the upper respiratory tract, administer 2 million u (50,000 u/kg for children) aqueous penicillin G, **except** penicillin G procaine suspension, intravenously or intramuscularly 30 to 60 minutes before the procedure and 1 million u (25,000 u/kg for children) six hours later. Doses for children should not exceed recommendations for adults for a single dose or for a 24-hour period.
Preparation of Solutions: Solutions of penicillin should be prepared as follows: Loosen powder. Hold vial horizontally and rotate it while *slowly* directing the stream of diluent against the wall of the vial. Shake vial vigorously after all the diluent has been added. Depending on the route of administration, use Sterile Water for Injection USP, Isotonic Sodium Chloride Injection USP, or Dextrose Injection USP. NOTE: Penicillins are rapidly inactivated in the presence of carbohydrate solutions at alkaline pH.
Reconstitute with 23 mL, 18 mL, 8 mL, or 3 mL diluent to provide concentrations of 200,000 u, 250,000 u, 500,000 u, or 1,000,000 u per mL, respectively.

HOW SUPPLIED

Penicillin G Sodium for Injection USP is available in vials providing 5 million u of crystalline penicillin G sodium.
Storage: The dry powder is relatively stable and may be stored at room temperature without significant loss of potency. Sterile solutions may be kept in the refrigerator one week without significant loss of potency. Solutions prepared for intravenous infusion are stable at room temperature for at least 24 hours.

REFERENCE

1. American Heart Association: Prevention of bacterial endocarditis. Circulation 70: 1123A–1127A, 1984

For information contact:
Squibb-Marsam, Inc., Cherry Hill, NJ 08034
(J4-067A)

PENTIDS® TABLETS ℞
[*pen'tidz*]
PENTIDS® '400' TABLETS ℞
PENTIDS® '800' TABLETS ℞
(Penicillin G Potassium Tablets USP)

PENTIDS® FOR SYRUP ℞
PENTIDS® '400' FOR SYRUP ℞
(Penicillin G Potassium for Oral Solution USP)

DESCRIPTION

Pentids Tablets (Penicillen G Potassium Tablets USP) contain crystalline penicillin G potassium for oral administration.

Pentids Tablets provide 125 mg (200,000 u) crystalline penicillin G potassium. Inactive ingredients: calcium carbonate, corn starch, lactose, magnesium stearate, and sodium benzoate.

Pentids '400' Tablets provide 250 mg (400,000 u) crystalline penicillin G potassium. Inactive ingredients: calcium carbonate, corn starch, lactose, magnesium stearate, and povidone.
Pentids '800' Tablets provide 500 mg (800,000 u) crystalline penicillin G potassium. Inactive ingredients: calcium carbonate, colorants [FD&C Blue No. 1 and Yellow No. 5 (tartrazine)], corn starch, magnesium stearate, povidone, and talc.
Pentids for Syrup and Pentids '400' for Syrup are flavored powders for constitution as syrups and oral administration; these liquid preparations are indicated especially for infants and children. Pentids for Syrup and Pentids '400' for Syrup provide 125 mg (200,000 u) and 250 mg (400,000 u) of penicillin G potassium, respectively, per 5 mL after constitution. Inactive ingredients: colorants [FD&C Yellow No. 5 (tartrazine) and Yellow No. 6], flavors, saccharin sodium, sodium phosphate, and sucrose.

CLINICAL PHARMACOLOGY

Penicillin G is bactericidal against penicillin-susceptible microorganisms during the stage of active multiplication. It acts by inhibiting biosynthesis of cell-wall mucopeptide. It is not active against the penicillinase-producing bacteria, which include many strains of staphylococci.
Penicillin G is highly active *in vitro* against staphylococci (except penicillinase-producing strains), streptococci (groups A, C, G, H, L, and M) and pneumococci. Other organisms susceptible *in vitro* to penicillin G are *Neisseria gonorrhoeae, Corynebacterium diphtheriae, Bacillus anthracis,* Clostridia, *Actinomyces bovis, Streptobacillus moniliformis, Listeria monocytogenes,* and Leptospira; *Treponema pallidum* is extremely susceptible. Some species of gram-negative bacilli are susceptible to moderate to high concentrations of penicillin G obtained with intravenous administration. These include most strains of *Escherichia coli,* all strains of *Proteus mirabilis,* Salmonella and Shigella and some strains of *Enterobacter aerogenes* (formerly *Aerobacter aerogenes*) and *Alcaligenes faecalis.*
Oral preparations of penicillin G are only slightly affected by normal gastric acidity (pH 2.0 to 3.5); however, a pH below 2.0 may partially or totally inactivate penicillin G. Oral penicillin G is absorbed in the upper small intestine, chiefly the duodenum; however, serum level and urinary excretion data indicate that only approximately 30 percent of the dose is absorbed. For this reason four to five times the dose of oral penicillin G must be given to obtain a blood level comparable to that obtained with parenteral penicillin G. Since gastric acidity, stomach emptying time, and other factors affecting absorption may vary considerably, serum levels may be appreciably reduced to nontherapeutic levels in certain individuals.
Approximately 60 percent of penicillin G is bound to serum protein. The drug is distributed throughout the body tissues in widely varying amounts. Highest levels are found in the kidneys with lesser amounts in the liver, skin, and intestines. Penicillin G penetrates into all other tissues to a lesser degree with very limited amounts found in the cerebrospinal fluid. The drug is excreted rapidly by tubular excretion in patients with normal kidney function. In neonates and young infants, and in individuals with impaired kidney function, excretion is considerably delayed. Normally, approximately 20 percent of a dose of oral penicillin G is excreted in the urine.

INDICATIONS AND USAGE

Pentids (Penicillin G Potassium) are indicated in the treatment of mild to moderately severe infections due to penicillin G-susceptible microorganisms. Therapy should be guided by bacteriological studies, including susceptibility tests, and by clinical response. Note: severe pneumonia, empyema, bacteremia, pericarditis, meningitis, and septic arthritis should not be treated with oral penicillin G during the acute stage.
Oral penicillin G is not recommended for short-term prevention of bacterial endocarditis in patients with valvular heart disease undergoing dental or surgical procedures.
Indicated surgical procedures should be performed.
The following infections will usually respond to adequate dosage:
Streptococcal infections Group A without bacteremia—Mild to moderate infections of the upper respiratory tract, skin and skin structures infections, scarlet fever, and mild erysipelas. Note: streptococci in groups A, C, G, H, L, and M are very susceptible to penicillin G. Other groups, including group D (enterococcus) are resistant.
Pneumococcal infections—Mild to moderately severe infections of the respiratory tract.
Staphylococcal infections — penicillin G-susceptible—Mild infections of the skin and skin structures. Note: reports indicate an increasing number of strains of staphylococci resistant to penicillin G, emphasizing the need for culture and susceptibility studies in treating suspected staphylococcal infections.
Vincent's gingivitis and pharyngitis (fusospirochetosis) —Mild to moderately severe infections of the oropharynx usually respond to oral penicillin G. Note: necessary dental care should be accomplished in infections involving gum tissue.
Medical conditions in which oral penicillin G therapy is indicated as prophylaxis: (A) *For the prevention of recurrence following rheumatic fever and/or chorea.* Prophylaxis with oral penicillin G on a continuing basis is effective in preventing recurrence of these conditions.
(B) *Prevention of bacteremia following tooth extraction.*

CONTRAINDICATIONS

Contraindicated in patients with a history of hypersensitivity to any penicillin.

WARNINGS

Serious and occasional fatal hypersensitivity (anaphylactoid) reactions have been reported in patients on penicillin therapy. Although anaphylaxis is more frequent following parenteral administration, it has occurred in patients on oral penicillins. These reactions are more apt to occur in individuals with a history of sensitivity to multiple allergens.
There have been well-documented reports of individuals with a history of penicillin hypersensitivity who have experienced severe hypersensitivity reactions when treated with cephalosporins. Before therapy with a penicillin, careful inquiry should be made concerning previous hypersensitivity reactions to penicillins, cephalosporins, and other allergens. If an allergic reaction occurs, the drug should be discontinued and the patient treated with the usual agents, e.g., pressor amines, antihistamines, and corticosteroids. Serious anaphylactoid reactions are not controlled by antihistamines alone, and require such emergency measures as the immediate use of epinephrine, aminophylline, oxygen, and intravenous corticosteroids.

PRECAUTIONS

Penicillin should be used with caution in individuals with histories of significant allergies and/or asthma.
The oral route of administration should not be relied upon in patients with severe illness, or with nausea, vomiting, gastric dilatation, cardiospasm or intestinal hypermotility.
Occasional patients will not absorb therapeutic amounts of orally administered penicillin.
In streptococcal infections, therapy must be sufficient to eliminate the organism (10 days minimum); otherwise the sequelae of streptococcal disease may occur. Cultures should be taken following completion of treatment to determine whether streptococci have been eradicated.
Prolonged use of antibiotics may promote the overgrowth of nonsusceptible organisms, including fungi. Should superinfection occur, appropriate measures should be taken.
In prolonged therapy with penicillin, and particularly with high dosage schedules, periodic evaluation of the renal and hematopoietic systems is recommended.
Pentids '800' Tablets (Penicillin G Potassium Tablets USP), Pentids for Syrup (Penicillin G Potassium for Oral Solution USP), and Pentids '400' for Syrup contain FD&C Yellow No. 5 (tartrazine) which may cause allergic-type reactions (including bronchial asthma) in certain susceptible individuals. Although the overall incidence of FD&C Yellow No. 5 (tartrazine) sensitivity in the general population is low, it is frequently seen in patients who also have aspirin hypersensitivity.

ADVERSE REACTIONS

Although the incidence of reactions to oral penicillins has been reported with much less frequency than following parenteral therapy, it should be remembered that all degrees of hypersensitivity, including fatal anaphylaxis, have been reported with oral penicillin.
The most common reactions to oral penicillin are nausea, vomiting, epigastric distress, diarrhea, and black hairy tongue. The hypersensitivity reactions reported are skin rashes ranging from maculopapular to exfoliative dermati-

tis; urticaria; serum sickness-like reactions including chills, fever, edema, arthralgia, and prostration; laryngeal edema; and anaphylaxis. Fever and eosinophilia may frequently be the only reactions observed. Hemolytic anemia, leukopenia, thrombocytopenia, neuropathy, and nephropathy are infrequent reactions usually associated with high doses of parenteral penicillin. Urticaria, other skin rashes, and serum sickness-like reactions may be controlled by antihistamines and, if necessary, corticosteroids. Whenever such reactions occur, penicillin should be discontinued unless, in the opinion of the physician, the condition being treated is life-threatening and amenable only to penicillin therapy. Serious anaphylactoid reactions require emergency measures (see WARNINGS).
An occasional patient may complain of sore mouth or tongue, as with any oral penicillin preparation.

DOSAGE AND ADMINISTRATION

The dosage of penicillin G should be determined according to the susceptibility of the causative microorganisms and the severity of infection, and adjusted to the clinical response of the patient.
Therapy for children under 12 years of age is calculated on the basis of body weight. For infants and small children the suggested dose is 15 to 56 mg (25,000 to 90,000 u) per kg/day in three to six divided doses.
For maximum absorption of penicillin, dosage should be given on an empty stomach. Thus, a dose of 200,000 units should be administered one-half hour before or at least two hours after meals. The blood concentration with a dose of 400,000 units is sufficiently high to inhibit susceptible bacteria when the antibiotic is given without regard to meals but, as can be expected, the resultant concentration will be higher when it is given before meals.
The usual dosage recommendation for adults and children 12 years and over is as follows:
Streptococcal infections—mild to moderately severe—of the upper respiratory tract and including otitis media, scarlet fever and mild erysipelas: 125 mg (200,000 u) tid or qid for 10 days for mild infections; 250 mg (400,000 u) tid for 10 days for moderately severe infections; alternatively, 500 mg (800,000 u) may be given bid.
Pneumococcal infections—mild to moderately severe—of the respiratory tract, including otitis media: 250 mg (400,000 u) qid until the patient has been afebrile for at least two days.
Staphylococcal infections—mild infections of skin and skin structures (culture and susceptibility tests should be performed): 125 to 250 mg (200,000 to 400,000 u) tid or qid until infection is cured.
Vincent's gingivitis and pharyngitis (fusospirochetosis) —mild to moderately severe infections of the oropharynx: 250 mg (400,000 u) tid or qid.
For the prevention of recurrence following rheumatic fever and/or chorea: 125 mg (200,000 u) twice daily on a continuing basis.

HOW SUPPLIED

•Pentids, •Pentids '400' and •Pentids '800' Tablets (Penicillin G Potassium Tablets USP) are available as scored, uncoated tablets which provide 125 mg (200,000 units), 250 mg (400,000 units) and 500 mg (800,000 units) crystalline penicillin G potassium, respectively. Pentids Tablets, in bottles of 100; Pentids '400' Tablets in bottles of 100 and Unimatic® cartons of 100; and Pentids '800' Tablets in bottles of 30 and 100.
Pentids for Syrup and Pentids '400' for Syrup (Penicillin G Potassium for Oral Solution USP) when constituted as directed on the container label, provide fruit-flavored syrups; Pentids for Syrup in 100 mL bottles, Pentids '400' for Syrup in 100 mL and 200 mL bottles.
Storage: Penicillin G Potassium Tablets USP— Store at room temperature; avoid excessive heat; keep bottle tightly closed. Dispense in tight containers.
Penicillin G Potassium for Oral Solution USP— Store at room temperature prior to preparation of syrup; store syrup in refrigerator; keep bottle tightly closed; discard unused portion after 14 days. Shake well before using.
(J2-282R/J3-311H)

PRINCIPEN® '250' CAPSULES ℞
[*prin'si-pen"*]
PRINCIPEN® '500' CAPSULES ℞
(Ampicillin Capsules USP)
PRINCIPEN® '125' FOR ORAL SUSPENSION ℞
PRINCIPEN® '250' FOR ORAL SUSPENSION ℞
(Ampicillin for Oral Suspension USP)

DESCRIPTION

Principen (Ampicillin Trihydrate), is a semisynthetic penicillin derived from the basic penicillin nucleus, 6-aminopenicillanic acid.
Principen '250' Capsules and Principen '500' Capsules (Ampicillin Capsules USP) are available for oral administration providing ampicillin trihydrate equivalent to 250 mg and 500 mg ampicillin, respectively. Inactive ingredients: gelatin, iron oxide colorant, lactose, magnesium stearate, and titanium dioxide.
Principen '125' for Oral Suspension and Principen '250' for Oral Suspension (Ampicillin for Oral Suspension USP) provide, after mixing, ampicillin trihydrate equivalent to 125 mg and 250 mg ampicillin, respectively, per 5 mL teaspoonful. Inactive ingredients: colorants (FD&C Red No. 3; Blue No. 1 in '250' only; Yellow No. 6 in '125' only), flavors, guar gum, saccharin, sodium citrate, and sucrose.

ACTIONS

Human Pharmacology: Ampicillin is bactericidal at low concentrations and is clinically effective not only against the gram-positive organisms usually susceptible to penicillin G but also against a variety of gram-negative organisms. It is stable in the presence of gastric acid and is well absorbed from the gastrointestinal tract. It diffuses readily into most body tissues and fluids; however, penetration into the cerebrospinal fluid and brain occurs only with meningeal inflammation. Ampicillin is excreted largely unchanged in the urine; its excretion can be delayed by concurrent administration of probenecid which inhibits the renal tubular secretion of ampicillin. In blood serum, ampicillin is the least bound of all the penicillins; an average of about 20 percent of the drug is bound to the plasma proteins as compared to 60 to 90 percent for the other penicillins. The administration of a 500 mg dose of ampicillin trihydrate capsules results in an average peak blood serum level of approximately 3.0 mcg/mL; the average peak serum level for the same dose of ampicillin trihydrate for oral suspension is approximately 3.4 mcg/mL.
Microbiology: The following microorganisms show *in vitro* sensitivity to ampicillin:
GRAM-POSITIVE—strains of alpha- and beta-hemolytic streptococci, *Diplococcus pneumoniae,* those strains of staphylococci which do not produce penicillinase, *Clostridium* sp., *Bacillus anthracis, Corynebacterium xerose,* and most strains of enterococci.
GRAM-NEGATIVE—*Hemophilus influenzae; Neisseria gonorrhoeae* and *N. meningitidis; Proteus mirabilis;* and many strains of Salmonella (including *S. typhosa),* Shigella, and *Escherichia coli.*
NOTE: Ampicillin is inactivated by penicillinase and therefore is ineffective against penicillinase-producing organisms including certain strains of staphylococci, *Pseudomonas aeruginosa, P. vulgaris, Klebsiella pneumoniae, Aerobacter aerogenes,* and some strains of *E. coli.* Ampicillin is not active against Rickettsia, Mycoplasma, and "large viruses" (Miyagawanella).
TESTING FOR SUSCEPTIBILITY: The invading organism should be cultured and its sensitivity demonstrated as a guide to therapy. If the Kirby-Bauer method of disc sensitivity is used, a 10 mcg ampicillin disc should be used to determine the relative *in vitro* susceptibility.

INDICATIONS

Principen Capsules (Ampicillin Capsules USP) and Principen for Oral Suspension (Ampicillin for Oral Suspension USP) are primarily indicated for the treatment of genitourinary, respiratory, and gastrointestinal tract infections caused by susceptible strains of gram-negative bacteria (including Shigella, *S. typhosa* and other Salmonella, *E. coli, H. influenzae, N. gonorrhoeae* and *N. meningitidis,* and *P. mirabilis).* Ampicillin may also be indicated in certain infections due to susceptible gram-positive bacteria: penicillin G-sensitive staphylococci, streptococci, pneumococci, and enterococci.
Bacteriology studies to determine the causative organisms and their sensitivity to ampicillin should be performed. Therapy may be instituted prior to the results of sensitivity testing.

CONTRAINDICATIONS

A history of a previous hypersensitivity reaction to any of the penicillins is a contraindication. Ampicillin is also contraindicated in infections caused by penicillinase-producing organisms.

WARNINGS

Serious and occasional fatal hypersensitivity (anaphylactoid) reactions have been reported in patients on penicillin therapy. Although anaphylaxis is more frequent following parenteral administration, it has occurred in patients on oral penicillins. These reactions are more apt to occur in individuals with a history of sensitivity to multiple allergens.
There have been well-documented reports of individuals with a history of penicillin hypersensitivity who have experienced severe hypersensitivity reactions when treated with cephalosporins. Before therapy with a penicillin, careful inquiry should be made concerning previous hypersensitivity reactions to penicillins, cephalosporins, and other allergens. If an allergic reaction occurs, the drug should be discontinued and the patient treated with the usual agents, e.g., pressor amines, antihistamines, and corticosteroids. **Serious anaphylactoid reactions require immediate emergency treatment with epinephrine. Oxygen, intravenous steroids and airway management, including intubation, should also be administered as indicated.**
Usage in Pregnancy: The safety of this drug for use in pregnancy has not been established.

PRECAUTIONS

Prolonged use of antibiotics may promote the overgrowth of nonsusceptible organisms, including fungi. Should superinfection occur, appropriate measures should be taken.
Cases of gonococcal infection with a suspected lesion of syphilis should have darkfield examinations ruling out syphilis before receiving ampicillin. Patients who do not have suspected lesions of syphilis and are treated with ampicillin should have a follow-up serologic test for syphilis each month for four months to detect syphilis that may have been masked by treatment for gonorrhea. Patients with gonorrhea who also have syphilis should be given additional appropriate parenteral penicillin treatment.
Treatment with ampicillin does not preclude the need for surgical procedures, particularly in staphylococcal infections.
In prolonged therapy, and particularly with high dosage schedules, periodic evaluation of the renal, hepatic, and hematopoietic systems is recommended.

ADVERSE REACTIONS

As with other penicillins, it may be expected that untoward reactions will be essentially limited to sensitivity phenomena. They are more likely to occur in individuals who have previously demonstrated hypersensitivity to penicillin and in those with a history of allergy, asthma, hay fever, or urticaria.
The following adverse reactions have been reported as associated with the use of ampicillin:
Gastrointestinal: glossitis, stomatitis, nausea, vomiting, enterocolitis, pseudomembranous colitis, and diarrhea. These reactions are usually associated with oral dosage forms of the drug.
Hypersensitivity Reactions: an erythematous, mildly pruritic, maculopapular skin rash has been reported fairly frequently. The rash, which usually does not develop within the first week of therapy, may cover the entire body including the soles, palms, and oral mucosa. The eruption usually disappears in 3 to 7 days. Other hypersensitivity reactions that have been reported are: skin rash, pruritus, urticaria, erythema multiforme, and an occasional case of exfoliative dermatitis. Anaphylaxis is the most serious reaction experienced and has usually been associated with the parenteral dosage form of the drug.
NOTE: Urticaria, other skin rashes, and serum sickness-like reactions may be controlled by antihistamines, and, if necessary, systemic corticosteroids. Whenever such reactions occur, ampicillin should be discontinued unless, in the opinion of the physician, the condition being treated is life-threatening and amenable only to ampicillin therapy. Serious anaphylactoid reactions require emergency measures (see WARNINGS).
Liver: moderate elevation in serum glutamic oxaloacetic transaminase (SGOT) has been noted, but the significance of this finding is unknown.
Hemic and Lymphatic Systems: anemia, thrombocytopenia, thrombocytopenic purpura, eosinophilia, leukopenia, and agranulocytosis have been reported during therapy with penicillins. These reactions are usually reversible on discontinuation of therapy and are believed to be hypersensitivity phenomena.
Other adverse reactions that have been reported with the use of ampicillin are laryngeal stridor and high fever. An occasional patient may complain of sore mouth or tongue as with any oral penicillin preparation.

DOSAGE AND ADMINISTRATION

Adults, and children weighing over 20 kg: **For genitourinary or gastrointestinal tract infections other than gonorrhea in men and women,** the usual dose is 500 mg qid in equally spaced doses; severe or chronic infections may require larger doses. For the treatment of gonorrhea in both men and women, a single oral dose of 3.5 grams of ampicillin administered simultaneously with 1.0 gram of probenecid is recommended. Physicians are cautioned to use no less than the above recommended dosage for the treatment of gonorrhea. Follow-up cultures should be obtained from the original site(s) of infection 7 to 14 days after therapy. In women, it is also desirable to obtain culture test-of-cure from both the endocervical and anal canals. Prolonged intensive therapy is needed for complications such as prostatitis and epididymitis. For **respiratory tract infections,** the usual dose is 250 mg qid in equally spaced doses.
Children weighing 20 kg or less: For **genitourinary or gastrointestinal tract infections,** the usual dose is 100 mg/kg/day total, qid in equally divided and spaced doses. For **respiratory infections,** the usual dose is 50 mg/kg/day total, in equally divided and spaced doses 3 to 4 times daily.
All patients, irrespective of age and weight: Larger doses may be required for severe or chronic infections. Although ampi-

Continued on next page

Squibb—Cont.

cillin is resistant to degradation by gastric acid, like all antibiotics given orally it should be administered at least two hours after or one-half hour before meals for maximal absorption. Except for the single dose regimen for gonorrhea referred to above, therapy should be continued for a minimum of 48 to 72 hours after the patient becomes asymptomatic or evidence of bacterial eradication has been obtained. In infections caused by hemolytic strains of streptococci, a minimum of 10 days' treatment is recommended to guard against the risk of rheumatic fever or glomerulonephritis. In the treatment of chronic urinary or gastrointestinal infections, frequent bacteriologic and clinical appraisal is necessary during therapy and may be necessary for several months afterwards. Stubborn infections may require treatment for several weeks. Smaller doses than those indicated above should not be used. Doses for children should not exceed doses recommended for adults.

HOW SUPPLIED

Principen is available for oral administration as *Principen '250' Capsules and *Principen '500' Capsules (Ampicillin Capsules USP) which provide ampicillin trihydrate equivalent to 250 mg and 500 mg ampicillin, respectively; the 250 mg potency in bottles of 100 and 500 and Unimatic® Unit-Dose Packs of 100; the 500 mg potency in bottles of 100, and 500 and Unimatic Unit-Dose Packs of 100. It is also available for oral administration as Principen '125' for Oral Suspension and Principen '250' for Oral Suspension (Ampicillin for Oral Suspension USP) which provide, after mixing, pleasantly flavored suspensions containing ampicillin trihydrate equivalent to 125 mg and 250 mg ampicillin, respectively, per 5 mL teaspoonful; both potencies in 80, 100, 150, and 200 mL bottles, and in Unimatic® cartons of 4 × 25 bottles (5 mL each bottle).

Storage: Principen Capsules—Store at room temperature; avoid excessive heat; keep bottle tightly closed. Dispense in tight containers.

Principen for Oral Suspension—Store at room temperature prior to preparation of suspension; after preparation of suspension, store at room temperature and discard unused portion after 7 days or store in refrigerator and discard unused portion after 14 days; keep bottle tightly closed. Shake well before using.

(J3-339E)

*Shown in Product Identification Section, page 431

PRINCIPEN® with PROBENECID ℞

[prin 'si-pen" with pro"ben'e-sid"]

(Ampicillin and Probenecid Capsules USP)

DESCRIPTION

Ampicillin trihydrate is a semisynthetic penicillin derived from the basic penicillin nucleus, 6-aminopenicillanic acid. Probenecid is a uricosuric and renal tubular blocking agent. Principen with Probenecid (Ampicillin and Probenecid Capsules) is provided in single-dose bottles containing nine capsules; each capsule contains ampicillin trihydrate equivalent to 389 mg ampicillin and 111 mg probenecid (9 capsules contain ampicillin trihydrate equivalent to 3.5 g ampicillin and 1 g probenecid). Inactive ingredients: colorants (D&C Red No. 33; D&C Yellow No. 10, FD&C Blue No. 1, FD&C Red No. 3, FD&C Yellow No. 6), gelatin, magnesium stearate, and titanium dioxide.

CLINICAL PHARMACOLOGY

Ampicillin is stable in the presence of gastric acid and is well absorbed from the gastrointestinal tract. It diffuses readily into most body tissues and fluids; however, penetration into the cerebrospinal fluid and brain occurs only with meningeal inflammation. Ampicillin is excreted largely unchanged in the urine; its excretion is delayed by concurrent administration of probenecid which inhibits the renal tubular secretion of ampicillin. In blood serum, ampicillin is the least bound of all the penicillins; an average of about 20 percent of the drug is bound to the plasma proteins as compared to 60 to 90 percent for the other penicillins. Probenecid inhibits the tubular reabsorption of urate, thus increasing the urinary excretion of uric acid and decreasing serum uric acid levels. It also inhibits the tubular secretion of penicillin and usually increases penicillin plasma levels by any route the antibiotic is given. A two-fold to four-fold elevation has been demonstrated for various penicillins.

Ampicillin is inactivated by penicillinase and therefore is ineffective against penicillinase-producing organisms.

INDICATIONS AND USAGE

Principen with Probenecid (Ampicillin and Probenecid Capsules) is indicated for the treatment of uncomplicated infection (urethral, endocervical, or rectal) caused by *Neisseria gonorrhoeae* in men and women.

Urethritis and the presence of gram-negative diplococci in urethral smears is strong presumptive evidence of gonorrhea. Culture or fluorescent antibody studies will confirm the diagnosis.

Susceptibility studies should be performed with recurrent infections or when resistant strains are encountered. Therapy may be instituted prior to obtaining results of susceptibility testing.

CONTRAINDICATIONS

A history of a previous hypersensitivity reaction to any of the penicillins or to probenecid is a contraindication.

Probenecid is not recommended in persons with known blood dyscrasias or uric acid kidney stones or during an acute attack of gout. It is not recommended in conjunction with ampicillin in the presence of known renal impairment.

WARNINGS

Serious and occasional fatal hypersensitivity (anaphylactoid) reactions have been reported in patients on penicillin therapy. Although anaphylaxis is more frequent following parenteral administration, it has occurred in patients on oral penicillins. These reactions are more apt to occur in individuals with a history of sensitivity to multiple allergens.

There have been well-documented reports of individuals with a history of penicillin hypersensitivity who have experienced severe hypersensitivity reactions when treated with cephalosporins. Before therapy with a penicillin, careful inquiry should be made concerning previous hypersensitivity reactions to penicillins, cephalosporins, and other allergens. If an allergic reaction occurs, the patient should be treated with the usual agents, e.g., pressor amines, antihistamines, and corticosteroids. **Serious anaphylactoid reactions require immediate emergency treatment with epinephrine. Oxygen, intravenous steroids, and airway management, including intubation, should also be administered as indicated.**

Usage in Pregnancy: The safety of these drugs for use in pregnancy has not been established.

PRECAUTIONS

Cases of gonococcal infection with a suspected lesion of syphilis should have darkfield examinations ruling out syphilis before receiving ampicillin. Patients who do not have suspected lesions of syphilis and are treated with ampicillin should have a follow-up serologic test for syphilis each month for four months to detect syphilis that may have been masked by treatment for gonorrhea. Patients with gonorrhea who also have syphilis should be given additional appropriate parenteral penicillin treatment.

ADVERSE REACTIONS

Ampicillin—As with other penicillins, it may be expected that untoward reactions will be essentially limited to sensitivity phenomena. They are more likely to occur in individuals who have previously demonstrated hypersensitivity to penicillin and in those with a history of allergy, asthma, hay fever, or urticaria.

The following adverse reactions have been reported as associated with the use of ampicillin:

Gastrointestinal: glossitis, stomatitis, nausea, vomiting, enterocolitis, pseudomembranous colitis, and diarrhea. These reactions are usually associated with oral dosage forms of the drug.

Hypersensitivity Reactions: An erythematous, mildly pruritic, maculopapular skin rash has been reported fairly frequently. The rash, which usually does not develop within the first week of therapy, may cover the entire body including the soles, palms, and oral mucosa. The eruption usually disappears in three to seven days. Other hypersensitivity reactions that have been reported are: skin rash, pruritus, urticaria, erythema multiforme, and an occasional case of exfoliative dermatitis. Anaphylaxis is the most serious reaction experienced and has usually been associated with the parenteral dosage form of the drug.

NOTE: Urticaria, other skin rashes, and serum sickness-like reactions may be controlled by antihistamines, and, if necessary, systemic corticosteroids. Serious anaphylactoid reactions require emergency measures (see WARNINGS).

Liver: Moderate elevation in serum glutamic oxaloacetic transaminase (SGOT) has been noted, but the significance of this finding is unknown.

Hemic and Lymphatic Systems: Anemia, thrombocytopenia, thrombocytopenic purpura, eosinophilia, leukopenia, and agranulocytosis have been reported during therapy with penicillins. These reactions are usually reversible on discontinuation of therapy and are believed to be hypersensitivity phenomena.

Probenecid—The following are the principal adverse reactions which have been reported as associated with the use of probenecid, generally with more prolonged or repeated administration: hypersensitivity reactions (including anaphylaxis), nephrotic syndrome, hepatic necrosis, aplastic anemia; also other anemias, including hemolytic anemia related to genetic deficiency of glucose-6-phosphate dehydrogenase.

DOSAGE AND ADMINISTRATION

For the treatment of gonorrhea in both men and women—3.5 g ampicillin and 1 g probenecid (9 capsules) is administered as a single dose.

Physicians are cautioned to use no less than the above recommended dosage.

Follow-up cultures should be obtained from the original site(s) of infection 7 to 14 days after therapy. In women, it is also desirable to obtain culture test-of-cure from both the endocervical and anal canals.

HOW SUPPLIED

Principen with Probenecid (Ampicillin and Probenecid Capsules USP) is provided in single-dose bottles containing nine capsules; each capsule contains ampicillin trihydrate equivalent to 389 mg ampicillin and 111 mg probenecid (9 capsules contain ampicillin trihydrate equivalent to 3.5 g ampicillin and 1 g probenecid).

Storage: Store at room temperature; avoid excessive heat.

(J3-335G)

SUMYCIN® '250' TABLETS ℞

[sū"mī'sin]

SUMYCIN® '500' TABLETS ℞

(Tetracycline Hydrochloride Tablets USP)

SUMYCIN® '250' CAPSULES ℞

SUMYCIN® '500' CAPSULES ℞

(Tetracycline Hydrochloride Capsules USP)

SUMYCIN® SYRUP ℞

(Tetracycline Oral Suspension USP)

DESCRIPTION

Sumycin '250' and Sumycin '500' Tablets (Tetracycline Hydrochloride Tablets) are available for oral administration as FILMLOK®* tablets providing 250 mg and 500 mg tetracycline, respectively. Inactive ingredients: cellulose, colorant (D&C Red No. 30), lactose, magnesium stearate, povidone, starch, stearic acid, and other ingredients.

Sumycin '250' and Sumycin '500' Capsules (Tetracycline Hydrochloride Capsules) contain 250 mg and 500 mg crystalline tetracycline hydrochloride, respectively. Inactive ingredients: colorants (FD&C Blue No. 1 and Red No. 3), gelatin, lactose, magnesium stearate, mineral oil, and titanium dioxide.

Symycin Syrup (Tetracycline Oral Suspension) is a suspension containing, in each 5 mL teaspoonful, tetracycline equivalent to 125 mg tetracycline hydrochloride. Inactive ingredients: citric acid, colorant (D&C Yellow No. 10), flavor, potassium citrate, potassium metaphosphate, purified water, saccharin sodium, sodium benzoate, sodium citrate, sodium metabisulfite, sorbitol solution, sucrose, and tragacanth.

CLINICAL PHARMACOLOGY

The tetracyclines are primarily bacteriostatic antibiotics and are thought to exert their antimicrobial effect by the inhibition of protein synthesis. Tetracyclines are active against a wide range of gram-negative and gram-positive organisms.

The drugs in the tetracycline class have closely similar antimicrobial spectra. Microorganisms that have become insensitive to one tetracycline invariably exhibit cross-resistance to other tetracyclines. In addition, gram-negative bacilli made tetracycline-resistant may also show cross-resistance to chloramphenicol. Microorganisms may be considered susceptible if the MIC (minimum inhibitory concentration) is not more than 4 mcg/mL and intermediate if the MIC is 4 to 12.5 mcg/mL.

Susceptibility plate testing: A tetracycline disc may be used to determine microbial susceptibility to drugs in the tetracycline class. If the Kirby-Bauer method of disc sensitivity is used, a 30 mcg tetracycline disc should give a zone of at least 19 mm when tested against a tetracycline-susceptible bacterial strain.

Tetracyclines are readily absorbed and are bound to plasma proteins in varying degree. They are concentrated by the liver in the bile and excreted in the urine and feces at high concentrations and in a biologically active form.

INDICATIONS AND USAGE

Tetracycline is indicated in infections caused by the following microorganisms.

Rickettsiae: Rocky mountain spotted fever, typhus fever and the typhus group, Q fever, rickettsialpox, tick fevers, *Mycoplasma pneumoniae* (PPLO, Eaton agent), agents of psittacosis and ornithosis, agents of *Lymphogranuloma venereum* and *Granuloma inguinale*, and the spirochetal agent of relapsing fever *(B. recurrentis)*.

The following gram-negative organisms: *H. ducreyi* (chancroid), *Pasteurella pestis* and *Past. tularensis*, *Bartonella bacilliformis*, Bacteroides, *Vibrio comma* and *V. fetus*, and Brucella organisms (in conjunction with streptomycin).

Because many strains of the following groups of microorganisms have been shown to be resistant to tetracyclines, culture and susceptibility testing are recommended.

The following gram-negative organisms, when bacteriologic testing indicates appropriate susceptibility to the drug: *E. coli, Enterobacter aerogenes* (formerly *A. aerogenes*), Shigella, *Mima, Herellea, H. influenzae* (respiratory infections), and Klebsiella infections (respiratory and urinary).
The following gram-positive organisms when bacteriologic testing indicates appropriate susceptibility to the drug:
1) Streptococcus species: Up to 44 percent of strains of *Streptococcus pyogenes* and 74 percent of *Streptococcus faecalis* have been found to be resistant to tetracycline drugs. Therefore, tetracyclines should not be used for streptococcal disease unless the organism has been demonstrated to be sensitive.
(For upper respiratory infections due to group A beta-hemolytic streptococci, penicillin is the usual drug of choice including prophylaxis of rheumatic fever.)
2) *D. pneumoniae.*
3) *Staphylococcus aureus* (skin and soft tissue infections). Tetracyclines are not the drugs of choice in the treatment of any type of staphylococcal infections.
When penicillin is contraindicated, tetracyclines are alternative drugs in the treatment of infections due to: *N. gonorrhoeae, T. pallidum* and *T. pertenue* (syphilis and yaws), *Listeria monocytogenes,* Clostridia, *B. anthracis, Fusobacterium fusiforme* (Vincent's infection), and *Actinomyces.*
Tetracycline hydrochloride is indicated for the treatment of uncomplicated urethral, endocervical, or rectal infections in adults caused by *Chlamydia trachomatis.*[1]
In acute intestinal amebiasis, the tetracyclines may be a useful adjunct to amebicides.
In severe acne the tetracyclines may be useful adjunctive therapy.
Tetracyclines are indicated in the treatment of trachoma, although the infectious agent is not always eliminated, as judged by immunofluorescence.
Inclusion conjunctivitis may be treated with oral tetracyclines or with a combination of oral and topical agents.

CONTRAINDICATIONS

This drug is contraindicated in persons who have shown hypersensitivity to any of the tetracyclines.

WARNINGS

THE USE OF DRUGS OF THE TETRACYCLINE CLASS DURING TOOTH DEVELOPMENT (LAST HALF OF PREGNANCY, INFANCY AND CHILDHOOD TO AGE OF EIGHT YEARS) MAY CAUSE PERMANENT DISCOLORATION OF THE TEETH (YELLOW-GRAY-BROWN). This reaction is more common during long-term use of the drugs but has been observed following repeated short-term courses. Enamel hypoplasia has also been reported. TETRACYCLINE DRUGS, THEREFORE, SHOULD NOT BE USED IN THIS AGE GROUP UNLESS OTHER DRUGS ARE NOT LIKELY TO BE EFFECTIVE OR ARE CONTRAINDICATED.
If renal impairment exists, even usual oral or parenteral doses may lead to excessive systemic accumulation of the drug and possible liver toxicity. Under such conditions, lower than usual doses are indicated and, if therapy is prolonged, serum level determinations of the drug may be advisable. The antianabolic action of tetracycline may cause an increase in BUN. While this is not a problem in those with normal renal function, in patients with significantly impaired function, higher serum levels of tetracycline may lead to azotemia, hyperphosphatemia, and acidosis.
Photosensitivity, manifested by an exaggerated sunburn reaction, has been observed in some individuals taking tetracyclines. Patients apt to be exposed to direct sunlight or ultra-violet light should be advised that this reaction can occur with tetracycline drugs, and treatment should be discontinued at the first evidence of skin erythema. NOTE: Photosensitization reactions have occurred most frequently with demeclocycline, less with chlortetracycline, and very rarely with oxytetracycline and tetracycline.
Usage in Pregnancy: (See WARNINGS about use during tooth development.)
Results of animal studies indicate that tetracyclines cross the placenta, are found in fetal tissues and can have toxic effects on the developing fetus (often related to retardation of skeletal development). Evidence of embryotoxicity has also been noted in animals treated early in pregnancy.
Usage in Newborns, Infants, and Children: (See WARNINGS about use during tooth development.)
Tetracyclines form a stable calcium complex in any bone-forming tissue. A decrease in the fibula growth rate has been observed in prematures given oral tetracycline in doses of 25 mg/kg every six hours. This reaction was shown to be reversible when the drug was discontinued.
Tetracyclines are present in the milk of lactating women who are taking a drug in this class.

PRECAUTIONS

As with other antibiotics, use of this drug may result in overgrowth of nonsusceptible organisms, including fungi. If superinfection occurs, the antibiotic should be discontinued and appropriate therapy instituted. Note: Superinfection of the bowel by staphylococci may be life-threatening.
In venereal diseases when coexistent syphilis is suspected, patients should have darkfield examinations before treatment is started and the blood serology should be repeated monthly for at least four months.
Because the tetracyclines have been shown to depress plasma prothrombin activity, patients who are on anticoagulant therapy may require downward adjustment of their anticoagulant dosage.
During long-term therapy, periodic laboratory evaluation of organ systems, including hematopoietic, renal and hepatic studies should be performed.
All infections due to group A beta-hemolytic streptococci should be treated for at least 10 days.
Since bacteriostatic drugs may interfere with the bactericidal action of penicillin, it is advisable to avoid giving tetracycline in conjunction with penicillin.
Since sensitivity reactions are more likely to occur in persons with a history of allergy, asthma, hay fever, or urticaria, the preparation should be used with caution in such individuals.

ADVERSE REACTIONS

Gastrointestinal: anorexia, epigastric distress, nausea, vomiting, diarrhea, bulky loose stools, stomatitis, sore throat, glossitis, black hairy tongue, dysphagia, hoarseness, enterocolitis, and inflammatory lesions (with candidal overgrowth) in the anogenital region, including proctitis and pruritus ani. These reactions have been caused by both the oral and parenteral administration of tetracyclines but are less frequent after parenteral use.
Skin: maculopapular and erythematous rashes. Exfoliative dermatitis has been reported but is uncommon. Onycholysis and discoloration of the nails have been reported rarely. Photosensitivity has occurred (see WARNINGS).
Renal toxicity: rise in BUN has been reported and is apparently dose-related (see WARNINGS).
Hepatic cholestasis has been reported rarely, and is usually associated with high dosage levels of tetracycline.
Hypersensitivity reactions: urticaria, angioneurotic edema, anaphylaxis, anaphylactoid purpura, pericarditis, exacerbation of systemic lupus erythematosus, and serum sickness-like reactions, as fever, rash, and arthralgia.
When given over prolonged periods, tetracyclines have been reported to produce brown-black microscopic discoloration of thyroid glands. No abnormalities of thyroid function studies are known to occur.
Bulging fontanels have been reported in young infants following full therapeutic dosage. This sign disappeared rapidly when the drug was discontinued.
Blood: anemia, hemolytic anemia, thrombocytopenia, thrombocytopenic purpura, neutropenia and eosinophilia have been reported.
Dizziness and headache have been reported.

DOSAGE AND ADMINISTRATION

Adults: usual daily dose is 1 to 2 g; for mild to moderate infections: 500 mg bid or 250 mg qid; higher dosages such as 500 mg qid may be required for severe infections.
For children above eight years of age: usual daily dose is 10 to 20 mg/lb (25 to 50 mg/kg) body weight divided in four equal doses.
Representative pediatric dosages for the syrup on a qid basis are as follows: 20 lbs—½ teaspoonful; 40 lbs—1 teaspoonful; 60 lbs—1½ teaspoonfuls; and 80 lbs—2 teaspoonfuls.
Therapy should be continued for at least 24 to 48 hours after symptoms and fever have subsided.
The treatment of brucellosis, 500 mg tetracycline four times daily for three weeks should be accompanied by streptomycin, 1 g intramuscularly twice daily the first week and once daily the second week.
For treatment of gonorrhea, the recommended dose is 1.5 g initially, then 0.5 g every six hours until a total of 9 g have been given.
For treatment of syphilis, a total of 30 to 40 g in equally divided doses over a period of 10 to 15 days should be given. Close followup, including laboratory tests, is recommended.
Uncomplicated urethral, endocervical, or rectal infection in adults caused by *Chlamydia trachomatis:* 500 mg, by mouth, four times a day for at least seven days.[1]
In cases of severe acne which, in the judgment of the clinician, require long-term treatment, the recommended initial dosage is 1 g daily in divided doses. When improvement is noted, usually within one week, dosage should be gradually reduced to maintenance levels ranging from 125 mg to 500 mg daily. In some patients it may be possible to maintain adequate remission of lesions with alternate-day or intermittent therapy. Tetracycline therapy of acne should augment the other standard measures known to be of value.
In patients with renal impairment (see WARNINGS) total dosage should be decreased by reduction of recommended individual doses and/or by extending time intervals between doses.
In the treatment of streptococcal infections, a therapeutic dose of tetracycline should be administered for at least 10 days.
Concomitant therapy: Antacids containing aluminum, calcium, or magnesium impair absorption and should not be given to patients taking oral tetracycline.
Foods and some dairy products also interfere with absorption. Oral forms of tetracycline should be given one hour before or two hours after meals. Pediatric oral dosage forms should not be given with milk formulas and should be given at least one hour prior to feeding.

HOW SUPPLIED

*Sumycin '250' Tablets (Tetracycline Hydrochloride Tablets USP) are available for oral administration as tablets containing 250 mg tetracycline hydrochloride in bottles of 100 and 1000. *Sumycin '500' Tablets are available for oral administration as tablets containing 500 mg tetracycline hydrochloride in bottles of 100 and 500. *Sumycin '250' Capsules (Tetracycline Hydrochloride Capsules USP) are available for oral administration as capsules containing 250 mg tetracycline hydrochloride in bottles of 100 (NSN 6505-00-655-8355) and 1000 and in Unimatic® Unit-Dose Packs of 100. *Sumycin '500' Capsules are available for oral administration as capsules containing 500 mg tetracycline hydrochloride in bottles of 100 and 500 and in Unimatic Unit-Dose Packs of 100.
Sumycin Syrup (Tetracycline Oral Suspension USP) is available as a fruit-flavored suspension containing, in each 5 mL teaspoonful, tetracycline equivalent to 125 mg tetracycline hydrochloride in bottles of 60 mL and 473 mL (1 pint). (NSN 6505-00-656-1344).
Storage: Store the tablets and capsules at room temperature; avoid excessive heat. Store the syrup below 30° C (86° F); avoid freezing; protect from light; keep bottle tightly closed.
Reference: 1. CDC Sexually Transmitted Diseases Guidelines 1982.
(J3-291F)

**Shown in Product Identification Section, page 431*

TESLAC® TABLETS ℞

[*tez 'lak*]
(Testolactone Tablets USP)

DESCRIPTION

Teslac (Testolactone) Tablets USP provides testolactone for oral administration. Each tablet contains 50 mg testolactone, which is chemically designated as D- Homo-17a-oxaandrosta-1, 4-diene-3, 17-dione (1-dehydrotestololactone, or Δ^1-testololactone). Inactive ingredients: calcium stearate, cornstarch, gelatin, and lactose.
Testolactone is a white, odorless, crystalline solid, soluble in ethanol and slightly soluble in water.

CLINICAL PHARMACOLOGY

The precise mechanism by which testolactone produces its clinical antineoplastic effects is unknown at present.
Although the chemical configuration of testolactone is similar to that of certain androgenic hormones, it is devoid of androgenic activity in the doses commonly employed.
Teslac was found to be effective in approximately 15% of patients with advanced or disseminated mammary cancer evaluated according to the following criteria: 1) those with a measurable decrease in size of all demonstrable tumor masses; 2) those in whom more than 50% of non-osseous lesions decreased in size although all bone lesions remained static; and 3) those in whom more than 50% of total lesions improved while the remainder were static.

INDICATIONS AND USAGE

Teslac Tablets (Testolactone Tablets USP) are recommended as adjunctive therapy in the palliative treatment of advanced or disseminated breast cancer in postmenopausal women when hormonal therapy is indicated. It may also be used in women who were diagnosed as having had disseminated breast carcinoma when premenopausal, in whom ovarian function has been subsequently terminated.

CONTRAINDICATIONS

Testolactone is contraindicated in the treatment of breast cancer in men.

WARNINGS

Usage in Pregnancy: Since safe use of testolactone has not been established with respect to adverse effects upon fetal development, and since this preparation is intended for use only in postmenopausal women, testolactone should not be used during pregnancy.

PRECAUTIONS

Plasma calcium levels should be routinely determined in any patient receiving therapy for mammary cancer, particularly during periods of active remission of bony metastases. If hypercalcemia occurs, appropriate measures should be instituted.

ADVERSE REACTIONS

Certain signs and symptoms have been reported in association with the use of this drug but, in these instances, it is

Continued on next page

Squibb—Cont.

often impossible to determine the relationship of the underlying disease and drug administration to the reported reaction. Such reactions include maculopapular erythema, increase in blood pressure, paresthesia, aches and edema of the extremities, glossitis, anorexia, and nausea and vomiting. Alopecia alone and with associated nail growth disturbance have been reported rarely; these side effects subsided without interruption of treatment.

DOSAGE AND ADMINISTRATION

The recommended oral dose is 250 mg qid.
In order to evaluate the response, therapy with testolactone should be continued for a minimum of three months unless there is active progression of the disease.

HOW SUPPLIED

Teslac is available for oral administration as tablets containing 50 mg testolactone in bottles of 100. Tablet identification number 690.
Storage: Store at room temperature; avoid excessive heat.
(J3-305C)

THERAGRAN HEMATINIC® ℞

[ther'ah-gran" hē mah-tin'ik]
(Therapeutic Formula Vitamin Tablets with Hematinics)

DESCRIPTION

Theragran Hematinic is a therapeutic iron-containing multivitamin with minerals tablet for oral administration.
Graphic formulas and physical/chemical information for the vitamins may be found in the US Pharmacopeia XX. Theragran Hematinic Tablets supply:

Active Ingredients	*Each Tablet*	*3 Tablets (usual daily dose)*
Vitamin A (as Acetate)	(8,333 IU) 2.5mg	25,000IU
Vitamin D (Ergocalciferol)	(133 IU) 3.3mcg	400IU
Thiamine Mononitrate	3.3mg	10mg
Riboflavin	3.3mg	10mg
Pyridoxine Hydrochloride	3.3mg	10mg
Niacinamide	33.3mg	100mg
Calcium Pantothenate	11.7mg	35mg
Vitamin E (dl-α-Tocopheryl Acetate)	(5 IU) 5mg	15IU
Copper (as Sulfate)	0.67mg	2mg
Magnesium (as Carbonate)	41.7mg	125mg
Iron, elemental (as Ferrous Fumarate)	66.7mg	200mg
Vitamin B_{12} (as Cyanocobalamin)	50mcg	150mcg
Folic Acid	0.33mg	1mg
Vitamin C (as Sodium Ascorbate)	100mg	300mg

Inactive ingredients: acacia, calcium carbonate, carnauba wax, castor oil, cellulose, colorants [FD&C Red No. 3 and Yellow No. 5 (tartrazine)], ethylcellulose, flavor, gelatin, lactose, magnesium stearate, povidone, shellac, sodium bisulfite, sodium starch glycolate, sucrose, talc, titanium dioxide, and white wax.

CLINICAL PHARMACOLOGY

Vitamins and dietary minerals are fundamentally involved in vital metabolic processes, where they usually serve as oxidizing and reducing agents and as factors in various enzyme systems. These essential micronutrients are so closely interrelated that the lack of any one may affect the body requirements of others.
Metabolic Functions of Inorganic Ions—*Iron* plays an important role in oxygen and electron transport. Iron may be functional (in hemoglobin, myoglobin, heme enzymes, and cofactor and transport iron) or stored as ferritin and hemosiderin in the liver, spleen, bone marrow, and reticuloendothelial system. The hemoglobin (0.34 percent iron) content of blood is about 14 to 17 g per 100 mL in adult males; in adult females it ranges between 12 and 14 g. Following ingestion, ferrous iron forms low molecular chelates with amino acids, ascorbic acid, and sugars which may be solubilized and absorbed before they reach the distal small intestine. Iron is probably absorbed passively into the mucosal layer of the small intestine, then transferred actively to transferrin where it is incorporated into red blood cells in bone marrow or into all body cells. Transferrin iron may also be stored in bone marrow, liver and spleen. Iron is removed from the body in the urine, bile, sweat, feces, and via desquamation of cells.
Copper: an essential enzyme cofactor in the utilization of iron in hemoglobin synthesis.
Magnesium: an enzyme activator—certain peptidases and phosphatases require magnesium for maximal activity as do virtually all reactions involving adenosine triphosphate.
Metabolic Functions of the Vitamins—***Fat Soluble Vitamins***—These tend to be stored in the body; their precise mode of action is largely unknown.
Vitamin A: essential to the production and regeneration of the visual purple of the retina; maintenance of the integrity of epithelial tissue; lysosome stability.
Vitamin D: functions in bone metabolism by regulating the intestinal absorption of calcium and phosphorus.
Vitamin E: intracellular antioxidant, important to the stability of biologic membranes.
Water Soluble Vitamins—except for vitamin B_{12}, these micronutrients are not stored in the body.
B Complex Vitamins (thiamine, riboflavin, pyridoxine, niacinamide, pantothenic acid, vitamin B_{12}, folic acid): these function, either alone or as structural components of more complex molecules, in catalytic systems where they usually function as coenzymes in carbohydrate, protein, or amino acid metabolism, synthesis of DNA and other molecules, maturation of RBCs, nerve cell function, or oxidation-reduction reactions.
Vitamin C: a coenzyme, essential to osteoid tissue; collagen formation; vascular function; tissue respiration and wound healing; facilitates absorption of iron.

INDICATIONS AND USAGE

Theragran Hematinic Tablets are indicated in the treatment of many of the common iron-deficiency anemias, particularly those associated with nutritional deficiency states or when nutritional requirements are high, and tropical and nontropical sprue. These iron-deficiency states include anemias associated with dietary inadequacy, convalescence, those frequently encountered in late childhood, early adolescence and old age, menorrhagia, and the anemias of women from menarche to menopause including macrocytic or microcytic anemia of pregnancy.
Iron deficiency may result in fatigue, palpitation, smooth and sore tongue, angular stomatitis, dysphagia, gastritis, enteropathy, and koilonychia, as well as anemia. In young children, depressed growth and impaired mental performance occur.

CONTRAINDICATIONS

Hemochromatosis and hemosiderosis are contraindications to iron therapy.

WARNINGS

Folic acid alone is improper therapy in the treatment of pernicious anemia and other megaloblastic anemias where vitamin B_{12} is deficient.

PRECAUTIONS

General—The use of niacin-containing preparations in patients with gastritis, peptic ulcer, or asthma should be undertaken carefully.
Since iron-deficiency anemia may be a manifestation of a basic systemic disturbance such as recurrent blood loss, the underlying cause of the anemia should be determined and corrected if possible.
The ingredients in Theragran Hematinic are not sufficient nor are they intended for the treatment of pernicious anemia. Folic acid in doses above 0.1 mg daily may obscure pernicious anemia in that hematologic remission can occur while neurological manifestations remain progressive; therefore, the possibility of pernicious anemia should be excluded before treatment with this preparation. Parenteral use of vitamin B_{12} is recommended to assure essential medical supervision of the patient (see WARNINGS).
This product contains FD&C Yellow No. 5 (tartrazine) which may cause allergic-type reactions (including bronchial asthma) in certain susceptible individuals. Although the overall incidence of FD&C Yellow No. 5 (tartrazine) sensitivity in the general population is low, it is frequently seen in patients who also have aspirin hypersensitivity.
Information for the Patient—Keep Theragran Hematinic and all other medication out of the reach of children.
Patients should be informed of symptoms of intolerance to components of this preparation; if any of these symptoms appear the patient should be advised to discontinue dosing, and to notify the physician.
Recommended dosage should not be exceeded unless directed by the physician.
Laboratory Tests—Periodic hematologic studies should be performed.
Drug Interactions—Since oral iron products interfere with absorption of oral tetracyclines, these products should not be taken within two hours of each other.
Mineral oil and bile-acid sequestrants such as cholestyramine and colestipol hydrochloride in long-term therapy have been shown to decrease the absorption of fat-soluble vitamins.
Pyridoxine hydrochloride may act as an antagonist to levodopa.
Hydralazine hydrochloride, penicillamine, isoniazid, and cycloserine may antagonize pyridoxine hydrochloride.
Phenytoin, methotrexate, and pyrimethamine may interfere with folic acid absorption.
Colestipol hydrochloride may decrease the bioavailability of niacin.
Vitamin C may decrease the hypoprothrombinemic effect of oral anticoagulants; prothrombin levels should be monitored.
Neomycin and colchicine may impair cyanocobalamin absorption.
Carcinogenesis, Mutagenesis, Impairment of Fertility—Long-term studies in animals have not been performed.
Pregnancy Category C—Animal reproduction studies have not been conducted with therapeutic formula vitamin tablets with hematinics. Controlled clinical studies have not been performed to determine if therapeutic formula vitamin tablets with hematinics can cause fetal harm when administered to a pregnant woman or can affect reproduction capacity. Theragran Hematinic should be given to a pregnant woman only if clearly needed.
Nursing Mothers—It is not known whether components of this product are excreted in human milk. Because many substances are excreted in human milk, caution should be exercised when Theragran Hematinic is administered to a nursing woman.
Pediatric Use—Safety and effectiveness in children have not been established.

ADVERSE REACTIONS

Allergic reactions, skin rashes, and gastrointestinal disturbances, such as nausea, vomiting, diarrhea, or constipation may occur.
A generalized flushing and a feeling of warmth has been reported following niacinamide therapy.
Allergic sensitization has been reported following both oral and parenteral administration of folic acid.

DOSAGE AND ADMINISTRATION

The usual adult dose is one Theragran Hematinic Tablet three times daily. When prescribed in late childhood and early adolescence, dosage reduction according to the size and weight of the child should be considered by the physician. Dosage may be adjusted according to the response of the patient. Since ferrous fumarate is not likely to cause gastric upsets, dosage need not be given at mealtime.

HOW SUPPLIED

Theragran Hematinic is supplied in bottles of 90 tablets.
Storage: Store at room temperature; avoid excessive heat.
(J2-574H)
Shown in Product Identification Section, page 431

THERAGRAN® LIQUID

[ther'ah-gran"]
(High Potency Vitamin Supplement)

(See PDR For Nonprescription Drugs)

THERAGRAN® TABLETS

[ther'ah-gran"]
(High Potency Multivitamin Formula)
ADVANCED FORMULA

(See PDR For Nonprescription Drugs)

THERAGRAN-M® TABLETS

[ther'ah-gran"em]
(High Potency Multivitamin Formula with Minerals)
ADVANCED FORMULA

(See PDR For Nonprescription Drugs)

THERAGRAN® STRESS FORMULA

(High Potency Multivitamin Formula with Iron and Biotin)

(See PDR For Nonprescription Drugs)

TRIMOX® '250' CAPSULES ℞

[trī'mokz]

TRIMOX® '500' CAPSULES ℞

(Amoxicillin Capsules USP)

TRIMOX® '125' FOR ORAL SUSPENSION ℞

TRIMOX® '250' FOR ORAL SUSPENSION ℞

(Amoxicillin for Oral Suspension USP)

DESCRIPTION

Trimox (amoxicillin) is a semisynthetic antibiotic, an analog of ampicillin, with a broad spectrum of bactericidal activity against many gram-positive and gram-negative microorganisms. Chemically it is D-(-)-alpha-amino-p-hydroxybenzyl penicillin trihydrate.
Trimox '250' and Trimox '500' Capsules (Amoxicillin Capsules) are available for oral administration as capsules providing amoxicillin trihydrate equivalent to 250 and 500 mg

amoxicillin, respectively. Inactive ingredients: colorants (D&C Yellow No. 10, FD&C Blue No. 1 and Yellow No. 6), gelatin, magnesium stearate, and titanium dioxide.
Trimox '125' and Trimox '250' for Oral Suspension (Amoxicillin for Oral Suspension) provide, after constitution, amoxicillin trihydrate equivalent to 125 mg and 250 mg amoxicillin per 5 mL, respectively. Inactive ingredients: calcium carrageenan, citric acid, colorant (FD&C Red. No. 3), flavor, potassium sorbate, silica gel, sucrose, and xanthan gum.

CLINICAL PHARMACOLOGY

Amoxicillin is stable in the presence of gastric acid and may be given without regard to meals. It is rapidly absorbed after oral administration. It diffuses readily into most body tissues and fluids, with the exception of brain and spinal fluid, except when meninges are inflamed. The half-life of amoxicillin is 61.3 minutes. Most of the amoxicillin is excreted unchanged in the urine; its excretion can be delayed by concurrent administration of probenecid. Amoxicillin is not highly protein-bound. In blood serum, amoxicillin is approximately 20 percent protein-bound as compared to 60 percent for penicillin G.
Orally administered doses of 250 mg and 500 mg amoxicillin capsules result in average peak blood levels one to two hours after administration in the range of 3.5 mcg/mL to 5.0 mcg/mL and 5.5 mcg/mL to 7.5 mcg/mL, respectively.
Orally administered doses of amoxicillin suspension 125 mg/5 mL and 250 mg/5 mL result in average peak blood levels one to two hours after administration in the range of 1.5 mcg/mL to 3.0 mcg/mL and 3.5 mcg/mL to 5.0 mcg/mL, respectively.
Detectable serum levels are observed up to 8 hours after an orally administered dose of amoxicillin. Following a 1 g dose and utilizing a special skin window technique to determine levels of the antibiotic, it was noted that therapeutic levels were found in the interstitial fluid. Approximately 60 percent of an orally administered dose of amoxicillin is excreted in the urine within six to eight hours.
Microbiology: Trimox (amoxicillin) is similar to ampicillin in its bactericidal action against susceptible organisms during the stage of active multiplication. It acts through the inhibition of biosynthesis of cell wall mucopeptides. *In vitro* studies have demonstrated the susceptibility of most strains of the following gram-positive bacteria: alpha- and beta-hemolytic streptococci, *Streptococcus pneumoniae* (formerly *Diplococcus pneumoniae*), nonpenicillinase-producing staphylococci, and *Streptococcus faecalis*. It is active *in vitro* against many strains of *Hemophilus influenzae, Neisseria gonorrhoeae, Escherichia coli* and *Proteus mirabilis*. Because it does not resist destruction by penicillinase, it is *not* effective against penicillinase-producing bacteria, particularly resistant staphylococci. All strains of Pseudomonas and most strains of Klebsiella and Enterobacter are resistant.
Disc Susceptibility Tests: Quantitative methods that require measurement of the diameters of zones of inhibition of microbial growth give the most precise estimates of antibiotic susceptibility. One recommended procedure (21 CFR Sec. 460.1) uses discs for testing susceptibility to ampicillin-class antibiotics. Interpretations correlate diameters of the disc test with MIC values for amoxicillin. With this procedure, a report from the laboratory of "susceptible" indicates that the infecting organism is likely to respond to therapy. A report of "resistant" indicates that the infecting organism is not likely to respond to therapy. A report of "intermediate susceptibility" suggests that the organism would be susceptible if high dosage is used, or if the infection is confined to tissues and fluids (e.g., urine) in which high antibiotic levels are attained.

INDICATIONS AND USAGE

Trimox (amoxicillin) is indicated in the treatment of infections due to susceptible strains of the following:
Gram-negative organisms — *H. influenzae, E. coli, P. mirabilis* and *N. gonorrhoeae.*
Gram-positive organisms — Streptococci (including *Streptococcus faecalis*), *S. pneumoniae* and nonpenicillinase-producing staphylococci.
Therapy may be instituted prior to obtaining results from bacteriological and susceptibility studies to determine the causative organisms and their susceptibility to amoxicillin. Indicated surgical procedures should be performed.

CONTRAINDICATIONS

The use of this drug is contraindicated in individuals with a history of an allergic reaction to any of the penicillins.

WARNINGS

Serious and occasionally fatal hypersensitivity (anaphylactoid) reactions have been reported in patients on penicillin therapy. Although anaphylaxis is more frequent following parenteral therapy, it has occurred in patients on oral penicillins. These reactions are more likely to occur in individuals with a history of sensitivity to multiple allergens. There have been reports of individuals with a history of penicillin hypersensitivity who have experienced severe reactions when treated with a cephalosporin. Before therapy with any penicillin, careful inquiry should be made concerning previous hypersensitivity reactions to penicillins, cephalosporins, or other allergens. If an allergic reaction occurs, appropriate therapy should be instituted and discontinuance of amoxicillin therapy considered. **Serious anaphylactoid reactions require immediate emergency treatment with epinephrine. Oxygen, intravenous steroids, and airway management, including intubation, should also be administered as indicated.**

PRECAUTIONS

As with any potent drug, periodic assessment of renal, hepatic and hematopoietic function should be made during prolonged therapy.
The possibility of superinfections with mycotic or bacterial pathogens should be kept in mind during therapy. If superinfections occur (usually involving Enterobacter, Pseudomonas or Candida), amoxicillin should be discontinued and/or appropriate therapy instituted.
Usage in Pregnancy: Safety for use in pregnancy has not been established.

ADVERSE REACTIONS

As with other penicillins, it may be expected that untoward reactions will be essentially limited to sensitivity phenomena. They are more likely to occur in individuals who have previously demonstrated hypersensitivity to penicillins and in those with a history of allergy, asthma, hay fever or urticaria. The following adverse reactions have been reported as associated with the use of the penicillins:
Gastrointestinal: Glossitis, stomatitis, black "hairy" tongue, nausea, vomiting and diarrhea.
Hypersensitivity Reactions: Erythematous maculopapular rashes, urticaria, and a few cases of exfoliative dermatitis and erythema multiforme have been reported. Anaphylaxis is the most serious reaction experienced and has usually been associated with parenteral dosage forms (See WARNINGS).
NOTE: Urticaria, other skin rashes and serum sickness-like reactions may be controlled with antihistamines and, if necessary, systemic corticosteroids. Whenever such reactions occur, amoxicillin should be discontinued unless, in the opinion of the physician, the condition being treated is life-threatening and amenable only to amoxicillin therapy.
Liver: A moderate rise in serum glutamic oxaloacetic transaminase (SGOT) has been noted, but the significance of this finding is unknown.
Hemic and Lymphatic Systems: Anemia, thrombocytopenia, thrombocytopenic purpura, eosinophilia, leukopenia and agranulocytosis have been reported during therapy with the penicillins. These reactions are usually reversible on discontinuation of therapy and are believed to be hypersensitivity phenomena.

DOSAGE AND ADMINISTRATION

Infections of the ear, nose and throat due to streptococci, pneumococci, nonpenicillinase-producing staphylococci and *H. influenzae;* **Infections of the genitourinary tract** due to *E. coli, P. mirabilis* and *S. faecalis;* **Infections of the skin and soft tissues** due to streptococci, susceptible staphylococci and *E. coli:*

USUAL DOSAGE:
Adults: 250 mg every 8 hours
Children: 20 mg/kg/day in divided doses every 8 hours
Children weighing 20 kg or more should be dosed according to the adult recommendations.

In severe infections or those caused by less susceptible organisms:
500 mg every 8 hours for adults and 40 mg/kg/day in divided doses every 8 hours for children may be needed.

Infections of the lower respiratory tract due to streptococci, pneumococci, nonpenicillinase-producing staphylococci and *H. influenzae:*

USUAL DOSAGE:
Adults: 500 mg every 8 hours
Children: 40 mg/kg/day in divided doses every 8 hours
Children weighing 20 kg or more should be dosed according to the adult recommendations.

Gonorrhea, acute uncomplicated ano-genital and urethral infections due to *N. gonorrhoeae* (males and females):
3 grams as a single oral dose

Cases of gonorrhea with a suspected lesion of syphilis should have darkfield examinations before receiving amoxicillin, and monthly serological tests for a minimum of four months.
General: Larger doses may be required for stubborn or severe infections.
The children's dosage is intended for individuals whose weight will not cause a dosage to be calculated greater than that recommended for adults.
It should be recognized that in the treatment of chronic urinary tract infections frequent bacteriological and clinical appraisals are necessary. Smaller doses than those recommended above should not be used. Even higher doses may be needed at times. In stubborn infections, therapy may be required for several weeks. It may be necessary to continue clinical and/or bacteriological follow-up for several months after cessation of therapy. Except for gonorrhea, treatment should be continued for a minimum of 48 to 72 hours beyond the time that the patient becomes asymptomatic or evidence of bacterial eradication has been obtained. It is recommended that there be at least 10 days' treatment for any infection caused by hemolytic streptococci to prevent the occurrence of acute rheumatic fever or glomerulonephritis.
Preparation and Storage of Oral Suspensions: Prepare the suspension at the time of dispensing. Follow the directions for constitution on the label of the package. Discard any unused suspension after 14 days. The suspension may be kept at room temperature; refrigeration is not required. **Shake well before using.**

HOW SUPPLIED

Trimox (amoxicillin) is available for oral administration as *Trimox '250' Capsules and *Trimox '500' Capsules (Amoxicillin Capsules USP). The 250 mg capsules are available in bottles of 100 and 500 and in Unimatic® cartons of 100. Each two-piece, green, hard gelatin capsule is imprinted with identification no. **230.** The 500 mg capsules are available in bottles of 50 and 500 and in Unimatic cartons of 100. Each two-piece, light green/dark green, hard gelatin capsule is imprinted with identification no. **231.** Trimox is also available as Trimox '125' for Oral Suspension and Trimox '250' for Oral Suspension (Amoxicillin for Oral Suspension USP) which provide, when constituted as directed on the container label, a pleasantly flavored suspension containing 125 mg/5mL teaspoonful and 250 mg/5mL teaspoonful, respectively. Available in bottles of 80, 100, and 150 mL and Unimatic® cartons of 100 unit-dose bottles.
Storage: Store Trimox Capsules (Amoxicillin Capsules USP) and Trimox for Oral Suspension (Amoxicillin for Oral Suspension USP) at room temperature. Dispense the capsules in tight containers.
(J4-440D)

**Shown in Product Identification Section, page 431*

VEETIDS® '250' TABLETS ℞
[*vē'tidz*]
VEETIDS® '500' TABLETS ℞
(Penicillin V Potassium Tablets USP)
VEETIDS® '125' FOR ORAL SOLUTION ℞
VEETIDS® '250' FOR ORAL SOLUTION ℞
(Penicillin V Potassium for Oral Solution USP)

DESCRIPTION

Veetids (Penicillin V Potassium) is the potassium salt of semisynthetically produced penicillin V.
Veetids '250' Tablets (Penicillin V Potassium Tablets) and Veetids '500' Tablets for oral administration provide penicillin V potassium equivalent to 250 mg (400,000 u) and 500 mg (800,000 u), respectively, of penicillin V. Inactive ingredients: carnauba wax, cellulose, colorants (for '250' only, D&C Red No. 30 and FD&C Yellow No. 6), flavor, lactose, magnesium stearate, povidone, talc, and other ingredients.
Veetids '125' for Oral Solution (Penicillin V Potassium for Oral Solution) and Veetids '250' for Oral Solution are powders that, when constituted as directed, provide flavored solutions containing penicillin V potassium equivalent to 125 mg (200,000 u) and 250 mg (400,000 u), respectively, of penicillin V per 5 mL teaspoonful. Inactive ingredients: colorants [FD&C Red No. 40, and, for '125' only, Yellow No. 5 (tartrazine)], flavors, saccharin sodium, sodium phosphate, and sucrose.

CLINICAL PHARMACOLOGY

Penicillin V is bactericidal against penicillin-susceptible microorganisms during the stage of active multiplication. It acts by inhibiting biosynthesis of cell-wall mucopeptide. It is not active against the penicillinase-producing bacteria, which include many strains of staphylococci. Penicillin V is highly active *in vitro* against staphylococci (except penicillinase-producing strains), streptococci (groups A, C, G, H, L, and M) and pneumococci. Other organisms susceptible *in vitro* to penicillin V are *Corynebacterium diphtheriae, Bacillus anthracis,* Clostridia, *Actinomyces bovis, Streptobacillus moniliformis, Listeria monocytogenes,* Leptospira and *Neisseria gonorrhoeae; Treponema pallidum* is extremely susceptible.
Penicillin V is more resistant to inactivation by gastric acid than penicillin G; however, it has the same bacterial spectrum as penicillin G. It may be given with meals; however, blood levels are slightly higher when the drug is given on an empty stomach. Average blood levels are two to five times higher than the levels following the same dose of oral penicillin G and also show much less individual variation.
Once absorbed, penicillin V is about 75 percent bound to serum protein. Highest levels are found in the kidneys, with lesser amounts in the liver, skin, and intestines. Penicillin V penetrates into all other tissues to a lesser degree with a very

Continued on next page

Squibb—Cont.

small level found in the cerebrospinal fluid. The drug is excreted rapidly by tubular excretion in patients with normal kidney function. In neonates and young infants, and in individuals with impaired kidney function, excretion is considerably delayed.

INDICATIONS AND USAGE

Veetids (Penicillin V Potassium) are indicated in the treatment of mild to moderately severe infections due to penicillin-susceptible microorganisms. Therapy should be guided by bacteriological studies, including susceptibility tests, and by clinical response. Note: severe pneumonia, empyema, bacteremia, pericarditis, meningitis, and septic arthritis should not be treated with penicillin V during the acute stage.

Indicated surgical procedures should be performed.

The following infections will usually respond to adequate oral dosage:

Streptococcal infections Group A without bacteremia—Mild to moderate infections of the upper respiratory tract (including otitis media), scarlet fever, and mild erysipelas. Note: streptococci in groups A, C, G, H, L, and M are very susceptible to penicillin. Other groups including group D (enterococcus) are resistant.

Pneumococcal infections—Mild to moderately severe infections of the respiratory tract, including otitis media.

Staphylococcal infections — penicillin-susceptible—Mild infections of the skin and skin structures. Note: reports indicate an increasing number of strains of staphylococci resistant to penicillin, emphasizing the need for culture and susceptibility studies in treating suspected staphylococcal infections.

Vincent's gingivitis and pharyngitis (fusospirochetosis) —Mild to moderately severe infections of the oropharynx usually respond to oral penicillin. Note: necessary dental care should be accomplished in infections involving gum tissue.

Medical conditions in which oral penicillin therapy is indicated as prophylaxis: *For the prevention of recurrence following rheumatic fever and/or chorea.* Prophylaxis with oral penicillin on a continuing basis is effective in preventing recurrence of these conditions. *To prevent bacterial endocarditis.* Although no controlled clinical efficacy studies have been conducted penicillin V has been suggested by the American Heart Association and the American Dental Association for use in a standard regimen (oral) and a special regimen (parenteral-oral) for prophylaxis against bacterial endocarditis in patients with congenital heart disease or rheumatic or other acquired valvular heart disease when they undergo dental procedures and surgical procedures of the respiratory tract.[1] Since it may happen that *alpha* hemolytic streptococci relatively resistant to penicillin may be found when patients are receiving continuous oral penicillin for secondary prevention of rheumatic fever, prophylactic agents other than penicillin may be chosen for these patients and prescribed in addition to their continuous rheumatic fever prophylactic regimen. Oral penicillin should not be used as adjunctive prophylaxis for genitourinary instrumentation or surgery, lower intestinal tract surgery, sigmoidoscopy, and childbirth. **NOTE: When selecting antibiotics for the prevention of bacterial endocarditis the physician or dentist should read the full joint statement of the American Heart Association and the American Dental Association.[1]**

CONTRAINDICATIONS

Contraindicated in patients with a history of hypersensitivity to any penicillin.

WARNINGS

Serious and occasional fatal hypersensitivity (anaphylactoid) reactions have been reported in patients on penicillin therapy. Although anaphylaxis is more frequent following parenteral administration, it has occurred in patients on oral penicillins. These reactions are more apt to occur in individuals with a history of sensitivity to multiple allergens.

There have been well-documented reports of individuals with a history of penicillin hypersensitivity who have experienced severe hypersensitivity reactions when treated with cephalosporins. Before therapy with a penicillin, careful inquiry should be made concerning previous hypersensitivity reactions to penicillins, cephalosporins, and other allergens. If an allergic reaction occurs, the drug should be discontinued and the patient treated with the usual agents, e.g., pressor amines, antihistamines, and corticosteroids. Serious anaphylactoid reactions are not controlled by antihistamines alone, and require such emergency measures as the immediate use of epinephrine, aminophylline, oxygen, and intravenous corticosteroids.

Concomitant use of oral neomycin therapy should be avoided since malabsorption of penicillin V potassium has been reported.

PRECAUTIONS

Penicillin should be used with caution in individuals with histories of significant allergies and/or asthma.

The oral route of administration should not be relied upon in patients with severe illness, or with nausea, vomiting, gastric dilatation, cardiospasm or intestinal hypermotility.

Occasional patients will not absorb therapeutic amounts of orally administered penicillin.

In streptococcal infections, therapy must be sufficient to eliminate the organism (10 days minimum); otherwise the sequelae of streptococcal disease may occur. Cultures should be taken following completion of treatment to determine whether streptococci have been eradicated.

Prolonged use of antibiotics may promote the overgrowth of nonsusceptible organisms, including fungi. Should superinfection occur, appropriate measures should be taken.

In prolonged therapy with penicillin, and particularly with high dosage schedules, periodic evaluation of the renal and hematopoietic systems is recommended.

Veetids '125' for Oral Solution (Penicillin V Potassium Oral Solution USP) contains FD&C Yellow No. 5 (tartrazine) which may cause allergic-type reactions (including bronchial asthma) in certain susceptible individuals. Although the overall incidence of FD&C Yellow No. 5 (tartrazine) sensitivity in the general population is low, it is frequently seen in patients who also have aspirin hypersensitivity.

ADVERSE REACTIONS

Although the incidence of reactions to oral penicillins has been reported with much less frequency than following parenteral therapy, it should be remembered that all degrees of hypersensitivity, including fatal anaphylaxis, have been reported with oral penicillin.

The most common reactions to oral penicillin are nausea, vomiting, epigastric distress, diarrhea, and black hairy tongue. The hypersensitivity reactions reported are skin rashes ranging from maculopapular to exfoliative dermatitis; urticaria; serum sickness-like reactions including chills, fever, edema, arthralgia, and prostration; laryngeal edema; and anaphylaxis. Fever and eosinophilia may frequently be the only reactions observed. Hemolytic anemia, leukopenia, thrombocytopenia, neuropathy, and nephropathy are infrequent reactions usually associated with high doses of parenteral penicillin. Urticaria, other skin rashes, and serum sickness-like reactions may be controlled by antihistamines and, if necessary, corticosteroids. Whenever such reactions occur, penicillin should be discontinued unless, in the opinion of the physician, the condition being treated is life-threatening and amenable only to penicillin therapy. Serious anaphylactoid reactions require emergency measures (see WARNINGS).

An occasional patient may complain of sore mouth or tongue, as with any oral penicillin preparation.

DOSAGE AND ADMINISTRATION

The dosage of Veetids (Penicillin V Potassium) should be determined according to the susceptibility of the causative microorganism and the severity of the infection, and adjusted to the clinical response of the patient.

For Therapeutic Use

Dosage for *children under 12 years* of age is calculated on the basis of body weight. For *infants and small children* the suggested dose is 15 to 56 mg (25,000 to 90,000 u) per kg/day in three to six divided doses.

The usual dosage recommendations for *adults and children 12 years and over* are as follows:

Streptococcal infections—mild to moderately severe—of the upper respiratory tract and including otitis media, scarlet fever and mild erysipelas: 125 mg (200,000 u) tid or qid for 10 days for mild infections; 250 mg (400,000 u) tid for 10 days for moderately severe infections; for mild to moderately severe streptococcal pharyngitis: 500 mg (800,000 u) bid may be used as an alternative regimen.

Pneumococcal infections—mild to moderately severe—of the respiratory tract, including otitis media: 250 to 500 mg (400,000 to 800,000 u) qid until the patient has been afebrile for at least two days.

Staphylococcal infections—mild infections of skin and skin structures (culture and susceptibility tests should be performed): 250 mg (400,000 u) tid or qid, or 500 mg (800,000 u) tid.

Vincent's gingivitis and pharyngitis (fusospirochetosis) —mild to moderately severe infections of the oropharynx: 250 mg (400,000 u) tid or qid, or 500 mg tid.

For Prophylactic Use

For the prevention of recurrence following rheumatic fever and/or chorea: *Adults*—125 mg (200,000 u) bid on a continuing basis. Dosage for *children under 12 years* of age is calculated on the basis of body weight. For *infants and small children* the suggested dose is 15 to 56 mg (25,000 to 90,000 u) per kg/day in three to six divided doses.

To prevent bacterial endocarditis. For prophylaxis against bacterial endocarditis[1] in patients with congenital heart disease or rheumatic or other acquired valvular heart disease when undergoing dental procedures or surgical procedures of the upper respiratory tract, one of two regimens may be selected:

(1) Standard regimen—administer 2 g of penicillin V orally (1 g for children under 60 lb) one hour before the procedure, and then 1 g (500 mg for children under 60 lb) six hours later.

(2) Special regimen—ampicillin 1 to 2 g (50 mg/kg for children) intramuscularly or intravenously, plus gentamicin 1.5 mg/kg (2 mg/kg for children) intramuscularly or intravenously, one-half hour before procedure, followed by 1 g (500 mg for children under 60 lb) oral penicillin V six hours later. Alternatively, omit the oral penicillin V and repeat the parenteral regimen eight hours later. Doses for children should not exceed recommendations for adults for a single dose or for a 24-hour period.

HOW SUPPLIED*Veetids '250' Tablets and *Veetids '500' Tablets (Penicillin V Potassium Tablets USP) are available as FILMLOK® tablets providing penicillin V potassium equivalent to 250 mg (400,000 u) and 500 mg (800,000 u), respectively, of penicillin V. (Filmlok is a Squibb trademark for veneer-coated tablets.) Bottles of 100 and 1000, and Unimatic® cartons of 100.

Veetids '125' for Oral Solution and Veetids '250' for Oral Solution (Penicillin V Potassium for Oral Solution USP) are available as powders that, when constituted as directed, provide pleasantly flavored solutions containing penicillin V potassium equivalent to 125 mg (200,000 u) and 250 mg (400,000 u), respectively, of penicillin V per 5 mL teaspoonful. Bottles of 100 mL (NSN 6505-00-080-0853) and 200 mL.

Storage: Store Veetids Tablets at room temperature; avoid excessive heat. Dispense in tight containers. Store Veetids for Oral Solution in dry form at room temperature; after preparation of the solution, store in refrigerator and discard unused portion after 14 days. Shake well before using. Keep tightly closed.

Reference: 1. American Heart Association: Prevention of bacterial endocarditis. Circulation 70:1123A–1127A, 1984.

(J3-392G)

**Shown in Product Identification Section, page 431*

VELOSEF® '250' CAPSULES ℞

[*vel 'ō-sef*]

VELOSEF® '500' CAPSULES ℞

(Cephradine Capsules USP)

VELOSEF® '125' FOR ORAL SUSPENSION ℞

VELOSEF® '250' FOR ORAL SUSPENSION ℞

(Cephradine for Oral Suspension USP)

DESCRIPTION

Velosef (Cephradine, Squibb) is a semisynthetic cephalosporin antibiotic; oral dosage forms include capsules containing 250 mg and 500 mg cephradine, and cephradine for oral suspension containing, after constitution, 125 mg and 250 mg per 5 mL dose. Cephradine is chemically designated as (6R,7R)-7-[(R)-2-amino-2-(1,4-cyclohexadien-1-yl) acetamido]-3-methyl-8-oxo-5-thia-1-azabicylo[4.2.0]oct-2-ene-2-carboxylic acid.

INACTIVE INGREDIENTS

Velosef Capsules—colorants (D&C Red No. 33 and Yellow No. 10; FD&C Blue No. 1, and, for '250' only, Red No. 3), gelatin, lactose, magnesium stearate, talc, and titanium dioxide. Velosef for Oral Suspension—citric acid, colorants (FD&C Red No. 40 for '250' only; FD&C Yellow No. 6 for '125' only), flavors, guar gum, methylcellulose, sodium citrate, and sucrose.

CLINICAL PHARMACOLOGY

Velosef (Cephradine, Squibb) is acid stable. It is rapidly absorbed after oral administration in the fasting state. Following single doses of 250 mg, 500 mg, and 1 g in normal adult volunteers, average peak serum concentrations within one hour were approximately 9 mcg/mL, 16.5 mcg/mL, and 24.2 mcg/mL, respectively.

In vitro studies by an ultracentrifugation technique show that at therapeutic serum antibiotic concentrations, cephradine is minimally bound (8 to 17 percent) to normal serum protein. Cephradine does not pass across the blood-brain barrier to any appreciable extent. The presence of food in the gastrointestinal tract delays absorption but does not affect the total amount of cephradine absorbed. Over 90 percent of the drug is excreted unchanged in the urine within six hours. Peak urine concentrations are approximately 1600 mcg/mL, 3200 mcg/mL, and 4000 mcg/mL following single doses of 250 mg, 500 mg, and 1 g, respectively.

Microbiology—In vitro tests demonstrate that the cephalosporins are bactericidal because of their inhibition of cell-wall synthesis. Cephradine is active against the following organisms *in vitro:*

- Group A beta-hemolytic streptococci
- Staphylococci, including coagulase-positive, coagulase-negative, and penicillinase-producing strains
- *Streptococcus pneumoniae* (formerly *Diplococcus pneumoniae*)

Escherichia coli
Proteus mirabilis
Klebsiella species
Hemophilus influenzae

Cephradine is not active against most strains of *Enterobacter* species, *P. morganii,* and *P. vulgaris.* It has no activity against *Pseudomonas* or *Herellea* species. When tested by *in vitro* methods, staphylococci exhibit cross-resistance between cephradine and methicillin-type antibiotics.

Note—Most strains of enterococci (*Streptococcus faecalis*) are resistant to cephradine.

Disc Susceptibility Tests—Quantitative methods that require measurement of zone diameters give the most precise estimates of antibiotic susceptibility. One recommended procedure (21 CFR Sec. 460.1) uses cephalosporin class discs for testing susceptibility; interpretations correlate zone diameters of this disc test with MIC values for cephradine. With this procedure, a report from the laboratory of "resistant" indicates that the infecting organism is not likely to respond to therapy. A report of "intermediate susceptibility" suggests that the organism would be susceptible if the infection is confined to the urinary tract, as high antibiotic levels can be obtained in the urine, or if high dosage is used in other types of infection.

INDICATIONS AND USAGE

Velosef Capsules (Cephradine Capsules USP), and Velosef for Oral Suspension (Cephradine for Oral Suspension USP) are indicated in the treatment of the following infections when caused by susceptible strains of the designated microorganisms:

RESPIRATORY TRACT INFECTIONS (e.g., tonsillitis, pharyngitis, and lobar pneumonia) caused by group A beta-hemolytic streptococci and *S. pneumoniae* (formerly *D. pneumoniae*).

[Penicillin is the usual drug of choice in the treatment and prevention of streptococcal infections, including the prophylaxis of rheumatic fever. Velosef is generally effective in the eradication of streptococci from the nasopharynx; substantial data establishing the efficacy of Velosef (Cephradine, Squibb) in the subsequent prevention of rheumatic fever are not available at present.]

OTITIS MEDIA caused by group A beta-hemolytic streptococci, *S. pneumoniae* (formerly *D. pneumoniae*), *H. influenzae,* and staphylococci.

SKIN AND SKIN STRUCTURE INFECTIONS caused by staphylococci (penicillin-susceptible and penicillin-resistant) and beta-hemolytic streptococci.

URINARY TRACT INFECTIONS, including prostatitis, caused by *E. coli, P. mirabilis, Klebsiella* species, and enterococci (*S. faecalis*). The high concentrations of cephradine achievable in the urinary tract will be effective against many strains of enterococci for which disc susceptibility studies indicate relative resistance. It is to be noted that among beta-lactam antibiotics, ampicillin is the drug of choice for enterococcal urinary tract (*S. faecalis*) infection.

Note—Culture and susceptibility tests should be initiated prior to and during therapy.

Following clinical improvement achieved with parenteral therapy, oral cephradine may be utilized for continuation of treatment of persistent or severe conditions where prolonged therapy is indicated.

CONTRAINDICATIONS

Cephradine is contraindicated in patients with known hypersensitivity to the cephalosporin group of antibiotics.

WARNINGS

In penicillin-sensitive patients, cephalosporin derivatives should be used with great caution. There is clinical and laboratory evidence of partial cross-allergenicity of the penicillins and the cephalosporins, and there are instances of patients who have had reactions to both drug classes (including anaphylaxis after parenteral use).

Any patient who has demonstrated some form of allergy, particularly to drugs, should receive antibiotics, including cephradine, cautiously and then only when absolutely necessary.

Pseudomembranous colitis has been reported with the use of cephalosporins (and other broad spectrum antibiotics); therefore, it is important to consider its diagnosis in patients who develop diarrhea in association with antibiotic use. Treatment with broad spectrum antibiotics alters normal flora of the colon and may permit overgrowth of clostridia. Studies indicate a toxin produced by *Clostridium difficile* is one primary cause of antibiotic-associated colitis. Cholestyramine and colestipol resins have been shown to bind the toxin *in vitro.* Mild cases of colitis may respond to drug discontinuance alone. Moderate to severe cases should be managed with fluid, electrolyte and protein supplementation as indicated. When the colitis is not relieved by drug discontinuance or when it is severe, oral vancomycin is the treatment of choice for antibiotic-associated pseudomembranous colitis produced by *C. difficile.* Other causes of colitis should also be considered.

PRECAUTIONS

General—Patients should be followed carefully so that any side effects or unusual manifestations of drug idiosyncrasy may be detected. If a hypersensitivity reaction occurs, the drug should be discontinued and the patient treated with the usual agents, e.g., pressor amines, antihistamines, or corticosteroids.

Administer cephradine with caution in the presence of markedly impaired renal function. In patients with known or suspected renal impairment, careful clinical observation and appropriate laboratory studies should be made prior to and during therapy as cephradine accumulates in the serum and tissues. See DOSAGE AND ADMINISTRATION section for information on treatment of patients with impaired renal function.

Cephradine should be prescribed with caution in individuals with a history of gastrointestinal disease, particularly colitis.

Prolonged use of antibiotics may promote the overgrowth of nonsusceptible organisms. Should superinfection occur during therapy, appropriate measures should be taken.

Indicated surgical procedures should be performed in conjunction with antibiotic therapy.

Information for Patients: Caution diabetic patients that false results may occur with urine glucose tests (see PRECAUTIONS, Drug/Laboratory Test Interactions).

Advise the patient to comply with the full course of therapy even if he begins to feel better and to take a missed dose as soon as possible. Inform the patient that this medication may be taken with food or milk since gastrointestinal upset may be a factor in compliance with the dosage regimen. The patient should report current use of any medicines and should be cautioned not to take other medications unless the physician knows and approves of their use (see PRECAUTIONS, Drug Interactions).

Laboratory Tests: In patients with known or suspected renal impairment, it is advisable to monitor renal function (see DOSAGE AND ADMINISTRATION).

Drug Interactions: When administered concurrently, the following drugs may interact with cephalosporins:

Other antibacterial agents—Bacteriostats may interfere with the bactericidal action of cephalosporins in acute infection; other agents, e.g., aminoglycosides, colistin, polymyxins, vancomycin, may increase the possibility of nephrotoxicity.

Diuretics (potent "loop diuretics," e.g., furosemide and ethacrynic acid)—Enhanced possibility for renal toxicity.

Probenecid—Increased and prolonged blood levels of cephalosporins, resulting in increased risk of nephrotoxicity.

Drug/Laboratory Test Interactions: After treatment with cephradine, a false-positive reaction for glucose in the urine may occur with Benedict's solution, Fehling's solution, or with Clinitest® tablets, but not with enzyme-based tests such as Clinistix® and Tes-Tape®.

False-positive Coombs test results may occur in newborns whose mothers received a cephalosporin prior to delivery.

Cephalosporins have been reported to cause false-positive reactions in tests for urinary proteins which use sulfosalicylic acid, false elevations of urinary 17-ketosteroid values, and prolonged prothrombin times.

Carcinogenesis, Mutagenesis: Long-term studies in animals have not been performed to evaluate carcinogenic potential or mutagenesis.

Pregnancy—Category B: Reproduction studies have been peformed in mice and rats at doses up to four times the maximum indicated human dose and have revealed no evidence of impaired fertility or harm to the fetus due to cephradine. There are, however, no adequate and well-controlled studies in pregnant women. Because animal reproduction studies are not always predictive of human response, this drug should be used during pregnancy only if clearly needed.

Nursing Mothers: Since cephradine is excreted in breast milk during lactation, caution should be exercised when cephradine is administered to a nursing woman.

Pediatric Use: See DOSAGE AND ADMINISTRATION. Adequate information is unavailable on the efficacy of b.i.d. regimens in children under nine months of age.

ADVERSE REACTIONS

As with other cephalosporins, untoward reactions are limited essentially to gastrointestinal disturbances and, on occasion, to hypersensitivity phenomena. The latter are more likely to occur in individuals who have previously demonstrated hypersensitivity and those with a history of allergy, asthma, hay fever, or urticaria.

The following adverse reactions have been reported following the use of cephradine:

Gastrointestinal: Symptoms of pseudomembranous colitis can appear during treatment. Nausea and vomiting have been reported rarely.

Skin and Hypersensitivity Reactions: Mild urticaria or skin rash, pruritus, and joint pains were reported by very few patients.

Hematologic: Mild, transient eosinophilia, leukopenia, and neutropenia have been reported.

Liver: Transient mild rise of SGOT, SGPT, and total bilirubin have been observed with no evidence of hepatocellular damage.

Renal: Transitory rises in BUN have been observed in some patients treated with cephalosporins; their frequency increases in patients over 50 years old. In adults for whom serum creatinine determinations were performed, the rise in BUN was not accompanied by a rise in serum creatinine.

Other adverse reactions have included dizziness and tightness in the chest and candidal vaginitis.

DOSAGE AND ADMINISTRATION

Velosef (Cephradine, Squibb) may be given without regard to meals.

Adults: *For respiratory tract infections (other than lobar pneumonia) and skin and skin structure infections,* the usual dose is 250 mg every 6 hours or 500 mg every 12 hours.

For lobar pneumonia, the usual dose is 500 mg every 6 hours or 1 g every 12 hours.

For uncomplicated urinary tract infections, the usual dose is 500 mg every 12 hours. In more serious urinary tract infections, including prostatitis, 500 mg every 6 hours or 1 g every 12 hours may be administered.

Larger doses (up to 1 g every 6 hours) may be given for severe or chronic infections.

Children: No adequate information is available on the efficacy of bid regimens in children under nine months of age. The usual dose in children over nine months of age is 25 to 50 mg/kg/day administered in equally divided doses every 6 or 12 hours. For otitis media due to *H. influenzae,* doses are from 75 to 100 mg/kg/day administered in equally divided doses every 6 or 12 hours, but should not exceed 4 g per day. Dosage for children should not exceed dosage recommended for adults.

All patients, regardless of age and weight: Larger doses (up to 1 gram qid) may be given for severe or chronic infections.

As with antibiotic therapy in general, treatment should be continued for a minimum of 48 to 72 hours after the patient becomes asymptomatic or evidence of bacterial eradication has been obtained. In infections caused by group A beta-hemolytic streptococci, a minimum of 10 days of treatment is recommended to guard against the risk of rheumatic fever or glomerulonephritis. In the treatment of chronic urinary tract infection, frequent bacteriologic and clinical appraisal is necessary during therapy and may be necessary for several months afterwards. Persistent infections may require treatment for several weeks. Prolonged intensive therapy is recommended for prostatitis. Doses smaller than those indicated are not recommended.

Patients With Impaired Renal Function

Not on Dialysis: The following initial dosage schedule is suggested as a guideline based on creatinine clearance. Further modification in the dosage schedule may be required because of individual variations in absorption.

Creatinine Clearance	Dose	Time Interval
> 20 mL/min.	500 mg	6 hours
15–20 mL/min.	250 mg	6 hours
< 5 mL/min.	250 mg	12 hours

On Chronic, Intermittent Hemodialysis:

250 mg Start
250 mg at 12 hours
250 mg 36–48 hours (after start)

Children may require dosage modification proportional to their weight and severity of infection.

HOW SUPPLIED

Velosef is available as *Velosef '250' Capsules and *Velosef '500' Capsules (Cephradine Capsules USP) providing 250 mg and 500 mg cephradine per capsule, respectively. The Capsules are available in bottles of 24 and 100 and Unimatic® cartons of 100. [Military/V.A. Depot Item: 250 mg capsules, 100's NSN 6505-01-009-9531; 500 mg capsules, 100's NSN 6505-01-023-8714; 500 mg Unimatic NSN 6505-01-023-1078.]

Velosef is also available as Velosef '125' for Oral Suspension and Velosef '250' for Oral Suspension (Cephradine for Oral Suspension USP) which, after constitution, provide 125 mg and 250 mg cephradine, respectively, per 5 mL teaspoonful in a pleasant fruit-flavored suspension. Bottles of 100 mL and 200 mL.

Storage: Velosef Capsules—Keep tightly closed. Do not store above 86°F.

Velosef for Oral Suspension— Prior to constitution, store at room temperature; avoid excessive heat. After constitution, when the suspension stored at room temperature, discard unused portion after seven days; when stored in refrigerator, discard unused portion after 14 days. Keep tightly closed. (J4-092)

**Shown in Product Identification Section, page 431*

Continued on next page

Squibb—Cont.

VELOSEF® for INJECTION ℞
[vel 'ō-sef]
(Cephradine for Injection USP)

DESCRIPTION

Velosef (Cephradine, Squibb) is a semisynthetic cephalosporin antibiotic. Cephradine is designated chemically as (6R, 7R)-7-[(R)- 2-amino-2-(1, 4-cyclohexadien-1-yl) acetamido]-3- methyl-8-oxo-5-thia-1-azabicyclo-[4.2.0] oct-2-ene-2-carboxylic acid.
Velosef for Injection is a sterile powder for constitution available in vials containing 250 mg, 500 mg, or 1 g cephradine; and bottles containing 2 g or 4 g cephradine; the preparations also contain 79 mg, 157 mg, 315 mg, 630 mg, or 1.26 g anhydrous sodium carbonate, respectively. The sodium content is approximately 136 mg (6 mEq) per gram of cephradine. At the time of manufacture, the air in the container is replaced by nitrogen.

CLINICAL PHARMACOLOGY

Table I indicates the blood levels following intramuscular administration of a 500 mg or 1 g dose to normal adults. [See table below].
Figure I depicts representative mean serum concentrations after administration of a 500 mg and 1 g IM dose, and a 500 mg oral dose of cephradine. Areas beneath the curves for the 500 mg oral and IM dose are equivalent.

Figure I
VELOSEF FOR INJECTION
(Cephradine for Injection USP)

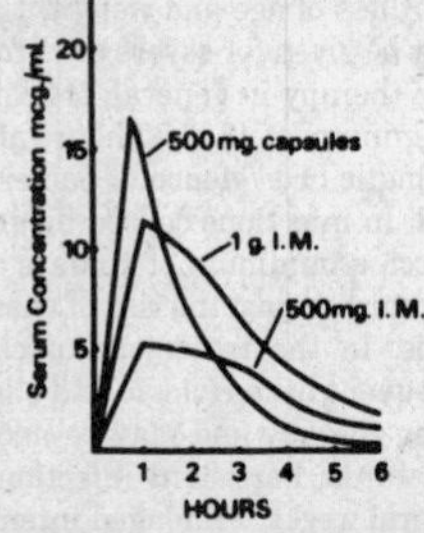

A single intravenous dose of 1 g cephradine resulted in serum levels of approximately 86 mcg/mL at 5 minutes, 50 mcg/mL at 15 minutes, 26 mcg/mL at 30 minutes, and 12 mcg/mL at 60 minutes; these levels declined to 1 mcg/mL at four hours.
In vitro studies by an ultracentrifugation technique show that, at therapeutic serum antibiotic concentrations, cephradine is minimally bound (8 to 17 percent) to normal human serum protein. Cephradine does not pass across the blood-brain barrier to any appreciable extent.
Velosef (Cephradine, Squibb) is excreted unchanged in the urine. The kidneys excrete 57 to 80 percent of an intramuscular dose in the first six hours; this results in a high urine concentration, e.g., a mean urine concentration of 313 mcg/mL within a six hour period following a 500 mg IM dose. Probenecid slows tubular excretion and increases serum concentration.
Assays of bone and cardiac tissue (atrial appendage) obtained at surgery have shown that cephradine penetrates these tissues.
Microbiology—In vitro tests demonstrate that the cephalosporins are bactericidal because of their inhibition of cell-wall synthesis. Cephradine is active against the following organisms *in vitro:* group A beta-hemolytic streptococci; staphylococci, including coagulase-positive, coagulase-negative, and penicillinase-producing strains; *Escherichia coli; Streptococcus pneumoniae* (formerly *Diplococcus pneumoniae); Proteus mirabilis; Klebsiella* species; and *Hemophilus influenzae.*
It is not active against most strains of Enterobacter species, *Proteus morganii,* and *Proteus vulgaris.* It has no activity against *Pseudomonas* or *Herellea* species. When tested by *in vitro* methods, staphylococci exhibit cross-resistance between cephradine and methicillin-type antibiotics.
NOTE—Most strains of enterococci (*Streptococcus faecalis*) are resistant to cephradine.
Disc Susceptibility Tests—Quantitative methods that require measurement of zone diameters give the most precise estimates of antibiotic susceptibility. One recommended procedure (21 CFR § 460.1) uses cephalosporin class discs for testing susceptibility; interpretations correlate zone diameters of this disc test with MIC values for cephradine. With this procedure, a report from the laboratory of "resistant" indicates that the infecting organism is not likely to respond to therapy. A report of "intermediate susceptibility" suggests that the organism would be susceptible if the infection is confined to the urinary tract, as high antibiotic levels can be obtained in the urine, or if high dosage is used in other types of infection.

INDICATIONS AND USAGE

Treatment—Velosef for Injection (Cephradine for Injection USP) is indicated in the treatment of the following serious infections when caused by susceptible strains of the designated microorganisms:
RESPIRATORY TRACT INFECTIONS due to *Streptococcus pneumoniae* (formerly *Diplococcus pneumoniae*), *Klebsiella* species, *H. influenzae, Staphylococcus aureus* (penicillin-susceptible and penicillin-resistant), and group A beta-hemolytic streptococci.
[Penicillin is the usual drug of choice in the treatment and prevention of streptococcal infections, including the prophylaxis of rheumatic fever. Velosef is generally effective in the eradication of streptococci from the nasopharynx; substantial data establishing the efficacy of Velosef in the subsequent prevention of rheumatic fever are not available at present.]
URINARY TRACT INFECTIONS due to *E. coli, P. mirabilis,* and *Klebsiella* species.
SKIN AND SKIN STRUCTURE INFECTIONS due to *S. aureus* (penicillin-susceptible and penicillin-resistant) and group A beta-hemolytic streptococci.
BONE INFECTIONS due to *S. aureus* (penicillin-susceptible and penicillin-resistant).
SEPTICEMIA due to *Streptococcus pneumoniae* (formerly *Diplococcus pneumoniae), S. aureus* (penicillin-susceptible and penicillin-resistant), *P. mirabilis,* and *E. coli.*
NOTE—Culture and susceptibility tests should be initiated prior to and during therapy.
Prevention: When compared to placebo in randomized controlled studies in patients undergoing vaginal hysterectomy and cesarean section, the prophylactic use of VELOSEF (cephradine) resulted in a significant reduction in the number of postoperative infections.
The prophylactic administration of VELOSEF perioperatively (preoperatively, intraoperatively, and postoperatively) may reduce the incidence of certain postoperative infections in patients undergoing surgical procedures (e.g., vaginal hysterectomy) that are classified as contaminated or potentially contaminated.
In patients undergoing cesarean section, intraoperative (after clamping the umbilical cord) and postoperative use of VELOSEF may reduce the incidence of certain postoperative infections.
Effective perioperative use depends on the time of administration. VELOSEF (Cephradine, Squibb) usually should be given 30 to 90 minutes before surgery, which is sufficient time to achieve effective tissue levels. Prophylactic administration should usually be stopped within 24 hours since continuing administration of any antibiotic increases the possibility of adverse reactions but, in the majority of surgical procedures, does not reduce the incidence of subsequent infection.
If there are signs of infection, specimens for culture should be obtained for identification of the causative organism so that appropriate therapy may be instituted.

CONTRAINDICATIONS

Cephradine is contraindicated in patients with known hypersensitivity to the cephalosporin group of antibiotics.

WARNINGS

In penicillin-sensitive patients, cephalosporin derivatives should be used with great caution. There is clinical and laboratory evidence of partial cross-allergenicity of the penicillins and the cephalosporins, and there are instances of patients who have had reactions to both drug classes (including fatal anaphylaxis after parenteral use).
Any patient who has demonstrated some form of allergy, particularly to drugs, should receive antibiotics, including cephradine, cautiously and then only when absolutely necessary. Serious anaphylactoid reactions require immediate emergency treatment with epinephrine. Oxygen, intravenous steroids, and airway management, including intubation, should also be administered as indicated.
Pseudomembranous colitis has been reported with the use of cephalosporins (and other broad spectrum antibiotics); therefore, it is important to consider its diagnosis in patients who develop diarrhea in association with antibiotic use. Treatment with broad spectrum antibiotics alters normal flora of the colon and may permit overgrowth of clostridia. Studies indicate a toxin produced by *Clostridium difficile* is one primary cause of antibiotic-associated colitis. Cholestyramine and colestipol resins have been shown to bind the toxin *in vitro.* Mild cases of colitis may respond to drug discontinuance alone. Moderate to severe cases should be managed with fluid, electrolyte and protein supplementation as indicated. When the colitis is not relieved by drug discontinuance or when it is severe, oral vancomycin is the treatment of choice for antibiotic-associated pseudomembranous colitis produced by *C. difficile.* Other causes of colitis should also be considered.

PRECAUTIONS

General—Prolonged use of antibiotics may promote the overgrowth of nonsusceptible organisms. Should superinfection occur during therapy, appropriate measures should be taken.
When cephradine is administered to patients with markedly impaired renal function lower daily dosage is required. (See DOSAGE AND ADMINISTRATION.) In patients with known or suspected renal impairment, careful clinical observation and appropriate laboratory studies should be conducted because cephradine in the usual recommended dosage will accumulate in the serum and tissues.
Cephradine should be prescribed with caution in individuals with a history of gastrointestinal disease, particularly colitis. Patients should be followed carefully so that any side effects or unusual manifestations of drug idiosyncrasy may be detected. If a hypersensitivity reaction occurs, the drug should be discontinued and the patient treated with the usual agents, e.g., pressor amines, antihistamines, or corticosteroids.
Velosef for Injection (Cephradine for Injection USP) is physically compatible with most commonly used intravenous fluids and electrolyte solutions (such as 5% Dextrose Injection or Sodium Chloride Injection or M/6 sodium lactate); however, it is *not* compatible with Lactated Ringer's Injection because of the incompatibility between calcium ions and the sodium carbonate present in Velosef for Injection.
Information for Patients: Caution diabetic patients that false test results may occur with urine glucose tests (see PRECAUTIONS, Drug/Laboratory Test Interactions). The patient should report current use of any medicines and should be cautioned not to take other medications unless the physician knows and approves of their use (see PRECAUTIONS, Drug Interactions).
Laboratory Tests: In patients with known or suspected renal impairment, it is advisable to monitor renal function (see DOSAGE AND ADMINISTRATION).
Drug Interactions: When administered concurrently, the following drugs may interact with cephalosporins:
Other antibacterial agents—Bacteriostats may interfere with the bactericidal action of cephalosporins in acute infection; other agents, e.g., aminoglycosides, colistin, polymyxins, vancomycin, may increase the possibility of nephrotoxicity.
Diuretics (potent "loop diuretics," e.g., furosemide and ethacrynic acid)—Enhanced possibility for renal toxicity.
Probenecid—Increased and prolonged blood levels of cephalosporins, resulting in increased risk of nephrotoxicity.
Drug/Laboratory Test Interactions: After treatment with cephradine, a false-positive reaction for glucose in the urine may occur with Benedict's solution, Fehling's solution, or with Clinitest® tablets, but not with enzyme-based tests such as Clinistix® and Tes-Tape®. False-positive Coombs test results may occur in newborns whose mothers received a cephalosporin prior to delivery.
Cephalosporins have been reported to cause false-positive reactions in tests for urinary proteins which use sulfosali-

TABLE I
VELOSEF FOR INJECTION
(Cephradine for Injection USP)

	MEAN TIME TO PEAK SERUM LEVELS Minutes		MEAN PEAK SERUM CONCENTRATION mcg/mL		MEAN SERUM CONCENTRATION AT 1 HR. - mcg/mL	
	500 mg IM	1 g IM	500 mg IM	1 g IM	500 mg IM	1 g IM
MALES	49 (41–59)*	52 (45–61)	6.3 (5.5–7.2)	13.6 (12.2–15.1)	6.2 (5.5–6.9)	12.4 (11.0–14.0)
FEMALES	98 (87–111)	128 (103–157)	5.8 (5.1–6.6)	9.9 (8.7–11.2)	4.3 (3.5–5.2)	6.0 (4.4–8.1)

*Figures in parentheses are 95% confidence limits.

cylic acid, false elevations of urinary 17-ketosteroid values, and prolonged prothrombin times.

Carcinogenesis, Mutagenesis: Long-term studies in animals have not been performed to evaluate carcinogenic potential or mutagenesis.

Pregnancy Category B: Reproduction studies have been performed in mice and rats at doses up to four times the maximum indicated human dose and have revealed no evidence of impaired fertility or harm to the fetus due to cephradine. There are, however, no adequate and well-controlled studies in pregnant women. Because animal reproduction studies are not always predictive of human response, this drug should be used during pregnancy only if clearly needed.

Nursing Mothers: Since cephradine is excreted in breast milk during lactation, caution should be exercised when cephradine is administered to a nursing woman.

Pediatric Use: See DOSAGE AND ADMINISTRATION. Cephradine has been effectively used in infants, but all laboratory parameters have not been extensively studied in infants one month to one year of age; therefore, in the treatment of children in this age group, the benefits of the drug to the risk involved must be considered.

Since safety for use in premature infants and in infants under one month of age has not been established, the use of cephradine by injection or infusion should be based on careful consideration of the benefits of the drug against the risk involved.

ADVERSE REACTIONS

As with other cephalosporins, untoward reactions are limited essentially to gastrointestinal disturbances and, on occasion, to hypersensitivity phenomena. The latter are more likely to occur in individuals who have previously demonstrated hypersensitivity and those with a history of allergy, asthma, hay fever, or urticaria.

The following adverse reactions have been reported following the use of cephradine:

Gastrointestinal: Symptoms of pseudomembranous colitis can appear during antibiotic treatment. Nausea and vomiting have been reported rarely.

Skin and Hypersensitivity Reactions: Mild urticaria or skin rash, edema, erythema, pruritus, joint pains and drug fever.

Hematologic: Mild, transient eosinophilia, leukopenia and neutropenia.

Liver: Instances of elevated SGOT and SGPT of approximately 10 percent and 2 percent of patients, respectively, have been observed; also, a few cases of elevated total bilirubin, alkaline phosphatase and LDH have been observed. In most patients, values tended to return to normal after the end of therapy.

Renal: Mild elevations in BUN have been observed in some patients treated with cephalosporins; their frequency increases in patients over 50 years old and in children under three. In adults for whom serum creatinine determinations were performed, the rise in BUN was not accompanied by a rise in serum creatinine.

Other adverse reactions are headache, dizziness, dyspnea, paresthesia, candidal overgrowth, candidal vaginitis, isolated instances of hepatomegaly, and thrombophlebitis at the site of injection.

Pain on intramuscular injection has been experienced by some patients. Since sterile abscesses have been reported following accidental subcutaneous injection, the preparation should be administered by deep intramuscular injection.

DOSAGE AND ADMINISTRATION

Adults— *Treatment:* The usual daily dosage of Velosef for Injection (Cephradine for Injection USP) is 2 to 4 g of cephradine given in equally divided doses four times a day intramuscularly or intravenously (e.g., 500 mg to 1 g qid). In bone infections the usual dosage is 1 g qid administered intravenously. A dosage of 500 mg qid is adequate in uncomplicated pneumonia, skin and skin structure and most urinary tract infections. In severe infections, the total daily dose may be increased by using a q 4 h dosage regimen or by increasing the dose given qid; the maximum dose should not exceed 8 g per day.

Prevention: To prevent postoperative infection in contaminated or potentially contaminated surgery, recommended doses are as follows:

a. 1 g IV or IM administered 30 to 90 minutes prior to start of surgery.

b. 1 g every 4 to 6 hours after the first dose for one or two doses, or for up to 24 hours postoperatively.

Cesarean Section Patients: The first dose of 1 g is administered intravenously as soon as the umbilical cord is clamped. The second and third doses should be given as 1 g intravenously or intramuscularly at 6 and 12 hours after the first dose.

Infants and Children—The usual dosage range of Velosef is 50 to 100 mg/kg/day (approximately 23 to 45 mg/lb/day) in equally divided doses four times a day and should be regulated by age, weight of the patient and severity of the infection being treated.

All laboratory parameters have not been extensively studied in infants under one year of age; therefore, in the treatment of children in this age group, the benefits of the drug to the risk involved must be considered. In newborn infants, accumulation of other cephalosporin-class antibiotics (with resultant prolongation of drug half-life) has been reported.

The maximum daily pediatric dose should not exceed doses recommended for adults.

[See table entitled "Pediatric Dosage Guide" above.]

VELOSEF FOR INJECTION
(Cephradine for Injection USP)

PEDIATRIC DOSAGE GUIDE

Weight lbs	Weight kg	50 mg/kg/day: Approx. single dose mg q 6 h	50 mg/kg/day: Volume needed @ 208 mg/mL dilution	100 mg/kg/day: Approx. single dose mg q 6 h	100 mg/kg/day: Volume needed @ 227 mg/mL
10	4.5	56 mg	0.27 mL	112 mg	0.5 mL
20	9.1	114 mg	0.55 mL	227 mg	1 mL
30	13.6	170 mg	0.82 mL	340 mg	1.5 mL
40	18.2	227 mg	1.1 mL	455 mg	2 mL
50	22.7	284 mg	1.4 mL	567 mg	2.5 mL

As with antibiotic therapy generally: therapy should be continued for a minimum of 48 to 72 hours after the patient becomes asymptomatic or evidence of bacterial eradication has been obtained; in infections caused by group A beta-hemolytic streptococci, a minimum of 10 days of treatment is recommended to guard against the risk of rheumatic fever or glomerulonephritis; in the treatment of chronic urinary tract infection, frequent bacteriologic and clinical appraisal is necessary during therapy and may be necessary for several months afterwards; persistent infections may require treatment for several weeks; doses smaller than those indicated above should not be used.

Parenteral therapy may be followed by oral Velosef either as capsules or as an oral suspension.

Velosef for Injection (Cephradine for Injection USP) may be given intravenously or by deep intramuscular injection. To minimize pain and induration, intramuscular injections should be made into a large muscle mass, such as the gluteus or lateral aspect of the thigh.

Patients With Impaired Renal Function

Not on Dialysis: The following initial dosage schedule is suggested as a guideline based on creatinine clearance. Further modification in the dosage schedule may be required because of individual variations in absorption.

Creatinine Clearance	Dose	Time Interval
> 20 mL/min	500 mg	6 hours
5–20 mL/min	250 mg	6 hours
< 5 mL/min	250 mg	12 hours

On Chronic Intermittent Hemodialysis:
250 mg Start
250 mg at 12 hours
250 mg 36–48 hours (after start)

Children may require dosage modification proportional to their weight and severity of infection.

Constitution and Storage:

Parenteral drug products should be inspected visually for particulate matter and discoloration prior to administration, whenever solution and container permit.

For I.M. Use.—Aseptically add Sterile Water for Injection or Bacteriostatic Water for Injection (containing 0.9% [w/v] benzyl alcohol, or 0.12% methylparaben and 0.014% propylparaben) according to the following table [i.e., the table entitled "IM Dilution Table"].

[See table below].

VELOSEF FOR INJECTION
(Cephradine for Injection USP)

IM DILUTION TABLE

Vial Size	Volume of Diluent	Approximate Available Volume	Approximate Available Concentration
250 mg	1.2 mL	1.2 mL	208 mg/mL
500 mg	2.0 mL	2.2 mL	227 mg/mL
1 g	4.0 mL	4.5 mL	222 mg/mL

Intramuscular solutions should be used within two hours at room temperature; if stored in the refrigerator at 5° C., solutions retain full potency for 24 hours. Constituted solutions may vary in color from light straw to yellow; however, this does not affect the potency.

For IV Use—Velosef (Cephradine for Injection USP) may also be administered by direct intravenous injection or by continuous or intermittent infusion. A 3 mcg/mL serum concentration can be maintained for each mg of cephradine per kg body weight per hour of infusion.

For Direct IV Administration: Suitable diluents are Sterile Water for Injection, 5% Dextrose Injection, or Sodium Chloride Injection. **Do not use Lactated Ringer's Injection.**

Aseptically add 5 mL of diluent to the 250 mg or 500 mg vials, 10 mL of diluent to the 1 g vial, or 20 mL of diluent to the 2 g bottle; withdraw entire contents. The solution may be slowly injected directly into a vein over a three to five minute period or may be given as a supplementary injection through the injection site on the administration set when the infusion solution is compatible with cephradine. These Velosef (Cephradine, Squibb) solutions should be used within two hours when held at room temperature; if stored at 5° C, the solutions retain full potency for 24 hours.

For Continuous or Intermittent IV Infusion: Suitable intravenous infusion solutions for Velosef are 5% or 10% Dextrose Injection; Sodium Chloride Injection; Sodium Lactate Injection (M/6 sodium lactate); Dextrose and Sodium Chloride Injection (5% : 0.9%) or (5% : 0.45%); 10% Invert Sugar in Water for Injection; Normosol®-R, and Ionosol® B with Dextrose 5%. Sterile Water for Injection may be used as an IV infusion solution for Velosef at a concentration of 30 to 50 mg/mL (30 mg/mL is approximately isotonic). **Do not use Lactated Ringer's Injection.**

a) To prepare a Velosef solution for transfer into an IV infusion bottle, aseptically add 10 mL, 20 mL, or 40 mL of Sterile Water for Injection or a suitable infusion solution, respectively, to the 1 g vial, or 2 g or 4 g bottles. Promptly withdraw the entire contents of the resulting solution and aseptically transfer to an IV infusion bottle. Intravenous infusion solutions containing Velosef at a concentration of five percent (50 mg/mL) or less retain potency as noted under (b) below. The choice of IV infusion solution and the volume to be employed are dictated by fluid and electrolyte management.

b) Velosef may be infused directly from the 2 g or 4 g IV bottle. Constitute the 2 g bottle with 40 mL and the 4 g bottle with 80 mL of a suitable intravenous infusion solution; attach an IV administration set directly to the Velosef IV infusion bottle. The 2 g and 4 g IV bottles are designed to be suspended from an IV stand.

Intravenous infusion solutions containing Velosef retain full potency for 10 hours at room temperature or 48 hours at 5° C; infusion solutions of Velosef in Sterile Water for Injection that are frozen immediately after reconstitution in the original container are stable for as long as six weeks when stored at −20° C.

For prolonged infusions, replace the infusion every 10 hours with a freshly prepared solution.

Extemporaneous mixtures of Velosef for Injection (Cephradine for Injection USP) with other antibiotics are not recommmended.

Protect solutions of Velosef from concentrated light or direct sunlight. Velosef for Injection may be stored at room temperature prior to constitution; avoid excessive heat; protect from light.

HOW SUPPLIED

Velosef for Injection (Cephradine for Injection USP) is available for intramuscular or intravenous use in vials containing 250 mg, 500 mg, or 1 g cephradine; and for intravenous use in 100 mL infusion bottles containing 2 g or 4 g cephradine.
(J3-508D)

Continued on next page

Squibb—Cont.

VIVOX™ ℞

[*vī-vox*]

Doxycycline Hyclate Capsules USP

Doxycycline Hyclate Tablets USP

DESCRIPTION

Doxycycline is a broad-spectrum antibiotic synthetically derived from oxytetracycline, and is available as doxycycline hydrochloride hemiethanolate hemihydrate. The chemical designation of this light-yellow crystalline powder is alpha-6-deoxy-5-oxytetracycline. Doxycycline has a high degree of lipoid solubility and a low affinity for calcium binding. It is highly stable in normal human serum. Doxycycline will not degrade into an epianhydro form.

Vivox (Doxycycline Hyclate Capsules) capsules contain doxycycline hyclate equivalent to 50 mg and 100 mg doxycycline. Inactive ingredients: cellulose, colorants (D&C Yellow No. 10 and Red No. 28; FD&C Blue No. 1), gelatin, magnesium stearate, and titanium dioxide.

Vivox (Doxycycline Hyclate Tablets) film coated tablets contain doxycycline hyclate equivalent to 100 mg doxycycline. Inactive ingredients- cellulose, colorants (FD&C Yellow No. 6 and Red No. 40), croscarmellose sodium, magnesium stearate, sodium lauryl sulfate, titanium dioxide, and other ingredients.

CLINICAL PHARMACOLOGY

Doxycycline is primarily bacteriostatic and is thought to exert its antimicrobial effect by the inhibition of protein synthesis. Doxycycline is active against a wide range of gram-positive and gram-negative organisms.

The drugs in the tetracycline class have closely similar antimicrobial spectra, and cross resistance among them is common. Microorganisms may be considered susceptible if the MIC (minimum inhibitory concentration) is less than 4.0 mcg/mL and intermediate if the MIC is 4.02-12.5 mcg/mL.

Susceptibility plate testing: If the Kirby-Bauer method of disc susceptibility testing is used, a 30 mcg doxycycline disc should give a zone of at least 16 mm when tested against a doxycycline-susceptible bacterial strain. A tetracycline disc may be used to determine microbial susceptibility to drugs in the tetracycline class. If the Kirby-Bauer method of disc susceptibility testing is used, a 30 mcg tetracycline disc should give a zone of at least 19 mm when tested against a tetracycline-susceptible bacterial strain.

Tetracyclines are readily absorbed and are bound to plasma proteins in varying degree. They are concentrated by the liver in the bile, and excreted in the urine and feces at high concentrations and in a biologically active form. Doxycycline is virtually completely absorbed after oral administration.

Following a 200 mg dose, normal adult volunteers averaged peak serum levels of 2.6 mcg/mL of doxycycline at two hours decreasing to 1.45 mcg/mL at 24 hours. Excretion of doxycycline by the kidney is about 40%/72 hours in individuals with normal function (creatinine clearance about 75 mL/min). This percentage excretion may fall as low as 1–5%/72 hours in individuals with severe renal insufficiency (creatinine clearance below 10 mL/min). Studies have shown no significant difference in serum half-life of doxycycline (range 18–22 hours) in individuals with normal and severely impaired renal function.

Hemodialysis does not alter serum half-life.

INDICATIONS

Doxycycline is indicated in infections caused by the following microorganisms:

Rickettsiae: Rocky Mountain spotted fever, typhus fever, and the typhus group. Q fever, rickettsialpox, and tick fevers.

Mycoplasma pneumoniae (PPLO, Eaton agent)

Agents of psittacosis and ornithosis

Agents of *Lymphogranuloma venereum* and *Granuloma inguinale*

The spirochetal agent of relapsing fever *(Borrelia recurrentis)*

The following gram-negative microorganisms:

Haemophilus ducreyi (chancroid)

Pasteurella pestis, and *Pasteurella tularensis*

Bartonella bacilliformis

Bacteroides species

Vibrio comma and *Vibrio fetus*

Brucella species (in conjunction with streptomycin)

Because many strains of the following groups of microorganisms have been shown to be resistant to tetracycline, culture and susceptibility testing are recommended.

Doxycycline is indicated for treatment of infections caused by the following gram-negative microorganisms, when bacteriologic testing indicates appropriate susceptibility to the drug:

Escherichia coli

Enterobacter aerogenes (formerly *Aerobacter aerogenes*)

Shigella species

Mima species and *Herellea*

Haemophilus influenzae (respiratory infections)

Klebsiella species (respiratory and urinary infections)

Doxycycline is indicated for treatment of infections caused by the following gram-positive microorganisms, when bacteriologic testing indicates appropriate susceptibility to the drug:

Streptococcus species: Up to 44 percent of strains of *Streptococcus pyogenes* and 74 percent of *Streptococcus faecalis* have been found to be resistant to tetracycline drugs. Therefore, tetracyclines should not be used for streptococcal disease unless the organism has been demonstrated to be sensitive. For upper respiratory infection due to group A beta-hemolytic streptococci, penicillin is the usual drug of choice, including prophylaxis of rheumatic fever.

Diplococcus pneumoniae

Staphylococcus aureus, respiratory, skin and soft-tissue infections.

Tetracyclines are not the drug of choice in the treatment of any type of staphylococcal infections.

When penicillin is contraindicated, doxycycline is an alternative drug in the treatment of infections due to:

Neisseria gonorrhoeae

Treponema pallidum and *Treponema pertenue* (syphilis and yaw)

Listeria monocytogenes

Clostridium species

Bacillus anthracis

Fusobacterium fusiforme (Vincent's infection)

Actinomyces species

In acute intestinal amebiasis doxycycline may be a useful adjunct to amebicides.

In severe acne doxycycline may be useful adjunctive therapy.

Doxycycline is indicated in the treatment of trachoma, although the infectious agent is not always eliminated, as judged by immunofluorescence.

Inclusion conjunctivitis may be treated with oral doxycycline alone, or with a combination of topical agents.

Doxycycline is indicated for the treatment of uncomplicated urethral, endocervical, or rectal infections in adults caused by *Chlamydia trachomatis*.[1]

CONTRAINDICATIONS

This drug is contraindicated in persons who have shown hypersensitivity to any of the tetracyclines.

WARNINGS

THE USE OF DRUGS OF THE TETRACYCLINE CLASS DURING TOOTH DEVELOPMENT (LAST HALF OF PREGNANCY, INFANCY AND CHILDHOOD TO THE AGE OF EIGHT YEARS) MAY CAUSE PERMANENT DISCOLORATION OF THE TEETH (YELLOW-GRAY-BROWN). This adverse reaction is more common during long-term use of the drugs, but has been observed following repeated short-term courses. Enamel hypoplasia has also been reported. TETRACYCLINE DRUGS, THEREFORE, SHOULD NOT BE USED IN THIS AGE GROUP UNLESS OTHER DRUGS ARE NOT LIKELY TO BE EFFECTIVE OR ARE CONTRAINDICATED.

Photosensitivity manifested by exaggerated sunburn reaction has been observed in some individuals taking tetracyclines. Patients apt to be exposed to direct sunlight or ultraviolet light should be advised that this reaction can occur with tetracycline drugs, and treatment should be discontinued at the first evidence of skin erythema.

The antianabolic action of the tetracyclines may cause an increase in BUN. Studies to date indicate that this does not occur with the use of doxycyline in patients with impaired renal function.

Usage in Pregnancy (See above WARNINGS about use during tooth development).

Results of animal studies indicate that tetracyclines cross the placenta, are found in fetal tissues, and can have toxic effects on the developing fetus (often related to retardation of skeletal development). Evidence of embryo-toxicity has also been noted in animals treated early in pregnancy.

Usage in Newborns, Infants, and Children (See above WARNINGS about use during tooth development.)

As with other tetracyclines, doxycycline forms a stable calcium complex in any bone-forming tissue. A decrease in the fibula growth rate has been observed in prematures given oral tetracycline in doses of 25 mg/kg every six hours. This reaction was shown to be reversible when the drug was discontinued.

Tetracyclines are present in the milk of lactating women who are taking a drug in this class.

PRECAUTIONS

As with other antibiotic preparations, use of this drug may result in overgrowth of nonsusceptible organisms, including fungi. If superinfection occurs, the antibiotic should be discontinued and appropriate therapy should be instituted.

In venereal disease when coexistent syphilis is suspected, a dark-field examination should be done before treatment is started and the blood serology repeated monthly for at least four months.

Because the tetracyclines have been shown to depress plasma prothrombin activity, patients who are on anticoagulant therapy may require downward adjustment of their anticoagulant dosage.

In long term therapy, periodic laboratory evaluation of organ systems, including hematopoietic, renal, and hepatic studies should be performed.

All infections due to group A beta-hemolytic streptococci should be treated for at least 10 days.

Since bacteriostatic drugs may interfere with the bactericidal action of penicillin, it is advisable to avoid giving tetracycline in conjunction with penicillin.

ADVERSE REACTIONS

Due to oral doxycycline's virtually complete absorption, side effects of the lower bowel, particularly diarrhea, have been infrequent. The following adverse reactions have been observed in patients receiving tetracyclines:

Gastrointestinal: anorexia, nausea, vomiting, diarrhea, glossitis, dysphagia, enterocolitis, and inflammatory lesions (with monilial overgrowth) in the anogenital region. These reactions have been caused by both the oral and parenteral administration of tetracyclines.

Rare instances of esophagitis and esophageal ulcerations have been reported in patients receiving capsule and tablet forms of the drugs in the tetracycline class. Most of these patients took medications immediately before going to bed (see DOSAGE AND ADMINISTRATION).

Skin: maculopapular and erythematous rashes. Exfoliative dermatitis has been reported but is uncommon. Photosensitivity is discussed above (see WARNINGS).

Renal toxicity: Rise in BUN has been reported and is apparently dose related (see WARNINGS).

Hypersensitivity reactions: urticaria, angioneurotic edema, anaphylaxis, anaphylactoid purpura, pericarditis, and exacerbation of systemic lupus erythematosus.

Bulging fontanels in infants and benign intracranial hypertension in adults have been reported in individuals receiving full therapeutic dosages. These conditions disappeared rapidly when the drug was discontinued.

Blood: hemolytic anemia, thrombocytopenia, neutropenia, and eosinophilia have been reported with tetracyclines.

When given over prolonged periods, tetracyclines have been reported to produce brown-black microscopic discoloration of thyroid glands. No abnormalities of thyroid function studies are known to occur.

DOSAGE AND ADMINISTRATION

THE USUAL DOSAGE AND FREQUENCY OF ADMINISTRATION OF DOXYCYCLINE DIFFERS FROM THAT OF THE OTHER TETRACYCLINES. EXCEEDING THE RECOMMENDED DOSAGE MAY RESULT IN AN INCREASED INCIDENCE OF SIDE EFFECTS.

Adults: The usual dose of doxycycline is 200 mg on the first day of treatment (administered 100 mg every 12 hours) followed by a maintenance dose of 100 mg/day. The maintenance dose may be administered as a single dose or as 50 mg every 12 hours. In the management of more severe infections (particularly chronic infections of the urinary tract), 100 mg every 12 hours is recommended.

For children above eight years of age: The recommended dosage schedule for children weighing 100 pounds or less is 2 mg/lb of body weight divided into two doses on the first day of treatment, followed by 1 mg/lb of body weight given as a single daily dose or divided into two doses, on subsequent days. For more severe infections up to 2 mg/lb of body weight may be used. For children over 100 lbs the usual adult dose should be used.

Acute gonococcal infections: 200 mg stat, and 100 mg at bedtime, the first day, followed by 100 mg bid for three days. As an alternate single visit dose, administer 300 mg stat followed in one hour by a second 300 mg dose. The dose may be administered with food, including milk or carbonated beverage, as required.

Primary and secondary syphilis: 300 mg a day in divided doses for at least 10 days.

The therapeutic antibacterial serum activity will usually persist for 24 hours following recommended dosage.

When used in streptococcal infections, therapy should be continued for 10 days.

Administration of adequate amounts of fluid along with capsule and tablet forms of drugs in the tetracycline class is recommended to wash down the drugs and reduce the risk of esophageal irritation and ulceration (see ADVERSE REACTIONS).

If gastric irritation occurs, it is recommended that doxycycline be given with food or milk. The absorption of doxycycline is not markedly influenced by simultaneous ingestion of food or milk.

Concomitant therapy: Antacids containing aluminum, calcium, or magnesium impair absorption and should not be given to patients taking oral doxycycline.

Studies to date have indicated that administration of doxycycline at the usual recommended doses does not lead to excessive accumulation of antibiotics in patients with renal impairment.

Uncomplicated urethral, endocervical, or rectal infection in adults caused by *Chlamydia trachomatis:* 100 mg by mouth, twice a day for at least seven days.[1]

HOW SUPPLIED

Vivox (Doxycycline Hyclate Capsules USP) is available in capsules containing doxycycline hyclate equivalent to 50 mg of doxycycline, in bottles of 50.

Vivox (Doxycycline Hyclate Capsules USP) is available in capsules containing doxycycline hyclate equivalent to 100 mg of doxycycline, in bottles of 50 and 500.

Vivox (Doxycycline Hyclate Tablets USP) is available in film coated tablets containing doxycycline hyclate equivalent to 100 mg of doxycycline, in bottles of 50 and 500.

Storage: Dispense in tight, light-resistant child-proof containers as defined in the USP. Store below 86°F (30°C).

Reference:

1. CDC Sexually Transmitted Diseases Treatment Guidelines 1982.

(J4-006A)

Shown in Product Identification Section, page 431

For information on Squibb products, write to: Squibb Professional Services Department, P.O. Box 4000, Princeton, N.J. 08540.

Squibb-Novo, Inc.

120 ALEXANDER STREET
PRINCETON, NJ 08540

STANDARD INSULIN

REGULAR INSULIN
Insulin Injection
USP (Pork) 100 units/ml

DESCRIPTION

Regular Insulin, Insulin Injection USP, 100 units of insulin per milliliter, is a clear, colorless solution which has a short duration of action. The effect of **Regular Insulin** begins approximately ½ hour after injection. The effect is maximal between 2½ and 5 hours and ends approximately 8 hours after injection. The time course of action of any insulin may vary considerably in different individuals, or at different times in the same individual. Because of this variation, the time periods listed here should be considered as general guidelines only.

SEMILENTE® INSULIN
Prompt Insulin Zinc Suspension
USP (Beef) 100 units/ml

DESCRIPTION

Semilente® Insulin, Prompt Insulin Zinc Suspension USP, 100 units of insulin per milliliter, is a cloudy or milky suspension of amorphous beef insulin. The insulin substance (the cloudy material) settles at the bottom of the vial, therefore, the vial must be gently agitated or rotated so that the contents are uniformly mixed before a dose is withdrawn. The effect of **Semilente® Insulin** begins approximately 1½ hours after injection. The effect is maximal between 5 and 10 hours and ends approximately 16 hours after injection. The time course of action of any insulin may vary considerably in different individuals, or at different times in the same individual. Because of this variation, the time periods listed here should be considered as general guidelines only.

LENTE® INSULIN
Insulin Zinc Suspension
USP (Beef) 100 units/ml

DESCRIPTION

LENTE® Insulin, Insulin Zinc Suspension USP, 100 units of insulin per milliliter, is a cloudy or milky suspension of 70% crystalline and 30% amorphous beef insulin. The Insulin substance (the cloudy material) settles at the bottom of the vial, therefore, the vial must be gently agitated or rotated so that the contents are uniformly mixed before a dose is withdrawn. **Lente® Insulin** has an intermediate duration of action. The effect of **Lente® Insulin** begins approximately 2½ hours after injection. The effect is maximal between 7 and 15 hours and ends approximately 24 hours after injection. The time course of action of any insulin may vary considerably in different individuals, or at different times in the same individual. Because of this variation, the time periods listed here should be considered as general guidelines only.

NPH INSULIN
Isophane Insulin Suspension USP (Beef) 100 units/ml

DESCRIPTION

NPH Insulin, Isophane Insulin Suspension USP, 100 units of insulin per milliliter, is a cloudy or milky suspension of beef insulin with protamine and zinc. The insulin substance (the cloudy material) settles at the bottom of the vial, therefore, the vial must be gently agitated or rotated so that the contents are uniformly mixed before a dose is withdrawn. **NPH Insulin** has an intermediate duration of action. The effect of **NPH Insulin** begins approximately 1½ hours after injection. The effect is maximal between 4 and 12 hours and ends approximately 24 hours after injection. The time course of action of any insulin may vary considerably in different individuals, or at different times in the same individual. Because of this variation, the time periods listed here should be considered as general guidelines only.

ULTRALENTE® INSULIN
Extended Insulin Zinc
Suspension USP (Beef) 100 units/ml

DESCRIPTION

Ultralente® Insulin, Extended Insulin Zinc Suspension USP, 100 units of insulin per milliliter, is a cloudy or milky suspension of crystalline beef insulin. The insulin substance (the cloudy material) settles at the bottom of the vial, therefore, the vial must be gently agitated or rotated so that the contents are uniformly mixed before a dose is withdrawn. The effect of **Ultralente® Insulin** begins approximately 4 hours after injection. The effect is maximal between 10 and 30 hours and ends approximately 36 hours after injection. The time course of action of any insulin may vary considerably in different individuals, or at different times in the same individual. Because of this variation, the time periods listed here should be considered as general guidelines only.

PURIFIED INSULIN

REGULAR PURIFIED PORK INSULIN
INJECTION USP 100 units/ml

DESCRIPTION

Regular Purified Pork Insulin Injection, USP, 100 units of insulin per milliliter, is a clear, colorless solution which has a short duration of action. The effect of Regular Purified Insulin begins approximately ½ hour after injection. The effect is maximal between 2½ and 5 hours and ends approximately 8 hours after injection. The time course of action of any insulin may vary considerably in different individuals, or at different times in the same individual. Because of this variation, the time periods listed here should be considered as general guidelines only.

The word "purified" on the label indicates that this insulin differs from standard insulin in that it has undergone additional purification steps (i.e., molecular sieve and ion-exchange chromatography).

SEMILENTE® PURIFIED PORK PROMPT INSULIN ZINC SUSPENSION USP 100 units/ml

DESCRIPTION

Semilente® Purified Pork Prompt Insulin Zinc Suspension, USP, 100 units of insulin per milliliter, is a cloudy or milky suspension of amorphous purified pork insulin. The insulin substance (the cloudy material) settles at the bottom of the vial, therefore, the vial must be gently agitated or rotated so that the contents are uniformly mixed before a dose is withdrawn. The effect of Semilente® Purified Insulin begins approximately 1½ hours after injection. The effect is maximal between 5 and 10 hours and ends approximately 16 hours after injection. The time course of action of any insulin may vary considerably in different individuals, or at different times in the same individual. Because of this variation, the time periods listed here should be considered as general guidelines only.

The word "purified" on the label indicates that this insulin differs from standard insulin in that it has undergone additional purification steps (i.e., molecular sieve and ion-exchange chromatography).

LENTE® PURIFIED PORK INSULIN
ZINC SUSPENSION USP 100 units/ml

DESCRIPTION

Lente® Purified Pork Insulin Zinc Suspension, USP, 100 units of insulin per milliliter, is a cloudy or milky suspension of 70% crystalline and 30% amorphous purified pork insulin. The insulin substance (the cloudy material) settles at the bottom of the vial, therefore, the vial must be gently agitated or rotated so that the contents are uniformly mixed before a dose is withdrawn. Lente® Purified Insulin has an intermediate duration of action. The effect of Lente® Purified Insulin begins approximately 2½ hours after injection. The effect is maximal between 7 and 15 hours and ends approximately 22 hours after injection. The time course of action of any insulin may vary considerably in different individuals, or at different times in the same individual. Because of this variation, the time periods listed here should be considered as general guidelines only. The word "purified" on the label indicates that this insulin differs from standard insulin in that it has undergone additional purification steps (i.e., molecular sieve and ion-exchange chromatography).

NPH PURIFIED PORK ISOPHANE INSULIN SUPSENSION USP 100 units/ml

DESCRIPTION

NPH Purified Pork Isophane Insulin Suspension, USP, 100 units of insulin per milliliter, is a cloudy or milky suspension of purified pork insulin with protamine and zinc. The insulin substance (the cloudy material) settles at the bottom of the vial, therefore, the vial must be gently agitated or rotated so that the contents are uniformly mixed before a dose is withdrawn. NPH Purified Insulin has an intermediate duration of action. The effect of NPH Purified Insulin begins approximately 1½ hours after injection. The effect is maximal between 4 and 12 hours and ends approximately 24 hours after injection. The time course of action of any insulin may vary considerably in different individuals, or at different times in the same individual. Because of this variation, the time periods listed here should be considered as general guidelines only.

The word "purified" on the label indicates that this insulin differs from standard insulin in that it has undergone additional purification steps (i.e., molecular sieve and ion-exchange chromatography).

ULTRALENTE® PURIFIED BEEF EXTENDED INSULIN ZINC SUSPENSION USP 100 units/ml

DESCRIPTION

Ultralente® Purified Beef Insulin Zinc Suspension, USP, 100 units of insulin per milliliter, is a cloudy or milky suspension of crystalline purified beef insulin. The insulin substance (the cloudy material) settles at the bottom of the vial, therefore, the vial must be gently agitated or rotated so that the contents are uniformly mixed before a dose is withdrawn. The effect of Ultralente® Purified Insulin begins approximately 4 hours after injection. The effect is maximal betwen 10 and 30 hours and ends approximately 36 hours after injection. The time course of action of any insulin may vary considerably in different individuals, or at different times in the same individual. Because of this variation, the time periods listed here should be considered as general guidelines only.

The word "purified" on the label indicates that this insulin differs from standard insulin in that it has undergone additional purification steps (i.e., molecular sieve and ion-exchange chromatography).

HUMAN INSULIN

NOVOLIN® R
Regular Human Insulin Injection (semi-synthetic) USP 100 units/ml

NOVOLIN® R is generically known as Regular Human Insulin Injection (semi-synthetic) USP. The concentration of this product is 100 Units per milliliter. It is a clear, colorless solution which has a short duration of action. The effects of NOVOLIN® R begins approximately ½ hour after injection. The effect is maximal between 2½ and 5 hours and ends approximately 8 hours after injection. The time course of action of any insulin may vary considerably in different individuals or a different times in the same individual. Because of this variation, the time periods listed here should be considered as general guidelines only.

This human insulin (semi-synthetic) is structurally identical to the insulin produced by the human pancreas and has undergone a special purification process. A naturally occurring enzyme is used in a process which converts pork insulin into human insulin. By this enzymatic transpeptidation process the amino acid alanine in pork insulin is selectively substituted by the amino acid threonine thus forming the human insulin molecule.

Shown in Product Identification Section, page 431

Continued on next page

Squibb-Novo—Cont.

NOVOLIN® L
Lente® Human Insulin Zinc Suspension (semi-synthetic)
100 units/ml

NOVOLIN® L is generically known as Lente® Human Insulin Zinc Suspension (semi-synthetic). The concentration of this product is 100 units of insulin per milliliter. It is a cloudy or milky suspension of 70% crystalline and 30% amorphous human insulin. The insulin substance (the cloudy material) settles at the bottom of the vial, therefore, the vial must be gently agitated or rotated so that the contents are uniformly mixed before a dose is withdrawn. NOVOLIN® L has an intermediate duration of action. The effect of NOVOLIN® L begins approximately 2½ hours after injection. The effect is maximal between 7 and 15 hours and ends approximately 22 hours after injection. The time course of action for any insulin may vary considerably in different individuals or at different times in the same individual. Because of this variation, the periods listed here should be considered as general guidelines only.
This human insulin (semi-synthetic) is structurally identical to the insulin produced by the human pancreas and has undergone a special purification process. A naturally occurring enzyme is used in a process which converts pork insulin into human insulin. By this enzymatic-transpeptidation process the amino acid alanine in pork insulin is selectively substituted by the amino acid threonine thus forming the human insulin molecule.
Shown in Product Identification Section, page 431

NOVOLIN® N
NPH Human Insulin Isophane Suspension (semi-synthetic)
100 units/ml

NOVOLIN® N is generically known as NPH Human Insulin Isophane Suspension (semi-synthetic). The concentration of this product is 100 units of insulin per milliliter. It is a cloudy or milky suspension of human insulin with protamine and zinc. The insulin substance (the cloudy material) settles at the bottom of the vial, therefore, the vial must be gently agitated or rotated so that the contents are uniformly mixed before a dose is withdrawn. NOVOLIN® N has an intermediate duration of action. The effect of NOVOLIN® N begins approximately 1½ hours after injection. The effect is maximal between 4 and 12 hours. The full duration of action may last up to 24 hours after injection. The time course of action for any insulin may vary considerably in different individuals, or at different times in the same individual. Because of this variation, the periods listed here should be considered as general guidelines only.
This human insulin (semi-synthetic) is structurally identical to the insulin produced by the human pancreas and has undergone a special purification process. A naturally occurring enzyme is used in a process which converts pork insulin into human insulin. By this enzymatic-transpeptidation process the amino acid alanine in pork insulin is selectively substituted by the amino acid threonine thus forming the human insulin molecule.
Shown in Product Identification Section, page 431

NOVOLIN® 70/30
70% NPH
Human Insulin Isophane Suspension &
30% Regular
Human Insulin Injection
(semi-synthetic)
100 units/ml

DESCRIPTION
Novolin® 70/30 is a mixture of 70% NPH Human Insulin Isophane Suspension (semi-synthetic) and 30% Regular Human Insulin Injection (semi-synthetic) USP. The concentration of this product is 100 units of insulin per milliliter. It is a cloudy or milky suspension of human insulin with protamine and zinc. The insulin substance (the cloudy material) settles at the bottom of the vial, therefore, the vial must be gently agitated or rotated so that the contents are uniformly mixed before a dose is withdrawn. **Novolin® 70/30** has an intermediate duration of action. The effect of **Novolin® 70/30** begins approximately ½ hour after injection. The effect is maximal between 2 and approximately 12 hours. The full duration of action may last up to 24 hours after injection. The time course of action of any insulin may vary considerably in different individuals, or at different times in the same individual. Because of this variation, the time periods listed here should be considered as general guidelines only.
This human insulin (semi-synthetic) is structurally identical to the insulin produced by the human pancreas and has undergone a special purification process. A naturally-occurring enzyme is used in a process which converts pork insulin into human insulin. By this enzymatic transpeptidation process the amino acid alanine in pork insulin is selectively substituted by the amino acid threonine thus forming the human insulin molecule.

EDUCATIONAL MATERIAL

Patient Education Materials
"Keeping Well With Diabetes"
A 36 page, four color booklet explaining the basics of diabetes and insulin therapy. Suitable for both Type I and Type II diabetics.
"Self-Monitoring Diary"
A 32 page log for keeping track of insulin injections, blood glucose test results and urine test results.
"Diabetes, Novolin® and You"
An 8 page, four color booklet explaining the different types of Novolin® Human Insulin (semi-synthetic) available, its time/action profile, as well as mixing, storing and traveling tips.
Free to patients and physicians

Standard Process Laboratories, Inc.
2023 WEST WISCONSIN AVENUE
MILWAUKEE, WI 53233

CHLOROPHYLL COMPLEX PERLES

COMPOSITION
Crude, natural chlorophyll extracted from Alfalfa and Tillandsia is a sterol rich source of fat soluble natural Vitamin K (2 Perles supply 1.1 mg. of Vitamin K). Vitamin K is indicated to be essential to the normal function of the liver and the formation of prothrombin, one of the normal constituents of the blood.

ACTION AND USES
Prothrombin is one of the several clotting agents in the blood. (Ref. #1) On the other hand, *water soluble* extracts of chlorophyll, being chemically altered from their natural form, contain no vitamins. Doses of synthetic Vitamin K have produced hemolytic anemia in rats and the toxicity of *synthetic* Vitamin K is attributed to increased breakdown of the red blood cells, (Ref. #2) whereas it is interesting to note, that administering *natural, fat soluble* Vitamin K, causes a prompt response by the body with the formation of prothrombin. The blood returns to its normal composition. (Ref. #3)

ADMINISTRATION
Two perles per day or as directed.

HOW SUPPLIED
CHLOROPHYLL COMPLEX PERLES in bottles of 60 and 350.

ALSO AVAILABLE
CHLOROPHYLL COMPLEX OINTMENT in 1½-oz. tube.

REFERENCES
(1) and (3) *Yearbook of Agriculture,* 1959, (U.S. Government Publication) pages 137-138. (2) *Recommended Dietary Allowances,* (Seventh Edition-1968), National Research Council Publication No. 1694, page 30.

ZYPAN TABLETS
An Enzymatic Digestive Supplement for Common Indigestion

DESCRIPTION
Each ZYPAN Tablet supplies 180 mg Betaine Hydrochloride, 65 mg Pancreatin (3X), 35 mg Bovine Pancreas Cytosol Extract, 25 mg Pepsin (1:10,000), and 10 mg Ammonium Chloride.
ZYPAN is a source of digestive enzymes as derived from fresh, frozen beef pancreas (as pancreatin), with betaine hydrochloride as a source of hydrochloric acid, and ammonium chloride as an acidifying agent. Pancreatin is a source of multiple digestive enzymes, notably as follows: (1) Trypsin, which breaks down *protein* into amino acids, (2) Diastase, which converts *starch* to an absorbable form, and (3) Lipase, which assists in the digestion of *fats.*

INDICATIONS
When intestinal fermentative processes result in such conditions as flatulence, bloating, and fullness after meals, a lack of digestive enzymes may be present. A long-term inability to absorb foods, because of incomplete digestion, may affect the general health. Deficient protein digestion should be a primary concern, and mere increase of protein in the diet may not correct a deficiency as efficiently as when aided by the proteolytic enzymes.

ADMINISTRATION
Two tablets with each meal, or as directed.

HOW SUPPLIED
Bottles of 90 tablets.

Star Pharmaceuticals, Inc.
1990 N.W. 44TH STREET
POMPANO BEACH, FL 33064-1278

URO-KP-NEUTRAL® OTC
[*ū 'ro-kp-nū 'tral*]
Phosphorous Supplement

Each peach capsule-shaped, film coated tablet contains:
Phosphorous .... 250 mg.
Potassium .... 49.25 mg.
Sodium .... 250 mg.
Derived from Disodium Phosphate Anhydrous, Dipotassium Phosphate Anhydrous, and Sodium Monobasic Anhydrous.

HOW SUPPLIED
Bottles of 100, 500.
NDC 0076-0109-03 & 04

UROLENE BLUE® ℞
[*ū 'ro-lene blue*]
Methylene Blue Tablets

Each blue coated tablet contains: Methylene blue USP 65 mg.

HOW SUPPLIED
Bottles of 100 and 1000.
NDC 0076-0501-03 & 04

VIRILON® ℞
[*vir 'i-lon*]
Methyltestosterone Macro-Beads Capsules
Oral Androgen Macro-Beads

Each capsule with black cap and clear body containing gray and white beads contains: Methyltestosterone Macro-Beads USP 10 mg.

HOW SUPPLIED
Bottles of 100 and 1000.
NDC 0076-0301-03 & 04

Write for complete prescribing information and samples.
Shown in Product Identification Section, page 431

Stellar Pharmacal Corp.
1990 N.W. 44TH STREET
POMPANO BEACH, FL 33064-1278

STAR-OTIC®

(See PDR For Nonprescription Drugs)

Stiefel Laboratories, Inc.
2801 PONCE DE LEON BLVD.
CORAL GABLES, FL 33134

DUOFILM® ℞
[*du 'ō-film*]

DESCRIPTION
Duofilm is a topical preparation containing 16.7% Salicyclic Acid, U.S.P., and 16.7% Lactic Acid, U.S.P., as the active ingredients in a base of Flexible Collodion, U.S.P.
Duofilm's pharmacologic activity is generally attributed to the keratolytic action of Salicylic Acid and Lactic Acid.

CLINICAL PHARMACOLOGY
The exact mode of action of Salicyclic Acid and Lactic Acid in the treatment of warts is not known. Their activity appears to be associated with keratolytic action which results in mechanical removal of epidermal cells infected with wart viruses.

INDICATIONS AND USAGE
Duofilm is indicated in the treatment of benign epithelial tumors such as common warts. See Dosage and Administration section for information on frequency and duration of use.

CONTRAINDICATIONS

Duofilm should not be used by diabetics or patients with impaired blood circulation. Do not use on moles, birthmarks, or unusual warts with hair growing from them.

PRECAUTIONS

Duofilm is for external use only. Do not permit Duofilm to contact eyes or mucosal membranes. If spilled in eyes or on mucosal membranes, flush with water, remove precipitated collodion, and flush with water for an additional 15 minutes. Duofilm should not be allowed to contact normal skin surrounding wart. Treatment should be discontinued if excessive irritation occurs. Duofilm is highly flammable and should be kept away from fire or flame. Keep bottle tightly capped when not in use. Store at controlled room temperature.

ADVERSE REACTIONS

A localized irritant reaction will occur if Duofilm is applied to the normal skin surrounding the wart. The irritation will normally be controlled by temporarily discontinuing use of Duofilm, and by applying the medication only to the wart site when treatment is resumed.

DOSAGE AND ADMINISTRATION

Prior to the application of Duofilm, soak affected area in hot water for at least five minutes. Dry thoroughly with a clean towel.

Apply a thin layer of Duofilm directly to wart once a day using the brush applicator. Duofilm should be applied with care to avoid contact with normal skin surrounding wart. Treated area should be covered by lightly applied Band-Aid.®

Clinically visible improvement will normally occur during the first two to four weeks of therapy. Maximum resolution may be expected after six to twelve weeks of drug use.

HOW SUPPLIED

Duofilm is supplied in a ½ oz. bottle with brush applicator, NDC 0145-6788-05.

See Precautions section for special handling and storage conditions.

LACTICARE®-HC Lotion 1%, 2½% ℞

[*lăk 'tĭ-kăr"*]

(hydrocortisone lotion, USP)

DESCRIPTION

Each ml of LactiCare-HC Lotion 1% and 2½% (hydrocortisone lotion, USP) contains 10 mg and 25 mg respectively of hydrocortisone in a vehicle consisting of carbomer 940, sodium PCA, lactic acid, sodium hydroxide, stearyl alcohol (and) ceteareth-20, glyceryl stearate (and) PEG-100 stearate, cetyl alcohol, isopropyl palmitate, light mineral oil, myristyl lactate, DMDM hydantoin, dehydroacetic acid, fragrance and purified water. Chemically, hydrocortisone is 11, 17, 20-trihydroxypregn-4-ene-3, 20-dione ($C_{21}H_{30}O_5$) and is represented by the following structural formula.

CH₂OH CO CH₃ OH HO H CH₃ H H H O

Its molecular weight is 362.47 and its CAS Registry Number is 50-23-7. The topical corticosteroids, including hydrocortisone, constitute a class of primarily synthetic steroids used as anti-inflammatory and antipruritic agents.

CLINICAL PHARMACOLOGY

Topical corticosteroids share anti-inflammatory, antipruritic and vasoconstrictive actions. The mechanism of anti-inflammatory activity of the topical corticosteroids is unclear. Various laboratory methods, including vasoconstrictor assays, are used to compare and predict potencies and/or clinical efficacies of the topical corticosteroids. There is some evidence to suggest that a recognizable correlation exists between vasoconstrictor potency and therapeutic efficacy in man.

PHARMACOKINETICS

The extent of percutaneous absorption of topical corticosteroids is determined by many factors including the vehicle, the integrity of the epidermal barrier, and the use of occlusive dressings.

Topical corticosteroids can be absorbed from normal intact skin. Inflammation and/or other disease processes in the skin increase percutaneous absorption. Occlusive dressings substantially increase the percutaneous absorption of topical corticosteroids. Thus, occlusive dressings may be a valuable therapeutic adjunct for treatment of resistant dermatoses. (See Dosage and Administration).

Once absorbed through the skin, topical corticosteroids are handled through pharmacokinetic pathways similar to systemically administered corticosteroids. Corticosteroids are bound to plasma proteins in varying degrees. Corticosteroids are metabolized primarily in the liver and are then excreted by the kidneys. Some of the topical corticosteroids and their metabolites are also excreted into the bile.

INDICATIONS AND USAGE

Topical corticosteroids are indicated for the relief of the inflammatory and pruritic manifestations of corticosteroid-responsive dermatoses.

CONTRAINDICATIONS

Topical corticosteroids are contraindicated in those patients with a history of hypersensitivity to any of the components of the preparation.

PRECAUTIONS

General—Systemic absorption of topical corticosteroids has produced reversible hypothalamic-pituitary- adrenal (HPA) axis suppression, manifestations of Cushing's syndrome, hyperglycemia, and glucosuria in some patients.

Conditions which augment systemic absorption include the application of the more potent steroids, use over large surface areas, prolonged use, and the addition of occlusive dressings.

Therefore, patients receiving a large dose of a potent topical steroid applied to a large surface area or under an oclusive dressing should be evaluated periodically for evidence of HPA axis suppression by using the urinary free cortisol and ACTH stimulation tests. If HPA axis suppression is noted, an attempt should be made to withdraw the drug, to reduce the frequency of application, or to substitute a less potent steroid.

Recovery of HPA axis function is generally prompt and complete upon discontinuation of the drug. Infrequently, signs and symptoms of steroid withdrawal may occur requiring supplemental systemic corticosteroids.

Children may absorb proportionally larger amounts of topical corticosteroids and thus be more susceptible to systemic toxicity (See PRECAUTIONS - Pediatric Use).

If irritation develops, topical corticosteroids should be discontinued and appropriate therapy instituted.

In the presence of dermatological infections, the use of an appropriate antifungal or antibacterial agent should be instituted. If a favorable response does not occur promptly, the corticosteroid should be discontinued until the infection has been adequately controlled.

Information for the Patient—Patients using topical corticosteroids should receive the following information and instructions.

1. This medication is to be used as directed by the physician. It is for external use only. Avoid contact with the eyes.
2. Patients should be advised not to use this medication for any disorder other than for which it was prescribed.
3. The treated skin area should not be bandaged or otherwise covered or wrapped as to be occlusive unless directed by the physician.
4. Patients should report any signs of local adverse reactions, especially under occlusive dressing.
5. Parents of pediatric patients should be advised not to use tight-fitting diapers or plastic pants on a child being treated in the diaper area, as these garments may constitute occlusive dressings.

Laboratory Tests—The following tests may be helpful in evaluating the HPA axis suppression:

Urinary free cortisol test

ACTH stimulation test

Carcinogenesis, Mutagenesis and Impairment of Fertility—Long-term animal studies have not been performed to evaluate the carcinogenic potential or the effect on fertility of topical corticosteroids.

Studies to determine mutagenicity with prednisolone and hydrocortisone have revealed negative results.

Pregnancy Category C—Corticosteroids are generally teratogenic in laboratory animals when administered systemically at relatively low dosage levels. The more potent corticosteroids have been shown to be teratogenic after dermal application on laboratory animals. There are no adequate and well-controlled studies in pregnant women on teratogenic effects from topically applied corticosteroids. Therefore, topical corticosteroids should be used during pregnancy only if the potential benefit justifies the potential risk to the fetus. Drugs of this class should not be used extensively on pregnant patients in large amounts or for prolonged periods of time.

Nursing Mothers—It is not known whether topical administration of corticosteroids could result in sufficient systemic absorption to produce detectable quantities in breast milk. Systemically administered corticosteroids are secreted into breast milk in quantities not likely to have a deleterious effect on the infant. Nevertheless, caution should be exercised when topical corticosteroids are administered to a nursing women.

Pediatric Use—Pediatric patients may demonstrate greater susceptibility to topical corticosteroid-induced HPA axis suppression and Cushing's syndrome than mature patients because of a larger skin surface area to body weight ratio. Hypothalamic-pituitary-adrenal (HPA) axis suppression, Cushing's syndrome, and intracranial hypertension have been reported in children receiving topical corticosteroids. Manifestations of adrenal suppression in children include linear growth retardation, delayed weight gain, low plasma cortisol levels, and absence of response to ACTH stimulation. Manifestations of intracranial hypertension include bulging fontanelles, headaches, and bilateral papilledema.

Administration of topical corticosteroids to children should be limited to the least amount compatible with an effective therapeutic regimen. Chronic corticosteroid therapy may interfere with the growth and development of children.

ADVERSE REACTIONS

The following local adverse reactions are reported infrequently with topical corticosteroids, but may occur more frequently with the use of occlusive dressings. These reactions are listed in an approximate decreasing order of occurrence:

Burning
Itching
Irritation
Dryness
Folliculitis
Hypertrichosis
Acneiform eruptions
Hypopigmentation
Perioral dermatitis
Allergic contact dermatitis
Maceration of the skin
Secondary infection
Skin atrophy
Striae
Miliaria

OVERDOSAGE

Topically applied corticosteroids can be absorbed in sufficient amounts to produce systemic effects (See PRECAUTIONS).

DOSAGE AND ADMINISTRATION

Shake well before using. Topical corticosteroids are generally applied to the affected area as a thin film from two to four times daily depending on the severity of the condition. Occlusive dressings may be used for the management of psoriasis or recalcitrant conditions.

If an infection develops, the use of occlusive dressings should be discontinued and appropriate antimicrobial therapy instituted.

HOW SUPPLIED

2½%—2 fl. oz. bottle NDC 0145-2538-02
1%—4 fl. oz. bottle NDC 0145-2537-04
Store at controlled room temperature, 15°-30°C (59°-86°F).

LASAN® 0.1 Cream ℞

[*lă-zan'*]

(Anthralin USP 0.1%)

LASAN® 0.2 Cream ℞

(Anthralin USP 0.2%)

LASAN® 0.4 Cream ℞

(Anthralin USP 0.4%)

LASAN® HP-1 Cream ℞

(Anthralin USP 1.0%)

LASAN® Ointment ℞

(Anthralin USP 0.4%)

DESCRIPTION

Lasan Cream and Lasan Ointment are topical preparations containing Anthralin as the active ingredient.

Lasan Cream contains: Anthralin USP, 0.1%, 0.2%, 0.4% or 1.0%, Aluminum Distearate, Ascorbyl Palmitate, BHT, Citric Acid, Disodium EDTA, Methylparaben, Mineral Oil, Octyldodecanol, Paraffin, Petrolatum, Polyglyceryl-4 Oleate, Propylparaben, Salicylic Acid, Sodium Bisulfite, Tocopherol, Water.

Lasan Ointment contains: Anthralin USP, 0.4%, Ascorbyl Palmitate, BHT, Cetyl Alcohol, Citric Acid, Magnesium Lauryl Sulfate, Mineral Oil, Petrolatum, Propylene Glycol, Salicylic Acid, Tocopherol, Water.

The structural formula of anthralin is:

OH OH OH

Continued on next page

Stiefel—Cont.

CLINICAL PHARMACOLOGY

The exact mode of action of anthralin in psoriasis is unknown. Anthralin is believed to exert a beneficial effect through its inhibitory effects on various enzyme systems or through its interaction with deoxyribonucleic acid which results in the reduction of cell turnover.

INDICATIONS AND USAGE

Lasan Cream and Lasan Ointment are indicated in the treatment of psoriasis.

CONTRAINDICATIONS

Lasan Cream and Lasan Ointment are contraindicated in persons who have shown hypersensitivity to anthralin or to any of the other ingredients in the products. Do not use in presence of renal disease. The drug should not be used in acute eruptions or on areas of the skin where inflammation is present.

PRECAUTIONS

Lasan Cream and Lasan Ointment are for external use only. Do not permit the drug to come in contact with the eyes since conjunctivitis may result. Exercise due care when applying to the face, scalp, or intertriginous skin areas. If irritation develops or redness is observed on adjacent normal skin, discontinue use and contact physician. Wash hands thoroughly and carefully after using. Anthralin may stain fabrics or skin and may temporarily discolor gray or white hair. Discoloration of hair fades slowly when drug use is reduced. Stained keratin at the scalp margins usually desquamates in four to seven days.

The use of plastic gloves when applying the drug will prevent fingernail staining. The use of a plastic cap over treated scalp at bedtime will prevent staining of the pillow.

Long-term studies utilizing mice have been performed to evaluate the carcinogenic potential of anthralin. Anthralin demonstrated co-carcinogenic activity in some of the studies. Anthralin has also demonstrated tumor promoting activity in these studies.

Pregnancy Category C: Animal reproduction studies have not been conducted with Lasan Cream or Lasan Ointment. It is also not known whether Lasan Cream or Lasan Ointment can cause fetal harm when administered to a pregnant woman or can affect reproduction capacity. Lasan Cream or Lasan Ointment should be given to a pregnant woman only if clearly needed.

It is not known whether this drug is excreted in human milk. Because of the tumor promoting and co-carcinogenic activities shown for anthralin in mouse studies a decision should be made whether to discontinue nursing or to discontinue the drug, taking into account the importance of the drug to the mother.

ADVERSE REACTIONS

A severe irritant reaction may occur if Lasan Cream or Lasan Ointment is applied to the normal skin surrounding the plaque site. The irritation may normally be controlled by temporarily discontinuing use of Lasan Cream or Lasan Ointment, and by carefully restricting application of the medication to the plaque site when treatment is resumed.

DOSAGE AND ADMINISTRATION

Lasan Cream and Lasan Ointment are suitable for skin and scalp treatment. The irritation potential of anthralin is related to drug concentration, duration of drug contact and individual patient tolerance. Therefore, where the response to anthralin therapy has not previously been established treatment should normally be initiated with the lowest (0.1%) concentration. When appropriate, treatment may continue with gradually increasing drug concentration until the desired clinical response is obtained.

Lasan Cream or Lasan Ointment is normally applied once daily. The optimal period of contact will vary according to the drug concentration used and patient response to treatment.

For use on the skin: Apply Lasan Cream or Lasan Ointment carefully to plaque sites, making certain the drug does not contact unaffected areas. A protective film of petrolatum applied to the areas surrounding the plaques may be helpful. At the conclusion of each treatment period any remaining Lasan Cream or Lasan Ointment should be removed by bathing.

For use on the scalp: Massage Lasan Cream or Lasan Ointment carefully into the affected areas of the scalp. Care should be taken to avoid scalp margins and the accumulation of excessive material behind the ears. Before using Lasan Cream or Lasan Ointment, a protective film of petrolatum may be applied to the uninvolved scalp margin and ears. At the conclusion of each treatment period, any remaining Lasan Cream or Lasan Ointment should be removed by shampooing.

HOW SUPPLIED

Lasan Cream is supplied in 65 gram sealed metal tubes.
Lasan 0.1 Cream NDC 0145-0946-04
Lasan 0.2 Cream NDC 0145-0947-04
Lasan 0.4 Cream NDC 0145-0948-04
Lasan HP-1 Cream NDC 0145-0949-04
Lasan Ointment is supplied in 60 gram sealed metal tubes.
Lasan Ointment NDC 0145-0950-04
Lasan Cream and Lasan Ointment should be stored at controlled room temperature 59–86°F (15–30°C).
Patient instruction sheets are available on request.

PANOXYL® 5 ℞

[*pan 'ăhx-il*]
(benzoyl peroxide 5%)

PANOXYL® 10 ℞

(benzoyl peroxide 10%)

DESCRIPTION

PanOxyl 5 and PanOxyl 10 are topical preparations containing benzoyl peroxide as the active ingredient.

PanOxyl 5 contains: 5% benzoyl peroxide in a gel base formulated with 20% alcohol, polyoxyethylene lauryl ether, colloidal magnesium aluminum silicate, hydroxypropylmethylcellulose, citric acid and purified water.

PanOxyl 10 contains: 10% benzoyl peroxide in a gel base formulated with 20% alcohol, polyoxyethylene lauryl ether, colloidal magnesium aluminum silicate, hydroxypropylmethylcellulose, citric acid and purified water.

PanOxyl 5 and PanOxyl 10 are members of the topical benzoyl peroxide class of drug whose pharmacologic activity is generally attributed to antimicrobial and keratolytic activity.

The structural formula of benzoyl peroxide is:

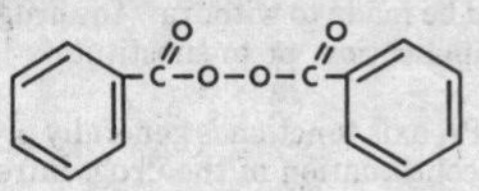

CLINICAL PHARMACOLOGY

The exact mode of action of benzoyl peroxide in acne vulgaris is unknown. Benzoyl Peroxide is believed to exert a beneficial effect because of its antimicrobial activity and its mild keratolytic action.

INDICATIONS AND USAGE

PanOxyl 5 and PanOxyl 10 are indicated in the treatment of acne vulgaris. See Dosage and Administration section for information on frequency and duration of drug use.

CONTRAINDICATIONS

PanOxyl 5 and PanOxyl 10 are contraindicated in persons who have shown hypersensitivity to benzoyl peroxide or to any of the other ingredients in the products.

PRECAUTIONS

PanOxyl 5 and PanOxyl 10 are for external use only. They should not be permitted to contact the eyes or mucosal membranes. These products may bleach hair, colored linens, towels and apparel.

Long-term studies utilizing rats and mice have been performed to evaluate the carcinogenic potential of benzoyl peroxide. Benzoyl Peroxide showed no carcinogenic activity in these studies.

Pregnancy Category C: Animal reproduction studies have not been conducted with PanOxyl 5 or PanOxyl 10. It is also not known whether PanOxyl 5 or PanOxyl 10 can cause fetal harm when administered to a pregnant woman or can affect reproduction capacity. PanOxyl 5 or PanOxyl 10 should be given to a pregnant woman only if clearly needed. It is not known whether this drug is excreted in human milk. Because many drugs are excreted in human milk, caution should be exercised when PanOxyl 5 or PanOxyl 10 is administered to a nursing woman.

ADVERSE REACTIONS

Contact sensitization reactions are associated with the use of topical benzoyl peroxide products and may be expected to occur in 10 to 25 of 1000 patients. The most frequent adverse reactions associated with benzoyl peroxide use are excessive erythema and peeling which may be expected to occur in 5 of 100 patients. Excessive erythema and peeling most frequently appear during the initial phase of drug use and may normally be controlled by reducing frequency of use.

DOSAGE AND ADMINISTRATION

It is recommended that therapy be initiated with PanOxyl 5, applying the medication to the affected areas once a day during the first week, and twice a day thereafter as tolerated. Frequency of use should be adjusted to obtain the desired clinical response. Therapy with PanOxyl 10 may be initiated in patients who demonstrate accommodation to PanOxyl 5. Gentle cleansing of the affected areas with a non-medicated soap prior to application of PanOxyl 5 or PanOxyl 10 may be beneficial.

Clinically visible improvement will normally occur by the third week of therapy. Maximum lesion reduction may be expected after approximately eight to twelve weeks of drug use. Continuing use of the drug is normally required to maintain a satisfactory clinical response.

HOW SUPPLIED

PanOxyl 5 and PanOxyl 10 are supplied in 2.0 ounce and 4.0 ounce plastic tubes.

PanOxyl 5
2.0 oz. tube NDC 0145-2372-06
4.0 oz. tube NDC 0145-2372-08
PanOxyl 10
2.0 oz. tube NDC 0145-2373-06
4.0 oz. tube NDC 0145-2373-08
PanOxyl 5 and PanOxyl 10 should be stored below 80°F.
U.S. Patent 4056611

PANOXYL® AQ 2½ ℞

[*pan 'ăhx-il*]
(benzoyl peroxide 2½%)

PANOXYL® AQ 5 ℞

(benzoyl peroxide 5%)

PANOXYL® AQ 10 ℞

(benzoyl peroxide 10%)

DESCRIPTION

PanOxyl AQ 2½, PanOxyl AQ 5, and PanOxyl AQ 10 are topical preparations containing benzoyl peroxide as the active ingredient.

PanOxyl AQ 2½ contains: 2½% benzoyl peroxide in a gel base formulated with purified water, polyoxyethylene lauryl ether, carbomer, sodium hydroxide and methyl paraben.

PanOxyl AQ 5 contains: 5% benzoyl peroxide in a gel base formulated with purified water, polyoxyethylene lauryl ether, carbomer, sodium hydroxide and methyl paraben.

PanOxyl AQ 10 contains: 10% benzoyl peroxide in a gel base formulated with purified water, polyoxyethylene lauryl ether, carbomer, sodium hydroxide and methyl paraben.

PanOxyl AQ 2½, PanOxyl AQ 5, and PanOxyl AQ 10 are members of the topical benzoyl peroxide class of drug whose pharmacologic activity is generally attributed to antimicrobial and keratolytic activity.

The structural formula of benzoyl peroxide is:

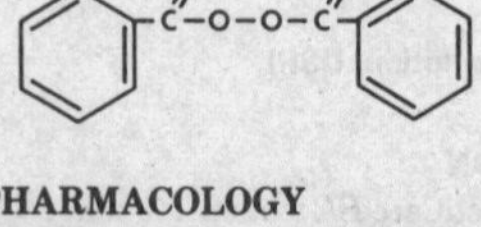

CLINICAL PHARMACOLOGY

The exact mode of action of benzoyl peroxide in acne vulgaris is unknown. Benzoyl Peroxide is believed to exert a beneficial effect because of its antimicrobial activity and its mild keratolytic action.

INDICATIONS AND USAGE

PanOxyl AQ 2½, PanOxyl AQ 5, and PanOxyl AQ 10 are indicated in the treatment of acne vulgaris. See Dosage and Administration section for information on frequency and duration of drug use.

CONTRAINDICATIONS

PanOxyl AQ 2½, PanOxyl AQ 5, and PanOxyl AQ 10 are contraindicated in persons who have shown hypersensitivity to benzoyl peroxide or to any of the other ingredients in the products.

PRECAUTIONS

PanOxyl AQ 2½, PanOxyl AQ 5, and PanOxyl AQ 10 are for external use only. They should not be permitted to contact the eyes or mucosal membranes. These products may bleach hair, colored linens, towels and apparel.

Long-term studies utilizing rats and mice have been performed to evaluate the carcinogenic potential of benzoyl peroxide. Benzoyl Peroxide showed no carcinogenic activity in these studies.

Pregnancy Category C: Animal reproduction studies have not been conducted with PanOxyl AQ 2½, PanOxyl AQ 5, or PanOxyl AQ 10. It is also not known whether PanOxyl AQ 2½, PanOxyl AQ 5, or PanOxyl AQ 10 can cause fetal harm when administered to a pregnant woman or can affect reproduction capacity. PanOxyl AQ 2½, PanOxyl AQ 5, or PanOxyl AQ 10 should be given to a pregnant woman only if clearly needed.

It is not known whether this drug is excreted in human milk. Because many drugs are excreted in human milk, caution should be exercised when PanOxyl AQ 2½, PanOxyl AQ 5, or PanOxyl AQ 10 is administered to a nursing woman.

ADVERSE REACTIONS

Contact sensitization reactions are associated with the use of topical benzoyl peroxide products and may be expected to occur in 10 to 25 of 1000 patients. The most frequent adverse reactions associated with benzoyl peroxide use are excessive erythema and peeling which may be expected to occur in 5 of 100 patients. Excessive erythema and peeling most frequently appear during the initial phase of drug use and may normally be controlled by reducing frequency of use.

DOSAGE AND ADMINISTRATION

It is recommended that therapy be initiated with PanOxyl AQ 2½, applying the medication to the affected areas once a day during the first week, and twice a day thereafter as tolerated. Frequency of use should be adjusted to obtain the desired clinical response. Therapy with PanOxyl AQ 5 or PanOxyl AQ 10 may be initiated in patients who demonstrate accommodation to PanOxyl AQ 2½.
Gentle cleansing of the affected areas with a non-medicated soap prior to application of PanOxyl AQ 2½, PanOxyl AQ 5, or PanOxyl AQ 10 may be beneficial.
Clinically visible improvement will normally occur by the third week of therapy. Maximum lesion reduction may be expected after approximately eight to twelve weeks of drug use. Continuing use of the drug is normally required to maintain a satisfactory clinical response.

HOW SUPPLIED

PanOxyl AQ 2½, PanOxyl AQ 5, and PanOxyl AQ 10 are supplied in 2.0 ounce and 4.0 ounce plastic tubes.

PanOxyl AQ 2½
2.0 oz. tube NDC 0145-2375-06
4.0 oz. tube NDC 0145-2375-08

PanOxyl AQ 5
2.0 oz. tube NDC 0145-2376-06
4.0 oz. tube NDC 0145-2376-08

PanOxyl AQ 10
2.0 oz. tube NDC 0145-2377-06
4.0 oz. tube NDC 0145-2377-08

PanOxyl AQ 2½, PanOxyl AQ 5, and PanOxyl AQ 10 should be stored away from heat.

SCABENE® LOTION ℞

[skā-bēn]
(lindane) 1%

DESCRIPTION

Scabene Lotion (lindane) 1% is an ectoparasiticide and ovicide effective against Sarcoptes scabiei (scabies). In addition to the active ingredient, lindane, it contains water, stearic acid, glyceryl stearate laureth-23, carrageenan, triethanolamine, cetyl alcohol, aminomethyl propanol, fragrance, butylparaben and methylparaben to form a non-greasy lotion.

CLINICAL PHARMACOLOGY

Scabene Lotion exerts its parasiticidal action by being directly absorbed into the parasites and their ova. Feldmann and Maibach[1] reported approximately 10% absorption of a lindane acetone solution applied to the forearm and left in place for 24 hours. Dale[2], et al reported a blood level of 290ng/ml associated with convulsions following the accidental ingestion of a lindane containing product. Ginsburg[3] found a mean peak blood level of 28ng/ml 6 hours after total body application of lindane lotion to scabietic infants and children. The half-life was determined to be 18 hours.

INDICATIONS AND USAGE

Scabene Lotion is indicated for the treatment of patients infested with Sarcoptes scabiei (scabies).

CONTRAINDICATIONS

Scabene Lotion is contraindicated for premature neonates because their skin may be more permeable than full term infants and their liver enzymes may not be sufficiently developed. It is also contraindicated for patients with known seizure disorders and for individuals with a known sensitivity to the product or any of its components.

WARNINGS

LINDANE PENETRATES HUMAN SKIN AND HAS THE POTENTIAL FOR CNS TOXICITY (SEE CLINICAL PHARMACOLOGY SECTION). SCABENE LOTION SHOULD BE USED ACCORDING TO RECOMMENDED DOSAGE (SEE DIRECTIONS FOR USE) ESPECIALLY ON INFANTS, PREGNANT WOMEN AND NURSING MOTHERS. ANIMAL STUDIES INDICATE THAT POTENTIAL TOXIC EFFECTS OF TOPICALLY APPLIED LINDANE ARE GREATER IN THE YOUNG. Seizures have been reported after excessive use or oral ingestion of lindane. No residual effects have been demonstrated, thus, it should not be used to ward off a possible infestation.
If accidental ingestion occurs prompt gastric lavage is indicated. Because oils may enhance absorption, saline rather than oily cathartics should be used. Central nervous excitation can be controlled by the administration of pentobarbital, phenobarbital or diazepam.

PRECAUTIONS

General: Care should be taken to avoid contact with the eyes. If such contact occurs, eyes should be immediately flushed with water. If irritation or sensitization occurs, the patient should be advised to consult a physician.
Information to Patients: Patient should be instructed on the proper use of the medication. Directions for Use should accompany the prescription.

LABORATORY TESTS

No laboratory tests are needed for the proper use of this medication.

DRUG INTERACTIONS

Oils may enhance absorption, therefore, simultaneous use of creams, ointments or oils should be avoided.

CARCINOGENESIS

Although no studies have been conducted with Scabene Lotion, numerous long term feeding studies have been conducted in mice and rats to evaluate the carcinogenic potential of the technical grade of hexachlorocyclohexane (BHC) as well as the alpha, beta, gamma (lindane) and delta isomers. Both oral and topical applications have been evaluated. Nagasaki[4], Goto[5] and Hanada[6] found varying amounts of benign and malignant hepatomas associated with BHC and the alpha, delta and epsilon isomers. None reported a carcinogenic potential for lindane. Tumors were found only in the animals which had received the alpha isomer. Weisse and Herbst[7] also evaluated the carcinogenic potential of lindane in mice but could find no evidence of lindane carcinogenicity. The National Cancer Institute[8] also found no evidence of carcinogenicity.
Thorpe and Walker[9] compared beta BHC with lindane, dieldrin, DDT and hexabarbital in mice. Despite the unusually high incidence of tumors in the control group, they concluded that 600 ppm of lindane was associated with a significant increase in the incidence of hepatoma and thus considered it a tumorigen.
Orr[10] and Kashyap et al[11] evaluated the carcinogenic potential in mice of topically applied BHC. In neither study was there any evidence of a tumorigenic or carcinogenic potential associated with topical application of BHC.
Mutagenicity tests have been used as predictive information about the carcinogenicity of various chemical compounds. Numerous types of mutagenicity tests have been performed with lindane. The results of these tests do not indicate that lindane is mutagenic.

PREGNANCY

Teratogenetic Effects: Pregnancy category B: Reproduction, including multigeneration, studies have been performed in mice, rats, rabbits, pigs, and dogs at doses up to 10 times the human dose and have revealed no evidence of impaired fertility or harm to the fetus due to orally administered lindane. There are, however, no adequate and well controlled studies in pregnant women. Because animal reproduction studies are not always predictive of human response, the recommended dosage should not be exceeded on pregnant women. They should be treated no more than twice during a pregnancy.

NURSING MOTHERS

Lindane is secreted in human milk in low concentrations. Studies conducted in the United States as well as Europe and South America found levels of lindane in human milk ranging from 0 to 113 ppb. as the result of ingestion of foods which had been treated with lindane. There appeared to be no difference in concentrations between country and urban dwellers. Although the levels of lindane found in blood after topical application with lindane lotion make it unlikely that amounts of lindane sufficient to cause serious adverse reactions will be excreted in the milk of nursing mothers who have used Scabene Lotion, if there is any concern, an alternate method of feeding may be used for 2 days.

PEDIATRIC USE

Refer to the Contraindications and Warnings sections.

ADVERSE REACTIONS

Lindane has been reported to cause central nervous stimulation ranging from dizziness to convulsions. Cases of convulsions have been reported in connection with lindane lotion therapy. However, these incidents were almost always associated with accidental oral ingestion or misuse of the product. Eczematous eruptions due to irritation from lindane lotion have also been reported. Incidence of these adverse reactions is relatively infrequent, occurring in less than 1 in 100,000 patients.

DRUG ABUSE AND DEPENDENCE

Scabene Lotion is not subject to abuse, nor is there any dependence on the drug.

OVERDOSAGE

Overdosage or oral ingestion of Scabene Lotion can cause central nervous system excitation and, if taken in sufficient quantities, convulsions may occur.
If accidental ingestion occurs, prompt gastric lavage should be instituted. However, since oils favor absorption, saline cathartics for intestinal evacuation should be given rather than oil laxatives. If central nervous system manifestations occur they can be antagonized by the administration of pentobarbital, phenobarbital or diazepam.

DOSAGE AND ADMINISTRATION

CAUTION: USE ONLY AS DIRECTED. DO NOT EXCEED RECOMMENDED DOSAGE.
No residual effects have been demonstrated, thus, it should not be used to ward off a possible infestation.
NOTE: PLEASE READ CAREFULLY.

DIRECTIONS FOR USE

Scabies (sarcoptes scabiei): The lotion should be applied to dry skin in a thin layer and rubbed in thoroughly. If crusted lesions are present, a tepid bath preceding the medication is helpful. If a bath is used, allow the skin to dry before applying the lotion. Usually two ounces are sufficient for an adult. A total body application should be made from the neck down including the soles of the feet. Scabies rarely affects the head of children or adults but may occur in infants. The lotion should be left on for 8–12 hours and should then be removed by thorough washing. ONE APPLICATION IS USUALLY CURATIVE.
Sexual contacts should be treated simultaneously.
Avoid unnecessary skin contact. Particularly when applying to more than one patient, those assisting in lindane therapy (especially pregnant and/or nursing women) should wear rubber gloves.
Avoid use on open cuts and extensive excoriations.
Many patients exhibit persistent pruritus after treatment; this is rarely a sign of treatment failure and is not an indication for retreatment unless living mites can be demonstrated.

HOW SUPPLIED

Scabene Lotion 2 fl. oz. (59 ml) Bottle NDC 0145-7064-02
Scabene Lotion 16 fl. oz. (472 ml) Bottle NDC 0145-7064-07

REFERENCES

1. Feldmann, R.J. and Maibach, H.I., *Toxicol. Appld. Pharmacol.*, 28:126, 1974.
2. Dale, W.E., Curly, A. and Cueto, C., *Life Sci.* 5:47, 1966.
3. Ginsburg, C.M., et al., *J. Pediatr.*, 91:6, 998–1000, 1977.
4. Nagasaki, T., Tomii, S., Mega, T., Marugami, M. and Ito, N. *Gann* (Cancer), 63(3):393, 1972.
5. Goto, M., Hattori, M., Miyagawa, T., and Enomoto, M., *Chemosphere* 6:279, 1972.
6. Hanada, M., Yatani, C., Miyaji, T, *Gann* 64:511, 1973.
7. Weisse, I. and Herbst, M., *Toxicol.*, 7:233, 1977.
8. Technical Report Series, NCI-CG-TR-14, *HEW PUBLICATIONS*, No. (NIH) 77–814.
9. Thorpe, E. and Walker, A.I.T., *Food Cosmetic Toxicol.*, 11:433, 1973.
10. Orr, J.W., *Nature* 162:189, 1948.
11. Kashyap, S.K. et al., *J. Environ. Sci. Health*, 14:305–318, 1979.

SCABENE® SHAMPOO ℞

[skā-bēn]
(lindane) 1%

DESCRIPTION

Scabene Shampoo (lindane) 1% is an ectoparasiticide and ovicide effective against Pediculosis capitis (head lice), Pediculosis pubis (crab lice) and their ova. In addition to the active ingredient, lindane, it contains polyoxyethylene sorbitan monostearate, triethanolamine lauryl sulfate, acetone, fragrance, citric acid and water to form a cosmetically pleasant shampoo.

CLINICAL PHARMACOLOGY

Scabene Shampoo exerts its parasiticidal action by being directly absorbed into the parasites and their ova. Dale et al.[1] reported a blood level of 290ng/ml associated with convulsions following the accidental ingestion of a lindane containing product. Analysis of blood taken from subjects before and after the use of lindane shampoo showed a mean peak blood level of only 3ng/ml which appeared at six hours and disappeared at eight hours after the shampoo was applied.[2]

INDICATIONS AND USAGE

Scabene Shampoo is indicated for the treatment of patients infested with Pediculus capitis (head lice), Pediculus pubis (crab lice) and their ova.

CONTRAINDICATIONS

Scabene Shampoo is contraindicated for premature neonates because their skin may be more permeable than full term infants and their liver enzymes may not be sufficiently developed. It is also contraindicated for patients with known seizure disorders and for individuals with a known sensitivity to the product or any of its components.

WARNINGS

LINDANE PENETRATES HUMAN SKIN AND HAS THE POTENTIAL FOR CNS TOXICITY (SEE CLINICAL PHARMACOLOGY SECTION). SCABENE SHAMPOO SHOULD BE USED ACCORDING TO RECOMMENDED DOSAGE (SEE DIRECTIONS FOR USE) ESPECIALLY ON INFANTS, PREGNANT WOMEN AND NURSING MOTHERS. ANIMAL STUDIES INDICATE THAT POTENTIAL TOXIC EFFECTS OF TOPICALLY APPLIED LINDANE ARE GREATER IN THE YOUNG. Seizures have been re-

Continued on next page

Stiefel—Cont.

ported after excessive use or oral ingestion of lindane. No residual effects have been demonstrated, thus, it should not be used to ward off a possible infestation.
If accidental ingestion occurs prompt gastric lavage is indicated. Because oils may enhance absorption, saline rather than oily cathartics should be used. Central nervous excitation can be controlled by the administration of pentobarbital, phenobarbital or diazepam.

PRECAUTIONS

General
Care should be taken to avoid contact with the eyes. If such contact occurs, eyes should be immediately flushed with water. If irritation or sensitization occurs, the patient should be advised to consult a physician.
Information to Patients
Patients should be instructed on the proper use of the medication.
Directions for use should accompany the prescription.

LABORATORY TESTS

No laboratory tests are needed for the proper use of this medication.

DRUG INTERACTIONS

Oils may enhance absorption, therefore, if an oil-based hair dressing is used, it is recommended that the hair be shampooed, rinsed and dried before application of Scabene Shampoo.

CARCINOGENESIS

Although no studies have been conducted with Scabene Shampoo, numerous long term feeding studies have been conducted in mice and rats to evaluate the carcinogenic potential of the technical grade of hexachlorocyclohexane (BHC) as well as the alpha, beta, gamma (lindane) and delta isomers. Both oral and topical applications have been evaluated. Nagasaki[3], Goto[4] and Hanada[5] found varying amounts of benign and malignant hepatomas associated with BHC and the alpha, delta and epsilon isomers. None reported a carcinogenic potential for lindane. Tumors were found only in the animals which had received the alpha isomer. Weisse and Herbst[6] also evaluated the carcinogenic potential of lindane in mice but could find no evidence of lindane carcinogenicity. The National Cancer Institute[7] had also found no evidence of carcinogenicity.
Thorpe and Walker[8] compared beta BHC with lindane, dieldrin, DDT and hexabarbital in mice. Despite the unusually high incidence of tumors in the control group, they concluded that 600 ppm of lindane was associated with a significant increase in the incidence of hepatoma and thus, considered it a tumorigen.
Orr[9] and Kashyap, et al[10] evaluated the carcinogenic potential in mice of topically applied BHC. In neither study was there any evidence of a tumorigenic or carcinogenic potential associated with topical application of BHC.
Mutagenicity tests have been used as predictive information about the carcinogenicity of various chemical compounds. Numerous types of mutagenicity tests have been performed with lindane. The results of these tests do not indicate that lindane is mutagenic.

PREGNANCY

Teratogenetic Effects
Pregnancy category B: Reproduction, including multigeneration studies have been performed in mice, rats, rabbits, pigs, and dogs at doses up to 10 times the human dose and have revealed no evidence of impaired fertility or harm to the fetus due to orally administered lindane. There are, however, no adequate and well controlled studies in pregnant women. Because animal reproduction studies are not always predictive of human response, the recommended dosage should not be exceeded on pregnant women. They should be treated no more than twice during a pregnancy.

NURSING MOTHERS

Lindane is secreted in human milk in low concentrations. Studies conducted in the United States as well as Europe and South America found levels of lindane in human milk ranging from 0 to 113 ppb, as the result of ingestion of foods which had been treated with lindane. There appeared to be no difference in concentrations between country and urban dwellers. Although the levels of lindane found in blood after topical application with lindane shampoo make it unlikely that amounts of lindane sufficient to cause serious adverse reactions will be excreted in the milk of nursing mothers who have used lindane shampoo, if there is any concern, an alternate method of feeding may be used for 2 days.

PEDIATRIC USE

Refer to the Contraindications and Warnings sections.

ADVERSE REACTIONS

Lindane has been reported to cause central nervous stimulation ranging from dizziness to convulsions. Cases of convulsions have been reported in connection with lindane shampoo therapy. However, these incidents were almost always associated with accidental oral ingestion or misuse of the product. Eczematous eruptions due to irritation from lindane shampoo have also been reported. Incidence of these adverse reactions is relatively infrequent, occurring in less than 1 in 100,000 patients.

DRUG ABUSE AND DEPENDENCE

Scabene Shampoo is not subject to abuse nor is there any dependence on the drug.

OVERDOSAGE

Overdosage or oral ingestion of Scabene Shampoo can cause central nervous system excitation and, if taken in sufficient quantities, convulsions may occur.
If accidental ingestion occurs, prompt gastric lavage should be instituted. However, since oils favor absorption, saline cathartics for intestinal evacuation should be given rather than oil laxatives. If central nervous system manifestations occur, they can be antagonized by the administration of pentobarbital, phenobarbital or diazepam.

DOSAGE AND ADMINISTRATION

CAUTION: USE ONLY AS DIRECTED. DO NOT EXCEED RECOMMENDED DOSAGE.
No residual effects have been demonstrated, thus, it should not be used to ward off a possible infestation.
NOTE: PLEASE READ CAREFULLY.

DIRECTIONS FOR USE

Pediculosis capitis (head lice)—1) Apply a sufficient quantity of the shampoo to the dry hair. Approximately 1 oz. (30 ml) for short, 1.5 oz. (45 ml) for medium and 2 oz. (60 ml) for long hair. 2) Work thoroughly into the hair and allow to remain in place four minutes. 3) Add small quantities of water until a good lather forms. 4) Rinse thoroughly. Towel briskly. Nits should be removed using a nit comb or tweezers.
Pediculosis pubis (crab lice)—1) Apply a sufficient quantity of the shampoo to the dry hair. 2) Work thoroughly into the hair and allow to remain in place four minutes. 3) Add small quantities of water until a good lather forms. 4) Rinse thoroughly. Towel briskly. Nits should be removed using a nit comb or tweezers.
Retreatment is usually not necessary. Demonstrable living organisms after 7 days indicate that retreatment is necessary.

NOTE

1. If person to be treated uses an oil-based hair dressing, it is recommended that their hair be shampooed and dried before applying Scabene Shampoo.
2. Avoid unnecessary skin contact. Particularly when applying to more than one patient, those assisting in lindane therapy (especially pregnant and/or nursing women) should wear rubber gloves.
3. Avoid use on open cuts and extensive excoriations. Sexual contacts should be treated simultaneously.

HOW SUPPLIED

SCABENE SHAMPOO 2 fl. oz. (59 ml.) bottle NDC 0145-7066-02
SCABENE SHAMPOO 16 fl. oz. (472 ml.) bottle NDC 0145-7066-07

REFERENCES

1. Dale, W.E., Curly, A. and Cueto, C. *Life Sci.* 5:47, 1966.
2. Data on File at Reed & Carnrick.
3. Nagasaki, T., Tomii, S., Mega, T., Marugami, M. and Ito, N. *Gann* (Cancer) 63(3):373, 1972.
4. Goto, M., Hattori, M., Miyagawa, T. and Enomoto, M., *Chemosphere* 6:279, 1972.
5. Hanada, M., Yatani, C., Miyaji, T., *Gann* 64:511, 1973.
6. Weisse, I. and Herbst, M., *Toxicol.* 7:233, 1977.
7. Technical Report Series, NCI-CG-TR-14, *HEW PUBLICATIONS*, No. (NIH) 77-814.
8. Thorpe, E., and Walker, A.I.T., *Food Cosmetic Toxicol.* 11:433, 1973.
9. Orr, J.W., *Nature* 162:189, 1948.
10. Kashyap, S.K. et al., *J. Environ. Sci. Health* 14:305-318, 1979.

Important Notice
Before prescribing or administering any product described in PHYSICIANS' DESK REFERENCE always consult the PDR Supplement for possible new or revised information

Stuart Pharmaceuticals
Div. of ICI Americas Inc.
WILMINGTON, DE 19897

ALternaGEL®
[all 'terna "jel]
Liquid
High-Potency Aluminum Hydroxide Antacid

DESCRIPTION

ALternaGEL is available as a white, pleasant-tasting, high-potency aluminum hydroxide liquid antacid. Each 5 ml. teaspoonful contains: Active: 600 mg. aluminum hydroxide (equivalent to dried gel, USP) providing 16 milliequivalents (mEq) of acid-neutralizing capacity (ANC), and less than 2.5 mg. (0.109 mEq) of sodium per teaspoonful (5 ml.). Inactive: butylparaben, flavors, propylparaben, purified water, simethicone, and other ingredients.

INDICATIONS

ALternaGEL is indicated for the symptomatic relief of hyperacidity associated with peptic ulcer, gastritis, peptic esophagitis, gastric hyperacidity, hiatal hernia, and heartburn.
ALternaGEL will be of special value to those patients for whom magnesium-containing antacids are undesirable, such as patients with renal insufficiency, patients requiring control of attendant G.I. complications resulting from steroid or other drug therapy, and patients experiencing the laxation which may result from magnesium or combination antacid regimens.

DIRECTIONS

One or two teaspoonfuls, as needed, between meals and at bedtime, or as directed by a physician. May be followed by a sip of water if desired.

WARNINGS

As with all medications, ALternaGEL should be kept out of the reach of children. ALternaGEL may cause constipation. Except under the advice and supervision of a physician, more than 18 teaspoonfuls should not be taken in a 24-hour period, or the maximum recommended dosage taken for more than two weeks.

DRUG INTERACTION PRECAUTION

ALternaGEL should not be taken concurrently with an antibiotic containing any form of tetracycline.

HOW SUPPLIED

ALternaGEL is available in bottles of 12 fluid ounces and 5 fluid ounces, and 1 fluid ounce hospital unit doses. NDC 0038-0860.

Shown in Product Identification Section, page 431

BUCLADIN®-S SOFTAB® Tablets ℞
[bu 'cla-din]
(buclizine hydrochloride)

DESCRIPTION

Buclizine hydrochloride is 1-(p-tert-Butylbenzyl) -4- (p-chloro- α -phenylbenzyl) piperazine dihydrochloride. Each tablet contains 50 mg. buclizine hydrochloride.
Inactive Ingredients: citric acid, flavor, magnesium stearate, mannitol, microcrystalline cellulose, povidone, Yellow 5 (tartrazine).

ACTIONS

BUCLADIN-S (buclizine hydrochloride) acts centrally to suppress nausea and vomiting.

INDICATIONS

BUCLADIN-S is effective in the management of nausea, vomiting, and dizziness associated with motion sickness.

CONTRAINDICATIONS

Buclizine hydrochloride, when administered to the pregnant rat, induced fetal abnormalities at doses above the human therapeutic range. Clinical data are not adequate to establish nonteratogenicity in early pregnancy. Until such data are available, buclizine hydrochloride is contraindicated for use in early pregnancy. Buclizine hydrochloride is contraindicated in individuals who have shown a previous hypersensitivity to it.

WARNINGS

Since drowsiness may occur with use of this drug, patients should be warned of this possibility and cautioned against engaging in activities requiring mental alertness, such as driving a car, or operating heavy machinery or appliances. Safe and effective dosage in children has not been established.

PRECAUTION

This product contains Yellow 5 (tartrazine) which may cause allergic-type reactions (including bronchial asthma) in certain susceptible individuals. Although the overall incidence of Yellow 5 (tartrazine) sensitivity in the general population is low, it is frequently seen in patients who also have aspirin hypersensitivity.

ADVERSE REACTIONS

Occasionally drowsiness, dryness of mouth, headache, and jitteriness are encountered.

DOSAGE AND ADMINISTRATION

BUCLADIN-S (buclizine hydrochloride) SOFTAB Tablets can be taken without swallowing water. Place the SOFTAB tablet in the mouth and allow it to dissolve, or the tablet may be chewed or swallowed whole.

Adults: One tablet usually serves to alleviate nausea. In severe cases, three tablets a day may be taken. The usual maintenance dosage is one tablet twice daily. In the prevention of motion sickness, one tablet taken at least ½ hour before beginning travel usually suffices. For extended travel, a second tablet may be taken after 4 to 6 hours.

HOW SUPPLIED

Bottles of 100 scored, yellow, SOFTAB Tablets, identified front "STUART", reverse "864". NDC 0038-0864.

Shown in Product Identification Section, page 431

C/11/85

CEFOTAN® ℞

[*cefo 'tan*]

(cefotetan disodium)

For Intravenous or Intramuscular Use

PRODUCT OVERVIEW

KEY FACTS

CEFOTAN® (cefotetan disodium) is a semisynthetic, broad-spectrum, beta-lactamase stable, cephalosporin (cephamycin) antibiotic for parenteral administration. The bactericidal action of cefotetan results from inhibition of cell wall synthesis. Therefore, CEFOTAN is exquisitely active against a wide range of gram-negative aerobes. Like other cephamycins, CEFOTAN exhibits good activity against *Bacteroides fragilis* and many other anaerobic organisms. The plasma elimination half-life of CEFOTAN is 3 to 4.6 hours after either intravenous or intramuscular administraion allowing twice-daily dosing for the treatment of indicated infections and single dose prophylaxis in appropriate surgical procedures.

MAJOR USES

CEFOTAN is indicated for the treatment of the following infections caused by susceptible organisms:

Gynecologic Infections
Intra-abdominal Infections
Skin and Skin Structure Infections

The preoperative administration of CEFOTAN may reduce the incidence of certain postoperative infections in patients undergoing surgical procedures that are classified as clean contaminated or potentially contaminated (eg, cesarean section, abdominal or vaginal hysterectomy, transurethral surgery, biliary tract surgery, and gastrointestinal surgery).

SAFETY INFORMATION

CEFOTAN is contraindicated in patients with known allergy to the cephalosporin group of antibiotics. In patients with renal impairment, dosage adjustment is necessary.

PRESCRIBING INFORMATION

CEFOTAN® ℞

[*cefo 'tan*]

(cefotetan disodium)

For Intravenous or Intramuscular Use

DESCRIPTION

CEFOTAN (cefotetan disodium) is a sterile, semisynthetic, broad-spectrum, beta-lactamase resistant, cephalosporin (cephamycin) antibiotic for parenteral administration. It is the disodium salt of [6*R*-(6α, 7α)]-7-[[[4-(2-amino-1-carboxy-2-oxoethylidene)-1,3-dithietan-2-yl]carbonyl]amino]-7-methoxy-3-[[(1-methyl-1*H*-tetrazol-5-yl)thio]methyl]-*8-oxo-5-thia-1-azabicyclo* [4.2.0]oct-2-ene-2-carboxylic acid. Its molecular formula is $C_{17}H_{15}N_7Na_2O_8S_4$ with a molecular weight of 619.56.

STRUCTURAL FORMULA

H_2NOC, NaOOC, OCH_3, CHCONH, S, N, O, CH_2S, COONa, CH_3

CEFOTAN contains approximately 80 mg (3.5 mEq) of sodium per gram of cefotetan activity. It is a white to pale yellow powder which is very soluble in water. The solution varies from colorless to yellow depending on the concentration. The pH of freshly reconstituted solutions is usually between 4.5 to 6.5.

CLINICAL PHARMACOLOGY

High plasma levels of cefotetan are attained after intravenous and intramuscular administration of single doses to normal volunteers.

PLASMA CONCENTRATIONS AFTER 1.0 GRAM IV* or IM DOSE
Mean Plasma Concentration (μg/mL)

Route	Time After Injection 15 min	30 min	1 h	2 h	4 h	8 h	12 h
IV	92	158	103	72	42	18	9
IM	34	56	71	68	47	20	9

*30-minute infusion

PLASMA CONCENTRATIONS AFTER 2.0 GRAM IV* or IM DOSE
Mean Plasma Concentration (μg/mL)

Route	Time After Injection 5 min	10 min	1 h	3 h	5 h	9 h	12 h
IV	237	223	135	74	48	22	12**
IM	–	20	75	91	69	33	19

*Injected over 3 minutes
**Concentrations estimated from regression line

The plasma elimination half-life of cefotetan is 3 to 4.6 hours after either intravenous or intramuscular administration.

Repeated administration of CEFOTAN does not result in accumulation of the drug in normal subjects.

Cefotetan is 88% plasma protein bound.

No active metabolites of cefotetan have been detected; however, small amounts (less than 7%) of cefotetan in plasma and urine may be converted to its tautomer, which has antimicrobial activity similar to the parent drug.

In normal patients, from 51% to 81% of an administered dose of CEFOTAN is excreted unchanged by the kidneys over a 24 hour period, which results in high and prolonged urinary concentrations. Following intravenous doses of 1 gram and 2 grams, urinary concentrations are highest during the first hour and reach concentrations of approximately 1700 and 3500 μg/mL respectively.

In patients with reduced renal function, the plasma half-life of cefotetan is prolonged.

Therapeutic levels of cefotetan are achieved in many body tissues and fluids including:

skin	ureter
muscle	bladder
fat	maxillary sinus mucosa
myometrium	tonsil
endometrium	bile
cervix	peritoneal fluid
ovary	umbilical cord serum
kidney	amniotic fluid

MICROBIOLOGY

The bactericidal action of cefotetan results from inhibition of cell wall synthesis. Cefotetan has in vitro activity against a wide range of gram-positive and gram-negative organisms. The methoxy group in the 7-alpha position provides cefotetan with a high degree of stability in the presence of betalactamases, both penicillinases and cephalosporinases of gram-negative bacteria. Cefotetan is usually active against the following organisms in vitro and in clinical infections:

GRAM-NEGATIVE:

Escherichia coli
Klebsiella species (including K pneumoniae)
Enterobacter aerogenes
Enterobacter agglomerans
Enterobacter cloacae
Proteus mirabilis
Proteus vulgaris
Morganella morganii (formerly *Proteus morganii*)
Providencia rettgeri (formerly *Proteus rettgeri*)
Providencia stuartii
Haemophilus influenzae (including ampicillin-resistant strains)
Neisseria gonorrhoeae

NOTE: Approximately one-half of the strains of *Enterobacter* species, and *Citrobacter* species are resistant to cefotetan. Most strains of *Pseudomonas aeruginosa* and *Acinetobacter* species are resistant to cefotetan.

GRAM-POSITIVE:

Staphylococcus aureus (including penicillinase- and nonpenicillinase-producing strains)
Staphylococcus epidermidis
Streptococcus pyogenes (group A beta-hemolytic streptococci)
Streptococcus agalactiae (group B beta-hemolytic streptococci)
Streptococcus pneumoniae (formerly *Diplococcus pneumoniae*)

NOTE: Methicillin-resistant staphylococci are resistant to cephalosporins. Some strains of *Staphylococcus epidermidis* and most strains of enterococci, e.g., *S faecalis,* are resistant to cefotetan.

ANAEROBES:

Bacteroides fragilis subsp *fragilis*
Bacteroides bivius
Bacteroides disiens
Bacteroides melaninogenicus
Bacteroides vulgatus
Fusobacterium species
Gram-positive bacilli (including *Clostridium* species)
Peptococcus and *Peptostreptococcus* species

NOTE: Most strains of *B distasonis, B ovatus,* and *B thetaiotaomicron* are resistant to cefotetan.

Cefotetan also demonstrates in vitro activity against the following microorganisms, although its clinical significance is unknown: *Citrobacter* species (including *C diversus* and *C freundii*), *Serratia* species (including *S marcescens*), *Salmonella* species, *Shigella* species, *Yersinia enterocolitica, Clostridium difficile, B asaccharolyticus, B oralis, B splanchnicus, Veillonella* species, and *Propionibacterium* species.

NOTE: Many strains of *C difficile* are resistant.

SUSCEPTIBILITY TESTS

Diffusion Technique: Quantitative methods that require measurement of zone diameters give the most precise estimate of antibiotic susceptibility. One such procedure[1] has been recommended for use with disks to test susceptibility to cefotetan. Organisms should be tested with the cefotetan 30 μg disk since cefotetan has been shown to be active in vitro against organisms which were found to be resistant to other beta-lactam antibiotics.

Reports from the laboratory with results of standardized single-disk susceptibility tests with a 30 μg cefotetan disk should be interpreted according to the following criteria:

Susceptible organisms produce zone sizes of 16 mm or greater, indicating that the tested organism is likely to respond to therapy.

Moderately susceptible organisms produce zones of 13 to 15 mm indicating the test organism would be susceptible if high dosage is used or if the infection is confined to tissues and fluids (e.g., urine) in which high antibiotic levels are attained.

Resistant organisms produce zones of 12 mm or less, indicating that other therapy should be selected.

Standardized procedures require the use of laboratory control organisms. The 30 μg cefotetan disk should give zone diameters between 17 and 22 mm for *S aureus* ATCC 25923. For *E coli* ATCC 25922, the zone diameters should be between 29 and 34 mm.

Dilution Techniques: Broth or agar dilution methods, e.g., ICS agar dilution[2] or an equivalent method such as that recommended by the National Committee for Clinical Laboratory Standards (NCCLS)[3], may be used to determine the minimal inhibitory concentration (MIC) of cefotetan.

Organisms inhibited by cefotetan at 16 μg/mL or less are considered susceptible. Organisms with MIC values 64 μg/mL or more are considered resistant to cefotetan.

As with standard diffusion methods, dilution procedures require the use of laboratory control organisms. Standard cefotetan powder should give MIC values in the range of 4 μg/mL and 16 μg/mL for *S aureus* ATCC 25923. For *E coli* ATCC 25922, the MIC range should be between 0.06 μg/mL and 0.25 μg/mL.

INDICATIONS AND USAGE

TREATMENT

CEFOTAN is indicated for the therapeutic treatment of the following infections when caused by susceptible strains of the designated organisms:

Urinary Tract Infections caused by *E coli, Klebsiella* species (including *K pneumoniae), Proteus mirabilis* and *Proteus spp* (which may include the organisms now called *Proteus vulgaris, Providencia rettgeri,* and *Morganella morganii*).

Lower Respiratory Tract Infections caused by *Streptococcus pneumoniae* (formerly *D pneumoniae*), Staphylococcus aureus (penicillinase- and nonpenicillinase-producing strains), *Haemophilus influenzae* (including ampicillin-resistant strains), *Klebsiella* species (including *K pneumoniae),* and *E coli.*

Skin and Skin Structure Infections caused by *Staphylococcus aureus* (penicillinase- and nonpenicillinase-producing strains), *Staphylococcus epidermidis, Streptococcus pyogenes* and *Streptococcus* species (excluding enterococci), and *E. coli.*

Gynecologic Infections caused by *Staphylococcus aureus** (including penicillinase- and nonpenicillinase-producing strains), *Staphylococcus epidermidis, Streptococcus* species (excluding enterococci), *E. coli, Proteus mirabilis, Neisseria gonorrhoeae, Bacteroides* species (excluding *B distasonis, B ovatus, B thetaiotaomicron*), *Fusobacterium* species*, and gram-positive anaerobic cocci (including *Peptococcus* and *Peptostreptococcus* species*).

Continued on next page

Stuart—Cont.

Intra-abdominal Infections caused by *E coli, Klebsiella* species (including *K pneumoniae**), *Streptococcus* species (excluding enterococci), and *Bacteroides* species (excluding *B distasonis, B ovatus, B thetaiotaomicron*).

Bone and Joint Infections caused by *Staphylococcus aureus.**

* Efficacy for this organism in this organ system was studied in fewer than ten infections.

Specimens for bacteriological examination should be obtained in order to isolate and identify causative organisms and to determine their susceptibilities to cefotetan. Therapy may be instituted before results of susceptibility studies are known; however, once these results become available, the antibiotic treatment should be adjusted accordingly.

In cases of confirmed or suspected gram-positive or gram-negative sepsis or in patients with other serious infections in which the causative organism has not been identified, it is possible to use CEFOTAN concomitantly with an aminoglycoside. Cefotetan combinations with aminoglycosides have been shown to be synergistic in vitro against many Enterobacteriaceae and also some other gram-negative bacteria. The dosage recommended in the labeling of both antibiotics may be given and depends on the severity of the infection and the patient's condition.

NOTE: If CEFOTAN and an aminoglycoside are used concomitantly, renal function should be carefully monitored, especially if higher dosages of the aminoglycoside are to be administered or if therapy is prolonged, because of the potential nephrotoxicity and ototoxicity of aminoglycosidic antibiotics. Although, to date, nephrotoxicity has not been noted when CEFOTAN was given alone, it is possible that nephrotoxicity may be potentiated if CEFOTAN is used concomitantly with an aminoglycoside.

PROPHYLAXIS

The preoperative administration of CEFOTAN may reduce the incidence of certain post-operative infections in patients undergoing surgical procedures that are classified as clean contaminated or potentially contaminated (e.g., cesarean section, abdominal or vaginal hysterectomy, transurethral surgery, biliary tract surgery, and gastrointestinal surgery).

The prophylactic dose of CEFOTAN should be administered 30 to 60 minutes prior to surgery. In patients undergoing cesarean section, CEFOTAN should be administered intravenously after the clamping of the umbilical cord.

If there are signs and symptoms of infection, specimens for culture should be obtained for identification of the causative organism so that appropriate therapeutic measures may be initiated.

CONTRAINDICATIONS

CEFOTAN is contraindicated in patients with known allergy to the cephalosporin group of antibiotics.

WARNINGS

Before therapy with CEFOTAN is instituted, careful inquiry should be made to determine whether the patient has had previous hypersensitivity reactions to cefotetan disodium, cephalosporins, penicillins, or other drugs. This product should be given cautiously to penicillin-sensitive patients. Antibiotics should be administered with caution to any patient who has demonstrated some form of allergy, particularly to drugs. If an allergic reaction to CEFOTAN occurs, discontinue the drug. Serious acute hypersensitivity reactions may require epinephrine and other emergency measures.

Pseudomembranous colitis has been reported with the use of cephalosporins (and other broad-spectrum antibiotics); therefore, it is important to consider its diagnosis in patients who develop diarrhea in association with antibiotic use.

Treatment with broad-spectrum antibiotics may alter normal flora of the colon and may permit overgrowth of clostridia. Studies indicate a toxin produced by *Clostridium difficile* is one primary cause of antibiotic-associated colitis. Cholestyramine and colestipol resins have been shown to bind the toxin in vitro.

Mild cases of colitis may respond to drug discontinuance alone. Moderate to severe cases should be managed with fluid, electrolyte, and protein supplementation as indicated. When the colitis is not relieved by drug discontinuance or when it is severe, oral vancomycin is the treatment of choice for antibiotic-associated pseudomembranous colitis produced by *C. difficile*. Other causes should also be considered.

DOSAGE GUIDELINES FOR PATIENTS WITH IMPAIRED RENAL FUNCTION

Creatinine Clearance mL/min	Dose	Frequency
>30	Usual Recommended Dose*	Every 12 hours
10–30	Usual Recommended Dose*	Every 24 hours
<10	Usual Recommended Dose*	Every 48 hours

*Dose determined by the type and severity of infection, and susceptibility of the causative organism.

PRECAUTIONS

General: As with other broad-spectrum antibiotics, prolonged use of CEFOTAN may result in overgrowth of nonsusceptible organisms. Careful observation of the patient is essential. If superinfection does occur during therapy, appropriate measures should be taken.

In common with many other broad-spectrum antibiotics, CEFOTAN may be associated with a fall in prothrombin activity. Those at risk include patients with renal or hepatic impairment, or poor nutritional state. Prothrombin times should be monitored in patients at risk and exogenous Vitamin K administered as indicated.

CEFOTAN should be used with caution in individuals with a history of gastrointestinal disease, particularly colitis.

Information for Patients: As with some other cephalosporins, a disulfiram-like reaction characterized by flushing, sweating, headache, and tachycardia may occur when alcohol (beer, wine, etc) is ingested within 72 hours after CEFOTAN administration. Patients should be cautioned about the ingestion of alcoholic beverages following the administration of CEFOTAN.

Drug Interactions: Although to date nephrotoxicity has not been noted when CEFOTAN was given alone, it is possible that nephrotoxicity may be potentiated if CEFOTAN is used concomitantly with an aminoglycoside.

Drug/Laboratory Test Interactions: A false positive reaction for glucose in urine may occur with Benedict's or Fehling's solution.

As with other cephalosporins, high concentrations of cefotetan may intefere with measurement of serum and urine creatinine levels of Jaffe reaction and produce false increases in the levels of creatinine reported.

Carcinogenesis, Mutagenesis, Impairment of Fertility: Although long-term studies in animals have not been performed to evaluate carcinogenic potential, no mutagenic potential of cefotetan was found in standard laboratory tests. Cefotetan has adverse effects on the testes of prepubertal rats. Subcutaneous administration of 500 mg/kg/day (approx. 8–16 times the usual adult human dose) on days 6–35 of life (thought to be developmentally analogous to late childhood and pre-puberty in humans) resulted in reduced testicular weight and seminiferous tubule degeneration in 10 of 10 animals. Affected cells included spermatogonia and spermatocytes; Sertoli and Leydig cells were unaffected. Incidence and severity of lesions were dose-dependent; at 120 mg/kg/day (approx. 2–4 times the usual human dose), only 1 of 10 treated animals was affected, and the degree of degeneration was mild.

Similar lesions have been observed in experiments of comparable design with other methylthiotetrazole-containing antibiotics and impaired fertility has been reported, particularly at high dose levels. No testicular effects were observed in 7-week-old rats treated with up to 1000 mg/kg/day SC for 5 weeks, or in infant dogs (3 weeks old) that received up to 300 mg/kg/day IV for 5 weeks. The relevance of these findings to humans is unknown.

Usage in Pregnancy: Pregnancy Category B: Reproduction studies have been performed in rats and monkeys at doses up to 20 times the human dose and have revealed no evidence of impaired fertility or harm to the fetus due to cefotetan. There are, however, no adequate and well-controlled studies in pregnant women. Because animal reproductive studies are not always predictive of human response, this drug should be used during pregnancy only if clearly needed.

Usage in Nursing Mothers: Cefotetan is excreted in human milk in very low concentrations. Caution should be exercised when cefotetan is administered to a nursing woman.

Pediatric Use: Safety and effectiveness in children have not been established.

ADVERSE REACTIONS

In clinical studies the following adverse effects were considered related to CEFOTAN therapy.

Gastrointestinal symptoms occurred in 1.5 percent of patients, the most frequent were diarrhea (1 in 80) and nausea (1 in 700).

Hematologic laboratory abnormalities occurred in 1.4 percent of patients and included eosinophilia (1 in 200), positive direct Coomb's test (1 in 250), and thrombocytosis (1 in 300).

Hepatic enzyme elevations occurred in 1.2 percent of patients and included a rise in SGPT (1 in 150), SGOT (1 in 300), alkaline phosphatase (1 in 700), and LDH (1 in 700).

Hypersensitivity reactions were reported in 1.2 percent of patients and included rash (1 in 150) and itching (1 in 700).

Local effects were reported in less than one percent of patients and included phlebitis at the site of injection (1 in 300), and discomfort (1 in 500).

DOSAGE AND ADMINISTRATION

TREATMENT

The usual adult dosage is 1 or 2 grams of CEFOTAN administered intravenously or intramuscularly every 12 hours for 5 to 10 days. Proper dosage and route of administration should be determined by the condition of the patient, severity of the infection, and susceptibility of the causative organism.

[See table below].

PROPHYLAXIS

To prevent postoperative infection in clean contaminated or potentially contaminated surgery in adults, the recommended dosage is 1 or 2 g of CEFOTAN administered once, intravenously 30 to 60 minutes prior to surgery. In patients undergoing cesarean section, the dose should be administered as soon as the umbilical cord is clamped.

IMPAIRED RENAL FUNCTION

When renal function is impaired, a reduced dosage schedule must be employed. the following dosage guidelines may be used.

[See table above].

Alternatively, the dosing interval may remain constant at 12 hour intervals, but the dose reduced to one-half the usual recommended dose for patients with a creatinine clearance of 10–30 mL/min, and one-quarter the usual recommended dose for patients with a creatinine clearance of less than 10 mL/min.

When only serum creatinine levels are available, creatinine clearance may be calculated from the following formula. The serum creatinine level should represent a steady state of renal function.

Males: $\dfrac{\text{Weight (kg)} \times (140 - \text{age})}{72 \times \text{serum creatinine (mg/100 mL)}}$

Females: $0.9 \times$ value for males

Cefotetan is dialyzable and it is recommended that for patients undergoing intermittent hemodialysis, one-quarter of the usual recommended dose be given every 24 hours on days between dialysis and one-half the usual recommended dose on the day of dialysis.

PREPARATION OF SOLUTION

For Intravenous Use: Reconstitute with Sterile Water for Injection. Shake to dissolve and let stand until clear.

Vial Size	Amount of Diluent To Be Added (mL)	Approximate Withdrawable Vol (mL)	Approximate Average Concentration (mg/mL)
1 gram	10	10.4	97.2
2 gram	10–20	11.0–21.0	179.8–98.4

Infusion bottles (100 mL) may be reconstituted with 50 to 100 mL of 5% Dextrose Solution or 0.9% Sodium Chloride Solution.

For Intramuscular Use: Reconstitute with Sterile Water for Injection; Bacteriostatic Water for Injection; Normal Saline, USP; 0.5% Lidocaine HCl; or 1.0% Lidocaine HCl. Shake to dissolve and let stand until clear.

Vial Size	Amount of Diluent To Be Added (mL)	Approximate Withdrawable Vol (mL)	Approximate Average Concentration (mg/mL)
1 gram	2	2.4	375.0
2 gram	3	3.9	471.5

GENERAL GUIDELINES FOR DOSAGE OF CEFOTAN

Type of Infection	Daily Dose	Frequency and Route
Urinary Tract	1–4 grams	500 mg every 12 hours IV or IM 1 or 2 g every 24 hours IV or IM 1 or 2 g every 12 hours IV or IM
Other Sites	2–4 grams	1 or 2 g every 12 hours IV or IM
Severe	4 grams	2 g every 12 hours IV
Life-Threatening	6* grams	3 g every 12 hours IV

*Maximum daily dosage should not exceed 6 grams.

INTRAVENOUS ADMINISTRATION

The intravenous route is preferable for patients with bacteremia, bacterial septicemia, or other severe or life-threatening infections, or for patients who may be poor risks because of lowered resistance resulting from such debilitating conditions as malnutrition, trauma, surgery, diabetes, heart failure, or malignancy, particularly if shock is present or impending.

For intermittent intravenous administration, a solution containing 1 gram or 2 grams of CEFOTAN in Sterile Water for Injection can be injected over a period of three to five minutes. Using an infusion system, the solution may also be given over a longer period of time through the tubing system by which the patient may be receiving other intravenous solutions. Butterfly® or scalp vein-type needles are preferred for this type of infusion. However, during infusion of the solution containing CEFOTAN, it is advisable to discontinue temporarily the administration of other solutions at the same site.

NOTE: Solutions of CEFOTAN must not be admixed with solutions containing aminoglycosides. If CEFOTAN and aminoglycosides are to be administered to the same patient, they must be administered separately and not as a mixed injection.

INTRAMUSCULAR ADMINISTRATION

As with all intramuscular preparations, CEFOTAN should be injected well within the body of a relatively large muscle such as the upper outer quadrant of the buttock (i.e., gluteus maximus); aspiration is necessary to avoid inadvertent injection into a blood vessel.

Compatability and Stability: CEFOTAN reconstituted as described above (Preparation of Solution) maintains satisfactory potency for 24 hours at room temperature (25°C), for 96 hours under refrigeration (5°C), and for at least 1 week in the frozen state. After reconstitution and subsequent storage in disposable glass or plastic syringes, CEFOTAN is stable for 24 hours at room temperature and 96 hours under refrigeration.

Frozen samples should be thawed at room temperature before use. After the periods mentioned above, any unused solutions or frozen materials should be discarded. Do not refreeze.

NOTE: Parenteral drug products should be inspected visually for particulate matter and discoloration prior to administration whenever solution and container permit.

HOW SUPPLIED

CEFOTAN is a dry, white to pale yellow powder supplied in vials containing cefotetan disodium equivalent to 1 g and 2 g cefotetan activity for intravenous and intramuscular administration. The 1 g dose is available in 10 mL and 100 mL vials, and the 2 g dose is available in 20 mL and 100 mL vials. The vials should not be stored at temperatures above 22°C and should be protected from light.

1 g in 10 mL vial (NDC 0038-0376-10)
2 g in 20 mL vial (NDC 0038-0377-20)
1 g in 100 mL vial (NDC 0038-0376-11)
2 g in 100 mL vial (NDC 0038-0377-21)

1. Am J Clin Pathol 1966:45:493.
   Federal Register 1974:39:19182–19184.
2. Ericson HM, Sherris JC: Acta Pathol Microbiol Immunol Scand (B) 1971; (suppl No. 217).
3. Thornsberry C, et al: Methods for Dilution: Antimicrobial Susceptibility Tests for Bacteria that Grow Aerobically. 1983, Vol 3, No. 2.

E/3/86

Shown in Product Identification Section, page 432

DIALOSE® Capsules

[di 'a-lose]

Stool Softener

DESCRIPTION

DIALOSE is a sodium-free, non-habit forming, stool softener containing docusate potassium in capsules of 100 mg.

The docusate in DIALOSE is a highly efficient surfactant which facilitates absorption of water by the stool to form a soft, easily evacuated mass. Unlike laxatives, DIALOSE does not interfere with normal peristalsis, neither does it cause griping nor sensations of urgency.

INGREDIENTS

Each capsule contains: Active: docusate potassium. Inactive: Blue 1, gelatin, lactose magnesium stearate, Red 28, Red 40, silicon dioxide, titanium dioxide.

INDICATIONS

DIALOSE is an effective aid to soften or prevent formation of hard stools in a wide range of conditions that may lead to constipation. DIALOSE helps to eliminate straining associated with obstetric, geriatric, cardiac, surgical, anorectal, or proctologic conditions. In cases of mild constipation, the fecal softening action of DIALOSE can prevent constipation from progressing and relieve painful defecation.

DIRECTIONS

Adults: Adjust dosage as needed, one capsule one to three times daily. *Children:* 6 years and over—One capsule at bedtime, or as directed by physician. *Children:* under 6 years —As directed by physician. It is helpful to increase the daily intake of fluids by taking a glass of water with each dose.

WARNINGS

As with any drug, if you are pregnant or nursing a baby, seek the advice of a health professional before using this product. Keep out of the reach of children.

HOW SUPPLIED

Bottles of 36, 100, and 500 pink capsules, identified "STUART 470". Also available in 100 capsule unit dose boxes (10 strips of 10 capsules each). NDC-0038-0470.

Shown in Product Identification Section, page 432

DIALOSE® PLUS Capsules

[di 'a-lose Plus]

Stool Softener
***plus* Peristaltic Activator**

DESCRIPTION

DIALOSE PLUS provides a sodium-free formulation of docusate potassium in capsules of 100 mg. and casanthranol, 30 mg.

INGREDIENTS

Each capsule contains: Active: docusate potassium, casanthranol. Inactive: gelatin, lactose, magnesium stearate, Red 33, silicon dioxide, titanium dioxide, Yellow 10.

INDICATIONS

DIALOSE PLUS is indicated for the treatment of constipation characterized by lack of moisture in the intestinal contents, resulting in hardness of stool and decreased intestinal motility.

DIALOSE PLUS combines the advantages of the stool softener, docusate potassium, with the peristaltic activating effect of casanthranol.

DIRECTIONS

Adults —Initially, one capsule two times a day. *Children* —As directed by physician. When adequate bowel function is restored, the dose may be adjusted to meet individual needs. It is helpful to increase the daily intake of fluids by taking a glass of water with each dose.

WARNINGS

As with any drug, if you are pregnant or nursing a baby, seek the advice of a health professional before using this product. And, as with any laxative, DIALOSE PLUS should not be used when abdominal pain, nausea, or vomiting are present. Frequent or prolonged use may result in dependence on laxatives. Keep out of the reach of children.

HOW SUPPLIED

Bottles of 36, 100, and 500 yellow capsules, identified "STUART 475". Also available in 100 capsule unit dose boxes (10 strips of 10 capsules each). NDC 0038-0475.

Shown in Product Identification Section, page 432

EFFER-SYLLIUM™

[ef'fer-sil'lium]

Natural Fiber Bulking Agent

DESCRIPTION

Each rounded teaspoonful, or individual packet (7 g.) contains psyllium hydrocolloid, 3 g.

INGREDIENTS

Active: psyllium hydrocolloid. Inactive: citric acid, ethyl vanillin, lemon and lime flavors, potassium bicarbonate, potassium citrate, saccharin calcium, sucrose.

EFFER-SYLLIUM contains less than 5 mg. sodium per rounded teaspoonful and is considered dietetically sodium free.

INDICATIONS

EFFER-SYLLIUM is indicated to restore normal bowel habits in chronic constipation, to promote normal elimination in irritable bowel syndrome, and to ease passage of stools in presence of anorectal disorders. EFFER- SYLLIUM produces a soft, lubricating bulk which promotes natural elimination. EFFER-SYLLIUM is not a one-dose, fast-acting bowel regulator. Administration for several days may be needed to establish regularity.

DIRECTIONS

Adults: One rounded teaspoonful, or one packet, in a glass of water one to three times a day, or as directed by physician. *Children, 6 years and over:* One level teaspoonful, or one-half packet (3.5 g.) in one-half glass of water at bedtime, or as directed by physician. *Children, under 6 years:* As directed by physician.

INSTRUCTIONS

Pour EFFER-SYLLIUM into a *dry* glass, add water and stir briskly. Drink immediately. To avoid caking, always use a *dry* spoon to remove EFFER-SYLLIUM from its container. Replace cap tightly. Keep in a dry place.

CAUTION

People sensitive to psyllium powder should avoid inhalation as it may cause an allergic reaction such as wheezing.

WARNING

As with all medications, keep out of the reach of children.

HOW SUPPLIED

Bottles of 9 oz. and 16 oz. tan, granular instant mix powder. Convenient pouch package 7 g. per packet in boxes of 12 or 24.

NDC 0038-0440.

Shown in Product Identification Section, page 432

FERANCEE®

[fer-an-see]

Chewable Hematinic

INGREDIENTS

Each tablet contains: Active: iron (from 200 mg. ferrous fumarate), 67 mg. and Vitamin C (as ascorbic acid, 49 mg. and sodium ascorbate, 114 mg.), 150 mg. Inactive: confectioner's sugar, flavors, magnesium stearate, mannitol, povidone, saccharin calcium, starch, Yellow 5 (tartrazine).

INDICATIONS

A pleasant-tasting hematinic for iron-deficiency anemias, well-tolerated FERANCEE is particularly useful when chronic blood loss, onset of menses, or pregnancy create additional demands for iron supplementation. Available information indicates a low incidence of staining of the teeth by ferrous fumarate, alone or in combination with ascorbic acid. The peach-cherry flavored chewable tablets dissolve quickly in the mouth and may be either chewed or swallowed.

DIRECTIONS

Adults: Two tablets daily, or as directed by physician.
Children over 6 years of age: One tablet daily, or as directed by physician.
Children under 6 years of age: As directed by physician.

WARNINGS

As with any drug, if you are pregnant or nursing a baby, seek the advice of a health professional before using this product. Keep out of the reach of children.

HOW SUPPLIED

Bottles of 100 brown and yellow, two-layer tablets identified "STUART 650" on brown layer. A childproof cap is standard on each bottle as a safeguard against accidental ingestion by children. Keep in a dry place. Replace cap tightly.

NDC 0038-0650.

Shown in Product Identification Section, page 432

FERANCEE®-HP Tablets

[fer-an-see-hp]

High Potency Hematinic

INGREDIENTS

Each tablet contains: Active: iron (from 330 mg. ferrous fumarate), 110 mg.; Vitamin C (as ascorbic acid, 350 mg. and sodium ascorbate, 281 mg.), 600 mg. Inactive: flavor, hydrogenated vegetable oil, microcrystalline cellulose, povidone, Red 40, and other ingredients.

INDICATIONS

FERANCEE-HP is a high potency formulation of iron and vitamin C and is intended for use as either:

(1) a maintenance hematinic for those patients needing a daily iron supplement to maintain normal hemoglobin levels, or
(2) intensive therapy for the acute and/or severe iron deficiency anemia where a high intake of elemental iron is required.

The use of well-tolerated ferrous fumarate provides high levels of elemental iron with a low incidence of gastric distress. The inclusion of 600 mg. of Vitamin C per tablet serves to maintain more of the iron in the absorbable ferrous state.

PRECAUTIONS

Because FERANCEE-HP contains 110 mg. of elemental iron per tablet, it is recommended that its use be limited to adults, i.e. over age 12 years. As with all medication, FERANCEE-HP should be kept out of the reach of children.

DIRECTIONS

One-tablet-a-day taken after a meal or as directed by a physician, should be sufficient to maintain normal hemoglobin levels in most patients with a history of recurring iron defi-

Continued on next page

Stuart—Cont.

ciency anemia. Not recommended for children under 12 years of age.

For acute and/or severe iron deficiency anemia, two or three tablets per day taken one tablet per dose after meals. (Each tablet provides 110 mg. elemental iron).

WARNINGS

As with all medications, keep out of the reach of children.

HOW SUPPLIED

FERANCEE-HP is supplied in bottles of 60 red, film coated, oval shaped tablets.
NDC 0038-0863.

Note: A childproof safety cap is standard on each bottle of 60 tablets as a safeguard against accidental ingestion by children.

Shown in Product Identification Section, page 432

HIBICLENS® Antiseptic Antimicrobial

[*hibi-klenz*]
Skin Cleanser
(chlorhexidine gluconate)

DESCRIPTION

HIBICLENS is an antiseptic antimicrobial skin cleanser possessing bactericidal activities. HIBICLENS contains 4% w/v HIBITANE (chlorhexidine gluconate) a chemically unique hexamethylenebis biguanide with inactive ingredients: fragrance, isopropyl alcohol 4%, purified water, Red 40, and other ingredients, in a mild, sudsing base adjusted to pH 5.0–6.5 for optimal activity and stability as well as compatability with the normal pH of the skin.

ACTION

HIBICLENS is bactericidal on contact. It has antiseptic activity and a persistent antimicrobial effect with rapid bactericidal activity against a wide range of microorganisms, including gram-positive bacteria, and gram-negative bacteria such as *Pseudomonas aeruginosa.* The effectiveness of HIBICLENS is not signficantly reduced by the presence of organic matter, such as blood.[1]

In a study[2] simulating surgical use, the immediate bactericidal effect of HIBICLENS after a single six-minute scrub resulted in a 99.9% reduction in resident bacterial flora, with a reduction of 99.98% after the eleventh scrub. Reductions on surgically gloved hands were maintained over the six-hour test period.

HIBICLENS displays persistent antimicrobial action. In one study[2], 93% of a radiolabeled formulation of HIBICLENS remained present on uncovered skin after five hours.

HIBICLENS prevents skin infection thereby reducing the risk of cross-infection.

INDICATIONS

HIBICLENS is indicated for use as a surgical scrub, as a health-care personnel handwash, for patient preoperative showering and bathing, as a patient preoperative skin preparation, and as a skin wound cleanser and general skin cleanser.

SAFETY

The extensive use of chlorhexidine gluconate for over 20 years outside the United States has produced no evidence of absorption of the compound through intact skin. The potential for producing skin reactions is extremely low. HIBICLENS can be used many times a day without causing irritation, dryness, or discomfort. Experimental studies indicate that when used for cleaning superficial wounds, HIBICLENS will neither cause additional tissue injury nor delay healing.

WARNINGS

For external use only. Keep out of eyes and ears and avoid contact with meninges. If HIBICLENS should get into the eyes or ears, rinse out promptly and thoroughly with water. Chlorhexidine has been reported to cause deafness when instilled in the middle ear through perforated eardrums. HIBICLENS should not be used by persons who have a sensitivity to it or its components. Adverse reactions such as dermatitis and photosensitivity are relatively rare; hypersensitivity and generalized allergic reactions have been reported, but very rarely. If any such reactions occur, discontinue use immediately. Keep this and all drugs out of the reach of children.

Avoid excessive heat (above 104°F).

Accidental ingestion: Chlorhexidine gluconate taken orally is poorly absorbed. Treat with gastric lavage using milk, egg white, gelatin or mild soap. Employ supportive measures as appropriate.

DIRECTIONS FOR USE

Patient preoperative skin preparation

Apply HIBICLENS liberally to surgical site and swab for at least two minutes. Dry with a sterile towel. Repeat procedure for an additional two minutes and dry with a sterile towel.

Preoperative showering and whole-body bathing

The patient should be instructed to wash the entire body, including the scalp, on two occasions immediately prior to surgery. Each procedure should consist of two consecutive thorough applications of HIBICLENS followed by thorough rinsing. If the patient's condition allows, showering is recommended for whole-body bathing. The recommended procedure is: Wet the body, including hair. Wash the hair using 25 ml. of HIBICLENS and the body with another 25 ml. of HIBICLENS. Rinse. Repeat. Rinse thoroughly after second application.

Skin wound and general skin cleansing

Thoroughly rinse area to be cleansed with water. Apply sufficient HIBICLENS and wash gently. Rinse again thoroughly.

Health-care personnel use

SURGICAL HAND SCRUB

Directions for use of HIBICLENS Liquid: Wet hands and forearms to the elbows with warm water. (Avoid using very cold or very hot water.) Dispense about 5 ml. of HIBICLENS into cupped hands. Spread over both hands. Scrub hands and forearms for 3 minutes without adding water, using a brush or sponge. (Avoid using extremely hard-bristled brushes.) While scrubbing, pay particular attention to fingernails, cuticles, and interdigital spaces. (Do not use excessive pressure to produce additional lather.) Rinse thoroughly with warm water. Dispense about 5 ml. of HIBICLENS into cupped hands. Wash for an additional 3 minutes. (No need to use brush or sponge.) Then rinse thoroughly. Dry thoroughly.

Directions for use of HIBICLENS® Sponge/Brush: Open package and remove nail cleaner. Wet hands. Use nail cleaner under fingernails and to clean cuticles. Wet hands and forearms to the elbow with warm water. (Avoid using very cold or very hot water.) Wet sponge side of sponge/brush. Squeeze and pump immediately to work up adequate lather. Apply lather to hands and forearms using *sponge* side of the product. *Start 3 minute scrub* by using the brush side of the product to scrub *only* nails, cuticles, and interdigital areas. Use sponge side for scrubbing hands and forearms. (Avoid using brush on these more sensitive areas.) Rinse thoroughly with warm water. Scrub for an additional 3 minutes *using sponge side* only. To produce additional lather, add a small amount of water and pump the sponge. (While scrubbing, do not use excessive pressure to produce lather—a small amount of lather is all that is required to adequately cleanse skin with HIBICLENS.) Rinse and dry thoroughly, blotting hands and forearms with a soft sterile towel.

HAND WASH

Wet hands with warm water. (Avoid using very cold or very hot water.) Dispense about 5 ml. of HIBICLENS into cupped hands. Wash for 15 seconds. (Do not use excessive pressure to produce additional lather.) Rinse thoroughly with warm water. Dry thoroughly.

IMPORTANT LAUNDERING ADVICE FOR HOSPITAL STAFF AND OTHER USERS OF ANTISEPTIC PATIENT SKIN PREPARATIONS CONTAINING CHLORHEXIDINE GLUCONATE

Chlorhexidine gluconate is a unique agent that most closely fits the definition of an ideal antimicrobial agent, having (among others) one of the most important characteristics of persistent activity. This persistence is due to chlorhexidine gluconate binding to the protein of the skin and, thus, being available for residual activity over a relatively long period of time.

Chlorhexidine gluconate, however, binds not only to protein of the skin but also to many fabrics, particularly cotton. Thus, special laundering procedures should be considered when such products contact these fabrics. As a result of such contact, chlorhexidine gluconate may become adsorbed onto the fabric and not be removed by washing. If sufficient available chlorine is present during the washing procedure, a fast brown stain may develop due to a chemical reaction between chlorhexidine gluconate and chlorine.

SUGGESTED LAUNDERING PROCEDURES TO LIMIT STAINING

1. **Not Aging.** Avoid allowing the product to age (set) on unwashed linens.
2. **Flushing and Washing.** A flush operation as the initial step in the wash process is helpful in the laundering of linen exposed to chlorhexidine gluconate. Such flushing is also important in the laundering of linen which contains organic materials such as blood or pus. For best results, warm water flushes (90°–100°F) are recommended. After a number of initial flushings followed by a washing with a low alkaline/nonchlorine detergent, most articles which come in contact with chlorhexidine gluconate should have an acceptable level of whiteness. If a rewash process using bleach is necessary to achieve a greater degree of whiteness, the bleach used should be a nonchlorine bleach.
3. **Not Using Chlorine Bleach.** Modern laundering methods often make the use of chlorine bleach unnecessary. It is worthwhile trying to wash without chlorine to ascertain if the resulting degree of whiteness is acceptable. Omission of chlorine from the laundering process can extend the useful life of cotton articles since oxidizing bleaches such as chlorine may cause some damage to cellulose even when used in low concentration.
4. **Changing to a Peroxide-Type Bleach, Such as Sodium Perborate, Sodium Percarbonate or Hydrogen Peroxide.** This should eliminate the reaction which could occur with the use of chlorine bleaches. If a chlorine bleach must be used, a concentration of less than 7 ppm available chlorine ($^1/_{10}$ the normal bleach level) is suggested to minimize possible staining.

A NOTE ON LAUNDERING OF PERSONAL CLOTHING

The laundering procedures set forth above using low alkaline, nonchlorinated laundry detergents are also applicable to laundering of uniforms and lab coats. Commercially available laundry detergents which do not contain chlorine include Borax, Borateem, Dreft, Oxydol, and Ivory Snow. These products, however, will not remove stains previously set into the fabric.

RECLAMATION OF STAINED LINENS

For those linens which previously have been stained due to the chemical reaction between chlorhexidine gluconate and chlorine, the following laundering procedure may be helpful in reducing the visible stain:
[See table below].

Operation	Water Level	Temperature	Time (Min)	Supplies/ 100 lb
Break	Low	180°F	20	1.5 lb oxalic acid
Flush	High	Cold	1	—
Emulsify	Low	160°F	5	18 oz emulsifier
Flush	High	Cold	1	—
Bleach	Low	180°F	20	2 lb alkali builder and 1 lb organic bleach
Rinse	High	Cold	1	—
Antichlor	High	Cold	2	4 oz antichlor
Rinse	High	Cold	1	—
Rinse	High	Cold	1	—
Sour	Low	Cold	4	2 oz rust removing sour

HOW SUPPLIED

For general handwashing locations: pocket-size, 15 ml. foil Packettes; plastic disposable bottles of 4 oz. and 8 oz. with dispenser caps; and 16 oz. filled globes. *For surgical scrub areas:* disposable, unit-of-use 22 ml. impregnated Sponge/-Brushes with nail cleaner; plastic disposable bottles of 32 oz. and 1 gal. The 32-oz. bottle is designed for a special foot-operated wall dispenser. A hand-operated wall dispenser is available for the 16-oz. globe. Hand pumps are available for 16 oz., 32 oz., and 1 gal. sizes. NDC 0038-0575.

REFERENCES

1. Lowbury, EJL, and Lilly, HA: The effect of blood on disinfection of surgeons' hands, Brit. J. Surg. 61:19–21 (Jan.) 1974.
2. Peterson AF, Rosenberg A, Alatary SD: Comparative evaluation of surgical scrub preparations, Surg. Gynecol. Obstet. 146:63–65 (Jan.) 1978.

Shown in Product Identification Section, page 432

HIBISTAT®
HIBISTAT® TOWELETTE

[*hi-bi-stat*]
(chlorhexidine gluconate)
Germicidal Hand Rinse

DESCRIPTION

HIBISTAT is a germicidal hand rinse which provides bactericidal action and has a persistent antimicrobial effect against a wide range of microorganisms. . HIBISTAT is a clear, colorless liquid containing 0.5% w/w HIBITANE® (chlorhexidine gluconate) with inactive ingredients: emollients, isopropanol 70%, purified water.

INDICATIONS

HIBISTAT is indicated for health-care personnel use as a germicidal hand rinse. HIBISTAT is for hand hygiene on physically clean hands. It is used in those situations where hands are physically clean, but in need of degerming, when routine handwashing is not convenient or desirable. HIBISTAT provides rapid germicidal action and has a persistent effect.

HIBISTAT should be used in-between patients and procedures where there are no sinks available or continued return to the sink area is inconvenient. HIBISTAT can be used as an alternative to detergent-based products when hands are physically clean. Also, HIBISTAT is an effective germicidal hand rinse following a soap and water handwash.

WARNINGS

Flammable. This product is alcohol based. Alcohol is extremely flammable. It should be kept away from flame or devices which may generate an electrical spark.

For external use only. Keep out of eyes and ears and avoid contact with meninges. If HIBISTAT should get into eyes or ears, rinse out promptly and thoroughly with water. Chlorhexidine has been reported to cause deafness when instilled in the middle ear through perforated eardrums. HIBISTAT should not be used by persons who have a sensitivity to it or its components. Adverse reactions such as dermatitis and photosensitivity are relatively rare; hypersensitivity and generalized allergic reactions have been reported, but very rarely. If any such reactions occur, discontinue use immediately. Keep this and all drugs out of the reach of children. In case of accidental ingestion, seek professional assistance or contact a Poison Control Center immediately.

Avoid excessive heat (above 104°F).

Accidental ingestion: Chlorhexidine gluconate taken orally is poorly absorbed. Treat with gastric lavage using milk, egg white, gelatin or mild soap avoiding pulmonary aspiration. Do not use apomorphine. Assist respiration if necessary and keep patient warm. Intravenous levulose can accelerate alcohol metabolism. In severe cases, hemodialysis or peritoneal dialysis may be appropriate.

DIRECTIONS FOR USE

HIBISTAT Towelette: Rub hands vigorously with the HIBISTAT Towelette for approximately 15 seconds, paying particular attention to nails and interdigital spaces. HIBISTAT dries rapidly in use. No water or towel drying are necessary. The emollients contained in the HIBISTAT Towelette protect the hands from the potential drying effect of alcohol.

HIBISTAT Liquid: Dispense about 5 ml. of HIBISTAT into cupped hands and rub vigorously until dry (about 15 seconds), paying particular attention to nails and interdigital spaces. HIBISTAT dries rapidly in use. No water or toweling are necessary. The emollients contained in HIBISTAT protect the hands from the potential drying effect of alcohol.

HOW SUPPLIED

In plastic disposable bottles of 4 oz. and 8 oz. with flip-top cap, and in disposable towelettes containing 5 ml., packaged 50 towelettes to a carton.

NDC 0038-0585 (bottles)

NDC 0038-0587 (towelettes)

Shown in Product Identification Section, page 432

KASOF® Capsules

[kay'sof]

High Strength Stool Softener

DESCRIPTION

KASOF provides a highly efficient wetting action to restore moisture to the bowel, thus softening the stool to prevent straining. The action of KASOF does not interfere with normal peristalsis and generally does not cause griping or extreme sensation of urgency: KASOF is sodium-free, containing a unique potassium formulation, without the problems associated with sodium intake.

INGREDIENTS

Each capsule contains: Active: docusate potassium, 240 mg. Inactive: Blue 1, gelatin, glycerin, methylparaben, polyethylene glycol, propylparaben, purified water, Red 40, Yellow 10.

INDICATIONS

KASOF is especially valuable for the severely constipated, as well for patients with anorectal disorders, such as hemorrhoids and anal fissures. KASOF is ideal for patients with any condition that can be complicated by straining at stool, for example, cardiac patients. The simple, one-a-day dosage helps assure patient compliance in maintaining normal bowel function.

DIRECTIONS

Adults: One KASOF capsule daily for several days, or until bowel movements are normal and gentle. It is helpful to increase the daily intake of fluids by drinking a glass of water with each dose.

WARNINGS

As with any drug, if you are pregnant or nursing a baby, seek the advice of a health professional before using this product. Keep out of the reach of children.

HOW SUPPLIED

KASOF is available in bottles of 30 and 60 brown, gelatin capsules, identified "Stuart 380".

NDC 0038-0380.

Shown in Product Identification Section, page 432

KINESED® Tablets ℞

[kin-e-sed]

(belladonna alkaloids and phenobarbital)

DESCRIPTION

Each chewable, fruit-flavored, scored, oval KINESED tablet contains:

Phenobarbital .... 16 mg.
(Warning: May be habit forming)
Hyoscyamine Sulfate
Atropine Sulfate .... 0.12 mg.
Scopolamine Hydrobromide .... 0.007 mg.

Inactive ingredients: calcium silicate, citric acid, confectioner's sugar, flavors, glyceryl monostearate, lactose, mannitol, povidone, saccharin calcium, sodium citrate, starch, stearic acid.

ACTIONS

This drug combination provides natural belladonna alkaloids in a specific, fixed ratio combined with phenobarbital to provide peripheral anticholinergic/antispasmodic action and mild sedation.

INDICATIONS

Based on a review of this drug by the National Academy of Sciences—National Research Council, and/or other information, FDA has classified the following indications as "possibly" effective:

For use as adjunctive therapy in the treatment of irritable bowel syndrome (irritable colon, spastic colon, mucous colitis) and acute enterocolitis.

May also be useful as adjunctive therapy in the treatment of duodenal ulcer. IT HAS NOT BEEN SHOWN CONCLUSIVELY WHETHER ANTICHOLINERGIC/ANTISPASMODIC DRUGS AID IN THE HEALING OF A DUODENAL ULCER, DECREASE THE RATE OF RECURRENCES, OR PREVENT COMPLICATIONS.

CONTRAINDICATIONS

Glaucoma, obstructive uropathy (for example, bladder neck obstruction due to prostatic hypertrophy); obstructive disease of the gastrointestinal tract (as in achalasia, pyloroduodenal stenosis, etc.); paralytic ileus, intestinal atony of the elderly or debilitated patient; unstable cardiovascular status in acute hemorrhage; severe ulcerative colitis especially if complicated by toxic megacolon; myasthenia gravis; hiatal hernia associated with reflux esophagitis.

KINESED is contraindicated in patients with known hypersensitivity to any of the ingredients. Phenobarbital is contraindicated in acute intermittent porphyria and in those patients in whom phenobarbital produces restlessness and/or excitement.

WARNINGS

In the presence of a high environmental temperature, heat prostration can occur with belladonna alkaloids (fever and heatstroke due to decreased sweating). Diarrhea may be an early symptom of incomplete intestinal obstruction, especially in patients with ileostomy or colostomy. In this instance treatment with this drug would be inappropriate and possibly harmful.

KINESED may produce drowsiness or blurred vision. The patient should be warned, should these occur, not to engage in activities requiring mental alertness, such as operating a motor vehicle or other machinery, and not to perform hazardous work.

Phenobarbital may decrease the effect of anticoagulants, and necessitate larger doses of the anticoagulant for optimal effect. When the phenobarbital is discontinued, the dose of the anticoagulant may have to be decreased.

Phenobarbital may be habit forming and should not be administered to individuals known to be addiction prone or those with a history of physical and/or psychological dependence upon drugs.

Since barbiturates are metabolized in the liver, they should be used with caution and initial doses should be small in patients with hepatic dysfunction.

PRECAUTIONS

Use with caution in patients with: autonomic neuropathy, hepatic or renal disease, hyperthyroidism, coronary heart disease, congestive heart failure, cardiac arrhythmias, tachycardia, and hypertension.

Belladonna alkaloids may produce a delay in gastric emptying (antral stasis) which would complicate the management of gastric ulcer. Theoretically, with overdosage, a curare-like action may occur.

Carcinogenesis, mutagenesis. Long-term studies in animals have not been performed to evaluate carcinogenic potential.

Pregnancy Category C. Animal reproduction studies have not been conducted with KINESED. It is not known whether KINESED can cause fetal harm when administered to a pregnant woman or can affect reproductive capacity. KINESED should be given to a pregnant woman only if clearly needed.

Nursing mothers. Because belladonna alkaloids and phenobarbital are excreted in human milk, caution should be exercised when KINESED is administered to a nursing mother.

ADVERSE REACTIONS

Adverse reactions may include xerostomia; urinary hesitancy and retention; blurred vision; tachycardia; palpitation; mydriasis; cycloplegia; increased ocular tension; loss of taste sense; headache; nervousness; drowsiness; weakness; dizziness; insomnia; nausea; vomiting; impotence; suppression of lactation; constipation; bloated feeling; severe allergic reaction or drug idiosyncrasies, including anaphylaxis, urticaria and other dermal manifestations; and decreased sweating. Elderly patients may react with symptoms of excitement, agitation, drowsiness, and other untoward manifestations to even small doses of the drug.

Phenobarbital may produce excitement in some patients, rather than a sedative effect. In patients habituated to barbiturates, abrupt withdrawal may produce delirium or convulsions.

DOSAGE AND ADMINISTRATION

The dosage of KINESED chewable tablets should be adjusted to the needs of the individual patient to assure symptomatic control with a minimum of adverse effects.

ADULTS: One or two KINESED tablets, three or four times daily, chewed or swallowed with liquids.

CHILDREN, 2 to 12 years: One-half to one KINESED tablet, three or four times daily, chewed or swallowed with liquids.

OVERDOSAGE

The signs and symptoms of overdose are headache, nausea, vomiting, blurred vision, dilated pupils, hot and dry skin, dizziness, dryness of the mouth, difficulty in swallowing and CNS stimulation. Treatment should consist of gastric lavage, emetics, and activated charcoal. If indicated, parenteral cholinergic agents such as physostigmine or bethanechol chloride should be added.

HOW SUPPLIED

Bottles of 100 white scored, oval, fruit-flavored, chewable tablets (embossed front "STUART," reverse "220"). Store at room temperature; avoid excess heat (above 104°F). Dispense in well-closed, light-resistant container. NDC 0038-0220.

Shown in Product Identification Section, page 432

C/10/85

MULVIDREN®–F SOFTAB® Tablets ℞

[mul'vi-dren"]

(fluoride with multivitamins)

DESCRIPTION

MULVIDREN-F SOFTAB Tablets are formulated to provide daily, oral supplementation of fluoride and multivitamins. The unique design of the tablet assures delivery of all ingredients whether swallowed whole, chewed, allowed to dissolve in the mouth or crushed and mixed with food.

EACH TABLET CONTAINS

Fluoride (as 2.2 mg sodium fluoride) .... 1 mg
Vitamin A (as palmitate) .... 4,000 USP units
Vitamin D (ergocalciferol) .... 400 USP units
Vitamin C (ascorbic acid and sodium ascorbate) .... 75 mg
Thiamine Mononitrate .... 2 mg
Riboflavin .... 2 mg
Vitamin B_6 (as pyridoxine hydrochloride) .... 1.2 mg
Vitamin B_{12} (cyanocobalamin) .... 3 mcg
Niacinamide .... 10 mg
Calcium Pantothenate .... 3 mg

Inactive ingredients: flavors, mannitol, saccharin calcium, starch, Yellow 6.

CLINICAL PHARMACOLOGY

Soluble fluorides such as sodium fluoride are efficiently absorbed from the gastrointestinal tract of man, and some topical absorption occurs on tooth surfaces. The major route of fluoride excretion is by way of the kidneys. Fluoride is also excreted in small amounts in sweat, breast milk and feces. Fluoride provides much of its protective action against dental caries by combining with apatite crystals in the tooth structure, thus, forming the less acid soluble compound fluorapatite.

Continued on next page

Stuart—Cont.

Controlled studies show a decrease in the incidence of dental caries in children receiving an optimal nutritional supply of fluoride. To achieve maximal anticariogenic effect, fluoride must be provided throughout the stages of tooth formation and calcification. Thus, fluoride should be provided in adequate amounts from birth through the first 15 years of life. If natural sources are deficient, Fluoride should be made available throughout this period by daily dietary supplementation. MULVIDREN-F SOFTAB is a well-accepted and convenient form of administering fluoride for both topical and systemic effects.

INDICATIONS AND USAGE
As an aid in promoting the development of caries-resistant teeth in children from birth through the first 15 years of life. MULVIDREN-F provides a source of daily fluoride supplementation in addition to full nutritional amounts of vitamins.

CONTRAINDICATIONS
Patients living in areas where the drinking water is fluoridated at a concentration of greater than 0.7 ppm and those persons with a known sensitivity to fluoride should not take MULVIDREN-F.

WARNINGS
Dental fluorosis (mottling) may result from exceeding the recommended dose (see Dosage and Administration).

PRECAUTIONS
When prescribing MULVIDREN-F, the physician should make sure the child is not receiving significant amounts of fluoride from other sources (ie, medications, drinking water) (see Dosage and Administration).

ADVERSE REACTIONS
In hypersensitive individuals, fluorides occasionally cause skin eruptions such as atropic dermatitis, eczema or urticaria. Gastric distress, headache and weakness have also been reported. These hypersensitivity reactions usually disappear promptly after discontinuation of the fluoride. In rare cases, a delay in the eruption of teeth has been reported.

DOSAGE AND ADMINISTRATION
The daily fluoride intake from dietary supplements such as MULVIDREN-F must be adjusted according to the fluoride intake from other sources such as drinking water. The following dosage schedules are recommended.
Less than 0.3 ppm fluoride in drinking water:
Infants, birth to 2 years of age—0.25 mg of fluoride daily.
Children 2 to 3 years of age—0.5 mg of fluoride daily or one-half MULVIDREN-F tablet daily.
Children 3 to 16 years of age—1.0 mg of fluoride daily or one MULVIDREN-F tablet daily.
0.3 to 0.7 ppm fluoride in drinking water:
Infants, birth to 2 years of age—no fluoride supplementation recommended.
Children 2 to 3 years of age—0.25 mg of fluoride daily
Children 3 to 16 years of age—0.5 mg of fluoride daily or one-half MULVIDREN-F tablet daily
Greater than 0.7 ppm fluoride in drinking water:
No fluoride supplementation recommended.
MULVIDREN-F tablets may be swallowed, chewed and swallowed, allowed to dissolve in the mouth or crushed and mixed with food.

HOW SUPPLIED
In bottles of 100 orange colored, scored SOFTAB tablets, identified front "Stuart," reverse "710" A childproof safety cap is standard on each 100 tablet bottle as a safeguard against accidental ingestion. NDC 0038-0710.
Shown in Product Identification Section, page 432

MYLANTA®
[my'lan"ta]
Liquid and Tablets
Antacid/Anti-Gas

INGREDIENTS
Each chewable tablet or each 5 ml. (one teaspoonful) of liquid contains:
Active: Aluminum hydroxide
(Dried Gel, USP in tablet and equiv.
to Dried Gel, USP in liquid) .... 200 mg.
Magnesium hydroxide .... 200 mg.
Simethicone .... 20 mg.
Inactive: Tablets: dextrates, flavors, magnesium stearate, mannitol, sorbitol, Yellow 10. Liquid: butylparaben, carboxymethylcellulose sodium, flavors, hydroxypropyl methylcellulose, microcrystalline cellulose, propylparaben, purified water, sorbitol solution.
Sodium Content: MYLANTA contains an insignificant amount of sodium per daily dose and is considered dietetically sodium free. Typical values are 0.68 mg. (0.03 mEq) sodium per 5 ml. teaspoonful of liquid; 0.77 mg. (0.03 mEq) per tablet.
Acid Neutralizing Capacity: Two teaspoonfuls of MYLANTA Liquid will neutralize 25.4 mEq of acid. Two MYLANTA tablets will neutralize 23.0 mEq.

INDICATIONS
MYLANTA, a well-balanced combination of two antacids and simethicone, provides consistently dependable relief of symptoms associated with gastric hyperacidity, and mucus-entrapped air or "gas". These indications include:
Common heartburn (pyrosis)
Hiatal hernia
Peptic esophagitis
Gastritis
Peptic ulcer
The exceptionally pleasant tasting liquid and soft, easy-to-chew tablets encourage patients' acceptance, thereby minimizing the skipping of prescribed doses. MYLANTA is appropriate whenever there is a need for effective relief of temporary gastric hyperacidity and mucus-entrapped gas.

DIRECTIONS
Liquid: Shake well, 2–4 teaspoonfuls between meals and at bedtime or as directed by a physician.
Tablets: 2–4 tablets, well chewed, between meals and at bedtime or as directed by a physician.

WARNINGS
Keep this and all other drugs out of the reach of children. Except under the advice and supervision of a physician: Do not take more than 24 tsps./tablets in a 24 hour period or use the maximum dose of this product for more than two weeks. Do not use this product if you have kidney disease.
Magnesium hydroxide and other magnesium salts, in the presence of renal insufficiency, may cause central nervous system depression and other symptoms of hypermagnesemia.

DRUG INTERACTION PRECAUTION
Do not use this product for any patient receiving a prescription antibiotic containing any form of tetracycline.

HOW SUPPLIED
MYLANTA is available as a white, pleasant tasting liquid suspension, and as a two-layer yellow and white chewable tablet, identified on yellow layer "STUART 620". Liquid supplied in bottles of 5 oz. and 12 oz. Tablets supplied in boxes of individually wrapped 40's and 100's, economy size bottles of 180, and consumer convenience pocket packs of 48. Also available for hospital use in liquid unit dose bottles of 1 oz., and bottles of 5 oz.
NDC 0038-0610 (liquid). NDC 0038-0620 (tablets).
Shown in Product Identification Section, page 432

MYLANTA®-II
[my'lan"ta]
Liquid and Tablets
Double Strength Antacid/Anti-Gas

INGREDIENTS
Each chewable tablet or each 5 ml. (one teaspoonful) of liquid contains:
Active: Aluminum hydroxide
(Dried Gel, USP in tablet and equiv.
to Dried Gel, USP in liquid) 400 mg.
Magnesium hydroxide 400 mg.
Simethicone 40 mg.
Inactive: Tablets: Blue 1, cereal solids, confectioner's sugar, flavors, glycerin, lactose, mannitol, starch, Yellow 10. Liquid: butylparaben, carboxymethylcellulose sodium, flavors, hydroxypropyl methylcellulose, microcrystalline cellulose, potassium citrate, propylparaben, purified water, sorbitol solution.
Sodium Content: MYLANTA-II contains an insignificant amount of sodium per daily dose. Typical values are 1.14 mg. (0.05 mEq) sodium per 5 ml. teaspoonful of liquid; 1.3 mg. (0.06 mEq) per tablet.
Acid Neutralizing Capacity: Two teaspoonfuls of MYLANTA-II liquid will neutralize 50.8 mEq of acid. Two MYLANTA-II tablets will neutralize 46.0 mEq.

INDICATIONS
MYLANTA-II is a double strength antacid with a double-strength antiflatulent. The exceptionally pleasant tasting liquid and soft, easy-to-chew tablets encourage patient acceptance, thereby minimizing the skipping of prescribed doses. MYLANTA-II provides consistently dependable relief of the symptoms of peptic ulcer and other problems related to acid hypersecretion. The high potency of MYLANTA-II is achieved through its concentration of noncalcium antacid ingredients. Thus MYLANTA-II can produce both rapid and long lasting neutralization without the acid rebound associated with calcium carbonate. The balanced formula of aluminum and magnesium hydroxides minimizes undesirable bowel effects. Simethicone is effective for the relief of concomitant distress caused by mucus-entrapped gas and swallowed air.

DIRECTIONS
Liquid: Shake well, 2–4 teaspoonfuls between meals and at bedtime or as directed by a physician.
Tablets: 2–4 tablets, well chewed, between meals and at bedtime or as directed by a physician.
Because patients with peptic ulcer vary greatly in both acid output and gastric emptying time, the amount and schedule of dosages should be varied accordingly.

WARNINGS
Keep this and all drugs out of the reach of children. Except under the advice and supervision of a physician: Do not take more than 12 tsps./tablets in a 24 hour period or use the maximum dose of this product for more than two weeks. Do not use this product if you have kidney disease.
Magnesium hydroxide and other magnesium salts, in the presence of renal insufficiency, may cause central nervous system depression and other symptoms of hypermagnesemia.

DRUG INTERACTION PRECAUTION
Do not use this product for any patient receiving a prescription antibiotic containing any form of tetracycline.

HOW SUPPLIED
MYLANTA-II is available as a white, pleasant tasting liquid suspension, and a two-layer green and white chewable tablet, identified on green layer "STUART 651". Liquid supplied in 2 oz., 5 oz. and 12 oz. bottles. Tablets supplied in boxes of 60 individually wrapped chewable tablets and consumer convenience pocket packs of 24. Also available for hospital use in liquid unit dose bottles of 1 oz., and bottles of 5 oz.
NDC 0038-0652 (liquid). NDC 0038-0651 (tablets).
Shown in Product Identification Section, page 432

MYLICON® Tablets and Drops
[my'li-con]
Antiflatulent

INGREDIENTS
Each tablet or 0.6 ml. of drops contains: Simethicone, 40 mg. Inactive ingredients: Tablets: calcium silicate, lactose, povidone, saccharin calcium. Drops: carbomer 934P, citric acid, flavors, hydroxypropyl methylcellulose, purified water, Red 3, saccharin calcium, sodium benzoate, sodium citrate.

INDICATIONS
For relief of the painful symptoms of excess gas in the digestive tract. Such gas is frequently caused by excessive swallowing of air or by eating foods that disagree. MYLICON is a valuable adjunct in the treatment of many conditions in which the retention of gas may be a problem, such as: postoperative gaseous distention, air swallowing, functional dyspepsia, peptic ulcer, spastic or irritable colon, diverticulitis. The defoaming action of MYLICON relieves flatulence by dispersing and preventing the formation of mucus-surrounded gas pockets in the gastrointestinal tract. MYLICON acts in the stomach and intestines to change the surface tension of gas bubbles enabling them to coalesce; thus the gas is freed and is eliminated more easily by belching or passing flatus.

DIRECTIONS
Tablets—One or two tablets four times daily after meals and at bedtime. May also be taken as needed up to 12 tablets daily or as directed by a physician. TABLETS SHOULD BE CHEWED THOROUGHLY.
Drops—0.6 ml. four times daily after meals and at bedtime. May also be taken as needed up to 500 mg. daily or as directed by a physician. Shake well before using.

WARNINGS
Keep this and all drugs out of the reach of chldren.

HOW SUPPLIED
Bottles of 100 and 500 white, scored, chewable tablets, identified front "STUART", reverse "450," and dropper bottles of 30 ml. (1 fl. oz.) pink, pleasant tasting liquid. Also available in 100 tablet unit dose boxes (10 strips of 10 tablets each).
NDC 0038-0450 (tablets).
NDC 0038-0630 (drops).
Shown in Product Identification Section, page 432

MYLICON®-80 Tablets
[my'li-con]
High-Capacity Antiflatulent

INGREDIENTS
Each tablet contains: Simethicone, 80 mg. Inactive ingredients: cereal solids, flavor, lactose, mannitol, povidone, Red 3, talc.

INDICATIONS

For relief of the painful symptoms of excess gas in the digestive tract. Such gas is frequently caused by excessive swallowing of air or by eating foods that disagree. MYLICON-80 is a high capacity antiflatulent for adjunctive treatment of many conditions in which the retention of gas may be a problem, such as the following: air swallowing, functional dyspepsia, postoperative gaseous distention, peptic ulcer, spastic or irritable colon, diverticulosis.

MYLICON-80 has a defoaming action that relieves flatulence by dispersing and preventing the formation of mucus-surrounded gas pockets in the gastrointestinal tract. MYLICON-80 acts in the stomach and intestines to change the surface tension of gas bubbles enabling them to coalesce; thus, the gas is freed and is eliminated more easily by belching or passing flatus.

DIRECTIONS

One tablet four times daily after meals and at bedtime. May also be taken as needed up to 6 tablets daily or as directed by a physician. TABLETS SHOULD BE CHEWED THOROUGHLY.

WARNINGS

Keep this and all drugs out of the reach of children.

HOW SUPPLIED

Economical bottles of 100 and convenience packages of individually wrapped 12 and 48 pink, scored, chewable tablets identified "STUART 858". Also available in 100 tablet unit dose boxes (10 strips of 10 tablets each).

NDC 0038-0858.

Shown in Product Identification Section, page 432

NOLVADEX® 10 mg. Tablets ℞

[nol 'va-dex]

(tamoxifen citrate)

DESCRIPTION

NOLVADEX (tamoxifen citrate) tablets for oral administration contain 15.2 mg of tamoxifen citrate, which is equivalent to 10 mg of tamoxifen. It is a nonsteroidal antiestrogen. Chemically, NOLVADEX is the trans-isomer of a triphenylethylene derivative. The chemical name is (Z) 2-[4-(1,2-diphenyl-1-butenyl) phenoxy]-N, N- dimethylethanamine 2-hydroxy-1, 2, 3-propanetricarboxylate (1:1).

Tamoxifen citrate has a molecular weight of 563.62, the pka' is 8.85, the equilibrium solubility in water at 37°C is 0.5mg/mL and in 0.02N HCl at 37°C it is 0.2 mg/mL.

NOLVADEX is intended only for oral administration; the tablets should be protected from heat and light.

Inactive ingredients: carboxymethylcellulose calcium, magnesium stearate, mannitol, starch.

CLINICAL PHARMACOLOGY

NOLVADEX is a nonsteroidal agent which has demonstrated potent antiestrogenic properties in animal test systems. The antiestrogenic effects may be related to its ability to compete with estrogen for binding sites in target tissues such as breast. Tamoxifen inhibits the induction of rat mammary carcinoma induced by dimethylbenzanthracene (DMBA), and causes the regression of already established DMBA-induced tumors. In this rat model tamoxifen appears to exert its antitumor effects by binding to estrogen receptors.

In cytosols derived from human breast adenocarcinomas, tamoxifen competes with estradiol for estrogen receptor protein.

Preliminary pharmacokinetics in women using radio-labeled tamoxifen has shown that most of the radioactivity is slowly excreted in the feces, with only small amounts appearing in urine. The drug is excreted mainly as conjugates, with unchanged drug and hydroxylated metabolites accounting for 30% of the total.

Blood levels of total radioactivity following single oral doses of approximately 0.3 mg/kg reached peak values of 0.06–0.14 μg/mL at 4–7 hours after dosing, with only 20–30% of the drug present as tamoxifen. There was an initial half-life of 7–14 hours with secondary peaks four or more days later. The prolongation of blood levels and fecal excretion is believed to be due to enterohepatic circulation.

Two studies (Hubay and NSABP B-09) demonstrated an improved disease-free survival following radical or modified radical mastectomy in postmenopausal women or women 50 years of age or older with surgically curable breast cancer with positive axillary nodes when NOLVADEX was added to adjuvant cytotoxic chemotherapy. In the Hubay study, NOLVADEX was added to 'low-dose' CMF (cyclophosphamide, methotrexate and fluorouracil). In the NSABP B-09 study, NOLVADEX was added to melphalan [L-phenylalanine mustard (P)] and fluorouracil (F).

Tumor hormone receptors may help predict which patients will benefit from the adjuvant therapy, but not all breast cancer adjuvant NOLVADEX studies have shown a clear relationship between hormone receptor status and treatment effect. In the Hubay study, patients with a positive (more than 3 fmols) estrogen receptor were more likely to benefit. In the NASBP B-09 study in women age 50–59 years, only women with both estrogen and progesterone receptor levels 10 fmols or greater clearly benefited, while there was a nonstatistically significant trend toward adverse effect in women with both estrogen and progesterone receptor levels less than 10 fmols. In women age 60–70 years, there was a trend toward a beneficial effect of NOLVADEX without any clear relationship to estrogen or progesterone receptor status.

INDICATIONS AND USAGE

NOLVADEX is effective in the treatment of metastatic breast cancer in postmenopausal women. Available evidence indicates that patients whose tumors are estrogen receptor positive are more likely to benefit from NOLVADEX therapy.

NOLVADEX in combination with cytotoxic chemotherapy following radical or modified radical mastectomy is effective in delaying recurrence of surgically curable breast cancer in postmenopausal women or women age 50 or older with positive axillary nodes. In the Hubay and NSABP studies most of the benefit to date has been in the subgroup with 4 or more positive axillary nodes. The contribution of the cytotoxic chemotherapy is uncertain. The estrogen and progesterone receptor values may help to predict whether the adjuvant therapy is likely to be beneficial.

CONTRAINDICATIONS

None known.

WARNINGS

Pregnancy Category D: NOLVADEX may cause fetal harm when administered to a pregnant woman. Individuals should not become pregnant while taking NOLVADEX. Effects on reproductive functions are expected from the antiestrogenic properties of the drug. In reproductive studies in rats at dose levels equal to or below the human dose, nonteratogenic developmental skeletal changes were seen and were found to be reversible. In addition, in fertility studies in rats and in teratology studies in rabbits using doses at or below those used in humans, a lower incidence of egg implantation and a higher incidence of fetal death or retarded in utero growth were observed with slower learning behavior in some rat pups. The impairment of learning behavior did not achieve statistical significance in one study, and, in another study where significance was reported, this was obtained by comparing dosed animals with controls of another study. Several pregnant marmosets were dosed during organogenesis or in the last half of pregnancy. No deformations, were seen, and although the dose was high enough to terminate pregnancy in some animals, those that did maintain pregnancy showed no evidence of teratogenic malformations. There are no adequate and well-controlled studies in pregnant women. There have been reports of spontaneous abortions, birth defects, fetal deaths, and vaginal bleeding. If this drug is used during pregnancy or the patient becomes pregnant while taking this drug, the patient should be apprised of the potential hazard to the fetus.

Ocular changes have been reported in a few patients who, as part of a clinical trial, were treated for periods greater than one year with NOLVADEX at doses at least four times the highest recommended daily dose of 40 mg. The ocular changes consist of retinopathy and, in some patients, there are also corneal changes and a decrease in visual acuity.

In addition, a few cases of ocular changes including visual disturbances, corneal changes, and/or retinopathy have been reported in patients treated with NOLVADEX at recommended doses. It is uncertain if these effects are due to NOLVADEX.

As with other additive hormonal therapy (estrogens and androgens), hypercalcemia has been reported in some breast cancer patients with bone metastases within a few weeks of starting treatment with NOLVADEX. If hypercalcemia does occur, appropriate measures should be taken, and if severe, NOLVADEX should be discontinued.

PRECAUTIONS

General: NOLVADEX should be used cautiously in patients with existing leukopenia or thrombocytopenia. Observations of leukopenia and thrombocytopenia occasionally have been made, but it is uncertain if these effects are due to NOLVADEX therapy. Transient decreases in platelet counts, usually to 50,000–100,000/mm^3, infrequently lower, have been occasionally reported in patients taking NOLVADEX for breast cancer. No hemorrhagic tendency has been recorded, and the platelet counts returned to normal levels even though treatment with NOLVADEX continued.

Laboratory Tests: Periodic complete blood counts, including platelet counts, may be appropriate.

Carcinogenesis: While no conventional bioassay has been conducted, endocrine changes in immature and mature mice were investigated in a 13-month study. Various tumors were found in all treated groups.

Mutagenesis: No genotoxic potential has been found in a battery of in vivo and in vitro tests with pro- and eukaryotic test systems with drug metabolizing systems present.

Impairment of Fertility: Fertility of male rats was decreased when doses of 0.96 mg/kg or greater were administered 11 weeks prior to mating and fertility in female rats was decreased following administration of 0.04 mg/kg for two weeks prior to mating through day 7 of pregnancy. There was a decreased number of implantations, and all fetuses were found dead.

Following administration to rats of 0.16 mg/kg from days 7–17 of pregnancy, there were increased numbers of fetal deaths. Administration of 0.125 mg/kg to rabbits during days 6–18 of pregnancy resulted in abortion or premature delivery. Fetal deaths occurred at higher doses. There were no teratogenic changes in either rat or rabbit segment II studies. Several pregnant marmosets were dosed with 10 mg/kg/day either during organogenesis or in the last half of pregnancy. No deformations were seen, and although the dose was high enough to terminate pregnancy in some animals, those that did maintain pregnancy showed no evidence of teratogenic malformations. Rats given 0.16 mg/kg from day 17 of pregnancy to 1 day before weaning demonstrated increased numbers of dead pups at parturition. It was reported that some rat pups showed slower learning behavior, but this did not achieve statistical significance in one study, and in another study where significance was reported, this was obtained by comparing dosed animals with controls of another study.

The recommended daily human dose of 20–40 mg corresponds to 0.4–0.8 mg/kg for an average 50 kg woman.

Pregnancy Category D: See WARNINGS.

Nursing Mothers: It is not known whether this drug is excreted in human milk. Because many drugs are excreted in human milk and because of the potential for serious adverse reactions in nursing infants from NOLVADEX, a decision should be made whether to discontinue nursing or to discontinue the drug, taking into account the importance of the drug to the mother.

ADVERSE REACTIONS

The most frequent adverse reactions to NOLVADEX are hot flashes, nausea, and vomiting. These may occur in up to one-fourth of patients, but are rarely severe enough to require discontinuation of treatment.

Less frequently reported adverse reactions are vaginal bleeding, vaginal discharge, menstrual irregularities, and skin rash. Usually these have not been of sufficient severity to require dosage reduction or discontinuation of treatment.

Increased bone and tumor pain, and also local disease flare have occurred which are sometimes associated with a good tumor response. Patients with increased bone pain may require additional analgesics. Patients with soft tissue disease may have sudden increases in the size of preexisting lesions, sometimes associated with marked erythema within and surrounding the lesions, and/or the development of new lesions. When they occur, the bone pain or disease flare are seen shortly after starting NOLVADEX and generally subside rapidly.

Other adverse reactions which are seen infrequently are hypercalcemia, peripheral edema, distaste for food, pruritus vulvae, depression, dizziness, light-headedness, and headache. There have been infrequent reports of thromboembolic events occurring during NOLVADEX therapy. Since for cancer patients in general, an increased incidence of thromboembolic events is known to occur, a causal relationship to NOLVADEX remains conjectural. An increased incidence has been reported when cytotoxins are combined with NOLVADEX.

If adverse reactions are severe, it is sometimes possible to control them by a simple reduction of dosage without loss of control of the disease.

OVERDOSAGE

Acute overdosage in humans has not been reported. Signs observed at the highest doses following studies to determine LD_{50} in animals were respiratory difficulties and convulsions. No specific treatment for overdosage is known; treatment must be symptomatic.

DOSAGE AND ADMINISTRATION

One or two 10 mg tablets twice a day (morning and evening).

HOW SUPPLIED

Tablets containing tamoxifen as the citrate in an amount equivalent to 10 mg of tamoxifen (round, biconvex, uncoated, white tablet identified with NOLVADEX 600 debossed on one side and a cameo debossed on the other side) are supplied in bottles of 60 tablets and 250 tablets. Protect from heat and light. NDC 0038-0600.

Shown in Product Identification Section, page 432

6/6/86

Continued on next page

Stuart—Cont.

OREXIN® SOFTAB® Tablets
[or 'ex-in]

INGREDIENTS

Each tablet contains: Vitamin B, (thiamine mononitrate) 10 mg.; Vitamin B_6 (as pyridoxine hydrochloride), 5 mg.; and Vitamin B_{12} (cyanocobalamin), 25 mcg. Inactive: flavor, mannitol, saccharin calcium, sodium chloride, starch.

INDICATIONS

OREXIN is a high-potency vitamin supplement providing vitamins B_1, B_6, and B_{12}.
OREXIN SOFTAB tablets are specially formulated to dissolve quickly in the mouth. They may be chewed or swallowed. Dissolve tablet in a teaspoonful of water or fruit juice if liquid is preferred.

DIRECTIONS

One tablet daily, or as directed by physician.

WARNINGS

Keep this and all drugs out of the reach of children.

HOW SUPPLIED

Bottles of 100 pale pink SOFTAB tablets, identified "STUART".
NDC 0038-0280.

PROBEC®-T Tablets
[pro 'bek-t]
Vitamin B Complex Supplement

INGREDIENTS

Each tablet contains: vitamin C (as ascorbic acid, 67 mg. and sodium ascorbate, 600 mg.), 600 mg.; thiamine mononitrate, 15 mg.; riboflavin, 10 mg.; vitamin B_6 (as pyridoxine hydrochloride), 5 mg.; vitamin B_{12} (cyanocobalamin), 5 mcg.; niacinamide, 100 mg.; calcium pantothenate, 20 mg.
Inactive: calcium sulfate, carnauba wax, magnesium oxide, pharmaceutical glaze, povidone, Red 30, sucrose, titanium dioxide, white wax, Yellow 10.

INDICATIONS

PROBEC-T is a high-potency B complex supplement with 600 mg. of Vitamin C in easy to swallow odorless tablets.

DIRECTIONS

One tablet a day with a meal, or as directed by physician.

WARNING

As with all medications, keep out of the reach of children.

HOW SUPPLIED

Bottles of 60, peach colored, capsule-shaped tablets.
NDC 0038-0840.
Shown in Product Identification Section, page 432

SORBITRATE® ℞
[sorb 'i-trate]
(Isosorbide Dinitrate)

DESCRIPTION

SORBITRATE (isosorbide dinitrate), an organic nitrate, is a vasodilator with effects on both arteries and veins.
SORBITRATE is available as:
SORBITRATE SUBLINGUAL
2.5 mg Sublingual Tablet. Each tablet contains 2.5 mg of isosorbide dinitrate.
Inactive ingredients: lactose, magnesium stearate, starch.
5 mg Sublingual Tablet. Each tablet contains 5 mg of isosorbide dinitrate.
Inactive ingredients: lactose, magnesium stearate, Red 3, starch.
10 mg Sublingual Tablet. Each tablet contains 10 mg of isosorbide dinitrate.
Inactive ingredients: lactose, magnesium stearate, starch, Yellow 10.
SORBITRATE CHEWABLE
5 mg Chewable Tablet. Each tablet contains 5 mg of isosorbide dinitrate.
Inactive ingredients: Blue 1, confectioner's sugar, flavor, hydrogenated vegetable oil, magnesium stearate, mannitol, povidone, starch, Yellow 10.
10 mg Chewable Tablet. Each tablet contains 10 mg of isosorbide dinitrate.
Inactive ingredients: confectioner's sugar, flavor, hydrogenated vegetable oil, magnesium stearate, mannitol, povidone, starch, Yellow 10.
SORBITRATE ORAL
5 mg Oral Tablet. Each tablet contains 5 mg of isosorbide dinitrate.
Inactive ingredients: Blue 1, lactose, magnesium stearate, starch, Yellow 10.
10 mg Oral Tablet. Each tablet contains 10 mg of isosorbide dinitrate.
Inactive ingredients: lactose, magnesium stearate, starch, Yellow 10.
20 mg Oral Tablet. Each tablet contains 20 mg of isosorbide dinitrate.
Inactive ingredients: Blue 1, lactose, magnesium stearate, starch.
30 mg Oral Tablet. Each tablet contains 30 mg of isosorbide dinitrate.
Inactive ingredients: lactose, magnesium stearate, starch.
40 mg Oral Tablet. Each tablet contains 40 mg of isosorbide dinitrate.
Inactive ingredients: Blue 1, lactose, magnesium stearate, starch.
SORBITRATE SA
Sustained Action Tablet. Each tablet contains 10 mg of isosorbide dinitrate in the outer coat and 30 mg in the inner core (sustained action base).
Inactive ingredients: carbomer 934P, ethylcellulose, lactose, magnesium stearate, polyethylene glycol, Yellow 10.
The chemical name for isosorbide dinitrate is 1,4,3,6-dianhydrosorbitol-2,5-dinitrate.
MOLECULAR WEIGHT: 236.14
Isosorbide dinitrate is a white, crystalline, odorless compound which is stable in air and in solution, has a melting point of 70°C and has an optical rotation of +134° c = 1.0, alcohol, 20°C). Isosorbide dinitrate is freely soluble in organic solvents such as acetone, alcohol, and ether; but is only sparingly soluble in water.

CLINICAL PHARMACOLOGY

The principal pharmacological action of isosorbide dinitrate is relaxation of vascular smooth muscle, producing a vasodilatory effect on both peripheral arteries and veins, with predominant effects on the latter. Dilation of the post-capillary vessels, including large veins, promotes peripheral pooling of blood and decreases venous return to the heart, thereby reducing left-ventricular end-diastolic pressure (preload). Arteriolar relaxation reduces systemic vascular resistance and arterial pressure (after-load).
The mechanism by which isosorbide dinitrate relieves angina pectoris is not fully understood. Myocardial oxygen consumption or demand (as measured by the pressure-rate product, tension-time index, and stroke-work index) is decreased by both the arterial and venous effects of isosorbide dinitrate and, presumably, a more favorable supply-demand ratio is achieved. While the large epicardial coronary arteries are also dilated by isosorbide dinitrate, the extent to which this contributes to relief of exertional angina is unclear.
Therapeutic doses of isosorbide dinitrate may reduce systolic, diastolic, and mean arterial blood pressures, especially in the upright posture. Effective coronary perfusion is usually maintained. The decrease in systemic blood pressure may result in reflex tachycardia, an effect which results in an unfavorable influence on myocardial oxygen demand. Hemodynamic studies indicate that isosorbide dinitrate may reduce the abnormally elevated left ventricular end-diastolic and pulmonary capillary wedge pressures that occur during an acute episode of angina pectoris.
Isosorbide dinitrate is metabolized by enzymatic denitration to the intermediate products isosorbide-2-mononitrate and isosorbide-5-mononitrate. Both metabolites have biological activity, especially the 5-mononitrate which is also the principal metabolite. The liver is a principal site of metabolism and isosorbide dinitrate is subject to a large first-pass effect. The systemic clearance of the drug following intravenous infusion is about 3.4 liters/min. Since the clearance exceeds hepatic blood flow, considerable extrahepatic metabolism must also occur.
The average bioavailability of isosorbide dinitrate is 59 and 22 percent following sublingual and oral administration, respectively. The terminal half-life is about 20 minutes, 60 minutes, and 4 hours following i.v., sublingual, and oral administration, respectively. The dependence of half-life on the route of administration is not understood. Over limited ranges of i.v. dosing, the pharmacokinetics of isosorbide dinitrate appear linear. However, both the 2- and 5-mononitrate metabolites have been shown to decrease the rate of disappearance of the dinitrate from the blood and the half-lives of isosorbide-5-mononitrate and isosorbide-2-mononitrate range from 4.0–5.6 and 1.5–3.1 hours, respectively.
The pharmacokinetics and/or bioavailability of isosorbide dinitrate during multiple dosing have not been well studied. Because the metabolites influence the clearance of isosorbide dinitrate, prediction of blood levels of parent compound or metabolites from single-dose studies is uncertain.

INDICATIONS AND USAGE

SORBITRATE (isosorbide dinitrate) is indicated for the treatment and prevention of angina pectoris. Controlled clinical trials have demonstrated that the sublingual, chewable, immediate release, and controlled release oral dosage forms of isosorbide dinitrate are effective in improving exercise tolerance in patients with angina pectoris. When single sublingual or chewable doses (5 mg) of isosorbide dinitrate were administered prophylactically to patients with angina pectoris in various clinical studies, duration of exercise until chest pain or fatigue was significantly improved for at least 45 minutes (and as long as 2 hours in some studies) following dosing. Similar studies after single oral (15 to 120 mg) and oral controlled-release (40 to 80 mg) doses of isosorbide dinitrate have shown significant improvement in exercise tolerance for up to 8 hours following dosing. The exercise electrocardiographic evidence suggests that improved exercise tolerance with isosorbide dinitrate is not at the expense of greater myocardial ischemia. All dosage forms of isosorbide dinitrate may therefore be used prophylactically to decrease frequency and severity of anginal attacks and can be expected to decrease the need for sublingual nitroglycerin.
The sublingual and chewable forms of the drug are indicated for acute prophylaxis of angina pectoris when taken a few minutes before situations likely to provoke anginal attacks. Because of a slower onset of effect, the oral forms of isosorbide dinitrate are not indicated for acute prophylaxis.
In controlled clinical trials, chewable and sublingual isosorbide dinitrate were effective in relieving an acute attack of angina pectoris. Relief occurred with a mean time of 2.9 and 3.4 minutes (chewable and sublingual respectively) compared to relief of angina with a mean time of 1.9 minutes following sublingual nitroglycerin. Because of the more rapid relief of chest pain with sublingual nitroglycerin, the use of sublingual or chewable isosorbide dinitrate for aborting an acute anginal attack should be limited to patients intolerant or unresponsive to sublingual nitroglycerin.

CONTRAINDICATIONS

SORBITRATE is contraindicated in patients who have shown purported hypersensitivity or idiosyncrasy to it or other nitrates or nitrites.

WARNINGS

The benefits of SORBITRATE during the early days of an acute myocardial infarction have not been established. If one elects to use organic nitrates in early infarction, hemodynamic monitoring and frequent clinical assessment should be used because of the potential deleterious effects of hypotension.

PRECAUTIONS

General: Severe hypotensive response, particularly with upright posture, may occur with even small doses of SORBITRATE. The drug should therefore be used with caution in subjects who may have blood volume depletion from diuretic therapy or in subjects who have low systolic blood pressure (e.g., below 90 mmHg). Paradoxical bradycardia and increased angina pectoris may accompany nitrate-induced hypotension.
Nitrate therapy may aggravate the angina caused by hypertrophic cardiomyopathy. Tolerance to this drug and cross-tolerance to other nitrates and nitrites may occur.
Marked symptomatic, orthostatic hypotension has been reported when calcium channel blockers and organic nitrates were used in combination. Dose adjustment of either class of agents may be necessary.
Tolerance to the vascular and antianginal effects of isosorbide dinitrate or nitroglycerin has been demonstrated in clinical trials, experience through occupational exposure, and in isolated tissue experiments in the laboratory. The importance of tolerance to the appropriate use of isosorbide dinitrate in the management of patients with angina pectoris has not been determined. However, one clinical trial using treadmill exercise tolerance (as an endpoint) found an 8-hour duration of action of oral isosorbide dinitrate following the first dose (after a 2-week placebo washout) and only a 2-hour duration of effect of the same dose after 1 week of repetitive dosing at conventional dosing intervals. On the other hand, several trials have been able to differentiate isosorbide dinitrate from placebo after 4 weeks of therapy, and in open trials, an effect seems detectable for as long as several months.
Tolerance clearly occurs in industrial workers continuously exposed to nitroglycerin. Moreover, physical dependence also occurs since chest pain, acute myocardial infarction, and even sudden death have occurred during temporary withdrawal of nitroglycerin from the workers. In clinical trials in angina patients, there are reports of anginal attacks being more easily provoked and of rebound in the hemodynamic effects soon after nitrate withdrawal. The relative importance of these observations to the routine, clinical use of isosorbide dinitrate is not known. However, it seems prudent to gradually withdraw patients from isosorbide dinitrate when the therapy is being terminated, rather than stopping the drug abruptly.
Information for Patients: Headache may occur during initial therapy with SORBITRATE. Headache is usually relieved by the use of standard headache remedies, or by lowering the dose, and tends to disappear after the first week or two of use.
Drug Interactions: Alcohol may enhance any marked sensitivity to the hypotensive effect of nitrates.

Isosorbide dinitrate acts directly on vascular smooth muscle; therefore, any other agent that depends on vascular smooth muscle as the final common path can be expected to have decreased or increased effect depending on the agent.

Carcinogenesis, Mutagenesis, Impairment of Fertility: No long-term studies in animals have been performed to evaluate the carcinogenic potential of this drug. A modified two-litter reproduction study in rats fed isosorbide dinitrate at 25 or 100 mg/kg/day did not reveal any effects on fertility or gestation or any remarkable gross pathology in any parent or offspring fed isosorbide dinitrate as compared with rats fed a basal-controlled diet.

Pregnancy Category C: Isosorbide dinitrate has been shown to cause a dose-related increase in embryotoxicity (increase in mummified pups) in rabbits at oral doses 35 and 150 times the maximum recommended human daily dose. There are no adequate and well-controlled studies in pregnant women. SORBITRATE should be used during pregnancy only if the potential benefit justifies the potential risk to the fetus.

Nursing Mothers: It is not known whether this drug is excreted in human milk. Because many drugs are excreted in human milk, caution should be exercised when SORBITRATE is administered to a nursing woman.

Pediatric Use: The safety and effectiveness of SORBITRATE in children has not been established.

ADVERSE REACTIONS

Adverse reactions, particularly headache and hypotension, are dose related. In clinical trials at various doses, the following have been observed.

Headache is the most common (reported incidence varies widely, apparently being dose related, with an average occurrence of about 25%) adverse reaction and may be severe and persistent. Cutaneous vasodilation with flushing may occur. Transient episodes of dizziness and weakness, as well as other signs of cerebral ischemia associated with postural hypotension, may occasionally develop (the incidence of reported symptomatic hypotension ranges from 2% to 36%). An occasional individual will exhibit marked sensitivity to the hypotensive effects of nitrates and severe responses (nausea, vomiting, weakness, restlessness, pallor, perspiration, and collapse) may occur even with the usual therapeutic dose. Drug rash and/or exfoliative dermatitis may occasionally occur. Nausea and vomiting appear to be uncommon.

OVERDOSAGE

Signs and Symptoms: These may include the following: a prompt fall in blood pressure, persistent and throbbing headache, vertigo, palpitation, visual disturbances, flushed and perspiring skin (later becoming cold and cyanotic), nausea and vomiting (possibly with colic and even bloody diarrhea), syncope (especially in the upright position), methemoglobinemia with cyanosis and anoxia, initial hyperpnea, dyspnea and slow breathing, slow pulse (dicrotic and intermittent), heart block, increased intracranial pressure with cerebral symptoms of confusion and moderate fever, paralysis and coma followed by clonic convulsions and possibly death due to circulatory collapse.

It is not known what dose of the drug is associated with symptoms of overdosing or what dose of the drug would be life-threatening. The acute oral LD_{50} of isosorbide dinitrate in rats was found to be approximately 1100 mg/kg of body weight. These animal experiments indicate that approximately 500 times the usual therapeutic dose would be required to produce such toxic symptoms in humans. It is not known whether the drug is dialyzable.

Treatment of Overdose: Prompt removal of the ingested material by gastric lavage is reasonable, but not documented to be useful. Keep the patient recumbent in a shock position and comfortably warm. Passive movements of the extremities may aid venous return. Administer oxygen and artificial respiration if necessary. If methemoglobinemia is present, administer methylene blue (1% solution), 1 to 2 mg/kg intravenously.

Methemoglobin: Case reports of clinically significant methemoglobinemia are rare at conventional doses of organic nitrates. The formation of methemoglobin is dose related and in the case of genetic abnormalities of hemoglobin that favor methemoglobin formulation, even conventional doses of organic nitrate could produce harmful concentrations of methemoglobin.

WARNING

Epinephrine is ineffective in reversing the severe hypotensive events associated with overdose. It and related compounds are contraindicated in this situation.

DOSAGE AND ADMINISTRATION

For the treatment of angina pectoris, the usual starting dose for sublingual SORBITRATE is 2.5 to 5 mg; and for chewable tablets, 5 mg.

SORBITRATE should be titrated upward until angina is relieved or side effects limit the dose. In ambulatory patients, the magnitude of the incremental dose increase should be guided by measurements of standing blood pressure.

The initial dosage of sublingual or chewable SORBITRATE for acute prophylactic therapy in angina pectoris patients is generally 5 or 10 mg every 2 to 3 hours. Adequate, controlled clinical studies demonstrating the effectiveness of chronic maintenance therapy with these dosage forms have not been reported.

For the treatment of chronic stable angina pectoris, the usual starting dose for immediate-release oral (swallowed) SORBITATE tablets is 5 to 20 mg; and for controlled-release forms, 40 mg. For maintenance therapy, oral doses of 10 to 40 mg given every 6 hours; or oral controlled-release doses of 40 to 80 mg given every 8 to 12 hours is generally recommended. The extent to which development of tolerance should modify the dosage program has not been defined. **The oral controlled release forms of isosorbide dinitrate should not be chewed.**

HOW SUPPLIED

SORBITRATE Sublingual

2.5 mg Sublingual Tablets. (NDC-0038-0853) White, round tablets (identified front "S", reverse "853") are supplied in bottles of 100, 500, and Unit Dose 100.

5 mg Sublingual Tablets. (NDC-0038-0760) Pink, round tablets (identified front "S", reverse "760") are supplied in bottles of 100, 500, and Unit Dose 100.

10 mg Sublingual Tablets. (NDC-0038-0761) Yellow, round tablets (identified front "S", reverse "761") are supplied in bottles of 100 and Unit Dose 100.

SORBITRATE Chewable

5 mg Chewable Tablets. (NDC-0038-0810) Green, round, scored tablets (identified front "STUART", reverse "810") are supplied in bottles of 100, 500, and Unit Dose 100.

10 mg Chewable Tablets. (NDC-0038-0815) Yellow, round, scored tablets (identified front "STUART", reverse "815") are supplied in bottles of 100 and Unit Dose 100.

SORBITRATE Oral

5 mg Oral Tablets. (NDC-0038-0770) Green, oval-shaped, scored tablets (identified front "STUART", reverse "770") are supplied in bottles of 100, 500, and Unit Dose 100.

10 mg Oral Tablets. (NDC-0038-0780) Yellow, oval-shaped, scored tablets (identified front "STUART", reverse "780") are supplied in bottles of 100, 500, and Unit Dose 100.

20 mg Oral Tablets. (NDC-0038-0820) Blue, oval-shaped, scored tablets (identified front "STUART", reverse "820") are supplied in bottles of 100 and Unit Dose 100.

30 mg Oral Tablets. (NDC-0038-0773) White, oval-shaped, scored tablets (identified front "STUART", reverse "773") are supplied in bottles of 100 and Unit Dose 100.

40 mg Oral Tablets. (NDC-0038-0774) Light blue, oval-shaped, scored tablets (identified front "STUART", reverse "774") are supplied in bottles of 100 and Unit Dose 100.

SORBITRATE SA

40 mg Sustained Action Tablets. (NDC-0038-0880) Yellow, round, compression-coated tablets (identified front "STUART", reverse "880") are supplied in bottles of 100 and Unit Dose 100.

All forms of SORBITRATE should be stored in a dry place at room temperature. Avoid excessive heat (over 104°F/40°C).

Shown in Product Identification Section, page 432

THE STUART FORMULA® Tablets

Multivitamin/Multimineral Supplement

INGREDIENTS

Each tablet contains:

Active:

<u>Vitamins:</u> vitamin A (as palmitate), 5000 I.U.; vitamin D (ergocalciferol), 400 I.U.; vitamin E (as dl-alpha tocopheryl acetate), 15 I.U.; vitamin C (as ascorbic acid), 60 mg.; folic acid, 0.4 mg.; thiamine (as thiamine mononitrate), 1.5 mg.; riboflavin, 1.7 mg.; niacin (as niacinamide), 20 mg.; vitamin B_6 (as pyridoxine hydrochloride), 2 mg.; vitamin B_{12} (cyanocobalamin), 6 mcg.

<u>Minerals:</u> calcium 160 mg.; phosphorus, 125 mg.; iodine, 150 mcg.; iron (from 54 mg. ferrous fumarate) 18 mg.; magnesium, 100 mg.

Inactive: calcium sulfate, carnauba wax, pharmaceutical glaze, povidone, sodium starch glycolate, sucrose, titanium dioxide, white wax.

INDICATIONS

The STUART FORMULA tablet provides a well-balanced multivitamin/multimineral formula intended for use as a daily dietary supplement for adults and children over age four.

DIRECTIONS

One tablet daily or as directed by a physician.

WARNINGS

Keep this and all drugs out of the reach of children.

HOW SUPPLIED

Bottles of 100 and 250 white round tablets. Childproof safety caps are standard on both bottles as a safeguard against accidental ingestion by children.

NDC 0038-0866.

Shown in Product Identification Section, page 432

STUART PRENATAL® Tablets

Multivitamin/Multimineral Supplement

INGREDIENTS

Each tablet contains:

Vitamins			**US RDA***
A	8,000	IU	100%
D	400	IU	100%
E	30	IU	100%
C	60	mg	100%
Folic Acid	0.8	IU	100%
Thiamine	1.7	IU	100%
Riboflavin	2	mg	100%
Niacin	20	mg	100%
B_4	4	mg	160%
B_{12}	8	mcg	100%
Minerals			
Calcium (from 679 mg calcium sulfate anhydrous)	200	mg	15%
Iodine	150	mcg	100%
Iron (from 182 mg ferrous fumarate)	60	mg	333%
Magnesium	100	mg	22%
Zinc	25	mg	165%

* US Recommended Daily Allowance

Iron Content of Various Iron Sources:

Ferrous Fumarate	33%
Ferrous Sulfate ex	30%
Ferrous Sulfate	20%
Ferrous Gluconate	12%

Calcium Content of Various Calcium Sources:

Calcium Carbonate*	40%
Calcium Sulfate Anhydrous	29%
Dicalcium Phosphate	23%
Calcium Gluconate	9%

* May have antacid effect

Ingredients: Each tablet contains:

Active: calcium sulfate, ferrous fumarate, magnesium oxide, ascorbic acid, dl-alpha tocopheryl acetate, zinc oxide, niacinamide, vitamin A acetate, pyridoxine hydrochloride, riboflavin, thiamine, mononitrate, folic acid, ergocalciferol, potassium iodide, cyanocobalamin. Inactive: carnauba wax, pharmaceutical glaze, povidone, Red 3, sodium starch glycolate, starch, sucrose, titanium dioxide, white wax.

INDICATIONS

STUART PRENATAL is a non-prescription multivitamin/multimineral supplement for use before, during, and after pregnancy. It provides vitamins equal to 100% or more of the U.S. RDA for pregnant and lactating women, plus essential minerals, including 60 mg. of elemental iron as well-tolerated ferrous fumarate, 200 mg. of elemental calcium (non-alkalizing and phosphorus-free), and 25 mg. zinc.

DIRECTIONS

Before, during and after pregnancy, one tablet daily after a meal, or as directed by a physician.

WARNINGS

As with all medications, keep out of the reach of children.

HOW SUPPLIED

Bottles of 100 pink capsule-shaped tablets. A childproof safety cap is standard on 100 tablet bottles as a safeguard against accidental ingestion by children.

NDC 0038-0073.

Shown in Product Identification Section, page 432

STUARTINIC® Tablets

[stu 'ar tin "ik]

Hematinic

INGREDIENTS

Each tablet contains: Active: iron (from 300 mg. ferrous fumarate), 100 mg.; vitamin C (as ascorbic acid, 300 mg. and sodium ascorbate, 225 mg.), 500 mg.; vitamin B_{12} (cyanocobalamin), 25 mcg.; thiamine mononitrate, 6 mg.; riboflavin, 6 mg.; vitamin B_6 (as pyridoxine hydrochloride), 1 mg.; niacinamide, 20 mg.; calcium pantothenate, 10 mg. Inactive: flavor, hydrogenated vegetable oil, microcrystalline cellulose, povidone, Yellow 10, and other ingredients.

INDICATIONS

STUARTINIC is a complete hematinic for patients with history of iron deficiency anemia who also lack proper amounts of vitamin C and B-complex vitamins due to inadequate diet.

The use of well-tolerated ferrous fumarate in STUARTINIC provides a high level of elemental iron with a low incidence of gastric distress. The inclusion of 500 mg. of Vitamin C per tablet serves to maintain more of the iron in the absorbable ferrous state. The B-complex vitamins improve nutrition where B-complex deficient diets contribute to the anemia.

Continued on next page

Stuart—Cont.

PRECAUTIONS
Because STUARTINIC contains 100 mg. of elemental iron per tablet, use should be confined to adults, i.e. over age 12 years.

WARNINGS
As with any drug, if you are pregnant or nursing a baby, seek the advice of a health professional before using this product. Keep out of the reach of children.

DIRECTIONS
One tablet daily taken after a meal to maintain normal hemoglobin levels in most patients with chronic iron deficiency anemia resulting from inadequate diet. Higher doses of STUARTINIC can be taken as directed by the physician.

HOW SUPPLIED
STUARTINIC is supplied in bottles of 60 yellow, film coated, oval shaped tablets. NDC 0038-0862.

Note: A childproof safety cap is standard on each 60 tablet bottle as a safeguard against accidental ingestion by children.

Shown in Product Identification Section, page 432

STUARTNATAL® 1+1 Tablets ℞
[stu 'art na 'tal]
Multivitamin/Multimineral Supplement

COMPOSITION
One tablet daily provides:

Vitamins		**US RDA***
A	8,000 IU	100%
D (ergocalciferol)	400 IU	100%
E	30 IU	100%
C (ascorbic acid)	90 mg	150%
Folic Acid	1 mg	125%
Thiamine (as thiamine mononitrate)	2.55 mg	150%
Riboflavin	3 mg	150%
Niacin (as niacinamide)	20 mg	100%
B_6 (as pyridoxine hydrochloride)	10 mg	400%
B_{12}	12 mcg	150%
Minerals		
Calcium (from 679 mg calcium sulfate anhydrous)	200 mg	15%
Iodine	150 mcg	100%
Iron (from 197 mg ferrous fumarate)	65 mg	361%
Magnesium	100 mg	22%
Zinc	25 mg	165%

*US Recommended Daily Allowance

Iron Content of Various Iron Sources:	
Ferrous Fumarate	33%
Ferrous Sulfate ex	30%
Ferrous Sulfate	20%
Ferrous Gluconate	12%
Calcium Content of Various Calcium Sources:	
Calcium Carbonate*	40%
Calcium Sulfate Anhydrous	29%
Dicalcium Phosphate	23%
Calcium Gluconate	9%

*May have antacid effect

INDICATIONS
STUARTNATAL 1+1 is indicated to provide potent vitamin and mineral supplementation throughout pregnancy and during the postnatal period—for both the lactating and nonlactating mother. It is also useful for improving nutritional status prior to conception.

Each tablet provides vitamins equal to 100% or more of U.S. RDA for pregnant and lactating women plus essential minerals, including 1 full grain of elemental iron and 200 mg. of elemental calcium (non-alkalizing and phosphorus-free), and 25 mg. zinc. STUARTNATAL 1+1 also offers 1 mg. folic acid to aid in the prevention of megaloblastic anemia.

PRECAUTION
Folic acid may partially correct the hematological damage due to Vitamin B_{12} deficiency of pernicious anemia, while the associated neurological damage progresses.

DIRECTIONS
Before, during and after pregnancy, one tablet daily after a meal, or as directed by a physician.

HOW SUPPLIED
Bottles of 100 and 500 light yellow capsule-shaped tablets identified "Stuart 023". A childproof safety cap is standard on 100 tablet bottles as a safeguard against accidental ingestion by children.
NDC 0038-0023.

Shown in Product Identification Section, page 432

TENORETIC® ℞
[ten 'or-et ik"]
(atenolol and chlorthalidone)

DESCRIPTION
TENORETIC (atenolol and chlorthalidone) is for the treatment of hypertension. It combines the antihypertensive activity of two agents: a $beta_1$-selective (cardioselective) hydrophilic blocking agent (atenolol, TENORMIN®) and a monosulfonamyl diuretic (chlorthalidone).

Atenolol is Benzeneacetamide, 4-[2'-hydroxy-3'-[(1-methylethyl) amino]propoxy]-.

Atenolol (free base) is a relatively polar hydrophilic compound with a water solubility of 26.5 mg/mL at 37°C. It is freely soluble in 1 N HCl (300 mg/mL at 25°C) and less soluble in chloroform (3 mg/mL at 25°C).

Chlorthalidone is 2-Chloro-5-(1-hydroxy-3-oxo-1-isoindolinyl) benzene sulfonamide.

Chlorthalidone has a water solubility of 12 mg/100 mL at 20°C.

Each TENORETIC 50 tablet contains:

Atenolol (TENORMIN)	50 mg
Chlorthalidone	25 mg

Each TENORETIC 100 tablet contains:

Atenolol (TENORMIN)	100 mg
Chlorthalidone	25 mg

Inactive ingredients: magnesium stearate, microcrystalline cellulose, povidone, sodium starch glycolate.

CLINICAL PHARMACOLOGY
Atenolol and chlorthalidone have been used singly and concomitantly for the treatment of hypertension. The antihypertensive effects of these agents are additive and studies have shown that there is no interference with bioavailability when these agents are given together in the single combination tablet. Therefore, this combination provides a convenient formulation for the concomitant administration of these two entities. In patients with more severe hypertension, TENORETIC may be administered with other antihypertensives such as vasodilators.

Atenolol: Atenolol is a $beta_1$-selective (cardioselective) beta-adrenergic receptor blocking agent without membrane stabilizing or intrinsic sympathomimetic (partial agonist) activities. This preferential effect is not absolute however and, at higher doses, atenolol inhibits $beta_2$-adrenoreceptors, chiefly located in the bronchial and vascular musculature.

Pharmacodynamics: In standard animal or human pharmacological tests, beta-adrenoreceptor blocking activity of atenolol has been demonstrated by: 1) reduction in resting and exercise heart rate and cardiac output, 2) reduction of systolic and diastolic blood pressure at rest and on exercise, 3) inhibition of isoproterenol induced tachycardia, and 4) reduction in reflex orthostatic tachycardia.

A significant beta-blocking effect of atenolol, as measured by reduction of exercise tachycardia, is apparent within 1 hour following oral administration of a single dose. This effect is maximal at about 2 to 4 hours and persists for at least 24 hours. The effect at 24 hours is dose-related and also bears a linear relationship to the logarithm of plasma atenolol concentration. However, as has been shown for all beta-blocking agents, the antihypertensive effect does not appear to be related to plasma level.

In normal subjects, the $beta_1$-selectivity of atenolol has been shown by its reduced ability to reverse the $beta_2$-mediated vasodilating effect of isoproterenol as compared to equivalent beta-blocking doses of propranolol. In asthmatic patients, a dose of atenolol producing a greater effect on resting heart rate than propranolol resulted in much less increase in airway resistance. In a placebo-controlled comparison of approximately equipotent oral doses of several beta blockers, atenolol produced a significantly smaller decrease of FEV_1 than nonselective beta blockers such as propranolol and unlike those agents did not inhibit bronchodilation in response to isoproterenol.

Consistent with its negative chronotropic effect due to beta blockade of the SA node, atenolol increases sinus cycle length and sinus node recovery time. Conduction in the AV node is also prolonged. Atenolol is devoid of membrane stabilizing activity, and increasing the dose well beyond that producing beta blockade does not further depress myocardial contractility. Several studies have demonstrated a moderate (approximately 10%) increase in stroke volume at rest and exercise.

In controlled clinical trials, atenolol given as a single daily dose, was an effective antihypertensive agent providing 24-hour reduction of blood pressure. Atenolol has been studied in combination with thiazide-type diuretics and the blood pressure effects of the combination are approximately additive. Atenolol is also compatible with methyldopa, hydralazine, and prazosin, the combination resulting in a larger fall in blood pressure than with the single agents. The dose range of atenolol is narrow, and increasing the dose beyond 100 mg once daily is not associated with increased antihypertensive effect. The mechanisms of the antihypertensive effects of beta-blocking agents have not been established. Several mechanisms have been proposed and include: 1) competitive antagonism of catecholamines at peripheral (especially cardiac) adrenergic neuron sites, leading to decreased cardiac output, 2) a central effect leading to reduced sympathetic outflow to the periphery, and 3) suppression of renin activity. The results from long-term studies have not shown any diminution of the antihypertensive efficacy of atenolol with prolonged use.

Pharmacokinetics and Metabolism: In man, absorption of an oral dose is rapid and consistent but incomplete. Approximately 50% of an oral dose is absorbed from the gastrointestinal tract, the remainder being excreted unchanged in the feces. Peak blood levels are reached between 2 and 4 hours after ingestion. Unlike propranolol or metoprolol, but like nadolol, hydrophilic atenolol undergoes little or no metabolism by the liver and the absorbed portion is eliminated primarily by renal excretion. Atenolol also differs from propranolol in that only a small amount (6-16%) is bound to proteins in the plasma. This kinetic profile results in relatively consistent plasma drug levels with about a fourfold interpatient variation. There is no information as to the pharmacokinetic effect of atenolol on chlorthalidone.

The elimination half-life of atenolol is approximately 6 to 7 hours, and there is no alteration of the kinetic profile of the drug by chronic administration. Following doses of 50 mg or 100 mg, both beta-blocking and antihypertensive effects persist for at least 24 hours. When renal function is impaired, elimination of atenolol is closely related to the glomerular filtration rate; but significant accumulation does not occur until the creatinine clearance falls below 35 mL/min/1.73 m^2. (See circular for atenolol [TENORMIN]).

Chlorthalidone: A monosulfonamyl diuretic which differs chemically from thiazide diuretics in that a double ring system is incorporated in its structure. It is an oral diuretic with prolonged action and low toxicity. The diuretic effect of the drug occurs within 2 hours of an oral dose. It produces diuresis with greatly increased excretion of sodium and chloride. At maximal therapeutic dosage, chlorthalidone is approximately equal in its diuretic effect to comparable maximal therapeutic doses of benzothiadiazine diuretics. The site of action appears to be the cortical diluting segment of the ascending limb of Henle's loop of the nephron.

INDICATIONS AND USAGE
TENORETIC is indicated for the treatment of hypertension. This fixed-dose combination drug is not indicated for initial therapy of hypertension. If the fixed-dose combination represents the dose appropriate to the individual patient's needs, it may be more convenient than the separate components.

CONTRAINDICATIONS
TENORETIC is contraindicated in patients with: sinus bradycardia, heart block greater than first degree, cardiogenic shock, overt cardiac failure (see WARNINGS), anuria, hypersensitivity to this product or to sulfonamide-derived drugs.

WARNINGS
Cardiac Failure: Sympathetic stimulation is necessary in supporting circulatory function in congestive heart failure, and beta blockade carries the potential hazard of further depressing myocardial contractility and precipitating more severe failure. In hypertensive patients who have congestive heart failure controlled by digitalis and diuretics, TENORETIC should be administered cautiously. Both digitalis and atenolol slow AV conduction.

IN PATIENTS WITHOUT A HISTORY OF CARDIAC FAILURE, continued depression of the myocardium with beta-blocking agents over a period of time can, in some cases, lead to cardiac failure. At the first sign or symptom of impending cardiac failure, patients receiving TENORETIC should be digitalized and/or be given additional diuretic therapy. Observe the patient closely. If cardiac failure continues despite adequate digitalization and diuretic therapy, TENORETIC therapy should be withdrawn.

Renal and Hepatic Disease and Electrolyte Disturbances: Since atenolol is excreted via the kidneys, TENORETIC should be used with caution in patients with impaired renal function.

In patients with renal disease, thiazides may precipitate azotemia. Since cumulative effects may develop in the presence of impaired renal function, if progressive renal impairment becomes evident TENORETIC should be discontinued.

In patients with impaired hepatic function or progressive liver disease, minor alterations in fluid and electrolyte balance may precipitate hepatic coma. TENORETIC should be used with caution in these patients.

Ischemic Heart Disease: Although not yet reported with atenolol following abrupt cessation of therapy with certain beta-blocking agents in patients with coronary artery disease, exacerbations of angina pectoris and, in some cases, myocardial infarction have been reported. Therefore, such patients should be cautioned against interruption of therapy without the physician's advice. Even in the absence of overt angina pectoris, when discontinuation of TENORETIC is planned, the patient should be carefully observed and should be advised to limit physical activity to a minimum.

TENORETIC should be reinstated if withdrawal symptoms occur.

Bronchospastic Diseases: PATIENTS WITH BRONCHOSPASTIC DISEASE SHOULD, IN GENERAL, NOT RECEIVE BETA BLOCKERS. Because of its relative beta$_1$-selectivity, however, TENORETIC may be used with caution in patients with bronchospastic disease who do not respond to, or cannot tolerate, other antihypertensive treatment. Since beta$_1$-selectivity is not absolute, the lowest possible dose of TENORETIC should be used and a beta$_2$-stimulating agent (bronchodilator) should be made available. If dosage must be increased, dividing the dose should be considered in order to achieve lower peak blood levels.

Anesthesia and Major Surgery: As with all beta-receptor blocking drugs, it may be decided to withdraw TENORETIC before surgery. In this case, 48 hours should be allowed to elapse between the last dose and anesthesia. If treatment is continued, care should be taken when using anesthetic agents because of the risk of further depression of the myocardium.

Beta blockers are competitive inhibitors of beta-receptor agonists and their effects on the heart can be reversed by administration of such agents; eg, dobutamine or isoproterenol with caution (see section on OVERDOSAGE). Manifestations of excessive vagal tone (eg, profound bradycardia, hypotension) may be corrected with atropine (1-2 mg I.V.).

Metabolic and Endocrine Effects: TENORETIC may be used with caution in diabetic patients. Beta blockers may mask tachycardia occurring with hypoglycemia, but other manifestations such as dizziness and sweating may not be significantly affected. Atenolol does not potentiate insulin-induced hypoglycemia and, unlike nonselective beta blockers, does not delay recovery of blood glucose to normal levels. Insulin requirements in diabetic patients may be increased, decreased, or unchanged, latent diabetes mellitus may become manifest during chlorthalidone administration.

Beta-adrenergic blockade may mask certain clinical signs (eg, tachycardia) of hyperthyroidism. Abrupt withdrawal of beta blockade might precipitate a thyroid storm; therefore, patients suspected of developing thyrotoxicosis and from whom TENORETIC therapy is to be withdrawn should be monitored closely.

Because calcium excretion is decreased by thiazides, TENORETIC should be discontinued before carrying out tests for parathyroid function. Pathologic changes in the parathyroid glands, with hypercalcemia and hypophosphatemia, have been observed in a few patients on prolonged thiazide therapy; however, the common complications of hyperparathyroidism such as renal lithiasis, bone resorption, and peptic ulceration have not been seen.

Hyperuricemia may occur or acute gout may be precipitated in certain patients receiving thiazide therapy.

PRECAUTIONS

General—Electrolyte and Fluid Balance Status: Periodic determination of serum electrolytes to detect possible electrolyte imbalance should be performed at appropriate intervals.

Patients should be observed for clinical signs of fluid or electrolyte imbalance, ie, hyponatremia, hypochloremic alkalosis, and hypokalemia. Serum and urine electrolyte determinations are particularly important when the patient is vomiting excessively or receiving parenteral fluids. Warning signs or symptoms of fluid and electrolyte imbalance include dryness of the mouth, thirst, weakness, lethargy, drowsiness, restlessness, muscle pains or cramps, muscular fatigue, hypotension, oliguria, tachycardia, and gastrointestinal disturbances such as nausea and vomiting.

Hypokalemia may develop, especially with brisk diuresis, when severe cirrhosis is present, or during concomitant use of corticosteroids or ACTH.

Interference with adequate oral electrolyte intake will also contribute to hypokalemia. Hypokalemia can sensitize or exaggerate the response of the heart to the toxic effects of digitalis (eg, increased ventricular irritability). Hypokalemia may be avoided or treated by use of potassium supplements or foods with a high potassium content.

Any chloride deficit during thiazide therapy is generally mild and usually does not require specific treatment except under extraordinary circumstances (as in liver disease or renal disease). Dilutional hyponatremia may occur in edematous patients in hot weather, appropriate therapy is water restriction rather than administration of salt except in rare instances when the hyponatremia is life-threatening. In actual salt depletion, appropriate replacement is the therapy of choice.

Drug Interactions: TENORETIC may potentiate the action of other antihypertensive agents used concomitantly. Patients treated with TENORETIC plus a catecholamine depletor (eg. reserpine) should be closely observed for evidence of hypotension and/or marked bradycardia which may produce vertigo, syncope, or postural hypotension.

Thiazides may decrease arterial responsiveness to norepinephrine. This diminution is not sufficient to preclude the therapeutic effectiveness of norepinephrine. Thiazides may increase the responsiveness to tubocurarine.

Lithium generally should not be given with diuretics because they reduce its renal clearance and add a high risk of lithium toxicity. Read circulars for lithium preparations before use of such preparations with TENORETIC.

Should it be decided to discontinue therapy in patients receiving TENORETIC and clonidine concurrently, the TENORETIC should be discontinued several days before the gradual withdrawal of clonidine.

Other Precautions: In patients receiving thiazides, sensitivity reactions may occur with or without a history of allergy or bronchial asthma. The possible exacerbation or activation of systemic lupus erythematosus has been reported. The antihypertensive effects of thiazides may be enhanced in the postsympathectomy patient.

Carcinogenesis, Mutagenesis, Impairment of Fertility: Two long-term (maximum dosing duration of 18 or 24 months) rat studies and one long-term (maximum dosing duration of 18 months) mouse study with atenolol, each employing dose levels as high as 300 mg/kg/day or 150 times the maximum recommended human dose, did not indicate a carcinogenic potential in rodents.

Atenolol was negative in the mouse dominant lethal test, the Chinese hamster in vivo cytogenetic test and the Salmonella typhimurium back mutation test (Ames test), with or without metabolic activation.

Fertility of male or female rats (evaluated at dose levels as high as 200 mg/kg/day or 100 times the maximum recommended human dose) was unaffected by atenolol administration.

Animal Toxicology: Six month oral studies were conducted in rats and dogs using TENORETIC dosages up to 12.5 mg/kg/day (approximately 5 times the proposed maximum therapeutic dose). There were no functional or morphological abnormalities resulting from dosing either compound alone or together other than minor changes in heart rate, blood pressure, and urine chemistry, which were attributed to the known pharmacologic properties of atenolol and/or chlorthalidone.

Chronic studies of atenolol performed in animals have revealed the occurrence of vacuolation of epithelial cells of Brunner's glands in the duodenum of both male and female dogs at all tested dose levels (starting at 15 mg/kg/day or 7.5 times the maximum recommended human dose) and increased incidence of atrial degeneration of hearts of male rats at 300 mg but not 150 mg atenolol/kg/day (150 and 75 times the maximum recommended human dose, respectively).

Use in Pregnancy: Pregnancy Category C. TENORETIC was studied for teratogenic potential in the rat and rabbit. Doses of 10, 100, and 300 mg/kg/day were administered orally to pregnant rats, with no teratologic effects observed. Two studies were conducted in rabbits. In the first study, pregnant rabbits were dosed with 10, 100, or 200 mg/kg/day. No teratologic changes were noted; embryonic resorptions were observed at all dose levels (ranging from approximately 5 times to 100 times the maximum recommended human dose). In a second rabbit study, dosages were 5, 10, and 25 mg/kg/day. No teratogenic or embryotoxic effects were demonstrated. It is concluded that the no-effect level for embryonic resorptions is 25 mg/kg/day (approximately 12.5 times the maximum recommended human dose) or greater. TENORETIC should be used during pregnancy only if the potential benefit justifies the potential risk to the fetus.

Atenolol—Atenolol has been shown to produce a dose-related increase in embryo/fetal resorptions in rats at doses equal to or greater than 50 mg/kg or 25 or more times the maximum recommended human dose. Although similar effects were not seen in rabbits, the compound was not evaluated in rabbits at doses above 25 mg/kg or 12.5 times the maximum recommended human dose. There are no adequate and well-controlled studies in pregnant women.

Chlorthalidone—Thiazides cross the placental barrier and appear in cord blood. The use of chlorthalidone and related drugs in pregnant women requires that the anticipated benefits of the drug be weighed against possible hazards to the fetus. These hazards include fetal or neonatal jaundice, thrombocytopenia, and possibly other adverse reactions which have occurred in the adult.

Nursing Mothers: It is not established to what extent this drug is excreted in human milk. Since most drugs are excreted in human milk, nursing should not be undertaken by mothers receiving TENORETIC.

Pediatric Use: Safety and effectiveness in children have not been established.

ADVERSE REACTIONS

TENORETIC is usually well tolerated in properly selected patients. Most adverse effects have been mild and transient. The adverse effects observed for TENORETIC are essentially the same as those seen with the individual components.

Atenolol: The frequency estimates that follow derive from controlled studies in which adverse reactions were either volunteered by the patient (U.S. studies) or elicited, eg, by checklist (foreign studies). The reported frequency of elicited adverse effects was higher for both atenolol and placebo-treated patients than when these reactions were volunteered. Where frequency of adverse effects for atenolol and placebo is similar, causal relationship to atenolol is uncertain.

The data present these estimates in terms of percentages: first from the U.S. studies (volunteered side effects) and then from both U.S. and foreign studies (volunteered and elicited side effects).

U.S. Studies (% Atenolol -% Placebo):

CARDIOVASCULAR: bradycardia (3%-0%), cold extremities (0%-0.5%), postural hypotension (2%-1%), leg pain (0%-0.5%).

CENTRAL NERVOUS SYSTEM / NEUROMUSCULAR: dizziness (4%-1%), vertigo (2%-0.5%), light-headedness (1%-0%), tiredness (0.6%-0.5%), fatigue (3%-1%), lethargy (1%-0%), drowsiness (0.6%-0%), depression (0.6%-0.5%), dreaming (0%-0%).

GASTROINTESTINAL: diarrhea (2%-0%), nausea (4%-1%).

RESPIRATORY (See WARNINGS): wheeziness (0%-0%), dyspnea (0.6%-1%).

Totals U.S. and Foreign Studies:

CARDIOVASCULAR: bradycardia (3%-0%), cold extremities (12%-5%), postural hypotension (4%-5%), leg pain (3%-1%).

CENTRAL NERVOUS SYSTEM / NEUROMUSCULAR: dizziness (13%-6%), vertigo (2%-0.2%), light-headedness (3%-0.7%), tiredness (26%-13%), fatigue (6%-5%), lethargy (3%-0.7%), drowsiness (2%-0.5%), depression (12%-9%), dreaming (3%-1%).

GASTROINTESTINAL: diarrhea (3%-2%), nausea (3%-1%).

RESPIRATORY (see WARNINGS): wheeziness (3%-3%), dyspnea (6%-4%).

MISCELLANEOUS: There have been reports of skin rashes and/or dry eyes associated with the use of beta-adrenergic blocking drugs. The reported incidence is small and, in most cases the symptoms have cleared when treatment was withdrawn. Discontinuance of the drug should be considered if any such reaction is not otherwise explicable. Patients should be closely monitored following cessation of therapy.

Chlorthalidone: Cardiovascular: orthostatic hypotension; Gastrointestinal: anorexia, gastric irritation, vomiting, cramping, constipation, jaundice (intrahepatic cholestatic jaundice), pancreatitis; CNS: vertigo, paresthesias, xanthopsia; Hematologic: leukopenia, agranulocytosis, thrombocytopenia, aplastic anemia; Hypersensitivity: purpura, photosensitivity, rash, urticaria, necrotizing angiitis (vasculitis), (cutaneous vasculitis), Lyell's syndrome (toxic epidermal necrolysis); Miscellaneous: hyperglycemia, glycosuria, hyperuricemia, muscle spasm, weakness, restlessness. Clinical trials of TENORETIC conducted in the United States (69 patients treated with TENORETIC) revealed no new or unexpected adverse effects.

Potential Adverse Effects: In addition, a variety of adverse effects not observed in clinical trials with atenolol but reported with other beta-adrenergic blocking agents, should be considered potential adverse effects of atenolol. Nervous System: reversible mental depression progressing to catatonia, hallucinations, an acute reversible syndrome characterized by disorientation for time and place, short-term memory loss, emotional lability, slightly clouded sensorium, decreased performance on neuropsychometrics; Cardiovascular: intensification of AV block (see CONTRAINDICATIONS); Gastrointestinal: mesenteric arterial thrombosis, ischemic colitis; Hematologic: agranulocytosis, nonthrombocytopenic purpura, thrombocytopenic purpura; Allergic: erythematous rash, fever combined with aching and sore throat, laryngospasm and respiratory distress; Miscellaneous: reversible alopecia, Peyronie's disease.

There have been reports of a syndrome comprising psoriasiform skin rash, conjunctivitis sicca, otitis, and sclerosing serositis attributed to the beta-adrenergic receptor blocking agent, practolol. This syndrome has not been reported with TENORETIC or TENORMIN (atenolol).

Clinical Laboratory Test Findings: Clinically important changes in standard laboratory parameters were rarely associated with the administration of TENORETIC. The changes in laboratory parameters were not progressive and usually were not associated with clinical manifestations. The most common changes were increases in uric acid and decreases in serum potassium.

OVERDOSAGE

No specific information is available with regard to overdosage with TENORETIC in humans. Treatment is symptomatic and supportive. Therapy with TENORETIC should be discontinued and the patient observed closely. Suggested measures include induction of emesis and /or gastric lavage, and correction of dehydration, electrolyte imbalance, and hypotension by established procedures.

Atenolol: To date, there is no known case of acute overdosage with atenolol. The most common effects expected with overdosage of a beta-adrenergic blocking agent are bradycardia, congestive heart failure, hypotension, bronchospasm, and hypoglycemia. Atenolol can be removed from the general circulation by hemodialysis. In addition to gastric la-

Continued on next page

Stuart—Cont.

vage, the following therapeutic measures are suggested if warranted.
BRADYCARDIA: atropine or another anticholinergic drug.
HEART BLOCK (second or third degree): isoproterenol or transvenous cardiac pacemaker.
CONGESTIVE HEART FAILURE: conventional therapy.
HYPOTENSION (depending on associated factors): epinephrine rather than isoproterenol or norepinephrine may be useful in addition to atropine and digitalis.
BRONCHOSPASM: aminophylline, isoproterenol, or atropine.
HYPOGLYCEMIA: intravenous glucose.
ELECTROLYTE IMBALANCE: supportive treatment; where necessary, intravenous dextrose-saline with potassium, administered with caution.
Chlorthalidone: Symptoms of chlorthalidone overdose include nausea, weakness, dizziness, and disturbances of electrolyte balance.

DOSAGE AND ADMINISTRATION

DOSAGE MUST BE INDIVIDUALIZED (SEE INDICATIONS): Chlorthalidone is usually given at a dose of 25 mg daily; the usual initial dose of atenolol is 50 mg daily. Therefore, the initial dose should be one TENORETIC 50 tablet given once a day. If an optimal response is not achieved, the dosage should be increased to one TENORETIC 100 tablet given once a day.
When necessary, another antihypertensive agent may be added gradually beginning with 50% of the usual recommended starting dose to avoid an excessive fall in blood pressure.
Since atenolol is excreted via the kidneys, dosage should be adjusted in cases of severe impairment of renal function. No significant accumulation of atenolol occurs until creatinine clearance falls below 35 mL/min/1.73 m^2 (normal range is 100–150 mL/min/1.73 m^2), therefore, the following maximum dosages are recommended for patients with renal impairment.

Creatinine Clearance (mL/min/1.73 m^2)	Atenolol Elimination Half-life (hrs)	Maximum Dosage
15–35	16–27	50 mg daily
< 15	> 27	50 mg every other day

HOW SUPPLIED

TENORETIC 50 Tablets (atenolol 50 mg and chlorthalidone 25 mg), NDC 0038-0115 (white, round, biconvex, uncoated tablets with TENORETIC 50 on one side and Stuart 115 on the other side) are supplied in bottles of 100 tablets. TENORETIC 100 Tablets (atenolol 100 mg and chlorthalidone 25 mg), NDC 0038-0117 (white, round, biconvex, uncoated tablets with TENORETIC 100 on one side and Stuart 117 on the other side) are supplied in bottles of 100 tablets.
Protect from heat, light, and moisture. Dispense in well-closed, light-resistant container.

Shown in Product Identification Section, page 432

E/1/85

TENORMIN® ℞

[ten 'or min"]
(atenolol)

DESCRIPTION

TENORMIN (atenolol), a synthetic, $beta_1$-selective (cardioselective) adrenoreceptor blocking agent, may be chemically described as benzeneacetamide, 4-[2'-hydroxy-3'-[(1-methylethyl) amino] propoxy]-.
Atenolol (free base) has a molecular weight of 266. It is a relatively polar hydrophilic compound with a water solubility of 26.5 mg/ml at 37°C and a log partition coefficient (octanol/-water) of 0.23. It is freely soluble in 1N HCl (300 mg/ml at 25°C) and less soluble in chloroform (3 mg/ml at 25°C).
TENORMIN is available as 50 mg. and 100 mg. tablets for oral administration.
Inactive ingredients: magnesium stearate, microcrystalline cellulose, povidone, sodium starch glycolate.

CLINICAL PHARMACOLOGY

TENORMIN is a $beta_1$-selective (cardioselective) beta-adrenergic receptor blocking agent without membrane-stabilizing or intrinsic sympathomimetic (partial agonist) activities. This preferential effect is not absolute, however and, at higher doses, TENORMIN inhibits $beta_2$ adrenoreceptors, chiefly located in the bronchial and vascular musculature.
Pharmacokinetics and Metabolism: In man, absorption of an oral dose is rapid and consistent but incomplete. Approximately 50% of an oral dose is absorbed from the gastrointestinal tract, the remainder being excreted unchanged in the feces. Peak blood levels are reached between 2 and 4 hours after ingestion. Unlike propranolol or metoprolol, but like nadolol, TENORMIN undergoes little or no metabolism by the liver and the absorbed portion is eliminated primarily by renal excretion. TENORMIN also differs from propranolol in that only a small amount (6%–16%) is bound to proteins in the plasma. This kinetic profile results in relatively consistent plasma drug levels with about a fourfold interpatient variation.
The elimination half-life of TENORMIN is approximately 6 to 7 hours and there is no alteration of the kinetic profile of the drug by chronic administration. Following doses of 50 mg or 100 mg, both beta-blocking and antihypertensive effects persist for at least 24 hours. When renal function is impaired, elimination of TENORMIN is closely related to the glomerular filtration rate; but, significant accumulation does not occur until the creatinine clearance falls below 35 ml/min/1.73 m^2 (see DOSAGE AND ADMINISTRATION).
By blocking the positive chronotropic and inotropic effects of catecholamines and by decreasing blood pressure, atenolol generally reduces the oxygen requirements of the heart at any given level of effort, making it useful for many patients in the long-term management of angina pectoris. On the other hand, atenolol can increase oxygen requirements by increasing left ventricular fiber length and end diastolic pressure, particularly in patients with heart failure.
Pharmacodynamics.: In standard animal or human pharmacological tests, beta-adrenoreceptor blocking activity of TENORMIN has been demonstrated by: (1) reduction in resting and exercise heart rate and cardiac output, (2) reduction of systolic and diastolic blood pressure at rest and on exercise, (3) inhibition of isoproterenol-induced tachycardia, and (4) reduction in reflex orthostatic tachycardia.
A significant beta-blocking effect of TENORMIN, as measured by reduction of exercise tachycardia, is apparent within 1 hour following oral administration of a single dose. This effect is maximal at about 2 to 4 hours, and persists for at least 24 hours. The effect at 24 hours is dose-related and also bears a linear relationship to the logarithm of plasma TENORMIN concentration. However, as has been shown for all beta-blocking agents, the antihypertensive effect does not appear to be related to plasma level.
In normal subjects, the $beta_1$ selectivity of TENORMIN has been shown by its reduced ability to reverse the $beta_2$-mediated vasodilating effect of isoproterenol as compared to equivalent beta-blocking doses of propranolol. In asthmatic patients, a dose of TENORMIN producing a greater effect on resting heart rate than propranolol resulted in much less increase in airway resistance. In a placebo-controlled comparison of approximately equipotent oral doses of several beta blockers, TENORMIN produced a significantly smaller decrease of FEV_1 than nonselective beta blockers such as propranolol and, unlike those agents, did not inhibit bronchodilation in response to isoproterenol.
Consistent with its negative chronotropic effect due to beta blockade of the SA node, TENORMIN increases sinus cycle length and sinus node recovery time. Conduction in the AV node is also prolonged. TENORMIN is devoid of membrane-stabilizing activity, and increasing the dose well beyond that producing beta blockade does not further depress myocardial contractility. Several studies have demonstrated a moderate (approximately 10%) increase in stroke volume at rest and exercise.
In controlled clinical trials TENORMIN given as a single daily dose was an effective antihypertensive agent providing 24-hour reduction of blood pressure. TENORMIN has been studied in combination with thiazide-type diuretics and the blood pressure effects of the combination are approximately additive. TENORMIN is also compatible with methyldopa, hydralazine, and prazosin, the combination resulting in a larger fall in blood pressure than with the single agents. The dose range of TENORMIN is narrow and increasing the dose beyond 100 mg. once daily is not associated with increased antihypertensive effect. The mechanisms of the antihypertensive effects of beta-blocking agents have not been established. Several possible mechanisms have been proposed and include: (1) competitive antagonism of catecholamines at peripheral (especially cardiac) adrenergic neuron sites, leading to decreased cardiac output, (2) a central effect leading to reduced sympathetic outflow to the periphery, and (3) suppression of renin activity. The results from long-term studies have not shown any diminution of the antihypertensive efficacy of TENORMIN with prolonged use.

INDICATIONS AND USAGE

Hypertension: TENORMIN is indicated in the management of hypertension. It may be used alone or concomitantly with other antihypertensive agents, particularly with a thiazide-type diuretic.
Angina Pectoris Due to Coronary Atherosclerosis: TENORMIN is indicated for the long-term management of patients with angina pectoris.

CONTRAINDICATIONS

TENORMIN is contraindicated in sinus bradycardia, heart block greater than first degree, cardiogenic shock, and overt cardiac failure (see WARNINGS).

WARNINGS

Cardiac Failure: Sympathetic stimulation is necessary in supporting circulatory function in congestive heart failure, and beta blockade carries the potential hazard of further depressing myocardial contractility and precipitating more severe failure. In hypertensive patients who have congestive heart failure controlled by digitalis and diuretics, TENORMIN should be administered cautiously. Both digitalis and atenolol slow AV conduction.
In Patients Without a History of Cardiac Failure: Continued depression of the myocardium with beta-blocking agents over a period of time can, in some cases, lead to cardiac failure. At the first sign or symptom of impending cardiac failure, patients should be fully digitalized and/or be given a diuretic and the response observed closely. If cardiac failure continues, despite adequate digitalization and diuresis, TENORMIN should be withdrawn. (See Dosage and Administration.)

Cessation of Therapy With TENORMIN: Patients with coronary artery disease, who are being treated with TENORMIN, should be advised against abrupt discontinuation of therapy. Severe exacerbation of angina and the occurrence of myocardial infarction and ventricular arrhythmias have been reported in angina patients following the abrupt discontinuation of therapy with other beta blockers. The last two complications may occur with or without preceding exacerbation of the angina pectoris. To date, there has been no report of myocardial infarction or severe angina upon withdrawal of TENORMIN, probably due to its long plasma half-life. Because of the problems encountered with other beta blockers, when discontinuation of TENORMIN is planned, the patients should be carefully observed and advised to limit physical activity to a minimum. If the angina worsens or acute coronary insufficiency develops, it is recommended that TENORMIN be promptly reinstituted, at least temporarily. (See Dosage and Administration).

Bronchospastic Diseases: PATIENTS WITH BRONCHOSPASTIC DISEASE SHOULD IN GENERAL NOT RECEIVE BETA BLOCKERS. Because of its relative $beta_1$ selectivity, however, TENORMIN may be used with caution in patients with bronchospastic disease who do not respond to, or cannot tolerate, other antihypertensive treatment. Since $beta_1$selectivity is not absolute, the lowest possible dose of TENORMIN should be used with therapy initiated at 50 mg. and a $beta_2$-stimulating agent (bronchodilator) should be made available. If dosage must be increased, dividing the dose should be considered in order to achieve lower peak blood levels.
Anesthesia and Major Surgery: As with all beta-receptor blocking drugs it may be decided to withdraw TENORMIN before surgery. In this case, 48 hours should be allowed to elapse between the last dose and anesthesia. If treatment is continued, care should be taken when using anesthetic agents which depress the myocardium such as ether, cyclopropane, and trichloroethylene.
TENORMIN, like other beta blockers, is a competitive inhibitor of beta-receptor agonists and its effects on the heart can be reversed by administration of such agents—(eg, dobutamine or isoproterenol with caution, see section on OVERDOSAGE). Manifestations of excessive vagal tone (eg, profound bradycardia, hypotension) may be corrected with atropine (1–2 mg. IV).
Diabetes and Hypoglycemia: TENORMIN should be used with caution in diabetic patients if a beta-blocking agent is required. Beta blockers may mask tachycardia occurring with hypoglycemia, but other manifestations such as dizziness and sweating may not be significantly affected. TENORMIN does not potentiate insulin-induced hypoglycemia and, unlike nonselective beta blockers, does not delay recovery of blood glucose to normal levels.
Thyrotoxicosis: Beta-adrenergic blockade may mask certain clinical signs (eg, tachycardia) of hyperthyroidism. Abrupt withdrawal of beta blockade might precipitate a thyroid storm; therefore, patients suspected of developing thyrotoxicosis from whom TENORMIN is to be withdrawn should be monitored closely. (See DOSAGE AND ADMINISTRATION).

PRECAUTIONS

Impaired Renal Function: The drug should be used with caution in patients with impaired renal function (see DOSAGE AND ADMINISTRATION).
Drug Interactions: Catecholamine-depleting drugs (eg, reserpine) may have an additive effect when given with beta-blocking agents. Patients treated with TENORMIN plus a catecholamine depletor should therefore be closely observed for evidence of hypotension and or marked bradycardia which may produce vertigo, syncope, or postural hypotension.
Should it be decided to discontinue therapy in patients receiving beta blockers and clonidine concurrently, the beta blocker should be discontinued several days before the gradual withdrawal of clonidine.

Carcinogenesis, Mutagenesis, Impairment of Fertility: Two long-term (maximum dosing duration of 18 or 24 months) rat studies and one long-term (maximum dosing duration of 18 months) mouse study, each employing dose levels as high as 300 mg./kg./day or 150 times the maximum recommended human dose, did not indicate a carcinogenic potential in rodents. Results of various mutagenicity studies support this finding.

Fertility of male or female rats (evaluated at dose levels as high as 200 mg./kg./day or 100 times the maximum recommended human dose) was unaffected by atenolol administration.

Animal Toxicology: Chronic studies performed in animals have revealed the occurrence of vacuolation of epithelial cells of Brunner's glands in the duodenum of both male and female dogs at all tested dose levels of atenolol (starting at 15 mg./kg./day or 7.5 times the maximum recommended human dose) and increased incidence of atrial degeneration of hearts of male rats at 300 mg. but not 150 mg. atenolol/kg./day (150 and 75 times the maximum recommended human dose, respectively).

USAGE IN PREGNANCY

Pregnancy Category C. Atenolol has been shown to produce a dose-related increase in embryo/fetal resorptions in rats at doses equal to or greater than 50 mg/kg/day or 25 or more times the maximum recommended human dose. Although similar effects were not seen in rabbits, the compound was not evaluated in rabbits at doses above 25 mg/kg/day or 12.5 times the maximum recommended human dose. There are no adequate and well-controlled studies in pregnant women. TENORMIN should be used during pregnancy only if the potential benefit justifies the potential risk to the fetus.

Nursing Mothers: Atenolol is excreted in human breast milk at a ratio of 1.5 to 6.8 when compared to the concentration in plasma. Caution should be exercised when TENORMIN is administered to a nursing woman.

Pediatric Use: Safety and effectiveness in children have not been established.

ADVERSE REACTIONS

Most adverse effects have been mild and transient. Frequency estimates were derived from controlled studies in which adverse reactions were either volunteered by the patient (U.S. studies) or elicited (eg, by checklist—foreign studies). The reported frequency of elicited adverse effects was higher for both TENORMIN and placebo-treated patients than when these reactions were volunteered. Where frequency of adverse effects for TENORMIN and placebo is similar, causal relationship is uncertain.

The following adverse-reaction data present frequency estimates in terms of percentages: first from the U.S. studies (volunteered side effects) and then from both U.S. and foreign studies (volunteered and elicited side effects):

U.S. STUDIES (% ATENOLOL—% PLACEBO):

CARDIOVASCULAR: bradycardia (3%–0%), cold extremities (0%–0.5%), postural hypotension (2%–1%), leg pain (0%–0.5%)

CENTRAL NERVOUS SYSTEM/NEUROMUSCULAR: dizziness (4%–1%), vertigo (2%–0.5%), light-headedness (1%–0%), tiredness (0.6%–0.5%), fatigue (3%–1%), lethargy (1%–0%), drowsiness (0.6%–0%), depression (0.6%–0.5%), dreaming (0%–0%)

GASTROINTESTINAL: diarrhea (2%–0%), nausea (4%–1%)

RESPIRATORY (See WARNINGS): wheeziness (0%–0%), dyspnea (0.6%–1%)

TOTALS U.S. AND FOREIGN STUDIES:

CARDIOVASCULAR: bradycardia (3%–0%), cold extremities (12%–5%), postural hypotension (4%–5%), leg pain (3%–1%)

CENTRAL NERVOUS SYSTEM/NEUROMUSCULAR: dizziness (13%–6%), vertigo (2%–0.2%), light-headedness (3%–0.7%), tiredness (26%–13%), fatigue (6%–5%), lethargy (3%–0.7%), drowsiness (2%–0.5%), depression (12%–9%), dreaming (3%–1%)

GASTROINTESTINAL: diarrhea (3%–2%), nausea (3%–1%)

RESPIRATORY (see WARNINGS): wheeziness (3%–3%), dyspnea (6%–4%)

MISCELLANEOUS: There have been reports of skin rashes and/or dry eyes associated with the use of beta-adrenergic blocking drugs. The reported incidence is small, and in most cases, the symptoms have cleared when treatment was withdrawn. Discontinuance of the drug should be considered if any such reaction is not otherwise explicable. Patients should be closely monitored following cessation of therapy.

POTENTIAL ADVERSE EFFECTS

In addition, a variety of adverse effects have been reported with other beta-adrenergic blocking agents and may be considered potential adverse effects of TENORMIN.

HEMATOLOGIC: Agranulocytosis, nonthrombocytopenic purpura, thrombocytopenic purpura.

ALLERGIC: Fever, combined with aching and sore throat, laryngospasm, respiratory distress.

CENTRAL NERVOUS SYSTEM: Reversible mental depression progressing to catatonia, visual disturbances, hallucinations, an acute reversible syndrome characterized by disorientation of time and place, short-term memory loss, emotional lability with slightly clouded sensorium, and decreased performance on neuropsychometrics.

GASTROINTESTINAL: Mesenteric arterial thrombosis, ischemic colitis.

OTHER: Reversible alopecia, Peyronie's disease, erythematous rash, Raynaud's phenomenon.

MISCELLANEOUS: The oculomucocutaneous syndrome associated with the beta blocker practolol has not been reported with TENORMIN during investigational use and foreign marketing experience. Furthermore, a number of patients who had previously demonstrated established practolol reactions were transferred to TENORMIN with subsequent resolution or quiescence of the reaction.

OVERDOSAGE

To date, there is no known case of acute overdosage, and no specific information on emergency treatment of overdosage is available. The most common effects expected with overdosage of a beta-adrenergic blocking agent are bradycardia, congestive heart failure, hypotension, bronchospasm, and hypoglycemia.

In the case of overdosage, treatment with TENORMIN should be stopped and the patient carefully observed. TENORMIN can be removed from the general circulation by hemodialysis. In addition to gastric lavage, the following therapeutic measures are suggested if warranted:

BRADYCARDIA: Atropine or another anticholinergic drug.

HEART BLOCK (SECOND OR THIRD DEGREE): Isoproterenol or transvenous cardiac pacemaker.

CONGESTIVE HEART FAILURE: Conventional therapy.

HYPOTENSION (DEPENDING ON ASSOCIATED FACTORS): Epinephrine rather than isoproterenol or norepinephrine may be useful in addition to atropine and digitalis.

BRONCHOSPASM: Aminophylline, isoproterenol, or atropine.

HYPOGLYCEMIA: Intravenous glucose.

DOSAGE AND ADMINISTRATION

Hypertension: The initial dose of TENORMIN is 50 mg. given as one tablet a day either alone or added to diuretic therapy. The full effect of this dose will usually be seen within one to two weeks. If an optimal response is not achieved, the dosage should be increased to TENORMIN 100 mg. given as one tablet a day. Increasing the dosage beyond 100 mg. a day is unlikely to produce any further benefit.

TENORMIN may be used alone or concomitantly with other antihypertensive agents including thiazide-type diuretics, hydralazine, prazosin, and alpha-methyldopa.

Angina Pectoris: The initial dose of TENORMIN (atenolol) is 50 mg. given as one tablet a day. If an optimal response is not achieved within one week, the dosage should be increased to TENORMIN 100 mg. given as one tablet a day. Some patients may require a dosage of 200 mg. once a day for optimal effect.

Twenty-four hour control with once daily dosing is achieved by giving doses larger than necessary to achieve an immediate maximum effect. The maximum early effect on exercise tolerance occurs with doses of 50 to 100 mg., but at these doses the effect at 24 hours is attenuated, averaging about 50% to 75% of that observed with once a day oral doses of 200 mg.

Patients with Renal Impairment: Since TENORMIN is excreted via the kidneys, dosage should be adjusted in cases of severe impairment of renal function. No significant accumulation of TENORMIN occurs until creatinine clearance falls below 35 ml./min./1.73 m^2 (normal range is 100–150 ml./min./1.73 m^2); therefore, the following maximum dosages are recommended for patients with renal impairment:

Creatinine Clearance (ml./min./1.73m^2)	Atenolol Elimination Half-life (hrs.)	Maximum Dosage
15–35	16–27	50 mg. daily
<15	>27	50 mg. every other day

Patients on hemodialysis should be given 50 mg. after each dialysis; this should be done under hospital supervision as marked falls in blood pressure can occur.

Cessation of Therapy: If withdrawal of TENORMIN therapy is planned, it should be achieved gradually over a period of about two weeks. Patients should be carefully observed and advised to limit physical activity to a minimum.

HOW SUPPLIED

Tablets of 50 mg. atenolol (round, flat, uncoated, white tablets identified with TENORMIN 50 debossed on one side and NDC number 105 debossed and scored on the other side) are supplied in bottles of 100 tablets and unit dose packages of 100 tablets. NDC 0038-0105.

Tablets of 100 mg. atenolol (round, flat, uncoated, white tablets identified with TENORMIN 100 debossed on one side and NDC number 101 debossed on the other side) are supplied in bottles of 100 tablets and unit dose packages of 100 tablets. NDC 0038-0101.

Protect from heat, light, and moisture.

Shown in Product Identification Section, page 432

C/7/85

Sween Corporation

SWEEN BUILDING
P.O. BOX 980
LAKE CRYSTAL, MN 56055

BEDSIDE-CARE™

Medicated, Antiseptic
No Rinse Shampoo and Body Wash

DESCRIPTION

BEDSIDE-CARE is a no-rinse shampoo and body wash consisting of Methylbenzethonium Chloride (a safe and effective non-irritating, antimicrobial agent) in a cleansing base of Water, Lauroamphoglycinate, Cocamidopropyl Betaine, Glycerin, Polysorbate 20, Quaternium-33, Ethyl Hexanediol, Isopropyl Alcohol, Citric Acid, Quaternium-15, Fragrance and D & C Green #5. National Drug Code (NDC) 11701-020.

INDICATIONS AND USAGES

BEDSIDE-CARE is a no-rinse formulation designed for daily, head-to-foot gentle cleansing of the nonambulatory patient. BEDSIDE-CARE is indicated for shampooing, applying it to DRY hair and requiring no rinsing. BEDSIDE-CARE eliminates the need for an elaborate procedure requiring a volume of water and equipment to accomplish the task. Cleansing the skin of the entire body is also easily accomplished with minimum of supplies and materials. Problem head and body odors are controlled with regular use of the product.

CONTRAINDICATIONS

Hypersensitivity to any components of the preparation.

PRECAUTIONS AND ADVERSE REACTIONS

For external use only. BEDSIDE-CARE is not toxic by oral ingestion and is not considered a primary eye or skin irritant under normal use conditions.

DOSAGE AND ADMINISTRATION

SHAMPOO

Note: Place towel under head before beginning shampoo.

1. Spray dry hair completely with BEDSIDE-CARE.
2. Work into lather, thoroughly massaging hair and scalp 30–60 seconds. Foaming action loosens dirt and oils.
3. Using a moist, warm washcloth, gently rub hair and scalp to remove loosened dirt and oils. Repeat if necessary.
4. Gently dry with towel which was placed under the head.

BODY WASH:

1. Add 3–4 sprays BEDSIDE-CARE to basin of water.
2. Beginning with face, gently wash with damp washcloth dipped in basin. Pat dry.

Note: Uncover only area being cleansed to avoid patient chills.

3. Continue with arms (one at a time) and upper part of body, washing gently with cloth rinsed in basin. Pat dry.
4. Wash each leg and foot in same manner and dry.
5. If the patient is unable to help himself, wash the genital area, being sure to cleanse all skin creases and folds with a freshly rinsed cloth. Pat dry.

Note: When the use of No-Rinse BEDSIDE-CARE is required for an extended period of time, a shampoo and bath using SWEEN GENTLE RAIN or SURGI-KLEEN is recommended every 7th or 8th day.

HOW SUPPLIED

8 fl. oz. bottles with spray fitment and one gallon containers.

FORDUSTIN'®

[fŏr-dŭs'tĭn]

Natural Corn Starch Body Powder

DESCRIPTION

A non-caking, natural Corn Starch based body powder with Sodium Bicarbonate, Silica, Methylbenzethonium Chloride and Fragrance. National Drug Code (NDC) 11701-005.

INDICATIONS AND USAGE

Lubrication of skin subject to excoriation from friction. Helps absorb perspiration to aid in the protection of the skin from perspiration irritation.

CONTRAINDICATIONS

Hypersensitivity to any components of the preparation.

PRECAUTIONS AND ADVERSE REACTIONS

Transmission electron microscopy and electron diffraction examinations of FORDUSTIN' powder found the product free of any form of fibrous material (asbestiform minerals

Continued on next page

Sweeen—Cont.

included) or inorganic materials. For External Use Only. Avoid contact with eyes. Fordustin' is not considered a primary eye or skin irritant under normal use conditions and is not toxic by oral ingestion.

DOSAGE AND ADMINISTRATION
Apply liberally to areas subject to friction and perspiration irritations.

HOW SUPPLIED
3 oz. and 8 oz. containers.

GENTLE RAIN™ Shampoo
[*gĕntle rāin*]
and Skin Cleanser

DESCRIPTION
A shampoo and skin cleanser consisting of Water, Sodium Lauryl Sulfate, Ammonium Lauryl Sulfate, Cocamidopropyl Betaine, Lauramide DEA, Glycol Stearate, Hydrolyzed Animal Protein, Quaternium-33, Ethyl Hexanediol, Citric Acid, Fragrance, Quaternium-15, Tetrasodium EDTA and FD&C Yellow #5.

INDICATIONS AND USAGE
GENTLE RAIN is a luxurious, non-alkaline formulation designed to condition hair as it cleans, plus cleanse sensitive skin gently and thoroughly. The pH has been carefully adjusted for compatibility with the normal range of hair and skin. The low pH, along with the benefits of the special protein and built-in conditioning ingredients, leave hair extremely manageable and easy to care for. This formulation is safe for color treated hair and gentle enough for daily use. Used as a skin cleanser, this same combination leaves the skin soft and supple.

CONTRAINDICATIONS
Hypersensitivity to any components of the preparation.

PRECAUTIONS AND ADVERSE REACTIONS
For External Use Only. May cause eye irritation. In case of eye contact, flush eyes with water. GENTLE RAIN is not toxic by oral ingestion and is not considered a primary skin irritant under normal use conditions.

DOSAGE AND ADMINISTRATION
Shampooing: Wet hair. Lather, rinse thoroughly and repeat.
Bathing: Apply liberally to a warm washcloth and gently wash skin. Rinse thoroughly and pat dry.

HOW SUPPLIED
2 fl.oz., 4 fl. oz. and 16 fl.oz. bottles with flip-top caps, 21 fl. oz. with pump dispenser, in addition to larger bulk sizes.

MICRO-GUARD™
[*mī'crō-gūard*]
Antimicrobial Skin Cream

DESCRIPTION
MICRO-GUARD Skin Cream contains the antimicrobial agent Chloroxylenol (PCMX) in a water washable, vanishing cream base. National Drug Code (NDC) 11701-012.

INDICATIONS AND USAGE
MICRO-GUARD is a soothing antiseptic and antifungal cream. MICRO-GUARD's antifungal action is effective treatment for conditions such as Athlete's Foot, Jock Itch and Ringworm, while its antiseptic activity helps prevent skin infection. MICRO-GUARD can be used for adjunctive topical treatment of superficial skin infections when oral antibiotic agents are concurrently being administered.

CONTRAINDICATIONS
Hypersensitivity to any components of the preparation.

WARNINGS
MICRO-GUARD is not for ophthalmic, otic or vaginal use.

PRECAUTIONS
For External Use Only. Do not use near eyes. If contact with eye occurs, rinse thoroughly with water and consult physician. Keep out of reach of children. If skin irritation occurs, or if there is no improvement within two weeks, discontinue use and consult physician.

ADVERSE REACTIONS
MICRO-GUARD is not considered a primary skin irritant or sensitizer, but occasional erythema, stinging and eczematous reactions have occurred following its use. If irritation or sensitivity develops with the use of MICRO-GUARD, treatment should be discontinued and appropriate therapy instituted.

DOSAGE AND ADMINISTRATION
Gently and thoroughly cleanse affected area and pat dry. Apply a thin layer of MICRO-GUARD over involved area. Repeat application 2 to 3 times daily or as directed by physician.

HOW SUPPLIED
½ oz. tube and 2 oz. jars.

PERI-CARE®
Moisture Barrier Ointment

DESCRIPTION
A soft petrolatum based ointment incorporating Petrolatum, Natural Vitamins A & D, Sodium Caseinate, Methylbenzethonium Chloride, Chloroxylenol, BHT and D & C Green #6. National Drug Code (NDC) 11701-010.

INDICATIONS AND USAGE
PERI-CARE provides a protective moisture barrier against urine and feces. This soothing ointment also contains casein which acts as a buffer between the skin and proteolytic enzymes present in feces and urine helping to eliminate skin breakdown and infection. The petrolatum base of PERI-CARE offers added protection through its physical barrier properties. PERI-CARE also provides a moisture barrier when uncontrollable drooling is a problem, plus gives added protection to hands often immersed in water.

CONTRAINDICATIONS
Hypersensitivity to any components of the preparation.

PRECAUTIONS AND ADVERSE REACTIONS
For External Use Only. Avoid contact with eyes. PERI-CARE ointment is not toxic by oral ingestion and is not considered a primary eye or skin irritant under normal use conditions.

DOSAGE AND ADMINISTRATION
Cleanse and rinse soiled perineal area thoroughly. Pat or air dry. Apply PERI-CARE ointment liberally to perineal area to be protected. Repeat cleansing procedure promptly whenever discharge occurs and re-apply PERI-CARE.

HOW SUPPLIED
½ oz., 1.75 oz. and 5 oz. tubes, 2-oz. and 8-oz. jars.

PERI-WASH®
[*pĕri-wăsh*]
Incontinent Cleanser

DESCRIPTION
A skin cleanser. A feces and urine emulsifier consisting of Water, TEA-Lauryl Sulfate, Cocoamphocarboxypropionate, Sodium Lauryl Sulfate, Propylene Glycol, PPG-12-PEG-65 Lanolin Oil, Citric Acid, Styrene/PVP Copolymer, PEG-8 Laurate, PEG-75 Lanolin, Laureth-23, PEG-4 Oleate, Glycol Stearate, Quaternium-15, Methylbenzethonium Chloride, PEG-90M, FD & C Yellow #5 and Other Ingredients. National Drug Code (NDC) 11701-014.

INDICATIONS AND USAGE
PERI-WASH is designed for daily cleansing and care of the perineal area. Sprayed directly on feces and urine, odors are stopped on contact. Through the process of emulsification, PERI-WASH loosens and softens feces for easier and safer removal from thin, sensitive skin, thereby reducing the irritation and formation of denuded skin around the anus. It is indicated for cleansing perineal areas afflicted with dermatitis and ammonia dermatitis associated with diarrhea. PERI-WASH reduces and eliminates the ammonia odors from urine or feces. When used during routine ostomy appliance change procedures, PERI-WASH stops odors and gently cleanses peristomal skin. It controls offensive odors when used in ostomy appliances and urine collecting bags. **Additional uses for odor control:** cleaning bed pans, urinals, wheelchairs, upholstery, vinyls, soiled linens/garments, and hands.

CONTRAINDICATIONS
Hypersensitivity to any components of the preparation.

PRECAUTIONS AND ADVERSE REACTIONS
For External Use Only. PERI-WASH is not toxic by oral ingestion and is not considered a primary skin irritant under normal use conditions. PERI-WASH is an eye irritant (Sodium Lauryl Sulfate) and should be rinsed thoroughly from eyes if accidental contact occurs.

DOSAGE AND ADMINISTRATION
Apply liberally to perineal area. Wash and rinse thoroughly with clean warm water in the normal manner.

HOW SUPPLIED
4 fl. oz. and 8 fl. oz. bottles with spray fitment, in addition to larger bulk sizes.

PERI-WASH® II
[*pĕri-wăsh*]
Medicated, Antiseptic
Incontinent Cleanser/Deodorizer

DESCRIPTION
PERI-WASH II, a skin cleanser, contains a safe and effective non-irritating, antimicrobial ingredient, Methylbenzethonium Chloride, in a combination of nonalkaline, soapless cleansers and wetting agents. National Drug Code (NDC) 11701-009.

INDICATIONS AND USAGE
PERI-WASH II, a non-rinse formulation with no added dyes or perfumes, is designed for daily gentle cleansing and care of the perineal area. PERI-WASH II is indicated for cleansing the perineal area by removing fecal matter easily from the skin through the process of emulsification, plus neutralizing and removing urine and odors. Also indicated for use as a gentle cleanser for areas afflicted with ammonia dermatitis associated with diarrhea. PERI-WASH II thoroughly cleanses without robbing the skin of essential moisture, is non-stinging and will not delay the skin's normal healing process.
The medicated, antiseptic quality is soothing to red, irritated skin. Through the incorporation of Methylbenzethonium Chloride, the antimicrobial ingredient, a protective "chemical barrier" is formed on the skin to provide residual protection between uses.
PERI-WASH II provides total elimination of odors associated with incontinent care.

CONTRAINDICATIONS
Hypersensitivity to any components of the preparation.

PRECAUTIONS AND ADVERSE REACTIONS
For External Use Only. If infection or other signs develop, discontinue use and consult a physician. PERI-WASH II is not toxic by oral ingestion and is not considered a primary eye or skin irritant under normal use conditions. Contains no perfumes or dyes.

DOSAGE AND ADMINISTRATION
No-rinse procedure. Spray PERI-WASH II on all feces on skin, pad, linens and clothing to STOP ODORS BEFORE STARTING THE CLEAN-UP PROCEDURE. Remove the bulk of feces. Spray additional PERI-WASH II on warm, wet cloth and cleanse skin of all remaining residue. Turn cloth to clean side and gently wipe entire area. Pat dry. **NOTE:** If area needing care is sizeable and fecal material massive, rinsing is advised. Debris and dead organisms unintentionally left behind can cause irritation.

HOW SUPPLIED
4 fl. oz. and 8 fl. oz. bottles with spray fitment, in addition to larger bulk sizes.

PURI-CLENS™
[*pūri-clĕns*]
Wound Deodorizer and Cleanser

DESCRIPTION
PURI-CLENS contains a safe and effective non-irritating antimicrobial ingredient, Methylbenzethonium Chloride, in a water washable, soothing base. National Drug Code (NDC) 11701-008.

INDICATIONS AND USAGE
PURI-CLENS deodorizes wounds and aids in the removal of foreign materials and exudates. Will not delay wound healing.

CONTRAINDICATIONS
Hypersensitivity to any components of the preparation.

PRECAUTIONS AND ADVERSE REACTIONS
For External Use Only. Do not use on animal bites or puncture wounds. Do not use for more than ten days without consulting physician. PURI-CLENS is not toxic by oral ingestion and is not considered a primary eye or skin irritant under normal use conditions.

DOSAGE AND ADMINISTRATION
Apply PURI-CLENS liberally to a sterile 4″ × 4″ pad. Gently and throughly cleanse wound and surrounding area. To aid in removing foreign material and exudates, dab wound carefully with clean 4″ × 4″ pad saturated with PURI-CLENS. May be rinsed with sterile saline, water or hydrogen peroxide solution.

DEODORIZATION
Apply PURI-CLENS directly to wound and cover with a sterile absorbent pad. Do not use solution with occlusive dressing. Repeat one to three times daily as necessary to control odors.

HOW SUPPLIED
2 fl. oz. unit dose and 8 fl. oz bottles with flip top caps.

SURGI-KLEEN™
[*sŭrgĭ-klēen*]
Skin cleanser and shampoo

DESCRIPTION
A skin cleanser consisting of Water, Sodium Lauryl Sulfate, TEA-Lauryl Sulfate, Cocoamphocarboxypropionate, Propylene Glycol, PPG-12-PEG-65 Lanolin Oil, Citric Acid, Styrene/PVP Copolymer, PEG-8 Laurate, PEG-75 Lanolin, Laureth-23, PEG-4 Oleate, Glycol Stearate, Quaternium-15, Fragrance, Methylbenzethonium Chloride, PEG-90M, FD & C Yellow #5, D & C Red #19 and Other Ingredients. National Drug Code (NDC) 11701-003

INDICATIONS AND USAGE
SURGI-KLEEN, a gentle and effective liquid skin cleanser and shampoo replaces the need for all bar soap and shampoos. One container for both tasks! Containing a special refined lanolin, SURGI-KLEEN, helps retain a soft and supple skin. This easy-to-use, low sudsing liquid rinses free, leaving no residue or film on the skin or hair. The convenient flip-top helps reduce the incidence of cross contamination. Problem head and body odors are controlled when using this one versatile cleanser.

CONTRAINDICATIONS
Hypersensitivity to any components of the preparation.

PRECAUTIONS AND ADVERSE REACTIONS
For External Use Only. SURGI-KLEEN is not toxic by oral ingestion and is not considered a primary skin irritant under normal use conditions. SURGI-KLEEN is an eye irritant (Sodium Lauryl Sulfate) and should be rinsed thoroughly from eyes if accidental contact occurs.

DOSAGE AND ADMINISTRATION
SURGI-KLEEN may be used full strength or diluted one part to three parts of water.
For Regular Bathing: Apply diluted product to moistened wash cloth and gently wash skin, rinse thoroughly and pat dry.
For Shampooing: Apply diluted or undiluted to moistened hair. Massage hair and scalp until lather develops. Then rinse thoroughly and lather again. A very small quantity of SURGI-KLEEN will develop a thick, rich lather when hair is clean.

HOW SUPPLIED
2 fl. oz., 8 fl. oz. and 16 fl. oz. bottles with flip-top caps, 21 fl. oz. with pump dispenser, in addition to larger bulk sizes.

SWEEN-A-PEEL™
Wafer Skin Protectant

DESCRIPTION
SWEEN-A-PEEL is a wafer skin protectant containing the following:
1. WA4 hydrophilic polymer—to provide moisture absorption.
2. High molecular weight synthetic rubber polymers—to provide elasticity and strength.
3. Low molecular weight synthetic rubber polymers—to provide adhesion to dry surfaces.
4. Karaya gum powder—to provide adhesion to moist surfaces.

INDICATIONS AND USAGE
SWEEN-A-PEEL wafers applied to the peristomal area in ostomy care or to the area surrounding draining wounds, aid in protecting the skin against contact with exudates. SWEEN-A-PEEL may also be applied to pressure points of immobile patients to help preserve skin integrity and reduce the possible occurrence of decubitus ulcers. SWEEN-A-PEEL has also proven effective when incorporated into a decubitus ulcer treatment procedure.

CONTRAINDICATIONS
Hypersensitivity to any components of the preparation.

PRECAUTIONS
Avoid excess heat and humidity. Store below 77°F (25°C). Reseal container after each use.

ADMINISTRATION
Preparation. 1. Cleanse entire area thoroughly. 2. A minimal amount of SWEEN CREAM® may be applied to soothe red, irritated skin and also to maintain healthy skin. Massage until completely absorbed and skin is dry to the touch. SWEEN CREAM will not interfere with adhesion of SWEEN-A-PEEL. 3. Remove any residue from weeping, excoriated areas as effectively as possible to assure maximum adherence of SWEEN-A-PEEL.
Ostomy Care: 1. **Important**—Use Measuring Guide to Trace and Cut Pattern of Stoma Base. No Area Skin Should Be Exposed. Transfer pattern to wafer using pencil, then cut. (Precision fit is a must to prevent body wastes from coming in contact with and excoriating unprotected skin). 2. Remove backing paper, and position wafer carefully onto skin. Take care not to touch adhesive surface any more than is necessary as this may impair effective adhesion. 3. Apply even, gentle pressure for 30–60 seconds to wafer with palm of hands, particularly the area immediately surrounding the aperture. This warming effect helps ensure even adhesion to body. If desired, porous tape may be used around edges.
Draining wound care: Use the same procedure as above to protect the area skin from contact with wound exudates. Trace pattern, cut, fit, apply gentle, warming hand pressure and follow prescribed wound care procedure.

HOW SUPPLIED
4″ x 4″ wafer in packets of 5 and tubs of 20 wafers each: 12″ x 12″ square in packages of 2 and 12 squares.

SWEEN CREAM®
[*Swēen Crēam*]
Protective Cream

DESCRIPTION
A vanishing cream consisting of Water, Lanolin Oil, Cetyl Alcohol, Propylene Glycol, Natural Vitamins A & D, Sodium Lauryl Sulfate, Beeswax, Fragrance, Quaternium-15, Methylbenzethonium Chloride and BHT. National Drug Code (NDC) 11701-002.

INDICATIONS AND USAGE
SWEEN CREAM is an effective preparation for use on skin conditions such as urine scald, diaper rash, rectal itch, psoriasis, minor burns, diarrheal breakdown, chafing and itching. Applied on skin before taping, SWEEN CREAM aids in the prevention of tape burns. SWEEN CREAM is used in long-term care of incontinent, geriatric and para/quadraplegic skin. Also apply to folds of skin subject to perspiration irritation, to dry or cracked skin and to pressure sensitive areas. For ostomy care, apply a small amount on peristomal skin for protection before attaching appliance. This relieves itching and improves adhesion.

CONTRAINDICATIONS
Hypersensitivity to any components of the preparation.

PRECAUTIONS AND ADVERSE REACTIONS
For External Use Only. Avoid contact with eyes. SWEEN CREAM is not toxic by oral ingestion and is not considered a primary eye or skin irritant under normal use conditions.

DOSAGE AND ADMINISTRATION
Apply liberally as required.

HOW SUPPLIED
½ oz., 2 oz. and 5 oz. tubes; 2-oz. and 9-oz. jars.

SWEEN KIND TOUCH™
[*swēen kīnd Tŏuch*]
Lotion Skin Cleanser

DESCRIPTION
SWEEN KIND TOUCH is a lotion skin cleanser consisting of Water, Sodium C14-16 Olefin Sulfonate, Cocamidopropyl Betaine, Sodium Chloride, Lauramide DEA, Glycerin, Glycol Stearate, Quaternium-33, Ethyl Hexanediol, Citric Acid, Fragrance, Quaternium-15, Tetrasodium EDTA and FD&C Blue #1.

INDICATIONS AND USAGE
SWEEN KIND TOUCH is a unique conditioning lotion skin cleanser formulated to incorporate richness, creaminess, quick sudsing action, easy rinsing, and a delightful light fragrance. Gentle enough for repeated daily use for all types of general skin cleansing. The pH has been carefully adjusted for compatibility with the normal range of the skin.

CONTRAINDICATIONS
Hypersensitivity to any components of the preparation.

PRECAUTIONS AND ADVERSE REACTIONS
For External Use Only. Avoid contact with eyes. If contact should occur, flush eyes with water. SWEEN KIND TOUCH is not toxic by oral ingestion and is not considered a primary skin irritant under normal use conditions.

DOSAGE AND ADMINISTRATION
Wet hands with warm water. Dispense a small amount of SWEEN KIND TOUCH into palm of hand. Wash thoroughly, rinse and dry.

HOW SUPPLIED
21 fl. oz. with pump dispensers, one gallon containers and 16 fl. oz. empties with flip top caps available.

SWEEN PREP™
[*Swēen Prĕp*]
Protective Skin Barrier Film

DESCRIPTION
SWEEN PREP is a medicated skin barrier which contains Chloroxylenol (PCMX), a well known antimicrobial agent, in a protective film forming base.

INDICATIONS AND USAGE
SWEEN PREP applies to the skin as a liquid, with the aid of the special "Dab-O-Matic" applicator, the non-aerosol sprayer or the single use wipe. It dries rapidly to form a tough film which provides a visible shield on the skin… a barrier between the skin and irritants. This protective film creates a surface other than the skin itself for the application of tapes, cements and doublefaced adhesives.

CONTRAINDICATIONS
Hypersensitivity to any components of the preparation.

PRECAUTIONS AND ADVERSE REACTIONS
If irritation or pain persists, discontinue use and consult physician. For External Use Only. If accidental ingestion occurs or if product comes into contact with the eyes, seek professional help. Flammable. Do not use near flame or while smoking. SWEEN PREP is not toxic by oral ingestion and is not considered a primary skin irritant under normal use conditions.

DOSAGE AND ADMINISTRATION
Wash the skin area thoroughly, rinse and pat dry. Apply SWEEN PREP liberally to the entire area to be protected (slight stinging may be experienced if the skin is excoriated). Allow to dry (approximately 2 minutes) and apply tapes, adhesives, etc., in the normal manner to the SWEEN PREPPED skin. SWEEN PREP may be removed from the skin with soap and water or for easier removal, with isopropyl alcohol. Removal is, however, not necessary and the skin may be recoated as frequently as required.

HOW SUPPLIED
Unit dose wipes (NDC 11701-007-20), 2 fl. oz. "Dab-O-Matic" applicator (NDC 11701-007-03) and 4 fl. oz. non-aerosol spray (NDC 11701-006-04).

SWEEN SOFT TOUCH™
[*Swēen Sŏft Tŏuch*]
Medicated, Antimicrobial Lotion Skin Cleanser

DESCRIPTION
SWEEN SOFT TOUCH is an antimicrobial lotion skin cleanser which contains Chloroxylenol (PCMX), a well known antimicrobial agent, in a mild, densely sudsing, soap-free base, adjusted to pH 5.0–5.5 for optimal activity and maintenance of the "acid-balanced" range for healthy skin. National Drug Code (NDC) 11701-015

INDICATIONS AND USAGE
SWEEN SOFT TOUCH is recommended for repeated daily use as a health care personnel handwash. It decreases bacteria on the skin, reducing the risk and/or chance of cross-infection.

CONTRAINDICATIONS
Hypersensitivity to any components of the preparation.

PRECAUTIONS AND ADVERSE REACTIONS
For External Use Only. Avoid contact with eyes. If accidental contact occurs, immediately flush eyes with water for 15 minutes and consult a physician. SWEEN SOFT TOUCH is not toxic by oral ingestion and is not considered a primary skin irritant under normal use conditions.

DOSAGE AND ADMINISTRATION
Wet skin with warm water. Spread a small amount on hands and forearms. Scrub well and rinse thoroughly with warm water after washing.

HOW SUPPLIED
2 fl. oz. and 16 fl. oz. bottles with flip-top caps, 21 fl. oz. and 32 fl. oz. with pump dispenser; in addition to larger bulk sizes.

WHIRL-SOL®
[*whĭrl-sŏl*]
Skin Conditioner

DESCRIPTION
Mineral Oil, Propylene Glycol Dipelargonate, Lanolin Oil, PEG-8 Dioleate, Fragrance, D&C Green #6. National Drug Code (NDC) 11701-001.

INDICATIONS AND USAGE
WHIRL-SOL provides total dispersion throughout the bathing water to aid in the relief of dry, pruritic conditions and to insure the entire body receives the benefits of this skin condi-

Continued on next page

Sween—Cont.

tioner. WHIRL-SOL's nongreasy protection locks in natural skin moisture to help maintain a healthy, elastic and pliable skin. WHIRL-SOL is an effective aid in treating problems such as soap dermatitis, pruritis senilis and hiemalis, chronic atopic dermatitis, asteatosis, xerosis, ichthyosis and psoriasis. It promotes a normal healthy skin with natural-like oils.

CONTRAINDICATIONS
Hypersensitivity to any components of the preparation.

PRECAUTIONS AND ADVERSE REACTIONS
For External Use Only. Avoid contact with eyes. WHIRL-SOL is not toxic by oral ingestion and is not considered a primary eye or skin irritant under normal use conditions. Guard against slipping in tub or shower.

DOSAGE AND ADMINISTRATION
WHIRL-SOL is always used with water. It is added, 1 to 2 capfuls to whirlpool bathing systems, regular bath tubs, or wash basins. Apply to washcloth for use in the shower.

HOW SUPPLIED
2 fl. oz., 8 fl. oz. and 16 fl. oz. bottles, with flip-top caps, 21 fl. oz. with pump dispenser; in addition to larger bulk sizes.

XTRACARE® II
[xtră-cāre]
Moisturizing Body Lotion

DESCRIPTION
A thick-bodied, high moisturizing lotion consisting of Water, Cetyl Alcohol, Propylene Glycol, Lanolin Oil, Beeswax, Sodium Lauryl Sulfate, Quaternium-15, Fragrance and Methylbenzethonium Chloride.
National Drug Code (NDC) 11701-004.

INDICATIONS AND USAGE
XTRACARE II is an unusually rich moisturizer which serves as an exceptional massage vehicle for the entire body. Its creamy consistency applies easily and uniformly to soothe and moisturize skin. The special emollient and humectant properties provide long lasting retardation of skin moisture evaporation. This leaves the skin feeling smooth, cool and comfortable without greasiness and tackiness or interference of normal skin respiration. Apply as needed for back rubs, dry skin problems and physical therapy. Especially suited for foot and lower leg care. Liberal application recommended before applying plaster casts.

CONTRAINDICATIONS
Hypersensitivity to any components of the preparation.

PRECAUTIONS AND ADVERSE REACTIONS
For External Use Only. Avoid contact with eyes. XTRACARE II is not toxic by oral ingestion and is not considered a primary eye or skin irritant under normal use conditions.

DOSAGE AND ADMINISTRATION
Apply liberally as often as needed for dry skin management. Use as a massage lubricant for back rubs and for therapeutic muscle massage.

HOW SUPPLIED
2 fl. oz., 4 fl. oz. and 8 fl. oz. bottles with flip top dispenser caps, 21 fl. oz. with pump dispenser, and 1 gallon containers.

IDENTIFICATION PROBLEM?
Consult PDR's
Product Identification Section
where you'll find over 1200
products pictured actual size
and in full color.

Syntex (F.P.) Inc.
HUMACAO, PUERTO RICO 00661

Syntex Laboratories, Inc
3401 HILLVIEW AVE.
P.O. BOX 10850
PALO ALTO, CA 94303

Syntex Puerto Rico, Inc.
HUMACAO, PUERTO RICO 00661

ANADROL®-50 ℞
[an 'ă-drawl]
(oxymetholone)
50 mg. Tablets
A product of Syntex Laboratories, Inc.

DESCRIPTION
ANADROL (oxymetholone) tablets for oral administration each contain 50 mg of the steroid oxymetholone, a potent anabolic and androgenic drug.
The chemical name for oxymetholone is 17β-hydroxy-2-(hydroxymethylene)-17-methyl-5α-androstan-3-one. The structural formula is:

Inactive Ingredients—lactose, magnesium stearate, povidone, starch

CLINICAL PHARMACOLOGY
Anabolic steroids are synthetic derivatives of testosterone. Nitrogen balance is improved with anabolic agents but only when there is sufficient intake of calories and protein. Whether this positive nitrogen balance is of primary benefit in the utilization of protein-building dietary substances has not been established. Oxymetholone enhances the production and urinary excretion of erythropoietin in patients with anemias due to bone marrow failure and often stimulates erythropoiesis in anemias due to deficient red cell production.
Certain clinical effects and adverse reactions demonstrate the androgenic properties of this class of drugs. Complete dissociation of anabolic and androgenic effects has not been achieved. The actions of anabolic steroids are therefore similar to those of male sex hormones with the possibility of causing serious disturbances of growth and sexual development if given to young children. They suppress the gonadotropic functions of the pituitary and may exert a direct effect upon the testes.

INDICATIONS AND USAGE
ANADROL-50 is indicated in the treatment of anemias caused by deficient red cell production. Acquired aplastic anemia, congenital aplastic anemia, myelofibrosis and the hypoplastic anemias due to the administration of myelotoxic drugs often respond.
ANADROL-50 should not replace other supportive measures such as transfusion, correction of iron, folic acid, vitamin B_{12} or pyridoxine deficiency, antibacterial therapy and the appropriate use of corticosteroids.

CONTRAINDICATIONS
1. Carcinoma of the prostate or breast in male patients.
2. Carcinoma of the breast in females with hypercalcemia; androgenic anabolic steroids may stimulate osteolytic resorption of bones.
3. Oxymetholone can cause fetal harm when administered to pregnant women. It is contraindicated in women who are or may become pregnant. If the patient becomes pregnant while taking the drug, she should be apprised of the potential hazard to the fetus.
4. Nephrosis or the nephrotic phase of nephritis.
5. Hypersensitivity to the drug.

WARNINGS
The following conditions have been reported in patients receiving androgenic, anabolic steroids as a general class of drugs:

Peliosis hepatis, a condition in which liver and sometimes splenic tissue is replaced with blood-filled cysts, has been reported in patients receiving androgenic anabolic steroid therapy. These cysts are sometimes present with minimal hepatic dysfunction, but at other times they have been associated with liver failure. They are often not recognized until life-threatening liver failure or intra-abdominal hemorrhage develops. Withdrawal of drug usually results in complete disappearance of lesions.
Liver cell tumors are also reported. Most often these tumors are benign and androgen-dependent, but fatal malignant tumors have been reported. Withdrawal of drug often results in regression or cessation of progression of the tumor. However, hepatic tumors associated with androgens or anabolic steroids are much more vascular than other hepatic tumors and may be silent until life-threatening intra-abdominal hemorrhage develops.
Blood lipid changes that are known to be associated with increased risk of atherosclerosis are seen in patients treated with androgens and anabolic steroids. These changes include decreased high density lipoprotein and sometimes increased low density lipoprotein. The changes may be very marked and could have a serious impact on the risk of atheroclerosis and coronary artery disease.

Cholestatic hepatitis and jaundice occur with 17-alpha-alkylated androgens at relatively low doses. If cholestatic hepatitis with jaundice appears, the anabolic steroid should be discontinued. If liver function tests become abnormal, the patient should be monitored closely and the etiology determined. Generally the anabolic steroid should be discontinued, although in cases of mild abnormalities, the physician may elect to follow the patient carefully at a reduced drug dosage.
In patients with breast cancer, anabolic steroid therapy may cause hypercalcemia by stimulating osteolysis. In this case, the drug should be discontinued.
Edema with or without congestive heart failure may be a serious complication in patients with pre-existing cardiac, renal or hepatic disease.
Geriatric male patients treated with androgenic anabolic steroids may be at an increased risk for the development of prostate hypertrophy and prostatic carcinoma.
Anabolic steroids have not been shown to enhance athletic ability.

PRECAUTIONS
General:
Women should be observed for signs of virilization (deepening of the voice, hirsutism, acne, and clitoromegaly). To prevent irreversible change, drug therapy must be discontinued, when mild virilism is first detected. Such virilization is usual following androgenic anabolic steroid use at high doses. Some virilizing changes in women are irreversible even after prompt discontinuance of therapy and are not prevented by concomitant use of estrogens. Menstrual irregularities may also occur.
The insulin or oral hypoglycemic dosage may need adjustment in diabetic patients who receive anabolic steroids.
Anabolic steroids may cause suppression of clotting factors II, V, VII, and X, and an increase in prothrombin time.
Information for the patient:
The physician should instruct patients to report any of the following side effects of androgens.
Adult or Adolescent Males: Too frequent or persistent erections of the penis, appearance or aggravation of acne.
Women: Hoarseness, acne, changes in menstrual periods, or more hair on the face.
All Patients: Any nausea, vomiting, changes in skin color or ankle swelling.
Laboratory Tests:
Women with disseminated breast carcinoma should have frequent determination of urine and serum calcium levels during the course of androgenic anabolic steroid therapy (see WARNINGS).
Because of the hepatotoxicity associated with the use of 17-alpha-alkylated androgens, liver function tests should be obtained periodically.
Periodic (every 6 months) x-ray examinations of bone age should be made during treatment of prepubertal patients to determine the rate of bone maturation and the effects of androgenic anabolic steroid therapy on the epiphyseal centers.
Anabolic steroids have been reported to lower the level of high-density lipoproteins and raise the level of low-density lipoproteins. These changes usually revert to normal on discontinuation of treatment. Increased low-density lipoproteins and decreased high-density lipro proteins are considered cardiovascular risk factors. Serum lipids and high-density lipoprotein cholesterol should be determined periodically.
Hemoglobin and hematocrit should be checked periodically for polycythemia in patients who are receiving high doses of anabolics.
Drug Interaction:
Anabolic steroids may increase sensitivity to anticoagulants; therefore dosage of an anticoagulant may have to be decreased in order to maintain the prothrombin time at the desired therapeutic level.

Drug/Laboratory Test Interferences: Therapy with androgenic anabolic steroids may decrease levels of thyroxine-binding globulin resulting in decreased total T_4 serum levels and increased resin uptake of T_3 and T_4. Free thyroid hormone levels remain unchanged and there is no clinical evidence of thyroid dysfunction.

Anabolic steroids may cause an increase in prothrombin time.

Carcinogenesis, Mutagenesis, Impairment of Fertility:

Long-term studies in animals have not been performed to evaluate the carcinogenic potential of oxymetholone. There are rare reports of hepatocellular carcinoma in patients receiving long-term therapy with anabolics in high doses. Withdrawal of the drugs did not lead to regression of the tumors in all cases.

Pregnancy:

Pregnancy category X. See CONTRAINDICATIONS.

Nursing Mothers:

It is not known whether anabolics are excreted in human milk. Because of the potential for serious adverse reactions in nursed infants from anabolics, women who take oxymetholone should not nurse.

Pediatric Use:

Anabolic/androgenic steroids should be used very cautiously in children and only by specialists who are aware of their effects on bone maturation.

Anabolic agents may accelerate epiphyseal maturation more rapidly than linear growth in children, and the effect may continue for 6 months after the drug has been stopped. Therefore, therapy should be monitored by x-ray studies at 6-month intervals in order to avoid the risk of compromising the adult height.

ADVERSE REACTIONS

Hepatic:

Cholestatic jaundice with, rarely, hepatic necrosis and death. Hepatocellular neoplasms and peliosis hepatis have been reported in association with long-term androgenic-anabolic steroid therapy (see WARNINGS).

Genitourinary System:

In Men:

Prepubertal: Phallic enlargement and increased frequency of erections.

Postpubertal: Inhibition of testicular function, testicular atrophy and oligospermia, impotence, chronic priapism, epididymitis and bladder irritability.

In Women:

Clitoral enlargement, menstrual irregularities.

In both sexes:

Increased or decreased libido.

CNS: Excitation, insomnia.

Gastrointestinal: Nausea, vomiting, diarrhea.

Hematologic: Bleeding in patients on concomitant anticoagulant therapy, iron-deficiency anemia.

Leukemia has been observed in patients with aplastic anemia treated with oxymetholone. The role, if any, of oxymetholone is unclear because malignant transformation has been seen in blood dyscrasias and leukemia has been reported in patients with aplastic anemia who have not been treated with oxymetholone.

Breast: Gynecomastia.

Larynx: Deepening of the voice in women.

Hair: Hirsutism and male-pattern baldness in women.

Skin: Acne (especially in women and prepubertal boys.)

Skeletal: Premature closure of epiphyses in children (see PRECAUTIONS, Pediatric Use.)

Fluid and Electrolytes: Edema, retention of serum electrolytes (sodium, chloride, potassium, phosphate, calcium).

Metabolic/Endocrine: Decreased glucose tolerance (see PRECAUTIONS), increased serum levels of low-density lipoproteins and decreased levels of high-density lipoproteins (see PRECAUTIONS, Laboratory tests), increased creatine and creatinine excretion, increased serum levels of creatinine phosphokinase (CPK). Reversible changes in liver function tests also occur including increased bromsulphalein (BSP) retention and increases in serum bilirubin, glutamic oxaloacetic transaminase (SGOT), and alkaline phosphatase.

OVERDOSAGE

There have been no reports of acute overdosage with anabolics.

DOSAGE AND ADMINISTRATION

The recommended daily dose in children and adults is 1–5 mg/kg body weight per day. The usual effective dose is 1–2 mg/kg/day but higher doses may be required and the dose should be individualized. Response is not often immediate and a minimum trial of three to six months should be given. Following remission, some patients may be maintained without the drug; others may be maintained on an established lower daily dosage. A continued maintenance dose is usually necessary in patients with congenital aplastic anemia.

HOW SUPPLIED

ANADROL-50 (oxymetholone) is supplied in bottles of 100 white scored tablets imprinted with "2902" and "SYNTEX" (NDC 0033-2902-42).

CAUTION: Federal law prohibits dispensing without prescription.

02-2902-42-5 © Revised April 1986

Shown in Product Identification Section, page 432

ANAPROX® ℞

[an 'ă-prox]

(naproxen sodium)

Tablets

A product of Syntex Puerto Rico, Inc.

DESCRIPTION

ANAPROX filmcoated tablets for oral administration each contain 275 mg of naproxen sodium, which is equivalent to 250 mg naproxen with 25 mg (about 1 mEq) sodium. It is a member of the arylacetic acid group of nonsteroidal anti-inflammatory drugs.

The chemical name of naproxen sodium is 2-naphthaleneacetic acid, 6-methoxy-α-methyl-, sodium salt, (—).

Naproxen sodium is a white to creamy white, crystalline solid, freely soluble in water.

Each ANAPROX tablet contains naproxen sodium, the active ingredient, with lactose, magnesium stearate, and microcrystalline cellulose. The coating suspension may contain hydroxypropyl methylcellulose, Opaspray® K-1-4210A, polyethylene glycol 8000 or Opadry® YS-1-4215.

CLINICAL PHARMACOLOGY

ANAPROX, the sodium salt of naproxen, has been developed as an analgesic because it is more rapidly absorbed. Naproxen is a nonsteroidal anti-inflammatory drug with analgesic and antipyretic properties. Naproxen anion inhibits prostaglandin synthesis but beyond this its mode of action is unknown.

Naproxen sodium is rapidly and completely absorbed from the gastrointestinal tract. After administration of naproxen sodium, peak plasma levels of naproxen anion are attained at 1–2 hours with steady-state conditions normally achieved after 4–5 doses. The mean biological half-life of the anion in humans is approximately 13 hours, and at therapeutic levels it is greater than 99% albumin bound. Approximately 95% of the dose is excreted in the urine, primarily as naproxen, 6-0-desmethyl naproxen or their conjugates. The rate of excretion has been found to coincide closely with the rate of drug disappearance from the plasma. The drug does not induce metabolizing enzymes.

The drug was studied in patients with mild to moderate pain, and pain relief was obtained within 1 hour. It is not a narcotic and is not a CNS-acting drug. Controlled double-blind studies have demonstrated the analgesic properties of the drug in, for example, post-operative, post-partum, orthopedic and uterine contraction pain and dysmenorrhea. In dysmenorrheic patients, the drug reduces the level of prostaglandins in the uterus, which correlates with a reduction in the frequency and severity of uterine contractions. Analgesic action has been shown by such measures as reduction of pain intensity scores, increase in pain relief scores, decrease in number of patients requiring additional analgesic medication, and delay in time for required remedication. The analgesic effect has been found to last for up to 7 hours.

The drug was studied in patients with rheumatoid arthritis, osteoarthritis, ankylosing spondylitis, tendinitis and bursitis, and acute gout. It is not a corticosteroid. Improvement in patients treated for rheumatoid arthritis has been demonstrated by a reduction in joint swelling, a reduction in pain, a reduction in duration of morning stiffness, a reduction in disease activity as assessed by both the investigator and patient, and by increased mobility as demonstrated by a reduction in walking time.

In patients with osteoarthritis, the therapeutic action of the drug has been shown by a reduction in joint pain or tenderness, an increase in range of motion in knee joints, increased mobility as demonstrated by a reduction in walking time, and improvement in capacity to perform activities of daily living impaired by the disease.

In clinical studies in patients with rheumatoid arthritis and osteoarthritis, the drug has been shown to be comparable to aspirin and indomethacin in controlling the aforementioned measures of disease activity, but the frequency and severity of the milder gastrointestinal adverse effects (nausea, dyspepsia, heartburn) and nervous system adverse effects (tinnitus, dizziness, lightheadedness) were less than in both the aspirin- and indomethacin-treated patients. It is not known whether the drug causes less peptic ulceration than aspirin.

In patients with ankylosing spondylitis, the drug has been shown to decrease night pain, morning stiffness and pain at rest. In double-blind studies the drug was shown to be as effective as aspirin, but with fewer side effects.

In patients with acute gout, a favorable response to the drug was shown by significant clearing of inflammatory changes (e.g., decrease in swelling, heat) within 24–48 hours, as well as by relief of pain and tenderness.

The drug may be used safely in combination with gold salts and/or corticosteroids; however, in controlled clinical trials, when added to the regimen of patients receiving corticosteroids it did not appear to cause greater improvement over that seen with corticosteroids alone. Whether the drug could be used in conjunction with partially effective doses of corticosteroid for a "steroid-sparing" effect has not been adequately studied. When added to the regimen of patients receiving gold salts, the drug did result in greater improvement. Its use in combination with salicylates is not recommended because data are inadequate to demonstrate that the drug produces greater improvement over that achieved with aspirin alone. Further, there is some evidence that aspirin increases the rate of excretion of the drug.

Generally, improvement due to the drug has not been found to be dependent on age, sex, severity or duration of disease.

In ^{51}Cr blood loss and gastroscopy studies with normal volunteers, daily administration of 1100 mg of ANAPROX (naproxen sodium) has been demonstrated to cause statistically significantly less gastric bleeding and erosion than 3250 mg of aspirin.

INDICATIONS AND USAGE

ANAPROX (naproxen sodium) is indicated in the relief of mild to moderate pain and for the treatment of primary dysmenorrhea.

It is also indicated for the treatment of rheumatoid arthritis, osteoarthritis, ankylosing spondylitis, tendinitis and bursitis, and acute gout.

CONTRAINDICATIONS

The drug is contraindicated in patients who have had allergic reactions to ANAPROX® (naproxen sodium) or to NAPROSYN® (naproxen). It is also contraindicated in patients in whom aspirin or other nonsteroidal anti-inflammatory/analgesic drugs induce the syndrome of asthma, rhinitis, and nasal polyps. Both types of reactions have the potential of being fatal.

WARNINGS

Gastrointestinal bleeding, sometimes severe, and occasionally fatal, has been reported in patients receiving the drug. Among 960 patients treated for rheumatoid arthritis or osteoarthritis during the course of clinical trials in the United States (260 treated for more than two years), 16 cases of peptic ulceration were reported. More than half were on concomitant corticosteroid and/or salicylate therapy and about a third had a prior history of peptic ulcer. Gastrointestinal bleeding, including nine potentially serious cases, was also reported in this population. These were not always preceded by premonitory gastrointestinal symptoms. Although most of the patients with serious bleeding were receiving concomitant therapy and had a history of peptic ulcer disease, it should be kept in mind that the drug also has the potential for causing gastrointestinal bleeding on its own. Therefore, it should not be given to patients with active peptic ulcer unless the potential benefit outweighs the potential risk. In such patients, and in other patients with a history of gastrointestinal disease, it should be given under close supervision.

PRECAUTIONS

General:

ANAPROX (NAPROXEN SODIUM) SHOULD NOT BE USED CONCOMITANTLY WITH THE RELATED DRUG NAPROSYN (NAPROXEN) SINCE THEY BOTH CIRCULATE IN PLASMA AS THE NAPROXEN ANION.

Anaphylactic reactions to ANAPROX or NAPROSYN, whether of the true allergic type or the pharmacologic idiosyncratic (e.g., aspirin syndrome) type, usually but not always occur in patients with a known history of such reactions. Therefore, careful questioning of patients for such things as asthma, nasal polyps, urticaria, and hypotension associated with nonsteroidal anti-inflammatory drugs before starting therapy is important. In addition, if such symptoms occur during therapy, treatment should be discontinued.

Renal Effects: As with other nonsteroidal anti-inflammatory drugs, long-term administration of naproxen to animals has resulted in renal papillary necrosis and other abnormal renal pathology. In humans, there have been reports of acute interstitial nephritis with hematuria, proteinuria, and occasionally nephrotic syndrome.

A second form of renal toxicity has been seen in patients with prerenal conditions leading to the reduction in renal blood flow or blood volume, where the renal prostaglandins have a supportive role in the maintenance of renal perfusion. In these patients, administration of a nonsteroidal anti-inflammatory drug may cause a dose-dependent reduction in prostaglandin formation and may precipitate overt renal decompensation. Patients at greatest risk of this reaction are those with impaired renal function, heart failure, liver dysfunction, those taking diuretics, and the elderly. Discontinuation of nonsteroidal anti-inflammatory therapy is typically followed by recovery to the pretreatment state.

ANAPROX and its metabolites are eliminated primarily by the kidneys, therefore the drug should be used with great caution in patients with significantly impaired renal function and the monitoring of serum creatinine and/or creati-

Continued on next page

Syntex—Cont.

nine clearance is advised in these patients. Caution should be used if the drug is given to patients with creatinine clearance of less than 20 mL/minute because accumulation of naproxen metabolites has been seen in such patients.
Chronic alcoholic liver disease and probably other forms of cirrhosis reduce the total plasma concentration of naproxen, but the plasma concentration of unbound naproxen is increased. Caution is advised when high doses are required and some adjustment of dosage may be required in these patients.
One study indicates that although total plasma concentration of naproxen is unchanged, the unbound plasma fraction of naproxen is increased in the elderly. Caution is advised when high doses are required and some adjustment of dosage may be required in elderly patients.
As with other nonsteroidal anti-inflammatory drugs, borderline elevations of one or more liver tests may occur in up to 15% of patients. These abnormalities may progress, may remain essentially unchanged, or may be transient with continued therapy. The SGPT (ALT) test is probably the most sensitive indicator of liver dysfunction. Meaningful (3 times the upper limit of normal) elevations of SGPT or SGOT (AST) occurred in controlled clinical trials in less than 1% of patients. A patient with symptoms and/or signs suggesting liver dysfunction, or in whom an abnormal liver test has occurred, should be evaluated for evidence of the development of more severe hepatic reaction while on therapy with this drug. Severe hepatic reactions, including jaundice and cases of fatal hepatitis, have been reported with this drug as with other nonsteroidal anti-inflammatory drugs. Although such reactions are rare, if abnormal liver tests persist or worsen, if clinical signs and symptoms consistent with liver disease develop, or if systemic manifestations occur (e.g. eosinophilia, rash, etc.), this drug should be discontinued.
If steroid dosage is reduced or eliminated during therapy, the steroid dosage should be reduced slowly and the patients must be observed closely for any evidence of adverse effects, including adrenal insufficiency and exacerbation of symptoms of arthritis.
Patients with initial hemoglobin values of 10 grams or less who are to receive long-term therapy should have hemoglobin values determined frequently.
Peripheral edema has been observed in some patients. Since each naproxen sodium tablet contains approximately 25 mg (about 1 mEq) of sodium, this should be considered in patients whose overall intake of sodium must be markedly restricted. For these reasons, the drug should be used with caution in patients with fluid retention, hypertension or heart failure.
The antipyretic and anti-inflammatory activities of the drug may reduce fever and inflammation, thus diminishing their utility as diagnostic signs in detecting complications of presumed non-infectious, non-inflammatory painful conditions.
Because of adverse eye findings in animal studies with drugs of this class it is recommended that ophthalmic studies be carried out within a reasonable period of time after starting therapy and at periodic intervals thereafter if the drug is to be used for an extended period of time.

Information for Patients:
Caution should be exercised by patients whose activities require alertness if they experience drowsiness, dizziness, vertigo or depression during therapy with the drug.

Drug Interactions:
In vitro studies have shown that naproxen anion, because of its affinity for protein, may displace from their binding sites other drugs which are also albumin-bound. Theoretically, the naproxen anion itself could likewise be displaced. Short-term controlled studies failed to show that taking the drug significantly affects prothrombin times when administered to individuals on coumarin-type anticoagulants. Caution is advised nonetheless, since interactions have been seen with other nonsteroidal agents of this class. Similarly, patients receiving the drug and a hydantoin, sulfonamide or sulfonylurea should be observed for signs of toxicity to these drugs.
The natriuretic effect of furosemide has been reported to be inhibited by some drugs of this class. Inhibition of renal lithium clearance leading to increases in plasma lithium concentrations has also been reported.
This and other nonsteroidal anti-inflammatory drugs can reduce the antihypertensive effect of propranolol and other beta-blockers.
Probenecid given concurrently increases naproxen anion plasma levels and extends its plasma half-life significantly.
Caution should be used if this drug is administered concomitantly with methotrexate. Naproxen and other nonsteroidal anti-inflammatory drugs have been reported to reduce the tubular secretion of methotrexate in an animal model, possibly enhancing the toxicity of that drug.

Drug/Laboratory Test Interactions:
The drug may decrease platelet aggregation and prolong bleeding time. This effect should be kept in mind when bleeding times are determined.
The administration of the drug may result in increased urinary values for 17-ketogenic steroids because of an interaction between the drug and/or its metabolites with m-dinitrobenzene used in this assay. Although 17-hydroxy-corticosteroid measurements (Porter-Silber test) do not appear to be artifactually altered, it is suggested that therapy with the drug be temporarily discontinued 72 hours before adrenal function tests are performed.
The drug may interfere with some urinary assays of 5-hydroxy indoleacetic acid (5HIAA).

Carcinogenesis:
A two-year study was performed in rats to evaluate the carcinogenic potential of the drug. No evidence of carcinogenicity was found.

Pregnancy:
Teratogenic Effects: Pregnancy Category B. Reproduction studies have been performed in rats, rabbits and mice at doses up to six times the human dose and have revealed no evidence of impaired fertility or harm to the fetus due to the drug. There are, however, no adequate and well-controlled studies in pregnant women. Because animal reproduction studies are not always predictive of human response, the drug should not be used during pregnancy unless clearly needed. Because of the known effect of drugs of this class on the human fetal cardiovascular system (closure of ductus arteriosus), use during late pregnancy should be avoided.
Non-teratogenic Effects: As with other drugs known to inhibit prostaglandin synthesis, an increased incidence of dystocia and delayed parturition occurred in rats.

Nursing Mothers:
The naproxen anion has been found in the milk of lactating women at a concentration of approximately 1% of that found in the plasma. Because of the possible adverse effects of prostaglandin-inhibiting drugs on neonates, use in nursing mothers should be avoided.

Pediatric Use:
Pediatric indications and dosage recommendations have not been established for ANAPROX® (naproxen sodium).

ADVERSE REACTIONS

Adverse reactions reported in controlled clinical trials in 960 patients treated for rheumatoid arthritis or osteoarthritis are listed below. In general, these reactions were reported 2 to 10 times more frequently than they were in studies in the 962 patients treated for mild to moderate pain or for dysmenorrhea.

Incidence greater than 1%

Gastrointestinal: The most frequent complaints reported related to the gastrointestinal tract. They were: constipation*, heartburn*, abdominal pain*, nausea*, dyspepsia, diarrhea, stomatitis.

Central Nervous System: Headache*, dizziness*, drowsiness*, lightheadedness, vertigo.

Dermatologic: Itching (pruritus)*, skin eruptions*, ecchymoses*, sweating, purpura.

Special Senses: Tinnitus*, hearing disturbances, visual disturbances.

Cardiovascular: Edema*, dyspnea*, palpitations.

General: Thirst.
*Incidence of reported reaction between 3% and 9%. Those reactions occurring in less than 3% of the patients are unmarked.

Incidence less than 1%

Probable Causal Relationship:
The following adverse reactions were reported less frequently than 1% during controlled clinical trials and through voluntary reports since marketing. The probability of a causal relationship exists between the drug and these adverse reactions.
Gastrointestinal: Abnormal liver function tests, gastrointestinal bleeding and/or perforation, hematemesis, jaundice, melena, peptic ulceration with bleeding and/or perforation, vomiting.
Renal: Glomerular nephritis, hematuria, interstitial nephritis, nephrotic syndrome, renal disease.
Hematologic: Eosinophilia, granulocytopenia, leukopenia, thrombocytopenia.
Central Nervous System: Depression, dream abnormalities, inability to concentrate, insomnia, malaise, myalgia and muscle weakness.
Dermatologic: Alopecia, photosensitive dermatitis, skin rashes.
Special Senses: Hearing impairment.
Cardiovascular: Congestive heart failure.
Respiratory: Eosinophilic pneumonitis.
General: Anaphylactoid reactions, menstrual disorders, pyrexia (chills and fever).

Causal Relationship Unknown:
Other reactions have been reported in circumstances in which a causal relationship could not be established. However, in these rarely reported events, the possibility cannot be excluded. Therefore these observations are being listed to serve as alerting information to the physicians.

Hematologic: Agranulocytosis, aplastic anemia, hemolytic anemia.

Central Nervous System: Cognitive dysfunction.

Dermatologic: Epidermal necrolysis, erythema multiforme, Stevens-Johnson syndrome, urticaria.

Gastrointestinal: Ulcerative stomatitis.

Cardiovascular: Vasculitis.

General: Angioneurotic edema, hyperglycemia, hypoglycemia.

OVERDOSAGE

Significant overdosage may be characterized by drowsiness, heartburn, indigestion, nausea or vomiting. Because naproxen sodium may be rapidly absorbed, high and early blood levels should be anticipated. No evidence of toxicity or late sequelae have been reported 5 to 15 months after ingestion for three to seven days of doses equivalent to up to 3,300 mg of naproxen sodium. One patient ingested a single dose equivalent to 27.5 g of naproxen sodium and experienced mild nausea and indigestion. It is not known what dose of the drug would be life threatening. The oral LD_{50} of the drug is 543 mg/kg in rats, 1234 mg/kg in mice, 4110 mg/kg in hamsters and greater than 1000 mg/kg in dogs.

Should a patient ingest a large number of tablets, accidentally or purposefully, the stomach may be emptied and usual supportive measures employed. Animal studies suggest that the prompt administration of 5 grams of activated charcoal would tend to reduce markedly the absorption of the drug. It is not known if the drug is dialyzable.

DOSAGE AND ADMINISTRATION

For Mild to Moderate Pain, Primary Dysmenorrhea, and Acute Tendinitis and Bursitis:

The recommended starting dose is two 275 mg tablets, followed by one 275 mg tablet every 6 to 8 hours, as required. The total daily dose should not exceed 5 tablets (1,375 mg).

For Rheumatoid Arthritis, Osteoarthritis, and Ankylosing Spondylitis:

The recommended starting dose in adults is one 275 mg tablet twice daily (morning and evening) or one 275 mg tablet in the morning and two 275 mg tablets in the evening. During long-term administration, the dose may be adjusted up or down depending on the clinical response of the patient. A lower daily dose may suffice for long-term administration. Daily doses higher than 1100 mg in these indications have not been studied. The morning and evening doses do not have to be equal in size and the administration of the drug more frequently than twice daily is not necessary. Symptomatic improvement in arthritis usually begins within two weeks. However, if improvement is not seen within this period, a trial for an additional two weeks should be considered.

For Acute Gout:

The recommended starting dose is three 275 mg tablets, followed by one 275 mg tablet every eight hours until the attack has subsided.

HOW SUPPLIED

ANAPROX® (naproxen sodium) is available in filmcoated tablets of 275 mg (light blue), in bottles of 100 tablets (NDC 18393-274-42) (NSN 6505-01-155-5157) and 500 tablets (NDC 18393-274-62) (NSN 6505-01-130-6832) or in cartons of 100 individually blister packed tablets (NDC 18393-274-53).
Store at room temperature in well-closed containers.
CAUTION: Federal law prohibits dispensing without prescription.
U.S. Patent Nos. 4,009,197; 3,998,966 and others.

Revised 10/85

Shown in Product Identification Section, page 432

BREVICON® Tablets ℞
[brev 'ĭ-kahn]
(norethindrone and ethinyl estradiol)

NORINYL® 1 + 35 Tablets ℞
[nor 'ĭ-nil]
(norethindrone and ethinyl estradiol)

NORINYL® 1 + 50 Tablets ℞
(norethindrone and mestranol)

NORINYL® 1 + 80 Tablets ℞
(norethindrone and mestranol)

NORINYL® 2 mg. Tablets ℞
(norethindrone and mestranol)

NOR–Q.D.® ℞
(norethindrone)
Tablets 0.35 mg.

TRI–NORINYL® Tablets
(norethindrone and ethinyl estradiol)
Oral Contraceptives

PRODUCT OVERVIEW

KEY FACTS

The Syntex line of oral contraceptives includes a triphasic "combination" oral contraceptive (TRI-NORINYL) in which the ethinyl estradiol dose is constant (0.035 mg.) but the norethindrone dose is 0.5 mg. on pill-taking days 1–7, increases to 1.0 mg. on days 8–16, and returns to 0.5 mg. on days 17–21, five constant-dose "combination" oral contraceptives (BREVICON, NORINYL 1 + 35, NORINYL 1 + 50, NORINYL 1 + 80, NORINYL 2 mg.) containing norethindrone (0.5 mg., 1.0 mg., or 2 mg.) and either ethinyl estradiol (0.035) or mestranol (0.05 mg., 0.08 mg., or 0.1 mg.), and a constant-dose oral contraceptive containing norethindrone (0.35 mg) alone (NOR-Q.D.). Except for NORINYL 2mg. and NOR-Q.D., each of the oral contraceptive products is available in both 28-day (including 7 days of inert tablets) and 21-day dosage regimens and is packaged in the Wallette™ pill dispenser.

MAJOR USES

Each of the Syntex oral contraceptive products is highly effective in the prevention of pregnancy. NORINYL 2 mg. is also indicated in the treatment of hypermenorrhea.

SAFETY INFORMATION

See complete safety information set forth below.

PRESCRIBING INFORMATION

BREVICON® Tablets ℞
[brev 'ĭ-kahn]
(norethindrone and ethinyl estradiol)

NORINYL® 1 + 35 Tablets ℞
[nor 'ĭ-nil]
(norethindrone and ethinyl estradiol)

NORINYL® 1 + 50 Tablets ℞
(norethindrone and mestranol)

NORINYL® 1 + 80 Tablets ℞
(norethindrone and mestranol)

NORINYL® 2 mg. Tablets ℞
(norethindrone and mestranol)

NOR–Q.D.® ℞
(norethindrone)
Tablets 0.35 mg.

TRI–NORINYL® Tablets
(norethindrone and ethinyl estradiol)
Oral Contraceptives
Products of Syntex (F.P.) Inc.

DESCRIPTION

BREVICON 21-DAY Tablets provide an oral contraceptive regimen consisting of 21 blue tablets containing norethindrone 0.5 mg. with ethinyl estradiol 0.035 mg.

BREVICON 28-DAY Tablets provide a continuous oral contraceptive regimen consisting of 21 blue tablets containing norethindrone 0.5 mg. with ethinyl estradiol 0.035 mg. and 7 orange tablets containing inert ingredients.

NORINYL 1 + 35 21-DAY Tablets provide an oral contraceptive regimen consisting of 21 green tablets containing norethindrone 1 mg. with ethinyl estradiol 0.035 mg.

NORINYL 1 + 35 28-DAY Tablets provide a continuous oral contraceptive regimen consisting of 21 green tablets containing norethindrone 1 mg. with ethinyl estradiol 0.035 mg. and 7 orange tablets containing inert ingredients.

NORINYL 1 + 50 21-DAY Tablets provide an oral contraceptive regimen consisting of 21 white tablets containing norethindrone 1 mg. with mestranol 0.05 mg.

NORINYL 1 + 50 28-DAY Tablets provide a continuous oral contraceptive regimen consisting of 21 white tablets containing norethindrone 1 mg. with mestranol 0.05 mg. and 7 orange tablets containing inert ingredients.

NORINYL 1 + 80 21-DAY Tablets provide an oral contraceptive regimen consisting of 21 yellow tablets containing norethindrone 1 mg. with mestranol 0.08 mg.

NORINYL 1 + 80 28-DAY Tablets provide a continuous oral contraceptive regimen consisting of 21 yellow tablets containing norethindrone 1 mg. with mestranol 0.08 mg. and 7 orange tablets containing inert ingredients.

NORINYL 2 mg. Tablets provide an oral contraceptive regimen consisting of 20 white tablets containing norethindrone 2 mg. with mestranol 0.1 mg.

NOR-Q.D. (norethindrone) Tablets provide a continuous oral contraceptive regimen of one yellow norethindrone 0.35 mg. tablet daily.

TRI-NORINYL 21-DAY Tablets provide an oral contraceptive regimen of 7 blue tablets followed by 9 green tablets and 5 more blue tablets. Each blue tablet contains norethindrone 0.5 mg with ethinyl estradiol 0.035 mg and each green tablet contains norethindrone 1.0 mg with ethinyl estradiol 0.035 mg.

TRI-NORINYL 28-DAY Tablets provide a continuous oral contraceptive regimen of 7 blue tablets, 9 green tablets, 5 more blue tablets, and then 7 orange tablets. Each blue tablet contains norethindrone 0.5 mg with ethinyl estradiol 0.035 mg, each green tablet contains norethindrone 1.0 mg with ethinyl estradiol 0.035 mg, and each orange tablet contains inert ingredients.

Norethindrone is a potent progestational agent with the chemical name 17-hydroxy-19-nor-17α-pregn-4-en-20-yn-3-one. Ethinyl estradiol is an estrogen with the chemical name 19-nor-17α-pregna-1, 3, 5(10) -trien-20-yne-3, 17-diol. Mestranol is an estrogen with the chemical name 3-methoxy-19-nor-17α-pregna-1, 3, 5(10) -trien-20-yn-17-ol.

Inactive Ingredients: Each tablet contains the following inactive ingredients: lactose, magnesium stearate, povidone, starch, and one or more of the following FDA certified dyes; D&C Green No. 5, D&C Yellow No. 10, FD&C Blue No. 1, FD&C Yellow No. 6.

CLINICAL PHARMACOLOGY

Combination oral contraceptives act primarily through the mechanism of gonadotrophin suppression due to the estrogenic and progestational activity of the ingredients. Although the primary mechanism of action is inhibition of ovulation, alterations in the genital tract including changes in the cervical mucus (which increase the difficulty of sperm penetration) and the endometrium (which reduce the likelihood of implantation) may also contribute to contraceptive effectiveness.

The primary mechanism through which NOR-Q.D. prevents conception is not known, but progestogen-only contraceptives are known to alter the cervical mucus, exert a progestational effect on the endometrium, interfering with implantation, and, in some patients, suppress ovulation.

INDICATIONS AND USAGE

Oral contraceptives are indicated for the prevention of pregnancy in women who elect to use oral contraceptives as a method of contraception. NORINYL 2 mg. is also indicated in the treatment of hypermenorrhea.

Oral contraceptives are highly effective. The pregnancy rate in women using conventional combination oral contraceptives (containing 0.035 mg. or more of ethinyl estradiol or 0.05 mg. or more of mestranol) is generally reported as less than one pregnancy per 100 woman-years of use. Slightly higher rates (somewhat more than 1 pregnancy per 100 woman-years of use) are reported for some combination products containing 0.035 mg. or less of ethinyl estradiol, and rates on the order of 3 pregnancies per 100 woman-years are reported for the progestogen-only oral contraceptives.

These rates are derived from separate studies conducted by different investigators in several population groups and cannot be compared precisely. Furthermore, pregnancy rates tend to be lower as clinical studies are continued, possibly due to selective retention in the longer studies of those patients who accept the treatment regimen and do not discontinue as a result of adverse reactions, pregnancy, or other reasons.

In clinical trials with BREVICON, 1,168 patients completed 16,345 cycles and a total of 3 pregnancies was reported. This represents a pregnancy rate of 0.22 per 100 woman-years. In clinical trials with NORINYL 1 + 35, 940 patients completed 14,366 cycles and a total of 2 pregnancies was reported. This represents a pregnancy rate of 0.17 per 100 woman-years.

The dropout rate for medical reasons, as observed in the clinical trials conducted with BREVICON and NORINYL 1 + 35, appears to be somewhat higher than observed with higher dose combination products. The dropout rate due to menstrual disorders and irregularities was also somewhat higher, dropouts being equally split between menstrual disorders and irregularities and other medical reasons attributable to the drug.

In clinical trials with NORINYL 1 + 50 21-DAY, 3,852 patients completed 45,937 cycles and a total of 10 pregnancies was reported. This represents a pregnancy rate of 0.26 per 100 woman-years. In clinical trials with NORINYL 1 + 50 28-DAY, 1,590 patients completed 7,330 cycles and a total of 3 pregnancies was reported. This represents a pregnancy rate of 0.5 per 100 woman-years. In clinical trials with NORINYL 1 + 80 21- and 28-DAY, 3,464 patients completed 34,068 cycles and a total of 5 pregnancies was reported. This represents a pregnancy rate of 0.18 per 100 woman-years. In clinical trials with NORINYL 2 mg. 6,097 patients completed 121,233 cycles and a total of 13 pregnancies was reported. This represents a pregnancy rate of 0.13 per 100 woman-years. In clinical trials with NOR-Q.D. (norethindrone) 2,963 patients completed 25,901 cycles of therapy and a total of 55 pregnancies was reported. This represents an average pregnancy rate of 2.54 per 100 woman-years. A higher pregnancy rate of 3.72 was recorded in "fresh" patients (those who had never taken oral contraceptives prior to starting NOR-Q.D. therapy) to a large extent because of incorrect tablet intake. This compares to the lower pregnancy rate of 1.95 recorded in "changeover" patients (those switched from other oral contraceptives). This difference was found to be statistically significant. Furthermore, an even greater statistically significant difference in pregnancy rates between these two groups was found during the first six months of NOR-Q.D. therapy. Therefore, it is especially important for "fresh" patients to strictly adhere to the regimen.

The TRI-NORINYL 21-DAY Tablet regimen is 7 blue tablets, 9 green tablets, and then 5 blue tablets. The TRI-NORINYL 28-DAY Tablet regimen is 7 blue tablets, 9 green tablets, 5 blue tablets, and then 7 orange placebo tablets.

Each blue tablet contains norethindrone 0.5 mg with ethinyl estradiol 0.035 mg. In clinical trials with this formulation, 1,168 patients completed 16,345 cycles and 3 pregnancies were reported. This represents a pregnancy rate of 0.22 per 100 woman-years.

Each green tablet contains norethindrone 1.0 mg with ethinyl estradiol 0.035 mg. In clinical trials with this formulation, 940 patients completed 14,366 cycles and 2 pregnancies were reported. This represents a pregnancy rate of 0.17 per 100 woman-years.

Table 1 gives ranges of pregnancy rates reported in the literature[1] for other means of contraception. The efficacy of these means of contraception (except the IUD) depends upon the degree of adherence to the method.

TABLE 1. *Pregnancies per 100 Woman-Years*

IUD, less than 1–6;
Diaphragm with spermicidal products (creams or jellies), 2–20;
Condom, 3–36;
Aerosol foams, 2–29;
Jellies and creams, 4–36;
Periodic abstinence (rhythm) all types, less than 1–47;
— Calendar method, 14–47;
— Temperature method, 1–20;
— Temperature method—intercourse only in post-ovulatory phase, less than 1–7;
— Mucus method, 1–25;
No contraception, 60–80.

Dose-Related Risk of Thromboembolism From Oral Contraceptives. Studies have shown a positive association between the dose of estrogens in oral contraceptives and the risk of thromboembolism[2,3,81,82]. For this reason, it is prudent and in keeping with good principles of therapeutics to minimize exposure to estrogen. The oral contraceptive product prescribed for any given patient should be that product which contains the least amount of estrogen that is compatible with an acceptable pregnancy rate and patient acceptance. It is recommended that new acceptors of oral contraceptives should be started on preparations containing 0.05 mg or less of estrogen.

CONTRAINDICATIONS

1. Known or suspected pregnancy (see Warning No. 5).
2. Thrombophlebitis or thromboembolic disorders.
3. A past history of deep vein thrombophlebitis or thromboembolic disorders.
4. Undiagnosed abnormal genital bleeding.
5. Oral contraceptives should not be used by women who have or have had any of the following conditions:
   a. Cerebral vascular or coronary artery disease, including myocardial infarction.
   b. Known or suspected carcinoma of the breast.
   c. Known or suspected estrogen dependent neoplasia.
   d. Benign or malignant liver tumor which developed during the use of oral contraceptives or other estrogen containing products.

Continued on next page

Syntex—Cont.

WARNINGS

Cigarette smoking increases the risk of serious cardiovascular side effects from oral contraceptive use. This risk increases with age and with heavy smoking (15 or more cigarettes per day) and is quite marked in women over 35 years of age. Women who use oral contraceptives should be strongly advised not to smoke.

The use of oral contraceptives is associated with increased risk of several serious conditions including thromboembolism, stroke, myocardial infarction, liver tumor, gall bladder disease, visual disturbances, fetal abnormalities, and hypertension. Practitioners prescribing oral contraceptives should be familiar with the following information relating to these risks.

1. *Thromboembolic Disorders and Other Vascular Problems:* An increased risk of thromboembolic and thrombotic disease associated with the use of oral contraceptives is well established. One British study[4] demonstrated an increased relative risk for fatal venous thromboembolism, several British[5,6,11,20,72] and three American[3,7,8,21] studies demonstrated an increased relative risk for non-fatal venous thromboembolism. These studies estimate that users of oral contraceptives are 4 to 11 times more likely than nonusers to develop these diseases without evident cause (Table 2). An analysis of deaths in one British study[73] reported an excess death rate of 40% in oral contraceptive users, most of which resulted from cardiovascular disease. A somewhat similar British study[74] showed a lower death rate in oral contraceptive users than controls; here an increase in cardiovascular deaths was seen although the findings were not statistically significant. A U.S. prospective study[75] failed to disclose increased mortality rates from cardiovascular disorders. However, a selected subset of this study, analyzed as a retrospective, case-control study[76] showed significant increases in venous thromboembolism.

Cerebrovascular Disorders. Two American studies[7,9,10] demonstrated an increased relative risk for stroke, which had not been shown in prior British studies[4–6]. In a collaborative American study[9,10] of cerebrovascular disorders in women with and without predisposing causes, it was estimated that the relative risk of hemorrhagic stroke was 2.0 times greater in users than nonusers and the relative risk of thrombotic stroke was 4 to 9.5 times greater in users than in nonusers (Table 2). A British long-term, follow-up study[11] reported in 1976 a highly significant association between oral contraceptive use and stroke, which was confirmed in a 1984 update.[93] Another British long-term, follow-up study[12] had suggested such an association in 1974, but the number of cases was too small to estimate the risk. Subarachnoid hemorrhage has been shown to be increased by oral contraceptive use in British[73] and American studies[75,77]. Smoking alone increases the incidence of these accidents and smoking and pill use appear to work together to produce a combined risk greater than either alone.

Myocardial Infarction. An increased relative risk of myocardial infarction associated with the use of oral contraceptives has been reported[13–15], confirming a previously suspected association[4]. One study[14,15] conducted in the United Kingdom found, as expected, that the greater the number of underlying risk factors for coronary artery disease (cigarette smoking, hypertension, hypercholesterolemia, obesity, diabetes, history of preeclamptic toxemia) the higher the risk of developing myocardial infarction, regardless of whether the patient was an oral contraceptive user or not. Oral contraceptives, however, were found to be an additional risk factor.

In terms of relative risk, it has been estimated[16,17] that oral contraceptive users who do not smoke (smoking is considered a major predisposing condition to myocardial infarction) are about twice as likely to have a fatal myocardial infarction as nonusers who do not smoke. Oral contraceptive users who are also smokers have about a 5-fold increased risk of fatal infarction compared to users who do not smoke, and about a 10- to 12-fold increased risk compared to nonusers who do not smoke. Furthermore, the number of cigarettes smoked is also an important factor. In determining the importance of these relative risks, however, the baseline rates for various age groups, as shown in Table 3, must be given serious consideration. (The estimates in Table 3 are based on British vital statistics which show acute myocardial infarction death rates 2- to 3-times less than in the U.S. for women in these age groups; consequently, actual U.S. death rates could be higher than those in Table 3[17].) The importance of other predisposing conditions mentioned above in determining relative and absolute risks has not been quantified; other synergistic actions may exist.

TABLE 2. *Summary of relative risk of thromboembolic disorders and other vascular problems in oral contraceptive users compared to nonusers*

	Relative risk, times greater
Idiopathic thromboembolic disease	4–11
Post surgery thromboembolic complications	4–6
Thrombotic stroke	4–9.5
Hemorrhagic stroke	2
Myocardial infarction	2–12
Subarachnoid hemorrhage	6–22

TABLE 3. *Estimated[16] annual mortality rate per 100,000 women from myocardial infarction by use of oral contraceptives, smoking habits, and age (in years)*

	Myocardial infarction			
	Women aged 30–39		Women aged 40–44	
Smoking habits	Users	Non-users	Users	Non-users
All smokers	10.2	2.6	62.0	15.9
Heavy*	13.0	5.1	78.7	31.3
Light	4.7	0.9	28.6	5.7
Nonsmokers	1.8	1.2	10.7	7.4
Smokers and nonsmokers	5.4	1.9	32.8	11.7

* Heavy smoker: 15 or more cigarettes per day.

Risk of Dose. In an analysis of data derived from several national adverse reaction reporting systems[2], British investigators concluded that the risk of thromboembolism including coronary thrombosis is directly related to the dose of estrogen used in oral contraceptives. Preparations containing 0.1 mg or more of estrogen were associated with a higher risk of thromboembolism than those containing 0.05–0.08 mg of estrogen. Their analysis did suggest, however, that the quantity of estrogen may not be the sole factor involved. This finding has been supported by a study in the United States[3]. A subsequent study in Great Britain[81] found a positive association between dose of progestogen or estrogen and certain thromboembolic conditions. Swedish authorities[82] noted decreased reporting of thromboembolic episodes when higher estrogen preparations were no longer prescribed. Careful epidemiological studies to determine the degree of thromboembolic risk associated with progestogen-only oral contraceptives have not been performed. Cases of thromboembolic disease have been reported in women using these products, and they should not be presumed to be free of excess risk.

Persistence of Risk: In confirmation of earlier reports,[18,73] two studies have suggested that an increased risk may persist for as long as 6 years after discontinuation of oral contraceptive use for cerebrovascular disease[87] and 9 years for myocardial infarction.[88] In addition, a prospective study suggested the persistence of risk for subarachnoid hemorrhage.[77]

Estimate of Excess Mortality from Circulatory Diseases. A large British prospective study[12,18] estimated[18] the mortality rate per 100,000 women per year from diseases of the circulatory system for users and nonusers of oral contraceptives according to age, smoking habits, and duration of use. The overall excess death rate annually from circulatory diseases for oral contraceptive users was estimated to be 20 per 100,000 (ages 15–34—5/100,000; ages 35–44—33/100,000; ages 45–49—140/100,000). The risk is concentrated in older women, in those with a long duration of use, and in cigarette smokers, and may persist after discontinuation of oral contraceptive use. It was not possible, however, to examine the interrelationships of age, smoking, and duration of use, nor to compare the effects of continuous vs. intermittent use. Although the study showed a 10-fold increase in death due to circulatory diseases in users for 5 or more years, all of these deaths occurred in women 35 or older. An update of this study[73] provided the following rates: ages 15–34—1/6700 for non-smokers and 1/2000 for smokers; ages 45 and over—1/2500 for non-smokers and 1/500 for smokers.

Risk appeared to increase with parity, but not with duration of use. Until larger numbers of women under 35 with continuous use for 5 or more years are available, it is not possible to assess the magnitude of the relative risk for this younger age group.

The available data from a variety of sources have been analyzed[19] to estimate the risk of death associated with various methods of contraception. The estimates of risk of death for each method include the combined risk of the contraceptive method (e.g., thromboembolic and thrombotic disease in the case of oral contraceptives) plus the risk attributable to pregnancy or abortion in the event of method failure. This latter risk varies with the effectiveness of the contraceptive method. The findings of this analysis are shown in Figure 1[19]. The study concluded that the mortality associated with all methods of birth control is low and below that of childbirth, with the exception of oral contraceptives in women over 40 who smoke. (The rates given for pill only/smokers for each age group are for smokers as a class. For "heavy" smokers (more than 15 cigarettes a day), the rates given would be about double; for "light" smokers (less than 15 cigarettes a day), about 50 percent.) The lowest mortality is associated with the condom or diaphragm backed up by early abortion. The study also concluded that oral contraceptive users who smoke, especially those over the age of 30, have a greater mortality risk than oral contraceptive users who do not smoke.

Figure 1. Annual number of deaths associated with control of fertility and no control per 100,000 nonsterile women, by regimen of control and age of woman

Annual deaths: 0–60

Age: 15–19, 20–24, 25–29, 30–34, 35–39, 40–44

Regimen of control: No method; Abortion only; Pill only/nonsmokers; Pill only/smokers; IUDS only; Traditional contraception only; Traditional contraception and abortion

The risk of thromboembolic and thrombotic disease associated with oral contraceptives increases with age after approximately age 30 and, for myocardial infarction, is further increased by hypertension, hyperlipidemias, obesity, diabetes, or history of preeclamptic toxemia and especially by cigarette smoking[16,17].

Based on the data currently available, the following chart gives a gross estimate of the risk of death from circulatory disorders associated with the use of oral contraceptives:

Smoking Habits and Other Predisposing Conditions—Risk Associated with Use of Oral Contraceptives

Age	Below 30	30–39	40+
Heavy smokers	C	B	A
Light smokers	D	C	B
Nonsmokers (no predisposing conditions)	D	C, D	C
Nonsmokers (other predisposing conditions)	C	C, B	B, A

A—Use associated with very high risk.
B—Use associated with high risk.
C—Use associated with moderate risk.
D—Use associated with low risk.

The physician and the patient should be alert to the earliest manifestations of thromboembolic and thrombotic disorders (e.g., thrombophlebitis, pulmonary embolism, cerebrovascular insufficiency, coronary occlusion, retinal thrombosis, and mesenteric thrombosis). Should any of these occur or be suspected, the drug should be discontinued immediately.

A four- to six-fold increased risk of post-surgery thromboembolic complications has been reported in oral contraceptive users[20,21]. If feasible, oral contraceptives should be discontinued at least 4 weeks before surgery of a type associated with an increased risk of thromboembolism or prolonged immobilization. The decision as to when to resume oral contraception following major surgery or bedrest should balance the recognized risks of post-surgery thromboembolic complications with the need to reinstate contraceptive practices.

Data[72] also suggest that the presence of varicose veins substantially increases the risk of superficial venous thrombosis of the leg, the risk depending on the severity of the varicosities.

2. *Ocular Lesions:* There have been reports of neuro-ocular lesions such as optic neuritis or retinal thrombosis associated with the use of oral contraceptives. Discontinue oral contraceptive medication if there is unexplained, sudden or gradual, partial or complete loss of vision; onset of proptosis or diplopia; papilledema; or retinal vascular lesions; and institute appropriate diagnostic and therapeutic measures.

3. *Carcinoma:* Long-term continuous administration of either natural or synthetic estrogen in certain animal species increases the frequency of certain tumors, benign or malignant, such as those of the breast, cervix, vagina, uterus, ovary, pituitary and liver. Certain synthetic progestogens, none currently contained in oral contraceptives, have been noted to increase the incidence of mammary nodules, benign and malignant, in dogs.

Several retrospective case-control studies[22–27] have reported an increased relative risk (3.1 to 13.9 times) associating endometrial carcinoma with the prolonged use of estrogens in postmenopausal women who took estrogen replacement medication to relieve menopausal symptoms. One publication[28] reported on the first 30 cases submitted by physicians to a registry of cases of adenocarcinoma of the endometrium in women under 40 on oral contraceptives. Of the adenocarcinomas found in women without predisposing risk factors for adenocarcinoma of the endometrium (e.g., irregular bleeding at the time oral contraceptives were first given, polycystic ovaries) nearly all occurred in women who had used a sequential oral contraceptive. These products are no longer marketed. No statistical association has been reported suggesting an increased risk of endometrial cancer in users of conventional combination or progestogen-only oral contraceptives, although individual cases have been reported.

Several studies[8,29–33] have shown no increased risk of breast cancer to women taking oral contraceptives or estrogens. In one study[34,35], however, while no overall increased risk of breast cancer was noted in women treated with oral contraceptives, a greater risk was suggested for the subgroups of oral contraceptive users with documented benign breast disease and for long-term (2–4 years) users. In one study, it was found that a history of breast cancer among grandmothers or aunts was significantly more frequent among breast cancer patients who had used an oral contraceptive continuously for one or more years than among non-users with breast cancer[83]. One other study[36] indicated an increasing risk of breast cancer in women taking menopausal estrogens, which increased with duration of follow-up. A reduced occurrence of benign breast tumors in users of oral contraceptives has been well documented[8,11,12,29,34,37,38]. In contrast, one author[79] suggests that extended (over 6 years) use of oral contraceptives prior to the first full term pregnancy was associated with a significant relative risk of breast cancer and other studies suggested an increased risk of breast cancer with long-term oral contraceptive use before the age of 25.[94,98]

One study[75] reported malignant melanoma more frequently in oral contraceptive users than in controls and suggests an increased incidence of urinary tract cancers and thyroid cancers.

In a prospective study[39] of women with cervical dysplasia, there was an increase in severity and of conversion to cancer *in situ* in oral contraceptive users compared with nonusers. This became statistically significant after 3 to 4 years of use. Nonreversal of dysplasia within the first 6 months of pill use was suggested to be predictive of progression after prolonged exposure. One study[75] disclosed an increased risk of cancer of the cervix (largely carcinoma-*in-situ*) in oral contraceptive users under 40, particularly those who had used these drugs for over four years. Two other studies suggested increasing incidence of cervical neoplasms with longer duration of oral contraceptive use.[95,99] There have been other reports of microglandular hyperplasia of the cervix in users of oral contraceptives.

One study reported an association between oral contraceptive use and endocervical adenocarcinoma.[89]

In summary, there is at present no confirmed evidence from human studies of an increased risk of cancer associated with oral contraceptives. Close clinical surveillance of all women taking oral contraceptives is, nevertheless, essential. In all cases of undiagnosed persistent or recurrent abnormal vaginal bleeding, appropriate diagnostic measures should be taken to rule out malignancy. Women with a strong family history of breast cancer or who have breast nodules, fibrocystic disease or abnormal mammograms should be monitored with particular care if they elect to use oral contraceptives instead of other methods of contraception.

4. *Liver Tumors:* Sudden severe abdominal pain or shock may be due to rupture and hemorrhage of a liver tumor. There have been reports associating benign or malignant liver tumors with oral contraceptive use[40–44]. This has been reported in short-term as well as long-term users of oral contraceptives. One study[44] reported that use of oral contraceptives with high hormonal potency and age over 30 years may further increase a woman's risk of hepatocellular adenoma. Two studies[41,44] relate risk with duration of use, the risk being much greater after 4 or more years of use. Long-term users of oral contraceptives have an estimated annual incidence of hepatocellular adenoma of 3-4 per 100,000.[44] Although it is an uncommon lesion, it should be considered in women presenting with an "acute abdomen". The tumor may cause serious or fatal hemorrhage. Patients with liver tumors have demonstrated variable clinical features which may make preoperative diagnosis difficult. Some cases presented because of right upper quadrant masses, while most had signs and symptoms of acute intraperitoneal hemorrhage. Routine radiological and laboratory studies may not be helpful. Liver scans may clearly show a focal defect. Hepatic arteriography may be a useful procedure in diagnosing primary liver neoplasm.

5. *Use in or Immediately Preceding Pregnancy, Birth Defects in Offspring, and Malignancy in Female Offspring:* The use of female sex hormones—both estrogenic and progestational agents—during early pregnancy may seriously damage the offspring. It has been shown that females exposed *in utero* to diethylstilbestrol, a nonsteroidal estrogen, have an increased risk of developing in later life a form of vaginal or cervical cancer that is ordinarily extremely rare[45,46]. This risk has been estimated to be of the order of 1 in 1,000 exposures or less[47,48]. Although there is no evidence at the present time that oral contraceptives further enhance the risk of developing this type of malignancy, such patients should be monitored with particular care if they elect to use oral contraceptives instead of other methods of contraception.

Furthermore, a high percentage of women exposed to diethylstilbestrol (from 30 to 90%) have been found to have epithelial changes of the vagina and cervix[49–53]. Although these changes are histologically benign, it is not known whether this condition is a precursor of vaginal malignancy. Male children so exposed may develop abnormalities of the urogenital tract[54–56]. Although similar data are not available with the use of other estrogens, it cannot be presumed that they would not induce similar changes.

An increased risk of congenital anomalies, including heart defects and limb defects, has been reported following use of sex hormones, including oral contraceptives, in pregnancy[57–61]. In one case-control study[60] it was estimated that there was a 4.7-fold increased relative risk of limb-reduction defects in infants exposed *in utero* to sex hormones (oral contraceptives, hormonal withdrawal tests for pregnancy or attempted treatment for threatened abortion). Some of these exposures were very short and involved only a few days of treatment. The data suggest that the risk of limb-reduction defects in exposed fetuses is somewhat less than 1 in 1,000 live births. In a large prospective study[61], cardiovascular defects in children born to women who received female hormones, including oral contraceptives, during early pregnancy occurred at a rate of 18.2 per 1,000 births, compared to 7.8 per 1,000 for children not so exposed *in utero*. These results are statistically significant. A Welsh study[80] identified a statistically significant excess of neural tube defects among offspring of prior users (within 3 months) of oral contraceptives than among controls. The incidence of twin births may be increased for women who conceive shortly after discontinuing use of the pill[11,60,84,85,86].

In the past, female sex hormones have been used during pregnancy in an attempt to treat threatened or habitual abortion. There is considerable evidence that estrogens are ineffective for these indications, and there is no evidence from well controlled studies that progestogens are effective for these uses.

There is some evidence that triploidy and possibly other types of polyploidy are increased among abortuses from women who become pregnant soon after ceasing oral contraceptives.[62]. Embryos with these anomalies are virtually always aborted spontaneously. Whether there is an overall increase in spontaneous abortion of pregnancies conceived soon after stopping oral contraceptives is unknown.

If the patient has not adhered to the prescribed schedule, the possibility of pregnancy should be considered at the time of the first missed period (or after 45 days from the last menstrual period if progestogen-only contraceptives are used) and further use of oral contraceptives should be withheld until pregnancy has been ruled out. It is recommended that for any patient who has missed two consecutive periods, pregnancy should be ruled out before continuing the contraceptive regimen. If pregnancy is confirmed, the patient should be apprised of the potential risks to the fetus and the advisability of continuation of the pregnancy should be discussed in the light of these risks.

It is also recommended that women who discontinue oral contraceptives with the intent of becoming pregnant use an alternate form of contraception for a period of time before attempting to conceive. Many clinicians recommend 3 months; this recommendation is supported by a study suggesting an increased frequency of neural tube defects in women impregnated during the first three months after cessation of pill use[80].

The administration of progestogen-only or progestogen-estrogen combinations to induce withdrawal bleeding should not be used as a test of pregnancy.

6. *Gall Bladder Disease:* Studies[3,8,11,12,31] report an increased risk of gall bladder disease in users of oral contraceptives or estrogens. In one study[12], an increased risk appeared after 2 years of use and doubled after 4 or 5 years of use. In another study[8], an increased risk was apparent between 6 and 12 months of use.

7. *Carbohydrate and Lipid Metabolic Effects:* A decrease in glucose tolerance has been observed in a significant percentage of patients on oral contraceptives. For this reason, prediabetic and diabetic patients should be carefully observed while receiving oral contraceptives. An increase in triglycerides and total phospholipids has been observed in patients receiving oral contraceptives[63]. The clinical significance of this finding is unknown.

8. *Elevated Blood Pressure:* An increase in blood pressure has been reported[12,64] with oral contraceptive use. In some women, hypertension may occur within a few months of beginning oral contraceptive use. In the first year of use, the prevalence of women with hypertension is low in users and may be no higher than that of a comparable group of nonusers. The prevalence in users increases, however, with longer exposure, and in the fifth year of use is two and a half to three times the reported prevalence in the first year. Age is also strongly correlated with the development of hypertension in oral contraceptive users. Women with a history of elevated blood pressure (hypertension), preexisting renal disease, a history of toxemia or elevated blood pressure during pregnancy, a familial tendency to hypertension or its consequences, or a history of excessive weight gain or fluid retention during the menstrual cycle may be more likely to develop elevation of blood pressure when given oral contraceptives and, therefore, should be monitored closely[65].

Even though elevated blood pressure may remain within the "normal" range, the clinical implications of elevations should not be ignored and close surveillance is indicated, particularly for women with other risk factors for cardiovascular disease or stroke[64]. High blood pressure may or may not persist after discontinuation of the oral contraceptive.

9. *Headache:* The onset or exacerbation of migraine or development of headache of a new pattern which is recurrent, persistent, or severe, requires discontinuation of oral contraceptives and evaluation of the cause.

10. *Bleeding Irregularities:* Breakthrough bleeding, spotting, and missed menses are frequent reasons for patients discontinuing oral contraceptives. In breakthrough bleeding, as in all cases of irregular bleeding from the vagina, nonfunctional causes should be borne in mind. In undiagnosed persistent or recurrent abnormal bleeding from the vagina, adequate diagnostic measures are indicated to rule out pregnancy or malig-

Continued on next page

Syntex—Cont.

nancy. If pathology has been excluded, time or a change to another formulation may solve the problem. Changing to an oral contraceptive with a higher estrogen content, while potentially useful in minimizing menstrual irregularity, should be done only if necessary since this may increase the risk of thromboembolic disease.

Women with a past history of oligomenorrhea or secondary amenorrhea or young women without regular cycles may have a tendency to remain anovulatory or to become amenorrheic after discontinuation of oral contraceptives. Women with these preexisting problems should be advised of this possibility and encouraged to use other contraceptive methods.

Post-use anovulation, possibly prolonged, may also occur in women without previous irregularities. A higher incidence of galactorrhea and of pituitary tumors (e.g., adenomas) has been associated with amenorrhea in former users compared with nonusers[66,67]. One study[67] reported a 16-fold increased prevalence of pituitary prolactin-secreting tumors among patients with postpill amenorrhea when galactorrhea was present.

11. *Infertility:* There is evidence of impairment of fertility in women discontinuing oral contraceptives in comparison with those discontinuing other methods of contraception. The impairment appears to be independent of the duration of use of the preparations. While the impairment diminishes with time, there is still an appreciable difference in the results in nulliparous women for the oral contraceptive and non-oral contraceptive groups 30 months after discontinuation of birth control. For parous women the difference is no longer apparent 30 months after cessation of contraception[11]. One study suggests that infection with *Chlamydia trachomatis,* the leading cause of nongonococcal pelvic inflammatory disease, is enhanced by oral contraceptives.[101]
12. *Ectopic Pregnancy:* Ectopic as well as intrauterine pregnancy may occur in contraceptive failures. However, in progestogen-only oral contraceptive failures, the ratio of ectopic to intrauterine pregnancies is higher than in women who are not receiving oral contraceptives, since the drugs are more effective in preventing intrauterine than ectopic pregnancies.
13. *Breast Feeding:* Oral contraceptives given in the postpartum period may interfere with lactation. There may be a decrease in the quantity and quality of the breast milk. Furthermore, a small fraction of the hormonal agents in oral contraceptives has been identified in the milk of mothers receiving these drugs[68]. The effects, if any, on the breast fed child have not been determined. If feasible, the use of oral contraceptives should be deferred until the infant has been weaned.

PRECAUTIONS

General

1. A complete medical and family history should be taken prior to the initiation of oral contraceptives. The pretreatment and periodic physical examinations should include special reference to blood pressure, breasts, abdomen and pelvic organs, including Papanicolaou smear and relevant laboratory tests. As a general rule, oral contraceptives should not be prescribed for longer than 1 year without another physical examination being performed.
2. Under the influence of estrogen-progestogen preparations, preexisting uterine leiomyomata may increase in size.
3. Patients with a history of psychic depression should be carefully observed and the drug discontinued if depression recurs to a serious degree. Patients becoming significantly depressed while taking oral contraceptives should stop the medication and use an alternate method of contraception in an attempt to determine whether the symptom is drug related.
4. Oral contraceptives may cause some degree of fluid retention. They should be prescribed with caution, and only with careful monitoring, in patients with conditions which might be aggravated by fluid retention, such as convulsive disorders, migraine syndrome, asthma or cardiac, hepatic or renal insufficiency.
5. Patients with a past history of jaundice during pregnancy have an increased risk of recurrence of jaundice while receiving oral contraceptive therapy. If jaundice develops in any patient receiving such drugs, the medication should be discontinued.
6. Steroid hormones may be poorly metabolized in patients with impaired liver function and should be administered with caution in such patients.
7. Oral contraceptive users may have disturbances in normal tryptophan metabolism which may result in a relative pyridoxine deficiency. The clinical significance of this is unknown.
8. Serum folate levels may be depressed by oral contraceptive therapy. Since the pregnant woman is predisposed to the development of folate deficiency and the incidence of folate deficiency increases with increasing gestation, it is possible that if a woman becomes pregnant shortly after stopping oral contraceptives, she may have a greater chance of developing folate deficiency and complications attributed to this deficiency.
9. The pathologist should be advised of oral contraceptive therapy when relevant specimens are submitted.
10. Certain endocrine and liver function tests and blood components may be affected by estrogen-containing oral contraceptives. For example:
    a. Increased sulfobromophthalein retention.
    b. Increased prothrombin and factors VII, VIII, IX, and X; decreased antithrombin 3; increased norepinephrine-induced platelet aggregability.
    c. Increased thyroid binding globulin (TBG) leading to increased circulating total thyroid hormone, as measured by protein-bound iodine (PBI), T4 by column, or T4 by radioimmunoassay. Free T3 resin uptake is decreased, reflecting the elevated TBG, free T4 concentration is unaltered.
    d. Decreased pregnanediol excretion.
    e. Reduced response to metyrapone test.
    f. Increased phospholipids and triglycerides.
    g. Temporarily decreased glucose tolerance.
11. Contact lens wearers who develop visual changes or changes in lens tolerance should be assessed by an ophthalmologist and temporary or permanent cessation of wear considered.

DRUG INTERACTIONS

Oral contraceptives may be rendered less effective and an increased incidence of breakthrough bleeding may occur by virtue of drug interaction with ampicillin[69,90], analgesics[69,90], antihistamines[69], antimigraine preparations[69], barbiturates[69,70], chloramphenicol[69], griseofulvin[96], isoniazid, neomycin[69], nitrofurantoin[69,70], penicillin V[69], phenytoin[69,70], primidone[69], rifampin[69,70], sulfonamides[70], tetracycline[92], and tranquilizers[69]. Oral contraceptives may alter the effectiveness of other types of drugs, such as anticonvulsants[69], antihypertensive agents (e.g., guanethidine)[69], beta blockers[97], hypnotic preparations[104], hypoglycemic agents[69], oral anticoagulants[69], theophylline[91], tranquilizers[78], tricyclic antidepressants[69], and vitamins[69].

Toxic liver effects have been reported with a combination of an oral contraceptive and Cyclosporin A.[100]

INFORMATION FOR THE PATIENT

See detailed patient labeling below.

CARCINOGENESIS

See Warnings section for information on the carcinogenic potential of oral contraceptives.

PREGNANCY

Pregnancy category X. See Contraindications and Warnings.

NURSING MOTHERS

See Warnings.

ADVERSE REACTIONS

An increased risk of the following serious adverse reactions has been associated with the use of oral contraceptives (see Warnings):

- Thrombophlebitis, thrombosis
- Pulmonary embolism
- Coronary thrombosis
- Cerebral thrombosis
- Mesenteric thrombosis
- Raynaud's disease
- Arterial thromboembolism
- Liver tumors
- Cerebral hemorrhage
- Hypertension
- Gall bladder disease
- Congenital anomalies
- Neuro-ocular lesions, e.g., retinal thrombosis and optic neuritis

The following adverse reactions have been reported in patients receiving oral contraceptives and are believed to be drug related:

- Bleeding irregularities
    - Breakthrough bleeding
    - Spotting
    - Missed menses during treatment
    - Amenorrhea after treatment
- Gastrointestinal symptoms
    - Nausea
    - Vomiting
    - Bloating
    - Abdominal cramps
    - Colitis
- Dysmenorrhea
- Infertility after discontinuance of treatment
- Edema
- Chloasma or melasma which may persist after drug is discontinued
- Breast changes: tenderness, enlargement, and secretion
- Intolerance to contact lenses
- Change in corneal curvature (steepening)
- Change in weight (increase or decrease)
- Change in cervical erosion and cervical secretion
- Possible diminution in lactation when given immediately postpartum
- Cholestatic jaundice
- Migraine
- Increase in size of uterine leiomyomata
- Rash (allergic)
- Mental depression
- Reduced tolerance to carbohydrates
- Vaginal candidiasis
- Prolaction-secreting pituitary tumors
- Chilblains

The following adverse reactions have been reported in users of oral contraceptives, and the association has been neither confirmed nor refuted:

- Premenstrual-like syndrome
- Cataracts
- Changes in libido
- Chorea
- Changes in appetite
- Cystitis-like syndrome
- Headache
- Nervousness
- Dizziness
- Hirsutism
- Loss of hair
- Erythema multiforme
- Erythema nodosum
- Hemorrhagic eruption
- Vaginitis
- Porphyria
- Impaired renal function
- Malignant nephrosclerosis (hemolytic uremic syndrome)
- Malignant hypertension
- Acute renal failure

ACUTE OVERDOSE

Serious ill effects have not been reported following acute ingestion of large doses of oral contraceptives by young children. Overdosage may cause nausea. Withdrawal bleeding may occur in females.

DOSAGE AND ADMINISTRATION

To achieve maximum contraceptive effectiveness, oral contraceptives must be taken exactly as directed and at intervals not exceeding 24 hours.

Important: The patient should be instructed to use an additional method of protection until after the first week of administration in the initial cycle. The possibility of ovulation and conception prior to initiation of use should be considered.

The patient should be instructed not to initiate treatment with oral contraceptives earlier than two weeks after delivery.[102] The patient should be instructed to start oral contraceptives immediately if a pregnancy of less than 12 weeks of gestation ends by abortion but to start two weeks after abortion for gestations lasting 12 weeks or longer.[103]

21-Day Regimen Dosage Schedule for BREVICON, NORINYL 1 + 35, NORINYL 1 + 50, NORINYL 1 + 80: For the initial cycle of therapy the first tablet may be taken on Day 5 of the menstrual cycle, counting the first day of menstrual flow as Day 1 (DAY 5 START), or the first tablet may be taken on the first Sunday after menstrual flow begins (SUNDAY START). For SUNDAY START when menstrual flow begins on Sunday, the first tablet is taken on that day. With either DAY 5 START or SUNDAY START, one tablet is taken each evening at bedtime for 21 days. No tablets are taken for 7 days, then, whether bleeding has stopped or not, a new course is started of one tablet a day for 21 days. This institutes a three weeks on, one week off dosage regimen.

28-Day Regimen Dosage Schedule for BREVICON, NORINYL 1 + 35, NORINYL 1 + 50, NORINYL 1 + 80: For the initial cycle of therapy the first tablet may be taken on Day 5 of the menstrual cycle, counting the first day of menstrual flow as Day 1 (DAY 5 START), or the first tablet may be taken on the first Sunday after menstrual flow begins (SUNDAY START). For SUNDAY START when menstrual flow begins on Sunday, the first tablet is taken on that day. With either DAY 5 START or SUNDAY START, one white, yellow, blue, or green tablet is taken each evening at bedtime for 21 days. Then the orange tablets are taken, one each evening at bedtime for 7 days. After all 28 tablets have been taken, whether bleeding has stopped or not, repeat the same dosage schedule beginning on the following day.

21-Day Regimen Dosage Schedule for TRI-NORINYL: The first blue tablet is taken on the first Sunday after menstrual flow begins. If menstrual flow begins on Sunday, the first blue tablet is taken on that day. One blue tablet is taken each evening at bedtime for 7 days, then one green tablet each evening for 9 days, then one blue tablet each evening for 5 days. No tablets are taken for 7 days; then, whether bleeding has stopped or not, a new sequence of tablets is started for 21 days. This institutes a three weeks on, one week off dosage regimen.

28-Day Regimen Dosage Schedule for TRI-NORINYL: The first blue tablet is taken on the first Sunday after menstrual flow begins. If menstrual flow begins on Sunday, the first blue tablet is taken on that day. One blue tablet is taken each evening at bedtime for 7 days, then one green tablet each evening for 9 days, then one blue tablet each evening for 5 days, then one orange (inert) tablet each evening for 7 days. After all 28 tablets have been taken, whether bleeding has stopped or not, the same dosage schedule is repeated beginning on the following day.

NORINYL 2 mg. Tablets: To prevent conception, one tablet is taken each evening at bedtime for 20 days beginning on DAY 5 of the menstrual cycle, counting the first day of menstrual flow as DAY 1. In the vast majority of women on this schedule menses occur within two to three days following the termination of each 20-day course, but tend to be scantier than normal menses. In those cases where withdrawal bleeding may be delayed until 4, 5 or 6 days after the 20-day course of therapy, the patient should start the next course of medication on the 7th day following completion of the previous 20-day course. For the treatment of hypermenorrhea, one tablet is taken each evening at bedtime from day 5 through day 24 of each menstrual cycle. Following three months of treatment of hypermenorrhea, medication may be discontinued to determine the need for further therapy.

20, 21, 28-Day Schedules for All Products: Even if spotting or breakthrough bleeding should occur, the patient should continue the medication according to the schedule. Should spotting or breakthrough bleeding persist, the patient should notify the physician.

Use of oral contraceptives in the event of a missed menstrual period:

1. If the patient has not adhered to the prescribed dosage regimen, the possibility of pregnancy should be considered after the first missed period and oral contraceptives should be withheld until pregnancy has been ruled out.
2. If the patient has adhered to the prescribed regimen and misses two consecutive periods, pregnancy should be ruled out before continuing the contraceptive regimen.

NOR-Q.D.® (norethindrone) is administered as a continuous daily dosage regimen starting on the first day of menstruation, i.e., one tablet each day, every day of the year. Tablets should be taken at the same time each day and continued daily, without interruption, whether bleeding occurs or not. This is especially important for patients new to progestogen alone oral contraception. The patient should be advised that if prolonged bleeding occurs, she should consult her physician.

The risk of pregnancy increases with each tablet missed. If the patient misses one tablet, she should be instructed to take it as soon as she remembers and also to take her next tablet at the regular time which means she will be taking two tablets on that day. If she misses two tablets in a row, she should take one of the missed tablets as soon as she remembers, discard the other missed tablet, and take her regular tablet for that day at the proper time. Furthermore, she should use an additional method of contraception in addition to taking NOR-Q.D. until menses has appeared or pregnancy has been excluded. If more than two tablets in a row have been missed, NOR-Q.D. should be discontinued immediately and an additional method of contraception should be used until menses has appeared or pregnancy has been excluded. Whether or not the patient has adhered to the prescribed schedule, if she does not have a period within 45 days of her last period, she should stop taking NOR-Q.D. and depend upon a method of nonhormonal contraception until pregnancy has been ruled out.

HOW SUPPLIED

BREVICON® 21-Day Tablets and BREVICON® 28-Day Tablets (norethindrone and ethinyl estradiol) are available in 21-pill or 28-pill blister cards with a WALLETTE™ pill dispenser. Each 28-pill card contains 7 orange inert pills.

NORINYL® 1 + 35 21-Day Tablets and NORINYL® 1 + 35 28-Day Tablets (norethindrone and ethinyl estradiol) are available in 21-pill or 28-pill blister cards with a WALLETTE™ pill dispenser. Each 28-pill card contains 7 orange inert pills.

NORINYL® 1 + 50 21-Day Tablets and NORINYL® 1 + 50 28-Day Tablets (norethindrone and mestranol) and NORINYL® 1 + 80 21-Day Tablets and NORINYL® 1 + 80 28-Day Tablets (norethindrone and mestranol) are available in 21-pill or 28-pill blister cards with a WALLETTE™ pill dispenser. Each 28-pill card contains 7 orange inert pills.

NORINYL® 2 mg. Tablets (norethindrone and mestranol) are available in MEMORETTE® Tablet Dispensers, each containing 20 tablets. Also supplied are 20-tablet refills.

NOR-Q.D.® (norethindrone) tablets are available in 42-tablet dispensers.

TRI-NORINYL® 21-DAY Tablets and TRI-NORINYL 28-DAY Tablets (northindrone and ethinyl estradiol) are each available in 21-pill or 28-pill blister cards with a WALLETTE pill dispenser. Each 28-pill card contains 7 orange inert pills.

CAUTION: Federal law prohibits dispensing without prescription.

REFERENCES

[1]Population Reports, Series H, Number 2, May 1974; Series I, Number 1, June 1974: Series B, Number 2, January 1975; Series H, Number 3, January 1975; Series H, Number 4, January 1976 (published by the Population Information Program, The George Washington University Medical Center, 2001 S St. NW, Washington, D. C.). [2]Inman, W., et al.: *Brit Med J* 2:203–209, 1970. [3]Stolley, P., et al.: *Am J Epidemiol* 102:197–208, 1975. [4]Inman, W., et al.: *Brit Med J* 2:193–199, 1968. [5]Royal College of General Practitioners: *J Coll Gen Pract* 13:267–279, 1967. [6]Vessey, M., et al.: *Brit Med J* 2:651–657, 1969. [7]Sartwell, P., et al.: *Am J Epidemiol* 90:365–380, 1969. [8]Boston Collaborative Drug Surveillance Program: *Lancet* 1:1399–1404, 1973. [9]Collaborative Group for the Study of Stroke in Young Women: *N Engl J Med* 288:871–878, 1973. [10]Collaborative Group for the Study of Stroke in Young Women: *JAMA* 231:718–722, 1975. [11]Vessey, M., et al.: *J Biosoc Sci* 8:373–427, (Oct.) 1976. [12]Royal College of General Practitioners: Oral Contraceptives and Health, London, Pitman, 1974. [13]Mann, J., et al.: *Brit Med J* 2:245–248, 1975. [14]Mann, J., et al.: *Brit Med J* 2:445–447, 1976. [15]Mann, J., et al.: *Brit Med J* 2:241–245, 1975. [16]Jain, A.: *Studies in Family Planning* 8:50–54, 1977. [17]Ory, H.: *JAMA* 237:2619–2622, (June 13) 1977. [18]Beral, V.: *Lancet* 2:727–731, 1977. [19]Tietze, C.: *Family Planning Perspectives* 9:74–76, 1977. [20]Vessey, M., et al.: *Brit Med J* 3:123–126, 1970. [21]Greene, G., et al.: *Am J Pub Health* 62:680–685, 1972. [22]Ziel, H., et al.: *N Engl J Med* 293:1167–1170, 1975. [23]Gordon, J., et al.: *N Engl J Med* 297:570–571, (Sept. 15) 1977. [24]Smith, D., et al.: *N Engl J Med* 293:1164–1167, 1975. [25]Mack, T., et al.: *N Engl J Med* 294:1262–1267, 1976. [26]Gray, L., et al.: *Obstet Gyncecol* 49:385–389, (April) 1977. [27]McDonald, T., et al.: *Am J Obstet Gynecol* 127:572–580, (Mar. 20) 1977. [28]Silverberg, S., et al.: *Cancer* 39:592–598, (Feb.) 1977). [29]Vessey, M., et al.: *Brit Med J* 3:719–724, 1972. [30]Vessey, M., et al.: *Lancet* 1:941–943, 1975. [31]Boston Collaborative Drug Surveillance Program: *N Engl J Med* 290:15–19, 1974. [32]Arthes, F., et al.: *Cancer* 28:1391–1394, 1971. [33]Casagrande, J., et al.: *J Natl Cancer Inst* 56:839–841, (April) 1976). [34]Fasal, E., et al.: *J Natl Cancer Inst* 55:767–773, 1975. [35]Paffenbarger, R., et al.: *Cancer* 49:1887–1891, (April Suppl.) 1977. [36]Hoover, R., et al.: *N Engl J Med* 295:401–405, (Aug. 19) 1976. [37]Kelsey, J., et al.: *Internat J Epidemiol* 3:333–340, 1974. [38]Ory, H., et al.: *N Engl J Med* 294:419–422, 1976. [39]Stern, E., et al.: *Science* 196:1460–1462, (June 24) 1977. [40]Mays, E., et al.: *JAMA* 235:730–732, 1976. [41]Edmondson, H., et al.: *N Engl J Med* 294:470–472, 1976. [42]Murphy, G.: *Am Col of Surg Bull*, (April) 1977. [43]Klatskin, G.: *Gastroent* 73:386–394, (Aug.) 1977. [44]Rooks, et al: *JAMA* 242:644, 1979. [45]Herbst, A., et al.: *N Engl J Med* 284:878–881, 1971. [46]Greenwald, P., et al.: *N Engl J Med* 285:390–392, 1971. [47]Lanier, A., et al.: *Mayo Clin Pro* 48:793–799, 1973. [48]Herbst, A., et al.: *Am J Obstet Gynecol* 128:43–50, 1977. [49]Herbst, A., et al.: *Obstet Gyncecol* 40:287–298, 1972. [50]Herbst, A., et al.: *Am J Obstet Gyncecol* 118:607–615, 1974. [51]Herbst, A., et al.: *N Engl J Med* 292:334–339, 1975. [52]Stafl, A., et al.: *Obstet Gynecol* 43:118–128, 1974. [53]Sherman, A., et al.: *Obstet Gynecol* 44:531–545, 1974. [54]Bibbo, M., et al.: *Jour of Repro Med* 15:29–32, 1975. [55]Gill, W., et al.: *Jour of Repro Med* 16:147–153, 1976. [56]Henderson, B., et al.: *Pediatrics* 58:505–507, 1976. [57]Gal, I., et al.: *Nature* 216:83, 1967. [58]Levy, E., et al.: *Lancet* 1:611, 1973. [59]Nora, J., et al.: *Lancet* 1:941–942, 1973. [60]Janerich, D., et al.: *N Engl J Med* 291:697–700, 1974. [61]Heinonen, O., et al.: *N Engl J Med* 296:67–70, 1977. [62]Carr, D.: *Canad Med Assoc J* 103:343–348, 1970. [63]Wynn, V., et al.: *Lancet* 2:720–723, 1966. [64]Fisch, I., et al.: *JAMA* 237:2499–2503, (June 6) 1977. [65]Laragh, J.: *Am J Obstet Gynecol* 126:141–147, (Sept.) 1976. [66]March, C., et al.: *Fertil and Steril* 28:346, (Mar.) 1977. [67]Van Campenhout, J., et al.: *Fertil and Steril* 28:728–732, (July) 1977. [68]Laumas, K., et al.: *Am J Obstet Gynecol* 98:411–413, 1967. [69]Stockley, I.: *Pharm J* 216:140–143, (Feb. 14) 1976. [70]Hempel, E., et al.: *Drugs* 12:442–448, (Dec.) 1976. [71]Bessot, J.-C., et al.: *Nouv* Press Med 6:1568, (Apr. 30) 1977. [72]Royal College of General Practitioners: *J Coll Gen Pract* 28:393–399, 1978. [73]Layde, P. M., et al.: *Lancet* 1:541–546, 1981. [74]Vessey, M. P., et al.: *Lancet* 1:549–550, 1981. [75]Ramcharan, S., et al.: *The Walnut Creek Contraceptive Drug Study*, Volume III, NIH Publication 81-564, 1981. [76]Petitti, D. B., et al.: *Am J Epidemiol* 108:480–485, 1978. [77]Petitti, D. B., et al.: *Lancet* 2:234, 1978. [78]Abernethy, D. R., et al.: *N Engl J Med* 306:791, 1982. [79]Pike, M. C., et al.: *Brit J Cancer* 43:72, 1981. [80]Kasan, P. N., et al.: *Brit J Obstet Gynecol* 87:545, 1980. [81]Meade, T. W., et al.: *Brit Med J* 280:1157, 1980. [82]Bottiger, L. E., et al.: *Lancet* 1:1097, 1980. [83]Black, M. M., et al.: *Cancer* 46:2747, 1980. [84]Rothman, E. J.: *N Engl J Med* 297:468, 1977. [85]Bracken, M. B.: *Am J Obstet Gynecol* 133:432, 1979. [86]Harlap, S., et al.: *Obstet Gynecol* 55:447, 1980. [87]Royal College of General Practitioners: *J Coll Gen Pract* 33:75, 1983. [88]Slone, D., et al.: *N Engl J Med* 305:420, 1981. [89]Dallenbach-Hellweg, G.: *Geburtsh u Fauenheilk* 42:249, 1982. [90]De Sano, E. A., et al.: *Fertil and Steril* 37:853, 1982. [91]Tornatore, K. M., et al.: *Eur J Clin Pharmacol* 23:129, 1982. [92]Bacon, J. F., et al.: *Brit Med J* 280:293, 1980. [93]Vessey, M. P., et al.: *Brit Med J* 289:530–531, 1984. [94]Vessey, M. P.: *J Roy Soc Med* 77:542–549, 1984. [95]Vessey, M. P., et al.: *Lancet* 2:930–934, 1983. [96]Van Dijke, C. P. H., et al.: *Brit Med J* 288:1125–1126, 1984. [97]Kendall, M. J., et al.: *Br J Clin Pharmac* 17:875–895, 1984. [98]Olsson, H., et al.: *Lancet* 1:748–749, 1985. [99]WHO Collaborative Study: *Brit Med J* 290:961–965, 1985. [100]Leimenstoll, G., et al.: *DMW* 109:1989–1990, 1984. [101]Washington, A.E., et al.: *JAMA* 253:2246–2250, 1985. [102]Mishell, D., et al.: *Reproductive Endocrinology, Infertility and Contraception:* F.A. Davis Co., Philadelphia, PA pub. 1979. [103]Dickey, R.P.: *Managing Contraceptive Pill Patients*, 4th ed.: Creative Infomatics Inc., Durant, OK pub. 1984. [104]Edgren, R.A.: *Experientia* Volume 13, No. 2:86, 1957.

Detailed Patient Labeling: Oral contraceptives ("the pill") are the most effective way (except for sterilization) to prevent pregnancy. They are also convenient and, for most women, free of serious or unpleasant side effects. Oral contraceptives must always be taken under the continuous supervision of a physician.

It is important that any woman who considers using an oral contraceptive understand the risks involved. Although the oral contraceptives have important advantages over the other methods of contraception, they have certain risks that no other method has, and some of these risks may continue after you have stopped using the pill. Only you can decide whether the advantages are worth these risks. This leaflet will tell you about the most important risks. It will explain how you can help your doctor prescribe the pill as safely as possible by telling him/her about yourself and being alert for the earliest signs of trouble. And it will tell you how to use the pill properly, so that it will be as effective as possible. There is more detailed information available in the leaflet prepared for doctors. If you need further help, ask your physician or pharmacist.

Who Should Not Use Oral Contraceptives:

A. If you have any of the following conditions you should not use the pill:
   1. Unusual vaginal bleeding that has not yet been diagnosed.
   2. Known or suspected pregnancy.

B. If you have or have had any of the following conditions you should not use the pill:
   1. Heart attack or stroke.
   2. Clots in the legs, lungs, brain, heart or elsewhere.
   3. Chest pain (angina pectoris).
   4. Known or suspected cancer of the breast or sex organs.
   5. Liver tumor associated with the use of the pill or other estrogen containing products.

C. Cigarette smoking increases the risk of serious adverse effects on the heart and blood vessels from oral contraceptive use. This risk increases with age and with heavy smoking (15 or more cigarettes per day) and is quite marked in women over 35 years of age. Women who use oral contraceptives should not smoke.

D. If you have scanty or irregular periods or are a young woman without a regular cycle, you should use another method of contraception because, if you use the pill, you may have difficulty becoming pregnant or may fail to have menstrual periods after discontinuing the pill.

What You Should Know About Oral Contraceptives: This leaflet describes the advantages and risks of oral contraceptives. Except for sterilization, the IUD and abortion, which have their own exclusive risks, the only risks of other methods of contraception are those due to pregnancy should the method fail or not be used conscientiously. Your doctor can answer questions you may have with respect to methods of contraception.

1. What Oral Contraceptives Are and How They Work. Oral contraceptives are of two types. The most common, often simply called "the pill", is a combination of an estrogen and a progestogen, the two kinds of female hormones. The amount of estrogen and progestogen can vary, but the amount of estrogen is most important because both the effectiveness and some of the dangers of oral contraceptives are related to the amount of estrogen. This kind of oral contraceptive works principally by preventing release of an egg from the ovary. When the amount of estrogen is 0.05 milligrams or more, and the pill is taken as directed, oral contraceptives are more than 99% effective (i.e., there would be less than one pregnancy if 100 women used the pill for 1 year). Pills that contain 0.02 to 0.035 milligrams of estrogen vary slightly in effectiveness, ranging from 98% to more than 99% effective.

The second type of oral contraceptive, often called the "mini-pill", contains only a progestogen. It works in part by preventing release of an egg from the ovary but also by keeping sperm from reaching the egg and by making the uterus (womb) less receptive to any fertilized egg that reaches it.

Continued on next page

Syntex—Cont.

The mini-pill is less effective than the combination oral contraceptive, about 97% effective. In addition, the progestogen-only pill has a tendency to cause irregular bleeding which may be quite inconvenient, or cessation of bleeding entirely. The progestogen-only pill is used despite its lower effectiveness in the hope that it will prove not to have some of the serious side effects of the estrogen-containing pill (see below) but it is not yet certain that the mini-pill does in fact have fewer serious side effects. The discussion below, while based mainly on information about the combination pills, should be considered to apply as well to the mini-pill.

2. Other Nonsurgical Ways to Prevent Pregnancy. As this leaflet will explain, oral contraceptives have several serious risks. Some other methods of contraception have lesser risks. They are usually less effective than oral contraceptives, but, used properly, may be effective enough for many women. The following table gives reported pregnancy rates (the number of women out of 100 who would become pregnant in 1 year) for these methods:

Pregnancies per 100 Women per Year
Intrauterine device (IUD), less than 1–6;
Diaphragm with spermicidal products (creams or jellies), 2–20;
Condom (rubber), 3–36;
Aerosol foams, 2–29;
Jellies and creams, 4–36;
Periodic abstinence (rhythm), all types, less than 1–47;
— Calendar method, 14–47;
— Temperature method, 1–20;
— Temperature method—intercourse only in post-ovulatory phase, less than 1–7;
— Mucus method, 1–25;
No contraception, 60–80.

The figures (except for the IUD) vary widely because people differ in how well they use each method. Very faithful users of the various methods, with the exception of the calendar method of periodic abstinence (rhythm), may achieve lower pregnancy rates than those given above, which are the average results for large groups of women. Except for the IUD, effective use of these methods requires somewhat more effort than simply taking a single pill every evening, but it is an effort that many couples undertake successfully. Your doctor can tell you a great deal more about these methods of contraception.

3. The Dangers of Oral Contraceptives

a. *Circulatory disorders (abnormal blood clots, strokes, and heart attacks).* Blood clots (in various blood vessels of the body) are the most common of the serious side effects of oral contraceptives. A clot can result in a stroke (if the clot is in the brain), a heart attack (if the clot is in a blood vessel of the heart), a pulmonary embolus (a clot which forms in the legs or pelvis, then breaks off and travels to the lungs), or loss of a limb (a clot in a blood vessel in or leading to an arm or leg). Any of these can cause death or disability. Clots also occur rarely in the blood vessels of the eye, resulting in blindness or impairment of vision in that eye. There is evidence that the risk of clotting increases with higher estrogen doses. It is therefore important to keep the dose of estrogen as low as possible, so long as the oral contraceptive used has an acceptable pregnancy rate and doesn't cause unacceptable changes in the menstrual pattern. The risk of abnormal clotting increases with age in both users and nonusers of oral contraceptives, but the increased risk from the contraceptive appears to be present at all ages.

In addition to blood-clotting disorders, it has been estimated that women taking oral contraceptives are twice as likely as nonusers to have a stroke due to rupture of a blood vessel in the brain.

Furthermore, cigarette smoking by oral contraceptive users increases the risk of serious adverse effects on the heart and blood vessels. This risk increases with age and with heavy smoking (15 or more cigarettes per day) and becomes quite marked in women over 35 years of age. For this reason, women who use oral contraceptives should not smoke.

For oral contraceptive users in general, it has been estimated that in women between the ages of 15 and 34 the risk of death due to a circulatory disorder is about 1 in 12,000 per year, whereas for nonusers the rate is about 1 in 50,000 per year. In the age group 35 to 44, the risk is estimated to be about 1 in 2,500 per year for oral contraceptive users and about 1 in 10,000 per year for nonusers. The risk is concentrated in older women, in those with a long duration of use, and in cigarette smokers. The effects on the circulatory system may persist after oral contraceptives are discontinued.

Even without the pill the risk of having a heart attack increases with age and is also increased by such heart attack risk factors as high blood pressure, high cholesterol, obesity, diabetes, and cigarette smoking. Without any risk factors present, the use of oral contraceptives alone may double the risk of heart attack. However, the combination of cigarette smoking, especially heavy smoking, and oral contraceptive use greatly increases the risk of heart attack. Oral contraceptive users who smoke are about 5 times more likely to have a heart attack than users who do not smoke and about 10 times more likely to have a heart attack than nonusers who do not smoke. It has been estimated that users between the ages of 30 and 39 who smoke have about a 1 in 10,000 chance each year of having a fatal heart attack compared to about a 1 in 50,000 chance in users who do not smoke, and about a 1 in 100,000 chance in nonusers who do not smoke. In the age group 40 to 44, the risk is about 1 in 1,700 per year for users who smoke compared to about 1 in 10,000 for users who do not smoke and to about 1 in 14,000 per year for nonusers who do not smoke. These are average figures for Great Britain; comparable estimates for the U.S. may be higher. Heavy smoking (about 15 cigarettes or more a day) further increases the risk. If you do not smoke and have none of the other heart attack risk factors described above, you will have a smaller risk than listed. If you have several heart attack risk factors, the risk may be considerably greater than listed.

b. *Formation of tumors.* Studies have found that when certain animals are given the female sex hormone estrogen, which is an ingredient of oral contraceptives, continuously for long periods, cancers may develop in the breast, cervix, vagina, uterus, ovary, pituitary and liver.

These findings suggest that oral contraceptives may cause cancer in humans. However, studies to date in women taking currently marketed oral contraceptives have not confirmed that oral contraceptives cause cancer in humans. Several studies have found no increase in breast cancer in users, although one study suggested oral contraceptives might cause an increase in breast cancer in women who already have benign breast disease (e.g., cysts) or who have used oral contraceptives for long periods (2–4 years) and other studies suggested an increased risk of breast cancer with long-term oral contraceptive use before the age of 25.

Women with a strong family history of breast cancer or who have breast nodules, fibrocystic disease, or abnormal mammograms or who were exposed to DES (diethylstilbestrol), an estrogen, during their mother's pregnancy must be followed very closely by their doctors if they choose to use oral contraceptives instead of another method of contraception. Many studies have shown that women taking oral contraceptives have less risk of getting benign breast disease than those who have not used oral contraceptives. Strong evidence has emerged that estrogens (one component of oral contraceptives) when given alone (unaccompanied by progestogen) for periods of more than one year to women after the menopause, increase the risk of cancer of the uterus (womb). There is also some evidence that a kind of oral contraceptive which is no longer marketed, the sequential oral contraceptive, may increase the risk of cancer of the uterus. There remains no evidence, however, that the oral contraceptives now available (containing estrogen and progestogen in combination or progestogen alone) increase the risk of this cancer. Cancer of the cervix may develop more readily in long-term (3–4 years) users of the pill with or without preexisting abnormal Pap smears. One study reported malignant melanoma (skin cancer), urinary tract cancers, and thyroid cancers more frequently in pill users than in non-users.

Benign or malignant liver tumors have been associated with short-term as well as long-term oral contraceptive use. The benign (non-malignant) tumors do not spread, but they may rupture and produce internal bleeding, which may cause death.

c. *Dangers to a developing child if oral contraceptives are used in or immediately preceding pregnancy.* Oral contraceptives should not be taken by pregnant women because they may damage the developing child. An increased risk of birth defects, including heart defects and limb defects, has been associated with the use of sex hormones, including oral contraceptives, in pregnancy. In addition, the developing female child whose mother has received DES (diethylstilbestrol), an estrogen, during pregnancy has a risk of getting cancer of the vagina or cervix in her teens or young adulthood. This risk is estimated to be about 1 in 1,000 exposures or less. Abnormalities of the urinary and sex organs have been reported in male offspring so exposed. It is possible that other estrogens, such as the estrogens in oral contraceptives, could have the same effect in the child if the mother takes them during pregnancy.

If you stop taking oral contraceptives to become pregnant, your doctor may recommend that you use another method of contraception for a short while. The reason for this is that there is evidence from studies in women who have had "miscarriages" soon after stopping the pill, that the lost fetuses are more likely to be abnormal. Whether there is an overall increase in "miscarriage" in women who become pregnant soon after stopping the pill as compared with women who do not use the pill is not known, but it is possible that there may be. If, however, you do become pregnant soon after stopping oral contraceptives, and do not have a miscarriage, there is no evidence that the baby has an increased risk of being abnormal.

d. *Gallbladder disease.* Women who use oral contraceptives have a greater risk than nonusers of having gallbladder disease requiring surgery. The increased risk may first appear within 1 year of use and may double after 4 to 5 years of use.

e. *Other side effects of oral contraceptives.* Some women using oral contraceptives experience unpleasant side effects that are not dangerous and are not likely to damage their health. Some of these may be temporary. Your breasts may feel tender, nausea and vomiting may occur, you may gain or lose weight, and your ankles may swell. A spotty darkening of the skin, particularly of the face, is possible and may persist. Many of these effects are seen more frequently with combination oral contraceptives containing 0.05 milligrams or more of estrogen. You may notice unexpected vaginal bleeding or changes in your menstrual period. Irregular bleeding is frequently seen when using the mini-pill or combination oral contraceptives containing less than 0.05 milligrams of estrogen. One study suggested that oral contraceptive use may predispose users to pelvic inflammatory disease caused by *Chlamydia trachomatis.*

More serious side effects include worsening of migraine, asthma, epilepsy, and kidney or heart disease because of a tendency for water to be retained in the body when oral contraceptives are used. Other side effects are growth of preexisting fibroid tumors of the uterus; mental depression; liver problems with jaundice (yellowing of the skin); and inflammation of the colon. Your doctor may find that levels of sugar and fatty substances in your blood are elevated; the long-term effects of these changes are not known. Some women develop high blood pressure while taking oral contraceptives, which may persist after discontinuation. High blood pressure may lead to serious disease of the kidney and circulatory system. Your physician may wish to check your blood pressure more frequently if you have a history of toxemia of pregnancy, kidney disease or increased blood pressure.

Other reactions have been reported occasionally. These include more frequent urination and some discomfort when urinating, kidney disease, blood cell breakdown with kidney failure, nervousness, dizziness, an increase in or loss of hair, an increase or decrease in sex drive, appetite changes, cataracts, and a need for a change in contact lens prescription or inability to use contact lenses.

After you stop using oral contraceptives, your ability to menstruate or become pregnant may be impaired. This impairment may be greater if you have never been pregnant.

As discussed previously, you should wait a few months after stopping the pill before you try to become pregnant. An increased incidence of twin births has been reported in women who have conceived soon after stopping the pill. During these few months, use another form of contraception. You should consult your physician before resuming use of oral contraceptives after childbirth, especially if you plan to nurse your baby. Drugs in oral contraceptives are known to appear in the milk, and the long-range effect on infants is not known. Furthermore, oral contraceptives may cause a decrease in your milk supply as well as in the quality of the milk.

4. Comparison of the Risks of Oral Contraceptives and Other Contraceptive Methods. The many studies on the risks and effectiveness of oral contraceptives and other methods of contraception have been analyzed to estimate the risk of death associated with various methods of contraception. This risk has two parts: (a) the risk associated with the method itself (e.g., the risk that an oral contraceptive user will die due to abnormal clotting), and (b) the risk associated with failure of the method (death due to pregnancy or abortion). The results of this analysis are shown in the bar graph (Figure 1). The height of the bars is the estimated number of deaths per 100,000 women each year. There are six sets of bars, each set referring to a specific age group of women. Within each set of bars, there are two bars for oral contraceptive users, one referring to users who smoke and one referring to users who do not smoke, and five bars for other contraceptive methods including one bar representing no method of contraception. ("Traditional contraception" means diaphragm or condom.)

This analysis is based on present knowledge and new information could, of course, alter it. The analysis shows that the risk of death from all methods of birth control is low compared to the risks of childbirth, *except for oral contraceptives in women over 40 who smoke.* It shows that the lowest risk of death is associated with the condom or diaphragm (traditional contraception) backed up by early abortion in case of failure of the condom or diaphragm to prevent pregnancy. Also, at any age the risk of death (due to unexpected pregnancy) from use of traditional contraception even without a backup of abortion is generally the same as, or less than, that from use of oral contraceptives.

Careful Use of Oral Contraceptives:

1. Tell Your Doctor About Any Of The Following:

a. Present or past conditions that mean you should not use oral contraceptives:

Clots in the legs, lungs, eyes, or elsewhere
A stroke, heart attack, or chest pain (angina pectoris)
Known or suspected cancer of the breast or sex organs

Irregular or scanty menstrual periods before starting to take the pill
Liver tumor associated with the use of the pill or other estrogen containing products.

b. Present conditions that mean you should not use oral contraceptives:
Unusual vaginal bleeding that has not yet been diagnosed.
Known or suspected pregnancy.

c. Conditions that your doctor will want to watch closely or which might cause him to suggest another method of contraception:
A family history of breast cancer
Breast nodules, fibrocystic disease of the breast, or an abnormal mammogram
Diabetes
High blood pressure
High cholesterol
Cigarette smoking
Migraine headaches
Heart or kidney disease
Epilepsy
Mental depression
Tingling of the fingers or toes
Fibroid tumors of the uterus
Gallbladder disease
Asthma
Problems during a prior pregnancy
Plans for elective surgery
History of jaundice or other liver disease

d. Use of any of the following kinds of drugs, which might interact with the pill: antibiotics, sulfa drugs, antifungal drugs, drugs for epilepsy or migraine, pain killers, tranquilizers, sedatives or sleeping pills, blood thinning drugs, vitamins, drugs being used for the treatment of depression, high blood pressure or other heart conditions, high blood sugar (diabetes), asthma, bronchitis, emphysema, or colds, or drugs used with organ transplants (e.g., cyclosporin A).

e. Once you are using oral contraceptives, you should be alert for signs of a serious adverse effect and call your doctor if they occur:
Sharp pain in the chest, coughing blood, or sudden shortness of breath (indicating possible clots in the lungs)
Pain in the calf (possible clot in the leg)
Crushing chest pain or heaviness (indicating possible heart attack)
Sudden severe headache or vomiting, dizziness or fainting, disturbance of vision or speech, or weakness or numbness in an arm or leg (indicating a possible stroke)
Sudden partial or complete loss of vision (indicating a possible clot in the eye)
Breast lumps (you should ask your doctor to show you how to examine your own breasts)
Severe pain or mass in the abdomen (indicating a possible tumor of the liver)
Severe depression
Yellowing of the skin (jaundice)
Unusual swelling.

2. How to Take the Pill So That It is Most Effective
Reduced effectiveness and an increased incidence of breakthrough bleeding have been associated with the use of oral contraceptives with antibiotics such as rifampicin, ampicillin, and tetracycline, with the antifungal griseofulvin, or with certain other drugs, such as barbiturates, phenylbutazone or phenytoin sodium. You should use an additional means of contraception during any cycle in which any of these drugs are taken.
When you first begin to use the pill, you should use an additional method of protection until you have taken your first seven pills.
Your physician has prescribed one of the following dosage schedules. Please follow the instructions appropriate for your schedule.
20-Day Schedule: Counting the onset of flow as day 1, take the first pill on day 5 of the menstrual cycle whether or not the flow has stopped. Take another pill the same time each day, preferably at bedtime, for 20 days. Then wait for 7 days, during which time a menstrual period usually occurs, and begin taking 1 pill every day on the 8th day after you took your last pill, whether or not the menstrual flow has stopped. This cycle is repeated 20 days on pills and 7 days off pills until time for the physician's examination and pill refill. If you are taking NORINYL® 2 mg Tablets for the control of excessive bleeding (hypermenorrhea), your physician may instruct you to stop taking the pills after 3 cycles to determine the need for further treatment. The information contained in this leaflet regarding who should not use the pill, the dangers of the pill and safe use of the pill applies to the use of the pill for hypermenorrhea, as well as for contraception.
21-Day Schedule for BREVICON, NORINYL 1 + 35, NORINYL 1 + 50, NORINYL 1 + 80 Tablets: You may start taking the pill on Day 5 of your menstrual cycle or on Sunday. To start on Day 5, count the first day of menstrual flow as Day 1 and take the first pill on Day 5 of the menstrual cycle whether or not the flow has stopped. To start on Sunday, take the first pill on the first Sunday after your menstrual period begins. If it begins on Sunday, take the first pill that day. Whether you start on day 5 or on Sunday, take another pill the same time each day, preferably at bedtime, for 21 days. Then wait for 7 days, during which time a menstrual period usually occurs, and begin taking 1 pill every day on the 8th day after you took your last pill, whether or not the menstrual flow has stopped. This cycle is repeated 21 days on pills and 7 days off pills until time for the physician's examination and pill refill.
28-Day Schedule for BREVICON, NORINYL 1 + 35, NORINYL 1 + 50, NORINYL 1 + 80 Tablets: You may start taking the pill on Day 5 of your menstrual cycle or on Sunday. To start on Day 5, count the first day of menstrual flow as Day 1 and take the first white, yellow, green, or blue pill on Day 5 of the menstrual cycle whether or not the flow has stopped. To start on Sunday, take the first white, yellow, green, or blue pill on the first Sunday after your menstrual period begins. If it begins on Sunday, take the first pill that day. Whether you start on Day 5 or on Sunday, follow the sequence around the card and continue taking another pill at the same time each day, preferably at bedtime, for 21 days. Then take an orange pill from the bottom of the card each day for seven days and expect a menstrual period during this week. The orange pills contain no active drug and are included simply for your convenience—to eliminate the need for counting days. After all 28 pills have been taken, whether bleeding has stopped or not, take the first white, yellow, green, or blue pill of the next cycle without any interruption. With the 28-day package, pills are taken every day of the year with no gap between cycles.
21-Day Schedule for TRI-NORINYL Tablets: Take the first blue pill on the first Sunday after menstrual flow begins. If menstrual flow begins on Sunday, take the first blue pill on that day. Take one blue pill the same time each day, preferably at bedtime, for the first 7 days, one green pill daily for the next 9 days, and then one blue pill each day for 5 days. Wait for 7 days, during which time a menstrual period usually occurs, then begin a new cycle of pills on the eighth day after you took your last pill, whether or not the menstrual flow has stopped. This cycle is repeated 21 days on pills and 7 days off pills until time for the physician's examination and pill refill.
28-Day Schedule for TRI-NORINYL Tablets: Take the first blue pill on the first Sunday after menstrual flow begins. If menstrual flow begins on Sunday, take the first blue pill on that day. Take one blue pill the same time each day, preferably at bedtime, for the first 7 days, one green pill daily for the next 9 days and then one blue pill each day for 5 days. Take one orange pill daily for the next 7 days and expect a menstrual period during this week. The orange pills contain no active drug and are included simply for your convenience —to eliminate the need of counting days. After all 28 pills have been taken, whether bleeding has stopped or not, take the first blue pill of the next cycle without any interruption. With the 28-day package, a pill is taken every day of the year with no gap between cycles.
Important Additional Instructions for the 20-Day, 21-Day and 28-Day Schedules
The prescribed dosage schedule must be followed exactly. The chance of becoming pregnant increases with each pill missed. If you miss one pill, you should take it as soon as you remember and also take your next pill at the regular time, which means you will be taking two pills on that day. If you miss two pills in a row, you should take one of the missed pills as soon as you remember, discard the other missed pill, and take your regular pill for that day at the proper time. Furthermore, you should use an additional method of contraception in addition to taking your pills for the remainder of the cycle. If more than 2 pills in a row have been missed, discontinue taking your pills immediately and use an additional method of contraception until you have a period or your doctor determines that you are not pregnant. Missing orange pills in the 28-day schedule does not increase your chances of becoming pregnant.
At times there may be no menstrual period after a cycle of pills. Therefore, if you miss one menstrual period but have taken the pills *exactly as you were supposed to,* continue as usual into the next cycle. If you have not taken the pills correctly, and have missed a menstrual period, *you may be pregnant* and should stop taking oral contraceptives until your doctor determines whether or not you are pregnant. Until you can get to your doctor, use another form of contraception. If two consecutive menstrual periods are missed, you should stop taking pills until it is determined whether you are pregnant. If you do become pregnant while using oral contraceptives, you should discuss the risks to the developing child with your doctor.
Even if spotting or breakthrough bleeding should occur, continue the medication according to the schedule. Should spotting or breakthrough bleeding persist you should notify your physician.
If you have just had a baby you should wait two weeks before starting to take oral contraceptives. If you have just had an abortion after a pregnancy of less than 12 weeks, you should start oral contraceptives immediately. If the pregnancy was 12 weeks or longer at the time of the abortion, wait two weeks before starting oral contraceptives.
NOR-Q.D.® (norethindrone) Tablets 0.35 mg. Schedule: Take the first pill on the first day of the menstrual flow, and take another pill each day, every day of the year. The pill should be taken at the same time of day, preferably at bedtime, and *continued daily, without interruption, whether bleeding occurs or not.* If prolonged bleeding occurs, you should consult your physician.
The chance of becoming pregnant increases with each pill missed. If you miss one pill, you should take it as soon as you remember and also take your next pill at the regular time, which means you will be taking two pills on that day. If you miss two pills in a row you should take one of the missed pills as soon as you remember, discard the other missed pill, and take your regular pill for that day at the proper time. Furthermore, you should use an additional method of contraception in addition to taking NOR-Q.D.® until you have a period or your doctor determines you are not pregnant. If more than 2 pills in a row have been missed, NOR-Q.D. should be discontinued immediately and an additional method of contraception should be used until you have a period or your doctor determines that you are not pregnant.
Whether or not you have missed a pill, if you have not had a period within 45 days of your last period, *you may be pregnant.* You should stop taking NOR-Q.D. until your doctor determines whether or not you are pregnant. Until you can get to your doctor, use another form of contraception. If you do become pregnant while using NOR-Q.D., you should discuss the risks to the developing child with your doctor.

3. Periodic Examination
Your doctor will take a complete medical and family history before prescribing oral contraceptives. At that time and about once a year thereafter, he will generally examine your blood pressure, breasts, abdomen, and pelvic organs (including a Papanicolaou smear).

SUMMARY

Oral contraceptives are the most effective method, except sterilization, for preventing pregnancy. Other methods, when used conscientiously, are also very effective and have fewer risks. Although the serious risks of oral contraceptives are uncommon, some of the risks may persist after you stop using the pill. On the other hand, the "pill" is a very convenient method of preventing pregnancy.
If you have certain conditions or have had these conditions in the past, you should not use oral contraceptives because the risk is too great. These conditions are listed in this leaflet. If you do not have these conditions, and decide to use the "pill", please read this leaflet carefully so that you can use the "pill" most safely and effectively.
Based on his or her assessment of your medical needs, your doctor has prescribed this drug for you. Do not give the drug to anyone else.

Revised 2/86

Shown in Product Identification Section, page 432

CARMOL® 10 OTC
[*kahr'mawl*]
10% urea lotion
for total body
dry skin care.

A product of Syntex Laboratories, Inc.
(See PDR For Nonprescription Drugs)

CARMOL® 20 OTC
[*kahr'mawl*]
20% Urea Cream
Extra strength for
rough, dry skin

A product of Syntex Laboratories, Inc.
(See PDR For Nonprescription Drugs)

CARMOL® HC ℞
[*kahr'mawl*]
(hydrocortisone acetate)
Cream 1%

Refer to entry under LIDEX® (fluocinonide) Cream 0.05%.

Continued on next page

Syntex—Cont.

FEMSTAT® ℞
[*fem 'stat*]
(butoconazole nitrate)
Vaginal Cream 2.0%

PRODUCT OVERVIEW

KEY FACTS

FEMSTAT Vaginal Cream contains as its active ingredient butoconazole nitrate 2.0%, an imidazole derivative that is clinically highly effective against vaginal infections induced by *Candida* species. The primary site of action of imidazoles appears to be the fungal cell membrane, although the exact mechanism of antifungal activity of butoconazole nitrate is unknown. FEMSTAT is unique in being a cream anticandidiasis preparation that is typically effective in 3 days (an additional 3 days of treatment is recommended for pregnant patients). It is packaged with three disposable applicators.

MAJOR USES

FEMSTAT Vaginal Cream is indicated for the local treatment of vulvovaginal mycotic infections caused by *Candida* species. It can be used concomitantly with oral contraceptives and antibiotics, and is effective in both non-pregnant and pregnant women (second and third trimesters). The recommended treatment regimen is 3 days in non-pregnant women and 6 days in pregnant women.

SAFETY INFORMATION

See complete safety information set forth below.

PRESCRIBING INFORMATION

FEMSTAT® ℞
[*fem 'stat*]
(butoconazole nitrate)
Vaginal Cream 2.0%

DESCRIPTION

FEMSTAT Vaginal Cream contains butoconazole nitrate 2.0%, an imidazole derivative with antifungal activity. Its chemical name is (±)-1-[4-(*p*-Chlorophenyl)-2-[(2,6-dichlorophenyl) thio]butyl] imidazole mononitrate and it has the following chemical structure:

$$Cl-C_6H_4-CH_2-CH_2-CH(S-C_6H_3Cl_2)-CH_2-N(C_3H_3N)\cdot HNO_3$$

Butoconazole nitrate is a white to off-white crystalline powder with a molecular weight of 474.79. It is sparingly soluble in methanol; slightly soluble in chloroform, methylene chloride, acetone and ethanol; very slightly soluble in ethyl acetate; and practically insoluble in water. It melts at about 159°C with decomposition.

FEMSTAT Vaginal Cream contains butoconazole nitrate 2.0% in a water-washable emollient cream of stearyl alcohol, propylene glycol, cetyl alcohol, sorbitan monostearate, glyceryl stearate (and) PEG-100 stearate, mineral oil, polysorbate 60, purified water, with methylparaben and propylparaben as preservatives.

CLINICAL PHARMACOLOGY

Butoconazole nitrate is an imidazole derivative that has fungicidal activity *in vitro* against *Candida, Trichophyton, Microsporum,* and *Epidermophyton*. It is also active against some gram positive bacteria. Clinically, it is highly effective against vaginal infections induced by strains of *Candida albicans, Candida tropicalis,* and other species of this genus. The primary site of action of imidazoles appears to be the cell membrane. The permeablilty of the cell membrane is altered, resulting in a reduced osmotic resistance and viability of the fungus. The exact mechanism of the antifungal activity of butoconazole nitrate is not known.

Following vaginal administration of butoconazole nitrate, 5.5% of the dose is absorbed on average. After vaginal administration peak plasma levels of the drug and its metabolites are attained at 24 hours and the plasma half-life is approximately 21–24 hours.

INDICATIONS AND USAGE

FEMSTAT Vaginal Cream is indicated for the local treatment of vulvovaginal mycotic infections caused by Candida species. The diagnosis should be confirmed by KOH smears and/or cultures.

FEMSTAT Vaginal Cream can be used in association with oral contraceptive and antibiotic therapy. FEMSTAT is effective in both non-pregnant and pregnant women, but in pregnant women it should be used only during the second and third trimesters.

CONTRAINDICATIONS

FEMSTAT Vaginal Cream 2.0% is contraindicated in patients with a history of hypersensitivity to any of the components of the cream.

PRECAUTIONS

General

If clinical symptoms persist, microbiological tests should be repeated to rule out other pathogens and to confirm the diagnosis.

If sensitization or irritation is reported during use, the treatment should be discontinued.

Information for the Patient

The patient should be cautioned against premature discontinuation of the medication during menstruation or in response to relief of symptoms.

Carcinogenesis

Long-term studies in animals have not been performed to evaluate the carcinogenic potential of this drug.

Mutagenesis

Butoconazole nitrate was not mutagenic when tested on microbial indicator organisms.

Impairment of Fertility

No impairment of fertility was seen in rabbits or rats administered butoconazole nitrate in oral doses up to 30 mg/kg/day or 100 mg/kg/day respectively.

Pregnancy

Pregnancy Category C.

In pregnant rats administered 6 mg/kg/day (3–7 times the human dose) butoconazole nitrate intravaginally during the period of organogenesis, there was an increase in resorption rate and decrease in litter size, but no teratogenicity. Butoconazole nitrate had no apparent adverse effect when administered orally to pregnant rats throughout organogenesis, at dose levels up to 50 mg/kg/day. Daily oral doses of 100, 300, or 750 mg/kg resulted in fetal malformations (abdominal wall defects, cleft palate), but maternal stress was evident at these higher dose levels. There were no adverse effects on litters of rabbits receiving butoconazole nitrate orally, even at maternally stressful dose levels (e.g., 150 mg/kg). There are no adequate and well-controlled studies in pregnant women during the first trimester.

Butoconazole nitrate, like other azole antimycotic agents, causes dystocia in rats when treatment is extended through parturition. However, this effect was not apparent in rabbits treated with as much as 100 mg/kg/day orally.

In clinical studies, over 200 pregnant patients have used butoconazole nitrate cream 2.0% for 3 or 6 days during the second or third trimester and the drug had no adverse effect on the course of pregnancy. Follow-up reports available on infants born to these women reveal no adverse effects or complications that were attributable to the drug.

Nursing Mothers

It is not known whether this drug is excreted in human milk. Because many drugs are excreted in human milk, caution should be exercised when butoconazole nitrate is administered to a nursing woman.

Pediatric Use

Safety and effectiveness in children have not been established.

ADVERSE REACTIONS

Of the 561 patients treated with butoconazole nitrate cream 2.0% for 3 or 6 days in controlled clinical trials, 13 (2.3%) reported complaints probably related to therapy. Vulvar/-vaginal burning occurred in 2.3%, vulvar itching in 0.9%, and discharge, soreness, swelling, and itching of the fingers each occurred in 0.2%. Nine patients (1.6%) discontinued because of these complaints.

DOSAGE AND ADMINISTRATION

Non-pregnant Patients: The recommended dose is one applicatorful of cream (approximately 5 grams) intravaginally at bedtime for three days. Treatment can be extended for an additional three days if necessary.

Pregnant Patients (2nd and 3rd trimesters only): The recommended dose is one applicatorful of cream (approximately 5 grams) intravaginally at bedtime for six days.

HOW SUPPLIED

FEMSTAT® (butoconazole nitrate) Vaginal Cream 2.0% is available in a 28-gram tube with 3 disposable measured-dose applicators (NDC 0033-2280-14).

Avoid excessive heat, above 40°C (104°F), and avoid freezing.

Caution: Federal law prohibits dispensing without prescription.

U.S. Patent No. 4,078,071 © JANUARY 1986

Shown in Product Identification Section, page 432

LIDEX® ℞
[*li 'dex*]
(fluocinonide)
Cream 0.05%
Gel 0.05%
Ointment 0.05%
Topical Solution 0.05%

LIDEX®-E ℞
(fluocinonide)
Cream 0.05%

CARMOL® HC ℞
(hydrocortisone acetate)
Cream 1%

NEO-SYNALAR® Cream ℞
[*ne "o sin 'ă-lahr*]
[neomycin sulfate 0.5% (0.35% neomycin base), fluocinolone acetonide 0.025%]

SYNACORT® ℞
[*sin 'ă-cort*]
(hydrocortisone)
Cream 1%
Cream 2.5%

SYNALAR® ℞
[*sin 'ă-lahr*]
(fluocinolone acetonide)
Cream 0.025%
Cream 0.01%
Ointment 0.025%
Topical Solution 0.01%

SYNALAR-HP® ℞
(fluocinolone acetonide)
Cream 0.2%

SYNEMOL® ℞
[*sin 'ĕ-mol*]
(fluocinolone acetonide)
Cream 0.025%

Products of Syntex Laboratories, Inc.

DESCRIPTION

These preparations are all intended for topical administration.

LIDEX preparations have as their active component the corticosteroid fluocinonide, which is the 21-acetate ester of fluocinolone acetonide and has the chemical name pregna-1,4-diene-3,20-dione, 21-(acetyloxy)-6, 9-difluoro-11-hydroxy-16,17- ((1-methylethylidene)bis(oxy))-, (6α,11β, 16α)-.

LIDEX cream contains fluocinonide 0.5 mg/g in FAPG® cream, a specially formulated cream base consisting of stearyl alcohol, polyethylene glycol 8000, propylene glycol, 1,2,6-hexanetriol and citric acid. This white cream vehicle is greaseless, non-staining, anhydrous and completely water miscible. The base provides emollient and hydrophilic properties. In this formulation the active ingredient is totally in solution.

LIDEX gel contains fluocinonide 0.5 mg/g in a specially formulated gel base consisting of propylene glycol, propyl gallate, edetate disodium, and carbomer 940, with NaOH and/or HCl added to adjust the pH. This clear, colorless thixotropic vehicle is greaseless, non-staining and completely water miscible. In this formulation the active ingredient is totally in solution.

LIDEX ointment contains fluocinonide 0.5 mg/g in a specially formulated ointment base consisting of Amerchol CAB (mixture of sterols and higher alcohols), white petrolatum, propylene carbonate and propylene glycol. It provides the occlusive and emollient effects desirable in an ointment. In this formulation the active ingredient is totally in solution.

LIDEX solution contains fluocinonide 0.5 mg/ml in a solution of propylene glycol, alcohol (35%), diisopropyl adipate, and citric acid. In this formulation the active ingredient is totally in solution.

LIDEX-E cream contains fluocinonide 0.5 mg/g in a water-washable aqueous emollient base of stearyl alcohol, cetyl alcohol, mineral oil, propylene glycol, sorbitan monostearate, polysorbate 60, citric acid and purified water.

CARMOL HC Cream has the corticosteroid hydrocortisone acetate, which has the chemical name pregn-4-ene-3,20-dione,21-(acetyloxy)-11,17-dihydroxy-,(11β)-, as its active component. CARMOL HC contains micronized hydrocortisone acetate, USP, 10 mg/g, in a water-washable vanishing cream containing urea (10%), purified water, stearic acid, isopropyl myristate, PPG-26 oleate, isopropyl palmitate, propylene glycol, trolamine, cetyl alcohol, carbomer 940, sodium bisulfite, sodium laureth sulfate, edetate disodium, xanthan gum; scented with hypoallergenic perfume.

CARMOL HC is non-lipid, non-occlusive and hypoallergenic; it contains no mineral oil, petrolatum, lanolin or parabens.

NEO-SYNALAR cream contains neomycin sulfate 5 mg/g (3.5 mg/g neomycin base) and fluocinolone acetonide 0.25

mg/g in a water-washable aqueous base of stearyl alcohol, propylene glycol, cetyl alcohol, polyoxyl 20 cetostearyl ether, mineral oil, white wax, simethicone, butylated hydroxytoluene, edetate disodium, citric acid, and purified water, with methylparaben and propylparaben as preservatives.

SYNACORT creams have as their active component the corticosteroid hydrocortisone, which has the chemical name pregn-4-ene-3,20-dione, 11,17,21-trihydroxy-,(11β)-.

SYNACORT creams contain hydrocortisone, USP, 10 mg/g or 25 mg/g in a cream containing propylene glycol, stearyl alcohol, mineral oil, cetyl alcohol, sorbitan monostearate, polysorbate 60, citric acid and purified water.

SYNALAR preparations, SYNALAR-HP cream, and SYNEMOL cream have as their active component the corticosteroid fluocinolone acetonide, which has the chemical name pregna-1,4-diene-3,20-dione,6,9-difluoro-11,21-dihydroxy-16,17-[(1-methylethylidene)bis(oxy)]-,(6α,11β,16α)-.

SYNALAR creams contains fluocinolone acetonide 0.25 mg/g or 0.1 mg/g in a water-washable aqueous base of stearyl alcohol, propylene glycol, cetyl alcohol, polyoxyl 20 cetostearyl ether, mineral oil, white wax, simethicone, butylated hydroxytoluene, edetate disodium, citric acid, and purified water, with methylparaben and propylparaben as preservatives.

SYNALAR ointment contains fluocinolone acetonide 0.25 mg/g in a white petrolatum USP vehicle.

SYNALAR solution contains fluocinolone acetonide 0.1 mg/ml in a water-washable base of propylene glycol with citric acid.

SYNALAR-HP cream contains fluocinolone acetonide 2 mg/g in a water-washable aqueous base of stearyl alcohol, cetyl alcohol, mineral oil, propylene glycol, sorbitan monostearate, polysorbate 60, purified water and citric acid with methylparaben and propylparaben as preservatives.

SYNEMOL cream contains fluocinolone acetonide 0.25 mg/g in a water-washable aqueous emollient base of stearyl alcohol, cetyl alcohol, mineral oil, propylene glycol, sorbitan monostearate, polysorbate 60, purified water and citric acid.

CLINICAL PHARMACOLOGY

Topical corticosteroids share anti-inflammatory, anti-pruritic and vasoconstrictive actions.

The mechanism of anti-inflammatory activity of the topical corticosteroids is unclear. Various laboratory methods, including vasoconstrictor assays, are used to compare and predict potencies and/or clinical efficacies of the topical corticosteroids. There is some evidence to suggest that a recognizable correlation exists between vasoconstrictor potency and therapeutic efficacy in man.

PHARMACOKINETICS

The extent of percutaneous absorption of topical corticosteroids is determined by many factors including the vehicle, the integrity of the epidermal barrier, and the use of occlusive dressings. A significantly greater amount of fluocinonide is absorbed from the solution than from the cream or gel formulations.

Topical corticosteroids can be absorbed from normal intact skin. Inflammation and/or other disease processes in the skin increase percutaneous absorption. Occlusive dressings substantially increase the percutaneous absorption of topical corticosteroids. Thus, occlusive dressings may be a valuable therapeutic adjunct for treatment of resistant dermatoses. (See DOSAGE AND ADMINISTRATION).

Once absorbed through the skin, topical corticosteroids are handled through pharmacokinetic pathways similar to systemically administered corticosteroids. Corticosteroids are bound to plasma proteins in varying degrees. Corticosteroids are metabolized primarily in the liver and are then excreted by the kidneys. Some of the topical corticosteroids and their metabolites are also excreted into the bile.

INDICATIONS AND USAGE

Relief of the inflammatory and pruritic manifestations of corticosteroid-responsive dermatoses.

NEO-SYNALAR is indicated for the treatment of corticosteroid-responsive dermatoses with secondary infection. It has not been demonstrated that this steroid-antibiotic combination provides greater benefit then the steroid component alone after 7 days of treatment (see WARNINGS).

CONTRAINDICATIONS

Topical corticosteroids are contraindicated in those patients with a history of hypersensitivity to any of the components of the preparation. NEO-SYNALAR should not be used in the external auditory canal if the eardrum is perforated.

Warnings for NEO-SYNALAR: If local infection should continue or become severe, or in the presence of systemic infection, appropriate systemic antibacterial therapy, based on susceptibility testing, should be considered.

Because of the concern of nephrotoxicity and ototoxicity associated with neomycin, this combination should not be used over a wide area or for extended periods of time.

There are articles in the current medical literature that indicate an increase in the prevalence of persons sensitive to neomycin.

Warnings for CARMOL HC: Contains sodium bisulfite, a sulfite that may cause serious allergic-type reactions (e.g., hives, itching, wheezing, anaphylaxis) in certain susceptible persons. Although the overall incidence of sulfite sensitivity in the general population is probably low, it is seen more frequently in asthmatics or in atopic nonasthmatic persons.

PRECAUTIONS

General: It is recommended that NEO-SYNALAR not be used under occlusive dressing.

Systemic absorption of topical corticosteroids has produced reversible hypothalamic-pituitary-adrenal (HPA) axis suppression, manifestations of Cushing's syndrome, hyperglycemia, and glucosuria in some patients.

Conditions which augment systemic absorption include the application of the more potent steroids, use over large surface areas, prolonged use, the addition of occlusive dressings, and dosage form.

Therefore, patients receiving a large dose of a potent topical steroid applied to a large surface area or under an occlusive dressing should be evaluated periodically for evidence of HPA axis suppression by using the urinary free cortisol and ACTH stimulation tests. If HPA axis suppression is noted, an attempt should be made to withdraw the drug, to reduce the frequency of application, or to substitute a less potent steroid.

Recovery of HPA axis function is generally prompt and complete upon discontinuation of the drug. Infrequently, signs and symptoms of steroid withdrawal may occur, requiring supplemental systemic corticosteroids.

Children may absorb proportionally larger amounts of topical corticosteroids and thus be more susceptible to systemic toxicity. (See PRECAUTIONS—Pediatric Use).

Not for ophthalmic use. Severe irritation is possible if fluocinonide solution contacts the eye. If that should occur, immediate flushing of the eye with a large volume of water is recommended.

If irritation develops, topical corticosteroids should be discontinued and appropriate therapy instituted.

In the presence of dermatological infections, the use of an appropriate antifungal or antibacterial agent should be instituted. If a favorable response does not occur promptly, the corticosteroid should be discontinued until the infection has been adequately controlled.

As with all antibiotics, prolonged use of NEO-SYNALAR may result in over-growth of nonsusceptible organisms. If superinfection occurs, appropriate measures should be taken.

SYNALAR-HP cream should not be used for prolonged periods and the quantity per day should not exceed 2 g. of formulated material.

Information for the Patient: Patients using topical corticosteroids should receive the following information and instructions:

1. This medication is to be used as directed by the physician. It is for external use only. Avoid contact with the eyes. If there is contact with the eyes and severe irritation occurs, immediately flush with a large volume of water.
2. Patients should be advised not to use this medication for any disorder other than for which it was prescribed.
3. The treated skin area should not be bandaged or otherwise covered or wrapped as to be occlusive unless directed by the physician.
4. Patients should report any signs of local adverse reactions especially under occlusive dressing.
5. Parents of pediatric patients should be advised not to use tight-fitting diapers or plastic pants on a child being treated in the diaper area, as these garments may constitute occlusive dressings.

Laboratory Tests: The following tests may be helpful in evaluating HPA axis suppression: Urinary free cortisol test and ACTH stimulation test.

Carcinogenesis, Mutagenesis, and Impairment of Fertility: Long-term animal studies have not been performed to evaluate the carcinogenic potential or the effect on fertility of topical corticosteroids.

Studies to determine mutagenicity with prednisolone and hydrocortisone have revealed negative results.

Pregnancy Category C: Corticosteroids are generally teratogenic in laboratory animals when administered systemically at relatively low dosage levels. The more potent corticosteroids have been shown to be teratogenic after dermal application in laboratory animals. There are no adequate and well-controlled studies in pregnant women on teratogenic effects from topically applied corticosteroids. Therefore, topical corticosteroids should be used during pregnancy only if the potential benefit justifies the potential risk to the fetus. Drugs of this class should not be used extensively on pregnant patients, in large amounts, or for prolonged periods of time.

Nursing Mothers: It is not known whether topical administration of corticosteroids could result in sufficient systemic absorption to produce detectable quantities in breast milk. Systemically administered corticosteroids are secreted into breast milk in quantities *not* likely to have a deleterious effect on the infant. Nevertheless, caution should be exercised when topical corticosteroids are administered to a nursing woman.

Pediatric Use: SYNALAR-HP® (fluocinolone acetonide) cream 0.2% should not be used on infants up to 2 years of age.

Pediatric patients may demonstrate greater susceptibility to topical corticosteroid-induced HPA axis suppression and Cushing's syndrome than mature patients because of a larger skin surface area to body weight ratio.

Hypothalamic-pituitary-adrenal (HPA) axis suppression, Cushing's syndrome, and intracranial hypertension have been reported in children receiving topical corticosteroids. Manifestations of adrenal suppression in children include linear growth retardation, delayed weight gain, low plasma cortisol levels, and absence of response to ACTH stimulation. Manifestations of intracranial hypertension include bulging fontanelles, headaches, and bilateral papilledema.

Administration of topical corticosteroids to children should be limited to the least amount compatible with an effective therapeutic regimen. Chronic corticosteroid therapy may interfere with the growth and development of children.

ADVERSE REACTIONS

The following local adverse reactions are reported infrequently with topical corticosteroids, but may occur more frequently with the use of occlusive dressings. These reactions are listed in an approximate decreasing order of occurrence: burning, itching, irritation, dryness, folliculitis, hypertrichosis, acneiform eruptions, hypopigmentation, perioral dermatitis, allergic contact dermatitis, maceration of the skin, secondary infection, skin atrophy, striae, miliaria. The following reactions have been reported with the topical use of neomycin: ototoxicity and nephrotoxicity.

OVERDOSAGE

Topically applied corticosteroids can be absorbed in sufficient amounts to produce systemic effects (See PRECAUTIONS).

DOSAGE AND ADMINISTRATION

Topical corticosteroids are generally applied to the affected area as a thin film from two to four times daily depending on the severity of the condition. In hairy sites, the hair should be parted to allow direct contact with the lesion.

Occlusive dressings may be used for the management of psoriasis or recalcitrant conditions. Some plastic films may be flammable and due care should be exercised in their use. Similarly, caution should be employed when such films are used on children or left in their proximity, to avoid the possibility of accidental suffocation.

If an infection develops, the use of occlusive dressings should be discontinued and appropriate antimicrobial therapy instituted.

HOW SUPPLIED

LIDEX® (fluocinonide) cream 0.05%—15 g Tube (NDC 0033-2511-13), 30 g Tube (NDC 0033-2511-14), 60 g Tube (NDC 0033-2511-17), and 120 g Tube (NDC 0033-2511-22). Store at room temperature. Avoid excessive heat, above 40°C (104°F).

LIDEX® (fluocinonide) gel 0.05%—15 g Tube (NDC 0033-2507-13), 30 g Tube (NDC 0033-2507-14), 60 g Tube (NDC 0033-2507-17), and 120 g Tube (NDC 0033-2507-22). Store at controlled room temperature, 15–30°C (59–86°F).

LIDEX® (fluocinonide) ointment 0.05%—15 g Tube (NDC 0033-2514-13), 30 g Tube (NDC 0033-2514-14), 60 g Tube (NDC 0033-2514-17), and 120 g Tube (NDC 0033-2514-22). Store at room temperature. Avoid excessive heat, above 40°C (104°F).

LIDEX® (fluocinonide) topical solution 0.05%—Plastic squeeze bottles: 20 cc (NDC 0033-2517-44) and 60 cc (NDC 0033-2517-46). Store at room temperature. Avoid excessive heat, above 40°C (104°F).

LIDEX-E® (fluocinonide) cream 0.05%—15 g Tube (NDC 0033-2513-13), 30 g Tube (NDC 0033-2513-14), 60 g Tube (NDC 0033-2513-17), and 120 g Tube (NDC 0033-2513-22). Store at room temperature. Avoid excessive heat, above 40°C (104°F).

CARMOL® HC (hydrocortisone acetate) cream 1%—1 oz. Tube (NDC 0033-2550-15) and 4 oz. Jar (NDC 0033-2550-11). Avoid excessive heat, above 40°C (104°F).

NEO-SYNALAR cream—15 g Tube (NDC 0033-2505-13), 30 g Tube (NDC 0033-2505-14), 60 g Tube (NDC 0033-2505-17). Store at room temperature. Avoid freezing and excessive heat, above 40°C (104°F).

SYNACORT® (hydrocortisone) cream 1%—15 g Tube (NDC 0033-2519-13), 30 g Tube (NDC 0033-2519-14), and 60 g Tube (NDC 0033-2519-17). SYNACORT® (hydrocortisone) cream 2.5%—30 g Tube (NDC 0033-2520-14). Store at room temperature. Avoid excessive heat, above 40°C (104°F).

SYNALAR® (fluocinolone acetonide) cream 0.025%—15 g Tube (NDC 0033-2501-13), 30 g Tube (NDC 0033-2501-14), 60 g Tube—(NDC 0033-2501-17), and 425 g Jar (NDC 0033-2501-23). Store tubes at room temperature. Avoid freezing and

Continued on next page

Syntex—Cont.

excessive heat, above 40°C (104°F). Store jars at controlled room temperature, 15°–30°C (59°–86°F).
SYNALAR® (fluocinolone acetonide) cream 0.01%—15 g Tube (NDC 0033-2502-13), 30 g Tube (NDC 0033-2502-14), 60 g Tube (NDC 0033-2502-17), and 425 g Jar (NDC 0033-2502-23). Store tubes at room temperature. Avoid freezing and excessive heat, above 40°C (104°F). Store jars at controlled room temperature, 15°–30°C (59°–86°F).
SYNALAR® (fluocinolone acetonide) ointment 0.025%—15 g Tube (NDC 0033-2504-13), 30 g Tube (NDC 0033-2504-14), 60 g Tube (NDC 0033-2504-17), 120 g Tube (NDC 0033-2504-22), and 425 g Jar (NDC 0033-2504-23). Store at room temperature. Avoid excessive heat, above 40°C (104°F).
SYNALAR® (fluocinolone acetonide) topical solution 0.01%—Plastic squeeze bottles: 20 cc (NDC 0033-2506-44) and 60 cc (NDC 0033-2506-46). Store at room temperature. Avoid freezing.
SYNALAR-HP® (fluocinolone acetonide) cream 0.2%—12 g Tube (NDC 0033-2503-12). Store at room temperature. Avoid excessive heat, above 40°C (104°F).
SYNEMOL® (fluocinolone acetonide) cream 0.025%—15 g Tube (NDC 0033-2509-13), 30 g Tube (NDC 0033-2509-14), 60 g Tube (NDC 0033-2509-17), and 120 g Tube (NDC 0033-2509-22). Store at room temperature. Avoid excessive heat, above 40°C (104°F).
CAUTION: Federal law prohibits dispensing without a prescription.
LIDEX ointment: U.S. Patent No. 4,017,615
LIDEX cream: U.S. Patent Nos. 3,592,930 and 3,888,995

Revised 2/86

NAPROSYN® ℞
[*nă 'pro-sin*]
(naproxen)
Tablets

PRODUCT OVERVIEW

KEY FACTS

NAPROSYN (naproxen) is an orally administered nonsteroidal anti-inflammatory drug (arylacetic acid group) with analgesic and antipyretic properties. The naproxen anion inhibits prostaglandin synthesis but beyond this its mode of action is unknown.

MAJOR USES

NAPROSYN has proved to be clinically effective for rheumatoid arthritis, osteoarthritis, ankylosing spondylitis, tendinitis and bursitis, and acute gout. It is also indicated in the relief of mild to moderate pain and the treatment of primary dysmenorrhea.

SAFETY INFORMATION

See complete safety information set forth below.

PRESCRIBING INFORMATION

NAPROSYN® ℞
[*nă 'pro-sin*]
(naproxen)
Tablets
A product of Syntex Puerto Rico, Inc.

DESCRIPTION

NAPROSYN® (naproxen) tablets for oral administration each contain 250 mg, 375 mg or 500 mg of naproxen. NAPROSYN is a member of the arylacetic acid group of nonsteroidal anti-inflammatory drugs.
The chemical name for naproxen is 2-naphthaleneacetic acid, 6-methoxy-α-methyl-,(+).
Naproxen is an odorless, white to off-white crystalline substance. It is lipid soluble, practically insoluble in water at low pH and freely soluble in water at high pH.
Each NAPROSYN tablet contains napoxen, the active ingredient, with D&C Yellow #10 (the 375 mg tablet does not contain this color additive), FD&C Yellow #6, lactose, magnesium stearate, povidone and starch.

CLINICAL PHARMACOLOGY

NAPROSYN (naproxen) is a nonsteroidal anti-inflammatory drug with analgesic and antipyretic properties. Naproxen sodium, the sodium salt of naproxen, has been developed as an analgesic because it is more rapidly absorbed. The naproxen anion inhibits prostaglandin synthesis but beyond this its mode of action is unknown.
Naproxen is rapidly and completely absorbed from the gastrointestinal tract. After administration of naproxen, peak plasma levels of naproxen anion are attained in 2 to 4 hours, with steady-state conditions normally achieved after 4–5 doses. The mean biological half-life of the anion in humans is approximately 13 hours, and at therapeutic levels it is greater than 99% albumin bound. Approximately 95% of the dose is excreted in the urine, primarily as naproxen, 6-0-desmethyl naproxen or their conjugates. The rate of excretion has been found to coincide closely with the rate of drug disappearance from the plasma. The drug does not induce metabolizing enzymes.
The drug was studied in patients with rheumatoid arthritis, osteoarthritis, ankylosing spondylitis, tendinitis and bursitis, and acute gout. It is not a corticosteroid. Improvement in patients treated for rheumatoid arthritis has been demonstrated by a reduction in joint swelling, a reduction in pain, a reduction in duration of morning stiffness, a reduction in disease activity as assessed by both the investigator and patient, and by increased mobility as demonstrated by a reduction in walking time.
In patients with osteoarthritis, the therapeutic action of the drug has been shown by a reduction in joint pain or tenderness, an increase in range of motion in knee joints, increased mobility as demonstrated by a reduction in walking time, and improvement in capacity to perform activities of daily living impaired by the disease.
In clinical studies in patients with rheumatoid arthritis and osteoarthritis, the drug has been shown to be comparable to aspirin and indomethacin in controlling the aforementioned measures of disease activity, but the frequency and severity of the milder gastrointestinal adverse effects (nausea, dyspepsia, heartburn) and nervous system adverse effects (tinnitus, dizziness, lightheadedness) were less than in both the aspirin- and indomethacin-treated patients. It is not known whether the drug causes less peptic ulceration than aspirin.
In patients with ankylosing spondylitis, the drug has been shown to decrease night pain, morning stiffness and pain at rest. In double-blind studies the drug was shown to be as effective as aspirin, but with fewer side effects.
In patients with acute gout, a favorable response to the drug was shown by significant clearing of inflammatory changes (e.g., decrease in swelling, heat) within 24–48 hours, as well as by relief of pain and tenderness.
The drug may be used safely in combination with gold salts and/or corticosteroids; however, in controlled clinical trials, when added to the regimen of patients receiving corticosteroids it did not appear to cause greater improvement over that seen with corticosteroids alone. Whether the drug could be used in conjunction with partially effective doses of corticosteroid for a "steroid-sparing" effect has not been adequately studied. When added to the regimen of patients receiving gold salts the drug did result in greater improvement. Its use in combination with salicylates is not recommended because data are inadequate to demonstrate that the drug produces greater improvement over that achieved with aspirin alone. Further, there is some evidence that aspirin increases the rate of excretion of the drug.
Generally, improvement due to the drug has not been found to be dependent on age, sex, severity or duration of disease.
The drug was studied in patients with mild to moderate pain, and pain relief was obtained within 1 hour. It is not a narcotic and is not a CNS-acting drug. Controlled double-blind studies have demonstrated the analgesic properties of the drug in, for example, post-operative, post-partum, orthopedic and uterine contraction pain and dysmenorrhea. In dysmenorrheic patients, the drug reduces the level of prostaglandins in the uterus, which correlates with a reduction in the frequency and severity of uterine contractions. Analgesic action has been shown by such measures as a reduction of pain intensity scores, increase in pain relief scores, decrease in numbers of patients requiring additional analgesic medication, and delay in time for required remedication. The analgesic effect has been found to last for up to 7 hours.
In ^{51}Cr blood loss and gastroscopy studies with normal volunteers, daily administration of 1000 mg of the drug has been demonstrated to cause statistically significantly less gastric bleeding and erosion than 3250 mg of aspirin.

INDICATIONS AND USAGE

NAPROSYN (naproxen) is indicated for the treatment of rheumatoid arthritis, osteoarthritis, ankylosing spondylitis, tendinitis and bursitis, and acute gout.
It is also indicated in the relief of mild to moderate pain and for the treatment of primary dysmenorrhea.

CONTRAINDICATIONS

The drug is contraindicated in patients who have had allergic reactions to NAPROSYN® (naproxen) or to ANAPROX® (naproxen sodium). It is also contraindicated in patients in whom aspirin or other nonsteroidal anti-inflammatory/analgesic drugs induce the syndrome of asthma, rhinitis, and nasal polyps. Both types of reactions have the potential of being fatal.

WARNINGS

Gastrointestinal bleeding, sometimes severe, and occasionally fatal, has been reported in patients receiving the drug. Among 960 patients treated for rheumatoid arthritis or osteoarthritis during the course of clinical trials in the United States (260 treated for more than two years), 16 cases of peptic ulceration were reported. More than half were on concomitant corticosteroid and/or salicylate therapy and about a third had a prior history of peptic ulcer. Gastrointestinal bleeding, including nine potentially serious cases, was also reported in this population. These were not always preceded by premonitory gastrointestinal symptoms. Although most of the patients with serious bleeding were receiving concomitant therapy and had a history of peptic ulcer disease, it should be kept in mind that the drug also has the potential for causing gastrointestinal bleeding on its own. Therefore, it should not be given to patients with active peptic ulcer unless the potential benefit outweighs the potential risk. In such patients, and in other patients with a history of gastrointestinal disease, it should be given under close supervision.

PRECAUTIONS

General:

***NAPROSYN* (NAPROXEN) SHOULD NOT BE USED CONCOMITANTLY WITH THE RELATED DRUG *ANAPROX* (NAPROXEN SODIUM) SINCE THEY BOTH CIRCULATE IN PLASMA AS THE NAPROXEN ANION.**
Anaphylactoid reactions to NAPROSYN or ANAPROX, whether of the true allergic type or the pharmacologic idiosyncratic (e.g., aspirin syndrome) type, usually but not always occur in patients with a known history of such reactions. Therefore, careful questioning of patients for such things as asthma, nasal polyps, urticaria, and hypotension associated with nonsteroidal anti-inflammatory drugs before starting therapy is important. In addition, if such symptoms occur during therapy, treatment should be discontinued.
Renal Effects: As with other nonsteroidal anti-inflammatory drugs, long-term administration of naproxen to animals has resulted in renal papillary necrosis and other abnormal renal pathology. In humans, there have been reports of acute interstitial nephritis with hematuria, proteinuria, and occasionally nephrotic syndrome.
A second form of renal toxicity has been seen in patients with prerenal conditions leading to the reduction in renal blood flow or blood volume, where the renal prostaglandins have a supportive role in the maintenance of renal perfusion. In these patients, administration of a nonsteroidal anti-inflammatory drug may cause a dose-dependent reduction in prostaglandin formation and may precipitate overt renal decompensation. Patients at greatest risk of this reaction are those with impaired renal function, heart failure, liver dysfunction, those taking diuretics, and the elderly. Discontinuation of nonsteroidal anti-inflammatory therapy is typically followed by recovery to the pretreatment state.
NAPROSYN and its metabolites are eliminated primarily by the kidneys, therefore the drug should be used with great caution in patients with significantly impaired renal function and the monitoring of serum creatinine and/or creatinine clearance is advised in these patients. Caution should be used if the drug is given to patients with creatinine clearance of less than 20 mL/minute because accumulation of naproxen metabolites has been seen in such patients.
Chronic alcoholic liver disease and probably other forms of cirrhosis reduce the total plasma concentration of naproxen, but the plasma concentration of unbound naproxen is increased. Caution is advised when high doses are required and some adjustment of dosage may be required in these patients.
One study indicates that although total plasma concentration of naproxen is unchanged, the unbound plasma fraction of naproxen is increased in the elderly. Caution is advised when high doses are required and some adjustment of dosage may be required in elderly patients.
As with other nonsteroidal anti-inflammatory drugs, borderline elevations of one or more liver tests may occur in up to 15% of patients. These abnormalities may progress, may remain essentially unchanged, or may be transient with continued therapy. The SGPT (ALT) test is probably the most sensitive indicator of liver dysfunction. Meaningful (3 times the upper limit of normal) elevations of SGPT or SGOT (AST) occurred in controlled clinical trials in less than 1% of patients. A patient with symptoms and/or signs suggesting liver dysfunction, or in whom an abnormal liver test has occurred, should be evaluated for evidence of the development of more severe hepatic reaction while on therapy with this drug. Severe hepatic reactions, including jaundice and cases of fatal hepatitis, have been reported with this drug as with other nonsteroidal anti-inflammatory drugs. Although such reactions are rare, if abnormal liver tests persist or worsen, if clinical signs and symptoms consistent with liver disease develop, or if systemic manifestations occur (e.g. eosinophilia, rash, etc.), this drug should be discontinued.
If steroid dosage is reduced or eliminated during therapy, the steroid dosage should be reduced slowly and the patients must be observed closely for any evidence of adverse effects, including adrenal insufficiency and exacerbation of symptoms of arthritis.
Patients with initial hemoglobin values of 10 grams or less who are to receive long-term therapy should have hemoglobin values determined frequently.
Peripheral edema has been observed in some patients. For this reason, the drug should be used with caution in patients with fluid retention, hypertension or heart failure.
The antipyretic and anti-inflammatory activities of the drug may reduce fever and inflammation, thus diminishing their utility as diagnostic signs in detecting complications of presumed non-infectious, non-inflammatory painful conditions.

Because of adverse eye findings in animal studies with drugs of this class it is recommended that ophthalmic studies be carried out within a reasonable period of time after starting therapy and at periodic intervals thereafter if the drug is to be used for an extended period of time.

Information for Patients:
Caution should be exercised by patients whose activities require alertness if they experience drowsiness, dizziness, vertigo or depression during therapy with the drug.

Drug Interactions:
In vitro studies have shown that naproxen anion, because of its affinity for protein, may displace from their binding sites other drugs which are also albumin-bound. Theoretically, the naproxen anion itself could likewise be displaced. Short-term controlled studies failed to show that taking the drug significantly affects prothrombin times when administered to individuals on coumarin-type anticoagulants. Caution is advised nonetheless, since interactions have been seen with other nonsteroidal agents of this class. Similarly, patients receiving the drug and a hydantoin, sulfonamide or sulfonylurea should be observed for signs of toxicity to these drugs.
The natriuretic effect of furosemide has been reported to be inhibited by some drugs of this class. Inhibition of renal lithium clearance leading to increases in plasma lithium concentrations has also been reported.
This and other nonsteroidal anti-inflammatory drugs can reduce the antihypertensive effect of propranolol and other beta-blockers.
Probenecid given concurrently increases naproxen anion plasma levels and extends its plasma half-life significantly.
Caution should be used if this drug is administered concomitantly with methotrexate. Naproxen and other nonsteroidal anti-inflammatory drugs have been reported to reduce the tubular secretion of methotrexate in an animal model, possibly enhancing the toxicity of that drug.

Drug/Laboratory Test Interactions:
The drug may decrease platelet aggregation and prolong bleeding time. This effect should be kept in mind when bleeding times are determined.
The administration of the drug may result in increased urinary values for 17-ketogenic steroids because of an interaction between the drug and/or its metabolites with m-dinitrobenzene used in this assay. Although 17-hydroxy-corticosteroid measurements (Porter-Silber test) do not appear to be artifactually altered, it is suggested that therapy with the drug be temporarily discontinued 72 hours before adrenal function tests are performed.
The drug may interfere with some urinary assays of 5-hydroxy indoleacetic acid (5HIAA).

Carcinogenesis:
A two-year study was performed in rats to evaluate the carcinogenic potential of the drug. No evidence of carcinogenicity was found.

Pregnancy:
Teratogenic Effects: Pregnancy Category B. Reproduction studies have been performed in rats, rabbits and mice at doses up to six times the human dose and have revealed no evidence of impaired fertility or harm to the fetus due to the drug. There are, however, no adequate and well-controlled studies in pregnant women. Because animal reproduction studies are not always predictive of human response, the drug should not be used during pregnancy unless clearly needed. Because of the known effect of drugs of this class on the human fetal cardiovascular system (closure of ductus arteriosus), use during late pregnancy should be avoided.
Non-teratogenic Effects: As with other drugs known to inhibit prostaglandin synthesis, an increased incidence of dystocia and delayed parturition occurred in rats.

Nursing Mothers:
The naproxen anion has been found in the milk of lactating women at a concentration of approximately 1% of that found in the plasma. Because of the possible adverse effects of prostaglandin-inhibiting drugs on neonates, use in nursing mothers should be avoided.

Pediatric Use:
Pediatric indications and dosage recommendations have not been established for NAPROSYN® (naproxen).

ADVERSE REACTIONS

Adverse reactions reported in controlled clinical trials in 960 patients treated for rheumatoid arthritis or osteoarthritis are listed below. In general, these reactions were reported 2 to 10 times more frequently than they were in studies in the 962 patients treated for mild to moderate pain or for dysmenorrhea.

Incidence greater than 1%

Gastrointestinal: The most frequent complaints reported related to the gastrointestinal tract. They were: constipation*, heartburn*, abdominal pain*, nausea*, dyspepsia, diarrhea, stomatitis.
Central Nervous System: Headache*, dizziness*, drowsiness*, lightheadedness, vertigo.
Dermatologic: Itching (pruritus)*, skin eruptions*, ecchymoses*, sweating, purpura.
Special Senses: Tinnitus*, hearing disturbances, visual disturbances.
Cardiovascular: Edema*, dyspnea*, palpitations.
General: Thirst.
* Incidence of reported reactions between 3% and 9%. Those reactions occurring in less than 3% of the patients are unmarked.

Incidence less than 1%

Probable Causal Relationship:
The following adverse reactions were reported less frequently than 1% during controlled clinical trials and through voluntary reports since marketing. The probability of a causal relationship exists between the drug and these adverse reactions:
Gastrointestinal: Abnormal liver function tests, gastrointestinal bleeding and/or perforation, hematemesis, jaundice, melena, peptic ulceration with bleeding and/or perforation, vomiting.
Renal: Glomerular nephritis, hematuria, interstitial nephritis, nephrotic syndrome, renal disease.
Hematologic: Eosinophilia, granulocytopenia, leukopenia, thrombocytopenia.
Central Nervous System: Depression, dream abnormalities, inability to concentrate, insomnia, malaise, myalgia and muscle weakness.
Dermatologic: Alopecia, photosensitive dermatitis, skin rashes.
Special Senses: Hearing impairment.
Cardiovascular: Congestive heart failure.
Respiratory: Eosinophilic pneumonitis.
General: Anaphylactoid reactions, menstrual disorders, pyrexia (chills and fever).

Causal Relationship Unknown:
Other reactions have been reported in circumstances in which a causal relationship could not be established. However, in these rarely reported events, the possibility cannot be excluded. Therefore these observations are being listed to serve as alerting information to the physicians:
Hematologic: Agranulocytosis, aplastic anemia, hemolytic anemia.
Central Nervous System: Cognitive dysfunction.
Dermatologic: Epidermal necrolysis, erythema multiforme, Stevens-Johnson syndrome, urticaria.
Gastrointestinal: Ulcerative stomatitis.
Cardiovascular: Vasculitis.
General: Angioneurotic edema, hyperglycemia, hypoglycemia.

OVERDOSAGE

Significant overdosage may be characterized by drowsiness, heartburn, indigestion, nausea or vomiting. No evidence of toxicity or late sequelae have been reported 5 to 15 months after ingestion for three to seven days of doses up to 3,000 mg of naproxen. One patient ingested a single dose of 25 g of naproxen and experienced mild nausea and indigestion. It is not known what dose of the drug would be life threatening. The oral LD_{50} of the drug is 543 mg/kg in rats, 1234 mg/kg in mice, 4110 mg/kg in hamsters and greater than 1000 mg/kg in dogs.
Should a patient ingest a large number of tablets, accidentally or purposefully, the stomach may be emptied and usual supportive measures employed. Animal studies suggest that the prompt administration of 5 grams of activated charcoal would tend to reduce markedly the absorption of the drug. It is not known if the drug is dialyzable.

DOSAGE AND ADMINISTRATION

For Rheumatoid Arthritis, Osteoarthritis, and Ankylosing Spondylitis:
The recommended starting dose in adults is one 250 mg tablet or one 375 mg tablet twice daily (morning and evening). During long-term administration, the dose may be adjusted up or down depending on the clinical response of the patient. A lower daily dose may suffice for long-term administration. Daily doses higher than 1000 mg in these indications have not been studied. The morning and evening doses do not have to be equal in size and the administration of the drug more frequently than twice daily is not necessary. Symptomatic improvement in arthritis usually begins within two weeks. However, if improvement is not seen within this period, a trial for an additional two weeks should be considered.

For Acute Gout:
The recommended starting dose is 750 mg, followed by 250 mg every eight hours until the attack has subsided.

For Mild to Moderate Pain, Primary Dysmenorrhea and Acute Tendinitis and Bursitis:
The recommended starting dose is 500 mg, followed by 250 mg every 6 to 8 hours, as required. The total daily dose should not exceed 1,250 mg.

HOW SUPPLIED

NAPROSYN (naproxen) is available in scored tablets of 250 mg (yellow) in bottles of 100 tablets (NDC 18393-272-42) (NSN 6505-01-026-9730) and 500 tablets (NDC 18393-272-62) (NSN 6505-01-046-0126) or in cartons of 100 individually blister packed tablets (NDC 18393-272-53) (NSN 6505-01-097-9611) and in 375 mg (peach) tablets in bottles of 100 tablets (NDC 18393-273-42) (NSN 6505-01-135-8462) and 500 tablets (NDC 18393-273-62) (NSN 6505-01-204-5297) or in cartons of 100 individually blister packed tablets (NDC 18393-273-53) (NSN 6505-01-204-5298). The 500 mg (yellow) tablets are available in bottles of 100 tablets (NDC 18393-277-42) (NSN 6505-01-200-2474) and 500 tablets (NDC 18393-277-62). Store at room temperature in well-closed containers; dispense in light-resistant containers.
CAUTION: Federal law prohibits dispensing without prescription.
U.S. Patent Nos. 3,904,682; 3,998,966 and others.
 Revised 11/85
Shown in Product Identification Section, page 432

NASALIDE® ℞
[na 'ză-lide]
(flunisolide)
Nasal Solution
0.025%
For Nasal Use Only

PRODUCT OVERVIEW

KEY FACTS

NASALIDE Nasal Solution, intended for administration as a spray to the nasal mucosa, contains the active ingredient flunisolide, an anti-inflammatory topical steroid. Clinical studies with flunisolide have shown local therapeutic activity on nasal mucous membranes, including reduction of symptoms of stuffy nose, runny nose and sneezing, with minimal evidence of systemic activity at the recommended doses.

MAJOR USES

NASALIDE is indicated for the topical treatment of the symptoms of seasonal or perennial rhinitis when effectiveness of or tolerance to conventional treatment is unsatisfactory. Symptomatic relief is usually seen within a few days after starting NASALIDE, but may not occur in some patients for as long as two weeks.

SAFETY INFORMATION

See complete safety information set forth below.

PRESCRIBING INFORMATION

NASALIDE® ℞
[na 'ză-lide]
(flunisolide)
Nasal Solution
0.025%
For Nasal Use Only

A product of Syntex Laboratories, Inc.

DESCRIPTION

NASALIDE® (flunisolide) nasal solution is intended for administration as a spray to the nasal mucosa. Flunisolide, the active component of NASALIDE nasal solution, is an anti-inflammatory steroid with the chemical name: 6α-fluoro-11β, 16α, 17,21-tetrahydroxypregna-1,4- diene-3,20-dione cyclic 16,17-acetal with acetone (USAN).
Flunisolide is a white to creamy white crystalline powder with a molecular weight of 434.49. It is soluble in acetone, sparingly soluble in chloroform, slightly soluble in methanol, and practically insoluble in water. It has a melting point of about 245°C.
Each 25 ml spray bottle contains flunisolide 6.25 mg (0.25 mg/ml) in a solution of propylene glycol, polyethylene glycol 3350, citric acid, sodium citrate, butylated hydroxyanisole, edetate disodium, benzalkonium chloride, and purified water, with NaOH and/or HCl added to adjust the pH to approximately 5.3. It contains no fluorocarbons.
After priming the delivery system for NASALIDE, each actuation of the unit delivers a metered droplet spray containing approximately 25 mcg of flunisolide. The size of the droplets produced by the unit is in excess of 8 microns to facilitate deposition on the nasal mucosa. The contents of one nasal spray bottle deliver at least 200 sprays.

CLINICAL PHARMACOLOGY

NASALIDE® (flunisolide) has demonstrated potent glucocorticoid and weak mineralocorticoid activity in classical animal test systems. As a glucocorticoid it is several hundred times more potent than the cortisol standard. Clinical studies with flunisolide have shown therapeutic activity on nasal mucous membranes with minimal evidence of systemic activity at the recommended doses.
A study in approximately 100 patients which compared the recommended dose of flunisolide nasal solution with an oral dose providing equivalent systemic amounts of flunisolide has shown that the clinical effectiveness of NASALIDE, whenused topically as recommended, is due to its direct local effect and not to an indirect effect through systemic absorption.
Following administration of flunisolide to man, approximately half of the administered dose is recovered in the urine and half in the stool; 65–70% of the dose recovered in urine is the primary metabolite, which has undergone loss of

Continued on next page

Syntex—Cont.

the 6α fluorine and addition of a 6β hydroxy group. Flunisolide is well absorbed but is rapidly converted by the liver to the much less active primary metabolite and to glucuronate and/or sulfate conjugates. Because of first-pass liver metabolism, only 20% of the flunisolide reaches the systemic circulation when it is given orally whereas 50% of the flunisolide administered intranasally reaches the systemic circulation unmetabolized. The plasma half-life of flunisolide is 1–2 hours.

The effects of flunisolide on hypothalamic-pituitary-adrenal (HPA) axis function have been studied in adult volunteers. NASALIDE was administered intranasally as a spray in total doses over 7 times the recommended dose (2200 mcg, equivalent to 88 sprays/day) in 2 subjects for 4 days, about 3 times the recommended dose (800 mcg, equivalent to 32 sprays/day) in 4 subjects for 4 days, and over twice the recommended dose (700 mcg, equivalent to 28 sprays/day) in 6 subjects for 10 days. Early morning plasma cortisol concentrations and 24-hour urinary 17-ketogenic steroids were measured daily. There was evidence of decreased endogenous cortisol production at all three doses.

In controlled studies, NASALIDE was found to be effective in reducing symptoms of stuffy nose, runny nose and sneezing in most patients. These controlled clinical studies have been conducted in 488 adult patients at doses ranging from 8 to 16 sprays (200–400 mcg) per day and 127 children at doses ranging from 6 to 8 sprays (150–200 mcg) per day for periods as long as 3 months. In 170 patients who had cortisol levels evaluated at baseline and after 3 months or more of flunisolide treatment, there was no unequivocal flunisolide-related depression of plasma cortisol levels.

The mechanisms responsible for the anti-inflammatory action of corticosteroids and for the activity of the aerosolized drug on the nasal mucosa are unknown.

INDICATIONS

NASALIDE® (flunisolide) is indicated for the topical treatment of the symptoms of seasonal or perennial rhinitis when effectiveness of or tolerance to conventional treatment is unsatisfactory.

Clinical studies have shown that improvement is based on a local effect rather than systemic absorption, and is usually apparent within a few days after starting NASALIDE. However, symptomatic relief may not occur in some patients for as long as two weeks. Although systemic effects are minimal at recommended doses, NASALIDE should not be continued beyond 3 weeks in the absence of significant symptomatic improvement.

NASALIDE should not be used in the presence of untreated localized infection involving nasal mucosa.

CONTRAINDICATIONS

Hypersensitivity to any of the ingredients.

WARNINGS

The replacement of a systemic corticosteroid with a topical corticoid can be accompanied by signs of adrenal insufficiency, and in addition some patients may experience symptoms of withdrawal, e.g., joint and/or muscular pain, lassitude and depression. Patients previously treated for prolonged periods with systemic corticosteroids and transferred to NASALIDE® (flunisolide) should be carefully monitored to avoid acute adrenal insufficiency in response to stress.

When transferred to NASALIDE, careful attention must be given to patients previously treated for prolonged periods with systemic corticosteroids. This is particularly important in those patients who have associated asthma or other clinical conditions, where too rapid a decrease in systemic corticosteroids may cause a severe exacerbation of their symptoms.

The use of NASALIDE with alternate-day prednisone systemic treatment could increase the likelihood of HPA suppression compared to a therapeutic dose of either one alone. Therefore, NASALIDE treatment should be used with caution in patients already on alternate-day prednisone regimens for any disease.

PRECAUTIONS

General: In clinical studies with flunisolide administered intranasally, the development of localized infections of the nose and pharynx with *Candida albicans* has occurred only rarely. When such an infection develops it may require treatment with appropriate local therapy or discontinuance of treatment with NASALIDE® (flunisolide).

Flunisolide is absorbed into the circulation. Use of excessive doses of NASALIDE may suppress hypothalamic-pituitary-adrenal function.

Flunisolide should be used with caution, if at all, in patients with active or quiescent tuberculosis infections of the respiratory tract or in untreated fungal, bacterial or systemic viral infections or ocular herpes simplex.

Because of the inhibitory effect of corticosteroids on wound healing, in patients who have experienced recent nasal septal ulcers, recurrent epistaxis, nasal surgery or trauma, a nasal corticosteroid should be used with caution until healing has occurred.

Although systemic effects have been minimal with recommended doses, this potential increases with excessive dosages. Therefore, larger than recommended doses should be avoided.

Information for Patients: Patients should use NASALIDE at regular intervals since its effectiveness depends on its regular use. The patient should take the medication as directed. It is not acutely effective and the prescribed dosage should not be increased. Instead, nasal vasoconstrictors or oral antihistamines may be needed until the effects of NASALIDE are fully manifested. One to two weeks may pass before full relief is obtained. The patient should contact the physician if symptoms do not improve, or if the condition worsens, or if sneezing or nasal irritation occurs.

For the proper use of this unit and to attain maximum improvement, the patient should read and follow the accompanying Patient Instructions carefully.

Carcinogenesis: A 22-month study was conducted in Swiss derived mice to evaluate the carcinogenic potential of the drug. There was an increase in the incidence of pulmonary adenomas within the range of adenomas previously reported in the literature for untreated or control Swiss derived mice. An additional study is being conducted in a species with a lower incidence of spontaneous pulmonary tumors.

Impairment of fertility: Female rats receiving high doses of flunisolide (200 mcg/kg/day) showed some evidence of impaired fertility. Reproductive performance in the low (8 mcg/kg/day) and mid-dose (40 mcg/kg/day) groups was comparable to controls.

Pregnancy: Teratogenic effects: Pregnancy Category C. As with other corticosteroids, flunisolide has been shown to be teratogenic in rabbits and rats at doses of 40 and 200 mcg/kg/day respectively. It was also fetotoxic in these animal reproductive studies. There are no adequate and well-controlled studies in pregnant women. Flunisolide should be used during pregnancy only if the potential benefit justifies the potential risk to the fetus.

Nursing Mothers: It is not known whether this drug is excreted in human milk. Because other corticosteroids are excreted in human milk, caution should be exercised when flunisolide is administered to nursing women.

ADVERSE REACTIONS

Adverse reactions reported in controlled clinical trials and long-term open studies in 595 patients treated with NASALIDE are described below. Of these patients, 409 were treated for 3 months or longer, 323 for 6 months or longer, 259 for 1 year or longer, and 91 for 2 years or longer.

In general, side effects elicited in the clinical studies have been primarily associated with the nasal mucous membranes. The most frequent complaints were those of mild transient nasal burning and stinging, which were reported in approximately 45% of the patients treated with NASALIDE in placebo-controlled and long-term studies. These complaints do not usually interfere with treatment; in only 3% of patients was it necessary to decrease dosage or stop treatment because of these symptoms. Approximately the same incidence of mild transient nasal burning and stinging was reported in patients on placebo as was reported in patients treated with NASALIDE in controlled studies, implying that these complaints may be related to the vehicle or the delivery system. The incidence of complaints of nasal burning and stinging decreased with increasing duration of treatment.

Other side effects reported at a frequency of 5% or less were: nasal congestion, sneezing, epistaxis and/or bloody mucus, nasal irritation, watery eyes, sore throat, nausea and/or vomiting, headaches and loss of sense of smell and taste. In rare instances, nasal septal perforations were observed during the studies but a causal relationship with NASALIDE was not established.

Systemic corticosteroid side effects were not reported during the controlled clinical trials. If recommended doses are exceeded, or if individuals are particularly sensitive, symptoms of hypercorticism, i.e., Cushing's syndrome, could occur.

OVERDOSAGE

I.V. flunisolide in animals at doses up to 4 mg/kg showed no effect. One spray bottle contains 6.25 mg of NASALIDE; therefore acute overdosage is unlikely.

DOSAGE AND ADMINISTRATION

The therapeutic effects of corticosteroids, unlike those of decongestants, are not immediate. This should be explained to the patient in advance in order to ensure cooperation and continuation of treatment with the prescribed dosage regimen. Full therapeutic benefit requires regular use, and is usually evident within a few days. However, a longer period of therapy may be required for some patients to achieve maximum benefit (up to 3 weeks). If no improvement is evident by that time, NASALIDE® (flunisolide) should not be continued.

Patients with blocked nasal passages should be encouraged to use a decongestant just before NASALIDE administration to ensure adequate penetration of the spray. Patients should also be advised to clear their nasal passages of secretions prior to use.

Adults: The recommended starting dose of NASALIDE is 2 sprays (50 mcg) in each nostril 2 times a day (total dose 200 mcg/day). If needed, this dose may be increased to 2 sprays in each nostril 3 times a day (total dose 300 mcg/day).

Children 6 to 14 years: The recommended starting dose of NASALIDE is one spray (25 mcg) in each nostril 3 times a day or two sprays (50 mcg) in each nostril 2 times a day (total dose 150-200 mcg/day). NASALIDE is not recommended for use in children less than 6 years of age as safety and efficacy studies, including possible adverse effects on growth, have not been conducted.

Maximum total daily doses should not exceed 8 sprays in each nostril for adults (total dose 400 mcg/day) and 4 sprays in each nostril for children under 14 years of age (total dose 200 mcg/day). Since there is no evidence that exceeding the maximum recommended dosage is more effective and increased systemic absorption would occur, higher doses should be avoided.

After the desired clinical effect is obtained, the maintenance dose should be reduced to the smallest amount necessary to control the symptoms. Approximately 15% of patients with perennial rhinitis may be maintained on as little as 1 spray in each nostril per day.

HOW SUPPLIED

Each 25 ml NASALIDE® (flunisolide) nasal solution spray bottle (NDC 0033-2906-40) (NSN 6505-01-132-9979) contains 6.25 mg (0.25 mg/ml) of flunisolide and is supplied with a nasal pump unit with dust cover and a patient leaflet of instructions.

Store at controlled room temperature, 15°–30°C (59°–86°F)

Revised 1/86

NORINYL® 1+35 Tablets ℞
(norethindrone and ethinyl estradiol tablets)
NORINYL® 1+50 Tablets ℞
(norethindrone and mestranol tablets)
NORINYL® 1+80 Tablets ℞
(norethindrone and mestranol tablets)
NORINYL® 2 mg. Tablets
(norethindrone and mestranol tablets)

Refer to entry under BREVICON® Tablets (norethindrone and ethinyl estradiol tablets).

Shown in Product Identification Section, page 432, 433

NOR-Q.D.® ℞
(norethindrone)
Tablets 0.35 mg.

Refer to entry under BREVICON® Tablets (norethindrone and ethinyl estradiol).

SYNACORT® ℞
(hydrocortisone)
Cream 1%
Cream 2.5%
SYNALAR® ℞
(fluocinolone acetonide)
Cream 0.025%
Cream 0.01%
Ointment 0.025%
Topical Solution 0.01%
SYNALAR-HP® ℞
(fluocinolone acetonide)
Cream 0.2%
SYNEMOL® ℞
(fluocinolone acetonide)
Cream 0.025%

Refer to entry under LIDEX® (fluocinonide) Cream 0.05%.

TAP Pharmaceuticals
NORTH CHICAGO, IL 60064

LUPRON® INJECTION ℞
[lu'pron]
leuprolide acetate

DESCRIPTION
LUPRON (leuprolide acetate) is a synthetic nonapeptide analog of naturally occurring gonadotropin releasing hormone (GnRH or LH-RH). The analog possesses greater potency than the natural hormone. The chemical name is 5-Oxo-L-prolyl-L-histidyl-L-tryptophyl-L-seryl-L-tyrosyl-D-leucyl-L-leucyl-L-arginyl-N-ethyl-L-prolinamide acetate (salt).
LUPRON is a sterile, aqueous solution intended for subcutaneous injection. It is available in a 2.8 ml multiple-dose vial containing 5 mg/ml of leuprolide acetate, sodium chloride for tonicity adjustment, 9 mg/ml of benzyl alcohol as a preservative and water for injection. The pH may have been adjusted with sodium hydroxide and/or acetic acid.

CLINICAL PHARMACOLOGY
Leuprolide acetate, an LH-RH agonist, acts as a potent inhibitor of gonadotropin secretion when given continuously and in therapeutic doses. Animal and human studies indicate that following an initial stimulation, chronic administration of leuprolide acetate results in suppression of ovarian and testicular steroidogenesis. This effect is reversible upon discontinuation of drug therapy. Administration of leuprolide acetate has resulted in inhibition of the growth of certain hormone dependent tumors (prostatic tumors in Noble and Dunning male rats and DMBA-induced mammary tumors in female rats) as well as atrophy of the reproductive organs.
In humans, subcutaneous administration of single daily doses of leuprolide acetate results in an initial increase in circulating levels of luteinizing hormone (LH) and follicle stimulating hormone (FSH), leading to a transient increase in levels of the gonadal steroids (testosterone and dihydrotestosterone in males, and estrone and estradiol in premenopausal females). However, continuous daily administration of leuprolide acetate results in decreased levels of LH and FSH in all patients. In males, testosterone is reduced to castrate levels. In pre-menopausal females, estrogens are reduced to post-menopausal levels. These decreases occur within two to four weeks after initiation of treatment, and castrate levels of testosterone in prostatic cancer patients have been demonstrated for periods of up to three years.
Leuprolide acetate is not active when given orally. Bioavailability by subcutaneous administration is comparable to that by intravenous administration. Leuprolide acetate has a plasma half-life of approximately three hours. The metabolism, distribution and excretion of leuprolide acetate in man have not been determined.

INDICATIONS AND USAGE
LUPRON is indicated in the palliative treatment of advanced prostatic cancer. It offers an alternative treatment of prostatic cancer when orchiectomy or estrogen administration are either not indicated or unacceptable to the patient.
In a controlled study comparing LUPRON 1 mg/day given subcutaneously to DES (diethylstilbestrol), 3 mg/day, the survival rate for the two groups was comparable after two years treatment. The objective response to treatment was also similar for the two groups.

CONTRAINDICATIONS
There are no known contraindications to the use of LUPRON.

WARNINGS
Isolated cases of worsening of signs and symptoms during the first few weeks of treatment have been reported. There is a report with another LH-RH analog where such worsening may have contributed to a rapid fatal outcome in two cases.

PRECAUTIONS
Patients with metastatic vertebral lesions and/or with urinary tract obstruction should be closely observed during the first few weeks of therapy (see "ADVERSE REACTIONS" section).
Patients with known allergies to benzyl alcohol, an ingredient of the drug's vehicle, may present symptoms of hypersensitivity, usually local, in the form of erythema and induration at the injection site.
Information for Patients: See Information for Patients which appears after the "HOW SUPPLIED" section.
Laboratory Tests: Response to leuprolide acetate should be monitored by measuring serum levels of testosterone and acid phosphatase. In the majority of patients, testosterone levels increased above baseline during the first week, declining thereafter to baseline levels or below by the end of the second week of treatment. Castrate levels were reached within two to four weeks and once attained were maintained for as long as drug administration continued. Transient increases in acid phosphatase levels occurred sometimes early in treatment. However, by the fourth week, the elevated levels usually decreased to values at or near baseline.
Drug Interactions: None have been reported.
Carcinogenesis, Mutagenesis, Impairment of Fertility: Two-year carcinogenicity studies were conducted in rats and mice. In rats, a dose-related increase of benign pituitary hyperplasia and benign pituitary adenomas was noted at 24 months when the drug was administered subcutaneously at high daily doses (0.6 to 4 mg/kg). In mice no pituitary abnormalities were observed at a dose as high as 60 mg/kg for two years. Patients have been treated with leuprolide acetate for up to three years with doses as high as 10 mg/day and for two years with doses as high as 20 mg/day without demonstrable pituitary abnormalities.
Mutagenicity studies have been performed with leuprolide acetate using bacterial and mammalian systems. These studies provided no evidence of a mutagenic potential.
Clinical and pharmacologic studies with analogs similar to leuprolide acetate have shown full reversibility of fertility suppression when the drug is discontinued after continuous administration for periods of up to 20 weeks. However, no clinical studies have been conducted with leuprolide acetate to assess the reversibility of fertility suppression.

ADVERSE REACTIONS
In the majority of patients testosterone levels increased above baseline during the first week, declining thereafter to baseline levels or below by the end of the second week of treatment. This transient increase was occasionally associated with a temporary worsening of signs and symptoms, usually manifested by an increase in bone pain (See "WARNINGS" section). In a few cases a temporary worsening of existing hematuria and urinary tract obstruction occurred during the first week. Temporary weakness and paresthesia of the lower limbs have been reported in a few cases.
Potential exacerbations of signs and symptoms during the first few weeks of treatment is a concern in patients with vertebral metastases and/or urinary obstruction which, if aggravated, may lead to neurological problems or increase the obstruction.
In a comparative trial of LUPRON (leuprolide acetate) versus DES, the following adverse reactions were reported in 3% or more of the patients:

	LUPRON (N = 98)	DES (N = 101)
	Number of Reports	
Cardiovascular		
Congestive Heart Failure	1	3
Edema (peripheral)	8	23
Thrombophlebitis/Phlebitis/ Pulmonary Emboli	1	7
Central Nervous System		
Anxiety	0	3
Dizziness	6	4
Pain	5	3
Headache	5	2
Paresthesia	3	0
Endocrine		
Gynecomastia/Breast Tenderness	3	49
Hot Flashes	51	11
Impotence	2	11
Gastrointestinal		
Anorexia	2	3
Constipation	3	1
Nausea/Vomiting	5	16
Musculoskeletal		
Bone Pain	3	1
Muscle Spasms	0	3

The following additional adverse reactions were reported in less than 3% of the patients in this study: *Cardiovascular*—cardiac arrhythmias, myocardial infarction; *Gastrointestinal*—gastrointestinal bleeding; *Hemic/Lymphatic*—decreased hematocrit and hemoglobin; *Integumentary*—erythema and ecchymosis at the injection site, rash, hair loss, itching; *Miscellaneous*—asthenia, increased BUN and creatinine, fatigue, fever, facial swelling; *Musculoskeletal*—myalgia; *Nervous System*—blurred vision, lethargy, insomnia, memory disorder, sour taste, numbness; *Respiratory*—difficulty breathing, pleural rub, worsening of pulmonary fibrosis; *Urogenital*—hematuria, decrease in testes size (probably due to the physiological/pharmacological action of the drug).

OVERDOSAGE
In rats subcutaneous administration of 250 to 500 times the recommended human dose, expressed on a per body weight basis, resulted in dyspnea, decreased activity, and local irritation at the injection site. There is no evidence at present that there is a clinical counterpart of this phenomenon. In early clinical trials with leuprolide acetate doses as high as 20 mg/day for up to two years caused no adverse effects differing from those observed with the 1 mg/day dose.

DOSAGE AND ADMINISTRATION
The recommended dose is 1 mg (0.2 ml) administered as a single daily subcutaneous injection. As with other drugs administered chronically by subcutaneous injection, the injection site should be varied periodically.
NOTE: As with all parenteral products, inspect container's solution for discoloration and particulate matter before each use.

HOW SUPPLIED
LUPRON (leuprolide acetate) is a sterile solution supplied in a 2.8 ml multiple-dose vial, NDC 0300-3626-28. Refrigerate until dispensed. Patient may store unrefrigerated below 86°F. Avoid freezing. Protect from light—store vial in carton until use.
Each 0.2 ml contains 1 mg of leuprolide acetate, sodium chloride for tonicity adjustment, 1.8 mg of benzyl alcohol as preservative and water for injection. The pH may have been adjusted with sodium hydroxide and/or acetic acid.

CAUTION
Federal (U.S.A.) law prohibits dispensing without a prescription.
Revised: Sept., 1985.
U.S. Patent Nos. 4,005,063 and 4,005,194.

INFORMATION FOR PATIENTS
NOTE: Be sure to consult your physician with any questions you may have or for information about LUPRON and its use.
What Is Cancer? Cancer is a disease characterized by uncontrolled growth and spread of abnormal body cells. Normally, the cells that make up all parts of the body reproduce themselves in an orderly manner so that growth occurs, worn out tissues are replaced and injuries repaired. Occasionally, certain cells grow into a mass of tissue called a tumor. Some tumors are benign; others are malignant, or cancerous.
Benign tumors may interfere with body function and may require surgical treatment but they do not invade neighboring tissue and seldom threaten life. However, malignant tumors invade and destroy normal tissue. By a process called metastasis, cells break away from a malignant tumor and spread through the blood and lymphatic systems to other parts of the body where they form new tumors. Sometimes cancer grows and spreads rapidly; sometimes the process takes years.
One very common place for cancer to develop in men is the prostate gland.
What Is The Prostate? The prostate is a male sex gland about the size of a chestnut. It lies just below the urinary bladder and surrounds the first inch of the urethra, the canal that carries urine from the bladder during urination. The secretion of the prostate provides part of the fluid for ejaculation.
Treatment Of Prostatic Cancer: Your doctor has a choice of treatments for prostatic cancer including surgery, radiation and drugs. The best choice for a particular patient usually depends on whether the cancer was found early or in an advanced stage.
The growth and function of the normal prostate gland is dependent upon the male hormone testosterone. If you have a prostatic tumor, its growth is usually stimulated by testosterone as well. For this reason, decreasing the body's supply of testosterone often controls tumor growth and relieves pain and difficulty in urinating.
The primary source of testosterone is the testes; therefore, one way to reduce production of testosterone is to remove the testes by surgery.
Another way is for men to take a female hormone, estrogen. This also causes the body to stop making testosterone. Estrogens have potential side effects such as swelling of the breasts, fluid retention, blood clotting problems, and decrease in libido and impotence.
Another choice is LUPRON (leuprolide acetate) which will also decrease testosterone production. LUPRON has potential side effects, such as hot flashes and decrease in libido and impotence. It may also initially aggravate signs and symptoms of your disease by temporary stimulation of the tumor during the first one to two weeks of treatment.
What Is LUPRON? LUPRON is chemically similar to gonadotropin releasing hormone (GnRH or LH-RH), a hormone which occurs naturally in your body.
Normally, your body releases small amounts of LH-RH, and this leads to events which stimulate the production of testosterone.
However, when you inject LUPRON, the normal events that lead to testosterone production are interrupted and testosterone is no longer produced by the testes.
LUPRON must be injected because, like insulin which is injected by diabetics, LUPRON is inactive when taken by mouth.
If you were to discontinue the drug for any reason, your body would begin making testosterone again.

Continued on next page

TAP Pharmaceuticals—Cont.

Directions For Using LUPRON:

1. Wash hands thoroughly with soap and water.
2. If using a new bottle for the first time, flip off the plastic cover to expose the gray rubber stopper. Wipe metal ring and rubber stopper with an alcohol wipe each time you use LUPRON. Check the liquid in the container. If it is not clear or has particles in it, DO NOT USE IT. Exchange it at your pharmacy for another container.
3. Remove outer wrapping from one syringe. Pull plunger back until the tip of the plunger is at the .2 mark.
4. Take cover off needle and push the cover into the appropriate hole in the Daily Dose Reminder area. Push the needle through the center of the rubber stopper on the LUPRON bottle.
5. Push the plunger all the way in to inject air into the bottle.
6. Keep the needle in the bottle and turn the bottle upside down. Check to make sure the tip of the needle is in the liquid. Slowly pull back on the plunger, until the syringe fills to the .2 mark.
7. Toward the end of a two-week period, the amount of LUPRON left in the bottle will be small. Take special care to hold the bottle straight and to keep the needle tip in liquid while pulling back on the plunger.
8. Keeping the needle in the bottle and the bottle upside down, check for air bubbles in the syringe. If you see any, push the plunger *slowly* in to push the air bubble back into the bottle. Keep the tip of the needle in the liquid and pull the plunger back again to fill to the .2 mark.
9. Do this again if necessary to eliminate air bubbles. Remove needle from bottle and lay syringe down on the syringe rest. DO NOT TOUCH THE NEEDLE OR ALLOW THE NEEDLE TO TOUCH ANY SURFACE.
10. To protect your skin, inject each daily dose at a different body spot.
11. Choose an injection spot. Cleanse the injection spot with another alcohol wipe.
12. Hold the syringe in one hand. Hold the skin taut, or pull up a little flesh with the other hand, as you were instructed.
13. Hold the syringe alongside the skin and slide the needle quickly just under the skin as far as it will go. Inject the drug by pushing in the plunger as far as it will go.
14. Hold an alcohol wipe down on your skin where the needle is inserted and withdraw the needle at the same angle it was inserted.
15. Use the disposable syringe only once and dispose of it properly as you were instructed. A waste area is provided in the LUPRON Patient Administration Kit. Needles thrown into a garbage bag could accidentally stick someone. NEVER LEAVE SYRINGES, NEEDLES OR DRUGS WHERE CHILDREN CAN REACH THEM.

Some Special Advice

- You may experience hot flashes when using LUPRON. During the first few weeks of treatment you may experience increased bone pain, increased difficulty in urinating, and less commonly but most importantly, you may experience the onset or aggravation of nerve symptoms. In any of these events, discuss the symptoms with your doctor.
- You may experience some irritation at the injection site, such as burning, itching or swelling. These reactions are usually mild and go away. If they do not, tell your doctor.
- Do not stop taking your injections because you feel better. You need an injection every day to make sure LUPRON (leuprolide acetate) keeps working for you.
- Use only the syringes provided in the kit, as other types may dispense an incorrect dose. If for any reason you cannot use one of the syringes, contact your doctor or pharmacist for advice.
- When the drug level gets low, take special care to hold the bottle straight up and down and to keep the needle tip in liquid while pulling back on the plunger.
- Do not try to get every last drop out of the bottle. This will increase the possibility of drawing air into the syringe and getting an incomplete dose. Some extra drug has been provided so that you can withdraw the recommended number of doses.
- Tell your pharmacist when you will need your next LUPRON kit so it will be at the pharmacy when you need it.
- This drug may be stored at room temperature (not above 86°F). Do not store near a radiator or other very warm place.
- Do not leave your drug or hypodermic syringes where anyone can pick them up.
- Keep this and all other medications out of reach of children.

Manufactured for TAP Pharmaceuticals
North Chicago, IL 60064, U.S.A.
by Abbott Laboratories
North Chicago, IL 60064

EDUCATIONAL MATERIAL

All Free to the medical profession
Product Monograph—"Introduction to Lupron® (leuprolide acetate) Injection".
"Information for Pharmacists" brochure will help pharmacists reinforce physician instruction, answer patients' questions, offer support and encourage compliance.
"Information for Patient Instruction" brochure will help professionals answer patients' questions about Lupron and teach the technique of self-injection.

Thompson Medical Company, Inc.

919 THIRD AVENUE
NEW YORK, NY 10022

MAXIMUM STRENGTH APPEDRINE® Tablets — OTC

[*ăpp-ĕ-drine*]
Anorectic for Weight Control

Each tablet contains:	
phenylpropanolamine HCl (immediate release)	25 mg
Each three tablets contain:	
Vitamin A	5000 IU
Vitamin D	400 IU
Vitamin E	30 IU
Vitamin C (Ascorbic Acid)	60 mg
Folic Acid	0.4 mg
Vitamin B_1 (Thiamine HCl)	1.5 mg
Vitamin B_2 (Riboflavin)	1.7 mg
Niacinamide	20 mg
Vitamin B_6 (Pyridoxine HCl)	2 mg
Vitamin B_{12} (Cyanocobalamin)	6 mcg
d-Calcium Pantothenate	10 mg
Iodine (as Potassium Iodide)	150 mcg
Iron (as Ferrous Sulfate)	12 mg
Copper (as Cupric Sulfate)	2 mg
Zinc (as Zinc Oxide)	15 mg

DESCRIPTION
Each tablet contains phenylpropanolamine HCl, an anorexiant and is fortified with 15 essential vitamins and minerals.

INDICATIONS
Maximum Strength APPEDRINE is indicated as adjunctive therapy in a regimen of weight reduction and control based on caloric restriction in the management of simple exogenous obesity.

CAUTION
READ BEFORE USING. For adult use only. Do not give this product to children under 12 years of age. Persons between the age of 12 and 18 or over 60 are advised to consult their doctor or pharmacist before using this or any drug. As with this or any drug, unwanted symptoms such as headaches, nervousness, rapid pulse, dizziness, sleeplessness, palpitations or other symptoms have occasionally been reported. Should any occur, discontinue use and consult your doctor.

WARNING
DO NOT EXCEED RECOMMENDED DOSAGE. Taking more of this or any other drug than is recommended can cause untoward health complications. It is sensible to check your blood pressure regularly. Do not use if you have high blood pressure, diabetes, heart, thyroid, kidney, or other disease or are being treated for high blood pressure or depression except under the advice and supervision of a doctor. As with any drug if you are pregnant or nursing a baby, seek the advice of a health professional before using this product. Do not use continuously for more than three months. When you have attained your desired weight loss or are able to control your appetite by yourself, use Appedrine only as needed.

DRUG INTERACTION PRECAUTION
Do not take if you are presently taking another medication containing phenylpropanolamine, or any type of nasal decongestant, or a prescription drug for high blood pressure or depression, or any other type of prescription medication except under the advice and supervision of a doctor.
KEEP THIS AND ALL MEDICATION OUT OF THE REACH OF CHILDREN. In case of accidental overdose seek professional assistance or contact a poison control center immediately.

ADVERSE REACTIONS
Side effects are rare when taken as directed. Nausea or nasal dryness may occasionally occur.

DOSAGE AND ADMINISTRATION
Adults: One tablet 30–60 minutes before each meal three times a day with one or two full glasses of water. Do not exceed 3 tablets in 24 hours.

HOW SUPPLIED
Maximum Strength APPEDRINE® packages of 30 and 60 tablets packaged with 1250 Calorie Maximum Strength Appedrine Diet Plan.

Reference: Griboff, Solomon, I., M.D., F.A.C.P. et al., A Double-Blind Clinical Evaluation of a Phenylpropanolamine-Caffeine Combination and a Placebo in the Treatment of Exogenous Obesity, Current Therapeutic Research 17, 6:535, (1975) June.
Silverman, H.I., D.Sc., Kreger, B.E., M.D., Lewis, G.P., M.D., et. al., Lack of Side Effects from Orally Administered Phenylpropanolamine and Phenylpropanolamine with Caffeine: A Controlled Three-Phase Study, Current Therapeutic Research 28, 2:185 (1980) August.
Altschuler, S., Conte, A., Sebok, M., Marlin, R., Winick, C., Three Controlled Trials of Weight Loss with Phenylpropanolamine, International Journal of Obesity (1982) 6, 549–556.

ASPERCREME®

[*ăs-per-crēme*]
External Analgesic Rub

DESCRIPTION
10% Trolamine Salicylate in a lotion and odorless creme. ASPERCREME is a rub that relieves pain effectively without stomach upset aspirin may cause.

OTHER INGREDIENTS
Lotion: Cetyl Alcohol, Fragrance, Glyceryl Stearate, Isopropyl Palmitate, Lanolin, Methylparaben, Potassium Phosphate, Propylene Glycol, Propylparaben, Sodium Lauryl Sulfate, Stearic Acid, Water.
Cream: Cetyl Alcohol, Glycerin, Methylparaben, Mineral Oil, Propylparaben, Stearic Acid, Water. May also Contain: Potassium Phosphate, Sodium Lauryl Sulfate.

ACTIONS
External analgesic with rapid penetration and absorption.

INDICATIONS
Salicylate analgesic for temporary relief of minor aches and pains of muscles and joints associated with arthritis, simple backaches, strains and sprains.

CONTRAINDICATIONS
Do not use in patients allergic to salicylates.

WARNINGS
Use only as directed. If prone to allergic reaction from aspirin or salicylate, consult your doctor before using. If redness or condition worsens or if pain persists for more than 7 days or clears up and occurs again within a few days, discontinue use and consult a doctor. Do not use on children under 10 years of age. Do not apply if skin is irritated or if irritation develops. Avoid getting into eyes or mucous membranes. As with any drug, if you are pregnant or nursing a baby, seek the advice of a health professional before using this product. For external use only. Avoid contact with eyes. Keep this and all medicines out of the reach of children. Protect from freezing and temperatures above 100°F. Close cap tightly after use.

PRECAUTIONS
Occasionally where this product has been used extensively, moderate peeling of the skin may occur. This is a normal reaction to salicylates on the skin, and should not warrant discontinuing use of the product.

DOSAGE AND ADMINISTRATION
Apply generously. Massage into painful area until thoroughly absorbed into skin, 3 or 4 times daily, especially before retiring.

HOW SUPPLIED
Lotion; 6 oz. plastic bottle. Cream; 1¼oz, 3 oz and 5 oz plastic tubes.

REFERENCES

Golden, Emanuel L., M.D., A Double-Blind Comparison of Orally Ingested Aspirin and a Topically Applied Salicylate Cream in the Relief of Rheumatic Pain, Current Therapeutic Research, Sept. 1978; 24(5):524.
Rabinowitz, J. L., Ph.D., "Comparative Tissue Absorption of Oral 14C Aspirin and Topical Triethanolamine 14C-Salicylate in Human and Canine Knee Joints," Journal of Clinical Pharmacology 1982, 22:42–48.
Rabinowitz, J. L., Ph.D., "Absorption of Labeled Triethanolamine Salicylate in Human and Canine Knee Joints. II," Journal of Clinical Pharmacology 1984; 24:537–539.

Politino, V., Ph.D., et al, "A Clinical Study of Topical 10% Trolamine Salicylate for Relief of Delayed-Onset Exercise-Induced Arthralgia/Myalgia," Current Therapeutic Research, August 1985; 38(2):321.
Shamszad, M., M.D. et al, "Two Double-Blind Comparisons of a Topically Applied Salicylate Cream and Orally Ingested Aspirin in the Relief of Chronic Musculoskeletal Pain," Current Therapeutic Research, April 1986; 39(4):470.

CONTROL Capsules OTC
Maximum Strength
Prolonged action anorectic for weight control containing
phenylpropanolamine HCl 75 mg

DESCRIPTION
Phenylpropanolamine HCl is a sympathomimetic with anorectic action.

INDICATION
CONTROL is indicated as adjunctive therapy in a regimen of weight reduction based on caloric restriction in the management and control of simple exogenous obesity.

CAUTION
READ BEFORE USING. For adult use only. Do not give this product to children under 12 years of age. Persons between the age of 12 and 18 or over 60 are advised to consult their doctor or pharmacist before using this or any drug. As with this or any drug, unwanted symptoms such as headaches, nervousness, rapid pulse, dizziness, sleeplessness, palpitations or other symptoms have occasionally been reported. Should any occur, discontinue use and consult your doctor.

WARNING
DO NOT EXCEED RECOMMENDED DOSAGE. Taking more of this or any other drug than is recommended can cause untoward health complications. It is sensible to check your blood pressure regularly. Do not use if you have high blood pressure, diabetes, heart, thyroid, kidney, or other disease or are being treated for high blood pressure or depression except under the advice and supervision of a doctor. As with any drug if you are pregnant or nursing a baby, seek the advice of a health professional before using this product. Do not use continuously for more than three months. When you have attained your desired weight loss or are able to control your appetite by yourself, use Control only as needed.

DRUG INTERACTION PRECAUTION
Do not take if you are presently taking another medication containing phenylpropanolamine, or any type of nasal decongestant, or a prescription drug for high blood pressure or depression, or any other type of prescription medication except under the advice and supervision of a doctor.
KEEP THIS AND ALL MEDICATION OUT OF THE REACH OF CHILDREN. In case of accidental overdose seek professional assistance or contact a poison control center immediately.

ADVERSE REACTIONS
Side effects are rare when taken as directed. Nausea or nasal dryness may occasionally occur.

DOSAGE AND ADMINISTRATION
One capsule with a full glass of water once a day at midmorning.

HOW SUPPLIED
CONTROL Capsules—Packages of 14, 28 and 56 capsules, packaged with 1250 Calorie CONTROL Diet Plan.

Reference: Griboff, Solomon, I., M.D., F.A.C.P. et al., A Double-Blind Clinical Evaluation of a Phenylpropanolamine-Caffeine Combination and a Placebo in the Treatment of Exogenous Obesity, Current Therapeutic Research 17, 6:535, (1975) June.
Silverman, H.I., D.Sc., Kreger, B.E., M.D., Lewis, G.P., M.D., et. al., Lack of Side Effects from Orally Administered Phenylpropanolamine and Phenylpropanolamine with Caffeine: A Controlled Three-Phase Study, Current Therapeutic Research 28, 2:185 (1980) August.
Altschuler, S., Conte, A., Sebok, M., Marlin, R., Winick, C., Three Controlled Trials of Weight Loss with Phenylpropanolamine, International Journal of Obesity (1982), 6, 549–556.

DEXATRIM® Capsules OTC
[dĕx-a-trĭm]
Prolonged action anorectic for weight control contains
phenylpropanolamine HCl 50 mg

DEXATRIM® Extra Strength OTC
Plus Vitamin C Capsules
phenylpropanolamine HCl 75 mg
Vitamin C 180 mg

Caffeine-Free DEXATRIM® OTC
Extra Strength Capsules
phenylpropanolamine HCl 75 mg

DEXATRIM® Extra Strength OTC
Plus Vitamins Capsules
phenylpropanolamine HCl 75 mg
Multi-vitamins

DEXATRIM® Maximum Strength OTC
Plus Vitamin C Caplets
phenylpropanolamine HCl 75 mg
Vitamin C 180 mg

Caffeine-Free DEXATRIM® OTC
Maximum Strength Caplets
phenylpropanolamine HCl 75 mg

DEXATRIM® Maximum Strength OTC
Pre-Meal Caplets (immediate release)
phenylpropanolamine HCl 25 mg

DESCRIPTION
Phenylpropanolamine hydrochloride is a sympathomimetic with anorectic action.

INDICATION
DEXATRIM is indicated as adjunctive therapy in a regimen of weight reduction based on caloric restriction in the management and control of simple exogenous obesity.
In a six week double-blind parallel study comparing phenylpropanolamine HCl to diethylpropion similar weight losses occurred in 62 clinically obese patients. Ninety-six percent of the patients receiving phenylpropanolamine HCl and 87% of the patients receiving diethylpropion lost weight.*

CAUTION
READ BEFORE USING. For adult use only. Do not give this product to children under 12 years of age. Persons between the age of 12 and 18 or over 60 are advised to consult their doctor or pharmacist before using this or any drug. As with this or any drug, unwanted symptoms such as headaches, nervousness, rapid pulse, dizziness, sleeplessness, palpitations or other symptoms have occasionally been reported. Should any occur, discontinue use and consult your doctor.

WARNING
DO NOT EXCEED RECOMMENDED DOSAGE. Taking more of this or any other drug than is recommended can cause untoward health complications. It is sensible to check your blood pressure regularly. Do not use if you have high blood pressure, diabetes, heart, thyroid, kidney, or other disease or are being treated for high blood pressure or depression except under the advice and supervision of a doctor. As with any drug if you are pregnant or nursing a baby, seek the advice of a health professional before using this product. Do not use continuously for more than three months. When you have attained your desired weight loss or are able to control your appetite by yourself, use DEXATRIM only as needed.

DRUG INTERACTION PRECAUTION
Do not take if you are presently taking another medication containing phenylpropanolamine, or any type of nasal decongestant, or a prescription drug for high blood pressure or depression, or any other type of prescription medication except under the advice and supervision of a doctor.
KEEP THIS AND ALL MEDICATION OUT OF THE REACH OF CHILDREN. In case of accidental overdose seek professional assistance or contact a poison control center immediately.

ADVERSE REACTIONS
Side effects are rare when taken as directed. Nasal dryness may occasionally occur.

DOSAGE AND ADMINISTRATION
DEXATRIM®, DEXATRIM Extra-Strength Plus Vitamin C, Caffeine-Free DEXATRIM Extra-Strength, DEXATRIM Extra Strength Plus Vitamins Capsules; DEXATRIM Maximum Strength Plus Vitamin C, Caffeine-Free DEXATRIM Maximum Strength Caplets: One capsule or caplet at midmorning (10 AM) with a full glass of water.
DEXATRIM Maximum Strength Pre-Meal Caplets: One caplet 30 minutes before each meal with one or two full glasses of water.

HOW SUPPLIED
DEXATRIM® Capsules: Packages of 28 or 56 with 1250 calorie DEXATRIM Diet Plan.
DEXATRIM® Extra Strength Plus Vitamin C Capsules: Packages of 10, 20, and 40 with 1250 calorie DEXATRIM Diet Plan.
Caffeine-Free DEXATRIM® Extra Strength Capsules: Packages of 10, 20, and 40 with 1250 calorie DEXATRIM Diet Plan.
DEXATRIM Extra Strength Plus Vitamins Capsules: Packages of 16 and 32 with 1250 calorie DEXATRIM Diet Plan.
DEXATRIM® Maximum Strength Plus Vitamin C Caplets: Packages of 20, and 40 with 1250 calorie DEXATRIM Diet Plan.
Caffeine-Free DEXATRIM® Maximum Strength Caplets: Packages of 20, and 40 with 1250 calorie DEXATRIM Diet Plan.
DEXATRIM Maximum Strength Pre-Meal Caplets: Packages of 30, and 60 with 1250 calorie DEXATRIM Diet Plan.

* Report on file, Professional Services, Thompson Medical Company, Inc. 919 Third Avenue, New York, New York 10022.

References: Griboff, Solomon, I., M.D., F.A.C.P. et. al., A Double-Blind Clinical Evaluation of a Phenylpropanolamine-Caffeine Combination and a Placebo in the Treatment of Exogenous Obesity, Current Therapeutic Research 17, 6:535, (1975) June.
Silverman, H.I., D.Sc., Kreger, B.E., M.D., Lewis, G.P., M.D., et. al., Lack of Side Effects from Orally Administered Phenylpropanolamine and Phenylpropanolamine with Caffeine: A Controlled Three-Phase Study, Current Therapeutic Research 28, 2:185 (1980) August.
Altschuler, S., Conte, A., Sebok, M., Marlin, R., Winick, C., Three Controlled Trials of Weight Loss with Phenylpropanolamine, International Journal of Obesity (1982) 6, 549–556.

Maximum Strength OTC
PROLAMINE™ Capsules
[prō-la-mine]
Continous Action Anorectic for Weight Control

Each capsule contains:
phenylpropanolamine HCl $37\frac{1}{2}$ mg

DESCRIPTION
Each capsule contains phenylpropanolamine hydrochloride an anorexiant.

INDICATION
Maximum Strength PROLAMINE is indicated as adjunctive therapy in the regimen of weight reduction based on caloric restriction in the management and control of simple exogenous obesity.

CAUTION
READ BEFORE USING. For adult use only. Do not give this product to children under 12 years of age. Persons between the age of 12 and 18 or over 60 are advised to consult their doctor or pharmacist before using this or any drug. As with this or any drug, unwanted symptoms such as headaches, nervousness, rapid pulse, dizziness, sleeplessness, palpitations or other symptoms have occasionally been reported. Should any occur, discontinue use and consult your doctor.

WARNING
DO NOT EXCEED RECOMMENDED DOSAGE. Taking more of this or any other drug than is recommended can cause untoward health complications. It is sensible to check your blood pressure regularly. Do not use if you have high blood pressure, diabetes, heart, thyroid, kidney, or other disease or are being treated for high blood pressure or depression except under the advice and supervision of a doctor. As with any drug if you are pregnant or nursing a baby, seek the advice of a health professional before using this product. Do not use continuously for more than three months. When you have attained your desired weight loss or are able to control your appetite by yourself, use Prolamine only as needed.

DRUG INTERACTION PRECAUTION
Do not take if you are presently taking another medication containing phenylpropanolamine, or any type of nasal decongestant, or a prescription drug for high blood pressure or depression, or any other type of prescription medication except under the advice and supervision of a doctor.
KEEP THIS AND ALL MEDICATION OUT OF THE REACH OF CHILDREN. In case of accidental overdose seek professional assistance or contact a poison control center immediately.

ADVERSE REACTIONS
Side effects are rare when taken as directed. Nausea and nasal dryness may occasionally occur.

DOSAGE AND ADMINISTRATION
One capsule with a full glass of water. at 10 A.M. and 1 capsule at 4 P.M. Do not exceed 2 capsules in 24 hours.

HOW SUPPLIED
Maximum Strength PROLAMINE™ Capsules: Packages of 20 and 50 packaged with 1250 Calorie PROLAMINE Diet Plan.

Reference: Griboff, Solomon, I., M.D., F.A.C.P. et. al., A Double-Blind Clinical Evaluation of a Phenylpropanolamine-Caffeine Combination and a Placebo in the Treatment of Exogenous Obesity, Current Therapeutic Research 17, 6:535, (1975) June.
Silverman, H.I., D.Sc., Kreger, B.E., M.D., Lewis, G.P., M.D., et. al., Lack of Side Effects from Orally Administered Phenylpropanolamine and Phenylpropanolamine with Caffeine:

Continued on next page

Thompson—Cont.

A Controlled Three-Phase Study, Current Therapeutic Research 28, 2:185 (1980) August.
Altschuler, S., Conte, A., Sebok, M., Marlin, R., Winick, C., Three Controlled Trials of Weight Loss with Phenylpropanolamine, International Journal of Obesity (1982) 6, 549–556.

Trimen Laboratories, Inc.

Pharmaceutical Division
80 TWENTY-SIXTH STREET
PITTSBURGH, PA 15222

AMACODONE™ TABLETS Ⓒ III
Acetaminophen/Hydrocodone

Each tablet contains:
Acetaminophen ....500 mg
Hydrocodone Bitartrate* ....5 mg
*(WARNING: May be habit forming)

HOW SUPPLIED
Bottles of 100's, capsule shaped, scored white tablet with blue specks embossed with TRIMEN.

AMAPHEN® CAPSULES ℞
(Non-Narcotic Analgesic)

Each Capsule contains:
50 mg .... Butalbital
(WARNING: May be habit forming)
40 mg .... Caffeine
325 mg .... Acetaminophen.

HOW SUPPLIED
Bottles of 100's; opaque white and opaque pink capsule, imprinted "TRIMEN".

AMAPHEN® with CODEINE #3 Ⓒ III
Analgesic

Each Amaphen with Codeine Capsule contains: 50 mg butalbital, U.S.P. (Warning: May be habit forming; 325 mg acetaminophen, U.S.P., and 40 mg caffeine, U.S.P.
In addition, Amaphen with Codeine also contains 30 mg of codeine phosphate, U.S.P. (Warning: May be habit forming).

HOW SUPPLIED
Bottles of 100's, pink and maroon capsules, imprinted TRIMEN.

DYREXAN™-OD Ⓒ III
Brand of Phendimetrazine Tartrate
Slow-Release Capsules 105 mg

HOW SUPPLIED
Bottles of 100's, clear yellow and opaque brown 105 mg capsules imprinted with TRIMEN.

KORIGESIC® TABLETS ℞
Analgesic Decongestant

Each Tablet contains: 4 mg. Chlorpheniramine Maleate, 14 mg. Phenylpropanolamine Hydrochloride, 5 mg. Phenylephrine Hydrochloride, 150 mg. Salicylamide, 200 mg. Acetaminophen, 30 mg. Caffeine.

HOW SUPPLIED
Bottles of 100's, two-layer, scored blue and white tablet, embossed with logo.

NATACOMP-FA® TABLETS ℞
Multivitamin, Multimineral supplement for pregnant or lactating women

HOW SUPPLIED
Bottles of 100's pink, oval, film coated tablet.

VIOPAN-T™ TABLETS
High Potency Vitamin Mineral Formula

HOW SUPPLIED
Red, film coated tablet, embossed with TRIMEN.

Tyson and Associates, Inc.

1661 LINCOLN BLVD.
SUITE 300
SANTA MONICA, CA 90404

ALPHA PLUS OTC
(Urea Cycle Intermediates)

DESCRIPTION
U.S.P. Crystalline Amino Acid Formulation. Contains 700 mg of the urea cycle intermediates.

COMPOSITION
L-Arginine, L-Aspartic Acid, L-Glutamic Acid, Alpha Ketoglutarate, L-Ornithine, Proline, Citric Acid, L-Citrulline.

DOSAGE AND ADMINISTRATION
One (1) to two (2) capsules with meals.

HOW SUPPLIED
700 mg capsules, bottles of 100's —NDC 53335-1232-1

REFERENCES
• Metabolic Role of Urea Cycle Intermediates: Nutritional and Clinical Aspects. J. of Nutr. Vol 115. No. 4 505–41, 1985.
• Disorders of the Urea Cycle. Hosp. Pract. 65–72. 1985.
• Ketoacids in the treatment of uremia. Clin. Neph. Vol. 3. No. 5, 180–86, 1975.

AMINOLETE OTC

DESCRIPTION
U.S.P. Crystalline Amino Acid Formulation. Formula contains 700 mg of 13 crystalline L-amino acids supplying 102 mg of Nitrogen per capsule.

COMPOSITION
L-Glutamine, L-Lysine, L-Methionine, Glycine, L-Leucine, L-Arginine, L-Phenylalanine, L-Valine, L-Isoleucine, L-Threonine, L-Tryptophan, L-Histidine, L-Tyrosine.

DOSAGE AND ADMINISTRATION
Two (2) to four (4) capsules t.i.d. or ¼ to ½ teaspoon of powder t.i.d.

HOW SUPPLIED
700 mg capsules, 100's—NDC 53335-1205-1, also available in bottles of 200 grams powder.

REFERENCES
Protein Metabolism during Endurance Exercise. Fed. Proc. 44:348–352, 1985.
Amino Acid Uptake and Levels: Influence of Endurance Training. Biochem. Med. 21:196–201, 1979.
Changes in Plasma Amino Acid Distribution and Urine Amino Acids Excretion During Prolonged Heavy Exercise. Scand. J. Clin. Lab. Invest. 39:407–413, 1979.

AMINOMINE OTC

DESCRIPTION
U.S.P. Crystalline Amino Acid Formulation. Formula contains 700 mg of 15 crystalline L-amino acids supplying 103 mg nitrogen per capsule. Source of excitatory neurotransmitters and L-glutamine.

COMPOSITION
L-Glutamine, Glycine, L-Alanine, L-Leucine, L-Lysine, L-Valine, L-Isoleucine, L-Arginine, L-Methionine, L-Histidine, L-Threonine, L-Phenylalanine, Proline, L-Tyrosine, L-Tryptophan.

DOSAGE AND ADMINISTRATION
Initially, it is recommended one (1) to two (2) capsules b.i.d. or ¼ to ½ teaspoon powder b.i.d.

HOW SUPPLIED
Bottles of 100's-NDC 53335-1129-1, also available in bottles of 200 grams powder.

REFERENCES
• Decrease in plasma amino acids in man after acute dose of ethanol. Studies on alcohol 44(2) 215–221, 1983.
• Glutamine in the treatment of alcoholism. J. Biol. Chem. 214:503–6, 1955.
• Changes in plasma amino acid patterns in chronic alcoholic patients during ethanol withdrawal syndrome: Their clinical implications. Medical Hypothesis 12:239–251, 1983.
• Effect of ethonal on amino acid absorption in vivo rat intestine. Am. J. Physiol., 241:176–181.

AMINOPLEX® OTC

DESCRIPTION
U.S.P. crystalline amino acid formulation. Formula contains 740 mg Anhydrous of 19 crystalline L-amino acids including neurotransmitter precursors and sulfur amino acids, and supplies 130 mg Nitrogen per capsule. Balanced formulation replacement based on quantitative Amino Acid Fractionation.

COMPOSITION
L-Lysine, L-Tryptophan, L-Arginine, L-Isoleucine, L-Leucine, L-Alanine, L-Threonine, L-Histidine, L-Cystine, L-Methionine, L-Glutamine, L-Tyrosine, L-Aspartic Acid, L-Valine, L-Glutamic Acid, L-Phenylalanine, Glycine, L-Serine, L-Cysteine.

DOSAGE AND ADMINISTRATION
Initially it is recommended two (2) to four (4) capsules t.i.d. or ¼ to ½ teaspoon t.i.d. Can be used in children over 4 years old.

HOW SUPPLIED
Bottles of 100's-NDC 53335-1116-1, also available in bottles of 50, 250 & 500 and bottles of 50 and 350 grams of powder. 370 mg capsules available in bottles of 100 and 250 capsules for pediatric use.

REFERENCES
Tryptophan and Tyrosine Availability: Relation to Clinical Response to Antidepressive Pharmacotherapy.
Frontiers Biochem. and Pharma Res. Depression. Raven Press, 319-26, 1984
Management of Depressions with Monoamine Precursors.
Adv. Biol. Psych., Vol. 10, 137-147, 1983
The Absence of Protein-Sparing Effects Utilizing Crystalline Aminos in Stressed Patients.
Ann. Sugr., 565-570, 1979
Dietary Enhancement of CNS Neurotransmitters
Integr. Psych. 149-155, 1984

AMINOSINE OTC
(Arginine-free Amino Acid Formula)

DESCRIPTION
U.S.P. crystalline amino acid formulation. Formula contains 700 mg of 19 crystalline L-amino acids supplying 85.5 mg Nitrogen per capsule. Source of essential amino acids without arginine.

COMPOSITION
L-Lysine, L-Tryptophan, L-Threonine, L-Isoleucine, L-Leucine, L-Alanine, L-Histidine, L-Tyrosine, L-Cystine, L-Glutamine, L-Aspartic Acid, L-Valine, L-Methionine, L-Citrulline, L-Glutamic Acid, L-Ornithine, Glycine, L-Serine, L-Phenylalanine.

DOSAGE AND ADMINISTRATION
Initially it is recommended two (2) to four (4) capsules t.i.d. or ¼ to ½ teaspoon powder t.i.d.

HOW SUPPLIED
Bottles of 100's-NDC 53335-1207-1, also available in bottles of 200 grams of powder.

REFERENCES
A Multicentered Study of Lysine Therapy in Herpes Simplex Infection
Dermatoloica 156:257-267, 1978
Lysine Malabsorption Syndrome: A New Type of Transport Defect
Pediatrics Vol. 57, No. 1, January 1976.

AMINOSTASIS™ OTC
(Branched Chain Amino Acid Formula)

DESCRIPTION
U.S.P. crystalline amino acid formulation. Formula contains 700 mg of 12 crystalline L-amino acids supplying 107 mg Nitrogen per capsule. Formula is a rich source of the branched chain amino acids.

COMPOSITION
L-Lysine, Glycine, L-Leucine, L-Methionine, L-Arginine, L-Phenylalanine, L-Valine, L-Isoleucine, L-Histidine, L-Threonine, L-Tyrosine, L-Tryptophan.

DOSAGE AND ADMINISTRATION
Initially it is recommended two (2) to four (4) capsules t.i.d. or ¼ to ½ teaspoon of powder t.i.d.

HOW SUPPLIED
Bottles of 100's-NCD 53335-1200-1, also available in bottles of 90 and 200 grams of powder.

REFERENCES
• Therapeutic Aspects of Branched Chain Amino and Keto Acids. Clinical Science 66:1–15 1984.

- Physiological Role of Branched Chain Amino and Keto Acids in Vivo. *Branched Chain Amino Acids in Health and Disease* pp. 162–181 (Karger, Basel 1984).
- Nutritional Intervention in Hepatic Encephalopathy by the use of Branched Chain enriched Amino Acid mixtures. *Metabolism and Clinical Implications of Branched Chain Amino and Keto Acids.* (Elsevier, North Holland 1981).
- Amino Acid Metabolism in Patients with Advanced Uremia and in Patients Undergoing Chronic Dialysis. *Advances in Nephrology* Volume 8 p.233–268.
- Plasma Amino Acid Levels and Amino Acid Losses During continuous Ambulatory Peritoneal Dialysis. Am. J. Clin. Nutr. Sept. 1982.
- Isotopic analysis of Leucine and Urea metabolism in Exercising Humans. J. Applied Physiol: 52 (2):458–466, 1982.

AMINOTATE® OTC
(Glycogenic Amino Acid Formula)

DESCRIPTION
U.S.P. crystalline amino acid formulation. Formula contains 700 mg of 15 crystalline L-amino acids supplying 102 mg Nitrogen per capsule. Formula is a rich source of the glycogenic amino acids.

COMPOSITION
Glycine, L-Alanine, L-Leucine, L-Lysine, L-Valine, L-Isoleucine, L-Arginine, L-Methionine, L-Histidine, L-Threonine, L-Phenylalanine, Proline, L-Glutamine, L-Tyrosine, L-Tryptophan.

DOSAGE AND ADMINISTRATION
Initially it is recommended 2–4 capsules b.i.d. in between meals. Powder ¼–½ teaspoon b.i.d.

HOW SUPPLIED
Bottles of 100's-NDC 53335-1209-1, also available in bottles of 90 & 200 grams powder.

REFERENCES
Hypoalanimenia: A concomitant of Ketotic Hypoglycemia. J. Clin. Invest., 51:73, 1440–9, 1971.
Amino Acid metabolism during prolonged starvation. J. Clin. Invest.,48:584
Ketotic Hypoglycemia: An Amino Acid Substrate limited Disorder. J. Clin. Endo & Metabol., 38 (4), 521–30, 1974.

AMINOXIN™ OTC
(Pyridoxal-5'-Phosphate)

DESCRIPTION
Each Aminoxin tablet contains 20 mg of pyridoxal-5'-phosphate, the co-enzymatic form of vitamin B_6. Enterically coated to protect the pyridoxal-5'-phosphate from dephosphorylization in the stomach acids, and enhancing molecular absorption.

ACTIONS AND USES
Required in transamination and decarboxylation reactions. Conversion of L-Tryptophan to Serotonin and L-Methionine to L-Cysteine, respectively. Reported useful in mitigating symptoms of PMS and nausea of pregnancy.

DOSAGE AND ADMINISTRATION
Daily dosage of 20–60 mg divided in parts and administered t.i.d. between meals.

HOW SUPPLIED
Bottles of 100's—NDC 53335-1120-1

L-CARNITINE U.S.P. OTC

DESCRIPTION
U.S.P. crystalline L-Carnitine containing 250 mg.

DOSAGE AND ADMINISTRATION
1–3 capsules t.i.d. between meals.

HOW SUPPLIED
250 mg capsules, bottles of 30's-NDC 53335-1124-1

REFERENCES
- Carnitine and its role in fatty acid metabolism. Adv. Lipid Res, 1:285–334, 1963.
- Role of carnitine in fatty acid metabolism of normal and ischemic myocardium Amer. Heart Journ., 1977.
- Improved Pacing Tolerance of the Ischemic Human Myocardium after Administration of Carnitine J. American Cardiology, Vol. 43, 304, 1978.
- Lipid Lowering Effect of Carnitine in Patients with Type IV Hyperlipoproteinemia. The Lancet, Oct. 14, 1978.
- Favorable Effects of L-Carnitine Treatment on Hypertriglyceridemia in Hemodialysis Patients: Decisive Role of Low Levels of High Density Lipoprotein Cholesterol. Am. J. Clin. Nutr. 38:October 1983 pp. 532–540.
- Carnitine Reduces Fasting Ketogenesis in Patients with Disorders of Propionate Metabolism. The Lancet, p. 289 Feb 8, 1986.
- Deficiency of Carnitine in Cachechtic Cirrhotic Patients. J. Clin. Invest 60:716, 1977.

ENDORPHENYL OTC
(D-Phenylalanine U.S.P.)

DESCRIPTION
U.S.P. crystalline D-Phenylalanine containing 500 mg or 200 mg.

ACTIONS AND USES
Enkephalinase inhibitor, psychiatry.

DOSAGE AND ADMINISTRATION
2–3 capsules t.i.d. upon arising, mid-a.m. & p.m.

HOW SUPPLIED
Bottles of 200 mg, 50's-NDC 3335-1225-1, and 500 mg 50's and 100's.

REFERENCES
- The Potential for the Use of Tryptophan and other Amine Precursors in the Treatment of Affective Disorders. Depressive Illness. Advances in Biolgical Psychiatry. Vol. 7. 1981.

MAX EPA™ OTC
(Omega 3 Fatty Acids)

DESCRIPTION
Omega 3 Fatty Acid formula. Capsules containing Eicosapentaenoic acid and docosahexaenoic acid.

COMPOSITION
Eicosapentaenoic acid 180 mg per gram Docosahexaenoic acid 120 mg per gram

DOSAGE AND ADMINISTRATION
2 capsules t.i.d.

HOW SUPPLIED
1g capsules in bottles of 100 capsules NDC #53335-1215-1

REFERENCES
- Reduction of Plasma Lipids, Lipoproteins, and Apoproteins by Dietary Fish Oils in Patients with Hypertriglyceridemia. N. Eng. J. Med 312(19): 1210–1216 1985.

MAXOVITE OTC
(PMS Multi-Vitamin/Mineral)

DESCRIPTION
A corn and yeast free multi-vitamin/mineral. Contains lipo and hydro soluble vitamins. Minerals are in amino acid chelated forms for maximum uptake.

HOW SUPPLIED
Bottle of 120 tablets NDC 53335-1142, also available in 240 tablet size.

REFERENCES
Effect of Oral Contraceptives on Vitamin Metabolism. Adv. Clin. Chem. 18:247–87, 1976
Premenstrual Tension: A Critical Study of the Syndrome J. Indian Med. Assoc. 24:82, 1959

L-TRYPTOPHAN U.S.P. OTC

DESCRIPTION
Encapsulated U.S.P. crystalline powder. Contains not less than 98.5% L-Tryptophan ($C_{11}H_{12}N_2O_2$)

ACTIONS AND USES
Precursor of Neurotransmitter, Serotonin (5-hydroxytryptamine). Medical research references listed under Tryptoplex.p.=

DOSAGE AND ADMINISTRATION
2–4 capsules with juice 30 minutes before retiring.

HOW SUPPLIED
Bottle of 400 mg. 100's—NDC 53335-1173-1, also available in bottles of 50 capsules, 75 and 150 grams of powder.

TRYPTOPLEX OTC
[tryp-toe-plex]
(Serotoninergic Precursor)

DESCRIPTION
Encapsulated pure U.S.P. crystalline powder of 400 mg L-Tryptophan, and the essential coenzymes. 4 mg nicotinic acid, 1 mg pyridoxine HCl.

ACTIONS AND USES
Biochemical precursor of neurotransmitter, serotonin. (5-hydroxytrptamine).

DOSAGE AND ADMINISTRATION
2–5 capsules with juice at bedtime or as directed by physician.

HOW SUPPLIED
Bottles of 60's—NDC 53335-1243-1
Bottles of 120's—NDC 53335-1243-3

REFERENCES
- L-Tryptophan in Drug-Induced Movement Disorders with Insomnia. N. Eng. J. Med. 314 (19):1257–1986
- The Pharmokinetics of Oral L-Tryptophan: Effects of Dose and of Concomitant Pyridoxine, Allopurinol or Nicotinamide Administration. Adv. Biol. Psych. Vol. 10: 67–81, 1983 (Karger)
- L-Tryptophan in Depression. Biol. Psych. Vol II. No. E 1976
- A Controlled Trial of L-Tryptophan in Mania. Brit. J. Psych 132 555-59, 1978.
- Effects of Long term Administration of L-Tryptophan on Human Sleep. Sleep Research. Vol. 4 1975.
- Depression and Serotonin Metabolism: Rational for Neurotransmitter Precursor Treatment. J. Clin. Psych Bol 5. No. 4 191–206, 1985.

UAD Laboratories, Inc.
6635 HIGHWAY 18 WEST
JACKSON, MS 39209

BUCET™ ℞
[bu 'set]

DESCRIPTION
Each capsule contains:
Butalbital .... 50 mg
(WARNING: May be habit forming.)
Acetaminophen .... 650 mg

HOW SUPPLIED
The capsules are opaque white imprinted with product name, ID number, UAD logo and supplied in bottles of 100 capsules. Each capsule contains Acetaminophen 650 mg, and Butalbital 50 mg. (WARNING: May be habit forming) The NDC number for 100 capsules is 0785-2307-01.

LORCET® Ⓒ ℞
[lōr-sĕt]

DESCRIPTION
Each film coated reddish-orange tablet contains:
Propoxyphene Hydrochloride ....65 mg.
Acetaminophen....................650 mg.

HOW SUPPLIED
In bottles of 100's—NDC 0785-1111-01.

LORCET-HD® Ⓒ ℞
[lōr-sĕt, h, d]

DESCRIPTION
Each Lorcet-HD capsule contains 5 mg. of Hydrocodone Bitartrate (WARNING: May be habit forming) and 500 mg. of Acetaminophen.

HOW SUPPLIED
Lorcet-HD Capsules are opaque maroon capsules and are supplied in bottles of 100 capsules. Each capsule contains Acetaminophen (APAP), 500 mg., and Hydrocodone Bitartrate, 5 mg. (WARNING: May be habit forming). The NDC number for containers of 100 capsules is 0785-1120-01.

TRIAD™ ℞
[trī 'ad]

DESCRIPTION
Each capsule contains
Butalbital .... 50 mg
(Warning: May be habit forming)
Acetaminophen .... 325 mg
Caffeine .... 40 mg

HOW SUPPLIED
Triad capsules are opaque red imprinted with product name, ID number, UAD logo and supplied in bottles of 100 capsules. Each capsule contains Acetaminophen 325 mg., Caffeine 40 mg., and Butalbital 50 mg. (WARNING: May be habit forming.) The NDC number for 100 capsules is 0785-2305-01.

Continued on next page

UAD—Cont.

ZONE-A CREAM 1% ℞

[zōn 'a]

DESCRIPTION

A topical preparation containing Hydrocortisone acetate 1% and Pramoxine HCL 1% in a hydrophilic cream base containing stearic acid, cetyl alcohol, aquaphor, isopropylpalmitate, polyoxyl-40-stearate, propylene glycol, potassium sorbate 0.1%, sorbic acid 0.1%, triethanolamine lauryl sulfate and water.

HOW SUPPLIED

1 oz. tube.

ZONE-A LOTION 1% ℞

[zōn 'ā]

DESCRIPTION

Zone-A Lotion is a topical preparation containing Hydrocortisone acetate 1% and Pramoxine HCL 1% in a hydrophylic lotion base containing stearic acid, cetyl alcohol, forlan-L glycerine, Triethanolamine, Myrj-52, Di-isopropyl adipate, polyvinyl-pyrrolidone, silicone, potassium sorbate 0.1% and sorbic acid 0.1% and water. Topical corticosteroids are anti-inflammatory and anti-pruritic agents.

CLINICAL PHARMACOLOGY

Topical corticosteroids share anti-inflammatory, anti-pruritic and vasoconstrictive actions.

The mechanism of anti-inflammatory activity of the topical corticosteroids is unclear. Various laboratory methods, including vasoconstrictor assays, are used to compare and predict potencies and/or clinical efficacies of the topical corticosteroids. There is some evidence to suggest that a recognizable correlation exists between vasoconstrictor potency and therapeutic efficacy in man.

Pramoxine hydrochloride is a topical anesthetic agent which provides temporary relief from itching and pain. It acts by stabilizing the neuronal membrane of nerve endings with which it comes into contact.

INDICATIONS AND USAGE

Topical corticosteroids are indicated for the relief of the inflammatory and pruritic manifestations of corticosteroid-responsive dermatoses.

CONTRAINDICATIONS

Topical corticosteroids are contraindicated in those patients with a history of hypersensitivity to any of the components of the preparation.

PRECAUTIONS

General: Systemic absorption of topical corticosteroids has produced reversible hypothalamic-pituitary-adrenal (HPA) axis suppression, manifestations of Cushing's syndrome, hyperglycemia, and glucosuria in some patients.

Conditions which augment systemic absorption include the application of the more potent steroids, use over large surface areas, prolonged use, and the addition of occlusive dressings.

Therefore, patients receiving a large dose of a potent topical steroid applied to a large surface area and under an occlusive dressing should be evaluated periodically for evidence of HPA axis suppression by using the urinary free cortisol and ACTH stimulation tests. If HPA axis suppression is noted, an attempt should be made to withdraw the drug, to reduce the frequency of application, or to substitute a less potent steroid.

Recovery of HPA axis function is generally prompt and complete upon discontinuation of the drug. Infrequently, signs and symptoms of steroid withdrawal may occur, requiring supplemental systemic corticosteroids.

Children may absorb proportionally larger amounts of topical corticosteroids and thus be more susceptible fo systemic toxicity. (See PRECAUTIONS—Pediatric Use).

If irritation develops topical corticosteroids should be discontinued and appropriate therapy instituted.

In the presence of dermatological infections, the use of an appropriate antifungal or antibacterial agent should be instituted. If a favorable response does not occur promptly, the corticosteroid should be discontinued until the infection has been adequately controlled.

Information for the Patient: Patients using topical corticosteroids should receive the following information and instructions:

1. This medication is to be used as directed by the physician. It is for external use only. Avoid contact with the eyes.
2. Patients should be advised not to use this medication for any disorder other than for which it was prescribed.
3. The treated skin area should not be bandaged or otherwise covered or wrapped as to be occlusive unless directed by the physician.
4. Patients should report any signs of local adverse reactions, especially under occlusive dressings.
5. Parents of pediatric patients should be advised not to use tight-fitting diapers or plastic pants on a child being treated in the diaper area, as these garments may constitute occlusive dressings.

Laboratory Tests: The following tests may be helpful in evaluating the HPA axis suppression:

Urinary free cortisol test
ACTH stimulation test

Carcinogenesis, Mutagenesis, and Impairment of Fertility: Long term animal studies have not been performed to evaluate the carcinogenic potential or the effect on fertility of topical corticosteroids.

Studies to determine mutagenicity with prednisolone and hydrocortisone have revealed negative results.

Pregnancy Category C: Corticosteroids are generally teratogenic in laboratory animals when administered systemically at relatively low dosage levels. The more potent corticosteroids have been shown to be teratogenic after dermal application in laboratory animals. There are no adequate and well-controlled studies in pregnant women on teratogenic effects from topically applied corticosteroids. Therefore topical corticosteroids should be used during pregnancy only if the potential benefit justifies the potential risk to the fetus. Drugs of this class should not be used extensively on pregnant patients, in large amounts, or for prolonged periods of time.

Nursing Mothers: It is not known whether topical administration of corticosteroids could result in sufficient systemic absorption to produce detectable amounts in breast milk. Systemically administered corticosteroids are secreted into breast milk in quantities NOT likely to have a deleterious effect on the infant. Nevertheless, caution should be exercised when topical corticosteroids are administered to a nursing woman.

Pediatric Use: Pediatric patients may demonstrate greater susceptibility to topical corticosteroid-induced HPA axis suppression and Cushing's syndrome than mature patients because of a larger skin surface area to body weight ratio.

Hypothalamic-pituitary-adrenal (HPA) axis suppression, Cushing's syndrome, and intracranial hypertension have been reported in children receiving topical corticosteroids. Manifestations of adrenal suppression in children include linear growth retardation, delayed weight gain, low plasma cortisol levels, and absence of response to ACTH stimulation. Manifestations of intracranial hypertension include bulging fontanelles, headaches, and bilateral papilledema.

Administration of topical corticosteroids to children should be limited to the least amount compatible with an effective therapeutic regimen. Chronic corticosteroids therapy may interfere with the growth and development of children.

ADVERSE REACTIONS

The following local adverse reactions are reported infrequently with topical corticosteroids, but may occur more frequently with the use of occlusive dressings. These reactions are listed in an approximate decreasing order of occurence: Burning, Itching, Irritation, Dryness, Folliculitis, Hypertrichosis, Acneiform eruptions, Hypopigmentation, Perioral dermatitis, Allergic contact dermatitis, Maceration of the skin, Secondary infection, Skin Atrophy, Striae and Miliaria.

OVERDOSAGE

Topically applied corticosteroids can be absorbed in sufficient amounts to produce systematic effects (See PRECAUTIONS).

DOSAGE AND ADMINISTRATION

Topical corticosteroids are generally applied to the affected area as a thin film three or four times daily depending on the severity of the condition.

Occlusive dressings may be used for the management of psoriasis or recalcitrant conditions.

If an infection develops, the use of occlusive dressings should be discontinued and appropriate antimicrobial therapy instituted.

HOW SUPPLIED

2 fl. oz.

CAUTION

Federal law prohibits dispensing without prescription.

Manufactured for:
UAD LABORATORIES, INC.
Jackson, Mississippi 39209

Products are cross-indexed by generic and chemical names in the **YELLOW SECTION**

U.S. Pharmaceutical Corporation

2500 PARK CENTRAL BLVD.
DECATUR, GA 30035

HEMOCYTE™ Tablets OTC

(ferrous fumarate 324 mg.)

HOW SUPPLIED

Bottles of 100 NDC 0184-0307-60

HEMOCYTE PLUS™ Tabules ℞

Iron-Vitamin-Mineral Complex

DESCRIPTION

Each tabule contains:

Ferrous Fumarate (anhydrous)	324	mg.
[Equivalent to about 106 mg. of Elemental Iron]		
Sodium Ascorbate (Vit. C)	200	mg.
Vit. B-1—Thiamine Mononitrate	10	mg.
Vit. B-2—Riboflavin	6	mg.
Vit. B-6—Pyridoxine HCl	5	mg.
Vit. B-12—Cyanocobalamin Concentrate	15	mcg.
Folic Acid	1	mg.
Niacinamide	30	mg.
Calcium Pantothenate	10	mg.
Zinc Sulfate	80	mg.
Magnesium Sulfate	70	mg.
Manganese Sulfate	4	mg.
Copper Sulfate	2	mg.

HOW SUPPLIED

Bottles of 100 NDC 0184-0308-60

HEMOCYTE-F TABLETS ℞

DESCRIPTION

Each tablet contains:

Ferrous Fumarate	324 mg.
Folic Acid	1 mg.

HOW SUPPLIED

Bottles of 100 NDC 0184-0306-60

ISOVEX® Capsules ℞

(ethaverine hydrochloride 100 mg.)

HOW SUPPLIED

Bottles of 100 NDC 52747-204-60
Bottles of 1000 NDC 52747-204-80

MAGSAL™ TABLETS ℞

DESCRIPTION

Each tablet contains:

Magnesium Salicylate	600 mg.
Phenyltoloxamine Citrate	25 mg.

HOW SUPPLIED

Bottles of 100
NDC 0184-0321-60

MEDIGESIC® PLUS Capsules ℞

DESCRIPTION

Each capsule contains:

Butalbital*	50 mg
*WARNING: May be habit forming.	
Acetaminophen	325 mg
Caffeine	40 mg

HOW SUPPLIED

Bottles of 100 NDC 0184-0212-60

IDENTIFICATION PROBLEM?
Consult PDR's
Product Identification Section
where you'll find over 1200 products pictured actual size and in full color.

USV Laboratories, Division
USV Pharmaceutical Corp.
FORT WASHINGTON, PA 19034

USV Laboratories Inc.
MANATI, P.R. 00701

USV (P.R.) Development Corp.
MANATI, P.R. 00701

ARLIDIN® ℞
[*ar'lĭ-dĭn"*]
nylidrin HCl
6 mg. tablets
12 mg. tablets

DESCRIPTION
A sympathomimetic agent, Arlidin is an original compound of organic synthesis, phenyl secondary butyl norhydroxyephedrine. It is related chemically to the epinephrine-ephedrine series.
The tablets also contain microcrystalline cellulose, corn starch, gelatin, lactose, magnesium stearate, and pregelatinized starch.

ACTIONS
Arlidin acts predominantly by beta-receptor stimulation. Beta stimulation with Arlidin has been demonstrated in a variety of isolated tissues from rabbits, guinea pigs and dogs. It has been shown to dilate arterioles in skeletal muscle and to increase cardiac output in the anesthetized dog and cat and in unanesthetized man.

INDICATIONS

Based on a review of this drug by the National Academy of Sciences—National Research Council and/or other information, FDA has classified the indications as follows:
"Possibly" effective whenever an increase in blood supply is desirable in vasospastic disorders such as:
peripheral vascular disease
- Arteriosclerosis Obliterans
- Thromboangiitis Obliterans
- Diabetic Vascular Disease
- Night Leg Cramps
- Raynaud's Phenomenon and Disease
- Ischemic Ulcer
- Frostbite
- Acrocyanosis
- Acroparesthesia
- Thrombophlebitis
- Cold Feet, Legs and Hands

circulatory disturbances of the inner ear
- Primary Cochlear Cell Ischemia
- Cochlear Stria Vascular Ischemia
- Macular or Ampullar Ischemia and other disturbances due to labyrinthine artery spasm or obstruction

"Lacks substantial evidence of effectiveness" for the indications:
cerebrovascular disorders
- Cerebral Ischemia
- Cerebral Arteriosclerosis and other circulatory insufficiencies of the brain

Final classification of the less-than-effective indications requires further investigation.

CONTRAINDICATIONS
Acute myocardial infarction, paroxysmal tachycardia, progressive angina pectoris and thyrotoxicosis.

WARNINGS
In patients with cardiac disease such as tachyarrhythmias and uncompensated congestive heart failure, the benefit/-risk ratio should be weighed prior to therapy and reconsidered at intervals during treatment.

ADVERSE REACTIONS
Trembling, nervousness, weakness, dizziness (not associated with labyrinthine artery insufficiency), palpitations, nausea and vomiting may occur. Postural hypotension, while not reported, may also occur.

DOSAGE
Orally, 3 to 12 mg three or four times a day.

HOW SUPPLIED
ARLIDIN (nylidrin HCl)— white, scored tablets, 6 mg and 12 mg: Bottles of 100 and 1000. Single-dose blister packs, boxes of 100 (10 x 10 strips).
CAUTION: Federal (U.S.A.) law prohibits dispensing without prescription.
NSN 6505-00-685-5435A, V.A. Depots (6 mg., 1000s).
Revised: May, 1986

Shown in Product Identification Section, page 433

CALCIMAR® ℞
[*kal'sĭ-mar*]
(calcitonin-salmon)
INJECTION, SYNTHETIC

DESCRIPTION
Calcitonin is a polypeptide hormone secreted by the parafollicular cells of the thyroid gland in mammals and by the ultimobranchial gland of birds and fish.
CALCIMAR® (calcitonin-salmon) Injection, Synthetic is a synthetic polypeptide of 32 amino acids in the same linear sequence that is found in calcitonin of salmon origin.
It is provided in sterile solution for subcutaneous or intramuscular injection. Each milliliter contains 200 I.U. (MRC) of Calcitonin-Salmon, 5 mg phenol (as preservative), with sodium chloride, sodium acetate, acetic acid, and sodium hydroxide to adjust tonicity and pH.
The activity of CALCIMAR® is stated in International Units (equal to MRC or Medical Research Council units) based on bioassay in comparison with the International Reference Preparation of Calcitonin, Salmon for Bioassay, distributed by the National Institute for Biological Standards and Control, Holly Hill, London.

CLINICAL PHARMACOLOGY
Calcitonin acts primarily on bone, but direct renal effects and actions on the gastrointestinal tract are also recognized. Salmon calcitonin appears to have actions essentially identical to calcitonins of mammalian origin, but its potency per mg is greater and it has a longer duration of action. The actions of calcitonin on bone and its role in normal human bone physiology are still incompletely understood.
Bone—Single injections of calcitonin cause a marked transient inhibition of the ongoing bone resorptive process. With prolonged use, there is a persistent, smaller decrease in the rate of bone resorption. Histologically this is associated with a decreased number of osteoclasts and an apparent decrease in their resorptive activity. Decreased osteocytic resorption may also be involved. There is some evidence that initially bone formation may be augmented by calcitonin through increased osteoblastic activity. However, calcitonin will probably not induce a long-term increase in bone formation.
Animal studies indicate that endogenous calcitonin, primarily through its action on bone, participates with parathyroid hormone in the homeostatic regulation of blood calcium. Thus, high blood calcium levels cause increased secretion of calcitonin which, in turn, inhibits bone resorption. This reduces the transfer of calcium from bone to blood and tends to return blood calcium to the normal level. The importance of this process in humans has not been determined. In normal adults, who have a relatively low rate of bone resorption, the administration of exogenous calcitonin results in only a slight decrease in serum calcium. In normal children and in patients with generalized Paget's disease, bone resorption is more rapid and decreases in serum calcium are more pronounced in response to calcitonin.
Paget's Disease of Bone (osteitis deformans)—Paget's disease is a disorder of uncertain etiology characterized by abnormal and accelerated bone formation and resorption in one or more bones. In most patients only small areas of bone are involved and the disease is not symptomatic. In a small fraction of patients, however, the abnormal bone may lead to bone pain and bone deformity, cranial and spinal nerve entrapment, or spinal cord compression. The increased vascularity of the abnormal bone may lead to high output congestive heart failure.
Active Paget's disease involving a large mass of bone may increase the urinary hydroxyproline excretion (reflecting breakdown of collagen-containing bone matrix) and serum alkaline phosphatase (reflecting increased bone formation).
Salmon calcitonin, presumably by an initial blocking effect on bone resorption, causes a decreased rate of bone turnover with a resultant fall in the serum alkaline phosphatase and urinary hydroxyproline excretion in approximately two thirds of patients treated. These biochemical changes appear to correspond to changes toward more normal bone, as evidenced by a small number of documented examples of: 1) radiologic regression of Pagetic lesions, 2) improvement of impaired auditory nerve and other neurologic function, 3) decreases (measured) in abnormally elevated cardiac output. These improvements occur extremely rarely, if ever, spontaneously (elevated cardiac output may disappear over a period of years when the disease slowly enters a sclerotic phase; in the cases treated with calcitonin, however, the decreases were seen in less than one year).
Some patients with Paget's disease who have good biochemical and/or symptomatic responses initially, later relapse. Suggested explanations have included the formation of neutralizing antibodies and the development of secondary hyperparathyroidism, but neither suggestion appears to explain adequately the majority of relapses.
Although the parathyroid hormone levels do appear to rise transiently during each hypocalcemic response to calcitonin, most investigators have been unable to demonstrate persistent hypersecretion of parathyroid hormone in patients treated chronically with calcitonin.
Circulating antibodies to calcitonin after 2–18 months' treatment have been reported in about half of the patients with Paget's disease in whom antibody studies were done, but calcitonin treatment remained effective in many of these cases. Occasionally patients with high antibody titers are found. These patients usually will have suffered a biochemical relapse of Paget's disease and are unresponsive to the acute hypocalcemic effects of calcitonin.
Hypercalcemia—In clinical trials, CALCIMAR® has been shown to lower the elevated serum calcium of patients with carcinoma (with or without demonstrated metastases), multiple myeloma or primary hyperparathyroidism (lesser response). Patients with higher values for serum calcium tend to show greater reduction during CALCIMAR® therapy. The decrease in calcium occurs about 2 hours after the first injection and lasts for about 6–8 hours. CALCIMAR® given every 12 hours maintained a calcium lowering effect for about 5–8 days, the time period evaluated for most patients during the clinical studies. The average reduction of 8-hour post-injection serum calcium during this period was about 9 percent.
Kidney—Calcitonin increases the excretion of filtered phosphate, calcium, and sodium by decreasing their tubular reabsorption. In some patients the inhibition of bone resorption by calcitonin is of such magnitude that the consequent reduction of filtered calcium load more than compensates for the decrease in tubular reabsorption of calcium. The result in these patients is a decrease rather than an increase in urinary calcium.
Transient increases in sodium and water excretion may occur after the initial injection of calcitonin. In most patients these changes return to pre-treatment levels with continued therapy.
Gastrointestinal tract—Increasing evidence indicates that calcitonin has significant actions on the gastrointestinal tract. Short-term administration results in marked transient decreases in the volume and acidity of gastric juice and in the volume and the trypsin and amylase content of pancreatic juice. Whether these effects continue to be elicited after each injection of calcitonin during chronic therapy has not been investigated.
Metabolism—The metabolism of salmon calcitonin has not yet been studied clinically. Information from animal studies with salmon calcitonin and from clinical studies with calcitonins of porcine and human origin suggests that salmon calcitonin is rapidly metabolized by conversion to smaller inactive fragments, primarily in the kidneys, but also in the blood and peripheral tissues. A small amount of unchanged hormone and its inactive metabolites are excreted in the urine.
It appears that salmon calcitonin cannot cross the placental barrier and its passage to the cerebrospinal fluid or to breast milk has not been determined.

INDICATIONS AND USAGE
CALCIMAR® (Calcitonin-Salmon) Injection, Synthetic is indicated for the treatment of symptomatic Paget's disease of bone, for the treatment of hypercalcemia, and for the treatment of postmenopausal osteoporosis.
Paget's Disease—At the present time effectiveness has been demonstrated principally in patients with moderate to severe disease characterized by polyostotic involvement with elevated serum alkaline phosphatase and urinary hydroxyproline excretion.
In these patients, the biochemical abnormalities were substantially improved (more than 30% reduction) in about two-thirds of patients studied, and bone pain was improved in a similar fraction. A small number of documented instances of reversal of neurologic deficits has occurred, including improvement in the basilar compression syndrome, and improvement of spinal cord and spinal nerve lesions. At present there is too little experience to predict the likelihood of improvement of any given neurologic lesion. Hearing loss, the most common neurologic lesion of Paget's disease is improved infrequently (4 of 29 patients studied audiometrically).
Patients with increased cardiac output due to extensive Paget's disease have had measured decreases in cardiac output while receiving calcitonin. The number of treated patients in this category is still too small to predict how likely such a result will be.
The large majority of patients with localized, especially monostotic disease do not develop symptoms and most patients with mild symptoms can be managed with analgesics. There is no evidence that the prophylactic use of calcitonin is beneficial in asymptomatic patients, although treatment may be considered in exceptional circumstances in which there is

Continued on next page

USV—Cont.

extensive involvement of the skull or spinal cord with the possibility of irreversible neurologic damage. In these instances treatment would be based on the demonstrated effect of calcitonin on Pagetic bone, rather than on clinical studies in the patient population in question.
Hypercalcemia—CALCIMAR® is indicated for early treatment of hypercalcemic emergencies, along with other appropriate agents, when a rapid decrease in serum calcium is required, until more specific treatment of the underlying disease can be accomplished. It may also be added to existing therapeutic regimens for hypercalcemia such as intravenous fluids and furosemide, oral phosphate or corticosteroids, or other agents.
Postmenopausal Osteoporosis—CALCIMAR® is indicated for the treatment of postmenopausal osteoporosis in conjunction with an adequate calcium and vitamin D intake to prevent the progressive loss of bone mass. The evidence of efficacy was based on an increase in total body calcium. No significant differences were observed in bone density measurements of the distal radius, and the clinical studies were not designed to detect differences in fracture rates.

CONTRAINDICATIONS
Clinical allergy to synthetic salmon calcitonin.

WARNINGS
Allergic Reactions
Because calcitonin is protein in nature, the possibility of a systemic allergic reaction cannot be overlooked. The usual provisions should be made for the emergency treatment of such a reaction should it occur. Patients with a positive skin test to CALCIMAR® were excluded from clinical trials.
Skin testing should be considered prior to treatment with calcitonin, particularly for patients with suspected sensitivity to calcitonin. The following procedure is suggested: Prepare a dilution at 10 I.U. per ml by withdrawing 1/20 ml (0.05 ml) in a tuberculin syringe and filling it to 1.0 ml with Sodium Chloride Injection, U.S.P. Mix well, discard 0.9 ml and inject intracutaneously 0.1 ml (approximately 1 I.U.) on the inner aspect of the forearm. Observe the injection site 15 minutes after injection. The appearance of more than mild erythema or wheal constitutes a positive response.
The incidence of osteogenic sarcoma is known to be increased in Paget's disease. Pagetic lesions, with or without therapy, may appear by x-ray to progress markedly, possibly with some loss of definition of periosteal margins. Such lesions should be evaluated carefully to differentiate these from osteogenic sarcoma.

PRECAUTIONS
1. General
The administration of calcitonin possibly could lead to hypocalcemic tetany under special circumstances although no cases have yet been reported. Provisions for parenteral calcium administration should be available during the first several administrations of calcitonin.
2. Laboratory Tests
Periodic examinations of urine sediment of patients on chronic therapy are recommended.
Coarse granular casts and casts containing renal tubular epithelial cells were reported in young adult volunteers at bed rest who were given salmon calcitonin to study the effect on immobilization osteoporosis. There was no other evidence of renal abnormality and the urine sediment became normal after calcitonin was stopped. Urine sediment abnormalities have not been reported by other investigators.
3. Instructions for the Patient
Careful instruction in sterile injection technique should be given to the patient, and to other persons who may administer CALCIMAR®.
4. Carcinogenesis
No long-term studies have been performed to evaluate carcinogenic potential of salmon calcitonin.
5. Pregnancy: *Teratogenic effects, Category C.*
Salmon calcitonin has been shown to cause decrease in fetal birth weights in rabbits when given in doses 14–56 times the dose recommended for human use. Since calcitonin does not cross the placental barrier, this finding may be due to metabolic effects of calcitonin on the pregnant animal. There are no adequate and well-controlled studies in pregnant women. CALCIMAR® should be used during pregnancy only if the potential benefit justifies the potential risk to the fetus.
6. Nursing Mothers
It is not known whether this drug is excreted in human milk. As a general rule, nursing should not be undertaken while a patient is on this drug since many drugs are excreted in human milk. Calcitonin has been shown to inhibit lactation in animals.
7. Pediatric Use
Disorders of bone in children referred to as juvenile Paget's disease have been reported rarely. The relationship of these disorders to adult Paget's disease has not been established and experience with the use of calcitonin in these disorders is very limited. There are no adequate data to support the use of CALCIMAR® in children.

ADVERSE REACTIONS
Gastrointestinal System—Nausea with or without vomiting has been noted in about 10% of patients treated with calcitonin. It is most evident when treatment is first initiated and tends to decrease or disappear with continued administration.
Dermatological Hypersensitivity—Local inflammatory reactions at the site of subcutaneous or intramuscular injection have been reported in about 10% of patients. Flushing of face or hands occurred in about 2% to 5% of patients. Skin rashes have been reported occasionally.

OVERDOSAGE
A dose of 1000 I.U. subcutaneously may produce nausea and vomiting as the only adverse effects. Doses of 32 units per kg per day for one or two days demonstrate no other adverse effects.
Data on chronic high dose administration are insufficient to judge toxicity.

DOSAGE AND ADMINISTRATION
Paget's Disease—The recommended starting dose of calcitonin in Paget's disease is 100 I.U. (0.5 ml) per day administered subcutaneously (preferred for outpatient self-administration) or intramuscularly. Drug effect should be monitored by periodic measurement of serum alkaline phosphatase and 24-hour urinary hydroxyproline (if available) and evaluation of symptoms. A decrease toward normal of the biochemical abnormalities is usually seen, if it is going to occur, within the first few months. Bone pain may also decrease during that time. Improvement of neurologic lesions, when it occurs, requires a longer period of treatment, often more than one year.
In many patients doses of 50 I.U. (0.25 ml) per day or every-other day are sufficient to maintain biochemical and clinical improvement. At the present time, however, there are insufficient data to determine whether this reduced dose will have the same effect as the higher dose on forming more normal bone structure. It appears preferable, therefore, to maintain the higher dose in any patient with serious deformity or neurological involvement.
In any patient with a good response initially who later relapses, either clinically or biochemically, the possibility of antibody formation should be explored.
The patient may be tested for antibodies by an appropriate specialized test or evaluated for the possibility of antibody formation by critical clinical evaluation.
Patient compliance should also be assessed in the event of relapse.
In patients who relapse, whether because of antibodies or for unexplained reasons, a dosage increase beyond 100 I.U. per day does not usually appear to elicit an improved response.
Hypercalcemia—The recommended starting dose of CALCIMAR® in hypercalcemia is 4 I.U./kg body weight every 12 hours by subcutaneous or intramuscular injection. If the response to this dose is not satisfactory after one or two days, the dose may be increased to 8 I.U./kg every 12 hours. If the response remains unsatisfactory after two more days, the dose may be further increased to a maximum of 8 I.U./kg every 6 hours.
Postmenopausal Osteoporosis—The recommended dose of calcitonin is 100 I.U. per day administered subcutaneously or intramuscularly. Patients also receive supplemental calcium such as calcium carbonate 1.5 g daily and an adequate vitamin D intake (400 units daily). An adequate diet is also essential.
If the volume of CALCIMAR® to be injected exceeds 2 ml, intramuscular injection is preferable and multiple sites of injection should be used.
Parenteral drug products should be inspected visually for particulate matter and discoloration prior to administration whenever solution and container permit.

HOW SUPPLIED
CALCIMAR® is available as a sterile solution in 2 ml vials containing 200 I.U. per ml.
Store in refrigerator—between 2°-8°C (36°-46°F)
CAUTION: FEDERAL (U.S.A.) LAW PROHIBITS DISPENSING WITHOUT PRESCRIPTION.
Revised: July, 1985
Shown in Product Identification Section, page 433

CALEL-D™

DESCRIPTION
Each tablet provides 500 mg of elemental Calcium (50% of U.S. RDA) from calcium carbonate and 200 I.U. of Vitamin D_3 (Cholecalciferol) (50% of U.S. RDA). The inactive ingredients are corn starch, croscarmellose sodium, hydroxypropyl methylcellulose, polyethylene glycol, calcium stearate.

INDICATIONS
Calel-D is indicated as a dietary supplement for those adults not receiving an adequate intake of calcium and Vitamin D.

USUAL DOSE
One or two tablets daily or as directed by a physician.
Store tablets at room temperature. Keep this and all drugs out of the reach of children.

HOW SUPPLIED
Bottles of 60 tablets.
Shown in Product Identification Section, page 433

CERESPAN® ℞
[sĕr 'ĕs-păn"]
(papaverine HCl)
in sustained-release micro-dialysis cells

COMPOSITION
Each capsule provides 150 mg papaverine hydrochloride in micro-dialysis cells, uniquely processed for sustained release of medication to provide prolonged therapeutic effect.
Each capsule also contains alcohol, microcrystalline cellulose, pharmaceutical glaze, povidone, sucrose, and talc.

ACTIONS AND USES
The main actions of papaverine are exerted on cardiac and various smooth muscles. It relaxes the smooth musculature of the larger blood vessels, especially coronary, systemic peripheral, cerebral and pulmonary arteries. This relaxation may be prominent if spasm exists. The muscle cell is not paralyzed by papaverine, and still responds to drugs and other stimuli causing contraction. The antispasmodic effect is a direct one, and unrelated to muscle innervation. Papaverine is practically devoid of effects on the central nervous system.
Perhaps by its direct vasodilating action on cerebral blood vessels, papaverine increases cerebral blood flow and decreases cerebral vascular resistance in normal subjects; oxygen consumption is unaltered. These effects may explain the benefit reported from the drug in cerebral vascular encephalopathy.
Like quinidine, papaverine acts directly on heart muscle to depress conduction and prolong the refractory period. These direct actions provide the basis for its clinical trial in abrogating atrial and ventricular premature systoles and ominous ventricular arrhythmias.
The coronary vasodilator action could be an additional factor of therapeutic value when such rhythms are secondary to insufficiency or occlusion of the coronary arteries.
In patients with acute coronary thrombosis, the occurrence of ventricular rhythms is serious and requires measures designed to decrease myocardial irritability. Papaverine may have advantages over quinidine, used for a similar purpose, in that it may be given in an emergency by the intravenous route, does not depress myocardial contraction or cause cinchonism, and produces coronary vasodilation.

INDICATIONS
For the relief of cerebral and peripheral ischemia associated with arterial spasm and myocardial ischemia complicated by arrhythmias.

PRECAUTIONS
Use with caution in patients with glaucoma. Hepatic hypersensitivity has been reported with gastrointestinal symptoms, jaundice, eosinophilia and altered liver function tests. Discontinue drug if these occur.

SIDE EFFECTS
Although occurring rarely, the reported side effects of papaverine include nausea, abdominal distress, anorexia, constipation or diarrhea, skin rash, malaise, drowsiness, vertigo, sweating, and headache.

ADMINISTRATION AND DOSAGE
One capsule every 12 hours. In difficult cases administration may be increased to one capsule every 8 hours, or two capsules every 12 hours.

HOW SUPPLIED
Bottles of 100 and 1000.
Revised: May, 1986

DDAVP® [intranasal] ℞
(desmopressin acetate)
DDAVP® Injection ℞
(desmopressin acetate)
Combined Product Information

DESCRIPTION
DDAVP® (desmopressin acetate) is an antidiuretic hormone affecting renal water conservation and is a synthetic analogue of 8-arginine vasopressin. It is chemically defined as follows:
Mol. Wt. 1183.2
1-(3-mercaptopropionic acid)-8-D-arginine vasopressin monoacetate (salt) trihydrate.
DDAVP® [intranasal] is provided as a sterile, aqueous solution for intranasal use. Each ml contains:

Desmopressin acetate	0.1 mg
Chlorobutanol	5.0 mg
Sodium chloride	9.0 mg

Hydrochloric acid to adjust pH to approximately 4

DDAVP® Injection is provided as a sterile, aqueous solution for injection. Each ml provides:

Desmopressin acetate	4.0 mcg
Chlorobutanol	5.0 mg
Sodium chloride	9.0 mg

Hydrochloric acid to adjust pH to 3.5

CLINICAL PHARMACOLOGY

DDAVP contains as active substance, 1-(3-mercaptopropionic acid)-8-D-arginine vasopressin, a synthetic analogue of the natural hormone arginine vasopressin. One ml (0.1 mg) of DDAVP® [intranasal] has an antidiuretic activity of about 400 IU; 10 mcg is equivalent to 40 IU. One ml (4 mcg) of DDAVP® Injection has an antidiuretic activity of about 16 IU; 1 mcg is equivalent to 4 IU.

DDAVP® Injection has been shown to be more potent than arginine vasopressin in increasing plasma levels of factor VIII activity in patients with hemophilia and von Willebrand's disease Type I.

Dose-response studies were performed in healthy persons, using doses of 0.1 to 0.4 mcg/kg body weight, infused over a 10-minute period. Maximal dose response occurred at 0.3 to 0.4 mcg/kg. The response to DDAVP® Injection of factor VIII activity and plasminogen activator is dose-related, with maximal plasma levels of 300 to 400 percent of initial concentrations obtained after infusion of 0.4 mcg/kg body weight. The increase is rapid and evident within 30 minutes, reaching a maximum at a point ranging from 90 minutes to two hours. The factor VIII related antigen and ristocetin cofactor activity were also increased to a smaller degree, but still dose-dependent.

The biphasic half-lives of DDAVP were 7.8 and 75.5 minutes for the fast and slow phases, respectively, compared with 2.5 and 14.5 minutes for lysine vasopressin, another form of the hormone. As a result, DDAVP provides a prompt onset of antidiuretic action with a long duration after each administration.

The change in structure of arginine vasopressin to DDAVP has resulted in a decreased vasopressor action and decreased actions on visceral smooth muscle relative to the enhanced antidiuretic activity, so that clinically effective antidiuretic doses are usually below the threshold levels for effects on vascular or visceral smooth muscle.

When administered by injection, DDAVP® Injection has an antidiuretic effect about ten times that of an equivalent dose administered intranasally.

The bioavailability of the subcutaneous route of administration of DDAVP® Injection was determined qualitatively using urine output data. The exact fraction of drug absorbed by that route of administration has not been quantitatively determined.

The percentage increase of factor VIII levels in patients with mild hemophilia A and von Willebrand's disease was not significantly different from that observed in normal healthy individuals when treated with 0.3 mcg/kg of DDAVP® Injection infused over 10 minutes.

Plasminogen activator activity increases rapidly after DDAVP® Injection infusion, but there has been no clinically significant fibrinolysis in patients treated with DDAVP.

The effect of repeated administration of DDAVP® Injection when doses were given every 12 to 24 hours has generally shown a gradual diminution of the factor VIII activity increase noted with a single dose. The initial response is reproducible in any particular patient if there are 2 or 3 days between administrations.

INDICATIONS AND USAGE

Diabetes Insipidus—DDAVP is indicated as antidiuretic replacement therapy in the management of central (cranial) diabetes insipidus and for the management of the temporary polyuria and polydipsia following head trauma or surgery in the pituitary region. DDAVP is ineffective for the treatment of nephrogenic diabetes insipidus.

The use of DDAVP® [intranasal] in patients with an established diagnosis will result in a reduction in urinary output with increase in urine osmolality and a decrease in plasma osmolality. This will allow the resumption of a more normal life style with a decrease in urinary frequency and nocturia.

There are reports of an occasional change in response to DDAVP® [intranasal] with time, usually greater than six months. Some patients may show a decreased responsiveness, others a shortened duration of effect. There is no evidence this effect is due to the development of binding antibodies but may be due to a local inactivation of the peptide.

Patients are selected for therapy by establishing the diagnosis by means of the water deprivation test, the hypertonic saline infusion test, and/or the response to antidiuretic hormone. Continued response to DDAVP® [intranasal] can be monitored by urine volume and osmolality.

DDAVP® [intranasal] delivery can be compromised by a variety of factors that can make nasal insufflation ineffective or inappropriate. These include poor intranasal absorption, nasal congestion and blockage, nasal discharge, atrophy of nasal mucosa, and severe atrophic rhinitis. Intranasal delivery may be inappropriate where there is an impaired level of consciousness. In addition, cranial surgical procedures, such as transphenoidal hypophysectomy, create situations where an alternative route of administration is needed as in cases of nasal packing or recovery from surgery. For such situations, DDAVP® Injection should be considered.

Hemophilia A—DDAVP® Injection is indicated for patients with hemophilia A with factor VIII coagulant activity levels greater than 5%.

DDAVP® Injection will often maintain hemostasis in patients with hemophilia A during surgical procedures and postoperatively when administered 30 minutes prior to the scheduled procedure.

DDAVP® Injection will also stop bleeding in hemophilia A patients with episodes of spontaneous or trauma-induced injuries such as hemarthroses, intramuscular hematomas, or mucosal bleeding.

DDAVP® Injection is not indicated for the treatment of hemophilia A with factor VIII coagulant activity levels equal to or less than 5%, or for the treatment of hemophilia B, or in patients who have factor VIII antibodies.

In certain clinical situations, it may be justified to try DDAVP® Injection in patients with factor VIII levels between 2–5%; however, these patients should be carefully monitored.

Von Willebrand 's Disease (Type I)—DDAVP® Injection is indicated for patients with mild to moderate classic von Willebrand's disease (Type I) with factor VIII levels greater than 5%. DDAVP® Injection will often maintain hemostasis in patients with mild to moderate von Willebrand's disease during surgical procedures and postoperatively when administered 30 minutes prior to the scheduled procedure.

DDAVP® Injection will usually stop bleeding in mild to moderate von Willebrand's patients with episodes of spontaneous or trauma-induced injuries such as hemarthroses, intramuscular hematomas, or mucosal bleeding.

Those von Willebrand's disease patients who are least likely to respond are those with severe homozygous von Willebrand's disease with factor VIII coagulant activity and factor VIII von Willebrand factor antigen levels less than 1%. Other patients may respond in a variable fashion depending on the type of molecular defect they have. Bleeding time and factor VIII coagulant activity, ristocetin cofactor activity, and von Willebrand factor antigen should be checked during administration of DDAVP® Injection to ensure that adequate levels are being achieved.

DDAVP® Injection is not indicated for the treatment of severe classic von Willebrand's disease (Type I) and when there is evidence of an abnormal molecular form of factor VIII antigen. See WARNING.

CONTRAINDICATIONS

Known hypersensitivity to DDAVP.

WARNING

Patients who do not have need of antidiuretic hormone for its antidiuretic effect, in particular those who are young or elderly, should be cautioned to ingest only enough fluid to satisfy thirst, in order to decrease the potential occurrence of water intoxication and hyponatremia.

DDAVP® is for intranasal use only. DDAVP® Injection is for injection use only.

DDAVP® Injection should not be used to treat patients with Type IIB von Willebrand's disease since platelet aggregation may be induced.

PRECAUTIONS

General: DDAVP® [intranasal] at high dosage or DDAVP® Injection has infrequently produced a slight elevation of blood pressure, which disappeared with a reduction in dosage. The drug should be used with caution in patients with coronary artery insufficiency and/or hypertensive cardiovascular disease, because of possible rise in blood pressure.

Since DDAVP® is used intranasally, changes in the nasal mucosa such as scarring, edema, or other disease may cause erratic, unreliable absorption in which case intranasal DDAVP should not be used. For such situations, DDAVP® Injection should be considered.

Severe allergic reactions have not been reported with DDAVP® Injection. It is not known whether antibodies to DDAVP® Injection are produced after repeated injections.

Diabetes Insipidus—Laboratory tests for monitoring the patient include urine volume and osmolality. In some cases, plasma osmolality may be required.

Hemophilia A —Laboratory tests for assessing patient status include levels of factor VIII coagulant, factor VIII antigen, factor VIII ristocetin cofactor (von Willebrand factor) as well as activated partial thromboplastin time. Factor VIII coagulant activity should be determined before giving DDAVP® Injection for hemostasis. If factor VIII coagulant activity is present at less than 5% of normal, DDAVP® Injection should not be relied on.

Von Willebrand 's Disease —Laboratory tests for assessing patient status include levels of factor VIII coagulant activity, factor VIII ristocetin cofactor activity, and factor VIII von Willebrand factor antigen. The skin bleeding time may be helpful in following these patients.

DRUG INTERACTIONS: Although the pressor activity of DDAVP is very low compared with the antidiuretic activity, use of large doses of DDAVP® [intranasal] or use of doses as large as 0.3 mcg/kg of DDAVP® Injection with other pressor agents should be done only with careful patient monitoring.

DDAVP® Injection has been used with epsilon aminocaproic acid without adverse effects.

CARCINOGENICITY, MUTAGENICITY, IMPAIRMENT OF FERTILITY: Teratology studies in rats have shown no abnormalities. No further data are available.

PREGNANCY CATEGORY B: Reproduction studies performed in rats and rabbits with subcutaneous doses up to 12.5 times the human dose when used for factor VIII stimulation and 125 times the human dose when used in diabetes insipidus have revealed no evidence of harm to the fetus due to DDAVP. There are several publications of management of diabetes insipidus in pregnant women with no harm to the fetus reported; however, there are no adequate and well-controlled studies in pregnant women. Published reports stress that, as opposed to preparations containing the natural hormones, DDAVP in antidiuretic doses has no uterotonic action, but the physician will have to weigh possible therapeutic advantages against possible danger in each case.

NURSING MOTHERS: There have been no controlled studies in nursing mothers. A single study in a post-partum woman demonstrated a marked change in plasma, but little if any change in assayable DDAVP in breast milk following an intranasal dose of 10 mg.

It is not known whether the drug is excreted in human milk. Because many drugs are excreted in human milk, caution should be exercised when DDAVP is administered to a nursing woman.

PEDIATRIC USE: DDAVP® [intranasal] has been used in children with diabetes insipidus. The dose must be individually adjusted to the patient with attention in the very young to the danger of an extreme decrease in plasma osmolality with resulting convulsions. Dose should start at 0.05 ml or less.

Use of DDAVP in infants and children will require careful fluid intake restriction to prevent possible hyponatremia and water intoxication.

DDAVP® Injection should not be used in infants younger than three months in the treatment of hemophilia A or von Willebrand 's disease; safety and effectiveness in children under 12 years of age with diabetes insipidus have not been established.

ADVERSE REACTIONS

Infrequently, high dosages of DDAVP® [intranasal] have produced transient headache and nausea. Nasal congestion, rhinitis and flushing have also been reported occasionally along with mild abdominal cramps. These symptoms disappeared with reduction in dosage.

Infrequently, DDAVP® Injection has produced transient headache, nausea, mild abdominal cramps, and vulval pain. These symptoms disappeared with reduction in dosage. Occasionally, injection of DDAVP has produced local erythema, swelling, or burning pain. Occasional facial flushing has been reported with the administration of DDAVP® Injection.

DDAVP® Injection has infrequently produced a slight elevation of blood pressure, which disappeared with a reduction in dosage. See WARNING for the possibility of water intoxication and hyponatremia.

OVERDOSAGE

See ADVERSE REACTIONS above. In case of overdosage, the dose should be reduced, frequency of administration decreased, or the drug withdrawn according to the severity of the condition.

There is no known specific antidote for DDAVP.

An oral LD_{50} has not been established. An intravenous dose of 2 mg/kg in mice demonstrated no effect.

DOSAGE AND ADMINISTRATION

DDAVP® is administered into the nose through a soft flexible plastic nasal tube which has four graduation marks on it that measure 0.2, 0.15, 0.1 and 0.05 ml. The dosage must be determined for each individual patient and adjusted according to the diurnal pattern of response. Response should be estimated by two parameters: adequate duration of sleep and adequate, not excessive, water turnover. Patients with nasal congestion and blockage have often responded well to DDAVP.® The usual dosage range in adults is 0.1 to 0.4 ml daily, either as a single dose or divided into two or three doses. Most adults require 0.2 ml daily in two divided doses. The morning and evening doses should be separately adjusted for an adequate diurnal rythm of water turnover. For children aged three months to 12 years, the usual dosage

Continued on next page

USV—Cont.

range is 0.05 to 0.3 ml daily, either as a single dose or divided into two doses.
About one-quarter to one-third of patients can be controlled by a single daily dose of DDAVP® [intranasal].
DDAVP® Injection for *Diabetes Insipidus*—DDAVP® Injection is administered subcutaneously or by direct intravenous injection. The dosage must be determined for each patient and adjusted according to the pattern of response. Response should be estimated by two parameters: adequate duration of sleep, and adequate, not excessive, water turnover.
The usual dosage range in adults is 0.5 ml (2.0 mcg) to 1 ml (4.0 mcg) daily, administered intravenously or subcutaneously, usually in two divided doses. The morning and evening doses should be separately adjusted for an adequate diurnal rhythm of water turnover. For patients who have been controlled on intranasal DDAVP and who must be switched to the injection form, either because of poor intranasal absorption, or because of the need for surgery, the comparable antidiuretic dose of the injection is about one-tenth the intranasal dose.
DDAVP® Injection for *Hemophilia A and von Willebrand's Disease (Type I)*—DDAVP® Injection is administered as an intravenous infusion at a dose of 0.3 mcg DDAVP/kg body weight diluted in sterile physiological saline and infused slowly over 15 to 30 minutes. In adults and children weighing more than 10 kg, 50 ml of diluent is used; in children weighing 10 kg or less, 10 ml of diluent is used. Blood pressure and pulse should be monitored during infusion. If DDAVP® Injection is used preoperatively, it should be administered 30 minutes prior to the scheduled procedure.
The necessity for repeat administration of DDAVP® Injection or use of any blood products for hemostasis should be determined by laboratory response as well as the clinical condition of the patient. The tendency toward tachyphylaxis (lessening of response) with repeated administration given more frequently than every 48 hours should be considered in treating each patient.
Parenteral drug products should be inspected visually for particulate matter and discoloration prior to administration whenever solution and container permit.

HOW SUPPLIED

DDAVP® [intranasal] 2.5 ml per vial, packaged with two applicator tubes per carton (NDC 0075-2450-01). Keep refrigerated at about 4°C. When traveling —controlled room temperature (22°C) closed sterile bottles will maintain stability for three weeks.
DDAVP® Injection is available as a sterile solution in cartons of ten 1 ml single-dose ampules (NDC 0075-2451-01) each containing 4.0 mcg DDAVP per ml. Keep refrigerated at about 4°C.

CAUTION

Federal (USA) law prohibits dispensing without prescription.
Revised: May, 1986

Shown in Product Identification Section, page 433

DEMI-REGROTON® ℞

[dĕm"ē-rĕg'rō-tōn]
Oral antihypertensive

See under Regroton®.
Shown in Product Identification Section, page 433

DORIDEN® Ⓒ

[dôr'ĭ-dĭn"]
glutethimide USP

0.5 g tablets
0.25 g tablets

DESCRIPTION

DORIDEN (glutethimide), an oral hypnotic, is a piperidinedione derivative that occurs as a white, crystalline powder and is practically insoluble in water, soluble in alcohol. Its chemical name is 2-ethyl-2-phenylglutarimide.
The tablets also contain corn starch, magnesium aluminum silicate, methylcellulose, colloidal silica, and stearic acid.

CLINICAL PHARMACOLOGY

Doriden is erratically absorbed from the gastrointestinal tract. Following single oral doses of 500 mg, wide variations in absorption of the drug were observed, and the peak plasma concentration occurred from one to six hours after administration. The average plasma half-life is 10–12 hours.
Glutethimide is a racemate; both isomers are hydroxylated; the d-isomer on the piperidinedione ring and the l-isomer on the phenyl substituent. Both hydroxylates are conjugated with glucuronic acid; the glucuronides pass into the enterohepatic circulation, and thence are excreted in the urine. Less than 2% of a usual dose is excreted in the urine unchanged. About 50% of the drug is bound to plasma proteins.
Glutethimide exhibits pronounced anticholinergic activity, which is manifested by mydriasis, inhibition of salivary secretions, and decreased intestinal motility.

INDICATIONS AND USAGE

Glutethimide has been shown to be effective as a hypnotic for three to seven days. It is not indicated for chronic administration. Should insomnia persist, a drug-free interval of one or more weeks should elapse before retreatment is considered. Attempts should be made to find alternative nondrug therapy in chronic insomnia.

CONTRAINDICATIONS

Glutethimide is contraindicated in patients with known hypersensitivity to the drug. It is also contraindicated in patients with porphyria.

WARNINGS

The concomitant use of alcohol or other CNS depressants may produce additive CNS depressant effects.

PRECAUTIONS

Information for Patients: The patient should be warned about the possible additive effects when glutethimide is taken concomitantly with other central nervous system depressants such as alcohol.
The patient on Doriden must be warned against driving a car or operating dangerous machinery while on the drug, since glutethimide may impair the ability to perform hazardous activities requiring mental alertness or physical coordination.
Drug Interactions: Glutethimide induces hepatic microsomal enzymes resulting in increased metabolism of coumarin anticoagulants and decreased anticoagulant response.
Carcinogenesis: No carcinogenicity studies in animals have been performed.
Pregnancy/Teratogenic Effects: *Pregnancy Category C.* Animal reproduction studies have not been conducted with glutethimide. It is also not known *whether glutethimide can cause fetal harm when administered to a pregnant woman or can affect reproduction capacity. Glutethimide should be given to a pregnant woman only if clearly needed.*
Nursing Mothers: Because of the potential for serious adverse reactions in nursing infants from glutethimide, a decision should be made whether to discontinue nursing or to discontinue the drug, taking into account the importance of the drug to the mother.
Pediatric Use: Glutethimide is not recommended for use in children, because its safety and effectiveness in the pediatric age group have not been established by clinical trials.

ADVERSE REACTIONS

In clinical studies in more than 796 patients 8.6% exhibited skin rash, 2.7% reported nausea, 1.1% hangover, and 1% reported drowsiness. The following reactions occurred in less than 1% of the patient population: vertigo, headache, depression, dizziness, ataxia, confusion, edema, indigestion, lightheadedness, nocturnal diaphoresis, vomiting, dry mouth, euphoria, impaired memory, slurred speech, and tinnitus. Paradoxical excitation, blurred vision, acute hypersensitivity, porphyria, and blood dyscrasia such as thrombocytopenic purpura, aplastic anemia, and leukopenia are rare.
In cases in which a generalized skin rash occurs, the medication should be withdrawn. This rash usually clears spontaneously within a few days after drug withdrawal.

DRUG ABUSE AND DEPENDENCE

Controlled Substance: This drug is controlled in Schedule III.
Dependence: Both physical and psychological dependence have occurred; therefore patients should be carefully evaluated before prescribing Doriden (glutethimide). Ordinarily, an amount adequate for one week is sufficient. The patient should be reevaluated before represcribing, after an interval of one or more weeks. Withdrawal symptoms include nausea, abdominal discomfort, tremors, convulsions, and delirium. Newborn infants of mothers dependent on glutethimide may also exhibit withdrawal symptoms. In the presence of dependence dosage should be reduced gradually.

OVERDOSAGE

Acute Overdosage: The single acute lethal dose of glutethimide in humans ranges from 10 g to 20 g. Although the majority of fatalities have resulted from single doses in this range, patients have died from single doses as low as 5 g and have recovered from single doses as high as 35 g. A single oral dose of 5 g usually produces severe intoxication. A plasma level of 3 mg/100 ml is indicative of severe poisoning, but the level may be higher if the patient is tolerant to the drug. However, the level may also be lower because of sequestration of the drug in body fat depots and in the gastrointestinal tract. A lower level does not preclude the possibility of severe poisoning; therefore, the extent of intoxication may not be accurately reflected by single glutethimide plasma level determinations. Serial determinations are mandatory for proper patient evaluation.
Ingestion of acutely excessive dosage of glutethimide can give rise to a life-threatening situation. The effects of glutethimide are exaggerated by concomitant ingestion of other hypnotics or sedatives such as alcohol, barbiturates, etc., and suicidal effects commonly involve multiple drugs of the sedative-hypnotic-tranquilizer types.
Signs and Symptoms: The principal signs and symptoms caused by glutethimide intoxication vary in severity in ratio to the ingested dosage, in general, and are indistinguishable from those caused by barbiturate intoxication. The degree of CNS depression often fluctuates, possibly due to irregular absorption of the drug and/or accumulation of an active toxic metabolite, 4-hydroxy-2-ethyl-2-phenyl-glutarimide (4-HG). They are: CNS depression, including coma *(profound and prolonged in severe intoxication)*; hypothermia, which may be followed by fever even without apparent infection; depressed or lost deep tendon reflexes; depression or absence of corneal and pupillary reflexes; dilation of pupils; depressed or absent response to painful stimuli; inadequate ventilation (even with relatively normal respiratory rate), sometimes with cyanosis; sudden apnea, especially with manipulation such as gastric lavage or endotracheal intubation; diminished or absent peristalsis. Severe hypotension unresponsive to volume expansion, tonic muscular spasms, twitching and convulsions may occur.
Treatment: As with all forms of acute intoxication, the sooner adequate treatment is instituted, the better the prognosis. Early and vigorous cardiopulmonary supportive measures should be employed and should include:
1) Maintenance of a patent airway with assisted ventilation if necessary.
2) Monitoring of vital signs and level of consciousness.
3) Continuous electrocardiogram to detect arrhythmias.
4) Maintenance of blood pressure with plasma volume expanders and, if absolutely essential, pressor drugs.
Blood for glutethimide levels and other chemical determinations should be obtained as well as arterial blood for blood gas determinations.
Vomiting should be induced if the patient is fully conscious. Gastric lavage should be done in all cases regardless of elapsed time since drug ingestion, with due caution to prevent aspiration of gastric contents or respiratory arrest during manipulation, including prior insertion of a cuffed endotracheal tube or employment of tracheostomy. Lavage with a 1:1 mixture of castor oil and water is capable of removing larger amounts of glutethimide from the stomach than with aqueous lavage. Fifty ml of castor oil should be left in the stomach as a cathartic.
Intestinal lavage is used to remove unabsorbed Doriden (glutethimide) from the intestines (100–250 ml of 20–40% sorbitol or mannitol). If emesis or gastric lavage cannot be effected in the fully conscious patient, delay absorption of Doriden by giving one pint of water, milk or fruit juice; flour or cornstarch suspension, or activated charcoal in water. Follow up as soon as possible with production of emesis or gastric lavage.
Adequate respiratory gas exchange must be maintained and may require tracheostomy and mechanical assistance. If coma is prolonged, urine output must be monitored and maintained while preventing overhydration which might contribute to pulmonary or cerebral edema.
In *Severe Intoxication*, in addition to intensive supportive measures and symptomatic care, consideration should be given to dialysis or hemoperfusion in the following circumstances: Grade III or Grade IV coma, but the level of coma per se is not a mandatory indication for the procedure. Hemodialysis may also be required when renal shutdown or impaired renal function are manifest and in life-threatening overdose situations complicated by (a) pulmonary edema, (b) heart failure, (c) circulatory collapse, (d) significant liver disease, (e) major metabolic disturbance, (f) uremia. While aqueous hemodialysis is less effective for glutethimide than for readily water-soluble compounds that are not bound by proteins or sequestered in body fat depots, glutethimide blood levels may decline more rapidly with hemodialysis and the duration of coma may be shortened; efficacy of the procedure, however, is largely controversial. As long as significant amounts of glutethimide remain in fat depots or as an unabsorbed bolus in the intestinal tract, the fall in serum level accelerated by hemodialysis may be followed by increased absorption into the bloodstream on termination of dialysis and may require further dialysis.
Recent clinical data indicate that use of pure food-grade soybean oil as the dialysate enhances removal of glutethimide and some other lipid-soluble substances by means of hemodialysis. Peritoneal dialysis, while able to remove some glutethimide, apparently is of minimal value.
Hemoperfusion appears to be a promising technique for eliminating glutethimide from the body. Charcoal hemoperfusion utilizing acrylic hydrogel microencapsulation of activated charcoal has been reported to be simpler and more effective than hemodialysis. Similarly, a microcapsule artificial kidney has been developed utilizing activated charcoal granules encapsulated with cellulose nitrate and albumin. *Resin* hemoperfusion utilizing a column containing Amberlite XAD-2 has demonstrated exceptionally high clear-

ance capabilities in glutethimide intoxication and has been reported to be clinically superior to hemodialysis in patients with profound life-threatening coma and potentially lethal blood concentrations of intoxicant drugs.
Drug extraction techniques should be continued for at least two hours after the patient regains consciousness. Glutethimide is highly lipid soluble and therefore, rapidly accumulated in lipoid tissue. As the drug is removed from the bloodstream by any technique, it is gradually released from fat storage depots back into the bloodstream. Even after substantial quantities of the drug have been extracted, this blood-level rebound can cause coma to persist or recur.
As in the case of any prolonged coma, appropriate antibiotic therapy is indicated if pulmonary or other infection intervenes.
Chronic Overdosage: Signs and symptoms of chronic glutethimide intoxication (and for all drugs producing barbiturate-alcohol type of dependence in chronic overdosage) include impairment of memory and ability to concentrate, impaired gait, ataxia, tremors, hyporeflexia, and slurring of speech. Abrupt discontinuance of glutethimide after prolonged overdosage will in most cases cause withdrawal reactions ranging from nervousness and anxiety to grand mal seizures, and may include abdominal cramping, chills, numbness of extremities and dysphagia.
Treatment: Chronic glutethimide intoxication may be treated by gradual, stepwise reduction of dosage over a period of days or weeks. Watch patient carefully. If withdrawal reactions occur, they can be controlled by readministration of glutethimide, or substitution of pentobarbital, and subsequent gradual withdrawal.

DOSAGE AND ADMINISTRATION

For use as a hypnotic, dosage should be individualized. The usual adult dosage is 0.25 to 0.5 g at bedtime. For elderly or debilitated patients, the initial daily dosage should not exceed 0.5 g at bedtime, in order to avoid oversedation.

HOW SUPPLIED

DORIDEN (glutethimide). Tablets, 0.5 g (white, scored); bottles of 100 (NDC 0105-0354-00), 500 (NDC 0105-0354-05), 1000 (NDC 0105-0354-99) and Strip Dispensers of 100 (NDC 0105-0354-61). Tablets, 0.25 g (white, scored); bottles of 100 (NDC 0105-0353-00).
Revised: 5/86

GASTROLYTE™

Oral Electrolyte Concentrate

DIRECTIONS FOR USE

Dissolve one packet of Gastrolyte™ in 7 fluid ounces (200 mL) of drinking water (to fill line). Only drinking water may be used to reconstitute Gastrolyte™. The solution should be made up immediately before use. If refrigerated, the solution may be stored for up to 24 hours, otherwise any solution remaining an hour after reconstitution should be discarded.
Each packet consumed provides: 18 mEq (410 mg) of sodium, 16 mEq of chloride, 6 mEq of citrate, and 4 mEq of potassium.
For children under 2 years: Consult your physician.
For children 2–12 years: Up to 2 fluid ounces/lb of body weight daily.
For adults: 7 fluid ounces (200 mL) of Gastrolyte™ solution after every loose bowel movement.

PRECAUTIONS

For oral use only. Each packet of Gastrolyte™ should always be dissolved in 7 fluid ounces of drinking water. Consult your physician if vomiting or fever is present or if diarrhea continues beyond 48 hours.

Shown in Product Identification Section, page 433

HISTASPAN-D® ℞

[*hĭst 'ŭ-spăn-dē "*]
in sustained-release micro-dialysis cells

COMPOSITION

Each Histaspan-D capsule provides 8 mg chlorpheniramine maleate, 20 mg phenylephrine hydrochloride, and 2.5 mg methscopolamine nitrate in sustained-release micro-dialysis cells, uniquely processed for sustained release of medication to provide prolonged therapeutic effect.
The capsules also contain alcohol, calcium silicate, pharmaceutical glaze, povidone, sucrose, and talc.

ACTION

Histaspan-D combines the highly effective and widely used antihistamine, chlorpheniramine maleate, with a decongestant, phenylephrine hydrochloride, and a drying agent, methscopolamine nitrate, for relief of rhinorrhea, sneezing, lacrimation, nasal congestion, and other respiratory symptoms accompanying the common cold, sinusitis, hay fever and similar allergic conditions. Prolonged therapeutic effect is obtained by sustained release of medication through the micro-dialysis process.

INDICATIONS

One capsule q. 12 h. usually provides relief of rhinorrhea, sneezing, lacrimation, itching of eyes and nose, and nasal congestion accompanying upper respiratory infections such as the common cold and sinusitis; and hay fever and similar allergic conditions.

CONTRAINDICATIONS

Hypersensitivity to any component of the drug, glaucoma, paralytic ileus, pyloric obstruction and prostatic hypertrophy.

PRECAUTIONS

Use with caution in diabetes mellitus, hyperthyroidism, hypertension, cardiovascular disease, debilitated patients with chronic lung disease, in the aged and in children under age 12. Since blurred vision, drowsiness and dizziness may occur, patients should be cautioned about driving or operating machinery.

ADVERSE REACTIONS

May include drowsiness, dizziness, blurred vision, and excessive dryness of the nose, throat and mouth. Other possible adverse reactions to individual components, infrequently seen, include photophobia, tachycardia, gastrointestinal symptoms, increased irritability or excitement, flushing, incoordination, headache, nervousness, weakness and urinary disturbances.

ADMINISTRATION AND DOSAGE

Adults and children over age 12, one capsule in the morning and one at night (q. 12 h.).

HOW SUPPLIED

Bottles of 100 and 1000 capsules.
Revised: May, 1986

HISTASPAN®-PLUS ℞

[*hĭst 'ŭ-spăn-plŭs "*]
in sustained-release micro-dialysis cells

COMPOSITION

Each Histaspan-Plus capsule provides 8 mg chlorpheniramine maleate and 20 mg phenylephrine hydrochloride in sustained-release micro-dialysis cells, uniquely processed for sustained release of medication to provide prolonged therapeutic effect.
The capsules also contain alcohol, calcium silicate, pharmaceutical glaze, povidone, sucrose, and talc.

INDICATIONS

Antihistaminic and decongestant for relief of nasal congestion and other respiratory symptoms accompanying the common cold, sinusitis, hay fever and similar allergic conditions.

CONTRAINDICATION

Hypersensitivity to any component of the drug.

PRECAUTIONS

Use with caution in diabetes mellitus, hyperthyroidism, hypertension and cardiovascular disease. Since blurred vision, drowsiness or dizziness may occur, patients should be cautioned about driving or operating machinery.

ADVERSE REACTIONS

May include drowsiness, dizziness, blurred vision, dry mouth, disturbed coordination, G.I. disturbance, tachycardia, headache, nervousness, weakness and urinary disturbances.

DOSAGE

Adults and children over age 12, one capsule every 12 hours.

HOW SUPPLIED

Bottles of 100.
5/86

HYGROTON® ℞

[*hī 'grō-tŏn "*]
(chlorthalidone USP)
Oral antihypertensive-diuretic

COMPOSITION

Each tablet provides 25 mg, 50 mg or 100 mg chlorthalidone.

DESCRIPTION

HYGROTON (chlorthalidone) is an oral antihypertensive/-diuretic. It is a monosulfamyl diuretic that differs chemically from thiazide diuretics in that a double-ring system is incorporated in its structure. It is 2-chloro-5-(1-hydroxy-3-oxo-1-isoindolinyl) benzenesulfonamide. Chlorthalidone is practically insoluble in water, in ether and in chloroform; soluble in methanol; slightly soluble in alcohol.
HYGROTON tablets also contain colloidal silica, corn starch, gelatin, glycerin, lactose, magnesium stearate, talc, and other ingredients. The 25 mg tablets also contain F.D.&C. Yellow #6, methylparaben, and propylparaben. The 50 mg tablets also contain F.D.&C. Blue #1, methylparaben, and propylparaben.

CLINICAL PHARMACOLOGY

HYGROTON is an oral diuretic with prolonged action (48–72 hours) and low toxicity. The major portion of the drug is excreted unchanged by the kidneys. The diuretic effect of the drug occurs in approximately 2.6 hours and continues for up to 72 hours. The mean half-life following a 50 to 200 mg dose is 40 hours. In the first order of absorption, the elimination half-life is 53 hours following a 50 mg dose, and 60 hours following a 100 mg dose. Approximately 75 percent of the drug is bound to plasma proteins, 58 percent of the drug being bound to albumin. This is caused by an increased affinity of the drug to erythrocyte carbonic anhydrase. Nonrenal routes of elimination have yet to be clarified. Data are not available regarding percentage of dose as unchanged drug and metabolites, concentration of the drug in body fluids, degree of uptake by a particular organ or in the fetus, or passage across the blood-brain barrier.
The drug produces copious diuresis with greatly increased excretion of sodium and chloride. At maximal therapeutic dosage, chlorthalidone is approximately equal in its diuretic effect to comparable maximal therapeutic doses of benzothiadiazine diuretics. The site of action appears to be the cortical diluting segment of the ascending limb of Henle's loop of the nephron.

INDICATIONS AND USAGE

Diuretics such as HYGROTON are indicated in the management of hypertension either as the sole therapeutic agent or to enhance the effect of other antihypertensive drugs in the more severe forms of hypertension.
HYGROTON is indicated as adjunctive therapy in edema associated with congestive heart failure, hepatic cirrhosis, and corticosteroid and estrogen therapy.
HYGROTON has also been found useful in edema due to various forms of renal dysfunction such as nephrotic syndrome, acute glomerulonephritis, and chronic renal failure.
USAGE IN PREGNANCY: The routine use of diuretics in an otherwise healthy woman is inappropriate and exposes mother and fetus to unnecessary hazard. Diuretics do not prevent development of toxemia of pregnancy, and there is no satisfactory evidence that they are useful in the treatment of developed toxemia.
Edema during pregnancy may arise from pathological causes or from the physiologic and mechnical consequences of pregnancy. Chlorthalidone is indicated in pregnancy when edema is due to pathologic causes, just as it is in the absence of pregnancy (however, see Warnings, below). Dependent edema in pregnancy, resulting from restriction of venous return by the expanded uterus, is properly treated through elevation of the lower extremities and use of support hose; use of diuretics to lower intravascular volume in this case is illogical and unnecessary. There is hypervolemia during normal pregnancy that is harmful to neither the fetus nor the mother (in the absence of cardiovascular disease), but that is associated with edema, including generalized edema, in the majority of pregnant women. If this edema produces discomfort, increased recumbency will often provide relief. In rare instances, this edema may cause extreme discomfort that is not relieved by rest. In these cases, a short course of diuretics may provide relief and may be appropriate.

CONTRAINDICATIONS

Anuria.
Known hypersensitivity to chlorthalidone or other sulfonamide-derived drugs.

WARNINGS

Chlorthalidone should be used with caution in severe renal disease. In patients with renal disease, chlorthalidone or related drugs may precipitate azotemia. Cumulative effects of the drug may develop in patients with impaired renal function.
Chlorthalidone should be used with caution in patients with impaired hepatic function or progressive liver disease, because minor alterations of fluid and electrolyte balance may precipitate hepatic coma.
Sensitivity reactions may occur in patients with a history of allergy or bronchial asthma.
The possibility of exacerbation or activation of systemic lupus erythematosus has been reported with thiazide diuretics, which are structurally related to chlorthalidone. However, systemic lupus erythematosus has not been reported following chlorthalidone administration.

PRECAUTIONS

GENERAL: Hypokalemia may develop with chlorthalidone as with any other potent diuretic, especially with brisk diuresis, when severe cirrhosis is present, or during concomitant use of corticosteroids or ACTH.
Interference with adequate oral electrolyte intake will also contribute to hypokalemia. Digitalis therapy may exaggerate metabolic effects of hypokalemia especially with reference to myocardial activity.

Continued on next page

USV—Cont.

Any chloride deficit is generally mild and usually does not require specific treatment except under extraordinary circumstances (as in liver disease or renal disease). Dilutional hyponatremia may occur in edematous patients in hot weather; appropriate therapy is water restriction, rather than administration of salt except in rare instances when the hyponatremia is life threatening. In actual salt depletion, appropriate replacement is the therapy of choice.
Hyperuricemia may occur or frank gout may be precipitated in certain patients receiving chlorthalidone.
The antihypertensive effects of the drug may be enhanced in the postsympathectomy patient.
If progressive renal impairment becomes evident, as indicated by a rising nonprotein nitrogen or blood urea nitrogen, a careful reappraisal of therapy is necessary with consideration given to withholding or discontinuing diuretic therapy.
INFORMATION FOR PATIENTS: Patients should inform their doctor if they have; 1) had an allergic reaction to HYGROTON or other diuretics or have asthma, 2) kidney disease 3) liver disease 4) gout 5) systemic lupus erythematosus, or 6) been taking other drugs such as cortisone, digitalis, lithium carbonate, or drugs for diabetes.
Patients should be cautioned to contact their physician if they experience any of the following symptoms of potassium loss: excess thirst, tiredness, drowsiness, restlessness, muscle pains or cramps, nausea, vomiting or increased heart rate or pulse.
Patients should also be cautioned that taking alcohol can increase the chance of dizziness occurring.
LABORATORY TESTS: Periodic determination of serum electrolytes to detect possible electrolyte imbalance should be performed at appropriate intervals.
All patients receiving chlorthalidone should be observed for clinical signs of fluid or electrolyte imbalance: namely, hyponatremia, hypochloremic alkalosis, and hypokalemia. Serum and urine electrolyte determinations are particularly important when the patient is vomiting excessively or receiving parenteral fluids.
DRUG INTERACTIONS: Chlorthalidone may add to or potentiate the action of other antihypertensive drugs. Potentiation occurs with ganglionic or peripheral adrenergic blocking drugs.
Medication such as digitalis may also influence serum electrolytes. Warning signs, irrespective of cause, are: Dryness of mouth, thirst, weakness, lethargy, drowsiness, restlessness, muscle pains or cramps, muscular fatigue, hypotension, oliguria, tachycardia, and gastrointestinal disturbances such as nausea and vomiting.
Insulin requirements in diabetic patients may be increased, decreased or unchanged. Higher dosage of oral hypoglycemic agents may be required. Latent diabetes mellitus may become manifest during chlorthalidone administration.
Chlorthalidone and related drugs may increase the responsiveness to tubocurarine.
Chlorthalidone and related drugs may decrease arterial responsiveness to norepinephrine. This diminution is not sufficient to preclude effectiveness of the pressor agent for therapeutic use.
DRUG/LABORATORY TEST INTERACTIONS: Chlorthalidone and related drugs may decrease serum PBI levels without signs of thyroid disturbance.
CARCINOGENESIS, MUTAGENESIS, IMPAIRMENT OF FERTILITY: No information is available.
PREGNANCY/TERATOGENIC EFFECTS: Pregnancy Category B: Reproduction studies have been performed in the rat and the rabbit at doses up to 420 times the human dose and have revealed no evidence of impaired fertility or harm to the fetus due to chlorthalidone. There are, however, no adequate and well-controlled studies in pregnant women. Because animal reproduction studies are not always predictive of human response, this drug should be used during pregnancy only if clearly needed.
PREGNANCY/NON-TERATOGENIC EFFECTS: Thiazides cross the placental barrier and appear in cord blood. The use of chlorthalidone and related drugs in pregnant women requires that the anticipated benefits of the drug be weighed against possible hazards to the fetus. These hazards include fetal or neonatal jaundice, thrombocytopenia, and possibly other adverse reactions that have occurred in the adult.
NURSING MOTHERS: Thiazides are excreted in human milk. Because of the potential for serious adverse reactions in nursing infants from chlorthalidone, a decision should be made whether to discontinue nursing or to discontinue the drug, taking into account the importance of the drug to the mother.
PEDIATRIC USE: Safety and effectiveness in children have not been established.

ADVERSE REACTIONS

The following adverse reactions have been observed, but there is not enough systematic collection of data to support an estimate of their frequency.

Gastrointestinal System Reactions:

anorexia	diarrhea
gastric irritation	constipation
nausea	jaundice (intrahepatic
vomiting	cholestatic jaundice)
cramping	pancreatitis

Central Nervous System Reactions:

dizziness	headache
vertigo	xanthopsia
paresthesias	

Hematologic Reactions:

leukopenia	thrombocytopenia
agranulocytosis	aplastic anemia

Dermatologic-Hypersensitivity Reactions:

purpura	necrotizing angiitis
photosensitivity	(vasculitis)
rash	(cutaneous vasculitis)
urticaria	Lyell's syndrome (toxic epidermal necrolysis)

Cardiovascular Reaction: Orthostatic hypotension may occur and may be aggravated by alcohol, barbiturates or narcotics.

Other Adverse Reactions:

hyperglycemia	muscle spasm
glycosuria	weakness
hyperuricemia	restlessness
	impotence

Whenever adverse reactions are moderate or severe, chlorthalidone dosage should be reduced or therapy withdrawn.

OVERDOSAGE

Symptoms of acute overdosage include nausea, weakness, dizziness, and disturbances of electrolyte balance. The oral LD_{50} of the drug in the mouse and the rat is more than 25,000 mg/kg body weight. The minimum lethal dose (MLD) in humans has not been established. There is no specific antidote, but gastric lavage is recommended, followed by supportive treatment. Where necessary, this may include intravenous dextrose-saline with potassium, administered with caution.

DOSAGE AND ADMINISTRATION

Therapy should be initiated with the lowest possible dose. This dose should be titrated according to individual patient response to gain maximal therapeutic benefit while maintaining the minimal dosage possible. A single dose given in the morning with food is recommended; divided doses are unnecessary.
Hypertension: *Initiation:* Therapy, in most patients, should be initiated with a single daily dose of 25 mg. If the response is insufficient after a suitable trial, the dosage may be increased to a single daily dose of 50 mg. If additional control is required, the dosage of HYGROTON (chlorthalidone) may be increased to 100 mg once daily or a second antihypertensive drug (step-2 therapy) may be added. Dosage above 100 mg daily usually does not increase effectiveness. Increases in serum uric acid and decreases in serum potassium are dose-related over the 25–100 mg day range.
Maintenance: Maintenance doses may be lower than initial doses and should be adjusted according to individual patient response. Effectiveness is well sustained during continued use.
Edema: *Initiation:* Adults, initially 50 to 100 mg daily, or 100 mg on alternate days. Some patients may require 150 to 200 mg at these intervals, or up to 200 mg daily. Dosages above this level, however, do not usually produce a greater response.
Maintenance: Maintenance doses may often be lower than initial doses and should be adjusted according to the individual patient. Effectiveness is well sustained during continued use.

HOW SUPPLIED

HYGROTON (chlorthalidone) is available as 25 mg peach-color, uniquely-shaped* tablets in bottles of 100 (NDC 0070-0022-00), 1000 (NDC 0070-0022-99), and unit-dose blister packs, boxes of 100 (10 × 10 strips) (NDC 0070-0022-62); 50 mg aqua, uniquely-shaped* tablets in bottles of 100 (NDC 0070-0020-00), 1000 (NDC 0070-0020-99), 5000 (NDC 0070-0020-65), and unit-dose blister packs, boxes of 100 (10 × 10 strips) (NDC 0070-0020-62); 100 mg white, single-scored tablets in bottles of 100 (NDC 0070-0021-00), 1000 (NDC 0070-0021-99), 5000 (NDC 0070-0021-65), and unit-dose blister packs, boxes of 100 (10 × 10 strips) (NDC 0070-0021-62).
Store at controlled room temperature between 15°–30°C (59°–86°F). Dispense in tight containers as defined in USP.
*Design patent pending. The appearance of HYGROTON 25 mg and 50 mg tablets is a trademark of USV Laboratories, Inc.
CAUTION: Federal (USA) law prohibits dispensing without prescription.

ANIMAL PHARMACOLOGY

Biochemical studies in animals have suggested reasons for the prolonged effect of chlorthalidone. Absorption from the gastrointestinal tract is slow, due to its low solubility. After passage to the liver, some of the drug enters the general circulation, while some is excreted in the bile, to be reabsorbed later. In the general circulation, it is distributed widely to the tissues, but is taken up in highest concentrations by the kidneys, where amounts have been found 72 hours after ingestion, long after it has disappeared from other tissues. The drug is excreted unchanged in the urine.
Revised: May 1985

Shown in Product Identification Section, page 433

LEVOTHROID® TABLETS ℞
(T_4 Thyroxine Sodium Tablets, USP)
for oral use

LEVOTHROID® FOR INJECTION ℞
(T_4 Thyroxine Sodium)
for parenteral use

DESCRIPTION

LEVOTHROID® Tablets (T_4 Thyroxine Sodium, USP) provides crystalline T_4 thyroxine sodium, a potent thyroid hormone, in nine different strengths to permit easy convenient dosage adjustment. The inactive ingredients are microcrystalline cellulose, lactose, magnesium stearate and silica. The tablets also contain the following dyes: 25 mcg—F.D.&C. Red No. 40 and F.D.&C. Yellow No. 10; 75 mcg—F.D.&C. Blue No. 1, F.D.&C. Red No. 40 and F.D.&C. Yellow No. 10; 100 mcg—F.D.&C. Red No. 40 and F.D.&C. Yellow No. 10; 125 mcg—F.D.&C. Blue No. 1 and F.D.&C. Red No. 40; 150 mcg—F.D.&C. Blue No. 1; 175 mcg—F.D.&C. Blue No. 1, F.D.&C. Red No. 40, and F.D.&C. Yellow No. 10; 200 mcg—F.D.&C. Red No. 40; 300 mcg—F.D.&C. Blue No. 1, F.D.&C. Red No. 40, and F.D.&C. Yellow No. 10.
LEVOTHROID FOR INJECTION (T_4 Thyroxine Sodium) is a sterile, lyophilized powder supplied in 6 mL vials containing 200 or 500 mcg of T_4 thyroxine sodium U.S.P. with 15 mg of mannitol.

CLINICAL PHARMACOLOGY

The major thyroid hormones are T_4 thyroxine and T_3 thyronine. The amounts of T_4 thyroxine and T_3 thyronine released into the circulation from the normally functioning thyroid gland are regulated by the amount of thyrotropin (TSH) secreted from the anterior pituitary gland. TSH secretion is in turn regulated by the levels of circulating T_4 thyroxine and T_3 thyronine and by secretion of thyrotropin releasing factor (TRH) from the hypothalamus. Recognition of this complex feedback system is important in the diagnosis and treatment of thyroid dysfunction.
The principal effect of exogenous thyroid hormones is to increase the metabolic rate of body tissues.
The thyroid hormones are also concerned with growth and differentiation of tissues. In deficiency states in the young there is retardation of growth and failure of maturation of the skeletal and other body systems, especially in failure of ossification in the epiphyses and in the growth and development of the brain.
The precise mechanism of action by which thyroid hormones affect thermogenesis and cellular growth and differentiation is not known. It is recognized that these physiologic effects are mediated at the cellular level primarily by T_3 thyronine, a large part of which is derived from T_4 thyroxine by deiodination in the peripheral tissues. T_4 thyroxine is the major component of normal secretions of the thyroid gland and is thus the primary determinant of normal thyroid function.
Depending on other factors, absorption has varied from 48 to 79 percent of the administered dose. Fasting increases absorption. Malabsorption syndromes, as well as dietary factors, (children's soybean formula, concomitant use of anionic exchange resins such as cholestyramine) cause excessive fecal loss.
More than 99 percent of circulating hormones are bound to serum proteins, including thyroid-binding globulin (TB_g), thyroid-binding prealbumin (TBPA), and albumin (TB_a), whose capacities and affinities vary for the hormones.
T_4 thyroxine displays greater binding affinity than T_3 thyronine, both in the circulation and at the cellular level, which explains its longer duration of action. The half-life of T_4 thyroxine in normal plasma is 6–7 days while that of T_3 thyronine is about 1 day. The plasma half-lives of T_4 thyroxine and T_3 thyronine are decreased in hyperthyroidism and increased in hypothyroidism.

INDICATIONS AND USAGE

LEVOTHROID (T_4 Thyroxine Sodium, USP) is indicated as replacement or substitution therapy for diminished or absent thyroid function (e.g., cretinism, myxedema, non-toxic goiter or hypothyroidism generally, including the hypothyroid state in children, in pregnancy and in the elderly) resulting from functional deficiency, primary atrophy, from partial or complete absence of the gland or from the effects of surgery, radiation or antithyroid agents. Therapy must be maintained continuously to control the symptoms of hypothyroidism.
It may also be used to suppress the secretion of thyrotropin (TSH) action which may be beneficial in simple nonendemic goiter and in chronic lymphocytic thyroiditis. This may cause a reduction in the goiter size.

Thyroid hormone drugs are indicated as a diagnostic agent in suppression tests to differentiate suspected mild hyperthyroidism or thyroid gland autonomy.
Thyroid hormones may also be used with antithyroid drugs to treat thyrotoxicosis. This combination has been used to prevent goitrogenesis and hypothyroidism. This may be particularly useful in the management of thyrotoxicosis during pregnancy.

CONTRAINDICATIONS

LEVOTHROID administration is contraindicated in untreated thyrotoxicosis and in acute myocardial infarction. LEVOTHROID is contraindicated in the presence of uncorrected adrenal insufficiency because it increases the tissue demands for adrenocortical hormones and may cause an acute adrenal crisis in such patients. (See Warnings)

WARNINGS

Drugs with thyroid hormone activity, alone or together with other therapeutic agents, have been used for the treatment of obesity. In euthyroid patients, doses within the range of daily hormonal requirements are ineffective for weight reduction. Larger doses may produce serious or even life-threatening manifestations of toxicity, particularly when given in association with sympathomimetic amines such as those used for their anorectic effects.

The use of thyroid hormones in the therapy of obesity, alone or combined with other drugs, is unjustified and has been shown to be ineffective. Neither is their use justified for the treatment of male or female infertility unless this condition is accompanied by hypothyroidism.

PRECAUTIONS

GENERAL—LEVOTHROID should be used with caution in patients with cardiovascular disease, including hypertension. The development of chest pain or other aggravation of cardiovascular disease will require a decrease in dosage.
Thyroid hormone therapy in patients with concomitant diabetes mellitus or insipidus or adrenal cortical insufficiency aggravates the intensity of their symptoms. Appropriate adjustments of the various therapeutic measures directed at these concomitant endocrine diseases are required. The therapy of myxedema coma requires simultaneous administration of glucocorticoids. (See DOSAGE AND ADMINISTRATION).

INFORMATION FOR THE PATIENT—Patients on thyroid preparations and parents of children on thyroid therapy should be informed that:

1. Replacement therapy is to be taken essentially for life, with the exception of cases of transient hypothyroidism, usually associated with thyroiditis, and in those patients receiving a therapeutic trial of the drug.
2. They should immediately report during the course of therapy any signs or symptoms of thyroid hormone toxicity, e.g., chest pain, increased pulse rate, palpitations, excessive sweating, heat intolerance, nervousness, or any other unusual event.
3. In case of concomitant diabetes mellitus, the daily dosage of antidiabetic medication may need readjustment as thyroid hormone replacement is achieved. If thyroid medication is stopped, a downward readjustment of the dosage of insulin or oral hypoglycemic agent may be necessary to avoid hypoglycemia. At all times, close monitoring of urinary glucose levels is mandatory in such patients.
4. In case of concomitant oral anticoagulant therapy, the prothrombin time should be measured frequently to determine if the dosage of oral anticoagulants is to be readjusted.
5. Partial loss of hair may be experienced by children in the first few months of thyroid therapy, but this is usually a transient phenomenon and later recovery is usually the rule.

LABORATORY TESTS—The patient's response to thyroid replacement therapy may be followed by laboratory tests such as serum T_4 thyroxine, serum T_3 thyronine, free thyroxine index and thyroid stimulating hormone (TSH) blood levels.

DRUG INTERACTIONS—In patients with diabetes mellitus, addition of thyroid hormone therapy may cause an increase in the required dosage of insulin or oral hypoglycemic agents. Conversely, decreasing the dose of thyroid hormone may possibly cause hypoglycemic reactions if the dosage of insulin or oral hypoglycemic agents is not adjusted.
Thyroid replacement may potentiate anticoagulant effects with agents such as warfarin or bishydroxycoumarin and reduction of one-third in anticoagulant dosage should be undertaken upon initiation of LEVOTHROID therapy. Subsequent anticoagulant dosage adjustment should be made on the basis of frequent prothrombin determinations.
Injection of epinephrine in patients with coronary artery disease may precipitate an episode of coronary insufficiency. This may be enhanced in patients receiving thyroid preparations. Careful observation is required if catecholamines are administered to patients in this category.
Cholestyramine binds both T_4 thyroxine and T_3 thyronine in the intestine, thus impairing absorption of these thyroid hormones. In vitro studies indicate that the binding is not easily removed. Therefore, four to five hours should elapse between administration of cholestyramine and thyroid hormones.
Estrogens tend to increase serum thyroxine-binding globulin (TBg). In a patient with a nonfunctioning thyroid gland who is receiving thyroid replacement therapy, free thyroxine may be decreased when estrogens are started thus increasing thyroid requirements. However, if the patient's thyroid gland has sufficient function the decreased free thyroxine will result in a compensatory increase in thyroxine output by the thyroid. Therefore, patients without a functioning thyroid gland who are on thyroid replacement therapy may need to increase their thyroid dose if estrogens or estrogen-containing oral contraceptives are given.

DRUG/LABORATORY TEST INTERACTIONS—The following drugs or moieties are known to interfere with laboratory tests performed in patients on thyroid hormone therapy: androgens, corticosteroids, estrogens, oral contraceptives containing estrogens, iodine-containing preparations, and the numerous preparations containing salicylates.

1. Changes in TBg concentration should be taken into consideration in the interpretation of T_4 thyroxine and T_3 thyronine values. In such cases, the unbound (free) hormone should be measured. Pregnancy, estrogens, and estrogen-containing oral contraceptives increase TBg concentrations. TBg may also be increased during infectious hepatitis. Decreases in TBg concentrations are observed in nephrosis, acromegaly, and after androgen or corticosteroid therapy. Familial hyper- or hypo-thyroxine-binding-globulinemias have been described. The incidence of TBg deficiency approximates 1 in 9000. The binding of thyroxine by thyroid-binding prealbumin (TBPA) is inhibited by salicylates.
2. Medical or dietary iodine interferes with all in vivo tests of radio-iodine uptake, producing low uptakes which may not be reflective of a true decrease in hormone synthesis.
3. The persistence of clinical and laboratory evidence of hypothyroidism in spite of adequate dosage replacement indicates either poor patient compliance, poor absorption, excessive fecal loss, or inactivity of the preparation. Intracellular resistance to thyroid hormone is quite rare.

CARCINOGENESIS, MUTAGENESIS, AND IMPAIRMENT OF FERTILITY—A reportedly apparent association between prolonged thyroid therapy and breast cancer has not been confirmed and patients on thyroid for established indications should not discontinue therapy. No confirmatory long-term studies in animals have been performed to evaluate carcinogenic potential, mutagenicity, or impairment of fertility in either males or females.

PREGNANCY-CATEGORY A—Thyroid hormones do not readily cross the placental barrier. The clinical experience to date does not indicate any adverse effect on fetuses when thyroid hormones are administered to pregnant women. On the basis of current knowledge, thyroid replacement therapy to hypothyroid women should not be discontinued during pregnancy.

NURSING MOTHERS—Minimal amounts of thyroid hormones are excreted in human milk. Thyroid is not associated with serious adverse reactions and does not have a known tumorigenic potential. However, caution should be exercised when thyroid is administered to a nursing woman.

PEDIATRIC USE—The diagnosis and institution of therapy for cretinism should be done as soon after birth as feasible to prevent developmental deficiency. Screening tests for serum T_4 thyroxine and TSH will identify this group of newborn patients.

ADVERSE REACTIONS

Patients who are sensitive to lactose may show intolerance to LEVOTHROID since this substance is used in the manufacture of the product.
Adverse reactions other than those indicative of hyperthyroidism because of therapeutic overdosage, either initially or during the maintenance period, are rare. (See OVERDOSAGE).

OVERDOSAGE

Excessive dosage of thyroid medication may result in symptoms of hyperthyroidism. Since, however, the effects do not appear at once, the symptoms may not appear for one to three weeks after the dosage regimen is begun. The most common signs and symptoms of overdosage are weight loss, palpitation, nervousness, diarrhea or abdominal cramps, sweating, tachycardia, cardiac arrhythmias, angina pectoris, tremors, headache, insomnia, intolerance to heat and fever. If symptoms of overdosage appear, discontinue medication for several days and reinstitute treatment at a lower dosage level.
Laboratory tests such as serum T_4 thyroxine, serum T_3 thyronine and the free thyroxine index will be elevated during the period of overdosage.
Complications as a result of the induced hypermetabolic state may include cardiac failure and death due to arrhythmia or failure.

TREATMENT OF OVERDOSAGE—Dosage should be reduced or therapy temporarily discontinued if signs and symptoms of overdosage appear. Treatment may be reinstituted at a lower dosage. In normal individuals, normal hypothalamic-pituitary-thyroid axis function is restored in 6 to 8 weeks after thyroid suppression.
Treatment of acute massive thyroid hormone overdosage is aimed at reducing gastrointestinal absorption of the drugs and counteracting central and peripheral effects, mainly those of increased sympathetic activity. Vomiting may be induced initially if further gastrointestinal absorption can reasonably be prevented and barring contraindications such as coma, convulsions, or loss of the gagging reflex. Treatment is symptomatic and supportive. Oxygen may be administered and ventilation maintained. Cardiac glycosides may be indicated if congestive heart failure develops. Measures to control fever, hypoglycemia, or fluid loss should be instituted if needed. Antiadrenergic agents, particularly propranolol, have been used advantageously in the treatment of increased sympathetic activity. Propranolol may be administered intravenously at a dosage of 1 to 3 mg over a 10 minute period or orally, 80 to 160 mg/day, especially when no contraindications exist for its use.

DOSAGE AND ADMINISTRATION

The goal of therapy should be the restoration of euthyroidism as judged by clinical response and confirmed by appropriate laboratory values. In adults with no complicating endocrine or cardiovascular disease, the predicted full maintenance dose may be achieved immediately with adjustments made as indicated by clinical evaluation. The usual maintenance dose of LEVOTHROID is 100 mcg to 200 mcg daily.
In patients with known complications or in case of doubt, individual dose titration at 2 to 4 week intervals is recommended. The usual starting dose is 50 mcg with increases of 50 mcg at 2 to 4 week intervals until the patient is euthyroid or symptoms ensue which preclude further dose increase.
In adult myxedema or hypothyroid patients with angina, the starting dose should be 25 mcg with increases at 2 to 4 week intervals of 25 to 50 mcg as determined by clinical response.
Myxedema coma is usually precipitated in the hypothyroid patient of long-standing by intercurrent illness or drugs such as sedatives and anesthetics and should be considered a medical emergency. Therapy should be directed at the correction of electrolyte disturbances and possible infection besides the administration of thyroid hormones. Corticosteroids should be administered routinely. T_4 thyroxine and T_3 thyronine may be administered via a nasogastric tube but the preferred route of administration of both hormones is intravenous. T_4 thyroxine sodium is given at a starting dose of 200–500 mcg (100 mcg/mL given rapidly), and is usually well tolerated, even in the elderly. This initial dose is followed by daily supplements of 100 to 200 mcg given intravenously. Normal T_4 thyroxine levels are achieved in 24 hours followed in 3 days by threefold elevation of T_3 thyronine. Oral therapy with LEVOTHROID tablets should be resumed as soon as the clinical situation has been stabilized and the patient is able to take oral medication.
In cretinism or severe hypothyroidism in children, the initial dosage should be 25 to 50 mcg with increases of 50 to 100 mcg at weekly intervals until the child is clinically euthyroid and laboratory values are in the normal range. In growing children, the usual maintenance dose may be as high as 300 to 400 mcg daily. It is essential in children to reach the euthyroid state as rapidly as possible because of the importance of thyroid in growth and maturation.

HOW SUPPLIED

LEVOTHROID (T_4 Thyroxine Sodium Tablets, USP) is available in bottles of 100 tablets and 1000 tablets. The 50 mcg, 75 mcg, 100 mcg, 125 mcg, 150 mcg, 175 mcg, 200 mcg, and 300 mcg potencies are also available in cartons of 100 (10 strips of 10 tablets) packaged in Unit Dose as Armadose®. Each LEVOTHROID is distinctively colored and bears identifying markings.

Strength (mcg)	Tablets Color	Markings
25	Orange	LK
50	White	LL
75	Grey	LT
100	Yellow	LM
125	Purple	LH
150	Blue	LN
175	Turquoise	LP
200	Pink	LR
300	Green	LS

Tablets should be stored at controlled room temperature—between 15°–30°C (59°–86°F) in capped bottles or unbroken plastic strip packaging.

Continued on next page

USV—Cont.

LEVOTHROID (T_4 Thyroxine Sodium) For Injection is supplied in 6 mL vials containing 200 or 500 mcg of drug lyophilized with 15 mg of Mannitol.
Store at room temperature, between 15°–30°C (59°–86°F). Directions for reconstitution: using aseptic technique add 2 mL, 0.9% Sodium Chloride Injection, U.S.P. to the 200 mcg vial and 5 mL, 0.9% Sodium Chloride Injection, U.S.P. to the 500 mcg vial. Note: Do not use Bacteriostatic Sodium Chloride Injection, U.S.P. Shake to dissolve the contents of the vial. Use immediately and discard the unused portion.

CAUTION

Federal (USA) law prohibits dispensing without prescription.
Revised: May, 1986
Shown in Product Identification Section, page 433

LOZOL® ℞
[lō 'zōl]
indapamide
2.5 mg tablets

DESCRIPTION

LOZOL (indapamide) is an oral antihypertensive/diuretic. Its molecule contains both a polar sulfamoyl chlorobenzamide moiety and a lipid-soluble methylindoline moiety. It differs chemically from the thiazides in that it does not possess the thiazide ring system and contains only one sulfonamide group. The chemical name of LOZOL is 1-(4-chloro-3-sulfamoylbenzamido)-2- methylindoline, and its molecular weight is 365.84. The compound is a weak acid, $pK_a = 8.8$, and is soluble in aqueous solutions of strong bases. It is a white to yellow-white crystalline (tetragonal) powder.
The tablets also contain microcrystalline cellulose, coloring agent, corn starch, hydroxypropyl methylcellulose, lactose, magnesium stearate, polyethylene glycol, and talc.

CLINICAL PHARMACOLOGY

Indapamide is the first of a new class of antihypertensive/diuretics, the indolines. The oral administration of 5 mg (two 2.5-mg tablets) of indapamide to healthy male subjects produced peak concentrations of approximately 260 ng/ml of the drug in the blood within two hours. A minimum of 70% of a single oral dose is eliminated by the kidneys and an additional 23% by the gastrointestinal tract, probably including the biliary route. The half-life of LOZOL in whole blood is approximately 14 hours.
LOZOL is preferentially and reversibly taken up by the erythrocytes in the peripheral blood. The whole blood/plasma ratio is approximately 6:1 at the time of peak concentration and decreases to 3.5:1 at eight hours. From 71 to 79% of the LOZOL in plasma is reversibly bound to plasma proteins.
LOZOL is extensively metabolized, unchanged drug accounting for approximately 7% of the total dose recovered in the urine during the first 48 hours after administration. The urinary elimination of ^{14}C-labeled indapamide and metabolites is biphasic with a terminal half-life of excretion of total radioactivity of 26 hours.
In parallel design, dose-ranging clinical trials in hypertension and edema, daily doses of indapamide between 0.5 and 5.0 mg produced dose-related effects. Generally, doses of 2.5 and 5.0 mg were not distinguishable from each other although each was differentiated from placebo and from 0.5 or 1.0 mg indapamide. At daily doses of 2.5 and 5.0 mg a mean decrease of serum potassium of 0.5 and 0.6 mEq/liter, respectively, was observed and uric acid increased by about 1.0 mg/100 ml.
Thus, at these doses, the effects of indapamide on blood pressure and edema are approximately equal to those obtained with conventional doses of other antihypertensive/diuretics. In hypertensive patients, daily doses of 2.5 and 5.0 mg of indapamide have no appreciable cardiac inotropic or chronotropic effect. The drug decreases peripheral resistance, with little or no effect on cardiac output, rate or rhythm. Chronic administration of indapamide to hypertensive patients has little or no effect on glomerular filtration rate or renal plasma flow.
LOZOL had an antihypertensive effect in patients with varying degrees of renal impairment, although in general, diuretic effects declined as renal function decreased.
In limited controlled studies adding LOZOL to other antihypertensive drugs such as hydralazine, propranolol, guanethidine, and methyldopa, indapamide appeared to have the additive effect typical of thiazide-type diuretics.

INDICATIONS

LOZOL is indicated for the treatment of hypertension, alone or in combination with other antihypertensive drugs.
LOZOL is also indicated for the treatment of salt and fluid retention associated with congestive heart failure.
Usage in Pregnancy: The routine use of diuretics in an otherwise healthy woman is inappropriate and exposes mother and fetus to unnecessary hazard (see PRECAUTIONS below).
Diuretics do not prevent development of toxemia of pregnancy, and there is no satisfactory evidence that they are useful in the treatment of developed toxemia.
Edema during pregnancy may arise from pathological causes or from the physiologic and mechanical consequences of pregnancy. Indapamide is indicated in pregnancy when edema is due to pathologic causes, just as it is in the absence of pregnancy (however, see PRECAUTIONS below). Dependent edema in pregnancy, resulting from restriction of venous return by the expanded uterus, is properly treated through elevation of the lower extremities and use of support hose; use of diuretics to lower intravascular volume in this case is illogical and unnecessary. There is hypervolemia during normal pregnancy which is not harmful to either the fetus or the mother (in the absence of cardiovascular disease), but which is associated with edema, including generalized edema in the majority of pregnant women. If this edema produces discomfort, increased recumbency will often provide relief. In rare instances, this edema may cause extreme discomfort which is not relieved by rest. In these cases, a short course of diuretics may provide relief and may be appropriate.

CONTRAINDICATIONS

Anuria. Known hypersensitivity to indapamide or to other sulfonamide-derived drugs.

WARNINGS

Hypokalemia occurs commonly with diuretics, and electrolyte monitoring is essential, particularly in patients who would be at increased risk from hypokalemia, such as those with cardiac arrhythmias or who are receiving concomitant cardiac glycosides.
In general, diuretics should not be given concomitantly with lithium because they reduce its renal clearance and add a high risk of lithium toxicity. Read prescribing information for lithium preparations before use of such concomitant therapy.

PRECAUTIONS

General:

1. *Hypokalemia and Other Fluid and Electrolyte Imbalances:* Periodic determinations of serum electrolytes should be performed at appropriate intervals. In addition, patients should be observed for clinical signs of fluid or electrolyte imbalance, such as hyponatremia, hypochloremic alkalosis, or hypokalemia. Warning signs include dry mouth, thirst, weakness, fatigue, lethargy, drowsiness, restlessness, muscle pains or cramps, hypotension, oliguria, tachycardia and gastrointestinal disturbance. Electrolyte determinations are particularly important in patients who are vomiting excessively or receiving parenteral fluids, in patients subject to electrolyte imbalance (including those with heart failure, kidney disease, and cirrhosis), and in patients on a salt-restricted diet.
The risk of hypokalemia secondary to diuresis and natriuresis is increased when larger doses are used, when the diuresis is brisk, when severe cirrhosis is present and during concomitant use of corticosteroids or ACTH. Interference with adequate oral intake of electrolytes will also contribute to hypokalemia. Hypokalemia can sensitize or exaggerate the response of the heart to the toxic effects of digitalis, such as increased ventricular irritability.
Dilutional hyponatremia may occur in edematous patients; the appropriate treatment is restriction of water rather than administration of salt, except in rare instances when the hyponatremia is life threatening. However, in actual salt depletion, appropriate replacement is the treatment of choice. Any chloride deficit that may occur during treatment is generally mild and usually does not require specific treatment except in extraordinary circumstances as in liver or renal disease.
2. *Hyperuricemia and Gout:* Serum concentrations of uric acid increased by an average of 1.0 mg/100 ml in patients treated with indapamide, and frank gout may be precipitated in certain patients receiving indapamide (see ADVERSE REACTIONS below). Serum concentrations of uric acid should therefore be monitored periodically during treatment.
3. *Renal Impairment:* Indapamide, like the thiazides, should be used with caution in patients with severe renal disease, as reduced plasma volume may exacerbate or precipitate azotemia. If progressive renal impairment is observed in a patient receiving indapamide, withholding or discontinuing diuretic therapy should be considered. Renal function tests should be performed periodically during treatment with indapamide.
4. *Impaired Hepatic Function:* Indapamide, like the thiazides, should be used with caution in patients with impaired hepatic function or progressive liver disease, since minor alterations of fluid and electrolyte balance may precipitate hepatic coma.
5. *Glucose Tolerance:* Latent diabetes may become manifest and insulin requirements in diabetic patients may be altered during thiazide administration. Serum concentrations of glucose should be monitored routinely during treatment with LOZOL.
6. *Calcium Excretion:* Calcium excretion is decreased by diuretics pharmacologically related to indapamide. In long-term studies of hypertensive patients, however, serum concentrations of calcium increased only slightly with indapamide. Prolonged treatment with drugs pharmacologically related to indapamide may in rare instances be associated with hypercalcemia and hypophosphatemia secondary to physiologic changes in the parathyroid gland; however, the common complications of hyperparathyroidism, such as renal lithiasis, bone resorption, and peptic ulcer, have not been seen. Treatment should be discontinued before tests for parathyroid function are performed. Like the thiazides, indapamide may decrease serum PBI levels without signs of thyroid disturbance.
7. *Interaction With Systemic Lupus Erythematosus:* Thiazides have exacerbated or activated systemic lupus erythematosus and this possibility should be considered with indapamide as well.

DRUG INTERACTIONS

1. *Other Antihypertensives:* LOZOL may add to or potentiate the action of other antihypertensive drugs. In limited controlled trials that compared the effect of indapamide combined with other antihypertensive drugs with the effect of the other drugs administered alone, there was no notable change in the nature or frequency of adverse reactions associated with the combined therapy.
2. *Lithium:* See WARNINGS.
3. *Post-Sympathectomy Patient:* The antihypertensive effect of the drug may be enhanced in the postsympathectomized patient.
4. *Norepinephrine:* Indapamide, like the thiazides, may decrease arterial responsiveness to norepinephrine, but this diminution is not sufficient to preclude effectiveness of the pressor agent for therapeutic use.

CARCINOGENESIS, MUTAGENESIS, IMPAIRMENT OF FERTILITY: Both mouse and rat life-time carcinogenicity studies were conducted. There was no significant difference in the incidence of tumors between the indapamide-treated animals and the control groups.
Pregnancy/Teratogenic Effects: Pregnancy Category B. Reproduction studies have been performed in rats, mice, and rabbits at doses up to 6,250 times the therapeutic human dose and have revealed no evidence of impaired fertility or harm to the fetus due to LOZOL (indapamide). Postnatal development in rats and mice was unaffected by pretreatment of parent animals during gestation. There are, however, no adequate and well-controlled studies in pregnant women. Moreover, diuretics are known to cross the placental barrier and appear in cord blood. Because animal reproduction studies are not always predictive of human response, this drug should be used during pregnancy only if clearly needed. There may be hazards associated with this use such as fetal or neonatal jaundice, thrombocytopenia, and possibly other adverse reactions that have occurred in the adult.
Nursing Mothers: It is not known whether this drug is excreted in human milk. Because most drugs are excreted in human milk, if use of this drug is deemed essential, the patient should stop nursing.

ADVERSE REACTIONS

Most adverse effects have been mild and transient.
The clinical adverse reactions listed in the following table represent data from Phase II placebo-controlled studies and long-term controlled clincial trials (426 patients given LOZOL 2.5 mg or 5.0 mg). The reactions are arranged into two groups: 1) a cumulative incidence equal to or greater than 5%; and 2) a cumulative incidence less than 5%. Reactions are counted regardless of relation to drug.

Incidence ≥ 5%	Incidence < 5%
CENTRAL NERVOUS SYSTEM/ NEUROMUSCULAR	
Headache	Lightheadedness
Dizziness	Drowsiness
Fatigue, weakness, loss of energy, lethargy, tiredness, or malaise	Vertigo Insomnia Depression
Muscle cramps or spasm or numbness of the extremities	Blurred Vision
Nervousness, tension, anxiety, irritability, or agitation	
GASTROINTESTINAL SYSTEM	
	Constipation
	Nausea
	Vomiting
	Diarrhea
	Gastric irritation
	Abdominal pain or cramps
	Anorexia

CARDIOVASCULAR SYSTEM
- Orthostatic hypotension
- Premature ventricular contractions
- Irregular heart beat
- Palpitations

GENITOURINARY SYSTEM
- Frequency of urination
- Nocturia
- Polyuria

DERMATOLOGIC/HYPERSENSITIVITY
- Rash
- Hives
- Pruritus
- Vasculitis

OTHER
- Impotence or reduced libido
- Rhinorrhea
- Flushing
- Hyperuricemia
- Hyperglycemia
- Hyponatremia
- Hypochloremia
- Increase in serum urea nitrogen (BUN) or creatinine
- Glycosuria
- Weight loss
- Dry mouth
- Tingling of extremities

Because most of these data are from long-term studies (up to 40 weeks of treatment), it is probable that many of the adverse experiences reported are due to causes other than the drug. Approximately 10% of patients given indapamide discontinued treatment in long-term trials because of reactions either related or unrelated to the drug.

Clinical hypokalemia (i.e., lowered serum potassium concentration with concomitant clinical signs or symptoms) occurred in 3% and 7% of patients given indapamide 2.5 mg and 5.0 mg respectively. In a long-term study of both doses (157 patients given indapamide), potassium supplementation was given to 12% of patients on indapamide 2.5 mg and 27% of patients on indapamide 5.0 mg.

As expected in long-term clinical trials, many patients experienced single instances of abnormal clinical laboratory test results. However, over time, the mean changes in selected values are slight, as shown in the table above.

Mean Changes from Baseline after 40 Weeks of Treatment

	Serum Electrolytes (mEq/l) Potassium	Sodium	Chloride	Serum Uric Acid (mg/dl)	BUN (mg/dl)
Indapamide 2.5 mg (n=76)	−0.4	−0.6	−3.6	0.7	−0.1
Indapamide 5.0 mg (n=81)	−0.6	−0.7	−5.1	1.1	1.4

Other adverse reactions reported with antihypertensive/diuretics are jaundice (intrahepatic cholestatic jaundice), sialadenitis, xanthopsia, photosensitivity, purpura, necrotizing angiitis, fever, respiratory distress (including pneumonitis), and anaphylactic reactions; also, agranulocytosis, leukopenia, thrombocytopenia, and aplastic anemia. However, these reactions have not been reported following LOZOL administration.

OVERDOSAGE

Symptoms of overdosage include nausea, vomiting, weakness, gastrointestinal disorders and disturbances of electrolyte balance. In severe instances, hypotension and depressed respiration may be observed. If this occurs, support of respiration and cardiac circulation should be instituted. There is no specific antidote. An evacuation of the stomach is recommended by emesis and gastric lavage after which the electrolyte and fluid balance should be evaluated carefully.

DOSAGE AND ADMINISTRATION

Hypertension and edema of congestive heart failure: The adult starting dose for hypertension or edema of congestive heart failure is 2.5 mg as a *single daily dose* taken in the morning. If the response to 2.5 mg is not satisfactory after one (edema) to four (hypertension) weeks, the daily dose may be increased to 5.0 mg taken once daily.

If the antihypertensive response to indapamide is insufficient, LOZOL may be combined with other antihypertensive drugs, with careful monitoring of blood pressure. It is recommended that the usual dose of other agents be reduced by 50% during initial combination therapy. As the blood pressure response becomes evident, further dosage adjustments may be necessary.

In general, doses of 5.0 mg and larger have not appeared to provide additional effects on blood pressure or heart failure, but are associated with a greater degree of hypokalemia. There is little clinical trial experience in patients with doses greater than 5.0 mg once a day.

HOW SUPPLIED

LOZOL (indapamide). White, round film-coated tablets of 2.5 mg in bottles of 100 (NDC 0075-0082-00), 1,000 (NDC 0075-0082-99), and 2,500 (NDC 0075-0082-70), and in unit-dose blister packs, boxes of 100 (10 × 10 strips) (NDC 0075-0082-62).

Revised: May, 1986

Shown in Product Identification Section, page 433

NICOBID® Tempules®
(niacin, USV)
TIMED-RELEASE NICOTINIC ACID SUPPLEMENT

DESCRIPTION

Each black-and-clear Tempule (timed-release capsule) contains 125 mg niacin (nicotinic acid); each green-and-clear Tempule (timed-release capsule) contains 250 mg niacin (nicotinic acid); and each opaque blue and white Tempule (timed-release capsule) contains 500 mg niacin (nicotinic acid). Nicobid Tempules® provides the full actions of niacin (nicotinic acid). Portions of the pellets contained in the Tempule are released immediately. The remainder is released over several hours.

The 125 mg and 250 mg capsules also contain sugar, starch, confectionary glaze, hydrogenated castor oil, povidone, artificial color, and synthetic calcium silicate. The 500 mg capsules also contain confectionary glaze, hydrogenated castor oil, povidone, and synthetic calcium silicate.

USES

Nicobid (niacin, USV) is used in all those conditions in which niacin (nicotinic acid) supplementation is indicated. It has the advantage of a slower release of niacin (nicotinic acid) than conventional tablet dosage forms. This may permit its use by those who do not tolerate the tablets.

CAUTIONS

Nicobid should not be used by persons with a known sensitivity to niacin (nicotinic acid) and by persons with arterial bleeding, glaucoma, severe diabetes, impaired liver function, peptic ulcer, or by pregnant women.

SIDE EFFECTS

Temporary flushing and feeling of warmth may be expected. These seldom reach levels so as to necessitate discontinuance. If these symptoms persist, discontinue use and consult a physician. Temporary headache, itching and tingling, gastric disturbances, skin rash and allergies may occur.

DOSAGE

Usual adult dose—one Tempule, 125 mg, 250 mg or 500 mg morning and evening.

KEEP OUT OF THE REACH OF CHILDREN

Revised: May, 1986.

Shown in Product Identification Section, page 433

NICOLAR® ℞
[nic'ō-lär"]
(niacin tablets, USV)

DESCRIPTION

Nicolar® (niacin tablets, USV) is a scored yellow colored tablet containing 500 mg of niacin (nicotinic acid).

The tablets also contain microcrystalline cellulose, F.D.&C. Yellow #5 (See PRECAUTIONS), magnesium stearate, povidone, and colloidal silica.

ACTIONS

Niacin functions in the body as a component of two hydrogen transporting coenzymes; Coenzyme I (Nicotinamide Adenine Dinucleotide [NAD], sometimes called Diphosphopyridine Nucleotide [DPN]) and Coenzyme II (Nicotinamide Adenine Dinucleotide Phosphate [NADP], sometimes called Triphosphopyridine Nucleotide [TPN]). Niacin in addition to its functions as a vitamin, exerts several distinctive pharmacologic effects which vary according to the dosage level employed.

Niacin, in large doses, causes a reduction in serum lipids. The exact mechanism of this action is unknown.

INDICATIONS

Nicolar® is indicated as adjunctive therapy in patients with significant hyperlipidemia (elevated cholesterol and/or triglycerides) who do not respond adequately to diet and weight loss.

Notice: It has not been established whether the drug-induced lowering of serum cholesterol or triglyceride levels has a beneficial effect, no effect, or a detrimental effect on the morbidity or mortality due to atherosclerosis including coronary heart disease. Investigations now in progress may yield an answer to this question.

CONTRAINDICATIONS

Niacin is contraindicated in patients with hepatic dysfunction or in patients with active acute peptic ulcer.

WARNINGS

Use of this drug in pregnancy, lactation or in women of child-bearing age requires that the potential benefits of the drug be weighed against its possible hazards to the mother and child. Although fetal abnormalities have not been reported with this drug, its use as an antilipidemic agent requires high dosages, and animal reproduction or teratology studies have not been done. There are insufficient studies done for usage in children.

PRECAUTIONS

Patients with gall bladder disease, or those with a past history of jaundice, liver disease or peptic ulcer should be observed closely while taking this medication.

Frequent monitoring of liver function tests and blood glucose should be performed in the initial stage of therapy until it is ascertained that the drug has no adverse effects on these organ systems.

Diabetic or potential diabetic patients should be observed closely in the event of decreased tolerance. Adjustment of diet and/or hypoglycemic therapy may be necessary.

Patients receiving antihypertensive drugs of the adrenal-blocking type may have an additive vasodilating effect and produce postural hypotension.

Elevated uric acid levels have occurred; therefore use with caution in patients predisposed to gout.

This product contains FD&C Yellow No. 5 (tartrazine) which may cause allergic-type reactions (including asthma) in certain susceptible individuals. Although the overall incidence of FD&C Yellow No. 5 (tartrazine) sensitivity in the general population is low, it is frequently seen in patients who also have aspirin hypersensitivity.

ADVERSE REACTIONS

- Severe generalized flushing
- Decreased glucose tolerance
- Activation of peptic ulcers
- Abnormalities of hepatic functional tests
- Jaundice
- Gastrointestinal disorders
- Dryness of the skin
- Keratosis nigricans
- Pruritus
- Hyperuricemia
- Toxic amblyopia
- Hypotension
- Transient headache

DOSAGE AND ADMINISTRATION

Two to four tablets (1–2 grams) three times a day with or following meals or as directed by physician.

Since flushing, pruritus and gastrointestinal distress appear frequently, begin therapy with small doses and slowly build up dose in gradual increments observing for adverse effects and efficacy. The usual maximum daily dose is 8 grams.

HOW SUPPLIED

Nicolar® (niacin tablets, USV) is available in bottles of 100 scored tablets, each containing 500 mg of nicotinic acid (identified by the code NE).

Revised: May, 1986

Shown in Product Identification Section, page 433

NITROSPAN® ℞
[nī'trō-span"]
(nitroglycerin)
in sustained-release capsules

DESCRIPTION

Nitroglycerin, an organic nitrate, is a vasodilator which has effects on both arteries and veins. The chemical name for nitroglycerin is 1,2,3 propanetriol trinitrate ($C_3H_5N_3O_9$). The compound has a molecular weight of 227.09.

Nitrospan® is provided in two strengths. Each Nitrospan® sustained-release capsule contains 2.5 mg or 6.5 mg nitroglycerin in a sustained-released vehicle.

Continued on next page

USV—Cont.

The inactive ingredients contained in both the 2.5 mg and the 6.5 mg capsules are: corn starch, ethylcellulose, lactose, pharmaceutical glaze, sucrose, and talc.

CLINICAL PHARMACOLOGY

The principal pharmacological action of nitroglycerin is relaxation of vascular smooth muscle, producing a vasodilator effect on both peripheral arteries and veins with more predominant effects on the latter. Dilation of the post-capillary vessels, including large veins, promotes peripheral pooling of blood and decreases venous return to the heart, thereby reducing left ventricular end-diastolic pressure (preload). Arteriolar relaxation reduces systemic vascular resistance and arterial pressure (afterload).

The mechanism by which nitroglycerin relieves angina pectoris is not fully understood. Myocardial oxygen consumption or demand (as measured by the pressure-rate product, tension-time index, and stroke work index) is decreased by both the arterial and venous effects of nitroglycerin and, presumably, a more favorable supply-demand ratio is achieved. While the large epicardial coronary arteries are also dilated by nitroglycerin, the extent to which this action contributes to relief of exertional angina is unclear.

Nitroglycerin is rapidly metabolized in vivo, with a liver reductase enzyme having primary importance in the formation of glycerol nitrate metabolites and inorganic nitrate. Two active major metabolites, 1–2 and 1–3 dinitroglycerols, the products of hydrolysis, although less potent as vasodilators, have longer plasma half-lives than the parent compound, and appear in substantial concentration. The dinitrates are further metabolized to mononitrates (considered biologically inactive with respect to cardiovascular effects) and ultimately glycerol and carbon dioxide. There is extensive first-pass deactivation by the liver of nitroglycerin following gastrointestinal absorption, but the hepatic reductase activity may be saturated by some doses of oral nitroglycerin, resulting in prolonged pharmacologic effects. Hemodynamic studies employing plethysmographic methods in human volunteers have demonstrated that oral nitroglycerin (single dose 6.5 mg) has biologic effects significantly different from placebo for up to 8 hours.

Adequate studies defining the pharmacokinetics of Nitrospan® have not been reported. The clinical relevance of nitroglycerin blood levels has not been established, since therapeutic levels of the drug and metabolites have not been defined. Therapeutic doses of nitroglycerin reduce systolic and mean arterial blood pressures, especially when the patient assumes upright posture. Systolic blood pressure is decreased for up to 4 hours after a single dose of 6.5 mg of swallowed controlled-release nitroglycerin.

Clinical studies indicate that oral controlled-release nitroglycerin may reduce abnormally elevated left ventricular end-diastolic pressure (LVEDP), a hemodynamic occurrence during acute episodes of angina pectoris. Although there have been no reported, invasively measured, hemodynamic studies of Nitrospan® in patients with angina pectoris, controlled clinical trials in patients with congestive heart failure have shown significant decreases in mean LVEDP for as long as 4 hours after a single dose (6.5–19.5 mg) of oral nitroglycerin. The onset of hemodynamic effect from the swallowed form of nitroglycerin is not sufficiently rapid to be of use in aborting an acute episode of angina pectoris.

INDICATIONS AND USAGE

Nitrospan® is indicated for the prevention of angina pectoris due to coronary artery disease. Controlled clinical trials have demonstrated that this form of nitroglycerin is effective in improving exercise tolerance in patients with exertional angina pectoris. Controlled clinical studies of 2.6 mg and larger (6.5–26 mg) doses in patients with angina pectoris have shown improvement in treadmill exercise time for at least 4 hours after dosing.

CONTRAINDICATIONS

Nitroglycerin is contraindicated in patients who have shown acute or recent myocardial infarction, severe anemia, closed-angle glaucoma, postural hypotension, increased intracranial pressure, hypersensitivity to nitroglycerin or other nitrates or nitrites.

WARNINGS

This form of nitroglycerin is not intended for immediate relief of anginal attacks. The use of any form of nitroglycerin during the early days of acute myocardial infarction requires particular attention to hemodynamic monitoring and clinical status. In general a long-acting dosage form such as Nitrospan® should not be used because its effects are difficult to terminate rapidly should excessive hypotension or tachycardia develop.

PRECAUTIONS

General: Intraocular pressure may be increased; therefore, caution is required in administering to patients with glaucoma. Severe hypotension, particularly with upright posture, may occur even with small doses of nitroglycerin. The drug therefore should be used with caution in subjects who may have volume depletion from diuretic therapy or in patients who have low systolic blood pressure (e.g., below 90 mm Hg). Paradoxical bradycardia and increased angina pectoris may accompany nitroglycerin-induced hypotension.

Nitrate therapy may aggravate the angina caused by hypertrophic cardiomyopathy.

If blurring of vision, dryness of mouth or lack of benefit occurs, the drug should be discontinued.

Tolerance to this drug and cross-tolerance to other nitrates and nitrites may occur. Tolerance to the vascular and antianginal effects of nitrates has been demonstrated in clinical trials, experience through occupational exposure, and in isolated tissue experiments in the Laboratory.

The importance of tolerance to the use of nitroglycerin in the management of patients with angina pectoris has not been determined. In controlled clinical trials in patients with angina pectoris, sustained therapy with some nitrate preparations resulted in significantly less and shorter duration of improvement in exercise time on stress testing than did acute therapy. However, a controlled study of repetitive doses of oral nitroglycerin showed treadmill performance to be significantly better with drug than with placebo in 18 patients with angina pectoris after 2 weeks of therapy.

In industrial workers continuously exposed to nitroglycerin, tolerance clearly occurs. Moreover, physical dependence also occurs since chest pain, acute myocardial infarction, and even sudden death have occurred during temporary withdrawal of nitroglycerin from the workers. In various clinical trials of angina patients, there are reports of anginal attacks being more easily provoked and of rebound in the hemodynamic effects soon after nitrate withdrawal. The relative importance of these observations to the routine, clinical use of nitroglycerin are not known. However, it seems prudent to gradually withdraw patients from nitroglycerin when the therapy is being terminated, rather than stopping the drug abruptly.

Drug Interactions: Alcohol may enhance sensitivity to the hypotensive effects of nitrates.

Adverse Reactions (see below) are enhanced by ingestion of alcohol, which appears to increase absorption from the gastrointestinal tract.

Nitroglycerin acts directly on vascular muscle. Therefore, any other agents that depend on vascular smooth muscle as the final common path can be expected to have decreased or increased effect depending on the agent.

Marked symptomatic orthostatic hypotension has been reported when calcium channel blockers and oral controlled-release nitroglycerin were used in combination. Dose adjustments of either class of agents may be necessary.

Carcinogenesis, Mutagenesis, Impairment of Fertility: No long-term studies in animals have been performed to evaluate carcinogenic potential of Nitrospan®.

Pregnancy: Pregnancy Category C. Animal reproduction studies have not been conducted with Nitrospan®. It is also not known whether nitroglycerin can cause fetal harm when administered to a pregnant woman or can affect reproduction capacity. Nitroglycerin should be given to a pregnant woman only if clearly needed.

Nursing Mothers: It is not known whether nitroglycerin is excreted in human milk. Because many drugs are excreted in human milk, caution should be exercised when Nitrospan® is administered to a nursing woman.

Pediatric Use: Safety and effectiveness in children have not been established.

ADVERSE REACTIONS

Adverse reactions to Nitrospan®, particularly headache and hypotension, are generally dose-related and may disappear with a reduction in dosage. In clinical trials at various doses of nitroglycerin, the following adverse effects have been observed:

Headache, which may be severe and persistent, is the most commonly reported side effect of nitroglycerin, with an incidence in the order of about 50% in some studies. Cutaneous vasodilation with flushing may occur. Transient episodes of dizziness and weakness, as well as other signs of cerebral ischemia associated with postural hypotension, may occasionally develop. An occasional individual may exhibit marked sensitivity to the hypotensive effects of nitrates and severe responses (nausea, vomiting, weakness, restlessness, pallor, perspiration, and collapse) may occur even with therapeutic doses of nitrates. Drug rash and/or exfoliative dermatitis have been reported in patients receiving nitrate therapy. Nausea and vomiting appear to be uncommon.

OVERDOSAGE

Signs and Symptoms: Nitrate overdosage may result in: Severe hypotension, persistent throbbing headache, vertigo, palpitation, visual disturbance, flushing and perspiring skin (later becoming cold and cyanotic), nausea and vomiting (possibly with colic and even bloody diarrhea), syncope (especially in the upright posture), methemoglobinemia with cyanosis and anorexia, initial hyperpnea, dyspnea and slow breathing, slow pulse (dicrotic and intermittent), heart block, increased intracranial pressure with cerebral symptoms of confusion and moderate fever, paralysis and coma followed by clonic convulsions, and possibly death due to circulatory collapse.

Treatment of Overdosage: Keep the patient recumbent in a shock position and comfortably warm. Gastric lavage may be of use if the medication has only recently been swallowed. Passive movement of the extremities may aid venous return. Administer oxygen and artificial ventilation if necessary. If methemoglobinemia is present, administration of methylene blue (1% solution), 1–2 mg/kg intravenously, may be required.

Methemoglobin: Case reports of clinically significant methemoglobinemia are rare at conventional doses of organic nitrates. The formation of methemoglobin is dose-related and in the case of genetic abnormalities of hemoglobin that favor methemoglobin formation, even conventional doses of organic nitrates could produce harmful concentrations of methemoglobin.

WARNING: Epinephrine is ineffective in reversing the severe hypotensive events associated with overdose. It and related compounds are contraindicated in this situation.

DOSAGE AND ADMINISTRATION

The usual starting dose for Nitrospan® (nitroglycerin) is 2.5 mg taken 3 to 4 times daily. Controlled trials have been carried out to 5 hours after dosing; therefore, it is not known whether the drug is effective in prevention of exertional angina beyond 5 hours after dosing.

Nitrospan® should be TITRATED upward until a dose effective in controlling angina is determined or until side effects limit the dose. The dose generally may be increased by 2.5 mg increments 2 to 4 times daily over a period of days or weeks. Doses as high as 26 mg given 4 times daily have been reported effective in angina pectoris patients.

Administer the smallest effective dose 3 to 4 times daily unless clinical response suggests a different regimen. Discontinue if not effective. At initiation of therapy or change in dosage, the blood pressure (patient standing) should be monitored.

Nitrospan® Capsules must be swallowed. They are NOT FOR CHEWING OR FOR SUBLINGUAL USE. Nitrospan® Capsules are not intended for immediate relief of anginal attacks.

HOW SUPPLIED

Nitrospan® (nitroglycerin) 2.5 mg Capsules are available in bottles of 100 (NDC 0075-0150-00), and 6.5 mg Capsules are available in bottles of 60 (NDC 0075-0151-60). [NSN 6505-00-998-5871A (2.5 mg), V.A. Depots]

Store capsules at controlled room temperature between 15°–30°C (59°–86°F).

Revised: January, 1986

PERTOFRANE® ℞

[*pert'ō-frān"*]

(desipramine hydrochloride USP)

COMPOSITION

Each capsule provides 25 mg or 50 mg desipramine hydrochloride. The capsules also contain lactose, magnesium stearate, and talc.

DESCRIPTION

PERTOFRANE is a metabolite of imipramine hydrochloride. It is a dibenzazepine derivative, representing the desmethyl analog of imipramine hydrochloride. Chemically, it is 10,11-dihydro-5-[3-(methylamino) propyl]-5H-dibenz [b,f] azepine Monohydrochloride, and differs from the parent substance by having only one methyl group on the side chain nitrogen.

Desipramine hydrochloride is a white, crystalline substance with a molecular weight of 302.8. It is soluble to the extent of about 10% w/v in water, and melts within a range of 5° between 208-218°C.

ACTIONS

PERTOFRANE has been found in some studies to have a more rapid onset of action than imipramine; antidepressant efficacy is similar though potency on a weight basis may be less. The earliest manifestations consist mainly of an increase in psychomotor activity. Full treatment benefit is seldom attained before the end of the second week.

PERTOFRANE is not a monoamine oxidase inhibitor and does not act primarily as a central nervous system stimulant. Like all tricyclic antidepressants, PERTOFRANE blocks the reuptake of norepinephrine by adrenergic nerve terminals. Demethylated analogs such as desipramine are more potent in increasing norepinephrine turnover rate than the methylated compounds. However, the exact mechanism of action of tricyclics in depression is still unknown.

A mechanism of action proposed for antidepressant drugs, the biogenic amine theory, postulates that some, if not all, depression is associated with a deficiency or depletion of catecholamines and that some antidepressant drugs increase the amount of amine available at the synaptic receptor.

Desipramine is metabolized in the liver and approximately 70% is excreted in the urine.

INDICATIONS

PERTOFRANE is indicated for the relief of mental depression (see Note before How Supplied section for additional information on depressive symptomatologies often responsive to this drug).

CONTRAINDICATIONS

The use of PERTOFRANE concomitantly or within two weeks of the administration of MAO inhibitors, is contraindicated. Hyperpyretic crises or severe convulsive seizures may occur in patients receiving such combinations. The potentiation of adverse reactions can be serious, or even fatal. When it is desired to substitute PERTOFRANE in patients receiving a monoamine oxidase inhibitor, as long an interval should elapse as the clinical situation allows, with a minimum of 14 days. Initial dosage should be low and increases should be gradual and cautiously prescribed.
The drug is contraindicated following recent myocardial infarction.
Patients with a known hypersensitivity to tricyclic antidepressants should not be given PERTOFRANE.

WARNINGS

As with other potent antidepressants, an activation of the psychosis may occasionally be observed in schizophrenic patients.
Due to the drug's atropine-like effects and sympathomimetic potentiation, PERTOFRANE should be used only with the greatest care in patients with narrow-angle glaucoma and with urethral or ureteral spasm.
Likewise, only when patient need outweighs the risk of serious adverse reactions should the drug be used in the presence of any of the following conditions: severe coronary heart disease with EKG abnormalities, progressive heart failure, angina pectoris, paroxysmal tachycardia and active seizure disorder (this agent has been shown to lower the seizure threshold).
In some instances, desipramine and the parent compound, imipramine, have been shown to block the pharmacologic action of the antihypertensive, guanethidine, and related adrenergic neuron-blocking agents.
Hypertensive episodes have been observed during surgery in patients on desipramine hydrochloride therapy.
The concurrent use of other central nervous system drugs or alcohol may potentiate the adverse effects of desipramine hydrochloride. Since many such drugs may be used during surgery, it is recommended that desipramine hydrochloride be discontinued for as long as the clinical situation will allow prior to elective surgery.
In patients who may use alcohol excessively, it should be borne in mind that the potentiation may increase the danger inherent in any suicide attempt or overdosage.
Patients should be cautioned about the possibility of impaired ability to operate a motor vehicle or other dangerous machinery.
Usage in Pregnancy: Although teratogenic studies in mice, rats and rabbits have revealed no adverse effects, safe use of this drug in women who are or may become pregnant has not been definitely established. Therefore, PERTOFRANE (desipramine hydrochloride USP) should be withheld from these women unless the clinical situation warrants the potential risk.
In view of the lack of experience in children, the drug is not recommended for use in patients under twelve years of age.
Elderly and adolescent patients can usually be managed on lower dosage than that recommended for other patients and may not tolerate higher doses as well because of an increased incidence of adverse reactions.

PRECAUTIONS

It should be kept in mind that the possibility of suicide in seriously depressed patients is inherent in the illness and may persist until remission occurs. These patients require careful supervision and protective measures during therapy.
Anxiety and increased agitation have been reported, particularly where depression is not the primary disorder. A shift to hypomanic or manic excitement may occur during therapy. Such reactions may necessitate discontinuation of the drug.
Although the anticholinergic activity of the drug is weak, in susceptible patients and in those receiving anticholinergic drugs (including antiparkinsonism agents), atropine-like effects may be more pronounced (e.g. paralytic ileus).
Caution should be observed in prescribing the drug in hyperthyroid patients and in those receiving thyroid medications.
Transient cardiac arrhythmias have occurred in rare instances.
Steady-state serum concentrations of tricyclic antidepressants are reported to fluctuate significantly as cimetidine is either added or deleted from the drug regimen. Serious anticholinergic symptoms (severe dry mouth, urinary retention, blurred vision) have been associated with elevations in serum levels of the tricyclic antidepressants when cimetidine is added to the drug regimen. Additionally, higher than expected steady-state serum concentrations of tricyclic antidepressant have been observed when therapy is initiated in patients already taking cimetidine. Alternatively, decreases in steady-state serum concentrations of tricyclic antidepressant have been reported in well-controlled patients on concurrent therapy, upon discontinuance of cimetidine. Therapeutic efficacy of the tricyclic antidepressant may be compromised in these patients.
In all patients undergoing extended courses of therapy, periodic blood and liver studies for signs of toxicity should supplement careful clinical observations.

ADVERSE REACTIONS

PERTOFRANE is well tolerated by most patients and severe complications or adverse reactions are infrequent. Those most often reported cause little discomfort and seldom require discontinuation of the drug.
Nervous System: Dizziness, drowsiness, insomnia, headache and disturbed visual accommodation have been reported with the drug. In addition, tremor, unsteadiness, tinnitus and paresthesias have been reported. Occasionally, mild extrapyramidal activity, falling, and neuromuscular incoordination have been seen. A confusional state (with such symptoms as hallucinations and disorientation) may be produced, particularly in older patients and at higher dosage, and may require discontinuation of the drug. Changes in EEG patterns have been observed. Epileptiform seizures may occur. The syndrome of inappropriate ADH (antidiuretic hormone) secretion may occur. A reduction in dosage may help control some of these adverse reactions.
Gastrointestinal Tract: Anorexia, dryness of the mouth, nausea, epigastric distress, constipation and diarrhea have been reported in patients receiving PERTOFRANE.
Skin: Skin rashes (including photosensitization), perspiration and flushing sensations have been reported during therapy.
Liver: Transient jaundice, apparently of an obstructive nature, and liver damage have been observed in rare cases. Elevation in transaminase and changes in alkaline phosphatase have occurred and should indicate repeated liver-function profiles. If progressive elevation occurs, the drug should be discontinued.
Blood Elements: Bone-marrow depression, agranulocytosis, thrombocytopenia and purpura have been reported. If these occur, the drug should be discontinued. Transient eosinophilia has been observed in some instances.
Cardiovascular System: Orthostatic hypotension and tachycardia have been observed but seldom require discontinuation of treatment. Patients who require concomitant vasodilating therapy should be carefully supervised, particularly during the initial phases.
Genitourinary System: Urinary frequency or retention and impotence have been reported.
Endocrine System: Occasional hormonal effects, including gynecomastia, galactorrhea and breast enlargement have been reported with PERTOFRANE (desipramine hydrochloride USP). In addition, decreased libido and estrogenic effect have been noted. The exact relationship of these adverse effects to the administration of the drug has not been established.
Sensitivity: Urticaria and rare instances of drug fever and cross-sensitivity with imipramine have been observed.
Withdrawal Symptoms: Abrupt cessation of treatment after prolonged administration may produce nausea, headache, and malaise. These are not indicative of addiction. Rare instances have been reported of mania or hypomania occurring within 2–7 days following cessation of chronic therapy with tricyclic antidepressants.

DOSAGE AND ADMINISTRATION

All Patients Except Geriatric and Adolescent: The usual dosage range is from 75 to 150 mg/day in divided doses or as a single daily dose. Titration to a maintenance dose should be based on clinical response and tolerance by starting in the low dose range and increasing dosage when required. When necessary, dosage may be increased, after initiation of therapy, up to 200 mg daily in divided doses. Continued therapy at the optimal dosage level should be maintained during the active phase of the depression.
It is recommended that a lower maintenance dosage be continued for at least two months after a satisfactory response has been achieved. This, too, may be given on a once-daily schedule for convenience and compliance.
In cases of relapse due to premature withdrawal of the drug, a prompt response may be obtained by immediate resumption of treatment.
Geriatric and Adolescent Patients: Elderly and adolescent patients can usually be managed on lower dosage and may not tolerate higher doses as well as other patients. Therapy in these age groups may be initiated with 25 to 50 mg daily. Dosage may be increased according to response and tolerance to a maximum of 100 mg daily. It is recommended that a lower maintenance dosage be continued for at least two months after a satisfactory response has been achieved. Therapy may be given in divided doses or as a single daily dose.

OVERDOSAGE

Signs and Symptoms: These may vary in severity depending on several factors, including the amount absorbed, age, interval between ingestion and start of treatment, etc. In infants and young children, especially, acute overdosage in any amount must be considered serious and potentially fatal.
CNS abnormalities may include drowsiness, stupor, coma, ataxia, restlessness, agitation, hyperactive reflexes, muscle rigidity, athetoid and choreiform movements, and convulsions.
Cardiac abnormalities may include arrhythmia, tachycardia, ECG evidence of impaired conduction, and signs of congestive failure.
Respiratory depression, cyanosis, hypotension, shock, vomiting, hyperpyrexia, mydriasis, and diaphoresis may also be present.
Treatment: Because CNS involvement, respiratory depression and cardiac arrhythmia can occur suddenly, hospitalization and close observation are necessary, even when the amount ingested is thought to be small or the initial degree of intoxication appears slight or moderate. All patients with ECG abnormalities should have continuous cardiac monitoring for at least 72 hours and be closely observed until well after cardiac status has returned to normal; relapses may occur after apparent recovery.
The *slow* intravenous administration of physostigmine salicylate has been reported to reverse most of the cardiovascular and CNS effects of overdosage with tricyclic antidepressants. In adults, 1 to 3 mg has been reported to be effective. In children, start with 0.5 mg and repeat at 5 minute intervals to determine the minimum effective dose; do not exceed 2 mg. Because of the short duration of action of physostigmine, repeat the effective dose at 30 to 50 minute intervals, as necessary. Avoid rapid injection to reduce the possibility of physostigmine-induced convulsions.
In the alert patient, empty the stomach promptly by induced emesis followed by lavage. In the obtunded patient, secure the airway with a cuffed endotracheal tube before beginning lavage (do not induce emesis). Continue lavage for 24 hours or longer, depending on the apparent severity of intoxication. Use normal or half-normal saline to avoid water intoxication, especially in children. Instillation of activated charcoal slurry may help reduce absorption of desipramine.
Minimize external stimulation to reduce the tendency to convulsions. If anticonvulsants are necessary, diazepam, short-acting barbiturates, paraldehyde or methocarbamol may be useful. Do not use barbiturates if MAO inhibitors have been taken recently.
Maintain adequate respiratory exchange. Do not use respiratory stimulants.
Shock should be treated with supportive measures, such as intravenous fluids, oxygen and corticosteroids. Digitalis may increase conduction abnormalities and further irritate an already sensitized myocardium. If congestive heart failure necessitates rapid digitalization, particular care must be exercised.
Hyperpyrexia should be controlled by whatever external means are available, including ice packs and cooling sponge baths, if necessary.
Hemodialysis, peritoneal dialysis, exchange transfusions and forced diuresis have been generally reported as ineffective because of the rapid fixation of desipramine in tissues. Blood desipramine levels may not correlate with the degree of intoxication, and are unreliable indicators in the clinical management of the patient.

NOTE

Depressions which are most responsive to PERTOFRANE (desipramine hydrochloride USP) may be described in terms of "target symptoms." These include:
Despondency, sadness and depressed mood
Fatigue
Lack of interest and emotional response
Helplessness, hopelessness, pessimism and despair
Feelings of incapacity and inferiority
Psychomotor retardation and inhibition
Delusions of guilt and unworthiness
Psychosomatic complaints
Insomnia
Anorexia and weight loss
Depression-related anxiety and agitation
Suicidal drive
It should be borne in mind that these "target symptoms" of depression assume their proper significance only after careful history, physical and mental evaluations and other investigative procedures have confirmed a diagnosis of one of the several types of depression.

HOW SUPPLIED

25 mg Capsules (pink), bottles of 100 and 1000 (NSN 6505-00-913-0382A—V.A. Depots); 50 mg Capsules (maroon and pink), bottles of 100 and 1000.

Continued on next page

USV—Cont.

CAUTION: Federal (U.S.A.) law prohibits dispensing without prescription.
Revised: May, 1986

REGROTON® ℞
[rĕ-grō-tŏn]
DEMI-REGROTON® ℞
Oral antihypertensives

COMPOSITION

Each REGROTON tablet provides 50 mg chlorthalidone USP and 0.25 mg reserpine USP. Each DEMI-REGROTON tablet provides 25 mg chlorthalidone USP and 0.125 mg reserpine USP.

DESCRIPTION

REGROTON and DEMI-REGROTON are drug combinations of two well-known antihypertensive agents, chlorthalidone and reserpine. DEMI-REGROTON provides one-half the amount of both agents as REGROTON, for flexibility of dosage in patient management. Chemistry: A monosulfamyl diuretic, chlorthalidone differs from thiazide diuretics in that a double-ring system is incorporated in its structure. Chemically, it is 2-Chloro-5-(1-hydroxy-3-oxo-1-isoindolinyl) benzenesulfonamide. Chlorthalidone is practically insoluble in water, in ether, and in chloroform; soluble in methanol; slightly soluble in alcohol.

Reserpine is a pure crystalline alkaloid from the root of Rauwolfia serpentina. Reserpine is insoluble in water; freely soluble in acetic acid and in chloroform; slightly soluble in benzene; very slightly soluble in alcohol and in ether.

REGROTON and DEMI-REGROTON contain the following inactive ingredients: corn starch, gelatin, glycerin, lactose, magnesium stearate, silica, talc, and other ingredients. REGROTON also contains FD&C Red No. 40 and FD&C Blue No. 1.

ACTIONS

The pharmacologic effects are those of the constituent drugs. Chlorthalidone produces a saluretic effect in humans, beginning within two hours after an oral dose and continuing for as long as 72 hours. Copious diuresis is produced, with greatly increased excretion of sodium and chloride.

Reserpine, because it reduces arterial blood pressure and exerts a sedative effect, is particularly useful in the therapy of hypertension with related emotional disturbance. Reserpine is characterized by slow onset of action and sustained effect. Both its cardiovascular and central nervous system effects may persist following withdrawal of the drug. (See Precautions.)

Both chlorthalidone and reserpine have prolonged action, and the combination is thus able to exert a smooth and concerted effect over a long period. The two drugs appear to enhance each other, and this gives the combination a high degree of effectiveness. When considered necessary the combination may be prescribed together with other antihypertensive agents, which may then be given in lower dosage with lessened chance of side reactions.

INDICATION

Treatment of hypertension. (See box warning.)

CONTRAINDICATIONS

Mental depression, demonstrated hypersensitivity, and most cases of severe renal or hepatic diseases are the only contraindications.

WARNINGS

> These fixed combination drugs are not indicated for initial therapy of hypertension. Hypertension requires therapy titrated to the individual patient. If the fixed combination represents the dosage so determined, its use may be more convenient in patient management. The treatment of hypertension is not static, but must be reevaluated as conditions in each patient warrant.

These drugs should be used with caution in severe renal disease, since products containing chlorthalidone or similar drugs may precipitate azotemia. Cumulative effects of the drug may develop in patients with impaired renal function.

They should be used with caution in patients with impaired hepatic function or progressive liver disease, since minor alterations of fluid and electrolyte balance may precipitate hepatic coma.

REGROTON or DEMI-REGROTON may add to or potentiate the action of other antihypertensive drugs. Potentiation occurs with ganglionic or peripheral adrenergic blocking drugs.

Sensitivity reactions may occur in patients with a history of allergy or bronchial asthma.

Discontinue the drug in patients in whom mental depression develops while on the drug (the possibility of suicide should be kept in mind). In patients who have had depression, the drug should not be started. Electroshock therapy should not be given to patients taking reserpine, since severe and even fatal reactions have occurred. The drug should be stopped at least seven days before giving electroshock therapy.

In susceptible patients, peptic ulcer may be precipitated or activated, in which case the drug should be discontinued.

Usage in Pregnancy: Reproduction studies with chlorthalidone in various animal species at multiples of the human dose showed no significant level of teratogenicity; no fetal or congenital abnormalities were observed. Animal data should not be extrapolated for clinical application.

Thiazides cross the placental barrier and appear in cord blood. The use of chlorthalidone and related drugs in pregnant women requires that the anticipated benefits of the drug be weighed against possible hazards to the fetus. These hazards include fetal or neonatal jaundice, thrombocytopenia, and possibly other adverse reactions which have occurred in the adult.

NURSING MOTHERS: Thiazides and reserpine cross the placental barrier and appear in cord blood and breast milk. Increased respiratory secretions, nasal congestion, cyanosis and anorexia may occur in infants born to reserpine-treated mothers. If use of the drug is deemed essential, the patient should stop nursing.

PRECAUTIONS

Antihypertensive therapy with chlorthalidone/reserpine combinations should always be initiated cautiously in postsympathectomy patients and in those receiving ganglionic blocking agents, other potent antihypertensive drugs, or curare. At least a one-half reduction in the usual dosage of such agents may be advisable. Careful and continuous supervision of patients on such multiple-drug regimens is necessary.

Since some patients receiving Rauwolfia preparations have experienced hypotension when undergoing surgery, it may be advisable to discontinue chlorthalidone/reserpine combination drugs therapy about two weeks prior to elective surgical procedures. Emergency surgery may be carried out by using, if necessary, anticholinergic or adrenergic drugs to prevent vagocirculatory responses; other supportive measures may be used as indicated.

Because of the possibility of progression of renal damage, periodic kidney function tests are indicated. In case of a rising BUN, the drug should be stopped.

The drug should be discontinued in cases of aggravated liver dysfunction (hepatic coma may be precipitated).

Periodic determination of serum electrolytes to detect possible electrolyte imbalance should be performed at appropriate intervals.

All patients receiving chlorthalidone should be observed for clinical signs of fluid or electrolyte imbalance; namely, hyponatremia, hypochloremic alkalosis, and hypokalemia. Serum and urine electrolyte determinations are particularly important when the patient is vomiting excessively or receiving parenteral fluids. Medication such as digitalis may also influence serum electrolytes. Warning signs, irrespective of cause, are: Dryness of mouth, thirst, weakness, lethargy, drowsiness, restlessness, muscle pains or cramps, muscular fatigue, hypotension, oliguria, tachycardia, and gastrointestinal disturbances such as nausea and vomiting.

Hypokalemia may develop with chlorthalidone as with any other potent diuretic, especially with brisk diuresis, when severe cirrhosis is present, or during concomitant use of corticosteroids or ACTH.

Interference with adequate oral electrolyte intake will also contribute to hypokalemia. Digitalis therapy may exaggerate metabolic effects of hypokalemia especially with reference to myocardial activity.

Any chloride deficit is generally mild and usually does not require specific treatment except under extraordinary circumstances (as in liver disease or renal disease). Dilutional hyponatremia may occur in edematous patients in hot weather; appropriate therapy is water restriction, rather than administration of salt except in rare instances when the hyponatremia is life threatening. In actual salt depletion, appropriate replacement is the therapy of choice.

Hyperuricemia may occur or frank gout may be precipitated in certain patients receiving chlorthalidone.

Insulin requirements in diabetic patients may be increased, decreased, or unchanged. Latent diabetes mellitus may become manifest during chlorthalidone administration.

Chlorthalidone and related drugs may decrease arterial responsiveness to norepinephrine. This diminution is not sufficient to preclude effectiveness of the pressor agent for therapeutic use.

Chlorthalidone and related drugs may decrease serum PBI levels without signs of thyroid disturbance.

Because reserpine increases gastrointestinal motility and secretion, REGROTON or DEMI-REGROTON should be used cautiously in patients with ulcerative colitis or gallstones, where biliary colic may be precipitated. In susceptible patients, bronchial asthma may occur.

Animal tumorigenicity: rodent studies have shown that reserpine is an animal tumorigen, causing an increased incidence of mammary fibroadenomas in female mice, malignant tumors of the seminal vesicles in male mice, and malignant adrenal medullary tumors in male rats. These findings arose in 2-year studies in which the drug was administered in the feed at concentrations of 5 and 10 ppm—about 100 to 300 times the usual human dose. The breast neoplasms are thought to be related to reserpine's prolactin-elevating effect. Several other prolactin-elevating drugs have also been associated with an increased incidence of mammary neoplasia in rodents.

The extent to which these findings indicate a risk to humans is uncertain. Tissue culture experiments show that about one third of human breast tumors are prolactin dependent in vitro, a factor of considerable importance if the use of the drug is contemplated in a patient with previously detected breast cancer. The possibility of an increased risk of breast cancer in reserpine users has been studied extensively; however, no firm conclusion has emerged. Although a few epidemiologic studies have suggested a slightly increased risk (less than twofold in all studies except one) in women who have used reserpine, other studies of generally similar design have not confirmed this. Epidemiologic studies conducted using other drugs (neuroleptic agents) that, like reserpine, increase prolactin levels and, therefore, would be considered rodent mammary carcinogens, have not shown an association between chronic administration of the drug and human mammary tumorigenesis. While long-term clinical observation has not suggested such an association, the available evidence is considered too limited to be conclusive at this time. An association of reserpine intake with pheochromocytoma or tumors of the seminal vesicles has not been explored.

ADVERSE REACTIONS

Clinical trials indicate that the combination of chlorthalidone with reserpine is generally well tolerated. The adverse reactions most frequently seen include anorexia, gastric irritation, nausea, vomiting, diarrhea, constipation, nasal congestion, muscle cramps, dizziness, weakness, headache, drowsiness, and mental depression. Skin rashes, urticaria, and a case of ecchymosis have been reported. (Other dermatologic manifestations may occur—see below.)

A decreased glucose tolerance evidenced by hyperglycemia and glycosuria may develop inconsistently. This condition —usually reversible on discontinuation of therapy—responds to control with antidiabetic treatment. Diabetics and those predisposed should be checked regularly.

Hyperuricemia may be observed on occasion and acute attacks of gout have been precipitated. In cases where prolonged and significant elevation of blood uric acid concentration is considered potentially deleterious, concomitant use of a uricosuric agent is effective in reversing hyperuricemia without loss of diuretic and/or antihypertensive activity.

In addition to the reactions listed above, certain adverse reactions attributable to the drugs' components are shown below. Since REGROTON and DEMI-REGROTON combine chlorthalidone and reserpine in relatively small doses, such reactions may be less than when those drugs are used in full dosage.

Chlorthalidone: Idiosyncratic drug reactions such as aplastic anemia, purpura, thrombocytopenia, leukopenia, agranulocytosis, necrotizing angiitis and Lyell's syndrome (toxic epidermal necrolysis) have occurred, but are rare.

The remote possibility of pancreatitis should be considered when epigastric pain or unexplained gastrointestinal symptoms develop after prolonged administration.

Other reported reactions include restlessness, transient myopia, impotence or dysuria, and orthostatic hypotension, which may be potentiated when chlorthalidone is combined with alcohol, barbiturates or narcotics. Since jaundice, xanthopsia, paresthesia, and photosensitization have been documented in related compounds, the possibility of these reactions should be kept in mind.

Reserpine: The sedative effect of reserpine may lead to drowsiness or lassitude in some patients. Frequently, this effect disappears with continued administration. Nasal stuffiness sometimes occurs. Gastrointestinal reactions include increased gastric secretions, loose stools, or increased bowel frequency.

Symptoms of mental depression may occur in a small percentage of patients, although the recommended dosage of REGROTON contains substantially less reserpine than that usually implicated in such reactions. The same is true of other rare side effects recorded for reserpine, which include bradycardia and ectopic cardiac rhythms (especially when used with digitalis), pruritus, eruptions and/or flushing of skin, angina pectoris, headache, dizziness, paradoxical anxiety, nightmare, dull sensorium, muscular aches, a reversible paralysis agitans-like syndrome, blurred vision, conjunctival injection, uveitis, optic atrophy and glaucoma, increased susceptibility to colds, dyspnea, weight gain, decreased libido or impotence, dryness of the mouth, deafness, and anorexia.

DOSAGE AND ADMINISTRATION

Selection of drug and dosage should be determined by individual titration. (See box warning.) According to the requirement, the recommended dose of either REGROTON or

DEMI-REGROTON is usually *one tablet once a day.* Some patients may require two tablets once a day. Divided doses are unnecessary, and a single dose given in the morning with food is recommended.
Maintenance: Maintenance dosage must be individually adjusted. Mild cases may be adequately controlled with one DEMI-REGROTON tablet daily. Optimal lowering of elevated blood pressure may require two weeks or more in some cases because of the slow onset of action of reserpine.
Combination With Other Drugs: In more severe cases, if the response to a chlorthalidone/reserpine combination alone is inadequate, potent antihypertensives may be added gradually in dosages at least 50% lower than those usually employed. Such patients should be supervised carefully and continuously. As soon as desired blood pressure levels have been attained, the lowest effective maintenance dosage should be followed.

OVERDOSAGE

Adverse reactions resulting from accidental acute overdosage may include nausea, weakness, dizziness, syncope, and disturbances of electrolyte balance. There is no specific antidote. However, the following is recommended: gastric lavage followed by supportive treatment, including intravenous dextrose-saline with potassium chloride if necessary, to be given with the usual caution. If marked hypotension results from overdosage, it can be treated with vasopressor drugs.

HOW SUPPLIED

REGROTON is available as pink, uniquely-shaped* tablets, in bottles of 100 (NDC 0070-0031-00) and 1000 (NDC 0070-0031-99); DEMI-REGROTON as white, uniquely-shaped* tablets, bottles of 100 (NDC 0070-0032-00) and 1000 (NDC 0070-0032-99). Store at controlled room temperature between 15°–30°C (59°–86°F). Dispense in tight, light-resistant containers as defined in USP.

*Design patent pending. The appearance of REGROTON and DEMI-REGROTON tablets is a trademark of USV Laboratories Inc.

CAUTION: Federal (USA) law prohibits dispensing without prescription.

ANIMAL PHARMACOLOGY

In animal biochemical studies, chlorthalidone is absorbed slowly from the gastrointestinal tract, due to low solubility. After passage to the liver, some of the drug enters the general circulation, while some is excreted in the bile, to be reabsorbed later. In the general circulation, the drug is distributed widely to the tissues, but is taken up in the highest concentrations in the kidneys, where amounts have been found 72 hours after ingestion, long after it has disappeared from other tissues. The drug is excreted unchanged in the urine. The high renal concentration of chlorthalidone may be causally associated with the prolonged saluretic effect of the drug. Chlorthalidone appears to inhibit sodium and chloride reabsorption in the cortical diluting segment of ascending limb of Henle's loop. The reduction of plasma volume following diuresis is a probable mechanism in the initial antihypertensive action of the drug.
Reserpine probably produces its sedative and hypotensive effects through a depletion in tissue stores of catecholamines. The antihypertensive action of reserpine is probably due to loss of epinephrine and norepinephrine from peripheral sites. By contrast, its sedative and tranquilizing properties are thought to be related to depletion of 5-hydroxytryptamine from the brain.
Revised: February, 1985

Shown in Product Identification Section, page 433

ARMOUR® THYROID Tablets ℞

[thī'roid]
(THYROID TABLETS, U.S.P.)

DESCRIPTION

Armour® Thyroid Tablets (Thyroid Tablets, USP) for oral use are derived from porcine thyroid glands. They provide 38 mcg T_4 thyroxine sodium (T_4 levothyroxine) and 9 mcg T_3 thyronine sodium (T_3 liothyronine) per grain of thyroid. The inactive ingredients are calcium stearate, dextrose and mineral oil.

CLINICAL PHARMACOLOGY

The steps in the synthesis of the thyroid hormones are controlled by thyrotropin (Thyroid Stimulating Hormone, TSH) secreted by the anterior pituitary. This hormone's secretion is in turn controlled by a feedback mechanism effected by the thyroid hormones themselves and by thyrotropin releasing hormone (TRH), a tripeptide of hypothalamic origin. Endogenous thyroid hormone secretion is suppressed when exogenous thyroid hormones are administered to euthyroid individuals in excess of the normal gland's secretion.
The mechanisms by which thyroid hormones exert their physiologic action are not well understood. These hormones enhance oxygen consumption by most tissues of the body, increase the basal metabolic rate, and the metabolism of carbohydrates, lipids, and proteins. Thus, they exert a profound influence on every organ system in the body and are of particular importance in the development of the central nervous system.
The normal thyroid gland contains approximately 200 mcg of T_4 thyroxine per gram of gland, and 15 mcg of T_3 thyronine per gram. The ratio of these two hormones in the circulation does not represent the ratio in the thyroid gland, since about 80 percent of peripheral T_3 thyronine comes from monodeiodination of T_4 thyroxine. Peripheral monodeiodination of T_4 thyroxine at the 5 position (inner ring) also results in the formation of reverse T_3 thyronine, which is calorigenically inactive.
T_3 thyronine levels are low in the fetus and newborn, in old age, in chronic caloric deprivation, hepatic cirrhosis, renal failure, surgical stress, and chronic illnesses representing what has been called the "T_3 thyronine syndrome."
Pharmacokinetics—Animal studies have shown that T_4 thyroxine is only partially absorbed from the gastrointestinal tract. The degree of absorption is dependent on the vehicle used for its administration and by the character of the intestinal contents, the intestinal flora, including plasma protein, soluble dietary factors, all of which bind thyroid and thereby make it unavailable for diffusion. Only 41 percent is absorbed when given in a gelatin capsule as opposed to a 74 percent absorption when given with an albumin carrier.
Depending on other factors, absorption has varied from 48 to 79 percent of the administered dose. Fasting increases absorption. Malabsorption syndromes, as well as dietary factors, (children's soybean formula, concomitant use of anionic exchange resins such as cholestyramine) cause excessive fecal loss. T_3 thyronine is almost totally absorbed, 95 percent in 4 hours. The hormones contained in the natural preparations are absorbed in a manner similar to the synthetic hormones.
More than 99 percent of circulating hormones are bound to serum proteins, including thyroid-binding globulin (TBg), thyroid-binding prealbumin (TBPA), and albumin (TBa), whose capacities and affinities vary for the hormones. The higher affinity of T_4 thyroxine for both TBg and TBPA as compared to T_3 thyronine partially explains the higher serum levels and longer half-life of the former hormone. Both protein-bound hormones exist in reverse equilibrium with minute amounts of free hormone, the latter accounting for the metabolic activity.
Deiodination of T_4 thyroxine occurs at a number of sites, including liver, kidney, and other tissues. The conjugated hormone, in the form of glucuronide or sulfate, is found in the bile and gut where it may complete an enterohepatic circulation. Eighty-five percent of T_4 thyroxine metabolized daily is deiodinated.

INDICATIONS AND USAGE

Armour® Thyroid Tablets are indicated:

1. As replacement or supplemental therapy in patients with hypothyroidism of any etiology, except transient hypothyroidism during the recovery phase of subacute thyroiditis. This category includes cretinism, myxedema, and ordinary hypothyroidism in patients of any age (children, adults, the elderly), or state (including pregnancy); primary hypothyroidism resulting from functional deficiency, primary atrophy, partial or total absence of thyroid gland, or the effects of surgery, radiation, or drugs, with or without the presence of goiter; and secondary (pituitary), or tertiary (hypothalamic) hypothyroidism (See WARNINGS).
2. As pituitary TSH suppressants, in the treatment or prevention of various types of euthyroid goiters, including thyroid nodules, sub-acute or chronic lymphocytic thyroiditis (Hashimoto's), multinodular goiter, and in the management of thyroid cancer.
3. As diagnostic agents in suppression tests to differentiate suspected mild hyperthyroidism or thyroid gland autonomy.

CONTRAINDICATIONS

Thyroid hormone preparations are generally contraindicated in patients with diagnosed but as yet uncorrected adrenal cortical insufficiency, untreated thyrotoxicosis, and apparent hypersensitivity to any of their active or extraneous constituents. There is no well documented evidence from the literature, however, of true allergic or idiosyncratic reactions to thyroid hormone.

WARNINGS

Drugs with thyroid hormone activity, alone or together with other therapeutic agents, have been used for the treatment of obesity. In euthyroid patients, doses within the range of daily hormonal requirements are ineffective for weight reduction. Larger doses may produce serious or even life-threatening manifestations of toxicity, particularly when given in association with sympathomimetic amines such as those used for their anorectic effects.

The use of thyroid hormones in the therapy of obesity, alone or combined with other drugs, is unjustified and has been shown to be ineffective. Neither is their use justified for the treatment of male or female infertility unless this condition is accompanied by hypothyroidism.

PRECAUTIONS

General—Thyroid hormones should be used with great caution in a number of circumstances where the integrity of the cardiovascular system, particularly the coronary arteries, is suspected. These include patients with angina pectoris or the elderly, in whom there is a greater likelihood of occult cardiac disease. In these patients therapy should be initiated with low doses, i.e. 15–30 mg Armour® Thyroid. When, in such patients, a euthyroid state can only be reached at the expense of an aggravation of the cardiovascular disease, thyroid hormone dosage should be reduced.
Thyroid hormone therapy in patients with concomitant diabetes mellitus or diabetes insipidus or adrenal cortical insufficiency aggravates the intensity of their symptoms. Appropriate adjustments of the various therapeutic measures directed at these concomitant endocrine diseases are required.
The therapy of myxedema coma requires simultaneous administration of glucocorticoids (See DOSAGE AND ADMINISTRATION).
Hypothyroidism decreases and hyperthyroidism increases the sensitivity to oral anticoagulants. Prothrombin time should be closely monitored in thyroid treated patients on oral anticoagulants and dosage of the latter agents adjusted on the basis of frequent prothrombin time determinations.
In infants, excessive doses of thyroid hormone preparations may produce craniosynostosis.
Information for the Patient—Patients on thyroid hormone preparations and parents of children on thyroid therapy should be informed that:

1. Replacement therapy is to be taken essentially for life, with the exception of cases of transient hypothyroidism, usually associated with thyroiditis, and in those patients receiving a therapeutic trial of the drug.
2. They should immediately report during the course of therapy any signs or symptoms of thyroid hormone toxicity, e.g., chest pain, increased pulse rate, palpitations, excessive sweating, heat intolerance, nervousness, or any other unusual event.
3. In case of concomitant diabetes mellitus, the daily dosage of antidiabetic medication may need readjustment as thyroid hormone replacement is achieved. If thyroid medication is stopped, a downward readjustment of the dosage of insulin or oral hypoglycemic agent may be necessary to avoid hypoglycemia. At all times, close monitoring of urinary glucose levels is mandatory in such patients.
4. In case of concomitant oral anticoagulant therapy, the prothrombin time should be measured frequently to determine if the dosage of oral anticoagulants is to be readjusted.
5. Partial loss of hair may be experienced by children in the first few months of thyroid therapy, but this is usually a transient phenomenon and later recovery is usually the rule.

Laboratory Tests—Treatment of patients with thyroid hormones requires the periodic assessment of thyroid status by means of appropriate laboratory tests besides the full clinical evaluation. The TSH suppression test can be used to test the effectiveness of any thyroid preparation bearing in mind the relative insensitivity of the infant pituitary to the negative feedback effect of thyroid hormones. Serum T_4 thyroxine levels can be used to test the effectiveness of all thyroid medications except T_3 thyronine. When the total serum T_4 thyroxine is low but TSH is normal, a test specific to assess unbound (free) T_4 thyroxine levels is warranted. Specific measurements of T_4 thyroxine and T_3 thyronine by competitive protein binding or radioimmunoassay are not influenced by blood levels of organic or inorganic iodine.
Drug Interactions—Oral Anticoagulants—Thyroid hormones appear to increase catabolism of vitamin K-dependent clotting factors. If oral anticoagulants are also being given, compensatory increases in clotting factor synthesis are impaired. Patients stabilized on oral anticoagulants who are found to require thyroid replacement therapy should be watched very closely when thyroid is started. If a patient is truly hypothyroid, it is likely that a reduction in anticoagulant dosage will be required. No special precautions appear to be necessary when oral anticoagulant therapy is begun in a patient already stabilized on maintenance thyroid replacement therapy.
Insulin or Oral Hypoglycemics—Initiating thyroid replacement therapy may cause increases in insulin or oral hypoglycemic requirements. The effects seen are poorly understood and depend upon a variety of factors such as dose and type of thyroid preparations and endocrine status of the patient. Patients receiving insulin or oral hypoglycemics should be closely watched during initiation of thyroid replacement therapy.

Continued on next page

USV—Cont.

Cholestyramine—Cholestyramine binds both T_4 thyroxine and T_3 thyronine in the intestine, thus impairing absorption of these thyroid hormones. *In vitro* studies indicate that the binding is not easily removed. Therefore, four to five hours should elapse between administration of cholestyramine and thyroid hormones.
Estrogen, Oral Contraceptives—Estrogens tend to increase serum thyroxine-binding globulin (TBg). In a patient with a nonfunctioning thyroid gland who is receiving thyroid replacement therapy, free T_4 thyroxine may be decreased when estrogens are started thus increasing thyroid requirements. However, if the patient's thyroid gland has sufficient function, the decreased free thyroxine will result in a compensatory increase in thyroxine output by the thyroid. Therefore, patients without a functioning thyroid gland who are on thyroid replacement therapy may need to increase their thyroid dose if estrogens or estrogen-containing oral contraceptives are given.
Drug/Laboratory Test Interactions—The following drugs or moieties are known to interfere with laboratory tests performed in patients on thyroid hormone therapy: androgens, corticosteroids, estrogens, oral contraceptives containing estrogens, iodine-containing preparations, and the numerous preparations containing salicylates.

1. Changes in TBg concentration should be taken into consideration in the interpretation of T_4 thyroxine and T_3 thyronine values. In such cases, the unbound (free) hormone should be measured. Pregnancy, estrogens, and estrogen-containing oral contraceptives increase TBg concentrations. TBg may also be increased during infectious hepatitis. Decreases in TBg concentrations are observed in nephrosis, acromegaly, and after androgen or corticosteroid therapy. Familial hyper- or hypo-thyroxine-binding-globulinemias have been described. The incidence of TBg deficiency approximates 1 in 9,000. The binding of thyroxine by TBPA is inhibited by salicylates.
2. Medicinal or dietary iodine interferes with all *in vivo* tests of radio-iodine uptake, producing low uptakes which may not be relative of a true decrease in hormone synthesis.
3. The persistence of clinical and laboratory evidence of hypothyroidism in spite of adequate dosage replacement indicates either poor patient compliance, poor absorption, excessive fecal loss, or inactivity of the preparation. Intracellular resistance to thyroid hormone is quite rare.

Carcinogenesis, Mutagenesis, and Impairment of Fertility—A reportedly apparent association between prolonged thyroid therapy and breast cancer has not been confirmed and patients on thyroid for established indications should not discontinue therapy. No confirmatory long-term studies in animals have been performed to evaluate carcinogenic potential, mutagenicity, or impairment of fertility in either males or females.
Pregnancy-Category A—Thyroid hormones do not readily cross the placental barrier. The clinical experience to date does not indicate any adverse effect on fetuses when thyroid hormones are administered to pregnant women. On the basis of current knowledge, thyroid replacement therapy to hypothyroid women should not be discontinued during pregnancy.
Nursing Mothers—Minimal amounts of thyroid hormones are excreted in human milk. Thyroid is not associated with serious adverse reactions and does not have a known tumorigenic potential. However, caution should be exercised when thyroid is administered to a nursing woman.
Pediatric Use—Pregnant mothers provide little or no thyroid hormone to the fetus. The incidence of congenital hypothyroidism is relatively high (1:4,000) and the hypothyroid fetus would not derive any benefit from the small amounts of hormone crossing the placental barrier. Routine determinations of serum T_4 thyroxine and/or TSH is strongly advised in neonates in view of the deleterious effects of thyroid deficiency on growth and development.
Treatment should be initiated immediately upon diagnosis, and maintained for life, unless transient hypothyroidism is suspected; in which case, therapy may be interrupted for 2 to 8 weeks after the age of 3 years to reassess the condition. Cessation of therapy is justified in patients who have maintained a normal TSH during those 2 to 8 weeks.

ADVERSE REACTIONS

Adverse reactions other than those indicative of hyperthyroidism because of therapeutic overdosage, either initially or during the maintenance period, are rare (See OVERDOSAGE).

OVERDOSAGE

Signs and Symptoms—Excessive doses of thyroid result in a hypermetabolic state resembling in every respect the condition of endogenous origin. The condition may be self-induced.
Treatment of Overdosage—Dosage should be reduced or therapy temporarily discontinued if signs and symptoms of overdosage appear.
Treatment may be reinstituted at a lower dosage. In normal individuals, normal hypothalamic-pituitary-thyroid axis function is restored in 6 to 8 weeks after thyroid suppression.
Treatment of acute massive thyroid hormone overdosage is aimed at reducing gastrointestinal absorption of the drugs and counteracting central and peripheral effects, mainly those of increased sympathetic activity. Vomiting may be induced initially if further gastrointestinal absorption can reasonably be prevented and barring contraindications such as coma, convulsions, or loss of the gagging reflex. Treatment is symptomatic and supportive. Oxygen may be administered and ventilation maintained. Cardiac glycosides may be indicated if congestive heart failure develops. Measures to control fever, hypoglycemia, or fluid loss should be instituted if needed. Antiadrenergic agents, particularly propranolol, have been used advantageously in the treatment of increased sympathetic activity. Propranolol may be administered intravenously at a dosage of 1 to 3 mg over a 10 minute period or orally, 80 to 160 mg/day, especially when no contraindications exist for its use.

DOSAGE AND ADMINISTRATION

The dosage of thyroid hormones is determined by the indication and must in every case be individualized according to patient response and laboratory findings.
Thyroid hormones are given orally. In acute, emergency conditions, injectable T_4 thyroxine sodium may be given intravenously when oral administration is not feasible or desirable, as in the treatment of myxedema coma, or during total parenteral nutrition. Intramuscular administration is not advisable because of reported poor absorption.
Hypothyroidism—Therapy is usually instituted using low doses, with increments which depend on the cardiovascular status of the patient. The usual starting dose is 30 mg Armour® Thyroid, with increments of 15 mg every 2 to 3 weeks. A lower starting dosage, 15 mg/day, is recommended in patients with long standing myxedema, particularly if cardiovascular impairment is suspected, in which case extreme caution is recommended. The appearance of angina is an indication for a reduction in dosage. Most patients require 60–120 mg/day. Failure to respond to doses of 180 mg suggests lack of compliance or malabsorption. Maintenance dosages 60–120 mg/day usually result in normal serum T_4 thyroxine and T_3 thyronine levels. Adequate therapy usually results in normal TSH and T_4 thyroxine levels after 2 to 3 weeks of therapy.
Readjustment of thyroid hormone dosage should be made within the first four weeks of therapy, after proper clinical and laboratory evaluations, including serum levels of T_4 thyroxine, bound and free, and TSH.
T_3 thyronine may be used in preference to T_4 thyroxine during radio-isotope scanning procedures, since induction of hypothyroidism in those cases is more abrupt and can be of shorter duration. It may also be preferred when impairment of peripheral conversion of T_4 thyroxine and T_3 thyronine is suspected.
Myxedema Coma—Myxedema coma is usually precipitated in the hypothyroid patient of long-standing by intercurrent illness or drugs such as sedatives and anesthetics and should be considered a medical emergency. Therapy should be directed at the correction of electrolyte disturbances and possible infection besides the administration of thyroid hormones. Corticosteroids should be administered routinely. T_4 thyroxine and T_3 thyronine may be administered via a nasogastric tube but the preferred route of administration of both hormones is intravenous. T_4 thyroxine sodium is given at a starting dose of 400 mcg (100 mcg/ml) given rapidly, and is usually well tolerated, even in the elderly. This initial dose is followed by daily supplements of 100 to 200 mcg given IV. Normal T_4 thyroxine levels are achieved in 24 hours followed in 3 days by threefold elevation of T_3 thyronine. Oral therapy with thyroid hormone would be resumed as soon as the clinical situation has been stabilized and the patient is able to take oral medication.
Thyroid Cancer—Exogenous thyroid hormone may produce regression of metastases from follicular and papillary carcinoma of the thyroid and is used as ancillary therapy of these conditions with radioactive iodine. TSH should be suppressed to low or undetectable levels. Therefore, larger amounts of thyroid hormone than those used for replacement therapy are required. Medullary carcinoma of the thyroid is usually unresponsive to this therapy.
Thyroid Suppression Therapy—Administration of thyroid hormone in doses higher than those produced physiologically by the gland results in suppression of the production of endogenous hormone. This is the basis for the thyroid suppression test and is used as an aid in the diagnosis of patients with signs of mild hyperthyroidism in whom base line laboratory tests appear normal, or to demonstrate thyroid gland autonomy in patients with Grave's ophthalmopathy. ^{131}I uptake is determined before and after the administration of the exogenous hormone. A fifty percent or greater suppression of uptake indicates a normal thyroid-pituitary axis and thus rules out thyroid gland autonomy.
For adults, the usual suppressive dose of T_4 thyroxine is 1.56 mg/kg of body weight per day given for 7 to 10 days. These doses usually yield normal serum T_4 thyroxine and T_3 thyronine levels and lack of response to TSH.
Thyroid hormones should be administered cautiously to patients in whom there is strong suspicion of thyroid gland autonomy, in view of the fact that the exogenous hormone effects will be additive to the endogenous source.
Pediatric Dosage—Pediatric dosage should follow the recommendations summarized in Table 1. In infants with congenital hypothyroidism, therapy with full doses should be instituted as soon as the diagnosis has been made.

Recommended Pediatric Dosage for Congenital Hypothyroidism

	Armour® Thyroid Tablets	
Age	**Dose per day**	**Daily dose per kg of body weight**
0–6 mos	15–30 mg	4.8–6 mg
6–12 mos	30–45 mg	3.6–4.8 mg
1–5 yrs	45–60 mg	3–3.6 mg
6–12 yrs	60–90 mg	2.4–3 mg
Over 12 yrs	Over 90 mg	1.2–1.8 mg

Table 1

HOW SUPPLIED

Armour® Thyroid Tablets (Thyroid Tablets, USP) are supplied as follows: 30 mg (½ gr) and 60 mg (1 gr) tablets in bottles of 100, 1000, and 5000; 120 mg (2 gr) tablets in bottles of 100, 1000, and 2500; 15 mg (¼ gr) and 180 mg (3 gr) tablets in bottles of 100 and 1000; and 90 mg (1½ gr), 240 mg (4 gr), and 300 mg (5 gr) tablets in bottles of 100.
The 15 mg (¼ gr), 30 mg (½ gr), 60 mg (1 gr), 90 mg (1½ gr), 120 mg (2 gr), 180 mg (3 gr), 240 mg (4 gr), and 300 mg (5 gr) potencies are available in special dispensing bottles of 100 tablets designated as Handy 100s® (child-resistant closure with tear-off label). The 30 mg (½ gr), 60 mg (1 gr), and 120 mg (2 gr) potencies are also available in cartons of 100 tablets (10 strips of 10 tablets) packaged in Unit Dose as Armadose.®
Tablets should be stored at controlled room temperature—between 15°–30°C (59°–86°F) in capped bottles or unbroken plastic strip packing.

CAUTION: Federal (U.S.A.) law prohibits dispensing without prescription.

Revised: March, 1985

Shown in Product Identification Section, page 433

THYROLAR® ℞

[*thī-rō-lär*]

(T_3/T_4 Liotrix Tablets, U.S.P.)

DESCRIPTION

Thyrolar® Tablets (T_3/T_4 Liotrix Tablets, U.S.P.) contain T_3 thyronine sodium (T_3 liothyronine) and T_4 thyroxine sodium (T_4 levothyroxine) in the amounts listed in the "How Supplied" section.
The inactive ingredients are calcium phosphate, microcrystalline cellulose, corn starch, lactose, and magnesium stearate. The tablets also contain the following dyes: Thyrolar® ¼—F.D.&C. Blue #1 and F.D.&C. Red #40; Thyrolar® ½—F.D.&C. Red #40 and F.D.&C. Yellow #10; Thyrolar® 1—F.D.&C. Red #40; Thyrolar® 2—F.D.&C. Blue #1, F.D.&C. Red #40, and F.D.&C. Yellow #10; Thyrolar® 3—F.D.&C. Red #40 and F.D.&C. Yellow #10.

CLINICAL PHARMACOLOGY

The steps in the synthesis of the thyroid hormones are controlled by thyrotropin (Thyroid Stimulating Hormone, TSH) secreted by the anterior pituitary. This hormone's secretion is in turn controlled by a feedback mechanism effected by the thyroid hormones themselves and by thyrotropin releasing hormone (TRH), a tripeptide of hypothalamic origin. Endogenous thyroid hormone secretion is suppressed when exogenous thyroid hormones are administered to euthyroid individuals in excess of the normal gland's secretion.
The mechanisms by which thyroid hormones exert their physiologic action are not well understood. These hormones enhance oxygen consumption by most tissues of the body, increase the basal metabolic rate, and the metabolism of carbohydrates, lipids, and proteins. Thus, they exert a profound influence on every organ system in the body and are of particular importance in the development of the central nervous system.
The normal thyroid gland contains approximately 200 mcg of T_4 thyroxine per gram of gland, and 15 mcg of T_3 thyronine per gram. The ratio of these two hormones in the circulation does not represent the ratio in the thyroid gland, since about 80 percent of peripheral T_3 thyronine comes from monodeiodination of T_4 thyroxine. Peripheral monodeiodination of T_4 thyroxine at the 5 position (inner ring) also re-

sults in the formation of reverse T_3 thyronine, which is calorigenically inactive.

T_3 thyronine levels are low in the fetus and newborn, in old age, in chronic caloric deprivation, hepatic cirrhosis, renal failure, surgical stress, and chronic illnesses representing what has been called the "T_3 thyronine syndrome."

Pharmacokinetics—Animal studies have shown that T_4 thyroxine is only partially absorbed from the gastrointestinal tract. The degree of absorption is dependent on the vehicle used for its administration and by the character of the intestinal contents, the intestinal flora, including plasma protein, soluble dietary factors, all of which bind thyroid and thereby make it unavailable for diffusion. Only 41 percent is absorbed when given in a gelatin capsule as opposed to a 74 percent absorption when given with an albumin carrier. Depending on other factors, absorption has varied from 48 to 79 percent of the administered dose. Fasting increases absorption. Malabsorption syndromes, as well as dietary factors, (children's soybean formula, concomitant use of anionic exchange resins such as cholestyramine) cause excessive fecal loss. T_3 thyronine is almost totally absorbed, 95 percent in 4 hours. The hormones contained in the natural preparations are absorbed in a manner similar to the synthetic hormones.

More than 99 percent of circulating hormones are bound to serum proteins, including thyroid-binding globulin (TBg), thyroid-binding prealbumin (TBPA), and albumin (TBa), whose capacities and affinities vary for the hormones. The higher affinity of T_4 thyroxine for both TBg and TBPA as compared to T_3 thyronine partially explains the higher serum levels and longer half-life of the former hormone. Both protein-bound hormones exist in reverse equilibrium with minute amounts of free hormone, the latter accounting for the metabolic activity.

Deiodination of T_4 thyroxine occurs at a number of sites, including liver, kidney, and other tissues. The conjugated hormone, in the form of glucuronide or sulfate, is found in the bile and gut where it may complete an enterohepatic circulation. Eighty-five percent of T_4 thyroxine metabolized daily is deiodinated.

INDICATIONS AND USAGE

Thyrolar® Tablets are indicated:

1. As replacement or supplemental therapy in patients with hypothyroidism of any etiology, except transient hypothyroidism during the recovery phase of subacute thyroiditis. This category includes cretinism, myxedema, and ordinary hypothyroidism in patients of any age (children, adults, the elderly), or state (including pregnancy); primary hypothyroidism resulting from functional deficiency, primary atrophy, partial or total absence of thyroid gland, or the effects of surgery, radiation, or drugs, with or without the presence of goiter; and secondary (pituitary), or tertiary (hypothalamic) hypothyroidism (See WARNINGS).
2. As pituitary TSH suppressants, in the treatment or prevention of various types of euthyroid goiters, including thyroid nodules, sub-acute or chronic lymphocytic thyroiditis (Hashimoto's), multinodular goiter, and in the management of thyroid cancer.
3. As diagnostic agents in suppression tests to differentiate suspected mild hyperthyroidism or thyroid gland autonomy.

CONTRAINDICATIONS

Thyroid hormone preparations are generally contraindicated in patients with diagnosed but as yet uncorrected adrenal cortical insufficiency, untreated thyrotoxicosis, and apparent hypersensitivity to any of their active or extraneous constituents. There is no well documented evidence from the literature, however, of true allergic or idiosyncratic reactions to thyroid hormone.

WARNINGS

> Drugs with thyroid hormone activity, alone or together with other therapeutic agents, have been used for the treatment of obesity. In euthyroid patients, doses within the range of daily hormonal requirements are ineffective for weight reduction. Larger doses may produce serious or even life-threatening manifestations of toxicity, particularly when given in association with sympathomimetic amines such as those used for their anorectic effects.

The use of thyroid hormones in the therapy of obesity, alone or combined with other drugs, is unjustified and has been shown to be ineffective. Neither is their use justified for the treatment of male or female infertility unless this condition is accompanied by hypothyroidism.

PRECAUTIONS

General—Thyroid hormones should be used with great caution in a number of circumstances where the integrity of the cardiovascular system, particularly the coronary arteries, is suspected. These include patients with angina pectoris or the elderly, in whom there is a greater likelihood of occult cardiac disease. In these patients therapy should be initiated with low doses, i.e. one tablet of Thyrolar® ¼ or Thyrolar® ½. When, in such patients, a euthyroid state can only be reached at the expense of an aggravation of the cardiovascular disease, thyroid hormone dosage should be reduced. Thyroid hormone therapy in patients with concomitant diabetes mellitus or diabetes insipidus or adrenal cortical insufficiency aggravates the intensity of their symptoms. Appropriate adjustments of the various therapeutic measures directed at these concomitant endocrine diseases are required. The therapy of myxedema coma requires simultaneous administration of glucocorticoids (See DOSAGE AND ADMINISTRATION).

Hypothyroidism decreases and hyperthyroidism increases the sensitivity to oral anticoagulants. Prothrombin time should be closely monitored in thyroid treated patients on oral anticoagulants and dosage of the latter agents adjusted on the basis of frequent prothrombin time determinations. In infants, excessive doses of thyroid hormone preparations may produce craniosynostosis.

Information for the Patient—Patients on thyroid hormone preparations and parents of children on thyroid therapy should be informed that:

1. Replacement therapy is to be taken essentially for life, with the exception of cases of transient hypothyroidism, usually associated with thyroiditis, and in those patients receiving a therapeutic trial of the drug.
2. They should immediately report during the course of therapy any signs or symptoms of thyroid hormone toxicity, e.g., chest pain, increased pulse rate, palpitations, excessive sweating, heat intolerance, nervousness, or any other unusual event.
3. In case of concomitant diabetes mellitus, the daily dosage of antidiabetic medication may need readjustment as thyroid hormone replacement is achieved. If thyroid medication is stopped, a downward readjustment of the dosage of insulin or oral hypoglycemic agent may be necessary to avoid hypoglycemia. At all times, close monitoring of urinary glucose levels is mandatory in such patients.
4. In case of concomitant oral anticoagulant therapy, the prothrombin time should be measured frequently to determine if the dosage of oral anticoagulants is to be readjusted.
5. Partial loss of hair may be experienced by children in the first few months of thyroid therapy, but this is usually a transient phenomenon and later recovery is usually the rule.

Laboratory Tests—Treatment of patients with thyroid hormones requires the periodic assessment of thyroid status by means of appropriate laboratory tests besides the full clinical evaluation. The TSH suppression test can be used to test the effectiveness of any thyroid preparation bearing in mind the relative insensitivity of the infant pituitary to the negative feedback effect of thyroid hormones. Serum T_4 thyroxine levels can be used to test the effectiveness of all thyroid medications except T_3 thyronine. When the total serum T_4 thyroxine is low but TSH is normal, a test specific to assess unbound (free) T_4 thyroxine levels is warranted. Specific measurements of T_4 thyroxine and T_3 thyronine by competitive protein binding or radioimmunoassay are not influenced by blood levels of organic or inorganic iodine.

Drug Interactions—Oral Anticoagulants—Thyroid hormones appear to increase catabolism of vitamin K-dependent clotting factors. If oral anticoagulants are also being given, compensatory increases in clotting factor synthesis are impaired. Patients stabilized on oral anticoagulants who are found to require thyroid replacement therapy should be watched very closely when thyroid is started. If a patient is truly hypothyroid, it is likely that a reduction in anticoagulant dosage will be required. No special precautions appear to be necessary when oral anticoagulant therapy is begun in a patient already stabilized on maintenance thyroid replacement therapy.

Insulin or Oral Hypoglycemics—Initiating thyroid replacement therapy may cause increases in insulin or oral hypoglycemic requirements. The effects seen are poorly understood and depend upon a variety of factors such as dose and type of thyroid preparations and endocrine status of the patient. Patients receiving insulin or oral hypoglycemics should be closely watched during initiation of thyroid replacement therapy.

Cholestyramine—Cholestyramine binds both T_4 thyroxine and T_3 thyronine in the intestine, thus impairing absorption of these thyroid hormones. *In vitro* studies indicate that the binding is not easily removed. Therefore, four to five hours should elapse between administration of cholestyramine and thyroid hormones.

Estrogen, Oral Contraceptives—Estrogens tend to increase serum thyroxine-binding globulin (TBg). In a patient with a nonfunctioning thyroid gland who is receiving thyroid replacement therapy, free T_4 thyroxine may be decreased when estrogens are started thus increasing thyroid requirements. However, if the patient's thyroid gland has sufficient function, the decreased free thyroxine will result in a compensatory increase in thyroxine output by the thyroid. Therefore, patients without a functioning thyroid gland who are on thyroid replacement therapy may need to increase their thyroid dose if estrogens or estrogen-containing oral contraceptives are given.

Drug/Laboratory Test Interactions—The following drugs or moieties are known to interfere with laboratory tests performed in patients on thyroid hormone therapy: androgens, corticosteroids, estrogens, oral contraceptives containing estrogens, iodine-containing preparations, and the numerous preparations containing salicylates.

1. Changes in TBg concentration should be taken into consideration in the interpretation of T_4 thyroxine and T_3 thyronine values. In such cases, the unbound (free) hormone should be measured. Pregnancy, estrogens, and estrogen-containing oral contraceptives increase TBg concentrations. TBg may also be increased during infectious hepatitis. Decreases in TBg concentrations are observed in nephrosis, acromegaly, and after androgen or corticosteroid therapy. Familial hyper- or hypo-thyroxine-binding-globulinemias have been described. The incidence of TBg deficiency approximates 1 in 9,000. The binding of thyroxine by TBPA is inhibited by salicylates.
2. Medicinal or dietary iodine interferes with all *in vivo* tests of radio-iodine uptake, producing low uptakes which may not be relative of a true decrease in hormone synthesis.
3. The persistence of clinical and laboratory evidence of hypothyroidism in spite of adequate dosage replacement indicates either poor patient compliance, poor absorption, excessive fecal loss, or inactivity of the preparation. Intracellular resistance to thyroid hormone is quite rare.

Carcinogenesis, Mutagenesis, and Impairment of Fertility—A reportedly apparent association between prolonged thyroid therapy and breast cancer has not been confirmed and patients on thyroid for established indications should not discontinue therapy. No confirmatory long-term studies in animals have been performed to evaluate carcinogenic potential, mutagenicity, or impairment of fertility in either males or females.

Pregnancy-Category A—Thyroid hormones do not readily cross the placental barrier. The clinical experience to date does not indicate any adverse effect on fetuses when thyroid hormones are administered to pregnant women. On the basis of current knowledge, thyroid replacement therapy to hypothyroid women should not be discontinued during pregnancy.

Nursing Mothers—Minimal amounts of thyroid hormones are excreted in human milk. Thyroid is not associated with serious adverse reactions and does not have a known tumorigenic potential. However, caution should be exercised when thyroid is administered to a nursing woman.

Pediatric Use—Pregnant mothers provide little or no thyroid hormone to the fetus. The incidence of congenital hypothyroidism is relatively high (1:4,000) and the hypothyroid fetus would not derive any benefit from the small amounts of hormone crossing the placental barrier. Routine determinations or serum T_4 thyroxine and/or TSH is strongly advised in neonates in view of the deleterious effects of thyroid deficiency on growth and development.

Treatment should be initiated immediately upon diagnosis, and maintained for life, unless transient hypothyroidism is suspected; in which case, therapy may be interrupted for 2 to 8 weeks after the age of 3 years to reassess the condition. Cessation of therapy is justified in patients who have maintained a normal TSH during those 2 to 8 weeks.

ADVERSE REACTIONS

Adverse reactions other than those indicative of hyperthyroidism because of therapeutic overdosage, either initially or during the maintenance period, are rare (See OVERDOSAGE).

OVERDOSAGE

Signs and Symptoms—Excessive doses of thyroid result in a hypermetabolic state resembling in every respect the condition of endogenous origin. The condition may be self-induced.

Treatment of Overdosage—Dosage should be reduced or therapy temporarily discontinued if signs and symptoms of overdosage appear.

Treatment may be reinstituted at a lower dosage. In normal individuals, normal hypothalamic-pituitary-thyroid axis function is restored in 6 to 8 weeks after thyroid suppression. Treatment of acute massive thyroid hormone overdosage is aimed at reducing gastrointestinal absorption of the drugs and counteracting central and peripheral effects, mainly those of increased sympathetic activity. Vomiting may be induced initially if further gastrointestinal absorption can reasonably be prevented and barring contraindications such as coma, convulsions, or loss of the gagging reflex. Treatment is symptomatic and supportive. Oxygen may be administered and ventilation maintained. Cardiac glycosides may be indicated if congestive heart failure develops. Measures to control fever, hypoglycemia, or fluid loss should be instituted if needed. Antiadrenergic agents, particularly propranolol, have been used advantageously in the treatment of increased sympathetic activity. Propranolol may be adminis-

Continued on next page

USV—Cont.

tered intravenously at a dosage of 1 to 3 mg over a 10 minute period or orally, 80 to 160 mg/day, especially when no contraindications exist for its use.

DOSAGE AND ADMINISTRATION

The dosage of Thyrolar® Tablets (T_3/T_4 Liotrix Tablets, U.S.P.) is determined by the indication and must in every case be individualized according to patient response and laboratory findings.

Thyroid hormones are given orally. In acute, emergency conditions, injectable T_4 thyroxine sodium may be given intravenously when oral administration is not feasible or desirable, as in the treatment of myxedema coma, or during total parenteral nutrition. Intramuscular administration is not advisable because of reported poor absorption.

Hypothyroidism—Therapy is usually instituted using low doses with increments which depend on the cardiovascular status of the patient. The usual starting dose is one tablet of Thyrolar® ½ with increments of one tablet of Thyrolar® ¼ every 2 to 3 weeks. A lower starting dose, one tablet of Thyrolar® ¼/day, is recommended in patients with long standing myxedema, particularly if cardiovascular impairment is suspected, in which case extreme caution is recommended. The appearance of angina is an indication for a reduction in dosage. Most patients require one tablet of Thyrolar® 1 to one tablet of Thyrolar® 2 per day. Failure to respond to doses of one tablet of Thyrolar® 3 suggests lack of compliance or malabsorption. Maintenance dosages one tablet of Thyrolar® 1 to one tablet of Thyrolar® 2 per day usually result in normal serum T_4 thyroxine and T_3 thyronine levels. Adequate therapy usually results in normal TSH and T_4 thyroxine levels after 2 to 3 weeks of therapy.

Readjustment of thyroid hormone dosage should be made within the first four weeks of therapy, after proper clinical and laboratory evaluations, including serum levels of T_4 thyroxine, bound and free, and TSH.

T_3 thyronine may be used in preference to T_4 thyroxine during radio-isotope scanning procedures, since induction of hypothyroidism in those cases is more abrupt and can be of shorter duration. It may also be preferred when impairment of peripheral conversion of T_4 thyroxine and T_3 thyronine is suspected.

Myxedema Coma—Myxedema coma is usually precipitated in the hypothyroid patient of long-standing by intercurrent illness or drugs such as sedatives and anesthetics and should be considered a medical emergency. Therapy should be directed at the correction of electrolyte disturbances and possible infection besides the administration of thyroid hormones. Corticosteroids should be administered routinely. T_4 thyroxine and T_3 thyronine may be administered via a nasogastric tube but the preferred route of administration of both hormones is intravenous. T_4 thyroxine is given at a starting dose of 400 mcg (100 mcg/ml) given rapidly, and is usually well tolerated, even in the elderly. This initial dose is followed by daily supplements of 100 to 200 mcg given IV. Normal T_4 thyroxine levels are achieved in 24 hours followed in 3 days by threefold elevation of T_3 thyronine. Oral therapy with thyroid hormone would be resumed as soon as the clinical situation has been stabilized and the patient is able to take oral medication.

Thyroid Cancer—Exogenous thyroid hormone may produce regression of metastases from follicular and papillary carcinoma of the thyroid and is used as ancillary therapy of these conditions with radioactive iodine. TSH should be suppressed to low or undetectable levels. Therefore, larger amounts of thyroid hormone than those used for replacement therapy are required. Medullary carcinoma of the thyroid is usually unresponsive to this therapy.

Thyroid Suppression Therapy—Administration of thyroid hormone in doses higher than those produced physiologically by the gland results in suppression of the production of endogenous hormone. This is the basis for the thyroid suppression test and is used as an aid in the diagnosis of patients with signs of mild hyperthyroidism in whom base line laboratory tests appear normal, or to demonstrate thyroid gland autonomy in patients with Grave's ophthalmopathy. ^{131}I uptake is determined before and after the administration of the exogenous hormone. A fifty percent or greater suppression of uptake indicates a normal thyroid-pituitary axis and thus rules out thyroid gland automomy.

For adults, the usual suppressive dose of T_4 thyroxine is 1.56 mg/kg of body weight per day given for 7 to 10 days. These doses usually yield normal serum T_4 thyroxine and T_3 thyronine levels and lack of response to TSH.

Thyroid hormones should be administered cautiously to patients in whom there is strong suspicion of thyroid gland autonomy, in view of the fact that the exogenous hormone effects will be additive to the endogenous source.

Pediatric Dosage—Pediatric dosage should follow the recommendations summarized in Table 1. In infants with congenital hypothyroidism, therapy with full doses should be instituted as soon as the diagnosis has been made.

Recommended Pediatric Dosage for Congenital Hypothyroidism

Age	Dose per day in mcg T_3/T_4	to	T_3/T_4
0–6 mos	3.1/12.5	to	6.25/25
6–12 mos	6.25/25	to	9.35/37.5
1–5 yrs	9.35/37.5	to	12.5/50
6–12 yrs	12.5/50	to	18.75/75
Over 12 yrs		over	18.75/75

Table 1

HOW SUPPLIED

Thyrolar® Tablets (T_3/T_4Liotrix Tablets, U.S.P.) are available in five potencies, coded as follows:
[See table below].

Supplied in bottles of 100, two-layered compressed tablets. Thyrolar®-½, Thyrolar®-1, Thyrolar®-2, and Thyrolar®-3 are also supplied in bottles of 1000.

Tablets should be stored at controlled room temperature—between 15°–30°C (59°–86°F) in capped bottles.

CAUTION: Federal (U.S.A.) law prohibits dispensing without prescription.

Revised: January, 1986

Shown in Product Identification Section, page 433

Name	Composition (T_3/T_4 per tablet)	Color	Armacode®
Thyrolar®—¼	3.1 mcg/12.5 mcg	Violet/White	YC
Thyrolar®—½	6.25 mcg/25 mcg	Peach/White	YD
Thyrolar®—1	12.5 mcg/50 mcg	Pink/White	YE
Thyrolar®—2	25 mcg/100 mcg	Green/White	YF
Thyrolar®—3	37.5 mcg/150 mcg	Yellow/White	YH

TUSSAR® DM — OTC

[*tŭs'är*]
Cough Syrup
Non-narcotic, Alcohol Free
Antitussive/Decongestant/Antihistaminic

Each 5 mL (one teaspoonful) contains:
Dextromethorphan
Hydrobromide, U.S.P. ....15 mg
Chlorpheniramine Maleate, U.S.P. ....2 mg
Phenylephrine Hydrochloride, U.S.P. ....5 mg
Methylparaben, N.F. ....5 mg

Also contains artifical flavor, citric acid, F.D.&C. Red. No. 40, glucose, glycerin, sodium citrate, and sucrose.

INDICATIONS

For relief of cough due to common cold and minor throat and bronchial irritations. TUSSAR DM provides relief of nasal congestion, running nose and watery eyes as may occur in allergic rhinitis (such as hay fever).

DIRECTIONS FOR USE

ADULTS—One or two teaspoonfuls (5 or 10 mL) every six to eight hours, not to exceed eight teaspoonfuls in any 24-hour period.

CHILDREN 6–12 YEARS—One teaspoonful (5 mL) every six to eight hours, not to exceed four teaspoonfuls in any 24-hour period.

CHILDREN UNDER 6 YEARS—Not to be administered unless directed by a physician.

WARNINGS

Do not take this product for persistent cough which may indicate a serious condition except under the supervision of a physician. Do not take this product if you have high blood pressure, heart disease or thyroid disease unless directed by a physician. Do not exceed recommended dosage. As with any drug, if you are pregnant or nursing a baby, seek the advice of a health professional before using this product.

CAUTIONS

If symptoms persist for more than 7 days or are accompanied by a high fever, rash or persistent headache, consult a physician. If drowsiness occurs, do not drive a car or operate machinery.

3/85

TUSSAR®-2 Ⓒ

[*tŭs-är*]
(exempt narcotic cough syrup)

Each 5 ml (one teaspoonful) contains:
Codeine Phosphate, USP ....10 mg

WARNINGS—MAY BE HABIT FORMING

As with any drug, if you are pregnant or nursing a baby, seek the advice of a health professional before using this product. DO NOT USE IF BAND IMPRINTED ***USV*** HAS BEEN BROKEN.

Carbetapentane Citrate ....7.5 mg
Chlorpheniramine Maleate, USP ....2.0 mg
Guaifenesin, USP ....50 mg
Sodium Citrate, USP ....130 mg
Citric Acid, USP ....20 mg
Methylparaben, N.F. 0.1%
Alcohol 5%

Also contains F.D.&C. Blue No. 1, F.D.&C. Yellow No. 10, glucose, methyl salicylate, synthetic peppermint oil, propylene glycol, saccharin, synthetic spearmint oil, and sucrose.

INDICATIONS

For relief of severe coughs due to respiratory conditions such as common cold, bronchitis, and influenza.

DIRECTIONS FOR USE

Adults—One teaspoonful 3 to 4 times a day as needed for cough, but no more than 8 teaspoonfuls in any 24-hour period.

CAUTIONS

Persistent cough may indicate the presence of a serious condition. Seek medical advice if there is a high fever or if relief does not occur within 3 days. Persons with a high fever or persistent cough should use only on advice of a physician. Not to be administered to infants or children unless directed by a physician. If drowsiness occurs, do not drive a car or operate machinery.

7/85

TUSSAR® SF (Sugar Free) Ⓒ

[*tŭs'är*]
(exempt narcotic cough syrup)

Formulation identical to Tussar®-2, except Tussar SF contains saccharin-sorbitol base and F.D.&C. Red No. 40 for patients who must limit sugar intake. Alcohol content 12 percent instead of 5 percent.

EDUCATIONAL MATERIAL

For further information, contact your local USV Sales Representative or USV Corporate Headquarters. Your request will be forwarded to the appropriate Sales Representative.

United

Division of Pfizer Hospital Products Group
11775 STARKEY ROAD
LARGO, FL 33543

SKIN-PREP™

Protective Dressing

DESCRIPTION

A flexible, plasticized protective dressing with n-butyl monoester of poly (methyl vinyl ether/maleic acid), and acetyl tributyl citrate dissolved in isopropyl alcohol.

INDICATIONS AND USAGE

Skin-Prep is formulated to coat and protect skin exposed to harmful organisms, adhesive trauma, chafing, irritation, urine, feces and digestive acids.

Skin-Prep also provides a water proof, artifact free, highly conductive skin surface for electronic monitoring and transcutaneous electronic nerve stimulation (TENS). Helps prevent and eliminate skin breakdown around stoma sites, under adhesives, around decubiti and abrasions.

CONTRAINDICATIONS

Hypersensitivity to any component of the preparation.

PRECAUTIONS AND ADVERSE REACTIONS

For external use only. Active ingredients indicate minimal animal toxicity but no toxicity reported throughout their long established use. Safe and convenient when used as directed. Allow to dry prior to application of tape or electrodes. Do not spray on or apply directly to open wounds or mucous membranes. Sting will be experienced if contacts cut or open wound. Flammable. When using aerosol can, do not spray near flame or while smoking.

DOSAGE AND ADMINISTRATION
Apply as needed.

HOW SUPPLIED
2 fl. oz. bottles with brush, 4.25 oz. wt. aerosol can, single wipes boxes of 50, swabs boxes of 50.

UNICARE™ Lotion

DESCRIPTION
An over-the-counter drug. A lotion specially formulated as a therapeutic aid in the prevention of skin irritation from dryness, itching, or exposure to weather and harsh environments.

INGREDIENTS
Active—Allantoin 0.5%, Dimethicone-1.0%
Cosmetic—Aloe vera gel, propylene glycol, isopropyl palmitate, stearic acid, lanolin oil, potassium hydroxide, carbomer 934, stearyl alcohol, methylparaben, propylparaben, titanium dioxide, fragrance, purified water.

INDICATIONS AND USE
UniCare soothes and helps heal dry, chapped and irritated skin. Formulated with allantoin to promote healing. Use UniCare daily. Cleanse skin, rinse and pat dry; apply liberally as needed.

CONTRAINDICATIONS
Hypersensitivity to any components of the preparation.

PRECAUTIONS AND ADVERSE REACTIONS
For external use only. Avoid contact with eyes. If irritation occurs or if symptoms persist for more than 7 days, discontinue use and consult a physician.

DOSAGE AND ADMINISTRATION
Apply liberally as needed.

HOW SUPPLIED
6 fl. oz. plastic bottle with flip-up cap.

UNI DERM® MOISTURIZER

DESCRIPTION
An over-the counter drug. A greaseless protective moisturizer which restores moisture and oils.

INGREDIENTS
Active—Lanolin anhydrous
Cosmetic—Isopropyl palmitate, Petrolatum, Sorbitan Sesquioleate, Paraffin, Mineral oil, Vitamin A and D_3 in vegetable oil, Benzethonium chloride, Edetate Disodium, Quaternium 15, Fragrances and water.

INDICATIONS AND USE
Uni Derm helps maintain skin integrity and prevent skin breakdown due to dryness, friction, pressure and incontinence, without affecting the holding power of adhesives. Formulated for long term use to prevent sensitive, dry or irritated skin.

CONTRAINDICATIONS
Hypersensitivity to any components of the preparation.

PRECAUTIONS AND ADVERSE REACTIONS
For external use only. Discontinue use if itching, burning or redness appears.

DOSAGE AND ADMINISTRATION
Apply liberally as needed.

HOW SUPPLIED
3 oz. wt. soft plastic tubes and 8.1 oz. wt. hard plastic jars.

UNI SALVE®
Protective Ointment

DESCRIPTION
An over-the-counter drug. A soothing, lubricating protective ointment.

INDGREDIENTS
Active—Petrolatum. Cosmetic—Chlorometaxylenol, Benzethonium Chloride, Propylparaben, Butylated Hydroxyanisole, Vitamins A & D_3 in vegetable oil, Fragrance, D & C Green #6.

INDICATIONS AND USE
Uni Salve provides a water-repellent shield to protect skin and retard moisture loss. Restores moisture and oils to help maintain proper skin integrity and prevent skin breakdown due to dryness, friction, pressure, and incontinence. Sooths minor skin irritations.

CONTRAINDICATIONS
Hypersensitivity to any components of the preparation.

PRECAUTIONS AND ADVERSE REACTIONS
For external use only. Avoid contact with eyes. Not to be applied over puncture wounds, infections or lacerations. If symptoms persist for more than seven days, discontinue use and consult a physician.

DOSAGE AND ADMINISTRATION
Apply liberally as needed.

HOW SUPPLIED
2.47 and 0.25 oz. wt. tubes.

UNI WASH®
Skin Cleanser

DESCRIPTION
A non-irritating pH balanced solution.

INGREDIENTS
Water, Propylene Glycol, Disodium Oleamido MEA-Sulfosuccinate, Octoxynol-9, Boric Acid, Lauramide DEA, Lauramidopropyl Betaine, Diazolidinyl Urea, Citric Acid, FD & C Yellow #5, Sodium Borate, Methyl Paraben, and Edetate Disodium.

INDICATIONS AND USAGE
UniWash cleanses and deodorizes affected areas, dissolving feces, urine and emesis residue for easy removal. It is soapless with a pH factor similar to skin. Use for gentle, meticulous care required in peristomal and perineal areas, around wounds and drainage tubes to prevent skin scald from urinary and fecal incontinence. UniWash helps reduce odor.

CONTRAINDICATIONS
Hypersensitivity to any components of the preparation.

PRECAUTIONS AND ADVERSE REACTIONS
For external use only. UniWash is not considered a primary skin irritant under normal use conditions. UniWash may cause eye irritation. Eyes should be rinsed thoroughly if accidental contact occurs. Should UniWash be accidentally ingested, induce vomiting.

DOSAGE AND ADMINISTRATION
Spray affected area, remove residue and rinse thoroughly.

HOW SUPPLIED
8.1 fl. oz. plastic bottles with hand pumps, one gallon plastic containers.

Products are listed alphabetically in the **PINK SECTION.**

Products are cross-indexed by product classifications in the **BLUE SECTION**

Products are cross-indexed by generic and chemical names in the **YELLOW SECTION**

The Upjohn Company
KALAMAZOO, MI 49001

UPJOHN PRODUCT IDENTIFICATION
Most capsules and tablets manufactured by The Upjohn Company are imprinted with one or a combination of the following: (1) Product trademark (2) Dosage strength (3) "Upjohn" or "U" (4) That portion of the National Drug Code (NDC) number which indicates product and strength.
A complete list of oral solid dosage forms with their assigned NDC numbers is provided below.

Code #	Product	Strength
10	**HALCION®** Tablets (Triazolam) *See Product Identification Section*	0.125 mg
11	**FEMINONE®** Tablets (ethinyl estradiol tablets, USP)	0.05 mg
12	**CORTEF®** Tablets (hydrocortisone tablets, USP)	5 mg
14	**HALOTESTIN®** Tablets (fluoxymesterone tablets, USP) *See Product Identification Section*	2 mg
15	**CORTISONE ACETATE** Tablets, USP	5 mg
17	**HALCION®** Tablets (triazolam) *See Product Identification Section*	0.25 mg
18	**DIDREX®** Tablets (benzphetamine hydrochloride) *See Product Identification Section*	Ⓒ III 25 mg
19	**HALOTESTIN®** Tablets (fluoxymesterone tablets, USP) *See Product Identification Section*	5 mg
22	**MEDROL®** Tablets (methylprednisolone tablets, USP) *See Product Identification Section*	8 mg
23	**CORTISONE ACETATE** Tablets, USP	10 mg
24	**DIDREX®** Tablets (benzphetamine hydrochloride) *See Product Identification Section*	50 mg
25	**DELTA-CORTEF®** Tablets (prednisolone tablets, USP)	5 mg
27	**HALCION®** Tablets (triazalam) *See Product Identification Section*	0.5 mg
29	**XANAX®** Tablets (alprazolam) *See Product Identification Section*	0.25 mg
31	**CORTEF®** Tablets (hydrocortisone tablets, USP)	10 mg
32	**DELTASONE®** Tablets (prednisone tablets, USP) *See Product Identification Section*	2.5 mg.
34	**CORTISONE ACETATE** Tablets, USP	25 mg
36	**HALOTESTIN®** Tablets (fluoxymesterone tablets, USP) *See Product Identification Section*	10 mg
38	**HALODRIN®** Tablets (fluoxymesterone and ethinyl estradiol)	
44	**CORTEF®** Tablets (hydrocortisone tablets, USP)	20 mg
45	**DELTASONE®** Tablets (prednisone tablets, USP) *See Product Identification Section*	5 mg
49	**MEDROL®** Tablets (methylprednisolone tablets, USP) *See Product Identification Section*	2 mg
50	**PROVERA®** Tablets (medroxyprogesterone acetate tablets, USP) *See Product Identification Section*	10 mg
55	**XANAX®** Tablets (alprazolam) *See Product Identification Section*	0.5 mg
56	**MEDROL®** Tablets (methylprednisolone tablets, USP) *See Product Identification Section*	4 mg
61	**PAMINE®** Tablets (methscopolamine bromide tablets, USP) *See Product Identification Section*	2.5 mg

Continued on next page

Information on these Upjohn products is based on labeling in effect August 15, 1986. Further information concerning these and other Upjohn products may be obtained by direct inquiry to Medical Information, The Upjohn Company, Kalamazoo, Michigan 49001.

Upjohn—Cont.

No.	Product	Strength
64	**PROVERA**® Tablets (medroxyprogesterone acetate tablets, USP) *See Product Identification Section*	2.5 mg
70	**TOLINASE**® Tablets (tolazamide tablets, USP) *See Product Identification Section*	100 mg
73	**MEDROL**® Tablets (methylprednisolone tablets, USP) *See Product Identification Section*	16 mg
81	**ADEFLOR CHEWABLE**® Tablets Fluoride and vitamins *See Product Identification Section*	0.5 mg
90	**XANAX**® Tablets (alprazolam) *See Product Identification Section*	1 mg
92	**ADEFLOR CHEWABLE**® Tablets Fluoride and vitamins *See Product Identification Section*	1 mg
100	**ORINASE**® Tablets (tolbutamide tablets, USP) *See Product Identification Section*	0.5 Gm
101	**ALBAMYCIN**® Capsules (novobiocin sodium)	250 mg
103	**E-MYCIN**® Tablets (erythromycin enteric-coated tablets) *See Product Identification Section*	250 mg
106	**DIOSTATE D**® Tablets Vitamin, calcium and phosphorus supplement	
114	**TOLINASE**® Tablets (tolazamide tablets, USP) *See Product Identification Section*	250 mg
115	**ADEFLOR M**® Tablets Vitamins and minerals with fluoride	
121	**LONITEN**® Tablets (minoxidil) *See Product Identification Section*	2.5 mg
122	**CEBENASE**® Tablets	
131	**MICRONASE**® Tablets (glyburide) *See Product Identification Section*	1.25 mg
137	**LONITEN**® Tablets (minoxidil) *See Product Identification Section*	10 mg
138	**UNICAP**® Capsules Multivitamin Supplement	
141	**MICRONASE**® Tablets (glyburide) *See Product Identification Section*	2.5 mg
155	**MEDROL**® Tablets (methylprednisolone tablets, USP) *See Product Identification Section*	24 mg
165	**DELTASONE**® Tablets (prednisone tablets, USP) *See Product Identification Section*	20 mg
171	**MICRONASE**® Tablets (glyburide) *See Product Identification Section*	5.0 mg
176	**MEDROL**® Tablets (methylprednisolone tablets, USP) *See Product Identification Section*	32 mg
193	**DELTASONE**® Tablets (prednisone tablets, USP) *See Product Identification Section*	10 mg
198	**UNICAP Jr**™ Chewable Tablets Multivitamin	
225	**CLEOCIN HCl**® Capsules (clindamycin HCl capsules, USP) *See Product Identification Section*	150 mg
243	**ALKETS**® Tablets	
251	**CALCIUM GLUCONATE** Tablets, USP	975 mg
272	**CALCIUM LACTATE** Tablets, USP	650 mg
285	**UNICAP**® Plus Iron Tablets	
286	**PROVERA**® Tablets (medroxyprogesterone acetate tablets, USP) *See Product Identification Section*	5 mg
331	**CLEOCIN HCl**® Capsules (clindamycin HCl capsules, USP) *See Product Identification Section*	75 mg
336	**LINCOCIN**® Pediatric Capsules (lincomycin hydrochloride capsules, USP)	250 mg
363	**ZYMACAP**® Capsules Multivitamins	
388	**DELTASONE**® Tablets (prednisone tablets, USP) *See Product Identification Section*	50 mg
412	**MAOLATE**® Tablets (chlorphenesin carbamate) *See Product Identification Section*	400 mg
461	**SIGTAB**® Tablets High potency vitamin supplement	
477	**TOLINASE**® Tablets (tolazamide tablets, USP) *See Product Identification Section*	500 mg
500	**LINCOCIN**® Capsules (lincomycin hydrochloride capsules, USP)	500 mg
521	**MYCIFRADIN**® Tablets (neomycin sulfate tablets, USP)	0.5 Gm
586	**UTICILLIN VK**® Tablets (penicillin V potassium tablets, USP)	250 mg
671	**UTICILLIN VK**® Tablets (penicillin V potassium tablets, USP)	500 mg
701	**ORINASE**® Tablets (tolbutamide tablets, USP) *See Product Identification Section*	250 mg
725	**MOTRIN**® Tablets (ibuprofen tablets, USP) *See Product Identification Section*	800 mg
730	**PHENOLAX**® Wafers (phenolphthalein)	
733	**MOTRIN**® Tablets (ibuprofen tablets, USP) *See Product Identification Section*	300 mg
742	**MOTRIN**® Tablets (ibuprofen tablets, USP) *See Product Identification Section*	600 mg
750	**MOTRIN**® Tablets (ibuprofen tablets, USP) *See Product Identification Section*	400 mg
782	**PANMYCIN**® Capsules (tetracycline hydrochloride capsules, USP)	250 mg
873	**SUPER D**® Perles (oleovitamins A and D capsules, N.F.)	
949	**URACIL MUSTARD** Capsules	1 mg
3176	**E-MYCIN**® Tablets (erythromycin base enteric-coated tablets) *See Product Identification Section*	333 mg
3212	**PYRROXATE**® Capsules	
3293	**KAOPECTATE**® Tablet Formula	
3300	**P-A-C**® Revised Formula Analgesic Tablets (aspirin and caffeine tablets)	
3336	**UNICAP M**® Tablets	
3338	**UNICAP T**® Tablets	
3340	**UNICAP**® Senior Tablets	
3342	**UNICAP**® Tablets	
3402	**HALTRAN**® Tablets (ibuprofen)	

ADEFLOR CHEWABLE® ℞
brand of fluoride with vitamins tablets

COMPOSITION
Each 0.5 mg or 1 mg tablet contains:

Fluoride (as sodium fluoride)	0.5 mg or 1 mg
Vitamin A	4000 Int. Units
Vitamin D (Cholecalciferol)	400 Int. Units
Ascorbic Acid (as sodium ascorbate)	75 mg
Thiamine Mononitrate	2 mg
Riboflavin	2 mg
Niacinamide	18 mg
Pyridoxine Hydrochloride	1 mg
Calcium Pantothenate	5 mg
Cyanocobalamin	2 mcg

INACTIVE INGREDIENTS
artificial flavors, calcium phosphate, corn starch, erythrosine sodium, FD & C Blue No. 1, lactose, mannitol, saccharin sodium, sorbitol.

The palatable cherry-flavored ADEFLOR CHEWABLE Tablets 0.5 mg or raspberry-flavored 1 mg tablets may be chewed, dissolved in the mouth or swallowed whole.

HOW SUPPLIED

0.5 mg	Bottles of 100	*NDC 0009-0081-01*
1 mg	Bottles of 100	*NDC 0009-0092-01*
	Bottles of 500	*NDC 0009-0092-02*

Shown in Product Identification Section, page 433

ADEFLOR® ℞
brand of fluoride with vitamins A, C, D and B_6 drops

COMPOSITION
Each 0.6 ml contains:

Fluoride (as sodium fluoride)	0.5 mg
Vitamin A	2000 Int. Units
Vitamin D (Cholecalciferol)	400 Int. Units
Ascorbic Acid (C)	50 mg
Pyridoxine Hydrochloride (B_6)	1 mg

INACTIVE INGREDIENTS
caramel, corn oil, flavors, glycerin, methylparaben, nonionic oxyalkene polymer, propylene glycol, propylparaben, saccharin sodium, sorbitan monooleate and pruified water.

HOW SUPPLIED
50 ml bottles with dropper calibrated for 0.3 and 0.6 ml.
NDC 0009-0211-02

BACIGUENT® Antibiotic Ointment

(See PDR For Nonprescription Drugs)

CHERACOL D® Cough Formula

(See PDR For Nonprescription Drugs)

CHERACOL PLUS® Head Cold/Cough Formula

(See PDR For Nonprescription Drugs)

CITROCARBONATE® Antacid

(See PDR For Nonprescription Drugs)

CLEOCIN HCl® ℞
brand of clindamycin hydrochloride capsules, USP

150 mg (100's):
NSN 6505-00-159-4892 (M & VA)

WARNING
Clindamycin therapy has been associated with severe colitis which may end fatally. Therefore, it should be reserved for serious infections where less toxic antimicrobial agents are inappropriate, as described in the Indications section. It should not be used in patients with nonbacterial infections, such as most upper respiratory tract infections. Studies indicate a toxin(s) produced by *Clostridia* is one primary cause of antibiotic associated colitis. Cholestyramine and colestipol resins have been shown to bind the toxin *in vitro*. See WARNINGS section. The colitis is usually characterized by severe, persistent diarrhea and severe abdominal cramps and may be associated with the passage of blood and mucus. Endoscopic examination may reveal pseudomembranous colitis.

When significant diarrhea occurs, the drug should be discontinued or, if necessary, continued only with close observation of the patient. Large bowel endoscopy has been recommended.

Antiperistaltic agents such as opiates and diphenoxylate with atropine (Lomotil) may prolong and/or worsen the condition. Vancomycin has been found to be effective in the treatment of antibiotic associated pseudomembranous colitis produced by *Clostridium difficile.* The usual adult dosage is 500 milligrams to 2 grams of vancomycin orally per day in three to four divided doses administered for 7 to 10 days. Cholestyramine or colestipol resins bind vancomycin *in vitro.* If both a resin and vancomycin are to be administered concurrently, it may be advisable to separate the time of administration of each drug.

Diarrhea, colitis, and pseudomembranous colitis have been observed to begin up to several weeks following cessation of therapy with clindamycin.

DESCRIPTION
Clindamycin hydrochloride is the hydrated hydrochloride salt of clindamycin. Clindamycin is a semisynthetic antibiotic produced by a 7(S)-chloro-substitution of the 7(R)-hydroxyl group of the parent compound lincomycin.

CLEOCIN HCL Capsules contain clindamycin hydrochloride equivalent to 75 mg or 150 mg of clindamycin.

Inactive ingredients: corn starch, erythrosine sodium, FD&C blue no. 1, FD&C yellow no. 5, gelatin, lactose and magnesium stearate.

The chemical name for clindamycin hydrochloride is Methyl 7-chloro-6, 7, 8-trideoxy-6-(1-methyl-*trans* -4-propyl-L-2-pyrrolidinecarboxamido)-1-thio-L-*threo* -*a* -D-*galacto* -octopyranoside monohydrochloride.

CLINICAL PHARMACOLOGY
Microbiology: Clindamycin has been shown to have *in vitro* activity against isolates of the following organisms:

Aerobic gram-positive cocci, including:
Staphylococcus aureus
Staphylococcus epidermidis
(penicillinase and nonpenicillinase producing strains). When tested by *in vitro* methods some staphylococcal strains originally resistant to erythromycin rapidly develop resistance to clindamycin.
Streptococci (except *Streptococcus faecalis*)
Pneumococci

Anaerobic gram-negative bacilli, including:
Bacteroides species (including *Bacteroides fragilis* group and *Bacteroides melaninogenicus* group)
Fusobacterium species

Anaerobic gram-positive nonsporeforming bacilli, including;
Propionibacterium
Eubacterium
Actinomyces species

Anaerobic and microaerophilic gram-positive cocci, including:
Peptococcus species
Peptostreptococcus species
Microaerophilic streptococci
Clostridia: Clostridia are more resistant than most anaerobes to clindamycin. Most *Clostridium perfringens* are susceptible, but other species, eg, *Clostridium sporogenes* and *Clostridium tertium,* are frequently resistant to clindamycin. Susceptibility testing should be done.

Cross resistance has been demonstrated between clindamycin and lincomycin.

Antagonism has been demonstrated between clindamycin and erythromycin.

Human Pharmacology. Serum level studies with a 150 mg oral dose of clindamycin hydrochloride in 24 normal adult volunteers showed that clindamycin was rapidly absorbed after oral administration. An average peak serum level of 2.50 mcg/ml was reached in 45 minutes; serum levels averaged 1.51 mcg/ml at 3 hours and 0.70 mcg/ml at 6 hours. Absorption of an oral dose is virtually complete (90%), and the concomitant administration of food does not appreciably modify the serum concentrations; serum levels have been uniform and predictable from person to person and dose to dose. Serum level studies following multiple doses of CLEOCIN HCL Capsules (clindamycin hydrochloride) for up to 14 days show no evidence of accumulation or altered metabolism of drug.

Serum half-life of clindamycin is increased slightly in patients with markedly reduced renal function. Hemodialysis and peritoneal dialysis are not effective in removing clindamycin from the serum.

Concentrations of clindamycin in the serum increased linearly with increased dose. Serum levels exceed the MIC (minimum inhibitory concentration) for most indicated organisms for at least six hours following administration of the usually recommended doses. Clindamycin is widely distributed in body fluids and tissues (including bones). The average biological half-life is 2.4 hours. Approximately 10% of the bio-activity is excreted in the urine and 3.6% in the feces; the remainder is excreted as bio-inactive metabolites.

Doses of up to 2 grams of clindamycin per day for 14 days have been well tolerated by healthy volunteers, except that the incidence of gastrointestinal side effects is greater with the higher doses.

No significant levels of clindamycin are attained in the cerebrospinal fluid, even in the presence of inflamed meninges.

INDICATIONS AND USAGE

Clindamycin is indicated in the treatment of serious infections caused by susceptible anaerobic bacteria.

Clindamycin is also indicated in the treatment of serious infections due to susceptible strains of streptococci, pneumococci, and staphylococci. Its use should be reserved for penicillin-allergic patients or other patients for whom, in the judgment of the physician, a penicillin is inappropriate. Because of the risk of colitis, as described in the WARNING box, before selecting clindamycin the physician should consider the nature of the infection and the suitability of less toxic alternatives (eg, erythromycin).

Anaerobes: Serious respiratory tract infections such as empyema, anaerobic pneumonitis and lung abscess; serious skin and soft tissue infections; septicemia; intra-abdominal infections such as peritonitis and intra-abdominal abscess (typically resulting from anaerobic organisms resident in the normal gastrointestinal tract); infections of the female pelvis and genital tract such as endometritis, nongonococcal tubo-ovarian abscess, pelvic cellulitis and postsurgical vaginal cuff infection.

Streptococci: Serious respiratory tract infections; serious skin and soft tissue infections.

Staphylococci: Serious respiratory tract infections; serious skin and soft tissue infections.

Pneumococci: Serious respiratory tract infections.

Bacteriologic studies should be performed to determine the causative organisms and their susceptibility to clindamycin.

In Vitro Susceptibility Testing: A standardized disk testing procedure* is recommended for determining susceptibility of aerobic bacteria to clindamycin. A description is contained in the CLEOCIN® Susceptibility Disk (clindamycin) insert. Using this method, the laboratory can designate isolates as resistant, intermediate, or susceptible. Tube or agar dilution methods may be used for both anaerobic and aerobic bacteria. When the directions in the CLEOCIN® Susceptibility Powder insert are followed, an MIC of 1.6 mcg/ml may be considered susceptible; MICs of 1.6 to 4.8 mcg/ml may be considered intermediate and MICs greater than 4.8 mcg/ml may be considered resistant.

CLEOCIN Susceptibility Disks 2 mcg. See package insert for use.

CLEOCIN Susceptibility Powder 20 mg. See package insert for use.

For anaerobic bacteria the minimal inhibitory concentration (MIC) of clindamycin can be determined by agar dilution and broth dilution (including microdilution) techniques. If MICs are not determined routinely, the disk broth method is recommended for routine use. THE KIRBY-BAUER DISK DIFFUSION METHOD AND ITS INTERPRETIVE STANDARDS ARE NOT RECOMMENDED FOR ANAEROBES.

*Bauer, A.W., Kirby, W.M.M., Sherris, J.C., Turck, M.; Antibiotic susceptibility testing by a standardized single disc method, *Am. J. Clin. Path.* 45:493-496, 1966. Standardized Disc Susceptibility Test, *Federal Register* 37:20527-29, 1972.

CONTRAINDICATIONS

CLEOCIN HCL Capsules (clindamycin hydrochloride) are contraindicated in individuals with a history of hypersensitivity to preparations containing clindamycin or lincomycin.

WARNINGS

See WARNING box. Studies indicate a toxin(s) produced by *Clostridia* is one primary cause of antibiotic associated colitis.[1–5] Cholestyramine and colestipol resins have been shown to bind the toxin *in vitro.* Mild cases of colitis may respond to drug discontinuance alone. Moderate to severe cases should be managed with fluid, electrolyte and protein supplementation as indicated. Vancomycin has been found to be effective in the treatment of antibiotic associated pseudomembranous colitis produced by *Clostridium difficile.* The usual adult dosage is 500 milligrams to 2 grams of vancomycin orally per day in three to four divided doses administered for 7 to 10 days. Cholestyramine or colestipol resins bind vancomycin *in vitro.* If both a resin and vancomycin are to be administered concurrently, it may be advisable to separate the time of administration of each drug. Systemic corticoids and corticoid retention enemas may help relieve the colitis. Other causes of colitis should also be considered.

A careful inquiry should be made concerning previous sensitivities to drugs and other allergens.

Usage in Pregnancy - Safety for use in pregnancy has not been established.

Usage in Newborns and Infants: When CLEOCIN HCL Capsules (clindamycin hydrochloride) are administered to newborns and infants, appropriate monitoring of organ system functions is desirable.

Nursing Mothers—Clindamycin has been reported to appear in breast milk in ranges of 0.7 to 3.8 mcg/ml.

Usage in Meningitis: Since clindamycin does not diffuse adequately into the cerebrospinal fluid, the drug should not be used in the treatment of meningitis.

Antagonism has been demonstrated between clindamycin and erythromycin *in vitro.* Because of possible clinical significance, these two drugs should not be administered concurrently.

1. Bartlett JG, et al: Antibiotic associated Pseudomembranous Colitis Due to Toxin-producing *Clostridia. N Engl J Med* 298(10):531-534, 1978.
2. George RH, et al: Identification of *Clostridium difficile* as a cause of Pseudomembranous Colitis. *Br Med J* 6114:669-671, 1978.
3. Larson HE, Price AB: Pseudomembranous Colitis Presence of Clostridial Toxin, *Lancet* 8052/3:1312-1314, 1977.
4. Rifkin GD, Fekety FR, Silva J: Antibiotic-induced Colitis Implication of a Toxin Neutralized by *Clostridium sordellii* Antitoxin. *Lancet* 8048:1103-1106, 1977.
5. Bailey WR, Scott EG: Diagnostic Microbiology. The CV Mosby Company, St. Louis, 1978.

PRECAUTIONS

Review of experience to date suggests that a subgroup of older patients with associated severe illness may tolerate diarrhea less well. When clindamycin is indicated in these patients, they should be carefully monitored for change in bowel frequency.

CLEOCIN HCL Capsules (clindamycin hydrochloride) should be prescribed with caution in individuals with a history of gastrointestinal disease, particularly colitis.

CLEOCIN HCL should be prescribed with caution in atopic individuals.

During prolonged therapy, periodic liver and kidney function tests and blood counts should be performed.

Indicated surgical procedures should be performed in conjunction with antibiotic therapy.

The use of CLEOCIN HCL occasionally results in overgrowth of nonsusceptible organisms—particularly yeasts. Should superinfections occur, appropriate measures should be taken as indicated by the clinical situation.

Patients with very severe renal disease and/or very severe hepatic disease accompanied by severe metabolic aberrations should be dosed with caution, and serum clindamycin levels monitored during high-dose therapy.

Clindamycin has been shown to have neuromuscular blocking properties that may enhance the action of other neuromuscular blocking agents. Therefore, it should be used with caution in patients receiving such agents.

This product contains FD&C Yellow No. 5 (tartrazine) which may cause allergic-type reactions (including bronchial asthma) in certain susceptible individuals. Although the overall incidence of FD&C Yellow No. 5 (tartrazine) sensitivity in the general population is low, it is frequently seen in patients who also have aspirin hypersensitivity.

ADVERSE REACTIONS

The following reactions have been reported with the use of clindamycin.

Gastrointestinal: Abdominal pain, esophagitis, nausea, vomiting and diarrhea. (See **Warning** Box)

Hypersensitivity Reactions: Maculopapular rash and urticaria have been observed during drug therapy. Generalized mild to moderate morbilliform-like skin rashes are the most frequently reported of all adverse reactions. Rare instances of erythema multiforme, some resembling Stevens-Johnson syndrome, have been associated with clindamycin. A few cases of anaphylactoid reactions have been reported. If a hypersensitivity reaction occurs, the drug should be discontinued. The usual agents (epinephrine, corticosteroids, antihistamines) should be available for emergency treatment of serious reactions.

Liver: Jaundice and abnormalities in liver function tests have been observed during clindamycin therapy.

Renal: Although no direct relationship of clindamycin to renal damage has been established, renal dysfunction as evidenced by azotemia, oliguria, and/or proteinuria has been observed in rare instances.

Hematopoietic: Transient neutropenia (leukopenia) and eosinophilia have been reported. Reports of agranulocytosis and thrombocytopenia have been made. No direct etiologic relationship to concurrent clindamycin therapy could be made in any of the foregoing.

Musculoskeletal: Rare instances of polyarthritis have been reported.

DOSAGE AND ADMINISTRATION

If significant diarrhea occurs during therapy, this antibiotic should be discontinued. (See **Warning** box).

Adults: *Serious infections* —150 to 300 mg every 6 hours. *More severe infections* —300 to 450 mg every 6 hours.

Children: *Serious infections* —8 to 16 mg/kg/day (4 to 8 mg/lb/day) divided into three or four equal doses. *More severe infections* —16 to 20 mg/kg/day (8 to 10 mg/lb/day) divided into three or four equal doses.

To avoid the possibility of esophageal irritation, CLEOCIN HCL Capsules (clindamycin hydrochloride) should be taken with a full glass of water.

Serious infections due to anaerobic bacteria are usually treated with CLEOCIN PHOSPHATE® Sterile Solution (clindamycin phosphate). However, in clinically appropriate circumstances, the physician may elect to initiate treatment or continue treatment with CLEOCIN HCl Capsules.

In cases of β-hemolytic streptococcal infections, treatment should continue for at least 10 days.

HOW SUPPLIED

CLEOCIN HCL Capsules (clindamycin hydrochloride) are available in the following strengths, colors and sizes:

75 mg Lavender:
Bottles of 100 *NDC 0009-0331-02*
150 mg Lavender and Maroon:
Bottles of 16 *NDC 0009-0225-01*
Bottles of 100 *NDC 0009-0225-02*
Unit Dose Package
(100) *NDC 0009-0225-03*

Store at controlled room temperature 15°–30°C (59°–86°F).

TOXICOLOGY

Animal toxicity studies showed the following:

LD_{50} I.P. Administration—
Mouse .... 361 mg/kg
LD_{50} I.V. Administration—
Mouse .... 245 mg/kg
LD_{50} Oral Administration—
Rat .... 2,618 mg/kg

Continued on next page

Information on these Upjohn products is based on labeling in effect August 15, 1986. Further information concerning these and other Upjohn products may be obtained by direct inquiry to Medical Information, The Upjohn Company, Kalamazoo, Michigan 49001.

Upjohn—Cont.

One year oral toxicity studies in Spartan Sprague-Dawley rats and Beagle dogs at levels of 30, 100 and 300 mg/kg/day (3 grams/day per dog) have shown CLEOCIN HCL to be well tolerated. No appreciable difference in pathological findings has been obtained in CLEOCIN HCL treated groups of animals from comparable control groups. Rats receiving CLEOCIN HCL Capsules (clindamycin hydrochloride) at 600 mg/kg/day for six months tolerated the drug well; however, dogs dosed at this level vomited, would not eat, and lost weight.

Code 810 570 210

Shown in Product Identification Section, page 433

CLEOCIN PEDIATRIC® ℞

brand of clindamycin palmitate hydrochloride flavored granules
(clindamycin palmitate hydrochloride for oral solution, USP)
Not for Injection

> **WARNING**
>
> Clindamycin therapy has been associated with severe colitis which may end fatally. Therefore, it should be reserved for serious infections where less toxic antimicrobial agents are inappropriate, as described in the Indications Section. It should not be used in patients with nonbacterial infections, such as most upper respiratory tract infections. Studies indicate a toxin(s) produced by *Clostridia* is one primary cause of antibiotic associated colitis. Cholestyramine and colestipol resins have been shown to bind the toxin *in vitro*. See WARNINGS section. The colitis is usually characterized by severe, persistent diarrhea and severe abdominal cramps and may be associated with the passage of blood and mucus. Endoscopic examination may reveal pseudomembranous colitis.
>
> When significant diarrhea occurs, the drug should be discontinued or, if necessary, continued only with close observation of the patient. Large bowel endoscopy has been recommended.
>
> Antiperistaltic agents such as opiates and diphenoxylate with atropine (Lomotil) may prolong and/or worsen the condition. Vancomycin has been found to be effective in the treatment of antibiotic associated pseudomembranous colitis produced by *Clostridium difficile*. The usual adult dosage is 500 milligrams to 2 grams of vancomycin orally per day in three to four divided doses administered for 7 to 10 days. Cholestyramine or colestipol resins bind vancomycin *in vitro*. If both a resin and vancomycin are to be administered concurrently, it may be advisable to separate the time of administration of each drug.
>
> Diarrhea, colitis, and pseudomembranous colitis have been observed to begin up to several weeks following cessation of therapy with clindamycin.

DESCRIPTION

Clindamycin palmitate hydrochloride is a water soluble hydrochloride salt of the ester of clindamycin and palmitic acid. Clindamycin is a semisynthetic antibiotic produced by a 7(S)-chloro-substitution of the 7(R)-hydroxyl group of the parent compound lincomycin.

The chemical name for clindamycin palmitate hydrochloride is Methyl 7-chloro-6,7,8-trideoxy-6-(1-methyl-*trans* -4-propyl-L-2-pyrrolindinecarboxamido) -1- thio-L-*threo* -*a* -D-*galacto* -octopyranoside 2-palmitate monohydrochloride.

CLEOCIN PEDIATRIC Flavored Granules contain clindamycin palmitate hydrochloride for reconstitution. Each 5 ml contains the equivalent of 75 mg clindamycin. Inactive ingredients: artificial cherry flavor, dextrin, ethylparaben, pluronic F68, polymethylsiloxane, sucrose.

CLINICAL PHARMACOLOGY

Microbiology: Although clindamycin palmitate HCl is inactive *in vitro*, rapid *in vivo* hydrolysis converts this compound to the antibacterially active clindamycin.

Clindamycin has been shown to have *in vitro* activity against isolates of the following organisms:

Aerobic gram positive cocci, including:

Staphylococcus aureus
Staphylococcus epidermidis
(penicillinase and non-penicillinase producing strains). When tested by *in vitro* methods some staphylococcal strains originally resistant to erythromycin rapidly develop resistance to clindamycin.
Streptococci (except *Streptococcus faecalis*)
Pneumococci

Anaerobic gram negative bacilli, including:

Bacteroides species (including *Bacteroides fragilis* group and *Bacteroides melaninogenicus* group)
Fusobacterium species

Anaerobic gram positive nonsporeforming bacilli, including:

Propionibacterium
Eubacterium
Actinomyces species

Anaerobic and microaerophilic gram positive cocci, including:

Peptococcus species
Peptostreptococcus species
Microaerophilic streptococci

Clostridia: Clostridia are more resistant than most anaerobes to clindamycin. Most *Clostridium perfringens* are susceptible, but other species, eg, *Clostridium sporogenes* and *Clostridium tertium* are frequently resistant to clindamycin. Susceptibility testing should be done.

Cross resistance has been demonstrated between clindamycin and lincomycin.

Antagonism has been demonstrated between clindamycin and erythromycin.

Human Pharmacology: Blood level studies comparing clindamycin palmitate HCl with clindamycin hydrochloride show that both products reach their peak active serum levels at the same time, indicating a rapid hydrolysis of the palmitate to the clindamycin.

Clindamycin is widely distributed in body fluids and tissues (including bones). Approximately 10% of the biological activity is excreted in the urine. The average biological half-life after doses of clindamycin is approximately two hours in children.

Serum half-life of clindamycin is increased slightly in patients with markedly reduced renal function. Hemodialysis and peritoneal dialysis do not appreciably affect the half-life of clindamycin in the serum.

Serum level studies with clindamycin palmitate HCl in normal children weighing 50-100 lbs given 2, 3 or 4 mg/kg every 6 hours (8, 12 or 16 mg/kg/day) demonstrated mean peak clindamycin serum levels of 1.24, 2.25 and 2.44 mcg/ml respectively, one hour after the first dose. By the fifth dose, the 6-hour serum concentration had reached equilibrium. Peak serum concentrations after this time would be about 2.46, 2.98 and 3.79 mcg/ml with doses of 8, 12, 16 mg/kg/day, respectively. Serum levels have been uniform and predictable from person to person and dose to dose. Multiple-dose studies in newborns and infants up to 6 months of age show that the drug does not accumulate in the serum and is excreted rapidly. Serum levels exceed the MICs for most indicated organisms for at least six hours following administration of the usually recommended doses of CLEOCIN PEDIATRIC in adults and children.

No significant levels of clindamycin are attained in the cerebrospinal fluid, even in the presence of inflamed meninges.

INDICATIONS AND USAGE

CLEOCIN PEDIATRIC Flavored Granules (clindamycin palmitate HCl) are indicated in the treatment of serious infections caused by susceptible anaerobic bacteria.

Clindamycin is also indicated in the treatment of serious infections due to susceptible strains of streptococci, pneumococci, and staphylococci. Its use should be reserved for penicillin-allergic patients or other patients for whom, in the judgment of the physician, a penicillin is inappropriate. Because of the risk of colitis, as described in the WARNING box, before selecting clindamycin the physician should consider the nature of the infection and the suitability of less toxic alternatives (eg, erythromycin).

Anaerobes: Serious respiratory tract infections such as empyema, anaerobic pneumonitis and lung abscess; serious skin and soft tissue infections; septicemia; intra-abdominal infections such as peritonitis and intra-abdominal abscess (typically resulting from anaerobic organisms resident in the normal gastrointestinal tract); infections of the female pelvis and genital tract such as endometritis, nongonococcal tubo-ovarian abscess, pelvic cellulitis and postsurgical vaginal cuff infection.

Streptococci: Serious respiratory tract infections; serious skin and soft tissue infections.

Staphylococci: Serious respiratory tract infections; serious skin and soft tissue infections.

Pneumococci: Serious respiratory tract infections.

Bacteriologic studies should be performed to determine the causative organisms and their susceptibility to clindamycin.

In Vitro Susceptibility Testing: A standardized disk testing procedure* is recommended for determining susceptibility of aerobic bacteria to clindamycin. A description is contained in the CLEOCIN® Susceptibility Disk (clindamycin) insert. Using this method, the laboratory can designate isolates as resistant, intermediate, or susceptible. Tube or agar dilution methods may be used for both anaerobic and aerobic bacteria. When the directions in the CLEOCIN Susceptibility Powder insert are followed, an MIC (minimal inhibitory concentration) of 1.6 mcg/ml may be considered susceptible; MICs of 1.6 to 4.8 mcg/ml may be considered intermediate and MICs greater than 4.8 mcg/ml may be considered resistant.

CLEOCIN Susceptibility Disks 2 mcg. See package insert for use.

CLEOCIN Susceptibility Powder 20 mg. See package insert for use.

For anaerobic bacteria the minimal inhibitory concentration (MIC) of clindamycin can be determined by agar dilution and broth dilution (including microdilution) techniques. If MICs are not determined routinely, the disk broth method is recommended for routine use. THE KIRBY-BAUER DISK DIFFUSION METHOD AND ITS INTERPRETIVE STANDARDS ARE NOT RECOMMENDED FOR ANAEROBES.

---

*Bauer, AW, Kirby, WMM, Sherris, JC, Turck, M.: Antibiotic susceptibility testing by a standardized single disc method, *Am J Clin Path,* **45**:493-496, 1966. Standardized Disc Susceptibility Test, *Federal Register* **37**:20527-29, 1972.

CONTRAINDICATIONS

This drug is contraindicated in individuals with a history of hypersensitivity to preparations containing clindamycin or lincomycin.

WARNINGS

See WARNING box. Studies indicate a toxin(s) produced by *Clostridia* is one primary cause of antibiotic associated colitis.[1-5] Cholestyramine and colestipol resins have been shown to bind the toxin *in vitro*. Mild cases of colitis may respond to drug discontinuance alone. Moderate to severe cases should be managed promptly with fluid, electrolyte and protein supplementation as indicated. Vancomycin has been found to be effective in the treatment of antibiotic associated pseudomembranous colitis produced by *Clostridium difficile*. The usual adult dosage is 500 milligrams to 2 grams of vancomycin orally per day in three to four divided doses administered for 7 to 10 days. Cholestyramine or colestipol resins bind vancomycin *in vitro*. If both a resin and vancomycin are to be administered concurrently, it may be advisable to separate the time of administration of each drug. Systemic corticoids and corticoid retention enemas may help relieve the colitis. Other causes of colitis should also be considered.

A careful inquiry should be made concerning previous sensitivities to drugs and other allergens.

Usage in Pregnancy—Safety for use in pregnancy has not been established.

Usage in Newborns and Infants: When CLEOCIN PEDIATRIC Flavored Granules (clindamycin palmitate HCl) are administered to newborns and infants, appropriate monitoring of organ system functions is desirable.

Nursing Mothers—Clindamycin has been reported to appear in breast milk in ranges of 0.7 to 3.8 mcg/ml.

Usage in Meningitis: Since clindamycin does not diffuse adequately into the cerebrospinal fluid, the drug should not be used in the treatment of meningitis.

Antagonism has been demonstrated between clindamycin and erythromycin *in vitro*. Because of possible clinical significance, these two drugs should not be administered concurrently.

1. Bartlett JG, et al: Antibiotic associated Pseudomembranous Colitis Due to Toxin-producing *Clostridia*. *N Engl J Med* 298(10):531-534, 1978.
2. George RH, et al: Identification of *Clostridium difficile* as a cause of Pseudomembranous Colitis. *Br Med J* 6114:669-671, 1978.
3. Larson HE, Price AB: Pseudomembranous Colitis Presence of Clostridial Toxin. *Lancet* 8052/3:1312-1314, 1977.
4. Rifkin GD, Fekety FR, Silva J: Antibiotic-induced Colitis Implication of a Toxin Neutralized by *Clostridium sordellii* Antitoxin. *Lancet* 8048:1103-1106, 1977.
5. Bailey WR, Scott EG: Diagnostic Microbiology. The CV Mosby Company, St. Louis, 1978.

PRECAUTIONS

Review of experience to date suggests that a subgroup of older patients with associated severe illness may tolerate diarrhea less well. When clindamycin is indicated in these patients, they should be carefully monitored for change in bowel frequency.

CLEOCIN PEDIATRIC Flavored Granules (clindamycin palmitate HCl) should be prescribed with caution in individuals with a history of gastrointestinal disease, particularly colitis.

CLEOCIN PEDIATRIC should be prescribed with caution in atopic individuals.

During prolonged therapy periodic liver and kidney function tests and blood counts should be performed.

Indicated surgical procedures should be performed in conjunction with antibiotic therapy.

The use of CLEOCIN PEDIATRIC may result in overgrowth of nonsusceptible organisms—particularly yeasts. Should superinfections occur, appropriate measures should be taken as indicated by the clinical situation.

Patients with very severe renal disease and/or very severe hepatic disease accompanied by severe metabolic aberra-

tions should be dosed with caution, and serum clindamycin levels monitored during high-dose therapy.
Clindamycin has been shown to have neuromuscular blocking properties that may enhance the action of other neuromuscular blocking agents. Therefore, it should be used with caution in patients receiving such agents.

ADVERSE REACTIONS

The following reactions have been reported with the use of clindamycin.
Gastrointestinal: Abdominal pain, nausea, vomiting and diarrhea. (See **Warning** box)
Hypersensitivity Reactions: Maculopapular rash and urticaria have been observed during drug therapy. Generalized mild to moderate morbilliform-like skin rashes are the most frequently reported of all adverse reactions. Rare instances of erythema multiforme, some resembling Stevens-Johnson syndrome, have been associated with clindamycin. A few cases of anaphylactoid reactions have been reported. If a hypersensitivity reaction occurs, the drug should be discontinued. The usual agents (epinephrine, corticosteroids, antihistamines) should be available for emergency treatment of serious reactions.
Liver: Jaundice and abnormalities in liver function tests have been observed during clindamycin therapy.
Renal: Although no direct relationship of clindamycin to renal damage has been established, renal dysfunction as evidenced by azotemia, oliguria, and/or proteinuria has been observed in rare instances.
Hematopoietic: Transient neutropenia (leukopenia) and eosinophilia have been reported. Reports of agranulocytosis and thrombocytopenia have been made. No direct etiologic relationship to concurrent clindamycin therapy could be made in any of the foregoing.
Musculoskeletal: Rare instances of polyarthritis have been reported.

DOSAGE AND ADMINISTRATION

If significant diarrhea occurs during therapy, this antibiotic should be discontinued. (See **Warning** box.) Concomitant administration of food does not adversely affect the absorption of clindamycin palmitate HCl contained in CLEOCIN PEDIATRIC Flavored Granules.
Serious infections: 8-12 mg/kg/day (4-6 mg/lb/day) divided into 3 or 4 equal doses.
Severe infections: 13-16 mg/kg/day (6.5-8 mg/lb/day) divided into 3 or 4 equal doses.
More severe infections: 17-25 mg/kg/day (8.5-12.5 mg/lb/day) divided into 3 or 4 equal doses.
In children weighing 10 kg or less, ½ teaspoon (37.5 mg) three times a day should be considered the minimum recommended dose.
Serious infections due to anaerobic bacteria are usually treated with CLEOCIN PHOSPHATE® Sterile Solution (clindamycin phosphate). However, in clinically appropriate circumstances, the physician may elect to initiate treatment or continue treatment with CLEOCIN PEDIATRIC.
NOTE: In cases of β-hemolytic streptococcal infections, treatment should be continued for at least 10 days.
Reconstitution instructions:
When reconstituted with water as follows, each 5 ml (teaspoon) of solution contains clindamycin palmitate HCl equivalent to 75 mg clindamycin.
Reconstitute bottles of 100 ml with **75 ml** of water. Add a large portion of the water and shake vigorously; add the remainder of the water and shake until the solution is uniform.
Storage conditions:
Store unreconstituted product at controlled room temperature 15°-30°C (59°-86°F).
Do **NOT** refrigerate the reconstituted solution; when chilled, the solution may thicken and be difficult to pour. The solution is stable for 2 weeks at room temperature.

HOW SUPPLIED

CLEOCIN PEDIATRIC Flavored Granules (clindamycin palmitate HCl) for oral solution is available in bottles of 100 ml *NDC 0009-0760-04*
When reconstituted as directed, each bottle yields a solution containing 75 mg of clindamycin per 5 ml.
Code 810 568 008

CLEOCIN PHOSPHATE® ℞

brand of clindamycin phosphate sterile solution
(clindamycin phosphate injection, USP)
For Intramuscular and Intravenous Use

2 ml vial 25's NSN 6505-01-185-3309 (M)
2 ml vial 100's NSN 6505-00-138-8474 (M & VA)
4 ml vial 25's NSN 6505-01-177-1982 (M)
4 ml vial 100's NSN 6505-00-139-1318 (M & VA)
6 ml vial 25's NSN 6505-01-187-5540 (M)
6 ml 100's NSN 6505-01-181-8688 (M & VA)

WARNING

Clindamycin therapy has been associated with severe colitis which may end fatally. Therefore, it should be reserved for serious infections where less toxic antimicrobial agents are inappropriate, as described in the Indications Section. It should not be used in patients with nonbacterial infections, such as most upper respiratory tract infections. Studies indicate a toxin(s) produced by *Clostridia* is one primary cause of antibiotic associated colitis. Cholestyramine and colestipol resins have been shown to bind the toxin *in vitro*. See WARNINGS section. The colitis is usually characterized by severe, persistent diarrhea and severe abdominal cramps and may be associated with the passage of blood and mucus. Endoscopic examination may reveal pseudomembranous colitis.
When significant diarrhea occurs, the drug should be discontinued or, if necessary, continued only with close observation of the patient. Large bowel endoscopy has been recommended.
Antiperistaltic agents such as opiates and diphenoxylate with atropine (Lomotil) may prolong and/or worsen the condition. Vancomycin has been found to be effective in the treatment of antibiotic associated pseudomembranous colitis produced by *Clostridium difficile*. The usual adult dosage is 500 milligrams to 2 grams of vancomycin orally per day in three to four divided doses administered for 7 to 10 days. Cholestyramine or colestipol resins bind vancomycin *in vitro*. If both a resin and vancomycin are to be administered concurrently, it may be advisable to separate the time of administration of each drug.
Diarrhea, colitis, and pseudomembranous colitis have been observed to begin up to several weeks following cessation of therapy with clindamycin.

DESCRIPTION

CLEOCIN PHOSPHATE Sterile Solution contains clindamycin phosphate, a water soluble ester of clindamycin and phosphoric acid. Each ml contains the equivalent of 150 mg clindamycin, 0.5 mg disodium edetate and 9.45 mg benzyl alcohol added as preservative in each ml. Clindamycin is a semisynthetic antibiotic produced by a 7(S)-chloro-substitution of the 7(R)-hydroxyl group of the parent compound lincomycin.

CLINICAL PHARMACOLOGY

Microbiology: Although clindamycin phosphate is inactive *in vitro*, rapid *in vivo* hydrolysis converts this compound to the antibacterially active clindamycin.
Clindamycin has been shown to have *in vitro* activity against isolates of the following organisms:
Aerobic gram positive cocci, including:
Staphylococcus aureus
Staphylococcus epidermidis
(penicillinase and nonpenicillinase producing strains). When tested by *in vitro* methods some staphylococcal strains originally resistant to erythromycin rapidly develop resistance to clindamycin.
Streptococci (except *S. faecalis*)
Pneumococci
Anaerobic gram negative bacilli, including:
Bacteroides species (including *Bacteroides fragilis* group and *Bacteroides melaninogenicus* group)
Fusobacterium species
Anaerobic gram positive nonsporeforming bacilli, including:
Propionibacterium
Eubacterium
Actinomyces species
Anaerobic and microaerophilic gram positive cocci, including:
Peptococcus species
Peptostreptococcus species
Microaerophilic streptococci
Clostridia: Clostridia are more resistant than most anaerobes to clindamycin. Most *Clostridium perfringens* are susceptible, but other species, eg, *Clostridium sporogenes* and *Clostridium Tertium* are frequently resistant to clindamycin. Susceptibility testing should be done.
Cross resistance has been demonstrated between clindamycin and lincomycin.
Antagonism has been demonstrated between clindamycin and erythromycin.
Human Pharmacology:
Biologically inactive clindamycin phosphate is rapidly converted to active clindamycin.
By the end of short-term intravenous infusion, peak serum levels of active clindamycin are reached. Biologically inactive clindamycin phosphate disappears rapidly from the serum; the average disappearance half-life is 6 minutes; however, the serum disappearance half-life of active clindamycin is about 3 hours in adults and 2 ½ hours in children.
After intramuscular injection of clindamycin phosphate, peak levels of active clindamycin are reached within 3 hours in adults and 1 hour in children. Serum level curves may be constructed from IV peak serum levels as given in Table 1 by application of disappearance half-lives listed above.
Serum levels of clindamycin can be maintained above the *in vitro* minimum inhibitory concentrations for most indicated organisms by administration of clindamycin phosphate every 8-12 hours in adults and every 6-8 hours in children, or by continuous intravenous infusion. An equilibrium state is reached by the third dose.
The disappearance half-life of clindamycin is increased slightly in patients with markedly reduced renal or hepatic function. Hemodialysis and peritoneal dialysis are not effective in removing clindamycin from the serum. Dosage schedules need not be modified in the presence of mild or moderate renal or hepatic disease.
No significant levels of clindamycin are attained in the cerebrospinal fluid, even in the presence of inflamed meninges.
Serum assays for active clindamycin require an inhibitor to prevent *in vitro* hydrolysis of clindamycin phosphate.
[See table above].

Table 1. Average Peak Serum Concentrations After Dosing with Clindamycin Phosphate

CLEOCIN PHOSPHATE Dosage Regimen	Clindamycin mcg/ml	Clindamycin Phosphate mcg/ml
Healthy Adult Males (Post equilibrium)		
300 mg IV in 10 min, q8h	7	15
600 mg IV in 20 min, q8h	10	23
900 mg IV in 30 min, q12h	11	29
1200 mg IV in 45 min, q12h	14	49
300 mg IM q8h	6	3
600 mg IM q12h*	9	3
Children (first dose)*		
5-7 mg/kg IV in 1 hr	10	
3-5 mg/kg IM	4	
5-7 mg/kg IM	8	

*Data in this group from patients being treated for infection

INDICATIONS AND USAGE

CLEOCIN PHOSPHATE Sterile Solution (clindamycin phosphate) is indicated in the treatment of serious infections caused by susceptible anaerobic bacteria.
CLEOCIN PHOSPHATE is also indicated in the treatment of serious infections due to susceptible strains of streptococci, pneumococci, and staphylococci. Its use should be reserved for penicillin-allergic patients or other patients for whom, in the judgment of the physician, a penicillin is inappropriate. Because of the risk of colitis, as described in the WARNING box, before selecting clindamycin the physician should consider the nature of the infection and the suitability of less toxic alternatives (e.g., erythromycin).
Anaerobes: Serious respiratory tract infections such as empyema, anaerobic pneumonitis and lung abscess; serious skin and soft tissue infections; septicemia; intra-abdominal infections such as peritonitis and intra-abdominal abscess (typically resulting from anaerobic organisms resident in the normal gastrointestinal tract); infections of the female pelvis and genital tract such as endometritis, nongonococcal tubo-ovarian abscess, pelvic cellulitis and postsurgical vaginal cuff infection.
Streptococci: Serious respiratory tract infections; serious skin and soft tissue infections; septicemia.
Staphylococci: Serious respiratory tract infections; serious skin and soft tissue infections; septicemia; acute hematogenous osteomyelitis.

Continued on next page

Information on these Upjohn products is based on labeling in effect August 15, 1986. Further information concerning these and other Upjohn products may be obtained by direct inquiry to Medical Information, The Upjohn Company, Kalamazoo, Michigan 49001.

Upjohn—Cont.

Pneumococci: Serious respiratory tract infections.
Adjunctive Therapy: In the surgical treatment of chronic bone and joint infections due to susceptible organisms.
Indicated surgical procedures should be performed in conjunction with antibiotic therapy.
Bacteriologic studies should be performed to determine the causative organisms and their susceptibility to clindamycin.
In Vitro Susceptibility Testing: A standardized disk testing procedure** is recommended for determining susceptibility of aerobic bacteria to clindamycin. A description is contained in the CLEOCIN® Susceptibility Disk (clindamycin) insert. Using this method, the laboratory can designate isolates as resistant, intermediate, or susceptible. Tube or agar dilution methods may be used for both anaerobic and aerobic bacteria. When the directions in the CLEOCIN Susceptibility Powder insert are followed, an MIC (minimal inhibitory concentration) of 1.6 mcg/ml may be considered susceptible; MICs of 1.6 to 4.8 mcg/ml may be considered intermediate and MICs greater than 4.8 mcg/ml may be considered resistant.
CLEOCIN Susceptibility Disks 2 mcg. See package insert for use.
CLEOCIN Susceptibility Powder 20 mg. See package insert for use.
For anaerobic bacteria the minimal inhibitory concentration (MIC) of clindamycin can be determined by agar dilution and broth dilution (including microdilution) techniques. If MICs are not determined routinely, the disk broth method is recommended for routine use. The KIRBY-BAUER DISK DIFFUSION METHOD AND ITS INTERPRETIVE STANDARDS ARE NOT RECOMMENDED FOR ANAEROBES.

Bauer, AW, Kirby, WMM, Sherris, JC, Turck, M: Antibiotic susceptibility testing by a standardized single disc method, *Am J Clin Path*, **45:493-496, 1966. Standardized Disc Susceptibility Test, *Federal Register* **37**:20527-29, 1972.

CONTRAINDICATIONS

This drug is contraindicated in individuals with a history of hypersensitivity to preparations containing clindamycin or lincomycin.

WARNINGS

See WARNING box. Studies indicate a toxin(s) produced by *Clostridia* is one primary cause of antibiotic associated colitis.[1-5] Cholestyramine and colestipol resins have been shown to bind the toxin *in vitro*. Mild cases of colitis may respond to drug discontinuance alone. Moderate to severe cases should be managed promptly with fluid, electrolyte and protein supplementation as indicated. Vancomycin has been found to be effective in the treatment of antibiotic associated pseudomembranous colitis produced by *Clostridium difficile*. The usual adult dosage is 500 milligrams to 2 grams of vancomycin orally per day in three to four divided doses administered for 7 to 10 days. Cholestyramine or colestipol resins bind vancomycin *in vitro*. If both a resin and vancomycin are to be administered concurrently, it may be advisable to separate the time of administration of each drug. Systemic corticoids and corticoid retention enemas may help relieve the colitis. Other causes of colitis should also be considered.
A careful inquiry should be made concerning previous sensitivities to drugs and other allergens.
Usage in Pregnancy—Safety for use in pregnancy has not been established.
Usage in Newborns and infants: When CLEOCIN PHOSPHATE Sterile Solution (clindamycin phosphate) is administered to newborns and infants, appropriate monitoring of organ system functions is desirable. This product contains benzyl alcohol which has been associated with a fatal gasping syndrome in infants.
Nursing Mothers—Clindamycin has been reported to appear in breast milk in ranges of 0.7 to 3.8 mcg/ml.
Usage in Meningitis: Since clindamycin does not diffuse adequately into the cerebrospinal fluid, the drug should not be used in the treatment of meningitis.
Antagonism has been demonstrated between clindamycin and erythromycin *in vitro*. Because of possible clinical significance, these two drugs should not be administered concurrently.
SERIOUS ANAPHYLACTOID REACTIONS REQUIRE IMMEDIATE EMERGENCY TREATMENT WITH EPINEPHRINE. OXYGEN AND INTRAVENOUS CORTICOSTEROIDS SHOULD ALSO BE ADMINISTERED AS INDICATED.

1. Bartlett JG, et al: Antibiotic associated Pseudomembranous Colitis Due to Toxin-producing *Clostridia*. *N Engl J Med* 298(10):531-534, 1978.
2. George RH, et al: Identification of *Clostridium difficile* as a cause of Pseudomembranous Colitis. *Br Med J* 6114:669-671, 1978.
3. Larson HE, Price AB: Pseudomembranous Colitis Presence of Clostridial Toxin. *Lancet* 8052/3:1312-1314, 1977.
4. Rifkin GD, Fekety FR, Silva J: Antibiotic-induced Colitis Implication of a Toxin Neutralized by *Clostridium sordellii* Antitoxin. *Lancet* 8048:1103-1106, 1977.
5. Bailey WR, Scott EG: Diagnostic Microbiology. The CV Mosby Company, St. Louis, 1978.

PRECAUTIONS

Review of experience to date suggests that a subgroup of older patients with associated severe illness may tolerate diarrhea less well. When clindamycin is indicated in these patients, they should be carefully monitored for change in bowel frequency.
CLEOCIN PHOSPHATE Sterile Solution (clindamycin phosphate) should be prescribed with caution in individuals with a history of gastrointestinal disease, particularly colitis.
CLEOCIN PHOSPHATE should be prescribed with caution in atopic individuals.
During prolonged therapy periodic liver and kidney function tests and blood counts should be performed.
Indicated surgical procedures should be performed in conjunction with antibiotic therapy.
The use of CLEOCIN PHOSPHATE may result in overgrowth of nonsusceptible organisms—particularly yeasts. Should superinfections occur, appropriate measures should be taken as indicated by the clinical situation.
CLEOCIN PHOSPHATE should not be injected intravenously undiluted as a bolus, but should be infused over at least 10-60 minutes as directed in the **Dosage and Administration** Section.
Patients with very severe renal disease and/or very severe hepatic disease accompanied by severe metabolic aberrations should be dosed with caution, and serum clindamycin levels monitored during high-dose therapy.
Clindamycin has been shown to have neuromuscular blocking properties that may enhance the action of other neuromuscular blocking agents. Therefore, it should be used with caution in patients receiving such agents.

ADVERSE REACTIONS

The following reactions have been reported with the use of clindamycin.
Gastrointestinal: Abdominal pain, nausea, vomiting and diarrhea (See **Warning** box). An unpleasant or metallic taste occasionally has been reported after intravenous administration of the higher doses of clindamycin phosphate.
Hypersensitivity Reactions: Maculopapular rash and urticaria have been observed during drug therapy. Generalized mild to moderate morbilliform-like skin rashes are the most frequently reported of all adverse reactions. Rare instances of erythema multiforme, some resembling Stevens-Johnson syndrome, have been associated with clindamycin. A few cases of anaphylactoid reactions have been reported.
If a hypersensitivity reaction occurs, the drug should be discontinued. The usual agents (epinephrine, corticosteroids, antihistamines) should be available for emergency treatment of serious reactions.
Liver: Jaundice and abnormalities in liver function tests have been observed during clindamycin therapy.
Renal: Although no direct relationship of clindamycin to renal damage has been established, renal dysfunction as evidenced by azotemia, oliguria, and/or proteinuria has been observed in rare instances.
Hematopoietic: Transient neutropenia (leukopenia) and eosinophilia have been reported. Reports of agranulocytosis and thrombocytopenia have been made. No direct etiologic relationship to concurrent clindamycin therapy could be made in any of the foregoing.
Local Reactions: Pain, induration and sterile abscess have been reported after intramuscular injection and thrombophlebitis after intravenous infusion. Reactions can be minimized or avoided by giving deep intramuscular injections and avoiding prolonged use of indwelling intravenous catheters.
Musculoskeletal: Rare instances of polyarthritis have been reported.
Cardiovascular: Rare instances of cardiopulmonary arrest and hypotension have been reported following too rapid intravenous administration. (See Dosage and Administration Section)

DOSAGE AND ADMINISTRATION

If significant diarrhea occurs during therapy, this antibiotic should be discontinued. (See **Warning** box).
Adults
Parenteral (IM or IV Administration):
Serious infections due to aerobic gram-positive cocci and the more sensitive anaerobes (NOT generally including *Bacteroides fragilis, Peptococcus* species and *Clostridium* species other than *Clostridium perfringens*):
600–1200 mg/day in 2, 3 or 4 equal doses
More severe infections, particularly those due to proven or suspected *Bacteroides fragilis, Peptococcus* species, or *Clostridium* species other than *Clostridium perfringens:*
1200–2700 mg/day in 2, 3 or 4 equal doses
For more serious infections, these doses may have to be increased. In life threatening situations due to aerobes or anaerobes, these doses may be increased. Doses of as much as 4800 mg daily have been given intravenously to adults. See **Dilution and Infusion Rates** section below.
Single IM injections of greater than 600 mg are not recommended.
Alternatively, drug may be administered in the form of a single rapid infusion of the first dose followed by continuous IV infusion as follows:
[See table below].
Children (over 1 month of age)
Parenteral (IM or IV Administration):
Serious infections:
15–25 mg/kg/day in 3 or 4 equal doses
More severe infections:
25–40 mg/kg/day in 3 or 4 equal doses
As an alternative to dosing on a body weight basis, children may be dosed on the basis of square meters body surface: 350 $mg/m^2/day$ for serious infections and 450 $mg/m^2/day$ for more severe infections.
Neonates (less than 1 month):
15 to 20 mg/kg/day in three to four equal doses. The lower dosage may be adequate for small prematures.
Children (over 1 month):
20 to 40 mg/kg/day in three to four equal doses. An equivalent dosage may be given based on body surface area calculation.
Parenteral therapy may be changed to oral CLEOCIN PEDIATRIC® Flavored Granules (clindamycin palmitate hydrochloride) or CLEOCIN HCl® Capsules (clindamycin hydrochloride) when the condition warrants and at the discretion of the physician.
In cases of β-hemolytic streptococcal infections, treatment should be continued for at least 10 days.
Dilution and Infusion Rates
Clindamycin phosphate must be diluted prior to IV administration. The concentration of clindamycin in diluent for infusion should not exceed 12 mg per ml and infusion rates should not exceed 30 mg per minute. The usual infusion dilutions and rates are as follows:

Dose	*Diluent*	*Time*
300 mg	50 ml	10 min
600 mg	50 ml	20 min
900 mg	100 ml	30 min
1200 mg	100 ml	40 min

Administration of more than 1200 mg in a single 1-hour infusion is not recommended.
Dilution and Compatibility
Physical and biological compatibility studies monitored for 24 hours at room temperature have demonstrated no inactivation or incompatibility with the use of CLEOCIN PHOSPHATE Sterile Solution (clindamycin phosphate) in IV solutions containing NaCl, glucose, calcium or potassium and solutions containing vitamin B complex in concentrations usually used clinically. No incompatibility has been demonstrated with the antibiotics cephalothin, kanamycin, gentamicin, penicillin or carbenicillin.
The following drugs are physically incompatible with CLEOCIN PHOSPHATE: ampicillin, phenytoin sodium, barbiturates, aminophylline, calcium gluconate, and magnesium sulfate.
Physico-Chemical Stability of 6, 9, and 12 mg/ml solutions of CLEOCIN PHOSPHATE
Room temperature: 6, 9 and 12 mg/ml (equivalent to clindamycin base) in dextrose 5% in water, sodium chloride 0.9%, or Lactated Ringers in glass bottles or minibags, demonstrated physical and chemical stability for at least 16 days at 25°C.
Refrigeration: 6, 9 and 12 mg/ml (equivalent to clindamycin base) in dextrose 5% in water, sodium chloride 0.9%, or Lactated Ringers in glass bottles or minibags, demonstrated physical and chemical stability for at least 32 days at 4°C.
Frozen: 6,9 and 12 mg/ml (equivalent to clindamycin base) in dextrose 5% in water, sodium chloride 0.9%, or Lactated Ringers in minibags demonstrated physical and chemical stability for at least eight weeks at −10°C.

CLEOCIN PHOSPHATE

To maintain serum clindamycin levels	Rapid infusion rate	Maintenance infusion rate
Above 4 mcg/ml	10 mg/min for 30 min	0.75 mg/min
Above 5 mcg/ml	15 mg/min for 30 min	1.00 mg/min
Above 6 mcg/ml	20 mg/min for 30 min	1.25 mg/min

HOW SUPPLIED

Each ml of CLEOCIN PHOSPHATE Sterile Solution contains clindamycin phosphate equivalent to 150 mg clindamycin; 0.5 mg disodium edetate; 9.45 mg benzyl alcohol added as preservative. When necessary, pH is adjusted with sodium hydroxide and/or hydrochloric acid.
CLEOCIN PHOSPHATE is available in the following packages:

25-2 ml ampoules	NDC 0009-0870-17
100-2 ml ampoules	NDC 0009-0870-03
100-4 ml ampoules	NDC 0009-0775-03
25-2 ml vials	NDC 0009-0870-21
100-2 ml vials	NDC 0009-0870-22
25-4 ml vials	NDC 0009-0775-20
100-4 ml vials	NDC 0009-0775-21
25-6 ml vials	NDC 0009-0902-11
100-6 ml vials	NDC 0009-0902-12

Code 810 020 117

Shown in Product Identification Section, page 433

CLEOCIN T® ℞

brand of clindamycin phosphate topical solution, USP
For External Use

30 ml bottle
NSN 6505-01-140-6450(M)
60 ml bottle
NSN 6505-01-116-5655 (M & VA)

DESCRIPTION

CLEOCIN T Topical Solution contains clindamycin phosphate, USP, at a concentration equivalent to 10 mg clindamycin per milliliter in an isopropyl alcohol and water solution.
Clindamycin phosphate is a water soluble ester of the semi-synthetic antibiotic produced by a 7(S)-chloro-substitution of the 7(R)-hydroxy group of the parent antibiotic lincomycin.
The solution contains isopropyl alcohol 50% v/v, propylene glycol, and water.
The chemical name for clindamycin phosphate is 7(S)-chloro-7-deoxylincomycin-2-phosphate.

CLINICAL PHARMACOLOGY

Although clindamycin phosphate is inactive *in vitro*, rapid *in vivo* hydrolysis converts this compound to the antibacterially active clindamycin.
Clindamycin has been shown to have *in vivo* activity against isolates of *Propionibacterium acnes*. This may account for its usefulness in acne.
Cross resistance has been demonstrated between clindamycin and lincomycin.
Antagonism has been demonstrated between clindamycin and erythromycin.
Studies of penetration into human skin with radiolabelled clindamycin have shown that approximately 10% of the dose is absorbed as indicated by concentration in the stratum corneum. Microbiological assay of urine has shown varying concentrations of clindamycin.
Clindamycin activity has been demonstrated in comedones from acne patients. The mean concentration of antibiotic activity in extracted comedones after application of CLEOCIN T for 4 weeks was 597 mcg/g of comedonal material (range 0–1490). Clindamycin *in vitro* inhibits all *Propionibacterium acnes* cultures tested (MICs 0.4 mcg/ml). Free fatty acids on the skin surface have been decreased from approximately 14% to 2% following application of clindamycin.

INDICATIONS AND USAGE

CLEOCIN T Topical Solution (clindamycin phosphate) is indicated in the treatment of acne vulgaris. In view of the potential for diarrhea, bloody diarrhea and pseudomembranous colitis, the physician should consider whether other agents are more appropriate. (See **Contraindications, Warnings and Adverse Reactions.)**

CONTRAINDICATIONS

CLEOCIN T Topical Solution (clindamycin phosphate) is contraindicated in individuals with a history of hypersensitivity to preparations containing clindamycin or lincomycin, a history of regional enteritis or ulcerative colitis, or a history of antibiotic-associated colitis.

WARNINGS

Orally and parenterally administered clindamycin has been associated with severe colitis which may end fatally. Use of the topical formulation results in absorption of the antibiotic from the skin surface. Diarrhea, bloody diarrhea, and colitis (including pseudomembranous colitis) have been reported with the use of topical and systemic clindamycin. Symptoms can occur after a few days, weeks or months following initiation of clindamycin therapy. They have also been observed to begin up to several weeks after cessation of therapy with clindamycin. Studies indicate a toxin(s) produced by *Clostridium difficile* is one primary cause of antibiotic-associated colitis. The colitis is usually characterized by severe persistent diarrhea and severe abdominal cramps and may be associated with the passage of blood and mucus. Endoscopic examination may reveal pseudomembranous colitis.
When significant diarrhea occurs, the drug should be discontinued. Large bowel endoscopy should be considered in cases of severe diarrhea.
Antiperistaltic agents such as opiates and diphenoxylate with atropine (Lomotil) may prolong and /or worsen the condition. Vancomycin has been found to be effective in the treatment of antibiotic-associated pseudomembranous colitis produced by *Clostridium difficile*. The usual adult dosage is 500 mg to 2 grams of vancomycin orally per day in three to four divided doses administered for 7 to 10 days.
Mild cases of colitis may respond to discontinuance of clindamycin. Moderate to severe cases should be managed promptly with fluid, electrolyte, and protein supplementation as indicated. Cholestyramine and colestipol resins have been shown to bind the toxin *in vitro*. If both a resin and vancomycin are to be administered concurrently, it may be advisable to separate the time of administration of each drug. Systemic corticoids and corticoid retention enemas may help relieve the colitis. Other causes of colitis should also be considered. A careful inquiry should be made concerning previous sensitivities to drugs and other allergens.

PRECAUTIONS

CLEOCIN T Topical Solution (clindamycin phosphate) contains an alcohol base which will cause burning and irritation of the eye. In the event of accidental contact with sensitive surfaces (eye, abraded skin, mucous membranes), bathe with copious amounts of cool tap water. The solution has an unpleasant taste and caution should be exercised when applying medication around the mouth.
CLEOCIN T Topical Solution should be prescribed with caution in atopic individuals.

Pregnancy Category B

Reproduction studies have been performed in rats and mice using subcutaneous and oral doses of clindamycin ranging from 100 to 600 mg/kg/day and have revealed no evidence of impaired fertility or harm to the fetus due to clindamycin. There are, however, no adequate and well-controlled studies in pregnant women. Because animal reproduction studies are not always predictive of human response, this drug should be used during pregnancy only if clearly needed.

Nursing Mothers

It is not known whether clindamycin is excreted in human milk following use of CLEOCIN T Topical Solution. However, orally and parenterally administered clindamycin has been reported to appear in breast milk. As a general rule, nursing should not be undertaken while a patient is on a drug since many drugs are excreted in human milk.

ADVERSE REACTIONS

Skin dryness is the most common adverse reaction.
Clindamycin has been associated with severe colitis which may end fatally (See WARNINGS).
Cases of diarrhea, bloody diarrhea and colitis (including pseudomembranous colitis) have been reported as adverse reactions in patients treated with topical formulations of clindamycin.
Other effects which have been reported in association with the use of topical formulations of clindamycin include:

- Abdominal pain
- Contact dermatitis
- Gastrointestinal disturbances
- Gram-negative folliculitis
- Irritation
- Oily skin
- Sensitization
- Stinging of the eye

DOSAGE AND ADMINISTRATION

Apply a thin film of CLEOCIN T Topical Solution (clindamycin phosphate) twice daily to affected area.

HOW SUPPLIED

CLEOCIN T Topical Solution containing clindamycin phosphate equivalent to 10 mg clindamycin per milliliter is available in the following sizes:

30 ml applicator bottle—NDC 0009-3116-01
60 ml applicator bottle—NDC 0009-3116-02
16 oz (473 ml) bottle—NDC 0009-3116-04

The applicator is designed so that the solution may be applied directly to the involved skin.
Code 811 373 111

Shown in Product Identification Section, page 433

COLESTID® ℞

brand of colestipol hydrochloride granules

Box of 30-5 gram packets
NSN 6505-01-051-4697 (M & VA)

DESCRIPTION

COLESTID Granules consist of colestipol hydrochloride, which is a hyperlipidemia agent for oral use. COLESTID is an insoluble, high molecular weight basic anion-exchange copolymer of diethylenetriamine and 1-chloro-2,3-epoxypropane, with approximately 1 out of 5 amine nitrogens protonated (chloride form). It is a light yellow resin which is hygroscopic and swells when placed in water or aqueous fluids. COLESTID is tasteless and odorless. Inactive ingredient: Silicon dioxide.

CLINICAL PHARMACOLOGY

Cholesterol is the major, and probably the sole precursor of bile acids. During normal digestion, bile acids are secreted via the bile from the liver and gall bladder into the intestines. Bile acids emulsify the fat and lipid materials present in food, thus facilitating absorption. A major portion of the bile acids secreted is reabsorbed from the intestines and returned via the portal circulation to the liver, thus completing the enterohepatic cycle. Only very small amounts of bile acids are found in normal serum.
COLESTID Granules (colestipol hydrochloride) bind bile acids in the intestine forming a complex that is excreted in the feces. This nonsystemic action results in a partial removal of the bile acids from the enterohepatic circulation, preventing their reabsorption. Since colestipol hydrochloride is an anion exchange resin, the chloride anions of the resin can be replaced by other anions, usually those with a greater affinity for the resin than chloride ion.
Colestipol hydrochloride is hydrophilic, but it is virtually water insoluble (99.75%) and it is not hydrolyzed by digestive enzymes. The high molecular weight polymer in COLESTID apparently is not absorbed. Less than 0.05% of ^{14}C-labeled colestipol hydrochloride is excreted in the urine.
The increased fecal loss of bile acids due to COLESTID administration leads to an increased oxidation of cholesterol to bile acids, a decrease in beta lipoprotein or low density lipoprotein serum levels, and a decrease in serum cholesterol levels. Although COLESTID produces an increase in the hepatic synthesis of cholesterol in man, serum cholesterol levels fall.
There is evidence to show that this fall in cholesterol is secondary to an increased rate of cholesterol rich lipoproteins (beta or low density lipoproteins) from the plasma. Serum triglyceride levels may increase or remain unchanged in colestipol treated patients.
The decline in serum cholesterol levels with treatment with COLESTID is usually evident by one month. When COLESTID is discontinued, serum cholesterol levels usually return to baseline levels within one month. Cholesterol may rise even with continued use of COLESTID, and serum levels should be determined periodically to confirm that a favorable initial response is maintained.
COLESTID is more effective than clofibrate in lowering total serum cholesterol and low density lipoprotein cholesterol in Frederickson type IIa hyperlipoproteinemia (pure hypercholesterolemia without hypertriglyceridemia) without affecting high density lipoprotein cholesterol.
In patients with heterozygous familial hypercholesterolemia who have not obtained an optimal response to colestipol hydrochloride alone in maximal doses, the combination of colestipol hydrochloride and nicotinic acid has been shown to provide effective further lowering of serum cholesterol, triglyceride, and LDL cholesterol values. Simultaneously, HDL cholesterol values increased significantly. In many such patients it is possible to normalize serum lipid values.[1–3]

INDICATIONS AND USAGE

Since no drug is innocuous, strict attention should be paid to the indications and contraindications, particularly when selecting drugs for chronic long-term use.
COLESTID Granules (colestipol hydrochloride) are indicated as adjunctive therapy to diet for the reduction of elevated serum cholesterol in patients with primary hypercholesterolemia (elevated low density lipoproteins). COLESTID has been shown to have no effect on or to increase triglyceride levels.
It has not been established whether the drug-induced lowering of serum colesterol or triglyceride levels has a beneficial effect, no effect, or a detrimental effect on the morbidity or mortality due to atherosclerosis including coronary heart disease. Investigations now in progress may yield an answer to this question.

CONTRAINDICATIONS

COLESTID Granules (colestipol hydrochloride) are contraindicated in those individuals who have shown hypersensitivity to any of its components.

WARNINGS

TO AVOID ACCIDENTAL INHALATION OR ESOPHAGEAL DISTRESS, COLESTID GRANULES (colestipol hydrochloride) SHOULD NOT BE TAKEN IN ITS DRY FORM.

Continued on next page

Information on these Upjohn products is based on labeling in effect August 15, 1986. Further information concerning these and other Upjohn products may be obtained by direct inquiry to Medical Information, The Upjohn Company, Kalamazoo, Michigan 49001.

Upjohn—Cont.

ALWAYS MIX COLESTID WITH WATER OR OTHER FLUIDS BEFORE INGESTING.

PRECAUTIONS

Before instituting therapy with COLESTID Granules (colestipol hydrochloride), a vigorous attempt should be made to control serum cholesterol by an appropriate dietary regimen and weight reduction; any underlying disorder that may contribute to the hypercholesterolemia should be treated.
Because it sequesters bile acids, COLESTID may interfere with normal fat absorption and thus may prevent absorption of fat soluble vitamins such as A, D, and K. If COLESTID resin is to be given for long periods of time, supplemental vitamin A and D should be considered.
Chronic use of COLESTID may be associated with an increased bleeding tendency due to hypoprothrombinemia from vitamin K deficiency. This will usually respond promptly to parenteral vitamin K_1 and recurrences can be prevented by oral administration of vitamin K_1.
Serum cholesterol and triglyceride levels should be measured periodically to detect significant changes. COLESTID may raise the serum triglycerides in long term use and, in some patients, the cholesterol levels return to baseline or rise above baseline.
COLESTID may produce or severely worsen pre-existing constipation. The dosage should be decreased in these patients since impaction may occur. Particular effort should be made to avoid constipation in patients with symptomatic coronary artery disease. Constipation associated with COLESTID may aggravate hemorrhoids.
While there have been no reports of hypothyroidism induced in individuals with normal thyroid function, the theoretical possibility exists, particularly in patients with limited thyroid reserve.

Use in Pregnancy
The use of COLESTID in pregnancy or lactation or by women of childbearing age requires that the potential benefits of drug therapy be weighed against the possible hazards to the mother and child. The safe use of COLESTID resin by pregnant women has not been established.

Use in Children
Safety and effectiveness in children have not been established.

DRUG INTERACTIONS

Since colestipol hydrochloride is an anion exchange resin, it may have a strong affinity for anions other than the bile acids. Therefore, colestipol hydrochloride resin may delay or reduce the absorption of concomitant oral medication. The interval between the administration of COLESTID and any other medication should be as long as possible. Patients should take other drugs at least one hour before or four hours after COLESTID to avoid impeding their absorption.
In vitro studies have indicated that COLESTID binds a number of drugs. Studies in humans show that the absorption of chlorothiazide as reflected in urinary excretion is markedly decreased even when administered one hour before COLESTID. The absorption of tetracycline and of penicillin G was significantly decreased when either one was given at the same time as COLESTID; these drugs were not tested to determine the effect of administration one hour before COLESTID.
No depressant effect on blood levels in humans was noted when COLESTID was administered with any of the following drugs: aspirin, clindamycin, clofibrate, methyldopa, tolbutamide or warfarin. Particular caution should be observed with digitalis preparations since there are conflicting results for the effect of COLESTID on the availability of digoxin and digitoxin. The potential for binding of these drugs if given concomitantly is present. Discontinuing COLESTID could pose a hazard to health if a potentially toxic drug that is significantly bound to the resin has been titrated to a maintenance level while the patient was taking COLESTID.

ADVERSE REACTIONS

1. *Gastrointestinal*
   The most common adverse reactions are confined to the gastrointestinal tract. Constipation, reported by about one patient in 10, is the major single complaint and at times is severe and occasionally accompanied by fecal impaction. Hemorrhoids may be aggravated. Most instances of constipation are mild, transient, and controlled with standard treatment. Some patients require decreased dosage or discontinuation of therapy.
   Less frequent gastrointestinal complaints occurring in about one in 30 to one in 100 patients, are abdominal discomfort (abdominal pain and distention), belching, flatulence, nausea, vomiting, and diarrhea. Peptic ulceration, gastrointestinal irritation and bleeding, cholecystitis, and cholelithiasis have been reported by fewer than one in 500 patients and are not necessarily drug related.
2. *Hypersensitivity*
   Urticaria and dermatitis were noted in fewer than one in 1,000 patients. Asthma and wheezing were not reported in the COLESTID studies but have been noted during treatment with other cholesterol-lowering agents.
3. *Musculoskeletal*
   Muscle and joint pains, and arthritis have had a reported incidence of less than one in 1,000 patients.
4. *Neurologic*
   Headache and dizziness were noted in about one in 300 patients; anxiety, vertigo, and drowsiness were reported in fewer than one in 1,000.
5. *Miscellaneous*
   Anorexia, fatigue, weakness, and shortness of breath have been seen in 1–3 patients in 1,000. Transient and modest elevations of serum glutamic oxaloacetic transaminase and of alkaline phosphatase were observed in one or more occasions in various patients treated with COLESTID Granules (colestipol hydrochloride). Some patients have shown an increase in serum phosphorus and chloride with a decrease in sodium and potassium.

OVERDOSE

Overdosage of COLESTID Granules (colestipol hydrochloride) has not been reported. Should overdosage occur, however, the chief potential harm would be obstruction of the gastrointestinal tract. The location of such potential obstruction, the degree of obstruction and the presence or absence of normal gut motility would determine treatment.

DOSAGE AND ADMINISTRATION

For adults, COLESTID Granules (colestipol hydrochloride) are recommended in doses of 15–30 grams/day taken in divided doses two to four times daily. To avoid accidental inhalation or esophageal distress, COLESTID should not be taken in its dry form. COLESTID should always be mixed with water or other fluids before ingesting. Patients should take other drugs at least one hour before or four hours after COLESTID to minimize possible interference with their absorption. (See DRUG INTERACTIONS).

Before COLESTID Administration
1. Define the type of hyperlipoproteinemia.
2. Institute a trial of diet and weight reduction.
3. Establish baseline serum cholesterol and triglyceride levels.

During COLESTID Administration
1. The patient should be carefully monitored clinically, including serum cholesterol and triglyceride levels.
2. Failure of cholesterol to fall or significant rise in triglyceride level should be considered as indications to discontinue medication.

Mixing and Administration Guide
COLESTID Granules (colestipol hydrochloride) should always be taken mixed in a liquid such as orange or tomato juice, water, milk, or carbonated beverage. It may also be taken in soups or with cereals or pulpy fruits. COLESTID should never be taken in its dry form.

With beverages
1. Add the prescribed amount of COLESTID to a glassful (three ounces or more) of water, milk, flavored drink, or a favorite juice (orange, tomato, pineapple, or other fruit juice).
2. Stir the mixture until the medication is completely mixed. (COLESTID will not dissolve in the liquid.) COLESTID may also be mixed with carbonated beverages, slowly stirred in a large glass.
   Rinse the glass with a small amount of additional beverage to make sure all the medication is taken.

With cereals, soups, and fruits
COLESTID may be taken mixed with milk in hot or regular breakfast cereals, or even mixed in soups that have a high fluid content (tomato or chicken noodle soup). It may also be added to fruits that are pulpy such as crushed pineapple, pears, peaches, or fruit cocktail.

HOW SUPPLIED

COLESTID Granules (colestipol hydrochloride) are available as follows:

Box of 30–5 gram packets	*NDC 0009-0260-01*
500 gram bottle	*NDC 0009-0260-02*

Each packet or each level scoop supplies 5 grams of COLESTID.
Store at controlled room temperature 15°-30°C (59°-86°F).

REFERENCES

1. Kane JP, Malloy MJ, Tun P et al: Normalization of low-density-lipoprotein levels in heterozygous familial hypercholesterolemia with a combined drug regimen. *N. Engl J Med* 304:251–258, 1981.
2. Illingworth DR, Phillipson BE, JH Rapp et al: Colestipol plus nicotinic acid in treatment of heterozygous familial hypercholesterolemia. *Lancet* 1:296–298, 1981.
3. Kuo PT, Kostis JB, Moreyra AE et al: Familial type II hyperlipoproteinemia with coronary heart disease: Effect of diet-colestipol-nicotinic acid treatment. *Chest* 79:286–291, 1981.

Code 810 307 002

CORTAID® Cream
(See PDR For Nonprescription Drugs)

CORTAID® Lotion
(See PDR For Nonprescription Drugs)

CORTAID® Ointment
(See PDR For Nonprescription Drugs)

CORTAID® Spray
(See PDR For Nonprescription Drugs)

CORTEF® Feminine Itch Cream
(See PDR For Nonprescription Drugs)

CYTOSAR-U® ℞

brand of cytarabine sterile powder
(sterile cytarabine, USP)
(ara-C)

For Intravenous and Subcutaneous Use Only

100 mg vial	**NSN 6505-00-434-0733 (M)**
500 mg vial	**NSN 6505-01-077-5690 (M)**

WARNING
Only physicians experienced in cancer chemotherapy should use CYTOSAR-U Sterile Powder.
For induction therapy patients should be treated in a facility with laboratory and supportive resources sufficient to monitor drug tolerance and protect and maintain a patient compromised by drug toxicity. The main toxic effect of CYTOSAR-U is bone marrow suppression with leukopenia, thrombocytopenia and anemia. Less serious toxicity includes nausea, vomiting, diarrhea and abdominal pain, oral ulceration, and hepatic dysfunction.
The physician must judge possible benefit to the patient against known toxic effects of this drug in considering the advisability of therapy with CYTOSAR-U. Before making this judgment or beginning treatment, the physician should be familiar with the following text.

DESCRIPTION

CYTOSAR-U Sterile Powder contains cytarabine (1-β-D-arabinofuranosylcytosine; β-cytosine arabinoside). Cytarabine is a synthetic nucleoside which differs from the normal nucleosides cytidine and deoxycytidine in that the sugar moiety is arabinose rather than ribose or deoxyribose.
CYTOSAR-U is an antineoplastic agent for parenteral administration. It is available as a sterile freeze-dried preparation in two sizes:

100 mg vials—when prepared as directed, each ml contains:
20 mg cytarabine (Supplied with 5 ml ampoule of Bacteriostatic Water for Injection with Benzyl Alcohol 0.945% w/v added as preservative. **Do not use this diluent for intrathecal use. See WARNINGS**).

500 mg vials—when prepared as directed, each ml contains:
50 mg cytarabine (Supplied with 10 ml ampoule of Bacteriostatic Water for Injection with Benzyl Alcohol 0.945% w/v added as preservative. **Do not use this diluent for intrathecal use. See WARNINGS**).

When necessary, the pH of CYTOSAR-U was adjusted with hydrochloric acid and/or sodium hydroxide.

PHARMACOLOGY

Cell Culture Studies
Cytarabine is cytotoxic to a wide variety of proliferating mammalian cells in culture. It exhibits cell phase specificity, primarily killing cells undergoing DNA synthesis (S-phase) and under certain conditions blocking the progression of cells from the G_1 phase to the S-phase. Although the mechanism of action is not completely understood, it appears that cytarabine acts through the inhibition of DNA polymerase. A limited, but significant, incorporation of cytarabine into both DNA and RNA has also been reported. Extensive chromosomal damage, including chromatoid breaks, have been produced by cytarabine and malignant transformation of rodent cells in culture has been reported. Deoxycytidine prevents or delays (but does not reverse) the cytotoxic activity. Cell culture studies have shown an antiviral effect.[1] However, efficacy against herpes zoster or smallpox could not be demonstrated in controlled clinical trials.[2–4]

TABLE I
ACUTE MYELOCYTIC LEUKEMIA
REMISSION INDUCTION
ADULTS

Drug-Dosage Schedule*	No. Patients Evaluated	Complete Remissions	Investigator
(CYTOSAR-U) SINGLE-DRUG THERAPY			
(infusion) 10 mg/m²/12 hrs/day 30 mg/m²/12 hrs/day 10 mg/m²/24 hrs/day 30 mg/m²/24 hrs/day	 12 41 9 36	 2 (17%) 10 (24%) 2 (22%) 2 (6%)	 Ellison[11] (1968)
(infusion) 200 mg/m²/24 hrs/5 days	36	9 (25%)	Bodey[12] (1969)
10 mg/m² IV injection initially, then infusions of 30 mg/m²/12 hrs or 60 mg/m²/day for 4 days	49	21 (43%)	Goodell[13] (1970)
(infusion therapy) 800 mg/m²/2 days 1000 mg/m²/5 days	 53 60	 12 (23%) 24 (40%)	Southwest Oncology Group[14] (1974)
100 mg/m²/day 1 hr infusion	49	7 (14%)	Carey[15] (1975)
5–12.5 mg/kg/12 hour infusion following IV synchronizing dose**	5	5 (100%)	Lampkin[16] (1976)
COMBINED THERAPY			
CYTOSAR-U, doxorubicin	41	30 (73%)	Preisler[17] (1979)
CYTOSAR-U, thioguanine, daunorubicin	28	22 (79%)	Gale[18] (1977)
CYTOSAR-U, doxorubicin, vincristine, prednisolone	35	23 (66%)	Weinstein[19] (1980)
CYTOSAR-U, daunorubicin, thioguanine, prednisone, vincristine	139	84 (60%)	Glucksberg[20] (1981)
CYTOSAR-U, daunorubicin	21	14 (67%)	Cassileth[21] (1977)

*Unless otherwise stated all doses given until drug effect—modifications then based on hematologic response. See references
**Highly experimental-requires ability to study mitotic indices

Cellular Resistance and Sensitivity
Cytarabine is metabolized by deoxycytidine kinase and other nucleotide kinases to the nucleotide triphosphate, an effective inhibitor of DNA polymerase; it is inactivated by a pyrimidine nucleoside deaminase which converts it to the nontoxic uracil derivative. It appears that the balance of kinase and deaminase levels may be an important factor in determining sensitivity or resistance of the cell to cytarabine.

Animal Studies
In experimental studies with mouse tumors, cytarabine was most effective in those tumors with a high growth fraction. The effect was dependent on the treatment schedule; optimal effects were achieved when the schedule (multiple closely spaced doses or constant infusion) ensured contact of the drug with the tumor cells when the maximum number of cells were in the susceptible S-phase. The best results were obtained when courses of therapy were separated by intervals sufficient to permit adequate host recovery.

Human Pharmacology
Cytarabine is rapidly metabolized and is not effective orally; less than 20 percent of the orally administered dose is absorbed from the gastrointestinal tract.
Following rapid intravenous injection of cytarabine with tritium, the disappearance from plasma is biphasic. There is an initial distributive phase with a half-life of about 10 minutes, followed by a second elimination phase with a half-life of about 1 to 3 hours. After the distributive phase, over 80 percent of plasma radioactivity can be accounted for by the inactive metabolite 1-β-D-arabino- furanosyluracil (ara-U). Within 24 hours about 80 percent of the administered radioactivity can be recovered in the urine, approximately 90 percent of which is excreted as ara-U.
Relatively constant plasma levels can be achieved by continuous intravenous infusion.
After subcutaneous or intramuscular administration of cytarabine labeled with tritium, peak-plasma levels of radioactivity are achieved about 20 to 60 minutes after injection and are considerably lower than those after intravenous administration.
Cerebrospinal fluid levels of cytarabine are low in comparison to plasma levels after single intravenous injection. However, in one patient in whom cerebrospinal levels were examined after 2 hours of constant intravenous infusion, levels approached 40 percent of the steady state plasma level. With intrathecal administration, levels of cytarabine in the cerebrospinal fluid declined with a first order half-life of about 2 hours. Because cerebrospinal fluid levels of deaminase are low, little conversion to ara-U was observed.

Immunosuppressive Action
CYTOSAR-U Sterile Powder (cytarabine) is capable of obliterating immune responses in man during administration with little or no accompanying toxicity.[5,6] Suppression of antibody responses to E-coli-VI antigen and tetanus toxoid have been demonstrated. This suppression was obtained during both primary and secondary antibody responses.
CYTOSAR-U also suppressed the development of cell-mediated immune responses such as delayed hypersensitivity skin reaction to dinitrochlorobenzene. However, it had no effect on already established delayed hypersensitivity reactions.
Following 5-day courses of intensive therapy with CYTOSAR-U the immune response was suppressed, as indicated by the following parameters: macrophage ingress into skin windows; circulating antibody response following primary antigenic stimulation; lymphocyte blastogenesis with phytohemagglutinin. A few days after termination of therapy there was a rapid return to normal.[7]

INDICATIONS AND USAGE

CYTOSAR-U Sterile Powder (cytarabine) is indicated primarily for induction and maintenance of remission in acute myelocytic leukemia of both adults and children. It has also been found useful in the treatment of other leukemias, such as acute lymphocytic leukemia, chronic myelocytic leukemia (blast phase) and erythroleukemia. CYTOSAR-U may be used alone or in combination with other antineoplastic agents; the best results are often obtained with combination therapy.
CYTOSAR-U has been used experimentally in a variety of neoplastic diseases. In general, few patients with solid tumors have benefited.
Children with non-Hodgkin's lymphoma have benefited from a combination drug program (LSA_2L_2) that includes CYTOSAR-U.[8,9,10]
Remissions induced by CYTOSAR-U not followed by maintenance treatment have been brief. Maintenance therapy has extended these and provided useful and comfortable remissions with relatively little toxicity.

Acute Myelocytic Leukemia
The following tables outline the results of treatment with CYTOSAR-U alone and in combination with other chemotherapeutic agents, in the treatment of acute myelocytic leukemia in adults and children.
The treatment regimens outlined in the tables should not be compared for efficacy. These were independent studies with a number of variables involved, such as patient population, duration of disease, and previous treatment.
[See Table I above].
The responsiveness and course of childhood acute myelocytic leukemia (AML) appears to be different from that in adults.[23-25] Numerous studies show response rates to be higher in children than in adults with similar treatment schedules. Experience indicates that at least with induction and initial drug responsiveness, childhood AML appears to be more similar to childhood acute lymphocytic leukemia (ALL) than to its adult variant.
[See Table II next page]

Acute Lymphocytic Leukemia
CYTOSAR-U has been used in the treatment of acute lymphocytic leukemia in both adults and children. When CYTOSAR-U was used with other antineoplastic agents as part of a total therapy program, results were equal to or better than those reported with such programs which did not include CYTOSAR-U.[26,27] Used singly, or in combination with other agents, CYTOSAR-U has also been effective in treating patients who had relapsed on other therapy. Table III summarizes the results obtained in previously treated patients. Since these are independent studies with such variables as patient population, duration of disease and previous

Continued on next page

Information on these Upjohn products is based on labeling in effect August 15, 1986. Further information concerning these and other Upjohn products may be obtained by direct inquiry to Medical Information, The Upjohn Company, Kalamazoo, Michigan 49001.

Upjohn—Cont.

treatment, results shown should not be used for comparing the efficacy of the outlined treatment programs.
[See Table III on next page].

Intrathecal Use in Meningeal Leukemia

CYTOSAR-U has been used intrathecally in acute leukemia in doses ranging from 5 mg/m^2 to 75 mg/m^2 of body surface area. The frequency of administration varied from once a day for 4 days to once every 4 days. The most frequently used dose was 30 mg/m^2 every 4 days until cerebrospinal fluid findings were normal, followed by one additional treatment.[36-40] The dosage schedule is usually governed by the type and severity of central nervous system manifestations and the response to previous therapy.

CYTOSAR-U has been used intrathecally with SOLU-CORTEF® Sterile Powder (hydrocortisone sodium succinate) and methotrexate, both as prophylaxis in newly diagnosed children with acute lymphocytic leukemia, as well as in the treatment of meningeal leukemia. Sullivan has reported that prophylactic triple therapy has prevented late CNS disease and given overall cure and survival rates similar to those seen in patients in whom CNS radiation and intrathecal methotrexate were used as initial CNS prophylaxis.[41] The dose of CYTOSAR-U was 30 mg/m^2 of cytarabine, SOLU-CORTEF 15 mg/m^2 of hydrocortisone sodium succinate, and methotrexate 15 mg/m^2. The physician should be familiar with this report before initiation of the regimen.

Prophylactic triple therapy following the successful treatment of the acute meningeal episode may be useful. The physician should familiarize himself with the current literature before instituting such a program.

CYTOSAR-U given intrathecally may cause systemic toxicity and careful monitoring of the hemopoietic system is indicated. Modification of other anti-leukemia therapy may be necessary. Major toxicity is rare. The most frequently reported reactions after intrathecal administration were nausea, vomiting and fever; these reactions are mild and self-limiting. Paraplegia has been reported.[42] Necrotizing leukoencephalopathy occurred in 5 children; these patients had also been treated with intrathecal methotrexate and hydrocortisone, as well as by central nervous system radiation.[43] Isolated neurotoxicity has been reported.[44] Blindness occurred in two patients in remission whose treatment had consisted of combination systemic chemotherapy, prophylactic central nervous system radiation and intrathecal CYTOSAR-U.[45]

Focal leukemic involvement of the central nervous system may not respond to intrathecal CYTOSAR-U and may better be treated with radiotherapy.

Non-Hodgkin's Lymphoma in Children

CYTOSAR-U has been used as part of a multi-drug program (LSA_2L_2) to treat non-Hodgkin's lymphoma in children.[8,9,10]

CONTRAINDICATIONS

CYTOSAR-U Sterile Powder (cytarabine) is contraindicated in those patients who are hypersensitive to the drug.

WARNINGS (See boxed WARNING)

Cytarabine is a potent bone marrow suppressant. Therapy should be started cautiously in patients with pre-existing drug-induced bone marrow suppression. Patients receiving this drug must be under close medical supervision and, during induction therapy, should have leukocyte and platelet counts performed daily. Bone marrow examinations should be performed frequently after blasts have disappeared from the peripheral blood. Facilities should be available for management of complications, possibly fatal, of bone marrow suppression (infection resulting from granulocytopenia and other impaired body defenses, and hemorrhage secondary to thrombocytopenia). One case of anaphylaxis that resulted in acute cardiopulmonary arrest and required resuscitation has been reported. This occurred immediately after the intravenous administration of CYTOSAR-U Sterile Powder.

Severe and at times fatal CNS, GI and pulmonary toxicity (different from that seen with conventional therapy regimens of CYTOSAR-U) has been reported following some experimental CYTOSAR-U dose schedules.[46-49] These reactions include reversible corneal toxicity, and hemorrhagic conjunctivitis, which may be prevented or diminished by prophylaxis with a local corticosteroid eye drop; cerebral and cerebellar dysfunction, including personality changes, somnolence and coma, usually reversible; severe gastrointestinal ulceration, including pneumatosis cystoides intestinalis leading to peritonitis; sepsis and liver abscess; pulmonary edema, liver damage with increased hyperbilirubinemia; bowel necrosis; and necrotizing colitis. Rarely, severe skin rash, leading to desquamation has been reported. Complete alopecia is more commonly seen with experimental high dose therapy than with standard CYTOSAR-U treatment programs. If experimental high dose therapy is used, do not use a diluent containing benzyl alcohol.

An increase in cardiomyopathy with subsequent death has been reported following experimental high dose therapy with cytarabine in combination with cyclophosphamide when used for bone marrow transplant preparation.[57]

A syndrome of sudden respiratory distress, rapidly progressing to pulmonary edema and radiographically pronounced cardiomegaly has been reported following experimental high dose therapy with cytarbine used for the treatment of relapsed leukemia from one institution in 16/72 patients. The outcome of this syndrome can be fatal.[58]

Benzyl alcohol is contained in the diluent for this product. Benzyl alcohol has been reported to be associated with a fatal "Gasping Syndrome" in premature infants.

If used intrathecally, do not use a diluent containing benzyl alcohol. Many clinicians reconstitute with preservative-free 0.9% sodium chloride for injection and use immediately.

Use in Pregnancy

Pregnancy Category C. CYTOSAR-U is known to be teratogenic in some animal species. Use of the drug in women who are or who may become pregnant should be undertaken only after due consideration of potential benefit and potential hazard to both mother and child.

A review of the literature has shown 32 reported cases where CYTOSAR-U was given during pregnancy, either alone or in combination with other cytotoxic agents.

Eighteen normal infants were delivered. Four of these had first trimester exposure. Five infants were premature or of low birth weight. Twelve of the 18 normal infants were followed up at ages ranging from six weeks to seven years, and showed no abnormalties. One apparently normal infant died at 90 days of gastroenteritis.

Two cases of congenital abnormalities have been reported, one with upper and lower distal limb defects,[50] and the other with extremity and ear deformities.[51] Both of these cases had first trimester exposure.

There were seven infants with various problems in the neonatal period, including pancytopenia; transient depression of WBC, hematocrit or platelets; electrolyte abnormalities; transient eosinophilia; and one case of increased IgM levels and hyperpyrexia possibly due to sepsis. Six of the seven infants were also premature. The child with pancytopenia died at 21 days of sepsis.

Therapeutic abortions were done in five cases. Four fetuses were grossly normal, but one had an enlarged spleen and another showed Trisomy C chromosome abnormality in the chorionic tissue.

Because of the potential for abnormalities with cytotoxic therapy, particularly during the first trimester, a patient who is or who may become pregnant while on CYTOSAR-U should be apprised of the potential risk to the fetus and the advisability of pregnancy continuation. There is a definite, but considerably reduced risk if therapy is initiated during the second or third trimester. Although normal infants have been delivered to patients treated in all three trimesters of pregnancy, follow-up of such infants would be advisable.

PRECAUTIONS

Patients receiving CYTOSAR-U Sterile Powder (cytarabine) must be monitored closely. Frequent platelet and leukocyte counts and bone marrow examinations are mandatory. Consider suspending or modifying therapy when drug-induced marrow depression has resulted in a platelet count under 50,000 or a polymorphonuclear granulocyte count under $1000/mm^3$. Counts of formed elements in the peripheral blood may continue to fall after the drug is stopped and reach lowest values after drug-free intervals of 12 to 24 days. When indicated, restart therapy when definite signs of marrow recovery appear (on successive bone marrow studies). Patients whose drug is withheld until "normal" peripheral blood values are attained may escape from control.

When large intravenous doses are given quickly, patients are frequently nauseated and may vomit for several hours post-injection. This problem tends to be less severe when the drug is infused.

The human liver apparently detoxifies a substantial fraction of an administered dose. Use the drug with caution and at reduced dose in patients whose liver function is poor.

Periodic checks of bone marrow, liver and kidney functions should be performed in patients receiving CYTOSAR-U.

Like other cytotoxic drugs, CYTOSAR-U may induce hyperuricemia secondary to rapid lysis of neoplastic cells. The clinician should monitor the patient's blood uric acid level and be prepared to use such supportive and pharmacologic measures as might be necessary to control this problem.

Acute pancreatitis has been reported to occur in patients being treated with CYTOSAR-U who have had prior treatment with L-asparaginase.[52]

ADVERSE REACTIONS

Expected Reactions

Because cytarabine is a bone marrow suppressant, anemia, leukopenia, thrombocytopenia, megaloblastosis and reduced reticulocytes can be expected as a result of administration with CYTOSAR-U Sterile Powder. The severity of these reactions are dose and schedule dependent.[53] Cellular changes in the morphology of bone marrow and peripheral smears can be expected.[54]

Following 5-day constant infusions or acute injections of 50 mg/m^2 to 600 mg/m^2, white cell depression follows a biphasic course. Regardless of initial count, dosage level, or schedule, there is an initial fall starting the first 24 hours with a nadir at days 7–9. This is followed by a brief rise which peaks around the twelfth day. A second and deeper fall reaches nadir at days 15–24. Then there is rapid rise to above baseline in the next 10 days. Platelet depression is noticeable at 5 days with a peak depression occurring between days 12–15. Thereupon, a rapid rise to above baseline occurs in the next 10 days.[55]

The Cytarabine (Ara-C) Syndrome

A cytarabine syndrome has been described by Castleberry.[56] It is characterized by fever, myalgia, bone pain, occasionally chest pain, maculopapular rash, conjunctivitis and malaise. It usually occurs 6-12 hours following drug administration. Corticosteroids have been shown to be beneficial in treating or preventing this syndrome. If the symptoms of the syndrome are deemed treatable, corticosteroids should be contemplated as well as continuation of therapy with CYTOSAR-U Sterile Powder (cytarabine).

Most Frequent Adverse Reactions

anorexia
nausea
vomiting
diarrhea
oral and anal inflammation or ulceration
hepatic dysfunction
fever
rash
thrombophlebitis
bleeding (all sites)

Nausea and vomiting are most frequent following rapid intravenous injection.

Less Frequent Adverse Reactions

sepsis
pneumonia
cellulitis at injection site
skin ulceration
urinary retention
renal dysfunction
neuritis
neural toxicity
sore throat
esophageal ulceration
esophagitis
chest pain
bowel necrosis
abdominal pain
freckling
jaundice
conjunctivitis (may occur with rash)
dizziness

TABLE II
ACUTE MYELOCYTIC LEUKEMIA
REMISSION INDUCTION
CHILDREN (21 and under)

Drug Therapy	No. Patients Evaluated	Complete Remissions	Investigator
CYTOSAR-U, (5–12.5 mg/kg following IV synchronizing dose**)	16	12 (75%)	Lampkin[16] (1976)
CYTOSAR-U, vincristine, doxorubicin, prednisolone	48	35 (73%)	Weinstein[19] (1980)
CYTOSAR-U, thioguanine-doxorubicin	11	8 (72%)	Hagbin[22] (1975)
CYTOSAR-U, thioguanine	47	20 (43%)	Pizzo[23] (1976)
CYTOSAR-U, cyclophosphamide	12	7 (58%)	

**Highly experimental-requires ability to study mitotic indices

TABLE III
ACUTE LYMPHATIC LEUKEMIA
REMISSION INDUCTION
PREVIOUSLY TREATED PATIENTS

ADULTS AND CHILDREN

Drug Therapy	No. of Patients Evaluated	Complete Remissions	Response	Investigator
CYTOSAR-U, 3–5 mg/kg/day (IV injection)	43	2 (5%)	15 (35%)	Howard[28] (1968)
CYTOSAR-U, asparaginase	9	8 (89%)	8 (89%)	McElwain[29] (1969)
CYTOSAR-U, cyclophosphamide	11	7 (64%)	9 (82%)	Bodey[30] (1970)
CYTOSAR-U, prednisone	83		(49%)	Nesbit[31] (1970)
CYTOSAR-U,-150–200 mg/m^2/5 days (infusion)	34	1 (3%)	4 (12%)	Wang[32] (1970)
CYTOSAR-U, L-asparaginase, prednisone, vincristine, doxorubicin	91	72 (79%)	—	Klemperer[33] (1978)
CYTOSAR-U, L-asparaginase, prednisone, vincristine, doxorubicin	55	42 (76%)	—	Klemperer[33] (1978)
CYTOSAR-U, asparaginase	22	13 (59%)	15 (68%)	Ortega[34] (1972)
CYTOSAR-U, thioguanine	19	9 (47%)	9 (47%)	Bryan[35] (1974)

alopecia
anaphylaxis (See WARNINGS)
allergic edema
pruritus
shortness of breath
urticaria
headache

Experimental Doses

Severe and at times fatal CNS, GI and pulmonary toxicity (different from that seen with conventional therapy regimens of CYTOSAR-U) has been reported following some experimental dose schedules of CYTOSAR-U.[46-49] These reactions include reversible corneal toxicity and hemorrhagic conjunctivitis, which may be prevented or diminished by prophylaxis with a local corticosteroid eye drop; cerebral and cerebellar dysfunction, including personality changes, somnolence and coma, usually reversible; severe gastrointestinal ulceration, including pneumatosis cystoides intestinalis leading to peritonitis; sepsis and liver abscess; pulmonary edema, liver damage with increased hyperbilirubinemia; bowel necrosis; and necrotizing colitis. Rarely, severe skin rash, leading to desquamation has been reported. Complete alopecia is more commonly seen with experimental high dose therapy than with standard CYTOSAR-U treatment programs. If experimental high dose therapy is used, do not use a diluent containing benzyl alcohol.

An increase in cardiomyopathy with subsequent death has been reported following experimental high dose therapy with cytarbine in combination with cyclophosphamide when used for bone marrow transplant preparation.[57]

A syndrome of sudden respiratory distress, rapidly progressing to pulmonary edema and radiographically pronounced cardiomegaly has been reported following experimental high dose therapy with cytarabine used for the treatment of relapsed leukemia from one institution in 16/72 patients. The outcome of this syndrome can be fatal.[58]

OVERDOSAGE

There is no antidote for CYTOSAR-U overdosage. Doses of 4.5 g/m^2 by intravenous infusion over 1 hour every 12 hours for 12 doses has caused an unacceptable increase in irreversible CNS toxicity and death.[47]

DOSAGE AND ADMINISTRATION

CYTOSAR-U Sterile Powder (cytarabine) is not active orally. The schedule and method of administration varies with the program of therapy to be used. CYTOSAR-U Sterile Powder may be given by intravenous infusion or injection or subcutaneously. Thrombophlebitis has occurred at the site of drug injection or infusion in some patients, and rarely patients have noted pain and inflammation at subcutaneous injection sites. In most instances, however, the drug has been well tolerated.

Patients can tolerate higher total doses when they receive the drug by rapid intravenous injection as compared with slow infusion. This phenomenon is related to the drug's rapid inactivation and brief exposure of susceptible normal and neoplastic cells to significant levels after rapid injection. Normal and neoplastic cells seem to respond in somewhat parallel fashion to these different modes of administration and no clear-cut clinical advantage has been demonstrated for either.

Clinical experience accumulated to date suggests that success with CYTOSAR-U is dependent more on adeptness in modifying day-to-day dosage to obtain maximum leukemic cell kill with tolerable toxicity than on the basic treatment schedule chosen at the outset of therapy. Toxicity necessitating dosage alteration almost always occurs.

In many chemotherapeutic programs, CYTOSAR-U is used in combination with other cytotoxic drugs. The addition of these cytotoxic drugs has necessitated changes and dose alterations. The dosage schedules for combination therapy outlined below have been reported in the literature (see **References**).

Dosage Schedules:

Acute myelocytic leukemia—induction remission, adults

CYTOSAR-U Sterile Powder (cytarabine)—200 mg/m^2 daily by continuous infusion for 5 days (120 hours)—total dose 1000 mg/m^2. This course is repeated approximately every 2 weeks. Modifications must be made and based on hematologic response.

Combined Chemotherapy

Before instituting a program of combined chemotherapy, the physician should be familiar with the literature, adverse reactions, precautions, contraindications, and warnings applicable to all the drugs involved in the program.

CYTOSAR-U, doxorubicin[17]

CYTOSAR-U: 100 mg/m^2/day, continuous IV infusion (Days 1–10)

Doxorubicin: 30 mg/m^2/day, IV infusion of 30 minutes (Days 1–3)

Additional (complete or modified) courses as necessary at 2–4 week intervals if leukemia is persistent.

CYTOSAR-U, thioguanine, daunorubicin[18]

CYTOSAR-U: 100 mg/m^2/day IV infusion over 30 minutes every 12 hours (Days 1–7)

Thioguanine: 100 mg/m^2, orally every 12 hours (Days 1–7)

Daunorubicin: 60 mg/m^2/day, IV infusion (Days 5–7)

Additional (complete or modified) courses as necessary at 2–4 week intervals if leukemia is persistent.

CYTOSAR-U, doxorubicin, vincristine, prednisolone[19]

CYTOSAR-U: 100 mg/m^2/day, continuous IV infusion (Days 1–7)

Doxorubicin: 30 mg/m^2/day, IV infusion (Days 1–3)

Vincristine: 1.5 mg/m^2/day, IV infusion (Days 1, 5)

Prednisolone: 40 mg/m^2/day, IV infusion every 12 hours (Days 1–5)

Additional (complete or modified) courses as necessary at 2–4 week intervals if leukemia is persistent.

CYTOSAR-U, daunorubicin, thioguanine, prednisone, vincristine[20]

CYTOSAR-U: 100 mg/m^2/day, IV every 12 hours (Days 1–7)

Daunorubicin: 70 mg/m^2/Day, IV infusion (Days 1–3)

Thioguanine: 100 mg/m^2, orally every 12 hours (Days 1–7)

Prednisone: 40 mg/m^2/day, orally (Days 1–7)

Vincristine: 1 mg/m^2/day, IV infusion (Days 1, 7)

Additional (complete or modified) courses as necessary at 2–4 week intervals if leukemia is persistent.

CYTOSAR-U, daunorubicin[21]

CYTOSAR-U: 100 mg/m^2/day, continuous IV infusion (Days 1–7)

Daunorubicin: 45 mg/m^2/day, IV push (Days 1–3)

Additional (complete or modified) courses as necessary at 2–4 week intervals if leukemia is persistent.

Acute myelocytic leukemia-maintenance, adults

Maintenance programs are modifications of induction programs and, in general, use similar schedules of drug therapy as were used during induction. Most programs have a greater time spacing between courses of therapy during remission maintenance.

Acute myelocytic leukemia-induction and maintenance in children

Numerous studies have shown that childhood AML responds better than adult AML given similar regimens. Where the adult dosage is stated in terms of body weight or surface area, the children's dosage may be calculated on the same basis. When specified amounts of a drug are indicated for the adult dosage, these should be adjusted for children on the basis of such factors as age, body weight or body surface area.

Acute lymphocytic leukemia

In general, dosage schedules are similar to those used in acute myelocytic leukemia with some modifications. For dosage recommendations see referenced literature in Table III under INDICATIONS AND USAGE.

Dosage Modification—The dosage of CYTOSAR-U must be modified or suspended when signs of serious hematologic depression appear. In general, consider discontinuing the drug if the patient has less than 50,000 platelets or 1000 polymorphonuclear granulocytes/mm^3 in his peripheral blood. These guidelines may be modified depending on signs of toxicity in other systems and on the rapidity of fall in formed blood elements. Restart the drug when there are signs of marrow recovery and the above platelet and granulocyte levels have been attained. Withholding therapy until the patient's blood values are normal may result in escape of the patient's disease from control by the drug.

Procedures for proper handling and disposal of anticancer drugs should be considered. Several guidelines on this subject have been published.[59-64] There is no general agreement that all of the procedures recommended in the guidelines are necessary or appropriate.

HOW SUPPLIED

Store unreconstituted product at controlled room temperature: 15°-30°C (59°-86°F). CYTOSAR-U Sterile Powder (cytarabine) is available as a freeze-dried preparation in multidose vials of two sizes:

100 mg* vial—Must be reconstituted with 5 ml of Bacteriostatic Water for Injection with Benzyl Alcohol 0.945% w/v added as preservative, the resulting solution contains 20 mg of cytarabine per ml. (Do not use this diluent for intrathecal use. See WARNINGS).

500 mg* vial—Must be reconstituted with 10 ml of Bacteriostatic Water for Injection with Benzyl Alcohol 0.945% w/v added as preservative, the resulting solution contains 50 mg of cytarabine per ml. (Do not use this diluent for intrathecal use. See WARNINGS).

*When necessary, the pH was adjusted with hydrochloric acid and/or sodium hydroxide.

In this form the drug is suitable for intravenous or subcutaneous administration. The pH of the reconstituted solution is about 5. THESE SOLUTIONS MAY BE STORED AT CONTROLLED ROOM TEMPERATURE 15°-30°C (59°-86°F) FOR 48 HOURS. DISCARD ANY SOLUTION IN WHICH A SLIGHT HAZE DEVELOPS.

Chemical Stability in Infusion Solutions

Chemical stability studies were performed by ultraviolet assay on CYTOSAR-U infusion solutions. These studies showed that when the reconstituted CYTOSAR-U Sterile Powder (cytarabine) was added to Water for Injection, 5% Dextrose in Water or Sodium Chloride Injection, 94 to 96

Continued on next page

Information on these Upjohn products is based on labeling in effect August 15, 1986. Further information concerning these and other Upjohn products may be obtained by direct inquiry to Medical Information, The Upjohn Company, Kalamazoo, Michigan 49001.

percent of the cytarabine was present after 192 hours storage at room temperature.

REFERENCES

1. Zaky DA, Betts RF, Douglas RG, et al: Varicella-Zoster Virus and Subcutaneous Cytarabine: Correlation of In Vitro Sensitivities to Blood Levels, Antimicrob Agents Chemother 7:229–232, 1975
2. Davis CM, VanDarsarl JV, Coltman CA Jr: Failure of Cytarabine in Varicella-Zoster Infections, JAMA *224*:122–123, 1973
3. Betts RF, Zaky DA, Douglas RG, et al: Ineffectiveness of Subcutaneous Cytosine Arabinoside in Localized Herpes Zoster, Ann Intern Med *82*:778–783, 1975
4. Dennis DT, Doberstyn EB, Awoke S, et al: Failure of Cytosine Arabinoside in Treating Smallpox; A Double-blind Study, Lancet *2*:377–379, 1974
5. Gray GD: ARA-C and Derivatives as Examples of Immunosuppressive Nucleoside Analogs, Ann NY Acad Sci *255*:372–379, 1975
6. Mitchell MS, Wade ME, DeConti RC, et al: Immunosuppressive Effects of Cytosine Arabinoside and Methotrexate in Man, Ann Intern Med *70*:535–547, 1969
7. Frei E, Ho DHW, Bodey GP, et al: Pharmacologic and Cytokinetic Studies of Arabinosyl Cytosine. In *Unifying Concepts of Leukemia*, Bibl. Hematol. No. 39. Karger, Basel 1973, pp 1085–1097
8. Wollner N, Burchenal JH, Lieberman PH, et al: Non-Hodgkin's Lymphoma in Children—A Comparative Study of Two Modalities of Therapy, Cancer *37*:123–134, 1976
9. Wollner N, Exelby PR, Lieberman PH: Non-Hodgkin's Lymphoma in Children—A Progress Report on the Original Patients Treated with the LSA_2-L_2 Protocol, Cancer *44*:1990–1999, 1979
10. Sullivan MP, Pullen J, Moore T, et al: Pediatric Oncology Group Trial of LSA_2-L_2 Therapy in Non-Hodgkin's Lymphoma, abstracted, Proc AACR and ASCO *22*:C-180, 1981
11. Ellison RR, Holland JF, Weil M, et al: Arabinosyl Cytosine: A Useful Agent in the Treatment of Acute Leukemia in Adults, Blood *32*:507–523, 1968
12. Bodey GP, Freireich EJ, Monto RW, et al: Cytosine Arabinoside (NSC-63878) Therapy for Acute Leukemia in Adults, Cancer Chemother Rep *53*:59–66, 1969
13. Goodell B, Leventhal B, Henderson E: Cytosine Arabinoside in Acute Granulocytic Leukemia, Clin Pharmacol Ther *12*:599–606, 1970
14. Southwest Oncology Group: Cytarabine for Acute Leukemia in Adults, Arch Intern Med *133*:251–259, 1974
15. Carey RW, Ribas-Mundo M, Ellison RR, et al: Comparative Study of Cytosine Arabinoside Therapy Alone and Combined with Thioguanine, Mercaptopurine or Daunorubicin in Acute Myelocytic Leukemia, Cancer *36*:1560–1566, 1975
16. Lampkin BC, McWilliam NB, Mauer AM, et al: Manipulation of the Mitotic Cycle in the Treatment of Acute Myelogenous Leukaemia, Brit J Haematol *32*:29–40, 1976
17. Preisler H, Bjornsson S, Henderson ES, et al: Remission Induction in Acute Nonlymphocytic Leukemia—Comparison of a Seven-Day and Ten-Day Infusion of Cytosine Arabinoside in Combination With Adriamycin, Med Pediatr Oncol 7:269–275, 1979
18. Gale RP, Cline MJ: High Remission- Induction Rate in Acute Myeloid Leukemia, Lancet *1*:497–499, 1977
19. Weinstein HJ, Mayer RJ, Rosenthal DS, et al: Treatment of Acute Myelogenous Leukemia In Children and Adults, N Eng J Med *303*:473–478, 1980
20. Glucksberg H, Cheever MA, Farewell UT, et al: High-Dose Combination Chemotherapy for Acute Nonlymphoblastic Leukemia in Adults, Cancer *48*:1073–1081, 1981
21. Cassileth PA, Katz ME: Chemotherapy for Adult Acute Nonlymphocytic Leukemia with Daunorubicin and Cytosine Arabinoside, Cancer Treat Rep *61*:1441–1445, 1977
22. Haghbin M: Acute Non-lymphoblastic Leukemia; Clinical and Morphological Characterization, Mod Prob Pediatr *16*:39–58, 1975
23. Pizzo PA, Henderson ES, Leventhal BG: Acute Myelogenous Leukemia in Children: A Preliminary Report of Combination Chemotherapy, J Pediatr *88*:125–130, 1976
24. Report of the Medical Research Council's Working Party on Leukaemia in Adults: Treatment of Acute Myeloid Leukaemia with Daunorubicin, Cytosine Arabinoside, Mercaptopurine, L-Asparaginase, Prednisone and Thioguanine: Results of Treatment with Five Multiple-Drug Schedules, Brit J Haematol *27*:373–389, 1974
25. Ansari BM, Thompson EN, Whittaker JA: A Comparative Study of Acute Myeloblastic Leukaemia in Children and Adults, Brit J Haematol *31*:269–277, 1975
26. Gee TS, Haghbin M, Dowling MD Jr, et al: Acute Lymphoblastic Leukemia in Adults and Children; Differences in Response with Similar Therapeutic Regimens, Cancer *37*:1256–1264, 1976
27. Spiers ASD, Roberts PD, Marsh GW, et al: Acute Lymphoblastic Leukaemia: Cyclical Chemotherapy with three Combinations of Four Drugs (COAP-POMP-CART Regimen). Brit Med J *4*:614–617, 1975
28. Howard JP, Albo V, Newton WA Jr: Cytosine Arabinoside: Results of a Cooperative Study in Acute Childhood Leukemia, Cancer *21*:341–345, 1968
29. McElwain TJ, Hardisty RM: Remission Induction with Cytosine Arabinoside and L-Asparaginase in Acute Lymphoblastic Leukaemia, Brit Med J *4*:596–598, 1969
30. Bodey GP, Rodriguez, V, Hart J, et al: Therapy of Acute Leukemia with the Combination of Cytosine Arabinoside (NSC-63878) and Cyclophosphamide (NSC-26271), Cancer Chemother Rep *54*:255–262, 1970
31. Nesbit ME Jr, Hammond D: Cytosine Arabinoside (ARAC) and Prednisone Therapy of Previously Treated Acute Lymphoblastic and Undifferentiated Leukemia (ALL/AUL) of Childhood, Proc Am Assoc Cancer Res *11*:59, 1970
32. Wang JJ, Selawry OS, Vietti TJ, et al: Prolonged Infusion of Arabinosyl Cytosine in Childhood Leukemia, Cancer *25*:1–6, 1970
33. Klemperer M, Coccia P, Albo V, et al: Reinduction of Remission After First Bone Marrow Relapse in Childhood Acute Lymphoblastic Leukemia, Proc Am Assoc Cancer Res *19*:414, 1978
34. Ortega JA, Finklestein JZ, Ertell, et al: Effective Combination Treatment of Advanced Acute Lymphocytic Leukemia with Cytosine Arabinoside (NSC-63878) and L-Asparaginase (NSC-109229), Cancer Chemother Rep *56*:363–368, 1972
35. Bryan JH, Henderson ES, Leventhal BG: Cytosine Arabinoside and 6- Thioguanine in Refractory Acute Lymphocytic Leukemia, Cancer *33*:539–544, 1974
36. Proceedings of the Chemotherapy Conference on ARA-C: Development and Application (Cytosine Arabinoside Hydrochloride—NSC 63878), Oct. 10, 1969
37. Lay HN, Colebatch JH, Ekert H: Experiences with Cytosine Arabinoside in Childhood Leukaemia and Lymphoma, Med J Aust *2*:187–192, 1971
38. Halikowski B, Cyklis R, Armata J, et al: Cytosine Arabinoside Administered Intrathecally in Cerebromeningeal Leukemia, Acta Paediat Scand *59*:164–168, 1970
39. Wang JJ, Pratt CB: Intrathecal Arabinosyl Cytosine in Meningeal Leukemia, Cancer *25*:531–534, 1970
40. Band PR, Holland JF, Bernard J, et al: Treatment of Central Nervous System Leukemia with Intrathecal Cytosine Arabinoside, Cancer *32*:744–748, 1973
41. Sullivan MP, Dyment P, Hvizdala E, et al: Favorable Comparison of All Out #2 with "Total" Therapy in the Treatment of Childhood Leukemia—The Equivalence of Intrathecal Chemotherapy and Radiotherapy as CNS
42. Saiki JH, Thompson S, Smith F, et al: Paraplegia Following Intrathecal Chemotherapy, Cancer *29*:370–374, 1972
43. Rubinstein LJ, Herman MM, Long TF, et al: Disseminated Necrotizing Leukoencephalopathy: A Complication of Treated Central System Leukemia and Lymphoma, Cancer *35*:291–305, 1975
44. Marmont Am, Damasio EE: Neurotoxicity of Intrathecal Chemotherapy for Leukaemia, Brit Med J *4*:47, 1973
45. Margileth DA, Poplack DG, Pizzo PA, et al: Blindness During Remission in Two Patients with Acute Lymphoblastic Leukemia, Cancer *39*:58–61, 1977
46. Hopen G, Mondino BJ, Johnson BL, et al: Corneal Toxicity with Systemic Cytarabine, *Am J Ophthalmol* 91:500–504, 1981
47. Lazarus HM, Herzig RH, Herzig GP, et al; Central Nervous System Toxicity of High-Dose Systemic Cytosine Arabinoside, *Cancer* 48:2577–2582, 1981.
48. Slavin RE, Dias MA, Soral R: Cytosine Arabinoside Induced Gastrointestinal Toxic Alterations in Sequential Chemotherapeutic Protocols—A Clinical Pathologic Study of 33 Patients, *Cancer* 42:1747–1759, 1978.
49. Haupt HM, Hutchins GM, Moore GW; Ara-C Lung: Noncardiogenic Pulmonary Edema Complicating Cytosine Arabinoside Therapy of Leukemia, *Am J Med* 70:256–261, 1981.
50. Shafer AI: Teratogenic Effects of Antileukemic Chemotherapy. *Arch Intern Med* 141:514–515, 1981.
51. Wagner VM, et al: Congenital Abnormalities in Baby Born to Cytarabine Treated Mother, *Lancet* 2:98–99, 1980.
52. Altman AJ, Dinndorf P, Quinn JJ: Acute Pancreatitis in Association with Cytosine Arabinoside Therapy, Cancer *49*:1384–1386, 1982
53. Frei E III, Bickers JN, Hewlett JS, et al: Dose Schedule and Antitumor Studies of Arabinosyl Cytosine (NSC 63878), Cancer Res *29*:1325–1332, 1969
54. Bell WR, Wang JJ, Carbone PP, et al: Cytogenetic and Morphologic Abnormalities in Human Bone Marrow Cells during Cytosine Arabinoside Therapy, J. Hematol *27*:771–781, 1966
55. Burke PJ, Serpick AA, Carbone PP, et al: A Clinical Evaluation of Dose and Schedule of Administration of Cytosine Arabinoside (NSC 63878), Cancer Res *28*:274–279, 1968
56. Castleberry RP, Crist WM, Holbrook T, et al: The Cytosine Arabinoside (Ara-C) Syndrome, *Med Pediatr Oncol* 9:257–264, 1981.
57. Takvorian T, Anderson K, Ritz J: A Fatal Cardiomyopathy Associated with High Dosage Ara-C (HIDAC) and Cyclophosphamide (CTX) in Bone Marrow Transplantation (BMTx). (Abstract submitted for 1985 AACR Meetings in Houston, Texas.)
58. Andersson BS, Cogan B, Keating MJ, Estey EH, et al: Subacute Pulmonary Failure Complicating Therapy with High-Dose Ara-C in Acute Leukemia. (Submitted for publication.)
59. Recommendations for the Safe Handling of Parenteral Antineoplastic Drugs. NIH Publication No. 83-2621. For sale by the Superintendent of Documents, US Government Printing Office, Washington, DC 20402.
60. AMA Council Report. Guidelines for Handling Parenteral Antineoplastics. JAMA, March 15, 1985.
61. National Study Commission on Cytotoxic Exposure-Recommendations for Handling Cytotoxic Agents. Available from Louis P. Jeffrey, ScD, Director of Pharmacy Services, Rhode Island Hospital, 593 Eddy Street, Providence, Rhode Island 02902.
62. Clinical Oncological Society of Australia: Guidelines and recommendations for safe handling of antineoplastic agents. Med J Australia *1*:426–428, 1983.
63. Jones, RB, et al. Safe handling of chemotherapeutic agents: A report from the Mount Sinai Medical Center CA-A Cancer Journal for Clinicians Sept/Oct., 1983, pp. 258–263.
64. American Society of Hospital Pharmacists Technical assistance bulletin on handling cytotoxic drugs in hospitals. AmJ Hosp Pharm *42*:131–137, 1985.

ANIMAL TOXICOLOGY

Toxicity of cytarabine in experimental animals, as well as activity, is markedly influenced by the schedule of administration. For example, in mice the LD_{10} for single intraperitoneal administration is greater than 6000 mg/m^2. However, when administered in 8 doses, each separated by 3 hours, the LD_{10} is less than 750 mg/m^2 total dose. Similarly, although a total dose of 1920 mg/m^2 administered as 12 injections at 6-hour intervals was lethal to beagle dogs (severe bone marrow hypoplasia with evidence of liver and kidney damage), dogs receiving the same total dose administered as 8 injections (again at 6-hour intervals) over a 48-hour period survived with minimal signs of toxicity. The most consistent observation in surviving dogs was elevated transaminase levels. In all experimental species the primary limiting toxic effect is marrow suppression with leukopenia. In addition, cytarabine causes abnormal cerebellar development in the neonatal hamster and is teratogenic to the rat fetus.

Code 810 126 110

DELTASONE® ℞

brand of prednisone tablets, USP

HOW SUPPLIED

Scored tablets in the following strength and sizes:

2.5 mg	Bottles of 100	*NDC 0009-0032-01*
5 mg	Bottles of 100	*NDC 0009-0045-01*
	Bottles of 500	*NDC 0009-0045-02*
Dosepak™	Unit of use (21)	*NDC 0009-0045-04*
	Unit Dose Package (100)	*NDC 0009-0045-05*
10 mg	Bottles of 100	*NDC 0009-0193-01*
	Bottles of 500	*NDC 0009-0193-02*
	Unit Dose Packages (100)	*NDC 0009-0193-03*
20 mg	Bottles of 100	*NDC 0009-0165-01*
	Bottles of 500	*NDC 0009-0165-02*
	Unit dose Packages (100)	*NDC 0009-0165-03*
50 mg	Bottles of 100	*NDC 0009-0388-01*
	Unit dose Packages (100)	*NDC 0009-0388-02*

Shown in Product Identification Section, page 433

DEPO-MEDROL® ℞

brand of methylprednisolone acetate sterile aqueous suspension (sterile methylprednisolone acetate suspension, USP)

Not for Intravenous Use

40 mg/ml (1 ml vial): NSN 6505-00-952-0267 (M)

DESCRIPTION

DEPO-MEDROL Sterile Aqueous Suspension contains methylprednisolone acetate which is the 6-methyl derivative of prednisolone. Methylprednisolone acetate is a white or practically white, odorless, crystalline powder which melts at about 215° with some decomposition. It is soluble in dioxane, sparingly soluble in acetone, in alcohol, in chloroform, and in methanol, and slightly soluble in ether. It is practically insoluble in water.

The chemical name for methylprednisolone acetate is pregna-1,4-diene-3,20-dione,21-(acetyloxy)- 11, 17-dihydroxy-6-methyl-,(6α, 11β)- and the molecular weight is 416.51.

DEPO-MEDROL is an anti-inflammatory glucocorticoid for intramuscular, intra-articular, soft tissue or intralesional injection. It is available in three strengths: 20 mg/ml; 40 mg/ml; 80 mg/ml.

[See table above].

DEPO-MEDROL Each ml of these preparations contains:	20 mg	40 mg	80 mg
Methylprednisolone Acetate	20 mg	40 mg	80 mg
Polyethylene Glycol 3350	29.6 mg	29 mg	28 mg
Sodium Chloride	8.9 mg	8.7 mg	8.5 mg
Myristyl-gamma-picolinium Chloride added as preservative	0.198 mg	0.195 mg	0.189 mg

When necessary, pH was adjusted with sodium hydroxide and/or hydrochloric acid.
The pH of the finished product remains within the USP specified range; ie, 3.5 to 7.0.

ACTIONS

Naturally occurring glucocorticoids (hydrocortisone), which also have salt retaining properties, are used in replacement therapy in adrenocortical deficiency states. Their synthetic analogs are used primarily for their potent anti-inflammatory effects in disorders of many organ systems.

Glucocorticoids cause profound and varied metabolic effects. In addition, they modify the body's immune response to diverse stimuli.

INDICATIONS

A. FOR INTRAMUSCULAR ADMINISTRATION

When oral therapy is not feasible and the strength, dosage form, and route of administration of the drug reasonably lend the preparation to the treatment of the condition, the intramuscular use of DEPO-MEDROL Sterile Aqueous Suspension (methylprednisolone acetate) is indicated as follows:

1. **Endocrine Disorders**
   Primary or secondary adrenocortical insufficiency (hydrocortisone or cortisone is the drug of choice; synthetic analogs may be used in conjunction with mineralocorticoids where applicable; in infancy, mineralocorticoid supplementation is of particular importance)
   Acute adrenocortical insufficiency (hydrocortisone or cortisone is the drug of choice; mineralocorticoid supplementation may be necessary, particularly when synthetic analogs are used)
   Preoperatively and in the event of serious trauma or illness, in patients with known adrenal insufficiency or when adrenocortical reserve is doubtful
   Congenital adrenal hyperplasia
   Hypercalcemia associated with cancer
   Nonsuppurative thyroiditis
2. **Rheumatic Disorders**
   As adjunctive therapy for short-term administration (to tide the patient over an acute episode or exacerbation) in:
   Post-traumatic osteoarthritis
   Synovitis of osteoarthritis
   Rheumatoid arthritis, including juvenile rheumatoid arthritis (selected cases may require low-dose maintenance therapy)
   Acute and subacute bursitis
   Epicondylitis
   Acute nonspecific tenosynovitis
   Acute gouty arthritis
   Psoriatic arthritis
   Ankylosing spondylitis
3. **Collagen Diseases**
   During an exacerbation or as maintenance therapy in selected cases of:
   Systemic lupus erythematosus
   Systemic dermatomyositis (polymyositis)
   Acute rheumatic carditis
4. **Dermatologic Diseases**
   Pemphigus
   Severe erythema multiforme (Stevens-Johnson syndrome)
   Exfoliative dermatitis
   Bullous dermatitis herpetiformis
   Severe seborrheic dermatitis
   Severe psoriasis
   Mycosis fungoides
5. **Allergic States**
   Control of severe or incapacitating allergic conditions intractable to adequate trials of conventional treatment in:
   Bronchial asthma
   Contact dermatitis
   Atopic dermatitis
   Serum sickness
   Seasonal or perennial allergic rhinitis
   Drug hypersensitivity reactions
   Urticarial transfusion reactions
   Acute noninfectious laryngeal edema (epinephrine is the drug of first choice)
6. **Ophthalmic Diseases**
   Severe acute and chronic allergic and inflammatory processes involving the eye, such as:
   Herpes zoster ophthalmicus
   Iritis, iridocyclitis
   Chorioretinitis
   Diffuse posterior uveitis and choroiditis
   Optic neuritis
   Sympathetic ophthalmia
   Anterior segment inflammation
   Allergic conjunctivitis
   Allergic corneal marginal ulcers
   Keratitis
7. **Gastrointestinal Diseases**
   To tide the patient over a critical period of the disease in:
   Ulcerative colitis (systemic therapy)
   Regional enteritis (systemic therapy)
8. **Respiratory Diseases**
   Symptomatic sarcoidosis
   Berylliosis
   Fulminating or disseminated pulmonary tuberculosis when used concurrently with appropriate antituberculous chemotherapy
   Loeffler's syndrome not manageable by other means
   Aspiration pneumonitis
9. **Hematologic Disorders**
   Acquired (autoimmune) hemolytic anemia
   Secondary thrombocytopenia in adults
   Erythroblastopenia (RBC anemia)
   Congenital (erythroid) hypoplastic anemia
10. **Neoplastic Diseases**
   For palliative management of:
   Leukemias and lymphomas in adults
   Acute leukemia of childhood
11. **Edematous States**
   To induce diuresis or remission of proteinuria in the nephrotic syndrome, without uremia, of the idiopathic type or that due to lupus erythematosus
12. **Nervous System**
   Acute exacerbations of multiple sclerosis
13. **Miscellaneous**
   Tuberculous meningitis with subarachnoid block or impending block when used concurrently with appropriate antituberculous chemotherapy
   Trichinosis with neurologic or myocardial involvement

B. FOR INTRA-ARTICULAR OR SOFT TISSUE ADMINISTRATION

DEPO-MEDROL is indicated as adjunctive therapy for short-term administration (to tide the patient over an acute episode or exacerbation) in:
Synovitis of osteoarthritis
Rheumatoid arthritis
Acute and subacute bursitis
Acute gouty arthritis
Epicondylitis
Acute nonspecific tenosynovitis
Post-traumatic osteoarthritis

C. FOR INTRALESIONAL ADMINISTRATION

DEPO-MEDROL is indicated for intralesional use in the following conditions:
Keloids
Localized hypertrophic, infiltrated, inflammatory lesions of:
lichen planus, psoriatic plaques, granuloma annulare, and lichen simplex chronicus (neurodermatitis)
Discoid lupus erythematosus
Necrobiosis lipodica diabeticorum
Alopecia areata
DEPO-MEDROL also may be useful in cystic tumors of an aponeurosis or tendon (ganglia).

CONTRAINDICATIONS

Systemic fungal infections.

WARNINGS

Multidose Use

Although initially sterile, any multidose use of vials may lead to contamination unless strict aseptic technique is observed. The preservative in DEPO-MEDROL Sterile Aqueous Suspension (methylprednisolone acetate) will prevent growth of most pathogenic organisms, but certain ones (eg *Serratia marcescens*) may remain viable. Particular care, such as use of disposable sterile syringes and needles, should be observed if intrasynovial use is intended.

While crystals of adrenal steroids in the dermis suppress inflammatory reactions, their presence may cause disintegration of the cellular elements and physiochemical changes in the ground substance of the connective tissue. The resultant infrequently occurring dermal and/or subdermal changes may form depressions in the skin at the injection site. The degree to which this reaction occurs will vary with the amount of adrenal steroid injected. Regeneration is usually complete within a few months or after all crystals of the adrenal steroid have been absorbed.

In order to minimize the incidence of dermal and subdermal atrophy, care must be exercised not to exceed recommended doses in injections. Multiple small injections into the area of the lesion should be made whenever possible. The technique of intra-articular and intramuscular injection should include precautions against injection or leakage into the dermis. Injection into the deltoid muscle should be avoided because of a high incidence of subcutaneous atrophy.

DEPO-MEDROL is Not Recommended For Intrathecal Administration.

In patients on corticosteroid therapy subjected to any unusual stress, increased dosage of rapidly acting corticosteroids before, during, and after the stressful situation is indicated.

Corticosteroids may mask some signs of infection, and new infections may appear during their use. There may be decreased resistance and inability to localize infection when corticosteroids are used. Do not use intra-articularly, intrabursally or for intratendinous administration for *local* effect in the presence of acute infection.

Prolonged use of corticosteroids may produce posterior subcapsular cataracts, glaucoma with possible damage to the optic nerves, and may enhance the establishment of secondary ocular infections due to fungi or viruses.

Usage in pregnancy. Since adequate human reproduction studies have not been done with corticosteroids, the use of these drugs in pregnancy, nursing mothers, or women of childbearing potential requires that the possible benefits of the drug be weighed against the potential hazards to the mother and embryo or fetus. Infants born of mothers who have received substantial doses of corticosteroids during pregnancy should be carefully observed for signs of hypoadrenalism.

Average and large doses of cortisone or hydrocortisone can cause elevation of blood pressure, salt and water retention, and increased excretion of potassium. These effects are less likely to occur with the synthetic derivatives except when used in large doses. Dietary salt restriction and potassium supplementation may be necessary. All corticosteroids increase calcium excretion.

While on corticosteroid therapy patients should not be vaccinated against smallpox. Other immunization procedures should not be undertaken in patients who are on corticosteroids, especially in high doses, because of possible hazards of neurological complications and lack of antibody response.

The use of DEPO-MEDROL in active tuberculosis should be restricted to those cases of fulminating or disseminated tuberculosis in which the corticosteroid is used for the management of the disease in conjunction with appropriate antituberculous regimen.

If corticosteroids are indicated in patients with latent tuberculosis or tuberculin reactivity, close observation is necessary as reactivation of the disease may occur. During prolonged corticosteroid therapy, these patients should receive chemoprophylaxis.

Because rare instances of anaphylactoid reactions have occurred in patients receiving parenteral corticosteroid ther-

Continued on next page

Information on these Upjohn products is based on labeling in effect August 15, 1986. Further information concerning these and other Upjohn products may be obtained by direct inquiry to Medical Information, The Upjohn Company, Kalamazoo, Michigan 49001.

Upjohn—Cont.

apy, appropriate precautionary measures should be taken prior to administration especially when the patient has a history of allergy to any drug.

PRECAUTIONS

Drug-induced secondary adrenocortical insufficiency may be minimized by gradual reduction of dosage. This type of relative insufficiency may persist for months after discontinuation of therapy; therefore, in any situation of stress occurring during that period, hormone therapy should be reinstituted. Since mineralocorticoid secretion may be impaired, salt and/or a mineralocorticoid should be administered concurrently.

When multidose vials are used, special care to prevent contamination of the contents is essential (See WARNINGS).

There is an enhanced effect of corticosteroids in patients with hypothyroidism and in those with cirrhosis.

Corticosteroids should be used cautiously in patients with ocular herpes simplex for fear of corneal perforation.

The lowest possible dose of corticosteroid should be used to control the condition under treatment, and when reduction in dosage is possible, the reduction must be gradual.

Psychic derangements may appear when corticosteroids are used, ranging from euphoria, insomnia, mood swings, personality changes, and severe depression to frank psychotic manifestations. Also, existing emotional instability or psychotic tendencies may be aggravated by corticosteroids.

Aspirin should be used cautiously in conjunction with corticosteroids in hypoprothrombinemia.

Steroids should be used with caution in nonspecific ulcerative colitis, if there is a probability of impending perforation, abscess or other pyogenic infection. Caution must also be used in diverticulitis, fresh intestinal anastomoses, active or latent peptic ulcer, renal insufficiency, hypertension, osteoporosis, and myasthenia gravis, when steroids are used as direct or adjunctive therapy.

Growth and development of infants and children on prolonged corticosteroid therapy should be carefully followed.

The following additional precautions apply for parenteral corticosteroids. Intra-articular injection of a corticosteroid may produce systemic as well as local effects.

Appropriate examination of any joint fluid present is necessary to exclude a septic process.

A marked increase in pain accompanied by local swelling, further restriction of joint motion, fever, and malaise are suggestive of septic arthritis. If this complication occurs and the diagnosis of sepsis is confirmed, appropriate antimicrobial therapy should be instituted.

Local injection of a steroid into a previously infected joint is to be avoided.

Corticosteroids should not be injected into unstable joints.

The slower rate of absorption by intramuscular administration should be recognized.

Although controlled clinical trials have shown corticosteroids to be effective in speeding the resolution of acute exacerbations of multiple sclerosis, they do not show that corticosteroids affect the ultimate outcome or natural history of the disease. The studies do show that relatively high doses of corticosteroids are necessary to demonstrate a significant effect. (See **Dosage And Administration**).

Since complications of treatment with glucocorticoids are dependent on the size of the dose and the duration of treatment, a risk/benefit decision must be made in each individual case as to dose and duration of treatment and as to whether daily or intermittent therapy should be used.

ADVERSE REACTIONS

Fluid and electrolyte disturbances:
- Sodium retention
- Fluid retention
- Congestive heart failure in susceptible patients
- Potassium loss
- Hypokalemic alkalosis
- Hypertension

Musculoskeletal:
- Muscle weakness
- Steroid myopathy
- Loss of muscle mass
- Osteoporosis
- Vertebral compression fractures
- Aseptic necrosis of femoral and humeral heads
- Pathologic fracture of long bones

Gastrointestinal:
- Peptic ulcer with possible subsequent perforation and hemorrhage
- Pancreatitis
- Abdominal distention
- Ulcerative esophagitis

Dermatologic:
- Impaired wound healing
- Thin fragile skin
- Petechiae and ecchymoses
- Facial erythema
- Increased sweating
- May suppress reactions to skin tests

Neurological:
- Convulsions
- Increased intracranial pressure with papilledema (pseudotumor cerebri) usually after treatment
- Vertigo
- Headache

Endocrine:
- Menstrual irregularities
- Development of Cushingoid state
- Suppression of growth in children
- Secondary adrenocortical and pituitary unresponsiveness, particularly in times of stress, as in trauma, surgery or illness
- Decreased carbohydrate tolerance
- Manifestations of latent diabetes mellitus
- Increased requirements for insulin or oral hypoglycemic agents in diabetes

Ophthalmic:
- Posterior subcapsular cataracts
- Increased intraocular pressure
- Glaucoma
- Exophthalmos

Metabolic:
- Negative nitrogen balance due to protein catabolism

The following *additional* adverse reactions are related to parenteral corticosteroid therapy:
- Rare instances of blindness associated with intralesional therapy around the face and head
- Anaphylactic reaction
- Allergic or hypersensitivity reactions
- Urticaria
- Hyperpigmentation or hypopigmentation
- Subcutaneous and cutaneous atrophy
- Sterile abscess
- Injection site infections following non-sterile administration (see WARNINGS)
- Postinjection flare, following intra-articular use
- Charcot-like arthropathy
- Arachnoiditis has been reported following intrathecal administration

DOSAGE AND ADMINISTRATION

Because of possible physical incompatibilities, DEPO-MEDROL Sterile Aqueous Suspension (methylprednisolone acetate) should not be diluted or mixed with other solutions.

A. Administration for Local Effect

Therapy with DEPO-MEDROL does not obviate the need for the conventional measures usually employed. Although this method of treatment will ameliorate symptoms, it is in no sense a cure and the hormone has no effect on the cause of the inflammation.

1. Rheumatoid and Osteoarthritis. The dose for intra-articular administration depends upon the size of the joint and varies with the severity of the condition in the individual patient. In chronic cases, injections may be repeated at intervals ranging from one to five or more weeks depending upon the degree of relief obtained from the initial injection. The doses in the following table are given as a general guide:

Size of Joint	*Examples*	*Range of Dosage*
Large	Knees Ankles Shoulders	20 to 80 mg
Medium	Elbows Wrists	10 to 40 mg
Small	Metacarpophalangeal Interphalangeal Sternoclavicular Acromioclavicular	4 to 10 mg

Procedure: It is recommended that the anatomy of the joint involved be reviewed before attempting intra-articular injection. In order to obtain the full anti-inflammatory effect it is important that the injection be made into the synovial space. Employing the same sterile technique as for a lumbar puncture, a sterile 20 to 24 gauge needle (on a dry syringe) is quickly inserted into the synovial cavity. Procaine infiltration is elective. The aspiration of only a few drops of joint fluid proves the joint space has been entered by the needle. *The injection site for each joint is determined by that location where the synovial cavity is most superficial and most free of large vessels and nerves.* With the needle in place, the aspirating syringe is removed and replaced by a second syringe containing the desired amount of DEPO-MEDROL Sterile Aqueous Suspension. The plunger is then pulled outward slightly to aspirate synovial fluid and to make sure the needle is still in the synovial space. After injection, the joint is moved gently a few times to aid mixing of the synovial fluid and the suspension. The site is covered with a small sterile dressing.

Suitable sites for intra-articular injection are the knee, ankle, wrist, elbow, shoulder, phalangeal, and hip joints. Since difficulty is not infrequently encountered in entering the hip joint, precautions should be taken to avoid any large blood vessels in the area. Joints not suitable for injection are those that are anatomically inaccessible such as the spinal joints and those like the sacroiliac joints that are devoid of synovial space. Treatment failures are most frequently the result of failure to enter the joint space. Little or no benefit follows injection into surrounding tissue. If failures occur when injections into the synovial spaces are certain, as determined by aspiration of fluid, repeated injections are usually futile. Local therapy does not alter the underlying disease process, and whenever possible comprehensive therapy including physiotherapy and orthopedic correction should be employed.

Following intra-articular steroid therapy, care should be taken to avoid overuse of joints in which symptomatic benefit has been obtained. Negligence in this matter may permit an increase in joint deterioration that will more than offset the beneficial effects of the steroid.

Unstable joints should not be injected. Repeated intra-articular injection may in some cases result in instability of the joint. X-ray follow-up is suggested in selected cases to detect deterioration.

If a local anesthetic is used prior to injection of DEPO-MEDROL the anesthetic package insert should be read carefully and all the precautions observed.

2. Bursitis. The area around the injection site is prepared in a sterile way and a wheal at the site made with 1 percent procaine hydrochloride solution. A 20 to 24 gauge needle attached to a dry syringe is inserted into the bursa and the fluid aspirated. The needle is left in place and the aspirating syringe changed for a small syringe containing the desired dose. After injection, the needle is withdrawn and a small dressing applied.

3. Miscellaneous: Ganglion, Tendinitis, Epicondylitis. In the treatment of conditions such as tendinitis or tenosynovitis, care should be taken, following application of a suitable antiseptic to the overlying skin, to inject the suspension into the tendon sheath rather than into the substance of the tendon. The tendon may be readily palpated when placed on a stretch. When treating conditions such as epicondylitis, the area of greatest tenderness should be outlined carefully and the suspension infiltrated into the area. For ganglia of the tendon sheaths, the suspension is injected directly into the cyst. In many cases, a single injection causes a marked decrease in the size of the cystic tumor and may effect disappearance. The usual sterile precautions should be observed, of course, with each injection.

The dose in the treatment of the various conditions of the tendinous or bursal structures listed above varies with the condition being treated and ranges from 4 to 30 mg. In recurrent or chronic conditions, repeated injections may be necessary.

4. Injections for Local Effect in Dermatologic Conditions. Following cleansing with an appropriate antiseptic such as 70% alcohol, 20 to 60 mg of the suspension is injected into the lesion. It may be necessary to distribute doses ranging from 20 to 40 mg by repeated local injections in the case of large lesions. Care should be taken to avoid injection of sufficient material to cause blanching since this may be followed by a small slough. One to four injections are usually employed, the intervals between injections varying with the type of lesion being treated and the duration of improvement produced by the initial injection.

When multidose vials are used, special care to prevent contamination of the contents is essential (See WARNINGS).

B. Administration for Systemic Effect

The intramuscular dosage will vary with the condition being treated. When employed as a temporary substitute for oral therapy, a single injection during each 24-hour period of a dose of the suspension equal to the total daily oral dose of MEDROL® Tablets (methylprednisolone) is usually sufficient. When a prolonged effect is desired, the weekly dose may be calculated by multiplying the daily oral dose by 7 and given as a single intramuscular injection.

Dosage must be individualized according to the severity of the disease and response of the patient. For infants and children, the recommended dosage will have to be reduced, but dosage should be governed by the severity of the condition rather than by strict adherence to the ratio indicated by age or body weight.

Hormone therapy is an adjunct to, and not a replacement for, conventional therapy. Dosage must be decreased or discontinued gradually when the drug has been administered for more than a few days. The severity, prognosis and expected duration of the disease and the reaction of the patient to medication are primary factors in determining dosage. If a period of spontaneous remission occurs in a chronic condition, treatment should be discontinued. Routine laboratory studies, such as urinalysis, two-hour postprandial blood sugar, determination of blood pressure and body weight, and a chest X-ray should be made at regular intervals during prolonged therapy. Upper GI X-rays are desirable in patients with an ulcer history or significant dyspepsia.

In patients with the **adrenogenital syndrome**, a single intramuscular injection of 40 mg every two weeks may be adequate. For maintenance of patients with **rheumatoid arthritis**, the weekly intramuscular dose will vary from 40 to 120 mg. The usual dosage for patients with **dermatologic lesions** benefited by systemic corticoid therapy is 40 to 120 mg of methylprednisolone acetate administered intramuscularly at weekly intervals for one to four weeks. In acute severe dermatitis due to poison ivy, relief may result within 8 to 12 hours following intramuscular administration of a single dose of 80 to 120 mg. In chronic contact dermatitis repeated injections at 5 to 10 day intervals may be necessary. In seborrheic dermatitis, a weekly dose of 80 mg may be adequate to control the condition.

Following intramuscular administration of 80 to 120 mg to asthmatic patients, relief may result within 6 to 48 hours and persist for several days to two weeks. Similarly in patients with allergic rhinitis (hay fever) an intramuscular dose of 80 to 120 mg may be followed by relief of coryzal symptoms within six hours persisting for several days to three weeks.

If signs of stress are associated with the condition being treated, the dosage of the suspension should be increased. If a rapid hormonal effect of maximum intensity is required, the intravenous administration of highly soluble methylprednisolone sodium succinate is indicated.

Multiple Sclerosis

In treatment of acute exacerbations of multiple sclerosis daily doses of 200 mg of prednisolone for a week followed by 80 mg every other day for 1 month have been shown to be effective (4 mg of methylprednisolone is equivalent to 5 mg of prednisolone).

HOW SUPPLIED

DEPO-MEDROL Sterile Aqueous Suspension (methylprednisolone acetate) is available in the following strengths and package sizes:

20 mg/ml	5 ml vial	*NDC 0009-0274-01*
	25–5 ml vials	*NDC 0009-0274-05*
40 mg/ml	1 ml vial	*NDC 0009-0280-01*
	25-1 ml vials	*NDC 0009-0280-23*
	5 ml vial	*NDC 0009-0280-02*
	25-5 ml vials	*NDC 0009-0280-32*
	10 ml vial	*NDC 0009-0280-03*
	25-10 vials	*NDC 0009-0280-33*
80 mg/ml	1 ml vial	*NDC 0009-0306-01*
	25-1 ml vials	*NDC 0009-0306-09*
	1 ml *U-Ject* ® Disposable Syringe	*NDC 0009-0306-04*
	5 ml vial	*NDC 0009-0306-02*
	25–5 ml vials	*NDC 0009-0306-10*

Store at controlled room temperature 15°–30° C (59°–86° F)

Code 810 341 008

Shown in Product Identification Section, page 433

DEPO-PROVERA® ℞

brand of medroxyprogesterone sterile aqueous suspension (sterile medroxyprogesterone acetate suspension, USP)

100 mg/ml, 5 ml NSN 6505-00-207-7965 (M)
400 mg/ml, 2.5 ml NSN 6505-01-059-9006 (M)

WARNING

THE USE OF PROGESTATIONAL AGENTS DURING THE FIRST FOUR MONTHS OF PREGNANCY IS NOT RECOMMENDED

Progestational agents have been used beginning with the first trimester of pregnancy in an attempt to prevent habitual abortion or treat threatened abortion. There is no adequate evidence that such use is effective and there is evidence of potential harm to the fetus when such drugs are given during the first four months of pregnancy. Furthermore, in the vast majority of women, the cause of abortion is a defective ovum, which progestational agents could not be expected to influence. In addition, the use of progestational agents, with their uterine-relaxant properties, in patients with fertilized defective ova may cause a delay in spontaneous abortion. Therefore, the use of such drugs during the first four months of pregnancy is not recommended.

Several reports suggest an association between intrauterine exposure to female sex hormones and congenital anomalies, including congenital heart defects and limb reduction defects[1–5]. One study[4] estimated a 4.7-fold increased risk of limb reduction defects in infants exposed in utero to sex hormones (oral contraceptives, hormone withdrawal tests for pregnancy, or attempted treatment for threatened abortion). Some of these exposures were very short and involved only a few days of treatment. The data suggest that the risk of limb reduction defects in exposed fetuses is somewhat less than 1 in 1000.

If the patient is exposed to DEPO-PROVERA Sterile Aqueous Suspension (medroxyprogesterone acetate) during the first four months of pregnancy or if she becomes pregnant while taking this drug, she should be apprised of the potential risks to the fetus.

DESCRIPTION

DEPO-PROVERA Sterile Aqueous Suspension contains medroxyprogesterone acetate which is a derivative of progesterone and is active by the parenteral and oral routes of administration. It is a white to off-white, odorless crystalline powder, stable in air, melting between 200 and 210° C. It is freely soluble in chloroform, soluble in acetone and dioxane, sparingly soluble in alcohol and methanol, slightly soluble in ether and insoluble in water.

The chemical name for medroxyprogesterone acetate is Pregn-4-ene-3,20-dione, 17-(acetyloxy)-6-methyl-, (6α)-.

DEPO-PROVERA for intramuscular injection is available in 2 strengths, 100 mg/ml and 400 mg/ml medroxyprogesterone acetate.

Each ml of the **100 mg/ml** suspension contains:

Medroxyprogesterone Acetate	100 mg
Also	
Polyethylene Glycol 3350	27.6 mg
Polysorbate 80	1.84 mg
Sodium Chloride	8.3 mg
with	
Methylparaben	1.75 mg
Propylparaben	0.194 mg
added as preservatives	

Each ml of the **400 mg/ml** suspension contains:

Medroxyprogesterone Acetate	400 mg
Polyethylene Glycol 3350	20.3 mg
Sodium Sulfate Anhydrous	11 mg
with	
Myristyl-gamma-picolinium Chloride	1.69 mg
added as preservative	

When necessary, pH was adjusted with sodium hydroxide and/or hydrochloric acid.

ACTIONS

Medroxyprogesterone acetate administered parenterally in the recommended doses to women with adequate endogenous estrogen transforms proliferative endometrium into secretory endometrium.

Medroxyprogesterone acetate inhibits (in the usual dose range) the secretion of pituitary gonadotropin which, in turn, prevents follicular maturation and ovulation.

Because of its prolonged action and the resulting difficulty in predicting the time of withdrawal bleeding following injection, medroxyprogesterone acetate is not recommended in secondary amenorrhea or dysfunctional uterine bleeding. In these conditions oral therapy is recommended.

INDICATIONS

Adjunctive therapy and palliative treatment of inoperable, recurrent, and metastatic endometrial carcinoma or renal carcinoma.

CONTRAINDICATIONS

1. Thrombophlebitis, thromboembolic disorders, cerebral apoplexy or patients with a past history of these conditions.
2. Carcinoma of the breast.
3. Undiagnosed vaginal bleeding.
4. Missed abortion.
5. As a diagnostic test for pregnancy.
6. Known sensitivity to DEPO-PROVERA Sterile Aqueous Suspension (medroxyprogesterone acetate).

WARNINGS

1. The physician should be alert to the earliest manifestations of thrombotic disorders (thrombophlebitis, cerebrovascular disorders, pulmonary embolism, and retinal thrombosis). Should any of these occur or be suspected, the drug should be discontinued immediately.
2. Long term toxicology studies in the monkey, dog and rat disclose:
   1) Beagle dogs receiving 75 mg/kg and 3 mg/kg every 90 days developed mammary nodules, as did some of the control animals. The nodules appearing in the control animals were intermittent in nature, whereas the nodules in the drug treated animals were larger, more numerous, persistent, and there were two high dose animals that developed breast malignancies.
   2) Two of the monkeys receiving 150 mg/kg every 90 days developed undifferentiated carcinoma of the uterus. No uterine malignancies were found in monkeys receiving 30 mg/kg, 3 mg/kg, or placebo every 90 days. Transient mammary nodules were found during the study in the control, 3 mg/kg and 30 mg/kg groups, but not in the 150 mg/kg group. At sacrifice, the only nodules extant were in three of the monkeys in the 30 mg/kg group. Upon histopathologic examination these nodules have been determined to be hyperplastic.
   3) No uterine or breast abnormalities were revealed in the rat.

   The relevance of any of these findings with respect to humans has not been established.
3. The use of DEPO-PROVERA Sterile Aqueous Suspension (medroxyprogesterone acetate) for contraception is investigational since there are unresolved questions relating to its safety for this indication. Therefore, this is not an approved indication.
4. Discontinue medication pending examination if there is sudden partial or complete loss of vision, or if there is a sudden onset of proptosis, diplopia or migraine. If examination reveals papilledema or retinal vascular lesions, medication should be withdrawn.
5. Usage in pregnancy (See WARNING Box).
6. Retrospective studies of morbidity and mortality in Great Britain and studies of morbidity in the United States have shown a statistically significant association between thrombophlebitis, pulmonary embolism, and cerebral thrombosis and embolism and the use of oral contraceptives.[6–9] The estimate of the relative risk of thromboembolism in the study by Vessey and Doll[8] was about sevenfold, while Sartwell and associates[9] in the United States found a relative risk of 4.4, meaning that the users are several times as likely to undergo thromboembolic disease without evident cause as non-users. The American study also indicated that the risk did not persist after discontinuation of administration, and that it was not enhanced by long continued administration. The American study was not designed to evaluate a difference between products.
7. Following repeated injections, amenorrhea and infertility may persist for periods up to 18 months and occasionally longer.
8. The physician should be alert to the earliest manifestations of impaired liver function. Should these occur or be suspected, the drug should be discontinued and the patient's status re-evaluated.

PRECAUTIONS

1. The pretreatment physical examination should include special reference to breast and pelvic organs, as well as Papanicolaou smear.
2. Because progestogens may cause some degree of fluid retention, conditions which might be influenced by this factor, such as epilepsy, migraine, asthma, cardiac or renal dysfunction, require careful observation.
3. In cases of breakthrough bleeding, as in all cases of irregular bleeding per vaginum, nonfunctional causes should be borne in mind. In cases of undiagnosed vaginal bleeding, adequate diagnostic measures are indicated.
4. Patients who have a history of psychic depression should be carefully observed and the drug discontinued if the depression recurs to a serious degree.
5. Any possible influence of prolonged progestin therapy on pituitary, ovarian, adrenal, hepatic or uterine functions awaits further study.
6. A decrease in glucose tolerance has been observed in a small percentage of patients on estrogen-progestin combination drugs. The mechanism of this decrease is obscure. For this reason, diabetic patients should be carefully observed while receiving progestin therapy.
7. The age of the patient constitutes no absolute limiting factor although treatment with progestins may mask the onset of the climacteric.
8. The pathologist should be advised of progestin therapy when relevant specimens are submitted.
9. Because of the occasional occurrence of thrombotic disorders, (thrombophlebitis, pulmonary embolism, retinal thrombosis, and cerebrovascular disorders) in patients taking estrogen-progestin combinations and since the mechanism is obscure, the physician should be alert to the earliest manifestation of these disorders.

Information for the Patient

See Patient Information at the end of the insert.

The patient insert should be given to all premenopausal women, except those in whom childbearing is impossible.

ADVERSE REACTIONS

(See WARNING Box for possible adverse effects on the fetus).

In a few instances there have been undesirable sequelae at the site of injection, such as residual lump, change in color of skin or sterile abscess.

The following adverse reactions have been associated with the use of DEPO-PROVERA Sterile Aqueous Suspension (medroxyprogesterone acetate).

Continued on next page

Information on these Upjohn products is based on labeling in effect August 15, 1986. Further information concerning these and other Upjohn products may be obtained by direct inquiry to Medical Information, The Upjohn Company, Kalamazoo, Michigan 49001.

Upjohn—Cont.

Breast—In a few instances, breast tenderness or galactorrhea have occurred.
Psychic—An occasional patient has experienced nervousness, insomnia, somnolence, fatigue or dizziness.
Thromboembolic Phenomena—Thromboembolic phenomena including thrombophlebitis and pulmonary embolism have been reported.
Skin and Mucous Membranes—Sensitivity reactions ranging from pruritus, urticaria, angioneurotic edema to generalized rash and anaphylaxis and/or anaphylactoid reactions have occasionally been reported. Acne, alopecia, or hirsutism have been reported in a few cases.
Gastrointestinal—Rarely, nausea has been reported. Jaundice, including neonatal jaundice, has been noted in a few instances.
Miscellaneous—Rare cases of headache and hyperpyrexia have been reported.
The following adverse reactions have been observed in women taking progestins including DEPO-PROVERA:
breakthrough bleeding
spotting
change in menstrual flow
amenorrhea
edema
change in weight
(increase or decrease)
changes in cervical erosion and
cervical secretions
cholestatic jaundice
rash (allergic) with and
without pruritus
melasma or chloasma
mental depression
A statistically significant association has been demonstrated between use of estrogen-progestin combination drugs and the following serious adverse reactions: thrombophlebitis; pulmonary embolism and cerebral thrombosis and embolism. For this reason patients on progestin therapy should be carefully observed.
Although available evidence is suggestive of an association, such a relationship has been neither confirmed nor refuted for the following serious adverse reactions: neuro-ocular lesions, eg, retinal thrombosis and optic neuritis.
The following adverse reactions have been observed in patients receiving estrogen-progestin combination drugs:
rise in blood pressure in susceptible individuals
premenstrual-like syndrome
changes in libido
changes in appetite
cystitis-like syndrome
headache
nervousness
dizziness
fatigue
backache
hirsutism
loss of scalp hair
erythema multiforme
erythema nodosum
hemorrhagic eruption
itching
In view of these observations, patients on progestin therapy should be carefully observed.
The following laboratory results may be altered by the use of estrogen-progestin combination drugs:
Increased sulfobromophthalein retention and other hepatic function tests.
Coagulation tests: increase in prothrombin factors VII, VIII, IX and X.
Metyrapone test.
Pregnanediol determination.
Thyroid function: increase in PBI, and butanol extractable protein bound iodine and decrease in T^3 uptake values.

DOSAGE AND ADMINISTRATION

The suspension is intended for intramuscular administration only.
This product must be vigorously shaken immediately before each use to ensure complete suspension of the drug.
Endometrial or renal carcinoma—doses of 400 mg to 1000 mg of DEPO-PROVERA Sterile Aqueous Suspension (medroxyprogesterone acetate) per week are recommended initially. If improvement is noted within a few weeks or months and the disease appears stabilized, it may be possible to maintain improvement with as little as 400 mg per month. Medroxyprogesterone acetate is not recommended as primary therapy, but as adjunctive and palliative treatment in advanced inoperable cases including those with recurrent or metastatic disease.

HOW SUPPLIED

DEPO-PROVERA Sterile Aqueous Suspension (medroxyprogesterone acetate) is available in 2 strengths:
100 mg/ml: 5 ml vials NDC 0009-0248-02
400 mg/ml:
1 ml U-JECT® Disposable Syringe NDC 0009-0626-03
2.5 ml vial NDC 0009-0626-01
10 ml vial NDC 0009-0626-02

REFERENCES

1. Gal I, Kirman B, Stern J: Hormonal pregnancy tests and congenital malformation. Nature *216*:83, 1967.
2. Levy EP, Cohen A, Fraser FC: Hormone treatment during pregnancy and congenital heart defects. Lancet *1*:611, 1973.
3. Nora JJ, Nora AH: Birth defects and oral contraceptives. Lancet *1*:941–942, 1973.
4. Janerich DT, Piper JM, Glebatis DM: Oral contraceptives and congenital limb-reduction defects. N Engl J Med *291*:697–700, 1974.
5. Heinonen OP, Slone D, Monson RR, et al: Cardiovascular birth defects and antenatal exposure to female sex hormones. N Engl J Med *296*:67–70, 1977.
6. Royal College of General Practitioners: Oral contraception and thromboembolic disease. J Coll Gen Pract *13*:267–279, 1967.
7. Inman WHW, Vessey MP: Investigation of deaths from pulmonary, coronary, and cerebral thrombosis and embolism in women of child-bearing age. Br Med J *2*:193–199, 1968.
8. Vessey MP, Doll R: Investigation of relation between use of oral contraceptives and thromboembolic disease. A further report. Br Med J *2*:651–657, 1969.
9. Sartwell PE, Masi AT, Arthes FG, et al: Thromboembolism and oral contraceptives: An epidemiological case-control study. Am J Epidemiol *90*:365–380, 1969.

The text of the patient insert for progesterone and progesterone-like drugs is set forth below.
Patient Information: DEPO-PROVERA Sterile Aqueous Suspension contains medroxyprogesterone acetate. The information below is that which the U.S. Food and Drug Administration requires be provided for all patients taking progesterones. The information below relates only to the risk to the unborn child associated with use of progesterone during pregnancy. For further information on the use, side effects and other risks associated with this product, ask your doctor.

WARNING FOR WOMEN

There is an increased risk of birth defects in children whose mothers take this drug during the first four months of pregnancy.
Medroxyprogesterone acetate is similar to the progesterone hormones naturally produced by the body. Progesterone and progesterone-like drugs are used to treat menstrual disorders, to test if the body is producing certain hormones, and to treat some forms of cancer in women.
They have been used as a test for pregnancy but such use is no longer considered safe because of possible damage to a developing baby. Also, more rapid methods for testing for pregnancy are now available.
These drugs have also been used to prevent miscarriage in the first few months of pregnancy. No adequate evidence is available to show that they are effective for this purpose. Furthermore, most cases of early miscarriage are due to causes which could not be helped by these drugs.
There is an increased risk of birth defects, such as heart or limb defects, if progesterone and progesterone-like drugs are taken during the first four months of pregnancy. The exact risk of taking this drug early in pregnancy and having a baby with a birth defect is not known. However, one study found that babies born to women who had taken sex hormones (such as progesterone-like drugs) during the first three months of pregnancy were 4 to 5 times more likely to have abnormalities of the arms or legs than if their mothers had not taken such drugs. Some of these women had taken these drugs for only a few days. The chance that an infant whose mother had taken this drug will have this type of defect is about 1 in 1,000.
If you take DEPO-PROVERA Sterile Aqueous Suspension and later find you were pregnant when you took it, be sure to discuss this with your doctor as soon as possible.
Code 810 597 004

DEPO®-TESTOSTERONE ℞

brand of testosterone cypionate sterile solution (testosterone cypionate injection, USP)
For Intramuscular Use Only

HOW SUPPLIED

DEPO-Testosterone Sterile Solution is available in the following packages:
50 mg per ml. Each ml contains 50 mg testosterone cypionate, also 5.4 mg chlorobutanol anhydrous (chloral deriv.), in 874 mg cottonseed oil.
10 ml vial *NDC 0009-0303-01*
100 mg per ml. Each ml contains 100 mg testosterone cypionate, also 0.1 ml benzyl benzoate, 9.45 mg benzyl alcohol in 736 mg cottonseed oil.
1 ml vial *NDC 0009-0347-01*
10 ml vial *NDC 0009-0347-02*
200 mg per ml. Each ml contains 200 mg testosterone cypionate, also 0.2 ml benzyl benzoate, 9.45 mg benzyl alcohol, in 560 mg cottonseed oil.
1 ml vial *NDC 0009-0417-01*
10 ml vial *NDC 0009-0417-02*

DIDREX® Ⓒ ℞

brand of benzphetamine hydrochloride tablets

DESCRIPTION

DIDREX Tablets contain the anorectic agent benzphetamine hydrochloride. Benzphetamine hydrochloride is a white crystalline powder readily soluble in water and 95% ethanol. The chemical name for benzphetamine hydrochloride is *d*-N,α-Dimethyl-N-(phenylmethyl)-benzeneethanamine hydrochloride and its molecular weight is 275.82.
Each DIDREX tablet, for oral administration, contains 25 or 50 mg of benzphetamine hydrochloride.
Inactive Ingredients
25 mg—Calcium Stearate, Corn Starch, FD & C Yellow #5, Lactose, Povidone, Sorbital.
50 mg—Calcium Stearate, Corn Starch, Erythrosine Sodium, FD & C Yellow #6, Lactose, Povidone, Sorbital.

CLINICAL PHARMACOLOGY

Benzphetamine hydrochloride is a sympathomimetic amine with pharmacologic activity similar to the prototype drugs of this class used in obesity, the amphetamines. Actions include central nervous system stimulation and elevation of blood pressure. Tachyphylaxis and tolerance have been demonstrated with all drugs of this class in which these phenomena have been looked for.
Drugs of this class used in obesity are commonly known as "anorectics" or "anorexigenics." It has not been established, however, that the action of such drugs in treating obesity is primarily one of appetite suppression. Other central nervous system actions, or metabolic effects, may be involved.
Adult obese subjects instructed in dietary management and treated with "anorectic" drugs, lose more weight on the average than those treated with placebo and diet, as determined in relatively short term clinical trials.
The magnitude of increased weight loss of drug treated patients over placebo treated patients is only a fraction of a pound a week. The rate of weight loss is greatest in the first weeks of therapy for both drug and placebo subjects and tends to decrease in succeeding weeks. The possible origins of the increased weight loss due to the various drug effects are not established. The amount of weight loss associated with the use of an "anorectic" drug varies from trial to trial, and the increased weight loss appears to be related in part to variables other than the drug prescribed, such as the physician-investigator, the population treated, and the diet prescribed. Studies do not permit conclusions as to the relative importance of the drug and nondrug factors on weight loss.
The natural history of obesity is measured in years, whereas the studies cited are restricted to a few weeks duration; thus, the total impact of drug induced weight loss over that of diet alone must be considered to be clinically limited.
Pharmacokinetic data in humans are not available.

INDICATIONS AND USAGE

DIDREX Tablets (benzphetamine hydrochloride) are indicated in the management of exogenous obesity as a short term adjunct (a few weeks) in a regimen of weight reduction based on caloric restriction. The limited usefulness of agents of this class (see **Clinical Pharmacology**) should be weighed against possible risks inherent in their use such as those described above.

CONTRAINDICATIONS

DIDREX Tablets (benzphetamine hydrochloride) are contraindicated in patients with advanced arteriosclerosis, symptomatic cardiovascular disease, moderate to severe hypertension, hyperthyroidism, known hypersensitivity or idiosyncrasy to sympathomimetic amines, and glaucoma. Benzphetamine should not be given to patients who are in an agitated state or who have a history of drug abuse.
Hypertensive crises have resulted when sympathomimetic amines have been used concomitantly or within 14 days following use of monamine oxidase inhibitors. DIDREX should not be used concomitantly with other CNS stimulants.
DIDREX may cause fetal harm when administered to a pregnant woman. Amphetamines have been shown to be teratogenic and embryotoxic in mammals at high multiples of the human dose. DIDREX is contraindicated in women who are or may become pregnant. If this drug is used during pregnancy, or if the patient becomes pregnant while taking this drug, the patient should be apprised of the potential hazard to the fetus.

WARNINGS

When tolerance to the anorectic effect develops, the recommended dose should not be exceeded in an attempt to increase the effect; rather, the drug should be discontinued.

PRECAUTIONS

General: Insulin requirements in diabetes mellitus may be altered in association with use of anorexigenic drugs and the concomitant dietary restrictions.

Psychological disturbances have been reported in patients who receive an anorectic agent together with a restrictive dietary regimen.

Caution is to be exercised in prescribing amphetamines for patients with even mild hypertension. The least amount feasible should be prescribed or dispensed at one time in order to minimize the possibility of overdosage.

DIDREX Tablets, 25 mg, contain FD&C Yellow No. 5 (tartrazine) which may cause allergic-type reactions (including bronchial asthma) in certain susceptible individuals. Although the overall incidence of FD&C Yellow No. 5 (tartrazine) sensitivity in the general population is low, it is frequently seen in patients who also have aspirin hypersensitivity.

INFORMATION FOR PATIENTS

Amphetamines may impair the ability of the patient to engage in potentially hazardous activities such as operating machinery or driving a motor vehicle; the patient should therefore be cautioned accordingly.

DRUG INTERACTIONS

Hypertensive crises have resulted when sympathomimetic amines have been used concomitantly or within 14 days following use of monoamine oxidase inhibitors. DIDREX should not be used concomitantly with other CNS stimulants.

Amphetamines may decrease the hypotensive effect of antihypertensives. Amphetamines may enhance the effects of tricyclic antidepressants.

Urinary alkalinizing agents increase blood levels and decrease excretion of amphetamines. Urinary acidifying agents decrease blood levels and increase excretion of amphetamines.

Carcinogenesis, Mutagenesis, Impairment of Fertility: Animal studies to evaluate the potential for carcinogenesis, mutagenesis or impairment of fertility have not been performed by the Upjohn Company.

Pregnancy: Pregnancy Category X. (See CONTRAINDICATIONS section).

Nursing Mothers: It is not known whether this drug is excreted in human milk. Because many drugs are excreted in human milk and because of the potential for serious adverse reactions from DIDREX in nursing infants, a decision should be made whether to discontinue nursing or to discontinue the drug taking into account the importance of the drug to the mother.

Pediatric Use: Use of benzphetamine hydrochloride is not recommended in children under 12 years of age.

ADVERSE REACTIONS

The following have been associated with the use of benzphetamine hydrochloride:

Cardiovascular

Palpitation, tachycardia, elevation of blood pressure.

CNS

Overstimulation, restlessness, dizziness, insomnia, tremor, sweating, headache; rarely, psychotic episodes at recommended doses; depression following withdrawal of the drug.

Gastrointestinal

Dryness of the mouth, unpleasant taste, nausea, diarrhea, other gastrointestinal disturbances.

Allergic

Urticaria and other allergic reactions involving the skin.

Endocrine

Changes in libido.

DRUG ABUSE AND DEPENDENCE

Benzphetamine is a controlled substance under the Controlled Substance Act by the Drug Enforcement Administration and has been assigned to Schedule III.

Benzphetamine hydrochloride is related chemically and pharmacologically to the amphetamines. Amphetamines and related stimulant drugs have been extensively abused and the possibility of abuse of DIDREX Tablets should be kept in mind when evaluating the desirability of including a drug as part of a weight reduction program. Abuse of amphetamines and related drugs may be associated with intense psychological dependence and severe social dysfunction. There are reports of patients who have increased the dosage to many times that recommended. Abrupt cessation following prolonged high dosage administration results in extreme fatigue and mental depression; changes are also noted on the sleep EEG. Manifestations of chronic intoxication with anorectic drugs include severe dermatoses, marked insomnia, irritability, hyperactivity, and personality changes. The most severe manifestation of chronic intoxication is psychosis, often clinically indistinguishable from schizophrenia.

OVERDOSAGE

Treatment of Overdosage:

(See **Warnings**) Information concerning the effects of overdosage with DIDREX Tablets (benzphetamine hydrochloride) is extremely limited. The following is based on experience with other anorexiants.

Management of acute amphetamine intoxication is largely symptomatic and includes sedation with a barbiturate. If hypertension is marked, the use of a nitrite or rapidly acting alpha receptor blocking agent should be considered. Experience with hemodialysis or peritoneal dialysis is inadequate to permit recommendations in this regard.

The oral LD_{50} is 174 mg/kg in mice and 104 mg/kg in rats. The intraperitoneal LD_{50} in mice is 153 mg/kg.

DOSAGE AND ADMINISTRATION

Dosage should be individualized according to the response of the patient. The suggested dosage ranges from 25 to 50 mg one to three times daily. Treatment should begin with 25 to 50 mg once daily with subsequent increase in individual dose or frequency according to response. A single daily dose is preferably given in mid-morning or mid-afternoon, according to the patient's eating habits. In an occasional patient it may be desirable to avoid late afternoon administration. Use of benzphetamine hydrochloride is not recommended in children under 12 years of age.

HOW SUPPLIED

DIDREX Tablets (benzphetamine hydrochloride) are available in the following strengths and colors:

25 mg (yellow)
Bottles of 100 *NDC 0009-0018-01*
50 mg (peach, scored)
Bottles of 100 *NDC 0009-0024-01*
Bottles of 500 *NDC 0009-0024-02*
Code 810 735 306

Shown in Product Identification Section, page 433

E-MYCIN® ℞

brand of erythromycin base enteric-coated tablets

Each E-MYCIN tablet contains erythromycin as the base

DESCRIPTION

Erythromycin is produced by a strain of *Streptomyces erythreus* and belongs to the macrolide group of antibiotics. It is basic and readily forms salts with acids. The base is a white to off-white crystals or powder slightly soluble in water, soluble in alcohol, in chloroform, and in ether. The chemical name for erythromycin is (3*R* *, 4*S* *, 5*S* *, 6*R* *, 7*R* *, 9*R* *, 11*R* *, 12*R* *, 13*S* *, 14*R* *)-4-[(2,6-Dideoxy-3-*C*-methyl-3-*O*-methyl-α-L-*ribo*-hexopyranosyl)-oxy]-14-ethyl-7, 12, 13-trihydroxy-3, 5, 7, 9, 11, 13-hexamethyl-6-[[3, 4, 6-trideoxy-3-(dimethylamino)-β-D-*xylo*-hexopyranosyl]oxy]oxacyclotetradecane-2,10-dione and the molecular weight is 733.94.

E-MYCIN Tablets (erythromycin), available in 250 mg and 333 mg strengths, are specially coated to protect the contents from the inactivating effects of gastric acidity and to permit efficient absorption of the antibiotic in the small intestine.

Inactive Ingredients: carboxymethylcellulose calcium, carnauba wax, cellulose acetate phthalate, corn starch, hydroxypropyl cellulose, lactose, magnesium stearate, mineral oil, propylene glycol, sorbic acid, sorbitan monooleate, sucrose, talc, titanium dioxide. The 250 mg tablet also contains erythrosine sodium and FD&C Yellow No. 6.

CLINICAL PHARMACOLOGY

The mode of action of erythromycin is inhibition of protein synthesis without affecting nucleic acid synthesis. Resistance to erythromycin of some strains of *Haemophilus influenzae* and staphylococci has been demonstrated. Culture and susceptibility testing should be done. If the Kirby-Bauer method of disk susceptibility is used, a 15 mcg erythromycin disk should give a zone diameter of at least 18 mm when tested against an erythromycin susceptible organism.

Bioavailability data are available from The Upjohn Company.

E-MYCIN Tablets (erythromycin base enteric-coated tablets) are well absorbed and may be given without regard to meals. After absorption, erythromycin diffuses readily into most body fluids. In the absence of meningeal inflammation, low concentrations are normally achieved in the spinal fluid but passage of the drug across the blood-brain barrier increases in meningitis. In the presence of normal hepatic function, erythromycin is concentrated in the liver and excreted in the bile; the effect of hepatic dysfunction on excretion of erythromycin by the liver into the bile is not known. After oral administration, less than 5 percent of the activity of the administered dose can be recovered in the urine.

Erythromycin crosses the placental barrier but fetal plasma levels are low.

INDICATIONS AND USAGE

Streptococcus pyogenes (Group A beta hemolytic streptococcus): For upper and lower respiratory tract, skin, and soft tissue infections of mild to moderate severity.

Injectable benzathine penicillin G is considered by the American Heart Association to be the drug of choice in the treatment and prevention of streptococcal pharyngitis and in long-term prophylaxis of rheumatic fever.

When oral medication is preferred for treatment of the above conditions, penicillin G, V, or erythromycin are alternate drugs of choice.

When oral medication is given, the importance of strict adherence by the patient to the prescribed dosage regimen must be stressed. A therapeutic dose should be administered for at least 10 days.

Alpha-hemolytic streptococci (viridans group): Although no controlled clinical efficacy trials have been conducted, oral erythromycin has been suggested by the American Heart Association and American Dental Association for use in a regimen for prophylaxis against bacterial endocarditis in patients hypersensitive to penicillin who have congenital heart disease or rheumatic or other acquired valvular heart disease when they undergo dental procedures and surgical procedures of the upper respiratory tract.[1] Erythromycin is not suitable prior to genitourinary or gastrointestinal tract surgery.

Note: When selecting antibiotics for the prevention of bacterial endocarditis the physician or dentist should read the full joint statement of the American Heart Association and the American Dental Association.[1]

Staphylococcus aureus: For acute infections of skin and soft tissue of mild to moderate severity. Resistant organisms may emerge during treatment.

Streptococcus pneumoniae (Diplococcus pneumoniae): For upper respiratory tract infections (eg, otitis media, pharyngitis) and lower respiratory tract infections (eg, pneumonia) of mild to moderate degree.

Mycoplasma pneumoniae (Eaton agent, PPLO): For respiratory infections due to this organism.

Hemophilus influenzae: For upper respiratory tract infections of mild to moderate severity when used concomitantly with adequate doses of sulfonamides. Not all strains of this organism are susceptible at the erythromycin concentrations ordinarily achieved (see appropriate sulfonamide labeling for prescribing information).

Treponema pallidum: Erythromycin is an alternate choice of treatment for primary syphilis in patients allergic to the penicillins. In treatment of primary syphilis, spinal fluid examinations should be done before treatment and as part of follow-up after therapy.

Corynebacterium diphtheriae and **C. minutissimum:** As an adjunct to antitoxin, to prevent establishment of carriers, and to eradicate the organism in carriers.

In the treatment of erythrasma.

Entamoeba histolytica: In the treatment of intestinal amebiasis only. Extraenteric amebiasis requires treatment with other agents.

Listeria monocytogenes: Infections due to this organism.

Neisseria gonorrhoeae: Erythromycin lactobionate for injection in conjunction with erythromycin base orally, as an alternative drug in treatment of acute pelvic inflammatory disease caused by *N. gonorrhoeae* in female patients with a history of sensitivity to penicillin. Before treatment of gonorrhea, patients who are suspected of also having syphilis should have a microscopic examination for *T. pallidum* (by immunofluorescence or darkfield) before receiving erythromycin, and monthly serologic tests for a minimum of 4 months.

Chlamydia trachomatis: Erythromycins are indicated for treatment of the following infections caused by *Chlamydia trachomatis:* conjunctivitis of the newborn, pneumonia of infancy, urogenital infections during pregnancy. When tetracyclines are contraindicated or not tolerated, erythromycin is indicated for the treatment of uncomplicated urethral, endocervical, or rectal infections in adults due to *Chlamydia trachomatis.*[2]

Bordetella pertussis: Erythromycin is effective in eliminating the organism from the nasopharynx of infected individuals, rendering them noninfectious. Some clinical studies suggest that erythromycin may be helpful in the prophylaxis of pertussis in exposed susceptible individuals.

Legionnaires Disease: Although no controlled clinical efficacy studies have been conducted, *in vitro* and limited preliminary clinical data suggest that erythromycin can be effective in treating Legionnaires Disease.

CONTRAINDICATIONS

Erythromycin is contraindicated in patients with known hypersensitivity to this antibiotic.

Continued on next page

Information on these Upjohn products is based on labeling in effect August 15, 1986. Further information concerning these and other Upjohn products may be obtained by direct inquiry to Medical Information, The Upjohn Company, Kalamazoo, Michigan 49001.

Upjohn—Cont.

WARNING

Usage in pregnancy: Safety for use in pregnancy has not been established.

PRECAUTIONS

Erythromycin is principally excreted by the liver. Caution should be exercised in administering the antibiotic to patients with impaired hepatic function.
There have been reports of hepatic dysfunction, with or without jaundice, occurring in patients receiving oral erythromycin products.
Surgical procedures should be performed when indicated.

DRUG INTERACTIONS

Recent data from studies of erythromycin reveal that its use in patients who are receiving high doses of theophylline may be associated with an increase of serum theophylline levels and potential theophylline toxicity. In cases of theophylline toxicity and/or elevated serum theophylline levels, the dose of theophylline should be reduced while the patient is receiving concomitant erythromycin therapy.
Erythromycin administration in children receiving carbamazepine has been reported to cause increased blood levels of carbamazepine with subsequent development of signs of carbamazepine toxicity (ataxia, dizziness, vomiting).
Erythromycin may decrease the clearance of warfarin and thus potentiate the hypoprothrombinemic effect of warfarin.

ADVERSE REACTIONS

The most frequent side effects of erythromycin preparations are gastrointestinal, such as abdominal cramping and discomfort, and are dose related. Nausea, vomiting, and diarrhea occur infrequently with usual oral doses.
During prolonged or repeated therapy, there is a possibility of overgrowth of nonsusceptible bacteria or fungi. If such infections occur, the drug should be discontinued and appropriate therapy instituted.
Mild allergic reactions such as urticaria and other skin rashes have occurred. Serious allergic reactions, including anaphylaxis, have been reported.
There have been isolated reports of reversible hearing loss occurring chiefly in patients with renal insufficiency and in patients receiving high doses of erythromycin.

DOSAGE AND ADMINISTRATION

E-MYCIN Tablets (erythromycin base enteric-coated tablets) are well absorbed and may be given without regard to meals.
Adults: The usual dose is 250 mg four times daily or 333 mg every 8 hours.
If twice a day dosage is desired, the recommended dose is 500 mg every 12 hours.
Dosage may be increased up to 4 or more grams per day according to the severity of the infection. Twice-a-day dosing is not recommended when doses larger than 1 gram daily are administered.
Children: Age, weight, and severity of the infection are important factors in determining the proper dosage. 30 to 50 mg/kg/day, in divided doses, is the usual dose. For more severe infections, this dose may be doubled.
In the treatment of streptococcal infections, a therapeutic dosage of erythromycin should be administered for at least 10 days. In continuous **prophylaxis** of streptococcal infections in persons with a history of rheumatic heart disease, the dose is 250 mg twice a day.
For prophylaxis against bacterial endocarditis[1] in patients with congenital heart disease or rheumatic, or other acquired valvular heart disease when undergoing dental procedures or surgical procedures of the upper respiratory tract, give 1.0 gram (20 mg/kg for children) orally 1 ½–2 hours before the procedure and then 500 mg (10 mg/kg for children) orally every 6 hours for 8 doses.
For treatment of primary syphilis: 30 to 40 grams given in divided doses over a period of 10 to 15 days.
For treatment of acute pelvic inflammatory disease caused by *N. gonorrhoeae:* After initial treatment with erythromycin lactobionate for injection (500 mg every 6 hours for 3 days), the oral dosage recommendation is 250 mg every 6 hours for 7 days or 333 mg every 8 hours for 7 days.
Urogenital infections during pregnancy due to *Chlamydia trachomatis:* Although the optimal dose and duration of therapy have not been established, the suggested treatment is erythromycin 500 mg, by mouth, four times a day or two 333 mg tablets every eight hours for at least seven days. For women who cannot tolerate this regimen, a decreased dose of 250 mg, by mouth, four times a day or one 333 mg tablet every eight hours should be used for at least 14 days.[2]
For adults with uncomplicated urethral, endocervical, or rectal infections caused by *Chlamydia trachomatis* in whom tetracyclines are contraindicated or not tolerated: 500 mg, by mouth, four times a day or two 333 mg tablets every eight hours for at least seven days.[2]
For dysenteric amebiasis: 250 mg four times daily or 333 mg every 8 hours for 10 to 14 days, for adults; 30 to 50 mg/kg/day in divided doses for 10 to 14 days, for children.
For use in pertussis: Although optimal dosage and duration have not been established, doses of erythromycin utilized in reported clinical studies were 40 to 50 mg/kg/day, given in divided doses for 5 to 14 days.
For treatment of Legionnaires Disease: Although optimal doses have not been established, doses utilized in reported clinical data were those recommended above (1 to 4 grams erythromycin base daily in divided doses).

TREATMENT OF OVERDOSAGE

Allergic reactions associated with acute overdosage should be handled in the usual manner—that is, by the administration of adrenalin, corticosteroids, and antihistamines as indicated and the prompt elimination of unabsorbed drug, in addition to all needed supportive measures.

HOW SUPPLIED

E-MYCIN Tablets (erythromycin base enteric-coated tablets) are available in the following strengths, colors and sizes:

250 mg, orange

Bottles of 100	*NDC 0009-0103-02*
Bottles of 500	*NDC 0009-0103-15*
Unit dose packages (100)	*NDC 0009-0103-03*
Bottles of 40, unit of use	*NDC 0009-0103-39*

333 mg, white

Bottles of 100	*NDC 0009-3176-01*
Unit dose packages (100)	*NDC* 0009-3176-03
Bottles of 500	*NDC* 0009-3176-04

[1] American Heart Association 1977. Prevention of bacterial endocarditis. Circulation *56*:139A–143A.
[2] CDC Sexually Transmitted Diseases Treatment Guidelines 1982.

Code 810 386 113

E-MYCIN E® ℞

brand of erythromycin ethylsuccinate liquid
(erythromycin ethylsuccinate oral suspension)

Each 5 ml (one teaspoon) of E-MYCIN E Liquid contains erythromycin ethylsuccinate equivalent to erythromycin 200 mg or 400 mg in a pleasant tasting oral suspension suitable for oral administration.

HOW SUPPLIED

E-MYCIN E Liquid (erythromycin ethylsuccinate oral suspension) is supplied in the following sizes and strengths:

200 mg/5 ml, 500 ml bottle	NDC 0009-0939-01
400 mg/5 ml, 500 ml bottle	NDC 0009-0940-01

GELFOAM®

brand of absorbable gelatin sterile sponge
(absorbable gelatin sponge, USP)

Size 12-7 mm:
NSN 6510-00-080-2053 (M & VA)
Size 100:
NSN 6510-00-080-2054 (M & VA)
Dental Packs, Size 4:
NSN 6510-00-064-4858 (M)

DESCRIPTION

GELFOAM Sterile Sponge is a sterile, pliable, surgical sponge prepared from specially treated, purified gelatin solution and capable of absorbing and holding within its meshes many times its weight of whole blood. It is used a as a hemostatic device.

ACTIONS

When implanted in tissues, GELFOAM Sterile Sponge (absorbable gelatin sponge) is absorbed completely in from four to six weeks without inducing excessive scar tissue. When applied to bleeding areas of nasal, rectal, or vaginal mucosa, it completely liquefies within two to five days.

INDICATIONS AND USAGE

Hemostasis: GELFOAM Sterile Sponge (absorbable gelatin sponge), dry or saturated with sodium chloride, is indicated in surgical procedures as an adjunct to hemostasis when control of bleeding by ligature or conventional procedures is ineffective or impractical.

DIRECTIONS FOR USE

Pieces of GELFOAM Sterile Sponge (absorbable gelatin sponge), cut to the desired size, may be applied dry or saturated with sodium chloride injection. When applied dry, pieces of GELFOAM should be compressed before application to the bleeding surface and should then be held in place with moderate pressure for 10 to 15 seconds. When used with saline, pieces of GELFOAM should be immersed in the solution, then withdrawn, squeezed between the gloved fingers to remove the air bubbles present in the meshes, replaced in the solution, and left there until needed. The GELFOAM should immediately swell to its original size and shape when dropped into the solution the second time. If it does not swell, it should be removed and kneaded vigorously until all air is expelled and it does expand to its original shape when dropped into the solution.
The piece of GELFOAM is then left wet or blotted to dampness on gauze and applied to the bleeding point. It should be held in place for 10 to 15 seconds with a pledget of cotton or small gauze sponge. Removal of the pledget of cotton or gauze is made easier by wetting it with a few drops of water to prevent pulling up the GELFOAM, which now encloses a firm clot. If desired, suction may be applied over the pledget of cotton or gauze to draw blood into the GELFOAM where it promptly clots. However, while suction hastens clotting, it is not essential, since GELFOAM will draw up blood by capillary attraction and cause clotting satisfactorily. Usually the first application of GELFOAM will control bleeding, but if not, additional applications should be made, using fresh pieces of GELFOAM prepared as previously described.
When bleeding is controlled, the pieces of GELFOAM should be left in place; otherwise bleeding may start again. Since GELFOAM causes but little more cellular infiltration than the blood clot, the wound may be closed over it. When applied to bleeding mucosa, GELFOAM will stay in place until it liquefies.

CONTRAINDICATIONS

GELFOAM Sterile Sponge (absorbable gelatin sponge) should not be used in the closure of skin incisions as it may interfere with the healing of skin edges.

WARNINGS

This product should not be resterilized by heat, because heating may change absorption time. Ethylene oxide is not recommended for resterilization since it may be trapped in the interstices of the foam. Although not reported for GELFOAM Sterile Sponge (absorbable gelatin sponge) the gas is toxic to tissue, and in trace amounts may cause burns or irritation.

PRECAUTIONS

Use of GELFOAM Sterile Sponge (absorbable gelatin sponge) is not recommended in the presence of frank infection. If signs of infection or abscess develop in an area where GELFOAM has been placed, reoperation may be necessary to remove the infected material and allow drainage.
GELFOAM should not be employed for controlling postpartum bleeding or menorrhagia.
By absorbing fluid, GELFOAM may expand and impinge on neighboring structures. Therefore, when placed into cavities or closed tissue spaces, minimal preliminary compression is advised and care should be exercised to avoid overpacking.

ADVERSE REACTIONS

GELFOAM Sterile Sponge (absorbable gelatin sponge) may form a nidus of infection and abscess formation. Giant cell granuloma has been reported at the site of absorbable gelatin product implantation in the brain, as has compression of the brain and spinal cord as a result of accumulation of sterile fluid. Excessive fibrosis and prolonged fixation of the tendon have been reported when absorbable gelatin products were used about a tendon juncture in repair of severed tendons.

HOW SUPPLIED

GELFOAM Sterile Sponge (absorbable gelatin sponge) is available in the following sizes:

Size 12—3 mm 20 mm × 60 mm (12 sq cm) × 3 mm [¾ in × 2⅜ in (1¾ sq in) × ⅛ in] *in boxes of 4 sponges in individual envelopes.*
NDC 0009-0301-01

Size 12—7 mm 20 mm × 60 mm (12 sq cm) × 7 mm [¾ in × 2⅜ in (1¾ sq in) × ¼ in] *in boxes of 12 sponges in individual envelopes, and in jars of 4 sponges.*
Box NDC 0009-0315-03
Jar NDC 0009-0315-02

Size 50, 80 mm × 62.5 mm (50 sq cm) × 10 mm [3⅛ in × 2½ in (7⅞ sq in) × ⅜in] *in boxes of 4 sponges in individual envelopes.*
NDC 0009-0323-01

Size 100, 80 mm × 125 mm (100 sq cm) × 10 mm [3⅛ in × 5 in (15⅝ sq in) × ⅜in] *in boxes of 6 sponges in individual envelopes.*
NDC 0009-0342-01

Size 200, 80 mm × 250 mm (200 sq cm) × 10 mm [3⅛ in × 10 in (31¼ sq in) × ⅜ in] *in boxes of 6 sponges in individual envelopes.*
NDC 0009-0349-01

Size 2 cm (approximately 40 cm × 2 cm) [15¾ in × ¾ in] *packaged in individual jars.*
NDC 0009-0364-01

Size 6 cm (approximately 40 cm × 6 cm) [15¾ in × 2⅜ in] *packaged in cartons of six sponges in individual envelopes.*
NDC 0009-0371-01

STORAGE AND HANDLING

GELFOAM Sterile Sponge (absorbable gelatin sponge) should be stored under normal conditions. Once the package is opened, contents are subject to contamination. It is recommended that GELFOAM be used as soon as the package is opened and unused contents discarded.

CAUTION

Federal law restricts this device to sale by or on the order of a physician.

Code 812 250 004

Also available:

Gelfoam Sterile Compressed Sponge (absorbable gelatin sponge, USP) Size 100. For application in dry state. Sponges measure 80 mm × 125 mm and are available in boxes of 6 sponges in individual envelopes.

NDC 0009-0353-01

Gelfoam Sterile Dental Packs (absorbable gelatin sponge, USP), Size 2 or 4. Each measures 10 × 20 × 7 mm or 20 × 20 × 7 mm, respectively; packaged in jars of 15 packs.

Size 2 NDC 0009-0379-01
Size 4 NDC 0009-0396-01

Gelfoam Sterile Prostatectomy Cones, (absorbable gelatin sponge, USP), Size 13 cm or 18 cm (for use with Foley bag catheter). Each cone diameter measures 13 cm or 18 cm, respectively; packaged in boxes of 6 cones in individual envelopes.

Size 13 cm NDC 0009-0449-01
Size 18 cm NDC 0009-0457-01

GELFOAM®

brand of absorbable gelatin sterile powder

HOW SUPPLIED

GELFOAM Sterile Powder (absorbable gelatin powder) is supplied in jars containing 1 gram.

NDC 0009-0433-01

HALCION® Ⓒ ℞

brand of triazolam tablets, USP

0.125 mg 100's
NSN 6505-01-220-5833 (VA)
0.25 mg 100's
NSN 6505-01-161-5036 (M&VA)
0.25 mg 100's Unit Dose
NSN 6505-01-184-1576 (VA)
0.5 mg 100's
NSN 6505-01-161-5034 (M)

DESCRIPTION

HALCION Tablets contain triazolam, a triazolobenzodiazepine hypnotic agent.

Triazolam is a white crystalline powder, soluble in alcohol and poorly soluble in water. It has a molecular weight of 343.21.

The chemical name for triazolam is 8-chloro- 6- (o-chlorophenyl) -1- methyl-4H-s-triazolo- [4,3-a] [1,4] benzodiazepine.

Each HALCION tablet, for oral administration, contains 0.125 mg, 0.25 mg or 0.5 mg of triazolam. Inactive ingredients: **0.125 mg**—cellulose, corn starch, docusate sodium, erythrosine sodium, FD&C blue no. 2, lactose, magnesium stearate, sodium benzoate; **0.25 mg**—cellulose, corn starch, docusate sodium, FD&C blue no. 2, lactose, magnesium stearate, silicon dioxide, sodium benzoate; **0.5 mg**—cellulose, corn starch, docusate sodium, lactose, magnesium stearate, silicon dioxide, sodium benzoate.

CLINICAL PHARMACOLOGY

Triazolam is a hypnotic with a short mean plasma half-life of 2.6 hours, and a range of 1.6–5.4 hours. Following oral administration, triazolam is readily absorbed. The mean peak concentration occurred at 1.3 hours following a single dose of triazolam ^{14}C. The nature of the relationship between dose and bioavailability of triazolam has not yet been established.

Triazolam and its metabolites, principally as conjugated glucuronides which are presumably inactive, are excreted primarily in the urine. Only small amounts of unmetabolized triazolam appear in the urine. The two primary metabolites accounted for 79.9% of urinary excretion. Urinary excretion appeared to be biphasic in its time course.

HALCION Tablets (triazolam) 0.5 mg, in two separate studies, did not affect the prothrombin times or plasma warfarin levels in male volunteers administered sodium warfarin orally.

Extremely high concentrations of triazolam do not displace bilirubin bound to human serum albumin *in vitro*.

Triazolam ^{14}C was administered orally to pregnant mice. Drug-related material appeared uniformly distributed in the fetus with ^{14}C concentrations approximately the same as in the brain of the mother.

In sleep laboratory studies, HALCION Tablets significantly decreased sleep latency, increased the duration of sleep and decreased the number of nocturnal awakenings. After two weeks of consecutive nightly administration, the drug's effect on total wake time is decreased, and the values recorded in the last third of the night approach baseline levels. On the first night after drug discontinuance (first post-drug night), total time asleep, percentage of time spent sleeping, and rapidity of falling asleep frequently were significantly less than on baseline (pre-drug) nights. This effect is often called "rebound" insomnia.

The type and duration of hypnotic effects and the profile of unwanted effects during administration of benzodiazepine drugs may be influenced by the biologic half-life of administered drug and any active metabolites formed. When half-lives are long, drug or metabolites may accumulate during periods of nightly administration and be associated with impairments of congnitive and motor performance during waking hours; the possibility of interaction with other psychoactive drugs or alcohol will be enhanced. In contrast, if half-lives are short, drug and metabolites will be cleared before the next dose is ingested, and carry-over effects related to excessive sedation or CNS depression should be minimal or absent. However, during nightly use for an extended period, pharmacodynamic tolerance or adaptation to some effects of benzodiazepine hypnotics may develop. If the drug has a short half-life of elimination, it is possible that a relative deficiency of the drug or its active metabolites (ie, in relationship to the receptor site) may occur at some point in the interval between each night's use. This sequence of events may account for two clinical findings reported to occur after several weeks of nightly use of rapidly eliminated benzodiazepine hypnotics: 1) increased wakefulness during the last third of the night, and 2) the appearance of increased signs of day-time anxiety reported by one author in a selected group of patients.

INDICATIONS AND USAGE

HALCION Tablets contain triazolam which is a hypnotic agent useful in the short-term management of insomnia characterized by difficulty in falling asleep, frequent nocturnal awakenings, and/or early morning awakenings.

In polysomnographic studies in man of 1 to 42 days duration, triazolam decreased sleep latency, increased duration of sleep, and decreased the number of nocturnal awakenings.

It is recommended that HALCION not be prescribed in quantities exceeding a one-month supply.

CONTRAINDICATIONS

HALCION Tablets (triazolam) are contraindicated in patients with known hypersensitivity to this drug or other benzodiazepines.

Benzodiazepines may cause fetal damage when administered during pregnancy. An increased risk of congenital malformations associated with the use of diazepam and chlordiazepoxide during the first trimester of pregnancy has been suggested in several studies. Transplacental distribution has resulted in neonatal CNS depression following the ingestion of therapeutic doses of a benzodiazepine hypnotic during the last weeks of pregnancy.

HALCION is contraindicated in pregnant women. If there is a likelihood of the patient becoming pregnant while receiving HALCION she should be warned of the potential risk to the fetus. Patients should be instructed to discontinue the drug prior to becoming pregnant. The possibility that a woman of childbearing potential may be pregnant at the time of institution of therapy should be considered.

WARNINGS

Overdosage may occur at four times the maximum recommended therapeutic dose (see DOSAGE AND ADMINISTRATION section). Patients should be cautioned *not* to exceed prescribed dosage.

Because of its depressant CNS effects, patients receiving triazolam should be cautioned against engaging in hazardous occupations requiring complete mental alertness such as operating machinery or driving a motor vehicle. For the same reason, patients should be cautioned about the simultaneous ingestion of alcohol and other CNS depressant drugs during treatment with HALCION Tablets (triazolam).

As with some but not all benzodiazepines, anterograde amnesia of varying severity and paradoxical reactions have been reported following therapeutic doses of HALCION.

PRECAUTIONS

General: In elderly and/or debilitated patients, it is recommended that treatment with HALCION Tablets (triazolam) be initiated at 0.125 mg to decrease the possibility of development of oversedation, dizziness, or impaired coordination. (See Dosage & Administration Section).

Caution should be exercised if HALCION is prescribed to patients with signs or symptoms of depression which could be intensified by hypnotic drugs. Suicidal tendencies may be present in such patients and protective measures may be required. Intentional overdosage is more common in these patients, and the least amount of drug that is feasible should be available to the patient at any one time.

The usual precautions should be observed in patients with impaired renal or hepatic function and chronic pulmonary insufficiency.

Information for Patients: To assure safe and effective use of HALCION Tablets (triazolam), the following information and instructions should be given to patients:

1. Inform your physician about any alcohol consumption and medicine you are taking now, including drugs you may buy without a prescription. Alcohol should generally not be used during treatment with hypnotics.
2. Inform your physician if you are planning to become pregnant, if you are pregnant, or if you become pregnant while you are taking this medicine.
3. Inform your physician if you are nursing.
4. Until you experience how this medication affects you, do not drive a car or operate potentially dangerous machinery, etc.
5. Do *not* increase prescribed dosage.
6. Patients should also be advised that they may experience an increase in sleep complaints (rebound insomnia) on the first night or two after discontinuing the drug.

Laboratory Tests: Laboratory tests are not ordinarily required in otherwise healthy patients.

Drug Interactions: The benzodiazepines, including triazolam, produce additive CNS depressant effects when co-administered with other psychotropic medications, anticonvulsants, anti-histaminics, ethanol, and other drugs which themselves produce CNS depression.

Pharmacokinetic interactions of benzodiazepines with other drugs have been reported. For example, the co-administration of triazolam and cimetidine in a controlled clinical trial in normal subjects resulted in a reduction of triazolam clearance and an increase in the elimination half-life from 2.2 to 3.7 hours. The plasma concentration of triazolam approximately doubled when co-administered with cimetidine. However, this did not result in any drug accumulation

Carcinogenesis, Mutagenesis,
Impairment of Fertility: No evidence of carcinogenic potential was observed in mice during a 24-month study with HALCION in doses up to 4000 times the human dose.

Pregnancy:

1. Teratogenic Effects: Pregnancy Category X. See CONTRAINDICATIONS.
2. Non-Teratogenic Effects: It is to be considered that the child born of a mother who is on benzodiazepines may be at some risk for withdrawal symptoms from the drug, during the postnatal period. Also, neonatal flaccidity has been reported in an infant born of a mother who had been receiving benzodiazepines.

Nursing Mothers: Human studies have not been performed; however, studies in rats have indicated that HALCION and its metabolites are secreted in milk. Therefore, administration of HALCION to nursing mothers is not recommended.

Pediatric Use: Safety and efficacy of HALCION in children below the age of 18 have not been established.

ADVERSE REACTIONS

During placebo-controlled clinical studies in which 1003 patients received HALCION Tablets (triazolam), the most troublesome side effects were extensions of the pharmacologic activity of triazolam, eg drowsiness, dizziness, or lightheadedness.

The figures cited below are estimates of untoward clinical event incidence among subjects who participated in the relatively short duration (ie, 1 to 42 days) placebo-controlled clinical trials of HALCION. The figures cannot be used to predict precisely the incidence of untoward events in the course of usual medical practice where patient characteristics and other factors often differ from those in the clinical trials. These figures cannot be compared with those obtained from other clinical studies involving related drug products and placebo as each group of drug trials are conducted under a different set of conditions.

Comparison of the cited figures, however, can provide the prescriber with some basis for estimating the relative contributions of drug and non-drug factors to the untoward event incidence rate in the population studied. Even this use must be approached cautiously, as a drug may relieve a symptom in one patient while inducing it in others. [For example, an anticholinergic, anxiolytic drug may relieve dry mouth (a sign of anxiety) in some subjects but induce it (an untoward event) in others.]

	HALCION	Placebo
Number of Patients	1003	997
% of Patients Reporting:		
Central Nervous System		
Drowsiness	14.0	6.4
Headache	9.7	8.4
Dizziness	7.8	3.1
Nervousness	5.2	4.5
Lightheadedness	4.9	0.9
Coordination Disorders/Ataxia	4.6	0.8
Gastrointestinal		
Nausea/Vomiting	4.6	3.7

Continued on next page

Information on these Upjohn products is based on labeling in effect August 15, 1986. Further information concerning these and other Upjohn products may be obtained by direct inquiry to Medical Information, The Upjohn Company, Kalamazoo, Michigan 49001.

Upjohn—Cont.

In addition to the relatively common (ie, 1% or greater) untoward events enumerated above, the following adverse events have been reported less frequently (ie, 0.9–0.5%): euphoria, tachycardia, tiredness, confusional states/memory impairment, cramps/pain, depression, visual disturbances.
Rare (ie, less than 0.5%) adverse reactions included constipation, taste alterations, diarrhea, dry mouth, dermatitis/allergy, dreaming/nightmares, insomnia, paresthesia, tinnitus, dysesthesia, weakness, congestion, death from hepatic failure in a patient also receiving diuretic drugs.
In addition to these untoward events, the following adverse events have been reported in association with the use of benzodiazepines: dystonia, irritability, anorexia, fatigue, sedation, slurred speech, jaundice, pruritus, dysarthria, changes in libido, menstrual irregularities, incontinence and urinary retention.
As with all benzodiazepines, paradoxical reactions such as stimulation, agitation, increased muscle spasticity, sleep disturbances, hallucinations and other adverse behavioral effects may occur in rare instances and in a random fashion. Should these occur, use of the drug should be discontinued.
Laboratory analyses were performed on all patients participating in the HALCION clinical program. The following incidences of abnormalities were observed in patients receiving HALCION and the corresponding placebo group. None of these changes were considered to be of physiological significance.
[See table below].
When treatment with HALCION is protracted, periodic blood counts, urinalysis and blood chemistry analyses are advisable.
Minor changes in EEG patterns, usually low-voltage fast activity have been observed in patients during therapy with HALCION and are of no known significance.

DRUG ABUSE AND DEPENDENCE

Controlled Substance: Triazolam is a controlled substance under the Controlled Substance Act and HALCION Tablets have been assigned to Schedule IV.
Abuse and Dependence: Withdrawal symptoms similar in character to those noted with barbiturates and alcohol have occurred following abrupt discontinuance of benzodiazepine drugs. These can range from mild dysphoria to a major syndrome which may include abdominal and muscle cramps, vomiting, sweating, tremor, and convulsions.
Patients with a history of seizures should not be abruptly withdrawn from any CNS depressant agent, including HALCION. Addiction-prone individuals, such as drug addicts and alcoholics, should be under careful surveillance when receiving triazolam because of the predisposition of such patients to habituation and dependence. As with all hypnotics, repeat prescriptions should be limited to those who are under medical supervision.

OVERDOSAGE

Because of the potency of triazolam, overdosage may occur at 2 mg, four times the maximum recommended therapeutic dose (0.5 mg).
Manifestations of overdosage with HALCION Tablets (triazolam) include somnolence, confusion, impaired coordination, slurred speech, and ultimately, coma. As in all cases of drug overdosage, respiration, pulse, and blood pressure should be monitored and supported by general measures when necessary. Immediate gastric lavage should be performed. An adequate airway should be maintained. Intravenous fluids may be administered.
Experiments in animals have indicated that cardiopulmonary collapse can occur with massive intravenous doses of HALCION (over 100 mg/kg, more than 10,000 times the maximum daily human dose). This could be reversed with positive mechanical respiration and the intravenous infusion of levarterenol or metaraminol. Hemodialysis and forced diuresis are probably of little value. As with the management of intentional overdosage with any drug, the physician should bear in mind that multiple agents may have been ingested by the patient.
The oral LD_{50} in mice is greater than 1000 mg/kg and in rats is greater than 5000 mg/kg.

DOSAGE AND ADMINISTRATION

It is important to individualize the dosage of HALCION Tablets (triazolam) for maximum beneficial effect and to help avoid significant adverse effects. The recommended dosage range for adults is 0.25 to 0.5 mg before retiring. A dose of 0.125 mg may be found to be sufficient for selected patients, however. As with all medications, the lowest effective dose should be used.
In geriatric and/or debilitated patients, the dosage range is 0.125 to 0.25 mg. Therapy should be initiated at 0.125 mg in this group until individual response is determined.

HOW SUPPLIED

HALCION Tablets (triazolam) scored, are available in the following strengths and package sizes:

0.125 mg (pale lavender):
- Bottles of 100 — NDC 0009-0010-01
- VISIPAK™ Reverse Numbered Pack (100) — NDC 0009-0010-04

0.25 mg (powder blue, scored):
- Bottles of 100 — NDC 0009-0017-01
- Unit Dose Pkg (100) — NDC 0009-0017-08
- VISIPAK™ Reverse Numbered Pack (100) — NDC 0009-0017-17
- Bottles of 500 — NDC 0009-0017-02

0.5 mg (white, scored)
- Bottles of 100 — NDC 0009-0027-01
- Unit Dose Pkg (100) — NDC 0009-0027-08
- Unit Dose Pkg (100) — NDC 0009-0027-18
- VISIPAK™ Reverse Numbered Pack (100) — NDC 0009-0027-18

Store at controlled room temperature 15°–30°C (59°–86°F).
Code 812 110 108

Shown in Product Identification Section, page 433

	HALCION 380		Placebo 361	
Number of patients	380		361	
% of Patients Reporting:	Low	High	Low	High
Hematology				
Hematocrit	*	*	*	*
Hemoglobin	*	*	*	*
Total WBC Count	1.7	2.1	*	1.3
Neutrophil Count	1.5	1.5	3.3	1.0
Lymphocyte Count	2.3	4.0	3.1	3.8
Monocyte Count	3.6	*	4.4	1.5
Eosinophil Count	10.2	3.2	9.8	3.4
Basophil Count	1.7	2.1	*	1.8
Urinalysis				
Albumin	—	1.1	—	*
Sugar	—	*	—	*
RBC/HPF	—	2.9	—	2.9
WBC/HPF	—	11.7	—	7.9
Blood Chemistry				
Creatinine	2.4	1.9	3.6	1.5
Bilirubin	*	1.5	1.0	*
SGOT	*	5.3	*	4.5
Alkaline Phosphatase	*	2.2	*	2.6

*Less than 1%

HALOTESTIN® ℞

brand of fluoxymesterone tablets, USP

10 mg-100s
NSN 6505-01-041-8165 (M & VA)

DESCRIPTION

HALOTESTIN Tablets contain fluoxymesterone, an androgenic hormone.
Fluoxymesterone is a white or practically white odorless, crystalline powder, melting at about 240° C. with some decomposition. It is practically insoluble in water, sparingly soluble in alcohol and slightly soluble in chloroform.
The chemical name for fluoxymesterone is androst-4-en-3-one, 9-fluoro -11, 17- dihydroxy-17- methyl-,(11β,17β). The molecular formula is $C_{20}H_{29}FO_3$ and the molecular weight 336.45.
Each HALOTESTIN tablet, for oral administration, contains 2 mg, 5 mg or 10 mg fluoxymesterone. Inactive ingredients: calcium stearate, corn starch, FD&C yellow no. 5, flavors, lactose, sorbic acid, sucrose, tragacanth. In addition, the **2 mg** tablet contains FD&C yellow no. 6 and the **5 mg** and **10 mg** contain FD&C blue no. 2.

CLINICAL PHARMACOLOGY

Endogenous androgens are responsible for normal growth and development of the male sex organs and for maintenance of secondary sex characteristics. These effects include growth and maturation of the prostate, seminal vesicles, penis, and scrotum; development of male hair distribution, such as beard, pubic, chest, and axillary hair; laryngeal enlargement, vocal cord thickening, and alterations in body musculature and fat distribution. Drugs in this class also cause retention of nitrogen, sodium, potassium, and phosphorus, and decreased urinary excretion of calcium. Androgens have been reported to increase protein anabolism and decrease protein catabolism. Nitrogen balance is improved only when there is sufficient intake of calories and protein.
Androgens are responsible for the growth spurt of adolescence and for eventual termination of linear growth, brought about by fusion of the epiphyseal growth centers. In children, exogenous androgens accelerate linear growth rates, but may cause disproportionate advancement in bone maturation. Use over long periods may result in fusion of the epiphyseal growth centers and termination of the growth process. Androgens have been reported to stimulate production of red blood cells by enhancing production of erythropoietic stimulation factor.
During exogenous administration of androgens, endogenous testosterone release is inhibited through feedback inhibition of pituitary luteinizing hormone (LH). At large doses of exogenous androgen, spermatogenesis may also be suppressed through feedback inhibition of pituitary follicle stimulating hormone (FSH).
Inactivation of testosterone occurs primarily in the liver.
The half-life of fluoxymesterone after oral administration is approximately 9.2 hours.

INDICATIONS AND USAGE

In the male—HALOTESTIN Tablets (fluoxymesterone) are indicated for:

1. Replacement therapy in conditions associated with symptoms of deficiency or absence of endogenous testosterone:
   a. Primary hypogonadism (congenital or acquired)—testicular failure due to cryptorchidism, bilateral torsion, orchitis, vanishing testis syndrome; or orchidectomy.
   b. Hypogonadotropic hypogonadism (congenital or acquired)—idiopathic gonadotropin or LHRH deficiency, or pituitary-hypothalamic injury from tumors, trauma, or radiation.
2. Delayed puberty, provided it has been definitely established as such, and is not just a familial trait.

In the female—HALOTESTIN Tablets are indicated for palliation of androgen-responsive recurrent mammary cancer in women who are more than one year but less than five years postmenopausal, or who have been proven to have a hormone-dependent tumor as shown by previous beneficial response to castration.

CONTRAINDICATIONS

1. Known hypersensitivity to the drug
2. Males with carcinoma of the breast
3. Males with known or suspected carcinoma of the prostate gland
4. Women known or suspected to be pregnant
5. Patients with serious cardiac, hepatic or renal disease

WARNINGS

Hypercalcemia may occur in immobilized patients and in patients with breast cancer. If this occurs, the drug should be discontinued.
Prolonged use of high doses of androgens (principally the 17-α alkyl-androgens) has been associated with development of hepatic adenomas, hepatocellular carcinoma, and peliosis hepatis—all potentially life-threatening complications.
Cholestatic hepatitis and jaundice may occur with 17-α-alkyl-androgens. Should this occur, the drug should be discontinued. This is reversible with discontinuation of the drug.
Geriatric patients treated with androgens may be at an increased risk of developing prostatic hypertrophy and prostatic carcinoma although conclusive evidence to support this concept is lacking.
Edema, with or without congestive heart failure, may be a serious complication in patients with pre-existing cardiac, renal or hepatic disease.
Gynecomastia may develop and occasionally persists in patients being treated for hypogonadism.
Androgen therapy should be used cautiously in males with delayed puberty. Androgens can accelerate bone maturation without producing compensatory gain in linear growth. The effect on bone maturation should be monitored by assessing bone age of the wrist and hand every six months.

PRECAUTIONS

General
Women should be observed for signs of virilization which is usual following androgen use at high doses. Discontinuation of drug therapy at the time of evidence of mild virilism is

necessary to prevent irreversible virilization. A decision may be made by the patient and the physician that some virilization will be tolerated during treatment for breast carcinoma. Patients with benign prostatic hypertrophy may develop acute urethral obstruction. Priapism or excessive sexual stimulation may develop. Oligospermia may occur after prolonged administration or excessive dosage. If any of these effects appear, the androgen should be stopped and if restarted, a lower dosage should be utilized.

This product contains FD&C Yellow No. 5 (tartrazine) which may cause allergic-type reactions (including bronchial asthma) in certain susceptible individuals. Although the overall incidence of FD&C Yellow No. 5 (tartrazine) sensitivity in the general population is low, it is frequently seen in patients who also have aspirin hypersensitivity.

Information for patients

Patients should be instructed to report any of the following: nausea, vomiting, changes in skin color, and ankle swelling. Males should be instructed to report too frequent or persistent erections of the penis and females any hoarseness, acne, changes in menstrual periods or increase in facial hair.

Laboratory tests

Women with disseminated breast carcinoma should have frequent determination of urine and serum calcium levels during the course of androgen therapy (See WARNINGS).

Because of the hepatotoxicity associated with the use of 17-alpha-alkylated androgens, liver function tests should be obtained periodically.

Periodic (every six months) x-ray examinations of bone age should be made during treatment of prepubertal males to determine the rate of bone maturation and the effects of androgen therapy on the epiphyseal centers.

Hemoglobin and hematocrit levels (to detect polycythemia) should be checked periodically in patients receiving long-term androgen administration.

Serum cholesterol may increase during androgen therapy.

DRUG INTERACTIONS

Androgens may increase sensitivity to oral anticoagulants. Dosage of the anticoagulant may require reduction in order to maintain satisfactory therapeutic hypoprothrombinemia.

Concurrent administration of oxyphenbutazone and androgens may result in elevated serum levels of oxyphenbutazone.

In diabetic patients, the metabolic effects of androgens may decrease blood glucose and, therefore, insulin requirements.

Drug/Laboratory test interferences

Androgens may decrease levels of thyroxine-binding globulin, resulting in decreased total T_4 serum levels and increased resin uptake of T_3 and T_4. Free thyroid hormone levels remain unchanged, however, and there is no clinical evidence of thyroid dysfunction.

Carcinogenesis

Animal data: Testosterone has been tested by subcutaneous injection and implantation in mice and rats. The implant induced cervical-uterine tumors in mice, which metastasized in some cases. There is suggestive evidence that injection of testosterone into some strains of female mice increases their susceptibility to hepatoma. Testosterone is also known to increase the number of tumors and decrease the degree of differentiation of chemically-induced carcinomas of the liver in rats.

Human data: There are rare reports of hepatocellular carcinoma in patients receiving long-term therapy with androgens in high doses. Withdrawal of the drugs did not lead to regression of the tumors in all cases.

Geriatric patients treated with androgens may be at an increased risk of developing prostatic hypertrophy and prostatic carcinoma although conclusive evidence to support this concept is lacking.

Pregnancy

Teratogenic effects: Pregnancy Category X. (See CONTRAINDICATIONS).

Nursing mothers

HALOTESTIN Tablets (fluoxymesterone) are not recommended for use in nursing mothers.

Pediatric use

Androgen therapy should be used very cautiously in children and only by specialists aware of the adverse effects on bone maturation. Skeletal maturation must be monitored every six months by an x-ray of the hand and wrist (See WARNINGS).

ADVERSE REACTIONS

Endocrine and urogenital

Female: The most common side effects of androgen therapy are amenorrhea and other menstrual irregularities; inhibition of gonadotropin secretion; and virilization, including deepening of the voice and clitoral enlargement. The latter usually is not reversible after androgens are discontinued. When administered to a pregnant woman, androgens can cause virilization of external genitalia of the female fetus.

Male: Gynecomastia, and excessive frequency and duration of penile erections. Oligospermia may occur at high dosage.

Skin and appendages

Hirsutism, male pattern of baldness, seborrhea, and acne.

Fluid and electrolyte disturbances

Retention of sodium, chloride, water, potassium, calcium, and inorganic phosphates.

Gastrointestinal

Nausea, cholestatic jaundice, alterations in liver function tests, rarely hepatocellular neoplasms and peliosis hepatis (see WARNINGS).

Hematologic

Suppression of clotting factors II, V, VII, and X, bleeding in patients on concomitant anticoagulant therapy, and polycythemia.

Nervous system

Increased or decreased libido, headache, anxiety, depression, and generalized paresthesia.

Allergic

Hypersensitivity, including skin manifestations and anaphylactoid reactions.

OVERDOSAGE

There have been no reports of acute overdosage with the androgens.

DOSAGE AND ADMINISTRATION

The dosage will vary depending upon the individual, the condition being treated, and its severity. The total daily oral dose may be administered singly or in divided (three or four) doses.

Male hypogonadism: For complete replacement in the hypogonadal male, a daily dose of 5 to 20 mg will suffice in the majority of patients. It is usually preferable to begin treatment with full therapeutic doses which are later adjusted to individual requirements. Priapism is indicative of excessive dosage and is indication for temporary withdrawal of the drug.

Delayed puberty: Dosage should be carefully titrated utilizing a low dose, appropriate skeletal monitoring, and by limiting the duration of therapy to four to six months.

Inoperable carcinoma of the breast in the female: The recommended total daily dose for palliative therapy in advanced inoperable carcinoma of the breast is 10 to 40 mg. Because of its short action, fluoxymesterone should be administered to patients in divided, rather than single, daily doses to ensure more stable blood levels. In general, it appears necessary to continue therapy for at least one month for a satisfactory subjective response, and for two to three months for an objective response.

HOW SUPPLIED

HALOTESTIN Tablets (fluoxymesterone), scored, are available in the following strengths and colors:

2 mg (peach)
Bottles of 100 NDC 0009-0014-01
5 mg (light green)
Bottles of 100 NDC 0009-0019-06
10 mg (green)
Bottles of 30 NDC 0009-0036-03
Bottles of 100 NDC 0009-0036-04
Code 810 804 202

Shown in Product Identification Section, page 433

HEPARIN SODIUM INJECTION, USP ℞

Sterile Solution

DESCRIPTION

Heparin Soldium Injection, USP is a heterogenous group of straight-chain anionic mucopolysaccharides, called glycosaminoglycans having anticoagulant properties. Although others may be present, the main sugars occurring in heparin are: (1) α-L-iduronic acid 2-sulfate, (2) 2-deoxy-2-sulfamino-α-D-glucose 6-sulfate, (3) β-D-glucoronic acid, (4) 2-acetamido-2-deoxy-α-D-glucose, and (5) α-L-iduronic acid. These sugars are present in decreasing amounts, usually in the order (2) > (1) > (4) > (3) > (5), and are joined by glycosidic linkages, forming polymers of varying sizes. Heparin is strongly acidic because of its content of covalently linked sulfate and carboxylic acid groups. In heparin sodium, the acidic protons of the sulfate units are partially replaced by sodium ions.

Heparin Sodium Injection, USP is a sterile solution of heparin sodium derived from bovine lung tissue, standardized for anticoagulant activity. It is to be administered by intravenous or deep subcutaneous routes. The potency is determined by a biological assay using a USP reference standard based on units of heparin activity per milligram.

Slight variations in the color of heparin sodium solutions do not affect the therapeutic efficiency. Each ml of the 1,000 and 5,000 USP Units per ml preparations contains: Heparin sodium 1,000 or 5,000 USP Units; 9 mg sodium chloride; 9.45 mg benzyl alcohol added as preservative. Each ml of the 10,000 USP Units per ml preparations contains: heparin sodium 10,000 USP Units; 9.45 mg benzyl alcohol added as preservative.

CLINICAL PHARMACOLOGY

Heparin inhibits reactions that lead to the clotting of blood and the formation of fibrin clots both *in vitro* and *in vivo*. Heparin acts at multiple sites in the normal coagulation system. Small amounts of heparin in combination with antithrombin III (heparin cofactor) can inhibit thrombosis by inactivating activated Factor X and inhibiting the conversion of prothrombin to thrombin. Once active thrombosis has developed, larger amounts of heparin can inhibit further coagulation by inactivating thrombin and preventing the conversion of fibrinogen to fibrin. Heparin also prevents the formation of a stable fibrin clot by inhibiting the activation of the fibrin stabilizing factor.

Bleeding time is usually unaffected by heparin. Clotting time is prolonged by full therapeutic doses of heparin; in most cases, it is not measurably affected by low doses of heparin.

Peak plasma levels of heparin are achieved 2–4 hours following subcutaneous administration, although there are considerable individual variations. Loglinear plots of heparin plasma concentrations with time for a wide range of dose levels are linear which suggests the absence of zero order processes. Liver and the reticulo-endothelial system are the site of biotransformation. The biphasic elimination curve, a rapidly declining alpha phase ($t\frac{1}{2}$ = 10 minutes) and after the age of 40 a slower beta phase, indicates uptake in organs. The absence of a relationship between anticoagulant half-life and concentration half-life may reflect factors such as protein binding of heparin.

Heparin does not have fibrinolytic activity; therefore, it will not lyse existing clots.

INDICATIONS AND USAGE

Heparin Sodium Injection is indicated for:

Anticoagulant therapy in prophylaxis and treatment of venous thrombosis and its extension;

(In a low-dose regimen) for prevention of postoperative deep venous thrombosis and pulmonary embolism in patients undergoing major abdomino-thoracic surgery or who for other reasons are at risk of developing thromboembolic disease (see DOSAGE AND ADMINISTRATION);

Prophylaxis and treatment of pulmonary embolism;

Atrial fibrillation with embolization;

Diagnosis and treatment of acute and chronic consumption coagulopathies (disseminated intravascular coagulation);

Prevention of clotting in arterial and heart surgery;

Prophylaxis and treatment of peripheral arterial embolism;

As an anticoagulant in blood transfusions, extracorporeal circulation, and dialysis procedures and in blood samples for laboratory purposes.

CONTRAINDICATIONS

Heparin sodium should not be used in patients:

With severe thrombocytopenia;

In whom suitable blood coagulation tests—e.g., the whole-blood clotting time, partial thromboplastin time, etc.—cannot be performed at appropriate intervals (this contraindication refers to full-dose heparin; there is usually no need to monitor coagulation parameters in patients receiving low-dose heparin);

With an uncontrollable active bleeding state (see WARNINGS), except when this is due to disseminated intravascular coagulation.

WARNINGS

Heparin is not intended for intramuscular use.

Hypersensitivity: Patients with documented hypersensitivity to heparin should be given the drug only in clearly life-threatening situations.

Hemorrhage: Hemorrhage can occur at virtually any site in patients receiving heparin. An unexplained fall in hematocrit, fall in blood pressure, or any other unexplained symptom should lead to serious consideration of a hemorrhagic event.

Heparin sodium should be used with extreme caution in disease states in which there is increased danger of hemorrhage. Some of the conditions in which increased danger of hemorrhage exists are:

Cardiovascular—Subacute bacterial endocarditis. Severe hypotension.

Surgical—During and immediately following (a) spinal tap or spinal anesthesia or (b) major surgery, especially involving the brain, spinal cord, or eye.

Hematologic—Conditions associated with increased bleeding tendencies, such as hemophilia, thrombocytopenia, and some vascular purpuras.

Gastrointestinal—Ulcerative lesions and continuous tube drainage of the stomach or small intestine.

Other—Menstruation, liver disease with impaired hemostasis.

Continued on next page

Information on these Upjohn products is based on labeling in effect August 15, 1986. Further information concerning these and other Upjohn products may be obtained by direct inquiry to Medical Information, The Upjohn Company, Kalamazoo, Michigan 49001.

Upjohn—Cont.

Coagulation Testing: When heparin sodium is administered in therapeutic amounts, its dosage should be regulated by frequent blood coagulation tests. If the coagulation test is unduly prolonged or if hemorrhage occurs, heparin sodium should be discontinued promptly (see OVERDOSAGE).

Thrombocytopenia: Thrombocytopenia has been reported to occur in patients receiving heparin with a reported incidence of 0 to 30%. Mild thrombocytopenia (count greater than 100,000/mm^3) may remain stable or reverse even if heparin is continued. However, thrombocytopenia of any degree should be monitored closely. If the count falls below 100,000/mm^3 or if recurrent thrombosis develops (see White Clot Syndrome, PRECAUTIONS), the heparin product should be discontinued. If continued heparin therapy is essential, administration of heparin from a different organ source can be reinstituted with caution.

Miscellaneous: This product contains benzyl alcohol as preservative: Benzyl alcohol has been reported to be associated with a fatal "Gasping Syndrome" in premature infants.

PRECAUTIONS

1. General

a. White Clot Syndrome

Rare patients on heparin may develop new thrombus formation in association with thrombocytopenia resulting from irreversible aggregation of platelets induced by heparin, the so-called "white clot syndrome." The process may lead to severe thromboembolic complications like skin necrosis, gangrene of the extremities, myocardial infarction, pulmonary embolism, and stroke. Therefore, heparin administration should be promptly discontinued if a patient develops new thrombosis in association with thrombocytopenia.

b. Heparin Resistance

Increased resistance to heparin is frequently encountered in fever, thrombosis, thrombophlebitis, infections with thrombosing tendencies, myocardial infarction, cancer and in postsurgical patients.

c. Increased Risk in Older Women:

A higher incidence of bleeding has been reported in women over 60 years of age.

2. Laboratory Tests: Periodic platelet counts, hematocrits, and tests for occult blood in stool are recommended during the entire course of heparin therapy, regardless of the route of administration (see DOSAGE AND ADMINISTRATION).

3. Drug Interactions:

Oral anticoagulants: Heparin sodium may prolong the one-stage prothrombin time. Therefore, when heparin sodium is given with dicumarol or warfarin sodium, a period of at least 5 hours after the last intravenous dose or 24 hours after the last subcutaneous dose should elapse before blood is drawn if a valid prothrombin time is to be obtained.

Platelet inhibitors: Drugs such as acetylsalicylic acid, dextran, phenylbutazone, ibuprofen, indomethacin, dipyridamole, hydroxychloroquine and others that interfere with platelet-aggregation reactions (the main hemostatic defense of heparinized patients) may induce bleeding and should be used with caution in patients receiving heparin sodium.

Other interactions: Digitalis, tetracyclines, nicotine, or antihistamines may partially counteract the anticoagulant action of heparin sodium.

4. Drug/Laboratory Tests Interactions:

Hyperaminotransferasemia: Significant elevations of aminotransferase (SGOT [S-AST] and SPT [S-ALT])levels have occurred in a high percentage of patients (and healthy subjects) who have received heparin. Since aminotransferase determinations are important in the differential diagnosis of myocardial infarction, liver disease, and pulmonary emboli, rises that might be caused by drugs (like heparin) should be interpreted with caution.

5. Carcinogenesis, Mutagenesis, Impairment of Fertility: No long-term studies in animals have been performed to evaluate carcinogenic potential of heparin. Also, no reproduction studies in animals have been performed concerning mutagenesis or impairment of fertility.

6. Pregnancy:

Teratogenic Effects: Pregnancy Category C. Animal reproduction studies have not been conducted with heparin sodium. It is also not known whether heparin sodium can cause fetal harm when administered to a pregnant woman or can affect reproduction capacity. Heparin sodium should be given to a pregnant woman only if clearly needed.

Nonteratogenic Effects: Heparin does not cross the placental barrier.

7. Nursing Mothers: Heparin is not excreted in human milk.

8. Pediatric Use: See DOSAGE AND ADMINISTRATION.

ADVERSE REACTIONS

1. Hemorrhage. Hemorrhage is the chief complication that may result from heparin therapy (see WARNINGS). An overly prolonged clotting time or minor bleeding during therapy can usually be controlled by withdrawing the drug (see OVERDOSAGE). **It should be appreciated that gastrointestinal or urinary tract bleeding during anticoagulant therapy may indicate the presence of an underlying occult lesion.** Bleeding can occur at any site but certain specific hemorrhagic complications may be difficult to detect.

a. Adrenal hemorrhage, with resultant acute adrenal insufficiency, has occurred during anticoagulant therapy. Therefore, such treatment should be discontinued in patients who develop signs and symptoms of acute adrenal hemorrhage and insufficiency. Initiation of corrective therapy should not depend on laboratory confirmation of the diagnosis, since any delay in an acute situation may result in the patient's death.

b. Ovarian (corpus luteum) hemorrhage developed in a number of women of reproductive age receiving short- or long-term anticoagulant therapy. This complication if unrecognized may be fatal.

c. Retroperitoneal hemorrhage.

2. Local irritation. Local irritation, erythema, mild pain, hematoma or ulceration may follow deep subcutaneous (intrafat) injection of heparin sodium. These complications are much more common after intramuscular use, and such use is not recommended.
3. Hypersensitivity. Generalized hypersensitivity reactions have been reported, with chills, fever, and urticaria as the most usual manifestations, and asthma, rhinitis, lacrimation, headache, nausea and vomiting, and anaphylactoid reactions, including shock, occurring more rarely. Itching and burning, especially on the plantar site of the feet, may occur.

Thrombocytopenia has been reported to occur in patients receiving heparin with a reported incidence of 0–30%. While often mild and of no obvious clinical significance, such thrombocytopenia can be accompanied by severe thromboembolic complications such as skin necrosis, gangrene of the extremities, myocardial infarction, pulmonary embolism, and stroke. (See WARNINGS, PRECAUTIONS.)

Certain episodes of painful, ischemic, and cyanosed limbs have in the past been attributed to allergic vasospastic reactions. Whether these are in fact identical to the thrombocytopenia associated complications remains to be determined.

4. Miscellaneous. Osteoporosis following long-term administration of high doses of heparin, cutaneous necrosis after systemic administration, supression of aldosterone synthesis, delayed transient alopecia, priapism, and rebound hyperlipemia on discontinuation of heparin sodium have also been reported.

Significant elevations of aminotransferase (SGOT [S-AST] and SGPT [S-ALT]) levels have occurred in a high percentage of patients (and healthy subjects) who have received heparin.

OVERDOSAGE

Symptoms: Bleeding is the chief sign of heparin overdosage. Nosebleeds, blood in urine or tarry stools may be noted as the first sign of bleeding. Easy bruising or petechial formations may precede frank bleeding.

Treatment: Neutralization of heparin effect. When clinical circumstances (bleeding) require reversal of heparinization, protamine sulfate (1% solution) by slow infusion will neutralize heparin sodium. **No more than 50 mg** should be administered, **very slowly,** in any 10 minute period. Each mg of protamine sulfate neutralizes approximately 100 USP heparin units. The amount of protamine required decreases over time as heparin is metabolized. Although the metabolism of heparin is complex, it may, for the purpose of choosing a protamine dose, be assumed to have a half-life of about ½ hour after intravenous injection.

Administration of protamine sulfate can cause severe hypotensive and anaphylactoid reactions. Because fatal reactions often resembling anaphylaxis have been reported, the drug should be given only when resuscitation techniques and treatment of anaphylactoid shock are readily available.

For additional information the labeling of Protamine Sulfate Injection, USP products should be consulted.

DOSAGE AND ADMINISTRATION

Parenteral drug products should be inspected visually for particulate matter and discoloration prior to administration, whenever solution and container permit. Slight discoloration does not alter potency.

When heparin is added to an infusion solution for continuous intravenous administration, the container should be inverted at least six times to insure adequate mixing and prevent pooling of the heparin in the solution.

Heparin sodium is not effective by oral administration and should be given by intermittent intravenous injection, intravenous infusion, or deep subcutaneous (intrafat, i.e., above the iliac crest or abdominal fat layer) injection. **The intramuscular route of administration should be avoided because of the frequent occurrence of hematoma at the injection site.**

The dosage of heparin soldium should be adjusted according to the patient's coagulation test results. When heparin is given by continuous intravenous infusion, the coagulation time should be determined approximately every 4 hours in the early stages of treatment. When the drug is administered intermittently by intravenous injection, coagulation tests should be performed before each injection during the early stages of treatment and at appropriate intervals thereafter. Dosage is considered adequate when the activated partial thromboplastin time (APTT) is 1.5 to 2 times normal or when the whole blood clotting time is elevated approximately 2.5 to 3 times the control value. After deep subcutaneous (intrafat) injections, tests for adequacy of dosage are best performed on samples drawn 4–6 hours after the injections.

Periodic platelet counts, hematocrits, and tests for occult blood in stool are recommended during the entire course of heparin therapy, regardless of the route of administration.

Converting to Oral Anticoagulant: When an oral anticoagulant of the coumarin or similar type is to be begun in patients already receiving heparin sodium, baseline and subsequent tests of prothrombin activity must be determined at a time when heparin activity is too low to affect the prothrombin time. This is about 5 hours after the last I.V. bolus and 24 hours after the last subcutaneous dose. If continuous I.V. heparin infusion is used, prothrombin time can usually be measured at any time.

In converting from heparin to an oral anticoagulant, the dose of the oral anticoagulant should be the usual initial amount and thereafter prothrombin time should be determined at the usual intervals. To ensure continuous anticoagulation, it is advisable to continue full heparin therapy for several days after the prothrombin time has reached the therapeutic range. Heparin therapy may then be discontinued without tapering.

Therapeutic Anticoagulant Effect with Full-Dose Heparin. Although dosage must be adjusted for the individual patient according to the results of suitable laboratory tests, the following dosage schedules may be used as guidelines:

[See table on top next page].

Pediatric Use: Follow recommendations of appropriate pediatric reference texts. In general, the following dosage schedule may be used as a guideline:

Initial Dose:	50 units/kg (I.V., drip)
Maintenance Dose:	100 units/kg (I.V., drip) every four hours, or 20,000 units/M^2/24 hours continuously

Surgery of the Heart and Blood Vessels: Patients undergoing total body perfusion for open-heart surgery should receive an initial dose of not less than 150 units of heparin sodium per kilogram of body weight. Frequently, a dose of 300 units per kilogram is used for procedures estimated to last less than 60 minutes or 400 units per kilogram for those estimated to last longer than 60 minutes.

Low-Dose Prophylaxis of Postoperative Thromboembolism: A number of well-controlled clinical trials have demonstrated that low-dose heparin prophylaxis, given just prior to and after surgery, will reduce the incidence of postoperative deep vein thrombosis in the legs (as measured by the I-125 fibrinogen technique and venography) and of clinical pulmonary embolism. The most widely used dosage has been 5,000 units 2 hours before surgery and 5,000 units every 8 to 12 hours thereafter for 7 days or until the patient is fully ambulatory, whichever is longer. The heparin is given by deep subcutaneous (intrafat, i.e., above the iliac crest or abdominal fat layer, arm or thigh) injection with a fine (25 to 26 - gauge) needle to minimize tissue trauma. A concentrated solution of heparin sodium is recommended. Such prophylaxis should be reserved for patients over the age of 40 who are undergoing major surgery. Patients with bleeding disorders and those having brain or spinal cord surgery, spinal anesthesia, eye surgery, or potentially sanguineous operations should be excluded, as should patients receiving oral anticoagulants or platelet-active drugs (see WARNINGS). The value of such prophylaxis in hip surgery has not been established. The possibility of increased bleeding during surgery or postoperatively should be borne in mind. If such bleeding occurs, discontinuance of heparin and neutralization with protamine sulfate are advisable. If clinical evidence of thromboembolism develops despite low-dose prophylaxis, full therapeutic doses of anticoagulants should be given unless contraindicated. Prior to initiating heparinization the physician should rule out bleeding disorders by appropriate history and laboratory tests, and appropriate coagulations tests should be repeated just prior to surgery. Coagulation tests values should be normal or only slightly elevated at these times.

Extracorporeal Dialysis: Follow equipment manufacturers' operating directions carefully.

Blood Transfusion: Addition of 400 to 600 USP units per 100 ml of whole blood is usually employed to prevent coagulation. Usually, 7,500 USP units of heparin sodium are added to 100 ml of 0.9% Sodium Chloride Injection, USP (or 75,000 USP units per 1,000 ml of 0.9% Sodium Chloride Injection, USP) and mixed; from this sterile solution, 6 to 8 ml are added per 100 ml of whole blood.

Laboratory Samples: Addition of 70 to 150 units of heparin sodium per 10 to 20 ml sample of whole blood is usually employed to prevent coagulation of the sample. Leukoycte

METHOD OF ADMINISTRATION	FREQUENCY	RECOMMENDED DOSE*
Deep Subcutaneous (Intrafat) Injection	Initial Dose	5,000 units by I.V. injection, followed by 10,000–20,000 units of a concentrated solution, subcutaneously
A different site should be used for each injection to prevent the development of massive hematoma.	Every 8 hours	8,000 –10,000 units of a concentrated solution
	or Every 12 hours	15,000–20,000 units of a concentrated solution
Intermittent Intravenous Injection	Initial Dose	10,000 units, either undiluted or in 50–100 ml of 0.9% Sodium Chloride Injection, USP
	Every 4 to 6 hours	5,000–10,000 units, either diluted or in 50–100 ml of 0.9% Sodium Chloride Injection, USP
Continuous intravenous Infusion	Initial Dose	5,000 units by I.V. injection
	Continuous	20,000–40,000 units/24 hours in 1,000 ml of 0.9% Sodium Chloride Injection, USP (or in any compatible solution) for infusion

*Based on 150-lb. (68-kg) patient.

counts should be performed on heparinized blood within 2 hours after addition of the heparin. Heparinized blood should not be used for isoagglutinin, complement, or erythrocyte fragility tests or platelet counts.

Clearing Intermittent Infusion (Heparin Lock) Sets: To prevent clot formation in a heparin lock set following its proper insertion, dilute heparin solution (Heparin Lock Flush Solution, USP) is injected via the injection hub in a quantity sufficient to fill the entire set to the needle tip. This solution should be replaced each time the heparin lock is used. Aspirate before administering any solution via the lock in order to confirm patency and location of needle or catheter tip. If the drug to be administered is incompatible with heparin, the entire heparin lock set should be flushed with sterile water or normal saline before and after the medication is administered; following the second flush, the dilute heparin solution may be reinstilled into the set. The set manufacturer's instructions should be consulted for specifics concerning the heparin lock set in use at a given time.

NOTE: Since repeated injections of small doses of heparin can alter tests for activated partial thromboplastin time (APTT), a baseline value for APTT should be obtained prior to insertion of a heparin lock set.

HOW SUPPLIED

Heparin Sodium Injection, USP derived **from beef lung** is available in the following strengths and package sizes:

1,000 units per ml	
10 ml vials	NDC 0009-0268-01
25–10 ml vials	NDC 0009-0268-07
30 ml vials	NDC 0009-0268-02
5,000 units per ml	
1 ml vials	NDC 0009-0291-02
10 ml vials	NDC 0009-0291-01
10,000 units per ml	
1 ml vials	NDC 0009-0317-01
25–1 ml vials	NDC 0009-0317-08
4 ml vials	NDC 0009-0317-02
25–4 ml vials	NDC 0009-0317-09

Code 810 670 011

KAOPECTATE® Anti-Diarrhea Medicine

(See PDR For Nonprescription Drugs)

KAOPECTATE CONCENTRATE®
Anti-Diarrhea Medicine

(See PDR For Nonprescription Drugs)

LINCOCIN® ℞

brand of lincomycin hydrochloride capsules and lincomycin hydrochloride sterile solution (lincomycin hydrochloride capsules, USP, and lincomycin hydrochloride injection, USP)

WARNING

Lincomycin therapy has been associated with severe colitis which may end fatally. Therefore, it should be reserved for serious infections where less toxic antimicrobial agents are inappropriate, as described in the Indications Section. It should not be used in patients with nonbacterial infections, such as most upper respiratory tract infections. Studies indicate a toxin(s) produced by *Clostridia* is one primary cause of antibiotic associated colitis. The colitis is usually characterized by severe, persistent diarrhea and severe abdominal cramps and may be associated with the passage of blood and mucus. Endoscopic examination may reveal pseudomembranous colitis.

When significant diarrhea occurs, the drug should be discontinued or, if necessary, continued only with close observation of the patient. Large bowel endoscopy has been recommended.

Antiperistaltic agents such as opiates and diphenoxylate with atropine (Lomotil) may prolong and/or worsen the condition. Vancomycin has been found to be effective in the treatment of antibiotic associated pseudomembranous colitis produced by *Clostridium difficile*. The usual adult dose is 500 milligrams to 2 grams of vancomycin orally per day in three to four divided doses administered for 7 to 10 days. Cholestyramine or colestipol resins bind vancomycin *in vitro*. If both a resin and vancomycin are to be administered concurrently, it may be advisable to separate the time of administration of each drug.

Diarrhea, colitis, and pseudomembranous colitis have been observed to begin up to several weeks following cessation of therapy with lincomycin.

DESCRIPTION

LINCOCIN Capsules and LINCOCIN Sterile Solution contain lincomycin hydrochloride which is the monohydrated salt of lincomycin, a substance produced by the growth of a member of the *lincolnensis* group of *Streptomyces lincolnensis* (Fam. *Streptomycetaceae*). It is a white, or practically white, crystalline powder and is odorless or has a faint odor. Its solutions are acid and are dextrorotatory. Lincomycin hydrochloride is freely soluble in water; soluble in dimethylformamide and very slightly soluble in acetone.

LINCOCIN Capsules contain the following inactive ingredients: erythrosine sodium, FD&C blue No. 1, gelatin, lactose, magnesium stearate, talc and titanium dioxide.

CLINICAL PHARMACOLOGY

Microbiology—Lincomycin has been shown to be effective against most of the common gram-positive pathogens. Depending on the sensitivity of the organism and concentration of the antibiotic, it may be either bactericidal or bacteriostatic. Cross resistance has not been demonstrated with penicillin, chloramphenicol, ampicillin, cephalosporins or the tetracyclines. Despite chemical differences, lincomycin exhibits antibacterial activity similar but not identical to the macrolide antibiotics (eg erythromycin). Some cross resistance (with erythromycin) including a phenomenon known as dissociated cross resistance or macrolide effect has been reported. Microorganisms have not developed resistance to lincomycin rapidly when tested by *in vitro* or *in vivo* methods. Staphylococci develop resistance to lincomycin in a slow, step-wise manner based on *in vitro*, serial subculture experiments. This pattern of resistance development is unlike that shown for streptomycin.

Studies indicate that lincomycin does not share antigenicity with penicillin compounds.

Biological Studies—*In vitro* studies indicate that the spectrum of activity includes *Staphylococcus aureus, Staphylococcus albus, β-hemolytic Streptococcus, Streptococcus viridans, Diplococcus pneumoniae, Clostridium tetani, Clostridium perfringens, Corynebacterium diphtheriae and Corynebacterium acnes.*

NOTE: The drug is not active against most strains of *Streptococcus faecalis,* nor against *Neisseria gonorrhoeae, Neisseria meningitidis, Hemophilus influenzae,* or other gram-negative organisms or yeasts.

Human Pharmacology—Lincomycin is absorbed rapidly after a 500 mg oral dose, reaching peak levels in 2 to 4 hours. Levels are maintained above the MIC (minimum inhibitory concentration) for most gram-positive organisms for 6 to 8 hours. Urinary recovery of drug in a 24-hour period ranges from 1.0 to 31 percent (mean: 4.0) after a single oral dose of 500 mg of lincomycin. Tissue level studies indicate that bile is an important route of excretion. Significant levels have been demonstrated in the majority of body tissues. Although the drug is not present in significant amounts in the spinal fluid of normal volunteers, it has been demonstrated in the spinal fluid of one patient with pneumococcal meningitis.

Intramuscular administration of a single dose of 600 mg produces a peak serum level at 30 minutes with detectable levels persisting for 24 hours. Urinary excretion after this dose ranges from 1.8 to 24.8 percent (mean: 17.3).

The intravenous infusion over a 2-hour interval of 600 mg of lincomycin hydrochloride in 500 ml of 5 percent glucose in distilled water yields therapeutic levels for 14 hours. Urinary excretion ranges from 4.9 to 30.3 percent (mean: 13.8).

The biological half-life, after oral, intramuscular or intravenous administration is 5.4 ± 1.0 hours.

Hemodialysis and peritoneal dialysis do not effectively remove lincomycin from the blood.

INDICATIONS AND USAGE

LINCOCIN preparations (lincomycin) are indicated in the treatment of serious infections due to susceptible strains of streptococci, pneumococci, and staphylococci. Its use should be reserved for penicillin-allergic patients or other patients for whom, in the judgment of the physician, a penicillin is inappropriate. Because of the risk of colitis, as described in the WARNING box, before selecting lincomycin the physician should consider the nature of the infection and the suitability of less toxic alternatives (eg, erythromycin).

Lincomycin has been demonstrated to be effective in the treatment of staphylococcal infections resistant to other antibiotics and susceptible to lincomycin. Staphylococcal strains resistant to LINCOCIN have been recovered; culture and susceptibility studies should be done in conjunction with therapy with LINCOCIN. In the case of macrolides, partial but not complete cross resistance may occur (see **Microbiology**). The drug may be administered concomitantly with other antimicrobial agents when indicated.

CONTRAINDICATIONS

This drug is contraindicated in patients previously found to be hypersensitive to lincomycin or clindamycin. It is not indicated in the treatment of minor bacterial infections or viral infections.

WARNINGS

See WARNING box. Studies indicate a toxin(s) produced by *Clostridia* is one primary cause of antibiotic associated colitis.[1–5] Mild cases of colitis may respond to drug discontinuance alone. Moderate to severe cases should be managed promptly with fluid, electrolyte and protein supplementation as indicated. Vancomycin has been found to be effective in the treatment of antibiotic associated pseudomembranous colitis produced by *Clostridium difficile.* The usual adult dosage is 500 milligrams to 2 grams of vancomycin orally per

Continued on next page

Information on these Upjohn products is based on labeling in effect August 15, 1986. Further information concerning these and other Upjohn products may be obtained by direct inquiry to Medical Information, The Upjohn Company, Kalamazoo, Michigan 49001.

Upjohn—Cont.

day in three to four divided doses administered for 7 to 10 days. Cholestyramine or colestipol resins bind vancomycin *in vitro.* If both a resin and vancomycin are to be administered concurrently, it may be advisable to separate the time of administration of each drug. Systemic corticoids and corticoid retention enemas may help relieve the colitis. Other causes of colitis should also be considered.
A careful inquiry should be made concerning previous sensitivities to drugs and other allergens.
Usage in Pregnancy—Safety for use in pregnancy has not been established.
Usage in Newborn—Until further clinical experience is obtained, LINCOCIN preparations (lincomycin) are not indicated in the newborn.
Nursing Mothers—LINCOCIN has been reported to appear in breast milk in ranges of 0.5 to 2.4 mcg/ml.
LINCOCIN Sterile Solution contains benzyl alcohol which has been associated with a fatal gasping syndrome in infants.

1. Bailey, WR, Scott, EG, *Diagnostic Microbiology* CV Mosby Company, St. Louis, 1978.
2. Bartlett, JG, et al, "Clindamycin-associated Colitis due to a Toxin-producing Species of *Clostridium* in Hamsters" *J. Inf. Dis.* **136**(5): 701–705, (November) 1977.
3. Larson, HE, Price, AB, "Pseudomembranous Colitis: Presence of Clostridial Toxin," *Lancet,* 1312–1314 (December) 24 and 31, 1977.
4. Lusk, RH, et al, "Clindamycin-Induced Enterocolitis in Hamsters", *J. Inf. Dis.* **137**(4): 464–474 (April) 1978.
5. "Antibiotic-associated Colitis: A Progress Report", *British Med. J.* **1**:669–671 (March 18) 1978.

PRECAUTIONS

Review of experience to date suggests that a subgroup of older patients with associated severe illness may tolerate diarrhea less well. When LINCOCIN preparations (lincomycin) are indicated in these patients, they should be carefully monitored for change in bowel frequency.
LINCOCIN should be prescribed with caution in individuals with a history of gastrointestinal disease, particularly colitis.
LINCOCIN, like any drug, should be used with caution in patients with a history of asthma or significant allergies.
The use of antibiotics occasionally results in overgrowth of nonsusceptible organisms—particularly yeasts. Should superinfections occur, appropriate measures should be taken. When patients with pre-existing monilial infections require therapy with LINCOCIN, concomitant antimonilial treatment should be given.
During prolonged therapy with LINCOCIN, periodic liver and renal function studies and blood counts should be performed.
Since adequate data are not yet available in patients with pre-existing liver disease, its use in such patients is not recommended at this time unless special clinical circumstances so indicate.
Lincomycin has been shown to have neuromuscular blocking properties that may enhance the action of other neuromuscular blocking agents. Therefore, it should be used with caution in patients receiving such agents.
Indicated surgical procedures should be performed in conjunction with antibiotic therapy.

ADVERSE REACTIONS

Gastrointestinal—Glossitis, stomatitis, nausea, vomiting. Persistent diarrhea, enterocolitis and pruritus ani. (See **Warning** box)
Hematopoietic: Neutropenia, leukopenia, agranulocytosis and thrombocytopenic purpura have been reported. There have been rare reports of aplastic anemia and pancytopenia in which LINCOCIN preparations (lincomycin hydrochloride) could not be ruled out as the causative agent.
Hypersensitivity Reactions—Hypersensitivity reactions such as angioneurotic edema, serum sickness and anaphylaxis have been reported, some of these in patients known to be sensitive to penicillin. Rare instances of erythema multiforme, some resembling Stevens-Johnson syndrome, have been associated with LINCOCIN. If an allergic reaction should occur, the drug should be discontinued and the usual agents (epinephrine, corticosteroids, antihistamines) should be available for emergency treatment.
Skin and Mucous Membranes—Skin rashes, urticaria and vaginitis and rare instances of exfoliative and vesiculobullous dermatitis have been reported.
Liver—Although no direct relationship of LINCOCIN to liver dysfunction has been established, jaundice and abnormal liver function tests (particularly elevations of serum transaminase) have been observed in a few instances.
Renal—Although no direct relationship of lincomycin to renal damage has been established, renal dysfunction as evidenced by azotemia, oliguria, and/or proteinuria has been observed in rare instances.
Cardiovascular—After too rapid intravenous administration, rare instances of cardiopulmonary arrest and hypotension have been reported. (See **Dosage and Administration**).
Special Senses—Tinnitus and vertigo have been reported occasionally.
Local Reactions—Patients have demonstrated excellent local tolerance to intramuscularly administered LINCOCIN. Reports of pain following injection have been infrequent. Intravenous administration of LINCOCIN in 250 to 500 ml of 5 percent glucose in distilled water or normal saline produced no local irritation or phlebitis.

DOSAGE AND ADMINISTRATION

If significant diarrhea occurs during therapy, this antibiotic should be discontinued. (See **Warning** box).
***Oral*—Adults:** *Serious infections*—500 mg 3 times per day (500 mg approximately every 8 hours). *More severe infections*—500 mg or more 4 times per day (500 mg or more approximately every 6 hours). **Children over 1 month of age:** *Serious infections*—30 mg/kg/day (15 mg/lb/day) divided into 3 or 4 equal doses. *More severe infections*—60 mg/kg/day (30 mg/lb/day) divided into 3 or 4 equal doses. With β-hemolytic streptococcal infections, treatment should continue for at least 10 days to diminish the likelihood of subsequent rheumatic fever or glomerulonephritis.
NOTE: For optimal absorption it is recommended that nothing be given by mouth except water for a period of one to two hours before and after oral administration of LINCOCIN preparations (lincomycin).
***Intramuscular*—Adults:** *Serious infections*—600 mg (2 ml) intramuscularly every 24 hours. *More severe infections*—600 mg (2 ml) intramuscularly every 12 hours or more often.
Children over 1 month of age: *Serious infections*—one intramuscular injection of 10 mg/kg (5 mg/lb) every 24 hours. *More severe infections*—one intramuscular injection of 10 mg/kg (5 mg/lb) every 12 hours or more often.
***Intravenous*—Adults:** The intravenous dose will be determined by the severity of the infection. For serious infections doses of 600 mg of lincomycin (2 ml of LINCOCIN Sterile Solution) to 1 gram are given every 8-12 hours. For more severe infections these doses may have to be increased. In life-threatening situations daily intravenous doses of as much as 8 grams have been given. **Intranvenous doses are given on the basis of 1 gram of lincomycin diluted in not less than 100 ml of appropriate solution (see PHYSICAL COMPATIBILITIES) and infused over a period of not less than one hour.**

Dose	Vol. Diluent	Time
600 mg	100 ml	1 hr
1 gram	100 ml	1 hr
2 grams	200 ml	2 hr
3 grams	300 ml	3 hr
4 grams	400 ml	4 hr

These doses may be repeated as often as required to the limit of the maximum recommended daily dose of 8 grams of lincomycin.
Children over 1 month of age: 10-20 mg/kg/day (5-10 mg/lb/day) depending on the severity of the infection may be infused in divided doses as described above for adults.
NOTE: Severe cardiopulmonary reactions have occurred when this drug has been given at greater than the recommended concentration and rate.
Subconjunctival Injection—0.25 ml (75 mg) injected subconjunctivally will result in ocular fluid levels of antibiotic (lasting for at least 5 hours) with MIC's sufficient for most susceptible pathogens.
Patients with diminished renal function: *When therapy with LINCOCIN is required in individuals with severe impairment of renal function, an appropriate dose is 25 to 30% of that recommended for patients with normally functioning kidneys.*

HOW SUPPLIED

LINCOCIN Capsules (lincomycin) are available in the following strengths and package sizes:
250 mg Pediatric (blue):
Bottles of 24 *NDC 0009-0336-01*
500 mg (powder blue and dark blue):
Bottles of 24 *NDC 0009-0500-01*
Bottles of 100 *NDC 0009-0500-02*
LINCOCIN Capsules contain lincomycin hydrochloride equivalent to 250 mg or 500 mg of lincomycin.
LINCOCIN Sterile Solution is available in the following strength and package sizes:
300 mg
2 ml Syringe—NDC 0009-0600-01
2 ml Vials—NDC 0009-0555-01
10 ml Vials—NDC 0009-0555-02
Each ml of LINCOCIN Sterile Solution contains lincomycin hydrochloride equivalent to lincomycin 300 mg; also benzyl alcohol, 9.45 mg added as preservative.
Store at controlled room temperature 15°-30°C (59°-86°F).

ANIMAL PHARMACOLOGY

In vivo experimental animal studies demonstrated the effectiveness of LINCOCIN preparations (lincomycin) in protecting animals infected with *Streptococcus viridans, β-hemolytic Streptococcus, Staphylococcus aureus, Diplococcus pneumoniae* and *Leptospira pomona.* It was ineffective in *Klebsiella, Pasteurella, Pseudomonas, Salmonella* and *Shigella* infections.

CLINICAL STUDIES

Experience with 345 obstetrical patients receiving this drug revealed no ill effects related to pregnancy.
Physical Compatibilities:
Physically compatible for 24 hours at room temperature unless otherwise indicated.
Infusion Solutions
Dextrose in Water, 5% and 10%
Dextrose in Saline, 5% and 10%
Ringer's Solution
Sodium Lactate 1/6 Molar
Travert 10%—Electrolyte No. 1
Dextran in Saline 6% w/v
Vitamins in Infusion Solutions
B-Complex
B-Complex with Ascorbic Acid
Antibiotics in Infusion Solutions
Penicillin G Sodium (Satisfactory for 4 hours)
Cephalothin
Tetracycline HCl
Cephaloridine
Colistimethate (Satisfactory for 4 hours)
Ampicillin
Methicillin
Chloramphenicol
Polymyxin B Sulfate
Physically Incompatible with:
Novobiocin
Kanamycin
IT SHOULD BE EMPHASIZED THAT THE COMPATIBLE AND INCOMPATIBLE DETERMINATIONS ARE PHYSICAL OBSERVATIONS ONLY, NOT CHEMICAL DETERMINATIONS. ADEQUATE CLINICAL EVALUATION OF THE SAFETY AND EFFICACY OF THESE COMBINATIONS HAS NOT BEEN PERFORMED.
Code 810 174 006

LONITEN® ℞

brand of minoxidil tablets

10 mg, 100's
NSN 6505-01-088-8120(M & VA)

2.5 mg, 100's
NSN 6505-01-088-8121(VA)

WARNINGS

LONITEN Tablets contain the powerful antihypertensive agent, minoxidil, which may produce serious adverse effects. It can cause pericardial effusion, occasionally progressing to tamponade, and angina pectoris may be exacerbated. LONITEN should be reserved for hypertensive patients who do not respond adequately to maximum therapeutic doses of a diuretic and two other antihypertensive agents.
In experimental animals, minoxidil caused several kinds of myocardial lesions as well as other adverse cardiac effects (see Cardiac Lesions in Animals).
LONITEN must be administered under close supervision, usually concomitantly with therapeutic doses of a beta-adrenergic blocking agent to prevent tachycardia and increased myocardial workload. It must also usually be given with a diuretic, frequently one acting in the ascending limb of the loop of Henle, to prevent serious fluid accumulation. Patients with malignant hypertension and those already receiving guanethidine (see Warnings) should be hospitalized when LONITEN is first administered so that they can be monitored to avoid too rapid, or large orthostatic, decreases in blood pressure.

DESCRIPTION

LONITEN Tablets contain minoxidil, an antihypertensive peripheral vasodilator. Minoxidil occurs as a white or off-white, odorless, crystalline solid that is soluble in water to the extent of approximately 2 mg/ml; is readily soluble in propylene glycol or ethanol; and is almost insoluble in acetone, chloroform or ethyl acetate. The chemical name for minoxidil is 2,4-pyrimidinediamine, 6-(1-piperidinyl)-, 3-oxide (mw = 209.25).
LONITEN Tablets for oral administration contain either 2.5 mg or 10 mg of minoxidil. Inactive ingredients: cellulose, corn starch, lactose, magnesium stearate, silicon dioxide.

CLINICAL PHARMACOLOGY

1. General Pharmacologic Properties
Minoxidil is an orally effective direct acting peripheral vasodilator that reduces elevated systolic and diastolic blood pressure by decreasing peripheral vascular resistance. Microcirculatory blood flow in animals is enhanced or maintained in all systemic vascular beds. In man, forearm and

renal vascular resistance decline; forearm blood flow increases while renal blood flow and glomerular filtration rate are preserved.
Because it causes peripheral vasodilation, minoxidil elicits a number of predictable reactions. Reduction of peripheral arteriolar resistance and the associated fall in blood pressure trigger sympathetic, vagal inhibitory, and renal homeostatic mechanisms, including an increase in renin secretion, that lead to increased cardiac rate and output and salt and water retention. These adverse effects can usually be minimized by concomitant administration of a diuretic and a beta-adrenergic blocking agent or other sympathetic nervous system suppressant.
Minoxidil does not interfere with vasomotor reflexes and therefore does not produce orthostatic hypotension. The drug does not enter the central nervous system in experimental animals in significant amounts, and it does not affect CNS function in man.

2. Effects on Blood Pressure and Target Organs
The extent and time-course of blood pressure reduction by minoxidil do not correspond closely to its concentration in plasma. After an effective single oral dose, blood pressure usually starts to decline within one-half hour, reaches a minimum between 2 and 3 hours and recovers at an arithmetically linear rate of about 30%/day. The total duration of effect is approximately 75 hours. When minoxidil is administered chronically, once or twice a day, the time required to achieve maximum effect on blood pressure with a given daily dose is inversely related to the size of the dose. Thus, maximum effect is achieved on 10 mg/day within 7 days, on 20 mg/day within 5 days, and on 40 mg/day within 3 days.
The blood pressure response to minoxidil is linearly related to the logarithm of the dose administered. The slope of this log-linear dose-response relationship is proportional to the extent of hypertension and approaches zero at a supine diastolic blood pressure of approximately 85 mmHg.
When used in severely hypertensive patients resistant to other therapy, frequently with an accompanying diuretic and beta-blocker, LONITEN Tablets (minoxidil) usually decreased the blood pressure and reversed encephalopathy and retinopathy."

3. Absorption and Metabolism
Minoxidil is at least 90% absorbed from the GI tract in experimental animals and man. Plasma levels of the parent drug reach maximum within the first hour and decline rapidly thereafter. The average plasma half-life in man is 4.2 hours. Approximately 90% of the administered drug is metabolized, predominantly by conjugation with glucuronic acid at the N-oxide position in the pyrimidine ring, but also by conversion to more polar products. Known metabolites exert much less pharmacologic effect than minoxidil itself; all are excreted principally in the urine. Minoxidil does not bind to plasma proteins, and its renal clearance corresponds to the glomerular filtration rate. In the absence of functional renal tissue, minoxidil and its metabolites can be removed by hemodialysis.

4. Cardiac Lesions in Animals
Minoxidil produced two types of cardiac lesions in non-primate species:

(a) Dog atrial lesion—
Daily oral doses of 0.5 mg/kg for several days to 1 month or longer produced a grossly visible hemorrhagic lesion of the right atrium of the dog. This lesion has not been seen in other species. Microscopic examination showed replacement of myocardial cells by proliferating fibroblasts and angioblasts; phagocytosis; and hemosiderin accumulation in macrophages.

(b) Papillary muscle lesion—
Short term treatment (about 3 days) in several species (dog, rat, minipig) produced necrosis of the papillary muscles, and, in some cases subendocardial areas of the left ventricle, lesions similar to those produced by other peripheral dilators and by beta-adrenergic receptor agonists such as isoproterenol and epinephrine. These are thought to result from myocardial ischemia resulting from reflex sympathetic or vagal withdrawal-induced tachycardia in combination with hypotension. These lesions were reduced in incidence and severity by beta-adrenergic receptor blockade.

(c) *Hemorrhagic lesions* were seen in many parts of the heart, mainly in the epicardium, endocardium, and walls of small coronary arteries and arterioles, after acute minoxidil treatment in dogs, and left atrial hemorrhagic lesions were seen in minipigs.

In addition to these lesions, longer term studies in rats, dogs, and monkeys showed cardiac hypertrophy and (in rats) cardiac dilation. In monkeys, hydrochlorothiazide partly reversed the increased heart weight, suggesting it may be related to fluid overload. In a one-year dog study, serosanguinous pericardial fluid was seen.
Autopsies of 79 patients who died from various causes and who had received minoxidil did not reveal right atrial or other hemorrhagic pathology of the kind seen in dogs. Instances of necrotic areas in the papillary muscles were seen, but these occurred in the presence of known pre-existing ischemic heart disease and did not appear different from, or more common than, lesions seen in patients never exposed to minoxidil. Studies to date cannot rule out the possibility that minoxidil can be associated with cardiac damage in humans.

INDICATIONS AND USAGE

Because of the potential for serious adverse effects, LONITEN Tablets (minoxidil) are indicated only in the treatment of hypertension that is symptomatic or associated with target organ damage and is not manageable with maximum therapeutic doses of a diuretic plus two other antihypertensive drugs. At the present time use in milder degrees of hypertension is not recommended because the benefit-risk relationship in such patients has not been defined.
LONITEN reduced supine diastolic blood pressure by 20 mm Hg or to 90 mm Hg or less in approximately 75% of patients, most of whom had hypertension that could not be controlled by other drugs.

CONTRAINDICATIONS

LONITEN Tablets (minoxidil) are contraindicated in pheochromocytoma, because minoxidil may stimulate secretion of catecholamines from the tumor through its antihypertensive action.

WARNINGS

1. Salt and Water Retention; Congestive Heart Failure—concomitant use of an adequate diuretic is required—LONITEN Tablets (minoxidil) must usually be administered concomitantly with a diuretic adequate to prevent fluid retention and possible congestive heart failure; a high ceiling (loop) diuretic is *almost always* required. Body weight should be monitored closely. If LONITEN is used without a diuretic, retention of several hundred milli-equivalents of salt and corresponding volumes of water can occur within a few days, leading to increased plasma and interstitial fluid volume and local or generalized edema. Diuretic treatment alone, or in combination with restricted salt intake, will usually minimize fluid retention, although reversible edema did develop in approximately 10% of nondialysis patients so treated. Ascites has also been reported. Diuretic effectiveness was limited mostly by disease-related impaired renal function. The condition of patients with preexisting congestive heart failure occasionally deteriorated in association with fluid retention although because of the fall in blood pressure (reduction of afterload), more than twice as many improved than worsened. Rarely, refractory fluid retention may require discontinuation of LONITEN. Provided that the patient is under close medical supervision, it may be possible to resolve refractory salt retention by discontinuing LONITEN for 1 or 2 days and then resuming treatment in conjunction with vigorous diuretic therapy.

2. Concomitant Treatment to Prevent Tachycardia is Usually Required—LONITEN increases the heart rate. Angina may worsen or appear for the first time during LONITEN treatment, probably because of the increased oxygen demands associated with increased heart rate and cardiac output. The increase in rate and the occurrence of angina generally can be prevented by the concomitant administration of a beta-adrenergic blocking drug or other sympathetic nervous system suppressant. The ability of beta-adrenergic blocking agents to minimize papillary muscle lesions in animals is further reason to utilize such an agent concomitantly. Round-the-clock effectiveness of the sympathetic suppressant should be ensured.

3. Pericardial Effusion and Tamponade—Pericardial effusion, occasionally with tamponade, has been observed in about 3% of treated patients not on dialysis, especially those with inadequate or compromised renal function. Although in many cases, the pericardial effusion was associated with a connective tissue disease, the uremic syndrome, congestive heart failure, or marked fluid retention, there have been instances in which these potential causes of effusion were not present. Patients should be observed closely for any suggestion of a pericardial disorder, and echocardiographic studies should be carried out if suspicion arises. More vigorous diuretic therapy, dialysis, pericardiocentesis, or surgery may be required. If the effusion persists, withdrawal of LONITEN should be considered in light of other means of controlling the hypertension and the patient's clinical status.

4. *Interaction with Guanethidine:*
Although minoxidil does not itself cause orthostatic hypotension, its administration to patients already receiving guanethidine can result in profound orthostatic effects. If at all possible, guanethidine should be discontinued well before minoxidil is begun. Where this is not possible, minoxidil therapy should be started in the hospital and the patient should remain institutionalized until severe orthostatic effects are no longer present or the patient has learned to avoid activities that provoke them.

5. *Hazard of Rapid Control of Blood Pressure:*
In patients with very severe blood pressure elevation, too rapid control of blood pressure, especially with intravenous agents, can precipitate syncope, cerebrovascular accidents, myocardial infarction and ischemia of special sense organs with resulting decrease or loss of vision or hearing. Patients with compromised circulation or cryoglobulinemia may also suffer ischemic episodes of the affected organs. Although such events have not been unequivocally associated with minoxidil use, total experience is limited at present.
Any patient with malignant hypertension should have initial treatment with minoxidil carried out in a hospital setting, both to assure that blood pressure is falling and to assure that it is not falling more rapidly than intended.

PRECAUTIONS

1. General Precautions—(a) **Monitor fluid and electrolyte balance and body weight** (see **Warnings:** Salt and Water Retention).
(b) **Observe patients for signs and symptoms of pericardial effusion** (see **Warnings:** Pericardial Effusion and Tamponade).
(c) Use after myocardial infarction—LONITEN Tablets (minoxidil) have not been used in patients who have had a myocardial infarction within the preceding month. It is possible that a reduction of arterial pressure with LONITEN might further limit blood flow to the myocardium, although this might be compensated by decreased oxygen demand because of lower blood pressure.
(d) **Hypersensitivity**—Possible hypersensitivity to LONITEN, manifested as a skin rash, has been seen in less than 1% of patients; whether the drug should be discontinued when this occurs depends on treatment alternatives.
(e) **Renal failure or dialysis patients** may require smaller doses of LONITEN and should have close medical supervision to prevent exacerbation of renal failure or precipitation of cardiac failure.

2. Information for patient—The patient should be made fully aware of the importance of continuing all of his antihypertensive medications and of the nature of symptoms that would suggest fluid overload. A patient brochure has been prepared and is included with each LONITEN package. The text of this brochure is reprinted at the end of the insert.

3. Laboratory tests
Those laboratory tests which are abnormal at the time of initiation of minoxidil therapy, such as urinalysis, renal function tests. EKG, chest x-ray, echocardiogram, etc., should be repeated at intervals to ascertain whether improvement or deterioration is occuring under minoxidil therapy. Initially, such tests should be performed frequently, eg, 1–3 month intervals; later as stabilization occurs, at intervals of 6–12 months.

4. Drug Interactions
See "Interaction with guanethidine" under **WARNINGS.**

5. Carcinogenesis, Mutagenesis and Impairment of Fertility—Twenty-two month carcinogenicity studies in rats at doses 15 times the human dose did not provide evidence of tumorigenicity. The drug was not mutagenic in the Salmonella (Ames) test.
Rats receiving up to five times the human dose of minoxidil had a reduction in conception rate, possibly related to drug treatment. There was no evidence of increased fetal resorptions in rats but they did occur in rabbits.

6. Pregnancy-Teratogenic Effects—Pregnancy Category C. Minoxidil has been shown to reduce the conception rate in rats and to show evidence of increased fetal absorption in rabbits when administered at five times the human dose. There was no evidence of teratogenic effects in rats and rabbits. There are no adequate and well controlled studies in pregnant women. LONITEN should be used during pregnancy only if the potential benefit justifies the potential risk to the fetus.

7. Labor and delivery
The effects on labor and delivery are unknown.

8. Nursing Mothers—Minoxidil has been reported to be secreted in human milk. As a general rule, nursing should not be undertaken while a patient is on LONITEN.

9. Pediatric Use—Use in children has been limited to date, particularly in infants. The recommendations under **Dosage and Administration** can be considered only a rough guide at present and careful titration is essential.

10. Unapproved Use—Use of LONITEN Tablets, in any formulation, to promote hair growth is not an approved indication. Clinical trials are in progress and are designed to determine efficacy, dosage, duration of treatment, and actual side effects. Pending completion and analysis of these trials, efficacy, dose and duration of the therapy are not known. Because systemic absorption of topically applied drug may occur and is dependent on vehicle and/or method of use, extemporaneous topical formulations made from LONITEN should be considered to share in the full range of CONTRAINDICATIONS, WARNINGS, PRECAUTIONS, and ADVERSE REACTIONS listed in this insert. In addition, skin intolerance to drug and/or vehicle may occur.

Continued on next page

Information on these Upjohn products is based on labeling in effect August 15, 1986. Further information concerning these and other Upjohn products may be obtained by direct inquiry to Medical Information, The Upjohn Company, Kalamazoo, Michigan 49001.

Upjohn—Cont.

ADVERSE REACTIONS

1. Salt and Water Retention (see **Warnings:** Concomitant Use of Adequate Diuretic is Required) —Temporary edema developed in 7% of patients who were not edematous at the start of therapy.

2. Pericardial Effusion and **Tamponade** (see **Warnings**).

3. Dermatologic - Hypertrichosis—Elongation, thickening, and enhanced pigmentation of fine body hair are seen in about 80% of patients taking LONITEN Tablets (minoxidil). This develops within 3 to 6 weeks after starting therapy. It is usually first noticed on the temples, between the eyebrows, between the hairline and the eyebrows, or in the side-burn area of the upper lateral cheek, later extending to the back, arms, legs, and scalp. Upon discontinuation of LONITEN, new hair growth stops, but 1 to 6 months may be required for restoration to pretreatment appearance. No endocrine abnormalities have been found to explain the abnormal hair growth; thus, it is hypertrichosis without virilism. Hair growth is especially disturbing to children and women and such patients should be thoroughly informed about this effect before therapy with LONITEN is begun.

Allergic—Rashes have been reported, including rare reports of bullous eruptions, and Stevens-Johnson Syndrome.

4. Hematologic—Thrombocytopenia and leukopenia (WBC < 3000/mm^3) have rarely been reported.

5. Gastrointestinal—Nausea and/or vomiting has been reported. In clinical trials the incidence of nausea and vomiting associated with the underlying disease has shown a decrease from pretrial levels.

6. Miscellaneous—Breast tenderness—This developed in less than 1% of patients.

7. Altered Laboratory Findings—(a) ECG changes—changes in direction and magnitude of the ECG T-waves occur in approximately 60% of patients treated with LONITEN. In rare instances a large negative amplitude of the T-wave may encroach upon the S-T segment, but the S-T segment is not independently altered. These changes usually disappear with continuance of treatment and revert to the pretreatment state if LONITEN is discontinued. No symptoms have been associated with these changes, nor have there been alterations in blood cell counts or in plasma enzyme concentrations that would suggest myocardial damage. Long-term treatment of patients manifesting such changes has provided no evidence of deteriorating cardiac function. At present the changes appear to be nonspecific and without identifiable clinical significance. (b) Effects of hemodilution—hematocrit, hemoglobin and erythrocyte count usually fall about 7% initially and then recover to pretreatment levels. (c) Other—Alkaline phosphatase increased varyingly without other evidence of liver or bone abnormality. Serum creatinine increased an average of 6% and BUN slightly more, but later declined to pretreatment levels.

OVERDOSAGE

There have been only a few instances of deliberate or accidental overdosage with LONITEN Tablets (minoxidil). One patient recovered after taking 50 mg of minoxidil together with 500 mg of a barbiturate. When exaggerated hypotension is encountered, it is most likely to occur in association with residual sympathetic nervous system blockade from previous therapy (guanethidine-like effects or alpha-adrenergic blockage), which prevents the usual compensatory maintenance of blood pressure. Intravenous administration of normal saline will help to maintain blood pressure and facilitate urine formation in these patients. Sympathomimetic drugs such as norepinephrine or epinephrine should be avoided because of their excessive cardiac stimulating action. Phenylephrine, angiotensin II, vasopressin, and dopamine all reverse hypotension due to LONITEN, but should only be used if underperfusion of a vital organ is evident.

Radioimmunoassay can be performed to determine the concentration of minoxidil in the blood. At the maximum adult dosage of 100 mg/day, peak blood levels of 1641 ng/ml and 2441 ng/ml were observed in two patients, respectively. Due to patient-to-patient variation in blood levels, it is difficult to establish an overdosage warning level. In general, a substantial increase above 2000 ng/ml should be regarded as overdosage, unless the physician is aware that the patient has taken no more than the maximum dose.

Oral LD_{50} in rats has ranged from 1321–3492 mg/kg; in mice, 2456-2648 mg/kg.

DOSAGE AND ADMINISTRATION

Patients over 12 years of age: The recommended initial dosage of LONITEN Tablets (minoxidil) is 5 mg given as a single daily dose. Daily dosage can be increased to 10, 20 and then to 40 mg in single or divided doses if required for optimum blood pressure control. The effective dosage range is usually 10 to 40 mg per day. The maximum recommended dosage is 100 mg per day.

Patients under 12 years of age: The initial dosage is 0.2 mg/kg minoxidil as a single daily dose. The dosage may be increased in 50 to 100% increments until optimum blood pressure control is achieved. The effective dosage range is usually 0.25 to 1.0 mg/kg/day. The maximum recommended dosage is 50 mg daily. (see **9. Pediatric Use** under **Precautions**).

Dose frequency: The magnitude of within-day fluctuation of arterial pressure during therapy with LONITEN is directly proportional to the extent of pressure reduction. If supine diastolic pressure has been reduced less than 30 mmHg, the drug need be administered only once a day; if supine diastolic pressure has been reduced more than 30 mmHg, the daily dosage should be divided into two equal parts.

Frequency of dosage adjustment: Dosage must be titrated carefully according to individual response. Intervals between dosage adjustments normally should be at least 3 days since the full response to a given dose is not obtained for at least that amount of time. **Where a more rapid management of hypertension is required, dose adjustments can be made every 6 hours if the patient is carefully monitored.**

Concomitant therapy: Diuretic and beta-blocker or other sympathetic nervous system supressant.

Diuretics: LONITEN must be used in conjunction with a diuretic in patients relying on renal function for maintaining salt and water balance. Diuretics have been used at the following dosages when starting therapy with LONITEN: hydrochlorothiazide (50 mg, b.i.d.) or other thiazides at equieffective dosage; chlorthalidone (50 to 100 mg, once daily); furosemide (40 mg, b.i.d.). If excessive salt and water retention results in a weight gain of more than 5 pounds, diuretic therapy should be changed to furosemide; if the patient is already taking furosemide, dosage should be increased in accordance with the patient's requirements.

Beta-blocker or other sympathetic nervous system suppressants: When therapy with LONITEN is begun, the dosage of a beta-adrenergic receptor blocking drug should be the equivalent of 80 to 160 mg of propranolol per day in divided doses.

If beta-blockers are contraindicated, methyldopa (250 to 750 mg, b.i.d.) may be used instead. Methyldopa must be given for at least 24 hours before starting therapy with LONITEN because of the delay in the onset of methyldopa's action. Limited clinical experience indicates that clonidine may also be used to prevent tachycardia induced by LONITEN; the usual dosage is 0.1 to 0.2 mg twice daily.

Sympathetic nervous system suppressants may not completely prevent an increase in heart rate due to LONITEN but usually do prevent tachycardia. Typically, patients receiving a beta-blocker prior to initiation of therapy with LONITEN have a bradycardia and can be expected to have an increase in heart rate toward normal when LONITEN is added. When treatment with LONITEN and beta-blocker or other sympathetic nervous system suppressant are begun simultaneously, their opposing cardiac effects usually nullify each other, leading to little change in heart rate.

HOW SUPPLIED

LONITEN Tablets (minoxidil) are available as round, scored, white tablets. Dosage strengths are imprinted on one convex surface. The following strengths and container sizes are available:

Strength	Container and Size	NDC Number
2.5 mg	Unit of Use bottles of 100,	0009-0121-01
10 mg	Unit of Use bottles of 100,	0009-0137-01
	bottles of 500	0009-0137-02

Store at controlled room temperature 15°–30°C (59°–86°F).

Patient Information: LONITEN Tablets contain minoxidil, a medicine for the treatment of high blood pressure in the patient who has not been controlled or is experiencing unacceptable side effects with other medications. It must usually be taken with other medicines.

Be absolutely sure to take all of your medicines for high blood pressure according to your doctor's instructions. Do not stop taking LONITEN unless your doctor tells you to. Do not give any of your medicine to other people.

It is important that you look for the warning signals of certain undesired effects of LONITEN. Call your doctor if they occur. Your doctor will need to see you regularly while you are taking LONITEN. Be sure to keep all your appointments or to arrange for new ones if you must miss one.

Do not hesitate to call your doctor if any discomforts or problems occur.

The information here is intended to help you take LONITEN properly. It does not tell you all there is to know about LONITEN. There is a more technical leaflet that you may request from the pharmacist; you may need your doctor's help in understanding parts of that leaflet.

What is LONITEN?

LONITEN Tablets contain minoxidil which is a drug for lowering the blood pressure. It works by relaxing and enlarging certain small blood vessels so that blood flows through them more easily.

Why lower blood pressure?

Your doctor has prescribed LONITEN to lower your blood pressure and protect vital parts of your body. Uncontrolled blood pressure can cause stroke, heart failure, blindness, kidney failure, and heart attacks.

Most people with high blood pressure need to take medicines to treat it for their whole lives.

Who should take LONITEN?

There are many people with high blood pressure, but most of them do not need LONITEN. LONITEN is used ONLY when your doctor decides that:

1. your high blood pressure is severe;
2. your high blood pressure is causing symptoms or damage to vital organs; and
3. other medicines did not work well enough or had very disturbing side effects.

LONITEN should be taken only when a doctor prescribes it. Never give any of your LONITEN Tablets, or any other high blood pressure medicine, to a friend or relative.

Pregnancy: In some cases doctors may prescribe LONITEN for women who are pregnant or who are planning to have children. However, its safe use in pregnancy has not been established. Laboratory animals had a reduced ability to become pregnant and a reduced survival of offspring while taking LONITEN. If you are pregnant or are planning to become pregnant, be sure to tell your doctor.

How to take LONITEN.

Usually, your doctor will prescribe two other medicines along with LONITEN. These will help lower blood pressure and will help prevent undesired effects of LONITEN.

Often, when a medicine like LONITEN lowers blood pressure, your body tries to return the blood pressure to the original, higher level. It does this by holding on to water and salt (so there will be more fluid to pump) and by making your heart beat faster. To prevent this, your doctor will usually prescribe a water tablet to remove the extra salt and water from your body (a diuretic dye-u-RET-tic) and another medicine to slow your heart beat.

You must follow your doctor's instructions exactly, taking all the prescribed medicines, in the right amounts, each day. These medicines will help keep your blood pressure down. The water tablet and heart beat medicine will help prevent the undesired effects of LONITEN.

LONITEN Tablets come in two strengths (2 ½ milligrams and 10 milligrams) that are marked on each tablet. Pay close attention to the tablet markings to be sure you are taking the correct strength. Your doctor may prescribe half a tablet; the tablets are scored (partly cut on one side) so that you can easily break them.

When you first start taking LONITEN, your doctor may need to see you often in order to adjust your dosage. Take all your medicine according to the schedule prescribed by your doctor. **Do not skip any doses. If you should forget a dose of LONITEN, wait until it is time for your next dose, then continue with your regular schedule. Remember: do not stop taking LONITEN, or any of your other high blood pressure medicines, without checking with your doctor.** Make sure that any doctor treating or examining you knows that you are taking high blood pressure medicines, including LONITEN.

WARNING SIGNALS

Even if you take all your medicines correctly, LONITEN Tablets may cause undesired effects. Some of these are serious and you should be on the lookout for them. **If any of the following warning signals occur, you must call your doctor immediately:**

1. Increase in heart rate —You should measure your heart rate by counting your pulse rate **while you are resting.** If you have an increase of 20 beats or more a minute over your normal pulse, contact your doctor immediately. If you do not know how to take your pulse rate, ask your doctor. Also ask your doctor how often to check your pulse.

2. Rapid weight gain of more than 5 pounds —You should weigh yourself daily. If you quickly gain five or more pounds, or if there is any swelling or puffiness in the face, hands, ankles, or stomach area, this could be a sign that you are retaining body fluids. Your doctor may have to change your drugs or change the dose of your drugs. You may also need to reduce the amount of salt you eat. A smaller weight gain (2 to 3 pounds) often occurs when treatment is started. You may lose this extra weight with continued treatment.

3. Increased difficulty in breathing, especially when lying down. This too may be due to an increase of body fluids. It can also happen because your high blood pressure is getting worse. In either case, you might require treatment with other medicines.

4. New or worsening of pain in the chest, arm, or shoulder or signs of severe indigestion — These could be signs of serious heart problems.

5. Dizziness, lightheadedness or fainting — These can be signs of high blood pressure or they may be side effects from one of the medicines. Your doctor may need to change or adjust the dosage of the medicines you are taking.

OTHER UNDESIRED EFFECTS

LONITEN Tablets can cause other undesired effects such as nausea and/or vomiting that are annoying but not dangerous. Do not stop taking the drug because of these other undesired effects without talking to your doctor.

Hair growth: About 8 out of every 10 patients who have taken LONITEN noticed that fine **body hair grew darker or longer** on certain parts of the body. This happened about three to six weeks after beginning treatment. The hair may first be noticed on the forehead and temples, between the eyebrows, or on the upper part of the cheeks. Later, hair may grow on the back, arms, legs, or scalp. Although hair growth may not be noticeable to some patients, it often is bothersome in women and children. **Unwanted hair can be controlled with a hair remover or by shaving.** The extra hair is not permanent, it disappears within 1 to 6 months of stopping LONITEN. Nevertheless, **you should not stop taking LONITEN without first talking to your doctor.**

A few patients have developed a rash or breast tenderness while taking LONITEN Tablets (minoxidil), but this is unusual.

Code 810 384 210

Shown in Product Identification Section, page 433

MAOLATE® ℞
brand of chlorphenesin carbamate tablets

500's
NSN 6505-00-998-7143 (M & VA)

HOW SUPPLIED
Scored tablets containing 400 mg chlorphenesin carbamate are available in the following packages.

Bottles of 50	*NDC 0009-0412-01*
Bottles of 500	*NDC 0009-0412-02*
Unit dose package (100)	*NDC 0009-0412-03*

Shown in Product Identification Section, page 433

MEDROL® ℞
brand of methylprednisolone acetate topical
For External Use Only

HOW SUPPLIED
In two concentrations-2.5 mg (0.25%) or 10 mg (1.0%) methylprednisolone acetate per gram.

0.25%	7.5 gram tubes	*NDC 0009-0483-01*
	30 gram tubes	*NDC 0009-0483-02*
1%	7.5 gram tubes	*NDC 0009-0505-01*
	30 gram tubes	*NDC 0009-0505-02*

MEDROL® ℞
brand of methylprednisolone tablets, USP

4 mg, 21's Dosepak	**NSN 6505-01-131-5619 (M)**
4 mg, 100's	**NSN 6505-01-134-6647 (M)**
4 mg, 500's	**NSN 6505-00-050-3068 (M&VA)**
16 mg, 50's	**NSN 6505-00-764-4358 (VA)**

DESCRIPTION
MEDROL Tablets contain methylprednisolone which is a glucocorticord. Glucocorticoids are adrenocortical steroids, both naturally occurring and synthetic, which are readily absorbed from the gastrointestinal tract. Methylprednisolone occurs as a white to practically white, odorless, crystalline powder. It is sparingly soluble in alcohol, in dioxane, and in methanol, slightly soluble in acetone, and in chloroform, and very slightly soluble in ether. It is practically insoluble in water.

The chemical name for methylprednisolone is pregna-1, 4-diene-3, 20-dione,11, 17, 21-trihydroxy-6-methyl-,(6α, 11β)- and the molecular weight is 374.48.

Each MEDROL tablet for oral administration contains 2 mg, 4 mg, 8 mg, 16 mg, 24 mg, or 32 mg of methylprednisolone.

Inactive ingredients:

2 mg	**4 and 16 mg**
Calcium Stearate	Calcium Stearate
Corn Starch	Corn Starch
Erythrosine Sodium	Lactose
F D & C Blue No. 1	Mineral Oil
Lactose	Sorbic Acid
Mineral Oil	Sucrose
Sorbic Acid	
Sucrose	
8 and 32 mg	**24 mg**
Calcium Stearate	Calcium Stearate
Corn Starch	Corn Starch
F D & C Yellow No. 6	F D & C Yellow No. 5
Lactose	Lactose
Mineral Oil	Mineral Oil
Sorbic Acid	Sorbic Acid
Sucrose	Sucrose

ACTIONS
Naturally occurring glucocorticoids (hydrocortisone and cortisone), which also have salt-retaining properties, are used as replacement therapy in adrenocortical deficiency states. Their synthetic analogs are primarily used for their potent anti-inflammatory effects in disorders of many organ systems.

Glucocorticoids cause profound and varied metabolic effects. In addition, they modify the body's immune responses to diverse stimuli.

INDICATIONS
MEDROL Tablets (methylprednisolone) are indicated in the following conditions:

1. **Endocrine Disorders**
   Primary or secondary adrenocortical insufficiency (hydrocortisone or cortisone is the first choice; synthetic analogs may be used in conjunction with mineralocorticoids where applicable; in infancy mineralocorticoid supplementation is of particular importance).
   Congenital adrenal hyperplasia
   Nonsuppurative thyroiditis
   Hypercalcemia associated with cancer
2. **Rheumatic Disorders**
   As adjunctive therapy for short-term administration (to tide the patient over an acute episode or exacerbation) in:
   Psoriatic arthritis
   Rheumatoid arthritis, including juvenile rheumatoid arthritis (selected cases may require low-dose maintenance therapy)
   Ankylosing spondylitis
   Acute and subacute bursitis
   Acute nonspecific tenosynovitis
   Acute gouty arthritis
   Post-traumatic osteoarthritis
   Synovitis of osteoarthritis
   Epicondylitis
3. **Collagen Diseases**
   During an exacerbation or as maintenance therapy in selected cases of:
   Systemic lupus erythematosus
   Acute rheumatic carditis
   Systemic dermatomyositis (polymyositis)
4. **Dermatologic Diseases**
   Pemphigus
   Bullous dermatitis herpetiformis
   Severe erythema multiforme (Stevens-Johnson syndrome)
   Exfoliative dermatitis
   Mycosis fungoides
   Severe psoriasis
   Severe seborrheic dermatitis
5. **Allergic States**
   Control of severe or incapacitating allergic conditions intractable to adequate trials of conventional treatment:
   Seasonal or perennial allergic rhinitis
   Serum sickness
   Bronchial asthma
   Drug hypersensitivity reactions
   Contact dermatitis
   Atopic dermatitis
6. **Ophthalmic Diseases**
   Severe acute and chronic allergic and inflammatory processes involving the eye and its adnexa such as:
   Allergic corneal marginal ulcers
   Herpes zoster ophthalmicus
   Anterior segment inflammation
   Diffuse posterior uveitis and choroiditis
   Sympathetic ophthalmia
   Allergic conjunctivitis
   Keratitis
   Chorioretinitis
   Optic neuritis
   Iritis and iridocyclitis
7. **Respiratory Diseases**
   Symptomatic sarcoidosis
   Loeffler's syndrome not manageable by other means
   Berylliosis
   Fulminating or disseminated pulmonary tuberculosis when used concurrently with appropriate antituberculous chemotherapy
   Aspiration pneumonitis
8. **Hematologic Disorders**
   Idiopathic thrombocytopenic purpura in adults
   Secondary thrombocytopenia in adults
   Acquired (autoimmune) hemolytic anemia
   Erythroblastopenia (RBC anemia)
   Congenital (erythroid) hypoplastic anemia
9. **Neoplastic Diseases**
   For palliative management of:
   Leukemias and lymphomas in adults
   Acute leukemia of childhood
10. **Edematous States**
    To induce a diuresis or remission of proteinuria in the nephrotic syndrome, without uremia, of the idiopathic type or that due to lupus erythematosus.
11. **Gastrointestinal diseases**
    To tide the patient over a critical period of the disease in:
    Ulcerative colitis
    Regional enteritis
12. **Nervous System**
    Acute exacerbations of multiple sclerosis
13. **Miscellaneous**
    Tuberculous meningitis with subarachnoid block or impending block when used concurrently with appropriate antituberculous chemotherapy.
    Trichinosis with neurologic or myocardial involvement

CONTRAINDICATIONS
Systemic fungal infections.

WARNINGS
In patients on corticosteroid therapy subjected to unusual stress, increased dosage of rapidly acting corticosteroids before, during, and after the stressful situation is indicated.

Corticosteroids may mask some signs of infection and new infections may appear during their use. There may be decreased resistance and inability to localize infection when corticosteroids are used.

Prolonged use of corticosteroids may produce posterior subcapsular cataracts, glaucoma with possible damage to the optic nerves, and may enhance the establishment of secondary ocular infections due to fungi or viruses.

Usage in pregnancy: Since adequate human reproduction studies have not been done with corticosteroids, the use of these drugs in pregnancy, nursing mothers or women of childbearing potential requires that the possible benefits of the drug be weighed against the potential hazards to the mother and embryo or fetus. Infants born of mothers who have received substantial doses of corticosteroids during pregnancy should be carefully observed for signs of hypoadrenalism.

Average and large doses of hydrocortisone or cortisone can cause elevation of blood pressure, salt and water retention, and increased excretion of potassium. These effects are less likely to occur with the synthetic derivatives except when used in large doses. Dietary salt restriction and potassium supplementation may be necessary. All corticosteroids increase calcium excretion.

While on corticosteroid therapy patients should not be vaccinated against smallpox. Other immunization procedures should not be undertaken in patients who are on corticosteroids, especially on high dose, because of possible hazards of neurological complications and a lack of antibody response.

The use of MEDROL Tablets (methylprednisolone) in active tuberculosis should be restricted to those cases of fulminating or disseminated tuberculosis in which the corticosteroid is used for the management of the disease in conjunction with an appropriate antituberculous regimen.

If corticosteroids are indicated in patients with latent tuberculosis or tuberculin reactivity, close observation is necessary as reactivation of the disease may occur. During prolonged corticosteroid therapy, these patients should receive chemoprophylaxis.

PRECAUTIONS
Drug-induced secondary adrenocortical insufficiency may be minimized by gradual reduction of dosage. This type of relative insufficiency may persist for months after discontinuation of therapy; therefore, in any situation of stress occurring during that period, hormone therapy should be reinstituted. Since mineralocorticoid secretion may be impaired, salt and/or a mineralocorticoid should be administered concurrently.

There is an enhanced effect of corticosteroids on patients with hypothyroidism and in those with cirrhosis.

Corticosteroids should be used cautiously in patients with ocular herpes simplex because of possible corneal perforation.

The lowest possible dose of corticosteroid should be used to control the condition under treatment, and when reduction in dosage is possible, the reduction should be gradual.

Psychic derangements may appear when corticosteroids are used, ranging from euphoria, insomnia, mood swings, personality changes and severe depression, to frank psychotic manifestations. Also, existing emotional instability or psychotic tendencies may be aggravated by corticosteroids.

Aspirin should be used cautiously in conjunction with corticosteroids in hypoprothrombinemia.

Steroids should be used with caution in nonspecific ulcerative colitis, if there is a probability of impending perforation, abscess or other pyogenic infection; diverticulitis; fresh

Continued on next page

Information on these Upjohn products is based on labeling in effect August 15, 1986. Further information concerning these and other Upjohn products may be obtained by direct inquiry to Medical Information, The Upjohn Company, Kalamazoo, Michigan 49001.

Upjohn—Cont.

intestinal anastomoses; active or latent peptic ulcer; renal insufficiency; hypertension; osteoporosis; and myasthenia gravis.

Growth and development of infants and children on prolonged corticosteroid therapy should be carefully observed.

Although controlled clinical trials have shown corticosteroids to be effective in speeding the resolution of acute exacerbations of multiple sclerosis, they do not show that corticosteroids affect the ultimate outcome or natural history of the disease. The studies do show that relatively high doses of corticosteroids are necessary to demonstrate a significant effect. (See **Dosage and Administration**)

Since complications of treatment with glucocorticoids are dependent on the size of the dose and the duration of treatment, a risk/benefit decision must be made in each individual case as to dose and duration of treatment and as to whether daily or intermittent therapy should be used.

The 24 mg tablet contains FD&C Yellow No. 5 (tartrazine) which may cause allergic-type reactions (including bronchial asthma) in certain susceptible individuals. Although the overall incidence of FD&C Yellow No. 5 (tartrazine) sensitivity in the general population is low, it is frequently seen in patients who also have aspirin hypersensitivity.

ADVERSE REACTIONS

Fluid and Electrolyte Disturbances

Sodium retention
Fluid retention
Congestive heart failure in susceptible patients
Potassium loss
Hypokalemic alkalosis
Hypertension

Musculoskeletal

Muscle weakness
Steroid myopathy
Loss of muscle mass
Osteoporosis
Vertebral compression fractures
Aseptic necrosis of femoral and humeral heads
Pathologic fracture of long bones

Gastrointestinal

Peptic ulcer with possible perforation and hemorrhage
Pancreatitis
Abdominal distention
Ulcerative esophagitis

Dermatologic

Impaired wound healing
Thin fragile skin
Petechiae and ecchymoses
Facial erythema
Increased sweating
May suppress reactions to skin tests

Neurological

Increased intracranial pressure with papilledema (pseudotumor cerebri) usually after treatment
Convulsions
Vertigo
Headache

Endocrine

Development of Cushingoid state
Suppression of growth in children
Secondary adrenocortical and pituitary unresponsiveness, particularly in times of stress, as in trauma, surgery or illness.
Menstrual irregularities
Decreased carbohydrate tolerance
Manifestations of latent diabetes mellitus
Increased requirements for insulin or oral hypoglycemic agents in diabetics

Ophthalmic

Posterior subcapsular cataracts
Increased intraocular pressure
Glaucoma
Exophthalmos

Metabolic

Negative nitrogen balance due to protein catabolism

The following additional reactions have been reported following oral as well as parenteral therapy: Urticaria and other allergic, anaphylactic or hypersensitivity reactions.

DOSAGE AND ADMINISTRATION

The initial dosage of MEDROL Tablets (methylprednisolone) may vary from 4 mg to 48 mg per day depending on the specific disease entity being treated. In situations of less severity lower doses will generally suffice while in selected patients higher initial doses may be required. The initial dosage should be maintained or adjusted until a satisfactory response is noted. If after a reasonable period of time there is a lack of satisfactory clinical response, MEDROL should be discontinued and the patient transferred to other appropriate therapy. **IT SHOULD BE EMPHASIZED THAT DOSAGE REQUIREMENTS ARE VARIABLE AND MUST BE INDIVIDUALIZED ON THE BASIS OF THE DISEASE UNDER TREATMENT AND THE RESPONSE OF THE PATIENT.** After a favorable response is noted, the proper maintenance dosage should be determined by decreasing the initial drug dosage in small decrements at appropriate time intervals until the lowest dosage which will maintain an adequate clinical response is reached. It should be kept in mind that constant monitoring is needed in regard to drug dosage. Included in the situations which may make dosage adjustments necessary are changes in clinical status secondary to remissions or exacerbations in the disease process, the patient's individual drug responsiveness, and the effect of patient exposure to stressful situations not directly related to the disease entity under treatment; in this latter situation it may be necessary to increase the dosage of MEDROL for a period of time consistent with the patient's condition. If after long-term therapy the drug is to be stopped, it is recommended that it be withdrawn gradually rather than abruptly.

Multiple Sclerosis

In treatment of acute exacerbations of multiple sclerosis daily doses of 200 mg of prednisolone for a week followed by 80 mg every other day for 1 month have been shown to be effective (4 mg of methylprednisolone is equivalent to 5 mg of prednisolone).

ADT® (Alternate Day Therapy)

Alternate day therapy is a corticosteroid dosing regimen in which twice the usual daily dose of corticoid is administered every other morning. The purpose of this mode of therapy is to provide the patient requiring long-term pharmacologic dose treatment with the beneficial effects of corticoids while minimizing certain undesirable effects, including pituitary-adrenal suppression, the Cushingoid state, corticoid withdrawal symptoms, and growth suppression in children.

The rationale for this treatment schedule is based on two major premises: (a) the anti-inflammatory or therapeutic effect of corticoids persists longer than their physical presence and metabolic effects and (b) administration of the corticosteroid every other morning allows for re-establishment of more nearly normal hypothalamic-pituitary-adrenal (HPA) activity on the off-steroid day.

A brief review of the HPA physiology may be helpful in understanding this rationale. Acting primarily through the hypothalamus a fall in free cortisol stimulates the pituitary gland to produce increasing amounts of corticotropin (ACTH) while a rise in free cortisol inhibits ACTH secretion. Normally the HPA system is characterized by diurnal (circadian) rhythm. Serum levels of ACTH rise from a low point about 10 pm to a peak level about 6 am. Increasing levels of ACTH stimulate adrenal cortical activity resulting in a rise in plasma cortisol with maximal levels occurring between 2 am and 8 am. This rise in cortisol dampens ACTH production and in turn adrenal cortical activity. There is a gradual fall in plasma corticoids during the day with lowest levels occurring about midnight.

The diurnal rhythm of the HPA axis is lost in Cushing's disease, a syndrome of adrenal cortical hyperfunction characterized by obesity with centripetal fat distribution, thinning of the skin with easy bruisability, muscle wasting with weakness, hypertension, latent diabetes, osteoporosis, electrolyte imbalance, etc. The same clinical findings of hyperadrenocorticism may be noted during long-term pharmacologic dose corticoid therapy administered in conventional daily divided doses. It would appear then, that a disturbance in the diurnal cycle with maintenance of elevated corticoid values during the night may play a significant role in the development of undesirable corticoid effects. Escape from these constantly elevated plasma levels for even short periods of time may be instrumental in protecting against undesirable pharmacologic effects.

During conventional pharmacologic dose corticosteroid therapy, ACTH production is inhibited with subsequent suppression of cortisol production by the adrenal cortex. Recovery time for normal HPA activity is variable depending upon the dose and duration of treatment. During this time the patient is vulnerable to any stressful situation. Although it has been shown that there is considerably less adrenal suppression following a single morning dose of prednisolone (10 mg) as opposed to a quarter of that dose administered every 6 hours, there is evidence that some suppressive effect on adrenal activity may be carried over into the following day when pharmacologic doses are used. Further, it has been shown that a single dose of certain corticosteroids will produce adrenal cortical suppression for two or more days. Other corticoids, including methylprednisolone, hydrocortisone, prednisone, and prednisolone, are considered to be short acting (producing adrenal cortical suppression for $1\frac{1}{4}$ to $1\frac{1}{2}$ days following a single dose) and thus are recommended for alternate day therapy.

The following should be kept in mind when considering alternate day therapy:

1) Basic principles and indications for corticosteroid therapy should apply. The benefits of ADT should not encourage the indiscriminate use of steroids.

2) ADT is a therapeutic technique primarily designed for patients in whom long-term pharmacologic corticoid therapy is anticipated.

3) In less severe disease processes in which corticoid therapy is indicated, it may be possible to initiate treatment with ADT. More severe disease states usually will require daily divided high dose therapy for initial control of the disease process. The initial suppressive dose level should be continued until satisfactory clinical response is obtained, usually four to ten days in the case of many allergic and collagen diseases. It is important to keep the period of initial suppressive dose as brief as possible particularly when subsequent use of alternate day therapy is intended.

Once control has been established, two courses are available: (a) change to ADT and then gradually reduce the amount of corticoid given every other day *or* (b) following control of the disease process reduce the daily dose of corticoid to the lowest effective level as rapidly as possible and then change over to an alternate day schedule. Theoretically, course (a) may be preferable.

4) Because of the advantages of ADT, it may be desirable to try patients on this form of therapy who have been on daily corticoids for long periods of time (eg, patients with rheumatoid arthritis). Since these patients may already have a suppressed HPA axis, establishing them on ADT may be difficult and not always successful. However, it is recommended that regular attempts be made to change them over. It may be helpful to triple or even quadruple the daily maintenance dose and administer this every other day rather than just doubling the daily dose if difficulty is encountered. Once the patient is again controlled, an attempt should be made to reduce this dose to a minimum.

5) As indicated above, certain corticosteroids, because of their prolonged suppressive effect on adrenal activity, are not recommended for alternate day therapy (eg, dexamethasone and betamethasone).

6) The maximal activity of the adrenal cortex is between 2 am and 8 am, and it is minimal between 4 pm and midnight. Exogenous corticosteroids suppress adrenocortical activity the least, when given at the time of maximal activity (am).

7) In using ADT it is important, as in all therapeutic situations, to individualize and tailor the therapy to each patient. Complete control of symptoms will not be possible in all patients. An explanation of the benefits of ADT will help the patient to understand and tolerate the possible flare-up in symptoms which may occur in the latter part of the off-steroid day. Other symptomatic therapy may be added or increased at this time if needed.

8) In the event of an acute flare-up of the disease process, it may be necessary to return to a full suppressive daily divided corticoid dose for control. Once control is again established alternate day therapy may be reinstituted.

9) Although many of the undesirable features of corticosteroid therapy can be minimized by ADT, as in any therapeutic situation, the physician must carefully weigh the benefit-risk ratio for each patient in whom corticoid therapy is being considered.

HOW SUPPLIED

MEDROL Tablets (methylprednisolone) are available in the following strengths and sizes:

2 mg	Bottles of 100	*NDC 0009-0049-02*
4 mg	Bottles of 30	*NDC 0009-0056-01*
	Bottles of 100	*NDC 0009-0056-02*
	Bottles of 500	*NDC 0009-0056-03*
	Unit Dose Package (100)	*NDC 0009-0056-05*
	Dosepak™ Unit of Use (21 tablets)	*NDC 0009-0056-04*
8 mg	Bottles of 25	*NDC 0009-0022-01*
16 mg	Bottles of 50	*NDC 0009-0073-01*
	ADT Pak ® (14 tablets) Unit of Use	*NDC 0009-0073-02*
24 mg	Bottles of 25	*NDC 0009-0155-01*
32 mg	Bottles of 25	*NDC 0009-0176-01*

Code 810 487 207

Shown in Product Identification Section, page 433

MICRONASE® ℞

brand of glyburide tablets
(1.25, 2.5, and 5 mg)

5 mg, 100's **NSN 6505-01-204-5417 (M)**

DESCRIPTION

MICRONASE Tablets contain glyburide, which is an oral blood-glucose-lowering drug of the sulfonylurea class. Glyburide is a white, crystalline compound, formulated as MICRONASE Tablets of 1.25, 2.5, and 5 mg strengths for oral administration. Inactive ingredients: colloidal silicon dioxide, dibasic calcium phosphate, magnesium stearate, microcrystalline cellulose, sodium alginate, talc. In addition, the **2.5 mg** contains aluminum oxide and FD&C red no. 40 and the **5 mg** contains aluminum oxide and FD&C blue no. 1. The chemical name for glyburide is 1-[[p-[2-(5-chloro-o-anisamido) ethyl]phenyl]-sulfonyl]-3-cyclohexylurea and the molecular weight is 493.99.

CLINICAL PHARMACOLOGY

Actions

Glyburide appears to lower the blood glucose acutely by stimulating the release of insulin from the pancreas, an effect dependent upon functioning beta cells in the pancreatic islets. The mechanism by which glyburide lowers blood glucose during long-term administration has not been clearly established. With chronic administration in Type II diabetic patients, the blood glucose lowering effect persists despite a gradual decline in the insulin secretory response to the drug. Extrapancreatic effects may be involved in the mechanism of action of oral sulfonylurea hypoglycemic drugs.

Some patients who are initially responsive to oral hypoglycemic drugs, including MICRONASE Tablets (glyburide), may become unresponsive or poorly responsive over time. Alternatively, MICRONASE may be effective in some patients who have become unresponsive to one or more other sulfonylurea drugs.

In addition to its blood glucose lowering actions, glyburide produces a mild diuresis by enhancement of renal free water clearance. Disulfiram-like reactions have very rarely been reported in patients treated with MICRONASE Tablets.

Pharmacokinetics

Single dose studies with MICRONASE Tablets in normal subjects demonstrate significant absorption of glyburide within one hour, peak drug levels at about four hours, and low but detectable levels at twenty-four hours. Mean serum levels of glyburide, as reflected by areas under the serum concentration-time curve, increase in proportion to corresponding increases in dose. Multiple dose studies with MICRONASE in diabetic patients demonstrate drug level concentration-time curves similar to single dose studies, indicating no buildup of drug in tissue depots. The decrease of glyburide in the serum of normal healthy individuals is biphasic; the terminal half-life is about 10 hours. In single dose studies in fasting normal subjects, the degree and duration of blood glucose lowering is proportional to the dose administered and to the area under the drug level concentration-time curve. The blood glucose lowering effect persists for 24 hours following single morning doses in nonfasting diabetic patients. Under conditions of repeated administration in diabetic patients, however, there is no reliable correlation between blood drug levels and fasting blood glucose levels. A one year study of diabetic patients treated with MICRONASE showed no reliable correlation between administered dose and serum drug level.

The major metabolite of glyburide is the 4-trans-hydroxy derivative. A second metabolite, the 3-cis-hydroxy derivative, also occurs. These metabolites probably contribute no significant hypoglycemic action in humans since they are only weakly active (1/400th and 1/40th as active, respectively, as glyburide) in rabbits.

Glyburide is excreted as metabolites in the bile and urine, approximately 50% by each route. This dual excretory pathway is qualitatively different from that of other sulfonylureas, which are excreted primarily in the urine.

Sulfonylurea drugs are extensively bound to serum proteins. Displacement from protein binding sites by other drugs may lead to enhanced hypoglycemic action. *In vitro*, the protein binding exhibited by glyburide is predominantly non-ionic, whereas that of other sulfonylureas (chlorpropamide, tolbutamide, tolazamide) is predominantly ionic. Acidic drugs such as phenylbutazone, warfarin, and salicylates displace the ionic-binding sulfonylureas from serum proteins to a far greater extent than the non-ionic binding glyburide. It has not been shown that this difference in protein binding will result in fewer drug-drug interactions with MICRONASE Tablets in clinical use.

INDICATIONS AND USAGE

MICRONASE Tablets (glyburide) are indicated as an adjunct to diet to lower the blood glucose in patients with non-insulin-dependent diabetes mellitus (type II) whose hyperglycemia cannot be satisfactorily controlled by diet alone.

In initiating treatment for non-insulin-dependent diabetes, diet should be emphasized as the primary form of treatment. Caloric restriction and weight loss are essential in the obese diabetic patient. Proper dietary management alone may be effective in controlling the blood glucose and symptoms of hyperglycemia. The importance of regular physical activity should also be stressed, and cardiovascular risk factors should be identified and corrective measures taken where possible. If this treatment program fails to reduce symptoms and/or blood glucose, the use of an oral sulfonylurea or insulin should be considered. Use of MICRONASE must be viewed by both the physician and patient as a treatment in addition to diet and not as a substitution or as a convenient mechanism for avoiding dietary restraint. Furthermore, loss of blood glucose control on diet alone may be transient, thus requiring only short-term administration of MICRONASE.

During maintenance programs, MICRONASE should be discontinued if satisfactory lowering of blood glucose is no longer achieved. Judgment should be based on regular clinical and laboratory evaluations.

In considering the use of MICRONASE in asymptomatic patients, it should be recognized that controlling blood glucose in non-insulin-dependent diabetes has not been definitely established to be effective in preventing the long-term cardiovascular or neural complications of diabetes.

CONTRAINDICATIONS

MICRONASE Tablets (glyburide) are contraindicated in patients with:

1. Known hypersensitivity or allergy to the drug.
2. Diabetic ketoacidosis, with or without coma. This condition should be treated with insulin.
3. Type I diabetes mellitus, as sole therapy.

Special Warning on Increased Risk of Cardiovascular Mortality: **The administration of oral hypoglycemic drugs has been reported to be associated with increased cardiovascular mortality as compared to treatment with diet alone or diet plus insulin. This warning is based on the study conducted by the University Group Diabetes Program (UGDP), a long-term prospective clinical trial designed to evaluate the effectiveness of glucose-lowering drugs in preventing or delaying vascular complications in patients with non-insulin-dependent diabetes. The study involved 823 patients who were randomly assigned to one of four treatment groups (*Diabetes,* 19 (Suppl. 2):747–830, 1970).**

UGDP reported that patients treated for 5 to 8 years with diet plus a fixed dose of tolbutamide (1.5 grams per day) had a rate of cardiovascular mortality approximately 2½ times that of patients treated with diet alone. A significant increase in total mortality was not observed, but the use of tolbutamide was discontinued based on the increase in cardiovascular mortality, thus limiting the opportunity for the study to show an increase in overall mortality. Despite controversy regarding the interpretation of these results, the findings of the UGDP study provide an adequate basis for this warning. The patient should be informed of the potential risks and advantages of MICRONASE and of alternative modes of therapy.

Although only one drug in the sulfonylurea class (tolbutamide) was included in this study, it is prudent from a safety standpoint to consider that this warning may also apply to other oral hypoglycemic drugs in this class, in view of their close similarities in mode of action and chemical structure.

PRECAUTIONS

General

Hypoglycemia: All sulfonylureas are capable of producing severe hypoglycemia. Proper patient selection and dosage and instructions are important to avoid hypoglycemic episodes. Renal or hepatic insufficiency may cause elevated drug levels of glyburide and the latter may also diminish gluconeogenic capacity, both of which increase the risk of serious hypoglycemic reactions. Elderly, debilitated or malnourished patients, and those with adrenal or pituitary insufficiency, are particularly susceptible to the hypoglycemic action of glucose-lowering drugs. Hypoglycemia may be difficult to recognize in the elderly and in people who are taking beta-adrenergic blocking drugs. Hypoglycemia is more likely to occur when caloric intake is deficient, after severe or prolonged exercise, when alcohol is ingested, or when more than one glucose lowering drug is used.

Loss of Control of Blood Glucose: When a patient stabilized on any diabetic regimen is exposed to stress such as fever, trauma, infection or surgery, a loss of control may occur. At such times it may be necessary to discontinue MICRONASE Tablets (glyburide) and administer insulin.

The effectiveness of any hypoglycemic drug, including MICRONASE, in lowering blood glucose to a desired level decreases in many patients over a period of time which may be due to progression of the severity of diabetes or to diminished responsiveness to the drug. This phenomenon is known as secondary failure, to distinguish it from primary failure in which the drug is ineffective in an individual patient when MICRONASE is first given. Adequate adjustment of dose and adherence to diet should be assessed before classifying a patient as a secondary failure.

Information for Patients: Patients should be informed of the potential risks and advantages of MICRONASE and of alternative modes of therapy. They also should be informed about the importance of adherence to dietary instructions, of a regular exercise program, and of regular testing of urine and/or blood glucose.

The risks of hypoglycemia, its symptoms and treatment, and conditions that predispose to its development should be explained to patients and responsible family members. Primary and secondary failure also should be explained.

Laboratory Tests

Therapeutic response to MICRONASE Tablets should be monitored by frequent urine glucose tests and periodic blood glucose tests. Measurement of glycosylated hemoglobin levels may be helpful in some patients.

Drug Interactions

The hypoglycemic action of sulfonylureas may be potentiated by certain drugs including nonsteroidal anti-inflammatory agents and other drugs that are highly protein bound, salicylates, sulfonamides, chloramphenicol, probenecid, coumarins, monoamine oxidase inhibitors, and beta adrenergic blocking agents. When such drugs are administered to a patient receiving MICRONASE, the patient should be observed closely for hypoglycemia. When such drugs are withdrawn from a patient receiving MICRONASE, the patient should be observed closely for loss of control.

Certain drugs tend to produce hyperglycemia and may lead to loss of control. These drugs include the thiazides and other diuretics, corticosteroids, phenothiazines, thyroid products, estrogens, oral contraceptives, phenytoin, nicotinic acid, sympathomimetics, calcium channel blocking drugs, and isoniazid. When such drugs are administered to a patient receiving MICRONASE, the patient should be closely observed for loss of control. When such drugs are withdrawn from a patient receiving MICRONASE, the patient should be observed closely for hypoglycemia.

A potential interaction between oral miconazole and oral hypoglycemic agents leading to severe hypoglycemia has been reported. Whether this interaction also occurs with the intravenous, topical or vaginal preparations of miconazole is not known.

Carcinogenesis, Mutagenesis, and Impairment of Fertility

Studies in rats at doses to 300 mg/kg/day for 18 months showed no carcinogenic effects. Glyburide is non-mutagenic when studied in the Salmonella microsome test (Ames test) and in the DNA damage/alkaline elution assay.

Pregnancy

Teratogenic Effects: Pregnancy Category B

Reproduction studies have been performed in rats and rabbits at doses up to 500 times the human dose and have revealed no evidence of impaired fertility or harm to the fetus due to glyburide. There are, however, no adequate and well controlled studies in pregnant women. Because animal reproduction studies are not always predictive of human response, this drug should be used during pregnancy only if clearly needed.

Because recent information suggests that abnormal blood glucose levels during pregnancy are associated with a higher incidence of congenital abnormalities, many experts recommend that insulin be used during pregnancy to maintain blood glucose as close to normal as possible.

Nonteratogenic Effects: Prolonged severe hypoglycemia (4 to 10 days) has been reported in neonates born to mothers who were receiving a sulfonylurea drug at the time of delivery. This has been reported more frequently with the use of agents with prolonged half-lives. If MICRONASE is used during pregnancy, it should be discontinued at least two weeks before the expected delivery date.

Nursing Mothers

Although it is not known whether glyburide is excreted in human milk, some sulfonylurea drugs are known to be excreted in human milk. Because the potential for hypoglycemia in nursing infants may exist, a decision should be made whether to discontinue nursing or to discontinue the drug, taking into account the importance of the drug to the mother. If the drug is discontinued, and if diet alone is inadequate for controlling blood glucose, insulin therapy should be considered.

Pediatric Use

Safety and effectiveness in children have not been established.

ADVERSE REACTIONS

Hypoglycemia: See Precautions and Overdosage Sections.

Gastrointestinal Reactions: Cholestatic jaundice may occur rarely; MICRONASE Tablets (glyburide) should be discontinued if this occurs.

Gastrointestinal disturbances, *e.g.,* nausea, epigastic fullness, and heartburn are the most common reactions, having occurred in 1.8% of treated patients during clinical trials. They tend to be dose related and may disappear when dosage is reduced.

Dermatologic Reactions: Allergic skin reactions, *e.g.,* pruritus, erythema, urticaria, and morbilliform or maculopapular eruptions occurred in 1.5% of treated patients during clinical trials. These may be transient and may disappear despite continued use of MICRONASE; if skin reactions persist, the drug should be discontinued.

Porphyria cutanea tarda and photosensitivity reactions have been reported with sulfonylureas.

Hematologic Reactions: Leukopenia, agranulocytosis, thrombocytopenia, hemolytic anemia, aplastic anemia, and pancytopenia have been reported with sulfonylureas.

Metabolic Reactions: Hepatic porphyria and disulfiram-like reactions have been reported with sulfonylureas; however, hepatic porphyria has not been reported with

Continued on next page

Information on these Upjohn products is based on labeling in effect August 15, 1986. Further information concerning these and other Upjohn products may be obtained by direct inquiry to Medical Information, The Upjohn Company, Kalamazoo, Michigan 49001.

Upjohn—Cont.

MICRONASE and disulfiram-like reactions have been reported very rarely.

OVERDOSAGE

Overdosage of sulfonylureas, including MICRONASE Tablets (glyburide), can produce hypoglycemia. Mild hypoglycemic symptoms, without loss of consciousness or neurological findings, should be treated aggressively with oral glucose and adjustments in drug dosage and/or meal patterns. Close monitoring should continue until the physician is assured that the patient is out of danger. Severe hypoglycemic reactions with coma, seizure, or other neurological impairment occur infrequently, but constitute medical emergencies requiring immediate hospitalization. If hypoglycemic coma is diagnosed or suspected, the patient should be given a rapid intravenous injection of concentrated (50%) glucose solution. This should be followed by a continuous infusion of a more dilute (10%) glucose solution at a rate which will maintain the blood glucose at a level above 100 mg/dL. Patients should be closely monitored for a minimum of 24 to 48 hours, since hypoglycemia may recur after apparent clinical recovery.

DOSAGE AND ADMINISTRATION

There is no fixed dosage regimen for the management of diabetes mellitus with MICRONASE Tablets (glyburide) or any other hypoglycemic agent. In addition to the usual monitoring of urinary glucose, the patient's blood glucose must also be monitored periodically to determine the minimum effective dose for the patient; to detect primary failure, *i.e.*, inadequate lowering of blood glucose at the maximum recommended dose of medication; and to detect secondary failure, *i.e.*, loss of adequate blood glucose lowering response after an initial period of effectiveness. Glycosylated hemoglobin levels may also be of value in monitoring the patient's response to therapy.

Short-term administration of MICRONASE may be sufficient during periods of transient loss of control in patients usually controlled well on diet.

Usual Starting Dose

The usual starting dose of MICRONASE Tablets is 2.5 to 5.0 mg daily, administered with breakfast or the first main meal. Those patients who may be more sensitive to hypoglycemic drugs should be started at 1.25 mg daily. (See Precautions Sections for patients at increased risk.) Failure to follow an appropriate dosage regimen may precipitate hypoglycemia. Patients who do not adhere to their prescribed dietary and drug regimen are more prone to exhibit unsatisfactory response to therapy.

Transfer From Other Hypoglycemic Therapy

Patients Receiving Other Oral Antidiabetic Therapy: Transfer of patients from other oral antidiabetic regimens to MICRONASE should be done conservatively and the initial daily dose should be 2.5 to 5 mg. When transferring patients from oral hypoglycemic agents other than chlorpropamide to MICRONASE, no transition period and no initial or priming dose are necessary. When transferring patients from chlorpropamide, particular care should be exercised during the first two weeks because the prolonged retention of chlorpropamide in the body and subsequent overlapping drug effects may provoke hypoglycemia.

Patients Receiving Insulin: Some type II diabetic patients being treated with insulin may respond satisfactorily to MICRONASE. If the insulin dose is less than 20 units daily, substitution of MICRONASE Tablets 2.5 to 5.0 mg as a single daily dose may be tried. If the insulin dose is between 20 and 40 units daily, the patient may be placed directly on MICRONASE Tablets 5.0 mg daily as a single dose. If the insulin dose is more than 40 units daily, a transition period is required for conversion to MICRONASE. In these patients, insulin dosage is decreased by 50% and MICRONASE Tablets 5 mg daily is started. Please refer to Titration to Maintenance Dose for further explanation.

Titration to Maintenance Dose

The usual maintenance dose is in the range of 1.25 to 20 mg daily, which may be given as a single dose or in divided doses (See Dosage Interval Section). Dosage increases should be made in increments of no more than 2.5 mg at weekly intervals based upon the patient's blood glucose response.

No exact dosage relationship exists between MICRONASE and the other oral hypoglycemic agents. Although patients may be transferred from the maximum dose of other sulfonylureas, the maximum starting dose of 5.0 mg of MICRONASE Tablets should be observed. A maintenance dose of 5 mg of MICRONASE Tablets provides approximately the same degree of blood glucose control as 250 to 375 mg chlorpropamide, 250 to 375 mg tolazamide, 500 to 750 mg acetohexamide, or 1000 to 1500 mg tolbutamide.

When transferring patients receiving more than 40 units of insulin daily, they may be started on a daily dose of MICRONASE Tablets 5 mg concomitantly with a 50% reduction in insulin dose. Progressive withdrawal of insulin and increase of MICRONASE in increments of 1.25 to 2.5 mg every 2 to 10 days is then carried out. During this conversion period when both insulin and MICRONASE are being used, hypoglycemia may rarely occur. During insulin withdrawal, patients should test their urine for glucose and acetone at least three times daily and report results to their physician. The appearance of persistent acetonuria with glycosuria indicates that the patient is a type I diabetic who requires insulin therapy.

Maximum Dose

Daily doses of more than 20 mg are not recommended.

Dosage Interval

Once-a-day therapy is usually satisfactory. Some patients, particularly those receiving more than 10 mg daily, may have a more satisfactory response with twice-a-day dosage.

Specific Patient Populations

MICRONASE is not recommended for use in pregnancy or for use in children.

In elderly patients, debilitated or malnourished patients, and patients with impaired renal or hepatic function, the initial and maintenance dosing should be conservative to avoid hypoglycemic reactions. (See Precautions Section.)

HOW SUPPLIED

MICRONASE Tablets (glyburide), scored, are available in the following strengths, colors and sizes:

1.25 mg	White	Bottles of 100	NDC 0009-0131-01
2.5 mg	Dark Pink	Bottles of 100	NDC 0009-0141-01
2.5 mg	Dark Pink	Unit Dose Pkg. of 100	NDC 0009-0141-01
5.0 mg	Blue	Bottles of 100	NDC 0009-0171-01
5.0 mg	Blue	Bottles of 500	NDC 0009-0171-02
5.0 mg	Blue	Unit Dose Pkg. of 100	NDC 0009-0171-03

Caution: Federal law prohibits dispensing without prescription. Store at controlled room temperature 15°–30° C (59°–86° F). Dispensed in well closed containers with safety closures. Keep container tightly closed.

Code 811 985 207

Shown in Product Identification Section, page 434

MOTRIN® ℞

brand of ibuprofen tablets, USP

400 mg, 120's	**NSN 6505-01-044-2566**
400 mg, 500's	**NSN 6505-00-128-8035**
400 mg, Unit Dose	**NSN 6505-01-041-6911**
600 mg, 90's	**NSN 6505-01-135-9655**
600 mg, 500's	**NSN 6505-01-098-0247**
600 mg, Unit Dose	**NSN 6505-01-115-3520**
800 mg, 100's	**NSN 6505-01-214-9061**
800 mg, 500's	**NSN 6505-01-214-9062**

DESCRIPTION

MOTRIN Tablets contain the active ingredient ibuprofen, which is (±)-2-(*p*-isobutylphenyl) propionic acid. Ibuprofen is a white powder with a melting point of 74–77°C and is very slightly soluble in water (<1 mg/ml) and readily soluble in organic solvents such as ethanol and acetone.

The structural formula is represented below:

MOTRIN, a nonsteroidal anti-inflammatory agent, is available in 400, 600, and 800 mg tablets for oral administration. Inactive ingredients: **300 mg**—acacia, acetylated monoglyceride, calcium sulfate, carboxymethylcellulose sodium, carnauba wax, colloidal silicon dioxide, corn starch, povidone, pregelatinized starch, sesame oil, shellac, stearic acid, sucrose, white wax; **400 mg**—acacia, acetylated monoglyceride, calcium sulfate, carboxymethylcellulose sodium, carnauba wax, colloidal silicon dioxide, corn starch, FD&C yellow no. 6, pregelatinized starch, povidone, sesame oil, shellac, sodium benzoate, stearic acid, sucrose, titanium dioxide, white wax; **600 mg**—carnauba wax, colloidal silicon dioxide, corn starch, FD&C yellow no. 6, hydroxypropyl cellulose, hydroxypropyl methylcellulose, pregelatinized starch, propylene glycol, stearic acid, titanium dioxide; **800 mg**—carnauba wax, colloidal silicon dioxide, croscarmellose sodium, FD&C yellow no. 6, hydroxypropyl methylcellulose, magnesium stearate, microcrystalline cellulose, propylene glycol, talc, titanium dioxide.

CLINICAL PHARMACOLOGY

MOTRIN Tablets contain ibuprofen which possesses analgesic and antipyretic activities. Its mode of action, like that of other nonsteroidal anti-inflammatory agents, is not completely understood, but may be related to prostaglandin synthetase inhibition.

In clinical studies in patients with rheumatoid arthritis and osteoarthritis, MOTRIN has been shown to be comparable to aspirin in controlling pain and inflammation and to be associated with a statistically significant reduction in the milder gastrointestinal side effects (see ADVERSE REACTIONS). MOTRIN may be well tolerated in some patients who have had gastrointestinal side effects with aspirin, but these patients when treated with MOTRIN should be carefully followed for signs and symptoms of gastrointestinal ulceration and bleeding. Although it is not definitely known whether MOTRIN causes less peptic ulceration than aspirin, in one study involving 885 patients with rheumatoid arthritis treated for up to one year, there were no reports of gastric ulceration with MOTRIN whereas frank ulceration was reported in 13 patients in the aspirin group (statistically significant $p < .001$).

Gastroscopic studies at varying doses show an increased tendency toward gastric irritation at higher doses. However, at comparable doses, gastric irritation is approximately half that seen with aspirin. Studies using ^{51}Cr-tagged red cells indicate that fecal blood loss associated with MOTRIN in doses up to 2400 mg daily did not exceed the normal range, and was significantly less than that seen in aspirin-treated patients.

In clinical studies in patients with rheumatoid arthritis, MOTRIN has been shown to be comparable to indomethacin in controlling the signs and symptoms of disease activity and to be associated with a statistically significant reduction of the milder gastrointestinal (see ADVERSE REACTIONS) and CNS side effects.

MOTRIN may be used in combination with gold salts and/or corticosteroids.

Controlled studies have demonstrated that MOTRIN is a more effective analgesic than propoxyphene for the relief of episiotomy pain, pain following dental extraction procedures, and for the relief of the symptoms of primary dysmenorrhea.

In patients with primary dysmenorrhea, MOTRIN has been shown to reduce elevated levels of prostaglandin activity in the menstrual fluid and to reduce resting and active intrauterine pressure, as well as the frequency of uterine contractions. The probable mechanism of action is to inhibit prostaglandin synthesis rather than simply to provide analgesia.

The ibuprofen in MOTRIN is rapidly absorbed when administered orally. Peak serum ibuprofen levels are generally attained one to two hours after administration. With single doses up to 800 mg, a linear relationship exists between amount of drug administered and the integrated area under the serum drug concentration vs time curve. Above 800 mg, however, the area under the curve increases less than proportional to increases in dose. There is no evidence of drug accumulation or enzyme induction.

The administration of MOTRIN Tablets either under fasting conditions or immediately before meals yields quite similar serum ibuprofen concentration-time profiles. When MOTRIN is administered immediately after a meal, there is a reduction in the rate of absorption but no appreciable decrease in the extent of absorption. The bioavailability of the drug is minimally altered by the presence of food.

A bioavailability study has shown that there was no interference with the absorption of ibuprofen when MOTRIN was given in conjunction with an antacid containing both aluminum hydroxide and magnesium hydroxide.

Ibuprofen is rapidly metabolized and eliminated in the urine. The excretion of ibuprofen is virtually complete 24 hours after the last dose. The serum half-life is 1.8 to 2.0 hours.

Studies have shown that following ingestion of the drug, 45% to 79% of the dose was recovered in the urine within 24 hours as metabolite A (25%), (+)-2-[*p*-(2hydroxymethyl-propyl)- phenyl] propionic acid and metabolite B (37%), (+)-2-[*p*-(2carboxypropyl)-phenyl] propionic acid; the percentages of free and conjugated ibuprofen were approximately 1% and 14%, respectively.

INDICATIONS AND USAGE

MOTRIN Tablets (ibuprofen) are indicated for relief of the signs and symptoms of rheumatoid arthritis and osteoarthritis.

MOTRIN is indicated for relief of mild to moderate pain.

MOTRIN is also indicated for the treatment of primary dysmenorrhea.

Since there have been no controlled clinical trials to demonstrate whether or not there is any beneficial effect or harmful interaction with the use of MOTRIN in conjunction with aspirin, the combination cannot be recommended (see **Drug Interactions**).

Controlled clinical trials to establish the safety and effectiveness of MOTRIN in children have not been conducted.

CONTRAINDICATIONS

MOTRIN Tablets (ibuprofen) should not be used in patients who have previously exhibited hypersensitivity to the drug, or in individuals with the syndrome of nasal polyps, angioedema and bronchospastic reactivity to aspirin or other nonsteroidal anti-inflammatory agents. Anaphylactoid reactions have occurred in such patients.

WARNINGS

Peptic ulceration and gastrointestinal bleeding, sometimes severe, have been reported in patients receiving MOTRIN

MOTRIN

	Incidence Greater than 1% (but less than 3%) Probable Causal Relationship	Precise Incidence Unknown (but less than 1%) Probable Causal Relationship**	Precise Incidence Unknown (but less than 1%) Causal Relationship Unknown**
GASTROINTESTINAL	Nausea*, epigastric pain*, heartburn*, diarrhea, abdominal distress, nausea and vomiting, indigestion, constipation, abdominal cramps or pain, fullness of GI tract (bloating and flatulence)	Gastric or duodenal ulcer with bleeding and/or perforation, gastrointestinal hemorrhage, melena, gastritis, hepatitis, jaundice, abnormal liver function tests; pancreatitis	
CENTRAL NERVOUS SYSTEM	Dizziness*, headache, nervousness	Depression, insomnia, confusion, emotional lability, somnolence, aseptic meningitis with fever and coma	Paresthesias, hallucinations, dream abnormalities, pseudotumor cerebri
DERMATOLOGIC	Rash* (including maculopapular type), pruritis	Vesiculobullous eruptions, urticaria, erythema multiforme, Stevens-Johnson syndrome, alopecia	Toxic epidermal necrolysis, photoallergic skin reactions
SPECIAL SENSES	Tinnitus	Hearing loss, amblyopia (blurred and/or diminished vision, scotomata and/or changes in color vision) (see PRECAUTIONS)	Conjunctivitis, diplopia, optic neuritis, cataracts
HEMATOLOGIC		Neutropenia, agranulocytosis, aplastic anemia, hemolytic anemia (sometimes Coombs positive), thrombocytopenia with or without purpura, eosinophilia, decreases in hemoglobin and hematocrit (see PRECAUTIONS)	Bleeding episodes (eg epistaxis, menorrhagia)
METABOLIC/ENDOCRINE	Decreased appetite		Gynecomastia, hypoglycemic reaction, acidosis
CARDIOVASCULAR	Edema, fluid retention (generally responds promptly to drug discontinuation; see PRECAUTIONS)	Congestive heart failure in patients with marginal cardiac function, elevated blood pressure, palpitations	Arrhythmias (sinus tachycardia, sinus bradycardia)
ALLERGIC		Syndrome of abdominal pain, fever, chills, nausea and vomiting; anaphylaxis; bronchospasm (see CONTRAINDICATIONS)	Serum sickness, lupus erythematosus syndrome, Henoch-Schönlein vasculitis, angioedema
RENAL		Acute renal failure in patients with pre-existing significantly impaired renal function, decreased creatinine clearance, polyuria, azotemia, cystitis, hematuria	Renal papillary necrosis
MISCELLANEOUS		Dry eyes and mouth, gingival ulcer, rhinitis	

* Reactions occurring in 3% to 9% of patients treated with MOTRIN. (Those reactions occurring in less than 3% of the patients are unmarked).

** Reactions are classified under "*Probable Causal Relationship (PCR)*" if there has been one positive rechallenge or if three or more cases occur which might be causally related. Reactions are classified under "*Causal Relationship Unknown*" if seven or more events have been reported but the criteria for PCR have not been met.

Tablets (ibuprofen). Peptic ulceration, perforation, or severe gastrointestinal bleeding can have a fatal outcome, and although a few such reports have been received with MOTRIN, a cause and effect relationship has not been established. MOTRIN should be given under close supervision to patients with a history of upper gastrointestinal tract disease, and only after consulting the ADVERSE REACTIONS section.

In patients with active peptic ulcer and active rheumatoid arthritis, attempts should be made to treat the arthritis with nonulcerogenic drugs, such as gold. If MOTRIN must be given, the patient should be under close supervision for signs of ulcer perforation or gastrointestinal bleeding.

PRECAUTIONS

Blurred and/or diminished vision, scotomata, and/or changes in color vision have been reported. If a patient develops such complaints while receiving MOTRIN Tablets (ibuprofen), the drug should be discontinued and the patient should have an ophthalmologic examination which includes central visual fields and color vision testing.

Fluid retention and edema have been reported in association with MOTRIN; therefore, the drug should be used with caution in patients with a history of cardiac decompensation or hypertension.

MOTRIN, like other nonsteroidal anti-inflammatory agents, can inhibit platelet aggregation but the effect is quantitatively less and of shorter duration than that seen with aspirin. MOTRIN has been shown to prolong bleeding time (but within the normal range) in normal subjects. Because this prolonged bleeding effect may be exaggerated in patients with underlying hemostatic defects, MOTRIN should be used with caution in persons with intrinsic coagulation defects and those on anticoagulant therapy.

Patients on MOTRIN should report to their physicians signs or symptoms of gastrointestinal ulceration or bleeding, blurred vision or other eye symptoms, skin rash, weight gain, or edema.

In order to avoid exacerbation of disease or adrenal insufficiency, patients who have been on prolonged corticosteroid therapy should have their therapy tapered slowly rather than discontinued abruptly when MOTRIN is added to the treatment program.

The antipyretic and anti-inflammatory activity of ibuprofen may reduce fever and inflammation, thus diminishing their utility as diagnostic signs in detecting complications of presumed noninfectious noninflammatory painful conditions.

As with other nonsteroidal anti-inflammatory drugs, borderline elevations of one or more liver tests may occur in up to 15% of patients. These abnormalities may progress, may remain essentially unchanged, or may be transient with continued therapy. The SGPT (ALT) test is probably the most sensitive indicator of liver dysfunction. Meaningful (3 times the upper limit of normal) elevations of SGPT or SGOT (AST) occurred in controlled clinical trials in less than 1% of patients. A patient with symptoms and/or signs suggesting liver dysfunction, or in whom an abnormal liver test has occurred, should be evaluated for evidence of the development of more severe hepatic reaction while on therapy with MOTRIN. Severe hepatic reactions, including jaundice and cases of fatal hepatitis, have been reported with ibuprofen as with other nonsteroidal anti-inflammatory drugs. Although such reactions are rare, if abnormal liver tests persist or worsen, if clinical signs and symptoms consistent with liver disease develop, or if systemic manifestations occur (eg, eosinophilia, rash, etc.), MOTRIN should be discontinued.

In cross-study comparisons with doses ranging from 1200 mg to 3200 mg daily for several weeks, a slight dose-response decrease in hemoglobin/hematocrit was noted. This has been observed with other nonsteroidal anti-inflammatory drugs; the mechanism is unknown. However, even with daily doses of 3200 mg, the total decrease in hemoglobin usually does not exceed 1 gram; if there are no signs of bleeding, it is probably not clinically important.

Renal Effects: As with other nonsteroidal anti-inflammatory drugs, long term administration of ibuprofen to animals has resulted in renal papillary necrosis and other abnormal renal pathology. In humans, there have been reports of acute interstitial nephritis with hematuria, proteinuria, and occasionally nephrotic syndrome.

A second form of renal toxicity has been seen in patients with prerenal conditions leading to a reduction in renal blood flow or blood volume, where the renal prostaglandins have a supportive role in the maintenance of renal perfusion. In these patients administration of a nonsteroidal anti-inflammatory drug may cause a dose dependent reduction in prostaglandin formation and may precipitate overt renal decompensation. Patients at greatest risk of this reaction are those with impaired renal function, heart failure, liver dysfunction, those taking diuretics and the elderly. Discontinuation of nonsteroidal anti-inflammatory drug therapy is typically followed by recovery to the pretreatment state.

Since ibuprofen is eliminated primarily by the kidneys, patients with significantly impaired renal function should be closely monitored; and a reduction in dosage should be anticipated to avoid drug accumulation. Prospective studies on the safety of ibuprofen in patients with chronic renal failure have not been conducted.

Drug Interactions: *Coumarin-type anticoagulants.* Several short-term controlled studies failed to show that MOTRIN significantly affected prothrombin times or a variety of other clotting factors when administered to individuals on coumarin-type anticoagulants. However, because bleeding has been reported when MOTRIN and other nonsteroidal anti-inflammatory agents have been administered to patients on coumarin-type anticoagulants, the physician should be cautious when administering MOTRIN to patients on anticoagulants.

Aspirin. Animal studies show that aspirin given with nonsteroidal anti-inflammatory agents, including MOTRIN, yields a net decrease in anti-inflammatory activity with lowered blood levels of the non-aspirin drug. Single dose bi-

Continued on next page

Information on these Upjohn products is based on labeling in effect August 15, 1986. Further information concerning these and other Upjohn products may be obtained by direct inquiry to Medical Information, The Upjohn Company, Kalamazoo, Michigan 49001.

Upjohn—Cont.

oavailability studies in normal volunteers have failed to show an effect of aspirin on ibuprofen blood levels. Correlative clinical studies have not been done.

Pregnancy: Reproductive studies conducted in rats and rabbits at doses somewhat less than the maximal clinical dose did not demonstrate evidence of developmental abnormalities. However, animal reproduction studies are not always predictive of human response. As there are no adequate and well-controlled studies in pregnant women, this drug should be used during pregnancy only if clearly needed. Because of the known effects of nonsteroidal anti-inflammatory drugs on the fetal cardiovascular system (closure of ductus arteriosus), use during late pregnancy should be avoided. As with other drugs known to inhibit prostaglandin synthesis, an increased incidence of dystocia and delayed parturition occurred in rats. Administration of MOTRIN is not recommended during pregnancy.

Nursing Mothers: In limited studies, an assay capable of detecting 1 mcg/ml did not demonstrate ibuprofen in the milk of lactating mothers. However, because of the limited nature of the studies, and the possible adverse effects of prostaglandin-inhibiting drugs on neonates, MOTRIN is not recommended for use in nursing mothers.

ADVERSE REACTIONS

The most frequent type of adverse reaction occurring with MOTRIN Tablets (ibuprofen) is gastrointestinal. In controlled clinical trials the percentage of patients reporting one or more gastrointestinal complaints ranged from 4% to 16%.

In controlled studies when MOTRIN was compared to aspirin and indomethacin in equally effective doses, the overall incidence of gastrointestinal complaints was about half that seen in either the aspirin- or indomethacin-treated patients.

Adverse reactions observed during controlled clinical trials at an incidence greater than 1% are listed in the following table. Those reactions listed in Column one encompass observations in approximately 3,000 patients. More than 500 of these patients were treated for periods of at least 54 weeks.

Still other reactions occurring less frequently than 1 in 100 were reported in controlled clinical trials and from marketing experience. These reactions have been divided into two categories: Column two of the following table lists reactions with therapy with MOTRIN where the probability of a causal relationship exists: for the reactions in Column three, a causal relationship with MOTRIN has not been established.

Reported side effects were higher at doses of 3200 mg/day than at doses of 2400 mg or less per day in clinical trials of patients with rheumatoid arthritis. The increases in incidence were slight and still within the ranges reported in the following table.

[See table on preceding page].

OVERDOSAGE

Approximately 1½ hours after the reported ingestion of from 7 to 10 MOTRIN Tablets (ibuprofen) (400 mg), a 19-month old child weighing 12 kg was seen in the hospital emergency room, apneic and cyanotic, responding only to painful stimuli. This type of stimulus, however, was sufficient to induce respiration. Oxygen and parenteral fluids were given; a greenish-yellow fluid was aspirated from the stomach with no evidence to indicate the presence of ibuprofen. Two hours after ingestion the child's condition seemed stable; she still responded only to painful stimuli and continued to have periods of apnea lasting from 5 to 10 seconds. She was admitted to intensive care and sodium bicarbonate was administered as well as infusions of dextrose and normal saline. By four hours post-ingestion she could be aroused easily, sit by herself and respond to spoken commands. Blood level of ibuprofen was 102.9 μg/ml approximately 8½ hours after accidental ingestion. At 12 hours she appeared to be completely recovered.

In two other reported cases where children (each weighing approximately 10 kg) accidentally, acutely ingested approximately 120 mg/kg, there were no signs of acute intoxication or late sequelae. Blood level in one child 90 minutes after ingestion was 700 μg/ml—about 10 times the peak levels seen in absorption-excretion studies.

A 19-year old male who had taken 8,000 mg of ibuprofen over a period of a few hours complained of dizziness, and nystagmus was noted. After hospitalization, parenteral hydration and three days' bed rest, he recovered with no reported sequelae.

In cases of acute overdosage, the stomach should be emptied by vomiting or lavage, though little drug will likely be recovered if more than an hour has elapsed since ingestion. Because the drug is acidic and is excreted in the urine, it is theoretically beneficial to administer alkali and induce diuresis.

DOSAGE AND ADMINISTRATION

Do not exceed 3200 mg total daily dose. If gastrointestinal complaints occur, administer MOTRIN Tablets (ibuprofen) with meals or milk.

Rheumatoid arthritis and osteoarthritis, including flare-ups of chronic disease:

Suggested Dosage: 1200 mg-3200 mg daily (300 mg qid; 400 mg, 600 mg or 800 mg tid or qid). Individual patients may show a better response to 3200 mg daily, as compared with 2400 mg, although in well-controlled clinical trials patients on 3200 mg did not show a better mean response in terms of efficacy. Therefore, when treating patients with 3200 mg/day, the physician should observe sufficient increased clinical benefits to offset potential increased risk.

The dose should be tailored to each patient, and may be lowered or raised depending on the severity of symptoms either at time of initiating drug therapy or as the patient responds or fails to respond.

In general, patients with rheumatoid arthritis seem to require higher doses of MOTRIN than do patients with osteoarthritis.

The smallest dose of MOTRIN that yields acceptable control should be employed. A linear blood level dose-response relationship exists with single doses up to 800 mg (See CLINICAL PHARMACOLOGY for effects of food on rate of absorption).

The availability of four tablet strengths facilitates dosage adjustment.

In chronic conditions, a therapeutic response to therapy with MOTRIN is sometimes seen in a few days to a week but most often is observed by two weeks. After a satisfactory response has been achieved, the patient's dose should be reviewed and adjusted as required.

Mild to moderate pain:

400 mg every 4 to 6 hours as necessary for relief of pain. In controlled analgesic clinical trials, doses of MOTRIN greater than 400 mg were no more effective than the 400 mg dose.

Dysmenorrhea:

For the treatment of dysmenorrhea, beginning with the earliest onset of such pain, MOTRIN should be given in a dose of 400 mg every 4 hours as necessary for the relief of pain.

HOW SUPPLIED

MOTRIN Tablets (ibuprofen) are supplied as follows:

MOTRIN Tablets, 300 mg (white)

Bottles of 500	NDC 0009-0733-02
Unit of Use bottles of 60	NDC 0009-0733-01

MOTRIN Tablets, 400 mg (orange)

Bottles of 500	NDC 0009-0750-02
Unit-dose package of 100	NDC 0009-0750-06
Unit of Use bottles of 100	NDC 0009-0750-25

MOTRIN Tablets, 600 mg (peach)

Unit-dose package of 100	NDC 0009-0742-05
Bottles of 500	NDC 0009-0742-02
Unit of Use bottles of 100	NDC 0009-0742-03

MOTRIN Tablets, 800 mg (apricot)

Bottles of 100	NDC 0009-0725-01
Bottles of 500	NDC 0009-0725-03
Unit of Use bottles of 30	NDC 0009-0725-06
Unit of Use bottles of 50	NDC 0009-0725-07

Code 810 015 20

Shown in Product Identification Section, page 434

MYCIGUENT® Antibiotic Ointment

(See PDR For Nonprescription Drugs)

MYCITRACIN® Triple Antibiotic Ointment

(See PDR For Nonprescription Drugs)

ORINASE® ℞

brand of tolbutamide tablets, USP

DESCRIPTION

ORINASE Tablets contain tolbutamide, an oral blood glucose lowering drug of the sulfonylurea category. Tolbutamide is a pure white crystalline compound practically insoluble in water but forming water-soluble salts with alkalies.

The chemical names for tolbutamide are (1) Benzenesulfonamide, N-[(butylamino) carbonyl]-4-methyl; (2) 1-Butyl-3-(p-tolylsulfonyl)urea and its molecular weight is 270.35.

ORINASE Tablets for oral administration are available as scored, white tablets containing 250 mg or 500 mg tolbutamide. Inactive ingredients: aluminum hydroxide, dibasic calcium phosphate, magnesium aluminum silicate, magnesium stearate.

CLINICAL PHARMACOLOGY

Actions

Tolbutamide appears to lower blood glucose acutely by stimulating the release of insulin from the pancreas, an effect dependent upon functioning beta cells in the pancreatic islets. The mechanism by which tolbutamide lowers blood glucose during long-term administration has not been clearly established. With chronic administration in Type II diabetic patients, the blood glucose lowering effect persists despite a gradual decline in the insulin secretory response to the drug. Extrapancreatic effects may be involved in the mechanism of action of oral sulfonylurea hypoglycemic drugs.

Some patients who are initially responsive to oral hypoglycemic drugs, including ORINASE, may become unresponsive or poorly responsive over time. Alternatively, ORINASE may be effective in some patients who have become unresponsive to one or more other sulfonylurea drugs.

Pharmacokinetics

When administered orally, the tolbutamide in ORINASE Tablets is readily absorbed from the gastrointestinal tract. Absorption is not impaired and glucose lowering and insulin releasing effects are not altered if the drug is taken with food. Detectable levels are present in the plasma within twenty minutes after oral ingestion of a 500 mg ORINASE tablet, with peak levels occurring at three to four hours and only small amounts detectable at 24 hours. The half-life of tolbutamide is 4.5 to 6.5 hours. As tolbutamide has no p-amino group, it cannot be acetylated, which is one of the common modes of metabolic degradation for the antibacterial sulfonamides. However, the presence of the p-methyl group renders tolbutamide susceptible to oxidation, and this appears to be the principal manner of its metabolic degradation in man. The p-methyl group is oxidized to form a carboxyl group, converting tolbutamide into the totally inactive metabolite 1-butyl-3-p-carboxy-phenylsulfonylurea, which can be recovered in the urine within 24 hours in amounts accounting for up to 75% of the administered dose.

The major tolbutamide metabolite has been found to have no hypoglycemic or other action when administered orally and IV to both normal and diabetic subjects. This tolbutamide metabolite is highly soluble over the critical acid range of urinary pH values, and its solubility increases with increase in pH. Because of the marked solubility of the tolbutamide metabolite, crystalluria does not occur. A second metabolite, 1-butyl-3-(p-hydroxymethyl) phenyl sulfonylurea also occurs to a limited extent. It is an inactive metabolite.

The administration of 3 grams of tolbutamide to either nondiabetic or tolbutamide-responsive diabetic subjects will, in both instances, occasion a gradual lowering of blood glucose. Increasing the dose to 6 grams does not usually cause a response which is significantly different from that produced by the 3 gram dose. Following the administration of a 3 gram dose of ORINASE solution, nondiabetic fasting adults exhibit a 30% or greater reduction in blood glucose within one hour, following which the blood glucose gradually returns to the fasting level over six to twelve hours. Following the administration of a 3 gram dose of ORINASE solution, tolbutamide responsive diabetic patients show a gradually progressive blood glucose lowering effect, the maximal response being reached between five to eight hours after ingestion of a single 3 gram dose. The blood glucose then rises gradually and by the 24th hour has usually returned to pretest levels. The magnitude of the reduction, when expressed in terms of percent of the protest blood glucose, tends to be similar to the response seen in the nondiabetic subject.

INDICATIONS AND USAGE

ORINASE Tablets (tolbutamide) are indicated as an adjunct to diet to lower the blood glucose in patients with noninsulin-dependent diabetes whose hyperglycemia cannot be satisfactorily controlled by diet alone. In initiating treatment for noninsulin-dependent diabetes, diet should be emphasized as the primary form of treatment. Caloric restriction and weight loss are essential in the obese diabetic patient. Proper dietary management alone may be effective in controlling the blood glucose and symptoms of hyperglycemia. The importance of regular physical activity should also be stressed and cardiovascular risk factors should be identified and corrective measures taken where possible.

If this treatment program fails to reduce symptoms and/or blood glucose, the use of an oral sulfonylurea or insulin should be considered. Use of ORINASE must be viewed by both the physician and patient as a treatment in addition to diet, and not as a substitute for diet or as a convenient mechanism for avoiding dietary restraint. Furthermore, loss of blood glucose control on diet alone may be transient, thus requiring only short-term administration of ORINASE.

During maintenance programs, ORINASE should be discontinued if satisfactory lowering of blood glucose is no longer achieved. Judgments should be based on regular clinical and laboratory evaluations.

In considering the use of ORINASE in asymptomatic patients, it should be recognized that controlling the blood glucose in noninsulin-dependent diabetes has not been definitely established to be effective in preventing the long-term cardiovascular or neural complications of diabetes.

CONTRAINDICATIONS

ORINASE Tablets (tolbutamide) are contraindicated in patients with: 1) known hypersensitivity or allergy to ORINASE; 2) diabetic ketoacidosis, with or without coma. This condition should be treated with insulin. 3) Type I diabetes, as sole therapy.

Special Warning on Increased Risk of Cardiovascular Mortality: The administration of oral hypoglycemic drugs has been reported to be associated with increased cardiovascular mortality as compared to treatment with diet alone or diet plus insulin. This warning is based on the study conducted by the University Group Diabetes Program (UGDP), a long-term prospective clinical trial designed to evaluate the effectiveness of glucose-lowering drugs in preventing or delaying vascular complications in patients with noninsulin-dependent diabetes. The study involved 823 patients who were randomly assigned to one of four treatment groups (Diabetes, 19 (supp. 2):747-830, 1970.)

UGDP reported that patients treated for five to eight years with diet plus a fixed dose of tolbutamide (1.5 grams per day) had a rate of cardiovascular mortality approximately 2½ times that of patients with diet alone. A significant increase in total mortality was not observed, but the use of tolbutamide was discontinued based on the increase in cardiovascular mortality, thus limiting the opportunity for the study to show an increase in overall mortality. Despite controversy regarding the interpretation of these results, the findings of the UGDP study provide an adequate basis for this warning. The patient should be informed of the potential risks and advantages of ORINASE and of alternative modes of therapy.

Although only one drug in the sulfonylurea class (tolbutamide) was included in this study, it is prudent from a safety standpoint to consider that this warning may also apply to other oral hypoglycemic drugs in this class, in view of their close similarities in mode of action and chemical structure.

PRECAUTIONS

General

Hypoglycemia—All sulfonylurea drugs are capable of producing severe hypoglycemia. Proper patient selection and dosage and instructions are important to avoid hypoglycemic episodes. Renal or hepatic insufficiency may cause elevated blood levels of tolbutamide and the latter may also diminish gluconeogenic capacity, both of which increase the risk of serious hypoglycemic reactions. Elderly, debilitated or malnourished patients and those with adrenal or pituitary insufficiency are particularly susceptible to the hypoglycemic action of glucose lowering drugs. Hypoglycemia may be difficult to recognize in the elderly and people who are taking beta-adrenergic blocking drugs. Hypoglycemia is more likely to occur when caloric intake is deficient, after severe or prolonged exercise, when alcohol is ingested, or when more than one glucose lowering drug is used.

Loss of Control of Blood Glucose—When a patient stabilized on any diabetic regimen is exposed to stress such as fever, trauma, infection, or surgery, loss of blood glucose control may occur. At such times it may be necessary to discontinue ORINASE and administer insulin.

The effectiveness of any hypoglycemic drug, including ORINASE, in lowering blood glucose to a desired level decreases in patients over a period of time, which may be due to progression of the severity of the diabetes or to diminished responsiveness to the drug. This phenomenon is known as secondary drug failure to distinguish it from primary failure in which the drug is ineffective in an individual patient when first given. Adequate adjustment of dose and adherence to diet should be assessed before classifying a patient as a secondary failure.

Information for Patients

Patients should be informed of the potential risks and advantages of ORINASE Tablets (tolbutamide) and of alternative modes of therapy. They should also be informed about the importance of adherence to dietary instructions, of a regular exercise program, and of regular testing of urine and/or blood glucose.

The risks of hypoglycemia, its symptoms and treatment, and conditions that predispose to its development should be explained to patients and responsible family members. Primary and secondary failure should also be explained.

Laboratory Tests

Blood and urine glucose should be monitored periodically. Measurement of glycosylated hemoglobin may be useful in some patients.

A metabolite of tolbutamide in urine may give a false positive reaction for albumin if measured by the acidification-after-boiling test, which causes the metabolite to precipitate. There is no interference with the sulfosalicylic acid test.

Drug Interactions

The hypoglycemic action of sulfonylureas may be potentiated by certain drugs including nonsteroidal anti-inflammatory agents and other drugs that are highly protein bound, salicylates, sulfonamides, chloramphenicol, probenecid, coumarins, monoamine oxidase inhibitors, and beta adrenergic blocking agents. When such drugs are administered to a patient receiving ORINASE, the patient should be closely observed for hypoglycemia. When such drugs are withdrawn from a patient receiving ORINASE, the patient should be observed closely for loss of control.

Certain drugs tend to produce hyperglycemia and may lead to loss of control. These drugs include the thiazides and other diuretics, corticosteroids, phenothiazines, thyroid products, estrogens, oral contraceptives, phenytoin, nicotinic acid, sympathomimetics, calcium channel blocking drugs and isoniazid. When such drugs are administered to a patient receiving ORINASE, the patient should be closely observed for loss of control of blood glucose. When such drugs are withdrawn from a patient receiving ORINASE, the patient should be observed closely for hypoglycemia.

A potential interaction between oral miconazole and oral hypoglycemic agents leading to severe hypoglycemia has been reported. Whether this interaction also occurs with the intravenous, topical or vaginal preparations of miconazole is not known.

Carcinogenesis, and Mutagenicity

Bioassay for carcinogenicity was performed in both sexes of rats and mice following ingestion of tolbutamide for 78 weeks. No evidence of carcinogenicity was found.

Tolbutamide has also been demonstrated to be nonmutagenic in the Ames salmonella/mammalian microsome mutagenicity test.

Pregnancy

Teratogenic Effects

Pregnancy Category C. ORINASE has been shown to be teratogenic in rats given in doses 25 to 100 times the human dose. In some studies, pregnant rats given high doses of tolbutamide have shown increased mortality in offspring and ocular and bony abnormalities. Repeat studies in other species (rabbits) have not demonstrated a teratogenic effect. There are no adequate and well controlled studies in pregnant women. ORINASE is not recommended for the treatment of pregnant diabetic patients. Serious consideration should also be given to the possible hazards of the use of ORINASE in women of child-bearing age and in those who might become pregnant while using the drug.

Because recent information suggests that abnormal blood glucose levels during pregnancy are associated with a higher incidence of congenital abnormalities, many experts recommend that insulin be used during pregnancy to maintain blood glucose levels as close to normal as possible.

Nonteratogenic Effects

Prolonged severe hypoglycemia (four to ten days) has been reported in neonates born to mothers who were receiving a sulfonylurea drug at the time of delivery. This has been reported more frequently with the use of agents with prolonged half lives. if ORINASE is used during pregnancy, it should be discontinued at least two weeks before the expected delivery date.

Nursing Mothers

Although it is not known whether tolbutamide is excreted in human milk, some sulfonylurea drugs are known to be excreted in human milk. Because the potential for hypoglycemia in nursing infants may exist, a decision should be made whether to discontinue nursing or to discontinue the drug, taking into account the importance of the drug to the mother. If the drug is discontinued and if diet alone is inadequate for controlling blood glucose, insulin therapy should be considered.

Pediatric Use

Safety and effectiveness in children have not been established.

ADVERSE REACTIONS

Hypoglycemia—See **Precautions** and **Overdosage** sections.

Gastrointestinal Reactions: Cholestatic jaundice may occur rarely; ORINASE Tablets (tolbutamide) should be discontinued if this occurs. Gastrointestinal disturbances, eg, nausea, epigastric fullness, and heartburn, are the most common reactions and occurred in 1.4% of patients treated during clinical trials. They tend to be dose-related and may disappear when dosage is reduced.

Dermatologic Reactions: Allergic skin reactions, eg, pruritus, erythema, urticaria, and morbilliform or maculopapular eruptions, occurred in 1.1% of patients treated during clinical trials. These may be transient and may disappear despite continued use of ORINASE; if skin reactions persist, the drug should be discontinued.

Porphyria cutanea tarda and photosensitivity reactions have been reported with sulfonylureas.

Hematologic Reactions: Leukopenia, agranulocytosis, thrombocytopenia, hemolytic anemia, aplastic anemia, and pancytopenia have been reported with sulfonylureas.

Metabolic Reactions: Hepatic porphria and disulfiram-like reactions have been reported with sulfonylureas.

Miscellaneous Reactions: Headache and taste alterations have occasionally been reported with tolbutamide administration.

OVERDOSAGE

Overdosage of sulfonylureas, including ORINASE Tablets, can produce symptoms of hypoglycemia.

Mild hypoglycemic symptoms without loss of consciousness or neurologic findings should be treated aggressively with oral glucose and adjustments in drug dosage and/or meal patterns. Close monitoring should continue until the physician is assured the patient is out of danger. Severe hypoglycemic reactions with coma, seizure, or other neurological impairment occur infrequently but constitute medical emergencies requiring immediate hospitalization. If hypoglycemic coma is suspected or diagnosed, the patient should be given a rapid intravenous injection of concentrated (50%) glucose solution. This should be followed by a continuous infusion of a more dilute (10%) glucose solution at a rate which will maintain the blood glucose level above 100 mg/dl. Patients should be closely monitored for a minimum of 24 to 48 hours, since hypoglycemia may recur after apparent clinical recovery.

DOSAGE AND ADMINISTRATION

There is no fixed dosage regimen for the management of diabetes mellitus with ORINASE Tablets (tolbutamide) or any other hypoglycemic agent. In addition to the usual monitoring of urinary glucose, the patient's blood glucose must also be monitored periodically to determine the minimum effective dose for the patient; to detect primary failure, ie, inadequate lowering of blood glucose at the maximum recommended dose of medication; and to detect secondary failure, ie, loss of adequate blood glucose response after an initial period of effectiveness. Glycosylated hemoglobin levels may also be of value in monitoring the patient's response to therapy.

Short-term administration of ORINASE may be sufficient during periods of transient loss of control in patients usually controlled well on diet.

Usual Starting Dose

The usual starting dose is 1 to 2 grams daily. This may be increased or decreased depending on individual patient response. Failure to follow an appropriate dosage regimen may precipitate hyoglycemia. Patients who do not adhere to their prescribed dietary regimens are more prone to exhibit unsatisfactory response to drug therapy.

Transfer From Other Hypoglycemic Therapy

Patients Receiving Other Oral Antidiabetic Therapy—Transfer of patients from other oral antidiabetes regimens to ORINASE should be done conservatively. When transferring patients from oral hypoglycemic agents other than chlorpropamide to ORINASE, no transition period and no initial or priming doses are necessary. When transferring patients from chlorpropamide, however, particular care should be exercised during the first two weeks because of the prolonged retention of chlorpropamide in the body and the possibility that subsequent overlapping drug effects might provoke hypoglycemia.

Patients Receiving Insulin—Patients requiring 20 units or less of insulin daily may be placed directly on ORINASE and insulin abruptly discontinued. Patients whose insulin requirement is between 20 and 40 units daily may be started on therapy with ORINASE with a concurrent 30 to 50% reduction in insulin dose, with further daily reduction of the insulin when response to tolbutamide is observed. In patients requiring more than 40 units of insulin daily, therapy with ORINASE may be initiated in conjunction with a 20% reduction in insulin dose the first day, with further careful reduction of insulin as response is observed. Occasionally, conversion to ORINASE in the hospital may be advisable in candidates who require more than 40 units of insulin daily. During this conversion period when both insulin and ORINASE are being used, hypoglycemia may rarely occur. During insulin withdrawal, patients should test their urine for glucose and acetone at least three times daily and report results to their physician. The appearance of persistent acetonuria with glycosuria indicates that the patient is a type 1 diabetic patient who requires insulin therapy.

Maximum Dose

Daily doses of greater than 3 grams are not recommended.

Usual Maintenance Dose

The maintenance dose is in the range of 0.25 - 3 grams daily. Maintenance doses above 2 grams are seldom required.

Dosage Interval

The total daily dose may be taken either in the morning or in divided doses through the day. While either schedule is usually effective, the divided dose system is preferred by some clinicians from the standpoint of digestive tolerance.

Continued on next page

Information on these Upjohn products is based on labeling in effect August 15, 1986. Further information concerning these and other Upjohn products may be obtained by direct inquiry to Medical Information, The Upjohn Company, Kalamazoo, Michigan 49001.

Upjohn—Cont.

In elderly, debilitated or malnourished patients and patients with impaired renal or hepatic function, the initial and maintenance dosing should be conservative to avoid hypoglycemic reactions (see **Precautions** section).

HOW SUPPLIED

ORINASE Tablets (tolbutamide) are available in the following strengths and package sizes:

250 mg (scored, round, white)

Unit-of-Use bottles of 100	NDC 0009-0701-01
0.5 gram (scored, round, white)	
Bottles of 200	NDC 0009-0100-02
Bottles of 500	NDC 0009-0100-03
Bottles of 1000	NDC 0009-0100-05
Unit-of-Use bottles of 50	NDC 0009-0100-01
Unit of Use bottles of 100	NDC 0009-0100-11
Unit-Dose package of 100	NDC 0009-0100-06

Store at controlled room temperature 15–30°C (59–86°F).
Code 811 646 004

Shown in Product Identification Section, page 434

PAMINE® ℞

brand of methscopolamine bromide tablets, USP

HOW SUPPLIED

Each tablet contains 2.5 mg methscopolamine bromide.
Bottles of 100 *NDC 0009-0061-01*
Bottles of 500 *NDC 0009-0061-02*

PROSTIN VR PEDIATRIC® ℞

brand of alprostadil sterile solution
(alprostadil injection, USP)
500 micrograms per ml

WARNING

Apnea is experienced by about 10 to 12% of neonates with congenital heart defects treated with PROSTIN VR PEDIATRIC Sterile Solution (alprostadil). Apnea is most often seen in neonates weighing less than 2 kg at birth and usually appears during the first hour of drug infusion. Therefore, respiratory status should be monitored throughout treatment, and PROSTIN VR PEDIATRIC should be used where ventilatory assistance is immediately available.

DESCRIPTION

PROSTIN VR PEDIATRIC Sterile Solution for intravascular infusion contains 500 micrograms alprostadil, more commonly known as prostaglandin E_1, in 1.0 ml dehydrated alcohol.

The chemical name for alprostadil is (11α, 13E, 15S)-11,15 dihydroxy-9-oxoprost-13-en-1-oic acid, and the molecular weight is 354.49.

Alprostadil is a white to off-white crystalline powder with a melting point between 110° and 116°C. Its solubility at 35°C is 8000 micrograms per 100 ml double distilled water.

CLINICAL PHARMACOLOGY

Alprostadil (prostaglandin E_1) is one of a family of naturally occurring acidic lipids with various pharmacologic effects. Vasodilation, inhibition of platelet aggregation, and stimulation of intestinal and uterine smooth muscle are among the most notable of these effects. Intravenous doses of 1 to 10 micrograms of alprostadil per kilogram of body weight lower the blood pressure in mammals by decreasing peripheral resistance. Reflex increases in cardiac output and rate accompany the reduction in blood pressure.

Smooth muscle of the ductus arteriosus is especially sensitive to alprostadil, and strips of lamb ductus markedly relax in the presence of the drug. In addition, administration of alprostadil reopened the closing ductus of newborn rats, rabbits, and lambs. These observations led to the investigation of alprostadil in infants who had congenital defects which restricted the pulmonary or systemic blood flow and who depended on a patent ductus arteriosus for adequate blood oxygenation and lower body perfusion.

In infants with restricted pulmonary blood flow, about 50% responded to alprostadil infusion with at least a 10 torr increase in blood pO_2 (mean increase about 14 torr and mean increase in oxygen saturation about 23%). In general, patients who responded best had low pretreatment blood pO_2 and were 4 days old or less.

In infants with restricted systemic blood flow, alprostadil often increased pH in those having acidosis, increased systemic blood pressure, and decreased the ratio of pulmonary artery pressure to aortic pressure.

Alprostadil must be infused continuously because it is very rapidly metabolized. As much as 80% of the circulating alprostadil may be metabolized in one pass through the lungs, primarily by β- and ω-oxidation. The metabolites are excreted primarily by the kidney, and excretion is essentially complete within 24 hours after administration. No unchanged alprostadil has been found in the urine, and there is no evidence of tissue retention of alprostadil or its metabolites.

INDICATIONS AND USAGE

PROSTIN VR PEDIATRIC Sterile Solution (alprostadil) is indicated for palliative, not definitive, therapy to temporarily maintain the patency of the ductus arteriosus until corrective or palliative surgery can be performed in neonates who have congenital heart defects and who depend upon the patent ductus for survival. Such congenital heart defects include pulmonary atresia, pulmonary stenosis, tricuspid atresia, tetralogy of Fallot, interruption of the aortic arch, coarctation of the aorta, or transposition of the great vessels with or without other defects.

In infants with restricted pulmonary blood flow, the increase in blood oxygenation is inversely proportional to pretreatment pO_2 values; that is, patients with low pO_2 values respond best, and patients with pO_2 values of 40 torr or more usually have little response.

PROSTIN VR PEDIATRIC should be administered only by trained personnel in facilities that provide pediatric intensive care.

CONTRAINDICATIONS

None.

WARNINGS

See WARNING box.

Note: PROSTIN VR PEDIATRIC Sterile Solution (alprostadil) must be diluted before it is administered. See dilution instructions in DOSAGE AND ADMINISTRATION section.

PRECAUTIONS

General Precautions

Cortical proliferation of the long bones, first observed in dogs, has also been observed in infants during long-term infusions of alprostadil. The cortical proliferation in infants regressed after withdrawal of the drug.

PROSTIN VR PEDIATRIC Sterile Solution (alprostadil) should be infused for the shortest time and at the lowest dose that will produce the desired effects. The risks of long-term infusion of PROSTIN VR PEDIATRIC should be weighed against the possible benefits that critically ill infants may derive from its administration.

Because alprostadil inhibits platelet aggregation, use PROSTIN VR PEDIATRIC cautiously in neonates with bleeding tendencies.

PROSTIN VR PEDIATRIC should not be used in neonates with respiratory distress syndrome. A differential diagnosis should be made between respiratory distress syndrome (hyaline membrane disease) and cyanotic heart disease (restricted pulmonary blood flow). If full diagnostic facilities are not immediately available, cyanosis (pO_2 less than 40 torr) and restricted pulmonary blood flow apparent on an X-ray are appropriate indicators of congenital heart defects.

Necessary Monitoring: In all neonates, arterial pressure should be monitored intermittently by umbilical artery catheter, auscultation, or with a Doppler transducer. *Should arterial pressure fall significantly, decrease the rate of infusion immediately.*

In infants with restricted pulmonary blood flow, measure efficacy of PROSTIN VR PEDIATRIC by monitoring improvement in blood oxygenation. In infants with restricted systemic blood flow, measure efficacy by monitoring improvement of systemic blood pressure and blood pH.

Drug Interactions: No drug interactions have been reported between PROSTIN VR PEDIATRIC and the therapy standard in neonates with restricted pulmonary or systemic blood flow. Standard therapy includes antibiotics, such as penicillin and gentamicin; vasopressors, such as dopamine and isoproterenol; cardiac glycosides; and diuretics, such as furosemide.

Carcinogenesis, Mutagenesis, and Impairment of Fertility: - Long-term carcinogenicity studies and fertility studies have not been done. The Ames and Alkaline Elution assays reveal no potential for mutagenesis.

ADVERSE REACTIONS

Central Nervous System: Apnea has been reported in about 12% of the neonates treated. (See WARNING box.) Other common adverse reactions reported have been fever in about 14% of the patients treated and seizures in about 4%. The following reactions have been reported in less than 1% of the patients: cerebral bleeding, hyperextension of the neck, hyperirritability, hypothermia, jitteriness, lethargy, and stiffness.

Cardiovascular System: The most common adverse reactions reported have been flushing in about 10% of patients (more common after intraarterial dosing), bradycardia in about 7%, hypotension in about 4%, tachycardia in about 3%, cardiac arrest in about 1%, and edema in about 1%. The following reactions have been reported in less than 1% of the patients: congestive heart failure, hyperemia, second degree heart block, shock, spasm of the right ventricle infundibulum, supraventricular tachycardia, and ventricular fibrillation.

Respiratory System: The following reactions have been reported in less than 1% of the patients: bradypnea, bronchial wheezing, hypercapnia, respiratory depression, respiratory distress, and tachypnea.

Gastrointestinal System: The most common adverse reaction reported has been diarrhea in about 2% of the patients. The following reactions have been reported in less than 1% of the patients; gastric regurgitation, and hyperbilirubinemia.

Hematologic System: The most common hematologic event reported has been disseminated intravascular coagulation in about 1% of the patients. The following events have been reported in less than 1% of the patients: anemia, bleeding, and thrombocytopenia.

Excretory System: Anuria and hematuria have been reported in less than 1% of the patients.

Skeletal System: Cortical proliferation of the long bones has been reported. See PRECAUTIONS.

Miscellaneous: Sepsis has been reported in about 2% of the patients. Peritonitis has been reported in less than 1% of the patients. Hypokalemia has been reported in about 1%, and hypoglycemia and hyperkalemia have been reported in less than 1% of the patients.

OVERDOSAGE

Apnea, bradycardia, pyrexia, hypotension, and flushing may be signs of drug overdosage. If apnea or bradycardia occurs, discontinue the infusion, and provide appropriate medical treatment. Caution should be used in restarting the infusion. If pyrexia or hypotension occurs, reduce the infusion rate until these symptoms subside. Flushing is usually a result of incorrect intraarterial catheter placement, and the catheter should be repositioned.

DOSAGE AND ADMINISTRATION

The preferred route of administration for PROSTIN VR PEDIATRIC Sterile Solution (alprostadil) is continuous intravenous infusion into a large vein. Alternatively, PROSTIN VR PEDIATRIC may be administered through an umbilical artery catheter placed at the ductal opening. Increases in blood pO_2 (torr) have been the same in neonates who received the drug by either route of administration.

Begin infusion with 0.1 micrograms alprostadil per kilogram of body weight per minute. After a therapeutic response is achieved (increased pO_2 in infants with restricted pulmonary blood flow or increased systemic blood pressure and blood pH in infants with restricted systemic blood flow), reduce the infusion rate to provide the lowest possible dosage that maintains the response. This may be accomplished by reducing the dosage from 0.1 to 0.05 to 0.025 to 0.01 micrograms per kilogram of body weight per minute. If response to 0.1 micrograms per kilogram of body weight per minute is inadequate, dosage can be increased up to 0.4 micrograms per kilogram of body weight per minute although, in general, higher infusion rates do not produce greater effects.

Dilution instructions: To prepare infusion solutions, dilute 1 ml of PROSTIN VR PEDIATRIC Sterile Solution with Sodium Chloride Injection USP or Dextrose Injection USP. Dilute to volumes appropriate for the pump delivery system available. Prepare fresh infusion solutions every 24 hours. *Discard any solution more than 24 hours old.*

Sample Dilutions and Infusion Rates to Provide a Dosage of 0.1 Micrograms per Kilogram of Body Weight per Minute

Add 1 ampoule (500 micrograms) alprostadil to:	Approximate concentration of resulting solution (micrograms/ml)	Infusion rate (ml/min per kg of body weight)
250 ml	2	0.05
100 ml	5	0.02
50 ml	10	0.01
25 ml	20	0.005

Example: To provide 0.1 micrograms/kilogram of body weight per minute to an infant weighing 2.8 kilograms using a solution of 1 ampoule PROSTIN VR PEDIATRIC in 100 ml of saline or dextrose: INFUSION RATE = 0.02 ml/min per kg × 2.8 kg = 0.056 ml/min or 3.36 ml/hr.

HOW SUPPLIED

PROSTIN VR PEDIATRIC Sterile Solution (alprostadil) is available in packages of 5—1 ml ampoules (NDC 0009-3169-01). Each ml contains 500 micrograms alprostadil in dehydrated alcohol.

Store PROSTIN VR PEDIATRIC Sterile Solution in a refrigerator at 2°–8°C (36°–46°F).
Code 811 987 002

PROVERA® ℞
brand of medroxyprogesterone acetate tablets, USP
2.5 mg, 25's
NSN 6505-01-184-1249 (M)
10 mg, Dosepak of 10, Box of 10
NSN 6505-01-071-5605 (M)
10 mg, 100's
NSN 6505-00-890-1355 (M & VA)

> WARNING:
> THE USE OF PROGESTATIONAL AGENTS DURING THE FIRST FOUR MONTHS OF PREGNANCY IS NOT RECOMMENDED
> Progestational agents have been used beginning with the first trimester of pregnancy in an attempt to prevent habitual abortion or treat threatened abortion. There is no adequate evidence that such use is effective and there is evidence of potential harm to the fetus when such drugs are given during the first four months of pregnancy. Furthermore, in the vast majority of women, the cause of abortion is a defective ovum, which progestational agents could not be expected to influence. In addition, the use of progestational agents with their uterine-relaxant properties, in patients with fertilized defective ova may cause a delay in spontaneous abortion. Therefore, the use of such drugs during the first four months of pregnancy is not recommended.
> Several reports suggest an association between intrauterine exposure to female sex hormones and congenital anomalies, including congenital heart defects and limb reduction defects[1-5]. One study[4] estimated a 4.7-fold increased risk of limb reduction defects in infants exposed in utero to sex hormones (oral contraceptives, hormone withdrawal tests for pregnancy, or attempted treatment for threatened abortion). Some of these exposures were very short and involved only a few days of treatment. The data suggest that the risk of limb reduction defects in exposed fetuses is somewhat less than 1 in 1,000.
> If the patient is exposed to PROVERA Tablets (medroxyprogesterone acetate) during the first four months of pregnancy or if she becomes pregnant while taking this drug, she should be apprised of the potential risks to the fetus.

DESCRIPTION

PROVERA Tablets contain medroxyprogesterone acetate, which is a derivative of progesterone. It is a white to off-white, odorless crystalline powder, stable in air, melting between 200 and 210° C. It is freely soluble in chloroform, soluble in acetone and in dioxane, sparingly soluble in alcohol and in methanol, slightly soluble in ether, and insoluble in water.
The chemical name for medroxyprogesterone acetate is Pregn-4-ene-3,20-dione, 17-(acetyloxy)-6-methyl-, (6α)-.
Each PROVERA tablet for oral administration contains 2.5 mg, 5 mg or 10 mg of medroxyprogesterone acetate. Inactive ingredients: calcium stearate, corn starch, lactose, mineral oil, sorbic acid, sucrose, talc. The 2.5 mg tablet contains FD&C Yellow no. 6.

ACTIONS

Medroxyprogesterone acetate, administered orally or parenterally in the recommended doses to women with adequate endogenous estrogen, transforms proliferative into secretory endometrium. Androgenic and anabolic effects have been noted, but the drug is apparently devoid of significant estrogenic activity. While parenterally administered medroxyprogesterone acetate inhibits gonadotropin production, which in turn prevents follicular maturation and ovulation, available data indicate that this does not occur when the usually recommended oral dosage is given as single daily doses.

INDICATIONS

Secondary amenorrhea; abnormal uterine bleeding due to hormonal imbalance in the absence of organic pathology, such as fibroids or uterine cancer.

CONTRAINDICATIONS

1. Thrombophlebitis, thromboembolic disorders, cerebral apoplexy or patients with a past history of these conditions.
2. Liver dysfunction or disease.
3. Known or suspected malignancy of breast or genital organs.
4. Undiagnosed vaginal bleeding.
5. Missed abortion.
6. As a diagnostic test for pregnancy.
7. Known sensitivity to PROVERA Tablets (medroxyprogesterone acetate).

WARNINGS

1. The physician should be alert to the earliest manifestations of thrombotic disorders (thrombophlebitis, cerebrovascular disorders, pulmonary embolism, and retinal thrombosis). Should any of these occur or be suspected, the drug should be discontinued immediately.
2. Beagle dogs treated with medroxyprogesterone acetate developed mammary nodules some of which were malignant. Although nodules occasionally appeared in control animals, they were intermittent in nature, whereas the nodules in the drug-treated animals were larger, more numerous, persistent, and there were some breast malignancies with metastases. Their significance with respect to humans has not been established.
3. Discontinue medication pending examination if there is sudden partial or complete loss of vision, or if there is a sudden onset of proptosis, diplopia or migraine. If examination reveals papilledema or retinal vascular lesions, medication should be withdrawn.
4. Detectable amounts of progestin have been identified in the milk of mothers receiving the drug. The effect of this on the nursing infant has not been determined.
5. Usage in pregnancy is not recommended (See WARNING Box).
6. Retrospective studies of morbidity and mortality in Great Britain and studies of morbidity in the United States have shown a statistically significant association between thrombophlebitis, pulmonary embolism, and cerebral thrombosis and embolism and the use of oral contraceptives.[6-9] The estimate of the relative risk of thromboembolism in the study by Vessey and Doll[8] was about sevenfold, while Sartwell and associates[9] in the United States found a relative risk of 4.4, meaning that the users are several times as likely to undergo thromboembolic disease without evident cause as nonusers. The American study also indicated that the risk did not persist after discontinuation of administration, and that it was not enhanced by long continued administration. The American study was not designed to evaluate a difference between products.

PRECAUTIONS

1. The pretreatment physical examination should include special reference to breast and pelvic organs, as well as Papanicolaou smear.
2. Because progestogens may cause some degree of fluid retention, conditions which might be influenced by this factor, such as epilepsy, migraine, asthma, cardiac or renal dysfunction, require careful observation.
3. In cases of breakthrough bleeding, as in all cases of irregular bleeding per vaginum, nonfunctional causes should be borne in mind. In cases of undiagnosed vaginal bleeding, adequate diagnostic measures are indicated.
4. Patients who have a history of psychic depression should be carefully observed and the drug discontinued if the depression recurs to a serious degree.
5. Any possible influence of prolonged progestin therapy on pituitary, ovarian, adrenal, hepatic or uterine functions awaits further study.
6. A decrease in glucose tolerance has been observed in a small percentage of patients on estrogen-progestin combination drugs. The mechanism of this decrease is obscure. For this reason, diabetic patients should be carefully observed while receiving progestin therapy.
7. The age of the patient constitutes no absolute limiting factor although treatment with progestins may mask the onset of the climacteric.
8. The pathologist should be advised of progestin therapy when relevant specimens are submitted.
9. Because of the occasional occurrence of thrombotic disorders, (thrombophlebitis, pulmonary embolism, retinal thrombosis, and cerebrovascular disorders) in patients taking estrogen-progestin combinations and since the mechanism is obscure, the physician should be alert to the earliest manifestation of these disorders.

Information for the Patient
See Patient Information at the end of insert.

ADVERSE REACTIONS

Pregnancy—(See WARNING Box for possible adverse effects on the fetus)
Breast—Breast tenderness or galactorrhea has been reported rarely.
Skin—Sensitivity reactions consisting of urticaria, pruritus, edema and generalized rash have occurred in an occasional patient. Acne, alopecia and hirsutism have been reported in a few cases.
Thromboembolic Phenomena—Thromboembolic phenomena including thrombophlebitis and pulmonary embolism have been reported.
The following adverse reactions have been observed in women taking progestins including PROVERA Tablets (medroxyprogesterone acetate):

- breakthrough bleeding
- spotting
- change in menstrual flow
- amenorrhea
- edema
- change in weight (increase or decrease)
- changes in cervical erosion and cervical secretions
- cholestatic jaundice
- anaphylactoid reactions and anaphylaxis
- rash (allergic) with and without pruritus
- mental depression
- pyrexia
- insomnia
- nausea
- somnolence

A statistically significant association has been demonstrated between use of estrogen-progestin combination drugs and the following serious adverse reactions: thrombophlebitis; pulmonary embolism and cerebral thrombosis and embolism. For this reason patients on progestin therapy should be carefully observed.
Although available evidence is suggestive of an association, such a relationship has been neither confirmed nor refuted for the following serious adverse reactions:

- neuro-ocular lesions, eg, retinal thrombosis and optic neuritis.

The following adverse reactions have been observed in patients receiving estrogen-progestin combination drugs:

- rise in blood pressure in susceptible individuals
- premenstrual-like syndrome
- changes in libido
- changes in appetite
- cystitis-like syndrome
- headache
- nervousness
- dizziness
- fatigue
- backache
- hirsutism
- loss of scalp hair
- erythema multiforme
- erythema nodosum
- hemorrhagic eruption
- itching

In view of these observations, patients on progestin therapy should be carefully observed.
The following laboratory results may be altered by the use of estrogen-progestin combination drugs:
Increased sulfobromophthalein retention and other hepatic function tests.
Coagulation tests: increase in prothrombin factors VII, VIII, IX and X.
Metyrapone test.
Pregnanediol determination.
Thyroid function: increase in PBI, and butanol extractable protein bound iodine and decrease in T^3 uptake values.

DOSAGE AND ADMINISTRATION

Secondary Amenorrhea—PROVERA Tablets (medroxyprogesterone acetate) may be given in dosages of 5 to 10 mg daily for from 5 to 10 days. A dose for inducing an optimum secretory transformation of an endometrium that has been adequately primed with either endogenous or exogenous estrogen is 10 mg of PROVERA Tablets daily for 10 days. In cases of secondary amenorrhea, therapy may be started at any time. Progestin withdrawal bleeding usually occurs within three to seven days after discontinuing therapy with PROVERA.
Abnormal Uterine Bleeding Due to Hormonal Imbalance in the Absence of Organic Pathology—Beginning on the calculated 16th or 21st day of the menstrual cycle, 5 to 10 mg of PROVERA Tablets may be given daily for from 5 to 10 days. To produce an optimum secretory transformation of an endometrium that has been adequately primed with either endogenous or exogenous estrogen, 10 mg of PROVERA Tablets daily for 10 days beginning on the 16th day of the cycle is suggested. Progestin withdrawal bleeding usually occurs within three to seven days after discontinuing therapy with PROVERA. Patients with a past history of recurrent episodes of abnormal uterine bleeding may benefit from planned menstrual cycling with PROVERA.

HOW SUPPLIED

PROVERA Tablets are available in the following strengths and package sizes:
2.5 mg (scored, round, orange)

Bottles of 25	NDC 0009-0064-01
Bottles of 100	NDC 0009-0064-04

5 mg (scored, hexagonal, white)

Bottles of 25	NDC 0009-0286-02
Bottles of 100	NDC 0009-0286-03

Continued on next page

Information on these Upjohn products is based on labeling in effect August 15, 1986. Further information concerning these and other Upjohn products may be obtained by direct inquiry to Medical Information, The Upjohn Company, Kalamazoo, Michigan 49001.

Upjohn—Cont.

10 mg (scored, round, white)

Bottles of 25	NDC 0009-0050-01
Bottles of 100	NDC 0009-0050-02
Bottles of 500	NDC 0009-0050-11
DOSEPAK™ Unit of Use (10)	NDC 0009-0050-12

Store at controlled room temperature 15°–30°C (59°–86°F).

REFERENCES

1. Gal I, Kirman B, Stern J: Hormonal pregnancy tests and congenital malformation. Nature *216*:83, 1967.
2. Levy EP, Cohen A, Fraser FC: Hormone treatment during pregnancy and congenital heart defects. Lancet *1*:611, 1973.
3. Nora JJ, Nora AH: Birth defects and oral contraceptives. Lancet *1*:941–942, 1973.
4. Janerich DT, Piper JM, Glebatis DM: Oral contraceptives and congenital limb-reduction defects. N Engl J Med *291*:697–700, 1974.
5. Heinonen OP, Slone D, Monson RR, et al: Cardiovascular birth defects and antenatal exposure to female sex hormones. N Engl J Med *296*:67–70, 1977.
6. Royal College of General Practitioners: Oral contraception and thromboembolic disease. J Coll Gen Pract *13*:267–279, 1967.
7. Inman WHW, Vessey MP: Investigation of deaths from pulmonary, coronary, and cerebral thrombosis and embolism in women of child-bearing age. Br Med J *2*:193–199, 1968.
8. Vessey MP, Doll R: Investigation of relation between use of oral contraceptives and thromboembolic disease. A further report. Br Med J *2*:651–657, 1969.
9. Sartwell PE, Masi AT, Arthes FG, et al: Thromboembolism and oral contraceptives: An epidemiological case-control study. Am J Epidemiol *90*:365–380, 1969.

The text of the patient insert for progesterone and progesterone-like drugs is set forth below.

Patient Information: PROVERA Tablets contain medroxyprogesterone acetate, a progesterone. The information below is that which the U.S. Food and Drug Administration requires be provided for all patients taking progesterones. The information below relates only to the risk to the unborn child associated with use of progesterone during pregnancy. For further information on the use, side effects and other risks associated with this product, ask your doctor.

WARNING FOR WOMEN

There is an increased risk of birth defects in children whose mothers take this drug during the first four months of pregnancy.

Medroxyprogesterone acetate is similar to the progesterone hormones naturally produced by the body. Progesterone and progesterone-like drugs are used to treat menstrual disorders, to test if the body is producing certain hormones, and to treat some forms of cancer in women.

They have been used as a test for pregnancy but such use is no longer considered safe because of possible damage to a developing baby. Also, more rapid methods for testing for pregnancy are now available.

These drugs have also been used to prevent miscarriage in the first few months of pregnancy. No adequate evidence is available to show that they are effective for this purpose. Furthermore, most cases of early miscarriage are due to causes which could not be helped by these drugs.

There is an increased risk of birth defects, such as heart or limb defects if progesterone and progesterone-like drugs are taken during the first four months of pregnancy. The exact risk of taking this drug early in pregnancy and having a baby with a birth defect is not known. However, one study found that babies born to women who had taken sex hormones (such as progesterone-like drugs) during the first three months of pregnancy were 4 to 5 times more likely to have abnormalities of the arms or legs than if their mothers had not taken such drugs. Some of these women had taken these drugs for only a few days. The chance that an infant whose mother had taken this drug will have this type of defect is about 1 in 1,000.

If you take PROVERA Tablets and later find you were pregnant when you took it, be sure to discuss this with your doctor as soon as possible.

Code 812 584 004

Shown in Product Identification Section, page 434

PYRROXATE® Capsules

(See PDR For Nonprescription Drugs)

SIGTAB® Tablets

(See PDR For Nonprescription Drugs)

SOLU–CORTEF® ℞

brand of hydrocortisone sodium succinate sterile powder (hydrocortisone sodium succinate for injection, USP)

For Intravenous or Intramuscular Administration

100 mg MIX-O-VIAL®:	**NSN 6505-00-753-9609**
250 mg MIX-O-VIAL:	**NSN 6505-00-951-5533**
500 mg MIX-O-VIAL:	**NSN 6505-00-116-5055**
1000 mg MIX-O-VIAL:	**NSN 6505-00-238-5222**

DESCRIPTION

SOLU-CORTEF Sterile Powder contains hydrocortisone sodium succinate as the active ingredient. Hydrocortisone sodium succinate is a white or nearly white, odorless, hygroscopic amorphous solid. It is very soluble in water and in alcohol, very slightly soluble in acetone and insoluble in chloroform. The chemical name is pregn-4-ene-3,20-dione,21-(3-carboxy-1-oxopropoxy)-11,17-dihydroxy-, monosodium salt, (11β)-and its molecular weight is 484.52.

Hydrocortisone sodium succinate is an anti-inflammatory adrenocortical steroid. This highly water-soluble sodium succinate ester of hydrocortisone permits the immediate intravenous administration of high doses of hydrocortisone in a small volume of diluent and is particularly useful where high blood levels of hydrocortisone are required rapidly.

SOLU-CORTEF Sterile Powder (hydrocortisone sodium succinate) is available in several packages for intravenous or intramuscular administration.

100 mg Plain—Vials containing hydrocortisone sodium succinate equivalent to 100 mg hydrocortisone, also 0.8 mg sodium biphosphate anhydrous, 8.73 mg dried sodium phosphate.

[See table below].

ACTIONS

Hydrocortisone sodium succinate has the same metabolic and anti-inflammatory actions as hydrocortisone. When given parenterally and in equimolar quantities, the two compounds are equivalent in biologic activity. Following the intravenous injection of hydrocortisone sodium succinate, demonstrable effects are evident within one hour and persist for a variable period. Excretion of the administered dose is nearly complete within 12 hours. Thus, if constantly high blood levels are required, injections should be made every 4 to 6 hours. This preparation is also rapidly absorbed when administered intramuscularly and is excreted in a pattern similar to that observed after intravenous injection.

INDICATIONS

When oral therapy is not feasible, and the strength, dosage form and route of administration of the drug reasonably lend the preparation to the treatment of the condition, SOLU-CORTEF Sterile Powder (hydrocortisone sodium succinate) is indicated for intravenous or intramuscular use in the following conditions:

1. **Endocrine Disorders**
   - Primary or secondary adrenocortical insufficiency (hydrocortisone or cortisone is the drug of choice; synthetic analogs may be used in conjunction with mineralocorticoids where applicable; in infancy, mineralocorticord supplementation is of particular importance)
   - Acute adrenocortical insufficiency (hydrocortisone or cortisone is the drug of choice; mineralocorticoid supplementation may be necessary, particularly when synthetic analogs are used)
   - Preoperatively and in the event of serious trauma or illness, in patients with known adrenal insufficiency or when adrenocortical reserve is doubtful
   - Shock unresponsive to conventional therapy if adrenocortical insufficiency exists or is suspected
   - Congenital adrenal hyperplasia
   - Hypercalcemia associated with cancer
   - Nonsuppurative thyroiditis
2. **Rheumatic Disorders**
   - As adjunctive therapy for short-term administration (to tide the patient over an acute episode or exacerbation) in:
   - Post-traumatic osteoarthritis
   - Synovitis of osteoarthritis
   - Rheumatoid arthritis, including juvenile rheumatoid arthritis (selected cases may require low-dose maintenance therapy)
   - Acute and subacute bursitis
   - Epicondylitis
   - Acute nonspecific tenosynovitis
   - Acute gouty arthritis
   - Psoriatic arthritis
   - Ankylosing spondylitis
3. **Collagen Diseases**
   - During an exacerbation or as maintenance therapy in selected cases of:
   - Systemic lupus erythematosus
   - Systemic dermatomyositis (polymyositis)
   - Acute rheumatic carditis
4. **Dermatologic Diseases**
   - Pemphigus
   - Severe erythema multiforme (Stevens-Johnson syndrome)
   - Exfoliative dermatitis
   - Bullous dermatitis herpetiformis
   - Severe seborrheic dermatitis
   - Severe psoriasis
   - Mycosis fungoides
5. **Allergic States**
   - Control of severe or incapacitating allergic conditions intractable to adequate trials of conventional treatment in:
   - Bronchial asthma
   - Contact dermatitis
   - Atopic dermatitis
   - Serum sickness
   - Seasonal or perennial allergic rhinitis
   - Drug hypersensitivity reactions
   - Urticarial transfusion reactions
   - Acute noninfectious laryngeal edema (epinephrine is the drug of first choice)
6. **Ophthalmic Diseases**
   - Severe acute and chronic allergic and inflammatory processes involving the eye, such as:
   - Herpes zoster ophthalmicus
   - Iritis, iridocyclitis
   - Chorioretinitis
   - Diffuse posterior uveitis and choroiditis
   - Optic neuritis
   - Sympathetic ophthalmia
   - Anterior segment inflammation
   - Allergic conjunctivitis
   - Allergic corneal marginal ulcers
   - Keratitis
7. **Gastrointestinal Diseases**
   - To tide the patient over a critical period of the disease in:
   - Ulcerative colitis (systemic therapy)
   - Regional enteritis (systemic therapy)
8. **Respiratory Diseases**
   - Symptomatic sarcoidosis
   - Berylliosis
   - Fulminating or disseminated pulmonary tuberculosis when used concurrently with appropriate antituberculous chemotherapy
   - Loeffler's syndrome not manageable by other means
   - Aspiration pneumonitis
9. **Hematologic Disorders**
   - Acquired (autoimmune) hemolytic anemia
   - Idiopathic thrombocytopenic purpura in adults (IV only; IM administration is contraindicated)
   - Secondary thrombocytopenia in adults
   - Erythroblastopenia (RBC anemia)
   - Congenital (erythroid) hypoplastic anemia

SOLU-CORTEF	**100 mg MIX-O-VIAL** Each 2 ml contains: (when mixed)	**250 mg MIX-O-VIAL** Each 2 ml contains: (when mixed)	**500 mg MIX-O-VIAL** Each 4 ml contains: (when mixed)	**1000 mg MIX-O-VIAL** Each 8 ml contains: (when mixed)
Hydrocortisone sodium succinate	equiv. to 100 mg hydrocortisone	equiv. to 250 mg hydrocortisone	equiv. to 500 mg hydrocortisone	equiv. to 1000 mg hydrocortisone
Monobasic sodium phosphate anhydrous	0.8 mg	2 mg	4 mg	8 mg
Diabasic sodium phosphate dried	8.76 mg	21.8 mg	44 mg	88 mg
Benzyl alcohol added as preservative	18.1 mg	16.4 mg	33.4 mg	66.9 mg

When necessary, the pH of each formula was adjusted with sodium hydroxide so that the pH of the reconstituted solution is within the USP specified range of 7 to 8.

10. **Neoplastic Diseases**
For palliative mangement of:
Leukemias and lymphomas in adults
Acute leukemia of childhood
11. **Edematous States**
To induce diuresis or remission of proteinuria in the nephrotic syndrome, without uremia, of the idiopathic type or that due to lupus erythematosus
12. **Nervous System**
Acute exacerbations of multiple sclerosis
13. **Miscellaneous**
Tuberculous meningitis with subarachnoid block or impending block when used concurrently with appropriate antituberculous chemotherapy
Trichinosis with neurologic or myocardial involvement

CONTRAINDICATIONS

Systemic fungal infections.

WARNINGS

In patients on corticosteroid therapy subjected to unusual stress, increased dosage of rapidly acting corticosteroids before, during, and after the stressful situation is indicated.
Corticosteroids may mask some signs of infection, and new infections may appear during their use. There may be decreased resistance and inability to localize infection when corticosteroids are used.
Prolonged use of corticosteroids may produce posterior subcapsular cataracts, glaucoma with possible damage to the optic nerves, and may enhance the establishment of secondary ocular infections due to fungi or viruses.
Usage in pregnancy. Since adequate human reproduction studies have not been done with corticosteroids, the use of these drugs in pregnancy, nursing mothers, or women of childbearing potential requires that the possible benefits of the drug be weighed against the potential hazards to the mother and embryo or fetus. Infants born of mothers who have received substantial doses of corticosteroids during pregnancy should be carefully observed for signs of hypoadrenalism.
Average and large doses of hydrocortisone can cause elevation of blood pressure, salt and water retention, and increased excretion of potassium. These effects are less likely to occur with the synthetic derivatives except when used in large doses. Dietary salt restriction and potassium supplementation may be necessary. All corticosteroids increase calcium excretion.
While on corticosteroid therapy patients should not be vaccinated against smallpox. Other immunization procedures should not be undertaken in patients who are on corticosteroids, especially on high dose, because of possible hazards of neurological complications and a lack of antibody response.
The use of SOLU-CORTEF Sterile Powder (hydrocortisone sodium succinate) in active tuberculosis should be restricted to those cases of fulminating or disseminated tuberculosis in which the corticosteroid is used for the management of the disease in conjunction with appropriate antituberculous regimen.
If corticosteroids are indicated in patients with latent tuberculosis or tuberculin reactivity, close observation is necessary as reactivation of the disease may occur. During prolonged corticosteroid therapy, these patients should receive chemoprophylaxis.
Because rare instances of anaphylactoid reactions (eg, bronchospasm) have occurred in patients receiving parenteral corticosteroid therapy, appropriate precautionary measures should be taken prior to administration, especially when the patient has a history of allergy to any drug.
The SOLU-CORTEF 100 mg, 250 mg, 500 mg and 1000 mg MIX-O-VIAL two-compartment vials contain benzyl alcohol. Benzyl alcohol has been reported to be associated with a fatal "Gasping Syndrome" in premature infants.

PRECAUTIONS

Drug-induced secondary adrenocortical insufficiency may be minimized by gradual reduction of dosage. This type of relative insufficiency may persist for months after discontinuation of therapy; therefore, in any situation of stress occurring during that period, hormone therapy should be reinstituted. Since mineralocorticoid secretion may be impaired, salt and/or a mineralocorticoid should be administered concurrently.
There is an enhanced effect of corticosteroids in patients with hypothyroidism and in those with cirrhosis.
Corticosteroids should be used cautiously in patients with ocular herpes simplex for fear of corneal perforation.
The lowest possible dose of corticosteroid should be used to control the condition under treatment, and when reduction in dosage is possible, the reduction must be gradual.
Psychic derangements may appear when corticosteroids are used, ranging from euphoria, insomnia, mood swings, personality changes, and severe depression to frank psychotic manifestations. Also, existing emotional instability or psychotic tendencies may be aggravated by corticosteroids.
Aspirin should be used cautiously in conjunction with corticosteroids in hypoprothrombinemia.
Steroids should be used with caution in nonspecific ulcerative colitis, if there is a probability of impending perforation, abscess or other pyogenic infection, also in diverticulitis, fresh intestinal anastomoses, active or latent peptic ulcer, renal insufficiency, hypertension, osteoporosis, and myasthenia gravis.
Growth and development of infants and children on prolonged corticosteroid therapy should be carefully followed.
Although controlled clinical trials have shown corticosteroids to be effective in speeding the resolution of acute exacerbations of multiple sclerosis, they do not show that corticosteroids affect the ultimate outcome or natural history of the disease. The studies do show that relatively high doses of corticosteroids are necessary to demonstrate a significant effect. (See **Administration and Dosage**).
Since complications of treatment with glucocorticoids are dependent on the size of the dose and the duration of treatment, a risk/benefit decision must be made in each individual case as to dose and duration of treatment and as to whether daily or intermittent therapy should be used.

ADVERSE REACTIONS

Fluid and Electrolyte Disturbances
Sodium retention
Fluid retention
Congestive heart failure in susceptible patients
Potassium loss
Hypokalemic alkalosis
Hypertension
Musculoskeletal
Muscle weakness
Steroid myopathy
Loss of muscle mass
Osteoporosis
Vertebral compression fractures
Aseptic necrosis of femoral and humeral heads
Pathologic fracture of long bones
Gastrointestinal
Peptic ulcer with possible perforation and hemorrhage
Pancreatitis
Abdominal distention
Ulcerative esophagitis
Dermatologic
Impaired wound healing
Thin fragile skin
Petechiae and ecchymoses
Facial erythema
Increased sweating
May suppress reactions to skin tests
Neurological
Convulsions
Increased intracranial pressure with papilledema (pseudotumor cerebri) usually after treatment
Vertigo
Headache
Endocrine
Menstrual irregularities
Development of Cushingoid state
Suppression of growth in children
Secondary adrenocortical and pituitary unresponsiveness, particularly in times of stress, as in trauma, surgery, or illness
Decreased carbohydrate tolerance
Manifestations of latent diabetes mellitus
Increased requirements for insulin or oral hypoglycemic agents in diabetics
Ophthalmic
Posterior subcapsular cataracts
Increased intraocular pressure
Glaucoma
Exophthalmos
Metabolic
Negative nitrogen balance due to protein catabolism
The following additional reactions are related to parenteral corticosteroid therapy:
Allergic, anaphylactic or other hypersensitivity reactions
Hyperpigmentation or hypopigmentation
Subcutaneous and cutaneous atrophy
Sterile abscess

ADMINISTRATION AND DOSAGE

This preparation may be administered by intravenous injection, by intravenous infusion, or by intramuscular injection, the preferred method for initial emergency use being intravenous injection. Following the initial emergency period, consideration should be given to employing a longer acting injectable preparation or an oral preparation.
Therapy is initiated by administering SOLU-CORTEF Sterile Powder (hydrocortisone sodium succinate) intravenously over a period of 30 seconds (eg, 100 mg) to 10 minutes (eg, 500 mg or more). In general, high dose corticosteroid therapy should be continued only until the patient's condition has stabilized—usually not beyond 48 to 72 hours. Although adverse effects associated with high dose, short-term corticoid therapy are uncommon, peptic ulceration may occur. Prophylactic anatacid therapy may be indicated.
When high dose hydrocortisone therapy must be continued beyond 48–72 hours, hypernatremia may occur. Under such circumstances it may be desirable to replace SOLU-CORTEF with a corticoid such as methylprednisolone sodium succinate which causes little or no sodium retention.
The initial dose of SOLU-CORTEF Sterile Powder is 100 mg to 500 mg, depending on the severity of the condition. This dose may be repeated at intervals of 2, 4 or 6 hours as indicated by the patient's response and clinical condition. While the dose may be reduced for infants and children, it is governed more by the severity of the condition and response of the patient than by age or body weight but should not be less than 25 mg daily.
Patients subjected to severe stress following corticosteroid therapy should be observed closely for signs and symptoms of adrenocortical insufficiency.
Corticoid therapy is an adjunct to, and not a replacement for, conventional therapy.

Preparation of Solutions

100 mg Plain—For intravenous or intramuscular injection, prepare solution by aseptically adding **not more than 2 ml** of Bacteriostatic Water for Injection or Bacteriostatic Sodium Chloride Injection to the contents of one vial. **For intravenous infusion,** first prepare solution by adding **not more than 2 ml** of Bacteriostatic Water for Injection to the vial; this solution may then be added to 100 to 1000 ml (but not less than 100 ml) of the following: 5% dextrose in water (or isotonic saline solution or 5% dextrose in isotonic saline solution if patient is not on sodium restriction).

Directions for using MIX-O-VIAL Two-Compartment Vial

1 Remove protective cap, give the plunger-stopper a quarter-turn and press to force diluent into the lower compartment.
2. Gently agitate to effect solution.
3. Sterilize top of plunger-stopper with a suitable germicide.
4. Insert needle **squarely through center** of plunger-stopper until tip is just visible. Invert vial and withdraw dose.

Further dilution is not necessary for intravenous or intramuscular injection. For intravenous infusion, first prepare solution as just described. The **100 mg** solution may then be added to 100 to 1000 ml of 5% dextrose in water (or isotonic saline solution or 5% dextrose in isotonic saline solution if patient is not on sodium restriction). The **250 mg** solution may be added to 250 to 1000 ml, the **500 mg** solution may be added to 500 to 1000 ml and the **1000 mg** solution to 1000 ml of the same diluents. In cases where administration of a small volume of fluid is desirable, 100 mg to 3000 mg of SOLU-CORTEF Sterile Powder may be added to 50 ml of the above diluents. The resulting solutions are stable for at least 4 hours and may be administered either directly or by IV piggyback.
When reconstituted as directed, pH's of the solutions range from 7 to 8 and the tonicities are: 100 mg MIX-O-VIAL, .36 osmolar; 250 mg MIX-O-VIAL, 500 mg MIX-O-VIAL, and the 1000 mg MIX-O-VIAL, .57 osmolar. (Isotonic saline =.28 osmolar.)

HOW SUPPLIED

SOLU-CORTEF Sterile Powder (hydrocortisone sodium succinate) is available in the following packages:
100 mg Plain—NDC 0009-0825-01
100 mg MIX-O-VIAL
2 ml—NDC 0009-0900-01
25-2 ml—NDC 0009-0900-12
250 mg MIX-O-VIAL
2 ml—NDC 0009-0909-01
25-2 ml—NDC 0009-0909-07
500 mg MIX-O-VIAL—NDC 0009-0912-01
1000 mg MIX-O-VIAL—NDC 0009-0920-01

STORAGE CONDITIONS

Store unreconstituted product at controlled room temperature 15°-30°C (59°-86°F).
Store solution at controlled room temperature 15°-30°C (59°-86°F) and protect from light. Use solution only if it is clear. Unused solution should be discarded after 3 days.
Code 810 379 008

Continued on next page

Information on these Upjohn products is based on labeling in effect August 15, 1986. Further information concerning these and other Upjohn products may be obtained by direct inquiry to Medical Information, The Upjohn Company, Kalamazoo, Michigan 49001.

Upjohn—Cont.

SOLU-MEDROL® ℞

brand of methylprednisolone sodium succinate sterile powder
(methylprednisolone sodium succinate for injection, USP)
For Intravenous or Intramuscular Administration

DESCRIPTION

SOLU-MEDROL Sterile Powder contains methylprednisolone sodium succinate as the active ingredient. Methylprednisolone sodium succinate, USP, occurs as a white, or nearly white, odorless hygroscopic, amorphous solid. It is very soluble in water and in alcohol; it is insoluble in chloroform and is very slightly soluble in acetone.

The chemical name for methylprednisolone sodium succinate is pregna-1,4-diene-3,20-dione,21-(3-carboxy-1-oxopropoxy)-11,17-dihydroxy-6-methyl-,monosodium salt, (6α, 11β), and the molecular weight is 496.53.

Methylprednisolone sodium succinate is so extremely soluble in water that it may be administered in a small volume of diluent and is especially well suited for intravenous use in situations in which high blood levels of methylprednisolone are required rapidly.

SOLU-MEDROL is available in several strengths and packages for intravenous or intramuscular administration. **40 mg ACT-O-VIAL® System and 40 mg MIX-O-VIAL® Two-Compartment Vial**—Each ml (when mixed) contains methylprednisolone sodium succinate equivalent to 40 mg methylprednisolone; also 1.6 mg monobasic sodium phosphate anhydrous; 17.46 mg dibasic sodium phosphate dried; 25 mg lactose hydrous; 8.8 mg benzyl alcohol added as preservative. **125 mg ACT-O-VIAL System and 125 MIX-O-VIAL Two-Compartment Vial**—Each 2 ml (when mixed) contains methylprednisolone sodium succinate equivalent to 125 mg methylprednisolone; also 1.6 mg monobasic sodium biphosphate anhydrous; 17.4 mg dibasic sodium phosphate dried; 17.6 mg benzyl alcohol added as preservative. **500 mg Vial**—Each 8 ml (when mixed as directed) contains methylprednisolone sodium succinate equivalent to 500 mg methylprednisolone; also 6.4 mg monobasic sodium biphosphate anhydrous; 69.6 mg dibasic sodium phosphate dried. **500 mg Vial with Diluent**—Each 8 ml (when mixed as directed) contains methylprednisolone sodium succinate equivalent to 500 mg methylprednisolone; also 6.4 mg monobasic sodium phosphate anhydrous; 69.6 mg dibasic sodium phosphate dried; 70.2 mg benzyl alcohol added as preservative. **1 gram Vial**—Each 16 ml (when mixed as directed) contains methylprednisolone sodium succinate equivalent to 1 gram methylprednisolone; also 12.8 mg monobasic sodium phosphate anhydrous; 139.2 mg dibasic sodium phosphate dried. **1 gram Vial with Diluent**—Each 16 ml (when mixed as directed) contains methylprednisolone sodium succinate equivalent to 1 gram methylprednisolone; also 12.8 mg monobasic sodium phosphate anhydrous; 139.2 mg dibasic sodium phosphate dried; 141 mg benzyl alcohol added as preservative. **2 gram Vial**—Each 30.6 ml (when mixed as directed) contains methylprednisolone sodium succinate equivalent to 2 grams methylprednisolone (62.5 mg per ml); also 25.6 mg monobasic sodium phosphate anhydrous; 278 mg dibasic sodium phosphate dried. **2 gram Vial with Diluent**—Each 30.6 ml (when mixed as directed) contains methylprednisolone sodium succinate equivalent to 2 grams methylprednisolone; also 25.6 mg monobasic sodium phosphate anhydrous; 278 mg dibasic sodium phosphate dried; 273 mg benzyl alcohol added as preservative.

When necessary, the pH of each formula was adjusted with sodium hydroxide so that the pH of the reconstituted solution is within the USP specified range of 7 to 8 and the tonicities are, for the 40 mg per ml solution, 0.50 osmolar; for the 125 mg per 2 ml, 500 mg per 8 ml and 1 gram per 16 ml solutions, 0.40 osmolar; for the 2 gram per 30.6 ml solutions, 0.42 osmolar. (Isotonic saline = 0.28 osmolar).

IMPORTANT—Use only the accompanying diluent or Bacteriostac Water For Injection with Benzyl Alcohol when reconstituting SOLU-MEDROL.

Use within 48 hours after mixing

ACTIONS

Methylprednisolone is a potent anti-inflammatory steroid synthesized in the Research Laboratories of The Upjohn Company. It has a greater anti-inflammatory potency than prednisolone and even less tendency than prednisolone to induce sodium and water retention.

Methylprednisolone sodium succinate has the same metabolic and anti-inflammatory actions as methylprednisolone. When given parenterally and in equimolar quantities, the two compounds are equivalent in biologic activity. The relative potency of SOLU-MEDROL Sterile Powder (methylprednisolone sodium succinate) and hydrocortisone sodium succinate, as indicated by depression of eosinophil count, following intravenous administration, is at least four to one. This is in good agreement with the relative oral potency of methylprednisolone and hydrocortisone.

INDICATIONS

When oral therapy is not feasible, and the strength, dosage form and route of administration of the drug reasonably lend the preparation to the treatment of the condition, SOLU-MEDROL Sterile Powder (methylprednisolone sodium succinate) is indicated for intravenous or intramuscular use in the following conditions:

1. **Endocrine Disorders**
   - Primary or secondary adrenocortical insufficiency (hydrocortisone or cortisone is the drug of choice; synthetic analogs may be used in conjunction with mineralocorticoids where applicable; in infancy, mineralocorticoid supplementation is of particular importance)
   - Acute adrenocortical insufficiency (hydrocortisone or cortisone is the drug of choice; mineralocorticoid supplementation may be necessary, particularly when synthetic analogs are used)
   - Preoperatively and in the event of serious trauma or illness, in patients with known adrenal insufficiency or when adrenocortical reserve is doubtful
   - Shock unresponsive to conventional therapy if adrenocortical insufficiency exists or is suspected
   - Congenital adrenal hyperplasia
   - Hypercalcemia associated with cancer
   - Nonsuppurative thyroiditis
2. **Rheumatic Disorders**
   - As adjunctive therapy for short-term administration (to tide the patient over an acute episode or exacerbation) in:
   - Post-traumatic osteoarthritis
   - Synovitis of osteoarthritis
   - Rheumatoid arthritis, including juvenile rheumatoid arthritis (selected cases may require low-dose maintenance therapy)
   - Acute and subacute bursitis
   - Epicondylitis
   - Acute nonspecific tenosynovitis
   - Acute gouty arthritis
   - Psoriatic arthritis
   - Ankylosing spondylitis
3. **Collagen Diseases**
   - During an exacerbation or as maintenance therapy in selected cases of:
   - Systemic lupus erythematosus
   - Systemic dermatomyositis (polymyositis)
   - Acute rheumatic carditis
4. **Dermatologic Diseases**
   - Pemphigus
   - Severe erythema multiforme (Stevens-Johnson syndrome)
   - Exfoliative dermatitis
   - Bullous dermatitis herpetiformis
   - Severe seborrheic dermatitis
   - Severe psoriasis
   - Mycosis fungoides
5. **Allergic States**
   - Control of severe or incapacitating allergic conditions intractable to adequate trials of conventional treatment in:
   - Bronchial asthma
   - Contact dermatitis
   - Atopic dermatitis
   - Serum sickness
   - Seasonal or perennial allergic rhinitis
   - Drug hypersensitivity reactions
   - Urticarial transfusion reactions
   - Acute noninfectious laryngeal edema (epinephrine is the drug of first choice)
6. **Ophthalmic Diseases**
   - Severe acute and chronic allergic and inflammatory processes involving the eye, such as:
   - Herpes zoster ophthalmicus
   - Iritis, iridocyclitis
   - Chorioretinitis
   - Diffuse posterior uveitis and choroiditis
   - Optic neuritis
   - Sympathetic ophthalmia
   - Anterior segment inflammation
   - Allergic conjunctivitis
   - Allergic corneal marginal ulcers
   - Keratitis
7. **Gastrointestinal Diseases**
   - To tide the patient over a critical period of the disease in:
   - Ulcerative colitis (systemic therapy)
   - Regional enteritis (systemic therapy)
8. **Respiratory Diseases**
   - Symptomatic sarcoidosis
   - Berylliosis
   - Fulminating or disseminated pulmonary tuberculosis when used concurrently with appropriate antituberculous chemotherapy
   - Loeffler's syndrome not manageable by other means
   - Aspiration pneumonitis
9. **Hematologic Disorders**
   - Acquired (autoimmune) hemolytic anemia
   - Idiopathic thrombocytopenic purpura in adults (IV only; IM administration is contraindicated)
   - Secondary thrombocytopenia in adults
   - Erythroblastopenia (RBC anemia)
   - Congenital (erythroid) hypoplastic anemia
10. **Neoplastic Diseases**
    - For palliative management of:
    - Leukemias and lymphomas in adults
    - Acute leukemia of childhood
11. **Edematous States**
    - To induce diuresis or remission of proteinuria in the nephrotic syndrome, without uremia, of the idiopathic type or that due to lupus erythematosus
12. **Nervous System**
    - Acute exacerbations of multiple sclerosis
13. **Miscellaneous**
    - Tuberculous meningitis with subarachnoid block or impending block when used concurrently with appropriate antituberculous chemotherapy
    - Trichinosis with neurologic or myocardial involvement

CONTRAINDICATIONS

Systemic fungal infections.

WARNINGS

In patients on corticosteroid therapy subjected to any unusual stress, increased dosage of rapidly acting corticosteroids before, during, and after the stressful situation is indicated.

Corticosteroids may mask some signs of infection, and new infections may appear during their use. There may be decreased resistance and inability to localize infection when corticosteroids are used.

A study has failed to establish the efficacy of SOLU-MEDROL in the treatment of sepsis syndrome and septic shock. The study also suggests that treatment of these conditions with SOLU-MEDROL may increase the risk of mortality in certain patients (ie, patients with elevated serum creatinine levels or patients who develop secondary infections after SOLU-MEDROL).

Prolonged use of corticosteroids may produce posterior subcapsular cataracts, glaucoma with possible damage to the optic nerves, and may enhance the establishment of secondary ocular infections due to fungi or viruses.

Usage in pregnancy. Since adequate human reproduction studies have not been done with corticosteroids, the use of these drugs in pregnancy, nursing mothers, or women of childbearing potential requires that the possible benefits of the drug be weighed against the potential hazards to the mother and embryo or fetus. Infants born of mothers who have received substantial doses of corticosteroids during pregnancy should be carefully observed for signs of hypoadrenalism.

Average and large doses of cortisone or hydrocortisone can cause elevation of blood pressure, salt and water retention, and increased excretion of potassium. These effects are less likely to occur with the synthetic derivatives except when used in large doses. Dietary salt restriction and potassium supplementation may be necessary. All corticosteroids increase calcium excretion.

While on corticosteroid therapy patients should not be vaccinated against smallpox. Other immunization procedures should not be undertaken in patients who are on corticosteroids, especially on high dose, because of possible hazards of neurological complications and a lack of antibody response.

The use of SOLU-MEDROL Sterile Powder (methylprednisolone sodium succinate) in active tuberculosis should be restricted to those cases of fulminating or disseminated tuberculosis in which the corticosteroid is used for the management of the disease in conjunction with appropriate antituberculous regimen.

If corticosteroids are indicated in patients with latent tuberculosis or tuberculin reactivity, close observation is necessary as reactivation of the disease may occur. During prolonged corticosteroid therapy, these patients should receive chemoprophylaxis.

Because rare instances of anaphylactic (eg, bronchospasm) reactions have occurred in patients receiving parenteral corticosteroid therapy, appropriate precautionary measures should be taken prior to administration, especially when the patient has a history of allergy to any drug.

There are reports of cardiac arrhythmias and/or circulatory collapse and/or cardiac arrest following the rapid administration of large IV doses of SOLU-MEDROL (greater than 0.5 gram administered over a period of less than 10 minutes).

Benzyl alcohol is contained in the 40 mg **MIX-O-VIAL, 40 mg ACT-O-VIAL, 125 mg MIX-O-VIAL,** and the **125 mg ACT-O-VIAL,** and in the accompanying diluent for the 500 mg and 1 gram vials. Benzyl alcohol has been reported to be associated with a fatal "Gasping Syndrome" in premature infants.

PRECAUTIONS

Drug-induced secondary adrenocortical insufficiency may be minimized by gradual reduction of dosage. This type of relative insufficiency may persist for months after discontinuation of therapy; therefore, in any situation of stress occurring during that period, hormone therapy should be reinstituted. Since mineralocorticoid secretion may be impaired, salt and/or a mineralocorticoid should be administered concurrently.

There is an enhanced effect of corticosteroids on patients with hypothyroidism and in those with cirrhosis.

Corticosteroids should be used cautiously in patients with ocular herpes simplex because of possible corneal perforation.

The lowest possible dose of corticosteroid should be used to control the condition under treatment, and when reduction in dosage is possible, the reduction should be gradual.

Psychic derangements may appear when corticosteroids are used, ranging from euphoria, insomnia, mood swings, personality changes and severe depression, to frank psychotic manifestations. Also, existing emotional instability or psychotic tendencies may be aggravated by corticosteroids.

Aspirin should be used cautiously in conjunction with corticosteroids in hypoprothrombinemia.

Steroids should be used with caution in nonspecific ulcerative colitis, if there is a probability of impending perforation, abscess or other pyogenic infection; diverticulitis; fresh intestinal anastomoses; active or latent peptic ulcer; renal insufficiency; hypertension; osteoporosis; and myasthenia gravis.

Growth and development of infants and children on prolonged corticosteroid therapy should be carefully observed.

Although controlled clinical trials have shown corticosteroids to be effective in speeding the resolution of acute exacerbations of multiple sclerosis, they do not show that corticosteroids affect the ultimate outcome or natural history of the disease. The studies do show that relatively high doses of corticosteroids are necessary to demonstrate a significant effect. (See DOSAGE AND ADMINISTRATION).

Since complications of treatment with glucocorticoids are dependent on the size of the dose and the duration of treatment, a risk/benefit decision must be made in each individual case as to dose and duration of treatment and as to whether daily or intermittent therapy should be used.

ADVERSE REACTIONS

Fluid and Electrolyte Disturbances

Sodium retention
Fluid retention
Congestive heart failure in susceptible patients
Potassium loss
Hypokalemic alkalosis
Hypertension

Musculoskeletal

Muscle weakness
Steroid myopathy
Loss of muscle mass
Severe arthralgia
Vertebral compression fractures
Aseptic necrosis of femoral and humeral heads
Pathologic fracture of long bones
Osteoporosis

Gastrointestinal

Peptic ulcer with possible perforation and hemorrhage
Pancreatitis
Abdominal distention
Ulcerative esophagitis

Dermatologic

Impaired wound healing
Thin fragile skin
Petechiae and ecchymoses
Facial erythema
Increased sweating
May suppress reactions to skin tests

Neurological

Increased intracranial pressure with papilledema (pseudotumor cerebri) usually after treatment
Convulsions
Vertigo
Headache

Endocrine

Development of Cushingoid state
Suppression of growth in children
Secondary adrenocortical and pituitary unresponsiveness, particularly in times of stress, as in trauma, surgery or illness
Menstrual irregularities
Decreased carbohydrate tolerance
Manifestations of latent diabetes mellitus
Increased requirements for insulin or oral hypoglycemic agents in diabetics

Ophthalmic

Posterior subcapsular cataracts
Increased intraocular pressure
Glaucoma
Exophthalmos

Metabolic

Negative nitrogen balance due to protein catabolism

The following *additional* adverse reactions are related to parenteral corticosteroid therapy:

Hyperpigmentation or hypopigmentation
Subcutaneous and cutaneous atrophy
Sterile abscess
Anaphylactic reaction with or without circulatory collapse, cardiac arrest, bronchospasm
Urticaria
Nausea and vomiting
Cardiac arrhythmias; hypotension or hypertension

DOSAGE AND ADMINISTRATION

When high dose therapy is desired, the recommended dose of SOLU-MEDROL Sterile Powder (methylprednisolone sodium succinate) is 30 mg/kg administered intravenously over a 10–20 minute period. This dose may be repeated every 4 to 6 hours for 48 hours.

Therapy is initiated by administering SOLU-MEDROL intravenously over a period of one to several minutes. In general, high dose corticosteroid therapy should be continued only until the patient's condition has stabilized; usually not beyond 48 to 72 hours.

Although adverse effects associated with high dose short-term corticoid therapy are uncommon, peptic ulceration may occur. Prophylactic antacid therapy may be indicated.

In other indications initial dosage will vary from 10 to 40 mg of methylprednisolone depending on the clinical problem being treated. The larger doses may be required for short-term management of severe, acute conditions. The initial dose usually should be given intravenously over a period of one to several minutes. Subsequent doses may be given intravenously or intramuscularly at intervals dictated by the patient's response and clinical condition. Corticoid therapy is an adjunct to, and not replacement for conventional therapy.

Dosage may be reduced for infants and children but should be governed more by the severity of the condition and response of the patient than by age or size. It should not be less than 0.5 mg per kg every 24 hours.

Dosage must be decreased or discontinued gradually when the drug has been administered for more than a few days. If a period of spontaneous remission occurs in a chronic condition, treatment should be discontinued. Routine laboratory studies, such as urinalysis, two-hour postprandial blood sugar, determination of blood pressure and body weight, and a chest X-ray should be made at regular intervals during prolonged therapy. Upper GI X-rays are desirable in patients with an ulcer history or significant dyspepsia.

SOLU-MEDROL may be administered by intravenous or intramuscular injection or by intravenous infusion, the preferred method for initial emergency use being intravenous injection. To administer by intravenous (or intramuscular) injection, prepare solution as directed. The desired dose may be administered intravenously over a period of approximately 60 seconds. Subsequent doses may be withdrawn and administered similarly. If desired, the medication may be administered in diluted solutions by adding Water for Injection or other suitable diluent (see below) to the **MIX-O-VIAL (ACT-O-VIAL)** and withdrawing the indicated dose.

To prepare solutions for intravenous infusion, first prepare the solution for injection as directed. This solution may then be added to indicated amounts of 5% dextrose in water, isotonic saline solution or 5% dextrose in isotonic saline solution.

Multiple Sclerosis

In treatment of acute exacerbations of multiple sclerosis, daily doses of 200 mg of prednisolone for a week followed by 80 mg every other day for 1 month have been shown to be effective (4 mg of methylprednisolone is equivalent to 5 mg of prednisolone).

Directions for Using the MIX-O-VIAL Two-Compartment Vial

1. Remove protective cap, give the plunger-stopper a quarter turn and press to force diluent into the lower compartment.
2. Gently agitate to effect solution. Use solution within 48 hours.
3. Sterilize top of plunger-stopper with a suitable germicide.
4. Insert needle **squarely through center** of plunger-stopper until the tip is just visible. Invert vial and withdraw dose.

Directions for Using the ACT-O-VIAL System

1. Press down on plastic activator to force diluent into the lower compartment.
2. Gently agitate to effect solution.
3. Remove plastic tab covering center of stopper.
4. Sterilize top of stopper with a suitable germicide.
5. Insert needle **squarely through center** of stopper until tip is just visible. Invert vial and withdraw dose.

STORAGE CONDITIONS

Store unreconstituted product at controlled room temperature 15°–30°C (59°– 86°F).

Store solution at controlled room temperature 15°–30°C (59°–86°F).

Use solution within 48 hours after mixing.

HOW SUPPLIED

SOLU-MEDROL Sterile Powder (methylprednisolone sodium succinate) is available in the following packages:

40 mg MIX-O-VIAL Two-Compartment Vial
1 ml NDC 0009-0113-01
25—1 ml NDC 0009-0113-11
40 mg ACT-O-VIAL System
1 ml NDC 0009-0113-12
25—1 ml NDC 0009-0113-13
125 mg MIX-O-VIAL Two-Compartment Vial
2 ml NDC 0009-0190-01
25—2 ml NDC 0009-0190-08
125 mg ACT-O-VIAL System
2 ml NDC 0009-0190-09
25—2 ml NDC 0009-0190-10
500 mg Vial NDC 0009-0758-01
500 mg Vial with Diluent NDC 0009-0887-01
1 gram Vial NDC 0009-0698-01
1 gram Vial with Diluent NDC 0009-0911-01
1 gram Vial with Diluent and IV Administration Set NDC 0009-0911-05
2 gram Vial NDC 0009-0988-01
2 gram Vial with Diluent NDC 0009-0796-01

Code 810 431 013

Shown in Product Identification Section, page 434

TOLINASE® ℞

brand of tolazamide tablets, USP

250 mg (100's):
NSN 6505-00-159-4990
250 mg (1000's):
NSN 6505-00-105-5842

DESCRIPTION

TOLINASE Tablets contain tolazamide, an oral blood glucose lowering drug of the sulfonylurea class. Tolazamide is a white or creamy-white powder with a melting point of 165° to 173° C. The solubility of tolazamide at pH 6.0 (mean urinary pH) is 27.8 mg per 100 ml.

The chemical names for tolazamide are (1) Benzenesulfonamide, N-[[(hexahydro-1H -azepin-1-yl)amino]-carbonyl]-4-methyl-; (2) 1-(Hexahydro-1H-azepin-1-yl)-3-(p-tolylsulfonyl)-urea and its molecular weight is 311.40.

TOLINASE Tablets for oral administration are available as scored, white tablets containing 100 mg, 250 mg or 500 mg tolazamide. Inactive ingredients: calcium sulfate, docusate sodium, magnesium stearate, methylcellulose, sodium alginate.

CLINICAL PHARMACOLOGY

Actions

Tolazamide appears to lower the blood glucose acutely by stimulating the release of insulin from the pancreas, an effect dependent upon functioning beta cells in the pancreatic islets. The mechanism by which tolazamide lowers blood glucose during long-term administration has not been clearly established. With chronic administration in type II diabetic patients, the blood glucose lowering effect persists despite a gradual decline in the insulin secretory response to the drug. Extrapancreatic effects may be involved in the mechanism of action of oral sulfonylurea hypoglycemic drugs.

Some patients who are initially responsive to oral hypoglycemic drugs, including TOLINASE Tablets (tolazamide), may become unresponsive or poorly responsive over time. Alternatively, TOLINASE may be effective in some patients who have become unresponsive to one or more sulfonylurea drugs.

In addition to its blood glucose lowering actions, tolazamide produces a mild diuresis by enhancement of renal free water clearance.

Pharmacokinetics

Tolazamide is rapidly and well absorbed from the gastrointestinal tract. Peak serum concentrations occur at three to four hours following a single oral dose of the drug. The average biological half-life of the drug is seven hours. The drug does not continue to accumulate in the blood after the first four to six doses are administered. A steady or equilibrium state is reached during which the peak and nadir values do not change from day to day after the fourth to sixth doses. Tolazamide is metabolized to five major metabolites ranging in hypoglycemic activity from 0–70%. They are excreted

Continued on next page

Information on these Upjohn products is based on labeling in effect August 15, 1986. Further information concerning these and other Upjohn products may be obtained by direct inquiry to Medical Information, The Upjohn Company, Kalamazoo, Michigan 49001.

Upjohn—Cont.

principally in the urine. Following a single oral dose of tritiated tolazamide, 85% of the dose was excreted in the urine and 7% in the feces over a five-day period. Most of the urinary excretion of the drug occurred within the first 24 hours postadministration.
When nomal fasting nondiabetic subjects are given a single 500 mg dose of tolazamide orally, a hypoglycemic effect can be noted within 20 minutes after ingestion with a peak hypoglycemic effect occurring in two to four hours. Following a single oral dose of 500 mg tolazamide, a statistically significant hypoglycemic effect was demonstrated in fasted nondiabetic subjects 20 hours after administration. With fasting diabetic patients, the peak hypoglycemic effect occurs at four to six hours. The duration of maximal hypoglycemic effect in fed diabetic patients is about ten hours, with the onset occurring at four to six hours and with the blood glucose levels beginning to rise at 14 to 16 hours. Single dose potency of tolazamide in normal subjects has been shown to be 6.7 times that of tolbutamide on a milligram basis. Clinical experience in diabetic patients has demonstrated tolazamide to be approximately five times more potent than tolbutamide on a milligram basis, and approximately equivalent in milligram potency to chlorpropamide.

INDICATIONS AND USAGE

TOLINASE Tablets (tolazamide) are indicated as an adjunct to diet to lower the blood glucose in patients with noninsulin dependent diabetes mellitus (type II) whose hyperglycemia cannot be satisfactorily controlled by diet alone.
In initiating treatment for noninsulin-dependent diabetes, diet should be emphasized as the primary form of treatment. Caloric restriction and weight loss are essential in the obese diabetic patient. Proper dietary management alone may be effective in controlling the blood glucose and symptoms of hyperglycemia. The importance of regular physical activity should also be stressed and cardiovascular risk factors should be identified and corrective measures taken where possible.
If this treatment program fails to reduce symptoms and/or blood glucose, the use of an oral sulfonylurea or insulin should be considered. Use of TOLINASE must be viewed by both the physician and patient as a treatment in addition to diet and not as a substitute for diet or as a convenient mechanism for avoiding dietary restraint. Furthermore, loss of blood glucose control on diet alone may be transient thus requiring only short-term administration of TOLINASE.
During maintenance programs, TOLINASE should be discontinued if satisfactory lowering of blood glucose is no longer achieved. Judgments should be based on regular clinical and laboratory evaluations.
In considering the use of TOLINASE in asymptomatic patients, it should be recognized that controlling the blood glucose in noninsulin-dependent diabetes has not been definitely established to be effective in preventing the long-term cardiovascular or neural complications of diabetes.

CONTRAINDICATIONS

TOLINASE Tablets (tolazamide) are contraindicated in patients with: 1) known hypersensitivity or allergy to TOLINASE; 2) diabetic ketoacidosis, with or without coma. This condition should be treated with insulin; 3) Type I diabetes, as sole therapy.
Special Warning on Increased Risk of Cardiovascular Mortality: The administration of oral hypoglycemic drugs has been reported to be associated with increased cardiovascular mortality as compared to treatment with diet alone or diet plus insulin. This warning is based on the study conducted by the University Group Diabetes Program (UGDP), a long-term prospective clinical trial designed to evaluate the effectiveness of glucose-lowering drugs in preventing or delaying vascular complications in patients with noninsulin-dependent diabetes. The study involved 823 patients who were randomly assigned to one of four treatment groups (DIABETES, 19 (supp. 2):747–830, 1970.)
UGDP reported that patients treated for five to eight years with diet plus a fixed dose of tolbutamide (1.5 grams per day) had a rate of cardiovascular mortality approximately 2½ times that of patients with diet alone. A significant increase in total mortality was not observed, but the use of tolbutamide was discontinued based on the increase on cardiovascular mortality, thus limiting the opportunity for the study to show an increase in overall mortality. Despite controversy regarding the interpretation of these results, the findings of the UGDP study provide an adequate basis for this warning. The patient should be informed of the potential risks and advantages of TOLINASE and of alternative modes of therapy.
Although only one drug in the sulfonylurea class (tolbutamide) was included in this study, it is prudent from a safety standpoint to consider that this warning may also apply to other oral hypoglycemic drugs in this class, in view of their close similarities in mode of action and chemical structure.

PRECAUTIONS

General

Hypoglycemia—All sulfonylurea drugs are capable of producing severe hypoglycemia. Proper patient selection and dosage and instructions are important to avoid hypoglycemic episodes. Renal or hepatic insufficiency may cause elevated blood levels of TOLINASE Tablets (tolazamide) and the latter may also diminish gluconeogenic capacity, both of which increase the risk of serious hypoglycemic reactions. Elderly, debilitated, or malnourished patients and those with adrenal or pituitary insufficiency are particularly susceptible to the hypoglycemic action of glucose lowering drugs. Hypoglycemia may be difficult to recognize in the elderly and in people who are taking beta-adrenergic blocking drugs. Hypoglycemia is more likely to occur when caloric intake is deficient, after severe or prolonged exercise, when alcohol is ingested, or when more than one glucose-lowering drug is used.
Loss of Control of Blood Glucose—When a patient stabilized on any diabetic regimen is exposed to stress such as fever, trauma, infection, or surgery, loss of control of blood glucose may occur. At such times it may be necessary to discontinue TOLINASE and administer insulin.
The effectiveness of any hypoglycemic drug, including TOLINASE, in lowering blood glucose to a desired level decreases in many patients over a period of time, which may be due to progression of the severity of the diabetes or to diminished responsiveness to the drug. This phenomenon is known as secondary failure to distinguish it from primary failure in which the drug is ineffective in an individual patient when first given. Adequate adjustment of dose and adherence to diet should be assessed before classifying a patient as a secondary failure.

Information for Patients

Patients should be informed of the potential risks and advantages of TOLINASE Tablets (tolazamide) and of alternative modes of therapy. They should also be informed about the importance of adherence to dietary instructions, of a regular exercise program, and of regular testing of urine and/or blood glucose.
The risks of hypoglycemia, its symptoms and treatment, and conditions that predispose to its development should be explained to patients and responsible family members. Primary and secondary failure should also be explained.

Laboratory Tests

Blood and urine glucose should be monitored periodically. Measurement of glycosylated hemoglobin may be useful in some patients.

Drug Interactions

The hypoglycemia action of sulfonylureas may be potentiated by certain drugs including nonsteroidal anti-inflammatory agents and other drugs that are highly protein bound, salicylates, sulfonamides, chloramphenicol, probenecid, coumarins, monoamine oxidase inhibitors, and beta-adrenergic blocking agents. When such drugs are administered to a patient receiving TOLINASE, the patient should be closely observed for hypoglycemia. When such drugs are withdrawn from a patient receiving TOLINASE, the patient should be observed closely for loss of control.
Certain drugs tend to produce hyperglycemia and may lead to loss of control. These drugs include the thiazides and other diuretics, corticosteroids, phenothiazines, thyroid products, estrogens, oral contraceptives, phenytoin, nicotinic acid, sympathomimetics, calcium channel blocking drugs, and isoniazid. When such drugs are administered to a patient receiving TOLINASE, the patient should be closely observed for loss of control. When such drugs are withdrawn from a patient receiving TOLINASE, the patient should be observed closely for hypoglycemia.
A potential interaction between oral miconazole and oral hypoglycemic agents leading to severe hypoglycemia has been reported. Whether this interaction also occurs with the intravenous, topical or vaginal preparations of miconazole is not known.

Carcinogenicity

In a bioassay for carcinogenicity, rats and mice of both sexes were treated with tolazamide for 103 weeks at low and high doses. No evidence of carcinogenicity was found.

Pregnancy

Teratogenic Effects:

Pregnancy Category C. TOLINASE, administered to pregnant rats at ten times the human dose, decreased litter size but did not produce teratogenic effects in the offspring. In rats treated at a daily dose of 14 mg/kg no reproductive aberrations or drug related fetal anomalies were noted. At an elevated dose of 100 mg/kg per day there was a reduction in the number of pups born and an increased perinatal mortality. There are, however, no adequate and well-controlled studies in pregnant women. Because animal reproduction studies are not always predictive of human response, TOLINASE is not recommended for the treatment of the pregnant diabetic patient. Serious consideration should also be given to the possible hazards of the use of TOLINASE in women of child bearing age and in those who might become pregnant while using the drug.
Because recent information suggests that abnormal blood glucose levels during pregnancy are associated with a higher incidence of congenital abnormalities, many experts recommend that insulin be used during pregnancy to maintain blood glucose levels as close to normal as possible.

Nonteratogenic Effects:

Prolonged severe hypoglycemia (four to ten days) has been reported in neonates born to mothers who were receiving a sulfonylurea drug at the time of delivery. This has been reported more frequently with the use of agents with prolonged half-lives. If TOLINASE is used during pregnancy, it should be discontinued at least two weeks before the expected delivery date.

Nursing Mothers

Although it is not known whether tolazamide is excreted in human milk, some sulfonylurea drugs are known to be excreted in human milk. Because the potential for hypoglycemia in nursing infants may exist, a decision should be made whether to discontinue nursing or to discontinue the drug, taking into account the importance of the drug to the mother. If the drug is discontinued and if diet alone is inadequate for controlling blood glucose, insulin therapy should be considered.

Pediatric Use

Safety and effectiveness in children have not been established.

ADVERSE REACTIONS

TOLINASE Tablets (tolazamide) have generally been well tolerated. In clinical studies in which more than 1,784 diabetic patients were specifically evaluated for incidence of side effects, only 2.1% were discontinued from therapy because of side effects.
Hypoglycemia: See **Precautions** and **Overdosage** sections.
Gastrointestinal Reactions: Cholestatic jaundice may occur rarely; TOLINASE Tablets should be discontinued if this occurs. Gastrointestinal disturbances, eg, nausea, epigastric fullness, and heartburn, are the most common reactions and occurred in 1% of patients treated during clinical trials. They tend to be dose-related and may disappear when dosage is reduced.
Dermatologic Reactions: Allergic skin reactions, eg, pruritus, erythema, urticaria, and morbilliform or maculopapular eruptions, occurred in 0.4% of patients treated during clinical trials. These may be transient and may disappear despite continued use of TOLINASE; if skin reactions persist, the drug should be discontinued.
Porphyria cutanea tarda and photosensitivity reactions have been reported with sulfonylureas.
Hematologic Reactions: Leukopenia, agranulocytosis, thrombocytopenia, hemolytic anemia, aplastic anemia, and pancytopenia have been reported with sulfonylureas.
Metabolic Reactions: Hepatic porphyria and disulfiram-like reactions have been reported with sulfonylureas; however, disulfiram-like reactions with TOLINASE have been reported very rarely.
Miscellaneous: Weakness, fatigue, dizziness, vertigo, malaise and headache were reported infrequently in patients treated during clinical trials. The relationship to therapy with TOLINASE is difficult to assess.

OVERDOSAGE

Overdosage of sulfonylureas, including TOLINASE Tablets (tolazamide), can produce hypoglycemia.
Mild hypoglycemic symptoms without loss of consciousness or neurologic findings should be treated aggressively with oral glucose and adjustment in drug dosage and/or meal patterns. Close monitoring should continue until the physician is assured the patient is out of danger. Severe hypoglycemic reactions with coma, seizure, or other neurological impairment occur infrequently, but constitute medical emergencies requiring immediate hospitalization. If hypoglycemic coma is suspected or diagnosed, the patient should be given a rapid intravenous injection of concentrated (50%) glucose solution. This should be followed by a continuous infusion of a more dilute (10%) glucose solution at a rate which will maintain the blood glucose at a level above 100 mg/dl. Patients should be closely monitored for a minimum of 24 to 48 hours since hypoglycemia may recur after apparent clinical recovery.

DOSAGE AND ADMINISTRATION

There is no fixed dosage regimen for the management of diabetes mellitus with TOLINASE Tablets (tolazamide) or any other hypoglycemic agent. In addition to the usual monitoring of urinary glucose, the patient's blood glucose must also be monitored periodically to determine the minimum effective dose for the patient; to detect primary failure, ie, inadequate lowering of blood glucose at the maximum recommended dose of medication; and to detect secondary failure, ie, loss of adequate blood glucose response after an initial period of effectiveness. Glycosylated hemoglobin levels may also be of value in monitoring the patient's response to therapy.

Short-term administration of TOLINASE may be sufficient during periods of transient loss of control in patients usually controlled well on diet.

Usual Starting Dose

The usual starting dose of TOLINASE Tablets for the mild to modertely severe type II diabetic patient is 100–250 mg daily administered with breakfast or the first main meal. Generally, if the fasting blood glucose is less than 200 mg/dl, the starting dose is 100 mg/day as a single daily dose. If the fasting blood glucose value is greater than 200 mg/dl, the starting dose is 250 mg/day as a single dose. If the patient is malnourished, underweight, elderly, or not eating properly, the initial therapy should be 100 mg once a day. Failure to follow an appropriate dosage regimen may precipitate hypoglycemia. Patients who do not adhere to their prescribed dietary regimen are more prone to exhibit unsatisfactory response to drug therapy.

Transfer From Other Hypoglycemic Therapy

Patients Receiving Other Oral Antidiabetic Therapy—Transfer of patients from other oral antidiabetes regimens to TOLINASE should be done conservatively. When transferring patients from oral hypoglycemic agents other than chlorpropamide to TOLINASE, no transition period or initial or priming dose is necessary. When transferring from chlorpropamide, particular care should be exercised to avoid hypoglycemia.

Tolbutamide: If receiving less than 1 gm/day, begin at 100 mg of tolazamide per day. If receiving 1 gm or more per day, initiate at 250 mg of tolazamide per day as a single dose.

Chlorpropamide: 250 mg of chlorpropamide may be considered to provide approximately the same degree of blood glucose control as 250 mg of tolazamide. The patient should be observed carefully for hypoglycemia during the transition period from chlorpropamide to TOLINASE (one to two weeks) due to the prolonged retention of chlorpropamide in the body and the possibility of a subsequent overlapping drug effect.

Acetohexamide: 100 mg of tolazamide may be considered to provide approximately the same degree of blood glucose control as 250 mg of acetohexamide.

Patients Receiving Insulin—Some type II diabetic patients who have been treated only with insulin may respond satisfactorily to therapy with TOLINASE. If the patient's previous insulin dosage has been less than 20 units, substitutioin of 100 mg of tolazamide per day as a single daily dose may be tried. If the previous insulin dosage was less than 40 units, but more than 20 units, the patient should be placed directly on 250 mg of tolazamide per day as a single dose. If the previous insulin dosage was greater than 40 units, the insulin dosage should be decreased by 50% and 250 mg of tolazamide per day started. The dosage of TOLINASE should be adjusted weekly (or more often in the group previously requiring more than 40 units of insulin). During this conversion period when both insulin and TOLINASE are being used, hypoglycemia may rarely occur. During insulin withdrawal, patients should test their urine for glucose and acetone at least three times daily and report results to their physician. The appearance of persistent acetonuria with glycosuria indicates that the patient is a type I diabetic who requires insulin therapy.

Maximum Dose

Daily doses of greater than 1000 mg are not recommended. Patients will generally have no further response to doses larger than this.

Usual Maintenance Dose

The usual maintenance dose is in the range of 100–1000 mg/day with the average maintenance dose being 250–500 mg/day. Following initiation of therapy, dosage adjustment is made in increments of 100 mg to 250 mg at weekly intervals based on the patient's blood glucose response.

Dosage Interval

Once a day therapy is usually satisfactory. Doses up to 500 mg/day should be given as a single dose in the morning. 500 mg once daily is as effective as 250 mg twice daily. When a dose of more than 500 mg/day is required, the dose may be divided and given twice daily.

In elderly patients, debilitated or malnourished patients, and patients with impaired renal or hepatic function, the initial and maintenance dosing should be conservative to avoid hypoglycemic reactions (see **PRECAUTIONS** section).

HOW SUPPLIED

TOLINASE Tablets (tolazamide) are available in the following strengths and package sizes:

100 mg (scored, round, white)
Unit-of-Use bottles of 100 NDC 0009-0070-02

250 mg (scored, round, white)
Bottles of 200 NDC 0009-0114-04
Bottles of 1000 NDC 0009-0114-02
Unit-of-Use bottles of 100 NDC 0009-0114-05
Unit-Dose package of 100 NDC 0009-0114-06

500 mg (scored, round, white)
Unit-of-Use bottles of 100 NDC 0009-0477-06

Store at controlled room temperature 15–30° C (59–86° F).
Code 811 417 105

Shown in Product Identification Section, page 434

TROBICIN® ℞

brand of spectinomycin hydrochloride sterile powder (sterile spectinomycin hydrochloride, USP)
For Intramuscular Injection

2 Gm vial NSN 6505-00-079-7611 (M)
4 Gm vial NSN 6505-00-079-7643 (M)

DESCRIPTION

TROBICIN Sterile Powder contains spectinomycin hydrochloride which is an aminocyclitol antibiotic produced by a species of soil microorganism designated as *Streptomyces spectabilis.* Sterile spectinomycin hydrochloride is the pentahydrated dihydrochloride salt of spectinomycin.

Spectinomycin hydrochloride is isolated as a white to pale buff crystalline dihydrochloride pentahydrate powder, molecular weight 495, and is stable in the dry state for 36 months.

ACTIONS

Spectinomycin hydrochloride is an inhibitor of protein synthesis in the bacterial cell; the site of action is the 30S ribosomal subunit.

In vitro studies have shown spectinomycin hydrochloride to be active against most strains of *Neisseria gonorrhoeae* (minimum inhibitory concentration < 7.5 to 20 mcg/ml).

Definitive *in vitro* studies have shown no cross-resistance of *N. gonorrhoeae* between streptinomycin hydrochloride and penicillin. The antibiotic is not significantly bound to plasma protein.

INDICATIONS

TROBICIN Sterile Powder (spectinomycin hydrochloride) is indicated in the treatment of acute gonorrheal urethritis and proctitis in the male and acute gonorrheal cervicitis and proctitis in the female when due to susceptible strains of *Neisseria gonorrhoeae.* Men and women with known recent exposure to gonorrhea should be treated as those known to have gonorrhea.

The *in vitro* susceptibility of *Neisseria gonorrhoeae* to spectinomycin hydrochloride can be tested by agar dilution methods. TROBICIN Susceptibility Powder is available for this purpose, and its package insert should be consulted for details.

CONTRAINDICATIONS

The use of TROBICIN Sterile Powder (spectinomycin hydrochloride) is contraindicated in patients previously found hypersensitive to it.

WARNINGS

Spectinomycin hydrochloride is not effective in the treatment of syphilis. Antibiotics used in high doses for short periods of time to treat gonorrhea may mask or delay the symptoms of incubating syphilis. Since the treatment of syphilis demands prolonged therapy with any effective antibiotic, patients being treated for gonorrhea should be closely observed clinically. All patients with gonorrhea should have a serologic test for syphilis at the time of diagnosis. Patients treated with spectinomycin hydrochloride should have a follow-up serologic test for syphilis after three months.

Usage in pregnancy: Safety for use in pregnancy has not been established.

Usage in infants and children: Safety for use in infants and children has not been established.

PRECAUTIONS

The usual precautions should be observed with atopic individuals.

The clinical effectiveness of TROBICIN Sterile Powder (spectinomycin hydrochloride) should be monitored to detect evidence of development of resistance by *Neisseria gonorrhoeae.*

ADVERSE REACTIONS

The following reactions were observed during the single dose clinical trials: soreness at the injection site, urticaria, dizziness, nausea, chills, fever and insomnia.

During multiple dose subchronic tolerance studies in normal human volunteers, the following were noted: a decrease in hemoglobin, hematocrit and creatinine clearance; elevation of alkaline phosphatase, BUN and SGPT. In single and multiple dose studies in normal volunteers, a reduction in urine output was noted. Extensive renal function studies demonstrated no consistent changes indicative of renal toxicity.

Although no clearly defined case of anaphylaxis has been reported with TROBICIN Sterile Powder, the possibility of such reactions should be considered particularly when using antibiotics.

DOSAGE AND ADMINISTRATION

Preparation of Drug for Intramuscular Injection

TROBICIN Sterile Powder, 2 grams (spectinomycin hydrochloride): reconstitute with 3.2 ml of the accompanying diluent.*

TROBICIN Sterile Powder, 4 grams: reconstitute with 6.2 ml of the accompanying diluent.*

*Bacteriostatic Water for Injection with Benzyl Alcohol 0.945% w/v added as preservative.

Shake vials vigorously immediately after adding diluent and before withdrawing dose. It is recommended that disposable syringes and needles be used to avoid contamination with penicillin residue, especially when treating patients known to be highly sensitive to penicillin. **Use of 20 gauge needle is recommended.**

Dosage

Intramuscular injections should be made deep into the upper outer quadrant of the gluteal muscle.

Adults (Men and Women)—Inject 5 ml intramuscularly for a 2 gram dose. This is also the recommended dose for patients being treated after failure of previous antibiotic therapy.

In geographic areas where antibiotic resistance is known to be prevalent, initial treatment with 4 grams (10 ml) intramuscularly is preferred. The 10 ml injection may be divided between two gluteal injection sites.

STORAGE CONDITIONS

Store unreconstituted product at controlled room temperature 15°- 30°C (59°-86°F). Store prepared suspension at controlled room temperature 15°-30°C (59°-86°F) and use within 24 hours.

HOW SUPPLIED

TROBICIN Sterile Powder (spectinomycin hydrochloride) is available as:

TROBICIN Sterile Powder, 2 gram vial—with one ampoule of Bacteriostatic Water for Injection with Benzyl Alcohol 0.945% w/v added as preservative. When reconstituted with 3.2 ml of the accompanying diluent, each vial yields a sufficient quantity for withdrawal of 5 ml of a suspension containing 400 mg spectinomycin per ml (as the hydrochloride). 5 ml provides 2 grams spectinomycin. For intramuscular use only.

NDC 0009-0566-01

TROBICIN Sterile Powder 4 gram vial—with one ampoule of Bacteriostatic Water for Injection with Benzyl Alcohol 0.945% w/v added as preservative. When reconstituted with 6.2 ml of the accompanying diluent, each vial yields a sufficient quantity for withdrawal of 10 ml of a suspension containing spectinomycin hydrochloride equivalent to 400 mg spectinomycin per ml. 10 ml provides 4 grams spectinomycin. For intramuscular use only.

NDC 0009-0592-01

TROBICIN Susceptibility Powder—100 mg. See package insert for *in vitro* testing procedure.

HUMAN PHARMACOLOGY

TROBICIN Sterile Powder (spectinomycin hydrochloride) is rapidly absorbed after intramuscular injection. A single, two gram injection produces peak serum concentrations averaging about 100 mcg/ml at one hour; a single, four gram injection produces peak serum concentrations averaging 160 mcg/ml at two hours. Average serum concentrations of 15 mcg/ml for the two gram dose and 31 mcg/ml for the four gram dose were present eight hours after dosing.
Code 810 130 005

UNICAP® Capsules/Tablets
(See PDR For Nonprescription Drugs)

UNICAP Jr™ Chewable Tablets
(See PDR For Nonprescription Drugs)

UNICAP M® Tablets
(See PDR For Nonprescription Drugs)

UNICAP® Plus Iron Tablets
(See PDR For Nonprescription Drugs)

UNICAP® Senior Tablets
(See PDR For Nonprescription Drugs)

UNICAP T® Tablets
(See PDR For Nonprescription Drugs)

Continued on next page

Information on these Upjohn products is based on labeling in effect August 15, 1986. Further information concerning these and other Upjohn products may be obtained by direct inquiry to Medical Information, The Upjohn Company, Kalamazoo, Michigan 49001.

Upjohn—Cont.

XANAX® Ⓒ ℞

brand of alprazolam tablets

0.25 mg, 100's Unit Dose	NSN 6505-01-188-7936
0.25 mg, 100's	NSN 6505-01-143-9269
0.25 mg, 500's	NSN 6505-01-197-3966
0.5 mg, 100's Unit Dose	NSN 6505-01-140-3201
0.5 mg, 100's	NSN 6505-01-140-3199
0.5 mg, 500's	NSN 6505-01-196-9501
1.0 mg, 100's Unit Dose	NSN 6505-01-140-3202
1.0 mg, 100's	NSN 6505-01-140-3200
1.0 mg, 500's	NSN 6505-01-197-9003

DESCRIPTION

XANAX Tablets contain alprazolam which is a triazolo analog of the 1,4 benzodiazepine class of central nervous system-active compounds.

The chemical name of alprazolam is 8- Chloro-1-methyl-6-phenyl-4H-s-triazolo[4,3-α] [1,4]benzodiazepine.

Alprazolam is a white crystalline powder, soluble in methanol or ethanol but with no appreciable solublity in water at physiological pH.

Each XANAX tablet, for oral administration, contains, 0.25, 0.5 or 1.0 mg of alprazolam.

Inactive ingredients: cellulose, corn starch, docusate sodium, lactose, magnesium stearate, silicon dioxide, sodium benzoate. In addition, the 0.5 mg tablet contains FD&C Yellow No. 6 and the 1 mg tablet contains FD&C Blue No. 2.

CLINICAL PHARMACOLOGY

CNS agents of the 1,4 benzodiazepine class presumably exert their effects by binding at stereo specific receptors at several sites within the central nervous system. Their exact mechanism of action is unknown. Clinically, all benzodiazepines cause a dose-related central nervous system depressant activity varying from mild impairment of task performance to hypnosis.

Following oral administration, alprazolam is readily absorbed. Peak concentrations in the plasma occur in one to two hours following administration. Plasma levels are proportionate to the dose given; over the dose range of 0.5 to 3.0 mg, peak levels of 8.0 to 37 ng/ml were observed. The mean elimination half-life of alprazolam is 12–15 hours. The predominant metabolites are α-hydroxy-alprazolam and a benzophenone derived from alprazolam. The biological activity of α-hydroxy-alprazolam is approximately one-half that of alprazolam. The benzophenone metabolite is essentially inactive. Plasma levels of these metabolites are extremely low, thus precluding precise pharmacokinetic description. However, their half-lives appear to be of the same order of magnitude as alprazolam. Alprazolam and its metabolites are excreted primarily in the urine.

The ability of alprazolam to induce human hepatic enzyme systems has not yet been determined. However, this is not a property of benzodiazepines in general. Further, alprazolam did not affect the prothrombin or plasma warfarin levels in male volunteers administered sodium warfarin orally.

In vitro, alprazolam is bound (80 percent) to human serum protein.

Changes in the absorption, distribution, metabolism and excretion of benzodiazepines have been reported in a variety of disease states including alcoholism, impaired hepatic function and impaired renal function. Changes have also been demonstrated in geriatric patients. It has not yet been determined if similar changes occur in the pharmacokinetics of alprazolam.

Because of its similarity to other benzodiazepines, it is assumed that alprazolam undergoes transplacental passage and is excreted in human milk.

INDICATIONS AND USAGE

XANAX Tablets (alprazolam) are indicated for the management of anxiety disorders or the short-term relief of the symptoms of anxiety. Anxiety or tension associated with the stress of everyday life usually does not require treatment with an anxiolytic.

Anxiety associated with depression is also responsive to XANAX.

The effectiveness of XANAX for long-term use, that is, more than four months, has not been established by systematic clinical trials. The physician should periodically reassess the usefulness of the drug for the individual patient.

CONTRAINDICATIONS

XANAX Tablets (alprazolam) are contraindicated in patients with known sensitivity to this drug or other benzodiazepines. XANAX may be used in patients with open angle glaucoma who are receiving appropriate therapy, but is contraindicated in acute narrow angle glaucoma.

WARNINGS

XANAX Tablets (alprazolam) are not of value in the treatment of psychotic patients and should not be employed in lieu of appropriate treatment for psychosis. Because of its depressant CNS effects, patients receiving XANAX should be cautioned against engaging in hazardous occupations requiring complete mental alertness such as operating machinery or driving a motor vehicle. For the same reason, patients should be cautioned about the simultaneous ingestion of alcohol and other CNS depressant drugs during treatment with XANAX.

Benzodiazepines can potentially cause fetal harm when administered to pregnant women. If XANAX is used during pregnancy, or if the patient becomes pregnant while taking this drug, the patient should be appraised of the potential hazard to the fetus. Because of experience with other members of the benzodiazepine class, XANAX is assumed to be capable of causing an increased risk of congenital abnormalities when administered to a pregnant woman during the first trimester. Because use of these drugs is rarely a matter of urgency, their use during the first trimester should almost always be avoided. The possibility that a woman of childbearing potential may be pregnant at the time of institution of therapy should be considered. Patients should be advised that if they become pregnant during therapy or intend to become pregnant they should communicate with their physicians about the desirability of discontinuing the drug.

PRECAUTIONS

General: In some patients receiving recommended (or higher) doses of XANAX Tablets (alprazolam) for relatively brief periods of time (eg, one week to four months), withdrawal seizures have been reported upon rapid decrease of dosage or abrupt discontinuation. Therefore, the dosage of XANAX should be reduced or withdrawn gradually (see DOSAGE AND ADMINISTRATION.)

If XANAX Tablets are to be combined with other psychotropic agents or anticonvulsant drugs, careful consideration should be given to the pharmacology of the agents to be employed—particularly with compounds which might potentiate the action of benzodiazepines (See Drug Interaction Section).

As with other psychotropic medications, the usual precautions with respect to administration of the drug and size of the prescription are indicated for severely depressed patients or those in whom there is reason to expect concealed suicidal ideation or plans.

In elderly and debilitated patients, it is recommended that the dosage be limited to the smallest effective amount to preclude the development of ataxia or oversedation (See Dosage and Administration Section). The usual precautions in treating patients with impaired renal or hepatic function should be observed.

Information for Patients: To assure safe and effective use of benzodiazepines, the following information and instructions should be given to patients:

1) Inform your physician about any alcohol consumption and medicine you are taking now, including drugs you may buy without a prescription. Alcohol should generally not be used during treatment with benzodiazepines.

2) Inform your physician if you are planning to become pregnant, if you are pregnant, or if you become pregnant while you are taking this medication.

3) Inform your physician if you are nursing.

4) Until you experience how this medication affects you, do not drive a car or operate potentially dangerous machinery, etc.

5) If benzodiazepines are used in large doses and/or for extended periods of time, they may produce habituation and emotional and physical dependence. Therefore, do not increase the dose even if you think the drug "does not work anymore."

6) Do not stop taking the drug abruptly without consulting your physician, since withdrawal symptoms can occur.

Laboratory Tests: Laboratory tests are not ordinarily required in otherwise healthy patients.

Drug interactions: The benzodiazepines, including alprazolam, produce additive CNS depressant effects when coadministered with other psychotropic medications, anticonvulsants, anti-histaminics, ethanol and other drugs which themselves produce CNS depression.

Pharmacokinetic interactions of benzodiazepines with other drugs have been reported. For example, the clearance of alprazolam and certain other benzodiazepines can be delayed by the co-administration of cimetidine. The clinical significance of this is unclear.

Drug/Laboratory Test Interactions: Although interactions between benzodiazepines and commonly employed clinical laboratory tests have occasionally been reported, there is no consistent pattern for a specific drug or specific test.

Carcinogenesis, Mutagenesis, Impairment of Fertility: No evidence of carcinogenic potential was observed in rats during a 24-month study with alprazolam in doses up to 375 times the human dose.

Alprazolam was not mutagenic in the rat micronucleus test at doses up to 1250 times the human dose.

Alprazolam produced no impairment of fertility in rats at doses up to 62.5 times the human dose.

Pregnancy: Teratogenic Effects: Pregnancy Category D: (See Warnings Section)

Nonteratogenic Effects: It is to be considered that the child born of a mother who is on benzodiazepines may be at some risk for withdrawal symptoms from the drug during the postnatal period. Also, neonatal flaccidity has been reported in children born of a mother who has been receiving benzodiazepines.

Labor and Delivery: XANAX has no established use in labor or delivery.

Nursing Mothers: Benzodiazepines are known to be excreted in human milk. It is to be assumed that alprazolam is as well. Chronic administration of diazepam to nursing mothers has been reported to cause their infants to become lethargic and lose weight. As a general rule, nursing should not be undertaken by mothers who must use XANAX.

Pediatric Use: Safety and effectiveness in children below the age of 18 have not been established.

ADVERSE REACTIONS

Side effects to XANAX Tablets (alprazolam), if they occur are generally observed at the beginning of therapy and usually disappear upon continued medication. In the usual patient, the most frequent side effects are likely to be an extension of the pharmacological activity of alprazolam, eg, drowsiness or lightheadedness.

The figures cited below are estimates of untoward clinical event incidence among subjects who participated in the relatively short duration (ie, four weeks) placebo-controlled clinical trials of XANAX. The figures cannot be used to predict precisely the incidence of untoward events in the course of usual medical practice where patient characteristics, and other factors often differ from those which obtained in the clinical trials. These figures cannot be compared with those obtained from other clinical studies involving related drug products and placebo as each group of drug trials are conducted under a different set of conditions.

Comparison of the cited figures, however, can provide the prescriber with some basis for estimating the relative contributions of drug and non-drug factors to the untoward event incidence rate in the population studied. Even this use must be approached cautiously, as a drug may relieve a symptom in one patient while inducing it in others. [For example, an anxiolytic drug may relieve dry mouth (a symptom of anxiety) in some subjects but induces (an untoward event) in others.]

Additionally, the cited figures can provide the prescriber with an indication as to the frequency with which physician intervention (eg increased surveillance, decreased dosage or discontinuation of drug therapy) may be necessary because of the untoward clinical event.

[See table on next page].

There have also been reports of withdrawal seizures upon rapid decrease or abrupt discontinuation of XANAX Tablets (See PRECAUTIONS—General).

In addition to the relatively common (i.e., greater than 1%) untoward events enumerated above, the following adverse events have been reported in association with the use of benzodiazepines: dystonia, irritability, concentration difficulties, anorexia, transient amnesia or memory impairment, loss of coordination, fatigue, sedation, slurred speech, jaundice, musculoskeletal weakness, pruritus, diplopia, dysarthria, changes in libido, menstrual irregularities, incontinence and urinary retention.

As with all benzodiazepines, paradoxical reactions such as stimulation, agitation, increased muscle spasticity, sleep disturbances, hallucinations and other adverse behavioral effects may occur in rare instances and in a random fashion. Should these occur, use of the drug should be discontinued.

Laboratory analyses were performed on all patients participating in the clinical program for XANAX. The following incidences of abnormalities were observed in patients receiving XANAX and the corresponding placebo group. None of these changes were considered to be of physiological significance.

	XANAX		Placebo	
	Low	**High**	**Low**	**High**
Hematology				
Hematocrit	*	*	*	*
Hemoglobin	*	*	*	*
Total WBC Count	1.4	2.3	1.0	2.0
Neutrophil Count	2.3	3.0	4.2	1.7
Lymphocyte Count	5.5	7.4	5.4	9.5
Monocyte Count	5.3	2.8	6.4	*
Eosinophil Count	3.2	9.5	3.3	7.2
Basophil Count	*	*	*	*
Urinalysis				
Albumin	—	*	—	*
Sugar	—	*	—	*
RBC/HPF	—	3.4	—	5.0
WBC/HPF	—	25.7	—	25.9
Blood Chemistry				
Creatinine	2.2	1.9	3.5	1.0
Bilirubin	*	1.6	*	*
SGOT	*	3.2	1.0	1.8
Alkaline Phosphatase	*	1.7	*	1.8

* Less than 1%

When treatment with XANAX is protracted, periodic blood counts, urinalysis and blood chemistry analyses are advisable.

Minor changes in EEG patterns, usually low-voltage fast activity have been observed in patients during therapy with XANAX and are of no known significance.

DRUG ABUSE AND DEPENDENCE

Physical and Psychological Dependence: Withdrawal symptoms (similar in character to those noted with barbiturates and alcohol) have occurred following abrupt discontinuance of benzodiazepines. (These can range from mild dysphoria and insomnia to a major syndrome which may include abdominal and muscle cramps, vomiting, sweating, tremor and convulsions). In addition, withdrawal seizures have occurred upon rapid decrease or abrupt discontinuation of therapy with XANAX Tablets (See PRECAUTIONS—General). It is recommended that all patients on XANAX who require a dosage reduction be gradually tapered under close supervision (See DOSAGE AND ADMINISTRATION).

Patients with a history of seizures or epilepsy, regardless of their concomitant anti-seizure drug therapy, should not be abruptly withdrawn from any CNS depressant agent, including XANAX Tablets (alprazolam). Addiction-prone individuals (such as drug addicts or alcoholics) should be under careful surveillance when receiving alprazolam or other psychotropic agents because of the predisposition of such patients to habituation and dependence.

Controlled Substance Class:

XANAX is a controlled substance under the Controlled Substance Act by the Drug Enforcement Administration and has been assigned to Schedule IV.

OVERDOSAGE

Manifestations of alprazolam overdosage include somnolence, confusion, impaired coordination, diminished reflexes and coma.

No delayed reactions (eg, organ toxicity) or clinical laboratory abnormalities have been reported.

The acute oral LD_{50} in rats is 331–2171 mg/kg. Other experiments in animals have indicated that cardiopulmonary collapse can occur following massive intravenous doses of alprazolam (over 195 mg/kg; 2000 times the maximum usual daily human dose). Animals could be resuscitated with positive mechanical ventilation and the intravenous infusion of levarterenol.

Animal experiments have suggested that forced diuresis or hemodialysis are probably of little value in treating overdosage.

General Treatment of Overdose: Overdosage reports with XANAX are limited. Respiration, pulse, and blood pressure should be monitored, as in all cases of drug overdosage. General supportive measures should be employed, along with immediate gastric lavage. Intravenous fluids should be administered and an adequate airway maintained. Hypotension may be combated by the use of Levophed (levarterenol) or Aramine (metaraminol). Dialysis is of limited value. As with the management of intentional overdosing with any drug, it should be borne in mind that multiple agents may have been ingested.

DOSAGE AND ADMINISTRATION

Dosage should be individualized for maximum beneficial effect. While the usual daily dosages given below will meet the needs of most patients, there will be some who require higher doses. In such cases, dosage should be increased cautiously to avoid adverse effects. Dosage should be reduced gradually when terminating therapy or decreasing the daily dose. It is suggested that the daily dosage be decreased no more than 0.5 milligram every three days.

DAILY DOSAGE SCHEDULE

The usual starting dose is 0.25 to 0.5 mg, given three times daily. This may be titrated according to the needs of the patient to a maximum total daily dose of 4 mg, given in divided doses.

In the elderly, or in the presence of debilitating disease, the usual starting dose is 0.25 mg, given two or three times daily. This may be gradually increased if needed and tolerated.

If side effects occur with the starting dose, the dose should be lowered.

HOW SUPPLIED

XANAX Tablets (alprazolam), ovoid-shaped and scored, are available as follows:

0.25 mg (white)
Bottles of 100 **NDC** 0009-0029-01
Unit-Dose Pkg (100) **NDC** 0009-0029-09
VISIPAK® Reverse Numbered Pack (100) **NDC** 0009-0029-20
Bottles of 500 **NDC** 0009-0029-02

0.5 mg (peach)
Bottles of 100 **NDC** 0009-0055-01
Unit-Dose Pkg (100) **NDC** 0009-0055-02
VISIPAK® Reverse Numbered Pack (100) **NDC** 0009-0055-22
Bottles of 500 **NDC** 0009-0055-03

XANAX

	Treatment Symptom XANAX	Emergent Incidence Placebo	Incidence of Intervention Because of Symptoms XANAX
Number of Patients	**565**	**505**	**565**
% of Patients Reporting:			
Central Nervous System			
Drowsiness	41.0	21.6	15.1
Light-headedness	20.8	19.3	1.2
Depression	13.9	18.1	2.4
Headache	12.9	19.6	1.1
Confusion	9.9	10.0	0.9
Insomnia	8.9	18.4	1.3
Nervousness	4.1	10.3	1.1
Syncope	3.1	4.0	*
Dizziness	1.8	0.8	2.5
Akathisia	1.6	1.2	*
Tiredness/Sleepiness	*	*	1.8
Gastrointestinal			
Dry Mouth	14.7	13.3	0.7
Constipation	10.4	11.4	0.9
Diarrhea	10.1	10.3	1.2
Nausea/Vomiting	9.6	12.8	1.7
Increased Salivation	4.2	2.4	*
Cardiovascular			
Tachycardia/Palpitations	7.7	15.6	0.4
Hypotension	4.7	2.2	*
Sensory			
Blurred Vision	6.2	6.2	0.4
Musculoskeletal			
Rigidity	4.2	5.3	
Tremor	4.0	8.8	0.4
Cutaneous			
Dermatitis/Allergy	3.8	3.1	0.6
Other			
Nasal Congestion	7.3	9.3	*
Weight Gain	2.7	2.7	*
Weight Loss	2.3	3.0	*

* None reported

1 mg (lavender)
Bottles of 100 **NDC** 0009-0090-01
Unit-Dose Pkg (100) **NDC** 0009-0090-02
VISIPAK® Reverse Numbered Pack (100) **NDC** 0009-0090-17
Bottles of 500 **NDC** 0009-0090-04

Store at controlled room temperature 15°–30°C (59°–86°F).

Caution: Federal law prohibits dispensing without prescription.

ANIMAL STUDIES

When rats were treated with alprazolam at 3, 10, and 30 mg/kg/day (37.5 to 375 times the maximum recommended human dose) orally for 2 years, a tendency for a dose related increase in the number of cataracts was observed in females and a tendency for a dose related increase in corneal vascularization was observed in males. These lesions did not appear until after 11 months of treatment.

CLINICAL STUDIES

XANAX Tablets (alprazolam) were compared to placebo in double blind clinical trials in patients with a diagnosis of anxiety or anxiety with associated depressive symptomatology. XANAX was significantly better than placebo at each of the evaluation periods of these four week studies as judged by the psychometric instruments: Physician's Global Impressions, Hamilton Anxiety Rating Scale Target Symptoms, Patient's Global Impressions and Self-Rating Symptom Scale.

Code 811 557 109

Shown in Product Identification Section, page 434

Products are listed alphabetically in the **PINK SECTION.**

Upsher-Smith Laboratories, Inc.

14905 23RD AVE., NORTH
MINNEAPOLIS, MN 55441

ACETAMINOPHEN UNISERTS® **OTC**
[*u'ni"sertz*]
Rectal Suppositories

DESCRIPTION

Acetaminophen Uniserts suppositories are supplied in 120 mg. (pediatric), 325 mg. and 650 mg. strengths. Acetaminophen Uniserts are foil strip-wrapped and unit dose labeled.

INDICATIONS

For the temporary relief of fever, minor aches, pains and headaches.

DOSAGE

Adults—One 650 mg. suppository every 4 to 6 hours. No more than a total of 6 suppositories in any 24-hour period.

Children (over 6)—One 325 mg. suppository every 4 to 6 hours. No more than a total of 8 suppositories in any 24-hour period.

Children (3 to 6)—One 120 mg. (pediatric) suppository every 4 to 6 hours. No more than a total of 6 suppositories in any 24-hour period. Children (under 3)—Consult a physician.

WARNING

Severe or recurrent pain or high or continued fever may be indicative of serious illness. Under these conditions, consult a physician. Do not use consistently for more than 2 days except on the advice of a physician. As with any drug, if you are pregnant or nursing a baby, seek the advice of a health professional before using this product.

HOW SUPPLIED

120 mg. 12's NDC 0245-0121-12
120 mg. 50's NDC 0245-0121-50
325 mg. 12's NDC 0245-0123-12
325 mg. 50's NDC 0245-0123-50
650 mg. 12's NDC 0245-0122-12
650 mg. 50's NDC 0245-0122-50
650 mg. 500's NDC 0245-0122-05

Continued on next page

Upsher-Smith—Cont.

KLOR-CON® Powder ℞

[*klōr 'kon*]
(Potassium Chloride for Oral Solution, U.S.P.)
20 mEq. (1.5g) per packet

DESCRIPTION
Each packet contains 1.5g potassium chloride providing potassium 20 mEq and chloride 20 mEq. Fruit-flavored with artificial color and sweetener (saccharin) added.

HOW SUPPLIED
KLOR-CON Powder 20 mEq (1.5g Potassium Chloride). In cartons of 30 and 100 packets.
30's NDC 0245-0035-30, 100's NDC 0245-0035-01

KLOR-CON®/25 Powder ℞

[*klōr 'kon*]
(Potassium Chloride for Oral Solution, U.S.P.)
25 mEq. (1.875 g) per packet

DESCRIPTION
Each packet contains 1.875 g potassium chloride providing potassium 25 mEq. and chloride 25 mEq. Fruit-flavored with artificial color and sweetener (saccharin) added.

HOW SUPPLIED
Cartons of 30, 100 and 250 packets.
30's NDC 0245-0037-30, 100's NDC 0245-0037-01
250's NDC 0245-0037-25

KLOR-CON® 8/KLOR-CON® 10 ℞

[*klōr 'kon*]
Potassium Chloride
Extended-release tablets, U.S.P.
8 mEq and 10 mEq

DESCRIPTION
KLOR-CON® Extended-release tablets are film coated (not enteric-coated) tablets containing 600 mg (equivalent to 8 mEq) or 750 mg (equivalent to 10 mEq) potassium chloride in an inert matrix. Potassium chloride has an empirical formula of KCl and its molecular weight is 74.55. This oral potassium supplement formulation is intended to provide a controlled release of potassium from the matrix to minimize the likelihood of producing high localized concentrations of potassium within the gastrointestinal tract. The expended matrix is not absorbed and may be excreted intact in the stool.

INACTIVE INGREDIENTS
Castor oil, D & C Yellow No. 10 (aluminum lake) or FD & C Blue No. 1 (aluminum lake), hydroxypropyl methylcellulose 2910, magnesium stearate, polyethylene glycol 3350, propylene glycol, synthetic iron oxide, and other ingredients.

CLINICAL PHARMACOLOGY
Potassium ion is the principal intracellular cation of most body tissues. Potassium ions participate in a number of essential physiological processes, including the maintenance of intracellular tonicity, the transmission of nerve impulses, the contraction of cardiac, skeletal, and smooth muscle and the maintenance of normal renal function.
Potassium depletion may occur whenever the rate of potassium loss through renal excretion and/or loss from the gastrointestinal tract exceeds the rate of potassium intake. Such depletion usually develops slowly as a consequence of prolonged therapy with oral diuretics, primary or secondary hyperaldosteronism, diabetic ketoacidosis, severe diarrhea, or inadequate replacement of potassium in patients on prolonged parenteral nutrition. Potassium depletion due to these causes is usually accompanied by a concomitant deficiency of chloride and is manifested by hypokalemia and metabolic alkalosis. Potassium depletion may produce weakness, fatigue, disturbances of cardiac rhythm (primarily ectopic beats), prominent U-waves in the electrocardiogram, and in advanced cases flaccid paralysis and/or impaired ability to concentrate urine.
Potassium depletion associated with metabolic alkalosis is managed by correcting the fundamental causes of the deficiency whenever possible and administering supplemental potassium chloride, in the form of high potassium food or potassium chloride solution or tablets.
In rare circumstances (e.g., patients with renal tubular acidosis) potassium depletion may be associated with metabolic acidosis and hyperchloremia. In such patients potassium replacement should be accomplished with potassium salts other than the chloride, such as potassium bicarbonate, potassium citrate, or potassium acetate.

INDICATIONS
BECAUSE OF REPORTS OF INTESTINAL AND GASTRIC ULCERATION AND BLEEDING WITH EXTENDED-RELEASE POTASSIUM CHLORIDE PREPARATIONS, THESE DRUGS SHOULD BE RESERVED FOR THOSE PATIENTS WHO CANNOT TOLERATE OR REFUSE TO TAKE LIQUID OR EFFERVESCENT POTASSIUM PREPARATIONS OR FOR PATIENTS IN WHOM THERE IS A PROBLEM OF COMPLIANCE WITH THESE PREPARATIONS.

1. For therapeutic use in patients with hypokalemia with or without metabolic alkalosis; in digitalis intoxication and patients with hypokalemic familial periodic paralysis.
2. For prevention of potassium depletion when the dietary intake of potassium is inadequate in the following conditions: Patients receiving digitalis and diuretics for congestive heart failure; hepatic cirrhosis with ascites; states of aldosterone excess with normal renal function; potassium-losing nephropathy, and certain diarrheal states.
3. The use of potassium salts in patients receiving diuretics for uncomplicated essential hypertension is often unnecessary when such patients have a normal dietary pattern. Serum potassium should be checked periodically, however, and, if hypokalemia occurs, dietary supplementation with potassium- containing foods may be adequate to control milder cases. In more severe cases supplementation with potassium salts may be indicated.

CONTRAINDICATIONS
Potassium supplements are contraindicated in patients with hyperkalemia since a further increase in serum potassium concentration is such patients can produce cardiac arrest. Hyperkalemia may complicate any of the following conditions: chronic renal failure, systemic acidosis such as diabetic acidosis, acute dehydration, extensive tissue breakdown as in severe burns, adrenal insufficiency, or the administration of a potassium-sparing diuretic (e.g., spironolactone, triamterene, or amiloride).
Wax-matrix potassium chloride preparations have produced esophageal ulceration in certain cardiac patients with esophageal compression due to an enlarged left atrium.
All solid dosage forms of potassium supplements are contraindicated in any patients in whom there is cause for arrest or delay in tablet passage through the gastrointestinal tract. In these instances, potassium supplementation should be with a liquid preparation.

WARNINGS
Hyperkalemia
In patients with impaired mechanisms for excreting potassium, the administration of potassium salts can produce hyperkalemia and cardiac arrest. This occurs most commonly in patients given potassium by the intravenous route but may also occur in patients given potassium orally. Potentially fatal hyperkalemia can develop rapidly and be asymptomatic.
The use of potassium salts in patients with chronic renal disease, or any other condition which impairs potassium excretion, requires particularly careful monitoring of the serum potassium concentration and appropriate dosage adjustment.
Interaction with Potassium-Sparing Diuretics
Hypokalemia should not be treated by the concomitant administration of potassium salts and a potassium-sparing diuretic (e.g., spironolactone, triamterene, or amiloride), since the simultaneous administration of these agents can produce severe hyperkalemia.
Gastrointestinal lesions
Potassium chloride tablets have produced stenotic and/or ulcerative lesions of the small bowel and deaths. These lesions are caused by a high localized concentration of potassium ion in the region of a rapidly dissolving tablet, which injures the bowel wall and thereby produces obstruction, hemorrhage, or perforation. Klor-Con® 8 and Klor-Con® 10 are extended-release tablets formulated to provide a controlled rate of release of potassium chloride and thus to minimize the possibility of high local concentration of potassium ion near the bowel wall. While the reported frequency of small-bowel lesions is much less with extended-release tablets (less than one per 100,000 patient-years) than with enteric-coated potassium chloride tablets (40-50 per 100,000 patient-years), cases associated with extended-release tablets have been reported both in foreign countries and the United States. In addition, perhaps because the extended-release preparations are not enteric-coated and release potassium in the stomach there have been reports of upper gastrointestinal bleeding associated with these products. The total number of gastrointestinal lesions remains less than one per 100,000 patient-years. Potassium chloride extended-release tablets should be discontinued immediately and the possibility of bowel obstruction or perforation considered if severe vomiting, abdominal pain, distention, or gastrointestinal bleeding occurs.
Metabolic acidosis
Hypokalemia in patients with metabolic acidosis should be treated with an alkalinizing potassium salt such as potassium bicarbonate, potassium citrate, or potassium acetate.

PRECAUTIONS
The diagnosis of potassium depletion is ordinarily made by demonstrating hypokalemia in a patient with a clinical history suggesting some cause for potassium depletion. In interpreting the serum potassium level, the physician should bear in mind that acute alkalosis per se can produce hypokalemia in the absence of a deficit in total body potassium, while acute acidosis per se can increase the serum potassium concentration into the normal range even in the presence of a reduced total body potassium. The treatment of potassium depletion, particularly in the presence of cardiac disease, renal disease, or acidosis, requires careful attention to acid-base balance and appropriate monitoring of serum electrolytes, the electrocardiogram, and the clinical status of the patient.
Pregnancy
Category C-Animal reproduction studies have not been conducted with potassium chloride products. It is also not known whether these products can cause fetal harm when administered to a pregnant woman or can affect reproduction capacity. They should be given to a pregnant woman only if clearly needed.
Nursing Mothers
Many drugs are excreted in human milk and because of the potential for serious adverse reactions in nursing infants from oral potassium supplements, a decision should be made whether to discontinue nursing or discontinue the drug, taking into account the importance of the drug to the mother.

ADVERSE REACTIONS
The most common adverse reactions to oral potassium salts are nausea, vomiting, abdominal discomfort, and diarrhea. These symptoms are due to irritation of the gastrointestinal tract and are best managed by diluting the preparation further, taking the dose with meals, or reducing the dose.
One of the most severe adverse effects is hyperkalemia (see Contraindications, Warnings and Overdosage). There also have been reports of upper and lower gastrointestinal conditions including obstruction, bleeding, ulceration and perforation (see Contraindications and Warnings); other factors known to be associated with such conditions were present in many of these patients. Skin rash has been reported rarely.

OVERDOSAGE
The administration of oral potassium salts to persons with normal excretory mechanisms for potassium rarely causes serious hyperkalemia. However, if excretory mechanisms are impaired or if potassium is administered too rapidly intravenously, potentially fatal hyperkalemia can result (see Contraindications and Warnings). It is important to recognize that hyperkalemia is usually asymptomatic and may be manifested only by an increased serum potassium concentration and characteristic electrocardiographic changes (peaking of T-waves, loss of P-wave, depression of S-T segment, and prolongation of the QT interval). Late manifestations include muscle paralysis and cardiovascular collapse from cardiac arrest.
Treatment measures for hyperkalemia include the following: (1) elimination of foods and medications containing potassium and of potassium-sparing diuretics; (2) intravenous administration of 300 to 500 ml/hr of 10% dextrose solution containing 10-20 units of insulin per 1,000 ml; (3) correction of acidosis, if present, with intravenous sodium bicarbonate; (4) use of exchange resins, hemodialysis, or peritoneal dialysis.
In treating hyperkalemia, it should be recalled that in patients who have been stabilized on digitalis, too rapid a lowering of the serum potassium concentration can produce digitalis toxicity.

DOSAGE AND ADMINISTRATION
The usual dietary intake of potassium by the average adult is 40 to 80 mEq per day. Potassium depletion sufficient to cause hypokalemia usually requires the loss of 200 mEq or more of potassium from the total body store. Dosage must be adjusted to the individual needs of each patient but is typically in the range of 20 mEq per day for the prevention of hypokalemia to 40- 100 mEq per day or more for the treatment of potassium depletion.
NOTE: Klor-Con® extended-release tablets must be swallowed whole and never crushed or chewed. Tablets should be taken with meals and with a glass of water or other liquid.

HOW SUPPLIED
Film Coated, Klor-Con® 8 (blue), Klor-Con® 10 (yellow), imprinted round tablets containing:
600 mg potassium chloride (equivalent to 8 mEq) in bottles of 100 (NDC 0245-0040-11) and bottles of 500 (NDC 0245-0040-15;
750 mg potassium chloride (equivalent to 10 mEq) in bottles of 100 (NDC 0245-0041-11) and bottles of 500 (NDC 0245- 0041-15).

Protect from light and moisture. Store at controlled room temperature 59°–86°F (15°–30°C). Dispense in container with child resistant closure.

KLOR-CON®/EF 25mEq ℞
[klōr'kon]
Potassium Bicarbonate Effervescent Tablets for Oral Solution, U.S.P.

DESCRIPTION
Each effervescent tablet in solution provides 25 mEq (978 mg) potassium as bicarbonate and citrate. KLOR-CON®/EF tablets are sugar free and orange flavored.

HOW SUPPLIED
KLOR-CON®/EF 25 mEq effervescent tablets in cartons of 30 and 100 individually wrapped tablets.
30's NDC 0245-0039-30, 100's NDC 0245-0039-01

LUBRIN® Vaginal Lubricating Inserts
[lu'brin]

List No. 0245-0118-19
(See PDR For Nonprescription Drugs)

RMS™ Suppositories Ⓒ ℞
(Rectal Morphine Sulfate)

WARNING—MAY BE HABIT FORMING

DESCRIPTION
Suppositories contain 5, 10 or 20 mg of morphine sulfate.

HOW SUPPLIED
RMS™ suppositories are individually sealed and unit dose labeled. 12 suppositories per carton.
5 mg NDC 0245-0160-12
10 mg NDC 0245-0161-12
20 mg NDC 0245-0162-12

SSKI® ℞
(potassium iodide oral solution, U.S.P.)

DESCRIPTION
SSKI® (potassium iodide oral solution, U.S.P.) is a saturated solution of potassium iodide containing 1 g of potassium iodide per ml.

HOW SUPPLIED
SSKI® (potassium iodide oral solution, U.S.P.) is supplied in 1 fluid ounce (30 ml) bottles (NDC 0245-0003-31) with a calibrated dropper marked to deliver 0.3 ml and 0.6 ml; and 8 fluid ounces (237 ml) bottles (NDC 0245-0003-08).

TROFAN
[tro'fan]
L-Tryptophan Tablets, 0.5 Gm.

COMPOSITION
Each capsule shaped tablet contains L-tryptophan, 0.5 Gm.

HOW SUPPLIED
Trofan® tablets 0.5 Gm. in bottles of 30 and 100 and unit dose 100's.
List No.—30's 0245-0095-30, 100's 0245-0095-11, UD 100's 0245-0095-01

TROFAN® DS
[tro'fan]
L-Tryptophan tablets, 1.0 gram

COMPOSITION
Each capsule shaped tablet contains L-tryptophan, 1 gram.

HOW SUPPLIED
Trofan® DS tablets 1.0 gram in bottles of 30 and 100 and unit dose 100.
List No.—30's 0245-0094-30, 100's 0245-0094-11, UD 100's 0245-0094-01

Products are cross-indexed
by product classifications
in the
BLUE SECTION

Vitaline Formulas

P.O. BOX 6757
INCLINE VILLAGE, NV 89450

BIOTIN FORTE
and
Extra Strength 5mg BIOTIN FORTE

Medical Food Products for physicians who want their patients supplemented with high potency biotin and folic acid.

BIOTIN FORTE

Each Tablet Provides:

BIOTIN	3000 mcg (3 mg)
FOLIC ACID	800 mcg
VITAMIN B-1 (thiamine mononitrate)	10 mg
VITAMIN B-2 (riboflavin)	10 mg
NIACINAMIDE	40 mg
PANTOTHENIC ACID	10 mg
VITAMIN B-6 (pyridoxine hydrochloride)	25 mg
VITAMIN B-12 (cyanocobalamine on ion exchange resin)	10 mcg
VITAMIN C (ascorbic acid)	200 mg
ZINC (zinc acetate)	30 mg

Extra Strength—No Zinc
5mg BIOTIN FORTE

Each Tablet Provides:

BIOTIN	(5000 mcg) 5 mg
FOLIC ACID	800 mcg
VITAMIN B-1 (thiamine mononitrate)	10 mg
VITAMIN B-2 (riboflavin)	10 mg
NIACINAMIDE	40 mg
PANTOTHENIC ACID	10 mg
VITAMIN B-6 (pyridoxine hydrochloride)	25 mg
VITAMIN B-12 (cyanocobalamine on ion exchange resin)	10 mcg
VITAMIN C (ascorbic acid)	100 mg

Biotin Forte is a medical food product for use only under medical supervision to meet nutritional requirements in specific medical conditions.

DOSAGE AND ADMINISTRATION
Adults and children as directed by physician.

SIDE EFFECTS
None reported

HOW SUPPLIED
Biotin Forte—yellow coated tablets in bottles of 60 and 1000 tablets. Extra Strength 5mg Biotin Forte—light green coated tablets in bottles of 60 and 1000 tablets.

LITERATURE AND SAMPLES
On request by physicians or Registered Dieticians.

BROMELAIN 500mg (2400mcu/gm)
(Proteolytic enzyme extracted from Ananas comosus)

DESCRIPTION
Each tablet contains 1200 milk clotting units of Bromelain, a proteolytic enzyme extracted from the pineapple plant (Ananus comosus).

INDICATIONS
As a source of proteolytic enzymes (protein digesting) to aid in the digestion of protein.

CONTRAINDICATIONS
Concomitant use with anticoagulants is contraindicated. Should not be used by patients with allergies to pineapple or pineapple products; by persons with bleeding tendencies, hemophilia, or any abnormality of the blood clotting system; or by persons with generalized systemic infections.

WARNING—USE IN PREGNANCY
Safe use of this product during pregnancy has not been established.

PRECAUTIONS
Bromelain should be used with caution in patients with severe renal or hepatic disease.

ADVERSE REACTIONS
Allergic reactions have been noted in persons sensitized to pineapple and/or pineapple products. Symptoms usually subside with discontinuance of Bromelain.

DOSAGE AND ADMINISTRATION
As a source of proteolytic enzymes to aid in the digestion of protein, 1 or 2 tablets with each meal.

HOW SUPPLIED
Bottles of 60 and 1000 tablets.

LITERATURE
On request by physician.

High Lipase
8X PANCREATIN 900mg USP
(non enteric coated)

Each Tablet Provides:

Lipase	22,500 USP Units
Protease	180,000 USP Units
Amylase	180,000 USP Units

Vitaline's 8X Pancreatin 900mg USP (High Lipase) tablets resist gastric inactivation and deliver predictable, high levels of biologically active enzymes into the duodenum. The enzymes catalyze the hydrolysis of fats into glycerol and fatty acids, proteoses and derived substances, and starch into dextrins and sugars. 8X Pancreatin 900mg USP tablets are effective in controlling steatorrhea and its consequences at low daily dosage levels.
Under conditions of the USP test method (in vitro) Vitaline's 8X Pancreatin 900mg USP has the following total digestive capacity:
Each Tablet

Dietary fat, grams	78gm
Dietary protein, grams	180gm
Dietary starch, grams	180gm

INDICATIONS AND USAGE
8X Pancreatin 900mg USP is indicated for patients with exocrine pancreatic enzyme deficiency as in:
- chronic pancreatitis
- pancreatectomy or gastrectomy
- cystic fibrosis

PRECAUTIONS
Use with caution in patients known to be allergic to pork protein.
Vitaline's 8X Pancreatin 900mg USP tablets contain no sugar, corn, wheat, soya, yeast, phenol, salicylates, preservatives or artificial coloring agents.

DOSAGE AND ADMINISTRATION
Usual dosage: One or two tablets during each meal and one tablet with snacks. Occasionally a third tablet with meals may be required depending upon individual requirements for control of steatorrhea.

HOW SUPPLIED
Uncoated tablets in bottles of 90, and 1000 tablets.

LITERATURE AVAILABLE
Complete literature available upon request by physician.

SELENIUM 200 MCG

DESCRIPTION
Each tablet contains: Selenium 200 mcg (organically bound in kelp)
Advantages of Kelp Bound Selenium Source
- Free of yeast protein allergens
- High bioavailability
- Uniformly distributed selenium
- Non toxic—not extractable
- Organic selenium—selenium is contained in a colloidal polymannuronate complex
- High trace element content

ACTION AND USES
A convenient source of selenium for patients deficient in this essential element.

ADMINISTRATION AND DOSAGE
As a dietary supplement, adults—1 tablet daily, or as directed by physician.

SIDE EFFECTS
None reported.

HOW SUPPLIED
Bottles of 90 and 1000.

LITERATURE AND SAMPLES
On request by physician.

TOTAL FORMULA®
(High Potency Multivitamin/Multimineral Supplement with micro-trace elements; Chromium, Selenium and Molybdenum)

DESCRIPTION
TOTAL FORMULA utilizes a unique technique of microspheres within the tablet to protect the delicate nutrients from moisture, air and the incompatibilities of certain minerals. Vitaline's microsphere technique also protects those nutrients that are susceptible to acid hydrolysis.
Each tablet provides:

Vitamins		**RDA %**
A (Water Soluble, Palmitate)	10,000 I.U.	200%

Continued on next page

Vitaline—Cont.

D-3	400	I.U.	100%
E (d-alpha tocopherol succinate) Water Soluble)	30	I.U.	100%
K (Water Soluble)	70	mcg	70%
C (Ascorbic Acid, from Sago Palm)	100	mg	166%
B-1 (Thiamine)	15	mg	1000%
B-2 (Riboflavin)	15	mg	882%
B-3 (Niacinamide)	25	mg	400%
B-5 (Pantothenic Acid)	25	mg	250%
B-6 (Pyridoxine HCL)	25	mg	1250%
B-12 (on ion exchange resin)	25	mcg	416%
Folic Acid	400	mcg	100%
Biotin	300	mcg	100%
Choline (Bitartrate)	10	mg	**
Hesperidin Complex	10	mg	***
Citrus Bioflavinoids	10	mg	***
Rutin	10	mg	***
Inositol	10	mg	***
PABA (para amino benzoic acid)	8	mg	***
Minerals			
Calcium (oyster shell)	100	mg	10%
Magnesium (chelate)	100	mg	25%
Phosphorus	52	mg	5%
Potassium (chelate)	25	mg	**
Iron (Fumarate)	20	mg	111%
Zinc (Gluconate)	30	mg	200%
Copper (Gluconate)	2	mg	100%
Manganese (Gluconate)	6	mg	**
Iodine (kelp)	100	mcg	66%
Chromium (GTF factor)	500	mcg	**
Selenium (organically bound chelate)	10	mcg	**
Molybdenum (chelate)	100	mcg	**
Silicon (kelp)	2.4	mg	**
Vanadium (chelate)	25	mcg	**

Chlorophyll coloring in coating. *RDA—recommended daily allowance. **Need in human nutrition established, RDA not determined. ***Need in human nutrition not determined.

TOTAL FORMULA contains no yeast, corn, wheat, soya, sugar, phenol, preservatives, dairy products, artificial colors, or added salicylates.

Directions: Adults, 1 tablet daily as a dietary supplement . . . children, as directed by physician.

HOW SUPPLIED

Bottles of 90 and 1000.

Literature and Samples: On request by physician.

Vivan Pharmacol, Inc.

1000 BENNETT BOULEVARD
LAKEWOOD, NJ 08701

ALPHADERM® Cream ℞
[āl-fā-derm']
(1% hydrocortisone)

PRODUCT OVERVIEW

KEY FACTS

Alphaderm is a novel cream formulation of 1% hydrocortisone in a self-stabilizing 10% urea base. Urea has been shown to increase the penetration of hydrocortisone into the epidermis. Alphaderm also possesses hydrating properties and can aid in the removal of surface scale.

MAJOR USES

Alphaderm cream is clinically effective in the management of mild to moderate eczema; where inflammation and itching are predominant features and where hydration of the skin is required. Apply a thin film of Alphaderm to the affected areas two to four times a day. Rub in well.

SAFETY INFORMATION

Alphaderm is indicated for topical use, with the exception of ophthalmic administration. Its use is contraindicated in patients who have a hypersensitivity to any of the components within the formulation. In keeping with all corticosteroids, the normal precautions should be observed.

PRESCRIBING INFORMATION

ALPHADERM® Cream ℞
[āl-fā-derm']
(1% hydrocortisone)

DESCRIPTION

Alphaderm Cream contains hydrocortisone 1% in a powder-in-cream base with urea 10% incorporated as a hypermolar solution, purified water, sorbitol, polyoxyethylene fatty glyceride, starch, white petrolatum, triglycerides of saturated fatty acids, isopropyl myristate, and sorbitan monolaurate. The near neutral pH of the formulation is made possible by the stabilized delivery system in which urea is absorbed by a polysaccharide powder matrix. Alphaderm (1% hydrocortisone) Cream is hypoallergenic and contains no parabens or lanolin.

HYDROCORTISONE
Molecular Weight: 362.47
Molecular Formula: $C_{21}H_{30}O_5$
CAS: 50-23-7

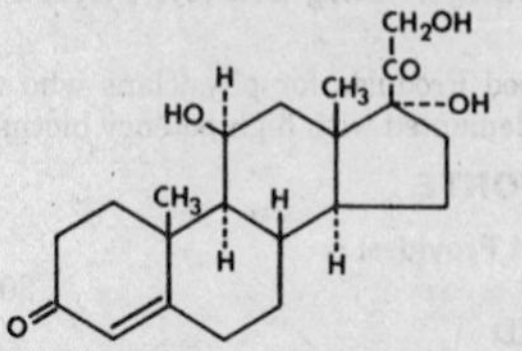

Pregn-4-ene-3,20-dione,11,17,21-trihydroxy-,(11β)-

CLINICAL PHARMACOLOGY

Topical corticosteroids are effective primarily because of their anti-inflammatory, antipruritic and vasoconstrictive actions.

The mechanisms of anti-inflammatory activity of the topical corticosteroids is unclear. Various laboratory methods, including vasoconstrictor assays, are used to compare and predict potencies and/or clinical efficacies of the topical corticosteroids. There is some evidence to suggest that a recognizable correlation exists between vasoconstrictor potency and therapeutic efficacy in man.

Pharmacokinetics: The extent of percutaneous absorption of topical corticosteroids is determined by many factors including the use of occlusive dressings, the integrity of the epidermal barrier and the vehicle itself. The Alphaderm Cream base contains 10% urea which has been shown to increase the penetration of the active ingredient, hydrocortisone 1%, into the epidermis.

Topical corticosteroids can be absorbed from normal intact skin. Inflammation and/or other disease processes in the skin increase percutaneous absorption. Occlusive dressings substantially increase the percutaneous absorption of topical corticosteroids. Thus, occlusive dressings may be a valuable therapeutic adjunct for treatment of resistant dermatoses. (See DOSAGE AND ADMINISTRATION.)

Once absorbed through the skin, topical corticosteroids are handled through pharmacokinetic pathways similar to systemically administered corticosteroids. Corticosteroids are bound to plasma proteins in varying degrees. Corticosteroids are metabolized primarily in the liver and are then excreted by the kidneys. Some of the topical corticosteroids and their metabolites are also excreted into the bile.

INDICATIONS AND USAGE

Alphaderm (1% hydrocortisone) Cream is indicated for the relief of the inflammatory and pruritic manifestations of corticosteroid-responsive dermatoses.

CONTRAINDICATIONS

Topical steroids are contraindicated in those patients with a history of hypersensitivity to any of the components of the preparation.

PRECAUTIONS

General: Systemic absorption of topical corticosteroids has produced reversible hypothalamic-pituitary-adrenal (HPA) axis suppression, manifestations of Cushing's syndrome, hyperglycemia, and glocosuria in some patients.

Conditions which augment systemic absorption include the application of the more potent steroids, use over large surface areas, prolonged use, and the addition of occlusive dressings.

Patients receiving a large dose of a potent topical steroid applied to a large surface area or under an occlusive dressing should be evaluated periodically for evidence of HPA axis suppression by using the urinary free cortisol and ACTH stimulation tests. If HPA axis suppression is noted, an attempt should be made to withdraw the drug, to reduce the frequency of application, or to substitute a less potent steroid.

Recovery of HPA axis function is generally prompt and complete upon discontinuation of the drug. Infrequently, signs and symptoms of steroid withdrawal may occur, requiring supplemental systemic corticosteroids.

Children may absorb proportionally larger amounts of topical corticosteroids and thus be more susceptible to systemic toxicity. (See Pediatric Use.) However, serious side effects secondary to topical 1% hydrocortisone are rare.

If irritation develops, topical corticosteroids should be discontinued and appropriate therapy instituted.

In the presence of dermatological infections, the use of an appropriate antifungal or antibacterial agent should be instituted. If a favorable response does not occur promptly, the corticosteroid should be discontinued until the infection has been adequately controlled.

Information for the Patient: Patients using topical corticosteroids should receive the following information and instructions:

1. This medication is to be used as directed by the physician. It is for external use only. Avoid contact with the eyes.
2. Patients should be advised not to use this medication for any disorder other than for which it was prescribed.
3. The treated skin area should not be bandaged or otherwise covered or wrapped as to be occlusive unless directed by the physician.
4. Patients should report any signs of local adverse reactions especially under occlusive dressing.
5. Parents of pediatric patients should be advised not to use tight-fitting diapers or plastic pants on a child being treated in the diaper area, as these garments may constitute occlusive dressings.

Laboratory Tests: The following tests may be helpful in evaluating the HPA axis suppression:
Urinary free cortisol test
ACTH stimulation test

Carcinogenesis, Mutagenesis, Impairment of Fertility: Long-term animal studies have not been performed to evaluate the carcinogenic potential or the effect on fertility of topical corticosteroids.

Studies to determine mutagenicity with prednisolone and hydrocortisone have revealed negative results.

Pregnancy: Pregnancy Category C: Corticosteroids are generally teratogenic in laboratory animals when administered systemically at relatively low dosage levels. The more potent corticosteroids have been shown to be teratogenic after dermal application in laboratory animals. There are no adequate and well-controlled studies in pregnant women on teratogenic effects from topically applied corticosteroids. Therefore, topical corticosteroids should be used during pregnancy only if the potential benefit justifies the potential risk to the fetus. Drugs of this class should be used extensively on pregnant patients, in large amounts, or for prolonged periods of time.

Nursing Mothers: It is not known whether topical administration of corticosteroids could result in sufficient systemic absorption to produce detectable quantities in breast milk. Systemically administered corticosteroids are secreted into breast milk in quantities *not* likely to have a deleterious effect on the infant. Nevertheless, caution should be exercised when topical corticosteroids are administered to a nursing woman.

Pediatric Use: *Pediatric patients may demonstrate greater susceptibility to topical corticosteroid-induced HPA axis suppression and Cushing's syndrome than mature patients because of a larger skin surface area to body weight ratio.*

Hypothalamic-pituitary-adrenal (HPA) axis suppression, Cushing's syndrome, and intracranial hypertension have been reported in children receiving topical corticosteroids. Manifestations of adrenal suppression in children include linear growth retardation, delayed weight gain, low plasma cortisol levels, and absence of response to ACTH stimulation. Manifestations of intracranial hypertension include bulging fontanelles, headaches, and bilateral papilledema.

Administration of topical corticosteroids to children should be limited to the least amount coompatible with an effective therapeutic regimen. Chronic corticosteroid therapy may interfere with the growth and development of children.

ADVERSE REACTIONS

The following local adverse reactions are reported infrequently with topical corticosteroids, but may occur more frequently with the use of occlusive dressings. These reactions are listed in an approximate decreasing order of occurrence:

1. Burning
2. Itching
3. Irritation
4. Dryness
5. Folliculitis
6. Hypertrichosis
7. Acneiform eruptions
8. Hypopigmentation
9. Perioral dermatitis
10. Allergic contact dermatitis
11. Maceration of the skin
12. Secondary infection
13. Skin atrophy
14. Striae
15. Miliaria

OVERDOSAGE

Topically applied corticosteroids can be absorbed in sufficient amounts to produce systemic effects (see PRECAUTIONS).

DOSAGE AND ADMINISTRATION

Apply a thin film of Alphaderm (1% hydrocortisone) Cream to affected areas two to four times a day, and rub in well. Occlusive dressings may be used for the management of recalcitrant conditions. If an infection develops, the use of occlusive dressings should be discontinued and appropriate antimicrobial therapy instituted.

HOW SUPPLIED

Alphaderm (1% hydrocortisone) Cream is available in:
NDC 54468-011-03 tube of 30 grams
NDC 54468-012-00 tube of 100 grams
Store below 59°F (15°C). Do not freeze.

CAUTION

Federal law prohibits dispensing without prescription.
REVISED: June, 1986

Wallace Laboratories
P.O. BOX 1
CRANBURY, NJ 08512

AQUATENSEN® ℞
(methyclothiazide, USP 5 mg)
Tablets

DESCRIPTION

AQUATENSEN (methyclothiazide) is a member of the benzothiadiazine (thiazide) family of drugs. It is an analogue of hydrochlorothiazide.
Clinically, AQUATENSEN is an oral diuretic-antihypertensive agent.

ACTIONS

The diuretic and saluretic effects of AQUATENSEN result from a drug-induced inhibition of the renal tubular reabsorption of electrolytes. The excretion of sodium and chloride is greatly enhanced. Potassium excretion is also enhanced to a variable degree, as it is with the other thiazides. Although urinary excretion of bicarbonate is increased slightly, there is usually no significant change in urinary pH. Methyclothiazide has a per mg natriuretic activity approximately 100 times that of the prototype thiazide, chlorothiazide. At maximal therapeutic dosages, all thiazides are approximately equal in their diuretic/natriuretic effects.
There is significant natriuresis and diuresis within two hours after administration of a single dose of methyclothiazide. These effects reach a peak in about six hours and persist for 24 hours following oral administration of a single dose.
Like other benzothiadiazines, AQUATENSEN also has antihypertensive properties, and may be used for this purpose either alone or to enhance the antihypertensive action of other drugs. The mechanism by which the benzothiadiazines, including methyclothiazide, produce a reduction of elevated blood pressure is not known. However, sodium depletion appears to be involved.
AQUATENSEN is readily absorbed from the gastrointestinal tract and is excreted unchanged by the kidneys.

INDICATIONS

AQUATENSEN is indicated in the management of hypertension either as the sole therapeutic agent or to enhance the effect of other antihypertensive drugs in the more severe forms of hypertension.
AQUATENSEN is indicated as adjunctive therapy in edema associated with congestive heart failure, hepatic cirrhosis, and corticosteroid and estrogen therapy.
AQUATENSEN has also been found useful in edema due to various forms of renal dysfunction such as the nephrotic syndrome, acute glomerulonephritis and chronic renal failure.
Usage in pregnancy: The routine use of diuretics in an otherwise healthy woman is inappropriate and exposes the mother and fetus to unnecessary hazard. Diuretics do not prevent development of toxemia of pregnancy, and there is no satisfactory evidence that they are useful in the treatment of developed toxemia.
Edema during pregnancy may arise from pathological causes or from the physiological and mechanical consequences of pregnancy. Thiazides are indicated in pregnancy when edema is due to pathologic causes, just as they are in the absence of pregnancy (however, see Warnings, below). Dependent edema in pregnancy, resulting from restriction of venous return by the expanded uterus, is properly treated through elevation of the lower extremities and use of support hose; use of diuretics to lower intravascular volume in this case is illogical and unnecessary. There is hypervolemia during normal pregnancy which is harmful to neither the fetus nor the mother (in the absence of cardiovascular disease), but which is associated with edema, including generalized edema, in the majority of pregnant women. If this edema produces discomfort, increased recumbency will often provide relief. In rare instances, this edema may cause extreme discomfort which is not relieved by rest. In these cases, a short course of diuretics may provide relief and may be appropriate.

CONTRAINDICATIONS

Renal decompensation.
Hypersensitivity to this or other sulfonamide derived drugs.

WARNINGS

Methyclothiazide shares with other thiazides the propensity to deplete potassium reserves to an unpredictable degree.
Thiazides should be used with caution in patients with renal disease or significant impairment of renal function, since azotemia may be precipitated and cumulative drug effects may occur.
Thiazides should be used with caution in patients with impaired hepatic function or progressive liver disease, since minor alterations of fluid and electrolyte balance may precipitate hepatic coma.
Thiazides may be additive or potentiative of the action of other antihypertensive drugs. Potentiation occurs with ganglionic or peripheral adrenergic blocking drugs.
Sensitivity reactions may occur in patients with a history of allergy or bronchial asthma.
The possibility of exacerbation or activation of systemic lupus erythematosus has been reported.
Usage in pregnancy: Thiazides cross the placental barrier and appear in cord blood. The use of thiazides in pregnant women requires that the anticipated benefit be weighed against possible hazards to the fetus. These hazards include fetal or neonatal jaundice, thrombocytopenia, and possibly other adverse reactions, that have occurred in the adult.
Nursing mothers: Thiazides appear in breast milk. If use of the drug is deemed essential, the patient should stop nursing.

PRECAUTIONS

Periodic determination of serum electrolytes should be performed at appropriate intervals for the purpose of detecting possible electrolyte imbalances such as hyponatremia, hypochloremic alkalosis, and hypokalemia. Serum and urine electrolyte determinations are particularly important when a patient is vomiting excessively or receiving parenteral fluids. All patients should be observed for other clinical signs of electrolyte imbalances such as dryness of mouth, thirst, weakness, lethargy, drowsiness, restlessness, muscle pains or cramps, muscular fatigue, hypotension, oliguria, tachycardia, and gastrointestinal disturbances such as nausea and vomiting.
Hypokalemia may develop with thiazides as with any other potent diuretic, especially when brisk diuresis occurs, severe cirrhosis is present, or when corticosteroids or ACTH are given concomitantly. Interference with the adequate oral intake of electrolytes will also contribute to the possible development of hypokalemia. Potassium depletion, even of a mild degree, resulting from thiazide use, may sensitize a patient to the effects of cardiac glycosides such as digitalis.
Any chloride deficit is generally mild and usually does not require specific treatment except under extraordinary circumstances (as in liver disease or renal disease). Dilutional hyponatremia may occur in edematous patients in hot weather; appropriate therapy is water restriction, rather than administration of salt except in rare instances when the hyponatremia is life threatening.
In actual salt depletion, appropriate replacement is the therapy of choice.
Hyperuricemia may occur or frank gout may be precipitated in certain patients receiving thiazide therapy.
Insulin requirements in diabetic patients may be increased, decreased, or unchanged. Latent diabetes mellitus may become manifest during thiazide administration.
Thiazide drugs may increase the responsiveness to tubocurarine.
The antihypertensive effects of the drug may be enhanced in the postsympathectomy patient.
Thiazides may decrease arterial responsiveness to norepinephrine. This diminution is not sufficient to preclude effectiveness of the pressor agent for therapeutic use.
If progressive renal impairment becomes evident as indicated by a rising nonprotein nitrogen or blood urea nitrogen, a careful reappraisal of therapy is necessary with consideration given to withholding or discontinuing diuretic therapy.
Thiazides may decrease serum PBI levels without signs of thyroid disturbance.
Thiazides have been reported, on rare occasions, to have elevated serum calcium to hypercalcemic levels. The serum calcium levels have returned to normal when the medication has been stopped. This phenomenon may be related to the ability of the thiazide diuretics to lower the amount of calcium excreted in the urine.

ADVERSE REACTIONS

Gastrointestinal system reactions: Anorexia, gastric irritation, nausea, vomiting, cramping, diarrhea, constipation, jaundice (intrahepatic cholestatic jaundice), pancreatitis.
Central nervous system reactions: Dizziness, vertigo, paresthesia, headache, xanthopsia.
Hematologic reactions: Leukopenia, agranulocytosis, thrombocytopenia, aplastic anemia.
Dermatologic-hypersensitivity reactions: Purpura, photosensitivity, rash, urticaria, necrotizing angiitis (vasculitis) (cutaneous vasculitis).
Cardiovascular reactions: Orthostatic hypotension may occur and may be aggravated by alcohol, barbiturates, or narcotics.
Other: Hyperglycemia, glycosuria, hypercalcemia, hyperuricemia, muscle spasm, weakness, restlessness.
There have been isolated reports that certain nonedematous individuals developed severe fluid and electrolyte derangements after only brief exposure to normal doses of thiazide and non-thiazide diuretics. The condition is usually manifested as severe dilutional hyponatremia, hypokalemia, and hypochloremia. It has been reported to be due to inappropriately increased ADH secretion and appears to be idiosyncratic. Potassium replacement is apparently the most important therapy in the treatment of this syndrome along with removal of the offending drug.
Whenever adverse reactions are severe, treatment should be discontinued.

DOSAGE AND ADMINISTRATION

AQUATENSEN (methyclothiazide) is administered orally. The usual adult dose ranges from 2.5 to 10 mg once daily.
Therapy should be individualized according to patient response. This therapy should be titrated to gain maximal therapeutic response as well as the minimal dose possible to maintain that therapeutic response.
To maintain an edema-free state or as an adjunct in the management of hypertension, 2.5 to 5.0 mg once daily is often adequate.
Maximum effective single dose is 10 mg; larger single doses do not accomplish greater diuresis, and are not recommended.
In the treatment of hypertension, methyclothiazide may be either employed alone or concurrently with other antihypertensive drugs. Combined therapy may provide adequate control of hypertension with lower dosage of the component drugs and fewer or less severe side effects.
For treatment of moderately severe or severe hypertension, supplemental use of other more potent antihypertensive agents may be indicated.
When other antihypertensive agents are to be added to the regimen, this should be accomplished gradually. Ganglionic blocking agents should be given at only half the usual dose since their effect is potentiated by pretreatment with AQUATENSEN.

OVERDOSAGE

Symptoms of overdosage include electrolyte imbalance and signs of potassium deficiency such as confusion, dizziness, muscular weakness, and gastrointestinal disturbances. General supportive measures including replacement of fluids and electrolytes may be indicated in treatment of overdosage.

HOW SUPPLIED

AQUATENSEN (methyclothiazide) is supplied as a 5 mg, peach-colored, monogrammed, grooved, rectangular-shaped tablet.
NDC 0037-0153-92, bottle of 100.
NDC 0037-0153-96, bottle of 500.
CAUTION: Federal law prohibits dispensing without prescription.

Rev. 4/83

Shown in Product Identification Section, page 434

BUTISOL SODIUM® Ⓒ ℞
(butabarbital sodium)
Tablets and Elixir

DESCRIPTION

BUTISOL SODIUM (butabarbital sodium) is a nonselective central nervous system depressant which is used as a sedative or hypnotic (WARNING: May be habit-forming). It is available for oral administration as *Tablets* containing 15 mg, 30 mg, 50 mg or 100 mg butabarbital sodium; and as *Elixir* containing 30 mg/5 mL, with alcohol (by volume) 7%. Other ingredients in the Tablets are: calcium stearate, corn starch, dibasic calcium phosphate, FD&C Blue No. 1 (15 mg and 30 mg only), FD&C Blue No. 2 (100 mg only); FD&C Red No. 3 (15 mg and 100 mg only), FD&C Yellow No. 5 (30 mg and 50 mg only)—see Precautions), FD&C Yellow No. 6 (100 mg only). Other ingredients in the Elixir are: D&C Green No. 5, edetate disodium, FD&C Yellow No. 5 (see Precautions), flavors (natural and artificial), propylene glycol, purified water, saccharin sodium, sodium benzoate. Butabarbital sodium occurs as a white, bitter powder which is freely soluble in water and alcohol, but practically insoluble in benzene and ether.
The structural formula for butabarbital sodium is:

Sodium 5-*sec*-butyl-5-ethylbarbiturate

Continued on next page

Wallace—Cont.

CLINICAL PHARMACOLOGY

BUTISOL SODIUM (butabarbital sodium), like other barbiturates, is capable of producing all levels of CNS mood alteration from excitation to mild sedation, to hypnosis, and deep coma. Overdosage can produce death. Barbiturates depress the sensory cortex, decrease motor activity, alter cerebellar function, and produce drowsiness, sedation, and hypnosis.

Barbiturate-induced sleep differs from physiological sleep. Sleep laboratory studies have demonstrated that barbiturates reduce the amount of time spent in the rapid eye movement (REM) phase of sleep or dreaming stage. Also, Stages III and IV sleep are decreased. Following abrupt cessation of barbiturates used regularly, patients may experience markedly increased dreaming, nightmares, and/or insomnia. Therefore, withdrawal of a single therapeutic dose over 5 or 6 days has been recommended to lessen the REM rebound and disturbed sleep which contribute to drug withdrawal syndrome (for example, decrease the dose from 3 to 2 doses a day for 1 week).

In studies, secobarbital sodium and pentobarbital sodium have been found to lose most of their effectiveness for both inducing and maintaining sleep by the end of 2 weeks of continued drug administration even with the use of multiple doses. As with secobarbital sodium and pentobarbital sodium, other barbiturates might be expected to lose their effectiveness for inducing and maintaining sleep after about 2 weeks. The short-, intermediate-, and, to a lesser degree, long-acting barbiturates have been widely prescribed for treating insomnia. Although the clinical literature abounds with claims that the short-acting barbiturates are superior for producing sleep while the intermediate-acting compounds are more effective in maintaining sleep, controlled studies have failed to demonstrate these differential effects. Therefore, as sleep medications, the barbiturates are of limited value beyond the short-term use.

Barbiturates are respiratory depressants. The degree of respiratory depression is dependent upon dose. With hypnotic doses, respiratory depression produced by barbiturates is similar to that which occurs during physiologic sleep with slight decrease in blood pressure and heart rate.

Barbiturates do not impair noraml hepatic function, but have been shown to induce liver microsomal enzymes, thus increasing and/or altering the metabolism of barbiturates and other drugs (see Precautions—*Drug interactions*).

Pharmacokinetics: BUTISOL SODIUM (butabarbital sodium) is the sodium salt of a weak acid. Barbiturates are weak acids that are absorbed and rapidly distributed to all tissues and fluids with high concentrations in the brain, liver, and kidneys. Barbiturates are bound to plasma and tissue proteins. The rate of absorption is increased if it is ingested as a dilute solution or taken on an empty stomach. Barbiturates are metabolized primarily by the hepatic microsomal enzyme system, and most metabolic products are excreted in the urine. The excretion of unchanged butabarbital in the urine is negligible. BUTISOL SODIUM (butabarbital sodium) is classified as an intermediate-acting barbiturate. The average plasma half-life for butabarbital is 100 hours in the adult.

Although variable from patient to patient, butabarbital has an onset of action of about ¾ to 1 hour, and a duration of action of about 6 to 8 hours.

INDICATIONS AND USAGE

BUTISOL SODIUM (butabarbital sodium) is indicated for use as a sedative or hypnotic.

Since barbiturates appear to lose their effectiveness for sleep induction and sleep maintenance after 2 weeks, use of BUTISOL SODIUM in treating insomnia should be limited to this time (see Clinical Pharmacology above).

CONTRAINDICATIONS

Barbiturates are contraindicated in patients with known barbiturate sensitivity. Barbiturates are also contraindicated in patients with a history of manifest or latent porphyria.

WARNINGS

Habit forming: Barbiturates may be habit forming. Tolerance, psychological and physical dependence may occur with continued use (see Drug Abuse and Dependence below). Patients who have psychological dependence on barbiturates may increase the dosage or decrease the dosage interval without consulting a physician and may subsequently develop a physical dependence on barbiturates. To minimize the possibility of overdosage or the development of dependence, the prescribing and dispensing of sedative-hypnotic barbiturates should be limited to the amount required for the interval until the next appointment. Abrupt cessation after prolonged use in the dependent person may result in withdrawal symptoms, including delirium, convulsions, and possibly death. Barbiturates should be withdrawn gradually from any patient known to be taking excessive dosage over long periods of time. (See Drug Abuse and Dependence below.)

Acute or chronic pain: Caution should be exercised when barbiturates are administered to patients with acute or chronic pain, because paradoxical excitement could be induced, or important symptoms could be masked. However, the use of barbiturates as sedatives in the postoperative surgical period, and as adjuncts to cancer chemotherapy, is well established.

Use in pregnancy: Barbiturates can cause fetal damage when administered to a pregnant woman. Retrospective, case-controlled studies have suggested a connection between the maternal consumption of barbiturates and a higher than expected incidence of fetal abnormalities. Following oral administration, barbiturates readily cross the placental barrier and are distributed throughout fetal tissues with highest concentrations found in the placenta, fetal liver, and brain. Withdrawal symptoms occur in infants born to mothers who receive barbiturates throughout the last trimester of pregnancy (see Drug Abuse and Dependence). If this drug is used during pregnancy, or if the patient becomes pregnant while taking this drug, the patient should be apprised of the potential hazard to the fetus.

PRECAUTIONS

General: Barbiturates should be administered with caution, if at all, to patients who are mentally depressed, have suicidal tendencies, or a history of drug abuse.

Elderly or debilitated patients may react to barbiturates with marked excitement, depression, and confusion. In some persons, barbiturates repeatedly produce excitement rather than depression.

In patients with hepatic damage, barbiturates should be administered with caution and initially in reduced doses. Barbiturates should not be administered to patients showing the premonitory signs of hepatic coma.

BUTISOL SODIUM (butabarbital sodium) Tablets, 30 mg and 50 mg, and Elixir contain FD&C Yellow No. 5 (tartrazine) which may cause allergic-type reactions (including bronchial asthma) in certain susceptible individuals. Although the overall incidence of FD&C Yellow No. 5 (tartrazine) sensitivity in the general population is low, it is frequently seen in patients who also have aspirin hypersensitivity.

Information for Patients: Practitioners should give the following information and instructions to patients receiving barbiturates.

The use of barbiturates carries with it an associated risk of psychological and/or physical dependence. The patient should be warned against increasing the dose of the drug without consulting a physician.

Barbiturates may impair mental and/or physical abilities required for the performance of potentially hazardous tasks, such as driving or operating machinery.

Alcohol should not be consumed while taking barbiturates. Concurrent use of the barbiturates with other CNS depressants, including other sedatives or hypnotics, alcohol, narcotics, tranquilizers, and antihistamines, may result in additional CNS depressant effects.

Laboratory tests: Prolonged therapy with barbiturates should be accompanied by periodic laboratory evaluation of organ systems, including hematopoietic, renal, and hepatic systems (see Precautions—*General* and Adverse Reactions).

Drug interactions: Most reports of clinically significant drug interactions occurring with the barbiturates have involved phenobarbital. However, the application of these data to other barbiturates appears valid and warrants serial blood level determinations of the relevant drugs when there are multiple therapies.

1. *Anticoagulants.* Phenobarbital lowers the plasma levels of dicumarol and causes a decrease in anticoagulant activity as measured by the prothrombin time. Barbiturates can induce hepatic microsomal enzymes resulting in increased metabolism and decreased anticoagulant response of oral anticoagulants (e.g., warfarin, acenocoumarol, dicumarol, and phenprocoumon). Patients stabilized on anticoagulant therapy may require dosage adjustments if barbiturates are added to or withdrawn from their dosage regimen.
2. *Corticosteroids.* Barbiturates appear to enhance the metabolism of exogenous corticosteroids probably through the induction of hepatic microsomal enzymes. Patients stabilized on corticosteroid therapy may require dosage adjustments if barbiturates are added to or withdrawn from their dosage regimen.
3. *Griseofulvin.* Phenobarbital appears to interfere with the absorption of orally administered griseofulvin, thus decreasing its blood level. The effect of the resultant decreased blood levels of griseofulvin on therapeutic response has not been established. However, it would be preferable to avoid concomitant administration of these drugs.
4. *Doxycycline.* Phenobarbital has been shown to shorten the half-life of doxycycline for as long as 2 weeks after barbiturate therapy is discontinued. The mechanism is probably through the induction of hepatic microsomal enzymes that metabolize the antibiotic. If phenobarbital and doxycycline are administered concurrently, the clinical response to doxycycline should be monitored closely.
5. *Phenytoin, sodium valproate, valproic acid.* The effect of barbiturates on the metabolism of phenytoin appears to be variable. Some investigators report an accelerating effect, while others report no effect. Because the effect of barbiturates on the metabolism of phenytoin is not predictable, phenytoin and barbiturate blood levels should be monitored more frequently if these drugs are given concurrently. Sodium valproate and valproic acid appear to decrease barbiturate metabolism; therefore, barbiturate blood levels should be monitored and appropriate adjustments made as indicated.
6. *Central nervous system.* The concomitant use of other central nervous system depressants, including other sedatives or hypnotics, antihistamines, tranquilizers, or alcohol, may produce additive depressant effects.
7. *Monoamine oxidase inhibitors (MAOI).* MAOI prolong the effects of barbiturates probably because metabolism of the barbiturate is inhibited.
8. *Estradiol, estrone, progesterone and other steroid hormones.* Pretreatment with or concurrent administration of phenobarbital may decrease the effect of estradiol by increasing its metabolism. There have been reports of patients treated with antiepileptic drugs (e.g. phenobarbital) who become pregnant while taking oral contraceptives. An alternate contraceptive method might be suggested to women taking phenobarbital.

Carcinogenesis, mutagenesis, impairment of fertility: No long-term studies in animals have been performed with butabarbital sodium to determine carcinogenic and mutagenic potential, or effects on fertility.

Pregnancy: Teratogenic effects—Pregnancy Category D (See Warnings—*Use in pregnancy* above).

Nonteratogenic effects—Infants suffering from long-term barbiturate exposure *in utero* may have an acute withdrawal syndrome of seizures and hyperirritability from birth to a delayed onset of up to 14 days (see Drug Abuse and Dependence).

Labor and delivery: Hypnotic doses of barbiturates do not appear to significantly impair uterine activity during labor. Administration of sedative-hypnotic barbiturates to the mother during labor may result in respiratory depression in the newborn. Premature infants are particularly susceptible to the depressant effects of barbiturates. If barbiturates are used during labor and delivery, resuscitation equipment should be available.

Nursing mothers: Caution should be exercised when a barbiturate is administered to a nursing woman since small amounts of some barbiturates are excreted in the milk.

ADVERSE REACTIONS

The following adverse reactions have been observed with the use of barbiturates in hospitalized patients. Because such patients may be less aware of certain of the milder adverse effects of barbiturates, the incidence of these reactions may be somewhat higher in fully ambulatory patients.

More than 1 in 100 patients. The most common adverse reaction, somnolence, is estimated to occur at a rate of 1 to 3 patients per 100.

Less than 1 in 100 patients. The most common adverse reactions estimated to occur at a rate of less than 1 in 100 patients listed below, grouped by organ system, and by decreasing order of occurrence are:

Central nervous system/psychiatric: Agitation, confusion, hyperkinesia, ataxia, CNS depression, nightmares, nervousness, psychiatric disturbance, hallucinations, insomnia, anxiety, dizziness, thinking abnormality.

Respiratory: Hypoventilation, apnea.

Cardiovascular: Bradycardia, hypotension, syncope.

Gastrointestinal: Nausea, vomiting, constipation.

Other reported reactions: Headache, hypersensitivity (angioedema, skin rashes, exfoliative dermatitis), fever, liver damage.

DRUG ABUSE AND DEPENDENCE

Controlled substance: Schedule III.

Abuse and dependence: Barbiturates may be habit-forming. Tolerance, psychological dependence, and physical dependence may occur especially following prolonged use of high doses of barbiturates. Daily administration in excess of 400 milligrams (mg) of pentobarbital or secobarbital for approximately 90 days is likely to produce some degree of physical dependence. A dosage of from 600 to 800 mg taken for at least 35 days is sufficient to produce withdrawal seizures. The average daily dose for the barbiturate addict is usually about 1.5 grams. As tolerance to barbiturates develops, the amount needed to maintain the same level of intoxication increases; tolerance to a fatal dosage, however, does not increase more than two-fold. As this occurs, the margin between an intoxicating dosage and fatal dosage becomes smaller.

Symptoms of acute intoxication with barbiturates include unsteady gait, slurred speech, and sustained nystagmus. Mental signs of chronic intoxication include confusion, poor judgment, irritability, insomnia, and somatic complaints.

Symptoms of barbiturate dependence are similar to those of chronic alcoholism.

If an individual appears to be intoxicated with alcohol to a degree that is radically disproportionate to the amount of alcohol in his or her blood, the use of barbiturates should be suspected. The lethal dose of a barbiturate is far less if alcohol is also ingested.

The symptoms of barbiturate withdrawal can be severe and may cause death. Minor withdrawal symptoms may appear 8 to 12 hours after the last dose of a barbiturate. These symptoms usually appear in the following order: anxiety, muscle twitching, tremor of hands and fingers, progressive weakness, dizziness, distortion in visual perception, nausea, vomiting, insomnia, and orthostatic hypotension. Major withdrawal symptoms (convulsions and delirium) may occur within 16 hours and last up to 5 days after abrupt cessation of these drugs. Intensity of withdrawal symptoms gradually declines over a period of approximately 15 days.

Drug dependence to barbiturates arises from repeated administration of a barbiturate or agent with barbiturate-like effect on a continuous basis, generally in amounts exceeding the therapeutic dose levels. The characteristics of drug dependence to barbiturates include: (a) a strong desire or need to continue taking the drug; (b) a tendency to increase the dose; (c) a psychic dependence on the effects of the drug related to subjective and individual appreciation for those effects; and (d) a physical dependence on the effects of the drug requiring its presence for maintenance of homeostasis and resulting in a definite, characteristic, and self-limited abstinence syndrome when the drug is withdrawn.

Treatment of barbiturate dependence consists of cautious and gradual withdrawal of the drug. Barbiturate-dependent patients can be withdrawn by using a number of different withdrawal regimens. In all cases, withdrawal takes an extended period of time. One method involves initiating treatment at the patient's regular dosage level, in 3 to 4 divided doses, and decreasing the daily dose by 10 percent if tolerated by the patient.

Infants physically dependent on barbiturates may be given phenobarbital 3 to 10 mg/kg/day. After withdrawal symptoms (hyperactivity, disturbed sleep, tremors, hyperreflexia) are relieved, the dosage of phenobarbital should be gradually decreased and completely withdrawn over a 2-week period.

OVERDOSAGE

Signs and symptoms: The toxic dose of barbiturates varies considerably. In general, an oral dose of 1 gram of most barbiturates produces serious poisoning in an adult. Death commonly occurs after 2 to 10 grams of ingested barbiturates. Symptoms of acute intoxication with barbiturates include unsteady gait, slurred speech, and sustained nystagmus. Mental signs of chronic intoxication include confusion, poor judgment, irritability, insomnia, and somatic complaints. Barbiturate intoxication may be confused with alcoholism, bromide intoxication, and with various neurological disorders.

Acute overdosage with barbiturates is manifested by CNS and respiratory depression which may progress to Cheyne-Stokes respiration, areflexia, constriction of the pupils to a slight degree (though in severe poisoning they may show paralytic dilation), oliguria, tachycardia, hypotension, lowered body temperature, and coma. Typical shock syndrome (apnea, circulatory collapse, respiratory arrest, and death) may occur.

In extreme overdose, all electrical activity in the brain may cease, in which case a "flat" EEG normally equated with clinical death cannot be accepted. This effect is fully reversible unless hypoxic damage occurs. Consideration should be given to the possibility of barbiturate intoxication even in situations that appear to involve trauma.

Complications: Pneumonia, pulmonary edema, cardiac arrhythmias, congestive heart failure, and renal failure may occur. Uremia may increase CNS sensitivity to barbiturates if renal function is impaired. Differential diagnosis should include hypoglycemia, head trauma, cerebrovascular accidents, convulsive states, and diabetic coma.

Treatment: Treatment of overdosage is mainly supportive and consists of the following:

1. Maintenance of an adequate airway, with assisted respiration and oxygen administration as necessary.
2. Monitoring of vital signs and fluid balance.
3. If the patient is conscious and has not lost the gag reflex, emesis may be induced with ipecac. Care should be taken to prevent pulmonary aspiration of vomitus. After completion of vomiting, 30 grams activated charcoal in a glass of water may be administered.
4. If emesis is contraindicated, gastric lavage may be performed with a cuffed endotracheal tube in place with the patient in the face down position. Activated charcoal may be left in the emptied stomach and a saline cathartic administered.
5. Fluid therapy and other standard treatment for shock, if needed.
6. If renal function is normal, forced diuresis may aid in the elimination of the barbiturate.
7. Although not recommended as a routine procedure, hemodialysis may be used in severe barbiturate intoxications or if the patient is anuric or in shock.
8. Appropriate nursing care, including rolling patients from side-to-side every 30 minutes, to prevent hypostatic pneumonia, decubiti, aspiration, and other complications of patients with altered states of consciousness.
9. Antibiotics should be given if pneumonia is suspected.

DOSAGE AND ADMINISTRATION

Usual adult dosage:

Daytime sedative—15 to 30 mg, 3 or 4 times daily.

Bedtime hypnotic—50 to 100 mg.

Preoperative sedative—50 to 100 mg, 60 to 90 minutes before surgery.

Usual pediatric dosage:

Preoperative sedative—2 to 6 mg/kg maximum 100 mg.

Special patient population:

Dosage should be reduced in the elderly or debilitated because these patients may be more sensitive to barbiturates. Dosage should be reduced for patients with impaired renal function or hepatic disease (see Precautions).

HOW SUPPLIED

BUTISOL SODIUM® (butabarbital sodium) Tablets:

15 mg—colored lavender, scored, imprinted "BUTISOL SODIUM" and $^{37}{}_{112}$ in bottles of 100 (NDC 0037-0112-60) and 1000 (NDC 0037-0112-80).

30 mg*—colored green, scored, imprinted "BUTISOL SODIUM" and $^{37}{}_{113}$ in bottles of 100 (NDC 0037-0113-60) and 1000 (NDC 0037-0113-80).

50 mg*—colored orange, scored, imprinted "BUTISOL SODIUM" and $^{37}{}_{114}$ in bottles of 100 (NDC 0037-0114-60).

100 mg—colored pink, scored, imprinted "BUTISOL SODIUM" and $^{37}{}_{115}$ in bottles of 100 (NDC 0037-0115-60).

BUTISOL SODIUM® (butabarbital sodium) Elixir*: 30 mg/5 mL, alcohol (by volume) 7%—colored green in bottles of one pint (NDC 0037-0110-16) and one gallon (NDC 0037-0110-28).

*Contains FD&C Yellow No. 5 (see Precautions).

Storage: *Tablets* and *Elixir*—Store at room temperature. Keep bottle tightly closed.

Rev. 2/85

Shown in Product Identification Section, page 434

DEPEN® ℞

(Penicillamine, Wallace)
Titratable Tablets

> Physicians planning to use penicillamine should thoroughly familiarize themselves with its toxicity, special dosage considerations, and therapeutic benefits. Penicillamine should never be used casually. Each patient should remain constantly under the close supervision of the physician. Patients should be warned to report promptly any symptoms suggesting toxicity.

DESCRIPTION

Penicillamine is 3-mercapto-D-valine. It is a white or practically white, crystalline powder, freely soluble in water, slightly soluble in alcohol, and insoluble in chloroform and ether. Although its configuration is D, it is levorotatory as usually measured:

$$[\alpha]^{25^\circ}_{D} = -62.5^\circ \pm 2^\circ \ (C = 0.05\%, 1N \text{ NaOH})$$

The empirical formula is $C_5H_{11}NO_2S$, giving it a molecular weight of 149.21.

It reacts readily with formaldehyde or acetone to form a thiazolidine-carboxylic acid.

Other ingredients: acetylated monoglycerides, edetate disodium, hydroxypropyl cellulose, hydroxypropyl methylcellulose, lactose, magnesium stearate, magnesium trisilicate, povidone, starch, stearic acid, titanium dioxide.

CLINICAL PHARMACOLOGY

Penicillamine is a chelating agent recommended for the removal of excess copper in patients with Wilson's disease. From *in vitro* studies which indicate that one atom of copper combines with two molecules of penicillamine, it would appear that one gram of penicillamine should be followed by the excretion of about 200 milligrams of copper; however, the actual amount excreted is about one percent of this.

Penicillamine also reduces excess cystine excretion in cystinuria. This is done, at least in part, by disulfide interchange between penicillamine and cystine, resulting in formation of penicillamine-cysteine disulfide, a substance that is much more soluble than cystine and is excreted readily.

Penicillamine interferes with the formation of cross-links between tropocollagen molecules and cleaves them when newly formed. The mechanism of action of penicillamine in rheumatoid arthritis is unknown, although it appears to suppress disease activity. Unlike cytotoxic immunosuppressants, penicillamine markedly lowers IgM rheumatoid factor but produces no significant depression in absolute levels of serum immunoglobulins. Also unlike cytotoxic immunosuppressants, which act on both, penicillamine *in vitro* depresses T-cell activity but not B-cell activity. *In vitro*, penicillamine dissociates macroglobulins (rheumatoid factor) although the relationship of the activity to its effect in rheumatoid arthritis is not known.

In rheumatoid arthritis, the onset of therapeutic response to DEPEN (Penicillamine, Wallace) may not be seen for two or three months. In those patients who respond, however, the first evidence of suppression of symptoms such as pain, tenderness, and swelling usually is apparent within three months. The optimum duration of therapy has not been determined. If remissions occur, they may last from months to years but usually require continued treatment (see DOSAGE AND ADMINISTRATION).

In patients with rheumatoid arthritis, it is important that DEPEN be given on an empty stomach, at least one hour before meals and at least one hour apart from any other drug, food or milk. This permits maximum absorption and reduces the likelihood of metal binding.

Methodology for determining the bioavailability of penicillamine is not available; however, penicillamine is known to be a very soluble substance.

INDICATIONS

DEPEN is indicated in the treatment of Wilson's disease, cystinuria, and in patients with severe, active rheumatoid arthritis who have failed to respond to an adequate trial of conventional therapy. Available evidence suggests that DEPEN is not of value in ankylosing spondylitis.

Wilson's Disease—Wilson's disease (hepatolenticular degeneration) results from the interaction of an inherited defect and an abnormality in copper metabolism. The metabolic defect, which is the consequence of the autosomal inheritance of one abnormal gene from each parent, manifests itself in a greater positive copper balance than normal. As a result, copper is deposited in several organs and appears eventually to produce pathologic effects most prominently seen in the brain, where degeneration is widespread; in the liver, where fatty infiltration, inflammation, and hepatocellular damage progress to postnecrotic cirrhosis; in the kidney, where tubular and glomerular dysfunction results; and in the eye, where characteristic corneal copper deposits are known as Kayser-Fleischer rings.

Two types of patients require treatment for Wilson's disease: (1) the symptomatic, and (2) the asymptomatic in whom it can be assumed the disease will develop in the future if the patient is not treated.

Diagnosis, suspected on the basis of family or individual history, physical examination, or a low serum concentration of ceruloplasmin*, is confirmed by the demonstration of Kayser-Fleischer rings or, particularly in the asymptomatic patient, by the quantitative demonstration in a liver biopsy specimen of a concentration of copper in excess of 250 mcg/g dry weight.

* For quantitative test for serum ceruloplasmin see: Morell, A. G.; Windsor, J.; Sternlieb, I.; Scheinberg, I. H.: Measurement of the concentration of ceruloplasmin in serum by determination of its oxidase activity, in "Laboratory Diagnosis of Liver Disease," F. W. Sunderman; F. W Sunderman, Jr. (eds.), St. Louis, Warren H. Green, Inc., 1968, pp. 193–195.

Treatment has two objectives:

(1) to minimize dietary intake and absorption of copper.
(2) to promote excretion of copper deposited in tissues.

The first objective is attained by a daily diet that contains no more than one or two milligrams of copper. Such a diet should exclude, most importantly, chocolate, nuts, shellfish, mushrooms, liver, molasses, broccoli, and cereals enriched with copper, and be composed to as great an extent as possible of foods with a low copper content. Distilled or demineralized water should be used if the patient's drinking water contains more than 0.1 mg of copper per liter.

For the second objective, a copper chelating agent is used. Penicillamine is the only one of these agents that is orally effective.

In symptomatic patients, this treatment usually produces marked neurologic improvement, fading of Kayser-Fleischer rings, and gradual amelioration of hepatic dysfunction and psychic disturbances.

Clinical experience to date suggests that life is prolonged with the above regimen.

Noticeable improvement may not occur for one to three months. Occasionally, neurologic symptoms become worse during initiation of therapy with DEPEN. Despite this, the drug should not be discontinued permanently, although temporary interruption may result in clinical improvement of the neurological symptoms but it carries an increased risk of developing a sensitivity reaction upon resumption of therapy (See WARNINGS).

Treatment of asymptomatic patients has been carried out for over ten years. Symptoms and signs of the disease appear to

Continued on next page

Wallace—Cont.

be prevented indefinitely if daily treatment with DEPEN can be continued.

Cystinuria—Cystinuria is characterized by excessive urinary excretion of the dibasic amino acids, arginine, lysine, ornithine, and cystine, and the mixed disulfide of cysteine and homocysteine. The metabolic defect that leads to cystinuria is inherited as an autosomal, recessive trait. Metabolism of the affected amino acids is influenced by at least two abnormal factors: (1) defective gastrointestinal absorption and (2) renal tubular dysfunction.

Arginine, lysine, ornithine, and cysteine are soluble substances, readily excreted. There is no apparent pathology connected with their excretion in excessive quantities.

Cystine, however, is so slightly soluble at the usual range of urinary pH that it is not excreted readily, and so crystallizes and forms stones in the urinary tract. Stone formation is the only known pathology in cystinuria.

Normal daily output of cystine is 40 to 80 mg. In cystinuria, output is greatly increased and may exceed 1 g/day. At 500 to 600 mg/day, stone formation is almost certain. When it is more than 300 mg/day, treatment is indicated. Conventional treatment is directed at keeping urinary cystine diluted enough to prevent stone formation, keeping the urine alkaline enough to dissolve as much cystine as possible, and minimizing cystine production by a diet low in methionine (the major dietary precursor of cystine). Patients must drink enough fluid to keep urine specific gravity below 1.010, take enough alkali to keep urinary pH at 7.5 to 8, and maintain a diet low in methionine. This diet is not recommended in growing children and probably is contraindicated in pregnancy because of its low protein content (see PRECAUTIONS).

When these measures are inadequate to control recurrent stone formation, DEPEN may be used as additional therapy. When patients refuse to adhere to conventional treatment, DEPEN may be a useful substitute. It is capable of keeping cystine excretion to near normal values, thereby hindering stone formation and the serious consequences of pyelonephritis and impaired renal function that develop in some patients.

Bartter and colleagues depict the process by which penicillamine interacts with cystine to form penicillamine-cysteine mixed disulfide as:

$$CSSC + PS' \rightleftharpoons CS' + CSSP$$
$$PSSP + CS' \rightleftharpoons PS' + CSSP$$
$$CSSC + PSSP \rightleftharpoons 2\ CSSP$$

CSSC = cystine
CS′ = deprotonated cysteine
PSSP = penicillamine
PS′ = deprotonated penicillamine sulfhydryl
CSSP = penicillamine-cysteine mixed disulfide

In this process, it is assumed that the deprotonated form of penicillamine, PS′, is the active factor in bringing about the disulfide interchange.

Rheumatoid Arthritis—Because DEPEN can cause severe adverse reactions, its use in rheumatoid arthritis should be restricted to patients who have severe, active disease and who have failed to respond to an adequate trial of conventional therapy. Even then, benefit-to-risk ratio should be carefully considered. Other measures, such as rest, physiotherapy, salicylates and corticosteroids should be used, when indicated, in conjunction with DEPEN (see PRECAUTIONS).

CONTRAINDICATIONS

Penicillamine should not be administered to patients with rheumatoid arthritis who are pregnant (see PRECAUTIONS).

Patients with a history of penicillamine-related aplastic anemia or agranulocytosis should not be restarted on penicillamine (see WARNINGS and ADVERSE REACTIONS).

Because of its potential for causing renal damage, penicillamine should not be administered to rheumatoid arthritis patients with a history or other evidence of renal insufficiency.

WARNINGS

The use of penicillamine has been associated with fatalities due to certain diseases, such as aplastic anemia, agranulocytosis, thrombocytopenia, Goodpasture's syndrome, and myasthenia gravis.

Because of the potential for serious hematological and renal adverse reactions, routine urinalysis, white and differential blood cell count, hemoglobin determination, and direct platelet count must be done every two weeks for the first six months of penicillamine therapy and monthly thereafter. Patients should be instructed to report promptly signs and symptoms of granulocytopenia and/or thrombocytopenia such as fever, sore throat, chills, bruising or bleeding and the above laboratory studies should be promptly repeated.

Leukopenia and thrombocytopenia have been reported to occur in up to 5% of patients during penicillamine therapy. Leukopenia is of the granulocytic series and may or may not be associated with an increase in eosinophils. A confirmed reduction in WBC below 3500 mandates discontinuance of penicillamine therapy. Thrombocytopenia may be on an idiosyncratic basis with decreased or absent megakaryocytes in the marrow, when it is part of an aplastic anemia. In other cases the thrombocytopenia is presumably on an immune basis since the number of megakaryocytes in the marrow has been reported to be normal or sometimes increased. The development of a platelet count below 100,000, even in the absence of clinical bleeding, requires at least temporary cessation of penicillamine therapy. A progressive fall in either platelet count or WBC in three successive determinations, even though values are still within the normal range, likewise requires at least temporary cessation.

Proteinuria and/or hematuria may develop during therapy and may be warning signs of membranous glomerulopathy which can progress to a nephrotic syndrome. Close observation of these patients is essential. In some patients the proteinuria disappears with continued therapy; in others penicillamine must be discontinued. When a patient develops proteinuria or hematuria the physician must ascertain whether it is a sign of drug-induced glomerulopathy or is unrelated to penicillamine.

Rheumatoid arthritis patients who develop moderate degrees of proteinuria may be continued cautiously on penicillamine therapy, provided that quantitative 24-hour urinary protein determinations are obtained at intervals of one to two weeks. Penicillamine dosage should not be increased under these circumstances. Proteinuria which exceeds 1 g/24 hours, or proteinuria which is progressively increasing requires either discontinuance of the drug or a reduction in the dosage. In some patients, proteinuria has been reported to clear following reduction in dosage.

In rheumatoid arthritis patients, penicillamine should be discontinued if unexplained gross hematuria or presistent microscopic hematuria develops.

In patients with Wilson's disease or cystinuria the risks of continued penicillamine therapy in patients manifesting potentially serious urinary abnormalities must be weighed against the expected therapeutic benefits.

When penicillamine is used in cystinuria, an annual x-ray for renal stones is advised. Cystine stones form rapidly, sometimes in six months.

Up to one year or more may be required for any urinary abnormalities to disappear after penicillamine has been discontinued.

Because of rare reports of intrahepatic cholestasis and toxic hepatitis, liver function tests are recommended every six months during therapy.

Goodpasture's syndrome has occurred rarely. The development of abnormal urinary findings associated with hemoptysis and pulmonary infiltrates on x-ray requires immediate cessation of penicillamine.

Myasthenic syndrome sometimes progressing to myasthenia gravis has been reported. In the majority of cases, symptoms of myasthenia have receded after withdrawal of penicillamine.

Pemphigoid-type reactions characterized by bullous lesions clinically indistinguishable from pemphigus have occurred and have required discontinuation of penicillamine and treatment with corticosteroids.

Once instituted for Wilson's disease or cystinuria, treatment with penicillamine should, as a rule, be continued on a daily basis. Interruptions for even a few days have been followed by sensitivity reactions after reinstitution of therapy.

PRECAUTIONS

Some patients may experience drug fever, a marked febrile response to penicillamine, usually in the second or third week following initiation of therapy. Drug fever may sometimes be accompanied by a macular cutaneous eruption.

In the case of drug fever in patients with Wilson's disease or cystinuria, because no alternative treatment is available, penicillamine should be temporarily discontinued until the reaction subsides. Then penicillamine should be reinstituted with a small dose that is gradually increased until the desired dosage is attained. Systemic steroid therapy may be necessary, and is usually helpful, in such patients in whom toxic reactions develop a second or third time.

In the case of drug fever in rheumatoid arthritis patients, because other treatments are available, penicillamine should be discontinued and another therapeutic alternative tried, since experience indicates that the febrile reaction will recur in a very high percentage of patients upon readministration of penicillamine.

The skin and mucous membranes should be observed for allergic reactions. Early and late rashes have occurred. Early rash occurs during the first few months of treatment and is more common. It is usually a generalized pruritic, erythematous, maculopapular or morbilliform rash and resembles the allergic rash seen with other drugs. Early rash usually disappears within days after stopping penicillamine and seldom recurs when the drug is restarted at a lower dosage. Pruritus and early rash may often be controlled by the concomitant administration of antihistamines. Less commonly, a late rash may be seen, usually after six months or more of treatment, and requires discontinuation of penicillamine. It is usually on the trunk, is accompanied by intense pruritus, and is usually unresponsive to topical corticosteroid therapy. Late rash may take weeks to disappear after penicillamine is stopped and usually recurs if the drug is restarted.

The appearance of drug eruption accompanied by fever, arthralgia, lymphadenopathy or other allergic manifestations usually requires discontinuation of penicillamine.

Certain patients will develop a positive antinuclear antibody (ANA) test and some of these may show a lupus erythematosus-like syndrome similar to drug-induced lupus associated with other drugs. The lupus erythematosus-like syndrome is not associated with hypocomplementemia and may be present without nephropathy. The development of a positive ANA test does not mandate discontinuance of the drug; however, the physician should be alerted to the possibility that a lupus erythematosus-like syndrome may develop in the future.

Some patients may develop oral ulcerations which in some cases have the appearance of aphthous stomatitis. The stomatitis usually recurs on rechallenge but often clears on a lower dosage. Although rare, cheilosis, glossitis and gingivostomatitis have also been reported. These oral lesions are frequently dose-related and may preclude further increase in penicillamine dosage or require discontinuation of the drug.

Hypogeusia (a blunting or diminution in taste perception) has occurred in some patients. This may last two to three months or more and may develop into a total loss of taste; however, it is usually self-limited, despite continued penicillamine treatment. Such taste impairment is rare in patients with Wilson's disease.

Penicillamine should not be used in patients who are receiving concurrent gold therapy, antimalarial or cytotoxic drugs, oxyphenbutazone or phenylbutazone because these drugs are also associated with similar serious hematologic and/or renal adverse reactions. Patients who have had gold salt therapy discontinued due to a major toxic reaction may be at greater risk of serious side effects with penicillamine, but not necessarily of the same type. Patients who are allergic to penicillin may theoretically have cross-sensitivity to penicillamine. The possibility of reactions from contamination of penicillamine by trace amounts of penicillin has been precluded now that penicillamine is being produced synthetically rather than as a degradation product of penicillin.

Because of their dietary restrictions, patients with Wilson's disease and cystinuria should be given 25 mg/day of pyridoxine during therapy, since penicillamine increases the requirement for this vitamin. Patients also may receive benefit from a multivitamin preparation, although there is no evidence that deficiency of any vitamin other than pyridoxine is associated with penicillamine. In Wilson's disease, multivitamin preparations must be copper-free.

Rheumatoid arthritis patients whose nutrition is impaired should also be given a daily supplement of pyridoxine. Mineral supplements should not be given, since they may block the response to penicillamine.

Iron deficiency may develop, especially in children and in menstruating women. In Wilson's disease, this may be a result of adding the effects of the low copper diet, which is probably also low in iron, and the penicillamine to the effects of blood loss or growth. In cystinuria, a low methionine diet may contribute to iron deficiency, since it is necessarily low in protein. If necessary, iron may be given in short courses, but a period of two hours should elapse between administration of penicillamine and iron, since orally administered iron has been shown to reduce the effects of penicillamine.

Penicillamine causes an increase in the amount of soluble collagen. In the rat this results in inhibition of normal healing and also a decrease in tensile strength of intact skin. In man this may be the cause of increased skin friability at sites especially subject to pressure or trauma, such as shoulders, elbows, knees, toes, and buttocks. Extravasations of blood may occur and may appear as purpuric areas, with external bleeding if the skin is broken, or as vesicles containing dark blood. Neither type is progressive. There is no apparent association with bleeding elsewhere in the body and no associated coagulation defect has been found. Therapy with penicillamine may be continued in the presence of these lesions. They may disappear if dosage is reduced. Other reported effects probably due to the action of penicillamine on collagen are excessive wrinkling of the skin and development of small, white papules at venipuncture and surgical sites.

The effects of penicillamine on collagen and elastin make it advisable to consider a reduction in dosage to 250 mg/day when surgery is contemplated. Reinstitution of full therapy should be delayed until wound healing is complete.

Caution patients to report immediately any abrupt onset of pulmonary symptoms, such as exertional dyspnea, wheezing, or cough and have appropriate pulmonary function studies done to rule out obstructive bronchiolitis.

Carcinogenesis—Long-term animal carcinogenicity studies have not been done with penicillamine. There is a report that 5 of 10 autoimmune disease-prone NZB Hybrid mice developed lymphocytic leukemia after 6 months' intraperitoneal treatment with a dose of 400 mg/kg penicillamine 5 days per week.

Usage in Pregnancy—Penicillamine has been shown to be teratogenic in rats when given in doses several times higher than the highest dose recommended for human use. Skeletal defects, cleft palates and fetal toxicity (resorptions) have been reported.

Wilson's disease—There are no controlled studies in pregnant women with Wilson's disease, but experience does not include any positive evidence of adverse effects to the fetus. Reported experience* shows that continued treatment with penicillamine throughout pregnancy protects the mother against relapse of the Wilson's disease, and that discontinuation of penicillamine has deleterious effects on the mother. It indicates that the drug does not increase the risk of fetal abnormalities, but it does not exclude the possibility of infrequent or subtle damage to the fetus.

* Scheinberg, I. H., Sternlieb, I.: *N Engl J Med 293:* 1300–1302, Dec. 18, 1975.

If penicillamine is administered during pregnancy to patients with Wilson's disease, it is recommended that the daily dosage be limited to 1 g. If Caesarean section is planned, the daily dosage should be limited to 250 mg during the last six weeks of pregnancy and postoperatively until wound healing is complete.

Cystinuria—If possible, penicillamine should not be given during pregnancy to women with cystinuria. There is a report of a woman with cystinuria treated with 2 g/day of penicillamine during pregnancy who gave birth to a child with a generalized connective tissue defect that may have been caused by penicillamine. If stones continue to form in these patients, the benefits of therapy to the mother must be evaluated against the risk to the fetus.

Rheumatoid Arthritis—Penicillamine should not be administered to rheumatoid arthritis patients who are pregnant (see CONTRAINDICATIONS) and should be discontinued promptly in patients in whom pregnancy is suspected or diagnosed. Penicillamine should be used in women of childbearing potential only when the expected benefits outweigh possible hazards. Women of childbearing potential should be informed of the possible hazards of penicillamine to the developing fetus and should be advised to report promptly any missed menstrual periods or other indications of possible pregnancy.

There is a report that a woman with rheumatoid arthritis treated with less than 1 g/day of penicillamine during pregnancy gave birth (Caesarean delivery) to an infant with growth retardation, flattened face with broad nasal bridge, low set ears, short neck with loose skin folds, and unusually lax body skin.

Usage in Children—The efficacy of DEPEN in juvenile rheumatoid arthritis has not been established.

ADVERSE REACTIONS

Penicillamine is a drug with a high incidence of untoward reactions, some of which are potentially fatal. Therefore, it is mandatory that patients receiving penicillamine therapy remain under close medical supervision throughout the period of drug administration (see WARNINGS and PRECAUTIONS).

Reported incidences (%) for the most commonly occurring adverse reactions in rheumatoid arthritis patients are noted, based on 17 representative clinical trials reported in the literature (1270 patients).

Allergic—Generalized pruritus, early and late rashes (5%), pemphigoid-type reactions and drug eruptions which may be accompanied by fever, arthralgia or lymphadenopathy have occurred (see WARNINGS and PRECAUTIONS). Some patients may show a lupus erythematosus-like syndrome similar to drug induced lupus produced by other pharmacological agents (see PRECAUTIONS).

Urticaria and exfoliative dermatitis have occurred.

Thyroiditis has been reported but is extremely rare.

Some patients may develop a migratory polyarthralgia, often with objective synovitis (see DOSAGE AND ADMINISTRATION).

Gastrointestinal—Anorexia, epigastric pain, nausea, vomiting or occasional diarrhea may occur (17%).

Isolated cases of reactivated peptic ulcer have occurred, as have hepatic dysfunction, cholestatic jaundice and pancreatitis. There have been a few reports of increased serum alkaline phosphatase, lactic dehydrogenase, and positive cephalin flocculation and thymol turbidity tests.

Some patients may report a blunting, diminution or total loss of taste perception (12%) or may develop oral ulcerations. Although rare, cheilosis, glossitis and gingivostomatitis have been reported (see PRECAUTIONS).

Gastrointestinal side effects are usually reversible following cessation of therapy.

Hematological—Penicillamine can cause bone marrow depression (see WARNINGS). Leukopenia (2%) and thrombocytopenia (4%) have occurred. Fatalities have been reported as a result of thrombocytopenia, agranulocytosis and aplastic anemia.

Thrombotic thrombocytopenic purpura, hemolytic anemia, red cell aplasia, monocytosis, leukocytosis, eosinophilia and thrombocytosis have also been reported.

Renal—Patients on penicillamine therapy may develop proteinuria (6%) and/or hematuria which, in some, may progress to the development of the nephrotic syndrome as a result of an immune complex membranous glomerulopathy (see WARNINGS)

Central Nervous System—Tinnitus has been reported. Reversible optic neuritis has been reported with the administration of penicillamine and may be related to pyridoxine deficiency.

Neuromuscular—Myasthenia gravis (see WARNINGS).

Other—Adverse reactions that have been reported rarely include thrombophlebitis; hyperpyrexia (see PRECAUTIONS); falling hair or alopecia; polymyositis; dermatomyositis; mammary hyperplasia; elastosis perforans serpiginosa; toxic epidermal necrolysis; anetoderma (cutaneous macular atrophy); Goodpasture's syndrome, a severe and ultimately fatal glomerulonephritis associated with intra-alveolar hemorrhage (see WARNINGS); and fatal renal vasculitis. Allergic alveolitis and obliterative bronchiolitis have been reported in patients with severe rheumatoid arthritis, some of whom were receiving penicillamine (see PRECAUTIONS).

Increased skin friability, excessive wrinkling of skin, and development of small, white papules at venipuncture and surgical sites have been reported (See PRECAUTIONS).

The chelating action of the drug may cause increased excretion of other heavy metals such as zinc, mercury and lead.

There have been reports associating penicillamine with leukemia. However, circumstances involved in these reports are such that a cause and effect relationship to the drug has not been established.

DOSAGE AND ADMINISTRATION

Wilson's Disease—DEPEN tablets should be given on an empty stomach, four times a day; one-half to one hour before meals and at bedtime—at least two hours after the evening meal.

Optimal dosage can be determined only by measurement of urinary copper excretion. The urine must be collected in copper-free glassware, and should be quantitatively analyzed for copper before and soon after initiation of therapy with DEPEN. Continued therapy should be monitored by doing a 24-hour urinary copper analysis every three months or so for the duration of therapy. Since a low copper diet should keep copper absorption down to less than one milligram a day, the patient probably will be in negative copper balance if 0.5 to one milligram of copper is present in a 24-hour collection of urine.

To achieve this, the suggested initial dosage of DEPEN in the treatment of Wilson's disease is 1 g/day for children or adults. This may be increased, as indicated by the urinary copper analyses, but it is seldom necessary to exceed a dosage of 2 g/day.

In patients who cannot tolerate as much as 1 g/day initially, initiating dosage with 250 mg/day, and increasing gradually to the requisite amount, gives closer control of the effects of the drug and may help to reduce the incidence of adverse reactions.

Cystinuria—It is recommended that DEPEN be used along with conventional therapy. By reducing urinary cystine, it decreases crystalluria and stone formation. In some instances, it has been reported to decrease the size of, and even to dissolve, stones already formed.

The usual dosage of DEPEN in the treatment of cystinuria is 2 g/day for adults; with a range of 1 to 4 g/day. For children, dosage can be based on 30 mg/kg/day. The total daily amount should be divided into four doses. If four equal doses are not feasible, give the larger portion at bedtime. If adverse reactions necessitate a reduction in dosage, it is important to retain the bedtime dose.

Initiating dosage with 250 mg/day, and increasing gradually to the requisite amount, gives closer control of the effects of the drug and may help to reduce the incidence of adverse reactions.

In addition to taking DEPEN, patients should drink copiously. It is especially important to drink about a pint of fluid at bedtime and another pint once during the night when urine is more concentrated and more acid than during the day. The greater the fluid intake, the lower the required dosage of DEPEN.

Dosage must be individualized to an amount that limits cystine excretion to 100–200 mg/day in those with no history of stones, and below 100 mg/day in those who have had stone formation and/or pain. Thus, in determining dosage, the inherent tubular defect, the patient's size, age, and rate of growth, and his diet and water intake all must be taken into consideration.

The standard nitroprusside cyanide test has been reported useful as a qualitative measure of the effective dose*: Add 2 ml of freshly prepared 5 percent sodium cyanide to 5 ml of a 24-hour aliquot of protein-free urine and let stand ten minutes. Add 5 drops of freshly prepared 5 percent sodium nitroprusside and mix. Cystine will turn the mixture magenta. If the result is negative, it can be assumed that cystine excretion is less than 100 mg/g creatinine.

* Lotz, M., Potts, J. T. and Bartter, F. C.: *Brit Med J 2*:521, Aug. 28, 1965 (in Medical Memoranda).

Although penicillamine is rarely excreted unchanged, it also will turn the mixture magenta. If there is any question as to which substance is causing the reaction, a ferric chloride test can be done to eliminate doubt: Add 3 percent ferric chloride dropwise to the urine. Penicillamine will turn the urine an immediate and quickly fading blue. Cystine will not produce any change in appearance.

Rheumatoid Arthritis—The principal rule of treatment with DEPEN in rheumatoid arthritis is patience. The onset of therapeutic response is typically delayed. Two or three months may be required before the first evidence of a clinical response is noted (see CLINICAL PHARMACOLOGY).

When treatment with DEPEN has been interrupted because of adverse reactions or other reasons, the drug should be reintroduced cautiously by starting with a lower dosage and increasing slowly.

Initial Therapy—

The currently recommended dosage regimen in rheumatoid arthritis begins with a single daily dose of 125 mg or 250 mg which is thereafter increased at one to three month intervals, by 125 mg or 250 mg/day, as patient response and tolerance indicate. If a satisfactory remission of symptoms is achieved, the dose associated with the remission should be continued (see **Maintenance Therapy**). If there is no improvement and there are no signs of potentially serious toxicity after two to three months of treatment with doses of 500–750 mg/day, increases of 250 mg/day at two to three month intervals may be continued until a satisfactory remission occurs (see **Maintenance Therapy**) or signs of toxicity develop (see WARNINGS and PRECAUTIONS). If there is no discernible improvement after three to four months of treatment with 1000 to 1500 mg penicillamine/day, it may be assumed the patient will not respond and DEPEN should be discontinued.

It is important that DEPEN be given on an empty stomach at least one hour before meals and at least one hour apart from any other drug, food or milk (see CLINICAL PHARMACOLOGY).

Maintenance Therapy—

The maintenance dosage of DEPEN must be individualized, and may require adjustment during the course of treatment. Many patients respond satisfactorily to a dosage within the 500–750 mg/day range. Some need less.

Changes in maintenance dosage levels may not be reflected clinically or in the erythrocyte sedimentation rate for two to three months after each dosage adjustment.

Some patients will subsequently require an increase in the maintenace dosage to achieve maximal disease suppression. In those patients who do respond, but who evidence incomplete suppression of their disease after the first six to nine months of treatment, the daily dosage of DEPEN may be increased by 125 mg or 250 mg/day at three-month intervals. It is unusual in current practice to employ a dosage in excess of 1 g/day, but up to 1.5 g/day has sometimes been required.

Management of Exacerbations—

During the course of treatment some patients may experience an exacerbation of disease activity following an initial good response. These may be self-limited and can subside within twelve weeks. They are usually controlled by the addition of nonsteroidal anti-inflammatory drugs, and only if the patient has demonstrated a true "escape" phenomenon (as evidenced by failure of the flare to subside within this time period) should an increase in the maintenance dose ordinarily be considered.

In the rheumatoid patient, migratory polyarthralgia due to penicillamine is extremely difficult to differentiate from an exacerbation of the rheumatoid arthritis. Discontinuance or a substantial reduction in the dosage of DEPEN for up to several weeks will usually determine which of these processes is responsible for the arthralgia.

Duration of Therapy—

The optimum duration of DEPEN therapy in rheumatoid arthritis has not been determined. If the patient has been in remission for six months or more, a gradual, stepwise dosage reduction in decrements of 125 mg or 250 mg/day at approximately three month intervals may be attempted.

Concomitant Drug Therapy—

DEPEN should not be used in patients who are receiving gold therapy, antimalarial or cytotoxic drugs, oxyphenbutazone or phenylbutazone (see PRECAUTIONS). Other measures, such as salicylates, other nonsteroidal anti-inflammatory drugs or systemic corticosteroids may be continued when DEPEN is initiated. After improvement commences, analgesic and anti-inflammatory drugs may be slowly discontinued as symptoms permit. Steroid withdrawal must be done gradually, and many months of DEPEN treatment may be required before steroids can be completely eliminated.

Continued on next page

Wallace—Cont.

Dosage Frequency—
Based on clinical experience, dosages up to 500 mg/day can be given as a single daily dose. Dosages in excess of 500 mg/day should be administered in divided doses.

HOW SUPPLIED

DEPEN® Titratable Tablets: 250 mg scored, oval, white tablets imprinted in red with 37-4401; available in bottles of 100 (NDC 0037-4401-01).

Manufactured under license from
HOMBURG (Degussa), West Germany.

Rev. 5/85

DEPROL® Ⓒ℞

(meprobamate 400 mg + benactyzine hydrochloride 1 mg)

DESCRIPTION

'Deprol' is available as light pink, scored tablets, each containing meprobamate, U.S.P., 400 mg and benactyzine hydrochloride 1 mg.
Other ingredients: alginic acid, D&C Red #30, FD&C Yellow #5, purified stearic acid, starch, talc.

ACTIONS

'Deprol'* (meprobamate + benactyzine hydrochloride) combines the tranquilizing action of meprobamate with the antidepressant action of benactyzine hydrochloride.

* U.S. Patent No. 3,090,726 covers the ingredients combination.

Benactyzine hydrochloride
Benactyzine hydrochloride is a mild antidepressant and anticholinergic agent which in animals has been shown to reduce the autonomic response to emotion-provoking stress.

Meprobamate
Meprobamate is a carbamate derivative which has been shown in animal studies to have effects at multiple sites in the central nervous system, including the thalamus and limbic system.

INDICATIONS

Based on a review of this drug by the National Academy of Sciences—National Research Council and/or other information, FDA has classified the indication as follows:
"Possibly" effective: in the management of depression, both acute (reactive) and chronic. It is particularly useful in the less severe depressions and where the depression is accompanied by anxiety, insomnia, agitation, or rumination. It is also useful for management of depression and associated anxiety accompanying or related to organic illnesses. Final classification of this indication requires further investigation.

CONTRAINDICATIONS

Benactyzine hydrochloride
Glaucoma and allergic or idiosyncratic reactions to benactyzine hydrochloride or related compounds.

Meprobamate
Acute intermittent porphyria as well as allergic or idiosyncratic reactions to meprobamate or related compounds such as carisoprodol, mebutamate, tybamate, or carbromal.

WARNINGS

The following information on meprobamate pertains to 'Deprol' (meprobamate + benactyzine hydrochloride):

Meprobamate
Drug Dependence—Physical dependence, psychological dependence, and abuse have occurred. When chronic intoxication from prolonged use occurs, it usually involves ingestion of greater than recommended doses and is manifested by ataxia, slurred speech, and vertigo. Therefore, careful supervision of dose and amounts prescribed is advised, as well as avoidance of prolonged administration, especially for alcoholics and other patients with a known propensity for taking excessive quantities of drugs.
Sudden withdrawal of the drug after prolonged and excessive use may precipitate recurrence of pre-existing symptoms, such as anxiety, anorexia, or insomnia, or withdrawal reactions, such as vomiting, ataxia, tremors, muscle twitching, confusional states, hallucinosis, and, rarely, convulsive seizures. Such seizures are more likely to occur in persons with central nervous system damage or pre-existent or latent convulsive disorders. Onset of withdrawal symptoms occurs usually within 12 to 48 hours after discontinuation of meprobamate; symptoms usually cease within the next 12 to 48 hours.
When excessive dosage has continued for weeks or months, dosage should be reduced gradually over a period of one or two weeks rather than abruptly stopped. Alternatively, a short-acting barbiturate may be substituted, then gradually withdrawn.

Potentially Hazardous Tasks—Patients should be warned that this drug may impair the mental and/or physical abilities required for the performance of potentially hazardous tasks such as driving a motor vehicle or operating machinery.

Additive Effects—Since the effects of meprobamate and alcohol or meprobamate and other CNS depressants or psychotropic drugs may be additive, appropriate caution should be exercised with patients who take more than one of these agents simultaneously.

Usage in Pregnancy and Lactation
An increased risk of congenital malformations associated with the use of minor tranquilizers (meprobamate, chlordiazepoxide, and diazepam) during the first trimester of pregnancy has been suggested in several studies. Because use of these drugs is rarely a matter of urgency, their use during this period should almost always be avoided. The possibility that a woman of childbearing potential may be pregnant at the time of institution of therapy should be considered. Patients should be advised that if they become pregnant during therapy or intend to become pregnant they should communicate with their physicians about the desirability of discontinuing the drug.
Meprobamate passes the placental barrier. It is present both in umbilical cord blood at or near maternal plasma levels and in breast milk of lactating mothers at concentrations two to four times that of maternal plasma. When use of meprobamate is contemplated in breast-feeding patients, the drug's higher concentrations in breast milk as compared to maternal plasma levels should be considered.

Usage in Children—This combination is not intended for use in children.

PRECAUTIONS

Meprobamate—The lowest effective dose should be administered, particularly to elderly and/or debilitated patients, in order to preclude oversedation.
The possibility of suicide attempts should be considered and the least amount of drug feasible should be dispensed at any one time.
Meprobamate is metabolized in the liver and excreted by the kidney; to avoid its excess accumulation, caution should be exercised in administration to patients with compromised liver or kidney function.
Meprobamate occasionally may precipitate seizures in epileptic patients.
This product contains FD&C Yellow No. 5 (tartrazine) which may cause allergic-type reactions (including bronchial asthma) in certain susceptible individuals. Although the overall incidence of FD&C Yellow No. 5 (tartrazine) sensitivity in the general population is low, it is frequently seen in patients who also have aspirin hypersensitivity.

ADVERSE REACTIONS

Side effects have included nausea, dryness of mouth, and other gastrointestinal symptoms; syncope; and one case each of severe nervousness and loss of power of concentration.
The following side effects, which have occurred after administration of its components alone, have either occurred or might occur when the combination is taken.

Benactyzine Hydrochloride
Benactyzine hydrochloride alone, particularly in high dosage, may produce dizziness, thought-blocking, a sense of depersonalization, aggravation of anxiety, or disturbance of sleep patterns, and a subjective feeling of muscle relaxation. There may also be anticholinergic effects such as blurred vision, dryness of mouth, or failure of visual accommodation. Other reported side effects have included gastric distress, allergic response, ataxia, and euphoria.

Meprobamate
Central Nervous System—Drowsiness, ataxia, dizziness, slurred speech, headache, vertigo, weakness, paresthesias, impairment of visual accommodation, euphoria, overstimulation, paradoxical excitement, fast EEG activity.
Gastrointestinal—Nausea, vomiting, diarrhea.
Cardiovascular—Palpitations, tachycardia, various forms of arrhythmia, transient ECG changes, syncope; also, hypotensive crises (including one fatal case).
Allergic or Idiosyncratic—Allergic or idiosyncratic reactions are usually seen within the period of the first to fourth dose in patients having had no previous contact with the drug. Milder reactions are characterized by an itchy, urticarial, or erythematous maculopapular rash which may be generalized or confined to the groin. Other reactions have included leukopenia, acute nonthrombocytopenic purpura, petechiae, ecchymoses, eosinophilia, peripheral edema, adenopathy, fever, fixed drug eruption with cross reaction to carisoprodol, and cross sensitivity between meprobamate/mebutamate and meprobamate/carbromal.
More severe hypersensitivity reactions, rarely reported, include hyperpyrexia, chills, angioneurotic edema, bronchospasm, oliguria, and anuria. Also, anaphylaxis, erythema multiforme, exfoliative dermatitis, stomatitis, proctitis, Stevens-Johnson syndrome, and bullous dermatitis, including one fatal case of the latter following administration of meprobamate in combination with prednisolone.
In case of allergic or idiosyncratic reactions to meprobamate, discontinue the drug and initiate appropriate symptomatic therapy, which may include epinephrine, antihistamines, and in severe cases corticosteroids. In evaluating possible allergic reactions, also consider allergy to excipients (information on excipients is available to physicians on request).
Hematologic (See also **Allergic or Idiosyncratic.**)—Agranulocytosis and aplastic anemia have been reported, although no causal relationship has been established. These cases rarely were fatal. Rare cases of thrombocytopenic purpura have been reported.
Other—Exacerbation of porphyric symptoms.

DOSAGE AND ADMINISTRATION

The usual adult starting dosage of 'Deprol' (meprobamate + benactyzine hydrochloride) is one tablet three or four times daily, which may be increased gradually to six tablets daily and gradually reduced to maintenance levels upon establishment of relief. Doses above six tablets daily are not recommended, even though higher doses have been used by some clinicians to control depression, and in chronic psychotic patients.

OVERDOSAGE

Overdosage of 'Deprol' (meprobamate + benactyzine hydrochloride) has not differed substantially from meprobamate overdosage:

Meprobamate
Suicidal attempts with meprobamate have resulted in drowsiness, lethargy, stupor, ataxia, coma, shock, vasomotor and respiratory collapse. Some suicidal attempts have been fatal.
The following data on meprobamate tablets have been reported in the literature and from other sources. These data are not expected to correlate with each case (considering factors such as individual susceptibility and length of time from ingestion to treatment), but represent the *usual ranges* reported.
Acute simple overdose (meprobamate alone): Death has been reported with ingestion of as little as 12 gm meprobamate and survival with as much as 40 gm.

Blood Levels:
0.5–2.0 mg% represents the usual blood level range of meprobamate after therapeutic doses. The level may occasionally be as high as 3.0 mg%.
3–10 mg% usually corresponds to findings of mild to moderate symptoms of overdosage, such as stupor or light coma.
10–20 mg% usually corresponds to deeper coma, requiring more intensive treatment. Some fatalities occur.
At levels greater than 20 mg%, more fatalities than survivals can be expected.

Acute combined overdose (meprobamate with alcohol or other CNS depressants or psychotropic drugs): Since effects can be additive, a history of ingestion of a low dose of meprobamate plus any of these compounds (or of a relatively low blood or tissue level) cannot be used as a prognostic indicator.
In cases where excessive doses have been taken, sleep ensues rapidly and blood pressure, pulse, and respiratory rates are reduced to basal levels. Any drug remaining in the stomach should be removed and symptomatic therapy given. Should respiration or blood pressure become compromised, respiratory assistance, central nervous system stimulants, and pressor agents should be administered cautiously as indicated. Meprobamate is metabolized in the liver and excreted by the kidney. Diuresis, osmotic (mannitol) diuresis, peritoneal dialysis, and hemodialysis have been used successfully. Careful monitoring of urinary output is necessary and caution should be taken to avoid overhydration. Relapse and death, after initial recovery, have been attributed to incomplete gastric emptying and delayed absorption. Meprobamate can be measured in biological fluids by two methods: colorimetric (Hoffman, A.J. and Ludwig, B.J.: *J Amer Pharm Assn 48:* 740, 1959) and gas chromatographic (Douglas, J.F. et al: *Anal Chem 39:* 956, 1967).

HOW SUPPLIED

Bottles of 100 (NDC 0037-3001-01). Bottles of 500 (NDC 0037-3001-03).

WALLACE LABORATORIES
Division of
CARTER-WALLACE, INC.
Cranbury, New Jersey 08512

Rev. 3/85

DIUTENSEN® ℞

Tablets

DESCRIPTION

DIUTENSEN® is a round, white-blue mottled tablet. Each tablet contains:

Cryptenamine (as tannate salts)	2 mg†
Methyclothiazide	2.5 mg

† Equivalent to 260 Carotid Sinus Reflex Units.

ACTIONS

Cryptenamine is an alkaloidal fraction obtained from *Veratrum viride* by a nonaqueous extraction procedure. The antihypertensive response to cryptenamine is widely documented. The principal mechanism of action of the drug in reducing the blood pressure involves widespread arteriolar dilatation mediated centrally, without peripheral adrenergic or ganglionic blockade. The major cardiovascular effects are reflex in nature and are mainly due to stimulation of afferent pressor receptors predominantly in the heart and carotid sinus area. These receptors initiate an increase in impulses which are interpreted by areas in the brain stem as denoting a pressure higher than that actually present. As a result, the mechanism concerned with blood pressure homeostasis is activated, sympathetic tone is decreased, vagal tone is increased, and the blood pressure is therefore reduced. Both systolic and diastolic pressure are decreased and the heart is slowed. Atropine abolishes the bradycrotic effect but only partially reverses the hypotensive effect.

Methyclothiazide is a synthetic saluretic-antihypertensive agent. It is a potent analogue of hydrochlorothiazide, being about 20 times as active, by weight, as the latter compound. The renal mechanism involved in the diuretic action of methyclothiazide is indistinguishable from that elicited by chlorothiazide or hydrochlorothiazide, but the duration of action of methyclothiazide is longer than that of either of these compounds. The principal mechanism of action of methyclothiazide is the production of diuresis by inhibition of renal tubular reabsorption of electrolytes, resulting in a marked increase in the urinary excretion of sodium, chloride, and water, and moderate increase in the excretion of potassium and bicarbonate.

INDICATIONS

Based on a review of this drug by the National Academy of Sciences—National Research Council and/or other information, FDA has classified the indications as follows:

Lacking substantial evidence of effectiveness as a fixed combination for use in basic hypertensive therapy and for essential hypertension of all grades of severity. (See box warning.)

Final classification of the less-than-effective indications requires further investigation.

CONTRAINDICATIONS

DIUTENSEN is contraindicated for patients with known idiosyncrasy to *Veratrum viride* or thiazide compounds and for those who have recently experienced either coronary artery occlusion or cerebral thrombosis. Treatment with thiazide diuretics (including methyclothiazide) is also contraindicated for patients with severe renal or hepatic disease.

WARNING

THIS FIXED COMBINATION DRUG IS NOT INDICATED FOR INITIAL THERAPY OF HYPERTENSION. HYPERTENSION REQUIRES THERAPY TITRATED TO THE INDIVIDUAL PATIENT. IF THE FIXED COMBINATION REPRESENTS THE DOSAGE SO DETERMINED, ITS USE MAY BE MORE CONVENIENT IN PATIENT MANAGEMENT. THE TREATMENT OF HYPERTENSION IS NOT STATIC, BUT MUST BE RE-EVALUATED AS CONDITIONS IN EACH PATIENT WARRANT.

WARNINGS

There have been several reports, published and unpublished, concerning non-specific small bowel lesions consisting of stenosis with or without ulceration, associated with the administration of enteric-coated thiazides with potassium salts. These lesions may occur with enteric-coated potassium tablets alone or when they are used with non-enteric-coated thiazides, or certain other oral diuretics. These small bowel lesions have caused obstruction, hemorrhage, and perforation. Surgery was frequently required and deaths have occurred. Available information tends to implicate enteric-coated potassium salts although lesions of this type also occur spontaneously. Therefore, coated potassium-containing formulations should be administered only when indicated, and should be discontinued immediately if abdominal pain, distention, nausea, vomiting, or gastrointestinal bleeding occur. Coated potassium tablets should be used only when adequate dietary supplementation is not practical.

USE IN PREGNANCY: USE OF ANY DRUG IN PREGNANCY, LACTATION, OR IN WOMEN OF CHILDBEARING AGE REQUIRES THAT THE POTENTIAL BENEFITS OF THE DRUG SHOULD BE WEIGHED AGAINST THE POSSIBLE HAZARDS TO THE MOTHER AND CHILD. DIUTENSEN SHOULD BE USED WITH CARE IN PREGNANT AND NURSING MOTHERS SINCE THIAZIDES CROSS THE PLACENTAL BARRIER AND APPEAR IN CORD BLOOD AND BREAST MILK. THIAZIDES MAY RESULT IN FETAL OR NEONATAL JAUNDICE, THROMBOCYTOPENIA, AND POSSIBLY OTHER ADVERSE REACTIONS WHICH HAVE OCCURRED IN THE ADULT.

Thiazides potentiate the action of other antihypertensive drugs. Therefore the dosage of these agents, especially the ganglion blockers, must be reduced by at least 50 percent as soon as thiazides are added to the regimen.

Exacerbation or activation of systemic lupus erythematosus has been reported with sulfonamide derived drugs, including thiazides.

PRECAUTIONS

Cryptenamine is a potent hypotensive and occasionally bradycrotic drug. Overdosage may produce nausea and vomiting, excessive hypotension and prostration and, rarely, bronchoconstriction. If necessary, atropine sulfate (0.5 to 1.0 mg) may be administered to reverse the bradycrotic effect. In the event of excessive fall in blood pressure, administer vasopressor drugs, such as ephedrine sulfate (30 to 50 mg) or phenylephrine hydrochloride (5 mg) subcutaneously. If left untended, the reaction will gradually disappear within 60 to 90 minutes.

Particular caution is warranted when treating patients with angina pectoris, coronary thrombosis, or cerebrovascular disease. Caution should also be exercised when treating hypertensive patients with chronic renal disease, since they adjust poorly to lowered blood pressure.

Special caution is warranted when treating patients with histories of bronchial asthma who may respond adversely to the cholinergic effect of cryptenamine.

The bradycrotic effect of veratrum alkaloids is additive to, but not synergistic with, that produced by morphine and related drugs.

Methyclothiazide is a potent saluretic drug. After initiation of therapy, the patient should be seen regularly to determine his individual response to therapy. Ordinarily, a total daily dose of 10 mg (4 DIUTENSEN tablets daily), or less, is not accompanied by significant untoward reactions. However, certain patients may be unusually responsive to the saluretic effect of methyclothiazide and they may experience disturbances in electrolyte balance with subsequent development of hypokalemia. Serum electrolytes should be checked periodically during treatment, particularly in patients receiving relatively large doses of the drug. Patients who are receiving simultaneous treatment either with DIUTENSEN and digitalis or DIUTENSEN and potassium-depleting corticosteroids and those with impending hepatic coma should be carefully watched for signs and symptoms of disturbances in serum electrolyte balance. In the event evidence of electrolyte imbalance with hypokalemia is seen, it may be necessary to give supplemental potassium therapy in the form of fruit juices or direct potassium supplements of one gram, two to four times daily. In severe cases not responding to supplemental potassium therapy, it may be necessary to withdraw the drug.

Hypochloremic alkalosis occurs infrequently with methyclothiazide. Nevertheless, it is a possibility and if this condition develops, it may be treated by the addition of ammonium chloride to the dosage schedule. However, ammonium chloride should not be administered concurrently with a thiazide compound to patients with liver disease because each may cause an elevation in serum ammonia and precipitate onset of coma.

Some elevation of the blood urea nitrogen has been noted occasionally in patients receiving methyclothiazide. This reaction occurs more frequently in patients with decreased renal function. If serum nitrogen (BUN, NPN, creatinine) increases progressively, thiazide therapy should be discontinued.

As with other thiazide diuretics, hyperglycemia has been noted during treatment with methyclothiazide. If a significant elevation in blood sugar is noted, the drug should be withdrawn.

As with thiazides in general, serum uric acid has been observed to rise in a few patients treated with methyclothiazide, with overt symptoms of gout appearing in some of these. Symptoms of gout are readily controlled by treatment with colchicine.

Because some patients receiving veratrum alkaloids have experienced marked hypotension when undergoing surgical procedures, it may be advisable to discontinue treatment with DIUTENSEN for a period of approximately two weeks prior to elective surgery. Thiazide drugs may increase the responsiveness of patients to tubocurarine. Thiazides may decrease arterial responsiveness to norepinephrine and therefore should be withdrawn 48 hours before elective surgery. If emergency surgery is indicated, preanesthetic and anesthetic agents should be administered in reduced dosage. Emergency surgery may be carried out with the use, if necessary, of anticholinergic or adrenergic drugs to prevent vagal circulatory responses and of other supportive measures, as indicated.

Thiazides may decrease serum protein bound iodine levels without signs of thyroid disturbance.

The antihypertensive effects of these drugs may be enhanced in the post-sympathectomy patient.

The concurrent use of DIUTENSEN with digitalis may increase the possibility of digitalis intoxication (due chiefly to the saluretic effects of methyclothiazide and perhaps to the vagotonic effects of cryptenamine). If there is evidence of myocardial irritability (extrasystoles, bigeminy, or AV block) dosage of DIUTENSEN should be reduced or discontinued.

ADVERSE REACTIONS

Thiazides—Varied reactions have been noted in patients treated with thiazides as follows:

Gastrointestinal: Anorexia, gastric irritation, nausea, vomiting, cramping, diarrhea, constipation, jaundice (intrahepatic cholestatic) and pancreatitis.

Central nervous system: Vertigo, paresthesia, headache and xanthopsia.

Dermatologic-hypersensitivity: Skin rash, photosensitivity, urticaria and cutaneous vasculitis.

Hematologic: Purpura, thrombocytopenia, leukopenia, agranulocytosis and aplastic anemia.

In addition, orthostatic hypotension (aggravated when thiazides were administered in combination with either alcohol, barbiturates or narcotics), hyperglycemia, glycosuria, muscle cramps, dizziness, weakness, and restlessness have been reported.

Cryptenamine—Patients treated with cryptenamine have experienced a variety of reactions as follows: excessive hypotension, prostration, anorexia, nausea and vomiting, epigastric and substernal burning, which may be mistaken for angina pectoris, unpleasant taste, salivation, sweating, hiccough, blurring of vision, mental confusion, cardiac arrhythmias, bradycardia, and, with excessive doses, bronchiolar construction and respiratory depression.

When adverse reactions occur during treatment with DIUTENSEN, they are usually reversible and disappear when treatment is discontinued.

DOSAGE AND ADMINISTRATION

As determined by individual titration (see box warning). The usual adult dosage of DIUTENSEN is one to four tablets a day depending on the individual patient response.

HOW SUPPLIED

NDC 0037-0272-92, bottle of 100.
NDC 0037-0272-96, bottle of 500.

CAUTION: Federal law prohibits dispensing without prescription.

WALLACE LABORATORIES
Division of
CARTER-WALLACE, INC.
Cranbury, New Jersey 08512

Rev. 1/84

Shown in Product Identification Section, page 434

DIUTENSEN®-R ℞
Tablets

WARNING

THIS FIXED COMBINATION DRUG IS NOT INDICATED FOR INITIAL THERAPY OF HYPERTENSION. HYPERTENSION REQUIRES THERAPY TITRATED TO THE INDIVIDUAL PATIENT. IF THE FIXED COMBINATION REPRESENTS THE DOSAGE SO DETERMINED, ITS USE MAY BE MORE CONVENIENT IN PATIENT MANAGEMENT. THE TREATMENT OF HYPERTENSION IS NOT STATIC, BUT MUST BE RE-EVALUATED AS CONDITIONS IN EACH PATIENT WARRANT.

DESCRIPTION

DIUTENSEN®-R is a two-component system of active ingredients containing 2.5 mg. methyclothiazide and 0.1 mg. reserpine per tablet. DIUTENSEN-R thus provides for easier titration of hypertensive patients than does a three-component system. DIUTENSEN-R tablets are round, white, pink-mottled tablets. NOTE: DIUTENSEN-R previously contained cryptenamine tannate as a third antihypertensive agent.

ACTIONS

Methyclothiazide—The predominant effects of methyclothiazide are diuresis, natriuresis, and chloruresis. The mechanism of action results in an interference with the renal tubular mechanism of electrolyte reabsorption. There is significant natriuresis and diuresis within two hours after administration of a single dose of methyclothiazide. These effects reach a peak in about six hours and persist for 24 hours following oral administration of a single dose.

Continued on next page

Wallace—Cont.

In nonedematous patients the "peak" (maximum effective) natriuretic single dose of methyclothiazide is 10 mg., whereas the peak kaliuretic dose is 5 mg. Thus, doubling a daily dose of 5 mg. results in an increase of sodium output without significantly increasing potassium excretion.
Like other benzothiadiazines, methyclothiazide also has antihypertensive properties. It also may be used to enhance the antihypertensive action of other drugs. The mechanism by which benzothiadiazines, including methyclothiazide, produce a reduction of elevated blood pressure has not been definitely established. Sodium depletion, however, appears to be of primary importance.
Methyclothiazide is readily absorbed from the gastrointestinal tract and is excreted unchanged by the kidneys.
Reserpine—Reserpine is a pure crystalline alkaloid from the root of *Rauwolfia serpentina.* The drug has mild antihypertensive and bradycrotic effects in addition to sedative and tranquilizing properties.
Reserpine probably produces its antihypertensive effects through depletion of tissue stores of catecholamines (epinephrine and norepinephrine) from peripheral sites. By contrast, its sedative and tranquilizing properties are thought to be due to a depletion of 5-hydroxytryptamine from the brain.
Reserpine is characterized by slow onset of action and sustained effect. Both its cardiovascular and central nervous system effects may persist following withdrawal of the drug.

INDICATIONS

Hypertension (see box warning).

CONTRAINDICATIONS

Methyclothiazide—This compound should not be used in anuric patients or those who exhibit a hypersensitivity to this or other sulfonamide derived drugs.
Reserpine—Reserpine is contraindicated in patients with known hypersensitivity, mental depression, especially with suicidal tendencies, active peptic ulcer, and ulcerative colitis. It is also contraindicated in patients receiving electroconvulsive therapy.

WARNINGS

Methyclothiazide—Thiazides should be used with caution in severe renal disease. In patients with renal disease, thiazides may precipitate azotemia. Cumulative effects of the drug may develop in patients with impaired renal function.
Thiazides should be used with caution in patients with impaired hepatic function or progressive liver disease, since minor alterations of fluid and electrolyte balance may precipitate hepatic coma.
Thiazides may be additive or potentiate the action of other antihypertensive drugs. Potentiation occurs with ganglionic or peripheral adrenergic blocking drugs.
Sensitivity reactions may occur in patients with a history of allergy or bronchial asthma. The possibility of exacerbation or activation of systemic lupus erythematosus has been reported.
Reserpine—Extreme caution should be exercised in treating patients with a history of mental depression. Discontinue the drug at the first sign of despondency, early morning insomnia, loss of appetite, impotence, or self-deprecation. Drug-induced depression may persist for several months after drug withdrawal and may be severe enough to result in suicide.
Electroshock therapy should not be given to patients under treatment with reserpine since severe and even fatal reactions to such therapy have been reported in patients receiving reserpine. Reserpine should be discontinued for two weeks before electroshock therapy is given.
Use in Pregnancy: USE OF ANY DRUG IN PREGNANCY, LACTATION, OR IN WOMEN OF CHILDBEARING AGE REQUIRES THAT THE POTENTIAL BENEFITS OF THE DRUG SHOULD BE WEIGHED AGAINST THE POSSIBLE HAZARDS TO THE MOTHER AND CHILD. DIUTENSEN-R SHOULD BE USED WITH CARE IN PREGNANT AND NURSING MOTHERS SINCE METHYCLOTHIAZIDE AND RESERPINE CROSS THE PLACENTAL BARRIER AND APPEAR IN CORD BLOOD AND BREAST MILK.
THE SAFETY OF RESERPINE FOR USE DURING PREGNANCY OR LACTATION HAS NOT BEEN ESTABLISHED. INCREASED RESPIRATORY SECRETIONS, NASAL CONGESTION, CYANOSIS, AND ANOREXIA MAY OCCUR IN INFANTS BORN TO RESERPINE-TREATED MOTHERS.
THIAZIDES MAY RESULT IN FETAL OR NEONATAL JAUNDICE, THROMBOCYTOPENIA, AND POSSIBLE OTHER ADVERSE REACTIONS WHICH HAVE OCCURRED IN THE ADULT.

PRECAUTIONS

Methyclothiazide—Periodic determinations of serum electrolytes to detect possible electrolyte imbalance should be performed at appropriate intervals.
All patients receiving thiazide therapy should be observed for clinical signs of fluid or electrolyte imbalance; namely, hyponatremia, hypochloremic alkalosis, and hypokalemia. Serum and urine electrolyte determinations are particularly important when the patient is vomiting excessively or receiving parenteral fluids. Medication such as digitalis may also influence serum electrolytes. Warning signs, irrespective of cause, are: Dryness of mouth, thirst, weakness, lethargy, drowsiness, restlessness, muscle pains or cramps, muscular fatigue, hypotension, oliguria, tachycardia, and gastrointestinal disturbances such as nausea and vomiting.
Hypokalemia may develop with thiazides as with any other potent diuretic, especially with brisk diuresis, when severe cirrhosis is present, or during concomitant use of corticosteroids or ACTH.
Interference with adequate oral electrolyte intake will also contribute to hypokalemia. Digitalis therapy may exaggerate metabolic effects of hypokalemia especially with reference to myocardial activity.
Any chloride deficit is generally mild and usually does not require specific treatment except under extraordinary circumstances (as in liver disease or renal disease). Dilutional hyponatremia may occur in edematous patients in hot weather; appropriate therapy is water restriction, rather than administration of salt except in rare instances when the hyponatremia is life threatening. In actual salt depletion, appropriate replacement is the therapy of choice.
Hyperuricemia may occur or frank gout may be precipitated in certain patients receiving thiazide therapy.
Insulin requirements in diabetic patients may be increased, decreased, or unchanged. Latent diabetes mellitus may become manifest during thiazide administration.
Thiazide drugs may increase the responsiveness of tubocurarine.
The antihypertensive effects of the drug may be enhanced in the postsympathectomy patient.
Thiazides may decrease arterial responsiveness to norepinephrine. This diminution is not sufficient to preclude effectiveness of the pressor agent for therapeutic use.
If progressive renal impairment becomes evident, as indicated by a rising non-protein nitrogen or blood urea nitrogen, a careful reappraisal of therapy is necessary with consideration given to withholding or discontinuing diuretic therapy.
Thiazides may decrease serum PBI levels without signs of thyroid disturbance.
Reserpine—Because reserpine preparations increase gastrointestinal motility and secretion, this drug should be used cautiously in patients with a history of peptic ulcer, ulcerative colitis, or gallstones, where biliary colic may be precipitated.
Caution should be exercised when treating hypertensive patients with renal insufficiency since they adjust poorly to lowered blood pressure levels.
Use reserpine cautiously with digitalis and quinidine since cardiac arrhythmias have occurred with the concurrent use of rauwolfia preparations.
Preoperative withdrawal of reserpine does not assure that circulatory instability will not occur. It is important that the anesthesiologist be aware of the patient's drug intake and consider this in the overall management, since hypotension has occurred in patients receiving rauwolfia preparations.
Anticholinergic and/or adrenergic drugs (metaraminol, norepinephrine) have been employed to treat adverse vagocirculatory effects.
Animal tumorigenicity: Rodent studies have shown that reserpine is an animal turmorigen, causing an increased incidence of mammary fibroadenomas in female mice, malignant tumors of the seminal vesicles in male mice, and malignant adrenal medullary tumors in male rats. These findings arose in 2 year studies in which the drug was administered in the feed at concentrations of 5 and 10 ppm—about 100 to 300 times the usual human dose. The breast neoplasms are thought to be related to reserpine's prolactin-elevating effect. Several other prolactin-elevating drugs have also been associated with an increased incidence of mammary neoplasia in rodents.
The extent to which these findings indicate a risk to humans is uncertain. Tissue culture experiments show that about one-third of human breast tumors are prolactin-dependent in vitro, a factor of considerable importance if the use of the drug is contemplated in a patient with previously detected breast cancer. The possibility of an increased risk of breast cancer in reserpine users has been studied extensively; however, no firm conclusion has emerged. Although a few epidemiologic studies have suggested a slightly increased risk (less than twofold in all studies except one) in women who have used reserpine, other studies of generally similar design have not confirmed this. Epidemiologic studies conducted using other drugs (neuroleptic agents) that, like reserpine, increase prolactin levels and therefore would be considered rodent mammary carcinogens, have not shown an association between chronic administration of the drug and human mammary tumorigenesis. While long-term clinical observation has not suggested such an association, the available evidence is considered too limited to be conclusive at this time. An association of reserpine intake with pheochromocytoma or tumors of the seminal vesicles has not been explored.

ADVERSE REACTIONS

Methyclothiazide—The following adverse reactions have been associated with the use of thiazide diuretics.
Gastrointestinal: Anorexia, gastric irritation, nausea, vomiting, cramping, diarrhea, constipation, jaundice (intrahepatic cholestatic jaundice), pancreatitis.
Central nervous system: Dizziness, vertigo, paresthesia, headache, xanthopsia.
Dermatologic-Hypersensitivity: Purpura, photosensitivity, rash, urticaria, necrotizing angiitis (vasculitis) (cutaneous vasculitis).
Hematologic: Leukopenia, agranulocytosis, thrombocytopenia, aplastic anemia.
Cardiovascular: Orthostatic hypotension may occur and may be aggravated by alcohol, barbiturates or narcotics.
Miscellaneous: Hyperglycemia, glycosuria, hyperuricemia, muscle spasm, weakness, restlessness.
Reserpine—Reserpine preparations have caused gastrointestinal reactions including hypersecretion, nausea and vomiting, anorexia, and diarrhea; cardiovascular reactions including angina-like symptoms, arrhythmias particularly when used concurrently with digitalis or quinidine, and bradycardia; and central nervous system reactions including drowsiness, depression, nervousness, paradoxical anxiety, nightmares, rare parkinsonian syndrome, CNS sensitization manifested by dull sensorium, deafness, glaucoma, uveitis, and optic atrophy. Nasal congestion is a frequent complaint, and pruritus, rash, dryness of mouth, dizziness, headache, dyspnea, purpura, impotence or decreased libido, dysuria, muscular aches, conjunctival injection, and weight gain have been reported. Extrapyramidal tract symptoms have also occurred. These reactions are usually reversible and disappear when the drug is discontinued.
Whenever DIUTENSEN-R therapy results in adverse reactions which are moderate or severe, dosage should be reduced or therapy withdrawn.

DOSAGE AND ADMINISTRATION

As determined by individual titration (see box warning). The usual adult dosage of DIUTENSEN-R is 1 to 4 tablets a day depending on the individual patient response.

HOW SUPPLIED

NDC 0037-0274-92, bottle of 100
NDC 0037-0274-96, bottle of 500

CAUTION

Federal law prohibits dispensing without prescription.

Rev. 5/83

Shown in Product Identification Section, page 434

LUFYLLIN® ℞

(dyphylline)
Elixir

DESCRIPTION

LUFYLLIN (dyphylline) Elixir is a bronchodilator available for oral administration as a clear red liquid. Each 15 ml (one tablespoonful) contains dyphylline, 100 mg, and alcohol, 20% (by volume).
Other ingredients: FD&C Blue No. 1, FD&C Red No. 40, saccharin sodium, white port wine.
Chemically, dyphylline is 7-(2,3-dihydroxypropyl)-theophylline, a white, extremely bitter, amorphous powder that is freely soluble in water and soluble in alcohol to the extent of 2 g/100 ml. Dyphylline forms a neutral solution that is stable in gastrointestinal fluids over a wide range of pH.
The molecular formula for dyphylline is $C_{10}H_{14}N_4O_4$ with a molecular weight of 254.25.

CLINICAL PHARMACOLOGY

Dyphylline is a xanthine derivative with pharmacologic actions similar to theophylline and other members of this class of drugs. Its primary action is that of bronchodilation, but it also exhibits peripheral vasodilatory and other smooth muscle relaxant activity to a lesser degree. The bronchodilatory action of dyphylline, as with other xanthines, is thought to be mediated through competitive inhibition of phosphodiesterase with a resulting increase in cyclic AMP producing relaxation of bronchial smooth muscle.
Dyphylline is well tolerated and produces less nausea than aminophylline and other alkaline theophylline compounds when administered orally. Unlike the hydrolyzable salts of theophylline, dyphylline is not converted to free theophylline *in vivo.* It is absorbed rapidly in therapeutically active form and in healthy volunteers reaches a mean peak plasma concentration of 17.1 mcg/ml in approximately 45 minutes following a single oral dose of 1000 mg.
Dyphylline exerts its bronchodilatory effects directly and, unlike theophylline, is excreted unchanged by the kidneys without being metabolized by the liver. Because of this, dyphylline pharmacokinetics and plasma levels are not influenced by various factors that affect liver function and hepatic enzyme activity, such as smoking, age, congestive heart

failure or concomitant use of drugs which effect liver function.

The elimination half-life of dyphylline is approximately two hours (1.8–2.1 hr) and approximately 88% of a single oral dose can be recovered from the urine unchanged. The renal clearance would be correspondingly reduced in patients with impaired renal function. In anuric patients, the half-life may be increased 3 to 4 times normal.

Dyphylline plasma levels are dose-related and generally predictable. The range of plasma levels within which dyphylline can be expected to produce effective bronchodilation has not been determined.

Dyphylline plasma concentrations can be accurately determined using high pressure liquid chromatography (HPLC)* or gas-liquid chromatography (GLC).

* *See* Valia, *et al, J Chromatogr 221*:170 (1980). Small quantities of pure dyphylline powder may be obtained from Wallace Laboratories, Cranbury, N.J. The internal standard, β-hydroxyethyltheophylline may be obtained from companies supplying analytic chemicals.

INDICATIONS AND USAGE

For relief of acute bronchial asthma and for reversible bronchospasm associated with chronic bronchitis and emphysema.

CONTRAINDICATIONS

Hypersensitivity to dyphylline or related xanthine compounds.

WARNINGS

LUFYLLIN Elixir is not indicated in the management of status asthmaticus which is a serious medical emergency.

Although the relationship between plasma levels of dyphylline and appearance of toxicity is unknown, excessive doses may be expected to be associated with an increased risk of adverse effects.

PRECAUTIONS

General: Use LUFYLLIN Elixir with caution in patients with severe cardiac disease, hypertension, hyperthyroidism, or acute myocardial injury or peptic ulcer.

Drug interactions: Synergism betwen xanthine bronchodilators (e.g., theophylline), ephedrine and other sympathomimetic bronchodilators has been reported. This should be considered whenever these agents are prescribed concomitantly. Concurrent administration of dyphylline and probenecid, which competes for tubular secretion, has been shown to increase the plasma half-life of dyphylline (see CLINICAL PHARMACOLOGY).

Carcinogenesis, mutagenesis, impairment of fertility: No long-term animal studies have been performed with LUFYLLIN Elixir.

Pregnancy: Teratogenic effects—Pregnancy category C. Animal reproduction studies have not been conducted with LUFYLLIN Elixir. It is also not known if 'Lufyllin' Elixir can cause fetal harm when administered to a pregnant woman or can affect reproduction capacity. LUFYLLIN Elixir should be given to a pregnant woman only if clearly needed.

Nursing mothers: Dyphylline is present in human milk at approximately twice the maternal plasma concentration. Caution should be exercised when 'Lufyllin' Elixir is administered to a nursing woman.

Pediatric use: Safety and effectiveness in children have not been established.

ADVERSE REACTIONS

Adverse reactions with the use of LUFYLLIN Elixir have been infrequent, relatively mild, and rarely required reduction in dosage or withdrawal of therapy.

The following adverse reactions which have been reported with other xanthine bronchodilators, and which have most often been related to excessive drug plasma levels, should be considered as potential adverse effects when dyphylline is administered:

Gastrointestinal: nausea, vomiting, epigastric pain, hematemesis, diarrhea.

Central nervous system: headache, irritability, restlessness, insomnia, hyperexcitability, agitation, muscle twitching, generalized clonic and tonic convulsions.

Cardiovascular: palpitation, tachycardia, extrasystoles, flushing, hypotension, circulatory failure, ventricular arrhythmias.

Respiratory: tachypnea.

Renal: albuminuria, gross and microscopic hematuria, diuresis.

Others: hyperglycemia, inappropriate ADH syndrome.

OVERDOSAGE

There have been no reports, in the literature, of overdosage with LUFYLLIN Elixir. However, the following information based on reports of theophylline overdosage are considered typical of the xanthine class of drugs and should be kept in mind.

Signs and symptoms: Restlessness, anorexia, nausea, vomiting, diarrhea, insomnia, irritability, and headache. Marked overdosage with resulting severe toxicity has produced agitation, severe vomiting, dehydration, excessive thirst, tinnitus, cardiac arrhythmias, hyperthermia, diaphoresis, and generalized clonic and tonic convulsions. Cardiovascular collapse has also occurred, with some fatalities. Seizures have occured in some cases associated with very high theophylline plasma concentrations, without any premonitory symptoms of toxicity.

Treatment: There is no specific antidote for overdosage with drugs of the xanthine class. Symptomatic treatment and general supportive measures should be instituted with careful monitoring and maintenance of vital signs, fluids and electrolytes. The stomach should be emptied by inducing emesis if the patient is conscious and responsive, or by gastric lavage, taking care to protect against aspiration, especially in stuporous or comatose patients. Maintenance of an adequate airway is essential in case oxygen or assisted respiration is needed. Symptomatic agents should be avoided but sedatives such as short-acting barbiturates may be useful. Dyphylline is dialyzable and, although not recommended as a routine procedure in overdosage cases, hemodialysis may be of some benefit when severe intoxication is present or when the patient has not responded to general supportive and symptomatic treatment.

DOSAGE AND ADMINISTRATION

Dosage should be individually titrated according to the severity of the condition and the response of the patient.

Usual adult dosage: 2 to 4 tablespoonfuls every six hours.

Appropriate dosage adjustments should be made in patients with impaired renal function (see CLINICAL PHARMACOLOGY).

HOW SUPPLIED

LUFYLLIN Elixir:

NDC 0037-0515-68, pint bottle.
NDC 0037-0515-69, gallon bottle.

Storage: Store below 30°C (86°F).

CAUTION: Federal law prohibits dispensing without prescription.

Rev. 2/85

LUFYLLIN® Injection ℞
(dyphylline injection USP)
FOR INTRAMUSCULAR USE ONLY

DESCRIPTION

Chemically, dyphylline is 7-(2,3-dihydroxypropyl)-theophylline, a white, extremely bitter, amorphous powder that is freely soluble in water and alcohol to the extent of 2 g/100 mL.

LUFYLLIN Injection is a clear, colorless, sterile aqueous solution of dyphylline, a xanthine derivative available as a bronchodilator *for intramuscular use only.*

Each mL of LUFYLLIN Injection contains 250 mg of dyphylline (pH adjusted with sodium hydroxide and/or hydrochloric acid).

The molecular formula for dyphylline is $C_{10}H_{14}N_4O_4$ with a molecular weight of 254.25. Its structural formula is:

OH
CH_2CHCH_2OH
H_3C O N N O N N CH_3

CLINICAL PHARMACOLOGY

Dyphylline is a xanthine derivative with pharmacologic actions similar to theophylline and other members of this class of drugs. Its primary action is that of bronchodilation, but it also exhibits peripheral vasodilatory and other smooth muscle relaxant activity to a lesser degree. The bronchodilatory action of dyphylline, as with other xanthines, is thought to be mediated through competitive inhibition of phosphodiesterase with a resulting increase in cyclic AMP producing relaxation of bronchial smooth muscle.

LUFYLLIN Injection is well tolerated and causes little or no discomfort, by the intramuscular route, and produces less nausea than aminophylline and other alkaline theophylline compounds. Unlike the hydrolyzable salts of theophylline, dyphylline is not converted to free theophylline *in vivo.* It is absorbed rapidly in therapeutically active form and in healthy volunteers reaches a mean peak plasma concentration comparable to that achieved with equivalent oral doses in approximately 45 minutes (17.1 mg following a single oral dose of 1000 mg).

Dyphylline exerts it bronchodilatory effects directly and, unlike theophylline, is excreted unchanged by the kidneys without being metabolized by the liver. Because of this, dyphylline pharmacokinetics and plasma levels are not influenced by various factors that affect liver function and hepatic enzyme activity, such as smoking, age, congestive heart failure or concomitant use of drugs which effect liver function. The renal clearance would be correspondingly reduced in patients with impaired renal function. In anuric patients, the half-life may be increased 3 to 4 times normal.

The range of plasma levels within which dyphylline can be expected to produce effective bronchodilation has not been determined.

Dyphylline plasma concentrations can be accurately determined using high pressure liquid chromatography (HPLC)* or gas-liquid chromatography (GLC).

* *See* Valia, *et al: J. Chromatogr.* **221**:170 (1980). Small quantities of pure dyphylline powder may be obtained from Wallace Laboratories, Cranbury, N.J. The internal standard, β-hydroxyethyltheophylline, may be obtained from companies supplying analytical chemicals.

INDICATIONS AND USAGE

For relief of acute bronchial asthma and for reversible bronchospasm associated with chronic bronchitis and emphysema.

CONTRAINDICATIONS

Hypersensitivity to dyphylline or related xanthine compounds.

WARNINGS

LUFYLLIN Injection is not indicated in the management of status asthmaticus or apnea in the newborn, which are serious medical emergencies.

Although the relationship between plasma levels of dyphylline and appearance of toxicity is unknown, excessive doses may be expected to be associated with an increased risk of adverse effects.

PRECAUTIONS

General: Use LUFYLLIN Injection with caution in patients with severe cardiac disease, hypertension, hyperthyroidism, acute myocardial injury or peptic ulcer.

Drug interactions: Synergism between xanthine bronchodilators (e.g., theophylline), ephedrine and other sympathomimetic bronchodilators has been reported. This should be considered whenever these agents are prescribed concomitantly.

Concurrent administration of dyphylline and probenecid, which competes for tubular secretion, has been shown to increase the plasma half-life of dyphylline (see Clinical Pharmacology).

Carcinogenesis, mutagenesis, impairment of fertility: No long-term animal studies have been performed with LUFYLLIN Injection.

Pregnancy: Teratogenic effects—Pregnancy Category C. Animal reproduction studies have not been conducted with LUFYLLIN Injection. It is also not known if LUFYLLIN Injection can cause fetal harm when administered to a pregnant woman or can affect reproduction capacity. LUFYLLIN Injection should be given to a pregnant woman only if clearly needed.

Nursing mothers: Dyphylline is present in human milk at approximately twice the maternal plasma concentration. Caution should be exercised when LUFYLLIN Injection is administered to a nursing woman.

Pediatric use: Safety and effectiveness in children have not been established.

ADVERSE REACTIONS

Adverse reactions with the use of LUFYLLIN Injection have been infrequent, relatively mild, and rarely required reduction in dosage or withdrawal of therapy.

The following adverse reactions which have been reported with other xanthine bronchodilators, and which have most often been related to excessive drug plasma levels, should be considered as potential adverse effects when dyphylline is administered:

Gastrointestinal: nausea, vomiting, epigastric pain, hematemesis, diarrhea.

Central nervous system: headache, irritability, restlessness, insomnia, hyperexcitability, agitation, muscle twitching, generalized clonic and tonic convulsions.

Cardiovascular: palpitation, tachycardia, extrasystoles, flushing, hypotension, circulatory failure, ventricular arrhythmias.

Respiratory: tachypnea.

Renal: albuminuria, gross and microscopic hematuria, diuresis.

Other: hyperglycemia, inappropriate ADH syndrome.

OVERDOSAGE

There have been no reports, in the literature, of overdosage with LUFYLLIN Injection. However, the following information based on reports of theophylline overdosage are considered typical of the xanthine class of drugs and should be kept in mind.

Signs and symptoms: Restlessness, anorexia, nausea, vomiting, diarrhea, insomnia, irritability, and headache. Marked overdosage with resulting severe toxicity has produced agitation, severe vomiting, dehydration, excessive thirst, tinnitus, cardiac arrhythmias, hyperthermia, diaphoresis, and generalized clonic and tonic convulsions. Cardiovascular collapse has also occurred, with some fatalities. Seizures have oc-

Continued on next page

Wallace—Cont.

curred in some cases associated with very high theophylline plasma concentrations, without any premonitory symptoms of toxicity.
Treatment: There is no specific antidote for overdosage with drugs of the xanthine class. Symptomatic treatment and general supportive measures should be instituted with careful monitoring and maintenance of vital signs, fluids and electrolytes. The stomach should be emptied by inducing emesis if the patient is conscious and responsive, or by gastric lavage, taking care to protect against aspiration, especially in stuporous or comatose patients. Maintenance of an adequate airway is essential in case oxygen or assisted respiration is needed. Sympathomimetic agents should be avoided but sedatives such as short-acting barbiturates may be useful.
Dyphylline is dialyzable and, although not recommended as a routine procedure in overdosage cases, hemodialysis may be of some benefit when severe intoxication is present or when the patient has not responded to general supportive and symptomatic treatment.

DOSAGE AND ADMINISTRATION

LUFYLLIN Injection is *for intramuscular use only.*
Usual adult dosage: 500 mg (2 mL) I.M. initially, followed by 250–500 mg (1 to 2 mL) every two to six hours, as indicated by the patient's response. Do not exceed total dosage of 15 mg/kg every six hours.

HOW SUPPLIED

Box of 25 × 2 mL ampuls (NDC 0037-0537-01).
Storage: Store below 40°C (104°F), preferably between 15° and 30°C (59° to 86°F). Excessive cold may cause formation of a precipitate. DO NOT USE if precipitate is present.
CAUTION: Federal law prohibits dispensing without prescription.

Distributed by
WALLACE LABORATORIES
Division of
CARTER-WALLACE, INC.
Cranbury, New Jersey 08512

Manufactured by:
Taylor Pharmacal Co.
Decatur, Illinois 62526

Rev. 2/85
Shown in Product Identification Section, page 434

LUFYLLIN® ℞
(Dyphylline Tablets, USP, 200 mg)
LUFYLLIN®-400 ℞
(Dyphylline Tablets, USP, 400 mg)

DESCRIPTION

LUFYLLIN (dyphylline), a xanthine derivative, is a bronchodilator available for oral administration as tablets containing 200 mg and 400 mg of dyphylline.
Other ingredients: magnesium stearate, microcrystalline cellulose.
Chemically, dyphylline is 7-(2,3-dihydroxypropyl)-theophylline, a white, extremely bitter, amorphous powder that is freely soluble in water and soluble in alcohol to the extent of 2 g/100 ml. Dyphylline forms a neutral solution that is stable in gastrointestinal fluids over a wide range of pH.
The molecular formula for dyphylline is $C_{10}H_{14}N_4O_4$ with a molecular weight of 254.25.

CLINICAL PHARMACOLOGY

Dyphylline is a xanthine derivative with pharmacologic actions similar to theophylline and other members of this class of drugs. Its primary action is that of bronchodilation, but it also exhibits peripheral vasodilatory and other smooth muscle relaxant activity to a lesser degree. The bronchodilatory action of dyphylline, as with other xanthines, is thought to be mediated through competitive inhibition of phosphodiesterase with a resulting increase in cyclic AMP producing relaxation of bronchial smooth muscle.
LUFYLLIN is well tolerated and produces less nausea than aminophylline and other alkaline theophylline compounds when administered orally. Unlike the hydrolyzable salts of theophylline, dyphylline is not converted to free theophylline *in vivo.* It is absorbed rapidly in therapeutically active form and in healthy volunteers reaches a mean peak plasma concentration of 17.1 mcg/ml in approximately 45 minutes following a single oral dose of 1000 mg of LUFYLLIN.
Dyphylline exerts its bronchodilatory effects directly and, unlike theophylline, is excreted unchanged by the kidneys without being metabolized by the liver. Because of this, dyphylline pharmacokinetics and plasma levels are not influenced by various factors that affect liver function and hepatic enzyme activity, such as smoking, age, congestive heart failure or concomitant use of drugs which affect liver function.
The elimination half-life of dyphylline is approximately two hours (1.8–2.1 hr) and approximately 88% of a single oral dose can be recovered from the urine unchanged. The renal clearance would be correspondingly reduced in patients with impaired renal function. In anuric patients, the half-life may be increased 3 to 4 times normal.
Dyphylline plasma levels are dose-related and generally predictable. The range of plasma levels within which dyphylline can be expected to produce effective bronchodilation has not been determined.
Dyphylline plasma concentrations can be accurately determined using high pressure liquid chromatography (HPLC)* or gas-liquid chromatography (GLC).

* *See* Valia, *et al, J. Chromatogr.* **221**:170 (1980). Small quantities of pure dyphylline powder may be obtained from Wallace Laboratories, Cranbury, N.J. The internal standard, β-hydroxyethyltheophylline, may be obtained from companies supplying analytical chemicals.

INDICATIONS AND USAGE

For relief of acute bronchial asthma and for reversible bronchospasm associated with chronic bronchitis and emphysema.

CONTRAINDICATIONS

Hypersensitivity to dyphylline or related xanthine compounds.

WARNINGS

LUFYLLIN is not indicated in the management of status asthmaticus, which is a serious medical emergency.
Although the relationship between plasma levels of dyphylline and appearance of toxicity is unknown, excessive doses may be expected to be associated with an increased risk of adverse effects.

PRECAUTIONS

General: Use LUFYLLIN with caution in patients with severe cardiac disease, hypertension, hyperthyroidism, acute myocardial injury or peptic ulcer.
Drug interactions: Synergism between xanthine bronchodilators (e.g., theophylline), ephedrine and other sympathomimetic bronchodilators has been reported. This should be considered whenever these agents are prescribed concomitantly.
Concurrent administration of dyphylline and probenecid, which competes for tubular secretion, has been shown to increase the plasma half-life of dyphylline (see CLINICAL PHARMACOLOGY).
Carcinogenesis, mutagenesis, impairment of fertility: No long-term animal studies have been performed with LUFYLLIN.
Pregnancy: Teratogenic effects—Pregnancy Category C. Animal reproduction studies have not been conducted with LUFYLLIN. It is also not known if LUFYLLIN can cause fetal harm when administered to a pregnant woman or can affect reproduction capacity. LUFYLLIN should be given to a pregnant woman only if clearly needed.
Nursing mothers: Dyphylline is present in human milk at approximately twice the maternal plasma concentration. Caution should be exercised when LUFYLLIN is administered to a nursing woman.
Pediatric use: Safety and effectiveness in children have not been established.

ADVERSE REACTIONS

Adverse reactions with the use of LUFYLLIN have been infrequent, relatively mild, and rarely required reduction in dosage or withdrawal of therapy.
The following adverse reactions which have been reported with other xanthine bronchodilators, and which have most often been related to excessive drug plasma levels, should be considered as potential adverse effects when dyphylline is administered:
Gastrointestinal: nausea, vomiting, epigastric pain, hematemesis, diarrhea.
Central nervous system: headache, irritability, restlessness, insomnia, hyperexcitability, agitation, muscle twitching, generalized clonic and tonic convulsions.
Cardiovascular: palpitation, tachycardia, extrasystoles, flushing, hypotension, circulatory failure, ventricular arrhythmias.
Respiratory: tachypnea.
Renal: albuminuria, gross and microscopic hematuria, diuresis.
Other: hyperglycemia, inappropriate ADH syndrome.

OVERDOSAGE

There have been no reports, in the literature, of overdosage with LUFYLLIN. However, the following information based on reports of theophylline overdosage are considered typical of the xanthine class of drugs and should be kept in mind.
Signs and symptoms: Restlessness, anorexia, nausea, vomiting, diarrhea, insomnia, irritability, and headache. Marked overdosage with resulting severe toxicity has produced agitation, severe vomiting, dehydration, excessive thirst, tinnitus, cardiac arrhythmias, hyperthermia, diaphoresis, and generalized clonic and tonic convulsions. Cardiovascular collapse has also occcurred, with some fatalities. Seizures have occurred in some cases associated with very high theophylline plasma concentrations, without any premonitory symptoms of toxicity.
Treatment: There is no specific antidote for overdosage with drugs of the xanthine class. Symptomatic treatment and general supportive measures should be instituted with careful monitoring and maintenance of vital signs, fluid and electrolytes. The stomach should be emptied by inducing emesis if the patient is conscious and responsive, or by gastric lavage, taking care to protect against aspiration, especially in stuporous or comatose patients. Maintenance of an adequate airway is essential in case oxygen or assisted respiration is needed. Sympathomimetic agents should be avoided but sedatives such as short-acting barbiturates may be useful.
Dyphylline is dialyzable and, although not recommended as a routine procedure in overdosage cases, hemodialysis may be of some benefit when severe intoxication is present or when the patient has not responded to general supportive and symptomatic treatment.

DOSAGE AND ADMINISTRATION

Dosage should be individually titrated according to the severity of the condition and the response of the patient.
Usual adult dosage: Up to 15 mg/kg every six hours.
Appropriate dosage adjustments should be made in patients with impaired renal function (see CLINICAL PHARMACOLOGY).

HOW SUPPLIED

LUFYLLIN Tablets: Available as white, rectangular, monogrammed tablets containing 200 mg dyphylline in bottles of 100 (NDC 0037-0521-92) and 1000 (NDC 0037-0521-97), and individually film-sealed tablets in unit-dose boxes of 100 (NDC 0037-0521-85).
LUFYLLIN-400 Tablets: Available as white, capsule-shaped, monogrammed tablets containing 400 mg dyphylline in bottles of 100 (NDC 0037-0731-92) and 1000 (NDC 0037-0731-97), and individually film-sealed tablets in unit-dose boxes of 100 (NDC 0037-0731-85).
Storage: Avoid excessive heat—above 40°C (104°F).
CAUTION: Federal law prohibits dispensing without prescription.

Rev. 2/85
Shown in Product Identification Section, page 434

LUFYLLIN®-GG ℞
Tablets and Elixir

DESCRIPTION

LUFYLLIN®-GG is a bronchodilator/expectorant combination available for oral administration as *Tablets* and *Elixir.*
Each Tablet contains:
Dyphylline .... 200 mg
Guaifenesin .... 200 mg
Other ingredients: corn starch, D&C Yellow No. 10, magnesium aluminium silicate, magnesium stearate, microcrystalline cellulose.
Each 15 mL (one tablespoonful) of Elixir contains:
Dyphylline .... 100 mg
Guaifenesin .... 100 mg
Alcohol (by volume) 17%
Other ingredients: citric acid, FD&C Yellow No. 6, flavor (artificial), purified water, saccharin sodium, sodium citrate, sucrose.
Dyphylline is 7-(2,3-dihydroxypropyl)-theophylline, a white, extremely bitter, amorphous powder that is fully soluble in water and soluble in alcohol to the extent of 2 g/100 mL. Dyphylline forms a neutral solution that is stable in gastrointestinal fluids over a wide range of pH.

CLINICAL PHARMACOLOGY

Dyphylline is a xanthine derivative with pharmacologic actions similar to theophylline and other members of this class of drugs. Its primary action is that of bronchodilation, but it also exhibits peripheral vasodilatory and other smooth muscle relaxant activity to a lesser degree. The bronchodilatory action of dyphylline, as with as other xanthines, is thought to be mediated through competitive inhibition of phosphodiesterase with a resulting increase in cyclic AMP producing relaxation of bronchial smooth muscle.
Dyphylline in LUFYLLIN-GG is well tolerated and produces less nausea than aminophylline and other alkaline theophylline compounds when administered orally. Unlike the hydrolyzable salts of theophylline, dyphylline is not converted to free theophylline *in vivo.* It is absorbed rapidly in therapeutically active form and in healthy volunteers reaches a mean peak plasma concentration of 17.1 mcg/mL in approximately 45 minutes following a single oral dose of 1000 mg of dyphylline.
Dyphylline exerts its bronchodilatory effects directly and, unlike theophylline, is excreted unchanged by the kidneys without being metabolized by the liver. Because of this, dyphylline pharmacokinetics and plasma levels are not influenced by various factors that affect liver function and he-

patic enzyme activity, such as smoking, age, or concomitant use of drugs which effect liver function.

The elimination half-life of dyphylline is approximately two hours (1.8–2.1 hr) and approximately 88% of a single oral dose can be recovered from the urine unchanged. The renal clearance would be correspondingly reduced in patients with impaired renal function. In anuric patients, the half-life may be increased 3 to 4 times normal.

Dyphylline plasma levels are dose-related and generally predictable. The therapeutic range of plasma levels within which dyphylline can be expected to produce effective bronchodilation has not been determined.

Dyphylline plasma concentrations can be accurately determined using high pressure liquid chromatography (HPLC)* or gas-liquid chromatography (GLC).

Guaifenesin is an expectorant whose action helps increase the output of thin respiratory tract fluid to facilitate mucociliary clearance and removal of inspissated mucus.

* *See* Valia, *et al*, *J Chromatogr.* **221**: 170 (1980). Small quantities of pure dyphylline powder may be obtained from Wallace Laboratories, Cranbury, N.J. The internal standard, β-hydroxyethyltheophylline, may be obtained from companies supplying analytical chemicals.

Guaifensin is an expectorant whose action helps increase the output of thin respiratory tract fluid to facilitate mucociliary clearance and removal of inspissated mucus.

INDICATIONS AND USAGE

For relief of acute bronchial asthma and for reversible bronchospasm associated with chronic bronchitis and emphysema.

CONTRAINDICATIONS

Hypersensitivity to any of the ingredients or related compounds.

WARNINGS

LUFYLLIN-GG is not indicated in the management of status asthmaticus, which is a serious medical emergency.

Although the relationship between plasma levels of dyphylline and appearance of toxicity is unknown, excessive doses may be expected to be associated with an increased risk of adverse effects.

PREACUTIONS

General: Use LUFYLLIN-GG with caution in patients with severe cardiac disease, hypertension, hyperthyroidism, acute myocardial injury or peptic ulcer.

Drug interactions: Synergism between xanthine bronchodilators (e.g., theophylline), ephedrine and other sympathomimetic bronchodilators has been reported. This should be considered whenever these agents are prescribed concomitantly. Concurrent administration of dyphylline and probenecid, which competes for tubular secretion, has been shown to increase plasma half-life of dyphylline (see Clinical Pharmacology).

Carcinogenesis, mutagenesis, impairment of fertility: No long-term animal studies have been performed with LUFYLLIN-GG.

Pregnancy: Teratogenic effects—Pregnancy Category C. Animal reproduction studies have not been conducted with LUFYLLIN-GG. It is also not known whether the product can cause fetal harm when administered to a pregnant woman or can affect reproduction capacity. LUFYLLIN-GG should be given to a pregnant woman only if clearly needed.

Nursing mothers: Dyphylline is present in human milk at approximately twice the maternal plasma concentration. Caution should be exercised when LUFYLLIN-GG is administered to a nursing woman.

Pediatric use: Safety and effectiveness in children below the age of six have not been established. Use caution when administering to children six years of age or older.

ADVERSE REACTIONS

LUFYLLIN-GG may cause nausea, headache, cardiac palpitation and CNS stimulation. Postprandial administration may help avoid gastric discomfort.

The following adverse reactions which have been reported with other xanthine bronchodilators, and which have most often been related to excessive drug plasma levels, should be considered as potential adverse effects when dyphylline is administered:

Gastrointestinal: nausea, vomiting, epigastric pain, hematemesis, diarrhea.

Central nervous system: headache, irritability, restlessness, insomnia, hyperexcitability, agitation, muscle twitching, generalized clonic and tonic convulsions.

Cardiovascular: palpitation, tachycardia, extrasystoles, flushing, hypotension, circulatory failure, ventricular arrhythmias.

Respiratory: tachypnea.

Renal: albuminuria, gross and microscopic hematuria, diuresis.

Other: hyperglycemia, inappropriate ADH syndrome.

OVERDOSAGE

There have been no reports, in the literature, of overdosage with LUFYLLIN-GG. However, the following information based on reports of theophylline overdosage are considered typical of the xanthine class of drugs and should be kept in mind.

Signs and symptoms: Restlessness, anorexia, nausea, vomiting, diarrhea, insomnia, irritability, and headache. Marked overdosage with resulting severe toxicity has produced agitation, severe vomiting, dehydration, excessive thirst, tinnitus, cardiac arrhythmias, hyperthermia, diaphoresis, and generalized clonic and tonic convulsions. Cardiovascular collapse has also occured, with some fatalities. Seizures have occured in some cases associated with very high theophylline plasma concentrations, without any premonitory symptoms of toxicity.

Treatment: There is no specific antidote for overdosage with drugs of the xanthine class. Symptomatic treatment and general supportive measures should be instituted with careful monitoring and maintenance of vital signs, fluids and electrolytes. The stomach should be emptied by inducing emesis if the patient is conscious and responsive, or by gastric lavage, taking care to protect against aspiration, especially in stuporous or comatose patients. Maintenance of an adequate airway is essential in case oxygen or assisted respiration is needed. Sympathomimetic agents should be avoided but sedatives such as short-acting barbiturates may be useful.

Dyphylline is dialyzable and, although not recommended as a routine procedure in overdosage cases, hemodialysis may be of some benefit when severe intoxication is present or when the patient has not responded to general supportive and symptomatic treatment.

DOSAGE AND ADMINISTRATION

Dosage should be individually titrated according to the severity of the condition and the response of the patient.

Usual adult dosage:

One tablet or 30 mL (2 tablespoonfuls) elixir, four times daily.

Children above age six:

One-half to one tablet or 15 to 30 mL (one to two tablespoonfuls) elixir, three to four times daily.

Not recommended for use in children below age six: (see Precautions).

HOW SUPPLIED

LUFYLLIN-GG Tablets: round, light yellow, monogrammed tablets, scored on one side, in bottles of 100 (NDC 0037-0541-92) and 1000 (NDC 0037-0541-97) and boxes of 100 unit-dose, individually film-sealed tablets (NDC 0037-0541-85).

LUFYLLIN-GG Elixir: clear, light yellow-orange liquid with a mild wine-like odor and taste, in bottles of one pint (NDC 0037-0545-68) and one gallon (NDC 0037-0545-69).

Storage:

Tablets—Avoid excessive heat—above 40°C (104°F).

Elixir—Store below 30°C (86°F).

CAUTION: Federal law prohibits dispensing without prescription.

WALLACE LABORATORIES
Division of
CARTER-WALLACE, INC.
Cranbury, New Jersey 08512

Rev. 2/85

Shown in Product Identification Section, page 434

MALTSUPEX® OTC

(malt soup extract)
Powder, Liquid, Tablets

(See PDR For Nonprescription Drugs)

MEPROSPAN® Ⓒ ℞

(meprobamate, sustained-release capsules)

DESCRIPTION

Meprobamate is a white powder with a characteristic odor and a bitter taste. It is slightly soluble in water, freely soluble in acetone and alcohol, and sparingly soluble in ether. The structural formula of meprobamate is

$$NH_2COOCH_2-\underset{CH_2CH_2CH_3}{\overset{CH_3}{C}}-CH_2OOCNH_2$$

'Meprospan' 400 contains 400 mg meprobamate per capsule. Other ingredients: corn starch, FD&C Blue #1, FD&C Yellow #6, gelatin, sucrose and other ingredients.

'Meprospan' 200 contains 200 mg meprobamate per capsule. Other ingredients: corn starch, FD&C Yellow #6, gelatin, sucrose and other ingredients.

ACTIONS

Meprobamate is a carbamate derivative which has been shown in animal studies to have effects at multiple sites in the central nervous system, including the thalamus and limbic system.

INDICATIONS

'Meprospan' (meprobamate) is indicated for the management of anxiety disorders or for the short-term relief of the symptoms of anxiety. Anxiety or tension associated with the stress of everyday life usually do not require treatment with an anxiolytic.

The effectiveness of 'Meprospan' in long-term use, that is, more than 4 months, has not been assessed by systematic clinical studies. The physician should periodically reassess the usefulness of the drug for the individual patient.

CONTRAINDICATIONS

Acute intermittent porphyria as well as allergic or idiosyncratic reactions to meprobamate or related compounds such as carisoprodol, mebutamate, tybamate, or carbromal.

WARNINGS

Drug Dependence—Physical dependence, psychological dependence, and abuse have occurred. When chronic intoxication from prolonged use occurs, it usually involves ingestion of greater than recommended doses and is manifested by ataxia, slurred speech, and vertigo. Therefore, careful supervision of dose and amounts prescribed is advised, as well as avoidance of prolonged administration, especially for alcoholics and other patients with a known propensity for taking excessive quantities of drugs.

Sudden withdrawal of the drug after prolonged and excessive use may precipitate recurrence of pre-existing symptoms, such as anxiety, anorexia, or insomnia, or withdrawal reactions, such as vomiting, ataxia, tremors, muscle twitching, confusional states, hallucinosis, and, rarely, convulsive seizures. Such seizures are more likely to occur in persons with central nervous system damage or pre-existent or latent convulsive disorders. Onset of withdrawal symptoms occurs usually within 12 to 48 hours after discontinuation of meprobamate; symptoms usually cease within the next 12 to 48 hours.

When excessive dosage has continued for weeks or months, dosage should be reduced gradually over a period of one or two weeks rather than abruptly stopped. Alternatively, a short-acting barbiturate may be substituted, then gradually withdrawn.

Potentially Hazardous Tasks—Patients should be warned that this drug may impair the mental and/or physical abilities required for the performance of potentially hazardous tasks such as driving a motor vehicle or operating machinery.

Additive Effects—Since the effects of meprobamate and alcohol or meprobamate and other CNS depressants or psychotropic drugs may be additive, appropriate caution should be exercised with patients who take more than one of these agents simultaneously.

USAGE IN PREGNANCY AND LACTATION—An increased risk of congenital malformations associated with the use of minor tranquilizers (meprobamate, chlordiazepoxide, and diazepam) during the first trimester of pregnancy has been suggested in several studies. Because use of these drugs is rarely a matter of urgency, their use during this period should almost always be avoided. The possibility that a woman of childbearing potential may be pregnant at the time of institution of therapy should be considered. Patients should be advised that if they become pregnant during therapy or intend to become pregnant they should communicate with their physicians about the desirability of discontinuing the drug.

Meprobamate passes the placental barrier. It is present both in umbilical cord blood at or near maternal plasma levels and in breast milk of lactating mothers at concentrations two or four times that of maternal plasma. When use of meprobamate is contemplated in breast-feeding patients, the drug's higher concentration in breast milk as compared to maternal plasma levels should be considered.

Usage in Children—Meprobamate should not be administered to children under age six, since there is a lack of documented evidence for safety and effectiveness in this age group.

PRECAUTIONS

The lowest effective dose should be administered, particularly to elderly and/or debilitated patients, in order to preclude oversedation.

The possibility of suicide attempts should be considered and the least amount of drug feasible should be dispensed at any one time.

Meprobamate is metabolized in the liver and excreted by the kidney; to avoid its excess accumulation, caution should be exercised in administration to patients with compromised liver or kidney function.

Meprobamate occasionally may precipitate seizures in epileptic patients.

Continued on next page

Wallace—Cont.

ADVERSE REACTIONS

Central Nervous System: Drowsiness, ataxia, dizziness, slurred speech, headache, vertigo, weakness, paresthesias, impairment of visual accommodation, euphoria, overstimulation, paradoxical excitement, fast EEG activity.
Gastrointestinal—Nausea, vomiting, diarrhea.
Cardiovascular—Palpitations, tachycardia, various forms of arrhythmia, transient ECG changes, syncope; also, hypotensive crises (including one fatal case).
Allergic or Idiosyncratic—Allergic or idiosyncratic reactions are usually seen within the period of the first to fourth dose in patients having had no previous contact with the drug. Milder reactions are characterized by an itchy, urticarial, or erythematous maculopapular rash which may be generalized or confined to the groin. Other reactions have included leukopenia, acute nonthrombocytopenic purpura, petechiae, ecchymoses, eosinophilia, peripheral edema, adenopathy, fever, fixed drug eruption with cross reaction to carisoprodol, and cross sensitivity between meprobamate/mebutamate and meprobamate/carbromal.
More severe hypersensitivity reactions, rarely reported, include hyperpyrexia, chills, angioneurotic edema, bronchospasm, oliguria, and anuria. Also, anaphylaxis, erythema multiforme, exfoliative dermatitis, stomatitis, proctitis, Stevens-Johnson syndrome, and bullous dermatitis, including one fatal case of the latter following administration of meprobamate in combination with prednisolone.
In case of allergic or idiosyncratic reactions to meprobamate, discontinue the drug and initiate appropriate symptomatic therapy, which may include epinephrine, antihistamines, and in severe cases corticosteroids. In evaluating possible allergic reactions, also consider allergy to excipients (information on excipients is available to physicians on request).
Hematologic—(See also *Allergic or Idiosyncratic.*) Agranulocytosis and aplastic anemia have been reported, although no causal relationship has been established. These cases rarely were fatal. Rare cases of thrombocytopenic purpura have been reported.
Other—Exacerbation of porphyric symptoms.

DOSAGE AND ADMINISTRATION

The usual adult dosage of 'Meprospan' (meprobamate, sustained-release capsules) is one to two 400 mg capsules in the morning and again at bedtime; doses above 2400 mg daily are not recommended. The usual dosage for children ages six to twelve is one 200 mg capsule in the morning and again at bedtime. Meprobamate is not recommended for children under age six.

OVERDOSAGE

Suicidal attempts with meprobamate have resulted in drowsiness, lethargy, stupor, ataxia, coma, shock, vasomotor and respiratory collapse. Some suicidal attempts have been fatal. Overdosage experience with 'Meprospan' (meprobamate, sustained-release capsules) is limited. However, the following data on meprobamate tablets have been reported in the literature and from other sources. These data are not expected to correlate with each case (considering factors such as individual susceptibility and length of time from ingestion to treatment), but represent the *usual ranges* reported.
Acute simple overdose (meprobamate alone): Death has been reported with ingestion of as little as 12 gm meprobamate and survival with as much as 40 gm.
Blood Levels:
0.5–2.0 mg% represents the usual blood level range of meprobamate after therapeutic doses. The level may occasionally be as high as 3.0 mg%.
3–10 mg% usually corresonds to findings of mild to moderate symptoms of overdosage, such as stupor or light coma.
10–20 mg% usually corresponds to deeper coma, requiring more intensive treatment. Some fatalities occur.
At levels greater than 20 mg%, more fatalities than survivals can be expected.
Acute combined overdose (meprobamate with alcohol or other CNS depressants or psychotropic drugs): Since effects can be additive, a history of ingestion of a low dose of meprobamate plus any of these compounds (or of a relatively low blood or tissue level) cannot be used as a prognostic indicator.
In cases where excessive doses have been taken, sleep ensues rapidly and blood pressure, pulse, and respiratory rates are reduced to basal levels. Any drug remaining in the stomach should be removed and symptomatic therapy given. Should respiration or blood pressure become compromised, respiratory assistance, central nervous system stimulants, and pressor agents should be administered cautiously as indicated. Meprobamate is metabolized in the liver and excreted by the kidney. Diuresis, osmotic (mannitol) diuresis, peritoneal dialysis, and hemodialysis have been used successfully. Careful monitoring of urinary output is necessary and caution should be taken to avoid overhydration. Relapse and death, after initial recovery, have been attributed to incomplete gastric emptying and delayed absorption. Meprobamate can be measured in biological fluids by two methods: colorimetric (Hoffman, A. J. and Ludwig, B. J.: *J Amer Pharm Assn 48:* 740, 1959) and gas chromatographic (Douglas, J. F. et al: *Anal Chem 39:* 956, 1967).

HOW SUPPLIED

'Meprospan' 400: Each sustained-release, blue-topped capsule contains meprobamate, U.S.P., 400 mg in bottles of 100 (NDC 0037-1301-01). 'Meprospan' 200: Each sustained-release, yellow-topped capsule contains meprobamate, U.S.P., 200 mg in bottles of 100 (NDC 0037-1401-01).

Distributed by WALLACE LABORATORIES
Division of CARTER-WALLACE, INC.
Cranbury, New Jersey 08512
Manufactured by KV Pharmacal, St. Louis, Mo. 63144
Rev. 8/85

MILTOWN® Ⓒ ℞
(meprobamate, U.S.P.)
Tablets
MILTOWN® 600 Ⓒ ℞
(meprobamate, U.S.P.)
Tablets

DESCRIPTION

Meprobamate is a white powder with a characteristic odor and a bitter taste. It is slightly soluble in water, freely soluble in acetone and alcohol, and sparingly soluble in ether.
'Miltown'-200 contain 200 mg meprobamate per tablet. Other ingredients: acacia, carnauba wax, gelatin, magnesium carbonate, magnesium stearate, methylcellulose, starch, sugar, talc, titanium dioxide, lac, white wax.
'Miltown'-400 contain 400 mg meprobamate per tablet. Other ingredients: magnesium stearate, methylcellulose, starch.
'Miltown'-600 contain 600 mg meprobamate per tablet. Other ingredients: alginic acid, ethylcellulose, magnesium stearate, purified stearic acid, starch.

ACTIONS

Meprobamate is a carbamate derivative which has been shown in animal studies to have effects at multiple sites in the central nervous system, including the thalamus and limbic system.

INDICATIONS

'Miltown' (meprobamate) is indicated for the management of anxiety disorders or for the short-term relief of the symptoms of anxiety. Anxiety or tension associated with the stress of everyday life usually do not require treatment with an anxiolytic.
The effectiveness of 'Miltown' in long-term use, that is, more than 4 months, has not been assessed by systematic clinical studies. The physician should periodically reassess the usefulness of the drug for the individual patient.

CONTRAINDICATIONS

Acute intermittent porphyria as well as allergic or idiosyncratic reactions to meprobamate or related compounds such as carisoprodol, mebutamate, tybamate, or carbromal.

WARNINGS

Drug Dependence
Physical dependence, psychological dependence, and abuse have occurred. When chronic intoxication from prolonged use occurs, it usually involves ingestion of greater than recommended doses and is manifested by ataxia, slurred speech, and vertigo. Therefore, careful supervision of dose and amounts prescribed is advised, as well as avoidance of prolonged administration, especially for alcoholics and other patients with a known propensity for taking excessive quantities of drugs.
Sudden withdrawal of the drug after prolonged and excessive use may precipitate recurrence of pre-existing symptoms, such as anxiety, anorexia, or insomnia, or withdrawal reactions, such as vomiting, ataxia, tremors, muscle twitching, confusional states, hallucinosis, and, rarely, convulsive seizures. Such seizures are more likely to occur in persons with central nervous system damage or pre-existent or latent convulsive disorders. Onset of withdrawal symptoms occurs usually within 12 to 48 hours after discontinuation of meprobamate; symptoms usually cease within the next 12 to 48 hours.
When excessive dosage has continued for weeks or months, dosage should be reduced gradually over a period of one or two weeks rather than abruptly stopped. Alternatively, a short-acting barbiturate may be substituted, then gradually withdrawn.
Potentially Hazardous Tasks
Patients should be warned that this drug may impair the mental and/or physical abilities required for the performance of potentially hazardous tasks such as driving a motor vehicle or operating machinery.
Additive Effects
Since the effects of meprobamate and alcohol or meprobamate and other CNS depressants or psychotropic drugs may be additive, appropriate caution should be exercised with patients who take more than one of these agents simultaneously.
USAGE IN PREGNANCY AND LACTATION
An increased risk of congenital malformations associated with the use of minor tranquilizers (meprobamate, chlordiazepoxide, and diazepam) during the first trimester of pregnancy has been suggested in several studies. Because use of these drugs is rarely a matter of urgency, their use during this period should almost always be avoided. The possibility that a woman of childbearing potential may be pregnant at the time of institution of therapy should be considered. Patients should be advised that if they become pregnant during therapy or intend to become pregnant they should communicate with their physicians about the desirability of discontinuing the drug.
Meprobamate passes the placental barrier. It is present both in umbilical cord blood at or near maternal plasma levels and in breast milk of lactating mothers at concentrations two to four times that of maternal plasma. When use of meprobamate is contemplated in breast-feeding patients, the drug's higher concentration in breast milk as compared to maternal plasma levels should be considered.
Usage in Children
'Miltown' (meprobamate)—Meprobamate should not be administered to children under age six, since there is a lack of documented evidence for safety and effectiveness in this age group.
'Miltown' 600 (meprobamate 600 mg)—This dosage form is not intended for use in children.

PRECAUTIONS

The lowest effective dose should be administered, particularly to elderly and/or debilitated patients, in order to preclude oversedation.
The possibility of suicide attempts should be considered and the least amount of drug feasible should be dispensed at any one time.
Meprobamate is metabolized in the liver and excreted by the kidney; to avoid its excess accumulation, caution should be exercised in administration to patients with compromised liver or kidney function.
Meprobamate occasionally may precipitate seizures in epileptic patients.

ADVERSE REACTIONS

Central Nervous System
Drowsiness, ataxia, dizziness, slurred speech, headache, vertigo, weakness, paresthesias, impairment of visual accommodation, euphoria, overstimulation, paradoxical excitement, fast EEG activity.
Gastrointestinal
Nausea, vomiting, diarrhea.
Cardiovascular
Palpitations, tachycardia, various forms of arrhythmia, transient ECG changes, syncope; also, hypotensive crises (including one fatal case).
Allergic or Idiosyncratic
Allergic or idiosyncratic reactions are usually seen within the period of the first to fourth dose in patients having had no previous contact with the drug. Milder reactions are characterized by an itchy, urticarial, or erythematous maculopapular rash which may be generalized or confined to the groin. Other reactions have included leukopenia, acute nonthrombocytopenic purpura, petechiae, ecchymoses, eosinophilia, peripheral edema, adenopathy, fever, fixed drug eruption with cross reaction to carisoprodol, and cross sensitivity between meprobamate/mebutamate and meprobamate/carbromal.
More severe hypersensitivity reactions, rarely reported, include hyperpyrexia, chills, angioneurotic edema, bronchospasm, oliguria, and anuria. Also, anaphylaxis, erythema multiforme, exfoliative dermatitis, stomatitis, proctitis, Stevens-Johnson syndrome, and bullous dermatitis, including one fatal case of the latter following administration of meprobamate in combination with prednisolone.
In case of allergic or idiosyncratic reactions to meprobamate, discontinue the drug and initiate appropriate symptomatic therapy, which may include epinephrine, antihistamines, and in severe cases corticosteroids. In evaluating possible allergic reactions, also consider allergy to excipients (information on excipients is available to physicians on request).
Hematologic
(See also **Allergic or Idiosyncratic.**) Agranulocytosis and aplastic anemia have been reported, although no causal relationship has been established. These cases rarely were fatal. Rare cases of thrombocytopenic purpura have been reported.
Other
Exacerbation of porphyric symptoms.

DOSAGE AND ADMINISTRATION

Doses of meprobamate above 2400 mg daily are not recommended.
'Miltown' (meprobamate)—**Adults:** the usual dosage is 1200 to 1600 mg daily, in three or four divided doses. **Children:** the usual dosage for children ages six to twelve is 100 to 200 mg two or three times daily. Meprobamate is not recommended for children under six.

'Miltown' 600 (meprobamate 600 mg)—**Adults:** the recommended dosage is one tablet twice a day. **Children:** not intended for use in children.

OVERDOSAGE

Suicidal attempts with meprobamate have resulted in drowsiness, lethargy, stupor, ataxia, coma, shock, vasomotor and respiratory collapse. Some suicidal attempts have been fatal. The following data on meprobamate tablets have been reported in the literature and from other sources. These data are not expected to correlate with each case (considering factors such as individual susceptibility and length of time from ingestion to treatment), but represent the *usual ranges* reported.

Acute simple overdose (meprobamate alone): Death has been reported with ingestion of as little as 12 gm meprobamate and survival with as much as 40 gm.

Blood levels:

0.5–2.0 mg% represents the usual blood level range of meprobamate after therapeutic doses. The level may occasionally be as high as 3.0 mg%.

3–10 mg% usually corresponds to findings of mild to moderate symptoms of overdosage, such as stupor or light coma.

10–20 mg% usually corresponds to deeper coma, requiring more intensive treatment. Some fatalities occur.

At levels greater than 20 mg%, more fatalities than survivals can be expected.

Acute combined overdose (meprobamate with alcohol or other CNS depressants or psychotropic drugs): Since effects can be additive, a history of ingestion of a low dose of meprobamate plus any of these compounds (or of a relatively low blood or tissue level) cannot be used as a prognostic indicator.

In cases where excessive doses have been taken, sleep ensues rapidly and blood pressure, pulse, and respiratory rates are reduced to basal levels. Any drug remaining in the stomach should be removed and symptomatic therapy given. Should respiration or blood pressure become compromised, respiratory assistance, central nervous system stimulants, and pressor agents should be administered cautiously as indicated. Meprobamate is metabolized in the liver and excreted by the kidney. Diuresis, osmotic (mannitol) diuresis, peritoneal dialysis, and hemodialysis have been used successfully. Careful monitoring of urinary output is necessary and caution should be taken to avoid overhydration. Relapse and death, after initial recovery, have been attributed to incomplete gastric emptying and delayed absorption. Meprobamate can be measured in biological fluids by two methods: colorimetric (Hoffman, A.J. and Ludwig, B.J.: *J Amer Pharm Assn 48:* 740, 1959) and gas chromatographic (Douglas, J.F. et al: *Anal Chem 39:* 956, 1967).

HOW SUPPLIED

'Miltown' (meprobamate, U.S.P.) is available as 400 mg white, scored tablets in bottles of:

100 (NDC 0037-1001-01)
500 (NDC 0037-1001-03)
1000 (NDC 0037-1001-02)

and 200 mg white, sugar-coated tablets in bottles of 100 (NDC 0037-1101-01).

'Miltown' 600 (meprobamate, U.S.P.) is available as 600 mg white, capsule-shaped tablets, in bottles of 100 (NDC 0037-1601-01).

WALLACE LABORATORIES
Division of
CARTER-WALLACE, INC.
Cranbury, New Jersey 08512

Rev. 6/85

Shown in Product Identification Section, page 434

ORGANIDIN® ℞

(iodinated glycerol)
Solution, Tablets, Elixir

DESCRIPTION

Organidin® (iodinated glycerol), a mucolytic-expectorant, is an isomeric mixture formed by the interaction of iodine and glycerol, whose active ingredient is thought to be iodopropylidene glycerol but whose structural and chemical formulas have not been precisely established. Iodinated glycerol is a viscous, amber liquid stable in acid media, including gastric juice, which contains virtually no inorganic iodide and no free iodine. ORGANIDIN is available for oral administration as:

Solution —5%, containing 50 mg ORGANIDIN (25 mg organically bound iodine) per mL. Other ingredients: caramel, glycerin, purified water.

Tablets —each containing 30 mg ORGANIDIN (15 mg organically bound iodine). Other ingredients: corn starch, dibasic calcium phosphate, FD&C Red No. 40, magnesium stearate, microcrystalline cellulose, tribasic calcium phosphate.

Elixir —1.2%, containing 60 mg ORGANIDIN (30 mg organically bound iodine) per 5 mL (teaspoonful); and alcohol, 21.75% by volume. Other ingredients: flavors (natural and artificial), liquid glucose, purified water, saccharin sodium.

CLINICAL PHARMACOLOGY

ORGANIDIN increases the output of thin respiratory tract fluid and helps liquefy tenacious mucus in the bronchial tree. Iodines are readily absorbed from the gastrointestinal tract and concentrated primarily in the secretions of the respiratory tract, but their mechanism of action as mucolytic-expectorants is not clear.

INDICATIONS AND USAGE

ORGANIDIN is indicated for adjunctive treatment as a mucolytic-expectorant in respiratory tract conditions such as bronchitis, bronchial asthma, pulmonary emphysema, cystic fibrosis, chronic sinusitis, or after surgery to help prevent atelectasis.

CONTRAINDICATIONS

History of marked sensitivity to inorganic iodides; hypersensitivity to any of the ingredients or related compounds; pregnancy; newborns; and nursing mothers.

The human fetal thyroid begins to concentrate iodine in the 12th to 14th week of gestation and the use of inorganic iodides in pregnant women during this period and thereafter has rarely been reported to induce fetal goiter (with or without hypothyroidism) with the potential for airway obstruction. If the patient becomes pregnant while taking ORGANIDIN, the drug should be discontinued and the patient should be apprised of the potential risk to the fetus.

WARNINGS

Discontinue use if rash or other evidence of hypersensitivity appears. Use with caution or avoid use in patients with history or evidence of thyroid disease.

PRECAUTIONS

General —Iodides have been reported to cause a flare-up of adolescent acne. Children with cystic fibrosis appear to have an exaggerated susceptibility to the goitrogenic effect of iodides.

Dermatitis and other reversible manifestations of iodism have been reported with chronic use of inorganic iodides. Although these have not been reported to be a problem clinically with ORGANIDIN, they should be kept in mind in patients receiving these preparations for prolonged periods.

Drug Interactions: Iodides may potentiate the hypothyroid effect of lithium and other antithyroid drugs.

Carcinogenesis, Mutagenesis, impairment of fertility: No long-term animal studies have been performed with ORGANIDIN.

Pregnancy Teratogenic Effects: Pregnancy Category X (see CONTRAINDICATIONS).

Nursing Mothers: ORGANIDIN should not be administered to a nursing woman.

ADVERSE REACTIONS

Reports of gastrointestinal irritation, rash, hypersensitivity, thyroid gland enlargement, and acute parotitis have been rare.

OVERDOSAGE

Acute overdosage experience with ORGANIDIN has been rare and there have been no reports of any serious problems.

DOSAGE AND ADMINISTRATION

Note: Add *Solution* to fruit juice or other liquid. One drop *Solution* equals approximately 3 mg ORGANIDIN.

Adults: *Solution* —20 drops 4 times a day.

Tablets —2 tablets 4 times a day, with liquid.

Elixir —1 teaspoonful 4 times a day.

Children: Up to one-half the adult dosage based on the child's weight.

HOW SUPPLIED

ORGANIDIN is available as—

Solution: 5%—clear amber liquid, in 30 ml dropper bottles (NDC 0037-4211-10).

Tablets: 30 mg—round, scored, rose-colored tablets, in bottles of 100 (NDC 0037-4224-40).

Elixir: 1.2%—clear amber liquid, in bottles of one pint (NDC 0037-4213-30) and one gallon (NDC 0037-4213-40).

Storage: Store at room temperature; avoid excessive heat. Keep bottle tightly closed.

ORGANIDIN *Solution* and *Elixir* are
distributed by
WALLACE LABORATORIES
Division of
CARTER-WALLACE, Inc.
Cranbury, New Jersey 08512
Manufactured by
DENVER CHEMICAL (Puerto Rico), Inc.
Humacao, Puerto Rico 00661
ORGANIDIN *Tablets* are manufactured by
WALLACE LABORATORIES
Division of
CARTER-WALLACE, Inc.
Cranbury, New Jersey 08512

Rev. 3/85

Shown in Product Identification Section, page 434

RONDOMYCIN® ℞

(methacycline HCl)

DESCRIPTION

'Rondomycin' (methacycline HCl) is a broad-spectrum antibiotic synthetically derived from oxytetracycline. Chemical dehydration at the 6-position yields a structural homologue which is a light-yellow crystalline powder with a chemical designation of 6-methylene-5-oxytetracycline.

'Rondomycin'-300 contains 300 mg methacycline HCl per capsule. Other ingredients: D&C Red #28. FD&C Blue #1, FD&C Red #40, gelatin. magnesium stearate, sodium lauryl sulfate, starch, titanium dioxide.

'Rondomycin'-150 contains 150 mg methacycline HCl per capsule.

Other ingredients: D&C Red #28. FD&C Blue #1, FD&C Red #40, gelatin. magnesium stearate, sodium lauryl sulfate, starch, titanium dioxide.

ACTIONS

The tetracyclines are primarily bacteriostatic and are thought to exert their antimicrobial effect by the inhibition of protein synthesis. Tetracyclines are active against a wide range of gram-negative and gram-positive organisms.

The drugs in the tetracycline class have closely similar antimicrobial spectra, and cross-resistance among them is common. Micro-organisms may be considered susceptible if the MIC (minimum inhibitory concentration) is not more than 4.0 mcg/ml and intermediate if the MIC is 4.0 to 12.5 mcg/ml.

Susceptibility plate testing: A tetracycline disc may be used to determine microbial susceptibility to drugs in the tetracycline class. If the Kirby-Bauer method of disc susceptibility testing is used, a 30 mcg tetracycline disc should give a zone of at least 19 mm when tested against a tetracycline-susceptible bacterial strain.

Tetracyclines are readily absorbed and are bound to plasma proteins in varying degree. They are concentrated by the liver in the bile and excreted in the urine and feces at high concentrations and in a biologically active form.

INDICATIONS

'Rondomycin' (methacycline HCl) is indicated in infections caused by the following micro-organisms:

Rickettsiae (Rocky Mountain spotted fever, typhus fever and the typhus group, Q fever, rickettsialpox and tick fevers),

Mycoplasma pneumoniae (PPLO, Eaton Agent),

Agents of psittacosis and ornithosis,

Agents of lymphogranuloma venereum and granuloma inguinale,

The spirochetal agent of relapsing fever *(Borrelia recurrentis).*

The following gram-negative micro-organisms:

Haemophilus ducreyi (chancroid),
Pasteurella pestis and *Pasteurella tularensis,*
Bartonella bacilliformis,
Bacteroides species,
Vibrio comma and *Vibrio fetus,*
Brucella species (in conjunction with streptomycin).

Because many strains of the following groups of micro-organisms have been shown to be resistant to tetracyclines, culture and susceptibility testing are recommended.

'Rondomycin' (methacycline HCl) is indicated for treatment of infections caused by the following gram-negative micro-organisms, when bacteriologic testing indicates appropriate susceptibility to the drug:

Escherichia coli,
Enterobacter aerogenes (formerly *Aerobacter aerogenes),*
Shigella species,
Mima species and *Herellea* species,
Haemophilus influenzae (respiratory infections),
Klebsiella species (respiratory and urinary infections).

'Rondomycin' (methacycline HCl) is indicated for treatment of infections caused by the following gram-positive micro-organisms when bacteriologic testing indicates appropriate susceptibility to the drug:

Streptococcus species: Up to 44 percent of strains of *streptococcus pyogenes* and 74 percent of *streptococcus faecalis* have been found to be resistant to tetracycline drugs. Therefore, tetracyclines should not be used for streptococcal disease unless the organism has been demonstrated to be sensitive.

For upper respiratory infections due to group A beta-hemolytic streptococci, penicillin is the usual drug of choice, including prophylaxis of rheumatic fever.

Diplococcus pneumoniae,

Staphylococcus aureus, skin and soft tissue infections. Tetracyclines are not the drugs of choice in the treatment of any type of staphylococcal infections.

Continued on next page

Wallace—Cont.

When penicillin is contraindicated, tetracyclines are alternative drugs in the treatment of infections due to:

Neisseria gonorrhoeae,
Treponema pallidum and *Treponema pertenue* (syphilis and yaws),
Listeria monocytogenes,
Clostridium species,
Bacillus anthracis,
Fusobacterium fusiforme (Vincent's infection),
Actinomyces species.

In acute intestinal amebiasis, the tetracyclines may be a useful adjunct to amebicides.

In severe acne, the tetracyclines may be useful adjunctive therapy.

Tetracyclines are indicated in the treatment of trachoma, although the infectious agent is not always eliminated, as judged by immunofluorescence.

Inclusion conjunctivitis may be treated with oral tetracyclines or with a combination of oral and topical agents.

CONTRAINDICATIONS

This drug is contraindicated in persons who have shown hypersensitivity to any of the tetracyclines.

WARNINGS

THE USE OF DRUGS OF THE TETRACYCLINE CLASS DURING TOOTH DEVELOPMENT (LAST HALF OF PREGNANCY, INFANCY, AND CHILDHOOD TO THE AGE OF 8 YEARS) MAY CAUSE PERMANENT DISCOLORATION OF THE TEETH (YELLOW-GRAY-BROWN). This adverse reaction is more common during long-term use of the drugs but has been observed following repeated short-term courses. Enamel hypoplasia has also been reported. TETRACYCLINE DRUGS, THEREFORE, SHOULD NOT BE USED IN THIS AGE GROUP UNLESS OTHER DRUGS ARE NOT LIKELY TO BE EFFECTIVE OR ARE CONTRAINDICATED.

If renal impairment exists, even usual oral or parenteral doses may lead to excessive systemic accumulation of the drug and possible liver toxicity. Under such conditions, lower than usual total doses are indicated, and, if therapy is prolonged, serum level determinations of the drug may be advisable.

Photosensitivity manifested by an exaggerated sunburn reaction has been observed in some individuals taking tetracyclines. Patients apt to be exposed to direct sunlight or ultraviolet light should be advised that this reaction can occur with tetracycline drugs, and treatment should be discontinued at the first evidence of skin erythema.

The anti-anabolic action of the tetracyclines may cause an increase in BUN. While this is not a problem in those with normal renal function, in patients with significantly impaired function, higher serum levels of tetracyclines may lead to azotemia, hyperphosphatemia, and acidosis.

Usage in pregnancy. (See above "Warnings" about use during tooth development.)

Results of animal studies indicate that tetracyclines cross the placenta, are found in fetal tissues and can have toxic effects on the developing fetus (often related to retardation of skeletal development). Evidence of embryotoxicity has also been noted in animals treated early in pregnancy.

Usage in newborns, infants, and children. (See above "Warnings" about use during tooth development.)

All tetracyclines form a stable calcium complex in any bone-forming tissue. A decrease in the fibula growth rate has been observed in prematures given oral tetracycline in doses of 25 mg/kg every 6 hours. This reaction was shown to be reversible when the drug was discontinued.

Tetracyclines are present in the milk of lactating women who are taking a drug in this class.

PRECAUTIONS

As with other antibiotic preparations, use of this drug may result in overgrowth of nonsusceptible organisms, including fungi. If superinfection occurs, the antibiotic should be discontinued and appropriate therapy instituted.

In venereal diseases when coexistent syphilis is suspected, darkfield examination should be done before treatment is started and the blood serology repeated monthly for at least 4 months.

Because tetracyclines have been shown to depress plasma prothrombin activity, patients who are on anticoagulant therapy may require downward adjustment of their anticoagulant dosage.

In long-term therapy, periodic laboratory evaluation of organ systems, including hematopoietic, renal and hepatic studies should be performed.

All infections due to Group A beta-hemolytic streptococci should be treated for at least 10 days.

Since bacteriostatic drugs may interfere with the bactericidal action of penicillin, it is advisable to avoid giving tetracycline in conjunction with penicillin.

ADVERSE REACTIONS

Gastrointestinal: Anorexia, nausea, vomiting, diarrhea, glossitis, dysphagia, enterocolitis, and inflammatory lesions (with monilial overgrowth) in the anogenital region. These reactions have been caused by both the oral and parenteral administration of tetracyclines.

Skin: Maculopapular and erythematous rashes. Exfoliative dermatitis has been reported but is uncommon. Photosensitivity is discussed above. (See "Warnings".)

Renal toxicity: Rise in BUN has been reported and is apparently dose related. (See "Warnings".)

Hypersensitivity reactions: Urticaria, angioneurotic edema, anaphylaxis, anaphylactoid purpura, pericarditis and exacerbation of systemic lupus erythematosus.

Bulging fontanels in infants and benign intracranial hypertension in adults have been reported in individuals receiving full therapeutic dosages. These conditions disappeared rapidly when the drug was discontinued.

Blood: Hemolytic anemia, thrombocytopenia, neutropenia and eosinophilia have been reported.

When given over prolonged periods, tetracyclines have been reported to produce brown-black microscopic discoloration of thyroid glands. No abnormalities of thyroid function studies are known to occur.

DOSAGE AND ADMINISTRATION

The usual adult dosage of 'Rondomycin' (methacycline HCl) is 600 mg daily. This may be given in four divided doses of 150 mg each or two divided doses of 300 mg each. An initial dose of 300 mg followed by 150 mg every six hours or 300 mg every 12 hours may be used in the management of more severe infections.

In uncomplicated gonorrhea, when penicillin is contraindicated, 'Rondomycin' (methacycline HCl) may be used for treating both males and females in the following clinical dosage schedule: 900 mg initially, followed by 300 mg q.i.d. for a total of 5.4 grams.

For treatment of syphilis, when penicillin is contraindicated, a total of 18 to 24 grams of 'Rondomycin' (methacycline HCl) in equally divided doses over a period of 10–15 days should be given. Close follow-up, including laboratory tests, is recommended.

In Eaton Agent pneumonia, the usual adult dosage is 900 mg daily for 6 days.

The recommended dosage schedule for children above eight years of age is 3 to 6 mg/lb of body weight per day divided into two or four equally spaced doses.

Therapy should be continued for at least 24–48 hours after symptoms and fever have subsided. It should be noted, however, that antibacterial serum levels may usually be present from 24 to 36 hours following the discontinuation of 'Rondomycin' (methacycline HCl).

Concomitant therapy: Antacids containing aluminum, calcium, or magnesium impair absorption and should no be given to patients taking oral tetracyclines.

Food and some dairy products also interfere with absorption. Oral forms of tetracycline should be given 1 hour before or 2 hours after meals. Pediatric oral dosage forms should not be given with milk formulas and should be given at least 1 hour prior to feeding.

In patients with renal impairment (see "Warnings"): Total dosage should be decreased by reduction of recommended individual doses and/or by extending time intervals between doses.

In the treatment of streptococcal infections, a therapeutic dose of tetracycline should be administered for at least 10 days.

HOW SUPPLIED

'Rondomycin'-300 is available as blue and white capsules, each containing 300 mg methacycline HCl equivalent to 280 mg methacycline base, supplied in bottles of 50 (NDC 0037-4101-06).

'Rondomycin'-150 is available as blue and white capsules, each containing 150 mg methacycline HCl equivalent to 140 mg methacycline base, supplied in bottles of 100 (NDC 0037-4001-01).

Rev. 4/85

WALLACE LABORATORIES
Division of
CARTER-WALLACE, INC.
Cranbury, New Jersey 08512

Shown in Product Identification Section, page 434

RYNA™(Liquid)
RYNA-C® Ⓒ
(Liquid)
RYNA-CX® Ⓒ
(Liquid)

(See PDR For Nonprescription Drugs)

RYNATAN® ℞
Tablets
Pediatric Suspension

DESCRIPTION

Rynatan® is an antihistaminic/decongestant combination available for oral administration as **Tablets** and as **Pediatric Suspension.** Each tablet contains:

Phenylephrine Tannate	25 mg
Chlorpheniramine Tannate	8 mg
Pyrilamine Tannate	25 mg

Other ingredients: corn starch, dibasic calcium phosphate, magnesium stearate, methylcellulose, polygalacturonic acid, talc.

Each 5 ml (teaspoonful) of the Pediatric Suspension contains:

Phenylephrine Tannate	5 mg
Chlorpheniramine Tannate	2 mg
Pyrilamine Tannate	12.5 mg

Other ingredients: benzoic acid, FD&C Red No. 3, flavors (natural and artificial), glycerin, kaolin, magnesium aluminum silicate, methylparaben, pectin, purified water, saccharin sodium, sucrose.

CLINICAL PHARMACOLOGY

Rynatan combines the sympathomimetic decongestant effect of phenylephrine with the antihistaminic actions of chlorpheniramine and pyrilamine.

INDICATIONS AND USAGE

Rynatan is indicated for symptomatic relief of the coryza and nasal congestion associated with the common cold, sinusitis, allergic rhinitis and other upper respiratory tract conditions. Appropriate therapy should be provided for the primary disease.

CONTRAINDICATIONS

Rynatan is contraindicated for newborns, nursing mothers and patients sensitive to any of the ingredients or related compounds.

WARNINGS

Use with caution in patients with hypertension, cardiovascular disease, hyperthyroidism, diabetes, narrow angle glaucoma or prostatic hypertrophy. Use with caution or avoid use in patients taking monoamine oxidase (MAO) inhibitors. This product contains antihistamines which may cause drowsiness and may have additive central nervous system (CNS) effects with alcohol or other CNS depressants (e.g., hypnotics, sedatives, tranquilizers).

PRECAUTIONS

General: Antihistamines are more likely to cause dizziness, sedation and hypotension in elderly patients. Antihistamines may cause excitation, particularly in children, but their combination with sympathomimetics may cause either mild stimulation or mild sedation.

Information for Patients: Caution patients against drinking alcoholic beverages or engaging in potentially hazardous activities requiring alertness, such as driving a car or operating machinery, while using this product.

Drug Interactions: MAO inhibitors may prolong and intensify the anticholinergic effects of antihistamines and the overall effects of sympathomimetic agents.

Carcinogenesis, Mutagenesis, Impairment of Fertility: No long-term animal studies have been performed with Rynatan.

Pregnancy: Teratogenic Effects: Pregnancy Category C. Animal reproduction studies have not been conducted with Rynatan. It is also not known whether Rynatan can cause fetal harm when administered to a pregnant woman or can affect reproduction capacity. Rynatan should be given to a pregnant woman only if clearly needed.

Nursing Mothers: Rynatan should not be administered to a nursing woman.

ADVERSE REACTIONS

Adverse effects associated with Rynatan at recommended doses have been minimal. The most common have been drowsiness, sedation, dryness of mucous membranes, and gastrointestinal effects. Serious side effects with oral antihistimines or sympathomimetics have been rare.

OVERDOSAGE

Signs & Symptoms—may vary from CNS depression to stimulation (restlessness to convulsions). Antihistamine overdosage in young children may lead to convulsions and death. Atropine-like signs and symptoms may be prominent.

Treatment—Induce vomiting if it has not occurred spontaneously. Precautions must be taken against aspiration especially in infants, children and comatose patients. If gastric lavage is indicated, isotonic or half-isotonic saline solution is preferred. Stimulants should not be used. If hypotension is a problem, vasopressor agents may be considered.

DOSAGE AND ADMINISTRATION

Administer the recommended dose every 12 hours.

Rynatan Tablets: Adults—1 or 2 tablets.

Rynatan Pediatric Suspension: Children over six years of age—5 to 10 ml (1 to 2 teaspoonfuls); **Children two to six**

years of age—2.5 to 5 ml (½ to 1 teaspoonful); **Children under two years of age**—Titrate dose individually.

HOW SUPPLIED

Rynatan® Tablets: buff, capsule-shaped, compressed tablets in bottles of 100 (NDC 0037-0713-92) and bottles of 500 (NDC 0037-0713-96)

Rynatan® Pediatric Suspension: dark-pink with strawberry-currant flavor, in pint bottles (NDC-0037-0715-68)

Storage: Rynatan Tablets—Store at room temperature; avoid excessive heat—(above 40°C/104°F).

Rynatan Pediatric Suspension—Store at controlled room temperature—between 15°C-30°C (59°F-86°F); protect from freezing.

Rev. 2/85

Shown in Product Identification Section, page 434

RYNATUSS® ℞
Tablets
Pediatric Suspension

DESCRIPTION

RYNATUSS® is an antitussive/ antihistaminic/decongestant/bronchodilator combination available for oral administration as *Tablets* and as *Pediatric Suspension.*

Each tablet contains:

Carbetapentane Tannate	60 mg
Chlorpheniramine Tannate	5 mg
Ephedrine Tannate	10 mg
Phenylephrine Tannate	10 mg

Other ingredients: corn starch, dibasic calcium phosphate, FD&C Blue No. 1, FD&C Red No. 40, magnesium stearate, methylcellulose, polygalacturonic acid, povidone, talc.

Each 5 ml (one teaspoonful) of the Pediatric Suspension contains:

Carbetapentane Tannate	30 mg
Chlorpheniramine Tannate	4 mg
Ephedrine Tannate	5 mg
Phenylephrine Tannate	5 mg

Other ingredients: benzoic acid, FD&C Blue No. 1, FD&C Red No. 3, FD&C Red No. 40, FD&C Yellow #5, flavors (natural and artificial), glycerin, kaolin, magnesium aluminum silicate, methylparaben, pectin, purified water, saccharin sodium, sucrose.

CLINICAL PHARMACOLOGY

RYNATUSS combines the antitussive action of carbetapentane, the sympathomimetic decongestant effect of phenylephrine, the antihistaminic action of chlorpheniramine, and the bronchodilator action of ephedrine.

INDICATIONS AND USAGE

RYNATUSS is indicated for the symptomatic relief of cough associated with respiratory tract conditions such as the common cold, bronchial asthma, acute and chronic bronchitis. Appropriate therapy should be provided for the primary disease.

CONTRAINDICATIONS

RYNATUSS is contraindicated for newborns, nursing mothers and patients who are sensitive to any of the ingredients or related compounds.

WARNINGS

Use with caution in patients with hypertension, cardiovascular disease, hyperthyroidism, diabetes, narrow angle glaucoma or prostatic hypertrophy. Use with caution or avoid use in patients taking monoamine oxidase (MAO) Inhibitors.

This product contains antihistamines which may cause drowsiness and may have additive central nervous system (CNS) effects with alcohol or other CNS depressants (e.g., hypnotics, sedatives, tranquilizers).

PRECAUTIONS

For RYNATUSS Pediatric Suspension only: This product contains FD&C Yellow No. 5 (tartrazine) which may cause allergic-type reactions (including bronchial asthma) in certain susceptible individuals. Although the overall incidence of FD&C Yellow No. 5 (tartrazine) sensitivity in the general population is low, it is frequently seen in patients who also have aspirin hypersensitivity.

General: Antihistamines are more likely to cause dizziness, sedation and hypotension in elderly patients. Antihistamines may cause excitation, particularly in children, but their combination with sympathomimetics may cause either mild stimulation or mild sedation.

Information for patients: Caution patients against drinking alcoholic beverages or engaging in potentially hazardous activities requiring alertness, such as driving a car or operating machinery, while using this product.

Drug interactions: MAO inhibitors may prolong and intensify the anticholinergic effects of antihistamines and the overall effects of sympathomimetic agents.

Carcinogenesis, mutagenesis, impairment of fertility: No long term animal studies have been performed with RYNATUSS.

Pregnancy: Teratogenic Effects: Pregnancy Category C. Animal reproduction studies have not been conducted with RYNATUSS. It is also not known whether RYNATUSS can cause fetal harm when administered to a pregnant woman or can affect reproduction capacity. RYNATUSS should be given to a pregnant woman only if clearly needed.

Nursing mothers: RYNATUSS should not be administered to a nursing woman.

ADVERSE REACTIONS

Adverse effects associated with RYNATUSS at recommended doses have been minimal. The most common have been drowsiness, sedation, dryness of mucous membranes, and gastrointestinal effects. Serious side effects with oral antihistamines or sympathomimetics have been rare.

OVERDOSAGE

Signs and Symptoms: May vary from CNS depression to stimulation (restlessness to convulsions). Antihistamine overdosage in young children may lead to convulsions and death. Atropine-like signs and symptoms may be prominent.

Treatment: Induce vomiting if it has not occurred spontaneously. Precautions must be taken against aspiration especially in infants, children and comatose patients. If gastric lavage is indicated, isotonic or half-isotonic saline solution is preferred. Stimulants should not be used. If hypotension is a problem, vasopressor agents may be considered.

DOSAGE AND ADMINISTRATION

Administer the recommended dose every 12 hours.

RYNATUSS Tablets: Adults—1 to 2 tablets.

RYNATUSS Pediatric Suspension: Children over six years of age—5 to 10 mL (1 to 2 teaspoonfuls); *Children two to six years of age*—2.5 to 5 mL (½ to 1 teaspoonful); *Children under two years of age*—Titrate dose individually.

HOW SUPPLIED

RYNATUSS® Tablets: mauve, capsule-shaped, compressed tablets in bottles of 100 (NDC 0037-0717-92) and bottles of 500 (NDC 0037-0717-96).

RYNATUSS® Pediatric Suspension: pink with strawberry-currant flavor, in bottles of 8 fl oz (NDC 0037-0718-67) and one pint (NDC 0037-0718-68).

STORAGE

RYNATUSS Tablets: Store at room temperature; avoid excessive heat—above 40°C (104°F).

RYNATUSS Pediatric Suspension: Store at controlled room temperature—between 15°C-30°C (59°F-86°F); protect from freezing.

WALLACE LABORATORIES
Division of
CARTER WALLACE, INC.
Cranbury, N.J. 08512 2/85

Shown in Product Identification Section, page 434

SOMA® ℞
(carisoprodol)

DESCRIPTION

'Soma' (carisoprodol) is available as 350 mg round, white tablets. Carisoprodol is N-isopropyl-2-methyl-2-propyl-1,3-propanediol dicarbamate.

Other ingredients: alginic acid, magnesium stearate, potassium sorbate, starch, tribasic calcium phosphate.

ACTIONS

Carisoprodol produces muscle relaxation in animals by blocking interneuronal activity in the descending reticular formation and spinal cord. The onset of action is rapid and effects last four to six hours.

INDICATIONS

Carisoprodol is indicated as an adjunct to rest, physical therapy, and other measures for the relief of discomfort associated with acute, painful musculo-skeletal conditions. The mode of action of this drug has not been clearly identified, but may be related to its sedative properties. Carisoprodol does not directly relax tense skeletal muscles in man.

CONTRAINDICATIONS

Acute intermittent porphyria as well as allergic or idiosyncratic reactions to carisoprodol or related compounds such as meprobamate, mebutamate, or tybamate.

WARNINGS

Idiosyncratic Reactions—On very rare occasions, the first dose of carisoprodol has been followed by idiosyncratic symptoms appearing within minutes or hours. Symptoms reported include: extreme weakness, transient quadriplegia, dizziness, ataxia, temporary loss of vision, diplopia, mydriasis, dysarthria, agitation, euphoria, confusion, and disorientation. Symptoms usually subside over the course of the next several hours. Supportive and symptomatic therapy, including hospitalization, may be necessary.

Usage in Pregnancy and Lactation—Safe usage of this drug in pregnancy or lactation has not been established. Therefore, use of this drug in pregnancy, in nursing mothers, or in women of childbearing potential requires that the potential benefits of the drug be weighed against the potential hazards to mother and child. Carisoprodol is present in breast milk of lactating mothers at concentrations two to four times that of maternal plasma. This factor should be taken into account when use of the drug is contemplated in breast-feeding patients.

Usage in Children—Because of limited clinical experience, 'Soma' is not recommended for use in patients under 12 years of age.

Potentially Hazardous Tasks—Patients should be warned that this drug may impair the mental and /or physical abilities required for the performance of potentially hazardous tasks such as driving a motor vehicle or operating machinery.

Additive Effects—Since the effects of carisoprodol and alcohol or carisoprodol and other CNS depressants or psychotropic drugs may be additive, appropriate caution should be exercised with patients who take more than one of these agents simultaneously.

Drug Dependence—In dogs, no withdrawal symptoms occurred after abrupt cessation of carisoprodol from dosages as high as 1 gm/kg/day. In a study in man, abrupt cessation of 100 mg/kg/day (about five times the recommended daily adult dosage) was followed in some subjects by mild withdrawal symptoms such as abdominal cramps, insomnia, chilliness, headache, and nausea. Delirium and convulsions did not occur. In clinical use, psychological dependence and abuse have been rare, and there have been no reports of significant abstinence signs. Nevertheless, the drug should be used with caution in addiction-prone individuals.

PRECAUTIONS

Carisoprodol is metabolized in the liver and excreted by the kidney; to avoid its excess accumulation, caution should be exercised in administration to patients with compromised liver or kidney function.

ADVERSE REACTIONS

Central Nervous System —Drowsiness and other CNS effects may require dosage reduction. Also observed: dizziness, vertigo, ataxia, tremor, agitation, irritability, headache, depressive reactions, syncope, and insomnia. (See also Idiosyncratic Reactions under "Warnings".)

Allergic or Idiosyncratic —Allergic or idiosyncratic reactions occasionally develop. They are usually seen within the period of the first to fourth dose in patients having had no previous contact with the drug. Skin rash, erythema multiforme, pruritus, eosinophilia, and fixed drug eruption with cross reaction to meprobamate have been reported with carisoprodol. Severe reactions have been manifested by asthmatic episodes, fever, weakness, dizziness, angioneurotic edema, smarting eyes, hypotension, and anaphylactoid shock. (See also Idiosyncratic Reactions under "Warnings".)

In case of allergic or idiosyncratic reactions to carisoprodol, discontinue the drug and initiate appropriate symptomatic therapy, which may include epinephrine, antihistamines, and in severe cases corticosteroids. In evaluating possible allergic reactions, also consider allergy to excipients (information on excipients is available to physicians on request).

Cardiovascular —Tachycardia, postural hypotension, and facial flushing.

Gastrointestinal —Nausea, vomiting, hiccup, and epigastric distress.

Hematologic —Leukopenia, in which other drugs or viral infection may have been responsible, and pancytopenia, attributed to phenylbutazone, have been reported. No serious blood dyscrasias have been attributed to carisoprodol.

DOSAGE AND ADMINISTRATION

The usual adult dosage of 'Soma' (carisoprodol) is one 350 mg tablet, three times daily and at bedtime. Usage in patients under age 12 is not recommended.

OVERDOSAGE

Overdosage of carisoprodol has produced stupor, coma, shock, respiratory depression, and, very rarely, death. The effects of an overdosage of carisoprodol and alcohol or other CNS depressants or psychotropic agents can be additive even when one of the drugs has been taken in the usual recommended dosage. Any drug remaining in the stomach should be removed and symptomatic therapy given. Should respiration or blood pressure become compromised, respiratory assistance, central nervous system stimulants, and pressor agents should be administered cautiously as indicated. Carisoprodol is metabolized in the liver and excreted by the kidney. Although carisoprodol overdosage experience is limited, the following types of treatment have been used successfully with the related drug meprobamate: diuresis, osmotic (mannitol) diuresis, peritoneal dialysis, and hemodialysis (carisoprodol is dialyzable). Careful monitoring of urinary output is necessary and caution should be taken to avoid overhydration. Observe for possible relapse due to incomplete gastric emptying and delayed absorption. Carisoprodol can be measured in biological fluids by gas chromatography (Douglas, J. F. et al: *J Pharm Sci 58:* 145, 1969).

Continued on next page

Wallace—Cont.

HOW SUPPLIED

'Soma': Bottles of 100 (NDC 0037-2001-01) and 500 (NDC 0037-2001-03).

Rev. 4/85

Shown in Product Identification Section, page 434

SOMA® ℞
COMPOUND TABLETS
(carisoprodol 200 mg + aspirin 325 mg)

DESCRIPTION

'Soma' Compound is a combination product containing carisoprodol, a centrally-acting muscle relaxant, plus aspirin, an analgesic with antipyretic and anti-inflammatory properties. It is available as a two-layered, white and orange, round tablet for oral administration. Each tablet contains carisoprodol 200 mg and aspirin 325 mg. Chemically, carisoprodol is N-isopropyl-2-methyl-2-propyl-1,3-propanediol dicarbamate. Its empirical formula is $C_{12}H_{24}N_2O_4$, with a molecular weight of 260.33. The structural formula is:

$$\begin{array}{c} CH_2CH_2CH_3 \\ | \\ H_2NCOOCH_2CCH_2OOCNHCH(CH_3)_2 \\ | \\ CH_3 \end{array}$$

Other ingredients: croscarmellose sodium, FD&C Red #40, FD&C Yellow #6, hydroxypropyl methylcellulose, magnesium stearate, microcrystalline cellulose, povidone, starch, stearic acid.

CLINICAL PHARMACOLOGY

Carisprodol: Carisprodol is a centrally-acting muscle relaxant that does not directly relax tense skeletal muscles in man. The mode of action of carisoprodol in relieving acute muscle spasm of local origin has not been clearly identified, but may be related to its sedative properties. In animals, carisoprodol has been shown to produce muscle relaxation by blocking interneuronal activity and depressing transmission of polysynaptic neurons in the spinal cord and in the descending reticular formation of the brain. The onset of action is rapid and lasts four to six hours.

Carisoprodol is metabolized in the liver and is excreted by the kidneys. It is dialyzable by peritoneal and hemodialysis.

Aspirin: Aspirin is a non-narcotic analgesic with anti-inflammatory and antipyretic activity. Inhibition of prostaglandin biosynthesis appears to account for most of its anti-inflammatory and for at least part of its analgesic and antipyretic properties.

Aspirin is rapidly absorbed and almost totally hydrolyzed to salicylic acid following oral administration. Although aspirin has a half-life of only about 15 minutes, the apparent biologic half-life of salicylic acid in the therapeutic plasma concentration range is between 6 and 12 hours. Salicylic acid is eliminated by renal excretion and by biotransformation to inactive metabolites. Clearance of salicylic acid in the high-dose range is sensitive to urinary pH (see ***Drug Interactions***) and is reduced by renal dysfunction.

INDICATIONS AND USAGE

'Soma' Compound is indicated as an adjunct to rest, physical therapy, and other measures for the relief of pain, muscle spasm, and limited mobility associated with acute, painful musculoskeletal conditions.

CONTRAINDICATIONS

Acute intermittent porphyria; bleeding disorders, allergic or idiosyncratic reactions to carisoprodol, aspirin or related compounds.

WARNINGS

On very rare occasions, the first dose of carisoprodol has been followed by an idiosyncratic reaction with symptoms appearing within minutes or hours. These may include extreme weakness, transient quadriplegia, dizziness, ataxia, temporary loss of vision, diplopia, mydriasis, dysarthria, agitation, euphoria, confusion, and disorientation. Although symptoms usually subside over the course of the next several hours, discontinue 'Soma' Compound and initiate appropriate supportive and symptomatic therapy, which may include epinephrine and/or antihistamines. In severe cases, corticosteroids may be necessary. Severe reactions have been manifested by asthmatic episodes, fever, weakness, dizziness, angioneurotic edema, smarting eyes, hypotension, and anaphylactoid shock.

The effects of carisoprodol with agents such as alcohol, other CNS depressants, or psychotropic drugs may be additive. Appropriate caution should be exercised with patients who may take one or more of these agents simultaneously with 'Soma' Compound.

PRECAUTIONS

General: To avoid excessive accumulation of carisoprodol, aspirin, or their metabolites, use 'Soma' Compound with caution in patients with compromised liver or kidney function, or in elderly or debilitated patients (see CLINICAL PHARMACOLOGY).

Use with caution in patients with history of gastritis or peptic ulcer, in patients on anticoagulant therapy, and in addiction-prone individuals.

Information for Patients: Caution patients that this drug may impair the mental and/or physical abilities required for the performance of potentially hazardous tasks such as driving a motor vehicle or operating machinery.

Caution patients with a predisposition for gastrointestinal bleeding that concomitant use of aspirin and alcohol may have an addictive effect in this regard.

Caution patients that dosage of medications used for gout, arthritis, or diabetes may have to be adjusted when aspirin is administered or discontinued (see ***Drug Interactions***).

Drug Interactions: Clinically important interactions may occur when certain drugs are administered concomitantly with aspirin or aspirin-containing drugs.

1. *Oral Anticoagulants*—By interfering with platelet function or decreasing plasma prothrombin concentration, aspirin enhances the potential for bleeding in patients on anticoagulants.
2. *Methotrexate*—aspirin enhances the toxic effects of this drug.
3. *Probenecid and Sulfinpyrazone*—large doses of aspirin reduce the uricosuric effect of both drugs. Renal excretion of salicylate may also be reduced.
4. *Oral Antidiabetic Drugs*—enhancement of hypoglycemia may occur.
5. *Antacids*—to the extent that they raise urinary pH, antacids may substantially decrease plasma salicylate concentrations; conversely, their withdrawal can result in a substantial increase.
6. *Ammonium Chloride*—this and other drugs that acidify a relatively alkaline urine can elevate plasma salicylate concentrations.
7. *Ethyl Alcohol*—enhanced aspirin-induced fecal blood loss has been reported.
8. *Corticosteroids*—salicylate plasma levels may be decreased when adrenal corticosteroids are given, and may be increased substantially when they are discontinued.

Carcinogenesis, Mutagenesis, Impairment of Fertility: No long-term studies have been done with 'Soma' Compound.

Pregnancy—Teratogenic Effects: **Pregnancy Category C.** Adequate animal reproduction studies have not been conducted with 'Soma' Compound. It is also not known whether 'Soma' Compound can cause fetal harm when administered to a pregnant woman or can affect reproduction capacity. 'Soma' Compound should be given to a pregnant woman only if clearly needed.

Studies in rodents have shown salicylates to be teratogenic when given in early gestation, and embryocidal when given in later gestation in doses considerably greater than usual therapeutic doses in humans. Studies in women who took aspirin during pregnancy have not demonstrated an increased incidence of congenital abnormalities in the offspring.

Labor and Delivery: Ingestion of aspirin near term or prior to delivery may prolong delivery or lead to bleeding in mother, fetus, or neonate.

Nursing Mothers: Carisoprodol is excreted in human milk in concentrations two-to-four times that in maternal plasma. Aspirin is excreted in human milk in moderate amounts and can produce a bleeding tendency in nursing infants. Because of the potential for serious adverse reactions in nursing infants, a decision should be made whether to discontinue nursing or the drug, taking into account the importance of the drug to the mother.

Pediatric Use: Safety and effectiveness in children below the age of twelve have not been established.

ADVERSE REACTIONS

If severe reactions occur, discontinue 'Soma' Compound and initiate appropriate symptomatic and supportive therapy.

The following side effects which have occurred with the administration of the individual ingredients alone may also occur with the combination.

Carisoprodol: *Central Nervous System*—Drowsiness is the most frequent complaint and along with other CNS effects may require dosage reduction. Observed less frequently are dizziness, vertigo and ataxia. Tremor, agitation, irritability, headache, depressive reactions, syncope, and insomnia have been infrequent or rare.

Idiosyncratic—Idiosyncratic reactions are very rare. They are usually seen within the period of the first to fourth dose in patients having had no previous contact with the drug (see WARNINGS).

Allergic—Skin rash, erythema multiforme, pruritus, eosinophilia, and fixed drug eruptions with cross-reaction to meprobamate have been reported. If allergic reactions occur, discontinue 'Soma' Compound and treat symptomatically. In evaluating possible allergic reactions, also consider allergy to excipients (information on excipients is available to physicians on request).

Cardiovascular—Tachycardia, postural hypotension, and facial flushing.

Gastrointestinal—Nausea, vomiting, epigastric distress and hiccup.

Hematologic—No serious blood dyscrasias have been attributed to carisoprodol alone. Leukopenia and pancytopenia have been reported, very rarely, in situations in which other drugs or viral infections may have been responsible.

Aspirin: The most common adverse reactions associated with the use of aspirin have been gastrointestinal, including nausea, vomiting, gastritis, occult bleeding, constipation and diarrhea. Gastric erosion, angioedema, asthma, rash, pruritus and urticaria have been reported less commonly. Tinnitus is a sign of high serum salicylate levels (see OVERDOSAGE).

Aspirin Intolerance—Allergic type reactions in aspirin-sensitive individuals may involve the respiratory tract or the skin. Symptoms of the former range from rhinorrhea and shortness of breath to severe asthma, and the latter may consist of urticaria, edema, rash, or angioedema (giant hives). These may occur independently or in combination.

DRUG ABUSE AND DEPENDENCE

Abuse: In clinical use, abuse has been rare.

Dependence: In clinical use, dependence with 'Soma' Compound has been rare and there have been no reports of significant abstinence signs. Nevertheless, the following information on the individual ingredients should be kept in mind.

Carisoprodol—In dogs, no withdrawal symptoms occurred after abrupt cessation of carisoprodol from dosages as high as 1 gm/kg/day. In a study in man, abrupt cessation of 100 mg/kg/day (about five times the recommended daily adult dosage) was followed in some subjects by mild withdrawal symptoms such as abdominal cramps, insomnia, chills, headache, and nausea. Delirium and convulsions did not occur (see PRECAUTIONS).

OVERDOSAGE

Signs and Symptoms: Any of the following which have been reported with the individual ingredients may occur and may be modified to a varying degree by the effects of the other ingredients present in 'Soma' Compound.

Carisoprodol—Stupor, coma, shock, respiratory depression and, very rarely, death. Overdosage with carisoprodol in combination with alcohol, other CNS depressants, or psychotropic agents can have additive effects, even when one of the agents has been taken in the usually recommended dosage.

Aspirin—Headache, tinnitus, hearing difficulty, dim vision, dizziness, lassitude, hyperpnea, rapid breathing, thirst, nausea, vomiting, sweating and occasionally diarrhea are characteristic of mild to moderate salicylate poisoning. Salicylate poisoning should be considered in children with symptoms of vomiting, hyperpnea, and hyperthermia.

Hyperpnea is an early sign of salicylate poisoning, but dyspnea supervenes at plasma levels above 50 mg/dl. These respiratory changes eventually lead to serious acid-base disturbances. Metabolic acidosis is a constant finding in infants but occurs in older children only with severe poisoning; adults usually exhibit respiratory alkalosis initially and acidosis terminally.

Other symptoms of severe salicylate poisoning include hyperthermia, dehydration, delirium, and mental disturbances. Skin eruptions, GI hemorrhage, or pulmonary edema are less common. Early CNS stimulation is replaced by increasing depression, stupor, and coma. Death is usually due to respiratory failure or cardiovascular collapse.

Treatment—*General:* Provide symptomatic and supportive treatment, as indicated. Any drug remaining in the stomach should be removed using appropriate procedures and caution to protect the airway and prevent aspiration, especially in the stuporous or comatose patient. Incomplete gastric emptying with delayed absorption of carisoprodol has been reported as a cause for relapse. Should respiration or blood pressure become compromised, respiratory assistance, central nervous system stimulants, and pressor agents should be administered cautiously, as indicated.

Carisoprodol: The following have been used successfully in overdosage with the related drug meprobamate: diuretics, osmotic (mannitol) diuresis, peritoneal dialysis, and hemodialysis (see CLINICAL PHARMACOLOGY). Careful monitoring of urinary output is necessary and caution should be taken to avoid overhydration. Carisoprodol can be measured in biological fluid by gas chromatography (Douglas, J.F., et al: *J Pharm Sci 58:* 145, 1969).

Aspirin—Since there are no specific antidotes for salicylate poisoning, the aim of treatment is to enhance elimination of salicylate and prevent or reduce further absorption; to correct any fluid electrolyte or metabolic imbalance; and to provide general and cardiorespiratory support. If acidosis is present, intravenous sodium bicarbonate must be given, along with adequate hydration, until salicylate levels decrease to within the therapeutic range. To enhance elimination, forced diuresis and alkalinization of the urine may be beneficial. The need for hemoperfusion or hemodialysis is rare and should be used only when other measures have failed.

DOSAGE AND ADMINISTRATION

Usual Adult Dosage: 1 or 2 tablets, four times daily.
Not recommended for use in children under age twelve (see PRECAUTIONS).

HOW SUPPLIED

'Soma' Compound Tablets: In bottles of 100 (NDC 0037-2103-01) and 500 (NDC 0037-2103-03) and Unit dose packages of 100 (NDC 0037-2103-85).
Storage: Store at room temperature. Keep bottle tightly closed.

WALLACE LABORATORIES
Division of
CARTER-WALLACE, Inc.
Cranbury, New Jersey 08512

Rev 3/85

Shown in Product Identification Section, page 434

SOMA® COMPOUND with CODEINE ©Ⓡ
(carisoprodol 200 mg + aspirin 325 mg + codeine phosphate 16 mg—
Warning: May be habit-forming)
Tablets

DESCRIPTION

'Soma' Compound with Codeine is a combination product containing carisprodol, a centrally-acting muscle relaxant, plus aspirin, an analgesic with antipyretic and anti-inflammatory properties and codeine phosphate, a centrally-acting narcotic analgesic. It is available as a two-layered, white and yellow, oval shaped tablet for oral administration. Each tablet contains carisoprodol 200 mg, aspirin 325 mg, and codeine phosphate 16 mg. Chemically, carisoprodol is N-isopropyl-2-methyl-2-propyl-1,3-propanediol dicarbamate. Its empirical formula is $C_{12}H_{24}N_2O_4$ with a molecular weight of 260.33. The structural formula is:

$$H_2NCOOCH_2\overset{\displaystyle CH_2CH_2CH_3}{\overset{|}{\underset{\underset{\displaystyle CH_3}{|}}{C}}}CH_2OOCNHCH(CH_3)_2$$

Other ingredients: croscarmellose sodium, D&C Yellow #10, hydroxypropyl methylcellulose, magnesium stearate, microcrystalline cellulose, povidone, sodium metabisulfite, starch, stearic acid.

CLINICAL PHARMACOLOGY

Carisoprodol: Carisoprodol is a centrally-acting muscle relaxant that does not directly relax tense skeletal muscles in man. The mode of action of carisoprodol in relieving acute muscle spasm of local origin has not been clearly identified, but may be related to its sedative properties. In animals, carisoprodol has been shown to produce muscle relaxation by blocking interneuronal activity and depressing transmission of polysynaptic neurons in the spinal cord and in the descending reticular formation of the brain. The onset of action is rapid and lasts four to six hours.
Carisoprodol is metabolized in the liver and is excreted by the kidneys. It is dialyzable by peritoneal and hemodialysis.
Aspirin: Aspirin is a non-narcotic analgesic with anti-inflammatory and antipyretic activity. Inhibition of prostaglandin biosynthesis appears to account for most of its anti-inflammatory and for at least part of this analgesic and antipyretic properties.
Aspirin is rapidly absorbed and almost totally hydrolyzed to salicylic acid following oral administration. Although aspirin has a half-life of only about 15 minutes, the apparent biologic half-life of salicylic acid in the therapeutic plasma concentration range is between 6 and 12 hours. Salicylic acid is eliminated by renal excretion and by biotransformation to inactive metabolite. Clearance of salicylic acid in the high-dose range is sensitive to urinary pH (see **Drug Interactions**) and is reduced by renal dysfunction.
Codeine Phosphate: Codeine phosphate is a centrally-acting narcotic-analgesic. Its actions are qualitatively similar to morphine, but its potency is substantially less.
Clinical studies have shown that combining aspirin and codeine produces a significant additive effect in analgesic efficacy.

INDICATIONS AND USAGE

'Soma' Compound with Codeine is indicated as an adjunct to rest, physical therapy, and other measures for relief of pain, muscle spasm, and limited mobility associated with acute, painful muscoloskeletal conditions when the additional action of codeine is desired.

CONTRAINDICATIONS

Acute intermittent porphyria; bleeding disorders; allergic or idiosyncratic reactions to carisoprodol, aspirin, codeine, or related compounds.

WARNINGS

On very rare occasions, the first dose of carisoprodol has been followed by idiosyncratic reactions with symptoms appearing within minutes or hours. These may include extreme weakness, transient quadriplegia, dizziness, ataxia, temporary loss of vision, diplopia, mydriasis, agitation, euphoria, confusion, and disorientation. Although symptoms usually subside over the course of the next several hours, discontinue 'Soma' Compound with Codeine and initiate appropriate supportive and symptomatic therapy, which may include epinephrine and/or antihistamines. In severe cases, corticosteroids may be necessary. Severe reactions have been manifested by asthmatic episodes, fever, weakness, dizziness, angioneurotic edema, smarting eyes, hypotension, and anaphylactoid shock.
The effects of carisoprodol with agents such as alcohol, other CNS depressants, or psychotropic drugs may be additive. Appropriate caution should be exercised with patients who take one or more of these agents simultaneously with 'Soma' Compound with Codeine.

PRECAUTIONS

General: To avoid excessive accumulation of carisoprodol, aspirin, or their metabolites, use 'Soma' Compound with Codeine with caution in patients with compromised liver or kidney function, or in elderly or debilitated patients (see CLINICAL PHARMACOLOGY.)
Use with caution in patients with history of gastritis or peptic ulcer, in patients on anticoagulant therapy, and in addiction-prone individuals.
Information for Patients: Caution patients that this drug may impair the mental and/or physical abilities required for the performance of potentially hazardous tasks such as driving a motor vehicle or operating machinery.
Caution patients with a predisposition for gastrointestinal bleeding that concomitant use of aspirin and alcohol may have an additive effect in this regard.
Caution patients that dosage of medications used for gout, arthritis, or diabetes may have to be adjusted when aspirin is administered or discontinued (see **Drug Interactions**).
Drug Interactions: Clinically important interactions may occur when certain drugs are administered concomitantly with aspirin or aspirin-containing drugs.

1. *Oral anticoagulants*—By interfering with platelet function or decreasing plasma prothrombin concentration, aspirin enhances the potential for bleeding in patients on anticoagulants.
2. *Methotrexate*—aspirin enhances the toxic effects of this drug.
3. *Probenecid and Sulfinpyrazone*—large doses of aspirin reduce the uricosuric effect of both drugs. Renal excretion of salicylate may also be reduced.
4. *Oral Antidiabetic Drugs*—enhancement of hypoglycemia may occur.
5. *Antacids*—to the extent that they raise urinary pH, antacids may substantially decrease plasma salicylate concentrations; conversely, their withdrawal can result in a substantial increase.
6. *Ammonium Chloride*—this and other drugs that acidify a relatively alkaline urine can elevate plasma salicylate concentrations.
7. *Ethyl Alcohol*—enhanced aspirin-induced fecal blood loss has been reported.
8. *Corticosteroids*—salicylate plasma levels may be decreased when adrenal corticosteroids are given, and may be increased substantially when they are discontinued.

Carcinogenesis, Mutagenesis, Impairment of Fertility: No long-term studies have been done with 'Soma' Compound with Codeine.
Pregnancy—Teratogenic Effects: Pregnancy Category C. Adequate animal reproduction studies have not been conducted with 'Soma' Compound with Codeine. It is also not known whether 'Soma' Compound with Codeine can cause fetal harm when administered to a pregnant woman or can affect reproduction capacity. 'Soma' Compound with Codeine should be given to a pregnant woman only if clearly needed. Studies in rodents have shown salicylates to be teratogenic when given in early gestation, and embryocidal when given in later gestation in doses considerably greater than usual therapeutic doses in humans. Studies in women who took aspirin during pregnancy have not demonstrated an increased incidence of congenital abnormalities in the offspring.
Labor and Delivery: Ingestion of aspirin near term or prior to delivery may prolong delivery or lead to bleeding in mother, fetus, or neonate.
Nursing Mothers: Carisoprodol is excreted in human milk in concentrations two-to-four times that in maternal plasma. Aspirin is excreted in human milk in moderate amounts and can produce a bleeding tendency in nursing infants. Because of the potential for serious adverse reactions in nursing infants, a decision should be made whether to discontinue nursing or the drug, taking into account the importance of the drug to the mother.
Pediatric Use: Safety and effectiveness in children below the age of twelve have not been established.

ADVERSE REACTIONS

If severe reactions occur, discontiue 'Soma' Compound with Codeine and initiate appropriate symptomatic and supportive therapy.
The following side effects which have occurred with the administration of the individual ingredients alone may also occur with the combination.
Carisoprodol: Central Nervous System—Drowsiness is the most frequent complaint and along with other CNS effects may require dosage reduction. Observed less frequently are dizziness, vertigo and ataxia. Tremor, agitation, irritability, headache, depressive reactions, syncope, and insomnia have been infrequent or rare.
Idiosyncratic—Idiosyncratic reactions are very rare. They are usually seen within the period of the first to fourth dose in patients having had no previous contact with the drug (see WARNINGS).
Allergic—Skin rash, erythema multiforme, pruritus, eosinophilia, and fixed drug eruptions with cross-reaction to meprobamate have been reported. If allergic reactions occur, discontinue 'Soma' Compound with Codeine and treat symptomatically. In evaluating possible allergic rections, also consider allergy to excipients (information on excipients is available to physicians on request).
Cardiovascular—Tachycardia, postural hypotension, and facial flushing.
Gastrointestinal—nausea, vomiting, epigastric distress and hiccup.
Hematologic—No serious blood dyscrasias have been attributed to carisoprodol alone. Leukopenia and pancytopenia have been reported, very rarely, in situations in which other drugs or viral infections may have been responsible.
Aspirin: The most common adverse reactions associated with the use of aspirin have been gastrointestinal, including nausea, vomiting, gastritis, occult bleeding, constipation and diarrhea. Gastric erosion, angioedema, asthma, rash, pruritus and urticaria have been reported less commonly. Tinnitus is a sign of high serum salicylate levels (see OVERDOSAGE).
Aspirin Intolerance—Allergic type reactions in aspirin-sensitive indiviuals may involve the respiratory tract or the skin. Symptoms of the former range from rhinorrhea and shortness of breath to severe asthma, and the latter may consist of urticaria, edema, rash, or angioedema (giant hives). These may occur independently or in combination.
Codeine Phosphate: Nausea, vomiting, constipation, miosis, sedation, and dizziness have been reported.

DRUG ABUSE AND DEPENDENCE

Controlled Substance: Schedule C-III (see PRECAUTIONS).
Abuse: In clincal use, abuse has been rare.
Dependence: In clinical use, dependence with 'Soma' Compound with Codeine has been rare and there have been no reports of significant abstinence signs. Nevertheless, the following information on the indiviual ingredients should be kept in mind.
Carisoprodol—In dogs, no withdrawal symptoms occurred after abrupt cessation of carisoprodol from dosages as high as 1 gm/kg/day. In a study in man, abrupt cessation of 100 mg/kg/day (about five times the recommended daily adult dosage) was followed in some subjects by mild withdrawal symptoms such as abdominal cramps, insomnia, chills, headache, and nausea. Delirium and convulsions did not occur (see PRECAUTIONS).
Codeine Phosphate—Drug dependence of the morphine type may result.

OVERDOSAGE

Signs and Symptoms: Any of the following which have been reported with the individual ingredients may occur and may be modified to a varying degree by the effects of the other ingredients present in 'Soma' Compound with Codeine.
Carisoprodol—Stupor, coma, shock, respiratory depression and, very rarely, death. Overdosage with carisoprodol in combination with alcohol, other CNS depressants, or psychotropic agents can have additive effects, even when one of the agents has been taken in the usually recommended dosage.
Aspirin—headache, tinnitus, hearing difficulty, dim vision, dizziness, lassitude, hyperpnea, rapid breathing, thirst, nausea, vomiting, sweating and occasionally diarrhea are characteristic of mild to moderate salicylate poisoning. Salicylate poisoning should be considered in children with symptoms of vomiting, hyperpnea, and hyperthermia.
Hyperpnea is an early sign of salicylate poisoning, but dyspnea supervenes at plasma levels above 50 mg/dl. These respiratory changes eventually lead to serious acid-base disturbances. Metabolic acidosis is a constant finding in infants but occurs in older children only with severe poisoning; adults usually exhibit respiratory alkalosis initially and acidosis terminally.

Continued on next page

Wallace—Cont.

Other symptoms of severe salicylate poisoning include hyperthermia, dehydration, delirium, and mental disturbances. Skin eruptions, GI hemorrhage, or pulmonary edema are less common. Early CNS stimulation is replaced by increasing depression, stupor, and coma. Death is usually due to respiratory failure or cardiovascular collapse.
Codeine Phosphate—pinpoint pupils, CNS depression, coma, respiratory depression, and shock.
Treatment: General:—Provide symptomatic and supportive treatment, as indicated. Any drug remaining in the stomach should be removed using appropriate procedures and caution to protect the airway and prevent aspiration, especially in the stuporous or comatose patient. Incomplete gastric emptying with delayed absorption of carisoprodol has been reported as a cause for relapse. Should respiration or blood pressure become compromised, respiratory assistance, central nervous system stimulants, and pressor agents should be administered cautiously, as indicated.
Carisoprodol—The following have been used successfully in overdosage with the related drug meprobamate: diuretics, osmotic (mannitol) diuresis, peritoneal dialysis, and hemodialysis (see CLINICAL PHARMACOLOGY). Careful monitoring of urinary output is necessary and caution should be taken to avoid overhydration. Carisoprodol can be measured in biological fluid by gas chromatography (Douglas, J.F., et al: *J Pharm Sci 58:* 145, 1969).
Aspirin—Since there are no specific antidotes for salicylate poisoning, the aim of treatment is to enhance elimination of salicylate and prevent or reduce further absorption; to correct any fluid electrolyte and metabolic imbalance; and to provide general and cardiorespiratory support. If acidosis is present, intravenous sodium bicarbonate must be given, along with adequate hydration, until salicylate levels decrease to within the therapeutic range. To enhance elimination, forced diuresis and alkalinization of the urine may be beneficial. The need for hemoperfusion or hemodialysis is rare and should be used only when other measures have failed.
Codeine Phosphate—Narcotic antagonists, such as nalorphine and levallorphan, may be indicated.

DOSAGE AND ADMINISTRATION

Usual Adult Dosage: 1 or 2 tablets, four times daily.
Not recommended for use in children under age twelve.

HOW SUPPLIED

'Soma' Compound with Codeine Tablets: In bottles of 100 (NDC 0037-2403-01).
Storage: Store at room temperature; avoid excessive heat and prolonged light exposure. Keep bottle tightly closed.

Rev. 3/85

Shown in Product Identification Section, page 434

THEO-ORGANIDIN® ℞
Elixir

DESCRIPTION

Theo-Organidin is a bronchodilator/mucolytic-expectorant combination available for oral administration as an *Elixir.* Each 15 ml (tablespoonful) contains theophylline (anhydrous), 120 mg; Organidin® (iodinated glycerol), 30 mg (15 mg organically bound iodine); and alcohol, 15% by volume. Other ingredients: citric acid, flavor, glycerin, purified water, saccharin sodium, sodium benzoate.

CLINICAL PHARMACOLOGY

Theo-Organidin combines the bronchodilator effects of theophylline, a xanthine derivative, and the mucolytic-expectorant action of Organidin. Therapeutic blood levels of theophylline are reached in approximately 15 minutes and peak blood levels in one hour.

INDICATIONS AND USAGE

Theo-Organidin is indicated for symptomatic treatment in bronchial asthma and other bronchospastic conditions such as bronchitis, bronchiolitis, and pulmonary emphysema; for the relief of wheezing and respiratory distress due to reversible bronchospasm and tenacious mucous secretions; and for daily maintenance therapy of patients with bronchial asthma and other chronic bronchospastic pulmonary disorders.

CONTRAINDICATIONS

History of marked sensitivity to inorganic iodides; hypersensitivity to any of the ingredients or related compounds; pregnancy; newborns; and nursing mothers.
The human fetal thyroid begins to concentrate iodine in the 12th to 14th week of gestation and the use of inorganic iodides in pregnant women during this period and thereafter has rarely been reported to induce fetal goiter (with or without hypothyroidism) with the potential for airway obstruction. If the patient becomes pregnant while taking Theo-Organidin, the drug should be discontinued and the patient should be apprised of the potential risk to the fetus.

WARNINGS

Discontinue use if rash or other evidence of hypersensitivity appears. Use with caution or avoid use in patients with history or evidence of thyroid disease. Do not exceed recommended dosage. Do not administer more often than every 6 hours or within 12 hours after rectal administration of any preparation containing theophylline or aminophylline. Use with caution or avoid use with other xanthine derivatives or CNS stimulants.

PRECAUTIONS

General—Children have been known to exhibit marked sensitivity to the CNS stimulant action of the xanthines. Toxic synergism (i.e., CNS stimulation) may occur with other sympathomimetic bronchodilator agents, particularly in children. Iodides have been reported to cause a flare-up of adolescent acne. Children with cystic fibrosis appear to have an exaggerated susceptibility to the goitrogenic effects of iodides.
Dermatitis and other reversible manifestations of iodism have been reported with chronic use of inorganic iodides. Although these have not been reported to be a problem clinically with Organidin formulations, they should be kept in mind in patients receiving these preparations for prolonged periods.
Drug Interactions—Iodides may potentiate the hypothyroid effect of lithium and other antithyroid drugs.
Carcinogenesis, Mutagenesis, Impairment of Fertility—No long-term animal studies have been performed with Theo-Organidin.
Pregnancy—Teratogenic Effects: Pregnancy Category X (see CONTRAINDICATIONS).
Nursing Mothers—Theo-Organidin should not be administered to a nursing woman.

ADVERSE REACTIONS

Side effects sometimes seen with individual ingredients may occur and may be modified as a result of their combination.
Theophylline—Gastric irritation, nausea, and vomiting may occur; these can be minimized by taking Theo-Organidin after meals. Palpitations and mild central nervous system stimulation (e.g., restlessness, sleeplessness) have been reported, particularly in children. *Organidin*—Reports of gastrointestinal irritation, rash, hypersensitivity, thyroid enlargement, and acute parotitis have been rare.

OVERDOSAGE

There have been no reports of any serious problems from overdosage with Theo-Organidin. However, overdosage with theophylline has been reported and the following may be expected if overdosage with Theo-Organidin should occur:
Signs and Symptoms—Toxic overdosage with theophylline may produce severe gastrointestinal adverse effects including nausea, vomiting, epigastric pain, hematemesis and diarrhea; CNS effects including insomnia, headache, irritability, restlessness, severe agitation and convulsions; cardiovascular effects including hypotension, circulatory failure, and life-threatening arrhythmias; renal effects including diuresis and hypokalemia; and respiratory arrest. Serious toxicity leading to seizures and death can occur with serum concentrations of 40 mcg/ml or more.
Treatment—There is no specific antidote for theophylline toxicity. Discontinue drug immediately. Avoid sympathomimetic agents. Emetics and gastric lavage may be of value. Provide general supportive measures to prevent hypotension, overcome hydration, and maintain adequate ventilation. Hemodialysis with the use of resin or charcoal hemoperfusion may be helpful in reducing theophylline serum levels.

DOSAGE AND ADMINISTRATION

Do not exceed recommended dosage. Acute attacks of asthma can usually be terminated fairly rapidly with the recommended dosage of Theo-Organidin; but in severe attacks, or when initiating treatment, the dose may be increased by ½ for up to 24 hours. The need for intravenous aminophylline and/or other regimens should also be considered in the management of severe episodes.
Usual Adult Dosage: For maintenance therapy: 1–2 tablespoonfuls 3 times a day (every 6–8 hours).
For the acute asthmatic attack: 3 tablespoonfuls initially, then reduce to maintenance dosage.
Children: 1 teaspoonful per 20 lbs. (9 kg) body weight, 2–3 times daily. Children over 99 lbs. (45 kg) may require adult dosage.

HOW SUPPLIED

Theo-Organidin Elixir—clear amber liquid, in bottles of one pint (NDC 0037-4611-10) and one gallon (NDC 0037-4611-20).
Storage: Store at room temperature; avoid excessive heat; protect from freezing. Keep bottle tightly closed.

Distributed by
WALLACE LABORATORIES
Division of
CARTER-WALLACE, INC.
Cranbury, New Jersey 08512
Manufactured by Denver Chemical (Puerto Rico), Inc.
Humacao, Puerto Rico 00661

Rev. 6/85

Shown in Product Identification Section, page 434

TUSSI-ORGANIDIN® Ⓒ ℞
TUSSI-ORGANIDIN® DM
Liquid

DESCRIPTION

Tussi-Organidin and *Tussi-Organidin DM* are antitussive/mucolytic-expectorant combinations available for oral administration as a *Liquid. Tussi-Organidin*—Each 5 ml (teaspoonful) contains: Organidin® (iodinated glycerol), 30 mg (15 mg organically bound iodine); and codeine phosphate (*Warning:* May be habit-forming), 10 mg.
Tussi-Organidin DM—Each 5 ml (teaspoonful) contains: Organidin (iodinated glycerol), 30 mg (15 mg organically bound iodine); dextromethorphan hydrobromide, 10 mg.

CLINICAL PHARMACOLOGY

Tussi-Organidin combines the antitussive action of codeine with the mucolytic-expectorant action of Organidin.
Tussi-Organidin DM combines the non-narcotic antitussive action of dextromethorphan with the mucolytic-expectorant action of Organidin.

INDICATIONS AND USAGE

Tussi-Organidin and *Tussi-Organidin DM* are indicated for the symptomatic relief of irritating, nonproductive cough associated with respiratory tract conditions such as chronic bronchitis, bronchial asthma, tracheobronchitis, and the common cold; also for the symptomatic relief of cough accompanying other respiratory tract conditions such as laryngitis, pharyngitis, croup, pertussis and emphysema. Appropriate therapy should be provided for the primary disease.

CONTRAINDICATIONS

History of marked sensitivity to inorganic iodides; hypersensitivity to any of the ingredients or related compounds; pregnancy; newborns; and nursing mothers.
The human fetal thyroid begins to concentrate iodine in the 12th to 14th week of gestation and the use of inorganic iodides in pregnant women during this period and thereafter has rarely been reported to induce fetal goiter (with or without hypothyroidism) with the potential for airway obstruction. If the patient becomes pregnant while taking any of these products, the drug should be discontinued and the patient should be apprised of the potential risk to the fetus.

WARNINGS

Discontinue use if rash or other evidence of hypersensitivity appears. Use with caution or avoid use in patients with history or evidence of thyroid disease.

PRECAUTIONS

General—Iodides have been reported to cause a flare-up of adolescent acne. Children with cystic fibrosis appear to have an exaggerated susceptibility to the goitrogenic effects of iodides.
Dermatitis and other reversible manifestations of iodism have been reported with chronic use of inorganic iodides. Although these have not been a problem clinically with Organidin formulations, they should be kept in mind in patients receiving these preparations for prolonged periods.
Drug Interactions—Iodides may potentiate the hypothyroid effect of lithium and other antithyroid drugs.
Carcinogenesis, Mutagenesis, Impairment of Fertility—No long-term animal studies have been performed with Tussi-Organidin or Tussi-Organidin DM.
Pregnancy—Teratogenic effects: Pregnancy Category X (see CONTRAINDICATIONS).
Nursing Mothers—Tussi-Organidin or Tussi-Organidin DM should not be administered to a nursing woman.

ADVERSE REACTIONS

Side effects with Tussi-Organidin and Tussi-Organidin DM have been rare, including those which may occur with the individual ingredients and which may be modified as a result of their combination:
Organidin—Rare side effects include gastrointestinal irritation, rash, hypersensitivity, thyroid gland enlargement, and acute parotitis.
Codeine—(Tussi-Organidin only): Nausea, vomiting, constipation, drowsiness, dizziness, and miosis have been reported.
Dextromethorphan—(Tussi-Organidin DM only): Rarely produces drowsiness or gastrointestinal disturbances.

DRUG ABUSE AND DEPENDENCE

(Tussi-Organidin only):
Controlled Substance—Schedule V.
Dependence—Codeine may be habit-forming.

OVERDOSAGE

There have been no reports of any serious problems from overdosage with Tussi-Organidin nor Tussi-Organidin DM.

DOSAGE AND ADMINISTRATION

Adults: 1 to 2 teaspoonfuls every 4 hours.
Children: ½ to 1 teaspoonful every 4 hours.

HOW SUPPLIED

Tussi-Organidin Liquid—clear red liquid, in bottles of one pint (NDC 0037-4811-10) and one gallon (NDC 0037-4811-20).
Tussi-Organidin DM Liquid—clear yellow liquid, in bottles of one pint (NDC 0037-4712-10) and one gallon (NDC 0037-4712-20).
Storage: Store at room temperature; avoid excessive heat. Keep bottle tightly closed.

Distributed by
WALLACE LABORATORIES
Division of
CARTER-WALLACE, INC.
Cranbury, New Jersey 08512
Manufactured by
Denver Chemical (Puerto Rico) Inc.
Humacao, Puerto Rico 00661

Rev. 4/84

Shown in Product Identification Section, page 434

VōSoL® Otic Solution ℞
(acetic acid-nonaqueous 2%)

VōSoL® HC Otic Solution ℞
(hydrocortisone 1%, acetic acid–nonaqueous 2%)

DESCRIPTION

VōSoL is a nonaqueous solution of acetic acid (2%), in a propylene glycol vehicle containing propylene glycol diacetate (3%), benzethonium chloride (0.02%), and sodium acetate (0.015%).
VōSoL HC also contains hydrocortisone (1%) and citric acid (0.2%).

ACTIONS

VōSoL is antibacterial, antifungal, and hydrophilic; it has an acid pH and a low surface tension.
VōSoL HC is, in addition, anti-inflammatory and anti-pruritic.

INDICATIONS

VōSoL: For the treatment of superficial infections of the external auditory canal caused by organisms susceptible to the action of the antimicrobial.
VōSol HC: For the treatment of superficial infections of the external auditory canal caused by organisms suspectible to the action of the antimicrobial, complicated by inflammation.

CONTRAINDICATIONS

These products are contraindicated in those individuals who have shown hypersensitivity to any of their components; perforated tympanic membranes are frequently considered a contraindication to the use of external ear canal medication.
VōSoL HC is contraindicated in vaccinia and varicella.

PRECAUTIONS

VōSol and VōSol HC: If sensitization or irritation occurs, medication should be discontinued promptly.
VōSoL HC : As safety of topical steroids during pregnancy has not been confirmed, they should not be used for an extended period during pregnancy. Systemic side effects may occur with extensive use of topical steroids.

DOSAGE AND ADMINISTRATION

Carefully remove all cerumen and debris to allow VōSoL (or VōSoL HC) to contact infected surfaces immediately. To promote continuous contact, insert a VōSoL (or VōSoL HC) saturated cotton wick in the ear with instructions to the patient to keep wick moist for the next 24 hours by occasionally adding a few drops on the wick. Remove wick after first 24 hours and continue to instill 5 drops of VōSoL (or VōSoL HC) three or four times daily thereafter.

HOW SUPPLIED

VōSoL Otic Solution, in 15 ml (NDC 0037-3611-10) and 30 ml (NDC 0037-3611-30) measured-drop, safety-tip plastic bottles.
VōSoL HC Otic Solution, in 10 ml measured-drop, safety-tip plastic bottle (NDC 0037-3811-12).

Distributed by
WALLACE LABORATORIES
Division of
CARTER-WALLACE, INC.
Cranbury, New Jersey 08512
Manufactured by
Denver Chemical (Puerto Rico), Inc.
Humacao, Puerto Rico 00661

Rev. 2/83

Shown in Product Identification Section, page 434

Webcon Pharmaceuticals

Division of
ALCON (Puerto Rico) INC.
P.O. BOX 3000
HUMACAO, PUERTO RICO 00661

SUPPRETTES®, Webcon's identifying trademark for suppository medication in the NEOCERA® BASE, a unique blend of water-soluble Carbowaxes* that release drugs by hydrophilic action.
*TM Union Carbide.

ANESTACON® ℞
[*ăne ′stăcon*]
(2% lidocaine hydrochloride viscous solution for topical use)

DESCRIPTION

A sterile anesthetic for endo-urethral use. Each ml contains: Active: Lidocaine Hydrochloride 20 mg (2%). Vehicle: Hydroxypropyl Methylcellulose 10 mg (1%). Preservative: Benzalkonium Chloride 0.1 mg (0.01%). Inactive: Sodium Chloride, Hydrochloric Acid and/or Sodium Hydroxide (to adjust pH), Purified Water.

CLINICAL PHARMACOLOGY

Lidocaine HCl acts on surface mucous membranes of the urethra to produce local anesthesia by altering the permeability of the nerve cell membrane to sodium and potassium ions, resulting in an increased threshold for electrical excitability and a decreased conduction of impulses whereby depolarization and ion exchanges are inhibited. The anesthetic effect usually begins within two to five minutes and lasts for at least 30 minutes.
Lidocaine is metabolized mainly in the liver and excreted via the kidneys. Approximately 90% of lidocaine administered is excreted in the form of various metabolites, while less than 10% is excreted unchanged.

INDICATIONS AND USAGE

For prevention and control of pain in procedures involving the male and female urethra and for topical treatment of painful urethritis.

CONTRAINDICATIONS

Contraindicated in patients with a known sensitivity (allergy) to lidocaine or other drugs of a similar chemical nature, or to other components of the formulation.

WARNINGS

RESUSCITATIVE EQUIPMENT AND DRUGS SHOULD BE IMMEDIATELY AVAILABLE WHEN ANY LOCAL ANESTHETIC IS USED. Lidocaine should be used with extreme caution on traumatized mucosa or in a region of sepsis. NOT FOR OPHTHALMIC USE.
NOTE: After initial use of the 15 ml single dose container, the remaining contents of the container should be discarded. The 240 ml container should be used for only an individual patient. See CAUTION under DOSAGE AND ADMINISTRATION.

PRECAUTIONS

The smallest volume that will produce effective anesthesia is recommended, and caution should be exercised to avoid overdosage. The safety and effectiveness are dependent on proper dosage, correct technique, adequate precautions, and readiness for emergencies. The debilitated, elderly, acutely ill, and children should be given reduced doses commensurate with their age and physical condition. Use cautiously in persons with known drug sensitivities or allergies.
PREGNANCY CATEGORY C: Animal reproduction studies have not been conducted with ANESTACON®. It is also not known whether ANESTACON can cause fetal harm when administered to a pregnant woman or can affect reproduction capacity. ANESTACON should be administered to a pregnant woman only if clearly needed.
NURSING MOTHERS: It is not known whether this drug is excreted in human milk. Because many drugs are excreted in human milk, caution should be exercised when ANESTACON is administered to a nursing mother.

ADVERSE REACTIONS

Adverse reactions result from high plasma levels due to excessive dosage, rapid absorption, or inadvertent intravascular injection. Hypersensitivity, idiosyncrasy, or diminished tolerance may also be the cause of reactions. Reactions due to overdosage (high plasma levels) are systemic and involve the central nervous system and the cardiovascular system.
Reactions involving the central nervous system are characterized by excitation and/or depression. Nervousness, dizziness, blurred vision or tremors may occur, followed by convulsions, unconsciousness, drowsiness, and possible respiratory arrest. Excitement may be transient or absent, and the first manifestations may be drowsiness, merging into unconsciousness and respiratory arrest.
Reactions involving the cardiovascular system include depression of the myocardium, hypotension, bradycardia, and even cardiac arrest. Treatment of a patient with toxic manifestations consists of maintaining an airway, and supporting ventilation using oxygen and assisted or controlled respiration as required. Supportive treatment of the cardiovascular system consists of using vasopressors, preferably those that stimulate the myocardium (e.g. ephedrine, metaraminol, etc.) and intravenous fluids. Convulsions may be controlled by the intravenous administration in small increments of an ultra-short-acting barbiturate (i.e. thiopental, thiamylal) or a short-acting muscle relaxant (succinylcholine), together with oxygen. Muscle relaxants and intravenous barbiturates should only be used by those familiar with their use.
Allergic reactions are characterized by cutaneous lesions of delayed onset, urticaria, edema, or other manifestations of allergy. The detection of sensitivity by skin testing is of doubtful value.

DOSAGE AND ADMINISTRATION

Dosage varies and depends upon the area to be anesthetized, vascularity of the tissues, individual tolerance, and the technique of anesthesia. The least volume of the drug needed to provide effective anesthesia should be administered. For specific techniques and procedures refer to standard texts. Avoid forceful injection in the presence of known stricture, as this may cause intravascular injection. THE USUAL DOSE SHOULD NOT EXCEED 600 mg or 30 ml OF ANESTACON IN ANY TWELVE HOUR PERIOD.
15 ML SINGLE-DOSE CONTAINER: ADULT MALES: Immediately before use, remove the label and cap and firmly insert the sterile tip into the urethral orifice. Slowly instill 5 ml to 15 ml by exerting pressure on opposite sides of the container - the full dose should be administered in a single action without removing the tip. While waiting two to five minutes for induction of anesthesia, the urethra should be occluded with a penile clamp or by manual compression. ADULT FEMALES: The sterile tip may be used to insert about 1 ml.
240 ml CONTAINER: Note: This is for use for an individual patient only. CAUTION: Care should be taken to prevent contamination of bottle contents (e.g., aspiration of urethral contents into the container when using insertion tip).
ADULT MALES: Instill slowly into the urethra 5 ml to 15 ml and allow two to five minutes for induction of anesthesia. Optimal anesthesia is attained after 5 minutes. The medication is retained in the urethra by means of a penile clamp or by manual compression of the distal urethra. ADULT FEMALES: Apply liberal amount of medication on a cotton swab and insert into urethra for two to five minutes, or a dropper may be employed to insert about 1 ml.

HOW SUPPLIED

In 15 ml single-dose (NDC 0998-0300-10) and 240 ml multiple-dose (NDC 0998-0300-20) disposable containers for single patient use.

B & O SUPPRETTES® Ⓒ ℞
No. 15A and No. 16A
(belladonna and opium rectal suppositories)

DESCRIPTION

Each B & O SUPPRETTE® contains (in the water-soluble Neocera® Suppository Base for rectal administration):
B & O No. 15A: powdered opium* 30 mg (½ gr.) and powdered belladonna extract 16.2 mg (equivalent to 0.21 mg or 0.0035 gr. alkaloid of belladonna).
B & O No. 16A: powdered opium* 60 mg (1 gr.) and powdered belladonna extract 16.2 mg (equivalent to 0.21 mg or 0.0035 gr. alkaloid of belladonna).
Neocera® Base is a blend of polyethylene glycol 400, 1450, 8000 and Polysorbate 60. This drug falls into the pharmacological/therapeutic class of narcotic analgesic/antispasmodic agents.
The pharmacologically active principles present in the belladonna extract component of B & O SUPPRETTES are Atropine and Scopolamine.
Opium contains more than a score of alkaloids, the principal ones being morphine (10%), narcotine (6%), papaverine (1%) and codeine (0.5%). The major pharmacologically active principle of the powdered opium component of B & O SUPPRETTES, however, is morphine.

CLINICAL PHARMACOLOGY

Through its parasympatholytic action, atropine relaxes smooth muscle resulting from parasympathetic stimulation. It is the *dl* isomer of *l*-hyoscyamine and therefore exhibits the same clinical effects. It is, however, approximately one-half as active peripherally as *l*-hyoscyamine, the latter being the major active plant principle. The *dl* isomer atropine is formed during the process of isolation of the belladonna extract.[1]
Morphine, the major active principle of powdered opium, is responsible for the action of powdered opium although the

Continued on next page

Webcon—Cont.

other alkaloids present also contribute to it. The sedative and analgesic action of morphine, the effect desired by inclusion in B & O SUPPRETTES of powdered opium, are thought to be due to its depressant effect on the cerebral cortex, hypothalamus and medullary centers. In large doses the opiates and their analogs also inhibit synaptic conduction in the spinothalamic tracts, depress the function of the reticular formation, the lemniscus and the thalamic relays, and inhibit spinal synaptic reflexes; but these inhibitor actions are not elicited with therapeutic doses of the drug. Moderate doses of powder opium do not alter the electroencephalogram.

The action of morphine consists mainly of a descending depression of the central nervous system. It exerts its analgesic action by increasing the pain threshold or the magnitude of stimulus required to evoke pain and by dulling the sensibility or reaction to pain. In addition to its action in abolishing pain, morphine induces a sense of well being (euphoria) facilitating certain mental processes while retarding others. Upon absorption of morphine, oxidative dealkylation to produce nor-compounds appears to be the first step in the reaction sequence which imparts analgesia. Morphine is conjugated in the liver to form the 3-glucuronide which passes into the bile and is reabsorbed and excreted in the urine.

The atropine effect of the belladonna extract serves to eliminate morphine induced smooth muscle spasm without affecting the sedative analgesic action of powdered opium.[2]

INDICATIONS AND USAGE

B & O SUPPRETTES are used for the relief of moderate to severe pain associated with ureteral spasm not responsive to non-narcotic analgesics and to space intervals between injections of opiates.

CONTRAINDICATIONS

Do not use B & O SUPPRETTES in patients suffering from glaucoma, severe hepatic or renal disease, bronchial asthma, narcotic idiosyncrasies, respiratory depression, convulsive disorders, acute alcoholism, delirium tremens and premature labor.

*WARNINGS

True addiction may result from opium usage. These preparations are not recommended for use in children.

PRECAUTIONS

Administer with caution to persons with a known idiosyncrasy to atropine or atropine-like compounds; to persons known to be sensitive to or addicted to morphine or morphine-like drugs; to persons with cardiac disease, incipient glaucoma or prostatic hypertrophy. Caution should be used in the administration of this drug to old and debilitated patients and patients with increased intracranial pressure, toxic psychosis and myxedema.

Pregnancy Category C. Animal studies have not been conducted with B & O SUPPRETTES No. 15A and No. 16A. It is also not known whether B & O SUPPRETTES No. 15A and No. 16A can affect reproduction capacity. The active principles of B & O SUPPRETTES, atropine and morphine, are known to enter the fetal circulation. Regular use of opium alkaloids during pregnancy has resulted in addiction of the fetus leading to withdrawal symptoms in the neonate. B & O SUPPRETTES No. 15A and No. 16A therefore should be used by a pregnant woman with caution and only when clearly indicated.

Nursing Mothers: It is not known whether this drug is excreted in human milk. Because many drugs are excreted in human milk, caution should be exercised when B & O SUPPRETTES are administered to a nursing woman.

ADVERSE REACTIONS

Belladonna may cause drowsiness, dry mouth, urinary retention, photophobia, rapid pulse, dizziness and blurred vision. Opium usage may result in constipation, nausea or vomiting. Pruritis and urticaria may occasionally occur.

DRUG ABUSE AND DEPENDENCE

Because of their content of opium, B & O SUPPRETTES No. 15A and No. 16A are considered as Schedule II drugs by the Drug Enforcement Agency. No data exists on chronic abuse effects or dependence characteristics of B & O SUPPRETTES No. 15A and No. 16A.

OVERDOSAGE

As with morphine and related narcotics, overdosage is characterized by respiratory depression, pinpoint pupils and coma. Respiratory depression may be reversed by intravenous administration of naloxone hydrochloride. In addition, supportive measures such as oxygenation, intravenous fluids and vasopressors should be used as indicated. As with atropine derivatives, hot, dry, flushed skin; dry mouth and hyperpyrexia may occur.

DOSAGE AND ADMINISTRATION

Adults: One B & O SUPPRETTE No. 15A or No. 16A rectally once or twice daily, not to exceed four doses daily, or as recommended by the physician. Moisten finger and SUPPRETTE with water before inserting. Not recommended for use in children. Absorption is dependent on body hydration and not on body temperature.

HOW SUPPLIED

In strip packaged units of 12 (scored for ½ dosage). DEA order required (Schedule II).

B & O SUPPRETTES No. 15A NDC 0998-5015-75.

B & O SUPPRETTES No. 16A NDC 0998-5016-75.

REFERENCES

1. Gilman, A. G., Goodman, L.S. & Gilman, A., 6th Edition, *The Pharmacological Basis of Therapeutics*, MacMillan Pub. Co., N.Y. 1980, pp. 121–127.
2. Ibid., pp. 494–513.

CYSTOSPAZ® ℞
(Hyoscyamine) Tablets
CYSTOSPAZ-M® ℞
(Hyoscyamine Sulfate) Timed-Release Capsules

DESCRIPTION

CYSTOSPAZ® is a pale blue uncoated compressed tablet for oral administration. It contains the parasympatholytic agent hyoscyamine as the free base. Each tablet contains hyoscyamine 0.15 mg.

CYSTOSPAZ-M® is a light blue timed-release capsule containing hyoscyamine sulfate 0.375 mg.

CLINICAL PHARMACOLOGY

Through its parasympatholytic action, hyoscyamine relaxes smooth muscle spasm resulting from parasympathetic stimulation. It is the λ-isomer of atropine and therefore exhibits the same clinical effects as atropine. It is, however, approximately twice as active peripherally as atropine, since the latter is the racemic (dλ) form of hyoscyamine and d-hyoscyamine possesses only a very weak anticholinergic action. Since only one-half the atropine dose is required for λ-hyoscyamine it has only one-half the unwanted central effects of atropine.[1]

INDICATIONS AND USAGE

In the management of disorders of the lower urinary tract associated with hypermotility. Although specific therapy is often required to remove the underlying cause of spasm, CYSTOSPAZ Tablets and CYSTOSPAZ-M Capsules are offered as antispasmodic agent dosage forms which may be combined with other forms of therapy where indicated.

CONTRAINDICATIONS

Glaucoma, urinary bladder neck or pyloric obstruction, duodenal obstruction and cardiospasm. Hypersensitivity to any of the ingredients.

PRECAUTIONS

Administer with caution to persons with known idiosyncrasy to atropine-like compounds and to patients suffering cardiac disease.

Pregnancy Category C. Animal reproduction studies have not been conducted with CYSTOSPAZ Tablets or CYSTOSPAZ-M Capsules. It is also not known whether CYSTOSPAZ Tablets or CYSTOSPAZ-M Capsules can cause fetal harm when administered to a pregnant woman or can affect reproduction capacity. CYSTOSPAZ Tablets and CYSTOSPAZ-M Capsules should be taken by a pregnant woman only if clearly needed.

Nursing Mothers: It is not known whether this drug is excreted in human milk. Because many drugs are excreted in human milk, caution should be exercised when CYSTOSPAZ Tablets or CYSTOSPAZ-M Capsules are administered to a nursing woman.

ADVERSE REACTIONS

Though rarely a problem, the side effects encountered with this class of antispasmodic-antisecretory agents (drowsiness, dryness of mouth, photophobia, constipation, urinary retention) may also be seen with this drug. If rapid pulse, dizziness or blurring of vision occurs, discontinue use immediately. Acute urinary retention may be precipitated in prostatic hypertrophy. **Note:** Slight dryness of mouth is an indication that parasympathetic blockage is effective. The patient should be warned that this may occur.

DRUG ABUSE AND DEPENDENCE

A dependence on the use of CYSTOSPAZ Tablets or CYSTOSPAZ-M Capsules has not been reported and due to the nature of their ingredients, abuse of CYSTOSPAZ Tablets or CYSTOSPAZ-M Capsules is not expected.

OVERDOSAGE

Symptoms of overdosage include severe dryness of mouth, nose throat, and hot dry flushed skin, hyperpyrexia (especially in children), difficulty or inability to swallow, difficult speech, dilated pupils until iris almost disappears, restlessness and garrulity indicating an irritability of the brain, marked tremors, convulsions, respiratory failure, death.[2] In adults, symptoms of overdosage may begin in the range of ingestion of 0.6 to 1 mg with doses exceeding 1–2 mg eliciting more profound toxicity.

DOSAGE AND ADMINISTRATION

Adults: CYSTOSPAZ® Tablets—One or two tablets four times daily or fewer if needed. CYSTOSPAZ-M® Capsules—One capsule every twelve hours.

Children (12 and under): Reduce dosage in proportion to age and weight.

HOW SUPPLIED

CYSTOSPAZ Tablets— Bottles of 100 light blue tablets NDC 0998-2225-10. Tablets are imprinted with a "**W** 2225".

CYSTOSPAZ-M Capsules—Bottles of 100 light blue timed-release capsules NDC 0998-2260-10. Capsules are identified with "**W** 2260" printed in black.

REFERENCES

1. Gilman, A. L., Goodman, L.S. & Gilman, A., *The Pharmacological Basis of Therapeutics*, 6th Edition, p. 125.
2. Ibid., p. 127.

CYSTOSPAZ-M Capsules are manufactured by:
K. V. Pharmaceutical Company
St. Louis, Mo. 63144

URISED® ℞

DESCRIPTION

URISED® is a purple, round, sugar coated tablet for oral administration. It is a combination of antiseptics (Methenamine, Methylene Blue, Phenyl Salicylate, Benzoic Acid) and parasympatholytics (Atropine Sulfate, Hyoscyamine). Each tablet contains: Methenamine 40.8 mg, Phenyl Salicylate 18.1 mg, Methylene Blue 5.4 mg, Benzoic Acid 4.5 mg, Atropine Sulfate 0.03 mg and Hyoscyamine 0.03 mg.

CLINICAL PHARMACOLOGY

Methenamine itself does not have antiseptic, irritant, or toxic properties in the urine. Methenamine, in an acid urine (pH 6 or below) hydrolyzes into formaldehyde within the urinary tract providing mild antiseptic activity[1]. When given as directed and the daily urine volume is 1000 to 1500 ml, a daily dose of 2 grams will yield a urinary concentration of 18–60 mcg/ml of free formaldehyde in the urine. This is more than the minimal inhibitory dose of formaldehyde which must be available for most urinary tract pathogens. Methenamine is readily absorbed from the gastrointestinal tract and is rapidly excreted almost entirely in the urine. Methylene Blue and Benzoic Acid are mild but effective antiseptics which contribute to the antiseptic properties of Methenamine. Phenyl Salicylate is a mild analgesic and antipyretic with weak antiseptic activity. All of these compounds are readily absorbed from the gastrointestinal tract and excreted in the urine. Through parasympatholytic action, atropine and hyoscyamine relax smooth muscle spasms resulting from parasympathetic stimulation.[2]

INDICATIONS AND USAGE

URISED is indicated for the relief of discomfort of the lower urinary tract caused by hypermotility resulting from inflammation or diagnostic procedures and in the treatment of cystitis, urethritis, and trigonitis when caused by organisms which maintain or produce an acid urine and are susceptible to formaldehyde.

CONTRAINDICATIONS

Glaucoma, urinary bladder neck obstruction, pyloric or duodenal obstruction, or cardiospasm. Hypersensitivity to any of the ingredients.

WARNINGS

Do not exceed recommended dose. Methenamine may combine with sulfonamides in the urine to give mutual antagonism and should not be used with sulfonamides.

PRECAUTIONS

Administer with caution to persons with known idiosyncrasy to atropine-like compounds and to patients suffering from cardiac disease. Bacteriological studies of the urine may be helpful in following the patient response. Methylene Blue interferes with the analysis for some urinary components such as free formaldehyde. Drugs and/or foods which produce an alkaline urine should be restricted.[3]

Patient should be advised that the urine may become blue to blue-green and the feces may be discolored as a result of excretion of Methylene Blue. Methenamine preparations should not be given to patients taking sulfonamides since insoluble precipitates may form with formaldehyde in the urine. No known long-term animal studies have been performed to evaluate carcinogenic potential.

Pregnancy Category C. Animal reproduction studies have not been conducted with URISED® tablets. It is also not known whether URISED tablets can cause fetal harm when administered to a pregnant woman or can affect reproduction capacity. URISED tablets should be given to a pregnant woman only if clearly needed.

Nursing Mothers: It is not known whether this drug is excreted in human milk. Because many drugs are excreted in human milk, caution should be exercised when URISED tablets are administered to a nursing woman.

ADVERSE REACTIONS

If pronounced dryness of the mouth, flushing, or difficulty in initiating micturition occurs, decrease dosage. If rapid pulse, dizziness or blurring of vision occurs, discontinue use immediately. Acute urinary retention may be precipitated in prostatic hypertrophy.

DRUG ABUSE AND DEPENDENCE

A dependence on the use of URISED has not been reported and due to the nature of its ingredients, abuse of URISED is not expected.

OVERDOSAGE

By exceeding the recommended dosage of URISED, symptomology related to the overdose of its individual active ingredients may be expected as follows:

Atropine Sulfate, Hyoscyamine: Symptoms associated with an overdosage of URISED will most probably be manifested in the symptoms related to overdosage of the alkaloids Atropine Sulfate and Hyoscyamine. Such symptoms as dryness of mucous membranes; dilatation of pupils, hot, dry, flushed skin; hyperpyrexa; tachycardia; palpitations; elevated blood pressure; coma; circulatory collapse and death from respiratory failure can occur due to overdosage of these alkaloids.

Methenamine: If large amounts of the drug (2-8 gm daily) are used over extended periods, (3-4 weeks), bladder and gastrointestinal irritation, painful and frequent micturition, albuminuria and gross hematuria may be expected.

Methylene Blue: Symptoms of Methylene Blue overdosage associated with the overdosage of URISED are not expected to be discernible from those associated with the other active ingredients in URISED.

Benzoic Acid: Symptoms of Benzoic Acid overdosage associated with the overdosage of URISED are not expected to be discernible from those associated with the other active ingredients in URISED.

Phenyl Salicylate: Symptoms of Phenyl Salicylate overdosage include burning pain in throat and mouth, white necrotic lesions in the mouth, abdominal pain, vomiting, bloody diarrhea, pallor, sweating, weakness, headache, dizziness and tinnitus. The symptoms, however, are not expected to be discernible from those associated with the other active ingredients in URISED.

DOSAGE AND ADMINISTRATION

Adults: Two tablets four times daily.

Children (12 years and older): Reduce dosage in proportion to age and weight.

HOW SUPPLIED

Bottles of 100 (NDC 0998-2183-10), 500 (NDC 0998-2183-20) and 1000 (NDC 0998-2183-30) tablets. Tablets are imprinted with a "**W 2183**".

REFERENCES

1. Stamey, T. A., *Urinary Infections.* Williams & Wilkins Co., Baltimore 1972.
2. Goodman, L. S. and Gilman, G., *The Pharmacological Basis of Therapeutics,* Sixth Edition, Macmillan Pub. Co. 121, 971, 980, 1119 (1980).
3. *AMA Drug Evaluation,* Fifth Edition, 1745 (1983).

Westwood Pharmaceuticals Inc.

100 FOREST AVENUE
BUFFALO, NY 14213

ALPHA KERI®
Therapeutic Shower and Bath Oil

COMPOSITION

Contains mineral oil, Hydroloc™ brand of Westwood's PEG-4 dilaurate, lanolin oil, fragrance, benzophenone-3, D&C green 6.

ACTION AND USES

ALPHA KERI is a water-dispersible, antipruritic oil for the care of dry skin. ALPHA KERI effectively deposits a thin, uniform, emulsified film of oil over the skin. This film helps relieve itching, lubricates and softens the skin. ALPHA KERI Shower and Bath Oil is an all-over skin moisturizer. Only Alpha Keri contains Hydroloc™ — the unique emulsifier that provides a more uniform distribution of the therapeutic oils to moisturize dry skin. ALPHA KERI is valuable as an aid in the treatment of dry, pruritic skin and mild skin irritations such as chronic atopic dermatitis; pruritus senilis and hiemalis; contact dermatitis; "bath-itch"; xerosis or asteatosis; ichthyosis; soap dermatitis; psoriasis.

ADMINISTRATION AND DOSAGE

ALPHA KERI *should always be used with water, either added to water or rubbed onto wet skin.* Because of its inherent cleansing properties it is not necessary to use soap when ALPHA KERI is being used.

For exact dosage, label directions should be followed.
BATH: Added as directed to bathtub of water. For optimum relief: 10 to 20 minute soak.
SHOWER: Dispense a small amount into hand and rub onto wet skin. Rinse as desired and pat dry.
SPONGE BATH: Added as directed to a basin of warm water then rubbed over entire body with washcloth.
SITZ BATH: Added as directed to tub water. Soak should last for 10 to 20 minutes.
INFANT BATH: Added as directed to basin or bathinette of water.
SKIN CLEANSING OTHER THAN BATH OR SHOWER: A small amount is rubbed onto wet skin. Rinse. Pat dry.

PRECAUTION

The patient should be warned to guard against slipping in tub or shower.

HOW SUPPLIED

4 fl. oz. (NDC 0072-3600-04), 8 fl. oz. (NDC 0072-3600-08) and 16 fl. oz. (NDC 0072-3600-16) plastic bottles. Also available in non-aerosol pump spray, 5.5 oz. (NDC 0072-3600-05)

ALPHA KERI® MOISTURIZING BAR
Non-detergent Soap

COMPOSITION

Sodium tallowate, sodium cocoate, water, mineral oil, fragrance, PEG-75, glycerin, titanium dioxide, lanolin oil, sodium chloride, BHT, trisodium HEDTA, D&C Green 5, D&C Yellow 10.

ACTION AND USES

ALPHA KERI Moisturizing Bar, rich in emollient oils, thoroughly cleanses as it soothes and softens the skin.

INDICATIONS

Adjunctive use in dry skin care.

ADMINISTRATION AND DOSAGE

To be used as any other soap.

HOW SUPPLIED

4 oz. (NDC 0072-3500-04) bar.

BALNETAR®
Water-dispersible Emollient Tar

COMPOSITION

Contains WESTWOOD® TAR (equivalent to 2.5% Coal Tar USP) in mineral oil, laureth-4, lanolin oil, PEG-4 dilaurate, fragrance, and sodium dioctyl sulfosuccinate.

ACTION AND USES

For temporary relief of itching and scaling due to psoriasis, eczema, and other tar-responsive dermatoses. Tar ingredient is chemically and biologically standardized to insure uniform therapeutic activity. BALNETAR exerts keratoplastic, antieczematous, antipruritic, and emollient actions. It deposits microfine particles of tar over the skin in a lubricant-moisturizing film that helps soften and remove scales and crusts, making the skin smoother and more supple. BALNETAR is an important adjunct in a wide range of dermatoses, including: atopic dermatitis; chronic eczematoid dermatitis; seborrheic dermatitis.

CONTRAINDICATIONS

Not indicated when acute inflammation is present.

ADMINISTRATION AND DOSAGE

BALNETAR *should always be used with water... either added to water or rubbed onto wet skin.* For exact dosage label directions are to be followed.
IN THE TUB—Add as directed to a bathtub of water. Soap is not used. The patient soaks for 10 to 20 minutes and then pats dry.
FOR DIRECT APPLICATION—A small amount is rubbed onto the wet skin. Excess is wiped off with tissue to help prevent staining of clothes or linens.
FOR SCALP APPLICATION —A small amount is rubbed onto the wet scalp with fingertips.

CAUTION

If irritation persists, discontinue use. May temporarily discolor blond, bleached or tinted hair. In rare cases BALNETAR may cause allergic sensitization attributable to coal tar. For external use only. Keep this and all drugs out of reach of children.

PRECAUTION

After use of BALNETAR, patient should avoid exposure to direct sunlight unless sunlight is being used therapeutically in a supervised, modified Goeckerman regimen. Contact with the eyes should be avoided. Patient should be cautioned against slipping when BALNETAR is used in bathtub. Also advise patient that use in a plastic or fiberglass tub may cause staining of the tub.

HOW SUPPLIED

8 fl. oz. (NDC 0072-4200-08) plastic shatterproof bottle.

CAPITROL® ℞
(chloroxine 2%)
Cream Shampoo

CAUTION

Federal law prohibits dispensing without prescription.

DESCRIPTION

CAPITROL is an antibacterial cream shampoo containing 2% chloroxine (each gram contains 20 mg chloroxine) suspended in a base of sodium octoxynol-3 sulfonate, PEG-6 lauramide, dextrin, stearyl alcohol/ceteareth-20, sodium lauryl sulfoacetate, dioctyl sodium sulfosuccinate, magnesium aluminum silicate, PEG-14M, EDTA, citric acid, water, color, fragrance and 1% benzyl alcohol. The pH of the shampoo is 7.0.
Chloroxine is a synthetic antibacterial compound that is effective in the treatment of dandruff and seborrheic dermatitis when incorporated in a shampoo.
The chemical name of chloroxine 5,7-dichloro-8-hydroxyquinoline. The chemical structure of chloroxine is:

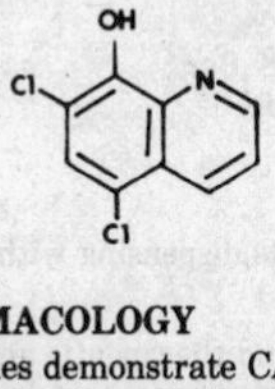

CLINICAL PHARMACOLOGY

Well controlled studies demonstrate CAPITROL effectively reduces the excess scaling in patients with dandruff or seborrheic dermatitis. Though the cause of dandruff is not known it is thought to be the result of accelerated mitotic activity in the epidermis. The presumed mechanism of action to reduce scaling would be to slow down the mitotic activity.
The role of microbes in seborrheic dermatitis is not known; however, *Staphylococcus aureus* and *Pityrosporon* species are often present in increased numbers during the course of the disease. Chloroxine is antibacterial, inhibiting the growth of Gram-positive as well as some Gram-negative organisms. Antifungal activity against some dermatophytes and yeasts also has been shown.
The absorption, metabolism and pharmacokinetics of CAPITROL in humans have not been studied.

INDICATIONS AND USAGE

CAPITROL is indicated in the treatment of dandruff and mild-to-moderately severe seborrheic dermatitis of the scalp. Clinical studies indicate that improvement may be observed after 14 days of therapy.

CONTRAINDICATIONS

CAPITROL is contraindicated in those patients with a history of hypersensitivity to any of the listed ingredients.

WARNINGS

CAPITROL should not be used on acutely inflamed (exudative) lesions of the scalp.

PRECAUTIONS

Information for patients: Exercise care to prevent CAPITROL from entering the eyes. If contact occurs, the patient should flush eyes with cool water. Discoloration of light-colored hair (e.g. blond, gray or bleached) may follow use of this preparation.
Irritation and a burning sensation on the scalp and adjacent areas have been reported.

Drug/Laboratory Test Interactions: There is no known interference of CAPITROL with laboratory tests.

Carcinogenesis, Mutagenesis: No long term studies in animals have been performed to evaluate the carcinogenic potential of CAPITROL.
Results of the *in vitro* Ames Salmonella/Microsome Plate test show that CAPITROL does not demonstrate genetic activity and is considered non-mutagenic.

Teratogenic Effects

Pregnancy Category C: Animal reproduction studies have not been conducted with CAPITROL. It is also not known whether CAPITROL can cause fetal harm when administered to a pregnant woman or can affect reproduction capacity. CAPITROL should be given to a pregnant woman only if clearly needed.

Nursing Mothers: It is not known whether this drug is excreted in human milk. Because many drugs are excreted in human milk, caution should be exercised when CAPITROL is administered to a nursing woman.

Pediatric Use: Specific studies to demonstrate the safety and effectiveness for use of CAPITROL in children have not been conducted.

Continued on next page

Westwood—Cont.

ADVERSE REACTION
One patient out of 225 in clinical studies was reported to have contact dermatitis.

OVERDOSAGE
The acute oral LD_{50} in mice was found to be 200 mg/kg and in rats 450 mg/kg. On the basis of these animal studies, CAPITROL may be considered practically non-toxic.

DOSAGE AND ADMINISTRATION
CAPITROL should be massaged thoroughly onto the wet scalp, avoiding contact with the eyes. Lather should remain on the scalp for approximately three minutes, then rinsed. The application should be repeated and the scalp rinsed thoroughly. Two treatments per week are usually sufficient.

HOW SUPPLIED
CAPITROL shampoo contains 2% chloroxine (20 mg chloroxine per gram) and is supplied in 85 g plastic tubes, (NDC 0072-6800-02).

DESQUAM-X10® Bar ℞
10% benzoyl peroxide

CAUTION
Federal law prohibits dispensing without prescription.

DESCRIPTION
DESQUAM-X10 brand therapeutic anti-acne BAR contains 10% benzoyl peroxide, boric acid, cellulose gum, dextrin (may contain wheat starch), disodium EDTA, docusate sodium, lactic acid, PEG-14M, sodium lauryl sulfoacetate (or sodium dodecyl benzene sulfonate and trisodium sulfosuccinate), sorbitol, urea and water.

O=C–O–O–C=O

Benzoyl Peroxide

CLINICAL PHARMACOLOGY
The effectiveness of benzoyl peroxide in the treatment of acne vulgaris is primarily attributable to its antibacterial activity, especially with respect to *Propionibacterium acnes*, the predominant organism in sebaceous follicles and comedones. The antibacterial activity of this compound is presumably due to the release of active or free-radical oxygen capable of oxidizing bacterial proteins. In acne patients treated topically with benzoyl peoxide, resolution of the acne usually coincides with reduction in the levels of *P. acnes* and free fatty acids (FFA). Mild desquamation is another observed action of topically applied benzoyl peroxide and may also play a role in the drug's effectiveness in acne. Studies also indicate that topical benzoyl peroxide may exert a sebostatic effect with a resultant reduction of skin surface lipids.
Benzoyl peroxide has been shown to be absorbed by the skin, where it is metabolized to benzoic acid and then excreted as benzoate in the urine.

INDICATIONS AND USAGE
DESQUAM-X10 BAR is indicated for the topical treatment of acne. It may be used as an adjunct in therapeutic regimens including benzoyl peroxide gels, antibiotics, retinoic acid products and sulfur/salicylic acid-containing preparations. The improvement of the treated condition is dependent on the degree and type of acne, the frequency of use of DESQUAM-X10 BAR and the nature of other therapies employed.

CONTRAINDICATIONS
This product should not be used in patients known to be sensitive to benzoyl peroxide or any other of the listed ingredients.

PRECAUTIONS
General: Avoid contact with eyes and other mucous membranes. For external use only. In patients known to be sensitive to the following substances, there is a possibility of cross-sensitization: benzoic acid derivatives (including certain topical anesthetics) and cinnamon.
Information for Patients: This product may bleach colored fabric or hair. Concurrent use with PABA-containing suncreens may result in transient discoloration of the skin.
Carcinogenesis, Mutagenesis, Impairment of Fertility: Based upon considerable evidence, benzoyl peroxide is not considered to be a carcinogen. However, in one study, using mice known to be highly susceptible to cancer, there was evidence for benzoyl peroxide as a tumor promoter. Benzoyl peroxide has been found to be inactive as a mutagen in the Ames Salmonella and other assays, including the mouse dominant lethal assay. This assay is frequently used to assess the effect of substances on spermatogenesis.
Pregnancy (Category C): Animal reproduction studies have not been conducted with benzoyl peroxide (DESQUAM-X10 BAR). It is also not known whether benzoyl peroxide can cause fetal harm when administered to a pregnant woman or can affect reproductive capacity. Benzoyl peroxide should be given to a pregnant woman only if clearly needed.
Nursing Mothers: It is not known whether this drug is excreted in human milk. Caution should be exercised when benzoyl peoxide is administered to a nursing woman.
Pediatric Use: Safety and effectiveness in children below the age of 12 have not been established.

ADVERSE REACTIONS
Adverse reactions which may be encountered with topical benzoyl peroxide include excessive drying (manifested by marked peeling, erythema and possible edema) and allergic contact sensitization.
Excessive dryness would appear to occur in approximately 2 patients in 50.
Pertinent literature would seem to indicate that allergic sensitization to benzoyl peroxide may occur in 10 to 25 patients in 1,000. There is one reference that reports an occurrence of sensitization in 5 of 100 patients.

OVERDOSAGE
In the event that excessive scaling, erythema or edema occur, the use of this preparation should be discontinued. If the reaction is judged to be due to excessive use and not allergenicity, after symptoms and signs subside, a reduced dosage schedule may be cautiously tried.
To hasten resolution of the adverse effects, emollients, cool compresses and/or topical corticosteroid preparations may be used.

DOSAGE AND ADMINISTRATION
Wash entire area gently with fingertips for 1 to 2 minutes 2 or 3 times daily or as physician directs. Rinse well. The desired degree of dryness and peeling may be obtained by regulating frequency of use.

HOW SUPPLIED
DESQUAM-X BAR (10%):

3.75 oz.	carton	NDC 0072-2000-04

Store at controlled room temperature (59°–86°F).

DESQUAM-X$^{2.5}$® Gel ℞
2.5% Benzoyl Peroxide, 6% Laureth-4

DESQUAM-X^{5}® Gel ℞
5% Benzoyl Peroxide, 6% Laureth-4

DESQUAM-X^{10}® Gel ℞
10% Benzoyl Peroxide, 6% Laureth-4

CAUTION
Federal law prohibits dispensing without prescription.

DESCRIPTION
DESQUAM-X2.5, DESQUAM-X5 and DESQUAM-X10 brand topical anti-acne gels contain benzoyl peroxide (2.5, 5 and 10%) and laureth-4 (6%), in a water-base vehicle of carbomer 940, diisopropanolamine and disodium edetate.

benzoyl peroxide

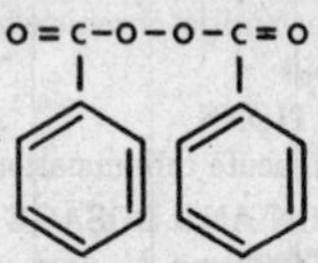

laureth-4

CLINICAL PHARMACOLOGY
The effectiveness of benzoyl peroxide in the treatment of acne vulgaris is primarily attributable to its antibacterial activity, especially with respect to *Propionibacterium acnes*, the predominant organism in sebaceous follicles and comedones. The antibacterial activity of this compound is presumably due to the release of active or free-radical oxygen capable of oxidizing bacterial proteins. In acne patients treated topically with benzoyl peroxide, resolution of the acne usually coincides with reduction in the levels of *P. acnes* and free fatty acids (FFA). Mild desquamation is another observed action of topically applied benzoyl peroxide and may also play a role in the drug's effectiveness in acne. Studies also indicate that topical benzoyl peroxide may exert a sebostatic effect with a resultant reduction of skin surface lipids.
Benzoyl peroxide has been shown to be absorbed by the skin, where it is metabolized to benzoic acid and then excreted as benzoate in the urine.
Laureth-4 is a non-toxic surfactant which exerts its action through cleansing and mild desquamation. The result of these actions is a drying and degreasing of the skin.

INDICATIONS AND USAGE
DESQUAM-X (2.5, 5 or 10) GEL is indicated for the topical treatment of mild to moderate acne vulgaris and as an adjunct in therapeutic regimens including antibiotics, retinoic acid products and sulfur/salicylic acid-containing preparations. DESQUAM-X GEL has been shown effective in the treatment of the following acne lesion types: papules, pustules, open and closed comedones. Clinical studies have demonstrated therapeutic response after two to three weeks. DESQUAM-X GEL may also be used as adjunctive treatment for nodulo-cystic acne (acne conglobata), although its effectiveness for this condition has not been proven.

CONTRAINDICATIONS
This product should not be used in patients known to be hypersensitive to benzoyl peroxide or any of the other listed ingredients.

PRECAUTIONS
General: Avoid contact with eyes and other mucous membranes. For external use only. In patients known to be sensitive to the following substances, there is a possibility of cross-sensitization: benzoic acid derivatives (including certain topical anesthetics) and cinnamon.
Information for Patients: This product may bleach colored fabric or hair. Concurrent use with PABA-containing sunscreens may result in transient discoloration of the skin.
Carcinogenesis, Mutagenesis, Impairment of Fertility: Based upon considerable evidence, benzyol peroxide is not considered to be a carcinogen. However, in one study, using mice known to be highly susceptible to cancer, there was evidence for benzoyl peroxide as a tumor promoter. Benzoyl peroxide has been found to be inactive as a mutagen in the *Ames Salmonella* and other assays, including the mouse dominant lethal assay. This assay is frequently used to assess the effect of substances on spermatogenesis.
Pregnancy (Category C): Animal reproduction studies have not been conducted with benzoyl peroxide (DESQUAM-X GEL). It is also not known whether benzoyl peroxide (DESQUAM-X GEL) can cause fetal harm when administered to a pregnant woman or can affect reproductive capacity. Benzoyl peroxide (DESQUAM-X GEL) should be given to a pregnant woman only if clearly needed.
Nursing Mothers: It is not known whether this drug is excreted in human milk. Caution should be exercised when benzoyl peroxide is administered to a nursing woman.
Pediatric Use: Safety and effectiveness in children below the age of 12 have not been established.

ADVERSE REACTIONS
Adverse reactions which may be encountered with topical benzoyl peroxide include excessive drying (manifested by marked peeling, erythema and possibly edema), and allergic contact sensitization.
Excessive dryness appears to occur in approximately 2 patients in 50.
Pertinent literature seems to indicate that allergic sensitization to benzoyl peroxide may occur in 10 to 25 patients in 1,000. There is one reference that reports an occurrence of sensitization in 5 of 100 patients.

OVERDOSAGE
In the event that excessive scaling, erythema or edema occur, the use of this preparation should be discontinued. If the reaction is judged to be due to excessive use and not allergenicity, after symptoms and signs subside, a reduced dosage schedule may be cautiously tried.
To hasten resolution of the adverse effects, emollients, cool compresses and/or topical corticosteroid preparations may be used.

DOSAGE AND ADMINISTRATION
DESQUAM-X GEL should be gently rubbed into all affected areas once or twice daily. Suitable cleansing of the affected area should precede application. In fair-skinned individuals or under excessively drying conditions, it is suggested that therapy be initiated with one application daily. The degree of drying or peeling may be controlled by modification of dose frequency or drug concentration. The use of DESQUAM-X GEL may be continued as long as deemed necessary.

HOW SUPPLIED

DESQUAM-X 2.5 GEL		
1.5 oz. (42.5 g)	Plastic Tubes	NDC 0072-6300-01
DESQUAM-X 5 GEL		
1.5 oz. (42.5 g)	Plastic Tubes	NDC 0072-6621-01
3 oz. (85 g)	Plastic Tubes	NDC 0072-6621-03
DESQUAM-X 10 GEL		
1.5 oz. (42.5 g)	Plastic Tubes	NDC 0072-6721-01
3 oz. (85 g)	Plastic Tubes	NDC 0072-6721-03

Store at controlled room temperature (59°–86° F).

WATER BASE
DESQUAM-X®5 WASH ℞
(5% benzoyl peroxide)
WATER BASE
DESQUAM-X®10 WASH ℞
(10% benzoyl peroxide)

CAUTION
Federal law prohibits dispensing without prescription.

DESCRIPTION
DESQUAM-X5 and DESQUAM-X10 brand topical therapeutic anti-acne cleansers contain benzoyl peroxide (5% and 10%) in a lathering water base of sodium octoxynol-3 sulfonate, dioctyl sodium sulfosuccinate, magnesium aluminum silicate, methylcellulose and EDTA.

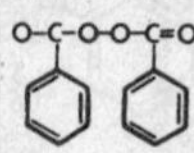

benzoyl peroxide

CLINICAL PHARMACOLOGY
The effectiveness of benzoyl peroxide in the treatment of acne vulgaris is primarily attributable to its antibacterial activity, especially with respect to *Propionibacterium acnes,* the predominant organism in sebaceous follicles and comedones. The antibacterial activity of this compound is presumably due to the release of active or free-radical oxygen capable of oxidizing bacterial proteins. In acne patients treated topically with benzoyl peroxide, resolution of the acne usually coincides with reduction in the levels of *P. acnes* and free fatty acids (FFA). Mild desquamation is another observed action of topically applied benzoyl peroxide and may also play a role in the drug's effectiveness in acne. Studies also indicate that topical benzoyl peroxide may exert a sebostatic effect with a resultant reduction of skin surface lipids.
Benzoyl peroxide has been shown to be absorbed by the skin, where it is metabolized to benzoic acid and then excreted as benzoate in the urine.

INDICATIONS AND USAGE
DESQUAM-X (5 or 10) WASH is indicated for the topical treatment of mild to moderate acne. In more severe cases, it may be used as an adjunct in therapeutic regimens including benzoyl peroxide gels, antibiotics, retinoic acid products and sulfur/salicylic acid-containing preparations. The improvement of the treated condition is dependent on the degree and type of acne, the frequency of use of DESQUAM-X WASH and the nature of other therapies employed.

CONTRAINDICATIONS
This product should not be used in patients known to be sensitive to benzoyl peroxide or any other of the listed ingredients.

PRECAUTIONS
General: Avoid contact with eyes and other mucous membranes. For external use only. In patients known to be sensitive to the following substances, there is a possibility of cross-sensitization: benzoic acid derivatives (including certain topical anesthetics) and cinnamon.
Information for Patients: This product may bleach colored fabric or hair. Concurrent use with PABA-containing sunscreens may result in transient discoloration of the skin.
Carcinogenesis, Mutagenesis, Impairment of Fertility: Based upon considerable evidence, benzoyl peroxide is not considered to be a carcinogen. However, in one study, using mice known to be highly susceptible to cancer, there was evidence for benzoyl peroxide as a tumor promoter. Benzoyl peroxide has been found to be inactive as a mutagen in the *Ames Salmonella* and other assays, including the mouse dominant lethal assay. This assay is frequently used to assess the effect of substances on spermatogenesis.
Pregnancy (Category C): Animal reproduction studies have not been conducted with benzoyl peroxide (DESQUAM-X WASH). It is also not known whether benzoyl peroxide can cause fetal harm when administered to a pregnant woman or can affect reproductive capacity. Benzoyl peroxide should be given to a pregnant woman only if clearly needed.
Nursing Mothers: It is not known whether this drug is excreted in human milk. Caution should be exercised when benzoyl peroxide is administered to a nursing woman.
Pediatric Use: Safety and effectiveness in children below the age of 12 have not been established.

ADVERSE REACTIONS
Adverse reactions which may be encountered with topical benzoyl peroxide include excessive drying (manifested by marked peeling, erythema and possible edema), and allergic contact sensitization.
Excessive dryness would appear to occur in approximately 2 patients in 50.
Pertinent literature would seem to indicate that allergic sensitization to benzoyl peroxide may occur in 10 to 25 patients in 1,000. There is one reference that reports an occurrence of sensitization in 5 of 100 patients.

OVERDOSAGE
In the event that excessive scaling, erythema or edema occur, the use of this preparation should be discontinued. If the reaction is judged to be due to excessive use and not allergenicity, after symptoms and signs subside, a reduced dosage schedule may be cautiously tried.
To hasten resolution of the adverse effects, emollients, cool compresses and/or topical corticosteroid preparations may be used.

DOSAGE AND ADMINISTRATION
Shake well before use. Wash affected areas once or twice daily, avoiding contact with eyes or mucous membranes. Wet skin areas to be treated prior to administration; apply DESQUAM-X WASH, work to a full lather, rinse thoroughly and pat dry. The amount of drying or peeling may be controlled by modification of dose frequency or drug concentration.

HOW SUPPLIED
Desquam-X Wash (5%): 5 oz. plastic bottle, NDC 0072-6905-05.
Desquam-X Wash (10%): 5 oz. plastic bottle, NDC 0072-7000-05.
Store at controlled room temperature (59°-86°F; 15°-30°C).

ESTAR®
Therapeutic Tar Gel

ACTIVE INGREDIENT
Westwood tar (biologically equivalent to 5% coal tar USP). Also contains: B-alanine, benzyl alcohol, carbomer 940, glycereth-7 coconate, polysorbate 80, 15.6% SD alcohol 40, simethicone, sorbitol and water.

ACTIONS AND USES
A therapeutic aid in the treatment of eczema, psoriasis, and other tar-responsive dermatoses such as atopic dermatitis, lichen simplex chronicus, and nummular eczema. ESTAR exerts keratoplastic, antieczematous, and antipruritic actions. It is equivalent in its photodynamic activity to 5% crude coal tar in either hydrophilic ointment or petrolatum. ESTAR provides the characteristic benefits of tar therapy in a form that is readily accepted by patients and nursing staff, due to its negligible tar odor and staining potential, and the superior cosmetic qualities of its gel base. ESTAR is suitable for use in a modified Goeckerman regimen, either in the hospital or on an outpatient basis; it also can be used in follow-up treatment to help maintain remissions. Substantivity to the skin can be demonstrated by examination with a Wood's light, which shows residual microfine particles of tar on the skin several days after application.

CONTRAINDICATIONS
ESTAR should not be applied to acutely inflamed skin or used by individuals who are known to be sensitive to coal tar.

ADMINISTRATION AND DOSAGE
Psoriasis: ESTAR can be applied at bedtime in the following manner: the patient should massage ESTAR into affected areas, allowing the gel to remain for five minutes, and then remove excess by patting with tissues. This procedure minimizes staining of skin and clothing, leaving behind an almost invisible layer of the active tar. If any staining of fabric should occur, it can be removed easily by standard laundry procedures.
The same technique of application may be used the following morning. If dryness occurs, an emollient may be applied one hour after ESTAR.
Because of ESTAR's superior substantivity and cosmetic qualities, patients who might otherwise be hospitalized for tar/UV therapy can now be treated as outpatients. The patient can easily apply ESTAR at bedtime and the following morning, then report for UV treatment that day. Laboratory tests and clinical experience to date suggest that it may be advisable to carefully regulate the length of UV exposure.
Chronic atopic dermatitis, lichen simplex chronicus, nummular eczema, and seborrheic dermatitis: One or two applications per day, as described above, are suggested. If dryness occurs, an emollient may be applied one hour after ESTAR and between applications as needed.

CAUTION
PROTECT TREATED AREAS FROM DIRECT SUNLIGHT, FOR AT LEAST 24 HOURS AFTER APPLICATION, UNLESS DIRECTED BY A PHYSICIAN. AVOID USE ON INFECTED, HIGHLY INFLAMED OR BROKEN SKIN. DO NOT APPLY TO GENITAL AREA. If used on the scalp, temporary discoloration of blond, bleached, or tinted hair may occur. If undue irritation develops or increases, the usage schedule should be changed or ESTAR discontinued. Contact with the eyes should be avoided. In case of contact, flush eyes with water.
Slight staining of clothing may occur. Standard laundry procedures will usually remove stains. For external use only.

HOW SUPPLIED
3 oz. (NDC 0072-7603-03) plastic tube.

EURAX® ℞
(crotamiton USP)
Lotion/Cream
Scabicide/Antipruritic

CAUTION
Federal law prohibits dispensing without prescription.

DESCRIPTION
EURAX, crotamiton USP, is a scabicidal and antipruritic agent available as a cream or lotion for topical use only. EURAX provides 10% of the synthetic, crotamiton USP, in a vanishing-cream or emollient-lotion base containing: glyceryl monostearate, anhydrous lanolin, PEG 6-32, glycerin, polysorbate 80, water, benzyl alcohol, quaternium-15 and fragrance. In addition, the cream contains mineral oil and white wax; the lotion, light mineral oil, carboxymethylcellulose sodium and simethicone. Crotamiton is N-ethyl-N-(o-methylphenyl)-2-butenamide and its structural formula is:

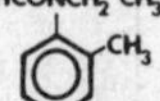

Crotamiton USP is a colorless to slightly yellowish oil, having a faint amine-like odor. It is miscible with alcohol and with methanol. The Crotamiton in EURAX is a mixture of the *cis* and *trans* isomers. Its molecular weight is 203.28.

CLINICAL PHARMACOLOGY
EURAX has scabicidal and antipruritic actions. The mechanisms of these actions are not known.

INDICATIONS AND USAGE
For eradication of scabies (*Sarcoptes scabiei*) and for symptomatic treatment of pruritic skin.

CONTRAINDICATIONS
EURAX should not be applied topically to patients who develop a sensitivity or are allergic to it or who manifest a primary irritation response to topical medications.

WARNINGS
If severe irritation or sensitization develops, treatment with this product should be discontinued and appropriate therapy instituted.

PRECAUTIONS
General: EURAX should not be applied in the eyes or mouth because it may cause irritation. It should not be applied to acutely inflamed skin or raw or weeping surfaces until the acute inflammation has subsided.
Information for Patients: See "Directions for patients with scabies".
Drug Interactions: None known.
Carcinogenesis, Mutagenesis, Impairment of Fertility: Long-term carcinogenicity studies in animals have not been conducted.
Pregnancy (Category C): Animal reproduction studies have not been conducted with EURAX. It is also not known whether Eurax can cause fetal harm when applied topically to a pregnant woman or can affect reproduction capacity. EURAX should be given to a pregnant woman only if clearly needed.
Pediatric Use: Safety and effectiveness in children have not been established.

ADVERSE REACTIONS
Allergic sensitivity or primary irritation reactions may occur in some patients.

OVERDOSAGE
There is no specific information on the effect of overtreatment with repeated topical applications in humans. Acute toxicity (after accidental oral administration in children): No deaths have occurred. Highest known doses ingested: Cream: small children—2g (age 1½ years): Lotion: small children—2.8g (age 2 years).
Oral LD_{50} in animals (mg/kg): rats, 2212; mice, 2011.
Signs and symptoms (of oral ingestion): Burning sensation in the mouth, irritation of the buccal, esophageal and gastric mucosa, nausea, vomiting, abdominal pain.
Treatment: There is no specific antidote if taken orally. General measures to eliminate the drug and reduce its absorption, combined with symptomatic treatment, are recommended.

DOSAGE AND ADMINISTRATION
LOTION Shake well before using—***In Scabies:*** Thoroughly massage into the skin of the whole body from the chin down, paying particular attention to all folds and creases. A second application is advisable 24 hours later.
Clothing and bed linen should be changed the next morning. A cleansing bath should be taken 48 hours after the last application.
In Pruritus: Massage gently into affected areas until medication is completely absorbed. Repeat as needed.

Continued on next page

Westwood—Cont.

Directions for Patients with Scabies:

1. Take a routine bath or shower. Thoroughly massage EURAX cream or lotion into the skin from the chin to the toes including folds and creases.
2. A second application is advisable 24 hours later.
3. This 60 gram tube or bottle is sufficient for two applications.
4. Clothing and bed linen should be changed the next day. Contaminated clothing and bed linen may be dry-cleaned, or washed in the hot cycle of the washing machine.
5. A cleansing bath should be taken 48 hours after the last application.

HOW SUPPLIED

Cream: 60 g tubes (NDC 0072-2100-60).
Lotion: 60 g (2 oz.) bottles (NDC 0072-2200-60).
454 g (16 oz.) bottles (NDC 0072-2200-16).

HALOTEX® ℞

(Haloprogin)
Cream 1%, Solution 1%
Antifungal Agent for Topical Use

CAUTION

Federal law prohibits dispensing without a prescription.

DESCRIPTION

HALOTEX (brand of haloprogin) Cream/Solution for topical use. Each gram of the cream contains 10 mg haloprogin in a water-dispersible base composed of polyethylene glycol 400, polyethylene glycol 4000, diethyl sebacate and polyvinylpyrrolidone.
Each ml of the solution contains 10 mg haloprogin in a clear, colorless vehicle composed of 75% alcohol and diethyl sebacate.
These preparations are effective topical antifungal agents. The chemical name for haloprogin is: 1,2,4-trichloro-5[(3-iodo-2-propynyl)oxy]benzene. The structure is:

Cl, $OCH_2C{\equiv}CI$, Cl, Cl

CLINICAL PHARMACOLOGY

The mechanism of antifungal activity for haloprogin in yeast cells is believed to be inhibition of respiration and disruption of the yeast cell membrane. The mechanism of antifungal activity in dermatophytes is unknown.
Dermal penetration studies utilizing single applications of ^{14}C ring-labeled haloprogin formulated as creams, or dissolved in acetone or alcoholic solutions, were performed in 18 male subjects. Urinary recovery from 3 subjects ranged from 9.47% (0.25% cream) to 14.89% (1% cream) over 5 days. The 0.25% and 1% alcoholic solutions were associated with lesser recoveries of 3% and 6%, respectively. Subtotal inunction studies have been conducted with both the cream and the solution. Fifteen grams of HALOTEX Cream (n=8) and 15 ml of HALOTEX Solution (n=14) were administered to the entire body for 10 consecutive days. Physical examinations and clinical laboratory tests conducted throughout the study showed no abnormalities. Repeat patch testing for contact sensitization and photosensitivity also were negative.
The following *in-vitro* data on haloprogin are available, but their clinical significance is not known.

Organism (# Strains Tested)	MIC[1] (μg/ml) Range Found
Microsporum audouini (2)	<0.0470 – 0.390
M. canis (2)	<0.0470 – 0.390
M. gypseum (2)	0.0950 – 0.190
Other *Microsporum* spp (3)	0.0030 – 0.190
Trichophyton mentagrophytes (5)	0.0950 – 0.780
T. rubrum (4)	0.0120 – 0.780
Other *Trichophyton* spp (9)	0.0015 – 0.095
Candida albicans (3)	0.0500 – 0.400
Other *Candida* spp (2)	0.4000 – 0.800
Other Yeasts/yeast-like fungi (8)	0.0500 – 0.400
Staphylococcus aureus (5)	1.5600 – 3.120
Streptococcus pyrogenes (3)	0.7800 –50.000
Other gram pos. organisms (6)	25.00 – >100.000
Gram neg. organisms	>100

[1]Minimal Inhibitory Concentration

INDICATIONS AND USAGE

HALOTEX Cream and Solution are indicated for the treatment of superficial mycotic infections including tinea pedis, tinea cruris, tinea corporis and tinea manuum due to infection with *Tricophyton rubrum, T. tonsurans, T. mentaprophytes, Microsporum canis* and *Epidermophyton floccosum.* HALOTEX also is indicated for the treatment of tinea versicolor caused by *Malassezia furfur.*

CONTRAINDICATIONS

HALOTEX Cream and Solution should not be used by patients known to have hypersensitivity to any of the listed ingredients.

WARNINGS

See Contraindications and Precautions.

PRECAUTIONS

General: Treatment with HALOTEX Cream or Solution should be discontinued in case of sensitization or persistent irritation and appropriate therapy instituted. The diagnosis in patients showing no improvement after four weeks of treatment with HALOTEX should be reconsidered.
In mixed infections, where bacteria or nonsusceptible fungi are present, supplementary antiinfective therapy may be indicated.
Information for Patients: HALOTEX is for topical use only. Contact of this drug with the eyes should be avoided.
Use of HALOTEX should be discontinued and a physician contacted in the event of increased irritation.
In order to minimize the risk of recurrence, use the prescribed medication for the full duration even if symptoms have abated.
Laboratory Tests: KOH preparations of the afflicted areas may be useful to verify the diagnosis of fungal infection prior to treatment. Periodic repeat KOH preparations at 2-week intervals during treatment and at 2–4 weeks after treatment will document the beneficial response to treatment. Cultures for bacteria or fungi of specimens from affected area, not responding to treatment may help to elucidate the lack of response.
In the event of a suspected irritation or sensitization, patch testing with components of the formulation used may help verify the reaction and identify its cause.
Carcinogenesis, Mutagenesis, Impairment of Fertility: The carcinogenic potential of haloprogin in laboratory animals has not been evaluated. HALOTEX was shown to be non-mutagenic in The Ames-Salmonella/Microsome Plate Assay.
Pregnancy: Pregnancy Category B: Reproduction studies have been performed in rats and rabbits, each group being given 10 daily topical applications, representing up to 3 times the estimated total human dose needed for a 30-day course of therapy. No evidence of impaired fertility or harm to the fetus due to haloprogin was revealed. There are, however, no adequate and well-controlled studies in pregnant women. Because animal reproduction studies are not always predictive of human response, this drug should be used during pregnancy only if clearly needed.
Nursing Mothers: It is not known whether this drug is excreted in human milk. Because many drugs are excreted in human milk, caution should be exercised when HALOTEX formulations are applied to a nursing mother.
Pediatric Use: Safety and efficacy studies in children have not been performed.

ADVERSE REACTIONS

In clinical studies with the cream and the solution 26 adverse reactions were noted out of a total 1796 patients treated. These reactions are tabulated below for each formulation.

	FORMULATION	
REACTION	Cream (n=977)	Solution (n=819)
Burning and/or irritation on application	8	14
Erythema and Scaling	1	—
Erythema and Itching	1	—
Folliculitis	1	—
Pruritus and Vesicle Formation	—	1

Reactions noted did not always require interruption of treatment.

OVERDOSAGE

The oral LD_{50} of haloprogin is >3000 mg/kg in mice, rats, dogs and rabbits. The maximum haloprogin in any single package is 300 mg total. There is no experience to allow extrapolation of acute toxicity and expected symptoms in man.

DOSAGE AND ADMINISTRATION

HALOTEX Cream and Solution should be applied liberally to the affected areas twice daily for 2–3 weeks. Intertriginous areas may require 4 weeks of treatment.

HOW SUPPLIED

HALOTEX (haloprogin) Cream 1% is supplied in 15 g (NDC 0072-7130-15) and 30 g (NDC 0072-7130-02) tubes. Store below 45°C (113°F). HALOTEX (haloprogin) Solution 1% is supplied in 10 ml (NDC 0072-7200-10) and 30 ml (NDC 0072-7200-30) bottles with controlled drop tip.

KERALYT® GEL ℞

6% Salicylic Acid

CAUTION

Federal law prohibits dispensing without prescription.

DESCRIPTION

KERALYT is a gel for topical administration containing 6% salicylic acid in a vehicle composed of propylene glycol, alcohol (19.4%), hydroxypropylcellulose and water. Salicylic acid is the 2-hydroxy derivative of benzoic acid having the following structure:

O, C–O–H, O–H

CLINICAL PHARMACOLOGY

Salicylic acid has been shown to produce desquamation of the horny layer of skin while not effecting qualitative or quantitative changes in the structure of the viable epidermis. The mechanism of action has been attributed to a dissolution of intercellular cement substance. In a study of the percutaneous absorption of salicylic acid from KERALYT GEL in four patients with extensive active psoriasis, Taylor and Halprin showed that the peak serum salicylate levels never exceeded 5 mg/100 ml even though more than 60% of the applied salicylic acid was absorbed. Systemic toxic reactions are usually associated with much higher serum levels (30 to 40 mg/100 ml). Peak serum levels occurred within 5 hours of the topical application under occlusion. The sites were occluded for 10 hours over the entire body surface below the neck. Since salicylates are distributed in the extracellular space, patients with a contracted extracellular space due to dehydration or diuretics have higher salicylate levels than those with a normal extracellular space. (See PRECAUTIONS.)
The major metabolites identified in the urine after topical administration are salicyluric acid (52%), salicylate glucuronides (42%) and free salicylic acid (6%). The urinary metabolites after percutaneous absorption differ from those after oral salicylate administration; those derived from percutaneous absorption contain more salicylate glucuronides and less salicyluric and salicylic acid. Almost 95% of a single dose of salicylate is excreted within 24 hours of its entrance into the extracellular space.
Fifty to eighty percent of salicylate is protein bound to albumin. Salicylates compete with the binding of several drugs and can modify the action of these drugs; by similar competitive mechanisms other drugs can influence the serum levels of salicylate. (See PRECAUTIONS.)

INDICATIONS AND USAGE

For Dermatologic Use: KERALYT GEL is a topical aid in the removal of excessive keratin in hyperkeratotic skin disorders, including verrucae, and the various ichthyoses (vulgaris, sex-linked and lamellar), keratosis palmaris and plantaris, keratosis pilaris, pityriasis rubra pilaris, psoriasis (including body, scalp, palms and soles).
For Podiatric Use: KERALYT GEL is a topical aid in the removal of excessive keratin on dorsal and plantar hyperkeratotic lesions. KERALYT has been reported to be useful adjunctive therapy for verrucae plantares.

CONTRAINDICATIONS

KERALYT GEL should not be used in any patient known to be sensitive to salicylic acid or any other listed ingredients. KERALYT should not be used in children under 2 years of age.

WARNINGS

Prolonged use over large areas, especially in children and those patients with significant renal or hepatic impairment, could result in salicylism. Concomitant use of other drugs which may contribute to elevated serum salicylate levels should be avoided where the potential for toxicity is present. In children under 12 years of age and those patients with renal or hepatic impairment, the area to be treated should be limited and the patient monitored closely for signs of salicylate toxicity: nausea, vomiting, dizziness, loss of hearing, tinnitus, lethargy, hyperpnea, diarrhea, psychic disturbances. In the event of salicylic acid toxicity, the use of KERALYT GEL should be discontinued. Fluids should be administered to promote urinary excretion. Treatment with sodium bicarbonate (oral or intravenous) should be instituted as appropriate.

PRECAUTIONS

For external use only. Avoid contact with eyes and other mucous membranes.

DRUG INTERACTIONS

(The following interactions are from a published review and include reports concerning both oral and topical salicylate administration. The relationship of these interactions to the use of KERALYT GEL is not known.)

I. Due to the competition of salicylate with other drugs for binding to serum albumin the following drug interactions may occur:

DRUG	DESCRIPTION OF INTERACTION
Tolbutamide	Hypoglycemia potentiated.
Methotrexate	Decreases tubular re- absorption; clinical toxicity from methotrexate can result.

II. Drugs changing salicylate levels by altering renal tubular reabsorption:

DRUG	DESCRIPTION
Corticosteroids	Decreases plasma salicylate level; tapering doses of steroids may promote salicylism
Ammonium Sulfate	Increases plasma salicylate level.

III. Drugs with Complicated Interactions with Salicylates

DRUG	DESCRIPTION
Heparin	Salicylate decreases platelet adhesiveness and interferes with hemostasis in heparin-treated patients.
Pyrazinamide	Inhibits pyrazinamide-induced hyperuricemia.
Uricosuric Agents	Effect of probenemide, sulfinpyrazone and phenylbutazone inhibited.

The following alterations of laboratory tests have been reported during salicylate therapy.

LABORATORY TESTS	EFFECT OF SALICYLATES
Thyroid Function	Decreased PBI; increased T_3 uptake.
Urinary Sugar	False negative with glucose oxidase; false positive with Clinitest with high-dose salicylate therapy (2-5g q.d.).
5-Hydroxyindole acetic acid	False negative with fluorometric test.
Acetone, ketone bodies	False positive $FeCl_3$ in Gerhardt reaction; red color persists with boiling.
17-OH corticosteroids	False reduced values with >4.8g q.d. salicylate.
Vanilmandelic acid	False reduced values.
Uric acid	May increase or decrease depending on dose.
Prothrombin	Decreased levels; slightly increased prothrombin time.

Pregnancy (Category C): Salicylic acid has been shown to be teratogenic in rats and monkeys. It is difficult to extrapolate from oral doses of acetylsalicylic acid used in these studies to topical administration as the oral dose to monkeys may represent 6 times the maximal daily human dose of salicylic acid (as supplied in one tube, 28 g, of Keralyt) when applied topically over a large body surface. There are no adequate and well-controlled studies in pregnant women. KERALYT GEL should be used during pregnancy only if the potential benefit justifies the potential risk to the fetus.

Nursing Mothers: Because of the potential for serious adverse reactions in nursing infants from the mother's use of KERALYT GEL, a decision should be made whether to discontinue nursing or to discontinue the drug, taking into account the importance of the drug to the mother.

Carcinogenesis, Mutagenesis, Impairment of Fertility: No data are available concerning potential carcinogenic or reproductive effects of KERALYT GEL. It has been shown to lack mutagenic potential in the Ames Salmonella test.

ADVERSE REACTIONS
Excessive erythema and scaling conceivably could result from use on open skin lesions.

OVERDOSAGE
See **Warnings.**

DOSAGE AND ADMINISTRATION
The preferable method of use is to apply KERALYT GEL thoroughly to the affected area and occlude the area at night. Preferably, the skin should be hydrated for at least five minutes prior to application. The medication is washed off in the morning and if excessive drying and/or irritation is observed a bland cream or lotion may be applied. Once clearing is apparent, the occasional use of KERALYT GEL will usually maintain the remission. In those areas where occlusion is difficult or impossible, application may be made more frequently; hydration by wet packs or baths prior to application apparently enhances the effect. Unless hands are being treated, hands should be rinsed thoroughly after application.

HOW SUPPLIED
1 oz. (28.4g) (NDC 0072-6500-01) plastic tube.

LAC-HYDRIN™ ℞
(ammonium lactate)
12%* Lactate Lotion

PRODUCT OVERVIEW

KEY FACTS
Lac-Hydrin™ is a therapeutic lotion which is active in the treatment of moderate to severe xerosis and ichthyosis vulgaris. The active ingredient, 12% ammonium lactate, helps improve the stratum corneum to provide a longer lasting effect in the treatment of dry skin.

MAJOR USES
Lac-Hydrin has been shown to be clinically effective for cases of moderate to severe xerosis and ichthyosis vulgaris.

SAFETY INFORMATION
Contact with eyes, lips or mucous membranes should be avoided. A mild transient stinging may occur on application to abraded or inflamed areas or in individuals with sensitive skin.

PRESCRIBING INFORMATION

LAC-HYDRIN™ ℞
(ammonium lactate)
12%* Lotion

CAUTION
Federal law prohibits dispensing without a prescription.

DESCRIPTION*
LAC-HYDRIN, specially formulates 12% lactic acid neutralized with ammonium hydroxide, as ammonium lactate to provide a lotion pH of 4.5–5.5. LAC-HYDRIN also contains light mineral oil, glyceryl stearate, PEG-100 stearate, propylene glycol, polyoxyl 40 stearate, glycerin, magnesium aluminum silicate, laureth-4, cetyl alcohol, methyl and propylparabens, methylcellulose, fragrance, quaternium-15 and water. Lactic acid is a racemic mixture of 2-hydroxypropanoic acid and has the following structural formula:

COOH
|
CHOH
|
CH_3

CLINICAL PHARMACOLOGY
It is generally accepted that the water content of the stratum corneum is a controlling factor in maintaining skin flexibility. When the stratum corneum contains more than 10% water it remains soft and pliable; however, when the water content drops below 10% the stratum corneum becomes less flexible and rough, and may exhibit scaling and cracking and the underlying skin may become irritated.

Symptomatic relief of dry skin is provided by skin protectants containing hygroscopic substances (humectants) which increase skin moisture. Lactic acid, an α-hydroxy acid, is reported to be one of the most effective naturally occurring humectants in the skin. The α-hydroxy acids (and their salts), in addition to having beneficial effects on dry skin, have also been shown to reduce excessive epidermal keratinization in patients with hyperkeratotic conditions (e.g., ichthyosis).

Pharmacokinetics: The mechanism of action of topically applied neutralized lactic acid is not yet known.

INDICATIONS AND USAGE
LAC-HYDRIN is indicated for the treatment of dry, scaly skin (xerosis) and ichthyosis vulgaris and for temporary relief of itching associated with these conditions.

CONTRAINDICATIONS
Known hypersensitivity to any of the label ingredients.

PRECAUTIONS
General: For external use only. Avoid contact with eyes, lips or mucous membranes. Caution is advised when used on the face of fair-skinned individuals since irritation may occur. A mild, transient stinging may occur on application to abraded or inflamed areas or in individuals with sensitive skin.

Carcinogenesis, Mutagenesis, Impairment of Fertility: LAC-HYDRIN was nonmutagenic in the Ames/Salmonella/Microsome Plate Assay. Reproductive studies in rats given lactic acid orally showed no effect on the sex ratio of the offspring.

Pregnancy (Category C): Animal reproduction studies have not been conducted with LAC-HYDRIN. It is also not known whether LAC-HYDRIN can cause fetal harm when administered to a pregnant woman or can affect reproduction capacity. LAC-HYDRIN should be given to a pregnant woman only if clearly needed.

Nursing Mothers: Although lactic acid is a normal constituent of blood and tissues, it is not known to what extent this drug affects normal lactic acid levels in human milk. Because many drugs are excreted in human milk, caution should be exercised when LAC-HYDRIN is administered to a nursing woman.

Pediatric Use: Safety and effectiveness of LAC-HYDRIN have been demonstrated in infants and children. No unusual toxic effects were reported.

ADVERSE REACTIONS
The most frequent adverse experiences in patients with xerosis are transient stinging (1 in 30 patients), burning (1 in 30 patients), erythema (1 in 50 patients) and peeling (1 in 60 patients). Other adverse reactions which occur less frequently are irritation, eczema, petechiae, dryness and hyperpigmentation.

Due to the more severe initial skin conditions associated with ichthyosis, there was a higher incidence of transient stinging, burning and erythema (each occurring in 1 in 10 patients).

OVERDOSAGE
The oral administration of LAC-HYDRIN to rats and mice showed this drug to be practically non-toxic ($LD_{50}>15$ ml/kg).

DOSAGE AND ADMINISTRATION
Apply to the affected areas and rub in thoroughly. Use twice daily or as directed by a physician.

HOW SUPPLIED
5 oz. (NDC 0072-5712-05) plastic tube.

LOWILA® CAKE
Soap-free Skin Cleanser

COMPOSITION
Contains dextrin, sodium lauryl sulfoacetate, water, boric acid, urea, sorbitol, mineral oil, PEG-14 M, lactic acid, dioctyl sodium sulfosuccinate, cellulose gum, fragrance.

ACTION AND USES
LOWILA CAKE is indicated when soap should not be used, for cleansing skin that is sensitive or irritated, or in dermatitic and eczematous conditions. Used for general bathing, infant bathing, routine washing of hands and face and shampooing. The pH of LOWILA CAKE helps protect the skin's normal acid mantle and create an environment favorable to therapy and healing.

ADMINISTRATION AND DOSAGE
LOWILA CAKE is used in place of soap. Lathers well in both hard and soft water.

HOW SUPPLIED
3¾ oz. (NDC 0072-2300-01) bar.

MAXIVATE™ ℞
(betamethasone dipropionate)
0.05%
For topical use. Not for use in eyes.

DESCRIPTION
Maxivate™ contains Betamethasone Dipropionate U.S.P. (Pregna-1, 4-diene-3, 20-dione, 9-fluoro-11-hydroxy-16-methyl-17, 21-bis (1-oxopropoxy)-,(11B, 16B)-); it has an empirical formula of $C_{28}H_{37}FO_7$ and a molecular weight of 504.59 (CAS Registry Number 5593-20-4).

Cream
Each gram of the 0.05% Cream contains 0.64 mg Betamethasone Dipropionate (equivalent to 0.5 mg Betamethasone) in a soft, white, hydrophilic cream of Purified Water, Mineral Oil, White Petrolatum, Polyethylene Glycol 1000 Monocetyl Ether, Cetostearyl Alcohol, Monobasic Sodium Phosphate and Phosphoric Acid or Sodium Hydroxide. Chlorocresol is present as a preservative. Maxivate™ Cream contains no parabens.

Ointment
Each gram of the 0.05% Ointment contains 0.64 mg Betamethasone Dipropionate (equivalent to 0.5 mg Betamethasone) in an ointment base of Mineral Oil and White Petrolatum. Maxivate™ Ointment contains no parabens.

Lotion
Each gram of the 0.05% Lotion contains 0.64 mg Betamethasone Dipropionate (equivalent to 0.5 mg Betamethasone) in a vehicle of Isopropyl Alcohol and Purified Water slightly thickened with Carbomer 934P. Phosphoric Acid or Sodium Hydroxide are used to adjust pH.

CLINICAL PHARMACOLOGY
Topical corticosteroids share anti-inflammatory, anti-pruritic and vasoconstrictive actions. The mechanism of anti-inflammatory activity of the topical corticosteroids is unclear. Various laboratory methods, including vasoconstrictor assays, are used to compare and predict potencies and/or clinical efficacies of the topical corticosteroids. There is some evidence to suggest that a recognizable correlation exists

Continued on next page

Westwood—Cont.

between vasoconstrictor potency and therapeutic efficacy in man.

Pharmacokinetics: The extent of percutaneous absorption of topical corticosteroids is determind by many factors including the vehicle, the integrity of the epidermal barrier, and the use of occlusive dressings. Topical corticosteroids can be absorbed from normal intact skin. Inflammation and/or other disease processes in the skin increase percutaneous absorption. Occlusive dressings substantially increase the percutaneous absorption of topical corticosteroids. Thus, occlusive dressings may be a valuable therapeutic adjunct for treatment of resistant dermatoses. (See DOSAGE AND ADMINISTRATION). Once absorbed through the skin, topical corticosteroids are handled through pharmacokinetic pathways similar to systemically administered corticosteroids. Corticosteroids are bound to plasma proteins in varying degrees. Corticosteroids are metabolized primarily in the liver and are then excreted by the kidneys. Some of the topical corticosteroids and their metabolites are also excreted into the bile.

INDICATIONS AND USAGE

Topical corticosteroids are indicated for the relief of the inflammatory and pruritic manifestations of corticosteroid-responsive dermatoses.

CONTRAINDICATIONS

Topical corticosteroids are contraindicated in those patients with a history of hypersensitivity to any of the components of the preparation.

PRECAUTIONS

General: Systemic absorption of topical corticosteroids has produced reversible hypothalamic-pituitary-adrenal (HPA) axis suppression, manifestations of Cushing's syndrome, hyperglycemia, and glucosuria in some patients. Conditions which augment systemic absorption include the application of the more potent steroids, use over large surface areas, prolonged use, and the addition of occlusive dressings. Therefore, patients receiving a large dose of a potent topical steroid applied to a large surface area or under an occlusive dressing should be evaluated periodically for evidence of HPA axis suppression by using the urinary free cortisol and ACTH stimulation tests. If HPA axis suppression is noted, an attempt should be made to withdraw the drug, to reduce the frequency of application, or to substitute a less potent steroid. Recovery of HPA axis function is generally prompt and complete upon discontinuation of the drug. Infrequently, signs and symptoms of steroid withdrawal may occur, requiring supplemental systemic corticosteroids. Children may absorb proportionally larger amounts of topical corticosteroids and thus be more susceptible to systemic toxicity. (See PRECAUTIONS—Pediatric Use). If irritation develops, topical corticosteroids should be discontinued and appropriate therapy instituted. In the presence of dermatological infections, the use of an appropriate antifungal or antibacterial agent should be instituted. If a favorable response does not occur promptly, the corticosteroid should be discontinued until the infection has been adequately controlled.

Information for the Patient: Patients using topical corticosteroids should receive the following information and instructions:

1. This medication is to be used as directed by the physician. It is for external use only. Avoid contact with the eyes.
2. Patients should be advised not to use this medication for any disorder other than for which it was prescribed.
3. The treated skin area should not be bandaged or otherwise covered or wrapped as to be occlusive unless directed by the physician.
4. Patients should report any signs of local adverse reactions especially under occlusive dressing.
5. Parents of pediatric patients should be advised not to use tight fitting diapers or plastic pants on a child being treated in the diaper area, as these garments may constitute occlusive dressings.

Laboratory Tests: The following test may be helpful in evaluating the HPA axis suppression: Urinary free cortisol test; ACTH stimulation test.

Carcinogenesis, Mutagenesis, and Impairment of Fertility: Long-term animal studies have not been performed to evaluate the carcinogenic potential or the effect on fertility of topical corticosteroids. Studies to determine mutagenicity with prednisolone and hydrocortisone have revealed negative results.

Pregnancy Category C: Corticosteroids are generally teratogenic in laboratory animals when administered systemically at relatively low dosage levels. The more potent corticosteroids have been shown to be teratogenic after dermal application in laboratory animals. There are no adequate and well-controlled studies in pregnant women on teratogenic effects from topically applied corticosteroids. Therefore, topical corticosteroids should be used during pregnancy only if the potential benefit justifies the potential risk to the fetus. Drugs of this class should not be used extensively on pregnant patients, in large amounts, or for prolonged periods of time.

Nursing Mothers: It is not known whether topical administration of corticosteroids could result in sufficient systemic absorption to produce detectable quantities in breast milk. Systemically administered corticosteroids are secreted into breast milk in quantities not likely to have a deleterious effect on the infant. Nevertheless, caution should be exercised when topical corticosteroids are administered to a nursing woman.

Pediatric Use: *Pediatric patients may demonstrate greater susceptibility to topical corticosteroid-induced HPA axis suppression and Cushing's syndrome than mature patients because of a larger skin surface area to body weight ratio.* Hypothalamic-pituitary-adrenal (HPA) axis suppression, Cushing's syndrome, and intracranial hypertension have been reported in children receiving topical corticosteroids. Manifestations of adrenal suppression in children include linear growth retardation, delayed weight gain, low plasma cortisol levels, and absence of response to ACTH stimulation. Manifestations of intracranial hypertension include bulging fontanelles, headaches, and bilateral papilledema. Administration of topical corticosteroids to children should be limited to the least amount compatible with an effective therapeutic regimen. Chronic corticosteroid therapy may interfere with the growth and development of children.

ADVERSE REACTIONS

The following local adverse reactions are reported infrequently with topical corticosteroids, but may occur more frequently with the use of occlusive dressings. These reactions are listed in an approximate decreasing order of occurrence; burning, itching, irritation, dryness, folliculitis, hypertrichosis, acneiform eruptions, hypopigmentation, perioral dermatitis, allergic contact dermatitis, maceration of the skin, secondary infection, skin atrophy, striae and miliaria.

OVERDOSAGE

Topically applied corticosteroids can be absorbed in sufficient amounts to produce systemic effects. (See PRECAUTIONS).

DOSAGE AND ADMINISTRATION

Topical corticosteroids are generally applied to the affected area as a thin film two or three times daily or as directed by a physician depending on the severity of the condition. Occlusive dressings may be used for the management of psoriasis or recalcitrant conditions. If an infection develops, the use of occlusive dressings should be discontinued and appropriate antimicrobial therapy instituted.

HOW SUPPLIED

Maxivate™ Ointment, 0.05% in 15 gram tubes, NDC 0072-9450-15 and 45 gram tubes, NDC 0072-9450-45.
Maxivate™ Cream, 0.05% in 15 gram tubes, NDC 0072-9410-15 and 45 gram tubes, NDC 0072-9410-45.
Maxivate™ Lotion, 0.05% in 60 ml bottles, NDC 0072-9490-60. Shake well before using.

CAUTION

Federal law prohibits dispensing without prescription.

MOISTUREL™
Skin Lubricant—Moisturizer

COMPOSITION

Water, petrolatum, glycerin, dimethicone, steareth-2, cetyl alcohol, benzyl alcohol, laureth-23, Mg Al silicate, carbomer-934, sodium hydroxide, quaternium-15.

ACTION AND USES

MOISTUREL is a non-greasy formula that leaves the skin feeling smooth and soft. Clinically proven to relieve dry skin. Free of parabens and fragrances that can sensitize or irritate skin. Indicated for generalized dry skin, chapped or chafed skin, diaper rash, sunburn, heat rash, itching and dryness associated with eczema.

ADMINISTRATION AND DOSAGES

Apply liberally as often as needed.

HOW SUPPLIED

8 oz. (NDC 0072-9100-08) and 12 oz. (NDC 0072-9100-12) plastic bottles.

PRESUN® 4 CREAMY SUNSCREEN
Moderate Sunscreen Protection

ACTIVE INGREDIENT

Octyl dimethyl PABA. Also contains: Dimethicone, fragrance, isopropyl myristate, stearic acid and water. May also contain: Acrylic-acrylate copolymer, ammonium hydroxide, benzyl alcohol, carbomer-934 or carbomer-940, cetyl alcohol, diazolidinyl urea, methylchloroisothiazolinone and methylisothiazolinone, petrolatum, quaternium-15, stearyl alcohol, titanium dioxide, triethanolamine, xanthan gum, and other ingredients.

ACTION AND USES

4 TIMES NATURAL PROTECTION: Used as directed, PRESUN 4 Creamy Sunscreen provides 4 times your natural *sunburn* protection and may help reduce the chance of premature aging and wrinkling of the skin as well as skin cancer caused by overexposure to the sun.

WATERPROOF: PRESUN 4 Creamy Sunscreen maintains its degree of protection even after 80 minutes in the water.

MOISTURIZING: Specially formulated creamy lotion that helps relieve skin from the drying effects of the sun.

ADMINISTRATION AND DOSAGE

Shake well. Smooth evenly onto dry skin before sun exposure. Massage in gently. Reapply to dry skin after prolonged swimming, excessive perspiration or towel drying. Repeated applications during prolonged sun exposure are recommended.

WARNINGS

Protect from freezing. For external use only. Do not use if sensitive to P-aminobenzoic acid (PABA) or related compounds. Discontinue use if irritation or rash appears. Avoid contact with eyes. In case of contact, flush eyes with water. Keep out of the reach of children.

HOW SUPPLIED

4 oz. (NDC 0072-5904-04) plastic bottle.

PRESUN® 8 LOTION AND CREAMY SUNSCREENS
Maximal Sunscreen Protection

COMPOSITION

Lotion: **Active Ingredients:** 7.3% (w/w) Octyl dimethyl PABA, 2.3% (w/w) oxybenzone. Also contains: Choleth-24, hydroxypropylcellulose, PG dioctanoate, PPG-15 stearyl ether, 60% (w/w) SD alcohol 40 and water.

Creamy: **Active Ingredients:** Octyl dimethyl PABA, oxybenzone. Also contains: Dimethicone, fragrance, isopropyl myristate, stearic acid and water. May also contain: Acrylic-acrylate copolymer, ammonium hydroxide, benzyl alcohol, carbomer-934 or carbomer-940, cetyl alcohol, diazolidinyl urea, methyl chloroisothiazolinone and methylisothiazolinone, petrolatum, quaternium-15, stearyl alcohol, titanium dioxide, triethanolamine, xanthan gum, and other ingredients.

ACTION AND USES

8 TIMES NATURAL PROTECTION: Used as directed, PRESUN 8 Sunscreen provides 8 times your natural *sunburn* protection and may help reduce the chance of premature aging and wrinkling of the skin as well as skin cancer caused by overexposure to the sun.

UVA/UVB PROTECTION: PRESUN 8 Suncreen is formulated to provide protection from the harmful effects of both UVA and UVB rays.

Lotion: PRESUN 8 Lotion Sunscreen is a clear formula containing a PABA ester—an ingredient widely recommended by physicians.

Creamy: PRESUN 8 Creamy Sunscreen maintains its degree of protection even after 80 minutes in the water.

WARNINGS

Lotion: For external use only. Do not use if sensitive to P-aminobenzoic acid (PABA) or related compounds. Discontinue use if irritation or rash appears. Transient facial stinging may occur in hot, humid weather. Avoid contact with eyes. In case of contact, flush eyes with water. Avoid flame. Keep out of the reach of children.

Creamy: Protect from freezing. For external use only. Do not use if sensitive to P-aminobenzoic acid (PABA) or related compounds. Discontinue use if irritation or rash appears. Avoid contact with eyes. In case of contact, flush eyes with water. Keep out of the reach of children.

ADMINISTRATION AND DOSAGE

Lotion: *Shake well.* Apply evenly to dry skin before sun exposure; let dry before dressing. Reapply to dry skin after swimming, excessive perspiration or towel drying. Repeated applications during prolonged sun exposure are recommended.

Creamy: *Shake well.* Smooth evenly onto dry skin before sun exposure. Massage in gently. Reapply to dry skin after prolonged swimming, excessive perspiration or towel drying. Repeated applications during prolonged sun exposure are recommended.

HOW SUPPLIED

Lotion: 4 fl. oz. (NDC 0072-5403-04) plastic bottles. Creamy: 4 oz. (NDC 0072-8504-04) plastic bottles.

PRESUN® 15 LOTION AND CREAMY SUNSCREENS
Ultra Sunscreen Protection

ACTIVE INGREDIENTS
Lotion: 5% Aminobenzoic acid (PABA), 5% Octyl dimethyl PABA, 3% oxybenzone. Also contains: hydroxypropylcellulose, PPG-15 stearyl ether, 58% SD alcohol 40 and water.

ACTIVE INGREDIENTS
Creamy: Octyl dimethyl PABA, oxybenzone. Also contains: Dimethicone, fragrance, isopropyl myristate, stearic acid and water. May also contain: Acrylic-acrylate copolymer, ammonium hydroxide, benzyl alcohol, carbomer-934 or carbomer-940, cetyl alcohol, diazolidinyl urea, methylchloroisothiazolinone and methylisothiazolinone, petrolatum, quaternium-15, stearyl alcohol, titanium dioxide, triethanolamine, xanthan gum, and other ingredients.

ACTION AND USES
15 TIMES NATURAL PROTECTION: Used as directed, PRESUN 15 Sunscreen provides 15 times your natural *sunburn* protection and may help reduce the chance of premature aging and wrinkling of the skin as well as skin cancer caused by overexposure to the sun.
UVA/UVB PROTECTION: PRESUN 15 Suncreen is formulated to provide protection from the harmful effects of both UVA and UVB rays.
Lotion: PRESUN 15 Lotion Sunscreen is a clear formula containing a PABA ester—an ingredient widely recommended by physicians.
Creamy: PRESUN 15 Creamy Sunscreen maintains its degree of protection even after 80 minutes in the water.

WARNINGS
Lotion: For external use only. Do not use if sensitive to P-aminobenzoic acid (PABA) or related compounds. Discontinue use if irritation or rash appears. Transient facial stinging may occur in hot, humid weather. Avoid contact with eyes. In case of contact, flush eyes with water. Avoid flame. Keep out of the reach of children.
Creamy: Protect from freezing. For external use only. Do not use if sensitive to P-aminobenzoic acid (PABA) or related compounds. Discontinue use if irritation or rash appears. Avoid contact with eyes. In case of contact, flush eyes with water. Keep out of the reach of children.

ADMINISTRATION AND DOSAGE
Lotion: *Shake well.* Apply evenly to dry skin before sun exposure; let dry before dressing. Reapply to dry skin after swimming, excessive perspiration or towel drying. Repeated applications during prolonged sun exposure are recommended.
Creamy: *Shake well.* Smooth evenly onto dry skin before sun exposure. Massage in gently. Reapply to dry skin after prolonged swimming, excessive perspiration or towel drying. Repeated applications during prolonged sun exposure are recommended.

HOW SUPPLIED
Lotion: 4 oz. (NDC 0072-8800-04) plastic bottle. Creamy: 4 oz. (NDC 0072-8904-04) plastic bottle.

PRESUN® 15 FACIAL STICK/LIP PROTECTOR SUNSCREEN

ACTIVE INGREDIENTS
8% Octyl dimethyl PABA, 3% oxybenzone. Also contains: Flavoring, lanolin oil, mineral oil, ozokerite, PEG-4 dilaurate, petrolatum and propylparaben.

ACTIONS AND USES
15 TIMES NATURAL PROTECTION: Used as directed, PRESUN 15 Facial Sunscreen Stick and Sunscreen Lip Protector provide 15 times your natural *sunburn* protection and may help reduce the chance of premature aging and wrinkling of the skin as well as skin cancer caused by overexposure to the sun.
UVA/UVB PROTECTION: PRESUN 15 Facial Sunscreen Stick and Sunscreen Lip Protector are formulated to provide protection from the harmful effects of both UVA and UVB rays.
MOISTURIZES: PRESUN 15 Facial Sunscreen Stick helps keep your skin soft and smooth—even after long hours in the sun.
PRESUN 15 Sunscreen Lip Protector helps prevent drying, cracking and chapping from the sun, wind or cold.

WARNINGS
For external use only. Do not use if sensitive to P-aminobenzoic acid (PABA) or related compounds. Discontinue use if irritation or rash appears. Avoid contact with eyes. In case of contact, flush eyes with water. Keep out of the reach of children.

ADMINISTRATION AND DOSAGE
Facial Stick: Apply evenly to dry skin before sun exposure. Reapply to dry skin after swimming, excessive perspiration or towel drying. Repeated applications during prolonged sun exposure are recommended.
Lip Protector: Apply to lips as needed. Repeated applications during prolonged exposure to the sun, wind or cold are recommended.

HOW SUPPLIED
.42 oz. (NDC 0072-8703-04) plastic Facial Stick, .15 oz. (NDC 0072-8703-01) plastic Lip Stick.

PRESUN® 15 FACIAL SUNSCREEN
Ultra Sunscreen Protection

ACTIVE INGREDIENTS
8% Octyl dimethyl PABA, 3% oxybenzone. Also contains: Benzyl alcohol, carbomer 934, cetyl alcohol, dimethicone, glyceryl stearate, laureth-23, magnesium aluminum silicate, petrolatum, propylene glycol dioctanoate, quaternium-15, sodium hydroxide, steareth-2 and water.

ACTION AND USES
15 TIMES NATURAL PROTECTION: Used as directed, PRESUN 15 Facial Sunscreen provides 15 times your natural *sunburn* protection and may help reduce the chance of premature aging and wrinkling of the skin as well as skin cancer caused by overexposure to the sun.
UVA/UVB PROTECTION: PRESUN 15 Facial Sunscreen is formulated to provide protection from the harmful effects of both UVA and UVB rays.
MOISTURIZES: PRESUN 15 Facial Sunscreen was developed especially for use on the face. The special moisturizers soften and smooth your skin while protecting it from the drying effects of the sun.
SUITABLE UNDER MAKE-UP: A non-greasy cream made especially for daily use under facial make-up and designed not to clog pores or cause acne or blemishes.

ADMINISTRATION AND DOSAGE
Gently smooth evenly onto dry skin before sun exposure. Reapply to dry skin after swimming, excessive perspiration or towel drying. Repeated applications during prolonged sun exposure are recommended.

WARNINGS
For external use only. Do not use if sensitive to p-aminobenzoic acid (PABA) or related compounds. Discontinue use if irritation or rash appears. Avoid contact with eyes. In case of contact, flush eyes with water. Keep out of reach of children.

HOW SUPPLIED
2 oz. (NDC 0072-9200-02) plastic tube.

SEBULEX® and SEBULEX® CREAM
Antiseborrheic Treatment Shampoo

ACTIVE INGREDIENTS
2% sulfur and 2% salicylic acid. Also contains: D&C yellow #10, docusate sodium, EDTA, FD&C blue #1, fragrance, PEG-6 lauramide, PEG-14M, sodium dodecyl benzene sulfonate, sodium octoxynol-2 ethane sulfonate and water. Cream also contains: Ceteareth-20, dextrin, magnesium aluminum silicate and stearyl alcohol.

ACTION AND USES
A penetrating therapeutic shampoo for the temporary relief of itchy scalp and the scaling of dandruff, SEBULEX helps relieve itching, remove dandruff, excess oil. It penetrates and softens the crusty, matted layers of scales adhering to the scalp, and leaves the hair soft and manageable.

ADMINISTRATION AND DOSAGE
SEBULEX liquid should be shaken before being used. SEBULEX or SEBULEX CREAM is massaged into wet scalp. Lather should be allowed to remain on scalp for about 5 minutes and then rinsed. Application is repeated, followed by a thorough rinse. Initially, SEBULEX or SEBULEX CREAM can be used daily, or every other day, or as directed, depending on the condition. Once symptoms are under control, one or two treatments a week usually will maintain control of itching, oiliness and scaling.

CAUTION
If undue skin irritation develops or increases, discontinue use. For external use only. Contact with eyes should be avoided. In case of contact, flush eyes thoroughly with water. Keep this and all drugs out of reach of children.

HOW SUPPLIED
SEBULEX in 4 oz. (NDC 0072-2700-04) and 8 oz. (NDC 0072-2700-08) plastic bottles. SEBULEX CREAM in 4 oz. (NDC 0072-2800-04) plastic tube.

SEBULEX® SHAMPOO WITH CONDITIONERS
Antiseborrheic Treatment and Conditioning Shampoo

COMPOSITION
Contains 2% sulfur, 2% salicylic acid, water, sodium octoxynol-3 sulfonate, sodium lauryl sulfate, lauramide DEA, acetamide MEA, amphoteric-2, hydrolyzed animal protein, magnesium aluminum silicate, propylene glycol, methylcellulose, PEG-14 M, fragrance, disodium EDTA, dioctyl sodium sulfosuccinate, FD & C blue 1, D & C yellow 10.

ACTION AND USES
SEBULEX SHAMPOO WITH CONDITIONERS provides effective temporary control of the scaling and itching of dandruff and seborrheic dermatitis, while adding protein to the hair shaft to increase its manageability.

ADMINISTRATION AND DOSAGE
SEBULEX SHAMPOO WITH CONDITIONERS should be shaken well before use. Shampoo five minutes. For optimum dandruff control and conditioning leave lather on scalp for the full five minutes. Rinse. Repeat. Use daily until control is achieved. Use two to three times weekly to maintain control, although daily use may be continued. Consult physician for severe or unresponsive scalp conditions.

CAUTION
If undue skin irritation develops or increases, discontinue use and consult physician. Contact with eyes should be avoided. In cases of contact, eyes should be flushed thoroughly with water. For external use only. Keep this and all drugs out of reach of children.

HOW SUPPLIED
4 oz. (NDC 0072-2600-04) and 8 oz. (NDC 0072-2600-08) plastic bottles.

SEBUTONE® and SEBUTONE® CREAM
Antiseborrheic Tar Shampoo

ACTIVE INGREDIENTS
Coal tar 0.5%, salicylic acid 2%, sulfur 2%. SEBUTONE also contains: D&C yellow #10, docusate sodium, EDTA, FD&C blue #1, fragrance, lanolin oil, PEG-6 lauramide, PEG-90M, sodium dodecyl benzene sulfonate, sodium octoxynol-2 ethane sulfonate, titanium dioxide, and water. SEBUTONE CREAM also contains: Ceteareth-20, D&C yellow #10, dextrin, docusate sodium, EDTA, FD&C blue #1, fragrance, laureth-4, lanolin oil, magnesium aluminum silicate, PEG-6 lauramide, PEG-14 M, sodium dodecyl benzene sulfonate, sodium octoxynol-2 ethane sulfonate, stearyl alcohol, titanium dioxide and water.

ACTION AND USES
A surface-active, penetrating therapeutic shampoo for the temporary relief of itchy scalp and the scaling of stubborn dandruff and psoriasis. Provides prompt and prolonged relief of itching, helps control oiliness and rid the scalp of scales and crust. Tar ingredient is chemically and biologically standardized to produce uniform therapeutic activity. Wood's light demonstrates residual microfine particles of tar on the scalp several days after a course of SEBUTONE shampoo. In addition to its antipruritic and antiseborrheic actions, SEBUTONE also helps offset excessive scalp dryness with a special moisturizing emollient.

ADMINISTRATION AND DOSAGE
SEBUTONE liquid should be well shaken before use. A liberal amount of SEBUTONE or SEBUTONE CREAM is massaged into the wet scalp for 5 minutes and the scalp is then rinsed. Application is repeated, followed by a thorough rinse. Use as often as necessary to keep the scalp free from itching and scaling or as directed. No other shampoo or soap washings are required.

CAUTION
If undue skin irritation develops or increases, discontinue use. In rare instances, temporary discoloration of white, blond, bleached or tinted hair may occur. Contact with the eyes is to be avoided. In case of contact flush eyes with water. For external use only. Keep this and all drugs out of reach of children.

HOW SUPPLIED
SEBUTONE in 4 oz. (NDC 0072-5000-04) and 8 oz. (NDC 0072-5000-08) plastic bottles.
SEBUTONE CREAM in 4 oz. (NDC 0072-5100-01) tubes.

TACARYL® Chewable Tablets ℞
(Methdilazine)
TACARYL® Tablets/Syrup ℞
(Methdilazine HCl)

CAUTION
FEDERAL LAW PROHIBITS DISPENSING WITHOUT PRESCRIPTION

DESCRIPTION
Tacaryl is an antihistamine antipruritic with the following chemical structure:

Continued on next page

Westwood—Cont.

10 [(1-methyl-3-pyrrolidinyl) methyl] phenothiazine

Methdilazine and its hydrochloride salt occur as light tan, crystalline powders with respectively poor and free solubility in water.

Tacaryl (methdilazine or methdilazine HCl) is a phenothiazine derivative available as

Tablets—Each tablet contains 8 mg methdilazine HCl. Also contains acacia, ascorbic acid, dibasic calcium phosphate, corn starch, D&C red #27 lake, ethyl cellulose, lactose, magnesium stearate and tablet brown;

Syrup—Each 5 ml (one teaspoonful) contains 4 mg methdilazine HCl in a syrup base of benzoic acid, citric acid, ethyl alcohol (7.37%), ethyl vanillin, flavoring, menthol, sodium bisulfite, sodium citrate, sorbitol, sucrose and water; and

Chewable Tablets—Each table contains methdilazine equivalent to 4 mg methdilazine HCl. Also contains acacia, D&C red #21 lake, D&C red #27 lake, flavoring, hydrogenated cottonseed oil, magnesium stearate, mannitol, sodium chloride, sodium saccharin and talc.

CLINICAL PHARMACOLOGY

No information is currently available which assesses the disposition of methdilazine.

INDICATIONS AND USAGE

Tacaryl and Tacaryl HCl are indicated for the treatment of pruritic symptoms in urticaria, symptomatic relief in the management of nasal allergies (hayfever, allergic rhinitis, etc.), relief of pruritic symptoms in a variety of allergic and non-allergic conditions including: atopic dermatitis, neurodermatitis, contact dermatitis, pityriasis rosea, poison ivy dermatitis, eczematous dermatitis, pruritus ani and vulvae, and drug rash.

CONTRAINDICATIONS

Tacaryl is contraindicated in patients who are comatose, those who have received large amounts of CNS depressants, patients with bone marrow depression, jaundice or those who have demonstrated an idiosyncrasy or hypersensitivity to methdilazine or other phenothiazines.

This drug is contraindicated in newborn or premature infants and nursing mothers as well as in children who are acutely ill and dehydrated, since there may be an increased susceptibility to dystonias.

WARNINGS

Phenothiazines with antihistaminic and anticholinergic effects, including methdilazine and methdilazine HCl, should be used with extreme caution in patients with: asthmatic attack, narrow-angle glaucoma, prostatic hypertrophy, stenosing peptic ulcer, pyloroduodenal obstruction, bladder neck obstruction, as well as in patients receiving monoamine oxidase inhibitors. Phenothiazine should **not** be used with alcohol ingestion.

Usage in Pregnancy: There are reports of jaundice and prolonged extrapyramidal symptoms in infants whose mothers received phenothiazines during pregnancy.

Hyperreflexia has been reported in the newborn when a phenothiazine was used during pregnancy.

Use in Children: Tacaryl should be used with caution, as administration in the young child may result in excitation. Overdosage may produce hallucinations, convulsions, and sudden death.

Use in the Elderly (60 years or older): The elderly are more prone to develop the following side effects from phenothiazines: hypotension, syncope, toxic confusional states, excessive sedation, extrapyramidal signs (especially parkinsonism), akathisia and persistent dyskinesia.

PRECAUTIONS

General: Phenothiazines may block and even reverse some of the actions of epinephrine. Tacaryl should be used cautiously in persons with acute or chronic respiratory impairment, particularly in children, as it may suppress the cough reflex.

The drug should be used cautiously in persons with cardiovascular disease, impairment of liver function or those with a history of ulcer disease.

Information for Patients: Patients should be cautioned that methdilazine HCl may impair the mental and/or physical ability required for the performance of potentially hazardous tasks, such as driving a vehicle or operating machinery. Similarly, it may impair mental alertness in children. The concomitant use of alcohol or other central nervous system depressants may have an additive effect.

DRUG INTERACTIONS

- CNS Depressants/Narcotics—Phenothiazines may increase, prolong or intensify the sedative action of nervous system depressants such as anesthetics, barbiturates or alcohol. The dose of a narcotic or barbiturate may be reduced to ¼ or ½ the usual amount when Tacaryl is administered concomitantly. Excessive amounts of Tacaryl, relative to a narcotic, may lead to restlessness and motor hyperactivity in the patient with pain.
- Epinephrine—Phenothiazines may block and even reverse some of the actions of epinephrine.
- MAO Inhibitors—Combined use of MAO inhibitors and phenthiazines may result in hypotension and extrapyramidal reactions.
- Thiazide Diuretics—The anticholinergic effects of phenothiazines may be prolonged and intensified by the concomitant use of thiazide diuretics.
- Oral Contraceptives, Progesterone, Reserpine, Nylidrin Hydrochloride—These drugs potentiate the effects of phenothiazines.

DRUG/LABORATORY TEST INTERACTIONS

The following changes in laboratory determinations have been reported in patients taking phenothiazines:

- increased serum cholesterol, blood glucose, spinal fluid protein, and urinary urobilinogen levels
- decreased protein bound iodine (PBI)
- false positives in urine bilirubin tests
- interference with urinary ketone determinations, pregnancy tests and steroid determinations.

Carcinogenesis/Mutagenesis/Impairment of Fertility: Mutagenicity and long-term carcinogenicity studies in animals have not been performed. Mutagenicity has been evaluated using the Ames Salmonella/Microsome Plate test. Tacaryl tablets and syrup were found to be non-mutagenic.

Pregnancy Category B: Reproduction studies have been performed in rats at doses up to 70 times the usual human dose and have revealed no evidence of impaired fertility or harm to the fetus due to Tacaryl. There are, however, no adequate and well controlled studies in pregnant women. Because animal reproduction studies are not always predictive of human response, this drug should be used during pregnancy only if clearly needed.

Nonteratogenic Effects: There are reports of jaundice and prolonged extrapyramidal symptoms in infants whose mothers received phenothiazines during pregnancy.

Nursing Mothers: It is not known whether this drug is excreted in human milk. Because many drugs are excreted in human milk, caution should be exercised when methdilazine is administered to a nursing woman. (See CONTRAINDICATIONS).

Pediatric Usage: Safety and effectiveness in children below the age of 3 years have not been established. (See CONTRAINDICATIONS, WARNINGS and DOSAGE and ADMINISTRATION.)

ADVERSE REACTIONS

This drug may produce adverse reactions common to both phenothiazines and antihistamines.

Note: Not all of the following adverse reactions have been reported with this specific drug; however, pharmacological similarities among the phenothiazine derivatives require that each be considered when Tacaryl is administered. There have been occasional reports of sudden death in patients receiving phenothiazine derivatives chronically.

CNS: Drowsiness is the most prominent CNS effect of this drug. Extrapyramidal reactions occur, particularly with high doses. Other reported reactions include dizziness, lassitude, tinnitus, incoordination, fatigue, blurred vision, euphoria, diplopia, nervousness, insomnia, tremors and grand mal seizures, excitation, catatonic-like states, neuritis and hysteria.

Cardiovascular: Postural hypotension is the most common cardiovascular effect of the phenothiazines. Reflex tachycardia may be seen. Bradycardia, faintness, dizziness and cardiac arrest have been reported. ECG changes, including blunting of T waves and prolongation of the Q-T interval may be seen.

Gastrointestinal: Anorexia, nausea, vomiting, epigastric distress, constipation and dry mouth may occur. Diarrhea has also been reported as well as increased appetite and weight gain.

Genitourinary: Urinary frequency, dysuria and urinary retention have been reported.

Respiratory: Thickening of bronchial secretions, tightness of the chest, wheezing and nasal stuffiness may occur.

Allergic Reactions: These include urticaria, dermatitis, asthma, laryngeal edema, angioneurotic edema, photosensitivity, lupus erythematosus-like syndrome and anaphylactoid reactions.

Other reported reactions: Leukopenia, agranulocytosis, thrombocytopenic purpura and jaundice of the obstructive type have been reported. The jaundice is usually reversible, but chronic jaundice has been reported.

Long-term therapy considerations: After prolonged administration at high dosage, pigmentation of the skin has occurred, chiefly in the exposed areas. Ocular changes consist of the appearance of lenticular and corneal opacities, epithelial keratopathies and pigmentary retinopathy. Vision may be impaired.

Endocrine: Early menses, induced lactation, gynecomastia, decreased libido and inhibition of ejaculation have been reported.

OVERDOSAGE

Signs and symptoms of overdosage range from mild depression of the central nervous system and cardiovascular system, to profound hypotension, respiratory depression and unconsciousness. Stimulation may be evident, especially in children and geratric patients. Atropine-like signs and symptoms—dry mouth, fixed dilated pupils, flushing, etc.—as well as gastrointestinal symptoms may occur. The treatment of overdosage is essentially symptomatic and supportive. Early gastric lavage may be beneficial. Centrally acting emetics are of little use.

Avoid analeptics, which may cause convulsions. Severe hypotension usually responds to the administration of levarterenol or phenylephrine. **EPINEPHRINE SHOULD NOT BE USED**, since its use in the patient with partial adrenergic blockade may further lower the blood pressure. Additional measures include oxygen and intravenous fluids. Limited experience with dialysis indicates that it is not helpful. The oral LD_{50} of methdilazine HCl is approximately 225 mg/kg in mice, 448 mg/kg in rats and 269 mg/kg in guinea pigs.

DOSAGE AND ADMINISTRATION

Tacaryl® Hydrochloride **Tablets** (methdilazine HCl) Adults: 1 tablet (8 mg) 2 to 4 times daily. Children over 3 years: ½ tablet (4 mg) 2 to 4 times daily.

Tacaryl® Hydrochloride **Syrup** (methdilazine HCl) Adults: 2 teaspoons (8 mg) 2 to 4 times daily. Children over 3 years: 1 teaspoon (4 mg) 2 to 4 times daily.

Tacaryl® **Chewable Tablets** (methdilazine) Adults: 2 tablets (7.2 mg) 2 to 4 times daily. Children over 3 years: 1 tablet (3.6 mg) 2 to 4 times daily. This product form should be chewed and swallowed promptly.

HOW SUPPLIED

Tacaryl® Hydrochloride (methdilazine HCl) Tablets 8 mg: a scored, peach colored tablet (W logo)

NDC 0072-7400-01 Bottles of 100 (with child-resistant closures)

Tacaryl® Hydrochloride (methdilazine HCl) Syrup 4 mg/5ml:

NDC 0072-7500-01 Bottles of 16 fl. oz. (1 pint) (with child-resistant closures)

Tacaryl® (methdilazine) Chewable Tablets 3.6 mg each (equivalent to 4 mg. methdilazine HCl) a pink unscored table (W logo)

NDC 0072-7300-01 Bottles of 100 (with child-resistant closures)

Dispense in tight, light-resistant container. Store at room temperature away from strong light.

Shown in Product Identification Section, page 434

T-STAT® 2.0% ℞
(erythromycin) Topical Solution

CAUTION

Federal law prohibits dispensing without prescription.

DESCRIPTION

T-STAT (erythromycin) 2.0% Topical Solution is a clear liquid antibiotic preparation formulated for the topical treatment of acne. It contains 20 mg of erythromycin per milliliter in a solution of alcohol 71.2%, propylene glycol and fragrance. May contain citric acid to adjust pH.

Erythromycin is a member of the macrolide class of antibiotics and is produced by the actinomycete *Streptomyces erythraeus*.

The chemical name of erythromycin is: (3*R* *,4*S* *,5*S* ,6*R* *,7*R* *,9*R* *,11*R* *,13*S* *,14*R* *)-4-[(2,6-Dideoxy-3-*C* -methyl-3-*O* -methyl-α-L-*ribo* -hexopyranosyl)oxy]-[14-ethyl-7,12,13-trihydroxy-3,5,7,9,11,13-hexamethyl-6-[[3,4,6-trideoxy-3-(dimethylamino)-β-D-*xylo* -hexopyranosyl] oxy]oxacyclotetradecane-2,10-dione.

The structural formula for erythromycin is:

CLINICAL PHARMACOLOGY

Topical erythromycin is effective in reducing inflammatory acne lesions and preventing the development of new acne lesions. The beneficial effects can be attributed to: 1) the reduction of *P. acnes*, the predominant bacterial species isolated from acne lesions (erythromycin inhibits protein synthesis in *P. acnes*, a Gram positive organism); and, 2) alleviating the inflammation associated with acne.

In well-controlled clinical studies, topical erythromycin has been shown to be effective in the treatment of acne vulgaris. In two separate studies, inflammatory lesion reductions ranged from 56%–64%, and 66%–76% of patients had good or excellent responses after 12 weeks of treatment with topical erythromycin.

The absorption, metabolism and excretion of topically applied erythromycin in humans are not known although they have been well studied for the much higher concentrations of systemically delivered erythromycin.

INDICATIONS AND USAGE

T-STAT is indicated for the topical control of acne vulgaris and the prevention of new inflammatory acne lesions.

CONTRAINDICATIONS

T-STAT is contraindicated in persons who have a known hypersensitivity to erythromycin or any of the other listed ingredients.

PRECAUTIONS

T-STAT is recommended for external use only and should be kept away from the eyes, mouth and other mucous membranes. Concomitant topical acne therapy should be used with caution because cumulative irritancy may occur especially with the use of peeling, desquamating or abrasive agents.

The prolonged use of antimicrobial agents may be associated with overgrowth of antibiotic-resistant organisms. If this occurs, therapy should be discontinued.

Drug/Laboratory Test Interactions:

Drug Interactions: Erythromycin is inactivated in the presence of acids due to hydrolysis. The activity of erythromycin is also reduced in the presence of sodium alginate, pectin, bentonite, calamine, silica, and polysorbate 80. Erythromycin is unstable in alkaline media having a pH greater than 10.5.

Interference with Laboratory Tests:

The effect on laboratory tests from topically applied erythromycin is not known.

Carcinogenesis/Mutagenesis/Impairment of Fertility:

Carcinogenesis—Long term carcinogenicity tests in animals have not been performed.

Mutagenesis—Erythromycin (2.0%) in a topical solution has been shown to be non-mutagenic in the Ames Salmonella/Microsome Plate Test.

Pregnancy Category B: Reproductive studies have been performed in rats and rabbits at 1.5, 4 and 13 times the estimated human dose and have revealed no evidence of impaired fertility or harm to the fetus due to erythromycin. There are however, no adequate and well-controlled studies in pregnant women. Because animal reproduction studies are not always predictive of human response, this drug should be used during pregnancy only if clearly needed.

Pediatric Use: Safety and effectiveness in children below the age of 12 have not been established.

ADVERSE REACTIONS

The most frequently reported adverse reactions to topical erythromycin are: dryness, peeling, erythema and irritation.

OVERDOSAGE

The acute oral LD_{50} in rats and mice is approximately 15 ml/kg of body weight; in rabbits it is greater than 5 ml/kg. The accidental ingestion of this formulation may cause nausea, vomiting and in small children, inebriation or sedation. Based on the amount ingested and the time elapsed since ingestion, induced emesis, gastric lavage or demulcent liquids and general support measures may be employed as treatment.

DOSAGE AND ADMINISTRATION

T-STAT should be applied each morning and evening to affected areas. These areas first should be washed, rinsed well, and patted dry. This medication should be applied with applicator top. If finger tips are used, wash hands after application. Drying and peeling may be controlled by reducing the frequency of applications.

HOW SUPPLIED

T-STAT Solution, 60 ml plastic bottle with optional applicator NDC 0072-8300-60.

STORAGE

Store at controlled room temperature 15°–30°C (59°–86°F) or lower.

WESTCORT® ℞

(hydrocortisone valerate)
Cream/Ointment, 0.2%

Caution: Federal law prohibits dispensing without a prescription.

DESCRIPTION

WESTCORT is a topical formulation containing hydrocortisone valerate, a non-fluorinated steroid. It has the chemical name Pregn-4-ene-3, 20-dione, 11, 21-dihydroxy-17-[(1-oxopentyl) oxy]-, (11β)-; the empirical formula is: $C_{26}H_{38}O_6$; the molecular weight is 446.58, and the CAS registry number is: 57524-89-7. The structural formula is:

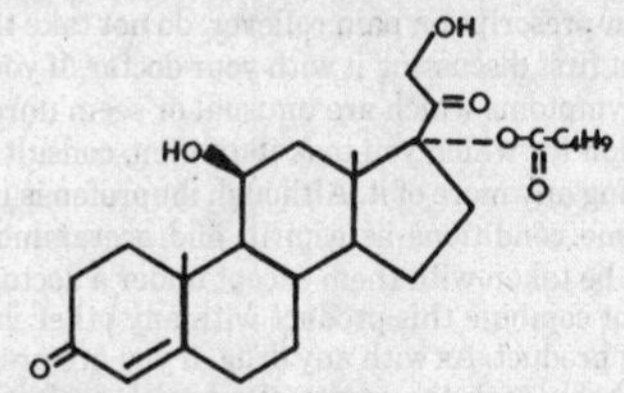

Each gram of WESTCORT CREAM contains 2.0 mg hydrocortisone valerate in a hydrophilic base composed of white petrolatum, stearyl alcohol, propylene glycol, amphoteric-9, carbomer 940, dried sodium phosphate, sodium lauryl sulfate, sorbic acid and water.

Each gram of Westcort Ointment contains 2.0 mg hydrocortisone valerate in a hydrophilic base composed of white petrolatum, stearyl alcohol, propylene glycol, sorbic acid, sodium lauryl sulfate, carbomer 934, dried sodium phosphate, mineral oil, steareth-2, steareth-100, and water.

CLINICAL PHARMACOLOGY

Topical corticosteroids share anti-inflammatory, anti-pruritic and vasoconstrictive actions.

The mechanism of anti-inflammatory activity of the topical corticosteroids is unclear. Various laboratory methods, including vasoconstrictor assays, are used to compare and predict potencies and/or clinical efficacies of the topical corticosteroids. There is some evidence to suggest that a recognizable correlation exists between vasoconstrictor potency and therapeutic efficacy in man.

Pharmacokinetics: The extent of percutaneous absorption of topical corticosteroids is determined by many factors including the vehicle, the integrity of the epidermal barrier, and the use of occlusive dressings.

Topical corticosteroids can be absorbed from normal intact skin. Inflammation and/or other disease processes in the skin increase percutaneous absorption. Occlusive dressings substantially increase the percutaneous absorption of topical corticosteroids. Thus, occlusive dressings may be a valuable therapeutic adjunct for treatment of resistant dermatoses (see DOSAGE AND ADMINISTRATION).

Once absorbed through the skin, topical corticosteroids are handled through pharmacokinetic pathways similar to systemically administered corticosteroids. Corticosteroids are bound to plasma proteins in varying degrees. Corticosteroids are metabolized primarily in the liver and are then excreted by the kidneys. Some of the topical corticosteroids and their metabolites are also excreted into the bile.

INDICATIONS AND USAGE

WESTCORT is indicated for the relief of the inflammatory and pruritic manifestations of the corticosteroid-responsive dermatoses.

CONTRAINDICATIONS

Topical corticosteroids are contraindicated in those patients with a history of hypersensitivity to any of the components of the preparation.

PRECAUTIONS

General: Systemic absorption of topical corticosteroids has produced reversible hypothalamic-pituitary-adrenal (HPA) axis suppression, manifestations of Cushing's syndrome, hyperglycemia, and glucosuria in some patients. Conditions which augment systemic absorption include the application of the more potent steroids, use over large surface areas, prolonged use, and the addition of occlusive dressings.

Therefore, patients receiving a large dose of a potent topical steroid applied to a large surface area or under an occlusive dressing should be evaluated periodically for evidence of HPA axis suppression by using the urinary free cortisol and ACTH stimulation tests. If HPA axis suppression is noted, an attempt should be made to withdraw the drug, to reduce the frequency of application, or to substitute a less potent steroid.

Recovery of HPA axis function is generally prompt and complete upon discontinuation of the drug. Infrequently, signs and symptoms of steroid withdrawal may occur, requiring supplemental systemic corticosteroids.

Children may absorb proportionally larger amounts of topical corticosteroids and thus be more susceptible to systemic toxicity (see PRECAUTIONS—Pediatric Use).

If irritation develops, topical corticosteroids should be discontinued and appropriate therapy instituted.

In the presence of dermatological infections, the use of an appropriate antifungal or antibacterial agent should be instituted. If a favorable response does not occur promptly, the corticosteroids should be discontinued until the infection has been adequately controlled.

Information for the Patient: Patients using topical corticosteroids should receive the following information and instructions:

1. This medication is to be used as directed by the physician. It is for external use only. Avoid contact with the eyes.
2. Patients should be advised not to use this medication for any disorder other than for which it was prescribed.
3. The treated skin area should not be bandaged or otherwise covered or wrapped as to be occlusive unless directed by the physician.
4. Patients should report any signs of local adverse reactions especially under occlusive dressing.
5. Parents of pediatric patients should be advised not to use tight-fitting diapers or plastic pants on a child being treated in the diaper area, as these garments may constitute occlusive dressing.

Laboratory Tests: The following tests may be helpful in evaluating the HPA axis suppression:

Urinary free cortisol test
ACTH stimulation test

Carcinogenesis, Mutagenesis, and Impairment of Fertility: Long-term animal studies have not been performed to evaluate the carcinogenic potential or the effect on fertility of topical corticosteroids.

Studies to determine mutagenicity with prednisolone and hydrocortisone have revealed negative results.

Pregnancy Category C: Corticosteroids are generally teratogenic in laboratory animals when administered systemically at relatively low dosage levels. The more potent corticosteroids have been shown to be teratogenic after dermal application in laboratory animals. There are no adequate and well-controlled studies in pregnant women on teratogenic effects from topically applied corticosteroids. Therefore, topical corticosteroids should be used during pregnancy only if the potential benefit justifies the potential risk to the fetus. Drugs of this class should not be used extensively on pregnant patients, in large amounts, or for prolonged periods of time.

Nursing Mothers: It is not known whether topical administration of corticosteroids could result in sufficient systemic absorption to produce detectable quantities in breast milk. Systemically administered corticosteroids are secreted into breast milk in quantities *not* likely to have a deleterious effect on the infant. Nevertheless, caution should be exercised when topical corticosteroids are administered to a nursing woman.

Pediatric Use: Pediatric patients may demonstrate greater susceptibility to topical corticosteroid-induced HPA axis suppression and Cushing's syndrome than mature patients because of a larger skin surface area to body weight ratio.

Hypothalamic-pituitary-adrenal (HPA) axis suppression, Cushing's syndrome, and intracranial hypertension have been reported in children receiving topical corticosteroids. Manifestations of adrenal suppression in children include linear growth retardation, delayed weight gain, low plasma cortisol levels, and absence of response to ACTH stimulation. Manifestations of intracranial hypertension include bulging fontanelles, headaches, and bilateral papilledema.

Administration of topical corticosteroids to children should be limited to the least amount compatible with an effective therapeutic regimen. Chronic corticosteroid therapy may interfere with the growth and development of children.

ADVERSE REACTIONS

The following local adverse reactions are reported infrequently with topical corticosteroids, but may occur more frequently with the use of occlusive dressings. These reactions are listed in an approximate decreasing order of occurrence: burning; itching; irritation; dryness; folliculitis; hypertrichosis; acneiform eruptions; hypopigmentation; perioral dermatitis; allergic contact dermatitis; maceration of the skin; secondary infection; skin atrophy; striae; miliaria.

OVERDOSAGE

Topically applied corticosteroids can be absorbed in sufficient amounts to produce systemic effects (see PRECAUTIONS).

DOSAGE AND ADMINISTRATION

WESTCORT should be applied to the affected area as a thin film two or three times daily depending on the severity of the condition.

Occlusive dressings may be used for the management of psoriasis or recalcitrant conditions.

If an infection develops, the use of occlusive dressings should be discontinued and appropriate antimicrobial therapy instituted.

Continued on next page

Westwood—Cont.

HOW SUPPLIED
WESTCORT CREAM, 0.2% is supplied in the following tube sizes:
15 g NDC 0072-8100-15.
45 g NDC 0072-8100-45.
60 g NDC 0072-8100-60.
120 g NDC 0072-8100-12.
WESTCORT OINTMENT, 0.2% is supplied in the following tube sizes:
15 g NDC 0072-7800-15
45 g NDC 0072-7800-45
60 g NDC 0072-7800-60
Store below 78°F (26°C).

Wharton Laboratories, Inc.
37-02 FORTY-EIGHTH AVE.
LONG ISLAND CITY, NY 11101

NITRONG® OINTMENT ℞
(Nitroglycerin 2%)

DESCRIPTION
NITRONG® Ointment provides 2% nitroglycerin in an absorptive base for topical administration. Each inch, as squeezed from the tube, provides approx. 15 mg nitroglycerin in controlled-release form.

HOW SUPPLIED
30 g tube (NDC 0195-280-50): 60 g tube (NDC 0195-280-51); Unit Dose (1" Equiv.) (NDC 0195-280-77)

NITRONG® 2.6 mg. Tablets ℞
(nitroglycerin, oral, controlled-release)

DESCRIPTION
Each NITRONG 2.6 mg. tablet for oral administration contains 2.6 mg. nitroglycerin in controlled-release form with light green granules.

NITRONG® 6.5 mg. Tablets ℞
(nitroglycerin, oral, controlled-release)

DESCRIPTION
Each NITRONG 6.5 mg. tablets for oral administration contains 6.5 mg. nitroglycerin in controlled-release form with light orange granules.

NITRONG® 9 mg. Tablets ℞
(nitroglycerin, oral, controlled-release)

DESCRIPTION
Each NITRONG 9.0 mg. tablet for oral administration contains 9.0 mg. nitroglycerin in controlled-release form with blue granules.

HOW SUPPLIED
NITRONG 2.6 mg (NDC 0195-0021-20), and 6.5 mg (NDC 0195-0274-20) in 100's; NITRONG 9.0 mg (NDC 0195-0300-17) in 60's.

Whitehall Laboratories Inc.
Division of American Home Products Corporation
685 THIRD AVENUE
NEW YORK, NY 10017

ADVIL®
Ibuprofen Tablets, USP
Ibuprofen Caplets, USP
Pain Reliever/Fever Reducer

Warning: ASPIRIN SENSITIVE PATIENTS. Do not take this product if you have had a severe allergic reaction to aspirin, e.g.—asthma, swelling, shock or hives, because even though this product contains no aspirin or salicylates, cross-reactions may occur in patients allergic to aspirin.

DOSAGE AND ADMINISTRATION
Adults: Take one tablet every 4 to 6 hours while symptoms persist. If pain or fever does not respond to one tablet, two tablets may be used but do not exceed six tablets in 24 hours unless directed by a doctor. The smallest effective dose should be used. Take with food or milk if occasional and mild heartburn, upset stomach, or stomach pain occurs with use. Consult a doctor if these symptoms are more than mild or if they persist. Children: Do not give this product to children under 12 except under the advice and supervision of a doctor.

WARNINGS
Do not take for pain for more than 10 days or for fever for more than 3 days unless directed by a doctor. If pain or fever persists or gets worse, if new symptoms occur, or if the painful area is red or swollen, consult a doctor. These could be signs of serious illness. If you are under a doctor's care for any serious condition, consult a doctor before taking this product. As with aspirin and acetaminophen, if you have any condition which requires you to take prescription drugs or if you have had any problems or serious side effects from taking any non-prescription pain reliever, do not take this product without first discussing it with your doctor. If you experience any symptoms which are unusual or seem unrelated to the condition for which you took ibuprofen, consult a doctor before taking any more of it. Although ibuprofen is indicated for the same conditions as aspirin and acetaminophen, it should not be taken with them except under a doctor's direction. Do not combine this product with any other ibuprofen-containing product. As with any drug, if you are pregnant or nursing a baby, seek the advice of a health professional before using this product. IT IS ESPECIALLY IMPORTANT NOT TO USE IBUPROFEN DURING THE LAST 3 MONTHS OF PREGNANCY UNLESS SPECIFICALLY DIRECTED TO DO SO BY A DOCTOR BECAUSE IT MAY CAUSE PROBLEMS IN THE UNBORN CHILD OR COMPLICATIONS DURING DELIVERY.
Keep this and all drugs out of the reach of children. In case of accidental overdose, seek professional assistance or contact a poison control center immediately.

ACTIVE INGREDIENT
Each tablet contains Ibuprofen 200 mg.

INACTIVE INGREDIENTS
Acacia, Acetylated Monoglycerides, Beeswax or Carnauba Wax, Calcium Sulfate, Colloidal Silicon Dioxide, Dimethicone, Iron Oxide, Lecithin, Pharmaceutical Glaze, Povidone, Sodium Benzoate, Sodium Carboxymethylcellulose, Starch, Stearic Acid, Sucrose, Titanium Dioxide.

INDICATIONS
For the temporary relief of minor aches and pains associated with the common cold, headache, toothache, muscular aches, backache, for the minor pain of arthritis, for the pain of menstrual cramps and for reduction of fever.

PROFESSIONAL LABELING
Same as stated under Indications.

HOW SUPPLIED
Coated tablets in bottles of 8, 24, 50, 100, 165 and 250.
Coated caplets in bottles of 8, 24, 50, 100 and 165.

STORAGE
Store at room temperature; avoid excessive heat 40°C (104°F).
Shown in Product Identification Section, page 434

ANACIN®
[an 'a-sin]
Analgesic Coated Tablets and Coated Caplets

ACTIVE INGREDIENTS
Each tablet or caplet contains: Aspirin 400 mg., Caffeine 32 mg.

INACTIVE INGREDIENTS
Tablets contain Hydroxypropyl Methylcellulose, Microcrystalline Cellulose, Polyethylene Glycol, Starch, Surfactant. Caplets contain Hydroxypropyl Methylcellulose, Iron Oxide, Microcrystalline Cellulose, Polyethylene Glycol, Starch, Surfactant.

INDICATIONS AND ACTIONS
Now Anacin® has a special protective coating that makes each tablet or caplet easy to swallow. Anacin provides relief from the pain of headaches, neuralgia, neuritis, sprains, muscular aches, sinus pressure... discomforts and fever of colds... pain caused by tooth extraction and toothache... menstrual discomfort. Anacin also temporarily relieves the minor aches and pains of arthritis and rheumatism.

WARNINGS
Children and teenagers should not use this medicine for chicken pox or flu symptoms before a doctor is consulted about Reye syndrome, a rare but serious illness. As with any drug, if you are pregnant or nursing a baby, seek the advice of a health professional before using this product. Keep this and all medicines out of children's reach. In case of accidental overdose, contact a physician immediately.

PRECAUTIONS
If pain persists for more than 10 days, or redness is present, or in arthritic or rheumatic conditions affecting children under 12 years of age, consult a physician immediately.

DOSAGE
Two tablets or caplets with water every 4 hours as needed. Do not exceed 10 tablets or 10 caplets daily. For children 6–12, half the adult dosage.

PROFESSIONAL LABELING
Same as those outlined under Indications.

HOW SUPPLIED
Tablets: In tins of 12's and bottles of 30's, 50's, 100's, 200's and 300's. Caplets: In bottles of 30's, 50's and 100's. Professional Samples: Available upon request. Write Whitehall Laboratories, PDR Department, New York, New York 10017.
Shown in Product Identification Section, page 434

Children's
ANACIN-3®
[an 'a-sin thre]
Acetaminophen
Chewable Tablets, Liquid, Drops

DESCRIPTION
Chewable Tablets: Each Children's ANACIN-3 Chewable Tablet is cherry flavored.
Liquid: Chidren's Anacin-3 Liquid is stable, cherry flavored, red in color. It contains no alcohol or saccharin.
Infant Drops: Infant Anacin-3 Drops are stable, fruit flavored, red in color and contain no alcohol.

ACTIVE INGREDIENTS
Chewable Tablets: Each chewable tablet contains 80 mg. acetaminophen.
Liquid: Each 5 ml. contains 160 mg. acetaminophen.
Infants' Drops: Each 0.8 ml. (one calibrated dropperful) contains 80 mg. acetaminophen.

INACTIVE INGREDIENTS
Chewable Tablets: Aspartame Cetyl Alcohol, Colloidal Silicon Dioxide, Dibutyl Sebacate, Ethyl Cellulose, FD&C Red No. 40 Lake, Flavor, Hydrogenated Vegetable Oil, Magnesium Stearate, Mannitol, Microcrystalline Cellulose, Simethicone, Sucrose and Surfactant.
Liquid: Citric Acid, D&C Red No. 33, Disodium Edetate, FD&C Red No. 40, Flavor, Glycerin, Methylparaben, Polyethylene Glycol, Propylene Glycol, Sorbitol, Sodium Benzoate, Sucrose and Water.
Infant Drops: FD&C Red No. 40, FD&C Yellow No. 6, Flavors, Glycerin, Polyethylene Glycol 1450, Propylene Glycol, Saccharin, Sodium Benzoate, Sorbitol and Water.

INDICATIONS AND ACTIONS
Children's Anacin-3 Chewable Tablets, Liquid and Infants' Drops are safe and effective 100% aspirin free products designed for treatment of infants and children with conditions requiring reduction of fever or relief of pain—such as mild upper respiratory infections (tonsillitis, common cold, "grippe"), headache, myalgia, post-immunization reactions, post-tonsillectomy discomfort and gastroenteritis. In conjunction with antibiotics or sulfanomides, Anacin-3 acetaminophen is useful as an analgesic and antipyretic in many bacterial or viral infections, such as bronchitis, pharyngitis, tracheobronchitis, sinusitis, pneumonia, otitis media, and cervical adenitis.

CAUTION
If fever persists for more than 3 days or recurs, or if pain continues for more than 5 days, consult your physician immediately.
Phenylketonurics: tablets contain Phenylalanine.

WARNINGS
Keep this and all medicines out of the reach of children. In case of accidental overdose contact a physician immediately.

DOSAGE
All dosages may be repeated every 4 hours. Do not exceed 5 dosages in any 24 hour period.
Children's Anacin-3 Chewable Tablets: 1–2 years, 18 to 23 lbs: one and one half tablets. 2–3 years, 24 to 35 lbs: two tablets. 4–5 years, 36 to 47 lbs: three tablets. 6–8 years, 48–59 lbs: four tablets. 9–10 years, 60 to 71 lbs: five tablets. 11–12 years, 72 to 95 lbs: six tablets.
Children's Anacin-3 Liquid: (Special cup for measuring dosage is provided) 4–11 months, 12 to 17 lbs: one-half teaspoon. 12–23 months, 18 to 23 lbs: three-quarters teaspoon. 2–3 years, 24 to 35 lbs: one teaspoon. 4–5 years, 36 to 47 lbs: one and one-half teaspoons. 6–8 years, 48 to 59 lbs: two teaspoons. 9–10 years, 60 to 71 lbs: two and one-half teaspoons. 11–12 years, 72 to 95 lbs: three teaspoons.
Infants' Anacin-3 Drops: 0–3 months, 6 to 11 lbs: one-half dropperful. 4–11 months, 12 to 17 lbs: one dropperful. 12–23 months, 18 to 23 lbs: one and one-half droppersful. 2–3 years, 24 to 35 lbs: 2 droppersful. 4–5 years, 36 to 47 lbs: 3 droppersful.

OVERDOSAGE

Acetaminophen in massive overdosage may cause hepatic toxicity in some patients. In all cases of suspected overdose, immediately call your regional poison center for assistance in diagnosis and for directions in the use of N-acetylcysteine as an antidote. Adverse effects are rare when acetaminophen is used as recommended.

HOW SUPPLIED

Chewable Tablets (colored pink, scored, imprinted "CHILDREN A-3")—Bottles of 30. Liquid (colored red)—bottles of 2 and 4 fl. oz. Drops (colored red)—bottles of ½ oz. (15 ml.) with calibrated plastic dropper.

All packages listed above have child-resistant safety caps and tamper resistant packaging.

Shown in Product Identification Section, page 435

MAXIMUM STRENGTH ANACIN®
Analgesic Coated Tablets

ACTIVE INGREDIENTS

Each tablet contains: Aspirin 500 mg., Caffeine 32 mg.

INACTIVE INGREDIENTS

Tablets contain Hydroxypropyl Methylcellulose, Microcrystalline Cellulose, Polyethylene Glycol, Starch, Surfactant.

INDICATIONS AND ACTIONS

Maximum Strength Anacin provides fast relief from the pain of headaches, neuralgia, neuritis, sprains, muscular aches, sinus pressure... discomforts and fever of colds... pain caused by tooth extraction and toothache... menstrual discomfort. Maximum strength Anacin also temporarily relieves the minor aches and pains of arthritis and rheumatism.

WARNINGS

Children and teenagers should not use this medicine for chicken pox or flu symptoms before a doctor is consulted about Reye syndrome, a rare but serious illness. As with any drug, if you are pregnant or nursing a baby, seek the advice of a health professional before using this product. Keep this and all medicines out of children's reach. In case of accidental overdose, contact a physician immediately.

PRECAUTIONS

If pain persists for more than 10 days, or redness is present, or in arthritic or rheumatic conditions affecting children under 12 years of age, consult a physician immediately.

DOSAGE

Adults: Two tablets with water 3 or 4 times a day. Do not exceed 8 tablets in any 24 hour period. Not recommended for children under 12 years of age.

PROFESSIONAL LABELING

Same as those outlined under Indications.

HOW SUPPLIED

Tablets: Tins of 12's and bottles of 20's, 40's, 75's and 150's.

Shown in Product Identification Section, page 435

Maximum Strength
ANACIN-3®
[an 'a-sin thre]
Film Coated Acetaminophen Tablets and Caplets

Regular Strength
ANACIN-3®
Film Coated Acetaminophen Tablets

ACTIVE INGREDIENTS

Maximum Strength Tablets and Caplets: Each film coated tablet and caplet contains acetetaminophen 500 mg.
Regular Strength: Each film coated tablet contains acetaminophen 325 mg.

INACTIVE INGREDIENTS

Maximum and Regular Strength Tablets:
Calcium Stearate, Croscarmellose Sodium, FD&C Blue No. 1 Lake, Hydroxypropyl Methylcellulose, Microcrystalline Cellulose, Polyethylene Glycol, Povidone, Propylene Gylcol, Starch, Stearic Acid and Titanium Dioxide.
Maximum Strength Caplets:
Calcium Stearate, Croscarmellose Sodium, D&C Red No. 7 Lake, FD&C Blue No. 1 Lake, Hydroxypropyl Methylcellulose, Microcrystalline Cellulose, Polyethylene Glycol, Povidone, Propylene Glycol, Starch, Stearic Acid and Titanium Dioxide.

INDICATIONS AND ACTIONS

Anacin-3 is a safe and effective 100% aspirin-free analgesic product that acts fast to provide temporary relief from pain of headache, colds or "flu", sinusitis, muscle aches, bursitis, sprains, overexertion, backache, menstrual discomfort, minor arthritis pain, toothaches and to reduce fever.

WARNINGS

Keep this and all medicines out of children's reach. In case of accidental overdose, contact a physician immediately. As with any drug, if you are pregnant or nursing a baby, seek the advice of a health professional before using this product.

CAUTION

If pain persists for more than 10 days or redness is present or in arthritic or rheumatic conditions affecting children under 12, consult a physician immediately.

DOSAGE AND ADMINISTRATION

Maximum Strength —Adults: Two tablets or caplets 3 or 4 times a day. Do not exceed 8 tablets or caplets in any 24-hour period. Regular Strength—Adults: 2 or 3 tablets every 4 hours not to exceed 12 tablets in a 24-hour period. Children (6-12): ½ to 1 tablet 3 to 4 times daily. Consult a physician for use by children under 6 or for use longer than 10 days.

OVERDOSAGE

Acetaminophen in massive overdosage may cause hepatic toxicity in some patients. In all cases of suspected overdose, immediately call your regional poison center for assistance in diagnosis and for directions in the use of N-acetylcysteine as an antidote. Adverse effects are rare when acetaminophen is used as recommended.

PROFESSIONAL LABELING

Same as those outlined under Indications.

HOW SUPPLIED

Maximum Strength Film Coated—Tablets (colored white, imprinted "A-3" and "500")—tins of 12 and bottles of 30, 60, and 100: Caplets (colored white, imprinted Anacin-3")—bottles of 24's, 50's, and 100's. Regular Strength Film Coated—Tablets (colored white, scored, imprinted "A-3") in bottles of 24, 50, and 100.

Shown in Product Identification Section, page 435

ANBESOL® Gel and Liquid
[an 'ba-sol"]
Antiseptic Anesthetic

DESCRIPTION

Anbesol is a safe and effective antiseptic-anesthetic that can be used by all family members for the temporary relief of minor mouth pain such as toothache, sore gums and denture irritation. Anbesol also soothes, relieves the pain and helps dry cold sores and fever blisters. Anbesol is also an excellent first-aid measure that provides fast, temporary pain relief and helps prevent infection from minor cuts, scrapes and burns.

ACTIVE INGREDIENTS

Gel: Benzocaine (6.3% w/v), Phenol (0.5 w/v), Alcohol (70%). Liquid: Benzocaine (6.3% w/v), Phenol (0.5%w/v), Alcohol (70%).

INACTIVE INGREDIENTS

Gel: Carbomer 934P, D&C Red #33 and Yellow #10, FD&C Blue #1 and Yellow #6, Flavor, Glycerin. Liquid: Camphor, Glycerin, Menthol, Povidone Iodine, Potassium Iodide.

INDICATIONS

For fast temporary pain relief of toothache, denture irritation, minor mouth irritations, cold sores, fever blisters, minor cuts, scrapes, and burns.

ACTIONS

Temporarily deadens sensations of nerve endings to provide relief of pain and discomfort; reduces oral bacterial flora temporarily as an aid in oral hygiene.

WARNINGS

Flammable. Keep away from fire or flame. Avoid smoking during application and until product has dried. Do not use near eyes. Keep this and all medicines out of the reach of children.

PRECAUTIONS

Not for prolonged use. If the condition persists or irritation develops, discontinue use and consult your physician or dentist. Not for use under dental work.

DOSAGE AND ADMINISTRATION

Apply topically to the affected area on or around the lips, or within the mouth. FOR DENTURE IRRITATION: Apply thin layer to affected area and do not reinsert dental work until irritation/pain is relieved. Rinse mouth before reinserting. If irritation/pain persists, contact your physician.

PROFESSIONAL LABELING

Same as outlined under Indications.

HOW SUPPLIED

Gel in .25 oz. (7.2 gram) tube. Liquid in two sizes—.31 fl. oz. (9 ml.) and .74 fl. oz. (22 ml.) bottles.

Shown in Product Identification Section, page 435

BABY ANBESOL®
[ăn 'bă-sōl"]
Anesthetic Gel

DESCRIPTION

Baby Anbesol Gel is a safe and effective anesthetic developed to soothe the sore gums of an infant by providing temporary relief from pain due to teething.

ACTIVE INGREDIENT

Benzocaine (7.5%).

INACTIVE INGREDIENTS

Carbomer 934, D&C Red No. 33, Disodium Edetate, Flavor, Glycerin, Polyethylene Glycol, Saccharin, Water.

INDICATIONS

For fast, temporary relief from the pain and irritation associated with teething.

ACTIONS

A topical anesthetic that temporarily inhibits the conduction of nerve impulses from sensory nerves in the gums to provide relief of pain and discomfort.

WARNING

Avoid getting into eyes. Keep this and all medicines out of the reach of children.

PRECAUTIONS

For persistent or excessive teething pain, consult your pediatrician.

DOSAGE AND ADMINISTRATION

Apply a small amount of Baby Anbesol on the infant's irritated gums with cotton swab or finger tip.

PROFESSIONAL LABELING

Baby Anbesol has been specially formulated to soothe your baby's sore gums and relieve teething pain on contact.

HOW SUPPLIED

Clear gel in .25 oz. (7.2 grams) tube.

Shown in Product Identification Section, page 435

ARTHRITIS PAIN FORMULA
[är 'thrīt-is 'pān 'for-mye-la]
By the Makers of Anacin® Analgesic Tablets

ACTIVE INGREDIENTS

Each tablet contains 500 mg. microfined aspirin. Also contains two buffers, 33 mg. Aluminum Hydroxide and 100 mg. Magnesium Hydroxide.

INACTIVE INGREDIENTS

Hydrogenated Vegetable Oil, Microcrystalline Cellulose, Starch, Surfactant.

INDICATIONS AND ACTIONS

Arthritis Pain Formula provides fast, temporary relief from minor aches and pain of arthritis and rheumatism and low back pain. Also relieves the pain of headache, neuralgia, neuritis, sprains, muscular aches, discomforts and fever of colds, pain caused by tooth extraction and toothache, and menstrual discomfort. Arthritis Pain Formula is a buffered analgesic and antipyretic that is formulated with microfined aspirin. The buffering agents help provide protection against stomach upset that could be associated with large antiarthritic doses of aspirin.

WARNINGS

Children and teenagers should not use this medicine for chicken pox or flu symptoms before a doctor is consulted about Reye syndrome, a rare but serious illness.
As with any drug, if you are pregnant or nursing a baby, seek the advice of a health professional before using this product. Keep this and all medications out of children's reach. In case of accidental overdose, contact a physician immediately.

CAUTION

If pain persists for more than 10 days, or redness is present or in arthritic or rheumatic conditions affecting children under 12, consult a physician immediately.

DOSAGE AND ADMINISTRATION

Adult Dosage: 2 tablets, 3 or 4 times a day. Do not exceed 8 tablets in any 24 hour period. For children under 12, consult a physician.

PROFESSIONAL LABELING

Same as stated under "Indications".

HOW SUPPLIED

In plastic bottles of 40, 100 and 175 tablets.

Shown in Product Identification Section, page 435

Continued on next page

Whitehall—Cont.

COMPOUND W®
[kam-paund w]
Solution and Gel

ACTIVE INGREDIENT
Salicylic Acid 17% w/w

INACTIVE INGREDIENTS
Solution: Acetone Collodion, Alcohol 2.2% w/w, Camphor, Castor Oil, Ether 63.5%, Menthol, Polysorbate 80. Gel: Alcohol 67.5% by vol., Camphor, Castor Oil, Collodion, Colloidal Silicon Dioxide, Hydroxypropyl Cellulose, Hypophosphorous Acid, Polysorbate 80.

INDICATIONS
Removes common warts safely and effectively.

ACTIONS
Warts are common benign skin lesions caused by an infectious virus which stimulates mitosis in the basal cell layer resulting in the production of elevated epithelial growths. The keratolytic action of salicylic acids in a flexible collodion vehicle causes the cornified epithelium to swell, soften, macerate and then desquamate.

WARNINGS
Highly Flammable. Keep away from fire or flame and store at room temperature. Avoid smoking during application and until product has dried. Do not use this product if you are a diabetic or have poor blood circulation as serious complications may result. Do not use on moles, birthmarks, unusual warts with hair growing from them, genital warts, or warts on the face or mucous membranes (inside mouth, nose, anus, genitals, or on lips). If pain should develop or if infection is present, consult your physician. Do not use near eyes. If product accidentally comes in contact with eyes flush with water to remove film and continue to flush with water for 15 minutes. Do not inhale. Keep bottle tightly capped. For external use only. In case of accidental ingestion, contact a physician or a Poison Control Center immediately. Keep this and all medicines out of the reach of children.

DOSAGE AND ADMINISTRATION
Use on common warts once daily. 1. Soak affected area in hot water for 5 minutes. If any tissue has loosened, remove by rubbing with a washcloth or soft brush. Do not rub hard enough to cause bleeding. Dry thoroughly. 2. Using the plastic rod provided with the solution or by squeezing the tube to apply, completely cover the wart with solution. To avoid irritating the skin surrounding the wart, confine the the solution to the wart only. To help achieve this, circle the wart with a ring of petrolatum. Allow the solution to dry, then reapply. The area covered with the medicine will appear white. 3. Follow this procedure once daily for the next 6 to 7 days. Most warts should clear within this time period. However, if the wart still remains, continue the treatment for up to 12 weeks. If the wart shows no improvement, see your physician.

PROFESSIONAL LABELING
Same as those outlined under Indications.

HOW SUPPLIED
Compound W is available in .31 fluid oz. clear bottles with plastic applicators. Compound W Gel is available in .25 oz. tubes.

DENOREX®
[dĕn 'ō-reks]
Medicated Shampoo
DENOREX®
Mountain Fresh Herbal Scent
Medicated Shampoo
DENOREX®
Medicated Shampoo and Conditioner

ACTIVE INGREDIENTS
Lotion: Coal Tar Solution 9.0%, Menthol 1.5%, Alcohol 7.5%. Also contains TEA-Lauryl Sulfate, Water, Lauramide DEA, Stearic Acid, Chloroxylenol.
Shampoo and Conditioner: Coal Tar Solution 9.0%, Menthol 1.5%, Alcohol 7.5%. Also contains TEA-Lauryl Sulfate, Water, Lauramide DEA, PEG-27 Lanolin, Quaterium 23, Fragrance, Chloroxylenol, Hydroxypropyl Methylcellulose, Citric Acid.
Gel: Coal Tar Solution 9.0%, Menthol 1.5%, Alcohol 7.5%. Also contains TEA-Lauryl Sulfate, Water, Hydroxypropyl Methylcellulose, Chloroxylenol.

INDICATIONS
Relieves scaling—itching—flaking of dandruff, seborrhea and psoriasis. Regular use promotes cleaner, healthier hair and scalp.

ACTIONS
Denorex Shampoo is antiseborrheic and antipruritic. Loosens and softens scales and crusts. Coal tar helps correct abnormalities of keratinization by decreasing epidermal proliferation and dermal infiltration. Denorex also contains the antipruritic agent, menthol, which is "one of the most widely used of antipruritics in dermatologic therapy of various diseases accompanied by itching". (The United States Dispensatory—27th Edition).

WARNINGS
For external use only. Discontinue treatment if irritation develops. Avoid contact with eyes. Keep this and all medicines out of children's reach.

DIRECTIONS
For best results, shampoo every other day. For severe scalp problems use daily. Wet hair thoroughly and briskly massage until you obtain a rich lather. Rinse thoroughly and repeat. Your scalp may tingle slightly during treatment.

PROFESSIONAL LABELING
Same as stated under Indications.

HOW SUPPLIED
Lotion: 4 oz. and 8 oz. and 12 oz. bottles in Regular Scent, Mountain Fresh Herbal Scent, and Shampoo and Conditioner.
Gel: 2 oz. Tube and 4 oz. Tube in Regular Scent
Shown in Product Identification Section, page 435

DRISTAN®
[drĭs 'tăn]
Nasal Spray
DRISTAN®
Menthol Nasal Spray

ACTIVE INGREDIENTS
Phenylephrine HCl 0.5%, Pheniramine Maleate 0.2%.

INACTIVE INGREDIENTS
Dristan Nasal Spray: Alcohol, Benzalkonium Chloride 1:5000 in buffered isotonic aqueous solution, Eucalyptol, Menthol, Sodium Chloride, Sodium Phosphate, Thimerosal Preservative 0.002% (loss is unavoidable), and Water.
Dristan Menthol Nasal Spray: Benzalkonium Chloride 1:5000 in buffered isotonic aqueous solution, aromatics consisting of Camphor, Eucalyptol, Menthol, Methyl Salicylate; Polysorbate 80, Sodium Chloride, Sodium Phosphate, Thimerosal Preservative 0.002% (loss is unavoidable), and Water.

INDICATIONS
For prompt temporary relief of nasal congestion due to the common cold, sinusitis, hay fever or other upper respiratory allergies.

ACTIONS
Phenylephrine HCI is a sympathomimetic agent that constricts the smaller arterioles of the nasal passages producing a gentle and predictable decongesting effect. Pheniramine Maleate is an antihistamine that controls rhinorrhea, sneezing, and lacrimation associated with elevated histamine levels in disorders of the respiratory tract.

WARNINGS
Do not exceed recommended dosage because symptoms may occur such as burning, stinging, sneezing, or increase of nasal discharge. Do not use this product for more than 3 days. If symptoms persist, consult a physician. The use of this dispenser by more than one person may spread infection. For adult use only. Do not give this product to children under 12 years except under the advice and supervision of a physician. Keep these and all medicines out of the reach of children. In case of accidental ingestion, seek professional assistance or contact a Poison Control Center immediately.

DOSAGE AND ADMINISTRATION
With head upright, insert nozzle in nostril. Spray quickly, firmly and sniff deeply. Adults: Spray 2 or 3 times into each nostril. Repeat every 4 hours as needed. Children under 12 years: As directed by a physician.

PROFESSIONAL LABELING
Same as those outlined under Indications.

HOW SUPPLIED
15 ml. and 30 ml. plastic squeeze bottles.
Shown in Product Identification Section, page 435

DRISTAN®
[drĭs 'tăn]
Long Lasting Nasal Spray
DRISTAN®
Long Lasting Menthol Nasal Spray

ACTIVE INGREDIENT
Oxymetazoline HCl 0.05%.

INACTIVE INGREDIENTS
Dristan Long Lasting Nasal Spray—Benzalkonium Chloride 1:5000 in buffered isotonic aqueous solution, Potassium Phosphate, Sodium Chloride, Sodium Phosphate, Thimerosal Preservative 0.002% (loss is unavoidable), and Water.
Dristan Long Lasting Menthol Nasal Spray—Alcohol, Benzalkonium Chloride 1:5000 in buffered isotonic aqueous solution, Aromatics consisting of Camphor, Eucalyptol, Menthol; Potassium Phosphate, Sodium Chloride, Sodium Phosphate, Thimerosal Preservative 0.002% (loss is unavoidable), and Water.

INDICATIONS
Dristan Long Lasting Nasal Spray and Dristan Long Lasting Menthol Nasal Spray are indicated for prompt temporary relief of nasal congestion due to the common cold, sinusitis, hay fever, or other upper respiratory allergies for up to 12 hours.

ACTIONS
The sympathomimetic action of Dristan Long Lasting Nasal Spray and Dristan Long Lasting Menthol Nasal Spray constricts the smaller arterioles of the nasal passages, producing a prolonged, up to 12 hours, gentle and predictable decongesting effect.

WARNINGS
Do not exceed recommended dosage because symptoms may occur, such as burning, stinging, sneezing, or an increase of nasal discharge. Do not use this product for more than 3 days. If symptoms persist, consult a physician. The use of the dispenser by more than one person may spread infection. Keep these and all medicines out of the reach of children. In case of accidental ingestion, seek professinal assistance or contact a Poison Control Center immediately.

DOSAGE AND ADMINISTRATION
With head upright, insert nozzle in nostril. Spray quickly, firmly and sniff deeply. Adults and children 6 years of age and over, spray 2 or 3 times into each nostril. Repeat twice daily—morning and evening. Not recommended for children under six.

PROFESSIONAL LABELING
Same as those outlined under Indications.

HOW SUPPLIED
Dristan Long Lasting Nasal Spray: 15 ml. and 30 ml. plastic squeeze bottles.
Dristan Long Lasting Menthol Nasal Spray: 15 ml. plastic squeeze bottle.
Shown in Product Identification Section, page 435

Advanced Formula
DRISTAN®
[drĭs 'tăn]
Decongestant/Antihistamine/Analgesic
Tablets and Coated Caplets

ACTIVE INGREDIENTS
Each Dristan Tablet or Coated Caplet contains: Phenylephrine HCl 5 mg., Chlorpheniramine Maleate 2 mg., Acetaminophen 325 mg.

INACTIVE INGREDIENTS
Tablets—Calcium Stearate, Croscarmellose Sodium, D&C Yellow #10 Lake, FD&C Yellow #6 Lake, Microcrystalline Cellulose, Povidone, Starch, Stearic Acid.
Caplets—Calcium Stearate, Croscarmellose Sodium, D&C Red #7 Lake, D&C Yellow #10 Lake, FD&C Yellow #6 Lake, Hydroxypropyl Methylcellulose, Microcrystalline Cellulose, Polyethylene Glycol, Povidone, Starch, Stearic Acid, Titanium Dioxide.

INDICATIONS
For hours of effective multi-symptom relief of colds/flu, sinusitis, hay fever, or other upper respiratory allergies: nasal congestion, sneezing, runny nose, fever, headache and minor aches and pains.

ACTIONS
Acetaminophen is both analgesic and antipyretic. Therapeutic doses of acetaminophen will effectively reduce an elevated body temperature. Also, acetaminophen is effective in reducing the discomfort of pain associated with headache. Phenylephrine HCl is an oral nasal decongestant (Sympathomimetic Amine), effective as a vasoconstrictor to help reduce nasal/sinus congestion. Phenylephrine produces little or no Central Nervous System stimulation.

Chlorpheniramine Maleate is an antihistamine effective in the control of rhinorrhea, sneezing and lacrimation associated with elevated histamine levels in disorders of the respiratory tract.

DOSAGE AND ADMINISTRATION

Adults: Two tablets or caplets every four hours, not to exceed 12 tablets or caplets in 24 hours. Children 6–12: One tablet or caplet every four hours, not to exceed six tablets or caplets in 24 hours.

WARNINGS

Avoid alcoholic beverages and driving a motor vehicle or operating heavy machinery while taking this product. May cause drowsiness or excitability, especially in children. Persons with asthma, glaucoma, high blood pressure, diabetes, heart or thyroid disease, difficulty in urination due to enlarged prostate gland, or taking an antidepressant drug, should use only as directed by a physician. Do not exceed recommended dosage because at higher doses nervousness, dizziness, or sleeplessness may occur. If symptoms do not improve within 7 days or are accompanied by high fever, discontinue use and see a physician. As with any drug, if you are pregnant or nursing a baby, seek the advice of a health professional before using this product.
Do not give to children under 6. Keep this and all medication out of children's reach. In case of accidental overdose contact a physician immediately.

PROFESSIONAL LABELING

Same as those outlined under Indications.

HOW SUPPLIED

Yellow/White uncoated tablets in tins of 12 and bottles of 24, 50, and 100, and physician dispensers of 100 2-tablet patient sample pouches. Yellow/White coated caplets in blister packages of 20 and 40.

Shown in Product Identification Section, page 435

PREPARATION H®

[prep-e 'rā-shen āch]

Hemorrhoidal Ointment

PREPARATION H®

Hemorrhoidal Suppositories

ACTIVE INGREDIENTS

Ointment—Live Yeast Cell Derivative supplying 2,000 units Skin Respiratory Factor per ounce of Ointment and Shark Liver Oil 3.0% in a specially prepared Rectal Petrolatum Base.
Suppositories—Live Yeast Cell Derivative supplying 2,000 units Skin Respiratory Factor per ounce of Cocoa Butter Suppository Base and Shark Liver Oil 3.0%.
Inactive Ingredients: Ointment—Beeswax, Glycerin, Lanolin, Lanolin Alcohol, Mineral Oil, Paraffin, Phenylmercuric Nitrate (1:10,000 as a preservative), Thyme Oil.
Suppositories—Beeswax, Glycerin, Phenylmercuric Nitrate 1:10,000 (as a preservative), Polyethylene Glycol 600 Dilaurate.

INDICATIONS

To help shrink swelling of hemorrhoidal tissues caused by inflammation and to give prompt, temporary relief in many cases from pain and itch in tissues.

ACTIONS

Live Yeast Cell Derivative acts by increasing the oxygen uptake of dermal tissues and facilitating collagen formation. Shark Liver Oil has been incorporated to act as a protectant which softens and soothes the tissues. Preparation H also lubricates inflamed, irritated surfaces to help make bowel movements less painful.

PRECAUTION

In case of bleeding, or if your condition persists, a physician should be consulted.

DOSAGE AND ADMINISTRATION

Ointment: Before applying, remove protective cover from applicator. Lubricate applicator before each application and thoroughly cleanse after use. It is recommended that Preparation H Hemorrhoidal ointment be applied freely to the affected rectal area whenever symptoms occur, from three to five times per day, especially at night, in the morning and after each bowel movement. Frequent application with Preparation H ointment provides continual therapy which leads to more rapid improvement of rectal conditions. Suppositories: Whenever symptoms occur, remove wrapper, insert rectally from three to five times per day, especially at night, in the morning and after each bowel movement. Frequent application with Preparation H suppositories provides continual therapy which leads to more rapid improvement of rectal conditions. Store at controlled room temperature in cool place but not over 80°F.

PROFESSIONAL LABELING

Same as those outlined under Indications.

HOW SUPPLIED

Ointment: Net Wt. 1 oz. and 2 oz.
Suppositories: 12's, 24's, 36's, and 48's.

Shown in Product Identification Section, page 435

PRIMATENE®

[prīm 'a-tēn]

Mist

(Epinephrine Inhalation Aerosol)

ACTIVE INGREDIENTS

Each spray delivers approximately 0.2 mg. Epinephrine. A 0.5% w/w (= 5.5 mg./cc.) solution of U.S.P. Epinephrine.

INACTIVE INGREDIENTS

Alcohol 34%, Ascorbic Acid, Fluorocarbons (propellant), water.
Contains No Sulfites.

INDICATIONS

Provides temporary relief from acute paroxysms of bronchial asthma.

WARNINGS

For INHALATION ONLY. Contents under pressure. Do not puncture or throw container into incinerator.
Using or storing near open flame or heating above 120° F may cause bursting.
Do not use unless a diagnosis of asthma has been established by a physician. Reduce dosage if bronchial irritation, nervousness, restlessness or sleeplessness occurs. Overdose may cause nervousness and rapid heartbeat. Use only on the advice of a physician if heart disease, high blood pressure, diabetes, or thyroid disease is present. If difficulty in breathing persists, or if relief does not occur within 20 minutes of inhalation, discontinue use and seek medical assistance immediately. As with any drug, if you are pregnant or nursing a baby, seek the advice of a health professional before using this product. Children under 6 years of age should use Primatene Mist only on the advice of a physician. KEEP THIS AND ALL MEDICINES OUT OF REACH OF CHILDREN.

DIRECTIONS

1. Take plastic cap off mouthpiece. (For refills, use mouthpiece from previous purchase).
2. Take plastic mouthpiece off bottle.
3. Place other end of mouthpiece on bottle.
4. Turn bottle upside down. Place thumb on bottom of mouthpiece over the circular button and forefinger on top of vial. Empty the lungs as completely as possible by exhaling.
5. Place mouthpiece in mouth with lips closed around opening. Inhale deeply while squeezing mouthpiece and bottle together. Release immediately and remove unit from mouth, then complete taking the deep breath, drawing medication into your lungs, holding breath as long as comfortable.
6. Then exhale slowly keeping lips nearly closed. This distributes the medication in the lungs.

DOSAGE

Start with one inhalation by squeezing mouthpiece and bottle together. Release immediately and remove unit from mouth. Then wait at least one minute. If not relieved, use Primatene Mist once more; do not repeat treatment for at least 4 hours.

PROFESSIONAL LABELING

Same as stated under Indications.

HOW SUPPLIED

½ fl. oz (15 cc) with mouthpiece.
½ fl. oz. (15 cc) refill
¾ fl. oz. (22.5 cc) refill

Shown in Product Identification Section, page 435

PRIMATENE®

[prīm 'a-tēn]

Mist Suspension

(Epinephrine Bitartrate Inhalation Aerosol)

ACTIVE INGREDIENTS

Each spray delivers 0.3 mg. Epinephrine Bitartrate equivalent to 0.16 mg. Epinephrine base. Contains Epinephrine Bitartrate 7.0 mg.

INACTIVE INGREDIENTS

Fluorocarbons (propellant), Sorbitan Trioleate.
Contains No Sulfites.

INDICATIONS

Provides temporary relief from acute paroxysms of bronchial asthma.

WARNINGS

For INHALATION ONLY. Contents under pressure. Do not puncture or throw container into incinerator. Using or storing near open flame or heating above 120°F may cause bursting.
Do not use unless a diagnosis of asthma has been established by a physician. Reduce dosage if bronchial irritation, nervousness, restlessness or sleeplessness occurs. Overdose may cause nervousness and rapid heartbeat. Use only on the advice of a physician if heart disease, high blood pressure, diabetes, or thyroid disease is present. If difficulty in breathing persists, or if relief does not occur within 20 minutes of inhalation, discontinue use and seek medical assistance immediately. As with any drug, if you are pregnant or nursing a baby, seek the advice of a health professional before using this product. Children under 6 years of age should use Primatene Mist only on the advice of a physician. KEEP THIS AND ALL MEDICINES OUT OF REACH OF CHILDREN.

ADMINISTRATION

Directions: 1. Shake well. 2. Hold inhaler with nozzle down while using. Empty the lungs as completely as possible by exhaling. 3. Purse the lips as in saying "o" and hold the nozzle up to the lips, keeping the tongue flat. As you start to take a deep breath, squeeze nozzle and can together, releasing one one full application. Complete taking deep breath, drawing medication into your lungs. 4. Hold breath for as long as comfortable. This distributes the medication in the lungs. Then exhale slowly, keeping the lips nearly closed. 5. Rinse nozzle daily with soap and hot water after removing from vial. Dry with clean cloth.

DOSAGE

Start with one inhalation—then wait at least one minute; if not relieved, use Primatene Mist Suspension once more; do not repeat treatment for at least 4 hours.

PROFESSIONAL LABELING

Same as stated under Indications.

HOW SUPPLIED

⅓ fl. oz. (10 cc.) pocket-size aerosol inhaler.

PRIMATENE®

[prīm 'a-tēn]

Tablets

Available in two formulas, "M" or "P", depending on state. See details below in section on "How Supplied".

ACTIVE INGREDIENTS

Theophylline 130 mg., Ephedrine Hydrochloride 24 mg., Phenobarbital 8 mg. (⅛ gr.) per tablet. In those states where Phenobarbital is ℞ only, Pyrilamine Maleate 16.6 mg. is substituted for the Phenobarbital.

INACTIVE INGREDIENTS

P Formula (Phenobarbital)—Colloidal Silicon Dioxide, D&C Yellow No. 10, FD&C Yellow No. 6, Magnesium Stearate, Sodium Starch Glycolate, Starch, Surfactant.
M Formula (Pyrilamine Maleate) D&C Yellow No. 10 Lake, FD&C Yellow No. 6 Lake, Hydrogenated Vegetable Oil, Magnesium Stearate, Microcrystalline Cellulose, Sodium Starch Glycolate, Surfactant.
Contains No Sulfites.

INDICATIONS

For relief and control of attacks of bronchial asthma and associated hay fever.

ACTIONS

Theophylline and ephedrine both produce bronchodilation through relaxation of bronchial muscle spasm, as occurs in attacks of bronchial asthma. Because theophylline is a methylxanthine and ephedrine is a sympathomimetic, they are believed to have different mechanisms of action.

WARNINGS

If symptoms persist, consult your physician. Some people are sensitive to ephedrine and, in such cases, temporary sleeplessness and nervousness may occur. These reactions will disappear if the use of the medication is discontinued. Do not exceed recommended dosage.
People who have heart disease, high blood pressure, diabetes or thyroid trouble should take this preparation only on the advice of a physician. People who have difficulty in urination due to enlarged prostate should take the "M" Formula only on advice of a Physician. "M" Formula, may cause drowsiness. People taking the "M" Formula should not drive or operate machinery. "P" Formula may be habit forming.

CAUTION

As with any drug, if you are pregnant or nursing a baby, seek the advice of a health professional before using this product. Keep all medicines out of reach of children.

DOSAGE AND ADMINISTRATION

Adults: 1 or 2 tablets initially and then one every 4 hours, as needed, not to exceed 6 tablets in 24 hours. Children (6–12): One half adult dose. For children under 6, consult a physician.

Continued on next page

Whitehall—Cont.

PROFESSIONAL LABELING
Same as stated under Indications.

HOW SUPPLIED
Available in two forms coded "M" or "P". "M" formula, containing pyrilamine maleate, is available in those states where phenobarbital is ℞ only. "P" formula, containing phenobarbital, is available in all other states. Both "M" and "P" formulas are supplied in glass bottles of 24 and 60 tablets.

Shown in Product Identification Section, page 435

SEMICID®
[sĕm 'ē-sĭd]
Vaginal Contraceptive Inserts

DESCRIPTION
Semicid is a safe, effective, vaginal contraceptive in insert form.
Convenient, Individually Wrapped, No Hormones, odorless, non-messy.

ACTIVE INGREDIENT
Each insert contains nonoxynol-9, 100 mg.

INACTIVE INGREDIENTS
Polyethylene Glycol, Benzethonium Chloride, Citric Acid, D&C Red #21, D&C Red #33, Methylparaben, Water.

INDICATION
For the prevention of pregnancy.

ACTIONS
Semicid dissolves in the vagina and blends with natural vaginal secretions to provide double birth control protection: a physical barrier, plus an effective sperm killing barrier that covers the cervical opening and adjoining vaginal walls. Each Semicid insert contains a fixed dosage of the maximum allowable amount of nonoxynol-9, the most widely used nonprescription spermicide.
Semicid requires no applicator and has no unpleasant taste or odor. Semicid is not messy and it does not drip or run like foams, creams and jellies. And it's not awkward to use like the diaphragm. As with all spermicides, some Semicid users experience irritation in using the product, but for years most women have used Semicid safely and effectively with full satisfaction. Also, Semicid does not effervesce like some inserts, so it is not as likely to cause a burning feeling.
Semicid is approximately as effective as vaginal foam contraceptives in actual use, but is not as effective as the Pill or IUD.
Semicid provides effective contraceptive protection when used properly. However, no contraceptive method or product can provide an absolute guarantee against becoming pregnant.

DOSAGE AND ADMINISTRATION
To use, just unwrap one insert and insert it deeply into the vagina. It is essential that Semicid be inserted at least 15 minutes before intercourse, however, Semicid is also effective when inserted up to 1 hour before intercourse. If intercourse is delayed for more than 1 hour after Semicid is inserted, or if intercourse is repeated, then another insert must be inserted. Semicid can be used as frequently as needed.

WARNINGS
Do not insert in urinary opening. Do not take orally. If irritation occurs, discontinue use. If irritation persists, consult your physician. Keep this and all contraceptives out of the reach of children.

HOW TO STORE
Keep Semicid at room temperature (not over 86°F or 30°C).

PRECAUTIONS
If douching is desired, one should wait at least six hours after intercourse before douching. If either partner experiences irritation, discontinue use. If irritation persists, consult a physician.
If your doctor has told you that you should not become pregnant, ask your doctor if you can use Semicid.
If menstrual period is missed, a physician should be consulted.

HOW SUPPLIED
Strip packaging of 10's and 20's.

Shown in Product Identification Section, page 435

TRENDAR®
Ibuprofen Tablets, USP
Menstrual Pain & Cramp Reliever

WARNING:
ASPIRIN SENSITIVE PATIENTS. Do not take this product if you have had a severe allergic reaction to aspirin, e.g. asthma, swelling, shock or hives, because even though this product contains no aspirin or salicylates cross-reacions may occur in patients allergic to aspirin.

INDICATIONS
For the temporary relief of painful menstrual cramps (Dysmenorrhea); also headaches, backaches and muscular aches and pains associated with Premenstrual Sydrome.

DOSAGE AND ADMINISTRATION
Adults: Take 1 tablet every 4 to 6 hours at the onset of menstrual symptoms and while pain persists. If pain does not respond to 1 tablet, 2 tablets may be used but do not exceed 6 tablets in 24 hours, unless directed by a doctor. The smallest effective dose should be used. Take with food or milk if occasional and mild heartburn, upset stomach, or stomach pain occurs with use. Consult a doctor if these symptoms are more than mild or if they persist. Children: Do not give this product to children under 12 except under the advice or supervision of a doctor.

WARNINGS
Do not take for pain for more than 10 days unless directed by a doctor. If pain persists or gets worse, or if new symptoms occur, consult a doctor. These could be signs of serious illness. If you are under a doctor's care for any serious condition, consult a doctor before taking this product. As with aspirin and acetaminophen, if you have any condition which requires you to take prescription drugs or if you have had any problems or serious side effects from taking any nonprescription pain reliever, do not take this product without first discussing it with your doctor. If you experience any symptoms which are unusual or seem unrelated to the condition for which you took ibuprofen, consult a doctor before taking any more of it. Although ibuprofen is indicated for the same conditions as aspirin and acetaminophen, it should not be taken with them except under a doctor's direction. Do not combine this product with any other ibuprofen-containing product. As with any drug, if you are pregnant or nursing a baby, seek the advice of a health professional before using this product. IT IS ESPECIALLY IMPORTANT NOT TO USE IBUPROFEN DURING THE LAST 3 MONTHS OF PREGNANCY UNLESS SPECIFICALLY DIRECTED TO DO SO BY A DOCTOR BECAUSE IT MAY CAUSE PROBLEMS IN THE UNBORN CHILD OR COMPLICATIONS DURING DELIVERY, Keep this and all drugs out of the reach of children. In case of accidental overdose, seek professional assistance or contact a poison control center immediately.

ACTIVE INGREDIENT
Each tablet contains Ibuprofen 200 mg.

INACTIVE INGREDIENTS
Acacia, Acetylated Monoglycerides, Beeswax, Calcium Sulfate, Colloidal Silicon Dioxide, Dimethicone, Iron Oxide, Lecithin, Pharmaceutical Glaze, Povidone, Sodium Benzoate, Sodium Carboxymethylcellulose, Starch, Stearic Acid, Sucrose, Titanium Dioxide.

PROFESSIONAL LABELING
Same as stated under Indications.

HOW SUPPLIED
Coated tablets in bottles of 20's & 40's.

STORAGE
Store at room temperature; avoid excessive heat 40°C (104°F).

Shown in Product Identification Section, page 435

Willen Drug Company
18 NORTH HIGH STREET
BALTIMORE, MD 21202

BICITRA®—Sugar-Free ℞
[bye "si-trah]
(Brand of Sodium Citrate & Citric Acid Oral Solution USP)

DESCRIPTION
BICITRA is a stable and pleasant tasting oral systemic alkalizer and neutralizing buffer composed of Sodium Citrate and Citric Acid in a sugar-free base. BICITRA is the USP formula for SHOHL's Solution.

COMPOSITION
BICITRA contains in each teaspoonful (5 ml):
SODIUM CITRATE-Dihydrate ....500 mg (0.34 Molar)
CITRIC ACID-Monohydrate ....334 mg (0.32 Molar)
Each ml contains 1 mEq Sodium and is equivalent to 1 mEq Bicarbonate (HCO_3).

ACTIONS
Sodium Citrate is absorbed and metabolized to sodium bicarbonate, thus acting as a systemic alkalizer. The effects are essentially those of chlorides before absorption and those of bicarbonates subsequently. BICITRA is useful for effectively buffering and neutralizing gastric acid, especially in preanesthesia medication.

INDICATIONS AND ADVANTAGES
BICITRA is an effective oral alkalizing agent and a non-particulate acid neutralizing buffer. BICITRA offers the advantage over particulate antacids by being absorbed and metabolized, since it is a systemic alkalizer. It is useful in those conditions where long term maintenance of an alkaline urine is desirable, and is of value in the alleviation of chronic metabolic acidosis such as results from chronic renal insufficiency or the syndrome of renal tubular acidosis, especially when the administration of potassium salts is undesirable or contraindicated. BICITRA is fast-acting and useful in raising the pH value of gastric acid. In vitro tests have shown that 15ml BICITRA plus 15ml water will neutralize and buffer 117ml of 0.1N HCl to a pH value of 2.5, with no alteration or changes in pH value after 2 hours elapsed time. BICITRA is concentrated, and when administered after meals and before bedtime, allows one to maintain an alkaline urine pH around the clock, usually without the necessity of a 2 A.M. dose. BICITRA alkalinizes the urine without producing a systemic alkalosis in the recommended dosage. BICITRA is pleasant tasting and tolerable, even when administered for long periods, and offers these advantages over SHOHL'S Solution, while supplying the equivalent sodium content. BICITRA is sugar-free.

CONTRAINDICATIONS
Patients on sodium-restricted diet or with severe renal impairment. In certain situations, Potassium Citrate, as contained in POLYCITRA-K may be preferable.

PRECAUTIONS
Should be used with caution by patients with low urinary output unless under the supervision of a physician. Patients should be directed to dilute adequately with water and preferably, to take each dose after meals to avoid saline laxative effect. Sodium salts should be used cautiously in patients with cardiac failure, hypertension, impaired renal function, peripheral and pulmonary edema and toxemia of pregnancy. Periodic examinations and determinations of serum electrolytes, particularly serum bicarbonate level, should be carried out in those patients with renal disease in order to avoid these complications.

ADVERSE REACTIONS
BICITRA is generally well tolerated without any unpleasant side effects when given in recommended doses to patients with normal renal function and urinary output. However, as with any alkalinizing agent, caution must be used in certain patients with abnormal renal mechanisms to avoid development of alkalosis, especially in the presence of hypocalcemia.

DOSAGE AND ADMINISTRATION
BICITRA should be taken diluted in water followed by additional water, if desired.
For Systemic Alkalization:
Usual Adult Dose: 10 to 30ml diluted in 1 to 3 ounces of water after meals and at bedtime, or as directed by physician.
As a Neutralizing Buffer: 15ml diluted with 15ml water, taken as a single dose, or as directed by physician.

OVERDOSAGE
Overdosage with sodium salts may cause diarrhea, nausea and vomiting, hypernoea, and convulsions.

HOW SUPPLIED
BICITRA—16 fl oz. (473ml) (NDC 11414-207-01); 1 gallon (NDC 11414-207-08); 4 fl oz (120ml) (NDC 11414-207-04); 15ml Unit-Dose (NDC 11414-207-15).

LITERATURE AVAILABLE
Yes

NEUTRA-PHOS® Powder & Capsules
NEUTRA-PHOS®-K Powder & Capsules
[new "trah foss ']
Oral Phosphorus Dietary Supplement

NEUTRA-PHOS and NEUTRA-PHOS-K supply the physiologically important element—PHOSPHORUS—as inorganic orthophosphate, in a well tolerated oral compound. Each contains a chemically balanced combination of readily soluble inorganic phosphates, affording a very high source of elemental Phosphorus. Both products supply equal concentration of elemental Phosphorus.

COMPOSITION
NEUTRA-PHOS is a stable powder combination of monobasic and dibasic Sodium and Potassium Phosphates. NEUTRA-PHOS-K is a stable sodium-free powder combination of monobasic and dibasic Potassium Phosphates intended for oral use in low sodium diets. Both products form an oral solution by reconstitution with water and are neutral (pH 7.3), isotonic, pleasant tasting sources of Phosphorus. There is less than 1 calorie per average dose.

INDICATIONS
NEUTRA-PHOS and NEUTRA-PHOS-K are recommended as oral Phosphorus supplements, particularly if the diet is low in mineral intake or if needs are increased.

ADVANTAGES
NEUTRA-PHOS and NEUTRA-PHOS-K, reconstituted to an oral liquid, provide rapid absorption and utilization from the alimentary tract. This is very advantageous compared to the use of coated or uncoated tablet dosage forms. (The patient ingests a liquid rather than a slowly dissolving tablet which may cause localized irritation or inflamation in sensitive individuals.) Both products are highly concentrated and thus economically provide inorganic Phosphate. They are especially useful for long term maintenance requirements. NEUTRA-PHOS also supplies Sodium and Potassium in equimolar proportions—a decided advantage over products which supply a high amount of sodium and a low amount of potassium per dose. NEUTRA-PHOS-K supplies only Potassium and is recommended when a low sodium diet is indicated.

ELECTROLYTES SUPPLIED
2-½ fluid ounces (75 ml) of the reconstituted solution or contents of 1 capsule* supplies:

NEUTRA-PHOS

Electrolyte	mg.	mEq
Phosphorus	250	14.25
Phosphate (PO_4)	765	—
Sodium	164	7.125
Potassium	278	7.125

NEUTRA-PHOS-K

Electrolyte	mg.	mEq
Phosphorus	250	14.25
Phosphate (PO_4)	765	—
Sodium	none	none
Potassium	556	14.25

(*reconstituted in water as per label directions. Refer to Capsules description.)

AVERAGE DIRECTIONS FOR ADULTS AND CHILDREN
4 or more years of age: 2-½ fl. oz. (75 ml) of the oral solution, or contents of 1 capsule, equivalent to 250 mg Phosphorus, taken 4 times a day. (See Capsules description).

PEDIATRIC DOSE
Infants and children under 4 years of age: 2 fl. oz. (60 ml) of the oral solution, equivalent to 200 mg of Phosphorus, taken 4 times a day.

USUAL DOSE RANGE
2-½ fl. oz. to 20 fl. oz. (75 ml to 600 ml) of the oral solution, or contents of 1 to 8 capsules (equivalent from 250 mg to 2 grams of Phosphorus) taken daily in divided doses, after meals and at bedtime.
2-½ fl. oz. (75 ml) or 1 capsule, 4 times a day supplies 1 gm. Phosphorus. 5 fl. oz. (150 ml) or 2 capsules, 3 times a day supplies 1.5 gm. Phosphorus. 5 fl. oz. (150 ml) or 2 capsules, 4 times a day supplies 2 gm. Phosphorus. (See Capsules description).

PRECAUTIONS AND SIDE EFFECTS
Reconstitute powder and contents of capsules as directed before taking. Occasionally some individuals may experience a mild laxative effect for the first day or two when beginning to use NEUTRA-PHOS. If this persists to an unpleasant degree, reduce the daily intake until this effect subsides or, if necessary, discontinue its use.

HOW SUPPLIED
Both products are supplied as powder concentrates, to be reconstituted with water by the patient, and are available in multiple dose or single dose capsule sizes.
Multiple Dose Powder Concentrate: For patient convenience, these powder concentrates are packaged in a size sufficient to make 1 gallon (3.785 Liters) and are intended for use while at home. This economical dosage form is prepared by the patient who is instructed to dissolve the entire contents of 1 bottle in sufficient water to make 1 gallon of solution. This solution is not to be diluted and can be stored for 60 days. It can be chilled if desired, to increase palatability. 2-½ fl. oz. (75 ml) of this solution supplies 250 mg Phosphorus (refer to electrolyte chart).
Capsules: For patient convenience, these products are supplied in premeasured capsules, which are intended for use, if difficult for patients to transport the reconstituted liquid prepared from the multiple dose powder concentrate. The contents of 1 capsule makes 2-½ fl. oz. (75 ml) of an oral suspension equal to the oral solution prepared above. To use, empty the contents of 1 capsule into ⅓ glass water (approx. 2-½ fl. oz.) and stir well and take promptly. Each capsule supplies 250 mg Phosphorus (refer to electrolyte chart).
NEUTRA-PHOS Powder Concentrate—2-¼ oz. (64 gm) bottle. Reconstitutes to 1 gallon Stock No. 201-01.
NEUTRA-PHOS Capsules—1.25 gm powder concentrate per capsule, 48 capsules per bottle Stock No. 202-01.
NEUTRA-PHOS-K Powder Concentrate— 2-½ oz. (71 gm) bottle. Reconstitutes to 1 gallon Stock No. 203-01.
NEUTRA-PHOS-K Capsules—1.45 gm powder concentrate per capsule, 48 capsules per bottle Stock No. 204-01.

IS THIS PRODUCT O.T.C.
Yes.

LITERATURE AVAILABLE
Yes.

POLYCITRA® Syrup ℞
POLYCITRA®-LC-Sugar-Free
[polly "si-trah]
(Brand of Tricitrates Oral Solution U.S.P.)

DESCRIPTION
Syrup POLYCITRA and POLYCITRA-LC are stable and pleasant-tasting oral systemic alkalizers containing Potassium Citrate, Sodium Citrate and Citric Acid. Syrup POLYCITRA is a sugar-base preparation. POLYCITRA-LC is a sugar-free solution, to be used by patients who desire a low-carbohydrate diet. Both products are non-alcoholic and contain identical amounts of active ingredients.

COMPOSITION
Syrup POLYCITRA and POLYCITRA-LC contains in each teaspoonful (5 ml):
POTASSIUM CITRATE-Monohydrate 550 mg (0.34 Molar)
SODIUM CITRATE-Dihydrate ....500 mg (0.34 Molar)
CITRIC ACID-Monohydrate...................334 mg (0.32 Molar)
Each ml contains 1 mEq. Potassium and 1 mEq. Sodium and is equivalent to 2 mEq. Bicarbonate (HCO_3).

ACTIONS
Potassium Citrate and Sodium Citrate are absorbed and metabolized to potassium bicarbonate and sodium bicarbonate, thus acting as systemic alkalizers. The effects are essentially those of chlorides before absorption and those of bicarbonates subsequently.

INDICATIONS AND ADVANTAGES
Syrup POLYCITRA and POLYCITRA-LC are effective alkalinizing agents useful in those conditions where long term maintenance of an alkaline urine is desirable, such as in patients with uric acid and cystine calculi of the urinary tract. In addition, they are valuable adjuvants when administered with uricosuric agents in gout therapy, since urates tend to crystallize out of an acid urine. They are also effective in correcting the acidosis of certain renal tubular disorders. Syrup POLYCITRA and POLYCITRA-LC are highly concentrated, and when administered after meals and before bedtime, allows one to maintain an alkaline urine pH around the clock, usually without the necessity of a 2 AM dose. Syrup POLYCITRA and POLYCITRA-LC alkalinize the urine without producing a systemic alkalosis in recommended dosage. They are highly palatable, pleasant tasting and tolerable, even when administered for long periods. POLYCITRA-LC is a fast-acting and effective non-particulate neutralizing buffer, useful in raising the pH value of gastric acid. In vitro tests have shown that 15 ml POLYCITRA-LC plus 15 ml water will neutralize and buffer 234 ml of 0.1N HCl to a pH value of 2.5, with no alteration or changes in pH value after 2 hours elapsed time.

CONTRAINDICATIONS
Severe renal impairment with oliguria or azotemia, untreated Addison's disease or severe myocardial damage. In certain situations, when patients are on a sodium-restricted diet, the use of Potassium Citrate, as contained in POLYCITRA-K, may be preferable; or when patients are on a potassium-restricted diet, the use of Sodium Citrate, as contained in BICITRA, may be preferable.

PRECAUTIONS AND WARNINGS
Should be used with caution by patients with low urinary output unless under the supervision of a physician. Patients should be directed to dilute adequately with water and preferably, to take each dose after meals, to minimize the possibility of gastrointestinal injury associated with oral ingestion of potassium salt preparations and to avoid saline laxative effect. Sodium salts should be used cautiously in patients with cardiac failure, hypertension, peripheral and pulmonary edema and toxemia of pregnancy. Concurrent administration of potassium-containing medication, potassium-sparing diuretics, or cardiac glycosides may lead to toxicity. Periodic examination and determinations of serum electrolytes, particularly serum bicarbonate level, should be carried out in those patients with renal disease in order to avoid these complications.

ADVERSE REACTIONS
Syrup POLYCITRA and POLYCITRA-LC are generally well tolerated without any unpleasant side effects when given in recommended doses to patients with normal renal function and urinary output. However, as with any alkalinizing agent, caution must be used in certain patients with abnormal renal mechanisms to avoid development of hyperkalemia or alkalosis, especially in the presence of hypocalcemia. Potassium intoxication causes listlessness, weakness, mental confusion and tingling of extremities.

DOSAGE AND ADMINISTRATION
Syrup POLYCITRA and POLYCITRA-LC should be taken diluted in water, followed by additional water if desired.
Usual Dosage: Adults: 15 to 30 ml diluted in water, four times a day after meals and at bedtime, or as directed by physician. Children: 5 to 15 ml diluted in water, four times a day after meals and at bedtime or as directed by physician.
Usual Dosage Range: 10 to 15 ml diluted with water, taken four times a day, will usually maintain a urine pH of 6.5–7.4. 15 to 20 ml diluted with water, taken four times a day, will usually maintain a urine pH of 7.0–7.6 throughout most of the 24 hours without unpleasant side effects.
As a Neutralizing Buffer: 15 ml diluted with 15 ml water, taken as a single dose, or as directed by physician.

OVERDOSAGE
Overdosage with sodium salts may cause diarrhea, nausea and vomiting, hypernoea, and convulsions. Overdosage with potassium salts may cause hyperkalemia and alkalosis, especially in the presence of renal disease.

HOW SUPPLIED
Syrup POLYCITRA—16 fl oz (473 ml) (NDC 11414-205-01) and 4 fl oz (120 ml) hospital size (NDC 11414-205-04).
POLYCITRA-LC—16 fl oz (473 ml) (NDC 11414-208-01) and 4 fl oz (120 ml) hospital size (NDC 11414-208-04)
Literature Available: Yes.

POLYCITRA®-K—Sugar Free ℞
[polly "si-trah-ka 'y]
(Brand of Potassium Citrate and Citric Acid Oral Solution USP)

DESCRIPTION
POLYCITRA-K is a stable and pleasant tasting oral systemic alkalizer containing Potassium Citrate and Citric Acid in a non-alcoholic sugar-free base.

COMPOSITION
POLYCITRA-K contains in each teaspoonful (5ml):
POTASSIUM CITRATE—Monohydrate .... 1100 mg (0.68 Molar)
CITRIC ACID—Monohydrate .... 334 mg (0.32 Molar).
Each ml contains 2 mEq. Potassium ion and is equivalent to 2 mEq. Bicarbonate (HCO_3).

ACTIONS
Potassium Citrate is absorbed and metabolized to potassium bicarbonate, thus acting as a systemic alkalizer. The effects are essentially those of chlorides before absorption and those of bicarbonates subsequently.

Continued on next page

Willen—Cont.

INDICATIONS AND ADVANTAGES

POLYCITRA-K is an effective alkalinizing agent useful in those conditions where long term maintenance of an alkaline urine is desirable, such as in patients with uric acid and cystine calculi of the urinary tract, especially when the administration of sodium salts is undesirable or contraindicated. In addition, it is a valuable adjuvant when administered with uricosuric agents in gout therapy, since urates tend to crystallize out of an acid urine. It is also effective in correcting the acidosis of certain renal tubular disorders where the administration of Potassium Citrate may be preferable. POLYCITRA-K is highly concentrated, and when administered after meals and before bedtime, allows one to maintain an alkaline urine pH around the clock, usually without the necessity of a 2 A.M. dose. POLYCITRA-K alkalinizes the urine without producing a systemic alkalosis in recommended dosage. It is highly palatable, pleasant tasting and tolerable, even when administered for long periods.- POLYCITRA-K is an oral liquid, providing rapid absorption and utilization from the alimentary tract. This is very advantageous compared to the use of tablet dosage forms. (The patient ingests a liquid rather than a slowly dissolving tablet, which may cause local irritation or inflammation in sensitive individuals).

CONTRAINDICATIONS

Severe renal impairment with oliguria or azotemia, untreated Addison's disease, adynamia episodica hereditaria, acute dehydration, heat cramps, anuria, severe myocardial damage, and hyperkalemia from any cause.

WARNING

Large doses may cause hyperkalemia and alkalosis, especially in the presence of renal disease. Concurrent administration of potassium-containing medication, potassium-sparing diuretics, or cardiac-glycosides may lead to toxicity.

PRECAUTIONS

Should be used with caution by patients with low urinary output unless under the supervision of a physician. As with all liquids containing a high concentration of potassium, patients should be directed to dilute adequately with water to minimize the possibility of gastrointestinal injury associated with the oral ingestion of concentrated potassium salt preparations; and preferably, to take each dose after meals to avoid saline laxative effect.

ADVERSE REACTIONS

POLYCITRA-K is generally well tolerated without any unpleasant side effects when given in recommended doses to patients with normal renal function and urinary output. However, as with any alkalinizing agent, caution must be used in certain patients with abnormal renal mechanisms to avoid development of hyperkalemia or alkalosis. Potassium intoxication causes listlessness, weakness, mental confusion, tingling of extremities, and other symptoms associated with a high concentration of potassium in the serum. Periodic determinations of serum electrolytes should be carried out in those patients with renal disease in order to avoid these complications. Hyperkalemia may exhibit the following electrocardiographic abnormalities; Disappearance of the P wave, widening and slurring of QRS complex, changes of the S-T segment, tall peaked T waves, etc.

DOSAGE AND ADMINISTRATION

POLYCITRA-K should be taken diluted in water according to directions, followed by additional water if desired.

Usual Adult Dose: 3 to 6 teaspoonfuls (15 to 30 ml), diluted with 1 glass of water, after meals and at bedtime, or as directed by physician.

Usual Pediatric Dose: 1 to 3 teaspoonfuls (5 to 15 ml), diluted with ½ glass of water, after meals and at bedtime, or as directed by physician.

Usual Dosage Range: 10 to 15 ml diluted with a glassful of water, taken four times a day, will usually maintain a urinary pH of 6.5–7.4. 15 to 20 ml diluted with a glassful of water, taken four times a day will usually maintain a urine pH of 7.0–7.6 throughout most of the 24 hours without unpleasant side effects.

OVERDOSAGE

The administration of oral potassium salts to persons with normal excretory mechanisms for potassium rarely causes serious hyperkalemia. However, if excretory mechanisms are impaired, hyperkalemia can result (see Contraindications and Warnings). Hyperkalemia, when detected, must be treated immediately because lethal levels can be reached in a few hours.

Treatment of Hyperkalemia: Should hyperkalemia occur, treatment measures include the following: (1) elimination of foods or medications containing potassium. (2) The intravenous administration of 300 to 500 ml/hr of dextrose solution (10 to 25%), containing 10 units of insulin/20 gm dextrose. (3) The use of exchange resins, hemodialysis, or peritoneal dialysis. In treating hyperkalemia, it should be recalled that in patients who have been stabilized on digitalis, too rapid a lowering of the plasma potassium concentration can produce digitalis toxicity.

HOW SUPPLIED

POLYCITRA-K—16 fl oz (473 ml) (NDC 11414-209-01) and 4 fl oz (120 ml) hospital size (NDC 11414-209-04)

Literature Available: Yes.

Winthrop-Breon Laboratories

90 PARK AVENUE
NEW YORK, NY 10016

AMIPAQUE® ℞
brand of metrizamide

(See Diagnostic Section.)

ARALEN® Hydrochloride ℞
brand of chloroquine hydrochloride injection, USP

For Malaria and Extraintestinal Amebiasis

WARNING: PHYSICIANS SHOULD COMPLETELY FAMILIARIZE THEMSELVES WITH THE COMPLETE CONTENTS OF THIS LEAFLET BEFORE PRESCRIBING ARALEN.

DESCRIPTION

Parenteral solution, each mL containing 50 mg of the dihydrochloride salt equivalent to 40 mg of chloroquine base. ARALEN hydrochloride, a 4-aminoquinoline compound, is chemically 7- (Chloro - 4 - [[4 - diethylamino) - 1 - methylbutyl] amino]-quinoline dihydrochloride, a white, crystalline substance, freely soluble in water.

ACTIONS

The compound is a highly active antimalarial and amebicidal agent.

ARALEN hydrochloride has been found to be highly active against the erythrocytic forms of *Plasmodium vivax* and *malariae* and most strains of *Plasmodium falciparum* (but not the gametocytes of *P. falciparum).* The precise mechanism of action of the drug is not known.

ARALEN hydrochloride does not prevent relapses in patients with vivax or malariae malaria because it is not effective against exoerythrocytic forms of the parasite, nor will it prevent vivax or malariae infection when administered as a prophylactic. It is highly effective as a suppressive agent in patients with vivax or malariae malaria, in terminating acute attacks, and significantly lengthening the interval between treatment and relapse. In patients with falciparum malaria it abolishes the acute attack and effects complete cure of the infection, unless due to a resistant strain of *P. falciparum.*

INDICATIONS

ARALEN hydrochloride is indicated for the treatment of extraintestinal amebiasis and for treatment of acute attacks of malaria due to *P. vivax, P. malariae, P. ovale,* and susceptible strains of *P. falciparum* when oral therapy is not feasible.

CONTRAINDICATIONS

Use of this drug is contraindicated in the presence of retinal or visual field changes either attributable to 4- aminoquinoline compounds or to any other etiology, and in patients with known hypersensitivity to 4-aminoquinoline compounds. However, in the treatment of acute attacks of malaria caused by susceptible strains of plasmodia, the physician may elect to use this drug after carefully weighing the possible benefits and risks to the patient.

WARNINGS

Children and infants are extremely susceptible to adverse effects from an overdose of parenteral ARALEN and sudden deaths have been recorded after such administration. In no instance should the single dose of parenteral ARALEN administered to infants or children exceed 5 mg base per kg.

In recent years it has been found that certain strains of *P. falciparum* have become resistant to 4-aminoquinoline compounds (including chloroquine and hydroxychloroquine) as shown by the fact that normally adequate doses have failed to prevent or cure clinical malaria or parasitemia. Treatment with quinine or other specific forms of therapy is therefore advised for patients infected with a resistant strain of parasites.

Use of ARALEN should be avoided in patients with psoriasis, for it may precipitate a severe attack of psoriasis. Some authors consider the use of 4-aminoquinoline compounds contraindicated in patients with porphyria since the condition may be exacerbated.

Irreversible retinal damage has been observed in some patients who had received long-term or high-dosage 4-aminoquinoline therapy. Retinopathy has been reported to be dose related.

If there is any indication (past or present) of abnormality in the visual acuity, visual field, or retinal macular areas (such as pigmentary changes, loss of foveal reflex), or any visual symptoms (such as light flashes and streaks) which are not fully explainable by difficulties of accommodation or corneal opacities, the drug should be discontinued immediately and the patient closely observed for possible progression. Retinal changes (and visual disturbances) may progress even after cessation of therapy.

Usage in Pregnancy. Usage of this drug during pregnancy should be avoided except in the suppression or treatment of malaria when in the judgment of the physician the benefit outweighs the possible hazard. It should be noted that radioactively tagged chloroquine administered intravenously to pregnant pigmented CBA mice passed rapidly across the placenta, accumulated selectively in the melanin structures of the fetal eyes and was retained in the ocular tissues for five months after the drug had been eliminated from the rest of the body.[1]

PRECAUTIONS

Since the drug is known to concentrate in the liver, it should be used with caution in patients with hepatic disease or alcoholism or in conjunction with known hepatotoxic drugs.

The drug should be administered with caution to patients having G-6-PD (glucose-6- phosphate dehydrogenase) deficiency.

ADVERSE REACTIONS

Respiratory depression, cardiovascular collapse, shock, convulsions, and death have been reported with overdoses of ARALEN hydrochloride, brand of chloroquine hydrochloride injection, especially in infants and children.

Any of the adverse reactions associated with short-term oral administration of chloroquine phosphate must be considered a possibility with chloroquine hydrochloride. Cardiovascular effects, such as hypotension and electrocardiographic changes (particularly inversion or depression of the T-wave, widening of the QRS complex), have rarely been noted in patients receiving usual antimalarial doses of the drug. Mild and transient headache, pruritus, psychic stimulation, visual disturbances (blurring of vision and difficulty of focusing or accommodation), pleomorphic skin eruptions, and gastrointestinal complaints (anorexia, nausea, vomiting, diarrhea, abdominal cramps) have been observed.

Instances of convulsive seizures associated with oral chloroquine therapy in patients with extraintestinal amebiasis have been reported.

A few cases of a nerve type of deafness have been reported after prolonged therapy, usually in high doses. Tinnitus and reduced hearing have been reported, in a patient with preexistent auditory damage, after administration of only 500 mg once a week for a few months. Since neuromyopathy, blood dyscrasias, lichen planus-like eruptions, and skin and mucosal pigmentary changes have been noted during prolonged oral therapy, their occurrence with this dosage form is possible.

Patients with retinal changes may be asymptomatic, especially in early cases, or may complain of nyctalopia and scotomatous vision with field defects of paracentral, pericentral ring types, and typically temporal scotomas, eg, difficulty in reading with words tending to disappear, seeing only half an object, misty vision, and fog before the eyes. Rarely scotomatous vision may occur without observable retinal changes.

DOSAGE AND ADMINISTRATION

Malaria —**Adult Dose.**An initial dose of 4 mL or 5 mL (160 mg to 200 mg chloroquine base) may be injected intramuscularly and repeated in 6 hours if necessary. The total parenteral dosage in the first 24 hours should not exceed 800 mg chloroquine base. Treatment by mouth should be started as soon as practicable and continued until a course of approximately 1.5 g of base in 3 days is completed.

Pediatric Dose. Infants and children are extremely susceptible to overdosage of parenteral ARALEN. Severe reactions and deaths have occurred. In the pediatric age range, parenteral ARALEN dosage should be calculated in proportion to the adult dose based upon body weight. The recommended single dose in infants and children is 5 mg base per kg. This dose may be repeated in 6 hours; however, the total dose in any 24 hour period should not exceed 10 mg base per kg of body weight. Parenteral administration should be terminated and oral therapy instituted as soon as possible.

Extraintestinal Amebiasis—In adult patients not able to tolerate oral therapy, from 4 mL to 5 mL (160 mg to 200 mg chloroquine base) may be injected daily for 10 to 12 days. Oral administration should be substituted or resumed as soon as possible.

OVERDOSAGE

Inadvertent toxic doses may produce respiratory depression or shock with hypotension. Respiratory depression is treated by artificial respiration and administration of oxygen. In shock with hypotension, a potent vasopressor, such as NEO-SYNEPHRINE® hydrochloride, brand of phenylephrine hydrochloride, USP, should be given intramuscularly in doses of 2 mg to 5 mg.

HOW SUPPLIED

Ampuls of 5 mL, box of 5 (NDC 0024-0074-01)

REFERENCE

Ullberg S, Lindquist N G, Sjostrand S E: Accumulation of chorio-retinotoxic drugs in the foetal eye. *Nature* 1970; 227:1257.

AW-100-G

ARALEN® Phosphate ℞

brand of chloroquine phosphate tablets, USP

For Malaria and Extraintestinal Amebiasis

WARNING: PHYSICIANS SHOULD COMPLETELY FAMILIARIZE THEMSELVES WITH THE COMPLETE CONTENTS OF THIS LEAFLET BEFORE PRESCRIBING ARALEN.

DESCRIPTION

ARALEN phosphate, a 4-aminoquinoline compound, is chemically 7-Chloro- 4-[[4- (diethylamino) -1-methylbutyl]amino]-quinoline phosphate (1:2), a white, crystalline substance, freely soluble in water.

Inactive Ingredients: Acacia, Carnauba Wax, Dibasic Calcium Phosphate, FD&C Red #3, Gelatin, Kaolin, Liquid Glucose, Magnesium Stearate, Pharmaceutical Glaze, Starch, Sucrose, Talc, Yellow Wax.

ACTIONS

ARALEN phosphate has been found to be highly active against the erythrocytic forms of *Plasmodium vivax* and *malariae* and most strains of *Plasmodium falciparum* (but not the gametocytes of *P. falciparum*). The precise mechanism of action of the drug is not known.

ARALEN phosphate does not prevent relapses in patients with vivax or malariae malaria because it is not effective against exo-erythrocytic forms of the parasite, nor will it prevent vivax or malariae infection when administered as a prophylactic. It is highly effective as a suppressive agent in patients with vivax or malariae malaria, in terminating acute attacks, and significantly lengthening the interval between treatment and relapse. In patients with falciparum malaria it abolishes the acute attack and effects complete cure of the infection, unless due to a resistant strain of *P. falciparum.*

In vitro studies with trophozoites of *Entamoeba histolytica* have demonstrated that ARALEN phosphate also possesses amebicidal activity comparable to that of emetine.

INDICATIONS

ARALEN phosphate is indicated for the suppressive treatment and for acute attacks of malaria due to *P. vivax, P. malariae, P. ovale,* and susceptible strains of *P. falciparum.* The drug is also indicated for treatment of extraintestinal amebiasis.

CONTRAINDICATIONS

Use of this drug is contraindicated in the presence of retinal or visual field changes either attributable to 4- aminoquinoline compounds or to any other etiology, and in patients with known hypersensitivity to 4-aminoquinoline compounds. However, in the treatment of acute attacks of malaria caused by susceptible strains of plasmodia, the physician may elect to use this drug after carefully weighing the possible benefits and risks to the patient.

WARNINGS

In recent years it has been found that certain strains of *P. falciparum* have become resistant to 4-aminoquinoline compounds (including chloroquine and hydroxychloroquine) as shown by the fact that normally adequate doses have failed to prevent or cure clinical malaria or parasitemia. Treatment with quinine or other specific forms of therapy is therefore advised for patients infected with a resistant strain of parasites.

Irreversible retinal damage has been observed in some patients who had received long-term or high-dosage 4-aminoquinoline therapy. Retinopathy has been reported to be dose related.

When prolonged therapy with any antimalarial compound is contemplated, initial (base line) and periodic ophthalmologic examinations (including visual acuity, expert slit-lamp, funduscopic, and visual field tests) should be performed.

If there is any indication (past or present) of abnormality in the visual acuity, visual field, or retinal macular areas (such as pigmentary changes, loss of foveal reflex), or any visual symptoms (such as light flashes and streaks) which are not fully explainable by difficulties of accommodation or corneal opacities, the drug should be discontinued immediately and the patient closely observed for possible progression. Retinal changes (and visual disturbances) may progress even after cessation of therapy.

All patients on long-term therapy with this preparation should be questioned and examined periodically, including testing knee and ankle reflexes, to detect any evidence of muscular weakness. If weakness occurs, discontinue the drug.

A number of fatalities have been reported following the accidental ingestion of chloroquine, sometimes in relatively small doses (0.75 or 1 g chloroquine phosphate in one 3-year-old child). Patients should be strongly warned to keep this drug out of the reach of children because they are especially sensitive to the 4- aminoquinoline compounds.

Use of ARALEN phosphate, brand of chloroquine phosphate tablets, in patients with psoriasis may precipitate a severe attack of psoriasis. When used in patients with porphyria the condition may be exacerbated. The drug should not be used in these conditions unless in the judgment of the physician the benefit to the patient outweighs the possible hazard.

Usage in Pregnancy. Usage of this drug during pregnancy should be avoided except in the suppression or treatment of malaria when in the judgment of the physician the benefit outweighs the possible hazard. It should be noted that radioactively tagged chloroquine administered intravenously to pregnant pigmented CBA mice passed rapidly across the placenta, accumulated selectively in the melanin structures of the fetal eyes and was retained in the ocular tissues for five months after the drug had been eliminated from the rest of the body.[1]

PRECAUTIONS

Since the drug is known to concentrate in the liver, it should be used with caution in patients with hepatic disease or alcoholism or in conjunction with known hepatotoxic drugs.

Complete blood cell counts should be made periodically if patients are given prolonged therapy. If any severe blood disorder appears which is not attributable to the disease under treatment, discontinuance of the drug should be considered. The drug should be administered with caution to patients having G-6-PD (glucose-6-phosphate dehydrogenase) deficiency.

ADVERSE REACTIONS

Following the administration of ARALEN phosphate in doses adequate for the treatment of an acute malarial attack or extraintestinal amebiasis, mild and transient headache, pruritus, gastrointestinal complaints (anorexia, nausea, vomiting, diarrhea, abdominal cramps), psychic stimulation, and rarely psychotic episodes or convulsions have been observed. Cardiovascular effects, such as hypotension and electrocardiographic changes (particularly inversion or depression of the T wave, widening of the QRS complex), have rarely been noted in patients receiving usual antimalarial doses of the drug. A few cases of a nerve type of deafness have been reported after prolonged therapy, usually in high doses. Tinnitus and reduced hearing have been reported, in a patient with preexistent auditory damage, after administration of only 500 mg once a week for a few months. Neuromyopathy, blood dyscrasias, lichen planus-like eruptions, and skin and mucosal pigmentary changes have also been noted during prolonged therapy.

When employed for the indications (malaria and extraintestinal amebiasis) and in the dosages recommended in this leaflet, visual disturbances, consisting of blurring of vision or difficulty in focusing or accommodation, occasionally may be noted; they are reversible and disappear on discontinuation of therapy. Other types of visual disturbances and ocular complications have been reported during the use of chloroquine for long-term therapy usually in daily doses exceeding 250 mg of chloroquine phosphate. These consisted of (1) reversible corneal changes (transient edema or opaque deposits in the epithelium) which may be asymptomatic or cause visual halos, focusing difficulties, or blurred vision and (2) generally irreversible, sometimes progressive, or, rarely delayed, retinal changes, such as narrowing of the arterioles, macular lesions (loss of foveal reflex, areas of edema, atrophy, and abnormal pigmentation), pallor of the optic disc, optic atrophy, and patchy retinal pigmentation.

Patients with retinal changes may be asymptomatic, especially in early cases, or may complain of nyctalopia and scotomatous vision with field defects of paracentral, pericentral ring types, and typically temporal scotomas, eg, difficulty in reading with words tending to disappear, seeing only half an object, misty vision, and fog before the eyes. Rarely scotomatous vision may occur without observable retinal changes.

DOSAGE AND ADMINISTRATION

The dosage of chloroquine phosphate is often expressed or calculated as the base. Each 500 mg tablet of ARALEN phosphate, brand of chloroquine phosphate tablets, is equivalent to 300 mg base. In infants and children the dosage is preferably calculated on the body weight.

Malaria: Suppression — **In adults**, 500 mg (= 300 mg base) on exactly the same day of each week. **In infants and children** the weekly suppressive dosage is 5 mg calculated as base, per kg of body weight, but should not exceed the adult dose regardless of weight.

If circumstances permit, suppressive therapy should begin two weeks prior to exposure. However, failing this in adults, an initial double (loading) dose of 1 g (= 600 mg base), or in children 10 mg base/kg may be taken in two divided doses, six hours apart. The suppressive therapy should be continued for eight weeks after leaving the endemic area.

Treatment of the acute attack—**In adults**, an initial dose of 1 g (= 600 mg base) followed by an additional 500 mg (= 300 mg base) after six to eight hours and a single dose of 500 mg (= 300 mg base) on each of two consecutive days. This represents a total dose of 2.5 g chloroquine phosphate or 1.5 g base in three days.

The dosage for adults may also be calculated on the basis of body weight; this method is preferred for infants and children. A total dose representing 25 mg of base per kg of body weight is administered in three days, as follows:

First dose: 10 mg base per kg (but not exceeding a single dose of 600 mg base).

Second dose: 5 mg base per kg (but not exceeding a single dose of 300 mg base) 6 hours after first dose.

Third dose: 5 mg base per kg 18 hours after second dose.

Fourth dose: 5 mg base per kg 24 hours after third dose.

For radical cure of *vivax* and *malariae* malaria concomitant therapy with an 8- aminoquinoline compound is necessary.

Extraintestinal Amebiasis: Adults, 1 g (600 mg base) daily for two days, followed by 500 mg (300 mg base) daily for at least two to three weeks. Treatment is usually combined with an effective intestinal amebicide.

OVERDOSAGE

Chloroquine is very rapidly and completely absorbed after ingestion, and in accidental overdosage, or rarely with lower doses in hypersensitive patients, toxic symptoms may occur within thirty minutes. These consist of headache, drowsiness, visual disturbances, cardiovascular collapse, and convulsions followed by sudden and early respiratory and cardiac arrest. The electrocardiogram may reveal atrial standstill, nodal rhythm, prolonged intraventricular conduction time, and progressive bradycardia leading to ventricular fibrillation and/or arrest. Treatment is symptomatic and must be prompt with immediate evacuation of the stomach by emesis (at home, before transportation to the hospital) or gastric lavage until the stomach is completely emptied. If finely powdered, activated charcoal is introduced by stomach tube, after lavage, and within 30 minutes after ingestion of the antimalarial, it may inhibit further intestinal absorption of the drug. To be effective, the dose of activated charcoal should be at least five times the estimated dose of chloroquine ingested.

Convulsions, if present, should be controlled before attempting gastric lavage. If due to cerebral stimulation, cautious administration of an ultrashort-acting barbiturate may be tried but, if due to anoxia, it should be corrected by oxygen administration, artificial respiration or, in shock with hypotension, by vasopressor therapy. Because of the importance of supporting respiration, tracheal intubation or tracheostomy, followed by gastric lavage, may also be necessary. Peritoneal dialysis and exchange transfusions have also been suggested to reduce the level of the drug in the blood.

A patient who survives the acute phase and is asymptomatic should be closely observed for at least six hours. Fluids may be forced, and sufficient ammonium chloride (8 g daily in divided doses for adults) may be administered for a few days to acidify the urine to help promote urinary excretion in cases of both overdosage or sensitivity.

HOW SUPPLIED

Tablets of 500 mg (= 300 mg base), bottle of 25 (NDC 0024-0077-01)

REFERENCE

1. Ullberg S, Lindquist N G, Sjostrand S E: Accumulation of chorio-retinotoxic drugs in the foetal eye. *Nature* 1970; 227:1257.

Shown in Product Identification Section, page 435

AW-123 F

Continued on next page

This product information was effective as of December 1, 1986. On these and other products of Winthrop-Breon Laboratories, detailed information may be obtained on a current basis by direct inquiry to the Professional Services Department, 90 Park Avenue, New York, NY 10016 (212) 907-2525.

Winthrop-Breon—Cont.

ARALEN® Phosphate ℞
brand of chloroquine phosphate, USP
with
PRIMAQUINE Phosphate, USP

For Malaria Prophylaxis Only

WARNING: PHYSICIANS SHOULD COMPLETELY FAMILIARIZE THEMSELVES WITH THE COMPLETE CONTENTS OF THIS LEAFLET BEFORE PRESCRIBING ARALEN PHOSPHATE WITH PRIMAQUINE PHOSPHATE.

DESCRIPTION

Each tablet contains ARALEN phosphate, brand of chloroquine phosphate, USP, 500 mg (equivalent to 300 mg base) and primaquine phosphate 79 mg (equivalent to 45 mg base).
Inactive Ingredients: Dibasic Calcium Phosphate, FD&C Yellow #6, Lactose, Magnesium Stearate, Povidone, Starch, Stearic Acid, Talc, Titanium Dioxide, Triacetin, Zein.

ACTIONS

ARALEN is a 4-aminoquinoline compound which is highly active against the erythrocytic forms of *Plasmodium vivax* and most strains of *Plasmodium falciparum* (but not the gametocytes of *P. falciparum).*
Primaquine is an 8-aminoquinoline compound which eliminates tissue (exo-erythrocytic) infection. Thereby, it prevents the development of the blood (erythrocytic) forms of the parasite which are responsible for relapses in vivax malaria. Primaquine phosphate is active against gametocytes of *P. falciparum.*
ARALEN phosphate with primaquine phosphate demonstrates antimalarial activity against all stages of human-malaria parasites, except for certain strains of *P. falciparum* resistant to chloroquine.

INDICATION

ARALEN phosphate with primaquine phosphate is intended solely for use in the prophylaxis of malaria, regardless of species, in all areas where this disease is endemic.

CONTRAINDICATIONS

The drug is contraindicated in acutely ill patients suffering from systemic disease manifested by tendency to granulocytopenia, such as rheumatoid arthritis and lupus erythematosus. The drug is also contraindicated in those patients receiving concurrently other potentially hemolytic drugs or depressants of myeloid elements of the bone marrow.
Primaquine should not be administered to patients who have received quinacrine recently, as toxicity is increased.

WARNINGS

Children are especially sensitive to 4-aminoquinoline compounds. A number of fatalities have been reported following the accidental ingestion of chloroquine, sometimes in relatively small doses (0.75 or 1 g in one 3- year-old child). Patients should be strongly warned to keep these drugs out of the reach of children.
Hemolytic reactions (moderate to severe) may occur after even a weekly dose of this preparation in glucose-6-phosphate dehydrogenase (G-6-PD) deficient Caucasians (particularly, in Sardinians and in individuals with a family or personal history of favism).
Usage in Pregnancy. Safe usage of this preparation in pregnancy has not been established. Therefore, use of it during pregnancy should be avoided except when in the judgment of the physician the benefit outweighs the possible hazard. It should be noted that radioactively tagged chloroquine administered intravenously to pregnant pigmented CBA mice passed rapidly across the placenta, accumulated selectively in the melanin structures of the fetal eyes and was retained in the ocular tissues for five months after the drug had been eliminated from the rest of the body.[1]

PRECAUTIONS

ARALEN phosphate, brand of chloroquine phosphate, with primaquine phosphate is intended for malaria prophylaxis only; it should not be used for the treatment of clinical malaria. The recommended dosage (one tablet weekly, on the same day each week) should not be exceeded. The drug should not be taken more often than once every seven days to minimize danger of toxicity.
If the combination is prescribed for (1) an individual who has shown a previous idiosyncrasy to either chloroquine or primaquine (as manifested by dermatitis, hemolytic anemia, methemoglobinemia, or leukopenia), (2) an individual with a family or personal history of favism, or (3) an individual with erythrocytic glucose-6-phosphate dehydrogenase (G-6-PD) deficiency or nicotinamide adenine dinucleotide (NADH) methemoglobin reductase deficiency, the person should be observed closely for tolerance. The drug should be discontinued immediately if marked darkening of the urine, sudden decrease in hemoglobin concentration or leukocyte count, or severe skin reaction occurs.
In areas with endemic falciparum malaria due to strains that are resistant to the 4-aminoquinolines (chloroquine, amodiaquine, hydroxychloroquine), chemoprophylaxis with this combination alone may not be effective.

ADVERSE REACTIONS

Gastrointestinal reactions: anorexia, nausea, vomiting, epigastric distress, and abdominal cramps. *Hematologic reactions:* leukopenia, hemolytic anemia in glucose-6-phosphate dehydrogenase (G-6-PD) deficient individuals, methemoglobinemia in nicotinamide adenine dinucleotide (NADH) methemoglobin reductase deficient individuals.
Cardiovascular effects, such as hypotension and electrocardiographic changes (particularly inversion or depression of the T wave, widening of the QRS complex), have rarely been noted in patients receiving usual antimalarial doses of the drug.
Visual disturbances, consisting of blurring of vision or difficulty in focusing or accommodation, have occasionally been noted when chloroquine has been employed for malaria. These symptoms are reversible and disappear on discontinuation of therapy. Other types of visual disturbances (reversible corneal changes) and ocular complications including retinal changes (narrowing of the arterioles, macular lesions, pallor of the optic disc, optic atrophy, and patchy retinal pigmentation) have been reported during the use of chloroquine for long-term therapy usually in daily doses exceeding 250 mg of chloroquine phosphate. These changes have not been reported with the use of ARALEN phosphate, brand of chloroquine phosphate, with primaquine phosphate for malaria prophylaxis.
Auditory disturbances: tinnitus and reduced hearing have been reported, in a patient with preexistent auditory damage, after administration of only 500 mg of ARALEN phosphate, brand of chloroquine phosphate, once a week for a few months.

DOSAGE AND ADMINISTRATION

Adults—Starting at least one day before entering the malarious area, one tablet weekly, taken on the same day each week. This schedule (one tablet weekly) should be continued for eight weeks after leaving the endemic area.
Children—Table 1 gives suggested dosage based on body weight.

Table 1

Weight (lb)	ARALEN base (mg)	Primaquine base (mg)	Dose* (mL)
10-15	20	3	2.5
16-25	40	6	5.0
26-35	60	9	7.5
36-45	80	12	10.0
46-55	100	15	12.5
56-100	150	22.5	½ tab
100†	300	45	1 tab

*Dose based on liquid containing approximately 40 mg of chloroquine base and 6 mg of primaquine base per 5 mL (1 teaspoon) prepared from ARALEN phosphate, brand of chloroquine phosphate, with primaquine phosphate tablets. Chocolate syrup could be used to prepare a suspension (one tablet crushed and suspended in 40 mL of liquid). Shake well before use.

OVERDOSAGE

Symptoms of overdosage are due to the two drug components.
Chloroquine is very rapidly and completely absorbed after ingestion, and in accidental overdosage, or rarely with lower doses in hypersensitive patients, toxic symptoms may occur within thirty minutes. These consist of headache, drowsiness, visual disturbances, cardiovascular collapse, and convulsions followed by sudden and early respiratory and cardiac arrest. The electrocardiogram may reveal atrial standstill, nodal rhythm, prolonged intraventricular conduction time, and progressive bradycardia leading to ventricular fibrillation and/or arrest.
Symptoms of overdosage of primaquine are similar to those seen after overdosage of pamaquine. They include abdominal cramps, vomiting, burning epigastric distress, central nervous system and cardiovascular disturbances, cyanosis, methemoglobinemia, moderate leukocytosis or leukopenia, and anemia. The most striking symptoms are granulocytopenia and acute hemolytic anemia in sensitive persons. Acute hemolysis occurs, but patients recover completely if the dosage is discontinued.
Treatment is symptomatic and must be prompt with immediate evacuation of the stomach by emesis (at home, before transportation to the hospital) or gastric lavage until the stomach is completely emptied. Finely powdered, activated charcoal in a dose not less than five times the estimated dose of chloroquine ingested, if introduced by the stomach tube after lavage within thirty minutes after ingestion of the antimalarial, may inhibit further intestinal absorption of the drug.
Convulsions, if present, should be controlled before attempting gastric lavage. If due to cerebral stimulation, cautious administration of an ultrashort-acting barbiturate may be tried but, if due to anoxia, it should be corrected by oxygen administration, artificial respiration or, in shock with hypotension, by vasopressor therapy. Because of the importance of supporting respiration, tracheal intubation or tracheostomy, followed by gastric lavage, may also be necessary. Exchange transfusions have also been suggested to reduce the level of the drug in the blood.
The patient should be kept in bed and warm. If methemoglobinemia and cyanosis occur, oxygen may be administered and use of methylene blue may be considered. If collapse and hypotension or shock occur, vasopressors may be used. The patient should be observed for the possible development of leukopenia or hemolytic anemia.
A patient who survives the acute stage and is asymptomatic should be closely observed for at least six hours. Fluids may be forced, and sufficient ammonium chloride (8 g daily in divided doses for adults) may be administered for a few days to acidify the urine to help promote urinary excretion in cases of both overdosage or sensitivity.

HOW SUPPLIED

Tablets, bottles of 100 (NDC 0024-0079-04)

CLINICAL STUDIES

On the basis of carefully controlled preliminary clinical trials, Alving and his associates[2] found that the weekly administration of 300 mg chloroquine base and 45 mg primaquine base (administered as the phosphate salts) proved highly effective as a prophylactic against severe *P. vivax* infections with the Chesson strain and did not produce clinical hemolysis even among primaquine-sensitive American Negro adult volunteers. A weekly dose of primaquine phosphate equivalent to 45 mg primaquine base cured 90 percent of infections. The studies of these workers indicate that the toxicity of primaquine phosphate, as regards the production of hemolysis, is markedly diminished when administered in weekly doses. When administered with standard suppressive doses of chloroquine phosphate, its therapeutic effectiveness in the radical cure of Chesson vivax malaria is increased. Thus, a weekly dose equivalent to 60 mg of primaquine base is less toxic than 15 mg base administered daily; and a dose equivalent to 45 mg base administered weekly was found to be practically without demonstrable toxicity. A dose equivalent to 45 mg base weekly for 8 weeks was more effective in the radical cure of infections than 15 mg base daily for 14 days.
Wittmer[3] conducted a double-blind study in 24 Caucasian male adults who received ARALEN phosphate, brand of chloroquine phosphate, with primaquine phosphate once each week (Friday) for 15 weeks to determine its safety and suitability for use in Armed Forces flying personnel. The author concluded that there appear to be no contraindications to the long-term use of the combination in flying personnel since there was no effect on vision, time of useful consciousness, or psychomotor performance. No deleterious synergistic effect of the two drugs was demonstrated.
Charles[4] investigated the effects of 5 weekly doses of primaquine phosphate (1 mg to 1.5 mg base per kg body weight) in combination with a 4-aminoquinoline antimalarial agent on the parasitemia and blood picture of 100 Ghanaian children from 2½ to 8 years old. Although the enzyme-deficiency trait (glucose-6-phosphate dehydrogenase deficiency) for primaquine sensitivity occurred in approximately 25 percent of the group, no general evidence of hemolysis was observed. Eight of the treated subjects were positive for the glucose-6-phosphate dehydrogenase deficiency test but maintained their pretreatment hemoglobin values.
However, Ziai and his associates[5] noted that serious hematologic reactions can occur in persons with a glucose-6-phosphate dehydrogenase (G-6-PD) deficiency with the small weekly doses of chloroquine-primaquine used for malaria suppressive therapy. This has been reported primarily in patients with a family history and/or personal history of favism.
Methemoglobinemia has been discovered in individuals with nicotinamide adenine dinucleotide methemoglobin reductase deficiency.[6]
The susceptibility of primaquine-sensitive children to hemolysis by primaquine phosphate is considered to be of the same order of magnitude as that of adults on an equal drug/body weight basis.

REFERENCES

1. Ullberg S, Lindquist N G, Sjostrand S E: Accumulation of chorio-retinotoxic drugs in the foetal eye. *Nature* 1970; 227:1257.
2. Alving A S, et al: Mitigation of the haemolytic effect of primaquine and enhancement of its action against exo-erythrocytic forms of the Chesson strain of *Plasmodium vivax* by intermittent regimens of drug administration. *Bull WHO* 1960; 22:621.

3. Wittmer J F: Aeromedical aspects of malaria prophylaxis with chloroquine-primaquine. *Aerospace Med* 1963; 34:944.
4. Charles L J: Observations on the haemolytic effect of primaquine in 100 Ghanaian children. *Ann Trop Med* 1960; 54:460.
5. Ziai M, et al: Malaria prophylaxis and treatment in G-6-PD deficiency. *Clin Pediat* 1967; 6:242.
6. Cohen R, et al: Methemoglobinemia provoked by malarial chemoprophylaxis in Vietnam. *New Eng J Med* 1968; 279:1127-1131.

AW-109-I

ATABRINE® Hydrochloride ℞
brand of quinacrine hydrochloride tablets, USP

DESCRIPTION
Each tablet contains 100 mg of quinacrine hydrochloride, a bright yellow, odorless, bitter crystalline powder that is water soluble (1:35), and bears identifying number A 82.
Inactive Ingredients: Pharmaceutical Glaze, Starch, Stearic Acid, Talc.

HOW SUPPLIED
Tablets of 100 mg (bright yellow, shellac-coated), bottle of 100 (NDC 0024-0082-04)
For complete prescribing information see package insert or contact Winthrop-Breon Medical Department.

AW-91-J

BREONESIN® OTC
brand of guaifenesin capsules, USP

(See PDR For Nonprescription Drugs)

BRONKEPHRINE® ℞
(ethylnorepinephrine hydrochloride injection, USP)
IN AQUEOUS SOLUTION

DESCRIPTION
BRONKEPHRINE is ethylnorepinephrine hydrochloride injection, USP. Each mL contains 2 mg ethylnorepinephrine HCl in a sterile isotonic solution of 0.7% sodium chloride with sodium acetone bisulfite 0.2% as preservative. The pH is adjusted to 2.9–4.5 with NaOH or HCl. BRONKEPHRINE is a synthetic sympathomimetic amine intended for subcutaneous or intramuscular injection. The chemical name is 1-(3, 4-dihydroxyphenyl)-2-amino-1-butanol hydrochloride.

CLINICAL PHARMACOLOGY
BRONKEPHRINE is primarily a beta-adrenergic agonist. Its actions are similar to those of isoproterenol, although it is less potent. Its bronchodilating properties closely simulate those of epinephrine but without significant pressor effects. It thus may be safer than epinephrine for hypertensive patients and severely ill patients in whom such effects are undesirable. It is particularly adapted for use in children because of its relative lack of adverse effects, especially central nervous system excitation. It also may be of value in diabetic asthmatics due to its lack of glycogenolytic activity.
Metabolic and pharmacokinetic data are unavailable.

INDICATIONS AND USAGE
BRONKEPHRINE is indicated for use as a bronchodilator for bronchial asthma and for reversible bronchospasm that may occur in association with bronchitis and emphysema.

CONTRAINDICATIONS
BRONKEPHRINE is contraindicated in patients who are hypersensitive to any of its ingredients or with idiosyncrasy to sympathomimetic drugs.

WARNINGS
BRONKEPHRINE should not be administered along with epinephrine or other sympathomimetic amines because these drugs are direct cardiac stimulants and may cause excessive tachycardia.

PRECAUTIONS
BRONKEPHRINE should be used with caution in persons with cardiovascular disease, a history of stroke or coronary artery disease. It is a potent drug and it may cause toxic symptoms through idiosyncratic response or overdosage.
Care should be taken in anatomical selection of injection sites to avoid inadvertent intraneural or intravascular injection.
Carcinogenesis, mutagenesis, impairment of fertility: Long-term animal studies of BRONKEPHRINE to evaluate carcinogenic potential and reproduction studies in animals have not been performed. There is no evidence from human data that BRONKEPHRINE may be carcinogenic or mutagenic or that it impairs fertility.
Pregnancy Category C: Animal reproduction studies have not been conducted with BRONKEPHRINE. It is not known whether BRONKEPHRINE can cause fetal harm when administered to a pregnant woman or can affect reproduction capacity. BRONKEPHRINE should be given to a pregnant woman only if clearly needed and the potential benefits outweigh the risk.
Nursing mothers: It is not known whether BRONKEPHRINE is excreted in human milk; however, because many drugs are excreted in human milk, caution should be exercised when BRONKEPHRINE is administered to a nursing woman.

ADVERSE REACTIONS
BRONKEPHRINE, brand of ethylnorepinephrine hydrochloride injection, is generally well tolerated. It may, however, produce changes in blood pressure (elevation or depression) or pulse rate (elevation), palpitation, headache, dizziness or nausea; as with other sympathomimetic amines.

OVERDOSAGE
The signs and symptoms of overdosage with BRONKEPHRINE are those typical of any sympathomimetic amine. Treatment should be symptomatic.

DOSAGE AND ADMINISTRATION
The usual adult dose by subcutaneous or intramuscular injection is 0.5 mL–1.0 mL. Depending on severity of the asthmatic attack, smaller doses (0.3 mL–0.5 mL) may suffice. Dosage in children varies according to age and weight; usually 0.1 mL to 0.5 mL is sufficient.

HOW SUPPLIED
1 mL sterile single-dose ampuls, UNI-NEST™ PAK of 25. **(NDC 0024-1001-25)**
PROTECT AMPULS FROM LIGHT.

BW-96

BRONKODYL® ℞
brand of theophylline anhydrous capsules
100 mg and 200 mg

DESCRIPTION
Each green and white hard gelatin capsule contains theophylline anhydrous, USP, 200 mg, in a micro-pulverized form. Each brown and white hard gelatin capsule contains 100 mg. Theophylline is a white, odorless crystalline powder having a bitter taste.
Inactive Ingredients: Benzyl Alcohol, Gelatin, Lactose, Magnesium Stearate, Parabens, Silicon Dioxide, Sodium Propionate, Sodium Starch Glycolate. Capsule **100 mg** contains FD&C Blue #1, Red #3, Yellow #6. Capsule **200 mg** contains D&C Yellow #10, FD&C Blue #1, Yellow #6.

HOW SUPPLIED
Capsules of 100 mg, bottles of 100 **NDC** 0024-1036-10
Capsules of 200 mg, bottles of 100 **NDC** 0024-1037-10
Distributed by
Winthrop-Breon Laboratories
Division of Sterling Drug Inc. New York, NY 10016
Mfd. by KV Pharmaceutical Co., St. Louis, Missouri 63144
For complete prescribing information, see package insert or contact Winthrop-Breon Laboratories Medical Department.

BW 98A

BRONKOLIXIR® OTC

(See PDR For Nonprescription Drugs)

BRONKOSOL® ℞
brand of isoetharine inhalation solution, USP, 1.0%
BRONCHODILATOR SOLUTION FOR ORAL INHALATION

DESCRIPTION
Isoetharine hydrochloride, USP, 1.0% also contains: Acetone Sodium Bisulfite, Glycerin, Parabens, Purified Water, Sodium Chloride, and Sodium Citrate.

BRONKOMETER® ℞
brand of isoetharine mesylate inhalation aerosol, USP

DESCRIPTION
BRONKOMETER is a complete pocket nebulizer containing isoetharine mesylate 0.61% (w/w). BRONKOMETER also contains: alcohol 30% (w/w), ascorbic acid 0.1% (w/w) as a preservative, dichlorodifluoromethane and dichlorotetrafluoroethane as propellants, menthol, and saccharin.
Isoetharine is 1-(3,4 dihydroxyphenyl)-2-isopropylamino-1-butanol. The BRONKOMETER unit delivers approximately 20 metered doses per mL of solution. Each average 56 mg delivery contains 340 mcg isoetharine.

CLINICAL PHARMACOLOGY
Isoetharine is a sympathomimetic amine with preferential affinity for Beta$_2$ adrenergic receptor sites of bronchial and certain arteriolar musculature, and a lower order of affinity for Beta$_1$ adrenergic receptors. Its activity in symptomatic relief of bronchospasm is rapid and of relatively long duration. By relieving bronchospasm, BRONKOSOL and BRONKOMETER help give prompt relief and significantly increase vital capacity.

INDICATIONS AND USAGE
BRONKOSOL and BRONKOMETER are indicated for use as bronchodilators for bronchial asthma and for reversible bronchospasm that may occur in association with bronchitis and emphysema.

CONTRAINDICATION
BRONKOSOL and BRONKOMETER should not be administered to patients who are hypersensitive to any of their ingredients.

WARNINGS
Excessive use of an adrenergic aerosol should be discouraged as it may lose its effectiveness. Occasional patients have been reported to develop severe paradoxical airway resistance with repeated excessive use of an aerosol adrenergic inhalation preparation. The cause of this refractory state is unknown. It is advisable that in such instances the use of the aerosol adrenergic be discontinued immediately and alternative therapy instituted, since in the reported cases the patients did not respond to other forms of therapy until the drug was withdrawn. Cardiac arrest has been noted in several instances.
BRONKOSOL and BRONKOMETER should not be administered along with epinephrine or other sympathomimetic amines, since these drugs are direct cardiac stimulants and may cause excessive tachycardia. They may, however, be alternated if desired.
Usage in Pregnancy: Although there has been no evidence of teratogenic effects with this drug, use of any drug in pregnancy, lactation, or in women of childbearing potential requires that the potential benefit of the drug be weighed against its possible hazard to the mother or child.

PRECAUTIONS
Dosage must be carefully adjusted in patients with hyperthyroidism, hypertension, acute coronary disease, cardiac asthma, limited cardiac reserve, and in individuals sensitive to sympathomimetic amines, since overdosage may result in tachycardia, palpitation, nausea, headache, or epinephrine-like side effects.

ADVERSE REACTIONS
Although BRONKOSOL and BRONKOMETER are relatively free of toxic side effects, too frequent use may cause tachycardia, palpitation, nausea, headache, changes in blood pressure, anxiety, tension, restlessness, insomnia, tremor, weakness, dizziness, and excitement, as is the case with other sympathomimetic amines.

DOSAGE AND ADMINISTRATION
BRONKOSOL can be administered by hand nebulizer, oxygen aerosolization, or intermittent positive pressure breathing (IPPB). Usually treatment need not be repeated more often than every four hours, although in severe cases more frequent administration may be necessary.

Method of Administration	Usual Dose	Range	Usual Dilution
Hand nebulizer	4 inhalations	3-7 inhalations	undiluted
Oxygen aerosolization*	½ mL	¼-½ mL	1:3 with saline or other diluent
IPPB†	½ mL	¼-1 mL	1:3 with saline or other diluent

* Administered with oxygen flow adjusted to 4 to 6 liters/minute over a period of 15 to 20 minutes.
† Usually an inspiratory flow rate of 15 liters/minute at a cycling pressure of 15 cm H_2O is recommended. It may be necessary, according to patient and type of IPPB apparatus, to adjust flow rate to 6 to 30 liters per minute, cycling pressure to 10 to 15 cm H_2O, and further dilution according to needs of patient.

BRONKOMETER®

DOSAGE AND ADMINISTRATION
The average adult dose is one or two inhalations. Occasionally, more may be required. It is important, however, to wait one full minute after the initial one or two inhalations in order to be certain whether another is necessary. In most

Continued on next page

This product information was effective as of December 1, 1986. On these and other products of Winthrop-Breon Laboratories, detailed information may be obtained on a current basis by direct inquiry to the Professional Services Department, 90 Park Avenue, New York, NY 10016 (212) 907-2525.

Winthrop-Breon—Cont.

cases, inhalations need not be repeated more often than every four hours, although more frequent administration may be necessary in severe cases.

HOW SUPPLIED

BRONKOMETER, brand of isoetharine mesylate inhalation aerosol
Vial of 10 mL, with oral nebulizer (NDC 0024-1040-01)
Refill only, 10 mL (NDC 0024-1041-01)
Vial of 15 mL, with oral nebulizer (NDC 0024-1040-03)
Refill only, 15 mL (NDC 0024-1041-03)
The bronchodilator isoetharine is also available in a convenient solution for use with conventional nebulizers, by oxygen aerosolization, and in IPPB machines as BRONKOSOL, brand of isoetharine hydrochloride, 1.0%. It is supplied as follows:
Bottle of 10 mL (NDC 0024-1071-10)
Bottle of 30 mL (NDC 0024-1071-30)
Distributed by Winthrop-Breon Laboratories
Division of Sterling Drug Inc
New York, NY 10016
Manufactured by
Sterling Pharmaceuticals Inc
Barceloneta, Puerto Rico 00617

BRONKOTABS® OTC

(See PDR For Nonprescription Drugs)

CARBOCAINE® Hydrochloride ℞
brand of mepivacaine hydrochloride injection, USP

THESE SOLUTIONS ARE NOT INTENDED FOR SPINAL ANESTHESIA OR DENTAL USE

DESCRIPTION

Mepivacaine hydrochloride is 1-methyl-2', 6'-pipecoloxylidide monohydrochloride.
It is a white crystalline, odorless powder, soluble in water, but very resistant to both acid and alkaline hydrolysis. Solutions may be stored for extended periods of time without decomposition and if without vasoconstrictors may be reautoclaved when necessary.
[See table below].

ACTIONS

Mepivacaine stabilizes the neuronal membrane and prevents the initiation and transmission of nerve impulses, thereby effecting local anesthesia.
Onset of anesthesia is rapid, the time of onset for sensory block ranging from about 3 to 20 minutes depending upon such factors as the anesthetic technique, the type of block, the concentration of the solution, and the individual patient. The degree of motor blockade produced is dependent on the concentration of the solution. A 0.5 percent solution will be effective in small superficial nerve blocks while the 1 percent concentration will block sensory and sympathetic conduction without loss of motor function. The 1.5 percent solution will provide extensive and often complete motor block and the 2 percent concentration of CARBOCAINE will produce complete sensory and motor block of any nerve group.
The duration of anesthesia also varies depending upon the technique and type of block, the concentration, and the individual. Mepivacaine will normally provide anesthesia which is adequate for 2 to 2½ hours of surgery. It has been reported that vasoconstrictors do not significantly prolong anesthesia with mepivacaine but epinephrine (1:200,000) may be added to the mepivacaine solution to promote local hemostasis and to delay systemic absorption of the anesthetic.
Mepivacaine, because of its amide structure, is not detoxified by the circulating plasma esterases. It is rapidly metabolized, with only a small percentage of the anesthetic (5 to 10 percent) being excreted unchanged in the urine. The liver is the principal site of metabolism, with over 50 percent of the administered dose being excreted into the bile as metabolites. Most of the metabolized mepivacaine is probably resorbed in the intestine and then excreted into the urine since only a small percentage is found in the feces. The principal route of excretion is via the kidney. Most of the anesthetic and its metabolites are eliminated within 30 hours. It has been shown that hydroxylation and N-demethylation, which are detoxification reactions, play important roles in the metabolism of the anesthetic. Three metabolites of mepivacaine have been identified from adult humans: two phenols, which are excreted almost exclusively as their glucuronide conjugates, and the N-demethylated compound (2', 6'-pipecoloxylidide).
Mepivacaine does not ordinarily produce irritation or tissue damage.

INDICATIONS

CARBOCAINE is indicated for the production of local anesthesia by infiltration injection, peripheral nerve block, and central neural blocks by the lumbar or caudal epidural route.

CONTRAINDICATION

Mepivacaine is contraindicated in patients with known hypersensitivity to the amide-type local anesthetics or to methylparaben, which is added to the multiple-dose vials.

WARNINGS

RESUSCITATIVE EQUIPMENT AND DRUGS SHOULD BE IMMEDIATELY AVAILABLE WHENEVER ANY LOCAL ANESTHETIC DRUG IS USED.
Large doses of local anesthetics should not be used in patients with heart block.
Reactions resulting in fatality have occurred on rare occasions with the use of local anesthetics, even in the absence of a history of hypersensitivity.
Solutions which contain a vasoconstrictor should be used with extreme caution in patients receiving drugs known to produce alterations in blood pressure (ie, monoamine oxidase (MAO) inhibitors, tricyclic antidepressants, phenothiazines, etc) as either severe sustained hypertension or hypotension may occur.
Usage in Children. Great care must be exercised in adhering to safe concentrations and dosages for pediatric administration (see Dosage and Administration).
Usage in Pregnancy. Safe use of mepivacaine has not been established with respect to adverse effects on fetal development. Careful consideration should be given to this fact before administering this drug to women of childbearing potential, particularly during early pregnancy. This does not exclude the use of the drug at term for obstetrical analgesia.
Vasopressor agents (administered for the treatment of hypotension related to caudal or other epidural blocks) should be used with extreme caution in the presence of oxytocic drugs as they are known to interact and may produce severe, persistent hypertension and/or rupture of cerebral blood vessels. CARBOCAINE, brand of mepivacaine hydrochloride, has been used for obstetrical analgesia by the peridural and paracervical routes without evidence of adverse effects on the fetus when no more than the maximum safe dosages are used and strict adherence to technique is followed.
Local anesthetic procedures should be used with caution when there is inflammation and/or sepsis in the region of the proposed injection.

PRECAUTIONS

Standard textbooks should be consulted for specific techniques and precautions for various regional anesthetic procedures.
The safety and effectiveness of a local anesthetic drug depend upon proper dosage, correct technique, adequate precautions, and readiness for emergencies.
The lowest dosage that results in effective anesthesia should be used to avoid high plasma levels and possible adverse effects. Injection of repeated doses of mepivacaine may cause significant increase in blood levels with each repeated dose due to slow accumulation of the drug or its metabolites or due to slower metabolic degradation than normal.
Tolerance varies with the status of the patient. Debilitated, elderly patients, or acutely ill patients should be given reduced doses commensurate with their weight and physical status.
Mepivacaine should be used with caution in patients with severe disturbances of cardiac rhythm, shock or heart block.
INJECTION SHOULD ALWAYS BE MADE SLOWLY AND WITH FREQUENT ASPIRATIONS TO AVOID INADVERTENT RAPID INTRAVASCULAR ADMINISTRATION WHICH CAN PRODUCE SYSTEMIC TOXICITY.
Fetal bradycardia which frequently follows paracervical block may be indicative of high fetal blood concentrations of CARBOCAINE with resultant fetal acidosis. Fetal heart rate should be monitored prior to and during paracervical block. Added risk appears to be present in prematurity, toxemia of pregnancy, and fetal distress. The physician should weigh the benefits against the risks in considering paracervical block in these conditions. Careful adherence to recommended dosage is of the utmost importance in paracervical block. Failure to achieve adequate analgesia with these doses should arouse suspicion of intravascular or fetal injection.
Case reports of maternal convulsions and cardiovascular collapse following use of mepivacaine for paracervical block in early pregnancy (as anesthesia for elective abortion) suggest that systemic absorption under these circumstances may be rapid. Therefore the recommended maximum dose of 100 mg per side should not be exceeded. Injection should be made slowly and with frequent aspiration. Allow a 5-minute interval between sides.
Vasoconstrictors. Solutions containing a vasoconstrictor should be used cautiously. The decision whether or not to use a vasoconstrictor with local anesthesia depends on the physician's appraisal of the benefits as opposed to the risk, eg, in injection of solutions containing a vasoconstrictor into areas where the blood supply is limited (eg, ears, nose, digits) or when peripheral vascular disease is present. Furthermore, serious cardiac arrhythmias may occur if preparations containing a vasoconstrictor are employed in patients during or immediately following the administration of halothane, cyclopropane, trichloroethylene, or other related agents.
MEPIVACAINE SHOULD BE USED WITH CAUTION IN PATIENTS WITH KNOWN DRUG ALLERGIES AND SENSITIVITIES. A thorough history of the patient's prior experience with CARBOCAINE or other local anesthetics as well as concomitant or recent drug use should be taken (see Contraindications). Patients allergic to methylparaben or para-aminobenzoic acid derivatives (procaine, tetracaine, benzocaine, etc) have not shown cross-sensitivity to agents of the amide-type such as mepivacaine. Since mepivacaine is metabolized in the liver and excreted by the kidneys, it should be used cautiously in patients with liver and renal disease.

ADVERSE REACTIONS

Systemic adverse reactions involving the central nervous system and the cardiovascular system usually result from high plasma levels due to excessive dosage, rapid absorption, or inadvertent intravascular injection.
A small number of reactions may result from hypersensitivity, idiosyncrasy, or diminished tolerance to normal dosage.
Excitatory CNS effects commonly represent the initial signs of local anesthetic systemic toxicity. However, these reactions may be very brief or absent in some patients in which case the first manifestation of toxicity may be drowsiness merging into unconsciousness and respiratory arrest.
Cardiovascular system reactions include depression of the myocardium, hypotension (or sometimes hypertension), bradycardia, and even cardiac arrest. In obstetrics, cases of fetal bradycardia have occurred (see Precautions).
Allergic reactions are characterized by cutaneous lesions of delayed onset, or urticaria, edema, and other manifestations of allergy. The detection of sensitivity by skin testing is of limited value. As with other local anesthetics, hypersensitivity, idiosyncrasy, and anaphylactoid reactions to CARBOCAINE, brand of mepivacaine hydrochloride, have occurred rarely. The reaction may be abrupt and severe, and is not usually dose related.
Sensitivity to methylparaben, a preservative added to multiple-dose vials, has been reported. Single-dose vials without methylparaben are also available.
Reactions following epidural or caudal anesthesia also may include: high or total spinal block, urinary retention; fecal incontinence; loss of perineal sensation and sexual function; persistent analgesia, paresthesia, and paralysis of the lower extremities; headache and backache; and slowing of labor and consequent increased incidence of forceps delivery.
Treatment of Reactions. Toxic effects of local anesthetics require symptomatic treatment; there is no specific cure. The physician should be prepared to maintain an airway and to support ventilation with oxygen and assisted or controlled respiration as required. Supportive treatment of the cardiovascular system includes intravenous fluids and, when appropriate, vasopressors (preferably those that stimulate the myocardium, such as ephedrine). *Convulsions* may be controlled with oxygen and by the intravenous administration of diazepam or short or ultrashort-acting barbiturates. Intravenous anticonvulsant agents should only be administered by those familiar with their use and only when ventilation and oxygenation are assured. In epidural anesthesia, sympathetic blockade also occurs as a pharmacological reaction, resulting in peripheral vasodilation and often *hypotension.*

Composition of Available Solutions

Each mL contains	Single-dose 1% vial	Multiple-dose 1% vial	Single-dose 1.5% vial	Single-dose 2% vial	Multiple-dose 2% vial
Mepivacaine hydrochloride	10 mg	10 mg	15 mg	20 mg	20 mg
Sodium chloride	6.6 mg	7 mg	5.6 mg	4.6 mg	5 mg
Potassium chloride	0.3 mg	——	0.3 mg	0.3 mg	——
Calcium chloride	0.33 mg	——	0.33 mg	0.33 mg	——
Methylparaben	——	1 mg	——	——	1 mg
Water for injection	30 mL	50 mL	30 mL	20 mL	50 mL

The pH of the solutions is adjusted between 4.5 and 6.8 with sodium hydroxide or hydrochloric acid.

The extent of the hypotension will usually depend on the number of dermatomes blocked. The blood pressure should therefore be monitored in the early phases of anesthesia. If hypotension occurs, it is readily controlled by vasoconstrictors administered either by the intramuscular or the intravenous route, the dosage of which would depend on the severity of the hypotension and the response to treatment.

DOSAGE AND ADMINISTRATION

As with all local anesthetics, the dose varies and depends upon the area to be anesthetized, the vascularity of the tissues, the number of neuronal segments to be blocked, individual tolerance, and the technique of anesthesia. The lowest dose needed to provide effective anesthesia should be administered. For specific techniques and procedures, refer to standard textbooks.

The recommended single adult dose (or the total of a series of doses given in one procedure) of CARBOCAINE, brand of mepivacaine hydrochloride, for unsedated, healthy, normal-sized individuals should not usually exceed 400 mg. The recommended dosage is based on requirements for the average adult and should be reduced for elderly or debilitated patients.

While maximum doses of 7 mg/kg (550 mg) have been administered without adverse effect, these are not recommended, except in exceptional circumstances and under no circumstances should the administration be repeated at intervals of less than 1½ hours. The total dose for any 24-hour period should not exceed 1000 mg because of a slow accumulation of the anesthetic or its derivatives or slower than normal metabolic degradation or detoxification with repeat administration (see Actions and Precautions).

Children tolerate the local anesthetic as well as adults. However, the pediatric dose should be carefully measured as a percentage of the total adult dose based on weight, and should not exceed 5 to 6 mg/kg (2.5 to 3 mg/lb) in children, especially those weighing less than 30 lbs. In children under 3 years of age or weighing less than 30 lbs concentrations less than 2 percent (eg, 0.5 to 1.5 percent) should be employed. [See table right].

HOW SUPPLIED

These solutions are not intended for spinal anesthesia or dental use.

1% single-dose vials of 30 mL (NDC 0024-0231-01)
1% multiple-dose vials of 50 mL (NDC 0024-0232-01)
1.5% single-dose vials of 30 mL (NDC 0024-0234-01)
2% single-dose vials of 20 mL (NDC 0024-0236-01)
2% multiple-dose vials of 50 mL (NDC 0024-0237-01)

For full prescribing information on the dental use of CARBOCAINE see Cook-Waite Laboratories, Inc. product listing in this publication.

CW-60-Q

Recommended Concentrations and Doses of CARBOCAINE

Procedure	Concentration	Total Dose mL	Total Dose mg	Comments
Cervical, brachial, intercostal, pudendal nerve block	1% 2%	5–40 5–20	50–400 100–400	Pudendal block; one half of total dose injected each side.
Transvaginal block (paracervical plus pudendal)	1%	up to 30 (both sides)	up to 300 (both sides)	One half of total dose injected each side. See Precautions.
Paracervical block	1%	up to 20 (both sides)	up to 200 (both sides)	One half of total dose injected each side. This is maximum recommended dose per 90 minute period in obstetrical and non-obstetrical patients. Inject slowly, 5 minutes between sides. See Precautions.
Caudal and Epidural block	1% 1.5% 2%	15–30 10–25 10–20	150–300 150–375 200–400	Use only single-dose vials which do not contain a preservative.
Infiltration	1%	up to 40	up to 400	An equivalent amount of a 0.5% solution (prepared by diluting the 1% solution with Sodium Chloride Injection, USP) may be used for large areas.
Therapeutic block	1% 2%	1–5 1–5	10–50 20–50	

Unused portions of solutions not containing preservatives should be discarded.

DANOCRINE® ℞

brand of danazol capsules, USP

DESCRIPTION

DANOCRINE, brand of danazol, is a synthetic androgen derived from ethisterone. Chemically, danazol is 17α-Pregna-2,4-dien-20-yno[2,3-*d*]-isoxazol-17-ol.

Inactive Ingredients: Benzyl Alcohol, Gelatin, Lactose, Magnesium Stearate, Parabens, Sodium Propionate, Starch, Talc. CAPSULES 50 mg and 200 mg contain D&C Yellow #10, FD&C Red #3. CAPSULE 100 mg contains D&C Yellow #10, FD&C Yellow #6.

CLINICAL PHARMACOLOGY

DANOCRINE suppresses the pituitary-ovarian axis by inhibiting the output of gonadotropins from the pituitary gland. The only other demonstrable hormonal effect is weak androgenic activity which is dose related. Studies have established that the drug is neither estrogenic nor progestational. DANOCRINE depresses the output of both follicle-stimulating hormone (FSH) and luteinizing hormone (LH).

Recent evidence suggests a direct inhibitory effect at gonadal sites and a binding of DANOCRINE to receptors of gonadal steroids at target organs.

Bioavailability studies indicate that blood levels do not increase proportionally with increases in the administered dose. When the dose of DANOCRINE is doubled the increase in plasma levels is only about 35% to 40%.

In the treatment of endometriosis, DANOCRINE alters the normal and ectopic endometrial tissue so that it becomes inactive and atrophic. Complete resolution of endometrial lesions occurs in the majority of cases.

Changes in vaginal cytology and cervical mucus reflect the suppressive effect of DANOCRINE on the pituitary-ovarian axis.

In the treatment of fibrocystic breast disease, DANOCRINE usually produces partial to complete disappearance of nodularity and complete relief of pain and tenderness. Changes in the menstrual pattern may occur.

Generally the pituitary-suppressive action of DANOCRINE is reversible. Ovulation and cyclic bleeding usually return within 60 to 90 days when therapy with DANOCRINE is discontinued.

In the treatment of hereditary angioedema, DANOCRINE at effective doses prevents attacks of the disease characterized by episodic edema of the abdominal viscera, extremities, face, and airway which may be disabling and, if the airway is involved, fatal. In addition, DANOCRINE corrects partially or completely the primary biochemical abnormality of hereditary angioedema by increasing the levels of the deficient C1 esterase inhibitor (C1EI). As a result of this action the serum levels of the C4 component of the complement system are also increased.

INDICATIONS AND USAGE

Endometriosis. DANOCRINE is indicated for the treatment of endometriosis amenable to hormonal management.

Fibrocystic Breast Disease. Most cases of symptomatic fibrocystic breast disease may be treated by simple measures (eg, padded brassieres and analgesics).

In infrequent patients, symptoms of pain and tenderness may be severe enough to warrant treatment by suppression of ovarian function. DANOCRINE is usually effective in decreasing nodularity, pain, and tenderness. It should be stressed to the patient that this treatment is not innocuous in that it involves considerable alterations of hormone levels and that recurrence of symptoms is very common after cessation of therapy.

Hereditary Angioedema. DANOCRINE is indicated for the prevention of attacks of angioedema of all types (cutaneous, abdominal, laryngeal) in males and females.

CONTRAINDICATIONS

DANOCRINE should not be administered to patients with:

1. Undiagnosed abnormal genital bleeding.
2. Markedly impaired hepatic, renal, or cardiac function.
3. Pregnancy.
4. Breast feeding.

WARNINGS

Safe use of the drug in pregnancy has not been established clinically. Therefore, a nonhormonal method of contraception should be recommended. If a patient becomes pregnant during treatment, administration of the drug should be discontinued. Continuing treatment may result in an androgenic effect on the fetus, which to date has been limited to clitoral hypertrophy and labial fusion of the external genitalia in the female fetus. If the patient becomes pregnant while taking DANOCRINE, she should be apprised of the potential risk to the fetus.

Before initiating therapy of fibrocystic breast disease with DANOCRINE, carcinoma of the breast should be excluded. However, nodularity, pain, tenderness due to fibrocystic breast disease may prevent recognition of underlying carcinoma before treatment is begun. Therefore, if any nodule persists or enlarges during treatment, carcinoma should be considered and ruled out.

Long-term experience with danazol is limited. Therapy with other steroids alkylated at the 17 position has been associated with serious toxicity (cholestatic jaundice, peliosis hepatis). The physician therefore should be alert to the possibility that similar toxicity may develop after therapy with danazol. Attempts should be made to determine the lowest dose that will provide adequate protection. If the drug was begun at a time of exacerbation of angioneurotic edema due to trauma, stress or other cause, periodic attempts to decrease or withdraw therapy should be considered.

Patients should be watched closely for signs of virilization. Some androgenic effects may not be reversible even when drug administration is stopped.

PRECAUTIONS

Because DANOCRINE may cause some degree of fluid retention, conditions that might be influenced by this factor, such as epilepsy, migraine, or cardiac or renal dysfunction, require careful observation.

Since hepatic dysfunction has been reported in patients treated with DANOCRINE, periodic liver function tests should be performed (see ADVERSE REACTIONS section).

Decreased high density lipoproteins and possibly increased low density lipoproteins have been reported during danazol therapy. While the clinical implications remain unclear, prescribers should consider this in accordance with the medical needs and related health concerns of the patient.

Check semen for volume, viscosity, sperm count and motility every 3 to 4 months, especially in adolescents.

ADVERSE REACTIONS

The following androgenic effects have occurred in patients receiving DANOCRINE: acne, edema, mild hirsutism, decrease in breast size, deepening of the voice, oiliness of the

Continued on next page

This product information was effective as of December 1, 1986. On these and other products of Winthrop-Breon Laboratories, detailed information may be obtained on a current basis by direct inquiry to the Professional Services Department, 90 Park Avenue, New York, NY 10016 (212) 907-2525.

Winthrop-Breon—Cont.

skin or hair, weight gain, and rarely, clitoral hypertrophy, or testicular atrophy.

Also hypoestrogenic manifestations such as flushing, sweating, vaginitis including itching, dryness, burning and vaginal bleeding, nervousness, and emotional lability have been reported.

Hepatic dysfunction, as evidenced by elevated serum enzymes and/or jaundice, has been reported in patients receiving a daily dosage of DANOCRINE of 400 mg or more. It is recommended that patients receiving DANOCRINE, brand of danazol capsules, be monitored for hepatic dysfunction by laboratory tests and clinical observation. Prolongation of prothrombin time in patients stabilized on warfarin has also been reported.

Although the following reactions have also been reported, a causal relationship to the administration of DANOCRINE has neither been confirmed nor refuted: *allergic:* urticaria and rarely, nasal congestion; *CNS effects:* headache, dizziness, depression, fatigue, sleep disorders, tremor, paresthesias, visual disturbances, and rarely, anxiety, changes in appetite, chills, and Guillain-Barré syndrome; *gastrointestinal:* gastroenteritis, nausea, vomiting, constipation, and rarely, pancreatitis; *musculoskeletal:* muscle cramps or spasms, joint lock-up, joint swelling, pain in back, neck, or extremities, and rarely, carpal tunnel syndrome; *genitourinary:* hematuria, prolonged posttherapy amenorrhea; *hematologic:* thrombocytopenia and rarely, eosinophilia, leukocytosis; *skin:* rashes (maculopapular, vesicular, papular, purpuric, petechial), hair loss, and rarely, sun sensitivity, Stevens-Johnson syndrome: *other:* abnormal glucose tolerance test and increased insulin requirements in diabetic patients, changes in libido, elevation in blood pressure, and rarely, cataracts, bleeding gums, fever, pelvic pain, nipple discharge.

DOSAGE AND ADMINISTRATION

Endometriosis. In moderate to severe disease, or in patients infertile due to endometriosis, a starting dose of 800 mg given in two divided doses is recommended. Amenorrhea and a rapid response to painful symptoms is best achieved at this dosage level. Gradual downward titration to a dose sufficient to maintain amenorrhea may be considered depending upon patient response. For mild cases, an initial daily dose of 200 mg to 400 mg given in two divided doses is recommended and may be adjusted depending on patient response. **Therapy should begin during menstruation. Otherwise, appropriate tests should be performed to ensure that the patient is not pregnant while on therapy with DANOCRINE.** (See **WARNINGS.**) **It is essential that therapy continue uninterrupted for 3 to 6 months but may be extended to 9 months if necessary.** After termination of therapy, if symptoms recur, treatment can be reinstituted.

Fibrocystic Breast Disease. The total daily dosage of DANOCRINE for fibrocystic breast disease ranges from 100 mg to 400 mg given in two divided doses depending upon patient response. **Therapy should begin during menstruation. Otherwise, appropriate tests should be performed to ensure that the patient is not pregnant while on therapy with DANOCRINE.** A nonhormonal method of contraception is recommended when DANOCRINE is administered at this dose, since ovulation may not be suppressed.

In most instances, breast pain and tenderness are significantly relieved by the first month and eliminated in 2 to 3 months. Usually elimination of nodularity requires 4 to 6 months of uninterrupted therapy. Regular menstrual patterns, irregular menstrual patterns, and amenorrhea each occur in approximately one-third of patients treated with 100 mg of DANOCRINE, brand of danazol capsules. Irregular menstrual patterns and amenorrhea are observed more frequently with higher doses. Clinical studies have demonstrated that 50% of patients may show evidence of recurrence of symptoms within one year. In this event, treatment may be reinstated.

Hereditary Angioedema. The dosage requirements for continuous treatment of hereditary angioedema with DANOCRINE should be individualized on the basis of the clinical response of the patient. It is recommended that the patient be started on 200 mg, two or three times a day. After a favorable initial response is obtained in terms of prevention of episodes of edematous attacks, the proper continuing dosage should be determined by decreasing the dosage by 50% or less at intervals of one to three months or longer if frequency of attacks prior to treatment dictates. If an attack occurs the daily dosage may be increased by up to 200 mg. During the dose adjusting phase, close monitoring of the patient's response is indicated, particularly if the patient has a history of airway involvement.

HOW SUPPLIED

Capsules of 200 mg (orange), bottles of 60 (NDC 0024-0305-60).

Capsules of 200 mg (orange), bottles of 100 (NDC 0024-0305-06).

Capsules of 200 mg (orange), bottles of 250 (NDC 0024-0305-25).

Capsules of 100 mg (yellow); bottles of 100 (NDC 0024-0304-06).

Capsules of 50 mg (orange and white), bottles of 100 (NDC 0024-0303-06).

Distributed by Winthrop-Breon Laboratories
Division of Sterling Drug Inc.
New York, NY 10016
Manufactured by
Sterling Pharmaceuticals Inc.
Barceloneta, Puerto Rico 00617

Shown in Product Identification Section, page 435

DW-254 O(O)

DEMEROL® Hydrochloride
brand of meperidine hydrochloride, USP

Ⓒ℞

DESCRIPTION

Meperidine hydrochloride is ethyl 1-methyl-4-phenylisonipecotate hydrochloride, a white crystalline substance with a melting point of 186°C to 189°C. It is readily soluble in water and has a neutral reaction and a slightly bitter taste. The solution is not decomposed by a short period of boiling.

The syrup is a pleasant-tasting, nonalcoholic, banana-flavored solution containing 50 mg of DEMEROL hydrochloride, brand of meperidine hydrochloride, per 5 mL teaspoon (25 drops contain 13 mg of DEMEROL hydrochloride). The tablets contain 50 mg or 100 mg of the analgesic.

DEMEROL hydrochloride, brand of meperidine hydrochloride, 5 percent solution has a specific gravity of 1.0086 at 20°C and 10 percent solution, a specific gravity of 1.0165 at 20°C.

Inactive Ingredients—TABLETS: Calcium Sulfate, Dibasic Calcium Phosphate, Starch, Stearic Acid, Talc.

SYRUP: Benzoic Acid, Flavor, Liquid Glucose, Purified Water, Saccharin Sodium.

CLINICAL PHARMACOLOGY

Meperidine hydrochloride is a narcotic analgesic with multiple actions qualitatively similar to those of morphine; the most prominent of these involve the central nervous system and organs composed of smooth muscle. The principal actions of therapeutic value are analgesia and sedation.

There is some evidence which suggests that meperidine may produce less smooth muscle spasm, constipation, and depression of the cough reflex than equianalgesic doses of morphine. Meperidine, in 60 mg to 80 mg parenteral doses, is approximately equivalent in analgesic effect to 10 mg of morphine. The onset of action is slightly more rapid than with morphine, and the duration of action is slightly shorter. Meperidine is significantly less effective by the oral than by the parenteral route, but the exact ratio of oral to parenteral effectiveness is unknown.

INDICATIONS AND USAGE

For the relief of moderate to severe pain (parenteral and oral forms)

For preoperative medication (parenteral form only)

For support of anesthesia (parenteral form only)

For obstetrical analgesia (parenteral form only)

CONTRAINDICATIONS

Hypersensitivity to meperidine.

Meperidine is contraindicated in patients who are receiving monoamine oxidase (MAO) inhibitors or those who have recently received such agents. Therapeutic doses of meperidine have occasionally precipitated unpredictable, severe, and occasionally fatal reactions in patients who have received such agents within 14 days. The mechanism of these reactions is unclear, but may be related to a preexisting hyperphenylalaninemia. Some have been characterized by coma, severe respiratory depression, cyanosis, and hypotension, and have resembled the syndrome of acute narcotic overdose. In other reactions the predominant manifestations have been hyperexcitability, convulsions, tachycardia, hyperpyrexia, and hypertension. Although it is not known that other narcotics are free of the risk of such reactions, virtually all of the reported reactions have occurred with meperidine. If a narcotic is needed in such patients, a sensitivity test should be performed in which repeated, small, incremental doses of morphine are administered over the course of several hours while the patient's condition and vital signs are under careful observation. (Intravenous hydrocortisone or prednisolone have been used to treat severe reactions, with the addition of intravenous chlorpromazine in those cases exhibiting hypertension and hyperpyrexia. The usefulness and safety of narcotic antagonists in the treatment of these reactions is unknown.)

Solutions of DEMEROL and barbiturates are chemically incompatible.

WARNINGS

Drug Dependence. Meperidine can produce drug dependence of the morphine type and therefore has the potential for being abused. Psychic dependence, physical dependence, and tolerance may develop upon repeated administration of meperidine, and it should be prescribed and administered with the same degree of caution appropriate to the use of morphine. Like other narcotics, meperidine is subject to the provisions of the Federal narcotic laws.

Interaction with Other Central Nervous System Depressants. MEPERIDINE SHOULD BE USED WITH GREAT CAUTION AND IN REDUCED DOSAGE IN PATIENTS WHO ARE CONCURRENTLY RECEIVING OTHER NARCOTIC ANALGESICS, GENERAL ANESTHETICS, PHENOTHIAZINES, OTHER TRANQUILIZERS (SEE DOSAGE AND ADMINISTRATION), SEDATIVE-HYPNOTICS (INCLUDING BARBITURATES), TRICYCLIC ANTIDEPRESSANTS, AND OTHER CNS DEPRESSANTS (INCLUDING ALCOHOL). RESPIRATORY DEPRESSION, HYPOTENSION, AND PROFOUND SEDATION OR COMA MAY RESULT.

Head Injury and Increased Intracranial Pressure. The respiratory depressant effects of meperidine and its capacity to elevate cerebrospinal fluid pressure may be markedly exaggerated in the presence of head injury, other intracranial lesions, or a preexisting increase in intracranial pressure. Furthermore, narcotics produce adverse reactions which may obscure the clinical course of patients with head injuries. In such patients, meperidine must be used with extreme caution and only if its use is deemed essential.

Intravenous Use. If necessary, meperidine may be given intravenously, but the injection should be given very slowly, preferably in the form of a diluted solution. Rapid intravenous injection of narcotic analgesics, including meperidine, increases the incidence of adverse reactions; severe respiratory depression, apnea, hypotension, peripheral circulatory collapse, and cardiac arrest have occurred. Meperidine should not be administered intravenously unless a narcotic antagonist and the facilities for assisted or controlled respiration are immediately available. When meperidine is given parenterally, especially intravenously, the patient should be lying down.

Asthma and Other Respiratory Conditions. Meperidine should be used with extreme caution in patients having an acute asthmatic attack, patients with chronic obstructive pulmonary disease or cor pulmonale, patients having a substantially decreased respiratory reserve, and patients with preexisting respiratory depression, hypoxia, or hypercapnia. In such patients, even usual therapeutic doses of narcotics may decrease respiratory drive while simultaneously increasing airway resistance to the point of apnea.

Hypotensive Effect. The administration of meperidine may result in severe hypotension in the postoperative patient or any individual whose ability to maintain blood pressure has been compromised by a depleted blood volume or the administration of drugs such as the phenothiazines or certain anesthetics.

Usage in Ambulatory Patients. Meperidine may impair the mental and/or physical abilities required for the performance of potentially hazardous tasks such as driving a car or operating machinery. The patient should be cautioned accordingly.

Meperidine, like other narcotics, may produce orthostatic hypotension in ambulatory patients.

Usage in Pregnancy and Lactation. Meperidine should not be used in pregnant women prior to the labor period, unless in the judgment of the physician the potential benefits outweigh the possible hazards, because safe use in pregnancy prior to labor has not been established relative to possible adverse effects on fetal development.

When used as an obstetrical analgesic, meperidine crosses the placental barrier and can produce depression of respiration and psychophysiologic functions in the newborn. Resuscitation may be required (see section on **OVERDOSAGE**).

Meperidine appears in the milk of nursing mothers receiving the drug.

PRECAUTIONS

As with all intramuscular preparations DEMEROL intramuscular injection should be injected well within the body of a large muscle.

Supraventricular Tachycardias. Meperidine should be used with caution in patients with atrial flutter and other supraventricular tachycardias because of a possible vagolytic action which may produce a significant increase in the ventricular response rate.

Convulsions. Meperidine may aggravate preexisting convulsions in patients with convulsive disorders. If dosage is escalated substantially above recommended levels because of tolerance development, convulsions may occur in individuals without a history of convulsive disorders.

Acute Abdominal Conditions. The administration of meperidine or other narcotics may obscure the diagnosis or clinical course in patients with acute abdominal conditions.

Special Risk Patients. Meperidine should be given with caution and the initial dose should be reduced in certain patients such as the elderly or debilitated, and those with severe impairment of hepatic or renal function, hypothyroidism, Addison's disease, and prostatic hypertrophy or urethral stricture.

ADVERSE REACTIONS

The major hazards of meperidine, as with other narcotic analgesics, are respiratory depression and, to a lesser degree, circulatory depression; respiratory arrest, shock, and cardiac arrest have occurred.

The most frequently observed adverse reactions include lightheadedness, dizziness, sedation, nausea, vomiting, and sweating. These effects seem to be more prominent in ambulatory patients and in those who are not experiencing severe pain. In such individuals, lower doses are advisable. Some adverse reactions in ambulatory patients may be alleviated if the patient lies down.

Other adverse reactions include:

Nervous System. Euphoria, dysphoria, weakness, headache, agitation, tremor, uncoordinated muscle movements, transient hallucinations and disorientation, visual disturbances. Inadvertent injection about a nerve trunk may result in sensory-motor paralysis which is usually, though not always, transitory.

Gastrointestinal. Dry mouth, constipation, biliary tract spasm.

Cardiovascular. Flushing of the face, tachycardia, bradycardia, palpitation, hypotension (see Warnings), syncope, phlebitis following intravenous injection.

Genitourinary. Urinary retention.

Allergic. Pruritus, urticaria, other skin rashes, wheal and flare over the vein with intravenous injection.

Other. Pain at injection site; local tissue irritation and induration following subcutaneous injection, particularly when repeated; antidiuretic effect.

DOSAGE AND ADMINISTRATION

For Relief of Pain

Dosage should be adjusted according to the severity of the pain and the response of the patient. While subcutaneous administration is suitable for occasional use, intramuscular administration is preferred when repeated doses are required. If intravenous administration is required, dosage should be decreased and the injection made very slowly, preferably utilizing a diluted solution. Meperidine is less effective orally than on parenteral administration. The dose of DEMEROL should be proportionately reduced (usually by 25 to 50 percent) when administered concomitantly with phenothiazines and many other tranquilizers since they potentiate the action of DEMEROL, brand of meperidine.

Adults. The usual dosage is 50 mg to 150 mg intramuscularly, subcutaneously, or orally, every 3 or 4 hours as necessary.

Children. The usual dosage is 0.5 mg/lb to 0.8 mg/lb intramuscularly, subcutaneously, or orally up to the adult dose, every 3 or 4 hours as necessary.

Each dose of the syrup should be taken in one-half glass of water, since if taken undiluted, it may exert a slight topical anesthetic effect on mucous membranes.

For Preoperative Medication

Adults. The usual dosage is 50 mg to 100 mg intramuscularly or subcutaneously, 30 to 90 minutes before the beginning of anesthesia.

Children. The usual dosage is 0.5 mg/lb to 1 mg/lb intramuscularly or subcutaneously up to the adult dose, 30 to 90 minutes before the beginning of anesthesia.

For Support of Anesthesia

Repeated slow intravenous injections of fractional doses (eg, 10 mg/mL) or continuous intravenous infusion of a more dilute solution (eg, 1 mg/mL) should be used. The dose should be titrated to the needs of the patient and will depend on the premedication and type of anesthesia being employed, the characteristics of the particular patient, and the nature and duration of the operative procedure.

For Obstetrical Analgesia

The usual dosage is 50 mg to 100 mg intramuscularly or subcutaneously when pain becomes regular, and may be repeated at 1- to 3-hour intervals.

OVERDOSAGE

Symptoms. Serious overdosage with meperidine is characterized by respiratory depression (a decrease in respiratory rate and/or tidal volume, Cheyne-Stokes respiration, cyanosis), extreme somnolence progressing to stupor or coma, skeletal muscle flaccidity, cold and clammy skin, and sometimes bradycardia and hypotension. In severe overdosage, particularly by the intravenous route, apnea, circulatory collapse, cardiac arrest, and death may occur.

Treatment. Primary attention should be given to the reestablishment of adequate respiratory exchange through provision of a patent airway and institution of assisted or controlled ventilation. The narcotic antagonist, naloxone hydrochloride, is a specific antidote against respiratory depression which may result from overdosage or unusual sensitivity to narcotics, including meperidine. Therefore, an appropriate dose of this antagonist should be administered, preferably by the intravenous route, simultaneously with efforts at respiratory resuscitation.

An antagonist should not be administered in the absence of clinically significant respiratory or cardiovascular depression.

Oxygen, intravenous fluids, vasopressors, and other supportive measures should be employed as indicated.

In cases of overdosage with DEMEROL, brand of meperidine, tablets, the stomach should be evacuated by emesis or gastric lavage.

NOTE: In an individual physically dependent on narcotics, the administration of the usual dose of a narcotic antagonist will precipitate an acute withdrawal syndrome. The severity of this syndrome will depend on the degree of physical dependence and the dose of antagonist administered. The use of narcotic antagonists in such individuals should be avoided if possible. If a narcotic antagonist must be used to treat serious respiratory depression in the physically dependent patient, the antagonist should be administered with extreme care and only one-fifth to one-tenth the usual initial dose administered.

HOW SUPPLIED

For Parenteral Use

Detecto-Seal ® — *Carpuject* ® **Sterile Cartridge-Needle Units**—*2.5 percent* (25 mg per 1 mL) **NDC** 0024-0324-02, *5 percent* (50 mg per 1 mL) **NDC** 0024-0325-02, *7.5 percent* (75 mg per 1 mL) **NDC** 0024-0326-02; and *10 percent* (100 mg per 1 mL) **NDC** 0024-0328-02 all in boxes of 10.

Each cartridge is only partially-filled based upon product volume to permit mixture with other sterile materials in accordance with the best judgment of the physician.

Uni-Amp ®—*5 percent solution;* ampuls of 0.5 mL (25 mg) **NDC** 0024-0361-04, 1 mL (50 mg) **NDC** 0024-0362-04, 1½ mL (75 mg) **NDC** 0024-0363-04, and 2 mL (100 mg) **NDC** 0024-0364-04 all in boxes of 25; and *10 percent solution,* ampuls of 1 mL (100 mg) **NDC** 0024-0365-04 in boxes of 25.

Uni-Nest ™—*5 percent solution;* ampuls of 0.5 mL (25 mg) **NDC** 0024-0371-04, 1 mL (50 mg) **NDC** 0024-0372-04, 1½ mL (75 mg) **NDC** 0024-0373-04, and 2 mL (100 mg) **NDC** 0024-0374-04 all in boxes of 25; and *10 percent solution,* ampuls of 1 mL (100 mg) **NDC** 0024-0375-04 in boxes of 25.

Vials—*5 percent* multiple-dose vials of 30 mL **NDC** 0024-0329-01, and *10 percent* multiple-dose vials of 20 mL **NDC** 0024-0331-01 all in boxes of 1.

Note: The pH of DEMEROL solutions is adjusted between 3.5 and 6.0 with sodium hydroxide or hydrochloric acid. Multiple-dose vials contain metacresol 0.1 percent as preservative. No preservatives are added to the ampuls or CARPUJECT Sterile Cartridge-Needle Units.

For Oral Use

Tablets of 50 mg, bottle of 100 **(NDC** 0024-0335-04) and 500 **(NDC** 0024-0335-06); Hospital Blister Pak of 25 **(NDC** 0024-0335-02); 100 mg, bottle of 100 **(NDC** 0024-0337-04) and 500 **(NDC** 0024-0337-06); Hospital Blister Pak of 25 **(NDC** 0024-0337-02).

Syrup, nonalcoholic, banana-flavored 50 mg per 5 mL teaspoon, bottles of 16 fl oz **(NDC** 0024-0332-06).

Shown in Product Identification Section, page 435

DW-55-FF(O)

INOCOR® LACTATE INJECTION ℞

brand of amrinone lactate
Sterile Intravenous Solution

DESCRIPTION

INOCOR lactate injection, brand of amrinone lactate, represents a new class of cardiac inotropic agents distinct from digitalis glycosides or catecholamines. Amrinone lactate is designated chemically as 5-Amino[3,4′-bipyridin]-6(1*H*)-one lactate.

Amrinone is a pale yellow crystalline compound with a molecular weight of 187.2 and an empirical formula of $C_{10}H_9N_3O$. Each mole of lactic acid has a molecular weight of 90.08 and an empirical formula of $C_3H_6O_3$. The solubilities of amrinone at pH's 4.1, 6.0, and 8.0 are 25, 0.9, and 0.7 mg/mL, respectively.

INOCOR lactate injection is available as a sterile solution in 20 mL ampuls for intravenous administration. Each mL contains INOCOR lactate equivalent to 5 mg of base and 0.25 mg of sodium metabisulfite added as a preservative in Water for Injection. All dosages expressed in the package insert are expressed in terms of the base, amrinone. The pH is adjusted to between 3.2 to 4.0 with lactic acid or sodium hydroxide. The total concentration of lactic acid can vary between 5.0 mg/mL and 7.5 mg/mL.

CLINICAL PHARMACOLOGY

INOCOR lactate injection is a positive inotropic agent with vasodilator activity, different in structure and mode of action from either digitalis glycosides or catecholamines.

The mechanism of its inotropic and vasodilator effects has not been fully elucidated.

With respect to its inotropic effect, experimental evidence indicates that it is not a beta-adrenergic agonist. It inhibits myocardial cyclic adenosine monophosphate (c-AMP) phosphodiesterase activity and increases cellular levels of c-AMP. Unlike digitalis, it does not inhibit sodium-potassium adenosine triphosphatase activity.

With respect to its vasodilatory activity, INOCOR reduces afterload and preload by its direct relaxant effect on vascular smooth muscle.

Pharmacokinetics

Following intravenous bolus (1 to 2 minutes) injection of 0.68 mg/kg to 1.2 mg/kg to normal volunteers, INOCOR had a volume of distribution of 1.2 liters/kg, and following a distributive phase half-life of about 4.6 minutes in plasma, had a mean apparent first-order terminal elimination half-life of about 3.6 hours. In patients with congestive heart failure receiving infusions of INOCOR the mean apparent first-order terminal elimination half-life was about 5.8 hours.

Amrinone has been shown in one study to be 10% to 22% bound to human plasma protein by ultrafiltration in vitro, and in another study 35% to 49% bound by either ultrafiltration or equilibrium dialysis.

The primary route of excretion in man is *via* the urine as both amrinone and several metabolites (N-glycolyl, N-acetate, O-glucuronide and N-glucuronide). In normal volunteers, approximately 63% of an oral dose of ^{14}C-labelled amrinone was excreted in the urine over a 96-hour period. In the first 8 hours, 51% of the radioactivity in the urine was amrinone with 5% as the N-acetate, 8% as the N-glycolate, and less than 5% for each glucuronide. Approximately 18% of the administered dose was excreted in the feces in 72 hours.

In a 24-hour nonradioactive intravenous study, 10% to 40% of the dose was excreted in urine as unchanged amrinone with the N-acetyl metabolite representing less than 2% of the dose.

In congestive heart failure patients, after a loading bolus dose, steady-state plasma levels of about 2.4 μg/mL were able to be maintained by an infusion of 5 μg/kg/min to 10 μg/kg/min. In some congestive heart failure patients, with associated compromised renal and hepatic perfusion, it is possible that plasma levels of amrinone may rise during the infusion period; therefore, in these patients, it may be necessary to monitor the hemodynamic response and/or drug level. The principal measures of patient response include cardiac index, pulmonary capillary wedge pressure, central venous pressure, and their relationship to plasma concentrations. Additionally, measurements of blood pressure, urine output, and body weight may prove useful, as may such clinical symptoms as orthopnea, dyspnea, and fatigue.

Pharmacodynamics

In patients with depressed myocardial function, INOCOR lactate injection produces a prompt increase in cardiac output due to its inotropic and vasodilator actions.

Following a single intravenous bolus dose of INOCOR of 0.75 mg/kg to 3 mg/kg in patients with congestive heart failure, dose-related maximum increases in cardiac output occur (of about 28% at 0.75 mg/kg to about 61% at 3 mg/kg). The peak effect occurs within 10 minutes at all doses. The duration of effect depends upon dose, lasting about ½ hour at 0.75 mg/kg and approximately 2 hours at 3 mg/kg.

Over the same range of doses, pulmonary capillary wedge pressure and total peripheral resistance show dose-related decreases (mean maximum decreases of 29% in pulmonary capillary wedge pressure and 29% in systemic vascular resistance). At doses up to 3.0 mg/kg dose-related decreases in diastolic pressure (up to 13%) have been observed. Mean arterial pressure decreases (9.7%) at a dose of 3.0 mg/kg. The heart rate is generally unchanged.

The changes in hemodynamic parameters are maintained during continuous intravenous infusion and for several hours thereafter.

INOCOR lactate injection, brand of amrinone lactate, is effective in fully digitalized patients without causing signs of cardiac glycoside toxicity. Its inotropic effects are additive to those of digitalis. In cases of atrial flutter/fibrillation, it is possible that INOCOR may increase ventricular response rate because of its slight enhancement of A/V conduction. In these cases, prior treatment with digitalis is recommended.

Improvement in left ventricular function and relief of congestive heart failure in patients with ischemic heart disease have been observed. The improvement has occurred without inducing symptoms or electrocardiographic signs of myocardial ischemia.

At constant heart rate and blood pressure, increases in cardiac output occur without measurable increases in myocardial oxygen consumption or changes in arterio-venous oxygen difference.

Inotropic activity is maintained following repeated intravenous doses of INOCOR. INOCOR administration produces hemodynamic and symptomatic benefits to patients not sat-

Continued on next page

This product information was effective as of December 1, 1986. On these and other products of Winthrop-Breon Laboratories, detailed information may be obtained on a current basis by direct inquiry to the Professional Services Department, 90 Park Avenue, New York, NY 10016 (212) 907-2525.

Winthrop-Breon—Cont.

isfactorily controlled by conventional therapy with diuretics and cardiac glycosides.

INDICATIONS AND USAGE

INOCOR lactate injection is indicated for the short-term management of congestive heart failure. Because of limited experience and potential for serious adverse effects (see ADVERSE REACTIONS), INOCOR should be used only in patients who can be closely monitored and who have not responded adequately to digitalis, diuretics, and/or vasodilators. Although most patients have been studied hemodynamically for periods only up to 24 hours, some patients were studied for longer periods and demonstrated consistent hemodynamic and clinical effects. The duration of therapy should depend on patient responsiveness.

CONTRAINDICATIONS

INOCOR lactate injection is contraindicated in patients who are hypersensitive to it.

It is also contraindicated in those patients known to be hypersensitive to bisulfites.

PRECAUTIONS

General: INOCOR lactate injection should not be used in patients with severe aortic or pulmonic valvular disease in lieu of surgical relief of the obstruction. Like other inotropic agents, it may aggravate outflow tract obstruction in hypertrophic subaortic stenosis.

During intravenous therapy with INOCOR lactate injection, blood pressure and heart rate should be monitored and the rate of infusion slowed or stopped in patients showing excessive decreases in blood pressure.

Patients who have received vigorous diuretic therapy may have insufficient cardiac filling pressure to respond adequately to INOCOR lactate injection, in which case cautious liberalization of fluid and electrolyte intake may be indicated.

Supraventricular and ventricular arrhythmias have been observed in the very high-risk population treated. While amrinone per se has not been shown to be arrhythmogenic, the potential for arrhythmia, present in congestive heart failure itself, may be increased by any drug or combination of drugs.

Thrombocytopenia and hepatotoxicity have been noted (see ADVERSE REACTIONS).

USE IN ACUTE MYOCARDIAL INFARCTION: No clinical trials have been carried out in patients in the acute phase of postmyocardial infarction. Therefore, INOCOR lactate injection, brand of amrinone lactate, is not recommended in these cases.

Laboratory Tests

Fluid and Electrolytes: Fluid and electrolyte changes and renal function should be carefully monitored during amrinone lactate therapy. Improvement in cardiac output with resultant diuresis may necessitate a reduction in the dose of diuretic. Potassium loss due to excessive diuresis may predispose digitalized patients to arrhythmias. Therefore, hypokalemia should be corrected by potassium supplementation in advance of or during amrinone use.

Drug Interactions

In a relatively limited experience, no untoward clinical manifestations have been observed in patients in which INOCOR lactate injection was used concurrently with the following drugs: digitalis glycosides; lidocaine, quinidine; metoprolol, propranolol; hydralazine, prazosin; isosorbide dinitrate, nitroglycerine, chlorthalidone, ethacrynic acid, furosemide, hydrochlorothiazide, spironolactone; captopril; heparin, warfarin; potassium supplements; insulin; diazepam.

One case report of excessive hypotension has been reported when amrinone was used concurrently with disopyramide.

Until additional experience is available, concurrent administration with NORPACE® (disopyramide) should be undertaken with caution.

Chemical Interactions

A chemical interaction occurs slowly over a 24-hour period when the intravenous solution of INOCOR lactate injection is mixed directly with dextrose(glucose)-containing solutions. **THEREFORE, INOCOR LACTATE INJECTION SHOULD NOT BE DILUTED WITH SOLUTIONS THAT CONTAIN DEXTROSE (GLUCOSE) PRIOR TO INJECTION.**

A chemical interaction occurs immediately, which is evidenced by the formation of a precipitate when furosemide is injected into an intravenous line of an infusion of amrinone. Therefore, furosemide should not be administered in intravenous lines containing amrinone.

Carcinogenesis, Mutagenesis, Impairment of Fertility

The 1-year interim evaluation of the 2-year oral carcinogenicity study on F344 rats indicated no tumor induction at that time.

The mouse micronucleus test (at 7.5 to 10 times the maximum human dose) and the Chinese hamster ovary chromosome aberration assay were positive indicating both clastogenic potential and suppression of the number of polychromatic erythrocytes. However, the Ames Salmonella assay, mouse lymphoma study, and cultured human lymphocyte metaphase analysis were all negative. The clastogenic effects are in contrast to negative results obtained in the rat male and female fertility studies, and a three-generation study in rats, both with oral dosing.

Slight prolongation of the rat gestation period was seen in these studies at dose levels of 50 mg/kg/day and 100 mg/kg/day. Dystocia occurred in dams receiving 100 mg/kg/day resulting in increased numbers of stillbirths, decreased litter size, and poor pup survival.

Pregnancy Category C

In New Zealand white rabbits, amrinone has been shown to produce fetal skeletal and gross external malformations at oral doses of 16 mg/kg and 50 mg/kg which were toxic for the rabbit. Studies in French Hy/Cr rabbits using oral doses up to 32 mg/kg/day did not confirm this finding. No malformations were seen in rats receiving amrinone intravenously at the maximum dose used, 15 mg/kg/day (approximately the recommended daily intravenous dose for patients with congestive heart failure). There are no adequate and well-controlled studies in pregnant women. Amrinone should be used during pregnancy only if the potential benefit justifies the potential risk to the fetus.

Nursing Mothers

Caution should be exercised when amrinone is administered to nursing women, since it is not known whether it is excreted in human milk.

Pediatric Use

Safety and effectiveness in children have not been established.

ADVERSE REACTIONS

Thrombocytopenia: Intravenous INOCOR lactate injection, brand of amrinone lactate, resulted in platelet count reductions to below 100,000/mm^3 or normal limits in 2.4 percent of the patients.

It is more common in patients receiving prolonged therapy. To date, in closely-monitored clinical trials, in patients whose platelet counts were not allowed to remain depressed, no bleeding phenomena have been observed.

Platelet reduction is dose dependent and appears due to a decrease in platelet survival time. Several patients who developed thrombocytopenia while receiving amrinone had bone marrow examinations which were normal. There is no evidence relating platelet reduction to immune response or to a platelet activating factor.

Gastrointestinal Effects: Gastrointestinal adverse reactions reported with INOCOR lactate injection during clinical use included nausea (1.7%), vomiting (0.9%), abdominal pain (0.4%), and anorexia (0.4%).

Cardiovascular Effects: Cardiovascular adverse reactions reported with INOCOR lactate injection include arrhythmia (3%) and hypotension (1.3%).

Hepatic Toxicity: In dogs, at IV doses between 9 mg/kg/day and 32 mg/kg/day, amrinone showed dose-related hepatotoxicity manifested either as enzyme elevation or hepatic cell necrosis or both. Hepatotoxicity has been observed in man following long-term oral dosing and has been observed, in a limited experience (0.2%), following intravenous administration of amrinone.

Hypersensitivity: There have been reports of several apparent hypersensitivity reactions in patients treated with oral amrinone for about two weeks. Signs and symptoms were variable but included pericarditis, pleuritis and ascites (1 case), myositis with interstitial shadowing on chest x-ray and elevated sedimentation rate (1 case) and vasculitis with nodular pulmonary densities, hypoxemia, and jaundice (1 case). The first patient died, not necessarily of the possible reaction, while the last two resolved with discontinuation of therapy. None of the cases were rechallenged so that attribution to amrinone is not certain, but possible hypersensitivity reactions should be considered in any patient maintained for a prolonged period on amrinone.

General: Additional adverse reactions observed in intravenous amrinone clinical studies include fever (0.9%), chest pain (0.2%), and burning at the site of injection (0.2%).

Management of Adverse Reactions

Platelet Count Reductions: Asymptomatic platelet count reduction (to <150,000/mm^3) may be reversed within one week of a decrease in drug dosage. Further, with no change in drug dosage, the count may stabilize at lower than predrug levels without any clinical sequelae. Pre-drug platelet counts and frequent platelet counts during therapy are recommended to assist in decisions regarding dosage modifications.

Should a platelet count less than 150,000/mm^3 occur, the following actions may be considered:

- Maintain total daily dose unchanged, since in some cases counts have either stabilized or returned to pretreatment levels.
- Decrease total daily dose.
- Discontinue amrinone if, in the clinical judgment of the physician, risk exceeds the potential benefit.

Gastrointestinal Side Effects: While gastrointestinal side effects were seen infrequently with intravenous therapy, should severe or debilitating ones occur, the physician may wish to reduce dosage or discontinue the drug based on the usual benefit-to-risk considerations.

Hepatic Toxicity: In clinical experience to date with intravenous administration, hepatotoxicity has been observed rarely. If acute marked alterations in liver enzymes occur together with clinical symptoms suggesting an idiosyncratic hypersensitivity reaction, amrinone therapy should be promptly discontinued.

If less than marked enzyme alterations occur without clinical symptoms, these nonspecific changes should be evaluated on an individual basis. The clinician may wish to continue amrinone, reduce dosage, or discontinue the drug based on the usual benefit/risk considerations.

OVERDOSAGE

A death has been reported with a massive accidental overdose of amrinone, although causal relation is uncertain. Diligence should be exercised during product preparation and administration.

Doses of INOCOR lactate injection may produce hypotension because of its vasodilator effect. If this occurs, amrinone administration should be reduced or discontinued. No specific antidote is known, but general measures for circulatory support should be taken.

In rats, the LD_{50} of amrinone, as the lactate salt, was 102 mg/kg or 130 mg/kg intravenously in two different studies and 132 mg/kg orally (intragastrically); as a suspension in aqueous gum tragacanth the oral LD_{50} was 239 mg/kg.

DOSAGE AND ADMINISTRATION

INOCOR lactate injection may be administered as supplied or diluted in normal, or half normal saline solution to a concentration of 1 mg/mL to 3 mg/mL. Diluted solutions should be used within 24 hours.

INOCOR lactate injection, brand of amrinone lactate, may be injected into running dextrose (glucose) infusions through a Y-Connector or directly into the tubing where preferable.

Chemical Interactions

A chemical interaction occurs slowly over a 24-hour period when the intravenous solution of INOCOR lactate injection is mixed directly with dextrose (glucose)-containing solutions. **THEREFORE, INOCOR LACTATE INJECTION SHOULD NOT BE DILUTED WITH SOLUTIONS THAT CONTAIN DEXTROSE (GLUCOSE) PRIOR TO INJECTION.**

A chemical interaction occurs immediately, which is evidenced by the formation of a precipitate when furosemide is injected into an intravenous line of an infusion of amrinone. Therefore, furosemide should not be administered in intravenous lines containing amrinone.

The following procedure is recommended for the administration of INOCOR lactate injection:

1. Initiate therapy with a 0.75 mg/kg bolus given slowly over 2 to 3 minutes.
2. Continue therapy with a maintenance infusion between 5 μg/kg/min and 10 μg/kg/min.
3. Based on clinical response, an additional bolus injection of 0.75 mg/kg may be given 30 minutes after the initiation of therapy.
4. The rate of infusion usually ranges from 5 μg/kg/min to 10 μg/kg/min such that the recommended total daily dose (including boluses) does not exceed 10 mg/kg. A limited number of patients studied at higher doses support a dosage regimen up to 18 mg/kg/day for shortened durations of therapy.
5. The rate of administration and the duration of therapy should be adjusted according to the response of the patient. The physician may wish to reduce or titrate the infusion downward based on clinical responsiveness or untoward effects.

The above dosing regimens can be expected to place most patient's plasma concentration of amrinone at approximately 3 μg/mL. Increases in cardiac index show a linear relationship to plasma concentration of a range of 0.5 μg/mL to 7 μg/mL. No observations have been made at greater plasma concentrations.

Patient improvement may be reflected by increases in cardiac output, reduction in pulmonary capillary wedge pressure, and such clinical responses as a lessening of dyspnea and an improvement in other symptoms of heart failure, such as orthopnea and fatigue.

Monitoring central venous pressure (CVP) may be valuable in the assessment of hypotension and fluid balance management. Prior correction or adjustment of fluid/electrolytes is essential to obtain satisfactory response with amrinone.

Parenteral drug products should be inspected visually and should not be used if particulate matter or discoloration is observed.

HOW SUPPLIED

Ampuls of 20 mL sterile, clear yellow solution containing INOCOR 5 mg/mL, box of 5 (NDC 0024-0888-20). Each 1 mL contains INOCOR lactate equivalent to 5 mg base and 0.25 mg sodium metabisulfite in Water for Injection. The pH of INOCOR lactate injection, brand of amrinone lactate, is adjusted to a range of 3.2 to 4.0 with lactic acid or sodium hydroxide.

Protect INOCOR lactate ampuls from light. Ampul packaging is light resistant for protection during storage.

Store at room temperature.

NOTE: Parenteral drug products should be inspected visually and should not be used if particulate matter or discoloration is observed.

NORPACE, trademark, G. D. Searle & Co.

IW-161 E

FOR MEDICAL INFORMATION ON INOCOR CALL TOLL FREE 1-800-446-6267

ISUPREL® ℞

brand of isoproterenol hydrochloride injection, USP

Sterile Injection 1:5000

DESCRIPTION

ISUPREL hydrochloride, brand of isoproterenol hydrochloride, is 3,4-Dihydroxy-α-[(isopropylamino) methyl] benzyl alcohol hydrochloride, a synthetic sympathomimetic amine that is structurally related to epinephrine but acts almost exclusively on beta receptors.

Each milliliter of the sterile 1:5000 solution contains 0.2 mg ISUPREL hydrochloride, brand of isoproterenol hydrochloride, 0.12 mg lactic acid, 1.8 mg sodium lactate, 7 mg sodium chloride, and not more than 1 mg sodium metabisulfite as preservative. The pH is adjusted with hydrochloric acid. The air in the ampuls has been displaced by nitrogen gas.

CLINICAL PHARMACOLOGY

The primary actions of ISUPREL are on the heart and on smooth muscle of bronchi, skeletal muscle vasculature, and alimentary tract. The positive inotropic and chronotropic actions of the drug increase cardiac output. There is also an increase in venous return to the heart. With usual therapeutic doses, the increase in cardiac output is generally sufficient to maintain or increase systolic blood pressure. ISUPREL also lowers peripheral vascular resistance; the diastolic pressure, therefore, may be expected to fall in normal individuals. Thus, the mean pressure may be reduced. The rate of discharge of cardiac pacemakers is increased with isoproterenol.

ISUPREL relaxes most smooth muscle, the most pronounced effect being on bronchial and gastrointestinal smooth muscle. It produces marked relaxation in the smaller bronchi and may even dilate the trachea and main bronchi past the resting diameter.

The acute toxicity of ISUPREL in animals is much less than that of epinephrine. Excessive doses in animals or man can cause a striking drop in blood pressure, and repeated large doses in animals may result in cardiac enlargement and focal myocarditis.

INDICATIONS AND USAGE

Parenteral isoproterenol hydrochloride is indicated as an adjunct in the management of shock (hypoperfusion syndrome) and in the treatment of cardiac standstill or arrest; carotid sinus hypersensitivity; Adams-Stokes syndrome; and ventricular tachycardia and ventricular arrhythmias that require increased inotropic cardiac activity for therapy. It may also be used in the management of bronchospasm during anesthesia.

SHOCK (HYPOPERFUSION SYNDROME)

Shock is a complex clinical syndrome characterized by inadequate tissue perfusion, which results from one or more of the following mechanisms: loss of effective blood volume, cardiac failure, peripheral vascular failure. Rational therapy must be aimed at correcting this perfusion deficit.

Since shock is often, but by no means always, associated with lowered blood pressure, administration of vasoactive drugs that increase blood pressure without increasing blood flow may not be in the best interest of the patient. However, in cases of shock characterized chiefly by peripheral vasodilatation and in shock following acute myocardial infarction, according to one group of investigators, a vasopressor such as norepinephrine bitartrate injection, USP, may be indicated. In addition to the routine monitoring of systemic blood pressure, heart rate, urine flow, and the use of the electrocardiogram, the shock state and the response to therapy should be monitored by frequent determinations of the central venous pressure, blood pH, and blood pCO_2 (or bicarbonate). Determinations of cardiac output and circulation time may also be helpful.

Adequate filling of the intravascular compartment by suitable volume expanders is of primary importance in most cases of shock, and should precede the administration of vasoactive drugs. Determination of central venous pressure is a reliable guide during volume replacement. If evidence of hypoperfusion persists after adequate volume replacement, ISUPREL may be given.

ISUPREL increases cardiac output by increasing the strength of cardiac contraction and, to a limited extent, the rate of contraction. ISUPREL also increases venous return to the heart by mobilizing blood from vascular reservoirs. In addition, the peripheral and coronary vasodilating effects of the drug may aid tissue perfusion. ISUPREL may be given to patients who are fully digitalized; in fact, ISUPREL may be particularly useful when cardiac competence cannot be restored by digitalization.

Appropriate measures should be taken to ensure adequate ventilation. Careful attention should be paid to acid-base balance and to the correction of electrolyte disturbance. In cases of shock associated with bacteremia, suitable antimicrobial therapy is, of course, imperative.

In a group of 10 patients with elevated central venous pressures who were in shock from cardiac failure, isoproterenol produced increases in cardiac output of 0.33 liters to 4.34 liters per minute in nine of the ten. Similarly, in a series of 12 patients with shock due to gram-negative bacteremia, Kardos found isoproterenol to be useful in correcting the hemodynamic alterations. (*N Engl J Med* 1966; 274:868).

Although the ultimate effect of ISUPREL on patient survival has not yet been documented, experimental studies in rats have shown that the fatal course of shock caused by transient hemorrhage was reversed by treatment with isoproterenol after replacement of blood volume. In addition, clinical studies have indicated that in a majority of patients in shock, administration of ISUPREL tends to correct the hemodynamic abnormalities.

CONTRAINDICATION

Administration of ISUPREL is contraindicated in patients with tachycardia caused by digitalis intoxication.

WARNING

Isoproterenol infusions may produce an increase in myocardial work and oxygen consumption. These effects may be detrimental to myocardial metabolism and functioning in patients who are in cardiogenic shock secondary to coronary artery occlusion and myocardial infarction.

PRECAUTIONS

ISUPREL and epinephrine should not be administered simultaneously, since both drugs are direct cardiac stimulants and their combined effects may induce serious arrhythmia. The drugs may, however, be administered alternately provided a proper interval has elapsed between doses.

Dosage of ISUPREL should be carefully adjusted, particularly in patients with coronary insufficiency, diabetes, or hyperthyroidism, and in patients sensitive to sympathomimetic amines.

Hypovolemia should be corrected by suitable volume expanders before treatment with ISUPREL. Patients in shock should be closely observed during isoproterenol administration. If the heart rate exceeds 110 beats per minute, it may be advisable to decrease the infusion rate or temporarily discontinue the infusion. Doses of ISUPREL sufficient to increase the heart rate to more than 130 beats per minute may induce ventricular arrhythmia.

There has been no clinical evidence of teratogenic effects attributable to ISUPREL in more than 20 years' use of the drug. However, before administration of any drug to pregnant women or women of childbearing potential, the expected benefit of the drug should be carefully weighed against the possible risk to the mother or child.

DOSAGE AND ADMINISTRATION

ISUPREL hydrochloride Solution 1:5000 should be diluted in 5 percent Dextrose Injection, USP, before it is administered to patients in shock.

- A convenient dilution is 1 mg ISUPREL (5 mL) in 500 mL diluent (final concentration, 1:500,000).
- Concentrations up to 10 times greater have been used. This may be important in patients in whom limitation of volume is essential.
- Infusion rates of 0.5 μg to 5 μg per minute (0.25 mL to 2.5 mL diluted solution 1:500,000) have been recommended.
- Rates over 30 μg per minute have been used in advanced stages of shock.

The speed of infusion should be adjusted on the basis of heart rate, central venous pressure, systemic blood pressure, and urine flow. If the heart rate exceeds 110 beats per minute, it may be advisable to decrease the infusion rate or temporarily discontinue the infusion.

CARDIAC STANDSTILL AND CARDIAC ARRHYTHMIAS

Because it has potent inotropic cardiac stimulant action with little or no pressor activity, ISUPREL hydrochloride, brand of isoproterenol hydrochloride, has been effective for the treatment of the following:

1. Adams-Stokes syndrome—atrioventricular heart block
2. Cardiac standstill (arrest)
3. Carotid sinus hypersensitivity
4. Ventricular arrhythmias, especially certain types of ventricular tachycardia and fibrillation occurring during the course of atrioventricular block.

It should be noted that in symptomatic heart block, electrical pacing is the preferred method of treatment for maintenance of an adequate ventricular rate. Moreover, in ventricular arrhythmias, especially certain types of ventricular tachycardia and fibrillation, electroshock may have to be used, and is usually the treatment of choice.

If, however, therapy with ISUPREL is elected in these conditions, intravenous administration, with constant monitoring, is preferred.

In patients with heart block and episodic ventricular tachycardia or fibrillation, ISUPREL stimulates the higher centers or nodal tissue without exciting the lower ventricular foci. In so doing, the normal idioventricular pacemaker function may take over, thereby abolishing ventricular acceleration. Epinephrine is contraindicated in patients with ventricular fibrillation because it may precipitate or prolong fibrillation by stimulation of multiple higher and lower foci. It also may further embarrass the cardiovascular system by its hypertensive action.

Intravenous administration of ISUPREL has been recommended for the management of patients with complete heart block following closure of ventricular septal defects. A 1:50,000 solution may be administered intravenously in doses ranging from 0.5 mL to 1.5 mL for infants and from 2 mL to 3 mL for adults. With such doses the heart rate accelerates and the effect often lasts for 15 or 20 minutes. Sinus rhythm sometimes occurs and persists for a variable period but often relapses again into complete block. In other cases, ISUPREL merely maintains an acceptable heart rate somewhere above 90 to 100 beats per minute. The patient must be monitored constantly by electrocardiography.

CONTRAINDICATIONS

Use of isoproterenol in patients with preexisting cardiac arrhythmias associated with tachycardia is generally considered contraindicated because the chronotropic effect of the drug on the heart may aggravate such disorders. Exceptions consist only of those ventricular tachycardias and ventricular arrhythmias which require increased inotropic cardiac activity for therapy.

Administration of ISUPREL, brand of isoproterenol, is contraindicated in patients with tachycardia caused by digitalis intoxication.

PRECAUTIONS

ISUPREL and epinephrine should not be administered simultaneously, since both drugs are direct cardiac stimulants and their combined effects may induce serious arrhythmia. The drugs may, however, be administered alternately provided a proper interval has elapsed between doses.

Dosage of ISUPREL should be carefully adjusted in patients with coronary insufficiency, diabetes, or hyperthyroidism, and in patients sensitive to sympathomimetic amines.

If the cardiac rate increases sharply, patients with angina pectoris may experience anginal pain until the cardiac rate decreases.

There has been no clinical evidence of teratogenic effects attributable to ISUPREL in more than 20 years' use of the drug. However, before administration of any drug to pregnant women or women of childbearing potential, the expected benefit of the drug should be carefully weighed against the possible risk to the mother or child.

ADVERSE REACTIONS

Serious reactions to ISUPREL are infrequent. The following reactions however, have been reported: flushing of the face, sweating, mild tremors, nervousness, headache, and tachycardia with palpitation manifested as a sensation of pounding in the chest. These reactions disappear quickly and usually do not require discontinuation of treatment with ISUPREL. No cumulative effects have been reported. Pulmonary edema has been reported in a patient extremely intolerant to all sympathomimetic drugs.

In a few patients, presumably with organic disease of the AV node and its branches, ISUPREL has been reported, paradoxically, to precipitate Adams-Stokes seizures during normal sinus rhythm or transient heart block.

DOSAGE AND ADMINISTRATION

In the treatment and prevention of cardiac standstill and cardiac arrhythmias, parenteral ISUPREL may be administered by intravenous injection, infusion, intramuscular and

Continued on next page

This product information was effective as of December 1, 1986. On these and other products of Winthrop-Breon Laboratories, detailed information may be obtained on a current basis by direct inquiry to the Professional Services Department, 90 Park Avenue, New York, NY 10016 (212) 907-2525.

Winthrop-Breon—Cont.

subcutaneous injection, and *in extremis*, by intracardiac injection.
The following table summarizes the dosage regimen suggested for various routes of administration in adults. Children may be given half the initial adult dose. In all patients, subsequent dosage and method of administration depend on the response of the ventricular rate and the rapidity with which the cardiac pacemaker can take over when the drug is gradually withdrawn.
The usual route of administration in emergency treatment of patients threatened with cardiac standstill or arrhythmia is by intravenous injection or infusion. Dosage must be regulated by monitoring of the electrocardiogram. If time is not of utmost importance, initial therapy by intramuscular or subcutaneous injection is preferred.
[See table below].

BRONCHOSPASM DURING ANESTHESIA

Parenteral ISUPREL hydrochloride, brand of isoproterenol hydrochloride, has been shown under experimental and clinical conditions to be a potent bronchodilating agent. However, when given in dosages to achieve this effect, it may also have a stimulating effect on the cardiovascular system. Like epinephrine, it may produce arrhythmias in patients anesthetized with cyclopropane, and should be used with caution. ISUPREL can be used for the management of bronchospasm by helping the patient to maintain adequate ventilation and a normally functioning circulatory system.

PRECAUTIONS AND ADVERSE REACTIONS
See corresponding sections under "Cardiac Standstill and Cardiac Arrhythmias."

DOSAGE AND ADMINISTRATION
For the management of bronchospasm during anesthesia, 1 mL of ISUPREL Solution 1:5000 is diluted to 10 mL with Sodium Chloride Injection, USP, or 5 percent Dextrose Injection, USP. An initial dose of 0.01 mg to 0.02 mg (0.5 mL to 1 mL of the diluted solution, 1:50,000) is administered intravenously, and may be repeated when necessary.

HOW SUPPLIED
Ampuls of 1 mL (0.2 mg)
UNI-NEST™ PAK of 25 NDC-0024-0866-25
Ampuls of 5 mL (1 mg) box of 10
NDC-0024-0866-02
Keep in a cool place. Protect from light–keep in opaque container until used.
Do not use the injection if it is pinkish to brownish in color or contains a precipitate.
IW-33-T

ISUPREL® ℞
brand of isoproterenol hydrochloride inhalation aerosol, USP
MISTOMETER®

Potent Bronchodilator

DESCRIPTION
ISUPREL MISTOMETER is a complete nebulizing unit consisting of a plastic-coated vial of aerosol solution, detachable plastic mouthpiece with built-in nebulizer, and protective cap. The vial contains isoproterenol hydrochloride with inert ingredients of alcohol 33 percent (w/w) and ascorbic acid and, as propellants dichlorodifluoromethane and dichlorotetrafluoroethane. The contents permit the delivery of not less than 200 actuations from the 11.2 g (10 mL) vial and not less than 300 actuations from the 16.8 g (15 mL) vial. The MISTOMETER unit delivers a measured dose of 131 μg of the bronchodilator in a fine, even mist for inhalation.

CLINICAL PHARMACOLOGY
ISUPREL relaxes bronchial spasm and facilitates expectoration of pulmonary secretions. It is frequently effective when epinephrine and other drugs fail, and it has a wide margin of safety. In dogs the toxic dose is 1000 times the therapeutic dose. Converted to the amount used clinically in man, this would be about 2500 times the therapeutic dose.

INDICATIONS AND USAGE
ISUPREL is indicated for the treatment of bronchospasm associated with acute and chronic bronchial asthma, pulmonary emphysema, bronchitis, and bronchiectasis.

CONTRAINDICATION
Use of isoproterenol in patients with preexisting cardiac arrhythmias associated with tachycardia is generally considered contraindicated because the cardiac stimulant effect of the drug may aggravate such disorders.

WARNINGS
Excessive use of an adrenergic aerosol should be discouraged as it may lose its effectiveness.
In patients with status asthmaticus and abnormal blood gas tensions, improvement in vital capacity and in blood gas tensions may not accompany apparent relief of bronchospasm. Facilities for administering oxygen mixtures and ventilatory assistance are necessary for such patients.
Occasional patients have been reported to develop severe paradoxical airway resistance with repeated, excessive use of isoproterenol inhalation preparations. The cause of this refractory state is unknown. It is advisable that in such instances the use of this preparation be discontinued immediately and alternative therapy instituted, since in the reported cases the patients did not respond to other forms of therapy until the drug was withdrawn.
Deaths have been reported following excessive use of isoproterenol inhalation preparations and the exact cause is unknown. Cardiac arrest was noted in several instances.

PRECAUTIONS
Epinephrine should not be administered concomitantly with ISUPREL, as both drugs are direct cardiac stimulants and their combined effects may induce serious arrhythmia. If desired they may, however, be alternated, provided an interval of at least four hours has elapsed.
Isoproterenol should be used with caution in patients with cardiovascular disorders including coronary insufficiency, diabetes, or hyperthyroidism, and in persons sensitive to sympathomimetic amines.
A single treatment with the ISUPREL MISTOMETER unit is usually sufficient for controlling isolated attacks of asthma. Any patient who requires more than three aerosol treatments within a 24-hour period should be under the close supervision of a physician. Further therapy with the bronchodilator aerosol alone is inadvisable when three to five treatments within six to twelve hours produce minimal or no relief.
During the course of over 30 years of use of ISUPREL (isoproterenol), there has been no clinical evidence of teratogenic effects. However, use of any drug in pregnancy, lactation, or in women of childbearing age requires that the potential benefit of the drug be weighed against its possible hazards to the mother or child.

ADVERSE REACTIONS
The mist from the ISUPREL MISTOMETER unit contains alcohol but is generally very well tolerated. An occasional patient may experience some transient throat irritation which has been attributed to the alcohol content.
Tachycardia, palpitation, nervousness, nausea, and vomiting may occur from overdosage. Rarely do headache, flushing of the skin, tremor, dizziness, weakness, sweating, precordial distress, or anginal-type pain occur. The inhalation route is usually accompanied by a minimum of side effects. These untoward reactions disappear quickly and do not, as a rule, inconvenience the patient to the extent that the drug must be discontinued. No cumulative effects have been reported.

DOSAGE AND ADMINISTRATION
Acute Bronchial Asthma: Hold the MISTOMETER unit in an inverted position. Close lips and teeth around open end of mouthpiece. Breathe out, expelling as much air from the lungs as possible; then inhale deeply while pressing down on the bottle to activate spray mechanism. Try to hold breath for a few seconds before exhaling. Wait one full minute in order to determine the effect before considering a second inhalation. A treatment may be repeated up to 5 times daily if necessary. (See Precautions.) If carefully instructed, children quickly learn to keep the stream of mist clear of the teeth and tongue, thereby assuring inhalation into the lungs. Occlusion of the nares of very young children may be advisable to make inhalation certain.
Warm water should be run through the mouthpiece once daily to wash it and prevent clogging.
The mouthpiece may also be sanitized by immersion in alcohol.
Bronchospasm in Chronic Obstructive Lung Disease: The MISTOMETER unit provides a convenient aerosol method for delivering ISUPREL, brand of isoproterenol hydrochloride inhalation aerosol. The preceding treatment described for Acute Bronchial Asthma may be repeated at not less than 3 to 4 hour intervals as part of a programmed regimen of treatment of obstructive lung disease complicated by a reversible bronchospastic component. One application from the MISTOMETER unit may be regarded as equivalent in effectiveness to 5 to 7 operations of a hand-bulb nebulizer using a 1:100 solution.
Children's Dosage. In general, the technique of ISUPREL MISTOMETER in administration to children is similar to that of adults, since children's smaller ventilatory exchange capacity automatically provides proportionally smaller aerosol intake.

HOW SUPPLIED
Vial of 11.2 g (10 mL) with oral nebulizer
(NDC 0024-0878-05)
Vial of 16.8 g (15 mL) with oral nebulizer
(NDC 0024-0878-01)
Refill only, 16.8 g (15 mL)
(NDC 0024-0879-01)
Distributed by Winthrop-Breon Laboratories
Division of Sterling Drug Inc.
New York, NY 10016
Manufactured by Sterling Pharmaceuticals Inc.
Barceloneta, Puerto Rico 00617
IW-67-BB

ISUPREL® Hydrochloride ℞
brand of isoproterenol
inhalation solution, USP
SOLUTION 1:200
SOLUTION 1:100

Potent Bronchodilator

DESCRIPTION
ISUPREL hydrochloride, brand of isoproterenol inhalation solution, is available as:
Solution 1:200 contains isoproterenol hydrochloride 5.0 mg/mL.
Inactive Ingredients: Chlorobutanol 0.5 percent and Sodium Metabisulfite 0.3 percent as preservatives, Citric Acid, Glycerin, Purified Water, and Sodium Chloride.
Solution 1:100 contains isoproterenol hydrochloride 10.0 mg/mL.
Inactive Ingredients: Chlorobutanol 0.5 percent and Sodium Metabisulfite 0.3 percent as preservatives, Citric Acid, Purified Water, Saccharin Sodium, Sodium Chloride, and Sodium Citrate.
The air in the bottles has been displaced by nitrogen gas.
Do not use the solutions if a precipitate or discoloration is observed. Although solutions of ISUPREL left in nebulizers will remain clear and potent for many days, for sanitary reasons it is recommended that they be changed daily.

CLINICAL PHARMACOLOGY
ISUPREL relaxes bronchial spasm and facilitates expectoration of pulmonary secretions. It is frequently effective when epinephrine and other drugs fail, and it has a wide margin of safety. In dogs the toxic dose is 1,000 times the therapeutic

Dosage of ISUPREL for Cardiac Standstill and Cardiac Arrhythmias in Adults

Route of Administration	Preparation of Dilution	Initial Dose	Subsequent Dose Range
Intravenous	Dilute 1 mL of Solution 1:5000 (0.2 mg) to 10 mL with Sodium Chloride Injection, USP, or 5% Dextrose Injection, USP.	0.02 to 0.06 mg (1 to 3 mL of diluted solution 1:50,000)	0.01 to 0.2 mg (0.5 to 10 mL of diluted solution)
Intravenous infusion	Dilute 10 mL of Solution 1:5000 (2 mg) in 500 mL of 5% Dextrose Injection, USP.	5 μg/min (1.25 mL of diluted solution 1:250,000 per minute)	
Intramuscular	Use Solution 1:5000 undiluted	0.2 mg (1 mL)	0.02 to 1 mg (0.1 to 5 mL)
Subcutaneous	Use Solution 1:5000 undiluted	0.2 mg (1 mL)	0.15 to 0.2 mg (0.75 to 1 mL)
Intracardiac	Use Solution 1:5000 undiluted	0.02 mg (0.1 mL)	

dose. Converted to the amount used clinically in man, this would be about 2,500 times the therapeutic dose.

INDICATIONS AND USAGE

ISUPREL is indicated for the treatment of bronchospasm associated with acute and chronic bronchial asthma, pulmonary emphysema, bronchitis, and bronchiectasis.

CONTRAINDICATION

Use of isoproterenol in patients with preexisting cardiac arrhythmias associated with tachycardia is generally considered contraindicated because the cardiac stimulant effect of the drug may aggravate such disorders.

WARNINGS

Excessive use of an adrenergic aerosol should be discouraged as it may lose its effectiveness.

In patients with status asthmaticus and abnormal blood gas tensions, improvement in vital capacity and in blood gas tensions may not accompany apparent relief of bronchospasm. Facilities for administering oxygen mixtures and ventilatory assistance are necessary for such patients.

Occasional patients have been reported to develop severe paradoxical airway resistance with repeated, excessive use of isoproterenol inhalation preparations. The cause of this refractory state is unknown. It is advisable that in such instances the use of this preparation be discontinued immediately and alternative therapy instituted, since in the reported cases the patients did not respond to other forms of therapy until the drug was withdrawn.

Deaths have been reported following excessive use of isoproterenol inhalation preparations and the exact cause is unknown. Cardiac arrest was noted in several instances.

PRECAUTIONS

Epinephrine should not be administered concomitantly with ISUPREL, as both drugs are direct cardiac stimulants and their combined effects may induce serious arrhythmia. If desired they may, however, be alternated, provided an interval of at least four hours has elapsed.

Isoproterenol should be used with caution in patients with cardiovascular disorders including coronary insufficiency, diabetes, or hyperthyroidism, and in persons sensitive to sympathomimetic amines.

Any patient who requires more than three aerosol treatments within a 24-hour period should be under the close supervision of his physician. Further therapy with the bronchodilator aerosol alone is inadvisable when three to five treatments within six to twelve hours produce minimal or no relief.

During the course of over 25 years of use of ISUPREL (isoproterenol) there has been no clinical evidence of teratogenic effects. However, use of any drug in pregnancy, lactation, or in women of childbearing age requires that the potential benefit of the drug be weighed against its possible hazards to the mother or child.

When compressed oxygen is employed as the aerosol propellant, the percentage of oxygen used should be determined by the patient's individual requirements to avoid depression of respiratory drive.

ADVERSE REACTIONS

Tachycardia, palpitation, nervousness, nausea, and vomiting may occur from overdosage. Rarely do headache, flushing of the skin, tremor, dizziness, weakness, sweating, precordial distress, or anginal-type pain occur. The inhalation route is usually accompanied by a minimum of side effects. These untoward reactions disappear quickly and do not, as a rule, inconvenience the patient to the extent that the drug must be discontinued. No cumulative effects have been reported.

DOSAGE AND ADMINISTRATION

ISUPREL hydrochloride solutions can be administered as an aerosol mist by hand-bulb nebulizer, compressed air or oxygen operated nebulizer, or by intermittent positive pressure breathing (IPPB) devices. The method of delivery, and the treatment regimen employed in the management of the reversible bronchospastic element accompanying bronchial asthma, chronic bronchitis, and chronic obstructive lung diseases, will depend on such factors as the severity of the bronchospasm, patient age, tolerance to the medication, complicating cardiopulmonary conditions, and whether therapy is for an intermittent acute attack of bronchospasm or is part of a programmed treatment regimen for constant bronchospasm.

Acute Bronchial Asthma. *Hand-Bulb Nebulizer*—Depending on the frequency of treatment and the type of nebulizer used, a volume of solution of ISUPREL, sufficient for not more than one day's treatment, should be placed in the nebulizer using the dropper provided. In time, the patient can learn to adjust the volume required. For adults and children, the 1:200 solution is administered by hand-bulb nebulization in a dosage of 5 to 15 deep inhalations (using an all glass or plastic nebulizer). In adults, the 1:100 solution may be used if a stronger solution seems to be indicated. The dose is 3 to 7 deep inhalations. If after about 5 to 10 minutes inadequate relief is observed, these doses may be repeated one more time. If the acute attack recurs, treatments may be repeated up to 5 times daily if necessary. (See PRECAUTIONS.)

Bronchospasm in Chronic Obstructive Lung Disease. *Hand-Bulb Nebulizer*—A solution of 1:200 or 1:100 of ISUPREL may be administered daily at not less than 3 to 4 hour intervals for subacute bronchospastic attacks or as part of a programmed treatment regimen in patients with chronic obstructive lung disease with a reversible bronchospastic component. An adequate dose is usually 5 to 15 deep inhalations, using the 1:200 solution. Some patients with severe attacks of bronchospasm may require 3 to 7 deep inhalations using the 1:100 solution of ISUPREL.

Nebulization by Compressed Air or Oxygen—A method often used in patients with severe chronic obstructive lung disease is to deliver the ISUPREL (isoproterenol) mist *in more dilute form over a longer period of time.* The purpose is, not so much to increase the dose supplied, as to achieve progressively deeper bronchodilatation and thus insure that the mist achieves maximum penetration of the finer bronchioles. In this method, 0.5 mL of a 1:200 solution of ISUPREL is diluted to 2 mL to 2.5 mL with water or isotonic saline to achieve a use concentration of 1:800 to 1:1000. If desired, 0.25 mL of the 1:100 solution may be similarly diluted to achieve the same use concentration. The diluted solution is placed in a nebulizer (eg, DeVilbiss #640 unit) connected to either a source of compressed air or oxygen. The flow rate is regulated to suit the particular nebulizer so that the diluted solution of ISUPREL will be delivered over approximately 10 to 20 minutes. A treatment may be repeated up to 5 times daily if necessary. Although the total delivered dose of ISUPREL is somewhat higher than with the treatment regimen employing the hand-bulb nebulizer, patients usually tolerate it well because of the greater dilution and longer application-time factors.

Intermittent Positive Pressure Breathing (IPPB)—Diluted solutions of 1:200 or 1:100 of ISUPREL are used in a programmed regimen for the treatment of reversible bronchospasm in patients with chronic obstructive lung disease who require intermittent positive pressure breathing therapy. These devices generally have a small nebulizer, usually of 3 mL to 5 mL capacity, on a patient-operated side arm. The effectiveness of IPPB therapy is greatly enhanced by the simultaneous use of aerosolized bronchodilators. As with compressed air or oxygen operated nebulizers, the usual regimen is to place 0.5 mL of 1:200 solution of ISUPREL diluted to 2 mL to 2.5 mL with water or isotonic saline in the nebulizer cup and follow the IPPB manufacturer's operating instructions. IPPB-bronchodilator treatments are usually administered over 15 to 20 minutes, up to 5 times daily if necessary.

Children's Dosage: In general, the technique of ISUPREL hydrochloride solution administration to children is similar to that of adults, since children's smaller ventilatory exchange capacity automatically provides proportionally smaller aerosol intake. However, it is generally recommended that the 1:200 solution (rather than the 1:100) be used for an acute attack of bronchospasm, and no more than 0.25 mL of the 1:200 solution should be used for each 10 to 15 minute programmed treatment in chronic bronchospastic disease.

HOW SUPPLIED

Solution 1:100
  bottle of 10 mL (**NDC** 0024-0873-01)
Solution 1:200
  bottle of 10 mL (**NDC** 0024-0871-01)
  bottle of 60 mL (**NDC** 0024-0871-03)

Do not use solutions if they are pinkish to brownish in color or contain a precipitate.

Distributed by Winthrop-Breon Laboratories
Division of Sterling Drug Inc.
New York, NY 10016
Manufactured by Sterling Pharmaceuticals Inc.
Barceloneta, Puerto Rico 00617

IW-154-C

ISUPREL® Hydrochloride ℞
brand of isoproterenol hydrochloride tablets, USP GLOSSETS®

DESCRIPTION

Each tablet contains 10 mg or 15 mg isoproterenol hydrochloride in a rapidly disintegrating base consisting of lactose, saccharin sodium, sodium metabisulfite 2 mg per tablet as antioxidant, starch, and talc.

HOW SUPPLIED

ISUPREL GLOSSETS 10 mg, bottle of 50
(NDC 0024-0875-02)
ISUPREL GLOSSETS 15 mg, bottle of 50
(NDC 0024-0877-02)

For complete prescribing information, see package insert or contact Winthrop-Breon Laboratories Medical Department.

1W-121-G

KAYEXALATE® ℞
brand of sodium polystyrene sulfonate, USP

Cation-Exchange Resin

DESCRIPTION

The drug is a light brown to brown, finely ground, powdered form of sodium polystyrene sulfonate, a cation-exchange resin prepared in the sodium phase with an *in vitro* exchange capacity of approximately 3.1 mEq (*in vivo* approximately 1 mEq) of potassium per gram. The sodium content is approximately 100 mg (4.1 mEq) per gram of the drug.

ACTION

As the resin passes along the intestine or is retained in the colon after administration by enema, the sodium ions are partially released and are replaced by potassium ions. For the most part, this action occurs in the large intestine, which excretes potassium ions to a greater degree than does the small intestine. The efficiency of this process is limited and unpredictably variable. It commonly approximates the order of 33 percent but the range is so large that definitive indices of electrolyte balance must be clearly monitored.

INDICATION

KAYEXALATE is indicated for the treatment of hyperkalemia.

WARNINGS

Since effective lowering of serum potassium with KAYEXALATE may take hours to days, treatment with this drug alone may be insufficient to rapidly correct severe hyperkalemia associated with states of rapid tissue breakdown (eg, burns and renal failure) or hyperkalemia so marked as to constitute a medical emergency. Therefore, other definitive measures, including dialysis, should always be considered and may be imperative.

Serious potassium deficiency can occur from KAYEXALATE therapy. The effect must be carefully controlled by frequent serum potassium determinations within each 24-hour period. Since intracellular potassium deficiency is not always reflected by serum potassium levels, the level at which treatment with KAYEXALATE should be discontinued must be determined individually for each patient. Important aids in making this determination are the patient's clinical condition and electrocardiogram. Early clinical signs of severe hypokalemia include a pattern of irritable confusion and delayed thought processes. Electrocardiographically, severe hypokalemia is often associated with a lengthened Q-T interval, widening, flattening, or inversion of the T wave, and prominent U waves. Also, cardiac arrhythmias may occur, such as premature atrial, nodal, and ventricular contractions, and supraventricular and ventricular tachycardias. The toxic effects of digitalis are likely to be exaggerated. Marked hypokalemia can also be manifested by severe muscle weakness, at times extending into frank paralysis.

Like all cation-exchange resins, KAYEXALATE is not totally selective (for potassium) in its actions, and small amounts of other cations such as magnesium and calcium can also be lost during treatment. Accordingly, patients receiving KAYEXALATE should be monitored for all applicable electrolyte disturbances. Systemic alkalosis has been reported after cation-exchange resins were administered orally in combination with nonabsorbable cation-donating antacids and laxatives such as magnesium hydroxide and aluminum carbonate. Magnesium hydroxide should not be administered with KAYEXALATE. One case of grand mal seizure has been reported in a patient with chronic hypocalcemia of renal failure who was given KAYEXALATE with magnesium hydroxide as laxative. Also, the simultaneous oral administration of KAYEXALATE with nonabsorbable cation-donating antacids and laxatives may reduce the resin's potassium exchange capability.

PRECAUTIONS

Caution is advised when KAYEXALATE is administered to patients who cannot tolerate even a small increase in sodium loads (ie, severe congestive heart failure, severe hypertension, or marked edema). In such instances compensatory restriction of sodium intake from other sources may be indicated.

If constipation occurs, patients should be treated with sorbitol (from 10 to 20 mL of 70 percent syrup every two hours or

Continued on next page

This product information was effective as of December 1, 1986. On these and other products of Winthrop-Breon Laboratories, detailed information may be obtained on a current basis by direct inquiry to the Professional Services Department, 90 Park Avenue, New York, NY 10016 (212) 907-2525.

Winthrop-Breon—Cont.

as needed to produce one or two watery stools daily), a measure which also reduces any tendency to fecal impaction.

ADVERSE REACTIONS

KAYEXALATE may cause some degree of gastric irritation. Anorexia, nausea, vomiting, and constipation may occur especially if high doses are given. Also, hypokalemia, hypocalcemia, and significant sodium retention may occur. Occasionally diarrhea develops. Large doses in elderly individuals may cause fecal impaction (see Precautions). This effect may be obviated through usage of the resin in enemas as described under Dosage and Administration. Intestinal obstruction due to concretions of aluminum hydroxide, when used in combination with KAYEXALATE, has been reported.

DOSAGE AND ADMINISTRATION

Suspension of this drug should be freshly prepared and not stored beyond 24 hours.

The average daily adult dose of the resin is 15 g to 60 g. This is best provided by administering 15 g (approximately 4 *level* teaspoons) of KAYEXALATE one to four times daily. One gram of KAYEXALATE contains 4.1 mEq of sodium; one level teaspoon contains approximately 3.5 g of KAYEXALATE and 15 mEq of sodium. (A heaping teaspoon may contain as much as 10 g to 12 g of KAYEXALATE, brand of sodium polystyrene sulfonate.) Since the *in vivo* efficiency of sodium-potassium exchange resins is approximately 33 percent, about one third of the resin's actual sodium content is being delivered to the body.

In smaller children and infants lower doses should be employed by using as a guide a rate of 1 mEq of potassium per gram of resin as the basis for calculation.

Each dose should be given as a suspension in a small quantity of water or, for greater palatability, in syrup. The amount of fluid usually ranges from 20 mL to 100 mL, depending on the dose, or may be simply determined by allowing 3 mL to 4 mL per gram of resin. Sorbitol may be administered in order to combat constipation.

The resin may be introduced into the stomach through a plastic tube and, if desired, mixed with a diet appropriate for a patient in renal failure.

The resin may also be given, although with less effective results, in an enema consisting (for adults) of 30 g to 50 g every six hours. Each dose is administered as a warm emulsion (at body temperature) in 100 mL of aqueous vehicle, such as sorbitol. The emulsion should be agitated gently during administration. The enema should be retained as long as possible and followed by a cleansing enema.

After an initial cleansing enema, a soft, large size (French 28) rubber tube is inserted into the rectum for a distance of about 20 cm, with the tip well into the sigmoid colon, and taped in place. The resin is then suspended in the appropriate amount of aqueous vehicle at body temperature and introduced by gravity, while the particles are kept in suspension by stirring. The suspension is flushed with 50 mL or 100 mL of fluid, following which the tube is clamped and left in place. If back leakage occurs, the hips are elevated on pillows or a knee-chest position is taken temporarily. A somewhat thicker suspension may be used, but care should be taken that no paste is formed, because the latter has a greatly reduced exchange surface and will be particularly ineffective if deposited in the rectal ampulla. The suspension is kept in the sigmoid colon for several hours, if possible. Then, the colon is irrigated with nonsodium containing solution at body temperature in order to remove the resin. Two quarts of flushing solution may be necessary. The returns are drained constantly through a Y tube connection.

The intensity and duration of therapy depend upon the severity and resistance of hyperkalemia.

KAYEXALATE, brand of sodium polystyrene sulfonate, should not be heated for to do so may alter the exchange properties of the resin.

HOW SUPPLIED

Jar of 1 pound (453.6 g)
NDC 0024-1075-01

KW 2-L

LEVOPHED® Bitartrate ℞

brand of norepinephrine bitartrate injection, USP

DESCRIPTION

Levarterenol (sometimes referred to as *l-arterenol* or as *l-norepinephrine*) is a primary amine which differs from epinephrine by the absence of a methyl group on the nitrogen atom.

LEVOPHED is supplied in sterile aqueous solution in the form of the bitartrate. Each 1 mL of norepinephrine bitartrate solution contains 1 mg of norepinephrine bitartrate base, sodium chloride for isotonicity, and not more than 2 mg of sodium metabisulfite as preservative. The air in the ampuls has been displaced by nitrogen gas.

CLINICAL PHARMACOLOGY

LEVOPHED functions as a powerful peripheral vasoconstrictor (alpha-adrenergic action) and as a potent inotropic stimulator of the heart and dilator of coronary arteries (beta-adrenergic action). Both of these actions result in an increase in systemic blood pressure and coronary artery blood flow. Cardiac output will vary reflexly in response to systemic hypertension but is usually increased in hypotensive man when the blood pressure is raised to an optimal level. In myocardial infarction accompanied by hypotension, LEVOPHED usually increases aortic blood pressure, coronary artery blood flow, and myocardial oxygenation, thereby helping to limit the area of myocardial ischemia and infarction. Venous return is increased and the heart tends to resume a more normal rate and rhythm than in the hypotensive state.

In hypotension that persists after correction of blood volume deficits, LEVOPHED helps raise the blood pressure to an optimal level and establish a more adequate circulation.

INDICATIONS AND USAGE

For the restoration of blood pressure in controlling certain acute hypotensive states (eg, pheochromocytomectomy, sympathectomy, poliomyelitis, spinal anesthesia, myocardial infarction, septicemia, blood transfusion, and drug reactions).

As an adjunct in the treatment of cardiac arrest and profound hypotension.

CONTRAINDICATIONS

LEVOPHED should not be given to patients who are hypotensive from blood volume deficits except as an emergency measure to maintain coronary and cerebral artery perfusion until blood volume replacement therapy can be completed. If LEVOPHED is continuously administered to maintain blood pressure in the absence of blood volume replacement, the following may occur: severe peripheral and visceral vasoconstriction, decreased renal perfusion and urine output, poor systemic blood flow despite "normal" blood pressure, tissue hypoxia, and lactate acidosis.

LEVOPHED should also not be given to patients with mesenteric or peripheral vascular thrombosis (because of the risk of increasing ischemia and extending the area of infarction) unless, in the opinion of the attending physician, the administration of LEVOPHED is necessary as a life-saving procedure.

Cyclopropane and halothane anesthetics increase cardiac autonomic irritability and therefore seem to sensitize the myocardium to the action of intravenously administered epinephrine or levarterenol. Hence, the use of LEVOPHED during cyclopropane and halothane anesthesia is generally considered contraindicated because of the risk of producing ventricular tachycardia or fibrillation. The same type of cardiac arrhythmias may result from the use of LEVOPHED in patients with profound hypoxia or hypercarbia.

WARNING

LEVOPHED should be used with extreme caution in patients receiving monoamine oxidase (MAO) inhibitors or antidepressants of the triptyline or imipramine types, because severe, prolonged hypertension may result.

PRECAUTIONS

Avoid Hypertension: Because of the potency of LEVOPHED and because of varying response to pressor substances, the possibility always exists that dangerously high blood pressure may be produced with overdoses of this pressor agent. It is desirable, therefore, to record the blood pressure every two minutes from the time administration is started until the desired blood pressure is obtained, then every five minutes if administration is to be continued. The rate of flow must be watched constantly, and the patient should never be left unattended while receiving LEVOPHED. Headache may be a symptom of hypertension due to overdosage.

Site of Infusion: Whenever possible, LEVOPHED should be given into a large vein, particularly an antecubital vein because, when administered into this vein, the risk of necrosis of the overlying skin from prolonged vasoconstriction is apparently very slight. Some authors have indicated that the femoral vein is also an acceptable route of administration. A catheter tie-in technique should be avoided, if possible, since the obstruction to blood flow around the tubing may cause stasis and increased local concentration of the drug. Occlusive vascular diseases (for example, atherosclerosis, arteriosclerosis, diabetic endarteritis, Buerger's disease) are more likely to occur in the lower than in the upper extremity. Therefore, one should avoid the veins of the leg in elderly patients or in those suffering from such disorders. Gangrene has been reported in a lower extremity when LEVOPHED was given in an ankle vein.

Extravasation: The infusion site should be checked frequently for free flow. Care should be taken to avoid extravasation of LEVOPHED (norepinephrine) into the tissues, as local necrosis might ensue due to the vasoconstrictive action of the drug. Blanching along the course of the infused vein, sometimes without obvious extravasation, has been attributed to vasa vasorum constriction with increased permeability of the vein wall, permitting some leakage. This also may progress on rare occasions to superficial slough, particularly during infusion into leg veins in elderly patients or in those suffering from obliterative vascular disease. Hence, if blanching occurs, consideration should be given to the advisability of changing the infusion site at intervals to allow the effects of local vasoconstriction to subside.

> **IMPORTANT—Antidote for Extravasation Ischemia:** To prevent sloughing and necrosis in areas in which extravasation has taken place, the area should be infiltrated as soon as possible with 10 mL to 15 mL of saline solution containing from 5 mg to 10 mg of **Regitine® (brand of phentolamine),** an adrenergic blocking agent. A syringe with a fine hypodermic needle is used, and the solution is infiltrated liberally throughout the area, which is easily identified by its cold, hard, and pallid appearance. Sympathetic blockade with phentolamine causes immediate and conspicuous local hyperemic changes if the area is infiltrated within 12 hours. Therefore, phentolamine should be given as soon as possible after the extravasation is noted.

Some investigators add phentolamine (5 mg to 10 mg) directly to the infusion flask because it is believed that the drug used in this manner is an effective antidote against sloughing should extravasation occur, whereas the systemic vasopressor activity of the LEVOPHED is not impaired.

Two investigators stated that, in the treatment of patients with severe hypotension following *myocardial infarction,* thrombosis in the infused vein and perivenous reactions and necrosis may usually be prevented if 10 mg of heparin are added to each 500 mL of infusion fluid (5 percent dextrose) containing LEVOPHED.

Sympathetic nerve block has also been suggested.

ADVERSE REACTIONS

When used as directed, LEVOPHED is more certain in action and better tolerated systemically than other pressor amines. Its therapeutic index is four times that of epinephrine. Bradycardia sometimes occurs, probably as a reflex result of a rise in blood pressure. Headache may indicate overdosage and extreme hypertension.

Overdosage with LEVOPHED may also result in severe hypertension, reflex bradycardia, marked increase in peripheral resistance, and decreased cardiac output.

Prolonged administration of any potent vasopressor may result in plasma volume depletion which should be continuously corrected by appropriate fluid and electrolyte replacement therapy. If plasma volumes are not corrected, hypotension may recur when LEVOPHED is discontinued, or blood pressure may be maintained at the risk of severe peripheral vasoconstriction with diminution in blood flow and tissue perfusion.

DOSAGE AND ADMINISTRATION

Restoration of Blood Pressure in Acute Hypotensive States

Blood volume depletion should always be corrected as fully as possible before any vasopressor is administered. When, as an emergency measure, intra-aortic pressures must be maintained to prevent cerebral or coronary artery ischemia, LEVOPHED bitartrate, brand of norepinephrine bitartrate injection, can be administered before and concurrently with blood volume replacement.

Diluent: Norepinephrine bitartrate solution should be administered in 5 percent dextrose solution in distilled water or 5 percent dextrose in saline solution. These fluids containing dextrose are protection against significant loss of potency due to oxidation. Administration in saline solution alone is not recommended. Whole blood or plasma, if indicated to increase blood volume, should be administered separately (for example, by use of a Y-tube and individual flasks if given simultaneously).

Average Dosage: Add 4 mL of norepinephrine bitartrate solution to 1000 mL of 5 percent dextrose solution. Each 1 mL of this dilution contains 4 μg of norepinephrine bitartrate base. Give this dilution intravenously. Insert a plastic intravenous catheter through a suitable bore needle well advanced centrally into the vein and securely fixed with adhesive tape, avoiding, if possible, a catheter tie-in technique as this promotes stasis. A drip bulb is necessary to permit an accurate estimation of the rate of flow in drops per minute. After observing the response to an initial dose of 2 mL to 3 mL (from 8 μg to 12 μg of base) per minute, adjust the rate of flow to establish and maintain a low normal blood pressure (usually 80 mm Hg to 100 mm Hg systolic) sufficient to maintain the circulation to vital organs. In previously hypertensive patients, it is recommended that the blood pressure should be raised no higher than 40 mm Hg below the preexisting systolic pressure. The average maintenance dose ranges from 0.5 mL to 1 mL per minute (from 2 μg to 4 μg of base).

High Dosage: Great individual variation occurs in the dose required to attain and maintain an adequate blood pressure. In all cases, dosage of LEVOPHED should be titrated according to the response of the patient. Occasionally much larger or even enormous daily doses (as high as 68 mg base or 17 ampuls) may be necessary if the patient remains hypotensive, but occult blood volume depletion should always be suspected and corrected when present. Central venous pressure monitoring is usually helpful in detecting and treating this situation.

Fluid Intake: The degree of dilution depends on clinical fluid volume requirements. If large volumes of fluid (dextrose) are needed at a flow rate that would involve an excessive dose of the pressor agent per unit of time, a more dilute solution than 4 µg per mL should be used. On the other hand, when large volumes of fluid are clinically undesirable, a concentration greater than 4 µg per mL may be used.

Duration of Therapy: The infusion should be continued until adequate blood pressure and tissue perfusion are maintained without therapy. Norepinephrine bitartrate infusion should be reduced gradually, avoiding abrupt withdrawal. In some of the reported cases of vascular collapse due to acute myocardial infarction, treatment was required for up to six days.

Adjunctive Treatment in Cardiac Arrest

LEVOPHED is usually administered intravenously during cardiac resuscitation to restore and maintain an adequate blood pressure after an effective heartbeat and ventilation have been established by other means. [The powerful beta-adrenergic stimulating action of LEVOPHED is also thought to increase the strength and effectiveness of systolic contractions once they occur.]

Average Dosage: To maintain systemic blood pressure during the management of cardiac arrest, LEVOPHED bitartrate, brand of norepinephrine bitartrate injection, is used in the same manner as described under Restoration of Blood Pressure in Acute Hypotensive States.

HOW SUPPLIED

Ampuls of 4 mL containing 4 mg norepinephrine bitartrate base, box of 10 (**NDC 0024-1123-02**)

Regitine, trademark, CIBA Pharmaceutical Company

LW-34-Q

LOTUSATE® Caplets® Ⓒ℞
brand of talbutal tablets, USP

DESCRIPTION

Each caplet contains 120 mg of 5-Allyl-5-*sec*-butylbarbituric acid, is white in color, and bears identifying number L 53.

Inactive Ingredients: Lactose, Magnesium Stearate, Starch, Talc.

HOW SUPPLIED

CAPLETS of 120 mg, bottle of 100 (NDC 0024-1150-01)

For complete prescribing information, see package insert or contact Winthrop-Breon Laboratories Medical Department.

LW-87-S

MARCAINE® HYDROCHLORIDE ℞
brand of bupivacaine hydrochloride injection, USP

MARCAINE® HYDROCHLORIDE ℞
WITH EPINEPHRINE 1:200,000 (AS BITARTRATE)
brand of bupivacaine and epinephrine injection, USP

DESCRIPTION

Bupivacaine hydrochloride is 2-Piperidinecarboxamide, 1-butyl-*N*-(2,6-dimethylphenyl)-, monohydrochloride, a white crystalline powder that is freely soluble in 95 percent ethanol, soluble in water, and slightly soluble in chloroform or acetone.

Epinephrine is (-)-3, 4-Dihydroxy-α-[(methylamino)methyl] benzyl alcohol.

MARCAINE hydrochloride is available in sterile isotonic solutions with and without epinephrine (as bitartrate) 1:200,000 for injection via local infiltration, peripheral nerve block, and caudal and lumbar epidural blocks. Solutions of MARCAINE may be autoclaved if they do not contain epinephrine.

Bupivacaine is related chemically and pharmacologically to the aminoacyl local anesthetics. It is a homologue of mepivacaine and is chemically related to lidocaine. All three of these anesthetics contain an amide linkage between the aromatic nucleus and the amino, or piperidine group. They differ in this respect from the procaine-type local anesthetics, which have an ester linkage.

MARCAINE hydrochloride—Sterile isotonic solutions containing sodium chloride. In multiple-dose vials, each 1 mL also contains 1 mg methylparaben as antiseptic preservative. The pH of these solutions is adjusted to between 4.0 and 6.5 with sodium hydroxide or hydrochloric acid.

MARCAINE hydrochloride with epinephrine 1:200,000 (as bitartrate)—Sterile isotonic solutions containing sodium chloride. Each 1 mL contains bupivacaine hydrochloride and 0.0091 mg epinephrine bitartrate, with 0.5 mg sodium metabisulfite, 0.001 mL monothioglycerol, and 2 mg ascorbic acid as antioxidants, 0.0017 mL 60% sodium lactate buffer, and 0.1 mg edetate calcium disodium as stabilizer. In multiple-dose vials, each 1 mL also contains 1 mg methylparaben as antiseptic preservative. The pH of these solutions is adjusted to between 3.4 and 4.5 with sodium hydroxide or hydrochloric acid. The specific gravity of MARCAINE 0.5% with epinephrine 1:200,000 (as bitartrate) at 25°C is 1.008 and at 37°C is 1.008.

CLINICAL PHARMACOLOGY

Local anesthetics block the generation and the conduction of nerve impulses, presumably by increasing the threshold for electrical excitation in the nerve, by slowing the propagation of the nerve impulse, and by reducing the rate of rise of the action potential. In general, the progression of anesthesia is related to the diameter, myelination, and conduction velocity of affected nerve fibers. Clinically, the order of loss of nerve function is as follows: (1) pain, (2) temperature, (3) touch, (4) proprioception, and (5) skeletal muscle tone.

Systemic absorption of local anesthetics produces effects on the cardiovascular and central nervous systems (CNS). At blood concentrations achieved with normal therapeutic doses, changes in cardiac conduction, excitability, refractoriness, contractility, and peripheral vascular resistance are minimal. However, toxic blood concentrations depress cardiac conduction and excitability, which may lead to atrioventricular block, ventricular arrhythmias, and cardiac arrest, sometimes resulting in fatalities. In addition, myocardial contractility is depressed and peripheral vasodilation occurs, leading to decreased cardiac output and arterial blood pressure. Recent clinical reports and animal research suggest that these cardiovascular changes are more likely to occur after unintended intravascular injection of bupivacaine. Therefore, incremental dosing is necessary.

Following systemic absorption, local anesthetics can produce central nervous system stimulation, depression, or both. Apparent central stimulation is manifested as restlessness, tremors and shivering progressing to convulsions, followed by depression and coma progressing ultimately to respiratory arrest. However, the local anesthetics have a primary depressant effect on the medulla and on higher centers. The depressed stage may occur without a prior excited state.

Pharmacokinetics: The rate of systemic absorption of local anesthetics is dependent upon the total dose and concentration of drug administered, the route of administration, the vascularity of the administration site, and the presence or absence of epinephrine in the anesthetic solution. A dilute concentration of epinephrine (1:200,000 or 5 mcg/mL) usually reduces the rate of absorption and peak plasma concentration of MARCAINE, permitting the use of moderately larger total doses and sometimes prolonging the duration of action.

The onset of action with MARCAINE is rapid and anesthesia is long lasting. The duration of anesthesia is significantly longer with MARCAINE than with any other commonly used local anesthetic. It has also been noted that there is a period of analgesia that persists after the return of sensation, during which time the need for strong analgesics is reduced.

The onset of action following dental injections is usually 2 to 10 minutes and anesthesia may last two or three times longer than lidocaine and mepivacaine for dental use, in many patients up to 7 hours. The duration of anesthetic effect is prolonged by the addition of epinephrine 1:200,000.

Local anesthetics are bound to plasma proteins in varying degrees. Generally, the lower the plasma concentration of drug the higher the percentage of drug bound to plasma proteins.

Local anesthetics appear to cross the placenta by passive diffusion. The rate and degree of diffusion is governed by (1) the degree of plasma protein binding, (2) the degree of ionization, and (3) the degree of lipid solubility. Fetal/maternal ratios of local anesthetics appear to be inversely related to the degree of plasma protein binding, because only the free, unbound drug is available for placental transfer. MARCAINE with a high protein binding capacity (95%) has a low fetal/maternal ratio (0.2 to 0.4). The extent of placental transfer is also determined by the degree of ionization and lipid solubility of the drug. Lipid soluble, nonionized drugs readily enter the fetal blood from the maternal circulation.

Depending upon the route of administration, local anesthetics are distributed to some extent to all body tissues, with high concentrations found in highly perfused organs such as the liver, lungs, heart, and brain.

Pharmacokinetic studies on the plasma profile of MARCAINE after direct intravenous injection suggest a three-compartment open model. The first compartment is represented by the rapid intravascular distribution of the drug. The second compartment represents the equilibration of the drug throughout the highly perfused organs such as the brain, myocardium, lungs, kidneys, and liver. The third compartment represents an equilibration of the drug with poorly perfused tissues, such as muscle and fat. The elimination of drug from tissue distribution depends largely upon the ability of binding sites in the circulation to carry it to the liver where it is metabolized.

After injection of MARCAINE for caudal, epidural, or peripheral nerve block in man, peak levels of bupivacaine in the blood are reached in 30 to 45 minutes, followed by a decline to insignificant levels during the next three to six hours.

Various pharmacokinetic parameters of the local anesthetics can be significantly altered by the presence of hepatic or renal disease, addition of epinephrine, factors affecting urinary pH, renal blood flow, the route of drug administration, and the age of the patient. The half-life of MARCAINE (bupivacaine) in adults is 2.7 hours and in neonates 8.1 hours.

Amide-type local anesthetics such as MARCAINE are metabolized primarily in the liver via conjugation with glucuronic acid. Patients with hepatic disease, especially those with severe hepatic disease, may be more susceptible to the potential toxicities of the amide-type local anesthetics. Pipecoloxylidine is the major metabolite of MARCAINE.

The kidney is the main excretory organ for most local anesthetics and their metabolites. Urinary excretion is affected by urinary perfusion and factors affecting urinary pH. Only 6% of bupivacaine is excreted unchanged in the urine.

When administered in recommended doses and concentrations, MARCAINE does not ordinarily produce irritation or tissue damage and does not cause methemoglobinemia.

INDICATIONS AND USAGE

MARCAINE is indicated for the production of local or regional anesthesia or analgesia for surgery, dental and oral surgery procedures, diagnostic and therapeutic procedures, and for obstetrical procedures. Only the 0.25% and 0.5% concentrations are indicated for obstetrical anesthesia. (See WARNINGS.)

Experience with nonobstetrical surgical procedures in pregnant patients is not sufficient to recommend use of 0.75% concentration of MARCAINE in these patients.

MARCAINE is not recommended for intravenous regional anesthesia (Bier Block). See WARNINGS.

The routes of administration and indicated MARCAINE concentrations are:

• local infiltration	0.25%
• peripheral nerve block	0.25% and 0.5%
• retrobulbar block	0.75%
• sympathetic block	0.25%
• lumbar epidural	0.25%, 0.5%, and 0.75% (0.75% not for obstetrical anesthesia)
• caudal	0.25% and 0.5%
• epidural test dose	0.5% with epinephrine 1:200,000
• dental blocks	0.5% with epinephrine 1:200,000

(See DOSAGE AND ADMINISTRATION for additional information.)

Standard textbooks should be consulted to determine the accepted procedures and techniques for the administration of MARCAINE.

CONTRAINDICATIONS

MARCAINE is contraindicated in obstetrical paracervical block anesthesia. Its use in this technique has resulted in fetal bradycardia and death.

MARCAINE (bupivacaine) is contraindicated in patients with a known hypersensitivity to it or to any local anesthetic agent of the amide type or to other components of MARCAINE solutions.

WARNINGS

THE 0.75% CONCENTRATION OF MARCAINE IS NOT RECOMMENDED FOR OBSTETRICAL ANESTHESIA. THERE HAVE BEEN REPORTS OF CARDIAC ARREST WITH DIFFICULT RESUSCITATION OR DEATH DURING USE OF MARCAINE FOR EPIDURAL ANESTHESIA IN OBSTETRICAL PATIENTS. IN MOST CASES, THIS HAS FOLLOWED USE OF THE 0.75% CONCENTRATION. RESUSCITATION HAS BEEN DIFFICULT OR IMPOSSIBLE DESPITE APPARENTLY ADEQUATE PREPARATION AND APPROPRIATE MANAGEMENT. CARDIAC ARREST HAS OCCURRED AFTER CONVULSIONS RESULTING FROM SYSTEMIC TOXICITY, PRESUMABLY FOLLOWING UNINTENTIONAL INTRAVASCULAR INJECTION. THE 0.75% CONCEN-

Continued on next page

This product information was effective as of December 1, 1986. On these and other products of Winthrop-Breon Laboratories, detailed information may be obtained on a current basis by direct inquiry to the Professional Services Department, 90 Park Avenue, New York, NY 10016 (212) 907-2525.

Winthrop-Breon—Cont.

TRATION SHOULD BE RESERVED FOR SURGICAL PROCEDURES WHERE A HIGH DEGREE OF MUSCLE RELAXATION AND PROLONGED EFFECT ARE NECESSARY.

LOCAL ANESTHETICS SHOULD ONLY BE EMPLOYED BY CLINICIANS WHO ARE WELL VERSED IN DIAGNOSIS AND MANAGEMENT OF DOSE-RELATED TOXICITY AND OTHER ACUTE EMERGENCIES WHICH MIGHT ARISE FROM THE BLOCK TO BE EMPLOYED, AND THEN ONLY AFTER INSURING THE *IMMEDIATE* AVAILABILITY OF OXYGEN, OTHER RESUSCITATIVE DRUGS, CARDIOPULMONARY RESUSCITATIVE EQUIPMENT, AND THE PERSONNEL RESOURCES NEEDED FOR PROPER MANAGEMENT OF TOXIC REACTIONS AND RELATED EMERGENCIES. (See also ADVERSE REACTIONS, PRECAUTIONS, and OVERDOSAGE.) DELAY IN PROPER MANAGEMENT OF DOSE-RELATED TOXICITY, UNDERVENTILATION FROM ANY CAUSE, AND/OR ALTERED SENSITIVITY MAY LEAD TO THE DEVELOPMENT OF ACIDOSIS, CARDIAC ARREST AND, POSSIBLY, DEATH.

Local anesthetic solutions containing antimicrobial preservatives, ie, those supplied in multiple-dose vials, should not be used for epidural or caudal anesthesia because safety has not been established with regard to intrathecal injection, either intentionally or unintentionally, of such preservatives.

It is essential that aspiration for blood or cerebrospinal fluid (where applicable) be done prior to injecting any local anesthetic, both the original dose and all subsequent doses, to avoid intravascular or subarachnoid injection. However, a negative aspiration does *not* ensure against an intravascular or subarachnoid injection.

MARCAINE with epinephrine 1:200,000 or other vasopressors should not be used concomitantly with ergot-type oxytocic drugs, because a severe persistent hypertension may occur. Likewise, solutions of MARCAINE containing a vasoconstrictor, such as epinephrine, should be used with extreme caution in patients receiving monoamine oxidase inhibitors (MAOI) or antidepressants of the triptyline or imipramine types, because severe prolonged hypertension may result.

Until further experience is gained in children younger than 12 years, administration of MARCAINE in this age group is not recommended.

Mixing or the prior or intercurrent use of any other local anesthetic with MARCAINE cannot be recommended because of insufficient data on the clinical use of such mixtures.

There have been reports of cardiac arrest and death during the use of MARCAINE for intravenous regional anesthesia (Bier Block). Information on safe dosages and techniques of administration of MARCAINE in this procedure is lacking. Therefore, MARCAINE is not recommended for use in this technique.

PRECAUTIONS

General: The safety and effectiveness of local anesthetics depend on proper dosage, correct technique, adequate precautions, and readiness for emergencies. Resuscitative equipment, oxygen, and other resuscitative drugs should be available for immediate use. (See WARNINGS, ADVERSE REACTIONS, and OVERDOSAGE.) During major regional nerve blocks, the patient should have IV fluids running via an indwelling catheter to assure a functioning intravenous pathway. The lowest dosage of local anesthetic that results in effective anesthesia should be used to avoid high plasma levels and serious adverse effects. The rapid injection of a large volume of local anesthetic solution should be avoided and fractional (incremental) doses should be used when feasible.

Epidural Anesthesia: During epidural administration of MARCAINE, 0.5% and 0.75% solutions should be administered in incremental doses of 3 mL to 5 mL with sufficient time between doses to detect toxic manifestations of unintentional intravascular or intrathecal injection. Injections should be made slowly, with frequent aspirations before and during the injection to avoid intravascular injection. Syringe aspirations should also be performed before and during each supplemental injection in continuous (intermittent) catheter techniques. An intravascular injection is still possible even if aspirations for blood are negative.

During the administration of epidural anesthesia, it is recommended that a test dose be administered initially and the effects monitored before the full dose is given. When using a "continuous" catheter technique, test doses should be given prior to both the original and all reinforcing doses, because plastic tubing in the epidural space can migrate into a blood vessel or through the dura. When clinical conditions permit, the test dose should contain epinephrine (10 mcg to 15 mcg have been suggested) to serve as a warning of unintended intravascular injection. If injected into a blood vessel, this amount of epinephrine is likely to produce a transient "epinephrine response" within 45 seconds, consisting of an increase in heart rate and/or systolic blood pressure, circumoral pallor, palpitations, and nervousness in the unsedated patient. The sedated patient may exhibit only a pulse rate increase of 20 or more beats per minute for 15 or more seconds. Therefore, following the test dose, the heart rate should be monitored for a heart rate increase. Patients on beta-blockers may not manifest changes in heart rate, but blood pressure monitoring can detect a transient rise in systolic blood pressure. The test dose should also contain 10 mg to 15 mg of MARCAINE or an equivalent amount of another local anesthetic to detect an unintended intrathecal administration. This will be evidenced within a few minutes by signs of spinal block (eg, decreased sensation of the buttocks, paresis of the legs, or, in the sedated patient, absent knee jerk). The MARCAINE Test Dose formulation contains 15 mg of bupivacaine and 15 mcg of epinephrine in a volume of 3 mL. An intravascular or subarachnoid injection is still possible even if results of the test dose are negative. The test dose itself may produce a systemic toxic reaction, high spinal or epinephrine-induced cardiovascular effects.

Injection of repeated doses of local anesthetics may cause significant increases in plasma levels with each repeated dose due to slow accumulation of the drug or its metabolites, or to slow metabolic degradation. Tolerance to elevated blood levels varies with the status of the patient. Debilitated, elderly patients and acutely ill patients should be given reduced doses commensurate with their age and physical status. Local anesthetics should also be used with caution in patients with hypotension or heart block.

Careful and constant monitoring of cardiovascular and respiratory (adequacy of ventilation) vital signs and the patient's state of consciousness should be performed after each local anesthetic injection. It should be kept in mind at such times that restlessness, anxiety, incoherent speech, lightheadedness, numbness and tingling of the mouth and lips, metallic taste, tinnitus, dizziness, blurred vision, tremors, twitching, depression, or drowsiness may be early warning signs of central nervous system toxicity.

Local anesthetic solutions containing a vasoconstrictor should be used cautiously and in carefully restricted quantities in areas of the body supplied by end arteries or having otherwise compromised blood supply such as digits, nose, external ear, or penis. Patients with hypertensive vascular disease may exhibit exaggerated vasoconstrictor response. Ischemic injury or necrosis may result.

Because amide-type local anesthetics such as MARCAINE (bupivacaine) are metabolized by the liver, these drugs, especially repeat doses, should be used cautiously in patients with hepatic disease. Patients with severe hepatic disease, because of their inability to metabolize local anesthetics normally, are at a greater risk of developing toxic plasma concentrations. Local anesthetics should also be used with caution in patients with impaired cardiovascular function because they may be less able to compensate for functional changes associated with the prolongation of A-V conduction produced by these drugs.

Serious dose-related cardiac arrhythmias may occur if preparations containing a vasoconstrictor such as epinephrine are employed in patients during or following the administration of potent inhalation anesthetics. In deciding whether to use these products concurrently in the same patient, the combined action of both agents upon the myocardium, the concentration and volume of vasoconstrictor used, and the time since injection, when applicable, should be taken into account.

Many drugs used during the conduct of anesthesia are considered potential triggering agents for familial malignant hyperthermia. Because it is not known whether amide-type local anesthetics may trigger this reaction and because the need for supplemental general anesthesia cannot be predicted in advance, it is suggested that a standard protocol for management should be available. Early unexplained signs of tachycardia, tachypnea, labile blood pressure, and metabolic acidosis may precede temperature elevation. Successful outcome is dependent on early diagnosis, prompt discontinuance of the suspect triggering agent(s) and prompt institution of treatment, including oxygen therapy, indicated supportive measures and dantrolene. (Consult dantrolene sodium intravenous package insert before using.)

Use in Head and Neck Area: Small doses of local anesthetics injected into the head and neck area, including retrobulbar, dental, and stellate ganglion blocks, may produce adverse reactions similar to systemic toxicity seen with unintentional intravascular injections of larger doses. The injection procedures require the utmost care. Confusion, convulsions, respiratory depression, and/or respiratory arrest, and cardiovascular stimulation or depression have been reported. These reactions may be due to intra-arterial injection of the local anesthetic with retrograde flow to the cerebral circulation. They may also be due to puncture of the dural sheath of the optic nerve during retrobulbar block with diffusion of any local anesthetic along the subdural space to the midbrain. Patients receiving these blocks should have their circulation and respiration monitored and be constantly observed. Resuscitative equipment and personnel for treating adverse reactions should be immediately available. Dosage recommendations should not be exceeded. (See DOSAGE AND ADMINISTRATION.)

Use in Ophthalmic Surgery: Clinicians who perform retrobulbar blocks should be aware that there have been reports of respiratory arrest following local anesthetic injection. Prior to retrobulbar block, as with all other regional procedures, the immediate availability of equipment, drugs, and personnel to manage respiratory arrest or depression, convulsions, and cardiac stimulation or depression should be assured (see also WARNINGS and USE IN HEAD AND NECK AREA, above). As with other anesthetic procedures, patients should be constantly monitored following ophthalmic blocks for signs of these adverse reactions, which may occur following relatively low total doses. A concentration of 0.75% bupivacaine is indicated for retrobular block; however, this concentration is not indicated for any other peripheral nerve block, including the facial nerve, and not indicated for local infiltration, including the conjunctiva (see INDICATIONS and PRECAUTIONS, ***General***). Mixing MARCAINE with other local anesthetics is not recommended because of insufficient data on the clinical use of such mixtures.

When MARCAINE 0.75% is used for retrobulbar block, complete corneal anesthesia usually precedes onset of clinically acceptable external ocular muscle akinesia. Therefore, presence of akinesia rather than anesthesia alone should determine readiness of the patient for surgery.

Use in Dentistry: Because of the long duration of anesthesia, when MARCAINE 0.5% with epinephrine is used for dental injections, patients should be cautioned about the possibility of inadvertent trauma to tongue, lips, and buccal mucosa and advised not to chew solid foods or test the anesthetized area by biting or probing.

Information for Patients: When appropriate, patients should be informed in advance that they may experience temporary loss of sensation and motor activity, usually in the lower half of the body, following proper administration of caudal or epidural anesthesia. Also, when appropriate, the physician should discuss other information including adverse reactions in the MARCAINE package insert.

Patients receiving dental injections of MARCAINE (bupivacaine) should be cautioned not to chew solid foods or test the anesthetized area by biting or probing until anesthesia has worn off (up to 7 hours).

Clinically Significant Drug Interactions: The administration of local anesthetic solutions containing epinephrine or norepinephrine to patients receiving monoamine oxidase inhibitors or tricyclic antidepressants may produce severe, prolonged hypertension. Concurrent use of these agents should generally be avoided. In situations when concurrent therapy is necessary, careful patient monitoring is essential.

Concurrent administration of vasopressor drugs and of ergot-type oxytocic drugs may cause severe, persistent hypertension or cerebrovascular accidents.

Phenothiazines and butyrophenones may reduce or reverse the pressor effect of epinephrine.

Carcinogenesis, Mutagenesis, Impairment of Fertility: Long-term studies in animals of most local anesthetics including bupivacaine to evaluate the carcinogenic potential have not been conducted. Mutagenic potential or the effect on fertility has not been determined. There is no evidence from human data that MARCAINE may be carcinogenic or mutagenic or that it impairs fertility.

Pregnancy Category C: Decreased pup survival in rats and an embryocidal effect in rabbits have been observed when bupivacaine hydrochloride was administered to these species in doses comparable to nine and five times respectively the maximum recommended daily human dose (400 mg). There are no adequate and well-controlled studies in pregnant women of the effect of bupivacaine on the developing fetus. Bupivacaine hydrochloride should be used during pregnancy only if the potential benefit justifies the potential risk to the fetus. This does not exclude the use of MARCAINE at term for obstetrical anesthesia or analgesia. (See ***Labor and Delivery.***)

Labor and Delivery: SEE BOXED WARNING REGARDING OBSTETRICAL USE OF 0.75% MARCAINE.

MARCAINE is contraindicated for obstetrical paracervical block anesthesia.

Local anesthetics rapidly cross the placenta, and when used for epidural, caudal, or pudendal block anesthesia, can cause varying degrees of maternal, fetal, and neonatal toxicity. (See *Pharmacokinetics* in **CLINICAL PHARMACOLOGY.**) The incidence and degree of toxicity depend upon the procedure performed, the type, and amount of drug used, and the technique of drug administration. Adverse reactions in the parturient, fetus, and neonate involve alterations of the central nervous system, peripheral vascular tone, and cardiac function.

Maternal hypotension has resulted from regional anesthesia. Local anesthetics produce vasodilation by blocking sympathetic nerves. Elevating the patient's legs and positioning her on her left side will help prevent decreases in blood pressure. The fetal heart rate also should be monitored continuously and electronic fetal monitoring is highly advisable.

Epidural, caudal, or pudendal anesthesia may alter the forces of parturition through changes in uterine contractility or maternal expulsive efforts. Epidural anesthesia has been reported to prolong the second stage of labor by removing the parturient's reflex urge to bear down or by interfering with motor function. The use of obstetrical anesthesia may increase the need for forceps assistance.

The use of some local anesthetic drug products during labor and delivery may be followed by diminished muscle strength and tone for the first day or two of life. This has not been reported with bupivacaine.

It is extremely important to avoid aortocaval compression by the gravid uterus during administration of regional block to parturients. To do this, the patient must be maintained in the left lateral decubitus position or a blanket roll or sandbag may be placed beneath the right hip and the gravid uterus displaced to the left.

Nursing Mothers: It is not known whether local anesthetic drugs are excreted in human milk. Because many drugs are excreted in human milk, caution should be exercised when local anesthetics are administered to a nursing woman.

Pediatric Use: Until further experience is gained in children younger than 12 years, administration of MARCAINE in this age group is not recommended.

ADVERSE REACTIONS

Reactions to MARCAINE (bupivacaine) are characteristic of those associated with other amide-type local anesthetics. A major cause of adverse reactions to this group of drugs is excessive plasma levels, which may be due to overdosage, unintentional intravascular injection, or slow metabolic degradation.

The most commonly encountered acute adverse experiences which demand immediate countermeasures are related to the central nervous system and the cardiovascular system. These adverse experiences are generally dose related and due to high plasma levels which may result from overdosage, rapid absorption from the injection site, diminished tolerance, or from unintentional intravascular injection of the local anesthetic solution. In addition to systemic dose-related toxicity, unintentional subarachnoid injection of drug during the intended performance of caudal or lumbar epidural block or nerve blocks near the vertebral column (especially in the head and neck region) may result in underventilation or apnea ("Total or High Spinal"). Also, hypotension due to loss of sympathetic tone and respiratory paralysis or underventilation due to cephalad extension of the motor level of anesthesia may occur. This may lead to secondary cardiac arrest if untreated. Factors influencing plasma protein binding, such as acidosis, systemic diseases which alter protein production, or competition of other drugs for protein binding sites, may diminish individual tolerance.

Central Nervous System Reactions: These are characterized by excitation and/or depression. Restlessness, anxiety, dizziness, tinnitus, blurred vision, or tremors may occur, possibly proceeding to convulsions. However, excitement may be transient or absent, with depression being the first manifestation of an adverse reaction. This may quickly be followed by drowsiness merging into unconsciousness and respiratory arrest. Other central nervous system effects may be nausea, vomiting, chills, and constriction of the pupils.

The incidence of convulsions associated with the use of local anesthetics varies with the procedure used and the total dose administered. In a survey of studies of epidural anesthesia, over toxicity progressing to convulsions occurred in approximately 0.1% of local anesthetic administrations.

Cardiovascular System Reactions: High doses or unintentional intravascular injection may lead to high plasma levels and related depression of the myocardium, decreased cardiac output, heart block, hypotension, bradycardia, ventricular arrhythmias, including ventricular tachycardia and ventricular fibrillation, and cardiac arrest. (See WARNINGS, PRECAUTIONS, and OVERDOSAGE sections.)

Allergic: Allergic-type reactions are rare and may occur as a result of sensitivity to the local anesthetic or to other formulation ingredients, such as the antimicrobial preservative methylparaben contained in multiple-dose vials or sulfites in epinephrine-containing solutions. These reactions are characterized by signs such as urticaria, pruritus, erythema, angioneurotic edema (including laryngeal edema), tachycardia, sneezing, nausea, vomiting, dizziness, syncope, excessive sweating, elevated temperature, and, possibly, anaphylactoid-like symptomatology (including severe hypotension). Cross sensitivity among members of the amide-type local anesthetic group has been reported. The usefulness of screening for sensitivity has not been definitely established.

Neurologic: The incidences of adverse neurologic reactions associated with the use of local anesthetics may be related to the total dose of local anesthetic administered and are also dependent upon the particular drug used, the route of administration, and the physical status of the patient. Many of these effects may be related to local anesthetic techniques, with or without a contribution from the drug.

In the practice of caudal or lumbar epidural block, occasional unintentional penetration of the subarachnoid space by the catheter or needle may occur. Subsequent adverse effects may depend partially on the amount of drug administered intrathecally and the physiological and physical effects of a dural puncture. A high spinal is characterized by paralysis of the legs, loss of consciousness, respiratory paralysis, and bradycardia.

Neurologic effects following epidural or caudal anesthesia may include spinal block of varying magnitude (including high or total spinal block); hypotension secondary to spinal block; urinary retention; fecal and urinary incontinence; loss of perineal sensation and sexual function; persistent anesthesia, paresthesia, weakness, paralysis of the lower extremities and loss of sphincter control all of which may have slow, incomplete, or no recovery; headache; backache; septic meningitis; meningismus; slowing of labor; increased incidence of forceps delivery; and cranial nerve palsies due to traction on nerves from loss of cerebrospinal fluid.

OVERDOSAGE

Acute emergencies from local anesthetics are generally related to high plasma levels encountered during therapeutic use of local anesthetics or to unintended subarachnoid injection of local anesthetic solution. (See ADVERSE REACTIONS, WARNINGS, and PRECAUTIONS.)

Management of Local Anesthetic Emergencies: The first consideration is prevention, best accomplished by careful and constant monitoring of cardiovascular and respiratory vital signs and the patient's state of consciousness after each local anesthetic injection. At the first sign of change, oxygen should be administered.

The first step in the management of systemic toxic reactions, as well as underventilation or apnea due to unintentional subarachnoid injection of drug solution, consists of ***immediate*** *attention to the establishment and maintenance of a patent airway and effective assisted or controlled ventilation with 100% oxygen with a delivery system capable of permitting immediate positive airway pressure by mask.* This may prevent convulsions if they have not already occurred.

If necessary, use drugs to control the convulsions. A 50 mg to 100 mg bolus IV injection of succinylcholine will paralyze the patient without depressing the central nervous or cardiovascular systems and facilitate ventilation. A bolus IV dose of 5 mg to 10 mg of diazepam or 50 mg to 100 mg of thiopental will permit ventilation and counteract central nervous system stimulation, but these drugs also depress central nervous system, respiratory, and cardiac function, add to postictal depression and may result in apnea. Intravenous barbiturates, anticonvulsant agents, or muscle relaxants should only be administered by those familiar with their use. Immediately after the institution of these ventilatory measures, the adequacy of the circulation should be evaluated. Supportive treatment of circulatory depression may require administration of intravenous fluids, and when appropriate, a vasopressor dictated by the clinical situation (such as ephedrine or epinephrine to enhance myocardial contractile force).

Endotracheal intubation, employing drugs and techniques familiar to the clinician, may be indicated after initial administration of oxygen by mask if difficulty is encountered in the maintenance of a patent airway, or if prolonged ventilatory support (assisted or controlled) is indicated.

Recent clinical data from patients experiencing local anesthetic-induced convulsions demonstrated rapid development of hypoxia, hypercarbia, and acidosis with bupivacaine within a minute of the onset of convulsions. These observations suggest that oxygen consumption and carbon dioxide production are greatly increased during local anesthetic convulsions and emphasize the importance of immediate and effective ventilation with oxygen which may avoid cardiac arrest.

If not treated immediately, convulsions with simultaneous hypoxia, hypercarbia, and acidosis plus myocardial depression from the direct effects of the local anesthetic may result in cardiac arrhythmias, bradycardia, asystole, ventricular fibrillation, or cardiac arrest. Respiratory abnormalities, including apnea, may occur. Underventilation or apnea due to unintentional subarachnoid injection of local anesthetic solution may produce these same signs and also lead to cardiac arrest if ventilatory support is not instituted. *If cardiac arrest should occur, successful outcome may require prolonged resuscitative efforts.*

The supine position is dangerous in pregnant women at term because of aortocaval compression by the gravid uterus. Therefore during treatment of systemic toxicity, maternal hypotension or fetal bradycardia following regional block, the parturient should be maintained in the left lateral decubitus position if possible, or manual displacement of the uterus off the great vessels be accomplished.

The mean seizure dosage of bupivacaine in rhesus monkeys was found to be 4.4 mg/kg with mean arterial plasma concentration of 4.5 mcg/mL. The intravenous and subcutaneous LD_{50} in mice is 6 mg/kg to 8 mg/kg and 38 mg/kg to 54 mg/kg respectively.

DOSAGE AND ADMINISTRATION

The dose of any local anesthetic administered varies with the anesthetic procedure, the area to be anesthetized, the vascularity of the tissues, the number of neuronal segments to be blocked, the depth of anesthesia and degree of muscle relaxation required, the duration of anesthesia desired, individual tolerance, and the physical condition of the patient. The smallest dose and concentration required to produce the desired result should be administered. Dosages of MARCAINE should be reduced for elderly and debilitated patients and patients with cardiac and/or liver disease. The rapid injection of a large volume of local anesthetic solution should be avoided and fractional (incremental) doses should be used when feasible.

For specific techniques and procedures, refer to standard textbooks.

In recommended doses, MARCAINE (bupivacaine) produces complete sensory block, but the effect on motor function differs among the three concentrations.

0.25%—when used for caudal, epidural, or peripheral nerve block, produces incomplete motor block. Should be used for operations in which muscle relaxation is not important, or when another means of providing muscle relaxation is used concurrently. Onset of action may be slower than with the 0.5% or 0.75% solutions.

0.5%—provides motor blockade for caudal, epidural, or nerve block, but muscle relaxation may be inadequate for operations in which complete muscle relaxation is essential.

0.75%—produces complete motor block. Most useful for epidural block in abdominal operations requiring complete muscle relaxation, and for retrobulbar anesthesia. Not for obstetrical anesthesia.

The duration of anesthesia with MARCAINE is such that for most indications, a single dose is sufficient.

Maximum dosage limit must be individualized in each case after evaluating the size and physical status of the patient, as well as the usual rate of systemic absorption from a particular injection site. Most experience to date is with single doses of MARCAINE up to 225 mg with epinephrine 1:200,000 and 175 mg without epinephrine; more or less drug may be used depending on individualization of each case.

These doses may be repeated up to once every three hours. In clinical studies to date, total daily doses have been up to 400 mg. Until further experience is gained, this dose should not be exceeded in 24 hours. The duration of anesthetic effect may be prolonged by the addition of epinephrine.

The dosages in Table 1 have generally proved satisfactory and are recommended as a guide for use in the average adult. These dosages should be reduced for elderly or debilitated patients. Until further experience is gained, MARCAINE (bupivacaine) is not recommended for children younger than 12 years. MARCAINE is contraindicated for obstetrical paracervical blocks, and is not recommended for intravenous regional anesthesia (Bier Block).

Use in Epidural Anesthesia: During epidural administration of MARCAINE, 0.5% and 0.75% solutions should be administered in incremental doses of 3 mL to 5 mL with sufficient time between doses to detect toxic manifestatons of unintentional intravascular or intrathecal injection. In obstetrics, only the 0.5% and 0.25% concentrations should be used; incremental doses of 3 mL to 5 mL of the 0.5% solution not exceeding 50 mg to 100 mg at any dosing interval are recommended. Repeat doses should be preceded by a test dose containing epinephrine if not contraindicated. Use only the single-dose ampuls and single-dose vials for caudal or epidural anesthesia; the multiple-dose vials contain a preservative and therefore should not be used for these procedures.

Test Dose for Caudal and Lumbar Epidural Blocks: MARCAINE Test Dose (0.5% bupivacaine with 1:200,000 epinephrine in a 3 mL ampul) is recommended for use as a test dose when clinical conditions permit prior to caudal and lumbar epidural blocks. This may serve as a warning of unintended intravascular or subarachnoid injection. (See PRECAUTIONS.) The pulse rate and other signs should be monitored carefully immediately following each test dose administration to detect possible intravascular injection, and adequate time for onset of spinal block should be allotted to detect possible intrathecal injection. An intravascular or subarachnoid injection is still possible even if results of the test dose are negative. The test dose itself may produce a systemic toxic reaction, high spinal or cardiovascular effects from the epinephrine. (See WARNINGS and OVERDOSAGE.)

Use in Dentistry: The 0.5% concentration with epinephrine is recommended for infiltration and block injection in the maxillary and mandibular area when a longer duration of local anesthetic action is desired, such as for oral surgical

Continued on next page

This product information was effective as of December 1, 1986. On these and other products of Winthrop-Breon Laboratories, detailed information may be obtained on a current basis by direct inquiry to the Professional Services Department, 90 Park Avenue, New York, NY 10016 (212) 907-2525.

Winthrop-Breon—Cont.

procedures generally associated with significant postoperative pain. The average dose of 1.8 mL (9 mg) per injection site will usually suffice; an occasional second dose of 1.8 mL (9 mg) may be used if necessary to produce adequate anesthesia after making allowance for 2 to 10 minutes onset time. (See CLINICAL PHARMACOLOGY.) The lowest effective dose should be employed and time should be allowed between injections; it is recommended that the total dose for all injection sites, *spread out* over a single dental sitting, should not ordinarily exceed 90 mg for a healthy adult patient (ten 1.8 mL injections of 0.5% MARCAINE with epinephrine, bupivacaine and epinephrine). Injections should be made slowly and with frequent aspirations. Until further experience is gained, MARCAINE in dentistry is not recommended for children younger than 12 years.

Unused portions of solutions not containing preservatives, ie, those supplied in single-dose ampuls and single-dose vials, should be discarded following initial use.

This product should be inspected visually for particulate matter and discoloration prior to administration whenever solution and container permit. Solutions which are discolored or which contain particulate matter should not be administered.

[See table below].

HOW SUPPLIED

These solutions are not for spinal anesthesia.

Store at controlled room temperature, between 15°C and 30°C (59°F and 86°F).

MARCAINE hydrochloride — Solutions of MARCAINE (bupivacaine) that do not contain epinephrine may be autoclaved. Autoclave at 15-pound pressure, 121°C (250°F) for 15 minutes.

0.25%—Contains 2.5 mg bupivacaine hydrochloride per mL.
Single-dose ampuls of 50 mL, box of 5
NDC 0024-1212-02
Single-dose vials of 10 mL, box of 10
NDC 0024-1212-10
Single-dose vials of 30 mL, box of 10
NDC 0024-1212-30
Multiple-dose vials of 50 mL, box of 1
NDC 0024-1217-01

0.5%—Contains 5 mg bupivacaine hydrochloride per mL.
Single-dose ampuls of 30 mL, box of 5
NDC 0024-1213-02
Single-dose vials of 10 mL, box of 10
NDC 0024-1213-10
Single-dose vials of 30 mL, box of 10
NDC 0024-1213-30
Multiple-dose vials of 50 mL, box of 1
NDC 0024-1218-01

0.75%—Contains 7.5 mg bupivacaine hydrochloride per mL.
Single-dose ampuls of 30 mL, box of 5
NDC 0024-1214-02
Single-dose vials of 10 mL, box of 10
NDC 0024-1214-10
Single-dose vials of 30 mL, box of 10
NDC 0024-1214-30

MARCAINE hydrochloride with epinephrine 1:200,000 (as bitartrate).—Solutions of MARCAINE that contain epinephrine should not be autoclaved and should be protected from light. Do not use if solution is discolored or contains a precipitate.

0.25%—with epinephrine 1:200,000
Contains 2.5 mg bupivacaine hydrochloride per mL.
Single-dose ampuls of 50 mL, box of 5
NDC 0024-1222-02
Single-dose vials of 10 mL, box of 10
NDC 0024-1222-10
Single-dose vials of 30 mL, box of 10
NDC 0024-1222-30
Multiple-dose vials of 50 mL, box of 1
NDC 0024-1227-01

0.5%—with epinephrine 1:200,000
Contains 5 mg bupivacaine hydrochloride per mL.
Single-dose ampuls of 3 mL, box of 10
NDC 0024-1223-03
Single-dose ampuls of 30 mL, box of 5
NDC 0024-1223-02
Single-dose vials of 10 mL, box of 10
NDC 0024-1223-10
Single-dose vials of 30 mL, box of 10
NDC 0024-1223-30
Multiple-dose vials of 50 mL, box of 1
NDC 0024-1228-01

0.75%—with epinephrine 1:200,000
Contains 7.5 mg bupivacaine hydrochloride per mL.
Single-dose ampuls of 30 mL, box of 5
NDC 0024-1224-02
MW-126-I

Table 1. Recommended Concentrations and Doses of MARCAINE

Type of Block	Conc.	Each Dose (mL)	Each Dose (mg)	Motor Block[1]
Local Infiltration	0.25%[4]	up to max.	up to max.	—
Epidural	0.75%[2,4]	10–20	75–150	complete
	0.5%[4]	10–20	50–100	moderate to complete
	0.25%[4]	10–20	25–50	partial to moderate
Caudal	0.5%[4]	15–30	75–150	moderate to complete
	0.25%[4]	15–30	37.5–75	moderate
Peripheral nerves	0.5%[4]	5 to max.	25 to max.	moderate to complete
	0.25%[4]	5 to max.	12.5 to max.	moderate to complete
Retrobulbar[3]	0.75%[4]	2–4	15–30	complete
Sympathetic	0.25%	20–50	50–125	—
Dental[3]	0.5% w/epi	1.8–3.6 per site	9–18 per site	—
Epidural[3] Test Dose	0.5% w/epi	2–3	10–15 (10–15 micrograms epinephrine)	—

[1]With continuous (intermittent) techniques, repeat doses increase the degree of motor block. The first repeat dose of 0.5% may produce complete motor block. Intercostal nerve block with 0.25% may also produce complete motor block for intraabdominal surgery.

[2]For single-dose use, not for intermittent (catheter) epidural technique. Not for obstetrical anesthesia.

[3]See PRECAUTIONS.

[4]Solutions with or without epinephrine.

MARCAINE® Spinal ℞

brand of bupivacaine in dextrose injection, USP

STERILE HYPERBARIC SOLUTION FOR SPINAL ANESTHESIA

DESCRIPTION

Bupivacaine hydrochloride is 2-Piperidinecarboxamide, 1-butyl-*N*-(2,6-dimethylphenyl)-, monohydrochloride, monohydrate, a white crystalline powder that is freely soluble in 95 percent ethanol, soluble in water, and slightly soluble in chloroform or acetone.

Dextrose is D-glucopyranose monohydrate.

MARCAINE Spinal is available in sterile hyperbaric solution for subarachnoid injection (spinal block).

Bupivacaine hydrochloride is related chemically and pharmacologically to the aminoacyl local anesthetics. It is a homologue of mepivacaine and is chemically related to lidocaine. All three of these anesthetics contain an amide linkage between the aromatic nucleus and the amino or piperidine group. They differ in this respect from the procaine-type local anesthetics, which have an ester linkage.

Each 1 mL of MARCAINE Spinal contains 7.5 mg bupivacaine hydrochloride and 82.5 mg dextrose. The pH of this solution is adjusted to between 4.0 and 6.5 with sodium hydroxide or hydrochloric acid.

The specific gravity of MARCAINE Spinal is between 1.030 and 1.035 at 25° C and 1.03 at 37° C.

MARCAINE Spinal does not contain any preservatives.

CLINICAL PHARMACOLOGY

Local anesthetics block the generation and the conduction of nerve impulses, presumably by increasing the threshold for electrical excitation in the nerve, by slowing the propagation of the nerve impulse, and by reducing the rate of rise of the action potential. In general, the progression of anesthesia is related to the diameter, myelination, and conduction velocity of affected nerve fibers. Clinically, the order of loss of nerve function is as follows: (1) pain, (2) temperature, (3) touch, (4) proprioception, and (5) skeletal muscle tone.

Systemic absorption of local anesthetics produces effects on the cardiovascular and central nervous systems (CNS). At blood concentrations achieved with normal therapeutic doses, changes in cardiac conduction, excitability, refractoriness, contractility, and peripheral vascular resistance are minimal. However, toxic blood concentrations depress cardiac conduction and excitability, which may lead to atrioventricular block, ventricular arrhythmias, and cardiac arrest, sometimes resulting in fatalities. In addition, myocardial contractility is depressed and peripheral vasodilation occurs, leading to decreased cardiac output and arterial blood pressure. Recent clinical reports and animal research suggest that these cardiovascular changes are more likely to occur after unintended direct intravascular injection of bupivacaine. Therefore, when epidural anesthesia with bupivacaine is considered, incremental dosing is necessary.

Following systemic absorption, local anesthetics can produce central nervous system stimulation, depression, or both. Apparent central stimulation is manifested as restlessness, tremors and shivering, progressing to convulsions, followed by depression and coma progressing ultimately to respiratory arrest. However, the local anesthetics have a primary depressant effect on the medulla and on higher centers. The depressed stage may occur without a prior excited stage.

Pharmacokinetics: The rate of systemic absorption of local anesthetics is dependent upon the total dose and concentration of drug administered, the route of administration, the vascularity of the administraton site, and the presence or absence of epinephrine in the anesthetic solution. A dilute concentration of epinephrine (1:200,000 or 5 μg/mL) usually reduces the rate of absorption and peak plasma concentration of MARCAINE, permitting the use of moderately larger total doses and sometimes prolonging the duration of action.

The onset of action with MARCAINE is rapid and anesthesia is long lasting. The duration of anesthesia is significantly longer with MARCAINE than with any other commonly used local anesthetic. It has also been noted that there is a period of analgesia that persists after the return of sensation, during which time the need for strong analgesics is reduced.

The onset of sensory blockade following spinal block with MARCAINE Spinal is very rapid (within one minute); maximum motor blockade and maximum dermatome level are achieved within 15 minutes in most cases. Duration of sensory blockade (time to return of complete sensation in the operative site or regression of two dermatomes) following a 12 mg dose averages 2 hours with or without 0.2 mg epinephrine. The time to return of complete motor ability with 12 mg MARCAINE Spinal averages 3½ hours without the addition of epinephrine and 4½ hours if 0.2 mg epinephrine is added. When compared to equal milligram doses of hyperbaric tetracaine, the duration of sensory blockade was the same but the time to complete motor recovery was significantly longer for tetracaine. Addition of 0.2 mg epinephrine significantly prolongs the motor blockade and time to first postoperative narcotic with MARCAINE Spinal.

Local anesthetics appear to cross the placenta by passive diffusion. The rate and degree of diffusion is governed by (1) the degree of plasma protein binding, (2) the degree of ionization, and (3) the degree of lipid solubility. Fetal/maternal ratios of local anesthetics appear to be inversely related to the degree of plasma protein binding, because only the free, unbound drug is available for placental transfer. MARCAINE with a high protein binding capacity (95%) has a low fetal/maternal ratio (0.2 to 0.4). The extent of placental transfer is also determined by the degree of ionization and lipid solubility of the drug. Lipid soluble, nonionized drugs readily enter the fetal blood from the maternal circulation.

Depending upon the route of administration, local anesthetics are distributed to some extent to all body tissues, with high concentrations found in highly perfused organs such as the liver, lungs, heart, and brain.

Pharmacokinetic studies on the plasma profiles of MARCAINE after direct intravenous injection suggest a three-compartment open model. The first compartment is represented by the rapid intravascular distribution of the drug. The second compartment represents the equilibration of the drug throughout the highly perfused organs such as the brain, myocardium, lungs, kidneys, and liver. The third compartment represents an equilibration of the drug with poorly perfused tissues, such as muscle and fat. The elimination of drug from tissue distribution depends largely upon the ability of binding sites in the circulation to carry it to the liver where it is metabolized.

Various pharmacokinetic parameters of the local anesthetics can be significantly altered by the presence of hepatic or renal disease, addition of epinephrine, factors affecting urinary pH, renal blood flow, the route of drug administration, and the age of the patient. The half-life of MARCAINE in adults is 2.7 hours and in neonates 8.1 hours.

Amide-type local anesthetics such as MARCAINE are metabolized primarily in the liver via conjugation with glucuronic acid. Patients with hepatic disease, especially those with severe hepatic disease, may be more susceptible to the potential toxicities of the amide-type local anesthetics. Pipecolylxylidine is the major metabolite of MARCAINE.

The kidney is the main excretory organ for most local anesthetics and their metabolites. Urinary excretion is affected by urinary perfusion and factors affecting urinary pH. Only 6% of bupivacaine is excreted unchanged in the urine.

When administered in recommended doses and concentrations, MARCAINE does not ordinarily produce irritation or tissue damage and does not cause methemoglobinemia.

INDICATIONS AND USAGE

MARCAINE Spinal, brand of bupivacaine in dextrose injection, is indicated for the production of subarachnoid block (spinal anesthesia).

Standard textbooks should be consulted to determine the accepted procedures and techniques for the administration of spinal anesthesia.

CONTRAINDICATIONS

MARCAINE Spinal is contraindicated in patients with a known hypersensitivity to it or to any local anesthetic agent of the amide-type.

The following conditions preclude the use of spinal anesthesia:

1. Severe hemorrhage, severe hypotension or shock and arrhythmias, such as complete heart block, which severely restrict cardiac output.
2. Local infection at the site of proposed lumbar puncture.
3. Septicemia.

WARNINGS

LOCAL ANESTHETICS SHOULD ONLY BE EMPLOYED BY CLINICIANS WHO ARE WELL VERSED IN DIAGNOSIS AND MANAGEMENT OF DOSE-RELATED TOXICITY AND OTHER ACUTE EMERGENCIES WHICH MIGHT ARISE FROM THE BLOCK TO BE EMPLOYED, AND THEN ONLY AFTER INSURING THE **IMMEDIATE** AVAILABILITY OF OXYGEN, OTHER RESUSCITATIVE DRUGS, CARDIOPULMONARY RESUSCITATIVE EQUIPMENT, AND THE PERSONNEL RESOURCES NEEDED FOR PROPER MANAGEMENT OF TOXIC REACTIONS AND RELATED EMERGENCIES. (See also ADVERSE REACTIONS and PRECAUTIONS.) DELAY IN PROPER MANAGEMENT OF DOSE-RELATED TOXICITY, UNDERVENTILATION FROM ANY CAUSE AND/OR ALTERED SENSITIVITY MAY LEAD TO THE DEVELOPMENT OF ACIDOSIS, CARDIAC ARREST, AND, POSSIBLY, DEATH.

Spinal anesthetics should not be injected during uterine contractions, because spinal fluid current may carry the drug further cephalad than desired.

A free flow of cerebrospinal fluid during the performance of spinal anesthesia is indicative of entry into the subarachnoid space. However, aspiration should be performed before the anesthetic solution is injected to confirm entry into the subarachnoid space and to avoid intravascular injection.

MARCAINE solutions containing epinephrine or other vasopressors should not be used concomitantly with ergot-type oxytocic drugs, because a severe persistent hypertension may occur. Likewise, solutions of MARCAINE containing a vasoconstrictor, such as epinephrine, should be used with extreme caution in patients receiving monoamine oxidase inhibitors (MAOI) or antidepressants of the triptyline or imipramine types, because severe prolonged hypertension may result.

Until further experience is gained in patients younger than 18 years, administration of MARCAINE in this age group is not recommended.

Mixing or the prior or intercurrent use of any other local anesthetic with MARCAINE cannot be recommended because of insufficient data on the clinical use of such mixtures.

PRECAUTIONS

General: The safety and effectiveness of spinal anesthetics depend on proper dosage, correct technique, adequate precautions, and readiness for emergencies. Resuscitative equipment, oxygen, and other resuscitative drugs should be available for immediate use. (See WARNINGS and ADVERSE REACTONS.) The patient should have IV fluids running via an indwelling catheter to assure a functioning intravenous pathway. The lowest dosage of local anesthetic that results in effective anesthesia should be used. Aspiration for blood should be performed before injection and injection should be made slowly. Tolerance varies with the status of the patient. Elderly patients and acutely ill patients may require reduced doses. Reduced doses may also be indicated in patients with increased intra-abdominal pressure (including obstetrical patients), if otherwise suitable for spinal anesthesia.

There should be careful and constant monitoring of cardiovascular and respiratory (adequacy of ventilation) vital signs and the patient's state of consciousness after local anesthetic injection. Restlessness, anxiety, incoherent speech, lightheadedness, numbness and tingling of the mouth and lips, metallic taste, tinnitus, dizziness, blurred vision, tremors, depression, or drowsiness may be early warning signs of central nervous system toxicity.

Spinal anesthetics should be used with caution in patients with severe disturbances of cardiac rhythm, shock, or heart block.

Sympathetic blockade occurring during spinal anesthesia may result in peripheral vasodilation and hypotension, the extent depending on the number of dermatomes blocked. Blood pressure should, therefore, be carefully monitored especially in the early phases of anesthesia. Hypotension may be controlled by vasoconstrictors in dosages depending on the severity of hypotension and response of treatment. The level of anesthesia should be carefully monitored because it is not always controllable in spinal techniques.

Because amide-type local anesthetics such as MARCAINE are metabolized by the liver, these drugs, especially repeat doses, should be used cautiously in patients with hepatic disease. Patients with severe hepatic disease, because of their inability to metabolize local anesthetics normally, are at a greater risk of developing toxic plasma concentrations.

Local anesthetics should also be used with caution in patients with impaired cardiovascular function because they may be less able to compensate for functional changes associated with the prolongation of AV conduction produced by these drugs. However, dosage recommendations for spinal anesthesia are much lower than dosage recommendations for other major blocks and most experience regarding hepatic and cardiovascular disease dose-related toxicity is derived from these other major blocks.

Serious dose-related cardiac arrhythmias may occur if preparations containing a vasoconstrictor such as epinephrine are employed in patients during or following the administration of potent inhalation agents. In deciding whether to use these products concurrently in the same patient, the combined action of both agents upon the myocardium, the concentration and volume of vasoconstrictor used, and the time since injection, when applicable, should be taken into account.

Many drugs used during the conduct of anesthesia are considered potential triggering agents for familial malignant hyperthermia. Because it is not known whether amide-type local anesthetics may trigger this reaction and because the need for supplemental general anesthesia cannot be predicted in advance, it is suggested that a standard protocol for management should be available. Early unexplained signs of tachycardia, tachypnea, labile blood pressure, and metabolic acidosis may precede temperature elevation. Successful outcome is dependent on early diagnosis, prompt discontinuance of the suspect triggering agent(s) and institution of treatment, including oxygen therapy, indicated supportive measures, and dantrolene. (Consult dantrolene sodium intravenous package insert before using.)

The following conditions may preclude the use of spinal anesthesia, depending upon the physician's evaluation of the situation and ability to deal with the complications or complaints which may occur:

- Preexisting diseases of the central nervous system, such as those attributable to pernicious anemia, poliomyelitis, syphilis, or tumor.
- Hematological disorders predisposing to coagulopathies or patients on anticoagulant therapy. Trauma to a blood vessel during the conduct of spinal anesthesia may, in some instances, result in uncontrollable central nervous system hemorrhage or soft tissue hemorrhage.
- Chronic backache and preoperative headache.
- Hypotension and hypertension.
- Technical problems (persistent paresthesias, persistent bloody tap).
- Arthritis or spinal deformity.
- Extremes of age.
- Psychosis or other causes of poor cooperation by the patient.

Information for Patients: When appropriate, patients should be informed in advance that they may experience temporary loss of sensation and motor activity, usually in the lower half of the body, following proper administration of spinal anesthesia. Also, when appropriate, the physician should discuss other information including adverse reactions in the MARCAINE Spinal package insert.

Clinically Significant Drug Interactions: The administration of local anesthetic solutions containing epinephrine or norepinephrine to patients receiving monoamine oxidase inhibitors or tricyclic antidepressants may produce severe, prolonged hypertension. Concurrent use of these agents should generally be avoided. In situations when concurrent therapy is necessary, careful patient monitoring is essential.

Concurrent administration of vasopressor drugs and of ergot-type oxytocic drugs may cause severe persistent hypertension or cerebrovascular accidents.

Phenothiazines and butyrophenones may reduce or reverse the pressor effect of epinephrine.

Carcinogenesis, Mutagenesis, and Impairment of Fertility: Long-term studies in animals of most local anesthetics including bupivacaine to evaluate the carcinogenic potential have not been conducted. Mutagenic potential or the effect on fertility have not been determined. There is no evidence from human data that MARCAINE Spinal, brand of bupivacaine in dextrose injection, may be carcinogenic or mutagenic or that it impairs fertility.

Pregnancy Category C: Decreased pup survival in rats and an embryocidal effect in rabbits have been observed when bupivacaine hydrochloride was administered to these species in doses comparable to 230 and 130 times respectively the maximum recommended human spinal dose. There are no adequate and well-controlled studies in pregnant women of the effect of bupivacaine on the developing fetus. Bupivacaine hydrochloride should be used during pregnancy only if the potential benefit justifies the potential risk to the fetus. This does not exclude the use of MARCAINE Spinal at term for obstetrical anesthesia. (See ***Labor and Delivery.***)

Labor and Delivery: Spinal anesthesia has a recognized use during labor and delivery. Bupivacaine hydrochloride, when administered properly, via the epidural route in doses 10 to 12 times the amount used in spinal anesthesia has been used for obstetrical analgesia and anesthesia without evidence of adverse effects on the fetus.

Maternal hypotension has resulted from regional anesthesia. Local anesthetics produce vasodilation by blocking sympathetic nerves. Elevating the patient's legs and positioning her on her left side will help prevent decreases in blood pressure. The fetal heart rate also should be monitored continuously and electronic fetal monitoring is highly advisable.

It is extremely important to avoid aortocaval compression by the gravid uterus during administrations of regional block to parturients. To do this, the patient must be maintained in the left lateral decubitus position or a blanket roll or sandbag may be placed beneath the right hip and the gravid uterus displaced to the left.

Spinal anesthesia may alter the forces of parturition through changes in uterine contractility or maternal expulsive efforts. Spinal anesthesia has also been reported to prolong the second stage of labor by removing the parturient's reflex urge to bear down or by interfering with motor function. The use of obstetrical anesthesia may increase the need for forceps assistance.

The use of some local anesthetic drug products during labor and delivery may be followed by diminished muscle strength and tone for the first day or two of life. This has not been reported with bupivacaine.

There have been reports of cardiac arrest during use of MARCAINE 0.75% solution for epidural anesthesia in obstetrical patients. The package insert for MARCAINE hydrochloride for epidural, nerve block, etc, has a more complete discussion of preparation for, and management of, this problem. These cases are compatible with systemic toxicity following unintended intravascular injection of the much larger doses recommended for epidural anesthesia and have not occurred within the dose range of bupivacaine hydrochloride 0.75% recommended for spinal anesthesia in obstetrics. The 0.75% concentration of MARCAINE is therefore not recommended for obstetrical epidural anesthesia. MARCAINE Spinal, brand of bupivacaine in dextrose injection, is recommended for spinal anesthesia in obstetrics.

Nursing Mothers: It is not known whether local anesthetic drugs are excreted in human milk. Because many drugs are excreted in human milk, caution should be exercised when local anesthetics are administered to a nursing woman.

Pediatric Use: Until further experience is gained in patients younger than 18 years, administration of MARCAINE Spinal in this age group is not recommended.

ADVERSE REACTIONS

Reactions to bupivacaine are characteristic of those associated with other amide-type local anesthetics.

The most commonly encountered acute adverse experiences which demand immediate countermeasures following the administration of spinal anesthesia are hypotension due to loss of sympathetic tone and respiratory paralysis or under-

Continued on next page

This product information was effective as of December 1, 1986. On these and other products of Winthrop-Breon Laboratories, detailed information may be obtained on a current basis by direct inquiry to the Professional Services Department, 90 Park Avenue, New York, NY 10016 (212) 907-2525.

Winthrop-Breon—Cont.

ventilation due to cephalad extension of the motor level of anesthesia. These may lead to cardiac arrest if untreated. In addition, dose-related convulsions and cardiovascular collapse may result from diminished tolerance, rapid absorption from the injection site, or from unintentional intravascular injection of a local anesthetic solution. Factors influencing plasma protein binding, such as acidosis, systemic diseases which alter protein production, or competition of other drugs for protein binding sites, may diminish individual tolerance.

Respiratory System: Respiratory paralysis or underventilation may be noted as a result of upward extension of the level of spinal anesthesia and may lead to secondary hypoxic cardiac arrest if untreated. Preanesthetic medication, intraoperative analgesics and sedatives, as well as surgical manipulation, may contribute to underventilation. This will usually be noted within minutes of the injection of spinal anesthetic solution, but because of differing maximal onset times, differing intercurrent drug usage and differing surgical manipulation, it may occur at any time during surgery or the immediate recovery period.

Cardiovascular System: Hypotension due to loss of sympathetic tone is a commonly encountered extension of the clinical pharmacology of spinal anesthesia. This is more commonly observed in patients with shrunken blood volume, shrunken interstitial fluid volume, cephalad spread of the local anesthetic, and/or mechanical obstruction of venous return. Nausea and vomiting are frequently associated with hypotensive episodes following the administration of spinal anesthesia. High doses, or inadvertent intravascular injection, may lead to high plasma levels and related depression of the myocardium, decreased cardiac output, bradycardia, heart block, ventricular arrhythmias, and, possibly, cardiac arrest. (See **WARNINGS, PRECAUTIONS,** and **OVERDOSAGE** sections.)

Central Nervous System: Respiratory paralysis or underventilation secondary to cephalad spread of the level of spinal anesthesia (See *Respiratory System*) and hypotension for the same reason (see *Cardiovascular System*) are the two most commonly encountered central nervous system-related adverse observations which demand immediate countermeasures.

High doses or inadvertent intravascular injection may lead to high plasma levels and related central nervous system toxicity characterized by excitement and/or depression. Restlessness, anxiety, dizziness, tinnitus, blurred vision, or tremors may occur, possibly proceeding to convulsions. However, excitement may be transient or absent, with depression being the first manifestation of an adverse reaction. This may quickly be followed by drowsiness merging into unconsciousness and respiratory arrest.

Neurologic: The incidences of adverse neurologic reactions associated with the use of local anesthetics may be related to the total dose of local anesthetic administered and are also dependent upon the particular drug used, the route of administration, and the physical status of the patient. Many of these effects may be related to local anesthetic techniques, with or without a contribution from the drug.

Neurologic effects following spinal anesthesia may include loss of perineal sensation and sexual function; persistent anesthesia, paresthesia, weakness and paralysis of the lower extremities, and loss of sphincter control all of which may have slow, incomplete, or no recovery; hypotension; high or total spinal block; urinary retention; headache; backache; septic meningitis; meningismus; arachnoiditis; slowing of labor; increased incidence of forceps delivery; shivering; cranial nerve palsies due to traction on nerves from loss of cerebrospinal fluid; and fecal and urinary incontinence.

Allergic: Allergic-type reactions are rare and may occur as a result of sensitivity to the local anesthetic. These reactions are characterized by signs such as urticaria, pruritus, erythema, angioneurotic edema (including laryngeal edema), tachycardia, sneezing, nausea, vomiting, dizziness, syncope, excessive sweating, elevated temperature, and, possibly, anaphylactoid-like symptomatology (including severe hypotension). Cross sensitivity among members of the amide-type local anesthetic group has been reported. The usefulness of screening for sensitivity has not been definitely established.

Other: Nausea and vomiting may occur during spinal anesthesia.

OVERDOSAGE

Acute emergencies from local anesthetics are generally related to high plasma levels encountered during therapeutic use or to underventilation (and perhaps apnea) secondary to upward extension of spinal anesthesia. Hypotension is commonly encountered during the conduct of spinal anesthesia due to relaxation of sympathetic tone, and sometimes, contributory mechanical obstruction of venous return.

Management of Local Anesthetic Emergencies: The first consideration is prevention, best accomplished by careful and constant monitoring of cardiovascular and respiratory vital signs and the patient's state of consciousness after each local anesthetic injection. At the first sign of change, oxygen should be administered.

The first step in the management of systemic toxic reactions, as well as underventilation or apnea due to a high or total spinal, consists of ***immediate*** *attention to the establishment and maintenance of a patent airway and effective assisted or controlled ventilation with 100% oxygen with a delivery system capable of permitting immediate positive airway pressure by mask.* This may prevent convulsions if they have not already occurred.

If necessary, use drugs to control the convulsions. A 50 mg to 100 mg bolus IV injection of succinylcholine will paralyze the patient without depressing the central nervous or cardiovascular systems and facilitate ventilation. A bolus IV dose of 5 mg to 10 mg of diazepam or 50 mg to 100 mg of thiopental will permit ventilation and counteract central nervous system stimulation, but these drugs also depress central nervous system, respiratory and cardiac function, add to postictal depression and may result in apnea. Intravenous barbiturates, anticonvulsant agents, or muscle relaxants should only be administered by those familiar with their use. Immediately after the institution of these ventilatory measures, the adequacy of the circulation should be evaluated. Supportive treatment of circulatory depression may require administration of intravenous fluids, and, when appropriate, a vasopressor dictated by the clinical situation (such as ephedrine or epinephrine to enhance myocardial contractile force).

Hypotension due to sympathetic relaxation may be managed by giving intravenous fluids (such as isotonic saline or lactated Ringer's solution), in an attempt to relieve mechanical obstruction of venous return, or by using vasopressors (such as ephedrine which increases the force of myocardial contractions) and, if indicated, by giving plasma expanders or whole blood.

Endotracheal intubation, employing drugs and techniques familiar to the clinician, may be indicated after initial administration of oxygen by mask if difficulty is encountered in the maintenance of a patent airway, or if prolonged ventilatory support (assisted or controlled) is indicated.

Recent clinical data from patients experiencing local anesthetic-induced convulsions demonstrated rapid development of hypoxia, hypercarbia, and acidosis with bupivacaine within a minute of the onset of convulsions. These observations suggest that oxygen consumption and carbon dioxide production are greatly increased during local anesthetic convulsions and emphasize the importance of immediate and effective ventilation with oxygen which may avoid cardiac arrest.

If not treated immediately, convulsions with simultaneous hypoxia, hypercarbia, and acidosis plus myocardial depression from the direct effects of the local anesthetic may result in cardiac arrhythmias, bradycardia, asystole, ventricular fibrillation, or cardiac arrest. Respiratory abnormalities, including apnea, may occur. Underventilation or apnea due to a high or total spinal may produce these same signs and also lead to cardiac arrest if ventilatory support is not instituted. If cardiac arrest should occur, standard cardiopulmonary resuscitative measures should be instituted and maintained for a prolonged period if necessary. Recovery has been reported after prolonged resuscitative efforts.

The supine position is dangerous in pregnant women at term because of aortocaval compression by the gravid uterus. Therefore during treatment of systemic toxicity, maternal hypotension, or fetal bradycardia following regional block, the parturient should be maintained in the left lateral decubitus position if possible, or manual displacement of the uterus off the great vessels be accomplished.

The mean seizure dosage of bupivacaine in rhesus monkeys was found to be 4.4 mg/kg with mean arterial plasma concentration of 4.5 μg/mL. The intravenous and subcutaneous LD_{50} in mice is 6 mg/kg to 8 mg/kg and 38 mg/kg to 54 mg/kg respectively.

DOSAGE AND ADMINISTRATION

The dose of any local anesthetic administered varies with the anesthetic procedure, the area to be anesthetized, the vascularity of the tissues, the number of neuronal segments to be blocked, the depth of anesthesia and degree of muscle relaxation required, the duration of anesthesia desired, individual tolerance, and the physical condition of the patient. The smallest dose and concentration required to produce the desired result should be administered. Dosages of MARCAINE Spinal, brand of bupivacaine in dextrose injection, should be reduced for elderly and debilitated patients and patients with cardiac and/or liver disease.

For specific techniques and procedures, refer to standard textbooks.

The extent and degree of spinal anesthesia depend upon several factors including dosage, specific gravity of the anesthetic solution, volume of solution used, force of injection, level of puncture, and position of the patient during and immediately after injection.

Seven and one-half mg (7.5 mg or 1.0 mL) MARCAINE Spinal has generally proven satisfactory for spinal anesthesia for lower extremity and perineal procedures including TURP and vaginal hysterectomy. Twelve mg (12.0 mg or 1.6 mL) has been used for lower abdominal procedures such as abdominal hysterectomy, tubal ligation, and appendectomy. These doses are recommended as a guide for use in the average adult and may be reduced for the elderly or debilitated patients. Because experience with MARCAINE Spinal is limited in patients below the age of 18 years, dosage recommendations in this age group cannot be made.

Obstetrical Use: Doses as low as 6 mg bupivacaine hydrochloride have been used for vaginal delivery under spinal anesthesia. The dose range of 7.5 mg to 10.5 mg (1 mL to 1.4 mL) bupivacaine hydrochloride has been used for Cesarean section under spinal anesthesia.

In recommended doses, MARCAINE Spinal produces complete motor and sensory block.

Unused portions of solutions should be discarded following initial use.

MARCAINE Spinal should be inspected visually for discoloration and particulate matter prior to administration; solutions which are discolored or which contain particulate matter should not be administered.

HOW SUPPLIED

Single-dose ampuls of 2 mL (15 mg bupivacaine hydrochloride with 165 mg dextrose), in Uni-Nest™ Unit Dose Pak of 10 (NDC 0024-1229-10)

Store at controlled room temperature, between 15° C and 30° C (59° F and 86° F).

MARCAINE Spinal solution may be autoclaved once at 15 pound pressure, 121° C (250° F) for 15 minutes. Do not administer any solution which is discolored or contains particulate matter.

MW-246-A

MEBARAL® Ⓒ ℞

brand of mephobarbital tablets, USP

DESCRIPTION

Mephobarbital, 5-Ethyl-1-methyl-5-phenylbarbituric acid, is a barbiturate with sedative, hypnotic, and anticonvulsant properties. It occurs as a white, nearly odorless, tasteless powder and is slightly soluble in water and in alcohol.

MEBARAL is available as tablets for oral administration.

Inactive Ingredients: Lactose, Starch, Stearic Acid, Talc.

CLINICAL PHARMACOLOGY

Barbiturates are capable of producing all levels of CNS mood alteration from excitation to mild sedation, to hypnosis, and deep coma. Overdosage can produce death. In high enough therapeutic doses, barbiturates induce anesthesia.

Barbiturates depress the sensory cortex, decrease motor activity, alter cerebellar function, and produce drowsiness, sedation, and hypnosis.

Barbiturates are respiratory depressants. The degree of respiratory depression is dependent upon dose. With hypnotic doses, respiratory depression produced by barbiturates is similar to that which occurs during physiologic sleep with slight decrease in blood pressure and heart rate.

Studies in laboratory animals have shown that barbiturates cause reduction in the tone and contractility of the uterus, ureters, and urinary bladder. However, concentrations of the drugs required to produce this effect in humans are not reached with sedative-hypnotic doses.

Barbiturates do not impair normal hepatic function, but have been shown to induce liver microsomal enzymes, thus increasing and/or altering the metabolism of barbiturates and other drugs. (See PRECAUTIONS—Drug Interactions.)

MEBARAL exerts a strong sedative and anticonvulsant action but has a relatively mild hypnotic effect. It reduces the incidence of epileptic seizures in grand mal and petit mal. MEBARAL usually causes little or no drowsiness or lassitude. Hence, when it is used as a sedative or anticonvulsant, patients usually become more calm, more cheerful, and better adjusted to their surroundings without clouding of mental faculties. MEBARAL is reported to produce less sedation than does phenobarbital.

Barbiturates are weak acids that are absorbed and rapidly distributed to all tissues and fluids with high concentrations in the brain, liver, and kidneys. Lipid solubility of the barbiturates is the dominant factor in their distribution within the body. Barbiturates are bound to plasma and tissue proteins to a varying degree with the degree of binding increasing directly as a function of lipid solubility.

Approximately 50% of an oral dose of mephobarbital is absorbed from the gastrointestinal tract. Therapeutic plasma concentrations for mephobarbital have not been established nor has the half-life been determined. Following oral administration, the onset of action of the drug is 30 to 60 minutes and the duration of action is 10 to 16 hours. The primary route of mephobarbital metabolism is N-demethylation by the microsomal enzymes of the liver to form phenobarbital. Phenobarbital may be excreted in the urine unchanged or further metabolized to *p*-hydroxyphenobarbital and excreted in the urine as glucuronide or sulfate conjugates.

About 75% of a single oral dose of mephobarbital is converted to phenobarbital in 24 hours.
Therefore, chronic administration of mephobarbital may lead to an accumulation of phenobarbital (not mephobarbital) in plasma. It has not been determined whether mephobarbital or phenobarbital is the active agent during long-time mephobarbital therapy.

INDICATIONS AND USAGE

MEBARAL is indicated for use as a sedative for the relief of anxiety, tension, and apprehension, and as an anticonvulsant for the treatment of grand mal and petit mal epilepsy.

CONTRAINDICATIONS

Hypersensitivity to any barbiturate. Manifest or latent porphyria.

WARNINGS

Habit Forming

Barbiturates may be habit forming. Tolerance, psychological, and physical dependence may occur with continued use. (See DRUG ABUSE AND DEPENDENCE and CLINICAL PHARMACOLOGY.) Patients who have psychological dependence on barbiturates may increase the dosage or decrease the dosage interval without consulting a physician and may subsequently develop a physical dependence on barbiturates. To minimize the possibility of overdosage or the development of dependence, the prescribing and dispensing of sedative-hypnotic barbiturates should be limited to the amount required for the interval until the next appointment. Abrupt cessation after prolonged use in the dependent person may result in withdrawal symptoms, including delirium, convulsions, and possibly death. Barbiturates should be withdrawn gradually from any patient known to be taking excessive dosage over long periods of time. (See DRUG ABUSE AND DEPENDENCE.)

Acute or Chronic Pain

Caution should be exercised when barbiturates are administered to patients with acute or chronic pain, because paradoxical excitement could be induced or important symptoms could be masked. However, the use of barbiturates as sedatives in the postoperative surgical period and as adjuncts to cancer chemotherapy is well established.

Use in Pregnancy

Barbiturates can cause fetal damage when administered to a pregnant woman. Retrospective, case-controlled studies have suggested a connection between the maternal consumption of barbiturates and a higher than expected incidence of fetal abnormalities. Following oral or parenteral administration, barbiturates readily cross the placental barrier and are distributed throughout fetal tissues with highest concentrations found in the placenta, fetal liver, and brain. Fetal blood levels approach maternal blood levels following parenteral administration.
Withdrawal symptoms occur in infants born to mothers who receive barbiturates throughout the last trimester of pregnancy. (See DRUG ABUSE AND DEPENDENCE.) If this drug is used during pregnancy, or if the patient becomes pregnant while taking this drug, the patient should be apprised of the potential hazard to the fetus.

Synergistic Effects

The concomitant use of alcohol or other CNS depressants may produce additive CNS depressant effects.

PRECAUTIONS

General

Barbiturates may be habit forming. Tolerance and psychological and physical dependence may occur with continuing use. (See DRUG ABUSE AND DEPENDENCE.) Barbiturates should be administered with caution, if at all, to patients who are mentally depressed, have suicidal tendencies, or a history of drug abuse.
Elderly or debilitated patients may react to barbiturates with marked excitement, depression, and confusion. In some persons, barbiturates repeatedly produce excitement rather than depression.
In patients with hepatic damage, barbiturates should be administered with caution and initially in reduced doses. Barbiturates should not be administered to patients showing the premonitory signs of hepatic coma.
Status epilepticus may result from the abrupt discontinuation of MEBARAL, even when administered in small daily doses in the treatment of epilepsy.
Caution and careful adjustment of dosage are required when MEBARAL, brand of mephobarbital tablets, is used in patients with impaired renal, cardiac, or respiratory function and in patients with myasthenia gravis and myxedema. The least quantity feasible should be prescribed or dispensed at any one time in order to minimize the possibility of acute or chronic overdosage.
Vitamin D Deficiency: MEBARAL may increase vitamin D requirements, possibly by increasing vitamin D metabolism via enzyme induction. Rarely, rickets and osteomalacia have been reported following prolonged use of barbiturates.
Vitamin K: Bleeding in the early neonatal period due to coagulation defects may follow exposure to anticonvulsant drugs *in utero;* therefore, vitamin K should be given to the mother before delivery or to the child at birth.

Information for the Patient

Practitioners should give the following information and instructions to patients receiving barbiturates.

1. The use of barbiturates carries with it an associated risk of psychological and/or physical dependence. The patient should be warned against increasing the dose of the drug without consulting a physician.
2. Barbiturates may impair mental and/or physical abilities required for the performance of potentially hazardous tasks (eg, driving, operating machinery, etc).
3. Alcohol should not be consumed while taking barbiturates. Concurrent use of the barbiturates with other CNS depressants (eg, alcohol, narcotics, tranquilizers, and antihistamines) may result in additional CNS depressant effects.

Laboratory Tests

Prolonged therapy with barbiturates should be accompanied by periodic laboratory evaluation of organ systems, including hematopoietic, renal, and hepatic systems. (See PRECAUTIONS [General] and ADVERSE REACTIONS.)

Drug Interactions

Most reports of clinically significant drug interactions occurring with the barbiturates have involved phenobarbital. However, the application of these data to other barbiturates appears valid and warrants serial blood level determinations of the relevant drugs when there are multiple therapies.

1. *Anticoagulants.* Phenobarbital lowers the plasma levels of dicumarol (name previously used: bishydroxycoumarin) and causes a decrease in anticoagulant activity as measured by the prothrombin time. Barbiturates can induce hepatic microsomal enzymes resulting in increased metabolism and decreased anticoagulant response of oral anticoagulants (eg, warfarin, acenocoumarol, dicumarol, and phenprocoumon). Patients stabilized on anticoagulant therapy may require dosage adjustments if barbiturates are added to or withdrawn from their dosage regimen.
2. *Corticosteroids.* Barbiturates appear to enhance the metabolism of exogenous corticosteroids probably through the induction of hepatic microsomal enzymes. Patients stabilized on corticosteroid therapy may require dosage adjustments if barbiturates are added to or withdrawn from their dosage regimen.
3. *Griseofulvin.* Phenobarbital appears to interfere with the absorption of orally administered griseofulvin, thus decreasing its blood level. The effect of the resultant decreased blood levels of griseofulvin on therapeutic response has not been established. However, it would be preferable to avoid concomitant administration of these drugs.
4. *Doxycycline.* Phenobarbital has been shown to shorten the half-life of doxycycline for as long as 2 weeks after barbiturate therapy is discontinued.
This mechanism is probably through the induction of hepatic microsomal enzymes that metabolize the antibiotic. If phenobarbital and doxycycline are administered concurrently, the clinical response to doxycycline should be monitored closely.
5. *Phenytoin, Sodium Valproate, Valproic Acid.* The effect of barbiturates on the metabolism of phenytoin appears to be variable. Some investigators report an accelerating effect, while others report no effect. Because the effect of barbiturates on the metabolism of phenytoin is not predictable, phenytoin and barbiturate blood levels should be monitored more frequently if these drugs are given concurrently. Sodium valproate and valproic acid appear to decrease barbiturate metabolism; therefore, barbiturate blood levels should be monitored and appropriate dosage adjustments made as indicated.
6. *Central Nervous System Depressants.* The concomitant use of other central nervous system depressants, including other sedatives or hypnotics, antihistamines, tranquilizers, or alcohol, may produce additive depressant effects.
7. *Monoamine Oxidase Inhibitors (MAOI).* MAOI prolong the effects of barbiturates probably because metabolism of the barbiturate is inhibited.
8. *Estradiol, Estone, Progesterone, and other Steroidal Hormones.* Pretreatment with or concurrent administration of phenobarbital may decrease the effect of estradiol by increasing its metabolism. There have been reports of patients treated with antiepileptic drugs (eg, phenobarbital) who become pregnant while taking oral contraceptives. An alternant contraceptive method might be suggested to women taking phenobarbital.

Carcinogenesis

Animal Data. Phenobarbital sodium is carcinogenic in mice and rats after lifetime administration. In mice, it produced benign and malignant liver cell tumors. In rats, benign liver cell tumors were observed very late in life. Phenobarbital is the major metabolite of MEBARAL.
Human Data. In a 29-year epidemiological study of 9,136 patients who were treated on an anticonvulsant protocol which included phenobarbital, results indicated a higher than normal incidence of hepatic carcinoma. Previously, some of these patients were treated with thorotrast, a drug which is known to produce hepatic carcinomas. Thus, this study did not provide sufficient evidence that phenobarbital sodium is carcinogenic in humans. Phenobarbital is the major metabolite of MEBARAL, brand of mephobarbital tablets.
A retrospective study of 84 children with brain tumors matched to 73 normal controls and 78 cancer controls (malignant disease other than brain tumors) suggested an association between exposure to barbiturates prenatally and an increased incidence of brain tumors.

Pregnancy

Teratogenic Effects. Pregnancy Category D—See WARNINGS—Use in Pregnancy.
Nonteratogenic Effects. Reports of infants suffering from long-term barbiturate exposure *in utero* included the acute withdrawal syndrome of seizures and hyperirritability from birth to a delayed onset of up to 14 days. (See DRUG ABUSE AND DEPENDENCE.)

Labor and Delivery.

Hypnotic doses of these barbiturates do not appear to significantly impair uterine activity during labor. Full anesthetic doses of barbiturates decrease the force and frequency of uterine contractions. Administration of sedative-hypnotic barbiturates to the mother during labor may result in respiratory depression in the newborn. Premature infants are particularly susceptible to the depressant effects of barbiturates. If barbiturates are used during labor and delivery, resuscitation equipment should be available.
Data are currently not available to evaluate the effect of these barbiturates when forceps delivery or other intervention is necessary. Also, data are not available to determine the effect of these barbiturates on the later growth, development, and functional maturation of the child.

Nursing Mothers.

Caution should be exercised when a barbiturate is administered to a nursing woman since small amounts of barbiturates are excreted in the milk.

ADVERSE REACTIONS

The following adverse reactions and their incidence were compiled from surveillance of thousands of hospitalized patients. Because such patients may be less aware of certain of the milder adverse effects of barbiturates, the incidence of these reactions may be somewhat higher in fully ambulatory patients.
More than 1 in 100 Patients. The most common adverse reaction estimated to occur at a rate of 1 to 3 patients per 100 is:
Nervous System: Somnolence.
Less than 1 in 100 Patients. Adverse reactions estimated to occur at a rate of less than 1 in 100 patients listed below, grouped by organ system, and by decreasing order of occurrence are:
Nervous System: Agitation, confusion, hyperkinesia, ataxia, CNS depression, nightmares, nervousness, psychiatric disturbance, hallucinations, insomnia, anxiety, dizziness, thinking abnormality.
Respiratory System: Hypoventilation, apnea.
Cardiovascular System: Bradycardia, hypotension, syncope.
Digestive System: Nausea, vomiting, constipation.
Other Reported Reactions: Headache, hypersensitivity reactions (angioedema, skin rashes, exfoliative dermatitis), fever, liver damage, megaloblastic anemia following chronic phenobarbital use.

DRUG ABUSE AND DEPENDENCE

Mephobarbital is a controlled substance in Narcotic Schedule IV. Barbiturates may be habit forming. Tolerance, psychological dependence, and physical dependence may occur especially following prolonged use of high doses of barbiturates. As tolerance to barbiturates develops, the amount needed to maintain the same level of intoxication increases; tolerance to a fatal dosage, however, does not increase more than two-fold. As this occurs, the margin between an intoxicating dosage and fatal dosage becomes smaller.
Symptoms of acute intoxication with barbiturates include unsteady gait, slurred speech, and sustained nystagmus. Mental signs of chronic intoxication include confusion, poor judgment, irritability, insomnia, and somatic complaints.
Symptoms of barbiturate dependence are similar to those of chronic alcoholism. If an individual appears to be intoxicated with alcohol to a degree that is radically disproportionate to the amount of alcohol in his or her blood the use of barbiturates should be suspected. The lethal dose of a barbiturate is far less if alcohol is also ingested.
The symptoms of barbiturate withdrawal can be severe and may cause death. Minor withdrawal symptoms may appear 8 to 12 hours after the last dose of a barbiturate. These symptoms usually appear in the following order: anxiety, muscle

Continued on next page

This product information was effective as of December 1, 1986. On these and other products of Winthrop-Breon Laboratories, detailed information may be obtained on a current basis by direct inquiry to the Professional Services Department, 90 Park Avenue, New York, NY 10016 (212) 907-2525.

Winthrop-Breon—Cont.

twitching, tremor of hands and fingers, progressive weakness, dizziness, distortion in visual perception, nausea, vomiting, insomnia, and orthostatic hypotension. Major withdrawal symptoms (convulsions and delirium) may occur within 16 hours and last up to 5 days after abrupt cessation of these drugs. Intensity of withdrawal symptoms gradually declines over a period of approximately 15 days. Individuals susceptible to a barbiturate abuse and dependence include alcoholics and opiate abusers, as well as other sedative-hypnotic and amphetamine abusers.
Drug dependence to barbiturates arises from repeated administration of a barbiturate or agent with barbiturate-like effect on a continuous basis, generally in amounts exceeding therapeutic dose levels. The characteristics of drug dependence to barbiturates include: (a) a strong desire or need to continue taking the drug; (b) a tendency to increase the dose; (c) a psychic dependence on the effects of the drug related to subjective and individual appreciation of those effects; and (d) a physical dependence on the effects of the drug requiring its presence for maintenance of homeostasis and resulting in a definite, characteristic, and self-limited abstinence syndrome when the drug is withdrawn.
Treatment of barbiturate dependence consists of cautious and gradual withdrawal of the drug. Barbiturate-dependent patients can be withdrawn by using a number of different withdrawal regimens. In all cases withdrawal takes an extended period of time. One method involves substituting a 30 mg dose of phenobarbital for each 100 mg to 200 mg dose of barbiturate that the patient has been taking. The total daily amount of phenobarbital is then administered in 3 to 4 divided doses, not to exceed 600 mg daily. Should signs of withdrawal occur on the first day of treatment, a loading dose of 100 mg to 200 mg of phenobarbital may be administered IM in addition to the oral dose. After stabilization on phenobarbital, the total daily dose is decreased by 30 mg a day as long as withdrawal is proceeding smoothly. A modification of this regimen involves initiating treatment at the patient's regular dosage level and decreasing the daily dosage by 10% if tolerated by the patient.
Infants physically dependent on barbiturates may be given phenobarbital 3 mg/kg/day to 10 mg/kg/day. After withdrawal symptoms (hyperactivity, disturbed sleep, tremors, hyperreflexia) are relieved, the dosage of phenobarbital should be gradually decreased and completely withdrawn over a 2-week period.

OVERDOSAGE

The toxic dose of barbiturates varies considerably. In general, an oral dose of 1 g of most barbiturates produces serious poisoning in an adult. Death commonly occurs after 2 g to 10 g of ingested barbiturate. Barbiturate intoxication may be confused with alcoholism, bromide intoxication, and with various neurological disorders.
Acute overdosage with barbiturates is manifested by CNS and respiratory depression which may progress to Cheyne-Stokes respiration, areflexia, constriction of the pupils to a slight degree (though in severe poisoning they may show paralytic dilation), oliguria, tachycardia, hypotension, lowered body temperature, and coma. Typical shock syndrome (apnea, circulatory collapse, respiratory arrest, and death) may occur.
In extreme overdose, all electrical activity in the brain may cease, in which case a "flat" EEG normally equated with clinical death cannot be accepted. This effect is fully reversible unless hypoxic damage occurs. Consideration should be given to the possibility of barbiturate intoxication even in situations that appear to involve trauma.
Complications such as pneumonia, pulmonary edema, cardiac arrhythmias, congestive heart failure, and renal failure may occur. Uremia may increase CNS sensitivity to barbiturates if renal function is impaired. Differential diagnosis should include hypoglycemia, head trauma, cerebrovascular accidents, convulsive states, and diabetic coma.
Treatment of overdosage is mainly supportive and consists of the following:

1. Maintenance of an adequate airway, with assisted respiration and oxygen administration as necessary.
2. Monitoring of vital signs and fluid balance.
3. If the patient is conscious and has not lost the gag reflex, emesis may be induced with ipecac. Care should be taken to prevent pulmonary aspiration of vomitus. After completion of vomiting, 30 g activated charcoal in a glass of water may be administered.
4. If emesis is contraindicated, gastric lavage may be performed with a cuffed endotracheal tube in place with the patient in the face down position. Activated charcoal may be left in the emptied stomach and a saline cathartic administered.
5. Fluid therapy and other standard treatment for shock, if needed.
6. If renal function is normal, forced diuresis may aid in the elimination of the barbiturate. Alkalinization of the urine increases renal excretion of some barbiturates, including mephobarbital (which is metabolized to phenobarbital).
7. Although not recommended as a routine procedure, hemodialysis may be used in severe barbiturate intoxications or if the patient is anuric or in shock.
8. Patient should be rolled from side to side every 30 minutes.
9. Antibiotics should be given if pneumonia is suspected.
10. Appropriate nursing care to prevent hypostatic pneumonia, decubiti aspiration, and other complications of patients with altered states of consciousness.

DOSAGE AND ADMINISTRATION

Epilepsy: Average dose for adults: 400 mg to 600 mg (6 grains to 9 grains) daily; children under 5 years: 16 mg to 32 mg (1/4 grain to 1/2 grain) three or four times daily; children over 5 years: 32 mg to 64 mg (1/2 grain to 1 grain) three or four times daily. MEBARAL is best taken at bedtime if seizures generally occur at night, and during the day if attacks are diurnal. Treatment should be started with a small dose which is gradually increased over four or five days until the optimum dosage is determined. If the patient has been taking some other antiepileptic drug, it should be tapered off as the doses of MEBARAL are increased, to guard against the temporary marked attacks that may occur when any treatment for epilepsy is changed abruptly. Similarly, when the dose is to be lowered to a maintenance level or to be discontinued, the amount should be reduced gradually over four or five days.
Special Patient Population. Dosage should be reduced in the elderly or debilitated because these patients may be more sensitive to barbiturates. Dosage should be reduced for patients with impaired renal function or hepatic disease.
Combination with Other Drugs: MEBARAL may be used in combination with phenobarbital, either in the form of alternating courses or concurrently. When the two drugs are used at the same time, the dose should be about one-half the amount of each used alone. The average daily dose for an adult is from 50 mg to 100 mg (3/4 grain to 1 1/2 grains) of phenobarbital and from 200 mg to 300 mg (3 grains to 4 1/2 grains) of MEBARAL, brand of mephobarbital tablets.
MEBARAL may also be used with phenytoin sodium; in some cases, combined therapy appears to give better results than either agent used alone, since phenytoin sodium is particularly effective for the psychomotor types of seizure but relatively ineffective for petit mal. When the drugs are employed concurrently, a reduced dose of phenytoin sodium is advisable, but the full dose of MEBARAL may be given. Satisfactory results have been obtained with an average daily dose of 230 mg (3 1/2 grains) of phenytoin sodium plus about 600 mg (9 grains) of MEBARAL.
Sedation: Adults: 32 mg to 100 mg (1/2 grain to 1 1/2 grains)—optimum dose, 50 mg (3/4 grain)—three or four times daily. Children: 16 mg to 32 mg (1/4 grain to 1/2 grain) three or four times daily.

HOW SUPPLIED

Tablets
32 mg (1/2 grain), bottle of 250
(NDC 0024-1231-05)
32 mg (1/2 grain), bottle of 1000
(NDC 0024-1231-08)
50 mg (3/4 grain), bottle of 250
(NDC 0024-1232-05)
100 mg (1 1/2 grains), bottle of 250
(NDC 0024-1233-05)

MW-86-U

NALOXONE HYDROCHLORIDE ℞
INJECTION, USP
NALOXONE HYDROCHLORIDE ℞
INJECTION, USP (NEONATAL)

DESCRIPTION

Naloxone hydrochloride, a narcotic antagonist, is a synthetic congener of oxymorphone. In structure it differs from oxymorphone in that the methyl group on the nitrogen atom is replaced by an allyl group. It is known chemically as 17-allyl-4,5α-epoxy-3, 14-dihydroxymorphinan-6-one-hydrochloride.
Naloxone hydrochloride occurs as a white to slightly off-white powder and is soluble in water, dilute acids, and strong alkali; slightly soluble in alcohol; practically insoluble in ether and in chloroform.
Naloxone hydrochloride is available as a sterile solution for intravenous, intramuscular, and subcutaneous administration in two concentrations. Each mL contains either 0.02 mg or 0.4 mg of naloxone hydrochloride. Each mL of either strength contains 8.9 mg of sodium chloride. The pH is adjusted between 3.0 to 4.5 with hydrochloric acid or sodium hydroxide.

CLINICAL PHARMACOLOGY

Naloxone hydrochloride prevents or reverses the effects of opioids including respiratory depression, sedation, and hypotension. Also, it can reverse the psychotomimetic and dysphoric effects of agonist-antagonists such as pentazocine.
Naloxone hydrochloride is an essentially pure narcotic antagonist, ie, it does not possess the agonistic or morphine-like properties characteristic of other narcotic antagonists; naloxone hydrochloride does not produce respiratory depression, psychotomimetic effects, or pupillary constriction. In the absence of narcotics or agonistic effects of other narcotic antagonists it exhibits essentially no pharmacologic activity.
In the presence of physical dependence on narcotics, naloxone hydrochloride will produce withdrawal symptoms; it has not been shown to produce tolerance nor to cause physical or psychological dependence.
The precise mechanism by which naloxone reverses most of the effects of opioid analgesics has not been fully determined. Evidence suggests that naloxone hydrochlorde antagonizes the opioid effects by competing for the same receptor sites.
When naloxone hydrochloride is administered intravenously the onset of action is generally apparent within two minutes; the onset of action is only slightly less rapid when it is administered subcutaneously or intramuscularly. The duration of action is dependent upon the dose and route of administration of naloxone hydrochloride. Intramuscular administration produces a more prolonged effect than intravenous administration.
The requirement for repeat doses of naloxone hydrochloride, however, will also be dependent upon the amount, type, and route of administration of the narcotic being antagonized.
Following parenteral administration naloxone hydrochloride is rapidly distributed in the body. It is metabolized by the liver, primarily by glucuronide conjugation and excreted in the urine. In one study the serum half-life in adults ranged from 30 to 81 minutes (mean 64 ± 12 minutes). In a neonatal study the mean plasma half-life was observed to be 3.1 ± 0.5 hours.

INDICATIONS AND USAGE

Naloxone hydrochloride is indicated for the complete or partial reversal of narcotic depression, including respiratory depression, induced by opioids including natural and synthetic narcotics, propoxyphene, methadone, and the narcotic-antagonist analgesics (nalbuphine, pentazocine, and butorphanol). Naloxone hydrochloride is also indicated for the diagnosis of suspected acute opioid overdosage.

CONTRAINDICATION

Naloxone hydrochloride is contraindicated in patients known to be hypersensitive to it.

WARNINGS

Naloxone hydrochloride should be administered cautiously to persons including newborns of mothers who are known or suspected to be physically dependent on opioids. In such cases an abrupt and complete reversal of narcotic effects may precipitate an acute abstinence syndrome.
The patient who has satisfactorily responded to naloxone hydrochloride should be kept under continued surveillance and repeated doses of naloxone hydrochloride should be administered, as necessary, since the duration of action of some narcotics may exceed that of naloxone hydrochloride.
Naloxone hydrochloride is not effective against respiratory depression due to nonopioid drugs.

PRECAUTIONS

In addition to naloxone hydrochloride, other resuscitative measures such as maintenance of a free airway, artifical ventilation, cardiac massage, and vasopressor agents should be available and employed when necessary to counteract acute narcotic poisoning.
Several instances of hypotension, hypertension, ventricular tachycardia and fibrillation, and pulmonary edema have been reported. These have occurred in postoperative patients most of whom had preexisting cardiovascular disorders or received other drugs which may have similar adverse cardiovascular effects.
Although a direct cause and effect relationship has not been established, naloxone hydrochloride should be used with caution in patients with preexisting cardiac disease or patients who have received potentially cardiotoxic drugs.
Carcinogenesis, Mutagenesis, Impairment of Fertility
Carcinogenicity and mutagenicity studies have not been performed with naloxone hydrochloride. Reproduction studies in mice and rats demonstrated no impairment of fertility.
Pregnancy Category B
Reproduction studies have been performed in mice and rats at doses up to 1,000 times the human dose and have revealed no evidence of impaired fertility or harm to the fetus due to naloxone hydrochloride. There are, however, no adequate and well-controlled studies in pregnant women. Because animal reproduction studies are not always predictive of human response, naloxone hydrochloride should be used during pregnancy only if clearly needed.
Nursing Mothers
It is not known whether naloxone hydrochloride is excreted in human milk. Because many drugs are excreted in human milk, caution should be exercised when naloxone hydrochloride is administered to a nursing woman.

ADVERSE REACTIONS

Abrupt reversal of narcotic depression may result in nausea, vomiting, sweating, tachycardia, increased blood pressure, and tremulousness. In postoperative patients, larger than necessary dosage of naloxone hydrochloride may result in significant reversal of analgesia, and in excitement. Hypotension, hypertension, ventricular tachycardia and fibrillation, and pulmonary edema have been associated with the use of naloxone hydrochloride postoperatively (see **PRECAUTIONS, DOSAGE AND ADMINISTRATION —Usage in Adults/*Postoperative Narcotic Depression***).
Seizures have been reported to occur infrequently after the administration of naloxone, however, a causal relationship has not been established.

OVERDOSAGE

There is no clinical experience with naloxone hydrochloride overdosage in humans.
In the mouse and rat the intravenous LD_{50} is 150 mg/kg $\pm$ 5 mg/kg and 109 mg/kg $\pm$ 4 mg/kg respectively. It has been reported that in acute subcutaneous toxicity studies in newborn rats the LD_{50} (95% CL) is 260 mg/kg (228 mg/kg to 296 mg/kg). Subcutaneous injection of 100 mg/kg/day in rats for 3 weeks produced only transient salivation and partial ptosis following injection; no toxic effects were seen at 10 mg/kg/day for 3 weeks.

DOSAGE AND ADMINISTRATION

Naloxone hydrochloride may be administered intravenously, intramuscularly, or subcutaneously. The most rapid onset of action is achieved by intravenous administration and it is recommended in emergency situations.
Since the duration of action of some narcotics may exceed that of naloxone hydrochloride, the patient should be kept under surveillance and repeated doses of naloxone hydrochloride should be administered, as necessary.

Intravenous Infusion
Naloxone hydrochloride may be diluted for intravenous infusion in normal saline or 5% dextrose solutions. The addition of 2 mg of naloxone hydrochloride in 500 mL of either solution provides a concentration of 0.004 mg/mL. Mixtures should be used within 24 hours. After 24 hours, the remaining unused solution must be discarded. The rate of administration should be titrated in accordance with the patient's response.

Parenteral drug products should be inspected visually for particulate matter and discoloration prior to administration, whenever solution and container permit.
Naloxone hydrochloride should not be mixed with preparations containing bisulfite, metabisulfite, long-chain or high molecular weight anions, or any solution having an alkaline pH. No drug or chemical agent should be added to naloxone hydrochloride unless its effect on the chemical and physical stability of the solution has first been established.

Usage in Adults
Narcotic Overdose—Known or Suspected. The usual initial adult dose is 0.4 mg to 2 mg naloxone hydrochloride administered intravenously. If the desired degree of counteraction and improvement in respiratory function is not obtained, it may be repeated intravenously at 2 to 3 minute intervals. Failure to obtain a response after 10 mg of naloxone hydrochloride have been administered suggests that the diagnosis of narcotic induced or partial narcotic induced toxicity should be questioned. Intramuscular or subcutaneous administration may be necessary if the intravenous route is not available.
Postoperative Narcotic Depression. For the partial reversal of narcotic depression following the use of narcotics during surgery, smaller doses of naloxone hydrochloride are usually sufficient. The dose of naloxone hydrochloride should be titrated according to the patient's response. For the initial reversal of respiratory depression, naloxone hydrochloride should be injected in increments of 0.1 mg to 0.2 mg intravenously at 2 to 3 minute intervals to the desired degree of reversal, ie, adequate ventilation and alertness without significant pain or discomfort. Larger than necessary dosage of naloxone hydrochloride may result in significant reversal of analgesia and increase in blood pressure. Similarly, too rapid reversal may induce nausea, vomiting, sweating, or circulatory stress.
Repeat doses of naloxone hydrochloride may be required within one to two hour intervals depending upon the amount, type (ie, short or long acting), and time interval since last administration of narcotic. Supplemental intramuscular doses have been shown to produce a longer lasting effect.

Usage in Children
Narcotic Overdose—Known or Suspected. The usual initial dose in children is 0.01 mg/kg body weight given IV. If this dose does not result in the desired degree of clinical improvement, a subsequent dose of 0.1 mg/kg body weight may be administered. If an IV route of administration is not available, naloxone hydrochloride may be administered IM or SC in divided doses. If necessary, naloxone hydrochloride can be diluted with Sterile Water for Injection, USP.
Postoperative Narcotic Depression. Follow the recommendations and cautions under **Usage in Adults/*Postoperative Narcotic Depression.*** For the initial reversal of respiratory depression, naloxone hydrochloride should be injected in increments of 0.005 mg to 0.01 mg intravenously at 2 to 3 minute intervals to the desired degree of reversal.

Usage in Neonates
Narcotic-Induced Depression. The usual initial dose is 0.01 mg/kg body weight administered IV, IM, or SC. This dose may be repeated in accordance with adult administration guidelines for postoperative narcotic depression.

HOW SUPPLIED

0.4 mg/mL (1 mL fill in 2 mL cartridge) CARPUJECT® Sterile Cartridge-Needle Units, (22-gauge, 1¼ inch needle) box of 10 (NDC 0024-1313-02).
Neonatal–0.04 mg/2 mL (0.02 mg/mL) (2 mL fill) CARPUJECT Sterile Cartridge-Needle Units, (25-gauge ⅝ inch needle) box of 10 (NDC 0024-1314-02).
Protect from light.
Store at controlled room temperature 15° C–30° C (59 °F–86° F).

NW-548-A

NegGram® Caplets® ℞
brand of nalidixic acid tablets, USP
NegGram® Suspension ℞
brand of nalidixic acid oral suspension, USP

DESCRIPTION

Nalidixic acid, an oral antibacterial agent, is 1-Ethyl-1,4-dihydro-7-methyl-4-oxo-1,8-naphthyridine-3-carboxylic acid. It is a pale yellow, crystalline substance and a very weak organic acid.
Inactive Ingredients.—SUSPENSION: Carbomer 934P, FD&C Red #40, Flavor, Parabens, Purified Water, Saccharin Sodium, Sodium Chloride, Sorbitol Solution. CAPLETS: Hydrogenated Vegetable Oil, Methylcellulose, Microcrystalline Cellulose, Sodium Lauryl Sulfate, Yellow Ferric Oxide.

CLINICAL PHARMACOLOGY

NegGram has marked antibacterial activity against gram-negative bacteria including *Proteus mirabilis, P. morganii, P. vulgaris,* and *P. rettgeri; Escherichia coli;* Enterobacter (Aerobacter), and Klebsiella. Pseudomonas strains are generally resistant to the drug. NegGram is bactericidal and is effective over the entire urinary pH range. Conventional chromosomal resistance to NegGram taken in full dosage has been reported to emerge in approximately 2 to 14 percent of patients during treatment; however, bacterial resistance to NegGram has not been shown to be transferable via R factor.

INDICATIONS AND USAGE

NegGram is indicated for the treatment of urinary tract infections caused by susceptible gram-negative microorganisms, including the majority of Proteus strains, Klebsiella, Enterobacter (Aerobacter), and *E. coli.* Disc susceptibility testing with the 30 μg disc should be performed prior to administration of the drug, and during treatment if clinical response warrants.

CONTRAINDICATIONS

NegGram is contraindicated in patients with known hypersensitivity to nalidixic acid and in patients with a history of convulsive disorders.

WARNINGS

CNS effects including brief convulsions, increased intracranial pressure, and toxic psychosis have been reported rarely. These have occurred in infants and children or in geriatric patients, usually from overdosage or in patients with predisposing factors, and have been completely and rapidly reversible upon discontinuation of the drug. If these reactions occur, NegGram should be discontinued and appropriate therapeutic measures instituted; only if rapid disappearance of CNS symptoms does not occur within 48 hours should diagnostic procedures involving risk to the patient be undertaken. (See ADVERSE REACTIONS and OVERDOSAGE.)

PRECAUTIONS

Blood counts and renal and liver function tests should be performed periodically if treatment is continued for more than two weeks. NegGram should be used with caution in patients with liver disease, epilepsy, or severe cerebral arteriosclerosis. While caution should be used in patients with severe renal failure, therapeutic concentrations of NegGram in the urine, without increased toxicity due to drug accumulation in the blood, have been observed in patients on full dosage with creatinine clearances as low as 2 mL/minute to 8 mL/minute.
Patients should be cautioned to avoid undue exposure to direct sunlight while receiving NegGram. Therapy should be discontinued if photosensitivity occurs.
If bacterial resistance to NegGram emerges during treatment, it usually does so within 48 hours, permitting rapid change to another antimicrobial. Therefore, if the clinical response is unsatisfactory or if relapse occurs, cultures and sensitivity tests should be repeated. Underdosage with NegGram during initial treatment (with less than 4 g per day for adults) may predispose to emergence of bacterial resistance. (See DOSAGE AND ADMINISTRATION.)
Drug Interactions. Nitrofurantoin interferes with the therapeutic action of nalidixic acid.
Cross resistance between NegGram and other antimicrobials has been observed only with oxolinic acid.
Nalidixic acid may enhance the effects of oral anticoagulants, warfarin or bishydroxycoumarin, by displacing significant amounts from serum albumin binding sites.
When Benedict's or Fehling's solutions or Clinitest® Reagent Tablets are used to test the urine of patients taking NegGram, a false-positive reaction for glucose may be obtained, due to the liberation of glucuronic acid from the metabolites excreted. However, a colorimetric test for glucose based on an enzyme reaction (eg, with Clinistix® Reagent Strips or Tes-Tape®) does not give a false-positive reaction to the liberated glucuronic acid.
Incorrect values may be obtained for urinary 17-keto and ketogenic steroids in patients receiving NegGram, brand of nalidixic acid, because of an interaction between the drug and the *m*-dinitrobenzene used in the usual assay method. In such cases, the Porter-Silber test for 17-hydroxycorticoids may be used.
Usage in Prepubertal Children. Recent toxicological studies have shown that nalidixic acid and related drugs can produce erosions of the cartilage in weight-bearing joints and other signs of arthropathy in immature animals of most species tested. No such joint lesions have been reported in man to date. Nevertheless, until the significance of this finding is clarified, care should be exercised when prescribing this product for prepubertal children.
Usage in Pregnancy. Safe use of NegGram during the first trimester of pregnancy has not been established. However, the drug has been used during the last two trimesters without producing apparent ill effects in mother or child.
Caution should be used in administering NegGram in the days prior to delivery because of the theoretical risk that exposure to maternal nalidixic acid *in utero* may lead to significant blood levels of nalidixic acid in the neonate immediately after birth. Patients using NegGram during pregnancy should be advised to discontinue use at the first sign of labor.

ADVERSE REACTIONS

Reactions reported after oral administration of NegGram include *CNS effects:* drowsiness, weakness, headache, and dizziness and vertigo. Reversible subjective visual disturbances without objective findings have occurred infrequently (generally with each dose during the first few days of treatment). These reactions include overbrightness of lights, change in color perception, difficulty in focusing, decrease in visual acuity, and double vision. They usually disappeared promptly when dosage was reduced or therapy was discontinued. Toxic psychosis or brief convulsions have been reported rarely, usually following excessive doses. In general, the convulsions have occurred in patients with predisposing factors such as epilepsy or cerebral arteriosclerosis. In infants and children receiving therapeutic doses of NegGram, increased intracranial pressure with bulging anterior fontanel, papilledema, and headache has occasionally been observed. A few cases of 6th cranial nerve palsy have been reported. Although the mechanisms of these reactions are unknown, the signs and symptoms usually disappeared rapidly with no sequelae when treatment was discontinued. *Gastrointestinal:* abdominal pain, nausea, vomiting, and diarrhea. *Allergic:* rash, pruritus, urticaria, angioedema, eosinophilia, arthralgia with joint stiffness and swelling, and rarely, anaphylactoid reaction. Photosensitivity reactions consisting of erythema and bullae on exposed skin surfaces usually resolve completely in 2 weeks to 2 months after NegGram is discontinued; however, bullae may continue to appear with successive exposures to sunlight or with mild skin trauma for up to 3 months after discontinuation of drug. (See PRECAUTIONS.) *Other:* rarely, cholestasis, paresthesia, metabolic acidosis, thrombocytopenia, leukopenia, or hemolytic anemia, sometimes associated with glucose-6-phosphate dehydrogenase deficiency.

DOSAGE AND ADMINISTRATION

Adults. The recommended dosage for initial therapy in adults is 1 g administered four times daily for one or two weeks (total daily dose, 4 g). For prolonged therapy, the total daily dose may be reduced to 2 g after the initial treatment period. Underdosage during initial treatment may predispose to emergence of bacterial resistance.

Continued on next page

This product information was effective as of December 1, 1986. On these and other products of Winthrop-Breon Laboratories, detailed information may be obtained on a current basis by direct inquiry to the Professional Services Department, 90 Park Avenue, New York, NY 10016 (212) 907-2525.

Winthrop-Breon—Cont.

Children. Until further experience is gained, NegGram should not be administered to infants younger than three months. Dosage in children 12 years of age and under should be calculated on the basis of body weight. The recommended total daily dosage for initial therapy is 25 mg/lb/day (55 mg/kg/day), administered in four equally divided doses. For prolonged therapy, the total daily dose may be reduced to 15 mg/lb/day (33 mg/kg/day). NegGram Suspension or NegGram CAPLETS of 250 mg may be used. One 250 mg tablet is equivalent to one teaspoon (5 mL) of the Suspension.

OVERDOSAGE

Manifestations: Toxic psychosis, convulsions, increased intracranial pressure, or metabolic acidosis may occur in patients taking more than the recommended dosage. Vomiting, nausea, and lethargy may also occur following overdosage.
Treatment: Reactions are short-lived (two to three hours) because the drug is rapidly excreted. If overdosage is noted early, gastric lavage is indicated. If absorption has occurred, increased fluid administration is advisable and supportive measures such as oxygen and means of artificial respiration should be available. Although anticonvulsant therapy has not been used in the few instances of overdosage reported, it may be indicated in a severe case.

HOW SUPPLIED

Suspension (250 mg/5 mL tsp), raspberry flavored, bottles of 1 pint (NDC 0024-1318-06)
CAPLETS of 1 g, scored, bottles of 100 (NDC 0024-1323-04)
Unit Dose Pack of 100 (NDC 0024-1323-14)—10 strips of ten—1 g CAPLETS each
CAPLETS of 500 mg, scored, bottles of 56 (NDC 0024-1322-03), 500 (NDC 0024-1322-06), and 1000 (NDC 0024-1322-08)
Unit Dose Pack of 100 (NDC 0024-1322-14)–10 strips of ten-500 mg CAPLETS each
CAPLETS of 250 mg, scored, bottles of 56 (NDC 0024-1321-03)

PHARMACOLOGY

Following oral administration, NegGram, brand of nalidixic acid, is rapidly absorbed from the gastrointestinal tract, partially metabolized in the liver, and rapidly excreted through the kidneys. Unchanged nalidixic acid appears in the urine along with an active metabolite, hydroxynalidixic acid, which has antibacterial activity similar to that of nalidixic acid. Other metabolites include glucuronic acid conjugates of nalidixic acid and hydroxynalidixic acid, and the dicarboxylic acid derivative. The hydroxy metabolite represents 30 percent of the biologically active drug in the blood and 85 percent in the urine. Peak serum levels of active drug average approximately 20 μg to 40 μg per mL (90 percent protein bound), one to two hours after administration of a 1 g dose to a fasting normal individual, with a half-life of about 90 minutes. Peak urine levels of active drug average approximately 150 μg to 200 μg per mL, three to four hours after administration, with a half-life of about six hours. Approximately four percent of NegGram is excreted in the feces. Traces of nalidixic acid were found in blood and urine of an infant whose mother had received the drug during the last trimester of pregnancy.

ANIMAL PHARMACOLOGY

NegGram (nalidixic acid) and related drugs have been shown to cause arthropathy in juvenile animals of most species tested. (See PRECAUTIONS.)
Hydroxynalidixic acid, the principal metabolite of NegGram, did not produce any oculotoxic effects at any dosage level in seven species of animals including three primate species. However, oral administration of this metabolite in high doses has been shown to have oculotoxic potential, namely in dogs and cats where it produced retinal degeneration upon prolonged administration leading, in some cases, to blindness.
In experiments with NegGram itself, little if any such activity could be elicited in either dogs or cats. Sensitivity to CNS side effects in these species limited the doses of NegGram that could be used; this factor, together with a low conversion rate to the hydroxy metabolite in these species, may explain the absence of these effects.

Shown in Product Identification Section, page 435

NW-375-L(O)

NEO-SYNEPHRINE® Hydrochloride ℞

brand of phenylephrine hydrochloride injection, USP
1% INJECTION

Well-Tolerated Vasoconstrictor and Pressor

WARNING: PHYSICIANS SHOULD COMPLETELY FAMILIARIZE THEMSELVES WITH THE COMPLETE CONTENTS OF THIS LEAFLET BEFORE PRESCRIBING NEO-SYNEPHRINE.

DESCRIPTION

NEO-SYNEPHRINE hydrochloride, brand of phenylephrine hydrochloride injection, is a vasoconstrictor and pressor drug chemically related to epinephrine and ephedrine.
NEO-SYNEPHRINE hydrochloride is a synthetic sympathomimetic agent in sterile form for parenteral injection. Chemically, phenylephrine hydrochloride is (−)-*m*-Hydroxy-α-[(methylamino) methyl] benzyl alcohol hydrochloride.

CLINICAL PHARMACOLOGY

NEO-SYNEPHRINE hydrochloride produces vasoconstriction that lasts longer than that of epinephrine and ephedrine. Responses are more sustained than those to epinephrine, lasting 20 minutes after intravenous and as long as 50 minutes after subcutaneous injection. Its action on the heart contrasts sharply with that of epinephrine and ephedrine, in that it slows the heart rate and increases the stroke output, producing no disturbance in the rhythm of the pulse.
Phenylephrine is a powerful postsynaptic alpha-receptor stimulant with little effect on the beta receptors of the heart. In therapeutic doses, it produces little if any stimulation of either the spinal cord or cerebrum. A singular advantage of this drug is the fact that repeated injections produce comparable effects.
The predominant actions of phenylephrine are on the cardiovascular system. Parenteral administration causes a rise in systolic and diastolic pressures in man and other species. Accompanying the pressor response to phenylephrine is a marked reflex bradycardia that can be blocked by atropine; after atropine, large doses of the drug increase the heart rate only slightly. In man, cardiac output is slightly decreased and peripheral resistance is considerably increased. Circulation time is slightly prolonged, and venous pressure is slightly increased; venous constriction is not marked. Most vascular beds are constricted; renal splanchnic, cutaneous, and limb blood flows are reduced but coronary blood flow is increased. Pulmonary vessels are constricted, and pulmonary arterial pressure is raised.
The drug is a powerful vasoconstrictor, with properties very similar to those of norepinephrine but almost completely lacking the chronotropic and inotropic actions on the heart. Cardiac irregularities are seen only very rarely even with large doses.

INDICATIONS AND USAGE

NEO-SYNEPHRINE is intended for the maintenance of an adequate level of blood pressure during spinal and inhalation anesthesia and for the treatment of vascular failure in shock, shocklike states, and drug-induced hypotension, or hypersensitivity. It is also employed to overcome paroxysmal supraventricular tachycardia, to prolong spinal anesthesia, and as a vasoconstrictor in regional analgesia.

CONTRAINDICATIONS

NEO-SYNEPHRINE hydrochloride should not be used in patients with severe hypertension, ventricular tachycardia, or in patients who are hypersensitive to it.

WARNINGS

If used in conjunction with oxytocic drugs, the pressor effect of sympathomimetic pressor amines is potentiated (see Drug Interaction). The obstetrician should be warned that some oxytocic drugs may cause severe persistent hypertension and that even a rupture of a cerebral blood vessel may occur during the postpartum period.

PRECAUTIONS

NEO-SYNEPHRINE hydrochloride should be employed only with extreme caution in elderly patients or in patients with hyperthyroidism, bradycardia, partial heart block, myocardial disease, or severe arteriosclerosis.
Drug Interactions—Vasopressors, particularly metaraminol, may cause serious cardiac arrhythmias during halothane anesthesia and therefore should be used only with great caution or not at all.
MAO Inhibitors—The pressor effect of sympathomimetic pressor amines is markedly potentiated in patients receiving monoamine oxidase inhibitors (MAOI). Therefore, when initiating pressor therapy in these patients, the initial dose should be small and used with due caution. The pressor response of adrenergic agents may also be potentiated by tricyclic antidepressants.
Carcinogenesis, Mutagenesis, Impairment of Fertility—No long-term animal studies have been done to evaluate the potential of NEO-SYNEPHRINE in these areas.
Pregnancy Category C—Animal reproduction studies have not been conducted with NEO-SYNEPHRINE. It is also not known whether NEO-SYNEPHRINE can cause fetal harm when administered to a pregnant woman or can affect reproduction capacity. NEO-SYNEPHRINE should be given to a pregnant woman only if clearly needed.
Labor and Delivery—If vasopressor drugs are either used to correct hypotension or added to the local anesthetic solution, the obstetrician should be cautioned that some oxytocic drugs may cause severe persistent hypertension and that even a rupture of a cerebral blood vessel may occur during the postpartum period (see WARNINGS).
Nursing Mother—It is not known whether this drug is excreted in human milk. Because many are excreted in human milk, caution should be exercised when NEO-SYNEPHRINE hydrochloride, brand of phenylephrine hydrochloride injection, is administered to a nursing woman.
Pediatric Use—To combat hypotension during spinal anesthesia in children, a dose of 0.5 mg to 1 mg per 25 pounds of body weight, administered subcutaneously or intramuscularly, is recommended.

ADVERSE REACTIONS

Headache, reflex bradycardia, excitability, restlessness, and rarely arrhythmias.

OVERDOSAGE

Overdosage may induce ventricular extrasystoles and short paroxysms of ventricular tachycardia, a sensation of fullness in the head and tingling of the extremities.
Should an excessive elevation of blood pressure occur, it may be immediately relieved by an α-adrenergic blocking agent, eg, phentolamine.
The oral LD_{50} in the rat is 350 mg/kg, in the mouse 120 mg/kg.

DOSAGE AND ADMINISTRATION

NEO-SYNEPHRINE is generally injected subcutaneously, intramuscularly, slowly intravenously, or in dilute solution as a continuous intravenous infusion. In patients with paroxysmal supraventricular tachycardia and, if indicated, in case of emergency, NEO-SYNEPHRINE is administered directly intravenously. The dose should be adjusted according to the pressor response.

Dosage Calculations

Dose Required	*Use* NEO-SYNEPHRINE *1%*
10 mg	1 mL
5 mg	0.5 mL
1 mg	0.1 mL

For convenience in intermittent intravenous administration, dilute 1 mL NEO-SYNEPHRINE 1% with 9 mL Sterile Water for Injection, USP, to yield 0.1% NEO-SYNEPHRINE.

Dose Required	*Use Diluted* NEO-SYNEPHRINE *(0.1%)*
0.1 mg	0.1 mL
0.2 mg	0.2 mL
0.5 mg	0.5 mL

Mild or Moderate Hypotension
Subcutaneously or Intramuscularly: Usual dose, from 2 mg to 5 mg. Range, from 1 mg to 10 mg. Initial dose should not exceed 5 mg.
Intravenously: Usual dose, 0.2 mg. Range, from 0.1 mg to 0.5 mg. Initial dose should not exceed 0.5 mg.
Injections should not be repeated more often than every 10 to 15 minutes. A 5 mg intramuscular dose should raise blood pressure for one to two hours. A 0.5 mg intravenous dose should elevate the pressure for about 15 minutes.

Severe Hypotension and Shock—Including Drug-Related Hypotension
Blood volume depletion should always be corrected as fully as possible before any vasopressor is administered. When, as an emergency measure, intraaortic pressures must be maintained to prevent cerebral or coronary artery ischemia, NEO-SYNEPHRINE hydrochloride, brand of phenylephrine hydrochloride injection, can be administered before and concurrently with blood volume replacement.
Hypotension and occasionally severe shock may result from overdosage or idiosyncrasy following the administration of certain drugs, especially adrenergic and ganglionic blocking agents, rauwolfia and veratrum alkaloids, and phenothiazine tranquilizers. Patients who receive a phenothiazine derivative as preoperative medication are especially susceptible to these reactions. As an adjunct in the management of such episodes, NEO-SYNEPHRINE hydrochloride is a suitable agent for restoring blood pressure.
Higher initial and maintenance doses of NEO-SYNEPHRINE are required in patients with persistent or untreated severe hypotension or shock. Hypotension produced by powerful peripheral adrenergic blocking agents, chlorpromazine, or pheochromocytomectomy may also require more intensive therapy.
Continuous Infusion—Add 10 mg of the drug (1 mL of 1 percent solution) to 500 mL of Dextrose Injection, USP, or Sodium Chloride Injection, USP (providing a 1:50,000 solution). To raise the blood pressure rapidly, start the infusion at about 100 μg to 180 μg per minute (based on 20 drops per mL this would be 100 to 180 drops per minute). When the blood pressure is stabilized (at a low normal level for the individual), a maintenance rate of 40 μg to 60 μg per minute usually suffices (based on 20 drops per mL this would be 40 to 60 drops per minute). If the drop size of the infusion system var-

ies from the 20 drops per mL, the dose must be adjusted accordingly.
If a prompt initial pressor response is not obtained, additional increments of NEO-SYNEPHRINE (10 mg or more) are added to the infusion bottle. The rate of flow is then adjusted until the desired blood pressure level is obtained. (In some cases, a more potent vasopressor, such as norepinephrine bitartrate, may be required.) Hypertension should be avoided. The blood pressure should be checked frequently. Headache and/or bradycardia may indicate hypertension. Arrhythmias are rare.

Spinal Anesthesia—Hypotension

Routine parenteral use of NEO-SYNEPHRINE has been recommended for the prophylaxis and treatment of hypotension during spinal anesthesia. It is best administered subcutaneously or intramuscularly three or four minutes before injection of the spinal anesthetic. The total requirement for high anesthetic levels is usually 3 mg, and for lower levels, 2 mg. For hypotensive emergencies during spinal anesthesia, NEO-SYNEPHRINE may be injected intravenously, using an initial dose of 0.2 mg. Any subsequent dose should not exceed the previous dose by more than 0.1 mg to 0.2 mg and no more than 0.5 mg should be administered in a single dose. To combat hypotension during spinal anesthesia in children, a dose of 0.5 mg to 1 mg per 25 pounds body weight, administered subcutaneously or intramuscularly, is recommended.

Prolongation of Spinal Anesthesia

The addition of 2 mg to 5 mg of NEO-SYNEPHRINE hydrochloride to the anesthetic solution increases the duration of motor block by as much as approximately 50 percent without any increase in the incidence of complications such as nausea, vomiting, or blood pressure disturbances.

Vasoconstrictor for Regional Analgesia

Concentrations about ten times those employed when epinephrine is used as a vasoconstrictor are recommended. The optimum strength is 1:20,000 (made by adding 1 mg of NEO-SYNEPHRINE hydrochloride to every 20 mL of local anesthetic solution). Some pressor responses can be expected when 2 mg or more are injected.

Paroxysmal Supraventricular Tachycardia

Rapid intravenous injection (within 20 to 30 seconds) is recommended; the initial dose should not exceed 0.5 mg, and subsequent doses, which are determined by the initial blood pressure response, should not exceed the preceding dose by more than 0.1 mg to 0.2 mg, and should never exceed 1 mg.

HOW SUPPLIED

Solution 1 percent

Each 1 mL contains 10 mg of NEO-SYNEPHRINE hydrochloride, 3.5 mg of sodium chloride, 4 mg of sodium citrate, 1 mg of citric acid monohydrate, and not more than 2 mg of sodium metabisulfite.
Uni-Nest™ ampuls of 1 mL, box of 25 (NDC 0024-1342-04).
CARPUJECT® Sterile Cartridge-Needle Units, 10 mg/mL (1 mL fill in 2 mL cartridge), 22-gauge, 1¼ inch needle, dispensing bins of 50 (NDC 0024-1340-02).
The air in all ampuls and Cartridge-Needle Units has been displaced by nitrogen gas.
Protect from light if removed from carton or dispensing bin.

NW-64-CC

NEO-SYNEPHRINE® Hydrochloride ℞

brand of phenylephrine hydrochloride ophthalmic solution, USP

Vasoconstrictor and Mydriatic

SOLUTIONS 2.5% AND 10%
VISCOUS SOLUTION 10%

For Use in Ophthalmology

WARNING: PHYSICIANS SHOULD COMPLETELY FAMILIARIZE THEMSELVES WITH THE COMPLETE CONTENTS OF THIS LEAFLET BEFORE PRESCRIBING NEO-SYNEPHRINE.

DESCRIPTION

NEO-SYNEPHRINE hydrochloride, brand of phenylephrine hydrochloride ophthalmic solution, is a sterile solution used as a vasoconstrictor and mydriatic for use in ophthalmology.
NEO-SYNEPHRINE hydrochloride is a synthetic sympathomimetic compound structurally similar to epinephrine and ephedrine.
Phenylephrine hydrochloride is (–)-*m*-Hydroxy- α- [(methylamino)methyl] benzyl alcohol hydrochloride.

CLINICAL PHARMACOLOGY

NEO-SYNEPHRINE possesses predominantly α-adrenergic effects. In the eye, phenylephrine acts locally as a potent vasoconstrictor and mydriatic, by constricting ophthalmic blood vessels and the radial muscle of the iris.
The ophthalmologic usefulness of NEO-SYNEPHRINE hydrochloride is due to its rapid effect and moderately prolonged action, as well as to the fact that it produces no compensatory vasodilatation.
The action of different concentrations of ophthalmic solutions of NEO-SYNEPHRINE hydrochloride is shown in the following table:

Strength of solution (%)	Mydriasis: Maximal (minutes)	Mydriasis: Recovery time (hours)	Paralysis of accommodation
2.5	15-60	3	trace
10	10-60	6	slight

Although rare, systemic absorption of sufficient quantities of phenylephrine may lead to systemic α-adrenergic effects, such as rise in blood pressure which may be accompanied by a reflex atropine-sensitive bradycardia.

INDICATIONS AND USAGE

NEO-SYNEPHRINE hydrochloride is recommended for use as a decongestant and vasoconstrictor and for pupil dilatation in uveitis (posterior synechiae), wide angle glaucoma, prior to surgery, refraction, ophthalmoscopic examination, and diagnostic procedures.

CONTRAINDICATIONS

Ophthalmic solutions of NEO-SYNEPHRINE hydrochloride are contraindicated in persons with narrow angle glaucoma (and in those individuals who are hypersensitive to NEO-SYNEPHRINE). NEO-SYNEPHRINE hydrochloride 10 percent ophthalmic solutions are contraindicated in infants and in patients with aneurysms.

WARNINGS

There have been rare reports associating the use of NEO-SYNEPHRINE 10 percent ophthalmic solutions with the development of serious cardiovascular reactions, including ventricular arrhythmias and myocardial infarctions. These episodes, some ending fatally, have usually occurred in elderly patients with preexisting cardiovascular diseases.

PRECAUTIONS

Exceeding recommended dosages or applying NEO-SYNEPHRINE hydrochloride ophthalmic solutions to the instrumented, traumatized, diseased or postsurgical eye or adnexa, or to patients with suppressed lacrimation, as during anesthesia, may result in the absorption of sufficient quantities of phenylephrine to produce a systemic vasopressor response.
A significant elevation in blood pressure is rare but has been reported following conjunctival instillation of recommended doses of NEO-SYNEPHRINE 10 percent ophthalmic solutions. Caution, therefore, should be exercised in administering the 10 percent solutions to children of low body weight, the elderly, and patients with insulin-dependent diabetes, hypertension, hyperthyroidism, generalized arteriosclerosis, or cardiovascular disease. The posttreatment blood pressure of these patients, and any patients who develop symptoms, should be carefully monitored.
Ordinarily, any mydriatic, including NEO-SYNEPHRINE hydrochloride, brand of phenylephrine hydrochloride ophthalmic solution, is contraindicated in patients with glaucoma, since it may occasionally raise intraocular pressure. However, when temporary dilatation of the pupil may free adhesions or when vasoconstriction of intrinsic vessels may lower intraocular tension, these advantages may temporarily outweigh the danger from coincident dilatation of the pupil.
Rebound miosis has been reported in older persons one day after receiving NEO-SYNEPHRINE hydrochloride ophthalmic solutions, and reinstillation of the drug produced a reduction in mydriasis. This may be of clinical importance in dilating the pupils of older subjects prior to retinal detachment or cataract surgery.
Due to a strong action of the drug on the dilator muscle, older individuals may also develop transient pigment floaters in the aqueous humor 30 to 45 minutes following the administration of NEO-SYNEPHRINE hydrochloride ophthalmic solutions. The appearance may be similar to anterior uveitis or to a microscopic hyphema.
To prevent pain, a drop of suitable topical anesthetic may be applied before using the 10 percent ophthalmic solution.
Drug Interaction: As with all other adrenergic drugs, when NEO-SYNEPHRINE 10 percent ophthalmic solutions or 2.5 percent ophthalmic solution is administered simultaneously with, or up to 21 days after, administration of monoamine oxidase (MAO) inhibitors, careful supervision and adjustment of dosages are required since exaggerated adrenergic effects may occur. The pressor response of adrenergic agents may also be potentiated by tricyclic antidepressants, propranolol, reserpine, guanethidine, methyldopa, and atropine-like drugs.
It has been reported that the concomitant use of NEO-SYNEPHRINE 10 percent ophthalmic solutions and systemic beta blockers has caused acute hypertension and, in one case, the rupture of a congenital cerebral aneurysm.
Carcinogenesis, Mutagenesis, Impairment of Fertility: No long-term animal studies have been done to evaluate the potential of NEO-SYNEPHRINE in these areas.
Pregnancy Category C: Animal reproduction studies have not been conducted with NEO-SYNEPHRINE. It is also not known whether NEO-SYNEPHRINE can cause fetal harm when administered to a pregnant woman or can affect reproduction capacity. NEO-SYNEPHRINE should be given to a pregnant woman only if clearly needed.
Nursing Mothers: It is not known whether this drug is excreted in milk; many are. Caution should be exercised when NEO-SYNEPHRINE hydrochloride ophthalmic solution is administered to a nursing woman.
Pediatric Use: NEO-SYNEPHRINE hydrochloride 10 percent ophthalmic solutions are contraindicated in infants. (See CONTRAINDICATIONS.) For use in older children see DOSAGE AND ADMINISTRATION.
Exceeding recommended dosages or applying NEO-SYNEPHRINE hydrochloride ophthalmic solutions to the instrumented, traumatized, diseased or postsurgical eye or adnexa, or to patients with suppressed lacrimation, as during anesthesia, may result in the absorption of sufficient quantities of phenylephrine to produce a systemic vasopressor response.
The hypertensive effects of phenylephrine may be treated with an alpha-adrenergic blocking agent such as phentolamine mesylate, 5 mg to 10 mg intravenously, repeated as necessary.
The oral LD_{50} of phenylephrine in the rat: 350 mg/kg, in the mouse: 120 mg/kg.

DOSAGE AND ADMINISTRATION

Prolonged exposure to air or strong light may cause oxidation and discoloration. Do not use if solution is brown or contains a precipitate.

Vasoconstriction and Pupil Dilatation

NEO-SYNEPHRINE hydrochloride 10 percent ophthalmic solutions is especially useful when rapid and powerful dilatation of the pupil and reduction of congestion in the capillary bed are desired. A drop of a suitable topical anesthetic may be applied, followed in a few minutes by 1 drop of the NEO-SYNEPHRINE hydrochloride 10 percent ophthalmic solution on the upper limbus. The anesthetic prevents stinging and consequent dilution of the solution by lacrimation. It may occasionally be necessary to repeat the instillation after one hour, again preceded by the use of the topical anesthetic.

Uveitis: Posterior Synechiae

NEO-SYNEPHRINE hydrochloride 10 percent ophthalmic solutions may be used in patients with uveitis when synechiae are present or may develop. The formation of synechiae may be prevented by the use of the 10 percent ophthalmic solutions and atropine to produce wide dilatation of the pupil. It should be emphasized, however, that the vasoconstrictor effect of NEO-SYNEPHRINE hydrochloride may be antagonistic to the increase of local blood flow in uveal infection.
To free recently formed posterior synechiae, 1 drop of the 10 percent ophthalmic solutions may be applied to the upper surface of the cornea. On the following day, treatment may be continued if necessary. In the interim, hot compresses should be applied for five or ten minutes three times a day, with 1 drop of a 1 or 2 percent solution of atropine sulfate before and after each series of compresses.

Glaucoma

In certain patients with glaucoma, temporary reduction of intraocular tension may be attained by producing vasoconstriction of the intraocular vessels; this may be accomplished by placing 1 drop of the 10 percent ophthalmic solutions on the upper surface of the cornea. This treatment may be repeated as often as necessary.
NEO-SYNEPHRINE hydrochloride, brand of phenylephrine hydrochloride ophthalmic solution, may be used with miotics in patients with wide angle glaucoma. It reduces the difficulties experienced by the patient because of the small field produced by miosis, and still it permits and often supports the effect of the miotic in lowering the intraocular pressure. Hence, there may be marked improvement in visual acuity after using NEO-SYNEPHRINE hydrochloride in conjunction with miotic drugs.

Surgery

When a short-acting mydriatic is needed for wide dilatation of the pupil before intraocular surgery, the 10 percent ophthalmic solutions or 2.5 percent ophthalmic solution may be applied topically from 30 to 60 minutes before the operation.

Continued on next page

This product information was effective as of December 1, 1986. On these and other products of Winthrop-Breon Laboratories, detailed information may be obtained on a current basis by direct inquiry to the Professional Services Department, 90 Park Avenue, New York, NY 10016 (212) 907-2525.

Winthrop-Breon—Cont.

Refraction
Prior to determination of refractive errors, NEO-SYNEPHRINE hydrochloride 2.5 percent ophthalmic solution may be used effectively with homatropine hydrobromide, atropine sulfate, or a combination of homatropine and cocaine hydrochloride.
For *adults,* a drop of the preferred cycloplegic is placed in each eye, followed in five minutes by 1 drop of NEO-SYNEPHRINE hydrochloride 2.5 percent ophthalmic solution and in ten minutes by another drop of the cycloplegic. In 50 to 60 minutes, the eyes are ready for refraction.
For *children,* a drop of atropine sulfate 1 percent is placed in each eye, followed in 10 to 15 minutes by 1 drop of NEO-SYNEPHRINE hydrochloride 2.5 percent ophthalmic solution and in five to ten minutes by a second drop of atropine sulfate 1 percent. In one to two hours, the eyes are ready for refraction.
For a "one application method," NEO-SYNEPHRINE hydrochloride 2.5 percent ophthalmic solution may be combined with a cycloplegic to elicit synergistic action. The additive effect varies depending on the patient. Therefore, when using a "one application method," it may be desirable to increase the concentration of the cycloplegic.
Ophthalmoscopic Examination
One drop of NEO-SYNEPHRINE hydrochloride 2.5 percent ophthalmic solution is placed in each eye. Sufficient mydriasis to permit examination is produced in 15 to 30 minutes. Dilatation lasts from one to three hours.
Diagnostic Procedures
Provocative Test for Angle Block in Patients with Glaucoma: The 2.5 percent ophthalmic solution may be used as a provocative test when latent increased intraocular pressure is suspected. Tension is measured before application of NEO-SYNEPHRINE hydrochloride and again after dilatation. A 3 to 5 mm of mercury rise in pressure suggests the presence of angle block in patients with glaucoma; however, failure to obtain such a rise does not preclude the presence of glaucoma from other causes.
Shadow Test (Retinoscopy): When dilatation of the pupil without cycloplegic action is desired for the shadow test, the 2.5 percent ophthalmic solution may be used alone.
Blanching Test: One or 2 drops of the 2.5 percent ophthalmic solution should be applied to the injected eye. After five minutes, examine for perilimbal blanching. If blanching occurs, the congestion is superficial and probably does not indicate iritis.

HOW SUPPLIED
In Mono-Drop ® (plastic dropper) bottle:
Low surface tension solutions
2.5 percent ophthalmic solution — NEO-SYNEPHRINE hydrochloride, brand of phenylephrine hydrochloride ophthalmic solution, 2.5 percent in a sterile, isotonic, buffered, low surface tension vehicle with sodium phosphate, sodium biphosphate, boric acid, and, as antiseptic preservative, benzalkonium chloride, NF, 1:7500. The pH is adjusted with phosphoric acid or sodium hydroxide.
Bottles of 15 mL (NDC 0024-1358-01)
10 percent ophthalmic solution — NEO-SYNEPHRINE hydrochloride
10 percent in a sterile, buffered, low surface tension vehicle with sodium phosphate, sodium biphosphate, and, as antiseptic preservative, benzalkonium chloride 1:10,000. The pH is adjusted with phosphoric acid or sodium hydroxide.
Bottles of 5 mL (NDC 0024-1359-01)
Viscous solution
10 percent ophthalmic solution — NEO-SYNEPHRINE hydrochloride
10 percent in a sterile, buffered, viscous vehicle with sodium phosphate, sodium biphosphate, methylcellulose, and, as antiseptic preservative, benzalkonium chloride 1:10,000. The pH is adjusted with phosphoric acid or sodium hydroxide.
Bottles of 5 mL (NDC 0024-1362-01)
NW-147-AA

NOVOCAIN® ℞
brand of procaine hydrochloride injection, USP

DESCRIPTION
Procaine hydrochloride is benzoic acid, 4-amino-, 2-(diethylamino)ethyl ester, monohydrochloride, the ester of diethylaminoethanol and para-aminobenzoic acid.
It is a white crystalline, odorless powder that is freely soluble in water, but less soluble in alcohol.

HOW SUPPLIED
NOVOCAIN Solution 1 percent
Ampuls of 2 mL UNI-NEST PAK of 25 **NDC** 0024-1381-25
Ampuls of 6 mL box of 50 **NDC** 0024-1381-05
Vials of 30 mL box of 100 **NDC** 0024-1385-01
NOVOCAIN Solution 2 percent
Vials of 30 mL box of 100 **NDC** 0024-1386-01
For complete prescribing information, see package insert or contact Winthrop-Breon Laboratories Medical Department
NW-63-S

NOVOCAIN® ℞
brand of procaine hydrochloride injection, USP
10% Solution for Spinal Anesthesia

DESCRIPTION
NOVOCAIN, brand of procaine hydrochloride, is benzoic acid, 4-amino-, 2-(diethylamino) ethyl ester, monohydrochloride, the ester of diethylaminoethanol and para-aminobenzoic acid.
It is a white crystalline, odorless powder that is freely soluble in water, but less soluble in alcohol. Each mL contains 100 mg procaine hydrochloride and 4 mg acetone sodium bisulfite as antioxidant. DO NOT USE SOLUTIONS IF CRYSTALS, CLOUDINESS, OR DISCOLORATION IS OBSERVED. EXAMINE SOLUTIONS CAREFULLY BEFORE USE. REAUTOCLAVING INCREASES LIKELIHOOD OF CRYSTAL FORMATION.

CLINICAL PHARMACOLOGY
NOVOCAIN stabilizes the neuronal membrane and prevents the initiation and transmission of nerve impulses, thereby effecting local anesthesia. NOVOCAIN lacks surface anesthetic activity. The onset of action is rapid (2 to 5 minutes) and the duration of action is relatively short (average 1 to 1½ hours), depending upon the anesthetic technique, the type of block, the concentration, and the individual patient.
NOVOCAIN is readily absorbed following parenteral administration and is rapidly hydrolyzed by plasma cholinesterase to para-aminobenzoic acid and diethylaminoethanol.
A vasoconstrictor may be added to the NOVOCAIN solution to promote local hemostasis, delay systemic absorption, and increase duration of anesthesia.

INDICATIONS AND USAGE
NOVOCAIN is indicated for spinal anesthesia.

CONTRAINDICATIONS
Spinal anesthesia with NOVOCAIN is contraindicated in patients with generalized septicemia: sepsis at the proposed injection site; certain diseases of the cerebrospinal system, eg, meningitis, syphilis; and a known hypersensitivity to the drug, drugs of a similar chemical configuration, or para-aminobenzoic acid or its derivatives.
The decision as to whether or not spinal anesthesia should be used in an individual case should be made by the physician after weighing the advantages with the risks and possible complications.

WARNINGS
RESUSCITATIVE EQUIPMENT AND DRUGS SHOULD BE IMMEDIATELY AVAILABLE WHENEVER ANY LOCAL ANESTHETIC DRUG IS USED. Spinal anesthesia should only be administered by those qualified to do so.
Large doses of local anesthetics should not be used in patients with heart block.
Reactions resulting in fatality have occurred on rare occasions with the use of local anesthetics, even in the absence of a history of hypersensitivity.
Usage in Pregnancy. Safe use of NOVOCAIN has not been established with respect to adverse effects on fetal development. Careful consideration should be given to this fact before administering this drug to women of childbearing potential particularly during early pregnancy. This does not exclude the use of the drug at term for obstetrical analgesia.
Vasopressor agents (administered for the treatment of hypotension or added to the anesthetic solution for vasoconstriction) should be used with extreme caution in the presence of oxytocic drugs as they may produce severe, persistent hypertension with possible rupture of a cerebral blood vessel.
Solutions which contain a vasoconstrictor should be used with extreme caution in patients receiving drugs known to produce alterations in blood pressure (ie, monoamine oxidase inhibitors (MAOI), tricyclic antidepressants, phenothiazines, etc), as either severe sustained hypertension or hypotension may occur.
Local anesthetic procedures should be used with caution when there is inflammation and/or sepsis in the region of the proposed injection.

PRECAUTIONS
Standard textbooks should be consulted for specific techniques and precautions for various spinal anesthetic procedures.
The safety and effectiveness of a spinal anesthetic depend upon proper dosage, correct technique, adequate precautions, and readiness for emergencies. The lowest dosage that results in effective anesthesia should be used to avoid high plasma levels and possible adverse effects. Tolerance varies with the status of the patient. Debilitated, elderly patients, or acutely ill patients should be given reduced doses commensurate with their weight and physical status. Reduced dosages are also indicated for obstetric delivery and patients with increased intraabdominal pressure.
The decision whether or not to use spinal anesthesia in the following disease states depends on the physician's appraisal of the advantages as opposed to the risk: cardiovascular disease (ie, shock, hypertension, anemia, etc), pulmonary disease, renal impairment, metabolic or endocrine disorders, gastrointestinal disorders (ie, intestinal obstruction, peritonitis, etc), or complicated obstetrical deliveries.
NOVOCAIN SHOULD BE USED WITH CAUTION IN PATIENTS WITH KNOWN DRUG ALLERGIES AND SENSITIVITIES. A thorough history of the patient's prior experience with NOVOCAIN or other local anesthetics as well as concomitant or recent drug use should be taken (see CONTRAINDICATIONS). NOVOCAIN should not be used in any condition in which a sulfonamide drug is being employed since para-aminobenzoic acid inhibits the action of sulfonamides.
Solutions containing a vasopressor should be used with caution in the presence of diseases which may adversely affect the cardiovascular system.
NOVOCAIN, brand of procaine hydrochloride injection, should be used with caution in patients with severe disturbances of cardiac rhythm, shock or heart block.

ADVERSE REACTIONS
Systemic adverse reactions involving the central nervous system and the cardiovascular system usually result from high plasma levels due to excessive dosage, rapid absorption, or inadvertent intravascular injection. In addition, use of inappropriate doses or techniques may result in extensive spinal blockade leading to hypotension and respiratory arrest.
A small number of reactions may result from hypersensitivity, idiosyncrasy, or diminished tolerance to normal dosage.
Excitatory CNS effects (nervousness, dizziness, blurred vision, tremors) commonly represent the initial signs of local anesthetic systemic toxicity. However, these reactions may be very brief or absent in some patients in which case the first manifestation of toxicity may be drowsiness or convulsions merging into unconsciousness and respiratory arrest.
Cardiovascular system reactions include depression of the myocardium, hypotension (or sometimes hypertension), bradycardia, and even cardiac arrest.
Allergic reactions are characterized by cutaneous lesions of delayed onset, or urticaria, edema, and other manifestations of allergy. The detection of sensitivity by skin testing is of limited value. As with other local anesthetics, hypersensitivity, idiosyncrasy and anaphylactoid reactions have occurred rarely. The reaction may be abrupt and severe and is not usually dose related.
The following adverse reactions may occur with spinal anesthesia: *Central Nervous System:* postspinal headache, meningismus, arachnoiditis, palsies, or spinal nerve paralysis. *Cardiovascular:* hypotension due to vasomotor paralysis and pooling of the blood in the venous bed. *Respiratory:* respiratory impairment or paralysis due to the level of anesthesia extending to the upper thoracic and cervical segments. *Gastrointestinal:* nausea and vomiting.
Treatment of Reactions. Toxic effects of local anesthetics require symptomatic treatment: there is no specific cure. The physician should be prepared to maintain an airway and to support ventilation with oxygen and assisted or controlled respiration as required. Supportive treatment of the cardiovascular system includes intravenous fluids and, when appropriate, vasopressors (preferably those that stimulate the myocardium, such as ephedrine). Convulsions may be controlled with oxygen and by the intravenous administration of diazepam or ultrashort-acting barbiturates or a short-acting muscle relaxant (succinylcholine). Intravenous anticonvulsant agents and muscle relaxants should only be administered by those familiar with their use and only when ventilation and oxygenation are assured. In spinal and epidural anesthesia, sympathetic blockade also occurs as a pharmacological reaction, resulting in peripheral vasodilation and often *hypotension.* The extent of the hypotension will usually depend on the number of dermatomes blocked. The blood pressure should therefore be monitored in the early phases of anesthesia. If hypotension occurs, it is readily controlled by vasoconstrictors administered either by the intramuscular or the intravenous route, the dosage of which would depend on the severity of the hypotension and the response to treatment.

DOSAGE AND ADMINISTRATION
As with all local anesthetics, the dose of NOVOCAIN, brand of procaine hydrochloride injection, varies and depends upon the area to be anesthetized, the vascularity of the tissues, the number of neuronal segments to be blocked, individual tolerance, and the technique of anesthesia. The lowest dose needed to provide effective anesthesia should be adminis-

tered. For specific techniques and procedures, refer to standard textbooks.
[See table right].
The diluent may be sterile normal saline, sterile distilled water, spinal fluid; and for hyperbaric technique, sterile dextrose solution.
The usual rate of injection is 1 mL per 5 seconds. Full anesthesia and fixation usually occur in 5 minutes.

STERILIZATION

The drug in intact ampuls is sterile. The preferred method of destroying bacteria on the exterior of ampuls before opening is heat sterilization (autoclaving). Immersion in antiseptic solution is not recommended.
Autoclave at 15-pound pressure, at 121°C (250°F), for 15 minutes. The diluent dextrose may show some brown discoloration due to caramelization.

HOW SUPPLIED

Ampuls of 2 mL (200 mg) UNI-NEST PAK of 25 (**NDC** 0024-1384-25).
Protect solutions from light.
The air in the ampuls has been displaced by nitrogen gas.
NW 62-O

RECOMMENDED DOSAGE FOR SPINAL ANESTHESIA

Extent of anesthesia	NOVOCAIN 10% Solution Volume of 10% Solution (mL)	Volume of Diluent (mL)	Total Dose (mg)	Site of Injection (lumbar interspace)
Perineum	0.5	0.5	50	4th
Perineum and lower extremities	1	1	100	3rd or 4th
Up to costal margin	2	1	200	2nd, 3rd or 4th

PEDIACOF® Ⓒ ℞

DESCRIPTION

Each teaspoon (5 mL) contains:
Codeine phosphate, USP .... 5.0 mg
(Warning: May be habit forming.)
Phenylephrine hydrochloride, USP .... 2.5 mg
Chlorpheniramine maleate, USP .... 0.75 mg
Potassium iodide, USP .... 75.0 mg
with sodium benzoate 0.2% as preservative and alcohol 5%.
Inactive Ingredients: Alcohol, Citric Acid, FD&C Red #40, Flavor, Glycerin, Liquid Glucose, Purified Water, Saccharin Sodium, Sodium Benzoate.

HOW SUPPLIED

Bottle of 16 fl oz (**NDC 0024-1509-06**)
Available on prescription only.
For complete prescribing information see package insert or contact Winthrop-Breon Medical Department.
PW-295-K

pHisoDerm® OTC

(See PDR For Nonprescription Drugs)

pHisoHex® ℞

brand of hexachlorophene detergent cleanser

sudsing antibacterial soapless skin cleanser

DESCRIPTION

pHisoHex, brand of hexachlorophene detergent cleanser, is an antibacterial sudsing emulsion for topical administration. pHisoHex contains a colloidal dispersion of hexachlorophene 3% (w/w) in a stable emulsion consisting of entsufon sodium, petrolatum, lanolin cholesterols, methylcellulose, polyethylene glycol, polyethylene glycol monostearate, lauryl myristyl diethanolamide, sodium benzoate, and water. pH is adjusted with hydrochloric acid. Entsufon sodium is a synthetic detergent.
Chemically, hexachlorophene is Phenol, 2, 2'-methylenebis[3,4,6-trichloro-.

CLINICAL PHARMACOLOGY

pHisoHex is a bacteriostatic cleansing agent. It cleanses the skin thoroughly and has bacteriostatic action against staphylococci and other gram-positive bacteria. Cumulative antibacterial action develops with repeated use. Cleansing with alcohol or soaps containing alcohol removes the antibacterial residue.
Detectable blood levels of hexachlorophene following absorption through intact skin have been found in subjects who regularly scrubbed with hexachlorophene emulsion 3%. (See **WARNINGS** for additional information.)
pHisoHex has the same slight acidity as normal skin (pH value 5.0 to 6.0).

INDICATIONS AND USAGE

pHisoHex is indicated for use as a surgical scrub and a bacteriostatic skin cleanser. It may also be used to control an outbreak of gram-positive infection where other infection control procedures have been unsuccessful. Use only as long as necessary for infection control.

CONTRAINDICATIONS

pHisoHex should not be used on burned or denuded skin.
It should not be used as an occlusive dressing, wet pack, or lotion.
It should not be used routinely for prophylactic total body bathing.
It should not be used as a vaginal pack or tampon, or on any mucous membranes.
pHisoHex should not be used on persons with sensitivity to any of its components. It should not be used on persons who have demonstrated primary light sensitivity to halogenated phenol derivatives because of the possibility of cross-sensitivity to hexachlorophene.

WARNINGS

RINSE THOROUGHLY AFTER EACH USE. Patients should be closely monitored and use should be immediately discontinued at the first sign of any of the symptoms described below.
Rapid absorption of hexachlorophene may occur with resultant toxic blood levels when preparations containing hexachlorophene are applied to skin lesions such as ichthyosis congenita, the dermatitis of Letterer-Siwe's syndrome, or other generalized dermatological conditions. Application to burns has also produced neurotoxicity and death.
PHISOHEX SHOULD BE DISCONTINUED PROMPTLY IF SIGNS OR SYMPTOMS OF CEREBRAL IRRITABILITY OCCUR.
Infants, especially premature infants or those with dermatoses, are particularly susceptible to hexachlorophene absorption. Systemic toxicity may be manifested by signs of stimulation (irritation) of the central nervous system, sometimes with convulsions.
Infants have developed dermatitis, irritability, generalized clonic muscular contractions and decerebrate rigidity following application of a 6 percent hexachlorophene powder. Examination of brainstems of those infants revealed vacuolization like that which can be produced in newborn experimental animals following repeated topical application of 3 percent hexachlorophene. Moreover, a study of histologic sections of premature infants who died of unrelated causes has shown a positive correlation between hexachlorophene baths and lesions in white matter of brains.

PRECAUTIONS

General—pHisoHex suds that get into the eyes accidentally during washing should be rinsed out promptly and thoroughly with water.
RINSE THOROUGHLY AFTER USE, especially from sensitive areas such as the scrotum and perineum.
pHisoHex is intended for external use only. If swallowed, pHisoHex is harmful, especially to infants and children. **pHisoHex should not be poured into measuring cups, medicine bottles, or similar containers since it may be mistaken for baby formula or other medications.**
Carcinogenesis, Mutagenesis, Impairment of Fertility
Carcinogenicity studies in animals: Hexachlorophene was tested in one experiment in rats by oral administration; it had no carcinogenic effect.
Hexachlorophene was not mutagenic in *Salmonella typhimurium* and was negative in a dominant lethal assay in male mice. Cytogenetic tests with cultured human lymphocytes were also negative.
Human data: No case reports or epidemiological studies were available.
Impairment of fertility: Topical exposure of neonatal rats to 3% hexachlorophene solution caused reduced fertility in 7-month-old males, due to inability to ejaculate.
Embryotoxicity and Teratogenicity
Placental transfer of hexachlorophene has been demonstrated in rats.
Hexachlorophene is embryotoxic and produces some teratogenic effects.
Pregnancy Category C
There are no adequate and well-controlled studies in pregnant women. Hexachlorophene should be used during pregnancy only if the potential benefit justifies potential risk to the fetus.
Hexachlorophene has been shown to be teratogenic and embryotoxic in rats when given by mouth or instilled into the vagina in large doses.
Administration of 500 mg/kg diet or 20 to 30 mg/kg bw/day by gavage to rats caused some malformations (angulated ribs, cleft palate, micro- and anophthalmia) and reduction in litter size.
Placental transfer and excretion in milk of hexachlorophene has been demonstrated in rats.
In another study, doses of up to 50 mg/kg diet failed to produce any effects in 3 generations of rats. Hexachlorophene did not interfere with reproduction in hamsters.
Nursing Mothers
It is not known whether this drug is excreted in human milk. Because many drugs are excreted in human milk and because of the potential for serious adverse reactions in nursing infants from hexachlorophene, a decision should be made whether to discontinue nursing or to discontinue the drug taking into account the importance of the drug to the mother.
Pediatric Use
pHisoHex, brand of hexachlorophene detergent cleanser, should not be used routinely for bathing infants. See **WARNINGS.** For premature infants: see **WARNINGS.**

ADVERSE REACTIONS

Adverse reactions to pHisoHex may include dermatitis and photosensitivity. Sensitivity to hexachlorophene is rare; however, persons who have developed photoallergy to similar compounds also may become sensitive to hexachlorophene.
In persons with highly sensitive skin the use of pHisoHex may at times produce a reaction characterized by redness and/or mild scaling or dryness, especially when it is combined with such mechanical factors as excessive rubbing or exposure to heat or cold.

OVERDOSAGE

The accidental ingestion of pHisoHex in amounts from 1 oz to 4 oz has caused anorexia, vomiting, abdominal cramps, diarrhea, dehydration, convulsions, hypotension, and shock, and in several reported instances, fatalities.
If patients are seen early, the stomach should be evacuated by emesis or gastric lavage. Olive oil or vegetable oil (60 mL or 2 fl oz) may then be given to delay absorption of hexachlorophene, followed by a saline cathartic to hasten removal. Treatment is symptomatic and supportive; intravenous fluids (5 percent dextrose in physiologic saline solution) may be given for dehydration. Any other electrolyte derangement should be corrected. If marked hypotension occurs, vasopressor therapy is indicated. Use of opiates may be considered if gastrointestinal symptoms (cramping, diarrhea) are severe. Scheduled medical or surgical procedures should be postponed until the patient's condition has been evaluated and stabilized.

DOSAGE AND ADMINISTRATION

Surgical Hand Scrub—
1. Wet hands and forearms with water. Apply approximately 5 mL of pHisoHex over the hands and rub into a copious lather by adding small amounts of water. Spread suds over hands and forearms and scrub well with a wet brush for 3 minutes. Pay particular attention to the nails and interdigital spaces. A separate nail cleaner may be used. *Rinse thoroughly* under running water.
2. Apply 5 mL of pHisoHex to hands again and scrub as above for another 3 minutes. *Rinse thoroughly* with running water and dry.
3. For repeat surgical scrubs during the day, scrub thoroughly with the same amount of pHisoHex for 3 minutes only. *Rinse thoroughly* with water and dry.
Bacteriostatic Cleansing—
Wet hands with water. Dispense approximately 5 mL of pHisoHex into the palm, work up a lather with water and apply to area to be cleansed.

Continued on next page

This product information was effective as of December 1, 1986. On these and other products of Winthrop-Breon Laboratories, detailed information may be obtained on a current basis by direct inquiry to the Professional Services Department, 90 Park Avenue, New York, NY 10016 (212) 907-2525.

Winthrop-Breon—Cont.

Rinse thoroughly after each washing.
INFANT CARE: pHisoHex should not be used routinely for bathing infants. See **WARNINGS.**
PREMATURE INFANTS: See **WARNINGS.**
Use of baby skin products containing alcohol may decrease the antibacterial action of pHisoHex, brand of hexachlorophene detergent cleanser.

HOW SUPPLIED

pHisoHex is available in plastic squeeze bottle of 5 ounces (NDC 0024-1535-02) and 1 pint (NDC 0024-1535-06); in plastic bottle of 1 gallon (NDC 0024-1535-08) and 1/4 oz (8 mL) unit packets, box of 50 (NDC 0024-1535-05).
The following, specially constructed, refillable dispensers made with metals and plastics compatible with pHisoHex can also be supplied: 16 oz hand operated wall dispensers; 30 oz pedal operated wall dispensers; 30 oz pedal operated wall dispenser with stand; portable stand with two 30 oz pedal operated dispensers.
Prolonged direct exposure of pHisoHex to strong light may cause brownish surface discoloration but does not affect its antibacterial or detergent properties. Shaking will disperse the color. If pHisoHex is spilled or splashed on porous surfaces, rinse off to avoid discoloration.

pHisoHex should not be dispensed from, or stored in, containers with ordinary metal parts. A special type of stainless steel must be used or undesirable discoloration of the product or oxidation of metal may occur. Specially designed dispensers for hospital or office use may be obtained through your local dealer.

Directions for Cleaning Dispensers: Before initial installation and use, run an antiseptic, such as an aqueous solution of benzalkonium chloride, NF, 1:500 to 1:750, or alcohol, through the working parts; rinse with sterile water. At weekly intervals thereafter, remove dispenser and pour off remainder of pHisoHex emulsion. Rinse empty dispenser with water. Run water through the working parts by operating the dispenser. Sanitize as described above. Rinse thoroughly with sterile water.

ANIMAL TOXICITY

The oral LD_{50} of hexachlorophene in male rats is 66 mg/kg bw, in females 56 mg/kg bw, and in weanling rats 120 mg/kg bw.
In suckling rats (10-days old), it is 9 mg/kg bw.

PW-61-CC

PLAQUENIL® Sulfate ℞
brand of hydroxychloroquine sulfate tablets, USP

WARNING
PHYSICIANS SHOULD COMPLETELY FAMILIARIZE THEMSELVES WITH THE COMPLETE CONTENTS OF THIS LEAFLET BEFORE PRESCRIBING HYDROXYCHLOROQUINE.

DESCRIPTION

The compound is a colorless crystalline solid, soluble in water to at least 20 percent; chemically the drug is 2-[[4-[(7-Chloro-4- quinolyl) amino] pentyl] ethylamino] ethanol sulfate (1:1).
Inactive Ingredients: Dibasic Calcium Phosphate, Magnesium Stearate, Starch.

ACTIONS

The drug possesses antimalarial actions and also exerts a beneficial effect in lupus erythematosus (chronic discoid or systemic) and acute or chronic rheumatoid arthritis. The precise mechanism of action is not known.

INDICATIONS

PLAQUENIL is indicated for the suppressive treatment and treatment of acute attacks of malaria due to *Plasmodium vivax, P. malariae, P. ovale,* and susceptible strains of *P. falciparum.* It is also indicated for the treatment of discoid and systemic lupus erythematosus, and rheumatoid arthritis.

CONTRAINDICATIONS

Use of this drug is contraindicated (1) in the presence of retinal or visual field changes attributable to any 4-aminoquinoline compound, (2) in patients with known hypersensitivity to 4-aminoquinoline compounds, and (3) for long-term therapy in children.

WARNINGS, General

PLAQUENIL is not effective against chloroquine-resistant strains of *P. falciparum.*
Children are especially sensitive to the 4-aminoquinoline compounds. A number of fatalities have been reported following the accidental ingestion of chloroquine, sometimes in relatively small doses (0.75 g or 1 g in one 3- year-old child). Patients should be strongly warned to keep these drugs out of the reach of children.
Use of PLAQUENIL in patients with psoriasis may precipitate a severe attack of psoriasis. When used in patients with porphyria the condition may be exacerbated. The preparation should not be used in these conditions unless in the judgment of the physician the benefit to the patient outweighs the possible hazard.
Usage in Pregnancy—Usage of this drug during pregnancy should be avoided except in the suppression or treatment of malaria when in the judgment of the physician the benefit outweighs the possible hazard. It should be noted that radioactively-tagged chloroquine administered intravenously to pregnant, pigmented CBA mice passed rapidly across the placenta. It accumulated selectively in the melanin structures of the fetal eyes and was retained in the ocular tissues for five months after the drug had been eliminated from the rest of the body.

PRECAUTIONS, General

Antimalarial compounds should be used with caution in patients with hepatic disease or alcoholism or in conjunction with known hepatotoxic drugs.
Periodic blood cell counts should be made if patients are given prolonged therapy. If any severe blood disorder appears which is not attributable to the disease under treatment, discontinuation of the drug should be considered. The drug should be administered with caution in patients having G-6-PD (glucose-6-phosphate dehydrogenase) deficiency.

OVERDOSAGE

The 4-aminoquinoline compounds are very rapidly and completely absorbed after ingestion, and in accidental overdosage, or rarely with lower doses in hypersensitive patients, toxic symptoms may occur within 30 minutes. These consist of headache, drowsiness, visual disturbances, cardiovascular collapse, and convulsions, followed by sudden and early respiratory and cardiac arrest. The electrocardiogram may reveal atrial standstill, nodal rhythm, prolonged intraventricular conduction time, and progressive bradycardia leading to ventricular fibrillation and/or arrest. Treatment is symptomatic and must be prompt with immediate evacuation of the stomach by emesis (at home, before transportation to the hospital) or gastric lavage until the stomach is completely emptied. If finely powdered, activated charcoal is introduced by the stomach tube, after lavage, and within 30 minutes after ingestion of the tablets, it may inhibit further intestinal absorption of the drug. To be effective, the dose of activated charcoal should be at least five times the estimated dose of hydroxychloroquine ingested. Convulsions, if present, should be controlled before attempting gastric lavage. If due to cerebral stimulation, cautious administration of an ultrashort-acting barbiturate may be tried but, if due to anoxia, it should be corrected by oxygen administration, artificial respiration or, in shock with hypotension, by vasopressor therapy. Because of the importance of supporting respiration, tracheal intubation or tracheostomy, followed by gastric lavage, may also be necessary. Exchange transfusions have been used to reduce the level of 4-aminoquinoline drug in the blood.
A patient who survives the acute phase and is asymptomatic should be closely observed for at least six hours. Fluids may be forced, and sufficient ammonium chloride (8 g daily in divided doses for adults) may be administered for a few days to acidify the urine to help promote urinary excretion in cases of both overdosage and sensitivity.

MALARIA

ACTIONS

Like chloroquine phosphate, USP, PLAQUENIL sulfate is highly active against the erythrocytic forms of *P. vivax* and *malariae* and most strains of *P. falciparum* (but not the gametocytes of *P. falciparum).*
PLAQUENIL sulfate does not prevent relapses in patients with *vivax* or *malariae* malaria because it is not effective against exo-erythrocytic forms of the parasite, nor will it prevent *vivax* or *malariae* infection when administered as a prophylactic. It is highly effective as a suppressive agent in patients with *vivax* or *malariae* malaria, in terminating acute attacks, and significantly lengthening the interval between treatment and relapse. In patients with *falciparum* malaria, it abolishes the acute attack and effects complete cure of the infection, unless due to a resistant strain of *P. falciparum.*

INDICATIONS

PLAQUENIL sulfate, brand of hydroxychloroquine sulfate tablets, is indicated for the treatment of acute attacks and suppression of malaria.

WARNING

In recent years, it has been found that certain strains of *P. falciparum* have become resistant to 4-aminoquinoline compounds (including hydroxychloroquine) as shown by the fact that normally adequate doses have failed to prevent or cure clinical malaria or parasitemia. Treatment with quinine or other specific forms of therapy is therefore advised for patients infected with a resistant strain of parasites.

ADVERSE REACTIONS

Following the administration in doses adequate for the treatment of an acute malarial attack, mild and transient headache, dizziness, and gastrointestinal complaints (diarrhea, anorexia, nausea, abdominal cramps and, on rare occasions, vomiting) may occur.

DOSAGE AND ADMINISTRATION

One tablet of 200 mg of hydroxychloroquine sulfate is equivalent to 155 mg base.
Malaria: Suppression—*In adults,* 400 mg (=310 mg base) on exactly the same day of each week. *In infants and children,* the weekly suppressive dosage is 5 mg, calculated as base, per kg of body weight, but should not exceed the adult dose regardless of weight.
If circumstances permit, suppressive therapy should begin two weeks prior to exposure. However, failing this, in adults an initial double (loading) dose of 800 mg (= 620 mg base), or in children 10 mg base/kg may be taken in two divided doses, six hours apart. The suppressive therapy should be continued for eight weeks after leaving the endemic area.
Treatment of the acute attack—*In adults,* an initial dose of 800 mg (= 620 mg base) followed by 400 mg (= 310 mg base) in six to eight hours and 400 mg (310 mg base) on each of two consecutive days (total 2 g hydroxychloroquine sulfate or 1.55 g base). An alternative method, employing a single dose of 800 mg (= 620 mg base), has also proved effective.
The dosage for adults may also be calculated on the basis of body weight; this method is preferred for infants and children. A total dose representing 25 mg of base per kg of body weight is administered in three days, as follows:
First dose: 10 mg base per kg (but not exceeding a single dose of 620 mg base).
Second dose: 5 mg base per kg (but not exceeding a single dose of 310 mg base) 6 hours after first dose.
Third dose: 5 mg base per kg 18 hours after second dose.
Fourth dose: 5 mg base per kg 24 hours after third dose.
For radical cure of *vivax* and *malariae* malaria concomitant therapy with an 8-aminoquinoline compound is necessary.

LUPUS ERYTHEMATOSUS AND RHEUMATOID ARTHRITIS

INDICATIONS

PLAQUENIL is useful in patients with the following disorders who have not responded satisfactorily to drugs with less potential for serious side effects: lupus erythematosus (chronic discoid and systemic) and acute or chronic rheumatoid arthritis.

WARNINGS

PHYSICIANS SHOULD COMPLETELY FAMILIARIZE THEMSELVES WITH THE COMPLETE CONTENTS OF THIS LEAFLET BEFORE PRESCRIBING PLAQUENIL.
Irreversible retinal damage has been observed in some patients who had received long-term or high-dosage 4-aminoquinoline therapy for discoid and systemic lupus erythematosus, or rheumatoid arthritis. Retinopathy has been reported to be dose related.
When prolonged therapy with any antimalarial compound is contemplated, initial (base line) and periodic (every three months) ophthalmologic examinations (including visual acuity, expert slit-lamp, funduscopic, and visual field tests) should be performed.
If there is any indication of abnormality in the visual acuity, visual field, or retinal macular areas (such as pigmentary changes, loss of foveal reflex), or any visual symptoms (such as light flashes and streaks) which are not fully explainable by difficulties of accommodation or corneal opacities, the drug should be discontinued immediately and the patient closely observed for possible progression. Retinal changes (and visual disturbances) may progress even after cessation of therapy.
All patients on long-term therapy with this preparation should be questioned and examined periodically, including the testing of knee and ankle reflexes, to detect any evidence of muscular weakness. If weakness occurs, discontinue the drug.
In the treatment of rheumatoid arthritis, if objective improvement (such as reduced joint swelling, increased mobility) does not occur within six months, the drug should be discontinued. Safe use of the drug in the treatment of juvenile arthritis has not been established.

PRECAUTIONS

Dermatologic reactions to PLAQUENIL sulfate, brand of hydroxychloroquine sulfate tablets, may occur and, therefore, proper care should be exercised when it is administered to any patient receiving a drug with a significant tendency to produce dermatitis.

The methods recommended for early diagnosis of "chloroquine retinopathy" consist of (1) funduscopic examination of the macula for fine pigmentary disturbances or loss of the foveal reflex and (2) examination of the central visual field with a small red test object for pericentral or paracentral scotoma or determination of retinal thresholds to red. Any unexplained visual symptoms, such as light flashes or streaks should also be regarded with suspicion as possible manifestations of retinopathy.

If serious toxic symptoms occur from overdosage or sensitivity, it has been suggested that ammonium chloride (8 g daily in divided doses for adults) be administered orally three or four days a week for several months after therapy has been stopped, as acidification of the urine increases renal excretion of the 4-aminoquinoline compounds by 20 to 90 percent. However, caution must be exercised in patients with impaired renal function and/or metabolic acidosis.

ADVERSE REACTIONS

Not all of the following reactions have been observed with every 4-aminoquinoline compound during long-term therapy, but they have been reported with one or more and should be borne in mind when drugs of this class are administered. Adverse effects with different compounds vary in type and frequency.

CNS Reactions: Irritability, nervousness, emotional changes, nightmares, psychosis, headache, dizziness, vertigo, tinnitus, nystagmus, nerve deafness, convulsions, ataxia.

Neuromuscular Reactions: Extraocular muscle palsies, skeletal muscle weakness, absent or hypoactive deep tendon reflexes.

Ocular Reactions:

A. *Ciliary body:* Disturbance of accommodation with symptoms of blurred vision. This reaction is dose related and reversible with cessation of therapy.

B. *Cornea:* Transient edema, punctate to lineal opacities, decreased corneal sensitivity. The corneal changes, with or without accompanying symptoms (blurred vision, halos around lights, photophobia), are fairly common, but reversible. Corneal deposits may appear as early as three weeks following initiation of therapy.

The incidence of corneal changes and visual side effects appears to be considerably lower with hydroxychloroquine than with chloroquine.

C. *Retina:*

Macula: Edema, atrophy, abnormal pigmentation (mild pigment stippling to a "bull's-eye" appearance), loss of foveal reflex, increased macular recovery time following exposure to a bright light (photo-stress test), elevated retinal threshold to red light in macular, paramacular and peripheral retinal areas.

Other fundus changes include optic disc pallor and atrophy, attenuation of retinal arterioles, fine granular pigmentary disturbances in the peripheral retina and prominent choroidal patterns in advanced stage.

D. *Visual field defects:* pericentral or paracentral scotoma, central scotoma with decreased visual acuity, rarely field constriction.

The most common visual symptoms attributed to the retinopathy are: reading and seeing difficulties (words, letters, or parts of objects missing), photophobia, blurred distance vision, missing or blacked out areas in the central or peripheral visual field, light flashes and streaks.

Retinopathy appears to be dose related and has occurred within several months (rarely) to several years of daily therapy; a small number of cases have been reported several years after antimalarial drug therapy was discontinued. It has not been noted during prolonged use of weekly doses of the 4-aminoquinoline compounds for suppression of malaria.

Patients with retinal changes may have visual symptoms or may be asymptomatic (with or without visual field changes). Rarely scotomatous vision or field defects may occur without obvious retinal change.

Retinopathy may progress even after the drug is discontinued. In a number of patients, early retinopathy (macular pigmentation sometimes with central field defects) diminished or regressed completely after therapy was discontinued. Paracentral scotoma to red targets (sometimes called "premaculopathy") is indicative of early retinal dysfunction which is usually reversible with cessation of therapy.

A small number of cases of retinal changes have been reported as occurring in patients who received only hydroxychloroquine. These usually consisted of alteration in retinal pigmentation which was detected on periodic ophthalmologic examination; visual field defects were also present in some instances. A case of delayed retinopathy has been reported with loss of vision starting one year after administration of hydroxychloroquine had been discontinued.

Dermatologic Reactions: Bleaching of hair, alopecia, pruritus, skin and mucosal pigmentation, skin eruptions (urticarial, morbilliform, lichenoid, maculopapular, purpuric, erythema annulare centrifugum and exfoliative dermatitis).

Hematologic Reactions: Various blood dyscrasias such as aplastic anemia, agranulocytosis, leukopenia, thrombocytopenia (hemolysis in individuals with glucose-6-phosphate dehydrogenase (G-6-PD) deficiency).

Gastrointestinal Reactions: Anorexia, nausea, vomiting, diarrhea, and abdominal cramps.

Miscellaneous Reactions: Weight loss, lassitude, exacerbation or precipitation of porphyria and nonlight-sensitive psoriasis.

DOSAGE AND ADMINISTRATION

One tablet of hydroxychloroquine sulfate, 200 mg, is equivalent to 155 mg base.

Lupus erythematosus—Initially, the average *adult* dose is 400 mg (=310 mg base) once or twice daily. This may be continued for several weeks or months, depending on the response of the patient. For prolonged maintenance therapy, a smaller dose, from 200 mg to 400 mg (=155 mg to 310 mg base) daily will frequently suffice.

The incidence of retinopathy has been reported to be higher when this maintenance dose is exceeded.

Rheumatoid arthritis—The compound is cumulative in action and will require several weeks to exert its beneficial therapeutic effects, whereas minor side effects may occur relatively early. Several months of therapy may be required before maximum effects can be obtained. If objective improvement (such as reduced joint swelling, increased mobility) does not occur within six months, the drug should be discontinued. Safe use of the drug in the treatment of juvenile rheumatoid arthritis has not been established.

Initial dosage—In ***adults,*** from 400 mg to 600 mg (=310 mg to 465 mg base) daily, each dose to be taken with a meal or a glass of milk. In a small percentage of patients, troublesome side effects may require temporary reduction of the initial dosage. Later (usually from five to ten days), the dose may gradually be increased to the optimum response level, often without return of side effects.

Maintenance dosage—When a good response is obtained (usually in four to twelve weeks), the dosage is reduced by 50 percent and continued at a usual maintenance level of 200 mg to 400 mg (=155 mg to 310 mg base) daily, each dose to be taken with a meal or a glass of milk. The incidence of retinopathy has been reported to be higher when this maintenance dose is exceeded.

Should a relapse occur after medication is withdrawn, therapy may be resumed or continued on an intermittent schedule if there are no ocular contraindications.

Corticosteroids and salicylates may be used in conjunction with this compound, and they can generally be decreased gradually in dosage or eliminated after the drug has been used for several weeks. When gradual reduction of steroid dosage is indicated, it may be done by reducing every four to five days the dose of cortisone by no more than from 5 mg to 15 mg; of hydrocortisone from 5 mg to 10 mg; of prednisolone and prednisone from 1 mg to 2.5 mg; of methylprednisolone and triamcinolone from 1 mg to 2 mg; and of dexamethasone from 0.25 mg to 0.5 mg.

HOW SUPPLIED

Tablets of 200 mg (equivalent to 155 mg of base), bottles of 100.

Distributed by Winthrop-Breon Laboratories
Division of Sterling Drug Inc.
New York, NY 10016
Manufactured by Sterling Pharmaceuticals Inc.
Barceloneta, Puerto Rico 00617

Shown in Product Identification Section, page 435

PW-306-P

PONTOCAINE® Hydrochloride ℞

brand of tetracaine hydrochloride, USP

Prolonged Spinal Anesthesia

DESCRIPTION

Tetracaine hydrochloride is 2-(dimethylamino) ethyl *p*-(butylamino) benzoate monohydrochloride. It is a white crystalline, odorless powder that is readily soluble in water, physiologic saline solution, and dextrose solution.

Tetracaine hydrochloride is a local anesthetic of the ester-linkage type, related to procaine.

PONTOCAINE hydrochloride is supplied in two forms for prolonged spinal anesthesia: Niphanoid® and 1% solution.

Niphanoid®: A sterile, instantly soluble form consisting of a network of extremely fine, highly purified particles, resembling snow.

1% solution: A sterile, isotonic, isobaric solution, each 1 mL containing 10 mg tetracaine hydrochloride, 6.7 mg sodium chloride, and not more than 2 mg acetone sodium bisulfite. The air in the ampuls has been displaced by nitrogen gas. The pH is 3.2 to 6.0.

These formulations do not contain preservatives.

CLINICAL PHARMACOLOGY

Parenteral administration of PONTOCAINE stabilizes the neuronal membrane and prevents initiation and transmission of nerve impulses thereby effecting local anesthesia.

The onset of action is rapid, and the duration prolonged (up to two or three hours or longer of surgical anesthesia).

PONTOCAINE is detoxified by plasma esterases to para-aminobenzoic acid and diethylaminoethanol.

INDICATIONS AND USAGE

PONTOCAINE is indicated for the production of spinal anesthesia for procedures requiring two to three hours.

CONTRAINDICATIONS

Spinal anesthesia with PONTOCAINE is contraindicated in patients with known hypersensitivity to tetracaine hydrochloride or to drugs of a similar chemical configuration (ester-type local anesthetics), or para- aminobenzoic acid or its derivatives; and in patients for whom spinal anesthesia as a technique is contraindicated.

The decision as to whether or not spinal anesthesia should be used for an individual patient should be made by the physician after weighing the advantages with the risks and possible complications. Contraindications to spinal anesthesia as a technique can be found in standard reference texts, and usually include generalized septicemia, infection at the site of injection, certain diseases of the cerebrospinal system, uncontrolled hypotension, etc.

WARNINGS

RESUSCITATIVE EQUIPMENT AND DRUGS SHOULD BE IMMEDIATELY AVAILABLE WHENEVER ANY LOCAL ANESTHETIC DRUG IS USED.

Large doses of local anesthetics should not be used in patients with heart block.

Reactions resulting in fatality have occurred on rare occasions with the use of local anesthetics, even in the absence of a history of hypersensitivity.

PRECAUTIONS

The safety and effectiveness of any spinal anesthetic depend upon proper dosage, correct technique, adequate precautions, and readiness for emergencies. The lowest dosage that results in effective anesthesia should be used to avoid high plasma levels and serious systemic side effects. Tolerance varies with the status of the patient; debilitated, elderly patients or acutely ill patients should be given reduced doses commensurate with their weight, age, and physical status. Reduced doses are also indicated for obstetric patients and those with increased intraabdominal pressure.

Caution should be used in administering PONTOCAINE to patients with abnormal or reduced levels of plasma esterases.

Blood pressure should be frequently monitored during spinal anesthesia and hypotension immediately corrected.

Spinal anesthetics should be used with caution in patients with severe disturbances of cardiac rhythm, shock or heart block.

Drug Interactions: PONTOCAINE should not be used if the patient is being treated with a sulfonamide because para-aminobenzoic acid inhibits the action of sulfonamides.

Carcinogenesis, mutagenesis, impairment of fertility: Long-term animal studies to evaluate carcinogenic potential and reproduction studies in animals have not been performed. There is no evidence from human data that PONTOCAINE may be carcinogenic or that it impairs fertility.

Pregnancy Category C: Animal reproduction studies have not been conducted with PONTOCAINE. It is not known whether PONTOCAINE can cause fetal harm when administered to a pregnant woman or can affect reproduction capacity. PONTOCAINE should be given to a pregnant woman only if clearly needed and the potential benefits outweigh the risk.

Labor and delivery: Vasopressor agents administered for the treatment of hypotension resulting from spinal anesthesia may result in severe persistent hypertension and/or rupture of cerebral blood vessels if oxytocic drugs have also been administered; therefore, vasopressors should be used with extreme caution in the presence of oxytocic drugs.

PONTOCAINE has a recognized use during labor and delivery; the effect of the drug on duration of labor, incidence of forceps delivery, status of the newborn, and later growth and development of the child have not been studied.

Nursing mothers: It is not known whether PONTOCAINE is excreted in human milk; however, it is rapidly metabolized following absorption into the plasma. Because many drugs are excreted in human milk, caution should be exercised when PONTOCAINE, brand of tetracaine hydrochloride, is administered to a nursing woman.

Pediatric use: Safety and effectiveness of PONTOCAINE in children have not been established.

Continued on next page

This product information was effective as of December 1, 1986. On these and other products of Winthrop-Breon Laboratories, detailed information may be obtained on a current basis by direct inquiry to the Professional Services Department, 90 Park Avenue, New York, NY 10016 (212) 907-2525.

Winthrop-Breon—Cont.

ADVERSE REACTIONS

Systemic adverse reactions to PONTOCAINE are characteristic of those associated with other local anesthetics and can involve the central nervous system and the cardiovascular system. Systemic reactions usually result from high plasma levels due to excessive dosage, rapid absorption, or inadvertent intravascular injection.

A small number of reactions to PONTOCAINE may result from hypersensitivity, idiosyncrasy or diminished tolerance to normal dosage.

Central nervous system effects are characterized by excitation or depression. The first manifestation may be nervousness, dizziness, blurred vision, or tremors, followed by drowsiness, convulsions, unconsciousness and possibly respiratory and cardiac arrest. Since excitement may be transient or absent, the first manifestation may be drowsiness, sometimes merging into unconsciousness and respiratory and cardiac arrest. Other central nervous system effects may be nausea, vomiting, chills, constriction of the pupils, or tinnitus.

Cardiovascular system reactions include depression of the myocardium, blood pressure changes (usually hypotension), and cardiac arrest.

Allergic reactions, which may be due to hypersensitivity, idiosyncrasy or diminished tolerance, are characterized by cutaneous lesions (eg, urticaria), edema, and other manifestations of allergy. Detection of sensitivity by skin testing is of limited value. Severe allergic reactions including anaphylaxis have occurred rarely and are not usually dose-related.

Reactions associated with spinal anesthesia techniques: Central nervous system: post-spinal headache, meningismus, arachnoiditis, palsies, or spinal nerve paralysis. Cardiovascular: hypotension due to vasomotor paralysis and pooling of the blood in the venous bed. Respiratory: respiratory impairment or paralysis due to the level of anesthesia extending to the upper thoracic and cervical segments. Gastrointestinal: nausea and vomiting.

Treatment of reactions: Toxic effects of local anesthetics require symptomatic treatment; there is no specific cure. **The most important measure is oxygenation of the patient by maintaining an airway and supporting ventilation.** Supportive treatment of the cardiovascular system includes intravenous fluids and, when appropriate, vasopressors (preferably those that stimulate the myocardium). Convulsions are usually controlled with adequate oxygenation alone but intravenous administration in small increments of a barbiturate (preferably an ultrashort-acting barbiturate such as thiopental and thiamylal) or diazepam can be utilized. Intravenous barbiturates or anticonvulsant agents should only be administered by those familiar with their use and only if ventilation and oxygenation have first been assured. In spinal anesthesia, sympathetic blockade also occurs as a pharmacological action, resulting in peripheral vasodilation and often hypotension. The extent of the hypotension will usually depend on the number of dermatomes blocked. The blood pressure should therefore be monitored in the early phases of anesthesia. If hypotension occurs, it is readily controlled by vasoconstrictors administered either by the intramuscular or the intravenous route, the dosage of which would depend on the severity of the hypotension and the response to treatment.

DOSAGE AND ADMINISTRATION

As with all anesthetics, the dosage varies and depends upon the area to be anesthetized, the number of neuronal segments to be blocked, individual tolerance, and the technique of anesthesia. The lowest dosage needed to provide effective anesthesia should be administered. For specific techniques and procedures, refer to standard textbooks.

[See table below].

The extent and degree of spinal anesthesia depend upon dosage, specific gravity of the anesthetic solution, volume of solution used, force of the injection, level of puncture, position of the patient during and immediately after injection, etc.

When spinal fluid is added to either the NIPHANOID or solution, some turbidity results, the degree depending on the pH of the spinal fluid, the temperature of the solution during mixing, as well as the amount of drug and diluent employed. This cloudiness is due to the release of the *base* from the hydrochloride. Liberation of base (which is completed within the spinal canal) is held to be essential for satisfactory results with any spinal anesthetic.

The specific gravity of spinal fluid at 25°/25°C varies under normal conditions from 1.0063 to 1.0075. A solution of the instantly soluble form (NIPHANOID) in spinal fluid has only a slightly greater specific gravity. The 1% concentration in saline solution has a specific gravity of 1.0060 to 1.0074 at 25°/25°C.

A hyperbaric solution may be prepared by mixing equal volumes of the 1% solution and Dextrose Solution 10% (which is available in ampuls of 3 mL).

If the NIPHANOID form is preferred, it is first dissolved in Dextrose Solution 10% in a ratio of 1 mL dextrose to 10 mg of the anesthetic. Further dilution is made with an equal volume of spinal fluid. The resulting solution now contains 5% dextrose with 5 mg of anesthetic agent per milliliter.

A hypobaric solution may be prepared by dissolving the NIPHANOID in Sterile Water for Injection, USP (1 mg per milliliter). The specific gravity of this solution is essentially the same as that of water, 1.000 at 25°/25°C.

Examine ampuls carefully before use. Do not use solution if crystals, cloudiness, or discoloration is observed.

These formulations of tetracaine hydrochloride do not contain preservatives; therefore, unused portions should be discarded and the reconstituted NIPHANOID should be used immediately.

STERILIZATION OF AMPULS: The drug in intact ampuls is sterile. The preferred method of destroying bacteria on the exterior of ampuls before opening is heat sterilization (autoclaving). Immersion in antiseptic solution is not recommended.

Autoclave at 15-pound pressure, at 121°C (250°F) for 15 minutes. The NIPHANOID form may also be autoclaved in the same way but may lose its snowlike appearance and tend to adhere to the sides of the ampul. This may slightly decrease the rate at which the drug dissolves but does not interfere with its anesthetic potency.

Autoclaving increases likelihood of crystal formation. Unused autoclaved ampuls should be discarded. In no case should unused autoclaved ampuls be placed back in stock for later use.

HOW SUPPLIED

Protect ampuls from light and store solution under refrigeration.

NIPHANOID (instantly soluble) ampuls of 20 mg, box of 100. **NDC** 0024-1577-06

1% isotonic isobaric solution: ampuls of 2 mL, UNI-NEST™ PAK of 25

NDC 0024-1574-25

PW-56-W

SULFAMYLON® Cream ℞

brand of mafenide acetate cream, USP

Topical Antibacterial Agent for Adjunctive Therapy in Second- and Third-Degree Burns

DESCRIPTION

SULFAMYLON Cream is a soft, white, nonstaining, water-miscible, anti-infective cream for topical administration to burn wounds.

SULFAMYLON Cream spreads easily, and can be washed off readily with water. It has a slight acetic odor. Each gram of SULFAMYLON Cream contains mafenide acetate equivalent to 85 mg of the base. The cream vehicle consists of cetyl alcohol, stearyl alcohol, cetyl esters wax, polyoxyl 40 stearate, polyoxyl 8 stearate, glycerin, and water, with methylparaben, propylparaben, sodium metabisulfite, and edetate disodium as preservatives.

Chemically, mafenide acetate is α-Amino-*p*-toluenesulfonamide monoacetate.

CLINICAL PHARMACOLOGY

SULFAMYLON Cream, applied topically, produces a marked reduction in the bacterial population present in the avascular tissues of second- and third-degree burns. Reduction in bacterial growth after application of SULFAMYLON Cream has also been reported to permit spontaneous healing of deep partial-thickness burns, and thus prevent conversion of burn wounds from partial thickness to full thickness. It should be noted, however, that delayed eschar separation has occurred in some cases.

Absorption and Metabolism. Applied topically, SULFAMYLON Cream diffuses through devascularized areas, is absorbed, and rapidly converted to a metabolite (*p*-carboxybenzenesulfonamide) which is cleared through the kidneys. SULFAMYLON is active in the presence of pus and serum, and its activity is not altered by changes in the acidity of the environment.

Antibacterial Activity. SULFAMYLON exerts bacteriostatic action against many gram-negative and gram-positive organisms, including *Pseudomonas aeruginosa* and certain strains of anaerobes.

INDICATIONS AND USAGE

SULFAMYLON Cream is a topical agent indicated for adjunctive therapy of patients with second- and third-degree burns.

CONTRAINDICATIONS

SULFAMYLON is contraindicated in patients who are hypersensitive to it. It is not known whether there is cross sensitivity to other sulfonamides.

WARNINGS

Fatal hemolytic anemia with disseminated intravascular coagulation, presumably related to a glucose-6-phosphate dehydrogenase deficiency, has been reported following SULFAMYLON Cream therapy.

PRECAUTIONS

SULFAMYLON and its metabolite, *p*-carboxybenzenesulfonamide, inhibit carbonic anhydrase, which may result in metabolic acidosis, usually compensated by hyperventilation. In the presence of impaired renal function, high blood levels of SULFAMYLON and its metabolite may exaggerate the carbonic anhydrase inhibition. Therefore, close monitoring of acid-base balance is necessary, particularly in patients with extensive second-degree or partial thickness burns and in those with pulmonary or renal dysfunction. Some burn patients treated with SULFAMYLON Cream have also been reported to manifest an unexplained syndrome of marked hyperventilation with resulting respiratory alkalosis (slightly alkaline blood pH, low arterial pCO_2, and decreased total CO_2); change in arterial pO_2 is variable. The etiology and significance of these findings are unknown.

Mafenide acetate cream should be used with caution in burn patients with acute renal failure.

SULFAMYLON Cream should be administered with caution to patients with history of hypersensitivity to mafenide. It is not known whether there is cross sensitivity to other sulfonamides.

Fungal colonization in and below the eschar may occur concomitantly with reduction of bacterial growth in the burn wound. However, fungal dissemination through the infected burn wound is rare.

Carcinogenesis, Mutagenesis, Impairment of Fertility. No long-term animal studies have been performed to evaluate the drug's potential in these areas.

Pregnancy Category C. Animal reproduction studies have not been conducted with SULFAMYLON. It is also not

SUGGESTED DOSAGE FOR SPINAL ANESTHESIA

	Using NIPHANOID		Using 1% solution		
Extent of anesthesia	Dose of NIPHANOID (mg)	Volume of spinal fluid (mL)	Dose of solution (mL)	Volume of spinal fluid (mL)	Site of injection (lumbar interspace)
Perineum	5*	1	0.5 (=5 mg)*	0.5	4th
Perineum and lower extremities	10	2	1.0 (=10 mg)	1.0	3d or 4th
Up to costal margin	15 to 20†	3	1.5 to 2.0 (=15 mg to 20 mg)†	1.5 to 2.0	2d, 3d, or 4th

*For vaginal delivery (saddle block), from 2 mg to 5 mg in dextrose.

† Doses exceeding 15 mg are rarely required and should be used only in exceptional cases. Inject solution at rate of about 1 mL per 5 seconds.

known whether SULFAMYLON can cause fetal harm when administered to a pregnant woman or can affect reproduction capacity. Therefore, the preparation is not recommended for the treatment of women of childbearing potential, unless the burned area covers more than 20% of the total body surface, or the need for the therapeutic benefit of SULFAMYLON Cream is, in the physician's judgment, greater than the possible risk to the fetus.

Nursing Mothers. It is not known whether mafenide acetate is excreted in human milk. Because many drugs are excreted in human milk and because of the potential for serious adverse reaction in nursing infants from SULFAMYLON, a decision should be made whether to discontinue nursing or to discontinue the drug, taking into account the importance of the drug to the mother.

Pediatric Use. Same as for adults. (See DOSAGE AND ADMINISTRATION.)

ADVERSE REACTIONS

It is frequently difficult to distinguish between an adverse reaction to SULFAMYLON Cream and the effect of a severe burn. A single case of bone marrow depression and a single case of an acute attack of porphyria have been reported following SULFAMYLON Cream therapy. Fatal hemolytic anemia with disseminated intravascular coagulation, presumably related to a glucose-6-phosphate dehydrogenase deficiency, has been reported following SULFAMYLON Cream therapy.

Dermatologic: The most frequently reported reaction was pain on application or a burning sensation. Rare occurrences are excoriation of new skin, and bleeding of skin.

Allergic: Rash, itching, facial edema, swelling, hives, blisters, erythema, and eosinophilia.

Respiratory: Tachypnea or hyperventilation, decrease in arterial pCO_2.

Metabolic: Acidosis, increase in serum chloride.

Accidental ingestion of SULFAMYLON Cream has been reported to cause diarrhea.

DOSAGE AND ADMINISTRATION

Prompt institution of appropriate measures for controlling shock and pain is of prime importance. The burn wounds are then cleansed and debrided, and SULFAMYLON Cream, brand of mafenide acetate cream, is applied with a sterile gloved hand. Satisfactory results can be achieved with application of the cream once or twice daily, to a thickness of approximately $\frac{1}{16}$ inch; thicker application is not recommended. The burned areas should be covered with SULFAMYLON Cream at all times. Therefore, whenever necessary, the cream should be reapplied to any areas from which it has been removed (eg, by patient activity). The routine of administration can be accomplished in minimal time, since dressings usually are not required. If individual patient demands make them necessary, however, only a thin layer of dressing should be used.

When feasible, the patient should be bathed daily, to aid in debridement. A whirlpool bath is particularly helpful, but the patient may be bathed in bed or in a shower.

The duration of therapy with SULFAMYLON Cream depends on each patient's requirements. Treatment is usually continued until healing is progressing well or until the burn site is ready for grafting. *SULFAMYLON Cream should not be withdrawn from the therapeutic regimen while there is the possibility of infection.* However, if allergic manifestations occur during treatment with SULFAMYLON Cream, discontinuation of treatment should be considered.

If acidosis occurs and becomes difficult to control, particularly in patients with pulmonary dysfunction, discontinuing SULFAMYLON Cream therapy for 24 to 48 hours while continuing fluid therapy may aid in restoring acid-base balance.

HOW SUPPLIED

Cans of 14.5 ounces (411 g)—NDC 0024-1884-09
Collapsible tubes of 4 ounces (113.4 g)
NDC 0024-1884-02
Collapsible tubes of 2 ounces (56.7 g)
NDC 0024-1884-01

SW-89-J

TALACEN® Ⓒ ℞

Pentazocine hydrochloride, USP, equivalent to 25 mg base and acetaminophen, USP, 650 mg

DESCRIPTION

TALACEN is a combination of pentazocine hydrochloride, USP, equivalent to 25 mg base and acetaminophen, USP, 650 mg.

Pentazocine is a member of the benzazocine series (also known as the benzomorphan series). Chemically, pentazocine is 1,2,3,4,5,6-hexahydro-6, 11-dimethyl-3-(3-methyl-2-butenyl)-2,6-methano-3-benzazocin-8-ol, a white, crystalline substance soluble in acidic aqueous solutions.

Chemically, acetaminophen is Acetamide, *N*- (4-hydroxyphenyl).

Pentazocine is an analgesic and acetaminophen is an analgesic and antipyretic.

TALACEN is a pale blue, scored caplet for oral administration.

Inactive Ingredients: Colloidal Silicon Dioxide, FD&C Blue #1, Gelatin, Microcrystalline Cellulose, Potassium Sorbate, Pregelatinized Starch, Sodium Lauryl Sulfate, Sodium Metabisulfite, Sodium Starch Glycolate, Stearic Acid.

CLINICAL PHARMACOLOGY

TALACEN is an analgesic possessing antipyretic actions.

Pentazocine is an analgesic with agonist/antagonist action which when administered orally is approximately equivalent on a mg for mg basis in analgesic effect to codeine.

Acetaminophen is an analgesic and antipyretic.

Onset of significant analgesia with pentazocine usually occurs between 15 and 30 minutes after oral administration, and duration of action is usually three hours or longer. Onset and duration of action and the degree of pain relief are related both to dose and the severity of pretreatment pain.

Pentazocine weakly antagonizes the analgesic effects of morphine, meperidine, and phenazocine; in addition, it produces incomplete reversal of cardiovascular, respiratory, and behavioral depression induced by morphine and meperidine.

Pentazocine has about 1/50 the antagonistic activity of nalorphine. It also has sedative activity.

Pentazocine is well absorbed from the gastrointestinal tract. Plasma levels closely correspond to the onset, duration, and intensity of analgesia. The mean peak concentration in 24 normal volunteers was 1.7 hours (range 0.5 to 4.0 hours) after oral administration and the mean plasma elimination half-life was 3.6 hours (range 1.5 to 10 hours).

The action of pentazocine is terminated for the most part by biotransformation in the liver with some free pentazocine excreted in the urine. The products of the oxidation of the terminal methyl groups and glucuronide conjugates are excreted by the kidney. Elimination of approximately 60% of the total dose occurs within 24 hours. Pentazocine passes the placental barrier.

Onset of significant analgesic and antipyretic activity of acetaminophen when administered orally occurs within 30 minutes and is maximal at approximately $2\frac{1}{2}$ hours. The pharmacological mode of action of acetaminophen is unknown at this time.

Acetaminophen is rapidly and almost completely absorbed from the gastrointestinal tract. In 24 normal volunteers the mean peak plasma concentration was 1 hour (range 0.25 to 3 hours) after oral administration and the mean plasma elimination half-life was 2.8 hours (range 2 to 4 hours).

The effect of pentazocine on acetaminophen plasma protein binding or vice versa has not been established. For acetaminophen there is little or no plasma protein binding at normal therapeutic doses. When toxic doses of acetaminophen are ingested and drug plasma levels exceed 90 μg/mL, plasma binding may vary from 8% to 43%.

Acetaminophen is conjugated in the liver with glucuronic acid and to a lesser extent with sulfuric acid. Approximately 80% of acetaminophen is excreted in the urine after conjugation and about 3% is excreted unchanged. The drug is also conjugated to a lesser extent with cysteine and additionally metabolized by hydroxylation.

If TALACEN is taken every 4 hours over an extended period of time, accumulation of pentazocine and to a lesser extent, acetaminophen, may occur.

INDICATIONS AND USAGE

TALACEN is indicated for the relief of mild to moderate pain.

CONTRAINDICATIONS

TALACEN should not be administered to patients who are hypersensitive to either pentazocine or acetaminophen.

WARNINGS

Head Injury and Increased Intracranial Pressure. As in the case of other potent analgesics, the potential of pentazocine for elevating cerebrospinal fluid pressure may be attributed to CO_2 retention due to the respiratory depressant effects of the drug. These effects may be markedly exaggerated in the presence of head injury, other intracranial lesions, or a preexisting increase in intracranial pressure. Furthermore, pentazocine can produce effects which may obscure the clinical course of patients with head injuries. In such patients, TALACEN must be used with extreme caution and only if its use is deemed essential.

Acute CNS Manifestations. Patients receiving therapeutic doses of pentazocine have experienced hallucinations (usually visual), disorientation, and confusion which have cleared spontaneously within a period of hours. The mechanism of this reaction is not known. Such patients should be closely observed and vital signs checked. If the drug is reinstituted, it should be done with caution since these acute CNS manifestations may recur.

There have been instances of psychological and physical dependence on parenteral pentazocine in patients with a history of drug abuse, and rarely, in patients without such a history. (See DRUG ABUSE AND DEPENDENCE.)

Due to the potential for increased CNS depressant effects, alcohol should be used with caution in patients who are currently receiving pentazocine.

Pentazocine may precipitate opioid abstinence symptoms in patients receiving courses of opiates for pain relief.

PRECAUTIONS

In prescribing TALACEN for chronic use, the physician should take precautions to avoid increases in dose by the patient.

Myocardial Infarction. As with all drugs, TALACEN should be used with caution in patients with myocardial infarction who have nausea or vomiting.

Certain Respiratory Conditions. Although respiratory depression has rarely been reported after oral administration of pentazocine, the drug should be administered with caution to patients with respiratory depression from any cause, severely limited respiratory reserve, severe bronchial asthma and other obstructive respiratory conditions, or cyanosis.

Impaired Renal or Hepatic Function. Decreased metabolism of the drug by the liver in extensive liver disease may predispose to accentuation of side effects. Although laboratory tests have not indicated that pentazocine causes or increases renal or hepatic impairment, the drug should be administered with caution to patients with such impairment. Since acetaminophen is metabolized by the liver, the question of the safety of its use in the presence of liver disease should be considered.

Biliary Surgery. Narcotic drug products are generally considered to elevate biliary tract pressure for varying periods following their administration. Some evidence suggests that pentazocine may differ from other marketed narcotics in this respect (ie, it causes little or no elevation in biliary tract pressures). The clinical significance of these findings, however, is not yet known.

CNS Effect. Caution should be used when TALACEN is administered to patients prone to seizures; seizures have occurred in a few such patients in association with the use of pentazocine although no cause and effect relationship has been established.

Information for Patients. Since sedation, dizziness, and occasional euphoria have been noted, ambulatory patients should be warned not to operate machinery, drive cars, or unnecessarily expose themselves to hazards. Pentazocine may cause physical and psychological dependence when taken alone and may have additive CNS depressant properties when taken in combination with alcohol or other CNS depressants.

Drug Interactions. Pentazocine is a mild narcotic antagonist. Some patients previously given narcotics, including methadone for the daily treatment of narcotic dependence, have experienced withdrawal symptoms after receiving pentazocine.

Carcinogenesis, Mutagenesis, Impairment of Fertility. Carcinogenesis, mutagenesis, and impairment of fertility studies have not been done with this combination product.

Pentazocine, when administered orally or parenterally, had no adverse effect on either the reproductive capabilities or the course of pregnancy in rabbits and rats. Embryotoxic effects on the fetuses were not shown.

The daily administration of 4 mg/kg to 20 mg/kg pentazocine subcutaneously to female rats during a 14 day pre-mating period and until the 13th day of pregnancy did not have any adverse effects on the fertility rate.

There is no evidence in long-term animal studies to demonstrate that pentazocine is carcinogenic.

Pregnancy Category C. Animal reproduction studies have not been conducted with TALACEN. It is also not known whether TALACEN can cause fetal harm when administered to pregnant women or can affect reproduction capacity. TALACEN should be given to pregnant women only if clearly needed. However, animal reproduction studies with pentazocine have not demonstrated teratogenic embryotoxic effects.

Nonteratogenic Effects. There has been no experience in this regard with the combination pentazocine and acetaminophen. However, there have been rare reports of possible abstinence syndromes in newborns after prolonged use of pentazocine during pregnancy.

Labor and Delivery. Patients receiving pentazocine during labor have experienced no adverse effects other than those that occur with commonly used analgesics. TALACEN should be used with caution in women delivering premature infants. The effect of TALACEN on the mother and fetus, the duration of labor or delivery, the possibility that forceps delivery or other intervention or resuscitation of the newborn

Continued on next page

This product information was effective as of December 1, 1986. On these and other products of Winthrop-Breon Laboratories, detailed information may be obtained on a current basis by direct inquiry to the Professional Services Department, 90 Park Avenue, New York, NY 10016 (212) 907-2525.

Winthrop-Breon—Cont.

may be necessary, or the effect of TALACEN, on the later growth, development, and functional maturation of the child are unknown at the present time.
Nursing Mothers. It is not known whether this drug is excreted in human milk. Because many drugs are excreted in human milk, caution should be exercised when TALACEN is administered to a nursing woman.
Pediatric Use. Safety and effectiveness in children below the age of 12 have not been established.

ADVERSE REACTIONS

Clinical experience with TALACEN has been insufficient to define all possible adverse reactions with this combination. However, reactions reported after oral administration of pentazocine hydrochloride in 50 mg dosage include *gastrointestinal:* nausea, vomiting, infrequently constipation; and rarely abdominal distress, anorexia, diarrhea. *CNS effects:* dizziness, lightheadedness, hallucinations, sedation, euphoria, headache, confusion, disorientation; infrequently weakness, disturbed dreams, insomnia, syncope, visual blurring and focusing difficulty, depression; and rarely tremor, irritability, excitement, tinnitus. *Autonomic:* sweating; infrequently flushing; and rarely chills. *Allergic:* infrequently rash; and rarely urticaria, edema of the face. *Cardiovascular:* infrequently decrease in blood pressure, tachycardia. *Hematologic:* rarely depression of white blood cells (especially granulocytes), which is usually reversible, moderate transient eosinophilia. *Other:* rarely respiratory depression, urinary retention, paresthesia, toxic epidermal necrolysis, and in one instance, an apparent anaphylactic reaction has been reported.
Numerous clinical studies have shown that acetaminophen, when taken in recommended doses, is relatively free of adverse effects in most age groups, even in the presence of a variety of disease states.
A few cases of hypersensitivity to acetaminophen have been reported, as manifested by skin rashes, thrombocytopenic purpura, rarely hemolytic anemia and agranulocytosis. Occasional individuals respond to ordinary doses with nausea and vomiting or diarrhea.

DRUG ABUSE AND DEPENDENCE

Controlled Substance. TALACEN is a Schedule IV controlled substance.
Abuse and Dependence. There have been some reports of dependence and of withdrawal symptoms with orally administered pentazocine. There have been recorded instances of psychological and physical dependence in patients using parenteral pentazocine. Abrupt discontinuance following the extended use of parenteral pentazocine has resulted in withdrawal symptoms. Patients with a history of drug dependence should be under close supervision while receiving TALACEN. There have been rare reports of possible abstinence syndromes in newborns after prolonged use of pentazocine during pregnancy.
Some tolerance to the analgesic and subjective effects of pentazocine develops with frequent and repeated use.
Drug addicts who are given closely spaced doses of pentazocine (eg, 60 mg to 90 mg every 4 hours) develop physical dependence which is demonstrated by abrupt withdrawal or by administration of naloxone. The withdrawal symptoms exhibited after chronic doses of more than 500 mg of pentazocine per day have similar characteristics, but to a lesser degree, of opioid withdrawal and may be associated with drug seeking behavior.

OVERDOSAGE

Manifestations. Clinical experience with TALACEN has been insufficient to define the signs of overdosage with this product. It may be assumed that signs and symptoms of TALACEN overdose would be a combination of those observed with pentazocine overdose and acetaminophen overdose.
For pentazocine alone in single doses above 60 mg there have been reports of the occurrence of nalorphine-like psychotomimetic effects such as anxiety, nightmares, strange thoughts, and hallucinations. Marked respiratory depression associated with increased blood pressure and tachycardia have also resulted from excessive doses as have dizziness, nausea, vomiting, lethargy, and paresthesias. The respiratory depression is antagonized by naloxone (see *Treatment*).
In acute acetaminophen overdosage, dose-dependent, potentially fatal hepatic necrosis is the most serious adverse effect. Renal tubular necrosis, hypoglycemic coma, and thrombocytopenia may also occur.
In adults, a single dose of 10 g to 15 g (200 mg/kg to 250 mg/kg) of acetaminophen may cause hepatotoxicity. A dose of 25 g or more is potentially fatal. The potential seriousness of the intoxication may not be evident during the first two days of acute acetaminophen poisoning. During the first 24 hours, nausea, vomiting, anorexia, and abdominal pain occur. These may persist for a week or more. Liver injury may become evident the second day, initial signs being elevation of serum transaminase and lactic dehydrogenase activity, increased serum bilirubin concentration, and prolongation of prothrombin time. Serum albumin concentration and alkaline phosphatase activity may remain normal. The hepatotoxicity may lead to encephalopathy, coma, and death. Transient azotemia is evident in a majority of patients and acute renal failure occurs in some.
There have been reports of glycosuria and impaired glucose tolerance, but hypoglycemia may also occur. Metabolic acidosis and metabolic alkalosis have been reported. Cerebral edema and nonspecific myocardial depression have also been noted. Biopsy reveals centrolobular necrosis with sparing of the periportal area. The hepatic lesions are reversible over a period of weeks or months in nonfatal cases.
The severity of the liver injury can be determined by measurement of the plasma half-time of acetaminophen during the first day of acute poisoning. If the half-time exceeds 4 hours, hepatic necrosis is likely and if the half-time is greater than 12 hours, hepatic coma will probably occur. Only minimal liver damage has developed when the serum concentration was below 120 μg/mL at 12 hours after ingestion of the drug. If serum bilirubin concentration is greater than 4 mg/100 mL during the first 5 days, encephalopathy may occur.
The seven day oral LD_{50} value for TALACEN in mice is 3,570 mg/kg.
Treatment. Oxygen, intravenous fluids, vasopressors, and other supportive measures should be employed as indicated. Assisted or controlled ventilation should also be considered. For respiratory depression due to overdosage or unusual sensitivity to TALACEN, parenteral naloxone is a specific and effective antagonist.
The toxic effects of acetaminophen may be prevented or minimized by antidotal therapy with N-acetylcysteine. In order to obtain the best possible results, N-acetylcysteine should be administered within approximately 16 hours of ingestion of the overdose.
The use of N-acetylcysteine as an antidote is currently restricted to investigational use. For information and directions for use, contact the Rocky Mountain Poison Center (800-525-6115).
Vigorous supportive therapy is required in severe intoxication. Procedures to limit the continuing absorption of the drug must be readily performed since the hepatic injury is dose dependent and occurs early in the course of intoxication. Induction of vomiting or gastric lavage, followed by oral administration of activated charcoal should be done in all cases.
If hemodialysis can be initiated within the first 12 hours, it is advocated for patients with a plasma acetaminophen concentration exceeding 120 μg/mL at 4 hours after ingestion of the drug.

DOSAGE AND ADMINISTRATION

Adult. The usual adult dose is 1 tablet every 4 hours as needed for pain relief, up to a maximum of 6 tablets per day. The usual duration of therapy is dependent upon the condition being treated but in any case should be reviewed regularly by the physician. The effect of meals on the rate and extent of bioavailability of both pentazocine and acetaminophen has not been documented.

HOW SUPPLIED

Caplets®, pale blue, scored, each containing pentazocine hydrochloride equivalent to 25 mg base and acetaminophen 650 mg.
Bottles of 100 (NDC 0024-1937-04).
Unit Dose Dispenser Package of 250 (NDC 0024-1937-14), 10 sleeves of 25 CAPLETS each.

Distributed by
Winthrop-Breon Laboratories
Division of Sterling Drug Inc
New York, NY 10016
Manufactured by
Sterling Pharmaceuticals Inc
Barceloneta, Puerto Rico 00617
Shown in Product Identification Section, page 435
TW-262-H

TALWIN® Injection
brand of pentazocine lactate injection, USP

Ⓒ℞

Analgesic for Parenteral Use

DESCRIPTION

TALWIN injection, brand of pentazocine lactate injection, is a member of the benzazocine series (also known as the benzomorphan series). Chemically, pentazocine lactate is 1, 2, 3, 4, 5, 6-hexahydro-6, 11-dimethyl-3-(3-methyl-2-butenyl)-2,6-methano-3- benzazocin-8-ol lactate, a white, crystalline substance soluble in acidic aqueous solutions.

CLINICAL PHARMACOLOGY

TALWIN is a potent analgesic and 30 mg is usually as effective an analgesic as morphine 10 mg or meperidine 75 mg to 100 mg; however, a few studies suggest the TALWIN to morphine ratio may range from 20 mg to 40 mg TALWIN to 10 mg morphine. The duration of analgesia may sometimes be less than that of morphine. Analgesia usually occurs within 15 to 20 minutes after intramuscular or subcutaneous injection and within 2 to 3 minutes after intravenous injection. TALWIN weakly antagonizes the analgesic effects of morphine, meperidine, and phenazocine; in addition, it produces incomplete reversal of cardiovascular, respiratory, and behavioral depression induced by morphine and meperidine. TALWIN has about 1/50 the antagonistic activity of nalorphine. It also has sedative activity.

INDICATIONS AND USAGE

For the relief of moderate to severe pain. TALWIN may also be used for preoperative or preanesthetic medication and as a supplement to surgical anesthesia.

CONTRAINDICATION

TALWIN should not be administered to patients who are hypersensitive to it.

WARNINGS

Drug Dependence. *Special care should be exercised in prescribing pentazocine for emotionally unstable patients and for those with a history of drug misuse. Such patients should be closely supervised when greater than 4 or 5 days of therapy is contemplated. There have been instances of psychological and physical dependence on TALWIN in patients with such a history and, rarely, in patients without such a history. Extended use of parenteral TALWIN may lead to physical or psychological dependence in some patients. When TALWIN is abruptly discontinued, withdrawal symptoms such as abdominal cramps, elevated temperature, rhinorrhea, restlessness, anxiety, and lacrimation may occur. However, even when these have occurred, discontinuance has been accomplished with minimal difficulty. In the rare patient in whom more than minor difficulty has been encountered, reinstitution of parenteral TALWIN with gradual withdrawal has ameliorated the patient's symptoms. Substituting methadone or other narcotics for TALWIN in the treatment of the pentazocine abstinence syndrome should be avoided. There have been rare reports of possible abstinence syndromes in newborns after prolonged use of TALWIN during pregnancy.*
In prescribing parenteral TALWIN for chronic use, particularly if the drug is to be self-administered, the physician should take precautions to avoid increases in dose and frequency of injection by the patient.
Just as with all medication, the oral form of TALWIN is preferable for chronic administration.
Tissue Damage at Injection Sites. Severe sclerosis of the skin, subcutaneous tissues, and underlying muscle have occurred at the injection sites of patients who have received multiple doses of pentazocine lactate. Constant rotation of injection sites is, therefore, essential. In addition, animal studies have demonstrated that TALWIN is tolerated less well subcutaneously than intramuscularly. (See DOSAGE AND ADMINISTRATION.)
Head Injury and Increased Intracranial Pressure. As in the case of other potent analgesics, the potential of TALWIN injection for elevating cerebrospinal fluid pressure may be attributed to CO_2 retention due to the respiratory depressant effects of the drug. These effects may be markedly exaggerated in the presence of head injury, other intracranial lesions, or a preexisting increase in intracranial pressure. Furthermore, TALWIN can produce effects which may obscure the clinical course of patients with head injuries. In such patients, TALWIN must be used with extreme caution and only if its use is deemed essential.
Usage in Pregnancy. Safe use of TALWIN during pregnancy (other than labor) has not been established. Animal reproduction studies have not demonstrated teratogenic or embryotoxic effects. However, TALWIN should be administered to pregnant patients (other than labor) only when, in the judgment of the physician, the potential benefits outweigh the possible hazards. Patients receiving TALWIN during labor have experienced no adverse effects other than those that occur with commonly used analgesics. TALWIN should be used with caution in women delivering premature infants.
Acute CNS Manifestations. Patients receiving therapeutic doses of pentazocine have experienced hallucinations (usually visual), disorientation, and confusion which have cleared spontaneously within a period of hours. The mechanism of this reaction is not known. Such patients should be closely observed and vital signs checked. If the drug is reinstituted, it should be done with caution since these acute CNS manifestations may recur.
Due to the potential for increased CNS depressant effects, alcohol should be used with caution in patients who are currently receiving pentazocine.
Usage in Children. Because clinical experience in children under twelve years of age is limited, the use of TALWIN in this age group is not recommended.
Ambulatory Patients. Since sedation, dizziness, and occasional euphoria have been noted, ambulatory patients should be warned not to operate machinery, drive cars, or unnecessarily expose themselves to hazards.

Myocardial Infarction. Caution should be exercised in the intravenous use of pentazocine for patients with acute myocardial infarction accompanied by hypertension or left ventricular failure. Data suggest that intravenous administration of pentazocine increases systemic and pulmonary arterial pressure and systemic vascular resistance in patients with acute myocardial infarction.

PRECAUTIONS

Certain Respiratory Conditions. The possibility that TALWIN may cause respiratory depression should be considered in treatment of patients with bronchial asthma. TALWIN injection, brand of pentazocine lactate injection, should be administered only with caution and in low dosage to patients with respiratory depression (eg, from other medication, uremia, or severe infection), severely limited respiratory reserve, obstructive respiratory conditions, or cyanosis.
Impaired Renal or Hepatic Function. Although laboratory tests have not indicated that TALWIN causes or increases renal or hepatic impairment, the drug should be administered with caution to patients with such impairment. Extensive liver disease appears to predispose to greater side effects (eg, marked apprehension, anxiety, dizziness, sleepiness) from the usual clinical dose, and may be the result of decreased metabolism of the drug by the liver.
Biliary Surgery. Narcotic drug products are generally considered to elevate biliary tract pressure for varying periods following their administration. Some evidence suggests that pentazocine may differ from other marketed narcotics in this respect (ie, it causes little or no elevation in biliary tract pressures). The clinical significance of these findings, however, is not yet known.
Patients Receiving Narcotics. TALWIN is a mild narcotic antagonist. Some patients previously given narcotics, including methadone for the daily treatment of narcotic dependence, have experienced withdrawal symptoms after receiving TALWIN.
CNS Effect. Caution should be used when TALWIN is administered to patients prone to seizures; seizures have occurred in a few such patients in association with the use of TALWIN although no cause and effect relationship has been established.
Use in Anesthesia. Concomitant use of CNS depressants with parenteral TALWIN may produce additive CNS depression. Adequate equipment and facilities should be available to identify and treat systemic emergencies should they occur.

ADVERSE REACTIONS

The most commonly occurring reactions are: nausea, dizziness or lightheadedness, vomiting, euphoria.
Dermatologic Reactions: Soft tissue induration, nodules, and cutaneous depression can occur at injection sites. Ulceration (sloughing) and severe sclerosis of the skin and subcutaneous tissues (and, rarely, underlying muscle) have been reported after multiple doses.
Infrequently occurring reactions are—*respiratory:* respiratory depression, dyspnea, transient apnea in a small number of newborn infants whose mothers received TALWIN during labor; *cardiovascular:* circulatory depression, shock, hypertension; *CNS effects:* dizziness, lightheadedness, hallucinations, sedation, euphoria, headache, confusion, disorientation; infrequently weakness, disturbed dreams, insomnia, syncope, visual blurring and focusing difficulty, depression; and rarely tremor, irritability, excitement, tinnitus. *Gastrointestinal:* constipation, dry mouth; *dermatologic including local:* diaphoresis, sting on injection, flushed skin including plethora, dermatitis including pruritus; *other:* urinary retention, headache, paresthesia, alterations in rate or strength of uterine contractions during labor.
Rarely reported reactions include—*neuromuscular and psychiatric:* muscle tremor, insomnia, disorientation, hallucinations; *gastrointestinal:* taste alteration, diarrhea and cramps; *ophthalmic:* blurred vision, nystagmus, diplopia, miosis; *hematologic:* depression of white blood cells (especially granulocytes), which is usually reversible, moderate transient eosinophilia; *other:* tachycardia, weakness or faintness, chills, allergic reactions including edema of the face, toxic epidermal necrolysis.
See **Acute CNS Manifestations** and **Drug Dependence** under **WARNINGS.**

DOSAGE AND ADMINISTRATION

Adults, Excluding Patients in Labor. The recommended single parenteral dose is 30 mg by intramuscular, subcutaneous, or intravenous route. This may be repeated every 3 to 4 hours. Doses in excess of 30 mg intravenously or 60 mg intramuscularly or subcutaneously are not recommended. Total daily dosage should not exceed 360 mg.
The subcutaneous route of administration should be used only when necessary because of possible severe tissue damage at injection sites (see WARNINGS). When frequent injections are needed, the drug should be administered intramuscularly. In addition, constant rotation of injection sites (eg, the upper outer quadrants of the buttocks, mid-lateral aspects of the thighs, and the deltoid areas) is essential.
Patients in Labor. A single, intramuscular 30 mg dose has been most commonly administered. An intravenous 20 mg dose has given adequate pain relief to some patients in labor when contractions become regular, and this dose may be given two or three times at two-to three-hour intervals, as needed.
Children Under 12 Years of Age. Since clinical experience in children under twelve years of age is limited, the use of TALWIN in this age group is not recommended.
CAUTION. TALWIN should not be mixed in the same syringe with soluble barbiturates because precipitation will occur.

OVERDOSAGE

Manifestations: Clinical experience with TALWIN overdosage has been insufficient to define the signs of this condition.
Treatment: Oxygen, intravenous fluids, vasopressors, and other supportive measures should be employed as indicated. Assisted or controlled ventilation should also be considered. For respiratory depression due to overdosage or unusual sensitivity to TALWIN, brand of pentazocine lactate injection, parenteral naloxone is a specific and effective antagonist.

HOW SUPPLIED

Uni-Amp ®—Individual unit dose ampuls of 1 mL (30 mg) **NDC 0024-1924-04,** *1.5 mL (45 mg)* **NDC 0024-1925-04,** *and 2 mL (60 mg)* **NDC 0024-1926-04** in box of 25.
Uni-Nest™ ampuls of 1 mL (30 mg) **NDC 0024-1924-14** *and 2 mL (60 mg)* **NDC 0024-1926-14** in box of 25.
Each 1 mL contains pentazocine lactate equivalent to 30 mg base and 2.8 mg sodium chloride, in Water for Injection.
Carpuject ® **Sterile Cartridge-Needle Units,** *1 mL (30 mg)* **NDC 0024-1917-02,** *1.5 mL (45 mg)* **NDC 0024-1918-02,** *and 2 mL (60 mg)* **NDC 0024-1919-02, all in 2 mL cartridges,** box of 10. Each 1 mL contains pentazocine lactate equivalent to 30 mg base, 1 mg acetone sodium bisulfite, and 2.2 mg sodium chloride, in Water for Injection.
Multiple-dose vials of 10 mL **NDC 0024-1916-01,** box of 1. Each 1 mL contains pentazocine lactate equivalent to 30 mg base, 2 mg acetone sodium bisulfite, 1.5 mg sodium chloride, and 1 mg methylparaben as preservative, in Water for Injection.
The pH of TALWIN solutions is adjusted between 4 and 5 with lactic acid or sodium hydroxide. The air in the ampuls, vials, and Cartridge-Needle Units has been displaced by nitrogen gas.

TW-109-EE

TALWIN® Compound ℂ ℞
brand of pentazocine hydrochloride and aspirin tablets, USP

DESCRIPTION

TALWIN Compound is a combination of pentazocine hydrochloride, USP, equivalent to 12.5 mg base and aspirin, USP, 325 mg.
Pentazocine is a member of the benzazocine series (also known as the benzomorphan series). Chemically, pentazocine is 1, 2, 3, 4, 5, 6 -hexahydro - 6, 11-dimethyl-3-(3-methyl-2-butenyl)-2, 6-methano-3-benzazocin-8-ol, a white, crystalline substance soluble in acidic aqueous solutions.
Chemically, aspirin is Benzoic acid, 2-(acetyloxy)-;.
Inactive Ingredients: Magnesium Stearate, Microcrystalline Cellulose, Sodium Lauryl Sulfate, Starch.

CLINICAL PHARMACOLOGY

Pentazocine is a potent analgesic which when administered orally is approximately equivalent, on a mg for mg basis, in analgesic effect to codeine. Two Caplets® of TALWIN Compound when administered orally have the additive analgesic effect equivalent to 25 mg of TALWIN plus 650 mg of aspirin. TALWIN Compound provides the analgesic effects of pentazocine and the analgesic, anti-inflammatory, and antipyretic actions of aspirin.
Onset of significant analgesia usually occurs between 15 and 30 minutes after oral administration, and duration of action is usually three hours or longer. Onset and duration of action and the degree of pain relief are related both to dose and the severity of pretreatment pain. Pentazocine weakly antagonizes the analgesic effects of morphine, meperidine, and phenazocine; in addition, it produces incomplete reversal of cardiovascular, respiratory, and behavioral depression induced by morphine and meperidine. Pentazocine has about $1/50$ the antagonistic activity of nalorphine. It also has sedative activity.

INDICATION AND USAGE

For the relief of moderate pain

CONTRAINDICATIONS

TALWIN Compound should not be administered to patients who are hypersensitive to either pentazocine or salicylates, or in any situation where aspirin is contraindicated.

WARNINGS

Drug Dependence. There have been instances of psychological and physical dependence on parenteral pentazocine in patients with a history of drug abuse, and rarely, in patients without such a history. Abrupt discontinuance following the extended use of parenteral pentazocine has resulted in withdrawal symptoms. There have been a few reports of dependence and of withdrawal symptoms with orally administered pentazocine. Patients with a history of drug dependence should be under close supervision while receiving TALWIN Compound orally. There have been rare reports of possible abstinence syndromes in newborns after prolonged use of pentazocine during pregnancy.
In prescribing TALWIN Compound for chronic use, the physician should take precautions to avoid increases in dose by the patient and to prevent the use of the drug in anticipation of pain rather than for the relief of pain.
Head Injury and Increased Intracranial Pressure. The respiratory depressant effects of pentazocine and its potential for elevating cerebrospinal fluid pressure may be markedly exaggerated in the presence of head injury, other intracranial lesions, or a preexisting increase in intracranial pressure. Furthermore, pentazocine can produce effects which may obscure the clinical course of patients with head injuries. In such patients, TALWIN Compound must be used with extreme caution and only if its use is deemed essential.
Usage in Pregnancy. Safe use of pentazocine during pregnancy (other than labor) has not been established. Animal reproduction studies have not demonstrated teratogenic or embryotoxic effects. However, TALWIN Compound should be administered to pregnant patients (other than labor) only when, in the judgment of the physician, the potential benefits outweigh the possible hazards. Patients receiving pentazocine during labor have experienced no adverse effects other than those that occur with commonly used analgesics. TALWIN Compound should be used with caution in women delivering premature infants.
Acute CNS Manifestations. Patients receiving therapeutic doses of pentazocine have experienced hallucinations (usually visual), disorientation, and confusion which have cleared spontaneously within a period of hours. The mechanism of this reaction is not known. Such patients should be closely observed and vital signs checked. If the drug is reinstituted it should be done with caution since these acute CNS manifestations may recur.
Due to the potential for increased CNS depressant effects, alcohol should be used with caution in patients who are currently receiving pentazocine.
Usage in Children. Because clinical experience in children under 12 years of age is limited, administration of TALWIN Compound in this age group is not recommended.
Ambulatory Patients. Since sedation, dizziness, and occasional euphoria have been noted, ambulatory patients should be warned not to operate machinery, drive cars, or unnecessarily expose themselves to hazards.
Other. Because of its aspirin content, TALWIN Compound should be used with caution in the presence of peptic ulcer, in conjunction with anticoagulant therapy, or in any situation where the effects of aspirin may be deleterious.

PRECAUTIONS

Certain Respiratory Conditions. Although respiratory depression has rarely been reported after oral administration of pentazocine, TALWIN Compound should be administered with caution to patients with respiratory depression from any cause, severely limited respiratory reserve, severe bronchial asthma and other obstructive respiratory conditions, or cyanosis.
Impaired Renal or Hepatic Function. Decreased metabolism of the drug by the liver in extensive liver disease may predispose to accentuation of side effects. Although laboratory tests have not indicated that pentazocine causes or increases renal or hepatic impairment, TALWIN Compound should be administered with caution to patients with such impairment.
Myocardial Infarction. As with all drugs, TALWIN Compound should be used with caution in patients with myocardial infarction who have nausea or vomiting.
Biliary Surgery. Narcotic drug products are generally considered to elevate biliary tract pressure for varying periods following administration. Some evidence suggests that pentazocine may differ in this respect (ie, it causes little or no elevation in biliary tract pressures). The clinical significance of these findings, however, is not yet known.
Patients Receiving Narcotics. Pentazocine is a mild narcotic antagonist. Some patients previously given narcotics, including methadone for the daily treatment of narcotic dependence, have experienced withdrawal symptoms after receiving pentazocine.

Continued on next page

This product information was effective as of December 1, 1986. On these and other products of Winthrop-Breon Laboratories, detailed information may be obtained on a current basis by direct inquiry to the Professional Services Department, 90 Park Avenue, New York, NY 10016 (212) 907-2525.

Winthrop-Breon—Cont.

CNS Effect. Caution should be used when pentazocine is administered to patients prone to seizures. Seizures have occurred in a few such patients in association with the use of pentazocine although no cause and effect relationship has been established.

ADVERSE REACTIONS

Reactions reported after oral administration of pentazocine or TALWIN Compound include *gastrointestinal:* nausea, vomiting; infrequently constipation; and rarely abdominal distress, anorexia, diarrhea. *CNS Effects:* dizziness, lightheadedness, hallucinations, sedation, euphoria, headache, confusion, disorientation; infrequently weakness, disturbed dreams, insomnia, syncope, visual blurring and focusing difficulty, depression; and rarely tremor, irritability, excitement, tinnitus. *Autonomic:* sweating; infrequently flushing; and rarely chills. *Allergic:* infrequently rash; and rarely urticaria, edema of the face. *Cardiovascular:* infrequently decrease in blood pressure, tachycardia. *Hematologic:* rarely depression of white blood cells (especially granulocytes), which is usually reversible, moderate transient eosinophilia. *Other:* rarely respiratory depression, urinary retention, paresthesia, toxic epidermal necrolysis.

DOSAGE AND ADMINISTRATION

Adults. The usual adult dose is 2 CAPLETS three or four times a day.

Children Under 12 Years of Age. Since clinical experience in children under 12 years of age is limited, administration of TALWIN Compound in this age group is not recommended.

Duration of Therapy. Patients with chronic pain who receive pentazocine orally for prolonged periods have only rarely been reported to experience withdrawal symptoms when administration was abruptly discontinued (see WARNINGS). Tolerance to the analgesic effect of pentazocine has also been reported only rarely. Significant abnormalities of liver and kidney function tests have not been reported, even after prolonged administration of pentazocine.

OVERDOSAGE

Manifestations: Clinical experience with pentazocine overdosage has been insufficient to define the signs of this condition. Signs of salicylate overdosage include headache, dizziness, confusion, tinnitus, diaphoresis, thirst, nausea, vomiting, diarrhea, tachycardia, tachypnea, Kussmaul breathing, convulsions, and coma. Death is usually from respiratory failure.

Treatment: Treatment for overdosage of TALWIN Compound should include treatment for salicylate poisoning as outlined in standard references.

Oxygen, intravenous fluids, vasopressors, and other supportive measures should be employed as indicated. Assisted or controlled ventilation should also be considered. For respiratory depression due to overdosage or unusual sensitivity to pentazocine, parenteral naloxone is a specific and effective antagonist.

HOW SUPPLIED

CAPLETS, white, each containing pentazocine hydrochloride equivalent to 12.5 mg base and aspirin 325 mg. Bottle of 100 (NDC 0024-1927-04).

Distributed by Winthrop-Breon Laboratories Division of Sterling Drug Inc., New York, NY 10016, Manufactured by Sterling Pharmaceuticals Inc., Barceloneta, Puerto Rico 00617

TW-225-I(O)

TALWIN® Nx Ⓒ℞

brand of pentazocine and naloxone hydrochlorides tablets, USP

Analgesic for Oral Use Only

> TALWIN® Nx is intended for oral use only. Severe, potentially lethal, reactions may result from misuse of TALWIN® Nx by injection either alone or in combination with other substances. (See **DRUG ABUSE AND DEPENDENCE** section.)

DESCRIPTION

TALWIN Nx contains pentazocine hydrochloride, USP, equivalent to 50 mg base and is a member of the benzazocine series (also known as the benzomorphan series), and naloxone hydrochloride, USP, equivalent to 0.5 mg base.

TALWIN Nx is an analgesic for oral administration.

Chemically, pentazocine hydrochloride is 1,2,3,4,5,6-Hexahydro -6,11 -dimethyl -3-(3-methyl-2-butenyl)-2, 6-methano-3-benzazocin-8-ol hydrochloride, a white, crystalline substance soluble in acidic aqueous solutions.

Chemically, naloxone hydrochloride is Morphinan-6-one, 4, 5-epoxy-3, 14-dihydroxy-17-(2-propenyl)-, hydrochloride, (5α)-. It is a slightly off-white powder, and is soluble in water and dilute acids.

Inactive Ingredients: Colloidal Silicon Dioxide, Dibasic Calcium Phosphate, D&C Yellow #10, FD&C Yellow #6, Magnesium Stearate, Microcrystalline Cellulose, Sodium Lauryl Sulfate, Starch.

CLINICAL PHARMACOLOGY

Pentazocine is a potent analgesic which when administered orally in a 50 mg dose appears equivalent in analgesic effect to 60 mg (1 grain) of codeine. Onset of significant analgesia usually occurs between 15 and 30 minutes after oral administration, and duration of action is usually three hours or longer. Onset and duration of action and the degree of pain relief are related both to dose and the severity of pretreatment pain. Pentazocine weakly antagonizes the analgesic effects of morphine and meperidine; in addition, it produces incomplete reversal of cardiovascular, respiratory, and behavioral depression induced by morphine and meperidine. Pentazocine has about 1/50 the antagonistic activity of nalorphine. It also has sedative activity.

Pentazocine is well absorbed from the gastrointestinal tract. Concentrations in plasma coincide closely with the onset, duration, and intensity of analgesia; peak values occur 1 to 3 hours after oral administration. The half-life in plasma is 2 to 3 hours.

Pentazocine is metabolized in the liver and excreted primarily in the urine. Pentazocine passes into the fetal circulation. Naloxone when administered orally at 0.5 mg has no pharmacologic activity. Naloxone hydrochloride administered parenterally at the same dose is an effective antagonist to pentazocine and a pure antagonist to narcotic analgesics.

TALWIN Nx is a potent analgesic when administered orally. However, the presence of naloxone in TALWIN Nx will prevent the effect of pentazocine if the product is misused by injection.

Studies in animals indicate that the presence of naloxone does not affect pentazocine analgesia when the combination is given orally. If the combination is given by injection the action of pentazocine is neutralized.

INDICATIONS AND USAGE

> TALWIN® Nx is intended for oral use only. Severe, potentially lethal, reactions may result from misuse of TALWIN® Nx by injection either alone or in combination with other substances. (See **DRUG ABUSE AND DEPENDENCE** section.)

TALWIN Nx is indicated for the relief of moderate to severe pain.

TALWIN Nx is indicated for oral use only.

CONTRAINDICATIONS

TALWIN Nx should not be administered to patients who are hypersensitive to either pentazocine or naloxone.

WARNINGS

> TALWIN® Nx is intended for oral use only. Severe, potentially lethal, reactions may result from misuse of TALWIN® Nx by injection either alone or in combination with other substances. (See **DRUG ABUSE AND DEPENDENCE** section.)

Drug Dependence. Pentazocine can cause a physical and psychological dependence. (See **DRUG ABUSE AND DEPENDENCE.**)

Head Injury and Increased Intracranial Pressure. As in the case of other potent analgesics, the potential of pentazocine for elevating cerebrospinal fluid pressure may be attributed to CO_2 retention due to the respiratory depressant effects of the drug. These effects may be markedly exaggerated in the presence of head injury, other intracranial lesions, or a preexisting increase in intracranial pressure. Furthermore, pentazocine can produce effects which may obscure the clinical course of patients with head injuries. In such patients, pentazocine must be used wth extreme caution and only if its use is deemed essential.

Usage with Alcohol. Due to the potential for increased CNS depressant effects, alcohol should be used with caution in patients who are currently receiving pentazocine.

Patients Receiving Narcotics. Pentazocine is a mild narcotic antagonist. Some patients previously given narcotics, including methadone for the daily treatment of narcotic dependence, have experienced withdrawal symptoms after receiving pentazocine.

Certain Respiratory Conditions. Although respiratory depression has rarely been reported after oral administration of pentazocine, the drug should be administered with caution to patients with respiratory depression from any cause, severely limited respiratory reserve, severe bronchial asthma, and other obstructive respiratory conditions, or cyanosis.

Acute CNS Manifestations. Patients receiving therapeutic doses of pentazocine have experienced hallucinations (usually visual), disorientation, and confusion which have cleared spontaneously within a period of hours. The mechanism of this reaction is not known. Such patients should be very closely observed and vital signs checked. If the drug is reinstituted, it should be done with caution since these acute CNS manifestations may recur.

PRECAUTIONS

CNS Effect. Caution should be used when pentazocine is administered to patients prone to seizures; seizures have occurred in a few such patients in association with the use of pentazocine though no cause and effect relationship has been established.

Impaired Renal or Hepatic Function. Decreased metabolism of pentazocine by the liver in extensive liver disease may predispose to accentuation of side effects. Although laboratory tests have not indicated that pentazocine causes or increases renal or hepatic impairment, the drug should be administered with caution to patients with such impairment.

In prescribing pentazocine for long-term use, the physician should take precautions to avoid increases in dose by the patient.

Biliary Surgery. Narcotic drug products are generally considered to elevate biliary tract pressure for varying periods following their administration. Some evidence suggests that pentazocine may differ from other marketed narcotics in this respect (ie, it causes little or no elevation in biliary tract pressures). The clinical significance of these findings, however, is not yet known.

Information for Patients. Since sedation, dizziness, and occasional euphoria have been noted, ambulatory patients should be warned not to operate machinery, drive cars, or unnecessarily expose themselves to hazards. Pentazocine may cause physical and psychological dependence when taken alone and may have additive CNS depressant properties when taken in combination with alcohol or other CNS depressants.

Myocardial Infarction. As with all drugs, pentazocine should be used with caution in patients with myocardial infarction who have nausea or vomiting.

Drug Interactions. Usage with Alcohol: See **WARNINGS.**

Carcinogenesis, Mutagenesis, Impairment of Fertility. No long-term studies in animals to test for carcinogenesis have been performed with the components of TALWIN Nx, brand of pentazocine and naloxone hydrochlorides tablets.

Pregnancy Category C. Animal reproduction studies have not been conducted with TALWIN Nx. It is also not known whether TALWIN Nx can cause fetal harm when administered to pregnant women or can affect reproduction capacity. TALWIN Nx should be given to pregnant women only if clearly needed. However, animal reproduction studies with pentazocine have not demonstrated teratogenic embryotoxic effects.

Labor and Delivery. Patients receiving pentazocine during labor have experienced no adverse effects other than those that occur with commonly used analgesics. TALWIN Nx should be used with caution in women delivering premature infants. The effect of TALWIN Nx on the mother and fetus, the duration of labor or delivery, the possibility that forceps delivery or other intervention or resuscitation of the newborn may be necessary, or the effect of TALWIN Nx on the later growth, development, and functional maturation of the child are unknown at the present time.

Nursing Mothers. It is not known whether this drug is excreted in human milk. Because many drugs are excreted in human milk, caution should be exercised when TALWIN Nx is administered to a nursing woman.

Pediatric Use. Safety and effectiveness in children below the age of 12 years have not been established.

ADVERSE REACTIONS

Cardiovascular: Hypotension, tachycardia, syncope.

Respiratory: Rarely, respiratory depression.

Acute CNS Manifestations: Patients receiving therapeutic doses of pentazocine have experienced hallucinations (usually visual), disorientation, and confusion which have cleared spontaneously within a period of hours. The mechanism of this reaction is not known. Such patients should be closely observed and vital signs checked. If the drug is reinstituted it should be done with caution since these acute CNS manifestations may recur.

Other CNS Effects: Dizziness, lightheadedness, hallucinations, sedation, euphoria, headache, confusion, disorientation; infrequently weakness, disturbed dreams, insomnia, syncope, visual blurring and focusing difficulty, depression; and rarely tremor, irritability, excitement, tinnitus.

Autonomic: Sweating; infrequently flushing; and rarely chills.

Gastrointestinal: Nausea, vomiting, constipation, diarrhea, anorexia, rarely abdominal distress.

Allergic: Edema of the face; dermatitis, including pruritus; flushed skin, including plethora; infrequently rash, and rarely urticaria.

Ophthalmic: Visual blurring and focusing difficulty.
Hematologic: Depression of white blood cells (especially granulocytes), which is usually reversible, moderate transient eosinophilia.
Other: Headache, chills, insomnia, weakness, urinary retention, paresthesia.

DRUG ABUSE AND DEPENDENCE

Controlled Substance. TALWIN Nx is a Schedule IV controlled substance.
There have been some reports of dependence and of withdrawal symptoms wth orally administered pentazocine. Patients with a history of drug dependence should be under close supervision while receiving pentazocine orally. There have been rare reports of possible abstinence syndromes in newborns after prolonged use of pentazocine during pregnancy.
There have been instances of psychological and physical dependence on parenteral pentazocine in patients with a history of drug abuse and rarely, in patients without such a history. Abrupt discontinuance following the extended use of parenteral pentazocine has resulted in withdrawal symptoms.
In prescribing pentazocine for chronic use, the physician should take precautions to avoid increases in dose by the patient.
The amount of naloxone present in TALWIN Nx (0.5 mg per tablet) has no action when taken orally and will not interfere with the pharmacologic action of pentazocine. However, this amount of naloxone given by injection has profound antagonistic action to narcotic analgesics.
Severe, even lethal, consequences may result from misuse of tablets by injection either alone or in combination with other substances, such as pulmonary emboli, vascular occlusion, ulceration and abscesses, and withdrawal symptoms in narcotic dependent individuals.
TALWIN Nx, brand of pentazocine and naloxone hydrochlorides tablets, contains an opioid antagonist, naloxone (0.5 mg). Naloxone is inactive when administered orally at this dose, and its inclusion in TALWIN Nx is intended to curb a form of misuse of oral pentazocine. Parenterally, naloxone is an active narcotic antagonist. Thus, TALWIN Nx has a lower potential for parenteral misuse than the previous oral pentazocine formulation TALWIN® 50, brand of pentazocine hydrochloride tablets, USP. However, it is still subject to patient misuse and abuse by the oral route.

OVERDOSAGE

Manifestations. Clinical experience of overdosage with this oral medication has been insufficient to define the signs of this condition.
Treatment. Oxygen, intravenous fluids, vasopressors, and other supportive measures should be employed as indicated. Assisted or controlled ventilation should also be considered. For respiratory depression due to overdosage or unusual sensitivity to pentazocine, parenteral naloxone is a specific and effective antagonist.

DOSAGE AND ADMINISTRATION

> TALWIN® Nx is intended for oral use only. Severe, potentially lethal, reactions may result from misuse of TALWIN® Nx by injection either alone or in combination with other substances. (See **DRUG ABUSE AND DEPENDENCE** section.)

Adults. The usual initial adult dose is 1 tablet every three or four hours. This may be increased to 2 tablets when needed. Total daily dosage should not exceed 12 tablets.
When anti-inflammatory or antipyretic effects are desired in addition to analgesia, aspirin can be administered concomitantly with this product.
Children Under 12 Years of Age. Since clinical experience in children under 12 years of age is limited, administration of this product in this age group is not recommended.
Duration of Therapy. Patients with chronic pain who receive TALWIN Nx orally for prolonged periods have only rarely been reported to experience withdrawal symptoms when administration was abruptly discontinued (see **WARNINGS**). Tolerance to the analgesic effect of pentazocine has also been reported only rarely. However, there is no long-term experience with the oral administration of TALWIN Nx.

HOW SUPPLIED

Tablets (oblong), yellow, scored, each containing pentazocine hydrochloride equivalent to 50 mg base and naloxone hydrochloride equivalent to 0.5 mg base.
Bottles of 100 (NDC 0024-1951-04).
Unit Dose Dispenser Package of 250 (NDC 0024-1951-24), 10 sleeves of 25 tablets each.

Distributed by
Winthrop-Breon Laboratories
Division of Sterling Drug Inc.
New York, NY 10016
Manufactured by
Sterling Pharmaceuticals Inc.
Barceloneta, Puerto Rico 00617
Shown in Product Identification Section, page 435
TW-267-G

TORNALATE® ℞
(bitolterol mesylate)
Metered Dose Inhaler
Bronchodilator for Oral Inhalation

DESCRIPTION

TORNALATE (bitolterol mesylate) is the di-*p*-toluate ester of the β-adrenergic bronchodilator *N-t*-butylarterenol (colterol). It has a molecular weight of 557.7. Bitolterol mesylate is known chemically as 4-[2-[(1,1-dimethylethyl) amino]-1-hydroxyethyl]-1,2-phenylene 4-methylbenzoate (ester) methanesulfonate (salt).
TORNALATE (bitolterol mesylate), Metered Dose Inhaler, is a complete aerosol unit for oral inhalation. It consists of a plastic-coated bottle of ready-to-use aerosol solution and a detachable plastic mouthpiece with built-in nebulizer. The bottle contains 16.4 g (15 mL) of 0.8% bitolterol mesylate in a vehicle containing 38% alcohol (w/w), inert propellants (dichlorodifluoromethane and dichlorotetrafluoroethane), ascorbic acid, saccharin, and menthol.
Each bottle provides at least 300 actuations. Each actuation delivers a measured dose of 0.37 mg of bitolterol mesylate as a fine, even mist.

CLINICAL PHARMACOLOGY

TORNALATE (bitolterol mesylate) is administered as a prodrug which is hydrolyzed by esterases in tissue and blood to the active moiety colterol. TORNALATE administered as an inhaled aerosol, has a rapid (3 to 4 minutes) onset of bronchodilator activity. The duration of action with TORNALATE is at least 5 hours in most patients and 8 or more hours in 25% to 35% of patients, based on 15% or greater increase in forced expiratory volume in one second (FEV_1), as demonstrated in 3 month isoproterenol controlled multicenter trials. Based on mean maximal expiratory flow (MMEF) measurements, the duration of action is 6 to 7 hours. The duration of bronchodilator action with TORNALATE in these trials is longer than that seen with isoproterenol, especially in steroid-dependent patients. Duration of effect was reduced over time in steroid-dependent asthmatic patients where the duration was 3.5 to 5 hours for FEV_1. The mean maximum increase in FEV_1 over baseline in the majority of patients was 39% to 42% and occurred by 30 to 60 minutes, similar to that seen in the isoproterenol group.
TORNALATE is a beta adrenergic agonist which has been shown by in vitro and in vivo pharmacological studies in animals to exert a preferential effect on $beta_2$ adrenergic receptors, such as those located in bronchial smooth muscle. However, controlled clinical trials in patients who were administered the drug have not revealed a preferential $beta_2$ adrenergic effect. At doses that produced long duration of bronchodilator activity (up to 8 hours in some patients) with a mean maximum bronchodilating effect of approximately 40% increase in FEV_1 (forced expiration volume in one second), a less than 10 beat per minute mean maximum increase in heart rate was seen. The effect on the heart rate was transient and similar to the increases seen in the isoproterenol treated patients in these studies.
Although blood levels of colterol formed by gradual release from the pro-drug (bitolterol) in the lungs are too low to be measured by currently available assay methods, data on disposition are available from oral studies in man. Following oral administration of 5.9 mg tritiated bitolterol mesylate to man, radioactivity measurements indicated mean maximum colterol concentration in blood of approximately 2.1 μg/mL one hour after medication. Urinary excretion data indicate that 83 percent of the radioactivity of this oral dose was excreted within the first 24 hours. By 72 hours, 85.6 percent of the tritium had been excreted in the urine and 8.1 percent in the feces. Most of the radioactivity was excreted as conjugated colterol; free colterol accounted for 2.1 to 3.7 percent of the total radioactivity excreted in the urine. No intact bitolterol was detected in urine.
The pharmacologic effects of β-adrenergic drugs including TORNALATE (bitolterol mesylate) are attributable to stimulation of adenyl cyclase, the enzyme which catalyzes the conversion of adenosine triphosphate (ATP) to cyclic-3′, 5′-adenosine monophosphate (c-AMP). Increased c-AMP levels are associated with relaxation of bronchial smooth muscle and with inhibition of release of mediators of immediate hypersensitivity.
In a six week clinical trial in which 24 asthmatic patients received TORNALATE and theophylline concurrently, improvement in pulmonary function was enhanced over that seen with either drug alone. No potentiation of side effects was observed, and 24-hour ECG recordings (Holter monitoring) indicated no greater degree of cardiac toxicity with TORNALATE alone or in combination with theophylline than that which occurred with theophylline alone.
TORNALATE did not adversely affect arterial oxygen tension in a blood-gas study in 24 asthmatic patients. However, a decrease in arterial oxygen tension has been reported with other adrenergic bronchodilators and could be anticipated to occur with TORNALATE as well.
In repetitive dosing studies, continued effectiveness was demonstrated throughout the 3 month period of treatment in the majority of patients. However, some overall decrease was observed in steroid dependent asthmatics.

INDICATIONS AND USAGE

TORNALATE (bitolterol mesylate) is indicated for both prophylactic and therapeutic use as a bronchodilator for bronchial asthma and for reversible bronchospasm. It may be used with or without concurrent theophylline and/or steroid therapy.

CONTRAINDICATIONS

TORNALATE (bitolterol mesylate) is contraindicated in patients who are hypersensitive to any of its ingredients.

WARNINGS

As with other β-adrenergic aerosols, TORNALATE (bitolterol mesylate) should not be used in excess. Use of aerosolized β-adrenergic drugs may have a deleterious cardiac effect. Paradoxical bronchoconstriction has been reported with administration of β-adrenergic agents. Immediate hypersensitivity (allergic) reactions can occur after the administration of TORNALATE. In such instances, the drug should be discontinued immediately and alternative therapy instituted.

PRECAUTIONS

General. As with all β-adrenergic stimulating agents, caution should be used when administering TORNALATE (bitolterol mesylate) to patients with cardiovascular disease such as ischemic heart disease or hypertension. Caution is also advised in patients with hyperthyroidism, diabetes mellitus, cardiac arrhythmias, convulsive disorders or unusual responsiveness to β-adrenergic agonists. Significant changes in systolic and diastolic blood pressure have been seen in individual patients and could be expected to occur in some patients after use of any β-adrenergic aerosol bronchodilator.
Information for Patients. The effects of TORNALATE may last up to eight hours or longer. It should not be used more often than recommended and the patient should not increase the number of inhalations or frequency of use without first asking the physician. If symptoms of asthma get worse, adverse reactions occur, or the patient does not respond to the usual dose, the patient should be instructed to contact the physician immediately. The patient should be advised to see the Illustrated Directions for Use.
Drug Interactions. Other sympathomimetic aerosol bronchodilators should not be used concomitantly with TORNALATE. If additional adrenergic drugs are to be administered by any route, they should be used with caution to avoid deleterious cardiovascular effects.
Carcinogenesis, Mutagenesis, and Impairment of Fertility. No tumorigenicity (and specifically no increase in leiomyomas) was observed in a two year oral study in Sprague-Dawley CD rats at doses of TORNALATE corresponding to 23 or 114 times the maximal daily human inhalational dose. TORNALATE was not tumorigenic in an 18 month oral study in Swiss-Webster mice at doses up to 568 times the maximal daily human inhalational dose.
Ames Salmonella and mouse lymphoma mutation assays in vitro revealed no mutagenesis due to TORNALATE. Reproductive studies in male and female rats revealed no significant effects on fertility at doses of TORNALATE up to 364 times the maximal daily human inhalational dose.
Teratogenic Effects—Pregnancy Category C. No teratogenic effects were seen in rats and rabbits after oral doses of TORNALATE up to 557 times the maximal daily human inhalational dose and in mice after oral doses up to 284 times the maximal daily human inhalational dose.
When TORNALATE was injected subcutaneously into mice at doses of 2 mg/kg, 10 mg/kg, and 20 mg/kg (corresponding to 23, 114, and 227 times the maximal daily human inhalational dose) cleft palate incidences of 5.7 percent, 3.8 percent, and 3.3 percent (compared with 0.9 percent in controls) were found. Cleft palate induction with isoproterenol at 10 mg/kg SC as the positive control was 10.7 percent. Since no well-controlled studies in pregnant women are available,

Continued on next page

This product information was effective as of December 1, 1986. On these and other products of Winthrop-Breon Laboratories, detailed information may be obtained on a current basis by direct inquiry to the Professional Services Department, 90 Park Avenue, New York, NY 10016 (212) 907-2525.

Winthrop-Breon—Cont.

TORNALATE should be used during pregnancy only if the potential benefit justifies the potential risk to the fetus.

Nursing Mothers. It is not known whether TORNALATE is excreted in human milk. Because many drugs are excreted in human milk, caution should be exercised when TORNALATE is administered to a nursing woman.

Pediatric Use. Safety and effectiveness of TORNALATE in children 12 years of age or younger has not been established.

ADVERSE REACTIONS

The results of all clinical trials with TORNALATE (bitolterol mesylate) in 492 patients showed the following side effects:

CNS: Tremors (14%), nervousness (5%), headache (4%), dizziness (3%), lightheadedness (3%), insomnia (<1%), hyperkinesia (<1%).

Gastrointestinal: Nausea (3%).

Oro-Pharyngeal: Throat irritation (5%).

Cardiovascular: The overall incidence of cardiovascular effects was approximately 5% of patients and these effects included palpitations (approximately 3%), and chest discomfort (approximately 1%). Tachycardia was seen in less than 1%. Premature ventricular contractions and flushing were rarely seen.

Respiratory: Coughing (4%), bronchospasm (<1%), dyspnea (<1%), chest tightness (<1%).

Clinical relevance or relationship to TORNALATE administration of rarely reported elevations of SGOT, decrease in platelets, decreases in WBC levels or proteinuria are not known.

In comparing the adverse reactions for bitolterol mesylate treated patients to those of isoproterenol treated patients, during three month clinical trials involving approximately 400 patients, the following moderate to severe reactions, as judged by the investigators, were reported for both steroid and non-steroid dependent patients. The table does not include mild reactions or those occurring only with the first dose.

PERCENT INCIDENCE OF MODERATE TO SEVERE ADVERSE REACTIONS

Reaction	Bitolterol N = 197	Isoproterenol N = 194
Central Nervous System		
Tremors	9.1%	1.5%
Nervousness	1.5%	1.0%
Headache	3.5%	6.1%
Dizziness	1.0%	1.5%
Insomnia	0.5%	0%
Cardiovascular		
Palpitations	1.5%	0%
PVC—Transient Increase	0.5%	0%
Chest Discomfort	0.5%	0%
Respiratory		
Cough	4.1%	1.0%
Bronchospasm	1.0%	0%
Dyspnea	1.0%	0%
Oro-Pharyngeal		
Throat Irritation	3.0%	3.1%
Gastrointestinal		
Nausea (Dyspepsia)	0.5%	0.5%

NOTE: In most patients, the total isoproterenol dosage was divided into three equally dosed inhalations, administered at three minute intervals. This procedure may have reduced the incidence of adverse reactions observed with isoproterenol.

OVERDOSAGE

Overdosage with TORNALATE (bitolterol mesylate) may be expected to result in exaggeration of those drug effects listed in the ADVERSE REACTIONS section. In such cases therapy with TORNALATE and all β-adrenergic stimulating drugs should be stopped, supportive therapy provided, and judicious use of a cardioselective β-adrenergic blocking agent should be considered bearing in mind the possibility that such agents can produce profound bronchospasm. As with all sympathomimetic aerosol medications, cardiac arrest and even death may be associated with abuse. The oral LD_{50} of TORNALATE in rats was greater than 5,000 mg/kg and in mice greater than 6,000 mg/kg.

DOSAGE AND ADMINISTRATION

The usual dose to relieve bronchospasm for adults and children over 12 years of age is two inhalations at an interval of at least one to three minutes followed by a third inhalation if needed. For prevention of bronchospasm, the usual dose is two inhalations every 8 hours. The dose of TORNALATE (bitolterol mesylate) should never exceed 3 inhalations every 6 hours or 2 inhalations every 4 hours. Medical consultation should be sought prior to an increase in the frequency of dosing because this may indicate a need for reevaluation of the patient's condition.

HOW SUPPLIED

TORNALATE (bitolterol mesylate), Metered Dose Inhaler, is supplied in 16.4 g (15 mL) self-contained aerosol units (NDC 0024-1060-01).

Refill of 16.4 g (15 mL) NDC 0024-1061-01.

Store at controlled room temperature between 15 °C and 30 °C (59 °F and 86 °F).

Distributed by Winthrop-Breon Laboratories
Division of Sterling Drug Inc. New York, NY 10016
Manufactured by Sterling Pharmaceuticals Inc.
Barceloneta, Puerto Rico 00617

Shown in Product Identification Section, page 435

TW 275 F

TRANCOPAL® ℞

brand of chlormezanone
Nonhypnotic Antianxiety Agent

DESCRIPTION

TRANCOPAL, brand of chlormezanone, is [2-(*p*-Chlorophenyl)tetrahydro-3-methyl-4*H*-1, 3-thiazin-4-one 1, 1-dioxide], a white, virtually tasteless, crystalline powder with a solubility of less than 0.25 percent w/v in water.

Inactive Ingredients—Caplets® **100 mg:** Dibasic Calcium Phosphate, FD&C Yellow #6, Magnesium Stearate, Saccharin Sodium, Starch; CAPLETS **200 mg:** Dibasic Calcium Phosphate, D&C Yellow #10, FD&C Blue #1, Magnesium Stearate, Saccharin Sodium, Starch.

CLINICAL PHARMACOLOGY

TRANCOPAL improves the emotional state by allaying mild anxiety, usually without impairing clarity of consciousness. The relief of symptoms is often apparent in fifteen to thirty minutes after administration and may last up to six hours or longer.

INDICATIONS AND USAGE

TRANCOPAL is indicated for the treatment of mild anxiety and tension states.

The effectiveness of chlormezanone in long-term use, that is, more than 4 months, has not been assessed by systematic clinical studies. The physician should periodically reassess the usefulness of the drug for the individual patient.

CONTRAINDICATION

Contraindicated in patients with a history of a previous hypersensitivity reaction to chlormezanone.

WARNINGS

Should drowsiness occur, the dose should be reduced. As with other CNS-acting drugs, patients receiving chlormezanone should be warned against performing potentially hazardous tasks which require complete mental alertness, such as operating a motor vehicle or dangerous machinery. Patients should also be warned of the possible additive effects which may occur when the drug is taken with alcohol or other CNS-acting drugs.

Usage in Pregnancy. Safe use of this preparation in pregnancy or lactation has not been established, as no animal reproduction studies have been performed; therefore, use of the drug in pregnancy, lactation, or in women of childbearing age requires that the potential benefit of the drug be weighed against its possible hazards to the mother and fetus.

ADVERSE REACTIONS

Adverse effects reported to occur with TRANCOPAL include drowsiness, drug rash, dizziness, flushing, nausea, depression, edema, inability to void, weakness, excitement, tremor, confusion, and headache. Medication should be discontinued or modified as the case demands.

Jaundice, apparently of the cholestatic type, has been reported as occurring rarely during the use of chlormezanone, but was reversible on discontinuance of therapy.

DOSAGE AND ADMINISTRATION

The usual **adult** dosage is 200 mg orally three or four times daily but in some patients 100 mg may suffice. The dosage for **children from 5 to 12 years** is 50 mg to 100 mg three or four times daily. Since the effect of CNS-acting drugs varies, treatment, particularly in children, should begin with the lowest dosage which may be increased as needed.

HOW SUPPLIED

100 mg (peach colored, scored CAPLETS)
bottle of 100 (NDC 0024-1973-04)
200 mg (green colored, scored CAPLETS)
bottle of 100 (NDC 0024-1974-04)
bottle of 1000 (NDC 0024-1974-08)

Shown in Product Identification Section, page 435

TW 72-L

WINSTROL® ℞

brand of stanozolol tablets, USP
For Oral Administration

DESCRIPTION

WINSTROL, brand of stanozolol tablets, is an anabolic steroid, a synthetic derivative of testosterone. Each tablet contains 2 mg of stanozolol. It is designated chemically as 17-methyl-2'*H*-5α-androst-2-eno[3,2-*c*]pyrazol-17β-ol.

Inactive Ingredients: Dibasic Calcium Phosphate, FD&C Red #3, Lactose, Magnesium Stearate, Starch.

CLINICAL PHARMACOLOGY

Anabolic steroids are synthetic derivatives of testosterone. Certain clinical effects and adverse reactions demonstrate the androgenic properties of this class of drugs. Complete dissociation of anabolic and androgenic effects has not been achieved. The actions of anabolic steroids are therefore similar to those of male sex hormones with the possibility of causing serious disturbances of growth and sexual development if given to young children. They suppress the gonadotropic functions of the pituitary and may exert a direct effect upon the testes.

WINSTROL has been found to increase low-density lipoproteins and decrease high-density lipoproteins. These changes are not associated with any increase in total cholesterol or triglyceride levels and revert to normal on discontinuation of treatment.

Hereditary angioedema (HAE) is an autosomal dominant disorder caused by a deficient or nonfunctional C1 esterase inhibitor (C1 INH) and clinically characterized by episodes of swelling of the face, extremities, genitalia, bowel wall, and upper respiratory tract.

In small scale clinical studies, stanozolol was effective in controlling the frequency and severity of attacks of angioedema and in increasing serum levels of C1 INH and C4. WINSTROL is not effective in stopping HAE attacks while they are under way. The effect of WINSTROL on increasing serum levels of C1 INH and C4 may be related to an increase in protein anabolism.

INDICATIONS AND USAGE

Hereditary Angioedema. WINSTROL is indicated prophylactically to decrease the frequency and severity of attacks of angioedema.

CONTRAINDICATIONS

The use of WINSTROL is contraindicated in the following:

1. Carcinoma of the prostate or breast in male patients.
2. Carcinoma of the breast in some females.
3. Nephrosis or the nephrotic phase of nephritis.
4. WINSTROL can cause fetal harm when administered to a pregnant woman.

WINSTROL is contraindicated in women who are or may become pregnant. If this drug is used during pregnancy, or if the patient becomes pregnant while taking this drug, the patient should be apprised of the potential hazard to the fetus.

WARNINGS

PELIOSIS HEPATIS, A CONDITION IN WHICH LIVER AND SOMETIMES SPLENIC TISSUE IS REPLACED WITH BLOOD-FILLED CYSTS, HAS BEEN REPORTED IN PATIENTS RECEIVING ANDROGENIC ANABOLIC STEROID THERAPY. THESE CYSTS ARE SOMETIMES PRESENT WITH MINIMAL HEPATIC DYSFUNCTION, BUT AT OTHER TIMES THEY HAVE BEEN ASSOCIATED WITH LIVER FAILURE. THEY ARE OFTEN NOT RECOGNIZED UNTIL LIFE-THREATENING LIVER FAILURE OR INTRA-ABDOMINAL HEMORRHAGE DEVELOPS. WITHDRAWAL OF DRUG USUALLY RESULTS IN COMPLETE DISAPPEARANCE OF LESIONS.

LIVER CELL TUMORS ARE ALSO REPORTED. MOST OFTEN THESE TUMORS ARE BENIGN AND ANDROGEN-DEPENDENT, BUT FATAL MALIGNANT TUMORS HAVE BEEN REPORTED. WITHDRAWAL OF DRUG OFTEN RESULTS IN REGRESSION OR CESSATION OF PROGRESSION OF THE TUMOR. HOWEVER, HEPATIC TUMORS ASSOCIATED WITH ANDROGENS OR ANABOLIC STEROIDS ARE MUCH MORE VASCULAR THAN OTHER HEPATIC TUMORS AND MAY BE SILENT UNTIL LIFE-THREATENING INTRA-ABDOMINAL HEMORRHAGE DEVELOPS.

BLOOD LIPID CHANGES THAT ARE KNOWN TO BE ASSOCIATED WITH INCREASED RISK OF ATHEROSCLEROSIS ARE SEEN IN PATIENTS TREATED WITH ANDROGENS AND ANABOLIC STEROIDS. THESE CHANGES INCLUDE DECREASED HIGH-DENSITY LIPOPROTEIN AND SOMETIMES INCREASED LOW-DENSITY LIPOPROTEIN. THE CHANGES MAY BE VERY MARKED AND COULD HAVE A SERIOUS IMPACT ON THE RISK OF ATH-

EROSCLEROSIS AND CORONARY ARTERY DISEASE.

Cholestatic hepatitis and jaundice occur with 17-alpha-alkylated androgens at relatively low doses. If cholestatic hepatitis with jaundice appears, the anabolic steroid should be discontinued. If liver function tests become abnormal, the patient should be monitored closely and the etiology determined. Generally, the anabolic steroid should be discontinued although in cases of mild abnormalities, the physician may elect to follow the patient carefully at a reduced drug dosage.
In patients with breast cancer, anabolic steroid therapy may cause hypercalcemia by stimulating osteolysis. In this case, the drug should be discontinued.
Edema with or without congestive heart failure may be a serious complication in patients with preexisting cardiac, renal, or hepatic disease.
Geriatric male patients treated with androgenic anabolic steroids may be at an increased risk for the development of prostatic hypertrophy and prostatic carcinoma.
Anabolic steroids have not been shown to enhance athletic ability.

PRECAUTIONS

General. Women should be observed for signs of virilization (deepening of the voice, hirsutism, acne, and clitoromegaly). To prevent irreversible change, drug therapy must be discontinued, or the dosage significantly reduced when mild virilism is first detected. Such virilization is usual following androgenic anabolic steroid use at high doses. Some virilizing changes in women are irreversible even after prompt discontinuance of therapy and are not prevented by concomitant use of estrogens. Menstrual irregularities may also occur.
The insulin or oral hypoglycemic dosage may need adjustment in diabetic patients who receive anabolic steroids.
Information for the Patient. The physician should instruct patients to report any of the following side effects of androgens:
Adult or Adolescent Males. Too frequent or persistent erections of the penis, appearance or aggravation of acne.
Women. Hoarseness, acne, changes in menstrual periods, or more hair on the face.
All Patients. Any nausea, vomiting, changes in skin color, or ankle swelling.
Laboratory Tests. Women with disseminated breast carcinoma should have frequent determination of urine and serum calcium levels during the course of androgenic anabolic steroid therapy (see WARNINGS).
Because of the hepatotoxicity associated with the use of 17-alpha-alkylated androgens, liver function tests should be obtained periodically.
Periodic (every 6 months) x-ray examinations of bone age should be made during treatment of prepubertal patients to determine the rate of bone maturation and the effects of androgenic anabolic steroid therapy on the epiphyseal centers.
In common with other anabolic steroids, WINSTROL, brand of stanozolol tablets, has been reported to lower the level of high-density lipoproteins and raise the level of low-density lipoproteins. These changes usually revert to normal on discontinuation of treatment. Increased low-density lipoproteins and decreased high-density lipoproteins are considered cardiovascular risk factors. Serum lipids and high-density lipoprotein cholesterol should be determined periodically.
Drug Interaction. Anabolic steroids may increase sensitivity to anticoagulants; therefore, dosage of an anticoagulant may have to be decreased in order to maintain the prothrombin time at the desired therapeutic level.
Drug/Laboratory Test Interferences. Therapy with androgenic anabolic steroids may decrease levels of thyroxine-binding globulin resulting in decreased total T_4 serum levels and increase resin uptake of T_3 and T_4. Free thyroid hormone levels remain unchanged and there is no clinical evidence of thyroid dysfunction.
Anabolic steroids may cause an increase in prothrombin time.
Carcinogenesis, Mutagenesis, Impairment of Fertility. WINSTROL has not been tested in laboratory animals for carcinogenic or mutagenic effects. No tumorigenic or cancer-inducing properties of WINSTROL, brand of stanozolol tablets, were seen in one-year toxicity studies in rats.
WINSTROL administered orally (intragastrically) to pregnant rats at dosages of 2.5 mg/kg/day to 20 mg/kg/day increased the ano-genital distance in rat fetuses, indicative of a masculinizing effect. WINSTROL prevented pregnancy when given orally to rats from the 1st to the 21st day of gestation.
No teratogenic effects or congenital malformation were observed in offspring of rabbits given 0.5 mg/day, 1.0 mg/day, or 5.0 mg/day of WINSTROL from the 8th through the 16th day of pregnancy, nor were there any adverse effects on the course of pregnancy at these dose levels.
Pregnancy Category X. See CONTRAINDICATIONS section.
Nursing Mothers. It is not known whether anabolic steroids are excreted in human milk. Many drugs are excreted in human milk and because of the potential for adverse reactions in nursing infants from WINSTROL, a decision should be made whether to discontinue nursing or discontinue the drug, taking into account the importance of the drug to the mother.
Pediatric Use. Anabolic agents may accelerate epiphyseal maturation more rapidly than linear growth in children, and the effect may continue for 6 months after the drug has been stopped. Therefore, therapy should be monitored by x-ray studies at 6 month intervals in order to avoid the risk of compromising the adult height. The safety and efficacy of WINSTROL in children with hereditary angioedema have not been established.

ADVERSE REACTIONS

Hepatic: Cholestatic jaundice with, rarely, hepatic necrosis and death. Hepatocellular neoplasms and peliosis hepatis have been reported in association with long-term androgenic-anabolic steroid therapy (see WARNINGS). Reversible changes in liver function tests also occur including increased bromsulphalein (BSP) retention and increases in serum bilirubin, glutamic oxaloacetic transaminase (SGOT), and alkaline phosphatase.
Genitourinary System: *In men. Prepubertal:* Phallic enlargement and increased frequency of erections.
Postpubertal: Inhibition of testicular function, testicular atrophy and oligospermia, impotence, chronic priapism, epididymitis and bladder irritability.
In women: Clitoral enlargement, menstrual irregularities.
In both sexes: Increased or decreased libido.
CNS: Habituation, excitation, insomnia, depression.
Gastrointestinal: Nausea, vomiting, diarrhea.
Hematologic: Bleeding in patients on concomitant anticoagulant therapy.
Breast: Gynecomastia.
Larynx: Deepening of the voice in women.
Hair: Hirsutism and male pattern baldness in women.
Skin: Acne (especially in women and prepubertal boys).
Skeletal: Premature closure of epiphyses in children (see PRECAUTIONS, **Pediatric Use**).
Fluid and Electrolytes: Edema, retention of serum electrolytes (sodium, chloride, potassium, phosphate, calcium).
Metabolic/Endocrine: Decreased glucose tolerance (see PRECAUTIONS), increased serum levels of low-density lipoproteins and decreased levels of high-density lipoproteins (see PRECAUTIONS, **Laboratory Tests**), increased creatine and creatinine excretion, increased serum levels of creatinine phosphokinase (CPK).

Some virilizing changes in women are irreversible even after prompt discontinuance of therapy and are not prevented by concomitant use of estrogens (see PRECAUTIONS).

DOSAGE AND ADMINISTRATION

The use of anabolic steroids may be associated with serious adverse reactions, many of which are dose related; therefore, patients should be placed on the lowest possible effective dose.
Hereditary Angioedema. The dosage requirements for continuous treatment of hereditary angioedema with WINSTROL should be individualized on the basis of the clinical response of the patient. It is recommended that the patient be started on 2 mg, three times a day. After a favorable initial response is obtained in terms of prevention of episodes of edematous attacks, the proper continuing dosage should be determined by decreasing the dosage at intervals of one to three months to a maintenance dosage of 2 mg a day. Some patients may be successfully managed on a 2 mg alternate day schedule. During the dose adjusting phase, close monitoring of the patient's response is indicated, particularly if the patient has a history of airway involvement.
The prophylactic dose of WINSTROL, brand of stanozolol tablets, to be used prior to dental extraction, or other traumatic or stressful situations has not been established and may be substantially larger.
Attacks of hereditary angioedema are generally infrequent in childhood and the risks from stanozolol administration are substantially increased. Therefore, long-term prophylactic therapy with this drug is generally not recommended in children, and should only be undertaken with due consideration of the benefits and risks involved (see PRECAUTIONS, **Pediatric Use**).

HOW SUPPLIED

Tablets of 2 mg, scored, bottle of 100 (NDC 0024-2253-04)
Distributed by Winthrop-Breon Laboratories
Division of Sterling Drug Inc
New York, NY 10016
Manufactured by Sterling Pharmaceuticals Inc
Barceloneta, Puerto Rico 00617
Shown in Product Identification Section, page 435
WW 5-V

ZEPHIRAN® CHLORIDE OTC
brand of benzalkonium chloride

(See PDR For Nonprescription Drugs)

Winthrop Consumer Products

Division of Sterling Drug Inc.
90 PARK AVENUE
NEW YORK, NY 10016

FERGON® CAPSULES
FERGON® TABLETS
brand of ferrous gluconate
FERGON® ELIXIR

COMPOSITION

FERGON (ferrous gluconate, USP) is stabilized to maintain a minimum of ferric ions. Each FERGON Capsule contains 435 mg of ferrous gluconate, yielding 50 mg of elemental iron. Also contains: Benzyl Alcohol, Calcium Stearate, D&C Red #7, Red #28, Red #36, FD&C Blue #1, Red #40, Gelatin, Glycerin, Hydroxypropyl Cellulose, Parabens, Pharmaceutical Glaze, Povidone, Sodium Propionate, Sucrose, Talc. Each FERGON tablet contains 320 mg (36 mg of elemental iron). Also contains: Acacia, Carnauba Wax, Cerelose Dextrose, FD & C Yellow #6, D & C Yellow #10, FD & C Blue #1, Gelatin, Kaolin, Magnesium Stearate, Parabens, Povidone, Precipitated Calcium Carbonate, Sodium Benzoate, Starch, Sucrose, Talc, Titanium Dioxide, Yellow Wax.
FERGON Elixir 6% contains 300 mg per teaspoon (34 mg of elemental iron). Also contains: Alcohol 7%, Flavor, Glycerin, Liquid Glucose, Purified Water, Saccharin Sodium.

ACTION AND USES

FERGON preparations produce rapid hemoglobin regeneration in patients with iron deficiency anemias. FERGON is better utilized and better tolerated than other forms of iron because of its low ionization constant and solubility in the entire pH range of the gastrointestinal tract. It does not precipitate proteins or have the astringency of more ionizable forms of iron, does not interfere with proteolytic or diastatic activities of the digestive system, and will not produce nausea, abdominal cramps, constipation or diarrhea in the great majority of patients. The pellets of ferrous gluconate contained in FERGON Capsules are coated to permit maximum availability of iron in the upper small bowel, the site of maximum absorption.
FERGON preparations are indicated in anemias amenable to iron therapy.

DOSAGE AND ADMINISTRATION

Adults—1 FERGON Capsule daily for mild to moderate iron deficiency anemia. For more severe anemia the dosage may be increased. One to two FERGON tablets or one to two teaspoons of FERGON Elixir daily. *For children and infants,* consult physician.

WARNINGS

Since oral iron products interfere with absorption of oral tetracycline antibiotics, these products should not be taken within two hours of each other. Keep this and all drugs out of the reach of children. As with any drug, if you are pregnant or nursing a baby, seek the advice of a health professional before using this product. In case of accidental overdose, seek professional assistance or contact a poison control center immediately.

HOW SUPPLIED

FERGON Capsules, bottle of 30 (NDC 0024-1016-03). FERGON Tablets, bottle of 100 (NDC 0024-1015-10), bottle of 500 (NDC 0024-1015-50), and bottle of 1,000 (NDC 0024-1015-00). FERGON Elixir, bottle of 16 oz. (NDC 0024-1019-16).

NEO-SYNEPHRINE®
phenylephrine hydrochloride

DESCRIPTION

This line of Nasal Spray and Nose Drops contain Phenylephrine Hydrochloride in strengths ranging from .125% (drops only) to 1%. Also contains: Benzalkonium Chloride and Thimerosal 0.001% as preservatives, Citric Acid, Purified Water, Sodium Chloride, Sodium Citrate.

ACTION

Rapid-acting nasal decongestant.

INDICATIONS

For temporary relief of nasal congestion due to common cold, hay fever or other upper respiratory allergies, or associated with sinusitis.

Continued on next page

Winthrop Consumer—Cont.

PRECAUTIONS

Some hypersensitive individuals may experience a mild stinging sensation. This is usually transient and often disappears after a few applications.

Do not exceed recommended dosage. Follow directions for use carefully. If symptoms are not relieved after several applications, a physician should be consulted. Frequent and continued usage of the higher concentrations (especially the 1% solution) occasionally may cause a rebound congestion of the nose. Therefore, long-term or frequent use of this solution is not recommended without the advice of a physician. Prolonged exposure to air or strong light will cause oxidation and some loss of potency. Do not use if brown in color or contains a precipitate.

ADVERSE REACTIONS

Generally very well tolerated; systemic side effects such as tremor, insomnia, or palpitation rarely occur.

WARNINGS

Keep these and all drugs out of the reach of children. In case of accidental ingestion seek professional assistance or contact a poison control center immediately. The use of this dispenser by more than one person may spread infection.

DOSAGE AND ADMINISTRATION

Topical—dropper or spray. The *0.25% solution* is adequate in most cases *(0.125% for infants)*. In resistant cases, or if more powerful decongestion is desired, the *0.5 or 1% solution* should be used. Also used as *0.5% jelly*.

HOW SUPPLIED

Nasal spray 0.25%—15 mL (for children and for adults who prefer a mild nasal spray)—NDC 0024-1348-03; nasal spray 0.5%—15 mL (for adults)—NDC 0024-1353-01 and 30 mL (1 fl oz) NDC 0024-1353-05; nasal spray 1%—15 mL (extra strength for adults)—NDC 0024-1352-02; nasal solution 0.125% (for infants and small children), ½ fl oz bottles—NDC 0024-1345-05; nasal solution 0.25% (for children and adults who prefer a mild solution), ½ fl oz bottles—NDC 0024-1347-05 and 16 fl oz bottles—NDC 0024-1347-06; nasal solution 0.5% (for adults), ½ fl oz bottles—NDC 0024-1351-05; nasal solution 1% (extra strength for adults), ½ fl oz bottles—NDC 0024-1355-05 and 16 fl oz bottles—NDC 0024-1355-06; and water soluble nasal jelly 0.5%, ⅝ oz tubes—NDC 0024-1367-01.

Also available—NEO-SYNEPHRINE Mentholated Nasal Spray 0.5% (for adults), ½ fl oz bottles—NDC 0024-1364-01.

NEO-SYNEPHRINE® 12 HOUR
oxymetazoline HCl

Nasal Spray 0.05%
Vapor Nasal Spray 0.05%
Nose Drops 0.05%
Children's Drops 0.025%

DESCRIPTION

Adult Strength Nasal Spray and *Nose Drops* contain Oxymetazoline Hydrochloride 0.05%. Also contains: Benzalkonium Chloride and Phenylmercuric Acetate 0.002% as preservatives, Glycine, Purified Water, Sorbitol, may also contain Sodium Chloride. *Adult Strength Vapor Nasal Spray* contains Oxymetazoline Hydrochloride 0.05%. Also contains: Benzalkonium Chloride and Thimerosal 0.001% as preservatives, Camphor, Citric Acid, Eucalyptol, Menthol, Methyl Salicylate, Purified Water, Sodium Chloride, Sodium Citrate, Tyloxapol. *Children's Nose* Drops contain Oxymetazoline Hydrochloride 0.025%. Also contains: Benzalkonium Chloride and Phenylmercuric Acetate 0.002% as preservatives, Glycine, Purified Water, Sorbitol, may also contain Sodium Chloride.

ACTION

12 HOUR Nasal Decongestant.

INDICATIONS

Provides temporary relief, for up to 12 HOURS, of nasal congestion due to colds, hay fever, sinusitis, or allergies. NEO-SYNEPHRINE 12-HOUR Nasal Sprays and Nose Drops contain oxymetazoline which provides the longest-lasting relief of nasal congestion available.

WARNINGS

Do not exceed recommended dosage because symptoms may occur such as burning, stinging, sneezing, or increase of nasal discharge. (Nasal Spray 0.05%, Vapor Nasal Spray 0.05%, Nose Drops 0.05% not recommended for children under 6; Children's Drops 0.025% not recommended for children under 2.) Do not use these products for more than 3 days. If symptoms persist, consult a physician. The use of this dispenser by more than one person may spread infection. Keep this and all drugs out of the reach of children. In case of accidental ingestion seek professional assistance or contact a poison control center immediately.

DOSAGE AND ADMINISTRATION

Adult Strength Nasal Spray and Vapor Nasal Spray—For adults and children 6 years of age and over: With head upright, spray two or three times in each nostril twice daily—morning and evening. To spray, squeeze bottle quickly and firmly.

Adult Strength Nose Drops—For adults and children 6 years of age and over: two or three drops in each nostril twice daily—morning and evening.

Children's Nose Drops—Specially formulated for children 2 through 5 years. Children 2 to under 6 years of age: two or three drops in each nostril twice daily— morning and evening.

HOW SUPPLIED

Nasal Spray Adult Strength—plastic squeeze bottles of 15 mL (½ fl oz) NDC 0024-1390-03 and 30 mL (1 fl oz) NDC 0024-1394-01; *Vapor Nasal Spray Adult Strength*—squeeze bottles of 15 mL (½ fl oz) NDC 0024-1391-03; *Nose Drops Adult Strength*—bottles of 15 mL (½ fl oz) with dropper (NDC 0024-1392-01); *Children's Strength 0.025%*—bottles of 15 mL (½ fl oz) with dropper (NDC 0024-1393-01).

Wyeth Laboratories
Division of American Home Products Corporation
P.O. BOX 8299
PHILADELPHIA, PA 19101

Product Identification Codes

All oral solid dosage forms manufactured by Wyeth are imprinted with their respective National Drug Code (NDC). The portion of the number indicating product and strength appears on each tablet and capsule, together with the name Wyeth. The process of imprinting "Wyeth" on all solid forms of former products of Ives Laboratories will be completed by the end of 1986. Because of the publisher's production deadlines, all newly imprinted tablets and/or capsules and corresponding product information were not available in time to be included in this edition's Product Identification and Product Information sections. The product code numbers of the National Drug Code for the former Ives products will remain the same.

The following is a numerical list of NDC code numbers with their corresponding product names for all oral solid dosage forms manufactured by Wyeth.

Numerical Listing

Product Ident. Code	Product
1	Equanil® (meprobamate) Tablet 400 mg. C-IV
2	Equanil® (meprobamate) Tablet 200 mg. C-IV
6	Serax® (oxazepam) Capsule 15 mg. C-IV
13	Amphojel® (dried aluminum hydroxide gel) Tablet 0.6 Gm. (10 gr.)
19	Phenergan® (promethazine HCl) Tablet 12.5 mg.
22	Aludrox® (alumina and magnesia) Tablet
27	Phenergan® (promethazine HCl) Tablet 25 mg.
28	Sparine® (promazine HCl) Tablet 50 mg.
29	Sparine® (promazine HCl) Tablet 25 mg.
33	Equanil® (meprobamate) Tablet, Wyseals® 400 mg. C-IV
51	Serax® (oxazepam) Capsule 10 mg. C-IV
52	Serax® (oxazepam) Capsule 30 mg. C-IV
53	Omnipen® (ampicillin) Capsule 250 mg.
56	Ovral® (each tablet contains 0.5 mg. norgestrel with 0.05 mg. ethinyl estradiol) Tablet, white
57	Unipen® [(nafcillin sodium) as the monohydrate] Capsule 250 mg.
59	Pen•Vee® K (penicillin V potassium) Tablet 250 mg. (400,000 units)
62	Ovrette® (norgestrel) Tablet
64	Ativan® (lorazepam) Tablet 1 mg. C-IV
65	Ativan® (lorazepam) Tablet 2 mg. C-IV
71	Mazanor® (mazindol) Tablet 1 mg. C-IV
73	Wytensin® (guanabenz acetate) Tablet 4 mg.
74	Wytensin® (guanabenz acetate) Tablet 8 mg.
75	Nordette-21® (each tablet contains 0.15 mg. levonorgestrel with 0.03 mg. ethinyl estradiol) Tablet
78	Lo/Ovral® (each tablet contains 0.3 mg. norgestrel with 0.03 mg. ethinyl estradiol) Tablet, white
81	Ativan® (lorazepam) Tablet 0.5 mg. C-IV
85	Wygesic® (each tablet contains 65 mg. propoxyphene HCl, U.S.P., and 650 mg. acetaminophen, U.S.P.) Tablet C-IV
91	Equagesic® (meprobamate with aspirin) Tablet
92	Wytensin® (guanabenz acetate) Tablet 16 mg.
119	Amphojel® (dried aluminum hydroxide gel) Tablet 0.3 Gm. (5 gr.)
165	Bicillin® (penicillin G benzathine) Tablet 200,000 units
200	Sparine® (promazine HCl) Tablet 100 mg.
227	Phenergan® (promethazine HCl) Tablet 50 mg.
261	Mepergan® Fortis (meperidine HCl and promethazine HCl) Capsule C-II
267	Phenobarbital Tablet 15 mg. (¼ gr.) C-IV
268	Phenobarbital Tablet 30 mg. (½ gr.) C-IV
269	Phenobarbital Tablet 100 mg. (1½ gr.) C-IV
308	Meperidine HCl Tablet 50 mg. C-II
309	Omnipen® (ampicillin) Capsule 500 mg.
313	Aspirin Tablet 300 mg. (5 gr.)
317	Serax® (oxazepam) Tablet 15 mg. C-IV
320	Phenobarbital Tablet 60 mg. (1 gr.) C-IV
326	Codeine Sulfate Tablet 30 mg. (½ gr.) C-II
327	Codeine Sulfate Tablet 60 mg. (1 gr.) C-II
360	Pathocil® (dicloxacillin sodium monohydrate) Capsule 250 mg.
389	Tetracycline HCl Capsule 250 mg.
390	Pen•Vee® K (penicillin V potassium) Tablet 500 mg. (800,000 units)
434	Phenergan®-D (promethazine HCl with pseudoephedrine HCl) Tablet
445	Ovral®-28 pink inert tablet
464	Unipen® [(nafcillin sodium) as the monohydrate] 500 mg. Tablet
471	Tetracycline HCl Capsule 500 mg.
472	Basaljel® (dried basic aluminum carbonate gel) Capsule
473	Basaljel® (dried basic aluminum carbonate gel) Swallow Tablet
486	Nordette®-28, Lo/Ovral®-28 pink inert tablet
559	Wymox® (amoxicillin) 250 mg. Capsule
560	Wymox® (amoxicillin) 500 mg. Capsule
576	Wyamycin®S (erythromycin stearate) Tablet, film coated, 250 mg.
578	Wyamycin®S (erythromycin stearate) Tablet, film coated, 500 mg.
593	Pathocil® (dicloxacillin sodium monohydrate) Capsule 500 mg
614	Cyclapen-W® (cyclacillin) Tablet 250 mg.
615	Cyclapen-W® (cyclacillin) Tablet 500 mg.
2511	Ovral®-28 Pilpak® (21 white tablets each containing 0.5 mg. norgestrel with 0.05 mg. ethinyl estradiol and 7 pink inert tablets)
2514	Lo/Ovral®-28 Pilpak® (21 white tablets each containing 0.3 mg. norgestrel with 0.03 mg. ethinyl estradiol and 7 pink inert tablets)
2533	Nordette®-28 Pilpak® (21 light-orange tablets each containing 0.15 mg. levonorgestrel with 0.03 mg ethinyl estradiol and 7 pink inert tablets)
2535	Triphasil®-21 Tablets (levonorgestrel and ethinyl estradiol tablets—triphasic regimen)
2536	Triphasil®-28 Tablets (levonorgestrel and ethinyl estradiol tablets—triphasic regimen)
4120	Cyclospasmol® Tablet 100 mg
4124	Cyclospasmol® Capsule 200 mg
4125	Isordil® Tembids® Tablet 40 mg
4126	Isordil® Sublingual Tablet 5 mg
4130	Trecator®-SC, Tablet 250 mg
4132	Surmontil® Capsule 25 mg
4133	Surmontil® Capsule 50 mg
4139	Isordil® Sublingual Tablet 2.5 mg
4140	Isordil® Tembids Capsule 40 mg
4148	Cyclospasmol® Capsule 400 mg
4152	Isordil® 5 Titradose Tablet 5 mg
4153	Isordil® 10 Titradose Tablet 10 mg
4154	Isordil® 20 Titradose Tablet 20 mg
4158	Surmontil® Capsule 100 mg
4159	Isordil® 30 Titradose Tablet 30 mg
4161	Isordil® Sublingual Tablet 10 mg
4164	Isordil® Chewable Tablet 10 mg
4177	Sectral® Capsule 200 mg
4179	Sectral® Capsule 400 mg
4181	Orudis® Capsule 50 mg
4187	Orudis® Capsule 75 mg
4188	Cordarone® Tablet
4190	Synalgos® Capsule
4191	Synalgos®-DC Capsule
4192	Isordil® 40 Titradose Tablet 40 mg

ALUDROX® OTC
[*al'u-drox*]
(alumina and magnesia)
ORAL SUSPENSION • TABLETS

COMPOSITION

Nonconstipating, noncathartic, effective and palatable antacid containing, in each 5 ml. teaspoonful of suspension, 307 mg. of aluminum hydroxide as a gel, and 103 mg. of magnesium hydroxide. The inactive ingredients present are artificial and natural flavors, benzoic acid, butylparaben, glycerin, hydroxypropyl methylcellulose, methylparaben, propylparaben, saccharin, simethicone, sorbitol solution, and water.

Each tablet contains 233 mg. aluminum hydroxide as a dried gel and 83 mg. magnesium hydroxide. Sodium content is 0.06 mEq per tablet and 0.10 mEq per 5 ml suspension.

INDICATIONS

For the symptomatic relief of hyperacidity associated with the diagnosis of peptic ulcer, gastritis, peptic esophagitis, gastric hyperacidity, and hiatal hernia.

DOSAGE AND ADMINISTRATION

Two tablets or 2 teaspoonfuls (10 ml.) of suspension every four hours, or as required. Suspension may be followed by a sip of water if desired. Tablets are designed to be chewed with or without water.

Two ALUDROX tablets have the capacity to neutralize 19 mEq of acid; 10 ml. of ALUDROX suspension have the capacity to neutralize 24 mEq of acid.

WARNINGS

Patients are advised not to take more than 12 teaspoonfuls (60 ml) or 16 tablets in a 24-hour period or use this maximum dosage for more than two weeks except under the advice and supervision of a physician. Pregnant women and nursing mothers are advised to seek the advice of a health professional before using this product.

DRUG INTERACTION PRECAUTIONS

This product must not be taken if the patient is presently taking a prescription antibiotic drug containing any form of tetracycline.

HOW SUPPLIED

Oral Suspension, bottles of 12 fluidounces.

Tablets, boxes of 100; each tablet is safety sealed in cellophane so that a day's supply can be conveniently carried.

AMPHOJEL® OTC

[am 'fo-jel]

(aluminum hydroxide gel)

SUSPENSION • TABLETS

COMPOSITION

Suspension—Each 5 ml. teaspoonful contains 320 mg. of aluminum hydroxide as a gel, and not more than 0.10 mEq of sodium. The inactive ingredients present are butylparaben, calcium benzoate, glycerin, hydroxypropyl methylcellulose, methylparaben, propylparaben, saccharin, simethicone, sorbitol solution, and water. *Tablets* contain a dried gel. The 0.3 Gm. (5 grain) strength is equivalent to about 1 teaspoonful of the suspension and the 0.6 Gm. (10 grain) strength is equivalent to about 2 teaspoonfuls. Each 0.3 Gm tablet contains 0.08 mEq of sodium and each 0.6 Gm tablet contains 0.13 mEq of sodium.

INDICATIONS

For the symptomatic relief of hyperacidity associated with the diagnosis of peptic ulcer, gastritis, peptic esophagitis, gastric hyperacidity, and hiatal hernia.

DOSAGE

Suspension—two teaspoonfuls followed by a sip of water if desired, five or six times daily, between meals and at bedtime. Two teaspoonfuls have the capacity to neutralize 20 mEq of acid. *Tablets*—Two tablets of the 0.3 Gm. strength, or one tablet of the 0.6 Gm. strength, five or six times daily between meals and at bedtime. Two tablets have the capacity to neutralize 16 mEq of acid.

WARNINGS

Patients are advised not to take more than 12 teaspoonfuls (60 ml) or 12 0.3 Gm tablets or 6 0.6 Gm tablets in a 24-hour period or use this maximum dosage for more than two weeks except under the advice and supervision of a physician. Pregnant women and nursing mothers are advised to seek the advice of a health professional before using this product.

PRECAUTION

May cause constipation.

DRUG INTERACTION PRECAUTIONS

This product must not be taken if the patient is presently taking a prescription antibiotic drug containing any form of tetracycline.

HOW SUPPLIED

Suspension—Peppermint flavored; without flavor—bottles of 12 fluidounces. *Tablets*—a convenient auxiliary dosage form—0.3 Gm. (5 gr.), bottles of 100; 0.6 Gm. (10 gr.), boxes of 100.

ANTIVENIN (CROTALIDAE) ℞

[an "te ven 'in]

POLYVALENT

(equine origin)

IMPORTANT

Pit viper bites may cause severe tissue damage or fatal envenomation, or both. The physician responsible for treatment of an envenomated patient should be familiar with the contents of this brochure and the pertinent medical literature concerning current concepts of first-aid and general supportive therapy as presented in the references listed at the end of this pamphlet.

COMPOSITION

Antivenin (Crotalidae) Polyvalent, Wyeth, is a refined and concentrated preparation of serum globulins obtained by fractionating blood from healthy horses immunized with the following venoms: *Crotalus adamanteus* (eastern diamond rattlesnake), *C. atrox* (western diamond rattlesnake), *C. durissus terrificus* (tropical rattlesnake, Cascabel), and Bothrops atrox ("Fer-de-lance"). Phenol, 0.25%, and thimerosal, 0.005%, are added as preservatives. The product is standardized by its ability to neutralize the lethal action of standard venoms by intravenous injection in mice.[1] Dried from the frozen state, the lyophilized serum has a moisture content of less than 1% and is soluble on addition of the diluent contained in each package (Bacteriostatic Water for Injection, USP, with preservative: 0.001% phenylmercuric nitrate).

Antivenin (Crotalidae) Polyvalent, Wyeth (hereinafter referred to as Antivenin) contains protective substances capable of neutralizing the toxic effects of venoms of crotalids (pit vipers) native to North, Central, and South America, including rattlesnakes *(Crotalus, Sistrurus);* copperhead and cottonmouth moccasins *(Agkistrodon),* including *A. halys* of Korea and Japan; the Fer-de-lance and other species of *Bothrops;* the tropical rattler (*Crotalus durissus* and similar species); the Cantil *(A. bilineatus);* and bushmaster *(Lachesis mutus)* of South and Central America.

INDICATION

Antivenin is indicated only for the treatment of envenomation caused by bites of those crotalids (pit vipers) specified in the immediately preceding paragraph.

Pit Viper Bites and Envenomation: The symptoms, signs, and severity of snake-venom poisoning resulting from pit viper bites depend on many factors, including, but not limited to, the following variables: species, age, and size of the biting snake; the number and location of bite(s); the depth of venom deposit by the snake's fangs; the condition of the snake's fangs and venom glands; the length of time the snake "hangs on"; the age, general health, and size of the victim; the type and efficacy of any first-aid treatment rendered in an attempt to remove venom and how soon such treatment was applied. In any venomous snake bite, the actual amount of venom introduced into the victim is always an unknown. Even the type of clothing or leg-footwear through which the snake's fangs pass may affect the amount of venom delivered by the bite. Although most North American pit vipers tend to bite and introduce venom superficially, their fangs may get hung-up in the subcutaneous tissues during the biting act and can penetrate deeper tissues during the attempt to release the bitten part. In some bites the fangs may penetrate into muscle. In such cases, the usual local superficial manifestations of envenomation may not appear early in the course of poisoning. In bites by some species, systemic evidence of envenomation may be present in the absence of significant local manifestations. It may be difficult to determine the severity of envenomation during the first several hours after a pit viper bite and estimates of severity may need to be revised as poisoning progresses. It must be remembered, too, that not all pit viper bites result in envenomation. In approximately 20% of rattlesnake bites, the snake may not inject any venom. The local and systemic symptoms and signs of envenomation include the following:

LOCAL:

Fang puncture(s).

Swelling—edema is usually seen around the site of bite within five minutes. It may progress rapidly and involve the entire extremity within an hour. More than 95% of all snakebites are inflicted on extremities.[2] Generally, however, edema spreads more slowly, usually over a period of 8 or more hours. Swelling is usually most severe following envenomation by the eastern diamondback; less severe after bites by the western diamondback, prairie, timber, red, Pacific, Mojave, and blacktailed rattlers, the sidewinder and cottonmouth moccasins; least severe after bites by copperheads, massasaugas, and pygmy rattlers.

Ecchymosis and discoloration of the skin —often appear in the area of the bite within a few hours. Vesicules may form within a few hours and are usually present at 24 hours. Hemorrhagic blebs and petechiae are common. Necrosis may develop, necessitating amputation of an extremity or a portion thereof.

Pain—frequently a complaint of the victim beginning shortly after the bite by most pit vipers. Pain may be absent after bites by Mojave rattlers.

SYSTEMIC:

Weakness; faintness; nausea; sweating; numbness or tingling around the mouth, tongue, scalp, fingers, toes, site of bite; muscle fasciculations; hypotension; prolongation of bleeding and clotting times; hemoconcentration, early followed by a decrease in erythrocytes; thrombocytopenia; hematuria; proteinuria; vomiting, including hematemesis; melena; hemoptysis; epistaxis. In fatal poisoning, a frequent cause of death is associated with destruction of erythrocytes and changes in capillary permeability, especially of the pulmonary vascular system, leading to pulmonary edema; hemoconcentration usually occurs early, probably as a result of plasma loss secondary to vascular permeability; the hemoglobin may fall, and bleeding may occur throughout the body as early as 6 hours after the bite. Renal involvement is not uncommon. Mojave rattler venom may cause neuromuscular changes leading to respiratory failure.

An estimate of the severity of envenomation should be made as soon as possible and before any Antivenin is administered. The amount (volume) of the first dose of Antivenin is determined on this estimate of severity. Every symptom, sign, laboratory-test result, and any other pertinent information should be considered in estimating severity—local manifestations; systemic manifestations, including abnormal laboratory findings; species and size of the biting snake, if known; number and location of bites(s); size and health of the patient; type of first-aid treatment rendered; and interval between bite and arrival for treatment. Russell et al,[3] and Wingert and Wainschel[4] grade severity as follows:

No envenomation—no local or systemic manifestations.

Minimal envenomation—local swelling and other local changes; no systemic manifestations; normal laboratory findings.

Moderate envenomation—swelling progressing beyond the site of bite and one or more systemic manifestations; abnormal laboratory findings, for example, a fall in hematocrit or platelets.

Severe envenomation—marked local response, severe systemic manifestations and significant alteration in laboratory findings.

Parrish and Hayes,[5] McCollough and Gennaro,[6] and Watt and Gennaro[7] have used a Grade 0 (no envenomation) through Grade IV (very severe) classification of severity which was developed for the most part in treatment of envenomation by the eastern diamondback and timber rattlers. This classification is more dependent on local manifestations, or the absence thereof, as the venoms of these species seem to be more consistent in inducing local tissue damage.

Any suspected envenomation should be treated as a medical emergency, and until careful observation provides clear evidence that envenomation has not occurred or is minimal, the following procedures are recommended:

Monitor vital signs at frequent intervals: Blood pressure, pulse, respiration.

Draw sufficient blood as soon as possible for baseline laboratory studies, including type and cross-match, CBC, hematocrit, platelet count, prothrombin time, clot retraction, bleeding and coagulation times, BUN, electrolytes, bilirubin. Some of these studies may need to be repeated at daily intervals, or less, depending on the severity of envenomation and the response to treatment. During the first 4 or 5 days of severe envenomations, hemoglobin, hematocrit, and platelet counts should be carried out several times a day.

Obtain urine samples at frequent intervals for analysis, with special attention to microscopic examination for presence of erythrocytes.

Chart fluid intake and urine output.

Measure and record the circumference of the bitten extremity just proximal to the bite and at one or more additional points each several inches closer to the trunk. Repeat measurements every 15-30 minutes to obtain information about progression of edema.

Have available and ready for immediate use:

Oxygen, resuscitation equipment including airway, tourniquet, epinephrine, injectable antihistaminic agents, and corticosteroids.

Start an intravenous infusion in one or two extremities: one line to be used for supportive therapy, if needed, such as whole blood, plasma, packed red cells, specific clotting factors, platelet transfusion, plasma expanders; the other line to be used for administration of Antivenin and electrolytes.

Carry out and interpret a skin test for horse-serum sensitivity. (See Precautions section below.)

DOSAGE AND ADMINISTRATION

Before administration, read Precautions and Systemic Reactions sections below. Since the possibility of a severe immediate reaction (anaphylaxis) exists whenever a horse-serum-containing product is administered, appropriate therapeutic agents, including a tourniquet, airway, oxygen, epinephrine, an injectable pressor amine, and corticosteroid, must be available and ready for immediate use. Constant attendance and observation of the patient for untoward reactions are mandatory when Antivenin is administered. Should any systemic reaction occur, administration should be discontinued immediately and appropriate treatment initiated.

The intravenous route of administration is preferred, and probably should always be used for moderate or severe envenomation. Intravenous administration is mandatory if venom-induced shock is present. To be most effective, Antivenin should be administered within 4 hours of the bite; it is less effective when given after 8 hours and may be of ques-

Continued on next page

Wyeth—Cont.

tionable value after 12 hours. However, it is recommended that Antivenin therapy be given in severe poisonings, even if 24 hours have elapsed since the time of the bite. It should be kept in mind that maximum blood levels of Antivenin may not be obtained for 8 or more hours after intramuscular administration.

For intravenous-drip use, prepare a 1:1 to 1:10 dilution of reconstituted Antivenin in Sodium Chloride Injection, USP, or 5% Dextrose Injection, USP. To avoid foaming, mix by gently swirling rather than shaking. Allow the initial 5 to 10 ml to infuse over a 3- to 5-minute period, with careful observation of the patient for evidence of untoward reaction. If no symptoms or signs of an immediate systemic reaction appear, continue the infusion with delivery at the maximum safe rate for intravenous fluid administration. The dilution of Antivenin to be used, the type of electrolyte solution used for dilution, and the rate of intravenous delivery of the diluted Antivenin must take into consideration the age, weight, and cardiac status of the patient; the severity of envenomation; the total amount and type of parenteral fluids it is anticipated will be given or are needed; and the interval between bite and initiation of specific therapy.

It is important to give as soon as possible the entire initial dose of Antivenin as based on the best estimate of the severity of envenomation at the time treatment is begun. The following initial doses are recommended:[3,4,8]

no envenomation—none
minimal envenomation—20-40 ml (contents of 2-4 vials)
moderate envenomation—50-90 ml (contents of 5-9 vials)
severe envenomation—100-150 ml or more (contents of 10-15 or more vials)

These recommended initial-dosage volumes are in general accord with those of others.[5-7,9]

The need for additional Antivenin must be based on the clinical response to the initial dose and continuing assessment of the severity of poisoning. If swelling continues to progress or if systemic symptoms or signs of envenomation increase in severity or if new manifestations appear, for example, fall in hematocrit or hypotension, administer an additional 10-50 ml (contents of 1-5 vials) intravenously.

Envenomation by large snakes in children or small adults requires larger doses of Antivenin. The amount administered to a child is not based on weight.

If Antivenin is given intramuscularly, it should be given into a large muscle mass, preferably the gluteal area, with care to avoid nerve trunks. Antivenin should never be injected into a finger or toe.

The effectiveness of corticosteroids in treatment of envenomation per se or venom shock is not resolved. Russell[3] and others[9,10] believe corticosteroids may mask the seriousness of hypovolemia in moderate or severe poisoning and have little, if any, effect on the local-tissue response to rattler venoms. Corticosteroids should not be given simultaneously with Antivenin on a routine basis or during the acute stage of envenomation; however, their use may be necessary to treat immediate allergic reactions to Antivenin, and corticosteroids are the agents of choice for treating serious delayed reactions to Antivenin.

Snakes' mouths do not harbor *Clostridium tetani.* However, appropriate tetanus prophylaxis is indicated, since tetanus spores may be carried into the fang puncture wounds by dirt present on skin at time of bite or by nonsterile first-aid procedures.

A broad-spectrum antibiotic in adequate dosage is indicated if local tissue damage is evident.

Shock following envenomation is treated like shock resulting from hypovolemia from any cause, including administration of whole blood, plasma, albumin, or other plasma expanders, as indicated.

Aspirin or codeine is usually adequate for relieving pain. Sedation with phenobarbital or mild tranquilizers may be used if indicated, but not in the presence of respiratory failure.

The bitten extremity should not be packed in ice, and so-called "cryotherapy" is contraindicated.

Compartment syndromes may complicate pit viper envenomations, especially those caused by bites on the lower extremities. Prompt surgical consultation is indicated whenever a closed-compartment syndrome is suspected.[3,12]

Defibrination and disseminated intravascular coagulation (DIC) syndromes have been associated with envenomation caused by some pit vipers native to the United States, and appropriate therapy may be indicated.[3,9,10,13–17]

TECHNIC FOR RECONSTITUTING THE DRIED ANTIVENIN

Pry off the small metal disc in the cap over the diaphragms of the vials of Antivenin and diluent. Swab the exposed surface of the rubber diaphragms of both vials with an appropriate germicide. With a sterile 10 ml syringe and needle, withdraw the diluent (Bacteriostatic Water for Injection, USP, containing phenylmercuric nitrate 1:100,000) from the vial of diluent and inject it into the vial of Antivenin. Gentle agitation will hasten complete dissolution of the lyophilized Antivenin.

PRECAUTIONS

Before administration of any product prepared from horse serum, appropriate measures must be taken in an effort to detect the presence of dangerous sensitivity: (1) A careful review of the patient's history, including any report of (a) asthma, hay fever, urticaria, or other allergic manifestations; (b) allergic reactions upon exposure to horses; and (c) prior injections of horse serum. (2) A suitable test for detection of sensitivity. A skin test should be performed in every patient prior to administration, regardless of clinical history.

Skin test—Inject intracutaneously 0.02 to 0.03 ml of a 1:10 dilution of Normal Horse Serum or Antivenin. A control test on the opposite extremity, using Sodium Chloride Injection, USP, facilitates interpretation. Use of larger amounts for the skin-test dose increases the likelihood of false-positive reactions, and in the exquisitely sensitive patient, increases the risk of a systemic reaction from the skin-test dose. A 1:100 or greater dilution should be used for preliminary skin testing if the history suggests sensitivity. A positive reaction to a skin test occurs within five to thirty minutes and is manifested by a wheal with or without pseudopodia and surrounding erythema. In general, the shorter the interval between injection and the beginning of the skin reaction, the greater the sensitivity.

If the history is negative for allergy and the result of a skin test is negative, proceed with administration of Antivenin as outlined above. If the history is positive and a skin test is strongly positive, administration may be dangerous, especially if the positive sensitivity test is accompanied by systemic allergic manifestations. In such instances, the risk of administering Antivenin must be weighed against the risk of withholding it, keeping in mind that severe envenomation can be fatal. (See last paragraph of this section.)

A negative allergic history and absence of reaction to a properly applied skin test do not rule out the possibility of an immediate reaction. Also, a negative skin test has no bearing on whether or not delayed serum reactions (serum sickness) will occur after administration of the full dose.

If the history is negative, and the skin test is mildly or questionably positive, administer as follows to reduce the risk of a severe immediate systemic reaction: (a) Prepare, in separate sterile vials or syringes, 1:100 and 1:10 dilutions of Antivenin. (b) Allow at least 15 minutes between injections and proceed with the next dose if no reaction follows the previous dose. (c) Inject subcutaneously, using a tuberculin-type syringe, 0.1, 0.2, and 0.5 ml of the 1:100 dilution at 15-minute intervals; repeat with the 1:10 dilution, and finally undiluted Antivenin. (d) If a systemic reaction occurs after any injection, place a tourniquet proximal to the site of injections and administer an appropriate dose of epinephrine, 1:1000, proximal to the tourniquet or into another extremity. Wait at least 30 minutes before injecting another dose. The amount of the next dose should be the same as the last that did not evoke a reaction. (e) If no reaction occurs after 0.5 ml of undiluted Antivenin has been administered, switch to the intramuscular route and continue doubling the dose at 15-minute intervals until the entire dose has been injected intramuscularly or proceed to the intravenous route as described above under Dosage and Administration.

Obviously, if the just-described schedule is used, 3 to 5 or more hours would be required to administer the initial dose suggested for a moderate or severe envenomation, and time is an important factor in neutralization of venom in a critically ill patient. Wingert and Wainschel[4] have described a procedure based on the experience of their group which they have used in some severely envenomated patients who have positive sensitivity tests: 50 to 100 mg of diphenhydramine hydrochloride is given intravenously, followed by slow intravenous infusion of diluted Antivenin for 15 to 20 minutes while carefully observing the patient for symptoms and signs of anaphylaxis; if anaphylaxis does not occur, Antivenin is continued maintaining close observation of the patient. Patients who require Antivenin but develop signs of impending anaphylaxis in spite of this or the procedure described earlier present a difficult problem, and consultation should be sought.

SYSTEMIC REACTIONS

A. The immediate reaction (shock, anaphylaxis) usually occurs within 30 minutes. Symptoms and signs may develop before the needle is withdrawn and may include apprehension, flushing, itching, urticaria; edema of the face, tongue, and throat; cough, dyspnea, cyanosis, vomiting, and collapse.

B. Serum sickness usually occurs 5 to 24 days after administration. The incubation period may be less than 5 days, especially in those who have received horse-serum-containing preparations in the past. The usual symptoms and signs are malaise, fever, urticaria, lymphadenopathy, edema, arthralgia, nausea, and vomiting. Occasionally, neurological manifestations develop, such as meningismus or peripheral neuritis. Peripheral neuritis usually involves the shoulders and arms. Pain and muscle weakness are frequently present, and permanent atrophy may develop.

REFERENCES

1. GINGRICH, W. & HOHENADEL, J.: Standardization of polyvalent antivenin. "Venoms", edited by E. Buckley and N. Porges. Publication No. 44, Amer. Assoc. for the Advancement of Science, Washington, D.C., 1956, Pages 337–80.
2. PARRISH, H.: Incidence of treated snakebite in the United States. Pub. Hlth. Rep. *81* :269, 1966.
3. RUSSELL, F., et al.: Snake venom poisoning in the United States. Experiences with 550 cases. JAMA *233* :341, 1975. RUSSELL, F.: Venomous bites and stings: Poisonous snakes. In The Merck Manual of Diagnosis and Therapy, pp. 2450–2456, 14th Ed., 1982.
4. WINGERT, W. and WAINSCHEL, J.: Diagnosis and management of envenomation by poisonous snakes. South. Med. J. *68* :1015, 1975.
5. PARRISH, H. & HAYES, R.: Hospital management of pit viper venenations. Clinical Toxicol. *3* :501, 1970.
6. McCOLLOUGH, N. & GENNARO, J.: Diagnosis, symptoms, treatment and sequelae of envenomation by *Crotalus adamanteus* and Genus *Agkistrodon.* J. Florida Med. Assoc. *55* :327, 1968.
7. WATT, C. & GENNARO, J.: Pit viper bites in South Georgia and North Florida. Tr. South. Surg. Assoc. 77 :378, 1966.
8. MINTON, S.: Venom Diseases: Snakebite. In Textbook of Medicine, P. Beeson and W. McDermott (Eds.), pp. 88–92; Saunders, Philadelphia, 1975.
9. VAN MIEROP, L.: Snakebite symposium. J. Florida Med. Assoc. *63* :101, 1976; Controversies and hazards in the treatment of pit viper bites. South. Med. J. *72* :902, 1979.
10. ARNOLD, R.: Treatment of snakebite. JAMA *236* :1843, 1976; Controversies and hazards in the treatment of pit viper bites. South Med. J. *72* :902, 1979.
11. Poisonous Snakes of the World. U.S. Government Printing Office, Washington, D.C., NAVMED, 1965.
12. GARFIN, S. et al.: Rattlesnake bites: Current concepts. Clin. Orthop. *140* :50, 1979; Role of surgical decompression in treatment of rattlesnake bites. Surg. Forum *30* :502, 1979.
13. VAN MIEROP, L. & KITCHENS, C.: Defibrination syndrome following bites by the eastern diamondback rattlesnake, J. Florida Med. Assoc. *67* :21, 1980.
14. HASIBA, U. et al.: DIC-like syndrome after envenomation by the snake, *Crotalus horridus horridus.* New Eng. J. Med. *292* :505, 1975.
15. WEISS, H. et al.: Afibrinogenemia in man following the bite of a rattlesnake *(Crotalus adamanteus).* Am. J. Med. *47* :625, 1969.
16. SIVAPRASAD, R. & CANTINI, E.: Western diamondback rattlesnake *(Crotalus atrox)* poisoning. Postgrad. Med. *71* :223, 1982.
17. SABBACK, M. et al.: A study of the treatment of pit viper envenomization in 45 patients. J. Trauma *17* :569, 1977.

HOW SUPPLIED

Each combination package contains one vacuum vial to yield 10 ml of serum—to be used immediately after reconstitution—(with preservatives: phenol 0.25% and thimerosal [mercury derivative] 0.005%). One vial containing 10 ml of Bacteriostatic Water for Injection, USP (with preservative: phenylmercuric nitrate 0.001%). One 1 ml vial of normal horse serum (diluted 1:10) as sensitivity testing material with preservatives: thimerosal (mercury derivative) 0.005% and phenol 0.35%. Not returnable.

ANTIVENIN (Micrurus fulvius) ℞

[an "te ven 'in]
(equine origin)
North American Coral Snake Antivenin

COMPOSITION

Each combination package contains one vial of lyophilized Antivenin (Micrurus fulvius) with 0.25% phenol and 0.005% thimerosal (mercury derivative) as preservatives (before lyophilization); one vial of diluent containing 10 ml. of Bacteriostatic Water for Injection, U.S.P., with phenylmercuric nitrate (1:100,000) as preservative.

HOW SUPPLIED

Combination packages as described (not returnable).
For prescribing information write to Professional Service, Wyeth Laboratories, Box 8299, Philadelphia, PA 19101, or contact your local Wyeth representative.

ATIVAN® Ⓒ ℞

[at 'i-van]
(lorazepam)
Injection

DESCRIPTION

Ativan (lorazepam) Injection, a benzodiazepine with anti-anxiety and sedative effects, is intended for intramuscular or intravenous route of administration. It has the chemical formula: 7-chloro-5-(*o*-chlorophenyl)-1,3-dihydro-3-hydroxy-

2*H*-1, 4-benzodiazepin-2-one. The molecular weight is 321.2 and the C.A.S. No. is [846-49-1].

Lorazepam is a nearly white powder almost insoluble in water. Each ml of sterile injection contains either 2.0 or 4.0 mg of lorazepam, 0.18 ml polyethylene glycol 400 in propylene glycol with 2.0% benzyl alcohol as preservative.

CLINICAL PHARMACOLOGY

Intravenous or intramuscular administration of the recommended dose of 2–4 mg of Ativan (lorazepam) Injection to adult patients is followed by dose-related effects of sedation (sleepiness or drowsiness), relief of preoperative anxiety, and lack of recall of events related to the day of surgery in the majority of patients. The clinical sedation (sleepiness or drowsiness) thus noted is such that the majority of patients are able to respond to simple instructions whether they give the appearance of being awake or asleep. The lack of recall is relative rather than absolute, as determined under conditions of careful patient questioning and testing using props designed to enhance recall. The majority of patients under these reinforced conditions had difficulty recalling perioperative events, or recognizing props from before surgery. The lack of recall and recognition was optimum within 2 hours following intramuscular administration and 15–20 minutes after intravenous injection.

The intended effects of the recommended adult dose of lorazepam injection usually last 6–8 hours. In rare instances and where patients received greater than the recommended dose, excessive sleepiness and prolonged lack of recall were noted. As with other benzodiazepines, unsteadiness, enhanced sensitivity to CNS-depressant effects of ethyl alcohol and other drugs were noted in isolated and rare cases for greater than 24 hours.

Studies in healthy adult volunteers reveal that intravenous lorazepam in doses up to 3.5 mg/70 kg does not alter sensitivity to the respiratory stimulating effect of carbon dioxide and does not enhance the respiratory depressant effects of doses of meperidine up to 100 mg/70 kg (also determined by carbon dioxide challenge) as long as patients remain sufficiently awake to undergo testing. Upper airway obstruction has been observed in rare instances where the patient received greater than the recommended dose, and was excessively sleepy and difficult to arouse. (See WARNINGS and ADVERSE REACTIONS.)

Clinically employed doses of lorazepam injectable do not greatly affect the circulatory system in the supine position or employing a 70-degree tilt test. Doses of 8–10 mg of intravenous lorazepam (2 to 2½ times the maximum recommended dosage) will produce loss of lid reflexes within 15 minutes.

Studies in six (6) healthy young adults who received lorazepam injection and no other drugs revealed that visual tracking (the ability to keep a moving line centered) was impaired for a mean of eight (8) hours following administration of 4 mg of intramuscular lorazepam and four (4) hours following administration of 2 mg intramuscularly with considerable subject variation. Similar findings were noted with pentobarbital, 150 and 75 mg. Although this study showed that both lorazepam and pentobarbital interfered with eye-hand coordination, the data are insufficient to predict when it would be safe to operate a motor vehicle or engage in a hazardous occupation or sport.

PHARMACOKINETICS

Injectable Ativan (lorazepam) is readily absorbed when given intramuscularly. Peak plasma concentrations occur approximately 60–90 minutes following administration and appear to be dose related, e.g., a 2.0 mg dose provides a level of approximately 20 ng/ml and a 4.0 mg dose aproximately 40 ng/ml in plasma. The mean half-life of lorazepam is about 16 hours when given intravenously or intramuscularly. Ativan (lorazepam) is rapidly conjugated at the 3-hydroxyl group into its major metabolite, lorazepam glucuronide, which is then excreted in the urine. Lorazepam glucuronide has no demonstrable CNS activity in animals. When 5 mg of intravenous lorazepam was administered to volunteers once a day for four consecutive days, a steady state of free lorazepam was achieved by the second day (approximately 52 ng/ml of plasma three hours after the first dose and approximately 62 ng/ml three hours after each subsequent dose, one day apart). At clinically relevant concentrations, lorazepam is bound 85% to plasma proteins.

INDICATIONS AND USAGE

Ativan (lorazepam) Injection is indicated in adult patients for preanesthetic medication, producing sedation (sleepiness or drowsiness), relief of anxiety, and a decreased ability to recall events related to the day of surgery. It is most useful in those patients who are anxious about their surgical procedure and who would prefer to have diminished recall of the events of the day of surgery. (see Information for Patients)

CONTRAINDICATIONS

Ativan (lorazepam) Injection is contraindicated in patients with a known sensitivity to benzodiazepines or its vehicle (polyethylene glycol, propylene glycol, and benzyl alcohol) and in patients with acute narrow-angle glaucoma. The use of Ativan (lorazepam) Injection intraarterially is contraindicated because, as with other injectable benzodiazepines, inadvertent intraarterial injection may produce arteriospasm resulting in gangrene which may require amputation (see Warnings).

WARNINGS

PRIOR TO INTRAVENOUS USE, ATIVAN INJECTION MUST BE DILUTED WITH AN EQUAL AMOUNT OF COMPATIBLE DILUENT (SEE DOSAGE AND ADMINISTRATION). INTRAVENOUS INJECTION SHOULD BE MADE SLOWLY AND WITH REPEATED ASPIRATION. CARE SHOULD BE TAKEN TO DETERMINE THAT ANY INJECTION WILL NOT BE INTRA-ARTERIAL AND THAT PERIVASCULAR EXTRAVASATION WILL NOT TAKE PLACE.

PARTIAL AIRWAY OBSTRUCTION MAY OCCUR IN HEAVILY SEDATED PATIENTS. INTRAVENOUS LORAZEPAM, WHEN GIVEN ALONE IN GREATER THAN THE RECOMMENDED DOSE, OR AT THE RECOMMENDED DOSE AND ACCOMPANIED BY OTHER DRUGS USED DURING THE ADMINISTRATION OF ANESTHESIA, MAY PRODUCE HEAVY SEDATION; THEREFORE, EQUIPMENT NECESSARY TO MAINTAIN A PATENT AIRWAY AND TO SUPPORT RESPIRATION/VENTILATION SHOULD BE AVAILABLE.

There is no evidence to support the use of lorazepam injection in coma, shock, or acute alcohol intoxication at this time. Since the liver is the most likely site of conjugation of lorazepam and since excretion of conjugated lorazepam (glucuronide) is a renal function, this drug is not recommended for use in patients with hepatic and/or renal *failure.* This does not preclude use of the drug in patients with mild to moderate hepatic or renal disease. When injectable lorazepam is selected for use in patients with mild to moderate hepatic or renal disease, the lowest effective dose should be considered since drug effect may be prolonged. Experience with other benzodiazepines and limited experience with parenteral lorazepam has demonstrated that tolerance to alcoholic beverages, and other central nervous system depressants is diminished when used concomitantly.

As is true of similar CNS-acting drugs, patients receiving injectable lorazepam should not operate machinery or engage in hazardous occupations or drive a motor vehicle for a period of 24–48 hours. Impairment of performance may persist for greater intervals because of extremes of age, concomitant use of other drugs, stress of surgery, or the general condition of the patient.

Clinical trials have shown that patients over the age of 50 years may have a more profound and prolonged sedation with intravenous lorazepam. Ordinarily, an initial dose of 2 mg may be adequate, unless a greater degree of lack of recall is desired.

As with all central-nervous- system depressant drugs, care should be exercised in patients given injectable lorazepam that premature ambulation may result in injury from falling.

There is no added beneficial effect to the addition of scopolamine to injectable lorazepam, and their combined effect may result in an increased incidence of sedation, hallucination, and irrational behavior.

PREGNANCY

ATIVAN® (LORAZEPAM) MAY CAUSE FETAL DAMAGE WHEN ADMINISTERED TO PREGNANT WOMEN.

An increased risk of congenital malformations associated with the use of minor tranquilizers (chlordiazepoxide, diazepam, and meprobamate) during the first trimester of pregnancy has been suggested in several studies. In humans, blood levels obtained from umbilical cord blood indicate placental transfer of lorazepam and lorazepam glucuronide.

Ativan Injection should not be used during pregnancy. There are insufficient data regarding obstetrical safety of parenteral lorazepam, including use in cesarean section. Such use, therefore, is not recommended.

Reproductive studies in animals were performed in mice, rats, and two strains of rabbits. Occasional anomalies (reduction of tarsals, tibia, metatarsals, malrotated limbs, gastroschisis, malformed skull, and microphthalmia) were seen in drug-treated rabbits without relationship to dosage. Although all of these anomalies were not present in the concurrent control group, they have been reported to occur randomly in historical controls. At doses of 40 mg/kg orally or 4 mg/kg intravenously and higher, there was evidence of fetal resorption and increased fetal loss in rabbits which was not seen at lower doses.

ENDOSCOPIC PROCEDURES

There are insufficient data to support the use of Ativan (lorazepam) Injection for outpatient endoscopic procedures. Inpatient endoscopic procedures require adequate recovery room observations.

Pharyngeal reflexes are not impaired when Ativan Injection is used for peroral endoscopic procedures; therefore, adequate topical or regional anesthesia is recommended to minimize reflex activity associated with such procedures.

PRECAUTIONS

GENERAL

The additive central-nervous-system effects of other drugs such as phenothiazines, narcotic analgesics, barbiturates, anti-depressants, scopolamine, and monoamine oxidase inhibitors should be borne in mind when these other drugs are used concomitantly with or during the period of recovery from Ativan (lorazepam) Injection. (See CLINICAL PHARMACOLOGY and WARNINGS.)

Extreme care must be used in administering Ativan Injection to elderly patients, very ill patients, and to patients with limited pulmonary reserve, because of the possibility that underventilation and/or hypoxic cardiac arrest may occur. Resuscitative equipment for ventilatory support should be readily available. (See WARNINGS and DOSAGE and ADMINISTRATION.)

When lorazepam injection is used IV as the premedicant prior to regional or local anesthesia, the possibility of excessive sleepiness or drowsiness may interfere with patient cooperation to determine levels of anesthesia. This is most likely to occur when greater than 0.05 mg/kg is given and when narcotic analgesics are used concomitantly with the recommended dose. (See ADVERSE REACTIONS.)

INFORMATION FOR PATIENTS

As appropriate, the patient should be informed of the pharmacological effects of the drug such as sedation, relief of anxiety, and lack of recall and the duration of these effects (about 8 hours) so that they may adequately perceive the risks as well as the benefits to be derived from its use.

Patients who receive Ativan Injection as a premedicant should be cautioned that driving an automobile or operating hazardous machinery, or engaging in a hazardous sport should be delayed for 24–48 hours following the injection. Sedatives, tranquilizers, and narcotic analgesics may produce a more prolonged and profound effect when administered along with injectable Ativan. This effect may take the form of excessive sleepiness or drowsiness, and on rare occasions, interfere with recall and recognition of events of the day of surgery and the day after.

Getting out of bed unassisted may result in falling and injury if undertaken within 8 hours of receiving lorazepam injection. Alcoholic beverages should not be consumed for at least 24–48 hours after receiving lorazepam injectable due to the additive effects on central-nervous-system depression seen with benzodiazepines in general. Elderly patients should be told that Ativan (lorazepam) Injection may make them very sleepy for a period longer than six (6) to eight (8) hours following surgery.

LABORATORY TESTS

In clinical trials no laboratory test abnormalities were identified with either single or multiple doses of Ativan (lorazepam) Injection. These tests included: CBC, urinalysis, SGOT, SGPT, bilirubin, alkaline phosphatase, LDH, cholesterol, uric acid, BUN, glucose, calcium, phosphorus, and total proteins.

DRUG INTERACTIONS

Ativan (lorazepam) Injection, like other injectable benzodiazepines, produces depression of the central nervous system when administered with ethyl alcohol, phenothiazines, barbiturates, MAO inhibitors, and other antidepressants. When scopolamine is used concomitantly with injectable lorazepam, an increased incidence of sedation, hallucinations, and irrational behavior has been observed.

DRUG/LABORATORY TEST INTERACTIONS

No laboratory test abnormalities were identified when lorazepam was given alone or concomitantly with another drug, such as narcotic analgesics, inhalation anesthetics, scopolamine, atropine, and a variety of tranquilizing agents.

CARCINOGENESIS, MUTAGENESIS, IMPAIRMENT OF FERTILITY

No evidence of carcinogenic potential emerged in rats and mice during an 18-month study with oral lorazepam. No studies regarding mutagenesis have been performed. Preimplantation study in rats was performed with oral lorazepam at a 20 mg/kg dose and showed no impairment of fertility.

PREGNANCY

Pregnancy Category D; See WARNINGS.

LABOR AND DELIVERY

There are insufficient data to support the use of Ativan (lorazepam) injection during labor and delivery, including cesarean section; therefore, its use in this situation is not recommended.

NURSING MOTHERS

Injectable lorazepam should not be administered to nursing mothers, because like other benzodiazepines, the possibility exists that lorazepam may be excreted in human milk and sedate the infant.

PEDIATRIC USE

There are insufficient data to support efficacy or make dosage recommendations for injectable lorazepam in patients less than 18 years of age; therefore, such use is not recommended.

Continued on next page

Wyeth—Cont.

ADVERSE REACTIONS

CENTRAL NERVOUS SYSTEM

The most frequent adverse effects seen with injectable lorazepam are an extension of the central-nervous-system depressant effects of the drug. The incidence varied from one study to another, depending on the dosage, route of administration, use of other central-nervous-system depressants, and the investigator's opinion concerning the degree and duration of desired sedation. Excessive sleepiness and drowsiness were the main side effects. This interfered with patient cooperation in approximately 6% (25/446) of patients undergoing regional anesthesia in that they were unable to assess levels of anesthesia in regional blocks or with caudal anesthesia. Patients over 50 years of age had a higher incidence of excessive sleepiness or drowsiness when compared with those under 50 (21/106 vs 24/245) when lorazepam was given intravenously (see DOSAGE and ADMINISTRATION). On rare occasion (3/1580) the patient was unable to give personal identification in the operating room on arrival, and one patient fell when attempting premature ambulation in the postoperative period.

Symptoms such as restlessness, confusion, depression, crying, sobbing, and delirium occurred in about 1.3% (20/1580). One patient injured himself by picking at his incision during the immediate postoperative period.

Hallucinations were present in about 1% (14/1580) of patients, and were visual and self-limiting.

An occasional patient complained of dizziness, diplopia, and/or blurred vision. Depressed hearing was infrequently reported during the peak-effect period.

An occasional patient had a prolonged recovery room stay, either because of excessive sleepiness or because of some form of inappropriate behavior. The latter was seen most commonly when scopolamine was given concomitantly as a premedicant.

Limited information derived from patients who were discharged the day after receiving injectable lorazepam showed one patient complained of some unsteadiness of gait and a reduced ability to perform complex mental functions. Enhanced sensitivity to alcoholic beverages has been reported more than 24 hours after receiving injectable lorazepam, similar to experience with other benzodiazepines.

LOCAL EFFECTS

Intramuscular injection of lorazepam has resulted in pain at the injection site, a sensation of burning, or observed redness in the same area in a very variable incidence from one study to another. The overall incidence of pain and burning was about 17% (146/859) in the immediate postinjection period, and about 1.4% (12/859) at the 24-hour observation time. Reactions at the injection site (redness) occurred in approximately 2% (17/859) in the immediate postinjection period, and were present 24 hours later in about 0.8% (7/859).

Intravenous administration of lorazepam resulted in painful responses in 13/771 patients or approximately 1.6% in the immediate postinjection period and 24 hours later 4/771 patients or about 0.5% still complained of pain. Redness did not occur immediately following intravenous injection, but was noted in 19/771 patients at the 24-hour observation period. This incidence is similar to that observed with an intravenous infusion before lorazepam is given.

CARDIOVASCULAR SYSTEM

Hypertension (0.1%) and hypotension (0.1%) have occasionally been observed after patients have received injectable lorazepam.

RESPIRATORY SYSTEM

Five patients (5/446) who underwent regional anesthesia were observed to have partial airway obstruction. This was believed due to excessive sleepiness at the time of the procedure, and resulted in temporary underventilation. Immediate attention to the airway, employing the usual countermeasures, will usually suffice to manage this condition (see also CLINICAL PHARMACOLOGY, WARNINGS, and PRECAUTIONS).

OTHER ADVERSE EXPERIENCES

Skin rash, nausea, and vomiting have occasionally been noted in patients who have received injectable lorazepam combined with other drugs during anesthesia and surgery.

DRUG ABUSE AND DEPENDENCE

As with other benzodiazepines, Ativan (lorazepam) Injection has a low potential for abuse and may lead to limited dependence. Although there are no clinical data available for injectable lorazepam in this respect, physicians should be aware that repeated doses over a prolonged period of time may result in limited physical and psychological dependence.

OVERDOSAGE

Overdosage of benzodiazepines is usually manifested by varying degrees of central-nervous-system depression ranging from drowsiness to coma. In mild cases symptoms include drowsiness, mental confusion and lethargy. In more serious examples, symptoms may include ataxia, hypotonia, hypotension, hypnosis, stages one (1) to three (3) coma, and very rarely death.

Treatment of overdosage is mainly supportive until the drug is eliminated from the body. Vital signs and fluid balance should be carefully monitored. An adequate airway should be maintained and assisted respiration used as needed. With normally functioning kidneys, forced diuresis with intravenous fluids and electrolytes may accelerate elimination of benzodiazepines from the body. In addition, osmotic diuretics such as mannitol may be effective as adjunctive measures. In more critical situations, renal dialysis and exchange blood transfusions may be indicated. Published reports indicate that intravenous infusion of 0.5 to 4 mg of physostigmine at the rate of 1 mg/minute may reverse symptoms and signs suggestive of central anticholinergic overdose (confusion, memory disturbance, visual disturbances, hallucinations, delirium); however, hazards associated with the use of physostigmine (i.e., induction of seizures) should be weighed against its possible clinical benefit.

DOSAGE AND ADMINISTRATION

INTRAMUSCULAR INJECTION

For the designated indications as a premedicant, the usual recommended dose of lorazepam for intramuscular injection is 0.05 mg/kg up to a maximum of 4 mg. As with all premedicant drugs, the dose should be individualized. (See also CLINICAL PHARMACOLOGY, WARNINGS, PRECAUTIONS, and ADVERSE REACTIONS.) Doses of other central-nervous-system depressant drugs should be ordinarily reduced (See PRECAUTIONS.) *For optimum effect, measured as lack of recall, intramuscular lorazepam should be administered at least 2 hours before the anticipated operative procedure.* Narcotic analgesics should be administered at their usual preoperative time. There are insufficient data to support efficacy to make dosage recommendations for intramuscular lorazepam in patients less than 18 years of age; therefore, such use is not recommended.

INTRAVENOUS INJECTION

For the primary purpose of sedation and relief of anxiety, the usual recommended initial dose of lorazepam for intravenous injection is 2 mg total, or 0.02 mg/lb (0.044 mg/kg), whichever is smaller. This dose will suffice for sedating most adult patients, and should not ordinarily be exceeded in patients over 50 years of age. In those patients in whom a greater likelihood of lack of recall for perioperative events would be beneficial, larger doses as high as 0.05 mg/kg up to a total of 4 mg may be administered. (See CLINICAL PHARMACOLOGY, WARNINGS, PRECAUTIONS, and ADVERSE REACTIONS.) Doses of other injectable central-nervous-system depressant drugs should ordinarily be reduced. (See PRECAUTIONS.) *For optimum effect, measured as lack of recall, intravenous lorazepam should be administered 15–20 minutes before the anticipated operative procedure.*

EQUIPMENT NECESSARY TO MAINTAIN A PATENT AIRWAY SHOULD BE IMMEDIATELY AVAILABLE PRIOR TO INTRAVENOUS ADMINISTRATION OF LORAZEPAM (See WARNINGS.)

There are insufficient data to support efficacy or make dosage recommendations for intravenous lorazepam in patients less than 18 years of age; therefore, such use is not recommended.

ADMINISTRATION

When given intramuscularly, Ativan Injection, undiluted, should be injected deep in the muscle mass.

Injectable Ativan (lorazepam) can be used with atropine sulfate, narcotic analgesics, other parenterally used analgesics, commonly used anesthetics, and muscle relaxants.

Immediately prior to intravenous use, Ativan (lorazepam) Injection must be diluted with an equal volume of compatible solution. When properly diluted the drug may be injected directly into a vein or into the tubing of an existing intravenous infusion. The rate of injection should not exceed 2.0 mg per minute.

Parenteral drug products should be inspected visually for particulate matter and discoloration prior to administration whenever solution and container permit. Do not use if solution is discolored or contains a precipitate.

Ativan (lorazepam) Injection is compatible for dilution purposes with the following solutions: Sterile Water for Injection, USP; Sodium Chloride Injection, USP; 5% Dextrose Injection, USP.

HOW SUPPLIED

Ativan® (lorazepam) Injection, Wyeth®, is available in the following dosage strengths in single-dose and multiple-dose vials and in TUBEX® Sterile Cartridge-Needle Units, packaged in boxes of 10 TUBEX:

2 mg per ml, NDC 0008-0581; 1 ml and 10 ml vials and 1 ml fill in 2 ml TUBEX.

4 mg per ml, NDC 0008-0570; 1 ml and 10 ml vials and 1 ml fill in 2 ml TUBEX.

For IM or IV injection.

Protect from light.

Keep in a refrigerator.

DIRECTIONS FOR DILUTION FOR IV USE

To dilute, adhere to the following procedure:

For TUBEX—

1. Extrude the entire amount of air in the half-filled TUBEX.
2. Slowly aspirate the desired volume of diluent.
3. Pull back slightly on the plunger to provide additional mixing space.
4. Immediately mix contents thoroughly by gently inverting TUBEX repeatedly until a homogenous solution results. Do not shake vigorously, as this will result in air entrapment.

For Vial—

Aspirate the desired amount of Ativan Injection into the syringe. Then proceed as described under TUBEX.

ATIVAN® ℂ ℞

[at'i-van]

(lorazepam)

Tablets

DESCRIPTION

Ativan (lorazepam), an antianxiety agent, has the chemical formula, 7-chloro-5-(o-chlorophenyl)-1,3-dihydro-3-hydroxy-2H-1,4- benzodiazepin-2-one.

It is a nearly white powder almost insoluble in water. Each Ativan (lorazepam) tablet, to be taken orally, contains 0.5 mg, 1 mg, or 2 mg of lorazepam. The inactive ingredients present are lactose and other ingredients.

CLINICAL PHARMACOLOGY

Studies in healthy volunteers show that in single high doses Ativan (lorazepam) has a tranquilizing action on the central nervous system with no appreciable effect on the respiratory or cardiovascular systems.

Ativan (lorazepam) is readily absorbed with an absolute bioavailability of 90 percent. Peak concentrations in plasma occur approximately 2 hours following administration. The peak plasma level of lorazepam from a 2 mg dose is approximately 20 ng/ml.

The mean half-life of unconjugated lorazepam in human plasma is about 12 hours and for its major metabolite, lorazepam glucuronide, about 18 hours. At clinically relevant concentrations, lorazepam is approximately 85% bound to plasma proteins. Ativan (lorazepam) is rapidly conjugated at its 3-hydroxy group into lorazepam glucuronide which is then excreted in the urine. Lorazepam glucuronide has no demonstrable CNS activity in animals.

The plasma levels of lorazepam are proportional to the dose given. There is no evidence of accumulation of lorazepam on administration up to six months.

Studies comparing young and elderly subjects have shown that the pharmacokinetics of lorazepam remain unaltered with advancing age.

INDICATIONS AND USAGE

Ativan (lorazepam) is indicated for the management of anxiety disorders or for the short-term relief of the symptoms of anxiety or anxiety associated with depressive symptoms. Anxiety or tension associated with the stress of everyday life usually does not require treatment with an anxiolytic.

The effectiveness of Ativan (lorazepam) in long-term use, that is, more than 4 months, has not been assessed by systematic clinical studies. The physician should periodically reassess the usefulness of the drug for the individual patient.

CONTRAINDICATIONS

Ativan (lorazepam) is contraindicated in patients with known sensitivity to the benzodiazepines or with acute narrow-angle glaucoma.

WARNINGS

Ativan (lorazepam) is not recommended for use in patients with a primary depressive disorder or psychosis. As with all patients on CNS-acting drugs, patients receiving lorazepam should be warned not to operate dangerous machinery or motor vehicles and that their tolerance for alcohol and other CNS depressants will be diminished.

PHYSICAL AND PSYCHOLOGICAL DEPENDENCE: Withdrawal symptoms similar in character to those noted with barbiturates and alcohol have occurred following abrupt discontinuance of benzodiazepine drugs. These symptoms include convulsions, tremor, abdominal and muscle cramps, vomiting and sweating. Addiction-prone individuals, such as drug addicts and alcoholics, should be under careful surveillance when receiving benzodiazepines because of the predisposition of such patients to habituation and dependence.

Withdrawal symptoms have also been reported following abrupt discontinuance of benzodiazepines taken continuously at therapeutic levels for several months.

PRECAUTIONS

In patients with depression accompanying anxiety, a possibility for suicide should be borne in mind.

For elderly or debilitated patients, the initial daily dosage should not exceed 2 mg in order to avoid oversedation.

Ativan® (lorazepam) dosage should be terminated gradually, since abrupt withdrawal of any anti-anxiety agent may result in symptoms similar to those for which patients are being treated: anxiety, agitation, irritability, tension, insomnia, and occasional convulsions.

The usual precautions for treating patients with impaired renal or hepatic function should be observed.

In patients where gastrointestinal or cardiovascular disorders coexist with anxiety, it should be noted that lorazepam has not been shown to be of significant benefit in treating the gastrointestinal or cardiovascular component.

Esophageal dilation occurred in rats treated with lorazepam for more than one year at 6 mg/kg/day. The no-effect dose was 1.25 mg/kg/day (approximately 6 times the maximum human therapeutic dose of 10 mg per day). The effect was reversible only when the treatment was withdrawn within two months of first observation of the phenomenon. The clinical significance of this is unknown. However, use of lorazepam for prolonged periods and in geriatric patients requires caution, and there should be frequent monitoring for symptoms of upper G.I. disease.

Safety and effectiveness of Ativan (lorazepam) in children of less than 12 years have not been established.

ESSENTIAL LABORATORY TESTS: Some patients on Ativan (lorazepam) have developed leukopenia, and some have had elevations of LDH. As with other benzodiazepines, periodic blood counts and liver-function tests are recommended for patients on long-term therapy.

CLINICALLY SIGNIFICANT DRUG INTERACTIONS: The benzodiazepines, including Ativan (lorazepam), produce CNS depressant effects when administered with such medications as barbiturates or alcohol.

CARCINOGENESIS AND MUTAGENESIS: No evidence of carcinogenic potential emerged in rats during an 18-month study with Ativan (lorazepam). No studies regarding mutagenesis have been performed.

PREGNANCY: Reproductive studies in animals were performed in mice, rats, and two strains of rabbits. Occasional anomalies (reduction of tarsals, tibia, metatarsals, malrotated limbs, gastroschisis, malformed skull, and microphthalmia) were seen in drug-treated rabbits without relationship to dosage. Although all of these anomalies were not present in the concurrent control group, they have been reported to occur randomly in historical controls. At doses of 40 mg/kg and higher, there was evidence of fetal resorption and increased fetal loss in rabbits which was not seen at lower doses.

The clinical significance of the above findings is not known. However, an increased risk of congenital malformations associated with the use of minor tranquilizers (chlordiazepoxide, diazepam, and meprobamate) during the first trimester of pregnancy has been suggested in several studies. Because the use of these drugs is rarely a matter of urgency, the use of lorazepam during this period should almost always be avoided. The possibility that a woman of childbearing potential may be pregnant at the time of institution of therapy should be considered. Patients should be advised that if they become pregnant, they should communicate with their physician about the desirability of discontinuing the drug.

In humans, blood levels obtained from umbilical cord blood indicate placental transfer of lorazepam and lorazepam glucuronide.

NURSING MOTHERS: It is not known whether oral lorazepam is excreted in human milk like the other benzodiazepine tranquilizers. As a general rule, nursing should not be undertaken while a patient is on a drug, since many drugs are excreted in human milk.

ADVERSE REACTIONS

Adverse reactions, if they occur, are usually observed at the beginning of therapy and generally disappear on continued medication or upon decreasing the dose. In a sample of about 3,500 anxious patients, the most frequent adverse reaction to Ativan® (lorazepam) is sedation (15.9%), followed by dizziness (6.9%), weakness (4.2%), and unsteadiness (3.4%). Less frequent adverse reactions are disorientation, depression, nausea, change in appetite, headache, sleep disturbance, agitation, dermatological symptoms, eye function disturbance, together with various gastrointestinal symptoms and autonomic manifestations. The incidence of sedation and unsteadiness increased with age.

Small decreases in blood pressure have been noted but are not clinically significant, probably being related to the relief of anxiety produced by Ativan (lorazepam).

Transient amnesia or memory impairment has been reported in association with the use of benzodiazepines.

OVERDOSAGE

In the management of overdosage with any drug, it should be borne in mind that multiple agents may have been taken.

Manifestations of Ativan (lorazepam) overdosage include somnolence, confusion, and coma. Induced vomiting and/or gastric lavage should be undertaken, followed by general supportive care, monitoring of vital signs, and close observation of the patient. Hypotension, though unlikely, usually may be controlled with Levarterenol Bitartrate Injection, USP. The usefulness of dialysis has not been determined.

DOSAGE AND ADMINISTRATION

Ativan® (lorazepam) is administered orally. For optimal results, dose, frequency of administration, and duration of therapy should be individualized according to patient response. To facilitate this, 0.5 mg, 1 mg, and 2 mg tablets are available.

The usual range is 2 to 6 mg/day given in divided doses, the largest dose being taken before bedtime, but the daily dosage may vary from 1 to 10 mg/day.

For anxiety, most patients require an initial dose of 2 to 3 mg/day given b.i.d. or t.i.d.

For insomnia due to anxiety or transient situational stress, a single daily dose of 2 to 4 mg may be given, usually at bedtime.

For elderly or debilitated patients, an initial dosage of 1 to 2 mg/day in divided doses is recommended, to be adjusted as needed and tolerated.

The dosage of Ativan (lorazepam) should be increased gradually when needed to help avoid adverse effects. When higher dosage is indicated, the evening dose should be increased before the daytime doses.

HOW SUPPLIED

Ativan® (lorazepam) Tablets, Wyeth®, are available in the following dosage strengths:

0.5 mg, NDC 0008-0081, white, five-sided tablet with a raised "A" on one side and "WYETH" and "81" on reverse side, in bottles of 100 and 500 tablets, in Redipak® Strip Pack cartons of 25 tablets, and in Redipak cartons of 100 tablets (20 strips of 5).

1 mg, NDC 0008-0064, white, five-sided tablet with a raised "A" on one side and "WYETH" and "64" on scored reverse side, in bottles of 100, 500, and 1000 tablets, in Redipak® Strip Pack cartons of 25 tablets, and in Redipak cartons of 100 tablets (20 strips of 5).

2 mg, NDC 0008-0065, white, five-sided tablet with a raised "A" on one side and "WYETH" and "65" on scored reverse side, in bottles of 100, 500, and 1000 tablets, in Redipak® Strip Pack cartons of 25 tablets, and in Redipak cartons of 100 tablets (20 strips of 5).

Store at controlled room temperature.
Keep bottles tightly closed.
Dispense in tight container.

The appearance of ATIVAN tablets is a registered trademark of Wyeth Laboratories.

Shown in Product Identification Section, page 435

BASALJEL® OTC

[*bā ′sel-jel*]
(basic aluminum carbonate gel)
SUSPENSION •CAPSULES •SWALLOW TABLETS

COMPOSITION

Suspension—each 5 ml teaspoonful contains basic aluminum carbonate gel equivalent to 400 mg aluminum hydroxide. Inactive ingredients are artificial and natural flavors, butylparaben, calcium benzoate, glycerin, hydroxypropyl methylcellulose, methylparaben, mineral oil, propylparaben, saccharin, simethicone, sorbitol solution, and water. Extra Strength Suspension—each 5 ml teaspoonful contains basic aluminum carbonate gel equivalent to 1000 mg aluminum hydroxide. Inactive ingredients are artificial and natural flavors, benzoic acid, butylparaben, methylparaben, propylparaben, saccharin, sorbitol solution, water, and other ingredients. Capsule contains dried basic aluminum carbonate gel equivalent to 608 mg of dried aluminum hydroxide gel or 500 mg aluminum hydroxide. Inactive ingredients are D&C Yellow 10, FD&C Blue 1, FD&C Red 40, FD&C Yellow 6, gelatin, polacrillin potassium, polyethylene glycol, talc, and titanium dioxide. Tablet contains dried basic aluminum carbonate gel equivalent to 608 mg of dried aluminum hydroxide gel or 500 mg aluminum hydroxide. Inactive ingredients are cellulose, hydrogenated vegetable oil, magnesium stearate, polacrillin potassium, starch, and talc.

INDICATIONS

Symptomatic relief of hyperacidity associated with peptic ulcer, gastritis, peptic esophagitis, gastric hyperacidity, and hiatal hernia. For the treatment, control, or management of hyperphosphatemia, or for use with a low phosphate diet to prevent formation of phosphate urinary stones, through the reduction of phosphates in the serum and urine.

WARNINGS

No more than 24 tablets/capsules/teaspoonfuls of BASALJEL, and no more than 12 teaspoonfuls of BASALJEL Extra Strength Suspension should be taken in a 24-hour period. Aluminum forms insoluble complexes with phosphate in the gastrointestinal tract, thus decreasing phosphate absorption. Prolonged use of aluminum-containing antacids by normophosphatemic patients may result in hypophosphatemia if phosphate intake is not adequate. In its more severe forms, hypophosphatemia can lead to anorexia, malaise, muscle weakness, and osteomalacia. A usually transient hypercalciuria of mild degree may be associated with the early weeks of therapy. Evidence suggests that elevated tissue aluminum levels have a role in development of the dialysis encephalopathy syndrome. A number of cases have been associated with elevated aluminum levels in the dialysate water. There is also evidence that small amounts of ingested aluminum are absorbed from the gastrointestinal tract, and it is likely that renal excretion of absorbed aluminum is impaired in renal failure. Prolonged use of aluminum-containing antacids in such patients may contribute to increased levels of aluminum. Pregnant women and nursing mothers are advised to seek the advice of a health professional before using this product.

PRECAUTIONS

May cause constipation. Adequate fluid intake should be maintained in addition to the specific medical or surgical management indicated by the patient's condition.

DRUG INTERACTIONS

Alumina-containing antacids should not be used concomitantly with any form of tetracycline therapy.

DOSAGE AND ADMINISTRATION

Suspension—2 teaspoonfuls (10 ml) in water or fruit juice taken as often as every 2 hours up to 12 times daily. Two teaspoonfuls have the capacity to neutralize 23 mEq of acid. Extra Strength Suspension—1 teaspoonful (5 ml) as often as every 2 hours up to 12 times daily. One teaspoonful is equivalent to 2 capsules or tablets and has the capacity to neutralize 22 mEq of acid. Capsules—2 capsules as often as every 2 hours up to 12 times daily. Two capsules have the capacity to neutralize 24 mEq of acid. Swallow Tablets—2 tablets as often as every 2 hours up to 12 times daily. Two tablets have the capacity to neutralize 25 mEq of acid.

Hyperphosphatemia: An initial dose of Basaljel equivalent to 1.0 gm aluminum hydroxide—2 capsules, 2 tablets, 2.5 teaspoonfuls (12 ml) suspension, or 1 teaspoonful (5 ml) extra strength suspension—taken 3 to 4 times per day with meals (total daily dose 3–4 gm) is recommended. After therapy is initiated, Basaljel dosage should be adjusted to the minimum required amount by carefully monitoring dietary phosphate intake (patients should be instructed on maintaining a low phosphate diet) and measurement of serum phosphorus levels on a regular basis. Sodium content is: 0.13 mEq/5 ml for the suspension, 1.0 mEq/5 ml for the extra strength suspension, 0.12 mEq per capsule, and 0.12 mEq per tablet.

HOW SUPPLIED

Suspension and Extra Strength Suspension—bottles of 12 fluidounces; Capsules—bottles of 100 and 500; Swallow Tablets (scored)—bottles of 100.

BICILLIN® C-R ℞

[*bī-sil ′in*]
(penicillin G benzathine and
penicillin G procaine suspension)
INJECTION

FOR DEEP INTRAMUSCULAR INJECTION ONLY

DESCRIPTION

Multiple-dose vials of 300,000 units per ml contain in each ml 150,000 units penicillin G benzathine and 150,000 units penicillin G procaine in a stabilized aqueous suspension with sodium citrate buffer, approximately 6 mg lecithin, 3 mg povidone, 1 mg carboxymethylcellulose, 0.5 mg sorbitan monopalmitate, 0.5 mg polyoxyethylene sorbitan monopalmitate, 1.2 mg methylparaben, and 0.14 mg propylparaben.

Each TUBEX® cartridge (1 ml size) contains 600,000 units of penicillin comprising: 300,000 units penicillin G benzathine and 300,000 units penicillin G procaine in a stabilized aqueous suspension with sodium citrate buffer; and as w/v, approximately 0.5% lecithin, 0.55% carboxymethylcellulose, 0.55% povidone, 0.1% methylparaben, and 0.01% propylparaben.

Each TUBEX cartridge (2 ml size) contains 1,200,000 units of penicillin comprising: 600,000 units penicillin G benzathine and 600,000 units penicillin G procaine in a stabilized aqueous suspension with sodium citrate buffer; and as w/v, approximately 0.5% lecithin, 0.55% carboxymethylcellulose, 0.55% povidone, 0.1% methylparaben, and 0.01% propylparaben.

Each disposable syringe (2 ml size) contains 1,200,000 units of penicillin comprising: 600,000 units penicillin G benzathine and 600,000 units penicillin G procaine in a stabilized aqueous suspension with sodium citrate buffer; and as w/v, approximately 0.5% lecithin, 0.55% carboxymethylcellulose, 0.55% povidone, 0.1% methylparaben, and 0.01% propylparaben.

Each disposable syringe (4 ml size) contains 2,400,000 units of penicillin comprising: 1,200,000 units penicillin G benza-

Continued on next page

Wyeth—Cont.

thine and 1,200,000 units penicillin G procaine in a stabilized aqueous suspension with sodium citrate buffer, and as w/v, approximately 0.5% lecithin, 0.55% carboxymethylcellulose, 0.55% povidone, 0.1% methylparaben, and 0.01% propylparaben.
Bicillin C-R suspension in the multiple-dose vial, TUBEX, and disposable syringe formulations is viscous and opaque. Read "Contraindications," "Warnings," "Precautions," and "Dosage and Administration" sections prior to use.

ACTIONS AND PHARMACOLOGY

Penicillin G exerts a bactericidal action against penicillin-sensitive microorganisms during the stage of active multiplication. It acts through the inhibition of biosynthesis of cell-wall mucopeptide. It is not active against the penicillinase-producing bacteria, which include many strains of staphylococci. Penicillin G exerts high *in vitro* activity against staphylococci (except penicillinase-producing strains) streptococci (Groups A, C, G, H, L, and M), and pneumococci. Other organisms sensitive to penicillin G are *Neisseria gonorrhoeae, Corynebacterium diphtheriae, Bacillus anthracis,* Clostridia, *Actinomyces bovis, Streptobacillus moniliformis, Listeria monocytogenes,* and Leptospira. *Treponema pallidum* is extremely sensitive to the bactericidal action for penicillin G.
Sensitivity plate testing: If the Kirby-Bauer method of disc sensitivity is used, a 10-unit penicillin disc should give a zone greater than 28 mm when tested against a penicillin-sensitive bacterial strain.
Intramuscular penicillin G benzathine is absorbed very slowly into the bloodstream from the intramuscular site and converted by hydrolysis to penicillin G. This combination of hydrolysis and slow absorption results in blood serum levels much lower but much more prolonged than other parenteral penicillins.
Penicillin G procaine is an equimolecular compound of procaine and penicillin G, administered intramuscularly as a suspension. It dissolves slowly at the site of injection, giving a plateau type of blood level at about 4 hours which falls slowly over a period of the next 15-20 hours.
Approximately 60% of penicillin G is bound to serum protein. The drug is distributed throughout the body tissues in widely varying amounts. Highest levels are found in the kidneys with lesser amounts in the liver, skin, and intestines. Penicillin G penetrates into all other tissues and the spinal fluid to a lesser degree. With normal kidney function the drug is excreted rapidly by tubular excretion. In neonates and young infants and in individuals with impaired kidney function, excretion is considerably delayed.

INDICATIONS

This drug is indicated in the treatment of moderately severe infections due to penicillin-G-susceptible microorganisms that are susceptible to serum levels common to this particular dosage form. Therapy should be guided by bacteriological studies (including susceptibility testing) and by clinical response. NOTE: When high, sustained serum levels are required, penicillin G sodium or potassium, either IM or IV, should be used. This drug should *not* be used in the treatment of venereal diseases, including syphilis, gonorrhea, yaws, bejel, and pinta.
The following infections will usually respond to adequate dosages of this drug:
Streptococcal infections Group A (without bacteremia). Moderately severe to severe infections of the upper respiratory tract, skin and soft-tissue infections, scarlet fever, and erysipelas.
NOTE: Streptococci in Groups A, C, G, H, L, and M are very sensitive to penicillin G. Other groups, including Group D (enterococci), are resistant. Penicillin G sodium or potassium is recommended for streptococcal infections with bacteremia.
Pneumococcal infections. Moderately severe pneumonia and otitis media.
NOTE: Severe pneumonia, empyema, bacteremia, pericarditis, meningitis, peritonitis, and arthritis of pneumococcal etiology are better treated with penicillin G sodium or potassium during the acute stage.

CONTRAINDICATIONS

A previous hypersensitivity reaction to any penicillin or to procaine is a contraindication.
Do not inject into or near an artery or nerve.

WARNINGS

Serious and occasionally fatal hypersensitivity (anaphylactoid) reactions have been reported in patients on penicillin therapy. Although anaphylaxis is more frequent following parenteral therapy, it has occurred in patients on oral penicillins. These reactions are more apt to occur in individuals with a history of sensitivity to multiple allergens.
There have been well-documented reports of individuals with a history of penicillin hypersensitivity reactions who have experienced severe hypersensitivity reactions when treated with a cephalosporin. Before therapy with a penicillin, careful inquiry should be made concerning previous hypersensitivity reactions to penicillins, cephalosporins, and other allergens. If an allergic reaction occurs, the drug should be discontinued and the patient treated with the usual agents, e.g., pressor amines, antihistamines, and corticosteroids.
Inadvertent intravascular administration, including inadvertent direct intraarterial injection or injection immediately adjacent to arteries, of Bicillin C-R and other penicillin preparations has resulted in severe neurovascular damage, including transverse myelitis with permanent paralysis, gangrene requiring amputation of digits and more proximal portions of extremities, and necrosis and sloughing at and surrounding the injection site. Such severe effects have been reported following injections into the buttock, thigh, and deltoid areas. Other serious complications of suspected intravascular administration which have been reported include immediate pallor, mottling or cyanosis of the extremity both distal and proximal to the injection site followed by bleb formation; severe edema requiring anterior and/or posterior compartment fasciotomy in the lower extremity. The above-described severe effects and complications have most often occurred in infants and small children. Prompt consultation with an appropriate specialist is indicated if any evidence of compromise of the blood supply occurs at, proximal to, or distal to the site of injection.[1-9] See "Contraindications," "Precautions," and "Dosage and Administration."
Quadriceps femoris fibrosis and atrophy have been reported following repeated intramuscular injections of penicillin preparations into the anterolateral thigh.
Injection into or near a nerve may result in permanent neurological damage.

PRECAUTIONS

Penicillin should be used with caution in individuals with histories of significant allergies and/or asthma.
Care should be taken to avoid intravenous or intraarterial administration, or injection into or near major peripheral nerves or blood vessels, since such injections may produce neurovascular damage. See "Contraindications," "Warnings," and "Dosage and Administration."
In streptococcal infections, therapy must be sufficient to eliminate the organism; otherwise the sequelae of streptococcal disease may occur. Cultures should be taken following completion of treatment to determine whether streptococci have been eradicated.
A small percentage of patients are sensitive to procaine. If there is a history of sensitivity make the usual test: Inject intradermally 0.1 ml of a 1 to 2 percent procaine solution. Development of an erythema, wheal, flare, or eruption indicates procaine sensitivity. Sensitivity should be treated by the usual methods, including barbiturates, and procaine penicillin preparations should not be used. Antihistaminics appear beneficial in treatment of procaine reactions.
The use of antibiotics may result in overgrowth of nonsusceptible organisms. Constant observation of the patient is essential. If new infections due to bacteria or fungi appear during therapy, the drug should be discontinued and appropriate measures taken.
Whenever allergic reactions occur, penicillin should be withdrawn unless, in the opinion of the physician, the condition being treated is life-threatening and amenable only to penicillin therapy.
In prolonged therapy with penicillin, and particularly with high-dosage schedules, periodic evaluation of the renal and hematopoietic systems is recommended.

ADVERSE REACTIONS

Penicillin is a substance of low toxicity but does possess a significant index of sensitization. The following hypersensitivity reactions associated with use of penicillin have been reported: Skin rashes, ranging from maculopapular eruptions to exfoliative dermatitis; urticaria; serum-sickness-like reactions, including chills, fever, edema, arthralgia, and prostration. Severe and often fatal anaphylaxis has been reported (see "Warnings").

DOSAGE AND ADMINISTRATION

Shake multiple-dose vial vigorously before withdrawing the desired dose.
Administer by DEEP, INTRAMUSCULAR INJECTION in the upper, outer quadrant of the buttock. In infants and small children, the midlateral aspect of the thigh may be preferable. When doses are repeated, vary the injection site.
When using the multiple-dose vial:
After selection of the proper site and insertion of the needle into the selected muscle, aspirate by pulling back on the plunger. While maintaining negative pressure for 2–3 seconds, carefully observe the neck of the syringe immediately proximal to the needle hub for appearance of blood or any discoloration. Blood or "typical blood color" may *not* be seen if a blood vessel has been entered —only a mixture of blood and Bicillin C-R. The appearance of any discoloration is reason to withdraw the needle and discard the syringe. If it is elected to inject at another site, a new syringe and needle should be used. If no blood or discoloration appears, inject the contents of the syringe slowly. Discontinue delivery of the dose if the subject complains of severe immediate pain at the injection site or if in infants and young children symptoms or signs occur suggesting onset of severe pain.
When using the TUBEX cartridge:
The Wyeth TUBEX® cartridge for this product incorporates several features that are designed to facilitate the visualization of blood on aspiration if a blood vessel is inadvertently entered.
The design of this cartridge is such that blood which enters its needle will be quickly visualized as a red or dark-colored "spot." This "spot" will appear on the barrel of the glass cartridge immediately proximal to the blue hub. Prior to injection, in order to determine where this "spot" can be seen, the operator should first insert and secure the cartridge in the Tubex syringe in the usual fashion. The needle cover should then be removed and the cartridge and syringe held in one hand with the needle pointing away from the operator. If the 2 ml metal syringe is used, the glass cartridge should then be rotated by turning the plunger of the syringe clockwise until the flat bevel at the tip of the needle is pointing upward and is horizontal when viewed directly from above. An imaginary straight line then drawn from the middle of the flat bevel to the back edge of the blue hub where it joins the glass will point to the area on the glass cartridge where the "spot" can be visualized. If the 1 ml metal syringe is used, it will not be possible to continue to rotate the glass cartridge clockwise once it is properly engaged and fully threaded; it can, however, then be rotated counterclockwise as far as necessary to properly orient the bevel of the needle and locate the observation area. (In this same area in some cartridges, a dark spot may sometimes be visualized prior to injection. This is the proximal end of the needle and does not represent a foreign body in, or other abnormality of, the suspension.)
Thus, before the needle is inserted into the selected muscle, it is important for the operator to orient the flat bevel of the needle so that any blood which might enter after its insertion and during aspiration can be visualized in the area of the cartridge where it will appear and not be obscured by the metal syringe or other obstructions.
After selection of the proper site and insertion of the needle into the selected muscle, aspirate by pulling back on the plunger. While maintaining negative pressure for 2 to 3 seconds, carefully observe the barrel of the cartridge in the area previously identified (see above) for the appearance of a red or dark-colored "spot."
Blood or "typical blood color" may *not* be seen if a blood vessel has been entered—only a mixture of blood and Bicillin C-R. The appearance of *any* discoloration is reason to withdraw the needle and discard the glass TUBEX cartridge. If it is elected to inject at another site, a new cartridge should be used. If no blood or discoloration appears, inject the contents of the cartridge slowly. Discontinue delivery of the dose if the subject complains of severe immediate pain at the injection site or if, especially in infants and young children, symptoms or signs occur suggesting onset of severe pain.
Some TUBEX cartridges may contain a small air bubble which may be disregarded since it does not affect administration of the product. Because of the high concentration of suspended material in this product, the needle may be blocked if the injection is not made at a slow, steady rate.
When using the disposable syringe:
The Wyeth disposable syringe for this product incorporates several new features that are designed to facilitate its use.
A single small indentation, or "dot," has been punched into the metal ring that surrounds the neck of the syringe near the base of the needle. It is important that this "dot" be placed in a position so that it can be easily visualized by the operator following the intramuscular insertion of the syringe needle.
After selection of the proper site and insertion of the needle into the selected muscle, aspirate by pulling back on the plunger. While maintaining negative pressure for 2 to 3 seconds, carefully observe the barrel of the syringe immediately proximal to the location of the "dot" for appearance of blood or any discoloration. Blood or "typical blood color" may *not* be seen if a blood vessel has been entered—only a mixture of blood and Bicillin C-R. The appearance of any discoloration is reason to withdraw the needle and discard the syringe. If it is elected to inject at another site, a new syringe should be used. If no blood or discoloration appears, inject the contents of the syringe slowly. Discontinue delivery of the dose if the subject complains of severe immediate pain at the injection site or if in infants and young children symptoms or signs occur suggesting onset of severe pain.
Streptococcal infections Group A —Infections of the upper-respiratory tract, skin and soft-tissue infections, scarlet fever, and erysipelas.
The following doses are recommended:
Adults and children over 60 lbs. in weight: 2,400,000 units.
Children from 30–60 lbs.: 900,000 units to 1,200,000 units.
Infants and children under 30 lbs.: 600,000 units.
NOTE: Treatment with the recommended dosage is usually given at a single session using multiple IM sites when indicated. An alternative dosage schedule may be used, giving one-half (½) the total dose on day 1 and one-half (½) on day 3. This will also insure the penicillinemia required over a

10-day period; however, this alternate schedule should be used only when the physician can be assured of the patient's cooperation.

Pneumococcal infections (except pneumococcal meningitis): 600,000 units in children and 1,200,000 units in adults, repeated every 2 or 3 days until the temperature is normal for 48 hours. Other forms of penicillin may be necessary for severe cases.

HOW SUPPLIED

300,000 units per ml—multiple-dose vials of 10 ml. *600,000 units per ml*—1 ml TUBEX® Sterile Cartridge-Needle Units, packages of 10; 2 ml TUBEX Sterile Cartridge-Needle Units (1,200,000 units per TUBEX), packages of 10; 4 ml single-dose (2,400,000 units) disposable syringes, packages of 10.

REFERENCES

1. SHAW, E.: Transverse myelitis from injection of penicillin. *Am. J. Dis. Child.,* *111*:548, 1966.
2. KNOWLES, J.: Accidental intra-arterial injection of penicillin. *Am. J. Dis. Child.,* *111*:552, 1966.
3. DARBY, C., et al: Ischemia following an intragluteal injection of benzathine-procaine penicillin G mixture in a one-year-old boy. *Clin. Pediatrics,* *12*:485, 1973.
4. BROWN, L. & NELSON, A.: Postinfectious intravascular thrombosis with gangrene. *Arch. Surg.,* *94*:652, 1967.
5. BORENSTINE, J.: Transverse myelitis and penicillin (Correspondence). *Am. J. Dis. Child.,* *112*:166, 1966.
6. ATKINSON, J.: Transverse myelopathy secondary to penicillin injection. *J. Pediatrics,* *75*:867, 1969.
7. TALBERT, J. et al: Gangrene of the foot following intramuscular injection in the lateral thigh: A case report with recommendations for prevention. *J. Pediatrics,* *70*:110, 1967.
8. FISHER, T.: Medicolegal affairs. *Canad. Med. Assoc. J.,* *112*:395, 1975.
9. SCHANZER, H. et al: Accidental intraarterial injection of penicillin G. *JAMA,* *242*:1289, 1979.

BICILLIN® C-R 900/300 ℞

[*bī-sil′in*]

(penicillin G benzathine and penicillin G procaine suspension)
INJECTION

FOR DEEP INTRAMUSCULAR INJECTION ONLY

DESCRIPTION

Each TUBEX® cartridge (2 ml size) contains 1,200,000 units of penicillin comprising: 900,000 units penicillin G benzathine and 300,000 units penicillin G procaine in a stabilized aqueous suspension with sodium citrate buffer; and as w/v, approximately 0.5% lecithin, 0.55% carboxymethylcellulose, 0.55% povidone, 0.1% methylparaben, and 0.01% propylparaben.

Bicillin C-R 900/300 suspension in the TUBEX formulation is viscous and opaque. Read "Contraindications," "Warnings," "Precautions," and "Dosage and Administration" sections prior to use.

ACTIONS AND PHARMACOLOGY

Penicillin G exerts a bactericidal action against penicillin-sensitive microorganisms during the stage of active multiplication. It acts through the inhibition of biosynthesis of cell-wall mucopeptide. It is not active against the penicillinase-producing bacteria, which include many strains of staphylococci. Penicillin G exerts high *in vitro* activity against staphylococci (except penicillinase-producing strains), streptococci (groups A, C, G, H, L, and M), and pneumococci.

Other organisms sensitive to penicillin G are *Neisseria gonorrhoeae, Corynebacterium diphtheriae, Bacillus anthracis,* Clostridia, *Actinomyces bovis, Streptobacillus moniliformis, Listeria monocytogenes,* and Leptospira. *Treponema pallidum* is extremely sensitive to the bactericidal action of penicillin G.

Sensitivity plate testing: If the Kirby-Bauer method of disc sensitivity is used, a 10-unit penicillin disc should give a zone greater than 28 mm when tested against a penicillin-sensitive bacterial strain.

Intramuscular penicillin G benzathine is absorbed very slowly into the bloodstream from the intramuscular site and converted by hydrolysis to penicillin G. This combination of hydrolysis and slow absorption results in blood serum levels much lower but much more prolonged than other parenteral penicillins.

Penicillin G procaine is an equimolecular compound of procaine and penicillin G, administered intramuscularly as a suspension. It dissolves slowly at the site of injection, giving a plateau type of blood level at about 4 hours which falls slowly over a period of the next 15–20 hours.

Approximately 60% of penicillin G is bound to serum protein. The drug is distributed throughout the body tissues in widely varying amounts. Highest levels are found in the kidneys with lesser amounts in the liver, skin, and intestines. Penicillin G penetrates into all other tissues and the spinal fluid to a lesser degree. With normal kidney function, the drug is excreted rapidly by tubular excretion. In neonates and young infants and in individuals with impaired kidney function, excretion is considerably delayed.

INDICATIONS

This drug is indicated for use in children of all ages in the treatment of moderately severe infections due to penicillin-G-susceptible microorganisms that are susceptible to serum levels common to this particular dosage form. Therapy should be guided by bacteriological studies (including susceptibility testing) and by clinical response.

NOTE: When high, sustained serum levels are required, penicillin G sodium or potassium, either IM or IV, should be used. This drug should *not* be used in the treatment of venereal diseases, including syphilis, gonorrhea, yaws, bejel, and pinta.

The following infections will usually respond to adequate dosages of this drug:

Streptococcal infections Group A (without bacteremia). Moderately severe to severe infections of the upper respiratory tract, skin and soft-tissue infections, scarlet fever, and erysipelas.

NOTE: Streptococci in groups A, C, G, H, L, and M are very sensitive to penicillin G. Other groups, including group D (enterococci), are resistant. Penicillin G sodium or potassium is recommended for streptococcal infections with bacteremia.

Pneumococcal infections. Moderately severe pneumonia and otitis media.

NOTE: Severe pneumonia, empyema, bacteremia, pericarditis, meningitis, peritonitis, and arthritis of pneumococcal etiology are better treated with penicillin G sodium or potassium during the acute stage.

CONTRAINDICATIONS

A previous hypersensitivity reaction to any penicillin or to procaine is a contraindication.

Do not inject into or near an artery or nerve.

WARNINGS

Serious and occasionally fatal hypersensitivity (anaphylactoid) reactions have been reported in patients on penicillin therapy. Although anaphylaxis is more frequent following parenteral therapy, it has occurred in patients on oral penicillins. These reactions are more apt to occur in individuals with a history of sensitivity to multiple allergens.

There have been well-documented reports of individuals with a history of penicillin hypersensitivity reactions who have experienced severe hypersensitivity reactions when treated with a cephalosporin. Before therapy with a penicillin, careful inquiry should be made concerning previous hypersensitivity reactions to penicillins, cephalosporins, and other allergens. If an allergic reaction occurs, the drug should be discontinued and the patient treated with the usual agents, e.g., pressor amines, antihistamines, and corticosteroids.

Inadvertent intravascular administration, including inadvertent direct intraarterial injection or injection immediately adjacent to arteries, of Bicillin C-R 900/300 and other penicillin preparations has resulted in severe neurovascular damage, including transverse myelitis with permanent paralysis, gangrene requiring amputation of digits and more proximal portions of extremities, and necrosis and sloughing at and surrounding the injection site. Such severe effects have been reported following injections into the buttock, thigh, and deltoid areas. Other serious complications of suspected intravascular administration which have been reported include immediate pallor, mottling or cyanosis of the extremity both distal and proximal to the injection site followed by bleb formation; severe edema requiring anterior and/or posterior compartment fasciotomy in the lower extremity. The above-described severe effects and complications have most often occurred in infants and small children. Prompt consultation with an appropriate specialist is indicated if any evidence of compromise of the blood supply occurs at, proximal to, or distal to the site of injection.[1-9] See "Contraindications," "Precautions," and "Dosage and Administration."

Quadriceps, femoris fibrosis and atrophy have been reported following repeated intramuscular injections of penicillin preparations into the anterolateral thigh.

Injection into or near a nerve may result in permanent neurological damage.

PRECAUTIONS

Penicillin should be used with caution in individuals with histories of significant allergies and/or asthma.

Care should be taken to avoid intravenous or intraarterial administration, or injection into or near major peripheral nerves or blood vessels, since such injections may produce neurovascular damage. See "Contraindications," "Warnings," and "Dosage and Administration."

In streptococcal infections, therapy must be sufficient to eliminate the organism; otherwise the sequelae of streptococcal disease may occur. Cultures should be taken following completion of treatment to determine whether streptococci have been eradicated.

A small percentage of patients are sensitive to procaine. If there is a history of sensitivity make the usual test: Inject intradermally 0.1 ml of a 1 to 2 percent procaine solution. Development of an erythema, wheal, flare, or eruption indicates procaine sensitivity. Sensitivity should be treated by the usual methods, including barbiturates, and procaine penicillin preparations should not be used. Antihistaminics appear beneficial in treatment of procaine reactions.

The use of antibiotics may result in overgrowth of nonsusceptible organisms. Constant observation of the patient is essential. If new infections due to bacteria or fungi appear during therapy, the drug should be discontinued and appropriate measures taken.

Whenever allergic reactions occur, penicillin should be withdrawn unless, in the opinion of the physician, the condition being treated is life-threatening and amenable only to penicillin therapy.

In prolonged therapy with penicillin, and particularly with high-dosage schedules, periodic evaluation of the renal and hematopoietic systems is recommended.

ADVERSE REACTIONS

Penicillin is a substance of low toxicity but does possess a significant index of sensitization. The following hypersensitivity reactions associated with use of penicillin have been reported: skin rashes, ranging from maculopapular eruptions to exfoliative dermatitis; urticaria; serum-sicknesslike reactions, including chills, fever, edema, arthralgia, and prostration. Severe and often fatal anaphylaxis has been reported (see "Warnings").

DOSAGE AND ADMINISTRATION

Administer by DEEP, INTRAMUSCULAR INJECTION in the upper, outer quadrant of the buttock. In infants and small children, the midlateral aspect of the thigh may be preferable. When doses are repeated, vary the injection site.

The Wyeth Tubex® cartridge for this product incorporates several features that are designed to facilitate the visualization of blood on aspiration if a blood vessel is inadvertently entered.

The design of this cartridge is such that blood which enters its needle will be quickly visualized as a red or dark-colored "spot." This "spot" will appear on the barrel of the glass cartridge immediately proximal to the blue hub. Prior to injection, in order to determine where this "spot" can be seen, the operator should first insert and secure the cartridge in the Tubex syringe in the usual fashion. The needle cover should then be removed and the cartridge and syringe held in one hand with the needle pointing away from the operator. If the 2 ml metal syringe is used, the glass cartridge should then be rotated by turning the plunger of the syringe clockwise until the flat bevel at the tip of the needle is pointing upward and is horizontal when viewed directly from above. An imaginary straight line then drawn from the middle of the flat bevel to the back edge of the blue hub where it joins the glass will point to the area on the glass cartridge where the "spot" can be visualized. If the 1 ml metal syringe is used, it will not be possible to continue to rotate the glass cartridge clockwise once it is properly engaged and fully threaded; it can, however, then be rotated counterclockwise as far as necessary to properly orient the bevel of the needle and locate the observation area. (In this same area in some cartridges, a dark spot may sometimes be visualized prior to injection. This is the proximal end of the needle and does not represent a foreign body in, or other abnormality of, the suspension.)

Thus, before the needle is inserted into the selected muscle, it is important for the operator to orient the flat bevel of the needle so that any blood which might enter after its insertion and during aspiration can be visualized in the area of the cartridge where it will appear and not be obscured by the metal syringe or other obstructions.

After selection of the proper site and insertion of the needle into the selected muscle, aspirate by pulling back on the plunger. While maintaining negative pressure for 2 to 3 seconds, carefully observe the barrel of the cartridge in the area previously identified (see above) for the appearance of a red or dark-colored "spot."

Blood or "typical blood color" may *not* be seen if a blood vessel has been entered—only a mixture of blood and Bicillin C-R 900/300. The appearance of *any* discoloration is reason to withdraw the needle and discard the glass TUBEX cartridge. If it is elected to inject at another site, a new cartridge should be used. If no blood or discoloration appears, inject the contents of the cartridge slowly. Discontinue delivery of the dose if the subject complains of severe immediate pain at the injection site or if, especially in infants and young children, symptoms or signs occur suggesting onset of severe pain.

Some TUBEX cartridges may contain a small air bubble which may be disregarded since it does not affect administration of the product. Because of the high concentration of suspended material in this product, the needle may be blocked if the injection is not made at a slow, steady rate.

Continued on next page

Wyeth—Cont.

Streptococcal infections Group A—Infections of the upper respiratory tract, skin and soft-tissue infections, scarlet fever, and erysipelas.
A single injection of Bicillin C-R 900/300 is usually sufficient for the treatment of Group A streptococcal infections in children of all ages.
Pneumococcal infections (except pneumococcal meningitis): One TUBEX Bicillin C-R 900/300 repeated at 2- or 3-day intervals until the temperature is normal for 48 hours. Other forms of penicillin may be necessary for severe cases.

HOW SUPPLIED

Bicillin® C-R 900/300 is supplied in 2 ml TUBEX® (Sterile Cartridge-Needle Unit) in packages of 10.

REFERENCES

1. SHAW, E.: Transverse myelitis from injection of penicillin. *Am. J. Dis. Child., 111:* 548, 1966.
2. KNOWLES, J.: Accidental intra-arterial injection of penicillin. *Am. J. Dis. Child., 111:* 552, 1966.
3. DARBY, C., et al: Ischemia following an intragluteal injection of benzathine-procaine penicillin G mixture in a one-year-old boy. *Clin. Pediatrics, 12:* 485, 1973.
4. BROWN, L. & NELSON, A.: Postinfectious intravascular thrombosis with gangrene. *Arch. Surg., 94:* 652, 1967.
5. BORENSTINE, J.: Transverse myelitis and penicillin (Correspondence). *Am. J. Dis. Child., 112:* 166, 1966.
6. ATKINSON, J.: Transverse myelopathy secondary to penicillin injection. *J. Pediatrics, 75:* 867, 1969.
7. TALBERT, J. et al: Gangrene of the foot following intramuscular injection in the lateral thigh: A case report with recommendations for prevention. *J. Pediatrics, 70:* 110, 1967.
8. FISHER, T.: Medicolegal affairs. *Canad. Med. Assoc. J., 112:* 395, 1975.
9. SCHANZER, H. et al: Accidental intra-arterial injection of penicillin G. *JAMA, 242:* 1289, 1979.

BICILLIN® L-A ℞

[*bī-sil'in*]
(sterile penicillin G benzathine suspension)
INJECTION
FOR DEEP INTRAMUSCULAR INJECTION ONLY

DESCRIPTION

Each TUBEX® Sterile Cartridge-Needle Unit or disposable syringe contains penicillin G benzathine in aqueous suspension with sodium citrate buffer; and as w/v, approximately 0.5% lecithin, 0.6% carboxymethylcellulose, 0.6% povidone, 0.1% methylparaben and, 0.01% propylparaben.
Each multiple-dose vial contains in each milliliter 300,000 units penicillin G benzathine with sodium citrate buffer and approx. 6 mg lecithin, 3 mg povidone, 1 mg carboxymethylcellulose, 0.5 mg sorbitan monopalmitate, 0.5 mg polyoxyethylene sorbitan monopalmitate, 1.2 mg methylparaben, and 0.14 mg propylparaben.
Bicillin L-A suspension in the multiple-dose vial, TUBEX, and disposable syringe formulations is viscous and opaque. Read "Contraindications," "Warnings," "Precautions," and "Dosage and Administration" sections prior to use.

ACTIONS AND PHARMACOLOGY

Penicillin G exerts a bactericidal action against penicillin-sensitive microorganisms during the stage of active multiplication. It acts through the inhibition of biosynthesis of cell-wall mucopeptide. It is not active against the penicillinase-producing bacteria, which include many strains of staphylococci. Penicillin G exerts high *in vitro* activity against staphylococci (except penicillinase-producing strains), streptococci (Groups A, C, G, H, L, and M), and pneumococci. Other organisms sensitive to penicillin G are: *Neisseria gonorrhoeae, Corynebacterium diphtheriae, Bacillus anthracis,* Clostridia, *Actinomyces bovis, Streptobacillus moniliformis, Listeria monocytogenes,* and Leptospira. *Treponema pallidum* is extremely sensitive to the bactericidal action of penicillin G.
Intramuscular penicillin G benzathine is absorbed very slowly into the bloodstream from the intramuscular site and converted by hydrolysis to penicillin G. This combination of hydrolysis and slow absorption results in blood serum levels much lower but much more prolonged than other parenteral penicillins.
Approximately 60% of penicillin G is bound to serum protein. The drug is distributed throughout the body tissues in widely varying amounts. Highest levels are found in the kidneys with lesser amounts in the liver, skin, and intestines. Penicillin G penetrates into all other tissues and the spinal fluid to a lesser degree. With normal kidney function the drug is excreted rapidly by tubular excretion. In neonates and young infants and in individuals with impaired kidney function, excretion is considerably delayed.

INDICATIONS

Intramuscular penicillin G benzathine is indicated in the treatment of infections due to penicillin-G-sensitive microorganisms that are susceptible to the low and very prolonged serum levels common to this particular dosage form. Therapy should be guided by bacteriological studies (including sensitivity tests) and by clinical response.
The following infections will usually respond to adequate dosage of intramuscular penicillin G benzathine:
Streptococcal infections (Group A—without bacteremia). Mild-to-moderate infections of the upper respiratory tract (e.g., pharyngitis).
Venereal infections—Syphilis, yaws, bejel, and pinta.
Medical Conditions in Which Penicillin G Benzathine Therapy Is Indicated as Prophylaxis: Rheumatic fever and/or chorea—Prophylaxis with penicillin G benzathine has proven effective in preventing recurrence of these conditions. It has also been used as follow-up prophylactic therapy for rheumatic heart disease and acute glomerulonephritis.

CONTRAINDICATIONS

A history of a previous hypersensitivity reaction to any of the penicillins is a contraindication.
Do not inject into or near an artery or nerve.

WARNINGS

Serious and occasionally fatal hypersensitivity (anaphylactoid) reactions have been reported in patients on penicillin therapy. Although anaphylaxis is more frequent following parenteral therapy, it has occurred in patients on oral penicillins. These reactions are more apt to occur in individuals with a history of sensitivity to multiple allergens.
There have been well-documented reports of individuals with a history of penicillin hypersensitivity reactions who have experienced severe hypersensitivity reactions when treated with a cephalosporin. Before therapy with a penicillin, careful inquiry should be made concerning previous hypersensitivity reactions to penicillins, cephalosporins, and other allergens. If an allergic reaction occurs, the drug should be discontinued and the patient treated with the usual agents, e.g., pressor amines, antihistamines, and corticosteroids.
Inadvertent intravascular administration, including inadvertent direct intraarterial injection or injection immediately adjacent to arteries, of Bicillin L-A and other penicillin preparations has resulted in severe neurovascular damage, including transverse myelitis with permanent paralysis, gangrene requiring amputation of digits and more proximal portions of extremities, and necrosis and sloughing at and surrounding the injection site. Such severe effects have been reported following injections into the buttock, thigh, and deltoid areas. Other serious complications of suspected intravascular administration which have been reported include immediate pallor, mottling or cyanosis of the extremity both distal and proximal to the injection site followed by bleb formation; severe edema requiring anterior and/or posterior compartment fasciotomy in the lower extremity. The above-described severe effects and complications have most often occurred in infants and small children. Prompt consultation with an appropriate specialist is indicated if any evidence of compromise of the blood supply occurs at, proximal to, or distal to the site of injection.[1-9] See "Contraindications," "Precautions," and "Dosage and Administration" sections.
Quadriceps femoris fibrosis and atrophy have been reported following repeated intramuscular injections of penicillin preparations into the anterolateral thigh.
Injection into or near a nerve may result in permanent neurological damage.

PRECAUTIONS

Penicillin should be used with caution in individuals with histories of significant allergies and/or asthma.
Care should be taken to avoid intravenous or intraarterial administration, or injection into or near major peripheral nerves or blood vessels, since such injection may produce neurovascular damage. See "Contraindications," "Warnings," and "Dosage and Administration" sections.
In streptococcal infections therapy must be sufficient to eliminate the organism; otherwise, the sequelae of streptococcal disease may occur. Cultures should be taken following completion of treatment to determine whether streptococci have been eradicated.
Prolonged use of antibiotics may promote the overgrowth of nonsusceptible organisms, including fungi. Should superinfection occur, appropriate measures should be taken.

ADVERSE REACTIONS

The hypersensitivity reactions reported are skin eruptions (maculopapular to exfoliative dermatitis), urticaria and other serum-sicknesslike reactions, laryngeal edema, and anaphylaxis. Fever and eosinophilia may frequently be the only reaction observed. Hemolytic anemia, leukopenia, thrombocytopenia, neuropathy, and nephropathy are infrequent reactions and usually associated with high doses of parenteral penicillin. As with other treatments for syphilis, the Jarisch-Herxheimer reaction has been reported.

DOSAGE AND ADMINISTRATION

Administer by DEEP INTRAMUSCULAR INJECTION in the upper, outer quadrant of the buttock. In infants and small children, the midlateral aspect of the thigh may be preferable. When doses are repeated, vary the injection site.
When using the multiple-dose vial:
Shake multiple-dose vial vigorously before withdrawing the desired dose.
After selection of the proper site and insertion of the needle into the selected muscle, aspirate by pulling back on the plunger. While maintaining negative pressure for 2–3 seconds, carefully observe the neck of the syringe immediately proximal to the needle hub for appearance of blood or any discoloration. Blood or "typical blood color" may *not* be seen if a blood vessel has been entered—only a mixture of blood and Bicillin L-A. The appearance of any discoloration is reason to withdraw the needle and discard the syringe. If it is elected to inject at another site, a new syringe and needle should be used. If no blood or discoloration appears, inject the contents of the syringe slowly. Discontinue delivery of the dose if the subject complains of severe immediate pain at the injection site or if in infants and young children symptoms or signs occur suggesting onset of severe pain.
When using the TUBEX cartridge:
The Wyeth TUBEX® cartridge for this product incorporates several features that are designed to facilitate the visualization of blood on aspiration if a blood vessel is inadvertently entered.
The design of this cartridge is such that blood which enters its needle will be quickly visualized as a red or dark-colored "spot." This "spot" will appear on the barrel of the glass cartridge immediately proximal to the blue hub. Prior to injection, in order to determine where this "spot" can be seen, the operator should first insert and secure the cartridge in the TUBEX syringe in the usual fashion. The needle cover should then be removed and the cartridge and syringe held in one hand with the needle pointing away from the operator. If the 2 ml metal syringe is used, the glass cartridge should then be rotated by turning the plunger of the syringe clockwise until the flat bevel at the tip of the needle is pointing upward and is horizontal when viewed directly from above. An imaginary straight line, then drawn from the middle of the flat bevel to the back edge of the blue hub where it joins the glass, will point to the area on the glass cartridge where the "spot" can be visualized. If the 1 ml metal syringe is used, it will not be possible to continue to rotate the glass cartridge clockwise once it is properly engaged and fully threaded; it can, however, then be rotated counterclockwise as far as necessary to properly orient the bevel of the needle and locate the observation area. (In this same area in some cartridges a dark spot may sometimes be visualized prior to injection. This is the proximal end of the needle and does not represent a foreign body in, or other abnormality of, the suspension.)
Thus, before the needle is inserted into the selected muscle, it is important for the operator to orient the flat bevel of the needle so that any blood which might enter after its insertion and during aspiration can be visualized in the area of the cartridge where it will appear and not be obscured by the metal syringe or other obstructions.
After selection of the proper site and insertion of the needle into the selected muscle, aspirate by pulling back on the plunger. While maintaining negative pressure for 2–3 seconds, carefully observe the barrel of the cartridge in the area previously identified (see above) for the appearance of a red or dark-colored "spot."
Blood or "typical blood color" may *not* be seen if a blood vessel has been entered—only a mixture of blood and Bicillin L-A. The appearance of *any* discoloration is reason to withdraw the needle and discard the glass TUBEX cartridge. If it is elected to inject at another site, a new cartridge should be used. If no blood or discoloration appears, inject the contents of the cartridge slowly. Discontinue delivery of the dose if the subject complains of severe immediate pain at the injection site or if, especially in infants and young children, symptoms or signs occur suggesting onset of severe pain.
Some TUBEX cartridges may contain a small air bubble which may be disregarded since it does not affect administration of the product. Because of the high concentration of suspended material in this product, the needle may be blocked if the injection is not made at a slow, steady rate.
When using the disposable syringe:
The Wyeth disposable syringe for this product incorporates several new features that are designed to facilitate its use.
A single small indentation, or "dot," has been punched into the metal ring that surrounds the neck of the syringe near the base of the needle. It is important that this "dot" be placed in a position so that it can be easily visualized by the operator following the intramuscular insertion of the syringe needle.
After selection of the proper site and insertion of the needle into the selected muscle, aspirate by pulling back on the plunger. While maintaining negative pressure for 2–3 seconds, carefully observe the barrel of the syringe immediately proximal to the location of the "dot" for appearance of blood

or any discoloration. Blood or "typical blood color" may *not* be seen if a blood vessel has been entered—only a mixture of blood and Bicillin L-A. The appearance of any discoloration is reason to withdraw the needle and discard the syringe. If it is elected to inject at another site, a new syringe should be used. If no blood or discoloration appears, inject the contents of the syringe slowly. Discontinue delivery of the dose if the subject complains of severe immediate pain at the injection site or if in infants and young children symptoms or signs occur suggesting onset of severe pain.
Some disposable syringes may contain a small air bubble which may be disregarded since it does not affect administration of the product. Because of the high concentration of suspended material in this product, the needle may be blocked if the injection is not made at a slow, steady rate.
Streptococcal (Group A) upper respiratory infections (for example, pharyngitis).
A single injection of 1,200,000 units for adults.
A single injection of 900,000 units for older children.
A single injection of 300,000 to 600,000 units for infants and for children under 60 pounds.
Venereal infections—
Syphilis—Primary, secondary, and latent—2.4 million units (1 dose). Late (tertiary and neurosyphilis)—2.4 million units at 7-day intervals for three doses.
Congenital—under 2 years of age: 50,000 units/kg/body weight; ages 2–12 years: adjust dosage based on adult dosage schedule.
Yaws, Bejel, and Pinta—1.2 million units (1 injection).
Prophylaxis—for rheumatic fever and glomerulonephritis. Following an acute attack, penicillin G benzathine (parenteral) may be given in doses of 1,200,000 units once a month or 600,000 units every 2 weeks.

HOW SUPPLIED

BICILLIN® L-A (sterile penicillin G benzathine suspension) Injection: *300,000 units per ml*—vials of 10 ml; *600,000 units per 1 ml* TUBEX® sterile cartridge-needle unit, packages of 10; *1,200,000 units per 2 ml* TUBEX, packages of 10; *2,400,000 units per 4 ml* disposable syringe, packages of 10.
Store in a refrigerator. Keep from freezing.

REFERENCES

1. SHAW, E.: Transverse myelitis from injection of penicillin. *Am. J. Dis. Child., 111:* 548, 1966.
2. KNOWLES, J.: Accidental intra-arterial injection of penicillin. *Am. J. Dis. Child., 111:* 552, 1966.
3. DARBY, C., et al: Ischemia following an intragluteal injection of benzathine-procaine penicillin G mixture in a one-year-old boy. *Clin. Pediatrics, 12:* 485, 1973.
4. BROWN, L. & NELSON, A.: Postinfectious intravascular thrombosis with gangrene. *Arch. Surg., 94:* 652, 1967.
5. BORENSTINE, J.: Transverse myelitis and penicillin (Correspondence). *Am. J. Dis. Child., 112:* 166, 1966.
6. ATKINSON, J.: Transverse myelopathy secondary to penicillin injection. *J. Pediatrics, 75:* 867, 1969.
7. TALBERT, J. et al: Gangrene of the foot following intramuscular injection in the lateral thigh: A case report with recommendations for prevention. *J. Pediatrics, 70:* 110, 1967.
8. FISHER, T.: Medicolegal affairs. *Canad. Med. Assoc. J., 112:* 395, 1975.
9. SCHANZER, H. et al: Accidental intra-arterial injection of penicillin G. *JAMA, 242:* 1289, 1979.

BIOLOGICALS

Each of Wyeth's biological products is listed separately in alphabetical order in Wyeth's Product Information Section. For prescribing information on the products listed—and for which information is not provided—write to Professional Service, Wyeth Laboratories, P.O. Box 8299, Philadelphia, PA 19101, or contact your local Wyeth representative.

CEROSE-DM® OTC

[se-rōs' DM]
Cough/Cold Preparation with Dextromethorphan
Sugar Free • Non-Narcotic

DESCRIPTION

Each teaspoonful (5 mL) contains 15 mg dextromethorphan hydrobromide, 4 mg chlorpheniramine maleate, and 10 mg phenylephrine hydrochloride. Alcohol 2.4%. The inactive ingredients present are artificial flavors, citric acid, edetate disodium, FD&C Yellow 6, glycerin, saccharin sodium, sodium benzoate, sodium citrate, sodium propionate, and water.

INDICATIONS

For the symptomatic control of cough due to colds.

DOSAGE AND ADMINISTRATION

Adults, and children 12 years and over, one to two teaspoonfuls 4 times daily. Children over 6 years, one teaspoonful 4 times daily. Children under 6, as directed by physician only.

CAUTION

Do not exceed recommended dosage. Individuals with high blood pressure, heart disease, diabetes, or thyroid disease should consult physician before using. If there is persistent cough or high fever which may indicate a serious condition, consult your physician. Drowsiness may occur; if so, do not drive or operate machinery or do not permit hazardous childhood activities.

WARNING

As with any drug, if you are pregnant or nursing a baby, seek the advice of a health professional before using this product.
Keep this and all drugs out of the reach of children. In case of accidental overdose, seek professional assistance or contact a Poison Control Center immediately.
Keep tightly closed below 77°F (25°C)

CERUBIDINE® ℞

[sĭ-rew "bĭ'dēan]
(daunorubicin hydrochloride)
For injection

WARNINGS

1. Cerubidine must be given into a rapidly flowing intravenous infusion. It must *never* be given by the intramuscular or subcutaneous route. Severe local tissue necrosis will occur if there is extravasation during administration.
2. Myocardial toxicity manifested in its most severe form by potentially fatal congestive heart failure may be encountered when total cumulative dosage exceeds 550 mg/m² in adults, 300 mg/m² in children more than 2 years of age, or 10 mg/kg in children less than two years of age.
   This may occur either during therapy or several months after termination of therapy. Treatment with digitalis, diuretics, sodium restriction, and bedrest is indicated.
3. Severe myelosuppression occurs when used in therapeutic doses.
4. It is recommended that Cerubidine be administered only by physicians who are experienced in leukemia chemotherapy and in facilities with laboratory and supportive resources adequate to monitor drug tolerance and protect and maintain a patient compromised by drug toxicity. The physician and institution must be capable of responding rapidly and completely to severe hemorrhagic conditions, and/or overwhelming infection.
5. Dosage should be reduced in patients with impaired hepatic or renal function.

DESCRIPTION

Cerubidine (daunorubicin hydrochloride) is the hydrochloride salt of an anthracycline cytotoxic antibiotic produced by a strain of *Streptomyces coeruleorubidus.* It is provided as a sterile reddish lyophilized powder in vials for intravenous administration only. Each vial contains 20 mg of base activity (21.4 mg as the hydrochloride salt) and 100 mg of mannitol. It is soluble in water when adequately agitated and produces a reddish solution. It has the following structural formula which may be described with the chemical name of 7-(3-amino-2,3,6-trideoxy-L-lyxohexosyloxy)-9-acetyl-7, 8, 9, 10-tetrahydro-6,9,11-trihydroxy-4-methoxy-5,12-naphthacenequinone hydrochloride. Its empirical formula is $C_{27}H_{29}NO_{10}HCl$ with a molecular weight of 563.99. It is a hygroscopic crystalline powder. The pH of a 5 mg/ml aqueous solution is 4.5 to 6.5.

STRUCTURAL FORMULA

O OH COCH₃ OH NH₂ OH OCH₃ O OH O—CH—CH₂—CH—CH—CH—CH₃ ·HCl O

ACTION

Cerubidine inhibits the synthesis of nucleic acids; its effect on deoxyribonucleic acid is particularly rapid and marked. Cerubidine has antimitotic and cytotoxic activity although the precise mode of action is unknown. Cerubidine displays an immunosuppressive effect. It has been shown to inhibit the production of heterohemagglutinins in mice. *In vitro,* it inhibits blast cell transformation of canine lymphocytes at 0.01 mcg/ml.
Cerubidine possesses a potent antitumor effect against a wide spectrum of animal tumors either grafted or spontaneous.

PHARMACOLOGY

Following intravenous injection of Cerubidine, plasma levels of daunorubicin decline rapidly indicating rapid tissue uptake and concentration. Thereafter, plasma levels decline slowly with a half-life of 18.5 hours. By one hour after drug administration, the predominant plasma species is daunorubicinol, an active metabolite, which disappears with a half-life of 26.7 hours. Further metabolism via reduction cleavage of the glycosidic bond, 4-0 demethylation, and conjugation with both sulfate and glucuronide have been demonstrated. Simple glycosidic cleavage of daunorubicin or daunorubicinol is not a significant metabolic pathway in man. Twenty-five percent of an administered dose of Cerubidine is eliminated in an active form by urinary excretion, and an estimated 40% by biliary excretion.
There is no evidence that Cerubidine crosses the blood-brain barrier.

INDICATIONS AND USAGE

Cerubidine has been successfully used for remission induction in acute nonlymphocytic leukemia (myelogenous, monocytic, erythroid) of adults and as part of a remission induction program in acute lymphocytic leukemia of children.
In the treatment of acute nonlymphocytic leukemia, Cerubidine used as a single agent has produced complete remission rates of 40 to 50%, and in combination with cytarabine, has produced complete remission rates of 53 to 65%.
The addition of Cerubidine to the two-drug induction regimen of vincristine-prednisone in the treatment of childhood acute lymphocytic leukemia does not increase the rate of complete remission. In children receiving only CNS prophylaxis and maintenance therapy (without consolidation) after induction, there is a prolongation of complete remission duration in those children induced with the three drug (Cerubidine-vincristine-prednisone) regimen as compared to two drugs (five-year disease-free survival 52% [three drugs] vs. 26% [two drugs], $p < 0.02$). There is no evidence of any impact of Cerubidine on the duration of complete remission when a consolidation (intensification) phase is employed as part of a total treatment program.

WARNINGS

Therapy with Cerubidine should not be started in patients with pre-existing drug-induced bone marrow suppression unless the benefit from such treatment warrants the risk.
Preexisting heart disease and previous therapy with doxorubicin are cofactors of increased risk of Cerubidine-induced cardiac toxicity and the benefit-to-risk ratio of Cerubidine therapy in such patients should be weighed before starting Cerubidine.
Bone Marrow—Cerubidine is a potent bone marrow suppressant. Suppression will occur in all patients given a therapeutic dose of this drug.
Cardiac Effects[1-6]—Special attention must be given to the potential cardiac toxicity of Cerubidine, particularly in infants and children. *In adults,* at total cumulative doses less than 550 mg/m², acute congestive heart failure is seldom encountered. However, rare instances of pericarditis-myocarditis, not dose-related, have been reported.
In adults, at cumulative doses exceeding 550 mg/m², there is an increased incidence of drug-induced congestive heart failure. Based on prior clinical experience with doxorubicin, this limit appears lower, namely 400 mg/m², in patients who received radiation therapy that encompassed the heart.
In infants and children, there appears to be a greater susceptibility to anthracycline-induced cardiotoxicity compared to that in adults, which is more clearly dose-related. However, there is very little risk for children over two years of age in developing Cerubidine-related cardiotoxicity below a cumulative dose of 300 mg/m² or in children less than two years of age (or < 0.5m² body surface area) below a cumulative dose of 10 mg/kg. In both children and adults, the total dose of Cerubidine administered should also take into account any previous or concomitant therapy with other potentially cardiotoxic agents or related compounds such as doxorubicin.
There is absolutely no reliable method of predicting the patients in whom acute congestive heart failure will develop as a result of the cardiac toxic effect of Cerubidine. However, certain changes in the electrocardiogram and a decrease in the systolic ejection fraction from pretreatment baseline may help to recognize those patients at greatest risk to develop congestive heart failure. On the basis of the electrocardiogram, a decrease equal to or greater than 30% in limb lead QRS voltage has been associated with a significant risk of drug-induced cardiomyopathy. Therefore, an electrocardiogram and/or determination of systolic ejection fraction should be performed before each course of Cerubidine. In the event that one or the other of these predictive parameters should occur, the benefit of continued therapy must be weighed against the risk of producing cardiac damage.
Early clinical diagnosis of drug-induced congestive heart failure appears to be essential for successful treatment with digitalis, diuretics, sodium restriction, and bed rest.

Continued on next page

Wyeth—Cont.

Evaluation of Hepatic and Renal Function— Significant hepatic or renal impairment can enhance the toxicity of the recommended doses of Cerubidine; therefore, prior to administration, evaluation of hepatic function and renal function using conventional clinical laboratory tests is recommended (see "Dosage and Administration").
Pregnancy—Cerubidine can cause fetal harm when administered to a pregnant woman because of its teratogenic potential. If this drug is used during pregnancy, or if the patient becomes pregnant while taking this drug, the patient should be apprised of the potential hazard to the fetus.
Extravasation at Injection Site—Extravasation of Cerubidine at the site of intravenous administration can cause severe local tissue necrosis.

PRECAUTIONS

Therapy with Cerubidine requires close observation of the patient and extensive chemical and laboratory monitoring.
Cerubidine may induce hyperuricemia secondary to rapid lysis of leukemic cells. Blood uric acid levels should be monitored and appropriate therapy initiated in the event that hyperuricemia develops.
Appropriate measures must be taken to control any systemic infection before beginning therapy with Cerubidine.
Cerubidine may transiently impart a red coloration to the urine after administration, and patients should be advised to expect this.
Carcinogenesis, Mutagenesis, Impairment of Fertility: Cerubidine, when injected subcutaneously into mice, causes fibrosarcomas to develop at the injection site. When administered to mice orally or intraperitoneally, no carcinogenic effect was noted after 22 months of observation.
In male dogs at a daily dose of 0.25 mg/kg administered intravenously, testicular atrophy was noted at autopsy. Histologic examination revealed total aplasia of the spermatocyte series in the seminiferous tubules with complete aspermatogenesis.
Pregnancy Category D. See Warnings Section.

ADVERSE REACTIONS

Dose-limiting toxicity includes myelosuppression and cardiotoxicity (see Warnings). Other reactions include:
Cutaneous—Reversible alopecia occurs in most patients.
Gastrointestinal—Acute nausea and vomiting occur but are usually mild. Antiemetic therapy may be of some help. Mucositis may occur three to seven days after administration. Diarrhea has occasionally been reported.
Local—If extravasation occurs during administration, tissue necrosis can result at the site.
Acute Reactions—Rarely fever, chills, and skin rash can occur.

DOSAGE AND ADMINISTRATION

Principles—In order to eradicate the leukemic cells and induce a complete remission, a profound suppression of the bone marrow is usually required. Evaluation of both the peripheral blood and bone marrow are mandatory in the formulation of appropriate treatment plans.
In the treatment of acute nonlymphocytic leukemia, Cerubidine is effective either alone or in combination with certain other antileukemic drugs. Combinations incorporating Cerubidine improve the complete remission frequency. Appropriate maintenance therapy should be instituted following the successful induction of a complete remission.
In the treatment of pediatric acute lymphocytic leukemia, induction of complete remission with Cerubidine-vincristine-prednisone (followed by maintenance therapy and appropriate central nervous system prophylaxis) increases the duration of continuous complete remission.
It is recommended that the dosage of Cerubidine be reduced in instances of hepatic or renal impairment. For example, usng serum bilirubin and serum creatinine as indicators of liver and kidney function, the following dose modifications are recommended:

Serum Bilirubin	Serum Creatinine	Recommended Dose
1.2 to 3.0 mg%		¾ normal dose
> 3 mg%	> 3 mg%	½ normal dose

Representative dose schedules and combinations for the approved indication of adult acute nonlymphocytic leukemia:
As a Single Agent[7]—Cerubidine (daunorubicin hydrochloride) 60 mg/m²/day IV on days 1,2,3 every 3 to 4 weeks.
In Combination[8,9]—Cerubidine 45 mg/m²/day IV on days 1,2,3 of the first course and on days 1,2 of subsequent courses **AND** cytosine arabinoside 100 mg/m²/day IV infusion daily for 7 days for the first course and for 5 days for subsequent courses.
The attainment of a normal appearing bone marrow may require up to three courses of induction therapy. Evaluation of the bone marrow following recovery from the previous course of induction therapy determines whether a further course of induction treatment is required.
Representative dose schedule, in combination, for the approved indication of remission induction in pediatric acute lymphocytic leukemia:
In Combination[10,11]—Cerubidine 25 mg/m² IV on day 1 every week, vincristine 1.5 mg/m² IV on day 1 every week, prednisone 40 mg/m² PO daily. Generally, a complete remission will be obtained within four such courses of therapy; however, if after four courses the patient is in partial remission, an additional one or, if necessary, two courses may be given in an effort to obtain a complete remission.
In children less than 2 years of age or below 0.5 m² body surface area, calculation of dosage should be made on the basis of weight (mg/kg) instead of body surface area.[5]
The contents of a vial should be reconstituted with 4 ml of Sterile Water for Injection, U.S.P., and agitated gently until the material has completely dissolved. The withdrawable vial contents provide 20 mg of daunorubicin activity, with 5 mg of daunorubicin activity per ml. The desired dose is withdrawn into a syringe containing 10 to 15 ml of normal saline and then injected into the tubing or sidearm of a rapidly flowing I.V. infusion of 5 percent glucose or normal saline solution. Cerubidine should not be administered mixed with other drugs or heparin. The reconstituted solution is stable for 24 hours at room temperature and 48 hours under refrigeration. It should be protected from exposure to sunlight.
Procedures for proper handling and disposal of anticancer drugs should be considered. Several guidelines on this subject have been published.[12–17] There is no general agreement that all of the procedures recommended in the guidelines are necessary or appropriate.

HOW SUPPLIED

Cerubidine (daunorubicin hydrochloride) for Injection, Wyeth®, is available in butyl-rubber-stoppered vials, each containing 20 mg of base activity (21.4 mg as the hydrochloride salt) and 100 mg of mannitol, as a sterile reddish lyophilized powder. When reconstituted with 4 ml of Sterile Water for Injection, U.S.P., each ml contains 5 mg of daunorubicin activity. Each package contains 10 vials. NDC 0008-4155-01.
Storage: (+15° to +25° C).

REFERENCES

1. Gilladoga AC, Manuel C Tan CTC, et al: The cardiotoxicity of adriamycin and daunomycin in children. Cancer 37:1070–1078, 1976.
2. Halzun JF, Wagner HR, Gaeta JF, et al: Daunorubicin cardiac toxicity in children with acute lymphocytic leukemia. Cancer 33:545–554, 1974.
3. Von Hoff DD, Rozencweig M, Layard M, et al: Daunomycin-induced cardiotoxicity in children and adults: a review of 110 cases. Am J Med 62:200–208, 1977.
4. Goorin AM, Borow KM, Goldman A, Williams RG, Henderson IC, Sallan SE, Cohen H, Jaffe N: Congestive heart failure due to adriamycin cardiotoxicity: its natural history in children. Cancer 47:2810–2816, 1981.
5. Sallan SE; Personal communication, 1981.
6. Praga C, Bretta G, Vigo PL, et al: Adriamycin cardiotoxicity: A survey of 1273 patients. Cancer Treat Rep 63:827–834, 1979.
7. Wiernik PH, Schimpff SC, Schiffer CA et al: Randomized clinical comparison of daunorubicin (NSC-82151) alone with a combination of daunorubicin, cytosine arabinoside (NSC-63878), 6-Thioguanine (NSC-752) and pyrimethamine (NSC-3061) for the treatment of acute non-lymphocytic leukemia. Cancer Treat Rep 60:41–53, 1979.
8. Yates JW, Wallace JH, Ellison RR, Holland JF: Cytosine arabinoside (NSC-63878) and daunorubicin (NSC-83142) therapy in acute non-lymphocytic leukemia. Cancer Chemo Rep 57:485–488, 1973.
9. Rai KR, Holland JF, Glidewell O: Improvement in remission induction therapy of acute myelocytic leukemia. Proc. Am. Assoc. Cancer Res., Am Soc. Clin. Oncol. 16:265, 1975.
10. Aur RJA, Simone JV, Hustu HO, Verzosa MS: A comparative study of central nervous system irradiation and intensive chemotherapy early in remission of childhood acute lymphocytic leukemia. Cancer 29:381–391, 1972.
11. Mauer AM: Therapy for acute lymphoblastic leukemia of childhood: Blood 56:1–10, 1980.
12. Recommendations for the Safe Handling of Parenteral Antineoplastic Drugs. NIH Publication No. 83-2621. For sale by the Superintendent of Documents, U.S. Government Printing Office, Washington, D.C. 20402.
13. AMA Council Report. Guidelines for Handling Parenteral Antineoplastics. JAMA, March 15, 1985.
14. National Study Commission on Cytotoxic Exposure—Recommendations for Handling Cytotoxic Agents. Available from Louis P. Jeffrey, Sc. D., Director of Pharmacy Services, Rhode Island Hospital, 593 Eddy Street, Providence, Rhode Island 02902.
15. Clinical Oncological Society of Australia: Guidelines and recommendations for safe handling of antineoplastic agents. Med J Australia *1*:426–428, 1983.
16. Jones RB, et al: Safe handling of chemotherapeutic agents: A report from the Mount Sinai Medical Center, Ca—A Cancer Journal for Clinicians Sept/Oct, 258–263, 1983.
17. American Society of Hospital Pharmacists technical assistance bulletin on handling cytotoxic drugs in hospitals. Am J Hosp Pharm *42*: 131–137, 1985.

Manufactured by SPECIA France
by arrangement with RHONE-POULENC France
Distributed by WYETH LABORATORIES INC., Philadelphia, PA 19101

CHOLERA VACCINE, U.S.P. ℞

[kol 'er-ah vak 'sēn]

DESCRIPTION

Each ml. contains 8 units each serotype antigen (Ogawa and Inaba). The preservative is 0.5% phenol.

HOW SUPPLIED

Vials of 1.5 ml. and 20 ml.
For prescribing information write to Professional Service, Wyeth Laboratories, Box 8299, Philadelphia, PA 19101, or contact your local Wyeth representative.

COLLYRIUM OTC

[ko-lir 'e-um]
a neutral borate solution
SOOTHING EYE LOTION

DESCRIPTION

A neutral borate solution containing boric acid and sodium borate as buffers, not more than 0.002% thimerosal as a preservative, and water.

INDICATIONS

For flushing or irrigating the eye to remove loose foreign material, air pollutants, or chlorinated water.

DOSAGE AND ADMINISTRATION

Patients are advised to rinse cup clean before each use and to avoid contamination of rim and inside surfaces of cup. The half-filled cup should be applied to the affected eye and pressed tightly to the eye to prevent the escape of the liquid, and the head tilted backward. Eyelids should be opened wide and the eyeball rotated to ensure thorough bathing with the wash or lotion. The cup should be rinsed with clean water after each use. After every use, the bottle can be reclosed by placing the threaded eyecup on the bottle which replaces the disposable top after opening.

WARNINGS

Patients are advised of the following. To avoid contamination of this product, do not touch tip of container to any other surface. Replace cap after using. Not for use in open wounds in or near the eyes. Consult a doctor if you experience eye pain, changes in vision, continued redness or irritation of the eye, or if the condition worsens or persists.
This product contains thimerosal as a preservative. Do not use this product if you are sensitive to mercury. Do not use if solution changes color or becomes cloudy, or with a wetting solution for contact lens or other eye lotions containing polyvinyl alcohol. Container should be kept tightly closed at room temperature, approx. 77°F (25°C).

HOW SUPPLIED

Bottles of 6 fl. oz. with eyecup.

COLLYRIUM OTC

[ko-lir 'e-um]
eye drops with tetrahydrozoline

DESCRIPTION

Collyrium Eye Drops contain tetrahydrozoline hydrochloride (0.05%) and glycerin (1.0%), with boric acid and sodium borate as buffering agents, hydrochloric acid to adjust pH, and benzalkonium chloride (0.01%) and edetate disodium (0.1%) as preservatives.

INDICATIONS

For the relief of redness of the eye due to minor irritations, temporary relief of burning and irritation due to dryness of the eye and/or discomfort due to minor irritations of the eye or to exposure to wind and sun.

DOSAGE AND ADMINISTRATION

One to two drops in the affected eye(s). Procedure may be repeated up to four times daily.

WARNINGS

Patients are advised of the following:
To avoid contamination of this product, do not touch tip of container to any other surface. Replace cap after using.
If you experience eye pain, changes in vision, continued redness or irritation of the eye, or if the condition worsens or persists for more than 72 hours, discontinue use and consult a doctor.
If you have glaucoma, do not use this product except under the advice and supervision of a doctor.
Overuse of this product may produce increased redness of the eye.
Do not use if solution changes color or becomes cloudy, or with povidone-containing contact lens wetting solutions.
Container should be kept tightly closed and stored at room temperature, approx. 77°F (25°C).

HOW SUPPLIED

Bottles of ½ fl. oz. with built-in eye dropper.

CORDARONE® ℞

[*kŏr 'dă-rōn*]
(amiodarone HCl)
Tablets

Caution: Federal law prohibits dispensing without prescription.

DESCRIPTION

Cordarone is a member of a new class of antiarrhythmic drugs with predominantly Class III (Vaughan Williams' classification) effects, available for oral administration as white, scored tablets containing 200 mg of amiodarone hydrochloride. The inactive ingredients present are colloidal silicon dioxide, lactose, magnesium stearate, povidone, and starch. Cordarone is a benzofuran derivative: 2-butyl-3-benzofuranyl 4-[2-(diethylamino)-ethoxy]-3-5-diiodophenyl ketone, hydrochloride. It is not chemically related to any other available antiarrhythmic drug.
The structural formula is as follows:

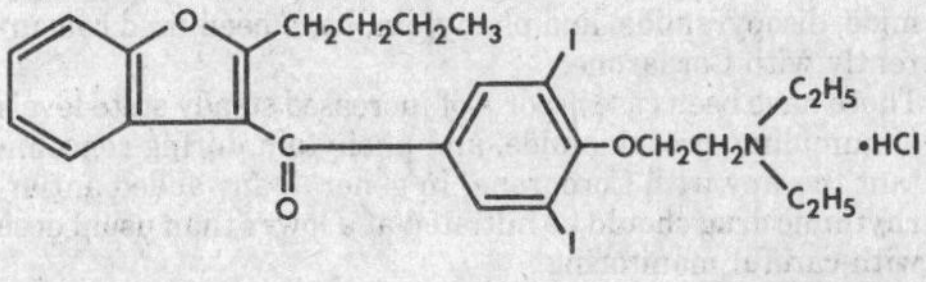

$C_{25}H_{29}I_2NO_3 \cdot HCl$

Molecular Weight: 681.8

Amiodarone HCl is a white to cream-colored crystalline powder. It is slightly soluble in water, soluble in alcohol, and freely soluble in chloroform. It contains 37.3% iodine by weight.

CLINICAL PHARMACOLOGY

ELECTROPHYSIOLOGY/MECHANISMS OF ACTION

In animals, Cordarone is effective in the prevention or suppression of experimentally induced arrhythmias. The antiarrhythmic effect of Cordarone may be due to at least two major properties: 1) a prolongation of the myocardial cell-action potential duration and refractory period and 2) noncompetitive alpha- and beta-adrenergic inhibition.
Cordarone prolongs the duration of the action potential of all cardiac fibers while causing minimal reduction of dV/dt (maximal upstroke velocity of the action potential). The refractory period is prolonged in all cardiac tissues. Cordarone increases the cardiac refractory period without influencing resting membrane potential, except in automatic cells where the slope of the prepotential is reduced, generally reducing automaticity. These electrophysiologic effects are reflected in a decreased sinus rate of 15 to 20%, increased PR and QT intervals of about 10%, the development of U-waves, and changes in T-wave contour. These changes should not require discontinuation of Cordarone as they are evidence of its pharmacological action, although Cordarone can cause marked sinus bradycardia or sinus arrest and heart block. On rare occasions QT prolongation has been associated with worsening of arrhythmia (see"WARNINGS").

HEMODYNAMICS

In animal studies and after intravenous administration in man, Cordarone relaxes vascular smooth muscle, reduces peripheral vascular resistance (afterload), and slightly increases cardiac index. After oral dosing, however, Cordarone produces no significant change in left ventrical ejection fraction (LVEF), even in patients with depressed LVEF. After acute intravenous dosing in man, Cordarone may have a mild negative inotropic effect.

PHARMACOKINETICS

Following oral administration in man, Cordarone is slowly and variably absorbed. The bioavailability of Cordarone is approximately 50%, but has varied between 35 and 65% in various studies. Maximum plasma concentrations are attained 3 to 7 hours after a single dose. Despite this, the onset of action may occur in 2 to 3 days, but more commonly takes 1 to 3 weeks, even with loading doses. Plasma concentrations with chronic dosing at 100 to 600 mg/day are approximately dose proportional, with a mean 0.5 mg/L increase for each 100 mg/day. These means, however, include considerable individual variability.
Cordarone has a very large but variable volume of distribution, averaging about 60 L/kg because of extensive accumulation in various sites, especially adipose tissue and highly perfused organs, such as the liver, lung, and spleen. One major metabolite of Cordarone, desethylamiodarone, has been identified in man. It accumulates to an even greater extent in almost all tissues. The pharmacological activity of this metabolite, however, is not known. During chronic treatment, the plasma ratio of metabolite to parent compound is approximately one.
The main route of elimination is via hepatic excretion into bile, and some enterohepatic recirculation may occur. However, its kinetics in patients with hepatic insufficiency have not been elucidated. Cordarone has a very low plasma clearance with negligible renal excretion, so that it does not appear necessary to modify the dose in patients with renal failure. In patients with renal impairment, the plasma concentration of Cordarone is not elevated. Neither Cordarone nor its metabolite is dialyzable.
In patients, following discontinuation of chronic oral therapy, Cordarone has been shown to have a biphasic elimination with an initial one-half reduction of plasma levels after 2.5 to 10 days. A much slower terminal plasma-elimination phase shows a half-life of the parent compound ranging from 26 to 107 days, with a mean of approximately 53 days and most patients in the 40- to 55-day range. In the absence of a loading-dose period, steady-state plasma concentrations, at constant oral dosing, would therefore be reached between 130 and 535 days, with an average of 265 days. For the metabolite, the mean plasma-elimination half-life was approximately 61 days. These data probably reflect an initial elimination of the drug from well-perfused tissue (the 2.5- to 10-day half-life phase), followed by a terminal phase representing extremely slow elimination from poorly perfused tissue compartments such as fat.
The considerable intersubject variation in both phases of elimination, as well as uncertainty as to what compartment is critical to drug effect, requires attention to individual responses once arrhythmia control is achieved with loading doses because the correct maintenance dose is determined, in part, by the elimination rates. Daily maintenance doses of Cordarone should be based on individual patient requirements (see "Dosage and Administration").
Cordarone and its metabolite have a limited transplacental transfer of approximately 10 to 50%. The parent drug and its metabolite have been detected in breast milk.
Cordarone is highly protein-bound (approximately 96%).
Although electrophysiologic effects, such as prolongation of QTc, can be seen within hours after a parenteral dose of Cordarone, effects on abnormal rhythms are not seen before 2 to 3 days and usually require 1 to 3 weeks, even when a loading dose is used. There may be a continued increase in effect for longer periods still. There is evidence that the time to effect is shorter when a loading-dose regimen is used.
Consistent with the slow rate of elimination, antiarrhythmic effects persist for weeks or months after Cordarone is discontinued, but the time of recurrence is variable and unpredictable. In general, when the drug is resumed after recurrence of the arrhythmia, control is established relatively rapidly compared to the initial response, presumably because tissue stores were not wholly depleted at the time of recurrence.

PHARMACODYNAMICS

There is no well-established relationship of plasma concentration to effectiveness, but it does appear that concentrations much below 1 mg/L are often ineffective and that levels above 2.5 mg/L are generally not needed. Within individuals dose reductions and ensuing decreased plasma concentrations can result in loss of arrhythmia control. Plasma-concentration measurements can be used to identify patients whose levels are unusually low, and who might benefit from a dose increase, or unusually high, and who might have dosage reduction in the hope of minimizing side effects. Some observations have suggested a plasma concentration, dose, or dose/duration relationship for side effects such as pulmonary fibrosis, liver-enzyme elevations, corneal deposits and facial pigmentation, peripheral neuropathy, gastrointestinal and central nervous system effects.

MONITORING EFFECTIVENESS

Predicting the effectiveness of any antiarrhythmic agent in long-term prevention of recurrent ventricular tachycardia and ventricular fibrillation is difficult and controversial, with highly qualified investigators recommending use of ambulatory monitoring, programmed electrical stimulation with various stimulation regimens, or a combination of these, to assess response. There is no present consensus on many aspects of how best to assess effectiveness, but there is a reasonable consensus on some aspects:

1. If a patient with a history of cardiac arrest does not manifest a hemodynamically unstable arrhythmia during electrocardiographic monitoring prior to treatment, assessment of the effectiveness of Cordarone requires some provocative approach, either exercise or programmed electrical stimulation (PES).
2. Whether provocation is also needed in patients who do manifest their life-threatening arrhythmia spontaneously is not settled, but there are reasons to consider PES or other provocation in such patients. In the fraction of patients whose PES-inducible arrhythmia can be made noninducible by Cordarone (a fraction that has varied widely in various series from less than 10% to almost 40%, perhaps due to different stimulation criteria) the prognosis has been almost uniformly excellent, with very low recurrence (ventricular tachycardia or sudden death) rates. More controversial is the meaning of continued inducibility. There has been an impression that continued inducibility in Cordarone patients may not foretell a poor prognosis but, in fact, many observers have found greater recurrence rates in patients who remain inducible than in those who do not. A number of criteria have been proposed, however, for identifying patients who remain inducible but who seem likely nonetheless to do well on Cordarone. These criteria include increased difficulty of Induction (more stimuli or more rapid stimuli), which has been reported to predict a lower rate of recurrence, and ability to tolerate the induced ventricular tachycardia without severe symptoms, a finding that has been reported to correlate with better survival but not with lower recurrence rates. While these criteria require confirmation and further study in general, *easier* inductibility or *poorer* tolerance of the induced arrhythmia should suggest consideration of a need to revise treatment.

Several predictors of success not based on PES have also been suggested, including complete elimination of all nonsustained ventricular tachycardia on ambulatory monitoring and very low premature ventricular-beat rates (less than 1 VPB/1,000 normal beats).
While these issues remain unsettled for Cordarone, as for other agents, the prescriber of Cordarone should have access to (direct or through referral), and familiarity with, the full range of evaluatory procedures used in the care of patients with life-threatening arrhythmias.
It is difficult to describe the effectiveness rates of Cordarone, as these depend on the specific arrhythmia treated, the success criteria used, the underlying cardiac disease of the patient, the number of drugs tried before resorting to Cordarone, the duration of follow-up, the dose of Cordarone, the use of additional antiarrhythmic agents, and many other factors. As Cordarone has been studied principally in patients with refractory life-threatening ventricular arrhythmias, in whom drug therapy must be selected on the basis of response and cannot be assigned arbitrarily, randomized comparisons with other agents or placebo have not been possible. Reports of series of treated patients with a history of cardiac arrest and mean follow-up of one year or more have given mortality (due to arrhythmia) rates that were highly variable, ranging from less than 5% to over 30%, with most series in the range of 10 to 15%. Overall arrhythmia-recurrence rates (fatal and nonfatal) also were highly variable (and, as noted above, depended on response to PES and other measures), and depend on whether patients who do not seem to respond initially are included. In most cases, considering only patients who seemed to respond well enough to be placed on long-term treatment, recurrence rates have ranged from 20 to 40% in series with a mean follow-up of a year or more.

INDICATIONS AND USAGE

Because of its life-threatening side effects and the substantial management difficulties associated with its use (see "Warnings" below), Cordarone is indicated only for the treatment of the following documented, life-threatening recurrent ventricular arrhythmias when these have not responded to documented adequate doses of other available antiarrhythmics or when alternative agents could not be tolerated.

1. Recurrent ventricular fibrillation.
2. Recurrent hemodynamically unstable ventricular tachycardia.

As is the case for other antiarrhythmic agents, there is no evidence from controlled trials that the use of Cordarone favorably affects survival.
Cordarone should be used only by physicians familiar with and with access to (directly or through referral) the use of all available modalities for treating recurrent life-threatening ventricular arrhythmias, and who have access to appropriate monitoring facilities, including in-hospital and ambulatory continuous electrocardiographic monitoring and electrophysiologic techniques. Because of the life-threatening nature of the arrhythmias treated, potential interactions with prior therapy, and potential exacerbation of the arrhythmia, initiation of therapy with Cordarone should be carried out in the hospital.

Continued on next page

Wyeth—Cont.

CONTRAINDICATIONS

Cordarone is contraindicated in severe sinus-node dysfunction, causing marked sinus bradycardia; second- and third-degree atrioventricular block; and when episodes of bradycardia have caused syncope (except when used in conjunction with a pacemaker).

WARNINGS

Cordarone is intended for use only in patients with the indicated life-threatening arrhythmias because its use is accompanied by substantial toxicity.

Cordarone has several potentially fatal toxicities, the most important of which is pulmonary toxicity (interstitial pneumonitis/alveolitis) that has resulted in clinically manifest disease at rates as high as 10 to 15% in some series of patients with ventricular arrhythmias given doses around 400 mg/day, and as abnormal diffusion capacity without symptoms in a much higher percentage of patients. Pulmonary toxicity has been fatal about 10% of the time. Liver injury is common with Cordarone, but is usually mild and evidenced only by abnormal liver enzymes. Overt liver disease can occur, however, and has been fatal in a few cases. Like other antiarrhythmics, Cordarone can exacerbate the arrhythmia, e.g., by making the arrhythmia less well tolerated or more difficult to reverse. This has occurred in 2 to 5% of patients in various series, and significant heart block or sinus bradycardia has been seen in 2 to 5%. All of these events should be manageable in the proper clinical setting in most cases. Although the frequency of such proarrhythmic events does not appear greater with Cordarone than with many other agents used in this population, the effects are prolonged when they occur.

Even in patients at high risk of arrhythmic death, in whom the toxicity of Cordarone is an acceptable risk, Cordarone poses major management problems that could be life-threatening in a population at risk of sudden death, so that every effort should be made to utilize alternative agents first.

The difficulty of using Cordarone effectively and safely itself poses a significant risk to patients. Patients with the indicated arrhythmias must be hospitalized while the loading dose of Cordarone is given, and a response generally requires at least one week, usually two or more. Because absorption and elimination are variable, maintenance-dose selection is difficult, and it is not unusual to require dosage decrease or discontinuation of treatment. In a retrospective survey of 192 patients with ventricular tachyarrhythmias, 84 required dose reduction and 18 required at least temporary discontinuation because of adverse effects, and several series have reported 15 to 20% overall frequencies of discontinuation due to adverse reactions. The time at which a previously controlled life-threatening arrhythmia will recur after discontinuation or dose adjustment is unpredictable, ranging from weeks to months. The patient is obviously at great risk during this time and may need prolonged hospitalization. Attempts to substitute other antiarrhythmic agents when Cordarone must be stopped will be made difficult by the gradually, but unpredictably, changing amiodarone body burden. A similar problem exists when Cordarone is not effective; it still poses the risk of an interaction with whatever subsequent treatment is tried.

PULMONARY TOXICITY

Cordarone causes a clinical syndrome of progressive dyspnea and cough accompanied by functional, radiographic, gallium-scan and pathological data showing a pulmonary interstitial process, sometimes called alveolitis. The frequency of pulmonary toxicity has generally been low, varying from 2 to 7% in most published reports, but recent preliminary reports have found rates of 11 to 15% in patients treated for more than a year on average and there is evidence of increasing frequency with time and/or daily or cumulative dose. Although the syndrome is usually reversible when Cordarone is discontinued, with or without steroid therapy, fatalities have occurred in about 10% of cases. Any new respiratory symptom in a patient receiving Cordarone should suggest the possibility of pulmonary toxicity and lead to clinical and radiographic evaluation, with gallium-scan and pulmonary-function evaluation if needed. Particular care should be taken not to presume that such symptoms are related to cardiac failure. Again, diffusion capacity appears to be the pulmonary-function test most likely to show abnormality. Evidence of toxicity should lead, at a minimum, to dose reduction, and preferably to withdrawal of the drug to establish reversibility. In some cases rechallenge at a lower dose has not resulted in return of toxicity.

Periodic chest X rays and clinical evaluation (every 3 to 6 months) are recommended and baseline pulmonary-function tests, including diffusion capacity, should be obtained.

WORSENED ARRHYTHMIA

Cordarone, like other antiarrhythmics, can cause serious exacerbation of the presenting arrhythmia, a risk that may be enhanced by the presence of concomitant antiarrhythmics. Exacerbation has been reported in about 2 to 5% in most series, and has included new ventricular fibrillation, incessant ventricular tachycardia, increased resistance to cardioversion, and polymorphic ventricular tachycardia associated with QT prolongation (Torsade de Pointes).

In addition, Cordarone has caused symptomatic bradycardia or sinus arrest with suppression of escape foci in 2 to 4% of patients.

LIVER INJURY

Elevations of hepatic enzyme levels are seen frequently in patients exposed to Cordarone and in most cases are asymptomatic. If the increase exceeds three times normal or doubles in a patient with an elevated baseline, discontinuation of Cordarone or dosage reduction should be considered. In a few cases in which biopsy has been done, the histology has resembled that of alcoholic hepatitis or cirrhosis. Hepatic failure has been a rare cause of death in patients treated with Cordarone.

PRECAUTIONS

CORNEAL MICRODEPOSITS; IMPAIRMENT OF VISION

Corneal microdeposits appear in the majority of adults treated with Cordarone. They are usually discernible only by slit-lamp examination, but give rise to symptoms such as visual halos or blurred vision in as many as 10% of patients. Corneal microdeposits are reversible upon reduction of dose or termination of treatment. Asymptomatic microdeposits are not a reason to reduce dose or discontinue treatment.

PHOTOSENSITIVITY

Cordarone has induced photosensitization in about 10% of patients; some protection may be afforded by the use of sun-barrier creams or protective clothing. During long-term treatment, a blue-gray discoloration of the exposed skin may occur. The risk may be increased in patients of fair complexion or those with excessive sun exposure, and may be related to cumulative dose and duration of therapy.

THYROID ABNORMALITIES

Cordarone inhibits peripheral conversion of thyroxine (T_4) to triiodothyronine (T_3), tending to cause somewhat increased thyroxine levels and increased levels of inactive reverse T_3, and somewhat decreased levels of T_3. It is also a potential source of large amounts of inorganic iodine. Because of its release of inorganic iodine, or perhaps for other reasons, Cordarone can cause both hypothyroidism or hyperthyroidism. Thyroid function should be monitored at baseline and periodically, particularly in any patient with a history of thyroid nodules, goiter, or other dysfunction.

Hyperthyroidism has been reported in 2 to 4% of patients in most series but in 8 to 10% in others and is probably best identified by a finding of elevated TSH. Careful supplementation with thyroid hormone can eliminate this problem.

A more difficult problem is hyperthyroidism, best identified by a serum T_3 of more than 200 mg/dL, presumably resulting from an increased supply of iodine to an autonomous nodule or gland, occurring in 1 to 3% of patients and potentially a reason for discontinuing drug.

HYPOTENSION POSTBYPASS

Rare occurrences of hypotension upon discontinuation of cardiopulmonary bypass during open-heart surgery in patients receiving Cordarone have been reported. The relationship of this event to Cordarone therapy is unknown.

LABORATORY TESTS

Elevations in liver enzymes (SGOT and SGPT) can occur. Liver enzymes in patients on relatively high maintenance doses should be monitored on a regular basis. Persistent significant elevations in the liver enzymes or hepatomegaly should alert the physician to consider reducing the maintenance dose of Cordarone or discontinuing therapy.

Cordarone alters the results of thyroid-function tests, causing an increase in serum T_4 and serum reverse T_3, and a decline in serum T_3 levels. Despite these biochemical changes, most patients remain clinically euthyroid.

DRUG INTERACTIONS

Although only a small number of drug-drug interactions with Cordarone have been explored formally, most of these have shown such an interaction. The potential for other interactions should be anticipated, particularly for drugs with potentially serious toxicity, such as other antiarrhythmics. If such drugs are needed, their dose should be reassessed and, where appropriate, plasma concentration measured.

In view of the long and variable half-life of Cordarone, potential for drug interactions exists not only with concomitant medication but also with drugs administered after discontinuation of Cordarone.

Digitalis

Administration of Cordarone to patients receiving digoxin therapy regularly results in an increase in the serum digoxin concentration that may reach toxic levels with resultant clinical toxicity. **On initiation of Cordarone, the need for digitalis therapy should be reviewed and the dose reduced by approximately 50% or discontinued.** If digitalis treatment is continued, serum levels should be closely monitored and patients observed for clinical evidence of toxicity. These precautions probably should apply to digitoxin administration as well.

Anticoagulants

Potentiation of warfarin-type anticoagulant response is almost always seen in patients receiving Cordarone and can result in serious or fatal bleeding. **The dose of the anticoagulant should be reduced by one-third to one-half, and prothrombin times should be monitored closely.**

Antiarrhythmic Agents

Other antiarrhythmic drugs, such as quinidine, procainamide, disopyramide, and phenytoin, have been used concurrently with Cordarone.

There have been case reports of increased steady-state levels of quinidine, procainamide, and phenytoin during concomitant therapy with Cordarone. In general, any added antiarrhythmic drug should be initiated at a lower than usual dose with careful monitoring.

In general, combination of Cordarone with other antiarrhythmic therapy should be reserved for patients with life-threatening ventricular arrhythmias who are incompletely responsive to a single agent or incompletely responsive to Cordarone. During transfer to Cordarone the dose levels of previously administered agents should be reduced by 30 to 50% several days after the addition of Cordarone, when arrhythmia suppression should be beginning. The continued need for the other antiarrhythmic agent should be reviewed after the effects of Cordarone have been established, and discontinuation ordinarily should be attempted. If the treatment is continued, these patients should be particularly carefully monitored for adverse effects, especially conduction disturbances and exacerbation of tachyarrhythmias, as Cordarone is continued. In Cordarone-treated patients who require additional antiarrhythmic therapy, the initial dose of such agents should be approximately half of the usual recommended dose.

Cordarone should be used with caution in patients receiving beta-blocking agents or calcium antagonists because of the possible potentiation of bradycardia, sinus arrest, and AV block; if necessary. Cordarone can continue to be used after insertion of a pacemaker in patients with severe bradycardia or sinus arrest.

[See table below left].

SUMMARY OF DRUG INTERACTIONS WITH CORDARONE

Concomitant Drug	Interaction: Onset (days)	Interaction: Magnitude	Recommended Dose Reduction of Concomitant Drug
Warfarin	3 to 4	Increases prothrombin time by 100%	1/3 to 1/2
Digoxin	1	Increases serum concentration by 70%	1/2
Quinidine	2	Increases serum concentration by 33%	1/3 to 1/2 (or discontinue)
Procainamide	<7	Increases plasma concentration by 55%, NAPA* concentration by 33%	1/3 (or discontinue)

*NAPA = n-acetyl procainamide.

ELECTROLYTE DISTURBANCES

Since antiarrhythmic drugs may be ineffective or may be arrhythmogenic in patients with hypokalemia, any potassium or magnesium deficiency should be corrected before instituting Cordarone therapy.

CARCINOGENESIS, MUTAGENESIS, IMPAIRMENT OF FERTILITY

Cordarone reduced fertility of male and female rats at a dose level of 90 mg/kg/day (8 × highest recommended human maintenance dose). Cordarone caused a statistically significant, dose-related increase in the incidence of thyroid tumors (follicular adenoma and/or carcinoma) in rats. The incidence of thyroid tumors was greater than control even at the lowest dose level of Cordarone tested, i.e., 5 mg/kg/day or approximately equal to 1/2 the highest recommended human maintenance dose. Mutagenicity studies (Ames, micronucleus, and lysogenic tests) with Cordarone were negative.

PREGNANCY: PREGNANCY CATEGORY C

Cordarone has been shown to be embryotoxic (increased fetal resorption and growth retardation) in the rat when given orally at a dose of 200 mg/kg/day (18 times the maximum recommended maintenance dose). Similar findings have been noted in one strain of mice at a dose of 5 mg/kg/day (approximately ½ the maximum recommended maintenance dose) and higher, but not in a second strain nor in the rabbit at doses up to 100 mg/kg/day (9 times the maximum recommended maintenance dose).

In general, Cordarone should be used during pregnancy only if the potential benefit to the mother justifies the unknown risk to the fetus.

LABOR AND DELIVERY

It is not know whether the use of Cordarone during labor or delivery has any immediate or delayed adverse effects. Preclinical studies in rodents have not shown any effect of Cordarone on the duration of gestation or on parturition.

NURSING MOTHERS

Cordarone is excreted in human milk, suggesting that breast-feeding could expose the nursing infant to a significant dose of the drug. Nursing offspring of lactating rats administered Cordarone have been shown to be less viable and have reduced body-weight gains. Therefore, when Cordarone therapy is indicated, the mother should be advised to discontinue nursing.

PEDIATRIC USE

The safety and effectiveness of Cordarone in children have not been established.

ADVERSE REACTIONS

Adverse reactions have been very common in virtually all series of patients treated with Cordarone for ventricular arrhythmias, with relatively large doses of drug (400 mg/day and above) occurring in about three-fourths of all patients and causing discontinuation in 7 to 18%. The most serious reactions are pulmonary toxicity, exacerbation of arrhythmia, and rare serious liver injury (see "Warnings"), but other adverse effects constitute important problems. They are often reversible with dose reduction and virtually always reversible with cessation of Cordarone treatment. Most of the adverse effects appear to become more frequent with continued treatment beyond six months, although rates appear to remain relatively constant beyond one year. The time and dose relationships of adverse effects are under continued study.

Neurologic problems are extremely common, occurring in 20 to 40% of patients and including malaise and fatigue, tremor and involuntary movements, poor coordination and gait, and peripheral neuropathy, they are rarely a reason to stop therapy and may respond to dose reductions.

Gastrointestinal complaints, most commonly nausea, vomiting, constipation, and anorexia, occur in about 25% of patients but rarely require discontinuation of drug. These commonly occur during high-dose administration (i.e., loading dose) and usually respond to dose reduction of divided doses.

Asymptomatic corneal microdeposits are present in virtually all adult patients who have been on drug for more than 6 months. Some patients develop eye symptoms of halos, photophobia, and dry eyes. Vision is rarely affected and drug discontinuation is rarely needed.

Dermatological adverse reactions occur in about 15% of patients, with photosensitivity being most common (about 10%). Sunscreen and protection from sun exposure may be helpful, and drug discontinuation is not usually necessary. Prolonged exposure to Cordarone occasionally results in a blue-gray pigmentation. This is slowly and occasionally incompletely reversible on discontinuation of drug but is of cosmetic importance only.

Cardiovascular adverse reactions, other than exacerbation of the arrhythmias, include the uncommon occurrences of congestive heart failure (3%) and bradycardia. Bradycardia usually responds to dosage reduction but may require a pacemaker for control. CHF rarely requires drug discontinuation. Cardiac conduction abnormalities occur infrequently and are reversible on discontinuation of drug.

The following side-effect rates are based on a retrospective study of 241 patients treated for 2 to 1,515 days (mean 441.3 days).

The following side effects were reported in 10 to 33% of patients:

Gastrointestinal: Nausea and vomiting

The following side effects were each reported in 4 to 9% of patients:

Dermatologic: Solar dermatitis/photosensitivity.

Neurologic: Malaise and fatigue, tremor/abnormal involuntary movements, lack of coordination, abnormal gait/ataxia, dizziness, paresthesias.

Gastrointestinal: Constipation, anorexia.

Ophthalmologic: Visual disturbances.

Hepatic: Abnormal liver-function tests.

Respiratory: pulmonary inflammation or fibrosis.

The following side effects were each reported in 1 to 3% of patients:

Thyroid: Hypothyroidism, hyperthyroidism.

Neurologic: Decreased libido, insomnia, headache, sleep disturbances.

Cardiovascular: Congestive heart failure, cardiac arrhythmias, SA node dysfunction.

	Loading Dose (Daily)	Adjustment and Maintenance Dose (Daily)	
Ventricular Arrhythmias	1 to 3 weeks	~1 month	usual maintenance
	800 to 1,600 mg	600 to 800 mg	400 mg

Gastrointestinal: Abdominal pain.

Hepatic: Nonspecific hepatic disorders.

Other: Flushing, abnormal taste and smell, edema, abnormal salivation, coagulation abnormalities.

The following side effects were each reported in less than 1% of patients: Blue skin discoloration, rash, spontaneous ecchymosis, alopecia, hypotension, and cardiac conduction abnormalities.

Rare occurrences of hepatitis and cirrhosis have been reported in patients receiving Cordarone. The relationship of these events to Cordarone therapy has not been definitively established.

In surveys of almost 5,000 patients treated in open U.S. studies and in published reports of treatment with Cordarone, the adverse reactions most frequently requiring discontinuation of Cordarone include pulmonary infiltrates or fibrosis, paroxysmal ventricular tachycardia, congestive heart failure, and elevation of liver enzymes. Other symptoms causing discontinuations less often included visual disturbances, solar dermatitis, blue skin discoloration, hyperthyroidism and hypothyroidism.

OVERDOSAGE

There have been 3 reported cases of Cordarone overdose in which 3 to 8 grams were taken. There were no deaths or permanent sequelae. Animal studies indicate that Cordarone has a high oral LD_{50} (> 3,000 mg/kg).

In addition to general supportive measures, the patient's cardiac rhythm and blood pressure should be monitored, and if bradycardia ensues, a β-adrenergic agonist or a pacemaker may be used. Hypotension with inadequate tissue perfusion should be treated with positive inotropic and/or vasopressor agents. Neither Cordarone nor its metabolite is dialyzable.

DOSAGE AND ADMINISTRATION

BECAUSE OF THE UNIQUE PHARMACOKINETIC PROPERTIES, DIFFICULT DOSING SCHEDULE, AND SEVERITY OF THE SIDE EFFECTS IF PATIENTS ARE IMPROPERLY MONITORED, CORDARONE SHOULD BE ADMINISTERED ONLY BY PHYSICIANS WHO ARE EXPERIENCED IN THE TREATMENT OF LIFE-THREATENING ARRHYTHMIAS WHO ARE THOROUGHLY FAMILIAR WITH THE RISK AND BENEFITS OF CORDARONE THERAPY, AND WHO HAVE ACCESS TO LABORATORY FACILITIES CAPABLE OF ADEQUATELY MONITORING THE EFFECTIVENESS AND SIDE EFFECTS OF TREATMENT.

In order to insure that an antiarrhythmic effect will be observed without waiting several months, loading doses are required. A uniform, optimal dosage schedule for administration of Cordarone has not been determined. Individual patient titration is suggested according to the following guidelines.

For life-threatening ventricular arrhythmias, such as ventricular fibrillation or hemodynamically unstable ventricular tachycardia: Close monitoring of the patients is indicated during the loading phase, particularly until risk of recurrent ventricular tachycardia or fibrillation has abated. Because of the serious nature of the arrhythmia and the lack of predictable time course of effect, loading should be performed in a hospital setting. Loading doses of 800 to 1,600 mg/day are required for 1 to 3 weeks (ocassionally longer) until initial therapeutic response occurs. (Administration of Cordarone in divided doses with meals is suggested for total daily doses of 1,000 mg or higher, or when gastrointestinal intolerance occurs.) If side effects become excessive, the dose should be reduced. Elimination of recurrence of ventricular fibrillation and tachycardia usually occurs within 1 to 3 weeks, along with reduction in complex and total ventricular ectopic beats.

Upon starting Cordarone therapy, an attempt should be made to gradually discontinue prior antiarrhythmic drugs (see section on "Drug Interactions"). When adequate arrhythmia control is achieved, or if side effects become prominent, Cordarone dose should be reduced to 600 to 800 mg/day for one month and then to the maintenance dose, usually 400 mg/day (see "Clinical Pharmacology"—"Monitoring Effectiveness"). Some patients may require larger maintenance doses, up to 600 mg/day, and some can be controlled on lower doses. Cordarone may be administered as a single daily dose, or in patients with severe gastrointestinal intolerance, as a b.i.d. dose. In each patient, the chronic maintenance dose should be determined according to antiarrhythmic effect as assessed by symptoms, Holter recordings, and/or programmed electrical stimulation and by patient tolerance. Plasma concentrations may be helpful in evaluating nonresponsiveness or unexpectedly severe toxicity (see "Clinical Pharmacology").

The lowest effective dose should be used to prevent the occurrence of side effects. In all instances, the physician must be guided by the severity of the individual patient's arrhythmia and response to therapy. When dosage adjustments are necessary, the patient should be closely monitored for an extended period of time because of the long and variable half-life of Cordarone and the difficulty in predicting the time required to attain a new steady-state level of drug. Dosage suggestions are summarized above:

[See table above].

HOW SUPPLIED

Cordarone® (amiodarone HCI) Tablets, Wyeth®, are available in bottles of 60 tablets and in Redipak® Strip Pack cartons containing 20 strips of 5 tablets each as follows:

200 mg, NDC 0008-4188, round, convex, white to slightly cream-colored tablets, scored on one side and marked "WYETH" and "4188" on the reverse side.

Protect from light

Manufactured for

Wyeth Laboratories, Inc., Philadelphia, PA 19101

by **Sanofi, S.A.**, Paris, France, by arrangement with

Sanofi Pharmaceuticals, Inc.

Shown in Product Identification Section, page 435

CYCLAPEN-W® ℞

[*si'klah-pen-w*]

(cyclacillin)

Tablets and Oral Suspension

HOW SUPPLIED

Cyclapen-W® (cyclacillin) Tablets, Wyeth®, are available in the following strengths:

250 mg, NDC 0008-0614, yellow capsule-shaped, scored tablet embossed with "WYETH" and "614", supplied in bottles of 100 tablets.

500 mg, NDC 0008-0615, yellow capsule-shaped, scored tablet embossed with "WYETH" and "615", supplied in bottles of 100 tablets.

Cyclapen-W (cyclacillin) Oral Suspension, Wyeth®, is available in the following strengths:

125 mg per 5 mL, NDC 0008-0599, white to pinkish-white powder in bottles to make 100 mL, 150 mL, and 200 mL of suspension.

250 mg per 5 mL, NDC 0008-0600, white to pinkish-white powder supplied in bottles to make 100 mL, 150 mL, and 200 mL of suspension.

For prescribing information write to Professional Service, Wyeth Laboratories, Box 8299, Philadelphia, PA 19101, or contact your local Wyeth representative.

Shown in Product Identification Section, page 435

CYCLOSPASMOL® ℞

[*cīclō'spas"mōl*]

(cyclandelate)

Capsules-Tablets

COMPOSITION

Each Cyclospasmol capsule contains 200 mg or 400 mg of cyclandelate. The inactive ingredients present are FD&C Blue 1, gelatin, magnesium stearate, methylcellulose, titanium dioxide, and other ingredients. The 200 mg strength also contains D&C Red 28. The 400 mg strength also contains FD&C Red 40 and FD&C Yellow 6.

Each Cyclospasmol tablet contains 100 mg of cyclandelate. The inactive ingredients present are acacia, calcium carbonate, calcium phosphate, confectioners sugar, D&C Yellow 10, FD&C Yellow 6, gelatin, magnesium stearate, methylparaben, pharmaceutical glaze, polacrilin potassium, povidone, propylparaben, sodium benzoate, starch, stearic acid, sucrose, talc, and titanium dioxide.

DESCRIPTION

Cyclandelate is a white amorphous powder having a faint menthol-like odor. It is slightly soluble in water and highly soluble in ethyl alcohol and organic solvents. Cyclandelate has the following formula: 3,5,5,-trimethylcyclohexyl mandelate.

ACTIONS

CYCLOSPASMOL is an orally acting vasodilator. The activity of this drug, as measured by pharmacological tests against various types of smooth-muscle spasm produced by acetylcholine, histamine, and barium chloride, exceeds that of papaverine, particularly in regard to the neurotropic component produced by the acetylcholine. Cyclandelate is musculotropic, acting directly on vascular smooth muscle, and

Continued on next page

Wyeth—Cont.

has no significant adrenergic stimulating or blocking actions.
The drug is not intended to substitute for other appropriate medical or surgical programs in the treatment of peripheral or cerebral vascular disease.

INDICATIONS

Based on a review of this drug by the National Academy of Sciences—National Research Council and/or other information, FDA has classified the indications as follows:
"Possibly" effective: CYCLOSPASMOL is indicated for adjunctive therapy in intermittent claudication; arteriosclerosis obliterans; thrombophlebitis (to control associated vasospasm and muscular ischemia); nocturnal leg cramps; Raynaud's phenomenon; and for selected cases of ischemic cerebral vascular disease.
Final classification of the less-than-effective indications requires further investigation.

CONTRAINDICATIONS

CYCLOSPASMOL is contraindicated in cases of known hypersensitivity to the drug.

WARNINGS

1. Cyclandelate should be used with extreme caution in patients with severe obliterative coronary-artery or cerebral-vascular disease, since there is a possibility that these diseased areas may be compromised by vasodilatory effects of the drug elsewhere. 2. **Use in Pregnancy:** The safety of cyclandelate for use during pregnancy or lactation has not been established; therefore, it should not be used in pregnant women or in women of childbearing age unless, in the judgment of the physician, its use is deemed absolutely essential to the welfare of the patient. 3. Although no prolongation of bleeding time has been demonstrated in humans in therapeutic dosages, it has been demonstrated in animals at very large doses. Therefore, the hazard of a prolonged bleeding time should be carefully considered when administering cyclandelate to a patient with active bleeding or a bleeding tendency.

PRECAUTIONS

Since CYCLOSPASMOL (cyclandelate) is a vasodilator, it should be used with caution in patients having glaucoma.

ADVERSE REACTIONS

Gastrointestinal distress (pyrosis, pain, and eructation) may occur with CYCLOSPASMOL. These symptoms occur infrequently and are usually mild. Relief can often be obtained by taking the medication with meals or by the concomitant use of antacids.
Mild flush, headache, feeling of weakness, or tachycardia may occur, especially during the first weeks of administration.

DOSAGE AND ADMINISTRATION

It is often advantageous to initiate therapy at higher dosage; e.g.: 1200-1600 mg. per day, given in divided doses before meals and at bedtime. When a clinical response is noted, the dosage can be decreased in 200-mg. decrements until the maintenance dosage is reached. The usual maintenance dosage of CYCLOSPASMOL (cyclandelate) is between 400 and 800 mg. per day given in two to four divided doses.
Although objective signs of therapeutic benefit may be rapid and dramatic, more often, this improvement occurs gradually over weeks of therapy. It is strongly recommended that the patient be educated to the fact that prolonged use may be necessary. Short-term use of CYCLOSPASMOL is rarely beneficial, nor is it likely to be of any permanent value.

HOW SUPPLIED

Cyclospasmol® (cyclandelate) Capsules, Wyeth®, are available in the following dosage strengths in bottles of 100 capsules:
200 mg, NDC 0008-4124, blue capsule marked "WYETH" and "4124".
400 mg, NDC 0008-4148, red and blue capsule marked "WYETH" and "4148".
Cyclospasmol® (cyclandelate) Tablets, Wyeth®, are available in the following dosage strength in bottles of 100 tablets:
100 mg, NDC 0008-4120, orange, coated tablet marked "WYETH" and "4120".
Keep tightly closed.
Protect from light.
Dispense in light-resistant, tight container.
Shown in Product Identification Section, page 435

DEPONIT® ℞

[dĕp'ō-nĭt]
(nitroglycerin transdermal delivery system)
5 mg/24 hours, 10 mg/24 hours

DESCRIPTION

Deponit is a unique nitroglycerin-containing transdermal delivery system. A multilayered self-adhesive film, the system contains nitroglycerin in a matrix composed of lactose, plasticizer, medical adhesive, polyisobutylene, and aluminized plastic for controlled release of the active agent through the skin into the systemic circulation. For the 24 hours during which the system is applied to the intact skin, its technology is intended to deliver an accurate dosage with no premature release of the nitroglycerin or undesired accumulation on the skin. Nitroglycerin (glyceryl trinitrate) is a vasodilator for the relief and prevention of anginal attacks.
Deponit is available in two strengths which release either 5 mg or 10 mg of nitroglycerin during a 24-hour period. The 5 mg/24 hr system has a 16 cm^2 releasing surface and contains 16 mg nitroglycerin. The 10 mg/24 hr system has a 32 cm^2 releasing surface and contains 32 mg nitroglycerin.
The Deponit system is approximately 0.3 mm thick, insoluble in water, and, as illustrated below, consists of two main elements:
1. A flexible, flesh-colored waterproof covering foil.
2. A multilayered adhesive film that constitutes simultaneously the drug reservoir and the release-control system.

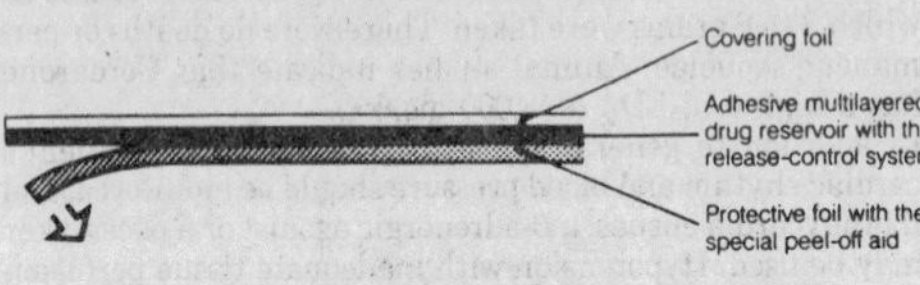

The system is protected by an aluminum foil which has a patented S-shaped opening to facilitate its removal prior to use of the system.

CLINICAL PHARMACOLOGY

When the Deponit system is applied to the skin, nitroglycerin is continuously released for absorption directly into the systemic circulation. Thus, active drug reaches the target organs (heart, extremities) before deactivation by the liver.
Nitroglycerin is a smooth-muscle relaxant with vascular effects manifested predominantly by venous dilatation and pooling. The major beneficial effect of nitroglycerin in angina pectoris is a reduction in myocardial oxygen consumption, secondary to vascular smooth-muscle relaxation with resultant reduction in cardiac preload and afterload. In recent years there has been increasing recognition of a direct vasodilator effect of nitroglycerin on the coronary vessels.
In a bioavailability study using healthy volunteers,[1] transdermal absorption of nitroglycerin from the Deponit system achieved steady-state venous plasma levels and maintained these levels for 24 hours. Detectable plasma levels were attained within 30 minutes after application of the system and were still detectable 30 minutes after removal of the system.
The amount of nitroglycerin released (5 mg/24 hr or 10 mg/24 hr) represents the mean release rate of nitroglycerin from the system as determined from healthy volunteers, and hence, the amount potentially available through the skin. Absorption will vary among individuals. Precise definition of "therapeutic plasma levels" is not known at this time.

INDICATIONS AND USAGE

This drug product has been conditionally approved by the FDA for the prevention and treatment of angina pectoris due to coronary artery disease. The conditional approval reflects a determination that the drug may be marketed while further investigation of its effectiveness is undertaken. A final evaluation of the effectiveness of the product will be announced by the FDA.

CONTRAINDICATIONS

Nitroglycerin is contraindicated in patients known to be intolerant of organic nitrate drugs and in patients with marked anemia.

WARNINGS

In patients with acute myocardial infarction or congestive heart failure, nitroglycerin should be used under careful clinical and/or hemodynamic monitoring.
In terminating treatment of patients with angina, both the dosage and frequency of application must be gradually reduced over a period of 4 to 6 weeks to prevent the sudden withdrawal reactions which are characteristic of vasodilators in the nitroglycerin class.
Transdermal nitroglycerin systems should be removed before attempting defibrillation or cardioversion because of the potential for altered electrical conductivity which may enhance the possibility of arcing, a phenomenon associated with the use of defibrillators.

PRECAUTIONS

Symptoms of hypotension, such as faintness, weakness, or dizziness, particularly orthostatic hypotension, may be due to overdosage. When these symptoms occur, the dosage should be reduced or use of the product discontinued.
Deponit is not intended for use in treatment of acute anginal attacks. For this purpose, occasional use of sublingual nitrates may be necessary.

PREGNANCY

Pregnancy Category C. Animal reproduction studies have not been conducted with nitroglycerin. It is not known whether nitroglycerin can cause fetal harm when administered to a pregnant woman or can affect reproduction capacity. Nitroglycerin should be given to a pregnant woman only if clearly needed.

NURSING MOTHERS

It is not known whether nitroglycerin is excreted in human milk. Because many drugs are excreted in human milk, caution should be exercised when the preparation is administered to a nursing woman.

ADVERSE REACTIONS

Transient headache is the most common side effect, especially when higher doses of the drug are used. These headaches should be treated with mild analgesics while Deponit therapy is continued. When such headaches are unresponsive to treatment, the dosage should be reduced or use of the product discontinued.
Adverse reactions reported less frequently include hypotension, increased heart rate, faintness, flushing, dizziness, nausea, vomiting, and dermatitis. Except for dermatitis these symptoms are attributable to the known pharmacologic effects of nitroglycerin, but may be symptoms of overdosage. When they persist, the Deponit dose should be reduced or use of the product discontinued.

DOSAGE AND ADMINISTRATION

Deponit can be applied as a single system or as multiples, depending upon the clinical requirements. Dosage should be titrated to achieve the optimal therapeutic effect by monitoring clinical response, side effects, heart rate, and the effect of therapy upon blood pressure.
Deponit should be removed from the single-unit package just prior to use. The protective aluminum precut S-shaped foil is removed according to the "Patient Instructions," and the system is applied with a firm pressure on a convenient skin site, preferably on the chest, innerside of the upper arm, or shoulders. Deponit should not be applied to the distal parts of extremities.
Each system is designed to remain in place for 24 hours; however, the treatment site should be changed daily to minimize skin irritation and should be intact, clean, and dry. If necessary, hair may be removed by clipping.
Therapy should be initiated with application of a single Deponit system, delivering 5 mg every 24 hours. Response in terms of satisfactory control of anginal symptoms without adverse effects should be evaluated to determine the optimal dose. Some patients may require adjustment of dosage to provide a better clinical response. This can be achieved by removing the system delivering 5 mg/24 hours, and applying a larger system delivering 10 mg/24 hours or a multiple of either system, depending on the dose required to achieve the desired effect.
After 24 hours, the system should be removed and discarded. Because no adhesive residue remains on the skin, there is no need to use a solvent.

STORAGE CONDITIONS

Store at room temperature not above 25°C (77°F). Do not refrigerate.
Patient Instructions for Application
Deponit® (nitroglycerin transdermal delivery system), Wyeth®, is packaged in cartons containing unit doses of 30 flesh-colored systems on aluminum backings. See table below.
[See table on next page].
Caution: Federal law prohibits dispensing without prescription.

REFERENCE

1. Data on file: Wyeth Laboratories Inc., Philadelphia, PA 19101.
U S Pat No. 4,524,095 and Patent Pending
Manufactured for
Wyeth Laboratories Inc., Philadelphia, PA 19101
by **Lohmann**, Neuwied, West Germany
under license from **Schwarz GmbH**, West Germany

DIPHTHERIA AND TETANUS TOXOIDS ADSORBED ℞
[dif-the're-ah and tet'ah-nus tok'soids]
aluminum phosphate adsorbed
ULTRAFINED®
PEDIATRIC

DESCRIPTION
Antigens adsorbed on aluminum phosphate. Preservative is 0.01% thimerosal (mercury derivative).

HOW SUPPLIED
Vials of 5 ml.; and 0.5-ml. TUBEX® Sterile Cartridge-Needle Units, packages of 10.
For prescribing information write to Professional Service, Wyeth Laboratories, Box 8299, Philadelphia, PA 19101, or contact your local Wyeth representative.

EQUAGESIC® ©IV ℞
[ek"wa-je'zik]
(meprobamate with aspirin)

DESCRIPTION
Each tablet of Equagesic contains 200 mg meprobamate and 325 mg aspirin. The inactive ingredients present are cellulose, D&C Yellow 10, FD&C Red 3, FD&C Yellow 6, hydrogenated vegetable oil, magnesium stearate, polacrilin potassium, and starch.

ACTIONS
Meprobamate is a carbamate derivative which has been shown (in animal and/or human studies) to have effects at multiple sites in the central nervous system, including the thalamus and limbic system.
Aspirin, acetylsalicylic acid, is a nonnarcotic analgesic with antipyretic and antiinflammatory properties.

INDICATIONS
As an adjunct in the short-term treatment of pain accompanied by tension and/or anxiety in patients with musculoskeletal disease. Clinical trials have demonstrated that in these situations relief of pain is somewhat greater than with aspirin alone.
The effectiveness of Equagesic in long-term use, that is, more than 4 months, has not been assessed by systematic clinical studies. The physician should periodically reassess the usefulness of the drug for the individual patient.

CONTRAINDICATIONS
ASPIRIN:
Allergic or idiosyncratic reactions to aspirin or related compounds.
MEPROBAMATE:
Acute intermittent porphyria and allergic or idiosyncratic reactions to meprobamate or related compounds, such as carisoprodol, mebutamate, or carbromal.

WARNINGS
ASPIRIN:
Salicylates should be used with extreme caution in patients with peptic ulcer, asthma, coagulation abnormalities, hypoprothrombinemia, vitamin K deficiency, or in those on anticoagulant therapy.
In rare instances, the use of aspirin in persons allergic to salicylates may result in life-threatening allergic episodes.
MEPROBAMATE:
DRUG DEPENDENCE: Physical dependence, psychological dependence, and abuse have occurred. Chronic intoxication from prolonged ingestion of, usually, greater-than-recommended doses is manifested by ataxia, slurred speech, and vertigo. Therefore, careful supervision of dose and amounts prescribed is advised, as well as avoidance of prolonged administration, especially for alcoholics and other patients with a known propensity for taking excessive quantities of drugs.
Sudden withdrawal of the drug after prolonged and excessive use may precipitate recurrence of preexisting symptoms such as anxiety, anorexia, or insomnia, or withdrawal reactions such as vomiting, ataxia, tremors, muscle twitching, confusional states, hallucinosis, and, rarely, convulsive seizures. Such seizures are more likely to occur in persons with central-nervous-system damage or preexistent or latent convulsive disorders. Onset of withdrawal symptoms occurs usually within 12 to 48 hours after discontinuation of meprobamate; symptoms usually cease within the next 12- to 48-hour period.
When excessive dosage has continued for weeks or months, dosage should be reduced gradually over a period of 1 to 2 weeks rather than abruptly stopped. Alternatively, a short-acting barbiturate may be substituted, then gradually withdrawn.
POTENTIALLY HAZARDOUS TASKS: Patients should be warned that meprobamate may impair the mental or physical abilities required for performance of potentially hazardous tasks, such as driving or operating machinery.

Nitroglycerin released *in vivo*	Total drug content/system	System size	Carton size
5 mg/24 hrs	16 mg	16 cm^2	30 Systems (**NDC** 0008-4195-01)
10 mg/24 hrs	32 mg	32 cm^2	30 Systems (**NDC** 0008-4196-01)

ADDITIVE EFFECTS: Since CNS-suppressant effects of meprobamate and alcohol or meprobamate and other psychotropic drugs may be additive, appropriate caution should be exercised with patients who take more than one of these agents simultaneously.

USAGE IN PREGNANCY AND LACTATION
An increased risk of congenital malformations associated with the use of minor tranquilizers (meprobamate, chlordiazepoxide, and diazepam) during the first trimester of pregnancy has been suggested in several studies. Because use of these drugs is rarely a matter of urgency, their use during this period should almost always be avoided. The possibility that a woman of childbearing potential may be pregnant at the time of institution of therapy should be considered. Patients should be advised that if they become pregnant during therapy or intend to become pregnant they should communicate with their physicians about the desirability of discontinuing the drug.
Meprobamate passes the placental barrier. It is present both in umbilical-cord blood at or near maternal plasma levels and in breast milk of lactating mothers at concentrations two to four times that of maternal plasma. When use of meprobamate is contemplated in breast-feeding patients, the drug's higher concentrations in breast milk as compared to maternal plasma levels should be considered.
USAGE IN CHILDREN: Preparations containing aspirin should be kept out of the reach of children. Equagesic (meprobamate with aspirin) is not recommended for patients 12 years of age and under.

PRECAUTIONS
ASPIRIN:
Salicylates antagonize the uricosuric activity of probenecid and sulfinpyrazone. Salicylates are reported to enhance the hypoglycemic effect of the sulfonylurea antidiabetic drugs.
MEPROBAMATE:
The lowest effective dose should be administered, particularly to elderly and/or debilitated patients, in order to preclude oversedation.
Meprobamate is metabolized in the liver and excreted by the kidney; to avoid its excess accumulation, caution should be exercised in the administration to patients with compromised liver or kidney function.
Meprobamate occasionally may precipitate seizures in epileptic patients.
The drug should be prescribed cautiously and in small quantities to patients with suicidal tendencies.

ADVERSE REACTIONS
ASPIRIN:
Aspirin may cause epigastric discomfort, nausea, and vomiting. Hypersensitivity reactions, including urticaria, angioneurotic edema, purpura, asthma, and anaphylaxis, may rarely occur.
Patients receiving large doses of salicylates may develop tinnitus.
MEPROBAMATE:
CENTRAL NERVOUS SYSTEM: Drowsiness, ataxia, dizziness, slurred speech, headache, vertigo, weakness, paresthesias, impairment of visual accommodation, euphoria, overstimulation, paradoxical excitement, fast EEG activity.
GASTROINTESTINAL: Nausea, vomiting, diarrhea.
CARDIOVASCULAR: Palpitation, tachycardia, various forms of arrhythmia, transient ECG changes, syncope, hypotensive crisis.
ALLERGIC OR IDIOSYNCRATIC: Milder reactions are characterized by an itchy, urticarial, or erythematous maculopapular rash which may be generalized or confined to the groin.
Other reactions have included leukopenia, acute nonthrombocytopenic purpura, petechiae, ecchymoses, eosinophilia, peripheral edema, adenopathy, fever, fixed drug eruption with cross-reaction to carisoprodol, and cross-sensitivity between meprobamate/mebutamate and meprobamate/carbromal.
More severe hypersensitivity reactions, rarely reported, include hyperpyrexia, chills, angioneurotic edema, bronchospasm, oliguria, and anuria. Also, anaphylaxis, exfoliative dermatitis, stomatitis, and proctitis, Stevens-Johnson syndrome and bullous dermatitis have occurred.
HEMATOLOGIC (SEE ALSO "ALLERGIC OR IDIOSYNCRATIC"): Agranulocytosis, aplastic anemia have been reported, although no causal relationship has been established, and thrombocytopenic purpura.
OTHER: Exacerbation of porphyric symptoms.

DOSAGE AND ADMINISTRATION
The usual dosage of Equagesic (meprobamate with aspirin) is one or two tablets, each tablet containing meprobamate, 200 mg, and aspirin, 325 mg, orally 3 to 4 times daily as needed for the relief of pain when tension or anxiety is present.
Equagesic is not recommended for patients 12 years of age and under.

OVERDOSAGE
Treatment of overdose with Equagesic is essentially symptomatic and supportive. Any drug remaining in the stomach should be removed. Induction of vomiting or gastric lavage may be indicated. Activated charcoal may reduce absorption of both aspirin and meprobamate.
Overdosage with aspirin produces the usual symptoms and signs of salicylate intoxication. Observation and treatment should include management of hyperthermia, specific parenteral electrolyte therapy for ketoacidosis and dehydration, watching for evidence of hemorrhagic manifestations due to hypoprothrombinemia which, if it occurs, usually requires whole-blood transfusions.
Suicidal attempts with meprobamate have resulted in drowsiness, lethargy, stupor, ataxia, coma, shock, vasomotor and respiratory collapse. Some suicidal attempts have been fatal.
The following data have been reported in the literature and from other sources. These data are not expected to correlate with each case (considering factors such as individual susceptibility and length of time from ingestion to treatment), but represent the usual ranges reported.
Acute simple overdose (meprobamate alone): Death has been reported with ingestion of as little as 12 grams meprobamate and survival with as much as 40 grams.
BLOOD LEVELS:
0.5 to 2.0 mg percent represents the usual blood-level range of meprobamate after therapeutic doses. The level may occasionally be as high as 3.0 mg percent.
3 to 10 mg percent usually corresponds to findings of mild-to-moderate symptoms of overdosage, such as stupor or light coma.
10 to 20 mg percent usually corresponds to deeper coma, requiring more intensive treatment. Some fatalities occur.
At levels greater than 20 mg percent, more fatalities than survivals can be expected.
Acute combined overdose (meprobamate with other psychotropic drugs or alcohol): Since effects can be additive, a history of ingestion of a low dose of meprobamate plus any of these compounds (or of a relatively low blood or tissue level) cannot be used as a prognostic indicator.
In cases where excessive doses have been taken, sleep ensues rapidly and blood pressure, pulse, and respiratory rates are reduced to basal levels. Any drug remaining in the stomach should be removed and symptomatic treatment given. Should respiration or blood pressure become compromised, respiratory assistance, central-nervous-system stimulants, and pressor agents should be administered cautiously as indicated. Diuresis, osmotic (mannitol) diuresis, peritoneal dialysis, and hemodialysis have been used successfully in removing both aspirin and meprobamate. Alkalinization of the urine increases the excretion of salicylates. Careful monitoring of urinary output is necessary, and caution should be taken to avoid overhydration. Relapse and death, after initial recovery, have been attributed to incomplete gastric emptying and delayed absorption.

HOW SUPPLIED
Equagesic® (meprobamate with aspirin) Tablets, Wyeth®, 200 mg meprobamate and 325 mg aspirin, are available as follows:
NDC 0008-0091, pink and yellow, double-layer, round, scored tablet marked "WYETH" and "91", in bottles of 100 tablets, in Redipak® Strip Pack cartons of 25 tablets, and in Redipak cartons of 100 individually wrapped tablets.
Keep tightly closed.
Protect from light.
Dispense in light-resistant, tight container.
The appearance of EQUAGESIC tablets is a registered trademark of Wyeth Laboratories.
Shown in Product Identification Section, page 435

Continued on next page

Wyeth—Cont.

EQUANIL® Ⓒ ℞
[ek 'wah-nil]
(meprobamate)
Tablets

HOW SUPPLIED

Equanil® (meprobamate) Tablets, Wyeth®, are available in the following dosage strengths:
200 mg, NDC 0008-0002, white, five-sided tablet marked "WYETH" and "2", in bottles of 100 tablets and in Redipak® Strip Pack cartons of 25 tablets.
400 mg, NDC 0008-0001, white, round, scored tablet marked "WYETH" and "1", in bottles of 100 and 500 tablets and in Redipak Strip Pack cartons of 25 tablets.
Equanil® (meprobamate) Wyseals® (film-coated tablets), 400 mg, are available in bottles of 50 tablets as follows:
NDC 0008-0033, yellow, round, film-coated tablet marked "WYETH" and "33".
For prescribing information write to Professional Service, Wyeth Laboratories, Box 8299, Philadelphia, PA 19101, or contact your local Wyeth representative.
Shown in Product Identification Section, page 435

HEPARIN ℞
[hep'ah-rin]
Lock Flush Solution, USP
anticoagulant for clearing intermittent infusion sets

DESCRIPTION

Wyeth's TUBEX® Heparin Lock Flush Solution, USP, is a sterile solution. Each mL contains either 10 or 100 USP units heparin sodium derived from porcine intestinal mucosa (standardized for use as an anticoagulant) in normal saline solution, and not more than 10 mg benzyl alcohol as a preservative.
The potency is determined by biological assay, using a USP reference standard based upon units of heparin activity per milligram.
Heparin is a heterogenous group of straight-chain anionic mucopolysaccharides, called glycosaminoglycans, having anticoagulant properties. Although others may be present, the main sugars occurring in heparin are: (1) α-L-iduronic acid 2-sulfate, (2) 2-deoxy-2-sulfamino-α-D-glucose 6-sulfate, (3) β-D-glucuronic acid, (4) 2-acetamido-2-deoxy-α-D-glucose, and (5) α-L-iduronic acid. These sugars are present in decreasing amounts, usually in the order (2) > (1) > (4) > (3) > (5), and are joined by glycosidic linkages, forming polymers of varying sizes. Heparin is strongly acidic because of its content of covalently linked sulfate and carboxylic acid groups. In heparin sodium, the acidic protons of the sulfate units are partially replaced by sodium ions.
STRUCTURE OF HEPARIN SODIUM (representative subunits):

(1) (2) (3) (4) (5)

CLINICAL PHARMACOLOGY

Heparin inhibits reactions that lead to the clotting of blood and the formation of fibrin clots both *in vitro* and *in vivo*. Heparin acts at multiple sites in the normal coagulation system. Small amounts of heparin in combination with antithrombin III (heparin cofactor) can inhibit thrombosis by inactivating activated Factor X and inhibiting the conversion of prothrombin to thrombin. Once active thrombosis has developed, larger amounts of heparin can inhibit further coagulation by inactivating thrombin and preventing the conversion of fibrinogen to fibrin. Heparin also prevents the formation of a stable fibrin clot by inhibiting the activation of the fibrin stabilizing factor.
Bleeding time is usually unaffected by heparin. Clotting time is prolonged by full therapeutic doses of heparin; in most cases, it is not measurably affected by low doses of heparin.
Peak plasma levels of heparin are achieved 2 to 4 hours following subcutaneous administration, although there are considerable individual variations. Loglinear plots of heparin plasma concentrations with time, for a wide range of dose levels, are linear which suggests the absence of zero order processes. Liver and the reticulo-endothelial system are the sites of biotransformation. The biphasic elimination curve, a rapidly declining alpha phase ($t_{1/2} = 10$ min.), and after the age of 40 a slower beta phase, indicates uptake in organs. The absence of a relationship between anticoagulant half-life and concentration half-life may reflect factors such as protein binding of heparin.
Heparin does not have fibrinolytic activity; therefore, it will not lyse existing clots.

INDICATIONS AND USAGE

Heparin Lock Flush Solution, USP, is intended to maintain patency of an indwelling venipuncture device designed for intermittent injection or infusion therapy, or blood sampling. Heparin Lock Flush Solution, USP, may be used following initial placement of the device in the vein, after each injection of a medication, or after withdrawal of blood for laboratory tests.
Heparin Lock Flush Solution, USP, is not to be used for anticoagulant therapy.
Heparin may also be employed as an anticoagulant in blood transfusions, extracorporeal circulation, dialysis procedures, and in blood samples for laboratory purposes.

CONTRAINDICATIONS

Heparin sodium should not be used in patients with the following conditons:
Severe thrombocytopenia;
An uncontrollable active bleeding state (see "Warnings"), except when this is due to disseminated intravascular coagulation.

WARNINGS

Heparin is not intended for intramuscular use.
HYPERSENSITIVITY
Patients with documented hypersensitivity to heparin should be given the drug only in clearly life-threatening situations.
HEMORRHAGE
Hemorrhage can occur at virtually any site in patients receiving heparin. An unexplained fall in hematocrit, fall in blood pressure, or any other unexplained symptom should lead to serious consideration of a hemorrhagic event.
Heparin sodium should be used with extreme caution in disease states in which there is increased danger of hemorrhage. Some of the conditions in which increased danger of hemorrhage exists are:
Cardiovascular—Subacute bacterial endocarditis. Severe hypertension.
Surgical—During and immediately following (a) spinal tap or spinal anesthesia or (b) major surgery, especially involving the brain, spinal cord, or eye.
Hematologic—Conditions associated with increased bleeding tendencies, such as hemophilia, thrombocytopenia, and some vascular purpuras.
Gastrointestinal—Ulcerative lesions and continuous tube drainage of the stomach or small intestine.
Other—Menstruation, liver disease with impaired hemostasis.
THROMBOCYTOPENIA
Thrombocytopenia has been reported to occur in patients receiving heparin with a reported incidence of 0 to 30%. Mild thrombocytopenia (count greater than 100,000/mm^3) may remain stable or reverse even if heparin is continued. However, thrombocytopenia of any degree should be monitored closely. If the count falls below 100,000/mm^3 or if recurrent thrombosis develops (see "White-clot Syndrome," "Precautions"), the heparin product should be discontinued. If continued heparin therapy is essential, administration of heparin from a different organ source can be reinstituted with caution.
MISCELLANEOUS
This product contains benzyl alcohol as preservative. Benzyl alcohol has been reported to be associated with a fatal "Gasping Syndrome" in premature infants.

PRECAUTIONS

GENERAL
White-clot Syndrome
Rare patients on heparin may develop new thrombus formation in association with thrombocytopenia, resulting from irreversible aggregation of platelets induced by heparin, the so-called "white-clot syndrome." The process may lead to severe thromboembolic complications like skin necrosis, gangrene of the extremities, myocardial infarction, pulmonary embolism, and stroke. Therefore, heparin administration should be promptly discontinued if a patient develops new thrombosis in association with thrombocytopenia.
Heparin Resistance
Increased resistance to heparin is frequently encountered in fever, thrombosis, thrombophlebitis, infections with thrombosing tendencies, myocardial infarction, cancer, and in postsurgical patients.
Increased Risk in Older Women
A higher incidence of bleeding has been reported in women over 60 years of age.
LABORATORY TESTS
Periodic platelet counts, hematocrits, and tests for occult blood in stool are recommended during the entire course of heparin therapy, regardless of the route of administration (see "Dosage and Administration").
DRUG INTERACTIONS
Platelet Inhibitors
Drugs such as acetylsalicylic acid, dextran, phenylbutazone, ibuprofen, indomethacin, dipyridamole, hydroxychloroquine, and others that interfere with platelet-aggregation reactions (the main hemostatic defense of heparinized patients) may induce bleeding and should be used with caution in patients receiving heparin sodium.
Other Interactions
Digitalis, tetracyclines, nicotine, or antihistamines may partially counteract the anticoagulant action of heparin sodium.
CARCINOGENESIS, MUTAGENESIS, IMPAIRMENT OF FERTILITY
No long-term studies in animals have been performed to evaluate carcinogenic potential of heparin. Also, no reproduction studies in animals have been performed concerning mutagenesis or impairment of fertility.
PREGNANCY
Teratogenic Effects—Pregnancy Category C
Animal reproduction studies have not been conducted with heparin sodium. It is also not known whether heparin sodium can cause fetal harm when administered to a pregnant woman or can affect reproduction capacity. Heparin sodium should be given to a pregnant woman only if clearly needed.
Nonteratogenic Effects
Heparin does not cross the placental barrier.
NURSING MOTHERS
Heparin is not excreted in human milk.

ADVERSE REACTIONS

HEMORRHAGE
Hemorrhage is the chief complication that may result from heparin therapy (see "Warnings"). An overly prolonged clotting time or minor bleeding during therapy can usually be controlled by withdrawing the drug (see "Overdosage"). It should be appreciated that gastrointestinal- or urinary-tract bleeding during anticoagulant therapy may indicate the presence of an underlying occult lesion. Bleeding can occur at any site but certain specific hemorrhagic complications may be difficult to detect:

a. Adrenal hemorrhage, with resultant acute adrenal insufficiency, has occurred during anticoagulant therapy. Therefore, such treatment should be discontinued in patients who develop signs and symptoms of acute adrenal hemorrhage and insufficiency. Initiation of corrective therapy should not depend on laboratory confirmation of the diagnosis, since any delay in an acute situation may result in the patient's death.
b. Ovarian (corpus luteum) hemorrhage developed in a number of women of reproductive age receiving short- or long-term anticoagulant therapy. This complication, if unrecognized, may be fatal.
c. Retroperitoneal hemorrhage.

LOCAL IRRITATION
Local irritation, erythema, mild pain, hematoma, or ulceration may follow deep, subcutaneous (intrafat) injection of heparin sodium. These complications are much more common after intramuscular use, and such use is not recommended.
HYPERSENSITIVITY
Generalized hypersensitivity reactions have been reported, with chills, fever, and urticaria as the most usual manifestations, and asthma, rhinitis, lacrimation, headache, nausea and vomiting, and anaphylactoid reactions, including shock, occurring more rarely. Itching and burning, especially on the plantar side of the feet, may occur.
Thrombocytopenia has been reported to occur in patients receiving heparin with a reported incidence of 0 to 30%. While often mild and of no obvious clinical significance, such thrombocytopenia can be accompanied by severe thromboembolic complications, such as skin necrosis, gangrene of the extremities, myocardial infarction, pulmonary embolism, and stroke. (See "Warnings," "Precautions.")
Certain episodes of painful, ischemic and cyanosed limbs have in the past been attributed to allergic vasospastic reactions. Whether these are, in fact, identical to the thrombocytopenia-associated complications remains to be determined.
MISCELLANEOUS
Osteoporosis following long-term administration of high doses of heparin, cutaneous necrosis after systemic administration, suppression of aldosterone synthesis, delayed transient alopecia, priapism, and rebound hyperlipemia on discontinuation of heparin sodium have also been reported.
Significant elevations of aminotransferase (SGOT [S-AST] and SGPT [S-ALT]) levels have occurred in a high percentage of patients (and healthy subjects) who have received heparin.

OVERDOSAGE

SYMPTOMS
Bleeding is the chief sign of heparin overdosage. Nosebleeds, blood in urine, or tarry stools may be noted as the first sign of

bleeding. Easy bruising or petechial formations may precede frank bleeding.

TREATMENT—Neutralization of Heparin Effect

When clinical circumstances (bleeding) require reversal of heparinization, protamine sulfate (1% solution) by slow infusion will neutralize heparin sodium. No more than 50 mg should be administered, very slowly, in any 10-minute period. Each mg of protamine sulfate neutralizes approximately 100 USP heparin units. The amount of protamine required decreases over time as heparin is metabolized. Although the metabolism of heparin is complex, it may, for the purpose of choosing a protamine dose, be assumed to have a half-life of about ½ hour after intravenous injection.

Administration of protamine sulfate can cause severe hypotensive and anaphylactoid reactions. Because fatal reactions, often resembling anaphylaxis, have been reported, the drug should be given only when resuscitation techniques and treatment of anaphylactoid shock are readily available.

For additional information consult the labeling of Protamine Sulfate Injection, USP, products.

DOSAGE AND ADMINISTRATION

Parenteral drug products should be inspected visually for particulate matter and discoloration prior to administration, whenever solution and container permit.

Slight discoloration does not alter potency.

CLEARING INTERMITTENT INFUSION (HEPARIN LOCK) SETS

To prevent clot formation in a heparin lock set following its proper insertion, Heparin Lock Flush Solution, USP, is injected via the injection hub in a quantity sufficient to fill the entire set to the needle tip. This solution should be replaced each time the heparin lock is used. Aspirate before administering any solution via the lock in order to confirm patency and location of needle or catheter tip. If the drug to be administered is incompatible with heparin, the entire heparin lock set should be flushed with normal saline before and after the medication is administered; following the second flush, Heparin Lock Flush Solution, USP, may be reinstilled into the set. The set manufacturer's instructions should be consulted for specifics concerning the heparin lock set in use at a given time.

Usually this dilute heparin solution will maintain anticoagulation within the device for up to 4 hours.

NOTE: Since repeated injections of small doses of heparin can alter tests for activated partial thromboplastin time (APTT), a baseline value for APTT should be obtained prior to insertion of a heparin lock set.

When heparin is added to an infusion solution for continuous intravenous administration, the container should be inverted at least six times to insure adequate mixing and prevent pooling of the heparin in the solution.

WITHDRAWAL OF BLOOD SAMPLES

Heparin Lock Flush Solution, USP, may also be used after each withdrawal of blood for laboratory tests. When heparin (or sodium chloride) would interfere with or alter the results of blood tests, the heparin solution should be cleared from the device by aspirating and discarding it before withdrawing the blood sample.

HOW SUPPLIED

Heparin Lock Flush Solution, USP, anticoagulant for clearing intermittent infusion sets, is supplied in TUBEX Sterile Cartridge-Needle Units which include 25 gauge × ⅝ inch needles.

Each 1 mL size TUBEX contains one of the following concentrations of heparin sodium, in packages of 50 TUBEX:

10 USP units per mL, NDC 0008-0523-01.

100 USP Units per mL, NDC 0008-0487-01.

Each 2.5 ml size TUBEX contains one of the following concentrations of heparin sodium, in packages of 50 TUBEX:

25 USP Units per TUBEX or 10 USP Units per mL, NDC 0008-0523-02.

250 USP Units per TUBEX or 100 USP Units per mL, NDC 0008-0487-03.

Do not Freeze

HEPARIN FLUSH KITS

All TUBEX® Sterile Cartridge-Needle Units in the following packages include 25 gauge × ⅝ inch needles.

10 USP UNITS HEPARIN SODIUM PER ML

Each Unit of Use Kit contains:

NDC 0008-2528-01; one TUBEX (1 mL) Heparin Lock Flush Solution, USP; two TUBEX (2.5 mL each) Bacteriostatic Sodium Chloride Injection, USP; in packages of 50 Kits.

NDC 0008-2528-02; one TUBEX (2.5 mL) Heparin Lock Flush Solution, USP (25 USP Units heparin sodium per TUBEX); two TUBEX (2.5 mL each) Bacteriostatic Sodium Chloride Injection, USP; in packages of 30 CVC (Central Venous Catheter) Kits.

NDC 0008-2528-03; one TUBEX (1 mL) Heparin Lock Flush Solution, USP; two TUBEX (1 mL each) Bacteriostatic Sodium Chloride Injection, USP; in packages of 50 Kits.

100 USP UNITS HEPARIN SODIUM PER ML

Each Unit of Use Kit contains:

NDC 0008-2529-01; one TUBEX (1 mL) Heparin Lock Flush Solution, USP; two TUBEX (2.5 mL each) Bacteriostatic Sodium Chloride Injection, USP; in packages of 50 Kits.

NDC 0008-2529-02; one TUBEX (2.5 mL) Heparin Lock Flush Solution, USP (250 USP Units heparin sodium per TUBEX); two TUBEX (2.5 mL each) Bacteriostatic Sodium Chloride Injection, USP; in packages of 30 CVC (Central Venous Catheter) Kits.

NDC 0008-2529-03; one TUBEX 81 mL) Heparin Lock Flush Solution, USP; two TUBEX (1 mL each) Bacteriostatic Sodium Chloride Injection, USP; in packages of 50 Kits.

Do not freeze

HEPARIN ℞

[hep'ah-rin]

Sodium Injection, USP

DESCRIPTION

Wyeth's TUBEX® Heparin Sodium Injection, USP, is a sterile solution. Each ml contains 1,000, 2,500, 5,000, 7,500, 10,000, 15,000, or 20,000 USP units heparin sodium, derived from porcine intestinal mucosa (standardized for use as an anticoagulant), in water for injection, and not more than 10 mg benzyl alcohol as a preservative.

The potency is determined by biological assay, using a USP reference standard based upon units of heparin activity per milligram.

Heparin is a heterogenous group of straight-chain anionic mucopolysaccharides, called glycosaminoglycans, having anticoagulant properties. Although others may be present, the main sugars occurring in heparin are: (1) α-L iduronic acid 2-sulfate, (2) 2-deoxy-2-sulfamino-α-D-glucose 6-sulfate, (3) β-D-glucuronic acid, (4) 2-acetamido-2-deoxy-α-D-glucose, and (5) α-L-iduronic acid. These sugars are present in decreasing amounts, usually in the order (2) > (1) > (4) > (3) > (5), and are joined by glycosidic linkages, forming polymers of varying sizes. Heparin is strongly acidic because of its content of covalently linked sulfate and carboxylic acid groups. In heparin sodium, the acidic protons of the sulfate units are partially replaced by sodium ions.

STRUCTURE OF HEPARIN SODIUM (representative subunits):

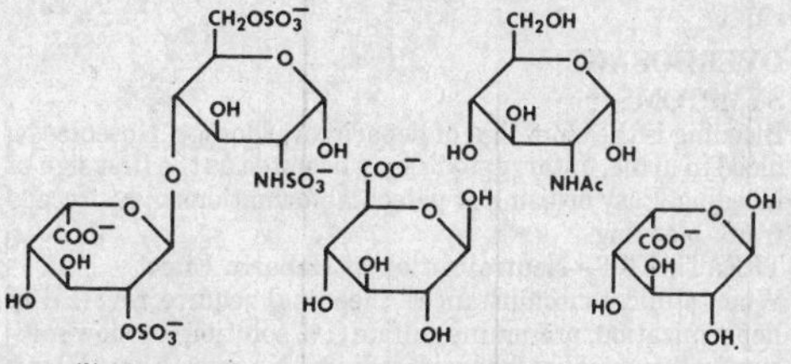

$CH_2OSO_3^-$ CH_2OH OH OH $NHSO_3^-$ COO^- HO OH NHAc COO^- OH HO OSO_3^- OH HO OH

(1) (2) (3) (4) (5)

CLINICAL PHARMACOLOGY:

Heparin inhibits reactions which lead to the clotting of blood and the formation of fibrin clots both *in vitro* and *in vivo.* Heparin acts at multiple sites in the normal coagulation system. Small amounts of heparin in combination with antithrombin III (heparin cofactor) can prevent the development of a hypercoagulable state by inactivating activated Factor X, preventing the conversion of prothrombin to thrombin. Once a hypercoagulable state exists, larger amounts of heparin in combination with antithrombin III can inhibit the coagulation process by inactivating thrombin and earlier clotting intermediates, thus preventing the conversion of fibrinogen to fibrin. Heparin also prevents the formation of a stable fibrin clot by inhibiting the activation of the fibrin stabilizing factor.

Bleeding time is usually unaffected by heparin. Clotting time is prolonged by full therapeutic doses of heparin; in most cases it is not measurably affected by low doses of heparin.

Peak plasma levels of heparin are achieved 2 to 4 hours following subcutaneous administration, although there are considerable individual variations. Loglinear plots of heparin plasma concentrations with time, for a wide range of dose levels, are linear which suggests the absence of zero order processes. Liver and the reticulo-endothelial system are the sites of biotransformation. The bophasic elimination curve, a rapidly declining alpha phase ($t_{1/2}$ = 10 min.), and after the age of 40 a slower beta phase, indicates uptake in organs. The absence of a relationship between anticoagulant half-life and concentration half-life may reflect factors such as protein binding of heparin.

Heparin does not have fibrinolytic activity; therefore, it will not lyse existing clots.

INDICATIONS AND USAGE

Heparin sodium injection is indicated for anticoagulant therapy in prophylaxis and treatment of venous thrombosis and its extension; in low-dose regimen for prevention of postoperative deep venous thrombosis and pulmonary embolism in patients undergoing major abdominothoracic surgery who are at risk of developing thromboembolic disease (see "Dosage and Administration"); for prophylaxis and treatment of pulmonary embolism; in atrial fibrillation with embolization; for diagnosis and treatment of acute and chronic consumptive coagulopathies (disseminated intravascular coagulation); for prevention of clotting in arterial and cardiac surgery; and for prophylaxis and treatment of peripheral arterial embolism.

Heparin may also be employed as an anticoagulant in blood transfusions, extracorporeal circulation, dialysis procedures, and in blood samples for laboratory purposes.

CONTRAINDICATIONS

Heparin sodium should not be used in patients:

with severe thrombocytopenia;

in whom suitable blood-coagulation tests—e.g., the whole-blood clotting time, partial thromboplastin time, etc.—cannot be performed at appropriate intervals (this contraindication refers to full-dose heparin; there is usually no need to monitor coagulation parameters in patients receiving low-dose heparin);

with an uncontrollable active bleeding state (see "Warnings"), except when this is due to disseminated intravascular coagulation.

WARNINGS

Heparin is not intended for intramuscular use.

HYPERSENSITIVITY

Patients with documented hypersensitivity to heparin should be given the drug only in clearly life-threatening situations.

HEMORRHAGE

Hemorrhage can occur at virtually any site in patients receiving heparin. An unexplained fall in hematocrit, fall in blood pressure, or any other unexplained symptom should lead to serious consideration of a hemorrhagic event.

Heparin sodium should be used with extreme caution in disease states in which there is increased danger of hemorrhage. Some of the conditions in which increased danger of hemorrhage exists are:

Cardiovascular—Subacute bacterial endocarditis. Severe hypertension.

Surgical—During and immediately following (a) spinal tap or spinal anesthesia or (b) major surgery, especially involving the brain, spinal cord, or eye.

Hematologic—Conditions associated with increased bleeding tendencies, such as hemophilia, thrombocytopenia, and some vascular purpuras.

Gastrointestinal—Ulcerative lesions and continuous tube drainage of the stomach or small intestine.

Other—Menstruation, liver disease with impaired hemostasis.

COAGULATION TESTING

When heparin sodium is administered in therapeutic amounts, its dosage should be regulated by frequent blood coagulation tests. If the coagulation test is unduly prolonged or if hemorrhage occurs, heparin sodium should be discontinued promptly (see "Overdosage").

THROMBOCYTOPENIA

Thrombocytopenia has been reported to occur in patients receiving heparin with a reported incidence of 0 to 30%. Mild thrombocytopenia (count greater than 100,000/mm^3) may remain stable or reverse even if heparin is continued. However, thrombocytopenia of any degree should be monitored closely. If the count falls below 100,000/mm^3 or if recurrent thrombosis develops (see "White-clot Syndrome," "Precautions"), the heparin product should be discontinued. If continued heparin therapy is essential, admistration of heparin from a different organ source can be reinstituted with caution.

MISCELLANEOUS

This product contains benzyl alcohol as preservative. Benzyl alcohol has been reported to be associated with a fatal "Gasping Syndrome" in premature infants.

PRECAUTIONS

GENERAL

White-clot Syndrome

Rare patients on heparin may develop new thrombus formation in association with thrombocytopenia, resulting from irreversible aggregation of platelets induced by heparin, the so-called "white-clot syndrome." The process may lead to severe thromboembolic complications like skin necrosis, gangrene of the extremities, myocardial infarction, pulmonary embolism, and stroke. Therefore, heparin administration should be promptly discontinued if a patient develops new thrombosis in association with thrombocytopenia.

Heparin Resistance

Increased resistance to heparin is frequently encountered in fever, thrombosis, thrombophlebitis, infactions with thrombosing tendencies, myocardial infarction, cancer, and in postsurgical patients.

Continued on next page

Wyeth—Cont.

Increased Risk in Older Women
A higher incidence of bleeding has been reported in women over 60 years of age.
LABORATORY TESTS
Periodic platelet counts, hematocrits, and tests for occult blood in stool are recommended during the entire course of heparin therapy, regardless of the route of administration (see "Dosage and Administration").
DRUG INTERACTIONS
Oral Anticoagulants
Heparin sodium may prolong the one-stage prothrombin time. Therefore, when heparin sodium is given with dicumarol or warfarin sodium, a period of at least 5 hours after the last intravenous dose or 24 hours after the last subcutaneous dose should elapse before blood is drawn if a valid prothrombin time is to be continued.
Platelet Inhibitors
Drugs such as acetylsalicylic acid, dextran, phenylbutazone, ibuprofen, indomethacin, dipyridamole, hydroxychloroquine, and others that interfere with platelet-aggregation reactions (the main hemostatic defense of heparinized patients) may induce bleeding and should be used with caution in patients receiving heparin sodium.
Other Interactions
Digitalis, tetracyclines, nicotine, or antihistamines may partially counteract the anticoagulant action of heparin sodium.
DRUG/LABORATORY TEST INTERACTIONS
Hyperaminotransferasemia
Significant elevations of aminotransferase (SGOT [S-AST] and SGPT [S-ALT]) levels have occured in a high percentage of patients (and healthy subjects) who have received heparin. Since aminotransferase determinations are important in the differential diagnosis of myocardial infarction, liver disease, and pulmonary emboli, rises that might be caused by drugs (like heparin) should be interpreted with caution.
CARCINOGENESIS, MUTAGENESIS, IMPAIRMENT OF FERTILITY
No long-term studies in animals hae been performed to evaluate carcinogenic potential of heparin. Also, no reproduction studies in animals have been performed concerning mutagenesis or impairment of fertility.
PREGNANCY
Teratogenic Effects—Pregnancy Category C
Animal reproduction studies have not been conducted with heparin sodium. It is also not known whether heparin sodium can cause fetal harm when administered to a pregnant woman or can affect reproduction capacity. Heparin sodium should be given to a pregnant woman only if clearly needed.
Nonteratogenic Effects
Heparin does not cross the placental barrier.
NURSING MOTHERS
Heparin is not excreted in human milk.
PEDIATRIC USE
See "Dosage and Administration."

ADVERSE REACTIONS

HEMORRHAGE
Hemorrhage is the chief complication that may result from heparin therapy (see "Warnings").
An overly prolonged clotting time or minor bleeding during therapy can usually be controlled by withdrawing the drug (see "Overdosage"). It should be appreciated that gastrointestinal- or urinary-tract bleeding during anticoagulant therapy may indicate the presence of an underlying occult lesion. Bleeding can occur at any site but certain specific hemorrhagic complications may be difficult to detect:
a. Adrenal hemorrhage, with resultant acute adrenal insufficiency, has occurred during anticoagulant therapy. Therefore, such treatment should be discontinued in patients who develop signs and symptoms of acute adrenal hemorrhage and insufficiency. Initiation of corrective therapy should not depend on laboratory confirmation of the diagnosis, since any delay in an acute situation may result in the patient's death.
b. Ovarian (corpus luteum) hemorrhage developed in a number of women of reproductive age receiving short- or long-term anticoagulant therapy. This complication, if unrecognized, may be fatal.
c. Retroperitoneal hemorrhage.

LOCAL IRRITATION
Local irritation, erythema, mild pain, hematoma, or ulceration may follow deep, subcutaneous (intrafat) injection of heparin sodium. These complications are much more common after intramuscular use, and such use is not recommended.
HYPERSENSITIVITY
Generalized hypersensitivity reactions have been reported, with chills, fever, and urticaria as the most usual manifestations, and asthma, rhinitis, lacrimation, headache, nausea and vomiting, and anaphylactoid reactions, including shock, occurring more rarely. Itching and burning, especially on the plantar side of the feet, may occur.
Thrombocytopenia has been reported to occur in patients receiving heparin with a reported incidence of 0 to 30%. While often mild and of no obvious clinical significance, such thrombocytopenia can be accompanied by severe thromboembolic complications, such as skin necrosis, gangrene of the extremities, myocardial infarction, pulmonary embolism, and stroke. (See "Warnings," "Precautions.")
Certain episodes of painful, ischemic and cyanosed limbs have in the past been attributed to allergic vasopastic reactions. Whether these are, in fact, identical to the thrombocytopenia-associated complications remains to be determined.
MISCELLANEOUS
Osteoporosis following long-term administration of high doses of heparin, cutaneous necrosis after systemic administration, suppression of aldosterone synthesis, delayed transient alopecia, priapism, and rebound hyperlipemia on discontinuation of heparin sodium have also been reported.
Significant elevations of aminotransferase (SGOT [S-AST] and SGPT [S-ALT]) levels have occurred in a high percentage of patients (and healthy subjects) who have received heparin.

OVERDOSAGE

SYMPTOMS
Bleeding is the chief sign of heparin overdosage. Nosebleeds, blood in urine, or tarry stools may be noted as the first sign of bleeding. Easy bruising or petechial formations may precede frank bleeding.
TREATMENT—Neutralization of Heparin Effect
When clinical circumstances (bleeding) require reversal of heparinization, protamine sulfate (1% solution) by slow infusion will neutralize heparin sodium. No more than 50 mg should be administered, very slowly, in any 10-minute period. Each mg of protamine sulfate neutralizes approximately 100 USP heparin units. The amount of protamine required decreases over time as heparin is metabolized. Although the metabolism of heparin is complex, it may, for the purpose of choosing a protamine dose, be assumed to have a half-life of about ½ hour after intravenous injection.
Administration of protamine sulfate can cause severe hypotensive and anaphylactoid reactions. Because fatal reactions, often resembling anaphylaxis, have been reported, the drug should be given only when resuscitation techniques and treatment of anaphylactoid shock are readily available.
For additional information consult the labeling of Protamine Sulfate Injection, USP, products.

DOSAGE AND ADMINISTRATION

Parenteral drug products should be inspected visually for particulate matter and discoloration prior to administration, whether solution and container permit. Slight discoloration does not alter potency.
When heparin is added to an infusion solution for continuous intravenous administration, the container should be inverted at lest six times to insure adequate mixing and prevent pooling of the heparin in the solution.
Heparin sodium is not effective by oral administration and should be given by intermittent intravenous injection, intravenous infusion, or deep, subcutaneous (intrafat, i.e., above the iliac crest or abdominal fat layer) injection. *The intramuscular route of administration should be avoided because of the frequent occurrence of hematoma at the injection site.*
The dosage of heparin sodium should be adjusted according to the patient's coagulation-test results. When heparin is given by continuous intravenous infusion, the coagulation time should be determined approximately every 4 hours in the early stages of treatment. When the drug is administered intermittently by intravenous injection, coagulation tests should be performed before each injection during the early stages of treatment and at appropriate intervals thereafter. Dosage is considered adequate when the activated partial thrombollastin time (APTT) is 1.5 to 2 times normal or when the whole-blood clotting time is elevated approximately 2.5 to 3 times the control value. After deep subcutaneous (intrafat) injections, tests for adequacy of dosage are best performed on samples drawn 4 to 6 hours after the injections.
Periodic platelet counts, hematocrits, and tests for occult blood in stool are recommended during the entire course of heparin therapy, regardless of the route of administration.
CONVERTING TO ORAL ANTICOAGULANT
When an oral anticoagulant of the coumarin or similar type is to be begun in patients already receiving heparin sodium, baseline and subsequent tests of prothrombin activity must be determined at a time when heparin activity is too low to affect the prothrombin time. This is about 5 hours after the last IV bolus and 24 hours after the last subcutaneous dose. If continuous IV heparin infusion is used, prothrombin time can usually be measured at any time.
In converting from heparin to an oral anticoagulant, the dose of the oral anticoagulant should be the usual initial amount, and thereafter prothrombin time should be determined at the usual intervals. To ensure continuous anticoagulation, it is advisable to continue full heparin therapy for several days after the prothrombin time has reached the therapeutic range. Heparin therapy may then be discontinued without tapering.
THERAPEUTIC ANTICOAGULANT EFFECT WITH FULL-DOSE HEPARIN
Although dosage must be adjusted for the individual patient according to the results of suitable laboratory tests, the following dosage schedules may be used as guidelines:
[See table below].
PEDIATRIC USE
Follow recommendations of appropriate pediatric reference tests. In general, the following dosage schedule may be used as a guideline.
Initial Dose: 50 units/kg (IV, drip).
Maintenance Dose: 100 units/kg (IV, drip) every four hours, or 20,000 units/M^2/24 hours continuously.
SURGERY OF THE HEART AND BLOOD VESSELS
Patients undergoing total body perfusion for open-heart surgery should receive an initial dose of not less than 150 units of heparin sodium per kilogram of body weight. Frequently, a dose of 300 units of heparin sodium per kilogram of body weight is used for procedures estimated to last less than 60 minutes; or 400 units per kilogram for those estimated to last longer than 60 minutes.
LOW-DOSE PROPHYLAXIS OF POSTOPERATIVE THROMBOEMBOLISM
A number of well-controlled clinical trials have demonstrated that low-dose heparin prophylaxis, given just prior to and after surgery, will reduce the incidence of postoperative deep-vein thrombosis in the legs, as measured by the I-125 fibrinogen technique and venography, and of clinical pulmonary embolism. The most widely used dosage has been 5,000 units 2 hours before surgery and 5,000 units every 8 to 12 hours thereafter for 7 days or until the patient is fully ambulatory, whichever is longer. The heparin is given by deep, subcutaneous injection in the arm or abdomen with a fine needle (25–26 gauge) to minimize tissue trauma. A concentrated solution of heparin sodium is recommended. Such prophylaxis should be reserved for patients over 40 undergoing major surgery. Patients with bleeding disorders, those having neurosurgery, spinal anesthesia, eye surgery, or potentially sanguineous operations should be excluded, as well as patients receiving oral anticoagulants or platelet-active drugs (see "Warnings"). The value of such prophylaxis in hip surgery has not been established. The possibility of increased bleeding during surgery or postoperatively should be borne in mind. If such bleeding occurs, discontinuance of heparin and neutralization with protamine sulfate is advisable. If clinical evidence of thromboembolism develops despite low-

Method of Administration	Frequency	Recommended Dose [based on 150 lb (68 kg) patient]
Deep, Subcutaneous (Intrafat) Injection A different site should be used for each injection to prevent the development of massive hematoma.	Initial Dose	5,000 units by IV injection followed by 10,000–20,000 units of a concentrated solution, subcutaneously
	Every 8 hours	8,000–10,000 units of a concentrated solution
	(or) Every 12 hours	15,000–20,000 units of a concentrated solution
Intermittent, Intravenous Injection	Initial Dose	10,000 units, either undiluted or in 50–100 ml isotonic sodium chloride injection
	Every 4 to 6 hours	5,000–10,000 units, either undiluted or in 50–100 ml isotonic sodium chloride injection
Intravenous Infusion	Initial Dose	5,000 units by IV injection
	Continuous	20,000–40,000 units in 1,000 ml of isotonic sodium chloride solution for infusion/day

dose prophylaxis, full therapeutic doses of anticoagulants should be given unless contraindicated. All patients should be screened prior to heparinization to rule out bleeding disorders, and monitoring should be performed with appropriate coagulation tests just prior to surgery. Coagulation-test values should be normal or only slightly elevated. There is usually no need for daily monitoring of the effect of low-dose heparin in patients with normal coagulation parameters.

EXTRACORPOREAL DIALYSIS USE

Follow equipment manufacturer's operating directions carefully.

BLOOD TRANSFUSION

Addition of 400 to 600 USP units per 100 ml of whole blood. Usually, 7,500 USP units of heparin sodium are added to 100 ml of Sterile Sodium Chloride Injection (or 75,000 USP units per 1,000 ml of Sterile Sodium Chloride Injection) and mixed, and from this sterile solution, 6 to 8 ml is added per 100 ml of whole blood. Leukocyte counts should be performed on heparinized blood within two hours after addition of the heparin. Heparinized blood should not be used for isoagglutinin, complement, erythrocyte fragility tests, or platelet counts.

LABORATORY SAMPLES

Addition of 70 to 150 units of heparin sodium per 10 to 20 ml sample of whole blood is usually employed to prevent coagulation of the sample. See comments under "Blood Transfusion."

HOW SUPPLIED

Heparin Sodium Injection, USP, is supplied in TUBEX® Sterile Cartridge-Needle Units.

Each 1l mL size TUBES contains one of the following concentrations of heparin sodium: 1,000 USP Units per mL (22 gauge × 1-1/4 inch needle), NDC 0008-0275-01, in packages of 10 TUBEX.

2,500 USP Units per mL (25 gauge × 5/8 inch needle), NDC 0008-0482-01, in packages of 10 TUBEX.

5,000 USP Units per 0.5 mL (10,000 USP Units per mL)(25 gauge = 5/8 inch needle), NDC 0008-0277-02, in packages of 10 TUBEX.

5,000 USP Units per 0.5 mL (10,000 USP Units per mL)(25 gauge = 5/8 inch needle), NDC 0008-0277-03, in packages of 50 TUBEX.

5,000 USP Units per mL (22 gauge = 1-1/4 inch needle), NDC 0008-0278-01, in packages of 10 TUBEX.

5,000 USP Units per mL (25 guage = 5/8 inch needle), NDC 0008-0278-02, in packages of 10 TUBEX.

7,500 USP Units per mL (25 gauge = 5/8 inch needle), NDC 0008-0293-01, in packages of 10 TUBEX.

10,000 USP Units per mL (25 gauge = 5/8 inch needle), NDC 0008-0277-01, in packages of 10 TUBEX.

15,000 USP Units per mL (25 gauge = 5/8 inch needle), NDC 0008-0279-01, in packages of 10 TUBEX.

20,000 USP Units per mL, (25 gauge = 5/8 inch needle), NDC 0008-0276-01, in packages of 10 TUBEX.

The 2.5 mL size TUBES or 1,000 USP Units per mL (25 gauge = 5/8 inch needle), NDC 0008-0275-02, in packages of 50 TUBEX.

Do not freeze

INFLUENZA VIRUS VACCINE, SUBVIRION TYPE ℞

[in "flu-en 'zah vi 'rus vak 'sēn sub vir 'ēon]

The formulation of influenza virus vaccine for use during each season is established by the office of Biologics Research and Review, Food and Drug Administration. For current information about formulation, dosage and recommended use, consult product direction circular which can be obtained by writing Professional Service, Wyeth Laboratories, P.O. Box 8299, Philadelphia, PA 19101, or through your local Wyeth representative.

ISORDIL® ℞

[ī 'sore "dĭl]

(isosorbide dinitrate)

(1,4,3,6-dianhydro-sorbitol-2,5-dinitrate)

DESCRIPTION

Isosorbide dinitrate, an organic nitrate, is a vasodilator with effects on both arteries and veins. Isordil is available as 2.5 mg, 5 mg, and 10 mg Sublingual tablets; 10 mg Chewable tablets; 5 mg, 10 mg, 20 mg, 30 mg, and 40 mg standard oral Titradose® tablets; and 40 mg controlled-release oral Tembids® capsules and tablets.

Isordil Sublingual tablets contain 2.5 mg, 5 mg, or 10 mg isosorbide dinitrate. The inactive ingredients present are cellulose, lactose, magnesium stearate, and starch. The 2.5 mg dosage strength also contains D&C Yellow 10 and FD&C Yellow 6, and the 5 mg dosage strength also contains FD&C Red 3.

Isordil Chewable tablets contain 10 mg isosorbide dinitrate. The inactive ingredients present are cellulose, D&C Yellow 10, FD&C Yellow 6, magnesium stearate, mannitol, natural flavors, and saccharin sodium.

Isordil Titradose tablets contain 5 mg, 10 mg, 20 mg, 30 mg, or 40 mg isosorbide dinitrate. The inactive ingredients present are lactose, magnesium stearate, and other ingredients. The 5 mg, 20 mg, 30 mg, and 40 mg dosage strengths also contain the following: 5 mg—FD&C Red 3; 20 mg and 40 mg—D&C Yellow 10, FD&C Blue 1, and FD&C Yellow 6; 30 mg—FD&C Blue 1.

Isordil Tembids capsules contain 40 mg isosorbide dinitrate. The inactive ingredients present are confectioners sugar, starch, gelatin capsule, and other ingredients.

Isordil Tembids tablets contain 40 mg isosorbide dinitrate. The inactive ingredients present are D&C Yellow 10, FD&C Blue 1, FD&C Yellow 6, lactose, magnesium stearate, sodium silicoaluminate, talc, and other ingredients.

The chemical name for isosorbide dinitrate is 1,4,3,6-dianhydro-sorbital-2,5-dinitrate, and compound has the following structural formula:

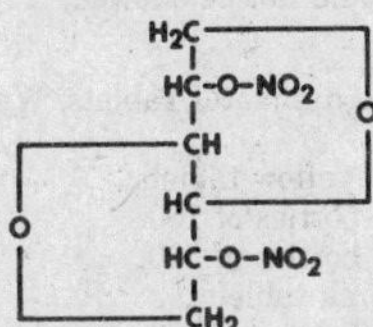

Molecular Weight 236.14

Isosorbide dinitrate is a white, crystalline, odorless compound which is stable in air and in solution, has a melting point of 70° C and has an optical rotation of +134° (c = 1.0, alcohol, 20° C). Isosorbide dinitrate is freely soluble in organic solvents such as acetone, alcohol, and ether, but is only sparingly soluble in water.

CLINICAL PHARMACOLOGY

The principal pharmacological action of Isordil is relaxation of vascular smooth muscle, producing a vasodilatory effect on both peripheral arteries and veins, with predominant effects on the latter. Dilation of the postcapillary vessels, including large veins, promotes peripheral pooling of blood and decreases venous return to the heart, thereby reducing left-ventricular end-diastolic pressure (preload). Arteriolar relaxation reduces systemic vascular resistance and arterial pressure (afterload).

The mechanism by which Isordil relieves angina pectoris is not fully understood. Myocardial oxygen consumption or demand (as measured by the pressure-rate product, tension-time index, and stroke-work index) is decreased by both the arterial and venous effects of Isordil, and, presumably, a more favorable supply-demand ratio is achieved. While the large epicardial coronary arteries are also dilated by Isordil, the extent to which this contributes to relief of exertional angina is unclear.

Therapeutic doses of Isordil may reduce systolic, diastolic, and mean arterial blood pressures, especially in the upright posture. Effective coronary perfusion is usually maintained. The decrease in systemic blood pressure may result in reflex tachycardia, an effect which could unfavorably influence myocardial oxygen demand. Hemodynamic studies indicate that Isordil may reduce the abnormally elevated left ventricular end-diastolic and pulmonary capillary wedge pressures that occur during an acute episode of angina pectoris.

Isordil is metabolized by enzymatic denitration to the intermediate products, isosorbide-2-mononitrate and isosorbide-5-mononitrate. Both metabolites have biological activity, especially the 5-mononitrate which is also the principal metabolite. The liver is a principal site of metabolism, and oral isosorbide dinitrate is subject to a large first pass effect. The systemic clearance of the drug following intravenous infusion is about 3.4 liters/min. Since the clearance exceeds hepatic blood flow, considerable extrahepatic metabolism must also occur.

The average bioavailability of Isordil is 59 and 22 percent following sublingual and oral administration, respectively. The terminal half-life is about 20 minutes, 60 minutes, and 4 hours following IV, sublingual, and oral administration, respectively. The dependence of half-life on the route of administration is not understood. Over limited ranges of IV dosing, the pharmacokinetics of isosorbide dinitrate appear linear. However, both the 2- and 5-mononitrate metabolites have been shown to decrease the rate of disappearance of the dinitrate from the blood. The half-lives of isosorbide-5-mononitrate and isosorbide-2-mononitrate range from 4.0–5.6 and 1.5–3.1 hours, respectively.

The pharmacokinetics and/or bioavailability of isosorbide dinitrate during multiple dosing have not been well studied. Because the metabolites influence the clearance of isosorbide dinitrate, prediction of blood levels of parent compound or metabolites from single-dose studies is uncertain.

INDICATIONS AND USAGE

Isordil is indicated for the treatment and prevention of angina pectoris. Controlled clinical trials have demonstrated that the sublingual, chewable, immediate release, and controlled-release oral dosage forms of Isordil are effective in improving exercise tolerance in patients with angina pectoris. When single sublingual or chewable doses (5 mg) of isosorbide dinitrate were administered prophylactically to patients with angina pectoris in various clinical studies, duration of exercise until chest pain or fatigue was significantly improved for at least 45 minutes (and as long as 2 hours in some studies) following dosing. Similar studies after single oral (15 to 120 mg) and oral controlled-release (40 to 80 mg) doses of isosorbide dinitrate have shown significant improvement in exercise tolerance for up to 8 hours following dosing. The exercise electrocardiographic evidence suggests that improved exercise tolerance with Isordil is not at the expense of greater myocardial ischemia. All dosage forms of Isordil may therefore be used prophylactically to decrease frequency and severity of anginal attacks and can be expected to decrease the need for sublingual nitroglycerin.

The sublingual and chewable forms of the drug are indicated for acute prophylaxis of angina pectoris when taken a few minutes before situations likely to provoke anginal attacks. Because of a slower onset of effect, the oral forms of Isordil are not indicated for acute prophylaxis.

In controlled clinical trials, chewable and sublingual isosorbide dinitrate were effective in relieving an acute attack of angina pectoris. Relief occurred with a mean time of 2.9 and 3.4 minutes (chewable and sublingual respectively) compared to relief of angina with a mean time of 1.9 minutes following sublingual nitroglycerin. Because of the more rapid relief of chest pain with sublingual nitroglycerin, the use of sublingual or chewable isosorbide dinitrate for aborting an acute anginal attack should be limited to patients intolerant or unresponsive to sublingual nitroglycerin.

CONTRAINDICATIONS

Isosorbide dinitrate is contraindicated in patients who have shown purported hypersensitivity or idiosyncrasy to it or other nitrates or nitrites.

WARNINGS

The benefits of isosorbide dinitrate during the early days of an acute myocardial infarction have not been established. If one elects to use organic nitrates in early infarction, hemodynamic monitoring and frequent clinical assessment should be used because of the potential deleterious effects of hypotension.

PRECAUTIONS

General. Severe hypotensive response, particularly with upright posture, may occur with even small doses of isosorbide dinitrate. The drug should therefore be used with caution in subjects who may have blood volume depletion from diuretic therapy or in subjects who have low systolic blood pressure (e.g., below 90 mm Hg). Paradoxical bradycardia and increased angina pectoris may accompany nitrate-induced hypotension.

Nitrate therapy may aggravate the angina caused by hypertrophic cardiomyopathy. Tolerance to this drug and cross-tolerance to other nitrates and nitrites may occur.

Marked symptomatic, orthostatic hypotension has been reported when calcium channel blockers and organic nitrates were used in combination. Dose adjustment of either class of agents may be necessary.

Tolerance to the vascular and antianginal effects of isosorbide dinitrate or nitroglycerin has been demonstrated in clinical trials, experience through occupational exposure, and in isolated tissue experiments in the laboratory. The importance of tolerance to the appropriate use of isosorbide dinitrate in the management of patients with angina pectoris has not been determined. However, one clinical trial using treadmill exercise tolerance (as an endpoint) found an 8-hour duration of action of oral isosorbide dinitrate following the first dose (after a 2-week placebo washout) and only a 2-hour duration of effect of the same dose after 1 week of repetitive dosing at conventional dosing intervals. On the other hand, several trials have been able to differentiate isosorbide dinitrate from placebo after 4 weeks of therapy, and in open trials an effect seems detectable for as long as several months.

Tolerance clearly occurs in industrial workers continuously exposed to nitroglycerin. Moreover, physical dependence also occurs, since chest pain, acute myocardial infarction, and even sudden death have occurred during temporary withdrawal of nitroglycerin from the workers. In clinical trials in angina patients, there are reports of anginal attacks being more easily provoked and of rebound in the hemodynamic effects soon after nitrate withdrawal. The relative importance of these observations to the routine, clinical use of isosorbide dinitrate is not known. However, it seems prudent to gradually withdraw patients from isosorbide dinitrate when the therapy is being terminated, rather than stopping the drug abruptly.

Information for Patients. Headache may occur during initial therapy with isosorbide dinitrate. Headache is usually relieved by the use of standard headache remedies, or by

Continued on next page

Wyeth—Cont.

lowering the dose, and tends to disappear after the first week or two of use.

Drug Interactions. Alcohol may enhance any marked sensitivity to the hypotensive effect of nitrates.

Isosorbide dinitrate acts directly on vascular smooth muscle; therefore, any other agent that depends on vascular smooth muscle as the final common path can be expected to have decreased or increased effect, depending on the agent.

Carcinogenesis, Mutagenesis, Impairment of Fertility. No long-term studies in animals have been performed to evaluate the carcinogenic potential of this drug. A modified two-liter reproduction study in rats fed isosorbide dinitrate at 25 or 100 mg/kg/day did not reveal any effects on fertility or gestation or any remarkable growth pathology in any parent or offspring fed isosorbide dinitrate as compared with rats fed a basal-controlled diet.

Pregnancy Category C. Isosorbide dinitrate has been shown to cause a dose-related increase in embryotoxicity (increase in mummified pups) in rabbits at oral doses 35 and 150 times the maximum recommended human daily dose. There are no adequate and well-controlled studies in pregnant women. Isosorbide dinitrate should be used during pregnancy only if the potential benefit justifies the potential risk to the fetus.

Nursing Mothers. It is not known whether this drug is excreted in human milk. Because many drugs are excreted in human milk, caution should be exercised when isosorbide dinitrate is administered to a nursing mother.

Pediatric Use. The safety and effectiveness of isosorbide dinitrate in children has not been established.

ADVERSE REACTIONS

Adverse reactions, particularly headache and hypotension, are dose related. In clinical trials at various doses, the following have been observed.

Headache is the most common (reported incidence varies widely, apparently being related, with an avergae occurrence of about 25%) adverse reaction and may be severe and persistent. Cutaneous vasodilation with flushing may occur. Transient episodes of dizziness and weakness, as well as other signs of cerebral ischemia associated with postural hypotension, may occasionally develop (the incidence of reported symptomatic hypotension ranges from 2% to 36%). An occasional individual will exhibit marked sensitivity to the hypotensive effects of nitrates, and severe responses (nausea, vomiting, weakness, restlessness, pallor, perspiration, and collapse) may occur even with the usual therapeutic dose. Drug rash and/or exfoliative dermatitis may occasionally occur. Nausea and vomiting appear to be uncommon.

OVERDOSAGE

Signs and Symptoms. These may include the following: a prompt fall in blood pressure, persistent and throbbing headache, vertigo, palpitation, visual disturbances, flushed and perspiring skin (later becoming cold and cyanotic), nausea and vomiting (possibly with colic and even bloody diarrhea), syncope (especially in the upright position), methemoglobinemia with cyanosis and anoxia, initial hyperpnea, dyspnea and slow breathing, slow pulse (dicrotic and intermittent), heart block, increased intracranial pressure with cerebral symptoms of confusion and moderate fever, paralysis and coma followed by clonic convulsions and possibly death due to circulatory collapse.

It is not known what dose of the drug is associated with symptoms of overdosing or what dose of the drug would be life-threatening. The acute oral LD_{50} of isosorbide dinitrate in rats was found to be approximately 1100 mg/kg of body weight. These animal experiments indicate that approximately 500 times the usual therapeutic dose would be required to produce such toxic symptoms in humans. It is not known whether the drug is dialyzable.

Treatment of Overdosage. Prompt removal of the ingested material by gastric lavage is reasonable but not documented to be useful. Keep the patient recumbent in a shock position and comfortably warm. Passive movements of the extremities may aid venous return. Administer oxygen and artificial respiration if necessary. If methemoglobinemia is present, administer methylene blue (1% solution), 1 to 2 mg/kg intravenously.

Methemoglobin. Case reports of clinically significant methemoglobinemia are rare at conventional doses of organic nitrates. The formation of methemoglobin is dose related, and in the case of genetic abnormalities of hemoglobin that favor methemoglobin formation, even conventional doses of organic nitrate could produce harmful concentrations of methemoglobin.

WARNING: Epinephrine is ineffective in reversing the severe hypotensive events associated with overdose. It and related compounds are contraindicated in this situation.

DOSAGE AND ADMINISTRATION

For the treatment of angina pectoris, the usual starting dose of sublingual Isordil is 2.5 to 5 mg; and for chewable tablets, 5 mg. Isordil should be titrated upward until angina is relieved or side effects limit the dose. In ambulatory patients, the magnitude of the incremental dose of increase should be guided by measurements of standing blood pressure.

The initial dosage of sublingual or chewable Isordil for acute prophylactic therapy in angina pectoris patients is generally 5 or 10 mg every 2 to 3 hours. Adequate, controlled clinical studies demonstrating the effectiveness of chronic maintenance therapy with these dosage forms have not been reported.

For the treatment of chronic stable angina pectoris, the usual starting dose for immediate-release (swallowed) tablets is 5 to 20 mg; and for controlled release forms, 40 mg. For maintenance therapy, oral doses of 10 to 40 mg given every 6 hours or oral controlled-release doses of 40 to 80 mg given every 8 to 12 hours are generally recommended. The extent to which development of tolerance should modify the dosage program has not been defined. The oral controlled-release forms of Isordil should not be chewed.

HOW SUPPLIED

Isordil® (isosorbide dinitrate) Tablets, Wyeth®, are available as follows:

Sublingual, 2.5 mg, yellow tablets:
NDC 0008-4139-01, bottles of 100.
NDC 0008-4139-03, bottles of 500.
Sublingual 5 mg, pink tablets:
NDC 0008-4126-01, bottles of 100.
NDC 0008-4126-03, bottles of 500.
Sublingual, 10 mg, white tablets:
NDC 0008-4161-01, bottles of 100.
Chewable, 10 mg, scored yellow tablets:
NDC 0008-4164-01, bottles of 100.
Oral Titradose®, 5 mg, scored pink tablets:
NDC 0008-4152-01, bottles of 100.
NDC 0008-4152-02, bottles of 500.
NDC 0008-4152-03, bottles of 1000.
Oral Titradose, 10 mg, scored white tablets:
NDC 0008-4153-01, bottles of 100.
NDC 0008-4153-02, bottles of 500.
NDC 0008-4153-03, bottles of 1000.
Oral Titradose, 20 mg, scored green tablets:
NDC 0008-4154-01, bottles of 100.
NDC 0008-4154-02, bottles of 500.
Oral Titradose, 30 mg, scored blue tablets:
NDC 0008-4159-01, bottles of 100.
NDC 0008-4159-02, bottles of 500.
Oral Titradose, 40 mg, scored light-green tablets:
NDC 0008-4192-01, bottles of 100.
Tembids®, 40 mg, scored green controlled-release tablets:
NDC 0008-4125-01, bottles of 100.
NDC 0008-4125-02, bottles of 500.
NDC 0008-4125-03, bottles of 1000.

ALSO AVAILABLE

Redipak® Strip Pack cartons of 100 tablets (20 strips of 5) as follows:
Sublingual, 2.5 mg, NDC 0008-4139-04.
Sublingual, 5 mg, NDC 0008-4126-06.
Sublingual, 10 mg, NDC 0008-4161-03.
Chewable, 10 mg, NDC 0008-4164-03.
Oral Titradose, 5 mg, NDC 0008-4152-04.
Oral Titradose, 10 mg, NDC 0008-4153-04.
Oral Titradose, 20 mg, NDC 0008-4154-04.
Oral Titradose, 30 mg, NDC 0008-4159-03.
Oral Titradose, 40 mg, NDC 0008-4192-04.

Isordil® (isosorbide dinitrate) Tembids® Capsules, Wyeth®, are available in 40 mg, controlled-release capsules (opaque, blue cap and colorless, transparent body):
NDC 0008-4140-01, bottles of 100.
NDC 0008-4140-02, bottles of 500.

US Pat. Nos. 3883647 and D224591 (Titradose®)

Shown in Product Identification Section, page 436

LO/OVRAL® ℞

[*lōh-ōh 'vral*]
Tablets
(norgestrel and ethinyl estradiol tablets)

DESCRIPTION

Each LO/OVRAL® tablet contains 0.3 mg of norgestrel (*dl*-13-beta-ethyl-17-alpha-ethinyl-17-beta-hydroxygon- 4-en-3-one), a totally synthetic progestogen, and 0.03 mg of ethinyl estradiol (19-nor-17α-pregna-1,3,5 (10)-trien-20-yne-3,17-diol). The inactive ingredients present are cellulose, lactose, magnesium stearate, and polacrilin potassium.

CLINICAL PHARMACOLOGY

Combination oral contraceptives act primarily through the mechanism of gonadotropin suppression due to the estrogenic and progestational activity of the ingredients. Although the primary mechanism of action is inhibition of ovulation, alterations in the genital tract, including changes in the cervical mucus (which increase the difficulty of sperm penetration) and the endometrium (which reduce the likelihood of implantation), may also contribute to contraceptive effectiveness.

INDICATIONS AND USAGE

LO/OVRAL is indicated for the prevention of pregnancy in women who elect to use oral contraceptives as a method of contraception.

Oral contraceptives are highly effective. The pregnancy rate in women using conventional combination oral contraceptives (containing 35 mcg or more of ethinyl estradiol or 50 mcg or more of mestranol) is generally reported as less than one pregnancy per 100 woman-years of use. Slightly higher rates (somewhat more than 1 pregnancy per 100 woman-years of use) are reported for some combination products containing 35 mcg or less of ethinyl estradiol, and rates on the order of 3 pregnancies per 100 woman-years are reported for the progestogen-only oral contraceptives.

These rates are derived from separate studies conducted by different investigators in several population groups and cannot be compared precisely. Furthermore, pregnancy rates tend to be lower as clinical studies are continued, possibly due to selective retention in the longer studies of those patients who accept the treatment regimen and do not discontinue as a result of adverse reactions, pregnancy, or other reasons.

In clinical trials with LO/OVRAL, 1,700 patients completed 22,489 cycles, and a total of two pregnancies were reported. This represents a pregnancy rate of 0.12 per 100 woman-years.

Table 1 gives ranges of pregnancy rates reported in the literature[1] for other means of contraception. The efficacy of these means of contraception (except the IUD) depends upon the degree of adherence to the method.

TABLE 1
PREGNANCIES PER 100 WOMAN-YEARS

IUD, less than 1–6; Diaphragm with spermicidal products (creams or jellies), 2–20; Condom, 3–36; Aerosol foams, 2–29; Jellies and creams, 4–36;

Periodic abstinence (rhythm) all types, less than 1–47:

1. Calendar method, 14–47;
2. Temperature method, 1–20;
3. Temperature method—intercourse only in postovulatory phase, less than 1–7;
4. Mucus method, 1–25;

No contraception, 60–80.

Dose-Related Risk of Thromboembolism from Oral Contraceptives: Two studies have shown a positive association between the dose of estrogens in oral contraceptives and the risk of thromboembolism.[2,3] For this reason, it is prudent and in keeping with good principles of therapeutics to minimize exposure to estrogen. The oral-contraceptive product prescribed for any given patient should be that product which contains the least amount of estrogen that is compatible with an acceptable pregnancy rate and patient acceptance. It is recommended that new acceptors of oral contraceptives be started on preparations containing 0.05 mg or less of estrogen.

CONTRAINDICATIONS

Oral contraceptives should not be used in women with any of the following conditions:

1. Thrombophlebitis or thromboembolic disorders.
2. A past history of deep-vein thrombophlebitis or thromboembolic disorders.
3. Cerebral-vascular or coronary-artery disease.
4. Known or suspected carcinoma of the breast.
5. Known or suspected estrogen-dependent neoplasia.
6. Undiagnosed abnormal genital bleeding.
7. Known or suspected pregnancy (see Warning No. 5).
8. Benign or malignant liver tumor which developed during the use of oral contraceptives or other estrogen-containing products.

WARNINGS

Cigarette smoking increases the risk of serious cardiovascular side effects from oral-contraceptive use. This risk increases with age and with heavy smoking (15 or more cigarettes per day) and is quite marked in women over 35 years of age. Women who use oral contraceptives should be strongly advised not to smoke.

The use of oral contraceptives is associated with increased risk of several serious conditions, including thromboembolism, stroke, myocardial infarction, hepatic adenoma, gallbladder disease, hypertension. Practitioners prescribing oral contraceptives should be familiar with the following information relating to these risks.

1. *Thromboembolic Disorders and Other Vascular Problems:* An increased risk of thromboembolic and thrombotic disease associated with the use of oral contraceptives is well-established. Three principal studies in Great Britain[4–6] and three in the United States[7–10] have demonstrated an increased risk of fatal and nonfatal venous thromboembolism and stroke, both hemorrhagic and thrombotic. These studies

estimate that users of oral contraceptives are 4 to 11 times more likely than nonusers to develop these diseases without evident cause (Table 2).

CEREBROVASCULAR DISORDERS

In a collaborative American study[9,10] of cerebrovascular disorders in women with and without predisposing causes, it was estimated that the risk of hemorrhagic stroke was 2.0 times greater in users than nonusers and the risk of thrombotic stroke was 4 to 9.5 times greater in users than in nonusers (Table 2).

TABLE 2

SUMMARY OF RELATIVE RISK OF THROMBOEMBOLIC DISORDERS AND OTHER VASCULAR PROBLEMS IN ORAL-CONTRACEPTIVE USERS COMPARED TO NONUSERS

	Relative risk, times greater
Idiopathic thromboembolic disease	4–11
Postsurgery thromboembolic complications	4–6
Thrombotic stroke	4–9.5
Hemorrhagic stroke	2
Myocardial infarction	2–12

MYOCARDIAL INFARCTION

An increased risk of myocardial infarction associated with the use of oral contraceptives has been reported,[11–13] confirming a previously suspected association. These studies, conducted in the United Kingdom, found, as expected, that the greater the number of underlying risk factors for coronary-artery disease (cigarette smoking, hypertension, hypercholesterolemia, obesity, diabetes, history of preeclamptic toxemia) the higher the risk of developing myocardial infarction, regardless of whether the patient was an oral-contraceptive user or not. Oral contraceptives, however, were found to be a clear additional risk factor.

In terms of relative risk, it has been estimated[52] that oral-contraceptive users who do not smoke (smoking is considered a major predisposing condition to myocardial infarction) are about twice as likely to have a fatal myocardial infarction as nonusers who do not smoke. Oral-contraceptive users who are also smokers have about a 5-fold increased risk of fatal infarction compared to users who do not smoke, but about a 10- to 12-fold increased risk compared to nonusers who do not smoke. Furthermore, the amount of smoking is also an important factor. In determining the importance of these relative risks, however, the baseline rates for various age groups, as shown in Table 3, must be given serious consideration. The importance of other predisposing conditions mentioned above in determining relative and absolute risks has not as yet been quantified; it is quite likely that the same synergistic action exists, but perhaps to a lesser extent.

TABLE 3

Estimated annual mortality rate per 100,000 women from myocardial infarction by use of oral contraceptives, smoking habits, and age (in years):

	Myocardial infarction			
	Women aged 30–39		Women aged 40–44	
Smoking habits	Users	Non-users	Users	Non-users
All smokers	10.2	2.6	62.0	15.9
Heavy*	13.0	5.1	78.7	31.3
Light	4.7	0.9	28.6	5.7
Nonsmokers	1.8	1.2	10.7	7.4
Smokers and nonsmokers	5.4	1.9	32.8	11.7

*Heavy smoker: 15 or more cigarettes per day.

From JAIN, A.K., *Studies in Family Planning, 8*:50, 1977

RISK OF DOSE

In an analysis of data derived from several national adverse-reaction reporting systems,[2] British investigators concluded that the risk of thromboembolism, including coronary thrombosis, is directly related to the dose of estrogen used in oral contraceptives. Preparations containing 100 mcg or more of estrogen were associated with a higher risk of thromboembolism than those containing 50–80 mcg of estrogen. Their analysis did suggest, however, that the quantity of estrogen may not be the sole factor involved. This finding has been confirmed in the United States.[3] Careful epidemiological studies to determine the degree of thromboembolic risk associated with progestogen-only oral contraceptives have not been performed. Cases of thromboembolic disease have been reported in women using these products, and they should not be presumed to be free of excess risk.

ESTIMATE OF EXCESS MORTALITY FROM CIRCULATORY DISEASES

A large prospective study[53] carried out in the U.K. estimated the mortality rate per 100,000 women per year from diseases of the circulatory system for users and nonusers of oral contraceptives according to age, smoking habits, and duration of use. The overall excess death rate annually from circulatory diseases for oral-contraceptive users was estimated to be 20 per 100,000 (ages 15–34—5/100,000; ages 35–44—33/100,000; ages 45–49—140/100,000), the risk being concentrated in older women, in those with a long duration of use, and in cigarette smokers. It was not possible, however, to examine the interrelationships of age, smoking, and duration of use, nor to compare the effects of continuous vs. intermittent use. Although the study showed a 10-fold increase in death due to circulatory diseases in users for 5 or more years, all of these deaths occurred in women 35 or older. Until larger numbers of women under 35 with continuous use for 5 or more years are available, it is not possible to assess the magnitude of the relative risk for this younger age group.

The available data from a variety of sources have been analyzed[14] to estimate the risk of death associated with various methods of contraception. The estimates of risk of death for each method include the combined risk of the contraceptive method (e.g., thromboembolic and thrombotic disease in the case of oral contraceptives) plus the risk attributable to pregnancy or abortion in the event of method failure. This latter risk varies with the effectiveness of the contraceptive method. The findings of this analysis are shown in the bar graph (Figure 1).[14] The study concluded that the mortality associated with all methods of birth control is low and below that associated with childbirth, with the exception of oral contraceptives in women over 40 who smoke. (The rates given for Pill only/smokers for each age group are for smokers as a class. For "heavy" smokers [more than 15 cigarettes a day], the rates given would be about double; for "light" smokers [less than 15 cigarettes a day], about 50 percent.) The lowest mortality is associated with the condom or diaphragm backed up by early abortion. The risk of thromboembolic and thrombotic disease associated with oral contraceptives increases with age after approximately age 30 and, for myocardial infarction, is further increased by hypertension, hypercholesterolemia, obesity, diabetes, or history of preeclamptic toxemia and especially by cigarette smoking.

Based on the data currently available, the following chart gives a gross estimate of the risk of death from circulatory disorders associated with the use of oral contraceptives:

SMOKING HABITS AND OTHER PREDISPOSING CONDITIONS—

RISK ASSOCIATED WITH USE OF ORAL CONTRACEPTIVES

Age	Below 30	30–39	40+
Heavy smokers	C	B	A
Light smokers	D	C	B
Nonsmokers (no predisposing conditions)	D	C,D	C
Nonsmokers (other predisposing conditions)	C	C,B	B,A

A—Use associated with very high risk.
B—Use associated with high risk.
C—Use associated with moderate risk.
D—Use associated with low risk.

The physician and the patient should be alert to the earliest manifestations of thromboembolic and thrombotic disorders (e.g., thrombophlebitis, pulmonary embolism, cerebrovascular insufficiency, coronary occlusion, retinal thrombosis, and mesenteric thrombosis). Should any of these occur or be suspected, the drug should be discontinued immediately.

A four- to six-fold increased risk of postsurgery thromboembolic complications has been reported in oral-contraceptive users.[15,16] If feasible, oral contraceptives should be discontinued at least 4 weeks before surgery of a type associated with an increased risk of thromboembolism or prolonged immobilization.

PERSISTENCE OF RISK OF VASCULAR DISORDERS

Findings from one study in Great Britain involving cerebrovascular disease[54] and another study in the United States concerning myocardial infarction[55] suggest that an increased risk of these conditions in users of oral contraceptives persists after discontinuation of the oral contraceptive. In the British study, the risk of cerebrovascular disease remained elevated in former oral-contraceptive users for at least six years after discontinuation. In the U.S. study, an increased risk of myocardial infarction persisted for at least 9 years in women 40- to 49-years-old who had used oral contraceptives for five or more years. The findings in both these studies require confirmation since they are inconsistent with other published information.[9,11,13,56–60]

2. *Ocular Lesions:*

There have been reports of neuro-ocular lesions such as optic neuritis or retinal thrombosis associated with the use of oral contraceptives. Discontinue oral-contraceptive medication if there is unexplained, sudden or gradual, partial or complete loss of vision; onset of proptosis or diplopia; papilledema; or retinal-vascular lesions, and institute appropriate diagnostic and therapeutic measures.

3. *Carcinoma:*

Long-term continuous administration of either natural or synthetic estrogen in certain animal species increases the frequency of carcinoma of the breast, cervix, vagina, and liver. Certain synthetic progestogens, none currently contained in oral contraceptives, have been noted to increase the incidence of mammary nodules, benign and malignant, in dogs.

Figure 1. Estimated annual number of deaths associated with control of fertility and no control per 100,000 nonsterile women, by regimen of control and age of woman.

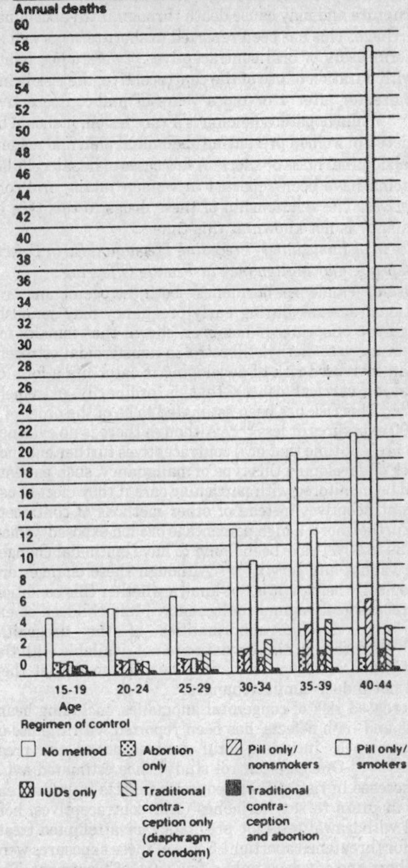

In humans, three case-control studies have reported an increased risk of endometrial carcinoma associated with the prolonged use of exogenous estrogen in postmenopausal women.[17–19] One publication[20] reported on the first 21 cases submitted by physicians to a registry of cases of adenocarcinoma of the endometrium in women under 40 on oral contraceptives. Of the cases found in women without predisposing risk factors for adenocarcinoma of the endometrium (e.g., irregular bleeding at the time oral contraceptives were first given, polycystic ovaries), nearly all occurred in women who had used a sequential oral contraceptive. These products are no longer marketed. No evidence has been reported suggesting an increased risk of endometrial cancer in users of conventional combination or progestogen-only oral contraceptives.

Several studies[8,21–24] have found no increase in breast cancer in women taking oral contraceptives or estrogen. One study,[25] however, while also noting no overall increased risk of breast cancer in women treated with oral contraceptives, found an excess risk in the subgroups of oral-contraceptive users with documented benign breast disease. A reduced occurrence of benign breast tumors in users of oral contraceptives has been well-documented.[8,21,25–27]

In summary, there is at present no confirmed evidence from human studies of an increased risk of cancer associated with oral contraceptives. Close clinical surveillance of all women taking oral contraceptives is, nevertheless, essential. In all cases of undiagnosed persistent or recurrent abnormal vaginal bleeding, appropriate diagnostic measures should be taken to rule out malignancy. Women with a strong family history of breast cancer or who have breast nodules, fibrocystic disease, or abnormal mammograms should be monitored with particular care if they elect to use oral contraceptives instead of other methods of contraception.

4. *Hepatic Tumors:*

Benign hepatic adenomas have been found to be associated with the use of oral contraceptives.[28–30,46] One study[46] showed that oral contraceptive formulations with high hormonal potency were associated with a higher risk than lower

Continued on next page

Wyeth—Cont.

potency formulations. Although benign, hepatic adenomas may rupture and may cause death through intra-abdominal hemorrhage. This has been reported in short-term as well as long-term users of oral contraceptives. Two studies relate risk with duration of use of the contraceptive, the risk being much greater after 4 or more years of oral-contraceptive use.[30,46] While hepatic adenoma is a rare lesion, it should be considered in women presenting abdominal pain and tenderness, abdominal mass or shock. A few cases of hepatocellular carcinoma have been reported in women taking oral contraceptives. The relationship of these drugs to this type of malignancy is not known at this time.

5. *Use in or Immediately Preceding Pregnancy, Birth Defects in Offspring, and Malignancy in Female Offspring:*
The use of female sex hormones—both estrogenic and progestational agents—during early pregnancy may seriously damage the offspring. It has been shown that females exposed in utero to diethylstilbestrol, a nonsteroidal estrogen, have an increased risk of developing in later life a form of vaginal or cervical cancer that is ordinarily extremely rare.[31,32] This risk has been estimated to be of the order of 1 in 1,000 exposures or less.[33,47] Although there is no evidence at the present time that oral contraceptives further enhance the risk of developing this type of malignancy, such patients should be monitored with particular care if they elect to use oral contraceptives instead of other methods of contraception. Furthermore, a high percentage of such exposed women (from 30 to 90%) have been found to have epithelial changes of the vagina and cervix.[34–38] Although these changes are histologically benign, it is not known whether this condition is a precursor of vaginal malignancy. Male children so exposed may develop abnormalities of the urogenital tract.[48–50] Although similar data are not available with the use of other estrogens, it cannot be presumed that they would not induce similar changes.

An increased risk of congenital anomalies, including heart defects and limb defects, has been reported with the use of sex hormones, including oral contraceptives, in pregnancy.[39–42,51] One case-control study[42] has estimated a 4.7-fold increase in risk of limb-reduction defects in infants exposed in utero to sex hormones (oral contraceptives, hormonal withdrawal tests for pregnancy, or attempted treatment for threatened abortion). Some of these exposures were very short and involved only a few days of treatment. The data suggest that the risk of limb-reduction defects in exposed fetuses is somewhat less than one in 1,000 live births.

In the past, female sex hormones have been used during pregnancy in an attempt to treat threatened or habitual abortion. There is considerable evidence that estrogens are ineffective for these indications, and there is no evidence from well-controlled studies that progestogens are effective for these uses.

There is some evidence that triploidy and possibly other types of polyploidy are increased among abortuses from women who become pregnant soon after ceasing oral contraceptives.[43] Embryos with these anomalies are virtually always aborted spontaneously. Whether there is an overall increase in spontaneous abortion of pregnancies conceived soon after stopping oral contraceptives is unknown. It is recommended that, for any patient who has missed two consecutive periods, pregnancy should be ruled out before continuing the contraceptive regimen. If the patient has not adhered to the prescribed schedule, the possibility of pregnancy should be considered at the time of the first missed period (or after 45 days from the last menstrual period if the progestogen-only oral contraceptives are used), and further use of oral contraceptives should be withheld until pregnancy has been ruled out. If pregnancy is confirmed, the patient should be apprised of the potential risks to the fetus, and the advisability of continuation of the pregnancy should be discussed in the light of these risks.

It is also recommended that women who discontinue oral contraceptives with the intent of becoming pregnant use an alternate form of contraception for a period of time before attempting to conceive. Many clinicians recommend 3 months, although no precise information is available on which to base this recommendation.

The administration of progestogen-only or progestogen-estrogen combinations to induce withdrawal bleeding should not be used as a test of pregnancy.

6. *Gallbladder Disease:*
Studies [8,23,26] report an increased risk of surgically confirmed gallbladder disease in users of oral contraceptives and estrogens. In one study, an increased risk appeared after 2 years of use and doubled after 4 or 5 years of use. In one of the other studies, an increased risk was apparent between 6 and 12 months of use.

7. *Carbohydrate and Lipid Metabolic Effects:*
A decrease in glucose tolerance has been observed in a significant percentage of patients on oral contraceptives. For this reason, prediabetic and diabetic patients should be carefully observed while receiving oral contraceptives.

An increase in triglycerides and total phospholipids has been observed in patients receiving oral contraceptives.[44] The clinical significance of this finding remains to be defined.

8. *Elevated Blood Pressure:*
An increase in blood pressure has been reported in patients receiving oral contraceptives.[26] In some women, hypertension may occur within a few months of beginning oral-contraceptive use. In the first year of use, the prevalence of women with hypertension is low in users and may be no higher than that of a comparable group of nonusers. The prevalence in users increases, however, with longer exposure, and in the fifth year of use is two-and-a-half to three times the reported prevalence in the first year. Age is also strongly correlated with the development of hypertension in oral-contraceptive users. Women who previously have had hypertension during pregnancy may be more likely to develop elevation of blood pressure when given oral contraceptives. Hypertension that develops as a result of taking oral contraceptives usually returns to normal after discontinuing the drug.

9. *Headache:*
The onset or exacerbation of migraine or development of headache of a new pattern which is recurrent, persistent, or severe, requires discontinuation of oral contraceptives and evaluation of the cause.

10. *Bleeding Irregularities:*
Breakthrough bleeding, spotting, and amenorrhea are frequent reasons for patients discontinuing oral contraceptives. In breakthrough bleeding, as in all cases of irregular bleeding from the vagina, nonfunctional causes should be borne in mind. In undiagnosed persistent or recurrent abnormal bleeding from the vagina, adequate diagnostic measures are indicated to rule out pregnancy or malignancy. If pathology has been excluded, time or a change to another formulation may solve the problem. Changing to an oral contraceptive with a higher estrogen content, while potentially useful in minimizing menstrual irregularity, should be done only if necessary, since this may increase the risk of thromboembolic disease.

Women with a past history of oligomenorrhea or secondary amenorrhea or young women without regular cycles may have a tendency to remain anovulatory or to become amenorrheic after discontinuation of oral contraceptives. Women with these preexisting problems should be advised of this possibility and encouraged to use other contraceptive methods. Post-use anovulation, possibly prolonged, may also occur in women without previous irregularities.

11. *Ectopic Pregnancy:*
Ectopic as well as intrauterine pregnancy may occur in contraceptive failures. However, in progestogen-only oral contraceptive failures, the ratio of ectopic to intrauterine pregnancies is higher than in women who are not receiving oral contraceptives, since the drugs are more effective in preventing intrauterine than ectopic pregnancies.

12. *Breast-feeding:*
Oral contraceptives given in the postpartum period may interfere with lactation. There may be a decrease in the quantity and quality of the breast milk. Furthermore, a small fraction of the hormonal agents in oral contraceptives has been identified in the milk of mothers receiving these drugs.[45] The effects, if any, on the breast-fed child have not been determined. If feasible, the use of oral contraceptives should be deferred until the infant has been weaned.

PRECAUTIONS

GENERAL

1. A complete medical and family history should be taken prior to initiation of oral contraceptives. The pretreatment and periodic physical examinations should include special reference to blood pressure, breasts, abdomen and pelvic organs, including Papanicolaou smear and relevant laboratory tests. As a general rule, oral contraceptives should not be prescribed for longer than 1 year without another physical examination being performed.
2. Under the influence of estrogen-progestogen preparations, preexisting uterine leiomyomata may increase in size.
3. Patients with a history of psychic depression should be carefully observed and the drug discontinued if depression recurs to a serious degree. Patients becoming significantly depressed while taking oral contraceptives should stop the medication and use an alternate method of contraception in an attempt to determine whether the symptom is drug-related.
4. Oral contraceptives may cause some degree of fluid retention. They should be prescribed with caution, and only with careful monitoring, in patients with conditions which might be aggravated by fluid retention, such as convulsive disorders, migraine syndrome, asthma, or cardiac or renal insufficiency.
5. Patients with a past history of jaundice during pregnancy have an increased risk of recurrence of jaundice while receiving oral-contraceptive therapy. If jaundice develops in any patient receiving such drugs, the medication should be discontinued.
6. Steroid hormones may be poorly metabolized in patients with impaired liver function and should be administered with caution in such patients.
7. Oral-contraceptive users may have disturbances in normal tryptophan metabolism which may result in a relative pyridoxine deficiency. The clinical significance of this is yet to be determined.
8. Serum folate levels may be depressed by oral-contraceptive therapy. Since the pregnant woman is predisposed to the development of folate deficiency and the incidence of folate deficiency increases with increasing gestation, it is possible that if a woman becomes pregnant shortly after stopping oral contraceptives, she may have a greater chance of developing folate deficiency and complications attributed to this deficiency.
9. The pathologist should be advised of oral-contraceptive therapy when relevant specimens are submitted.
10. Certain endocrine- and liver-function tests and blood components may be affected by estrogen-containing oral contraceptives:

a. Increased sulfobromophthalein retention.
b. Increased prothrombin and factors VII, VIII, IX, and X; decreased antithrombin 3; increased norepinephrine-induced platelet aggregability.
c. Increased thyroid-binding globulin (TBG) leading to increased circulating total-thyroid hormone, as measured by protein-bound iodine (PBI), T4 by column, or T4 by radioimmunoassay. Free T3 resin uptake is decreased, reflecting the elevated TBG; free T4 concentration is unaltered.
d. Decreased pregnanediol excretion.
e. Reduced response to metyrapone test.

INFORMATION FOR THE PATIENT

(See Patient Labeling Printed Below.)

DRUG INTERACTIONS

Reduced efficacy and increased incidence of breakthrough bleeding have been associated with concomitant use of rifampin. A similar association has been suggested with barbiturates, phenylbutazone, phenytoin sodium, ampicillin, and tetracycline.

CARCINOGENESIS

See Warnings section for information on the carcinogenic potential of oral contraceptives.

PREGNANCY

Pregnancy Category X. See Contraindications and Warnings.

NURSING MOTHERS

See Warnings.

ADVERSE REACTIONS

An increased risk of the following serious adverse reactions has been associated with the use of oral contraceptives (see Warnings):

- Thrombophlebitis.
- Pulmonary embolism.
- Coronary thrombosis.
- Cerebral thrombosis.
- Cerebral hemorrhage.
- Hypertension.
- Gallbladder disease.
- Benign hepatomas.
- Congenital anomalies.

There is evidence of an association between the following conditions and the use of oral contraceptives, although additional confirmatory studies are needed:

- Mesenteric thrombosis.
- Neuro-ocular lesions, e.g., retinal thrombosis and optic neuritis.

The following adverse reactions have been reported in patients receiving oral contraceptives and are believed to be drug-related:

- Nausea and/or vomiting, usually the most common adverse reactions, occur in approximately 10% or less of patients during the first cycle. Other reactions, as a general rule, are seen much less frequently or only occasionally.
- Gastrointestinal symptoms (such as abdominal cramps and bloating).
- Breakthrough bleeding.
- Spotting.
- Change in menstrual flow.
- Dysmenorrhea.
- Amenorrhea during and after treatment.
- Temporary infertility after discontinuance of treatment.
- Edema.
- Chloasma or melasma which may persist.
- Breast changes: tenderness, enlargement, and secretion.
- Change in weight (increase or decrease).
- Change in cervical erosion and cervical secretion.
- Possible diminution in lactation when given immediately postpartum.
- Cholestatic jaundice.
- Migraine.
- Increase in size of uterine leiomyomata.

Rash (allergic).
Mental depression.
Reduced tolerance to carbohydrates.
Vaginal candidiasis.
Change in corneal curvature (steepening).
Intolerance to contact lenses.

The following adverse reactions have been reported in users of oral contraceptives, and the association has been neither confirmed nor refuted:

Premenstrual-like syndrome.
Cataracts.
Changes in libido.
Chorea.
Changes in appetite.
Cystitis-like syndrome.
Headache.
Nervousness.
Dizziness.
Hirsutism.
Loss of scalp hair.
Erythema multiforme.
Erythema nodosum.
Hemorrhagic eruption.
Vaginitis.
Porphyria.
Hemolytic uremic syndrome.

ACUTE OVERDOSE

Serious ill effects have not been reported following acute ingestion of large doses of oral contraceptives by young children. Overdosage may cause nausea, and withdrawal bleeding may occur in females.

DOSAGE AND ADMINISTRATION

To achieve maximum contraceptive effectiveness, LO/OVRAL must be taken exactly as directed and at intervals not exceeding 24 hours. The dosage of LO/OVRAL is one tablet daily for 21 consecutive days per menstrual cycle according to prescribed schedule. Tablets are then discontinued for 7 days (three weeks on, one week off).

It is recommended that LO/OVRAL tablets be taken at the same time each day, preferably after the evening meal or at bedtime.

During the first cycle of medication, the patient is instructed to take one LO/OVRAL tablet daily for twenty-one consecutive days beginning on day five of her menstrual cycle. (The first day of menstruation is day one.) The tablets are then discontinued for one week (7 days). Withdrawal bleeding should usually occur within three days following discontinuation of LO/OVRAL.

(If LO/OVRAL is first taken later than the fifth day of the first menstrual cycle of medication or postpartum, contraceptive reliance should not be placed on LO/OVRAL until after the first seven consecutive days of administration. The possibility of ovulation and conception prior to initiation of medication should be considered.) The patient begins her next and all subsequent 21-day courses of LO/OVRAL tablets on the same day of the week that she began her first course, following the same schedule: 21 days on—7 days off. She begins taking her tablets on the 8th day after discontinuance regardless of whether or not a menstrual period has occurred or is still in progress. Any time a new cycle of LO/OVRAL is started later than the 8th day the patient should be protected by another means of contraception until she has taken a tablet daily for seven consecutive days.

If spotting or breakthrough bleeding occurs, the patient is instructed to continue on the same regimen. This type of bleeding is usually transient and without significance; however, if the bleeding is persistent or prolonged, the patient is advised to consult her physician. Although the occurrence of pregnancy is highly unlikely if LO/OVRAL is taken according to directions, if withdrawal bleeding does not occur, the possibility of pregnancy must be considered. If the patient has not adhered to the prescribed schedule (missed one or more tablets or started taking them on a day later than she should have) the probability of pregnancy should be considered at the time of the first missed period and appropriate diagnostic measures taken before the medication is resumed. If the patient has adhered to the prescribed regimen and misses two consecutive periods, pregnancy should be ruled out before continuing the contraceptive regimen.

The patient should be instructed to take a missed tablet as soon as it is remembered. If two consecutive tablets are missed they should both be taken as soon as remembered. The next tablet should be taken at the usual time.

Any time the patient misses one or two tablets she should also use another method of contraception until she has taken a tablet daily for seven consecutive days. If breakthrough bleeding occurs following missed tablets it will usually be transient and of no consequence. While there is little likelihood of ovulation occurring if only one or two tablets are missed, the possibility of ovulation increases with each successive day that scheduled tablets are missed. If three consecutive tablets are missed, all medication should be discontinued and the remainder of the package discarded. A new tablet cycle should be started on the 8th day after the last tablet was taken, and an alternate means of contraception should be prescribed during the seven days without tablets and until the patient has taken a tablet daily for seven consecutive days. In the nonlactating mother, LO/OVRAL may be prescribed in the postpartum period either immediately or at the first postpartum examination whether or not menstruation has resumed.

HOW SUPPLIED

LO/OVRAL® tablets (0.3 mg norgestrel and 0.03 mg ethinyl estradiol), Wyeth®, are available in packages of 6 PIL-PAK® dispensers with 21 tablets each and in 3-PAK packages containing 63 tablets each as follows:
NDC 0008-0078, white, round tablet marked "WYETH" and "78".

ALSO AVAILABLE

LO/OVRAL®-28 tablets in containers of 28 tablets, consisting of 21 white LO/OVRAL® tablets (0.3 mg norgestrel and 0.03 mg ethinyl estradiol) and 7 pink inert tablets.

REFERENCES

1. "Population Reports," Series H, Number 2, May 1974; Series I, Number 1, June 1974; Series B, Number 2, January 1975; Series H, Number 3, 1975; Series H, Number 4, January 1976 (published by the Population Information Program, The George Washington University Medical Center, 2001 S St. NW., Washington, D.C.).
2. Inman, W. H. W., Vessey, M. P., Westerholm, B., and Engelund, A., "Thromboembolic disease and the steroidal content of oral contraceptives. A report to the Committee on Safety of Drugs," Brit Med J *2*:203–209, 1970.
3. Stolley, P. D., Tonascia, J. A., Tockman, M. S., Sartwell, P. E., Rutledge, A. H., and Jacobs, M. P., "Thrombosis with low-estrogen oral contraceptives," Am J Epidemiol *102*:197–208, 1975.
4. Royal College of General Practitioners, "Oral contraception and thromboembolic disease," J Coll Gen Pract *13*:267–279, 1967.
5. Inman, W. H. W., and Vessey, M. P., "Investigation of deaths from pulmonary, coronary and cerebral thrombosis and embolism in women of childbearing age," Brit Med J *2*:193–199, 1968.
6. Vessey, M. P., and Doll, R., "Investigation of relation between use of oral contraceptives and thromboembolic disease. A further report," Brit Med J *2*:651–657, 1969.
7. Sartwell, P. E., Masi, A. T., Arthes, F. G., Greene, G. R., and Smith, H. E., "Thromboembolism and oral contraceptives: an epidemiological case control study," Am J Epidemiol *90*:365–380, 1969.
8. Boston Collaborative Drug Surveillance Program, "Oral contraceptives and venous thromboembolic disease, surgically confirmed gallbladder disease and breast tumors," Lancet *1*:1399–1404, 1973.
9. Collaborative Group for the Study of Stroke in Young Women, "Oral contraception and increased risk of cerebral ischemia or thrombosis," N Engl J Med *288*:871–878, 1973.
10. Collaborative Group for the Study of Stroke in Young Women, "Oral contraceptives and stroke in young women: associated risk factors," JAMA *231*:718–722, 1975.
11. Mann, J. I., and Inman, W. H. W., "Oral contraceptives and death from myocardial infarction," Brit Med J *2*:245–248, 1975.
12. Mann, J. I., Inman, W. H. W., and Thorogood, M., "Oral contraceptive use in older women and fatal myocardial infarction," Brit Med J *2*:445–447, 1976.
13. Mann, J. I., Vessey, M. P., Thorogood, M., and Doll, R., "Myocardial infarction in young women with special reference to oral contraceptive practice," Brit Med J *2*:241–245, 1975.
14. Tietze, C., "New Estimates of Mortality Associated with Fertility Control," Family Planning Perspectives, *9*:74–76, 1977.
15. Vessey, M. P., Doll, R., Fairbairn, A. S., and Glober, G., "Post-operative thromboembolism and the use of oral contraceptives," Brit Med J *3*:123–126, 1970.
16. Greene, G. R., Sartwell, P. E., "Oral contraceptive use in patients with thromboembolism following surgery, trauma, or infection," Am J Pub Health *62*:680–685, 1972.
17. Smith, D. C., Prentice, R., Thompson, D. J., and Herrmann, W. L., "Association of exogenous estrogen and endometrial carcinoma," N Engl J Med *293*:1164–1167, 1975.
18. Ziel, H. K., and Finkle, W. D., "Increased risk of endometrial carcinoma among users of conjugated estrogens," N Engl J Med *293*:1167–1170, 1975.
19. Mack, T. N., Pike, M. C., Henderson, B. E., Pfeffer, R. I., Gerkins, V. R., Arthur, M., and Brown, S. E., "Estrogens and endometrial cancer in a retirement community," N Engl J Med *294*:1262–1267, 1976.
20. Silverberg, S. G., and Makowski, E. L., "Endometrial carcinoma in young women taking oral contraceptive agents," Obstet Gynecol *46*:503–506, 1975.
21. Vessey, M. P., Doll, R., and Sutton, P. M., "Oral contraceptives and breast neoplasia: a retrospective study," Brit Med J *3*:719–724, 1972.
22. Vessey, M. P., Doll, R., and Jones K., "Oral contraceptives and breast cancer. Progress report of an epidemiological study," Lancet *1*:941–943, 1975.
23. Boston Collaborative Drug Surveillance Program, "Surgically confirmed gallbladder disease, venous thromboembolism and breast tumors in relation to postmenopausal estrogen therapy," N Engl J Med *290*:15–19, 1974.
24. Arthes, F. G., Sartwell, P. E., and Lewison, E. F., "The pill, estrogens, and the breast. Epidemiologic aspects," Cancer *28*:1391–1394, 1971.
25. Fasal, E., and Paffenbarger, R. S., "Oral contraceptives as related to cancer and benign lesions of the breast," J Natl Cancer Inst *55*:767–773, 1975.
26. Royal College of General Practitioners, "Oral Contraceptives and Health," London, Pitman, 1974.
27. Ory, H., Cole P., MacMahon, B., and Hoover, R., "Oral contraceptives and reduced risk of benign breast diseases," N Engl J Med *294*:419–422, 1976.
28. Baum, J., Holtz, F., Bookstein, J. J., and Klein, E. W., "Possible association between benign hepatomas and oral contraceptives," Lancet *2*:926–928, 1973.
29. Mays, E. T., Christopherson, W. M., Mahr, M. M., and Williams, H. C., "Hepatic changes in young women ingesting contraceptive steroids. Hepatic hemorrhage and primary hepatic tumors," JAMA *235*:730–732, 1976.
30. Edmondson, H. A., Henderson, B., and Benton, B., "Liver-cell adenomas associated with use of oral contraceptives," N Engl J Med *294*:470–472, 1976.
31. Herbst, A. L., Ulfedler, H., and Poskanzer, D. C., "Adenocarcinoma of the vagina," N Engl J Med *284*:878–881, 1971.
32. Greenwald, P., Barlow, J. J., Nasca, P. C., and Burnett, W., "Vaginal cancer after maternal treatment with synthetic estrogens," N Engl J Med *285*:390–392, 1971.
33. Lanier, A. P., Noller, K. L., Decker, D. G., Elveback, L., and Kurland, L. T., "Cancer and stilbestrol. A follow-up of 1719 persons exposed to estrogens in utero and born 1943–1959," Mayo Clin Pro *48*:793–799, 1973.
34. Herbst, A. L., Kurman, R. J., and Scully, R. E., "Vaginal and cervical abnormalities after exposure to stilbestrol in utero," Obstet Gynecol *40*:287–298, 1972.
35. Herbst, A. L., Robboy, S. J., Macdonald, G. J., and Scully, R. E., "The effects of local progesterone on stilbestrol-associated vaginal adenosis," Am J Obstet Gynecol *118*:607–615, 1974.
36. Herbst, A. L., Poskanzer, D. C., Robboy, S. J., Friedlander, L., and Scully, R. E., "Prenatal exposure to stilbestrol: a prospective comparison of exposed female offspring with unexposed controls," N Engl J Med *292*:334–339, 1975.
37. Stafl, A., Mattingly, R. F., Foley, D. V., Fetherston, W., "Clinical diagnosis of vaginal adenosis," Obstet Gynecol *43*:118–128, 1974.
38. Sherman, A. I., Goldrath, M., Berlin, A., Vakhariya, V., Banooni, F., Michaels, W., Goodman, P., and Brown, S., "Cervical-vaginal adenosis after in utero exposure to synthetic estrogens," Obstet Gynecol *44*:531–545, 1974.
39. Gal, I., Kirman, B., and Stern, J., "Hormone pregnancy tests and congenital malformation," Nature *216*:83, 1967.
40. Levy, E. P., Cohen, A., and Fraser, F. C., "Hormone treatment during pregnancy and congenital heart defects," Lancet *1*:611, 1973.
41. Nora, J. J., and Nora, A. H., "Birth defects and oral contraceptives," Lancet *1*:941–942, 1973.
42. Janerich, D. T., Piper, J. M., and Glebatis, D. M., "Oral contraceptives and congenital limb-reduction defects," N Engl J Med *291*:697–700, 1974.
43. Carr, D. H., "Chromosome studies in selected spontaneous abortions: I. Conception after oral contraceptives," Canad Med Assoc J *103*:343–348, 1970.
44. Wynn, V., Doar, J. W. H., and Mills, G. L., "Some effects of oral contraceptives on serum-lipid and lipoprotein levels," Lancet *2*:720–723, 1966.
45. Laumas, K. R., Malkani, P. K., Bhatnagar, S., and Laumas, V., "Radioactivity in the breast milk of lactating women after oral administration of 3 H-norethynodrel," Amer J Obstet Gynecol *98*:411–413, 1967.
46. Center for Disease Control, "Increased Risk of Hepatocellular Adenoma in Women with Long-term use of Oral Contraceptives," Morbidity and Mortality Weekly Report, *26*:293–294, 1977.
47. Herbst, A. L., Cole, P., Colton, T., Robboy, S. J., Scully, R. E., "Age-incidence and Risk of Diethylstilbestrol-related Clear Cell Adenocarcinoma of the Vagina and Cervix," Am. J. Obstet. Gynecol., *128*:43–50, 1977.
48. Bibbo, M., Al-Naqeeb, M., Baccarini, I., Gill, W., Newton, M., Sleeper, K. M., Sonek, M., Wied, G. L., "Follow-up Study of Male and Female Offspring of DES-treated Mothers. A Preliminary Report," Jour. of Repro. Med., *15*:29–32, 1975.
49. Gill, W. B., Schumacher, G. F. B., Bibbo, M., "Structural and Functional Abnormalities in the Sex Organs of Male Offspring of Mothers Treated with Diethylstilbestrol (DES)," Jour. of Repro. Med., *16*:147–153, 1976.
50. Henderson, B. E., Senton, B., Cosgrove, M., Baptista, J., Aldrich, J., Townsend, D., Hart, W., Mack, T., "Urogenital

Continued on next page

Wyeth—Cont.

Tract Abnormalities in Sons of Women Treated with Diethylstilbestrol," Pediatrics, *58*:505–507, 1976.

51. Heinonen, O. P., Slone, D., Nonson, R. R., Hook, E. B., Shapiro, S., "Cardiovascular Birth Defects and Antenatal Exposure to Female Sex Hormones," N. Engl. J. Med., *296*:67–70, 1977.

52. Jain, A. K., "Mortality Risk Associated with the Use of Oral Contraceptives," Studies in Family Planning, *8*:50–54, 1977.

53. Beral, V., "Mortality Among Oral Contraceptive Users," Lancet, *2*:727–731, 1977.

54. Royal College of General Practitioners' Oral contraception study, "Incidence of arterial disease among oral contraceptive users," J Royal Col Gen Pract *33*:75-82, 1983.

55. Slone, D., Shapiro, S., Kaufman, D. W., Rosenberg, L., Miettinen, O., and Stolley, P., "Risk of myocardial infarction in relation to current and discontinued use of oral contraceptives," N Engl J Med *305*:420-424, 1981.

56. Inman, W.H.W., "Oral contraceptives and fatal subarachnoid haemorrhage," Brit Med J 2:1468-1470, 1979.

57. Petitti, D. B., and Wingerd, J., "Use of oral contraceptives, cigarette smoking and risk of subarachnoid haemorrhage," Lancet *2*:234-236, 1978.

58. Thorogood, M., Adam, S. A., and Mann, J. I., "Fatal subarachnoid haemorrhage in young women: role of oral contraceptives," Brit Med J *283*:762, 1981.

59. Rosenberg, L., Hennekens, C.H., Rosner, B., Belanger, C., Rothman, K. J., and Speizer, F. E., "Oral contraceptive use in relation to nonfatal myocardial infarction," Am J Epidemiol *111*:59-66, 1980.

60. Adam, S. A., Thorogood, M., and Mann, J. I., "Oral contraception and myocardial infarction revisited: the effects of new preparations and prescribing patterns," Brit J Obstet Gynaecol *88*:838-845, 1981.

The patient labeling for oral-contraceptive drug products is set forth below:

Brief Summary Patient Package Insert

Cigarette smoking increases the risk of serious adverse effects on the heart and blood vessels from oral-contraceptive use. This risk increases with age and with heavy smoking (15 or more cigarettes per day) and is quite marked in women over 35 years of age. Women who use oral contraceptives should not smoke.

Oral contraceptives taken as directed are about 99% effective in preventing pregnancy. (The mini-pill, however, is somewhat less effective.) Forgetting to take your pills increases the chance of pregnancy. Women who have or have had clotting disorders, cancer of the breast or sex organs, unexplained vaginal bleeding, a stroke, heart attack, angina pectoris, or who suspect they may be pregnant should not use oral contraceptives. Various drugs, such as some antibiotics, may also decrease the effectiveness of oral contraceptives.

Most side effects of the pill are not serious. The most common side effects are nausea, vomiting, bleeding between menstrual periods, weight gain, and breast tenderness. However, proper use of oral contraceptives requires that they be taken under your doctor's continuous supervision, because they can be associated with serious side effects which may be fatal. Fortunately, these occur very infrequently. The serious side effects are:

1. Blood clots in the legs, lungs, brain, heart, or other organs, and hemorrhage into the brain due to bursting of a blood vessel. Certain of these effects may occur after pill use has been stopped.
2. Liver tumors, which may rupture and cause severe bleeding.
3. Birth defects if the pill is taken while you are pregnant.
4. High blood pressure.
5. Gallbladder disease.

The symptoms associated with these serious side effects are discussed in the detailed leaflet given you with your supply of pills. Notify your doctor if you notice any unusual physical disturbance while taking the pill.

The estrogen in oral contraceptives has been found to cause breast cancer and other cancers in certain animals. These findings suggest that oral contraceptives may also cause cancer in humans. However, studies to date in women taking currently marketed oral contraceptives have not confirmed that oral contraceptives cause cancer in humans.

The detailed leaflet describes more completely the benefits and risks of oral contraceptives. It also provides information on other forms of contraception. Read it carefully. If you have any questions, consult your doctor.

CAUTION

Oral contraceptives are of no value in the prevention or treatment of venereal disease.

DETAILED PATIENT LABELING

WHAT YOU SHOULD KNOW ABOUT ORAL CONTRACEPTIVES

Oral contraceptives ("the pill") are the most effective way (except for sterilization) to prevent pregnancy. They are also convenient and, for most women, free of serious or unpleasant side effects. Oral contraceptives must always be taken under the continuous supervision of a physician.

It is important that any woman who considers using an oral contraceptive understand the risks involved. Although the oral contraceptives have important advantages over other methods of contraception, they have certain risks that no other method has. Only you can decide whether the advantages are worth these risks. This leaflet will tell you about the most important risks. It will explain how you can help your doctor prescribe the pill as safely as possible by telling him about yourself and being alert for the earliest signs of trouble. And it will tell you how to use the pill properly, so that it will be as effective as possible. There is more detailed information available in the leaflet prepared for doctors. Your pharmacist can show you a copy; you may need your doctor's help in understanding parts of it.

WHO SHOULD NOT USE ORAL CONTRACEPTIVES

A. If you have any of the following conditions, you should not use the pill:

1. Clots in the legs or lungs.
2. Angina pectoris.
3. Known or suspected cancer of the breast or sex organs.
4. Unusual vaginal bleeding that has not yet been diagnosed.
5. Known or suspected pregnancy.

B. If you have had any of the following conditions, you should not use the pill:

1. Heart attack or stroke.
2. Clots in the legs or lungs.

C. Cigarette smoking increases the risk of serious adverse effects on the heart and blood vessels from oral-contraceptive use. This risk increases with age and with heavy smoking (15 or more cigarettes per day) and is quite marked in women over 35 years of age. Women who use oral contraceptives should not smoke.

D. If you have scanty or irregular periods or are a young woman without a regular cycle, you should use another method of contraception because, if you use the pill, you may have difficulty becoming pregnant or may fail to have menstrual periods after discontinuing the pill.

DECIDING TO USE ORAL CONTRACEPTIVES

If you do not have any of the conditions listed above and are thinking about using oral contraceptives, to help you decide, you need information about the advantages and risks of oral contraceptives and of other contraceptive methods as well. This leaflet describes the advantages and risks of oral contraceptives. Except for sterilization, the IUD, and abortion, which have their own inherent risks, the only risks of other methods of contraception are those due to pregnancy should the method fail. Your doctor can answer questions you may have with respect to other methods of contraception. He can also answer any questions you may have after reading this leaflet on oral contraceptives.

1. What Oral Contraceptives Are and How They Work. Oral contraceptives are of two types. The most common, often simply called "the pill," is a combination of an estrogen and a progestogen, the two kinds of female hormones. The amount of estrogen and progestogen can vary, but the amount of estrogen is most important because both the effectiveness and some of the dangers of oral contraceptives are related to the amount of estrogen. This kind of oral contraceptive works principally by preventing release of an egg from the ovary. When the amount of estrogen is 50 micrograms or more, and the pill is taken as directed, oral contraceptives are more than 99% effective (i.e., there would be less than 1 pregnancy if 100 women used the pill for 1 year). Pills that contain 20 to 35 micrograms of estrogen vary slightly in effectiveness, ranging from 98% to more than 99% effective.

The second type of oral contraceptive, often called the "mini-pill", contains only a progestogen. It works in part by preventing release of an egg from the ovary but also by keeping sperm from reaching the egg and by making the uterus (womb) less receptive to any fertilized egg that reaches it. The mini-pill is less effective than the combination oral contraceptive, about 97% effective. In addition, the progestogen-only pill has a tendency to cause irregular bleeding which may be quite inconvenient, or cessation of bleeding entirely. The progestogen-only pill is used despite its lower effectiveness in the hope that it will prove not to have some of the serious side effects of the estrogen-containing pill (see below), but it is not yet certain that the mini-pill does in fact have fewer serious side effects. The discussion below, while based mainly on information about the combination pills, should be considered to apply as well to the mini-pill.

2. Other Nonsurgical Ways to Prevent Pregnancy. As this leaflet will explain, oral contraceptives have several serious risks. Other methods of contraception have lesser risks or none at all. They are also less effective than oral contraceptives, but, used properly, may be effective enough for many women.

The following table gives reported pregnancy rates (the number of women out of 100 who would become pregnant in 1 year) for these methods.

PREGNANCIES PER 100 WOMEN PER YEAR

Intrauterine device (IUD), less than 1-6; Diaphragm with spermicidal products (creams or jellies), 2-20; Condom (rubber), 3-36; Aerosol foams, 2-29; Jellies and creams, 4-36;

Periodic abstinence (rhythm) all types, less than 1-47:

1. Calendar method, 14-47;
2. Temperature method, 1-20;
3. Temperature method—intercourse only in postovulatory phase, less than 1-7;
4. Mucus method, 1-25;

No contraception, 60-80.

The figures (except for the IUD) vary widely because people differ in how well they use each method. Very faithful users of the various methods obtain very good results, except for users of the calendar method of periodic abstinence (rhythm). Except for the IUD, effective use of these methods requires somewhat more effort than simply taking a single pill every day, but it is an effort that many couples undertake successfully. Your doctor can tell you a great deal more about these methods of contraception.

3. The Dangers of Oral Contraceptives.

a. *Circulatory disorders (abnormal blood clotting and stroke due to hemorrhage).*

Blood clots (in various blood vessels of the body) are the most common of the serious side effects of oral contraceptives. A clot can result in a stroke (if the clot is in the brain), a heart attack (if the clot is in a blood vessel of the heart), or a pulmonary embolus (a clot which forms in the legs or pelvis, then breaks off and travels to the lungs). Any of these can be fatal. Clots also occur rarely in the blood vessels of the eye, resulting in blindness or impairment of vision in that eye. There is evidence that the risk of clotting increases with higher estrogen doses. It is therefore important to keep the dose of estrogen as low as possible, so long as the oral contraceptive used has an acceptable pregnancy rate and doesn't cause unacceptable changes in the menstrual pattern. Furthermore, cigarette smoking by oral-contraceptive users increases the risk of serious adverse effects on the heart and blood vessels. This risk increases with age and with heavy smoking (15 or more cigarettes per day) and begins to become quite marked in women over 35 years of age. For this reason, women who use oral contraceptives should not smoke.

The risk of abnormal clotting increases with age in both users and nonusers of oral contraceptives, but the increased risk from the oral contraceptive appears to be present at all ages.

Figure 1. Estimated annual number of deaths associated with control of fertility and no control per 100,000 nonsterile women, by regimen of control and age of woman.

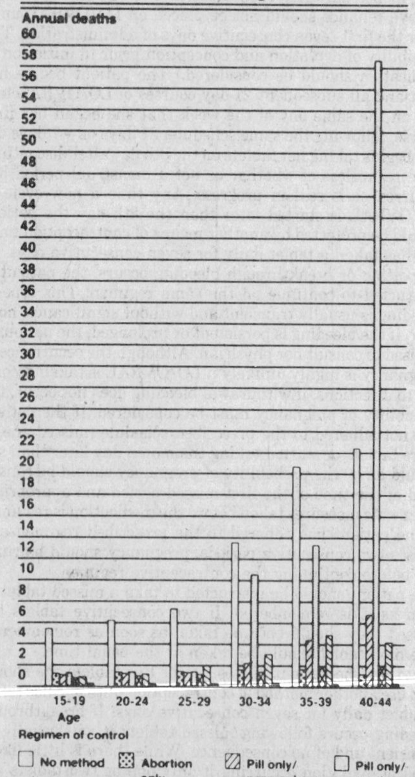

For oral-contraceptive users in general, it has been estimated that in women between the ages of 15 and 34 the risk of death due to a circulatory disorder is about 1 in 12,000 per year, whereas for nonusers the risk is about 1 in 50,000 per year. In the age group 35 to 44, the risk is estimated to be about 1 in 2,500 per year for oral-contraceptive users and about 1 in 10,000 per year for nonusers.

Even without the pill the risk of having a heart attack increases with age and is also increased by such heart attack risk factors as high blood pressure, high cholesterol, obesity, diabetes, and cigarette smoking. Without any risk factors present, the use of oral contraceptives alone may double the risk of heart attack. However, the combination of cigarette smoking, especially heavy smoking, and oral contraceptive use greatly increases the risk of heart attack. Oral-contraceptive users who smoke are about 5 times more likely to have a heart attack than users who do not smoke and about 10 times more likely to have a heart attack than nonusers who do not smoke. It has been estimated that users between the ages of 30 and 39 who smoke have about a 1 in 10,000 chance each year of having a fatal heart attack compared to about a 1 in 50,000 chance in users who do not smoke, and about a 1 in 100,000 chance in nonusers who do not smoke. In the age group 40 to 44, the risk is about 1 in 1,700 per year for users who smoke compared to about 1 in 10,000 for users who do not smoke and to about 1 in 14,000 per year for nonusers who do not smoke. Heavy smoking (about 15 cigarettes or more a day) further increases the risk. If you do not smoke and have none of the other heart attack risk factors described above, you will have a smaller risk than listed. If you have several heart attack risk factors, the risk may be considerably greater than listed. In addition to blood-clotting disorders, it has been estimated that women taking oral contraceptives are twice as likely as nonusers to have a stroke due to rupture of a blood vessel in the brain. There is evidence that patients who stop taking oral contraceptives after using them continuously for five or more years may continue to have an increased risk of stroke or heart attack for at least six to nine years after discontinuation.

b. *Formation of tumors.* Studies have found that when certain animals are given the female sex hormone, estrogen, which is an ingredient of oral contraceptives, continuously for long periods, cancers may develop in the breast, cervix, vagina, and liver.

These findings suggest that oral contraceptives may cause cancer in humans. However, studies to date in women taking currently marketed oral contraceptives have not confirmed that oral contraceptives cause cancer in humans. Several studies have found no increase in breast cancer in users, although one study suggested oral contraceptives might cause an increase in breast cancer in women who already have benign breast disease (e.g., cysts).

Women with a strong family history of breast cancer or who have breast nodules, fibrocystic disease, or abnormal mammograms or who were exposed to DES (Diethylstilbestrol), an estrogen, during their mother's pregnancy must be followed very closely by their doctors if they choose to use oral contraceptives instead of another method of contraception. Many studies have shown that women taking oral contraceptives have less risk of getting benign breast disease than those who have not used oral contraceptives. Recently, strong evidence has emerged that estrogens (one component of oral contraceptives), when given for periods of more than one year to women after the menopause, increase the risk of cancer of the uterus (womb). There is also some evidence that a kind of oral contraceptive which is no longer marketed, the sequential oral contraceptive, may increase the risk of cancer of the uterus. There remains no evidence, however, that the oral contraceptives now available increase the risk of this cancer. Oral contraceptives do cause, although rarely, a benign (nonmalignant) tumor of the liver. These tumors do not spread, but they may rupture and cause internal bleeding, which may be fatal. A few cases of cancer of the liver have been reported in women using oral contraceptives, but it is not yet known whether the drug caused them.

c. *Dangers to a developing child if oral contraceptives are used in or immediately preceding pregnancy.* Oral contraceptives should not be taken by pregnant women because they may damage the developing child. An increased risk of birth defects, including heart defects and limb defects, has been associated with the use of sex hormones, including oral contraceptives, in pregnancy. In addition, the developing female child whose mother has received DES (diethylstilbestrol), an estrogen, during pregnancy has a risk of getting cancer of the vagina or cervix in her teens or young adulthood. This risk is estimated to be about 1 in 1,000 exposures or less. Abnormalities of the urinary and sex organs have been reported in male offspring so exposed. It is possible that other estrogens, such as the estrogens in oral contraceptives, could have the same effect in the child if the mother takes them during pregnancy.

If you stop taking oral contraceptives to become pregnant, your doctor may recommend that you use another method of contraception for a short while. The reason for this is that there is evidence from studies in women who have had "miscarriages" soon after stopping the pill, that the lost fetuses are more likely to be abnormal. Whether there is an overall increase in "miscarriage" in women who become pregnant soon after stopping the pill as compared with women who do not use the pill is not known, but it is possible that there may be. If, however, you do become pregnant soon after stopping oral contraceptives, and do not have a miscarriage, there is no evidence that the baby has an increased risk of being abnormal.

d. *Gallbladder disease.* Women who use oral contraceptives have a greater risk than nonusers of having gallbladder disease requiring surgery. The increased risk may first appear within 1 year of use and may double after 4 or 5 years of use.

e. *Other side effects of oral contraceptives.* Some women using oral contraceptives experience unpleasant side effects that are not dangerous and are not likely to damage their health. Some of these may be temporary. Your breasts may feel tender, nausea and vomiting may occur, you may gain or lose weight, and your ankles may swell. A spotty darkening of the skin, particularly of the face, is possible and may persist. You may notice unexpected vaginal bleeding or changes in your menstrual period. Irregular bleeding is frequently seen when using the mini-pill or combination oral contraceptives containing less than 50 micrograms of estrogen.

More serious side effects include worsening of migraine, asthma, epilepsy, and kidney or heart disease because of a tendency for water to be retained in the body when oral contraceptives are used. Other side effects are growth of preexisting fibroid tumors of the uterus; mental depression, and liver problems with jaundice (yellowing of the skin). Your doctor may find that levels of sugar and fatty substances in your blood are elevated; the long-term effects of these changes are not known. Some women develop high blood pressure while taking oral contraceptives, which ordinarily returns to the original levels when the oral contraceptive is stopped.

Other reactions, although not proved to be caused by oral contraceptives, are occasionally reported. These include more frequent urination and some discomfort when urinating, blood-cell breakdown with kidney failure, nervousness, dizziness, some loss of scalp hair, an increase in body hair, an increase or decrease in sex drive, appetite changes, cataracts, and a need for a change in contact lens prescription, or inability to use contact lenses.

After you stop using oral contraceptives, there may be a delay before you are able to become pregnant or before you resume having menstrual periods. This is especially true of women who had irregular menstrual cycles prior to the use of oral contraceptives. As discussed previously, your doctor may recommend that you wait a short while after stopping the pill before you try to become pregnant. During this time, use another form of contraception. You should consult your physician before resuming use of oral contraceptives after childbirth, especially if you plan to nurse your baby. Drugs in oral contraceptives are known to appear in the milk, and the long-range effect on infants is not known at this time. Furthermore, oral contraceptives may cause a decrease in your milk supply as well as in the quality of the milk.

4. Comparison of the Risks of Oral Contraceptives and Other Contraceptive Methods. The many studies on the risks and effectiveness of oral contraceptives and other methods of contraception have been analyzed to estimate the risk of death associated with various methods of contraception. This risk has two parts: (a) the risk of the method itself (e.g., the risk that oral contraceptives will cause death due to abnormal clotting), and (b) the risk of death due to pregnancy or abortion in the event the method fails. The results of this analysis are shown in the bar graph (Figure 1). The height of the bars is the number of deaths per 100,000 women each year. There are six sets of bars, each set referring to a specific age group of women. Within each set of bars, there is a single bar for each of the different contraceptive methods. For oral contraceptives, there are two bars—one for smokers and the other for nonsmokers. The analysis is based on present knowledge, and new information could, of course, alter it. The analysis shows that the risk of death from all methods of birth control is low and below that associated with childbirth, except for oral contraceptives in women over 40 who smoke. It shows that the lowest risk of death is associated with the condom or diaphragm (traditional contraception) backed up by early abortion in case of failure of the condom or diaphragm to prevent pregnancy. Also, at any age the risk of death (due to unexpected pregnancy) from the use of traditional contraception, even without a backup of abortion, is generally the same as or less than that from use of oral contraceptives.

HOW TO USE ORAL CONTRACEPTIVES AS SAFELY AND EFFECTIVELY AS POSSIBLE, ONCE YOU HAVE DECIDED TO USE THEM

1. What to Tell your Doctor.

You can make use of the pill as safely as possible by telling your doctor if you have any of the following:

a. Conditions that mean you should not use oral contraceptives:

Clots in the legs or lungs.
Clots in the legs or lungs in the past.
A stroke, heart attack, or angina pectoris.
Known or suspected cancer of the breast or sex organs.
Unusual vaginal bleeding that has not yet been diagnosed.
Known or suspected pregnancy.

b. Conditions that your doctor will want to watch closely or which might cause him to suggest another method of contraception:

A family history of breast cancer.
Breast nodules, fibrocystic disease of the breast, or an abnormal mammogram.

Diabetes.	Heart or kidney disease.
High blood pressure.	Epilepsy.
High cholesterol.	Mental depression.
Cigarette smoking.	Fibroid tumors of the uterus.
Migraine headaches.	Gallbladder disease.

c. Once you are using oral contraceptives, you should be alert for signs of a serious adverse effect and call your doctor if they occur.

Sharp pain in the chest, coughing blood, or sudden shortness of breath (indicating possible clots in the lungs).
Pain in the calf (possible clot in the leg).
Crushing chest pain or heaviness (indicating possible heart attack).
Sudden severe headache or vomiting, dizziness or fainting, disturbance of vision or speech, or weakness or numbness in an arm or leg (indicating a possible stroke).
Sudden partial or complete loss of vision (indicating a possible clot in the eye).
Breast lumps (you should ask your doctor to show you how to examine your own breasts).
Severe pain in the abdomen (indicating a possible ruptured tumor of the liver).
Severe depression.
Yellowing of the skin (jaundice).

2. How to Take the Pill So That It is Most Effective.

Reduced effectiveness and an increased incidence of breakthrough bleeding have been associated with the use of oral contraceptives with antibiotics such as rifampin, ampicillin, and tetracycline or with certain other drugs such as barbiturates, phenylbutazone or phenytoin sodium. You should use an additional means of contraception during any cycle in which any of these drugs are taken.

To achieve maximum contraceptive effectiveness, oral contraceptives must be taken exactly as directed and at intervals not exceeding 24 hours. It is recommended that tablets be taken at the same time each day, preferably after the evening meal or at bedtime. Taking them on a definite schedule will decrease the chance of forgetting a tablet and also help keep the proper amount of medication in your system. See detailed instructions below for Nordette-21, Ovral® and Lo/Ovral®, Nordette-28, Ovral®-28 and Lo/Ovral®-28, and for Ovrette®.

NORDETTE®-21,OVRAL®, LO/OVRAL®

The dosage of Nordette-21,Ovral and Lo/Ovral is one tablet daily for 21 days in a row per menstrual cycle. Tablets are then discontinued for 7 days.

The basic schedule is 21 days on—7 days off.

During the first month, you should begin taking Nordette-21, Ovral or Lo/Ovral on Day 5 of your menstrual cycle whether or not you still have your period. (Day 1 is the first day of menstruation, even if it is almost midnight when you start.)

Note: During your first month on Nordette-21, Ovral or Lo/Ovral, if you start taking tablets later than Day 5 of your menstrual cycle, you should protect yourself by also using another method of birth control until you have taken a tablet daily for seven consecutive days. Thereafter, if you follow directions carefully you will obtain the full contraceptive benefit. If you begin taking tablets later than the proper day, the possibility of ovulation and pregnancy occurring before beginning medication should be considered.

Take one tablet every day until you finish all 21 tablets. No tablets are then taken for one week (7 days). Your period will usually begin about three days after you take the last tablet. Don't be alarmed if the amount of bleeding is not the same as before. On the 8th day, start a new Pilpak®, even if you still have your period. If, for example, you took Nordette-21, Ovral or Lo/Ovral for the first time on a Tuesday, the 8th day will also be a Tuesday. Thus, you will always begin a new cycle on the same day of the week as long as you do not interrupt your original schedule. If you start taking tablets later than the 8th day, you should protect yourself by also using another method of birth control until you have taken a tablet daily for seven days in a row.

NORDETTE®-28, OVRAL®-28, LO/OVRAL®-28

The dosage of Nordette-28, Ovral-28 and Lo/Ovral-28 is one white or light-orange active tablet daily for 21 consecutive days followed by one pink inactive tablet daily for 7 consecutive days. The basic schedule is 21 days on white or light-orange active tablets—7 days on pink inactive tablets. Always take all 21 white or light-orange tablets in each Pilpak before taking the pink tablets.

You should begin taking Nordette-28, Ovral-28 or Lo/Ovral-28 on the first Sunday after your menstrual period

Continued on next page

Wyeth—Cont.

begins, whether or not you are still bleeding. If your period begins on a Sunday, take your first tablet that very same day. Your first white or light-orange tablet is marked with a large arrow and the word "Start". Note: During your first month on Nordette-28, Ovral-28 or Lo/Ovral-28, you should protect yourself by also using another method of birth control until you have taken a white or light-orange tablet daily for seven consecutive days. Thereafter, if you follow directions carefully, you will obtain the full contraceptive benefit.
If you begin taking tablets later than the proper day, the possibility of ovulation and pregnancy occurring before beginning medication should be considered. Take one tablet every day until you finish all 21 white or light-orange tablets in a Pilpak, followed by all seven pink tablets. Your period will usually begin about three days after you take the last white or light-orange tablet, which will be during the time you are taking the pink tablets. Don't be alarmed if the amount of bleeding is not the same as before. The day after you have taken your last pink tablet, begin a new Pilpak of tablets (taking all 21 white or light-orange tablets first, just as you did before) so that you will take a tablet every day without interruption. The starting day for each new Pilpak will always be Sunday. If in any cycle you start tablets later than the proper day, you should also use another method of birth control until you have taken a white or light-orange tablet daily for 7 days in a row.
Spotting or Breakthrough Bleeding:
Spotting is slight staining between menstrual periods which may not even require a pad. Breakthrough bleeding is a flow much like a regular period, requiring sanitary protection. Spotting is more common than breakthrough bleeding, and both occur more often in the first few cycles than in later cycles. These types of bleeding are usually temporary and without significance. It is important to continue taking your pills on schedule. If the bleeding persists for more than a few days, consult your doctor.
Forgotten Pills:
Nordette-21, Ovral and Lo/Ovral each contain 21 active white or light-orange tablets per Pilpak. Nordette-28, Ovral-28 and Lo/Ovral -28 each contain 21 active white or light-orange tablets plus 7 pink inactive tablets per Pilpak.
The chance of becoming pregnant is probably quite small if you miss only one white or light-orange tablet in a cycle. Of course, with each additional one you skip, the chance increases. If you miss one or more pink tablets (Nordette-28, Ovral-28, Lo/Ovral-28) you are still protected against pregnancy as long as you begin taking your next white or light-orange tablet on the proper day. It is important to take a missed white or light-orange tablet as soon as it is remembered. If two consecutive white or light-orange tablets are missed they should both be taken as soon as remembered. The next tablet should then be taken at the usual time. Any time you miss one or two white or light-orange tablets, or begin a new Pilpak after the proper starting day, you should also use another method of birth control until you have taken a white or light-orange tablet daily for seven consecutive days. If breakthrough bleeding occurs following missed tablets, it will usually be temporary and of no consequence. While there is little likelihood of pregnancy occurring if only one or two white or light-orange tablets are missed, the possibility of pregnancy increases with each successive day that scheduled white or light-orange tablets are missed.
If you are taking Nordette-21, Ovral or Lo/Ovral and forget to take three white or light-orange tablets in a row, do not take them when you remember. Wait four more days—which makes a whole week without tablets. Then begin a new Pilpak on the 8th day after the last tablet was taken. During the seven days without tablets, and until you have taken a white or light-orange tablet daily for seven consecutive days, you should protect yourself from pregnancy by also using another method of birth control.
If you are taking Nordette-28, Ovral-28 or Lo/Ovral-28 and forget to take three white or light-orange tablets in a row, do not take them when you remember. Stop taking all medication until the first Sunday following the last missed tablet. Then, whether or not you have had your period, and even if you are still bleeding, start a new Pilpak. During the days without tablets, and until you have taken a white or light-orange tablet daily for seven consecutive days, you should protect yourself from pregnancy by also using another method of birth control.
OVRETTE®
Ovrette is administered on a continuous daily dosage schedule, one tablet each day, every day of the year. Take the first tablet on the first day of your menstrual period. Tablets should be taken at the same time every day, without interruption, whether bleeding occurs or not. If bleeding is prolonged (more than 8 days) or unusually heavy, you should contact your doctor.
Forgotten Pills:
The risk of pregnancy increases with each tablet missed. Therefore, it is very important that you take one tablet daily as directed. If you miss one tablet, take it as soon as you remember and also take your next tablet at the regular time. If you miss two tablets, take one of the missed tablets as soon as you remember, as well as your regular tablet for that day at the proper time. Furthermore, you should use another method of birth control in addition to taking Ovrette until you have taken fourteen days (2 weeks) of medication.
If more than two tablets have been missed, Ovrette should be discontinued immediately and another method of birth control used until the start of your next menstrual period. Then you may resume taking Ovrette.

At times there may be no menstrual period after a cycle of pills. Therefore, if you miss one menstrual period but have taken the pills *exactly as you were supposed to,* continue as usual into the next cycle. If you have not taken the pills correctly and miss a menstrual period, or if you are taking mini-pills and it is 45 days or more from the start of your last menstrual period, you may be pregnant and should stop taking oral contraceptives until your doctor determines whether or not you are pregnant. Until you can get to your doctor, use another form of contraception. If two consecutive menstrual periods are missed, you should stop taking pills until it is determined whether you are pregnant. If you do become pregnant while using oral contraceptives, you should discuss the risks to the developing child with your doctor.
3. Periodic Examination.
Your doctor will take a complete medical and family history before prescribing oral contraceptives. At that time and about once a year thereafter, he will generally examine your blood pressure, breasts, abdomen, and pelvic organs (including a Papanicolaou smear, i.e., test for cancer).
SUMMARY
Oral contraceptives are the most effective method, except sterilization, for preventing pregnancy. Other methods when used conscientiously, are also very effective and have fewer risks. The serious risks of oral contraceptives are uncommon, and the "pill" is a very convenient method of preventing pregnancy.
If you have certain conditions or have had these conditions in the past, you should not use oral contraceptives, because the risk is too great. These conditions are listed in the leaflet. If you do not have these conditions, and decide to use the "pill", please read the leaflet carefully so that you can use the "pill" most safely and effectively.
Based on his or her assessment of your medical needs, your doctor has prescribed this drug for you. Do not give the drug to anyone else.

Shown in Product Identification Section, page 436

LO/OVRAL®-28 ℞

[*lōh-oh 'vral-28*]
Tablets
(norgestrel and ethinyl estradiol tablets)

DESCRIPTION
21 white LO/OVRAL® tablets, each containing 0.3 mg of norgestrel (*dl* -13-beta-ethyl-17-alpha-ethinyl-17-beta-hydroxygon-4-en-3-one), a totally synthetic progestogen, and 0.03 mg of ethinyl estradiol (19-nor-17α-pregna-1,3,5(10)-trien-20-yne-3,17-diol), and 7 pink inert tablets. The inactive ingredients present are cellulose, FD&C Red 3, lactose, magnesium stearate, and polacrilin potassium.

CLINICAL PHARMACOLOGY
See Lo/Ovral®.

INDICATIONS AND USAGE
See Lo/Ovral.
Dose-Related Risk of Thromboembolism from Oral Contraceptives: See Lo/Ovral.

CONTRAINDICATIONS
See Lo/Ovral.

WARNINGS
See Lo/Ovral.

PRECAUTIONS
See Lo/Ovral.
Information for the Patient: See Lo/Ovral.
Drug Interactions: See Lo/Ovral.
Carcinogenesis: See Lo/Ovral.
Pregnancy: See Lo/Ovral.
Nursing Mothers: See Lo/Ovral.

ADVERSE REACTIONS
See Lo/Ovral.
Acute Overdosage: See Lo/Ovral.

DOSAGE AND ADMINISTRATION
To achieve maximum contraceptive effectiveness, LO/OVRAL-28 must be taken exactly as directed and at intervals not exceeding 24 hours.
The dosage of LO/OVRAL-28 is one white tablet daily for 21 consecutive days followed by one pink inert tablet daily for 7 consecutive days according to prescribed schedule. It is recommended that tablets be taken at the same time each day, preferably after the evening meal or at bedtime.
During the first cycle of medication, the patient is instructed to begin taking LO/OVRAL-28 on the first Sunday after the onset of menstruation. If menstruation begins on a Sunday, the first tablet (white) is taken that day. One white tablet should be taken daily for 21 consecutive days followed by one pink inert tablet daily for 7 consecutive days. Withdrawal bleeding should usually occur within three days following discontinuation of white tablets.
During the first cycle, contraceptive reliance should not be placed on LO/OVRAL-28 until a white tablet has been taken daily for 7 consecutive days. The possibility of ovulation and conception prior to initiation of medication should be considered.
The patient begins her next and all subsequent 28-day courses of tablets on the same day of the week (Sunday) on which she began her first course, following the same schedule: 21 days on white tablets—7 days on pink inert tablets. If in any cycle the patient starts tablets later than the proper day, she should protect herself by using another method of birth control until she has taken a white tablet daily for 7 consecutive days.
If spotting or breakthrough bleeding occurs, the patient is instructed to continue on the same regimen. This type of bleeding is usually transient and without significance; however, if the bleeding is persistent or prolonged the patient is advised to consult her physician. Although the occurrence of pregnancy is highly unlikely if LO/OVRAL-28 is taken according to directions, if withdrawal bleeding does not occur, the possibility of pregnancy must be considered. If the patient has not adhered to the prescribed schedule (missed one or more tablets or started taking them on a day later than she should have) the probability of pregnancy should be considered at the time of the first missed period and appropriate diagnostic measures taken before the medication is resumed. If the patient has adhered to the prescribed regimen and misses two consecutive periods, pregnancy should be ruled out before continuing the contraceptive regimen.
The patient should be instructed to take a missed white tablet as soon as it is remembered. If two consecutive white tablets are missed they should both be taken as soon as remembered. The next tablet should be taken at the usual time. Any time the patient misses one or two white tablets she should also use another method of contraception until she has taken a white tablet daily for seven consecutive days. If the patient misses one or more pink tablets she is still protected against pregnancy *provided* she begins taking white tablets again on the proper day.
If breakthrough bleeding occurs following missed white tablets it will usually be transient and of no consequence. While there is little likelihood of ovulation occurring if only one or two white tablets are missed, the possibility of ovulation increases with each successive day that scheduled white tablets are missed. (If three consecutive days white LO/OVRAL tablets are missed, all medication should be discontinued and the remainder of the 28-day package discarded. A new tablet cycle should be started on the first Sunday following the last missed tablet, and an alternate means of contraception should be prescribed during the days without tablets and until the patient has taken a white tablet daily for 7 consecutive days.) In the nonlactating mother, LO/OVRAL may be prescribed in the postpartum period either immediately or at the first postpartum examination whether or not menstruation has resumed.

HOW SUPPLIED
LO/OVRAL®-28 Tablets (0.3 mg norgestrel and 0.03 mg ethinyl estradiol), Wyeth®, are available in packages of 6 PILPAK® dispensers, each containing 28 tablets as follows:
21 active tablets, NDC 0008-0078, white, round tablet marked "WYETH" and "78".
7 inert tablets, NDC 0008-0486, pink, round tablet marked "WYETH" and "486".

REFERENCES
See Lo/Ovral.
Brief Summary Patient Package Insert: See Lo/Ovral.
DETAILED PATIENT LABELING: See Lo/Ovral.

Shown in Product Identification Section, page 436

MAZANOR® Ⓒ ℞

[*maz 'a-nor*]
(mazindol)

DESCRIPTION
Mazanor (mazindol) is an imidazoisoindole anorectic agent. It is chemically designated as 5-p-chloro-phenyl-5-hydroxy-2,3-dihydro-5H-imidazo (2,1-a)isoindole, a tautomeric form of 2-[2'-(p-chlorobenzoyl)phenyl]-2-imidazoline. Mazanor tablets contain 1 mg mazindol. The inactive ingredients present are calcium sulfate, cellulose, lactose, magnesium stearate, povidone, and talc.

ACTIONS

Mazanor (mazindol), although an isoindole, has pharmacologic activity similar in many ways to the prototype drugs used in obesity, the amphetamines. Actions include central-nervous-system stimulation in humans and animals, as well as such amphetamine-like effects in animals as the production of stereotyped behavior. Animal experiments also suggest certain differences from phenethylamine anorectic drugs, e.g., amphetamine, with respect to site and mechanism of action; for example, mazindol appears to exert its primary effects on the limbic system. The significance of these differences for humans is uncertain. It does not cause brain norepinephrine depletion in animals; on the other hand, it does appear to inhibit storage-site uptake of norepinephrine as is suggested by its marked potentiation of the effect of exogenous norepinephrine on blood pressure in dogs (see "Warnings") and on smooth-muscle contraction *in vitro.*
Tolerance has been demonstrated with all drugs of this class in which this phenomenon has been studied.
Drugs used in obesity are commonly known as "anorectics" or "anorexigenics." It has not been established, however, that the action of such drugs in treating obesity is exclusively one of appetite suppression. Other central-nervous-system actions or metabolic effects may be involved as well.
Adult obese subjects, instructed in dietary management and treated with anorectic drugs, lose more weight on the average than those treated with placebo and diet, as determined in relatively short-term clinical trials.
The average magnitude of increased weight loss of drug-treated patients over placebo-treated patients in studies of anorectics in general is ordinarily only a fraction of a pound a week. The rate of weight loss is greatest in the first weeks of therapy for both drug and placebo subjects and tends to decrease in succeeding weeks.
The amount of weight loss associated with the use of Mazanor (mazindol), as with other anorectic drugs, varies from trial to trial, and the increased weight loss appears to be related in part to variables other than the drugs prescribed, such as the interaction between physician-investigator and the patient, the population treated, and the diet prescribed. The importance of non-drug factors in such weight loss has not been elucidated.
The natural history of obesity is measured in years, whereas, most studies cited are restricted to a few weeks duration; thus, the total impact of drug-induced weight loss over that of diet alone must be considered clinically limited.

INDICATION

Mazanor (mazindol) is indicated in the management of exogenous obesity as a short-term (a few weeks) adjunct in a regimen of weight reduction based on caloric restriction. The limited usefulness of agents of this class (see "Actions") should be measured against possible risk factors inherent in their use, such as those described below.

CONTRAINDICATIONS

Glaucoma, hypersensitivity or idiosyncrasy to Mazanor (mazindol).
Agitated states.
Patients with a history of drug abuse.
During or within 14 days following the administration of monoamine oxidase inhibitors (hypertensive crises may result).

WARNINGS

Tolerance to the effect of many anorectic drugs may develop within a few weeks; if this occurs, the recommended dose should not be exceeded in an attempt to increase the effect; rather, the drug should be discontinued.
Mazanor (mazindol) may impair the ability of the patient to engage in potentially hazardous activities, such as operating machinery or driving a motor vehicle; the patient should therefore be cautioned accordingly.
DRUG INTERACTIONS
Mazanor (mazindol) may decrease the hypotensive effect of guanethidine; patients should be monitored accordingly.
Mazanor (mazindol) may markedly potentiate the pressor effect of exogenous catecholamines. If it should be necessary to give a pressor amine agent (e.g., levarterenol or isoproterenol) to a patient in shock (e.g., from a myocardial infarction) who has recently been taking Mazanor (mazindol), extreme care should be taken in monitoring blood pressure at frequent intervals and initiating pressor therapy with a low initial dose and careful titration.
DRUG DEPENDENCE
Mazanor (mazindol) shares important pharmacologic properties with amphetamines. Amphetamines and related stimulant drugs have been extensively abused and can produce tolerance and severe psychologic dependence. In this regard, the manifestations of chronic overdosage or withdrawal of Mazanor (mazindol) have not been determined in humans. Abstinence effects have been observed in dogs after abrupt cessation for prolonged periods. There was some self-administration of the drug in monkeys. EEG studies and "liking" scores in human studies yielded equivocal results. While the abuse potential of Mazanor (mazindol) has not been further defined, the possibility of dependence should be kept in mind when evaluating the desirability of including Mazanor (mazindol) as part of a weight-reduction program.
USAGE IN PREGNANCY
Mazanor (mazindol) was studied in reproduction experiments in rats and rabbits, and an increase in neonatal mortality and a possible increased incidence of rib anomalies in rats were observed at relatively high doses. Although these studies have not indicated important adverse effects, use of mazindol by women who are or may become pregnant requires that the potential benefit be weighed against the possible hazard to mother and infant.
USAGE IN CHILDREN
Mazanor (mazindol) is not recommended for use in children under 12 years of age.

PRECAUTIONS

Insulin requirements in diabetes mellitus may be altered in association with the use of mazindol and the concomitant dietary regimen.
The least amount feasible should be prescribed or dispensed at one time in order to minimize the possibility of overdosage.
Use only with caution in hypertension with monitoring of blood pressure, since evidence is insufficient to rule out a possible adverse effect on blood pressure in some hypertensive patients. The drug is not recommended in severely hypertensive patients. The drug is not recommended for patients with symptomatic cardiovascular disease including arrhythmias.

ADVERSE REACTIONS

The most common adverse effects of Mazanor (mazindol) are: dry mouth, tachycardia, constipation, nervousness, and insomnia.
Cardiovascular: Palpitation, tachycardia.
Central Nervous System: Overstimulation, restlessness, dizziness, insomnia, dysphoria, tremor, headache, depression, drowsiness, weakness.
Gastrointestinal: Dryness of the mouth, unpleasant taste, diarrhea, constipation, nausea, other gastrointestinal disturbances.
Skin: Rash, excessive sweating, clamminess.
Endocrine: Impotence, changes in libido have rarely been observed with Mazanor (mazindol).
Eye: Treatment of dogs with high doses of Mazanor (mazindol) for long periods resulted in some corneal opacities, reversible on cessation of medication. No such effect has been observed in humans.

DOSAGE AND ADMINISTRATION

Usual dosage is 1 mg three times daily, one hour before meals, or 2 mg once daily, one hour before lunch. The lowest effective dose should be used. To determine the lowest effective dose, therapy with Mazanor may be initiated at 1 mg once a day, and adjusted to the need and response of the patient. Should G.I. discomfort occur, Mazanor may be taken with meals.

OVERDOSAGE

There are no data as yet on acute overdosage with Mazanor (mazindol) in humans.
Manifestations of acute overdosage with amphetamines and related substances include restlessness, tremor, rapid respiration, dizziness. Fatigue and depression may follow the stimulatory phase of overdosage. Cardiovascular effects include tachycardia, hypertension, and circulatory collapse. Gastrointestinal symptoms include nausea, vomiting, and abdominal cramps. While similar manifestations of overdosage may be seen with Mazanor (mazindol), their exact nature has yet to be determined. The management of acute intoxication is largely symptomatic. Data are not available on the treatment of acute intoxication with Mazanor (mazindol) by hemodialysis or peritoneal dialysis, but the substance is poorly soluble except at very acid pH.

HOW SUPPLIED

Mazanor® (mazindol) Tablets, Wyeth®, are available in the following dosage strength in bottles of 30 tablets:
1 mg, NDC 0008-0071, white, round, scored tablet marked "WYETH" and "71".
Keep bottles tightly closed.
Store below 25° C (77° F).
Dispense in tight containers.
Shown in Product Identification Section, page 436

MEPERGAN® Ⓒ℞

[mep'er-gan]
(meperidine HCl and promethazine HCl) Injection

DESCRIPTION

This product is available in concentration providing 25 mg each of meperidine hydrochloride and promethazine hydrochloride per ml with 0.1 mg edetate disodium, 0.04 mg calcium chloride, and not more than 0.75 mg sodium formaldehyde sulfoxylate, 0.25 mg sodium metabisulfite, and 5 mg phenol with sodium acetate buffer.

ACTIONS

Meperidine hydrochloride is a narcotic analgesic with multiple actions qualitatively similar to those of morphine. Phenergan® (promethazine HCl) is a phenothiazine derivative that has several different pharmacologic properties including antihistaminic, sedative, and antiemetic actions.

INDICATIONS

As a preanesthetic medication when analgesia and sedation are indicated. As an adjunct to local and general anesthesia.

CONTRAINDICATIONS

Hypersensitivity to meperidine or promethazine.
Under no circumstances should Mepergan be given by intra-arterial injection, due to the likelihood of severe arteriospasm and the possibility of resultant gangrene (see Warnings).
Mepergan should not be given by the subcutaneous route; evidence of chemical irritation has been noted and necrotic lesions have resulted on rare occasions following subcutaneous injection. The preferred parenteral route of administration is by deep intramuscular injection.
Meperidine is contraindicated in patients who are receiving monoamine oxidase inhibitors (MAOI) or those who have received such agents within 14 days.
Therapeutic doses of meperidine have inconsistently precipitated unpredictable, severe, and occasionally fatal reactions in patients who have received such agents within 14 days. The mechanism of these reactions is unclear. Some have been characterized by coma, severe respiratory depression, cyanosis, and hypotension, and have resembled the syndrome of acute narcotic overdose. In other reactions the predominant manifestations have been hyperexcitability, convulsions, tachycardia, hyperpyrexia, and hypertension. Although it is not known that other narcotics are free of the risk of such reactions, virtually all of the reported reactions have occurred with meperidine. If a narcotic is needed in such patients, a sensitivity test should be performed in which repeated, small, incremental doses of morphine are administered over the course of several hours while the patient's condition and vital signs are under careful observation.
(Intravenous hydrocortisone or prednisolone have been used to treat severe reactions, with the addition of intravenous chlorpromazine in those cases exhibiting hypertension and hyperpyrexia. The usefulness and safety of narcotic antagonists in the treatment of these reactions is unknown.)

WARNINGS

Tolerance and Addiction Liability
Warning—may be habit forming
DRUG DEPENDENCE: Meperidine can produce drug dependence of the morphine type and therefore has the potential for being abused. Psychic dependence, physical dependence, and tolerance may develop upon repeated administration of meperidine, and it should be prescribed and administered with the same degree of caution appropriate to the use of morphine. Like other narcotics, meperidine is subject to the provisions of the Federal narcotic laws.
INTERACTION WITH OTHER CENTRAL-NERVOUS-SYSTEM DEPRESSANTS: Meperidine should be used with great caution and in reduced dosage in patients who are concurrently receiving other narcotic analgesics, general anesthetics, phenothiazines, other tranquilizers, sedative-hypnotics, tricyclic antidepressants, and other CNS depressants (including alcohol). Respiratory depression, hypotension, and profound sedation or coma may result.
The sedative action of promethazine hydrochloride is additive to the sedative effects of central-nervous-system depressants; therefore, agents such as alcohol, barbiturates, and narcotic analgesics should either be eliminated or given in reduced dosage in the presence of promethazine hydrochloride. When given concomitantly with promethazine hydrochloride the dose of barbiturates should be reduced by at least one-half and the dose of analgesic depressants, such as morphine or meperidine, should be reduced by one-quarter to one-half.
HEAD INJURY AND INCREASED INTRACRANIAL PRESSURE: The respiratory depressant effects of meperidine and its capacity to elevate cerebrospinal-fluid pressure may be markedly exaggerated in the presence of head injury, other intracranial lesions, or a preexisting increase in intracranial pressure. Furthermore, narcotics produce adverse reactions which may obscure the clinical course of patients with head injuries. In such patients, meperidine must be used with extreme caution and only if its use is deemed essential.
INADVERTENT INTRA-ARTERIAL INJECTION: Due to the close proximity of arteries and veins in the areas most commonly used for intravenous injection, extreme care should be exercised to avoid perivascular extravasation or inadvertent intra-arterial injection of Mepergan. Reports compatible with inadvertent intra-arterial injection suggest

Continued on next page

Wyeth—Cont.

that pain, severe chemical irritation, severe spasm of distal vessels, and resultant gangrene requiring amputation is likely under such circumstances. Intravenous injection was intended in all the cases reported, but perivascular extravasation or arterial placement of the needle is now suspect. There is no proven successful management of this condition after it occurs, although sympathetic block and heparinization are commonly employed during the acute management because of the results of animal experiments with other known arteriolar irritants. Aspiration of dark blood does not preclude intra-arterial needle placement, because blood is discolored upon contact with promethazine. Use of syringes with rigid plungers or of small bore needles might obscure typical arterial backflow if this is relied upon alone.
INTRAVENOUS USE: If necessary, meperidine may be given intravenously, but the injection should be given very slowly, preferably in the form of a diluted solution. Rapid intravenous injection of narcotic analgesics, including meperidine, increases the incidence of adverse reactions; severe respiratory depression, apnea, hypotension, peripheral circulatory collapse, and cardiac arrest have occurred. Meperidine should not be administered intravenously unless a narcotic antagonist and the facilities for assisted or controlled respiration are immediately available. When meperidine is given parenterally, especially intravenously, the patient should be lying down.
When used intravenously, Mepergan® (meperidine hydrochloride and promethazine hydrochloride) should be given at a rate not to exceed 1 ml (25 mg of each component) per minute. When administering any irritant drug intravenously it is usually preferable to inject it through the tubing of an intravenous infusion set that is known to be functioning satisfactorily. In the event that a patient complains of pain during intended intravenous injection of Mepergan, the injection should immediately be stopped to provide for evaluation of possible arterial placement or perivascular extravasation.
ASTHMA AND OTHER RESPIRATORY CONDITIONS: Meperidine should be used with extreme caution in patients having an acute asthmatic attack, patients with chronic obstructive pulmonary disease or cor pulmonale, patients having a substantially decreased respiratory reserve, and patients with preexisting respiratory depression, hypoxia, or hypercapnia. In such patients, even usual therapeutic doses of narcotics may decrease respiratory drive while simultaneously increasing airway resistance to the point of apnea.
HYPOTENSIVE EFFECT: The administration of meperidine may result in severe hypotension in an individual whose ability to maintain his blood pressure has already been compromised by a depleted blood volume or concurrent administration of drugs such as the phenothiazines or certain anesthetics.
USAGE IN AMBULATORY PATIENTS: Meperidine may impair the mental and/or physical abilities required for the performance of potentially hazardous tasks such as driving a car or operating machinery. The patient should be cautioned accordingly.
Meperidine, like other narcotics, may produce orthostatic hypotension in ambulatory patients.
USAGE IN PREGNANCY AND LACTATION: Meperidine should not be used in pregnant women prior to the labor period, unless in the judgment of the physician the potential benefits outweigh the possible hazards, because safe use in pregnancy prior to labor has not been established relative to possible adverse effects on fetal development.
When used as an obstetrical analgesic, meperidine crosses the placental barrier and can produce respiratory depression in the newborn; resuscitation may be required (see section on Overdosage).
Meperidine appears in the milk of nursing mothers receiving the drug.

PRECAUTIONS

SUPRAVENTRICULAR TACHYCARDIAS: Meperidine should be used with caution in patients with atrial flutter and other supraventricular tachycardias because of a possible vagolytic action which may produce a significant increase in the ventricular response rate.
CONVULSIONS: Meperidine may aggravate preexisting convulsions in patients with convulsive disorders. If dosage is escalated substantially above recommended levels because of tolerance development, convulsions may occur in individuals without a history of convulsive disorders.
ACUTE ABDOMINAL CONDITIONS: The administration of meperidine or other narcotics may obscure the diagnosis or clinical course in patients with acute abdominal conditions.
SPECIAL-RISK PATIENTS: Meperidine should be given with caution and the initial dose should be reduced in certain patients such as the elderly or debilitated, and those with severe impairment of hepatic or renal function, hypothyroidism, Addison's disease, and prostatic hypertrophy or urethral stricture.
Antiemetics may mask the symptoms of an unrecognized disease and thereby interfere with diagnosis.
Patients in pain who have received inadequate or no analgesia have been noted to develop "athetoid-like" movements of the upper extremities following the parenteral administration of promethazine. These symptoms usually disappear upon adequate control of the pain.
Ambulatory patients should be cautioned against driving automobiles or operating dangerous machinery until it is known that they do not become drowsy or dizzy from promethazine hydrochloride therapy.

ADVERSE REACTIONS

The major hazards of meperidine, as with other narcotic analgesics, are respiratory depression and, to a lesser degree, circulatory depression; respiratory arrest, shock, and cardiac arrest have occurred.
The most frequently observed adverse reactions include light-headedness, dizziness, sedation, nausea, vomiting, and sweating. These effects seem to be more prominent in ambulatory patients and in those who are not experiencing severe pain. In such individuals, lower doses are advisable. Some adverse reactions in ambulatory patients may be alleviated if the patient lies down.
Other adverse reactions include:
CENTRAL NERVOUS SYSTEM: Euphoria, dysphoria, weakness, headache, agitation, tremor, uncoordinated muscle movements, transient hallucinations and disorientation, visual disturbances and, rarely, extrapyramidal reactions.
GASTROINTESTINAL: Dry mouth, constipation, biliary-tract spasm.
CARDIOVASCULAR: Flushing of the face, tachycardia, bradycardia, palpitation, faintness, syncope.
Cardiovascular effects from promethazine have been rare. Minor increases in blood pressure and occasional mild hypotension have been reported. Venous thrombosis at the injection site has been reported. Intra-arterial injection of Mepergan may result in gangrene of the affected extremity (see Warnings).
GENITOURINARY: Urinary retention.
ALLERGIC: Pruritus, urticaria, other skin rashes, wheal and flare over the vein with IV injection.
Photosensitivity, although extremely rare, has been reported. Occurrence of photosensitivity may be a contraindication to further treatment with promethazine or related drugs.
OTHER: Pain at injection site; local tissue irritation and induration following subcutaneous injection, particularly when repeated; antidiuretic effect.
Patients may occasionally complain of autonomic reactions such as dryness of the mouth, blurring of vision and, rarely, dizziness following the use of promethazine.
Very rare cases have been reported where patients receiving promethazine have developed leukopenia. In one instance agranulocytosis has been reported. In nearly every instance reported, other toxic agents known to have caused these conditions have been associated with the administration of promethazine.

DOSAGE AND ADMINISTRATION

WARNING —BARBITURATES ARE NOT CHEMICALLY COMPATIBLE IN SOLUTION WITH MEPERGAN® (MEPERIDINE HYDROCHLORIDE AND PROMETHAZINE HYDROCHLORIDE), AND SHOULD NOT BE MIXED IN THE SAME SYRINGE.
The TUBEX® (Sterile Cartridge-Needle Unit) is designed for single-dose use. VIALS should be used when required doses are fractions of a milliliter, as indicated below.
Mepergan® is usually administered intramuscularly. However, in certain specific situations, the intravenous route may be employed. INADVERTENT INTRA-ARTERIAL INJECTION CAN RESULT IN GANGRENE OF THE AFFECTED EXTREMITY (see Warnings). SUBCUTANEOUS ADMINISTRATION IS CONTRAINDICATED, AS IT MAY RESULT IN TISSUE NECROSIS (see Contraindications). INJECTION INTO OR NEAR PERIPHERAL NERVES MAY RESULT IN PERMANENT NEUROLOGICAL DEFICIT.
When used intravenously, the rate should not be greater than 1 ml of Mepergan (25 mg of each component) per minute; it is preferable to inject through the tubing of an intravenous infusion set that is known to be functioning satisfactorily.
ADULT DOSE: 1-2 ml (25-50 mg of each component) per single injection, which can be repeated every 3 to 4 hours.
CHILDREN 12 YEARS OF AGE AND UNDER: 0.5 mg of each component per pound of body weight. The dosage may be repeated every 3 to 4 hours as necessary. For preanesthetic medication the usual adult dose is 2 ml (50 mg of each component) intramuscularly with or without appropriate atropine-like drug. Atropine sulfate 0.3 to 0.4 mg or scopolamine hydrobromide 0.25 to 0.4 mg in sterile solution may be mixed in the same syringe with Mepergan. Repeat doses of 50 mg or less of both promethazine and meperidine may be administered by either route at 3- to 4-hour intervals, as necessary. As an adjunct to local or general anesthesia the usual dose is 2 ml (50 mg each of meperidine and promethazine).

OVERDOSAGE

SYMPTOMS: Serious overdose with meperidine is characterized by respiratory depression (a decrease in respiratory rate and/or tidal volume, Cheyne-Stokes respiration, cyanosis), extreme somnolence progressing to stupor or coma, skeletal muscle flaccidity, cold and clammy skin, and sometimes bradycardia and hypotension. In severe overdosage, particularly by the intravenous route, apnea, circulatory collapse, cardiac arrest, and death may occur.
TREATMENT: Primary attention should be given to the reestablishment of adequate respiratory exchange through provision of a patent airway and institution of assisted or controlled ventilation. The narcotic antagonists, naloxone hydrochloride, nalorphine hydrochloride, and levallorphan tartrate, are specific antidotes against respiratory depression which may result from overdosage or unusual sensitivity to narcotics, including meperidine. Therefore, an appropriate dose of one of these antagonists should be administered, preferably by the intravenous route, simultaneously with efforts at respiratory resuscitation.
An antagonist should not be administered in absence of clinically significant respiratory or cardiovascular depression.
Oxygen, intravenous fluids, vasopressors, and other supportive measures should be employed as indicated.
NOTE: In an individual physically dependent on narcotics, the administration of the usual dose of a narcotic antagonist will precipitate an acute withdrawal syndrome. The severity of this syndrome will depend on the degree of physical dependence and the dose of antagonist administered. The use of narcotic antagonists in such individuals should be avoided if possible. If a narcotic antagonist must be used to treat serious respiratory depression in the physically dependent patient, the antagonist should be administered with extreme care and only one-fifth to one-tenth the usual initial dose administered.
Attempted suicides with promethazine have resulted in deep sedation, coma, rarely convulsions and cardiorespiratory symptoms compatible with the depth of sedation present. Extrapyramidal reactions may be treated with anticholinergic antiparkinson agents, diphenhydramine, or barbiturates.
If severe hypotension occurs, levarterenol or phenylephrine may be indicated. Epinephrine is probably best avoided, since it has been suggested that promethazine overdosage could produce a partial alpha-adrenergic blockade.
A paradoxical reaction, characterized by hyperexcitability and nightmares, has been reported in children receiving large single doses of promethazine.

HOW SUPPLIED

Mepergan® (meperidine hydrochloride and promethazine hydrochloride) is supplied in 10 ml vials and TUBEX® Sterile Cartridge-Needle Units.
Subject to Regulations of Federal Bureau Narcotics and Dangerous Drugs.

NORDETTE®-21 ℞

[nor-det '-21]
TABLETS
(levonorgestrel and ethinyl estradiol tablets)

DESCRIPTION

ORAL CONTRACEPTIVE

Each Nordette® tablet contains 0.15 mg of levonorgestrel (*d* (-)-13 beta-ethyl-17-alpha-ethinyl-17-beta-hydroxygon-4-en-3-one), a totally synthetic progestogen, and 0.03 mg of ethinyl estradiol (19-nor-17α-pregna-1,3,5 (10)-trien-20-yne-3,17-diol). The inactive ingredients present are cellulose, FD&C Yellow 6, lactose, magnesium stearate, and polacrilin potassium.

CLINICAL PHARMACOLOGY

Combination oral contraceptives act primarily through the mechanism of gonadotropin suppression due to the estrogenic and progestational activity of the ingredients. Although the primary mechanism of action is inhibition of ovulation, alterations in the genital tract, including changes in the cervical mucus (which increase the difficulty of sperm penetration) and the endometrium (which reduce the likelihood of implantation), may also contribute to contraceptive effectiveness.

INDICATIONS AND USAGE

Nordette is indicated for the prevention of pregnancy in women who elect to use oral contraceptives as a method of contraception.
Oral contraceptives are highly effective. The pregnancy rate in women using conventional combination oral contraceptives (containing 35 mcg or more of ethinyl estradiol or 50 mcg or more of mestranol) is generally reported as less than one pregnancy per 100 woman-years of use. Slightly higher rates (somewhat more than 1 pregnancy per 100 woman-years of use) are reported for some combination products

containing 35 mcg or less of ethinyl estradiol, and rates on the order of 3 pregnancies per 100 woman-years are reported for the progestogen-only oral contraceptives.

These rates are derived from separate studies conducted by different investigators in several population groups and cannot be compared precisely. Furthermore, pregnancy rates tend to be lower as clinical studies are continued, possibly due to selective retention in the longer studies of those patients who accept the treatment regimen and do not discontinue as a result of adverse reactions, pregnancy, or other reasons.

In clinical trials with Nordette, 1,084 patients completed 8,186 cycles, and a total of three pregnancies were reported. This represents a pregnancy rate of 0.48 per 100 woman-years.

Table 1 gives ranges of pregnancy rates reported in the literature[1] for other means of contraception. The efficacy of these means of contraception (except the IUD) depends upon the degree of adherence to the method.

TABLE 1

PREGNANCIES PER 100 WOMAN-YEARS

IUD, less than 1–6; Diaphragm with spermicidal products (creams or jellies), 2–20; Condom, 3–36; Aerosol foams, 2–29; Jellies and creams, 4–36;

Periodic abstinence (rhythm) all types, less than 1–47:

1. Calendar method, 14–47;
2. Temperature method, 1–20;
3. Temperature method—intercourse only in postovulatory phase, less than 1–7;
4. Mucus method, 1–25;

No contraception, 60–80.

Dose-Related Risk of Thromboembolism from Oral Contraceptives: Two studies have shown a positive association between the dose of estrogens in oral contraceptives and the risk of thromboembolism.[2,3] For this reason, it is prudent and in keeping with good principles of therapeutics to minimize exposure to estrogen. The oral-contraceptive product prescribed for any given patient should be that product which contains the least amount of estrogen that is compatible with an acceptable pregnancy rate and patient acceptance. It is recommended that new acceptors of oral contraceptives be started on preparations containing 0.05 mg or less of estrogen.

CONTRAINDICATIONS

Oral contraceptives should not be used in women with any of the following conditions:

1. Thrombophlebitis or thromboembolic disorders.
2. A past history of deep-vein thrombophlebitis or thromboembolic disorders.
3. Cerebral-vascular or coronary-artery disease.
4. Known or suspected carcinoma of the breast.
5. Known or suspected estrogen-dependent neoplasia.
6. Undiagnosed abnormal genital bleeding.
7. Known or suspected pregnancy (see Warning No. 5).
8. Benign or malignant liver tumor which developed during the use of oral contraceptives or other estrogen-containing products.

WARNINGS

Cigarette smoking increases the risk of serious cardiovascular side effects from oral-contraceptive use. This risk increases with age and with heavy smoking (15 or more cigarettes per day) and is quite marked in women over 35 years of age. Women who use oral contraceptives should be strongly advised not to smoke.

The use of oral contraceptives is associated with increased risk of several serious conditions, including thromboembolism, stroke, myocardial infarction, hepatic adenoma, gallbladder disease, hypertension. Practitioners prescribing oral contraceptives should be familiar with the following information relating to these risks.

1. *Thromboembolic Disorders and Other Vascular Problems:* An increased risk of thromboembolic and thrombotic disease associated with the use of oral contraceptives is well-established. Three principal studies in Great Britain[4-6] and three in the United States[7-10] have demonstrated an increased risk of fatal and nonfatal venous thromboembolism and stroke, both hemorrhagic and thrombotic. These studies estimate that users of oral contraceptives are 4 to 11 times more likely than nonusers to develop these diseases without evident cause (Table 2).

CEREBROVASCULAR DISORDERS

In a collaborative American study[9,10] of cerebrovascular disorders in women with and without predisposing causes, it was estimated that the risk of hemorrhagic stroke was 2.0 times greater in users than nonusers and the risk of thrombotic stroke was 4 to 9.5 times greater in users than in nonusers (Table 2).

TABLE 2

SUMMARY OF RELATIVE RISK OF THROMBOEMBOLIC DISORDERS AND OTHER VASCULAR PROBLEMS IN ORAL-CONTRACEPTIVE USERS COMPARED TO NONUSERS

	Relative risk, times greater
Idiopathic thromboembolic disease	4-11
Postsurgery thromboembolic complications	4-6
Thrombotic stroke	4-9.5
Hemorrhagic stroke	2
Myocardial infarction	2-12

MYOCARDIAL INFARCTION

An increased risk of myocardial infarction associated with the use of oral contraceptives has been reported,[11-13] confirming a previously suspected association. These studies, conducted in the United Kingdom, found, as expected, that the greater the number of underlying risk factors for coronary-artery disease (cigarette smoking, hypertension, hypercholesterolemia, obesity, diabetes, history of preeclamptic toxemia) the higher the risk of developing myocardial infarction, regardless of whether the patient was an oral-contraceptive user or not. Oral contraceptives, however, were found to be a clear additional risk factor.

In terms of relative risk, it has been estimated[52] that oral-contraceptive users who do not smoke (smoking is considered a major predisposing condition to myocardial infarction) are about twice as likely to have a fatal myocardial infarction as nonusers who do not smoke. Oral-contraceptive users who are also smokers have about a 5-fold increased risk of fatal infarction compared to users who do not smoke, but about a 10- to 12-fold increased risk compared to nonusers who do not smoke. Furthermore, the amount of smoking is also an important factor. In determining the importance of these relative risks, however, the baseline rates for various age groups, as shown in Table 3, must be given serious consideration. The importance of other predisposing conditions mentioned above in determining relative and absolute risks has not as yet been quantified; it is quite likely that the same synergistic action exists, but perhaps to a lesser extent.

TABLE 3

Estimated annual mortality rate per 100,000 women from myocardial infarction by use of oral contraceptives, smoking habits, and age (in years):

[See table next page].

RISK OF DOSE

In an analysis of data derived from several national adverse-reaction reporting systems,[2] British investigators concluded that the risk of thromboembolism, including coronary thrombosis, is directly related to the dose of estrogen used in oral contraceptives. Preparations containing 100 mcg or more of estrogen were associated with a higher risk of thromboembolism than those containing 50-80 mcg of estrogen. Their analysis did suggest, however, that the quantity of estrogen may not be the sole factor involved. This finding has been confirmed in the United States.[3] Careful epidemiological studies to determine the degree of thromboembolic risk associated with progestogen-only oral contraceptives have not been performed. Cases of thromboembolic disease have been reported in women using these products, and they should not be presumed to be free of excess risk.

ESTIMATE OF EXCESS MORTALITY FROM CIRCULATORY DISEASES

A large prospective study[53] carried out in the U.K. estimated the mortality rate per 100,000 women per year from diseases of the circulatory system for users and nonusers of oral contraceptives according to age, smoking habits, and duration of use. The overall excess death rate annually from circulatory diseases for oral-contraceptive users was estimated to be 20 per 100,000 (ages 15-34—5/100,000; ages 35-44—33/100,000; ages 45-49—140/100,000), the risk being concentrated in older women, in those with a long duration of use, and in cigarette smokers. It was not possible, however, to examine the interrelationships of age, smoking, and duration of use, nor to compare the effects of continuous vs. intermittent use. Although the study showed a 10-fold increase in death due to circulatory diseases in users for 5 or more years, all of these deaths occurred in women 35 or older. Until larger numbers of women under 35 with continuous use for 5 or more years are available, it is not possible to assess the magnitude of the relative risk for this younger age group.

The available data from a variety of sources have been analyzed[14] to estimate the risk of death associated with various methods of contraception. The estimates of risk of death for each method include the combined risk of the contraceptive method (e.g., thromboembolic and thrombotic disease in the case of oral contraceptives) plus the risk attributable to pregnancy or abortion in the event of method failure. This latter risk varies with the effectiveness of the contraceptive method. The findings of this analysis are shown in the bar graph (Figure 1).[14] The study concluded that the mortality associated with all methods of birth control is low and below that associated with childbirth, with the exception of oral contraceptives in women over 40 who smoke. (The rates given for Pill only/smokers for each age group are for smokers as a class. For "heavy" smokers [more than 15 cigarettes a day], the rates given would be about double; for "light" smokers [less than 15 cigarettes a day], about 50 percent.)

The lowest mortality is associated with the condom or diaphragm backed up by early abortion. The risk of thromboembolic and thrombotic disease associated with oral contraceptives increases with age after approximately age 30 and, for myocardial infarction, is further increased by hypertension, hypercholesterolemia, obesity, diabetes, or history of preeclamptic toxemia and especially by cigarette smoking.

Based on the data currently available, the following chart gives a gross estimate of the risk of death from circulatory disorders associated with the use of oral contraceptives:

SMOKING HABITS AND OTHER PREDISPOSING CONDITIONS—RISK ASSOCIATED WITH USE OF ORAL CONTRACEPTIVES

Age	Below 30	30-39	40+
Heavy smokers	C	B	A
Light smokers	D	C	B
Nonsmokers (no predisposing conditions)	D	C,D	C
Nonsmokers (other predisposing conditions)	C	C,B	B,A

A—Use associated with very high risk.
B—Use associated with high risk.
C—Use associated with moderate risk.
D—Use associated with low risk.

The physician and the patient should be alert to the earliest manifestations of thromboembolic and thrombotic disorders (e.g., thrombophlebitis, pulmonary embolism, cerebrovascular insufficiency, coronary occlusion, retinal thrombosis, and mesenteric thrombosis). Should any of these occur or be suspected, the drug should be discontinued immediately.

A four- to six-fold increased risk of postsurgery thromboembolic complications has been reported in oral-contraceptive users.[15,16] If feasible, oral contraceptives should be discontinued at least 4 weeks before surgery of a type associated with an increased risk of thromboembolism or prolonged immobilization.

Figure 1. Estimated annual number of deaths associated with control of fertility and no control per 100,000 nonsterile women, by regimen of control and age of woman.

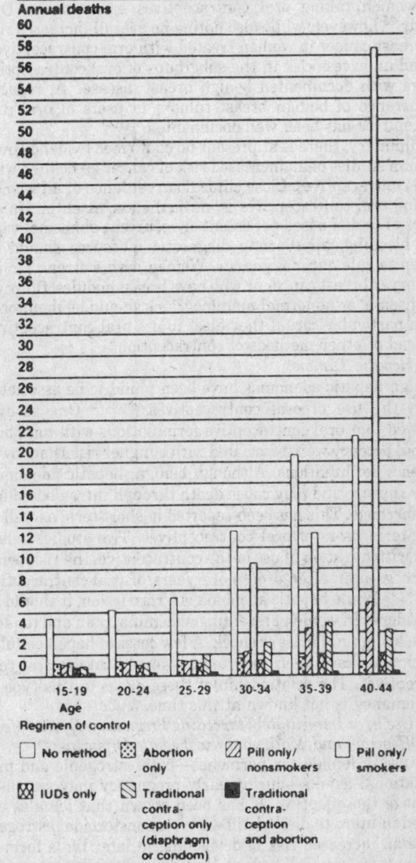

PERSISTENCE OF RISK OF VASCULAR DISORDERS

Findings from one study in Great Britain involving cerebro-

Continued on next page

Wyeth—Cont.

	Myocardial infarction			
	Women aged 30-39		Women aged 40-44	
Smoking habits	Users	Nonusers	Users	Nonusers
All smokers	10.2	2.6	62.0	15.9
Heavy*	13.0	5.1	78.7	31.3
Light	4.7	0.9	28.6	5.7
Nonsmokers	1.8	1.2	10.7	7.4
Smokers and nonsmokers	5.4	1.9	32.8	11.7

* Heavy smoker: 15 or more cigarettes per day.
From JAIN, A.K., *Studies in Family Planning, 8*:50, 1977.

vascular disease[56] and another study in the United States concerning myocardial infarction[57] suggest that an increased risk of these conditions in users of oral contraceptives persists after discontinuation of the oral contraceptive. In the British study, the risk of cerebrovascular disease remained elevated in former oral-contraceptive users for at least six years after discontinuation. In the U. S. study, an increased risk of myocardial infarction persisted for at least 9 years in women 40- to 49-years-old who had used oral contraceptives for five or more years. The findings in both these studies require confirmation since they are inconsistent with other published information.[9,11,13,58–62]

2. *Ocular Lesions:*
There have been reports of neuro-ocular lesions such as optic neuritis or retinal thrombosis associated with the use of oral contraceptives. Discontinue oral-contraceptive medication if there is unexplained, sudden or gradual, partial or complete loss of vision; onset of proptosis or diplopia; papilledema; or retinal-vascular lesions, and institute appropriate diagnostic and therapeutic measures.

3. *Carcinoma:*
Long-term continuous administration of either natural or synthetic estrogen in certain animal species increases the frequency of carcinoma of the breast, cervix, vagina, and liver. Certain synthetic progestogens, none currently contained in oral contraceptives, have been noted to increase the incidence of mammary nodules, benign and malignant, in dogs.

In humans, three case-control studies have reported an increased risk of endometrial carcinoma associated with the prolonged use of exogenous estrogen in postmenopausal women.[17–19] One publication[20] reported on the first 21 cases submitted by physicians to a registry of cases of adenocarcinoma of the endometrium in women under 40 on oral contraceptives. Of the cases found in women without predisposing risk factors for adenocarcinoma of the endometrium (e.g., irregular bleeding at the time oral contraceptives were first given, polycystic ovaries), nearly all occurred in women who had used a sequential oral contraceptive. These products are no longer marketed. No evidence has been reported suggesting an increased risk of endometrial cancer in users of conventional combination or progestogen-only oral contraceptives.

Several studies[8,21–24] have found no increase in breast cancer in women taking oral contraceptives or estrogens. One study,[25] however, while also noting no overall increased risk of breast cancer in women treated with oral contraceptives, found an excess risk in the subgroups of oral-contraceptive users with documented benign breast disease. A reduced occurrence of benign breast tumors in users of oral contraceptives has been well-documented.[8,21,25–27]

In summary, there is at present no confirmed evidence from human studies of an increased risk of cancer associated with oral contraceptives. Close clinical surveillance of all women taking oral contraceptives is, nevertheless, essential. In all cases of undiagnosed persistent or recurrent abnormal vaginal bleeding, appropriate diagnostic measures should be taken to rule out malignancy. Women with a strong family history of breast cancer or who have breast nodules, fibrocystic disease, or abnormal mammograms should be monitored with particular care if they elect to use oral contraceptives instead of other methods of contraception.

4. *Hepatic Tumors:*
Benign hepatic adenomas have been found to be associated with the use of oral contraceptives.[28–30,46] One study[46] showed that oral contraceptive formulations with high hormonal potency were associated with a higher risk than lower potency formulations. Although benign, hepatic adenomas may rupture and may cause death through intra-abdominal hemorrhage. This has been reported in short-term as well as long-term users of oral contraceptives. Two studies relate risk with duration of use of the contraceptive, the risk being much greater after 4 or more years of oral-contraceptive use.[30,46] While hepatic adenoma is a rare lesion, it should be considered in women presenting abdominal pain and tenderness, abdominal mass or shock. A few cases of hepatocellular carcinoma have been reported in women taking oral contraceptives. The relationship of these drugs to this type of malignancy is not known at this time.

5. *Use in or Immediately Preceding Pregnancy, Birth Defects in Offspring, and Malignancy in Female Offspring:*
The use of female sex hormones—both estrogenic and progestational agents—during early pregnancy may seriously damage the offspring. It has been shown that females exposed in utero to diethylstilbestrol, a nonsteroidal estrogen, have an increased risk of developing in later life a form of vaginal or cervical cancer that is ordinarily extremely rare.[31,32] This risk has been estimated to be of the order of 1 in 1,000 exposures or less.[33,47] Although there is no evidence at the present time that oral contraceptives further enhance the risk of developing this type of malignancy, such patients should be monitored with particular care if they elect to use oral contraceptives instead of other methods of contraception. Furthermore, a high percentage of such exposed women (from 30 to 90%) have been found to have epithelial changes of the vagina and cervix.[34–38] Although these changes are histologically benign, it is not known whether this condition is a precursor of vaginal malignancy. Male children so exposed may develop abnormalities of the urogenital tract.[48–50] Although similar data are not available with the use of other estrogens, it cannot be presumed that they would not induce similar changes.

An increased risk of congenital anomalies, including heart defects and limb defects, has been reported with the use of sex hormones, including oral contraceptives, in pregnancy.[39–42,51] One case-control study[42] has estimated a 4.7-fold increase in risk of limb-reduction defects in infants exposed in utero to sex hormones (oral contraceptives, hormonal withdrawal tests for pregnancy, or attempted treatment for threatened abortion). Some of these exposures were very short and involved only a few days of treatment. The data suggest that the risk of limb-reduction defects in exposed fetuses is somewhat less than one in 1,000 live births.

In the past, female sex hormones have been used during pregnancy in an attempt to treat threatened or habitual abortion. There is considerable evidence that estrogens are ineffective for these indications, and there is no evidence from well-controlled studies that progestogens are effective for these uses.

There is some evidence that triploidy and possibly other types of polyploidy are increased among abortuses from women who become pregnant soon after ceasing oral contraceptives.[43] Embryos with these anomalies are virtually always aborted spontaneously. Whether there is an overall increase in spontaneous abortion of pregnancies conceived soon after stopping oral contraceptives is unknown. It is recommended that, for any patient who has missed two consecutive periods, pregnancy should be ruled out before continuing the contraceptive regimen. If the patient has not adhered to the prescribed schedule, the possibility of pregnancy should be considered at the time of the first missed period (or after 45 days from the last menstrual period if the progestogen-only oral contraceptives are used), and further use of oral contraceptives should be withheld until pregnancy has been ruled out. If pregnancy is confirmed, the patient should be apprised of the potential risks to the fetus, and the advisability of continuation of the pregnancy should be discussed in the light of these risks.

It is also recommended that women who discontinue oral contraceptives with the intent of becoming pregnant use an alternate form of contraception for a period of time before attempting to conceive. Many clinicians recommend 3 months, although no precise information is available on which to base this recommendation.

The administration of progestogen-only or progestogen-estrogen combinations to induce withdrawal bleeding should not be used as a test of pregnancy.

6. *Gallbladder Disease:*
Studies[8,23,26] report an increased risk of surgically confirmed gallbladder disease in users of oral contraceptives and estrogens. In one study, an increased risk appeared after 2 years of use and doubled after 4 or 5 years of use. In one of the other studies, an increased risk was apparent between 6 and 12 months of use.

7. *Carbohydrate and Lipid Metabolic Effects:*
A decrease in glucose tolerance has been observed in a significant percentage of patients on oral contraceptives. For this reason, prediabetic and diabetic patients should be carefully observed while receiving oral contraceptives.

An increase in triglycerides and total phospholipids has been observed in patients receiving oral contraceptives.[44] The clinical significance of this finding remains to be defined.

8. *Elevated Blood Pressure:*
An increase in blood pressure has been reported in patients receiving oral contraceptives.[26] In some women, hypertension may occur within a few months of beginning oral-contraceptive use. In the first year of use, the prevalence of women with hypertension is low in users and may be no higher than that of a comparable group of nonusers. The prevalence in users increases, however, with longer exposure, and in the fifth year of use is two-and-a-half to three times the reported prevalence in the first year. Age is also strongly correlated with the development of hypertension in oral-contraceptive users. Women who previously have had hypertension during pregnancy may be more likely to develop elevation of blood pressure when given oral contraceptives. Hypertension that develops as a result of taking oral contraceptives usually returns to normal after discontinuing the drug.

9. *Headache:*
The onset or exacerbation of migraine or development of headache of a new pattern which is recurrent, persistent, or severe, requires discontinuation of oral contraceptives and evaluation of the cause.

10. *Bleeding Irregularities:*
Breakthrough bleeding, spotting, and amenorrhea are frequent reasons for patients discontinuing oral contraceptives. In breakthrough bleeding, as in all cases of irregular bleeding from the vagina, nonfunctional causes should be borne in mind. In undiagnosed persistent or recurrent abnormal bleeding from the vagina, adequate diagnostic measures are indicated to rule out pregnancy or malignancy. If pathology has been excluded, time or a change to another formulation may solve the problem. Changing to an oral contraceptive with a higher estrogen content, while potentially useful in minimizing menstrual irregularity, should be done only if necessary, since this may increase the risk of thromboembolic disease.

Women with a past history of oligomenorrhea or secondary amenorrhea or young women without regular cycles may have a tendency to remain anovulatory or to become amenorrheic after discontinuation of oral contraceptives. Women with these preexisting problems should be advised of this possibility and encouraged to use other contraceptive methods. Post-use anovulation, possibly prolonged, may also occur in women without previous irregularities.

11. *Ectopic Pregnancy:*
Ectopic as well as intrauterine pregnancy may occur in contraceptive failures. However, in progestogen-only oral contraceptive failures, the ratio of ectopic to intrauterine pregnancies is higher than in women who are not receiving oral contraceptives, since the drugs are more effective in preventing intrauterine than ectopic pregnancies.

12. *Breast-feeding:*
Oral contraceptives given in the postpartum period may interfere with lactation. There may be a decrease in the quantity and quality of the breast milk. Furthermore, a small fraction of the hormonal agents in oral contraceptives has been identified in the milk of mothers receiving these drugs.[45,54,55] The effects, if any, on the breast-fed child have not been determined. If feasible, the use of oral contraceptives should be deferred until the infant has been weaned.

PRECAUTIONS

GENERAL

1. A complete medical and family history should be taken prior to initiation of oral contraceptives. The pretreatment and periodic physical examinations should include special reference to blood pressure, breasts, abdomen and pelvic organs, including Papanicolaou smear and relevant laboratory tests. As a general rule, oral contraceptives should not be prescribed for longer than 1 year without another physical examination being performed.
2. Under the influence of estrogen-progestogen preparations, preexisting uterine leiomyomata may increase in size.
3. Patients with a history of psychic depression should be carefully observed and the drug discontinued if depression recurs to a serious degree. Patients becoming significantly depressed while taking oral contraceptives should stop the medication and use an alternate method of contraception in an attempt to determine whether the symptom is drug-related.
4. Oral contraceptives may cause some degree of fluid retention. They should be prescribed with caution, and only with careful monitoring, in patients with conditions which might be aggravated by fluid retention, such as convulsive disorders, migraine syndrome, asthma, or cardiac or renal insufficiency.
5. Patients with a past history of jaundice during pregnancy have an increased risk of recurrence of jaundice while receiving oral-contraceptive therapy. If jaundice develops in any patient receiving such drugs, the medication should be discontinued.

6. Steroid hormones may be poorly metabolized in patients with impaired liver function and should be administered with caution in such patients.
7. Oral-contraceptive users may have disturbances in normal tryptophan metabolism which may result in a relative pyridoxine deficiency. The clinical significance of this is yet to be determined.
8. Serum folate levels may be depressed by oral-contraceptive therapy. Since the pregnant woman is predisposed to the development of folate deficiency and the incidence of folate deficiency increases with increasing gestation, it is possible that if a woman becomes pregnant shortly after stopping oral contraceptives, she may have a greater chance of developing folate deficiency and complications attributed to this deficiency.

INFORMATION FOR THE PATIENT
(See Patient Labeling which follows.)

LABORATORY TESTS
1. The pathologist should be advised of oral-contraceptive therapy when relevant specimens are submitted.
2. Certain endocrine- and liver-function tests and blood components may be affected by estrogen-containing oral contraceptives:
a. Increased sulfobromophthalein retention.
b. Increased prothrombin and factors VII, VIII, IX, and X; decreased antithrombin 3; increased norepinephrine-induced platelet aggregability.
c. Increased thyroid-binding globulin (TBG) leading to increased circulating total-thyroid hormone, as measured by protein-bound iodine (PBI), T4 by column, or T4 by radioimmunoassay. Free T3 resin uptake is decreased, reflecting the elevated TBG; free T4 concentration is unaltered.
d. Decreased pregnanediol excretion.
e. Reduced response to metyrapone test.

DRUG INTERACTIONS
Reduced efficacy and increased incidence of breakthrough bleeding have been associated with concomitant use of rifampin. A similar association has been suggested with barbiturates, phenylbutazone, phenytoin sodium, ampicillin, and tetracycline.

CARCINOGENESIS, MUTAGENESIS, IMPAIRMENT OF FERTILITY
See WARNINGS section #3, 4, and 5 for information on carcinogenesis, mutagenesis, and impairment of fertility.

PREGNANCY
Pregnancy Category X. See Contraindications and Warnings.

NURSING MOTHERS
See WARNINGS. Because of the potential for adverse reactions in nursing infants from oral-contraceptive tablets, a decision should be made whether to discontinue the drug, taking into account the importance of the drug to the mother.

ADVERSE REACTIONS

An increased risk of the following serious adverse reactions has been associated with the use of oral contraceptives (see Warnings):

Thrombophlebitis
Pulmonary embolism.
Coronary thrombosis.
Cerebral thrombosis.
Cerebral hemorrhage.
Hypertension.
Gallbladder disease.
Benign hepatomas.
Congenital anomalies.

There is evidence of an association between the following conditions and the use of oral contraceptives, although additional confirmatory studies are needed:

Mesenteric thrombosis.
Neuro-ocular lesions, e.g., retinal thrombosis and optic neuritis.

The following adverse reactions have been reported in patients receiving oral contraceptives and are believed to be drug-related:

Nausea and/or vomiting, usually the most common adverse reactions, occur in approximately 10 percent or less of patients during the first cycle. Other reactions, as a general rule, are seen much less frequently or only occasionally.
Gastrointestinal symptoms (such as abdominal cramps and bloating).
Breakthrough bleeding.
Spotting.
Change in menstrual flow.
Dysmenorrhea.
Amenorrhea during and after treatment.
Temporary infertility after discontinuance of treatment.
Edema.
Chloasma or melasma which may persist.
Breast changes: tenderness, enlargement, and secretion.
Change in weight (increase or decrease).
Change in cervical erosion and cervical secretion.
Possible diminution in lactation when given immediately postpartum.
Cholestatic jaundice.
Migraine.
Increase in size of uterine leiomyomata.
Rash (allergic).
Mental depression.
Reduced tolerance to carbohydrates.
Vaginal candidiasis.
Change in corneal curvature (steepening).
Intolerance to contact lenses.

The following adverse reactions have been reported in users of oral contraceptives, and the association has been neither confirmed nor refuted:

Premenstrual-like syndrome.
Cataracts.
Changes in libido.
Chorea.
Changes in appetite.
Cystitis-like syndrome.
Headache.
Nervousness
Dizziness.
Hirsutism.
Loss of scalp hair.
Erythema multiforme.
Erythema nodosum.
Hemorrhagic eruption.
Vaginitis.
Porphyria.
Hemolytic uremic syndrome.

ACUTE OVERDOSE

Serious ill effects have not been reported following acute ingestion of large doses of oral contraceptives by young children. Overdosage may cause nausea, and withdrawal bleeding may occur in females.

DOSAGE AND ADMINISTRATION

To achieve maximum contraceptive effectiveness, Nordette-21 must be taken exactly as directed and at intervals not exceeding 24 hours. The dosage of Nordette-21 is one tablet daily for 21 consecutive days per menstrual cycle according to prescribed schedule. Tablets are then discontinued for 7 days (three weeks on, one week off). It is recommended that Nordette-21 tablets be taken at the same time each day, preferably after the evening meal or at bedtime.

During the first cycle of medication, the patient is instructed to take one Nordette-21 tablet daily for twenty-one consecutive days beginning on day five of her menstrual cycle. (The first day of menstruation is day one.) The tablets are then discontinued for one week (7 days). Withdrawal bleeding should usually occur within three days following discontinuation of Nordette-21.

(If Nordette-21 is first taken later than the fifth day of the first menstrual cycle of medication or postpartum, contraceptive reliance should not be placed on Nordette-21 until after the first seven consecutive days of administration. The possibility of ovulation and conception prior to initiation of medication should be considered.)

The patient begins her next and all subsequent 21-day courses of Nordette-21 tablets on the same day of the week that she began her first course, following the same schedule: 21 days on—7 days off. She begins taking her tablets on the 8th day after discontinuance regardless of whether or not a menstrual period has occurred or is still in progress. Any time a new cycle of Nordette-21 is started later than the 8th day the patient should be protected by another means of contraception until she has taken a tablet daily for seven consecutive days.

If spotting or breakthrough bleeding occurs, the patient is instructed to continue on the same regimen. This type of bleeding is usually transient and without significance; however, if the bleeding is persistent or prolonged the patient is advised to consult her physician. Although the occurrence of pregnancy is highly unlikely if Nordette-21 is taken according to directions, if withdrawal bleeding does not occur, the possibility of pregnancy must be considered. If the patient has not adhered to the prescribed schedule (missed one or more tablets or started taking them on a day later than she should have) the probability of pregnancy should be considered at the time of the first missed period and appropriate diagnostic measures taken before the medication is resumed. If the patient has adhered to the prescribed regimen and misses two consecutive periods, pregnancy should be ruled out before continuing the contraceptive regimen.

The patient should be instructed to take a missed tablet as soon as it is remembered. If two consecutive tablets are missed they should both be taken as soon as remembered. The next tablet should be taken at the usual time.

Any time the patient misses one or two tablets she should also use another method of contraception until she has taken a tablet daily for seven consecutive days. If breakthrough bleeding occurs following missed tablets it will usually be transient and of no consequence. While there is little likelihood of ovulation occurring if only one or two tablets are missed, the possibility of ovulation increases with each successive day that scheduled tablets are missed. If three consecutive tablets are missed, all medication should be discontinued and the remainder of the package discarded. A new tablet cycle should be started on the 8th day after the last tablet was taken, and an alternate means of contraception should be prescribed during the seven days without tablets and until the patient has taken a tablet daily for seven consecutive days. In the nonlactating mother Nordette may be prescribed in the postpartum period either immediately or at the first postpartum examination whether or not menstruation has resumed.

HOW SUPPLIED

Nordette®-21 Tablets (0.15 mg levonorgestrel and 0.03 mg ethinyl estradiol tablets), Wyeth®, are available in 6 PIL-PAK® dispensers of 21 tablets each as follows: NDC 0008-0075, light-orange, round tablet marked "WYETH" and "75".

REFERENCES

1. "*Population Reports,*" Series H, Number 2, May 1974; Series I, Number 1, June 1974; Series B, Number 2, January 1975; Series H, Number 3, 1975; Series H, Number 4, January 1976 (published by the Population Information Program, The George Washington University Medical Center, 2001 S St. NW., Washington, D.C.).
2. Inman, W. H. W., Vessey, M. P., Westerholm, B., and Engelund, A., "Thromboembolic disease and the steroidal content of oral contraceptives. A report to the Committee on Safety of Drugs," Brit Med J *2:* 203-209, 1970.
3. Stolley, P. D., Tonascia, J. A., Tockman, M. S., Sartwell, P. E., Rutledge, A. H., and Jacobs, M. P., "Thrombosis with low-estrogen oral contraceptives," Am J Epidemiol *102:* 197-208, 1975.
4. Royal College of General Practitioners, "Oral contraception and thromboembolic disease," J Coll Gen Pract *13:* 267-279, 1967.
5. Inman, W. H. W., and Vessey, M. P., "Investigation of deaths from pulmonary, coronary and cerebral thrombosis and embolism in women of childbearing age," Brit Med J *2:* 193-199, 1968.
6. Vessey, M. P., and Doll, R., "Investigation of relation between use of oral contraceptives and thromboembolic disease. A further report," Brit Med J *2:* 651-657, 1969.
7. Sartwell, P. E., Masi, A. T., Arthes, F. G., Greene, G. R., and Smith, H. E., "Thromboembolism and oral contraceptives: an epidemiological case control study," Am J Epidemiol *90:* 365-380, 1969.
8. Boston Collaborative Drug Surveillance Program, "Oral contraceptives and venous thromboembolic disease, surgically confirmed gallbladder disease and breast tumors," Lancet *1:* 1399-1404, 1973.
9. Collaborative Group for the Study of Stroke in Young Women, "Oral contraception and increased risk of cerebral ischemia or thrombosis," N Engl J Med *288:* 871–878, 1973.
10. Collaborative Group for the Study of Stroke in Young Women, "Oral contraceptives and stroke in young women: associated risk factors," JAMA *231:* 718-722, 1975.
11. Mann, J. I., and Inman, W. H. W., "Oral contraceptives and death from myocardial infarction," Brit Med J *2:* 245-248, 1975.
12. Mann, J. I., Inman, W. H. W., and Thorogood, M., "Oral contraceptive use in older women and fatal myocardial infarction," Brit Med J *2:* 445-447, 1976.
13. Mann, J. I., Vessey, M. P., Thorogood, M., and Doll, R., "Myocardial infarction in young women with special reference to oral contraceptive practice," Brit Med J *2:* 241-245, 1975.
14. Tietze, C., "New Estimates of Mortality Associated with Fertility Control," Family Planning Perspectives, *9:* 74-76, 1977.
15. Vessey, M. P., Doll, R., Fairbairn, A. S., and Glober, G., "Post-operative thromboembolism and the use of oral contraceptives," Brit Med J *3:* 123-126, 1970.
16. Greene, G. R., Sartwell, P. E., "Oral contraceptive use in patients with thromboembolism following surgery, trauma, or infection," Am J Pub Health *62:* 680-685, 1972.
17. Smith, D. C., Prentice, R., Thompson, D. J., and Herrmann, W. L., "Association of exogenous estrogen and endometrial carcinoma," N Engl J Med *293:* 1164-1167, 1975.
18. Ziel, H. K., and Finkle, W. D., "Increased risk of endometrial carcinoma among users of conjugated estrogens," N Engl J Med *293:* 1167-1170, 1975.
19. Mack, T. N., Pike, M. C., Henderson, B. E., Pfeffer, R. I., Gerkins, V. R., Arthur, M., and Brown, S. E., "Estrogens and endometrial cancer in a retirement community," N Engl J Med *294:* 1262-1267, 1976.
20. Silverberg, S. G., and Makowski, E. L., "Endometrial carcinoma in young women taking oral contraceptive agents," Obstet Gynecol *46:* 503-506, 1975.

Continued on next page

Wyeth—Cont.

21. Vessey, M. P., Doll, R., and Sutton, P. M., "Oral contraceptives and breast neoplasia: a retrospective study," Brit Med J *3:* 719-724, 1972.
22. Vessey, M. P., Doll, R., and Jones K., "Oral contraceptives and breast cancer. Progress report of an epidemiological study," Lancet *1:* 941-943, 1975.
23. Boston Collaborative Drug Surveillance Program, "Surgically confirmed gallbladder disease, venous thromboembolism and breast tumors in relation to postmenopausal estrogen therapy," N Engl J Med *290:* 15-19, 1974.
24. Arthes, F. G., Sartwell, P. E., and Lewison, E. F., "The pill, estrogens, and the breast. Epidemiologic aspects," Cancer *28:* 1391-1394, 1971.
25. Fasal, E., and Paffenbarger, R. S., "Oral contraceptives as related to cancer and benign lesions of the breast," J Natl Cancer Inst *55:* 767-773, 1975.
26. Royal College of General Practitioners, "Oral Contraceptives and Health," London, Pitman, 1974.
27. Ory, H., Cole, P., MacMahon, B., and Hoover, R., "Oral contraceptives and reduced risk of benign breast diseases," N Engl J Med *294:* 419-422, 1976.
28. Baum, J., Holtz, F., Bookstein, J. J., and Klein, E. W., "Possible association between benign hepatomas and oral contraceptives," Lancet *2:* 926-928, 1973.
29. Mays, E. T., Christopherson, W. M., Mahr, M. M., and Williams, H. C., "Hepatic changes in young women ingesting contraceptive steroids. Hepatic hemorrhage and primary hepatic tumors," JAMA *235:* 730-732, 1976.
30. Edmondson, H. A., Henderson, B., and Benton, B., "Liver-cell adenomas associated with use of oral contraceptives," N Engl J Med *294:* 470-472, 1976.
31. Herbst, A. L., Ulfedler, H., and Poskanzer, D. C., "Adenocarcinoma of the vagina," N Engl J Med *284:* 878-881, 1971.
32. Greenwald, P., Barlow, J. J., Nasca, P. C., and Burnett, W., "Vaginal cancer after maternal treatment with synthetic estrogens," N Engl J Med *285:* 390-392, 1971.
33. Lanier, A. P., Noller, K. L., Decker, D. G., Elveback, L., and Kurland, L. T., "Cancer and stilbestrol. A follow-up of 1719 persons exposed to estrogens in utero and born 1943-1959," Mayo Clin Pro *48:* 793-799, 1973.
34. Herbst, A. L., Kurman, R. J., and Scully, R. E., "Vaginal and cervical abnormalities after exposure to stilbestrol in utero," Obstet Gynecol *40:* 287-298, 1972.
35. Herbst, A. L. Robboy, S. J., Macdonald, G. J., and Scully, R. E., "The effects of local progesterone on stilbestrol-associated vaginal adenosis." Am J Obstet Gynecol *118:* 607:615, 1974.
36. Herbst, A. L., Poskanzer, D. C., Robboy, S. J., Friedlander, L., and Scully, R. E., "Prenatal exposure to stilbestrol: a prospective comparison of exposed female offspring with unexposed controls," N Engl J Med *292:* 334-339, 1975.
37. Stafl, A., Mattingly, R. F., Foley, D. V., Fetherston, W., "Clinical diagnosis of vaginal adenosis," Obstet Gynecol *43:* 118-128, 1974.
38. Sherman, A. I., Goldrath, M., Berlin, A., Vakhariya, V., Banooni, F., Michaels, W., Goodman, P., and Brown S., "Cervical-vaginal adenosis after in utero exposure to synthetic estrogens," Obstet Gynecol *44:* 531-545, 1974.
39. Gal, I., Kirman, B., and Stern, J., "Hormone pregnancy tests and congenital malformation," Nature *216:* 83, 1967.
40. Levy, E. P., Cohen, A., and Fraser, F. C., "Hormone treatment during pregnancy and congenital heart defects," Lancet *1:* 611, 1973.
41. Nora, J. J., and Nora, A. H., "Birth defects and oral contraceptives," Lancet *1:* 941-942, 1973.
42. Janerich, D. T., Piper, J. M., and Glebatis, D. M., "Oral contraceptives and congenital limb-reduction defects," N Engl J Med *291:* 697-700, 1974.
43. Carr, D. H., "Chromosome studies in selected spontaneous abortions: I. Conception after oral contraceptives," Canad Med Assoc J *103:* 343-348, 1970.
44. Wynn, V., Doar, J. W. H., and Mills, G. L., "Some effects of oral contraceptives on serum-lipid and lipoprotein levels," Lancet *2:* 720-723, 1966.
45. Laumas, K. R., Malkani, P. K., Bhatnagar, S., and Laumas, V., "Radioactivity in the breast milk of lactating women after oral administration of 3 H-norethynodrel," Amer J Obstet Gynecol *98:* 411-413, 1967.
46. Center for Disease Control, "Increased Risk of Hepatocellular Adenoma in Women with Long-term use of Oral Contraceptives," Morbidity and Mortality Weekly Report, *26:* 293-294, 1977.
47. Herbst, A. L., Cole, P., Colton, T., Robboy, S. J., Scully, R. E., "Age-incidence and Risk of Diethylstilbestrol-related Clear Cell Adenocarcinoma of the Vagina and Cervix," Am J Obstet Gynecol, *128:* 43-50, 1977.
48. Bibbo, M., Al-Naqeeb, M., Baccarini, I., Gill, W., Newton, M., Sleeper, K. M., Sonek, M., Wied, G. L., "Follow-up Study of Male and Female Offspring of DES-treated Mothers. A Preliminary Report," J of Repro Med, *15:* 29-32, 1975.
49. Gill, W. B., Schumacher, G. F. B., Bibbo, M., "Structural and Functional Abnormalities in the Sex Organs of Male Offspring of Mothers Treated with Diethylstilbestrol (DES)," J of Repro Med, *16:* 147-153, 1976.
50. Henderson, B. E., Senton, B., Cosgrove, M., Baptista, J., Aldrich, J., Townsend, D., Hart, W., Mack, T., "Urogenital Tract Abnormalities in Sons of Women Treated with Diethylstilbestrol," Pediatrics, *58:* 505-507, 1976.
51. Heinonen, O. P., Slone, D., Nonson, R. R., Hook, E. B., Shapiro, S., "Cardiovascular Birth Defects and Antenatal Exposure to Female Sex Hormones," N Engl J Med *296:* 67-70, 1977.
52. Jain, A. K., "Mortality Risk Associated with the Use of Oral Contraceptives," Studies in Family Planning *8:* 50-54, 1977.
53. Beral, V., "Mortality Among Oral Contraceptive Users," Lancet, *2:* 727-731, 1977.
54. Nilsson, S., Nygren, K., and Johansson, E., "Ethinyl Estradiol in Human Milk and Plasma after Oral Administration," Contraception *17:* 131-139, 1978.
55. Nilsson, S., Nygren, K., and Johansson, E., "d-Norgestrel Concentrations in Maternal Plasma, Milk and Child Plasma During Administration of Oral Contraceptives to Nursing Women," Am J Obstet Gynecol, *129:* 178, 1977.
56. Royal College of General Practioners' Oral contraception study, "Incidence of arterial disease among oral contraceptive users," J Royal Col Gen Pract *33:* 75–82, 1983.
57. Slone, D., Shapiro, S., Kaufman, D. W., Rosenberg, L., Miettinen, O., and Stolley, P., "Risk of myocardial infarction in relation to current and discontinued use of oral contraceptives," N Engl J Med *305:* 420–424, 1981.
58. Inman, W.H.W., "Oral contraceptives and fatal subarachnoid haemorrhage," Brit Med J *2:* 1468–1470, 1979.
59. Petitti, D. B., and Wingerd, J., "Use of oral contraceptives, cigarette smoking and risk of subarachnoid haemorrhage," Lancet *2:* 234–236, 1978.
60. Thorogood, M., Adam, S. A., and Mann, J. I., "Fatal subarachnoid haemorrhage in young women: role of oral contraceptives," Brit Med J *283:* 762, 1981.
61. Rosenberg, L., Hennekens, C. H., Rosner, B., Belanger, C., Rothman, K. J., and Speizer, F. E., "Oral contraceptive use in relation to nonfatal myocardial infarction," Am J Epidemiol *111:* 59–66, 1980.
62. Adam, S. A., Thorogood, M., and Mann, J. I., "Oral contraception and myocardial infarction revisited: the effects of new preparations and prescribing patterns," Brit J Obstet Gynaecol *88:* 838–845, 1981.

Brief Summary Patient Package Insert: See Lo/Ovral.
DETAILED PATIENT LABELING: See Lo/Ovral.

Shown in Product Identification Section, page 436

NORDETTE®-28 ℞

[*nor-det'-28*]
TABLETS
(levonorgestrel and ethinyl estradiol tablets)

DESCRIPTION

ORAL CONTRACEPTIVE

21 light-orange Nordette® tablets, each containing 0.15 mg of levonorgestrel (*d* (-)-13 beta-ethyl -17-alpha-ethinyl-17-beta-hydroxygon-4-en-3-one), a totally synthetic progestogen, and 0.03 mg of ethinyl estradiol (19-nor-17α-pregna-1,3,5 (10)-trien-20-yne-3,17-diol), and 7 pink inert tablets. The inactive ingredients present are cellulose, FD&C Red 3, FD&C Yellow 6, lactose, magnesium stearate, and polacrilin potassium.

CLINICAL PHARMACOLOGY

See NORDETTE®-21

INDICATIONS AND USAGE

See NORDETTE-21

Dose-Related Risk of Thromboembolism from Oral Contraceptives: See NORDETTE-21

CONTRAINDICATIONS

See NORDETTE-21

WARNINGS

See NORDETTE-21

PRECAUTIONS

See NORDETTE-21

ADVERSE REACTIONS

See NORDETTE-21

Acute Overdosage: See NORDETTE-21

DOSAGE AND ADMINISTRATION

To achieve maximum contraceptive effectiveness, Nordette-28 must be taken exactly as directed and at intervals not exceeding 24 hours. The dosage of Nordette-28 is one light-orange tablet daily for 21 consecutive days followed by one pink inert tablet daily for 7 consecutive days according to prescribed schedule. It is recommended that tablets be taken at the same time each day, preferably after the evening meal or at bedtime.

During the first cycle of medication, the patient is instructed to begin taking Nordette-28 on the first Sunday after the onset of menstruation. If menstruation begins on a Sunday, the first tablet (light-orange) is taken that day. One light-orange tablet should be taken daily for 21 consecutive days followed by one pink inert tablet daily for 7 consecutive days. Withdrawal bleeding should usually occur within three days following discontinuation of light-orange tablets.

During the first cycle, contraceptive reliance should not be placed on Nordette-28 until a light-orange tablet has been taken daily for 7 consecutive days. The possibility of ovulation and conception prior to initiation of medication should be considered.

The patient begins her next and all subsequent 28-day courses of tablets on the same day of the week (Sunday) on which she began her first course, following the same schedule: 21 days on light-orange tablets—7 days on pink inert tablets. If in any cycle the patient starts tablets later than the proper day, she should protect herself by using another method of birth control until she has taken a light-orange tablet daily for 7 consecutive days.

If spotting or breakthrough bleeding occurs, the patient is instructed to continue on the same regimen. This type of bleeding is usually transient and without significance; however, if the bleeding is persistent or prolonged, the patient is advised to consult her physician. Although the occurrence of pregnancy is highly unlikely if Nordette-28 is taken according to directions, if withdrawal bleeding does not occur, the possibility of pregnancy must be considered. If the patient has not adhered to the prescribed schedule (missed one or more tablets or started taking them on a day later than she should have), the probability of pregnancy should be considered at the time of the first missed period and appropriate diagnostic measures taken before the medication is resumed. If the patient has adhered to the prescribed regimen and misses two consecutive periods, pregnancy should be ruled out before continuing the contraceptive regimen. The patient should be instructed to take a missed light-orange tablet as soon as it is remembered. If two consecutive light-orange tablets are missed, they should both be taken as soon as remembered. The next tablet should be taken at the usual time. Any time the patient misses one or two light-orange tablets she should also use another method of contraception until she has taken a light-orange tablet daily for seven consecutive days. If the patient misses one or more pink tablets, she is still protected against pregnancy *provided* she begins taking light-orange tablets again on the proper day.

If breakthrough bleeding occurs following missed light-orange tablets, it will usually be transient and of no consequence. While there is little likelihood of ovulation occurring if only one or two light-orange tablets are missed, the possibility of ovulation increases with each successive day that scheduled light-orange tablets are missed. (If three consecutive light-orange Nordette tablets are missed, all medication should be discontinued and the remainder of the 28-day package discarded. A new tablet cycle should be started on the first Sunday following the last missed tablet, and an alternate means of contraception should be prescribed during the days without tablets and until the patient has taken a light-orange tablet daily for 7 consecutive days.) In the non-lactating mother, Nordette may be prescribed in the postpartum period either immediately or at the first postpartum examination whether or not menstruation has resumed.

HOW SUPPLIED

Nordette®-28 Tablets (0.15 mg levonorgestrel and 0.03 mg ethinyl estradiol tablets), Wyeth®, are available in 6 PIL-PAK® dispensers, each containing 28 tablets as follows: 21 active tablets, NDC 0008-2533, light-orange, round tablet marked "WYETH" and "75". 7 inert tablets, NDC 0008-0486, pink, round tablet marked "WYETH" and "486".

REFERENCES

See NORDETTE-21.

Brief Summary Patient Package Insert: See LO/OVRAL.
DETAILED PATIENT LABELING: See LO/OVRAL.

Shown in Product Identification Section, page 436

NURSOY®

[*nur-soy*]
Soy protein formula
READY-TO-FEED
CONCENTRATED LIQUID
POWDER

NURSOY® milk free formula is intended to meet the nutritional needs of infants and children who are not breast-fed and are allergic to cow's milk protein or intolerant to lactose. NURSOY Ready-to-Feed and Concentrated Liquid contain sucrose as their carbohydrate. NURSOY Powder contains corn syrup solids as its carbohydrate. Professional advice should be followed.

INGREDIENTS

(in normal dilution supplying 20 calories per fluidounce): 87% water; 6.7% sucrose; 3.4% oleo, coconut, oleic (safflower) and soybean oils; 2.3% soy protein isolate; 0.10% potassium citrate; 0.09% monobasic sodium phosphate; 0.04% calcium carbonate; 0.04% dibasic calcium phosphate;

0.03% magnesium chloride; 0.03% calcium chloride; 0.03% soy lecithin; 0.03% calcium carrageenan; 0.03% calcium hydroxide; 0.03% l-methionine; 0.01% sodium chloride; 0.01% potassium bicarbonate; ferrous, zinc and cupric sulfates; (68ppb) potassium iodide; ascorbic acid; choline chloride; alpha tocopheryl acetate; niacinamide; calcium pantothenate; riboflavin; vitamin A palmitate; thiamine hydrochloride; pyridoxine hydrochloride; beta-carotene; phytonadione; folic acid; biotin; activated 7-dehydrocholesterol; cyanocobalamin. NURSOY Powder contains corn syrup solids. NURSOY Ready-to-Feed and Concentrated Liquid contain sucrose.

PROXIMATE ANALYSIS

at 20 calories per fluidounce

READY-TO-FEED, CONCENTRATED LIQUID and POWDER

	(W/V)
Protein	2.1%
Fat	3.6%
Carbohydrate	6.9%
Ash	0.35%
Water	87.0%
Crude fiber	not more than 0.01%
Calories/fl. oz.	20

Vitamins, Minerals: In normal dilution, each quart contains:

A	2,500	IU
D_3	400	IU
E	9	IU
K_1	0.1	mg
C (ascorbic acid)	55	mg
B_1 (thiamine)	0.67	mg
B_2 (riboflavin)	1	mg
B_6	0.4	mg
B_{12}	2	mcg
Niacin mg equivalents	9.5	
Pantothenic acid	3	mg
Folic acid	50	mcg
Choline	85	mg
Inositol	26	mg
Biotin	35	mcg
Calcium	600	mg
Phosphorus	420	mg
Sodium	190	mg
Potassium	700	mg
Chloride	355	mg
Magnesium	65	mg
Manganese	0.2	mg
Iron	12	mg
Copper	0.45	mg
Zinc	3.5	mg
Iodine	65	mcg

PREPARATION

Ready-to-Feed (32 fl. oz. cans of 20 calories per fluidounce formula)—shake can, open and pour into previously sterilized nursing bottle; attach nipple and feed. Cover opened can and immediately store in refrigerator. Use contents of can within 48 hours of opening.

Concentrated Liquid—For normal dilution supplying 20 calories per fluidounce, use equal amounts of Nursoy® liquid and cooled, previously boiled water. *Note: Prepared formula should be used within 24 hours.*

Powder—For normal dilution supplying 20 calories per fluid ounce, use 7 fluidounces of cooled, previously boiled water and 1 unit-of-use packet of NURSOY Powder. *Note: Prepared formula should be used within 24 hours.*

HOW SUPPLIED

Ready-to-Feed—presterilized and premixed, 32 fluidounce (1 quart) cans, cases of 6; *Concentrated Liquid*—13 fluidounce cans, cases of 24; *Powder*—1 pound cans, cases of 6.

Also available to hospitals only:

Ready-to-Feed 4 oz. disposable bottles (48 bottles/case) as part of the Wyeth Hospital Infant Feeding System.

OMNIPEN® ℞

[*om 'nī-pen*]
(ampicillin)
CAPSULES

HOW SUPPLIED

Omnipen® (ampicillin) Capsules—250 mg ampicillin anhydrous, bottles of 100 and 500 capsules; 500 mg, bottles of 100 and 500 capsules.

For prescribing information write to Professional Service, Wyeth Laboratories, Box 8299, Philadelphia, PA 19101, or contact your local Wyeth representative.

Shown in Product Identification Section, page 436

OMNIPEN® ℞

[*om 'nī-pen*]
(ampicillin)
ORAL SUSPENSION

HOW SUPPLIED

Omnipen® (ampicillin) for Oral Suspension in bottles of powder for reconstitution. When reconstituted with water they will make a palatable suspension containing 125 mg, 250 mg, or 500 mg ampicillin per 5 ml.

For prescribing information write to Professional Service, Wyeth Laboratories, Box 8299, Philadelphia, PA 19101, or contact your local Wyeth representative.

OMNIPEN® Pediatric Drops ℞

[*om 'nī-pen*]
(ampicillin)
ORAL SUSPENSION

HOW SUPPLIED

One bottle of powder for reconstitution with water to make 20 ml suspension. When reconstituted according to instructions on label, each ml contains 100 mg of ampicillin.

For prescribing information write to Professional Service, Wyeth Laboratories, Box 8299, Philadelphia, PA 19101, or contact your local Wyeth representative.

OMNIPEN®-N ℞

[*om 'nī-pen-N*]
(ampicillin sodium)
INJECTION

HOW SUPPLIED

Omnipen®-N (ampicillin sodium) for Injection: Ampicillin sodium equivalent to 125 mg, 250 mg, 500 mg, 1 gram, or 2 gram ampicillin per standard vial; 10 gram per pharmacy bulk vial. Piggyback Units: Supplied in single units equivalent to 500 mg, 1 gram or 2 gram ampicillin per unit, packed in 10 vials per package.

For prescribing information write to Professional Service, Wyeth Laboratories, Box 8299, Philadelphia, PA 19101, or contact your local Wyeth representative.

ORUDIS® ℞

[*ō "roo 'dĭs*]
(ketoprofen)
Capsules

DESCRIPTION

Orudis (ketoprofen) is a nonsteroidal antiinflammatory drug. The chemical name for ketoprofen is 2-(3-benzoylphenyl)-propionic acid with the following structural formula:

[structural formula: O, C, CHCOOH, CH3]

Its empirical formula is $C_{16}H_{14}O_3$, with a molecular weight of 254.29.

Ketoprofen is a white or off-white, odorless, nonhygroscopic, fine to granular powder, melting at about 95°C. It is freely soluble in ethanol, chloroform, acetone, and ether; soluble in benzene and strong alkali, but practically insoluble in water at 20°C.

Orudis capsules contain 50 mg or 75 mg of ketoprofen for oral administration. The inactive ingredients present are D&C Yellow 10, FD&C Blue 1, FD&C Yellow 6, gelatin, lactose, magnesium stearate, and titanium dioxide.

CLINICAL PHARMACOLOGY

Orudis (ketoprofen) is a nonsteroidal antiinflammatory drug with analgesic and antipyretic properties.

The antiinflammatory, analgesic, and antipyretic properties of Orudis have been demonstrated in classical animal and *in vitro* test systems. In antiinflammatory models Orudis has been shown to have inhibitory effects on prostaglandin and leukotriene synthesis, to have antibradykinin activity, as well as to have lysosomal membrane-stabilizing action. However, its mode of action, like that of other nonsteroidal antiinflammatory drugs, is not fully understood.

Orudis is rapidly and completely absorbed from the gastrointestinal tract. Mean Orudis peak plasma levels are reached in 0.5 to 2 hours. The total absolute bioavailability of Orudis, as demonstrated by area under the plasma concentration-time curve (AUC), is approximately 90% for capsule formulations tested when compared to IV administration and is linear for 75 to 200 mg single doses. The plasma clearance of ketoprofen is approximately 0.08 L/kg/hr with a V_d of 0.1 L/kg after IV administration. The mean plasma elimination half-life of Orudis ranged from 2 to 4 hours in 14 pharmacokinetic studies which included 6 to 24 normal volunteers.

Following absorption, Orudis can be detected in plasma as the unchanged compound, hydroxylated metabolites and their respective glucuronides. There are no known active metabolites of Orudis. The drug is 99% bound to plasma proteins, mainly to the albumin fraction. Approximately 60% of an administered dose of Orudis is excreted in the urine primarily as the glucuronide metabolite in the first 24 hours. Enterohepatic recirculation of the drug has been postulated to account for the other 40% of the absorbed ketoprofen, although biliary levels have never been measured to confirm this.

Orudis has been shown to not induce drug-metabolizing enzymes.

Steady-state concentrations of Orudis are attained within 24 hours after commencing treatment.

When ketoprofen is administered with food, its total bioavailability (AUC) is not altered; however, the rate of absorption is slowed resulting in delayed and reduced peak concentrations (C_{max}). Following a single 50 mg dose of Orudis while fasting, the mean C_{max} is 4.1 mg/L (at 1.1 hours); when administered after food, it decreases to 2.4 mg/L (at 2.0 hours).

To date, studies of the effects of age and renal-function impairment have been small, generally involving 5 to 8 subjects per group, but they indicate modest decrease in clearance in the elderly and in patients with impaired renal function. In normal elderly volunteers (mean age 73 years), the plasma and renal clearance and protein-binding were reduced while the V_d increased when compared to a younger normal population (mean age 27 years). (Plasma clearance and V_d were 0.05 L/kg/hr and 0.4 L/kg in elderly and 0.06 L/kg/hr and 0.3 L/kg in young subjects, respectively.) The mean half-life of Orudis in this normal geriatric population, as well as in a rheumatoid elderly population (mean age 64 years), was about 5 hours as compared to 3 hours in the younger population.

Patients with impaired renal function (mean age 44 years) also demonstrate decreases in plasma clearance (0.04 L/kg/hr) of drug, with the mean half-life increasing to about 3.5 hours.

For patients with alcoholic cirrhosis, no significant changes in the kinetic disposition of Orudis were observed relative to age-matched normal subjects; the plasma clearance of drug was 0.07 L/kg/hr) in both groups (N=8 for each group) and total bioavailability was comparable. However, the protein unbound (biologically active) fraction was increased from 0.85% to 1.15%, probably due to hypoalbuminemia, and high variability was observed in the pharmacokinetics in cirrhotic patients. Therefore, these patients should be carefully monitored and daily doses kept at the minimum levels providing the desired therapeutic effect.

In healthy men, the average blood loss in stool, measured over a one-week period during administration of 200 mg per day of Orudis, was 50% lower than that resulting from administration of 3,900 mg per day of aspirin. In addition, a double-blind crossover trial using gastroscopy in 13 normal volunteers demonstrated fewer mucosal lesions with Orudis than aspirin.

The efficacy of Orudis has been demonstrated in patients with rheumatoid arthritis and osteoarthritis. Using standard assessment of therapeutic response, Orudis demonstrated effectiveness comparable to aspirin, ibuprofen, and indomethacin.

In studies in patients with rheumatoid arthritis, Orudis was administered in combination with gold salts, antimalarials, and/or corticosteroids with results comparable to those seen with the control nonsteroidal drugs.

INDICATIONS AND USAGE

Orudis is indicated for the acute or long-term treatment of the signs and symptoms of rheumatoid arthritis and osteoarthritis.

CONTRAINDICATIONS

Orudis is contraindicated in patients who have shown hypersensitivity to it. Orudis should not be given to patients in whom aspirin or other nonsteroidal antiinflammatory drugs induce asthma, urticaria, or other allergic-type reactions because severe, rarely fatal, anaphylactic reactions to Orudis have been reported in such patients.

WARNINGS

As with other steroidal and nonsteroidal antiinflammatory drugs, peptic ulcerations and gastrointestinal bleeding have been reported in patients receiving Orudis. Unlike most adverse reactions, which usually manifest themselves in the first month if they are going to occur in an individual, new peptic ulcers keep appearing in patients under treatment with ketoprofen at a rate of greater than 1% per year (see "Adverse Reactions"). In patients with evidence of gastrointestinal bleeding or an active peptic ulcer, an appropriate anti-ulcer regimen should be instituted, and the physician must weigh the benefits of treatment with Orudis against

Continued on next page

Wyeth—Cont.

possible hazards, and closely monitor the patient's progress. When the drug is given to patients with a history of gastrointestinal-tract disease, it should be given under careful supervision, and only after consulting the "Adverse Reactions" section.

GENERAL PRECAUTIONS

Orudis and other nonsteroidal antiinflammatory drugs cause nephritis in mice and rats associated with chronic administration. Cases of interstitial nephritis and nephrotic syndrome have been reported with Orudis since it has been marketed abroad.

A second form of renal toxicity has been seen in patients with conditions leading to a reduction in renal blood flow or blood volume, where renal prostaglandins have a supportive role in the maintenance of renal blood flow. In these patients administration of a nonsteroidal antiinflammatory drug results in a dose-dependent decrease in prostaglandin synthesis and, secondarily, in renal blood flow which may precipitate overt renal failure. Patients at greatest risk of this reaction are those with impaired renal function, heart failure, liver dysfunction, those taking diuretics, and the elderly. Discontinuation of nonsteroidal antiinflammatory drug therapy is typically followed by recovery to the pretreatment state.

Since ketoprofen is primarily eliminated by the kidneys and its pharmacokinetics are altered by renal failure (see "Clinical Pharmacology"), patients with significantly impaired renal function should be closely monitored, and a reduction of dosage should be anticipated to avoid accumulation of ketoprofen and/or it metabolites.

As with other nonsteroidal antiinflammatory drugs, borderline elevations of one or more liver-function tests may occur in up to 15% of patients. These abnormalities may progress, may remain essentially unchanged, or may disappear with continued therapy. The SGPT (AL) test is probably the most sensitive indicator of liver dysfunction. Meaningful (3 times the upper limit of normal) elevations of SGPT or SGOT (AST) occurred in controlled clinical trials in less than 1% of patients. A patient with symptoms and/or signs suggesting liver dysfunction, or whom an abnormal liver test has occurred, should be evaluated for evidence of the development of a more severe hepatic reaction while on therapy with ketoprofen. Serious hepatic reactions, including jaundice, have been reported from postmarketing experience with ketoprofen as well as with other nonsteroidal antiinflammatory drugs.

If steroid dosage is reduced or eliminated during therapy, it should be reduced slowly and the patients observed closely for any evidence of adverse effects, including adrenal insufficiency and exacerbation of symptoms of arthritis.

Anemia is commonly observed in rheumatoid arthritis and is sometimes aggravated by nonsteroidal antiinflammatory drugs, which may produce fluid retention or minor gastrointestinal blood loss in some patients. Therefore, patients with initial hemoglobin values of 10 g/dL or less who are to receive long- term therapy should have hemoglobin values determined frequently.

Peripheral edema has been observed in approximately 2% of patients taking ketoprofen. Therefore, as with other nonsteroidal antiinflammatory drugs, ketoprofen should be used with caution in patients with fluid retention, hypertension, or heart failure.

INFORMATION FOR PATIENTS

Because aspirin causes an increase in the level of unbound ketoprofen, patients should be advised not to take aspirin while taking Orudis (see "Drug Interactions"). It is possible that minor adverse symptoms of gastric intolerance may be prevented by administering Orudis with antacids, food, or milk. Because antacids do not affect bioavailability (see "Drug Interactions") but food and milk do affect the rate but not the extent of absorption (see "Clinical Pharmacology"), physicians may want to make specific recommendations to patients about when they should take Orudis in relation to food and/or what patients should do if they experience minor GI symptoms associated with Orudis therapy.

DRUG INTERACTIONS

The following drug interactions were studied with Orudis doses of 200 mg per day (50 mg q.i.d.). The possibility of increased interaction should be kept in mind when Orudis doses greater than 50 mg as a single dose or 200 mg per day are used concomitantly with highly bound drugs.

1. *Antacids*

Concomitant administration of magnesium hydroxide and aluminum hydroxide does not interfere with the rate or extent of the absorption of ketoprofen.

2. *Aspirin*

Orudis does not alter aspirin absorption; however, in a study of 12 normal subjects, concurrent administration of aspirin decreased ketoprofen protein-binding and increased ketoprofen plasma clearance from 0.07 L/kg/hr without aspirin to 0.11 L/kg/hr with aspirin. The clinical significance of these changes has not been adequately studied. Therefore, concurrent use of aspirin and ketoprofen is not recommended.

3. *Diuretic*

Hydrochlorothiazide, given concomitantly with Orudis, produces a reduction in urinary potassium and chloride excretion compared to hydrochlorothiazide alone. Patients taking diuretics are at greater risk of developing renal failure secondary to a decrease in renal blood flow caused by prostaglandin inhibition (see "General Precautions").

4. *Digoxin*

In a study in 12 patients with congestive heart failure where Orudis and digoxin were concomitantly administered, Orudis did not alter the serum levels of digoxin.

5. *Warfarin*

In a short-term controlled study in 14 normal volunteers, Orudis did not significantly interfere with the effect of warfarin on prothrombin time. Bleedng from a number of sites may be a complication of warfarin treatment and GI bleeding a complication of Orudis treatment. Because prostaglandins play an important role in hemostasis and ketoprofen has an effect on platelet function as well (see "Blood Coagulation"), concurrent therapy with Orudis and warfarin requires close monitoring of patients on both drugs.

6. *Probenecid*

Probenecid increases both free and bound ketoprofen through reducing the plasma clearance of ketoprofen to about one-third, as well as decreasing its protein-binding. Therefore, the combination of Orudis and probenecid is not recommended.

DRUG/LABORATORY TEST INTERACTIONS: EFFECT ON BLOOD COAGULATION

Orudis decreases platelet adhesion and aggregation. Therefore, it can prolong bleeding time by approximately 3 to 4 minutes from baseline values. There is no significant change in platelet count, prothrombin time, partial thromboplastin time, or thrombin time.

CARCINOGENESIS, MUTAGENESIS, IMPAIRMENT OF FERTILITY

Chronic oral toxicity studies in mice (up to 32 mg/kg/day) did not indicate a carcinogenic potential for Orudis (maximum recommended human therapeutic dose for a 50 kg man is 6 mg/kg/day). A chronic oral toxicity study was also performed in rats (up to 12.5 mg/kg/day) with no statistically significant increase in any tumor type; however, this study was unacceptable because of poor survival. Orudis did not show mutagenic potential in the Ames Test. Orudis administered to male rats (up to 9 mg/kg/day) had no significant effect on reproductive performance or fertility. In female rats administered 6 or 9 mg/kg/day, a decrease in the number of implantation sites has been noted.

TERATOGENIC EFFECTS: PREGNANCY CATEGORY B

In teratology studies Orudis administered to mice at doses up to 12 mg/kg/day and rats at doses up to 9 mg/kg/day, the approximate equivalent of 1.5 times the maximum recommended therapeutic dose in (a 50 kg) man, showed no teratogenic or embryotoxic effects. In separate studies in rabbits, maternally toxic doses were associated with embryotoxicity but not teratogenicity.

There are no adequate and well-controlled studies in pregnant women. Because animal teratology studies are not always predictive of the human response, Orudis should be used during pregnancy only if the potential benefit justifies the risk.

LABOR AND DELIVERY

The effects of Orudis on labor and delivery in pregnant women are unknown. Studies in rats have shown Orudis at doses of 6 mg/kg (approximately equal to the maximum recommended human dose) prolong pregnancy when given before the onset of labor. Because of the known effects of prostaglandin-inhibiting drugs on the fetal cardiovascular system (closure of ductus arteriosus), use of Orudis during late pregnancy should be avoided.

NURSING MOTHERS

In rats, Orudis at doses of 9 mg/kg (approximately 1.5 times the maximum human therapeutic dose) did not affect perinatal development. Upon administration to lactating dogs, the milk concentration of Orudis was found to be 4 to 5% of the plasma drug level. Data on secretion in human milk after ingestion of ketoprofen do not exist. As with other drugs that are excreted in milk, Orudis is not recommended for use in nursing mothers.

PEDIATRIC USE

Orudis is not recommended for use in children because its safety and effectiveness have not been studied in children.

ADVERSE REACTIONS

The incidence of common adverse reactions (above 1%) was obtained from a population of 835 ketoprofen-treated patients in double-blind trials lasting from 4 to 54 weeks.

Minor gastrointestinal side effects predominated; upper gastrointestinal symptoms were more common than lower gastrointestinal symptoms. Peptic ulcer or GI bleeding occurred in controlled clinical trials in less than 1% of 1,076 patients; however, in open label continuation studies in 1,292 patients the rate was greater than 2%. The incidence of peptic ulceration in patients on NSAIDs is dependent on many risk factors including age, sex, smoking, alcohol use, diet, stress, concomitant drugs such as aspirin and corticoids, as well as the dose and duration of treatment with NSAIDs (see "Warnings"). These were followed in frequency by central nervous system side effects, such as headache, dizziness, or drowsiness. The incidence of some adverse reactions appears to be dose-related (see "Dosage and Administration"). Those rare adverse reactions (incidence less than 1%) were collected from foreign reports to manufacturers and regulatory agencies, publications, and U.S. clinical trials.

In double-blind trials, 233 ketoprofen-treated patients had fewer minor gastrointestinal complaints, tinnitus and hearing impairment, fluid retention, and minor abnormalities in liver- function tests than 228 aspirin-tested patients.

INCIDENCE GREATER THAN 1%
(PROBABLE CAUSAL RELATIONSHIP)

Digestive: Dyspepsia (11.5%), nausea*, abdominal pain*, diarrhea*, constipation*, flatulence*, anorexia, vomiting, stomatitis.

Central Nervous System: Headache*, dizziness, CNS inhibition (i.e., pooled reports of somnolence, malaise, depression, etc.) or excitation (i.e., insomnia, nervousness, dreams, etc.).*

Special Senses: Tinnitus, visual disturbance.

Skin and Appendages: Rash.

Urogenital: Impairment of renal function (edema, increased BUN)*, signs or symptoms of urinary-tract irritation.

*Side effects with incidence greater than 3%.

INCIDENCE LESS THAN 1%
(PROBABLE CAUSAL RELATIONSHIP)

Digestive: Appetite increased, dry mouth, eructation, gastritis, rectal hemorrhage, melena, fecal occult blood, salivation, peptic ulcer, gastrointestinal perforation, hematemesis, intestinal ulceration.

Central Nervous System: Amnesia, confusion, impotence, migraine, paresthesia, vertigo.

Special Senses: Conjunctivitis, conjunctivitis sicca, eye pain, hearing impairment, retinal hemorrhage and pigmentation change, taste perversion.

Skin and Appendages: Alopecia, eczema, pruritus, purpuric rash, sweating, urticaria, bullous rash, exfoliative dermatitis, photosensitivity, skin discoloration, onycholysis.

Body as a Whole: Chills, facial edema, infection, pain, allergic raction, anaphylaxis.

Cardiovascular: Hypertension, palpitation, tachycardia, congestive heart failure, peripheral vascular disease, vasodilation.

Hemic: Hypocoagulability, agranulocytosis, anemia, hemolysis, purpura, thrombocytopenia.

Metabolic and Nutritional: Thirst, weight gain, weight loss, hepatic dysfunction, hyponatremia.

Musculoskeletal: Myalgia.

Respiratory: Dyspnea, hemoptysis, epistaxis, pharyngitis, rhinitis, bronchospasm, laryngeal edema.

Urogenital: Menometrorrhagia, hematuria, renal failure, interstitial nephritis, nephrotic syndrome.

CAUSAL RELATIONSHIP UNKNOWN

The following rare adverse reactions, whose causal relationship to ketoprofen is uncertain, are being listed to serve as alerting information to the physician.

Digestive: Buccal necrosis, ulcerative colitis.

Central Nervous System: Dysphoria, hallucination, libido disturbance, nightmares, personality disorder.

Body as a Whole: Septicemia, shock.

Cardiovascular: Arrhythmias, myocardial infarction.

Endocrine: Diabetes mellitus (aggravated).

Metabolic and Nutritional: Jaundice.

Urogenital: Acute tubulopathy, gynecomastia.

OVERDOSAGE

The reports of overdosage with Orudis are rare. Of the 20 subjects reported in Great Britain (5 children, 14 adolescents or young adults, and 1 man 80-years-old), only 4 had mild symptoms (vomiting in 3, drowsiness in 1 child). The highest reported dose was 5,000 mg in the elderly man who displayed no symptoms.

Should a patient ingest a large number of capsules, the stomach should be emptied by gastric lavage or induction of vomiting and usual supportive measures employed. The drug is dialyzable; therefore, hemodialysis may be useful to remove circulating drug and to assist in case of renal failure.

DOSAGE AND ADMINISTRATION

The recommended daily dose of Orudis is 150 to 300 mg, divided in three or four doses. The recommended starting dose is 75 mg three times or 50 mg four times a day. If minor side effects appear, they may disappear at a lower dose which may still have an adequate therapeutic effect. If well tolerated but not optimally effective, the dosage my be increased. Individual patients may show a better response to 300 mg daily as compared to 200 mg, although in well-controlled clinical trials patients on 300 mg did not show greater mean effectiveness. They did, however, show an increased frequency of upper- and lower-GI distress and headaches. It is of interest that women also had an increased frequency of these adverse effects compared to men. When treating patients

with 300 mg a day, the physician should observe sufficient increased clinical benefit to offset potential increased risk. Dosages higher than 300 mg per day are not recommended because they have not been adequately studied. Relatively small people may need smaller doses.
Orudis is eliminated primarily by renal excretion; therefore, initial dosage should be reduced by ½ to ⅓ in patients with impaired renal function, including the elderly who normally have decreased renal function even with normal serum creatinine and/or BUN, because the lean body weight of older patients results in less creatinine formation.
Because hypoalbuminemia and reduced renal function both increase the fraction of free drug (biologically active form), patients who have both conditions may be at greater risk of adverse effects. Therefore, it is recommended that such patients also be started on lower doses and closely monitored.
As with other nonsteroidal antiinflammatory drugs, the predominant adverse effects of ketoprofen are gastrointestinal. To attempt to minimize these effects, physicians may wish to prescribe that Orudis be taken with antacids, food, or milk. Although food affects the bioavailability of Orudis (see "Clinical Pharmacology"), in most of the clinical trials Orudis was taken with food or milk.

HOW SUPPLIED

Orudis® (ketoprofen) Capsules, Wyeth®, are available in bottles of 100 capsules in the following dosage strengths.
50 mg. NDC 0008-4181, opaque dark-green and light-green capsule marked "WYETH" and "4181".
75 mg. NDC 0008-4187, opaque dark-green and white capsule marked "WYETH" "4187".
Keep tightly closed.
Dispense in tight container.
The appearance of these capsules is a trademark of Wyeth Laboratories.

Shown in Product Identification Section, page 436

OVRAL® TABLETS ℞

[oh 'vral]
(norgestrel and ethinyl estradiol tablets)

DESCRIPTION

Each Ovral® tablet contains 0.5 mg of norgestrel (*dl*-13-beta-ethyl-17-alpha-ethinyl-17-beta-hydroxygon-4-en-3-one), a totally synthetic progestogen, and 0.05 mg of ethinyl estradiol (19-nor-17α-pregna-1,3,5(10)-trien-20-yne-3, 17-diol). The inactive ingredients present are cellulose, lactose, magnesium stearate, and polacrilin potassium.

CLINICAL PHARMACOLOGY

See LO/OVRAL®.

INDICATIONS AND USAGE

Ovral® is indicated for the prevention of pregnancy in women who elect to use oral contraceptives as a method of contraception. Oral contraceptives are highly effective. The pregnancy rate in women using conventional combination oral contraceptives (containing 35 mcg or more of ethinyl estradiol or 50 mcg or more of mestranol) is generally reported as less than one pregnancy per 100 woman-years of use. Slightly higher rates (somewhat more than 1 pregnancy per 100 woman-years of use) are reported for some combination products containing 35 mcg or less of ethinyl estradiol, and rates on the order of 3 pregnancies per 100 woman-years are reported for the progestogen-only oral contraceptives.
These rates are derived from separate studies conducted by different investigators in several population groups and cannot be compared precisely. Furthermore, pregnancy rates tend to be lower as clinical studies are continued possibly due to selective retention in the longer studies of those patients who accept the treatment regimen and do not discontinue as a result of adverse reactions, pregnancy, or other reasons.
In clinical trials with Ovral, 6,806 patients completed 127,872 cycles, and a total of 19 pregnancies were reported. This represents a pregnancy rate of 0.19 per 100 woman-years. All of the pregnancies reported in these trials were the result of patient failure.
Table 1 gives ranges of pregnancy rates reported in the literature[1] for other means of contraception. The efficacy of these means of contraception (except the IUD) depends upon the degree of adherence to the method.
TABLE 1
PREGNANCIES PER 100 WOMAN-YEARS
IUD, less than 1–6; Diaphragm with spermicidal products (creams or jellies), 2–20; Condom, 3–36; Aerosol foams, 2–29; Jellies and creams, 4–36;
Periodic abstinence (rhythm) all types, less than 1–47:

1. Calendar method, 14–47;
2. Temperature method, 1–20;
3. Temperature method—intercourse only in postovulatory phase, less than 1–7;
4. Mucus method, 1–25;

No contraception, 60–80.
Dose-Related Risk of Thromboembolism from Oral Contraceptives: See LO/OVRAL.

CONTRAINDICATIONS

See LO/OVRAL.

WARNINGS

See LO/OVRAL.

PRECAUTIONS

See LO/OVRAL.

INFORMATION FOR THE PATIENT

See LO/OVRAL.

DRUG INTERACTIONS

See LO/OVRAL.

CARCINOGENESIS

See LO/OVRAL.

PREGNANCY

See LO/OVRAL.

NURSING MOTHERS

See LO/OVRAL.

ADVERSE REACTIONS

See LO/OVRAL.

ACUTE OVERDOSE

See LO/OVRAL.

DOSAGE AND ADMINISTRATION

To achieve maximum contraceptive effectiveness, Ovral must be taken exactly as directed and at intervals not exceeding 24 hours. The dosage of Ovral is one tablet daily for 21 consecutive days per menstrual cycle according to prescribed schedule. Tablets are then discontinued for 7 days (three weeks on, one week off).
It is recommended that Ovral tablets be taken at the same time each day, preferably after the evening meal or at bedtime.
During the first cycle of medication, the patient is instructed to take one Ovral tablet daily for twenty-one consecutive days beginning on day five of her menstrual cycle. (The first day of menstruation is day one.) The tablets are then discontinued for one week (7 days). Withdrawal bleeding should usually occur within three days following discontinuation of Ovral. (If Ovral is first taken later than the fifth day of the first menstrual cycle of medication or postpartum, contraceptive reliance should not be placed on Ovral until after the first seven consecutive days of administration. The possibility of ovulation and conception prior to initiation of medication should be considered.) The patient begins her next and all subsequent 21-day courses of Ovral tablets on the same day of the week that she began her first course, following the same schedule: 21 days on—7 days off.
She begins taking her tablets on the 8th day after discontinuance regardless of whether or not a menstrual period has occurred or is still in progress. Any time a new cycle of Ovral is started later than the 8th day, the patient should be protected by another means of contraception until she has taken a tablet daily for seven consecutive days.
If spotting or breakthrough bleeding occurs, the patient is instructed to continue on the same regimen. This type of bleeding is usually transient and without significance; however, if the bleeding is persistent or prolonged, the patient is advised to consult her physician. Although the occurrence of pregnancy is highly unlikely if Ovral is taken according to directions, if withdrawal bleeding does not occur, the possibility of pregnancy must be considered. If the patient has not adhered to the prescribed schedule (missed one or more tablets or started taking them on a day later than she should have) the probability of pregnancy should be considered at the time of the first missed period and appropriate diagnostic measures taken before the medication is resumed. If the patient has adhered to the prescribed regimen and misses two consecutive periods, pregnancy should be ruled out before continuing the contraceptive regimen.
The patient should be instructed to take a missed tablet as soon as it is remembered. If two consecutive tablets are missed, they should both be taken as soon as remembered. The next tablet should be taken at the usual time.
Any time the patient misses one or two tablets she should also use another method of contraception until she has taken a tablet daily for seven consecutive days. If breakthrough bleeding occurs following missed tablets, it will usually be transient and of no consequence. While there is little likelihood of ovulation occurring if only one or two tablets are missed, the possibility of ovulation increases with each successive day that scheduled tablets are missed. If three consecutive tablets are missed, all medication should be discontinued and the remainder of the package discarded. A new tablet cycle should be started on the 8th day after the last tablet was taken, and an alternate means of contraception should be prescribed during the seven days without tablets and until the patient has taken a tablet daily for seven consecutive days. In the nonlactating mother, Ovral may be prescribed in the postpartum period either immediately or at the first postpartum examination whether or not menstruation has resumed.

HOW SUPPLIED

Ovral® Tablets (0.5 mg norgestrel and 0.05 mg ethinyl estradiol), Wyeth®, are available in packages of 6 PILPAK® dispensers with 21 tablets each and in 3-PAK packages containing 63 tablets each as follows: NDC 0008-0056, white, round tablet marked "WYETH" and "56".

REFERENCES

See LO/OVRAL.
Brief Summary Patient Package Insert: See LO/OVRAL.
DETAILED PATIENT LABELING: See LO/OVRAL.

Shown in Product Identification Section, page 436

OVRAL®-28 ℞

[oh 'vral-28]
Tablets
(norgestrel and ethinyl estradiol tablets)

DESCRIPTION

21 white Ovral® tablets, each containing 0.5 mg of norgestrel (*dl* -13-beta-ethyl-17-alpha-ethinyl-17-beta-hydroxygon-4-en-3-one), a totally synthetic progestogen, and 0.05 mg of ethinyl estradiol (19-nor-17α-pregna-1,3,5 (10)-trien-20-yne-3,17-diol), and 7 pink inert tablets. The inactive ingredients present are cellulose, FD&C Red 3, lactose, magnesium stearate, and polacrilin potassium.

CLINICAL PHARMACOLOGY

See LO/OVRAL®.

INDICATIONS AND USAGE

See OVRAL®.
Dose-Related Risk of Thromboembolism from Oral Contraceptives: See LO/OVRAL.

CONTRAINDICATIONS

See LO/OVRAL.

WARNINGS

See LO/OVRAL.

PRECAUTIONS

See LO/OVRAL.
Information for the Patient: See LO/OVRAL.
Drug Interactions: See LO/OVRAL.
Carcinogenesis: See LO/OVRAL.
Pregnancy: See LO/OVRAL.
Nursing Mothers: See LO/OVRAL.

ADVERSE REACTIONS

See LO/OVRAL.
Acute Overdosage: See LO/OVRAL.

DOSAGE AND ADMINISTRATION

To achieve maximum contraceptive effectiveness, Ovral-28 must be taken exactly as directed and at intervals not exceeding 24 hours. The dosage of Ovral-28 is one white tablet daily for 21 consecutive days followed by one pink inert tablet for 7 consecutive days according to prescribed schedule. It is recommended that tablets be taken at the same time each day, preferably after the evening meal or at bedtime. During the first cycle of medication, the patient is instructed to begin taking Ovral-28 on the first Sunday after the onset of menstruation. If menstruation begins on a Sunday, the first tablet (white) is taken that day. One white tablet should be taken daily for 21 consecutive days followed by one pink inert tablet daily for 7 consecutive days. Withdrawal bleeding should usually occur within three days following discontinuation of white tablets.
During the first cycle, contraceptive reliance should not be placed on Ovral-28 until a white tablet has been taken daily for 7 consecutive days. The possibility of ovulation and conception prior to initiation of medication should be considered.
The patient begins her next and all subsequent 28-day courses of tablets on the same day of the week (Sunday) on which she began her first course, following the same schedule: 21 days on white tablets—7 days on pink inert tablets. If in any cycle the patient starts tablets later than the proper day, she should protect herself by using another method of birth control until she has taken a white tablet daily for 7 consecutive days.
If spotting or breakthrough bleeding occurs, the patient is instructed to continue on the same regimen. This type of bleeding is usually transient and without significance; however, if the bleeding is persistent or prolonged, the patient is advised to consult her physician. Although the occurrence of pregnancy is highly unlikely if Ovral-28 is taken according to directions, if withdrawal bleeding does not occur, the possibility of pregnancy must be considered. If the patient has not adhered to the prescribed schedule (missed one or more tablets or started taking them on a day later than she should have) the probability of pregnancy should be considered at the time of the first missed period and appropriate diagnostic measures taken before the medication is resumed. If the patient has adhered to the prescribed regimen and misses two

Continued on next page

Wyeth—Cont.

consecutive periods, pregnancy should be ruled out before continuing the contraceptive regimen. The patient should be instructed to take a missed white tablet as soon as it is remembered. If two consecutive white tablets are missed they should both be taken as soon as remembered. The next tablet should be taken at the usual time.
Any time the patient misses one or two white tablets she should also use another method of contraception until she has taken a white tablet daily for seven consecutive days. If the patient misses one or more pink tablets she is still protected against pregnancy *provided* she begins taking white tablets again on the proper day.
If breakthrough bleeding occurs following missed white tablets, it will usually be transient and of no consequence. While there is little likelihood of ovulation occurring if only one or two white tablets are missed, the possibility of ovulation increases with each successive day that scheduled white tablets are missed. If three consecutive white Ovral tablets are missed, all medication should be discontinued and the remainder of the 28-day package discarded. A new tablet cycle should be started on the first Sunday following the last missed tablet, and an alternate means of contraception should be prescribed during the days without tablets and until the patient has taken a white tablet daily for 7 consecutive days. In the nonlactating mother, Ovral-28 may be prescribed in the postpartum period either immediately or at the first postpartum examination whether or not menstruation has resumed.

HOW SUPPLIED

Ovral®-28 Tablets (0.5 mg norgestrel and 0.05 mg ethinyl estradiol), Wyeth®, are available in packages of 6 PILPAK® dispensers, each containing 28 tablets as follows:
21 active tablets, NDC 0008-0056, white, round tablet marked "WYETH" and "56".
7 inert tablets, NDC 0008-0445, pink, round tablet marked "WYETH" and "445".

REFERENCES

See LO/OVRAL.
Brief Summary Patient Package Insert: See LO/OVRAL.
DETAILED PATIENT LABELING: See LO/OVRAL.
Shown in Product Identification Section, page 436

OVRETTE® TABLETS ℞

[*oh-vret'*]
(norgestrel tablets)

Each OVRETTE® tablet contains 0.075 mg of norgestrel (*dl*-13-beta-ethyl-17-alpha-ethinyl-17-beta-hydroxygon-4-en-3-one). The inactive ingredients present are cellulose, FD&C Yellow 5, lactose, magnesium stearate, and polacrilin potassium.

DESCRIPTION

Each OVRETTE tablet contains 0.075 mg of a single active steroid ingredient, norgestrel, a totally synthetic progestogen. The available data suggest that the *d* (-)enantiomeric form of norgestrel is the biologically active portion. This form amounts to 0.0375 mg per OVRETTE tablet.

CLINICAL PHARMACOLOGY

The primary mechanism through which OVRETTE prevents conception is not known, but progestogen-only contraceptives are known to alter the cervical mucus, exert a progestational effect on the endometrium, interfering with implantation, and, in some patients, suppress ovulation.

INDICATIONS AND USAGE

OVRETTE is indicated for the prevention of pregnancy in women who elect to use oral contraceptives as a method of contraception. Oral contraceptives are highly effective. The pregnancy rate in women using conventional combination oral contraceptives (containing 35 mcg or more of ethinyl estradiol or 50 mcg or more of mestranol) is generally reported as less than one pregnancy per 100 woman-years of use. Slightly higher rates (somewhat more than 1 pregnancy per 100 woman-years of use) are reported for some combination products containing 35 mcg or less of ethinyl estradiol, and rates on the order of 3 pregnancies per 100 woman-years are reported for the progestogen-only oral contraceptives.
These rates are derived from separate studies conducted by different investigators in several population groups and cannot be compared precisely. Furthermore, pregnancy rates tend to be lower as clinical studies are continued, possibly due to selective retention in the longer studies of those patients who accept the treatment regimen and do not discontinue as a result of adverse reactions, pregnancy, or other reasons.
In clinical trials with OVRETTE, 2,752 patients completed 38,245 cycles, and a total of 78 pregnancies were reported. This represents a pregnancy rate of 2.45 per 100 woman-years. Approximately one-half of the pregnancies reported in these trials were due to method failure, and the other half were due to patient failure.
Table 1 gives ranges of pregnancy rates reported in the literature[1] for other means of contraception. The efficacy of these means of contraception (except the IUD) depends upon the degree of adherence to the method.
TABLE 1
PREGNANCIES PER 100 WOMAN-YEARS
IUD, less than 1–6; Diaphragm with spermicidal products (creams or jellies), 2–20; Condom, 3–36; Aerosol foams, 2–29; Jellies and creams, 4–36;
Periodic abstinence (rhythm) all types, less than 1–47:

1. Calendar method, 14–47;
2. Temperature method, 1–20;
3. Temperature method—intercourse only in postovulatory phase, less than 1–7;
4. Mucus method, 1–25;

No contraception, 60–80.
Dose-Related Risk of Thromboembolism from Oral Contraceptives: See LO/OVRAL®.

CONTRAINDICATIONS

See LO/OVRAL.

WARNINGS

See LO/OVRAL.

PRECAUTIONS

See LO/OVRAL.

INFORMATION FOR THE PATIENT

See LO/OVRAL.

DRUG INTERACTIONS

See LO/OVRAL.

CARCINOGENESIS

See LO/OVRAL.

PREGNANCY

See LO/OVRAL.

NURSING MOTHERS

See LO/OVRAL.

ADVERSE REACTIONS

See LO/OVRAL.

ACUTE OVERDOSE

See LO/OVRAL.

DOSAGE AND ADMINISTRATION

To achieve maximum contraceptive effectiveness, OVRETTE (norgestrel) must be taken exactly as directed and at intervals not exceeding 24 hours. OVRETTE is administered on a continuous daily dosage regimen starting on the first day of menstruation, i.e., one tablet each day, every day of the year.
Tablets should be taken at the same time each day and continued daily, without interruption, whether bleeding occurs or not. The patient should be advised that, if prolonged bleeding occurs, she should consult her physician. In the non-nursing mother, OVRETTE may be prescribed in the postpartum period either immediately or at the first postpartum examination whether or not menstruation has resumed.
The risk of pregnancy increases with each tablet missed. If the patient misses one tablet, she should be instructed to take it as soon as she remembers and to also take her next tablet at the regular time. If she misses two tablets, she should take one of the missed tablets as soon as she remembers, as well as taking her regular tablet for that day at the proper time. Furthermore, she should use a method of non-hormonal contraception in addition to taking OVRETTE until fourteen tablets have been taken. If more than 2 tablets have been missed, OVRETTE should be discontinued immediately and a method of nonhormonal contraception should be used until menses has appeared or pregnancy has been excluded. If menses does not appear within 45 days from the last period, a method of nonhormonal contraception should be substituted until the start of the next menstrual period or an appropriate diagnostic procedure is performed to rule out pregnancy.

HOW SUPPLIED

OVRETTE® tablets (0.075 mg norgestrel), Wyeth®, are available in packages of 6 PILPAK® dispensers with 28 tablets each as follows: NDC 0008-0062, yellow, round tablet marked "WYETH" and "62".

REFERENCES

See LO/OVRAL.
Brief Summary Patient Package Insert: See LO/OVRAL
DETAILED PATIENT LABELING: See LO/OVRAL.

OXYTOCIN ℞

[*ok"se-to'sin*]
Injection, USP
(synthetic)

DESCRIPTION

Each ml of TUBEX® Oxytocin Injection sterile solution contains an oxytocic activity equivalent to 10 USP Posterior Pituitary Units, chlorobutanol (a chloroform derivative), 0.5%, as a preservative, and acetic acid to adjust pH (2.5 to 4.5). Wyeth Oxytocin is intended for IM or IV use. Oxytocin is a synthetic polypeptide; it occurs as a white powder and is soluble in water.

CLINICAL PHARMACOLOGY

The pharmacologic and clinical properties of oxytocin are identical with those of the naturally occurring oxytocin principle of the posterior lobe of the pituitary. Oxytocin exerts a selective action on the smooth musculature of the uterus, particularly toward the end of pregnancy, during labor, and immediately following delivery. Oxytocin stimulates rhythmic contractions of the uterus, increases the frequency of existing contractions, and raises the tone of the uterine musculature.
When given in appropriate doses during pregnancy, oxytocin is capable of eliciting graded increases in uterine motility from a moderate increase in the rate and force of spontaneous motor activity to sustained tetanic contraction. The sensitivity of the uterus to oxytocic activity increases progressively throughout pregnancy until term when it is maximal.
Oxytocin is distributed throughout the extracellular fluid. Small amounts of this drug probably reach the fetal circulation. Oxytocin has a plasma half-life of about 3 to 5 minutes. Following parenteral administration, uterine response occurs within 3 to 5 minutes and persists for 2 to 3 hours. Its rapid removal from plasma is accomplished largely by the kidney and the liver. Only small amounts of oxytocin are excreted in the urine unchanged.

INDICATIONS AND USAGE

IMPORTANT NOTICE
Oxytocin is indicated for the medical rather than the elective induction of labor. Available data and information are inadequate to define the benefits-to-risks considerations in the use of the drug product for elective induction. Elective induction of labor is defined as the initiation of labor for convenience in an individual with a term pregnancy who is free of medical indications.

ANTEPARTUM: Oxytocin is indicated for the initiation or improvement of uterine contractions, where this is desirable and considered suitable for reasons of fetal or maternal concern, in order to achieve early vaginal delivery. It is indicated for (1) induction of labor in patients with a medical indication for the initiation of labor, such as Rh problems, maternal diabetes, preeclampsia at or near term, when delivery is in the best interest of mother and fetus or when membranes are prematurely ruptured and delivery is indicated; (2) stimulation or reinforcement of labor, as in selected cases of uterine inertia; (3) as adjunctive therapy in the management of incomplete or inevitable abortion. In the first trimester, curettage is generally considered primary therapy. In second trimester abortion, oxytocin infusion will often be successful in emptying the uterus. Other means of therapy, however, may be required in such cases.
POSTPARTUM: Oxytocin is indicated to produce uterine contractions during the third stage of labor and to control postpartum bleeding or hemorrhage.

CONTRAINDICATIONS

Oxytocin is contraindicated in any of the following conditions:
significant cephalopelvic disproportion;
unfavorable fetal positions or presentations which are undeliverable without conversion prior to delivery, e.g., transverse lies;
in obstetrical emergencies where the benefit-to-risk ratio for either the fetus or the mother favors surgical intervention;
in cases of fetal distress where delivery is not imminent;
hypertonic uterine patterns;
hypersensitivity to the drug.
Prolonged use in uterine inertia or severe toxemia is contraindicated.
Oxytocin should not be used in cases where vaginal delivery is not indicated, such as cord presentation or prolapse, total placenta previa, and vasa previa.

WARNINGS

Oxytocin, when given for induction or stimulation of labor, must be administered only by intravenous infusion (drip method) and with adequate medical supervision in a hospital.

PRECAUTIONS

GENERAL:

1. All patients receiving intravenous infusions of oxytocin must be under continuous observation by trained personnel with a thorough knowledge of the drug and qualified to identify complications. A physician qualified to manage any complications should be immediately available.

2. When properly administered, oxytocin should stimulate uterine contractions similar to those seen in normal labor. Overstimulation of the uterus by improper administration can be hazardous to both mother and fetus. Even with proper administration and adequate supervision, hypertonic contractions can occur in patients whose uteri are hypersensitive to oxytocin.

3. Except in unusual circumstances, oxytocin should not be administered in the following conditions: prematurity, borderline cephalopelvic disproportion, previous major surgery on the cervix or uterus, including cesarean section, overdistention of the uterus, grand multiparity, or invasive cervical carcinoma. Because of the variability of the combinations of factors which may be present in the conditions listed above, the definition of "unusual circumstances" must be left to the judgment of the physician. The decision can only be made by carefully weighing the potential benefits which oxytocin can provide in a given case against the rare occurrence of hypertonicity or tetanic spasm with this drug.

4. Maternal deaths due to hypertensive episodes, subarachnoid hemorrhage, rupture of the uterus, fetal deaths and permanent CNS or brain damage of the infant due to various causes have been reported to be associated with the use of parenteral oxytocic drugs for induction of labor or for augmentation in the first and second stages of labor.

5. Oxytocin has been shown to have an intrinsic antidiuretic effect, acting to increase water reabsorption from the glomerular filtrate. Consideration should, therefore, be given to the possibility of water intoxication, particularly when oxytocin is administered continuously by infusion and the patient is receiving fluids by mouth.

6. Oxytocin should be considered for use only in patients who have been carefully selected. Pelvic adequacy must be considered and maternal and fetal conditions thoroughly evaluated before use of the drug.

DRUG INTERACTIONS

Severe hypertension has been reported when oxytocin was given 3 to 4 hours following prophylactic administration of a vasoconstrictor in conjunction with caudal block anesthesia. Cyclopropane anesthesia may modify oxytocin's cardiovascular effects, so as to produce unexpected results such as hypotension. Maternal sinus bradycardia with abnormal atrioventricular rhythms has also been noted when oxytocin was used concomitantly with cyclopropane anesthesia.

CARCINOGENESIS, MUTAGENESIS, IMPAIRMENT OF FERTILITY

There are no animal or human studies on the carcinogenicity and mutagenicity of this drug, nor is there any information on its effect on fertility.

PREGNANCY

See "Indications and Usage."

Nonteratogenic Effects.

See "Adverse Reactions" in the fetus or infant.

LABOR AND DELIVERY

See "Indications and Usage."

ADVERSE REACTIONS

The following adverse reactions have been reported in the mother:

anaphylactic reaction
postpartum hemorrhage
cardiac arrhythmia
fatal afibrinogenemia
nausea
vomiting
premature ventricular contractions
pelvic hematoma

Excessive dosage or hypersensitivity to the drug may result in uterine hypertonicity, spasm, tetanic contraction, or rupture of the uterus.

The possibility of increased blood loss and afibrinogenemia should be kept in mind when administering the drug.

Severe water intoxication with convulsions and coma has occurred, associated with a slow oxytocin infusion over a 24-hour period. Maternal death due to oxytocin-induced water intoxication has been reported.

The following adverse reactions have been reported in the fetus or infant:

(Due to induced uterine motility)
Bradycardia
Premature ventricular contractions and other arrhythmias
Permanent CNS or brain damage
Fetal death
(Due to use of oxytocin in the mother)
Low Apgar scores at five minutes
Neonatal jaundice

OVERDOSAGE

Overdosage with oxytocin depends essentially on uterine hyperactivity whether or not due to hypersensitivity to this agent. Hyperstimulation with strong (hypertonic) or prolonged (tetanic) contractions, or a resting tone of 15 to 20 mmH_2O or more between contractions can lead to tumultuous labor, uterine rupture, cervical and vaginal lacerations, postpartum hemorrhage, utero-placental hypoperfusion, and variable deceleration of fetal heart, fetal hypoxia, hypercapnia or death. Water intoxication with convulsions, which is caused by the inherent antidiuretic effect of oxytocin, is a serious complication that may occur if large doses (40 to 50 milliunits/minute) are infused for long periods. Management consists of immediate discontinuation of oxytocin, and symptomatic and supportive therapy.

DOSAGE AND ADMINISTRATION

Parenteral drug products should be inspected visually for particulate matter and discoloration prior to administration, whenever solution and container permit. Dosage of oxytocin is determined by uterine response. The following dosage information is based upon the various regimens and indications in general use.

A. INDUCTION OR STIMULATION OF LABOR

Intravenous infusion (drip method) is the only acceptable method of administration for the induction or stimulation of labor.

Accurate control of the rate of infusion flow is essential. An infusion pump or other such device and frequent monitoring of strength of contractions and fetal heart rate are necessary for the safe administration of oxytocin for the induction or stimulation of labor. If uterine contractions become too powerful, the infusion can be abruptly stopped, and oxytocic stimulation of the uterine musculature will soon wane.

1. An intravenous infusion of nonoxytocin-containing solution should be started. Physiologic electrolyte solution should be used except under unusual circumstances.

2. To prepare the usual solution for infusion, the contents of one 1-ml TUBEX® (10 units) is combined aseptically with 1,000 ml of nonhydrating diluent (physiologic electrolyte solution). The combined solution, rotated in the infusion bottle to insure thorough mixing, contains 10 mU/ml. Add the container with dilute oxytocic solution to the system through use of a constant infusion pump or other such device, to control accurately the rate of infusion.

3. The initial dose should be no more than 1–2 mU/min. The dose may be gradually increased in increments of no more than 1 to 2 mU/min. until a contraction pattern has been established which is similar to normal labor.

4. The fetal heart rate, resting uterine tone, and the frequency, duration, and force of contractions should be monitored.

5. The oxytocin infusion should be discontinued immediately in the event of uterine hyperactivity or fetal distress. Oxygen should be administered to the mother. The mother and the fetus must be evaluated by the responsible physician.

B. CONTROL OF POSTPARTUM UTERINE BLEEDING

1. Intravenous infusion (Drip Method):

To control postpartum bleeding, 10 to 40 units of oxytocin may be added to 1,000 ml of a nonhydrating diluent (physiologic electrolyte solution) and run at a rate necessary to control uterine atony.

2. Intramuscular Administration:

1 ml (10 units) of oxytocin can be given after delivery of the placenta.

C. TREATMENT OF INCOMPLETE OR INEVITABLE ABORTION

Intravenous infusion with physiologic saline solution, 500 ml, or 5% dextrose in physiologic saline solution to which 10 units of oxytocin have been added should be infused at a rate of 20 to 40 drops per minute.

HOW SUPPLIED

Oxytocin Injection, USP (synthetic), 10 USP units in 1 ml TUBEX® Sterile Cartridge-Needle Unit, is supplied as follows:

NDC 0008-0406-1, package of 10 TUBEX.

Keep in a refrigerator, do not freeze.

When stored out of refrigeration at temperatures of up to 26° C (79° F), this product has exhibited acceptable data for a period not exceeding three (3) months.

PATHOCIL® ℞

[path 'o-sil]

(dicloxacillin sodium monohydrate)
CAPSULES • ORAL SUSPENSION

DESCRIPTION

Dicloxacillin sodium monohydrate is an isoxazolyl penicillin which resists destruction by the enzyme penicillinase (beta-lactamase). It is the monohydrate sodium salt of 6-[3-(2,6-Dichlorophenyl) -5- methyl -4- isoxazole- carboxamido] -3,3-dimethyl -7- oxo -4- thia -1- azabicyclo- [3.2.0] heptane-2-carboxylic acid.

Pathocil capsules contain 250 mg or 500 mg dicloxacillin sodium monohydrate. The inactive ingredients present are D&C Red 28, FD&C Blue 1, FD&C Red 40, gelatin, lactose, stearic acid, talc, and titanium dioxide.

Pathocil oral suspension is a powder which when reconstituted as directed yields a suspension with a concentration of 62.5 mg dicloxacillin sodium monohydrate per 5 mL. The inactive ingredients present are artificial and natural flavors, carboxymethylcellulose sodium, citric acid, colloidal silicon dioxide, edetate disodium, FD&C Red 3, saccharin sodium, sodium benzoate, sodium citrate, sucrose, and water.

ACTIONS

Pharmacology

Dicloxacillin sodium monohydrate is resistant to destruction by acid and is exceptionally well absorbed from the gastrointestinal tract. Oral administration of dicloxacillin sodium monohydrate gives blood levels considerably higher than those obtained with equivalent doses of any other presently available oral penicillin.

Microbiology

In vitro dicloxacillin is active against certain gram-positive cocci, including most strains of beta-hemolytic streptococci, pneumococci, penicillin-G-sensitive staphylococci and, because of its resistance to penicillinase, penicillin-G-resistant staphylococci. Dicloxacillin has less intrinsic antibacterial activity and a narrower spectrum than penicillin G.

Disc Susceptibility Tests

Quantitative methods that require measurement of zone diameters give the most precise estimates of antibiotic susceptibility. One such procedure* has been recommended for use with discs for testing susceptibility to penicillinase-resistant penicillin-class antibiotics. Interpretations correlate diameters on the disc test with MIC values for penicillinase-resistant penicillins. With this procedure, a report from the laboratory of "susceptible" indicates that the infecting organism is likely to respond to therapy. A report of "resistant" indicates that the infecting organism is not likely to respond to therapy. A report of "intermediate susceptibility" suggests that the organism would be susceptible if high dosage is used, or if the infection is confined to tissues and fluids (e.g., urine), in which high antibiotic levels are attained.

INDICATIONS

Although the principal indication for dicloxacillin is in the treatment of infections due to penicillinase-producing staphylococci, it may be used to initiate therapy in such patients in whom a staphylococcal infection is suspected. (See Important Note.)

Bacteriologic studies to determine the causative organisms and their sensitivity to dicloxacillin should be performed.

In serious, life-threatening infections, oral preparations of the penicillinase-resistant penicillins should not be relied on for initial therapy.

IMPORTANT NOTE

When it is judged necessary that treatment be initiated before definitive culture and sensitivity results are known, the choice of dicloxacillin should take into consideration the fact that it has been shown to be effective only in the treatment of infections caused by pneumococci, Group A beta-hemolytic streptococci, and penicillin-G-resistant and penicillin-G-sensitive staphylococci. If the bacteriology report later indicates the infection is due to an organism other than a penicillin-G-resistant staphylococcus sensitive to dicloxacillin, the physician is advised to continue therapy with a drug other than dicloxacillin or any other penicillinase-resistant penicillin.

Recent studies have reported that the percentage of staphylococcal isolates resistant to penicillin G outside the hospital is increasing, approximating the high percentage of resistant staphylococcal isolates found in the hospital. For this reason, it is recommended that a penicillinase-resistant penicillin be used as initial therapy for any suspected staphylococcal infection until culture and sensitivity results are known.

Dicloxacillin acts through a mechanism similar to that of methicillin against penicillin-G-resistant staphylococci. Strains of staphylococci resistant to methicillin have existed in nature, and it is known that the number of these strains reported has been increasing. Such strains of staphylococci have been capable of producing serious disease, in some instances resulting in fatality. Because of this, there is concern that widespread use of the penicillinase-resistant penicillins may result in the appearance of an increasing number of staphylococcal strains which are resistant to these penicillins.

Methicillin-resistant strains are almost always resistant to all other penicillinase-resistant penicillins (cross-resistance with cephalosporin derivatives also occurs frequently). Resistance to any penicillinase-resistant penicillin should be interpreted as evidence of clinical resistance to all in spite of the fact that minor variations in *in vitro* sensitivity may be

Continued on next page

Wyeth—Cont.

encountered when more than one penicillinase-resistant penicillin is tested against the same strain of staphylococcus.

CONTRAINDICATIONS

A history of a previous hypersensitivity reaction to any of the penicillins is a contraindication.

WARNINGS

Serious and occasionally fatal hypersensitivity (anaphylactoid) reactions have been reported in patients on penicillin therapy. Although anaphylaxis is more frequent following parenteral therapy, it has occurred in patients on oral penicillins. These reactions are more apt to occur in individuals with a history of sensitivity to multiple allergens.
There have been reports of individuals with a history of penicillin hypersensitivity reactions who experienced severe hypersensitivity reactions when treated with cephalosporins. Before therapy with a penicillin, careful inquiry should be made concerning previous hypersensitivity reactions to penicillins, cephalosporins, and other allergens. If an allergic reaction occurs, appropriate therapy should be instituted and discontinuance of dicloxacillin therapy considered. The usual agents (antihistamines, pressor amines, corticosteroids) should be readily available.

Usage in pregnancy
Safety for use in pregnancy has not been established.

PRECAUTIONS

As with any potent drug, periodic assessment of organ-system function, including renal, hepatic, and hematopoietic, should be made during prolonged therapy.
The possibility of bacterial and fungal superinfection should be kept in mind during long-term therapy. If overgrowth of resistant organisms occurs, appropriate measures should be taken.
This oral preparation should not be relied upon in patients with severe illness or with nausea, vomiting, gastric dilatation, cardiospasm, or intestinal hypermotility.
Since experience in neonates is limited, a dose for the newborn is not recommended at this time.

ADVERSE REACTIONS

Gastrointestinal disturbances such as nausea, vomiting, epigastric discomfort, flatulence, and loose stools have been noted in some patients receiving dicloxacillin. As with other penicillins, pruritus, urticaria, skin rashes, eosinophilia, anaphylactic reactions, and other allergic symptoms have been occasionally encountered.
Minor changes in the results of liver-function tests such as transient elevation of SGOT and changes in cephalin flocculation tests have been reported. The clinical significance of these changes is unknown.

DOSAGE AND ADMINISTRATION

For mild-to-moderate upper-respiratory and localized skin and soft-tissue infections due to sensitive organisms:
Adults and children weighing 40 kg (88 lbs.) or more: 125 mg q. 6h.
Children weighing less than 40 kg (88 lbs.): 12.5 mg/kg/day in equally divided doses q. 6h.
For more severe infections such as those of the lower-respiratory tract or disseminated infections:
Adults and children weighing 40 kg (88 lbs.) or more: 250 mg q. 6h or higher.
Children weighing less than 40 kg (88 lbs.): 25 mg/kg/day or higher in equally divided doses q. 6h.
Since experience in neonates is limited, a dose for the newborn is not recommended at this time.
Dicloxacillin sodium monohydrate is best absorbed when taken on an empty stomach, preferably one to two hours before meals.

N.B.: INFECTIONS CAUSED BY GROUP A BETA-HEMOLYTIC STREPTOCOCCI SHOULD BE TREATED FOR AT LEAST 10 DAYS TO HELP PREVENT THE OCCURRENCE OF ACUTE RHEUMATIC FEVER OR ACUTE GLOMERULONEPHRITIS.

HOW SUPPLIED

Pathocil® (dicloxacillin sodium monohydrate), Wyeth®, is available in capsules of the following dosage strengths:
250 mg, NDC 0008-0360, purple and white capsule marked "WYETH" and "360" in bottles of 100 capsules.
500 mg, NDC 0008-0593, purple and white capsule marked "WYETH" and "593" in bottles of 50 capsules.
Keep bottles tightly closed.
Dispense in tight containers.
The appearance of Pathocil capsules is a registered trademark of Wyeth Laboratories.
Pathocil® (dicloxacillin sodium monohydrate) for Oral Suspension, Wyeth®, is available as a light-pink powder which when reconstituted as directed yields a palatable, pink suspension in the following dosage strength:
62.5 mg per 5 mL, NDC 0008-0361, in bottles to make 100 mL.
Shake well before using.
Keep bottles of suspension tightly closed.
After reconstitution store suspension in refrigerator. Discard unused portion after 14 days.
Bibliography: A bibliography is available upon request.

*Bauer, A.W., Kirby, W.M.M., Sherris, J.C., and Turck, M.: Antibiotic Testing by a Standardized Single Discs Method, Am. J. Clin. Pathol., 45:493, 1966; Standardized Disc Susceptibility Test, FEDERAL REGISTER *37*:20527-29, 1972.

Shown in Product Identification Section, page 436

PEN•VEE® K ℞

[pen-vee-kay]
(penicillin V potassium)
TABLETS • FOR ORAL SOLUTION

HOW SUPPLIED

Pen-Vee® K (penicillin V potassium) Tablets, Wyeth®, are available as white, round, scored tablets in the following dosage strengths:
250 mg (400,000 units), NDC 0008-0059, marked "WYETH" and "59", in bottles of 100 or 500 tablets, and in Redipak® cartons of 100 individually wrapped tablets.
500 mg (800,000 units), NDC 0008-0390, marked "WYETH" and "390", in bottles of 100 or 500 tablets, and in Redipak cartons of 100 individually wrapped tablets.
Pen-Vee® K (penicillin V potassium) for Oral Suspension, Wyeth®, is available as a powder which when reconstituted as directed yields a palatable solution in the following dosage strengths:
125 mg (200,000 units) per 5 mL, NDC 0008-0004, faint pink powder, in bottles to make 100 mL or 200 mL of red solution.
250 mg (400,000 units) per 5 mL, NDC 0008-0036, light peach-colored powder, in bottles to make 100 mL, 150 mL, or 200 mL of light-orange solution.
For prescribing information write to Professional Service, Wyeth Laboratories, Box 8299, Philadelphia, PA, 19101, or contact your local Wyeth representative.

Shown in Product Identification Section, page 436

PHENERGAN® ℞

[fen'er-gan]
(promethazine HCl)
INJECTION

DESCRIPTION

Promethazine HCl (10*H*-phenothiazine-10-ethanamine, *N,N*,α-trimethyl-, monohydrochloride). Each ml of TUBEX® Sterile Cartridge-Needle Unit contains either 25 or 50 mg promethazine hydrochloride with 0.1 mg edetate disodium, 0.04 mg calcium chloride, not more than 5 mg monothioglycerol and 5 mg phenol with sodium acetate-acetic acid buffer. Each Ampul of injection contains either 25 mg or 50 mg promethazine hydrochloride with 0.1 mg edetate disodium, 0.04 mg calcium chloride, not more than 0.25 mg sodium metabisulfite and 5 mg phenol with sodium acetate-acetic acid buffer.

ACTIONS

Promethazine hydrochloride, a phenothiazine derivative, possesses antihistaminic, sedative, antimotion-sickness, antiemetic, and anticholinergic effects. The duration of action is generally from four to six hours. The major side reaction of this drug is sedation. As an antihistamine it acts by competitive antagonism, but does not block the release of histamine. It antagonizes in varying degrees most but not all of the pharmacological effects of histamine.

INDICATIONS

The injectable form of promethazine hydrochloride is indicated for the following conditions:
1. Amelioration of allergic reactions to blood or plasma.
2. In anaphylaxis as an adjunct to epinephrine and other standard measures after the acute symptoms have been controlled.
3. For other uncomplicated allergic conditions of the immediate type when oral therapy is impossible or contraindicated.
4. Active treatment of motion sickness.
5. Preoperative, postoperative, and obstetric (during labor) sedation.
6. Prevention and control of nausea and vomiting associated with certain types of anesthesia and surgery.
7. As an adjunct to analgesics for the control of postoperative pain.
8. For sedation and relief of apprehension and to produce light sleep from which the patient can be easily aroused.
9. Intravenously in special surgical situations, such as repeated bronchoscopy, ophthalmic surgery, and poor-risk patients, with reduced amounts of meperidine or other narcotic analgesic as an adjunct to anesthesia and analgesia.

CONTRAINDICATIONS

Promethazine is contraindicated in comatose states, in patients who have received large amounts of central-nervous-system depressants (alcohol, sedative hypnotics, including barbiturates, general anesthetics, narcotics, narcotic analgesics, tranquilizers, etc.), and in patients who have demonstrated an idiosyncrasy or hypersensitivity to promethazine.
Under no circumstances should promethazine be given by intra-arterial injection due to the likelihood of severe arteriospasm and the possibility of resultant gangrene (see Warnings).
Phenergan injection should not be given by the subcutaneous route; evidence of chemical irritation has been noted and necrotic lesions have resulted on rare occasions following subcutaneous injection. The preferred parenteral route of administration is by deep intramuscular injection.

WARNINGS

Promethazine may impair the mental and/or physical abilities required for the performance of potentially hazardous tasks, such as driving a vehicle or operating machinery. The concomitant use of alcohol, sedative hypnotics (including barbiturates), general anesthetics, narcotics, narcotic analgesics, tranquilizers or other central-nervous-system depressants may have an additive sedative effect. Patients should be warned accordingly.
USAGE IN PREGNANCY: The safe use of promethazine has not been established with respect to the possible adverse effects upon fetal development. Therefore, the need for the use of this drug during pregnancy should be weighed against the possible but unknown hazards to the developing fetus.
USE IN CHILDREN: Excessively large dosages of antihistamines, including promethazine, in children may cause hallucinations, convulsions, and sudden death. In children who are acutely ill associated with dehydration, there is an increased susceptibility to dystonias with the use of promethazine hydrochloride injection.
CAUTION SHOULD BE EXERCISED WHEN ADMINISTERING PHENERGAN TO CHILDREN. ANTIEMETICS ARE NOT RECOMMENDED FOR TREATMENT OF UNCOMPLICATED VOMITING IN CHILDREN, AND THEIR USE SHOULD BE LIMITED TO PROLONGED VOMITING OF KNOWN ETIOLOGY. THE EXTRAPYRAMIDAL SYMPTOMS WHICH CAN OCCUR SECONDARY TO PHENERGAN® ADMINISTRATION MAY BE CONFUSED WITH THE CNS SIGNS OF UNDIAGNOSED PRIMARY DISEASE, e.g., ENCEPHALOPATHY OR REYE'S SYNDROME. THE USE OF PHENERGAN SHOULD BE AVOIDED IN CHILDREN WHOSE SIGNS AND SYMPTOMS MAY SUGGEST REYE'S SYNDROME, OR OTHER HEPATIC DISEASES.
USE IN THE ELDERLY (APPROXIMATELY 60 YEARS OR OLDER): Since therapeutic requirements for sedative drugs tend to be less in elderly patients, the dosage of Phenergan should be reduced for these patients.
OTHER CONSIDERATIONS: Drugs having anticholinergic properties should be used with caution in patients with asthmatic attack, narrow-angle glaucoma, prostatic hypertrophy, stenosing peptic ulcer, pyloroduodenal obstruction, and bladder-neck obstruction.
Phenergan should be used with caution in patients with bone-marrow depression. Leukopenia and agranulocytosis have been reported, usually when Phenergan has been used in association with other known toxic agents.
INADVERTENT INTRA-ARTERIAL INJECTION: Due to the close proximity of arteries and veins in the areas most commonly used for intravenous injection, extreme care should be exercised to avoid perivascular extravasation or inadvertent intra-arterial injection. Reports compatible with inadvertent intra-arterial injection of promethazine, usually in conjunction with other drugs intended for intravenous use, suggest that pain, severe chemical irritation, severe spasm of distal vessels, and resultant gangrene requiring amputation are likely under such circumstances. Intravenous injection was intended in all the cases reported, but perivascular extravasation or arterial placement of the needle is now suspect. There is no proven successful management of this condition after it occurs, although sympathetic block and heparinization are commonly employed during the acute management because of the results of animal experiments with other known arteriolar irritants. Aspiration of dark blood does not preclude intra-arterial needle placement, because blood is discolored upon contact with promethazine. Use of syringes with rigid plungers or of small bore needles might obscure typical arterial backflow if this is relied upon alone.
When used intravenously, promethazine hydrochloride should be given in a concentration no greater than 25 mg per ml and at a rate not to exceed 25 mg per minute. When administering any irritant drug intravenously, it is usually preferable to inject it through the tubing of an intravenous infusion set that is known to be functioning satisfactorily. In the event that a patient complains of pain during intended intravenous injection of promethazine, the injection should immediately be stopped to provide for evaluation of possible arterial placement or perivascular extravasation.

PRECAUTIONS

Promethazine may significantly affect the actions of other drugs. It may increase, prolong, or intensify the sedative action of central-nervous-system depressants, such as alcohol, sedative hypnotics (including barbiturates), general anesthetics, narcotics, narcotic analgesics, tranquilizers, etc. When given concomitantly with promethazine hydrochloride, the dose of barbiturates should be reduced by at least one-half, and the dose of narcotics should be reduced by one-quarter to one-half. Dosage must be individualized. Excessive amounts of promethazine relative to a narcotic may lead to restlessness and motor hyperactivity in the patient with pain; these symptoms usually disappear with adequate control of the pain. Promethazine should be used cautiously in persons with cardiovascular disease or impairment of liver funtion.

Although reversal of the vasopressor effect of epinephrine has not been reported with promethazine, the possibility should be considered in case of promethazine overdose.

ADVERSE REACTIONS

CNS EFFECTS: Drowsiness is the most prominent CNS effect of this drug. Extrapyramidal reactions may occur with high doses; this is almost always responsive to a reduction in dosage. Other reported reactions include dizziness, lassitude, tinnitus, incoordination, fatigue, blurred vision, euphoria, diplopia, nervousness, insomnia, tremors, convulsive seizures, oculogyric crises, excitation, catatonic-like states, and hysteria.

CARDIOVASCULAR EFFECTS: Tachycardia, bradycardia, faintness, dizziness, and increases and decreases in blood pressure have been reported following the use of promethazine hydrochloride injection. Venous thrombosis at the injection site has been reported. INTRA-ARTERIAL INJECTION MAY RESULT IN GANGRENE OF THE AFFECTED EXTREMITY (see Warnings).

GASTROINTESTINAL: Nausea and vomiting have been reported, usually in association with surgical procedures and combination drug therapy.

ALLERGIC REACTIONS: These include urticaria, dermatitis, asthma, and photosensitivity. Angioneurotic edema has been reported.

OTHER REPORTED REACTIONS: Leukopenia and agranulocytosis, usually when Phenergan has been used in association with other known toxic agents, have been reported. Thrombocytopenic purpura and jaundice of the obstructive type have been associated with the use of promethazine. The jaundice is usually reversible on discontinuation of the drug. Subcutaneous injection has resulted in tissue necrosis. Nasal stuffiness may occur. Dry mouth has been reported.

LABORATORY TESTS: The following laboratory tests may be affected in patients who are receiving therapy with promethazine hydrochloride:

Pregnancy Tests—Diagnostic pregnancy tests based on immunological reactions between HCG and anti-HCG may result in false-negative or false-positive interpretations.

Glucose Tolerance Test—An increase in glucose tolerance has been reported in patients receiving promethazine hydrochloride.

PARADOXICAL REACTIONS (OVERDOSAGE): Hyperexcitability and abnormal movements which have been reported in children following a single administration of promethazine may be manifestations of relative overdosage, in which case, consideration should be given to the discontinuation of the promethazine and to the use of other drugs. Respiratory depression, nightmares, delirium, and agitated behavior have also been reported in some of these patients.

DRUG INTERACTIONS

NARCOTICS AND BARBITURATES: The CNS-depressant effects of narcotics and barbiturates are additive with promethazine hydrochloride.

MAO INHIBITORS: Drug interactions, including an increased incidence of extra-pyramidal effects, have been reported when some MAO inhibitors and phenothiazines are used concomitantly. Although such a reaction has not been reported with promethazine, the possibility should be considered.

DOSAGE AND ADMINISTRATION

The preferred parenteral route of administration for promethazine hydrochloride is by deep, intramuscular injection. The proper intravenous administration of this product is well tolerated, but use of this route is not without some hazard.

INADVERTENT INTRA-ARTERIAL INJECTION CAN RESULT IN GANGRENE OF THE AFFECTED EXTREMITY (see Warnings). SUBCUTANEOUS INJECTION IS CONTRAINDICATED AS IT MAY RESULT IN TISSUE NECROSIS (see Contraindications). When used intravenously, promethazine hydrochloride should be given in concentration no greater than 25 mg/ml at a rate not to exceed 25 mg per minute; it is preferable to inject through the tubing of an intravenous infusion set that is known to be functioning satisfactorily.

ALLERGIC CONDITIONS: The average adult dose is 25 mg. This dose may be repeated within two hours if necessary, but continued therapy, if indicated, should be via the oral route as soon as existing circumstances permit. After initiation of treatment, dosage should be adjusted to the smallest amount adequate to relieve symptoms. The average adult dose for amelioration of allergic reactions to blood or plasma is 25 mg.

SEDATION: In hospitalized adult patients, nighttime sedation may be achieved by a dose of 25 to 50 mg of promethazine hydrochloride.

PRE- AND POSTOPERATIVE USE:

As an adjunct to pre- or postoperative medication, 25 to 50 mg of promethazine hydrochloride in adults may be combined with appropriately reduced doses of analgesics and atropine-like drugs as desired. Dosage of concomitant analgesic or hypnotic medication should be reduced accordingly.

NAUSEA AND VOMITING: For control of nausea and vomiting the usual adult dose is 12.5 to 25 mg, not to be repeated more frequently than every four hours. When used for control of postoperative nausea and vomiting, the medication may be administered either intramuscularly or intravenously and dosage of analgesics and barbiturates reduced accordingly.

OBSTETRICS: Phenergan (promethazine hydrochloride) in doses of 50 mg will provide sedation and relieve apprehension in the early stages of labor. When labor is definitely established, 25 to 75 mg (average dose, 50 mg) promethazine hydrochloride may be given intramuscularly or intravenously with an appropriately reduced dose of any desired narcotic. Amnesic agents may be administered as necessary. If necessary, Phenergan with a reduced dose of analgesic may be repeated once or twice at four-hour intervals in the course of a normal labor. A maximum total dose of 100 mg of Phenergan may be administered during a 24-hour period to patients in labor.

CHILDREN: In children under the age of 12 years, the dosage should not exceed half that of the suggested adult dose. As an adjunct to premedication, the suggested dose is 0.5 mg per lb. of body weight in combination with an equal dose of narcotic or barbiturate and the appropriate dose of an atropine-like drug. Antiemetics should not be used in vomiting of unknown etiology in children.

MANAGEMENT OF OVERDOSAGE

Signs and symptoms of overdosage range from mild depression of the central nervous system and cardiovascular system, to profound hypotension, respiratory depression, and unconsciousness. Stimulation may be evident, especially in children and geriatric patients. Atropine-like signs and symptoms—dry mouth, fixed, dilated pupils, flushing, etc., as well as gastrointestinal symptoms, may occur. The treatment of overdosage is essentially symptomatic and supportive. Early gastric lavage may be beneficial if promethazine has been taken orally. Centrally acting emetics are of little use.

Avoid analeptics, which may cause convulsions. Severe hypotension usually responds to the administration of levarterenol or phenylephrine. EPINEPHRINE SHOULD NOT BE USED, since its use in a patient with partial adrenergic blockade may further lower the blood pressure. Extrapyramidal reactions may be treated with anticholinergic antiparkinson agents, diphenhydramine, or barbiturates. Additional measures include oxygen and intravenous fluids. Limited experience with dialysis indicates that it is not helpful.

HOW SUPPLIED

Phenergan® (promethazine hydrochloride) Injection as TUBEX® (Sterile Cartridge-Needle Unit), either 25 or 50 mg per ml, in packages of 10 TUBEX, and Ampuls of 1 ml, either 25 or 50 mg per ml, in packages of 5 and 25 Ampuls.

PHENERGAN® ℞
[fen 'er-gan]
Syrup Plain and
PHENERGAN® ℞
Syrup Fortis
(promethazine HCl)

DESCRIPTION

Each teaspoon (5 mL) of Phenergan Syrup Plain contains 6.25 mg promethazine hydrochloride in a flavored syrup base with a pH between 4.7 and 5.2. Alcohol 7%. The inactive ingredients present are artificial and natural flavors, citric acid, D&C Red 33, D&C Yellow 10, FD&C Blue 1, FD&C Yellow 6, glycerin, saccharin sodium, sodium benzoate, sodium citrate, sodium propionate, water, and other ingredients.

Each teaspoonful (5mL) of Phenergan Syrup Fortis contains 25 mg promethazine hydrochloride in a flavored syrup base with a pH between 5.0 and 5.5. Alcohol 1.5%. The inactive ingredients present are artificial and natural flavors, citric acid, saccharin sodium, sodium benzoate, sodium propionate, water, and other ingredients.

Promethazine hydrochloride, a phenothiazine derivative, is designated chemically as N,N,α-trimethyl-10*H*-phenothiazine-10-ethanamine monohydrochloride with the following structural formula:

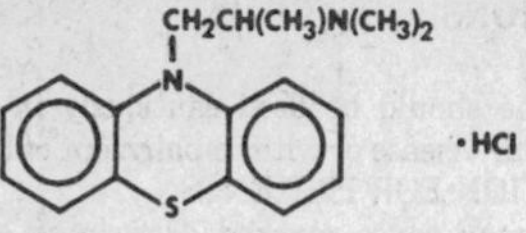

Promethazine hydrochloride occurs as a white to faint yellow, practically odorless, crystalline powder which slowly oxidizes and turns blue on prolonged exposure to air. It is soluble in water and freely soluble in alcohol.

CLINICAL PHARMACOLOGY

Promethazine is a phenothiazine derivative which differs structurally from the antipsychotic phenothiazines by the presence of a branched side chain and no ring substitution. It is thought that this configuration is responsible for its relative lack (1/10 that of chlorpromazine) of dopaminergic (CNS) action.

Promethazine is an H_1 receptor blocking agent. In addition to its antihistaminic action, it provides clinically useful sedative and antiemetic effects. In therapeutic dosage, promethazine produces no significant effects on the cardiovascular system.

Promethazine is well absorbed from the gastrointestinal tract. Clinical effects are apparent within 20 minutes after oral administration and generally last four to six hours, although they may persist as long as 12 hours. Promethazine is metabolized by the liver to a variety of compounds; the sulfoxides of promethazine and N-demethylpromethazine are the predominant metabolites appearing in the urine.

INDICATIONS AND USAGE

Phenergan is useful for:
Perennial and seasonal allergic rhinitis.
Vasomotor rhinitis.
Allergic conjunctivitis due to inhalant allergens and foods.
Mild, uncomplicated allergic skin manifestations of urticaria and angioedema.
Amelioration of allergic reactions to blood or plasma.
Dermographism.
Anaphylactic reactions, as adjunctive therapy to epinephrine and other standard measures, after the acute manifestations have been controlled.
Preoperative, postoperative, or obstetric sedation.
Prevention and control of nausea and vomiting associated with certain types of anesthesia and surgery.
Therapy adjunctive to meperidine or other analgesics for control of postoperative pain.
Sedation in both children and adults, as well as relief of apprehension and production of light sleep from which the patient can be easily aroused.
Active and prophylactic treatment of motion sickness.
Antiemetic therapy in postoperative patients.

CONTRAINDICATIONS

Promethazine is contraindicated in individuals known to be hypersensitive or to have had an idiosyncratic reaction to promethazine or to other phenothiazines.

Antihistamines are contraindicated for use in the treatment of lower respiratory tract symptoms including asthma.

WARNINGS

Promethazine may cause marked drowsiness. Ambulatory patients should be cautioned against such activities as driving or operating dangerous machinery until it is known that they do not become drowsy or dizzy from promethazine therapy.

The sedative action of promethazine hydrochloride is additive to the sedative effects of central nervous system depressants; therefore, agents such as alcohol, narcotic analgesics, sedatives, hypnotics, and tranquilizers should either be eliminated or given in reduced dosage in the presence of promethazine hydrochloride. When given concomitantly with promethazine hydrochloride, the dose of barbiturates should be reduced at least one-half, and the dose of analgesic depressants, such as morphine or meperidine, should be reduced by one-quarter to one-half.

Promethazine may lower seizure threshold. This should be taken into consideration when adminstering to persons with known seizure disorders or when giving in combination with narcotics or local anesthetics which may also affect seizure threshold.

Sedative drugs or CNS depressants should be avoided in patients with a history of sleep apnea.

Antihistamines should be used with caution in patients with narrow-angle glaucoma, stenosing peptic ulcer, pyloroduodenal obstruction, and urinary bladder obstruction due to symptomatic prostatic hypertrophy and narrowing of the bladder neck.

Administration of promethazine has been associated with reported cholestatic jaundice.

Continued on next page

Wyeth—Cont.

PRECAUTIONS
GENERAL
Promethazine should be used cautiously in persons with cardiovascular disease or with impairment of liver function.
INFORMATION FOR PATIENTS
Phenergan may cause marked drowsiness or impair the mental and/or physical abilities required for the performance of potentially hazardous tasks, such as driving a vehicle or operating machinery. Ambulatory patients should be told to avoid engaging in such activities until it is known that they do not become drowsy or dizzy from Phenergan therapy. Children should be supervised to avoid potential harm in bike riding or in other hazardous activities.
The concomitant use of alcohol or other central nervous system depressants, including narcotic analgesics, sedatives, hypnotics, and tranquilizers, may have an additive effect and should be avoided or their dosage reduced.
Patients should be advised to report any involuntry muscle movements or unusual sensitivity to sunlight.
DRUG INTERACTIONS
The sedative action of promethazine is additive to the sedative effects of other central nervous system depressants, including alcohol, narcotic analgesics, sedatives, hypnotics, tricyclic antidepressants, and tranquilizers; therefore, these agents should be avoided or administered in reduced dosage to patients receiving promethazine.
DRUG/LABORATORY TEST INTERACTIONS
The following laboratory tests may be affected in patients who are receiving therapy with promethazine hydrochloride:
Pregnancy Tests
Diagnostic pregnancy tests based on immunological reactions between HCG and anti-HCG may result in false-negative or false-positive interpretations.
Glucose Tolerance Test
An increase in blood glucose has been reported in patients receiving promethazine.
CARCINOGENESIS, MUTAGENESIS, IMPAIRMENT OF FERTILITY
Long-term animal studies have not been performed to assess the carcinogenic potential of promethazine, nor are there other animal or human data concerning carcinogenicity, mutagenicity, or impairment of fertility with this drug. Promethazine was nonmutagenic in the *Salmonella* test system of Ames.
PREGNANCY
Teratogenic Effects —Pregnancy Category C
Teratogenic effects have not been demonstrated in rat-feeding studies at doses of 6.25 and 12.5 mg/kg of promethazine. These doses are from approximately 6 to 16.7 times the maximum recommended total daily dose of promethazine for a 50-kg subject, depending upon the indication for which the drug is prescribed. Specific studies to test the action of the drug on parturition, lactation, and development of the animal neonate were not done, but a general preliminary study in rats indicated no effect on these parameters. Although antihistamines, including promethazine, have been found to produce fetal mortality in rodents, the pharmacological effects of histamine in the rodent do not parallel those in man. There are no adequate and well-controlled studies of promethazine in pregnant women. Phenergan should be used during pregnancy only if the potential benefit justifies the potential risk to the fetus.
Nonteratogenic Effects
Promethazine taken within two weeks of delivery my inhibit platelet aggregation in the newborn.
LABOR AND DELIVERY
Phenergan, in appropriate dosage form, may be used alone or an an adjunct to narcotic analgesics during labor and delivery. (See "Indications and Usage" and "Dosage and Administration.")
See also "Nonteratogenic Effects."
NURSING MOTHERS
It is not known whether promethazine is excreted in human milk. Caution should be exercised when promethazine is administered to a nursing woman.
PEDIATRIC USE
This product should not be used in children under 2 years of age because safety for such use has not been established.

ADVERSE REACTIONS
Nervous System —Sedation, sleepiness, occasional blurred vision, dryness of mouth, dizziness; rarely confusion, disorientation, and extrapyramidal symptoms such as oculogyric crisis, torticollis, and tongue protrusion (usually in association with parenteral injection or excessive dosage).
Cardiovascular —Increased or decreased blood pressure.
Dermatologic —Rash, rarely photosensitivity.
Hematologic —Rarely leukopenia, thrombocytopenia; agranulocytosis (1 case).
Gastrointestinal —Nausea and vomiting.

OVERDOSAGE
Signs and symptoms of overdosage with promethazine range from mild depression of the central nervous system and cardiovascular system to profound hypotension, respiratory depression, and unconsciousness.
Stimulation may be evident, especially in children and geriatric patients. Convulsions may rarely occur. A paradoxical reaction has been reported in children receiving single doses of 75 mg to 125 mg orally, characterized by hyperexcitability and nightmares.
Atropine-like signs and symptoms—dry mouth, fixed, dilated pupils, flushing, as well as gastrointestinal symptoms, may occur.
TREATMENT
Treatment of overdosage is essentially symptomatic and supportive. Only in cases of extreme overdosage or individual sensitivity do vital signs including respiration, pulse, blood pressure, temperature, and EKG need to be monitored. Activated charcoal orally or by lavage may be given, or sodium or magnesium sulfate orally as a cathartic. Attention should be given to the reestablishment of adequate respiratory exchange through provision of a patent airway and institution of assisted or controlled ventilation. Diazepam may be used to control convulsions. Acidosis and electrolyte losses should be corrected. Note that any depressant effects of promethazine are not reversed by naloxone. Avoid analeptics which may cause convulsions.
Severe hypotension usually responds to the administration of norepinephrine or phenylephrine. EPINEPHRINE SHOULD NOT BE USED, since its use in patients with partial adrenergic blockade may further lower the blood pressure.
Limited experience with dialysis indicates that it is not helpful.

DOSAGE AND ADMINISTRATION
ALLERGY
The average oral dose is 25 mg taken before retiring; however, 12.5 mg may be taken before meals and on retiring, if necessary. Children tolerate this product well. Single 25-mg doses at bedtime or 6.25 to 12.5 mg taken three times daily will usually suffice. After initiation of treatment in children or adults, dosage should be adjusted to the smallest amount adequate to relieve symptoms. The administration of promethazine hydrochloride in 25-mg doses will control minor transfusion reactions of an allergic nature.
MOTION SICKNESS
The average adult dose is 25 mg taken twice daily. The initial dose should be taken one-half to one hour before anticipated travel and be repeated 8 to 12 hours later, if necessary. On succeeding days of travel, it is recommended that 25 mg be given on arising and again before the evening meal. For children, Phenergan Tablets, Syrup, or Rectal Suppositories, 12.5 to 25 mg, twice daily, may be administered.
NAUSEA AND VOMITING
The average effective dose of Phenergan for the active therapy of nausea and vomiting in children or adults is 25 mg. When oral medication cannot be tolerated, the dose should be given parenterally (cf. Phenergan Injection) or by rectal suppository. 12.5 to 25-mg doses may be repeated, as necessary, at 4- to 6-hour intervals.
For nausea and vomiting in children, the usual dose is 0.5 mg per pound of body weight, and the dose should be adjusted to the age and weight of the patient and the severity of the condition being treated.
For prophylaxis of nausea and vomiting, as during surgery and the postoperative period, the average dose is 25 mg repeated at 4- to 6-hour intervals, as necessary.
SEDATION
This product relieves apprehension and induces a quiet sleep from which the patient can be easily aroused. Administration of 12.5 to 25 mg Phenergan by the oral route or by rectal suppository at bedtime will provide sedation in children. Adults usually require 25 to 50 mg for nighttime, presurgical, or obsterical sedation.
PRE- AND POSTOPERATIVE USE
Phenergan in 12.5- to 25-mg doses for children and 50-mg doses for adults the night before surgery relieves apprehension and produces a quiet sleep.
For preoperative medication children require doses of 0.5 mg per pound of body weight in combination with an equal dose of meperidine and the appropriate dose of an atropine-like drug.
Usual adult dosage is 50 mg Phenergan with an equal amount of meperidine and the required amount of a belladonna alkaloid.
Postoperative sedation and adjunctive use with analgesics may be obtained by the administration of 12.5 to 25 mg in children and 25- to 50-mg doses in adults.
Phenergan Syrup Plain and Phenergan Syrup Fortis are not recommended for children under 2 years of age.

HOW SUPPLIED
Phenergan® (promethazine HCl) Syrup Plain, Wyeth®, is a clear, green solution supplied as follows:
NDC 0008-0549-02, case of 24 bottles of 4 fl. oz.
NDC 0008-0549-06, case of 16 bottles of 6 fl. oz.
NDC 0008-0549-08, case of 12 bottles of 8 fl. oz.
NDC 0008-0549-03, bottle of 1 pint.
NDC 0008-0549-04, bottle of 1 gallon.
Phenergan® (promethazine HCl) Syrup Fortis, Wyeth®, is a clear, light straw-colored solution supplied as follows:
NDC 0008-0231-01, bottle of 1 pint.
Keep bottles tightly closed at Room Temperature, Approx. 25°C (77°F).
Protect from light.
Dispense in light-resistant, glass, tight containers.

PHENERGAN® ℞
[fen 'er-gan]
(promethazine HCl)
TABLETS •
SUPPOSITORIES

DESCRIPTION
Each tablet of Phenergan contains 12.5 mg, 25 mg, or 50 mg promethazine hydrochloride. The inactive ingredients present are lactose, magnesium stearate, and methylcellulose.
Each dosage strength also contains the following:
12.5 mg—FD&C Yellow 6 and saccharin sodium;
25 mg—saccharin sodium;
50 mg—FD&C Red 3 and FD&C Yellow 6.
Each rectal suppository of Phenergan contains 12.5 mg, 25 mg, or 50 mg promethazine hydrochloride with ascorbyl palmitate, silicon dioxide, white wax, and cocoa butter.
Promethazine hydrochloride, a phenothiazine derivative, is designated chemically as N,N,α-trimethyl-10H-phenothiazine-10-ethanamine monohydrochloride.
Promethazine hydrochloride occurs as a white to faint yellow, practically odorless, crystalline powder which slowly oxidizes and turns blue on prolonged exposure to air. It is soluble in water and freely soluble in alcohol.

CLINICAL PHARMACOLOGY
Promethazine is a phenothiazine derivative which differs structurally from the antipsychotic phenothiazines by the presence of a branched side chain and no ring substitution. It is thought that this configuration is responsible for its relative lack ($^1/_{10}$ that of chlorpromazine) of dopaminergic (CNS) action.
Promethazine is an H_1 receptor blocking agent. In addition to its antihistaminic action, it provides clinically useful sedative and antiemetic effects. In therapeutic dosage, promethazine produces no significant effects on the cardiovascular system.
Promethazine is well absorbed from the gastrointestinal tract. Clinical effects are apparent within 20 minutes after oral administration and generally last four to six hours, although they may persist as long as 12 hours. Promethazine is metabolized by the liver to a variety of compounds; the sulfoxides of promethazine and N-demethylpromethazine are the predominant metabolites appearing in the urine.

INDICATIONS AND USAGE
Phenergan, either orally or by suppository, is useful for:
Perennial and seasonal allergic rhinitis.
Vasomotor rhinitis.
Allergic conjunctivitis due to inhalant allergens and foods.
Mild, uncomplicated allergic skin manifestations of urticaria and angioedema.
Amelioration of allergic reactions to blood or plasma.
Dermographism.
Anaphylactic reactions, as adjunctive therapy to epinephrine and other standard measures, after the acute manifestations have been controlled.
Preoperative, postoperative, or obstetric sedation.
Prevention and control of nausea and vomiting associated with certain types of anesthesia and surgery.
Therapy adjunctive to meperidine or other analgesics for control of postoperative pain.
Sedation in both children and adults, as well as relief of apprehension and production of light sleep from which the patient can be easily aroused.
Active and prophylactic treatment of motion sickness.
Antiemetic therapy in postoperative patients.

CONTRAINDICATIONS
Promethazine is contraindicated in individuals known to be hypersensitive or to have an idiosyncratic reaction to promethazine or to other phenothiazines.
Antihistamines are contraindicated for use in the treatment of lower respiratory tract symptoms including asthma.

WARNINGS
Promethazine may cause marked drowsiness. Ambulatory patients should be cautioned against such activities as driving or operating dangerous machinery until it is known that they do not become drowsy or dizzy from promethazine therapy.
The sedative action of promethazine hydrochloride is additive to the sedative effects of central nervous system depres-

sants; therefore, agents such as alcohol, narcotic analgesics, sedatives, hypnotics, and tranquilizers should either be eliminated or given in reduced dosage in the presence of promethazine hydrochloride. When given concomitantly with promethazine hydrochloride, the dose of barbiturates should be reduced by at least one-half, and the dose of analgesic depressants, such as morphine or meperidine, should be reduced by one-quarter to one-half.

Promethazine may lower seizure threshold. This should be taken into consideration when administering to persons with known seizure disorders or when giving in combination with narcotics and local anesthetics which may also affect seizure threshold.

Sedative drugs or CNS depressants should be avoided in patients with a history of sleep apnea.

Antihistamines should be used with caution in patients with narrow-angle glaucoma, stenosing peptic ulcer, pyloroduodenal obstruction, and urinary bladder obstruction due to symptomatic prostatic hypertrophy and narrowing of the bladder neck.

Administration of promethazine has been associated with reported cholestatic jaundice.

PRECAUTIONS

GENERAL

Promethazine should be used cautiously in persons with cardiovascular disease or with impairment of liver function.

INFORMATION FOR PATIENTS

Phenergan may cause marked drowsiness or impair the mental and/or physical abilities required for the performance of potentially hazardous tasks, such as driving a vehicle or operating machinery. Ambulatory patients should be told to avoid engaging in such activities until it is known that they do not become drowsy or dizzy from Phenergan therapy. Children should be supervised to avoid potential harm in bike riding or in other hazardous activities.

The concomitant use of alcohol or other central nervous system depressants, including narcotic analgesics, sedatives, hypnotics, and tranquilizers, may have an additive effect and should be avoided or their dosage reduced.

Patients should be advised to report any involuntary muscle movements or unusual sensitivity to sunlight.

DRUG INTERACTIONS

The sedative action of promethazine is additive to the sedative effects of other central nervous system depressants, including alcohol, narcotic analgesics, sedatives, hypnotics, tricyclic antidepressants, and tranquilizers; therefore, these agents should be avoided or administered in reduced dosage to patients receiving promethazine.

DRUG/LABORATORY TEST INTERACTIONS

The following laboratory tests may be affected in patients who are receiving therapy with promethazine hydrochloride:

Pregnancy Tests

Diagnostic pregnancy tests based on immunological reactions between HCG and anti-HCG may result in false-negative or false-positive interpretations.

Glucose Tolerance Test

An increase in blood glucose has been reported in patients receiving promethazine.

CARCINOGENESIS, MUTAGENESIS, IMPAIRMENT OF FERTILITY

Long-term animal studies have not been performed to assess the carcinogenic potential of promethazine, nor are there other animal or human data concerning carcinogenicity, mutagenicity, or impairment of fertility with this drug. Promethazine was nonmutagenic in the *Salmonella* test system of Ames.

PREGNANCY

Teratogenic Effects—Pregnancy Category C

Teratogenic effects have not been demonstrated in rat-feeding studies at doses of 6.25 and 12.5 mg/kg of promethazine. These doses are from approximately 6 to 16.7 times the maximum recommended total daily dose of promethazine for a 50-kg subject, depending upon the indication for which the drug is prescribed. Specific studies to test the action of the drug on parturition, lactation, and development of the animal neonate were not done, but a general preliminary study in rats indicated no effect on these parameters. Although antihistamines, including promethazine, have been found to produce fetal mortality in rodents, the pharmacological effects of histamine in the rodent do not parallel those in man. There are no adequate and well-controlled studies of promethazine in pregnant women. Phenergan should be used during pregnancy only if the potential benefit justifies the potential risk to the fetus.

Nonteratogenic Effects

Promethazine taken within two weeks of delivery may inhibit platelet aggregation in the newborn.

LABOR AND DELIVERY

Phenergan, in appropriate dosage form, may be used alone or as an adjunct to narcotic analgesics during labor and delivery. (See "Indications and Usage" and "Dosage and Administration.")

See also "Nonteratogenic Effects."

NURSING MOTHERS

It is not known whether promethazine is excreted in human milk. Caution should be exercised when promethazine is administered to a nursing woman.

PEDIATRIC USE

This product should not be used in children under 2 years of age because safety for such use has not been established.

ADVERSE REACTIONS

Nervous System—Sedation, sleepiness, occasional blurred vision, dryness of mouth, dizziness; rarely confusion, disorientation, and extrapyramidal symptoms such as oculogyric crisis, torticollis, and tongue protrusion (usually in association with parenteral injection or excessive dosage).

Cardiovascular—Increased or decreased blood pressure.

Dermatologic—Rash, rarely photosensitivity.

Hematologic—Rarely leukopenia, thrombocytopenia; agranulocytosis (1 case).

Gastrointestinal—Nausea and vomiting.

OVERDOSAGE

Signs and symptoms of overdosage with promethazine range from mild depression of the central nervous system and cardiovascular system to profound hypotension, respiratory depression, and unconsciousness.

Stimulation may be evident, especially in children and geriatric patients. Convulsions may rarely occur. A paradoxical reaction has been reported in children receiving single doses of 75 mg to 125 mg orally, characterized by hyperexcitability and nightmares.

Atropine-like signs and symptoms—dry mouth, fixed, dilated pupils, flushing, as well as gastrointestinal symptoms, may occur.

TREATMENT

Treatment of overdosage is essentially symptomatic and supportive. Only in cases of extreme overdosage or individual sensitivity do vital signs including respiration, pulse, blood pressure, temperature, and EKG need to be monitored. Activated charcoal orally or by lavage may be given, or sodium or magnesium sulfate orally as a cathartic. Attention should be given to the re-establishment of adequate respiratory exchange through provision of a patent airway and institution of assisted or controlled ventilation. Diazepam may be used to control convulsions. Acidosis and electrolyte losses should be corrected. Note that any depressant effects of promethazine are not reversed by naloxone. Avoid analeptics which may cause convulsions.

Severe hypotension usually responds to the administration of norepinephrine or phenylephrine. EPINEPHRINE SHOULD NOT BE USED, since its use in patients with partial adrenergic blockade may further lower the blood pressure.

Limited experience with dialysis indicates that it is not helpful.

DOSAGE AND ADMINISTRATION

Allergy: The average oral dose is 25 mg. taken before retiring; however, 12.5 mg. may be taken before meals and on retiring, if necessary. Children tolerate this product well. Single 25-mg. doses at bedtime or 6.25 to 12.5 mg. taken three times daily will usually suffice. After initiation of treatment, in children or adults, dosage should be adjusted to the smallest amount adequate to relieve symptoms. The administration of promethazine hydrochloride in 25-mg. doses will control minor transfusion reactions of an allergic nature.

Motion Sickness: The average adult dose is 25 mg. taken twice daily. The initial dose should be taken one-half to one hour before anticipated travel and be repeated eight to twelve hours later if necessary. On succeeding days of travel, it is recommended that 25 mg. be given on arising and again before the evening meal. For children, Phenergan Tablets, Syrup, or Rectal Suppositories, 12.5 to 25 mg., twice daily, may be administered.

Nausea and Vomiting: The average effective dose of Phenergan for the active therapy of nausea and vomiting in children or adults is 25 mg. When oral medication cannot be tolerated, the dose should be given parenterally (cf. Phenergan Injection) or by rectal suppository. 12.5- to 25-mg. doses may be repeated as necessary at four- to six-hour intervals.

For nausea and vomiting in children, the usual dose is 0.5 mg per pound of body weight, and the dose should be adjusted to the age and weight of the patient and the severity of the condition being treated.

For prophylaxis of nausea and vomiting, as during surgery and the postoperative period, the average dose is 25 mg. repeated at four- to six-hour intervals, as necessary.

Sedation: This product relieves apprehension and induces a quiet sleep from which the patient can be easily aroused. Administration of 12.5 to 25 mg. Phenergan by the oral route or by rectal suppository at bedtime will provide sedation in children. Adults usually require 25 to 50 mg. for nighttime, presurgical or obstetrical sedation.

Pre- and Postoperative Use: Phenergan in 12.5- to 25-mg. doses for children and 50-mg. doses for adults the night before surgery relieves apprehension and produces a quiet sleep.

For preoperative medication, children require doses of 0.5 mg. per pound of body weight in combination with an equal dose of meperidine and the appropriate dose of an atropine-like drug.

Usual adult dosage is 50 mg. Phenergan with an equal amount of meperidine and the required amount of a belladonna alkaloid.

Postoperative sedation and adjunctive use with analgesics may be obtained by the administration of 12.5 to 25 mg. in children and 25- to 50-mg. doses in adults.

Phenergan tablets and Phenergan suppositories are not recommended for children under 2 years of age.

HOW SUPPLIED

Phenergan® (promethazine HCl) Tablets, Wyeth®, are available as follows:

12.5 mg, orange tablet with "WYETH" on one side and "19" on the scored reverse side.

NDC 0008-0019-01, bottle of 100 tablets.

NDC 0008-0019-05, Redipak® carton of 100 individually wrapped tablets.

25 mg, white tablet with "WYETH" and "27" on one side and scored on the reverse side.

NDC 0008-0027-02, bottle of 100 tablets.

NDC 0008-0027-01, Redipak carton of 25 tablets.

NDC 0008-0027-05, Redipak carton of 100 individually wrapped tablets.

50 mg, pink tablet with "WYETH" on one side and "227" on the other side.

NDC 0008-0227-01, bottle of 100 tablets.

Keep tablets in tightly closed bottles at Room Temperature, Approx. 25°C (77°F).

Protect from light.

Dispense in light-resistant, tight container.

Phenergan® (promethazine HCl) Suppositories, Wyeth®, are available as follows:

12.5 mg, ivory, cone-shaped suppository wrapped in copper-colored foil.

NDC 0008-0498-01, box of 12 suppositories.

25 mg, ivory, cone-shaped suppository wrapped in light-green foil.

NDC 0008-0212-01, box of 12 suppositories.

NDC 0008-0212-02, Redipak Unit of Use Suppository Pack carton of 25 suppositories.

50 mg, ivory, torpedo-shaped suppository wrapped in light-green foil

NDC 0008-0229-01, box of 12 suppositories.

NDC 0008-0229-02, Redipak Unit of Use Suppository Pack carton of 25 suppositories.

Refrigerate suppositories.

Dispense in well-closed container.

Shown in Product Identification Section, page 436

PHENERGAN® Ⓒ ℞

[fen 'er-gan]

with codeine

DESCRIPTION

Each teaspoon (5 ml) of Phenergan with codeine contains 10 mg (1/6 grain) codeine phosphate (Warning—may be habit-forming) and 6.25 mg promethazine hydrochloride in a flavored syrup base with pH between 4.7 and 5.2. Alcohol 7%. The inactive ingredients present are artificial and natural flavors, citric acid, D&C Red 33, FD&C Blue 1, FD&C Yellow 6, glycerine, saccharin sodium, sodium benzoate, sodium citrate, sodium propionate, water, and other ingredients.

Codeine is one of the naturally occurring phenanthrene alkaloids of opium derived from the opium poppy; it is classified pharmacologically as a narcotic analgesic. Codeine phosphate may be chemically named as (5α,6α)-7,8-didehydro-4,5-epoxy-3-methoxy-17-methylmorphinan-6-ol phosphate (1:1) (salt) hemihydrate with the following structural formula:

$\cdot H_3PO_4 \cdot \frac{1}{2}H_2O$

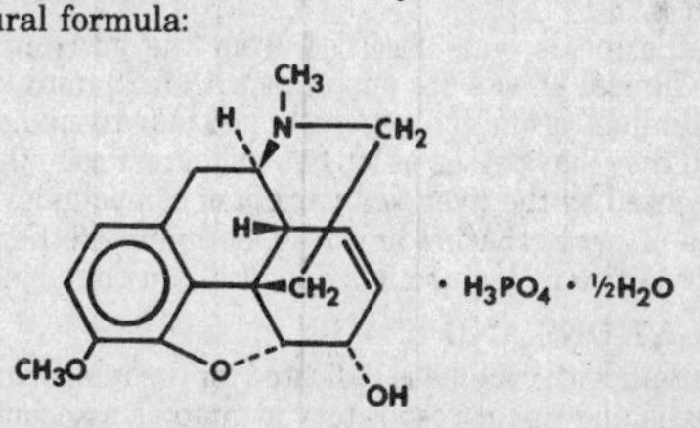

The phosphate salt of codeine occurs as white, needle-shaped crystals or white crystalline powder. Codeine phosphate is freely soluble in water and slightly soluble in alcohol.

Promethazine hydrochloride, a phenothiazine derivative, is designated chemically as N,N,α-trimethyl-10*H*-phenothiazine-10-ethanamine monohydrochloride with the following structural formula:

[See Chemical Formula at top of next page].

Continued on next page

Wyeth—Cont.

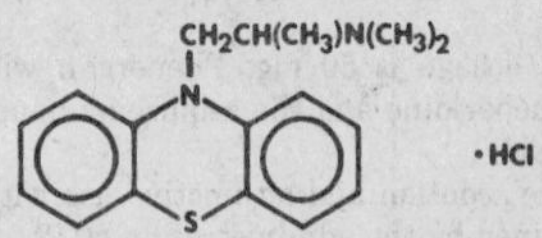

Promethazine hydrochloride occurs as a white to faint yellow, practically odorless, crystalline powder which slowly oxidizes and turns blue on prolonged exposure to air. It is soluble in water and freely soluble in alcohol.

CLINICAL PHARMACOLOGY

CODEINE

Narcotic analgesics, including codeine, exert their primary effects on the central nervous system and gastrointestinal tract. The analgesic effects of codeine are due to its central action; however, the precise sites of action have not been determined, and the mechanisms involved appear to be quite complex. Codeine resembles morphine both structurally and pharmacologically, but its actions at the doses of codeine used therapeutically are milder, with less sedation, respiratory depression, and gastrointestinal, urinary, and pupillary effects. Codeine produces an increase in biliary tract pressure, but less than morphine or meperidine. Codeine is less constipating than morphine.

Codeine has good antitussive activity, although less than that of morphine at equal doses. It is used in preference to morphine, because side effects are infrequent at the usual antitussive dose of codeine.

Codeine in oral therapeutic dosage does not usually exert major effects on the cardiovascular system.

Narcotic analgesics may cause nausea and vomiting by stimulating the chemoreceptor trigger zone (CTZ); however, they also depress the vomiting center, so that subsequent doses are unlikely to produce vomiting. Nausea is minimal after usual oral doses of codeine.

Narcotic analgesics cause histamine release, which appears to be responsible for wheals or urticaria sometimes seen at the site of injection on parenteral administration. Histamine release may also produce dilation of cutaneous blood vessels, with resultant flushing of the face and neck, pruritus, and sweating.

Codeine and its salts are well absorbed following both oral and parenteral administration. Codeine is about 2/3 as effective orally as parenterally. Codeine is metabolized primarily in the liver by enzymes of the endoplasmic reticulum, where it undergoes O-demethylation, N-demethylation, and partial conjugation with glucuronic acid. The drug is excreted primarily in the urine, largely as inactive metabolites and small amounts of free and conjugated morphine. Negligible amounts of codeine and its metabolites are found in the feces.

Following oral or subcutaneous administration of codeine, the onset of analgesia occurs within 15 to 30 minutes and lasts for four to six hours.

The cough-depressing action, in animal studies, was observed to occur 15 minutes after oral administration of codeine, peak action at 45 to 60 minutes after ingestion. The duration of action, which is dose-dependent, usually did not exceed 3 hours.

PROMETHAZINE

Promethazine is a phenothiazine derivative which differs structurally from the antipsychotic phenothiazines by the presence of a branched side chain and no ring substitution. It is thought that this configuration is responsible for its lack (1/10 that of chlorpromazine) of dopaminergic (CNS) action.

Promethazine is an H_1 receptor blocking agent. In addition to its antihistaminic action, it provides clinically useful sedative and antiemetic effects. In therapeutic dosages, promethazine produces no significant effects on the cardiovascular system.

Promethazine is well absorbed from the gastrointestinal tract. Clinical effects are apparent within 20 minutes after oral administration and generally last four to six hours, although they may persist as long as 12 hours. Promethazine is metabolized by the liver to a variety of compounds; the sulfoxides of promethazine and N-demethylpromethazine are the predominant metabolites appearing in the urine.

INDICATIONS AND USAGE

Phenergan with codeine is indicated for the temporary relief of coughs and upper respiratory symptoms associated with allergy or the common cold.

CONTRAINDICATIONS

Codeine is contraindicated in patients with a known hypersensitivity to the drug.

Promethazine is contraindicated in individuals known to be hypersensitive or to have had an idiosyncratic reaction to promethazine or to other phenothiazines.

Antihistamines and codeine are both contraindicated for use in the treatment of lower respiratory tract symptoms, including asthma.

WARNINGS

CODEINE

Dosage of codeine SHOULD NOT BE INCREASED if cough fails to respond; an unresponsive cough should be reevaluated in 5 days or sooner for possible underlying pathology, such as foreign body or lower respiratory tract disease.

Codeine may cause or aggravate constipation.

Respiratory depression leading to arrest, coma, and death has occurred with the use of codeine antitussives in young children, particularly in the under-one-year infants whose ability to deactivate the drug is not fully developed.

Administration of codeine may be accompanied by histamine release and should be used with caution in atopic children.

Head Injury and Increased Intracranial Pressure

The respiratory-depressant effects of narcotic analgesics and their capacity to elevate cerebrospinal fluid pressure may be markedly exaggerated in the presence of head injury, intracranial lesions, or a preexisting increase in intracranial pressure. Narcotics may produce adverse reactions which may obscure the clinical course of patients with head injuries.

Asthma and Other Respiratory Conditions

Narcotic analgesics or cough suppressants, including codeine, should not be used in asthmatic patients (see "Contraindications"). Nor should they be used in acute febrile illness associated with productive cough or in chronic respiratory disease where interference with ability to clear the tracheobronchial tree of secretions would have a deleterious effect on the patient's respiratory function.

Hypotensive Effect

Codeine may produce orthostatic hypotension in ambulatory patients.

PROMETHAZINE

Promethazine may cause marked drowsiness. Ambulatory patients should be cautioned against such activities as driving or operating dangerous machinery until it is known that they do not become drowsy or dizzy from promethazine therapy.

The sedative action of promethazine hydrochloride is additive to the sedative effects of central nervous system depressants; therefore, agents such as alcohol, narcotic analgesics, sedatives, hypnotics, and tranquilizers should either be eliminated or given in reduced dosage in the presence of promethazine hydrochloride. When given concomitantly with promethazine hydrochloride, the dose of barbiturates should be reduced by at least one-half, and the dose of analgesic depressants, such as morphine or meperidine, should be reduced by one-quarter to one-half.

Promethazine may lower seizure threshold. This should be taken into consideration when administering to persons with known seizure disorders or when giving in combination with narcotics or local anesthetics which may also affect seizure threshold.

Sedative drugs or CNS depressants should be avoided in patients with a history of sleep apnea.

Antihistamines should be used with caution in patients with narrow-angle glaucoma, stenosing peptic ulcer, pyloroduodenal obstruction, and urinary bladder obstruction due to symptomatic prostatic hypertrophy and narrowing of the bladder neck.

Administration of promethazine has been associated with reported cholestatic jaundice.

PRECAUTIONS

Animal reproduction studies have not been conducted with the drug combination—promethazine and codeine. It is not known whether this drug combination can cause fetal harm when administered to a pregnant woman or can affect reproduction capacity. Phenergan with codeine should be given to a pregnant woman only if clearly needed.

GENERAL

Narcotic analgesics, including codeine, should be administered with caution and the initial dose reduced in patients with acute abdominal conditions, convulsive disorders, significant hepatic or renal impairment, fever, hypothyroidism, Addison's disease, ulcerative colitis, prostatic hypertrophy, in patients with recent gastrointestinal or urinary tract surgery, and in the very young or elderly or debilitated patients.

Promethazine should be used cautiously in persons with cardiovascular disease or with impairment of liver function.

INFORMATION FOR PATIENTS

Phenergan with codeine may cause marked drowsiness or may impair the mental and/or physical abilities required for the performance of potentially hazardous tasks, such as driving a vehicle or operating machinery. Ambulatory patients should be told to avoid engaging in such activities until it is known that they do not become drowsy or dizzy from Phenergan with codeine therapy. Children should be supervised to avoid potential harm in bike riding or in other hazardous activities.

The concomitant use of alcohol or other central nervous system depressants, including narcotic analgesics, sedatives, hypnotics, and tranquilizers, may have an additive effect and should be avoided or their dosage reduced.

Patients should be advised to report any involuntary muscle movements or unusual sensitivity to sunlight.

Codeine, like other narcotic analgesics, may produce orthostatic hypotension in some ambulatory patients. Patients should be cautioned accordingly.

DRUG INTERACTIONS

CODEINE

In patients receiving MAO inhibitors, an initial small test dose is advisable to allow observation of any excessive narcotic effects or MAOI interaction.

PROMETHAZINE

The sedative action of promethazine is additive to the effects of other central nervous system depressants, including alcohol, narcotic analgesics, sedatives, hypnotics, tricyclic antidepressants, and tranquilizers; therefore, these agents should be avoided or administered in reduced dosage to patients receiving promethazine.

DRUG/LABORATORY TEST INTERACTIONS

Because narcotic analgesics may increase biliary tract pressure, with resultant increases in plasma amylase or lipase levels, determination of these enzyme levels may be unreliable for 24 hours after a narcotic analgesic has been given.

The following laboratory tests may be affected in patients who are receiving therapy with promethazine hydrochloride:

Pregnancy Tests

Diagnostic pregnancy tests based on immunological reactions between HCG and anti-HCG may result in false-negative or false-positive interpretations.

Glucose Tolerance Test

An increase in blood glucose has been reported in patients receiving promethazine.

CARCINOGENESIS, MUTAGENESIS, IMPAIRMENT OF FERTILITY

Long-term animal studies have not been performed to assess the carcinogenic potential of codeine or of promethazine, nor are there other animal or human data concerning carcinogenicity, mutagenicity, or impairment of fertility with these agents. Codeine has been reported to show no evidence of carcinogenicity or mutagenicity in a variety of test systems, including the micronucleus and sperm abnormality assays and the *Salmonella* assay. Promethazine was nonmutagenic in the *Salmonella* test system of Ames.

PREGNANCY

Teratogenic Effects —Pregnancy Category C

CODEINE

A study in rats and rabbits reported no teratogenic effect of codeine administered during the period of organogenesis in doses ranging from 5 to 120 mg/kg. In the rat, doses at the 120-mg/kg level, in the toxic range for the adult animal, were associated with an increase in embryo resorption at the time of implantation. In another study a single 100-mg/kg dose of codeine administered to pregnant mice reportedly resulted in delayed ossification in the offspring.

There are no studies in humans, and the significance of these findings to humans, if any, is not known.

PROMETHAZINE

Teratogenic effects have not been demonstrated in rat-feeding studies at doses of 6.25 and 12.5 mg/kg of promethazine. These doses are 8.3 and 16.7 times the maximum recommended total daily dose of promethazine for a 50-kg subject. Specific studies to test the action of the drug on parturition, lactation, and development of the animal neonate were not done, but a general preliminary study in rats indicated no effect on these parameters. Although antihistamines, including promethazine, have been found to produce fetal mortality in rodents, the pharmacological effects of histamine in the rodent do not parallel those in man. There are no adequate and well-controlled studies of promethazine in pregnant women.

Phenergan with codeine should be used during pregnancy only if the potential benefit justifies the potential risk to the fetus.

Nonteratogenic Effects

Dependence has been reported in newborns whose mothers took opiates regularly during pregnancy. Withdrawal signs include irritability, excessive crying, tremors, hyperreflexia, fever, vomiting, and diarrhea. Signs usually appear during the first few days of life.

Promethazine taken within two weeks of delivery may inhibit platelet aggregation in the newborn.

LABOR AND DELIVERY

Narcotic analgesics cross the placental barrier. The closer to delivery and the larger the dose used, the greater the possibility of respiratory depression in the newborn. Narcotic analgesics should be avoided during labor if delivery of a premature infant is anticipated. If the mother has received narcotic analgesics during labor, newborn infants should be observed closely for signs of respiratory depression. Resuscitation may be required (see "Overdosage"). The effect of codeine, if any, on the later growth, development, and functional maturation of the child is unknown.

See also "Nonteratogenic Effects."

NURSING MOTHERS

Some studies, but not others, have reported detectable amounts of codeine in breast milk. The levels are probably not clinically significant after usual therapeutic dosage. The possibility of clinically important amounts being excreted in breast milk in individuals abusing codeine should be considered.

It is not known whether promethazine is excreted in human milk.

Caution should be exercised when Phenergan with codeine is administered to a nursing woman.

PEDIATRIC USE

This product should not be used in children under 2 years of age because safety for such use has not been established.

ADVERSE REACTIONS

CODEINE

Nervous System—CNS depression, particularly respiratory depression, and to a lesser extent circulatory depression; light-headedness, dizziness, sedation, euphoria, dysphoria, headache, transient hallucination, disorientation, visual disturbances, and convulsions.

Cardiovascular—Tachycardia, bradycardia, palpitation, faintness, syncope, orthostatic hypotension (common to narcotic analgesics).

Gastrointestinal—Nausea, vomiting, constipation, and biliary tract spasm. Patients with chronic ulcerative colitis may experience increased colonic motility; in patients with acute ulcerative colitis, toxic dilation has been reported.

Genitourinary—Oliguria, urinary retention; antidiuretic effect has been reported (common to narcotic analgesics).

Allergic—Infrequent pruritus, giant urticaria, angioneurotic edema, and laryngeal edema.

Other—Flushing of the face, sweating and pruritus (due to opiate-induced histamine release); weakness.

PROMETHAZINE

Nervous System—Sedation, sleepiness, occasional blurred vision, dryness of mouth, dizziness; rarely confusion, disorientation, and extrapyramidal symptoms such as oculogyric crisis, torticollis, and tongue protrusion (usually in association with parenteral injection or excessive dosage).

Cardiovascular—Increased or decreased blood pressure.

Dermatologic—Rash, rarely photosensitivity.

Hematologic—Rarely leukopenia, thrombocytopenia; agranulocytosis (1 case).

Gastrointestinal—Nausea and vomiting.

DRUG ABUSE AND DEPENDENCE

CONTROLLED SUBSTANCE

Phenergan with codeine is a Schedule V Controlled Substance.

ABUSE

Codeine is known to be subject to abuse; however, the abuse potential of oral codeine appears to be quite low. Even parenteral codeine does not appear to offer the psychic effects sought by addicts to the same degree as heroin or morphine. However, codeine must be administered only under close supervision to patients with a history of drug abuse or dependence.

DEPENDENCE

Psychological dependence, physical dependence, and tolerance are known to occur with codeine.

OVERDOSAGE

CODEINE

Serious overdose with codeine is characterized by respiratory depression (a decrease in respiratory rate and/or tidal volume, Cheyne-Stokes respiration, cyanosis), extreme somnolence progressing to stupor or coma, skeletal muscle flaccidity, cold and clammy skin, and sometimes bradycardia and hypotension. The triad of coma, pinpoint pupils, and respiratory depression is strongly suggestive of opiate poisoning. In severe overdosage, particularly by the intravenous route, apnea, circulatory collapse, cardiac arrest, and death may occur. Promethazine is additive to the depressant effects of codeine.

It is difficult to determine what constitutes a standard toxic or lethal dose. However, the lethal oral dose of codeine in an adult is reported to be in the range of 0.5 to 1.0 gram. Infants and children are believed to be relatively more sensitive to opiates on a bodyweight basis. Elderly patients are also comparatively intolerant to opiates.

PROMETHAZINE

Signs and symptoms of overdosage with promethazine range from mild depression of the central nervous system and cardiovascular system to profound hypotension, respiratory depression, and unconsciousness.

Stimulation may be evident, especially in children and geriatric patients. Convulsions may rarely occur. A paradoxical reaction has been reported in children receiving single doses of 75 mg to 125 mg orally, characterized by hyperexcitability and nightmares.

Atropine-like signs and symptoms—dry mouth, fixed, dilated pupils, flushing, as well as gastrointestinal symptoms, may occur.

TREATMENT

The treatment of overdosage with Phenergan with codeine is essentially symptomatic and supportive. Only in cases of extreme overdosage or individual sensitivity do vital signs including respiration, pulse, blood pressure, temperature,

Adults	1 teaspoon (5 ml) every 4 to 6 hours, not to exceed 30.0 ml in 24 hours.
Children 6 years to under 12 years	1/2 to 1 teaspoon (2.5 to 5 ml) every 4 to 6 hours, not to exceed 30.0 ml in 24 hours.
Children under 6 years (weight: 18 kg or 40 lbs)	1/4 to 1/2 teaspoon (1.25 to 2.5 ml) every 4 to 6 hours, not to exceed 9.0 ml in 24 hours.
Children under 6 years (weight: 16 kg or 35 lbs)	1/4 to 1/2 teaspoon (1.25 to 2.5 ml) every 4 to 6 hours, not to exceed 8.0 ml in 24 hours.
Children under 6 years (weight: 14 kg or 30 lbs)	1/4 to 1/2 teaspoon (1.25 to 2.5 ml) every 4 to 6 hours, not to exceed 7.0 ml in 24 hours.
Children under 6 years (weight: 12 kg or 25 lbs)	1/4 to 1/2 teaspoon (1.25 to 2.5 ml) every 4 to 6 hours, not to exceed 6.0 ml in 24 hours.

Phenergan with codeine is not recommended for children under 2 years of age.

and EKG need to be monitored. Activated charcoal orally or by lavage may be given, or sodium or magnesium sulfate orally as a cathartic. Attention should be given to the reestablishment of adequate respiratory exchange through provision of a patent airway and institution of assisted or controlled ventilation. The narcotic antagonist, naloxone hydrochloride, may be administered when significant respiratory depression occurs with Phenergan with codeine; any depressant effects of promethazine are not reversed with naloxone. Diazepam may be used to control convulsions. Avoid analeptics, which may cause convulsions. Acidosis and electrolyte losses should be corrected. A rise in temperature or pulmonary complications may signal the need for institution of antibiotic therapy.

Severe hypotension usually responds to the administration of norepinephrine or phenylephrine. EPINEPHRINE SHOULD NOT BE USED, since its use in a patient with partial adrenergic blockade may further lower the blood pressure.

Limited experience with dialysis indicates that it is not helpful.

DOSAGE AND ADMINISTRATION

The average effective dose is given in the following table: [See table above].

HOW SUPPLIED

Phenergan® with codeine, Wyeth®, is a clear, purple solution supplied as follows:

NDC 0008-0550-02, case of 24 bottles of 4 fl. oz.
NDC 0008-0550-06, case of 16 bottles of 6 fl. oz.
NDC 0008-0550-08, case of 12 bottles of 8 fl. oz.
NDC 0008-0550-03, bottle of 1 pint.
NDC 0008-0550-04, bottle of 1 gallon.

Keep bottles tightly closed at Room Temperature, Approx. 25° C (77° F).

Protect from light.

Dispense in light-resistant, glass, tight containers.

PHENERGAN® ℞

[fen ′er-gan]

with dextromethorphan

DESCRIPTION

Each teaspoon (5 ml) of Phenergan with dextromethorphan contains 6.25 mg promethazine hydrochloride and 15 mg dextromethorphan hydrobromide in a flavored syrup base with a pH between 4.7 and 5.2. Alcohol 7%. The inactive ingredients present are artificial and natural flavors, citric acid, D&C Yellow 10, FD&C Yellow 6, glycerin, saccharin sodium, sodium benzoate, sodium citrate, sodium propionate, water, and other ingredients.

Promethazine hydrochloride, a phenothiazine derivative, is designated chemically as N,N,α-trimethyl-10*H*-phenothiazine-10-ethanamine monohydrochloride with the following structural formula:

$CH_2CH(CH_3)N(CH_3)_2$ · HCl

Promethazine hydrochloride occurs as a white to faint yellow, practically odorless, crystalline powder which slowly oxidizes and turns blue on prolonged exposure to air. It is soluble in water and freely soluble in alcohol.

Dextromethorphan hydrobromide is a salt of the methyl ether of the dextrorotatory isomer of levorphanol, a narcotic analgesic. It is chemically named as 3-methoxy-17-methyl-9α, 13α, 14α-morphinan hydrobromide monohydrate with the following structural formula:

CH_3 · HBr · H_2O · CH_3O

Dextromethorphan hydrobromide occurs as white crystals sparingly soluble in water and freely soluble in alcohol.

CLINICAL PHARMACOLOGY

PROMETHAZINE

Promethazine is a phenothiazine derivative which differs structurally from the antipsychotic phenothiazines by the presence of a branched side chain and no ring substitution. It is thought that this configuration is responsible for its relative lack (1/10 that of cholrpromazine) of dopaminergic (CNS) action.

Promethazine is an H_1 receptor blocking agent. In addition to its antihistaminic action, it provides clinically useful sedative and antiemetic effects. In therapeutic dosages, promethazine produces no significant effects on the cardiovascular system.

Promethazine is well absorbed from the gastrointestinal tract. Clinical effects are apparent within 20 minutes after oral administration and generally last four to six hours, although they may persist as long as 12 hours. Promethazine is metabolized by the liver to a variety of compounds; the sulfoxides of promethazine and N-demethylpromethazine are the predominant metabolites appearing in the urine.

DEXTROMETHORPHAN

Dextromethorphan is an antitussive agent and, unlike the isomeric levorphanol, it has no analgesic or addictive properties.

The drug acts centrally and elevates the threshold for coughing. It is about equal to codeine in depressing the cough reflex. In therapeutic dosage dextromethorphan does not inhibit ciliary activity.

Dextromethorphan is rapidly absorbed from the gastrointestinal tract and exerts its effect in 15 to 30 minutes. The duration of action after oral administration is approximately three to six hours. Dextromethorphan is metabolized primarily by liver enzymes undergoing O-demethylation, N-demethylation, and partial conjugation with glucuronic acid and sulfate. In humans, (+)-3-hydroxy-N-methylmorphinan, (+)-3-hydroxymorphinan, and traces of unmetabolized drug were found in urine after oral administration.

INDICATIONS AND USAGE

Phenergan with dextromethorphan is indicated for the temporary relief of coughs and upper respiratory symptoms associated with allergy or the common cold.

CONTRAINDICATIONS

Promethazine is contraindicated in individuals known to be hypersensitive or to have had an idiosyncratic reaction to promethazine or to other phenothiazines.

Antihistamines are contraindicated for use in the treatment of lower respiratory tract symptoms, including asthma.

Dextromethorphan should not be used in patients receiving a monoamine oxidase inhibitor (MAOI).

WARNINGS

PROMETHAZINE

Promethazine may cause marked drowsiness. Ambulatory patients should be cautioned against such activities as driving or operating dangerous machinery until it is known that they do not become drowsy or dizzy from promethazine therapy.

The sedative action of promethazine hydrochloride is additive to the sedative effects of central nervous system depressants; therefore, agents such as alcohol, narcotic analgesics, sedatives, hypnotics, and tranquilizers should either be eliminated or given in reduced dosage in the presence of promethazine hydrochloride. When given concomitantly with promethazine hydrochloride, the dose of barbiturates should be reduced by at least one-half, and the dose of analgesic depressants, such as morphine or meperidine, should be reduced by one-quarter to one-half.

Promethazine may lower seizure threshold. This should be taken into consideration when administering to persons with known seizure disorders or when giving in combination with narcotics or local anesthetics which may also affect seizure threshold.

Continued on next page

Wyeth—Cont.

Sedative drugs or CNS depressants should be avoided in patients with a history of sleep apnea.
Antihistamines should be used with caution in patients with narrow-angle glaucoma, stenosing peptic ulcer, pyloroduodenal obstruction, and urinary bladder obstruction due to symptomatic prostatic hypertrophy and narrowing of the bladder neck.
Administration of promethazine has been associated with reported cholestatic jaundice.
DEXTROMETHORPHAN
Administration of dextromethorphan may be accompanied by histamine release and should be used with caution in atopic children.

PRECAUTIONS

Animal reproduction studies have not been conducted with the drug combination—promethazine and dextromethorphan. It is not known whether this drug combination can cause fetal harm when administered to a pregnant woman or can affect reproduction capacity. Phenergan with dextromethorphan should be given to a pregnant woman only if clearly needed.
GENERAL
Promethazine should be used cautiously in persons with cardiovascular disease or with impairment of liver function.
Dextromethorphan should be used with caution in sedated patients, in the debilitated, and in patients confined to the supine position.
INFORMATION FOR PATIENTS
Phenergan with dextromethorphan may cause marked drowsiness or impair the mental and/or physical abilities required for the performance of potentially hazardous tasks, such as driving a vehicle or operating machinery. Ambulatory patients should be told to avoid engaging in such activities until is it known that they do not become drowsy or dizzy from Phenergan with dextromethorphan therapy. Children should be supervised to avoid potential harm in bike riding or in other hazardous activities.
The concomitant use of alcohol or other central nervous system depressants, including narcotic analgesics, sedatives, hypnotics, and tranquilizers, may have an additive effect and should be avoided or their dosage reduced.
Patients should be advised to report any involuntary muscle movements or unusual sensitivity to sunlight.
DRUG INTERACTIONS
The sedative action of promethazine is additive to the sedative effects of other central nervous system depressants, including alcohol, narcotic analgesics, sedatives, hypnotics, tricyclic antidepressants, and tranquilizers; therefore, these agents should be avoided or administered in reduced dosage to patients receiving promethazine.
DRUG/LABORATORY TEST INTERACTIONS
The following laboratory tests may be affected in patients who are receiving therapy with promethazine hydrochloride:
Pregnancy Tests
Diagnostic pregnancy tests based on immunological reactions between HCG and anti-HCG may result in false-negative or false-positive interpretations.
Glucose Tolerance Test
An increase in blood glucose has been reported in patients receiving promethazine.
CARCINOGENESIS, MUTAGENESIS, IMPAIRMENT OF FERTILITY
Long-term animal studies have not been performed to assess the carcinogenic potential of promethazine or of dextromethorphan. There are no animal or human data concerning the carcinogenicity, mutagenicity, or impairment of fertility with these drugs. Promethazine was nonmutagenic in the *Salmonella* test system of Ames.
PREGNANCY
Teratogenic Effects—Pregnancy Category C
Teratogenic effects have not been demonstrated in rat-feeding studies at doses of 6.25 and 12.5 mg/kg of promethazine. These doses are 8.3 and 16.7 times the maximum recommended total daily dose for a 50-kg subject. Specific studies to test the action of the drug on parturition, lactation, and development of the animal neonate were not done, but a general preliminary study in rats indicated no effect on these parameters. Although antihistamines, including promethazine, have been found to produce fetal mortality in rodents, the pharmacological effects of histamine in the rodent do not parallel those in man. There are no adequate and well-controlled studies of promethazine in pregnant women.
Phenergan with dextromethorphan should be used during pregnancy only if the potential benefit justifies the potential risk to the fetus.
Nonteratogenic Effects
Promethazine taken within two weeks of delivery may inhibit platelet aggregation in the newborn.
LABOR AND DELIVERY
See "Nonteratogenic Effects."
NURSING MOTHERS
It is not known whether promethazine or dextromethorphan is excreted in human milk. Caution should be exercised when Phenergan with dextromethorphan is administered to a nursing woman.
PEDIATRIC USE
This product should not be used in children under 2 years of age because safety for that use has not been established.

ADVERSE REACTIONS

PROMETHAZINE
Nervous System—Sedation, sleepiness, occasional blurred vision, dryness of mouth, dizziness; rarely confusion, disorientation, and extrapyramidal symptoms such as oculogyric crisis, torticollis, and tongue protrusion (usually in association with parenteral injection or excessive dosage).
Cardiovascular—Increased or decreased blood pressure.
Dermatologic—Rash, rarely photosensitivity.
Hematologic—Rarely leukopenia, thrombocytopenia; agranulocytosis (1 case).
Gastrointestinal—Nausea and vomiting.
DEXTROMETHORPHAN
Dextromethorphan hydrobromide occasionally causes slight drowsiness, dizziness, and gastrointestinal disturbances.

DRUG ABUSE AND DEPENDENCE

According to the WHO Expert Committee on Drug Dependence, dextromethorphan could produce very slight psychic dependence but no physical dependence.

OVERDOSAGE

PROMETHAZINE
Signs and symptoms of overdosage with promethazine range from mild depression of the central nervous system and cardiovascular system to profound hypotension, respiratory depression, and unconsciousness.
Stimulation may be evident, especially in children and geriatric patients. Convulsions may rarely occur. A paradoxical reaction has been reported in children receiving single doses of 75 mg to 125 mg orally, characterized by hyperexcitability and nightmares.
Atropine-like signs and symptoms—dry mouth, fixed, dilated pupils, flushing, as well as gastrointestinal symptoms, may occur.
DEXTROMETHORPHAN
Dextromethorphan may produce central excitement and mental confusion. Very high doses may produce respiratory depression. One case of toxic psychosis (hyperactivity, marked visual and auditory hallucinations) after ingestion of a single dose of 20 tables (300 mg) of dextromethorphan has been reported.
TREATMENT
Treatment of overdosage with Phenergan with dextromethorphan is essentially symptomatic and supportive. Only in cases of extreme overdosage or individual sensitivity do vital signs including respiration, pulse, blood pressure, temperature, and EKG need to be monitored. Activated charcoal orally or by lavage may be given, or sodium or magnesium sulfate orally as a cathartic. Attention should be given to the reestablishment of adequate respiratory exchange through provision of a patent airway and institution of assisted or controlled ventilation. Diazepam may be used to control convulsions. Acidosis and electrolyte losses should be corrected. The antidotal efficacy of narcotic antagonists to dextromethorphan has not been established; note that any of the depressant effects of promethazine are not reversed by naloxone. Avoid analeptics, which may cause convulsions.
Severe hypotension usually responds to the administration of norepinephrine or phenylephrine. EPINEPHRINE SHOULD NOT BE USED, since its use in a patient with partial adrenergic blockade may further lower the blood pressure.
Limited experience with dialysis indicates that it is not helpful.

DOSAGE AND ADMINISTRATION

The average effective dose for adults is one teaspoon (5 ml) every 4 to 6 hours, not to exceed 30.0 ml in 24 hours. For children 6 years to under 12 years of age, the dose is one-half to one teaspoon (2.5 to 5.0 ml) every 4 to 6 hours, not to exceed 20.0 ml in 24 hours. For children 2 years to under 6 years of age, the dose is one-quarter to one-half teaspoon (1.25 to 2.5 ml) every 4 to 6 hours, not to exceed 10.0 ml in 24 hours. Phenergan with dextromethorphan is not recommended for children under 2 years of age.

HOW SUPPLIED

Phenergan® with dextromethorphan, Wyeth®, is a clear, yellow solution supplied as follows:
NDC 0008-0548-02, case of 24 bottles of 4 fl. oz.
NDC 0008-0548-06, case of 16 bottles of 6 fl. oz.
NDC 0008-0548-03, bottle of 1 pint.
NDC 0008-0548-04, bottle of 1 gallon.

Keep bottles tightly closed at Room Temperature, Approx. 25° C (77° F).
Protect from light.
Dispense in light-resistant, glass, tight containers.

PHENERGAN®-D ℞

[fen 'er-gan-D]

DESCRIPTION

Phenergan-D Tablets for oral administration each contain 6.25 mg of the antihistamine promethazine hydrochloride and 60 mg of the sympathomimetic pseudoephedrine hydrochloride. The inactive ingredients present are cellulose, edetate disodium, FD&C Yellow 6, lactose, magnesium stearate, methylcellulose, and saccharin sodium.
Phenergan (promethazine hydrochloride) may be designated chemically as 10-[2-(dimethylamino)propyl] phenothiazine monohydrochloride with the following structural formula:

$CH_2CH(CH_3)N(CH_3)_2$ N S •HCl

Pseudoephedrine hydrochloride may be designated chemically as benzenemethanol, α-[1-(methylamino)ethyl]-, [S-(R*,R*)]-, hydrochloride with the following structural formula:

H NHCH3 —C—C—CH3 •HCl OH H

CLINICAL PHARMACOLOGY

Phenergan is an antihistaminic drug useful in the management of all allergic conditions amenable to antihistamine therapy. In addition to its antihistaminic effects, promethazine has both antiemetic and anti-motion sickness activity. Promethazine exhibits clinically useful sedative properties. In therapeutic dosage, promethazine exerts no signficant effects on the cardiovascular system. In contrast to the antipsychotic phenothiazine, promethazine has a branched side chain, which appears to be responsible for its markedly different pharmacological properties.
Promethazine is well absorbed from the gastrointestinal tract. Antihistaminic effects are apparent within 20 minutes after oral administration and generally last four to six hours, although they may persist as long as 12 hours. Promethazine is metabolized by the liver to a variety of compounds; the sulfoxides of promethazine and N-desmethylpromethazine are the predominant metabolites appearing in the urine.
Pseudoephedrine is an orally effective nasal decongestant and bronchodilator. Pseudoephedrine acts directly on both *alpha* (α)- and, to a lesser degree, *beta* (β)-adrenergic receptors. It also has an indirect effect by releasing norepinephrine from storage sites. Pseudoephedrine has nasopharyngeal vasoconstrictor and bronchodilator actions of relatively the same degree as its diastereoisomer, ephedrine, but relatively weaker pressor, cardiac, mydriatic, and central-stimulant actions. Pseudoephedrine may produce mild central stimulation, especially in patients sensitive to sympathomimetic drugs. In usual dosage, pseudoephedrine generally has negligible effects on blood pressure in normotensive individuals.
After oral administration of pseudoephedrine, nasal decongestion occurs within 30 minutes and generally lasts for four to six hours. Pseudoephedrine is partially metabolized in the liver by N-demethylation. The drug and its inactive metabolite are excreted in the urine; between 55 and 75% of a dose is excreted unchanged. The urinary excretion of unchanged drug varies with the pH of the urine, more being excreted in acid urine and less in alkaline urine.

INDICATIONS AND USAGE

Phenergan-D is recommended for the symptomatic relief of upper-respiratory mucosal congestion associated with perennial and seasonal nasal allergies, vasomotor rhinitis, sinusitis, and hay fever.

CONTRAINDICATIONS

Phenergan-D is contraindicated in patients known to be hypersensitive or to exhibit an idiosyncratic reaction to promethazine or pseudoephedrine, or other antihistamines or sympathomimetics.
Phenergan-D is contraindicated in patients with severe hypertension or coronary-artery disease or in those who are taking MAO inhibitors (see "Precautions—Drug Interactions").

WARNINGS

Pseudoephedrine causes virtually no pressor effect in normotensive patients but should be used with caution in those patients who are hypertensive. Pseudoephedrine should also be used with caution in patients having cardiovascular disease, diabetes, hyperthyroidism, narrow-angle glaucoma, and prostatic hypertrophy.

Promethazine may cause sedation. Ambulatory patients should be cautioned against such activities as driving or operating dangerous machinery until it is known that they do not become drowsy or dizzy from promethazine therapy. The concomitant use of alcohol or other central nervous system depressants may have an additive effect. Patients should be warned accordingly.

PRECAUTIONS

GENERAL

Elderly patients may be particularly sensitive to the effects of sympathomimetic drugs, including pseudoephedrine.

Phenergan-D should be considered an adjunct to other means of therapy when bacterial infections complicate sinusitus.

INFORMATION FOR PATIENTS

Promethazine may impair the mental and/or physical abilities required for the performance of potentially hazardous tasks such as driving a vehicle or operating machinery. Ambulatory patients should be cautioned against engaging in such activities until it is known that they do not become drowsy or dizzy from promethazine therapy. The concomitant use of alcohol or other central nervous system depressants, including sedatives, hypnotics, tranquilizers, phenothiazines, and antihistamines, may have an additive effect and should be avoided or their dosage reduced.

DRUG INTERACTIONS

Monoamine oxidase (MAO) inhibitors, by increasing the quantity of norepinephrine in adrenergic nerve tissue, can greatly increase the pressor effect of indirectly acting sympathomimetic drugs, including pseudoephedrine. A hypertensive crisis may result. Pseudoephedrine is contraindicated in patients taking MAO inhibitors, or who have taken such drugs within the past two weeks.

Because of the possibility of additive effects and increased toxicity, pseudoephedrine should not be administered concomitantly with other sympathomimetic drugs.

The sedative action of promethazine is additive to the sedative effects of other central nervous system depressants, including alcohol, narcotic analgesics, barbiturates, tricyclic antidepressants, tranquilizers, and phenothiazines; therefore, these agents should be avoided or administered in reduced dosage to patients receiving promethazine.

DRUG/LABORATORY TEST INTERACTIONS

The following laboratory tests may be affected in patients who are receiving therapy with promethazine hydrochloride.

Pregnancy Tests—Diagnostic pregnancy tests based on immunological reactions between HCG and anti-HCG may result in false-negative or false-positive interpretations.

Glucose Tolerance Test—An increase in glucose tolerance has been reported in patients receiving promethazine hydrochloride.

CARCINOGENESIS, MUTAGENESIS, IMPAIRMENT OF FERTILITY

Long-term animal studies have not been performed to assess the carcinogenic potential of promethazine or pseudoephedrine, nor are there other animal or human data concerning carcinogenicity, mutagenicity, or impairment of fertility with these drugs. Promethazine was nonmutagenic in the *Salmonella* test system of Ames.

PREGNANCY

Teratogenic Effects—Pregnancy Category C. Teratogenic effects have not been demonstrated in rat-feeding studies at doses of 6.25 and 12.5 mg/kg of promethazine. While antihistamines, including promethazine, have been found to produce fetal mortality in rodents, the pharmacological effects of histamine in the rodent do not parallel those in man. There are no data concerning teratogenicity of pseudoephedrine in animals or man. There are no adequate and well-controlled studies of Phenergan-D in pregnant women.

Phenergan-D should be used during pregnancy only if the potential benefit justifies the potential risk to the fetus.

NURSING MOTHERS

It is not known whether promethazine or pseudoephedrine are excreted in human milk. Because many drugs are excreted in human milk, caution should be exercised when Phenergan-D is administered to a nursing woman.

PEDIATRIC USE

Phenergan-D is not recommended for use in children under 12 years of age.

ADVERSE REACTIONS

Patients taking Phenergan-D may be subject to any of the adverse reactions which have commonly been observed with sympathomimetic and antihistaminic drugs. Because of the sedative action attendant to the use of promethazine hydrochloride in full therapeutic doses, it should be administered with caution to ambulatory patients. Ambulatory patients may occasionally complain of autonomic reactions such as dryness of the mouth, blurring of vision and, rarely, dizziness, confusion, or disorientation. As with other antihistamines, nausea and vomiting, as well as skin rash, may occasionally be seen. Very rare cases have been reported where patients receiving promethazine have developed leukopenia and thrombocytopenia. In one instance agranulocytosis has been reported. In nearly every instance reported, other toxic agents known to have caused these conditions have been associated with the administration of promethazine. Rare cases of obstructive jaundice have been reported with promethazine. Attempted suicides with promethazine have resulted in deep sedation, coma, rarely convulsions and cardiorespiratory symptoms compatible with the depth of sedation present. Extrapyramidal symptoms have rarely been reported, usually in association with excessive dosage; this almost always responds to a reduction in dosage.

Although pseudoephedrine is less apt to produce stimulation than other sympathomimetic agents, it may be associated with such symptoms as restlessness, palpitation, tachycardia, insomnia, weakness, anxiety, sweating, nausea, vomiting, headache, or anorexia.

OVERDOSAGE

PROMETHAZINE

Signs and symptoms of overdosage with promethazine range from mild depression of the central nervous system and cardiovascular system, to profound hypotension, respiratory depression, and unconsciousness. Stimulation may be evident, especially in children and geriatric patients. Atropinelike signs and symptoms—dry mouth, fixed, dilated pupils, flushing, etc., as well as gastrointestinal symptoms, may occur. The treatment of overdosage is essentially symptomatic and supportive. Early gastric lavage may be beneficial. Centrally acting emetics are of little use.

Avoid analeptics, which may cause convulsions. Severe hypotension usually responds to the administration of levarterenol or phenylephrine. EPINEPHRINE SHOULD NOT BE USED, since its use in a patient with partial adrenergic blockade may further lower the blood pressure. Extrapyramidal reactions may be treated with anticholinergic antiparkinson agents, diphenhydramine, or barbiturates. Additional measures include oxygen and intravenous fluids. Limited experience with dialysis indicates that it is not helpful.

PSEUDOEPHEDRINE

There have been few reported cases of overdosage with pseudoephedrine. Like other sympathomimetic drugs, symptoms of excessive pseudoephedrine dosage would probably include CNS stimulation: restlessness, tremor, irritability, excitement, agitation, and convulsions. Cardiovascular symptoms, including hypertension, tachycardia, and other arrhythmias, might also be expected to occur. There is no specific antidote to pseudoephedrine; treatment should be symptomatic and supportive.

DOSAGE AND ADMINISTRATION

ADULTS

One tablet 3 or 4 times daily as needed during normal waking hours is recommended. If symptoms are mild or signs of excessive drug activity develop, this dose may be reduced.

HOW SUPPLIED

Phenergan®-D Tablets, Wyeth®, are available in bottles of 100;

NDC 0008-0434, white and orange, double layer, round, scored tablet marked "WYETH" and "434".

Keep tightly closed.

Protect from light.

Dispense in light-resistant, tight container.

Shown in Product Identification Section, page 436

PHENERGAN® VC ℞

[fen 'er-gan]

DESCRIPTION

Each teaspoon (5 ml) of Phenergan VC contains 6.25 mg promethazine hydrochloride and 5 mg phenylephrine hydrochloride in a flavored syrup base with a pH between 4.7 and 5.2. Alcohol 7%. The inactive ingredients present are artificial and natural flavors, citric acid, FD&C Yellow 6, glycerin, saccharin sodium, sodium benzoate, sodium citrate, sodium propionate, water, and other ingredients.

Promethazine hydrochloride, a phenothiazine derivative, is designated chemically as N,N,α-trimethyl-10*H*-phenothiazine-10-ethanamine monohydrochloride with the following structural formula:

$CH_2CH(CH_3)N(CH_3)_2$ · HCl

Promethazine hydrochloride occurs as white to faint yellow, practically odorless, crystalline powder which slowly oxidizes and turns blue on prolonged exposure to air. It is soluble in water and freely soluble in alcohol.

Phenylephrine hydrochloride is a sympathomimetic amine salt. It may be chemically named as 3-hydroxy-α-[(methylamino)methyl]-benzenemethanol hydrochloride and has the following chemical formula:

[See Chemical Formula at top of next column].

OH — C — CH_2NHCH_3 · HCl, OH

Phenylephrine hydrochloride occurs as white or nearly white crystals, having a bitter taste. It is freely soluble in water and alcohol. Phenylephrine hydrochloride is subject to oxidation and must be protected from light and air.

CLINICAL PHARMACOLOGY

PROMETHAZINE

Promethazine is a phenothiazine derivative which differs structurally from the antipsychotic phenothiazines by the presence of a branched side chain and no ring substitution. It is thought that this configuration is responsible for its relative lack (1/10 that of chlorpromazine) of dopaminergic (CNS) action.

Promethazine is an H_1 receptor blocking agent. In addition to its antihistaminic action, it provides clinically useful sedative and antiemetic effects. In therapeutic dosages, promethazine produces no significant effects on the cardiovascular system.

Promethazine is well absorbed from the gastrointestinal tract. Clinical effects are apparent within 20 minutes after oral administration and generally last four to six hours, although they may persist as long as 12 hours. Promethazine is metabolized by the liver to a variety of compounds; the sulfoxides of promethazine and N-demethylpromethazine are the predominant metabolites appearing in the urine.

PHENYLEPHRINE

Phenylephrine is a potent postsynaptic α-receptor agonist with little effect on β receptors of the heart. Phenylephrine has no effect on β-adrenergic receptors of the bronchi or peripheral blood vessels. A direct action at receptors accounts for the greater part of its effects, only a small part being due to its ability to release norepinephrine.

Therapeutic doses of phenylephrine mainly cause vasoconstriction. Phenylephrine increases resistance and, to a lesser extent, decreases capacitance of blood vessels. Total peripheral resistance is increased, resulting in increased systolic and diastolic blood pressure. Pulmonary arterial pressure is usually increased, and renal blood flow is usually decreased. Local vasoconstriction and hemostasis occur following topical application or infiltration of phenylephrine into tissues. The main effect of phenylephrine on the heart is bradycardia; it produces a positive inotropic effect on the myocardium in doses greater than those usually used therapeutically. Rarely, the drug may increase the irritability of the heart, causing arrhythmias. Cardiac output is decreased slightly. Phenylephrine increases the work of the heart by increasing peripheral arterial resistance.

Phenylephrine has a mild central stimulant effect.

Following oral administration or topical application of phenylephrine to the mucosa, constriction of blood vessels in the nasal mucosa relieves nasal congestion associated with allergy or head colds. Following oral administration, nasal decongestion may occur within 15 or 20 minutes and may persist for up to 4 hours.

Phenylephrine is irregularly absorbed from and readily metabolized in the gastrointestinal tract. Phenylephrine is metabolized in the liver and intestine by monoamine oxidase. The metabolites and their route and rate of excretion have not been identified. The pharmacologic action of phenylephrine is terminated at least partially by uptake of the drug into tissues.

INDICATIONS AND USAGE

Phenergan VC is indicated for the temporary relief of upper respiratory symptoms, including nasal congestion, associated with allergy or the common cold.

CONTRAINDICATIONS

Promethazine is contraindicated in individuals known to be hypersensitive or to have had an idiosyncratic reaction to promethazine or to other phenothiazines.

Antihistamines are contraindicated for use in the treatment of lower respiratory tract symptoms or asthma.

Phenylephrine is contraindicated in patients with hypertension or with peripheral vascular insufficiency (ischemia may result with risk of gangrene or thrombosis of compromised vascular beds). Phenylephrine should not be used in patients known to be hypersensitive to the drug or in those receiving a monoamine oxidase inhibitor (MAOI).

WARNINGS

PROMETHAZINE

Promethazine may cause marked drowsiness. Ambulatory patients should be cautioned against such activities as driving or operating dangerous machinery until it is known that they do not become drowsy or dizzy from promethazine therapy.

The sedative action of promethazine hydrochloride is additive to the sedative effects of central nervous system depres-

Continued on next page

Wyeth—Cont.

sants; therefore, agents such as alcohol, narcotic analgesics, sedatives, hypnotics, and tranquilizers should either be eliminated or given in reduced dosage in the presence of promethazine hydrochloride. When given concomitantly with promethazine hydrochloride, the dose of barbiturates should be reduced by at least one-half, and the dose of analgesic depressants, such as morphine or meperidine, should be reduced by one-quarter to one-half.
Promethazine may lower seizure threshold. This should be taken into consideration when administering to persons with known seizure disorders or when giving in combination with narcotics or local anesthetics which may also affect seizure threshold.
Sedative drugs or CNS depressants should be avoided in patients with a history of sleep apnea.
Antihistamines should be used with caution in patients with narrow-angle glaucoma, stenosing peptic ulcer, pyloroduodenal obstrucition, and urinary bladder obstruction due to symptomatic prostatic hypertrophy and narrowing of the bladder neck.
Administration of promethazine has been associated with reported cholestatic jaundice.
PHENYLEPHRINE
Because phenylephrine is an adrenergic agent, it should be given with caution to patients with thyroid diseases, diabetes mellitus, and heart diseases or those receiving tricyclic antidepressants.
Men with symptomatic, benign prostatic hypertrophy can experience urinary retention when given oral nasal decongestants.
Phenylephrine can cause a decrease in cardiac output, and extreme caution should be used when administering the drug, parenterally or orally, to patients with arteriosclerosis, to elderly individuals, and/or to patients with initially poor cerebral or coronary circulation.
Phenylephrine should be used with caution in patients taking diet preparations, such as amphetamines or phenylpropanolamine, because synergistic adrenergic effects could result in serious hypertensive response and possible stroke.

PRECAUTIONS

Animal reproduction studies have not been conducted with the drug combination—promethazine and phenylephrine. It is not known whether this drug combination can cause fetal harm when administered to a pregnant woman or can affect reproduction capacity. Phenergan VC should be given to a pregnant woman only if clearly needed.
GENERAL
Promethazine should be used cautiously in persons with cardiovascular disease or impairment of liver function.
Phenylephrine should be used with caution in patients with cardiovascular disease, particularly hypertension.
INFORMATION FOR PATIENTS
Phenergan VC may cause marked drowsiness or impair the mental and/or physical abilities required for the performance of potentially hazardous tasks, such as driving a vehicle or operating machinery. Ambulatory patients should be told to avoid engaging is such activities until it is known that they do not become drowsy or dizzy from Phenergan VC therapy. Children should be supervised to avoid potential harm in bike riding or other hazardous acitvities.
The concomitant use of alcohol or other central nervous system depressants, including narcotic analgesics, sedatives, hypnotics, and tranquilizers, may have an additive effect and should be avoided or their dosage reduced.
Patients should be advised to report any involuntary muscle movements or unusual sensitivity to sunlight.

DRUG INTERACTIONS
PROMETHAZINE
The sedative action of promethazine is additive to the sedative effects of other central nervous system depressants, including alcohol, narcotic analgesics, sedatives, hypnotics, tricyclic antidepressants, and tranquilizers; therefore, these agents should be avoided or administered in reduced dosage to patients receiving promethazine.
[See table below].
DRUG/LABORATORY TEST INTERACTIONS
The following laboratory tests may be affected in patients who are receiving therapy with promethazine hydrochloride:
Pregnancy Tests
Diagnostic pregnancy tests based on immunological reactions between HCG and anti-HCG may result in false-negative or false-positive interpretations.
Glucose Tolerance Test
An increase in blood glucose has been reported in patients receiving promethazine.
CARCINOGENESIS, MUTAGENESIS, IMPAIRMENT OF FERTILITY
PROMETHAZINE
Long-term animal studies have not been performed to assess the carcinogenic potential of promethazine, nor are there other animal or human data concerning carcinogenicity, mutagenicity, or impairment of fertility with this drug. Promethazine was nonmutagenic in the *Salmonella* test system of Ames.
PHENYLEPHRINE
A study which followed the develpment of cancer in 143,574 patients over a four-year period indicated that in 11,981 patients who received phenylephrine (systemic or topical), there was no statistically significant association between the drug and cancer at any or all sites.
Long-term animal studies have not been performed to assess the carcinogenic potential of phenylephrine, nor are there other animal or human data concerning mutagenicity.
A study of the effects of adrenergic drugs on ovum transport in rabbits indicated that treatment with phenylephrine did not alter incidence of pregnancy; the number of implantations was significantly reduced when high doses of the drug were used.
PREGNANCY
Teratogenic Effects —Pregnancy Category C
PROMETHAZINE
Teratogenic effects have not been demonstrated in rat-feeding studies at doses of 6.25 and 12.5 mg/kg of promethazine. These doses are 8.3 and 16.7 times the maximum recommended total daily dose of promethazine for a 50-kg subject. Specific studies to test the action of the drug on parturition, lactation, and development of the animal neonate were not done, but a general preliminary study in rats indicated no effect on these parameters. Although antihistamines, including promethazine, have been found to produce fetal mortality in rodents, the pharmacological effects of histamine in the rodent do not parallel those in man. There are no adequate and well-controlled studies of promethazine in pregnant women.
PHENYLEPHRINE
A study in rabbits indicated that continued moderate overexposure to phenylephrine (3 mg/day) during the second half of pregnancy (22nd day of gestation to delivery) may contribute to perinatal wastage, prematurity, premature labor, and possibly fetal anomalies; when phenylephrine (3 mg/day) was given to rabbits during the first half of pregnancy (3rd day after mating for seven days), a significant number gave birth to litters of low birth weight. Another study showed that phenylephrine was associated with anomalies of aortic arch and with ventricular septal defect in the chick embryo.

PHENYLEPHRINE

Drug	Effect
Phenylephrine with prior administration of monoamine oxidase inhibitors (MAOI).	Cardiac pressor response potentiated. May cause acute hypertensive crisis.
Phenylephrine with tricyclic antidepressants.	Pressor response increased.
Phenylephrine with ergot alkaloids.	Excessive rise in blood pressure.
Phenylephrine with bronchodilator sympathomimetic agents and with epinephrine or other sympathomimetics.	Tachycardia or other arrhythmias may occur.
Phenylephrine with prior administration of propranolol or other β-adrenergic blockers.	Cardiostimulating effects blocked.
Phenylephrine with atropine sulfate.	Reflex bradycardia blocked; pressor response enhanced.
Phenylephrine with prior administration of phentolamine or other α-adrenergic blockers.	Pressor response decreased.
Phenylephrine with diet preparations, such as amphetamines or phenylpropanolamine.	Synergistic adrenergic response.

Phenergan VC should be used during pregnancy only if the potential benefit justifies the potential risk to the fetus.
Nonteratogenic Effects
Promethazine taken within two weeks of delivery may inhibit platelet aggregation in the newborn.
LABOR AND DELIVERY
Administration of phenylephrine to patients in late pregnancy or labor may cause fetal anoxia or bradycardia by increasing contractility of the uterus and decreasing uterine blood flow.
See also "Nonteratogenic Effects."
NURSING MOTHERS
It is not known whether promethazine or phenylephrine are excreted in human milk.
Caution should be exercised when Phenergan VC is administered to a nursing woman.
PEDIATRIC USE
This product should not be used in children under 2 years of age because safety for such use has not been established.

ADVERSE REACTIONS

PROMETHAZINE
Nervous System—Sedation, sleepiness, occasional blurred vision, dryness of mouth, dizziness; rarely confusion, disorientation, and extrapyramidal symptoms such as oculogyric crisis, torticollis, and tongue protrusion (usually in association with parenteral injection or excessive dosage).
Cardiovascular—Increased or decreased blood pressure.
Dermatologic—Rash, rarely photosensitivity.
Hematologic—Rarely leukopenia, thrombocytopenia; agranulocytosis (1 case).
Gastrointestinal—Nausea and vomiting.
PHENYLEPHRINE
Nervous System—Restlessness, anxiety, nervousness, and dizziness.
Cardiovascular—Hypertension (see "Warnings").
Other—Precordial pain, respiratory distress, tremor, and weakness.

OVERDOSAGE

PROMETHAZINE
Signs and symptoms of overdosage with promethazine range from mild depression of the central nervous system and cardiovascular system to profound hypotension, respiratory depression, and unconsciousness.
Stimulation may be evident, especially in children and geriatric patients. Convulsions may rarely occur. A paradoxical reaction has been reported in children receiving single doses of 75 mg to 125 mg orally, characterized by hyperexcitability and nightmares.
Atropine-like signs and symptoms—dry mouth, fixed, dilated pupils, flushing, as well as gastrointestinal symptoms, may occur.
PHENYLEPHRINE
Signs and symptoms of overdosage with phenylephrine include hypertension, headache, convulsions, cerebral hemorrhage, and vomiting. Ventricular premature beats and short paroxysms of ventricular tachycardia may also occur. Headache may be a symptom of hypertension. Bradycardia may also be seen early in phenylephrine overdosage through stimulation of baroreceptors.
TREATMENT
Treatment of overdosage with Phenergan VC is essentially symptomatic and supportive. Only in cases of extreme overdosage or individual sensitivity do vital signs including respiration, pulse, blood pressure, temperature, and EKG need to be monitored. Activated charcoal orally or by lavage may be given, or sodium or magnesium sulfate orally as a cathartic. Attention should be given to the reestablishment of adequate respiratory exchange through provision of a patent airway and institution of assisted or controlled ventilation. Diazepam may be used to control convulsions. Acidosis and electrolyte losses should be corrected. Note that any depressant effects of promethazine are not reversed by naloxone. Avoid analeptics which may cause convulsions.
Severe hypotension usually responds to the administration of norepinephrine or phenylephrine. EPINEPHRINE SHOULD NOT BE USED, since its use in patients with partial adrenergic blockade may further lower the blood pressure.
Limited experience with dialysis indicates that it is not helpful.

DOSAGE AND ADMINISTRATION

The recommended adult dose is one teaspoon (5 ml) every 4 to 6 hours, not to exceed 30.0 ml in 24 hours. For children 6 years to under 12 years of age, the dose is one-half to one teaspoon (2.5 to 5.0 ml) repeated at 4- to 6-hour intervals, not to exceed 30.0 ml in 24 hours. For children 2 years to under 6 years of age, the dose is one-quarter to one-half teaspoon (1.25 to 2.5 ml) every 4 to 6 hours.
Phenergan VC is not recommended for children under 2 years of age.

HOW SUPPLIED

Phenergan® VC, Wyeth®, is a clear, orange-yellow solution supplied as follows:

NDC 0008-0551-02, case of 24 bottles of 4 fl. oz.
NDC 0008-0551-06, case of 16 bottles of 6 fl. oz.
NDC 0008-0551-08, case of 12 bottles of 8 fl. oz.
NDC 0008-0551-03, bottle of 1 pint.
NDC 0008-0551-04, bottle of 1 gallon.

Keep bottles tightly closed below 25°C (77°F).
Protect from light.
Dispense in light-resistant, glass, tight containers.

PHENERGAN® VC ℭ ℞

[fen 'er-gan]
with codeine

DESCRIPTION

Each teaspoon (5 ml) of Phenergan VC with codeine contains 10 mg (1/6 grain) codeine phosphate (Warning—may be habit-forming), 6.25 mg promethazine hydrochloride, and 5 mg phenylephrine hydrochloride in a flavored syrup base with a pH between 4.7 and 5.2. Alcohol 7%. The inactive ingredients present are artificial and natural flavors, citric acid, D&C Red 33, FD&C Yellow 6, glycerin, saccharin sodium, sodium benzoate, sodium citrate, sodium propionate, water, and other ingredients. Codeine is one of the naturally occurring phenanthrene alkaloids of opium derived from the opium poppy; it is classified pharmacologically as a narcotic analgesic. Codeine phosphate may be chemically named as (5α,6α)-7,8-didehydro-4,5-epoxy-3-methoxy-17-methylmorphinan-6-ol phosphate (1:1) (salt) hemihydrate with the following structural formula:

$\cdot H_3PO_4 \cdot \frac{1}{2}H_2O$

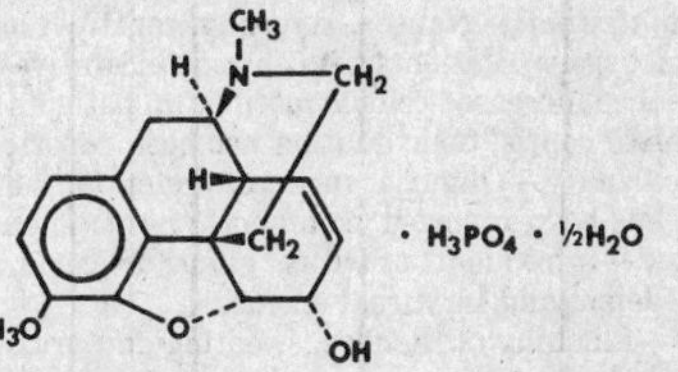

The phosphate salt of codeine occurs as white, needle-shaped crystals or white crystalline powder. Codeine phosphate is freely soluble in water and slightly soluble in alcohol.

Promethazine hydrochloride, a phenothiazine derivative, is designated chemically as N,N,α-trimethyl-10*H*-phenothiazine-10-ethanamine monohydrochloride with the following structural formula:

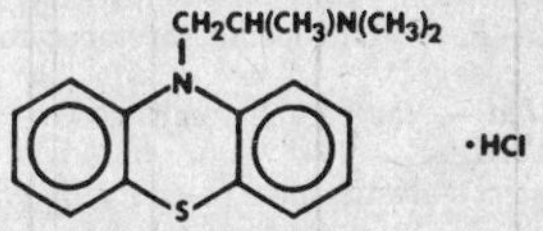

$CH_2CH(CH_3)N(CH_3)_2 \cdot HCl$

Promethazine hydrochloride occurs as a white to faint yellow, practically odorless, crystalline powder which slowly oxidizes and turns blue on prolonged exposure to air. It is soluble in water and freely soluble in alcohol. Phenylephrine hydrochloride is a sympathomimetic amine salt. It may be chemically named as 3-hydroxy-α-[(methylamino)methyl]-benzenemethanol hydrochloride and has the following chemical formula:

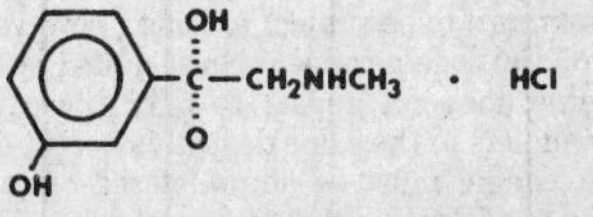

$-CH_2NHCH_3 \cdot HCl$

Phenylephrine hydrochloride occurs as white or nearly white crystals, having a bitter taste. It is freely soluble in water and alcohol. Phenylephrine hydrochloride is subject to oxidation and must be protected from light and air.

CLINICAL PHARMACOLOGY

CODEINE: Narcotic analgesics, including codeine, exert their primary effects on the central nervous system and gastrointestinal tract. The analgesic effects of codeine are due to its central action; however, the precise sites of action have not been determined, and the mechanisms involved appear to be quite complex. Codeine resembles morphine both structurally and pharmacologically, but its actions at the doses of codeine used therapeutically are milder, with less sedation, respiratory depression, and gastrointestinal, urinary, and pupillary effects. Codeine produces an increase in biliary tract pressure, but less than morphine or meperidine. Codeine is less constipating than morphine.

Codeine has good antitussive activity, although less than that of morphine at equal doses. It is used in preference to morphine, because side effects are infrequent at the usual antitussive dose of codeine.

Codeine in oral therapeutic dosage does not usually exert major effects on the cardiovascular system. Narcotic analgesics may cause nausea and vomiting by stimulating the chemoreceptor trigger zone (CTZ); however, they also depress the vomiting center, so that subsequent doses are unlikely to produce vomiting. Nausea is minimal after usual oral doses of codeine.

Narcotic analgesics cause histamine release, which appears to be responsible for wheals or urticaria sometimes seen at the site of injection on parenteral administration. Histamine release may also produce dilation of cutaneous blood vessels, with resultant flushing of the face and neck, pruritus, and sweating.

Codeine and its salts are well absorbed following both oral and parenteral administration. Codeine is about 2/3 as effective orally as parenterally. Codeine is metabolized primarily in the liver by enzymes of the endoplasmic reticulum, where it undergoes O-demethylation, N-demethylation, and partial conjugation with glucuronic acid. The drug is excreted primarily in the urine, largely as inactive metabolites and small amounts of free and conjugated morphine. Negligible amounts of codeine and its metabolites are found in the feces.

Following oral or subcutaneous administration of codeine, the onset of analgesia occurs within 15 to 30 minutes and lasts for four to six hours.

The cough-depressing action, in animal studies, was observed to occur 15 minutes after oral administration of codeine, peak action at 45 to 60 minutes after ingestion. The duration of action, which is dose-dependent, usually did not exceed 3 hours.

PROMETHAZINE: Promethazine is a phenothiazine derivative which differs structurally from the antipsychotic phenothiazines by the presence of a branched side chain and no ring substitution. It is thought that this configuration is responsible for its relative lack (1/10 that of chlorpromazine) of dopaminergic (CNS) action.

Promethazine is an H_1 receptor blocking agent. In addition to its antihistaminic action, it provides clinically useful sedative and antiemetic effects. In therapeutic dosages, promethazine produces no significant effects on the cardiovascular system.

Promethazine is well absorbed from the gastrointestinal tract. Clinical effects are apparent within 20 minutes after oral adminstration and generally last four to six hours, although they may persist as long as 12 hours. Promethazine is metabolized by the liver to a variety of compounds; the sulfoxides of promethazine and N-demethylpromethazine are the predominant metabolites appearing in the urine.

PHENYLEPHRINE: Phenylephrine is a potent postsynaptic α-receptor agonist with little effect on β receptors of the heart. Phenylephrine has no effect on β-adrenergic receptors of the bronchi or peripheral blood vessels. A direct action at receptors accounts for the greater part of its effects, only a small part being due to its ability to release norepinephrine.

Therapeutic doses of phenylephrine mainly cause vasoconstriction. Phenylephrine increases resistance and, to a lesser extent, decreases capacitance of blood vessels. Total peripheral resistance is increased, resulting in increased systolic and diastolic blood pressure. Pulmonary arterial pressure is usually increased, and renal blood flow is usually decreased. Local vasoconstriction and hemostasis occur following topical application or infiltration of phenylephrine into tissues. The main effect of phenylephrine on the heart is bradycardia; it produces a positive inotropic effect on the myocardium in doses greater than those usually used therapeutically. Rarely, the drug may increase the irritability of the heart, causing arrhythmias. Cardiac output is decreased slightly. Phenylephrine increases the work of the heart by increasing peripheral arterial resistance. Phenylephrine has a mild central stimulant effect.

Following oral administration or topical application of phenylephrine to the mucosa, constriction of blood vessels in the nasal mucosa relieves nasal congestion associated with allergy or head colds. Following oral administration, nasal decongestion may occur within 15 or 20 minutes and may persist for up to 4 hours.

Phenylephrine is irregularly absorbed from and readily metabolized in the gastrointestinal tract. Phenylephrine is metabolized in the liver and intestine by monoamine oxidase. The metabolites and their route and rate of excretion have not been identified. The pharmacologic action of phenylephrine is terminated at least partially by uptake of the drug into tissues.

INDICATIONS AND USAGE

Phenergan VC with codeine is indicated for the temporary relief of coughs and upper respiratory symptoms, including nasal congestion, associated with allergy or the common cold.

CONTRAINDICATIONS

Codeine is contraindicated in patients with a known hypersensitivity to the drug.

Promethazine is contraindicated in individuals known to be hypersensitive or to have had an idiosyncratic reaction to promethazine or to other phenothiazines.

Phenylephrine is contraindicated in patients with hypertension or with peripheral vascular insufficiency (ischemia may result wtih risk of gangrene or thrombosis of compromised vascular beds). Phenylephrine should not be used in patients known to be hypersensitive to the drug or in those receiving a monoamine oxidase inhibitor (MAOI).

Antihistamines and codeine are both contraindicated for use in the treatment of lower respiratory tract symptoms, including asthma.

WARNINGS

CODEINE: Dosage of codeine SHOULD NOT BE INCREASED if cough fails to respond; an unresponsive cough should be reevaluated in 5 days or sooner for possible underlying pathology, such as foreign body or lower respiratory tract disease.

Codeine may cause or aggravate constipation.

Respiratory depression leading to arrest, coma, and death has occurred with the use of codeine antitussives in young children, particularly in the under-one-year infants whose ability to deactivate the drug is not fully developed.

Administration of codeine may be accompanied by histamine release and should be used with caution in atopic children.

Head Injury and Increased Intracranial Pressure

The respiratory-depressant effects of narcotic analgesics and their capacity to elevate cerebrospinal fluid pressure may be markedly exaggerated in the presence of head injury, intracranial lesions, or a preexisting increase in intracranial pressure. Narcotics may produce adverse reactions which may obscure the clinical course of patients with head injuries.

Asthma and Other Respiratory Conditions

Narcotic analgesics or cough suppressants, including codeine, should not be used in asthmatic patients (see "Contraindications"). Nor should they be used in acute febrile illness associated with productive cough or in chronic respiratory disease where interference with ability to clear the tracheobronchial tree of secretions would have a deleterious effect on the patient's respiratory function.

Hypotensive Effect

Codeine may produce orthostatic hypotension in ambulatory patients.

PROMETHAZINE: Promethazine may cause marked drowsiness. Ambulatory patients should be cautioned against such activities as driving or operating dangerous machinery until it is known that they do not become drowsy or dizzy from promethazine therapy.

The sedative action of promethazine hydrochloride is additive to the sedative effects of central nervous system depressants; therefore, agents such as alcohol, narcotic analgesics, sedatives, hypnotics, and tranquilizers should either be eliminated or given in reduced dosage in the presence of promethazine hydrochloride. When given concomitantly with promethazine hydrochloride, the dose of barbiturates should be reduced by at least one-half, and the dose of analgesic depressants, such as morphine or meperidine, should be reduced by one-quarter to one-half.

Promethazine may lower seizure threshold. This should be taken into consideration when administering to persons with known seizure disorders or when giving in combination with narcotics or local anesthetics which may also affect seizure threshold.

Sedative drugs or CNS depressants should be avoided in patients with a history of sleep apnea. Antihistamines should be used with caution in patients with narrow-angle glaucoma, stenosing peptic ulcer, pyloroduodenal obstruction, and urinary bladder obstruction due to symptomatic prostatic hypertrophy and narrowing of the bladder neck.

Administration of promethazine has been associated with reported cholestatic jaundice.

PHENYLEPHRINE: Because phenlephrine is an adrenergic agent, it should be given with caution to patients with thyroid diseases, diabetes mellitus, and heart diseases or those receiving tricyclic antidepressants.

Men with symptomatic, benign prostatic hypertrophy can experience urinary retention when given oral nasal decongestants.

Phenylephrine can cause a decrease in cardiac output, and extreme caution should be used when administering the drug, parenterally or orally, to patients with arteriosclerosis, to elderly individuals, and/or to patients with initially poor cerebral or coronary circulation.

Phenylephrine should be used with caution in patients taking diet preparations, such as amphetamines or phenylpropanolamine, because synergistic adrenergic effects could result in serious hypertensive response and possible stroke.

PRECAUTIONS

Animal reproduction studies have not been conducted with the drug combination—promethazine, phenylephrine, and codeine. It is not known whether this drug combination can cause fetal harm when administered to a pregnant woman or can affect reproduction capacity. Phenergan VC with codeine should be given to a pregnant woman only if clearly needed.

GENERAL

Narcotic analgesics, including codeine, should be administered with caution and the initial dose reduced in patients

Continued on next page

Wyeth—Cont.

with acute abdominal conditions, convulsive disorders, significant hepatic or renal impairment, fever, hypothyroidism, Addison's disease, ulcerative colitis, prostatic hypertrophy, in patients with recent gastrointestinal or urinary tract surgery, and in the very young or elderly or debilitated patients. Promethazine should be used cautiously in persons with cardiovascular disease or with impairment of liver function.
Phenylephrine should be used with caution in patients with cardiovascular disease, particulary hypertension.
INFORMATION FOR PATIENTS
Phenergan VC with codeine may cause marked drowsiness or impair the mental and/or physical abilities required for the performance of potentially hazardous tasks, such as driving a vehicle or operating machinery. Ambulatory patients should be told to avoid engaging in such activities until it is known that they do not become drowsy or dizzy from Phenergan VC with codeine therapy. Children should be supervised to avoid potential harm in bike riding or in other hazardous activities. The concomitant use of alcohol or other central nervous system depressants, including narcotic analgesics, sedatives, hypnotics, and tranquilizers, may have an additive effect and should be avoided or their dosage reduced.
Patients should be advised to report any involuntary muscle movements or unusual sensitivity to sunlight.
Codeine, like other narcotic analgesics, may produce orthostatic hypotension is some ambulatory patients. Patients should be cautioned accordingly.
DRUG INTERACTIONS
CODEINE: In patients receiving MAO inhibitors, an initial small test dose is advisable to allow observation of any excessive narcotic effects or MAOI interaction.
PROMETHAZINE: The sedative action of promethazine is additive to the effects of other central nervous system depressants, including alcohol, narcotic analgesics, sedatives, hypnotics, tricyclic antidepressants, and tranquilizers; therefore, these agents should be avoided or administered in reduced dosage to patients receiving promethazine.
[See table below].
DRUG/LABORATORY TEST INTERACTIONS
Because narcotic analgesics may increase biliary tract pressure, with resultant increases in plasma amylase or lipase levels, determination of these enzyme levels may be unreliable for 24 hours after a narcotic analgesic has been given.
The following laboratory tests may be affected in patients who are receiving therapy with promethazine hydrochloride:
Pregnancy Tests
Diagnostic pregnancy tests based on immunological reactions between HCG and anti-HCG may result in false-negative or false-positive interpretations.
Glucose Tolerance Test
An increase in blood glucose has been reported in patients receiving promethazine.
CARCINOGENESIS, MUTAGENESIS, IMPAIRMENT OF FERTILITY
CODEINE AND PROMETHAZINE
Long-term animal studies have not been performed to assess the carcinogenic potential of codeine or of promethazine, nor are there other animal or human data concerning carcinogenicity, mutagenicity, or impairment of fertility with these agents. Codeine has been reported to show no evidence of carcinogencity or mutagenicity in a variety of test systems, including the micronucleus and sperm abnormality assays and the *Salmonella* assay. Promethazine was nonmutagenic in the *Salmonella* test system of Ames.
PHENYLEPHRINE
A study which followed the development of cancer in 143,574 patients over a four-year period indicated that in 11,981 patients who received phenylephrine (systemic or topical), there was no statistically significant association between the drug and cancer at any or all sites.
Long-term animal studies have not been performed to assess the carcinogenic potential of phenylephrine, nor are there other animal or human data concerning mutagenicity.
A study of the effects of adrenergic drugs on ovum transport in rabbits indicated that treatment with phenylephrine did not alter incidence of pregnancy; the number of implantations was significantly reduced when high doses of the drug were used.
PREGNANCY
Teratogenic Effects—Pregnancy Category C
CODEINE: A study in rats and rabbits reported no teratogenic effect of codeine administered during the period of organogenesis in doses ranging from 5 to 120 mg/kg. In the rat, doses at the 120-mg/kg level, in the toxic range for the adult animal, were associated with an increase in embryo resorption at the time of implantation. In another study a single 100-mg/kg dose of codeine administered to pregnant mice reportedly resulted in delayed ossification in the offspring.
There are no studies in humans, and the significance of these findings to humans, if any, is not known.
PROMETHAZINE: Teratogenic effects have not been demonstrated in rat-feeding studies at doses of 6.25 and 12.5 mg/kg of promethazine. These doses are 8.3 and 16.7 times the maximum recommended total daily dose for a 50-kg subject. Specific studies to test the action of the drug on parturition, lactation, and development of the animal neonate were not done, but a general preliminary study in rats indicated no effect on these parameters. Although antihistamines, including promethazine, have been found to produce fetal mortality in rodents, the pharmacological effects of histamine in the rodent do not parallel those in man. There are no adequate and well-controlled studies of promethazine in pregnant women.
PHENYLEPHRINE: A study in rabbits indicated that continued moderate overexposure to phenylephrine (3 mg/day) during the second half of pregnancy (22nd day of gestation to delivery) may contribute to perinatal wastage, prematurity, premature labor, and possibly fetal anomalies; when phenylephrine (3 mg/day) was given to rabbits during the first half of pregnancy (3rd day after mating for seven days), a significant number gave birth to litters of low birth weight. Another study showed that phenylephrine was associated with anomalies of aortic arch and with ventricular septal defect in the chick embryo.
Phenergan VC with codeine should be used during pregnancy only if the potential benefit justifies the potential risk to the fetus.
Nonteratogenic Effects
Dependence has been reported in newborns whose mothers took opiates regularly during pregnancy. Withdrawal signs include irritability, excessive crying, tremors, hyperreflexia, fever, vomiting, and diarrhea. Signs usually appear during the first few days of life.
Promethazine taken within two weeks of delivery may inhibit platelet aggregation in the newborn.
LABOR AND DELIVERY
Narcotic analgesics cross the placental barrier. The closer to delivery and the larger the dose used, the greater the possibility of respiratory depression in the newborn. Narcotic analgesics should be avoided during labor if delivery of a premature infant is anticipated. If the mother has received narcotic analgesics during labor, newborn infants should be observed closely for signs of respiratory depression. Resuscitation may be required (see "Overdosage"). The effect of codeine, if any, on the later growth, development, and functional maturation of the child is unknown.

PHENYLEPHRINE Drug	Effect
Phenylephrine with prior administration of monoamine oxidase inhibitors (MAOI).	Cardiac pressor response potentiated. May cause acute hypertensive crisis.
Phenylephrine with tricyclic antidepressants.	Pressor response increased.
Phenylephrine with ergot alkaloids.	Excessive rise in blood pressure.
Phenylephrine with bronchodilator sympathomimetic agents and with epinephrine or other sympathomimetics.	Tachycardia or other arrhythmias may occur.
Phenylephrine with prior administration of propranolol or other β-adrenergic blockers.	Cardiostimulating effects blocked.
Phenylephrine with atropine sulfate.	Reflex bradycardia blocked; pressor response enhanced.
Phenylephrine with prior administration of phentolamine or other α-adrenergic blockers.	Pressor response decreased.
Phenylephrine with diet preparations, such as amphetamines or phenylpropanolamine.	Synergistic adrenergic response.

Administration of phenylephrine to patients in late pregnancy or labor may cause fetal anoxia or bradycardia by increasing contractility of the uterus and decreasing uterine blood flow.
See also "Nonteratogenic Effects."
NURSING MOTHERS
Some studies, but not others, have reported detectable amounts of codeine in breast milk. The levels are probably not clinically significant after usual therapeutic dosage. The possibility of clinically important amounts being excreted in breast milk in individuals abusing codeine should be considered.
It is not known whether either phenylephrine or promethazine is excreted in human milk.
Caution should be exercised when Phenergan VC with codeine is administered to a nursing woman.
PEDIATRIC USE
This product should not be used in children under 2 years of age because safety for such use has not been established.

ADVERSE REACTIONS

CODEINE
Nervous System—CNS depression, particularly respiratory depression, and to a lesser extent circulatory depression; light-headedness, dizziness, sedation, euphoria, dysphoria, headache, transient hallucination, disorientation, visual disturbances, and convulsions.
Cardiovascular—Tachycardia, bradycardia, palpitation, faintness, syncope, orthostatic hypotension (common to narcotic analgesics).
Gastrointestinal—Nausea, vomiting, constipation, and biliary tract spasm. Patients with chronic ulcerative colitis may experience increased colonic motility; in patients with acute ulcerative colitis, toxic dilation has been reported.
Genitourinary—Oliguria, urinary retention; antidiuretic effect has been reported (common to narcotic analgesics).
Allergic—Infrequent pruritus, giant urticaria, angioneurotic edema, and laryngeal edema.
Other—Flushing of the face, sweating and pruritus (due to opiate-induced histamine release); weakness.
PROMETHAZINE
Nervous System—Sedation, sleepiness, occasional blurred vision, dryness of mouth, dizziness; rarely confusion, disorientation, and extrapyramidal symptoms such as oculogyric crisis, torticollis, and tongue protrusion (usually in association with parenteral injection or excessive dosage).
Cardiovascular—Increased or decreased blood pressure.
Dermatologic—Rash, rarely photosensitivity.
Hematologic—Rarely leukopenia, thrombocytopenia; agranulocytosis (1 case).
Gastrointestinal—Nausea and vomiting.
PHENYLEPHRINE
Nervous System—Restlessness, anxiety, nervousness, and dizziness.
Cardiovascular—Hypertension (see "Warnings").
Other—Precordial pain, respiratory distress, tremor, and weakness.

DRUG ABUSE AND DEPENDENCE

CONTROLLED SUBSTANCE
Phenergan VC with codeine is a Schedule V Controlled Substance.
ABUSE
Codeine is known to be subject to abuse; however, the abuse potential of oral codeine appears to be quite low. Even parenteral codeine does not appear to offer the psychic effects sought by addicts to the same degree as heroin or morphine. However, codeine must be administered only under close supervision to patients with a history of drug abuse or dependence.
DEPENDENCE
Psychological dependence, physical dependence, and tolerance are known to occur with codeine.

OVERDOSAGE

CODEINE: Serious overdose with codeine is characterized by respiratory depression (a decrease in respiratory rate and/or tidal volume, Cheyne-Stokes respiration, cyanosis), extreme somnolence progressing to stupor or coma, skeletal muscle flaccidity, cold and clammy skin, and sometimes bradycardia and hypotension. The triad of coma, pinpoint pupils, and respiratory depression is strongly suggestive of opiate poisoning. In severe overdosage, particularly by the intravenous route, apnea, circulatory collapse, cardiac arrest, and death may occur. Promethazine is additive to the depressant effects of codeine.
It is difficult to determine what constitutes a standard toxic or lethal dose. However, the lethal oral dose of codeine in an adult is reported to be in the range of 0.5 to 1.0 gram. Infants and children are believed to be relatively more sensitive to opiates on a body-weight basis. Elderly patients are also comparatively intolerant to opiates.
PROMETHAZINE: Signs and symptoms of overdosage with promethazine range from mild depression of the central nervous system and cardiovascular system to profound hypotension, respiratory depression, and unconsciousness.

Stimulation may be evident, especially in children and geriatric patients. Convulsions may rarely occur. A paradoxical reaction has been reported in children receiving single doses of 75 mg to 125 mg orally, characterized by hyperexcitability and nightmares.

Atropine-like signs and symptoms—dry mouth, fixed, dilated pupils, flushing, as well as gastrointestinal symptoms, may occur.

PHENYLEPHRINE: Signs and symptoms of overdosage with phenylephrine include hypertension, headache, convulsions, cerebral hemorrhage, and vomiting. Ventricular premature beats and short paroxysms of ventricular tachycardia may also occur. Headache may be a symptom of hypertension. Bradycardia may also be seen early in phenylephrine overdosage through stimulation of baroreceptors.

TREATMENT

Treatment of overdosage with Phenergan VC with codeine is essentially symptomatic and supportive. Only in cases of extreme overdosage or individual sensitivity do vital signs including respiration, pulse, blood pressure, temperature, and EKG need to be monitored. Activated charcoal orally or by lavage may be given, or sodium or magnesium sulfate orally as a cathartic. Attention should be given to the reestablishment of adequate respiratory exchange through provision of a patent airway and institution of assisted or controlled ventilation. The narcotic antagonist, naloxone hydrochloride, may be administered when significant respiratory depression occurs with Phenergan VC with codeine; any depressant effects of promethazine are not reversed by naloxone. Diazepam may be used to control convulsions. Avoid analeptics, which may cause convulsions. Acidosis and electrolyte losses should be corrected. A rise in temperature or pulmonary complications may signal the need for institution of antibiotic therapy.

Severe hypotension usually responds to the administration of norepinephrine or phenylephrine. EPINEPHRINE SHOULD NOT BE USED, since its use in a patient with partial adrenergic blockade may further lower the blood pressure.

Limited experience with dialysis indicates that it is not helpful.

DOSAGE AND ADMINISTRATION

The average effective dose is given in the following table:
[See table above right].

Adults	1 teaspoon (5 ml) every 4 to 6 hours, not to exceed 30.0 ml in 24 hours.
Children 6 years to under 12 years	½ to 1 teaspoon (2.5 to 5 ml) every 4 to 6 hours, not to exceed 30.0 ml in 24 hours.
Children under 6 years (weight: 18 kg or 40 lbs)	¼ to ½ teaspoon (1.25 to 2.5 ml) every 4 to 6 hours, not to exceed 9.0 ml in 24 hours.
Children under 6 years (weight: 16 kg or 35 lbs)	¼ to ½ teaspoon (1.25 to 2.5 ml) every 4 to 6 hours, not to exceed 8.0 ml in 24 hours.
Children under 6 years (weight: 14 kg or 30 lbs)	¼ to ½ teaspoon (1.25 to 2.5 ml) every 4 to 6 hours, not to exceed 7.0 ml in 24 hours.
Children under 6 years (weight: 12 kg or 25 lbs)	¼ to ½ teaspoon (1.25 to 2.5 ml) every 4 to 6 hours, not to exceed 6.0 ml in 24 hours.

Phenergan VC with codeine is not recommended for children under 2 years of age.

HOW SUPPLIED

Phenergan ® VC with codeine, Wyeth®, is a clear, reddish-orange solution supplied as follows:

NDC 0008-0552-02, case of 24 bottles of 4 fl. oz.
NDC 0008-0552-06, case of 16 bottles of 6 fl. oz.
NDC 0008-0552-08, case of 12 bottles of 8 fl. oz.
NDC 0008-0552-03, bottle of 1 pint.
NDC 0008-0552-04, bottle of 1 gallon.

Keep bottles tightly closed below 25°C (77°F).
Protect from light.
Dispense in light-resistance, glass, tight containers.

RESOL® OTC

[ree 'sol]
Oral Electrolyte Rehydration and Maintenance Solution

RESOL® is intended for replacement and maintenance of water and electrolytes in diarrhea with mild to moderate dehydration. RESOL is ready to feed and presterilized, and water should not be added. Sterilized nipples should be used.

INGREDIENTS

Water, glucose, sodium chloride, potassium citrate, citric acid, disodium phosphate, magnesium chloride, calcium chloride, and sodium citrate.

PROXIMATE ANALYSIS

One fluidounce supplies about 2.5 Calories.

	mEq/liter	Approximate mEq/8 fl. oz. (237 mL)
Sodium	50	12
Potassium	20	4.7
Calcium	4	0.95
Magnesium	4	0.95
Chloride	50	12
Citrate	34	8.0
Phosphate (HPO_4^{-2})	5	1.2
	gram/liter	
Glucose	20	

HOW SUPPLIED

Ready to feed—presterilized, 8 fluidounce bottles, cartons of 6 bottles.

SMA®

[ess-em-ay]
Iron fortified infant formula
READY-TO-FEED
CONCENTRATED LIQUID
POWDER

Breast milk is the preferred feeding for newborns. Infant formula is intended to replace or supplement breast milk when breast feeding is not possible or is insufficient, or when mothers elect not to breast feed.

Good maternal nutrition is important for the preparation and maintenance of breast feeding. Extensive or prolonged use of partial bottle feeding, before breast feeding has been well established, could make breast feeding difficult to maintain. A decision not to breast feed could be difficult to reverse.

Professional advice should be followed on all matters of infant feeding. Infant formula should always be prepared and used as directed. Unnecessary or improper use of infant formula could present a health hazard. Social and financial implications should be considered when selecting the method of infant feeding.

SMA® is unique among prepared formulas for its fat blend, whey-dominated protein composition, amino acid pattern and mineral content.

SMA, utilizing a hybridized safflower (oleic) oil, became the first infant formula offering fat and calcium absorption equal to that of human milk, with a physiologic level of linoleic acid. Thus, the fat blend in SMA provides a ready source of energy, helps protect infants against neonatal tetany and produces a ratio of vitamin E to polyunsaturated fatty acids (linoleic acid) more than adequate to prevent hemolytic anemia.

By combining reduced minerals whey with skimmed cow's milk, SMA adjusts the protein content to within the range of human milk, reverses the whey-protein to casein ratio of cow's milk so that it is like that of human milk, and reduces the mineral content to a physiologic level.

The resultant 60:40 whey-protein to casein ratio provides protein nutrition superior to a casein-dominated formula. In addition, the essential amino acids, including cystine, are present in amounts close to those of human milk. So the protein in SMA is of high biologic value.

The physiologic mineral content makes possible a low renal solute load which helps protect the functionally immature infant kidney, increases expendable water reserves and helps protect against dehydration.

Use of lactose as the carbohydrate results in a physiologic stool flora and a low stool pH, decreasing the incidence of perianal dermatitis.

INGREDIENTS

SMA® Concentrated Liquid or Ready-to-Feed. Water; nonfat milk; reduced minerals whey; lactose; oleo, coconut, oleic (safflower), and soybean oils; soy lecithin; calcium carrageenan. *Minerals:* Potassium bicarbonate; calcium chloride and citrate; potassium chloride; sodium citrate; ferrous sulfate; sodium bicarbonate; zinc, cupric, and manganese sulfates. *Vitamins:* Ascorbic acid, alpha tocopheryl acetate, niacinamide, vitamin A palmitate, calcium pantothenate, thiamine hydrochloride, riboflavin, pyridoxine hydrochloride, beta-carotene, folic acid, phytonadione, activated 7-dehydrocholesterol, biotin, cyanocobalamin.

SMA® Powder. Nonfat milk; reduced minerals whey; lactose; oleo, coconut, oleic (safflower), and soybean oils; soy lecithin.

Minerals: Calcium chloride; sodium bicarbonate; calcium hydroxide; ferrous sulfate; potassium hydroxide and bicarbonate; potassium chloride; zinc, cupric, and manganese sulfates.

Vitamins: Ascorbic acid, alpha tocopheryl acetate, niacinamide, vitamin A palmitate, calcium pantothenate, thiamine hydrochloride, riboflavin, pyridoxine hydrochloride, beta-carotene, folic acid, phytonadione, activated 7-dehydrocholesterol, biotin, cyanocobalamin.

PROXIMATE ANALYSIS
at 20 calories per fluidounce
READY-TO-FEED, POWDER, and CONCENTRATED LIQUID:

	(w/v)
Fat	3.6%
Carbohydrate	7.2%
Protein	1.5%
60% Lactalbumin (whey protein)	0.9%
40% Casein	0.6%
Ash	0.25%
Crude Fiber	None
Total Solids	12.6%
Calories/fl. oz.	20

Vitamins, Minerals: In normal dilution, each quart contains 2500 IU vitamin A, 400 IU vitamin D_3, 9 IU vitamin E, 55 mcg vitamin K_1, 0.67 mg vitamin B_1 (thiamine), 1 mg vitamin B_2 (riboflavin), 55 mg vitamin C (ascorbic acid), 0.4 mg vitamin B_6 (pyridoxine hydrochloride), 1 mcg vitamin B_{12}, 9.5 mg equivalents niacin, 2 mg pantothenic acid, 50 mcg folic acid, 14 mcg biotin, 100 mg choline, 420 mg calcium, 312 mg phosphorus, 50 mg magnesium, 142 mg sodium, 530 mg potassium, 355 mg chloride, 12 mg iron, 0.45 mg copper, 3.5 mg zinc, 150 mcg manganese, 65 mcg iodine.

PREPARATION

Ready-to-Feed (8 and 32 fl. oz. cans of 20 calories per fluidounce formula)— shake can, open and pour into previously sterilized nursing bottle; attach nipple and feed. Cover opened can and immediately store in refrigerator. Use contents of can within 48 hours of opening.

Powder—(1 pound can)—For normal dilution supplying 20 calories per fluidounce, use 1 scoop (or 1 standard tablespoonful) of powder, packed and leveled, to 2 fluidounces of cooled, previously boiled water. For larger amount of formula, use ¼ standard measuring cup of powder, packed and leveled, to 8 fluidounces (1 cup) of water. Three of these portions make 26 fluidounces of formula.

Concentrated Liquid—For normal dilution supplying 20 calories per fluidounce, use equal amounts of SMA liquid and cooled, previously boiled water.

Note: Prepared formula should be used within 24 hours.

HOW SUPPLIED

Ready-to-Feed—presterilized and premixed, 32 fluidounce (1 quart) cans, cases of 6; 8 fluidounce cans, cases of 24 (4 carriers of 6 cans). *Powder*—1 pound cans with measuring scoop, cases of 6. *Concentrated Liquid* — 13 fluidounce cans, cases of 24.

For Hospital Nursery Use—an infant feeding system which provides premixed, presterilized, ready-to-feed items, thus saving space, time and equipment. It eliminates washing, measuring, mixing, sterilizing, refrigerating and heating.

The system is offered in a choice of two forms:

1. Prefilled and presterilized 4 oz. glass bottles for which sterile nipple assemblies are available, to be attached before feeding. These units may be used again after resterilizing or may be discarded, as desired.
2. The E-Z NURSER® (single unit nurser), also prefilled and presterilized, consists of a 4 oz. glass bottle with sterile nipple already attached; the entire unit is designed to be discarded after use.

The following items are supplied in both the forms described above:

SMA® Ready-to-Feed	
13 calories/oz.	48 bottles of 4 fl. oz.
20 calories/oz.	48 bottles of 4 fl. oz.
24 calories/oz.	48 bottles of 4 fl. oz.
27 calories/oz.	48 bottles of 4 fl. oz.
SMA® lo-iron Ready-to-Feed	
13 calories/oz.	48 bottles of 4 fl. oz.
20 calories/oz.	48 bottles of 4 fl. oz.
24 calories/oz.	48 bottles of 4 fl. oz.
"preemie" SMA® Ready-to-Feed	
24 calories/oz.	48 bottles of 4 fl. oz.
(Not available in the E-Z NURSER®)	
Distilled Water	48 bottles of 4 fl. oz.
Glucose, 5% in Distilled Water, 6 calories/oz.	48 bottles of 4 fl. oz.
Glucose, 10% in Distilled Water, 12 calories/oz.	48 bottles of 4 fl. oz.

Continued on next page

Wyeth—Cont.

NURSOY® (soy protein formula)

20 calories/oz. 48 bottles of 4 fl. oz.

(Not available in the E-Z NURSER®)

Supplied in 8 oz. bottles, to which sterile nipple assemblies must be attached before feeding, are the following:

SMA® Ready-to-Feed

20 calories/oz.	24 bottles of 8 fl. oz.
Oral Electrolyte Solution	24 bottles of 8 fl. oz.
Distilled Water	24 bottles of 8 fl. oz.

NIPPLE ASSEMBLIES—presterilized, for both premature and term infants, single-hole and cross-cut, suitable for use with all ready-to-feed products requiring them, cartons of 288 nipple units. Single-hole, cross cut and orthodontic nipples.

ACCUFEED™, Wyeth Graduated Nursers—presterilized, disposable nursers (60 ml capacity) for accurately measured feedings, packages of 200.

Also Available: SMA® lo-iron. For those who appreciate the particular advantages of SMA®, the infant formula closest in composition nutritionally to mother's milk, but who sometimes need or wish to recommend a formula that does not contain a high level of iron, now there is SMA lo-iron with all the benefits of regular SMA but with a reduced level of iron of 1.4 mg per quart. Infants should receive supplemental dietary iron from an outside source to meet daily requirements.

Concentrated Liquid, 13 fl. oz. cans, cases of 24. Powder, 1 pound cans with measuring scoop, cases of 6. Ready-to-Feed, 32 fl. oz. cans, cases of 6.

Preparation of the standard 20 calories per fluidounce formula of SMA lo-iron is the same as SMA iron fortified given above.

SECTRAL® ℞

[*sek 'tral*]

(acebutolol hydrochloride)

Capsules

DESCRIPTION

SECTRAL® (acebutolol HCl) is a selective, hydrophilic beta-adrenoreceptor blocking agent with mild intrinsic sympathomimetic activity for use in treating patients with hypertension and ventricular arrhythmias. It is marketed in capsule form for oral administration. SECTRAL capsules are provided in two dosage strengths which contain 200 or 400 mg of acebutolol as the hydrochloride salt. The inactive ingredients present are D&C Red 22, FD&C Blue 1, FD&C Yellow 6, gelatin, povidone, starch, stearic acid, and titanium dioxide. The 200 mg dosage strength also contains D&C Red 28 and the 400 mg dosage strength also contains FD&C Red 40.

Acebutolol HCl has the following structural formula:

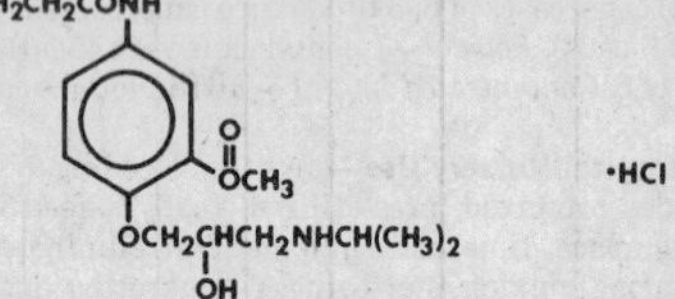

$C_{18}H_{28}N_2O_4 \cdot HCl$ M.W. 372.9

Acebutolol HCl is a white or slightly off-white powder freely soluble in water, and less soluble in alcohol. Chemically it is defined as Butanamide, N-[3-acetyl-4-[2-hydroxy-3-[(1-methylethyl)amino]propoxy]phenyl]-, (±)-or (±)-3'-Acetyl-4'-[2-hydroxy-3-(isopropylamino)propoxy] butyranilide.

CLINICAL PHARMACOLOGY

SECTRAL is a cardioselective, β-adrenoreceptor blocking agent, which possesses mild intrinsic sympathomimetic activity (ISA) in its therapeutically effective dose range.

PHARMACODYNAMICS

β_1-cardioselectivity has been demonstrated in experimental animal studies. In anesthetized dogs and cats, SECTRAL is more potent in antagonizing isoproterenol-induced tachycardia (β_1) than in antagonizing isoproterenol-induced vasodilatation (β_2). In guinea pigs and cats, it is more potent in antagonizing this tachycardia than in antagonizing isoproterenol-induced bronchodilatation (β_2). ISA of SECTRAL has been demonstrated in catecholamine-depleted rats by tachycardia induced by intravenous administration of this agent. A membrane stabilizing effect has been detected in animals, but only with high concentrations of SECTRAL.

Clinical studies have demonstrated β_1-blocking activity at the recommended doses by: a) reduction in the resting heart rate and decrease in exercise-induced tachycardia; b) reduction in cardiac output at rest and after exercise; c) reduction of systolic and diastolic blood pressures at rest and post-exercise; d) inhibition of isoproterenol-induced tachycardia.

The β_1-selectivity of SECTRAL has also been demonstrated on the basis of the following vascular and bronchial effects:

Vascular Effects: SECTRAL has less antagonistic effects on peripheral vascular β_2-receptors at rest and after epinephrine stimulation than non-selective β-antagonists.

Bronchial Effects: In single dose studies in asthmatics examining effects of various beta-blockers on pulmonary function, low doses of acebutolol produce less evidence of bronchoconstriction and less reduction of beta$_2$ agonist, bronchodilating effects, than non-selective agents like propranolol but more than atenolol.

ISA has been observed with SECTRAL in man, as shown by a slightly smaller (about 3 beats per minute) decrease in resting heart rate when compared to equivalent β-blocking doses of propranolol, metoprolol or atenolol. Chronic therapy with SECTRAL induced no significant alteration in the blood lipid profile.

SECTRAL has been shown to delay AV conduction time and to increase the refratoriness of the AV node without significantly affecting sinus node recovery time, atrial refractory period, or the HV conduction time. The membrane stabilizing effect of SECTRAL is not manifest at the doses used clinically.

Significant reductions in resting and exercise heart rates and systolic blood pressures have been observed 1.5 hours after SECTRAL administration with maximal effects occurring between 3 and 8 hours post-dosing in normal volunteers. SECTRAL has demonstrated a significant effect on exercise-induced tachycardia 24–30 hours after drug administration.

There are significant correlations between plasma levels of acebutolol and both the reduction in resting heart rate and the percent of β-blockade of exercise-induced tachycardia.

The antihypertensive effect of SECTRAL has been shown in double-blind controlled studies to be superior to placebo and similar to propranolol and hydrochlorothiazide. In addition, patients responding to SECTRAL administered twice daily had a similar response whether the dosage regimen was changed to once daily administration or continued on a b.i.d. regimen. Most patients responded to 400–800 mg per day in divided doses.

The antiarrhythmic effect of SECTRAL was compared with placebo, propranolol and quinidine. Compared with placebo, SECTRAL significantly reduced mean total ventricular ectopic beats (VEB), paired VEB, multiform VEB, R-on-T beats and ventricular tachycardia (VT). Both SECTRAL and propranolol significantly reduced mean total and paired VEB and VT. SECTRAL and quinidine significantly reduced resting total and complex VEB; the antiarrhythmic efficacy of SECTRAL was also observed during exercise.

PHARMACOKINETICS AND METABOLISM

SECTRAL is well-absorbed from the GI tract. It is subject to extensive first-pass hepatic biotransformation, with an absolute bioavailability of approximately 40% for the parent compound. The major metabolite, an N-acetyl derivative (diacetolol), is pharmacologically active. This metabolite is equipotent to SECTRAL and in cats is more cardioselective than SECTRAL; therefore, this first-pass phenomenon does not attenuate the therapeutic effect of SECTRAL. Food intake does not have a significant effect on the area under the plasma concentration-time curve (AUC) of SECTRAL although the rate of absorption and peak concentration decreased slightly.

The plasma elimination half-life of SECTRAL is approximately 3 to 4 hours, while that of its metabolite, diacetolol, is 8 to 13 hours. The time to reach peak concentration for SECTRAL is 2.5 hours and for diacetolol, after oral administration of SECTRAL, 3.5 hours.

Within the single oral dose range of 200 to 400 mg, the kinetics are dose proportional. However, this linearity is not seen at higher doses, probably due to saturation of hepatic biotransformation sites. In addition, after multiple dosing the lack of linearity is also seen by AUC increases of approximately 100% as compared to single oral dosing. Elimination via renal excretion is approximately 30% to 40% and by non-renal mechanisms 50% to 60%, which includes excretion into the bile and direct passage through the intestinal wall.

SECTRAL has a low binding affinity for plasma proteins (about 26%). SECTRAL and its metabolite, diacetolol, are relatively hydrophilic and therefore only minimal quantities have been detected in the cerebrospinal fluid (CSF).

Drug interaction studies with tolbutamide and warfarin indicated no influence on the therapeutic effects of these compounds. Digoxin and hydrochlorothiazide plasma levels were not affected by concomitant SECTRAL administration. The kinetics of SECTRAL were not significantly altered by concomitant administration of hydrochlorothiazide, hydralazine, sulfinpyrazone or oral contraceptives.

In patients with renal impairment, there is no effect on the elimination half-life of SECTRAL, but there is decreased elimination of the metabolite, diacetolol, resulting in a two- to three-fold increase in its half-life. For this reason, the drug should be administered with caution in patients with renal insufficiency (see PRECAUTIONS). SECTRAL and its major metabolite are dialyzable.

SECTRAL crosses the placental barrier, and is secreted in breast milk.

In geriatric patients, the bioavailability of SECTRAL and its metabolite is increased, approximately two-fold, probably due to decreases in the first-pass metabolism and renal function in the elderly.

INDICATIONS AND USAGE

HYPERTENSION: SECTRAL is indicated for the management of hypertension in adults. It may be used alone or in combination with other anti-hypertensive agents, especially thiazide-type diuretics.

VENTRICULAR ARRHYTHMIAS: SECTRAL is indicated in the management of ventricular premature beats; it reduces the total number of premature beats, as well as the number of paired and multiform ventricular ectopic beats, and R-on-T beats.

CONTRAINDICATIONS

SECTRAL is contraindicated in: 1) persistently severe bradycardia; 2) second- and third-degree heart block; 3) overt cardiac failure; and 4) cardiogenic shock. (See WARNINGS)

WARNINGS

CARDIAC FAILURE: Sympathetic stimulation may be essential for support of the circulation in individuals with diminished myocardial contractility, and its inhibition by β-adrenergic receptor blockade may precipitate more severe failure. Although β-blockers should be avoided in overt cardiac failure, SECTRAL can be used with caution in patients with a history of heart failure who are controlled with digitalis and/or diuretics. Both digitalis and SECTRAL impair AV conduction. If cardiac failure persists, therapy with SECTRAL should be withdrawn.

IN PATIENTS WITHOUT A HISTORY OF CARDIAC FAILURE: In patients with aortic or mitral valve disease or compromised left ventricular function, continued depression of the myocardium with β-blocking agents over a period of time may lead to cardiac failure. At the first signs of failure, patients should be digitalized and/or be given a diuretic and the response observed closely. If cardiac failure continues despite adequate digitalization and/or diuretic, SECTRAL therapy should be withdrawn.

EXACERBATION OF ISCHEMIC DISEASE FOLLOWING ABRUPT WITHDRAWAL: Following abrupt cessation of therapy with certain β-blocking agents in patients with coronary artery disease, exacerbation of angina pectoris and, in some cases, myocardial infarction and death have been reported. Therefore, such patients should be cautioned against interruption of therapy without a physician's advice. Even in the absence of overt ischemic heart disease, when discontinuation of SECTRAL is planned, the patient should be carefully observed, and should be advised to limit physical activity to a minimum. SECTRAL should be reinstated if withdrawal symptoms occur.

PERIPHERAL VASCULAR DISEASE: Treatment with β-antagonists reduces cardiac output and can precipitate or aggravate the symptoms of arterial insufficiency in patients with peripheral or mesenteric vascular disease. Caution should be exercised with such patients and they should be observed closely for evidence of progression of arterial obstruction.

BRONCHOSPASTIC DISEASES: PATIENTS WITH BRONCHOSPASTIC DISEASE SHOULD, IN GENERAL, NOT RECEIVE A β-BLOCKER. Because of its relative β_1-selectivity, however, low doses of SECTRAL may be used with caution in patients with bronchospastic disease who do not respond to, or who cannot tolerate, alternative treatment. Since β_1-selectivity is not absolute and is dose-dependent, the lowest possible dose of SECTRAL should be used initially, preferably in divided doses to avoid the higher plasma levels associated with the longer dose-interval. A bronchodilator, such as a theophylline or a β_2-stimulant, should be made available in advance with instructions concerning its use.

ANESTHESIA AND MAJOR SURGERY: The necessity, or desirability, of withdrawal of a β-blocking therapy prior to major surgery is controversial. β-adrenergic receptor blockade impairs the ability of the heart to respond to β-adrenergically mediated reflex stimuli. While this might be of benefit in preventing arrhythmic response, the risk of excessive myocardial depression during general anesthesia may be enhanced and difficulty in re-starting and maintaining the heart beat has been reported with beta-blockers. If treatment is continued, particular care should be taken when using anesthetic agents which depress the myocardium, such as ether, cyclopropane and trichlorethylene, and it is prudent to use the lowest possible dose of SECTRAL. Like other β-blockers, is a competitive inhibitor of β-receptor agonists and its effect on the heart can be reversed by cautious administration of such agents (e.g. dobutamine or isoproterenol—see OVERDOSE). Manifestations of excessive vagal tone (e.g. profound bradycardia, hypotension) may be corrected with atropine 1–3 mg i.v. in divided doses.

DIABETES AND HYPOGLYCEMIA: β-blockers may potentiate insulin-induced hypoglycemia and mask some of its manifestations such as tachycardia; however, dizziness and sweating are usually not significantly affected. Diabetic patients should be warned of the possibility of masked hypoglycemia.

THYROTOXICOSIS: β-adrenergic blockade may mask certain clinical signs (tachycardia) of hyperthyroidism. Abrupt withdrawal of β-blockade may precipitate a thryoid storm; therefore, patients suspected of developing thryotoxicosis from whom SECTRAL therapy is to be withdrawn should be monitored closely.

PRECAUTIONS

IMPAIRED RENAL OR HEPATIC FUNCTION: Studies on the effect of acebutolol in patients with renal insufficiency have not been performed in the U.S. Foreign published experience shows that acebutolol has been used successfully in chronic renal insufficiency. Acebutolol is excreted through the G.I. tract, but the active metabolite, diacetolol, is eliminated predominantly by the kidney. There is a linear relationship between renal clearance of diacetolol and creatinine clearance. Therefore, the daily dose of acebutolol should be reduced by 50% when the creatinine clearance is less than 50 ml/min and by 75% when it is less than 25 ml/min. SECTRAL should be used cautiously in patients with impaired hepatic function.

SECTRAL has been used successfully and without problems in elderly patients in the U.S. clinical trials without specific adjustment of dosage. However, elderly patients may require lower maintenance doses because the bioavailability of both SECTRAL and its metabolite are approximately doubled in this age group.

CLINICAL LABORATORY FINDINGS: SECTRAL, like other β-blockers, has been associated with the development of antinuclear antibodies (ANA). In prospective clinical trials, patients receiving SECTRAL had a dose dependent increase in the development of positive ANA titers and the overall incidence was higher than that observed with propranolol. Symptoms (generally persistent arthralgias and myalgias) related to this laboratory abnormality were infrequent (less than 1% with both drugs). Symptoms and ANA titers were reversible upon discontinuation of treatment.

INFORMATION FOR PATIENTS: Patients, especially those with evidence of coronary artery disease, should be warned against interruption or discontinuation of SECTRAL therapy without a physician's supervision. Although cardiac failure rarely occurs in properly selected patients, those being treated with β-adrenergic blocking agents should be advised to consult a physician if they develop signs or symptoms suggestive of impending CHF, or unexplained respiratory symptoms.

Patients should also be warned of possible severe hypertensive reactions from concomitant use of α-adrenergic stimulants such as the nasal decongestants commonly used in OTC cold preparations and nasal drops.

DRUG INTERACTIONS: Catecholamine-depleting drugs, such as reserpine, may have an additive effect when given with β-blocking agents. Patients treated with SECTRAL plus catecholamine depletors should, therefore, be observed closely for evidence of marked bradycardia or hypotension which may present as vertigo, syncope/pre-syncope, or orthostatic changes in blood pressure without compensatory tachycardia. Exaggerated hypertensive responses have been reported from the combined use of β-adrenergic antagonists and α-adrenergic stimulants, including those contained in proprietary cold remedies and vasoconstrictive nasal drops. Patients receiving β-blockers should be warned of this potential hazard. No significant interactions with digoxin, hydrochlorothiazide, hydralazine, sulfinpyrazone, oral contraceptives, tolbutamide or warfarin have been observed.

CARCINOGENESIS, MUTAGENESIS, IMPAIRMENT OF FERTILITY: Chronic oral toxicity studies in rats and mice, employing dose levels as high as 300 mg/kg/day, which is equivalent to 15 times the maximum recommended (60 kg) human dose, did not indicate a carcinogenic potential for SECTRAL. Diacetolol, the major metabolite of SECTRAL in man, was without carcinogenic potential in rats when tested at doses as high as 1800 mg/kg/day. SECTRAL and diacetolol were also shown to be devoid of mutagenic potential in the Ames Test. SECTRAL, administered orally to two generations of male and female rats at doses of up to 240 mg/kg/day [equivalent to 12 times the maximum recommended therapeutic dose in (a 60 kg) man] and diacetolol, administered to two generations of male and female rats at doses of up to 1000 mg/kg/day, had no significant impact on reproductive performance or fertility.

TERATOGENIC EFFECTS

Pregnancy Category B: Reproduction studies have been performed with SECTRAL in rats and rabbits at doses of up to 60 mg/kg/day, the equivalent of 3 times the maximum recommended therapeutic dose in (a 60 kg) man. Studies have also been performed in these species with diacetolol (at doses of up to 450 mg/kg/day in rabbits and up to 1800 mg/kg/day in rats). Other than a significant elevation in post-implantation loss with 450 mg/kg/day diacetolol, a level at which food consumption and body weight gain was reduced in rabbit dams and a non-statistically significant increase in incidence of bilateral cataract in rat fetuses from

TOTAL VOLUNTEERED AND ELICITED (U.S. STUDIES)

Body System/ Adverse Reaction	SECTRAL (N = 1002) %	Propranolol (N = 424) %	Hydrochlorothiazide (N = 178) %	Placebo (N = 314) %
Cardiovascular				
Chest Pain	2	4	4	1
Edema	2	2	4	1
Central Nervous System				
Depression	2	1	3	1
Dizziness	6	7	12	2
Fatigue	11	17	10	4
Headache	6	9	13	4
Insomnia	3	6	5	1
Abnormal dreams	2	3	0	1
Dermatologic				
Rash	2	2	4	1
Gastrointestinal				
Constipation	4	2	7	0
Diarrhea	4	5	5	1
Dyspepsia	4	6	3	1
Flatulence	3	4	7	1
Nausea	4	6	3	0
Genitourinary				
Micturition (frequency)	3	1	9	<1
Musculoskeletal				
Arthralgia	2	1	3	2
Myalgia	2	1	4	0
Respiratory				
Cough	1	1	2	0
Dyspnea	4	6	4	2
Rhinitis	2	1	4	<1
Special Senses				
Abnormal Vision	2	2	3	0

dams treated with 1800 mg/kg/day diacetolol, there was no evidence of harm to the fetus with either drug. There are no adequate and well-controlled trials in pregnant women in the U.S.; however, studies have shown that both acebutolol and diacetolol cross the placenta. Because animal teratology studies are not always predictive of the human response, SECTRAL should be used during pregnancy only if the potential benefit justifies the risk to the fetus.

Labor and Delivery: The effect of SECTRAL on labor and delivery in pregnant women is unknown. Studies in animals have not shown any effect of SECTRAL on the usual course of labor and delivery.

Nursing Mothers: Acebutolol and diacetolol also appear in breast milk with a milk: plasma ratio of 7.1 and 12.2, respectively. Use in nursing mothers is not recommended.

Pediatric Use: Safety and effectiveness in children have not been established.

ADVERSE REACTIONS

SECTRAL is well tolerated in properly selected patients. Most adverse reactions have been mild, not required discontinuation of therapy, and tended to decrease as duration of treatment increases.

The following table shows the frequency of treatment-related side effects derived from controlled clinical trials in patients with hypertension, angina pectoris, and arrhythmia. These patients received SECTRAL, propranolol, or hydrochlorothiazide as monotherapy, or placebo.

[See table above].

The following selected (potentially important) side effects were seen in up to 2% of SECTRAL patients:

Cardiovascular: hypotension, bradycardia, heart failure.

Central Nervous System: anxiety, hyper/hypoesthesia, impotence.

Dermatological: pruritus.

Gastrointestinal: vomiting, abdominal pain.

Genitourinary: dysuria, nocturia.

Musculoskeletal: back pain, joint pain.

Respiratory: pharyngitis, wheezing, cough.

Special Senses: conjunctivitis, dry eye, eye pain.

The incidence of drug-related adverse effects (volunteered and solicited) according to SECTRAL dose is shown below. (Data from 266 hypertensive patients treated for 3 months on a constant dose.)

Body System	400 mg/day (N = 132)	800 mg/day (N = 63)	1200 mg/day (N = 71)
Cardiovascular	5%	2%	1%
Gastrointestinal	3%	3%	7%
Musculoskeletal	2%	3%	4%
Central Nervous System	9%	13%	17%
Respiratory	1%	5%	6%
Skin	1%	2%	1%
Special Senses	2%	2%	6%
Genitourinary	2%	3%	1%

POTENTIAL ADVERSE EFFECTS

In addition, certain adverse effects not listed above have been reported with other β-blocking agents and should also be considered as potential adverse effects of SECTRAL.

Central Nervous System: Reversible mental depression progressing to catatonia (an acute syndrome characterized by disorientation for time and place), short-term memory loss, emotional lability, slightly clouded sensorium, and decreased performance (neuropsychometrics).

Cardiovascular: Intensification of AV block (see CONTRAINDICATIONS).

Allergic: Erythematous rash, fever combined with aching and sore throat, laryngospasm, and respiratory distress.

Hematologic: Agranulocytosis, non-thrombocytopenic, and thrombocytopenic purpura.

Gastrointestinal: Mesenteric arterial thrombosis and ischemic colitis.

Miscellaneous: Reversible alopecia and Peyronie's disease. The oculomucocutaneous syndrome associated with the β-blocker practolol has not been reported with SECTRAL during investigational use and extensive foreign clinical experience.

OVERDOSAGE

No specific information on emergency treatment of overdosage is available for SECTRAL. However, overdosage with other β-blocking agents has been accompanied by extreme bradycardia, advanced atrio-ventricular block, intraventricular conduction defects, hypotension, severe congestive heart failure, seizures, and in susceptible patients, bronchospasm and hypoglycemia. Although specific information on the emergency treatment of SECTRAL overdose is not available, on the basis of the pharmacological actions and the observations in treating overdoses with other β-blockers, the following general measures should be considered:

1. Empty stomach by emesis or lavage.
2. Bradycardia: i.v. atropine (1 to 3 mg. in divided doses). If antivagal response is inadequate, administer isoproterenol cautiously since larger than usual doses of isoproterenol may be required.
3. Persistent hypotension in spite of correction of bradycardia: Administer vasopressor (e.g. epinephrine, levarterenol, dopamine, or dobutamine) with frequent monitoring of blood pressure and pulse rate.
4. Bronchospasm: A theophylline derivative, such as aminophylline and/or parenteral β_2-stimulant, such as terbutaline.
5. Cardiac failure: Digitalize the patient and/or administer a diuretic. It has been reported that glucagon is useful in this situation.

SECTRAL is dialyzable.

DOSAGE AND ADMINISTRATION

HYPERTENSION: The initial dosage of SECTRAL in uncomplicated mild-to-moderate hypertension is 400 mg. This can be given as a single daily dose, but in occasional patients twice daily dosing (200 mg b.i.d.) may be required for adequate 24 hour blood pressure control. An optimal response is

Continued on next page

Wyeth—Cont.

usually achieved with dosages of 400 to 800 mg per day, although some patients have been maintained on as little as 200 mg per day. Patients with more severe hypertension or who have demonstrated inadequate control may respond to a total of 1200 mg daily (administered b.i.d.), or to the addition of a second antihypertensive agent. Beta-1 selectivity diminishes as dosage is increased.
VENTRICULAR ARRHYTHMIA: The usual initial dose of SECTRAL is 400 mg daily given as 200 mg b.i.d. Dosage should be increased gradually until an optimal clinical response is obtained, generally at 600 to 1200 mg per day.
USE IN OLDER PATIENTS: Older patients have an approximately 2-fold increase in bioavailability and may require lower maintenance doses. Doses above 800 mg/day should be avoided in the elderly.

HOW SUPPLIED

Sectral® (acebutolol HCl), Wyeth®, is available in the following dosage strengths:
200 mg, opaque purple and orange capsule marked "WYETH 4177" and "Sectral 200"
NDC 0008-4177-01, in bottles of 100 capsules.
NDC 0008-4177-02, in Redipak® cartons of 100 capsules (20 strips of 5).
400 mg, opaque brown and orange capsule marked "WYETH 4179" and "Sectral 400"
NDC 0008-4179-01, in bottles of 100 capsules.
NDC 0008-4179-02, in Redipak cartons of 100 capsules (20 strips of 5).
Keep at Room Temperature, Approx. 25° C (77° F).
The appearance of these capsules is a trademark of Wyeth Laboratories.

Shown in Product Identification Section, page 436

SERAX® Ⓒ℞

[ser'aks]
(oxazepam)
CAPSULES • TABLETS

DESCRIPTION

Serax is the first of a chemically new series of compounds, the 3-hydroxybenzodiazepinones. A new therapeutic agent providing versatility and flexibility in control of common emotional disturbances, this product exerts prompt action in a wide variety of disorders associated with anxiety, tension, agitation, and irritability, and anxiety associated with depression. In tolerance and toxicity studies on several animal species, this product reveals significantly greater safety factors than related compounds (chlordiazepoxide and diazepam) and manifests a wide separation of effective doses and doses inducing side effects.
Serax capsules contain 10 mg, 15 mg, or 30 mg oxazepam. The inactive ingredients present are FD&C Red 40, gelatin, lactose, titanium dioxide, and other ingredients. Each dosage strength also contains the following:
10 mg—D&C Red 22, D&C Red 28, and FD&C Blue 1;
15 mg—FD&C Yellow 6;
30 mg—D&C Red 28 and FD&C Blue 1.
Serax tablets contain 15 mg oxazepam. The inactive ingredients present are FD&C Yellow 5, lactose, magnesium stearate, methylcellulose, and polacrilin potassium.
Serax is 7 chloro-1,3-dihydro-3- hydroxy-5-phenyl-2*H*-1,4-benzodiazepin-2-one, a white crystalline powder with a molecular weight of 286.7.

ANIMAL PHARMACOLOGY AND TOXICOLOGY

In mice, SERAX exerts an anticonvulsant (anti-Metrazol®) activity at 50 percent effective doses of about 0.6 mg/kg orally. (Such anticonvulsant activity of benzodiazepines correlates with their tranquilizing properties.) To produce ataxia (rotabar test) and sedation (abolition of spontaneous motor activity), the 50 percent effective doses of this product are greater than 5 mg/kg orally. Thus, about ten times the therapeutic (anticonvulsant) dose must be given before ataxia ensues, indicating a wide separation of effective doses and doses inducing side effects.
In evaluation of antianxiety activity of compounds, conflict behavioral tests in rats differentiate continuous response for food in the presence of anxiety-provoking stress (shock) from drug-induced motor incoordination. This product shows significant separation of doses required to relieve anxiety and doses producing sedation or ataxia. Ataxia-producing doses exceed those of related CNS-acting drugs.
Acute oral LD_{50} in mice is greater than 5000 mg/kg, compared to 800 mg/kg for a related compound (chlordiazepoxide).
Subacute toxicity studies in dogs for four weeks at 480 mg/kg daily showed no specific changes; at 960 mg/kg two out of eight died with evidence of circulatory collapse. This wide margin of safety is significant compared to chlordiazepoxide HCl, which showed nonspecific changes in six dogs at 80 mg/kg. On chlordiazepoxide, two out of six died with evidence of circulatory collapse at 127 mg/kg, and six out of six died at 200 mg/kg daily. Chronic toxicity studies of Serax in dogs at 120 mg/kg/day for 52 weeks produced no toxic manifestation.
Fatty metamorphosis of the liver has been noted in six-week toxicity studies in rats given this product at 0.5% of the diet. Such accumulations of fat are considered reversible as there is no liver necrosis or fibrosis.
Breeding studies in rats through two successive litters did not produce fetal abnormality.
This product has a single major metabolite in man, a glucuronide excreted in the urine.

INDICATIONS

SERAX (oxazepam) is indicated for the management of anxiety disorders or for the short-term relief of the symptoms of anxiety. Anxiety or tension associated with the stress of everyday life usually does not require treatment with an anxiolytic.
Anxiety associated with depression is also responsive to SERAX (oxazepam) therapy.
This product has been found particularly useful in the management of anxiety, tension, agitation, and irritability in older patients.
Alcoholics with acute tremulousness, inebriation, or with anxiety associated with alcohol withdrawal are responsive to therapy.
The effectiveness of SERAX in long-term use, that is, more than 4 months, has not been assessed by systematic clinical studies. The physician should reassess periodically the usefulness of the drug for the individual patient.

CONTRAINDICATIONS

History of previous hypersensitivity reaction to oxazepam. Oxazepam is not indicated in psychoses.

WARNINGS

As with other CNS-acting drugs, patients should be cautioned against driving automobiles or operating dangerous machinery until it is known that they do not become drowsy or dizzy on oxazepam therapy.
Patients should be warned that the effects of alcohol or other CNS-depressant drugs may be additive to those of Serax, possibly requiring adjustment of dosage or elimination of such agents.

USE IN PREGNANCY

An increased risk of congenital malformations associated with the use of minor tranquilizers (chlordiazepoxide, diazepam, and meprobamate) during the first trimester of pregnancy has been suggested in several studies. Serax, a benzodiazepine derivative, has not been studied adequately to determine whether it, too, may be associated with an increased risk of fetal abnormality. Because use of these drugs is rarely a matter of urgency, their use during this period should almost always be avoided. The possibility that a woman of childbearing potential may be pregnant at the time of institution of therapy should be considered. Patients should be advised that if they become pregnant during therapy or intend to become pregnant they should communicate with their physician about the desirability of discontinuing the drug.

PRECAUTIONS

Although hypotension has occurred only rarely, oxazepam should be administered with caution to patients in whom a drop in blood pressure might lead to cardiac complications. This is particularly true in the elderly patient.
In some patients exhibiting drug dependency through chronic overdose with SERAX (oxazepam), withdrawal symptoms have been noted on discontinuance of drug administration. Withdrawal symptoms have also been reported following abrupt discontinuance of benzodiazepines taken continuously at therapeutic levels for several months. Careful supervision of dose and amounts prescribed for patients is advised, especially with those patients with a known propensity for taking excessive quantities of drugs. Excessive and prolonged use in susceptible persons, for example, alcoholics, former addicts, and others, may result in dependence on or habituation to the drug. Where excessive dosage is continued for weeks or months, dosage should be reduced gradually rather than abruptly stopped. Abrupt discontinuance of doses in excess of the recommended dose may result in some cases in the occurrence of epileptiform seizures. Withdrawal symptoms following abrupt discontinuance are similar to those seen with barbiturates.
SERAX 15 mg tablets, *but none of the other available dosage forms of this product,* contain FD&C Yellow No. 5 (tartrazine) which may cause allergic-type reactions (including bronchial asthma) in certain susceptible individuals. Although the overall incidence of FD&C Yellow No. 5 (tartrazine) sensitivity in the general population is low, it is frequently seen in patients who also have aspirin hypersensitivity.

ADVERSE REACTIONS

The necessity for discontinuation of therapy due to undesirable effects has been rare. Transient mild drowsiness is commonly seen in the first few days of therapy. If it persists, the dosage should be reduced. In few instances, dizziness, vertigo, headache, and rarely syncope have occurred either alone or together with drowsiness. Mild paradoxical reactions, i.e., excitement, stimulation of affect, have been reported in psychiatric patients; these reactions may be secondary to relief of anxiety and usually appear in the first two weeks of therapy.
Other side effects occurring during oxazepam therapy include rare instances of minor diffuse skin rashes—morbilliform, urticarial and maculopapular—nausea, lethargy, edema, slurred speech, tremor, and altered libido. Such side effects have been infrequent and are generally controlled with reduction of dosage.
Although rare, leukopenia and hepatic dysfunction including jaundice have been reported during therapy. Periodic blood counts and liver-function tests are advisable.
Ataxia with oxazepam has been reported in rare instances and does not appear to be specifically related to dose or age.
Although the following side reactions have not as yet been reported with oxazepam, they have occurred with related compounds (chlordiazepoxide and diazepam): paradoxical excitation with severe rage reactions, hallucinations, menstrual irregularities, change in EEG pattern, blood dyscrasias including agranulocytosis, blurred vision, diplopia, incontinence, stupor, disorientation, fever, and euphoria.
Transient amnesia or memory impairment has been reported in association with the use of benzodiazepines.

DOSAGE AND ADMINISTRATION

Because of the flexibility of this product and the range of emotional disturbances responsive to it, dosage should be individualized for maximum beneficial effects.
[See table below left].

SERAX (oxazepam)

	Usual Dose
Mild-to moderate-anxiety, with associated tension, irritability, agitation, or related symptoms of functional origin or secondary to organic disease.	10 to 15 mg, 3 or 4 times daily
Severe anxiety syndromes, agitation, or anxiety associated with depression.	15 to 30 mg, 3 or 4 times daily
Older patients with anxiety, tension, irritability, and agitation.	Initial dosage: 10 mg, 3 times daily. If necessary, increase cautiously to 15 mg, 3 or 4 times daily
Alcoholics with acute inebriation, tremulousness, or anxiety on withdrawal.	15 to 30 mg, 3 or 4 times daily

This product is not indicated in children under 6 years of age. Absolute dosage for children 6–12 years of age is not established.

HOW SUPPLIED

Serax® (oxazepam) Capsules and Tablets, Wyeth® are available in the following dosage strengths:
10 mg, NDC 0008-0051, white and pink capsule banded with Wyeth logo and marked "SERAX", "10", and "51", in bottles of 100 and 500 capsules and in Redipak® Strip Pack in cartons of 25 capsules, and in Redipak® cartons of 100 capsules (10 strips of 10).
15 mg, NDC 0008-0006, white and red capsule banded with Wyeth logo and marked "SERAX", "15", and "6", in bottles of 100 and 500 capsules, in Redipak® Strip Pack in cartons of 25 capsules, and in Redipak® cartons of 100 capsules (10 strips of 10).
30 mg. NDC 0008-0052, white and maroon capsule banded with Wyeth logo and marked "SERAX", "30", and "52", in bottles of 100 and 500 capsules, in Redipak® Strip Pack in cartons of 25 capsules, and in Redipak® cartons of 100 capsules (10 strips of 10).
15 mg, NDC 0008-0317, yellow, five-sided tablet with a raised "S" and a "15" on one side and "WYETH" and "317" on reverse side, in bottles of 100 tablets.

The appearance of SERAX capsules and tablets is a trademark of Wyeth Laboratories.
Keep bottles tightly closed.
Dispense in tight containers.
Shown in Product Identification Section, page 436

SIMECO® OTC

[sim 'e-ko]
(aluminum hydroxide gel, magnesium hydroxide, simethicone)
SUSPENSION

COMPOSITION

Each teaspoonful (5 ml) contains aluminum hydroxide gel equivalent to 365 mg of dried gel, USP, 300 mg of magnesium hydroxide and 30 mg of simethicone. Sodium content is 0.53 mEq per teaspoonful. The inactive ingredients are artificial and natural flavors, butylparaben, glycerin, methylparaben, propylparaben, saccharin, sorbitol solution, and water. High potency and low dose are provided by high concentration of antacid per teaspoonful.

INDICATIONS

For the symptomatic relief of hyperacidity associated with the diagnosis of peptic ulcer, gastritis, peptic esophagitis, gastric hyperacidity and hiatal hernia. To relieve the symptoms of gas.

DOSAGE AND ADMINISTRATION

Usually: 1 or 2 teaspoonfuls undiluted or with a little water to be taken 3 or 4 times daily between meals and at bedtime. Five ml SIMECO suspension neutralizes 22 mEq of acid.

WARNINGS

Patients are advised not to take more than 8 teaspoonfuls (40 ml) in a 24-hour period or use the maximum dosage for more than two weeks except under the advice and supervision of a physician. Not to be used except under the advice and supervision of a physician if patient has kidney disease. Pregnant women and nursing mothers are advised to seek the advice of a health professional before using this product.

DRUG INTERACTION PRECAUTIONS

Alumina-containing antacids should not be used concomitantly with any form of tetracycline therapy.

HOW SUPPLIED

Suspension—Cool mint flavor available in 12 fl. oz. plastic bottles.

SURMONTIL® ℞

[sir 'mon "til]
(trimipramine maleate)

DESCRIPTION

Surmontil (trimipramine maleate) is 5-(3-dimethylamino-2-methylpropyl)-10,11-dihydro-5H-dibenz (b,f) azepine acid maleate (racemic form).

$\cdot C_4H_4O_4$

$CH_2—\overset{*}{C}H(CH_3)—CH_2—N(CH_3)_2$

MOLECULAR FORMULA: $C_{20}H_{26}N_2 \cdot C_4H_4O_4$
MOLECULAR WEIGHT: 410.5

Surmontil capsules contain 25 mg, 50 mg, or 100 mg trimipramine maleate. The inactive ingredients present are FD&C Blue 1, gelatin, lactose, magnesium stearate, and titanium dioxide. The 25 mg dosage strength also contains D&C Yellow 10 and FD&C Yellow 6; the 50 mg dosage strength also contains D&C Red 28, FD&C Red 40, and FD&C Yellow 6.

Trimipramine maleate is prepared as a racemic mixture which can be resolved into levorotatory and dextrorotatory isomers. The asymmetric center responsible for optical isomerism is marked in the formula by an asterisk. Trimipramine maleate is an almost odorless, white or slightly cream-colored, crystalline substance, melting at 140–144°C. It is very slightly soluble in ether and water, is slightly soluble in ethyl alcohol and acetone, and freely soluble in chloroform and methanol at 20°C.

CLINICAL PHARMACOLOGY

Surmontil is an antidepressant with an anxiety-reducing sedative component to its action. The mode of action of Surmontil on the central nervous system is not known. However, unlike amphetamine-type compounds it does not act primarily by stimulation of the central nervous system. It does not act by inhibition of the monoamine oxidase system.

INDICATIONS

Surmontil is indicated for the relief of symptoms of depression. Endogenous depression is more likely to be alleviated than other depressive states. In studies with neurotic outpatients, the drug appeared to be equivalent to amitriptyline in the less-depressed patients but somewhat less effective than amitriptyline in the more severely depressed patients. In hospitalized depressed patients, trimipramine and imipramine were equally effective in relieving depression.

CONTRAINDICATIONS

Surmontil is contraindicated in cases of known hypersensitivity to the drug. The possibility of cross-sensitivity to other dibenzazepine compounds should be kept in mind. Surmontil should not be given in conjunction with drugs of the monoamine oxidase inhibitor class (e.g., tranylcypromine, isocarboxazid or phenelzine sulfate). The concomitant use of monoamine oxidase inhibitors (MAOI) and tricyclic compounds similar to Surmontil has caused severe hyperpyretic reactions, convulsive crises, and death in some patients. At least two weeks should elapse after cessation of therapy with MAOI before instituting therapy with Surmontil. Initial dosage should be low and increased gradually with caution and careful observation of the patient. The drug is contraindicated during the acute recovery period after a myocardial infarction.

WARNINGS

Use in Children—This drug is not recommended for use in children, since safety and effectiveness in the pediatric age group have not been established.

General Consideration for Use—Extreme caution should be used when this drug is given to patients with any evidence of cardiovascular disease because of the possibility of conduction defects, arrhythmias, myocardial infarction, strokes, and tachycardia.

Caution is advised in patients with increased intraocular pressure, history of urinary retention, or history of narrow-angle glaucoma because of the drug's anticholinergic properties; hyperthyroid patients or those on thyroid medication because of the possibility of cardiovascular toxicity; patients with a history of seizure disorder, because this drug has been shown to lower the seizure threshold; patients receiving guanethidine or similar agents, since Surmontil may block the pharmacologic effects of these drugs.

Since the drug may impair the mental and/or physical abilities required for the performance of potentially hazardous tasks, such as operating an automobile or machinery, the patient should be cautioned accordingly.

PRECAUTIONS

The possibility of suicide is inherent in any severely depressed patient and persists until a significant remission occurs. When a patient with a serious suicidal potential is not hospitalized, the prescription should be for the smallest amount feasible.

In schizophrenic patients activation of the psychosis may occur and require reduction of dosage or the addition of a major tranquilizer to the therapeutic regime.

Manic or hypomanic episodes may occur in some patients, in particular those with cyclic-type disorders. In some cases therapy with Surmontil must be discontinued until the episode is relieved, after which therapy may be reinstituted at lower dosages if still required.

Concurrent administration of Surmontil (trimipramine maleate) and electroshock therapy may increase the hazards of therapy. Such treatment should be limited to those patients for whom it is essential. When possible, discontinue the drug for several days prior to elective surgery.

Patients should be warned that the concomitant use of alcoholic beverages may be associated with exaggerated effects.

It has been reported that tricyclic antidepressants can potentiate the effects of catecholamines. Similarly, atropinelike effects may be more pronounced in patients receiving anticholinergic therapy. Therefore, particular care should be exercised when it is necessary to administer tricyclic antidepressants with sympathomimetic amines, local decongestants, local anesthetics containing epinephrine, atropine or drugs wih an anticholinergic effect. In resistant cases of depression in adults, a dose of 2.5 mg/kg/day may have to be exceeded. If a higher dose is needed, ECG monitoring should be maintained during the initiation of therapy and at appropriate intervals during stabilization of dose.

Usage in Pregnancy—Pregnancy Category C. Surmontil has shown evidence of embryotoxicity and /or increased incidence of major anomalies in rats or rabbits at doses 20 times the human dose. There are no adequate and well-controlled studies in pregnant women. Surmontil should be used during pregnancy only if the potential benefit justifies the potential risk to the fetus.

Semen studies in man (four schizophrenics and nine normal volunteers) revealed no significant changes in sperm morphology. It is recognized that drugs having a parasympathetic effect including tricyclic antidepressants, may alter the ejaculatory response.

Chronic animal studies showed occasional evidence of degeneration of seminiferous tubules at the highest dose of 60 mg/kg/day.

Surmontil should be used with caution in patients with impaired liver function.

Chronic animal studies showed occasional occurrence of hepatic congestion, fatty infiltration, or increased serum liver enzymes at the highest dose of 60 mg/kg/day.

Both elevation and lowering of blood sugar have been reported with tricyclic antidepressants.

ADVERSE REACTIONS

Note: The pharmacological similarities among the tricyclic antidepressants require that each of the reactions be considered when Surmontil (trimipramine maleate) is administered. Some of the adverse reactions included in this listing have not in fact been reported with Surmontil.

Cardiovascular—Hypotension, hypertension, tachycardia, palpitation, myocardial infarction, arrhythmias, heart block, stroke.

Psychiatric—Confusional states (especially the elderly) with hallucinations, disorientation, delusions; anxiety, restlessness, agitation; insomnia and nightmares; hypomania; exacerbation of psychosis.

Neurological—Numbness, tingling, paresthesias of extremities; incoordination, ataxia, tremors, peripheral neuropathy; extrapyramidal symptoms; seizures, alterations in EEG patterns; tinnitus; syndrome of inappropriate ADH (antidiuretic hormone) secretion.

Anticholinergic—Dry mouth and, rarely, associated sublingual adenitis; blurred vision, disturbances of accommodation, mydriasis, constipation, paralytic ileus; urinary retention, delayed micturition, dilation of the urinary tract.

Allergic—Skin rash, petechiae, urticaria, itching, photosensitization, edema of face and tongue.

Hematologic—Bone-marrow depression including agranulocytosis, eosinophilia; purpura; thrombocytopenia. Leukocyte and differential counts should be performed in any patient who develops fever and sore throat during therapy; the drug should be discontinued if there is evidence of pathological neutrophil depression.

Gastrointestinal—Nausea and vomiting, anorexia, epigastric distress, diarrhea, peculiar taste, stomatitis, abdominal cramps, black tongue.

Endocrine—Gynecomastia in the male; breast enlargement and galactorrhea in the female; increased or decreased libido, impotence; testicular swelling; elevation or depression of blood-sugar levels.

Other—Jaundice (simulating obstructive); altered liver function; weight gain or loss; perspiration; flushing; urinary frequency; drowsiness, dizziness, weakness, and fatigue; headache; parotid swelling; alopecia.

Withdrawal Symptoms—Though not indicative of addiction, abrupt cessation of treatment after prolonged therapy may produce nausea, headache, and malaise.

DOSAGE AND ADMINISTRATION

Dosage should be initiated at a low level and increased gradually, noting carefully the clinical response and any evidence of intolerance.

Lower dosages are recommended for elderly patients and adolescents. Lower dosages are also recommended for outpatients as compared to hospitalized patients who will be under close supervision. It is not possible to prescribe a single dosage schedule of Surmontil that will be therapeutically effective in all patients. The physical psychodynamic factors contributing to depressive symtomatology are very complex; spontaneous remissions or exacerbations of depressive symptoms may occur with or without drug therapy. Consequently, the recommended dosage regimens are furnished as a guide which may be modified by factors such as the age of the patient, chronicity and severity of the disease, medical condition of the patient, and degree of psychotherapeutic support.

Most antidepressant drugs have a lag period of ten days to four weeks before a therapeutic response is noted. Increasing the dose will not shorten this period but rather increase the incidence of adverse reactions.

Usual Adult Dose:

Outpatients and Office Patients—Initially, 75 mg/day in divided doses, increased to 150 mg/day. Dosages over 200 mg/day are not recommended. Maintenance therapy is in the range of 50 to 150 mg/day. For convenient therapy and to facilitate patient compliance, the total dosage requirement may be given at bedtime.

Hospitalized Patients—Initially, 100 mg/day in divided doses. This may be increased gradually in a few days to 200 mg/day, depending upon individual response and tolerance. If improvement does not occur in 2–3 weeks, the dose may be increased to the maximum recommended dose of 250–300 mg/day.

Adolescent and Geriatric Patients—Initially, a dose of 50 mg/day is recommended, with gradual increments up to 100 mg/day, depending upon patient response and tolerance.

Maintenance—Following remission, maintenance medication may be required for a longer period of time, at the lowest dose that will maintain remission. Maintenance therapy is preferably administered as a single dose at bedtime. To minimize relapse, maintenance therapy should be continued for about three months.

Continued on next page

Wyeth—Cont.

OVERDOSAGE

Signs and Symptoms—The response of the patient to toxic overdosage of tricyclic antidepressants may vary in severity and is conditioned by factors such as age, amount ingested, amount absorbed, interval between ingestion and start of treatment. Surmontil (trimipramine maleate) is not recommended for infants or young children. Should accidental ingestion occur in any amount, it should be regarded as serious and potentially fatal.

CNS abnormalities may include drowsiness, stupor, coma, ataxia, restlessness, agitation, hyperactive reflexes, muscle rigidity, athetoid and choreiform movements, and convulsions. Cardiac abnormalities may include arrhythmia, tachycardia, ECG evidence of impaired conduction, and signs of congestive failure. Other symptoms may include respiratory depression, cyanosis, hypotension, shock, vomiting, hyperpyrexia, mydriasis, and diaphoresis.

Treatment is supportive and symptomatic as no specific antidote is known. Depending upon need the following measures can be considered:

1. Surmontil is not recommended for use in infants and children. Hospitalization with continuous cardiac monitoring for up to 4 days is recommended for children who have ingested Surmontil in any amount. This is based on the reported greater sensitivity of children to acute overdosage with tricyclic antidepressants.
2. Blood and urine levels may not reflect the severity of the poisoning and are mostly of diagnostic value.
3. CNS involvement, respiratory depression, or cardiac arrhythmia can occur suddenly; hospitalization and close observation are necessary, even when the amount ingested is thought to be small or initial toxicity appears slight. Patients with any alteration of ECG should have continuous cardiac monitoring for at least 72 hours and be observed until well after the cardiac status has returned to normal; relapses may occur after apparent recovery.
4. The slow intravenous administration of physostigmine salicylate has been reported to reverse most of the cardiovascular and CNS effects of overdosage with tricyclic antidepressants. In adults, 1 to 3 mg has been reported to be effective. In children, start with 0.5 mg and repeat at 5-minute intervals to determine the minimum effective dose; do not exceed 2.0 mg. Avoid rapid injection, to reduce the possibility of physostigmine-induced convulsions. Because of the short duration of action of physostigmine, it may be necessary to repeat doses to 30- to 60-minute intervals as necessary.
5. In the alert patient, empty the stomach rapidly by induced emesis, followed by lavage. In the obtunded patient, secure the airway with a cuffed endotracheal tube before beginning lavage (do not induce emesis). Instillation of activated-charcoal slurry may help reduce absorption of trimipramine.
6. Minimize external stimulation to reduce the tendency to convulsions. If anticonvulsants are necessary, diazepam, short-acting barbiturates, paraldehyde, or methocarbamol may be useful. Do not use barbiturates if MAO inhibitors have been taken recently.
7. Maintain adequate respiratory exchange. Do not use respiratory stimulants.
8. Shock should be treated with supportive measures, such as intravenous fluids, oxygen, and corticosteroids. Digitalis may increase conduction abnormalities and further irritate an already sensitized myocardium. If congestive heart failure necessitates rapid digitalization, particular care must be exercised.
9. Hyperpyrexia should be controlled by whatever external means available, including ice packs and cooling sponge baths if necessary.
10. Hemodialysis, peritoneal dialysis, exchange transfusions, and forced diuresis have been generally reported as ineffective in tricyclic poisoning.

HOW SUPPLIED

Surmontil® (trimipramine maleate) Capsules, Wyeth®, are available in the following dosage strengths:

25 mg, NDC 0008-4132, opaque blue and yellow capsule marked "WYETH" and "4132", in bottles of 100 capsules and in Redipak® cartons of 100 capsules (20 strips of 5).

50 mg, NDC 0008-4133, opaque blue and orange capsule marked "WYETH" and "4133", in bottles of 100 capsules and in Redipak cartons of 100 capsules (20 strips of 5).

100 mg, NDC 0008-4158, opaque blue and white capsule marked "WYETH" and "4158", in bottles of 100 capsules.

Keep tightly closed.

Dispense in tight container.

The appearance of these capsules is a trademark of Wyeth Laboratories.

Shown in Product Identification Section, page 436

SYNALGOS®-DC Capsules Ⓒ ℞

[*sĭn 'al "gōs*]

DESCRIPTION

Each blue and gray capsule contains:

Drocode (dihydrocodeine) bitartrate .... 16 mg
Warning—May be habit forming

Aspirin .... 356.4 mg

Caffeine .... 30 mg

The inactive ingredients present are alginic acid, cellulose, D&C Red 28, FD&C Blue 1, gelatin, iron oxides, stearic acid, and titanium dioxide.

ACTIONS

Dihydrocodeine is a semisynthetic narcotic analgesic, related to codeine, with multiple actions qualitatively similar to those of codeine; the most prominent of these involve the central nervous system and organs with smooth-muscle components. The principal action of therapeutic value is analgesia.

Synalgos-DC also contains the non-narcotic antipyretic-analgesic, aspirin.

INDICATIONS

For the relief of moderate to moderately severe pain.

CONTRAINDICATIONS

Hypersensitivity to dihydrocodeine, codeine, or aspirin.

WARNINGS

Salicylates should be used with extreme caution in the presence of peptic ulcer or coagulation abnormalities.

Drug Dependence: Dihydrocodeine can produce drug dependence of the codeine type and therefore has the potential of being abused. Psychic dependence, physical dependence, and tolerance may develop upon repeated administration of dihydrocodeine, and it should be prescribed and administered with the same degree of caution appropriate to the use of other oral narcotic containing medications.

Like other narcotic-containing medications, dihydrocodeine is subject to the provisions of the Federal Controlled Substances Act.

Usage in Ambulatory Patients: Dihydrocodeine and may impair the mental and/or physical abilities required for the performance of potentially hazardous tasks such as driving a car or operating machinery. The patient using Synalgos-DC should be cautioned accordingly.

Interactions with other Central-Nervous-System Depressants: Patients receiving other narcotic analgesics, general anesthetics, tranquilizers, sedative-hypnotics or other CNS depressants (including alcohol) concomitantly with Synalgos-DC may exhibit an additive CNS depression. When such combined therapy is contemplated, the dose of one or both agents should be reduced.

Usage in Pregnancy: Reproduction studies have not been performed in animals. There is no adequate information on whether this drug may affect fertility in human males and females or has a teratogenic potential or other adverse effect on the fetus.

Usage in Children: Since there is no experience in children who have received this drug, safety and efficacy in children have not been established.

PRECAUTIONS

Synalgos-DC should be given with caution to certain patients such as the elderly or debilitated.

ADVERSE REACTIONS

The most frequently observed reactions include light-headedness, dizziness, drowsiness, sedation, nausea, vomiting, constipation, pruritus, and skin reactions.

DOSAGE AND ADMINISTRATION

Dosage should be adjusted according to the severity of the pain and the response of the patient. Synalgos-DC is given orally. The usual adult dose is two capsules every 4 hours as needed for pain.

DRUG INTERACTIONS

The CNS depressant effects of Synalgos-DC may be additive with that of other CNS depressants.

See Warnings.

Aspirin may enhance the effects of anticoagulants and inhibit the uricosuric effects of uricosuric agents.

HOW SUPPLIED

Synalgos®-DC Capsules, Ives®, are supplied in bottles of 100 and 500 capsules and in Clinipak® Unit Dose dispenser cartons of 25 capsules (DEA Schedule III):

NDC 0082-4191, blue and gray capsule marked "Ives" and "4191".

Store capsules below 25°C (77°F).

Keep bottles tightly closed.

Dispense in tight containers.

Shown in Product Identification Section, page 436

TETANUS AND DIPHTHERIA TOXOIDS ADSORBED for Adult Use ℞

[*tet 'ah-nus and dif-the 're-ah tok 'soids*]

aluminum phosphate adsorbed

ULTRAFINED®

DESCRIPTION

A combination of refined tetanus and diphtheria toxoids for adult use, in which the fully potent antigens are adsorbed on aluminum phosphate. The preservative is 0.01% thimerosal (mercury derivative). Each dose contains no more than 2 Lf of purified diphtheria toxoid.

HOW SUPPLIED

Tetanus and Diphtheria Toxoids Adsorbed **for Adult Use**, Aluminum Phosphate Adsorbed, Ultrafined®, is available in vials of 5 mL and 0.5 mL TUBEX® Sterile Cartridge-Needle Units, packaged in cartons of 10 TUBEX.

For prescribing information write to Professional Service, Wyeth Laboratories, Box 8299, Philadelphia, PA 19101, or contact your local Wyeth representative.

TETANUS TOXOID ADSORBED ℞

[*tet 'ah-nus tok 'soid*]

aluminum phosphate adsorbed,

ULTRAFINED®

DESCRIPTION

A refined toxoid, in which the antigen is adsorbed on aluminum phosphate. The preservative is 0.01% thimerosal (mercury derivative).

HOW SUPPLIED

Vials of 5 ml.; and 0.5-ml. TUBEX ® Sterile Cartridge-Needle Units, packages of 10.

For prescribing information write to Professional Service, Wyeth Laboratories, Box 8299, Philadelphia, PA 19101, or contact your local Wyeth representative.

TETANUS TOXOID ℞

[*tet 'ahnus tok 'soid*]

fluid, purified

ULTRAFINED®

DESCRIPTION

A refined tetanus toxoid. The preservative is 0.01% thimerosal (mercury derivative).

HOW SUPPLIED

Vials of 7.5 ml.; and 0.5-ml. TUBEX® Sterile Cartridge-Needle Units, packages of 10.

For prescribing information write to Professional Service, Wyeth Laboratories, Box 8299, Philadelphia, PA 19101, or contact your local Wyeth representative.

TRECATOR®-SC ℞

[*trek "ă 'tōre*]

(ethionamide)

Sugar-Coated Tablets

DESCRIPTION

Ethionamide is a yellow crystalline substance that is practically insoluble in water. It has a faint-to-moderate sulfide odor and is stable at all ordinary temperatures and levels of humidity.

Trecator-SC tablets contain 250 mg ethionamide. The inactive ingredients present are acacia, calcium carbonate, confectioners sugar, FD&C Red 3, FD&C Yellow 6, gelatin, lactose, magnesium stearate, methylcellulose, pharmaceutical glaze, polacrilin potassium, sucrose, talc, and titanium dioxide.

Trecator has the following structural formula:

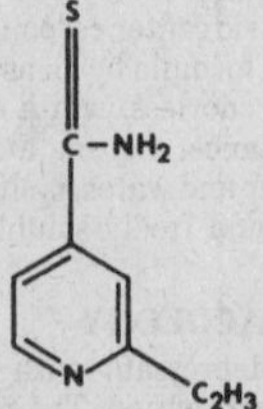

ACTION

Bacteriostatic against *Mycobacterium tuberculosis.*

INDICATIONS

Failure after adequate treatment with primary drugs (i.e., isoniazid, streptomycin, aminosalicylic acid) in any form of active tuberculosis. Ethionamide should only be given with other effective antituberculous agents.

CONTRAINDICATIONS
Severe hypersensitivity.
Severe hepatic damage.

WARNING
USE IN PREGNANCY: Teratogenic effects have been demonstrated in animals (rabbits, rats) receiving doses in excess of those recommended in humans. Use of the drug should be avoided during pregnancy or in women of childbearing potential, unless the benefits outweigh its possible hazard.
USE IN CHILDREN: Optimum dosage for children has not been established. This, however, does not preclude use of the drug when its use is crucial to therapy.

PRECAUTIONS
Pretreatment examinations should include *in vitro* susceptibility tests of recent cultures of *M. tuberculosis* from the patient as measured against ethionomide and the usual primary antituberculous drugs.
Determinations of serum transaminase (SGOT, SGPT) should be made prior to and every 2 to 4 weeks during therapy.
In patients with diabetes mellitus, management may be more difficult and hepatitis occurs more frequently.
Ethionamide may intensify the adverse effects of the other antituberculous drugs administered concomitantly. Convulsions have been reported and special care should be taken, particularly when ethionamide is administered with cycloserine.

ADVERSE REACTIONS
The most common side effect is gastrointestinal intolerance.
Other adverse effects similar to those seen with isoniazid have been reported: peripheral neuritis, optic neuritis, psychic disturbances (including mental depression), postural hypotension, skin rashes, thrombocytopenia, pellagra-like syndrome, jaundice and/or hepatitis, increased difficulty in management of diabetes mellitus, stomatitis, gynecomastia, and impotence.

DOSAGE AND ADMINISTRATION
Ethionamide should be administered with at least one other effective antituberculous drug.
Average adult dose: 0.5 gram to 1.0 gram/day in divided doses.
Concomitant administration of pyridoxine is recommended.

HOW SUPPLIED
Trecator®-SC (ethionamide) Tablets, Wyeth®, are supplied in bottles of 100 tablets as follows:
250 mg, NDC 0008-4130, orange, sugar-coated tablet marked "WYETH" and "4130".
Keep tightly closed
Dispense in tight container.

TRIPHASIL®-21 ℞
[tri-fa'sil]
Tablets
(levonorgestrel and ethinyl estradiol tablets—triphasic regimen)

DESCRIPTION
Each Triphasil cycle of 21 tablets consists of three different drug phases as follows: Phase 1 comprised of 6 brown tablets, each containing 0.050 mg of levonorgestrel (d(-)-13 beta-ethyl-17-alpha-ethinyl-17-beta-hydroxygon-4-en-3-one), a totally synthetic progestogen, and 0.030 mg of ethinyl estradiol (19-nor-17α-pregna-1,3,5(10)-trien-10-yne-3,17-diol); phase 2 comprised of 5 white tablets, each containing 0.075 mg levonorgestrel and 0.040 mg ethinyl estradiol; and, phase 3 comprised of 10 light-yellow tablets, each containing 0.125 mg levonorgestrel and 0.030 mg ethinyl estradiol. The inactive ingredients present are calcium carbonate, glycerin, iron oxides, lactose, magnesium stearate, methylparaben, polyethylene glycol, povidone, propylparaben, sodium benzoate, starch, sucrose, talc, and titanium dioxide.

Levonorgestrel

Ethinyl Estradiol

CLINICAL PHARMACOLOGY
Combination oral contraceptives act primarily through the mechanism of gonadotropin suppression due to the estrogenic and progestational activity of the ingredients. Although the primary mechanism of action is inhibition of ovulation, alterations in the genital tract, including changes in the cervical mucus (which increase the difficulty of sperm penetration) and the endometrium (which reduce the likelihood of implantation), may also contribute to contraceptive effectiveness.

INDICATIONS AND USAGE
Triphasil Tablets are indicated for the prevention of pregnancy in women who elect to use oral contraceptives as a method of contraception.
Oral contraceptives are highly effective. The pregnancy rate in women using conventional combination oral contraceptives (containing 35 mcg or more of ethinyl estradiol or 50 mcg or more of mestranol) is generally reported as less than one pregnancy per 100 woman-years of use. Slightly higher rates (somewhat more than 1 pregnancy per 100 woman-years of use) are reported for some combination products containing 35 mcg or less of ethinyl estradiol, and rates on the order of 3 pregnancies per 100 woman-years are reported for the progestogen-only oral contraceptives.
These rates are derived from separate studies conducted by different investigators in several population groups and cannot be compared precisely. Furthermore, pregnancy rates tend to be lower as clinical studies are continued, possibly due to selective retention in the longer studies of those patients who accept the treatment regimen and do not discontinue as a result of adverse reactions, pregnancy, or other reasons.
In clinical trials with Triphasil Tablets, 3,546 patients completed 35,036 cycles, and a total of nine pregnancies were reported. This represents a pregnancy rate of 0.33 per 100 woman-years. When used as directed, two pregnancies resulted for a corrected pregnancy rate of 0.07 per 100 woman-years.
Table 1 gives ranges of pregnancy rates reported in the literature[1] for other means of contraception. The efficacy of these means of contraception (except the IUD) depends upon the degree of adherence to the method.
TABLE 1
PREGNANCIES PER 100 WOMAN-YEARS
IUD, less than 1–6; Diaphragm with spermicidal products (creams or jellies), 2–20; Condom, 3–36; Aerosol foams, 2–29; Jellies and creams, 4–36;
Periodic abstinence (rhythm) all types, less than 1–47:
1. Calendar method, 14–47;
2. Temperature method, 1–20;
3. Temperature method—intercourse only in postovulatory phase, less than 1–7;
4. Mucus method, 1–25;

No contraception, 60–80.
Dose-Related Risk of Thromboembolism from Oral Contraceptives: Two studies have shown a positive association between the dose of estrogens in oral contraceptives and the risk of thromboembolism.[2,3] For this reason, it is prudent and in keeping with good principles of therapeutics to minimize exposure to estrogen. The oral-contraceptive product prescribed for any given patient should be that product which contains the least amount of estrogen that is compatible with an acceptable pregnancy rate and patient acceptance. It is recommended that new acceptors of oral contraceptives be started on preparations containing 0.05 mg or less of estrogen.

CONTRAINDICATIONS
Oral contraceptives should not be used in women with any of the following conditions:
1. Thrombophlebitis or thromboembolic disorders.
2. A past history of deep-vein thrombophlebitis or thromboembolic disorders.
3. Cerebral-vascular or coronary-artery disease.
4. Known or suspected carcinoma of the breast.
5. Known or suspected estrogen-dependent neoplasia.
6. Undiagnosed abnormal genital bleeding.
7. Known or suspected pregnancy (see Warning No. 5).
8. Benign or malignant liver tumor which developed during the use of oral contraceptives or other estrogen-containing products.

WARNINGS
Cigarette smoking increases the risk of serious cardiovascular side effects from oral-contraceptive use. This risk increases with age and with heavy smoking (15 or more cigarettes per day) and is quite marked in women over 35 years of age. Women who use oral contraceptives should be strongly advised not to smoke.
The use of oral contraceptives is associated with increased risk of several serious conditions, including thromboembolism, stroke, myocardial infarction, hepatic adenoma, gallbladder disease, hypertension. Practitioners prescribing oral contraceptives should be familiar with the following information relating to these risks.

1. *Thromboembolic Disorders and Other Vascular Problems:* An increased risk of thromboembolic and thrombotic disease associated with the use of oral contraceptives is well-established. Three principal studies in Great Britain[4–6] and three in the United States[7–10] have demonstrated an increased risk of fatal and nonfatal venous thromboembolism and stroke, both hemorrhagic and thrombotic. These studies estimate that users of oral contraceptives are 4 to 11 times more likely than nonusers to develop these diseases without evident cause (Table 2).
CEREBROVASCULAR DISORDERS
In a collaborative American study[9,10] of cerebrovascular disorders in women with and without predisposing causes, it was estimated that the risk of hemorrhagic stroke was 2.0 times greater in users than nonusers and the risk of thrombotic stroke was 4 to 9.5 times greater in users than in nonusers (Table 2).
TABLE 2
SUMMARY OF RELATIVE RISK OF THROMBOEMBOLIC DISORDERS AND OTHER VASCULAR PROBLEMS IN ORAL-CONTRACEPTIVE USERS COMPARED TO NONUSERS

	Relative risk, times greater
Idiopathic thromboembolic disease	4–11
Postsurgery thromboembolic complications	4–6
Thrombotic stroke	4–9.5
Hemorrhagic stroke	2
Myocardial infarction	2–12

MYOCARDIAL INFARCTION
An increased risk of myocardial infarction associated with the use of oral contraceptives has been reported,[11–13] confirming a previously suspected association. These studies, conducted in the United Kingdom, found, as expected, that the greater the number of underlying risk factors for coronary-artery disease (cigarette smoking, hypertension, hypercholesterolemia, obesity, diabetes, history of preeclamptic toxemia) the higher the risk of developing myocardial infarction, regardless of whether the patient was an oral-contraceptive user or not. Oral contraceptives, however, were found to be a clear additional risk factor.
In terms of relative risk, it has been estimated[52] that oral-contraceptive users who do not smoke (smoking is considered a major predisposing condition to myocardial infarction) are about twice as likely to have a fatal myocardial infarction as nonusers who do not smoke. Oral-contraceptive users who are also smokers have about a 5-fold increased risk of fatal infarction compared to users who do not smoke, but about a 10- to 12-fold increased risk compared to nonusers who do not smoke. Furthermore, the amount of smoking is also an important factor. In determining the importance of these relative risks, however, the baseline rates for various age groups, as shown in Table 3, must be given serious consideration. The importance of other predisposing conditions mentioned above in determining relative and absolute risks has not as yet been quantified; it is quite likely that the same synergistic action exists, but perhaps to a lesser extent.
TABLE 3
Estimated annual mortality rate per 100,000 women from myocardial infarction by use of oral contraceptives, smoking habits, and age (in years):

	Myocardial infarction			
	Women aged 30–39		Women aged 40–44	
Smoking habits	Users	Non-users	Users	Non-users
All smokers	10.2	2.6	62.0	15.9
Heavy*	13.0	5.1	78.7	31.3
Light	4.7	0.9	28.6	5.7
Nonsmokers	1.8	1.2	10.7	7.4
Smokers and nonsmokers	5.4	1.9	32.8	11.7

*Heavy smoker: 15 or more cigarettes per day.
From JAIN, A.K., *Studies in Family Planning, 8*:50, 1977
RISK OF DOSE
In an analysis of data derived from several national adverse-reaction reporting systems,[2] British investigators concluded that the risk of thromboembolism, including coronary thrombosis, is directly related to the dose of estrogen used in oral contraceptives. Preparations containing 100 mcg or more of estrogen were associated with a higher risk of thromboembolism than those containing 50–80 mcg of estrogen. Their analysis did suggest, however, that the quantity of estrogen may not be the sole factor involved. This finding has been confirmed in the United States.[3] Careful epidemiologi-

Continued on next page

Wyeth—Cont.

cal studies to determine the degree of thromboembolic risk associated with progestogen-only oral contraceptives have not been performed. Cases of thromboembolic disease have been reported in women using these products, and they should not be presumed to be free of excess risk.

ESTIMATE OF EXCESS MORTALITY FROM CIRCULATORY DISEASES

A large prospective study[53] carried out in the U.K. estimated the mortality rate per 100,000 women per year from diseases of the circulatory system for users and nonusers of oral contraceptives according to age, smoking habits, and duration of use. The overall excess death rate annually from circulatory diseases for oral-contraceptive users was estimated to be 20 per 100,000 (ages 15–34—5/100,000; ages 35–44—33/100,000; ages 45–49—140/100,000), the risk being concentrated in older women, in those with a long duration of use, and in cigarette smokers. It was not possible, however, to examine the interrelationships of age, smoking, and duration of use, nor to compare the effects of continuous vs. intermittent use. Although the study showed a 10-fold increase in death due to circulatory diseases in users for 5 or more years, all of these deaths occurred in women 35 or older. Until larger numbers of women under 35 with continuous use for 5 or more years are available, it is not possible to assess the magnitude of the relative risk for this younger age group.

The available data from a variety of sources have been analyzed[14] to estimate the risk of death associated with various methods of contraception. The estimates of risk of death for each method include the combined risk of the contraceptive method (e.g., thromboembolic and thrombotic disease in the case of oral contraceptives) plus the risk attributable to pregnancy or abortion in the event of method failure. This latter risk varies with the effectiveness of the contraceptive method. The findings of this analysis are shown in the bar graph (Figure 1).[14] The study concluded that the mortality associated with all methods of birth control is low and below that associated with childbirth, with the exception of oral contraceptives in women over 40 who smoke. (The rates given for Pill only/smokers for each age group are for smokers as a class. For "heavy" smokers [more than 15 cigarettes a day], the rates given would be about double; for "light" smokers [less than 15 cigarettes a day], about 50 percent.) The lowest mortality is associated with the condom or diaphragm backed up by early abortion. The risk of thromboembolic and thrombotic disease associated with oral contraceptives increases with age after approximately age 30 and, for myocardial infarction, is further increased by hypertension, hypercholesterolemia, obesity, diabetes, or history of preeclamptic toxemia and especially by cigarette smoking.

Figure 1. Estimated annual number of deaths associated with control of fertility and no control per 100,000 nonsterile women, by regimen of control and age of woman.

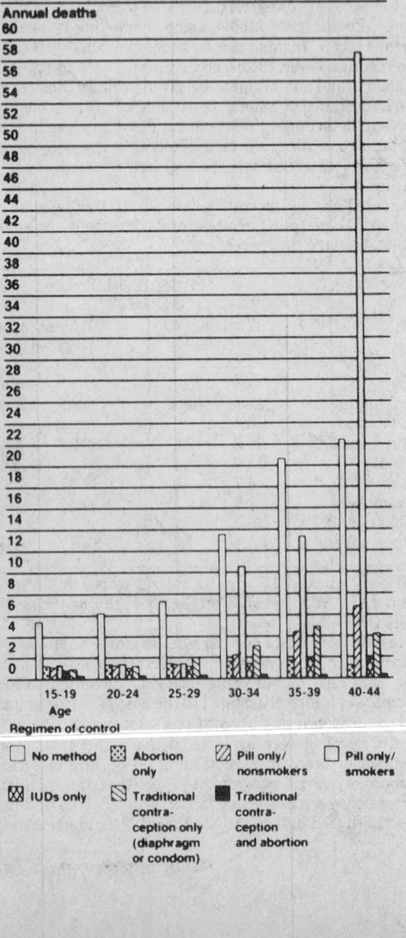

Annual deaths (0–60); Age: 15-19, 20-24, 25-29, 30-34, 35-39, 40-44

Regimen of control: No method; Abortion only; Pill only/nonsmokers; Pill only/smokers; IUDs only; Traditional contraception only (diaphragm or condom); Traditional contraception and abortion

Based on the data currently available, the following chart gives a gross estimate of the risk of death from circulatory disorders associated with the use of oral contraceptives:

SMOKING HABITS AND OTHER PREDISPOSING CONDITIONS—RISK ASSOCIATED WITH USE OF ORAL CONTRACEPTIVES

Age	Below 30	30–39	40+
Heavy smokers	C	B	A
Light smokers	D	C	B
Nonsmokers (no predisposing conditions)	D	C,D	C
Nonsmokers (other predisposing conditions)	C	C,B	B,A

A—Use associated with very high risk.
B—Use associated with high risk.
C—Use associated with moderate risk.
D—Use associated with low risk.

The physician and the patient should be alert to the earliest manifestations of thromboembolic and thrombotic disorders (e.g., thrombophlebitis, pulmonary embolism, cerebrovascular insufficiency, coronary occlusion, retinal thrombosis, and mesenteric thrombosis). Should any of these occur or be suspected, the drug should be discontinued immediately.

A four- to six-fold increased risk of postsurgery thromboembolic complications has been reported in oral-contraceptive users.[15,16] If feasible, oral contraceptives should be discontinued at least 4 weeks before surgery of a type associated with an increased risk of thromboembolism or prolonged immobilization.

PERSISTENCE OF RISK OF VASCULAR DISORDERS

Findings from one study in Great Britain involving cerebrovascular disease[54] and another study in the United States concerning myocardial infarction[55] suggest that an increased risk of these conditions in users of oral contraceptives persists after discontinuation of the oral contraceptive. In the British study, the risk of cerebrovascular disease remained elevated in former oral-contraceptive users for at least six years after discontinuation. In the U.S. study, an increased risk of myocardial infarction persisted for at least 9 years in women 40- to 49-years-old who had used oral contraceptives for five or more years. The findings in both these studies require confirmation since they are inconsistent with other published information.[9,11,13,56–60]

2. *Ocular Lesions:*

There have been reports of neuro-ocular lesions such as optic neuritis or retinal thrombosis associated with the use of oral contraceptives. Discontinue oral-contraceptive medication if there is unexplained, sudden or gradual, partial or complete loss of vision; onset of proptosis or diplopia; papilledema; or retinal-vascular lesions, and institute appropriate diagnostic and therapeutic measures.

3. *Carcinoma:*

Long-term continuous administration of either natural or synthetic estrogen in certain animal species increases the frequency of carcinoma of the breast, cervix, vagina, and liver. Certain synthetic progestogens, none currently contained in oral contraceptives, have been noted to increase the incidence of mammary nodules, benign and malignant, in dogs.

In humans, three case-control studies have reported an increased risk of endometrial carcinoma associated with the prolonged use of exogenous estrogen in postmenopausal women.[17–19] One publication[20] reported on the first 21 cases submitted by physicians to a registry of cases of adenocarcinoma of the endometrium in women under 40 on oral contraceptives. Of the cases found in women without predisposing risk factors for adenocarcinoma of the endometrium (e.g., irregular bleeding at the time oral contraceptives were first given, polycystic ovaries), nearly all occurred in women who had used a sequential oral contraceptive. These products are no longer marketed. No evidence has been reported suggesting an increased risk of endometrial cancer in users of conventional combination or progestogen-only oral contraceptives.

Several studies[8,21–24] have found no increase in breast cancer in women taking oral contraceptives or estrogens. One study,[25] however, while also noting no overall increased risk of breast cancer in women treated with oral contraceptives, found an excess risk in the subgroups of oral-contraceptive users with documented benign breast disease. A reduced occurrence of benign breast tumors in users of oral contraceptives has been well-documented.[8,21,25–27]

In summary, there is at present no confirmed evidence from human studies of an increased risk of cancer associated with oral contraceptives. Close clinical surveillance of all women taking oral contraceptives is, nevertheless, essential. In all cases of undiagnosed persistent or recurrent abnormal vaginal bleeding, appropriate diagnostic measures should be taken to rule out malignancy. Women with a strong family history of breast cancer or who have breast nodules, fibrocystic disease, or abnormal mammograms should be monitored with particular care if they elect to use oral contraceptives instead of other methods of contraception.

4. *Hepatic Tumors:*

Benign hepatic adenomas have been found to be associated with the use of oral contraceptives.[28–30,46] One study[46] showed that oral contraceptive formulations with high hormonal potency were associated with a higher risk than lower potency formulations. Although benign, hepatic adenomas may rupture and may cause death through intra-abdominal hemorrhage. This has been reported in short-term as well as long-term users of oral contraceptives. Two studies relate risk with duration of use of the contraceptive, the risk being much greater after 4 or more years of oral-contraceptive use.[30,46] While hepatic adenoma is a rare lesion, it should be considered in women presenting abdominal pain and tenderness, abdominal mass or shock. A few cases of hepatocellular carcinoma have been reported in women taking oral contraceptives. The relationship of these drugs to this type of malignancy is not known at this time.

5. *Use in or Immediately Preceding Pregnancy, Birth Defects in Offspring, and Malignancy in Female Offspring:*

The use of female sex hormones—both estrogenic and progestational agents—during early pregnancy may seriously damage the offspring. It has been shown that females exposed in utero to diethylstilbestrol, a nonsteroidal estrogen, have an increased risk of developing in later life a form of vaginal or cervical cancer that is ordinarily extremely rare.[31,32] This risk has been estimated to be of the order of 1 in 1,000 exposures or less.[33,47] Although there is no evidence at the present time that oral contraceptives further enhance the risk of developing this type of malignancy, such patients should be monitored with particular care if they elect to use oral contraceptives instead of other methods of contraception. Furthermore, a high percentage of such exposed women (from 30 to 90%) have been found to have epithelial changes of the vagina and cervix.[34–38] Although these changes are histologically benign, it is not known whether this condition is a precursor of vaginal malignancy. Male children so exposed may develop abnormalities of the urogenital tract.[48–50] Although similar data are not available with the use of other estrogens, it cannot be presumed that they would not induce similar changes.

An increased risk of congenital anomalies, including heart defects and limb defects, has been reported with the use of sex hormones, including oral contraceptives, in pregnancy.[39–42,51] One case-control study[42] has estimated a 4.7-fold increase in risk of limb-reduction defects in infants exposed in utero to sex hormones (oral contraceptives, hormonal withdrawal tests for pregnancy, or attempted treatment for threatened abortion). Some of these exposures were very short and involved only a few days of treatment. The data suggest that the risk of limb-reduction defects in exposed fetuses is somewhat less than one in 1,000 live births.

In the past, female sex hormones have been used during pregnancy in an attempt to treat threatened or habitual abortion. There is considerable evidence that estrogens are ineffective for these indications, and there is no evidence from well-controlled studies that progestogens are effective for these uses.

There is some evidence that triploidy and possibly other types of polyploidy are increased among abortuses from women who become pregnant soon after ceasing oral contraceptives.[43] Embryos with these anomalies are virtually always aborted spontaneously. Whether there is an overall increase in spontaneous abortion of pregnancies conceived soon after stopping oral contraceptives is unknown. It is recommended that, for any patient who has missed two consecutive periods, pregnancy should be ruled out before continuing the contraceptive regimen. If the patient has not adhered to the prescribed schedule, the possibility of pregnancy should be considered at the time of the first missed period (or after 45 days from the last menstrual period if the progestogen-only oral contraceptives are used), and further use of oral contraceptives should be withheld until pregnancy has been ruled out. If pregnancy is confirmed, the patient should be apprised of the potential risks to the fetus, and the advisability of continuation of the pregnancy should be discussed in the light of these risks.

It is also recommended that women who discontinue oral contraceptives with the intent of becoming pregnant use an alternate form of contraception for a period of time before attempting to conceive. Many clinicians recommend 3 months, although no precise information is available on which to base this recommendation.

The administration of progestogen-only or progestogen-estrogen combinations to induce withdrawal bleeding should not be used as a test of pregnancy.

6. *Gallbladder Disease:*

Studies[8,23,26] report an increased risk of surgically confirmed gallbladder disease in users of oral contraceptives and estrogens. In one study, an increased risk appeared after 2 years of use and doubled after 4 or 5 years of use. In one of the other studies, an increased risk was apparent between 6 and 12 months of use.

7. *Carbohydrate and Lipid Metabolic Effects:*
A decrease in glucose tolerance has been observed in a significant percentage of patients on oral contraceptives. For this reason, prediabetic and diabetic patients should be carefully observed while receiving oral contraceptives.
An increase in triglycerides and total phospholipids has been observed in patients receiving oral contraceptives.[44] Three studies[61,62,63] have been performed with the Triphasil Tablets (Levonorgestrel and Ethinyl Estradiol Tablets—Triphasic Regimen) formulation and no significant alterations in lipid metabolism were noted with the exception of a slight increase in triglyceride levels in one study.[62] The clinical significance of these findings remains to be defined.

8. *Elevated Blood Pressure:*
An increase in blood pressure has been reported in patients receiving oral contraceptives.[26] In some women, hypertension may occur within a few months of beginning oral-contraceptive use. In the first year of use, the prevalence of women with hypertension is low in users and may be no higher than that of a comparable group of nonusers. The prevalence in users increases, however, with longer exposure, and in the fifth year of use is two-and-a-half to three times the reported prevalence in the first year. Age is also strongly correlated with the development of hypertension in oral-contraceptive users. Women who previously have had hypertension during pregnancy may be more likely to develop elevation of blood pressure when given oral contraceptives. Hypertension that develops as a result of taking oral contraceptives usually returns to normal after discontinuing the drug.

9. *Headache:*
The onset or exacerbation of migraine or development of headache of a new pattern which is recurrent, persistent, or severe, requires discontinuation of oral contraceptives and evaluation of the cause.

10. *Bleeding Irregularities:*
Breakthrough bleeding, spotting, and amenorrhea are frequent reasons for patients discontinuing oral contraceptives. In breakthrough bleeding, as in all cases of irregular bleeding from the vagina, nonfunctional causes should be borne in mind. In undiagnosed persistent or recurrent abnormal bleeding from the vagina, adequate diagnostic measures are indicated to rule out pregnancy or malignancy. If pathology has been excluded, time or a change to another formulation may solve the problem. Changing to an oral contraceptive with a higher estrogen content, while potentially useful in minimizing menstrual irregularity, should be done only if necessary, since this may increase the risk of thromboembolic disease.
Women with a past history of oligomenorrhea or secondary amenorrhea or young women without regular cycles may have a tendency to remain anovulatory or to become amenorrheic after discontinuation of oral contraceptives. Women with these preexisting problems should be advised of this possibility and encouraged to use other contraceptive methods. Post-use anovulation, possibly prolonged, may also occur in women without previous irregularities.

11. *Ectopic Pregnancy:*
Ectopic as well as intrauterine pregnancy may occur in contraceptive failures. However, in progestogen-only oral contraceptive failures, the ratio of ectopic to intrauterine pregnancies is higher than in women who are not receiving oral contraceptives, since the drugs are more effective in preventing intrauterine than ectopic pregnancies.

12. *Breast-feeding:*
Oral contraceptives given in the postpartum period may interfere with lactation. There may be a decrease in the quantity and quality of the breast milk. Furthermore, a small fraction of the hormonal agents in oral contraceptives has been identified in the milk of mothers receiving these drugs.[45,64,65] The effects, if any, on the breast-fed child have not been determined. If feasible, the use of oral contraceptives should be deferred until the infant has been weaned.

PRECAUTIONS

GENERAL

1. A complete medical and family history should be taken prior to initiation of oral contraceptives. The pretreatment and periodic physical examinations should include special reference to blood pressure, breasts, abdomen and pelvic organs, including Papanicolaou smear and relevant laboratory tests. As a general rule, oral contraceptives should not be prescribed for longer than 1 year without another physical examination and PAP smear being performed.
2. Under the influence of estrogen-progestogen preparations, preexisting uterine leiomyomata may increase in size.
3. Patients with a history of psychic depression should be carefully observed and the drug discontinued if depression recurs to a serious degree.
Patients becoming significantly depressed while taking oral contraceptives should stop the medication and use an alternate method of contraception in an attempt to determine whether the symptom is drug-related.
4. Oral contraceptives may cause some degree of fluid retention. They should be prescribed with caution, and only with careful monitoring, in patients with conditions which might be aggravated by fluid retention, such as convulsive disorders, migraine syndrome, asthma, or cardiac or renal insufficiency.
5. Patients with a past history of jaundice during pregnancy have an increased risk of recurrence of jaundice while receiving oral-contraceptive therapy. If jaundice develops in any patient receiving such drugs, the medication should be discontinued.
6. Steroid hormones may be poorly metabolized in patients with impaired liver function and should be administered with caution in such patients.
7. Oral-contraceptive users may have disturbances in normal tryptophan metabolism which may result in a relative pyridoxine deficiency. The clinical significance of this is yet to be determined.
8. Serum folate levels may be depressed by oral-contraceptive therapy. Since the pregnant woman is predisposed to the development of folate deficiency and the incidence of folate deficiency increases with increasing gestation, it is possible that if a woman becomes pregnant shortly after stopping oral contraceptives, she may have a greater chance of developing folate deficiency and complications attributed to this deficiency.
9. The pathologist should be advised of oral-contraceptive therapy when relevant specimens are submitted.
10. Certain endocrine- and liver-function tests and blood components may be affected by estrogen-containing oral contraceptives:
a. Increased sulfobromophthalein retention.
b. Increased prothrombin and factors VII, VIII, IX, and X; decreased antithrombin 3; increased norepinephrine-induced platelet aggregability.
c. Increased thyroid-binding globulin (TBG) leading to increased circulating total-thyroid hormone, as measured by protein-bound iodine (PBI), T4 by column, or T4 by radioimmunoassay. Free T3 resin uptake is decreased, reflecting the elevated TBG; free T4 concentration is unaltered.
d. Decreased pregnanediol excretion.
e. Reduced response to metyrapone test.

INFORMATION FOR THE PATIENT

(See patient labeling which follows.)

DRUG INTERACTIONS

Reduced efficacy and increased incidence of breakthrough bleeding have been associated with concomitant use of rifampin. A similar association has been suggested with barbiturates, phenylbutazone, phenytoin sodium, ampicillin, and tetracycline.

CARCINOGENESIS

See "Warnings" section for information on the carcinogenic potential of oral contraceptives.

PREGNANCY

Pregnancy Category X. See "Contraindications" and "Warnings."

NURSING MOTHERS

See "Warnings."

ADVERSE REACTIONS

An increased risk of the following serious adverse reactions has been associated with the use of oral contraceptives (see "Warnings"):

Thrombophlebitis.
Pulmonary embolism.
Coronary thrombosis.
Cerebral thrombosis.
Cerebral hemorrhage.
Hypertension.
Gallbladder disease.
Benign hepatomas.
Congenital anomalies.

There is evidence of an association between the following conditions and the use of oral contraceptives, although additional confirmatory studies are needed:

Mesenteric thrombosis.
Neuro-ocular lesions, e.g., retinal thrombosis and optic neuritis.

The following adverse reactions have been reported in patients receiving oral contraceptives and are believed to be drug-related:

Nausea and/or vomiting, usually the most common adverse reactions, occur in approximately 10% or less of patients during the first cycle. Other reactions, as a general rule, are seen much less frequently or only occasionally.
Gastrointestinal symptoms (such as abdominal cramps and bloating).
Breakthrough bleeding.
Spotting.
Change in menstrual flow.
Dysmenorrhea.
Amenorrhea during and after treatment.
Temporary infertility after discontinuance of treatment.
Edema.
Chloasma or melasma which may persist.
Breast changes: tenderness, enlargement, and secretion.
Change in weight (increase or decrease).
Change in cervical erosion and cervical secretion.
Possible diminution in lactation when given immediately postpartum.
Cholestatic jaundice.
Migraine.
Increase in size of uterine leiomyomata.
Rash (allergic).
Mental depression.
Reduced tolerance to carbohydrates.
Vaginal candidiasis.
Change in corneal curvature (steepening).
Intolerance to contact lenses.

The following adverse reactions have been reported in users of oral contraceptives, and the association has been neither confirmed nor refuted:

Premenstrual-like syndrome.
Cataracts.
Changes in libido.
Chorea.
Changes in appetite.
Cystitis-like syndrome.
Headache.
Nervousness.
Dizziness.
Hirsutism.
Loss of scalp hair.
Erythema multiforme.
Erythema nodosum.
Hemorrhagic eruption.
Vaginitis.
Porphyria.
Hemolytic uremic syndrome.

ACUTE OVERDOSE

Serious ill effects have not been reported following acute ingestion of large doses of oral contraceptives by young children. Overdosage may cause nausea, and withdrawal bleeding may occur in females.

DOSAGE AND ADMINISTRATION

To achieve maximum contraceptive effectiveness, Triphasil-21 Tablets (Levonorgestrel and Ethinyl Estradiol Tablets—Triphasic Regimen) must be taken exactly as directed and at intervals not exceeding 24 hours. Triphasil-21 Tablets are a three-phase preparation. The dosage of Triphasil-21 Tablets is **one tablet daily** for 21 consecutive days per menstrual cycle in the following order: 6 brown tablets (phase 1), followed by 5 white tablets (phase 2), and then followed by the last 10 light-yellow tablets (phase 3), according to the prescribed schedule. Tablets are then discontinued for 7 days (three weeks on, one week off).
It is recommended that Triphasil-21 Tablets be taken at the same time each day, preferably after the evening meal or at bedtime. During the first cycle of medication, the patient should be instructed to take one Triphasil-21 Tablet daily in the order of 6 brown, 5 white and, finally, 10 light-yellow tablets for twenty-one (21) consecutive days, beginning on day one (1) of her menstrual cycle. (The first day of menstruation is day one.) The tablets are then discontinued for one week (7 days). Withdrawal bleeding usually occurs within 3 days following discontinuation of Triphasil-21 Tablets. (If Triphasil-21 Tablets is first taken later than the first day of the first menstrual cycle of medication or postpartum, contraceptive reliance should not be placed on Triphasil-21 Tablets until after the first 7 consecutive days of administration. The possibility of ovulation and conception prior to initiation of medication should be considered.)
When switching from another oral contraceptive, Triphasil-21 Tablets should be started on the first day of bleeding following the last tablet taken of the previous oral contraceptive.
The patient begins her next and all subsequent 21-day courses of Triphasil-21 Tablets on the same day of the week that she began her first course, following the same schedule: 21 days on—7 days off. She begins taking her brown tablets on the 8th day after discontinuance regardless of whether or not a menstrual period has occurred or is still in progress. Any time the next cycle of Triphasil-21 Tablets are started later than the 8th day, the patient should be protected by another means of contraception until she has taken a tablet daily for seven consecutive days.
If spotting or breakthrough bleeding occurs, the patient is instructed to continue on the same regimen. This type of bleeding is usually transient and without significance; however, if the bleeding is persistent or prolonged, the patient is advised to consult her physician. Although the occurrence of pregnancy is highly unlikely if Triphasil-21 Tablets are taken according to directions, if withdrawal bleeding does not occur, the possibility of pregnancy must be considered. If the patient has not adhered to the prescribed schedule

Continued on next page

Wyeth—Cont.

(missed one or more tablets or started taking them on a day later than she should have), the probability of pregnancy should be considered at the time of the first missed period and appropriate diagnostic measures taken before the medication is resumed. If the patient has adhered to the prescribed regimen and misses two consecutive periods, pregnancy should be ruled out before continuing the contraceptive regimen.

The patient should be instructed to take a missed tablet as soon as it is remembered. If two consecutive tablets are missed they should both be taken as soon as remembered. The next tablet should be taken at the usual time.

Any time the patient misses one or two tablets she should also use another method of contraception until she has taken a tablet daily for seven consecutive days. If breakthrough bleeding occurs following missed tablets it will usually be transient and of no consequence. While there is little likelihood of ovulation occurring if only one or two tablets are missed, the possibility of ovulation increases with each successive day that scheduled tablets are missed. If three consecutive tablets are missed, all medication should be discontinued and the remainder of the package discarded. A new package of Triphasil-21 Tablets should be started on the first day of the patient's next bleed after the last tablet was taken. An alternate means of contraception should be prescribed during the days without tablets and continued until the patient has taken a tablet daily for seven consecutive days. In the nonlactating mother, Triphasil-21 Tablets may be prescribed in the postpartum period either immediately or at the first postpartum examination whether or not menstruation has resumed.

HOW SUPPLIED

Triphasil®-21 Tablets (Levonorgestrel and Ethinyl Estradiol Tablets—Triphasic Regimen), Wyeth®, NDC 0008-2535, are available in packages of 3 compacts, and in packages of 6 compact refills; packages of 12 Pilpak® dispensers are also available for clinic use only. Each cycle contains 21 coated tablets as follows:

NDC 0008-0641, six brown tablets, each containing 0.050 mg levonorgestrel and 0.030 mg ethinyl estradiol;

NDC 0008-0642, five white tablets, each containing 0.075 mg levonorgestrel and 0.040 mg ethinyl estradiol; and

NDC 0008-0643, ten light-yellow tablets, each containing 0.125 mg levonorgestrel and 0.030 mg ethinyl estradiol.

REFERENCES

1. "*Population Reports,*" Series H, Number 2, May 1974; Series I, Number 1, June 1974; Series B, Number 2, January 1975; Series H, Number 3, 1975; Series H, Number 4, January 1976 (published by the Population Information Program, The George Washington University Medical Center, 2001 S St. NW., Washington, D.C.).
2. Inman, W. H. W., Vessey, M. P., Westerholm, B., and Engelund, A., "Thromboembolic disease and the steroidal content of oral contraceptives. A report to the Committee on Safety of Drugs," Brit Med J *2*:203–209, 1970.
3. Stolley, P. D., Tonascia, J. A., Tockman, M. S., Sartwell, P. E., Rutledge, A. H., and Jacobs, M. P., "Thrombosis with low-estrogen oral contraceptives," Am J Epidemiol *102*:197–208, 1975.
4. Royal College of General Practitioners, "Oral contraception and thromboembolic disease," J Coll Gen Pract *13*:267–279, 1967.
5. Inman, W. H. W., and Vessey, M. P., "Investigation of deaths from pulmonary, coronary and cerebral thrombosis and embolism in women of childbearing age," Brit Med J *2*:193–199, 1968.
6. Vessey, M. P., and Doll, R., "Investigation of relation between use of oral contraceptives and thromboembolic disease. A further report," Brit Med J *2*:651–657, 1969.
7. Sartwell, P. E., Masi, A. T., Arthes, F. G., Greene, G. R., and Smith, H. E., "Thromboembolism and oral contraceptives: an epidemiological case control study," Am J Epidemiol *90*:365–380, 1969.
8. Boston Collaborative Drug Surveillance Program, "Oral contraceptives and venous thromboembolic disease, surgically confirmed gallbladder disease and breast tumors," Lancet *1*:1399–1404, 1973.
9. Collaborative Group for the Study of Stroke in Young Women, "Oral contraception and increased risk of cerebral ischemia or thrombosis," N Engl J Med *288*:871–878, 1973.
10. Collaborative Group for the Study of Stroke in Young Women, "Oral contraceptives and stroke in young women: associated risk factors," JAMA *231*:718–722, 1975.
11. Mann, J. I., and Inman, W. H. W., "Oral contraceptives and death from myocardial infarction," Brit Med J *2*:245–248, 1975.
12. Mann, J. I., Inman, W. H. W., and Thorogood, M., "Oral contraceptive use in older women and fatal myocardial infarction," Brit Med J *2*:445–447, 1976.
13. Mann, J. I., Vessey, M. P., Thorogood, M., and Doll, R., "Myocardial infarction in young women with special reference to oral contraceptive practice," Brit Med J *2*:241–245, 1975.
14. Tietze, C., "New Estimates of Mortality Associated with Fertility Control," Family Planning Perspectives, *9*:74–76, 1977.
15. Vessey, M. P., Doll, R., Fairbairn, A. S., and Glober, G., "Post-operative thromboembolism and the use of oral contraceptives," Brit Med J *3*:123–126, 1970.
16. Greene, G. R., and Sartwell, P. E., "Oral contraceptive use in patients with thromboembolism following surgery, trauma, or infection," Am J Pub Health *62*:680–685, 1972.
17. Smith, D. C., Prentice, R., Thompson, D. J., and Herrmann, W. L., "Association of exogenous estrogen and endometrial carcinoma," N Engl J Med *293*:1164–1167, 1975.
18. Ziel, H. K., and Finkle, W. D., "Increased risk of endometrial carcinoma among users of conjugated estrogens," N Engl J Med *293*:1167–1170, 1975.
19. Mack, T. N., Pike, M. C., Henderson, B. E., Pfeffer, R. I., Gerkins, V. R., Arthur, M., and Brown, S. E., "Estrogens and endometrial cancer in a retirement community," N Engl J Med *294*:1262–1267, 1976.
20. Silverberg, S. G., and Makowski, E. L., "Endometrial carcinoma in young women taking oral contraceptive agents," Obstet Gynecol *46*:503–506, 1975.
21. Vessey, M. P., Doll, R., and Sutton, P. M., "Oral contraceptives and breast neoplasia: a retrospective study," Brit Med J *3*:719–724, 1972.
22. Vessey, M. P., Doll, R., and Jones K., "Oral contraceptives and breast cancer. Progress report of an epidemiological study," Lancet *1*:941–943, 1975.
23. Boston Collaborative Drug Surveillance Program, "Surgically confirmed gallbladder disease, venous thromboembolism and breast tumors in relation to postmenopausal estrogen therapy," N Engl J Med *290*:15–19, 1974.
24. Arthes, F. G., Sartwell, P. E., and Lewison, E. F., "The pill, estrogens, and the breast. Epidemiologic aspects," Cancer *28*:1391–1394, 1971.
25. Fasal, E., and Paffenbarger, R. S., "Oral contraceptives as related to cancer and benign lesions of the breast," J Natl Cancer Inst *55*:767–773, 1975.
26. Royal College of General Practitioners, "Oral Contraceptives and Health," London, Pitman, 1974.
27. Ory, H., Cole P., MacMahon, B., and Hoover, R., "Oral contraceptives and reduced risk of benign breast diseases," N Engl J Med *294*:419–422, 1976.
28. Baum, J., Holtz, F., Bookstein, J. J., and Klein, E. W., "Possible association between benign hepatomas and oral contraceptives," Lancet *2*:926–928, 1973.
29. Mays, E. T., Christopherson, W. M., Mahr, M. M., and Williams, H. C., "Hepatic changes in young women ingesting contraceptive steroids. Hepatic hemorrhage and primary hepatic tumors," JAMA *235*:730–732, 1976.
30. Edmondson, H. A., Henderson, B., and Benton, B., "Liver-cell adenomas associated with use of oral contraceptives," N Engl J Med *294*:470–472, 1976.
31. Herbst, A. L., Ulfedler, H., and Poskanzer, D. C., "Adenocarcinoma of the vagina," N Engl J Med *284*:878–881, 1971.
32. Greenwald, P., Barlow, J. J., Nasca, P. C., and Burnett, W., "Vaginal cancer after maternal treatment with synthetic estrogens," N Engl J Med *285*:390–392, 1971.
33. Lanier, A. P., Noller, K. L., Decker, D. G., Elveback, L., and Kurland, L. T., "Cancer and stilbestrol. A follow-up of 1719 persons exposed to estrogens in utero and born 1943–1959," Mayo Clin Pro *48*:793–799, 1973.
34. Herbst, A. L., Kurman, R. J., and Scully, R. E., "Vaginal and cervical abnormalities after exposure to stilbestrol in utero," Obstet Gynecol *40*:287–298, 1972.
35. Herbst, A. L., Robboy, S. J., Macdonald, G. J., and Scully, R. E., "The effects of local progesterone on stilbestrol-associated vaginal adenosis," Am J Obstet Gynecol *118*:607–615, 1974.
36. Herbst, A. L., Poskanzer, D. C., Robboy, S. J., Friedlander, L., and Scully, R. E., "Prenatal exposure to stilbestrol: a prospective comparison of exposed female offspring with unexposed controls," N Engl J Med *292*:334–339, 1975.
37. Stafl, A., Mattingly, R. F., Foley, D. V., Fetherston, W., "Clinical diagnosis of vaginal adenosis," Obstet Gynecol *43*:118–128, 1974.
38. Sherman, A. I., Goldrath, M., Berlin, A., Vakhariya, V., Banooni, F., Michaels, W., Goodman, P., and Brown, S., "Cervical-vaginal adenosis after in utero exposure to synthetic estrogens," Obstet Gynecol *44*:531–545, 1974.
39. Gal, I., Kirman, B., and Stern, J., "Hormone pregnancy tests and congenital malformation," Nature *216*:83, 1967.
40. Levy, E. P., Cohen, A., and Fraser, F. C., "Hormone treatment during pregnancy and congenital heart defects," Lancet *1*:611, 1973.
41. Nora, J. J., and Nora, A. H., "Birth defects and oral contraceptives," Lancet *1*:941–942, 1973.
42. Janerich, D. T., Piper, J. M., and Glebatis, D. M., "Oral contraceptives and congenital limb-reduction defects," N Engl J Med *291*:697–700, 1974.
43. Carr, D. H., "Chromosome studies in selected spontaneous abortions: I. Conception after oral contraceptives," Canad Med Assoc J *103*:343–348, 1970.
44. Wynn, V., Doar, J. W. H., and Mills, G. L., "Some effects of oral contraceptives on serum-lipid and lipoprotein levels," Lancet *2*:720–723, 1966.
45. Laumas, K. R., Malkani, P. K., Bhatnagar, S., and Laumas, V., "Radioactivity in the breast milk of lactating women after oral administration of 3 H-norethynodrel," Am J Obstet Gynecol *98*:411–413, 1967.
46. Center for Disease Control, "Increased Risk of Hepatocellular Adenoma in Women with Long-term use of Oral Contraceptives," Morbidity and Mortality Weekly Report, *26*:293–294, 1977.
47. Herbst, A. L., Cole, P., Colton, T., Robboy, S. J., and Scully, R. E., "Age-incidence and Risk of Diethylstilbestrol-related Clear Cell Adenocarcinoma of the Vagina and Cervix," Am J Obstet Gynecol *128*:43–50, 1977.
48. Bibbo, M., Al-Naqeeb, M., Baccarini, I., Gill, W., Newton, M., Sleeper, K. M., Sonek, M., and Wied, G. L., "Follow-up Study of Male and Female Offspring of DES-treated Mothers. A Preliminary Report," J of Repro Med *15*:29–32, 1975.
49. Gill, W. B., Schumacher, G. F. B., and Bibbo, M., "Structural and Functional Abnormalities in the Sex Organs of Male Offspring of Mothers Treated with Diethylstilbestrol (DES)," J of Repro Med *16*:147–153, 1976.
50. Henderson, B. E., Senton, B., Cosgrove, M., Baptista, J., Aldrich, J., Townsend, D., Hart, W., and Mack, T., "Urogenital Tract Abnormalities in Sons of Women Treated with Diethylstilbestrol," Pediatrics, *58*:505–507, 1976.
51. Heinonen, O. P., Slone, D., Nonson, R. R., Hook, E. B., and Shapiro, S., "Cardiovascular Birth Defects and Antenatal Exposure to Female Sex Hormones," N Engl J Med *296*:67–70, 1977.
52. Jain, A. K., "Mortality Risk Associated with the Use of Oral Contraceptives," Studies in Family Planning, *8*:50–54, 1977.
53. Beral, V., "Mortality Among Oral Contraceptive Users," Lancet, *2*:727–731, 1977.
54. Royal College of General Practitioners' Oral contraception study, "Incidence of arterial disease among oral contraceptive users," J Royal Col Gen Pract *33*:75–82, 1983.
55. Slone, D., Shapiro, S., Kaufman, D. W., Rosenberg, L., Miettinen, O., and Stolley, P., "Risk of myocardial infarction in relation to current and discontinued use of oral contraceptives," N Engl J Med *305*:420–424, 1981.
56. Inman, W.H.W., "Oral contraceptives and fatal subarachnoid haemorrhage," Brit Med J *2*:1468–1470, 1979.
57. Petitti, D. B., and Wingerd, J., "Use of oral contraceptives, cigarette smoking and risk of subarachnoid haemorrhage," Lancet *2*:234–236, 1978.
58. Thorogood, M., Adam, S. A., and Mann, J. I., "Fatal subarachnoid haemorrhage in young women: role of oral contraceptives," Brit Med J *283*:762, 1981.
59. Rosenberg, L., Hennekens, C.H., Rosner, B., Belanger, C., Rothman, K. J., and Speizer, F. E., "Oral contraceptive use in relation to nonfatal myocardial infarction," Am J Epidemiol *111*:59–66, 1980.
60. Adam, S. A., Thorogood, M., and Mann, J. I., "Oral contraception and myocardial infarction revisited: the effects of new preparations and prescribing patterns," Brit J Obstet Gynaecol *88*:838–845, 1981.
61. Data on file.
62. Briggs, M. H., "Implications and assessment of metabolic effects of oral contraceptives." New considerations in oral contraception. Proceedings of an international symposium, Catholic University-Leuven, Leuven, Belgium. September, 1981 Ed. I. Brosens.
63. Vermeulen, A., and Thiery, M., "Metabolic effects of the triphasic oral contraceptive Trigynon®." Contraception *26*:505–513, 1982.
64. Nilsson, S., Nygren, K., and Johansson, E., "Ethinyl Estradiol in Human Milk and Plasma after Oral Administration." Contraception *17*:131–139, 1978.
65. Nilsson, S., Nygren, K., and Johansson, E., "d-Norgestrel Concentrations in Maternal Plasma, Milk, and Child Plasma During Administration of Oral Contraceptives to Nursing Women." Am J Obstet Gynecol *129*:178, 1977.

The patient labeling for oral-contraceptive drug products is set forth below:

Brief Summary Patient Package Insert

Cigarette smoking increases the risk of serious adverse effects on the heart and blood vessels from oral-contraceptive use. This risk increases with age and with heavy smoking (15 or more cigarettes per day) and is quite marked in women over 35 years of age. Women who use oral contraceptives should not smoke.

Oral contraceptives taken as directed are about 99% effective in preventing pregnancy. (The mini-pill, however, is somewhat less effective.) Forgetting to take your pills increases the chance of pregnancy. Women who have or have had clotting disorders, cancer of the breast or sex organs, unexplained vaginal bleeding, a stroke, heart attack, angina pectoris, or who suspect they may be pregnant should not use oral contraceptives. Various drugs, such as some antibiotics, may also decrease the effectiveness of oral contraceptives.

Most side effects of the pill are not serious. The most common side effects are nausea, vomiting, bleeding between menstrual periods, weight gain, and breast tenderness. However, proper use of oral contraceptives requires that they be taken under your doctor's continuous supervision, because they can be associated with serious side effects which may be fatal. Fortunately, these occur very infrequently. The serious side effects are:

1. Blood clots in the legs, lungs, brain, heart, or other organs, and hemorrhage into the brain due to bursting of a blood vessel. Certain of these effects may occur after pill use has been stopped.
2. Liver tumors, which may rupture and cause severe bleeding.
3. Birth defects if the pill is taken while you are pregnant.
4. High blood pressure.
5. Gallbladder disease.

The symptoms associated with these serious side effects are discussed in the detailed leaflet given you with your supply of pills. Notify your doctor if you notice any unusual physical disturbance while taking the pill.

The estrogen in oral contraceptives has been found to cause breast cancer and other cancers in certain animals. These findings suggest that oral contraceptives may also cause cancer in humans. However, studies to date in women taking currently marketed oral contraceptives have not confirmed that oral contraceptives cause cancer in humans.

The detailed leaflet describes more completely the benefits and risks of oral contraceptives. It also provides information on other forms of contraception. Read it carefully. If you have any questions, consult your doctor.

CAUTION

Oral contraceptives are of no value in the prevention or treatment of venereal disease.

DETAILED PATIENT LABELING

WHAT YOU SHOULD KNOW ABOUT ORAL CONTRACEPTIVES

Oral contraceptives ("the pill") are the most effective way (except for sterilization) to prevent pregnancy. They are also convenient and, for most women, free of serious or unpleasant side effects. Oral contraceptives must always be taken under the continuous supervision of a physician.

It is important that any woman who considers using an oral contraceptive understand the risks involved. Although the oral contraceptives have important advantages over other methods of contraception, they have certain risks that no other method has. Only you can decide whether the advantages are worth these risks. This leaflet will tell you about the most important risks. It will explain how you can help your doctor prescribe the pill as safely as possible by telling him about yourself and being alert for the earliest signs of trouble. And it will tell you how to use the pill properly, so that it will be as effective as possible. There is more detailed information available in the leaflet prepared for doctors. Your pharmacist can show you a copy; you may need your doctor's help in understanding parts of it.

WHO SHOULD NOT USE ORAL CONTRACEPTIVES

A. If you have any of the following conditions, you should not use the pill:

1. Clots in the legs or lungs.
2. Angina pectoris.
3. Known or suspected cancer of the breast or sex organs.
4. Unusual vaginal bleeding that has not yet been diagnosed.
5. Known or suspected pregnancy.

B. If you have had any of the following conditions, you should not use the pill:

1. Heart attack or stroke.
2. Clots in the legs or lungs.

C. Cigarette smoking increases the risk of serious adverse effects on the heart and blood vessels from oral-contraceptive use. This risk increases with age and with heavy smoking (15 or more cigarettes per day) and is quite marked in women over 35 years of age. Women who use oral contraceptives should not smoke.

D. If you have scanty or irregular periods or are a young woman without a regular cycle, you should use another method of contraception because, if you use the pill, you may have difficulty becoming pregnant or may fail to have menstrual periods after discontinuing the pill.

DECIDING TO USE ORAL CONTRACEPTIVES

If you do not have any of the conditions listed above and are thinking about using oral contraceptives, to help you decide, you need information about the advantages and risks of oral contraceptives and of other contraceptive methods as well. This leaflet describes the advantages and risks of oral contraceptives. Except for sterilization, the IUD, and abortion, which have their own inherent risks, the only risks of other methods of contraception are those due to pregnancy should the method fail. Your doctor can answer questions you may have with respect to other methods of contraception. He can also answer any questions you may have after reading this leaflet on oral contraceptives.

1. What Oral Contraceptives Are and How They Work. Oral contraceptives are of two types. The most common, often simply called "the pill," is a combination of an estrogen and a progestogen, the two kinds of female hormones. The amount of estrogen and progestogen can vary, but the amount of estrogen is most important because both the effectiveness and some of the dangers of oral contraceptives are related to the amount of estrogen. This kind of oral contraceptive works principally by preventing release of an egg from the ovary. When the amount of estrogen is 50 micrograms or more, and the pill is taken as directed, oral contraceptives are more than 99% effective (i.e., there would be less than 1 pregnancy if 100 women used the pill for 1 year). Pills that contain 20 to 35 micrograms of estrogen vary slightly in effectiveness, ranging from 98% to more than 99% effective.

The second type of oral contraceptive, often called the "mini-pill", contains only a progestogen. It works in part by preventing release of an egg from the ovary but also by keeping sperm from reaching the egg and by making the uterus (womb) less receptive to any fertilized egg that reaches it. The mini-pill is less effective than the combination oral contraceptive, about 97% effective. In addition, the progestogen-only pill has a tendency to cause irregular bleeding which may be quite inconvenient, or cessation of bleeding entirely. The progestogen-only pill is used despite its lower effectiveness in the hope that it will prove not to have some of the serious side effects of the estrogen-containing pill (see below), but it is not yet certain that the mini-pill does in fact have fewer serious side effects. The discussion below, while based mainly on information about the combination pills, should be considered to apply as well to the mini-pill.

2. Other Nonsurgical Ways to Prevent Pregnancy. As this leaflet will explain, oral contraceptives have several serious risks. Other methods of contraception have lesser risks or none at all. They are also less effective than oral contraceptives, but, used properly, may be effective enough for many women.

The following table gives reported pregnancy rates (the number of women out of 100 who would become pregnant in 1 year) for these methods.

PREGNANCIES PER 100 WOMEN PER YEAR

Intrauterine device (IUD), less than 1–6; Diaphragm with spermicidal products (creams or jellies), 2–20; Condom (rubber), 3–36; Aerosol foams, 2–29; Jellies and creams, 4–36; Periodic abstinence (rhythm) all types, less than 1–47:

1. Calendar method, 14–47;
2. Temperature method, 1–20;
3. Temperature method—intercourse only in postovulatory phase, less than 1–7;
4. Mucus method, 1–25;

No contraception, 60–80.

The figures (except for the IUD) vary widely because people differ in how well they use each method. Very faithful users of the various methods obtain very good results, except for users of the calendar method of periodic abstinence (rhythm). Except for the IUD, effective use of these methods requires somewhat more effort than simply taking a single pill every day, but it is an effort that many couples undertake successfully. Your doctor can tell you a great deal more about these methods of contraception.

3. The Dangers of Oral Contraceptives.

a. *Circulatory disorders (abnormal blood clotting and stroke due to hemorrhage).* Blood clots (in various blood vessels of the body) are the most common of the serious side effects of oral contraceptives. A clot can result in a stroke (if the clot is in the brain), a heart attack (if the clot is in a blood vessel of the heart), or a pulmonary embolus (a clot which forms in the legs or pelvis, then breaks off and travels to the lungs). Any of these can be fatal. Clots also occur rarely in the blood vessels of the eye, resulting in blindness or impairment of vision in that eye. There is evidence that the risk of clotting increases with higher estrogen doses. It is therefore important to keep the dose of estrogen as low as possible, so long as the oral contraceptive used has an acceptable pregnancy rate and doesn't cause unacceptable changes in the menstrual pattern. Furthermore, cigarette smoking by oral-contraceptive users increases the risk of serious adverse effects on the heart and blood vessels. This risk increases with age and with heavy smoking (15 or more cigarettes per day) and begins to become quite marked in women over 35 years of age. For this reason, women who use oral contraceptives should not smoke.

The risk of abnormal clotting increases with age in both users and nonusers of oral contraceptives, but the increased risk from the contraceptive appears to be present at all ages. For oral-contraceptive users in general, it has been estimated that in women between the ages of 15 and 34 the risk of death due to a circulatory disorder is about 1 in 12,000 per year, whereas for nonusers the risk is about 1 in 50,000 per year. In the age group 35 to 44, the risk is estimated to be about 1 in 2,500 per year for oral-contraceptive users and about 1 in 10,000 per year for nonusers.

Even without the pill, the risk of having a heart attack increases with age and is also increased by such heart attack risk factors as high blood pressure, high cholesterol, obesity, diabetes, and cigarette smoking. Without any risk factors present, the use of oral contraceptives alone may double the risk of heart attack. However, the combination of cigarette smoking, especially heavy smoking, and oral contraceptive use greatly increases the risk of heart attack. Oral-contraceptive users who smoke are about 5 times more likely to have a heart attack than users who do not smoke and about 10 times more likely to have a heart attack than nonusers who do not smoke. It has been estimated that users between the ages of 30 and 39 who smoke have about a 1 in 10,000 chance each year of having a fatal heart attack compared to about a 1 in 50,000 chance in users who do not smoke, and about a 1 in 100,000 chance in nonusers who do not smoke. In the age group 40 to 44, the risk is about 1 in 1,700 per year for users who smoke compared to about 1 in 10,000 for users who do not smoke and to about 1 in 14,000 per year for nonusers who do not smoke. Heavy smoking (about 15 cigarettes or more a day) further increases the risk. If you do not smoke and have none of the other heart attack risk factors described above, you will have a smaller risk than listed. If you have several heart attack risk factors, the risk may be considerably greater than listed.

In addition to blood-clotting disorders, it has been estimated that women taking oral contraceptives are twice as likely as nonusers to have a stroke due to rupture of a blood vessel in the brain. There is evidence that patients who stop taking oral contraceptives after using them continuously for five or more years may continue to have an increased risk of stroke or heart attack for at least six to nine years after discontinuation.

b. *Formation of tumors.* Studies have found that when certain animals are given the female sex hormone, estrogen, which is an ingredient of oral contraceptives, continuously for long periods, cancers may develop in the breast, cervix, vagina, and liver.

These findings suggest that oral contraceptives may cause cancer in humans. However, studies to date in women taking currently marketed oral contraceptives have not confirmed that oral contraceptives cause cancer in humans. Several studies have found no increase in breast cancer in users, although one study suggested oral contraceptives might cause an increase in breast cancer in women who already have benign breast disease (e.g., cysts).

Women with a strong family history of breast cancer or who have breast nodules, fibrocystic disease, or abnormal mammograms or who were exposed to DES (diethylstilbestrol), an estrogen, during their mother's pregnancy must be followed very closely by their doctors if they choose to use oral contraceptives instead of another method of contraception. Many studies have shown that women taking oral contraceptives have less risk of getting benign breast disease than those who have not used oral contraceptives. Recently, strong evidence has emerged that estrogens (one component of oral contraceptives), when given for periods of more than one year to women after the menopause, increase the risk of cancer of the uterus (womb). There is also some evidence that a kind of oral contraceptive which is no longer marketed, the sequential oral contraceptive, may increase the risk of cancer of the uterus. There remains no evidence, however, that the oral contraceptives now available increase the risk of this cancer. Oral contraceptives do cause, although rarely, a benign (nonmalignant) tumor of the liver. These tumors do not spread, but they may rupture and cause internal bleeding, which may be fatal. A few cases of cancer of the liver have been reported in women using oral contraceptives, but it is not yet known whether the drug caused them.

c. *Dangers to a developing child if oral contraceptives are used in or immediately preceding pregnancy.* Oral contraceptives should not be taken by pregnant women because they may damage the developing child. An increased risk of birth defects, including heart defects and limb defects, has been associated with the use of sex hormones, including oral contraceptives, in pregnancy. In addition, the developing female child whose mother has received DES (diethylstilbestrol), an estrogen, during pregnancy has a risk of getting cancer of the vagina or cervix in her teens or young adulthood. This risk is estimated to be about 1 in 1,000 exposures or less. Abnormalities of the urinary and sex organs have been reported in male offspring so exposed. It is possible that other estrogens, such as the estrogens in oral contraceptives, could have the same effect in the child if the mother takes them during pregnancy.

If you stop taking oral contraceptives to become pregnant, your doctor may recommend that you use another method of contraception for a short while. The reason for this is that there is evidence from studies in women who have had "miscarriages" soon after stopping the pill, that the lost fetuses are more likely to be abnormal. Whether there is an overall increase in "miscarriage" in women who become pregnant soon after stopping the pill as compared with women who do not use the pill is not known, but it is possible that there may be. If, however, you do become pregnant soon after stopping

Continued on next page

Wyeth—Cont.

oral contraceptives, and do not have a miscarriage, there is no evidence that the baby has an increased risk of being abnormal.

d. *Gallbladder disease.* Women who use oral contraceptives have a greater risk than nonusers of having gallbladder disease requiring surgery. The increased risk may first appear within 1 year of use and may double after 4 or 5 years of use.

e. *Other side effects of oral contraceptives.* Some women using oral contraceptives experience unpleasant side effects that are not dangerous and are not likely to damage their health. Some of these may be temporary. Your breasts may feel tender, nausea and vomiting may occur, you may gain or lose weight, and your ankles may swell. A spotty darkening of the skin, particularly of the face, is possible and may persist. You may notice unexpected vaginal bleeding or changes in your menstrual period. Irregular bleeding is frequently seen when using the mini-pill or combination oral contraceptives containing less than 50 micrograms of estrogen.

More serious side effects include worsening of migraine, asthma, epilepsy, and kidney or heart disease because of a tendency for water to be retained in the body when oral contraceptives are used.

Other side effects are growth of preexisting fibroid tumors of the uterus; mental depression, and liver problems with jaundice (yellowing of the skin). Your doctor may find that levels of sugar and fatty substances in your blood are elevated; the long-term effects of these changes are not known. Some women develop high blood pressure while taking oral contraceptives, which ordinarily returns to the original levels when the oral contraceptive is stopped.

Other reactions, although not proved to be caused by oral contraceptives, are occasionally reported. These include more frequent urination and some discomfort when urinating, blood cell breakdown with kidney failure, nervousness, dizziness, some loss of scalp hair, an increase in body hair, an increase or decrease in sex drive, appetite changes, cataracts, and a need for a change in contact lens prescription, or inability to use contact lenses.

After you stop using oral contraceptives, there may be a delay before you are able to become pregnant or before you resume having menstrual periods. This is especially true of women who had irregular menstrual cycles prior to the use of oral contraceptives. As discussed previously, your doctor may recommend that you wait a short while after stopping the pill before you try to become pregnant. During this time, use another form of contraception. You should consult your physician before resuming use of oral contraceptives after childbirth, especially if you plan to nurse your baby. Drugs in oral contraceptives are known to appear in the milk, and the long-range effect on infants is not known at this time. Furthermore, oral contraceptives may cause a decrease in your milk supply as well as in the quality of the milk.

4. Comparison of the Risks of Oral Contraceptives and Other Contraceptive Methods. The many studies on the risks and effectiveness of oral contraceptives and other methods of contraception have been analyzed to estimate the risk of death associated with various methods of contraception. This risk has two parts: (a) the risk of the method itself (e.g., the risk that oral contraceptives will cause death due to abnormal clotting), and (b) the risk of death due to pregnancy or abortion in the event the method fails. The results of this analysis are shown in the bar graph (Figure 1). The height of the bars is the number of deaths per 100,000 women each year. There are six sets of bars, each set referring to a specific age group of women. Within each set of bars, there is a single bar for each of the different contraceptive methods. For oral contraceptives, there are two bars—one for smokers and the other for nonsmokers. The analysis is based on present knowledge, and new information could, of course, alter it. The analysis shows that the risk of death from all methods of birth control is low and below that associated with childbirth, except for oral contraceptives in women over 40 who smoke. It shows that the lowest risk of death is associated with the condom or diaphragm (traditional contraception) backed up by early abortion in case of failure of the condom or diaphragm to prevent pregnancy. Also, at any age the risk of death (due to unexpected pregnancy) from the use of traditional contraception, even without a backup of abortion, is generally the same as or less than that from use of oral contraceptives.

HOW TO USE ORAL CONTRACEPTIVES AS SAFELY AND EFFECTIVELY AS POSSIBLE, ONCE YOU HAVE DECIDED TO USE THEM

1. What to Tell your Doctor.

You can make use of the pill as safely as possible by telling your doctor if you have any of the following:

a. Conditions that mean you should not use oral contraceptives:

Clots in the legs or lungs.
Clots in the legs or lungs in the past.
A stroke, heart attack, or angina pectoris.
Known or suspected cancer of the breast or sex organs.
Unusual vaginal bleeding that has not yet been diagnosed.
Known or suspected pregnancy.

b. Conditions that your doctor will want to watch closely or which might cause him to suggest another method of contraception:

A family history of breast cancer.
Breast nodules, fibrocystic disease of the breast, or an abnormal mammogram.
Diabetes.
High blood pressure.
High cholesterol.
Cigarette smoking.
Migraine headaches.
Heart or kidney disease.
Epilepsy.
Mental depression.
Fibroid tumors of the uterus.
Gallbladder disease.

c. Once you are using oral contraceptives, you should be alert for signs of a serious adverse effect and call your doctor if they occur.

Sharp pain in the chest, coughing blood, or sudden shortness of breath (indicating possible clots in the lungs).

Figure 1. Estimated annual number of deaths associated with control of fertility and no control per 100,000 nonsterile women, by regimen of control and age of woman.

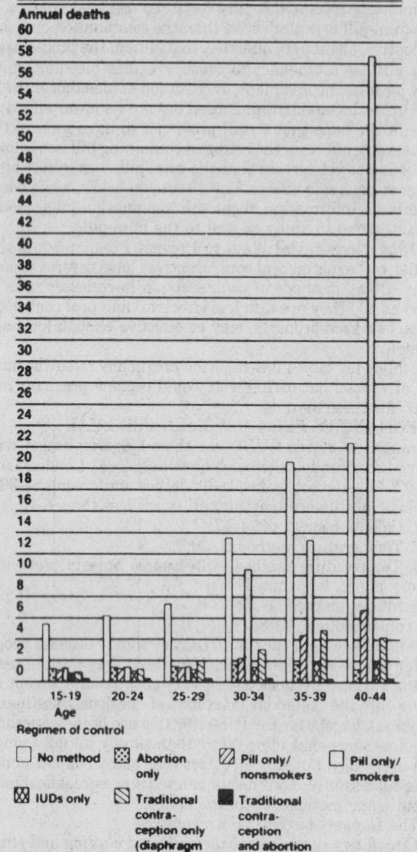

Pain in the calf (possible clot in the leg).
Crushing chest pain or heaviness (indicating possible heart attack).
Sudden severe headache or vomiting, dizziness or fainting, disturbance of vision or speech, or weakness or numbness in an arm or leg (indicating a possible stroke).
Sudden partial or complete loss of vision (indicating a possible clot in the eye).
Breast lumps (you should ask your doctor to show you how to examine your own breasts).
Severe pain in the abdomen (indicating a possible ruptured tumor of the liver).
Severe depression.
Yellowing of the skin (jaundice).

2. How to Take the Pill So That It is Most Effective.

Reduced effectiveness and an increased incidence of breakthrough bleeding have been associated with the use of oral contraceptives with antibiotics such as rifampin, ampicillin, and tetracycline or with certain other drugs such as barbiturates, phenylbutazone or phenytoin sodium. You should use an additional means of contraception during any cycle in which any of these drugs are taken.

To achieve maximum contraceptive effectiveness, oral contraceptives must be taken exactly as directed and at intervals not exceeding 24 hours. It is recommended that tablets be taken at the same time each day, preferably after the evening meal or at bedtime. Taking them on a definite schedule will decrease the chance of forgetting a tablet and also help keep the proper amount of medication in your system. See detailed instructions below for Triphasil-21 Tablets (Levonorgestrel and Ethinyl Estradiol Tablets—Triphasic Regimen) and Triphasil-28 Tablets (Levonorgestrel and Ethinyl Estradiol Tablets—Triphasic Regimen).

For specific instructions on **how to use your particular package,** refer to the Brief Summary Patient Package insert provided with your pill package.

TRIPHASIL®-21 TABLETS (LEVONORGESTREL AND ETHINYL ESTRADIOL TABLETS—TRIPHASIC REGIMEN)

Triphasil is a three-phased contraceptive, different from the usual same-dose-every-day combination oral contraceptive. Triphasil-21 Tablets contain 21 active pills divided among 6 brown pills, 5 white pills, and 10 light-yellow pills in each package.

The dosage of Triphasil-21 Tablets is **one pill daily** for 21 days in a row in your menstrual cycle beginning with the first brown pill, continuing through the white pills and finishing the cycle with the light-yellow pills, **in that order.** Pills are then discontinued for 7 days. The basic schedule is 21 days on—7 days off.

In the first month, you should begin taking Triphasil-21 Tablets on day one (1) of your menstrual cycle, which is the first day of your menstruation regardless of the amount of bleeding or spotting. (Day 1 is the first day of menstruation, even if it is almost midnight when you start.) Note: During the first month on Triphasil-21 Tablets, if you start taking pills later than day 1 of your menstrual cycle, you should protect yourself by also using another method of birth control until you have taken a pill daily for seven days in a row (6 brown pills followed by 1 white pill). Thereafter, if you follow directions carefully you will obtain the full contraceptive benefit. If you begin taking pills later than the proper day, the possibility of ovulation and pregnancy occurring before or during the taking of the brown pills should be considered.

Take one pill every day until you finish all 21 pills. No pills are then taken for one week (7 days). Your period will usually begin about three days after you take the last light-yellow pill. Don't be alarmed if the amount of bleeding is not the same as before. On the 8th day, start with a brown pill from a new package, even if you still have your period. If, for example, you took Triphasil-21 Tablets for the first time on a Tuesday, the 8th day will also be a Tuesday. **If you have taken the pills as directed,** you will begin the next cycle on the same day of the week. If you start taking pills later than the 8th day, you should protect yourself by also using another method of birth control until you have taken a pill daily for seven days in a row.

When switching from another oral contraceptive, Triphasil-21 Tablets should be started on the first day of bleeding following the last pill taken of the previous oral contraceptive.

TRIPHASIL®-28 TABLETS (LEVONORGESTREL AND ETHINYL ESTRADIOL TABLETS—TRIPHASIC REGIMEN)

Triphasil is a three-phased contraceptive, different from the usual same-dose-every-day combination oral contraceptive. Triphasil-28 Tablets contain active pills divided among 6 brown pills, 5 white pills, and 10 light-yellow pills plus 7 light-green inactive pills per package.

The dosage of Triphasil-28 Tablets is one active pill daily for 21 days in a row beginning with the 6 brown pills, followed by the 5 white pills, followed by the 10 light-yellow pills, and then one of the 7 light-green inactive pills daily for the next 7 days, **in that order,** for a total of 28 days or 4 weeks. The basic schedule is 21 days on active pills (brown, white, and light-yellow)—7 days on light-green inactive pills. Always take all of the 21 active pills (brown, white, and light-yellow) in each package before taking the light-green pills.

When you start your **first** cycle of Triphasil-28 Tablets, you should begin taking your pills on the **first** day of your next menstrual period, regardless of the day of the week or the amount of the bleeding or spotting. Note: During the first month on Triphasil-28 Tablets, if you start taking pills later than day 1 of your menstrual cycle, you should protect yourself by also using another method of birth control until you have taken a pill daily for seven days in a row (6 brown pills followed by 1 white pill). Thereafter, if you follow directions carefully you will obtain the full contraceptive benefit. If you begin taking pills later than the proper day, the possibility of ovulation and pregnancy occurring before or during the taking of the brown pills should be considered. Take one pill every day until you finish all 6 brown, 5 white, and 10 light-yellow pills in a package followed by all 7 light-green pills. Your period will usually begin about three days after you take the last light-yellow pill, which will be during the time you are taking the light-green pills. Don't be alarmed if the amount of bleeding is not the same as before.

The day after you have taken your last light-green pill, begin a new package of pills (first taking the 6 brown, then the 5 white, and then the 10 light-yellow pills one a day just as you did before) so that you will take a pill every day without interruption. **If you have taken the pills as directed,** the starting day for each new package will always be the same day as in the previous cycle. When switching from another oral contraceptive, Triphasil-28 Tablets should be started on the first day of bleeding following the last pill taken of the previous oral contraceptive.

Spotting or Breakthrough Bleeding:
Spotting is slight staining between menstrual periods which may not even require a pad. Breakthrough bleeding is a flow much like a regular period, requiring sanitary protection. Spotting is more common than breakthrough bleeding, and both occur more often in the first few cycles than in later cycles. These types of bleeding are usually temporary and without significance. It is important to continue taking your pills on schedule. If the bleeding persists for more than a few days, consult your doctor.
MISSED PILLS
There is a chance of becoming pregnant if you miss one brown, white, or light-yellow pill, and that chance increases with each additional brown, white, or light-yellow pill missed. If you miss any one of these pills, it is important it be taken as soon as remembered. If you miss any two of these pills consecutively, it is important both be taken as soon as remembered. The next pill should then be taken at the usual time. Any time you miss one or two brown, white, or light-yellow pills, **or begin a new package later than directed,** you should also use another method of birth control until you have taken a brown, white, or light-yellow pill daily for seven consecutive days. If you miss one or more light-green inactive pills (Triphasil-28 Tablets only), you are still protected against pregnancy **provided** you begin taking your next brown pill on the proper day. If breakthrough bleeding occurs following missed pills, it will usually be temporary and of no consequence.
If you forget to take brown, white, or light-yellow pills three days in a row, do not take them when you remember but stop the medication and discard the package. Begin a new package, as directed above, on the first day of bleeding of your next period. During the days without pills, and until you have taken 6 brown and a white pill daily for seven consecutive days, you should protect yourself from pregnancy by also using another method of birth control.

At times there may be no menstrual period after a cycle of pills. Therefore, if you miss one menstrual period but have taken the pills **exactly as you were supposed to,** continue as usual into the next cycle. If you have not taken the pills correctly and miss a menstrual period, you may be pregnant and should stop taking oral contraceptives until your doctor determines whether or not you are pregnant. Until you can get to your doctor, use another form of contraception. If two consecutive menstrual periods are missed, you should stop taking pills until it is determined whether you are pregnant. If you do become pregnant while using oral contraceptives, you should discuss the risks to the developing child with your doctor.
3. Periodic Examination.
Your doctor will take a complete medical and family history before prescribing oral contraceptives. At that time and about once a year thereafter, he will generally examine your blood pressure, breasts, abdomen, and pelvic organs (including a Papanicolaou smear, i.e., test for cancer).
SUMMARY
Oral contraceptives are the most effective method, except sterilization, for preventing pregnancy. Other methods when used conscientiously, are also very effective and have fewer risks. The serious risks of oral contraceptives are uncommon, and the "pill" is a very convenient method of preventing pregnancy. If you have certain conditions or have had these conditions in the past, you should not use oral contraceptives, because the risk is too great. These conditions are listed in the leaflet. If you do not have these conditions, and decide to use the "pill", please read the leaflet carefully so that you can use the "pill" most safely and effectively. Based on his or her assessment of your medical needs, your doctor has prescribed this drug for you. Do not give the drug to anyone else.

Shown in Product Identification Section, page 437

TRIPHASIL®-28 ℞
[*tri-fa 'sil*]
Tablets
(levonorgestrel and ethinyl estradiol tablets—triphasic regimen)

DESCRIPTION

Each Triphasil cycle of 28 tablets consists of three different drug phases as follows: Phase 1 comprised of 6 brown tablets, each containing 0.050 mg of levonorgestrel (d(-)-13-beta-ethyl-17-alpha-ethinyl-17-beta-hydroxygon-4-en-3-one), a totally synthetic progestogen, and 0.030 mg of ethinyl estradiol (19-nor-17α-pregna-1,3,5(10)-trien-20-yne-3,17-diol); phase 2 comprised of 5 white tablets, each containing 0.075 mg levonorgestrel and 0.040 mg ethinyl estradiol; and, phase 3 comprised of 10 light-yellow tablets, each containing 0.125 mg levonorgestrel and 0.030 mg ethinyl estradiol; then followed by 7 light-green inert tablets.
[See Chemical Formula at top of next column].

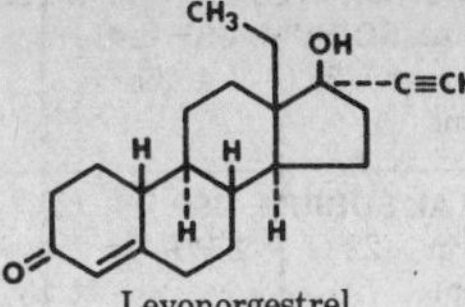

Levonorgestrel

Ethinyl Estradiol

CLINICAL PHARMACOLOGY

See Triphasil®-21.

INDICATIONS AND USAGE

See Triphasil-21.

Dose-Related Risk of Thromboembolism from Oral Contraceptives: See Triphasil-21.

CONTRAINDICATIONS

See Triphasil-21.

WARNINGS

See Triphasil-21.

PRECAUTIONS

See Triphasil-21.

INFORMATION FOR THE PATIENT

See Triphasil-21.

DRUG INTERACTIONS

See Triphasil-21.

CARCINOGENESIS

See Triphasil-21.

PREGNANCY

See Triphasil-21.

NURSING MOTHERS

See Triphasil-21.

ADVERSE REACTIONS

See Triphasil-21.

ACUTE OVERDOSE

See Triphasil-21.

DOSAGE AND ADMINISTRATION

To achieve maximum contraceptive effectiveness, Triphasil-28 Tablets (Levonorgestrel and Ethinyl Estradiol Tablets—Triphasic Regimen) must be taken exactly as directed and at intervals not exceeding 24 hours. Triphasil-28 Tablets are a three-phase preparation plus 7 inert tablets. The dosage of Triphasil-28 Tablets is **one tablet daily** for 28 consecutive days per menstrual cycle in the following order: 6 brown tablets (phase 1), followed by 5 white tablets (phase 2), followed by 10 light-yellow tablets (phase 3), plus 7 light-green inert tablets, according to the prescribed schedule.
It is recommended that Triphasil-28 tablets be taken at the same time each day, preferably after the evening meal or at bedtime. During the first cycle of medication, the patient should be instructed to take one Triphasil-28 Tablet daily in the order of 6 brown, 5 white, 10 light-yellow tablets, and then 7 light-green inert tablets for twenty-eight (28) consecutive days, beginning on day one (1) of her menstrual cycle. (The first day of menstruation is day one.) Withdrawal bleeding usually occurs within 3 days following the last light-yellow tablet. (If Triphasil-28 Tablets are first taken later than the first day of the first menstrual cycle of medication or postpartum, contraceptive reliance should not be placed on Triphasil-28 Tablets until after the first 7 consecutive days of administration. The possibility of ovulation and conception prior to initiation of medication should be considered.)
When switching from another oral contraceptive, Triphasil-28 Tablets should be started on the first day of bleeding following the last tablet taken of the previous oral contraceptive.
The patient begins her next and all subsequent 28-day courses of Triphasil-28 Tablets on the same day of the week that she began her first course, following the same schedule. She begins taking her brown tablets on the next day after ingestion of the last light-green tablet, regardless of whether or not a menstrual period has occurred or is still in progress. Any time a subsequent cycle of Triphasil-28 Tablets is started later than the next day, the patient should be protected by another means of contraception until she has taken a tablet daily for seven consecutive days.
If spotting or breakthrough bleeding occurs, the patient is instructed to continue on the same regimen. This type of bleeding is usually transient and without significance; however, if the bleeding is persistent or prolonged, the patient is advised to consult her physician. Although the occurrence of pregnancy is highly unlikely if Triphasil-28 Tablets are taken according to directions, if withdrawal bleeding does not occur, the possibility of pregnancy must be considered. If the patient has not adhered to the prescribed schedule (missed one or more tablets or started taking them on a day later than she should have), the probability of pregnancy should be considered at the time of the first missed period and appropriate diagnostic measures taken before the medication is resumed. If the patient has adhered to the prescribed regimen and misses two consecutive periods, pregnancy should be ruled out before continuing the contraceptive regimen.
The patient should be instructed to take a missed brown, white, or light-yellow tablet as soon as it is remembered. If two consecutive brown, white, or light-yellow tablets are missed they should both be taken as soon as remembered. The next tablet should be taken at the usual time.
Any time the patient misses one or two brown, white, or light-yellow tablets, she should also use another method of contraception until she has taken a brown, white, or light-yellow tablet daily for seven consecutive days. If the patient misses one or more light-green tablets, she is still protected against pregnancy provided she begins taking brown tablets again on the proper day. If breakthrough bleeding occurs following missed brown, white, or light-yellow tablets, it will usually be transient and of no consequence.
While there is little likelihood of ovulation occurring if only one or two brown, white, or light-yellow tablets are missed, the possibility of ovulation increases with each successive day that scheduled tablets are missed. If three consecutive brown, white, or light-yellow tablets are missed, all medication should be discontinued and the remainder of the package discarded. A new package of Triphasil-28 Tablets should be started on the first day of the patient's next bleed after the last tablet was taken. An alternate means of contraception should be prescribed during the days without tablets and continued until the patient has taken a tablet daily for seven consecutive days. In the nonlactating mother, Triphasil-28 Tablets may be prescribed in the postpartum period either immediately or at the first postpartum examination whether or not menstruation has resumed.

HOW SUPPLIED

Triphasil®-28 Tablets (Levonorgestrel and Ethinyl Estradiol Tablets—Triphasic Regimen), Wyeth®, NDC 0008-2536, are available in packages of 3 compacts, and in packages of 6 compact refills; packages of 12 Pilpak® dispensers are also available for clinic use only. Each cycle contains 28 coated tablets as follows:
NDC 0008-0641, six brown tablets, each containing 0.050 mg levonorgestrel and 0.030 mg ethinyl estradiol;
NDC 0008-0642, five white tablets, each containing 0.075 mg levonorgestrel and 0.040 mg ethinyl estradiol;
NDC 0008-0643, ten light-yellow tablets, each containing 0.125 mg levonorgestrel and 0.030 mg ethinyl estradiol; and
NDC 0008-0650, seven light-green inert tablets.

REFERENCES

See Triphasil-21.

Brief Summary Patient Package Insert: See Triphasil-21.

CAUTION

See Triphasil-21.

DETAILED PATIENT LABELING: See Triphasil-21.

Shown in Product Identification Section, page 437

TUBEX® Closed Injection System
[*tū 'beks*]
The TUBEX® closed injection system delivers injectable medication in accurately machine-measured doses with each sterile, prefilled cartridge-needle unit permanently identified up to the moment of injection. Precisely calibrated single-use cartridge-needle units eliminate cross contamination and minimize dosage errors. Super-sharp, siliconized needles minimize penetration pressure. Medication is easily delivered via the sturdy, stainless TUBEX hypodermic syringe, or the improved Tubex® Fast-Trak® syringe.
TUBEX sterile cartridge-needle units are ready for instant use, fit easily into the physician's bag, and are readily stored and inventoried in the office.
TAMP-R-TEL® (tamper resistant package) — a clear, sturdy plastic package for all TUBEX narcotics and barbiturates — adds a new dimension to the handling and record keeping of these controlled drugs. In TAMP-R-TEL, each TUBEX® sterile cartridge-needle unit is locked into an individual slot within the package by its own end-lock tab, which is easily broken to release the unit for use. Once the end-lock tab is broken, it is almost impossible to replace it. TAMP-R-TEL thus enhances package integrity, discourages pilferage and facilitates "at a glance" drug count.
The following products are currently available in TUBEX closed injection system. *For prescribing information on products listed write to Professional Service, Wyeth Laboratories, P.O. Box 8299, Philadelphia, PA 19101, or contact your local Wyeth representative.*

Continued on next page

Wyeth—Cont.

Product and Needle Size Units Per Pkg	NDC 0008-
NARCOTICS in TAMP-R-TEL® **(tamper resistant package)**	
CODEINE PHOSPHATE, USP Ⓒ II ●	
30 mg (½ gr.) (25 G × ⅝″) 10—1 ml	0608-01
60 mg (1 gr.) (25 G × ⅝″) 10—1 ml	0609-01
HYDROMORPHONE HYDROCHLORIDE, USP Ⓒ II ●	
1 mg (1/60 gr.) (25 G × ⅝″) 10—1 ml fill in 2 ml	0387-01
1 mg (1/60 gr.) (22 G × 1¼″) 10—1 ml fill in 2 ml	0387-03
2 mg (1/30 gr.) (25 G × ⅝″) 10—1 ml fill in 2 ml	0295-02
2 mg (1/30 gr.) (22 G × 1¼″) 10—1 ml fill in 2 ml	0295-01
3 mg (1/20 gr.) (25 G × ⅝″) 10—1 ml fill in 2 ml	0388-01
4 mg (1/15 gr.) (25 G × ⅝″) 10—1 ml fill in 2 ml	0296-02
4 mg (1/15 gr.) (22 G × 1¼″) 10—1 ml fill in 2 ml	0296-01
MEPERGAN® (Meperidine HCl and Promethazine HCl) 25 mg each/ml Ⓒ II ●	
(22 G × 1¼″) 10—2 ml	0235-01
MEPERIDINE HYDROCHLORIDE, USP Ⓒ II ●	
25 mg (25 G × ⅝″) 10—1 ml fill in 2 ml	0601-03
25 mg (22 G × 1¼″) 10—1 ml fill in 2 ml	0601-02
50 mg (25 G × ⅝″) 10—1 ml fill in 2 ml	0602-03
50 mg (22 G × 1¼″) 10—1 ml fill in 2 ml	0602-02
75 mg (25 G × ⅝″) 10—1 ml fill in 2 ml	0605-03
75 mg (22 G × 1¼″) 10—1 ml fill in 2 ml	0605-02
100 mg (25 G × ⅝″) 10—1 ml fill in 2 ml	0613-03
100 mg (22 G × 1¼″) 10—1 ml fill in 2 ml	0613-02
MORPHINE SULFATE, USP Ⓒ II ●	
2 mg (1/30 gr.) (25 G × ⅝″) 10—1 ml	0649-01
4 mg (1/15 gr.) (25 G × ⅝″) 10—1 ml	0653-01
8 mg (1/8 gr.) (25 G × ⅝″) 10—1 ml fill in 2 ml	0655-01
8 mg (1/8 gr.) (22 G × 1¼″) 10—1 ml fill in 2 ml	0655-03
10 mg (1/6 gr.) (25 G × ⅝″) 10—1 ml fill in 2 ml	0656-02
10 mg (1/6 gr.) (22 G × 1¼″) 10—1 ml fill in 2 ml	0656-01
15 mg (¼ gr.) (25 G × ⅝″) 10—1 ml fill in 2 ml	0657-02
15 mg (¼ gr.) (22 G × 1¼″) 10—1 ml fill in 2 ml	0657-01
BARBITURATES in TAMP-R-TEL®	
PENTOBARBITAL SODIUM, USP Ⓒ II ●	
100 mg (1½ gr.) (22 G × 1¼″) 10—2 ml	0303-02
PHENOBARBITAL SODIUM, USP Ⓒ IV	
30 mg (½ gr.) (22 G × 1¼″) 10—1 ml	0499-01
60 mg (1 gr.) (22 G × 1¼″) 10—1 ml	0457-01
130 mg (2 gr.) (22 G × 1¼″) 10—1 ml	0304-01
SECOBARBITAL SODIUM, USP Ⓒ II ●	
100 mg (1½ gr.) (22 G × 1¼″) 10—2 ml	0305-02

● Narcotic order blank required.

ANTIBIOTICS	
BICILLIN® C-R (Penicillin G Benzathine and Penicillin G Procaine Suspension) 300,000 U each/ml	
600,000 U (20 G × 1¼″) 10—1 ml	0026-17
1,200,000 U (20 G × 1¼″) 10—2 ml	0026-16
2,400,000 U (18 G × 2″) 10—4 ml (disposable syringe)	0026-22
BICILLIN C-R 900/300 (900,000 units Penicillin G Benzathine and 300,000 units Penicillin G Procaine in suspension)	
1,200,000 U (20 G × 1¼″) 10—2 ml	0079-01
BICILLIN LONG-ACTING (Sterile Penicillin G Benzathine Suspension)	
600,000 U (20 G × 1¼″) 10—1 ml	0021-08
1,200,000 U (20 G × 1¼″) 10—2 ml	0021-07
2,400,000 U (18 G × 2″) 10—4 ml (disposable syringe)	0021-12
WYCILLIN® (Sterile Penicillin G Procaine Suspension)	
600,000 U (20 G × 1¼″) 10—1 ml	0018-10
1,200,000 U (20 G × 1¼″) 10—2 ml	0018-08
2,400,000 U (18 G × 2″) 10—4 ml (disposable syringe)	0018-12
WYCILLIN Injection and PROBENECID Tablets (Sterile Penicillin G Procaine Suspension and Probenecid Tablets)	
2,400,000 U (18 G × 2″) 2—4 ml (package contains two disposable syringes and two 0.5 gram Probenecid tablets)	2517-01
BIOLOGICALS	
DIPHTHERIA and TETANUS TOXOIDS ADSORBED (PEDIATRIC)	
(25 G × ⅝″) 10—0.5 ml	0338-01
INFLUENZA VIRUS VACCINE (purified subvirion)	
1986-1987 Formula (25 G × ⅝″) 10—0.5 ml	0647-02
TETANUS and DIPHTHERIA TOXOIDS ADSORBED (ADULT)	
(25 G × ⅝″) 10—0.5 ml	0341-01
TETANUS TOXOID ADSORBED	
(25 G × ⅝″) 10—0.5 ml	0339-01
TETANUS TOXOID FLUID	
(25 G × ⅝″) 10—0.5 ml	0340-01
VITAMINS	
CYANOCOBALAMIN, USP	
100 mcg (22 G × 1¼″) 10—1 ml	0265-01
1,000 mcg (25 G × ⅝″) 10—1 ml	0264-03
1,000 mcg (22 G × 1¼″) 10—1 ml	0264-01
1,000 mcg (22 G × 1¼″) 10—1 ml fill in 2 ml	0264-02
THIAMINE HYDROCHLORIDE, USP	
100 mg (22 G × 1¼″) 10—1 ml fill in 2 ml	0302-01
CARDIOVASCULAR AGENTS	
DIGOXIN, USP	
0.25 mg (22 G × 1¼″) 10—1 ml	0480-02
0.5 mg (22 G × 1¼″) 10—2 ml	0480-01
EPINEPHRINE, USP (1:1000)	
(25 G × ⅝″) 10—1 ml	0263-01
HEPARIN SODIUM, USP	
1,000 USP units (22 G × 1¼″) 10—1 ml	0275-01
2,500 USP units (25 G × ⅝″) 10—1 ml	0482-01
5,000 USP units (25 G × ⅝″) 10—0.5 ml	0277-02
5,000 USP units (25 g × ⅝″) 50—0.5 ml	0277-03
5,000 USP units (25 G × ⅝″) 10—1 ml	0278-02
5,000 USP units (22 G × 1¼″) 10—1 ml	0278-01
7,500 USP units (25 G × ⅝″) 10—1 ml	0293-01
10,000 USP units (25 G × ⅝″) 10—1 ml	0277-01
15,000 USP units (25 G × ⅝″) 10—1 ml	0279-01
20,000 USP units (25 G × ⅝″) 10—1 ml	0276-01
SPECIAL AGENTS	
ATIVAN® (Lorazepam) Ⓒ IV	
2 mg/ml (22 G × 1¼″) 10—1 ml fill in 2 ml	0581-02
4 mg/ml (22 G × 1¼″) 10—1 ml fill in 2 ml	0570-02
DIMENHYDRINATE, USP	
50 mg (22 G × 1¼″) 10—1 ml	0485-01
DIPHENHYDRAMINE HYDROCHLORIDE, USP	
50 mg (22 G × 1¼″) 10—1 ml	0384-01
CVC HEPARIN FLUSH KITS	
25 USP units (25 G × ⅝″) 30 Kits	2528-02

Each Unit of Use Kit contains:
One 2.5 ml size (25 G × ⅝″) TUBEX Heparin Lock Flush Solution, USP, 10 USP units per ml and two 2.5 ml size (25 G × ⅝″) TUBEX Bacteriostatic Sodium Chloride Injection, USP.

250 USP units (25 G × ⅝″) 30 Kits	2529-02

Each Unit of Use Kit contains:
One 2.5 ml size (25 G × ⅝″) TUBEX Heparin Lock Flush Solution, USP, 100 USP units per ml and two 2.5 ml size (25

G × 5/8") TUBEX Bacteriostatic Sodium Chloride Injection, USP.

HEPARIN FLUSH KITS
10 USP units
(25 G × 5/8")
50 Kits 2528-01
Each Unit of Use Kit contains:
One 1 ml size (25 G × 5/8") TUBEX Heparin Lock Flush Solution, USP, 10 USP units per ml and two 2.5 ml size (25 G × 5/8") TUBEX Bacteriostatic Sodium Chloride Injection, USP.

100 USP units
(25 G × 5/8")
50 Kits 2529-01
Each Unit of Use Kit contains:
One 1 ml size (25 G × 5/8") TUBEX Heparin Lock Flush Solution, USP, 100 USP units per ml and two 2.5 ml size (25 G × 5/8") TUBEX Bacteriostatic Sodium Chloride Injection, USP.

HEPARIN FLUSH 1 ml KITS
10 USP units
(25 G × 5/8")
50 Kits 2528-03
Each Unit of Use Kit contains:
One 1 ml size (25 G × 5/8") TUBEX Heparin Lock Flush Solution, USP, 10 USP units per ml and two 1 ml size (25 G × 5/8") TUBEX Bacteriostatic Sodium Chloride Injection, USP.

100 USP units
(25 G × 5/8")
50 Kits 2529-03
Each Unit of Use Kit contains:
One 1 ml size (25 G × 5/8") TUBEX Heparin Lock Flush Solution, USP, 100 USP units per ml and two 1 ml size (25 G × 5/8") TUBEX Bacteriostatic Sodium Chloride Injection, USP.

HEPARIN LOCK FLUSH Solution, USP
10 USP units per ml (25 G × 5/8")
50—1 ml 0523-01

100 USP units per ml (25 G × 5/8")
50—1 ml 0487-01

10 USP units per ml—25 USP units
(25 G × 5/8")
50—2.5 ml 0523-02

100 USP units per ml—250 USP units
(25 G × 5/8")
50—2.5 ml 0487-03

HYDROXYZINE HCl, USP
100 mg (22 G × 1¼")
10—2 ml 0541-02

OXYTOCIN, USP (Synthetic)
10 USP units (22 G × 1¼")
10—1 ml 0406-01

PHENERGAN® (Promethazine HCl)
25 mg (22 G × 1¼")
10—1 ml 0416-01

50 mg (22 G × 1¼")
10—1 ml 0417-01

PROCHLORPERAZINE EDISYLATE, USP
5 mg (22 G × 1¼")
10—1 ml 0542-01

10 mg (22 G × 1¼")
10—2 ml 0542-02

SODIUM CHLORIDE, USP (Bacteriostatic)
(25 G × 5/8")
50—1 ml 0333-08

(22 G × 1¼")
50—2.5 ml 0333-05

(25 G × 5/8")
50—2.5 ml 0333-02

SPARINE® (Promazine HCl)
50 mg (22 G × 1¼")
10—1 ml 0236-01

100 mg (22 G × 1¼")
10—2 ml 0236-02

TUBEX, EMPTY, STERILE CARTRIDGE-NEEDLE UNITS
(25 G × 5/8")
50—2 ml 9103-04

(22 G × 1¼")
50—2 ml 9103-03

Shown in Product Identification Section, page 436

Wyeth®
TUBEX®
Fast-Trak® Syringe
QUICK-LOADING
1 and 2 mL size

DIRECTIONS FOR USE
NOTE: The TUBEX Fast-Trak Syringe is reusable: do not discard after use.

To load the TUBEX Fast-Trak Syringe

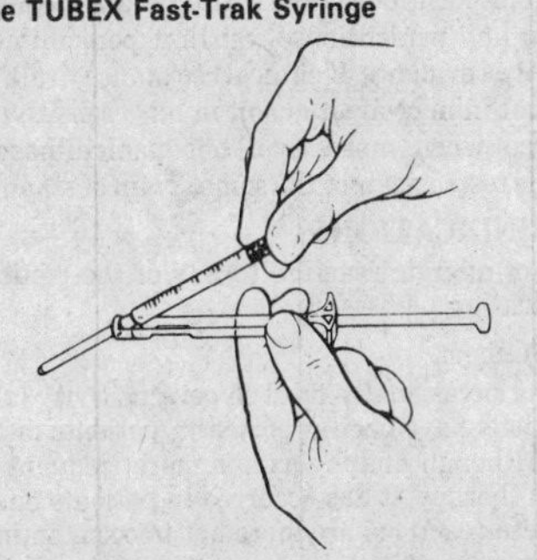

1. With plunger rod fully withdrawn, insert TUBEX Sterile Cartridge-Needle Unit, needle end first, into the barrel. Rotate the cartridge clockwise to engage the threads on the needle hub with the threads at front end of syringe (a clicking sound will be heard when fully engaged).

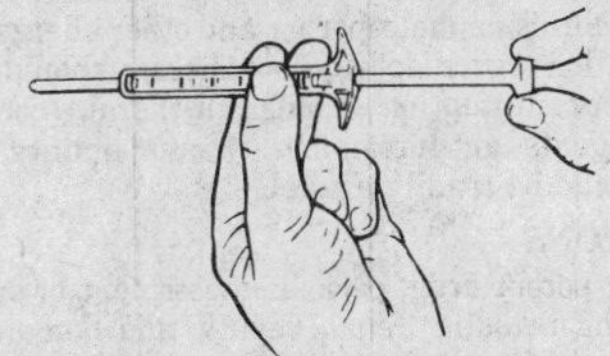

2. After engaging the TUBEX cartridge in the TUBEX Fast-Trak Syringe, hold the syringe barrel with one hand and thread the plunger rod to the rubber plunger by gently rotating the plunger rod. Both ends of the TUBEX Sterile Cartridge-Needle Unit should be fully, but lightly, engaged.

To maintain sterility, leave rubber needle sheath in place until just before use.

To administer
Method of administration is the same as with conventional syringe. Remove rubber sheath by grasping securely at the tip and pulling firmly. Do not discard sheath. Introduce needle into patient, aspirate by pulling back slightly on the plunger, and inject.

To remove the empty TUBEX Cartridge-Needle Unit

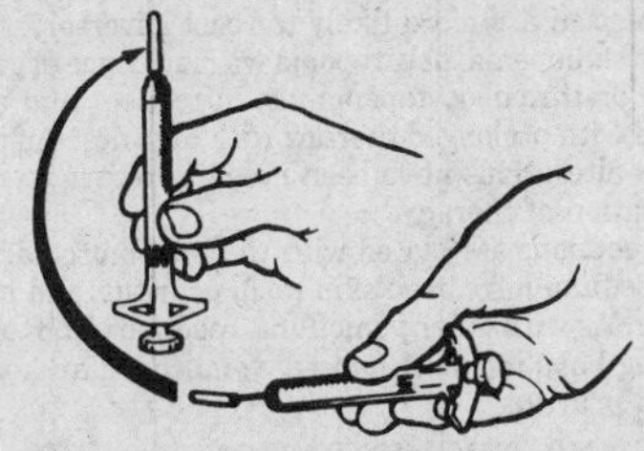

Place sheath on a flat surface with opening facing the operator. Do not hold or touch sheath with hand. Hold syringe in one hand and insert needle into the opening of the sheath. Lift the sheath onto the needle with a sweeping motion of the syringe. Bring syringe into a vertical (needle-up) position, allowing the sheath to drop over the needle. Then carefully pull down on the proximal (open) end of the sheath to fully cover the needle base.[1]

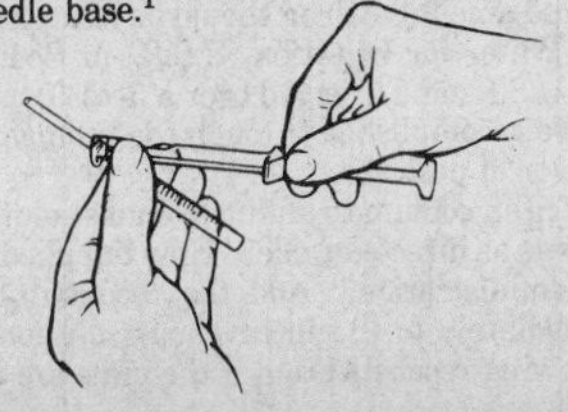

Unscrew and withdraw the plunger rod. Rotate cartridge counterclockwise to disengage at front end of syringe. Remove the used TUBEX Cartridge-Needle Unit and discard in a efficient needle-disposal system.
Used TUBEX Cartridge-Needle Units should not be employed for successive injections or as multiple-dose containers. They are intended to be used only once and discarded.
NOTE: Any graduated markings on TUBEX Sterile Cartridge-Needle Units are to be used only as a guide in mixing, withdrawing, or administering measured doses.
Wyeth does not recommend and will not accept any responsibility for the use of any cartridge-needle unit other than TUBEX® in the TUBEX® Fast-Trak® Syringe.

Reference
1. GREEN, S. T.: Avoiding needle sticks. Lancet *1(8489)*: 1096, 1986.

TYPHOID VACCINE, U.S.P. ℞
[ti 'foid vak 'sēn]

DESCRIPTION
Each ml. contains not more than 1000 million Salmonella typhosa (Ty-2 strain) organisms, killed and suspended in buffered sodium chloride injection. The preservative is 0.5% phenol. Contains 8 units per ml.

HOW SUPPLIED
Vials of 5 ml., 10 ml., and 20 ml., each containing 8 units per ml.
For prescribing information write to Professional Service, Wyeth Laboratories, Box 8299, Philadelphia, PA 19101, or contact your local Wyeth representative.

UNIPEN® ℞
[ū 'ni-pen]
(nafcillin sodium) as the monohydrate
INJECTION • CAPSULES • POWDER FOR ORAL SOLUTION • TABLETS

DESCRIPTION
UNIPEN (nafcillin sodium) is a semisynthetic penicillin developed by Wyeth research. Although primarily designed as an antistaphylococcal penicillin, in limited clinical trials it has been shown to be effective in the treatment of infections caused by pneumococci and Group A beta-hemolytic streptococci. Because of this wide gram-positive spectrum, this product is particularly suitable for *Initial Therapy* in severe or potentially severe infections before definitive culture results are known and in which staphylococci are suspected.
This product is readily soluble and can be conveniently administered in both oral and parenteral dosage forms. It is resistant to inactivation by staphylococcal penicillinase. Following intramuscular administration in humans, it rapidly appears in the plasma, penetrates body tissues in high concentration, and diffuses well into pleural, pericardial, and synovial fluids.
Unipen capsules contain 250 mg nafcillin sodium as the monohydrate. The inactive ingredients present are calcium carbonate, D&C Yellow 10, FD&C Blue 1, FD&C Yellow 6, gelatin, mineral oil, and titanium dioxide.
Unipen tablets contain 500 mg nafcillin sodium as the monohydrate. The inactive ingredients present are calcium carbonate, cellulose, hydroxypropyl methylcellulose, lactose, magnesium stearate, polacrilin potassium, starch, and talc.
Unipen for oral suspension is a powder which when reconstituted as directed yields a suspension of 250 mg nafcillin sodium per 5 mL. The inactive ingredients present are artificial and natural flavors, citric acid, edetate disodium, FD&C Red 40, FD&C Yellow 6, saccharin sodium, sodium benzoate, sodium citrate, sodium propionate, sucrose, and water.
Unipen injection is available in vial sizes of 500 mg, 1 gram, and 2 gram nafcillin sodium as the monohydrate. When reconstituted as directed each vial contains, respectively, 2 mL, 4 mL, or 8 mL of sodium. Each mL contains nafcillin sodium equivalent to 250 mg nafcillin buffered with 10 mg sodium citrate.
NOTE: Unipen contains 2.9 milliequivalents of sodium per gram of nafcillin as the sodium salt.

MICROBIOLOGY
UNIPEN is a bactericidal penicillin which has shown activity *in vitro* against both penicillin-G-sensitive and penicillin-G-resistant strains of *Staphylococcus aureus* as well as against pneumococcus, beta-hemolytic streptococcus, and alpha streptococcus (viridans).
In experimental mouse infections induced with pneumococci, beta-hemolytic streptococci, and both penicillin-G-susceptible and penicillin-G-resistant strains of *Staph. aureus,* nafcillin sodium was compared with methicillin and oxacillin. Regardless of the route of drug administration

Continued on next page

Wyeth—Cont.

(intramuscular or oral), nafcillin sodium was consistently and significantly more effective than the other two penicillins.

The fate of a penicillin-G-resistant strain of *Staph. aureus* was determined in the kidneys of mice treated with penicillin G, methicillin, and nafcillin sodium. Animals injected with the nafcillin sodium showed negative cultures after the fourteenth day, whereas positive kidney cultures were obtained during the entire 28-day period from mice treated with penicillin G and methicillin.

PHARMACOLOGY

UNIPEN is relatively nontoxic for animals. The acute LD_{50} of this product by oral administration in rats and mice was greater than 5 g/kg; by intramuscular administration in rats, 2800 mg/kg; by intraperitoneal administration in rats, 1240 mg/kg; and by intravenous administration in mice, 1140 mg/kg. The intraperitoneal LD_{50} in dogs is 600 mg/kg. Animal studies indicated that local tissue responses following intramuscular administration of 25% solutions were minimal and resembled those of penicillin G rather than methicillin.

Animal studies indicate that antibacterial amounts are concentrated in the bile, kidney, lung, heart, spleen, and liver. Eighty-four percent of an intravenously administered dose can be recovered by biliary cannulation and 13 percent by renal excretion in 24 hours. High and prolonged tissue levels can be demonstrated by both biological activity assays and C^{14} distribution patterns.

At comparable dosage, intramuscular absorption of this product is nearly equivalent to that of intramuscular methicillin, and oral absorption to that of oral oxacillin. Blood concentrations may be tripled by the concurrent use of probenecid. Clinical studies with nafcillin sodium monohydrate in infants under three days of age and prematures have revealed higher blood levels and slower rates of urinary excretion than in older children and adults.

Studies of the effect of this product on reproduction in rats and rabbits have been completed and reveal no fetal or maternal abnormalities. These studies include the observation of the effects of administration of the drug before conception and continuously through weaning (one generation).

Disc Susceptibility Tests: Quantitative methods that require measurement of zone diameters give the most precise estimates of antibiotic susceptibility. One such procedure* has been recommended for use with discs for testing susceptibility to penicillinase-resistant penicillin-class antibiotics. Interpretations correlate diameters on the disc test with MIC values for penicillinase-resistant penicillins. With this procedure, a report from the laboratory of "susceptible" indicates that the infecting organism is likely to respond to therapy. A report of "resistant" indicates that the infecting organism is not likely to respond to therapy. A report of "intermediate susceptibility" suggests that the organism would be susceptible if high dosage is used, or if the infection is confined to tissues and fluids (e.g., urine) in which high antibiotic levels are attained.

*Bauer, A.W., Kirby, W.M.M., Sherris, J.C., and Turck, M.: Antibiotic Testing by a Standardized Single-Discs Method, Am. J. Clin. Pathol., *45*:493, 1966; Standardized Disc Susceptibility Test, FEDERAL REGISTER *37*:20527–29, 1972.

INDICATIONS

Although the principal indication for nafcillin sodium is in the treatment of infections due to penicillinase-producing staphylococci, it may be used to initiate therapy in such patients in whom a staphylococcal infection is suspected. (See Important Note below.)

Bacteriologic studies to determine the causative organisms and their sensitivity to nafcillin sodium should be performed.

In serious, life-threatening infections, oral preparations of the penicillinase-resistant penicillins should not be relied on for initial therapy.

IMPORTANT NOTE

When it is judged necessary that treatment be initiated before definitive culture and sensitivity results are known, the choice of nafcillin sodium should take into consideration the fact that it has been shown to be effective only in the treatment of infections caused by pneumococci, Group A beta-hemolytic streptococci, and penicillin-G-resistant and penicillin-G-sensitive staphylococci. If the bacteriology report later indicates the infection is due to an organism other than a penicillin-G-resistant staphylococcus sensitive to nafcillin sodium, the physician is advised to continue therapy with a drug other than nafcillin sodium or any other penicillinase-resistant, semisynthetic penicillin.

Recent studies have reported that the percentage of staphylococcal isolates resistant to penicillin G outside the hospital is increasing, approximating the high percentage of resistant staphylococcal isolates found in the hospital. For this reason, it is recommended that a penicillinase-resistant penicillin be used as initial therapy for any suspected staphylococcal infection until culture and sensitivity results are known.

Methicillin is a compound that acts through a mechanism similar to that of nafcillin sodium against penicillin-G-resistant staphylococci. Strains of staphylococci resistant to methicillin have existed in nature, and it is known that the number of these strains reported has been increasing. Such strains of staphylococci have been capable of producing serious disease, in some instances resulting in fatality. Because of this there is concern that widespread use of the penicillinase-resistant penicillins may result in the appearance of an increasing number of staphylococcal strains which are resistant to these penicillins.

Methicillin-resistant strains are almost always resistant to all other penicillinase-resistant penicillins (cross-resistance with cephalosporin derivatives also occurs frequently). Resistance to any penicillinase-resistant penicillin should be interpreted as evidence of clinical resistance to all, in spite of the fact that minor variations in *in vitro* sensitivity may be encountered when more than one penicillinase-resistant penicillin is tested against the same strain of staphylococcus.

CONTRAINDICATIONS

A history of allergic reaction to any of the penicillins is a contraindication.

WARNINGS

Serious and occasionally fatal hypersensitivity (anaphylactoid) reactions have been reported in patients on penicillin therapy. Although anaphylaxis is more frequent following parenteral therapy, it has occurred in patients on oral penicillins. These reactions are more apt to occur in individuals with a history of sensitivity to multiple allergens.

There have been reports of individuals with a history of penicillin hypersensitivity reactions who have experienced severe hypersensitivity reactions when treated with a cephalosporin. Before therapy with a penicillin, careful inquiry should be made concerning previous hypersensitivity reactions to penicillins, cephalosporins, and other allergens. If an allergic reaction occurs, appropriate therapy should be instituted, and discontinuation of nafcillin therapy considered. The usual agents (antihistamines, pressor amines, corticosteroids) should be readily available.

PRECAUTIONS

As with any potent drug, periodic assessment of organ-system function, including renal, hepatic and hematopoietic, should be made during prolonged therapy.

The possibility of bacterial and fungal overgrowth should be kept in mind during long-term therapy. If overgrowth of resistant organisms occurs, appropriate measures should be taken.

The oral route of administration should not be relied upon in patients with severe illness, or with nausea, vomiting, gastric dilatation, cardiospasm, or intestinal hypermotility.

Safety for use in pregnancy has not been established.

Particular care should be taken with intravenous administration because of the possibility of thrombophlebitis.

ADVERSE REACTIONS

Reactions to nafcillin sodium have been infrequent and mild in nature. As with other penicillins, the possibility of an anaphylactic reaction or serum-sickness-like reactions should be considered. A careful history should be taken. Patients with histories of hay fever, asthma, urticaria, or previous sensitivity to penicillin are more likely to react adversely.

Transient leukopenia, neutropenia with evidence of granulocytopenia or thrombocytopenia are infrequent and usually associated with prolonged therapy with high doses of penicillin. These alterations have been noted to return to normal after cessation of therapy.

The few reactions associated with the intramuscular use of nafcillin sodium have been skin rash, pruritus, and possible drug fever. As with other penicillins, reactions from oral use of the drug have included nausea, vomiting, diarrhea, urticaria, and pruritus.

DOSAGE AND ADMINISTRATION

It is recommended that parenteral therapy be used initially in severe infections. The patient should be placed on oral therapy with this product as soon as the clinical condition warrants. Very severe infections may require very high doses.

Intravenous Route: 500 mg every 4 hours in adults; double the dose if necessary in very severe infections.

The required amount of drug should be diluted in 15 to 30 ml of Sterile Water for Injection, U.S.P., or Sodium Chloride Injection, U.S.P., and injected over a 5- to 10-minute period. This may be accomplished through the tubing of an intravenous infusion if desirable.

To add nafcillin sodium to an intravenous solution, reconstitute the vials as directed under "How Supplied"—"For Parenteral Administration." Add the reconstituted vial contents immediately to the intravenous solution or within 8 hours following reconstitution if the vials are kept at room temperature (25° C) or within 48 hours following reconstitution if the vials are kept at refrigeration (2°-8° C).

Stability studies on nafcillin sodium at concentrations of 2 mg/ml to 40 mg/ml in the following intravenous solutions indicate the drug will lose less than 10% activity at room temperature (70° F) or, if kept under refrigeration, during the time period stipulated:

STABILITY OF	ROOM TEMPERATURE	REFRIGERATED
Sterile Water for Injection	24 hours	96 hours
Isotonic sodium chloride	24 hours	96 hours
5% dextrose in water	24 hours	96 hours
5% dextrose in 0.4% sodium chloride solution	24 hours	96 hours
Ringer's solution	24 hours	96 hours
M/6 sodium lactate solution	24 hours	96 hours

Discard any unused portions of intravenous solutions after 24 hours if kept at room temperature or after 96 hours if kept under refrigeration.

Only those solutions listed above should be used for the intravenous infusion of UNIPEN (nafcillin sodium). The concentration of the antibiotic should fall within the range of 2 to 40 mg/ml. The drug concentrate and the rate and volume of the infusion should be adjusted so that the total dose of nafcillin is administered before the drug loses its stability in the solution in use.

There is no clinical experience available on the use of this agent in neonates or infants for this route of administration.

This route of administration should be used for relatively short-term therapy (24-48 hours) because of the occasional occurrence of thrombophlebitis, particularly in elderly patients.

PIGGYBACK UNITS (for Intravenous Drip Use)—

As diluents, use the following solutions: Sterile Water for Injection, Isotonic Sodium Chloride, 5% dextrose in water, 5% dextrose in 0.4% sodium chloride solution, Ringer's solution, or M/6 sodium lactate solution.

1-GRAM BOTTLE:

Add a minimum of 49 ml diluent and shake well. If lower concentrations are desired, the solution could be further diluted with up to a total of 99 ml of diluent.

Amount of Diluent	Concentration of Solution
49 ml	20 mg/ml
99 ml	10 mg/ml

1.5-GRAM BOTTLE:

Add a minimum of 49 ml diluent and shake well. If lower concentrations are desired, the solution could be further diluted with up to a total of 99 ml of diluent.

Amount of Diluent	Concentration of Solution
49 ml	30 mg/ml
99 ml	15 mg/ml

2-GRAM BOTTLE:

Add a minimum of 49 ml diluent and shake well. If lower concentrations are desired, the solution could be further diluted with up to a total of 99 ml of diluent.

Amount of Diluent	Concentration of Solution
49 ml	40 mg/ml
99 ml	20 mg/ml

4-GRAM BOTTLE:

Add 97 ml diluent and shake well. The resulting solution will contain 40 mg/ml.

The resulting solutions may then be administered alone or with the intravenous solutions listed above. Discard unused solution after 24 hours at room temperature (70°F) or 96 hours if kept under refrigeration. Administer piggyback through an IV tubing very slowly (at least 30–60 minutes) to avoid vein irritation.

At times it may be desired to use the contents of the piggyback bottles for addition to large-volume IV fluids. In this case the entire vial contents should be dissolved in not less than 25 ml of Sterile Water for Injection. Use the resulting concentration within 24 hours when kept at room temperature or within 96 hours when kept under refrigeration.

Intramuscular Route: 500 mg every 6 hours in adults; decrease the interval to 4 hours if necessary in severe infections. In infants and children, a dose of 25 mg/kg (about 12 mg per pound) twice daily is usually adequate.

For neonates 10 mg/kg is recommended twice daily.

To reconstitute see directions and table below.

The clear solution should be administered by deep intragluteal injection immediately after reconstitution. After reconstitution, keep refrigerated (2°–8° C) and use within 7 days, keep at room temperature (25° C) and use within 3 days, or keep frozen (−20° C) for up to 3 months.

Oral Route: In adults a dose of 250 to 500 mg every 4 to 6 hours is sufficient for mild-to-moderate infections. In severe infections 1 gram every 4 to 6 hours may be necessary.
In children, streptococcal pharyngitis cases have responded to a dosage of 250 mg t.i.d. Beta-hemolytic streptococcal infections should be treated for at least ten days to prevent development of acute rheumatic fever or glomerulonephritis.
Children and infants with scarlet fever and pneumonia should receive 25 mg/kg/day in four divided doses. For staphylococcal infections, 50 mg/kg/day in four divided doses is recommended. For neonates, 10 mg/kg three to four times daily is recommended. If inadequate, resort to parenteral UNIPEN® (nafcillin sodium) Wyeth.
To reconstitute the powder for oral solution, add the water in two separate portions. Shake well after each addition. After reconstitution the solution must be refrigerated. Discard any unused portion after seven days.

HOW SUPPLIED

FOR ORAL ADMINISTRATION

Capsules

Supplied as capsules containing nafcillin sodium, as the monohydrate, equivalent to 250 mg nafcillin buffered with calcium carbonate as follows:
NDC 0008-0057, green and yellow capsule marked "WYETH" and "57", in bottles of 100 capsules, and in REDIPAK® cartons of 100 individually wrapped capsules.
Keep tightly closed.
Dispense in tight container.

Tablets

Supplied as tablets containing nafcillin sodium, as the monohydrate, equivalent to 500 mg nafcillin buffered with calcium carbonate as follows:
NDC 0008-0464, white, capsule-shaped, scored, film-coated tablet marked "WYETH" and "464", in bottles of 50 tablets.
Keep tightly closed.
Protect from light.
Dispense in light-resistant tight container.

Oral Solution

Supplied as a powder for oral solution as follows. When reconstituted with water, each 5 mL will contain nafcillin sodium equivalent to 250 mg nafcillin.
NDC 0008-0513, white powder in bottles to make 100 mL of solution.
Keep tightly closed.

FOR PARENTERAL ADMINISTRATION (intravenous or intramuscular)

Vials

Supplied in vial sizes of 500 mg, 1 gram, and 2 gram nafcillin sodium as the monohydrate, buffered as follows:
NDC 0008-0431, in packages of 10 vials.
When reconstituted as recommended (see table below) with Sterile Water for Injection, USP, Sodium Chloride Injection, USP, Bacteriostatic Water for Injection, USP (TUBEX®), or Bacteriostatic Water for Injection, USP, with parabens or with benzyl alcohol, each vial contains, respectively, 2 mL, 4 mL, or 8 mL of solution. Each mL contains nafcillin sodium equivalent to 250 mg nafcillin buffered with 10 mg sodium citrate.

Vial Size	Amount of Diluent	Nafcillin Sodium Solution
500 mg	1.7 mL	2 mL
1 gram	3.4 mL	4 mL
2 gram	6.8 mL	8 mL

FOR INTRAVENOUS USE ONLY

Piggyback Units: Supplied in single units equivalent to 1 gram, 1.5 gram, 2 gram, or 4 gram nafcillin per unit buffered with 40 mg sodium citrate per gram as follows:
NDC 0008-0431, in packages of 10 PIGGYBACK vials.
ALSO AVAILABLE (for IV stock solution only)
Bulk Vial: Supplied in vial size of 10 gram nafcillin per vial buffered with 40 mg sodium citrate per gram as follows:
NDC 0008-0431, as single vials.
Shake vial well after adding diluent and before using.
Use solution within 8 hours if kept at room temperature or 48 hours if kept under refrigeration.

BIBLIOGRAPHY

A bibliography is available upon request.

Shown in Product Identification Section, page 437

WYAMYCIN® E ℞

[*wi-a-mi'sin*]
Liquid
(erythromycin ethylsuccinate oral suspension)

HOW SUPPLIED

Wyamycin® E Liquid (erythromycin ethylsuccinate oral suspension), Wyeth®, is available in the following dosage strengths in bottles of one pint:
200 mg per 5 mL, NDC 0008-0555, pink suspension.
400 mg per 5 mL, NDC 0008-0556, orange suspension.

ALSO AVAILABLE:
Wyamycin® S (erythromycin stearate) Tablets, Wyeth®, containing the equivalent of 250 mg or 500 mg erythromycin, are available as follows:
250 mg, NDC 0008-0576, pink, round, film-coated tablet marked "WYETH" and "576", in bottles of 100 and 500 tablets.
500 mg, NDC 0008-0578, pink, elliptical, film-coated tablet marked "WYETH" and "578", in bottles of 100 tablets.
For prescribing information write to Professional Service, Wyeth Laboratories, Box 8299, Philadelphia, PA 19101, or contact your local Wyeth representative.

WYANOIDS® OTC

[*wi'a-noids*]
Hemorrhoidal Suppositories

DESCRIPTION

Each suppository contains 15 mg extract belladonna (0.19 mg equiv. total alkaloids), 3 mg ephedrine sulfate, zinc oxide, boric acid, bismuth oxyiodide, bismuth subcarbonate, and peruvian balsam in cocoa butter and beeswax. Wyeth Wyanoids have an unusual "torpedo" design which facilitates insertion and insures retention.

INDICATIONS

For the temporary relief of pain and itching of hemorrhoidal tissue in many cases.

WARNING

Not to be used by persons having glaucoma or excessive pressure within the eye, by elderly persons (where undiagnosed glaucoma or excessive pressure within the eye occurs most frequently), or by children under 6 years of age, unless directed by a physician. Discontinue use if blurring of vision, rapid pulse, or dizziness occurs. Do not exceed recommended dosage. Not for frequent or prolonged use. If dryness of the mouth occurs, decrease dosage. If eye pain occurs, discontinue use and see your physician immediately as this may indicate undiagnosed glaucoma. In case of rectal bleeding, consult physician promptly.

USUAL DOSAGE

One suppository twice daily for six days.

DIRECTIONS

Remove wrapper of suppository and insert suppository rectally with gentle pressure, pointed end first. Use preferably upon arising and at bedtime.

HOW SUPPLIED

Boxes of 12.

Shown in Product Identification Section, page 437

WYCILLIN® ℞

[*wi-sil'in*]
(sterile penicillin G procaine suspension)
INJECTION
FOR DEEP INTRAMUSCULAR INJECTION ONLY

DESCRIPTION

This product is designed to provide a stable aqueous suspension of sterile penicillin G procaine, ready for immediate use. This eliminates the necessity for addition of any diluent, required for the usual dry formulation of injectable penicillin.
Each TUBEX® (Sterile Cartridge-Needle Unit, Wyeth), 1,200,000 units (2 ml size) or 600,000 units (1 ml size) or disposable syringe 2,400,000 units (4 ml size) contains penicillin G procaine in a stabilized aqueous suspension with sodium citrate buffer; and as w/v, approximately 0.5% lecithin, 0.5% carboxymethylcellulose, 0.5% povidone, 0.1% methylparaben, and 0.01% propylparaben.
Each TUBEX, 300,000 units (1 ml size), contains penicillin G procaine in a stabilized aqueous suspension with sodium citrate buffer; and as w/v, approximately 0.3% lecithin, 0.9% carboxymethylcellulose, 0.9% povidone, 0.14% methylparaben, and 0.015% propylparaben.
Wycillin (sterile penicillin G procaine suspension) must be stored in a refrigerator. Keep from freezing. This will prevent deterioration and assure that no significant loss of potency occurs within the expiration date.
Wycillin suspension in the TUBEX and disposable syringe formulations is viscous and opaque. Read "Contraindications," "Warnings," "Precautions," and "Dosage and Administration" sections prior to use.

ACTIONS AND PHARMACOLOGY

Penicillin G exerts a bactericidal action against penicillin-sensitive microorganisms during the stage of active multiplication. It acts through the inhibition of biosynthesis of cell-wall mucopeptide. It is not active against the penicillinase-producing bacteria, which include many strains of staphylococci. Penicillin G exerts high *in vitro* activity against staphylococci (except penicillinase-producing strains), streptococci (Groups A, C, G, H, L, and M), and pneumococci. Other organisms sensitive to penicillin G are *Neisseria gonorrhoeae, Corynebacterium diphtheriae, Bacillus anthracis,* Clostridia, *Actinomyces bovis, Streptobacillus moniliformis, Listeria monocytogenes,* and Leptospira. *Treponema pallidum* is extremely sensitive to the bactericidal action of penicillin G.
Sensitivity plate testing: If the Kirby-Bauer method of disc sensitivity is used, a 10-unit penicillin disc should give a zone greater than 28 mm when tested against a penicillin-sensitive bacterial strain.
Penicillin G procaine is an equimolecular compound of procaine and penicillin G, administered intramuscularly as a suspension. It dissolves slowly at the site of injection, giving a plateau type of blood level at about 4 hours which falls slowly over a period of the next 15–20 hours.
Approximately 60% of penicillin G is bound to serum protein. The drug is distributed throughout the body tissues in widely varying amounts. Highest levels are found in the kidneys with lesser amounts in the liver, skin, and intestines. Penicillin G penetrates into all other tissues to a lesser degree with a very small level found in the cerebrospinal fluid. With normal kidney function, the drug is excreted rapidly by tubular excretion. In neonates and young infants and in individuals with impaired kidney functions, excretion is considerably delayed. Approximately 60 to 90 percent of a dose of parenteral penicillin G is excreted in the urine within 24 to 36 hours.

INDICATIONS

Penicillin G procaine is indicated in the treatment of moderately severe infections due to penicillin-G-sensitive microorganisms that are sensitive to the low and persistent serum levels common to this particular dosage form. Therapy should be guided by bacteriological studies (including sensitivity tests) and by clinical response.
NOTE: When high, sustained serum levels are required, aqueous penicillin G, either IM or IV, should be used.
The following infections will usually respond to adequate dosages of intramuscular penicillin G procaine:
Streptococcal infections (Group A—without bacteremia). Moderately severe to severe infections of the upper respiratory tract, skin and soft-tissue infections, scarlet fever, and erysipelas.
NOTE: Streptococci in Groups A, C, G, H, L, and M are very sensitive to penicillin G. Other groups, including Group D (enterococcus), are resistant. Aqueous penicillin is recommended for streptococcal infections with bacteremia.
Pneumococcal infections. Moderately severe infections of the respiratory tract.
NOTE: Severe pneumonia, empyema, bacteremia, pericarditis, meningitis, peritonitis, and arthritis of pneumococcal etiology are better treated with aqueous penicillin G during the acute stage.
Staphylococcal infections—penicillin-G-sensitive. Moderately severe infections of the skin and soft tissues.
NOTE: Reports indicate an increasing number of strains of staphylococci resistant to penicillin G, emphasizing the need for culture and sensitivity studies in treating suspected staphylococcal infections.
Indicated surgical procedures should be performed.
Fusospirochetosis (Vincent's gingivitis and pharyngitis). Moderately severe infections of the oropharynx respond to therapy with penicillin G procaine.
NOTE: Necessary dental care should be accomplished in infections involving the gum tissue.
Treponema pallidum (syphilis); all stages.
N. gonorrhoeae; acute and chronic (without bacteremia).
Yaws, Bejel, Pinta.
C. diphtheriae —penicillin G procaine as an adjunct to antitoxin for prevention of the carrier stage.
Anthrax.
Streptobacillus moniliformis and *Spirillum minus* infections (rat-bite fever).
Erysipeloid.
Subacute bacterial endocarditis (Group A streptococcus), only in extremely sensitive infections.
Although no controlled clinical efficacy studies have been conducted, aqueous crystalline penicillin G for injection and penicillin G procaine suspension have been suggested by the American Heart Association and the American Dental Association for use as part of a combined parenteral-oral regimen for prophylaxis against bacterial endocarditis in patients who have congenital heart disease or rheumatic or other acquired valvular heart disease when they undergo dental procedures and surgical procedures of the upper respiratory tract.[1]
Since it may happen that *alpha* -hemolytic streptococci relatively resistant to penicillin may be found when patients are receiving continuous oral penicillin for secondary prevention of rheumatic fever, prophylactic agents other than penicillin may be chosen for these patients and prescribed in ad-

Continued on next page

Wyeth—Cont.

dition to their continuous rheumatic fever prophylactic regimen.

NOTE: When selecting antibiotics for the prevention of bacterial endocarditis, the physician or dentist should read the full joint statement of the American Heart Association and the American Dental Association.[1]

CONTRAINDICATIONS

A previous hypersensitivity reaction to any penicillin is a contraindication.

Do not inject into or near an artery or nerve.

WARNINGS

Serious and occasionally fatal hypersensitivity (anaphylactoid) reactions have been reported in patients on penicillin therapy.

Serious anaphylactoid reactions require immediate emergency treatment with epinephrine. Oxygen and intravenous corticosteroids should also be administered as indicated.

Although anaphylaxis is more frequent following parenteral therapy, it has occurred in patients on oral penicillins. These reactions are more apt to occur in individuals with a history of sensitivity to multiple allergens.

There have been well-documented reports of individuals with a history of penicillin hypersensitivity reactions who have experienced severe hypersensitivity reactions when treated with a cephalosporin. Before therapy with a penicillin, careful inquiry should be made concerning previous hypersensitivity reactions to penicillins, cephalosporins, and other allergens. If an allergic reaction occurs, the drug should be discontinued and the patient treated with the usual agents, e.g., pressor amines, antihistamines, and corticosteroids.

Immediate toxic reactions to procaine may occur in some individuals, particularly when a large single dose is administered in the treatment of gonorrhea (4.8 million units). These reactions may be manifested by mental disturbances, including anxiety, confusion, agitation, depression, weakness, seizures, hallucinations, combativeness, and expressed "fear of impending death." The reactions noted in carefully controlled studies occurred in approximately one in 500 patients treated for gonorrhea. Reactions are transient, lasting from 15 to 30 minutes.

Inadvertent intravascular administration, including inadvertent direct intraarterial injection or injection immediately adjacent to arteries, of Wycillin (sterile penicillin G procaine suspension) and other penicillin preparations has resulted in severe neurovascular damage, including transverse myelitis with permanent paralysis, gangrene requiring amputation of digits and more proximal portions of extremities, and necrosis and sloughing at and surrounding the injection site. Such severe effects have been reported following injections into the buttock, thigh, and deltoid areas. Other serious complications of suspected intravascular administration which have been reported include immediate pallor, mottling or cyanosis of the extremity both distal and proximal to the injection site followed by bleb formation; severe edema requiring anterior and/or posterior compartment fasciotomy in the lower extremity. The above described severe effects and complications have most often occurred in infants and small children. Prompt consultation with an appropriate specialist is indicated if any evidence of compromise of the blood supply occurs at, proximal to, or distal to the site of injection.[2-10] See "Contraindications," "Precautions," and "Dosage and Administration" sections.

Quadriceps femoris fibrosis and atrophy have been reported following repeated intramuscular injections of penicillin preparations into the anterolateral thigh.

Injection into or near a nerve may result in permanent neurological damage.

PRECAUTIONS

Penicillin should be used with caution in individuals with histories of significant allergies and/or asthma.

Care should be taken to avoid intravenous or intraarterial administration, or injection into or near major peripheral nerves or blood vessels, since such injections may produce neurovascular damage. See "Contraindications," "Warnings," and "Dosage and Administration" sections.

In suspected staphylococcal infections, proper laboratory studies, including sensitivity tests, should be performed.

A small percentage of patients are sensitive to procaine. If there is a history of sensitivity, make the usual test: Inject intradermally 0.1 ml of a 1 to 2 percent procaine solution. Development of an erythema, wheal, flare, or eruption indicates procaine sensitivity. Sensitivity should be treated by the usual methods, including barbiturates, and procaine penicillin preparations should not be used. Antihistaminics appear beneficial in treatment of procaine reactions.

The use of antibiotics may result in overgrowth of nonsusceptible organisms. Constant observation of the patient is essential. If new infections due to bacteria or fungi appear during therapy, the drug should be discontinued and appropriate measures taken.

Whenever allergic reactions occur, penicillin should be withdrawn unless, in the opinion of the physician, the condition being treated is life-threatening and amenable only to penicillin therapy.

In prolonged therapy with penicillin, and particularly with high-dosage schedules, periodic evaluation of the renal and hematopoietic systems is recommended.

When treating gonococcal infections in which primary or secondary syphillis may be suspected, proper diagnostic procedures, including dark-field examinations, should be done. In all cases in which concomitant syphilis is suspected, monthly serological tests should be made for at least four months.

ADVERSE REACTIONS

Penicillin is a substance of low toxicity but does possess a significant index of sensitization. The following hypersensitivity reactions associated with use of penicillin have been reported: Skin rashes, ranging from maculopapular eruptions to exfoliative dermatitis; urticaria; serum-sickness-like reactions, including chills, fever, edema, arthralgia, and prostration. Severe and often fatal anaphylaxis has been reported (see "Warnings"). As with other treatments for syphilis, the Jarisch-Herxheimer reaction has been reported. Procaine toxicity manifestations have been reported (see "Warnings"). Although procaine hypersensitivity reactions have not been reported with this drug, there are patients who are sensitive to procaine (see "Precautions").

DOSAGE AND ADMINISTRATION

Penicillin G procaine (aqueous) is for intramuscular injection only.

Administer by DEEP, INTRAMUSCULAR INJECTION in the upper, outer quadrant of the buttock. In infants and small children, the midlateral aspect of the thigh may be preferable. When doses are repeated, vary the injection site.

When using the TUBEX cartridge:

The Wyeth TUBEX cartridge for this product incorporates several features that are designed to facilitate the visualization of blood on aspiration if a blood vessel is inadvertently entered.

The design of this cartridge is such that blood which enters its needle will be quickly visualized as a red or dark-colored "spot." This "spot" will appear on the barrel of the glass cartridge immediately proximal to the blue hub. Prior to injection, in order to determine where this "spot" can be seen, the operator should first insert and secure the cartridge in the TUBEX syringe in the usual fashion. The needle cover should then be removed and the cartridge and syringe held in one hand with the needle pointing away from the operator. If the 2 ml metal syringe is used the glass cartridge should then be rotated by turning the plunger of the syringe clockwise until the flat bevel at the tip of the needle is pointing upward and is horizontal when viewed directly from above. An imaginary straight line then drawn from the middle of the flat bevel to the back edge of the blue hub where it joins the glass will point to the area on the glass cartridge where the "spot" can be visualized. If the 1 ml metal syringe is used, it will not be possible to continue to rotate the glass cartridge clockwise once it is properly engaged and fully threaded; it can, however, then be rotated counterclockwise as far as necessary to properly orient the bevel of the needle and locate the observation area. (In this same area in some cartridges a dark spot may sometimes be visualized prior to injection. This is the proximal end of the needle and does not represent a foreign body in, or other abnormality of, the suspension.)

Thus, before the needle is inserted into the selected muscle, it is important for the operator to orient the flat bevel of the needle so that any blood which might enter after its insertion and during aspiration can be visualized in the area of the cartridge where it will appear and not be obscured by the metal syringe or other obstructions.

After selection of the proper site and insertion of the needle into the selected muscle, aspirate by pulling back on the plunger. While maintaining negative pressure for 2 to 3 seconds, carefully observe the barrel of the cartridge in the area previously identified (see above) for the appearance of a red or dark-colored "spot."

Blood or "typical blood color" may not be seen if a blood vessel has been entered—only a mixture of blood and Wycillin. The appearance of *any* discoloration is reason to withdraw the needle and discard the glass TUBEX cartridge. If it is elected to inject at another site, a new cartridge should be used. If no blood or discoloration appears, inject the contents of the cartridge slowly. Discontinue delivery of the dose if the subject complains of severe immediate pain at the injection site or if, especially in infants and young children, symptoms or signs occur suggesting onset of severe pain.

Some TUBEX cartridges may contain a small air bubble which may be disregarded, since it does not affect administration of the product.

Because of the high concentration of suspended material in this product, the needle may be blocked if the injection is not made at a slow, steady rate.

When using the disposable syringe:

The Wyeth disposable syringe for this product incorporates several new features that are designed to facilitate its use.

A single small indentation, or "dot", has been punched into the metal ring that surrounds the neck of the syringe near the base of the needle. It is important that this "dot" be placed in a position so that it can be easily visualized by the operator following the intramuscular insertion of the syringe needle.

After selection of the proper site and insertion of the needle into the selected muscle, aspirate by pulling back on the plunger. While maintaining negative pressure for 2 to 3 seconds, carefully observe the barrel of the syringe immediately proximal to the location of the "dot" for appearance of blood or any discoloration. Blood or "typical blood color" may *not* be seen if a blood vessel has been entered—only a mixture of blood and Wycillin. The appearance of any discoloration is reason to withdraw the needle and discard the syringe. If it is elected to inject at another site, a new syringe should be used. If no blood or discoloration appears, inject the contents of the syringe slowly. Discontinue delivery of the dose if the subject complains of severe immediate pain at the injection site or if in infants and young children symptoms or signs occur suggesting onset of severe pain.

Pneumonia (pneumococcal), moderately severe (uncomplicated): 600,000–1,000,000 units daily.

Streptococcal infections (Group A), moderately severe to severe tonsillitis, erysipelas, scarlet fever, upper respiratory tract, skin and soft tissue: 600,000–1,000,000 units daily for 10-day minimum.

Staphylococcal infections, moderately severe to severe: 600,000–1,000,000 units daily.

In pneumonia, streptococcal (Group A) and staphylococcal infections in children under 60 pounds: 300,000 units daily.

Bacterial endocarditis (Group A streptococci) only in extremely sensitive infections: 600,000–1,000,000 units daily.

For prophylaxis against bacterial endocarditis[1] in patients with congenital heart disease or rheumatic or other acquired valvular heart disease when undergoing dental procedures or surgical procedures of the upper respiratory tract, use a combined parenteral-oral regimen. One million units of aqueous crystalline penicillin G (30,000 units/kg in children) intramuscularly mixed with 600,000 units penicillin G procaine (600,000 units for children) should be given one-half to one hour before the procedure. Oral penicillin V (phenoxymethyl penicillin), 500 mg for adults or 250 mg for children less than 60 lbs., should be given every 6 hours for 8 doses. Doses for children should not exceed recommendations for adults for a single dose or for a 24-hour period.

Syphilis—

Primary, secondary, and latent with a negative spinal fluid in adults and children over 12 years of age: 600,000 units daily for 8 days—total 4,800,000 units.

Late (tertiary, neurosyphilis, and latent syphilis with positive spinal-fluid examination or no spinal-fluid examination): 600,000 units daily for 10–15 days—total 6–9 million units.

Congenital syphilis under 70-lb. body weight: 10,000 units/kg/day for 10 days.

Yaws, Bejel, and Pinta: Treatment as syphilis in corresponding stage of disease.

Although some isolates of *Neisseria gonorrhoeae* have decreased susceptibility to penicillin, this inherent resistance is relative, not absolute, and penicillin in large doses remains the drug of choice for these strains. Strains producing penicillinase, however, are resistant to penicillin G, and a drug other than penicillin G should be used. Physicians are cautioned not to use less than the recommended doses.

Gonorrheal infections (uncomplicated)—Men or Women: Aqueous penicillin G procaine, 4.8 million units intramuscularly, divided into at least two doses and injected at different sites at one visit, together with 1 gram of oral probenecid, preferably given just before the injection.

NOTE: Treatment of severe complications of gonorrhea should be individualized, using large amounts of short-acting penicillin.

Gonorrheal endocarditis should be treated intensively with aqueous penicillin G. Prophylactic or epidemiologic treatment for gonorrhea (male and female) is accomplished with the same treatment schedules as for the uncomplicated gonorrhea.

Retreatment

The National Center for Disease Control, Venereal Disease Branch, U.S. Department of Health and Human Services, Atlanta, Georgia, recommends:

Test of cure procedures at approximately 7–14 days after therapy. In the male, a gram-stained smear is adequate if positive; otherwise, a culture specimen should be obtained from the anterior urethra. In the female, culture specimens should be obtained from both the endocervical and anal canal sites.

Retreatment in the male is indicated if the urethral discharge persists for three or more days following initial therapy and the smear or culture remains positive. Follow-up treatment consists of 4,800,000 units of aqueous penicillin G procaine intramuscularly, divided in two injection sites at a single visit.

In uncomplicated gonorrhea in the female, retreatment is indicated if follow-up cervical or rectal cultures remain positive for *N. gonorrhoeae.* Follow-up treatment consists of 4,800,000 units of aqueous penicillin G procaine daily on two successive days.

Syphilis: All gonorrhea patients should have a serologic test for syphilis at the time of diagnosis. Patients with gonorrhea who also have syphilis should be given additional treatment appropriate to the stage of syphilis.

Diphtheria—adjunctive therapy with antitoxin: 300,000–600,000 units daily.

Diphtheria carrier state: 300,000 units daily for 10 days.

Anthrax-cutaneous: 600,000–1,000,000 units/day.

Vincent's infection (fusospirochetosis): 600,000–1,000,000 units/day.

Erysipeloid: 600,000–1,000,000 units/day.

Streptobacillus moniliformis and *Spirillum minus* (rat-bite fever): 600,000–1,000,000 units/day.

HOW SUPPLIED

600,000 units per ml—1 ml TUBEX sterile cartridge-needle unit, packages of 10; *1,200,000 units in 2 ml* TUBEX, packages of 10; *2,400,000 units in 4 ml* single-dose disposable syringe, packages of 10.

REFERENCES

1. American Heart Association: Prevention of bacterial endocarditis. *Circulation, 56:* 139A-143A, 1977.
2. SHAW, E.: Transverse myelitis from injection of penicillin. *Am. J. Dis. Child., 11:* 548, 1966.
3. KNOWLES, J.: Accidental intra-arterial injection of penicillin. *Am. J. Dis. Child., 111:* 552, 1966.
4. DARBY, C., et al: Ischemia following an intragluteal injection of benzathine-procaine penicillin G mixture in a one-year-old boy. *Clin. Pediatrics, 12:* 485, 1973.
5. BROWN, L. & NELSON, A.: Postinfectious intravascular thrombosis with gangrene. *Arch. Surg., 94:* 652, 1967.
6. BORENSTINE, J.: Transverse myelitis and penicillin (Correspondence). *Am. J. Dis. Child., 112:* 166, 1966.
7. ATKINSON, J.: Transverse myelopathy secondary to penicillin injection. *J. Pediatrics, 75:* 867, 1969.
8. TALBERT, J. et al: Gangrene of the foot following intramuscular injection in the lateral thigh: A case report with recommendations for prevention. *J. Pediatrics, 79:* 110, 1967.
9. FISHER, T.: Medicolegal affairs. *Canad. Med. Assoc. J., 112:* 395, 1975.
10. SCHANZER, H. et al: Accidental intraarterial injection of penicillin G. *JAMA, 242:* 1289, 1979.

WYCILLIN® and PROBENECID ℞

[wi-sil 'in and pro-ben 'is-id]
(sterile penicillin G procaine suspension and probenecid tablets)
Disposable Syringe and Tablets
Wycillin is for deep IM injection only.

DESCRIPTION

The Wycillin disposable syringe is designed to provide a stable aqueous suspension of sterile penicillin G procaine, ready for immediate use. This eliminates the necessity for addition of any diluent, required for the usual dry formulation of injectable penicillin.

Each syringe, 2,400,000 units (4 ml size), contains penicillin G procaine in a stabilized aqueous suspension with sodium citrate buffer; and as w/v, approximately 0.5% lecithin, 0.5% carboxymethylcellulose, 0.5% povidone, 0.1% methylparaben, and 0.01% propylparaben.

Wycillin must be stored in a refrigerator. Keep from freezing. This will prevent deterioration and assure that no significant loss of potency occurs within the expiration date.

Probenecid is a uricosuric and renal tubular-blocking agent. Probenecid tablets contain 0.5 gram probenecid. The inactive ingredients present are calcium stearate, D&C Yellow 10, gelatin, hydroxypropyl methylcellulose, iron oxide, magnesium carbonate, polyethylene glycol, starch, talc, and titanium dioxide.

Wycillin suspension in the disposable syringe formulation is viscous and opaque. Read "Contraindications," "Warnings," "Precautions," and "Dosage and Administration" sections prior to use.

ACTIONS AND PHARMACOLOGY

Penicillin G exerts a bactericidal action against penicillin-sensitive microorganisms during the stage of active multiplication. It acts through the inhibition of biosynthesis of cell-wall mucopeptide. It is not active against the penicillinase-producing bacteria, which include many strains of staphylococci. Neisseria gonorrhoeae are included among the various organisms which are sensitive to penicillin G. Penicillin G procaine is an equimolecular salt of procaine and penicillin G, administered intramuscularly as a suspension. It dissolves slowly at the site of injection, giving a plateau type of blood level at about 4 hours which falls slowly over a period of the next 15–20 hours. Approximately 60% to 90% of a dose of penicillin G is excreted in the urine within 24 to 36 hours. Approximately 60% of penicillin G is bound to serum protein. The drug is distributed throughout the body tissues in widely varying amounts, with highest levels found in the kidneys and lesser amounts in the liver, skin, and intestines. Penicillin G penetrates into all other tissues to a lesser degree, with a very small level found in the cerebrospinal fluid. With normal kidney function the drug is excreted rapidly by tubular excretion. In neonates and young infants and in individuals with impaired kidney function, excretion is considerably delayed.

Probenecid inhibits the tubular reabsorption of urate, thus increasing the urinary excretion of uric acid and decreasing serum uric acid levels. It also inhibits the tubular excretion of penicillin and usually increases penicillin plasma levels, regardless of the route by which the antibiotic is given. A 2-fold to 4-fold elevation has been demonstrated for various penicillins. Probenecid does not influence plasma concentrations of salicylates, nor the excretion of streptomycin, chloramphenicol, chlortetracycline, oxytetracycline, or neomycin.

INDICATIONS

Wycillin and Probenecid is indicated for the single-dose treatment of uncomplicated (without bacteremia) urethral, cervical, rectal, or pharyngeal infections caused by *Neisseria gonorrhoeae* (gonorrhea) in men and women.

Susceptibility studies should be performed when recurrent infections or resistant strains are encountered. Urethritis and the presence of gram-negative diplococci in urethral smears are strong presumptive evidence of gonorrhea. Culture or fluorescent antibody studies will confirm the diagnosis. Therapy may be instituted prior to obtaining results of susceptibility testing.

CONTRAINDICATIONS

A history of a previous hypersensitivity reaction to any of the penicillins or to Probenecid is a contraindication.

Probenecid is not recommended in persons with known blood dyscrasias or uric kidney stones or during an acute attack of gout. It is not recommended in conjunction with penicillin G procaine suspension in the presence of known renal impairment.

Do not inject into or near an artery or nerve.

WARNINGS

PENICILLIN G PROCAINE: Serious and occasionally fatal hypersensitivity (anaphylactoid) reactions have been reported in patients on penicillin therapy. Serious anaphylactoid reactions require immediate emergency treatment with epinephrine. Oxygen and intravenous corticosteroids should also be administered as indicated. Although anaphylaxis is more frequent following parenteral therapy, it has occurred in patients on oral penicillins. These reactions are more apt to occur in individuals with a history of sensitivity to multiple allergens.

There have been well-documented reports of individuals with a history of penicillin-hypersensitivity reactions who have experienced severe hypersensitivity reactions when treated with a cephalosporin. Before therapy with a penicillin, careful inquiry should be made concerning previous hypersensitivity reactions to penicillins, cephalosporins, and other allergens. If an allergic reaction occurs, the drug should be discontinued and the patient treated with the usual agents, e.g., pressor amines, antihistamines, and corticosteroids.

Immediate toxic reactions to procaine may occur in some individuals, particularly when a large single dose is administered in the treatment of gonorrhea (4.8 million units). These reactions may be manifested by mental disturbances, including anxiety, confusion, agitation, depression, weakness, seizures, hallucinations, combativeness, and expressed "fear of impending death." The reactions noted in carefully controlled studies occurred in approximately one in 500 patients treated for gonorrhea. Reactions are transient, lasting from 15–30 minutes.

Inadvertent intravascular administration, including inadvertent direct intraarterial injection or injection immediately adjacent to arteries, of Wycillin (sterile penicillin G procaine suspension) and other penicillin preparations has resulted in severe neurovascular damage, including transverse myelitis with permanent paralysis, gangrene requiring amputation of digits and more proximal portions of extremities, and necrosis and sloughing at and surrounding the injection site. Such severe effects have been reported following injections into the buttock, thigh, and deltoid areas. Other serious complications of suspected intravascular administration which have been reported include immediate pallor, mottling or cyanosis of the extremity both distal and proximal to the injection site followed by bleb formation; severe edema requiring anterior and/ or posterior compartment fasciotomy in the lower extremity. The above-described severe effects and complications have most often occurred in infants and small children. Prompt consultation with an appropriate specialist is indicated if any evidence of compromise of the blood supply occurs at, proximal to, or distal to the site of injection.[1-9] See "Contraindications," "Precautions," and "Dosage and Administration" sections.

Quadriceps femoris fibrosis and atrophy have been reported following repeated intramuscular injections of penicillin preparations into the anterolateral thigh.

Injection into or near a nerve may result in permanent neurological damage.

PROBENECID: Exacerbation of gout following therapy with Probenecid may occur; in such cases colchicine therapy is advisable.

In patients on Probenecid, the use of salicylates in either small or large doses is not recommended because it antagonizes the uricosuric action of Probenecid. Patients on Probenecid who require a mild analgesic agent should receive acetaminophen rather than salicylates, even in small doses.

USAGE IN PREGNANCY: The safety of these drugs for use in pregnancy has not been established.

PRECAUTIONS

PENICILLIN G PROCAINE: When treating gonococcal infections in which primary or secondary syphilis may be suspected, proper diagnostic procedures, including dark-field examinations, should be done. In all cases in which concomitant syphilis is suspected, monthly serological tests should be made for at least four months. Patients with gonorrhea, who also have syphilis, should be given additional appropriate parenteral penicillin treatment.

Penicillin should be used with caution in individuals with histories of significant allergies and/or asthma. When administering Wycillin, care should be taken to avoid intravenous or intraarterial administration, or injection into or near major peripheral nerves or blood vessels, since such injections may produce neurovascular damage. See "Contraindications," "Warnings," and "Dosage and Administration" sections.

A small percentage of patients are sensitive to procaine. If there is a history of sensitivity, make the usual test: Inject intradermally 0.1 ml of a 1- to 2-percent procaine solution. Development of an erythema, wheal, flare, or eruption indicates procaine sensitivity. Sensitivity should be treated by the usual methods, including barbiturates, and procaine penicillin preparations should not be used. Antihistaminics appear beneficial in treatment of procaine reactions.

PROBENECID: Use Probenecid with caution in patients with a history of peptic ulcer. A reducing substance may appear in the urine of patients receiving Probenecid. Although this disappears with discontinuance of therapy, a false diagnosis of glycosuria may be made because of a false-positive Benedict's test.

ADVERSE REACTIONS

WYCILLIN: Penicillin is a substance of low toxicity but does possess a significant index of sensitization. The following hypersensitivity reactions associated with use of penicillin have been reported: skin rashes, ranging from maculopapular eruptions to exfoliative dermatitis; urticaria; serum-sickness-like reactions, including chills, fever, edema, arthralgia, and prostration. Severe and often fatal anaphylaxis has been reported (see "Warnings"). As with other treatments for syphilis, the Jarisch-Herxheimer reaction has been reported.

Procaine toxicity manifestations have been reported (see "Warnings"). Although procaine hypersensitivity reactions have not been reported with this drug, there are patients who are sensitive to procaine (see "Precautions").

PROBENECID: The following are the principal adverse reactions which have been reported as associated with the use of Probenecid, generally with more prolonged or repeated administration: Hypersensitivity reactions (including anaphylaxis), nephrotic syndrome, hepatic necrosis, aplastic anemia; also other anemias, including hemolytic anemia related to genetic deficiency of glucose-6-phosphate dehydrogenase.

DOSAGE AND ADMINISTRATION

Penicillin G procaine (aqueous) is for intramuscular injection only.

Administer by DEEP INTRAMUSCULAR INJECTION in the upper, outer quadrant of the buttock. When doses are repeated, vary the injection site.

The Wyeth disposable syringe for this product incorporates several new features that are designed to facilitate its use. A single small indentation, or "dot", has been punched into the metal ring that surrounds the neck of the syringe near the base of the needle. It is important that this "dot" be placed in a position so that it can be easily visualized by the operator following the intramuscular insertion of the syringe needle.

After selection of the proper site and insertion of the needle into the selected muscle, aspirate by pulling back on the plunger. While maintaining negative pressure for 2–3 seconds, carefully observe the barrel of the syringe immediately proximal to the location of the "dot" for appearance of blood or any discoloration. Blood or "typical blood color" may *not* be seen if a blood vessel has been entered—only a mixture of blood and Wycillin. The appearance of any discoloration is

Continued on next page

Wyeth—Cont.

reason to withdraw the needle and discard the syringe. If it is elected to inject at another site, a new syringe should be used. If no blood or discoloration appears, inject the contents of the syringe slowly. Discontinue delivery of the dose if the subject complains of severe immediate pain at the injection site or if in infants and young children symptoms or signs occur suggesting onset of severe pain.

Although some isolates of *Neisseria gonorrhoeae* have decreased susceptibility to penicillin, this inherent resistance is relative, not absolute, and penicillin in large doses remains the drug of choice for these strains. Strains producing penicillinase, however, are resistant to penicillin G, and a drug other than penicillin G should be used.

GONORRHEAL INFECTIONS (UNCOMPLICATED) MEN OR WOMEN: Aqueous penicillin G procaine, 4.8 million units intramuscularly, divided into at least two doses and injected at different sites at one visit, together with 1 gram (2 tablets, 0.5 gram each) of Probenecid orally, given just before the injections. Physicians are cautioned to use no less than the recommended dosages.

NOTE: Treatment of severe complications of gonorrhea should be individualized, using large amounts of short-acting penicillin. Gonorrheal endocarditis should be treated intensively with aqueous penicillin G. Prophylactic or epidemiologic treatment for gonorrhea (male and female) is accomplished with the same treatment schedules as for the uncomplicated gonorrhea.

RETREATMENT: The National Center for Disease Control, Venereal Disease Branch, U.S. Department of Health and Human Services, Atlanta, Georgia, recommends:

Test of cure procedures at approximately 7–14 days after therapy. In the male, a gram-stained smear is adequate if positive; otherwise, a culture specimen should be obtained from the anterior urethra. In the female, culture specimens should be obtained from both the endocervical and anal canal sites.

Retreatment in the male is indicated if the urethral discharge persists for three or more days following initial therapy and the smear or culture remains positive. Follow-up treatment consists of 4,800,000 units of aqueous penicillin G procaine, intramuscular, divided in two injection sites at a single visit.

In uncomplicated gonorrhea in the female, retreatment is indicated if follow-up cervical or rectal cultures remain positive for *N. gonorrhoeae.* Follow-up treatment consists of 4,800,000 units of aqueous penicillin G procaine daily on two successive days.

Syphilis: All gonorrhea patients should have a serologic test for syphilis at the time of diagnosis. Patients with gonorrhea who also have syphilis should be given additional treatment appropriate to the stage of syphilis.

HOW SUPPLIED

Wycillin® (sterile penicillin G procaine suspension) Injection and Probenecid Tablets is supplied as a combination package, NDC 0008-2517, containing the following:

Two disposable syringes of Wycillin (2,400,000 units each), 4 mL size (18 gauge × 2 inch needle, and

Two tablets Probenecid, Benemid® (0.5 gram each).

Store in a refrigerator—Keep from freezing.

Wycillin® Disposable Syringes manufactured by **Wyeth Laboratories Inc.,** Philadelphia, PA 19101

Probenecid Tablets (Benemid®) manufactured by **Merck, Sharp and Dohme,** Division of Merck & Co., West Point, PA 19486

REFERENCES

1. SHAW, E.: Transverse myelitis from injection of penicillin, *Am. J. Dis. Child., 111:* 548, 1966.
2. KNOWLES, J.: Accidental intra-arterial injection of penicillin. *Am. J. Dis. Child., 111:* 552, 1966.
3. DARBY, C., et al: Ischemia following an intragluteal injection of benzathine-procaine penicillin G mixture in a one-year-old boy. *Clin. Pediatrics, 12:* 485, 1973.
4. BROWN, L. & NELSON, A.: Postinfectious intravascular thrombosis with gangrene, *Arch. Surg., 94:* 652, 1967.
5. BORENSTINE, J.: Transverse myelitis and penicillin (Correspondence), *Am. J. Dis. Child., 112:* 166, 1966.
6. ATKINSON, J.: Transverse myelopathy secondary to penicillin injection. *J. Pediatrics, 75:* 867, 1969.
7. TALBERT, J. et al: Gangrene of the foot following intramuscular injection in the lateral thigh: A case report with recommendations for prevention. *J. Pediatrics, 70:* 110, 1967.
8. FISHER, T.: Medicolegal affairs, *Canad. Med. Assoc. J., 112:* 395, 1975.
9. SCHANZER, H. et al: Accidental intraarterial injection of penicillin G. *JAMA, 242:* 1289, 1979.

WYDASE® ℞

[*wi-dās*]

(hyaluronidase)

INJECTION

DESCRIPTION

Wydase, a protein enzyme, is a preparation of highly purified bovine testicular hyaluronidase. The exact chemical structure of this enzyme is unknown. Wydase is available in two dosage forms:

WYDASE LYOPHILIZED

Hyaluronidase, dehydrated in the frozen state under high vacuum, with lactose and thimerosal (mercury derivative), is supplied as a sterile, white, odorless, amorphous solid and is to be reconstituted with Sodium Chloride Injection, USP, before use, usually in the proportion of one mL per 150 USP units of hyaluronidase (Wydase Lyophilized).

Each vial of 1,500 USP units contains 1.0 mg thimerosal (mercury derivative), added as a preservative, and 13.3 mg lactose. Each vial of 150 USP units contains 0.075 mg thimerosal (mercury derivative), added as a preservative, and 2.66 mg lactose.

WYDASE STABILIZED SOLUTION

A hyaluronidase injection solution ready for use, colorless and odorless, containing 150 USP units of hyaluronidase per mL with 8.5 mg sodium chloride, 1 mg edetate disodium, 0.4 mg calcium chloride, monobasic sodium phosphate buffer, and not more than 0.1 mg thimerosal (mercury derivative).

The USP and the NF hyaluronidase units are equivalent to the turbidity-reducing (TR) unit and to the International Unit.

CLINICAL PHARMACOLOGY

Hyaluronidase is a spreading or diffusing substance which modifies the permeability of connective tissue through the hydrolysis of hyaluronic acid, a polysaccharide found in the intracellular ground substance of connective tissue, and of certain specialized tissues, such as the umbilical cord and vitreous humor. Hyaluronic acid is also present in the capsules of type A and C hemolytic streptococci. Hyaluronidase hydrolyzes hyaluronic acid by splitting the glucosaminidic bond between C_1 of the glucosamine moiety and C_4 of glucuronic acid. This temporarily decreases the viscosity of the cellular cement and promotes diffusion of injected fluids or of localized transudates or exudates, thus facilitating their absorption.

When no spreading factor is present, material injected subcutaneously spreads very slowly, but hyaluronidase causes rapid spreading, provided local interstitial pressure is adequate to furnish the necessary mechanical impulse. Such an impulse is normally initiated by injected solutions. The rate of diffusion is proportionate to the amount of enzyme, and the extent is proportionate to the volume of solution.

Animal studies indicated that in dogs, given 160,000 U/kg hyaluronidase intravenously, peak protein excretion in the urine occurred in the first hour and accounted for most of the 82 mg of protein recovered from the urine. The recovery represents 5% of the total amount of protein injected. One hour after the intravenous administration of 160,000 U/kg of hyaluronidase to rabbits, the agent could no longer be detected in the blood (mucin clot assay). It was also noted that the sojourn of hyaluronidase in the blood, as measured by the spreading technique, is considerably longer than the sojourn determined by the mucin clot assay. Rabbits and dogs were given 80,000 to 160,000 U/kg hyaluronidase intravenously, plasma and urine samples were collected and were injected into the shaven skin of another rabbit. The spreading activity (trypan blue as indicator) of the plasma reached a maximum within 5 minutes, remained constant for the first hour, and then declined slowly over 5 hours. The spreading activity of the urine reached a maximum within the first hour and paralleled that of the plasma thereafter.

A study in rats, sacrificed 3 hours after 2,400–3,000 U of radiolabeled hyaluronidase was administered intraperitoneally, indicated that all organs and tissues investigated displayed radioactivity, and that particularly high radioactivity was observed in the thymus, pancreas, kidneys, and ovaries.

Knowledge of the mechanisms involved in the disappearance of injected hyaluronidase is limited. It is known, however, that the blood of a number of mammalian species brings about the inactivation of hyaluronidase. Studies have demonstrated that hyaluronidase is antigenic; repeated injections of relatively large amounts of this enzyme may result in the formation of neutralizing antibodies. The reconstitution of the dermal barrier removed by intradermal injection of hyaluronidase (20.2, 0.2, 0.02, and 0.002 U/mL) to adult humans indicated that at 24 hours the restoration of the barrier is incomplete and inversely related to the dosage of enzyme; at 48 hours the barrier is completely restored in all treated areas.

Results from an experimental study, in humans, on the influence of hyaluronidase in bone repair support the conclusion that this enzyme alone, in the usual clinical dosage, does not deter bone healing.

INDICATIONS AND USAGE

Wydase is indicated as an adjuvant to increase the absorption and dispersion of other injected drugs; for hypodermoclysis; and as an adjunct in subcutaneous urography for improving resorption of radiopaque agents.

CONTRAINDICATIONS

Hypersensitivity to hyaluronidase. A preliminary test for sensitivity should be conducted. (See "Precautions"—'Laboratory Tests.")

Because of the danger of spreading a localized infection, Wydase should not be injected into or around an infected or acutely inflamed area. Similarly, Wydase should not be injected into an area that is known or suspected to be cancerous.

PRECAUTIONS

GENERAL

When considering the administration of any other drug with hyaluronidase, it is recommended that appropriate references first be consulted to determine the usual precautions for the use of the other drug; e.g., when epinephrine is injected along with hyaluronidase, the precautions for the use of epinephrine in cardiovascular disease, thyroid disease, diabetes, digital nerve block, ischemia of the fingers and toes, etc., should be observed.

LABORATORY TESTS

A preliminary skin test for sensitivity to hyaluronidase should be performed with an intradermal injection of approximately 0.02 mL of the solution. A positive reaction consists of a wheal with pseudopods appearing within five minutes and persisting for 20 to 30 minutes and accompanied by localized itching. Transient vasodilation at the site of the test, i.e., erythema, is not a positive reaction.

DRUG INTERACTIONS

When hyaluronidase is added to a local anesthetic agent, it hastens the onset of analgesia and tends to reduce the swelling caused by local infiltration, but the wider spread of the local anesthetic solution increases its absorption; this shortens its duration of action and tends to increase the incidence of systemic reaction.

CARCINOGENESIS, MUTAGENESIS, IMPAIRMENT OF FERTILITY

Long-term animal studies have not been performed to assess the carcinogenic or mutagenic potential of hyaluronidase. It has been observed that intravenous administration of as much as 75,000 U (500 times the therapeutic dose) of hyaluronidase in animals caused no histological changes in the tissues.

Long-term animal studies have not been performed to assess whether hyaluronidase impaired fertility; however, it has been reported that testicular degeneration may occur with the production of organ-specific antibodies against this enzyme following repeated injections. Human studies on the effect of intravaginal hyaluronidase in sterility due to oligospermia indicated that Wydase may have aided conception. Thus, it appears that hyaluronidase may not adversely affect fertility in females.

PREGNANCY

Teratogenic Effects—Pregnancy Category C

Animal reproductive studies have not been conducted with Wydase. It is also not known whether hyaluronidase can cause fetal harm when administered to a pregnant woman. Wydase should be given to a pregnant woman only if clearly needed.

LABOR AND DELIVERY

Administration of hyaluronidase during labor was reported to cause no complications: no increase in blood loss or differences in cervical trauma were observed. It is not known whether Wydase has an effect on the fetus if used during labor; the effect of hyaluronidase on the later growth, development, and functional maturation of the infant is unknown.

NURSING MOTHERS

It is not known whether hyaluronidase is excreted in human milk. Because many drugs are excreted in human milk, caution should be exercised when Wydase is administered to a nursing woman.

PEDIATRIC USE

Hyaluronidase may be added to small volumes of solution (up to 200 mL), such as a small clysis for infants or solutions of drugs for subcutaneous injection. The potential for chemical or physical incompatibilities should be kept in mind. (See "Dosage and Administration.")

ADVERSE REACTIONS

The subcutaneous administration of hyaluronidase has been associated with very few adverse reactions. Allergic reactions (urticaria) are rare. Anaphylacticlike reactions following retrobulbar block or intravenous injections have occurred in isolated cases. Cardiac fibrillation has been encountered once.

OVERDOSAGE

Symptoms of toxicity consist of local edema or urticaria, erythema, chills, nausea, vomiting, dizziness, tachycardia. and hypotension. The enzyme should be discontinued and supportive measures initiated immediately. Agents such as epinephrine, corticosteroids, and antihistamines should always be available for emergency treatment.

DOSAGE AND ADMINISTRATION

Wydase (hyaluronidase) should be administered only as discussed below, since its effects relative to absorption and dispersion of other drugs are not produced when it is administered intravenously.

RECONSTITUTION

If the lyophilized powder for injection is used, 1 mL of 0.9% sodium chloride should be added to a vial containing 150 U of hyaluronidase, and 10 mL of 0.9% sodium chloride to a vial containing 1,500 U of hyaluronidase, respectively, to provide a solution containing approximately 150 U/mL.

ABSORPTION AND DISPERSION OF INJECTED DRUGS

Absorption and dispersion of other injected drugs may be enhanced by adding 150 U hyaluronidase to the injection solution. In order to prepare a solution containing epinephrine, add 0.5 mL epinephrine [Wyeth Epinephrine Hydrochloride Injection, USP (1:1000)] to the above solution.

Before adding Wydase to a solution containing another drug, it is recommended that appropriate references be consulted regarding physical or chemical incompatibilities.

HYPODERMOCLYSIS

Insert needle with aseptic precautions. With tip lying free and movable between skin and muscle, begin clysis; fluid should start in readily without pain or lump. Then inject Solution Wydase into rubber tubing close to needle.

An alternate method is to inject Wydase under skin prior to clysis. 150 U will facilitate absorption of 1,000 mL or more of solution. As with all parenteral fluid therapy, observe effect closely, with same precautions for restoring fluid and electrolyte balance as in intravenous injections. The dose, the rate of injection, and the type of solution (saline, glucose, Ringer's, etc.) must be adjusted carefully to the individual patient. When solutions devoid of inorganic electrolytes are given by hypodermoclysis, hypovolemia may occur. This may be prevented by using solutions containing adequate amounts of inorganic electrolytes and/or controlling the volume and speed of administration.

Hyaluronidase may be added to small volumes of solution (up to 200 mL), such as small clysis for infants or solutions of drugs for subcutaneous injection. *For children less than 3 years old, the volume of a single clysis should be limited to 200 mL; and in premature infants or during the neonatal period, the daily dosage should not exceed 25 mL/kg of body weight; the rate of administration should not be greater than 2 mL per minute. For older patients, the rate and volume of administration should not exceed those employed for intravenous infusion.*

SUBCUTANEOUS UROGRAPHY

The subcutaneous route of administration of urographic contrast media is indicated when intravenous administration cannot be successfully accomplished, particularly in infants and small children. With the patient prone, 75 U of Wydase (hyaluronidase, Wyeth) is injected subcutaneously over each scapula, followed by injection of the contrast medium at the same sites.

NOTE: Parenteral drug products should be inspected visually for particulate matter and discoloration prior to administration, whenever solution and container permit.

HOW SUPPLIED

Wydase®, Lyophilized, Wyeth®, is supplied as follows:
150 USP (TR) units of hyaluronidase
NDC 0008-0121-01, 1 mL vial, as single vials
1,500 USP (TR) units of hyaluronidase
NDC 0008-0149-01, 10 mL vial, as single vials.

Not Recommended for IV Use.

Keep at controlled room temperature in a dry place. Sterile reconstituted solution may be stored below 30°C (86°F) for two weeks without significant loss of potency.

Wydase®, Stabilized Solution, Wyeth®, is supplied as follows:
150 USP (TR) units of hyaluronidase per mL
NDC 0008-0170-01, 1 mL vial, as single vials.
NCD 0008-0170-02, 10 mL vial, as single vials.

Not Recommended for IV Use.

Must be refrigerated.

Do not use if solution is discolored or contains a precipitate.

WYGESIC® Ⓒ℞

[wi-je 'zik]

(propoxyphene HCl and acetaminophen)

DESCRIPTION

Wygesic tablets contain 65 mg propoxyphene HCl and 650 mg acetaminophen. The inactive ingredients present are cellulose, D&C Yellow 10, FD&C Blue 1, FD&C Yellow 6, hydrogenated vegetable oil, hydroxypropyl cellulose, hydroxypropyl methylcellulose, methylcellulose, polacrilin potassium, and titanium dioxide.

Propoxyphene hydrochloride is an odorless white crystalline powder with a bitter taste. It is freely soluble in water. Chemically, it is [S-(R*,S*)]-α[2-(dimethylamino)-1-methylethyl]-α-phenylbenzeneethanol, propanoate (ester), hydrochloride.

Acetaminophen is a white, crystalline powder, possessing a slightly bitter taste. It is soluble in boiling water and freely soluble in alcohol. Chemically, it is N-Acetyl-p-aminophenol.

CLINICAL PHARMACOLOGY

Propoxyphene is a centrally acting narcotic analgesic agent. Repeated doses of propoxyphene at 6-hour intervals lead to increasing plasma concentrations, with a plateau after the ninth dose at 48 hours.

Propoxyphene is metabolized in the liver to yield norpropoxyphene. Propoxyphene has a half-life of 6 to 12 hours, whereas that of norpropoxyphene is 30 to 36 hours.

Norpropoxyphene has substantially less central-nervous-system-depressant effect than propoxyphene, but a greater local anesthetic effect, which is similar to that of amitriptyline and antiarrhythmic agents, such as lidocaine and quinidine.

In animal studies in which propoxyphene and norpropoxyphene were continuously infused in large amounts, intracardiac conduction time (P-R and QRS intervals) was prolonged. Any intracardiac conduction delay attributable to high concentrations of norpropoxyphene may be of relatively long duration.

ACTIONS

Propoxyphene is a mild narcotic analgesic structurally related to methadone.

The combination of propoxyphene and acetaminophen produces greater analgesia than that produced by either propoxyphene or acetaminophen administered alone.

INDICATIONS

These products are indicated for the relief of mild-to-moderate pain, either when pain is present alone or when it is accompanied by fever.

CONTRAINDICATIONS

Hypersensitivity to propoxyphene or to acetaminophen.

WARNINGS

Do not prescribe propoxyphene for patients who are suicidal or addiction-prone.

Prescribe propoxyphene with caution for patients taking tranquilizers or antidepressant drugs and patients who use alcohol in excess.

Tell your patients not to exceed the recommended dose and to limit their intake of alcohol.

Propoxyphene products in excessive doses, either alone or in combination with other CNS depressants, including alcohol, are a major cause of drug-related deaths. Fatalities within the first hour of overdosage are not uncommon. In a survey of deaths due to overdosage conducted in 1975, in approximately 20% of the fatal cases, death occurred within the first hour (5% occurred within 15 minutes). Propoxyphene should not be taken in doses higher than those recommended by the physician. The judicious prescribing of propoxyphene is essential to the safe use of this drug. With patients who are depressed or suicidal, consideration should be given to the use of nonnarcotic analgesics. Patients should be cautioned about the concomitant use of propoxyphene products and alcohol because of potentially serious CNS-additive effects of these agents. Because of its added depressant effects, propoxyphene should be prescribed with caution for those patients whose medical condition requires the concomitant administration of sedatives, tranquilizers, muscle relaxants, antidepressants, or other CNS-depressant drugs. Patients should be advised of the additive depressant effects of these combinations.

Many of the propoxyphene-related deaths have occurred in patients with previous histories of emotional disturbances or suicidal ideation or attempts as well as histories of misuse of tranquilizers, alcohol, and other CNS-active drugs. Some deaths have occurred as a consequence of the accidental ingestion of excessive quantities of propoxyphene alone or in combination with other drugs. Patients taking propoxyphene should be warned not to exceed the dosage recommended by the physician.

DRUG DEPENDENCE: Propoxyphene, when taken in higher-than-recommended doses over long periods of time, can produce drug dependence characterized by psychic dependence and, less frequently, physical dependence and tolerance. Propoxyphene will only partially suppress the withdrawal syndrome in individuals physically dependent on morphine or other narcotics. The abuse liability of propoxyphene is qualitatively similar to that of codeine although quantitatively less, and propoxyphene should be prescribed with the same degree of caution appropriate to the use of codeine.

USAGE IN AMBULATORY PATIENTS: Propoxyphene may impair the mental and/or physical abilities required for the performance of potentially hazardous tasks, such as driving a car or operating machinery. The patient should be cautioned accordingly.

PRECAUTIONS

DRUG INTERACTIONS: The CNS-depressant effect of propoxyphene is additive with that of other CNS depressants, including alcohol.

USAGE IN PREGNANCY: Safe use in pregnancy has not been established relative to possible adverse effects on fetal development. Instances of withdrawal symptoms in the neonate have been reported following usage during pregnancy. Therefore, propoxyphene should not be used in pregnant women unless, in the judgment of the physician, the potential benefits outweigh the possible hazards.

USAGE IN NURSING MOTHERS: Low levels of propoxyphene have been detected in human milk. In postpartum studies involving nursing mothers who were given propoxyphene, no adverse effects were noted in infants receiving mother's milk.

USAGE IN CHILDREN: Propoxyphene is not recommended for use in children, because documented clinical experience has been insufficient to establish safety and a suitable dosage regimen in the pediatric age group.

Patient Information is available for this product. See text following "How Supplied" section below.

ADVERSE REACTIONS

In a survey conducted in hospitalized patients, less than 1% of patients taking propoxyphene hydrochloride at recommended doses experienced side effects. The most frequently reported have been dizziness, sedation, nausea, and vomiting. Some of these adverse reactions may be alleviated if the patient lies down.

Other adverse reactions include constipation, abdominal pain, skin rashes, light-headedness, headache, weakness, euphoria, dysphoria, and minor visual disturbances.

Cases of liver dysfunction have been reported.

DOSAGE AND ADMINISTRATION

This product is given orally. The usual dose is 65 mg propoxyphene HCl and 650 mg acetaminophen every 4 hours as needed for pain. The maximum recommended dose of propoxyphene HCl is 390 mg per day.

MANAGEMENT OF OVERDOSAGE

Initial consideration should be given to the management of the CNS effects of propoxyphene overdosage. Resuscitative measures should be initiated promptly.

SYMPTOMS OF PROPOXYPHENE OVERDOSAGE: The manifestations of acute overdosage with propoxyphene are those of narcotic overdosage. The patient is usually somnolent, but may be stuporous or comatose and convulsing. Respiratory depression is characteristic. The ventilatory rate and/or tidal volume is decreased, which results in cyanosis and hypoxia. Pupils, initially pinpoint, may become dilated as hypoxia increases. Cheyne-Stokes respiration and apnea may occur. Blood pressure and heart rate are usually normal initially, but blood pressure falls and cardiac performance deteriorates, which ultimately results in pulmonary edema and circulatory collapse unless the respiratory depression is corrected and adequate ventilation is restored promptly. Cardiac arrhythmias and conduction delay may be present. A combined respiratory-metabolic acidosis occurs, owing to retained CO_2 (hypercapnea) and to lactic acid formed during anaerobic glycolysis. Acidosis may be severe if large amounts of salicylates have also been ingested. Death may occur.

TREATMENT OF PROPOXYPHENE OVERDOSAGE: Attention should be directed first to establishing a patent airway and to restoring ventilation. Mechanically assisted ventilation, with or without oxygen, may be required, and positive-pressure respiration may be desirable if pulmonary edema is present. The narcotic antagonist naloxone will markedly reduce the degree of respiratory depression and should be administered promptly, preferably intravenously, 0.4 mg to 2.0 mg, and carefully repeated as necessary at 2- to 3-minute intervals.

The duration of action of the antagonist may be brief. If no response is observed after 10 mg of naloxone have been administered, the diagnosis of propoxyphene toxicity should be questioned. (Nalorphine may be used if naloxone is not available, but this agent is not as satisfactory as naloxone).

Blood gases, pH, and electrolytes should be monitored in order that acidosis and any electrolyte disturbance present may be corrected promptly. Acidosis, hypoxia, and generalized CNS depression predispose to the development of cardiac arrhythmias. Ventricular fibrillation or cardiac arrest may occur and necessitate the full complement of cardiopulmonary resuscitation (CPR) measures. Respiratory acidosis rapidly subsides as ventilation is restored and hypercapnea eliminated, but lactic acidosis may require intravenous bicarbonate for prompt correction.

Electrocardiographic monitoring is essential. Prompt correction of hypoxia, acidosis, and electrolyte disturbance (when present) will help prevent these cardiac complications and

Continued on next page

Wyeth—Cont.

will increase the effectiveness of agents administered to restore normal cardiac function.
In addition to the use of a narcotic antagonist, the patient may require careful titration with an anticonvulsant to control convulsions. Analeptic drugs (for example, caffeine or amphetamine) should not be used because of their tendency to precipitate convulsions.
General supportive measures, in addition to oxygen, include, when necessary, intravenous fluids, vasopressor-inotropic compounds, and, when infection is likely, anti-infective agents.
Gastric lavage may be useful, and activated charcoal can adsorb a significant amount of ingested propoxyphene. Dialysis is of little value in poisoning due to propoxyphene. Efforts should be made to determine whether other agents, such as alcohol, barbiturates, tranquilizers, or other CNS depressants, were also ingested, since these increase CNS depression as well as cause specific toxic effects.
SYMPTOMS OF ACETAMINOPHEN OVERDOSAGE: Acetaminophen in massive overdosage may cause hepatic toxicity in some patients. In case of suspected overdose, you may wish to call your regional poison center for assistance in diagnosis and for directions in the use of N-acetylcysteine as an antidote.
In adults, hepatic toxicity has rarely been reported with acute overdoses of less than 10 grams and fatalities with less than 15 grams. Importantly, young children seem to be more resistant than adults to the hepatotoxic effect of an acetaminophen overdose. Despite this, the measures outlined below should be initiated in any adult or child suspected of having ingested an acetaminophen overdose.
Early symptoms following a potentially hepatotoxic overdose may include: nausea, vomiting, diaphoresis, and general malaise. Clinical and laboratory evidence of hepatic toxicity may not be apparent until 48 to 72 hours postingestion.
After the initial symptoms, the patient may feel less ill; however, laboratory determinations are likely to show a rapid rise in liver enzymes, including serum transaminase and lactic dehydrogenase and bilirubin. In case of serious hepatotoxicity, jaundice, coagulation defects, hypoglycemia, encephalopathy, and coma may follow.
Death from hepatic failure may result 3 to 7 days after overdose.
TREATMENT OF ACETAMINOPHEN OVERDOSAGE: The stomach should be emptied promptly by lavage or by induction of emesis with syrup of ipecac. Patients' estimates of the quantity of a drug ingested are notoriously unreliable. Therefore, if an acetaminophen overdose is suspected, a serum acetaminophen assay should be obtained as early as possible, but no sooner than four hours following ingestion. Liver-function studies should be obtained initially and repeated at 24-hour intervals.
The antidote, N-acetylcysteine, should be administered as early as possible, and within 16 hours of the overdose ingestion for optimal results. Following recovery, there are no residual, structural, or functional hepatic abnormalities.

HOW SUPPLIED

Wygesic® (propoxyphene HCl and acetaminophen) Tablets, Wyeth®, are available as follows:
NDC 0008-0085, green, capsule-shaped, scored, film-coated tablet marked "WYETH" and "85", in bottles of 100 and 500 tablets, and in REDIPAK® cartons of 100 tablets (10 strips of 10).
Keep tightly closed.
Protect from light.
Dispense in light-resistant, tight container.

PATIENT INFORMATION

YOUR PRESCRIPTION FOR A PROPOXYPHENE PRODUCT
Your doctor has chosen to prescribe a medicine containing propoxyphene. Propoxyphene is used for the relief of pain. It is important that you read and understand the information in this leaflet. If you have any questions, ask your doctor or pharmacist.

GENERAL CAUTIONS

OTHER DRUGS: Combinations of excessive doses of propoxyphene, alcohol, and tranquilizers may be dangerous. Make sure your doctor knows that you are taking tranquilizers, sleep aids, antidepressant drugs, antihistamines, or any other drugs that make you sleepy. The use of these drugs with propoxyphene increases their sedative effects and may lead to overdosage symptoms, including death (see "Overdosage" below).
ALCOHOL: Heavy use of alcohol with propoxyphene is hazardous and may lead to overdosage symptoms (see "Overdosage" below). THEREFORE, LIMIT YOUR INTAKE OF ALCOHOL WHILE TAKING PROPOXYPHENE.
REGULAR ACTIVITIES: Propoxyphene may cause drowsiness or impair your mental and/or physical abilities; therefore, use caution when driving a vehicle or operating dangerous machinery. DO NOT perform any hazardous task until you have seen your response to this drug.
PREGNANCY: Do not take propoxyphene or other drugs during pregnancy unless your doctor knows you are pregnant and specifically recommends their use.
CHILDREN: Propoxyphene is not recommended for use in children under 12 years of age.
ALLERGY: Do not take propoxyphene if you have had an allergic reaction to any drug containing propoxyphene.
DEPENDENCE: Propoxyphene, when taken in higher-than-recommended doses over a long period of time, has produced physical and psychologic dependence (a craving for the drug or an inability to function normally without the drug).
Side Effects: When propoxyphene is taken as directed, side effects are infrequent. Among those reported are drowsiness, dizziness, nausea, and vomiting. If these effects occur, some of them may go away if you lie down.
Less frequently reported side effects include constipation, abdominal pain, skin rashes, light-headedness, headache, weakness, minor visual disturbances, and feelings of elation or discomfort.
If one of these side effects occurs and becomes severe, contact your physician.

DOSAGE

Your prescription should be taken as directed by your doctor. Do not exceed the maximum daily dose shown below. Always follow dosage recommendations carefully—do *not* increase the dosage without your doctor's approval. If you miss a dose of the drug, do *not* take twice as much the next time.

Propoxyphene HCl	with Acetaminophen	MAXIMUM DAILY DOSE
65 mg	650 mg	6

OVERDOSAGE

An overdosage of propoxyphene, alone or in combination with other drugs, including alcohol, may cause weakness, difficulty in breathing, confusion, anxiety, and more severe drowsiness and dizziness. Extreme overdosage may lead to unconsciousness and death.
In *any* suspected overdosage situation, GET EMERGENCY HELP IMMEDIATELY.
Other Information: This medication was prescribed specifically for you. It should not be given to anyone else even if his/her condition appears to be similar to yours. If you want more information or have any questions about propoxyphene, ask your doctor or pharmacist. There is a more detailed leaflet available from them. You may need their help in understanding parts of the detailed leaflet.
Keep this and all other drugs out of the reach of children.

Shown in Product Identification Section, page 437

WYMOX® ℞

[*wi'moks*]
(amoxicillin)
Capsules and Oral Suspension

HOW SUPPLIED

Wymox® (amoxicillin) Capsules, Wyeth®, contain 250 mg or 500 mg amoxicillin as the trihydrate and are supplied as follows:
250 mg, NDC 0008-0559, grey and green capsule marked "WYETH" and "559", in bottles of 100 and 500 capsules.
500 mg, NDC 0008-0560, grey and green capsule marked "WYETH" and "560", in bottles of 50 and 500 capsules.
Wymox® (amoxicillin) Oral Suspension, Wyeth®, is available as a pink powder which when reconstituted as directed yields a palatable, pink suspension of amoxicillin trihydrate in the following dosage strengths:
125 mg per 5 mL, NDC 0008-0557, in bottles to make 80 mL, 100 mL, or 150 mL.
250 mg per 5 mL, NDC 0008-0558, in bottles to make 80 mL, 100 mL, or 150 mL.
For prescribing information write to Professional Service, Wyeth Laboratories, Box 8299, Philadelphia, PA 19101, or contact your local Wyeth representative.

Shown in Product Identification Section, page 437

WYTENSIN® ℞

[*wi-ten'sin*]
(guanabenz acetate)

DESCRIPTION

Wytensin (guanabenz acetate), an antihypertensive agent for oral administration, is an aminoguanidine derivative, 2,6-dichlorobenzylideneaminoguanidine acetate.
It is an odorless, white to off-white, crystalline substance, sparingly soluble in water and soluble in alcohol, with a molecular weight of 291.14. Each tablet of Wytensin is equivalent to 4 mg, 8 mg, or 16 mg of free guanabenz base. The inactive ingredients present are cellulose, lactose, and magnesium stearate.
Wytensin is available as 4 mg, 8 mg, or 16 mg tablets for oral administration.

CLINICAL PHARMACOLOGY

Wytensin is an orally active central alpha-2 adrenergic agonist. Its antihypertensive action appears to be mediated via stimulation of central alpha adrenergic receptors, resulting in a decrease of sympathetic outflow from the brain at the bulbar level to the peripheral circulatory sytem.
PHARMACOKINETICS
In human studies, about 75% of an orally administered dose of Wytensin is absorbed and metabolized with less than 1% of unchanged drug recovered from the urine. Peak plasma concentrations of unchanged drug occur between two and five hours after a single oral dose. The average half-life for Wytensin is about 6 hours. The site or sites of metabolism of Wytensin and the consequences of renal or hepatic insufficiency on excretion of Wytensin or its metabolites have not been determined. The effect of meals on the absorption of Wytensin has not been studied.
PHARMACODYNAMICS
The onset of the antihypertensive action of Wytensin begins within 60 minutes after a single oral dose and reaches a peak effect within two to four hours. The effect of an acute single dose is reduced appreciably six to eight hours after administration, and blood pressure approaches baseline values within 12 hours of administration.
The acute antihypertensive effect of Wytensin occurs without major changes in peripheral resistance, but its chronic effect appears to be a decrease in peripheral resistance. A decrease in blood pressure is seen in both the supine and standing positions without alterations of normal postural mechanisms, so that postural hypotension has not been observed. Wytensin decreases pulse rate by about 5 beats per minute. Cardiac output and left ventricular ejection fraction are unchanged during long-term therapy.
With effective control of blood pressure in hypertensive patients, Wytensin has not demonstrated any significant effect on glomerular filtration rate, renal blood flow, renal sodium or potassium excretion, renal concentrating ability, body fluid volume, or body weight. In clinical trials of six to thirty months, hypertensive patients whose blood pressure was controlled with Wytensin lost one to four pounds of body weight. The mechanism of this weight loss has not been established. Tolerance to the antihypertensive effect of Wytensin has not been observed.
During long-term administration of Wytensin, there is a small decrease in serum cholesterol and total triglycerides without any change in the high-density lipoprotein fraction. Plasma norepinephrine, serum dopamine beta-hydroxylase and plasma renin activity are decreased during chronic administration of Wytensin. No changes in serum electrolytes, uric acid, blood-urea nitrogen, calcium, or glucose have been observed.
Wytensin and hydrochlorothiazide have been shown to have at least partially additive effects in patients not responding adequately to either drug alone.

INDICATIONS AND USAGE

Wytensin (guanabenz acetate) is indicated in the treatment of hypertension. It may be employed alone or in combination with a thiazide diuretic.

CONTRAINDICATION

Wytensin is contraindicated in patients with a known sensitivity to the drug.

PRECAUTIONS

1. Sedation: Wytensin causes sedation or drowsiness in a large fraction of patients. When Wytensin is used with centrally active depressants, such as phenothiazines, barbiturates, and benzodiazepines, the potential for additive sedative effects should be considered.
2. Patients with vascular insufficiency: Wytensin, like other antihypertensive agents, should be used with caution in patients with severe coronary insufficiency, recent myocardial infarction, cerebrovascular disease, or severe hepatic or renal failure.
3. Rebound: Sudden cessation of therapy with central alpha agonists like Wytensin may rarely result in "overshoot" hypertension and more commonly produces an increase in serum catecholamines and subjective symptomatology.

INFORMATION FOR PATIENTS
Patients who receive Wytensin should be advised to exercise caution when operating dangerous machinery or driving motor vehicles until it is determined that they do not become drowsy or dizzy from the medication. Patients should be warned that their tolerance for alcohol and other CNS depressants may be diminished. Patients should be advised not to discontinue therapy abruptly.
LABORATORY TESTS
In clinical trials, no clinically significant laboratory test abnormalities were identified during either acute or chronic therapy with Wytensin. Tests carried out included CBC, urinalysis, electrolytes, SGOT, bilirubin, alkaline phosphatase, uric acid, BUN, creatinine, glucose, calcium, phosphorus, total protein, and Coombs' test. During long-term adminis-

tration of Wytensin, there was a small decrease in serum cholesterol and total triglycerides without any change in the high-density lipoprotein fraction. In rare instances an occasional nonprogressive increase in liver enzymes has been observed. However, no clinical evidence of hepatic disease has been found.

DRUG INTERACTIONS

Wytensin has not been demonstrated to cause any drug interactions when administered with other drugs, such as digitalis, diuretics, analgesics, anxiolytics, and antiinflammatory or antiinfective agents, in clinical trials. However, the potential for increased sedation when Wytensin is administered concomitantly with CNS-depressant drugs should be noted.

DRUG/LABORATORY TEST INTERACTIONS

No laboratory test abnormalities were identified with the use of Wytensin.

CARCINOGENESIS, MUTAGENESIS, IMPAIRMENT OF FERTILITY

No evidence of carcinogenic potential emerged in rats during a two-year oral study with Wytensin at doses up to 9.5 mg/kg/day, i.e., about 10 times the maximum recommended human dose. In the Salmonella microsome mutagenicity (Ames) test system, Wytensin at 200-500 mcg per plate or at 30-50 mcg/ml in suspension gave dose-related increases in the number of mutants in one (TA 1537) of five *Salmonella typhimurium* strains with or without inclusion of rat liver microsomes. No mutagenic activity was seen at doses up to those which inhibit growth in the eukaryotic microorganism, *Schizosaccharomyces pombe*, or in Chinese hamster ovary cells at doses up to those which were lethal to the cells in culture. In another eukaryotic system, *Saccharomyces cerevisiae*, Wytensin produced no activity in an assay measuring induction of repairable DNA damage. Reproductive studies showed a decreased pregnancy rate in rats administered high oral doses (9.6 mg/kg) of Wytensin, suggesting an impairment of fertility. The fertility of treated males (9.6 mg/kg) may also have been affected, as suggested by the decreased pregnancy rate of their mates, even though the females received Wytensin only during the last third of pregnancy.

PREGNANCY

Pregnancy Category C

WYTENSIN MAY HAVE ADVERSE EFFECTS ON THE FETUS WHEN ADMINISTERED TO PREGNANT WOMEN. A teratology study in mice has indicated a possible increase in skeletal abnormalities when Wytensin is given orally at doses of 3 to 6 times the maximum recommended human dose of 1.0 mg/kg. These abnormalities, principally costal and vertebral, were not noted in similar studies in rats and rabbits. However, increased fetal loss has been observed after oral Wytensin administration to pregnant rats (14 mg/kg) and rabbits (20 mg/kg). Reproductive studies of Wytensin in rats have shown slightly decreased live-birth indices, decreased fetal survival rate, and decreased pup body weight at oral doses of 6.4 and 9.6 mg/kg. There are no adequate, well-controlled studies in pregnant women. Wytensin should be used during pregnancy only if the potential benefit justifies the potential risk to the fetus.

NURSING MOTHERS

Because no information is available on the excretion of Wytensin in human milk, it should not be administered to nursing mothers.

PEDIATRIC USE

The safety and effectiveness of Wytensin in children less than 12 years of age have not been demonstrated. Therefore, its use in this age group cannot be recommended at this time.

ADVERSE REACTIONS

The incidence of adverse effects has been ascertained from controlled clinical studies conducted in the United States and is based on data from 859 patients who received Wytensin for up to 3 years. There is some evidence that the side effects are dose-related.

The following table shows the incidence of adverse effects occurring in at least 5% of patients in a study comparing Wytensin (guanabenz acetate) to placebo, at a starting dose of 8 mg b.i.d.

Adverse Effect	Placebo (%) n=102	Wytensin (%) n=109
Dry mouth	7	28
Drowsiness or sedation	12	39
Dizziness	7	17
Weakness	7	10
Headache	6	5

In other controlled clinical trials at the starting dose of 16 mg/day in 476 patients, the incidence of dry mouth was slightly higher (38%) and that of dizziness was slightly lower (12%), but the incidence of the most frequent adverse effects was similar to the placebo-controlled trial. Although these side effects were not serious, they led to discontinuation of treatment about 15% of the time. In more recent studies using an initial dose of 8 mg/day in 274 patients, the incidence of drowsiness or sedation was lower, about 20%.

Other adverse effects were reported during clinical trials with Wytensin but are not clearly distinguished from placebo effects and occurred with a frequency of 3% or less:

Cardiovascular—chest pain, edema, arrhythmias, palpitations.

Gastrointestinal—nausea, epigastric pain, diarrhea, vomiting, constipation, abdominal discomfort.

Central nervous system—anxiety, ataxia, depression, sleep disturbances.

ENT disorders—nasal congestion.

Eye disorders—blurring of vision.

Musculoskeletal—aches in extremities, muscle aches.

Respiratory—dyspnea.

Dermatologic—rash, pruritus.

Urogenital—urinary frequency, disturbances of sexual function.

Other—gynecomastia, taste disorders.

DRUG ABUSE AND DEPENDENCE

No reported dependence or abuse has been associated with the administration of Wytensin.

OVERDOSAGE

Accidental ingestion of Wytensin caused hypotension, somnolence, lethargy, irritability, miosis, and bradycardia in two children aged one and three years. Gastric lavage and administration of pressor substances, fluids, and oral activated charcoal resulted in complete and uneventful recovery within 12 hours in both patients.

Since experience with accidental overdosage is limited, the suggested treatment is mainly supportive while the drug is being eliminated from the body and until the patient is no longer symptomatic. Vital signs and fluid balance should be carefully monitored. An adequate airway should be maintained and, if indicated, assisted respiration instituted. There are no data available on the dialyzability of Wytensin.

DOSAGE AND ADMINISTRATION

Dosage with Wytensin should be individualized. A starting dose of 4 mg twice a day is recommended, whether Wytensin is used alone or with a thiazide diuretic. Dosage may be increased in increments of 4 to 8 mg per day every one to two weeks, depending on the patient's response. The maximum dose studied to date has been 32 mg twice daily, but doses as high as this are rarely needed.

HOW SUPPLIED

Wytensin® (guanabenz acetate) Tablets, Wyeth®, are available in the following dosage strengths:

4 mg, NDC 0008-0073, white, five-sided tablet with a raised "W" and a "4" under the "W" on one side and "WYETH 73" on reverse side, in bottles of 100 and 500 tablets and in Redipak® cartons of 100 individually wrapped tablets.

8 mg, NDC 0008-0074, white, five-sided tablet with a raised "W" and an "8" under the "W" on one side and "WYETH 74" on scored reverse side, in bottles of 100 tablets.

16 mg, NDC 0008-0092, white, five-sided tablet with a raised "W" and a "16" on one side and "WYETH 92" on scored reverse side, in bottles of 100 tablets.

The appearance of these tablets is a registered trademark of Wyeth Laboratories.

Keep bottles of Wytensin Tablets tightly closed.
Dispense in tight containers.
Protect from light.

Shown in Product Identification Section, page 437

EDUCATIONAL MATERIAL

Films—Slides—Videos

The Wyeth Film and Audiovisual Catalog, listing films, audiovisual and slide programs available through the Wyeth Film Library or on loan through the local Wyeth representative, can be obtained by writing Professional Service, Wyeth Laboratories. Box 8299, Philadelphia, PA 19101.

Products are cross-indexed by generic and chemical names in the **YELLOW SECTION**

Zenith Laboratories, Inc.

50 WILLIAMS DRIVE
RAMSEY, NJ 07446

COMPLETE LISTING OF ZENITH PRODUCTS

Following is a complete listing of Zenith's products. Each tablet or capsule may be identified by the letter Z on its surface along with the middle 4 digits of the product's NDC number as listed below. The sole exceptions are Propranolol HCl tablets which are engraved with the letter M and their respective strengths. Each product comes in a variety of package configurations, with the most common being 100s, 500s and 1000s.

NDC # 0172-	PRODUCT	
3915	Acetaminophen and Codeine Phosphate 30 mg Tablets, No. 3*	C-III
3916	Acetaminophen and Codeine Phosphate 60 mg Tablets, No. 4*	C-III
3984	Aspirin and Codeine Phosphate 30 mg Tablets USP No. 3	C-III
3985	Aspirin and Codeine Phosphate 60 mg Tablets USP No. 4	C-III
3747	Azpan Tablets	OTC
3996	Butalbital Compound Tablets	C-III
2960	Chloramphenicol Capsules, USP 250 mg	℞
2013	Chlordiazepoxide HCl Capsules, USP 5 mg*	C-IV
3977	Chlordiazepoxide HCl Capsules, USP 10 mg*	C-IV
2015	Chlordiazepoxide HCl Capsules, USP 25 mg*	C-IV
2982	Chlordiazepoxide HCl and Clidinium Capsules, 5 mg/2.5 mg	℞
3657	Chlorpropamide Tablets, USP 100 mg*	℞
2902	Chlorpropamide Tablets, USP 250 mg*	℞
2974	Chlorthalidone Tablets, USP 25 mg, yellow	℞
2999	Chlorthalidone Tablets, USP 50 mg, green	℞
2904	Chlorthalidone Tablets, USP 100 mg	℞
2812	Chlorzoxazone and Acetaminophen Tablets, USP 250 mg/300 mg	℞
2047	Colchicine Tablets, USP 0.6 mg	℞
3636	Conjugated Estrogens Tablets, USP 0.3 mg	℞
2042	Conjugated Estrogens Tablets, USP 0.625 mg	℞
2045	Conjugated Estrogens Tablets, USP 1.25 mg	℞
2160	Conjugated Estrogens Tablets, USP 2.5 mg	℞
2814	Cyclandelate Capsules, 200 mg	℞
2815	Cyclandelate Capsules, 400 mg	℞
2929	Cyproheptadine Tablets, USP 4 mg*	℞
2945	Decontabs Tablets	℞
3006	Detuss Capsules (Formula Modified)	℞
3925	Diazepam Tablets, USP 2 mg.	C-IV
3926	Diazepam Tablets, USP 5 mg	C-IV
3927	Diazepam Tablets, USP 10 mg.	C-IV
2058	Digoxin Tablets, USP 0.25 mg	℞
2055	Diphenhydramine HCl Capsules, USP 25 mg	℞
2056	Diphenhydramine HCl Capsules, USP 50 mg	℞
3966	Diphenoxylate HCl and Atropine Sulfate Tablets USP*	C-V
2994	Dipyridamole Tablets, USP 25 mg	℞
2976	Dipyridamole Tablets, USP 50 mg	℞
2977	Dipyridamole Tablets, USP 75 mg	℞
4051	Disopyramide Phosphate Capsules, USP 100 mg	℞
4052	Disopyramide Phosphate Capsules, USP 150 mg	℞
2984	Doxycycline Hyclate Capsules, USP 50 mg*	℞
2985	Doxycycline Hyclate Capsules, USP 100 mg*	℞
3626	Doxycycline Hyclate Tablets, USP 100 mg	℞
2958	Ergoloid Mesylates Sublingual Tablets, USP 0.5 mg	℞
2959	Ergoloid Mesylates Sublingual Tablets, USP 1 mg	℞
2458	Erythromycin Stearate Tablets, USP 250 mg	℞
2823	Erythromycin Stearate Tablets, USP 500 mg	℞
2908	Furosemide Tablets, USP 20 mg*	℞
2907	Furosemide Tablets, USP 40 mg*	℞
2338	Hydralazine HCl Tablets, USP 10 mg	℞
2339	Hydralazine HCl Tablets, USP 25 mg	℞
2493	Hydralazine HCl Tablets, USP 50 mg	℞
3633	Hydralazine and Hydrochlorothiazide Capsules, 25 mg/25 mg*	℞
3632	Hydralazine and Hydrochlorothiazide Capsules, 50 mg/50 mg*	℞
2083	Hydrochlorothiazide Tablets, USP 25 mg*	℞
2089	Hydrochlorothiazide Tablets, USP 50 mg,* orange	℞
2205	Hydrochlorothiazide Tablets, USP 50 mg, yellow	℞
2169	Hydroserpine Tablets, USP No. 1*	℞
2168	Hydroserpine Tablets, USP No. 2*	℞

Continued on next page

Zenith—Cont.

2335	Hydroserpine Plus Tablets (R.H.H.) USP*	℞
2962	Hydroxy Compound Tablets	℞
6100	Hydroxyzine HCl Tablets USP 10 mg.*	
6200	Hydroxyzine HCl Tablets USP 25 mg.*	
6300	Hydroxyzine HCl Tablets USP 50 mg.*	
2911	Hydroxyzine Pamoate Capsules, USP 25 mg*	℞
2909	Hydroxyzine Pamoate Capsules, USP 50 mg*	℞
4029	Indomethacin Capsules, USP 25 mg	℞
4030	Indomethacin Capsules, USP 50 mg	℞
2151	Isosorbide Dinitrate Tablets, 10 mg Oral*	℞
2342	Isosorbide Dinitrate Tablets, USP 2.5 mg* Sublingual	℞
2343	Isosorbide Dinitrate Tablets, USP 5 mg Sublingual	℞
2387	Isoxsuprine HCl Tablets, USP 10 mg	℞
2388	Isoxsuprine HCl Tablets, USP 20 mg	℞
5600	Lorazepam Tablets, 0.5 mg	C-IV
5800	Lorazepam Tablets, 1 mg	C-IV
6000	Lorazepam Tablets, 2 mg	C-IV
2384	Meclizine HCl Tablets USP 12.5 mg.*	℞
2350	Meclizine HCl Tablets USP 25 mg.*	℞
3905	Meprobamate Tablets, USP 200 mg*	C-IV
3904	Meprobamate Tablets, USP 400 mg*	C-IV
2364	Methocarbamol Tablets, USP 500 mg*	℞
2365	Methocarbamol Tablets, USP 750 mg*	℞
2813	Methocarbamol and Aspirin Tablets,* 400 mg/325 mg	℞
2987	Methyclothiazide Tablets, USP 5 mg*	℞
2931	Methyldopa Tablets, USP 250 mg	℞
2932	Methyldopa Tablets, USP 500 mg	℞
2971	Metronidazole Tablets, USP 250 mg	℞
3007	Metronidazole Tablets, USP 500 mg	℞
2963	Nitroglycerin Capsules 2.5 mg T.D.	℞
2964	Nitroglycerin Capsules 6.5 mg T.D.	℞
2348	Nylidrin HCl Tablets, USP 6 mg	℞
2349	Nylidrin HCl Tablets, USP 12 mg	℞
2180	Papaverine HCl Capsules, 150 mg	℞
2936	Perphenezine and Amitriptyline HCl Tablets, 2–10 mg.	℞

2937	Perphenazine and Amitriptyline HCl Tablets, 2–25 mg.	℞
2938	Perphenazine and Amitriptyline HCl Tablets 4–10 mg.	℞
2939	Perphenazine and Amitriptyline HCl Tablets, 4–25 mg.	℞
3671	Perphenazine and Amitriptyline HCl Tablets, 4–50 mg.	℞
3921	Phentermine HCl Capsules, USP 30 mg, yellow*	C-IV
3991	Phentermine HCl Capsules, USP 30 mg, blue*	C-IV
4038	Phenylbutazone Capsules, 100 mg	℞
2057	Phenytoin Sodium Capsules Prompt, USP 100 mg*	℞
2190	Probenecid Tablets, USP 500 mg	℞
2193	Probenecid and Colchicine Tablets, USP 500 mg/0.5 mg*	℞
2345	Procainamide HCl Capsules, USP 250 mg	℞
2346	Procainamide HCl Capsules, USP 375 mg	℞
2347	Procainamide HCl Capsules, USP 500 mg	℞
2186	Propoxyphene HCl Capsules, USP 65 mg*	C-IV
4811	Propoxyphene Compound Capsules, USP 65*	C-IV
3981	Propoxyphene Napsylate and Acetaminophen Tablets, USP 100 mg/650 mg	C-IV
3614	Propranolol Hydrochloride Tablets, USP 10 mg	℞
3615	Propranolol Hydrochloride Tablets, USP 20 mg	℞
3616	Propranolol Hydrochloride Tablets, USP 40 mg	℞
3638	Propranolol Hydrochloride Tablets, USP 60 mg*	℞
3617	Propranolol Hydrochloride Tablets, USP 80 mg	℞
2173	Propylthiouracil Tablets, USP 50 mg*	℞
2201	Quinidine Sulfate Tablets, USP 200 mg*	℞
2359	Quinine Sulfate Capsules, USP 200 mg	OTC
2184	Quinine Sulfate Capsules, USP 325 mg	OTC
3001	Quinine Sulfate Tablets, 260 mg	℞
2507	Reserpine and Hydroflumethiazide Tablets, 0.125 mg/50 mg	℞
2903	Spironolactone Tablets, USP 25 mg*	℞
2819	Spironolactone and Hydrochlorothiazide* Tablets, 25 mg/25 mg	℞
2970	Sulfinpyrazone Tablets, USP 100 mg*	℞
2969	Sulfinpyrazone Capsules, USP 200 mg	℞
2218	Sulfisoxazole Tablets, USP 500 mg	℞
2416	Tetracycline HCl Capsules, USP 250 mg, orange*	℞

2430	Tetracycline HCl Capsules, USP 250 mg	℞
2407	Tetracycline HCl Capsules, USP 500 mg	℞
3606	Thioridazine HCl Tablets, USP 10 mg*	℞
3607	Thioridazine HCl Tablets, USP 15 mg*	℞
3608	Thioridazine HCl Tablets, USP 25 mg*	℞
3609	Thioridazine HCl Tablets, USP 50 mg*	℞
3610	Thioridazine HCl Tablets, USP 100 mg*	℞
2978	Tolazamide Tablets, USP 100 mg	℞
2979	Tolazamide Tablets, USP 250 mg	℞
2980	Tolazamide Tablets, USP 500 mg	℞
2245	Tolbutamide Tablets, USP 500 mg*	℞
2916	Trifluoperazine HCl Tablets, USP 1 mg*	℞
2940	Trifluoperazine HCl Tablets, USP 2 mg*	℞
2941	Trifluoperazine HCl Tablets, USP 5 mg*	℞
2942	Trifluoperazine HCl Tablets, USP 10 mg*	℞
2484	Triprolidine HCl and Pseudoephedrine HCl Tablets, USP 2.5 mg/60 mg*	℞

*Available soon

EDUCATIONAL MATERIAL

Books-Booklets-Brochures

Complimentary product catalogs and bioequivalency studies are available upon request. They are useful in deciding which of Zeniths products are most suitable for specification to patients. Please write to us at the above address for complete prescribing information.

Samples

Product samples are available upon written request to Zenith Laboratories at the above address.

SECTION 7

Diagnostic Product Information

Products described in PHYSICIANS' DESK REFERENCE® which have official package circulars must be in full compliance with Food & Drug Administration regulations pertaining to labeling for prescription drugs. These regulations require that for PDR copy, "indications, effects, dosages, routes, methods, and frequency and duration of administration, and any relevant warnings, hazards, contraindications, side effects, and precautions" must be the *"same in language and emphasis"* as the approved labeling for the product. FDA regards the words *"same in language and emphasis"* as requiring VERBATIM use of the approved labeling providing such information. Furthermore, information in the approved labeling that is emphasized by the use of type set in a box or in capitals, bold face, or italics must also be given the same emphasis in PDR. For products which do not have official package circulars, the Publisher emphasized to manufacturers the necessity of describing such products comprehensively so that physicians would have access to all information essential for intelligent and informed prescribing. In organizing and presenting the material in PHYSICIANS' DESK REFERENCE, the Publisher is providing all the information made available to PDR by manufacturers.

This edition of PHYSICIANS' DESK REFERENCE contains the latest product information available at press-time. During the year, however, new and revised information about the products described herein may be furnished us. This information will be published in the PDR Supplement. Therefore, before prescribing or administering any product described in the following pages, you should first consult the PDR Supplement.

In presenting the following material to the medical profession, the Publisher is not necessarily advocating the use of any product listed.

Abbott Laboratories
DIAGNOSTICS DIVISION
ABBOTT PARK 6C4, DEPT. 49B
ABBOTT PARK, IL 60064

THYPINONE® Injection ℞
[*thī'pĭ-nōn*]
(Protirelin)

DESCRIPTION

Chemically, Thypinone (protirelin) is identified as 5-oxo-L-prolyl-L-histidyl-L-proline amide. It is a synthetic tripeptide which is believed to be structurally identical with the naturally-occurring thyrotropin-releasing hormone produced by the hypothalamus.

Thypinone (protirelin) is supplied as 1 ml ampules. Each ampule contains 500 mcg protirelin in a sterile non-pyrogenic isotonic saline solution having a pH of 5.5 to 7.5. In addition, each ampule contains sodium chloride, 9.0 mg, water for injection, and hydrochloric acid as needed to adjust pH. Thypinone (protirelin) is intended for intravenous administration.

CLINICAL PHARMACOLOGY

Pharmacologically, Thypinone increases the release of the thyroid stimulating hormone (TSH) from the anterior pituitary. Prolactin release is also increased. It has recently been observed that approximately 65% of acromegalic patients tested respond with a rise in circulating growth hormone levels; the clinical significance is as yet not clear. Following intravenous administration, the mean plasma half-life of protirelin in normal subjects is approximately five minutes. TSH levels rise rapidly and reach a peak at 20 to 30 minutes. The decline in TSH levels takes place more slowly, approaching baseline levels after approximately three hours.

INDICATIONS AND USAGE

Thypinone (protirelin) is indicated as an adjunctive agent in the diagnostic assessment of thyroid function. As an adjunct to other diagnostic procedures, testing with Thypinone may yield useful information in patients with pituitary or hypothalamic dysfunction.

Thypinone (protirelin) is indicated as an adjunct to evaluate the effectiveness of thyrotropin suppression with a particular dose of T4 in patients with nodular or diffuse goiter. A normal TSH baseline value and a minimal difference between the 30 minute and baseline response to Thypinone (protirelin) injection would indicate adequate suppression of the pituitary secretion of TSH.

Thypinone (protirelin) may be used, adjunctively, for adjustment of thyroid hormone dosage given to patients with primary hypothyroidism. A normal or slightly blunted TSH response, thirty minutes following Thypinone (protirelin) injection, would indicate adequate replacement therapy.

WARNINGS

Transient changes in blood pressure, either increases or decreases, frequently occur immediately following administration of Thypinone (protirelin). BLOOD PRESSURE SHOULD THEREFORE BE MEASURED BEFORE THYPINONE (PROTIRELIN) IS ADMINISTERED AND AT FREQUENT INTERVALS DURING THE FIRST 15 MINUTES AFTER ITS ADMINISTRATION.

Increases in systolic pressure (usually less than 30 mm Hg) and/or increases in diastolic pressure (usually less than 20 mm Hg) have been observed more frequently than decreases in pressure. These changes have not ordinarily persisted for more than 15 minutes nor have they required therapy. MORE SEVERE DEGREES OF HYPERTENSION OR HYPOTENSION WITH OR WITHOUT SYNCOPE, HAVE BEEN REPORTED IN A FEW PATIENTS.

To minimize the incidence and/or severity of hypotension, THE PATIENT SHOULD BE SUPINE BEFORE, DURING AND AFTER THYPINONE (PROTIRELIN) ADMINISTRATION. IF A CLINICALLY IMPORTANT CHANGE IN BLOOD PRESSURE OCCURS, MONITORING OF BLOOD PRESSURE SHOULD BE CONTINUED UNTIL IT RETURNS TO BASELINE LEVELS.

THYPINONE (PROTIRELIN) SHOULD NOT BE ADMINISTERED TO PATIENTS IN WHOM MARKED RAPID CHANGES IN BLOOD PRESSURE WOULD BE DANGEROUS UNLESS THE POTENTIAL BENEFIT CLEARLY OUTWEIGHS THE POTENTIAL RISK.

PRECAUTIONS

Thyroid hormones reduce the TSH response to Thypinone (protirelin). Accordingly, patients in whom Thypinone is to be used diagnostically should be taken off liothyronine (T3) approximately seven days prior to testing and should be taken off thyroid medications containing levothyroxine (T4), e.g., desiccated thyroid, thyroglobulin, or liotrix, at least 14 days before testing. Hormone therapy is NOT to be discontinued when the test is used to evaluate the effectiveness of thyroid suppression with a particular dose of T4 in patients with nodular or diffuse goiter, or for adjustment of thyroid hormone dosage given to patients with primary hypothyroidism.

Figure 1
Mean ± One Standard Deviation of TSH levels Observed at Baseline and 30 Minutes After Thypinone (μU/ml)

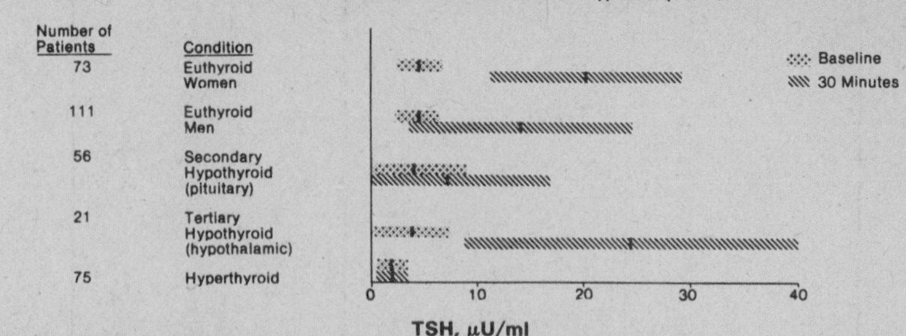

Chronic administration of levodopa has been reported to inhibit the TSH response to Thypinone.

It is not advisable to withdraw maintenance doses of adrenocortical drugs used in the therapy of known hypopituitarism. Several published reports have shown that prolonged treatment with glucocorticoids at physiologic doses has no significant effect on the TSH response to thyrotropin releasing hormone, but that the administration of pharmacologic doses of steroids reduces the TSH response.

Therapeutic doses of acetylsalicylic acid (2 to 3.6 g/day) have been reported to inhibit the TSH response to protirelin. The ingestion of acetylsalicylic acid caused the peak level of TSH to decrease approximately 30% as compared to values obtained without acetylsalicylic acid administration. In both cases, the TSH peak occurred 30 minutes post-administration of protirelin.

Pregnancy

Reproduction studies have been performed in rats and rabbits. At doses 1-½ and 6 times the human dose, there was an increase in the number of resorption sites in the pregnant rabbit. There are no studies in pregnant women which bear on the safety of Thypinone for the human fetus. Thypinone should be used in pregnant women only when clearly needed.

ADVERSE REACTIONS

Side effects have been reported in about 50% of the patients tested with Thypinone (protirelin). Generally, the side effects were minor, have occurred promptly, and have persisted for only a few minutes following injection.

Cardiovascular Reactions

MARKED CHANGES IN BLOOD PRESSURE INCLUDING BOTH HYPERTENSION AND HYPOTENSION WITH OR WITHOUT SYNCOPE, HAVE BEEN REPORTED IN A SMALL NUMBER OF PATIENTS.

Endocrine Reaction

Breast enlargement and leakage in lactating women for up to two or three days.

Other Reactions

Headaches, sometimes severe, and transient amaurosis in patients with pituitary tumors. Rarely, convulsions may occur in patients with presdisposing conditions, e.g. epilepsy, brain damage. Nausea; urge to urinate; flushed sensation; lightheadedness; bad taste; abdominal discomfort; headache; and dry mouth. Less frequently reported were: anxiety; sweating; tightness in the throat; pressure in the chest; tingling sensation; and drowsiness.

DOSAGE AND ADMINISTRATION

Thypinone (protirelin) is intended for intravenous administration with the patient in the supine position. The drug is administered as a bolus over a period of 15 to 30 seconds, with the patient remaining supine for an additional 15 minutes during which time the blood pressure is monitored.

Dosage

Adults: 500 mcg. Doses between 200 and 500 mcg have been used. 500 mcg is considered the optimum dose to give the maximum response in the greatest number of patients. Doses greater than 500 mcg are unlikely to elicit a greater TSH response.

Children age 6 to 16 years: 7 mcg/kg body weight up to 500 mcg.

Infants and children up to 6 years: Experience is limited in this age group; doses of 7 mcg/kg have been administered.

One blood sample for TSH assay should be drawn immediately prior to the injection of Thypinone, and a second sample should be obtained 30 minutes after injection.

The TSH response to Thypinone (protirelin) is reduced by repetitive administration of the drug. Accordingly, if the Thypinone test is repeated, an interval of seven days before testing is recommended.

Elevated serum lipids may interfere with the TSH assay. Thus, fasting (except in patients with hypopituitarism) or a low-fat meal is recommended prior to the test.

Interpretation of Test Results: Interpretation of the TSH response to Thypinone (protirelin) requires an understanding of thyroid-pituitary-hypothalamic physiology and knowledge of the clinical status of the individual patient. Because the TSH test results may vary with the laboratory, the physician should be familiar with the TSH assay method used and the normal range for the laboratory performing the assay.

TSH response 30 minutes after Thypinone administration in normal subjects and in patients with hyperthyroidism and hypothyroidism are presented in Figure 1. The diagnoses were established prior to the administration of Thypinone on the basis of the clinical history, physical examination, and the results of other thyroid and/or pituitary function tests.

Among the normal euthyroid subjects, women and children were found to have higher levels of TSH at 30 minutes than men. Among the patients with hyperthyroidism or primary (thyroidal), secondary (pituitary) or tertiary (hypothalamic) hypothyroidism, no significant differences in TSH levels by age or sex were found.

Normal: Baseline TSH levels of less than 10 microunits/ml (μU/ml) were observed in 97% of euthyroid normal subjects tested. Thirty minutes after Thypinone (protirelin), the serum TSH increased by 2.0 μU/ml or more in 95% of euthyroid subjects.

Hyperthyroidism: All hyperthyroid patients tested had baseline TSH levels of less than 10 μU/ml and a rise of less than 2 μU/ml 30 minutes after Thypinone.

Primary (thyroidal) hypothyroidism: The diagnosis of primary hypothyroidism is frequently supported by finding clearly elevated baseline TSH levels; 93% of patients tested had levels above 10 μU/ml. Thypinone (protirelin) administration to these patients generally would not be expected to yield additional useful information. Ninety-four percent of patients with primary hypothyroidism given Thypinone in clinical trials responded with a rise in TSH of 2.0 μU/ml or greater; since this response is also found in normal subjects, Thypinone testing does not differentiate primary hypothyroidism from normal.

Secondary (pituitary) and tertiary (hypothalamic) hypothyroidism: In the presence of clinical and other laboratory evidence of hypothyroidism, the finding of a baseline TSH level less than 10 μU/ml should suggest secondary or tertiary hypothyroidism. In this situation, a response to Thypinone of less than 2 μU/ml suggests secondary hypothyroidism since this response was observed in about 60% of patients with secondary hypothyroidism and only approximately 5% of patients with tertiary hypothyroidism. A TSH response to Thypinone greater than 2 μU/ml is not helpful in differentiating between secondary and tertiary hypothyroidism since this response was noted in about 40% of the former and about 95% of the latter.

Establishing the diagnosis of secondary or tertiary hypothyroidism requires a careful history and physical examination along with appropriate tests of anterior pituitary and or target gland function. The Thypinone test should not be used as the only laboratory determinant for establishing these diagnoses.

[See table on top next page].

HOW SUPPLIED

As 1 ml ampules—boxes of 5 (NDC 0074-8971-05). Each ml contains Thypinone (protirelin) 0.50 mg (500 mcg), sodium chloride 9.0 mg for isotonicity, and pH adjusted with hydrochloric acid.

Products are cross-indexed by generic and chemical names in the **YELLOW SECTION**

Table 1
Characterization Based on Serum TSH Levels at Baseline and 30 Minutes after Thypinone

	Baseline Serum TSH (µU/ml)	Change of Serum TSH (µU/ml) at 30 Minutes
Euthyroidism (normal thyroid function)	10 or less (usually 6 or less; 20% have < 1.5 µU/ml)	2 or more (usually 6 to 30)
Hyperthyroidism	10 or less (usually 4 or less)	less than 2
Primary Hypothyroidism (thyroidal)	more than 10 (usually 15 to 200)	2 or more (usually 20 or more)
Secondary Hypothyroidism (pituitary)	10 or less (usually 6 or less)	less than 2 (59%) 2 to 50 (41%)
Tertiary Hypothyroidism (hypothalamic)	10 or less (often less than 2)	2 or more

Ayerst Laboratories
Division of American Home Products Corporation
685 THIRD AVE.
NEW YORK, NY 10017-4071

FACTREL® ℞
[făc'trel]
(gonadorelin hydrochloride)
Synthetic Luteinizing Hormone Releasing Hormone (LH-RH)
DIAGNOSTIC USE ONLY

CAUTION: Federal law prohibits dispensing without prescription.

DESCRIPTION

An agent for use in evaluating hypothalamic-pituitary gonadotropic function. FACTREL (gonadorelin hydrochloride) injectable is available as a sterile lyophylized powder for reconstitution and administration by subcutaneous or intravenous routes.

Chemical Name: 5-oxo-L-prolyl-L-histidyl-L-tryptophyl-L-seryl -L- tyrosyl-glycyl -L- leucyl-L-arginyl-L-prolyl glycinamide hydrochloride
[See structural formula below].

FACTREL is $C_{55}H_{75}N_{17}O_{13}HCl$, as the mono- or dihydrochloride, or their mixture. The gonadorelin base has a molecular weight of 1182.33. It is a white powder, soluble in alcohol and water, hygroscopic and moisture-sensitive, and stable at room temperature. The synthetic decapeptide, FACTREL, has a chemical composition and structure identical to the natural hormone, identified from porcine or ovine hypothalami.

Each vial of FACTREL contains 100 or 500 mcg gonadorelin as the hydrochloride, with 100 mg lactose, USP. Each ampul of sterile diluent contains 2% benzyl alcohol and Water for Injection, USP.

CLINICAL PHARMACOLOGY

FACTREL has been shown to have gonadotropin-releasing effects upon the anterior pituitary. The range for normal baseline LH levels, as determined from the literature, is 5–25 mIU/mL in postpubertal males, and postpubertal and premenopausal females. The standard used is the Second International Reference Preparation—HMC. This range may not correspond in each laboratory performing the assay since the concentration of LH in normal individuals varies with different assay methods. The normal responses to FACTREL analyzed from the results of clinical studies included:

(1) LH peak (mIU/mL)
(highest LH value post-FACTREL administration)

(2) Maximum LH increase (mIU/mL)
(peak LH value—LH baseline value)

(3) LH percent response
$$\frac{\text{peak LH—baseline LH}}{\text{baseline LH}} \times 100\%$$

(4) Time to peak (minutes)
(time required to reach LH peak value)

Normal adult subjects were shown to have these LH responses following FACTREL administration by subcutaneous or intravenous routes.

I. MALE ADULTS:

A) Subcutaneous Administration
The results are based on 18 tests in males between the ages of 18–42 years, inclusive:
(1) LH peak: mean 60.3 ± 26.2 mIU/mL
100% ≥ 24.0 mIU/mL
90% ≥ 32.8 mIU/mL
(2) Maximum LH increase: mean 46.7 ± 20.8 mIU/mL
100% ≥ 12.3 mIU/mL
90% ≥ 20.9 mIU/mL
(3) LH percent response: mean 437 ± 243% range: 66–1853%
90% ≥ 188%
(4) Time to peak: mean 34 ± 13 min.

B) Intravenous Administration
The results are based on 26 tests in males between the ages of 19–58 years, inclusive:
(1) LH peak: mean 63.8 ± 40.3 mIU/mL
100% ≥ 12.6 mIU/mL
90% ≥ 26.0 mIU/mL
(2) Maximum LH increase: mean 51.3 ± 35.2 mIU/mL
100% ≥ 7.4 mIU/mL
90% ≥ 14.8 mIU/mL
(3) LH percent response: mean 481 ± 184% range: 67–2139%
90% ≥ 142%
(4) Time to peak: mean 27 ± 14 min.

In males older than 50 years, the LH baseline and peak levels tend to be higher; however, the maximum LH increases do not differ in regard to age.

II. FEMALE ADULTS:

A) Subcutaneous Administration
The results are based on 38 tests in females between the ages of 19–36 years, inclusive:
(1) LH peak: mean 67.9 ± 27.5 mIU/mL
100% ≥ 12.5 mIU/mL
90% ≥ 39.0 mIU/mL
(2) Maximum LH increase: mean 52.8 ± 26.4 mIU/mL
100% ≥ 7.5 mIU/mL
90% ≥ 23.8 mIU/mL
(3) LH percent response: mean 374 ± 221% range: 108–981%
90% ≥ 185%
(4) Time to peak: mean 71.5 ± 49.6 min.

B) Intravenous Administration
The results are based on 31 tests in females between the ages of 20–35 years inclusive:
(1) LH peak: mean 57.6 ± 36.7 mIU/mL
100% ≥ 20.0 mIU/mL
90% ≥ 24.6 mIU/mL
(2) Maximum LH increase: mean 44.5 ± 31.8 mIU/mL
100% ≥ 7.5 mIU/mL
90% ≥ 16.2 mIU/mL
(3) LH percent response: mean 356 ± 282% range: 60–1300%
90% ≥ 142%
(4) Time to peak: mean 36 ± 24 min.

The FACTREL (gonadorelin hydrochloride) tests on which the normal female responses are based were performed in the early follicular phase of the menstrual cycle (Days 1–7). In menopausal and postmenopausal females, the baseline LH levels are elevated and the maximum LH increases are exaggerated when compared with the premenopausal levels. Patients with clinically diagnosed or suspected pituitary and/or hypothalamic dysfunction were often shown to have subnormal or no LH responses following FACTREL administration. For example, in clinical tests of 6 patients with known postpubertal panhypopituitarism, and 11 patients with Prader-Willi syndrome, 100% showed subnormal responses or no rise in LH. Subnormal responses to the FACTREL test also were observed in 21 (95%) of 22 patients with prepubertal panhypopituitarism. In 19 patients with Sheehan's syndrome, 16 (84%) had a subnormal response. In the FACTREL test in 44 patients with Kallmann's syndrome, 33 (77%) had subnormal LH responses.

INDICATIONS AND USAGE

FACTREL as a single injection is indicated for evaluating the functional capacity and response of the gonadotropes of the anterior pituitary. This single injection test does not measure pituitary gonadotropic reserve for which more prolonged or repeated administration may be required. The LH response is useful in testing patients with suspected gonadotropin deficiency, whether due to the hypothalamus alone or in combination with anterior pituitary failure. FACTREL is also indicated for evaluating residual gonadotropic function of the pituitary following removal of a pituitary tumor by surgery and/or irradiation. In clinical studies to date, however, the single injection test has not been useful in differentiating pituitary disorders from hypothalamic disorders. The FACTREL test can be performed concomitantly with other post-treatment evaluations.

The results of the FACTREL test complement the clinical examination and other laboratory tests used to confirm or substantiate hypogonadotropic hypogonadism.

In cases where there is a normal response, it indicates the presence of functional pituitary gonadotropes. The single injection test does not measure pituitary gonadotropic reserve.

CONTRAINDICATIONS

Hypersensitivity to gonadorelin hydrochloride or any of the components.

PRECAUTIONS

Antibody formation has been rarely reported after chronic administration of large doses of FACTREL.

The FACTREL test should be conducted in the absence of other drugs which directly affect the pituitary secretion of the gonadotropins. These would include a variety of preparations which contain androgens, estrogens, progestins, or glucocorticoids. The gonadotropin levels may be transiently elevated by spironolactone, minimally elevated by levodopa, and suppressed by oral contraceptives and digoxin. The response to FACTREL may be blunted by phenothiazines and dopamine antagonists which cause a rise in prolactin.

Pregnancy Category B. Reproduction studies have been performed in mice, rats, and rabbits at doses up to 50 times the human dose, and have revealed no evidence of harm to the fetus due to FACTREL. There are, however, no adequate and well-controlled studies in pregnant women. Because animal reproduction studies are not always predictive of human response, this drug should be used during pregnancy only if clearly needed.

Appropriate precautions should be taken because the effects of LH-RH on the fetus and developing offspring have not been adequately evaluated. Repetitive, high doses of FACTREL may cause luteolysis and inhibition of spermatogenesis.

ADVERSE REACTIONS

Systemic complaints such as headaches, nausea, lightheadedness, abdominal discomfort, and flushing have been re-

Continued on next page

Structural Formula:

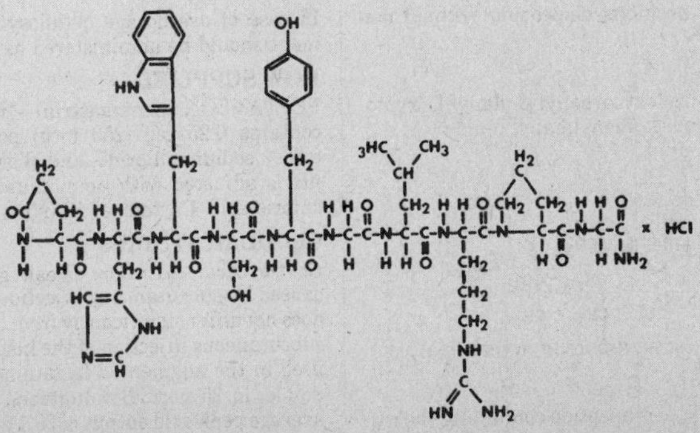

Ayerst—Cont.

ported rarely following administration of 100 mcg of FACTREL (gonadorelin hydrochloride). Local swelling, occasionally with pain and pruritus, at the injection site may occur if FACTREL is administered subcutaneously. Local and generalized skin rash have been noted after chronic subcutaneous administration.

Rare instances of hypersensitivity reaction (bronchospasm, tachycardia, flushing, urticaria, induration at injection site) have been reported following multiple-dose administration.

OVERDOSAGE

FACTREL has been administered parenterally in doses up to 3 mg BID for 28 days without any signs or symptoms of overdosage. In case of overdosage or idiosyncrasy, symptomatic treatment should be administered as required.

DOSAGE AND ADMINISTRATION

Adults: 100 mcg dose, subcutaneously or intravenously. In females for whom the phase of the menstrual cycle can be established, the test should be performed in the early follicular phase (Days 1–7).

TEST METHODOLOGY

To determine the status of the gonadotropin secretory capacity of the anterior pituitary, a test procedure requiring seven venous blood samples for LH is recommended.

PROCEDURE:

1. Venous blood samples should be drawn at -15 minutes and immediately prior to FACTREL administration. The LH baseline is obtained by averaging the LH values of the two samples.
2. Administer a bolus of 100 mcg of FACTREL subcutaneously or intravenously.
3. Draw venous blood samples at 15, 30, 45, 60, and 120 minutes after administration.
4. Blood samples should be handled as recommended by the laboratory that will determine the LH content. It must be emphasized that the reliability of the test is directly related to the inter-assay and intra-assay reliability of the laboratory performing the assay.

INTERPRETATION OF TEST RESULTS

Interpretation of the LH response to FACTREL requires an understanding of the hypothalamic-pituitary physiology, knowledge of the clinical status of the individual patient, and familiarity with the normal ranges and the standards used in the laboratory performing the LH assays.

Figures 1 through 4 represent the LH response curves after FACTREL administration in normal subjects. The normal LH response curves were established between the 10th percentile (B line) and 90th percentile (A line) of all LH responses in normal subjects analyzed from the results of clinical studies. LH values are reported in units of mIU/mL and time is displayed in minutes. Individual patient responses should be plotted on the appropriate curve. A subnormal response in patients is defined as three or more LH values which fall below the B line of the normal LH response curve.

Fig. 1:
Normal Male LH Response After FACTREL 100 mcg, Subcutaneous Administration 10th and 90th percentiles.

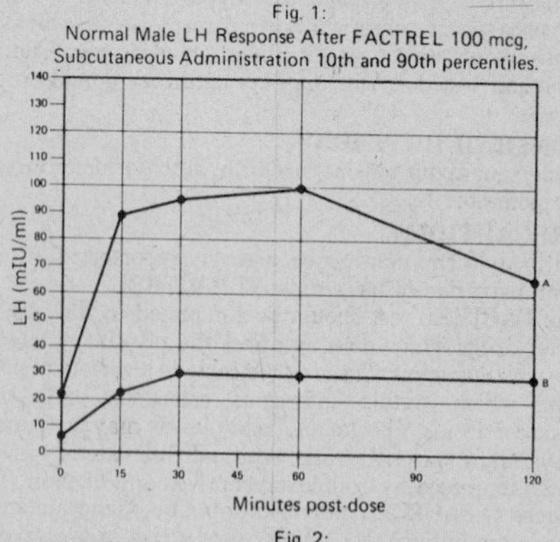

Fig. 2:
Normal Male LH Response After FACTREL 100 mcg, Intravenous Administration 10th and 90th percentiles.

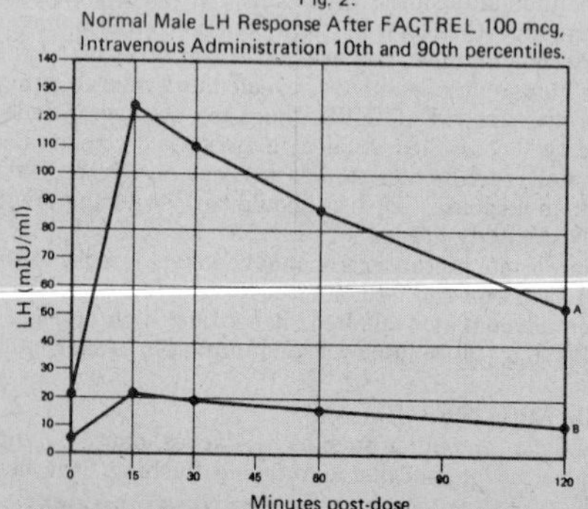

Fig. 3:
Normal Female LH Response After FACTREL 100 mcg Subcutaneous Administration 10th and 90th percentiles

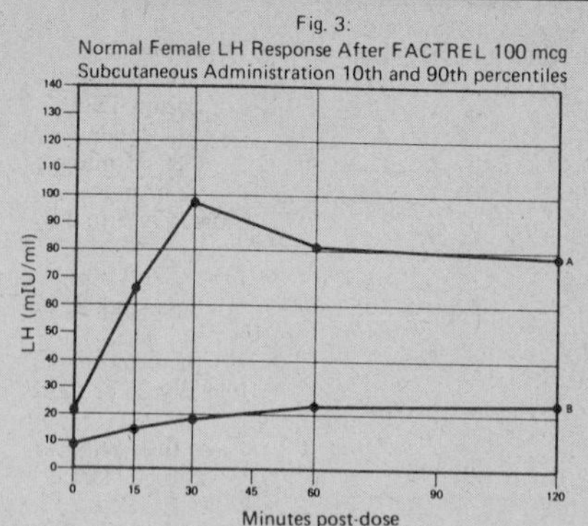

Fig. 4:
Normal Female LH Response After FACTREL 100 mcg, Intravenous Administration 10th and 90th percentiles.

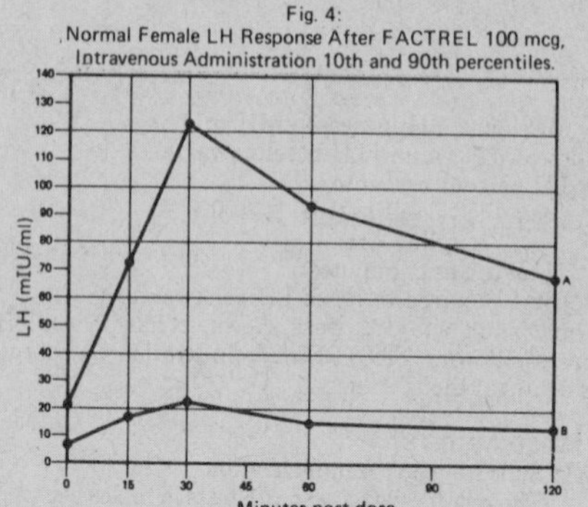

In cases where there is a blunted or borderline response, the FACTREL (gonadorelin hydrochloride) test should be repeated.

The FACTREL (gonadorelin hydrochloride) test complements the clinical assessment of patients with a variety of endocrine disorders involving the hypothalamic-pituitary axis. In cases where there is a normal response, it indicates the presence of functional pituitary gonadotropes. The single injection test does not determine the pathophysiological cause for the subnormal response and does not measure pituitary gonadotropic reserve.

HOW SUPPLIED

LYOPHILIZED POWDER—
in single-dose vials containing 100 mcg (NDC 0046-0507-05) and 500 mcg (NDC 0046-0509-05) gonadorelin as the hydrochloride with 100 mg lactose, USP. Each vial is accompanied by one ampul containing 2 mL sterile diluent of 2% benzyl alcohol in Water for Injection, USP.

DIRECTIONS

Store at room temperature (approximately 25°C).
Reconstitute 100 mcg vial with 1.0 mL of the accompanying sterile diluent.
Reconstitute 500 mcg vial with 2.0 mL of the accompanying sterile diluent.
Prepare solution immediately before use.
After reconstitution, store at room temperature and use within 1 day.
Discard unused reconstituted solution and diluent.
Diagnostic Method of Use Patent 3,947,569

Shown in Product Identification Section, page 404

PEPTAVLON® ℞

[pĕp-tăv ′lon]
Brand of pentagastrin
A diagnostic agent for evaluation of gastric acid secretory function.

CAUTION: Federal law prohibits dispensing without prescription.

DESCRIPTION

Chemical name: N-t-butyloxycarbonyl-β-alanyl-L-tryptophyl-L-methionyl-L-aspartyl-L-phenylalanyl amide.
Structural formula:

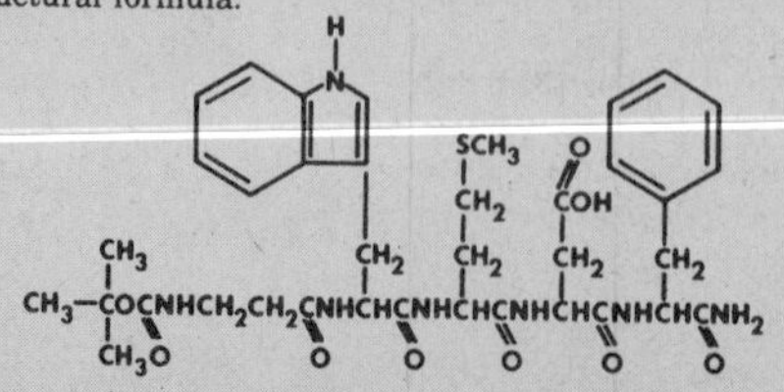

Pentagastrin is a synthetic pentapeptide containing the carboxyl terminal tetrapeptide, the active portion found in all natural gastrins. Pentagastrin is a colorless crystalline solid. It is soluble in dimethylformamide and dimethylsulfoxide; it is almost insoluble in water, ethanol, ether, benzene, chloroform, and ethyl acetate.

ACTIONS

PEPTAVLON (pentagastrin) contains the C-terminal tetrapeptide responsible for the actions of the natural gastrins and, therefore, acts as a physiologic gastric acid secretagogue. The recommended dose of 6 mcg/kg subcutaneously produces a peak acid output which is reproducible when used in the same individual.

PEPTAVLON stimulates gastric acid secretion approximately ten minutes after subcutaneous injection, with peak responses occurring in most cases twenty to thirty minutes after administration. Duration of activity is usually between sixty and eighty minutes.

INDICATIONS

PEPTAVLON (pentagastrin) is used as a diagnostic agent to evaluate gastric acid secretory function. It is useful in testing for:

Anacidity:—as a diagnostic aid in patients with suspected pernicious anemia, atrophic gastritis, or gastric carcinoma.
Hypersecretion:—as a diagnostic aid in patients with suspected duodenal ulcer or postoperative stomal ulcer, and for the diagnosis of Zollinger-Ellison tumor.

PEPTAVLON (pentagastrin) is also useful in determining the adequacy of acid-reducing operations for peptic ulcer.

CONTRAINDICATIONS

Hypersensitivity or idiosyncrasy to pentagastrin.

WARNINGS

Use in Pregnancy—The use of pentagastrin in pregnancy has NOT been studied, and the benefit of administration of the drug must be weighed against any possible risk to the mother and/or fetus.

Use in Children—There are insufficient data to recommend the use of, or establish a dosage, in children.

****

In amounts in excess of the recommended dose, pentagastrin may cause inhibition of gastric acid secretion.

PRECAUTIONS

Use with caution in patients with pancreatic, hepatic, or biliary disease. Like gastrin, pentagastrin could, in some cases, have the physiologic effect of stimulating pancreatic enzyme and bicarbonate secretion, as well as biliary flow.

ADVERSE REACTIONS

Pentagastrin causes fewer and less severe cardiovascular and other adverse reactions than histamine or betazole. The majority of reactions to pentagastrin are related to the gastrointestinal tract.

The following reactions associated with the use of pentagastrin have been reported.

Gastrointestinal: Abdominal pain, desire to defecate, nausea, vomiting, borborygmi, blood-tinged mucus
Cardiovascular: Flushing, tachycardia
Central Nervous System: Dizziness, faintness or lightheadedness, drowsiness, sinking feeling, transient blurring of vision, tiredness, headache
Allergic and Hypersensitivity Reactions: May occur in some patients.
Miscellaneous: Shortness of breath, heavy sensation in arms and legs, tingling in fingers, chills, sweating, generalized burning sensation, warmth, pain at site of injection, bile in collected specimens

DOSAGE AND ADMINISTRATION

Adults: 6 mcg/kg subcutaneously. Effect begins in about ten minutes; peak response usually occurs in twenty to thirty minutes. (For discussion of the test and explicit directions, consult Baron, JH: Gastric function tests, in Wastell, C: *Chronic Duodenal Ulcer,* New York, Appleton-Century-Crofts, 1972, pp 82–114.)

Note: Data are inadequate to recommend the use of, or establish a dosage, in children.

OVERDOSAGE

In case of overdosage or idiosyncrasy, symptomatic treatment should be administered as required.

HOW SUPPLIED

PEPTAVLON (pentagastrin)—In 2 mL ampuls. Each mL contains 0.25 mg (250 mcg) pentagastrin. Also contains 0.88% sodium chloride, and Water for Injection, USP. The pH is adjusted with ammonium hydroxide and/or hydrochloric acid. Cartons of 10 (NDC 0046-3290-10).

CLINICAL STUDIES

Gastric Acid Secretion: Peak gastric output in mEq/hr caused by subcutaneous injection of 6 mcg/kg pentagastrin does not differ significantly from that caused by the standard subcutaneous injection of the histamine acid phosphate dose used in the augmented histamine test (40 mcg/kg). For example, in 25 normal volunteers, pentagastrin produced an average peak acid output of 28.4 mEq/hr compared with 24.7 mEq/hr by histamine. In 45 patients with duodenal ulcer, or suspected duodenal ulcer, pentagastrin produced an average peak gastric acid output of 39.7 mEq/hr compared with 33.7 mEq/hr by histamine. In 18 patients with gastric ulcer, or suspected gastric ulcer, pentagastrin produced an average peak acid output of 17.4 mEq/hr compared with 19.4 mEq/hr by histamine. The overall mean for peak acid secretion by pentagastrin was 24.8 mEq/hr compared with 22.6 mEq/hr by histamine. No biochemical abnormality which might indicate specific organ toxicity has been encountered following the administration of pentagastrin.

Boehringer Mannheim Diagnostics

9115 HAGUE ROAD
INDIANAPOLIS, IN 46250

CHEMSTRIP bG®

[kim 'strip bee-jee ']

BLOOD GLUCOSE TEST

Test Strips for Semi-Quantitative Determination of Glucose in Whole Blood

SUMMARY AND EXPLANATION

CHEMSTRIP bG is a sensitive and specific test strip which facilitates accurate semi-quantitative determination of blood glucose within 2 minutes.

CHEMSTRIP bG is a glucose test strip with 2 separate test zones whose different reagent concentrations optimize sensitivity and colorimetric accuracy of semi-quantitative values from 20 mg/dl to 800 mg/dl. A wide range of test values permits wide use of CHEMSTRIP bG—for **stat** semi-quantitative assays of hypo- and hyperglycemia, as well as in emergency diagnosis of coma, mass screening of metabolic status, monitoring of diabetes mellitus and in home blood glucose monitoring programs.

SPECIMEN COLLECTION AND PREPARATION

CHEMSTRIP bG is free from interference when used with fresh capillary blood. It is specific for D-glucose in whole blood and nonreactive to fructose, lactose, galactose, and pentose sugars. Hematocrit values between 30–70% have no significant effect, and neither physiologic concentrations of uric or ascorbic acid, nor therapy with heparin, EDTA or the usual plasma expanders, affect test results with CHEMSTRIP bG. Do not use preservatives that contain fluoride.

PROCEDURE FOR *IN VITRO* DIAGNOSTIC USE

Two-minute test procedure with CHEMSTRIP bG requires only 3 steps: (1) Place a large enough drop of whole blood on the reagent area to cover both test zones completely. (2) After 60 seconds, wipe off the blood with a dry cotton ball and then rewipe the strip 2 more times. **Do not use water;** unlike other strips, CHEMSTRIP bG needs no washing. (3) After another 60 seconds, read test results by comparing test-zone colors with the vial label's color values for 20, 40, 80, 120, 180, and 240 mg/dl. (For colors **darker** than those for 240 mg/dl, wait an extra minute before reading 400 or 800 mg/dl.) The 8 distinct, precalibrated color values facilitate reproducible reading and permit practical estimation of intermediate values.

HOW SUPPLIED

Nonbreakable aluminum vials of 25 test strips, moisture-protected by drying agent in vial cap. Cat. No. 00501. Vial of 50 test strips with calibration strip included, may be read visually or may be used with Accu-chek bG blood glucose monitor. Cat. No. 00503. Vial of 50 test strips with calibration strip included, may be read visually or may be used with Accu-Chek® II blood glucose monitor. Cat. No. 00502.

Complete self-testing system also available. Kit includes 25 test strips, lancets, cotton balls, alcohol wipes, illustrated "How-to-Use" card and diabetic information guide. Cat. No. 00505.

ORDERING/PRICING/TECHNICAL INFORMATION

Call (800) 428-5076/(800) 858-8072.

CHEMSTRIP®

[kim ' strip]

URINE TESTING SYSTEM

Dip-and-Read Test Strips for Nitrite-pH-Protein-Glucose-Ketones-Urobilinogen-Bilirubin-Blood-Leukocytes in Urine

SUMMARY AND EXPLANATION

CHEMSTRIP is a uniquely constructed test strip of inert plastic to which a nylon mesh bonds, without glue, 1 to 9 reagent papers to determine nitrite, pH, protein, glucose, ketones, urobilinogen, bilirubin, blood and leukocytes in urine. The nylon mesh holds each reagent paper in place, protects it and promotes rapid and even urine-diffusion in each complete test area. To prevent the "run-over" phenomenon, certain test papers also have an inert absorbent paper between the reagent paper and the plastic strip.

[See table above].

Chemstrip Test Parameters

	Nitrite	Blood	Protein	Glucose	Ketones	Urobilinogen	Bilirubin	pH	Leukocytes	Catalog No.	Strips Per Vial
CHEMSTRIP® 9	X	X	X	X	X	X	X	X	X	417109	100
CHEMSTRIP® 7L		X	X	X	X	X	X	X	X	417117	100
CHEMSTRIP® 6L		X	X	X	X		X	X	X	417126	100
CHEMSTRIP® 5L		X	X	X	X			X	X	417135	100
CHEMSTRIP® GP			X	X						200743	100
CHEMSTRIP® uGK				X	X					00513 or 00514	100 or 50
CHEMSTRIP® K					X					00515 or 00516	100 or 25
CHEMSTRIP® uG				X						00511	100
CHEMSTRIP® LN	X								X	417152	100

CHEMSTRIPS are packaged in an aluminum vial with a tight-fitting cap which contains a drying agent. Each CHEMSTRIP is stable and ready for use when removed from the vial. No additional equipment or instrumentation is required.

SPECIMEN COLLECTION AND PREPARATION

CHEMSTRIPS may be used on any freshly voided urine specimen or on urines collected under special conditions, such as first-morning specimens and postprandial urines. The urine must be collected in a clean container and should be tested as soon as possible after collection (do not centrifuge). It is of particular importance to use fresh urine to obtain the best results with the test for urine bilirubin because this compound is very unstable when exposed to room temperature and daylight. If testing cannot be performed within an hour after collection, the specimen should be refrigerated immediately at 2 to 8° C and returned to room temperature before testing. Mix thoroughly before use.

PROCEDURE FOR *IN VITRO* DIAGNOSTIC USE

For convenience, all values on the strip may be read at 60 seconds (during the second minute) after immersion in the urine. Color changes occurring more than 2 minutes after strip immersion are not of diagnostic value. (Semi-quantitative assay of abnormally high glucose concentrations may require 4–5 minutes.) Color changes that occur only along the edge of the test area should be ignored. Careful removal of excess urine should eliminate this effect.

Calibration of the CHEMSTRIP during use is not required. Color blocks on vial label are previously calibrated by use of precise standards during the manufacturing process.

ORDERING/PRICING/TECHNICAL INFORMATION

Call (800) 428-5076/(800) 858-8072.

EDUCATIONAL MATERIAL

Books-Booklets-Brochures

"Merchandising to The Diabetic Consumer", R. Hitchens and G. Morris

Discusses the potential market for blood glucose monitoring products, and tells the pharmacist how to enter the market. Free to pharmacists.

Diabetes Product Brochure

Presents the complete line of Boehringer Mannheim diabetes monitoring products. Free.

"The New Role of The Pharmacist in the Management of Diabetes Mellitus", Dr. Nick Popovich

A pharmacist continuing education program offering 5 hours of C.E. credit, $6.00 processing fee.

Diabetes Merchandising Plan-o-grams

Suggested merchandising plan-o-grams for creating a "modern" diabetic department. Free to pharmacists.

Products are listed alphabetically in the **PINK SECTION.**

C. B. Fleet Co., Inc.

4615 MURRAY PL.
LYNCHBURG, VA. 24502-2235

FLEET DETECATEST® OTC

Home use test for determination of presence of fecal occult blood.

Fleet Detecatest contains all the necessary materials to test for occult blood at home. Included are: complete instructions regarding diet, medications, preparation of specimens, development, and reading results; three guaiac impregnated paper slides for two samples from each of three consecutive stools with Control Dots to indicate proper activity of paper and developer; Fleet Detecatest Developing Solution 2 ml.; three stool collection applicator sticks.

When a small stool sample that has blood in it is placed on the Detecatest paper, hemoglobin will come in contact with the guaiac. The addition of Fleet Detecatest Developing Solution causes oxidation of the guaiac resulting in a blue color.

Important: Reading the instructions thoroughly before beginning the test is important in performing the test and understanding the results.

Important: This test is not intended to replace a physician's diagnosis: If a patient reports a positive test, he should be questioned concerning diet, medication intake, and testing procedures. The person should then be tested under physician's supervision.

HOW SUPPLIED

One dozen test kits per case.

IS THIS PRODUCT OTC

Yes.

LITERATURE AVAILABLE

Yes.

Helena Laboratories

1530 LINDBERGH DRIVE
P.O. BOX 752
BEAUMONT, TX 77704

COLOSCREEN SELF-TEST (CS-T™)

Fecal Occult Blood Test

DESCRIPTION

ColoScreen Self-Test (CS-T™) is a simple, sanitary, one-step test for the detection of occult blood in the stool. No stool sample collection or color development reagents are needed. The patient simply places a test pad in the toilet, watches for a color change and records the results. No dietary fruit or vegetable restrictions are necessary. Red meat and vitamin C dietary restrictions should be followed.

ORDER INFORMATION

CS-T Office Packs contain an instruction sheet for the physician and 25 or 50 patient kits. Each patient kit consists of 3 CS-T test pads, instructions for the patient, and a reply card for return of results to the physician.

CS-T™ 50 Patient Kit Office Pack — Cat. No. 5176
CS-T™ 25 Patient Kit Office Pack — Cat. No. 5170

COLOSCREEN

Fecal Occult Blood Test

DESCRIPTION

ColoScreen is the standard guaiac slide test for the detection of occult blood in the stool. The patient smears a small fecal sample on the slide and then returns the slide to the physician's office or lab for testing. ColoScreen is identical in specificity and sensitivity to Hemoccult® (a registered trade-

Continued on next page

Helena—Cont.

mark of SmithKline Diagnostics, Inc.). As with other guaiac slide tests, certain fruits and vegetables, red meats and vitamin C should be restricted from the diet.

ORDER INFORMATION

ColoScreen Kits contain all materials necessary for complete testing, including developer and instructions. (Lab packs are also available in cartons of 1000 tests.)

ColoScreen III Office Pack **Cat. No. 5071**
100 Patient Kits (300 Tests). Each patient kit consists of one ColoScreen triple slide with monitors and applicators in a mail-back envelope printed with instructions for the patient.

ColoScreen Lab Pack **Cat. No. 5072**
100 Single Slides with Monitors (100 Tests)

ColoScreen III Lab Pack **Cat. No. 5082**
34 Triple Slides with Monitors (102 Tests)

COLOSCREEN/VPI™
Fecal Occult Blood Test

DESCRIPTION

ColoScreen/VPI™ is a guaiac slide for the detection of occult blood in the stool. A small fecal sample is collected by the patient and smeared onto the slide. The slide is returned to the physician's office or lab for testing. Unlike standard guaiac slide tests, ColoScreen/VPI is unaffected by fruit and vegetable peroxidase. There are fewer dietary restrictions and fewer false positives with ColoScreen/VPI.

ORDER INFORMATION

Available in the same packaging configuration as listed above for ColoScreen.

To Order or for Technical Information: 800-231-5663
In Texas 800-392-3126

Hoechst-Roussel Pharmaceuticals Inc.
SOMERVILLE, NJ 08876

RELEFACT® TRH ℞
(protirelin)
Injection IV

DESCRIPTION

Chemically, Relefact® TRH (protirelin) is identified as 5-oxo-L-prolyl-L-histidyl-L-proline amide. It is a synthetic tripeptide which is believed to be structurally identical with the naturally-occurring thyrotropin-releasing hormone produced by the hypothalamus.
Relefact TRH is supplied as 1 mL ampuls. Each ampul contains 500 mcg protirelin in a sterile non-pyrogenic isotonic saline solution having a pH of approximately 6.5. In addition, each ampul contains sodium chloride, 9.0 mg, Water for Injection, and hydrochloric acid as needed to adjust pH. Relefact TRH is intended for intravenous administration.

CLINICAL PHARMACOLOGY

Pharmacologically, Relefact TRH increases the release of the thyroid stimulating hormone (TSH) from the anterior pituitary. Prolactin release is also increased. It has recently been observed that approximately 65% of acromegalic patients tested respond with a rise in circulating growth hormone levels; the clinical significance is as yet not clear. Following intravenous administration, the mean plasma half-life of protirelin in normal subjects is approximately five minutes. TSH levels rise rapidly and reach a peak at 20 to 30 minutes. The decline in TSH levels takes place more slowly, approaching baseline levels after approximately three hours.

INDICATIONS AND USAGE

Relefact® TRH (protirelin) is indicated as an adjunctive agent in the diagnostic assessment of thyroid function. As an adjunct to other diagnostic procedures, testing with Relefact TRH may yield useful information in patients with pituitary or hypothalamic dysfunction.
Relefact TRH is indicated as an adjunct to evaluate the effectiveness of thyrotropin suppression with a particular dose of T4 in patients with nodular or diffuse goitre. A normal TSH baseline value and a minimal difference between the 30 minute and baseline response to Relefact TRH injection would indicate adequate suppression of the pituitary secretion of TSH.
Relefact TRH may be used, adjunctively, for adjustment of thyroid hormone dosage given to patients with primary hypothyroidism. A normal or slightly blunted TSH response, thirty minutes following Relefact TRH injection, would indicate adequate replacement therapy.

WARNINGS

Transient changes in blood pressure, either increases or decreases, frequently occur immediately following administration of Relefact TRH (protirelin). Blood pressure should therefore be measured before Relefact TRH is administered and at frequent intervals during the first 15 minutes after its administration.
Increases in systolic pressure (usually less than 30 mm Hg) and/or increases in diastolic pressure (usually less than 20 mm Hg) have been observed more frequently than decreases in pressure. These changes have not ordinarily persisted for more than 15 minutes nor have they required therapy. More severe degrees of hypertension or hypotension with or without syncope have been reported in a few patients. To minimize the incidence and /or severity of hypotension, the patient should be supine before, during, and after Relefact TRH administration. If a clinically important change in blood pressure occurs, monitoring of blood pressure should be continued until it returns to baseline levels.
Relefact® TRH (protirelin) should not be administered to patients in whom marked, rapid changes in blood pressure would be dangerous unless the potential benefit clearly outweighs the potential risk.

PRECAUTIONS

Thyroid hormones reduce the TSH response to Relefact TRH. Accordingly, patients in whom Relefact TRH is to be used diagnostically should be taken off liothyronine (T3) approximately seven days prior to testing and should be taken off thyroid medications containing levothyroxine (T4), e.g., desiccated thyroid, thyroglobulin, or liatrix, at least 14 days before testing. Hormone therapy is NOT to be discontinued when the test is used to evaluate the effectiveness of thyroid suppression with a particular dose of T4 in patients with nodular or diffuse goitre, or for adjustment of thyroid hormone dosage given to patients with primary hypothyroidism.
Chronic administration of levodopa has been reported to inhibit the TSH response to Relefact TRH.
It is not advisable to withdraw maintenance doses of adrenocortical drugs used in the therapy of known hypopituitarism. Several published reports have shown that prolonged treatment with glucocorticoids at physiologic doses has no significant effect on the TSH response to thyrotropin releasing hormone, but that the administration of pharmacologic doses of steroids reduces the TSH response.
Therapeutic doses of acetylsalicylic acid (2 to 3.6 g/day) have been reported to inhibit the TSH response to protirelin. The ingestion of acetylsalicylic acid caused the peak level of TSH to decrease approximately 30% as compared to values obtained without acetylsalicylic acid administration. In both cases, the TSH peak occurred 30 minutes post-administration of protirelin.
Pregnancy: Reproduction studies have been performed in rats and rabbits. At doses 1½ and 6 times the human dose, there was an increase in the number of resorption sites in the pregnant rabbit. There are no studies in pregnant women which bear on the safety of Relefact® TRH (protirelin) for the human fetus. Relefact TRH should be used in pregnant women only when clearly needed.

ADVERSE REACTIONS

Side effects have been reported in about 50% of the patients tested with Relefact TRH. Generally, the side effects are minor, have occurred promptly, and have persisted for only a few minutes following injection.
Cardiovascular reactions:
Marked changes in blood pressure, including both hypertension and hypotension with or without syncope, have been reported in a small number of patients.
Endocrine reaction: Breast enlargement and leakage in lactating women for up to two or three days.
Rarely, convulsions may occur in patients with predisposing conditions, e.g. epilepsy, brain damage.
Other reactions: Headaches, sometimes severe, and transient amaurosis in patients with pituitary tumors.
Nausea; urge to urinate; flushed sensation; lightheadedness; bad taste; abdominal discomfort; and dry mouth. Less frequently reported were: anxiety; sweating; tightness in the throat; pressure in the chest; tingling sensation; and drowsiness.

DOSAGE AND ADMINISTRATION

Relefact TRH is intended for intravenous administration with the patient in the supine position. The drug is administered as a bolus over a period of 15 to 30 seconds, with the patient remaining supine until all scheduled postinjection blood samples have been taken. Blood pressure should be measured before Relefact TRH is administered and at frequent intervals during the first 15 minutes thereafter (see **Warnings**).
Dosage: Adults: 500 mcg. Doses between 200 and 500 mcg have been used. 500 mcg is considered the optimum dose to give the maximum response in the greatest number of patients. Doses greater than 500 mcg are unlikely to elicit a greater TSH response.
Children age 6 to 16 years: 7 mcg/kg body weight up to a dose of 500 mcg.
Infants and children up to 6 years: Experience is limited in this age group; doses of 7 mcg/kg have been administered.
One blood sample for TSH assay should be drawn immediately prior to the injection of Relefact® TRH (protirelin), and a second sample should be obtained 30 minutes after injection.
The TSH response to Relefact TRH is reduced by repetitive administration of the drug. Accordingly, if the Relefact TRH test is repeated, an interval of seven days before testing is recommended.
Elevated serum lipids may interfere with the TSH assay. Thus, fasting (except in patients with hypopituitarism) or a low-fat meal is recommended prior to the test.

INTERPRETATION OF TEST RESULTS

Interpretation of the TSH response to Relefact TRH requires an understanding of thyroid-pituitary-hypothalamic physiology and knowledge of the clinical status of the individual patient.
Because the TSH test results may vary with the laboratory, the physician should be familiar with the TSH assay method used and the normal range for the laboratory performing the assay.
TSH response 30 minutes after Relefact TRH administration in normal subjects and in patients with hyperthyroidism and hypothyroidism are presented in Figure 1. The diagnoses were established prior to the administration of Relefact TRH on the basis of the clinical history, physical examination, and the results of other thyroid and/or pituitary function tests.
Among the normal euthyroid subjects, women and children were found to have higher levels of TSH at 30 minutes than men. Among the patients with hyperthyroidism or primary (thyroidal), secondary (pituitary), or tertiary (hypothalamic) hypothyroidism, no significant differences in TSH levels by age or sex were found.
[See table left].
Normal: Baseline TSH levels of less than 10 microunits/mL (μU/mL) were observed in 97% of euthyroid normal subjects tested. Thirty minutes after Relefact® TRH (protirelin), the serum TSH increased by 2.0 μU/mL or more in 95% of euthyroid subjects.
Hyperthyroidism: All hyperthyroid patients tested had baseline TSH levels of less than 10 μU/mL and a rise of less than 2 μU/mL 30 minutes after Relefact TRH.

Figure 1
Mean ± One Standard Deviation of TSH Levels (μU/mL)
Observed at Baseline and 30 Minutes After Relefact® TRH (protirelin)

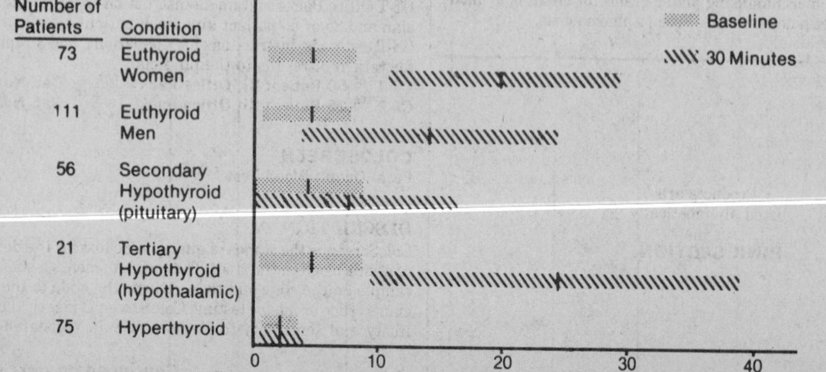

Primary (thyroidal) hypothyroidism: The diagnosis of primary hypothyroidism is frequently supported by finding clearly elevated baseline TSH levels; 93% of patients tested had levels above 10 μU/mL. Relefact TRH administration to these patients generally would not be expected to yield additional useful information. Ninety-four percent of patients with primary hypothyroidism given Relefact TRH in clinical trials responded with a rise in TSH of 2.0 μU/mL or greater, since this response is also found in normal subjects. Relefact TRH testing does not differentiate primary hypothyroidism from normal.

Table 1
Characterization Based on Serum TSH Levels at Baseline and 30 Minutes after Relefact TRH

	Baseline Serum TSH (μU/mL)	Change of Serum TSH (μU/mL) at 30 minutes
Euthyroidism (normal thyroid function)	10 or less (usually 6 or less: 20% have < 1.5 μU/mL)	2 or more (usually 6 to 30)
Hyperthyroidism	10 or less (usually 4 or less)	less than 2
Primary Hypothyroidism (thyroidal)	more than 10 (usually 15 to 100)	2 or more (usually 20 or more)
Secondary Hypothyroidism (pituitary)	10 or less (usually 6 or less)	less than 2 (59%) 2 to 50 (41%)
Tertiary Hypothyroidism (hypothalamic)	10 or less (often less than 2)	2 or more

Secondary (pituitary) and tertiary (hypothalamic) hypothyroidism: In the presence of clinical and other laboratory evidence of hypothyroidism, the finding of a baseline TSH level less than 10 μU/mL should suggest secondary or tertiary hypothyroidism. In this situation, a response to Relefact® TRH (protirelin) of less than 2 μU/mL suggests secondary hypothyroidism since this response was observed in about 60% of patients with secondary hypothyroidism and only approximately 5% of patients with tertiary hypothyroidism. A TSH response to Relefact TRH greater than 2 μU/mL is not helpful in differentiating between secondary and tertiary hypothyroidism since this response was noted in about 40% of the former and about 95% of the latter.

Establishing the diagnosis of secondary or tertiary hypothyroidism requires a careful history and physical examination along with appropriate tests of anterior pituitary and/or target gland function. The Relefact TRH test should not be used as the only laboratory determinant for establishing these diagnoses.

HOW SUPPLIED

As 1 mL ampuls - boxes of 5 (NDC 0039-0081-08). Each mL contains Relefact TRH 0.50 mg (500 mcg), sodium chloride 9.0 mg for isotonicity, and hydrochloric acid for pH adjustment.

* RELEFACT® REG TM HOECHST AG

78100 - 6/85

Lederle Laboratories

A Division of American Cyanamid Co.
ONE CYANAMID PLAZA
WAYNE, NJ 07470

TUBERCULIN, OLD, TINE TEST® ℞

[*to-ber-cu-lĭn*]

DESCRIPTION

The Tuberculin, Old, TINE TEST® is a sterile, simple, multiple-puncture, disposable intradermal test device for the detection of tuberculin reactivity. These convenient devices are especially useful in mass tuberculosis screening programs.

Each test unit consists of a stainless steel disc attached to a plastic handle. Projecting from the disc are four triangular-shaped prongs (tines) which are 2 mm long and approximately 4 mm apart. The tines have been mechanically dipped in a solution of Old Tuberculin, containing 7% Acacia (Gum Arabic) and 8.5% lactose as stabilizers, and then dried. The entire unit has been sterilized by Colbalt 60 irradiation. No preservative has been added. The unit is disposable and there is no need for syringes, needles, and other equipment necessary for the standard intradermal tests.

Tuberculin, Old, TINE TEST® UNITS have been standardized by clinical evaluation in human subjects to give reactions equivalent to or more potent than 5 T.U.* of standard old tuberculin administered intradermally in the Mantoux test. However, all multiple puncture-type devices must be regarded as screening tools and other appropriate diagnostic procedures such as the Mantoux test should be utilized for retesting reactors.

*US (International) tuberculin units.

CLINICAL PHARMACOLOGY

Tuberculin deposited in the skin of tuberculin reactive individuals reacts with sensitized lymphocytes to effect the release of mediators of cellular hypersensitivity. Some of these indicators (eg, skin reactive factor) induce an inflammatory response in the skin causing the edema and erythema characteristic of "positive" reactions.[1,2]

INDICATIONS AND USAGE

Tuberculin, Old, TINE TEST® is indicated to detect tuberculin-sensitive individuals. TINE TEST units are also useful in programs to determine priorities for additional testing (ie, chest x-rays) and in epidemiological surveys to identify those areas having high levels of infection.

In clinical studies covering various geographical areas of the US and all age groups, with a total of 30,588 test subjects, there were 911 (4%) false positive reactors among 26,236 subjects who were Mantoux negative, and 342 (8%) false negative reactors among 4,352 subjects who were Mantoux positive.

The frequency of repeated tuberculin tests depends on the risk of exposure of the child and on the prevalence of tuberculosis in the population group. For the pediatrician's office or outpatient clinic, an annual or biennial tuberculin test, unless local circumstances clearly indicate otherwise, is appropriate. The initial test should be done at the time of, or preceding, the measles immunization.[3] The repeated testing of uninfected individuals does not sensitize to tuberculin. Among individuals with waning sensitivity to homologous or heterologous mycobacterial antigens, however, the stimulus of a tuberculin test may "boost" or increase the size of the reaction to a second test, even causing an apparent development of sensitivity in some cases.[4]

Tuberculin testing should be done with caution in individuals with active tuberculosis. (See PRECAUTIONS).

CONTRAINDICATIONS

There are no known contraindications for use of Tuberculin, Old, TINE TEST®. See PRECAUTIONS section for information regarding special care to be exercised for safe and effective use.

WARNINGS

There are no known serious adverse reactions or potential safety hazards associated with the use of Tuberculin, Old, TINE TEST®. However, as with the use of any biological product, the possibility of anaphylactic reaction should be considered. See PRECAUTION section for information regarding special care to be exercised for safe and effective use.

PRECAUTIONS

Tuberculin testing should be done with caution in individuals with active tuberculosis. Although activation of quiescent lesions is rare, if a patient has a history of occurrence of vesiculation and necrosis with a previous tuberculin test by any method, tuberculin testing should be avoided.

Although clinical allergy to acacia is very rare, this product contains some acacia as stabilizer and should be used with caution in patients with known allergy to this component. In this instance remedial measures for anaphylactoid reactions, including epinephrine injection (1:1000), must be available for immediate use.

Reactivity to the test may be suppressed in patients who are receiving corticosteroids or immunosuppressive agents, or those who have recently been vaccinated with live virus vaccines such as measles, mumps, rubella, polio, etc.

With a positive reaction further diagnostic procedures must be considered. These may include x-ray of the chest, microbiologic examinations of sputa and other specimens, and confirmation of the positive TINE TEST reaction (except vesiculation reactions) using the Mantoux method. In general, the TINE TEST does not need to be repeated.

Antituberculous chemotherapy should not be instituted solely on the basis of a single positive TINE TEST.

When vesiculation occurs, the reaction is to be interpreted as strongly positive and a repeat test by the Mantoux method must not be attempted. Similar or more severe vesiculation with or without necrosis is likely to occur.

Pregnancy Category C. Animal reproduction studies have not been conducted with Tuberculin, Old, TINE TEST®. It is also not known whether Tuberculin, Old, TINE TEST can cause fetal harm when administered to a pregnant woman or can affect reproduction capacity. Tuberculin, Old, TINE TEST should be given to a pregnant woman only if clearly needed.

During pregnancy, known positive reactors may demonstrate a negative response to a Tuberculin TINE TEST.

Tuberculin, Old, TINE TEST® units must never be reused.

ADVERSE REACTIONS

Vesiculation (positive reaction), ulceration, or necrosis may occur at the test site in highly sensitive persons. Pain, pruritus, and discomfort at the test site may be relieved by cold packs or by topical glucocorticoid ointment or cream. Transient bleeding may be observed at a puncture site and is of no significance.

DOSAGE AND ADMINISTRATION

Tuberculin, Old, TINE TEST® UNITS have been standardized by clinical evaluation in human subjects to give reactions equivalent to or more potent than 5 T.U.* of standard old tuberculin administered intradermally in the Mantoux test. However, all multiple puncture-type devices must be regarded as screening tools and other appropriate diagnostic procedures such as the Mantoux test should be utilized for retesting reactors.

The volar surface of the upper one-third of the forearm, over a muscle belly, is the preferred site. Hairy areas, and areas without adequate subcutaneous tissue, eg, concavities over a tendon or bone should be avoided.

*US (International) tuberculin units.

Alcohol, acetone, ether, or soap and water may be used to cleanse the skin. The area must be clean and thoroughly dry before application of the Tuberculin, Old, TINE TEST®.

Expose the four coated tines by removing the protective cap while holding the plastic handle. Grasp the patient's forearm firmly, since the sharp momentary sting may cause the patient to jerk his or her arm, resulting in scratching. Stretch the skin of the forearm tightly and apply the disc with the other hand. **Hold at least one second.** Release tension grip on forearm. Withdraw tine unit.

Sufficient pressure should be exerted so that the four puncture sites, and circular depression of the skin from the plastic base are visible.

Local care of the skin is not necessary.

Tuberculin, Old, TINE TEST® Unit must never be reused.

Reading Reactions. Tests should be read at 48 to 72 hours. Vesiculation or the extent of induration are the determining factors; erythema without induration is of no significance. Readings should be made in good light with the forearm slightly flexed. The size of the induration in millimeters should be determined by inspection, measuring, and palpation with gentle finger stroking. Identification of the application site is usually easy because of the distinct four-point pattern. The diameter of the largest single reaction around one of the puncture sites should be measured. With pronounced reactions, the areas of induration around the puncture sites may coalesce.

Interpretation:

Positive Reactions

A. Vesiculation. If vesiculation is present, the test may be interpreted as positive, in which case the management of the patient is the same as that for one classified as positive to the Mantoux test.[5]

B. Induration, 2mm or greater. The test may be interpreted as positive but further diagnostic procedures must be considered. These may include x-ray of the chest, microbiologic examination of sputa and other specimens, and confirmation of the positive TINE TEST reaction using the Mantoux Method.

Negative Reaction. Induration less than 2mm. With a negative reaction there is no need for retesting unless the person is a contact of a patient with tuberculosis or there is clinical evidence suggestive of the disease.[5]

Descriptive literature illustrating typical reactions is available upon request.

HOW SUPPLIED

Tuberculin, Old, TINE TEST® is supplied as follows:

NDC 0005-2722-25 25 individual tests in a jar
NDC 0005-2722-28 100 individual tests
NDC 0005-2722-34 250 individual tests

Military Depot: NSN 6505-00-890-1534—Jar 25
USPHS: NSN 6505-00-890-1534

STORAGE

Tuberculin, Old, TINE TEST® UNITS should be stored unrefrigerated below 30° C (86° F).

REFERENCES

1. Comstock, CW, et al: The Tuberculin Skin Test, *Amer Rev Respir Dis* 1981;124:356–363.
2. Burrows W: *Immunity and Hypersensitivity: Textbook of Microbiology* 1979, 369–424.

Continued on next page

The information on each product appearing here is based on labelling effective in August, 1986 and is either the entire official brochure or an accurate condensation therefrom. Information concerning all Lederle products may be obtained from the Professional Services Department, Lederle Laboratories, Pearl River, New York, 10965.

Lederle—Cont.

3. Report of the Committee on the Control of Infectious Diseases. American Academy of Pediatrics, 1977.
4. Comstock, CW, et al: The Tuberculin Skin Test, *Amer Rev Respir Dis 1971;104(5):769–775.*
5. Committee on Diagnostic Skin Testing of the American Thoracic Society: The Tuberculin Test (rev). New York, American Lung Association, 1974.

LEDERLE LABORATORIES DIVISION
American Cyanamid Company, Pearl River, NY 10965

TINE TEST® PPD ℞

[*tīne těst*]

Tuberculin, Purified Protein Derivative

DESCRIPTION

THE TUBERCULIN, PURIFIED PROTEIN DERIVATIVE (PPD) TINE TEST® is a sterile, simple, multiple-puncture, disposable intradermal test device for the detection of tuberculin reactivity. These convenient devices are especially useful in mass tuberculosis screening programs.

Each test unit consists of a stainless steel disc attached to a light blue plastic handle. Projecting from the disc are four triangular-shaped prongs (tines) which are 2 mm long and approximately 4 mm apart. The tines have been mechanically dipped into a concentrated solution of PPD. The PPD concentrate is prepared by the Seibert Process[1,2] and is stabilized with seven percent acacia (gum Arabic), thirty percent dextrose and five percent glycerol. The glycerol also acts as a humectant preventing the film on the tines from becoming brittle-dry. The final PPD concentrate is standardized against U.S. Standard PPD. The tines are dipped into concentrated PPD, capped and sterilized with ethylene oxide. No preservative has been added. The TINE TEST (PPD) unit is disposable, and there is no need for syringes, needles, and other equipment necessary for the standard intradermal tests.

The Tine Test (PPD) units have been standardized by clinical evaluation in human subjects to give reactions equivalent to or more potent than 5 T.U.* of standard PPD administered intradermally in the Mantoux test. However, all multiple puncture-type devices must be regarded as screening tools and other appropriate diagnostic procedures such as the Mantoux test should be utilized for retesting reactors.

* US (International) tuberculin units.

CLINICAL PHARMACOLOGY

Tuberculin deposited in the skin of tuberculin reactive individuals reacts with sensitized lymphocytes to effect the release of mediators of cellular hypersensitivity. Some of these indicators (eg, skin reactive factor) induce an inflammatory response in the skin causing the edema and erythema characteristic of a "positive" reaction.[3,4]

INDICATIONS AND USAGE

TUBERCULIN, PURIFIED PROTEIN DERIVATIVE TINE TEST® PPD is indicated to detect tuberculin-sensitive individuals. Tine Test units are also useful in programs to determine priorities for additional testing (ie, chest x-rays) and in epidemiological surveys to identify those areas having high levels of infection.

Data obtained from clinical studies with a total of 3,062 volunteer subjects (males and females), ranging in age from 4 to 96 years, of which 47.5% (1,443) were Mantoux positive, clearly demonstrates that TINE TEST PPD, when used as a screening test to determine tuberculin reactivity is associated with very little, if any, adverse reactivity. Other than the skin test reaction itself, slight vesiculation and slight ulceration were the only adverse experiences reported. The slight to mild vesiculation was equally divided between the two tests (TINE TEST, 54/3062, 1.78%, and PPD-T Mantoux, 55/3062, 1.81%). The slight ulceration observed with one subject at 72 hours was associated with the TINE TEST site. Of the subjects classified as positive or intermediate by PPD-T Mantoux, 93.8% were classified similarly with the TINE TEST. The results of the clinical trials revealed a 72-hour false positive rate of 10.9% and a false negative rate of 6.2%. In clinical studies of more than 1,800 PPD-S Mantoux positive subjects only 6.3% gave negative TINE TEST PPD reactions at 72 hours; of more than 1,900 TINE TEST PPD positive tests, less than 11% gave negative Mantoux results.

The frequency of repeated tuberculin tests depends on risk of exposure of the child and on the prevalence of tuberculosis in the population group. For the pediatrician's office or outpatient clinic, an annual or biennial tuberculin test, unless local circumstances clearly indicate otherwise, is appropriate. The initial test should be done at the time of, or preceding, the measles immunization.[5] The repeated testing of uninfected individuals does not sensitize to tuberculin. Among individuals with waning sensitivity to homologous or heterologous mycobacterial antigens, however, the stimulus of a tuberculin test may "boost" or increase the size of the reaction to a second test, even causing an apparent development of sensitivity in some cases.[6]

Tuberculin testing should be done with caution in individuals with active tuberculosis. (See PRECAUTIONS).

CONTRAINDICATIONS

There are no known contraindications for use of Tuberculin, Purified Protein Derivative (PPD) TINE TEST®. See PRECAUTIONS section for information regarding special care to be exercised for safe and effective use.

WARNINGS

There are no known serious adverse reactions or potential safety hazards associated with the use of Tuberculin, Purified, Protein Derivative (PPD) TINE TEST®. However, as with the use of any biological product, the possibility of anaphylactic reaction should be considered. See PRECAUTION section for information regarding special care to be exercised for safe and effective use.

PRECAUTIONS

Tuberculin testing should be done with caution in individuals with active tuberculosis. However, activation of quiescent lesions is rare. If a patient has a history of occurrence of vesiculation and necrosis with a previous tuberculin test by any method, tuberculin testing should be avoided.

Although clinical allergy to acacia is very rare, this product contains some acacia as stabilizer and should be used with caution in patients with known allergy to this component. In these instances remedial measures for anaphylactoid reactions, including epinephrine injection (1:1000), must be available for immediate use.

Reactivity to the test may be suppressed in patients who are receiving corticosteroids or immunosuppressive agents, or those who have recently been vaccinated with live virus vaccines such as measles, mumps, rubella, polio, etc.

With a positive reaction further diagnostic procedures must be considered. These may include x-ray of the chest, microbiologic examinations of sputa and other specimens, and confirmation of the positive TINE TEST reaction (except vesiculation reactions) using the Mantoux method. In general, the TINE TEST does not need to be repeated.

Antituberculous chemotherapy should not be instituted solely on the basis of a single positive TINE TEST.

When vesiculation occurs, the reaction is to be interpreted as strongly positive and a repeat test by the Mantoux method must not be attempted. Similar or more severe vesiculation with or without necrosis is likely to occur.

Pregnancy Category C. Animal reproduction studies have not been conducted with Tuberculin, Purified Protein Derivative (PPD) TINE TEST®. It is also not known whether Tuberculin, Purified Protein Derivative (PPD) Tine Test can cause fetal harm when administered to a pregnant woman or can affect reproduction capacity. Tuberculin, Purified Protein Derivative (PPD) TINE TEST should be given to a pregnant woman only if clearly needed.

During pregnancy, known positive reactors may demonstrate a negative response to a Tuberculin (PPD) TINE TEST.

Tuberculin, Purified Protein Derivative TINE TEST® PPD units must never be reused.

ADVERSE REACTIONS

Vesiculation (positive reaction), ulceration, or necrosis may occur at the test site in highly sensitive persons. Pain, pruritus, and discomfort at the test site may be relieved by cold packs or by topical glucocorticoid ointment or cream. Transient bleeding may be observed at a puncture site and is of no significance.

DOSAGE AND ADMINISTRATION

TUBERCULIN, OLD, TINE TEST® UNITS have been standardized by clinical evaluation in human subjects to give reactions equivalent to or more potent than 5 T.U.* of standard PPD administered intradermally in the Mantoux test. However, all multiple puncture-type devices must be regarded as screening tools and other appropriate diagnostic procedures such as the Mantoux test should be utilized for retesting reactors.

The volar surface of the upper one-third of the forearm, over a muscle belly, is the preferred site. Hairy areas, and areas without adequate subcutaneous tissue, eg, concavities over a tendon or bone should be avoided.

* US (International) tuberculin units.

Alcohol, acetone, ether, or soap and water may be used to cleanse the skin. The area must be clean and thoroughly dry before application of the TINE TEST PPD.

Expose the four coated tines by removing the protective cap while holding the plastic handle. Grasp the patient's forearm firmly, since the sharp momentary sting may cause the patient to jerk his or her arm, resulting in scratching. Stretch the skin of the forearm tightly and apply the disc with the other hand. **Hold at least one second.** Release tension grip on forearm. Withdraw tine unit. **Sufficient pressure should be exerted so that the four puncture sites, and circular depression of the skin from the plastic base are visible.**

Local care of the skin is not necessary.

TUBERCULIN, PURIFIED PROTEIN DERIVATIVE TINE TEST® PPD Unit *must never be re-used.*

READING REACTIONS

Tests should be read at 48–72 hours. Vesiculation or the extent of induration are the determining factors; erythema without induration is of no significance. Readings should be made in good light with the forearm slightly flexed. The size of the induration in millimeters should be determined by inspection, measuring, and palpation with gentle finger stroking. Identification of the application site is usually easy because of the distinct four-point pattern. The diameter of the largest single reaction around one of the puncture sites should be measured. With pronounced reactions, the areas of induration around the puncture sites may coalesce.

INTERPRETATION

Positive Reactions

A. **Vesiculation.** If vesiculation is present, the test may be interpreted as positive, in which case the management of the patient is the same as that for one classified as positive to the Mantoux Test.[7]

B. **Induration, 2mm or Greater.** The test may be interpreted as positive but further diagnostic procedures must be considered. These may include x-ray of the chest, microbiologic examination of sputa and other specimens, and confirmation of the positive TINE TEST reaction using the Mantoux Method.

Negative Reaction

Induration Less Than 2mm. With a negative reaction there is no need for retesting unless the person is a contact of a patient with tuberculosis or there is clinical evidence suggestive of the disease.[7]

Descriptive literature illustrating typical reactions is available upon request.

HOW SUPPLIED

TUBERCULIN, PURIFIED PROTEIN DERIVATIVE TINE TEST® PPD is supplied as follows:
NDC 0005-2720-25 25 individual tests in a jar
NDC 0005-2720-28 100 individual tests

STORAGE

Tine Test PPD Units should be stored unrefrigerated below 30° C (86° F.)

REFERENCES

1. Seibert, FB: Isolation and Properties of Purified Protein Derivative of Tuberculin. *Am Rev Tuberc,* 1934;30:713.
2. Seibert, FB, Glenn, JF: Tuberculin Purified Protein Derivative—Preparation and Analysis of a Large Quantity for Standard. *Amer Rev Tuberc* 1941;44:9.
3. Comstock, CW, et al: The Tuberculin Skin Test, *Amer Rev Resp Dis* 1981;124:356–363.
4. Burrows, W: Immunity and Hypersensitivity: Textbook of Microbiology 1979, 369–424.
5. Report of the Committee on the Control of Infectious Diseases. American Academy of Pediatrics, 1977.
6. Comstock, GW, et al: The Tuberculin Skin Test, *Amer Rev Resp Dis* 1971;104(5):769–775.
7. Committee on Diagnostic Skin Testing of the American Thoracic Society, The Tuberculin Test (rev). New York, American Lung Association, 1974.

Eli Lilly and Company

LILLY CORPORATE CENTER
INDIANAPOLIS, IN 46285

TES-TAPE® OTC

[*těs 'tāp*]

(glucose enzymatic test strip)
USP

For In Vitro Diagnostic Use in Testing for the Presence and Semiquantitative Measurement of Glucose in Human Urine

Tes-Tape has been used since 1956, when Dr. A. S. Keston described the novel idea of using two enzymes simultaneously to test for glucose and Dr. J. P. Comer published data on the specificity and accuracy of Tes-Tape for the semiquantitative analysis of urine glucose.

During the development and testing of this urine test method, Tes-Tape was found to be an accurate and reliable semiquantitative method for determining urine glucose. To date, relatively few instances of faulty results have occurred with the use of Tes-Tape. Problems associated with the product are usually due to improper techniques or exposure of the tape to adverse conditions or due to drugs which have an inhibitory effect on the enzyme reaction. Considerable data may be found in the published scientific documents.

Tes-Tape is impregnated with the enzymes glucose oxidase and peroxidase and an oxidizable substrate, orthotolidine. When the tape is dipped into urine containing glucose, the glucose oxidase catalyzes the reaction of glucose in the urine with oxygen from the air to form gluconic acid and hydrogen peroxide. The enzyme peroxidase (from horseradish) then catalyzes the reaction of hydrogen peroxide and orthotolidine to form a blue color. With the addition of a yellow dye (FDC Yellow No. 5) to the paper, the possible color range of the test is extended from yellow to light green to deep blue. If no glucose is present, the tape maintains its yellow color.

Reactive Ingredient	Approximate Amount per 1.5 Inches of Tape
Glucose oxidase	3.78 units
Horseradish peroxidase	2.82 PZ units
O-tolidine	0.136 mg

Nonreactive ingredients include filter paper, FDC Yellow No. 5 coloring, buffers, stabilizers, and wetting agents.
For in vitro diagnostic use. Store below 86°F (30°C). Protect from high humidity and light.
Do not use if the tape becomes dark yellow or yellowish-brown or if a 2 percent reading is not obtained when the reliability is tested, as described under the heading **IMPORTANT.**
The urine should be collected in a container free of chemicals and glucose.
If the freshly voided specimen is not to be tested within four hours, it should be refrigerated.
Drugs that are known to have an inhibitory effect on the enzyme reactions include ascorbic acid (vitamin C), dipyrone, gentisic acid (a metabolite of aspirin), homogentisic acid (present in alkaptonuria), levodopa, meralluride injection, and methyldopa. The inhibiting effect is notable on the dipped part of the tape, but accurate readings may be obtained by observing the narrow band of color at the junction of the dry and wet portions. A separation of glucose from the inhibitory substances occurs as the urine travels along the dry portion of the tape. Ingestion of more than 1.5 g of ascorbic acid may produce urine with inhibitory action on Tes-Tape.
Specimens for storage or shipment should be refrigerated or preserved with up to 0.37 percent formaldehyde.
All materials are provided for the test and include dispenser, tape, and color chart.
Results on the color chart are expressed in percent of glucose (urine sugar) and by a corresponding arbitrary system of 0, +, + +, + + +, + + + +, representing 0, 1/10, 1/4, 1/2, 2 (or more) percent of glucose respectively.
When testing, do not place the tape on the lavatory or on paper or allow moistened portion to contact fingers. Contamination of the tape by glucose from other sources (e.g., perspiration, tears, and saliva) or with a residue of chlorine from lavatory cleansing agents can cause false-positive results.
Patients who are receiving high doses of ascorbic acid or whose urine contains dipyrone, meralluride, homogentisic acid, gentisic acid, levodopa, or methyldopa should read only the very narrow band of color in the moist portion of the tape above the level to which it was dipped into the specimen.
Very high doses of ascorbic acid may cause a false-negative test even with the above precaution. (Urinary levels of ascorbic acid in excess of 0.1 percent are necessary to block the test completely. This concentration is most likely to appear within three to seven hours after a single dose of 1.5 g or more.)
Normal urine should test 0 percent with Tes-Tape. Persons using Tes-Tape for a screening test should report all values above 0 percent to their physician. Diabetic urine values in the range of the color chart should also be recorded and reported to the patient's physician. Measured values of 2 percent should be reported as 2 percent or more.
The overall semiquantitative accuracy of Tes-Tape originally reported in 1956 on 1000 determinations was 96 percent. This was confirmed in 1973 on 14,000 determinations over a two-year period. These data were obtained on urine samples containing concentrations of glucose at each increment shown to be measurable on the color chart. The color chart provided is based on the average color perception of many observers. Patients who have difficulty in differentiating color should seek the advice of their physician before using Tes-Tape.
Numerous other clinical and laboratory studies have shown that Tes-Tape is accurate in qualitative and semiquantitative determination of urine sugar. Tes-Tape is specific for glucose in urine sugar testing. Except for instances involving contamination of the tape or urine receptacle with glucose from other sources (e.g., perspiration, tears, and saliva) or with a residue of chlorine from cleansing agents, there is no known clinical situation in which a false-positive test for glucose occurs with Tes-Tape. The sensitivity of Tes-Tape is such that it will react with concentrations of 0.05 percent glucose or more. Trace reactions shown by the development of a very light yellow-green color may be observed with less than this amount of glucose.
After opening plastic wrapper, use tape within four months. It must be used prior to expiration date.

IMPORTANT

The reliability of a roll of Tes-Tape may easily be checked by dipping a piece into a properly prepared glucose solution.* The tape should be removed immediately, as one would when testing a urine specimen. After two minutes have elapsed, the reading obtained when the tape is compared with the color chart should be approximately + + + + (2 percent). If such a reading is not obtained, the tape has apparently deteriorated and should not be used.
Measurements for the amount of glucose present (semiquantitative) should not be made after two minutes because the colors gradually change as the tape dries. Screening tests for the presence of glucose (qualitative) in urine may be made for several hours after the tape has dried.
The patient should consult the package insert in regard to Procedure, What to Do If Tape Breaks, and a record chart for urine sugar tests with Tes-Tape.

*If a properly prepared glucose solution is not available, any nationally known *sugar (glucose)-containing* beverage from a freshly opened bottle or can is satisfactory. (Diet cola beverages would not be satisfactory.)

HOW SUPPLIED

M-73, Tes-Tape® (Glucose Enzymatic Test Strip, USP), dispenser package, approximately 100 tests, in single packages. (NDC 0002-2344-41) [080583]
M-73—100 tests—6505-00-559-6859

Marion Scientific

A Division of Marion Laboratories, Inc.
P.O. BOX 8480
KANSAS CITY, MO 64114

CULTURETTE Brand 10-MINUTE GROUP A STREP ID

DESCRIPTION

The CULTURETTE Brand 10-MINUTE GROUP A STREP ID is a latex slide agglutination test for the detection of group A streptococcal antigen directly from throat swabs. When the exposed group A streptococcal antigen reacts with the specific antibody-coated latex beads, a macroscopically visible agglutination occurs.
Principles of the Procedure: The CULTURETTE Brand 10-MINUTE GROUP A STREP ID does not depend upon growth of the organism. This screening test allows the identification of group A *Streptococcus* within minutes of taking the specimen.
In essence, a throat swab is subjected to a 5-min extraction procedure in a plastic microtube. If group A antigen is present, it is exposed during this time. The exposed antigen is then mixed with both specific and negative control latex agglutination reagents on two separate circles of an agglutination slide. If agglutination is observed in the circle in which the extract has been mixed with specific latex reagent and it is not observed in the circle with the negative control reagent, it is a positive test.
Sterilization of the specimen is achieved during the extraction procedure, resulting in easy and safe disposal. No incubation or centrifugation is required during the procedure.

Cat. No. 26-30-00 CULTURETTE Brand 10-MINUTE GROUP A STREP ID Sterile Dacron-Tipped Swabs—100 per carton
Cat. No. 26-30-01 CULTURETTE Brand 10-MINUTE GROUP A STREP ID—55 Determinations
Cat. No. 26-30-02 CULTURETTE Brand 10-MINUTE GROUP A STREP ID—Complete In-Office Kit—55 Determinations
Cat. No. 26-30-04 CULTURETTE Brand 10-MINUTE GROUP A STREP ID—200 Determinations

Issued 5/85

CULTURETTE® FAMILY

Cat. No.	Product/Description
26-02-10	CULTURETTE®—Single Swab, Sterile Culture collection system with modified Stuart's transport medium, 0.5 ml. Packaged: 100 per carton/10 cartons per case
26-02-19	CULTURETTE II®—Dual Swab, Sterile Culture collection system with modified Stuart's transport medium, 1.0 ml. Packaged: 100 per carton/10 cartons per case
26-02-15	MINI-TIP CULTURETTE®—Single Swab, Sterile Culture collection system with flexible/extendable wire swab and modified Stuart's transport medium, 0.5 ml. Packaged: 100 per carton/10 cartons per case
26-02-18	ANAEROBIC CULTURETTE®—Single Swab Sterile culture collection system designed for collection and transport of anaerobic bacteria. Packaged: 10 per carton/10 cartons per case
26-15-14	VIRAL CULTURETTE®—Single Swab, Sterile Culture collection and transport system for viral specimens with modified Hanks balanced salt solution, 0.5 ml. Packaged: 100 per carton/10 cartons per case

Issued 5/85

Merieux Institute, Inc.

P. O. BOX 52-3980
MIAMI, FL 33152-3980

MULTITEST® CMI™ ℞

[mul 'tĭ-test]
(Skin Test Antigens for Cellular Hypersensitivity)

NDC 50361-780-80

DESCRIPTION

Skin Test Antigens for Cellular Hypersensitivity, MULTITEST® CMI™ is a disposable, plastic applicator consisting of eight sterile test heads preloaded with the following seven delayed hypersensitivity skin test antigens and glycerin negative control for precutaneous administration: Tetanus Toxoid Antigen, Diphtheria Toxoid Antigen, Streptococcus Antigen, Old Tuberculin, Candida Antigen, Trichophyton Antigen, and Proteus Antigen.
MULTITEST® CMI™ provides a quick, convenient and uniform procedure for delayed cutaneous hypersensitivity testing.
Supplied in box of 10 individual cartons containing one preloaded MULTITEST® CMI™ per carton.

TUBERCULIN, MONO-VACC® TEST (O.T.) ℞

[tu-ber 'ku-lin]
(old tuberculin)
Multiple Puncture Device

NDC 50361-770-40 25 tests per box
Supplied in plastic tamper proof box of 25 tests per box; test reading cards in English or Spanish also available.

Parke-Davis

DIVISION OF WARNER-LAMBERT COMPANY
201 TABOR ROAD
MORRIS PLAINS, NEW JERSEY 07950

APLISOL® ℞

[ă 'plĭ-sōl "]
(Tuberculin Purified Protein Derivative, Diluted [Stabilized Solution])

DESCRIPTION

Aplisol (tuberculin PPD, diluted) is a sterile aqueous solution of a purified protein fraction for intradermal administration as an aid in the diagnosis of tuberculosis. The solution is stabilized with polysorbate (Tween) 80, buffered with potassium and sodium phosphates and contains approximately 0.35% phenol as a preservative.
The product is clinically equivalent in potency to the standard PPD-S* (5 TU** per 0.1 ml) of the U.S. Public Health Service, National Center for Disease Control, and is ready for immediate use without further dilution. This product meets all applicable standards.

CLINICAL PHARMACOLOGY

The purified protein fraction is isolated from culture filtrates of human type strains of *Mycobacterium tuberculosis* by the method of F.B. Seibert.[1,2] This product is made from a single master lot (No. 924994) to eliminate lot to lot variation inherent in manufacturing.
The 5 TU dose of Tuberculin PPD intradermally (Mantoux) is recommended as the standard tuberculin test, and Tuberculin PPD is recommended by the American Lung Association as an aid in the detection of infection with *Mycobacterium tuberculosis.*
Reactions to the Mantoux test are interpreted on the basis of a quantitative measurement of the response to a specific dose (5 TU PPD-S or equivalent) of Tuberculin PPD. Other dosages are regarded as having no demonstrable usefulness in ordinary practice.[3]Accordingly, Aplisol is available in only one potency (5 TU equivalent) and the use of this potency

This product information was prepared in August 1986. On these and other Parke-Davis Products, information may be obtained by addressing PARKE-DAVIS, Division of Warner-Lambert Company, Morris Plains, New Jersey 07950.

Continued on next page

Parke-Davis—Cont.

only is recommended. The selection of 5 TU as the test dose is based upon data indicating that (1) the 5 TU dose gives measurable reactions in over 95 percent of the known tuberculous infected; (2) doses larger than 5 TU might elicit reactions not caused by tuberculosis infection; and (3) nonreactors to doses considerably less than 5 TU are not accepted as negative but are retested with a stronger dose.[3]

INDICATIONS AND USAGE

Tuberculin PPD is recommended by the American Lung Association as an aid in the detection of infection with *Mycobacterium tuberculosis.* The standard tuberculin test recommended employs the intradermal (Mantoux) test using a 5 TU dose of tuberculin PPD.[3] The 0.1 ml test dose of Aplisol (tuberculin PPD, diluted) is equivalent to the 5 TU dose recommended as clinically established and standardized with PPD-S.

CONTRAINDICATIONS

None known.

WARNINGS

Tuberculin should not be administered to known tuberculin-positive reactors because of the severity of reactions (e.g., vesiculation, ulceration or necrosis) that may occur at the test site in very highly sensitive individuals.

Avoid injecting tuberculin subcutaneously. If this occurs, no local reaction develops, but a general febrile reaction and/or acute inflammation around old tuberculous lesions may occur in highly sensitive individuals.

PRECAUTIONS

General

A separate heat sterilized syringe and needle, or a sterile disposable unit, should be used for each individual patient to prevent possible transmission of homologous serum hepatitis virus and other infectious agents from one person to another.

Syringes that have previously been used with histoplasmin, blastomycin and other antigens should not be used for tuberculin.

As with any biological product, epinephrine should be immediately available in case an anaphylactoid or acute hypersensitivity reaction occurs.

Pregnancy

Teratogenic effects: Pregnancy Category C. Animal reproduction studies have not been conducted with Aplisol. It is also not known whether Aplisol can cause fetal harm when administered to a pregnant woman or can affect the reproduction capacity. Aplisol should be given to a pregnant woman only if clearly needed.

However, the risk of unrecognized tuberculosis and the close postpartum contact between a mother with active disease and an infant leaves the infant in grave danger of tuberculosis and complications such as tuberculous meningitis. Although there have been not been reported any adverse effects upon the fetus recognized as being due to tuberculosis skin testing, the prescribing physician will want to consider if the potential benefits outweigh the possible risks for performing the tuberculin test on a pregnant woman or woman of childbearing age, particularly in certain high risk populations.

ADVERSE REACTIONS

In highly sensitive individuals, strongly positive reactions including vesiculation, ulceration or necrosis may occur at the test site. Cold packs or topical steroid preparations may be employed for symptomatic relief of the associated pain, pruritus, and discomfort.

Strongly positive test reactions may result in scarring at the test site.

DOSAGE AND ADMINISTRATION

Standard Method (Mantoux Test)

The Mantoux test is performed by intradermally injecting with a syringe and needle exactly 0.1 ml of tuberculin PPD, diluted. The result is read 48 to 72 hours later and induration only is considered in interpreting the test. The standard test is performed as follows:

1. The site of the test is usually the flexor or dorsal surface of the forearm about 4″ below the elbow. Other skin sites may be used, but the flexor surface of the forearm is preferred.
2. The skin at the injection site is cleansed with 70% alcohol and allowed to dry.
3. The test material is administered with a tuberculin syringe (0.5 or 1.0 ml) fitted with a short (½″) 26 or 27 gauge needle.
4. The syringe and needle should be of a sterile disposable, single use type or should have been sterilized by autoclaving, boiling or by the use of dry heat. A separate sterile unit should be used for each person tested.
5. The diaphragm of the vial-stopper should be wiped with 70% alcohol.
6. The needle is inserted through the stopper diaphragm of the inverted vial. Exactly 0.1 ml is filled into the syringe, with care being taken to exclude air bubbles and to maintain the lumen of the needle filled.
7. The point of the needle is inserted into the most superficial layers of the skin with the needle bevel pointing upward. As the tuberculin solution is injected, a pale bleb 6 to 10 mm in size (⅜″) will rise over the point of the needle. This is quickly absorbed and no dressing is required.

In the event the injection is delivered subcutaneously (ie, no bleb will form), or if a significant part of the dose leaks from the injection site, the test should be repeated immediately at another site at least 5 cm (2″) removed.

Aplisol vials should be inspected visually for particulate matter and discoloration prior to administration.

The Mantoux test is the standard of comparison for all other tuberculin tests.

Aplisol is a stabilized solution of Tuberculin PPD. Data indicate that Aplisol is stable when prefilled into syringes and stored in a refrigerator for up to 30 days.

However, the practice of storing such prefilled syringes is not recommended as good practice because of the increased potential for contamination.

Interpretation of Tuberculin Reaction

Readings of Mantoux reactions should be made during the period from 48 to 72 hours after the injection. Induration only should be considered in interpreting the test. The diameter of induration should be measured transversely to the long axis of the forearm and recorded in millimeters. Erythema of less than 10 mm should be disregarded. If the area of erythema is greater than 10 mm and induration is absent the injection may have been made too deeply and retesting is indicated.

Reactions should be interpreted as follows:

Positive—Induration measuring 10 mm or more. This indicates hypersensitivity to tuberculoprotein and should be interpreted as positive for past or present infection with *M. tuberculosis.*

Doubtful—Induration measuring 5 to 9 mm. Retesting is indicated using a different site of injection. Evaluation to rule out cross-reaction from other mycobacterial infection should be considered.

Negative—Induration of less than 5 mm. This indicates a lack of hypersensitivity to tuberculoprotein and tuberculous infection is highly unlikely.

It should be noted that reactivity to tuberculin may be depressed or suppressed for as long as four weeks by viral infections, live virus vaccines (i.e., measles, smallpox, polio, rubella and mumps), or by the administration of corticosteroids. Malnutrition may also have a similar effect. When of diagnostic importance, a negative test should be accepted as proof that hypersensitivity is absent only after normal reactivity to nonspecific irritants has been demonstrated. A primary injection of tuberculin may possibly have a boosting effect on subsequent tuberculin reactions.

A child who is known to have been exposed to a tuberculous adult must not be adjudged free of infection until he has a negative tuberculin reaction at least ten weeks after contact with the tuberculous person has ceased.[4]

A positive tuberculin reaction does not necessarily signify the presence of active disease. Further diagnostic procedures should be carried out before a diagnosis of tuberculosis is made. A small percentage of responders may not have been infected with *M. tuberculosis* but by some other mycobacterium.

HOW SUPPLIED

N 0071-4525-03 (Bio. 1525)

1 ml (10 tests)—rubber-diaphragm-capped vial

N 0071-4525-08 (Bio. 1607)

5 ml (50 tests)—rubber-diaphragm-capped vial

This product should be stored at 2° to 8°C (36° to 46°F), and protected from light.

REFERENCES

1. Seibert, F.B.: Am. Rev. Tuberc. 30:713, 1934.
2. Seibert, F.B., and Glenn, J.T.: Am. Rev. Tuberc. 44:9, 1941.
3. Diagnostic Standards and Classification of Tuberculosis and Other Mycobacterial Diseases, American Lung Association, New York, 1974.
4. Sewell, E.M., O'Hare, D., and Kendig, E.L., Jr.: The Tuberculin Test, Pediatrics, Vol. 54, No. 5, Nov. 1974.

* PPD-S (No. 49608) World Health Organization International PPD-Tuberculin Standard (PPD-S is a dried powder from which WHO and U.S. Standard tuberculin solutions are made.)

** U.S. Tuberculin Unit

4525G032

APLITEST® ℞

[ă′plĭ-tĕst″]

Tuberculin Purified Protein Derivative
Multiple-Puncture Device

DESCRIPTION

Aplitest (tuberculin PPD) is a sterile, single-use, multiple-puncture type device for percutaneous administration for use in determining the tuberculin sensitivity status of individuals. Aplitest, a diagnostic aid, has been clinically compared with 5 US Tuberculin Units of PPD-S administered intradermally.

These disposable devices are useful in mass tuberculosis screening programs. The product packaging facilitates the use of Aplitest units for testing of individual patients in office, ward, or clinic settings.

Each Aplitest unit consists of a cylindrical plastic holder bearing four equally spaced stainless steel tines at one end. The tines have been coated by dipping in a solution of tuberculin PPD and dried. The tuberculin solution applied to the tines is buffered with potassium and sodium phosphates and contains approximately 0.5% phenol as a preservative. The narrow (tine-bearing) end of each unit fits into a protective cap to protect the tines and maintain their sterility.

The purified tuberculin protein fraction is isolated from culture filtrates of human-type strains of *Mycobacterium tuberculosis* by the method of F.B. Seibert.[1,2] Purified tuberculin protein solution is prepared from a single master lot (No. 975302) to eliminate lot to lot variation.

CLINICAL PHARMACOLOGY

Tuberculin deposited in the skin of tuberculin-reactive individuals reacts with sensitized lymphocytes to effect the release of mediators of cellular hypersensitivity. Some of these mediators, eg, skin reactive factor, induce an inflammatory response to the skin, causing the induration characteristic of a "positive" or "significant" reaction.

Aplitest has been standardized by clinical studies in human subjects against 5 TU* of PPD-S administered intradermally by the Mantoux test, and guidelines relating response to the two treatments have been formulated. (See "Interpretation of Response" section.)

INDICATIONS AND USAGE

Aplitest is indicated to detect tuberculin-sensitive individuals. Aplitest units are also useful in programs to establish priorities for additional testing (ie, chest x-rays) and in epidemiological surveys to identify areas with high levels of infection.

All multiple-puncture type devices should be regarded as screening tools, and appropriate diagnostic procedures (eg, Mantoux test with tuberculin PPD diluted, Aplisol®) should be employed for retesting "doubtful" reactors.

Regular periodic (annual or biennial)[3] testing of tuberculin-negative persons is recommended and is especially valuable because the conversion of an individual from negative to positive is highly indicative of recent tuberculosis infection. Repeated testing of the uninfected individual does not sensitize to tuberculin. In persons with waning sensitivity to homologous or heterologous mycobacterial antigens, however, the stimulus of a tuberculin test may "boost" or increase the size of reaction to a second test, even causing an apparent development of sensitivity in some instances.

CONTRAINDICATIONS

None known.

WARNINGS

Tuberculin should not be administered to known tuberculin-positive reactors because of the severity of reactions (eg, vesiculation, ulceration or necrosis) that may occur at the test site in very highly sensitive individuals.

As with any biological product, epinephrine should be immediately available in case an anaphylactoid or acute hypersensitivity reaction occurs.

PRECAUTIONS

General: A separate, sterile unit must be used for each individual patient and disposed of after use.

Sensitivity may decrease or disappear temporarily during or immediately following severe febrile illness, measles, and other exanthemas, live virus vaccination, sarcoidosis, overwhelming miliary or pulmonary tuberculosis, and the administration of corticosteroids or immunosuppressive drugs. Severe malnutrition may also have a similar effect.

A positive tuberculin reaction does not necessarily signify the presence of active disease. Further diagnostic procedures should be carried out before a diagnosis of tuberculosis is made.

Simultaneous application of two or more multiple-puncture devices is not recommended. The response of an individual to a single multiple-puncture device may be altered by the simultaneous administration of additional tuberculin tests (multiple-puncture or Mantoux).[4]

Pregnancy: Teratogenic effects: Pregnancy Category C. Animal reproduction studies have not been conducted with Aplitest. It is also not known whether Aplitest can

cause fetal harm when administered to a pregnant woman or can affect reproduction capacity. Aplitest should be given to a pregnant woman only if clearly needed.
However, the risk of unrecognized tuberculosis and the close postpartum contact between a mother with active disease and an infant leaves the infant in grave danger of tuberculosis and complications such as tuberculous meningitis. Although there have not been reported any adverse effects upon the fetus recognized as being due to tuberculosis skin testing, the prescribing physician will want to consider if the potential benefits outweigh the possible risks for performing the tuberculin test on a pregnant woman or a woman of childbearing age, particularly in certain high risk populations.

ADVERSE REACTIONS

In highly sensitive individuals, strongly positive reactions, including vesiculation, ulceration or necrosis, may occur at the test site. Cold packs or topical steroid preparations may be employed for symptomatic relief of the associated pain, pruritus and discomfort.
Strongly positive test reactions may result in scarring at the test site.
Minimal bleeding may be experienced at a puncture site. This occurs infrequently and does not affect the interpretation of the test.

DOSAGE AND ADMINISTRATION

Each Aplitest unit provides for the intradermal administration of one test-dose of tuberculin PPD.

Method of Application

1. The preferred site of the test is the flexor surface of the forearm about 4 inches below the elbow. Other suitable skin sites, such as the dorsal surface of the forearm, may be used. Areas without adequate subcutaneous tissue, such as over a tendon, should be avoided.
2. The skin at the test site should be cleaned with 70% alcohol, or other suitable agent, and allowed to dry thoroughly.
3. To expose the four impregnated tines, grasp the device and twist to break the perforated label seal.
4. Grasp the patient's forearm firmly to stretch the skin taut at the test site and to prevent any jerking motion of the arm that could cause scratching with the tines.
5. Apply the Aplitest unit firmly and without twisting to the test area for approximately one second. Sufficient pressure should be exerted to assure that all four tines have penetrated the skin of the test area.
6. Dispose of used units in a manner to avoid accidents. Do not reuse.

Interpretation of Response

Selection of the appropriate criteria for interpretation of response to the tuberculin PPD Aplitest should be made in accordance with the objectives of the specific testing program and with consideration of the history and clinical status of the individuals.
Reading of reactions should be made during the period from 48 to 72 hours after application of Aplitest and should be conducted under good lighting conditions. Induration only should be considered in interpreting the test. Erythema should be disregarded. The diameter of the induration of the greatest response at any of the four puncture points should be determined by visual inspection and palpation. If there is coalescence of reaction, the largest diameter of coalescent induration should be measured and recorded.
The American Thoracic Society recommends that all multiple-puncture tuberculin skin test devices be interpreted as follows: If vesiculation is present, the test may be interpreted as positive. If vesiculation is not present, induration of 2 mm or more is considered as a doubtful reaction and a Mantoux test for diagnostic evaluation should be given. Decisions concerning management should be based on the reaction to the Mantoux test and relevant diagnostic criteria. Induration of less than 2 mm and/or erythema of any size is a negative test and there is no need for retesting.[5]
In clinical studies with Aplitest, it has been determined that coalescence of the induration around two or more puncture sites corresponds more than 90% of the time to 10 mm or more of induration in the same individual tested by Mantoux test at the 5 TU level with PPD-S.†
Thus, the following criteria of interpretation have been established.

1. Vesiculation—Positive Reaction

The test should be interpreted as positive and the management of the subject is the same as that for one classified as positive by Mantoux test.

2. Coalescence of induration from two or more puncture points—Doubtful Reaction

A subject with a coalescent reaction may be considered for Mantoux retest. However, more than 90% of the time this reaction was equivalent to a reaction of 10 mm or more of induration with PPD-S (5 TU) administered by Mantoux test.[6] Other criteria, such as contact with tuberculosis patients and case history, should be considered to determine the likelihood that such a reaction is considered positive.

3. 2 mm or more of induration without coalescence—Doubtful Reaction

Reactions of this size range reflect sensitivity that can result from infection with either atypical mycobacteria or *M tuberculosis;* hence, they are classified as doubtful.
A standard Mantoux test should be done on all subjects in this group. Management should be based on the reaction to the Mantoux test, as well as other clinical considerations.

4. Less than 2 mm of induration—Negative Reaction

There is no need for retesting unless the individual is in contact with a case of tuberculosis or there is clinical evidence suggestive of the disease.

HOW SUPPLIED

N 0071-4589-13 (Bio. 1590) 25-test package. Twenty-five individually capped Aplitest units in a dispensing package.
Aplitest (tuberculin PPD, multiple-puncture device) units should be stored at no warmer than 30°C (86°F).

REFERENCES

1. Seibert, F.B.: Am. Rev. Tuberc. 30:713, 1934.
2. Seibert, F.B., and Glenn J.T.: Am. Rev. Tuberc. 44:9, 1941.
3. Report of the Committee on Infectious Diseases, American Academy of Pediatrics, 1982.
4. Rosenthal, S.R., and Libby, J.E.P.: Bull. Wld. Hlth. Org. 23:689, 1960.
5. Diagnostic Standards and Classification of Tuberculosis and Other Mycobacterial Diseases, American Lung Association, 1974.
6. Unpublished data from Warner-Lambert Co. available upon request.

* U.S. (International) tuberculin units.
† Purified Protein Derivative (Seibert). Lot No. 49608, the standard adopted by the World Health Organization in 1952 as International PPD Tuberculin and used to prepare the official U.S. Public Health Service 5 TU solution of tuberculin for skin testing known as PPD-S.

4589G022

Roche Laboratories

Division of Hoffmann-La Roche Inc.
NUTLEY, NJ 07110

TENSILON®

℞

[*ten 'sill-on*]
(edrophonium chloride/Roche)
Injectable Solution
ampuls • vials

The following text is complete prescribing information based on official labeling in effect June 1, 1986.

DESCRIPTION

Tensilon is a short and rapid-acting cholinergic drug. Chemically, edrophonium chloride is ethyl(*m*-hydroxyphenyl)-dimethylammonium chloride.
10-ml vials: Each ml contains, in a sterile solution, 10 mg edrophonium chloride/Roche compounded with 0.45% phenol and 0.2% sodium sulfite as preservatives, buffered with sodium citrate and citric acid, and pH adjusted to approximately 5.4.
1-ml ampuls: Each ml contains, in a sterile solution, 10 mg edrophonium chloride/Roche compounded with 0.2% sodium sulfite, buffered with sodium citrate and citric acid, and pH adjusted to approximately 5.4.

ACTIONS

Tensilon is an anticholinesterase drug. Its pharmacological action is due primarily to the inhibition or inactivation of acetylcholinesterase at sites of cholinergic transmission. Its effect is manifest within 30 to 60 seconds after injection and lasts an average of 10 minutes.

INDICATIONS

Tensilon is recommended for the differential diagnosis of myasthenia gravis and as an adjunct in the evaluation of treatment requirements in this disease. It may also be used for evaluating emergency treatment in myasthenic crises. Because of its brief duration of action, it is not recommended for maintenance therapy in myasthenia gravis.
Tensilon is also useful whenever a curare antagonist is needed to reverse the neuromuscular block produced by curare, tubocurarine, gallamine triethiodide or dimethyl-tubocurarine. It is *not* effective against decamethonium bromide and succinylcholine chloride. It may be used adjunctively in the treatment of respiratory depression caused by curare overdosage.

CONTRAINDICATIONS

Known hypersensitivity to anticholinesterase agents; intestinal and urinary obstructions of mechanical type.

WARNINGS

Whenever anticholinesterase drugs are used for testing, a syringe containing 1 mg of atropine sulfate should be immediately available to be given in aliquots intravenously to counteract severe cholinergic reactions which may occur in the hypersensitive individual, whether he is normal or myasthenic. Tensilon should be used with caution in patients with bronchial asthma or cardiac dysrhythmias. The transient bradycardia which sometimes occurs can be relieved by atropine sulfate. Isolated instances of cardiac and respiratory arrest following administration of Tensilon have been reported. It is postulated that these are vagotonic effects.
Usage in Pregnancy: The safety of Tensilon during pregnancy or lactation in humans has not been established. Therefore, use of Tensilon in women who may become pregnant requires weighing the drug's potential benefits against its possible hazards to mother and child.

PRECAUTIONS

Patients may develop "anticholinesterase insensitivity" for brief or prolonged periods. During these periods the patients should be carefully monitored and may need respiratory assistance. Dosages of anticholinesterase drugs should be reduced or withheld until patients again become sensitive to them.

ADVERSE REACTIONS

Careful observation should be made for severe cholinergic reactions in the hyperreactive individual. The myasthenic patient in crisis who is being tested with Tensilon should be observed for bradycardia or cardiac standstill and cholinergic reactions if an overdose is given. The following reactions common to anticholinesterase agents may occur, although not all of these reactions have been reported with the administration of Tensilon, probably because of its short duration of action and limited indications: **Eye:** Increased lacrimation, pupillary constriction, spasm of accommodation, diplopia, conjunctival hyperemia. **CNS:** Convulsions, dysarthria, dysphonia, dysphagia. **Respiratory:** Increased tracheobronchial secretions, laryngospasm, bronchiolar constriction, paralysis of muscles of respiration, central respiratory paralysis. **Cardiac:** Arrhythmias (especially bradycardia), fall in cardiac output leading to hypotension. **G.I.:** Increased salivary, gastric and intestinal secretion, nausea, vomiting, increased peristalsis, diarrhea, abdominal cramps. **Skeletal Muscle:** Weakness, fasciculations. **Miscellaneous:** Increased urinary frequency and incontinence, diaphoresis.

DOSAGE AND ADMINISTRATION

Tensilon Test in the Differential Diagnosis of Myasthenia Gravis:[1-8]
Intravenous Dosage (Adults): A tuberculin syringe containing 1 ml (10 mg) of Tensilon is prepared with an intravenous needle, and 0.2 ml (2 mg) is injected intravenously within 15 to 30 seconds. The needle is left *in situ. Only* if no reaction occurs after 45 seconds is the remaining 0.8 ml (8 mg) injected. If a cholinergic reaction (muscarinic side effects, skeletal muscle fasciculations and increased muscle weakness) occurs after injection of 0.2 ml (2 mg), the test is discontinued and atropine sulfate 0.4 mg to 0.5 mg is administered intravenously. After one-half hour the test may be repeated.
Intramuscular Dosage (Adults): In adults with inaccessible veins, dosage for intramuscular injection is 1 ml (10 mg) of Tensilon. Subjects who demonstrate hyperreactivity to this injection (cholinergic reaction), should be retested after one-half hour with 0.2 ml (2 mg) of Tensilon intramuscularly to rule out false-negative reactions.
Dosage (Children): The intravenous testing dose of Tensilon in children weighing up to 75 lbs is 0.1 ml (1 mg); above this weight, the dose is 0.2 ml (2 mg). If there is no response after 45 seconds, it may be titrated up to 0.5 ml (5 mg) in children under 75 lbs, given in increments of 0.1 ml (1 mg) every 30 to 45 seconds and up to 1 ml (10 mg) in heavier children. In infants, the recommended dose is 0.05 ml (0.5 mg). Because of technical difficulty with intravenous injection in children, the intramuscular route may be used. In children weighing up to 75 lbs, 0.2 ml (2 mg) is injected intramuscularly. In children weighing more than 75 lbs, 0.5 ml (5 mg) is injected intramuscularly. All signs which would appear with the intravenous test appear with the intramuscular test except that there is a delay of two to ten minutes before a reaction is noted.
Tensilon Test for Evaluation of Treatment Requirements in Myasthenia Gravis: The recommended dose is 0.1 ml to 0.2 ml (1 mg to 2 mg) of Tensilon, administered intravenously one hour after oral intake of the drug being used in treatment.[1-5] Response will be myasthenic in the undertreated patient, adequate in the controlled patient, and cholinergic in the overtreated patient. Responses to Tensilon in myasthenic and nonmyasthenic individuals are summarized in the accompanying chart.[2]
[See table on next page].
Tensilon Test in Crisis: The term *crisis* is applied to the myasthenic whenever severe respiratory distress with objective ventilatory inadequacy occurs and the response to medication is not predictable. This state may be secondary to a sudden increase in severity of myasthenia gravis (myasthenic crisis), or to overtreatment with anticholinesterase drugs (cholinergic crisis).

Continued on next page

Roche—Cont.

When a patient is apneic, controlled ventilation must be secured immediately in order to avoid cardiac arrest and irreversible central nervous system damage. No attempt is made to test with Tensilon until respiratory exchange is adequate. *Dosage used at this time is most important:* If the patient is cholinergic, Tensilon will cause increased oropharyngeal secretions and further weakness in the muscles of respiration. If the crisis is myasthenic, the test clearly improves respiration and the patient can be treated with longer-acting intravenous anticholinesterase medication. When the test is performed, there should not be more than 0.2 ml (2 mg) Tensilon in the syringe. An intravenous dose of 0.1 ml (1 mg) is given initially. The patient's heart action is carefully observed. If, after an interval of one minute, this dose does not further impair the patient, the remaining 0.1 ml (1 mg) can be injected. If no clear improvement of respiration occurs after 0.2 ml (2 mg) dose, it is usually wisest to discontinue all anticholinesterase drug therapy and secure controlled ventilation by tracheostomy with assisted respiration.[5]

For Use as a Curare Antagonist: Tensilon should be administered by intravenous injection in 1 ml (10 mg) doses given slowly over a period of 30 to 45 seconds so that the onset of cholinergic reaction can be detected. This dosage may be repeated whenever necessary. The maximal dose for any one patient should be 4 ml (40 mg). Because of its brief effect, Tensilon should not be given prior to the administration of curare, tubocurarine, gallamine triethiodide or dimethyltubocurarine; it should be used at the time when its effect is needed. When given to counteract curare overdosage, the effect of each dose on the respiration should be carefully observed before it is repeated, and assisted ventilation should always be employed.

DRUG INTERACTIONS

Care should be given when administering this drug to patients with symptoms of myasthenic weakness who are also on anticholinesterase drugs. Since symptoms of anticholinesterase overdose (cholinergic crisis) may mimic underdosage (myasthenic weakness), their condition may be worsened by the use of this drug. (See OVERDOSAGE section for treatment.)

OVERDOSAGE

With drugs of this type, muscarine-like symptoms (nausea, vomiting, diarrhea, sweating, increased bronchial and salivary secretions and bradycardia) often appear with overdosage (cholinergic crisis). An important complication that can arise is obstruction of the airway by bronchial secretions. These may be managed with suction (especially if tracheostomy has been performed) and by the use of atropine. Many experts have advocated a wide range of dosages of atropine *(for Tensilon, see atropine dosage below),* but if there are copious secretions, up to 1.2 mg intravenously may be given initially and repeated every 20 minutes until secretions are controlled. Signs of atropine overdosage such as dry mouth, flush and tachycardia should be avoided as tenacious secretions and bronchial plugs may form. A total dose of atropine of 5 to 10 mg or even more may be required. The following steps should be taken in the management of overdosage of Tensilon:

1. Adequate respiratory exchange should be maintained by assuring an open airway, and the use of assisted respiration augmented by oxygen.
2. Cardiac function should be monitored until complete stabilization has been achieved.
3. Atropine sulfate in doses of 0.4 to 0.5 mg should be administered intravenously. This may be repeated every 3 to 10 minutes. Because of the short duration of action of Tensilon the total dose required will seldom exceed 2 mg.
4. Pralidoxime chloride (a cholinesterase reactivator) may be given intravenously at the rate of 50 to 100 mg per minute; usually the total dose does not exceed 1000 mg. Extreme caution should be exercised in the use of pralidoxime chloride when the cholinergic symptoms are induced by double-bond phosphorous anticholinesterase drugs.[9]
5. If convulsions or shock is present, appropriate measures should be instituted.

HOW SUPPLIED

Multiple Dose Vials, 10 ml, boxes of 10. *Ampuls,* 1 ml, boxes of 10.

REFERENCES

1. Osserman, K.E. and Kaplan, L.I., *J.A.M.A., 150:* 265, 1952.
2. Osserman, K.E., Kaplan, L.I. and Besson, G., *J. Mt. Sinai Hosp., 20:* 165, 1953.
3. Osserman, K.E. and Kaplan, L.I., *Arch. Neurol. & Psychiat., 70:* 385, 1953.
4. Osserman, K.E. and Teng, P., *J.A.M.A., 160:* 153, 1956.
5. Osserman, K.E. and Genkins, G., *Ann. N.Y. Acad. Sci., 135:* 312, 1966.
6. Tether, J.E., Second International Symposium Proceedings, Myasthenia Gravis, 1961, p. 444.
7. Tether, J.E., in H.F. Conn: *Current Therapy 1960,* Philadelphia, W. B. Saunders Company, p. 551.
8. Tether, J.E., in H.F. Conn: *Current Therapy 1965,* Philadelphia, W. B. Saunders Company, p. 556.
9. Grob, D. and Johns, R.J., *J.A.M.A., 166:* 1855, 1958.

Responses to Tensilon in Myasthenic and Nonmyasthenic Individuals

	Myasthenic*	Adequate†	Cholinergic‡
Muscle Strength (ptosis, diplopia, dysphonia, dysphagia, dysarthria, respiration, limb strength)	Increased	No change	Decreased
Fasciculations (orbicularis oculi, facial muscles, limb muscles)	Absent	Present or absent	Present or absent
Side reactions (lacrimation, diaphoresis, salivation, abdominal cramps, nausea, vomiting, diarrhea)	Absent	Minimal	Severe

* Myasthenic Response—occurs in untreated myasthenics and may serve to establish diagnosis; in patients under treatment, indicates that therapy is inadequate.

† Adequate Response—observed in treated patients when therapy is stabilized; a typical response in normal individuals. In addition to this response in nonmyasthenics, the phenomenon of forced lid closure is often observed in psychoneurotics.[1]

‡ Cholinergic Response—seen in myasthenics who have been overtreated with anticholinesterase drugs.

Sclavo Inc.

5 MANSARD COURT
WAYNE, NJ 07470

SclavoTest®–PPD ℞

Tuberculin Purified Protein Derivative (PPD)
Multiple Puncture Device

COMPOSITION/DESCRIPTION

SclavoTest-PPD is a sterile multiple-puncture device containing a tuberculin PPD used for the identification of individuals who have a delayed hypersensitivity to tuberculin. SclavoTest-PPD is an easy-to-use, self-contained, unit-dose disposable system which minimizes waste and can be stored at room temperature. No needles, syringes, or vials are needed.

The SclavoTest-PPD device is composed of a plastic handle with four sharp stainless steel points to which has been affixed and dried a tuberculin PPD solution. The retracted points are projected, after the device is placed upon the skin, by gentle pressure applied through a spring inside the handle. SclavoTest-PPD is stored at room temperature until the moment of use in a hermetically sealed unit-dose blister pack, which is designed to impede the passage of moisture and maintain sterility.

ADVERSE REACTIONS

Vesiculation, occasionally necrosis, ulceration.

HOW SUPPLIED

20 or 250 units individually blister-sealed in strips of 1.

Products are cross-indexed
by product classifications
in the
BLUE SECTION

SmithKline Diagnostics, Inc.

A SmithKline Beckman Company
POST OFFICE BOX 61947
SUNNYVALE, CA 94086

GASTROCCULT®

[gas 'trō-cult]
Test for Gastric Occult Blood and pH

To meet the need for a reliable test for detecting occult blood in gastric samples (both aspirates and vomitus), SKD has developed Gastroccult®, the only test specifically designed for this purpose.

The test is as easy to run as Hemoccult®, but is not affected by the low pH frequently encountered in gastric samples. Also, it is not affected by oral cimetidine (Tagamet®). Further, it also features a convenient test for pH right on the slide.

Gastroccult® slides are available from leading distributors in economical boxes of 40 slides, SKD product number 66000.

HEMOCCULT®

[hē 'mō-cult]

INTENDED USES

The Hemoccult® test is a rapid, convenient, and virtually odorless method for detecting the presence of fecal occult blood, as an aid to diagnosis of various gastrointestinal conditions:

- during routine physical examinations
- in newly admitted hospital patients
- in postoperative patients
- in newborn infants
- in screening programs for colorectal cancer

Because Hemoccult® tests require only a small stool specimen, offensive odors are minimized and storage or transport of large stool specimens is unnecessary.

Hemoccult® Single Slides are convenient for use when single stool specimens are to be tested.

Hemoccult II® Slides, in cards of three tests, are designed so your patient can collect serial specimens at home over the course of three bowel movements. After the patient collects the specimens, the Hemoccult II® test may be returned to a laboratory, a hospital, or a medical office for developing and evaluation. Serial fecal specimen analysis is recommended when screening asymptomatic patients.[1]

Hemoccult® Tape is designed to complement Hemoccult® slides and is best suited for "on-the-spot" testing for occult blood during rectal or sigmoidoscopic examinations.

The Hemoccult® test and other unmodified guaiac tests are not recommended for use with gastric specimens.[2]

SUMMARY AND EXPLANATION OF THE TEST

The Hemoccult® test is a simplified, standardized variation of the guaiac test for occult blood. It contains specially treated guaiac paper and is ready for use without additional preparation.

When a small stool specimen containing occult blood is applied to Hemoccult® test paper, the hemoglobin comes in contact with the guaiac. Application of Hemoccult® Developer (a stabilized hydrogen peroxide solution) creates a guaiac/peroxidase-like reaction which turn the test paper blue within 60 seconds if occult blood is present. The test reacts with hemoglobin released from lysed cells. When blood is present, hemolysis is promoted by substances in the stool, primarily water and salts. As with any occult blood test, results with the Hemoccult® test cannot be considered conclusive evidence of the presence or absence of gastrointestinal bleeding or pathology. Hemoccult® tests are designed for preliminary screening as a diagnostic aid and are not intended to replace other diagnostic procedures such as proctosigmoidoscopic examination, barium enema, or other x-ray studies. (See LIMITATIONS OF PROCEDURE).

REAGENTS

High-quality filter paper treated with natural guaiac resin.
A developing solution containing a stabilized dilute mixture of hydrogen peroxide (less than 6%) and 75% denatured ethyl alcohol in aqueous solution.

PERFORMANCE MONITORS®

The function and stability of the slides and Developer can be tested using the on-slide Performance Monitors®. Both a positive and negative Performance Monitor® are located under the flap and below the specimen windows on the back of the Hemoccult II® and Hemoccult® single slides.

The positive Performance Monitor® contains a hemoglobin-derived catalyst which, upon application of Developer, will turn blue within 10 seconds.

The negative Performance Monitor® contains no such catalyst and should not turn blue upon application of Developer.

The Performance Monitors® provide additional assurance that the guaiac-treated paper and Developer are functional.

In the unlikely event that the Performance Monitors® do not react as expected after application of Developer, the test results should be regarded as invalid. The Product Support Department at SmithKline Diagnostics will provide further assistance should this occur.

PRECAUTIONS

Slides and Tape

For *In Vitro* Diagnostic Use. Do not use after expiration date which appears on each Slide or Tape Dispenser.

Prolonged exposure to some air pollutants and light may cause slides to turn blue. This does not affect the performance of the test and results can be read in the usual manner.

Developer

Hemoccult® Developer should be protected from heat and the bottle kept tightly capped when not in use. It is flammable and subject to evaporation.

Hemoccult® Developer is an irritant. Avoid contact with the skin.

Do Not Use in Eyes. Should such contact occur, solution should be rinsed out promptly with water.

Do not use after expiration date on bottle.

STORAGE AND STABILITY

Do not refrigerate. Store at controlled room temperature 15°–30°C (59°–86°F) in original packaging. Protect from heat. Do not store with volatile chemicals (eg. iodine, chlorine, bromine or ammonia). The Hemoccult® test, stored as recommended, will maintain its sensitivity until the expiration date on the slide. The expiration date appears on each slide and tape dispenser.

Hemoccult® Developer, stored as recommended, will remain stable until the expiration date on the bottle. The expiration date appears on each bottle.

SPECIMEN COLLECTION

Only a very small stool sample, about the size of a matchhead, thinly applied is necessary in preparing either slide or tape. When specimen is to be collected from toilet bowl, the patient should flush the toilet before defecating. The slides may be prepared and developed immediately or prepared and stored for up to 12 days.[3]

Patients with bleeding from other conditions which may affect test results (e.g., hemorrhoids, menstrual bleeding, hematuria) are not appropriate test subjects while such bleeding is active.

Since bleeding from gastrointestinal lesions may be intermittent, it is recommended that stool smears for testing be collected from three consecutive bowel movements. To increase the probability of detecting occult blood, Greegor recommends that samples be taken from two different sections of each stool.[4,5]

PATIENT PREPARATION

Whenever practicable, patients should be placed on a meat-free, high residue diet[4,5] starting two days before and continuing through the test period. Such a diet may increase the accuracy of the test and at the same time provide roughage to help uncover "silent" lesions which may bleed only intermittently.

An alternative procedure is to omit the special diet initially. Then if a patient has one or more positive tests in the initial three-slide series, he should be placed on the special diet and retested for three days.[6]

INTERFERING SUBSTANCES

Some oral medications (e.g. aspirin, indomethacin, phenylbutazone, corticosteroids, reserpine, etc.) can cause g.i. irritation and occult bleeding in some patients.[7,8]

These substances should be discontinued two days prior to and during testing.

Ascorbic acid (Vitamin C) in excess of 250 mg/day may cause false-negative results[9] and should also be eliminated before testing.

Therapeutic dosages of iron can yield false-positive fecal occult blood test reactions. Use of iron preparations should be suspended before and during testing for fecal occult blood.[10]

SATISFACTORY LIMITS OF PERFORMANCE; EXPECTED RESULTS

Results with the Hemoccult® test are visually determined. The Hemoccult® guaiac test paper should be observed for color change within 60 seconds after Developer has been applied. This reading time is important, because the color reaction may fade after two to four minutes.

If any trace of blue on or at the edge of the smear is seen, the test is positive for occult blood.

NOTE

Because this test is visually read and requires color differentiation, it should not be read by the visually impaired.

The function and stability of the Hemoccult® slides and Developer can be tested using the on-slide Performance Monitors®. The Hemoccult® Tape may be tested by applying a drop of diluted whole blood (1:5,000 in distilled water) to an unused portion of the tape. Add Developer to opposite side. If any blue appears, the specially treated guaiac paper and Developer are functional.

LIMITATIONS OF PROCEDURE

As with any occult blood test, results with the Hemoccult® test cannot be considered conclusive evidence of the presence or absence of gastrointestinal bleeding or pathology. Hemoccult® tests are designed for preliminary screening as an aid to diagnosis and are not intended to replace other diagnostic procedures such as proctosigmoidoscopic examination, barium enema, or other x-ray studies. Hemoccult® tests are designed to detect fecal blood which normally contains enough water and salts to hemolyze the blood cells so that they will release hemoglobin.

Hemoccult®, as well as other fecal occult blood tests, should not be used to test gastric specimens.

Summary of the Hemoccult® test's performance based on reported experience to date:

1. The positive rate in screening situations has been approximately 3% to 5%.
2. False-positive rate in patients receiving adequate preparation has been between 1% and 2%.

A bibliography on the Hemoccult® test is available on request from the Product Support Department, SmithKline Diagnostics, Inc.

HEMOCCULT® TEST ORDERING INFORMATION

(Please order by product number)

Hemoccult® guaiac paper tests for fecal occult blood are available as follows:

Product	Product Number
HEMOCCULT II® DISPENSAPAK™ with on-slide Performance Monitors®	
• **100 Patients Kits** (300 Hemoccult II® slides) Each kit contains 3 Hemoccult II® slides and applicators in a dispensing envelope printed with diet and test instructions. Six 15 ml. bottles of Developer also included.	61100
HEMOCCULT II® Two-Specimen Units of Three with on-slide Performance Monitors®	
• **Boxes of 102** 34 units of 3 Hemoccult II® slides, two 15 ml. bottles of Developer and applicators	61200
• **Cartons of 1020** 10 boxes, each containing 34 units of 3 Hemoccult II® slides; twenty 15 ml. bottles of Developer and applicators	61300
HEMOCCULT® 2-Hole Single Slides with on-slide Performance Monitors®	
• **Boxes of 100** 100 single slides, two 15 ml. bottles of Developer and applicators	60151
• **Cartons of 1000** 10 boxes, each containing 100 single slides; twenty 15 ml. bottles of Developer and applicators	60152
HEMOCCULT® TAPE	
• **2 Tape Kits** Each kit contains one plastic tape dispenser with 100-test capacity and one 15 ml. bottle of Developer.	63202
HEMOCCULT® DEVELOPER	
• **Twenty 15 ml. bottles**	62115

References:

[1]Winawer, S.L. et al: "Screening for Colon Cancer," Gastroenterology 70:783 (May) 1976

[2]Layne, E.A., et al.: "Insensitivity of Guaiac Slide Tests for Detection of Blood in Gastric Juice," Annals of Int. Med. 94:774–776, 1981

[3]Data on file, SmithKline Diagnostics, Inc.

[4]Greegor, D.H.: "Detection of Silent Colon Cancer in Routine Examination," Ca 19:330, 1969

[5]Greegor, D.H.: "Occult Blood Testing for Detection of Asymptomatic Colon Cancer," Cancer 28:131, 1971

[6]Ross, T.H. and Johnson, J.C.M.: "Preliminary Report of a Cancer Screening Program by Physicians in Maricopa County (Ariz.) Arizona Med. 33:445 (June) 1976.

[7]Ostrow, J.D., Mulvaney, C.A., Hansell, J.R. and Rhodes, R.S.: "Sensitivity and Reproducibility of Chemical Tests for Fecal Occult Blood with an Emphasis on False-Positive Reactions," Am. J. Digest Dis. 18:930–40 (Nov.) 1973

[8]Grossman, M.I.; Matsumoto, K.K., and Lichter, R.J.: "Fecal Blood Loss Produced by Oral and Intravenous Administration of Various Salicylates," Gastroenterology 40:383–388 1961

[9]Jaffe, R.M. et al.: "False-Negative Stool Occult Blood Tests Caused by Ingestion of Ascorbic Acid (Vitamin C)," Ann. Int. Med. 83:824 (Dec.) 1975

[10]Lifton, L.J., Kreiser, J.: "False-Positive Stool Occult Blood Tests Caused by Iron Preparations," Gastroenterology 83:860–3 1982.

ISOCULT®

[ī'sō-cult]

The Isocult® Diagnostic Culturing System is a fast, accurate, cost-effective way to culture certain medically important organisms as an aid to diagnosis. Clinical studies show Isocult® results are equivalent or superior to standard laboratory procedures. All Isocult® tests are ready to use. Media are contained on the culture paddle (or in the bottom of the culture tube for the *T. vaginalis* test) and are specially formulated to encourage the growth of specific micro-organisms and, when necessary, to suppress or inhibit others. Media are usually modified to enhance the visibility of colonies or to increase the contrast between colonies and the surrounding medium.

A color-coded plastic collar identifies each Isocult® test. Patented tines in the collar streak the specimen along the medium to separate the organisms and isolate colonies when the paddle is inserted through the collar into the tube.

CO_2 generating tablets are supplied with some tests to supply an optimal growth environment.

The Isocult® prodecure includes three simple steps:

Inoculate Collect specimens, inoculate, and insert paddle into tube.

Incubate Incubate Isocult® culture test at 35–37° C for the time recommended in each test's product instructions.

Interpret Interpret results by comparing appearance of Isocult® culture test with color photographs on the Organism Identification Chart.

Isocult® culture tests are available for:

- Throat Streptococci
- Bacteriuria
- *Neisseria gonorrhoeae*
- Candida
- *N. gonorrhoeae* / Candida combination
- *Trichomonas vaginalis*
- *T. vaginalis* / Candida combination
- *Pseudomonas aeruginosa*
- *Staphylococcus aureus*

RAPIDTEST–STREP™

RapidTest-Strep™ is a latex slide agglutination test for detecting group A streptococcal antigen directly from pharyngeal swabs. This test depends on the reaction of the test latex reagent, composed of anti-group A streptococcal antibodies affixed to latex particles, and the bacterial extract, containing the group A streptococcal antigen. RapidTest-Strep™ offers better than 96% accuracy, provides results within seven minutes, and contains all necessary components (e.g., swabs, tubes and patient identification pad). RapidTest-Strep™ is easy to use and does not require special training or additional instrumentation. RapidTest-Strep™ is available from local distributors in two kit sizes: 25-test kit (Product No. 70025), and 100-test kit (Product No. 70100).

EDUCATIONAL MATERIAL

Patient Education Information and Poster Display

Questions & Answers about Colorectal Cancer/Fecal Occult Blood Testing

Reprint Folder

Selected Articles on Colorectal Cancer and Fecal Occult Blood Testing

Winthrop-Breon Laboratories
90 PARK AVENUE
NEW YORK, NY 10016

AMIPAQUE® ℞
brand of metrizamide
SECTION I. Intrathecal Use
SECTION II. Intravascular Use

DESCRIPTION

Metrizamide, 2-[3-Acetamido-2, 4, 6-triiodo-5-(*N*-methylacetamido) benzamido]-2- deoxy-D-glucopyranose, is a compound derived from metrizoic acid and glucosamine. It is a nonionic water-soluble contrast medium with a molecular weight of 789 (iodine content: 48.25%).

The viscosity in centipoise of the "use" concentration ranges from 2.9 at 170 mgI/mL to 12.7 at 300 mgI/mL at room temperature (20°C) and from 1.8 to 6.2 at body temperature (37°C) respectively. Osmolality in mosm/kg at 37°C ranges from 300 at 170 mgI/mL concentration to 484 at 300 mgI/mL. CSF is approximately 301. Specific gravity ranges from 1.184 at 170 mgI/mL to 1.329 at 300 mgI/mL. (CSF normal range is 1.005 to 1.009.) The pH of the solution reconstituted from the diluent is approximately 7.4.

AMIPAQUE is provided as a sterile, white lyophilized powder under vacuum. Each 2.5 g/20 mL vial contains 2.5 g metrizamide (1.21 g organically bound iodine) and 0.8 mg edetate calcium disodium. Each 3.75 g/20 mL vial contains 3.75 g metrizamide (1.81 g organically bound iodine) and 1.2 mg edetate calcium disodium. Each 6.75 g/50 mL vial contains 6.75 g metrizamide (3.26 g organically bound iodine) and 2.16 mg edetate calcium disodium.

Each 20 mL vial and 40 mL vial of sterile aqueous diluent contains 0.05 mg/mL sodium bicarbonate in water for injection. pH is adjusted with Carbon Dioxide, USP, if necessary.

AMIPAQUE solution and powder is sensitive to heat or light and, therefore, should be protected from exposure.

SECTION I

CLINICAL PHARMACOLOGY—Intrathecal

AMIPAQUE is absorbed from cerebrospinal fluid into the bloodstream in adults. Approximately 60 percent of the administered dose is excreted unchanged through the kidneys within 48 hours.

The initial concentration and volume of the medium, in conjunction with appropriate patient manipulation, will determine the extent of the diagnostic contrast that can be achieved. This can be monitored by fluoroscopy.

Following subarachnoid injection conventional radiography will continue to provide good diagnostic contrast for at least 30 minutes. At about 1 hour diagnostic degree of contrast will not usually be available. However, sufficient contrast for CT myelography will be available for several hours. CT myelography, following conventional myelography, should be deferred for at least 4 hours to reduce the degree of contrast.

In a multi-centered study, AMIPAQUE was used in 502 pediatric patients for a variety of procedures. The results and effects of the medium were similar to that in adults.

Following subarachnoid placement, irrespective of the position in which the patient is later maintained, slow upward diffusion of AMIPAQUE takes place through the CSF. After introduction into the lumbar subarachnoid space, without special positioning of the patient, computerized tomography (CT) shows CSF contrast enhancement in the thoracic region in about 1 hour, in the cervical region in about 2 hours, and in the basal cisterns in 3 to 4 hours.

When low doses (4 mL to 6 mL of 170 mgI/mL to 190 mgI/mL) of AMIPAQUE are introduced into the lumbar CSF and moved cephalad under gravity control and examined by CT scanning, they will provide immediate CSF contrast in the basal cisterns. Depending on the specific technique used, the lateral, third, and fourth ventricles may also be visualized. The contrast in this area will markedly diminish at 6 hours and disappear by 24 hours. CSF enhancement will be evident at the cortical sulci and interhemispheric fissures at 6 hours.

Between 12 and 24 hours the surfaces of the cerebrum and cerebellum, in contact with the subarachnoid spaces, will develop a "blush" effect on the scan which will normally disappear in 36 to 48 hours. The rate, time, extent of diffusion, and the disappearance or stasis of AMIPAQUE as demonstrated with CT scanning, can be used to detect or infer the presence of CNS or CSF circulation abnormalities.

[illegible]ATIONS AND USAGE—Intrathecal

[illegible]ted in adults and pediatric patients for [illegible]al, and total columnar myelography [illegible]ized tomography of the intracranial [illegible]ollowing spinal subarachnoid injec-[illegible]

[illegible]MIPAQUE is also indicated for cister[illegible]culography by direct injection using [illegible]echniques.

CONTRAINDICATIONS—Intrathecal

AMIPAQUE should not be administered to patients with a known hypersensitivity to metrizamide.

Intrathecal administration of corticosteroids with AMIPAQUE, brand of metrizamide, is contraindicated.

Immediate repeat myelography, in the event of technical failure, is contraindicated because of overdosage considerations. (See interval recommendation under DOSAGE AND ADMINISTRATION.)

Lumbar puncture should not be performed in the presence of significant local or systemic infection where bacteremia is likely.

WARNINGS—Intrathecal

If grossly bloody CSF is encountered, the possible benefits of a myelographic procedure should be considered in terms of the risk to the patient.

Fatal reactions have been associated with the administration of water-soluble contrast media. Therefore, it is of utmost importance that a course of action be carefully planned in advance for the immediate treatment of serious reactions, and that adequate and appropriate facilities and personnel be readily available in case of a severe reaction.

Caution is advised in patients with a history of epilepsy, severe cardiovascular disease, chronic alcoholism or multiple sclerosis.

Elderly patients may present a greater risk following myelography. The need for the procedure in these patients should be evaluated carefully. Special attention must be paid to dose and concentration of the medium, hydration, and technique used.

Patients who are receiving anticonvulsants should be maintained on this therapy. Should a seizure occur, intravenous diazepam or phenobarbital sodium is recommended. In patients with a history of seizure activity who are not on anticonvulsant therapy, premedication with barbiturates or phenytoin should be considered.

Prophylactic anticonvulsant treatment with barbiturates should be considered in patients with evidence of inadvertent intracranial entry of a large or concentrated bolus of the contrast medium since there is an increased risk of seizures in such cases.

Drugs which lower the seizure threshold, especially phenothiazine derivatives, including those used for their antihistamine properties should not be used with AMIPAQUE. Others include MAO inhibitors, tricyclic antidepressants, CNS stimulants, psychoactive drugs described as analeptics, major tranquilizers, or antipsychotic drugs. Such medication should be discontinued at least 48 hours before myelography, should not be used for the control of nausea and vomiting, and should not be resumed for at least 24 hours postprocedure.

Care is required in patient management to prevent inadvertent intracranial entry of a large dose or concentrated bolus of the medium. Also, effort should be directed to avoid rapid dispersion of the medium causing inadvertent rise to intracranial levels (eg, by active patient movement). Direct intracisternal or ventricular administration for standard radiography (not CT) is not recommended.

In most reported cases of major motor seizures one or more of the following factors were present. Therefore avoid:

- Deviations from recommended procedure or in myelographic management.
- Use in patients with a history of epilepsy.
- Inadvertent overdosage.
- Intracranial entry of a bolus or premature diffusion of a high concentration of the medium.
- Medication with neuroleptic drugs or phenothiazine antinauseants.
- Failure to maintain elevation of the head during the procedure, on the stretcher, or in bed.
- Excessive and particularly active patient movement or straining.

At concentrations of 200 mgI/mL or less, these seizures have been noted only very rarely.

Treatment with intravenous diazepam or administration of phenobarbital sodium has provided rapid control of seizures. (See PATIENT MANAGEMENT.)

PRECAUTIONS—Intrathecal

Before a contrast medium is injected, the patient should be questioned for a history of allergy. Although a history of allergy, including asthma, may imply a greater than usual risk, it does not arbitrarily contraindicate the use of the medium. No conclusive relationship between severe reactions and antigen-antibody reactions or other manifestations of allergy has been established.

In patients with severe renal insufficiency or failure, the drug is excreted by the liver into the bile at a much slower rate. Patients with hepatorenal insufficiency should not be examined unless the possibility of benefit clearly outweighs the additional risk.

For Repeat Procedure see DOSAGE AND ADMINISTRATION.

If nondisposable equipment is used, scrupulous care should be taken to prevent residual contamination with traces of cleansing agents.

Pregnancy Category B. Reproduction studies have been performed in rats and rabbits up to 70 times the human dose and have revealed no evidence of impaired fertility or harm to the fetus due to AMIPAQUE, brand of metrizamide. There are, however, no adequate and well controlled studies in pregnant women. Because animal reproduction studies are not always predictive of human response, this drug should be used during pregnancy only if clearly needed.

Nursing Mothers. Caution should be exercised when AMIPAQUE is administered to a nursing woman. AMIPAQUE is excreted in milk to the extent of 1 mg of the injected myelographic dose over 2 days.

ADVERSE REACTIONS—Intrathecal

The most frequently occurring adverse reactions are headache, nausea, and vomiting. These reactions occur 3 to 8 hours postinjection, almost all occurring within 24 hours. They are usually mild to moderate in degree lasting for a few hours and usually disappearing within 24 hours. Rarely, headaches may be severe or persist for days. The reported incidence of headaches varies from 20 to over 60 percent and they are often accompanied by nausea and vomiting. Headaches tend to be more frequent and persistent in patients not optimally hydrated. (See PATIENT MANAGEMENT.)

Backache, neck stiffness, numbness and paresthesias, leg or sciatic-type pain occurred less frequently, often in the form of a transient exacerbation of preexisting symptomatology. Temperature elevations constitute the fourth most common reaction in individuals under 18 years of age. Dizziness has also been reported.

The incidence and nature of adverse reactions in pediatric patients is similar to adult patients except for the occurrence of a higher incidence of fever (19%) and occasional incidence of croup, breast feeding problems, and crying spells. Of the 42 percent of pediatric patients who received general anesthesia, the incidence of nausea and vomiting was generally higher.

Cardiovascular: Chest pain, tachycardia, bradycardia and other arrhythmias, hypertension or hypotension, cardiac arrest, vasculitis, hemorrhage, collapse, and shock have also been reported.

Transient alterations in **vital signs** may occur. Their significance must be assessed on an individual basis.

Other rarely occurring adverse reactions include the following:

Major motor seizures: Focal or generalized grand mal seizures have occurred with an incidence reported between 0.1 and 0.3 percent. They have usually occurred 4 to 12 hours following injection, and have consisted of one or two episodes 1 or more hours apart, which have responded promptly to the intravenous injection of diazepam. For prolonged prophylaxis barbiturates have been recommended.

Early onset of seizures (less than 2 hours) is indicative of early substantial intracranial entry.

Transitory EEG changes are frequent and usually take the form of slow wave activity, although sharp activity and paroxysmal activity have been reported up to 24 hours after the procedure, the incidence of EEG changes may be as high as 30 percent.

An **aseptic meningitis** syndrome, has been reported rarely (less than 0.1%). It was usually preceded by pronounced headaches, nausea and vomiting. Onset usually occurred about 12 to 18 hours postprocedure. Prominent features were meningismus, fever, sometimes with oculomotor signs and mental confusion. Lumbar puncture revealed a high white cell count, high protein content often with a low glucose level and with absence of organisms. The condition usually started to clear spontaneously about 10 hours after onset, with complete recovery over 2 to 3 days.

Allergy or idiosyncrasy: Chills, fever, profuse diaphoresis, pruritus, urticaria, nasal congestion, dyspnea, and a case of Guillain-Barré syndrome.

CNS irritation: Mild and transitory perceptual aberrations such as hallucinations, depersonalization, amnesia, hostility, amblyopia, diplopia, photophobia, psychosis, insomnia, anxiety, depression, hyperesthesia, visual, auditory or speech disturbances, confusion and disorientation. In addition, malaise, weakness, EEG changes, meningismus, hyperreflexia or areflexia, hypertonia or flaccidity, hemiplegia, paralysis, quadriplegia, restlessness, tremor, echoacousia, echolalia, asterixis or dysphasia have occurred.

Profound mental disturbances have also rarely been reported. They have usually consisted of various forms and degrees of aphasia, mental confusion or disorientation. The onset is usually at 8 to 10 hours and lasts for about 24 hours, without aftereffects. However, occasionally they have been manifest as apprehension, agitation, or progressive withdrawal in several instances to the point of somnolence, stupor and coma. In a few cases these have been accompanied by transitory hearing loss or other auditory symptoms and visual disturbances (believed subjective or delusional), including unilateral or bilateral loss of vision which may last for hours. In one case persistent cortical loss of vision has been reported in association with convulsions. Ventricular block has been reported in two cases, amnesia of varying degrees may be present for the reaction event.

Rarely, persistent though transitory weakness in the leg or ocular muscles has been reported.

Neuropathies: Neuropathies have been rare and almost always transitory. They include sensory and/or motor or nerve root disturbances, myelitis, persistent leg muscle pain or weakness, or 6th nerve palsy, or cauda equina syndrome. Muscle cramps, fasciculation or myoclonia, spinal convulsion, or spasticity are unusual and have responded promptly to a small intravenous dose of diazepam.

Respiratory: Apnea and pulmonary edema have been reported.

Body-General: Asthenia, cellulitis, hyponatremia, hemolytic anemia, generalized angioedema with marked dyspnea and stridor, and deaths have been reported.

Urogenital: Renal failure, polyuria, hematuria, and urinary retention have been reported.

OVERDOSAGE—Intrathecal

There is clinical evidence that reactions, particularly seizures and mental aberrations, following the administration of myelographic doses in excess of those recommended tend to be dose related. Even use of a recommended dose can produce effects tantamount to overdosage, if incorrect management of the patient during or immediately following the procedure permits inadvertent early intracranial entry of a large portion of the medium.

Treatment: See ADVERSE REACTIONS—Major motor seizures.

The subarachnoid LD_{50} in mice is greater than 1,500 mgI/kg.

DOSAGE AND ADMINISTRATION—Intrathecal

See also PATIENT MANAGEMENT

The dosage and concentration of AMIPAQUE will depend on the degree and extent of contrast required in the area(s) under examination and on the equipment and technique employed. Concentrations which are approximately isotonic (170 mgI/mL to 190 mgI/mL) are recommended for examination in the lumbar region. For movement of the medium to distant target areas, higher concentrations are recommended to compensate for dilution of AMIPAQUE with CSF. A total dose of 3000 mg iodine or a concentration of 300 mgI/mL should not be exceeded. As in all diagnostic procedures, the least amount to produce adequate visualization should be used. Most procedures do not require either maximum dose or concentration. The incidence of serious adverse reactions is considerably less with concentrations of 200 mgI/mL or less. The dose and concentration used in the spinal area influence ultimate intracranial concentrations.

Anesthesia is not necessary. Premedication sedatives or tranquilizers are usually not needed (see PRECAUTIONS). Patients should be well hydrated. Epileptic patients should be maintained on their anticonvulsant medication.

As with any lumbar puncture, sterile technique must be employed. The lumbar puncture is usually made between L3 and L4, but if pathology is suspected at this level the interspace immediately above or below may be selected. A lateral cervical puncture may also be used.

Rate of Injection: To avoid excessive mixing with CSF and consequent loss of contrast as well as premature dispersion upward, injection must be made slowly over 1 to 2 minutes. The lumbar puncture needle is removed immediately following injection since it is not necessary to remove AMIPAQUE after injection into subarachnoid spaces.

Repeat Procedure: An interval of at least 48 hours should be allowed before repeat examination; however, whenever possible 5 to 7 days is recommended.

The recommended usual and maximum doses of AMIPAQUE, brand of metrizamide, are summarized in the following tables:

[See table above].

ADULT DOSAGE TABLE—Iodine Content

Procedure	Conc. of Solution (mgI/mL)	Usual Recommended Dose* (mL)	Max. Dose Total (mgI)
Lumbar myelogram	170–190	10–15	2850
Thoracic myelogram	220	12	2640
Cervical myelogram (lumbar injection)	250–300	10	3000
Cervical myelogram (lateral cervical injection)	220	10	2200
Total columnar myelography	250–280	10	2800
CT cisternography (lumbar injection)	170–190	4–6	1140

* Refer to DILUTION TABLE FOR INTRATHECAL USE for preparation of Solution

The pediatric doses, intended as guidelines, are based on age range rather than weight because brain or CSF capacity is independent of weight. Variations will depend on such factors as height, nature of pathology, condition of the patient, technique used, etc (eg, whether for CSF contrast for CT scan or for standard radiography, or whether movement of the medium is to be directed to an area distal to the site of injection). Direct intracranial placement will require particular care in planning to maintain total dose and concentration as low as practical to avoid convulsive response. Whenever possible (eg, for CT scan) the use of the isotonic concentration (170 mgI/mL) is preferable. In children, loss of contrast due to mixing on movement of the medium is less apt to occur because of their shorter spinal cord. Therefore, the use of relatively lower dosages may be feasible.

[See table left].

PEDIATRIC DOSAGE TABLE—Iodine Content

Conventional Radiography

Procedure	Age	Conc. of Solution (mgI/mL)	Usual Recommended Dose* (mL)
Lumbar, thoracic myelography (lumbar injection)	Less than 2 months	170–190	2–3
	2 months to 2 years	170–190	2–4
	3 to 7 years	170–190	4–8
	8 to 12 years	170–190	7–9
	13 to 18 years	170–190	8–10
Cervical myelography (lumbar injection)	Less than 2 months	170–210	2–3
	2 months to 2 years	170–200	2–4
	3 to 7 years	170–210	4–8
	8 to 12 years	170–230	7–9
	13 to 18 years	170–230	8–10
Cervical myelography (lateral cervical injection)	8 to 18 years	200–220	3–5
Cisternography (direct injection)	Less than 2 months	170–220	2–3
	8 to 18 years	170–220	2–5
Cisternography (lumbar injection)	2 months to 2 years	170–220	2–3
	3 to 7 years	170–190	3–5
	8 to 12 years	170–190	5–6
Ventriculography (direct injection)	Less than 2 months	170–220	2–3
	2 months to 2 years	170–220	2–3
	3 to 12 years	170–220	2–4
	13 to 18 years	190–220	2–5
Ventriculography (lumbar injection)	2 months to 2 years	170–220	2–3
CT Radiography			
CT cisternography (lumbar injection)	3 to 7 years	170–190	3–5
	8 to 12 years	180–190	3–5
	13 to 18 years	170–190	3–5
CT ventriculography (direct injection)	Less than 2 months	170–220	2
	2 months to 2 years	170–220	2
	3 to 7 years	170–220	3
CT ventriculography (lumbar injection)	3 to 7 years	170–220	3

* Refer to DILUTION TABLE FOR INTRATHECAL USE for preparation of Solution

The medium disperses in about 60 minutes following direct ventricular placement.

Young children may require general anesthesia for technical reasons.

Convulsions occurred in a few patients, only one attributable to the medium, at these dosage schedules.

Prophylactic barbiturates are suggested for inadvertent overdosage. Parenteral diazepam or barbiturates is suggested for treatment of seizures and barbiturates and/or phenytoin for continued suppression.

PREPARATION OF THE SOLUTION—Intrathecal

1. Select the correct iodine concentration recommended for the procedure in the DOSAGE TABLES.
2. The volume of diluent required to obtain that iodine concentration can be obtained from the DILUTION TABLE.
3. Using a sterile technique with a small gauge transfer needle (approximately 22 gauge to help prevent coring), withdraw the required amount of diluent.
4. Insert this volume of diluent into the lyophil vial also using the fine needle. Contents under vacuum. Use only if vacuum is present as evidenced by diluent being drawn into vial when stopper is punctured. Leave syringe and needle in place.
5. Gently swirl the vial (without shaking) until its contents are dissolved (approximately 3 to 10 minutes) to insure complete dissolution of the lyophil. The resulting solution should be clear and colorless to slightly yellow. Do not use if undissolved particulate matter or bubbles are present.
6. Withdraw the volume of AMIPAQUE, brand of metrizamide, recommended for the procedure in the DOSAGE TABLES.

Continued on next page

This product information was effective as of December 1, 1986. On these and other products of Winthrop-Breor Laboratories, detailed information may be obtained on current basis by direct inquiry to the Professional Serv Department, 90 Park Avenue, New York, NY 10016 907-2525.

Winthrop-Breon—Cont.

7. Detach syringe and attach to myelographic injection unit. Use immediately after reconstitution. Discard any unused portion. (See INDIVIDUAL INDICATIONS AND USAGE—Intravascular section/PREPARATION OF THE SOLUTION—Intravascular Use #7.)
[See table below].

PATIENT MANAGEMENT—Intrathecal

Suggestions for Usual Patient Management

Preprocedure

- Discontinue neuroleptic drugs (including phenothiazines, eg, chlorpromazine, prochlorperazine, and promethazine) 48 hours beforehand.
- Maintain normal diet up to 2 hours before.
- Ensure hydration—fluids up to procedure.

During Procedure

- Use minimum dose and concentration required for satisfactory contrast. (See DOSAGE AND ADMINISTRATION.)
- In all positioning techniques keep the patient's head elevated above highest level of spine.
- Do not lower head of table more than 15° during thoracocervical procedures.
- In patients with excessive lordosis consider lateral position for injection and movement of the medium cephalad.
- Avoid intracranial entry of a bolus.
- Avoid early and high cephalad dispersion of the medium.
- Inject slowly over 1 to 2 minutes to avoid excessive mixing.
- Abrupt or active patient movement causes excessive mixing with CSF. Instruct patient to remain passive. Move patient slowly and only as necessary.
- To maintain as a bolus, move medium to distal area very slowly under fluoroscopic control.
- At completion of direct cervical or lumbo-cervical procedures, raise head of table steeply (45°) for about 2 minutes to restore medium to lower levels.

Postprocedure

- Raise head of stretcher to at least 15° before moving patient onto it.
- Movement onto stretcher, and off the stretcher to bed, should be done slowly with patient completely passive, maintaining head up position.
- Before moving patient onto bed, raise head of bed 15° to 30°.
- Advise patient to remain still in bed, in head up position, especially in first few hours.
- Maintain close observation for at least 12 hours after myelogram.
- After 8 hours, patient may be lowered to a horizontal position for further 16 hours.
- Obtain visitors' cooperation in keeping the patient quiet and in head up position, especially in first few hours.
- Encourage oral fluids and diet as tolerated.
- If nausea or vomiting occurs, do not use phenothiazine antinauseants. Persistent nausea and vomiting will result in dehydration. Therefore, prompt consideration of replacement by intravenous fluids is recommended.

Alternative Postprocedure Method

- Recent evidence suggests that maintaining the patient postmyelography in an upright position (via wheelchair or ambulation) may help minimize adverse effects. The upright position may help to delay upward dispersion of the medium and to maximize the spinal arachnoid absorption.

SECTION II

CLINICAL PHARMACOLOGY—Intravascular

Intravascular injection of a radiopaque diagnostic agent opacifies those vessels in the path of flow of the contrast medium permitting radiographic visualization of the internal structures of the human body until significant hemodilution occurs. The pharmacokinetics of the intravenously administered radiopaque contrast media are usually best described by a two compartment model with a rapid alpha phase for drug distribution and a slow beta phase for drug elimination. In patients with renal functional impairment, the elimination half-life for the beta phase may be prolonged for up to several days.
Following intravenous injection, AMIPAQUE is distributed and excreted in a manner similar to the diatrizoates, ie, following initial high serum levels, the level falls rapidly as the medium becomes distributed throughout the extravascular compartment. Thereafter, it is excreted unchanged principally by glomerular filtration. It is not metabolized. About 94% of the medium is excreted in this manner in 24 hours and a further 5% by hepatobiliary excretion via the bowel.

INDICATIONS AND USAGE—Intravascular

AMIPAQUE is indicated for intravenous digital arteriography for head and neck, adult peripheral arteriography, and pediatric angiocardiography.

CONTRAINDICATIONS—Intravascular

Known hypersensitivity to AMIPAQUE, brand of metrizamide.

WARNINGS—Intravascular

In patients with myelomatosis the effects of nonionic media on renal function is unknown. If a decision to use AMIPAQUE is made, the patient should be well hydrated beforehand, a minimal diagnostic dose used, and renal function and extent of urinary precipitation of the myeloma protein checked for a few days afterwards.
Contrast media may promote sickling in individuals who are homozygous for sickle cell disease when the material is injected intravenously or intra-arterially.
Administration of radiopaque materials to patients known or suspected of having pheochromocytoma should be performed with extreme caution. If, in the opinion of the physician, the possible benefits of such procedures outweigh the considered risks, the procedures may be performed; however, the amount of radiopaque medium injected should be kept to an absolute minimum. The blood pressure should be assessed throughout the procedure and measures for treatment of a hypertensive crisis should be available.
Recent reports of thyroid storm occurring following the intravascular use of iodinated radiopaque diagnostic agents in patients with hyperthyroidism or with an autonomously functioning thyroid nodule suggest that this additional risk be evaluated in such patients before use of these drugs.
Arteriography should be performed with caution in patients with severely impaired renal function and patients with combined renal and hepatic disease.

DILUTION TABLE FOR INTRATHECAL USE

Conc. of Solution (mgI/mL)	Volume of Diluent to be Added: 2.5 g vial (mL)	3.75 g vial (mL)	6.75 g vial (mL)
170	6.0	8.9	16.1
180	5.6	8.3	15.0
190	5.3	7.8	14.0
200	4.9	7.3	13.2
210	4.7	6.9	12.4
220	4.4	6.5	11.7
230	4.2	6.1	11.1
240	3.9	5.8	10.5
250	3.7	5.5	10.0
260	3.6	5.2	9.4
270	3.4	5.0	9.0
280	3.2	4.7	8.5
290	3.1	4.5	8.1
300	2.9	4.3	7.8
	The volume of the final solution will equal the volume of …e diluent + 1.1 mL	The volume of the final solution will equal the volume of the diluent + 1.7 mL	The volume of the final solution will equal the volume of the diluent + 3.1 mL

…solution will exceed the amount required to achieve the recommended dosage. For volume for injec- …TABLES.

PRECAUTIONS—Intravascular

Diagnostic procedures which involve the use of radiopaque diagnostic agents should be carried out under the direction of personnel with the prerequisite training and with a thorough knowledge of the particular procedure to be performed. Appropriate facilities should be available for coping with any complication of the procedure, as well as for emergency treatment of severe reactions to the contrast agent itself. After parenteral administration of a radiopaque agent, competent personnel and emergency facilities should be available for at least 30 to 60 minutes since severe delayed reactions have occurred (see ADVERSE REACTIONS).
Since allergic response can occur with the nonionic media, similar preparations to those recommended for ionic media should be planned to handle severe or potentially fatal complications. These measures are to ensure the ready availability of appropriate resuscitative drugs, equipment, and personnel.
A history of allergy to the intravascular use of metrizamide, or other contrast agents, may indicate a greater likelihood of allergic response. However, such history is not a contraindication but calls for caution in use.
The possibility of an idiosyncratic reaction in susceptible patients should always be considered (see ADVERSE REACTIONS). The susceptible population includes patients with a history of a previous reaction to a contrast media, patients with a known sensitivity to iodine per se, and patients with a known clinical hypersensitivity: bronchial asthma, hay fever and food allergies.
The occurrence of severe idiosyncratic reactions has prompted the use of several pretesting methods. However, pretesting cannot be relied upon to predict severe reactions and may itself be hazardous for the patient. It is suggested that a thorough medical history with emphasis on allergy and hypersensitivity, prior to the injection of any contrast media, may be more accurate than pretesting in predicting potential adverse reactions.
A positive history of allergies or hypersensitivity does not arbitrarily contraindicate the use of a contrast agent, where a diagnostic procedure is thought essential, but caution should be exercised (see ADVERSE REACTIONS). Premedication with antihistamines or corticosteroids to avoid or minimize possible allergic reactions in such patients should be considered. Recent reports indicate that such pretreatment does not prevent serious life-threatening reactions, but may reduce both their incidence and severity.
Azotemia is not a contraindication. Care should be taken regarding dosage and hydration status and the patient's renal status should be monitored for days afterwards.
Acute renal failure has been reported in diabetic patients with diabetic nephropathy and in susceptible nondiabetic patients (often elderly with preexisting renal disease) following intravascular use of contrast media. Therefore, careful consideration of the potential risks should be given before performing this radiographic procedure in these patients.
Preparatory dehydration is dangerous and may contribute to acute renal failure in infants, young children, elderly, patients with preexisting renal insufficiency, and patients with advanced vascular disease. Dehydration in these patients seems to be enhanced by the osmotic diuretic action of contrast agents. It is believed that overnight fluid restriction prior to angiography does not provide better visualization in normal patients. Therefore, preparatory dehydration is unnecessary, and is usually contraindicated, in association with the angiographic use of AMIPAQUE, brand of metrizamide.
Angiography should be avoided whenever possible in patients with homocystinuria, because of the risk of inducing thrombosis and embolism.
The inhibitory effects of nonionic contrast media on mechanisms of hemostasis have been shown, in vitro, to be less than ionic contrast media at comparable concentrations. For this reason, standard angiographic procedures should always be followed: angiographic catheters should be flushed frequently, and prolonged contact of blood with contrast media in syringes and catheters should be avoided.

Drug/Laboratory Test Interactions

It is expected that the results of thyroid function tests, which depend on iodine estimations, will not reflect true function for about 16 days. Tests which directly determine thyroxine levels should not be affected.

Pregnancy Category B. See Intrathecal Uses. Precautions.

Nursing Mothers. Caution should be exercised when AMIPAQUE is administered to a nursing woman. AMIPAQUE is excreted in milk to the extent of 1 mg of the injected myelographic dose over 2 days.
The nature of the adverse effects which occur following intravascular administration of AMIPAQUE is similar to that following corresponding ionic media although their incidence and severity may be less.
The following is based on general vascular experience with both ionic and nonionic media.

ADVERSE REACTIONS—Intravascular

Reactions which have been observed are similar in nature to those following the use of ionic media.
Cardiovascular: Various arrhythmias, bradycardia being the most frequent, as well as peripheral vasodilation with brief hypotension have occurred.
Hemodynamic: A feeling of heat, usually mild but which may be moderate in degree, may be evident particularly following selective arterial procedures. Frank pain is very unusual.
Renal: Mild diuresis and transitory mild increase in urine osmolarity.
Allergic: Dermal urticaria or erythemata have occurred. Therefore, other allergic manifestations such as rigors, broncho or laryngospastic attacks with serious cardiopulmonary complications resulting in fatality must be considered a possibility.
Respiratory: Pulmonary or laryngeal edema, dyspnea.
Nervous System: Restlessness, tremors.
Technical Factors: Hematoma, ecchymosis, extravasation of the medium particularly on mechanical high pressure injection, venous rupture or hemorrhage from arterial injection sites (observe areas for at least 24 hours).

INDIVIDUAL INDICATIONS AND USAGE—Intravascular

INTRAVENOUS DIGITAL ARTERIOGRAPHY FOR THE HEAD AND NECK

AMIPAQUE solution can be injected intravenously as a rapid bolus to provide arterial visualization using digital subtraction radiography. Preprocedural medications are not considered necessary. AMIPAQUE will provide diagnostic arterial radiographs in about 90% of patients. In almost all cases in which poor arterial visualization occurs (10%), it can be attributed to patient movement. AMIPAQUE is very well tolerated in the vascular system. There is very little subjective or objective evidence of patient discomfort (general sensation of heat) following the injection as compared with ionic media. Very few of the reactions are moderate to severe in degree. In about 87% of patients discomfort is either absent or is mild. Some patients exhibit mild nausea which does not appear to be dose related.
Precautions: Since the dose is usually administered mechanically under high pressure, rupture of smaller peripheral veins has occurred. It has been suggested that this can be avoided by using an intravenous catheter threaded proximally beyond larger tributaries or in the case of the antecubital vein, into the superior vena cava. Sometimes the femoral vein is used.
Dosage and Administration: The maximum total dose administered to the patient should not exceed 87.5 g of iodine. See DESCRIPTION section for iodine content.
AMIPAQUE is administered intravenously as a bolus injection in a concentration of 370 mgI/mL.
The usual individual volume is about 40 mL (range 30 mL to 60 mL).
Frequently three injections may be required, up to a total volume of about 120 mL (range 40 mL to 165 mL).
The patient is urged not to move during, or immediately after, the injection. In the case of carotid-cerebral arteriography, the patient is also asked not to swallow during this period. AMIPAQUE is usually administered via 16–18 gauge catheter by mechanical injection at a rate of about 12 mL/sec.
A dextrose solution may be layered over the contrast medium in the injector with the purpose of pushing the remnant of the bolus forward into the main circulation, and to flush out the vein.

ADULT PERIPHERAL ARTERIOGRAPHY

AMIPAQUE, brand of metrizamide, solution in a concentration of 370 mgI/mL is recommended for arteriography of the lower limbs. The injection is usually through a catheter introduced into the femoral artery with the tip placed as to achieve lower aortic or aorto-iliac runoff or visualization of individual femoral artery or its distribution throughout the lower limb. When necessary, the catheter tip may be advanced to the level of the renal artery. Pressure injection is usually employed. Visualization is similar to that achieved with ionic media of similar dose and concentration. Sedative premedication may be employed with AMIPAQUE, however, anesthesia is usually not considered necessary.
Adverse Reactions: Very brief (seconds to minutes) nausea immediately following the injection or mild urticaria starting within minutes and of a few hours duration, has been reported in about 3% of patients; these reactions have not interfered with the procedure. Patient discomfort during and immediately following the injection is substantially less than the discomfort which follows injection of ionic media of similar volume and concentrations. Severe discomfort is very unusual.
Dosage and Administration: The maximum total dose administered to the patient should not exceed 87.5 g of iodine. See DESCRIPTION section for iodine content.
The volume required will depend on the size, flow rate and disease status of the injected artery, and on the size and condition of the patient as well as the imaging technique used. The usual individual volume is about 50 mL (range 25 mL to 65 mL). Two injections are usually required, sometimes three, and rarely up to five.

PEDIATRIC ANGIOCARDIOGRAPHY

AMIPAQUE at a maximum concentration of 370 mgI/mL may be used for angiocardiography in infants and young children.
Dosage and Administration: The recommended single dose of AMIPAQUE in 370 mgI/mL concentration is about 1.5 mL/kg (range 1 mL/kg to 2 mL/kg). In addition, small test volumes of about 2 mL may be used for catheter placement.
The usual total dose of AMIPAQUE per procedure, which includes diagnostic and test doses, is about 4 mL/kg (range 1.5 mL/kg to 6 mL/kg).
Analgesics and/or sedative tranquilizers may be required in these young patients.

PREPARATION OF THE SOLUTION—Intravascular Use

1. Determine the concentration required for the vascular procedure.
2. The volume of diluent required to obtain that iodine concentration can be obtained from the DILUTION TABLE.
3. Using a sterile technique with a small gauge transfer needle (approximately 22 gauge to help prevent coring), withdraw the required amount of diluent.
4. Insert this volume of diluent into the lyophil vial also using the fine needle. Contents under vacuum. Use only if vacuum is present as evidenced by diluent being drawn into vial when stopper is punctured. Leave syringe and needle in place.
5. Gently swirl the vial (without shaking) until its contents are dissolved (approximately 3 to 22 minutes) to insure complete dissolution of the lyophil. The resulting solution should be clear and colorless to slightly yellow. Do not use if undissolved particulate matter or bubbles are present.
6. Withdraw the volume of AMIPAQUE, brand of metrizamide, required.
7. Do not prefill plastic syringes with AMIPAQUE for prolonged periods (ie, for several hours or longer) before use. Use immediately after reconstitution. Discard any unused portion.

DILUTION TABLE FOR INTRAVASCULAR USE

Conc. of Solution (mgI/mL)	Volume of Diluent to be Added 6.75 g vial (mL)
300	7.8
310	7.4
320	7.1
330	6.8
340	6.5
350	6.2
360	6.0
370	5.7

The volume of the final solution will equal the volume of the diluent + 3.1 mL

The volume of the final solution will exceed the amount required to achieve the recommended dosage. For volume for injection refer to individual Dosage and Administration sections.

HOW SUPPLIED

Kits, each containing
One 3.75 g/20 mL single-dose vial of AMIPAQUE with 1 (20 mL) vial of diluent (NDC 0024-0044-01); or
One 6.75 g/50 mL single-dose vial of AMIPAQUE with 1 (20 mL) vial of diluent (NDC 0024-0046-01).
Combination packs, each containing
Five 2.5 g/20 mL single-dose vials of AMIPAQUE with 5 (20 mL) vials of diluent (NDC 0024-0047-12); or
Five 3.75 g/20 mL single-dose vials of AMIPAQUE with 5 (20 mL) vials of diluent (NDC 0024-0044-12); or
Five 6.75 g/50 mL single-dose vials of AMIPAQUE with 5 (20 mL) vials of diluent (NDC 0024-0046-12).
Protect vials of AMIPAQUE, brand of metrizamide, from light or excessive heat 40°C (104°F).

AW-144-O

OMNIPAQUE® 180 240 300 350 ℞
INJECTION (IOHEXOL)
Section I—Intrathecal
Section II—Intravascular

DESCRIPTION

Iohexol, *N,N'*-Bis(2,3-dihydroxypropyl)-5-[*N*-(2,3-dihydroxypropyl)-acetamido]-2,4,6-triiodoisophthalamide, is a nonionic, water-soluble radiographic contrast medium with a molecular weight of 821.14 (iodine content 46.36%). In aqueous solution each triiodinated molecule remains undissociated.
OMNIPAQUE is provided as a sterile, colorless to pale yellow solution, in the following iodine concentrations: 180, 240, 300, and 350 mgI/mL. Each milliliter of iohexol solution contains 1.21 mg tromethamine and 0.1 mg edetate calcium disodium with the pH adjusted between 6.8 and 7.7 with hydrochloric acid or sodium hydroxide. All solutions are sterilized by autoclaving and contain no preservatives. Unused portions must be discarded. Iohexol solution is sensitive to light and therefore should be protected from exposure.
The four available concentrations have the following physical properties:
[See table above].

Concentration (mgI/mL)	Osmolality* (mOsm/kg water)	Osmolarity (mOsm/L)	Absolute Viscosity (cp) 20°C	37°C	Specific Gravity (g/mL) 37°C
180	408	331	3.1	2.0	1.209
240	520	391	5.8	3.4	1.280
300	672	465	11.8	6.3	1.349
350	844	541	20.4	10.4	1.406

*By vapor-pressure osmometry.

OMNIPAQUE 180, OMNIPAQUE 240, OMNIPAQUE 300, and OMNIPAQUE 350 have osmolalities from approximately 1.5 to 3.0 times that of plasma (285 mOsm/kg water) or cerebrospinal fluid (301 mOsm/kg water) as shown in the above table and are hypertonic under conditions of use.

SECTION I

CLINICAL PHARMACOLOGY—Intrathecal

Iohexol is absorbed from cerebrospinal fluid (CSF) into the bloodstream and is eliminated by renal excretion. No significant metabolism, deiodination, or biotransformation occurs.
In five adult patients receiving 16 to 18 milliliters of iohexol (180 mgI/mL) by lumbar intrathecal injection, approximately 88 (73.1–98.2) percent of the injected dose was excreted in the urine within the first 24 hours after administration. The renal and body clearances were 99 (47–137) milliliters per minute and 109 (52–138) milliliters per minute. The mean maximal plasma concentration was 119 (72–177) micrograms of iohexol per milliliter and occurred after 3.8 (2–6) hours. The volume of distribution was 557 (350–849) milliliters per kilogram. In one patient with a large spinal cord tumor, excretion was delayed (67 percent of the dose appeared in urine within the first 24 hours) with no difference in the total overall recovery in the urine after 48 hours. The delay in excretion appeared to be related to a decrease in the rate of transfer of iohexol from the cerebrospinal fluid to the blood (plasma maximal concentration was approximately 30 micrograms/mL).
The initial concentration and volume of the medium, in conjunction with appropriate patient manipulation and the volume of CSF into which the medium is placed, will determine the extent of the diagnostic contrast that can be achieved.
Following intrathecal injection in conventional radiography, OMNIPAQUE 180 and OMNIPAQUE 240 will continue to provide good diagnostic contrast for at least 30 minutes. Slow diffusion of iohexol takes place throughout the CSF with subsequent absorption into the bloodstream. Once in the systemic circulation, iohexol displays little tendency to bind to serum or plasma proteins. At approximately 1 hour following injection, contrast of diagnostic quality will no longer be available for conventional myelography. If computerized tomographic (CT) myelography is to follow, consid-

Continued on next page

This product information was effective as of December 1 1986. On these and other products of Winthrop-B Laboratories, detailed information may be obtained current basis by direct inquiry to the Professional Se Department, 90 Park Avenue, New York, NY 1001 907-2525.

Winthrop-Breon—Cont.

eration should be given to a delay of several hours to allow the degree of contrast to decrease.

After administration into the lumbar subarachnoid space, computerized tomography shows the presence of contrast medium in the thoracic region in about 1 hour, in the cervical region in about 2 hours, and in the basal cisterns in 3 to 4 hours.

In patients with renal impairment, depending on the degree of impairment, prolonged plasma iohexol levels may be anticipated due to decreased renal elimination.

INDICATIONS AND USAGES—Intrathecal

OMNIPAQUE 180 and OMNIPAQUE 240 are indicated for intrathecal administration in adults including myelography (lumbar and thoracic) and in contrast enhancement for computerized tomography.

CONTRAINDICATIONS—Intrathecal

OMNIPAQUE should not be administered to patients with a known hypersensitivity to iohexol.

Myelography should not be performed in the presence of significant local or systemic infection where bacteremia is likely.

Intrathecal administration of corticosteroids with OMNIPAQUE (iohexol) is contraindicated.

Because of the possibility of overdosage, immediate repeat myelography in the event of technical failure is contraindicated (see DOSAGE AND ADMINISTRATION).

WARNINGS—General

If grossly bloody CSF is encountered, the possible benefits of a myelographic procedure should be considered in terms of the risk to the patient.

Caution is advised in patients with a history of epilepsy, severe cardiovascular disease, chronic alcoholism, or multiple sclerosis.

Elderly patients may present a greater risk following myelography. The need for the procedure in these patients should be evaluated carefully. Special attention must be paid to dose and concentration of the medium, hydration, and technique used.

Patients who are receiving anticonvulsants should be maintained on this therapy. Should a seizure occur, intravenous diazepam or phenobarbital sodium is recommended. In patients with a history of seizure activity who are not on anticonvulsant therapy, premedication with barbiturates should be considered.

Prophylactic anticonvulsant treatment with barbiturates should be considered in patients with evidence of inadvertent intracranial entry of a large or concentrated bolus of the contrast medium since there may be an increased risk of seizure in such cases.

Drugs which lower the seizure threshold, especially phenothiazine derivatives, including those used for their antihistamine properties, should not be used with OMNIPAQUE. Others include MAO inhibitors, tricyclic antidepressants, CNS stimulants, and psychoactive drugs described as analeptics, major tranquilizers, or antipsychotic drugs. Such medication should be discontinued at least 48 hours before myelography, should not be used for the control of nausea and vomiting, and should not be resumed for at least 24 hours postprocedure.

Care is required in patient management to prevent inadvertent intracranial entry of a large dose or concentrated bolus of the medium. Also, effort should be directed to avoid rapid dispersion of the medium causing inadvertent rise to intracranial levels (eg, by active patient movement). Direct intracisternal or ventricular administration for standard radiography (not CT) is not recommended.

In most reported cases of major motor seizures with other nonionic myelographic media, one or more of the following factors were present. Therefore avoid:

- Deviations from recommended procedure or in myelographic management.
- Use in patients with a history of epilepsy.
- Overdosage.
- Intracranial entry of a bolus or premature diffusion of a high concentration of the medium.
- Medication with neuroleptic drugs or phenothiazine antinauseants.
- Failure to maintain elevation of the head during the procedure, on the stretcher, or in bed.
- Excessive and particularly active patient movement or straining.

...CAUTIONS—General

...cedures which involve the use of radiopaque ...uld be carried out under the direction ...equisite training and with a thor... ...ticular procedure to be performed. ...ould be available for coping with ...procedure, as well as for emergency ...actions to the contrast agent itself. ...istration of a radiopaque agent, competent personnel and emergency facilities should be available for at least 30 to 60 minutes since severe delayed reactions have occurred. (See ADVERSE REACTIONS.)

Preparatory dehydration is dangerous and may contribute to acute renal failure in patients with advanced vascular disease, diabetic patients, and in susceptible nondiabetic patients (often elderly with pre-existing renal disease). Dehydration in these patients seems to be enhanced by the osmotic diuretic action of contrast agents. *Patients should be well hydrated prior to and following iohexol administration.*

The possibility of a reaction, including serious, life-threatening, fatal, anaphylactoid or cardiovascular reactions should always be considered (see ADVERSE REACTIONS). Therefore, it is of utmost importance that a course of action be carefully planned in advance for the immediate treatment of serious reactions, and that adequate and appropriate facilities and personnel be readily available in case of a severe reaction.

The possibility of an idiosyncratic reaction in susceptible patients should always be considered (see ADVERSE REACTIONS). The susceptible population includes patients with a history of a previous reaction to contrast media, patients with a known sensitivity to iodine per se, and patients with a known clinical hypersensitivity: bronchial asthma, hay fever, and food allergies.

The occurrence of severe idiosyncratic reactions has prompted the use of several pretesting methods. However, pretesting cannot be relied upon to predict severe reactions and may itself be hazardous for the patient. It is suggested that a thorough medical history with emphasis on allergy and hypersensitivity, prior to the injection of any contrast media, may be more accurate than pretesting in predicting potential adverse reactions.

A positive history of allergies or hypersensitivity does not arbitrarily contraindicate the use of a contrast agent where a diagnostic procedure is thought essential, but caution should be exercised (see ADVERSE REACTIONS). Premedication with antihistamines or corticosteroids to avoid or minimize possible allergic reactions in such patients should be considered. Recent reports indicate that such pretreatment does not prevent serious life-threatening reactions, but may reduce both their incidence and severity.

In patients with severe renal insufficiency or failure, compensatory biliary excretion of the drug is anticipated to occur, with a slow clearance into the bile. Patients with hepatorenal insufficiency should not be examined unless the possibility of benefit clearly outweighs the additional risk.

Administration of contrast media should be performed by qualified personnel familiar with the procedure and appropriate patient management (see PATIENT MANAGEMENT). Sterile technique must be used with any spinal puncture.

When OMNIPAQUE (iohexol) is to be injected using plastic disposable syringes, the contrast medium should be drawn into the syringe and used immediately.

If nondisposable equipment is used, scrupulous care should be taken to prevent residual contamination with traces of cleansing agents.

Parenteral products should be inspected visually for particulate matter and discoloration prior to administration. If particulate matter or discoloration is present, do not use.

Repeat Procedures. If in the clinical judgment of the physician sequential or repeat examinations are required, a suitable interval of time between administrations should be observed to allow for normal clearance of the drug from the body (see DOSAGE AND ADMINISTRATION and CLINICAL PHARMACOLOGY).

Information for Patients

Patients receiving injectable radiopaque diagnostic agents should be instructed to:

1. Inform your physician if you are pregnant (see CLINICAL PHARMACOLOGY).
2. Inform your physician if you are diabetic or if you have multiple myeloma, pheochromocytoma, homozygous sickle cell disease or known thyroid disorder (see WARNINGS).
3. Inform your physician if you are allergic to any drugs, food, or if you had any reactions to previous injections of dyes used for x-ray procedures (see PRECAUTIONS—GENERAL).
4. Inform your physician about any other medications you are currently taking, including nonprescription drugs, before you are administered this drug.

Drug Interactions

Drugs which lower seizure threshold, especially phenothiazine derivatives including those used for their antihistaminic or antinauseant properties, should not be used with OMNIPAQUE 180 or OMNIPAQUE 240. Others include monoamine oxidase (MAO) inhibitors, tricyclic antidepressants, CNS stimulants, psychoactive drugs described as analeptics, major tranquilizers, or antipsychotic drugs. Such medications should be discontinued at least 48 hours before myelography, should not be used for the control of nausea or vomiting during or after myelography, and should not be resumed for at least 24 hours postprocedure. In nonelective procedures in patients on these drugs, consider prophylactic use of anticonvulsants.

Carcinogensis, Mutagenesis, Impairment of Fertility

No long-term animal studies have been performed to evaluate carcinogenic potential, mutagenesis, or whether OMNIPAQUE (iohexol) can affect fertility in men or women.

Pregnancy Category B

Reproduction studies have been performed in rats and rabbits with up to 100 times the recommended human dose. No evidence of impaired fertility or harm to the fetus has been demonstrated due to OMNIPAQUE. There are, however, no studies in pregnant women. Because animal reproduction studies are not always predictive of human response, this drug should be used during pregnancy only if clearly needed.

Nursing Mothers

It is not known to what extent iohexol is excreted in human milk. However, many injectable contrast agents are excreted unchanged in human milk. Although it has not been established that serious adverse reactions occur in nursing infants, caution should be exercised when intravascular contrast media are administered to nursing women. Bottle feedings may be substituted for breast feedings for 24 hours following administration of OMNIPAQUE.

Pediatric Use

Safety and effectiveness in children have not been established.

ADVERSE REACTIONS—Intrathecal

The most frequently reported adverse reactions with OMNIPAQUE 180 and OMNIPAQUE 240 are headache, mild pain including backache and stiffness, nausea, and vomiting. These reactions usually occur 1 to 10 hours after injection, and almost all occur within 24 hours. They are usually mild to moderate in degree, lasting for a few hours, and usually disappearing within 24 hours. Rarely, headaches may be severe or persist for days. Headache is often accompanied by nausea and vomiting and tends to be more frequent and persistent in patients not optimally hydrated.

Transient alterations in vital signs may occur and their significance must be assessed on an individual basis. Those reactions reported in clinical studies with OMNIPAQUE are listed below in decreasing order of occurrence, based on clinical studies of 584 patients.

Headaches: The most frequently occurring adverse reaction following myelography has been headache, with an incidence of less than 20%. Headache may be caused by either a direct effect of the contrast medium or by CSF leakage at the dural puncture site. However, in managing the patient, it is considered more important to minimize intracranial entry of contrast medium by postural management than attempting to control possible CSF leakage (see PATIENT MANAGEMENT).

Pain: Mild pain including backache, stiffness, and neuralgia occurred following injection, with an incidence of about 8%.

Nausea and Vomiting: Nausea was reported with an incidence of about 6%, and vomiting about 3%, based on clinical studies of 584 patients (see PATIENT MANAGEMENT). Maintaining normal hydration is very important. The use of phenothiazine antinauseants is contraindicated. Reassurance to the patient that the nausea will clear usually is all that is required.

Dizziness: Transient dizziness was reported in about 2% of the patients.

Other Reactions: Other reactions occurring with an individual incidence of less than 0.1% included: feeling of heaviness, hypotension, hypertonia, sensation of heat, sweating, vertigo, loss of appetite, drowsiness, hypertension, photophobia, tinnitus, neuralgia, paresthesia, difficulty in micturition, and neurological changes. All were transient and mild with no clinical sequelae.

General Adverse Reactions to Contrast Media

Physicians should remain alert for the occurrence of adverse effects in addition to those discussed above, particularly the following reactions which have been reported in the literature for other nonionic, water-soluble myelographic media. These have included, but are not limited to, aseptic and bacterial meningitis, and CNS and other neurological disturbances.

An aseptic meningitis syndrome has been reported rarely (less than 0.01%). It was usually preceded by pronounced headaches, nausea and vomiting. Onset usually occurred about 12 to 18 hours postprocedure. Prominent features were meningismus, fever, sometimes with oculomotor signs and mental confusion. Lumbar puncture revealed a high white cell count, high protein content often with a low glucose level and with absence of organisms. The condition usually started to clear spontaneously about 10 hours after onset, with complete recovery over 2 to 3 days.

Allergy or Idiosyncrasy: Chills, fever, profuse diaphoresis, pruritus, urticaria, nasal congestion, dyspnea, and a case of Guillain-Barré syndrome.

CNS Irritation: Mild and transitory perceptual aberrations such as hallucinations, depersonalization, amnesia, hostility, amblyopia, diplopia, photophobia, psychosis, insomnia, anxiety, depression, hyperesthesia, visual or auditory or speech disturbances, confusion and disorientation. In addition, malaise, weakness, EEG changes, meningismus, hyperreflexia or areflexia, hypertonia or flaccidity, hemiplegia, paralysis, quadriplegia, restlessness, tremor, echoacousia, echolalia, asterixis, and dysphasia have occurred.

Profound mental disturbances have also rarely been reported. They have usually consisted of various forms and degrees of aphasia, mental confusion, or disorientation. The onset is usually at 8 to 10 hours and lasts for about 24 hours, without aftereffects. However, occasionally they have been manifest as apprehension, agitation, or progressive withdrawal in several instances to the point of somnolence, stupor, and coma. In a few cases these have been accompanied by transitory hearing loss or other auditory symptoms and visual disturbances (believed subjective or delusional), including unilateral or bilateral loss of vision which may last for hours. In one case, persistent cortical loss of vision has been reported in association with convulsions. Ventricular block has been reported in two cases; amnesia of varying degrees may be present for the reaction event.

Rarely, persistent though transitory weakness in the leg or ocular muscles has been reported.

Peripheral neuropathies have been rare and transitory. They include sensory and/or motor or nerve root disturbances, myelitis, persistent leg muscle pain or weakness, 6th nerve palsy, or cauda equina syndrome. Muscle cramps, fasciculation or myoclonia, spinal convulsion, or spasticity is unusual and have responded promptly to a small intravenous dose of diazepam.

In general, the reactions which are known to occur upon parenteral administration of iodinated contrast agents are possible with any nonionic agent. Approximately 95 percent of adverse reactions accompanying the use of water-soluble contrast agents are mild to moderate in degree. However, severe, life-threatening, anaphylactoid and fatal reactions, mostly of cardiovascular origin, have occurred.

Adverse reactions to injectable contrast media fall into two categories: chemotoxic reactions and idiosyncratic reactions. Chemotoxic reactions result from the physicochemical properties of the contrast media, the dose and speed of injection. All hemodynamic disturbances and injuries to organs or vessels perfused by the contrast medium are included in this category.

Idiosyncratic reactions include all other reactions. They occur more frequently in patients 20 to 40 years old. Idiosyncratic reactions may or may not be dependent on the amount of dose injected, the speed of injection, and the radiographic procedure. Idiosyncratic reactions are subdivided into minor, intermediate, and severe. The minor reactions are self-limited and of short duration; the severe reactions are life-threatening and treatment is urgent and mandatory.

The reported incidence of adverse reactions to contrast media in patients with a history of allergy is twice that of the general population. Patients with a history of previous reactions to a contrast medium are three times more susceptible than other patients. However, sensitivity to contrast media does not appear to increase with repeated examinations.

Most adverse reactions to injectable contrast media appear within 1 to 3 minutes after the start of injection, but delayed reactions may occur.

OVERDOSAGE

Clinical consequences of overdosage with OMNIPAQUE (iohexol) have not been reported. However, based on experience with other nonionic myelographic media, physicians should be alert to a potential increase in frequency and severity of CNS-mediated reactions. Even use of a recommended dose can produce effects tantamount to overdosage, if incorrect management of the patient during or immediately following the procedure permits inadvertent early intracranial entry of a large portion of the medium.

The intracisternal LD_{50} value of OMNIPAQUE (in grams of iodine per kilogram body weight) is greater than 2.0 in mice.

DOSAGE AND ADMINISTRATION—Intrathecal

The volume and concentration of OMNIPAQUE 180 or OMNIPAQUE 240 to be administered will depend on the degree and extent of contrast required in the area(s) under examination and on the equipment and technique employed.

OMNIPAQUE 180 at a concentration of 180 mgI/mL or OMNIPAQUE 240 at a concentration of 240 mgI/mL is recommended for the examination of the lumbar and thoracic regions in adults and is slightly hypertonic to CSF.

A total dose of 3,060 mg iodine or a concentration of 240 mgI/mL should not be exceeded in a single myelographic examination. This is based on clinical trial evaluation to date in the United States. As in all diagnostic procedures, the minimum volume and dose to produce adequate visualization should be used. Most procedures do not require either maximum dose or concentration.

Anesthesia is not necessary. Premedication sedatives or tranquilizers are usually not needed (see PRECAUTIONS). Patients should be well hydrated prior to and following contrast administration. Seizure-prone patients should be maintained on anticonvulsant medication.

Many radiopaque contrast agents are incompatible in vitro with some antihistamines and many other drugs; therefore, concurrent drugs should not be physically admixed with contrast agents.

Rate of Injection: To avoid excessive mixing with CSF and consequent dilution of contrast, injection should be made slowly over 1 to 2 minutes.

Depending on the estimated volume of contrast medium which may be required for the procedure a small amount of CSF may be removed to minimize distention of the subarachnoid spaces.

The lumbar puncture needle may be removed immediately following injection since it is not necessary to remove OMNIPAQUE (iohexol) after injection into the subarachnoid space.

The usual recommended total doses for use in lumbar and thoracic myelography are 1.70 gI to 3.06 gI:

OMNIPAQUE 180

(180 mgI/mL) 10 mL to 17 mL 1.8 gI to 3.06 gI

OMNIPAQUE 240

(240 mgI/mL) 7 mL to 12.5 mL 1.7 gI to 3.00 gI

Withdrawal of contrast agents from their containers should be accomplished under aseptic conditions with sterile syringes. Spinal puncture must always be performed under sterile conditions.

Parenteral products should be inspected visually for particulate matter or discoloration prior to administration. If particulate matter or discoloration is present, do not use.

Repeat Procedures: If in the clinical judgment of the physician sequential or repeat examinations are required, a suitable interval of time between administrations should be observed to allow for normal clearance of the drug from the body. An interval of at least 48 hours should be allowed before repeat examination; however, whenever possible, 5 to 7 days is recommended.

PATIENT MANAGEMENT—Intrathecal

Suggestions for Usual Patient Management

Good patient management should be exercised at all times to minimize the potential for procedurally related complications.

Preprocedure

- Discontinue neuroleptic drugs (including phenothiazines, eg, chlorpromazine, prochlorperazine, and promethazine) at least 48 hours beforehand.
- Maintain normal diet up to 2 hours before procedure.
- Ensure hydration—fluids up to procedure.

During Procedure

- Use minimum dose and concentration required for satisfactory contrast (see DOSAGE AND ADMINISTRATION).
- In all positioning techniques keep the patient's head elevated above highest level of spine.
- Do not lower head of table more than 15° in moving contrast medium cranially.
- In patients with excessive lordosis, consider lateral position for injection and movement of the medium cephalad.
- Inject slowly (over 1 to 2 minutes) to avoid excessive mixing.
- To maintain as a bolus, move medium to distal area very slowly. Use fluoroscopic monitoring.
- Avoid intracranial entry of a bolus.
- Avoid early and high cephalad dispersion of the medium.
- Avoid abrupt or active patient movement to minimize excessive mixing of medium with CSF. Instruct patient to remain passive. Move patient slowly and only as necessary.

Postprocedure

- Raise head of stretcher to at least 30° before moving patient onto it.
- Movement onto and off the stretcher should be done slowly with the patient completely passive, maintaining head-up position.
- Before moving patient onto bed, raise head of bed 30° to 45°.
- Advise patient to remain still in bed, in a sitting or semisitting position, especially in the first few hours.
- Maintain close observation for at least 12 hours after myelogram.
- Obtain visitors' cooperation in keeping the patient quiet and in head-up position, especially in first few hours.
- Encourage oral fluids. Diet as tolerated.
- If nausea or vomiting occurs, do not use phenothiazine antinauseants. Persistent nausea and vomiting will result in dehydration. Therefore, prompt consideration of replacement by intravenous fluids is recommended.

Alternative Postprocedure Method

- Recent evidence with nonionic, water-soluble contrast media suggests that maintaining the patient postmyelography in an upright position (via wheelchair or ambulation) may help minimize adverse effects. The upright position may help to delay upward dispersion of the medium and to maximize the spinal arachnoid absorption.

HOW SUPPLIED

OMNIPAQUE 180

Vials of 10 mL, 180 mgI/mL, boxes of 10 (NDC 0024-1411-10)

Vials of 20 mL, 180 mgI/mL, boxes of 10 (NDC 0024-1411-20)

OMNIPAQUE 240

Vials of 10 mL, 240 mgI/mL, boxes of 10 (NDC 0024-1412-10)

MYELO-KIT™ containing: One 10 mL vial of OMNIPAQUE 180, 180 mgI/mL, and one sterile myelogram tray, boxes of 5 (NDC 0024-1411-05)

MYELO-KIT containing: One 20 mL vial of OMNIPAQUE 180, 180 mgI/mL, and one sterile myelogram tray, boxes of 5 (NDC 0024-1411-51)

MYELO-KIT containing: One 10 mL vial of OMNIPAQUE 240, 240 mgI/mL, and one sterile myelogram tray, boxes of 5 (NDC 0024-1412-05)

STORAGE

Protect vials of OMNIPAQUE from strong daylight and direct exposure to sunlight. Do not freeze. Store at 59°F to 86°F (15°C to 30°C).

SECTION II

CLINICAL PHARMACOLOGY—Intravascular

Following intravascular injection, iohexol is distributed in the extracellular fluid compartment and is excreted unchanged by glomerular filtration. It will opacify those vessels in the path of flow of the contrast medium permitting radiographic visualization of the internal structures until significant hemodilution occurs.

Approximately 90% or more of the injected dose is excreted within the first 24 hours, with the peak urine concentrations occurring in the first hour after administration. Plasma and urine iohexol levels indicate that the iohexol body clearance is due primarily to renal clearance. An increase in the dose from 500 mgI/kg to 1500 mgI/kg does not significantly alter the clearance of the drug. The following pharmacokinetic values were observed following the intravenous administration of iohexol (between 500 mgI/kg to 1500 mgI/kg) to 16 human subjects: renal clearance—120 (86-162) mL/min; total body clearance—131 (98-165) mL/min; and volume of distribution—165 (108-219) mL/kg.

Renal accumulation is sufficiently rapid that the period of maximal opacification of the renal passages may begin as early as 1 minute after intravenous injection. Urograms become apparent in about 1 to 3 minutes with optimal contrast occurring between 5 to 15 minutes. In nephropathic conditions, particularly when excretory capacity has been altered, the rate of excretion may vary unpredictably, and opacification may be delayed after injection. Severe renal impairment may result in a lack of diagnostic opacification of the collecting system and, depending on the degree of renal impairment, prolonged plasma iohexol levels may be anticipated. In these patients, the route of excretion through the gallbladder and into the small intestine may increase.

Iohexol displays a low affinity for serum or plasma proteins and is poorly bound to serum albumin. No significant metabolism, deiodination or biotransformation occurs.

Animal studies indicate that iohexol does not cross the blood-brain barrier to any significant extent following intravascular administration.

OMNIPAQUE (iohexol) probably crosses the placental barrier in humans by simple diffusion. It is not known to what extent iohexol is excreted in human milk.

INDICATIONS AND USAGE, GENERAL — Intravascular

OMNIPAQUE 350 is indicated in adults for angiocardiography (ventriculography, selective coronary arteriography), aortography including studies of the aortic root, aortic arch, ascending aorta, abdominal aorta and its branches, digital subtraction angiography, peripheral arteriography, and excretory urography.

OMNIPAQUE 300 is indicated in adults for aortography including studies of the aortic arch, abdominal aorta and its branches, cerebral arteriography, peripheral venography (phlebography), and excretory urography.

OMNIPAQUE 240 is indicated in adults for peripheral venography (phlebography).

CONTRAINDICATIONS

OMNIPAQUE should not be administered to patients with a known hypersensitivity to iohexol.

WARNINGS—General

OMNIPAQUE should be used with extreme care in patients with severe functional disturbances of the liver and kidneys, severe thyrotoxicosis, or myelomatosis. Diabetics with a

Continued on next page

This product information was effective as of December 1986. On these and other products of Winthrop-Br Laboratories, detailed information may be obtained current basis by direct inquiry to the Professional S Department, 90 Park Avenue, New York, NY 10 907-2525.

Winthrop-Breon—Cont.

serum creatinine level above 3 mg/dL should not be examined unless the possible benefits of the examination clearly outweigh the additional risk. OMNIPAQUE (iohexol) is not recommended for use in patients with anuria.

Radiopaque contrast agents are potentially hazardous in patients with multiple myeloma or other paraproteinemia, particularly in those with therapeutically resistant anuria. Although neither the contrast agent nor dehydration has separately proven to be the cause of anuria in myeloma, it has been speculated that the combination of both may be causative factors. The risk in myelomatous patients is not a contraindication; however, special precautions are necessary. Partial dehydration in the preparation of these patients prior to injection is not recommended since this may predispose the patient to precipitation of the myeloma protein in the renal tubules. No form of therapy, including dialysis, has been successful in reversing the effect. Myeloma, which occurs most commonly in persons over age 40, should be considered before instituting intravascular administration of contrast agents.

Ionic contrast media, when injected intravenously or intraarterially, may promote sickling in individuals who are homozygous for sickle cell disease.

Administration of radiopaque materials to patients known or suspected of having pheochromocytoma should be performed with extreme caution. If, in the opinion of the physician, the possible benefits of such procedures outweigh the considered risks, the procedures may be performed; however, the amount of radiopaque medium injected should be kept to an absolute minimum. The patient's blood pressure should be assessed throughout the procedure and measures for the treatment of hypertensive crisis should be readily available.

Reports of thyroid storm following the use of iodinated, ionic radiopaque contrast media in patients with hyperthyroidism or with an autonomously functioning thyroid nodule suggest that this additional risk be evaluated in such patients before use of any contrast medium.

Urography should be performed with caution in patients with severely impaired renal function and patients with combined renal and hepatic disease.

PRECAUTIONS—General

Diagnostic procedures which involve the use of radiopaque diagnostic agents should be carried out under the direction of personnel with the prerequisite training and with a thorough knowledge of the particular procedure to be performed. Appropriate facilities should be available for coping with any complication of the procedure, as well as for emergency treatment of severe reactions to the contrast agent itself. After parenteral administration of a radiopaque agent, competent personnel and emergency facilities should be available for at least 30 to 60 minutes since severe delayed reactions have occurred (see ADVERSE REACTIONS).

Preparatory dehydration is dangerous and may contribute to acute renal failure in patients with advanced vascular disease, diabetic patients, and in susceptible nondiabetic patients (often elderly with pre-existing renal disease). Dehydration in these patients seems to be enhanced by the osmotic diuretic action of urographic agents. It is believed that overnight fluid restriction prior to excretory urography generally does not provide better visualization in normal patients. *Patients should be well hydrated prior to and following iohexol administration.*

Acute renal failure has been reported in diabetic patients with diabetic nephropathy and in susceptible nondiabetic patients (often elderly with preexisting renal disease) following excretory urography. Therefore, careful consideration of the potential risks should be given before performing this radiographic procedure in these patients.

Immediately following surgery, excretory urography should be used with caution in renal transplant recipients.

The possibility of a reaction, including serious, life-threatening, fatal, anaphylactoid or cardiovascular reactions should always be considered (see ADVERSE REACTIONS). It is of utmost importance that a course of action be carefully planned in advance for immediate treatment of serious reactions, and that adequate and appropriate personnel be readily available in case a severe reaction should occur.

The possibility of an idiosyncratic reaction in susceptible patients should always be considered (see ADVERSE REACTIONS). The susceptible population includes patients with a history of a previous reaction to contrast media, patients with a known sensitivity to iodine per se, and patients with a [illegible] clinical hypersensitivity: bronchial asthma, hay fe[illegible]d allergies.

[illegible] severe idiosyncratic reactions has [illegible]l pretesting methods. However, [illegible] upon to predict severe reactions [illegible]us for the patient. It is suggested [illegible] history with emphasis on allergy [illegible]or to the injection of any contrast [illegible]curate than pretesting in predicting [illegible]ions.

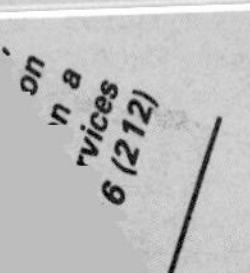

A positive history of allergies or hypersensitivity does not arbitrarily contraindicate the use of a contrast agent where a diagnostic procedure is thought essential, but caution should be exercised (see ADVERSE REACTIONS). Premedication with antihistamines or corticosteroids to avoid or minimize possible allergic reactions in such patients should be considered. Recent reports indicate that such pretreatment does not prevent serious life-threatening reactions, but may reduce both their incidence and severity.

Even though the osmolality of OMNIPAQUE is low compared to diatrizoate- or iothalamate-based ionic agents of comparable iodine concentration, the potential transitory increase in the circulatory osmotic load in patients with congestive heart failure requires caution during injection. These patients should be observed for several hours following the procedure to detect delayed hemodynamic disturbances.

General anesthesia may be indicated in the performance of some procedures in selected adult patients; however, a higher incidence of adverse reactions has been reported in these patients, and may be attributable to the inability of the patient to identify untoward symptoms, or to the hypotensive effect of anesthesia which can reduce cardiac output and increase the duration of exposure to the contrast agent.

Angiography should be avoided whenever possible in patients with homocystinuria, because of the risk of inducing thrombosis and embolism.

In angiographic procedures, the possibility of dislodging plaques or damaging or perforating the vessel wall should be borne in mind during the catheter manipulations and contrast medium injection. Test injections to ensure proper catheter placement are recommended.

Selective coronary arteriography should be performed only in those patients in whom the expected benefits outweigh the potential risk. The inherent risks of angiocardiography in patients with chronic pulmonary emphysema must be weighed against the necessity for performing this procedure.

When OMNIPAQUE (iohexol) is to be injected using plastic disposable syringes, the contrast medium should be drawn into the syringe and used immediately.

The inhibitory effects of nonionic contrast media on mechanisms of hemostasis have been shown, in vitro, to be less than ionic contrast media at comparable concentrations. For this reason, standard angiographic procedures should always be followed: angiographic catheters should be flushed frequently, and prolonged contact of blood with contrast media in syringes and catheters should be avoided.

If nondisposable equipment is used, scrupulous care should be taken to prevent residual contamination with traces of cleansing agents.

Parenteral products should be inspected visually for particulate matter and discoloration prior to administration. If particulate matter or discoloration is present, do not use.

Information for Patients

Patients receiving injectable radiopaque diagnostic agents should be instructed to:

1. Inform your physician if you are pregnant (see CLINICAL PHARMACOLOGY).
2. Inform your physician if you are diabetic or if you have multiple myeloma, pheochromocytoma, homozygous sickle cell disease, or known thyroid disorder (see WARNINGS).
3. Inform your physician if you are allergic to any drugs, food, or if you had any reactions to previous injections of dyes used for x-ray procedures (see PRECAUTIONS—GENERAL).
4. Inform your physician about any other medications you are currently taking, including nonprescription drugs, before you are administered this drug.

Drug/Laboratory Test Interaction

If iodine-containing isotopes are to be administered for the diagnosis of thyroid disease, the iodine-binding capacity of thyroid tissue may be reduced for up to 2 weeks after contrast medium administration. Thyroid function tests which do not depend on iodine estimation, eg, T_3 resin uptake or direct thyroxine assays, are not affected.

Carcinogenesis, Mutagenesis, Impairment of Fertility

No long-term animal studies have been performed to evaluate carcinogenic potential, mutagenesis, or whether OMNIPAQUE (iohexol) can affect fertility in men or women.

Pregnancy Category B

Reproduction studies have been performed in rats and rabbits with up to 100 times the recommended human dose. No evidence of impaired fertility or harm to the fetus has been demonstrated due to OMNIPAQUE. There are, however,no studies in pregnant women. Because animal reproduction studies are not always predictive of human response, this drug should be used during pregnancy only if clearly needed.

Nursing Mothers

It is not known to what extent iohexol is excreted in human milk. However, many injectable contrast agents are excreted unchanged in human milk. Although it has not been established that serious adverse reactions occur in nursing infants, caution shoul[illegible]e exercised when intravascular contrast media are [illegible]red to nursing women. Bottle feedings may be substituted for breast feedings for 24 hours following administration of OMNIPAQUE.

Pediatric Use

Safety and effectiveness in children have not been established.

ADVERSE REACTIONS

Adverse reactions following the use of OMNIPAQUE 240, OMNIPAQUE 300, and OMNIPAQUE 350 are usually of mild to moderate severity. However, serious, life-threatening and fatal reactions, mostly of cardiovascular origin, have been associated with the administration of iodine-containing contrast media, including OMNIPAQUE. The injection of contrast media is frequently associated with the sensation of warmth and pain, especially in peripheral angiography; pain and warmth are less frequent and less severe with OMNIPAQUE than with many contrast media.

Cardiovascular System: Arrhythmias including PVCs and PACs (3%), angina/chest pain (2%), and hypotension (1%). Others including cardiac failure, asystole, bradycardia, tachycardia, and vasovagal reaction were reported with an individual incidence of less than 0.8%. In controlled clinical trials involving 900 patients, one fatality occurred. In widespread clinical use, the incidence of fatality is estimated at 0.0003%.

Nervous System: Pain (6%), photomas (3%), headache (2%), and metallic taste (0.8%). Others including anxiety, blurred vision, dizziness, fever, motor and speech dysfunction, convulsion, lightheadness, paresthesia, somnolence, vertigo, stiff neck, hemiparesis, and nystagmus were reported, with an individual incidence of less than 0.3%.

Respiratory System: Dyspnea and laryngitis, with an individual incidence of 0.1%.

Gastrointestinal System: Nausea (2%) and vomiting (0.5%). Others including diarrhea, dyspepsia, and dry mouth were reported, with an individual incidence of 0.1%.

Skin and Appendages: Urticaria (0.3%) and purpura (0.1%).

Individual adverse reactions which occurred to a significantly greater extent for a specific procedure are listed under that indication.

General Adverse Reactions to Contrast Media

Physicians should remain alert for the occurrence of adverse effects in addition to those discussed above.

The following reactions have been reported after administration of other intravascular iodinated contrast media. *Reactions due to technique:* hematomas and ecchymoses. *Hemodynamic reactions:* vein cramp and thrombophlebitis following intravenous injection. *Cardiovascular reactions:* rare cases of cardiac arrhythmias, reflex tachycardia, chest pain, cyanosis, hypertension, hypotension, peripheral vasodilatation, shock, and cardiac arrest. *Renal reactions:* occasionally, transient proteinuria, and rarely, oliguria or anuria. *Allergic reactions:* asthmatic attacks, nasal and conjunctival symptoms, dermal reactions such as urticaria with or without pruritus, as well as pleomorphic rashes, sneezing and lacrimation and, rarely, anaphylactic reactions. Rare fatalities have occurred, due to this or unknown causes. *Signs and symtpoms related to the respiratory system:* pulmonary or laryngeal edema, bronchospasm, dyspnea; *or to the nervous system:* restlessness, tremors, convulsions. *Other reactions:* flushing, pain, warmth, metallic taste, nausea, vomiting, anxiety, headache, confusion, pallor, weakness, sweating, localized areas of edema, especially facial cramps, neutropenia, and dizziness. Rarely, immediate or delayed rigors can occur, sometimes accompanied by hyperpyrexia. Infrequently, "iodism" (salivary gland swelling) from organic iodinated compounds appears two days after exposure and subsides by the sixth day.

In general, the reactions which are known to occur upon parenteral administration of iodinated contrast agents are possible with any nonionic agent. Approximately 95 percent of adverse reactions accompanying the use of water-soluble intravascularly administered contrast agents are mild to moderate in degree. However, severe, life-threatening anaphylactoid reactions, mostly of cardiovascular origin, have occurred. Reported incidences of death range from 6.6 per 1 million (0.00066 percent) to 1 in 10,000 (0.01 percent). Most deaths occur during injection or 5 to 10 minutes later; the main feature being cardiac arrest with cardiovascular disease as the main aggravating factor. Isolated reports of hypotensive collapse and shock are found in the literature. The incidence of shock is estimated to be 1 out of 20,000 (0.005 percent) patients.

Adverse reactions to injectable contrast media fall into two categories: chemotoxic reactions and idiosyncratic reactions. Chemotoxic reactions result from the physicochemical properties of the contrast media, the dose and speed of injection. All hemodynamic disturbances and injuries to organs or vessels perfused by the contrast medium are included in this category.

Idiosyncratic reactions include all other reactions. They occur more frequently in patients 20 to 40 years old. Idiosyncratic reactions may or may not be dependent on the amount of dose injected, the speed of injection and the radiographic procedure. Idiosyncratic reactions are subdivided into mi-

nor, intermediate, and severe. The minor reactions are self-limited and of short duration; the severe reactions are life-threatening and treatment is urgent and mandatory.
The reported incidence of adverse reactions to contrast media in patients with a history of allergy are twice that of the general population. Patients with a history of previous reactions to a contrast medium are three times more susceptible than other patients. However, sensitivity to contrast media does not appear to increase with repeated examinations.
Most adverse reactions to injectable contrast media appear within 1 to 3 minutes after the start of injection, but delayed reactions may occur.
Regardless of the contrast agent employed, the overall estimated incidence of serious adverse reactions is higher with angiocardiography than with other procedures. Cardiac decompensation, serious arrhythmias, angina pectoris, or myocardial ischemia or infarction may occur during angiocardiography and left ventriculography. Electrocardiographic and hemodynamic abnormalities occur less frequently with OMNIPAQUE than with diatrizoate meglumine and diatrizoate sodium injection.

OVERDOSAGE

Overdosage may occur. The adverse effects of overdosage are life-threatening and affect mainly the pulmonary and cardiovascular systems. The symptoms included: cyanosis, bradycardia, acidosis, pulmonary hemorrhage, convulsions, coma, and cardiac arrest. Treatment of an overdosage is directed toward the support of all vital functions, and prompt institution of symptomatic therapy.
The intravenous LD_{50} values of OMNIPAQUE (iohexol) (in grams of iodine per kilogram body weight) are 24.2 in mice and 15.0 in rats.

INDIVIDUAL INDICATIONS AND USAGE

ANGIOCARDIOGRAPHY

Pharmacology—Hemodynamic Changes
OMNIPAQUE 350 at a concentration of 350 mgI/mL is indicated in adults for angiocardiography (ventriculography, aortic root injections, and selective coronary arteriography).
After both ventricular and coronary injection, decreases in systolic pressure were less pronounced and returned to baseline values earlier with OMNIPAQUE 350 than with diatrizoate meglumine and diatrizoate sodium injection.
OMNIPAQUE 350 produced less Q-T interval prolongation than seen with diatrizoate meglumine and diatrizoate sodium injection.
If repeat injections are made in rapid succession, all these changes are likely to be more pronounced. (See DOSAGE AND ADMINISTRATION.)
Precautions: During administration of large doses of OMNIPAQUE 350, continuous monitoring of vital signs is desirable. Caution is advised in the administration of large volumes to patients with incipient heart failure because of the possibility of aggravating the preexisting condition. Hypotension should be corrected promptly since it may induce serious arrhythmias.
Special care regarding dosage should be observed in patients with right ventricular failure, pulmonary hypertension, or stenotic pulmonary vascular beds because of the hemodynamic changes which may occur after injection into the right heart outflow tract. (See PRECAUTIONS—GENERAL.)
Adverse Reactions: Cardiovascular system reactions in angiocardiography included angina (8%), hypotension (2.5%), bradycardia (1.0%), and tachycardia (1.0%). (See ADVERSE REACTIONS—GENERAL.)
Dosage and Administration: The individual dose or volume is determined by the size of the structure to be visualized, the anticipated degree of hemodilution, and valvular competence. Weight is a minor consideration in adults. The volume of each individual injection is a more important consideration than the total dosage used. When large individual volumes are administered, as in ventriculography and aortography, it has been suggested that several minutes be permitted to elapse between each injection to allow for subsidence of possible hemodynamic disturbances.
The recommended single injection volume of OMNIPAQUE 350 at a concentration of 350 mgI/mL for angiocardiographic procedures is as follows:
Ventriculography
The usual adult volume for a single injection is 40 mL with a range of 30 mL to 60 mL. This may be repeated as necessary. When combined with selective coronary arteriography, the total administered volume should not exceed 250 mL (87.5 gI).
Selective Coronary Arteriography
The usual adult volume for right or left coronary arteriography is 5 mL (range 3 mL to 14 mL) per injection.
Aortic Root and Arch Study When Used Alone
The usual adult single injection volume is 50 mL, with a range of 20 mL to 75 mL.

Combined Angiocardiographic Procedures
Multiple Procedures
The visualization of multiple vascular systems and target organs is possible during a single radiographic examination of the patient.
Large doses of OMNIPAQUE 350 were well tolerated in angiographic procedures requiring multiple injections.
The maximum total volume for multiple procedures should not exceed 250 mL of 350 mgI/mL (87.5 gI).

AORTOGRAPHY

OMNIPAQUE 300 at a concentration of 300 mgI/mL or OMNIPAQUE (iohexol) 350 at a concentration of 350 mgI/mL is indicated in adults for use in aortography including aortic arch studies, ascending aorta, and abdominal aorta and its branches.
Precautions: Under conditions of slowed aortic circulation there is an increased likelihood for aortography to cause muscle spasm. Occasional serious neurologic complications, including paraplegia, have also been reported in patients with aortoiliac obstruction, femoral artery obstruction, abdominal compression, hypotension, hypertension, spinal anesthesia, and injection of vasopressors to increase contrast. In these patients the concentration, volume, and number of repeat injections of the medium should be maintained at a minimum with appropriate intervals between injections. The position of the patient and catheter tip should be carefully monitored.
Entry of a large aortic dose into the renal artery may cause, even in the absence of symptoms, albuminuria, hematuria, and an elevated creatinine and urea nitrogen. Rapid and complete return of function usually follows. (See PRECAUTIONS—GENERAL.)
Adverse Reactions: See ADVERSE REACTIONS—GENERAL, and ADVERSE REACTIONS—ANGIOCARDIOGRAPHY.
Dosage and Administration: The usual adult volume as a single injection is 50 mL to 80 mL, repeated if indicated, but not to exceed a total volume which contains 87.5 gI.

CEREBRAL ARTERIOGRAPHY

OMNIPAQUE 300 at a concentration of 300 mgI/mL is indicated in adults for use in cerebral arteriography.
The degree of pain and flushing as the result of the use of OMNIPAQUE 300 in cerebral arteriography is less than that seen with comparable injections of many contrast media.
In cerebral arteriography, patients should be appropriately prepared consistent with existing or suspected disease states.
Precautions: Cerebral arteriography should be undertaken with extreme care with special caution in elderly patients, patients in poor clinical condition, advanced arteriosclerosis, severe arterial hypertension, recent cerebral embolism or thrombosis, and cardiac decompensation.
Since the contrast medium is given by rapid injection, the patient should be monitored for possible untoward reactions. (See PRECAUTIONS—GENERAL.)
Adverse Reactions: Cerebral arteriography with water-soluble contrast media has been associated with temporary neurologic complications including seizures, drowsiness, transient paresis, and mild disturbances in vision such as photomas of 1-second or less duration.
Central nervous system reactions in cerebral arteriography included photomas (15%), headache (5.5%), and pain (4.5%). (See ADVERSE REACTIONS—GENERAL.)
Dosage and Administration: OMNIPAQUE 300 is recommended for cerebral arteriography at the following volumes: common carotid artery (6 mL to 12 mL), internal carotid artery (8 mL to 10 mL), external carotid artery (6 mL to 9 mL), and vertebral artery (6 mL to 20 mL).

DIGITAL SUBTRACTION ANGIOGRAPHY

OMNIPAQUE 350 at a concentration of 350 mgI/mL is indicated in adults for use in intravenous digital arteriography of the vessels of the head and neck.
Arteriograms of diagnostic quality can be obtained following the intravenous administration of contrast media employing digital subtraction and computer imaging enhancement techniques. The intravenous route of administration using these techniques has the advantage of being less invasive than the corresponding selective catheter placement of medium. The dose is administered into a peripheral vein or the superior vena cava usually by mechanical injection although sometimes by rapid manual injection. The technique has been used to visualize the ventricles, aorta and most of its larger branches, including the carotids, cerebrals, vertebrals, renal, celiac, mesenterics, and the major peripheral vessels of the limbs. Radiographic visualization of these structures is possible until significant hemodilution occurs.
OMNIPAQUE 350 can be injected intravenously as a rapid bolus to provide arterial visualization using digital subtraction radiography. Preprocedural medications are not considered necessary. OMNIPAQUE 350 has provided diagnostic arterial radiographs in about 95% of patients. In some cases, poor arterial visualization has been attributed to patient movement. OMNIPAQUE 350 is very well tolerated in the vascular system. Patient discomfort (general sensation of heat and/or pain) following injection is less than with various other contrast media.
Precautions: Since the contrast medium is usually administered mechanically under high pressure, rupture of smaller peripheral veins can occur. It has been suggested that this can be avoided by using an intravenous catheter threaded proximally beyond larger tributaries or, in the case of the antecubital vein, into the superior vena cava. Sometimes the femoral vein is used. (See PRECAUTIONS—GENERAL.)
Adverse Reactions: Cardiovascular system reactions in digital arteriography included transient PVCs (16%) and PACs (6.5%). (See ADVERSE REACTIONS—GENERAL.)
Dosage and Administration: The usual injection volume of OMNIPAQUE 350 for the intravenous digital technique is 30 mL to 50 mL of a 350 mgI/mL solution. This is administered as a bolus at 7.5 to 30 mL/second using a pressure injector. The volume and rate of injection will depend primarily on the type of equipment and technique used.
Frequently three or more injections may be required, up to a total volume not to exceed 250 mL (87.5 gI).

PERIPHERAL ANGIOGRAPHY

OMNIPAQUE (iohexol) 300 at a concentration of 300 mgI/mL or OMNIPAQUE 350 at a concentration of 350 mgI/mL is indicated in adults for use in peripheral arteriography. OMNIPAQUE 240 at a concentration of 240 mgI/mL or OMNIPAQUE 300 at a concentration of 300 mgI/mL is indicated in adults for use in peripheral venography.
Sedative medication may be employed prior to use. Anesthesia is not considered necessary.
Patient discomfort during and immediately following injection is substantially less than that following injection of various other contrast media. Moderate to severe discomfort is very unusual.
Precautions: Pulsation should be present in the artery to be injected. In thromboangiitis obliterans, or ascending infection associated with severe ischemia, angiography should be performed with extreme caution, if at all. (See PRECAUTIONS—GENERAL.)
Adverse Reactions: A transient sensation of mild warmth is usual, immediately following injection. This has not interfered with the procedure.
In phlebography the incidence of leg pain was 21%. This usually was mild and lasted a short time after injection. (See ADVERSE REACTIONS—GENERAL.)
Dosage and Administration: The volume required will depend on the size, flow rate, and disease state of the injected vessel and on the size and condition of the patient, as well as the imaging technique used.
The dosage recommended for use in peripheral angiography is as follows:

Aortofemoral runoffs:
- 20 mL to 70 mL of OMNIPAQUE 350 (350 mgI/mL)
- 30 mL to 90 mL of OMNIPAQUE 300 (300 mgI/mL)

Selective arteriograms (femoral/iliac):
- 10 mL to 30 mL of OMNIPAQUE 350 (350 mgI/mL)
- 10 mL to 60 mL of OMNIPAQUE 300 (300 mgI/mL)

Venography (per leg):
- 20 mL to 150 mL of OMNIPAQUE 240 (240 mgI/mL)
- 40 mL to 100 mL of OMNIPAQUE 300 (300 mgI/mL)

EXCRETORY UROGRAPHY

OMNIPAQUE 300 at a concentration of 300 mgI/mL or OMNIPAQUE 350 at a concentration of 350 mgI/mL is indicated for use in adults in excretory urography to provide diagnostic contrast of the urinary tract.
For pharmacokinetics of excretion: See CLINICAL PHARMACOLOGY—INTRAVASCULAR.
Precautions: Preparatory dehydration is not recommended in the elderly, diabetic, or azotemic patients, or in patients with suspected myelomatosis.
Since there is a possibility of temporary suppression of urine formation, it is recommended that a suitable interval elapse before excretory urography is repeated, especially in patients with unilateral or bilateral reduction in renal func[tion]. (See PRECAUTIONS—GENERAL.)
Adverse Reactions: See ADVERSE REACTIONS—GE[N]ERAL.
Dosage and Administration: OMNIPAQUE 300 ... OMNIPAQUE 350 at dosages from 200 mgI/kg body ... to 350 mgI/kg body weight has produced diagnosti... cation of the excretory system in patients with no... function.

HOW SUPPLIED

OMNIPAQUE 240
Vials of 10 mL, 240 mgI/mL, boxes of 1...
(NDC 0024-1412-10)
Vials of 100 mL, 240 mgI/mL, boxes ...
(NDC 0024-1412-15)
Bottles of 200 mL, 240 mgI/mL, b...
(NDC 0024-1412-25)

This product information was e... ber 1, 1986. On these and other p... p-Breon Laboratories, detailed inform... ned on a current basis by direct inqu... nal Services Department, 90 Park Ave... 10016 (212) 907-2525.

...ed on next page

Winthrop-Breon—Cont.

OMNIPAQUE 300
- Vials of 10 mL, 300 mgI/mL, boxes of 10 (NDC 0024-1413-10)
- Vials of 30 mL, 300 mgI/mL, boxes of 10 (NDC 0024-1413-30)
- Vials of 50 mL, 300 mgI/mL, boxes of 10 (NDC 0024-1413-50)
- Vials of 100 mL, 300 mgI/mL, boxes of 5 (NDC 0024-1413-15)

OMNIPAQUE 350
- Vials of 50 mL, 350 mgI/mL, boxes of 10 (NDC 0024-1414-50)
- Vials of 100 mL, 350 mgI/mL, boxes of 5 (NDC 0024-1414-15)
- Bottles of 200 mL, 350 mgI/mL, boxes of 5 (NDC 0024-1414-25)

STORAGE

Protect vials and bottles of OMNIPAQUE (iohexol) from strong daylight and direct exposure to sunlight. Do not freeze. Store at 59°F to 86°F (15°C to 30°C).

OW-57 C

Key to Controlled Substances Categories

Products listed with the symbols shown below are subject to the Controlled Substances Act of 1970. These drugs are categorized according to their potential for abuse. The greater the potential, the more severe the limitations on their prescription.

CATEGORY	INTERPRETATION
C II	**High potential for abuse.** Use may lead to severe physical or psychological dependence. Prescriptions must be written in ink, or typewritten and signed by the practitioner. Verbal prescriptions must be confirmed in writing within 72 hours, and may be given only in a genuine emergency. No renewals are permitted.
C III	**Some potential for abuse.** Use may lead to low-to-moderate physical dependence or high psychological dependence. Prescriptions may be oral or written. Up to 5 renewals are permitted within 6 months.
C IV	**Low potential for abuse.** Use may lead to limited physical or psychological dependence. Prescriptions may be oral or written. Up to 5 renewals are permitted within 6 months.
C V	**Subject to state and local regulation.** Abuse potential is low; a prescription may not be required.

Key to FDA Use-in-pregnancy Ratings

~~he Food and Drug Administration's Pregnancy Categories are based on the degree to which available information ...led out risk to the fetus, balanced against the drug's potential benefits to the patient. Ratings range from "A," for ...t have been tested for teratogenicity under controlled conditions without showing evidence of damage to the ...D" and "X" for drugs that are definitely teratogenic. The "D" rating is generally reserved for drugs with no ...atives. The "X" rating means there is absolutely no reason to risk using the drug in pregnancy.

CATEGORY	INTERPRETATION
B	**Controlled studies show no risk.** Adequate, well-controlled studies in pregnant women have ...ailed to demonstrate risk to the fetus.
C	**...evidence of risk in humans.** Either animal findings show risk, but human findings do not; or, if ...dequate human studies have been done, animal findings are negative.
D	**...annot be ruled out.** Human studies are lacking, and animal studies are either positive for ... or lacking as well. However, potential benefits may justify the potential risk.
X	**...vidence of risk.** Investigational or post-marketing data show risk to the fetus. Never- ...ential benefits may outweigh the potential risk.
	...ed in pregnancy. Studies in animals or human, or investigational or post-marketing ...own fetal risk which clearly outweighs any possible benefit to the patient.

Conversion Tables

Metric Doses With Approximate Apothecary Equivalents

The approximate dose equivalents represent the quantities usually prescribed by physicians using, respectively, the metric and apothecary system of weights and measures. When prepared dosage forms such as tablets, capsules, etc. are prescribed in the metric system, the pharmacist may dispense the corresponding approximate equivalent in the apothecary system and vice versa. (Note: A milliliter [mL] is the approximate equivalent of a cubic centimeter [cc]). Exact equivalents, which appear in the United States Pharmacopeia and the National Formulary, must be used to calculate quantities in pharmaceutical formulas and prescription compounding:

LIQUID MEASURE		LIQUID MEASURE		LIQUID MEASURE		LIQUID MEASURE	
Metric	Approximate Apothecary Equivalents	Metric	Approximate Apothecary Equivalents	Metric	Approximate Apothecary Equivalents	Metric	Approximate Apothecary Equivalents
1000 mL	1 quart	3 mL	45 minims	30 mL	1 fluid ounce	0.25 mL	4 minims
750 mL	1½ pints	2 mL	30 minims	15 mL	4 fluid drams	0.2 mL	3 minims
500 mL	1 pint	1 mL	15 minims	10 mL	2½ fluid drams	0.1 mL	1½ minims
250 mL	8 fluid ounces	0.75 mL	12 minims	8 mL	2 fluid drams	0.06 mL	1 minim
200 mL	7 fluid ounces	0.6 mL	10 minims	5 mL	1¼ fluid drams	0.05 mL	¾ minim
100 mL	3½ fluid ounces	0.5 mL	8 minims	4 mL	1 fluid dram	0.03 mL	½ minim
50 mL	1¾ fluid ounces	0.3 mL	5 minims				

WEIGHT		WEIGHT		WEIGHT		WEIGHT	
Metric	Approximate Apothecary Equivalents	Metric	Approximate Apothecary Equivalents	Metric	Approximate Apothecary Equivalents	Metric	Approximate Apothecary Equivalents
30g	1 ounce	30mg	1/2 grain	500mg	7½ grains	1.2 mg	1/50 grain
15g	4 drams	25mg	3/8 grain	400mg	6 grains	1 mg	1/60 grain
10g	2½ drams	20mg	1/3 grain	300mg	5 grains	800 µg	1/80 grain
7.5g	2 drams	15mg	1/4 grain	250mg	4 grains	600 µg	1/100 grain
6g	90 grains	12mg	1/5 grain	200mg	3 grains	500 µg	1/120 grain
5g	75 grains	10mg	1/6 grain	150mg	2½ grains	400 µg	1/150 grain
4g	60 grains (1 dram)	8mg	1/8 grain	125mg	2 grains	300 µg	1/200 grain
3g	45 grains	6mg	1/10 grain	100mg	1½ grains	250 µg	1/250 grain
2g	30 grains (½ dram)	5mg	1/12 grain	75mg	1¼ grains	200 µg	1/300 grain
1.5g	22 grains	4mg	1/15 grain	60mg	1 grain	150 µg	1/400 grain
1g	15 grains	3mg	1/20 grain	50mg	¾ grain	120 µg	1/500 grain
750mg	12 grains	2mg	1/30 grain	40mg	⅔ grain	100 µg	1/600 grain
600mg	10 grains	1.5mg	1/40 grain				

Approximate Household Equivalents

For household purposes, an American Standard Teaspoon is defined by the American National Standards Institute as containing 4.93 ± 0.24 mL. The USP states that in view of the almost universal practice of employing teaspoons ordinarily available in the household for administration of medicine, the teaspoon may be regarded as representing 5 mL. Household units of measure often are used to inform patients of the size of a liquid dose. Because of difficulties involved in measuring liquids under normal conditions of use, household spoons are not appropriate when accurate measurement of a liquid dose is required. When accurate measurement of a liquid dose is required, the USP recommends that a calibrated oral syringe or dropper be used.

1 fluid dram = 1 teaspoonful = 5 mL
2 fluid drams = 1 dessertspoonful = 10 mL
4 fluid drams = 1 tablespoonful = 15 mL
2 fluid ounces = 1 wineglassful = 60 mL
4 fluid ounces = 1 teacupful = 120 mL
8 fluid ounces = 1 tumblerful = 240 mL

Pounds—Kilograms (kg) Conversion

1 pound = 0.453592 kg
1 kg = 2.2 pounds

Temperature Conversion Table:

9 × °C = (5 × °F) − 160

Centigrade to Fahrenheit = (°C × 9/5) + 32 = °F

Fahrenheit to Centigrade = (°F − 32) × 5/9 = °C

Milliequivalents per Liter (mEq/L)

$$\text{mEq/L} = \frac{\text{weight of salt (g)} \times \text{valence of ion} \times 1000}{\text{molecular weight of salt}}$$

$$\text{weight of salt (g)} = \frac{\text{mEq/L} \times \text{molecular weight of salt}}{\text{valence of ion} \times 1000}$$

GUIDE TO MANAGEMENT OF DRUG OVERDOSE

Prepared by:
Eric G. Comstock, M.D.
and
Eugene V. Boisaubin, M.D.
Department of Medicine
Baylor College of Medicine
Houston, Texas

INTRODUCTION: The following discussion is designed for use in adult patients. In the pediatric age group, general principles apply, but the volumes of fluid or suggested medication must be adjusted for body size. Symptomatic and supportive care is the basis for treatment of drug overdose. All other approaches are secondary. Procedures directed toward the offending substance, such as the performance of gastric lavage or the administration of a specific pharmacologic antagonist, should be undertaken only after adequate vital function has been assured. Procedures to facilitate excretion of toxic substances, such as peritoneal or extracorporeal dialysis and forced diuresis are required infrequently, and should never be relied upon as the primary approach to treatment. For sedative, hypnotic, and tranquilizer drugs, alone or in combination, supportive care is sufficient as outlined in the following discussion.

INITIAL ASSESSMENT: If the patient is symptomatic, determine the adequacy of respiration and cardiac function and note reflex activity, such as pupillary, corneal, gag and deep tendon. If vital function is compromised, or consciousness is impaired, proceed immediately to supportive measures.

THE ASYMPTOMATIC PATIENT: The drug overdosed patient may be asymptomatic because he has not ingested a sufficient dose of the drugs, or because a sufficient quantity has not been absorbed to produce symptoms. After the ingestion of a life threatening quantity of drugs, symptoms may be delayed as long as six hours, although ordinarily symptoms are manifested within thirty (30) minutes to two (2) hours. Ingestion of alcohol simultaneoulsy with drugs may shorten the time for symptoms to appear. Vomiting should be induced only during the asymptomatic interval. If significant central nervous system depression intervenes between the administration of emetic and the occurrence of vomiting, then the airway should be protected by insertion of a cuffed endotracheal tube. Fluids must be forced orally to obtain satisfactory results from any effort to induce vomiting. An alternate approach to the asymptomatic patient alleged to have ingested drugs, is the administration by mouth of a slurry of no less than 100 grams of activated charcoal powder (USP) in water. Gastric lavage with a large caliber tube (34 French) may be performed in the asymptomatic patient. Any patient whose consciousness is impaired to the point where a cuffed endotracheal tube will be tolerated should be intubated prior to the performance of gastric lavage.

THE SYMPTOMATIC PATIENT: If the patient is symptomatic all treatment procedures directed toward the toxic substance are secondary to the support of vital function. If the patient is in coma, attention to respiratory support and cardiac function should proceed immediately.

RESPIRATORY SUPPORT: Examine the mouth. Remove all foreign material including dentures. Position the head so that respiration is not sonorous and so that regurgitated stomach contents are not readily aspirated. If respiration is not present, provide ventilation by mouth-to-mouth, ambu bag, or positive pressure respirator until the patient is adequately oxygenated. Insert an oropharyngeal airway and suction excess secretions while preparing to insert an endotracheal tube. A cuffed endotracheal tube should be inserted and inflated. Bronchial suction should be administered to clear mucus and foreign material. Determine that the chest is being inflated symmetrically and that breath sounds are audible bilaterally. After the acute emergency, determine placement of the endotracheal tube by x-ray. Monitor adequacy of ventilation using arterial blood gases.

IV ACCESS AND CARDIAC FUNCTION: While one member of the treatment team is assuring adequate ventilation, a second member of the team should be assuring adequate IV access by insertion of an 18 gauge venous catheter and initiation of IV fluid administration such as Ringers Lactate or ½ normal saline at a maintenance rate in adults of 150 ml. per hour. Since hypotension from sedative drug intoxication results from relative hypovolemia complicated frequently by dehydration, the rate of intravenous infusion should be increased to 10-20 cc per minute if the systolic pressure is under 80 mm of mercury. Placing the patient in the Trendelenburg position may quickly correct small to moderate degrees of hypotension. A central venous pressure catheter or a Swan-Ganz catheter is required if the continuous high rate infusion reaches one (1) liter within one hour or if the positive fluid balance exceeds two (2) liters during the first two hours. Intermittent monitoring of central venous pressure should continue throughout the period of intensive supportive care. A baseline electrocardiogram should be obtained as soon as vital functions have been supported. The appearance of conduction defects should lead to suspicion of drugs with direct cardiac effects, such as the tricyclic antidepressants. In uncomplicated sedative drug overdose, the central venous pressure will be under ten centimeters of water and will not change appreciably with high volume fluid infusion. If the central venous pressure increases abruptly in excess of five centimeters of water, or if the CVP exceeds 16 centimeters of water, high rate fluid infusion should be stopped pending evaluation of cardiac status. Adequate tissue perfusion is obtained with a systolic pressure in the range of 80 to 100 milliliters of mercury. A systolic pressure higher than this is required only in the patient with pre-existing hypertension. The formation of urine is an indication that tissue perfusion is adequate.

URINARY CATHETERIZATION: An in-dwelling urinary catheter should be inserted early in the course of treatment of any unconscious drug overdose patient. Upon insertion of the catheter, the volume of residual urine should be measured and the specimen should be saved separately for urinalysis including specific gravity, labeled for drug analysis, and sent to the laboratory to be retained for 24 hours. Recording of urine output hourly is necessary to maintain fluid balance records. Abrupt cessation of urine output most frequently is due to an obstructed catheter, but deserves immediate appraisal. Anuria for a period in excess of one hour should lead to reduction of high rate intravascular volume infusion until cardiac and renal status has been reappraised. Failure to achieve adequate urinary output after initial emptying of the bladder may reflect uncompensated dehydration and relative hypovolemia, each of which must be corrected before balanced fluid intake and output plus insensible loss can be achieved. The immediate or automatic use of diuretics at this stage only aggravates the basic defect and may result in intractable hypotension. Addition of vasopressor drugs at this stage may precipitate renal failure. Electrolyte solutions as transient volume expanders are preferred to whole blood or plasma to avoid congestive heart failure when normal vascular tone is re-established. A positive fluid balance of 2 to 4 liters may be required before fluid intake and output are in equilibrium. As vascular tone returns, urine output may increase abruptly exceeding one liter per hour. Profound diuresis may precede recurrence of deep tendon reflexes and heralds reduction in CNS depression.

GASTRIC LAVAGE: Gastric lavage should be performed only after vital function has been determined to be adequate or procedures for support have been implemented. Gastric lavage should be undertaken only after a cuffed endotracheal tube is protecting the airway. If corrosive substances are thought to have been ingested, lavage should not be performed until examination demonstrates there is no destruction of the mucous membranes of the mouth or of the esophagus as determined by esophagoscopy. Gastric lavage should be performed if the ingestion of drugs is estimated to have been within the preceding six hours. If there are no audible bowel sounds, gastric lavage should be performed regardless of the time lapse between ingestion and treatment. A 34 French lavage tube should be used. Smaller tubes do not permit sufficiently rapid fluid flow to remove particulate material. Gastric contents should be aspirated prior to lavage and saved in the event subsequent laboratory analysis is required. In an adult, lavage should be performed in cyles of 300 to 500 milliliters of fluid instilled over one to two minutes, left in place for about one minute, and drained by gravity over a period of approximately three to four minutes. If these time intervals cannot be maintained, then the lavage system is defective. The total fluid volume to be used in lavage should be three liters beyond that volume required to obtain a clear return. Lavage may be performed with tap water or normal saline solution.

ACTIVATED CHARCOAL: Powdered activated charcoal effectively adsorbs the vast majority of drugs, thereby limiting their bio-availability. One hundred (100) grams of activated charcoal suspended in six ounces of water should be instilled through the lavage tube after initial gastric aspiration and prior to lavage. The activated charcoal forms an effective barrier between any remaining particulate material and the gastrointestinal mucosa. Drugs adsorbed on activated charcoal are not desorbed to any practical extent in the lower intestinal tract. When an enteroenteric circulation of the active drug exists, excess activated charcoal in the intestine effectively prevents reabsorption thereby facilitating excretion. This appears effective with the tricyclic antidepressants and the cardiac glycosides. Activated charcoal is not effective with cyanide or small electrolytes such as sodium, potassium or mineral acids or bases.

SPECIFIC ANTIDOTES: Specific antidotal substances effective in the treatment of drug overdose are few. They should be used only with specific indications and never should be used prophyllactically or in quantities sufficient to return the comatose patient to consciousness. They should be used only to improve adequacy of vital function and never be relied upon to the exclusion of supportive care. When specific antidotes are used, special attention must be given to duration of action of the antidote as compared with the duration of action of the primary drug. Release of a patient after administration of a relatively short acting antidote may result in serious compromise of clinical status after the patient has been released from medical care.

AVOID UNNECESSARY DRUGS: Central nervous system depression and coma should be treated by the supportive means described above and should not be treated by central nervous system stimulant drugs. Shortening of coma with CNS stimulant drugs may result in hyperpyrexia and convulsions which otherwise might be avoided. Hypotension resulting from sedative or tranquilizer drug overdose is due to relative hypovolemia properly corrected by increasing the intravascular volume. Vasopressor drugs are not helpful and should be avoided. Body temperature outside of the normal range should be controlled by heat exchangers which warm or cool the body mechanically. Anti-pyretic drugs should be avoided. Anti-pyretic drugs in overdose cause hyperpyrexia. Alkaline diuresis is effective in removing phenobarbital and barbital, but only rarely is it an essential part of treatment of overdose due to these drugs. Except for salicylate, the risk benefit ratio of forced diuresis in the treatment of other drugs does not favor its use. Diuretic drugs should not be used routinely in the treatment of drug overdose.

CONTINUING CARE: Coma from sedative drug intoxication may persist for many days. Total apnea for five days and an isoelectric electroencephalogram for intervals up to 36 hours have been recorded with drug overdose patients who have survived without apparent neurologic sequelae. Continuing care should be provided in a medical intensive care unit with monitoring of temperature, blood pressure, pulse, respiratory rate, tidal volume, electrocardiogram, central venous pressure, fluid balance, electrolytes, and arterial blood gases with appropriate compensatory treatment of abnormalities. Intensive respiratory care should include frequent tracheal suction, and repositioning, and frequent chest x-rays. Endotracheal tubes should be changed under supervision of a critical care specialist. Tracheostomy should be performed only for surgical indications. Carefully attentive continuous nursing care is essential.

COMPLICATIONS: Aspiration pneumonia and subsequent infection is the most commonly occuring complication of coma secondary to drug overdose. Treatment consists of vigorous tracheal suction and antibiotic coverage. Interstitial edema is common in profound coma and usually represents increased capillary permeability rather than overhydration. Parenteral steroids may be helpful in this situation. Always be mindful that the patient may have sustained traumatic injury especially to the head, so be watchful for lateralizing neurologic signs.

TOXICOLOGIC ANALYSIS: Any ingested material, initial gastric aspirate, and the first catheterized urine specimen all should be saved and labeled for laboratory examination with instructions to hold at least twenty-four (24) hours prior to discarding. Analysis of these fluids for drugs occasionally will change fundamental approach to treatment. Frequently multiple drugs are involved. Interpretation of quantitative findings is extremely difficult and usually is helpful only to follow the clearance of substances from the body. Previous drug use may result in tolerance which prevents meaningful interpretation of absolute concentrations. Instructions for management of specific drugs identified should be consulted once symptomatic and supportive care is under way.

CHARCOAL HEMOPERFUSION: During the past decade interest has increased in the insertion of innert adsorbent material into the blood stream of poisoned patients to improve clearance of the toxic substance. The most popular current technique utilizes adsorbent hemoperfusion cartridges containing activated charcoal. Extremely high clearance occurs of virtually all commonly ingested intoxicants and several life-saving case reports utilizing this procedure have appeared. Despite the theoretical virtues of this new technique there are problems associated with its use. First, aggressive but simpler comprehensive supportive management as outlined above has already reduced mortality of even severely intoxicated hospitalized patients to 2% or less. Side effects may occur and include hypotension, thrombocytopenia and the complications of systemic heparinization. The system requires additional skilled personnel and concern with the hemoperfusion technique may distract attention from the more proven supportive measures. Hemoperfusion may have a role in select, severely poisoned patients where supportive therapy is insufficient, but it is not currently recommended for routine use.

This form is published by PDR in conjunction with pharmaceutical manufacturers and FDA as a public service. Health professionals are encouraged to send reports of adverse events associated with drugs and biological products to the manufacturer or to the Food and Drug Administration, Division of Epidemiology and Surveillance, HFN-730, 5600 Fishers Lane, Rockville, MD 20857. Manufacturers are required by law to submit all such reports of adverse events to FDA.

For new drugs all suspected, serious events should be reported. For other drugs, serious reactions not listed in the current product information are of interest. Patient and initial reporter identification are held in confidence by the FDA and are not subject to release under the Freedom of Information Act.

Do not remove this Form. Please photocopy for use.

Form Approved: OMB No 0910-0230

ADVERSE EVENT REPORT
(Drugs and Biologics)

1 PATIENT INITIALS *(Optional)*	2. AGE *(Years)*	3. SEX ☐ MALE ☐ FEMALE	4. DATE OF EVENT ONSET

5. DESCRIBE EVENT

6. CHECK ALL APPROPRIATE:
- ☐ PATIENT DIED
- ☐ EVENT TREATED WITH Rx DRUG
- ☐ RESULTED IN, OR PROLONGED, INPATIENT HOSPITALIZATION
- ☐ RESULTED IN PERMANENT DISABILITY
- ☐ NONE OF THE ABOVE

7 SUSPECT DRUG(S): *(Give Manufacturer and Trade Name)*

8 REASON FOR USE OF DRUG(S)	9. ROUTE	10. TOTAL DAILY DOSE	11. DATES OF ADMINISTRATION

12. OTHER DRUGS TAKEN CONCOMITANTLY AND DATES OF ADMINISTRATION *(Exclude Those Used to Treat Event)*

13. RELEVANT TESTS/LABORATORY DATA/MEDICAL HISTORY/DECHALLENGE/RECHALLENGE

14. HEALTH PROFESSIONAL'S NAME, ADDRESS AND TELEPHONE NUMBER

Note: Submission of a report does not necessarily constitute an admission that the drug caused the adverse event.

15. ALSO REPORTED TO MANUFACTURER? ☐ YES ☐ NO

FORM FDA 1639b (10/86)